DRUG INFORMATION HANDBOOK

A Comprehensive Resource for all Clinicians and Healthcare Professionals

American Pharmacists Association®
Improving medication use. Advancing patient care.

APhA

Lexicomp is the official drug reference for the American Pharmacists Association

21st Edition

Lexicomp®

NOTICE

This data is intended to serve the user as a handy reference and not as a complete drug information resource. It does not include information on every therapeutic agent available. The publication covers over 1450 commonly used drugs and is specifically designed to present important aspects of drug data in a more concise format than is typically found in medical literature or product material supplied by manufacturers.

The nature of drug information is that it is constantly evolving because of ongoing research and clinical experience and is often subject to interpretation. While great care has been taken to ensure the accuracy of the information and recommendations presented, the reader is advised that the authors, editors, reviewers, contributors, and publishers cannot be responsible for the continued currency of the information or for any errors, omissions, or the application of this information, or for any consequences arising therefrom. Therefore, the author(s) and/or the publisher shall have no liability to any person or entity with regard to claims, loss, or damage caused, or alleged to be caused, directly or indirectly, by the use of information contained herein. Because of the dynamic nature of drug information, readers are advised that decisions regarding drug therapy must be based on the independent judgment of the clinician, changing information about a drug (eg, as reflected in the literature and manufacturer's most current product information), and changing medical practices. Therefore, this data is designed to be used in conjunction with other necessary information and is not designed to be solely relied upon by any user. The user of this data hereby and forever releases the authors and publishers of this data from any and all liability of any kind that might arise out of the use of this data. The editors are not responsible for any inaccuracy of quotation or for any false or misleading implication that may arise due to the text or formulas as used or due to the quotation of revisions no longer official.

Certain of the authors, editors, and contributors have written this book in their private capacities. No official support or endorsement by any federal or state agency or pharmaceutical company is intended or inferred.

The publishers have made every effort to trace any third party copyright holders, if any, for borrowed material. If they have inadvertently overlooked any, they will be pleased to make the necessary arrangements at the first opportunity.

If you have any suggestions or questions regarding any information presented in this data, please contact our drug information pharmacists at (330) 650-6506. Book revisions are available at our website at http://www.lexi.com/home/revisions/.

This manual was produced using Lexi-Comp's Information Management System™ (LIMS) — a complete publishing service of Lexi-Comp Inc.

Lexicomp

1100 Terex Road • Hudson, Ohio 44236
(330) 650-6506

ISBN 978-1-59195-307-4 (North American Edition)

TABLE OF CONTENTS

DRUG INFORMATION HANDBOOK EDITORIAL ADVISORY PANEL

William J. Dana, PharmD, FASHP
Pharmacy Quality Assurance
Harris County Hospital District

Matthew A. Fuller, PharmD, BCPS, BCPP, FASHP
Clinical Pharmacy Specialist, Psychiatry
Cleveland Department of Veterans Affairs Medical Center
Associate Clinical Professor of Psychiatry and *Clinical Instructor of Psychology*
Case Western Reserve University
Adjunct Associate Professor of Clinical Pharmacy
University of Toledo

Morton P. Goldman, RPh, PharmD, BCPS, FCCP
Senior Editor
Lexi-Comp, Inc

Julie A. Golembiewski, PharmD
Clinical Associate Professor and *Clinical Pharmacist, Anesthesia/Pain*
Colleges of Pharmacy and Medicine
University of Illinois

Jeffrey P. Gonzales, PharmD, BCPS
Critical Care Clinical Pharmacy Specialist
University of Maryland Medical Center

Jennifer Fisher Lowe, PharmD, BCOP
Pharmacotherapy Contributor
Lexi-Comp, Inc

Joseph Snoke, RPh, BCPS
Manager
Core Pharmacology Group
Lexi-Comp, Inc

EDITORIAL ADVISORY PANEL

Julie J. Kelsey, PharmD
Clinical Specialist
Women's Health and Family Medicine
Department of Pharmacy Services
University of Virginia Health System

Patrick J. Kiel, PharmD, BCPS, BCOP
Clinical Pharmacy Specialist
Hematology and Stem Cell Transplant
Indiana University Simon Cancer Center

Polly E. Kintzel, PharmD, BCPS, BCOP
Clinical Pharmacy Specialist-Oncology
Spectrum Health

Michael Klepser, PharmD, FCCP
Professor of Pharmacy
Department of Pharmacy Practice
Ferris State University

Daren Knoell, PharmD
Associate Professor of Pharmacy Practice and Internal Medicine
Davis Heart and Lung Research Institute
The Ohio State University

David Knoppert, MScPhm, FCCP, MSc, FCSHP
Clinical Leader - Paediatrics
Pharmacy Services
London Health Sciences Centre
Children's Health Research Institute

Sandra Knowles, RPh, BScPhm
Drug Safety Pharmacist
Sunnybrook and Women's College HSC

Jill M. Kolesar, PharmD, FCCP, BCPS
Associate Professor
School of Pharmacy
University of Wisconsin Paul P. Carbone Comprehensive Cancer Center

Susannah E. Koontz, PharmD, BCOP
Principal and Consultant
Pediatric Hematology/Oncology and Stem Cell Transplantation/Cellular Therapy
Koontz Oncology Consulting, LLC

Donna M. Kraus, PharmD, FAPhA, FPPAG
Associate Professor of Pharmacy Practice and *Pediatric Clinical Pharmacist*
Departments of Pharmacy Practice and Pediatrics
University of Illinois

Daniel L. Krinsky, RPh, MS
Manager, MTM Services
Giant Eagle Pharmacy
Assistant Professor
Department of Pharmacy Practice
Northeast Ohio Medical University (NEOMED)

Tim T.Y. Lau, PharmD, ACPR, FCSHP
Pharmacotherapeutic Specialist in Infectious Diseases
Pharmaceutical Sciences
Vancouver General Hospital

Mandy C. Leonard, PharmD, BCPS
Assistant Professor
Cleveland Clinic Lerner College of Medicine of Case Western University
Assistant Director, Drug Information Services
The Cleveland Clinic Foundation

John J. Lewin III, PharmD, BCPS
Clinical Specialist, Neurosciences Critical Care
The Johns Hopkins Hospital

Jeffrey D. Lewis, PharmD, MACM
Assistant Dean and Associate Professor of Pharmacy Practice
Cedarville University School of Pharmacy

John Lindsley, PharmD, BCPS
Cardiology Clinical Pharmacy Specialist
The Johns Hopkins Hospital

Nicholas A. Link, PharmD, BCOP
Clinical Specialist, Oncology
Hillcrest Hospital

Jennifer Fisher Lowe, PharmD, BCOP
Pharmacotherapy Contributor
Lexi-Comp, Inc

Sherry Luedtke, PharmD
Associate Professor
Department of Pharmacy Practice
Texas Tech University HSC School of Pharmacy

Melissa Makii, PharmD, BCPS
Clinical Pharmacy Specialist
Pediatric Oncology
Rainbow Babies & Children's Hospital

Vincent F. Mauro, BS, PharmD, FCCP
Professor of Clinical Pharmacy and *Adjunct Professor of Medicine*
Colleges of Pharmacy and Medicine
The University of Toledo

Barrie McCombs, MD, FCFP
Medical Information Service Coordinator
The Alberta Rural Physician Action Plan

Christopher McPherson, PharmD
Clinical Pharmacist
Neonatal Intensive Care Unit
St. Louis Children's Hospital

Timothy F. Meiller, DDS, PhD
Professor
Oncology and Diagnostic Sciences
Baltimore College of Dental Surgery
Professor of Oncology
Marlene and Stewart Greenebaum Cancer Center
University of Maryland Medical System

Geralyn M. Meny, MD
Medical Director
American Red Cross, Penn-Jersey Region

Charla E. Miller, RPh, PharmD
Neonatal Clinical Pharmacy Specialist
Wolfson Children's Hospital

Julie Miller, PharmD
Pharmacy Clinical Specialist, Cardiology
Columbus Children's Hospital

Katherine Mills, PharmD
Pharmacotherapy Contributor
Lexi-Comp, Inc

Leah Millstein, MD
Assistant Professor
Division of General Internal Medicine
University of Maryland School of Medicine

Kristin Watson, PharmD, BCPS
Assistant Professor, Cardiology
and *Clinical Pharmacist, Cardiology Service*
Heart Failure Clinic
University of Maryland Medical Center

David M. Weinstein, PhD, RPh
Manager
Metabolism, Interactions, and Genomics Group
Lexi-Comp, Inc

Anne Marie Whelan, PharmD
Associate Professor
College of Pharmacy
Dalhouise University

Sherri J. Willard Argyres, MA, PharmD
Medical Science Pharmacist
Lexi-Comp, Inc

John C. Williamson, PharmD, BCPS
Pharmacy Clinical Coordinator, Infectious Diseases
Wake Forest Baptist Health

Nathan Wirick, PharmD
Infectious Disease and Antibiotic Management Clinical Specialist
Hillcrest Hospital

Richard L. Wynn, BSPharm, PhD
Professor of Pharmacology
Baltimore College of Dental Surgery
University of Maryland

Monica Yoshinaga, PharmD
Pharmacist Evidence Analyst and Strategist
Kaiser Permanente Drug Information Services

Sallie Young, PharmD, BCPS, AQ Cardiology
Clinical Pharmacy Specialist, Cardiology
Penn State Milton S. Hershey Medical Center

Jennifer Zimmer-Young, PharmD, CCRP
Educator, Clinical Pharmacist
ThedaCare

DESCRIPTION OF SECTIONS AND FIELDS USED IN THIS HANDBOOK

The *Drug Information Handbook, 21st Edition* is divided into four sections.

The first section is a compilation of introductory text pertinent to the use of this book.

The drug information section of the handbook, in which all drugs are listed alphabetically, details information pertinent to each drug. Extensive cross-referencing is provided by U.S. brand names, Canadian brand names, and index terms.

The third section is an invaluable appendix which offers a compilation of tables, guidelines, nomograms, algorithms, and conversion information which can be helpful when considering patient care.

The last section of this handbook contains a Pharmacologic Category Index which lists all drugs in this handbook in their unique pharmacologic class.

The **Alphabetical Listing of Drugs** is presented in a consistent format and provides the following fields of information:

Generic Name	U.S. adopted name
Pronunciation	Phonetic pronunciation guide
Brand Names: U.S.	Trade names (manufacturer-specific) found in the United States. The symbol [DSC] appears after trade names that have been recently discontinued.
Brand Names: Canada	Trade names found in Canada
Index Terms	Includes names or accepted abbreviations of the generic drug; may include common brand names no longer available; this field is used to create cross-references to monographs
Pharmacologic Category	Unique systematic classification of medications
Additional Appendix Information	Cross-reference to other pertinent drug information found in the appendix section of this handbook
Use	Information pertaining to appropriate FDA-approved indications of the drug.
Unlabeled Use	Information pertaining to non-FDA approved indications of the drug.
Pregnancy Risk Factor	Five categories established by the FDA to indicate the potential of a systemically absorbed drug for causing risk to fetus.
Pregnancy Considerations	A summary of human and/or animal information pertinent to or associated with the use of the drug as it relates to clinical effects on the fetus, newborn, or pregnant women.
Lactation	Indicates if the drug listed in the monograph is present in breast milk and the manufacturers' recommendation for use while breast-feeding (where recommendation of American Academy of Pediatrics differs, notation is made).
Prescribing and Access Restrictions	Provides information on any special requirements regarding the prescribing, obtaining or dispensing of drugs, including access restrictions pertaining to drugs with REMS elements and those drugs whose access restrictions are not REMS-related.
Medication Guide Available	Identifies drugs that have an FDA-approved Medication Guide.
Contraindications	Information pertaining to inappropriate use of the drug as dictated by approved labeling.
Warnings/Precautions	Precautionary considerations, hazardous conditions related to use of the drug, and disease states or patient populations in which the drug should be cautiously used. Boxed warnings, when present, are clearly identified and are adapted from the FDA approved labeling. Consult the product labeling for the exact black box warning through the manufacturer's or the FDA website.
Adverse Reactions	Side effects are grouped by percentage of incidence (if known) and/or body system; in the interest of saving space, <1% effects are grouped only by percentage
Drug Interactions	
Metabolism/Transport Effects	If a drug has demonstrated involvement with cytochrome P450 enzymes, or other metabolism or transport proteins, this field will identify the drug as an inhibitor, inducer, or substrate of the specific enzyme(s) (eg, CYP1A2 or UGT1A1). CYP450 isoenzymes are identified as substrates (minor or major), inhibitors (weak, moderate, or strong), and inducers (weak or strong).
Avoid Concomitant Use	Designates drug combinations which should not be used concomitantly, due to an unacceptable risk:benefit assessment. Frequently, the concurrent use of the agents is explicitly prohibited or contraindicated by the product labeling.
Increased Effect/Toxicity	Drug combinations that result in a increased or toxic therapeutic effect between the drug listed in the monograph and other drugs or drug classes.
Decreased Effect	Drug combinations that result in a decreased therapeutic effect between the drug listed in the monograph and other drugs or drug classes.

Ethanol/Nutrition/Herb Interactions	Presents a description of the interaction between the drug listed in the monograph and ethanol, food, or herb/nutraceuticals.
Stability	Information regarding storage of product or steps for reconstitution. Provides the time and conditions for which a solution or mixture will maintain full potency. For example, some solutions may require refrigeration after reconstitution while stored at room temperature prior to preparation. Also includes compatibility information. **Note:** Professional judgment of the individual pharmacist in application of this information is imperative. While drug products may exhibit stability over longer durations of time, it may not be appropriate to utilize the drug product due to concerns in sterility.
Mechanism of Action	How the drug works in the body to elicit a response
Pharmacodynamics/ Kinetics	The magnitude of a drug's effect depends on the drug concentration at the site of action. The pharmacodynamics are expressed in terms of onset of action and duration of action. Pharmacokinetics are expressed in terms of absorption, distribution (including appearance in breast milk and crossing of the placenta), protein binding, metabolism, bioavailability, half-life, time to peak serum concentration, and elimination.
Dosage	The amount of the drug to be typically given or taken during therapy for children and adults; also includes any dosing adjustment/comments for renal impairment or hepatic impairment and other suggested dosing adjustments (eg, hematological toxicity)
Dietary Considerations	Includes information on how the medication should be taken relative to meals or food.
Administration	Information regarding the recommended final concentrations, rates of administration for parenteral drugs, or other guidelines when giving the medication
Monitoring Parameters	Laboratory tests and patient physical parameters that should be monitored for safety and efficacy of drug therapy
Reference Range	Therapeutic and toxic serum concentrations listed including peak and trough levels
Test Interactions	Listing of assay interferences when relevant; (B) = Blood; (S) = Serum; (U) = Urine
Additional Information	Information about sodium content and/or pertinent information about specific brands
Product Availability	Provides availability information on products that have been approved by the FDA, but not yet available for use. Estimates for when a product may be available are included, when this information is known. May also provide any unique or critical drug availability issues.
Dosage Forms	Information with regard to form, strength, and availability of the drug in the United States. **Note:** Additional formulation information (eg, excipients, preservatives) is included when available. Please consult labeling for further information.
Dosage Forms: Canada	Information with regard to form, strength, and availability of products that are uniquely available in Canada, but currently not available in the United States.
Controlled Substance	Contains controlled substance schedule information as assigned by the United States Drug Enforcement Administration (DEA) or Canadian Controlled Substance Act (CDSA). CDSA information is only provided for drugs available in Canada and not available in the U.S.
Extemporaneous Preparations	Directions for preparing liquid formulations from solid drug products. May include stability information and references.

PREGNANCY CATEGORIES

Pregnancy Categories (sometimes referred to as pregnancy risk factors) are a letter system currently required under the *Teratogenic Effects* subsection of the product labeling. The system was initiated in 1979. The categories are required to be part of the package insert for prescription drugs that are systemically absorbed.

The categories are defined as follows:

A Adequate and well-controlled studies in pregnant women have not shown that the drug increases the risk of fetal abnormalities.

B Animal reproduction studies show no evidence of impaired fertility or harm to the fetus; however, no adequate and well-controlled studies have been conducted in pregnant women.
or
Animal reproduction studies have shown adverse events; however, studies in pregnant women have not shown that the drug increases the risk of abnormalities.

C Animal reproduction studies have shown an adverse effect on the fetus. There are no adequate and well-controlled studies in humans and the benefits from the use of the drug in pregnant women may be acceptable, despite its potential risks.
or
Animal reproduction studies have not been conducted.

D Based on human data, the drug can cause fetal harm when administered to pregnant women, but the potential benefits from the use of the drug may be acceptable, despite its potential risks.

X Studies in animals or humans have demonstrated fetal abnormalities (or there is positive evidence of fetal risk based on reports and/or marketing experience) and the risk of using the drug in pregnant women clearly outweighs any possible benefit (for example, safer drugs or other forms of therapy are available).

The categories do not take into consideration nonteratogenic effects (that information is currently presented separately). In 2008, the Food and Drug Administration (FDA) proposed new labeling requirements which would eliminate the use of the pregnancy category system and replace it with scientific data and other information specific to the use of the drug in pregnant women. These proposed changes were suggested because the current category system may be misleading. For instance, some practitioners may believe that risk increases from category A to B to C to D to X, which is not the intent. In addition, practitioners may not be aware that some medications are categorized based on animal data, while others are based on human data. When the new labeling requirements are approved, product labeling will contain pregnancy and lactation subsections, each describing a risk summary, clinical considerations, and section for specific data.

For full descriptions of the current and proposed labeling requirements, refer to the following websites:

Labeling Requirements for Prescription Drugs and/or Insulin (Code of Federal Regulations, Title 21, Volume 4, Revised April 1, 2010). Available at http://www.accessdata.fda.gov/scripts/cdrh/cfdocs/cfCFR/CFRSearch.cfm?fr=201.57

Content and Format of Labeling for Human Prescription Drug and Biological Products; Requirements for Pregnancy and Lactation Labeling (Federal Register, May 29, 2008). Available at http://frwebgate.access.gpo.gov/cgi-bin/getdoc.cgi?dbname=2008_register&docid=fr29my08-33.pdf

PREVENTING PRESCRIBING ERRORS

Prescribing errors account for the majority of reported medication errors and have prompted healthcare professionals to focus on the development of steps to make the prescribing process safer. Prescription legibility has been attributed to a portion of these errors and legislation has been enacted in several states to address prescription legibility. However, eliminating handwritten prescriptions and ordering medications through the use of technology [eg, computerized prescriber order entry (CPOE)] has been the primary recommendation. Whether a prescription is electronic, typed, or hand-printed, additional safe practices should be considered for implementation to maximize the safety of the prescribing process. Listed below are suggestions for safer prescribing:

- Ensure correct patient by using at least 2 patient identifiers on the prescription (eg, full name, birth date, or address). Review prescription with the patient or patient's caregiver.
- If pediatric patient, document patient's birth date or age and most recent weight. If geriatric patient, document patient's birth date or age.
- Prevent drug name confusion:
  - Use TALLman lettering (eg, buPROPion, busPIRone, predniSONE, prednisoLONE). For more information see http://www.fda.gov/Drugs/DrugSafety/MedicationErrors/ucm164587.htm.
  - Avoid abbreviated drug names (eg, MSO_4, $MgSO_4$, MS, HCT, 6MP, MTX), as they may be misinterpreted and cause error.
  - Avoid investigational names for drugs with FDA approval (eg, FK-506, CBDCA).
  - Avoid chemical names such as 6-mercaptopurine or 6-thioguanine, as sixfold overdoses have been given when these were not recognized as chemical names. The proper names of these drugs are mercaptopurine or thioguanine.
  - Use care when prescribing drugs that look or sound similar (eg, look- alike, sound-alike drugs). Common examples include: Celebrex® vs Celexa®, hydroxyzine vs hydralazine, Zyprexa® vs Zyrtec®.
- Avoid dangerous, error-prone abbreviations (eg, regardless of letter-case: U, IU, QD, QOD, µg, cc, @). Do not use apothecary system or symbols. Additionally, text messaging abbreviations (eg, "2Day") should never be used.
  - For more information see http://www.ismp.org/Tools/errorproneabbreviations.pdf
- Always use a leading zero for numbers less than 1 (0.5 mg is correct and .5 mg is **incorrect**) and never use a trailing zero for whole numbers (2 mg is correct and 2.0 mg is **incorrect**).
- Always use a space between a number and its units as it is easier to read. There should be no periods after the abbreviations mg or mL (10 mg is correct and 10mg is **incorrect**).
- For doses that are greater than 1,000 dosing units, use properly placed commas to prevent 10-fold errors (100,000 units is correct and 100000 units is **incorrect**).
- Do not prescribe drug dosage by the type of container in which the drug is available (eg, do not prescribe "1 amp", "2 vials", etc).
- Do not write vague or ambiguous orders which have the potential for misinterpretation by other healthcare providers. Examples of vague orders to avoid: "Resume pre-op medications," "give drug per protocol," or "continue home medications."
- Review each prescription with patient (or patient's caregiver) including the medication name, indication, and directions for use.
- Take extra precautions when prescribing *high alert drugs* (drugs that can cause significant patient harm when prescribed in error). Common examples of these drugs include: Anticoagulants, chemotherapy, insulins, opiates, and sedatives.
  - For more information see http://www.ismp.org/Tools/highalertmedications.pdf

To Err Is Human: Building a Safer Health System, Kohn LT, Corrigan JM, and Donaldson MS, eds, Washington, D.C.: National Academy Press, 2000.

A Complete Outpatient Prescription[1]

A complete outpatient prescription can prevent the prescriber, the pharmacist, and/or the patient from making a mistake and can eliminate the need for further clarification. The complete outpatient prescription should contain:

- Patient's full name
- Medication indication
- Allergies
- Prescriber name and telephone or pager number
- For pediatric patients: Their birth date or age and current weight
- For geriatric patients: Their birth date or age
- Drug name, dosage form and strength
- For pediatric patients: Intended daily weight-based dose so that calculations can be checked by the pharmacist (ie, mg/kg/day or units/kg/day)
- Number or amount to be dispensed
- Complete instructions for the patient or caregiver, including the purpose of the medication, directions for use (including dose), dosing frequency, route of administration, duration of therapy, and number of refills.
- Dose should be expressed in convenient units of measure.
- When there are recognized contraindications for a prescribed drug, the prescriber should indicate knowledge of this fact to the pharmacist (ie, when prescribing a potassium salt for a patient receiving an ACE inhibitor, the prescriber should write "K serum leveling being monitored").

Upon dispensing of the final product, the pharmacist should ensure that the patient or caregiver can effectively demonstrate the appropriate administration technique. An appropriate measuring device should be provided or recommended. Household teaspoons and tablespoons should not be used to measure liquid medications due to their variability and inaccuracies in measurement; oral medication syringes are recommended.

For additional information see http://www.ppag.org/attachments/files/111/Guidelines_Peds.pdf

[1]Levine SR, Cohen MR, Blanchard NR, et al, "Guidelines for Preventing Medication Errors in Pediatrics," *J Pediatr Pharmacol Ther*, 2001, 6:426-42.

FDA NAME DIFFERENTIATION PROJECT: THE USE OF TALL-MAN LETTERS

Confusion between similar drug names is an important cause of medication errors. For years, The Institute For Safe Medication Practices (ISMP), has urged generic manufacturers to use a combination of large and small letters as well as bolding (ie, chlorpro**MAZINE** and chlorpro**PAMIDE**) to help distinguish drugs with look-alike names, especially when they share similar strengths. Recently the FDA's Division of Generic Drugs began to issue recommendation letters to manufacturers suggesting this novel way to label their products to help reduce this drug name confusion. Although this project has had marginal success, the method has successfully eliminated problems with products such as diphenhydr**AMINE** and dimenhy**DRINATE**. Hospitals should also follow suit by making similar changes in their own labels, preprinted order forms, computer screens and printouts, and drug storage location labels.

Lexi-Comp, Inc. Medical Publishing will use "Tall-Man" letters for the drugs suggested by the FDA or recommended by ISMP.

The following is a list of generic and brand name product names and recommended revisions.

Drug Product	Recommended Revision
acetazolamide	aceta**ZOLAMIDE**
alprazolam	**ALPRAZ**olam
amiloride	a**MIL**oride
amlodipine	am**LODIP**ine
aripiprazole	**ARIP**iprazole
Avinza	**AVIN**za
azacitidine	aza**CITID**ine
azathioprine	aza**THIO**prine
bupropion	bu**PROP**ion
buspirone	bus**PIR**one
carbamazepine	car**BAM**azepine
carboplatin	**CARBO**platin
cefazolin	ce**FAZ**olin
cefotetan	cefo**TE**tan
cefoxitin	cef**OX**itin
ceftazidime	cef**TAZ**idime
ceftriaxone	cef**TRIAX**one
Celebrex	Cele**BREX**
Celexa	Cele**XA**
chlordiazepoxide	chlordiaze**POXIDE**
chlorpromazine	chlorpro**MAZINE**
chlorpropamide	chlorpro**PAMIDE**
cisplatin	**CIS**platin
clomiphene	clomi**PHENE**
clomipramine	clomi**PRAMINE**
clonazepam	clonaze**PAM**
clonidine	clo**NID**ine
clozapine	clo**ZAP**ine
cycloserine	cyclo**SERINE**
cyclosporine	cyclo**SPORINE**
dactinomycin	**DACTIN**omycin
daptomycin	**DAPTO**mycin
daunorubicin	**DAUNO**rubicin
dimenhydrinate	dimenhy**DRINATE**
diphenhydramine	diphenhydr**AMINE**
dobutamine	**DOBUT**amine
docetaxel	**DOCE**taxel
dopamine	**DOP**amine
doxorubicin	**DOXO**rubicin
duloxetine	**DUL**oxetine
ephedrine	e**PHED**rine
epinephrine	**EPINEPH**rine
fentanyl	fenta**NYL**

Drug Product	Recommended Revision
flavoxate	flavox**ATE**
fluoxetine	**FLU**oxetine
fluphenazine	flu**PHENAZ**ine
fluvoxamine	fluvoxa**MINE**
glipizide	glipi**ZIDE**
glyburide	gly**BURIDE**
guaifenesin	guai**FEN**esin
guanfacine	guan**FACINE**
Humalog	Huma**LOG**
Humulin	Humu**LIN**
hydralazine	hydr**ALAZINE**
hydrocodone	**HYDRO**codone
hydromorphone	**HYDRO**morphone
hydroxyzine	hydr**OXY**zine
idarubicin	**IDA**rubicin
infliximab	in**FLIX**imab
Invanz	**INV**anz
isotretinoin	**ISO**tretinoin
Klonopin	Klono**PIN**
Lamictal	La**MIC**tal
Lamisil	Lam**ISIL**
lamivudine	lami**VUD**ine
lamotrigine	lamo**TRI**gine
levetiracetam	Lev**ETIRA**cetam
levocarnitine	lev**OCARN**itine
lorazepam	**LOR**azepam
medroxyprogesterone	medroxy**PROGESTER**one
metformin	met**FORMIN**
methylprednisolone	methyl**PREDNIS**olone
methyltestosterone	methyl**TESTOSTER**one
metronidazole	metro**NIDAZOLE**
mitomycin	mito**MY**cin
mitoxantrone	Mito**XAN**trone
Nexavar	Nex**AVAR**
Nexium	Nex**IUM**
nicardipine	ni**CAR**dipine
nifedipine	**NIFE**dipine
nimodipine	ni**MOD**ipine
Novolin	Novo**LIN**
Novolog	Novo**LOG**
olanzapine	**OLANZ**apine
oxcarbazepine	**OX**carbazepine
oxycodone	oxy**CODONE**
Oxycontin	Oxy**CONTIN**
paclitaxel	**PACL**itaxel
paroxetine	**PAR**oxetine
pemetrexed	**PEME**trexed
penicillamine	penicill**AMINE**
pentobarbital	**PENT**obarbital
phenobarbital	**PHEN**obarbital
pralatrexate	**PRALA**trexate
prednisolone	predniso**LONE**
prednisone	predni**SONE**
Prilosec	Pri**LOSEC**
Prozac	**PRO**zac
quetiapine	**QUE**tiapine
quinidine	qui**NID**ine

Drug Product	Recommended Revision
quinine	qui**NINE**
rabeprazole	**RABE**prazole
Risperdal	Risper**DAL**
risperidone	risperi**DONE**
rituximab	ri**TUX**imab
romidepsin	romi**DEP**sin
romiplostim	romi**PLOS**tim
ropinirole	r**OPINIR**ole
Sandimmune	sand**IMMUNE**
Sandostatin	Sando**STATIN**
Seroquel	**SERO**quel
Sinequan	**SINE**quan
sitagliptin	sita**GLIP**tin
Solu-Cortef	Solu-**CORTEF**
Solu-Medrol	Solu-**MEDROL**
sorafenib	**SORA**fenib
sufentanil	**SUF**entanil
sulfadiazine	sulf**ADIAZINE**
sulfasalazine	sulfa**SALA**zine
sumatriptan	**SUMA**triptan
sunitinib	**SUNI**tinib
Tegretol	**TEG**retol
tiagabine	tia**GAB**ine
tizanidine	ti**ZAN**idine
tolazamide	**TOLAZ**amide
tolbutamide	**TOLBUT**amide
tramadol	tra**MAD**ol
trazodone	tra**ZOD**one
Trental	**TREN**tal
valacyclovir	val**ACY**clovir
valganciclovir	val**GAN**ciclovir
vinblastine	vin**BLAS**tine
vincristine	vin**CRIS**tine
zolmitriptan	**ZOLM**itriptan
Zyprexa	Zy**PREXA**
Zyrtec	Zyr**TEC**

"FDA and ISMP Lists of Look-Alike Drug Names with Recommended Tall Man Letter." Available at http://www.ismp.org/tools/tallmanletters.pdf. Last accessed January 6, 2011.
"Name Differentiation Project." Available at http://www.fda.gov/Drugs/DrugSafety/MedicationErrors/ucm164587.htm. Last accessed January 6, 2011.
U.S. Pharmacopeia, "USP Quality Review: Use Caution-Avoid Confusion," March 2001, No. 76. Available at http://www.usp.org

ALPHABETICAL LISTING OF DRUGS

- ◆ **A-25 [OTC]** *see* Vitamin A *on page 1795*
- ◆ **A200® Lice [OTC]** *see* Permethrin *on page 1336*
- ◆ **A-200® Lice Treatment Kit [OTC]** *see* Pyrethrins and Piperonyl Butoxide *on page 1435*
- ◆ **A-200® Maximum Strength [OTC]** *see* Pyrethrins and Piperonyl Butoxide *on page 1435*
- ◆ **A and D® Original [OTC]** *see* Vitamin A and Vitamin D *on page 1796*

Abacavir (a BAK a veer)

Brand Names: U.S. Ziagen®

Brand Names: Canada Ziagen®

Index Terms Abacavir Sulfate; ABC

Pharmacologic Category Antiretroviral Agent, Reverse Transcriptase Inhibitor (Nucleoside)

Additional Appendix Information

Management of Healthcare Worker Exposures to HBV, HCV, and HIV *on page 1935*

Perinatal HIV Guidelines *on page 1946*

Use Treatment of HIV infections in combination with other antiretroviral agents

Pregnancy Risk Factor C

Pregnancy Considerations Adverse events have been observed in some animal reproduction studies. Abacavir crosses the human placenta. No increased risk of overall birth defects has been observed following first trimester exposure according to data collected by the antiretroviral pregnancy registry. Cases of lactic acidosis/hepatic steatosis syndrome related to mitochondrial toxicity have been reported in pregnant women with prolonged use of nucleoside analogues. It is not known if pregnancy itself potentiates this known side effect; however, women may be at increased risk of lactic acidosis and liver damage. In addition, these adverse events are similar to other rare but life-threatening syndromes which occur during pregnancy (eg, HELLP syndrome). Hepatic enzymes and electrolytes should be monitored in women receiving nucleoside analogues and clinicians should watch for early signs of the syndrome. In addition, mitochondrial dysfunction may develop in infants following *in utero* exposure. The pharmacokinetics of abacavir are not significantly changed by pregnancy and dose adjustment is not needed for pregnant women. The DHHS Perinatal HIV Guidelines consider abacavir to be an alternative NRTI in dual nucleoside combination regimens.

Regardless of CD4 count or HIV RNA copy number, all HIV-infected pregnant women should receive a combination antepartum antiretroviral (ARV) drug regimen; this includes women who require therapy for their own health, as well as women who do not yet require therapy for their own health. ARV therapy should be started as soon as possible if required for the woman's health or immediately after the first trimester if not needed for the mother's health (although earlier initiation may be considered). Long-term follow-up is recommended for all infants exposed to ARV medications.

Healthcare providers are encouraged to enroll pregnant women exposed to antiretroviral medications in the Antiretroviral Pregnancy Registry (1-800-258-4263 or www.APRegistry.com). Healthcare providers caring for HIV-infected women and their infants may contact the National Perinatal HIV Hotline (888-448-8765) for clinical consultation (DHHS [perinatal], 2011).

Lactation Excretion in breast milk unknown/contraindicated

Medication Guide Available Yes

Contraindications Hypersensitivity to abacavir or any component of the formulation (do not rechallenge patients who have experienced hypersensitivity to abacavir regardless of *HLA-B*5701* status); moderate-to-severe hepatic impairment

Warnings/Precautions Abacavir should always be used as a component of a multidrug regimen. **[U.S. Boxed Warning]: Serious and sometimes fatal hypersensitivity reactions have occurred.** Patients testing positive for the presence of the *HLA-B*5701* allele are at an increased risk for hypersensitivity reactions. Screening for *HLA-B*5701* allele status is recommended prior to initiating therapy or reinitiating therapy in patients of unknown status, including patients who previously tolerated therapy. Therapy is **not** recommended in patients testing positive for the *HLA-B*5701* allele. An allergy to abacavir should be reported in the patient's medical record (DHHS, 2011). Reactions usually occur within 9 days of starting abacavir; ~90% occur within 6 weeks. Patients exhibiting symptoms from two or more of the following: Fever, skin rash, constitutional symptoms (malaise, fatigue, aches), respiratory symptoms (eg, pharyngitis, dyspnea, cough), and GI symptoms (eg, abdominal pain, diarrhea, nausea, vomiting) should discontinue therapy immediately and call for medical attention. Abacavir should be permanently discontinued if hypersensitivity cannot be ruled out, even when other diagnoses are possible and regardless of *HLA-B*5701* status. Abacavir SHOULD NOT be restarted because more severe symptoms may occur within hours, including LIFE-THREATENING HYPOTENSION AND DEATH. Fatal hypersensitivity reactions have occurred following the reintroduction of abacavir in patients whose therapy was interrupted (ie, interruption in drug supply, temporary discontinuation while treating other conditions). In some cases, signs of hypersensitivity may have been previously present, but attributed to other medical conditions (eg, acute onset respiratory diseases, gastroenteritis, reactions to other medications). If abacavir is restarted following an interruption in therapy, evaluate the patient for previously unsuspected symptoms of hypersensitivity. To report these events on abacavir hypersensitivity, a registry has been established (1-800-270-0425). A higher incidence of severe hypersensitivity reactions may be associated with a 600 mg once daily dosing regimen.

[U.S. Boxed Warning]: Lactic acidosis and severe hepatomegaly with steatosis (sometimes fatal) have occurred with antiretroviral nucleoside analogues. Female gender, prior liver disease, obesity, and prolonged treatment may increase the risk of hepatotoxicity. May be associated with fat redistribution. Immune reconstitution syndrome may develop; further evaluation and treatment may be required. Use has been associated with an increased risk of myocardial infarction (MI) in observational studies; however, based on a meta-analysis of 26 randomized trials, the FDA has concluded there is not an increased risk. Consider using with caution in patients with risks for coronary heart disease and minimizing modifiable risk factors (eg, hypertension, hyperlipidemia, diabetes mellitus, and smoking) prior to use. Products may contain propylene glycol. Safety and efficacy in children <3 months of age have not been established.

Adverse Reactions Hypersensitivity reactions (which may be fatal) occur in ~5% of patients. Symptoms may include anaphylaxis, fever, rash (including erythema multiforme), fatigue, diarrhea, abdominal pain; respiratory symptoms (eg, pharyngitis, dyspnea, cough, adult respiratory distress syndrome, or respiratory failure); headache, malaise, lethargy, myalgia, myolysis, arthralgia, edema, paresthesia, nausea and vomiting, mouth ulcerations, conjunctivitis, lymphadenopathy, hepatic failure, and renal failure.

Note: Rates of adverse reactions were defined during combination therapy with other antiretrovirals (lamivudine and efavirenz **or** lamivudine and zidovudine). Only reactions which occurred at a higher frequency in adults (except where noted) than in the comparator group are noted. Adverse reaction rates attributable to abacavir alone are not available.

>10%:

Central nervous system: Headache (7% to 13%)
Gastrointestinal: Nausea (7% to 19%, children 9%)

1% to 10%:

Central nervous system: Depression (6%), fever/chills (6%, children 9%), anxiety (5%)
Dermatologic: Rash (5% to 6%, children 7%)
Endocrine & metabolic: Triglycerides increased (2% to 6%)
Gastrointestinal: Diarrhea (7%), vomiting (children 9%), amylase increased (2%)
Hematologic: Thrombocytopenia (1%)
Hepatic: AST increased (6%)
Neuromuscular & skeletal: Musculoskeletal pain (5% to 6%)
Miscellaneous: Hypersensitivity reactions (2% to 9%; may include reactions to other components of antiretroviral regimen), infection (ENT 5%)

<1% (Limited to important or life-threatening): Erythema multiforme, fat redistribution, GGT increased, hepatic steatosis, hepatomegaly, hepatotoxicity, lactic acidosis, MI, pancreatitis, Stevens-Johnson syndrome, toxic epidermal necrolysis

Drug Interactions

Metabolism/Transport Effects None known.

Avoid Concomitant Use There are no known interactions where it is recommended to avoid concomitant use.

Increased Effect/Toxicity

The levels/effects of Abacavir may be increased by: Ganciclovir-Valganciclovir; Ribavirin

Decreased Effect

The levels/effects of Abacavir may be decreased by: Protease Inhibitors

Ethanol/Nutrition/Herb Interactions Ethanol: Ethanol may increase the risk of toxicity.

Stability Store oral solution and tablets at controlled room temperature of 20°C to 25°C (68°F to 77°F). Oral solution may be refrigerated; do not freeze.

Mechanism of Action Nucleoside reverse transcriptase inhibitor. Abacavir is a guanosine analogue which is phosphorylated to carbovir triphosphate which interferes with HIV viral RNA-dependent DNA polymerase resulting in inhibition of viral replication.

Pharmacodynamics/Kinetics

Absorption: Rapid and extensive absorption
Distribution: V_d: 0.86 L/kg
Protein binding: 50%
Metabolism: Hepatic via alcohol dehydrogenase and glucuronyl transferase to inactive carboxylate and glucuronide metabolites
Bioavailability: 83%
Half-life elimination: 1.5 hours
Time to peak: 0.7-1.7 hours
Excretion: Primarily urine (as metabolites, 1.2% as unchanged drug); feces (16% total dose)

Dosage Oral:

Infants and Children ≥3 months to <16 years: 8 mg/kg body weight twice daily (maximum: 300 mg twice daily) in combination with other antiretroviral agents. **Note:** May consider 16-20 mg/kg once daily dosing (maximum: 600 mg/day) in stable patients with undetectable viral load and stable CD4 count (DHHS [Pediatric], 2011)

U.S. manufacturer labeling: Alternative dosing to be considered for pediatric patients ≥14 kg who are able to swallow tablets:
14-21 kg: 150 mg (1/2 tablet) twice daily
>21 kg to <30 kg: 150 mg (1/2 tablet) in the morning and 300 mg (1 tablet) in the evening
≥30 kg: 300 mg (1 tablet) twice daily

Adolescents ≥16 years and Adults: 300 mg twice daily or 600 mg once daily in combination with other antiretroviral agents (DHHS, 2011; DHHS [Pediatric], 2011)

Canadian labeling:
Infants and Children ≥3 months to 12 years: 8 mg/kg body weight twice daily (maximum: 300 mg twice daily) in combination with other antiretroviral agents
Adolescents >12 years and Adults: 300 mg twice daily in combination with other antiretroviral agents

Dosage adjustment in renal impairment: Canadian labeling (not in U.S. labeling): Use in ESRD or use of 600 mg once daily dosing is not recommended.

Dosage adjustment in hepatic impairment:
Mild impairment (Child-Pugh score 5-6): 200 mg twice daily (oral solution is recommended)
Moderate-to-severe impairment (Child-Pugh score >6): Use is contraindicated by the manufacturer

Dietary Considerations May be taken with or without food.

Administration May be administered with or without food.

Monitoring Parameters CBC with differential, serum creatine kinase, CD4 count, HIV RNA plasma levels, serum transaminases, triglycerides, serum amylase; *HLA-B*5701* genotype status prior to initiation of therapy and prior to reinitiation of therapy in patients of unknown *HLA-B*5701* status; signs and symptoms of hypersensitivity, particularly in patients untested for the *HLA-B*5701* allele

Additional Information A high rate of early virologic nonresponse was observed when abacavir, lamivudine, and tenofovir were used as the initial regimen in treatment-naive patients. Use of this combination is not recommended; patients currently on this regimen should be closely monitored for modification of therapy. Use regimens of abacavir and nevirapine with caution; both agents cause hypersensitivity reactions early in therapy (DHHS, 2011).

Hypersensitivity testing (*HLA-B*5701*): Prevalence of hypersensitivity reactions has been estimated at 5% to 8% in Caucasians and 2% to 3% in African-Americans. Pretherapy identification of *HLA-B*5701*-positive patients, and subsequent avoidance of abacavir therapy in these patients has been shown to reduce the occurrence of abacavir-mediated hypersensitivity reactions. An allergy to abacavir should be reported in the patient's medical record (DHHS, 2011). A skin patch test is in development for clinical screening purposes; however, only PCR-mediated genotyping methods are currently in clinical practice use for documentation of this susceptibility marker.

Dosage Forms Excipient information presented when available (limited, particularly for generics); consult specific product labeling. [DSC] = Discontinued product

Solution, oral:
Ziagen®: 20 mg/mL (240 mL [DSC]) [strawberry-banana flavor]
Ziagen®: 20 mg/mL (240 mL) [contains propylene glycol; strawberry-banana flavor]

Tablet, oral:
Ziagen®: 300 mg [DSC]
Ziagen®: 300 mg [scored]

Abacavir and Lamivudine

(a BAK a veer & la MI vyoo deen)

Brand Names: U.S. Epzicom®
Brand Names: Canada Kivexa™
Index Terms Abacavir Sulfate and Lamivudine; Lamivudine and Abacavir
Pharmacologic Category Antiretroviral Agent, Reverse Transcriptase Inhibitor (Nucleoside)
Use Treatment of HIV infections in combination with other antiretroviral agents
Pregnancy Risk Factor C
Medication Guide Available Yes
Dosage Oral: Adults: HIV: One tablet (abacavir 600 mg and lamivudine 300 mg) once daily
Dosage adjustment in renal impairment: Cl_{cr} <50 mL/minute: Use not recommended
Dosage adjustment in hepatic impairment: Use contraindicated.
Additional Information Complete prescribing information for this medication should be consulted for additional detail.
Dosage Forms Excipient information presented when available (limited, particularly for generics); consult specific product labeling.
Tablet:
Epzicom®: Abacavir 600 mg and lamivudine 300 mg

Abacavir, Lamivudine, and Zidovudine

(a BAK a veer, la MI vyoo deen, & zye DOE vyoo deen)

Brand Names: U.S. Trizivir®
Brand Names: Canada Trizivir®
Index Terms 3TC, Abacavir, and Zidovudine; Azidothymidine, Abacavir, and Lamivudine; AZT, Abacavir, and Lamivudine; Compound S, Abacavir, and Lamivudine; Lamivudine, Abacavir, and Zidovudine; ZDV, Abacavir, and Lamivudine; Zidovudine, Abacavir, and Lamivudine
Pharmacologic Category Antiretroviral Agent, Reverse Transcriptase Inhibitor (Nucleoside)
Use Treatment of HIV infection (either alone or in combination with other antiretroviral agents) in patients whose regimen would otherwise contain the components of Trizivir®
Pregnancy Risk Factor C
Medication Guide Available Yes
Dosage Oral:
Adolescents ≥40 kg and Adults: 1 tablet twice daily
Dosage adjustment in renal impairment: Because lamivudine and zidovudine require dosage adjustment in renal impairment, Trizivir® should not be used in patients with Cl_{cr} <50 mL/minute
Dosage adjustment in hepatic impairment: Use contraindicated.
Additional Information Complete prescribing information for this medication should be consulted for additional detail.
Dosage Forms Excipient information presented when available (limited, particularly for generics); consult specific product labeling.
Tablet, oral:
Trizivir®: Abacavir sulfate 300 mg, lamivudine 150 mg, and zidovudine 300 mg

◆ **Abacavir Sulfate** *see* Abacavir *on page 18*
◆ **Abacavir Sulfate and Lamivudine** *see* Abacavir and Lamivudine *on page 20*

Abatacept

(ab a TA sept)

Brand Names: U.S. Orencia®
Brand Names: Canada Orencia®
Index Terms BMS-188667; CTLA-4Ig
Pharmacologic Category Antirheumatic, Disease Modifying; Selective T-Cell Costimulation Blocker
Use
Treatment of moderately- to severely-active adult rheumatoid arthritis (RA); may be used as monotherapy or in combination with other DMARDs
Treatment of moderately- to severely-active juvenile idiopathic arthritis (JIA); may be used as monotherapy or in combination with methotrexate
Note: Abatacept should **not** be used in combination with anakinra or TNF-blocking agents
Pregnancy Risk Factor C
Pregnancy Considerations Teratogenic effects were not observed in animal studies. There are no adequate and well-controlled studies in pregnant women. Due to the potential risk for development of autoimmune disease in the fetus, use during pregnancy only if clearly needed. A pregnancy registry has been established to monitor outcomes of women exposed to abatacept during pregnancy (1-877-311-8972).
Lactation Excretion in breast milk unknown/not recommended
Contraindications There are no contraindications listed within the FDA-approved labeling.
Warnings/Precautions Serious and potentially fatal infections (including tuberculosis and sepsis) have been reported, particularly in patients receiving concomitant immunosuppressive therapy. RA patients receiving a concomitant TNF antagonist experienced an even higher rate of serious infection. Caution should be exercised when considering the use of abatacept in any patient with a history of recurrent infections, with conditions that predispose them to infections, or with chronic, latent, or localized infections. Patients who develop a new infection while undergoing treatment should be monitored closely. If a patient develops a serious infection, abatacept should be discontinued. Screen patients for latent tuberculosis infection prior to initiating abatacept; safety in tuberculosis-positive patients has not been established. Treat patients testing positive according to standard therapy prior to initiating abatacept. Adult patients receiving abatacept in combination with TNF-blocking agents had higher rates of infections (including serious infections) than patients on TNF-blocking agents alone. The manufacturer does not recommend concurrent use with anakinra or TNF-blocking agents. Monitor for signs and symptoms of infection when transitioning from TNF-blocking agents to abatacept. Due to the effect of T-cell inhibition on host defenses, abatacept may affect immune responses against infections and malignancies; impact on the development and course of malignancies is not fully defined.

Use caution with chronic obstructive pulmonary disease (COPD), higher incidences of adverse effects (COPD exacerbation, cough, rhonchi, dyspnea) have been observed; monitor closely. Rare cases of hypersensitivity, anaphylaxis, or anaphylactoid reactions have been reported; medications for the treatment of hypersensitivity reactions should be available for immediate use. Patients should be screened for viral hepatitis prior to use; antirheumatic therapy may cause reactivation of hepatitis B. Patients should be brought up to date with all immunizations before initiating therapy. Live vaccines should not be given concurrently or within 3 months of discontinuation of therapy; there is no data available concerning secondary transmission of live vaccines in patients receiving therapy. Powder for injection may contain maltose, which may result in falsely-elevated serum glucose readings on the day of infusion. Higher incidences of infection and malignancy were observed in the elderly; use with caution.

Adverse Reactions Note: Percentages not always reported; COPD patients experienced a higher frequency of COPD-related adverse reactions (COPD exacerbation, cough, dyspnea, pneumonia, rhonchi)

>10%:

Central nervous system: Headache (≤18%)
Gastrointestinal: Nausea
Respiratory: Nasopharyngitis (12%), upper respiratory tract infection
Miscellaneous: Infection (adults 54%; children 36%), antibody formation (2% to 41%)

1% to 10%:

Cardiovascular: Hypertension (7%)
Central nervous system: Dizziness (9%), fever
Dermatologic: Rash (4%)
Gastrointestinal: Dyspepsia (6%), abdominal pain, diarrhea
Genitourinary: Urinary tract infection (6%)
Local: Injection site reaction (3%)
Neuromuscular & skeletal: Back pain (7%), limb pain (3%)
Respiratory: Cough (8%), bronchitis, pneumonia, rhinitis, sinusitis
Miscellaneous: Infusion-related reactions (≤9%), herpes simplex, immunogenicity (1% to 2%), influenza

<1% (Limited to important or life-threatening): Acute lymphocytic leukemia, anaphylaxis, anaphylactoid reactions, cellulitis, COPD exacerbation, disease flare, diverticulitis, dyspnea, flushing, hypersensitivity, hypotension, joint wear, lung cancer, lymphoma; malignancies (including bile duct, bladder, breast, cervical, melanoma, myelodysplastic syndrome, prostate, renal, skin, thyroid and uterine); ovarian cyst, pruritus, pyelonephritis, rhonchi, urticaria, varicella infection, vasculitis (including cutaneous vasculitis and leukocytoclastic vasculitis), wheezing

Drug Interactions

Metabolism/Transport Effects None known.

Avoid Concomitant Use

Avoid concomitant use of Abatacept with any of the following: Anti-TNF Agents; BCG; Belimumab; Natalizumab; Pimecrolimus; Tacrolimus (Topical); Vaccines (Live)

Increased Effect/Toxicity

Abatacept may increase the levels/effects of: Belimumab; Leflunomide; Natalizumab; Vaccines (Live)

The levels/effects of Abatacept may be increased by: Anti-TNF Agents; Denosumab; Pimecrolimus; Roflumilast; Tacrolimus (Topical); Trastuzumab

Decreased Effect

Abatacept may decrease the levels/effects of: BCG; Coccidioidin Skin Test; Sipuleucel-T; Vaccines (Inactivated); Vaccines (Live)

The levels/effects of Abatacept may be decreased by: Echinacea

Ethanol/Nutrition/Herb Interactions Herb/Nutraceutical: Avoid echinacea (has immunostimulant properties; consider therapy modifications).

Stability

Prefilled syringe: Store at 2°C to 8°C (36°F to 46°F); do not freeze. Protect from light.

Powder for injection: Prior to reconstitution, store at 2°C to 8°C (36°F to 46°F); do not freeze. Protect from light. Reconstitute each vial with 10 mL SWFI using the provided silicone-free disposable syringe (discard solutions accidentally reconstituted with siliconized syringe as they may develop translucent particles). Inject SWFI down the side of the vial to avoid foaming. The reconstituted solution contains 25 mg/mL abatacept. Further dilute (using a silicone-free syringe) in 100 mL NS to a final concentration of ≤10 mg/mL. Prior to adding abatacept to the 100 mL bag, the manufacturer recommends withdrawing a volume of NS equal to the abatacept volume required, resulting in a final volume of 100 mL. Mix gently; do not shake.

After dilution, may be stored for up to 24 hours at room temperature or refrigerated at 2°C to 8°C (36°F to 46°F). Must be used within 24 hours of reconstitution.

Mechanism of Action Selective costimulation modulator; inhibits T-cell (T-lymphocyte) activation by binding to CD80 and CD86 on antigen presenting cells (APC), thus blocking the required CD28 interaction between APCs and T cells. Activated T lymphocytes are found in the synovium of rheumatoid arthritis patients.

Pharmacodynamics/Kinetics

Bioavailability: SubQ: 78.6% (relative to I.V. administration)
Distribution: V_{ss}: 0.02-0.13 L/kg
Half-life elimination: 8-25 days

Dosage

Children 6-17 years: JIA: I.V.:

<75 kg: 10 mg/kg, repeat dose at 2 and 4 weeks after initial infusion, and every 4 weeks thereafter
≥75 kg: Refer to adult I.V. dosing; maximum dose: 1000 mg

Adults: RA:

I.V.: Dosing is according to body weight:

<60 kg: 500 mg
60-100 kg: 750 mg
>100 kg: 1000 mg

I.V. regimen: Following the initial I.V. infusion, repeat I.V. dose (using the same weight-based dosing) at 2 weeks and 4 weeks after the initial infusion, and every 4 weeks thereafter.

SubQ regimen: Following the initial I.V. infusion (using the weight-based dosing), administer 125 mg subcutaneously within 24 hours of the infusion, followed by 125 mg subcutaneously once weekly thereafter. **Note:** Patients unable to receive I.V. infusions may omit the initial I.V. loading dose and initiate once weekly SubQ therapy directly.

Transitioning from I.V. therapy to SubQ therapy: Administer the first SubQ dose instead of the next scheduled I.V. dose.

Elderly: Refer to adult dosing; due to potential for higher rates of infections and malignancies, use caution.

Dosage adjustment for toxicity: Discontinue in patients who develop a serious infection.

Administration

I.V.: Infuse over 30 minutes. Administer through a 0.2-1.2 micron low protein-binding filter

SubQ: Allow prefilled syringe to warm to room temperature (for 30-60 minutes) prior to administration. Inject into the front of the thigh (preferred), abdomen (except for 2-inch area around the navel), or the outer area of the upper arms (if administered by a caregiver). Rotate injection sites (≥1 inch apart); do not administer into tender, bruised, red, or hard skin.

Monitoring Parameters Signs and symptoms of infection, signs and symptoms of hypersensitivity reaction; hepatitis and TB screening prior to therapy initiation

Test Interactions Contains maltose; may result in falsely elevated blood glucose levels with dehydrogenase pyrroloquinolinequinone or glucose-dye-oxidoreductase testing methods on the day of infusion. Glucose monitoring methods which utilize glucose dehydrogenase nicotine adenine dinucleotide (GDH-NAD), glucose oxidase, or glucose hexokinase are recommended.

Dosage Forms Excipient information presented when available (limited, particularly for generics); consult specific product labeling.

Injection, powder for reconstitution [preservative free]:
Orencia®: 250 mg [contains maltose]

Injection, solution [preservative free]:
Orencia®: 125 mg/mL (1 mL) [contains sucrose 170 mg/mL]

- **Abbott-43818** *see* Leuprolide *on page 989*
- **ABC** *see* Abacavir *on page 18*
- **ABCD** *see* Amphotericin B Cholesteryl Sulfate Complex *on page 108*

Abciximab (ab SIK si mab)

Brand Names: U.S. Reopro®
Brand Names: Canada ReoPro®
Index Terms 7E3; C7E3
Pharmacologic Category Antiplatelet Agent, Glycoprotein IIb/IIIa Inhibitor
Use Prevention of cardiac ischemic complications in patients undergoing percutaneous coronary intervention (PCI); prevention of cardiac ischemic complications in patients with unstable angina not responding to conventional therapy when PCI is scheduled within 24 hours

Note: Intended for use with aspirin and heparin, at a minimum.

Unlabeled Use To support PCI during ST-elevation myocardial infarction (STEMI) (administered at the time of primary PCI); STEMI as an adjunct to half-dose thrombolysis (eg, tenecteplase). **Note:** The 2004 ACC/AHA STEMI guidelines state that combination of abciximab and half-dose thrombolysis may be considered in selected patients (ie, anterior location of MI, age <75 years, and no risk factors for bleeding). However, given similar mortality between treatment groups and higher incidence of bleeding especially in the elderly in clinical trials, the 2008 ACCP guidelines recommend against the use of combination therapy for any patient with acute STEMI.
Pregnancy Risk Factor C
Pregnancy Considerations Animal reproduction studies have not been conducted. *In vitro* studies have shown only small amounts of abciximab to cross the placenta. It is not known whether abciximab can cause fetal harm when administered to a pregnant woman or can affect reproduction capacity.
Lactation Excretion in breast milk unknown/use caution
Contraindications Hypersensitivity to abciximab, murine proteins, or any component of the formulation; active internal hemorrhage or recent (within 6 weeks) clinically-significant GI or GU bleeding; history of cerebrovascular accident within 2 years or with significant neurological deficit; clotting abnormalities or administration of oral anticoagulants within 7 days unless prothrombin time (PT) is ≤1.2 times control PT value; thrombocytopenia (<100,000 cells/µL); recent (within 6 weeks) major surgery or trauma; intracranial tumor, arteriovenous malformation, or aneurysm; severe uncontrolled hypertension; history of vasculitis; use of dextran before PTCA or intent to use dextran during PTCA; concomitant use of another parenteral GP IIb/IIIa inhibitor
Warnings/Precautions Administration of abciximab is associated with increased frequency of major bleeding complications, including retroperitoneal bleeding, pulmonary bleeding, spontaneous GI or GU bleeding, and bleeding at the arterial access. Risk may be increased with patients weighing <75 kg, elderly patients (>65 years of age), history of previous GI disease, and recent thrombolytic therapy. When attempting I.V. access, avoid non-compressible sites (eg, subclavian or jugular veins).

The risk of major bleeds may increase with concurrent use of thrombolytics. Anticoagulation, such as with heparin, may contribute to the risk of bleeding. In serious, uncontrolled bleeding, abciximab and heparin should be stopped. Increased risk of hemorrhage during or following angioplasty is associated with unsuccessful PTCA, PTCA procedure >70 minutes duration, or PTCA performed within 12 hours of symptom onset for acute myocardial infarction. Prior to pulling the sheath, heparin should be discontinued for 3-4 hours and ACT ≤175 seconds or aPTT ≤50 seconds. Use standard compression techniques after sheath removal. Watch the site closely afterwards for further bleeding.

Administration of abciximab may result in human antichimeric antibody formation that can cause hypersensitivity reactions (including anaphylaxis), thrombocytopenia, or diminished efficacy. Readministration of abciximab within 30 days or in patients with human antichimeric antibodies (HACA) increases the incidence and severity of thrombocytopenia.
Adverse Reactions As with all drugs which may affect hemostasis, bleeding is associated with abciximab. Hemorrhage may occur at virtually any site. Risk is dependent on multiple variables, including the concurrent use of multiple agents which alter hemostasis and patient susceptibility.

>10%:
- Cardiovascular: Hypotension (14.4%), chest pain (11.4%)
- Gastrointestinal: Nausea (13.6%)
- Hematologic: Minor bleeding (4.0% to 16.8%)
- Neuromuscular & skeletal: Back pain (17.6%)

1% to 10%:
- Cardiovascular: Bradycardia (4.5%), peripheral edema (1.6%)
- Central nervous system: Headache (6.45)
- Gastrointestinal: Vomiting (7.3%), abdominal pain (3.1%)
- Hematologic: Major bleeding (1.1% to 14%), thrombocytopenia: <100,000 cells/mm^3 (2.5% to 5.6%); <50,000 cells/mm^3 (0.4% to 1.7%)
- Local: Injection site pain (3.6%)

<1% (Limited to important or life-threatening): Abnormal thinking, allergic reactions/anaphylaxis (possible), AV block, bronchospasm, bullous eruption, coma, confusion, diabetes mellitus, embolism, hyperkalemia, ileus, inflammation, intracranial hemorrhage, myalgia, nodal arrhythmia, pleural effusion, pulmonary embolism, prostatitis, pruritus, stroke, urinary retention, ventricular tachycardia, xerostomia
Drug Interactions
Metabolism/Transport Effects None known.
Avoid Concomitant Use
Avoid concomitant use of Abciximab with any of the following: Belimumab; Dextran
Increased Effect/Toxicity
Abciximab may increase the levels/effects of: Anticoagulants; Antiplatelet Agents; Belimumab; Collagenase (Systemic); Drotrecogin Alfa (Activated); Ibritumomab; Monoclonal Antibodies; Rivaroxaban; Salicylates; Thrombolytic Agents; Tositumomab and Iodine I 131 Tositumomab

The levels/effects of Abciximab may be increased by: Dasatinib; Dextran; Glucosamine; Herbs (Anticoagulant/Antiplatelet Properties); Nonsteroidal Anti-Inflammatory Agents; Omega-3-Acid Ethyl Esters; Pentosan Polysulfate Sodium; Pentoxifylline; Prostacyclin Analogues; Vitamin E
Decreased Effect
The levels/effects of Abciximab may be decreased by: Nonsteroidal Anti-Inflammatory Agents
Stability Vials should be stored at 2°C to 8°C (36°F to 46°F). Do not freeze or shake. After admixture, the prepared solution is stable for 12 hours.

The following stability information has also been reported: May store intact vials at 24°C to 28°C (76°F to 82°F) for up to 8 days (data on file [Eli Lilly, 2011]). However, the manufacturer recommends storage under refrigeration. Room temperature stability information should only be utilized in situations where the drug has been inadvertently exposed to prolonged room temperature.

Mechanism of Action Fab antibody fragment of the chimeric human-murine monoclonal antibody 7E3; this agent binds to platelet IIb/IIIa receptors, resulting in steric hindrance, thus inhibiting platelet aggregation

Pharmacodynamics/Kinetics

Onset: Rapid; platelet aggregation reduced to <20% of baseline at 10 minutes

Duration: Up to 72 hours for restoration of normal hemostasis (Schror, 2003)

Distribution: V_d: 0.07 L/kg (Schror, 2003)

Protein binding: Mostly bound to GP IIb/IIIa receptors on platelet surface

Metabolism: Unbound abciximab metabolized via proteolytic cleavage (Schror, 2003)

Half-life elimination: Plasma: ~30 minutes; dissociation half-life from GP IIb/IIIa receptors: up to 4 hours (Schror, 2003). **Note:** 29% and 13% of abciximab estimated to remain on GP IIb/IIIa receptors at 8 and 15 days, respectively (Mascelli, 1998). Platelet function may remain abnormal for up to 7 days post infusion (Osende, 2001).

Time to peak: Platelet inhibition: ~30 minutes (Mascelli, 1998)

Dosage

Percutaneous coronary intervention (PCI): I.V.: 0.25 mg/kg bolus administered 10-60 minutes prior to start of PCI followed by an infusion of 0.125 mcg/kg/minute (maximum: 10 mcg/minute) for 12 hours

Patients with unstable angina not responding to conventional medical therapy with planned PCI within 24 hours: I.V.: 0.25 mg/kg bolus followed by an 18- to 24-hour infusion of 10 mcg/minute, concluding 1 hour after PCI.

ST-elevation myocardial infarction (STEMI) undergoing primary percutaneous coronary intervention (PCI) (unlabeled use; Kushner, 2009): I.V.:

Loading dose: 0.25 mg/kg bolus administered at the time of PCI

Maintenance infusion: 0.125 mcg/kg/minute (maximum: 10 mcg/minute) continued for up to 12 hours

Administration Abciximab is intended for coadministration with aspirin postangioplasty and heparin infused and weight adjusted to maintain a therapeutic bleeding time (eg, ACT 300-500 seconds). Solution must be filtered prior to administration. Do not shake the vial.

Bolus dose: Aseptically withdraw the necessary amount of abciximab for the bolus dose into a syringe using a 0.2 or 5 micron low protein-binding syringe filter (or equivalent); the bolus should be administered 10-60 minutes before the procedure.

Continuous infusion: Aseptically withdraw amount required of abciximab for the infusion through a 0.2 or 5 micron low protein-binding syringe filter into a syringe; inject this into 250 mL of NS or D_5W to make solution. If a syringe filter was not used when preparing the infusion, administer using an in-line 0.2 or 0.22 micron low protein-binding filter. **Note:** Alternatively, a standard concentration of 7.2 mg in 250 mL of NS or D_5W may also be prepared for all patients and administered at the standard dose (0.125 mcg/kg/minute; maximum: 10 mcg/minute) with a variable rate in mL/hour. Infuse for 12-24 hours via pump after bolus dose; length of therapy dependent on indication.

Monitoring Parameters Prothrombin time, activated partial thromboplastin time (aPTT), hemoglobin, hematocrit, platelet count, fibrinogen, fibrin split products, transfusion requirements, signs of hypersensitivity reactions, guaiac stools, Hemastix® urine. Platelet count should be monitored at baseline, 2-4 hours following bolus infusion, and at 24 hours (or prior to discharge, if before 24 hours). To minimize risk of bleeding:

Abciximab initiated 18-24 hours prior to PCI: Maintain aPTT between 60-85 seconds during the heparin/abciximab infusion period

During PCI: Maintain ACT between 200-300 seconds

Following PCI (if anticoagulation is maintained): Maintain aPTT between 50-75 seconds

Sheath removal should not occur until aPTT is ≤50 seconds or ACT ≤175 seconds.

Maintain bleeding precautions, avoid unnecessary arterial and venous punctures, use saline or heparin lock for blood drawing, assess sheath insertion site and distal pulses of affected leg every 15 minutes for the first hour and then every 1 hour for the next 6 hours. Arterial access site care is important to prevent bleeding. Care should be taken when attempting vascular access that only the anterior wall of the femoral artery is punctured, avoiding a Seldinger (through and through) technique for obtaining sheath access. Femoral vein sheath placement should be avoided unless needed. While the vascular sheath is in place, patients should be maintained on complete bedrest with the head of the bed at a 30° angle and the affected limb restrained in a straight position.

Observe patient for mental status changes, hemorrhage; assess nose and mouth mucous membranes, puncture sites for oozing, ecchymosis, and hematoma formation; and examine urine, stool, and emesis for presence of occult or frank blood; gentle care should be provided when removing dressings.

Dosage Forms Excipient information presented when available (limited, particularly for generics); consult specific product labeling.

Injection, solution [preservative free]:

Reopro®: 2 mg/mL (5 mL) [contains polysorbate 80]

◆ **Abelcet®** *see* Amphotericin B (Lipid Complex) *on page 112*
◆ **Abenol® (Can)** *see* Acetaminophen *on page 27*
◆ **ABI-007** *see* PACLitaxel (Protein Bound) *on page 1275*
◆ **Abilify®** *see* ARIPiprazole *on page 142*
◆ **Abilify Discmelt®** *see* ARIPiprazole *on page 142*
◆ **Abiraterone** *see* Abiraterone Acetate *on page 23*

Abiraterone Acetate (a bir A ter one AS e tate)

Brand Names: U.S. Zytiga™

Brand Names: Canada Zytiga™

Index Terms Abiraterone; CB7630

Pharmacologic Category Antiandrogen; Antineoplastic Agent, Antiandrogen

Use Treatment of metastatic, castration-resistant prostate cancer (in combination with prednisone) in patients previously treated with docetaxel

Pregnancy Risk Factor X

Pregnancy Considerations Animal reproduction studies have not been conducted. Adverse effects were observed in the reproductive system of animals during toxicology and pharmacology studies. Abiraterone is not indicated for use in women and is specifically contraindicated in women who are or may become pregnant. It is not known if abiraterone is excreted in semen, therefore, men should use a condom and another method of birth control during treatment and for 1 week following therapy if having intercourse with a woman of reproductive age. Pregnant women should wear gloves if contact with tablets may occur.

Lactation Excretion in breast milk unknown/not recommended

Contraindications Use in women who are or may become pregnant

Canadian labeling: Additional contraindication (not in U.S. labeling): Hypersensitivity to abiraterone acetate or any component of the formulation or container

Warnings/Precautions Hazardous agent; use appropriate precautions for handling and disposal. Significant increases in liver enzymes have been reported; may require dosage reduction or discontinuation. ALT, AST, and bilirubin should be monitored prior to treatment, every 2 weeks for 3 months and monthly thereafter; patients with hepatic impairment, elevations in liver function tests, or experiencing hepatotoxicity require more frequent monitoring (see dosage adjustment for hepatic impairment and Monitoring Parameters). Evaluate liver function promptly with signs or symptoms of hepatotoxicity. The safety of retreatment after significant elevations (ALT or AST >20 times the upper limit of normal [ULN] or total bilirubin >10 times ULN) has not been evaluated. Avoid use in patients with pre-existing severe hepatic impairment; dosage reduction is recommended in patients with baseline moderate impairment. Canadian labeling (not in U.S. labeling) also recommends avoiding use in patients with pre-existing moderate hepatic impairment.

Concurrent infection, stress, or interruption of daily corticosteroids is associated with reports of adrenocortical insufficiency. Monitor closely for signs and symptoms of adrenocorticoid insufficiency, which could be masked by adverse events associated with mineralocorticoid excess. Diagnostic testing for insufficiency may be clinically indicated. Increased corticosteroid doses may be required before, during, and after stress. May cause increased mineralocorticoid levels, which may result in hypertension, hypokalemia and fluid retention. Concomitant administration with corticosteroids reduces the incidence and severity of these adverse events. Due to potential for hypertension, hypokalemia, or fluid retention, use with caution in patients with cardiovascular disease (particularly heart failure, recent MI, or ventricular arrhythmia); patients with left ventricular ejection fraction (LVEF) <50% or NYHA class III or IV heart failure were excluded from clinical trials. Monitor at least monthly for hypertension, hypokalemia, and fluid retention.

Must be administered on an empty stomach (administer at least 1 hour before and 2 hours after any food). Avoid (or use caution) with concomitant CYP3A4 strong inhibitors and inducers. Avoid concurrent administration with CYP2D6 substrates with a narrow therapeutic index (eg, thioridazine); if concurrent administration cannot be avoided, consider a dose reduction of the CYP2D6 substrate.

Adverse Reactions Note: Adverse reactions reported for use in combination with prednisone.

>10%:

Cardiovascular: Edema (27%)

Endocrine & metabolic: Triglycerides increased (63%), hypokalemia (28%; grades 3/4: 5%), hypophosphatemia (24%; grades 3/4: 7%), hot flush (19%)

Gastrointestinal: Diarrhea (18%)

Genitourinary: Urinary tract infection (12%)

Hepatic: AST increased (31%; grades 3/4: 2%), ALT increased (11%; grades 3/4: 1%)

Neuromuscular & skeletal: Joint swelling/discomfort (30%), muscle discomfort (26%)

Respiratory: Cough (11%)

1% to 10%:

Cardiovascular: Hypertension (9%; grades 3/4: 1%), arrhythmia (7%), chest pain/discomfort (4%), heart failure (2%)

Gastrointestinal: Dyspepsia (6%)

Genitourinary: Polyuria (7%), nocturia (6%)

Hepatic: Bilirubin increased (7%; grades 3/4: <1%)

Respiratory: Upper respiratory infection (5%)

<1% (Limited to important or life-threatening): Adrenal insufficiency

Drug Interactions

Metabolism/Transport Effects Substrate of CYP3A4 (major); **Note:** Assignment of Major/Minor substrate status based on clinically relevant drug interaction potential; **Inhibits** CYP1A2 (strong), CYP2C19 (moderate), CYP2C9 (moderate), CYP2D6 (strong), CYP3A4 (moderate), P-glycoprotein

Avoid Concomitant Use

Avoid concomitant use of Abiraterone Acetate with any of the following: Clopidogrel; Conivaptan; Pimozide; Silodosin; Tamoxifen; Thioridazine; Topotecan

Increased Effect/Toxicity

Abiraterone Acetate may increase the levels/effects of: ARIPiprazole; Atomoxetine; Bendamustine; Budesonide (Systemic, Oral Inhalation); Citalopram; Colchicine; CYP1A2 Substrates; CYP2C19 Substrates; CYP2C9 Substrates; CYP2D6 Substrates; CYP3A4 Substrates; Dabigatran Etexilate; Eplerenone; Everolimus; FentaNYL; Fesoterodine; Halofantrine; Iloperidone; Lurasidone; Nebivolol; P-glycoprotein/ABCB1 Substrates; Pimecrolimus; Pimozide; Propafenone; Rivaroxaban; Salmeterol; Silodosin; Tamoxifen; Tetrabenazine; Thioridazine; Topotecan; Vilazodone; Zuclopenthixol

The levels/effects of Abiraterone Acetate may be increased by: Conivaptan; CYP3A4 Inhibitors (Moderate); CYP3A4 Inhibitors (Strong); Dasatinib

Decreased Effect

Abiraterone Acetate may decrease the levels/effects of: Clopidogrel; Codeine; Iloperidone; TraMADol

The levels/effects of Abiraterone Acetate may be decreased by: CYP3A4 Inducers (Strong); Deferasirox; Herbs (CYP3A4 Inducers); Tocilizumab

Ethanol/Nutrition/Herb Interactions Food: Do not administer with food (will increase systemic exposure).

Stability Store at 20°C to 25°C (68°F to 77°F); excursions permitted to 15°C to 30°C (59°F to 86°F).

Mechanism of Action Selectively and irreversibly inhibits CYP17 (17 alpha-hydroxylase/C17,20-lyase), an enzyme required for androgen biosynthesis which is expressed in testicular, adrenal, and prostatic tumor tissues. Inhibits the formation of the testosterone precursors dehydroepiandrosterone (DHEA) and androstenedione.

Pharmacodynamics/Kinetics

Distribution: V_{dss}: 19,669 ± 13,358 L

Protein binding: >99%; to albumin and $alpha_1$-acid glycoprotein

Metabolism: Abiraterone acetate is hydrolyzed to the active metabolite abiraterone; further metabolized to inactive metabolites abiraterone sulphate and N-oxide abiraterone sulphate via CYP3A4 and SULT2A1

Bioavailability: Systemic exposure is increased by food

Half-life elimination: 12 ± 5 hours

Time to peak: 2 hours

Excretion: Feces (~88%); urine (~5%)

Dosage Oral: Adults: Prostate cancer, metastatic, castration-resistant: 1000 mg once daily (in combination with prednisone 5 mg twice daily)

Dosing adjustment in renal impairment: No adjustment required

Dosing adjustment in hepatic impairment:

Hepatic impairment ***prior to*** treatment initiation:

Mild (Child-Pugh class A): No adjustment required

Moderate (Child-Pugh class B): 250 mg once daily (**Note:** Canadian labeling does not recommend use). Permanently discontinue treatment if ALT and/or AST >5 times the upper limit of normal (ULN) or total bilirubin >3 times ULN.

Severe (Child-Pugh class C): Avoid use

Hepatotoxicity ***during*** treatment:

U.S. labeling:

ALT and/or AST >5 times ULN or total bilirubin >3 times ULN: Withhold treatment until liver function tests return to baseline or ALT and AST ≤2.5 times ULN and total bilirubin ≤1.5 times ULN, then reinitiate at 750 mg once daily.

Recurrent hepatotoxicity on 750 mg/day: Withhold treatment until liver function tests return to baseline or ALT and AST ≤2.5 times ULN and total bilirubin ≤1.5 times ULN, then reinitiate at 500 mg once daily.

Recurrent hepatotoxicity on 500 mg/day: Discontinue treatment

Canadian labeling:

ALT and/or AST >5 times ULN or total bilirubin >3 times ULN:

Withhold treatment until liver function tests return to baseline, then reinitiate at 500 mg once daily

Recurrent hepatotoxicity on 500 mg/day: Discontinue treatment

ALT >20 times ULN (any time during treatment): Discontinue permanently.

Dietary Considerations Must be taken on an empty stomach, at least 1 hour before and 2 hours after food.

Administration Administer orally on an empty stomach, at least 1 hour before and 2 hours after food. Swallow tablets whole with water.

Monitoring Parameters ALT, AST, and bilirubin prior to treatment, every 2 weeks for 3 months and monthly thereafter; if baseline moderate hepatic impairment (Child-Pugh class B), monitor ALT, AST, and bilirubin prior to treatment, weekly for the first month, every 2 weeks for 2 months then monthly thereafter. If hepatotoxicity develops during treatment (and only after therapy is interrupted and liver function tests have returned to safe levels), monitor ALT, AST, and bilirubin every 2 weeks for 3 months and monthly thereafter. Monitoring of testosterone levels is not necessary.

Monitor for signs and symptoms of adrenocorticoid insufficiency; monthly for hypertension, hypokalemia, and fluid retention.

Dosage Forms Excipient information presented when available (limited, particularly for generics); consult specific product labeling.

Tablet, oral:

Zytiga™: 250 mg

◆ **ABLC** *see* Amphotericin B (Lipid Complex) *on page 112*

AbobotulinumtoxinA

(aye bo BOT yoo lin num TOKS in aye)

Brand Names: U.S. Dysport™

Index Terms Botulinum Toxin Type A

Pharmacologic Category Neuromuscular Blocker Agent, Toxin

Use Treatment of cervical dystonia in both toxin-naive and previously treated patients; temporary improvement in the appearance of moderate-severe glabellar lines associated with procerus and corrugator muscle activity

Pregnancy Risk Factor C

Medication Guide Available Yes

Dosage

Adults:

Cervical dystonia: I.M.: Initial: 500 units divided among affected muscles in toxin-naïve or toxin-experienced patients. May re-treat at intervals of ≥12 weeks

Dosage adjustments: Adjust dosage in 250-unit increments; do not administer at intervals <12 weeks; dosage range used in studies: 250-1000 units

Glabellar lines: Adults <65 years: I.M.: Inject 10 units (0.05 mL or 0.08 mL) into each of 5 sites (2 injections in each corrugator muscle and 1 injection in the procerus muscle) for a total dose of 50 units; do not administer at intervals <3 months; efficacy has been demonstrated up to 4 repeated administrations

Elderly:

Cervical dystonia: Refer to adult dosing.

Glabellar lines: Not recommended in patients ≥65 years of age

Dosage adjustment in renal impairment: No adjustment necessary

Dosage adjustment in hepatic impairment: No adjustment necessary

Additional Information Complete prescribing information for this medication should be consulted for additional detail.

Dosage Forms Excipient information presented when available (limited, particularly for generics); consult specific product labeling.

Injection, powder for reconstitution:

Dysport™: 500 units [contains albumin (human), lactose 2.5 mg]

◆ **Abraxane®** *see* PACLitaxel (Protein Bound) *on page 1275*

◆ **Abreva® [OTC]** *see* Docosanol *on page 537*

◆ **Abstral®** *see* FentaNYL *on page 697*

◆ **Abstral™ (Can)** *see* FentaNYL *on page 697*

◆ **ABT-335** *see* Fenofibric Acid *on page 695*

◆ **ABX-EGF** *see* Panitumumab *on page 1288*

◆ **AC 2993** *see* Exenatide *on page 678*

◆ **ACAM2000®** *see* Smallpox Vaccine *on page 1563*

Acamprosate (a kam PROE sate)

Brand Names: U.S. Campral®

Brand Names: Canada Campral®

Index Terms Acamprosate Calcium; Calcium Acetylhomotaurinate

Pharmacologic Category GABA Agonist/Glutamate Antagonist

Use Maintenance of alcohol abstinence

Pregnancy Risk Factor C

Dosage Oral: Adults: Alcohol abstinence: 666 mg 3 times/day (a lower dose may be effective in some patients). **Note:** Treatment should be initiated as soon as possible following the period of alcohol withdrawal, when the patient has achieved abstinence and should be maintained if patient relapses.

Dosage adjustment in renal impairment:

Cl_{cr} 30-50 mL/minute: 333 mg 3 times/day

Cl_{cr} <30 mL/minute: Contraindicated in severe renal impairment.

Dosage adjustment in renal impairment:

Mild-to-moderate impairment: No dosage adjustments are recommended

Severe impairment: There are no dosage adjustments provided in manufacturer's labeling.

Additional Information Complete prescribing information for this medication should be consulted for additional detail.

Dosage Forms Excipient information presented when available (limited, particularly for generics); consult specific product labeling.

Tablet, delayed release, enteric coated, oral, as calcium:
Campral®: 333 mg [contains calcium 33 mg/tablet, sulfites]

◆ **Acamprosate Calcium** *see* Acamprosate *on page 25*

Acarbose (AY car bose)

Brand Names: U.S. Precose®

Brand Names: Canada Glucobay™

Pharmacologic Category Antidiabetic Agent, Alpha-Glucosidase Inhibitor

Additional Appendix Information

Diabetes Mellitus Management, Adults *on page 1983*

Use Adjunct to diet and exercise to lower blood glucose in patients with type 2 diabetes mellitus (noninsulin dependent, NIDDM)

Pregnancy Risk Factor B

Pregnancy Considerations Adverse events have not been reported in animal reproduction studies; therefore, acarbose is classified as pregnancy category B. Low amounts of acarbose are absorbed systemically which should limit fetal exposure. Maternal hyperglycemia can be associated with adverse effects in the fetus, including macrosomia, neonatal hyperglycemia, and hyperbilirubinemia; the risk of congenital malformations is increased when the Hb A_{1c} is above the normal range. Diabetes can also be associated with adverse effects in the mother. Poorly-treated diabetes may cause end-organ damage that may in turn negatively affect obstetric outcomes. Physiologic glucose levels should be maintained prior to and during pregnancy to decrease the risk of adverse events in the mother and the fetus. Acarbose has been studied for its potential role in treating GDM; however, only limited information is available describing pregnancy outcomes. Until additional safety and efficacy data are obtained, the use of oral agents is generally not recommended as routine management of GDM or type 2 diabetes mellitus during pregnancy. Insulin is the drug of choice for the control of diabetes mellitus during pregnancy.

Lactation Excretion in breast milk unknown/not recommended

Contraindications Hypersensitivity to acarbose or any component of the formulation; patients with diabetic ketoacidosis or cirrhosis; patients with inflammatory bowel disease, colonic ulceration, partial intestinal obstruction, or in patients predisposed to intestinal obstruction; patients who have chronic intestinal diseases associated with marked disorders of digestion or absorption, and in patients who have conditions that may deteriorate as a result of increased gas formation in the intestine

Warnings/Precautions Acarbose given in combination with a sulfonylurea or insulin will cause a further lowering of blood glucose and may increase the hypoglycemic potential of the sulfonylurea or insulin. Treatment-emergent elevations of serum transaminases (AST and/or ALT) occurred in up to 14% of acarbose-treated patients in long-term studies. These serum transaminase elevations appear to be dose related and were asymptomatic, reversible, more common in females, and, in general, were not associated with other evidence of liver dysfunction. Fulminant hepatitis has been reported rarely. It may be necessary to discontinue acarbose and administer insulin if the patient is exposed to stress (ie, fever, trauma, infection, surgery). Use not recommended in patients with significant impairment (S_{cr} >2 mg/dL); use with caution in other patients with renal impairment.

Adverse Reactions

>10%:

Gastrointestinal: Diarrhea (31%) and abdominal pain (19%) tend to return to pretreatment levels over time; frequency and intensity of flatulence (74%) tend to abate with time

Hepatic: Transaminases increased (≤4%)

Postmarketing and/or case reports: Edema, erythema, exanthema, hepatitis, ileus/subileus, jaundice, liver damage, pneumatosis cystoides intestinalis, rash, thrombocytopenia, urticaria

Drug Interactions

Metabolism/Transport Effects None known.

Avoid Concomitant Use There are no known interactions where it is recommended to avoid concomitant use.

Increased Effect/Toxicity

Acarbose may increase the levels/effects of: Hypoglycemic Agents

The levels/effects of Acarbose may be increased by: Herbs (Hypoglycemic Properties); Neomycin; Pegvisomant

Decreased Effect

Acarbose may decrease the levels/effects of: Digoxin

The levels/effects of Acarbose may be decreased by: Corticosteroids (Orally Inhaled); Corticosteroids (Systemic); Luteinizing Hormone-Releasing Hormone Analogs; Somatropin; Thiazide Diuretics

Ethanol/Nutrition/Herb Interactions Ethanol: Limit ethanol.

Stability Store at <25°C (77°F). Protect from moisture.

Mechanism of Action Competitive inhibitor of pancreatic α-amylase and intestinal brush border α-glucosidases, resulting in delayed hydrolysis of ingested complex carbohydrates and disaccharides and absorption of glucose; dose-dependent reduction in postprandial serum insulin and glucose peaks; inhibits the metabolism of sucrose to glucose and fructose

Pharmacodynamics/Kinetics

Absorption: <2% as active drug; ~35% as metabolites

Metabolism: Exclusively via GI tract, principally by intestinal bacteria and digestive enzymes; 13 metabolites identified (major metabolites are sulfate, methyl, and glucuronide conjugates)

Bioavailability: Low systemic bioavailability of parent compound; acts locally in GI tract

Half-life elimination: ~2 hours

Time to peak: Active drug: ~1 hour

Excretion: Urine (~34% as inactive metabolites, <2% parent drug and active metabolite); feces (~51% as unabsorbed drug)

Dosage Oral:

Adults: Dosage must be individualized on the basis of effectiveness and tolerance while not exceeding the maximum recommended dose

Initial dose: 25 mg 3 times/day with the first bite of each main meal; to reduce GI effects, some patients may benefit from initiating at 25 mg once daily with gradual titration to 25 mg 3 times/day as tolerated

Maintenance dose: Should be adjusted at 4- to 8-week intervals based on 1-hour postprandial glucose levels and tolerance until maintenance dose is reached. Dosage may be increased from 25 mg 3 times/day to 50 mg 3 times/day. Some patients may benefit from increasing the dose to 100 mg 3 times/day.

Maintenance dose ranges: 50-100 mg 3 times/day.

Maximum dose:

≤60 kg: 50 mg 3 times/day

>60 kg: 100 mg 3 times/day

Patients receiving sulfonylureas or insulin: Acarbose given in combination with a sulfonylurea or insulin will cause a further lowering of blood glucose and may increase the hypoglycemic potential of the sulfonylurea or insulin. If hypoglycemia occurs, appropriate adjustments in the dosage of these agents should be made.

Dosing adjustment in renal impairment:

Cl_{cr} <25 mL/minute: Peak plasma concentrations were 5 times higher and AUCs were 6 times larger than in volunteers with normal renal function.

Significant renal dysfunction (S_{cr} >2 mg/dL): Use is not recommended.

Dietary Considerations Take with food (first bite of meal).

Administration Should be administered with the first bite of each main meal.

Monitoring Parameters Postprandial glucose, glycosylated hemoglobin levels, serum transaminase levels should be checked every 3 months during the first year of treatment and periodically thereafter, renal function (serum creatinine); blood pressure

Reference Range Recommendations for glycemic control in adults with diabetes:

Hb A_{1c}: <7%

Preprandial capillary plasma glucose: 70-130 mg/dL

Peak postprandial capillary blood glucose: <180 mg/dL

Dosage Forms Excipient information presented when available (limited, particularly for generics); consult specific product labeling.

Tablet, oral: 25 mg, 50 mg, 100 mg

Precose®: 25 mg, 50 mg, 100 mg

- ◆ **A-Caro-25 [OTC]** *see* Beta-Carotene *on page 207*
- ◆ **Accel-Amlodipine (Can)** *see* AmLODIPine *on page 97*
- ◆ **Accel-Pioglitazone (Can)** *see* Pioglitazone *on page 1355*
- ◆ **Accolate®** *see* Zafirlukast *on page 1808*
- ◆ **AccuNeb®** *see* Albuterol *on page 52*
- ◆ **Accupril®** *see* Quinapril *on page 1444*
- ◆ **Accutane® (Can)** *see* ISOtretinoin *on page 939*
- ◆ **ACE** *see* Captopril *on page 277*

Acebutolol (a se BYOO toe lole)

Brand Names: U.S. Sectral®

Brand Names: Canada Apo-Acebutolol®; Mylan-Acebutolol; Mylan-Acebutolol (Type S); Novo-Acebutolol; Nu-Acebutolol; Rhotral; Sandoz-Acebutolol; Sectral®; Teva-Acebutolol

Index Terms Acebutolol Hydrochloride

Pharmacologic Category Antiarrhythmic Agent, Class II; Beta Blocker With Intrinsic Sympathomimetic Activity

Additional Appendix Information

Beta-Blockers *on page 1884*

Use Treatment of hypertension; management of ventricular arrhythmias

Unlabeled Use Treatment of chronic stable angina (**Note:** Not recommended for patients with prior MI)

Pregnancy Risk Factor B

Dosage Oral:

Adults:

Ventricular arrhythmias: Initial: 400 mg/day in 2 divided doses; maintenance: 600-1200 mg/day in divided doses; maximum: 1200 mg/day

Hypertension: 400-800 mg/day (larger doses may be divided); maximum: 1200 mg/day; usual dose range (JNC 7): 200-800 mg/day in 2 divided doses

Chronic stable angina (unlabeled use): Usual dose: 400-1200 mg/day in 2 divided doses (Gibbons, 2002); low doses (ie, 400 mg/day) may also be given as once daily (Pina, 1988)

Elderly: Consider dose reduction due to age-related increase in bioavailability; do not exceed 800 mg/day. In the management of hypertension, consider lower initial dose (eg, 200-400 mg/day) and titrate to response (Aronow, 2011).

Dosing adjustment in renal impairment:

Cl_{cr} 25-49 mL/minute: Reduce dose by 50%.

Cl_{cr} <25 mL/minute: Reduce dose by 75%.

Dosing adjustment in hepatic impairment: There are no dosage adjustments provided in manufacturer's labeling; use with caution.

Additional Information Complete prescribing information for this medication should be consulted for additional detail.

Dosage Forms Excipient information presented when available (limited, particularly for generics); consult specific product labeling.

Capsule, oral, as hydrochloride: 200 mg, 400 mg

Sectral®: 200 mg, 400 mg

- ◆ **Acebutolol Hydrochloride** *see* Acebutolol *on page 27*
- ◆ **Aceon®** *see* Perindopril Erbumine *on page 1334*
- ◆ **Acephen™ [OTC]** *see* Acetaminophen *on page 27*
- ◆ **Acerola [OTC]** *see* Ascorbic Acid *on page 149*
- ◆ **Acetadote®** *see* Acetylcysteine *on page 34*

Acetaminophen (a seet a MIN oh fen)

Brand Names: U.S. Acephen™ [OTC]; APAP 500 [OTC]; Aspirin Free Anacin® Extra Strength [OTC]; Cetafen® Extra [OTC]; Cetafen® [OTC]; Excedrin® Tension Headache [OTC]; Feverall® [OTC]; Infantaire [OTC]; Little Fevers™ [OTC]; Mapap® Arthritis Pain [OTC]; Mapap® Children's [OTC]; Mapap® Extra Strength [OTC]; Mapap® Infant's [OTC]; Mapap® Junior Rapid Tabs [OTC]; Mapap® [OTC]; Non-Aspirin Pain Reliever [OTC]; Nortemp Children's [OTC]; Ofirmev™; Pain & Fever Children's [OTC]; Pain Eze [OTC]; Silapap Children's [OTC]; Silapap Infant's [OTC]; Triaminic™ Children's Fever Reducer Pain Reliever [OTC]; Tylenol® 8 Hour [OTC]; Tylenol® Arthritis Pain Extended Relief [OTC]; Tylenol® Children's Meltaways [OTC]; Tylenol® Children's [OTC]; Tylenol® Extra Strength [OTC]; Tylenol® Infant's Concentrated [OTC]; Tylenol® Jr. Meltaways [OTC]; Tylenol® [OTC]; Valorin Extra [OTC]; Valorin [OTC]

Brand Names: Canada Abenol®; Apo-Acetaminophen®; Atasol®; Novo-Gesic; Pediatrix; Tempra®; Tylenol®

Index Terms APAP (abbreviation is not recommended); N-Acetyl-P-Aminophenol; Paracetamol

Pharmacologic Category Analgesic, Miscellaneous

Use Treatment of mild-to-moderate pain and fever (analgesic/antipyretic)

I.V.: Additional indication: Management of moderate-to-severe pain when combined with opioid analgesia

Pregnancy Risk Factor C (intravenous)

Pregnancy Considerations Animal reproduction studies have not been conducted with intravenous acetaminophen, therefore, acetaminophen I.V. is classified as pregnancy category C. Acetaminophen crosses the placenta and can be detected in cord blood, newborn serum, and urine immediately after delivery. An increased risk of teratogenic effects has not been observed following maternal use of acetaminophen during pregnancy. Prenatal constriction of the ductus arteriosus has been noted in case reports following maternal use during the third trimester. The use of acetaminophen in normal doses during pregnancy is not associated with an increased risk of miscarriage or still birth; however, an increase in fetal death or spontaneous abortion may be seen following maternal overdose if treatment is delayed. Frequent maternal use of acetaminophen during pregnancy may be ▶

associated with wheezing and asthma in early childhood. The absorption may be delayed and the bioavailability of acetaminophen may be decreased in some women during pregnancy due to delayed gastric emptying.

Lactation Enters breast milk/use caution (AAP rates "compatible"; AAP 2001 update pending)

Contraindications Hypersensitivity to acetaminophen or any component of the formulation; severe hepatic impairment or severe active liver disease (Ofirmev™)

Warnings/Precautions Limit dose to <4 g/day. May cause severe hepatotoxicity on acute overdose; in addition, chronic daily dosing in adults has resulted in liver damage in some patients. Use with caution in patients with alcoholic liver disease; consuming ≥3 alcoholic drinks/day may increase the risk of liver damage. Use caution in patients with hepatic impairment or active liver disease. Use of intravenous formulation is contraindicated in patients with severe hepatic impairment or severe active liver disease. Use caution in patients with known G6PD deficiency; rare reports of hemolysis have occurred. Use caution in patients with chronic malnutrition and hypovolemia (intravenous formulation). Use caution in patients with severe renal impairment; consider dosing adjustments. Hypersensitivity and anaphylactic reactions have been reported; discontinue immediately if symptoms of allergic or hypersensitivity reactions occur.

OTC labeling: When used for self-medication, patients should be instructed to contact healthcare provider if used for fever lasting >3 days or for pain lasting >10 days in adults or >5 days in children.

Adverse Reactions Oral, Rectal: Frequency not defined:

Dermatologic: Rash

Endocrine & metabolic: May increase chloride, uric acid, glucose; may decrease sodium, bicarbonate, calcium

Hematologic: Anemia, blood dyscrasias (neutropenia, pancytopenia, leukopenia)

Hepatic: Bilirubin increased, alkaline phosphatase increased

Renal: Ammonia increased, nephrotoxicity with chronic overdose, analgesic nephropathy

Miscellaneous: Hypersensitivity reactions (rare)

I.V.:

>10%: Gastrointestinal: Nausea (adults 34%; children ≥5%), vomiting (adults 15%; children ≥5%)

1% to 10%:

Cardiovascular: Edema (peripheral), hypervolemia, hypo/hypertension, tachycardia

Central nervous system: Headache (adults 10%; children ≥1%), insomnia (adults 7%; children ≥1%), agitation (children ≥5%), anxiety, fatigue

Dermatologic: Pruritus (children ≥5%), rash

Endocrine & metabolic: Hypoalbuminemia, hypokalemia, hypomagnesemia, hypophosphatemia

Gastrointestinal: Constipation (children ≥5%), abdominal pain, diarrhea

Hematologic: Anemia

Hepatic: Transaminases increased

Local: Infusion site pain

Neuromuscular & skeletal: Muscle spasms, pain in extremity, trismus

Ocular: Periorbital edema

Renal: Oliguria (children ≥1%)

Respiratory: Atelectasis (children ≥5%), breath sounds abnormal, dyspnea, hypoxia, pleural effusion, pulmonary edema, stridor, wheezing

All formulations: <1% (Limited to important or life-threatening): Anaphylaxis (rare), hypersensitivity reactions

Drug Interactions

Metabolism/Transport Effects Substrate of CYP1A2 (minor), CYP2A6 (minor), CYP2C9 (minor), CYP2D6 (minor), CYP2E1 (minor), CYP3A4 (minor); **Note:** Assignment of Major/Minor substrate status based on clinically relevant drug interaction potential; **Inhibits** CYP3A4 (weak)

Avoid Concomitant Use

Avoid concomitant use of Acetaminophen with any of the following: Pimozide

Increased Effect/Toxicity

Acetaminophen may increase the levels/effects of: Busulfan; Dasatinib; Imatinib; Pimozide; Prilocaine; SORAfenib; Vitamin K Antagonists

The levels/effects of Acetaminophen may be increased by: Conivaptan; Dasatinib; Imatinib; Isoniazid; Metyrapone; Probenecid; SORAfenib

Decreased Effect

The levels/effects of Acetaminophen may be decreased by: Anticonvulsants (Hydantoin); Barbiturates; CarBAMazepine; Cholestyramine Resin; Cyproterone; Peginterferon Alfa-2b; Tocilizumab

Ethanol/Nutrition/Herb Interactions

Ethanol: Excessive intake of ethanol may increase the risk of acetaminophen-induced hepatotoxicity. Avoid ethanol or limit to <3 drinks/day.

Food: Rate of absorption may be decreased when given with food.

Herb/Nutraceutical: St John's wort may decrease acetaminophen levels.

Stability

Injection: Store intact vials at room temperature of 20°C to 25°C (68°F to 77°F); do not refrigerate or freeze. Injectable solution may be administered directly from the vial without further dilution. For doses <1000 mg, withdraw the appropriate volume and transfer to a separate sterile container (eg, glass bottle, plastic I.V. container, syringe) for administration. Use within 6 hours of opening vial or transferring to another container. Discard any unused portion; single use vials only.

Oral formulations: Store at controlled room temperature.

Suppositories: Store at <27°C (80°F); do not freeze.

Mechanism of Action Although not fully elucidated, believed to inhibit the synthesis of prostaglandins in the central nervous system and work peripherally to block pain impulse generation; produces antipyresis from inhibition of hypothalamic heat-regulating center

Pharmacodynamics/Kinetics

Onset of action:

Oral: <1 hour

I.V.: Analgesia: 5-10 minutes; Antipyretic: Within 30 minutes

Peak effect: I.V.: Analgesic: 1 hour

Duration:

I.V., Oral: Analgesia: 4-6 hours

I.V.: Antipyretic: ≥6 hours

Absorption: Primarily absorbed in small intestine (rate of absorption dependent upon gastric emptying); minimal absorption from stomach; varies by dosage form

Distribution: ~1 L/kg at therapeutic doses

Protein binding: 10% to 25% at therapeutic concentrations; 8% to 43% at toxic concentrations

Metabolism: At normal therapeutic dosages, primarily hepatic metabolism to sulfate and glucuronide conjugates, while a small amount is metabolized by CYP2E1 to a highly reactive intermediate, N-acetyl-p-benzoquinone imine (NAPQI), which is conjugated rapidly with glutathione and inactivated to nontoxic cysteine and mercapturic acid conjugates. At toxic doses (as little as 4 g daily) glutathione conjugation becomes insufficient to meet the metabolic demand causing an increase in NAPQI concentrations, which may cause hepatic cell necrosis. Oral administration is subject to first pass metabolism.

Half-life elimination: Prolonged following toxic doses

Neonates: 7 hours (range: 4-10 hours)

Infants: ~4 hours (range: 1-7 hours)

Children: 3 hours (range: 2-5 hours)

Adolescents: ~3 hours (range: 2-4 hours)

Adults: ~2 hours (range: 2-3 hours); may be slightly prolonged in severe renal insufficiency (Cl_{cr}<30 mL/minute): 2-5.3 hours

Time to peak, serum: Oral: Immediate release: 10-60 minutes (may be delayed in acute overdoses); I.V.: 15 minutes

Excretion: Urine (<5% unchanged; 60% to 80% as glucuronide metabolites; 20% to 30% as sulphate metabolites; ~8% cysteine and mercapturic acid metabolites)

Dosage Note: No dose adjustment required if converting between different acetaminophen formulations.

Oral, rectal:

Children <12 years: 10-15 mg/kg/dose every 4-6 hours as needed; do **not** exceed 5 doses (2.6 g) in 24 hours; alternatively, the following age-based doses may be used; see table.

Acetaminophen Dosing (Oral and Rectal Formulations)

Age	Dosage (mg)	Age	Dosage (mg)
0-3 mo	40	4-5 y	240
4-11 mo	80	6-8 y	320
1-2 y	120	9-10 y	400
2-3 y	160	11 y	480

Note: Higher rectal doses have been studied for use in preoperative pain control in children. However, specific guidelines are not available and dosing may be product dependent. The safety and efficacy of alternating acetaminophen and ibuprofen dosing has not been established.

Adults: 325-650 mg every 4-6 hours or 1000 mg 3-4 times/day; do **not** exceed 4 g/day

I.V.:

Children 2-12 years: 15 mg/kg every 6 hours **or** 12.5 mg/kg every 4 hours; maximum single dose: 15 mg/kg/dose; maximum daily dose: 75 mg/kg/day (≤3.75 g/day)

Adolescents >12 years and Adults:

<50 kg: 15 mg/kg every 6 hours or 12.5 mg/kg every 4 hours; maximum single dose: 750 mg/dose; maximum daily dose: 75 mg/kg/day (≤3.75 g/day)

≥50 kg: 650 mg every 4 hours or 1000 mg every 6 hours; maximum single dose: 1000 mg/dose; maximum daily dose: 4 g/day

Dosing interval in renal impairment:

Oral (Aronoff, 2007):

Children:

Cl_{cr} <10 mL/minute: Administer every 8 hours

Intermittent hemodialysis or peritoneal dialysis: Administer every 8 hours

CRRT: No adjustments necessary

Adults:

Cl_{cr} 10-50 mL/minute: Administer every 6 hours

Cl_{cr} <10 mL/minute: Administer every 8 hours

Intermittent hemodialysis or peritoneal dialysis: No adjustment necessary

CRRT: Administer every 8 hours

I.V.: Cl_{cr} ≤30 mL/minute: Use with caution; consider decreasing daily dose and extending dosing interval

Dosing adjustment/comments in hepatic impairment: Use with caution. Limited, low-dose therapy is usually well tolerated in hepatic disease/cirrhosis. However, cases of hepatotoxicity at daily acetaminophen dosages <4 g/day have been reported. Avoid chronic use in hepatic impairment.

Dietary Considerations Some products may contain phenylalanine.

Administration

Suspension, oral: Shake well before pouring a dose.

Injection: For I.V. infusion only. May administer undiluted over 15 minutes.

Doses <1000 mg (<50 kg): Withdraw appropriate dose from vial and place into separate empty, sterile container prior to administration. Small volume pediatric doses (up to 60 mL) may be placed in a syringe and infused over 15 minutes via syringe pump.

Doses of 1000 mg (≥50 kg): Insert vented I.V. set through vial stopper.

Monitoring Parameters Relief of pain or fever

Dosage Forms Excipient information presented when available (limited, particularly for generics); consult specific product labeling. [DSC] = Discontinued product

Caplet, oral: 500 mg

Cetafen® Extra: 500 mg

Mapap® Extra Strength: 500 mg

Mapap® Extra Strength: 500 mg [scored]

Pain Eze: 650 mg

Tylenol®: 325 mg

Tylenol® Extra Strength: 500 mg

Caplet, extended release, oral:

Mapap® Arthritis Pain: 650 mg

Tylenol® 8 Hour: 650 mg

Tylenol® Arthritis Pain Extended Relief: 650 mg

Capsule, oral:

Mapap® Extra Strength: 500 mg

Captab, oral: 500 mg

Elixir, oral:

Mapap® Children's: 160 mg/5 mL (118 mL, 480 mL) [ethanol free; contains benzoic acid, propylene glycol, sodium benzoate; cherry flavor]

Gelcap, oral: 500 mg

Mapap®: 500 mg

Gelcap, rapid release, oral: 500 mg

Tylenol® Extra Strength: 500 mg

Geltab, oral: 500 mg

Excedrin® Tension Headache: 500 mg [contains caffeine 65 mg/geltab]

Injection, solution [preservative free]:

Ofirmev™: 10 mg/mL (100 mL)

Liquid, oral: 160 mg/5 mL (120 mL, 473 mL); 500 mg/5 mL (240s)

APAP 500: 500 mg/5 mL (237 mL) [ethanol free, sugar free; cherry flavor]

Silapap Children's: 160 mg/5 mL (118 mL, 237 mL, 473 mL) [ethanol free, sugar free; contains propylene glycol, sodium benzoate; cherry flavor]

Tylenol® Extra Strength: 500 mg/15 mL (240 mL) [ethanol free; contains propylene glycol, sodium benzoate; cherry flavor]

Solution, oral: 160 mg/5 mL (5 mL, 10 mL, 20 mL)

Pain & Fever Children's: 160 mg/5 mL (118 mL, 473 mL) [ethanol free; contains benzoic acid, propylene glycol, sodium benzoate; cherry flavor]

Solution, oral [drops]: 80 mg/0.8 mL (15 mL)

Infantaire: 80 mg/0.8 mL (15 mL, 30 mL)

Little Fevers™: 80 mg/mL (30 mL) [dye free, ethanol free, gluten free; contains propylene glycol, sodium benzoate; berry flavor]

Mapap®: 80 mg/0.8 mL (15 mL) [fruit flavor]

Silapap Infant's: 80 mg/0.8 mL (15 mL, 30 mL) [ethanol free; contains propylene glycol, sodium benzoate; cherry flavor]

Suppository, rectal: 120 mg (12s); 325 mg (12s); 650 mg (12s)
Acephen™: 120 mg (12s, 50s, 100s); 325 mg (6s, 12s, 50s, 100s); 650 mg (12s, 50s, 100s, 500s [DSC])
Feverall®: 80 mg (6s, 50s); 120 mg (6s, 50s); 325 mg (6s, 50s); 650 mg (50s)
Suspension, oral: 160 mg/5 mL (5 mL, 10 mL [DSC], 10.15 mL, 20 mL [DSC], 20.3 mL)
Mapap® Children's: 160 mg/5 mL (118 mL) [ethanol free; contains propylene glycol, sodium benzoate; cherry flavor]
Nortemp Children's: 160 mg/5 mL (118 mL) [ethanol free; contains propylene glycol, sodium benzoate; cotton candy flavor]
Tylenol® Children's: 160 mg/5 mL (120 mL) [dye free, ethanol free; contains propylene glycol, sodium benzoate; cherry flavor]
Tylenol® Children's: 160 mg/5 mL (120 mL) [ethanol free; contains propylene glycol, sodium 2 mg/5 mL, sodium benzoate; bubblegum flavor]
Tylenol® Children's: 160 mg/5 mL (60 mL, 120 mL) [ethanol free; contains propylene glycol, sodium 2 mg/5 mL, sodium benzoate; cherry flavor]
Tylenol® Children's: 160 mg/5 mL (120 mL) [ethanol free; contains propylene glycol, sodium 2 mg/5 mL, sodium benzoate; grape flavor]
Tylenol® Children's: 160 mg/5 mL (120 mL) [ethanol free; contains propylene glycol, sodium 2 mg/5 mL, sodium benzoate; strawberry flavor]
Suspension, oral [drops]: 80 mg/0.8 mL (0.8 mL, 2 mL)
Mapap® Infant's: 80 mg/0.8 mL (15 mL, 30 mL) [ethanol free; contains propylene glycol, sodium benzoate; cherry flavor]
Tylenol® Infant's Concentrated: 80 mg/0.8 mL (30 mL) [dye free; contains propylene glycol; cherry flavor]
Tylenol® Infant's Concentrated: 80 mg/0.8 mL (15 mL, 30 mL) [ethanol free; contains sodium benzoate; cherry flavor]
Tylenol® Infant's Concentrated: 80 mg/0.8 mL (15 mL, 30 mL) [ethanol free; contains sodium benzoate; grape flavor]
Syrup, oral:
Triaminic™ Children's Fever Reducer Pain Reliever: 160 mg/5 mL (118 mL) [contains benzoic acid, sodium 6 mg/5 mL; bubblegum flavor]
Triaminic™ Children's Fever Reducer Pain Reliever: 160 mg/5 mL (118 mL) [contains sodium 5 mg/5 mL, sodium benzoate; grape flavor]
Tablet, oral: 325 mg, 500 mg
Aspirin Free Anacin® Extra Strength: 500 mg
Cetafen®: 325 mg
Mapap®: 325 mg
Non-Aspirin Pain Reliever: 325 mg
Tylenol®: 325 mg
Valorin: 325 mg [sugar free]
Valorin Extra: 500 mg [sugar free]
Tablet, chewable, oral: 80 mg
Mapap® Children's: 80 mg [fruit flavor]
Tablet, orally disintegrating, oral: 80 mg, 160 mg
Mapap® Children's: 80 mg [bubblegum flavor]
Mapap® Children's: 80 mg [grape flavor]
Mapap® Junior Rapid Tabs: 160 mg [bubblegum flavor]
Tylenol® Children's Meltaways: 80 mg [scored; bubblegum flavor]
Tylenol® Children's Meltaways: 80 mg [scored; grape flavor]
Tylenol® Jr. Meltaways: 160 mg [bubblegum flavor]
Tylenol® Jr. Meltaways: 160 mg [grape flavor]

◆ **Acetaminophen and Butalbital** *see* Butalbital and Acetaminophen *on page 255*

◆ **Acetaminophen and Chlorpheniramine** *see* Chlorpheniramine and Acetaminophen *on page 344*

Acetaminophen and Codeine

(a seet a MIN oh fen & KOE deen)

Brand Names: U.S. Capital® and Codeine; Tylenol® with Codeine No. 3; Tylenol® with Codeine No. 4

Brand Names: Canada ratio-Emtec; ratio-Lenoltec; Triatec-30; Triatec-8; Triatec-8 Strong; Tylenol Elixir with Codeine; Tylenol No. 1; Tylenol No. 1 Forte; Tylenol No. 2 with Codeine; Tylenol No. 3 with Codeine; Tylenol No. 4 with Codeine

Index Terms Codeine and Acetaminophen; Tylenol #2; Tylenol #3; Tylenol Codeine

Pharmacologic Category Analgesic, Opioid

Use Relief of mild-to-moderate pain

Pregnancy Risk Factor C

Dosage Doses should be adjusted according to severity of pain and response of the patient. Adult doses ≥60 mg codeine fail to give commensurate relief of pain but merely prolong analgesia and are associated with an appreciably increased incidence of side effects. Oral:

Children: Analgesic:
Codeine: 0.5-1 mg codeine/kg/dose every 4-6 hours
Acetaminophen: 10-15 mg/kg/dose every 4 hours up to a maximum of 2.6 g/24 hours for children <12 years; **alternatively, the following can be used:**
3-6 years: 5 mL 3-4 times/day as needed of elixir
7-12 years: 10 mL 3-4 times/day as needed of elixir
>12 years: 15 mL every 4 hours as needed of elixir

Adults:
Antitussive: Based on codeine (15-30 mg/dose) every 4-6 hours (maximum: 360 mg/24 hours based on codeine component)
Analgesic: Based on codeine (30-60 mg/dose) every 4-6 hours (maximum: 4000 mg/24 hours based on acetaminophen component)
1-2 tablets every 4 hours to a maximum of 12 tablets/24 hours

Dosing adjustment in renal impairment: See individual agents.

Dosing adjustment in hepatic impairment: Use with caution. Limited, low-dose therapy is usually well tolerated in hepatic disease/cirrhosis; however, cases of hepatotoxicity at daily acetaminophen dosages <4 g/day have been reported. Avoid chronic use in hepatic impairment.

Additional Information Complete prescribing information for this medication should be consulted for additional detail.

Dosage Forms Excipient information presented when available (limited, particularly for generics); consult specific product labeling.
Solution, oral [C-V]: Acetaminophen 120 mg and codeine phosphate 12 mg per 5 mL (5 mL, 10 mL, 12.5 mL, 15 mL, 120 mL, 480 mL) [contains alcohol 7%]
Suspension, oral [C-V] (Capital® and Codeine): Acetaminophen 120 mg and codeine phosphate 12 mg per 5 mL (480 mL) [alcohol free; contains propylene glycol, sodium benzoate; fruit punch flavor]
Tablet [C-III]: Acetaminophen 300 mg and codeine phosphate 15 mg; acetaminophen 300 mg and codeine phosphate 30 mg; acetaminophen 300 mg and codeine phosphate 60 mg
Tylenol® with Codeine No. 3: Acetaminophen 300 mg and codeine phosphate 30 mg [contains sodium metabisulfite]
Tylenol® with Codeine No. 4: Acetaminophen 300 mg and codeine phosphate 60 mg [contains sodium metabisulfite]

Dosage Forms: Canada Excipient information presented when available (limited, particularly for generics); consult specific product labeling. **Note:** In countries outside of the U.S., some formulations of Tylenol® with Codeine include caffeine.

Caplet:

ratio-Lenoltec No. 1, Tylenol No. 1: Acetaminophen 300 mg, codeine phosphate 8 mg, and caffeine 15 mg

Tylenol No. 1 Forte: Acetaminophen 500 mg, codeine phosphate 8 mg, and caffeine 15 mg

Solution, oral:

Tylenol Elixir with Codeine: Acetaminophen 160 mg and codeine phosphate 8 mg per 5 mL (500 mL) [contains alcohol 7%, sucrose 31%; cherry flavor]

Tablet:

ratio-Emtec, Triatec-30: Acetaminophen 300 mg and codeine phosphate 30 mg

ratio-Lenoltec No. 1: Acetaminophen 300 mg, codeine phosphate 8 mg, and caffeine 15 mg

ratio-Lenoltec No. 2, Tylenol No. 2 with Codeine: Acetaminophen 300 mg, codeine phosphate 15 mg, and caffeine 15 mg

ratio-Lenoltec No. 3, Tylenol No. 3 with Codeine: Acetaminophen 300 mg, codeine phosphate 30 mg, and caffeine 15 mg

ratio-Lenoltec No. 4, Tylenol No. 4 with Codeine: Acetaminophen 300 mg and codeine phosphate 60 mg

Triatec-8: Acetaminophen 325 mg, codeine phosphate 8 mg, and caffeine 30 mg

Triatec-8 Strong: Acetaminophen 500 mg, codeine phosphate 8 mg, and caffeine 30 mg

Controlled Substance C-III; C-V

Acetaminophen and Diphenhydramine

(a seet a MIN oh fen & dye fen HYE dra meen)

Brand Names: U.S. Excedrin PM® [OTC]; Goody's PM® [OTC]; Legatrin PM® [OTC]; Mapap PM [OTC]; Percogesic® Extra Strength [OTC]; TopCare® Pain Relief PM [OTC]; Tylenol® PM [OTC]; Tylenol® Severe Allergy [OTC]

Index Terms Diphenhydramine and Acetaminophen

Pharmacologic Category Analgesic, Miscellaneous

Use Aid in the relief of insomnia accompanied by minor pain

Dosage Oral: Adults: 50 mg of diphenhydramine HCl (76 mg diphenhydramine citrate) at bedtime or as directed by physician; do not exceed recommended dosage; not for use in children <12 years of age

Dosing adjustment in hepatic impairment: Use with caution. Limited, low-dose therapy is usually well tolerated in hepatic disease/cirrhosis; however, cases of hepatotoxicity at daily acetaminophen dosages <4 g/day have been reported. Avoid chronic use in hepatic impairment.

Additional Information Complete prescribing information for this medication should be consulted for additional detail.

Dosage Forms Excipient information presented when available (limited, particularly for generics); consult specific product labeling.

Caplet, oral:

Excedrin PM®: Acetaminophen 500 mg and diphenhydramine citrate 38 mg

Legatrin PM®: Acetaminophen 500 mg and diphenhydramine hydrochloride 50 mg

Mapap PM: Acetaminophen 500 mg and diphenhydramine hydrochloride 25 mg

Percogesic® Extra Strength: Acetaminophen 500 mg and diphenhydramine hydrochloride 12.5 mg

TopCare® Pain Relief PM: Acetaminophen 500 mg and diphenhydramine citrate 25 mg

Tylenol® PM: Acetaminophen 500 mg and diphenhydramine hydrochloride 25 mg

Tylenol® Severe Allergy: Acetaminophen 500 mg and diphenhydramine hydrochloride 12.5 mg

Captab, oral: Acetaminophen 500 mg and diphenhydramine hydrochloride 25 mg

Gelcap, rapid release, oral:

Tylenol® PM: Acetaminophen 500 mg and diphenhydramine hydrochloride 25 mg

Geltab, oral: Acetaminophen 500 mg and diphenhydramine hydrochloride 25 mg

Excedrin® PM: Acetaminophen 500 mg and diphenhydramine citrate 38 mg

Tylenol® PM: Acetaminophen 500 mg and diphenhydramine hydrochloride 25 mg

Liquid, oral:

Tylenol® PM: Acetaminophen 500 mg and diphenhydramine hydrochloride 25 mg per 15 mL (240 mL) [contains sodium benzoate; vanilla flavor]

Powder for solution, oral:

Goody's PM®: Acetaminophen 500 mg and diphenhydramine citrate 38 mg [contains potassium 41.9 mg and sodium 3.15 mg per powder]

Tablet, oral: Acetaminophen 500 mg and diphenhydramine hydrochloride 25 mg

Excedrin® PM: Acetaminophen 500 mg and diphenhydramine citrate 38 mg

◆ **Acetaminophen and Hydrocodone** *see* Hydrocodone and Acetaminophen *on page 837*

◆ **Acetaminophen and Oxycodone** *see* Oxycodone and Acetaminophen *on page 1269*

Acetaminophen and Pseudoephedrine

(a seet a MIN oh fen & soo doe e FED rin)

Brand Names: U.S. Ornex® Maximum Strength [OTC]; Ornex® [OTC]

Brand Names: Canada Contac® Cold and Sore Throat, Non Drowsy, Extra Strength; Dristan® N.D.; Dristan® N.D., Extra Strength; Sinutab® Non Drowsy; Sudafed® Head Cold and Sinus Extra Strength; Tylenol® Decongestant; Tylenol® Sinus

Index Terms Pseudoephedrine and Acetaminophen; Pseudoephedrine Hydrochloride and Acetaminophen

Pharmacologic Category Alpha/Beta Agonist; Analgesic, Miscellaneous

Use Temporary relief of nasal congestion, and minor aches and pains associated with colds, flu, sinusitis, or allergies

Dosage Oral:

Children 6-11 years (Ornex®): One caplet every 4-6 hours as needed (maximum: 4 caplets/day)

Children ≥12 years and Adults (Ornex®, Ornex® Maximum Strength): Two caplets every 4-6 hours as needed (maximum: 8 caplets/day)

Dosing adjustment in hepatic impairment: Use with caution. Limited, low-dose therapy is usually well tolerated in hepatic disease/cirrhosis; however, cases of hepatotoxicity at daily acetaminophen dosages <4 g/day have been reported. Avoid chronic use in hepatic impairment.

Additional Information Complete prescribing information for this medication should be consulted for additional detail.

Dosage Forms Excipient information presented when available (limited, particularly for generics); consult specific product labeling.

Caplet:

Ornex®: Acetaminophen 325 mg and pseudoephedrine hydrochloride 30 mg

Ornex® Maximum Strength: Acetaminophen 500 mg and pseudoephedrine hydrochloride 30 mg

Acetaminophen and Tramadol

(a seet a MIN oh fen & TRA ma dole)

Brand Names: U.S. Ultracet®

Brand Names: Canada Apo-Tramadol/Acet®; Tramacet

Index Terms Tramadol Hydrochloride and Acetaminophen

Pharmacologic Category Analgesic, Miscellaneous; Analgesic, Opioid

Use Short-term (≤5 days) management of acute pain

Pregnancy Risk Factor C

Dosage Oral: Adults: Acute pain: Two tablets every 4-6 hours as needed for pain relief (maximum: 8 tablets/day); treatment should not exceed 5 days

Dosage adjustment in renal impairment: Cl_{cr} <30 mL/minute: Maximum of 2 tablets every 12 hours; treatment should not exceed 5 days

Dosage adjustment in hepatic impairment: Use is not recommended.

Additional Information Complete prescribing information for this medication should be consulted for additional detail.

Dosage Forms Excipient information presented when available (limited, particularly for generics); consult specific product labeling.

Tablet: Acetaminophen 325 mg and tramadol hydrochloride 37.5 mg

Ultracet®: Acetaminophen 325 mg and tramadol hydrochloride 37.5 mg

Acetaminophen, Aspirin, and Caffeine

(a seet a MIN oh fen, AS pir in, & KAF een)

Brand Names: U.S. Anacin® Advanced Headache Formula [OTC]; Excedrin® Extra Strength [OTC]; Excedrin® Migraine [OTC]; Fem-Prin® [OTC]; Goody's® Extra Strength Headache Powder [OTC]; Goody's® Extra Strength Pain Relief [OTC]; Pain-Off [OTC]; Vanquish® Extra Strength Pain Reliever [OTC]

Index Terms Aspirin, Acetaminophen, and Caffeine; Aspirin, Caffeine and Acetaminophen; Caffeine, Acetaminophen, and Aspirin; Caffeine, Aspirin, and Acetaminophen

Pharmacologic Category Analgesic, Miscellaneous

Use Relief of mild-to-moderate pain; mild-to-moderate pain associated with migraine headache

Pregnancy Risk Factor D

Dosage Oral: Adults:

Analgesic:

Based on **acetaminophen** component:

Mild-to-moderate pain: 325-650 mg every 4-6 hours as needed; do **not** exceed 4 g/day

Mild-to-moderate pain associated with migraine headache: 500 mg/dose (in combination with 500 mg aspirin and 130 mg caffeine) every 6 hours while symptoms persist; do not use for longer than 48 hours

Based on **aspirin** component:

Mild-to-moderate pain: 325-650 mg every 4-6 hours as needed; do **not** exceed 4 g/day

Mild-to-moderate pain associated with migraine headache: 500 mg/dose (in combination with 500 mg acetaminophen and 130 mg caffeine) every 6 hours while symptoms persist; do not use for longer than 48 hours

Product labeling:

Excedrin® Extra Strength, Excedrin® Migraine: Children >12 years and Adults: 2 doses every 6 hours (maximum: 8 doses/24 hours)

Note: When used for migraine, do not use for longer than 48 hours

Goody's® Extra Strength Headache Powder: Children >12 years and Adults: 1 powder, placed on tongue or dissolved in water, every 4-6 hours (maximum: 4 powders/24 hours)

Goody's® Extra Strength Pain Relief Tablets: Children >12 years and Adults: 2 tablets every 4-6 hours (maximum: 8 tablets/24 hours)

Vanquish® Extra Strength Pain Reliever: Children >12 years and Adults: 2 tablets every 4 hours (maximum: 12 tablets/24 hours)

Dosing adjustment in hepatic impairment: Use with caution. Limited, low-dose therapy is usually well tolerated in hepatic disease/cirrhosis; however, cases of hepatotoxicity at daily acetaminophen dosages <4 g/day have been reported. Avoid chronic use in hepatic impairment.

Additional Information Complete prescribing information for this medication should be consulted for additional detail.

Dosage Forms Excipient information presented when available (limited, particularly for generics); consult specific product labeling.

Caplet:

Excedrin® Extra Strength, Excedrin® Migraine: Acetaminophen 250 mg, aspirin 250 mg, and caffeine 65 mg

Vanquish® Extra Strength Pain Reliever: Acetaminophen 194 mg, aspirin 227 mg, and caffeine 33 mg

Geltab (Excedrin® Extra Strength, Excedrin® Migraine): Acetaminophen 250 mg, aspirin 250 mg, and caffeine 65 mg

Powder (Goody's® Extra Strength Headache Powder): Acetaminophen 260 mg, aspirin 520 mg, and caffeine 32.5 mg [contains lactose]

Tablet:

Anacin® Advanced Headache Formula: Acetaminophen 250 mg, aspirin 250 mg, and caffeine 65 mg

Excedrin® Extra Strength, Excedrin® Migraine, Pain-Off: Acetaminophen 250 mg, aspirin 250 mg, and caffeine 65 mg

Fem-Prin®: Acetaminophen 194.4 mg, aspirin 226.8 mg, and caffeine 32.4 mg

Goody's® Extra Strength Pain Relief: Acetaminophen 130 mg, aspirin 260 mg, and caffeine 16.25 mg

◆ **Acetaminophen, Butalbital, and Caffeine** *see* Butalbital, Acetaminophen, and Caffeine *on page* 255

◆ **Acetasol® HC** *see* Acetic Acid, Propylene Glycol Diacetate, and Hydrocortisone *on page* 33

◆ **Acetazolam (Can)** *see* AcetaZOLAMIDE *on page* 32

AcetaZOLAMIDE

(a set a ZOLE a mide)

Brand Names: U.S. Diamox® Sequels®

Brand Names: Canada Acetazolam; Diamox®

Pharmacologic Category Anticonvulsant, Miscellaneous; Carbonic Anhydrase Inhibitor; Diuretic, Carbonic Anhydrase Inhibitor; Ophthalmic Agent, Antiglaucoma

Use Treatment of glaucoma (chronic simple open-angle, secondary glaucoma, preoperatively in acute angle-closure); drug-induced edema or edema due to congestive heart failure (adjunctive therapy; I.V. and immediate release dosage forms); centrencephalic epilepsies (I.V. and immediate release dosage forms); prevention or amelioration of symptoms associated with acute mountain sickness (immediate and extended release dosage forms)

Unlabeled Use Metabolic alkalosis; respiratory stimulant in stable hypercapnic COPD

Pregnancy Risk Factor C

Dosage Note: I.M. administration is not recommended because of pain secondary to the alkaline pH

Children:

Altitude illness:

Prevention: Oral: 2.5 mg/kg/dose every 12 hours started either the day before (preferred) or on the day of ascent and may be discontinued after staying at the same elevation for 2-3 days or if descent initiated; maximum dose: 125 mg/dose (Luks, 2010). **Note:** The International Society for Mountain Medicine does not recommend prophylaxis in children except in the rare circumstance of unavoidable rapid ascent or in children with known previous susceptibility to acute mountain sickness (Pollard, 2001).

Treatment: Oral: 2.5 mg/kg/dose every 8-12 hours; maximum dose: 250 mg/dose. **Note:** With high altitude cerebral edema, dexamethasone is the primary treatment; however, acetazolamide may be used adjunctively with the same treatment dose (Luks, 2010; Pollard, 2001).

Epilepsy: Oral: 8-30 mg/kg/day in divided doses. A lower dosing range of 4-16 mg/kg/day in 1-4 divided doses has also been recommended; maximum dose: 30 mg/kg/day or 1 g/day (Oles, 1989; Reiss, 1996). **Note:** Minimal additional benefit with doses >16 mg/kg/day. **Extended release capsule is not recommended for treatment of epilepsy.**

Adults:

Altitude illness: Oral: Manufacturer's labeling: 500-1000 mg/day in divided doses every 8-12 hours (immediate release tablets) or divided every 12-24 hours (extended release capsules). These doses are associated with more frequent and/or increased side effects. Alternative dosing has been recommended:

Prevention: 125 mg twice daily; beginning either the day before (preferred) or on the day of ascent; may be discontinued after staying at the same elevation for 2-3 days or if descent initiated (Basnyat, 2006; Luks, 2010). **Note:** In situations of rapid ascent (such as rescue or military operations), 1000 mg/day is recommended by the manufacturer. The Wilderness Medical Society recommends consideration of using dexamethasone in addition to acetazolamide in these situations (Luks, 2010).

Treatment: 250 mg twice daily. **Note:** With high altitude cerebral edema, dexamethasone is the primary treatment; however, acetazolamide may be used adjunctively with the same treatment dose (Luks, 2010).

Edema: Oral, I.V.: 250-375 mg once daily

Epilepsy: Oral: 8-30 mg/kg/day in divided doses. A lower dosing range of 4-16 mg/kg/day in 1-4 divided doses has also been recommended; maximum dose: 30 mg/kg/day or 1 g/day (Oles, 1989; Reiss, 1996). **Note:** Minimal additional benefit with doses >16 mg/kg/day. **Extended release capsule is not recommended for treatment of epilepsy.**

Glaucoma:

Chronic simple (open-angle): Oral, I.V.: 250 mg 1-4 times/day or 500 mg extended release capsule twice daily

Secondary or acute (closed-angle): Oral, I.V.: Initial: 250-500 mg; maintenance: 125-250 mg every 4 hours (250 mg every 12 hours has been effective in short-term treatment of some patients)

Metabolic alkalosis (unlabeled use): I.V.: 500 mg as a single dose; reassess need based upon acid-base status (Marik, 1991; Mazur, 1999)

Respiratory stimulant in stable hypercapnic COPD (unlabeled use): Oral: 250 mg twice daily (Wagenaar, 2003)

Elderly: Oral: Initial doses should begin at the low end of the dosage range.

Dosing adjustment in renal impairment: Note: Use is contraindicated in marked renal impairment; creatinine clearance cutoff not specified in manufacturer's labeling.

Cl_{cr} 10-50 mL/minute: Administer every 12 hours

Cl_{cr} <10 mL/minute: Avoid use

Hemodialysis: Moderately dialyzable (20% to 50%)

Peritoneal dialysis: Supplemental dose is not necessary (Schwenk, 1994)

Additional Information Complete prescribing information for this medication should be consulted for additional detail.

Dosage Forms Excipient information presented when available (limited, particularly for generics); consult specific product labeling.

Capsule, extended release, oral: 500 mg

Capsule, sustained release, oral:

Diamox® Sequels®: 500 mg

Injection, powder for reconstitution: 500 mg

Tablet, oral: 125 mg, 250 mg

Acetic Acid (a SEE tik AS id)

Brand Names: U.S. VoSoL®

Index Terms Ethanoic Acid

Pharmacologic Category Otic Agent, Anti-infective; Topical Skin Product

Use Irrigation of the bladder; periodic irrigation of indwelling catheters; treatment of superficial bacterial infections of the external auditory canal

Pregnancy Risk Factor C

Dosage

Irrigation: Adults: (**Note:** Dosage of an irrigating solution depends on the capacity or surface area of the structure being irrigated):

For continuous irrigation of the urinary bladder with 0.25% acetic acid irrigation, the rate of administration will approximate the rate of urine flow; usually 500-1500 mL/24 hours

For periodic irrigation of an indwelling urinary catheter to maintain patency, about 50 mL of 0.25% acetic acid irrigation is required

Otic:

Children ≥3 years: Otitis externa: Insert saturated wick; keep moist 24 hours; remove wick and instill 5 drops 3-4 times/day. **Note:** 3-4 drops may be sufficient in children due to the smaller capacity of the ear canal.

Adults: Otitis externa: Insert saturated wick; keep moist 24 hours; remove wick and instill 5 drops 3-4 times/day

Additional Information Complete prescribing information for this medication should be consulted for additional detail.

Dosage Forms Excipient information presented when available (limited, particularly for generics); consult specific product labeling.

Solution, for irrigation: 0.25% (1000 mL)

Solution, for irrigation [preservative free]: 0.25% (250 mL, 500 mL, 1000 mL)

Solution, otic [drops]: 2% (15 mL, 60 mL)

VoSoL®: 2% (15 mL) [contains benzethonium chloride]

◆ **Acetic Acid, Hydrocortisone, and Propylene Glycol Diacetate** *see* Acetic Acid, Propylene Glycol Diacetate, and Hydrocortisone *on page* 33

Acetic Acid, Propylene Glycol Diacetate, and Hydrocortisone

(a SEE tik AS id, PRO pa leen GLY kole dye AS e tate, & hye droe KOR ti sone)

Brand Names: U.S. Acetasol® HC; VoSol® HC

Index Terms Acetic Acid, Hydrocortisone, and Propylene Glycol Diacetate; Hydrocortisone, Acetic Acid, and Propylene Glycol Diacetate; Propylene Glycol Diacetate, Acetic Acid, and Hydrocortisone

Pharmacologic Category Otic Agent, Anti-infective

Use Treatment of superficial infections of the external auditory canal caused by organisms susceptible to the action of the antimicrobial, complicated by swelling

Dosage Children ≥3 years and Adults: Otic: Instill 3-5 drops in ear(s) every 4-6 hours

Additional Information Complete prescribing information for this medication should be consulted for additional detail.

Dosage Forms Excipient information presented when available (limited, particularly for generics); consult specific product labeling.

Solution, otic [drops]: Acetic acid 2%, propylene glycol diacetate 3%, and hydrocortisone 1% (10 mL)

Acetasol® HC: Acetic acid 2%, propylene glycol diacetate 3%, and hydrocortisone 1% (10 mL) [contains benzethonium chloride]

VoSol® HC: Acetic acid 2%, propylene glycol diacetate 3%, and hydrocortisone 1% (10 mL) [contains benzethonium chloride]

◆ **Acetoxymethylprogesterone** *see* MedroxyPROGESTERone *on page 1058*

Acetylcholine (a se teel KOE leen)

Brand Names: U.S. Miochol®-E

Brand Names: Canada Miochol®-E

Index Terms Acetylcholine Chloride

Pharmacologic Category Cholinergic Agonist; Ophthalmic Agent, Miotic

Use Produces complete miosis in cataract surgery, keratoplasty, iridectomy, and other anterior segment surgery where rapid miosis is required

Contraindications Hypersensitivity to acetylcholine chloride or any component of the formulation

Warnings/Precautions During cataract surgery, use only after lens is in place. Open under aseptic conditions only; do not gas sterilize. Systemic effects rarely occur but can cause problems for patients with acute cardiac failure, bronchial asthma, peptic ulcer, hyperthyroidism, GI spasm, urinary tract obstruction, and Parkinson's disease.

Adverse Reactions Frequency not defined.

Cardiovascular: Bradycardia, flushing, hypotension

Ocular: Clouding, corneal edema, decompensation

Respiratory: Dyspnea

Miscellaneous: Diaphoresis

Drug Interactions

Metabolism/Transport Effects None known.

Avoid Concomitant Use There are no known interactions where it is recommended to avoid concomitant use.

Increased Effect/Toxicity

The levels/effects of Acetylcholine may be increased by: Acetylcholinesterase Inhibitors; Beta-Blockers

Decreased Effect There are no known significant interactions involving a decrease in effect.

Stability Store unopened vial at 4°C to 25°C (39°F to 77°F); prevent from freezing. Prepare solution in an aseptic environment immediately before use and discard unused portion. Acetylcholine solutions are unstable; reconstitute immediately before use. Only use if solution is clear and colorless.

Mechanism of Action Causes contraction of the sphincter muscles of the iris, resulting in miosis and contraction of the ciliary muscle, leading to accommodation spasm

Pharmacodynamics/Kinetics

Onset of action: Rapid

Duration: ~6 hours

Dosage Adults: Intraocular: 0.5-2 mL of 1% injection (5-20 mg) instilled into anterior chamber before or after securing one or more sutures

Administration Ophthalmic: Open under aseptic conditions only. Attach filter before irrigating eye. Instill into anterior chamber before or after securing one or more sutures; instillation should be gentle and parallel to the iris face and tangential to the pupil border; in cataract surgery, acetylcholine should be used only after delivery of the lens.

Dosage Forms Excipient information presented when available (limited, particularly for generics); consult specific product labeling.

Powder for solution, intraocular, as chloride:

Miochol®-E: 20 mg (2 mL) [supplied with diluent; reconstitution results in 1:100 solution]

◆ **Acetylcholine Chloride** *see* Acetylcholine *on page 34*

Acetylcysteine (a se teel SIS teen)

Brand Names: U.S. Acetadote®

Brand Names: Canada Acetylcysteine Solution; Mucomyst®; Parvolex®

Index Terms *N* Acetylcysteine; *N*-Acetyl-L-cysteine; *N*-Acetylcysteine; Acetylcysteine Sodium; Mercapturic Acid; Mucomyst; NAC

Pharmacologic Category Antidote; Mucolytic Agent

Use Antidote for acute acetaminophen poisoning; repeated supratherapeutic ingestion (RSTI) of acetaminophen; adjunctive mucolytic therapy in patients with abnormal or viscid mucous secretions in acute and chronic bronchopulmonary diseases; pulmonary complications of surgery and cystic fibrosis; diagnostic bronchial studies

Unlabeled Use Prevention of contrast-induced renal dysfunction (oral, I.V.); distal intestinal obstruction syndrome (DIOS, previously referred to as meconium ileus equivalent)

Pregnancy Risk Factor B

Pregnancy Considerations Based on limited reports using acetylcysteine to treat acetaminophen poisoning in pregnant women, acetylcysteine has been shown to cross the placenta and may provide protective levels in the fetus.

Lactation Excretion in breast milk unknown/use caution

Contraindications Hypersensitivity to acetylcysteine or any component of the formulation

Warnings/Precautions

Inhalation: Since increased bronchial secretions may develop after inhalation, percussion, postural drainage, and suctioning should follow. If bronchospasm occurs, administer a bronchodilator; discontinue acetylcysteine if bronchospasm progresses.

Intravenous: Acute flushing and erythema have been reported; usually occurs within 30-60 minutes and may resolve spontaneously. Serious anaphylactoid reactions have also been reported and are more commonly associated with I.V. administration, but may also occur with oral administration (Mroz, 1997). When used for acetaminophen poisoning, the incidence is reduced when the initial loading dose is administered over 60 minutes. The acetylcysteine infusion may be interrupted until treatment of allergic symptoms is initiated; the infusion can then be carefully restarted. Treatment for anaphylactoid reactions should be immediately available. Use caution in patients with asthma or history of bronchospasm as these patients may be at increased risk. Conversely, patients with high acetaminophen levels (>150 mg/dL) may be at a reduced risk for anaphylactoid reactions (Pakravan, 2008; Waring, 2008; Sandilands, 2009).

Acute acetaminophen poisoning: Acetylcysteine is indicated in patients with a serum acetaminophen level that indicates they are at "possible" risk or greater for hepatotoxicity when plotted on the Rumack-Matthew nomogram. There are several situations where the nomogram is of limited use. Serum acetaminophen levels obtained <4 hours postingestion are not interpretable; patients presenting late may have undetectable serum concentrations, despite having received a toxic dose. The nomogram is less predictive of hepatic injury following an acute overdose with an extended release acetaminophen product. The nomogram also does not take into account patients who may be at higher risk of acetaminophen toxicity (eg, alcoholics, malnourished patients). Nevertheless, acetylcysteine should be administered to any patient with signs of hepatotoxicity, even if the serum acetaminophen level is low or undetectable. Patients who present >24 hours after an acute ingestion or patients who present following an acute ingestion at an unknown time may be candidates for acetylcysteine therapy; consultation with a poison control center or clinical toxicologist is highly recommended.

Repeated supratherapeutic ingestion (RSTI) of acetaminophen: The Rumack-Matthew nomogram is not designed to be used following RSTIs. In general, an accurate past medical history, including a comprehensive acetaminophen ingestion history, in conjunction with AST concentrations and serum acetaminophen levels, may give the clinician insight as to the patient's risk of acetaminophen toxicity. Some experts recommend that acetylcysteine be administered to any patient with "higher than expected" serum acetaminophen levels or serum acetaminophen level >10 mcg/mL, even in the absence of hepatic injury; others recommend treatment for patients with laboratory evidence and/or signs and symptoms of hepatotoxicity (Hendrickson, 2006; Jones, 2000). Consultation with a poison control center or a clinical toxicologist is highly recommended.

Adverse Reactions

Inhalation: Frequency not defined.

Central nervous system: Drowsiness, chills, fever

Gastrointestinal: Vomiting, nausea, stomatitis

Local: Irritation, stickiness on face following nebulization

Respiratory: Bronchospasm, rhinorrhea, hemoptysis

Miscellaneous: Acquired sensitization (rare), clamminess, unpleasant odor during administration

Intravenous:

>10%: Miscellaneous: Anaphylactoid reaction (8% to 18%; shorter infusion periods [eg, <60 minutes] associated with increased incidence)

1% to 10%:

Cardiovascular: Flushing (1% to 8%), tachycardia (1% to 4%), edema (1% to 2%)

Dermatologic: Urticaria (6% to 8%), rash (2% to 4%), pruritus (1% to 4%)

Gastrointestinal: Vomiting (2% to 10%), nausea (1% to 6%)

Respiratory: Pharyngitis (≤1%), rhinorrhea (≤1%), rhonchi (≤1%), throat tightness (≤1%)

<1% (Limited to important or life-threatening): Anaphylaxis, angioedema, bronchospasm, chest tightness, cough, dizziness, dyspnea, headache, hypotension, respiratory distress, stridor, wheezing

Drug Interactions

Metabolism/Transport Effects None known.

Avoid Concomitant Use There are no known interactions where it is recommended to avoid concomitant use.

Increased Effect/Toxicity There are no known significant interactions involving an increase in effect.

Decreased Effect There are no known significant interactions involving a decrease in effect.

Stability

Solution for injection (Acetadote®): Store unopened vials at room temperature, 20°C to 25°C (68°F to 77°F). Following reconstitution with D_5W, solution is stable for 24 hours at room temperature. A color change may occur in opened vials (light purple) and does not affect the safety or efficacy.

Loading dose: Dilute 150 mg/kg in D_5W 200 mL.

Second dose: Dilute 50 mg/kg in D_5W 500 mL.

Third dose: Dilute 100 mg/kg in D_5W 1000 mL.

Note: To avoid fluid overload in patients <40 kg and those requiring fluid restriction, decrease volume of D_5W proportionally (see table on next page). Discard unused portion.

Solution for inhalation: Store unopened vials at room temperature; once opened, store under refrigeration and use within 96 hours. The 20% solution may be diluted with sodium chloride or sterile water; the 10% solution may be used undiluted. A color change may occur in opened vials (light purple) and does not affect the safety or efficacy.

Intravenous administration of solution for inhalation (unlabeled route): Using D_5W, dilute acetylcysteine 20% oral solution to a 3% solution.

Mechanism of Action Exerts mucolytic action through its free sulfhydryl group which opens up the disulfide bonds in the mucoproteins thus lowering mucous viscosity.

In patients with acetaminophen toxicity, acetylcysteine acts as a hepatoprotective agent by restoring hepatic glutathione, serving as a glutathione substitute, and enhancing the nontoxic sulfate conjugation of acetaminophen.

The presumed mechanism in preventing contrast-induced nephropathy is its ability to scavenge oxygen-derived free radicals and improve endothelium-dependent vasodilation.

Pharmacodynamics/Kinetics

Onset of action: Inhalation: 5-10 minutes

Duration: Inhalation: >1 hour

Distribution: 0.47 L/kg

Protein binding: 83%

Half-life elimination:

Reduced acetylcysteine: 2 hours

Total acetylcysteine: Adults: 5.6 hours; Newborns: 11 hours

Time to peak, plasma: Oral: 1-2 hours

Excretion: Urine

Dosage

Acetaminophen poisoning: **Note:** Only the 72-hour oral and 21-hour I.V. regimens are FDA-approved. Ideally, in patients with an acute acetaminophen ingestion, treatment should begin within 8 hours of ingestion or as soon as possible after ingestion. In patients who present following RSTI and treatment is deemed appropriate, acetylcysteine should be initiated immediately.

Children and Adults:

Oral: **Note:** Consultation with a poison control center or clinical toxicologist is highly recommended when considering the discontinuation of oral acetylcysteine prior to the conclusion of a full 18-dose course of therapy.

72-hour regimen: Consists of 18 doses; total dose delivered: 1330 mg/kg

Loading dose: 140 mg/kg

Maintenance dose: 70 mg/kg every 4 hours; repeat dose if emesis occurs within 1 hour of administration

I.V. (Acetadote®):

21-hour regimen: Consists of 3 doses; total dose delivered: 300 mg/kg

Loading dose: 150 mg/kg (maximum: 15 g) infused over 60 minutes

Second dose: 50 mg/kg (maximum: 5 g) infused over 4 hours

Third dose: 100 mg/kg (maximum: 10 g) infused over 16 hours

Note: The fluid volume should be reduced in patients weighing <40 kg according to the following table:

Acetadote® Dosing / Fluid Volume Guidelines for Patients <40 kg

Body Weight (kg)	Loading Dose 150 mg/kg over 1 h		Second Dose 50 mg/kg over 4 h		Third Dose 100 mg/kg over 16 h	
	Acetadote® (mL)	D_5W (mL)	Acetadote® (mL)	D_5W (mL)	Acetadote® (mL)	D_5W (mL)
30	22.5	100	7.5	250	15	500
25	18.75	100	6.25	250	12.5	500
20	15	60	5	140	10	280
15	11.25	45	3.75	105	7.5	210
10	7.5	30	2.5	70	5	140

Adjuvant therapy in respiratory conditions: **Note:** Patients should receive an aerosolized bronchodilator 10-15 minutes prior to acetylcysteine.

Inhalation, nebulization (face mask, mouth piece, tracheostomy): Acetylcysteine 10% and 20% solution (dilute 20% solution with sodium chloride or sterile water for inhalation); 10% solution may be used undiluted

Infants: 1-2 mL of 20% solution or 2-4 mL of 10% solution until nebulized given 3-4 times/day

Children and Adults: 3-5 mL of 20% solution or 6-10 mL of 10% solution until nebulized given 3-4 times/day; dosing range: 1-10 mL of 20% solution or 2-20 mL of 10% solution every 2-6 hours

Inhalation, nebulization (tent, croupette): Children and Adults: Dose must be individualized; may require up to 300 mL solution/treatment

Direct instillation: Adults:

Into tracheostomy: 1-2 mL of 10% to 20% solution every 1-4 hours

Through percutaneous intratracheal catheter: 1-2 mL of 20% or 2-4 mL of 10% solution every 1-4 hours via syringe attached to catheter

Diagnostic bronchogram: Nebulization or intratracheal: Adults: 1-2 mL of 20% solution or 2-4 mL of 10% solution administered 2-3 times prior to procedure

Prevention of contrast-induced nephropathy (CIN) (unlabeled use): Adults: Oral: 600-1200 mg twice daily for 2 days (beginning the day before the procedure); may be given as powder in capsules (some centers use solution, diluted in cola beverage or juice). **Note:** No longer recommended for use prior to percutaneous coronary intervention; instead adequate hydration is preferred (Levine, 2011).

Administration

Inhalation: Acetylcysteine is incompatible with tetracyclines, erythromycin, amphotericin B, iodized oil, chymotrypsin, trypsin, and hydrogen peroxide. Administer separately. Intermittent aerosol treatments are commonly given when patient arises, before meals, and just before retiring at bedtime.

Oral: Treatment of acetaminophen poisoning, administer orally as a 5% solution. Dilute the 20% solution 1:3 with a cola, orange juice, or other soft drink. Use within 1 hour of preparation. The unpleasant odor (sulfur-like) becomes less noticeable as treatment progresses. If patient vomits within 1 hour of dose, readminister. (**Note:** It is helpful to put the acetylcysteine on ice, in a cup with a cover, and drink through a straw; alternatively, administer via an NG tube).

I.V. (Acetadote®): Acetaminophen poisoning:

Loading dose: Dilute in D_5W 200 mL; administer over 60 minutes.

Second dose: Dilute in D_5W 500 mL; administer over 4 hours.

Third dose: Dilute in D_5W 1000 mL; administer over 16 hours.

Note: To avoid fluid overload in patients <40 kg and those requiring fluid restriction, decrease volume of D_5W proportionally (see table in Dosage). Discard unused portion.

If the commercial I.V. form is unavailable, the solution for inhalation has been used; each dose should be infused through a 0.2 micron Millipore filter (in-line) over 60 minutes (Yip, 1998); intravenous administration of the solution for inhalation is not USP 797-compliant.

Monitoring Parameters Acetaminophen poisoning: Monitor patient for the development of anaphylaxis or anaphylactoid reactions; monitor serum acetaminophen levels, AST, ALT, bilirubin, PT, INR, serum creatinine, BUN, serum glucose, hemoglobin, hematocrit, and electrolytes. Assess patient for nausea, vomiting, and skin rash following oral administration. Reassess LFTs for possible hepatotoxicity every 4-6 hours. An early elevation in the INR may be related to acetylcysteine therapy (Schmidt, 2002).

Acute ingestion: Obtain the first acetaminophen level 4 hours postingestion (or as soon as possible thereafter); plot on the Rumack-Matthew nomogram. In patients who have ingested an extended release formulation of acetaminophen or have coingested an agent known to delay gastric emptying, obtain a repeat serum acetaminophen measurement 4-6 hours following the first measurement if the original level (taken at 4-8 hours postingestion) when plotted on the Rumack-Matthew nomogram indicated that treatment was not necessary.

Dosage Forms Excipient information presented when available (limited, particularly for generics); consult specific product labeling. [DSC] = Discontinued product

Injection, solution:

Acetadote®: 20% [200 mg/mL] (30 mL [DSC]) [contains edetate disodium]

Injection, solution [preservative free]:

Acetadote®: 20% [200 mg/mL] (30 mL)

Solution, for inhalation/oral: 10% [100 mg/mL] (10 mL, 30 mL); 20% [200 mg/mL] (10 mL, 30 mL)

Solution, for inhalation/oral [preservative free]: 10% [100 mg/mL] (4 mL, 10 mL); 20% [200 mg/mL] (4 mL, 10 mL, 30 mL)

◆ **Acetylcysteine, Methylcobalamin, and Methylfolate** *see* Methylfolate, Methylcobalamin, and Acetylcysteine *on page 1106*

◆ **Acetylcysteine, Methylfolate, and Methylcobalamin** *see* Methylfolate, Methylcobalamin, and Acetylcysteine *on page 1106*

◆ **Acetylcysteine Sodium** *see* Acetylcysteine *on page 34*

◆ **Acetylcysteine Solution (Can)** *see* Acetylcysteine *on page 34*

◆ **Acetylsalicylic Acid** *see* Aspirin *on page 154*

◆ **Achromycin** *see* Tetracycline *on page 1661*

◆ **Aciclovir** *see* Acyclovir (Systemic) *on page 39*

◆ **Aciclovir** *see* Acyclovir (Topical) *on page 42*

◆ **Acid Control (Can)** *see* Famotidine *on page 688*

◆ **Acid Gone [OTC]** *see* Aluminum Hydroxide and Magnesium Carbonate *on page 79*

◆ **Acid Gone Extra Strength [OTC]** *see* Aluminum Hydroxide and Magnesium Carbonate *on page 79*

◆ **Acid Reducer (Can)** *see* Ranitidine *on page 1462*

◆ **Acidulated Phosphate Fluoride** *see* Fluoride *on page 728*

◆ **Acilac (Can)** *see* Lactulose *on page 964*

◆ **AcipHex®** *see* RABEprazole *on page 1451*

Acitretin (a si TRE tin)

Brand Names: U.S. Soriatane®
Brand Names: Canada Soriatane®
Pharmacologic Category Retinoid-Like Compound
Use Treatment of severe psoriasis
Pregnancy Risk Factor X
Pregnancy Considerations [U.S. Boxed Warning]: Not for use by women who are pregnant or intend to become pregnant. Acitretin is teratogenic in humans. Severe birth defects have been reported when conception occurred during treatment or after therapy was complete. Patients should not get pregnant for at least 3 years after discontinuation. In addition, because ethanol forms a teratogenic metabolite and would increase the duration of teratogenic potential, ethanol should not be consumed during treatment or for 2 months after discontinuation. The Do Your P.A.R.T. (Pregnancy Prevention Actively Required During and After Treatment) program explains teratogenic risks and requirements expected of females of childbearing potential. Limited amounts of acitretin are found in seminal fluid; although it appears this poses little risk to a fetus, the actual risk of teratogenicity is not known. Any pregnancy which occurs during treatment, or within 3 years after treatment is discontinued, should be reported to the manufacturer at 1-888-784-3335 or to the FDA at 1-800-FDA-1088.
Lactation Enters breast milk/not recommended
Medication Guide Available Yes
Contraindications Hypersensitivity to acitretin, other retinoids, or any component of the formulation; patients who are pregnant or intend on becoming pregnant; severe hepatic or renal dysfunction; chronically-elevated blood lipid levels; concomitant use with methotrexate or tetracyclines

Acitretin is contraindicated in females of childbearing potential unless all of the following conditions apply.

1) Patient has severe psoriasis unresponsive to other therapy or if clinical condition contraindicates other treatments.
2) Patient must have two negative urine or serum pregnancy tests prior to therapy.
3) Patient must have pregnancy test repeated monthly during therapy. After discontinuation of therapy, a pregnancy test must be repeated every 3 months for at least 3 years.
4) Patient must commit to using two effective forms of birth control starting 1 month prior to acitretin treatment and for 3 years after discontinuation. Prescriber must counsel patient about contraception every month during therapy and every 3 months following discontinuation for at least 3 years.
5) Patient is reliable in understanding and carrying out instructions.
6) Patient has received, and acknowledged, understanding of a careful oral and printed explanation of the hazards of fetal exposure to acitretin and the risk of possible contraception failure. Patient must sign an agreement/informed consent document stating that she understands these risks and that she should not consume ethanol during therapy or for 2 months after discontinuation.

Warnings/Precautions [U.S. Boxed Warning]: Not for use by women who want to become pregnant; patient should not get pregnant for at least 3 years after discontinuation. The Do Your P.A.R.T. (Pregnancy Prevention Actively Required During and After Treatment) program explains teratogenic risks and requirements expected of females of childbearing potential to prevent pregnancies from occurring during use and 3 years following discontinuation; this should be used to educate patients and healthcare providers. **[U.S. Boxed Warning]: Female patients should abstain from ethanol or ethanol-containing products during therapy and for 2 months after discontinuation. [U.S. Boxed Warning]: All patients should be advised not to donate blood during therapy or for 3 years following completion of therapy. [U.S. Boxed Warning]: Changes in transaminases occur in up to 1/3 of patients.** Monitor for hepatotoxicity; discontinue if significant elevations of liver enzymes occur. Use with caution in patients at risk of hypertriglyceridemias. Lipid changes including, increased triglycerides, increased cholesterol, and decreased HDL are common (up to 66%). Pseudotumor cerebri has been reported (rarely); may occur with the use of tetracyclines and acitretin independently. Discontinue if visual changes occur. May cause adverse effects to the eyes and vision, including a decrease in night vision or decreased tolerance to contact lenses. Use caution when operating vehicles at night; discontinue if visual changes occur. Patients receiving long-term treatment should be periodically examined for bony abnormalities; risk vs benefit of therapy should be considered if abnormalities occur. Depression, including thoughts of self-harm have been reported; use with caution in patients with a history of mental illness. May be photosensitizing; minimize sun or other UV exposure to treated areas. The risk of burning is increased with phototherapy; decreased doses are required. Transient worsening of psoriasis may initially occur; patients should be advised that it may take 2-3 months to achieve the full benefits of treatment. Not indicated for the treatment of acne. **[U.S. Boxed Warning]: All patients must be provided with a medication guide each time acitretin is dispensed. Female patients must also sign an informed consent prior to therapy.** Safety and efficacy for pediatric patients have not been established; growth potential may be affected.

Adverse Reactions
>10%:
Central nervous system: Hyperesthesia (10% to 25%)
Dermatologic: Cheilitis (>75%), alopecia (50% to 75%), skin peeling (50% to 75%), dry skin (25% to 50%), nail disorder (25% to 50%), pruritus (25% to 50%), erythematous rash (10% to 25%), paronychia (10% to 25%), skin atrophy (10% to 25%), sticky skin (10% to 25%)
Endocrine & metabolic: Hypertriglyceridemia (50% to 75%), fasting blood sugar increased (25% to 50%), HDL decreased (25% to 50%), hypercholesterolemia (25% to 50%), fasting blood sugar decreased (10% to 25%), magnesium increased/decreased (10% to 25%), phosphorus increased (10% to 25%), potassium increased (10% to 25%), sodium increased (10% to 25%)
Gastrointestinal: Xerostomia (10% to 25%)
Hematologic: Reticulocytes increased (25% to 50%), haptoglobin increased (10% to 25%), hematocrit decreased (10% to 25%), hemoglobin decreased (10% to 25%), neutrophils increased (10% to 25%), WBC increased/decreased (10% to 25%)
Hepatic: Liver function tests increased (25% to 50%), alkaline phosphatase increased (10% to 25%), direct bilirubin increased (10% to 25%), GGTP increased (10% to 25%)
Neuromuscular & skeletal: CPK increased (25% to 50%), arthralgia (10% to 25%), paresthesia (10% to 25%), rigors (10% to 25%), spinal hyperostosis progression (10% to 25%)
Ocular: Xerophthalmia (10% to 25%)
Renal: WBC in urine (25% to 50%), acetonuria (10% to 25%), hematuria (10% to 25%), RBC in urine (10% to 25%), uric acid increased (10% to 25%)
Respiratory: Rhinitis (25% to 50%), epistaxis (10% to 25%)

1% to 10%:
- Cardiovascular: Edema, flushing
- Central nervous system: Depression, fatigue, headache, insomnia, pain, somnolence
- Dermatologic: Bullous eruption, cold/clammy skin, dermatitis, fissures, hair texture change, psoriasiform rash, purpura, pyogenic granuloma, rash, seborrhea, skin odor, sunburn, ulcers
- Endocrine & metabolic: Calcium increased or decreased, chloride increased or decreased, hot flashes, iron increased/decreased, phosphorus decreased, potassium decreased, sodium decreased
- Gastrointestinal: Abdominal pain, anorexia, appetite increased, diarrhea, gingival bleeding, gingivitis, nausea, saliva increased, stomatitis, taste disturbance, thirst, tongue disorder, ulcerative stomatitis
- Hematologic: Haptoglobin decreased, hematocrit increased, hemoglobin increased, neutrophils decreased, RBC increased/decreased, reticulocytes decreased
- Hepatic: Total bilirubin increased
- Neuromuscular & skeletal: Arthritis, arthrosis, back pain, Bell's palsy, hypertonia, myalgia, osteodynia, peripheral joint hyperostosis
- Ocular: Blepharitis, blurred vision, cataract, conjunctivitis, corneal epithelial abnormality, diplopia, eye pain, eyebrow or eyelash loss, night blindness, photophobia
- Otic: Earache, tinnitus
- Renal: Albumin decreased/increased, BUN increased, creatinine increased, glycosuria, proteinuria
- Respiratory: Sinusitis
- Miscellaneous: Diaphoresis increased

<1% (Limited to important or life-threatening): Abnormal gait, acne, aggression, anal disorder, anxiety, bleeding time increased, bone disorder, breast pain, chalazion, chest pain, ceruminosis, cirrhosis, conjunctival hemorrhage, constipation, corneal lesions, corneal ulceration, cough, cyanosis, cyst, deafness, diplopia, dizziness, dyspepsia, dysphonia, dysuria, ectropion, eczema, esophagitis, ethanol intolerance, fever, flu-like syndrome, fungal infection, furunculosis, gastritis, gastroenteritis, glossitis, gum hyperplasia, hair discoloration, healing impaired, hemorrhage, hemorrhoids, hepatic dysfunction, hepatitis, herpes simplex, hyperkeratosis, hypertrichosis, hypoesthesia, intermittent claudication, itchy eyes, jaundice, lacrimation abnormal, laryngitis, leukorrhea, libido decreased, malaise, melena, MI, migraine, moniliasis, muscle weakness, myopathy with peripheral neuropathy, nail fragility, nervousness, neuritis, olecranon bursitis, otitis media, pancreatitis, papilledema, peripheral ischemia, pharyngitis, photosensitivity, pseudotumor cerebri, recurrent sties, scaling of skin, scleroderma, skin fragility or thinning, skin hypertrophy, skin nodule, spinal hyperostosis (new lesion), sputum increased, suicidal thoughts, taste loss, tendonitis, tenesmus, thromboembolism, tongue ulceration, urticaria, vaginitis, vulvovaginitis, wart, weight gain

Drug Interactions

Metabolism/Transport Effects None known.

Avoid Concomitant Use

Avoid concomitant use of Acitretin with any of the following: Alcohol (Ethyl); Methotrexate; Tetracycline Derivatives; Vitamin A

Increased Effect/Toxicity

Acitretin may increase the levels/effects of: Methotrexate; Porfimer; Vitamin A

The levels/effects of Acitretin may be increased by: Alcohol (Ethyl); Tetracycline Derivatives; Vitamin A

Decreased Effect

Acitretin may decrease the levels/effects of: Contraceptives (Estrogens); Contraceptives (Progestins)

Ethanol/Nutrition/Herb Interactions Ethanol: Use leads to formation of etretinate, a teratogenic metabolite with a prolonged half-life; concomitant use of ethanol or ethanol-containing products is contraindicated.

Stability Store between 15°C to 25°C (59°F to 77°F). Avoid high temperatures and humidity. Protect from light.

Pharmacodynamics/Kinetics Etretinate has been detected in serum for up to 3 years following therapy, possibly due to storage in adipose tissue.

Onset of action: May take 2-3 months for full effect; improvement may be seen within 8 weeks.

Absorption: Oral: ~72% absorbed when given with food

Protein binding: >99% bound, primarily to albumin

Metabolism: Metabolized to *cis*-acitretin; both compounds are further metabolized. Concomitant ethanol use leads to the formation of etretinate (active).

Half-life elimination: Acitretin: 49 hours (range: 33-96); *cis*-acitretin: 63 hours (range: 28-157); etretinate: 120 days (range: up to 168 days)

Time to peak: 2-5 hours

Excretion: Feces (34% to 54%); urine (16% to 53%)

Dosage Oral: Adults: Individualization of dosage is required to achieve maximum therapeutic response while minimizing side effects

Initial therapy: Therapy should be initiated at 25-50 mg/day, given as a single dose with the main meal

Maintenance doses of 25-50 mg/day may be given after initial response to treatment; the maintenance dose should be based on clinical efficacy and tolerability

American Academy of Dermatology recommends: 10-50 mg/day as a single dose; doses ≤25 mg/day are used to decrease side effects (Menter, 2009)

Dosing adjustment in renal impairment: There are no dosage adjustments provided in manufacturer's labeling.

Hemodialysis: Not removed by hemodialysis

Dosing adjustment in hepatic impairment: There are no dosage adjustments provided in manufacturer's labeling.

Dietary Considerations Take with food. Avoid ingestion of additional sources of exogenous vitamin A (in excess of RDA); use of ethanol and ethanol-containing products is contraindicated.

Administration Administer with food, preferably with the main meal of the day.

Monitoring Parameters Lipid profile (baseline and at 1- to 2-week intervals for 4-8 weeks); liver function tests (baseline, and at 1- to 2-week intervals until stable, then as clinically indicated); blood glucose in patients with diabetes; bone abnormalities (with long-term use); pregnancy tests (2 negative tests prior to therapy initiation, monthly during treatment, and every 3 months for ≥3 years after discontinuation of therapy)

The American Academy of Dermatology recommends: CBC and renal function tests (baseline and then every 12 weeks); liver function tests (every 2 weeks for the first 8 weeks, then every 6-12 weeks thereafter) (Menter, 2009)

Additional Information Female patients are required to use two forms of birth control, at least one of which is a primary form, unless they have undergone a hysterectomy or are postmenopausal. Both forms of birth control must be used simultaneously for at least 1 month prior to therapy and for at least 3 years after discontinuation. Primary forms of birth control include tubal ligation, partner's vasectomy, IUD, or hormonal birth control products. Microdosed progestin products, referred to as "mini-pills," have been shown to be less effective when used with acitretin, and are not recommended. Secondary forms of contraception include diaphragms, latex condoms and cervical caps, all if used with a spermicide.

Dosage Forms Excipient information presented when available (limited, particularly for generics); consult specific product labeling.
Capsule, oral:
Soriatane®: 10 mg, 17.5 mg, 25 mg

- ◆ **Aclaro®** *see* Hydroquinone *on page 846*
- ◆ **Aclaro PD®** *see* Hydroquinone *on page 846*
- ◆ **Aclasta® (Can)** *see* Zoledronic Acid *on page 1821*
- ◆ **Aclovate®** *see* Alclometasone *on page 54*

Acrivastine and Pseudoephedrine

(AK ri vas teen & soo doe e FED rin)

Brand Names: U.S. Semprex®-D

Index Terms Pseudoephedrine Hydrochloride and Acrivastine

Pharmacologic Category Alkylamine Derivative; Alpha/Beta Agonist; Decongestant; Histamine H_1 Antagonist; Histamine H_1 Antagonist, Second Generation

Use Relief of symptoms associated with seasonal allergic rhinitis

Pregnancy Risk Factor B

Dosage Oral: Children ≥12 years and Adults: One capsule every 4-6 hours (maximum: 4 doses/24 hours); treatment for >14 days has not been evaluated

Dosing adjustment in renal impairment: Avoid use in patients with Cl_{cr} ≤48 mL/minute.

Dosing adjustment in hepatic impairment: There are no dosage adjustments recommended in manufacturer's labeling.

Additional Information Complete prescribing information for this medication should be consulted for additional detail.

Dosage Forms Excipient information presented when available (limited, particularly for generics); consult specific product labeling.
Capsule:
Semprex®-D: Acrivastine 8 mg and pseudoephedrine hydrochloride 60 mg

- ◆ **Act® [OTC]** *see* Fluoride *on page 728*
- ◆ **ACT-D** *see* DACTINomycin *on page 439*
- ◆ **Actemra®** *see* Tocilizumab *on page 1700*
- ◆ **ActHIB®** *see Haemophilus* b Conjugate Vaccine *on page 815*
- ◆ **Acthrel®** *see* Corticorelin *on page 413*
- ◆ **Actidose®-Aqua [OTC]** *see* Charcoal, Activated *on page 335*
- ◆ **Actidose® with Sorbitol [OTC]** *see* Charcoal, Activated *on page 335*
- ◆ **Actifed® (Can)** *see* Triprolidine and Pseudoephedrine *on page 1741*
- ◆ **Actifed® Cold & Allergy [OTC]** ***[reformulation]*** *see* Chlorpheniramine and Phenylephrine *on page 345*
- ◆ **Actigall®** *see* Ursodiol *on page 1751*
- ◆ **Actimmune®** *see* Interferon Gamma-1b *on page 919*
- ◆ **Actinomycin** *see* DACTINomycin *on page 439*
- ◆ **Actinomycin D** *see* DACTINomycin *on page 439*
- ◆ **Actinomycin CI** *see* DACTINomycin *on page 439*
- ◆ **Actiq®** *see* FentaNYL *on page 697*
- ◆ **Activase®** *see* Alteplase *on page 76*
- ◆ **Activase® rt-PA (Can)** *see* Alteplase *on page 76*
- ◆ **Activated Carbon** *see* Charcoal, Activated *on page 335*
- ◆ **Activated Charcoal** *see* Charcoal, Activated *on page 335*
- ◆ **Activated Ergosterol** *see* Ergocalciferol *on page 610*
- ◆ **Activated Factor XIII** *see* Factor XIII Concentrate (Human) *on page 686*
- ◆ **Activated Protein C, Human, Recombinant** *see* Drotrecogin Alfa (Activated) *on page 564*
- ◆ **Activella®** *see* Estradiol and Norethindrone *on page 635*
- ◆ **Act® Kids [OTC]** *see* Fluoride *on page 728*
- ◆ **Actonel®** *see* Risedronate *on page 1494*
- ◆ **Actonel® DR (Can)** *see* Risedronate *on page 1494*
- ◆ **Actoplus Met®** *see* Pioglitazone and Metformin *on page 1357*
- ◆ **Actoplus Met® XR** *see* Pioglitazone and Metformin *on page 1357*
- ◆ **Actos®** *see* Pioglitazone *on page 1355*
- ◆ **Act® Restoring™ [OTC]** *see* Fluoride *on page 728*
- ◆ **Act® Total Care™ [OTC]** *see* Fluoride *on page 728*
- ◆ **Acular®** *see* Ketorolac (Ophthalmic) *on page 959*
- ◆ **Acular LS®** *see* Ketorolac (Ophthalmic) *on page 959*
- ◆ **Acuvail®** *see* Ketorolac (Ophthalmic) *on page 959*
- ◆ **ACV** *see* Acyclovir (Systemic) *on page 39*
- ◆ **ACV** *see* Acyclovir (Topical) *on page 42*
- ◆ **Acycloguanosine** *see* Acyclovir (Systemic) *on page 39*
- ◆ **Acycloguanosine** *see* Acyclovir (Topical) *on page 42*

Acyclovir (Systemic) (ay SYE kloe veer)

Brand Names: U.S. Zovirax®

Brand Names: Canada Apo-Acyclovir®; Gen-Acyclovir; Mylan-Acyclovir; Novo-Acyclovir; Nu-Acyclovir; ratio-Acyclovir; Teva-Acyclovir; Zovirax®

Index Terms Aciclovir; ACV; Acycloguanosine

Pharmacologic Category Antiviral Agent

Use Treatment of genital herpes simplex virus (HSV) and HSV encephalitis

Unlabeled Use Prevention of HSV reactivation in HIV-positive patients; prevention of HSV reactivation in hematopoietic stem cell transplant (HSCT); prevention of HSV reactivation during periods of neutropenia in patients with cancer; prevention of varicella zoster virus (VZV) reactivation in allogenic HSCT; prevention of CMV reactivation in low-risk allogeneic HSCT; treatment of disseminated HSV or VZV in immunocompromised patients with cancer; empiric treatment of suspected encephalitis in immunocompromised patients with cancer; treatment of initial and prophylaxis of recurrent mucosal and cutaneous herpes simplex (HSV-1 and HSV-2) infections in immunocompromised patients

Pregnancy Risk Factor B

Pregnancy Considerations Teratogenic effects were not observed in animal studies. Acyclovir has been shown to cross the human placenta. There are no adequate and well-controlled studies in pregnant women. Results from a pregnancy registry, established in 1984 and closed in 1999, did not find an increase in the number of birth defects with exposure to acyclovir when compared to those expected in the general population. However, due to the small size of the registry and lack of long-term data, the manufacturer recommends using during pregnancy with caution and only when clearly needed. Data from the pregnancy registry may be obtained from GlaxoSmithKline.

Lactation Enters breast milk/use with caution (AAP rates "compatible"; AAP 2001 update pending)

Contraindications Hypersensitivity to acyclovir, valacyclovir, or any component of the formulation

Warnings/Precautions Use with caution in immunocompromised patients; thrombocytopenic purpura/hemolytic uremic syndrome (TTP/HUS) has been reported. Use caution in the elderly, pre-existing renal disease (may require dosage modification), or in those receiving other nephrotoxic drugs. Renal failure (sometimes fatal) has been reported. Maintain adequate hydration during oral or intravenous therapy. Use I.V. preparation with caution in patients with underlying neurologic abnormalities, serious hepatic or electrolyte abnormalities, or substantial hypoxia.

Varicella-zoster: Treatment should begin within 24 hours of appearance of rash; oral route not recommended for routine use in otherwise healthy children with varicella, but may be effective in patients at increased risk of moderate-to-severe infection (>12 years of age, chronic cutaneous or pulmonary disorders, long-term salicylate therapy, corticosteroid therapy).

Adverse Reactions

Oral:

>10%: Central nervous system: Malaise (≤12%)

1% to 10%:

Central nervous system: Headache (≤2%)

Gastrointestinal: Nausea (2% to 5%), vomiting (≤3%), diarrhea (2% to 3%)

Parenteral:

1% to 10%:

Dermatologic: Hives (2%), itching (2%), rash (2%)

Gastrointestinal: Nausea/vomiting (7%)

Hepatic: Liver function tests increased (1% to 2%)

Local: Inflammation at injection site or phlebitis (9%)

Renal: BUN increased (5% to 10%), creatinine increased (5% to 10%), acute renal failure

All forms: <1% (Limited to important or life-threatening): Abdominal pain, aggression, agitation, anemia, anorexia, ataxia, coma, confusion, consciousness decreased, delirium, desquamation, disseminated intravascular coagulopathy (DIC), dizziness, dysarthria, encephalopathy, fatigue, fever, gastrointestinal distress, hallucinations, hematuria, hemolysis, hepatitis, hyperbilirubinemia, hypotension, insomnia, jaundice, leukocytoclastic vasculitis, leukocytosis, leukopenia, lymphadenopathy, mental depression, myalgia, neutrophilia, pain, psychosis, renal failure, renal pain, seizure, somnolence, sore throat, thrombocytopenia, thrombocytopenic purpura/hemolytic uremic syndrome (TTP/HUS), thrombocytosis, visual disturbances

Drug Interactions

Metabolism/Transport Effects None known.

Avoid Concomitant Use

Avoid concomitant use of Acyclovir (Systemic) with any of the following: Zoster Vaccine

Increased Effect/Toxicity

Acyclovir (Systemic) may increase the levels/effects of: Mycophenolate; Tenofovir; Zidovudine

The levels/effects of Acyclovir (Systemic) may be increased by: Mycophenolate

Decreased Effect

Acyclovir (Systemic) may decrease the levels/effects of: Zoster Vaccine

Ethanol/Nutrition/Herb Interactions Food: Does not affect absorption of oral acyclovir.

Stability

Capsule, tablet: Store at controlled room temperature of 15°C to 25°C (59°F to 77°F); protect from moisture.

Injection: Store powder at controlled room temperature of 15°C to 25°C (59°F to 77°F). Reconstitute acyclovir 500 mg powder with SWFI 10 mL; do not use bacteriostatic water containing benzyl alcohol or parabens. For intravenous infusion, dilute in D_5W, D_5NS, $D_5\frac{1}{4}NS$, $D_5\frac{1}{2}NS$, LR, or NS to a final concentration ≤7 mg/mL. Concentrations >10 mg/mL increase the risk of phlebitis. Reconstituted solutions remain stable for 12 hours at room temperature. Do not refrigerate reconstituted solutions or solutions diluted for infusion as they may precipitate. Once diluted for infusion, use within 24 hours.

Mechanism of Action Acyclovir is converted to acyclovir monophosphate by virus-specific thymidine kinase then further converted to acyclovir triphosphate by other cellular enzymes. Acyclovir triphosphate inhibits DNA synthesis and viral replication by competing with deoxyguanosine triphosphate for viral DNA polymerase and being incorporated into viral DNA.

Pharmacodynamics/Kinetics

Absorption: Oral: 15% to 30%

Distribution: V_d: 0.8 L/kg (63.6 L): Widely (eg, brain, kidney, lungs, liver, spleen, muscle, uterus, vagina, CSF)

Protein binding: 9% to 33%

Metabolism: Converted by viral enzymes to acyclovir monophosphate, and further converted to diphosphate then triphosphate (active form) by cellular enzymes

Bioavailability: Oral: 10% to 20% with normal renal function (bioavailability decreases with increased dose)

Half-life elimination: Terminal: Neonates: 4 hours; Children 1-12 years: 2-3 hours; Adults: 3 hours

Time to peak, serum: Oral: Within 1.5-2 hours

Excretion: Urine (62% to 90% as unchanged drug and metabolite)

Dosage Note: Obese patients should be dosed using ideal body weight

Genital herpes simplex virus (HSV) infection:

I.V.: Children ≥12 years and Adults (immunocompetent): Initial episode, severe: 5 mg/kg/dose every 8 hours for 5-7 days **or** 5-10 mg/kg/dose every 8 hours for 2-7 days, follow with oral therapy to complete at least 10 days of therapy (CDC, 2010)

Oral:

Children, immunocompetent:

Initial episode (unlabeled use): 40-80 mg/kg/day divided into 3-4 doses for 5-10 days (maximum: 1 g/day)

Chronic suppression (unlabeled use; limited data): 80 mg/kg/day in 3 divided doses (maximum: 1 g/day), re-evaluate after 12 months of treatment

Children, immunocompromised (unlabeled use; CDC, 2009): Initial episode:

Children <45 kg: 60 mg/kg/day divided into 3 doses for 5-14 days (maximum: 1.2 g/day)

Adolescents: 400 mg twice daily for 5-14 days

Adults:

Initial episode: 200 mg every 4 hours while awake (5 times/day) for 10 days **or** 400 mg 3 times/day for 7-10 days (CDC, 2010)

Recurrence: 200 mg every 4 hours while awake (5 times/day) for 5 days (per manufacturer's labeling; begin at earliest signs of disease)

Alternatively, the following regimens are also recommended by the CDC: 400 mg 3 times/day for 5 days; 800 mg twice daily for 5 days; 800 mg 3 times/day for 2 days (CDC, 2010)

Chronic suppression: 400 mg twice daily or 200 mg 3-5 times/day, for up to 12 months followed by re-evaluation (per manufacturer's labeling)

Herpes zoster (shingles):

Oral: Adults (immunocompetent): 800 mg every 4 hours (5 times/day) for 7-10 days

I.V.:

Children <12 years (immunocompromised): 20 mg/kg/dose every 8 hours for 7 days

Children ≥12 years and Adults (immunocompromised): 10 mg/kg/dose or 500 mg/m²/dose every 8 hours for 7 days

HSV encephalitis: I.V.:

Children 3 months to 12 years: 20 mg/kg/dose every 8 hours for 10 days (per manufacturer's labeling); dosing for 14-21 days also reported

Children ≥12 years and Adults: 10 mg/kg/dose every 8 hours for 10 days (per manufacturer's labeling); 10-15 mg/kg/dose every 8 hours for 14-21 days also reported

Mucocutaneous HSV:

I.V.:

Children <12 years (immunocompromised): Treatment: 10 mg/kg/dose every 8 hours for 7 days

Children ≥12 years and Adults (immunocompromised): Treatment: 5-10 mg/kg/dose every 8 hours for 7 days (Leflore, 2000); dosing for up to 14 days also reported

Oral (unlabeled use): Adults (immunocompromised): 400 mg 5 times/day for 7 days (Leflore, 2000)

Neonatal HSV: I.V.: Infants: Birth to 3 months: 10 mg/kg/dose every 8 hours for 10 days (manufacturer's labeling); 20 mg/kg/dose every 8 hours for 14 (skin and mucous membrane disease) to 21 days (CNS disease) (CDC, 2010)

Orolabial HSV (unlabeled use): Oral:

Children 1-6 years (immunocompetent, gingivostomatitis): Treatment of primary infection: 15 mg/kg/dose (maximum: 200 mg/dose) 5 times/day for 7 days, initiated within 72 hours of symptom onset (Amir, 1997)

Adults (immunocompetent):

Treatment: 200-400 mg 5 times/day for 5 days (Cernik, 2008; Leflore, 2000; Spruance, 1990) for episodic/recurrent treatment; for initial treatment, limited data are available, 200 mg 5 times/day or 400 mg 3 times/day for 7-10 days has been recommended by some clinicians.

Chronic suppression: 400 mg 2 times/day (has been clinically evaluated for up to 1 year) (Cernik, 2008; Rooney, 1993)

Varicella-zoster (chickenpox): Begin treatment within the first 24 hours of rash onset:

Oral: **Note:** The CDC HIV guidelines recommended duration of therapy is 7-10 days or until no new lesions for 48 hours (for patients with mild varicella and no or moderate immune suppression).

Children ≥2 years and ≤40 kg (immunocompetent): 20 mg/kg/dose (up to 800 mg/dose) 4 times/day for 5 days

Children >40 kg and Adults (immunocompetent): 800 mg/dose 4 times/day for 5 days

I.V.:

Manufacturer's labeling (immunocompromised):

Children <12 years: 20 mg/kg/dose every 8 hours for 7 days

Children ≥12 years and Adults: 10 mg/kg/dose every 8 hours for 7 days

CDC HIV guidelines (immunocompromised):

Children <1 year: 10 mg/kg/dose every 8 hours for 7-10 days or until no new lesions for 48 hours

Children ≥1 year: 10 mg/kg/dose or 500 mg/m²/dose every 8 hours for 7-10 days or until no new lesions for 48 hours

Adolescents and Adults: 10-15 mg/kg/dose every 8 hours for 7-10 days

Varicella-zoster acute retinal necrosis infection in HIV-exposed/-positive (unlabeled use; CDC, 2009): I.V.: Infants and Children: 10-15 mg/kg/dose every 8 hours for 10-14 days, followed by valacyclovir for 4-6 weeks

Prevention of HSV reactivation in HIV-positive patient (unlabeled use): Oral:

Children: 20 mg/kg/dose twice daily (maximum: 400 mg/dose) (CDC, 2009)

Adults: 400-800 mg 2-3 times/day (CDC, 2010)

Prevention of HSV reactivation in HSCT (unlabeled use): *CDC recommendations:* **Note:** Start at the beginning of conditioning therapy and continue until engraftment or until mucositis resolves (~30 days)

Oral: Adults: 200 mg 3 times/day

I.V.:

Children: 250 mg/m²/dose every 8 hours or 125 mg/m²/dose every 6 hours

Adults: 250 mg/m²/dose every 12 hours

Prevention of VZV reactivation in allogeneic HSCT (unlabeled use): *NCCN guidelines:* Oral: Adults: 800 mg twice a day

Prevention of CMV reactivation in low-risk allogeneic HSCT (unlabeled use): *NCCN guidelines:* **Note:** Requires close monitoring (due to weak activity); not for use in patients at high risk for CMV disease: Oral: Adults: 800 mg 4 times/day

Treatment of disseminated HSV or VZV or empiric treatment of suspected encephalitis in immunocompromised patients with cancer: (unlabeled use): *NCCN guidelines:* I.V.: Adults: 10-12 mg/kg/dose every 8 hours

Treatment of episodic HSV infection in HIV-positive patient (unlabeled use): Oral: Adults: 400 mg 3 times/day for 5-10 days (CDC, 2010)

Dosing adjustment in renal impairment:

Oral:

Cl_{cr} 10-25 mL/minute/1.73 m²: Normal dosing regimen 800 mg every 4 hours: Administer 800 mg every 8 hours

Cl_{cr} <10 mL/minute/1.73 m²:

Normal dosing regimen 200 mg every 4 hours or 400 mg every 12 hours: Administer 200 mg every 12 hours

Normal dosing regimen 800 mg every 4 hours: Administer 800 mg every 12 hours

I.V.:

Cl_{cr} 25-50 mL/minute/1.73 m²: Administer recommended dose every 12 hours

Cl_{cr} 10-25 mL/minute/1.73 m²: Administer recommended dose every 24 hours

Cl_{cr} <10 mL/minute/1.73 m²: Administer 50% of recommended dose every 24 hours

Intermittent hemodialysis (IHD) (administer after hemodialysis on dialysis days): Dialyzable (60% reduction following a 6-hour session): I.V.: 2.5-5 mg/kg every 24 hours (Heintz, 2009). **Note:** Dosing dependent on the assumption of 3 times/week, complete IHD sessions.

Peritoneal dialysis (PD): Administer 50% of normal dose once daily; no supplemental dose needed

Continuous renal replacement therapy (CRRT) (Heintz, 2009; Trotman, 2005): Drug clearance is highly dependent on the method of renal replacement, filter type, and flow rate. Appropriate dosing requires close monitoring of pharmacologic response, signs of adverse reactions due to drug accumulation, as well as drug concentrations in relation to target trough (if appropriate). The following are general recommendations only (based on dialysate flow/ultrafiltration rates of 1-2 L/hour and minimal residual renal function) and should not supersede clinical judgment:

CVVH: I.V.: 5-10 mg/kg every 24 hours

CVVHD/CVVHDF: I.V.: 5-10 mg/kg every 12-24 hours

Note: The higher end of dosage range (eg, 10 mg/kg every 12 hours for CVVHDF) is recommended for viral meningoencephalitis and varicella-zoster virus infections.

Dietary Considerations May be taken with or without food. Some products may contain sodium.

Administration

Oral: May be administered with or without food.

I.V.: Avoid rapid infusion; infuse over 1 hour to prevent renal damage; maintain adequate hydration of patient; check for phlebitis and rotate infusion sites. Avoid I.M. or SubQ administration.

Monitoring Parameters Urinalysis, BUN, serum creatinine, liver enzymes, CBC

Dosage Forms Excipient information presented when available (limited, particularly for generics); consult specific product labeling.

Capsule, oral: 200 mg
 Zovirax®: 200 mg

Injection, powder for reconstitution, as sodium [strength expressed as base]: 500 mg, 1000 mg

Injection, solution, as sodium [strength expressed as base, preservative free]: 50 mg/mL (10 mL, 20 mL)

Suspension, oral: 200 mg/5 mL (473 mL)
 Zovirax®: 200 mg/5 mL (473 mL) [banana flavor]

Tablet, oral: 400 mg, 800 mg
 Zovirax®: 400 mg
 Zovirax®: 800 mg [scored]

Acyclovir (Topical) (ay SYE kloe veer)

Brand Names: U.S. Zovirax®

Brand Names: Canada Zovirax®

Index Terms Aciclovir; ACV; Acycloguanosine

Pharmacologic Category Antiviral Agent, Topical

Use Treatment of herpes labialis (cold sores), mucocutaneous HSV in immunocompromised patients

Pregnancy Risk Factor B

Dosage Topical:

Genital HSV: Adults (immunocompromised): Ointment: Initial episode: 1/2" ribbon of ointment for a 4" square surface area every 3 hours (6 times/day) for 7 days

Herpes labialis (cold sores): Children ≥12 years and Adults: Cream: Apply 5 times/day for 4 days

Mucocutaneous HSV: Ointment: Adults (non-life-threatening, immunocompromised): 1/2" ribbon of ointment for a 4" square surface area every 3 hours (6 times/day) for 7 days

Additional Information Complete prescribing information for this medication should be consulted for additional detail.

Dosage Forms Excipient information presented when available (limited, particularly for generics); consult specific product labeling.

Cream, topical:
 Zovirax®: 5% (2 g, 5 g)

Ointment, topical:
 Zovirax®: 5% (15 g, 30 g)

◆ **ACZ885** *see* Canakinumab *on page 272*

◆ **AD32** *see* Valrubicin *on page 1760*

◆ **Adacel®** *see* Diphtheria and Tetanus Toxoids, and Acellular Pertussis Vaccine *on page 523*

◆ **Adagen®** *see* Pegademase Bovine *on page 1305*

◆ **Adalat® XL® (Can)** *see* NIFEdipine *on page 1202*

◆ **Adalat® CC** *see* NIFEdipine *on page 1202*

Adalimumab (a da LIM yoo mab)

Brand Names: U.S. Humira®; Humira® Pen

Brand Names: Canada Humira®

Index Terms Antitumor Necrosis Factor Alpha (Human); D2E7; Human Antitumor Necrosis Factor Alpha

Pharmacologic Category Antirheumatic, Disease Modifying; Gastrointestinal Agent, Miscellaneous; Monoclonal Antibody; Tumor Necrosis Factor (TNF) Blocking Agent

Use

Treatment of active rheumatoid arthritis (moderate-to-severe) and active psoriatic arthritis; may be used alone or in combination with disease-modifying antirheumatic drugs (DMARDs); treatment of ankylosing spondylitis

Treatment of moderately- to severely-active Crohn's disease in patients with inadequate response to conventional treatment, or patients who have lost response to or are intolerant of infliximab

Treatment of moderate-to-severe plaque psoriasis

Treatment of moderately- to severely-active juvenile idiopathic arthritis

Pregnancy Risk Factor B

Pregnancy Considerations Teratogenic effects were not observed in animal studies, however, there are no adequate and well-controlled studies in pregnant women. Use during pregnancy only if clearly needed. A pregnancy registry has been established to monitor outcomes of women exposed to adalimumab during pregnancy (877-311-8972).

Lactation Excretion in breast milk unknown/not recommended

Medication Guide Available Yes

Contraindications There are no contraindications listed within the FDA-approved labeling.

Canadian labeling: Additional contraindications (not in U.S. labeling): Hypersensitivity to adalimumab or any component of the formulation; severe infection (eg, sepsis, tuberculosis, opportunistic infection)

Warnings/Precautions [U.S. Boxed Warnings]: Patients should be evaluated for latent tuberculosis infection with a tuberculin skin test prior to therapy. Treatment of latent tuberculosis should be initiated before adalimumab is used. Tuberculosis (disseminated or extrapulmonary) has been reactivated while on adalimumab. Most cases have been reported within the first 8 months of treatment. Doses higher than recommended are associated with an increased risk for tuberculosis reactivation. **Patients with initial negative tuberculin skin tests should receive continued monitoring for tuberculosis throughout treatment; active tuberculosis has developed in this population during treatment.** Rare reactivation of hepatitis B virus (HBV) has occurred in chronic virus carriers; use with caution; evaluate prior to initiation and during treatment.

[U.S. Boxed Warning]: Patients receiving adalimumab are at increased risk for serious infections which may result in hospitalization and/or fatality; infections usually developed in patients receiving concomitant immunosuppressive agents (eg, methotrexate or corticosteroids) and may present as disseminated (rather than local) disease. Active tuberculosis (or reactivation of latent tuberculosis), invasive fungal (including aspergillosis, blastomycosis, candidiasis, coccidioidomycosis, histoplasmosis, and pneumocystosis) and bacterial, viral or other opportunistic infections (including legionellosis and listeriosis) have been reported in patients receiving TNF-blocking agents, including adalimumab. Monitor closely for signs/symptoms of infection. Discontinue for serious infection or sepsis. Consider risks versus benefits prior to use in patients with a history of chronic or recurrent infection. Consider empiric antifungal therapy in patients who are at risk for invasive fungal infection and develop severe systemic illness. Caution should be exercised when considering use in the elderly or in patients with conditions that predispose them to infections (eg, diabetes) or residence/travel from areas of endemic mycoses (blastomycosis, coccidioidomycosis, histoplasmosis), or with latent or localized infections. Do not initiate adalimumab therapy with clinically important active infection. Patients who develop a new infection while undergoing treatment should be monitored closely. **[U.S. Boxed Warning]: Lymphoma and other malignancies have been reported in children and adolescent patients receiving other TNF-blocking agents.** Half the cases are lymphomas (Hodgkin's and non-Hodgkin's) and the other cases are varied, but include malignancies not typically observed in this population. Most patients were receiving concomitant immunosuppressants. **[U.S. Boxed Warning]: Hepatosplenic T-cell lymphoma (HSTCL), a rare T-cell lymphoma, has also been reported primarily in patients with Crohn's disease or ulcerative colitis treated with adalimumab and who received concomitant azathioprine or mercaptopurine; reports occurred predominantly in adolescent and young adult males.** Rare cases of lymphoma have also been reported in association with adalimumab. A higher incidence of nonmelanoma skin cancers was noted in adalimumab treated patients, when compared to the control group. Impact on the development and course of malignancies is not fully defined. May exacerbate pre-existing or recent-onset central or peripheral nervous system demyelinating disorders. Consider discontinuing use in patients who develop peripheral or central nervous system demyelinating disorders during treatment.

May exacerbate pre-existing or recent-onset demyelinating CNS disorders. Worsening and new-onset heart failure (HF) has been reported; use caution in patients with decreased left ventricular function. Use caution in patients with HF. Patients should be brought up to date with all immunizations before initiating therapy. No data are available concerning the effects of adalimumab on vaccination. Live vaccines should not be given concurrently. No data are available concerning secondary transmission of live vaccines in patients receiving adalimumab. Rare cases of pancytopenia (including aplastic anemia) have been reported with TNF-blocking agents; with significant hematologic abnormalities, consider discontinuing therapy. Positive antinuclear antibody titers have been detected in patients (with negative baselines) treated with adalimumab. Rare cases of autoimmune disorder, including lupus-like syndrome, have been reported; monitor and discontinue adalimumab if symptoms develop. May cause hypersensitivity reactions, including anaphylaxis; monitor. Infection and malignancy has been reported at a higher incidence in elderly patients compared to younger adults; use caution in elderly patients. The packaging (needle cover of prefilled syringe) may contain latex. Product may contain polysorbate 80.

Adverse Reactions

>10%:

Central nervous system: Headache (12%)

Dermatologic: Rash (6% to 12%)

Local: Injection site reaction (12% to 20%; includes erythema, itching, hemorrhage, pain, swelling)

Neuromuscular & skeletal: CPK increased (15%)

Respiratory: Upper respiratory tract infection (17%), sinusitis (11%)

Miscellaneous: Antibodies to adalimumab (3% to 26%; significance unknown), positive ANA (12%)

5% to 10%:

Cardiovascular: Hypertension (5%)

Endocrine & metabolic: Hyperlipidemia (7%), hypercholesterolemia (6%)

Gastrointestinal: Nausea (9%), abdominal pain (7%)

Genitourinary: Urinary tract infection (8%)

Hepatic: Alkaline phosphatase increased (5%)

Local: Injection site reaction (8%; other than erythema, itching, hemorrhage, pain, swelling)

Neuromuscular & skeletal: Back pain (6%)

Renal: Hematuria (5%)

Miscellaneous: Accidental injury (10%), flu-like syndrome (7%)

<5%:

Cardiovascular: Arrhythmia, atrial fibrillation, chest pain, CHF, coronary artery disorder, heart arrest, MI, palpitation, pericardial effusion, pericarditis, peripheral edema, syncope, tachycardia, thrombosis (leg), vascular disorder

Central nervous system: Confusion, fever, hypertensive encephalopathy, multiple sclerosis, subdural hematoma

Dermatologic: Cellulitis, erysipelas

Endocrine & metabolic: Dehydration, menstrual disorder, parathyroid disorder

Gastrointestinal: Diverticulitis, esophagitis, gastroenteritis, gastrointestinal hemorrhage, vomiting

Genitourinary: Cystitis, pelvic pain

Hematologic: Agranulocytosis, granulocytopenia, leukopenia, pancytopenia, paraproteinemia, polycythemia

Hepatic: Cholecystitis, cholelithiasis, hepatic necrosis

Neuromuscular & skeletal: Arthralgia, arthritis, bone fracture, bone necrosis, joint disorder, muscle cramps, myasthenia, pain in extremity, paresthesia, pyogenic arthritis, synovitis, tendon disorder, tremor

Ocular: Cataract

Renal: Kidney calculus, pyelonephritis

Respiratory: Asthma, bronchospasm, dyspnea, lung function decreased, pleural effusion, pneumonia

Miscellaneous: Adenoma, allergic reactions (1%), carcinoma (including breast, gastrointestinal, skin, urogenital), healing abnormality, herpes zoster, ketosis, lupus erythematosus syndrome, lymphoma, melanoma, post-surgical infection, sepsis, tuberculosis (reactivation of latent infection; miliary, lymphatic, peritoneal and pulmonary)

Postmarketing and/or case reports: Anaphylactoid reaction, anaphylaxis, angioneurotic edema, aplastic anemia, appendicitis, cutaneous vasculitis, cytopenia, erythema multiforme, fixed drug eruption, Guillain-Barré syndrome, infections (bacterial, viral, fungal and protozoal), interstitial lung disease (eg, pulmonary fibrosis), intestinal perforation, leukemias, pancreatitis, psoriasis (including new onset, palmoplantar, pustular, or exacerbation), septic arthritis, Stevens-Johnson syndrome, systemic vasculitis, thrombocytopenia, transaminases increased, urticaria

Drug Interactions

Metabolism/Transport Effects None known.

Avoid Concomitant Use

Avoid concomitant use of Adalimumab with any of the following: Abatacept; Anakinra; BCG; Belimumab; Canakinumab; Certolizumab Pegol; Natalizumab; Pimecrolimus; Rilonacept; Tacrolimus (Topical); Vaccines (Live)

Increased Effect/Toxicity

Adalimumab may increase the levels/effects of: Abatacept; Anakinra; Belimumab; Canakinumab; Certolizumab Pegol; Leflunomide; Natalizumab; Rilonacept; Vaccines (Live)

The levels/effects of Adalimumab may be increased by: Abciximab; Denosumab; Pimecrolimus; Roflumilast; Tacrolimus (Topical); Trastuzumab

Decreased Effect

Adalimumab may decrease the levels/effects of: BCG; Coccidioidin Skin Test; Sipuleucel-T; Vaccines (Inactivated); Vaccines (Live)

The levels/effects of Adalimumab may be decreased by: Echinacea

Ethanol/Nutrition/Herb Interactions Herb/nutraceutical: Echinacea may decrease the therapeutic effects of adalimumab; avoid concurrent use.

Stability Store under refrigeration at 2°C to 8°C (36°F to 46°F); do not freeze. Protect from light.

Mechanism of Action Adalimumab is a recombinant monoclonal antibody that binds to human tumor necrosis factor alpha (TNF-alpha), thereby interfering with binding to TNFα receptor sites and subsequent cytokine-driven inflammatory processes. Elevated TNF levels in the synovial fluid are involved in the pathologic pain and joint destruction in immune-mediated arthritis. Adalimumab decreases signs and symptoms of psoriatic arthritis, rheumatoid arthritis, and ankylosing spondylitis. It inhibits progression of structural damage of rheumatoid and psoriatic arthritis. Reduces signs and symptoms and maintains clinical remission in Crohn's disease; reduces epidermal thickness and inflammatory cell infiltration in plaque psoriasis.

Pharmacodynamics/Kinetics

Distribution: V_d: 4.7-6 L; Synovial fluid concentrations: 31% to 96% of serum

Bioavailability: Absolute: 64%

Half-life elimination: Terminal: ~2 weeks (range: 10-20 days)

Time to peak, serum: SubQ: 131 ± 56 hours

Excretion: Clearance increased in the presence of anti-adalimumab antibodies; decreased in patients ≥40 years of age

Dosage SubQ:

Children ≥4 years: Juvenile idiopathic arthritis (JIA):
- 15 kg to <30 kg: 20 mg every other week
- ≥30 kg: 40 mg every other week

Adults:
- Rheumatoid arthritis: 40 mg every other week; may be administered with other DMARDs; patients not taking methotrexate may increase dose to 40 mg every week
- Ankylosing spondylitis, psoriatic arthritis: 40 mg every other week
- Crohn's disease: Initial: 160 mg (given as 4 injections on day 1 or as 2 injections/day over 2 consecutive days), then 80 mg 2 weeks later (day 15); maintenance: 40 mg every other week beginning day 29. **Note:** Some patients may require 40 mg every week as maintenance therapy (Lichtenstein, 2009).
- Plaque psoriasis: Initial: 80 mg as a single dose; maintenance: 40 mg every other week beginning 1 week after initial dose

Administration For SubQ injection; rotate injection sites. Do not use if solution is discolored. Do not administer to skin which is red, tender, bruised, or hard. Needle cap of the prefilled syringe may contain latex.

Monitoring Parameters Monitor improvement of symptoms and physical function assessments. Latent TB screening prior to initiating and during therapy; signs/symptoms of infection (prior to, during, and following therapy); CBC with differential; signs/symptoms/worsening of heart failure; HBV screening prior to initiating (all patients), HBV carriers (during and for several months following therapy); signs and symptoms of hypersensitivity reaction; symptoms of lupus-like syndrome.

Dosage Forms Excipient information presented when available (limited, particularly for generics); consult specific product labeling.

Injection, solution [preservative free]:
- Humira®: 40 mg/0.8 mL (0.8 mL) [contains natural rubber/natural latex in packaging, polysorbate 80; prefilled syringe]
- Humira® Pen: 40 mg/0.8 mL (0.8 mL) [contains natural rubber/natural latex in packaging, polysorbate 80]

Injection, solution [pediatric, preservative free]:
- Humira®: 20 mg/0.4 mL (0.4 mL) [contains natural rubber/natural latex in packaging, polysorbate 80; prefilled syringe]

◆ **Adamantanamine Hydrochloride** *see* Amantadine *on page 82*

Adapalene (a DAP a leen)

Brand Names: U.S. Differin®

Brand Names: Canada Differin®; Differin® XP

Pharmacologic Category Acne Products; Topical Skin Product, Acne

Use Treatment of acne vulgaris

Pregnancy Risk Factor C

Dosage Topical: Children >12 years and Adults: Apply once daily at bedtime

Additional Information Complete prescribing information for this medication should be consulted for additional detail.

Dosage Forms Excipient information presented when available (limited, particularly for generics); consult specific product labeling.

Cream, topical: 0.1% (45 g)
- Differin®: 0.1% (45 g)

Gel, topical: 0.1% (45 g)
- Differin®: 0.1% (45 g); 0.3% (45 g) [ethanol free]

Lotion, topical:
- Differin®: 0.1% (59 mL)

Adapalene and Benzoyl Peroxide
(a DAP a leen & BEN zoe il peer OKS ide)

Brand Names: U.S. Epiduo®

Brand Names: Canada Tactuo™

Index Terms Benzoyl Peroxide and Adapalene

Pharmacologic Category Acne Products; Topical Skin Product; Topical Skin Product, Acne

Use Topical treatment of acne vulgaris

Pregnancy Risk Factor C

Dosage Topical: Children ≥12 years and Adults: Apply once daily to affected areas after skin has been cleaned and dried

Additional Information Complete prescribing information for this medication should be consulted for additional detail.

Dosage Forms Excipient information presented when available (limited, particularly for generics); consult specific product labeling.

Gel, topical:
- Epiduo®: Adapalene 0.1% and benzoyl peroxide 2.5% (45 g)

◆ **Adcetris™** *see* Brentuximab Vedotin *on page 234*

◆ **Adcirca®** *see* Tadalafil *on page 1621*

◆ **ADD 234037** *see* Lacosamide *on page 963*

◆ **Addaprin [OTC]** *see* Ibuprofen *on page 860*

◆ **Adderall® [DSC]** *see* Dextroamphetamine and Amphetamine *on page 488*

◆ **Adderall XR®** *see* Dextroamphetamine and Amphetamine *on page 488*

Adefovir (a DEF o veer)

Brand Names: U.S. Hepsera®

Brand Names: Canada Hepsera™

Index Terms Adefovir Dipivoxil; Bis-POM PMEA

Pharmacologic Category Antiretroviral Agent, Reverse Transcriptase Inhibitor (Nucleotide)

Use Treatment of chronic hepatitis B with evidence of active viral replication (based on persistent elevation of ALT/AST or histologic evidence), including patients with lamivudine-resistant hepatitis B

Pregnancy Risk Factor C

Pregnancy Considerations Teratogenic effects were not observed in animal studies. There are no adequate and well-controlled studies in pregnant women. Use in pregnancy only when clearly needed. Pregnant women exposed to adefovir should be registered with the pregnancy registry (800-258-4263).

Lactation Excretion in breast milk unknown/not recommended

Contraindications Hypersensitivity to adefovir or any component of the formulation

Warnings/Precautions [U.S. Boxed Warning]: Use with caution in patients with renal dysfunction or in patients at risk of renal toxicity (including concurrent nephrotoxic agents or NSAIDs). Chronic administration may result in nephrotoxicity. Dosage adjustment is required in adult patients with renal dysfunction or in patients who develop renal dysfunction during therapy; no data available for use in children ≥12 years or adolescents with renal impairment. Not recommended as first line therapy of chronic HBV due to weak antiviral activity and high rate of resistance after first year. May be more appropriate as second-line agent in treatment-naïve patients. Combination therapy with lamivudine in nucleoside-naïve patients has not been shown to provide synergistic antiviral effects. In patients with lamivudine-resistant HBV, switching to adefovir monotherapy was associated with a higher risk of adefovir resistance compared to adding adefovir to lamivudine therapy (Lok, 2009).

Calculate creatinine clearance before initiation of therapy. Consider alternative therapy in patients who do not respond to adefovir monotherapy treatment. **[U.S. Boxed Warning]: May cause the development of HIV resistance in patients with unrecognized or untreated HIV infection.** Determine HIV status prior to initiating treatment with adefovir. **[U.S. Boxed Warning]: Fatal cases of lactic acidosis and severe hepatomegaly with steatosis have been reported with the use of nucleoside analogues alone or in combination with other antiretrovirals.** Female gender, obesity, and prolonged treatment may increase the risk of hepatotoxicity. Treatment should be discontinued in patients with lactic acidosis or signs/symptoms of hepatotoxicity (which may occur without marked transaminase elevations). **[U.S. Boxed Warning]: Acute exacerbations of hepatitis may occur (in up to 25% of patients) when antihepatitis therapy is discontinued.** Exacerbations typically occur within 12 weeks and may be self-limited or resolve upon resuming treatment; risk may be increased with advanced liver disease or cirrhosis. Monitor patients following discontinuation of therapy. Safety and efficacy in children <12 years of age have not been established. Do not use concurrently with tenofovir (Viread®) or any product containing tenofovir (eg, Truvada®, Atripla®).

Adverse Reactions

>10%:

Central nervous system: Headache (24% to 25%)

Gastrointestinal: Abdominal pain (15%), diarrhea (up to 13%)

Hepatic: Hepatitis exacerbation (up to 25% within 12 weeks of adefovir discontinuation)

Neuromuscular & skeletal: Weakness (up to 25%)

Renal: Hematuria (grade ≥3: 11%)

1% to 10%:

Dermatologic: Rash, pruritus

Endocrine & metabolic: Hypophosphatemia (<2 mg/dL: 1% and 3% in pre-/post-liver transplant patients, respectively)

Gastrointestinal: Flatulence (up to 8%), dyspepsia (5% to 9%), nausea, vomiting

Neuromuscular & skeletal: Back pain (up to 10%)

Renal: Serum creatinine increased (≥0.5 mg/dL: 2% to 3% in compensated liver disease; incidence may be higher in patients with decompensated cirrhosis or in liver transplant recipients), renal failure

Note: In liver transplant patients with baseline renal dysfunction, frequency of increased serum creatinine has been observed to be as high as 32% to 51% at 48 and 96 weeks post-transplantation, respectively; considering the concomitant use of other potentially nephrotoxic medications, baseline renal insufficiency, and predisposing comorbidities, the role of adefovir in these changes could not be established.

Respiratory: Cough (6% to 8%), rhinitis (up to 5%)

Postmarketing and/or case reports: Fanconi syndrome, hepatitis, myopathy, nephrotoxicity, osteomalacia, pancreatitis, proximal renal tubulopathy

Drug Interactions

Metabolism/Transport Effects None known.

Avoid Concomitant Use

Avoid concomitant use of Adefovir with any of the following: Tenofovir

Increased Effect/Toxicity

Adefovir may increase the levels/effects of: Tenofovir

The levels/effects of Adefovir may be increased by: Ganciclovir-Valganciclovir; Ribavirin; Tenofovir

Decreased Effect

Adefovir may decrease the levels/effects of: Tenofovir

Ethanol/Nutrition/Herb Interactions

Ethanol: Should be avoided in hepatitis B infection due to potential hepatic toxicity.

Food: Does not have a significant effect on adefovir absorption.

Stability Store controlled room temperature of 25°C (77°F).

Mechanism of Action Acyclic nucleotide reverse transcriptase inhibitor (adenosine analog) which interferes with HBV viral RNA-dependent DNA polymerase resulting in inhibition of viral replication.

Pharmacodynamics/Kinetics

Distribution: 0.35-0.39 L/kg

Protein binding: ≤4%

Metabolism: Prodrug; rapidly converted to adefovir (active metabolite) in intestine

Bioavailability: 59%

Half-life elimination: 7.5 hours; prolonged in renal impairment

Time to peak: 1.75 hours

Excretion: Urine (45% as active metabolite within 24 hours)

Dosage Oral: Children ≥12 years and Adults: 10 mg once daily

Treatment duration (AASLD practice guidelines): Adults:

Hepatitis Be antigen (HBeAg) positive chronic hepatitis: Treat ≥1 year until HBeAg seroconversion and undetectable serum HBV DNA; continue therapy for ≥6 months after HBeAg seroconversion

HBeAg negative chronic hepatitis: Treat >1 year until hepatitis B surface antigen (HBsAg) clearance

Note: Patients not achieving a <2 log decrease in serum HBV DNA after at least 6 months of therapy should either receive additional treatment or be switched to an alternative therapy (Lok, 2009).

Dosage adjustment in renal impairment: Adult recommendations only (no dosage adjustment recommendations available for patients <18 years with renal impairment):

Cl_{cr} ≥50 mL/minute: No dosage adjustment necessary

Cl_{cr} 20-49 mL/minute: 10 mg every 48 hours

Cl_{cr} 10-19 mL/minute: 10 mg every 72 hours

Hemodialysis: 10 mg every 7 days (following dialysis)

Dosage adjustment in hepatic impairment: No adjustment required

Dietary Considerations May be taken without regard to food.

Administration May be administered without regard to food.

Monitoring Parameters HIV status (prior to initiation of therapy); serum creatinine (prior to initiation and during therapy; every 3 months in patients with medical conditions which predispose to renal insufficiency and in all patients treated for >1 year; more frequent monitoring required if pre-existing real insufficiency detected [Lok, 2009]); LFTs for several months following discontinuation of adefovir; HBV DNA (every 3-6 months during therapy); HBeAg and anti-HBe

Additional Information Adefovir dipivoxil is a prodrug, rapidly converted to the active component (adefovir). It was previously investigated as a treatment for HIV infections (at dosages substantially higher than the approved dose for hepatitis B). The NDA was withdrawn, and no further studies in the treatment of HIV are anticipated (per manufacturer).

Dosage Forms Excipient information presented when available (limited, particularly for generics); consult specific product labeling.

Tablet, oral, as dipivoxil:

Hepsera®: 10 mg

◆ **Adefovir Dipivoxil** *see* Adefovir *on page 44*

◆ **Adenocard® (Can)** *see* Adenosine *on page 46*

◆ **Adenocard® IV** *see* Adenosine *on page 46*

◆ **Adenoscan®** *see* Adenosine *on page 46*

Adenosine (a DEN oh seen)

Brand Names: U.S. Adenocard® IV; Adenoscan®

Brand Names: Canada Adenocard®; Adenoscan®; Adenosine Injection, USP; PMS-Adenosine

Index Terms 9-Beta-D-Ribofuranosyladenine

Pharmacologic Category Antiarrhythmic Agent, Miscellaneous; Diagnostic Agent

Use

Adenocard®: Treatment of paroxysmal supraventricular tachycardia (PSVT) including that associated with accessory bypass tracts (Wolff-Parkinson-White syndrome); when clinically advisable, appropriate vagal maneuvers should be attempted prior to adenosine administration; **not effective for conversion of atrial fibrillation, atrial flutter, or ventricular tachycardia**

Adenoscan®: Pharmacologic stress agent used in myocardial perfusion thallium-201 scintigraphy

Unlabeled Use

ACLS/PALS Guidelines (2010): Stable, narrow-complex regular tachycardias; unstable narrow-complex regular tachycardias while preparations are made for synchronized direct-current cardioversion; stable regular monomorphic, wide-complex tachycardia as a therapeutic (if SVT) and diagnostic maneuver

Adenoscan®: Acute vasodilator testing in pulmonary artery hypertension

Pregnancy Risk Factor C

Pregnancy Considerations Animal reproduction studies have not been conducted. Adenosine is an endogenous substance and adverse fetal effects would not be anticipated. Case reports of administration during pregnancy have indicated no adverse effects on fetus or newborn attributable to adenosine. ACLS guidelines suggest use is safe and effective in pregnancy.

Lactation Excretion in breast milk unknown

Contraindications Hypersensitivity to adenosine or any component of the formulation; second- or third-degree AV block, sick sinus syndrome, or symptomatic bradycardia (except in patients with a functioning artificial pacemaker); use in patients with atrial fibrillation/flutter with underlying Wolff-Parkinson-White (WPW) syndrome (Fuster, 2006); asthma (ACLS, 2010)

In addition to the above, Adenoscan® should be avoided in patients with known or suspected bronchoconstrictive or bronchospastic lung disease.

Warnings/Precautions ECG monitoring required during use. Equipment for resuscitation and trained personnel experienced in handling medical emergencies should always be immediately available. Adenosine decreases conduction through the AV node and may produce first-, second-, or third-degree heart block. Patients with pre-existing S-A nodal dysfunction may experience prolonged sinus pauses after adenosine; use caution in patients with first-degree AV block or bundle branch block. Use is contraindicated in patients with high-grade AV block, sinus node dysfunction or symptomatic bradycardia (unless a functional artificial pacemaker is in place). Rare, prolonged episodes of asystole have been reported, with fatal outcomes in some cases. Use caution in patients receiving other drugs which slow AV node conduction (eg, digoxin, verapamil).

There have been reports of atrial fibrillation/flutter after adenosine administration in patients with PSVT associated with accessory conduction pathways; has also been reported in patients with or without a history of atrial fibrillation undergoing myocardial perfusion imaging with adenosine infusion. Adenosine may also produce profound vasodilation with subsequent hypotension. When used as a bolus dose (PSVT), effects are generally self-limiting (due to the short half-life of adenosine). However, when used as a continuous infusion (pharmacologic stress testing), effects may be more pronounced and persistent, corresponding to continued exposure; discontinue infusion in patients who develop persistent or symptomatic hypotension. Adenosine infusions should be used with caution in patients with autonomic dysfunction, stenotic valvular heart disease, pericarditis, pleural effusion, carotid stenosis (with cerebrovascular insufficiency), or uncorrected hypovolemia. Use caution in elderly patients; may be at increased risk of hemodynamic effects, bradycardia, and/or AV block.

Avoid use in patients with bronchoconstriction or bronchospasm (eg, asthma); mild-to-moderate exacerbations have been reported following use in a limited number of patients with asthma. Per the ACLS guidelines, use considered contraindicated in patients with asthma. Use caution in patients with obstructive lung disease not associated with bronchoconstriction (eg, emphysema, bronchitis); respiratory compromise has occurred during use.

Adenocard®: Transient AV block is expected. Administer as a rapid bolus, either directly into a vein or (if administered into an I.V. line), as close to the patient as possible (followed by saline flush). Dose reduction recommended when administered via central line (ACLS, 2010). When used in PSVT, at the time of conversion to normal sinus rhythm, a variety of new rhythms may appear on the ECG. Watch for proarrhythmic effects (eg, polymorphic ventricular tachycardia) during and shortly after administration/termination of arrhythmia. Benign transient occurrence of atrial and ventricular ectopy is common upon termination of arrhythmia. Adenosine does not convert atrial fibrillation/flutter to normal sinus rhythm; however, may be used diagnostically in these settings if the underlying rhythm is not apparent. Use in patients with atrial fibrillation/flutter with underlying WPW syndrome is considered to be contraindicated since ventricular fibrillation may result (Fuster, 2006). Use with extreme caution in heart transplant recipients; adenosine may cause prolonged asystole; reduction of initial adenosine dose is recommended (ACLS, 2010); considered by some to be contraindicated in this setting (Delacrétaz, 2006). Avoid use in irregular or polymorphic wide-complex tachycardias; may cause degeneration to ventricular fibrillation (ACLS, 2010). When used for PSVT, dosage reduction recommended when used with concomitant drugs which potentiate the effects of adenosine (carbamazepine, dipyridamole)

Adenoscan®: Drugs which antagonize adenosine (theophylline [includes aminophylline], caffeine) should be withheld for five half-lives prior to adenosine use. Avoid dietary caffeine for at least 12 hours prior to pharmacologic stress testing (Henzlova, 2006). Withhold dipyridamole-containing medications for at least 24 hours prior to pharmacologic stress testing (Henzlova, 2006).

Pulmonary artery hypertension: Acute vasodilator testing (not an approved use): Use with extreme caution in patients with concomitant heart failure (LV systolic dysfunction with significantly elevated left heart filling pressures) or pulmonary veno-occlusive disease/pulmonary capillary hemangiomatosis; significant decompensation has occurred with other highly selective pulmonary vasodilators resulting in acute pulmonary edema.

Adverse Reactions Note: Frequency varies based on use; higher frequency of infusion-related effects, such as flushing and lightheadedness, were reported with continuous infusion (Adenoscan®).

>10%:

Cardiovascular: Transient new arrhythmia (eg, atrial premature contractions, atrial fibrillation, PVCs) after cardioversion (55%), facial flushing (18% to 44%)

Central nervous system: Headache (2% to 18%), dizziness/lightheadedness (2% to 12%)

Gastrointestinal: GI discomfort (13%)

Neuromuscular & skeletal: Discomfort of neck, throat, jaw (<1% to 15%)

Respiratory: Chest pressure/discomfort (7% to 40%), dyspnea (12% to 28%)

1% to 10%:

Cardiovascular: AV block (infusion 6%; third-degree <1%), ST segment depression (3%), hypotension (<1% to 2%), chest pain, palpitation

Central nervous system: Nervousness (2%), apprehension

Gastrointestinal: Nausea (3%)

Neuromuscular & skeletal: Upper extremity discomfort (≤4%), numbness (≤2%), paresthesia (≤2%)

Respiratory: Hyperventilation

Miscellaneous: Diaphoresis

<1% (Limited to important or life-threatening): Asystole (prolonged), atrial fibrillation, bradycardia, bronchospasm, burning sensation, blurred vision, hypertension (transient), injection site reaction, intracranial pressure increased, loss of consciousness, metallic taste, MI, respiratory arrest, seizure, torsade de pointes, ventricular fibrillation, ventricular tachycardia

Drug Interactions

Metabolism/Transport Effects None known.

Avoid Concomitant Use There are no known interactions where it is recommended to avoid concomitant use.

Increased Effect/Toxicity

The levels/effects of Adenosine may be increased by: CarBAMazepine; Digoxin; Dipyridamole; Nicotine

Decreased Effect

The levels/effects of Adenosine may be decreased by: Caffeine; Theophylline Derivatives

Ethanol/Nutrition/Herb Interactions Food: Avoid food or drugs with caffeine. Adenosine's therapeutic effect may be decreased if used concurrently with caffeine. Avoid dietary caffeine for at least 12 hours prior to pharmacologic stress testing.

Stability Store at controlled room temperature of 15°C to 30°C (59°F to 86°F). Do **not** refrigerate; crystallization may occur (may dissolve by warming to room temperature).

Mechanism of Action

Antiarrhythmic actions: Slows conduction time through the AV node, interrupting the re-entry pathways through the AV node, restoring normal sinus rhythm

Myocardial perfusion scintigraphy: Adenosine also causes coronary vasodilation and increases blood flow in normal coronary arteries with little to no increase in stenotic coronary arteries; thallium-201 uptake into the stenotic coronary arteries will be less than that of normal coronary arteries revealing areas of insufficient blood flow.

Pharmacodynamics/Kinetics

Onset of action: Rapid

Duration: Very brief

Metabolism: Blood and tissue to inosine then to adenosine monophosphate (AMP) and hypoxanthine

Half-life elimination: <10 seconds

Dosage

Adenocard®: **Rapid I.V. push (over 1-2 seconds) via peripheral line, followed by a normal saline flush:**

Infants and Children:

Paroxysmal supraventricular tachycardia: Manufacturer's recommendation: I.V.:

<50 kg: Initial: 0.05-0.1 mg/kg (maximum initial dose: 6 mg). If conversion of PSVT does not occur within 1-2 minutes, may increase dose by 0.05-0.1 mg/kg. May repeat until sinus rhythm is established or to a maximum single dose of 0.3 mg/kg or 12 mg. Follow each dose with normal saline flush.

≥50 kg: Refer to Adult dosing

Pediatric advanced life support (PALS, 2010): Treatment of SVT: I.V., I.O.: Initial: 0.1 mg/kg (maximum initial dose: 6 mg); if not effective within 1-2 minutes, administer 0.2 mg/kg (maximum single dose: 12 mg). Follow each dose with ≥5 mL normal saline flush.

Adults: Paroxysmal supraventricular tachycardia: I.V. (peripheral line; see **"Note"**): Initial: 6 mg; if not effective within 1-2 minutes, 12 mg may be given; may repeat 12 mg bolus if needed (maximum single dose: 12 mg). Follow each dose with 20 mL normal saline flush. **Note:** Initial dose of adenosine should be reduced to 3 mg if patient is currently receiving carbamazepine or dipyridamole, has a transplanted heart or if adenosine is administered via central line (ACLS, 2010).

Adenoscan®:

Pharmacologic stress testing: Continuous I.V. infusion via peripheral line: 140 mcg/kg/minute for 6 minutes using syringe or volumetric infusion pump; total dose: 0.84 mg/kg. Thallium-201 is injected at midpoint (3 minutes) of infusion.

Acute vasodilator testing in pulmonary artery hypertension (unlabeled use): I.V.: Initial: 50 mcg/kg/minute increased by 50 mcg/kg/minute every 2 minutes to a maximum dose of 500 mcg/kg/minute (Schrader, 1992) **or** to a maximum dose of 250 mcg/kg/minute (McLaughlin, 2009); acutely assess vasodilator response

Dietary Considerations Avoid dietary caffeine for at least 12 hours prior to pharmacologic stress testing.

Administration

Adenocard®: For rapid bolus I.V. use only; administer I.V. push over 1-2 seconds at a peripheral I.V. site as proximal as possible to trunk (not in lower arm, hand, lower leg, or foot); follow each bolus with a rapid normal saline flush (infants and children ≥5 mL; adults 20 mL). Use of 2 syringes (one with adenosine dose and the other with NS flush) connected to a T-connector or stopcock is recommended. If administered via **central line** in adults, reduce initial dose (ACLS, 2010).

Adenoscan®: For I.V. infusion only via peripheral line

Monitoring Parameters ECG, heart rate, blood pressure

Dosage Forms Excipient information presented when available (limited, particularly for generics); consult specific product labeling.

Injection, solution [preservative free]: 3 mg/mL (2 mL, 4 mL)

Adenocard® IV: 3 mg/mL (2 mL, 4 mL)

Adenoscan®: 3 mg/mL (20 mL, 30 mL)

- **Adenosine Injection, USP (Can)** *see* Adenosine *on page 46*
- **ADH** *see* Vasopressin *on page 1775*
- **Adipex-P®** *see* Phentermine *on page 1341*
- **ADL-2698** *see* Alvimopan *on page 81*
- **Adoxa®** *see* Doxycycline *on page 557*
- **Adoxa® Pak™ 1/75 [DSC]** *see* Doxycycline *on page 557*
- **Adoxa® Pak™ 1/150 [DSC]** *see* Doxycycline *on page 557*
- **Adrenalin®** *see* EPINEPHrine (Systemic, Oral Inhalation) *on page 594*
- **Adrenaline** *see* EPINEPHrine (Systemic, Oral Inhalation) *on page 594*
- **ADR (error-prone abbreviation)** *see* DOXOrubicin *on page 552*
- **AdreView™** *see* Iobenguane I 123 *on page 920*
- **Adria** *see* DOXOrubicin *on page 552*
- **Adriamycin®** *see* DOXOrubicin *on page 552*
- **Adrucil®** *see* Fluorouracil (Systemic) *on page 730*
- **Adsorbent Charcoal** *see* Charcoal, Activated *on page 335*
- **Advagraf® (Can)** *see* Tacrolimus (Systemic) *on page 1615*
- **Advair® (Can)** *see* Fluticasone and Salmeterol *on page 741*
- **Advair Diskus®** *see* Fluticasone and Salmeterol *on page 741*
- **Advair® HFA** *see* Fluticasone and Salmeterol *on page 741*
- **Advate** *see* Antihemophilic Factor (Recombinant) *on page 127*
- **Advicor®** *see* Niacin and Lovastatin *on page 1197*
- **Advil® [OTC]** *see* Ibuprofen *on page 860*
- **Advil® (Can)** *see* Ibuprofen *on page 860*
- **Advil® Children's [OTC]** *see* Ibuprofen *on page 860*
- **Advil® Cold & Sinus [OTC]** *see* Pseudoephedrine and Ibuprofen *on page 1432*
- **Advil® Cold & Sinus (Can)** *see* Pseudoephedrine and Ibuprofen *on page 1432*
- **Advil® Cold & Sinus Daytime (Can)** *see* Pseudoephedrine and Ibuprofen *on page 1432*
- **Advil® Infants' [OTC]** *see* Ibuprofen *on page 860*
- **Advil® Migraine [OTC]** *see* Ibuprofen *on page 860*
- **Aerius® (Can)** *see* Desloratadine *on page 475*
- **Aerius® Kids (Can)** *see* Desloratadine *on page 475*
- **Afeditab® CR** *see* NIFEdipine *on page 1202*
- **Afinitor®** *see* Everolimus *on page 673*

Aflibercept (a FLIB er sept)

Brand Names: U.S. Eylea™

Index Terms AVE 0005; AVE 005; AVE-0005; VEGF Trap; VEGF Trap-Eye

Pharmacologic Category Ophthalmic Agent; Vascular Endothelial Growth Factor (VEGF) Inhibitor

Use Treatment of neovascular (wet) age-related macular degeneration (AMD)

Pregnancy Risk Factor C

Pregnancy Considerations Adverse events were observed in animal reproduction studies.

Lactation Excretion in breast milk unknown/not recommended

Contraindications Hypersensitivity to aflibercept or any component of the formulation; current ocular or periocular infection; active intraocular inflammation

Warnings/Precautions Administer injection using proper aseptic technique. Intravitreal injections may be associated with endophthalmitis, retinal detachment, increased intraocular pressure, infections, or thromboembolic events (eg, nonfatal stroke/MI, vascular death); postprocedure monitoring for these adverse effects should be completed.

Adverse Reactions

>10%: Ocular: Conjunctival hemorrhage (25%)

1% to 10%:

Local: Injection site pain (3%), injection site hemorrhage (1%)

Ocular: Eye pain (9%), cataract (7%), vitreous detachment (6%), vitreous floaters (6%), intraocular pressure increased (5%), conjunctival hyperemia (4%), corneal erosion (4%), foreign body sensation (3%), lacrimation increased (3%), retinal pigment epithelium detachment (3%), blurred vision (2%), retinal pigment epithelium tear (2%), eyelid edema (1%), corneal edema (1%)

Miscellaneous: Aflibercept antibodies (1% to 3%)

<1% (Limited to important or life-threatening): Endophthalmitis, hypersensitivity, thromboembolic events, traumatic cataract

Drug Interactions

Metabolism/Transport Effects None known.

Avoid Concomitant Use There are no known interactions where it is recommended to avoid concomitant use.

Increased Effect/Toxicity There are no known significant interactions involving an increase in effect.

Decreased Effect There are no known significant interactions involving a decrease in effect.

Stability Store at 2°C to 8°C (36°F to 46°F); do not freeze. Store in original container prior to use; protect from light.

Mechanism of Action Aflibercept is a recombinant fusion protein that acts as a decoy receptor for vascular endothelial growth factor-A (VEGF-A) and placental growth factor (PIGF). Decoy receptor binding prevents VEGF-A and PIGF from binding and activating endothelial cell receptors, thereby suppressing neovascularization and slowing vision loss.

Pharmacodynamics/Kinetics

Absorption: Low levels are detected in the serum following intravitreal injection

Half-life elimination: Plasma: 5-6 days

Dosage

Intravitreal: Adults: 2 mg (0.05 mL) every 4 weeks for 3 months, then every 8 weeks thereafter

Dosage adjustment in renal impairment: No dosage adjustment necessary

Dosage adjustment in hepatic impairment: No dosage adjustment provided in manufacturer's labeling (has not been studied); however, no adjustment expected due to minimal systemic absorption

Administration For ophthalmic intravitreal injection only. Remove contents from vial using a 5 micron, 19-gauge 1 1/2 inch filter needle (supplied) attached to a 1 mL syringe (supplied). Discard filter needle and replace with a sterile 30 gauge 1/2 inch needle (supplied) for intravitreal injection procedure (do not use filter needle for intravitreal injection). Depress plunger to expel excess air and medication (plunger tip should align with the 0.05 mL marking on syringe). Adequate anesthesia and a broad-spectrum antimicrobial agent should be administered prior to the procedure.

Monitoring Parameters Intraocular pressure immediately following injection; signs of infection/inflammation (for first week following injection); retinal perfusion; endophthalmitis; visual acuity

Dosage Forms Excipient information presented when available (limited, particularly for generics); consult specific product labeling.

Injection, solution, intravitreal [preservative free]:

Eylea™: 40 mg/mL (0.05 mL) [derived from or manufactured using Chinese hamster ovary cells]

◆ **Afluria®** *see* Influenza Virus Vaccine (Inactivated) *on page 897*

Agalsidase Beta (aye GAL si days BAY ta)

Brand Names: U.S. Fabrazyme®

Brand Names: Canada Fabrazyme®

Index Terms Alpha-Galactosidase-A (Recombinant); r-h α-GAL

Pharmacologic Category Enzyme

Use Replacement therapy for Fabry disease

Pregnancy Risk Factor B

Dosage I.V.: Children ≥8 years and Adults: 1 mg/kg every 2 weeks

Dosage adjustment in toxicity: Patient with IgE antibodies to agalsidase beta (rechallenge): 0.5 mg/kg every 2 weeks at an initial maximum infusion rate of 0.01 mg/minute; may gradually escalate dose (to maximum of 1 mg/kg every 2 weeks) and/or infusion rate (doubling the infusion rate every 30 minutes to a maximum rate of 0.25 mg/minute) as tolerated.

Dosage adjustment in renal impairment: No dosage adjustment required

Additional Information Complete prescribing information for this medication should be consulted for additional detail.

Dosage Forms Excipient information presented when available (limited, particularly for generics); consult specific product labeling.

Injection, powder for reconstitution:

Fabrazyme®: 5 mg [contains mannitol; derived from or manufactured using Chinese hamster ovary cells]

Fabrazyme®: 35 mg [contains mannitol; derived from or manufactured using Chinese hamster ovary cells]

◆ **Aggrastat®** *see* Tirofiban *on page 1694*
◆ **Aggrenox®** *see* Aspirin and Dipyridamole *on page 157*
◆ **AGN 1135** *see* Rasagiline *on page 1466*
◆ **$AgNO_3$** *see* Silver Nitrate *on page 1554*
◆ **Agriflu™ (Can)** *see* Influenza Virus Vaccine (Inactivated) *on page 897*
◆ **Agrylin®** *see* Anagrelide *on page 119*
◆ **AHF (Human)** *see* Antihemophilic Factor (Human) *on page 125*
◆ **AHF (Human)** *see* Antihemophilic Factor/von Willebrand Factor Complex (Human) *on page 128*
◆ **AHF (Recombinant)** *see* Antihemophilic Factor (Recombinant) *on page 127*
◆ **A-hydroCort** *see* Hydrocortisone (Systemic) *on page 839*
◆ **A-Hydrocort®** *see* Hydrocortisone (Systemic) *on page 839*
◆ **A-hydroCort** *see* Hydrocortisone (Topical) *on page 841*
◆ **AICC** *see* Anti-inhibitor Coagulant Complex *on page 130*
◆ **Airomir (Can)** *see* Albuterol *on page 52*
◆ **AK Cide Oph (Can)** *see* Sulfacetamide and Prednisolone *on page 1600*
◆ **AK-Con™** *see* Naphazoline (Ophthalmic) *on page 1176*
◆ **AK-Fluor®** *see* Fluorescein *on page 727*
◆ **Akne-mycin®** *see* Erythromycin (Topical) *on page 619*
◆ **AK-Pentolate™** *see* Cyclopentolate *on page 420*
◆ **AK-Poly-Bac™** *see* Bacitracin and Polymyxin B *on page 186*
◆ **AK Sulf Liq (Can)** *see* Sulfacetamide (Ophthalmic) *on page 1599*
◆ **AK-Tob™** *see* Tobramycin (Ophthalmic) *on page 1700*
◆ **ALA** *see* Aminolevulinic Acid *on page 90*
◆ **5-ALA** *see* Aminolevulinic Acid *on page 90*
◆ **Ala-Cort** *see* Hydrocortisone (Topical) *on page 841*
◆ **Alagesic LQ** *see* Butalbital, Acetaminophen, and Caffeine *on page 255*
◆ **Alamag [OTC]** *see* Aluminum Hydroxide and Magnesium Hydroxide *on page 80*
◆ **Alamag Plus [OTC]** *see* Aluminum Hydroxide, Magnesium Hydroxide, and Simethicone *on page 80*
◆ **Alamast®** *see* Pemirolast *on page 1319*
◆ **Ala-Scalp** *see* Hydrocortisone (Topical) *on page 841*
◆ **Alavert® Allergy 24 Hour [OTC]** *see* Loratadine *on page 1031*
◆ **Alavert™ Allergy and Sinus [OTC]** *see* Loratadine and Pseudoephedrine *on page 1032*
◆ **Alavert® Children's Allergy [OTC]** *see* Loratadine *on page 1031*
◆ **Alaway™ [OTC]** *see* Ketotifen (Ophthalmic) *on page 959*

Albendazole (al BEN da zole)

Brand Names: U.S. Albenza®

Pharmacologic Category Anthelmintic

Use Treatment of parenchymal neurocysticercosis caused by *Taenia solium* and cystic hydatid disease of the liver, lung, and peritoneum caused by *Echinococcus granulosus*

Unlabeled Use Albendazole has activity against *Ascaris lumbricoides* (roundworm); *Ancylostoma caninum*; *Ancylostoma duodenale* and *Necator americanus* (hookworms); cutaneous larva migrans; *Enterobius vermicularis* (pinworm); *Giardia duodenalis* (giardiasis); *Gnathostoma spinigerum*; *Gongylonema* sp; *Mansonella perstans* (filariasis); *Oesophagostomum bifurcum*; *Opisthorchis sinensis* (liver fluke); *Trichinella spiralis* (Trichinellosis); visceral larva migrans (toxocariasis); activity has also been shown against the liver fluke *Clonorchis sinensis*, *Giardia lamblia*, *Cysticercus cellulosae*, and *Echinococcus multilocularis*. Albendazole has also been used for the treatment of intestinal microsporidiosis (*Encephalitozoon intestinalis*), disseminated microsporidiosis (*E. hellem*, *E. cuniculi*, *E. intestinalis*, *Pleistophora* sp, *Trachipleistophora* sp, *Brachiola vesicularum*), and ocular microsporidiosis (*E. hellem*, *E. cuniculi*, *Vittaforma corneae*).

Pregnancy Risk Factor C

Pregnancy Considerations Albendazole has been shown to be teratogenic in laboratory animals and should not be used during pregnancy, if at all possible. Women should be advised to avoid pregnancy for at least 1 month following therapy. Discontinue if pregnancy occurs during treatment.

Lactation Excretion in breast milk unknown/use caution

Contraindications Hypersensitivity to albendazole, benzimidazoles, or any component of the formulation

Warnings/Precautions Reversible elevations in hepatic enzymes have been reported; patients with abnormal LFTs and hepatic echinococcosis are at an increased risk of hepatotoxicity. Discontinue therapy if LFT elevations are >2 times the upper limit of normal; may consider restarting treatment with frequent monitoring of LFTs when hepatic enzymes return to pretreatment values. Agranulocytosis, aplastic anemia, granulocytopenia, leukopenia, and pancytopenia have occurred leading to fatalities (rare); use with caution in patients with hepatic impairment (more susceptible to hematologic toxicity). Discontinue therapy in all patients who develop clinically significant decreases in blood cell counts.

Neurocysticercosis: Corticosteroids should be administered before or upon initiation of albendazole therapy to minimize inflammatory reactions and prevent cerebral hypertension. Anticonvulsant therapy should be used concurrently during the first week of therapy to prevent seizures. These measures are important to minimize neurological symptoms which may result from uncovering of pre-existing neurocysticercosis when using albendazole to treat other conditions. If retinal lesions exist, weigh risk of further retinal damage due to albendazole-induced changes to the retinal lesion vs benefit of disease treatment.

Adverse Reactions

>10%:
- Central nervous system: Headache (11% neurocysticercosis; 1% hydatid)
- Hepatic: LFTs increased (16% hydatid; <1% neurocysticercosis)

1% to 10%:
- Central nervous system: Intracranial pressure increased (≤2%), dizziness (≤1%), fever (≤1%), vertigo (≤1%), meningeal signs (1%)
- Dermatologic: Alopecia (<1% to 2%)
- Gastrointestinal: Abdominal pain (≤6%), nausea/vomiting (4% to 6%)

<1% (Limited to important or life-threatening symptoms): Acute liver failure, acute renal failure, aplastic anemia, agranulocytosis, erythema multiforme, granulocytopenia, hepatitis, hypersensitivity reaction, leukopenia, neutropenia, pancytopenia, rash, Stevens-Johnson syndrome, thrombocytopenia, urticaria

Drug Interactions

Metabolism/Transport Effects Substrate of CYP1A2 (minor), CYP3A4 (minor); **Note:** Assignment of Major/Minor substrate status based on clinically relevant drug interaction potential

Avoid Concomitant Use There are no known interactions where it is recommended to avoid concomitant use.

Increased Effect/Toxicity

The levels/effects of Albendazole may be increased by: Conivaptan

Decreased Effect

The levels/effects of Albendazole may be decreased by: Aminoquinolines (Antimalarial); Cyproterone; Tocilizumab

Ethanol/Nutrition/Herb Interactions Food: Albendazole serum levels may be increased if taken with a fatty meal (increases the oral bioavailability by up to 5 times).

Stability Store between 20°C and 25°C (68°F to 77°F)

Mechanism of Action Active metabolite, albendazole sulfoxide, causes selective degeneration of cytoplasmic microtubules in intestinal and tegmental cells of intestinal helminths and larvae; glycogen is depleted, glucose uptake and cholinesterase secretion are impaired, and desecratory substances accumulate intracellulary. ATP production decreases causing energy depletion, immobilization, and worm death.

Pharmacodynamics/Kinetics

Absorption: Poor; may increase up to 5 times when administered with a fatty meal

Distribution: Well inside hydatid cysts and CSF

Protein binding: 70%

Metabolism: Hepatic; extensive first-pass effect; pathways include rapid sulfoxidation to active metabolite (albendazole sulfoxide [major]), hydrolysis, and oxidation

Half-life elimination: 8-12 hours

Time to peak, serum: 2-5 hours

Excretion: Urine (<1% as active metabolite); feces

Dosage Oral:

Infants and Children: Microsporidiosis (other than *Enterocytozoon bienuesi* or *V. corneae*), disseminated or intestinal infection (HIV-positive, unlabeled use): 15 mg/kg/day (maximum: 800 mg/day) in 2 divided doses continued until immune reconstitution after HAART initiation (CDC, 2009)

Children:

- *Cysticercus cellulosae* (unlabeled use): 15 mg/kg/day (maximum: 800 mg/day) in 2 divided doses for 8-30 days; may be repeated as necessary
- *Echinococcus granulosus* (tapeworm) (unlabeled use): 15 mg/kg/day (maximum: 800 mg) divided twice daily for 1-6 months
- *Giardia duodenalis* (giardiasis) (unlabeled use): 10 mg/kg/day for 5 days (Yereli, 2004)

Children and Adults:

Neurocysticercosis:
- <60 kg: 15 mg/kg/day in 2 divided doses (maximum: 800 mg/day) for 8-30 days
- ≥60 kg: 800 mg/day in 2 divided doses for 8-30 days
- **Note:** Give concurrent anticonvulsant and steroid therapy during first week.

Hydatid:
- <60 kg: 15 mg/kg/day in 2 divided doses (maximum: 800 mg/day)
- ≥60 kg: 800 mg/day in 2 divided doses
- **Note:** Administer dose for three 28-day cycles with a 14-day drug-free interval in between each cycle.

Ancylostoma caninum, Ascaris lumbricoides (roundworm), *Ancylostoma duodenale* (hookworm), and *Necator americanus* (hookworm) (unlabeled use): 400 mg as a single dose

Clonorchis sinensis (Chinese liver fluke) (unlabeled use): 10 mg/kg/day for 7 days

Cutaneous larva migrans (unlabeled use): 400 mg once daily for 3 days

Enterobius vermicularis (pinworm) (unlabeled use): 400 mg as a single dose; repeat in 2 weeks

Gnathostoma spinigerum (unlabeled use): 800 mg/day in 2 divided doses for 21 days

Gongylonemiasis (unlabeled use): 400 mg once daily for 3 days

Mansonella perstans (unlabeled use): 800 mg/day in 2 divided doses for 10 days

Oesophagostomum bifurcum (unlabeled use): 400 mg as a single dose (Ziem, 2004)

Trichinella spiralis (Trichinellosis) (unlabeled use): 800 mg/day in 2 divided doses for 8-14 days plus steroids for severe symptoms

Visceral larva migrans (toxocariasis) (unlabeled use): 800 mg/day in 2 divided doses for 5 days

Adults:

- *Cysticercus cellulosae* (unlabeled use): 800 mg/day in 2 divided doses for 8-30 days; may be repeated as necessary
- Disseminated microsporidiosis (unlabeled use): 800 mg/day in 2 divided doses

Echinococcus granulosus (tapeworm) (unlabeled use): 800 mg/day in 2 divided doses for 1-6 months

Giardia duodenalis (giardiasis) (unlabeled use): 400 mg once daily for 5 days

Intestinal microsporidiosis (*E. intestinalis*) (unlabeled use): 800 mg/day in 2 divided doses for 21 days

Ocular microsporidiosis (unlabeled use): 800 mg/day in 2 divided doses, in combination with fumagillin

Dietary Considerations Should be taken with a high-fat meal.

Administration Should be administered with a high-fat meal. Administer anticonvulsant and steroid therapy during first week of neurocysticercosis therapy. If patients have difficulty swallowing, tablets may be crushed or chewed, then swallowed with a drink of water.

Monitoring Parameters Monitor fecal specimens for ova and parasites for 3 weeks after treatment; if positive, retreat; LFTs and CBC with differential at start of each 28-day cycle and every 2 weeks during therapy (more frequent monitoring for patients with liver disease); ophthalmic exam (patients with neurocysticercosis); pregnancy test

Dosage Forms Excipient information presented when available (limited, particularly for generics); consult specific product labeling.

Tablet, oral:

Albenza®: 200 mg

◆ **Albenza®** *see* Albendazole *on page 49*

◆ **Albert® Pentoxifylline (Can)** *see* Pentoxifylline *on page 1333*

◆ **Albuked™ 5** *see* Albumin *on page 51*

◆ **Albuked™ 25** *see* Albumin *on page 51*

Albumin (al BYOO min)

Brand Names: U.S. Albuked™ 25; Albuked™ 5; Albuminar®-25; Albuminar®-5; AlbuRx® 25; AlbuRx® 5; Albutein®; Buminate; Flexbumin 25%; Human Albumin Grifols® 25%; Kedbumin™; Plasbumin®-25; Plasbumin®-5

Brand Names: Canada Plasbumin®-25; Plasbumin®-5

Index Terms Albumin (Human); Normal Human Serum Albumin; Normal Serum Albumin (Human); Salt Poor Albumin; SPA

Pharmacologic Category Blood Product Derivative; Plasma Volume Expander, Colloid

Use Plasma volume expansion and maintenance of cardiac output in the treatment of certain types of shock or impending shock; may be useful for burn patients, ARDS, and cardiopulmonary bypass; other uses considered by some investigators (but not proven) are retroperitoneal surgery, peritonitis, and ascites; unless the condition responsible for hypoproteinemia can be corrected, albumin can provide only symptomatic relief or supportive treatment

Note: Nutritional supplementation is not an appropriate indication.

Unlabeled Use In patients with cirrhosis, administered with diuretics to help facilitate diuresis; large volume paracentesis; volume expansion in dehydrated, mildly hypotensive patients with cirrhosis; to prevent renal impairment and reduce mortality associated with spontaneous bacterial peritonitis (SBP) in patients with cirrhosis

Pregnancy Risk Factor C

Pregnancy Considerations Animal reproduction studies have not been conducted. Albumin is used for the treatment of ovarian hyperstimulation syndrome (ASRM, 2008). Use for other indications may be considered in pregnant women when contraindications to nonprotein colloids exist (Liumbruno, 2009).

Contraindications Hypersensitivity to albumin or any component of the formulation; patients with severe anemia or cardiac failure

Warnings/Precautions Use with caution in patients with hepatic or renal failure because of added protein load; rapid infusion of albumin solutions may cause vascular overload. All patients should be observed for signs of hypervolemia such as pulmonary edema. Use with caution in those patients for whom sodium restriction is necessary. Avoid 25% concentration in preterm infants due to risk of intraventricular hemorrhage. Packaging may contain natural latex rubber.

Adverse Reactions Frequency not defined.

Cardiovascular: CHF precipitation, edema, hyper-/hypotension, hypervolemia, tachycardia

Central nervous system: Chills, fever, headache

Dermatologic: Pruritus, rash, urticaria

Gastrointestinal: Nausea, vomiting

Respiratory: Bronchospasm, pulmonary edema

Miscellaneous: Anaphylaxis

Drug Interactions

Metabolism/Transport Effects None known.

Avoid Concomitant Use There are no known interactions where it is recommended to avoid concomitant use.

Increased Effect/Toxicity There are no known significant interactions involving an increase in effect.

Decreased Effect There are no known significant interactions involving a decrease in effect.

Stability Store at a temperature ≤30°C (86°F); do not freeze. Do not use solution if it is turbid or contains a deposit; use within 4 hours after opening vial; discard unused portion.

If 5% human albumin is unavailable, it may be prepared by diluting 25% human albumin with 0.9% sodium chloride or 5% dextrose in water. Do not use sterile water to dilute albumin solutions, as this has been associated with hypotonic-associated hemolysis.

Mechanism of Action Provides increase in intravascular oncotic pressure and causes mobilization of fluids from interstitial into intravascular space

Dosage I.V.:

5% should be used in hypovolemic patients or intravascularly-depleted patients

25% should be used in patients in whom fluid and sodium intake must be minimized

Dose depends on condition of patient:

Children: Hypovolemia: 0.5-1 g/kg/dose (10-20 mL/kg/dose of albumin 5%); maximum dose: 6 g/kg/day

Adults: Usual dose: 25 g; initial dose may be repeated in 15-30 minutes if response is inadequate; no more than 250 g should be administered within 48 hours

Hypovolemia: 5% albumin: 0.5-1 g/kg/dose; repeat as needed. **Note:** May be considered after inadequate response to crystalloid therapy and when nonprotein colloids are contraindicated. The volume administered and the speed of infusion should be adapted to individual response.

Large-volume paracentesis (>5 L) (unlabeled use): 25% albumin: 5-8 g for every liter removed (Garcia-Compeán, 1993; Moore, 2003) **or** 50 g total for paracentesis >5 L (ATS, 2004). **Note:** Administer soon after the procedure to avoid postprocedural complications (eg, hypovolemia, hyponatremia, renal impairment) (Moore, 2003).

SBP in patients with cirrhosis (unlabeled use): 25% albumin: Initial: 1.5 g/kg, followed by 1 g/kg on day 3 (in conjunction with appropriate antimicrobial therapy) (ATS, 2004; Sort, 1999). **Note:** Clinical trial employed albumin 20%; however, the difference in concentration compared with 25% albumin is deemed to be clinically inconsequential.

Dietary Considerations Some products may contain potassium and/or sodium.

Administration For I.V. administration only. Use within 4 hours after opening vial; discard unused portion. In emergencies, may administer as rapidly as necessary to improve clinical condition. After initial volume replacement:

5%: Do not exceed 2-4 mL/minute in patients with normal plasma volume; 5-10 mL/minute in patients with hypoproteinemia

25%: Do not exceed 1 mL/minute in patients with normal plasma volume; 2-3 mL/minute in patients with hypoproteinemia

Do not dilute 5% solution. Rapid infusion may cause vascular overload. Albumin 25% may be given undiluted or diluted in normal saline. May give in combination or through the same administration set as saline or carbohydrates. Do not use with ethanol or protein hydrolysates, precipitation may form.

Monitoring Parameters Blood pressure, pulmonary edema, hematocrit

Additional Information Albumin 5% and 25% solutions contain 130-160 mEq/L sodium and are considered isotonic with plasma. Dilution of albumin 25% solution with sterile water produces a hypotonic solution; administration of such can cause hemolysis and/or renal failure. An albumin 5% solution is osmotically equivalent to an equal volume of plasma, whereas a 25% solution is osmotically equivalent to 5 times its volume of plasma. Albumin solutions are heated to 60°C for 10 hours, decreasing any possible risk of viral hepatitis transmission. To date, there have been no reports of viral transmission using these products.

Dosage Forms Excipient information presented when available (limited, particularly for generics); consult specific product labeling.

Injection, solution [human, preservative free]: 5% [50 mg/mL] (250 mL, 500 mL); 20% [200 mg/mL] (50 mL, 100 mL); 25% [250 mg/mL] (50 mL, 100 mL)

Albuked™ 5: 5% [50 mg/mL] (250 mL) [contains sodium 145 mEq/L]

Albuked™ 25: 25% [250 mg/mL] (50 mL) [contains sodium 145 mEq/L]

Albuminar®-5: 5% [50 mg/mL] (250 mL, 500 mL) [contains potassium ≤1 mEq/L, sodium 130-160 mEq/L]

Albuminar®-25: 25% [250 mg/mL] (50 mL, 100 mL) [contains potassium ≤1 mEq/L, sodium 130-160 mEq/L]

Buminate: 5% [50 mg/mL] (250 mL, 500 mL); 25% [250 mg/mL] (20 mL) [contains natural rubber/natural latex in packaging, potassium ≤2 mEq/L, sodium 130-160 mEq/L]

Flexbumin 25%: 25% [250 mg/mL] (50 mL, 100 mL) [contains potassium ≤2 mEq/L, sodium 130-160 mEq/L]

Plasbumin®-5: 5% [50 mg/mL] (50 mL, 250 mL) [contains sodium 145 mEq/L]

Plasbumin®-25: 25% [250 mg/mL] (20 mL, 50 mL, 100 mL) [contains potassium ≤2 mEq/L, sodium ~145 mEq/L]

Injection, solution [human/low aluminum formulation, preservative free]:

AlbuRx® 5: 5% [50 mg/mL] (250 mL, 500 mL) [contains potassium ≤2 mEq/L, sodium 130-160 mEq/L]

AlbuRx® 25: 25% [250 mg/mL] (50 mL, 100 mL) [contains potassium ≤2 mEq/L, sodium 130-160 mEq/L]

Albutein®: 5% [50 mg/mL] (250 mL, 500 mL); 25% [250 mg/mL] (50 mL, 100 mL) [contains potassium ≤2 mEq/L, sodium 130-160 mEq/L]

Human Albumin Grifols® 25%: 25% [250 mg/mL] (50 mL, 100 mL) [contains potassium ≤2 mEq/L, sodium 130-160 mEq/L]

Kedbumin™: 25% [250 mg/mL] (50 mL) [contains sodium 130-160 mEq/L]

Plasbumin®-5: 5% [50 mg/mL] (50 mL, 250 mL) [contains potassium ≤2 mEq/L, sodium ~145 mEq/L]

Plasbumin®-25: 25% [250 mg/mL] (20 mL, 50 mL, 100 mL) [contains potassium ≤2 mEq/L, sodium ~145 mEq/L]

- ◆ **Albuminar®-5** *see* Albumin *on page 51*
- ◆ **Albuminar®-25** *see* Albumin *on page 51*
- ◆ **Albumin-Bound Paclitaxel** *see* PACLitaxel (Protein Bound) *on page 1275*
- ◆ **Albumin (Human)** *see* Albumin *on page 51*
- ◆ **Albumin-Stabilized Nanoparticle Paclitaxel** *see* PACLitaxel (Protein Bound) *on page 1275*
- ◆ **AlbuRx® 5** *see* Albumin *on page 51*
- ◆ **AlbuRx® 25** *see* Albumin *on page 51*
- ◆ **Albutein®** *see* Albumin *on page 51*

Albuterol (al BYOO ter ole)

Brand Names: U.S. AccuNeb®; ProAir® HFA; Proventil® HFA; Ventolin® HFA; VoSpire ER®

Brand Names: Canada Airomir; Apo-Salvent®; Apo-Salvent® AEM; Apo-Salvent® CFC Free; Apo-Salvent® Sterules; Dom-Salbutamol; Med-Salbutamol; Mylan-Salbutamol Respirator Solution; Mylan-Salbutamol Sterinebs P.F.; Novo-Salbutamol HFA; Nu-Salbutamol; PHL-Salbutamol; PMS-Salbutamol; ratio-Ipra-Sal; ratio-Salbutamol; Sandoz-Salbutamol; Ventolin®; Ventolin® Diskus; Ventolin® HFA; Ventolin® I.V. Infusion; Ventolin® Nebules P.F.

Index Terms Albuterol Sulfate; Salbutamol; Salbutamol Sulphate

Pharmacologic Category $Beta_2$-Adrenergic Agonist

Additional Appendix Information

Bronchodilators *on page 1886*

Use Treatment or prevention of bronchospasm in patients with reversible obstructive airway disease; prevention of exercise-induced bronchospasm

Pregnancy Risk Factor C

Pregnancy Considerations Albuterol crosses the placenta; tocolytic effects, fetal tachycardia, fetal hypoglycemia secondary to maternal hyperglycemia with oral or intravenous routes reported. Available evidence suggests safe use as an inhalation during pregnancy, and albuterol is the preferred short-acting beta agonist for use in asthma according to the NHLBI 2007 Guidelines for the Diagnosis and Management of Asthma.

Lactation Excretion in breast milk unknown/use caution

Contraindications Hypersensitivity to albuterol or any component of the formulation

Injection formulation (Canadian labeling; product not available in U.S.): Hypersensitivity to albuterol or any component of the formulation; tachyarrhythmias; risk of abortion during first or second trimester

Warnings/Precautions Optimize anti-inflammatory treatment before initiating maintenance treatment with albuterol. Do not use as a component of chronic therapy without an anti-inflammatory agent. Only the mildest forms of asthma (Step 1 and/or exercise-induced) would not require concurrent use based upon asthma guidelines. Patient must be instructed to seek medical attention in cases where acute symptoms are not relieved or a previous level of response is diminished. The need to increase frequency of use may indicate deterioration of asthma, and treatment must not be delayed.

Use caution in patients with cardiovascular disease (arrhythmia or hypertension or HF), convulsive disorders, diabetes, glaucoma, hyperthyroidism, or hypokalemia. Beta-agonists may cause elevation in blood pressure, heart rate, and result in CNS stimulation/excitation. $Beta_2$-agonists may increase risk of arrhythmia, increase serum glucose, or decrease serum potassium.

Immediate hypersensitivity reactions (urticaria, angioedema, rash, bronchospasm) have been reported. Do not exceed recommended dose; serious adverse events, including fatalities, have been associated with excessive use of inhaled sympathomimetics. Rarely, paradoxical bronchospasm may occur with use of inhaled bronchodilating agents; this should be distinguished from inadequate response. All patients should utilize a spacer device or valved holding chamber when using a metered-dose inhaler; in addition, face masks should be used in children <4 years of age.

Adverse Reactions Incidence of adverse effects is dependent upon age of patient, dose, and route of administration.

Cardiovascular: Angina, atrial fibrillation, arrhythmias, chest discomfort, chest pain, extrasystoles, flushing, hyper-/hypotension, palpitation, supraventricular tachycardia, tachycardia

Central nervous system: CNS stimulation, dizziness, drowsiness, headache, insomnia, irritability, lightheadedness, migraine, nervousness, nightmares, restlessness, seizure

Dermatologic: Angioedema, rash, urticaria

Endocrine & metabolic: Hyperglycemia, hypokalemia, lactic acidosis

Gastrointestinal: Diarrhea, dry mouth, dyspepsia, gastroenteritis, nausea, unusual taste, vomiting

Genitourinary: Micturition difficulty

Local: Injection: Pain, stinging

Neuromuscular & skeletal: Muscle cramps, musculoskeletal pain, tremor, weakness

Otic: Otitis media, vertigo

Respiratory: Asthma exacerbation, bronchospasm, cough, epistaxis, laryngitis, oropharyngeal drying/irritation, oropharyngeal edema, pharyngitis, rhinitis, upper respiratory inflammation, viral respiratory infection

Miscellaneous: Allergic reaction, anaphylaxis, diaphoresis, lymphadenopathy

Postmarketing and/or case reports: Anxiety, glossitis, hoarseness, metabolic acidosis, myocardial ischemia, pulmonary edema, throat irritation, tongue ulceration

Drug Interactions

Metabolism/Transport Effects None known.

Avoid Concomitant Use

Avoid concomitant use of Albuterol with any of the following: Beta-Blockers (Nonselective); Iobenguane I 123

Increased Effect/Toxicity

Albuterol may increase the levels/effects of: Loop Diuretics; Sympathomimetics; Thiazide Diuretics

The levels/effects of Albuterol may be increased by: Atomoxetine; Cannabinoids; MAO Inhibitors; Tricyclic Antidepressants

Decreased Effect

Albuterol may decrease the levels/effects of: Iobenguane I 123

The levels/effects of Albuterol may be decreased by: Alpha-/Beta-Blockers; Beta-Blockers (Beta1 Selective); Beta-Blockers (Nonselective); Betahistine

Ethanol/Nutrition/Herb Interactions

Food: Avoid or limit caffeine (may cause CNS stimulation).

Herb/Nutraceutical: Avoid ephedra, yohimbe (may cause CNS stimulation). Avoid St John's wort (may decrease the levels/effects of albuterol).

Stability

HFA aerosols: Store at 15°C to 25°C (59°F to 77°F).

Ventolin® HFA: Discard when counter reads 000 or 12 months after removal from protective pouch, whichever comes first. Store with mouthpiece down.

Infusion solution (Canadian labeling; product not available in U.S.): Ventolin® I.V.: Store at 15°C to 30°C (59°F to 86°F). Protect from light. After dilution, discard unused portion after 24 hours.

Inhalation solution: Solution for nebulization (0.5%): Store at 2°C to 25°C (36°F to 77°F). To prepare a 2.5 mg dose, dilute 0.5 mL of solution to a total of 3 mL with normal saline; also compatible with cromolyn or ipratropium nebulizer solutions.

AccuNeb®: Store at 2°C to 25°C (36°F to 77°F). Do not use if solution changes color or becomes cloudy. Use within 1 week of opening foil pouch.

Syrup: Store at 20°C to 25°C (68°F to 77°F).

Tablet: Store at 20°C to 25°C (68°F to 77°F).

Tablet, extended release: Store at 20°C to 25°C (68°F to 77°F)

Mechanism of Action Relaxes bronchial smooth muscle by action on $beta_2$-receptors with little effect on heart rate

Pharmacodynamics/Kinetics

Onset of action: Peak effect:

Nebulization/oral inhalation: 0.5-2 hours

CFC-propelled albuterol: 10 minutes

Ventolin® HFA: 25 minutes

Oral: 2-3 hours

Duration: Nebulization/oral inhalation: 3-4 hours; Oral: 4-6 hours

Metabolism: Hepatic to an inactive sulfate

Half-life elimination: Inhalation: 3.8 hours; Oral: 3.7-5 hours

Excretion: Urine (30% as unchanged drug)

Dosage

Oral:

Children: Bronchospasm:

2-6 years: 0.1-0.2 mg/kg/dose 3 times/day; maximum dose not to exceed 12 mg/day (divided doses)

6-12 years: 2 mg/dose 3-4 times/day; maximum dose not to exceed 24 mg/day (divided doses)

Extended release: 4 mg every 12 hours; maximum dose not to exceed 24 mg/day (divided doses)

Children >12 years and Adults: Bronchospasm (treatment): 2-4 mg/dose 3-4 times/day; maximum dose not to exceed 32 mg/day (divided doses)

Extended release: 8 mg every 12 hours; maximum dose not to exceed 32 mg/day (divided doses). A 4 mg dose every 12 hours may be sufficient in some patients, such as adults of low body weight.

Elderly: Bronchospasm (treatment): 2 mg 3-4 times/day; maximum: 8 mg 4 times/day

Metered-dose inhaler (90 mcg/puff):

Children ≤4 years *(NIH Guidelines, 2007)*:

Quick relief: 2 puffs every 4-6 hours as needed

Exacerbation of asthma (acute, severe): 4-8 puffs every 20 minutes for 3 doses, then every 1-4 hours as needed

Exercise-induced bronchospasm (prevention): 1-2 puffs 5 minutes prior to exercise

Children 5-11 years *(NIH Guidelines, 2007)*:

Bronchospasm, quick relief: 2 puffs every 4-6 hours as needed

Exacerbation of asthma (acute, severe): 4-8 puffs every 20 minutes for 3 doses, then every 1-4 hours as needed

Exercise-induced bronchospasm (prevention): 2 puffs 5-30 minutes prior to exercise

Children ≥12 years and Adults:

Bronchospasm, quick relief *(NIH Guidelines, 2007)*: 2 puffs every 4-6 hours as needed

Exacerbation of asthma (acute, severe) *(NIH Guidelines, 2007)*: 4-8 puffs every 20 minutes for up to 4 hours, then every 1-4 hours as needed

Exercise-induced bronchospasm (prevention) *(NIH Guidelines, 2007)*: 2 puffs 5-30 minutes prior to exercise

Solution for nebulization:

Children 2-12 years (AccuNeb®): Bronchospasm: 0.63-1.25 mg 3-4 times daily as needed

Children ≤4 years *(NIH Guidelines, 2007)*:

Quick relief: 0.63-2.5 mg every 4-6 hours as needed

Exacerbation of asthma (acute, severe): 0.15 mg/kg (minimum: 2.5 mg) every 20 minutes for 3 doses, then 0.15-0.3 mg/kg (maximum: 10 mg) every 1-4 hours as needed **or** 0.5 mg/kg/hour by continuous nebulization

Children 5-11 years *(NIH Guidelines, 2007)*:

Quick relief: 1.25-5 mg every 4-8 hours as needed

Exacerbation of asthma (acute, severe): 0.15 mg/kg (minimum: 2.5 mg) every 20 minutes for 3 doses, then 0.15-0.3 mg/kg (maximum: 10 mg) every 1-4 hours as needed **or** 0.5 mg/kg/hour by continuous nebulization

Children ≥12 years and Adults:

Bronchospasm: 2.5 mg 3-4 times daily as needed

Quick relief *(NIH Guidelines, 2007)*: 1.25-5 mg every 4-8 hours as needed

Exacerbation of asthma (acute, severe) *(NIH Guidelines, 2007)*: 2.5-5 mg every 20 minutes for 3 doses then 2.5-10 mg every 1-4 hours as needed, **or** 10-15 mg/hour by continuous nebulization

I.V. continuous infusion: Adults (Canadian labeling; product not available in U.S.): Severe bronchospasm and status asthmaticus: Initial: 5 mcg/minute; may increase up to 10-20 mcg/minute at 15- to 30-minute intervals if needed

Dosage adjustment in renal impairment: Use with caution in patients with renal impairment. No dosage adjustment required (including patients on hemodialysis, peritoneal dialysis, or CRRT; Aronoff, 2007).

Dietary Considerations Oral forms should be taken with water 1 hour before or 2 hours after meals.

Administration

Metered-dose inhaler: Shake well before use; prime prior to first use, and whenever inhaler has not been used for >2 weeks or when it has been dropped, by releasing 3-4 test sprays into the air (away from face). HFA inhalers should be cleaned with warm water at least once per week; allow to air dry completely prior to use. A spacer device or valved holding chamber is recommended for use with metered-dose inhalers.

Solution for nebulization: Concentrated solution should be diluted prior to use. Blow-by administration is not recommended, use a mask device if patient unable to hold mouthpiece in mouth for administration.

Infusion solution (Canadian labeling; product not available in U.S.): Do not inject undiluted. Reduce concentration by at least 50% before infusing. Administer as a continuous infusion via infusion pump.

Oral: Do not crush or chew extended release tablets.

Monitoring Parameters FEV_1, peak flow, and/or other pulmonary function tests; blood pressure, heart rate; CNS stimulation; serum glucose, serum potassium; asthma symptoms; arterial or capillary blood gases (if patients condition warrants)

Test Interactions Increased renin (S), increased aldosterone (S)

Additional Information The 2007 National Heart, Lung, and Blood Institute Guidelines for the Diagnosis and Management of Asthma do not recommend the use of oral systemic albuterol as a quick-relief medication and do not recommend regularly scheduled daily, chronic use of inhaled beta-agonists for long-term control of asthma.

Dosage Forms Excipient information presented when available (limited, particularly for generics); consult specific product labeling.

Aerosol, for oral inhalation:

ProAir® HFA: 90 mcg/inhalation (8.5 g) [chlorofluorocarbon free; 200 metered actuations]

Proventil® HFA: 90 mcg/inhalation (6.7 g) [chlorofluorocarbon free; 200 metered actuations]

Ventolin® HFA: 90 mcg/inhalation (18 g) [chlorofluorocarbon free; 200 metered actuations]

Ventolin® HFA: 90 mcg/inhalation (8 g) [chlorofluorocarbon free; 60 metered actuations]

Solution, for nebulization: 0.083% [2.5 mg/3 mL] (25s, 30s, 60s); 0.5% [100 mg/20 mL] (1s)

Solution, for nebulization [preservative free]: 0.021% [0.63 mg/3 mL] (25s); 0.042% [1.25 mg/3 mL] (25s, 30s); 0.083% [2.5 mg/3 mL] (3 mL, 25s, 30s, 60s); 0.5% [2.5 mg/0.5 mL] (30s)

AccuNeb®: 0.021% [0.63 mg/3 mL] (25s); 0.042% [1.25 mg/3 mL] (25s)

Syrup, oral: 2 mg/5 mL (473 mL)

Tablet, oral: 2 mg, 4 mg

Tablet, extended release, oral: 4 mg, 8 mg

VoSpire ER®: 4 mg, 8 mg

Dosage Forms: Canada Excipient information presented when available (limited, particularly for generics); consult specific product labeling.

Injection, solution, as sulphate:

Ventolin® I.V.: 1 mg/1mL (5 mL)

◆ **Albuterol and Ipratropium** *see* Ipratropium and Albuterol *on page 924*

◆ **Albuterol Sulfate** *see* Albuterol *on page 52*

◆ **Alcaine®** *see* Proparacaine *on page 1421*

◆ **Alcalak [OTC]** *see* Calcium Carbonate *on page 266*

Alclometasone (al kloe MET a sone)

Brand Names: U.S. Aclovate®

Index Terms Alclometasone Dipropionate

Pharmacologic Category Corticosteroid, Topical

Additional Appendix Information

Corticosteroids *on page 1888*

Use Treatment of inflammation of corticosteroid-responsive dermatosis (low to medium potency topical corticosteroid)

Pregnancy Risk Factor C

Dosage Note: Therapy should be discontinued when control is achieved; if no improvement is seen within 2 weeks, reassessment of diagnosis may be necessary.

Topical:

Children ≥1 year: Apply thin film to affected area 2-3 times/day; do not use for >3 weeks

Adults: Apply a thin film to the affected area 2-3 times/day

Additional Information Complete prescribing information for this medication should be consulted for additional detail.

Dosage Forms Excipient information presented when available (limited, particularly for generics); consult specific product labeling.

Cream, topical, as dipropionate: 0.05% (15 g, 45 g, 60 g)

Aclovate®: 0.05% (15 g, 60 g)

Ointment, topical, as dipropionate: 0.05% (15 g, 45 g, 60 g)

Aclovate®: 0.05% (15 g, 60 g)

◆ **Alclometasone Dipropionate** *see* Alclometasone *on page 54*

◆ **Alcortin® A** *see* Iodoquinol and Hydrocortisone *on page 921*

◆ **Aldactone®** *see* Spironolactone *on page 1590*

◆ **Aldara®** *see* Imiquimod *on page 879*

Aldesleukin (al des LOO kin)

Brand Names: U.S. Proleukin®

Brand Names: Canada Proleukin®

Index Terms IL-2; Interleukin 2; Interleukin-2; Lymphocyte Mitogenic Factor; Recombinant Human Interleukin-2; T-Cell Growth Factor; TCGF; Thymocyte Stimulating Factor

Pharmacologic Category Antineoplastic Agent, Miscellaneous; Biological Response Modulator

Use Treatment of metastatic renal cell cancer, metastatic melanoma

Unlabeled Use Treatment of acute myeloid leukemia (AML)

Pregnancy Risk Factor C

Pregnancy Considerations Maternal toxicity and embryocidal effects were noted in animal studies. There are no adequate and well-controlled studies in pregnant women; use during pregnancy only if benefits to the mother outweigh potential risk to the fetus. Contraception is recommended for fertile males or females using this medication.

Lactation Excretion in breast milk unknown/not recommended

Contraindications Hypersensitivity to aldesleukin or any component of the formulation; patients with abnormal thallium stress or pulmonary function tests; patients who have had an organ allograft. **Retreatment is contraindicated** in patients who have experienced sustained ventricular tachycardia (≥5 beats), uncontrolled or unresponsive cardiac arrhythmias, chest pain with ECG changes consistent with angina or MI, cardiac tamponade, intubation >72 hours, renal failure requiring dialysis for >72 hours, coma or toxic psychosis lasting >48 hours, repetitive or refractory seizures, bowel ischemia/perforation, or GI bleeding requiring surgery.

Warnings/Precautions Hazardous agent - use appropriate precautions for handling and disposal.

[U.S. Boxed Warning]: High-dose aldesleukin therapy has been associated with capillary leak syndrome (CLS), characterized by vascular tone loss and extravasation of plasma proteins and fluid into extravascular space. CLS results in significant hypotension and reduced organ perfusion which may be severe and can result in death; CLS onset is immediately after treatment initiation. Cardiac arrhythmia, angina, MI, respiratory insufficiency (requiring intubation), gastrointestinal bleeding or infarction, renal insufficiency, edema and mental status changes are also associated with CLS. Monitor fluid status and organ perfusion status carefully; consider fluids and/or pressor agents to maintain organ perfusion. **[U.S. Boxed Warning]: Therapy should be restricted to patients with normal cardiac and pulmonary functions as defined by thallium stress and formal pulmonary function testing.** Extreme caution should be used in patients with a history of prior cardiac or pulmonary disease and in patients who are fluid-restricted or where edema may be poorly tolerated. Withhold treatment for signs of organ hypoperfusion, including altered mental status, reduced urine output, systolic BP <90 mm Hg or cardiac arrhythmia. Once blood pressure is normalized, may consider diuretics for excessive weight gain/edema. Recovery from CLS generally begins soon after treatment cessation. Perform a thorough clinical evaluation prior to treatment initiation; exclude patients with significant cardiac, pulmonary, renal, hepatic, or central nervous system impairment from treatment. Patients with a more favorable performance status prior to treatment initiation are more likely to respond to aldesleukin treatment, with a higher response rate and generally lower toxicity.

[U.S. Boxed Warning]: Should be administered under the supervision of an experienced cancer chemotherapy physician in a facility with cardiopulmonary or intensive specialists and intensive care facilities available. Adverse effects are frequent and sometimes fatal. May exacerbate pre-existing or initial presentation of autoimmune diseases and inflammatory disorders; exacerbation and/or new onset have been reported with aldesleukin and interferon alfa combination therapy. Patients should be evaluated and treated for CNS metastases and have a negative scan prior to treatment; new neurologic symptoms and lesions have been reported in patients without pre-existing evidence of CNS metastases (symptoms generally improve upon discontinuation, however, cases with permanent damage have been reported). Mental status changes (irritability, confusion, depression) can occur and may indicate bacteremia, sepsis, hypoperfusion, CNS malignancy, or CNS toxicity. May cause seizure; use with caution in patients with seizure disorder.

[U.S. Boxed Warning]: Impaired neutrophil function is associated with treatment; patients are at risk for disseminated infection (including sepsis and bacterial endocarditis), and central line-related gram-positive infections. Treat pre-existing bacterial infection appropriately prior to treatment initiation. Monitor for signs of infection or sepsis during treatment. Antibiotic prophylaxis which has been associated with a reduced incidence of staphylococcal infections in aldesleukin studies includes the use of oxacillin, nafcillin, ciprofloxacin, or vancomycin.

[U.S. Boxed Warning]: Withhold treatment for patients developing moderate-to-severe lethargy or somnolence; continued treatment may result in coma. Standard prophylactic supportive care during high-dose aldesleukin treatment includes acetaminophen to relieve constitutional symptoms and an H_2 antagonist to reduce the risk of GI ulceration and/or bleeding. May impair renal or hepatic function; patients must have a serum creatinine ≤1.5 mg/dL prior to treatment. Concomitant nephrotoxic or hepatotoxic agents may increase the risk of renal or hepatic toxicity. Enhancement of cellular immune function may increase the risk of allograft rejection in transplant patients. An acute array of symptoms resembling aldesleukin adverse reactions (fever, chills, nausea, rash, pruritus, diarrhea, hypotension, edema, and oliguria) were observed within 1-4 hours after iodinated contrast media administration, usually when given within 4 weeks after aldesleukin treatment, although has been reported several months after aldesleukin treatment. The incidence of dyspnea and severe urogenital toxicities is potentially increased in elderly patients.

Adverse Reactions

>10%:

Cardiovascular: Hypotension (71%; grade 4: 3%), peripheral edema (28%), tachycardia (23%), edema (15%), vasodilation (13%), supraventricular tachycardia (12%; grade 4: 1%), cardiovascular disorder (11%; includes blood pressure changes, HF and ECG changes)

Central nervous system: Chills (52%), confusion (34%; grade 4: 1%), fever (29%; grade 4: 1%), malaise (27%), somnolence (22%), anxiety (12%), pain (12%), dizziness (11%)

Dermatologic: Rash (42%), pruritus (24%), exfoliative dermatitis (18%)

Endocrine & metabolic: Acidosis (12%; grade 4: 1%), hypomagnesemia (12%), hypocalcemia (11%)

Gastrointestinal: Diarrhea (67%; grade 4: 2%), vomiting (19% to 50%; grade 4: 1%), nausea (19% to 35%), stomatitis (22%), anorexia (20%), weight gain (16%), abdominal pain (11%)

Hematologic: Thrombocytopenia (37%; grade 4: 1%), anemia (29%), leukopenia (16%)

Hepatic: Hyperbilirubinemia (40%; grade 4: 2%), AST increased (23%; grade 4: 1%)

Neuromuscular & skeletal: Weakness (23%)

Renal: Oliguria (63%; grade 4: 6%), creatinine increased (33%; grade 4: 1%)

Respiratory: Dyspnea (43%; grade 4: 1%), lung disorder (24%; includes pulmonary congestion, rales, and rhonchi), cough (11%), respiratory disorder (11%; includes acute respiratory distress syndrome, infiltrates and pulmonary changes)

Miscellaneous: Infection (13%; grade 4: 1%)

1% to 10%:

Cardiovascular: Arrhythmia (10%), cardiac arrest (grade 4: 1%), MI (grade 4: 1%), ventricular tachycardia (grade 4: 1%)

Central nervous system: Coma (grade 4: 2%), stupor (grade 4: 1%), psychosis (grade 4: 1%)

Gastrointestinal: Abdomen enlarged (10%)

Hematologic: Coagulation disorder (grade 4: 1%)

Hepatic: Alkaline phosphatase increased (10%)

Renal: Anuria (grade 4: 5%), acute renal failure (grade 4: 1%)

Respiratory: Rhinitis (10%), apnea (grade 4: 1%)

Miscellaneous: Sepsis (grade 4: 1%)

<1% (Limited to important or life-threatening): Acute tubular necrosis, allergic interstitial nephritis, anaphylaxis, atrial arrhythmia, AV block, blindness (transient or permanent), bowel infarction/necrosis/perforation, bradycardia, bullous pemphigoid, BUN increased, capillary leak syndrome, cardiomyopathy, cellulitis, cerebral edema, cerebral lesions, cerebral vasculitis, cholecystitis, colitis, crescentic IgA glomerulonephritis, Crohn's disease exacerbation, delirium, depression (severe; leading to suicide), diabetes mellitus, duodenal ulcer, encephalopathy, endocarditis, extrapyramidal syndrome, gastritis, hematemesis, hemoptysis, hemorrhage (including cerebral, gastrointestinal, retroperitoneal), hepatic failure, hepatitis, hepatosplenomegaly, hypertension, hyperuricemia, hyper-/hypoventilation, hypothermia, hyperthyroidism, hypoxia, inflammatory arthritis, injection site necrosis, insomnia, intestinal obstruction, intestinal perforation, leukocytosis, malignant hyperthermia, meningitis, myocardial ischemia, myocarditis, myopathy, myositis, neuralgia, neuritis, neuropathy, neutropenia, NPN increased, oculobulbar myasthenia gravis, optic neuritis, organ perfusion decreased, pancreatitis, pericardial effusion, pericarditis, peripheral gangrene, phlebitis, pneumonia, pneumothorax, pulmonary edema, pulmonary embolus, respiratory acidosis, respiratory arrest, respiratory failure, rhabdomyolysis, scleroderma, seizure, shock, Stevens-Johnson syndrome, stroke, syncope, thrombosis, thyroiditis, tracheoesophageal fistula, transient ischemic attack, urticaria, ventricular extrasystoles

Drug Interactions

Metabolism/Transport Effects None known.

Avoid Concomitant Use

Avoid concomitant use of Aldesleukin with any of the following: CloZAPine; Corticosteroids

Increased Effect/Toxicity

Aldesleukin may increase the levels/effects of: CloZAPine; Hypotensive Agents

The levels/effects of Aldesleukin may be increased by: Contrast Media (Non-ionic); Interferons (Alfa)

Decreased Effect

The levels/effects of Aldesleukin may be decreased by: Corticosteroids

Ethanol/Nutrition/Herb Interactions Ethanol: May increase CNS adverse effects.

Stability Store intact vials under refrigeration at 2°C to 8°C (36°F to 46°F). Protect from light. Reconstitute vials with 1.2 mL SWFI (preservative free) to a concentration of 18 million units (1.1 mg)/1 mL (sterile water should be injected towards the side of the vial). Gently swirl; do not shake. Further dilute with 50 mL of D_5W. Smaller volumes of D_5W should be used for doses ≤1.5 mg; avoid concentrations <30 mcg/mL and >70 mcg/mL (an increased variability in drug delivery has been seen). Plastic (polyvinyl chloride) bags result in more consistent drug delivery and are recommended. According to the manufacturer, reconstituted vials and solutions diluted for infusion are stable for 48 hours at room temperature or refrigerated; however, refrigeration is preferred because they do not contain preservatives. Do not freeze. Solution diluted with D_5W to a concentration of 220 mcg/mL and repackaged into tuberculin syringes was reported to be stable for 14 days refrigerated. Filtration may result in loss of bioactivity. Addition of 0.1% albumin has been used to increase stability and decrease the extent of sorption if low final concentrations cannot be avoided.

Mechanism of Action Aldesleukin is a human recombinant interleukin-2 product which promotes proliferation, differentiation, and recruitment of T and B cells, natural killer (NK) cells, and thymocytes; causes cytolytic activity in a subset of lymphocytes and subsequent interactions between the immune system and malignant cells; can stimulate lymphokine-activated killer (LAK) cells and tumor-infiltrating lymphocytes (TIL) cells.

Pharmacodynamics/Kinetics

Distribution: V_d: 4-7 L; primarily in plasma and then in the lymphocytes

Metabolism: Renal (metabolized to amino acids)

Half-life elimination: I.V.: Initial: 6-13 minutes; Terminal: 80-120 minutes

Excretion: Urine (primarily as metabolites)

Dosage Consider premedication with an antipyretic to reduce fever, an H_2 antagonist for prophylaxis of gastrointestinal irritation/bleeding, antiemetics, and antidiarrheals; continue for 12 hours after the last aldesleukin dose. Antibiotic prophylaxis is recommended to reduce the incidence of infection.

Children: I.V.: AML (unlabeled use): 9 million int. units (9×10^6 int. units)/m^2/day continuous infusion over 24 hours daily for 4 days; repeat 4 days later with 1.6 million int. units (1.6×10^6 int. units)/m^2/day continuous infusion over 24 hours daily for 10 days (Lange, 2008)

Adults: I.V.:

Renal cell carcinoma: 600,000 int. units/kg every 8 hours for a maximum of 14 doses; repeat after 9 days for a total of 28 doses per course; retreat if tumor shrinkage observed (and if no contraindications) at least 7 weeks after hospital discharge date

or

Unlabeled dosing: 720,000 int. units/kg every 8 hours for up to 12 doses; repeat with a second cycle 10-15 days later (Klapper, 2008)

Melanoma:

Single-agent use: 600,000 int. units/kg every 8 hours for a maximum of 14 doses; repeat after 9 days for a total of 28 doses per course; retreat if tumor shrinkage observed (and if no contraindications) at least 7 weeks after hospital discharge date

or

Unlabeled dosing: 720,000 int. units/kg every 8 hours for 12-15 doses; repeat with a second cycle ~14 days after the first dose of the initial cycle (Smith, 2008)

Combination biochemotherapy (unlabeled use): 9 million int. units/m^2/day continuous infusion over 24 hours for 4 days every 3 weeks for up to 4 cycles (Atkins, 2008) **or** 9 million int. units/m^2/day continuous infusion over 24 hours days 5 to 8, 17 to 20, and 26 to 29 every 42 days for up to 5 cycles (Eton, 2002) **or** 9 million int. units/m^2/day continuous infusion over 24 hours for 4 days every 3 weeks for 6 cycles (Legha, 1998)

Dosage adjustment in renal impairment: No specific recommendations by manufacturer. Use with caution.

Dosage adjustment for toxicity: Withhold or interrupt a dose for toxicity; do not reduce the dose.

Cardiovascular toxicity:

Atrial fibrillation, supraventricular tachycardia, or bradycardia that is persistent, recurrent, or requires treatment: Withhold dose; may resume when asymptomatic with full recovery to normal sinus rhythm.

Systolic BP <90 mm Hg (with increasing pressor requirements): Withhold dose; may resume treatment when systolic BP ≥90 mm Hg and stable or pressor requirements improve.

Any ECG change consistent with MI, ischemia or myocarditis (with or without chest pain), or suspected cardiac ischemia: Withhold dose; may resume when asymptomatic, MI/myocarditis have been ruled out, suspicion of angina is low, or there is no evidence of ventricular hypokinesia.

CNS toxicity: Mental status change, including moderate confusion or agitation: Withhold dose; may resume when resolved completely.

Dermatologic toxicity: Bullous dermatitis or marked worsening of pre-existing skin condition: Withhold dose; may treat with antihistamines or topical products (do not use topical steroids); may resume with resolution of all signs of bullous dermatitis.

Gastrointestinal: Stool guaiac repeatedly >3-4+: Withhold dose; may resume with negative stool guaiac.

Hepatotoxicity: Signs of hepatic failure, encephalopathy, increasing ascites, liver pain, hypoglycemia: Withhold dose and discontinue treatment for balance of cycle; may initiate a new course if indicated only after at least 7 weeks past resolution of all signs of hepatic failure (including hospital discharge).

Infection: Sepsis syndrome, clinically unstable: Withhold dose; may resume when sepsis syndrome has resolved, patient is clinically stable, and infection is under treatment.

Renal toxicity:

Serum creatinine >4.5 mg/dL (or ≥4 mg/dL with severe volume overload, acidosis or hyperkalemia): Withhold dose; may resume when <4 mg/dL and fluid/electrolyte status is stable.

Persistent oliguria or urine output <10 mL/hour for 16-24 hours with rising serum creatinine: Withhold dose; may resume when urine output >10 mL/hour with serum creatinine decrease of >1.5 mg/dL or normalization.

Respiratory toxicity: Oxygen saturation <90%: Withhold dose; may resume when >90%.

Retreatment with aldesleukin is contraindicated with the following toxicities: Sustained ventricular tachycardia (≥5 beats), uncontrolled or unresponsive cardiac arrhythmias, chest pain with ECG changes consistent with angina or MI, cardiac tamponade, intubation >72 hours, renal failure requiring dialysis for >72 hours, coma or toxic psychosis lasting >48 hours, repetitive or refractory seizures, bowel ischemia/perforation, or GI bleeding requiring surgery

Administration Administer as I.V. infusion over 15 minutes (do not administer with an inline filter). Allow solution to reach room temperature prior to administration. Flush before and after with D_5W, particularly if maintenance I.V. line contains sodium chloride. May also be administered by SubQ injection (unlabeled route)

Monitoring Parameters

Baseline and periodic: CBC with differential and platelets, blood chemistries including electrolytes, renal and hepatic function tests, and chest x-ray; pulmonary function tests and arterial blood gases (baseline), thallium stress test (prior to treatment)

Monitoring during therapy should include daily (hourly if hypotensive) vital signs (temperature, pulse, blood pressure, and respiration rate), weight and fluid intake and output; in a patient with a decreased blood pressure, especially systolic BP <90 mm Hg, cardiac monitoring for rhythm should be conducted. If an abnormal complex or rhythm is seen, an ECG should be performed; vital signs in these hypotension patients should be taken hourly and central venous pressure (CVP) checked; monitor for change in mental status, and for signs of infection.

Additional Information 18 x 10^6 int. units = 1.1 mg protein

Dosage Forms Excipient information presented when available (limited, particularly for generics); consult specific product labeling.

Injection, powder for reconstitution:

Proleukin®: 22 x 10^6 int. units [18 million int. units/mL = 1.1 mg/mL when reconstituted]

- **Aldex® CT** *see* Diphenhydramine and Phenylephrine *on page 518*
- **Aldomet** *see* Methyldopa *on page 1104*
- **Aldroxicon I [OTC]** *see* Aluminum Hydroxide, Magnesium Hydroxide, and Simethicone *on page 80*
- **Aldroxicon II [OTC]** *see* Aluminum Hydroxide, Magnesium Hydroxide, and Simethicone *on page 80*
- **Aldurazyme®** *see* Laronidase *on page 977*

Alefacept (a LE fa sept)

Brand Names: U.S. Amevive®
Brand Names: Canada Amevive®
Index Terms B 9273; BG 9273; Human LFA-3/IgG(1) Fusion Protein; LFA-3/IgG(1) Fusion Protein, Human
Pharmacologic Category Monoclonal Antibody
Use Treatment of moderate-to-severe chronic plaque psoriasis in adults who are candidates for systemic therapy or phototherapy
Pregnancy Risk Factor B
Pregnancy Considerations Teratogenic effects have not been observed in animal reproduction studies. Patients who become pregnant during therapy or within 8 weeks of treatment are advised to enroll in pregnancy registry (866-834-7223).
Lactation Excretion in breast milk unknown/not recommended
Prescribing and Access Restrictions Alefacept will be distributed directly to physician offices or to a specialty pharmacy; injections are intended to be administered in the physician's office. Contact Amevive® Start Assistance Program (ASAP) at 1-800-477-6472 to initiate treatment.
Contraindications Hypersensitivity to alefacept or any component of the formulation; patients with HIV infection
Warnings/Precautions Hazardous agent - use appropriate precautions for handling and disposal. Has been associated with hypersensitivity reactions; discontinue if anaphylaxis or severe reaction occurs. Alefacept induces a decline in circulating T-lymphocytes ($CD4^+$ and $CD8^+$); $CD4^+$ lymphocyte counts should be monitored every 2 weeks throughout therapy. Do not initiate in pre-existing depression of $CD4^+$ lymphocytes; withhold treatment in any patient who develops a depressed $CD4^+$ lymphocyte count (<250 cells/µL) during treatment and monitor $CD4^+$ lymphocyte counts weekly; permanently discontinue if $CD4^+$ lymphocyte counts remain <250 cells/µL for 1 month.

Alefacept may increase the risk of malignancies; avoid use in patients with a history of systemic malignancy; use caution in patients at high risk for malignancy. Discontinue if malignancy develops during therapy. Alefacept may increase the risk of infection and may reactivate latent infection; monitor for new infections. Avoid use in patients with clinically important infections or a history of recurrent infections; not recommended for use in patients receiving other immunosuppressant drugs or phototherapy. Discontinue if a serious infection occurs. In postmarketing reports, significant transaminase elevations, as well as rare cases of hepatitis, fatty liver, decompensation of cirrhosis, and acute hepatic failure (a causal relationship not established). Discontinue if signs and symptoms of hepatic injury occur. Safety and efficacy of live or attenuated vaccines have not been evaluated.

Adverse Reactions

≥10%:

Hematologic: Lymphopenia (up to 10% of patients required temporary discontinuation, up to 17% during a second course of therapy)

Local: Injection site reactions (up to 16% of patients; includes pain, inflammation, bleeding, edema, or other reaction)

1% to 10%:

Central nervous system: Chills (6%; primarily during intravenous administration), dizziness (≥2%)

Dermatologic: Pruritus (≥2%)

Gastrointestinal: Nausea (≥2%)

Hepatic: Transaminases increased (2%; AST and ALT ≥3 times ULN)

Neuromuscular & skeletal: Myalgia (≥2%)

Respiratory: Pharyngitis (≥2%), cough (≥2%)

Miscellaneous: Antibodies to alefacept (3%; significance unknown), infection (1% requiring hospitalization), malignancies (1%)

<1% (Limited to important or life-threatening): Anaphylaxis, allergic reaction, angioedema, headache, hepatitis, hepatic failure, MI, urticaria

Drug Interactions

Metabolism/Transport Effects None known.

Avoid Concomitant Use

Avoid concomitant use of Alefacept with any of the following: BCG; Belimumab; Natalizumab; Pimecrolimus; Tacrolimus (Topical); Vaccines (Live)

Increased Effect/Toxicity

Alefacept may increase the levels/effects of: Belimumab; Leflunomide; Natalizumab; Vaccines (Live)

The levels/effects of Alefacept may be increased by: Denosumab; Pimecrolimus; Roflumilast; Tacrolimus (Topical); Trastuzumab

Decreased Effect

Alefacept may decrease the levels/effects of: BCG; Coccidioidin Skin Test; Sipuleucel-T; Vaccines (Inactivated); Vaccines (Live)

The levels/effects of Alefacept may be decreased by: Echinacea

Ethanol/Nutrition/Herb Interactions Ethanol: Avoid ethanol (may increase risk of liver toxicity).

Stability Store under refrigeration at 2°C to 8°C (36°F to 46°F). Protect from light. Reconstitute 15 mg vial for I.M. solution with 0.6 mL of SWFI (supplied); reconstituted solution contains 15 mg/0.5 mL of alefacept. Gently swirl to avoid excessive foaming. Do not filter reconstituted solutions. Following reconstitution, may be stored for up to 4 hours at 2°C to 8°C (36°F to 46°F). Discard any unused solution within 4 hours of reconstitution.

Mechanism of Action Binds to CD2, a receptor on the surface of lymphocytes, inhibiting their interaction with leukocyte functional antigen 3 (LFA-3). Interaction between CD2 and LFA-3 is important for the activation of T lymphocytes in psoriasis. Activated T lymphocytes secrete a number of inflammatory mediators, including interferon gamma, which are involved in psoriasis. Since CD2 is primarily expressed on T lymphocytes, treatment results in a reduction in $CD4^+$ and $CD8^+$ T lymphocytes, with lesser effects on other cell populations (NK and B lymphocytes).

Pharmacodynamics/Kinetics

Distribution: I.V.: V_d: 0.094 L/kg

Bioavailability: I.M.: 63%

Half-life elimination: I.V.: 270 hours

Excretion: Clearance: I.V.: 0.25 mL/hour/kg

Dosage

Adults:

I.M.: 15 mg once weekly; duration of treatment: 12 weeks

A second 12- week course of treatment may be initiated at least 12 weeks after completion of the initial course of treatment, provided $CD4^+$ T-lymphocyte counts are within the normal range.

Elderly: Refer to adult dosing; use with caution since elderly patients may be at an increased risk for infections and malignancies.

Dosage adjustment in renal impairment: Use has not been evaluated in patients with renal impairment; there are no dosage adjustments provided in manufacturer's labeling.

Dosage adjustment in hepatic impairment: Use has not been evaluated in patients with hepatic impairment; there are no dosage adjustments provided in manufacturer's labeling.

Dietary Considerations Some products may contain sucrose.

Administration I.M. injections should be administered at least 1 inch from previous administration sites.

Monitoring Parameters Baseline $CD4^+$ T-lymphocyte counts prior to initiation and every 2 weeks during treatment course; weekly $CD4^+$ T-lymphocyte counts if $CD4^+$ counts are <250 cells/μL during therapy; severity of psoriatic lesions; signs and symptoms of infection

Dosage Forms Excipient information presented when available (limited, particularly for generics); consult specific product labeling.

Injection, powder for reconstitution:

Amevive®: 15 mg [contains sucrose 12.5 mg; for I.M. administration]

Alemtuzumab (ay lem TU zoo mab)

Brand Names: U.S. Campath®

Brand Names: Canada MabCampath®

Index Terms Anti-CD52 Monoclonal Antibody; Campath-1H; Humanized IgG1 Anti-CD52 Monoclonal Antibody; MoAb CD52; Monoclonal Antibody Campath-1H; Monoclonal Antibody CD52

Pharmacologic Category Antineoplastic Agent, Monoclonal Antibody

Use Treatment of B-cell chronic lymphocytic leukemia (B-CLL)

Unlabeled Use Treatment of cutaneous T-cell lymphoma, peripheral T-cell lymphoma, refractory T-cell prolymphocytic leukemia, refractory or resistant autoimmune cytopenias; preconditioning regimen and prophylaxis of graft-versus-host disease (GVHD) in allogeneic stem cell transplant; immunosuppressant in solid organ transplant (induction and rejection)

Pregnancy Risk Factor C

Pregnancy Considerations Human IgG is known to cross the placental barrier; therefore, alemtuzumab may also cross the barrier and cause fetal B- and T-lymphocyte depletion. Well-controlled human trials have not been done. Use during pregnancy only if the benefit to the mother outweighs the potential risk to the fetus. Effective contraception is recommended during and for 6 months after treatment for women of childbearing potential and men of reproductive potential.

Lactation Excretion in breast milk unknown/not recommended

Contraindications There are no contraindications listed in the manufacturer's labeling

Warnings/Precautions Hazardous agent - use appropriate precautions for handling and disposal. **[U.S. Boxed Warning]: Serious infections (bacterial, viral, fungal, and protozoan) have been reported. Prophylactic medications against PCP pneumonia and herpes viral infections are recommended upon initiation of therapy** and for at least 2 months following last dose or until $CD4^+$ counts are ≥200 cells/µL (whichever is later). Severe and prolonged lymphopenia may occur; $CD4^+$ counts usually return to ≥200 cells/µL within 2-6 months; however, $CD4^+$ and $CD8^+$ lymphocyte counts may not return to baseline levels for more than 1 year. Monitor for CMV infection (during and for at least 2 months after completion of therapy). Withhold treatment during serious infections; may be reinitiated upon resolution of infection. Monitor for CMV infection (during and for at least 2 months after completion of therapy); initiate appropriate antiviral treatment and withhold alemtuzumab for CMV infection or confirmed CMV viremia (withhold alemtuzumab during CMV antiviral treatment).

[U.S. Boxed Warning]: Serious and potentially fatal infusion-related reactions may occur; withhold treatment for grade 3 or 4 infusion reactions. Gradual escalation to the recommended maintenance dose is required at initiation and with therapy interruption (for ≥7 days) to minimize infusion-related reactions. Infusion reaction symptoms may include acute respiratory distress syndrome, anaphylactic shock, angioedema, bronchospasm, cardiac arrest, cardiac arrhythmias, chills, dyspnea, fever, hypotension, myocardial infarction, pulmonary infiltrates, rash, rigors, syncope, or urticaria. The incidence of infusion reaction is highest during the first week of treatment. Premedication with acetaminophen and an oral antihistamine is recommended. Medications for the treatment of reactions should be available for immediate use. Use caution and carefully monitor blood pressure in patients with ischemic heart disease and patients on antihypertensive therapy. Reinitiate with gradual dose escalation if treatment is withheld ≥7 days.

[U.S. Boxed Warning]: Serious and fatal cytopenias (including pancytopenia, bone marrow hypoplasia, autoimmune hemolytic anemia, and autoimmune idiopathic thrombocytopenia) have occurred. Single doses >30 mg or cumulative weekly doses >90 mg are associated with an increased incidence of pancytopenia. Severe prolonged myelosuppression, hemolytic anemia, pure red cell aplasia, and bone marrow aplasia have also been reported. Discontinue therapy during serious hematologic or other serious toxicity (except lymphopenia) until the event resolves. Permanently discontinue if autoimmune anemia or autoimmune thrombocytopenia occurs. Patients receiving blood products should only receive irradiated blood products due to the potential for transfusion-associated GVHD during lymphopenia.

Patients should not be immunized with live, viral vaccines during or recently after treatment. The ability to respond to any vaccine following therapy is unknown. Women of childbearing potential and men of reproductive potential should use effective contraceptive methods during treatment and for a minimum of 6 months following therapy. Safety and efficacy have not been established in pediatric patients.

Adverse Reactions

>10%:

Cardiovascular: Hypotension (15% to 32%), peripheral edema (13%), hypertension (11% to 15%), dysrhythmia/tachycardia/SVT (10% to 14%)

Central nervous system: Fever (69% to 85%), chills (53%), fatigue (22% to 34%), headache (13% to 24%), dysthesias (15%), dizziness (12%)

Dermatologic: Rash (13% to 40%), urticaria (16% to 30%), pruritus (14% to 24%)

Gastrointestinal: Nausea (47% to 54%), vomiting (33% to 41%), anorexia (20%), diarrhea (10% to 22%), stomatitis/mucositis (14%), abdominal pain (11%)

Hematologic: Lymphopenia (grades 3/4: 97%), neutropenia (77% to 85%; grade 3/4: 42% to 70% [median onset: 31 days, median duration: 28-37 days]), anemia (76% to 80%; grade 3/4: 12% to 47% [median onset: 31 days, median duration 8 days]), thrombocytopenia (71% to 72%; grade 3/4: 13% to 52% [median onset: 9 days; median duration: 14-21 days])

Local: Injection site reaction (SubQ administration: 90%)

Neuromuscular & skeletal: Rigors (86% to 89%), skeletal pain (24%), weakness (13%), myalgia (11%)

Respiratory: Dyspnea (14% to 26%), cough (25%), bronchitis/pneumonitis (21%), pneumonia (16%), pharyngitis (12%)

Miscellaneous: Infection (43% to 74%; grades 3/4: 21% to 37%; incidence is lower if prophylactic anti-infectives are utilized), CMV viremia (55%), infusion reactions (grades 3/4: 10% to 35%), diaphoresis (19%), CMV infection (6% to 16%), sepsis (15%; grades 3/4: 3% to 10%), herpes viral infections (1% to 11%)

1% to 10%:

Cardiovascular: Chest pain (10%)

Central nervous system: Insomnia (10%), malaise (9%), anxiety (8%), depression (7%), temperature change sensation (5%), somnolence (5%)

Dermatologic: Purpura (8%), erythema (4%)

Gastrointestinal: Dyspepsia (10%), constipation (9%)

Hematologic: Neutropenic fever (10%; grades 3/4: 5% to 10%), pancytopenia/marrow hypoplasia (5% to 6%; grade 3/4: 3%), positive Coombs' test without hemolysis (2%), autoimmune thrombocytopenia (2%), autoimmune hemolytic anemia (1%)

Neuromuscular & skeletal: Back pain (10%), tremor (3% to 7%)

Respiratory: Bronchospasm (9%), epistaxis (7%), rhinitis (7%)

Miscellaneous: Moniliasis (8%)

<1% (Limited to important or life-threatening): Acidosis, acute renal failure, acute respiratory distress syndrome, agranulocytosis, alkaline phosphatase increased, allergic reactions, anaphylactoid reactions, angina pectoris, angioedema, anuria, aphasia, aplastic anemia, arrhythmia, ascites, asthma, atrial fibrillation, bacterial infection, biliary pain, bone marrow aplasia, bullous eruption, capillary fragility, cardiac arrest, cardiac failure, cardiac insufficiency, cardiomyopathy, cellulitis, cerebral hemorrhage, cerebrovascular disorder, chronic inflammatory demyelinating polyradiculoneuropathy (CIDP), coagulation abnormality, colitis, coma, COPD, coronary artery disorder, cyanosis, deep vein thrombosis, dehydration, diabetes mellitus exacerbation, disseminated intravascular coagulation (DIC), duodenal ulcer, ejection fraction decreased, endophthalmitis, Epstein-Barr virus associated lymphoproliferative disorder, esophagitis, fluid overload, flu-like syndrome, gastrointestinal hemorrhage, Goodpasture's syndrome, Graves' disease, Guillain-Barré syndrome, hallucinations, hematemesis, hematoma, hematuria, hemolysis, hemolytic anemia, hemoptysis, hepatic failure, hepatocellular damage, HF, hyperbilirubinemia, hyper-/hypoglycemia, hyper-/hypokalemia, hypersensitivity, hyperthyroidism, hypoalbuminemia, hyponatremia, hypovolemia, hypoxia, idiopathic thrombocytopenic purpura (ITP), interstitial pneumonitis, intestinal obstruction, intestinal perforation, intracranial hemorrhage, *Legionella* pneumonia, *Listeria* meningitis, lymphadenopathy, marrow depression, melena, MI,

mouth edema, myositis, optic neuropathy, osteomyelitis, pancreatitis, paralysis, paralytic ileus, paroxysmal nocturnal hemoglobinuria-like monocytes, peptic ulcer, pericarditis, peritonitis, plasma cell dyscrasia, phlebitis, pleural effusion, pleurisy, *Pneumocystis jirovecii* pneumonia, pneumothorax, polymyositis, progressive multifocal leukoencephalopathy, pseudomembranous colitis, pulmonary edema, pulmonary embolism, pulmonary fibrosis, pulmonary infiltration, pure red cell aplasia, purpuric rash, renal dysfunction, respiratory alkalosis, respiratory arrest, respiratory depression, respiratory insufficiency, seizure (grand mal), serum sickness, sinus bradycardia, splenic infarction, splenomegaly, stridor, subarachnoid hemorrhage, syncope, toxic nephropathy, thrombocythemia, thrombophlebitis, throat tightness, transfusion-associated GVHD, tuberculosis, tumor lysis syndrome, ureteric obstruction, urinary retention, urinary tract infection, ventricular arrhythmia, ventricular tachycardia, viral meningitis, virus reactivation (latent)

Drug Interactions

Metabolism/Transport Effects None known.

Avoid Concomitant Use

Avoid concomitant use of Alemtuzumab with any of the following: BCG; Belimumab; CloZAPine; Natalizumab; Pimecrolimus; Tacrolimus (Topical); Vaccines (Live)

Increased Effect/Toxicity

Alemtuzumab may increase the levels/effects of: Belimumab; CloZAPine; Leflunomide; Natalizumab; Vaccines (Live)

The levels/effects of Alemtuzumab may be increased by: Abciximab; Denosumab; Pimecrolimus; Roflumilast; Tacrolimus (Topical); Trastuzumab

Decreased Effect

Alemtuzumab may decrease the levels/effects of: BCG; Coccidioidin Skin Test; Sipuleucel-T; Vaccines (Inactivated); Vaccines (Live)

The levels/effects of Alemtuzumab may be decreased by: Echinacea

Ethanol/Nutrition/Herb Interactions Herb/Nutraceutical: Echinacea may diminish the therapeutic effect of alemtuzumab.

Stability Prior to dilution, store at 2°C to 8°C (36°F to 46°F); do not freeze (if accidentally frozen, thaw in refrigerator prior to administration). Do not shake; protect from light. Following dilution, store at room temperature or refrigerate; protect from light; use within 8 hours. Dilute with 100 mL NS or D_5W. Gently invert the bag to mix the solution. Do not shake prior to use.

Mechanism of Action Binds to CD52, a nonmodulating antigen present on the surface of B and T lymphocytes, a majority of monocytes, macrophages, NK cells, and a subpopulation of granulocytes. After binding to $CD52^+$ cells, an antibody-dependent lysis of leukemic cells occurs.

Pharmacodynamics/Kinetics

Distribution: V_d: I.V.: 0.1-0.4 L/kg

Metabolism: Clearance decreases with repeated dosing (due to loss of CD52 receptors in periphery), resulting in a sevenfold increase in AUC.

Half-life elimination: I.V.: 11 hours (following first 30 mg dose; range: 2-32 hours); 6 days (following the last 30 mg dose; range: 1-14 days)

Dosage Note: Dose escalation is required; usually accomplished in 3-7 days. Single doses >30 mg or cumulative doses >90 mg/week increase the incidence of pancytopenia. Pretreatment (with acetaminophen and diphenhydramine) is recommended prior to the first dose, with dose escalations, and as clinically indicated; I.V. hydrocortisone may be used for severe infusion-related reactions. Reinitiate with gradual dose escalation if treatment is withheld ≥7 days.

I.V. infusion: Adults:

B-cell CLL: Initial: 3 mg/day beginning on day 1; if tolerated (infusion reaction ≤grade 2), increase to 10 mg/day; if tolerated (infusion reaction ≤grade 2), increase to maintenance of 30 mg/dose 3 times/week on alternate days for a total duration of therapy of up to 12 weeks

Cutaneous T-cell lymphoma (unlabeled use): 3 mg on day 1; if tolerated increase the next dose to 10 mg; if tolerated increase the next dose to 30 mg; Maintenance dose: 30 mg/dose 3 times/week for up to 12 weeks (Lundin, 2003)

Peripheral T-cell lymphoma (unlabeled use): 3 mg on day 1; 10 mg on day 3, followed by 30 mg/dose 3 times/week for a duration of therapy of up to 12 weeks (Enblad, 2004)

T-cell prolymphocytic leukemia (unlabeled use): Initial test dose 3 mg or 10 mg, followed by dose escalation to 30 mg/dose 3 times/week as tolerated (Dearden, 2001)

or

Week 1: 3 mg on day 1; 10 mg on day 2; 30 mg on day 3, followed in subsequent weeks by 30 mg/dose on alternate days 3 times/week for a total of 4-12 weeks (Ferrajoli, 2003)

or

Initial dose: 3 mg day 1, if tolerated increase to 10 mg day 2, if tolerated increase to 30 mg on day 3 (days 1, 2, and 3 are consecutive days), followed by 30 mg/dose every Monday, Wednesday, Friday for a total of 4-12 weeks (Keating, 2002)

SubQ (unlabeled route): Adults: B-cell CLL: Initial: 3 mg on day 1; if tolerated 10 mg on day 3; if tolerated increase to 30 mg on day 5; maintenance: 30 mg/dose 3 times/week for a maximum of 18 weeks (Lundin, 2002) **or** 3 mg on day 1; if tolerated 10 mg on day 2; if tolerated 30 mg on day 3, followed by 30 mg/dose 3 times/week for 4-12 weeks (Stilgenbauer, 2009)

Dosage adjustment for nonhematologic toxicity:

Grade 3 or 4 infusion reaction: Withhold infusion

Serious infection or other serious adverse reaction: Withhold alemtuzumab until resolution

Autoimmune anemia or autoimmune thrombocytopenia: Discontinue alemtuzumab

Dosage adjustment for hematologic toxicity (severe neutropenia or thrombocytopenia, not autoimmune):

First occurrence: ANC <250/µL and/or platelet count ≤25,000/µL: Hold therapy; resume at 30 mg/dose when ANC ≥500/µL and platelet count ≥50,000/µL

Second occurrence: ANC <250/µL and/or platelet count ≤25,000/µL: Hold therapy; resume at 10 mg/dose when ANC ≥500/µL and platelet count ≥50,000/µL

Third occurrence: ANC <250/µL and/or platelet count ≤25,000/µL: Discontinue alemtuzumab

Patients with a baseline ANC ≤250/µL and/or a baseline platelet count ≤25,000/µL at initiation of therapy: If ANC and/or platelet counts decrease to ≤50% of the baseline value, hold therapy

First occurrence: When ANC and/or platelet count return to baseline, resume therapy at 30 mg/dose

Second occurrence: When ANC and/or platelet count return to baseline, resume therapy at 10 mg/dose

Third occurrence: Discontinue alemtuzumab

Administration Administer by I.V. infusion over 2 hours. Consider premedicating with diphenhydramine 50 mg and acetaminophen 500-1000 mg 30 minutes before initiation of infusion. Hydrocortisone 200 mg has been effective in decreasing severe infusion-related events. Start anti-infective prophylaxis. Other drugs should not be added to or simultaneously infused through the same I.V. line. Do not give I.V. push.

SubQ (unlabeled route): SubQ administration has been studied (Lundin, 2002; Stilgenbauer, 2009); an increased rate of injection site reactions has been observed, with only rare incidences of chills or infusion-like reactions typically observed with I.V. infusion. A longer dose escalation time (1-2 weeks) may be needed due to injection site reactions (Lundin, 2002). Premedication and anti-infective prophylaxis regimens should be given as are recommended with I.V. administration.

Monitoring Parameters Vital signs; carefully monitor BP especially in patient with ischemic heart disease or on antihypertensive medications; CBC with differential and platelets (weekly, more frequent if worsening); signs and symptoms of infection; $CD4^+$ lymphocyte counts (after treatment until recovery); CMV antigen (every 1-2 weeks). Monitor closely for infusion reactions (including hypotension, rigors, fever, shortness of breath, bronchospasm, chills, and/or rash).

Test Interactions May interfere with diagnostic serum tests that utilize antibodies.

Dosage Forms Excipient information presented when available (limited, particularly for generics); consult specific product labeling.

Injection, solution [preservative free]:

Campath®: 30 mg/mL (1 mL) [contains edetate disodium, polysorbate 80]

Alendronate (a LEN droe nate)

Brand Names: U.S. Fosamax®

Brand Names: Canada Alendronate-FC; Apo-Alendronate®; CO Alendronate; Dom-Alendronate; Fosamax®; Mylan-Alendronate; Novo-Alendronate; PHL-Alendronate; PMS-Alendronate; PMS-Alendronate-FC; ratio-Alendronate; Riva-Alendronate; Sandoz-Alendronate; Teva-Alendronate

Index Terms Alendronate Sodium; Alendronic Acid Monosodium Salt Trihydrate; MK-217

Pharmacologic Category Bisphosphonate Derivative

Use Treatment and prevention of osteoporosis in postmenopausal females; treatment of osteoporosis in males; Paget's disease of the bone in patients who are symptomatic, at risk for future complications, or with alkaline phosphatase ≥2 times the upper limit of normal; treatment of glucocorticoid-induced osteoporosis in males and females with low bone mineral density who are receiving a daily dosage ≥7.5 mg of prednisone (or equivalent)

Pregnancy Risk Factor C

Pregnancy Considerations Safety and efficacy have not been established in pregnant women. Animal studies have shown delays in delivery and fetal/neonatal death (secondary to hypocalcemia). Bisphosphonates are incorporated into the bone matrix and gradually released over time. Theoretically, there may be a risk of fetal harm when pregnancy follows the completion of therapy. Based on limited case reports with pamidronate, serum calcium levels in the newborn may be altered if administered during pregnancy.

Lactation Excretion in breast milk unknown/use caution

Medication Guide Available Yes

Contraindications Hypersensitivity to alendronate, other bisphosphonates, or any component of the formulation; hypocalcemia; abnormalities of the esophagus which delay esophageal emptying such as stricture or achalasia; inability to stand or sit upright for at least 30 minutes; oral solution should not be used in patients at risk of aspiration

Warnings/Precautions Use caution in patients with renal impairment (not recommended for use in patients with Cl_{cr} <35 mL/minute); hypocalcemia must be corrected before therapy initiation; ensure adequate calcium and vitamin D intake. May cause irritation to upper gastrointestinal mucosa. Esophagitis, dysphagia, esophageal ulcers, esophageal erosions, and esophageal stricture (rare) have been reported; risk increases in patients unable to comply with dosing instructions. Use with caution in patients with dysphagia, esophageal disease, gastritis, duodenitis, or ulcers (may worsen underlying condition). Discontinue use if new or worsening symptoms develop.

Osteonecrosis of the jaw (ONJ) has been reported in patients receiving bisphosphonates. Risk factors include invasive dental procedures (eg, tooth extraction, dental implants, boney surgery); a diagnosis of cancer, with concomitant chemotherapy or corticosteroids; poor oral hygiene, ill-fitting dentures; and comorbid disorders (anemia, coagulopathy, infection, pre-existing dental disease). Most reported cases occurred after I.V. bisphosphonate therapy; however, cases have been reported following oral therapy. A dental exam and preventative dentistry should be performed prior to placing patients with risk factors on chronic bisphosphonate therapy. The manufacturer's labeling states that discontinuing bisphosphonates in patients requiring invasive dental procedures may reduce the risk of ONJ. However, other experts suggest that there is no evidence that discontinuing therapy reduces the risk of developing ONJ (Assael, 2009). The benefit/risk must be assessed by the treating physician and/or dentist/surgeon prior to any invasive dental procedure. Patients developing ONJ while on bisphosphonates should receive care by an oral surgeon.

Atypical femur fractures have been reported in patients receiving bisphosphonates for treatment/prevention of osteoporosis. The fractures include subtrochanteric femur (bone just below the hip joint) and diaphyseal femur (long segment of the thigh bone). Some patients experience prodromal pain weeks or months before the fracture occurs. It is unclear if bisphosphonate therapy is the cause for these fractures, although the majority have been reported in patients taking bisphosphonates. Patients receiving long-term (>3-5 years) therapy may be at an increased risk. Discontinue bisphosphonate therapy in patients who develop a femoral shaft fracture.

Severe (and occasionally debilitating) bone, joint, and/or muscle pain have been reported during bisphosphonate treatment. The onset of pain ranged from a single day to several months. Consider discontinuing therapy in patients who experience severe symptoms; symptoms usually resolve upon discontinuation. Some patients experienced recurrence when rechallenged with same drug or another bisphosphonate; avoid use in patients with a history of these symptoms in association with bisphosphonate therapy.

Adverse Reactions Note: Incidence of adverse effects (mostly GI) increases significantly in patients treated for Paget's disease at 40 mg/day.

>10%: Endocrine & metabolic: Hypocalcemia (transient, mild, 18%); hypophosphatemia (transient, mild, 10%)

1% to 10%:

Central nervous system: Headache (up to 3%)

Gastrointestinal: Abdominal pain (1% to 7%), acid reflux (1% to 4%), dyspepsia (1% to 4%), nausea (1% to 4%), flatulence (up to 4%), diarrhea (1% to 3%), gastroesophageal reflux disease (1% to 3%), constipation (up to 3%), esophageal ulcer (up to 2%), abdominal distension (up to 1%), gastritis (up to 1%), vomiting (up to 1%), dysphagia (up to 1%), gastric ulcer (1%), melena (1%)

Neuromuscular & skeletal: Musculoskeletal pain (up to 6%), muscle cramps (up to 1%)

<1% (Limited to important or life-threatening): Alopecia, anastomotic ulcer, angioedema, atrial fibrillation; bone, muscle, or joint pain (occasionally severe, considered incapacitating in rare cases); diaphyseal femur fracture, dizziness, duodenal ulcer, episcleritis, erythema,

esophageal cancer, esophageal erosions, esophageal perforation, esophageal stricture, esophageal ulcers, esophagitis, fever, flu-like syndrome, hypersensitivity reactions, hypocalcemia (symptomatic), joint swelling, low-energy femoral shaft and subtrochanteric fractures, lymphocytopenia, malaise, myalgia, oropharyngeal ulceration, osteonecrosis (jaw), peripheral edema, photosensitivity (rare), pruritus, rash, scleritis (rare), Stevens-Johnson syndrome, taste perversion, toxic epidermal necrolysis, urticaria, uveitis (rare), vertigo, weakness

Drug Interactions

Metabolism/Transport Effects None known.

Avoid Concomitant Use There are no known interactions where it is recommended to avoid concomitant use.

Increased Effect/Toxicity

Alendronate may increase the levels/effects of: Deferasirox; Phosphate Supplements

The levels/effects of Alendronate may be increased by: Aminoglycosides; Aspirin; Nonsteroidal Anti-Inflammatory Agents

Decreased Effect

The levels/effects of Alendronate may be decreased by: Antacids; Calcium Salts; Iron Salts; Magnesium Salts; Proton Pump Inhibitors

Ethanol/Nutrition/Herb Interactions

Ethanol: Avoid ethanol (may increase risk of osteoporosis and gastric irritation).

Food: All food and beverages interfere with absorption. Coadministration with caffeine may reduce alendronate efficacy. Coadministration with dairy products may decrease alendronate absorption. Beverages (especially orange juice and coffee) and food may reduce the absorption of alendronate as much as 60%.

Stability Store tablets and oral solution at room temperature of 15°C to 30°C (59°F to 86°F). Keep in well-closed container.

Mechanism of Action A bisphosphonate which inhibits bone resorption via actions on osteoclasts or on osteoclast precursors; decreases the rate of bone resorption, leading to an indirect increase in bone mineral density. In Paget's disease, characterized by disordered resorption and formation of bone, inhibition of resorption leads to an indirect decrease in bone formation; but the newly-formed bone has a more normal architecture.

Pharmacodynamics/Kinetics

Distribution: 28 L (exclusive of bone)

Protein binding: ~78%

Metabolism: None

Bioavailability: Fasting: 0.6%; reduced up to 60% with food or drink

Half-life elimination: Exceeds 10 years

Excretion: Urine; feces (as unabsorbed drug)

Dosage Oral: Adults: **Note:** Patients should receive supplemental calcium and vitamin D if dietary intake is inadequate.

Osteoporosis in postmenopausal females:

Prophylaxis: 5 mg once daily **or** 35 mg once weekly

Treatment: 10 mg once daily **or** 70 mg once weekly

Osteoporosis in males: 10 mg once daily **or** 70 mg once weekly

Osteoporosis secondary to glucocorticoids in males and females: Treatment: 5 mg once daily; a dose of 10 mg once daily should be used in postmenopausal females who are not receiving estrogen.

Paget's disease of bone in males and females: 40 mg once daily for 6 months

Retreatment: Relapses during the 12 months following therapy occurred in 9% of patients who responded to treatment. Specific retreatment data are not available. Following a 6-month post-treatment evaluation period, retreatment with alendronate may be considered in patients who have relapsed based on increases in serum alkaline phosphatase, which should be measured periodically. Retreatment may also be considered in those who failed to normalize their serum alkaline phosphatase.

Elderly: No dosage adjustment is necessary

Dosage adjustment in renal impairment:

Cl_{cr} 35-60 mL/minute: None necessary

Cl_{cr} <35 mL/minute: Alendronate is not recommended due to lack of experience

Dosage adjustment in hepatic impairment: None necessary

Dietary Considerations Ensure adequate calcium and vitamin D intake; women and men >50 years of age should consume 1200-1500 mg/day of elemental calcium and 800-1000 int. units/day of vitamin D. Wait at least 30 minutes after taking alendronate before taking any supplement. Alendronate must be taken with plain water first thing in the morning and at least 30 minutes before the first food or beverage of the day. Do not take with mineral water or with other beverages.

Administration Alendronate must be taken with plain water (tablets 6-8 oz; oral solution follow with 2 oz) first thing in the morning and ≥30 minutes before the first food, beverage, or other medication of the day. Do not take with mineral water or with other beverages. Patients should be instructed to stay upright (not to lie down) for at least 30 minutes **and** until after first food of the day (to reduce esophageal irritation).

Monitoring Parameters

Osteoporosis: Bone mineral density as measured by central dual-energy x-ray absorptiometry (DXA) of the hip or spine (prior to initiation of therapy and at least every 2 years; after 6-12 months of combined glucocorticoid and alendronate treatment); annual measurements of height and weight, assessment of chronic back pain; serum calcium and 25(OH)D; may consider monitoring biochemical markers of bone turnover

Paget's disease: Alkaline phosphatase; pain; serum calcium and 25(OH)D

Reference Range Calcium (total): Adults: 9.0-11.0 mg/dL (2.05-2.54 mmol/L), may slightly decrease with aging; phosphorus: 2.5-4.5 mg/dL (0.81-1.45 mmol/L)

Test Interactions Bisphosphonates may interfere with diagnostic imaging agents such as technetium-99m-diphosphonate in bone scans.

Dosage Forms Excipient information presented when available (limited, particularly for generics); consult specific product labeling. [DSC] = Discontinued product

Solution, oral:

Fosamax®: 70 mg/75 mL (75 mL [DSC]) [raspberry flavor]

Tablet, oral: 5 mg, 10 mg, 35 mg, 40 mg, 70 mg

Fosamax®: 5 mg [DSC], 10 mg, 35 mg [DSC], 40 mg [DSC], 70 mg

Alendronate and Cholecalciferol

(a LEN droe nate & kole e kal SI fer ole)

Brand Names: U.S. Fosamax Plus D®

Brand Names: Canada Fosavance

Index Terms Alendronate Sodium and Cholecalciferol; Cholecalciferol and Alendronate; Vitamin D_3 and Alendronate

Pharmacologic Category Bisphosphonate Derivative; Vitamin D Analog

Use Treatment of osteoporosis in postmenopausal females; increase bone mass in males with osteoporosis

Pregnancy Risk Factor C

Medication Guide Available Yes

Dosage Oral: Adults: One tablet (alendronate 70 mg/cholecalciferol 2800 int. units **or** alendronate 70 mg/cholecalciferol 5600 int. units) once weekly. Appropriate dose in most osteoporotic women or men: Alendronate 70 mg/ cholecalciferol 5600 int. units once weekly. Supplemental calcium and vitamin D may be necessary if dietary intake is inadequate.

Dosage adjustment in renal impairment:
Cl_{cr} 35-60 mL/minute: No adjustment needed
Cl_{cr} <35 mL/minute: Not recommended

Dosage adjustment in hepatic impairment: Alendronate: None necessary. Cholecalciferol: May not be adequately absorbed in patients who have malabsorption due to inadequate bile production.

Additional Information Complete prescribing information for this medication should be consulted for additional detail.

Dosage Forms Excipient information presented when available (limited, particularly for generics); consult specific product labeling.

Tablet:
Fosamax Plus D® 70/2800: Alendronate 70 mg and cholecalciferol 2800 int. units
Fosamax Plus D® 70/5600: Alendronate 70 mg and cholecalciferol 5600 int. units

- ◆ **Alendronate-FC (Can)** *see* Alendronate *on page* 61
- ◆ **Alendronate Sodium** *see* Alendronate *on page* 61
- ◆ **Alendronate Sodium and Cholecalciferol** *see* Alendronate and Cholecalciferol *on page* 62
- ◆ **Alendronic Acid Monosodium Salt Trihydrate** *see* Alendronate *on page* 61
- ◆ **Aler-Cap [OTC]** *see* DiphenhydrAMINE (Systemic) *on page* 516
- ◆ **Aler-Dryl [OTC]** *see* DiphenhydrAMINE (Systemic) *on page* 516
- ◆ **Aler-Tab [OTC]** *see* DiphenhydrAMINE (Systemic) *on page* 516
- ◆ **Alertec® (Can)** *see* Modafinil *on page* 1147
- ◆ **Alesse® (Can)** *see* Ethinyl Estradiol and Levonorgestrel *on page* 656
- ◆ **Aleve® [OTC]** *see* Naproxen *on page* 1177
- ◆ **Alfenta®** *see* Alfentanil *on page* 63

Alfentanil (al FEN ta nil)

Brand Names: U.S. Alfenta®

Brand Names: Canada Alfentanil Injection, USP; Alfenta®

Index Terms Alfentanil Hydrochloride

Pharmacologic Category Analgesic, Opioid; Anilidopiperidine Opioid

Use Analgesic adjunct for the induction and maintenance of general anesthesia; analgesic component for monitored anesthesia care (MAC)

Pregnancy Risk Factor C

Pregnancy Considerations Alfentanil is known to cross the placenta, which may result in respiratory or CNS depression in the newborn. Use during labor and delivery is not recommended.

Contraindications Hypersensitivity to alfentanil hydrochloride, to narcotics, or any component of the formulation; increased intracranial pressure, severe respiratory depression

Warnings/Precautions Use with caution in patients with drug dependence, head injury, morbid obesity, acute asthma and respiratory conditions; hypotension has occurred in neonates with respiratory distress syndrome; use caution when administering to patients with bradyarrhythmias; inject slowly over 3-5 minutes (rapid I.V. infusion may result in skeletal muscle and chest wall rigidity, impaired ventilation, or respiratory distress/arrest); use of a nondepolarizing skeletal muscle relaxant may be required. Alfentanil may produce more hypotension compared to fentanyl, therefore, administer slowly and ensure patient has adequate hydration. Shares the toxic potentials of opiate agonists, and precautions of opiate agonist therapy should be observed. Should be administered by trained individuals. Safety and efficacy have not been established in children <12 years old.

Adverse Reactions

>10%:
Cardiovascular: Bradycardia, peripheral vasodilation
Central nervous system: Drowsiness, sedation, intracranial pressure increased
Endocrine & metabolic: Antidiuretic hormone release
Gastrointestinal: Nausea, vomiting, constipation
Ocular: Miosis

1% to 10%:
Cardiovascular: Cardiac arrhythmia, orthostatic hypotension
Central nervous system: Confusion, CNS depression
Ocular: Blurred vision

<1% (Limited to important or life-threatening): Convulsions, mental depression, paradoxical CNS excitation or delirium, dizziness, dysesthesia, rash, urticaria, itching, biliary tract spasm, urinary tract spasm, respiratory depression, bronchospasm, laryngospasm, physical and psychological dependence with prolonged use; cold, clammy skin

Drug Interactions

Metabolism/Transport Effects Substrate of CYP3A4 (major); **Note:** Assignment of Major/Minor substrate status based on clinically relevant drug interaction potential

Avoid Concomitant Use

Avoid concomitant use of Alfentanil with any of the following: Conivaptan; Crizotinib; MAO Inhibitors

Increased Effect/Toxicity

Alfentanil may increase the levels/effects of: Alcohol (Ethyl); Alvimopan; Beta-Blockers; Calcium Channel Blockers (Nondihydropyridine); CNS Depressants; Desmopressin; Fospropofol; MAO Inhibitors; Propofol; Selective Serotonin Reuptake Inhibitors; Thiazide Diuretics

The levels/effects of Alfentanil may be increased by: Amphetamines; Antifungal Agents (Azole Derivatives, Systemic); Antipsychotic Agents (Phenothiazines); Cimetidine; Conivaptan; Crizotinib; CYP3A4 Inhibitors (Moderate); CYP3A4 Inhibitors (Strong); Dasatinib; Diltiazem; Droperidol; Fluconazole; HydrOXYzine; Macrolide Antibiotics; MAO Inhibitors; Succinylcholine

Decreased Effect

Alfentanil may decrease the levels/effects of: Pegvisomant

The levels/effects of Alfentanil may be decreased by: Ammonium Chloride; Mixed Agonist / Antagonist Opioids; Rifamycin Derivatives; Tocilizumab

Stability Store unopened ampuls at 20°C to 25°C (68°F to 77°F). Protect from light. For infusion, dilute in D_5W, NS, LR, or D_5NS to a concentration of 25-80 mcg/mL.

Mechanism of Action Binds with stereospecific receptors at many sites within the CNS, increases pain threshold, alters pain perception, inhibits ascending pain pathways; is an ultra short-acting narcotic

Pharmacodynamics/Kinetics

Onset of action: Rapid
Duration (dose dependent): 30-60 minutes
Distribution: V_d: Newborns, premature: 1 L/kg; Children: 0.163-0.48 L/kg; Adults: 0.46 L/kg
Half-life elimination: Newborns, premature: 5.33-8.75 hours; Children: 40-60 minutes; Adults: 83-97 minutes

Dosage Doses should be titrated to appropriate effects; wide range of doses is dependent upon desired degree of analgesia/anesthesia

Children <12 years: Dose not established

Adults: Dose should be based on ideal body weight as follows (see table):

Alfentanil

Indication	Approx Duration of Anesthesia (min)	Induction Period (Initial Dose) (mcg/kg)	Maintenance Period (Increments/ Infusion)	Total Dose (mcg/kg)	Effects
Incremental injection	≤30	8-20	3-5 mcg/kg or 0.5-1 mcg/kg/min	8-40	Spontaneously breathing or assisted ventilation when required.
	30-60	20-50	5-15 mcg/kg	Up to 75	Assisted or controlled ventilation required. Attenuation of response to laryngoscopy and intubation.
Continuous infusion	>45	50-75	0.5-3 mcg/kg/min; average infusion rate 1-1.5 mcg/kg/min	Dependent on duration of procedure	Assisted or controlled ventilation required. Some attenuation of response to intubation and incision, with intraoperative stability.
Anesthetic induction	>45	130-245	0.5-1.5 mcg/kg/min or general anesthetic	Dependent on duration of procedure	Assisted or controlled ventilation required. Administer slowly (over 3 minutes). Concentration of inhalation agents reduced by 30% to 50% for initial hour.

Administration Administer I.V. slowly over 3-5 minutes or by I.V. continuous infusion.

Monitoring Parameters Respiratory rate, blood pressure, heart rate

Reference Range 100-340 ng/mL (depending upon procedure)

Additional Information Alfentanil may produce more muscle rigidity compared to fentanyl; therefore, be sure to administer slowly.

Dosage Forms Excipient information presented when available (limited, particularly for generics); consult specific product labeling. [DSC] = Discontinued product

Injection, solution [preservative free]: 500 mcg/mL (2 mL, 5 mL)

Alfenta®: 500 mcg/mL (2 mL, 5 mL, 10 mL [DSC], 20 mL [DSC])

Controlled Substance C-II

◆ **Alfentanil Hydrochloride** *see* Alfentanil *on page 63*

◆ **Alfentanil Injection, USP (Can)** *see* Alfentanil *on page 63*

◆ **Alferon® N** *see* Interferon Alfa-n3 *on page 916*

Alfuzosin (al FYOO zoe sin)

Brand Names: U.S. Uroxatral®

Brand Names: Canada Apo-Alfuzosin®; Sandoz-Alfuzosin; Teva-Alfuzosin PR; Xatral

Index Terms Alfuzosin Hydrochloride

Pharmacologic Category $Alpha_1$ Blocker

Use Treatment of the functional symptoms of benign prostatic hyperplasia (BPH)

Unlabeled Use Facilitation of expulsion of ureteral stones

Pregnancy Risk Factor B

Pregnancy Considerations Teratogenic effects were not observed in animal studies.

Contraindications Hypersensitivity to alfuzosin or any component of the formulation; moderate or severe hepatic insufficiency (Child-Pugh class B and C); concurrent use with potent CYP3A4 inhibitors (eg, itraconazole, ketoconazole, ritonavir) or other $alpha_1$-blocking agents

Warnings/Precautions Not intended for use as an antihypertensive drug. May cause significant orthostatic hypotension and syncope, especially with first dose; anticipate a similar effect if therapy is interrupted for a few days, if dosage is rapidly increased, or used with antihypertensives (particularly vasodilators), PDE-5 inhibitors, nitrates or other medications which may result in hypotension. Discontinue if symptoms of angina occur or worsen. Alfuzosin has been shown to prolong the QT interval alone (minimal) and with other drugs with comparable effects on the QT interval (additive); use with caution in patients with known QT prolongation (congenital or acquired). Patients should be cautioned about performing hazardous tasks when starting new therapy or adjusting dosage upward. Discontinue if symptoms of angina occur or worsen. Rule out prostatic carcinoma before beginning therapy. Use caution with severe renal or mild hepatic impairment; contraindicated in moderate-to-severe hepatic impairment. Intraoperative floppy iris syndrome has been observed in cataract surgery patients who were on or were previously treated with $alpha_1$-blockers. Causality has not been established and there appears to be no benefit in discontinuing alpha-blocker therapy prior to surgery. May cause priapism. Contraindicated in patients taking strong CYP3A4 inhibitors or other $alpha_1$-blockers.

Adverse Reactions

1% to 10%:

Central nervous system: Dizziness (6%), fatigue (3%), headache (3%), pain (1% to 2%)

Gastrointestinal: Abdominal pain (1% to 2%), constipation (1% to 2%), dyspepsia (1% to 2%), nausea (1% to 2%)

Genitourinary: Impotence (1% to 2%)

Respiratory: Upper respiratory tract infection (3%), bronchitis (1% to 2%), pharyngitis (1% to 2%), sinusitis (1% to 2%)

<1% (Limited to important or life-threatening): Angina pectoris (pre-existing CAD), angioedema, atrial fibrillation, chest pain, cholestatic liver injury, diarrhea, edema, flushing, hepatocellular injury, intraoperative floppy iris syndrome (with cataract surgery), jaundice, priapism, pruritus, rash, rhinitis, tachycardia, urticaria

Drug Interactions

Metabolism/Transport Effects **Substrate** of CYP3A4 (major); **Note:** Assignment of Major/Minor substrate status based on clinically relevant drug interaction potential

Avoid Concomitant Use

Avoid concomitant use of Alfuzosin with any of the following: Alpha1-Blockers; CYP3A4 Inhibitors (Strong); Protease Inhibitors; Telaprevir

Increased Effect/Toxicity

Alfuzosin may increase the levels/effects of: Alpha1-Blockers; Antihypertensives; Calcium Channel Blockers; Nitroglycerin; QTc-Prolonging Agents

The levels/effects of Alfuzosin may be increased by: Beta-Blockers; CYP3A4 Inhibitors (Moderate); CYP3A4 Inhibitors (Strong); MAO Inhibitors; Phosphodiesterase 5 Inhibitors; Protease Inhibitors; Telaprevir

Decreased Effect

The levels/effects of Alfuzosin may be decreased by: CYP3A4 Inducers (Strong); Deferasirox; Herbs (CYP3A4 Inducers); Tocilizumab

Ethanol/Nutrition/Herb Interactions

Food: Food increases the extent of absorption.

Herb/Nutraceutical: Avoid St John's wort (may decrease alfuzosin levels).

Stability Store at room temperature of 25°C (77°F); excursions permitted to 15°C to 30°C (59°F to 86°F). Protect from light and moisture.

Mechanism of Action An antagonist of alpha$_1$-adrenoreceptors in the lower urinary tract. Smooth muscle tone is mediated by the sympathetic nervous stimulation of alpha$_1$-adrenoreceptors, which are abundant in the prostate, prostatic capsule, prostatic urethra, and bladder neck. Blockade of these adrenoreceptors can cause smooth muscles in the bladder neck and prostate to relax, resulting in an improvement in urine flow rate and a reduction in BPH symptoms.

Pharmacodynamics/Kinetics

Absorption: Decreased 50% under fasting conditions

Distribution: V_d: 3.2 L/kg

Protein binding: 82% to 90%

Metabolism: Hepatic, primarily via CYP3A4; metabolism includes oxidation, O-demethylation, and N-dealkylation; forms metabolites (inactive)

Bioavailability: 49% following a meal

Half-life elimination: 10 hours

Time to peak, plasma: 8 hours following a meal

Excretion: Feces (69%); urine (24%; 11% as unchanged drug)

Dosage Oral: Adults:

Benign prostatic hyperplasia (BPH): 10 mg once daily

Ureteral stones, expulsion (unlabeled use): 10 mg once daily, discontinue after successful expulsion (average time to expulsion 1-2 weeks) (Agrawal, 2009; Ahmed, 2010; Gurbuz, 2011). **Note:** Patients with stones >10 mm were excluded from studies.

Dosage adjustment in renal impairment: Bioavailability and maximum serum concentrations are increased by ~50% with mild (Cl_{cr} 60-80 mL/minute), moderate (Cl_{cr} 30-59 mL/minute), or severe (Cl_{cr} <30 mL/minute) renal impairment.

Note: Safety data is limited in patients with severe renal impairment (Cl_{cr} <30 mL/minute). Use with caution.

Dosage adjustment in hepatic impairment:

Mild hepatic impairment: Use has not been studied; use caution

Moderate or severe hepatic impairment (Child-Pugh class B and C): Clearance is decreased 1/3 to 1/4 and serum concentration is increased three- to fourfold; use is contraindicated

Dietary Considerations Take immediately following a meal at the same time each day.

Administration Tablet should be swallowed whole; do not crush or chew. Administer once daily (immediately following a meal); should be taken at the same time each day.

Monitoring Parameters Urine flow, blood pressure, PSA

Dosage Forms Excipient information presented when available (limited, particularly for generics); consult specific product labeling.

Tablet, extended release, oral, as hydrochloride: 10 mg

Uroxatral®: 10 mg

◆ **Alfuzosin Hydrochloride** *see* Alfuzosin *on page 64*

Alglucerase (al GLOO ser ase)

Brand Names: U.S. Ceredase®

Index Terms Glucocerebrosidase

Pharmacologic Category Enzyme

Use Replacement therapy for Gaucher's disease (type 1)

Pregnancy Risk Factor C

Dosage I.V.: Children and Adul' Initial: 30-60 units/kg every 2 weeks; dosing is individualized based on disease severity; average dose: 60 units/kg every 2 weeks. Range: 2.5 units/kg 3 times/week to 60 units/kg once weekly to every 4 weeks. Once patient response is well established, dose may be reduced every 3-6 months to determine maintenance therapy.

Additional Information Complete prescribing information for this medication should be consulted for additional detail.

Dosage Forms Excipient information presented when available (limited, particularly for generics); consult specific product labeling.

Injection, solution [preservative free]:

Ceredase®: 80 units/mL (5 mL) [contains albumin (human)]

◆ **Alglucosidase** *see* Alglucosidase Alfa *on page 65*

Alglucosidase Alfa (al gloo KOSE i dase AL fa)

Brand Names: U.S. Lumizyme®; Myozyme®

Brand Names: Canada Myozyme®

Index Terms Alglucosidase; GAA; rhGAA

Pharmacologic Category Enzyme

Use

Lumizyme™: Replacement therapy for late-onset (non-infantile) Pompe disease without evidence of cardiac hypertrophy in patients 8 years and older

Myozyme®: Replacement therapy for infantile-onset Pompe disease

Pregnancy Risk Factor B

Prescribing and Access Restrictions As a requirement of the REMS program, access to this medication is restricted. Lumizyme™ is available only through Lumizyme ACE (Alglucosidase Alfa Control and Education) program; only trained and certified prescribers and healthcare facilities enrolled in the program may prescribe, dispense, or administer Lumizyme™. Patients must be enrolled in and meet all the conditions of the program to receive therapy. For enrollment, call 1-800-745-4447.

Access to Myozyme® is restricted by the manufacturer, and allowed only to patients <8 years of age with infantile-onset or late-onset Pompe disease (who are restricted from access to Lumizyme™) or to patients of any age with a diagnosis of infantile-onset Pompe disease or evidence of cardiac hypertrophy. To obtain Myozyme®, call 1-800-745-4447; no formal distribution program is established, but availability is controlled by Genzyme.

Dosage I.V.: Replacement therapy for Pompe disease:

Infantile-onset (Myozyme®):

Children 1 month to 3.5 years (at first infusion): 20 mg/kg over ~4 hours every 2 weeks

Children >3.5 years and Adults (unlabeled use): 20 mg/kg over ~4 hours every 2 weeks

Noninfantile, late-onset (Lumizyme™):

Children <8 years: Not recommended

Children ≥8 years and Adults: 20 mg/kg over ~4 hours every 2 weeks

Additional Information Complete prescribing information for this medication should be consulted for additional detail.

Dosage Forms Excipient information presented when available (limited, particularly for generics); consult specific product labeling.

Injection, powder for reconstitution:

Lumizyme®: 50 mg [contains mannitol, polysorbate 80; derived from or manufactured using Chinese hamster ovary cells]

Myozyme®: 50 mg [contains mannitol, polysorbate 80; derived from or manufactured using Chinese hamster ovary cells]

◆ **Alimta®** *see* PEMEtrexed *on page 1317*

◆ **Alinia®** *see* Nitazoxanide *on page 1209*

Aliskiren (a lis KYE ren)

Brand Names: U.S. Tekturna®

Brand Names: Canada Rasilez®

Index Terms Aliskiren Hemifumarate; SPP100

Pharmacologic Category Renin Inhibitor

Additional Appendix Information

Angiotensin Agents *on page 1869*

Use Treatment of hypertension, alone or in combination with other antihypertensive agents

Unlabeled Use Treatment of persistent proteinuria in patients with type 2 diabetes mellitus, hypertension, and nephropathy despite administration of optimized recommended renoprotective therapy (eg, angiotensin II receptor blocker)

Pregnancy Risk Factor C (1st trimester); D (2nd and 3rd trimesters)

Pregnancy Considerations Medications which act on the renin-angiotensin system are reported to have the following fetal/neonatal effects: Hypotension, neonatal skull hypoplasia, anuria, renal failure, and death; oligohydramnios is also reported. These effects are reported to occur with exposure during the second and third trimesters. There are no adequate and well-controlled studies in pregnant women. Women who use aliskiren during pregnancy or become pregnant during therapy should be warned of the potential risks to the fetus. **[U.S. Boxed Warning]: Based on human data, drugs that act on the renin-angiotensin system can cause injury and death to the developing fetus when used in the second and third trimesters. Aliskiren should be discontinued as soon as possible once pregnancy is detected.**

Lactation Excretion in breast milk unknown/not recommended

Contraindications

U.S. labeling: There are no contraindications listed in manufacturer's labeling.

Canada labeling: Hypersensitivity to aliskiren or any component of the formulation

Warnings/Precautions [U.S. Boxed Warning]: Based on human data, drugs that act on the renin-angiotensin system can cause injury and death to the developing fetus when used in the second and third trimesters. Aliskiren should be discontinued as soon as possible once pregnancy is detected. Since the effect of aliskiren on bradykinin levels is unknown, the risk of kinin-mediated etiologies of angioedema occurring is also unknown. Use with caution in any patient with a history of angioedema (of any etiology) as angioedema, some cases necessitating hospitalization and intubation, has been observed (rarely) with aliskiren use. Discontinue immediately following any signs and symptoms of angioedema; do not readminister. Prolonged frequent monitoring may be required especially if tongue, glottis, or larynx are involved as they are associated with airway obstruction. Patients with a history of airway surgery may have a higher risk of airway obstruction. Early, aggressive, and appropriate management is critical. Hyperkalemia may occur (rarely) during monotherapy; risk may increase in patients with predisposing factors (eg, renal dysfunction, diabetes mellitus or concomitant use with ACE inhibitors, potassium-sparing diuretics, potassium supplements, and/or potassium-containing salts). Symptomatic hypotension may occur (rarely) during the initiation of therapy, particularly in patients with an activated renin-angiotensin system (ie, volume or salt-depleted patients). Use with caution in patients with severe renal impairment; not studied in patients with severe renal impairment (eGFR <30 mL/minute and/or S_{cr} ≥1.7 mg/dL [women]; S_{cr} ≥2 mg/dL [men]), history of dialysis, nephrotic syndrome, or renovascular hypertension. Use with caution or avoid in patients with deteriorating renal function or renal artery stenosis (bilateral or unilateral). Avoid concurrent use with strong inhibitors of P-glycoprotein (eg, cyclosporine, itraconazole).

Adverse Reactions

1% to 10%:

Dermatologic: Rash (1%)

Endocrine & metabolic: Hyperkalemia (monotherapy ≤1%; concurrent with ACE inhibitor in patients with diabetes 6%)

Gastrointestinal: Diarrhea (2%)

Hematologic: Creatine kinase increased (>300%: 1%)

Renal: BUN increased (≤7%), serum creatinine increased (≤7%)

Respiratory: Cough (1%)

<1% (Limited to important or life-threatening): Angioedema, gastroesophageal reflux, hypotension (severe), myositis, periorbital edema, rhabdomyolysis, seizure, uric acid increased

Drug Interactions

Metabolism/Transport Effects Substrate of CYP3A4 (minor), P-glycoprotein; **Note:** Assignment of Major/Minor substrate status based on clinically relevant drug interaction potential

Avoid Concomitant Use

Avoid concomitant use of Aliskiren with any of the following: CycloSPORINE; CycloSPORINE (Systemic); Itraconazole

Increased Effect/Toxicity

Aliskiren may increase the levels/effects of: Amifostine; Antihypertensives; Hypotensive Agents; RiTUXimab

The levels/effects of Aliskiren may be increased by: Alfuzosin; Atorvastatin; Conivaptan; CycloSPORINE; CycloSPORINE (Systemic); Diazoxide; Herbs (Hypotensive Properties); Itraconazole; Ketoconazole; Ketoconazole (Systemic); MAO Inhibitors; Pentoxifylline; P-glycoprotein/ABCB1 Inhibitors; Phosphodiesterase 5 Inhibitors; Prostacyclin Analogues; Verapamil

Decreased Effect

Aliskiren may decrease the levels/effects of: Furosemide

The levels/effects of Aliskiren may be decreased by: Grapefruit Juice; Herbs (Hypertensive Properties); Methylphenidate; P-glycoprotein/ABCB1 Inducers; Tocilizumab; Yohimbine

Ethanol/Nutrition/Herb Interactions

Food: High-fat meals decrease absorption.

Herb/Nutraceutical: Avoid herbs with *hypertensive* properties (bayberry, blue cohosh, cayenne, ephedra, ginger, ginseng [American], kola, licorice). Avoid herbs with *hypotensive* properties (black cohosh, California poppy, coleus, garlic, goldenseal, hawthorn, mistletoe, periwinkle, quinine, shepherd's purse).

Stability Store at 25°C (77°F); excursions permitted to 15°C to 30°C (59°F to 86°F). Protect from moisture.

Mechanism of Action Aliskerin is a direct renin inhibitor, resulting in blockade of the conversion of angiotensinogen to angiotensin I. Angiotensin I suppression decreases the formation of angiotensin II (Ang II), a potent blood pressure-elevating peptide (via direct vasoconstriction, aldosterone release, and sodium retention). Ang II also functions within the Renin-Angiotensin-Aldosterone System (RAAS) as a negative inhibitory feedback mediator within the renal parenchyma to suppress the further release of renin. Thus, reductions in Ang II levels suppress this feedback loop, leading to further increased plasma renin concentrations (PRC) and subsequent activity (PRA). This disinhibition effect can be potentially problematic for ACE inhibitor and ARB therapy, as increased PRA could partially overcome the pharmacologic inhibition of the RAAS. As aliskiren is a direct inhibitor of renin activity, blunting of PRA despite the increased PRC (from loss of the negative feedback) may be clinically advantageous. The effect of aliskiren on bradykinin levels is unknown.

Pharmacodynamics/Kinetics

Onset of action: Maximum antihypertensive effect: Within 2 weeks

Absorption: Poor; absorption decreased by high-fat meal. Aliskiren is a substrate of P-glycoprotein; concurrent use of P-glycoprotein inhibitors may increase absorption.

Metabolism: Extent of metabolism unknown; *in vitro* studies indicate metabolism via CYP3A4

Bioavailability: ~3%

Half-life elimination: ~24 hours (range: 16-32 hours)

Time to peak, plasma: 1-3 hours

Excretion: Urine (~25% of absorbed dose excreted unchanged in urine); feces (unchanged via biliary excretion)

Dosage Oral:

Adults: Initial: 150 mg once daily; may increase to 300 mg once daily (maximum: 300 mg/day). **Note:** Prior to initiation, correct hypovolemia and/or closely monitor volume status in patients on concurrent diuretics during treatment initiation.

Elderly: No initial dosage adjustment required

Dosage adjustment in renal impairment:

Mild-to-moderate impairment (eGFR ≥30 mL/minute and/or S_{cr} <1.7 mg/dL [women]; S_{cr} <2 mg/dL [men]): No dose adjustment required

Severe impairment (eGFR <30 mL/minute and/or S_{cr} ≥1.7 mg/dL [women]; S_{cr} ≥2 mg/dL [men]): Use caution; not studied in severe renal impairment

Dosage adjustment in hepatic impairment: No dosage adjustment required

Dietary Considerations May be taken with or without food; however, a high-fat meal reduces absorption. Consistent administration with regards to meals is recommended.

Administration Administer at the same time daily; may take with or without a meal, but consistent administration with regards to meals is recommended.

Monitoring Parameters Blood pressure; serum potassium, BUN, serum creatinine

Dosage Forms Excipient information presented when available (limited, particularly for generics); consult specific product labeling.

Tablet, oral:

Tekturna®: 150 mg, 300 mg

Aliskiren, Amlodipine, and Hydrochlorothiazide

(a lis KYE ren, am LOE di peen, & hye droe klor oh THYE a zide)

Brand Names: U.S. Amturnide™

Index Terms Aliskiren, Hydrochlorothiazide, and Amlodipine; Amlodipine Besylate, Aliskiren Hemifumarate, and Hydrochlorothiazide; Amlodipine, Aliskiren, and Hydrochlorothiazide; Amlodipine, Hydrochlorothiazide, and Aliskiren; Hydrochlorothiazide, Aliskiren, and Amlodipine; Hydrochlorothiazide, Amlodipine, and Aliskiren

Pharmacologic Category Antianginal Agent; Calcium Channel Blocker; Calcium Channel Blocker, Dihydropyridine; Diuretic, Thiazide; Renin Inhibitor

Use Treatment of hypertension (not for initial therapy)

Pregnancy Risk Factor D

Dosage Note: Not for initial therapy. Dose is individualized; combination product may be substituted for individual components in patients currently maintained on all three agents separately, used to switch a patient on any dual combination of the components who is experiencing dose-limiting adverse reactions from an individual component (to a lower dose of that component), or used as add-on therapy in patients not adequately controlled with any two of the following: Aliskiren, dihydropyridine calcium channel blockers, and thiazide diuretics.

Oral: Hypertension: Add-on/switch therapy/replacement therapy:

Adults: Aliskiren 150-300 mg and amlodipine 5-10 mg and hydrochlorothiazide 12.5-25 mg once daily; dose may be titrated after 2 weeks of therapy. Maximum recommended daily dose: Aliskiren 300 mg; amlodipine 10 mg; hydrochlorothiazide 25 mg

Elderly:

Patients ≥65 and <75 years: Refer to adult dosing

Patients ≥75 years: Initial: Amlodipine 2.5 mg (strength not available in combination product)

Dosage adjustment in renal impairment: Cl_{cr} ≤30 mL/minute: Use of combination product is not recommended

Dosage adjustment in hepatic impairment: Severe hepatic impairment: Initial: Amlodipine 2.5 mg daily (strength not available in combination product)

Additional Information Complete prescribing information for this medication should be consulted for additional detail.

Dosage Forms Excipient information presented when available (limited, particularly for generics); consult specific product labeling.

Tablet, oral:

Amturnide™: Aliskiren 150 mg, amlodipine 5 mg, and hydrochlorothiazide 12.5 mg

Amturnide™: Aliskiren 300 mg, amlodipine 5 mg, and hydrochlorothiazide 12.5 mg

Amturnide™: Aliskiren 300 mg, amlodipine 5 mg, and hydrochlorothiazide 25 mg

Amturnide™: Aliskiren 300 mg, amlodipine 10 mg, and hydrochlorothiazide 12.5 mg

Amturnide™: Aliskiren 300 mg, amlodipine 10 mg, and hydrochlorothiazide 25 mg

Aliskiren and Hydrochlorothiazide

(a lis KYE ren & hye droe klor oh THYE a zide)

Brand Names: U.S. Tekturna HCT®

Brand Names: Canada Rasilez HCT

Index Terms Aliskiren Hemifumarate and Hydrochlorothiazide; Hydrochlorothiazide and Aliskiren

Pharmacologic Category Diuretic, Thiazide; Renin Inhibitor

Use Treatment of hypertension, including use as initial therapy in patients likely to need multiple antihypertensives for adequate control

Pregnancy Risk Factor D

Dosage Oral: **Note:** Dosage must be individualized. Combination product may be used as initial therapy or substituted for individual components in patients currently maintained on both agents separately or in patients not adequately controlled with monotherapy (using one of the agents or an agent within same antihypertensive class).

Adults: Hypertension:

Initial therapy: Aliskiren 150 mg and hydrochlorothiazide 12.5 mg once daily, dose may be titrated at 2- to 4-week intervals; maximum recommended daily doses: Aliskiren 300 mg; hydrochlorothiazide 25 mg

Add-on therapy: Initiate by adding the lowest available dose of the alternative component (aliskiren 150 mg or hydrochlorothiazide 12.5 mg); titrate to effect; maximum recommended daily doses: Aliskiren 300 mg; hydrochlorothiazide 25 mg

Replacement therapy: Substitute for the individually titrated components

Elderly: No initial dosage adjustment required

Dosage adjustment in renal impairment:

Mild-to-moderate impairment (Cl_{cr} >30 mL/minute): No adjustment required

Severe impairment (Cl_{cr} ≤30 mL/minute): Use not recommended

Dosage adjustment in hepatic impairment: No initial dosage adjustment required; titrate slowly

Additional Information Complete prescribing information for this medication should be consulted for additional detail.

Dosage Forms Excipient information presented when available (limited, particularly for generics); consult specific product labeling.

Tablet:

Tekturna HCT®:

150/12.5: Aliskiren 150 mg and hydrochlorothiazide 12.5 mg

150/25: Aliskiren 150 mg and hydrochlorothiazide 25 mg

300/12.5: Aliskiren 300 mg and hydrochlorothiazide 12.5 mg

300/25: Aliskiren 300 mg and hydrochlorothiazide 25 mg

Aliskiren and Valsartan (a lis KYE ren & val SAR tan)

Brand Names: U.S. Valturna®

Index Terms Aliskiren Hemifumarate and Valsartan; Valsartan and Aliskiren

Pharmacologic Category Angiotensin II Receptor Blocker; Renin Inhibitor

Use Treatment of hypertension, including use as initial therapy in patients likely to need multiple antihypertensives for adequate control

Pregnancy Risk Factor D

Dosage Oral: Dose is individualized; combination product may be used as initial therapy or substituted for individual components in patients currently maintained on both agents separately or in patients not adequately controlled with monotherapy (using one of the agents or an agent within same antihypertensive class). Titrate at 2- to 4-week intervals as necessary.

Adults: Hypertension:

Initial therapy: Aliskiren 150 mg and valsartan 160 mg once daily; titrate to effect (maximum daily aliskiren dose: 300 mg; maximum daily valsartan dose: 320 mg)

Patients not controlled with single-agent therapy: Aliskiren 150 mg and valsartan 160 mg once daily; titrate to effect (maximum daily aliskiren dose: 300 mg; maximum daily valsartan dose: 320 mg)

Dosing adjustment in renal impairment:

Mild-to-moderate impairment (Cl_{cr} ≥30 mL/minute): No dose adjustment required

Severe impairment (Cl_{cr} <30 mL/minute): Use caution; not studied in severe renal impairment

Dosing adjustment in hepatic impairment: In mild-to-moderate liver disease no adjustment is needed. Use caution in patients with severe hepatic impairment; clinical experience is limited.

Additional Information Complete prescribing information for this medication should be consulted for additional detail.

Dosage Forms Excipient information presented when available (limited, particularly for generics); consult specific product labeling.

Tablet:

Valturna®:

150/160: Aliskiren 150 mg and valsartan 160 mg

300/320: Aliskiren 300 mg and valsartan 320 mg

◆ **Aliskiren Hemifumarate** *see* Aliskiren *on page 66*

◆ **Aliskiren Hemifumarate and Hydrochlorothiazide** *see* Aliskiren and Hydrochlorothiazide *on page 67*

◆ **Aliskiren Hemifumarate and Valsartan** *see* Aliskiren and Valsartan *on page 68*

◆ **Aliskiren, Hydrochlorothiazide, and Amlodipine** *see* Aliskiren, Amlodipine, and Hydrochlorothiazide *on page 67*

◆ **Alka-Mints® [OTC]** *see* Calcium Carbonate *on page 266*

◆ **Alkeran®** *see* Melphalan *on page 1065*

◆ **All Day Allergy [OTC]** *see* Cetirizine *on page 330*

◆ **Allegra®** *see* Fexofenadine *on page 708*

◆ **Allegra-D® (Can)** *see* Fexofenadine and Pseudoephedrine *on page 709*

◆ **Allegra-D® 12 Hour** *see* Fexofenadine and Pseudoephedrine *on page 709*

◆ **Allegra-D® 24 Hour** *see* Fexofenadine and Pseudoephedrine *on page 709*

◆ **Allegra® Allergy 12 Hour [OTC]** *see* Fexofenadine *on page 708*

◆ **Allegra® Allergy 24 Hour [OTC]** *see* Fexofenadine *on page 708*

◆ **Allegra® Children's Allergy [OTC]** *see* Fexofenadine *on page 708*

◆ **Allegra® Children's Allergy ODT [OTC]** *see* Fexofenadine *on page 708*

◆ **Allegra® ODT [DSC]** *see* Fexofenadine *on page 708*

◆ **Allerdryl® (Can)** *see* DiphenhydrAMINE (Systemic) *on page 516*

◆ **Allerest** *see* Chlorpheniramine and Pseudoephedrine *on page 346*

◆ **Allerfrim [OTC]** *see* Triprolidine and Pseudoephedrine *on page 1741*

◆ **AllerMax® [OTC]** *see* DiphenhydrAMINE (Systemic) *on page 516*

◆ **Allernix (Can)** *see* DiphenhydrAMINE (Systemic) *on page 516*

◆ **AlleRx™-D [DSC]** *see* Pseudoephedrine and Methscopolamine *on page 1432*

◆ **Allfen [OTC]** *see* GuaiFENesin *on page 809*

◆ **Allfen CD** *see* Guaifenesin and Codeine *on page 810*

◆ **Allfen CDX** *see* Guaifenesin and Codeine *on page 810*

◆ **Allfen DM [OTC] [DSC]** *see* Guaifenesin and Dextromethorphan *on page 810*

◆ **Alli® [OTC]** *see* Orlistat *on page 1251*

◆ **Alloprin® (Can)** *see* Allopurinol *on page 68*

Allopurinol (al oh PURE i nole)

Brand Names: U.S. Aloprim®; Zyloprim®

Brand Names: Canada Alloprin®; Apo-Allopurinol®; Novo-Purol; Zyloprim®

Index Terms Allopurinol Sodium

Pharmacologic Category Antigout Agent; Xanthine Oxidase Inhibitor

Use

Oral: Management of primary or secondary gout (acute attack, tophi, joint destruction, uric acid lithiasis, and/or nephropathy); management of hyperuricemia associated with cancer treatment for leukemia, lymphoma, or solid tumor malignancies; management of recurrent calcium oxalate calculi (with uric acid excretion >800 mg/day in men and >750 mg/day in women)

I.V.: Management of hyperuricemia associated with cancer treatment for leukemia, lymphoma, or solid tumor malignancies

Pregnancy Risk Factor C

Pregnancy Considerations There are few reports describing the use of allopurinol during pregnancy; no adverse fetal outcomes attributable to allopurinol have been reported in humans; use only if potential benefit outweighs the potential risk to the fetus.

Lactation Enters breast milk/use caution (AAP rates "compatible"; AAP 2001 update pending)

Contraindications Hypersensitivity to allopurinol or any component of the formulation

Warnings/Precautions Do not use to treat asymptomatic hyperuricemia. Has been associated with a number of hypersensitivity reactions, including severe reactions (vasculitis and Stevens-Johnson syndrome); discontinue at first sign of rash. Reversible hepatotoxicity has been reported; use with caution in patients with pre-existing hepatic impairment. Bone marrow suppression has been reported; use caution with other drugs causing myelosuppression. Caution in renal impairment, dosage adjustments needed. Use with caution in patients taking diuretics concurrently. Risk of skin rash may be increased in patients receiving amoxicillin or ampicillin. The risk of hypersensitivity may be increased in patients receiving thiazides, and possibly ACE inhibitors. Use caution with mercaptopurine or azathioprine; dosage adjustment necessary. Full effect on serum uric acid levels in chronic gout may take several weeks to become evident; gradual titration is recommended.

Adverse Reactions

Dermatologic: Rash

Endocrine & metabolic: Gout (acute)

Gastrointestinal: Diarrhea, nausea

Hepatic: Alkaline phosphatase increased, liver enzymes increased

<1% (Limited to important or life-threatening): Abdominal pain, agranulocytosis, alopecia, angioedema, aplastic anemia, arthralgia, bronchospasm, cataracts, cholestatic jaundice, dermatitis (eczematoid, exfoliative, vascular bullous), dyspepsia, ecchymosis, eosinophilia, epistaxis, fever, gastritis, granuloma annulare, hepatitis, gynecomastia, headache, hepatic necrosis, hepatomegaly, hyperbilirubinemia, hypersensitivity reactions, leukocytosis, leukopenia, lichen planus, loss of taste perception, macular retinitis, myopathy, necrotizing angiitis, nephritis, neuritis, neuropathy, onycholysis, pancreatitis, paresthesia, purpura, pruritus, renal failure, somnolence, Stevens-Johnson syndrome, taste perversion, thrombocytopenia, toxic epidermal necrolysis, toxic pustuloderma, uremia, vasculitis, vomiting

Drug Interactions

Metabolism/Transport Effects None known.

Avoid Concomitant Use

Avoid concomitant use of Allopurinol with any of the following: Didanosine

Increased Effect/Toxicity

Allopurinol may increase the levels/effects of: Amoxicillin; Ampicillin; Anticonvulsants (Hydantoin); AzaTHIOprine; CarBAMazepine; ChlorproPAMIDE; Cyclophosphamide; Didanosine; Mercaptopurine; Theophylline Derivatives; Vitamin K Antagonists

The levels/effects of Allopurinol may be increased by: ACE Inhibitors; Loop Diuretics; Thiazide Diuretics

Decreased Effect

The levels/effects of Allopurinol may be decreased by: Antacids

Ethanol/Nutrition/Herb Interactions

Ethanol: May decrease effectiveness.

Iron supplements: Hepatic iron uptake may be increased.

Vitamin C: Large amounts of vitamin C may acidify urine and increase kidney stone formation.

Stability

Powder for injection: Store at controlled room temperature of 20°C to 25°C (68°F to 77°F). Reconstitute powder for injection with SWFI. Further dilution with NS or D_5W (50-100 mL) to ≤6 mg/mL is recommended. Following preparation, intravenous solutions should be stored at 20°C to 25°C (68°F to 77°F). Do not refrigerate reconstituted and/or diluted product. Must be administered within 10 hours of solution preparation.

Tablet: Store at controlled room temperature of 20°C to 25°C (68°F to 77°F). Protect from moisture and light.

Mechanism of Action Allopurinol inhibits xanthine oxidase, the enzyme responsible for the conversion of hypoxanthine to xanthine to uric acid. Allopurinol is metabolized to oxypurinol which is also an inhibitor of xanthine oxidase; allopurinol acts on purine catabolism, reducing the production of uric acid without disrupting the biosynthesis of vital purines.

Pharmacodynamics/Kinetics

Onset of action: Peak effect: 1-2 weeks

Absorption: Oral: ~80%; Rectal: Poor and erratic

Distribution: V_d: ~1.6 L/kg; V_{ss}: 0.84-0.87 L/kg; enters breast milk

Protein binding: <1%

Metabolism: ~75% to active metabolites, chiefly oxypurinol

Bioavailability: 49% to 53%

Half-life elimination:

Normal renal function: Parent drug: 1-3 hours; Oxypurinol: 18-30 hours

End-stage renal disease: Prolonged

Time to peak, plasma: Oral: 30-120 minutes

Excretion: Urine (76% as oxypurinol, 12% as unchanged drug)

Allopurinol and oxypurinol are dialyzable

Dosage Oral: **Note:** Doses >300 mg should be given in divided doses.

Management of hyperuricemia associated with chemotherapy:

Manufacturer's labeling:

Children <6 years: 150 mg/day

Children 6-10 years: 300 mg/day

Children >10 years and Adults: 600-800 mg/day in 2-3 divided doses

Alternative recommendations (unlabeled dosing; intermediate-risk for tumor lysis syndrome): Children and Adults: Intermediate-risk for tumor lysis syndrome: 10 mg/kg/day (maximum dose/day: 800 mg) in 3 divided doses **or** 50-100 mg/m^2 every 8 hours (maximum dose: 300 mg/m^2/day), begin 1-2 days before initiation of induction chemotherapy; may continue for 3-7 days after chemotherapy (Coiffier, 2008)

Gout (chronic): Adults:

Manufacturer's labeling: Mild: 200-300 mg/day; Severe: 400-600 mg/day; to reduce the possibility of acute gouty attacks, initiate dose at 100 mg/day and increase weekly to recommended dosage, also consider using low-dose colchicine or an NSAID to reduce the risk of a gouty attack. Maximum daily dose: 800 mg/day.

Alternative recommendations (unlabeled dosing): Initial: 100 mg/day, increasing the dose gradually every 4 weeks, while monitoring plasma uric acid levels to achieve a goal of <6 mg/dL; dosages of 600 mg/day and rarely, 900 mg/day may be required (McGill, 2010) **or** Initial: 100 mg/day, increasing the dose by 100 mg/day at 2-4 weeks intervals as required to achieve desired uric acid level of ≤6 mg/dL (EULAR gout guidelines; Zhang, 2006).

Recurrent calcium oxalate stones: Adults: 200-300 mg/day in single or divided doses

I.V.:

Management of hyperuricemia associated with chemotherapy: Note: Intravenous daily dose can be given as a single infusion or in equally divided doses at 6-, 8-, or 12-hour intervals.

Manufacturer's labeling:

Children: Starting dose: 200 mg/m^2/day beginning 1-2 days before chemotherapy

Adults: 200-400 mg/m^2/day (maximum: 600 mg/day) beginning 1-2 days before chemotherapy

Alternative recommendations (unlabeled dosing; intermediate-risk for tumor lysis syndrome): Children and Adults: 200-400 mg/m^2/day (maximum dose/day: 600 mg) in 1-3 divided doses beginning 1-2 days before the start of induction chemotherapy; may continue for 3-7 days after chemotherapy (Coiffier, 2008)

Note: Adequate fluid intake is desirable. A fluid intake sufficient to yield a daily urinary output of at least 2 L in adults is desirable.

Dosing adjustment in renal impairment:

Manufacturer's labeling: Oral, I.V.: Lower doses are required in renal impairment due to potential for accumulation of allopurinol and metabolites.

Cl_{cr} 10-20 mL/minute: 200 mg/day

Cl_{cr} 3-10 mL/minute: ≤100 mg/day

Cl_{cr} <3 mL/minute: 100 mg/dose at extended intervals

Alternative recommendations (unlabeled dosing):

Management of hyperuricemia associated with chemotherapy: Dosage reduction of 50% is recommended in renal impairment (Coiffier, 2008)

Gout: Oral:

Initiate therapy with 50-100 mg daily, and gradually increase to a maintenance dose to achieve a serum uric acid level of ≤6 mg/dL (with close monitoring of serum uric acid levels and for hypersensitivity) (Dalbeth, 2007).

Hemodialysis: Initial: 100 mg alternate days given postdialysis, increase cautiously to 300 mg based on response. If dialysis is on a daily basis, an additional 50% of the dose may be required postdialysis (Dalbeth, 2007)

Dietary Considerations Should take oral forms after meals with plenty of fluid. Fluid intake should be administered to yield neutral or slightly alkaline urine and an output of ~2 L (in adults).

Administration

Oral: Do not initiate or discontinue allopurinol during an acute gout attack. Should administer oral forms after meals with plenty of fluid.

I.V.: The rate of infusion depends on the volume of the infusion. Whenever possible, therapy should be initiated at 24-48 hours before the start of chemotherapy known to cause tumor lysis (including adrenocorticosteroids). I.V. daily dose can be administered as a single infusion or in equally divided doses at 6-, 8-, or 12-hour interval.

Monitoring Parameters CBC, serum uric acid levels, I & O, hepatic and renal function, especially at start of therapy; signs and symptoms of hypersensitivity

Reference Range Uric acid, serum: An increase occurs during childhood

Adults:

Males: 3.4-7 mg/dL or slightly more

Females: 2.4-6 mg/dL or slightly more

Target: ≤6 mg/dL

Values >7 mg/dL are sometimes arbitrarily regarded as hyperuricemia, but there is no sharp line between normals on the one hand, and the serum uric acid of those with clinical gout. Normal ranges cannot be adjusted for purine ingestion, but high purine diet increases uric acid. Uric acid may be increased with body size, exercise, and stress.

Dosage Forms Excipient information presented when available (limited, particularly for generics); consult specific product labeling.

Injection, powder for reconstitution, as sodium: 500 mg (base)

Aloprim®: 500 mg (base)

Tablet, oral: 100 mg, 300 mg

Zyloprim®: 100 mg, 300 mg [scored]

Extemporaneous Preparations A 20 mg/mL oral suspension may be made with tablets and either a 1:1 mixture of Ora-Sweet® and Ora-Plus® or a 1:1 mixture of Ora-Sweet® SF and Ora-Plus® or a 1:4 mixture of cherry syrup concentrate and simple syrup, NF. Crush eight 300 mg tablets in a mortar and reduce to a fine powder. Add small portions of chosen vehicle and mix to a uniform paste; mix while adding the vehicle in incremental proportions to **almost** 120 mL; transfer to a calibrated bottle, rinse mortar with vehicle, and add quantity of vehicle sufficient to make 120 mL. Label "shake well". Stable for 60 days refrigerated or at room temperature (Allen, 1996; Nahata, 2004).

Allen LV Jr and Erickson MA 3rd, "Stability of Acetazolamide, Allopurinol, Azathioprine, Clonazepam, and Flucytosine in Extemporaneously Compounded Oral Liquids," *Am J Health Syst Pharm*, 1996, 53(16):1944-9.

Nahata MC, Pai VB, and Hipple TF, *Pediatric Drug Formulations*, 5th ed, Cincinnati, OH: Harvey Whitney Books Co, 2004.

◆ **Allopurinol Sodium** *see* Allopurinol *on page 68*

◆ **All-*trans* Retinoic Acid** *see* Tretinoin (Systemic) *on page 1729*

◆ **All-*trans* Vitamin A Acid** *see* Tretinoin (Systemic) *on page 1729*

◆ **Almacone® [OTC]** *see* Aluminum Hydroxide, Magnesium Hydroxide, and Simethicone *on page 80*

◆ **Almacone Double Strength® [OTC]** *see* Aluminum Hydroxide, Magnesium Hydroxide, and Simethicone *on page 80*

Almotriptan (al moh TRIP tan)

Brand Names: U.S. Axert®

Brand Names: Canada Axert®

Index Terms Almotriptan Malate

Pharmacologic Category Antimigraine Agent; Serotonin $5\text{-}HT_{1B,\ 1D}$ Receptor Agonist

Additional Appendix Information

Antimigraine Drugs: $5\text{-}HT_1$ Receptor Agonists *on page 1878*

Use Acute treatment of migraine with or without aura in adults (with a history of migraine) and adolescents (with a history of migraine lasting ≥4 hours when left untreated)

Pregnancy Risk Factor C

Pregnancy Considerations There are no adequate and well-controlled studies in pregnant women. Use in pregnancy should be limited to situations where benefit outweighs risk to fetus. In some (but not all) animal studies, administration was associated with embryolethality, fetal malformations, and decreased pup weight.

Lactation Excretion in breast milk unknown/use caution

Contraindications Hypersensitivity to almotriptan or any component of the formulation; hemiplegic or basilar migraine; known or suspected ischemic heart disease (eg, angina pectoris, MI, documented silent ischemia, coronary artery vasospasm, Prinzmetal's variant angina); cerebrovascular syndromes (eg, stroke, transient ischemic attacks); peripheral vascular disease (eg, ischemic bowel disease); uncontrolled hypertension; use within 24 hours of another $5\text{-}HT_1$ agonist; use within 24 hours of ergotamine derivatives and/or ergotamine-containing medications (eg, dihydroergotamine, ergotamine)

Warnings/Precautions Almotriptan is only indicated for the treatment of acute migraine headache; not indicated for migraine prophylaxis, or the treatment of cluster headaches, hemiplegic migraine, or basilar migraine. If a patient does not respond to the first dose, the diagnosis of acute migraine should be reconsidered.

Almotriptan should not be given to patients with documented ischemic or vasospastic CAD. Patients with risk factors for CAD (eg, hypertension, hypercholesterolemia, smoker, obesity, diabetes, strong family history of CAD, menopause, male >40 years of age) should undergo adequate cardiac evaluation prior to administration; if the cardiac evaluation is "satisfactory," the first dose of almotriptan should be given in the healthcare provider's office (consider ECG monitoring). All patients should undergo periodic evaluation of cardiovascular status during treatment. Cardiac events (coronary artery vasospasm, transient ischemia, myocardial infarction, ventricular tachycardia/fibrillation, cardiac arrest, and death), cerebral/subarachnoid hemorrhage, stroke, peripheral vascular ischemia, and colonic ischemia have been reported with 5-HT_1 agonist administration. Patients who experience sensations of chest pain/pressure/tightness or symptoms suggestive of angina following dosing should be evaluated for coronary artery disease or Prinzmetal's angina before receiving additional doses; if dosing is resumed and similar symptoms recur, monitor with ECG. Significant elevation in blood pressure, including hypertensive crisis, has also been reported on rare occasions following 5-HT_1 agonist administration in patients with and without a history of hypertension.

Transient and permanent blindness and partial vision loss have been reported (rare) with 5-HT_1 agonist administration. Almotriptan contains a sulfonyl group which is structurally different from a sulfonamide. Cross-reactivity in patients with sulfonamide allergy has not been evaluated; however, the manufacturer recommends that caution be exercised in this patient population. Use with caution in liver or renal dysfunction. Symptoms of agitation, confusion, hallucinations, hyper-reflexia, myoclonus, shivering, and tachycardia (serotonin syndrome) may occur with concomitant proserotonergic drugs (ie, SSRIs/SNRIs or triptans) or agents which reduce almotriptan's metabolism. Concurrent use of serotonin precursors (eg, tryptophan) is not recommended. If concomitant administration with SSRIs is warranted, monitor closely, especially at initiation and with dose increases. Efficacy has not been demonstrated in improvement of migraine-associated symptoms (eg, phonophobia, nausea, photophobia) in patients aged 12-17 years (Linder, 2008).

Adverse Reactions

1% to 10%:

Central nervous system: Somnolence (≤5%), dizziness (≤4%), headache (≤2%)

Gastrointestinal: Nausea (1% to 3%), vomiting (≤2%), xerostomia (1%)

Neuromuscular & skeletal: Paresthesia (≤1%)

<1% (Limited to important or life-threatening): Anaphylactic shock, angina, angioedema, breast pain, colitis, coronary artery vasospasm, hemiplegia, hypertension, myocardial ischemia, MI, neuropathy, rash, seizure, syncope, tachycardia, ventricular fibrillation, ventricular tachycardia, vertigo

Drug Interactions

Metabolism/Transport Effects Substrate of CYP2D6 (minor), CYP3A4 (minor); **Note:** Assignment of Major/Minor substrate status based on clinically relevant drug interaction potential

Avoid Concomitant Use

Avoid concomitant use of Almotriptan with any of the following: Ergot Derivatives; MAO Inhibitors

Increased Effect/Toxicity

Almotriptan may increase the levels/effects of: Ergot Derivatives; Metoclopramide; Serotonin Modulators

The levels/effects of Almotriptan may be increased by: Antipsychotics; CYP3A4 Inhibitors (Strong); Ergot Derivatives; MAO Inhibitors

Decreased Effect

The levels/effects of Almotriptan may be decreased by: Peginterferon Alfa-2b; Tocilizumab

Stability Store at 25°C (77°F); excursions permitted to 15°C to 30°C (59°F to 86°F).

Mechanism of Action Selective agonist for serotonin (5-HT_{1B} and 5-HT_{1D} receptors) in cranial arteries; causes vasoconstriction and reduces sterile inflammation associated with antidromic neuronal transmission correlating with relief of migraine

Pharmacodynamics/Kinetics

Absorption: Well absorbed

Distribution: V_d: ~180-200 L

Protein binding: ~35%

Metabolism: Via MAO type A oxidative deamination (~27% of dose) and CYP3A4 and 2D6 (~12% of dose) to inactive metabolites

Bioavailability: ~70%

Half-life elimination: 3-4 hours

Time to peak, plasma: 1-3 hours

Excretion: Urine (~75%; ~40% of total dose as unchanged drug); feces (~13% of total dose as unchanged drug and metabolites)

Dosage Oral: Children ≥12 years and Adults: Migraine: Initial: 6.25-12.5 mg in a single dose; if the headache returns, repeat the dose after 2 hours (maximum daily dose: 25 mg)

Note: The safety of treating more than 4 migraines/month has not been established.

Dosage adjustment with concomitant use of an enzyme inhibitor:

Patients receiving a potent CYP3A4 inhibitor: Initial: 6.25 mg in a single dose; maximum daily dose: 12.5 mg

Patients with renal impairment and concomitant use of a potent CYP3A4 inhibitor: Avoid use

Patients with hepatic impairment and concomitant use of a potent CYP3A4 inhibitor: Avoid use

Dosage adjustment in renal impairment: Severe renal impairment (Cl_{cr} ≤30 mL/minute): Initial: 6.25 mg in a single dose; maximum daily dose: 12.5 mg

Dosage adjustment in hepatic impairment: Initial: 6.25 mg in a single dose; maximum daily dose: 12.5 mg

Dietary Considerations May be taken without regard to meals.

Administration Administer without regard to meals.

Dosage Forms Excipient information presented when available (limited, particularly for generics); consult specific product labeling.

Tablet, oral, as maleate:

Axert®: 6.25 mg, 12.5 mg

◆ **Almotriptan Malate** *see* Almotriptan *on page 70*

◆ **Alocril®** *see* Nedocromil *on page 1184*

◆ **Alodox™** *see* Doxycycline *on page 557*

◆ **Aloe Vesta® Antifungal [OTC]** *see* Miconazole (Topical) *on page 1126*

◆ **Alomide®** *see* Lodoxamide *on page 1025*

◆ **Alophen® [OTC]** *see* Bisacodyl *on page 219*

◆ **Aloprim®** *see* Allopurinol *on page 68*

◆ **Alora®** *see* Estradiol (Systemic) *on page 627*

◆ **Aloxi®** *see* Palonosetron *on page 1281*

Alpha-Galactosidase (AL fa ga lak TOE si days)

Brand Names: U.S. beano® Meltaways [OTC]; beano® [OTC]

Index Terms *Aspergillus niger*

Pharmacologic Category Enzyme

Use Prevention of flatulence and bloating attributed to a variety of grains, cereals, nuts, and vegetables

Dosage Oral: Children ≥12 years and Adults: Adjust dose according to the number of problem foods per meal:

Tablet, chewable (beano®): Usual dose: 2-3 tablets/meal

Tablet, orally disintegrating (beano® Meltaways): One tablet per meal

Additional Information Complete prescribing information for this medication should be consulted for additional detail.

Dosage Forms Excipient information presented when available (limited, particularly for generics); consult specific product labeling.

Tablet, chewable, oral:
beano®: 150 Galactosidase units [scored]

Tablet, orally disintegrating, oral:
beano® Meltaways: 300 Galactosidase units [strawberry flavor]

- ◆ **Alpha-Galactosidase-A (Recombinant)** *see* Agalsidase Beta *on page 49*
- ◆ **Alphagan® (Can)** *see* Brimonidine *on page 235*
- ◆ **Alphagan® P** *see* Brimonidine *on page 235*
- ◆ **1α-Hydroxyergocalciferol** *see* Doxercalciferol *on page 552*
- ◆ **Alphanate®** *see* Antihemophilic Factor/von Willebrand Factor Complex (Human) *on page 128*
- ◆ **AlphaNine® SD** *see* Factor IX *on page 683*
- ◆ **Alphaquin HP®** *see* Hydroquinone *on page 846*
- ◆ **Alph-E [OTC]** *see* Vitamin E *on page 1796*
- ◆ **Alph-E-Mixed [OTC]** *see* Vitamin E *on page 1796*

ALPRAZolam (al PRAY zoe lam)

Brand Names: U.S. Alprazolam Intensol™; Niravam™; Xanax XR®; Xanax®

Brand Names: Canada Apo-Alpraz®; Apo-Alpraz® TS; Mylan-Alprazolam; Nu-Alpraz; Teva-Alprazolam; Xanax TS™; Xanax®

Pharmacologic Category Benzodiazepine

Additional Appendix Information

Beers Criteria – Potentially Inappropriate Medications for Geriatrics *on page 1973*

Benzodiazepines *on page 1882*

Use Treatment of anxiety disorder (GAD); short-term relief of symptoms of anxiety; panic disorder, with or without agoraphobia; anxiety associated with depression

Unlabeled Use Anxiety in children

Pregnancy Risk Factor D

Pregnancy Considerations Benzodiazepines have the potential to cause harm to the fetus. Alprazolam and its metabolites cross the human placenta. Teratogenic effects have been observed with some benzodiazepines; however, additional studies are needed. The incidence of premature birth and low birth weights may be increased following maternal use of benzodiazepines; hypoglycemia and respiratory problems in the neonate may occur following exposure late in pregnancy. Neonatal withdrawal symptoms may occur within days to weeks after birth and "floppy infant syndrome" (which also includes withdrawal symptoms) has been reported with some benzodiazepines.

Lactation Enters breast milk/not recommended (AAP rates "of concern"; AAP 2001 update pending)

Contraindications Hypersensitivity to alprazolam or any component of the formulation (cross-sensitivity with other benzodiazepines may exist); narrow-angle glaucoma; concurrent use with ketoconazole or itraconazole

Warnings/Precautions Rebound or withdrawal symptoms, including seizures, may occur following abrupt discontinuation or large decreases in dose (more common in patients receiving >4 mg/day or prolonged treatment); the risk of seizures appears to be greatest 24-72 hours following discontinuation of therapy. Breakthrough anxiety may occur at the end of dosing interval. Use with caution in patients receiving concurrent CYP3A4 inhibitors, moderate or strong CYP3A4 inducers, and major CYP3A4 substrates; consider alternative agents that avoid or lessen the potential for CYP-mediated interactions. Use with caution in renal impairment or predisposition to urate nephropathy; has weak uricosuric properties. Use with caution in elderly; due to increased sensitivity in this age group, smaller doses of benzodiazepines may be safer and as effective. Avoid using doses >2 mg daily of alprazolam (Beers Criteria) Use with caution in or debilitated patients, patients with hepatic disease (including alcoholics) or respiratory disease, or obese patients.

Causes CNS depression (dose related) which may impair physical and mental capabilities. Patients must be cautioned about performing tasks that require mental alertness (eg, operating machinery or driving). Effects with other sedative drugs or ethanol may be potentiated. Benzodiazepines have been associated with falls and traumatic injury and should be used with extreme caution in patients who are at risk of these events.

Use caution in patients with depression, particularly if suicidal risk may be present. Episodes of mania or hypomania have occurred in depressed patients treated with alprazolam. May cause physical or psychological dependence. Acute withdrawal may be precipitated in patients after administration of flumazenil.

Benzodiazepines have been associated with anterograde amnesia. Paradoxical reactions have been reported with benzodiazepines, particularly in adolescent/pediatric or psychiatric patients. Does not have analgesic, antidepressant, or antipsychotic properties.

Adverse Reactions

>10%:

Central nervous system: Abnormal coordination, cognitive disorder, depression, drowsiness, fatigue, irritability, lightheadedness, memory impairment, sedation, somnolence

Endocrine & metabolic: Libido decreased

Gastrointestinal: Appetite increased/decreased, constipation, weight gain/loss, xerostomia

Genitourinary: Micturition difficulty

Neuromuscular & skeletal: Dysarthria

Respiratory: Nasal congestion

1% to 10%:

Cardiovascular: Chest pain, hypotension, palpitation, sinus tachycardia

Central nervous system: Agitation, akathisia, ataxia, attention disturbance, confusion, depersonalization, derealization, disorientation, disinhibition, dizziness, dream abnormalities, fear, hallucination, headache, hypersomnia, hypoesthesia, insomnia, lethargy, malaise, mental impairment, nervousness, nightmares, restlessness, seizure, syncope, talkativeness, vertigo

Dermatologic: Dermatitis, rash

Endocrine & metabolic: Dysmenorrhea, libido increased, menstrual disorders, sexual dysfunction

Gastrointestinal: Abdominal pain, anorexia, diarrhea, dyspepsia, nausea, salivation increased, vomiting

Genitourinary: Incontinence

Hepatic: Bilirubin increased, jaundice, liver enzymes increased

Neuromuscular & skeletal: Arthralgia, back pain, dyskinesia, dystonia, muscle cramps, muscle twitching, myalgia, paresthesia, tremor, weakness

Ocular: Blurred vision

Respiratory: Allergic rhinitis, dyspnea, hyperventilation, upper respiratory infection

Miscellaneous: Diaphoresis

<1% (Limited to important or life-threatening): Amnesia, angioedema, bilirubin increased, diplopia, falls, homicidal ideation, galactorrhea, gynecomastia, hepatic failure, hepatitis, hyperprolactinemia, hypomania, jaundice, liver enzymes increased, mania, peripheral edema, sleep apnea syndrome, Stevens-Johnson syndrome, suicidal ideation, syncope, tinnitus

Drug Interactions

Metabolism/Transport Effects Substrate of CYP3A4 (major); **Note:** Assignment of Major/Minor substrate status based on clinically relevant drug interaction potential

Avoid Concomitant Use

Avoid concomitant use of ALPRAZolam with any of the following: Conivaptan; Indinavir; OLANZapine

Increased Effect/Toxicity

ALPRAZolam may increase the levels/effects of: Alcohol (Ethyl); CloZAPine; CNS Depressants; Methotrimeprazine; Selective Serotonin Reuptake Inhibitors

The levels/effects of ALPRAZolam may be increased by: Antifungal Agents (Azole Derivatives, Systemic); Aprepitant; Boceprevir; Calcium Channel Blockers (Nondihydropyridine); Cimetidine; Conivaptan; Contraceptives (Estrogens); Contraceptives (Progestins); CYP3A4 Inhibitors (Moderate); CYP3A4 Inhibitors (Strong); Dasatinib; Droperidol; Fluconazole; Fosaprepitant; Grapefruit Juice; HydrOXYzine; Indinavir; Isoniazid; Macrolide Antibiotics; Methotrimeprazine; Nefazodone; OLANZapine; Protease Inhibitors; Proton Pump Inhibitors; Selective Serotonin Reuptake Inhibitors; Telaprevir

Decreased Effect

The levels/effects of ALPRAZolam may be decreased by: CarBAMazepine; CYP3A4 Inducers (Strong); Deferasirox; Rifamycin Derivatives; St Johns Wort; Theophylline Derivatives; Tocilizumab; Yohimbine

Ethanol/Nutrition/Herb Interactions

Cigarette smoking: May decrease alprazolam concentrations up to 50%.

Ethanol: May increase CNS depression; monitor for increased effects with coadministration. Caution patients about effects.

Food: Alprazolam serum concentration is unlikely to be increased by grapefruit juice because of alprazolam's high oral bioavailability. The C_{max} of the extended release formulation is increased by 25% when a high-fat meal is given 2 hours before dosing. T_{max} is decreased 33% when food is given immediately prior to dose. T_{max} is increased by 33% when food is given ≥1 hour after dose.

Herb/Nutraceutical: St John's wort may decrease alprazolam levels. Avoid valerian, St John's wort, kava kava, gotu kola (may increase CNS depression).

Stability

Immediate release tablets: Store at 20°C to 25°C (68°F to 77°F).

Extended release tablets: Store at 25°C (77°F); excursions permitted to 15°C to 30°C (59°F to 86°F).

Orally-disintegrating tablet: Store at room temperature of 20°C to 25°C (68°F to 77°F). Protect from moisture. Seal bottle tightly and discard any cotton packaged inside bottle.

Mechanism of Action Binds to stereospecific benzodiazepine receptors on the postsynaptic GABA neuron at several sites within the central nervous system, including the limbic system, reticular formation. Enhancement of the inhibitory effect of GABA on neuronal excitability results by increased neuronal membrane permeability to chloride ions. This shift in chloride ions results in hyperpolarization (a less excitable state) and stabilization.

Pharmacodynamics/Kinetics

Onset of action: Immediate release and extended release formulations: 1 hour

Duration: Immediate release: 5.1 ± 1.7 hours; Extended release: 11.3 ± 4.2 hours

Absorption: Extended release: Slower relative to immediate release formulation resulting in a concentration that is maintained 5-11 hours after dosing

Distribution: V_d: 0.9-1.2 L/kg

Protein binding: 80%; primarily to albumin

Metabolism: Hepatic via CYP3A4; forms two active metabolites (4-hydroxyalprazolam and α-hydroxyalprazolam)

Bioavailability: 90%

Half-life elimination:

- Adults: 11.2 hours (Immediate release range: 6.3-26.9 hours; Extended release range: 10.7-15.8 hours); Orally-disintegrating tablet range: 7.9-19.2 hours)
- Elderly: 16.3 hours (range: 9-26.9 hours)
- Alcoholic liver disease: 19.7 hours (range: 5.8-65.3 hours)
- Obesity: 21.8 hours (range: 9.9-40.4 hours)
- Race: Asians: Increased by ~25% (as compared to Caucasians)

Time to peak, serum:

- Immediate release: 1-2 hours
- Extended release: ~9 hours (Glue, 2006); decreased by 1 hour when administered at bedtime (as compared to morning administration); decreased by 33% when administered with a high-fat meal; increased by 33% when administered ≥1 hour after a high-fat meal
- Orally-disintegrating tablet: 1.5-2 hours; occurs ~15 minutes earlier when administered with water; decreased by 2 hours when administered with a high-fat meal

Excretion: Urine (as unchanged drug and metabolites)

Dosage Oral: **Note:** Treatment >4 months should be reevaluated to determine the patient's continued need for the drug

Children: Anxiety (unlabeled use): Immediate release: Initial: 0.005 mg/kg/dose or 0.125 mg/dose 3 times/day; increase in increments of 0.125-0.25 mg, up to a maximum of 0.02 mg/kg/dose or 0.06 mg/kg/day (range of doses reported in one study: 0.375-3 mg/day) (Pfefferbaum, 1987). See "dose reduction" comment.

Adults:

Anxiety: Immediate release: Initial: 0.25-0.5 mg 3 times/day; titrate dose upward every 3-4 days; usual maximum: 4 mg/day. Patients requiring doses >4 mg/day should be increased cautiously. Periodic reassessment and consideration of dosage reduction is recommended.

Panic disorder:

- Immediate release: Initial: 0.5 mg 3 times/day; dose may be increased every 3-4 days in increments ≤1 mg/day. Mean effective dosage: 5-6 mg/day; some patients may require much as 10 mg/day
- Extended release: 0.5-1 mg once daily; may increase dose every 3-4 days in increments ≤1 mg/day (range: 3-6 mg/day)
- Switching from immediate release to extended release: Patients may be switched to extended release tablets by taking the total daily dose of the immediate release tablets and giving it once daily using the extended release preparation.

Preoperative anxiety (unlabeled use): 0.5 mg 60-90 minutes before procedure (De Witte, 2002)

Dose reduction: Abrupt discontinuation should be avoided. Daily dose may be decreased by 0.5 mg every 3 days; however, some patients may require a slower reduction. If withdrawal symptoms occur, resume previous dose and discontinue on a less rapid schedule.

Elderly: **Note:** Elderly patients may be more sensitive to the effects of alprazolam including ataxia and oversedation. The elderly may also have impaired renal function leading to decreased clearance. Titrate gradually, if needed and tolerated.

Immediate release: Initial: 0.25 mg 2-3 times/day

Extended release: Initial: 0.5 mg once daily

Dosing adjustment in renal impairment: No dosage adjustment provided in manufacturer's labeling; however, use caution

Dosing adjustment in hepatic impairment: Advanced liver disease:

Immediate release: 0.25 mg 2-3 times/day; titrate gradually if needed and tolerated

Extended release: 0.5 mg once daily; titrate gradually if needed and tolerated

Dietary Considerations Extended release tablet should be taken once daily in the morning.

Administration

Immediate release preparations: Can be administered sublingually if oral administration is not possible; absorption and onset of effect are comparable to oral administration (Scavone,1987; Scavone, 1992)

Extended release tablet: Should be taken once daily in the morning; do not crush, break, or chew.

Orally-disintegrating tablets: Using dry hands, place tablet on top of tongue and allow to disintegrate. If using one-half of tablet, immediately discard remaining half (may not remain stable). Administration with water is not necessary.

Monitoring Parameters Respiratory and cardiovascular status

Additional Information Not intended for management of anxieties and minor distresses associated with everyday life. Treatment longer than 4 months should be re-evaluated to determine the patient's need for the drug. Patients who become physically dependent on alprazolam tend to have a difficult time discontinuing it; withdrawal symptoms may be severe. To minimize withdrawal symptoms, taper dosage slowly; do not discontinue abruptly. Abrupt discontinuation after sustained use (generally >10 days) may cause withdrawal symptoms.

Dosage Forms Excipient information presented when available (limited, particularly for generics); consult specific product labeling.

Solution, oral [concentrate]:

Alprazolam Intensol™: 1 mg/mL (30 mL) [dye free, ethanol free, sugar free; contains propylene glycol]

Tablet, oral: 0.25 mg, 0.5 mg, 1 mg, 2 mg

Xanax®: 0.25 mg, 0.5 mg, 1 mg, 2 mg [scored]

Tablet, extended release, oral: 0.5 mg, 1 mg, 2 mg, 3 mg

Xanax XR®: 0.5 mg, 1 mg, 2 mg, 3 mg

Tablet, orally disintegrating, oral: 0.25 mg, 0.5 mg, 1 mg, 2 mg

Niravam™: 0.25 mg, 0.5 mg, 1 mg, 2 mg [scored; orange flavor]

Controlled Substance C-IV

Extemporaneous Preparations Note: Commercial oral solution is available (Alprazolam Intensol™: 1 mg/mL [dye free, ethanol free, sugar free; contains propylene glycol])

A 1 mg/mL oral suspension may be made with tablets and one of three different vehicles (a 1:1 mixture of Ora-Sweet® and Ora-Plus®, a 1:1 mixture of Ora-Sweet® SF and Ora-Plus®, or a 1:4 mixture of cherry syrup with Simple Syrup, NF). Crush sixty 2 mg tablets in a mortar and reduce to a fine powder. Add 40 mL of vehicle and mix to a uniform paste; mix while adding the vehicle in incremental proportions to **almost** 120 mL; transfer to a calibrated bottle, rinse mortar with vehicle, and add a quantity of vehicle sufficient to make 120 mL. Label "shake well" and "refrigerate". Stable for 60 days.

Nahata MC, Pai VB, and Hipple TF, *Pediatric Drug Formulations*, 5th ed, Cincinnati, OH: Harvey Whitney Books Co, 2004.

◆ **Alprazolam Intensol™** *see* ALPRAZolam *on page* 72

Alprostadil (al PROS ta dill)

Brand Names: U.S. Caverject Impulse®; Caverject®; Edex®; Muse®; Prostin VR Pediatric®

Brand Names: Canada Caverject®; Muse® Pellet; Prostin® VR

Index Terms PGE_1; Prostaglandin E_1

Pharmacologic Category Prostaglandin; Vasodilator

Use

Prostin VR Pediatric®: Temporary maintenance of patency of ductus arteriosus in neonates with ductal-dependent congenital heart disease until surgery can be performed. These defects include cyanotic (eg, pulmonary atresia, pulmonary stenosis, tricuspid atresia, Fallot's tetralogy, transposition of the great vessels) and acyanotic (eg, interruption of aortic arch, coarctation of aorta, hypoplastic left ventricle) heart disease.

Caverject®: Treatment of erectile dysfunction of vasculogenic, psychogenic, or neurogenic etiology; adjunct in the diagnosis of erectile dysfunction

Edex®, Muse®: Treatment of erectile dysfunction of vasculogenic, psychogenic, or neurogenic etiology

Unlabeled Use Treatment of pulmonary hypertension in infants and children with congenital heart defects with left-to-right shunts

Pregnancy Risk Factor X/C (Muse®)

Pregnancy Considerations Alprostadil is embryotoxic in animal studies. It is not indicated for use in women. The manufacturer of Muse® recommends a condom barrier when being used during sexual intercourse with a pregnant women.

Lactation Not indicated for use in women

Contraindications Hypersensitivity to alprostadil or any component of the formulation; hyaline membrane disease or persistent fetal circulation and when a dominant left-to-right shunt is present; respiratory distress syndrome; conditions predisposing patients to priapism (sickle cell anemia, multiple myeloma, leukemia); patients with anatomical deformation of the penis, penile implants; use in men for whom sexual activity is inadvisable or contraindicated; pregnancy

Warnings/Precautions Use cautiously in neonates with bleeding tendencies. **[U.S. Boxed Warning]: Apnea may occur in 10% to 12% of neonates with congenital heart defects, especially in those weighing <2 kg at birth.** Apnea usually appears during the first hour of drug infusion. When used for patency of ductus arteriosus infuse for the shortest time at the lowest dose consistent with good patient care. Use for >120 hours has been associated with antral hyperplasia and gastric outlet obstruction.

When used in erectile dysfunction, priapism may occur; treat proloonged priapism (erection persisting for >4 hours) immediately to avoid penile tissue damage and permanent loss of potency; discontinue therapy if signs of penile fibrosis develop (penile angulation, cavernosal fibrosis, or Peyronie's disease). When used in erectile dysfunction (Muse®), syncope occurring within 1 hour of administration has been reported. The potential for drug-drug interactions may occur when Muse® is prescribed concomitantly with antihypertensives.

Adverse Reactions

Intraurethral:

>10%: Genitourinary: Penile pain, urethral burning

2% to 10%:

Central nervous system: Headache, dizziness, pain

Genitourinary: Vaginal itching (female partner), testicular pain, urethral bleeding (minor)

<2% (Limited to important or life-threatening): Tachycardia, perineal pain, leg pain

Intracavernosal injection:
>10%: Genitourinary: Penile pain
1% to 10%:
Cardiovascular: Hypertension
Central nervous system: Headache, dizziness
Genitourinary: Prolonged erection (>4 hours, 4%), penile fibrosis, penis disorder, penile rash, penile edema
Local: Injection site hematoma and/or bruising
<1% (Limited to important or life-threatening): Balanitis, injection site hemorrhage, priapism (0.4%)

Intravenous:
>10%:
Cardiovascular: Flushing
Central nervous system: Fever
Respiratory: Apnea
1% to 10%:
Cardiovascular: Bradycardia, hyper-/hypotension, tachycardia, cardiac arrest, edema
Central nervous system: Seizure, headache, dizziness
Endocrine & metabolic: Hypokalemia
Gastrointestinal: Diarrhea
Hematologic: Disseminated intravascular coagulation
Neuromuscular & skeletal: Back pain
Respiratory: Upper respiratory infection, flu syndrome, sinusitis, nasal congestion, cough
Miscellaneous: Sepsis, localized pain in structures other than the injection site
<1% (Limited to important or life-threatening): Anemia, anuria, bleeding, bradypnea, bronchial wheezing, cerebral bleeding, CHF, gastric regurgitation, hematuria, hyperbilirubinemia, hyperemia, hyperextension of neck, hyperirritability, hyperkalemia, hypoglycemia, hypothermia, jitteriness, lethargy, peritonitis, second-degree heart block, shock, stiffness, supraventricular tachycardia, thrombocytopenia, ventricular fibrillation

Drug Interactions

Metabolism/Transport Effects None known.

Avoid Concomitant Use There are no known interactions where it is recommended to avoid concomitant use.

Increased Effect/Toxicity There are no known significant interactions involving an increase in effect.

Decreased Effect There are no known significant interactions involving a decrease in effect.

Ethanol/Nutrition/Herb Interactions Ethanol: Avoid concurrent use (vasodilating effect).

Stability

Caverject® Impulse™: Store at controlled room temperature of 15°C to 30°C (59°F to 86°F). Provided as a dual-chamber syringe with diluent in one chamber. To mix, hold syringe with needle pointing upward and turn plunger clockwise; turn upside down several times to mix. Device can be set to deliver specified dose, each device can be set at various increments. Following reconstitution, use within 24 hours and discard any unused solution.

Caverject® powder: The 5 mcg, 10 mcg, and 20 mcg vials should be stored at or below 25°C (77°F). The 40 mcg vial should be stored at 2°C to 8°C until dispensed. After dispensing, stable for up to 3 months at or below 25°C. Use only the supplied diluent for reconstitution (ie, bacteriostatic/sterile water with benzyl alcohol 0.945%). Following reconstitution, all strengths should be stored at or below 25°C (77°F); do not refrigerate or freeze; use within 24 hours.

Caverject® solution: Prior to dispensing, store frozen at -20°C to -10°C (-4°F to -14°F); once dispensed, may be stored frozen for up to 3 months, or under refrigeration at 2°C to 8°C (36°F to 46°F) for up to 7 days. Do not refreeze. Once removed from foil wrap, solution may be allowed to warm to room temperature prior to use. If not used immediately, solution should be discarded. Shake well prior to use.

Edex®: Store at controlled room temperature of 15°C to 30°C (59°F to 86°F); following reconstitution with NS, use immediately and discard any unused solution.

Muse®: Refrigerate at 2°C to 8°C (36°F to 46°F); may be stored at room temperature for up to 14 days.

Prostin VR Pediatric®: Refrigerate at 2°C to 8°C (36°F to 46°F). The following stability information has also been reported: may be stored at 20°C for up to 34 days or 30°C for up to 26 days (Cohen, 2007). Prior to infusion, dilute with D_5W or NS; use within 24 hours.

Mechanism of Action Causes vasodilation by means of direct effect on vascular and ductus arteriosus smooth muscle; relaxes trabecular smooth muscle by dilation of cavernosal arteries when injected along the penile shaft, allowing blood flow to and entrapment in the lacunar spaces of the penis (ie, corporeal veno-occlusive mechanism)

Pharmacodynamics/Kinetics
Onset of action: Rapid
Duration: <1 hour
Distribution: Insignificant following penile injection
Protein binding, plasma: 81% to albumin
Metabolism: ~75% by oxidation in one pass via lungs
Half-life elimination: 5-10 minutes
Excretion: Urine (90% as metabolites) within 24 hours

Dosage

Patent ductus arteriosus (Prostin VR Pediatric®):

I.V. continuous infusion into a large vein, or alternatively through an umbilical artery catheter placed at the ductal opening: 0.05-0.1 mcg/kg/minute with therapeutic response, rate is reduced to lowest effective dosage; with unsatisfactory response, rate is increased gradually; maintenance: 0.01-0.4 mcg/kg/minute

PGE_1 is usually given at an infusion rate of 0.1 mcg/kg/minute, but it is often possible to reduce the dosage to 1/2 or even 1/10 without losing the therapeutic effect.

Therapeutic response is indicated by increased pH in those with acidosis or by an increase in oxygenation (PO_2) usually evident within 30 minutes

Erectile dysfunction:

Caverject®, Edex®: Intracavernous: Individualize dose by careful titration; doses >40 mcg (Edex®) or >60 mcg (Caverject®) are not recommended: Initial dose must be titrated in physician's office. Patient must stay in the physician's office until complete detumescence occurs; if there is no response, then the next higher dose may be given within 1 hour; if there is still no response, a 1-day interval before giving the next dose is recommended; increasing the dose or concentration in the treatment of impotence results in increasing pain and discomfort

Vasculogenic, psychogenic, or mixed etiology: Initiate dosage titration at 2.5 mcg, increasing by 2.5 mcg to a dose of 5 mcg and then in increments of 5-10 mcg depending on the erectile response until the dose produces an erection suitable for intercourse, not lasting >1 hour; if there is absolutely no response to initial 2.5 mcg dose, the second dose may be increased to 7.5 mcg, followed by increments of 5-10 mcg

Neurogenic etiology (eg, spinal cord injury): Initiate dosage titration at 1.25 mcg, increasing to a dose of 2.5 mcg and then 5 mcg; increase further in increments 5 mcg until the dose is reached that produces an erection suitable for intercourse, not lasting >1 hour

Maintenance: Once appropriate dose has been determined, patient may self-administer injections at a frequency of no more than 3 times/week with at least 24 hours between doses

Muse® Pellet: Intraurethral:
Initial: 125-250 mcg
Maintenance: Administer as needed to achieve an erection; duration of action is about 30-60 minutes; use only two systems per 24-hour period

Elderly: Elderly patients may have a greater frequency of renal dysfunction; lowest effective dose should be used. In clinical studies with Edex®, higher minimally effective doses and a higher rate of lack of effect were noted.

Administration

Patent ductus arteriosus (Prostin VR Pediatric®): I.V. continuous infusion into a large vein or alternatively through an umbilical artery catheter placed at the ductal opening; manufacturer recommended maximum concentration for I.V. infusion: 20 mcg/mL

Erectile dysfunction: Use a 1/2 inch, 27- to 30-gauge needle. Inject into the dorsolateral aspect of the proximal third of the penis, avoiding visible veins; alternate side of the penis for injections.

Monitoring Parameters Arterial pressure, respiratory rate, heart rate, temperature, degree of penile pain, length of erection, signs of infection

Dosage Forms Excipient information presented when available (limited, particularly for generics); consult specific product labeling.

Injection, powder for reconstitution:
Caverject Impulse®: 10 mcg, 20 mcg [contains benzyl alcohol (in diluent), lactose 45.4 mg; cartridge; supplied with diluent]
Caverject®: 20 mcg, 40 mcg [contains benzyl alcohol (in diluent), lactose 172 mg; supplied with diluent]
Edex®: 10 mcg, 20 mcg, 40 mcg [contains lactose 51.06 mg; cartridge; supplied with diluent]

Injection, solution: 500 mcg/mL (1 mL)
Prostin VR Pediatric®: 500 mcg/mL (1 mL) [contains dehydrated ethanol]

Pellet, urethral:
Muse®: 125 mcg (1s, 6s); 250 mcg (1s, 6s); 500 mcg (1s, 6s); 1000 mcg (1s, 6s)

◆ **Alrex®** *see* Loteprednol *on page* *1037*
◆ **Alsuma™** *see* SUMAtriptan *on page* *1609*
◆ **Altabax™** *see* Retapamulin *on page* *1475*
◆ **Altacaine** *see* Tetracaine (Ophthalmic) *on page* *1661*
◆ **Altace®** *see* Ramipril *on page* *1459*
◆ **Altachlore [OTC]** *see* Sodium Chloride *on page* *1567*
◆ **Altamist [OTC]** *see* Sodium Chloride *on page* *1567*
◆ **Altaryl [OTC]** *see* DiphenhydrAMINE (Systemic) *on page* *516*

Alteplase (AL te plase)

Brand Names: U.S. Activase®; Cathflo® Activase®

Brand Names: Canada Activase® rt-PA; Cathflo® Activase®

Index Terms Alteplase, Recombinant; Alteplase, Tissue Plasminogen Activator, Recombinant; tPA

Pharmacologic Category Thrombolytic Agent

Use Management of ST-elevation myocardial infarction (STEMI) for the lysis of thrombi in coronary arteries; management of acute ischemic stroke (AIS); management of acute pulmonary embolism (PE)

Recommended criteria for treatment:

STEMI: Chest pain ≥20 minutes duration, onset of chest pain within 12 hours of treatment (or within prior 12-24 hours in patients with continuing ischemic symptoms), and ST-segment elevation >0.1 mV in at least two contiguous precordial leads or two adjacent limb leads on ECG or new or presumably new left bundle branch block (LBBB)

AIS: Onset of stroke symptoms within 3 hours of treatment

Acute pulmonary embolism: Age ≤75 years: Documented massive PE (defined as acute PE with sustained hypotension [SBP <90 mm Hg for ≤15 minutes or requiring inotropic support], persistent profound bradycardia [HR <40 bpm with signs or symptoms of shock], or pulselessness); alteplase may be considered for submassive PE with clinical evidence of adverse prognosis (eg, new hemodynamic instability, worsening respiratory insufficiency, severe RV dysfunction, or major myocardial necrosis) and low risk of bleeding complications. **Note:** Not recommended for patients with low-risk PE (eg, normotensive, no RV dysfunction, normal biomarkers) or submassive acute PE with minor RV dysfunction, minor myocardial necrosis, and no clinical worsening (Jaff, 2011).

Cathflo® Activase®: Restoration of central venous catheter function

Unlabeled Use Acute ischemic stroke presenting 3-4.5 hours after symptom onset; acute peripheral arterial occlusive disease; pediatric parapneumonic effusion (chest tube instillation)

Pregnancy Risk Factor C

Pregnancy Considerations Teratogenic effects were not observed in animal studies. There are no adequate and well-controlled studies in pregnant women. The risk of bleeding may be increased in pregnant women. Use during pregnancy is limited; administer to pregnant women only if the potential benefits justify the risk to the fetus.

Lactation Excretion in breast milk unknown/use caution

Contraindications Hypersensitivity to alteplase or any component of the formulation

Treatment of STEMI or PE: Active internal bleeding; history of CVA; ischemic stroke within 3 months (Antman, 2004; Jaff, 2011); recent intracranial or intraspinal surgery or trauma; intracranial neoplasm; prior intracranial hemorrhage (Antman, 2004; Jaff, 2011); arteriovenous malformation or aneurysm; known bleeding diathesis; severe uncontrolled hypertension (listed as a relative contraindication in STEMI [Antman, 2004] and PE [Jaff, 2011] guidelines); suspected aortic dissection (Antman, 2004; Jaff, 2011); significant closed head or facial trauma (Antman, 2004; Jaff, 2011) within 3 months with radiographic evidence of bony fracture or brain injury (Jaff, 2011)

Treatment of acute ischemic stroke: Evidence of intracranial hemorrhage or suspicion of subarachnoid hemorrhage on pretreatment evaluation; intracranial or intraspinal surgery within 3 months; stroke or serious head injury within 3 months; history of intracranial hemorrhage; uncontrolled hypertension at time of treatment (eg, >185 mm Hg systolic or >110 mm Hg diastolic); seizure at the onset of stroke; active internal bleeding; intracranial neoplasm; arteriovenous malformation or aneurysm; multilobar cerebral infarction (hypodensity >1/3 cerebral hemisphere; Adams, 2007); clinical presentation suggesting post-MI pericarditis; known bleeding diathesis including but not limited to current use of oral anticoagulants producing an INR >1.7, an INR >1.7, administration of heparin within 48 hours preceding the onset of stroke with an elevated aPTT at presentation, platelet count <100,000/mm^3.

Additional exclusion criteria within clinical trials:

Presentation <3 hours after initial symptoms (NINDS, 1995): Time of symptom onset unknown, rapidly improving or minor symptoms, major surgery within 2 weeks, GI or urinary tract hemorrhage within 3 weeks, aggressive treatment required to lower blood pressure, glucose level <50 or >400 mg/dL, and arterial puncture at a noncompressible site or lumbar puncture within 1 week.

Presentation 3-4.5 hours after initial symptoms (ECASS-III; Hacke, 2008): Age >80 years, time of symptom onset unknown, rapidly improving or minor symptoms, current use of anticoagulants regardless of INR, glucose level <50 or >400 mg/dL, aggressive intravenous treatment required to lower blood pressure, major surgery or severe trauma within 3 months, baseline National Institutes of Health Stroke Scale (NIHSS) score >25, and history of both stroke and diabetes.

Warnings/Precautions Concurrent heparin anticoagulation may contribute to bleeding. In the treatment of acute ischemic stroke, concurrent use of anticoagulants was not permitted during the initial 24 hours of the <3 hour window trial (NINDS, 1995). Initiation of SubQ heparin (≤10,000 units) or equivalent doses of low molecular weight heparin for prevention of DVT during the first 24 hours of the 3-4.5 hour window trial was permitted and did not increase the incidence of intracerebral hemorrhage (Hacke, 2008). For acute PE, withhold heparin during the 2-hour infusion period. Monitor all potential bleeding sites. Do not use doses >150 mg; associated with increased risk of intracranial hemorrhage. Intramuscular injections and nonessential handling of the patient should be avoided. Venipunctures should be performed carefully and only when necessary. If arterial puncture is necessary, use an upper extremity vessel that can be manually compressed. If serious bleeding occurs, the infusion of alteplase and heparin should be stopped. Avoid aspirin for 24 hours following administration of alteplase; administration within 24 hours increases the risk of hemorrhagic transformation.

For the following conditions, the risk of bleeding is higher with use of thrombolytics and should be weighed against the benefits of therapy: Recent major surgery (eg, CABG, obstetrical delivery, organ biopsy, pregnancy, previous puncture of noncompressible vessels), prolonged CPR with evidence of thoracic trauma, lumbar puncture within 1 week, cerebrovascular disease, recent gastrointestinal or genitourinary bleeding, recent trauma, hypertension (systolic BP >175 mm Hg and/or diastolic BP >110 mm Hg), high likelihood of left heart thrombus (eg, mitral stenosis with atrial fibrillation), acute pericarditis, subacute bacterial endocarditis, hemostatic defects including ones caused by severe renal or hepatic dysfunction, significant hepatic dysfunction, pregnancy, diabetic hemorrhagic retinopathy or other hemorrhagic ophthalmic conditions, septic thrombophlebitis or occluded AV cannula at seriously infected site, advanced age (eg, >75 years), any other condition in which bleeding constitutes a significant hazard or would be particularly difficult to manage because of location. When treating acute MI or pulmonary embolism, use with caution in patients receiving oral anticoagulants. In the treatment of acute ischemic stroke within 3 hours of stroke symptom onset, the current use of oral anticoagulants producing an INR >1.7 is contraindicated.

Coronary thrombolysis may result in reperfusion arrhythmias. Patients who present **within 3 hours** of stroke symptom onset should be treated with alteplase unless contraindications exist. A longer time window (**3-4.5 hours** after symptom onset) has now been formally evaluated and shown to be safe and efficacious for select individuals (del Zoppo, 2009; Hacke, 2008). Treatment of patients with minor neurological deficit or with rapidly improving symptoms is not recommended. Follow standard management for STEMI while infusing alteplase.

Cathflo® Activase®: When used to restore catheter function, use Cathflo® cautiously in those patients with known or suspected catheter infections. Evaluate catheter for other causes of dysfunction before use. Avoid excessive pressure when instilling into catheter.

Adverse Reactions As with all drugs which may affect hemostasis, bleeding is the major adverse effect associated with alteplase. Hemorrhage may occur at virtually any site. Risk is dependent on multiple variables, including the dosage administered, concurrent use of multiple agents which alter hemostasis, and patient predisposition. Rapid lysis of coronary artery thrombi by thrombolytic agents may be associated with reperfusion-related atrial and/or ventricular arrhythmia. **Note:** Lowest rate of bleeding complications expected with dose used to restore catheter function.

1% to 10%:
- Cardiovascular: Hypotension
- Central nervous system: Fever
- Dermatologic: Bruising (1%)
- Gastrointestinal: GI hemorrhage (5%), nausea, vomiting
- Genitourinary: GU hemorrhage (4%)
- Hematologic: Bleeding (0.5% major, 7% minor: GUSTO trial)
- Local: Bleeding at catheter puncture site (15.3%, accelerated administration)

<1% (Limited to important or life-threatening): Angioedema (orolingual), intracranial hemorrhage (0.4% to 0.87% when dose is ≤100 mg), retroperitoneal hemorrhage, pericardial hemorrhage, gingival hemorrhage, epistaxis, allergic reaction (anaphylaxis, anaphylactoid reactions, laryngeal edema, rash, and urticaria [<0.02%])

Additional cardiovascular events associated **with use in STEMI:** AV block, cardiogenic shock, heart failure, cardiac arrest, recurrent ischemia/infarction, myocardial rupture, electromechanical dissociation, pericardial effusion, pericarditis, mitral regurgitation, cardiac tamponade, thromboembolism, pulmonary edema, asystole, ventricular tachycardia, bradycardia, ruptured intracranial AV malformation, seizure, hemorrhagic bursitis, cholesterol crystal embolization

Additional events associated **with use in pulmonary embolism:** Pulmonary re-embolization, pulmonary edema, pleural effusion, thromboembolism

Additional events associated **with use in stroke:** Cerebral edema, cerebral herniation, seizure, new ischemic stroke

Drug Interactions

Metabolism/Transport Effects None known.

Avoid Concomitant Use There are no known interactions where it is recommended to avoid concomitant use.

Increased Effect/Toxicity

Alteplase may increase the levels/effects of: Anticoagulants; Drotrecogin Alfa (Activated)

The levels/effects of Alteplase may be increased by: Antiplatelet Agents; Herbs (Anticoagulant/Antiplatelet Properties); Nonsteroidal Anti-Inflammatory Agents; Salicylates

Decreased Effect

The levels/effects of Alteplase may be decreased by: Aprotinin; Nitroglycerin

Ethanol/Nutrition/Herb Interactions Herb/Nutraceutical: Avoid cat's claw, dong quai, evening primrose, feverfew, red clover, horse chestnut, garlic, green tea, ginseng, ginkgo (all have additional antiplatelet activity).

Stability

Activase®: The lyophilized product may be stored at room temperature (not to exceed 30°C/86°F), or under refrigeration. Once reconstituted, it should be used within 8 hours. Reconstitution:

50 mg vial: Use accompanying diluent; mix by gentle swirling or slow inversion; do not shake. Vacuum is present in 50 mg vial. Final concentration: 1 mg/mL.

100 mg vial: Use transfer set with accompanying diluent (100 mL vial of sterile water for injection). No vacuum is present in 100 mg vial. Final concentration: 1 mg/mL.

Cathflo® Activase®: Store lyophilized product under refrigeration. The following stability information has also been reported: Intact vials may be stored at room temperature for up to 4 months (Cohen, 2007).

To reconstitute, add 2.2 mL SWFI to vial; do not shake. Final concentration: 1 mg/mL. Once reconstituted, store at 2°C to 30°C (36°F to 86°F) and use within 8 hours. Do not mix other medications into infusion solution.

Mechanism of Action Initiates local fibrinolysis by binding to fibrin in a thrombus (clot) and converts entrapped plasminogen to plasmin

Pharmacodynamics/Kinetics

Duration: >50% present in plasma cleared ~5 minutes after infusion terminated, ~80% cleared within 10 minutes

Excretion: Clearance: Rapidly from circulating plasma (550-650 mL/minute), primarily hepatic; >50% present in plasma is cleared within 5 minutes after the infusion is terminated, ~80% cleared within 10 minutes

Dosage

I.V. (Activase®):

ST-elevation myocardial infarction (STEMI): Front loading dose (weight-based):

Patients >67 kg: Total dose: 100 mg over 1.5 hours; infuse 15 mg over 1-2 minutes. Infuse 50 mg over 30 minutes. Infuse remaining 35 mg of alteplase over the next hour. See **"Note."**

Patients ≤67 kg: Infuse 15 mg I.V. bolus over 1-2 minutes, then infuse 0.75 mg/kg (not to exceed 50 mg) over next 30 minutes, followed by 0.5 mg/kg over next 60 minutes (not to exceed 35 mg). See **"Note."**

Note: All patients should receive 162-325 mg of chewable nonenteric coated aspirin as soon as possible and then daily. Administer concurrently with heparin 60 units/kg bolus (maximum: 4000 units) followed by continuous infusion of 12 units/kg/hour (maximum: 1000 units/hour) and adjust to aPTT target of 50-70 seconds (or 1.5-2 times the upper limit of control).

Acute massive or submassive pulmonary embolism (PE): 100 mg over 2 hours; may be administered as a 10 mg bolus followed by 90 mg over 2 hours as was done in patients with submassive PE (Konstantinides, 2002). **Note:** Not recommended for submassive PE with minor RV dysfunction, minor myocardial necrosis, and no clinical worsening or low-risk PE (ie, normotensive, no RV dysfunction, normal biomarkers) (Jaff, 2011).

Acute ischemic stroke: Within 3 hours of the onset of symptom onset (labeled use) **or** within 3-4.5 hours of symptom onset (unlabeled use; del Zoppo, 2009; Hacke, 2008): **Note:** Initiation of anticoagulants (eg, heparin) or antiplatelet agents (eg, aspirin) within 24 hours after starting alteplase is not recommended; however, initiation of aspirin between 24-48 hours after stroke onset is recommended (Adams, 2007). Initiation of SubQ heparin (≤10,000 units) or equivalent doses of low molecular weight heparin for prevention of DVT during the first 24 hours of the 3-4.5 hour window trial did not increase incidence of intracerebral hemorrhage (Hacke, 2008).

Recommended total dose: 0.9 mg/kg (maximum total dose: 90 mg)

Patients ≤100 kg: Load with 0.09 mg/kg (10% of 0.9 mg/kg dose) as an I.V. bolus over 1 minute, followed by 0.81 mg/kg (90% of 0.9 mg/kg dose) as a continuous infusion over 60 minutes.

Patients >100 kg: Load with 9 mg (10% of 90 mg) as an I.V. bolus over 1 minute, followed by 81 mg (90% of 90 mg) as a continuous infusion over 60 minutes.

Intracatheter: Central venous catheter clearance (Cathflo® Activase® 1 mg/mL):

Patients <30 kg: 110% of the internal lumen volume of the catheter, not to exceed 2 mg/2 mL; retain in catheter for 0.5-2 hours; may instill a second dose if catheter remains occluded

Patients ≥30 kg: 2 mg (2 mL); retain in catheter for 0.5-2 hours; may instill a second dose if catheter remains occluded

Intra-arterial: Acute peripheral arterial occlusive disease (unlabeled use): 0.02-0.1 mg/kg/hour for up to 36 hours Advisory Panel to the Society for Cardiovascular and Interventional Radiology on Thrombolytic Therapy recommendation: ≤2 mg/hour and subtherapeutic heparin (aPTT <1.5 times baseline)

Intrapleural: Parapneumonic effusion (unlabeled use; IDSA/PIDS, 2011): Children >3 months: 4 mg in 40 mL NS, first dose at time of chest tube placement with 1 hour dwell time, repeat every 24 hours for 3 days (total of 3 doses); **or** 0.1 mg/kg (maximum: 3 mg) in 10-30 mL NS, first dose after pigtail catheter (chest tube) placement, 0.75-1 hour dwell time, repeat every 8 hours for 3 days (total of 9 doses)

Administration

Activase®: ST-elevation MI: Accelerated infusion: Bolus dose may be prepared by one of three methods:

1) Removal of 15 mL reconstituted (1 mg/mL) solution from vial
2) Removal of 15 mL from a port on the infusion line after priming
3) Programming an infusion pump to deliver a 15 mL bolus at the initiation of infusion

Activase®: Acute ischemic stroke: Bolus dose (10% of total dose) may be prepared by one of three methods:

1) Removal of the appropriate volume from reconstituted solution (1 mg/mL)
2) Removal of the appropriate volume from a port on the infusion line after priming
3) Programming an infusion pump to deliver the appropriate volume at the initiation of infusion

Note: Remaining dose for STEMI, AIS, or total dose for acute pulmonary embolism may be administered as follows: Any quantity of drug not to be administered to the patient must be removed from vial(s) prior to administration of remaining dose.

50 mg vial: Either PVC bag or glass vial and infusion set

100 mg vial: Insert spike end of the infusion set through the same puncture site created by transfer device and infuse from vial

If further dilution is desired, may be diluted in equal volume of 0.9% sodium chloride or D_5W to yield a final concentration of 0.5 mg/mL.

Cathflo® Activase®: Intracatheter: Instill dose into occluded catheter. Do not force solution into catheter. After a 30-minute dwell time, assess catheter function by attempting to aspirate blood. If catheter is functional, aspirate 4-5 mL of blood in patients ≥10 kg or 3 mL in patients <10 kg to remove Cathflo® Activase® and residual clots. Gently irrigate the catheter with NS. If catheter remains nonfunctional, let Cathflo® Activase® dwell for another 90 minutes (total dwell time: 120 minutes) and reassess function. If catheter function is not restored, a second dose may be instilled.

Pediatric parapneumonic effusion (unlabeled use): Intrapleural: Instill dose into chest tube at time of chest tube placement and clamp drain. After 1 hour dwell time, release clamp and connect chest tube to continuous suction (-20 cm H_2O) (St. Peter, 2009); or instill dose into chest tube after pigtail catheter (chest tube) placement and clamp drain. After 0.75-1 hour dwell time, release clamp and connect chest tube to continuous suction (-20 to -25 cm H_2O) (Hawkins, 2004).

Monitoring Parameters

Acute ischemic stroke: In addition to monitoring for bleeding complications, the 2007 AHA/ASA Guidelines for the early management of acute ischemic stroke recommends the following:

Perform neurological assessments every 15 minutes during infusion and every 30 minutes thereafter for the next 6 hours, then hourly until 24 hours after treatment.

If severe headache, acute hypertension, nausea, or vomiting occurs, discontinue the infusion and obtain emergency CT scan.

Measure BP every 15 minutes for the first 2 hours then every 30 minutes for the next 6 hours, then hourly until 24 hours after initiation of alteplase. Increase frequency if a systolic BP is ≥180 mm Hg or if a diastolic BP is ≥105 mm Hg; administer antihypertensive medications to maintain BP at or below these levels.

Obtain a follow-up CT scan at 24 hours before starting anticoagulants or antiplatelet agents.

Central venous catheter clearance: Assess catheter function by attempting to aspirate blood.

ST-elevation MI: Assess for evidence of cardiac reperfusion through resolution of chest pain, resolution of baseline ECG changes, preserved left ventricular function, cardiac enzyme washout phenomenon, and/or the appearance of reperfusion arrhythmias; assess for bleeding potential through clinical evidence of GI bleeding, hematuria, gingival bleeding, fibrinogen levels, fibrinogen degradation products, prothrombin times, and partial thromboplastin times.

Reference Range Not routinely measured; literature supports therapeutic levels of 0.52-1.8 mcg/mL

Fibrinogen: 200-400 mg/dL

Activated partial thromboplastin time (aPTT): 22.5-38.7 seconds

Prothrombin time (PT): 10.9-12.2 seconds

Test Interactions Altered results of coagulation and fibrinolytic agents

Dosage Forms Excipient information presented when available (limited, particularly for generics); consult specific product labeling.

Injection, powder for reconstitution [recombinant]:

Activase®: 50 mg [29 million int. units], 100 mg [58 million int. units] [contains polysorbate 80; derived from or manufactured using Chinese hamster ovary cells; supplied with diluent]

Cathflo® Activase®: 2 mg [contains polysorbate 80; derived from or manufactured using Chinese hamster ovary cells]

- ◆ **Alteplase, Recombinant** *see* Alteplase *on page 76*
- ◆ **Alteplase, Tissue Plasminogen Activator, Recombinant** *see* Alteplase *on page 76*
- ◆ **ALternaGel® [OTC]** *see* Aluminum Hydroxide *on page 79*
- ◆ **Alti-Clindamycin (Can)** *see* Clindamycin (Systemic) *on page 378*
- ◆ **Alti-Clonazepam (Can)** *see* ClonazePAM *on page 390*
- ◆ **Alti-Desipramine (Can)** *see* Desipramine *on page 473*
- ◆ **Alti-Doxazosin (Can)** *see* Doxazosin *on page 548*
- ◆ **Alti-Flurbiprofen (Can)** *see* Flurbiprofen (Systemic) *on page 737*
- ◆ **Alti-Fluvoxamine (Can)** *see* FluvoxaMINE *on page 746*
- ◆ **Alti-Ipratropium (Can)** *see* Ipratropium (Nasal) *on page 924*
- ◆ **Alti-MPA (Can)** *see* MedroxyPROGESTERone *on page 1058*
- ◆ **Alti-Nadolol (Can)** *see* Nadolol *on page 1169*
- ◆ **Alti-Nortriptyline (Can)** *see* Nortriptyline *on page 1220*
- ◆ **Alti-Sulfasalazine (Can)** *see* SulfaSALAzine *on page 1605*
- ◆ **Altoprev®** *see* Lovastatin *on page 1038*

Aluminum Hydroxide

(a LOO mi num hye DROKS ide)

Brand Names: U.S. ALternaGel® [OTC]; Dermagran® [OTC]

Brand Names: Canada Amphojel®; Basaljel®

Pharmacologic Category Antacid; Antidote; Protectant, Topical

Use Treatment of hyperacidity; hyperphosphatemia; temporary protection of minor cuts, scrapes, and burns

Pregnancy Risk Factor C

Dosage

Oral:

Hyperphosphatemia:

Children: 50-150 mg/kg/24 hours in divided doses every 4-6 hours, titrate dosage to maintain serum phosphorus within normal range

Adults: Initial: 300-600 mg 3 times/day with meals

Antacid: Adults: 600-1200 mg between meals and at bedtime

Topical: Apply to affected area as needed; reapply at least every 12 hours

Dosage adjustment in renal impairment: Aluminum may accumulate in renal impairment.

Additional Information Complete prescribing information for this medication should be consulted for additional detail.

Dosage Forms Excipient information presented when available (limited, particularly for generics); consult specific product labeling. [DSC] = Discontinued product

Ointment, topical:

Dermagran®: 0.275% (113 g)

Suspension, oral: 320 mg/5 mL (30 mL, 355 mL [DSC], 360 mL, 473 mL, 480 mL); 600 mg/5 mL (355 mL)

ALternaGel®: 600 mg/5 mL (360 mL) [sugar free]

Aluminum Hydroxide and Magnesium Carbonate

(a LOO mi num hye DROKS ide & mag NEE zhum KAR bun nate)

Brand Names: U.S. Acid Gone Extra Strength [OTC]; Acid Gone [OTC]; Gaviscon® Extra Strength [OTC]; Gaviscon® Liquid [OTC]; Genaton™ [OTC] [DSC]

Index Terms Magnesium Carbonate and Aluminum Hydroxide

Pharmacologic Category Antacid

Use Temporary relief of symptoms associated with gastric acidity

Dosage Oral: Adults:

Liquid:

Gaviscon® Regular Strength: 15-30 mL 4 times/day after meals and at bedtime

Gaviscon® Extra Strength: 15-30 mL 4 times/day after meals

Tablet (Gaviscon® Extra Strength): Chew 2-4 tablets 4 times/day

Dosage adjustment in renal impairment: Aluminum and/or magnesium may accumulate in renal impairment.

Additional Information Complete prescribing information for this medication should be consulted for additional detail.

Dosage Forms Excipient information presented when available (limited, particularly for generics); consult specific product labeling. [DSC] = Discontinued product

Liquid:

Acid Gone: Aluminum hydroxide 31.7 mg and magnesium carbonate 119.3 mg per 5 mL (360 mL)

Gaviscon®: Aluminum hydroxide 31.7 mg and magnesium carbonate 119.3 mg per 5 mL (355 mL) [contains sodium 0.57 mEq/5 mL and benzyl alcohol; cool mint flavor]

Gaviscon® Extra Strength: Aluminum hydroxide 84.6 mg and magnesium carbonate 79.1 mg per 5 mL (355 mL) [contains sodium 0.9 mEq/5 mL and benzyl alcohol; cool mint flavor]

Genaton™: Aluminum hydroxide 31.7 mg and magnesium carbonate 119.3 mg per 5 mL (360 mL) [DSC]

Tablet, chewable:

Acid Gone Extra Strength: Aluminum hydroxide 160 mg and magnesium carbonate 105 mg

Gaviscon® Extra Strength: Aluminum hydroxide 160 mg and magnesium carbonate 105 mg [contains sodium 19 mg/tablet (1.3 mEq/tablet); cherry and original flavors]

Aluminum Hydroxide and Magnesium Hydroxide

(a LOO mi num hye DROKS ide & mag NEE zhum hye DROK side)

Brand Names: U.S. Alamag [OTC]; Mag-Al Ultimate [OTC]; Mag-Al [OTC]

Brand Names: Canada Diovol®; Diovol® Ex; Gelusil® Extra Strength; Mylanta™

Index Terms Magnesium Hydroxide and Aluminum Hydroxide

Pharmacologic Category Antacid

Use Antacid for symptoms related to hyperacidity associated with heartburn, hiatal hernia, upset stomach, peptic ulcer, peptic esophagitis, or gastritis

Dosage Oral: Children ≥12 years and Adults: OTC labeling:

Liquid (aluminum hydroxide 200 mg and magnesium hydroxide 200 mg per 5 mL): 10-20 mL 4 times/day (maximum:80 mL/day)

Suspension (aluminum hydroxide 500 mg and magnesium hydroxide 500 mg per 5 mL): 10-20 mL 4 times/day, between meals and at bedtime (maximum: 45 mL/day)

Tablet (aluminum hydroxide 300 mg and magnesium hydroxide 150 mg): 1-2 tablets after meals or at bedtime, or as needed (maximum: 16 tablets/day)

Dosage adjustment in renal impairment: Aluminum and/or magnesium may accumulate in severe renal impairment.

Additional Information Complete prescribing information for this medication should be consulted for additional detail.

Dosage Forms Excipient information presented when available (limited, particularly for generics); consult specific product labeling. [DSC] = Discontinued product

Liquid, oral:

Mag-Al: Aluminum hydroxide 200 mg and magnesium hydroxide 200 mg per 5 mL (30 mL) [dye free, ethanol free, sugar free; contains propylene glycol, sodium 4 mg/5 mL; peppermint flavor]

Suspension, oral:

Mag-Al Ultimate: Aluminum hydroxide 500 mg and magnesium hydroxide 500 mg per 5 mL (20 mL) [contains propylene glycol, sodium 4 mg/5 mL; peppermint flavor]

Tablet, chewable:

Alamag: Aluminum hydroxide 300 mg and magnesium hydroxide 150 mg [contains phenylalanine 2.63 mg; wild cherry flavor]

Aluminum Hydroxide and Magnesium Trisilicate

(a LOO mi num hye DROKS ide & mag NEE zhum trye SIL i kate)

Brand Names: U.S. Gaviscon® Tablet [OTC]

Index Terms Magnesium Trisilicate and Aluminum Hydroxide

Pharmacologic Category Antacid

Use Temporary relief of hyperacidity

Pregnancy Risk Factor C

Dosage Oral: Adults: Chew 2-4 tablets 4 times/day or as directed by healthcare provider

Dosage adjustment in renal impairment: Aluminum and/or magnesium may accumulate in renal impairment.

Additional Information Complete prescribing information for this medication should be consulted for additional detail.

Dosage Forms Excipient information presented when available (limited, particularly for generics); consult specific product labeling. [DSC] = Discontinued product

Tablet, chewable: Aluminum hydroxide 80 mg and magnesium trisilicate 20 mg

Gaviscon®: Aluminum hydroxide 80 mg and magnesium trisilicate 20 mg [contains sodium 0.8 mEq/tablet; butterscotch flavor]

Aluminum Hydroxide, Magnesium Hydroxide, and Simethicone

(a LOO mi num hye DROKS ide, mag NEE zhum hye DROKS ide, & sye METH i kone)

Brand Names: U.S. Alamag Plus [OTC]; Aldroxicon I [OTC]; Aldroxicon II [OTC]; Almacone Double Strength® [OTC]; Almacone® [OTC]; Gelusil® [OTC]; Maalox® Advanced Maximum Strength [OTC]; Maalox® Advanced Regular Strength [OTC]; Mi-Acid Maximum Strength [OTC] [DSC]; Mi-Acid [OTC]; Mintox Plus [OTC]; Mylanta® Classic Maximum Strength Liquid [OTC]; Mylanta® Classic Regular Strength Liquid [OTC]; Rulox [OTC]

Brand Names: Canada Diovol Plus®; Gelusil®; Mylanta® Double Strength; Mylanta® Extra Strength; Mylanta® Regular Strength

Index Terms Magnesium Hydroxide, Aluminum Hydroxide, and Simethicone; Simethicone, Aluminum Hydroxide, and Magnesium Hydroxide

Pharmacologic Category Antacid; Antiflatulent

Use Temporary relief of hyperacidity associated with gas; may also be used for indications associated with other antacids

Pregnancy Risk Factor C

Dosage Oral: Adults: 10-20 mL or 2-4 tablets 4-6 times/day between meals and at bedtime; may be used every hour for severe symptoms

Dosage adjustment in renal impairment: Aluminum and/or magnesium may accumulate in renal impairment.

Additional Information Complete prescribing information for this medication should be consulted for additional detail.

Dosage Forms Excipient information presented when available (limited, particularly for generics); consult specific product labeling. [DSC] = Discontinued product

Liquid, oral: Aluminum hydroxide 200 mg, magnesium hydroxide 200 mg, and simethicone 20 mg per 5 mL (360 mL); aluminum hydroxide 400 mg, magnesium hydroxide 400 mg, and simethicone 40 mg per 5 mL (360 mL)

Aldroxicon I: Aluminum hydroxide 200 mg, magnesium hydroxide 200 mg, and simethicone 20 mg per 5 mL (30 mL)

Aldroxicon II: Aluminum hydroxide 400 mg, magnesium hydroxide 400 mg, and simethicone 40 mg per 5 mL (30 mL)

Almacone®: Aluminum hydroxide 200 mg, magnesium hydroxide 200 mg, and simethicone 20 mg per 5 mL (360 mL)

Almacone Double Strength®: Aluminum hydroxide 400 mg, magnesium hydroxide 400 mg, and simethicone 40 mg per 5 mL (360 mL)

Maalox® Advanced Maximum Strength: Aluminum hydroxide 400 mg, magnesium hydroxide 400 mg, and simethicone 40 mg per 5 mL (355 mL, 769 mL) [contains magnesium 167 mg/5 mL; cherry flavor]
Maalox® Advanced Maximum Strength: Aluminum hydroxide 400 mg, magnesium hydroxide 400 mg, and simethicone 40 mg per 5 mL (355 mL, 769 mL) [contains magnesium 167 mg/5 mL; lemon flavor]
Maalox® Advanced Maximum Strength: Aluminum hydroxide 400 mg, magnesium hydroxide 400 mg, and simethicone 40 mg per 5 mL (355 mL) [contains magnesium 167 mg/5 mL; mint flavor]
Maalox® Advanced Maximum Strength: Aluminum hydroxide 400 mg, magnesium hydroxide 400 mg, and simethicone 40 mg per 5 mL (355 mL) [contains magnesium 167 mg/5 mL; vanilla crème flavor]
Maalox® Advanced Regular Strength: Aluminum hydroxide 200 mg, magnesium hydroxide 200 mg, and simethicone 20 mg per 5 mL (360 mL, 780 mL) [contains magnesium 75 mg/5 mL, potassium 5 mg/5 mL, propylene glycol; mint flavor]
Mi-Acid: Aluminum hydroxide 200 mg, magnesium hydroxide 200 mg, and simethicone 20 mg per 5 mL (360 mL)
Mi-Acid Maximum Strength: Aluminum hydroxide 400 mg, magnesium hydroxide 400 mg, and simethicone 40 mg per 5 mL (360 mL)
Mylanta® Classic Maximum Strength: Aluminum hydroxide 400 mg, magnesium hydroxide 400 mg, and simethicone 40 mg per 5 mL (360 mL, 720 mL) [original, cherry, orange creme, and mint flavors]
Mylanta® Classic Regular Strength: Aluminum hydroxide 200 mg, magnesium hydroxide 200 mg, and simethicone 20 mg per 5 mL (360 mL) [original and mint flavors]

Suspension, oral: Aluminum hydroxide 225 mg, magnesium hydroxide 200 mg, and simethicone 25 mg per 5 mL (360 mL)
Rulox: Aluminum hydroxide 200 mg, magnesium hydroxide 200 mg, and simethicone 25 mg per 5 mL (355 mL) [contains magnesium 85 mg/5 mL; mint flavor]

Tablet, chewable: Aluminum hydroxide 200 mg, magnesium hydroxide 200 mg, and simethicone 25 mg
Alamag Plus: Aluminum hydroxide 200 mg, magnesium hydroxide 200 mg, and simethicone 25 mg [contains magnesium 83 mg/tablet, phenyalanine 2.6 mg/tablet; cherry flavor]
Almacone®: Aluminum hydroxide 200 mg, magnesium hydroxide 200 mg, and simethicone 20 mg [dye free; contains magnesium 82 mg/tablet; peppermint flavor]
Gelusil®: Aluminum hydroxide 200 mg, magnesium hydroxide 200 mg, and simethicone 25 mg [peppermint flavor]
Mintox Plus: Aluminum hydroxide 200 mg, magnesium hydroxide 200 mg, and simethicone 25 mg [lemon crème flavor]

◆ **Aluminum Sucrose Sulfate, Basic** *see* Sucralfate *on page 1598*

Aluminum Sulfate and Calcium Acetate

(a LOO mi num SUL fate & KAL see um AS e tate)

Brand Names: U.S. Domeboro® [OTC]; Gordon Boro-Packs [OTC]; Pedi-Boro® [OTC]
Index Terms Calcium Acetate and Aluminum Sulfate
Pharmacologic Category Topical Skin Product
Use Astringent wet dressing for relief of inflammatory conditions of the skin; reduce weeping that may occur in dermatitis
Dosage Topical: Soak affected area in the solution 2-4 times/day for 15-30 minutes or apply wet dressing soaked in the solution for more extended periods; rewet dressing with solution 2-4 times/day every 15-30 minutes
Additional Information Complete prescribing information for this medication should be consulted for additional detail.
Dosage Forms Excipient information presented when available (limited, particularly for generics); consult specific product labeling.
Powder, for topical solution:
Domeboro®: Aluminum sulfate 1191 mg and calcium acetate 839 mg per packet (12s, 100s)
Gordon Boro-Packs: Aluminum sulfate 49% and calcium acetate 51% per packet (100s)
Pedi-Boro®: Aluminum sulfate 1191 mg and calcium acetate 839 mg per packet (12s, 100s)

◆ **Alupent** *see* Metaproterenol *on page 1085*

◆ **Alvesco®** *see* Ciclesonide (Systemic) *on page 354*

Alvimopan (al VI moe pan)

Brand Names: U.S. Entereg®
Index Terms ADL-2698; LY246736
Pharmacologic Category Gastrointestinal Agent, Miscellaneous; Opioid Antagonist, Peripherally-Acting
Use Accelerate the time to upper and lower GI recovery following partial large or small bowel resection surgery with primary anastomosis
Pregnancy Risk Factor B
Pregnancy Considerations Animal studies have not shown teratogenic effects to the fetus. However, there are no adequate and well-controlled studies in pregnant women; use during pregnancy only if clearly needed.
Lactation Excretion in breast milk unknown/use caution
Prescribing and Access Restrictions As a requirement of the REMS program, access to this medication is restricted. Only hospitals enrolled in the ENTEREG Access Support and Education (E.A.S.E.™) Program may administer this medication. Hospital staff must be educated on the need to limit to short-term (no more than 15 doses) and inpatient use. Hospitals may contact the E.A.S.E.™ program at 1-866-423-6567 (1-866-4ADOLOR).
Contraindications Patients who have taken therapeutic doses of opioids for more than 7 consecutive days immediately prior to alvimopan
Warnings/Precautions [U.S. Boxed Warning]: For short-term (≤15 doses) hospital use only. Only hospitals that have registered through the ENTEREG Access Support and Education (E.A.S.E.™) Program and met all requirements may use. It will not be dispensed to patients who have been discharged from the hospital. Use not recommended in patients with complete bowel obstruction. Use with caution in patients with hepatic or renal impairment; use not recommended in patients with severe hepatic impairment or ESRD. Use with caution is patients recently exposed to opioids; may be more sensitive to gastrointestinal adverse effects (eg, abdominal pain, diarrhea, nausea and vomiting). Contraindicated in patients who have received therapeutic opioids for >7 consecutive days immediately prior to use. A trend towards an increased incidence of MI was observed in alvimopan (low dose) treated patients compared to placebo in a 12-month study in patients treated with opioids for chronic pain. MI was generally observed more frequently in the initial 1-4 months of treatment. Other studies have not observed this trend and a causal relationship has not been found. Patients of Japanese descent should be monitored closely for gastrointestinal side effects (eg, abdominal pain, cramping, diarrhea) due to possibility of greater drug exposure; discontinue use if side effects occur.

Adverse Reactions Note: Incidence reported limited to bowel resection patients only.

1% to 10%:
Endocrine & metabolic: Hypokalemia (10%)
Gastrointestinal: Dyspepsia (7%)
Genitourinary: Urinary retention (3%)
Hematologic: Anemia (5%)
Neuromuscular & skeletal: Back pain (3%)

Drug Interactions

Metabolism/Transport Effects None known.

Avoid Concomitant Use There are no known interactions where it is recommended to avoid concomitant use.

Increased Effect/Toxicity
The levels/effects of Alvimopan may be increased by: Analgesics (Opioid)

Decreased Effect There are no known significant interactions involving a decrease in effect.

Ethanol/Nutrition/Herb Interactions Food: When administered with a high-fat meal, extent and rate of absorption may be reduced (C_{max} and AUC decreased by ~38% and 21%, respectively).

Stability Store at 25°C (77°F); excursions permitted to 15°C to 30°C (59°F to 86°F).

Mechanism of Action An opioid receptor antagonist which blocks opioid binding at the mu receptor; alvimopan has restricted ability to cross the blood-brain barrier at therapeutic doses. It selectively and competitively binds to the GI tract mu opioid receptors and antagonizes the peripheral effects of opioids on gastrointestinal motility and secretion. Does not affect opioid analgesic effects or induce opioid withdrawal symptoms.

Pharmacodynamics/Kinetics
Distribution: V_d: 20-40 L
Protein binding: Parent drug: 80%; metabolite: 94% (both primarily to albumin)
Metabolism: Hydrolyzed to an amide hydrolysis compound (active metabolite) by gut microflora; further metabolism of active metabolite to glucuronide conjugates and other minor metabolites.
Bioavailability: ~6% (range: 1% to 19%)
Half-life elimination: 10-17 hours
Time to peak, plasma: Parent drug: ~2 hours; Metabolite: 36 hours
Excretion: Urine (~35% as unchanged drug and metabolites); feces (via biliary excretion)

Dosage Note: For hospital use only
Oral: Adults:
Initial: 12 mg administered 30 minutes to 5 hours prior to surgery
Maintenance: 12 mg twice daily beginning the day after surgery for a maximum of 7 days or until discharged from hospital (maximum total treatment: 15 doses)

Dosage adjustment in renal impairment:
Mild-to-severe impairment: No adjustment needed; use caution
ESRD: Use not recommended

Dosage adjustment in hepatic impairment:
Mild-to-moderate impairment (Child-Pugh class A and B): No adjustment needed; use caution
Severe impairment (Child-Pugh class C): Use not recommended

Dietary Considerations Take with or without food; high-fat meals may decrease the rate and extent of absorption

Administration Patient must be hospitalized. Initial dose should be administered 30 minutes to 5 hours prior to surgery. May be administered with or without food.

Dosage Forms Excipient information presented when available (limited, particularly for generics); consult specific product labeling.
Capsule, oral:
Entereg®: 12 mg

Amantadine (a MAN ta deen)

Brand Names: Canada Endantadine®; Mylan-Amantadine; PMS-Amantadine; Symmetrel®

Index Terms Adamantanamine Hydrochloride; Amantadine Hydrochloride; Symmetrel

Pharmacologic Category Anti-Parkinson's Agent, Dopamine Agonist; Antiviral Agent; Antiviral Agent, Adamantane

Additional Appendix Information
Antiparkinsonian Agents *on page 1879*

Use Prophylaxis and treatment of influenza A viral infection (per manufacturer labeling; also refer to current ACIP guidelines for recommendations during current flu season); treatment of parkinsonism; treatment of drug-induced extrapyramidal symptoms

Pregnancy Risk Factor C

Pregnancy Considerations Teratogenic effects were observed in animal studies and in case reports in humans.

Influenza infection may be more severe in pregnant women. Untreated influenza infection is associated with an increased risk of adverse events to the fetus and an increased risk of complications or death to the mother. Oseltamivir and zanamivir are currently recommended for the treatment or prophylaxis influenza in pregnant women and women up to 2 weeks postpartum. Antiviral agents are currently recommended as an adjunct to vaccination and should not be used as a substitute for vaccination in pregnant women (consult current CDC guidelines).

Healthcare providers are encouraged to refer women exposed to influenza vaccine, or who have taken an antiviral medication during pregnancy to the Vaccines and Medications in Pregnancy Surveillance System (VAMPSS) by contacting The Organization of Teratology Information Specialists (OTIS) at (877) 311-8972

Lactation Enters breast milk/not recommended

Contraindications Hypersensitivity to amantadine or any component of the formulation

Warnings/Precautions May cause CNS depression, which may impair physical or mental abilities; patients must be cautioned about performing tasks which require mental alertness (eg, operating machinery or driving). There have been reports of suicidal ideation/attempt in patients with and without a history of psychiatric illness. Use with caution in patients with liver disease, a history of recurrent and eczematoid dermatitis, uncontrolled psychosis or severe psychoneurosis, seizures and in those receiving CNS stimulant drugs; reduce dose in renal disease; when treating Parkinson's disease, do not discontinue abruptly. In many patients, the therapeutic benefits of amantadine are limited to a few months. Abrupt discontinuation may cause agitation, anxiety, delirium, delusions, depression, hallucinations, paranoia, parkinsonian crisis, slurred speech, or stupor. Upon discontinuation of amantadine therapy, gradually taper dose. Elderly patients may be more susceptible to the CNS effects (using 2 divided daily doses may minimize this effect); may require dosage reductions based on renal function. Use with caution in patients with HF, peripheral edema, or orthostatic hypotension; dosage reduction may be required. Avoid in untreated angle closure glaucoma.

Dopamine agonists have been associated with compulsive behaviors and/or loss of impulse control, which has manifested as pathological gambling, libido increases (hypersexuality), and/or binge eating. Causality has not been established, and controversy exists as to whether this phenomenon is related to the underlying disease, prior behaviors/addictions, and/or drug therapy. Dose reduction or discontinuation of therapy has been reported to reverse these behaviors in some, but not all cases. Risk for melanoma development is increased in Parkinson's disease patients; drug causation or factors contributing to risk have not been established. Patients should be monitored closely and periodic skin examinations should be performed.

Due to increased resistance, the ACIP has recommended that rimantadine and amantadine no longer be used for the treatment or prophylaxis of influenza A in the United States until susceptibility has been re-established; consult current guidelines. Safety and efficacy have not been established in children <1 year of age.

Adverse Reactions

1% to 10%:

Cardiovascular: Orthostatic hypotension, peripheral edema

Central nervous system: Agitation, anxiety, ataxia, confusion, delirium, depression, dizziness, dream abnormality, fatigue, hallucinations, headache, insomnia, irritability, lightheadedness, nervousness, somnolence

Dermatologic: Livedo reticularis

Gastrointestinal: Anorexia, constipation, diarrhea, nausea, xerostomia

Respiratory: Dry nose

<1% (Limited to important or life-threatening): Aggressive behavior, agranulocytosis, alkaline phosphatase increased, allergic reaction, ALT increased, AST increased, amnesia, anaphylaxis, arrhythmia, bilirubin increased, BUN increased, cardiac arrest, coma, CPK increased, creatinine increased, delusions, diaphoresis, dysphagia, dyspnea, eczematoid dermatitis, euphoria, GGT increased, heart failure, hyperkinesis, LDH increased, leukopenia, mania, neutropenia, neuroleptic malignant syndrome (NMS; associated with dosage reduction or abrupt withdrawal of amantadine), oculogyric episodes, paresthesia, photosensitivity, psychosis, pulmonary edema, rash, respiratory failure (acute), seizures, suicidal ideation, suicide, urinary retention, withdrawal reactions (may include delirium, hallucinations, and psychosis), visual disturbances

Reported with dopamine agonists: Impulsive/compulsive behaviors (eg, pathological gambling, hypersexuality, binge eating)

Drug Interactions

Metabolism/Transport Effects None known.

Avoid Concomitant Use There are no known interactions where it is recommended to avoid concomitant use.

Increased Effect/Toxicity

Amantadine may increase the levels/effects of: Glycopyrrolate; Trimethoprim

The levels/effects of Amantadine may be increased by: Antipsychotics (Typical); MAO Inhibitors; Methylphenidate; Trimethoprim

Decreased Effect

Amantadine may decrease the levels/effects of: Antipsychotics (Typical); Influenza Virus Vaccine (Live/Attenuated)

The levels/effects of Amantadine may be decreased by: Antipsychotics (Atypical); Metoclopramide

Ethanol/Nutrition/Herb Interactions Ethanol: Avoid ethanol (may increase CNS adverse effects).

Stability Store at 25°C (77°F); excursions permitted to 15°C to 30°C (59°F to 86°F).

Mechanism of Action As an antiviral, blocks the uncoating of influenza A virus preventing penetration of virus into host; antiparkinsonian activity may be due to its blocking the reuptake of dopamine into presynaptic neurons or by increasing dopamine release from presynaptic fibers

Pharmacodynamics/Kinetics

Onset of action: Antidyskinetic: Within 48 hours

Absorption: Well absorbed

Distribution: V_d: Normal: 1.5-6.1 L/kg; Renal failure: 5.1 ± 0.2 L/kg; in saliva, tear film, and nasal secretions; in animals, tissue (especially lung) concentrations higher than serum concentrations; crosses blood-brain barrier

Protein binding: Normal renal function: ~67%; Hemodialysis: ~59%

Metabolism: Not appreciable; small amounts of an acetyl metabolite identified

Bioavailability: 86% to 90%

Half-life elimination: Normal renal function: 16 ± 6 hours (9-31 hours); Healthy, older (≥60 years) males: 29 hours (range: 20-41 hours); End-stage renal disease: 7-10 days

Time to peak, plasma: 2-4 hours

Excretion: Urine (80% to 90% unchanged) by glomerular filtration and tubular secretion

Dosage Oral:

Children: Influenza A treatment/prophylaxis: **Note:** Due to issues of resistance, amantadine is no longer recommended for the treatment or prophylaxis of influenza A. Please refer to the current ACIP recommendations.

Influenza A treatment:

1-9 years: 5 mg/kg/day in 2 divided doses (manufacturers range: 4.4-8.8 mg/kg/day); maximum dose: 150 mg/day

≥10 years and <40 kg: 5 mg/kg/day in 2 divided doses (CDC, 2011)

≥10 years and ≥40 kg: 100 mg twice daily (CDC, 2011)

Note: Initiate within 24-48 hours after onset of symptoms; continue for 24-48 hours after symptom resolution (duration of therapy is generally 3-5 days)

Influenza A prophylaxis: Refer to "Influenza A treatment" dosing. **Note:** Continue prophylaxis throughout the peak influenza activity in the community or throughout the entire influenza season in patients who cannot be vaccinated. Development of immunity following vaccination takes ~2 weeks; amantadine therapy should be considered for high-risk patients from the time of vaccination until immunity has developed. For children <9 years receiving influenza vaccine for the first time, amantadine prophylaxis should continue for 6 weeks (4 weeks after the first dose and 2 weeks after the second dose).

Adults:

Drug-induced extrapyramidal symptoms: 100 mg twice daily; may increase to 300 mg/day in divided doses, if needed

Parkinson's disease: Usual dose: 100 mg twice daily as monotherapy; may increase to 400 mg/day in divided doses, if needed, with close monitoring. **Note:** Patients with a serious concomitant illness or those receiving high doses of other anti-parkinson drugs should be started at 100 mg/day; may increase to 100 mg twice daily, if needed, after one to several weeks.

Influenza A treatment/prophylaxis: **Note:** Due to issues of resistance, amantadine is no longer recommended for the treatment or prophylaxis of influenza A. Please refer to the current ACIP recommendations. The following is based on the manufacturer's labeling:

Influenza A treatment: 200 mg once daily **or** 100 mg twice daily (may be preferred to reduce CNS effects); **Note:** Initiate within 24-48 hours after onset of symptoms; continue for 24-48 hours after symptom resolution (duration of therapy is generally 3-5 days).

Influenza A prophylaxis: 200 mg once daily **or** 100 mg twice daily (may be preferred to reduce CNS effects). **Note:** Continue prophylaxis throughout the peak influenza activity in the community or throughout the entire influenza season in patients who cannot be vaccinated. Development of immunity following vaccination takes ~2 weeks; amantadine therapy should be considered for high-risk patients from the time of vaccination until immunity has developed.

Elderly (≥65 years): Adjust dose based on renal function; some patients tolerate the drug better when it is given in 2 divided daily doses (to avoid adverse neurologic reactions).

Influenza A treatment/prophylaxis: 100 mg once daily

Dosing interval in renal impairment:

Cl_{cr} 30-50 mL/minute: Administer 200 mg on day 1, then 100 mg/day

Cl_{cr} 15-29 mL/minute: Administer 200 mg on day 1, then 100 mg on alternate days

Cl_{cr} <15 mL/minute: Administer 200 mg every 7 days

Hemodialysis: Administer 200 mg every 7 days

Peritoneal dialysis: No supplemental dose is needed

Continuous arteriovenous or venous-venous hemofiltration: No supplemental dose is needed

Monitoring Parameters Renal function, Parkinson's symptoms, mental status, influenza symptoms, blood pressure

Test Interactions May interfere with urine detection of amphetamines/methamphetamines (false-positive).

Dosage Forms Excipient information presented when available (limited, particularly for generics); consult specific product labeling.

Capsule, oral, as hydrochloride: 100 mg

Capsule, softgel, oral, as hydrochloride: 100 mg

Solution, oral, as hydrochloride: 50 mg/5 mL (473 mL)

Syrup, oral, as hydrochloride: 50 mg/5 mL (10 mL, 473 mL, 480 mL)

Tablet, oral, as hydrochloride: 100 mg

- **Amantadine Hydrochloride** *see* Amantadine *on page* 82
- **Amaryl®** *see* Glimepiride *on page* 793
- **Amatine® (Can)** *see* Midodrine *on page* 1130
- **Ambi 10PEH/400GFN [OTC]** *see* Guaifenesin and Phenylephrine *on page* 812
- **Ambien®** *see* Zolpidem *on page* 1826
- **Ambien CR®** *see* Zolpidem *on page* 1826
- **Ambifed [OTC] [DSC]** *see* Guaifenesin and Pseudoephedrine *on page* 813
- **Ambifed DM** *see* Guaifenesin, Pseudoephedrine, and Dextromethorphan *on page* 814
- **Ambifed-G [OTC]** *see* Guaifenesin and Pseudoephedrine *on page* 813
- **Ambifed-G DM** *see* Guaifenesin, Pseudoephedrine, and Dextromethorphan *on page* 814
- **AmBisome®** *see* Amphotericin B (Liposomal) *on page* 113

Ambrisentan (am bri SEN tan)

Brand Names: U.S. Letairis®

Brand Names: Canada Volibris®

Index Terms BSF208075

Pharmacologic Category Endothelin Antagonist; Vasodilator

Use Treatment of pulmonary artery hypertension (PAH) World Health Organization (WHO) Group I to improve exercise ability and decrease the rate of clinical deterioration

Pregnancy Risk Factor X

Pregnancy Considerations [U.S. Boxed Warning]: Use in pregnancy is contraindicated. Based on animal studies, ambrisentan is likely to produce major birth defects if used by pregnant women. Pregnancy must be excluded prior to initiation of therapy and follow-up pregnancy tests should be obtained monthly. Two reliable methods of contraception must be used throughout treatment and for one month after stopping treatment unless the patient has undergone a tubal ligation or the insertion of an intrauterine device (Copper T 380A or LNg 20). No other contraceptive measures are required for these patients.

Lactation Excretion in breast milk unknown/not recommended

Prescribing and Access Restrictions As a requirement of the REMS program, access to this medication is restricted. Ambrisentan (Letairis®) is only available through Letairis Education and Access Program (LEAP). Only prescribers and pharmacies registered with LEAP may prescribe and dispense ambrisentan. Further information may be obtained from the manufacturer, Gilead Sciences, Inc (1-866-664-5327).

Medication Guide Available Yes

Contraindications Pregnancy

Canadian labeling: Additional contraindications (not in U.S. labeling): Hypersensitivity to ambrisentan or any component of the formulation

Warnings/Precautions [U.S. Boxed Warning]: Use in pregnancy is contraindicated; may cause birth defects. Exclude pregnancy prior to initiation of therapy and monthly thereafter. Two reliable methods of contraception must be used in women of childbearing potential during therapy and for one month after stopping treatment except in patients with tubal ligation or an implanted IUD (Copper T 380A or LNg 20). No other contraceptive measures are required for these patients. A missed menses should be reported to healthcare provider and prompt immediate pregnancy testing. Women should also be educated on the appropriate use of emergency contraception if failure of contraceptive is known or suspected or in the event of unprotected sex.

[U.S. Boxed Warning]: Because of the high likelihood of teratogenic effects, ambrisentan is only available through the LEAP restricted distribution program. Patients, prescribers, and pharmacies must be registered with and meet conditions of LEAP. Call 1-866-664-5327 for more information.

Use caution in patients with low hemoglobin levels. May cause decreases in hemoglobin and hematocrit (monitoring of hemoglobin is recommended. Use not recommended in patients with clinically significant anemia. Development of peripheral edema due to treatment and/or disease state (pulmonary arterial hypertension) may occur; a higher incidence is seen in elderly patients. Sperm count may be reduced in men during treatment (as observed with bosentan). No changes in sperm function or hormone levels have been noted. Fertility issues may require discussion with patient. Increases in serum liver aminotransferases have been reported during postmarketing use; however, in the majority of the cases, alternative causes of hepatotoxicity could be identified. Perform liver enzyme testing only when clinically indicated. Discontinue therapy if signs/symptoms of hepatic injury appear, if serum liver aminotransferases >5 times ULN are observed, or if aminotransferases are increased in the presence of bilirubin >2 times ULN. Hepatotoxicity has been reported with other endothelin receptor antagonists (eg, bosentan); however, ambrisentan may be tried in patients that have experienced asymptomatic increases in liver enzymes caused by another endothelin receptor antagonist after the liver enzymes have returned to normal. Use caution in patients with mild hepatic impairment; use not recommended in patients with moderate-to-severe impairment. There have also been postmarketing reports of fluid retention requiring treatment (eg, diuretics, fluid management, hospitalization). Further evaluation may be necessary to determine cause and appropriate treatment or discontinuation of therapy. Discontinue in any patient with pulmonary edema suggestive of pulmonary veno-occlusive disease (PVOD).

Adverse Reactions
>10%:
Cardiovascular: Peripheral edema (17%)
Central nervous system: Headache (15%)
1% to 10%:
Cardiovascular: Palpitation (5%), flushing (4%)
Gastrointestinal: Constipation (4%), abdominal pain (3%)
Hematologic: Hemoglobin decreased (7% to 10%)
Respiratory: Nasal congestion (6%), dyspnea (4%), nasopharyngitis (3%), sinusitis (3%)
Postmarketing and/or case reports: Anemia, angioedema, fluid retention, heart failure, hypersensitivity, liver enzymes increased, nausea, rash, vomiting

Drug Interactions
Metabolism/Transport Effects Substrate of CYP2C19 (minor), CYP3A4 (minor), P-glycoprotein, UGT1A3, UGT1A9, UGT2B7; **Note:** Assignment of Major/Minor substrate status based on clinically relevant drug interaction potential
Avoid Concomitant Use There are no known interactions where it is recommended to avoid concomitant use.
Increased Effect/Toxicity
The levels/effects of Ambrisentan may be increased by: Conivaptan; CycloSPORINE; CycloSPORINE (Systemic)
Decreased Effect
The levels/effects of Ambrisentan may be decreased by: Tocilizumab

Ethanol/Nutrition/Herb Interactions
Food: Grapefruit/grapefruit juice may increase levels/effects of ambrisentan.
Herb/Nutraceutical: Avoid St John's wort (concurrent use may decrease levels/effects of ambrisentan).

Stability Store in original packaging at 25°C (77°F); excursions permitted to 15°C to 30°C (59°F to 86°F).

Mechanism of Action Blocks endothelin receptor subtypes ET_A and ET_B on vascular endothelium and smooth muscle. Stimulation of ET_A receptors, located primarily in pulmonary vascular smooth muscle cells is associated with vasoconstriction and cellular proliferation. Stimulation of ET_B receptors, located in both pulmonary vascular endothelial cells and smooth muscle cells is associated with vasodilation, antiproliferative effects, and endothelin clearance. Although ambrisentan blocks both ET_A and ETB receptors, the affinity is greater for the ET_A receptor (>4000 fold higher affinity).

Pharmacodynamics/Kinetics
Protein binding: 99%
Metabolism: Hepatic via CYP3A4, CYP2C19, and uridine 5'-diphosphate glucuronosyltransferases (UGTs) 1A9S, 2B7S, and 1A3S; *in vitro* studies also suggest it is a substrate of organic anion transporting polypeptides (OATP) 1B1 and 1B3 and P-glycoprotein (P-gp)
Half-life elimination: ~9 hours
Time to peak, plasma: ~2 hours
Excretion: Primarily nonrenal

Dosage Oral: Adults: Initial: 5 mg once daily; if tolerated, may increase to maximum 10 mg once daily
Coadministration with cyclosporine: Ambrisentan dose should not exceed 5 mg/day

Dosage adjustment in renal impairment:
Mild-to-moderate renal impairment: No dosage adjustments are recommended.
Severe renal impairment: There is no data available for use in severe renal impairment.

Dosage adjustment in hepatic impairment:
Mild hepatic impairment: There is no data available for use in mild hepatic impairment; exposure may be increased.
Moderate-to-severe hepatic impairment: Use not recommended

Dietary Considerations May be taken with or without food. Avoid grapefruit and grapefruit juice.

Administration Swallow tablet whole. Do not split, crush, or chew tablets. May be administered with or without food.

Monitoring Parameters Monitor for significant peripheral edema and evaluate etiology if it occurs; liver enzyme testing when clinically appropriate

A woman of childbearing potential must have a negative pregnancy test prior to the initiation of therapy and monthly thereafter. Hemoglobin and hematocrit should be measured at baseline, at 1 month, and periodically thereafter (generally stabilizes after the first few weeks of treatment).

Dosage Forms Excipient information presented when available (limited, particularly for generics); consult specific product labeling.
Tablet, oral:
Letairis®: 5 mg, 10 mg

- ◆ **AMD3100** *see* Plerixafor *on page* 1361
- ◆ **Amerge®** *see* Naratriptan *on page* 1180
- ◆ **Americaine® Hemorrhoidal [OTC]** *see* Benzocaine *on page* 202
- ◆ **A-Methapred** *see* MethylPREDNISolone *on page* 1110
- ◆ **A-Methapred®** *see* MethylPREDNISolone *on page* 1110
- ◆ **Amethia™** *see* Ethinyl Estradiol and Levonorgestrel *on page* 656
- ◆ **Amethia™ Lo** *see* Ethinyl Estradiol and Levonorgestrel *on page* 656
- ◆ **Amethocaine Hydrochloride** *see* Tetracaine (Ophthalmic) *on page* 1661
- ◆ **Amethocaine Hydrochloride** *see* Tetracaine (Systemic) *on page* 1660
- ◆ **Amethocaine Hydrochloride** *see* Tetracaine (Topical) *on page* 1661
- ◆ **Amethopterin** *see* Methotrexate *on page* 1098
- ◆ **Amethyst™** *see* Ethinyl Estradiol and Levonorgestrel *on page* 656
- ◆ **Ametop™ (Can)** *see* Tetracaine (Topical) *on page* 1661
- ◆ **Amevive®** *see* Alefacept *on page* 57
- ◆ **Amfepramone** *see* Diethylpropion *on page* 502
- ◆ **AMG 073** *see* Cinacalcet *on page* 360
- ◆ **AMG-162** *see* Denosumab *on page* 471
- ◆ **AMG 531** *see* RomiPLOStim *on page* 1516
- ◆ **Amicar®** *see* Aminocaproic Acid *on page* 89
- ◆ **Amidate®** *see* Etomidate *on page* 668

Amifostine (am i FOS teen)

Brand Names: U.S. Ethyol®
Brand Names: Canada Ethyol®
Index Terms Ethiofos; Gammaphos; WR-2721; YM-08310
Pharmacologic Category Adjuvant, Chemoprotective Agent (Cytoprotective); Antidote
Use Reduce the incidence of moderate-to-severe xerostomia in patients undergoing postoperative radiation treatment for head and neck cancer, where the radiation port includes a substantial portion of the parotid glands; reduce the cumulative renal toxicity associated with repeated administration of cisplatin
Unlabeled Use Prevention of radiation proctitis in patients with rectal cancer
Pregnancy Risk Factor C
Pregnancy Considerations Animal studies have demonstrated embryotoxicity. There are no adequate and well-controlled studies in pregnant women.
Lactation Excretion in breast milk unknown/not recommended
Contraindications Hypersensitivity to aminothiol compounds or any component of the formulation

Warnings/Precautions Patients who are hypotensive or dehydrated should not receive amifostine. Interrupt antihypertensive therapy for 24 hours before treatment; patients who cannot safely stop their antihypertensives 24 hours before, should not receive amifostine. Adequately hydrated prior to treatment and keep in a supine position during infusion. Monitor blood pressure every 5 minutes during the infusion. If hypotension requiring interruption of therapy occurs, patients should be placed in the Trendelenburg position and given an infusion of normal saline using a separate I.V. line; subsequent infusions may require a dose reduction. Infusions >15 minutes are associated with a higher incidence of adverse effects. Use caution in patients with cardiovascular and cerebrovascular disease and any other patients in whom the adverse effects of hypotension may have serious adverse events.

Serious cutaneous reactions, including erythema multiforme, Stevens-Johnson syndrome, toxic epidermal necrolysis, toxoderma and exfoliative dermatitis have been reported with amifostine. May be delayed, developing up to weeks after treatment initiation. Cutaneous reactions have been reported more frequently when used as a radioprotectant. Discontinue treatment for severe/serious cutaneous reaction, or with fever. Withhold treatment and obtain dermatologic consultation for rash involving lips or mucosa (of unknown etiology outside of radiation port) and for bullous, edematous or erythematous lesions on hands, feet, or trunk; reinitiate only after careful evaluation.

It is recommended that antiemetic medication, including dexamethasone 20 mg I.V. and a serotonin 5-HT_3 receptor antagonist be administered prior to and in conjunction with amifostine. Rare hypersensitivity reactions, including anaphylaxis and allergic reaction, have been reported; discontinue if allergic reaction occurs; do not rechallenge. Medications for the treatment of hypersensitivity reactions should be available.

Reports of clinically-relevant hypocalcemia are rare, but serum calcium levels should be monitored in patients at risk of hypocalcemia, such as those with nephrotic syndrome; may require calcium supplementation. Should not be used (in patients receiving chemotherapy for malignancies other than ovarian cancer) where chemotherapy is expected to provide significant survival benefit or in patients receiving definitive radiotherapy, unless within the context of a clinical trial. Safety and efficacy in children have not been established.

Adverse Reactions

>10%:

Cardiovascular: Hypotension (15% to 61%; grades 3/4: 3% to 8%; dose dependent)

Gastrointestinal: Nausea/vomiting (53% to 96%; grades 3/4: 8% to 30%; dose dependent)

1% to 10%: Endocrine & metabolic: Hypocalcemia (clinically significant: 1%)

<1% (Limited to important or life-threatening): Apnea, anaphylactoid reactions, anaphylaxis, arrhythmia, atrial fibrillation, atrial flutter, back pain, bradycardia, cardiac arrest, chest pain, chest tightness, chills, cutaneous eruptions, dizziness, erythema multiforme, exfoliative dermatitis, extrasystoles, dyspnea, fever, flushing, hiccups, hypersensitivity reactions (fever, rash, hypoxia, dyspnea, laryngeal edema), hypertension (transient), hypoxia, malaise, MI, myocardial ischemia, pruritus, rash (mild), renal failure, respiratory arrest, rigors, seizure, sneezing, somnolence, Stevens-Johnson syndrome, supraventricular tachycardia, syncope, tachycardia, toxic epidermal necrolysis, toxoderma, urticaria

Drug Interactions

Metabolism/Transport Effects None known.

Avoid Concomitant Use There are no known interactions where it is recommended to avoid concomitant use.

Increased Effect/Toxicity

The levels/effects of Amifostine may be increased by: Antihypertensives

Decreased Effect There are no known significant interactions involving a decrease in effect.

Stability Store intact vials of lyophilized powder at room temperature of 20°C to 25°C (68°F to 77°F). For I.V. infusion, reconstitute intact vials with 9.7 mL 0.9% sodium chloride injection and dilute in 0.9% sodium chloride to a final concentration of 5-40 mg/mL. For SubQ administration, reconstitute with 2.5 mL NS or SWFI. Reconstituted solutions (500 mg/10 mL) and solutions for infusion are chemically stable for up to 5 hours at room temperature (25°C) or up to 24 hours under refrigeration (2°C to 8°C).

Mechanism of Action Prodrug that is dephosphorylated by alkaline phosphatase in tissues to a pharmacologically-active free thiol metabolite. The free thiol is available to bind to, and detoxify, reactive metabolites of cisplatin; and can also act as a scavenger of free radicals that may be generated (by cisplatin or radiation therapy) in tissues.

Pharmacodynamics/Kinetics

Distribution: V_d: 3.5 L

Metabolism: Hepatic dephosphorylation to two metabolites (active-free thiol and disulfide)

Half-life elimination: ~8-9 minutes

Excretion: Urine

Clearance, plasma: 2.17 L/minute

Dosage Note: Antiemetic medication, including dexamethasone 20 mg I.V. and a serotonin 5-HT_3 receptor antagonist, is recommended prior to and in conjunction with amifostine.

Adults:

Cisplatin-induced renal toxicity, reduction: I.V.: 910 mg/m^2 over 15 minutes once daily 30 minutes prior to cisplatin

For 910 mg/m^2 doses, the manufacturer suggests the following blood pressure-based adjustment schedule:

The infusion of amifostine should be interrupted if the systolic blood pressure decreases significantly from baseline, as defined below:

Decrease of 20 mm Hg if baseline systolic blood pressure <100

Decrease of 25 mm Hg if baseline systolic blood pressure 100-119

Decrease of 30 mm Hg if baseline systolic blood pressure 120-139

Decrease of 40 mm Hg if baseline systolic blood pressure 140-179

Decrease of 50 mm Hg if baseline systolic blood pressure ≥180

If blood pressure returns to normal within 5 minutes (assisted by fluid administration and postural management) and the patient is asymptomatic, the infusion may be restarted so that the full dose of amifostine may be administered. If the full dose of amifostine cannot be administered, the dose of amifostine for subsequent cycles should be 740 mg/m^2.

Xerostomia from head and neck cancer, reduction:

I.V.: 200 mg/m^2 over 3 minutes once daily 15-30 minutes prior to radiation therapy **or**

SubQ (unlabeled route): 500 mg once daily prior to radiation therapy

Prevention of radiation proctitis in rectal cancer (unlabeled use): I.V.: 340 mg/m^2 once daily prior to radiation therapy (Keefe, 2007; Peterson, 2008)

Administration I.V.: Administer over 3 minutes (prior to radiation therapy) or 15 minutes (prior to cisplatin); administration as a longer infusion is associated with a higher incidence of side effects. Patients should be kept in supine position during infusion. **Note:** SubQ administration (unlabeled) has been used.

Monitoring Parameters Blood pressure should be monitored every 5 minutes during the infusion and after administration if clinically indicated; serum calcium levels (in patients at risk for hypocalcemia). Evaluate for cutaneous reactions prior to each dose.

Additional Information Oncology Comment: The American Society of Clinical Oncology (ASCO) guidelines for the use of protectants for chemotherapy and radiation (Hensley, 2008) recommend the use of amifostine for prevention of nephrotoxicity due to cisplatin-based chemotherapy and to decrease the incidence of acute and delayed radiation therapy-induced xerostomia. The ASCO guidelines do not recommend the use of amifostine to reduce the incidence of neutropenia or thrombocytopenia associated with chemotherapy or radiation therapy, neurotoxicity or ototoxicity associated with platinum-based chemotherapy, radiation therapy-induced mucositis associated with head and neck cancer, or esophagitis due to chemotherapy in patients with nonsmall cell lung cancer. Additionally, the guidelines do not support the use of amifostine in patients with head and neck cancer receiving concurrent platinum-based chemotherapy.

Dosage Forms Excipient information presented when available (limited, particularly for generics); consult specific product labeling.

Injection, powder for reconstitution: 500 mg

Ethyol®: 500 mg

◆ **Amigesic® (Can)** *see* Salsalate *on page* 1534

Amikacin (am i KAY sin)

Brand Names: Canada Amikacin Sulfate Injection, USP; Amikin®

Index Terms Amikacin Sulfate

Pharmacologic Category Antibiotic, Aminoglycoside

Use Treatment of serious infections (bone infections, respiratory tract infections, endocarditis, and septicemia) due to organisms resistant to gentamicin and tobramycin, including *Pseudomonas*, *Proteus*, *Serratia*, and other gram-negative bacilli; documented infection of mycobacterial organisms susceptible to amikacin

Unlabeled Use Bacterial endophthalmitis

Pregnancy Risk Factor D

Pregnancy Considerations Adverse events were not observed in the initial animal reproduction studies; however, renal toxicity has been reported in additional studies. Amikacin crosses the placenta, produces detectable serum levels in the fetus, and concentrates in the fetal kidneys. Because of several reports of total irreversible bilateral congenital deafness in children whose mothers received another aminoglycoside (streptomycin) during pregnancy, the manufacturer classifies amikacin as pregnancy risk factor D. Although serious side effects to the fetus have not been reported following maternal use of amikacin, a potential for harm exists.

Due to pregnancy-induced physiologic changes, some pharmacokinetic parameters of amikacin may be altered. Pregnant women have an average-to-larger volume of distribution which may result in lower peak serum levels than for the same dose in nonpregnant women. Serum half-life may also be shorter.

Lactation Enters breast milk/not recommended

Contraindications Hypersensitivity to amikacin sulfate or any component of the formulation; cross-sensitivity may exist with other aminoglycosides

Warnings/Precautions [U.S. Boxed Warning]: Amikacin may cause neurotoxicity, nephrotoxicity, and/or neuromuscular blockade and respiratory paralysis; usual risk factors include pre-existing renal impairment, concomitant neuro-/nephrotoxic medications, advanced age and dehydration. Dose and/or frequency of administration must be monitored and modified in patients with renal impairment. Drug should be discontinued if signs of ototoxicity, nephrotoxicity, or hypersensitivity occur. Ototoxicity is proportional to the amount of drug given and the duration of treatment. Tinnitus or vertigo may be indications of vestibular injury and impending bilateral irreversible damage. Renal damage is usually reversible. Use with caution in patients with neuromuscular disorders, hearing loss and hypocalcemia. Prolonged use may result in fungal or bacterial superinfection, including *C. difficile*-associated diarrhea (CDAD) and pseudomembranous colitis; CDAD has been observed >2 months postantibiotic treatment. Solution contains sodium metabisulfate; use caution in patients with sulfite allergy.

Adverse Reactions

1% to 10%:

Central nervous system: Neurotoxicity

Otic: Ototoxicity (auditory), ototoxicity (vestibular)

Renal: Nephrotoxicity

<1% (Limited to important or life-threatening): Allergic reaction, dyspnea, eosinophilia

Drug Interactions

Metabolism/Transport Effects None known.

Avoid Concomitant Use

Avoid concomitant use of Amikacin with any of the following: BCG; Gallium Nitrate

Increased Effect/Toxicity

Amikacin may increase the levels/effects of: AbobotulinumtoxinA; Bisphosphonate Derivatives; CARBOplatin; Colistimethate; CycloSPORINE; CycloSPORINE (Systemic); Gallium Nitrate; Neuromuscular-Blocking Agents; OnabotulinumtoxinA; RimabotulinumtoxinB

The levels/effects of Amikacin may be increased by: Amphotericin B; Capreomycin; Cephalosporins (2nd Generation); Cephalosporins (3rd Generation); Cephalosporins (4th Generation); CISplatin; Loop Diuretics; Nonsteroidal Anti-Inflammatory Agents; Vancomycin

Decreased Effect

Amikacin may decrease the levels/effects of: BCG; Typhoid Vaccine

The levels/effects of Amikacin may be decreased by: Penicillins

Stability Store at controlled room temperature. Following admixture at concentrations of 0.25-5 mg/mL, amikacin is stable for 24 hours at room temperature and 2 days at refrigeration when mixed in D_5W, NS, and LR.

Mechanism of Action Inhibits protein synthesis in susceptible bacteria by binding to 30S ribosomal subunits

Pharmacodynamics/Kinetics

Absorption:

I.M.: Rapid

Oral: Poorly absorbed

Distribution: V_d: 0.25 L/kg; primarily into extracellular fluid (highly hydrophilic); penetrates blood-brain barrier when meninges inflamed

Relative diffusion of antimicrobial agents from blood into CSF: Good only with inflammation (exceeds usual MICs)

CSF:blood level ratio: Normal meninges: 10% to 20%; Inflamed meninges: 15% to 24%

Protein-binding: 0% to 11%

Half-life elimination (renal function and age dependent):

Infants: Low birth weight (1-3 days): 7-9 hours; Full-term >7 days: 4-5 hours

Children: 1.6-2.5 hours

Adults: Normal renal function: 1.4-2.3 hours; Anuria/end-stage renal disease: 28-86 hours

Time to peak, serum: I.M.: 45-120 minutes

Excretion: Urine (94% to 98%)

Dosage Note: Individualization is critical because of the low therapeutic index

Use of ideal body weight (IBW) for determining the mg/kg/dose appears to be more accurate than dosing on the basis of total body weight (TBW)

In morbid obesity, dosage requirement may best be estimated using a dosing weight of IBW + 0.4 (TBW - IBW)

Initial and periodic peak and trough plasma drug levels should be determined, particularly in critically-ill patients with serious infections or in disease states known to significantly alter aminoglycoside pharmacokinetics (eg, cystic fibrosis, burns, or major surgery). Manufacturer recommends a maximum daily dose of 15 mg/kg/day (or 1.5 g/day in heavier patients). Higher doses may be warranted based on therapeutic drug monitoring or susceptibility information.

Usual dosage range:

Infants and Children: I.M., I.V.: 5-7.5 mg/kg/dose every 8 hours

Adults:

I.M., I.V.: 5-7.5 mg/kg/dose every 8 hours; **Note:** Some clinicians suggest a daily dose of 15-20 mg/kg for all patients with normal renal function. This dose is at least as efficacious with similar, if not less, toxicity than conventional dosing.

Intrathecal/intraventricular (unlabeled route): Meningitis (susceptible gram-negative organisms): 5-50 mg/day

Indication-specific dosing:

Adults:

Endophthalmitis, bacterial (unlabeled use): Intravitreal: 0.4 mg/0.1 mL NS in combination with vancomycin

Hospital-acquired pneumonia (HAP): I.V.: 20 mg/kg/day with antipseudomonal beta-lactam or carbapenem (American Thoracic Society/ATS guidelines)

Meningitis (susceptible gram-negative organisms):

I.V.: 5 mg/kg every 8 hours (administered with another bacteriocidal drug)

Intrathecal/intraventricular (unlabeled route): Usual dose: 30 mg/day (IDSA, 2004); Range: 5-50 mg/day (with concurrent systemic antimicrobial therapy) (Gilbert, 1986; Guardado, 2008; IDSA, 2004; Kasiakou, 2005)

Mycobacterium fortuitum, M. chelonae, or M. abscessus: I.V.: 10-15 mg/kg daily for at least 2 weeks with high dose cefoxitin

Dosing interval in renal impairment: Some patients may require larger or more frequent doses if serum levels document the need (ie, cystic fibrosis or febrile granulocytopenic patients).

Cl_{cr} ≥60 mL/minute: Administer every 8 hours

Cl_{cr} 40-60 mL/minute: Administer every 12 hours

Cl_{cr} 20-40 mL/minute: Administer every 24 hours

Cl_{cr} <20 mL/minute: Loading dose, then monitor levels

Intermittent hemodialysis (IHD) (administer after hemodialysis on dialysis days): Dialyzable (20%; variable; dependent on filter, duration, and type of HD): 5-7.5 mg/kg every 48-72 hours. Follow levels. Redose when pre-HD concentration <10 mg/L; redose when post-HD concentration <6-8 mg/L (Heintz, 2009). **Note:** Dosing dependent on the assumption of 3 times/week, complete IHD sessions.

Peritoneal dialysis (PD): Dose as Cl_{cr} <20 mL/minute: Follow levels

Continuous renal replacement therapy (CRRT) (Heintz, 2009; Trotman, 2005): Drug clearance is highly dependent on the method of renal replacement, filter type, and flow rate. Appropriate dosing requires close monitoring of pharmacologic response, signs of adverse reactions due to drug accumulation, as well as drug concentrations in relation to target trough (if appropriate). The following are general recommendations only (based on dialysate flow/ultrafiltration rates of 1-2 L/hour and minimal residual renal function) and should not supersede clinical judgment:

CVVH/CVVHD/CVVHDF: Loading dose of 10 mg/kg followed by maintenance dose of 7.5 mg/kg every 24-48 hours

Note: For severe gram-negative rod infections, target peak concentration of 15-30 mg/L; redose when concentration <10 mg/L (Heintz, 2009).

Dietary Considerations Some products may contain sodium.

Administration Administer around-the-clock to promote less variation in peak and trough serum levels. Do not mix with other drugs, administer separately.

I.M.: Administer I.M. injection in large muscle mass.

I.V.: Infuse over 30-60 minutes.

Some penicillins (eg, carbenicillin, ticarcillin, and piperacillin) have been shown to inactivate *in vitro*. This has been observed to a greater extent with tobramycin and gentamicin, while amikacin has shown greater stability against inactivation. Concurrent use of these agents may pose a risk of reduced antibacterial efficacy *in vivo*, particularly in the setting of profound renal impairment. However, definitive clinical evidence is lacking. If combination penicillin/aminoglycoside therapy is desired in a patient with renal dysfunction, separation of doses (if feasible), and routine monitoring of aminoglycoside levels, CBC, and clinical response should be considered.

Intrathecal/Intraventricular (unlabeled route): Reserved solely for meningitis due to susceptible gram-negative organisms. Available formulation contains sodium metabisulfite. If possible, consider alternative therapy with gentamicin or tobramycin as both of these agents are available as preservative-free formulations.

Monitoring Parameters Urinalysis, BUN, serum creatinine, appropriately timed peak and trough concentrations, vital signs, temperature, weight, I & O, hearing parameters

Some penicillin derivatives may accelerate the degradation of aminoglycosides *in vitro*. This may be clinically-significant for certain penicillin (ticarcillin, piperacillin, carbenicillin) and aminoglycoside (gentamicin, tobramycin) combination therapy in patients with significant renal impairment. Close monitoring of aminoglycoside levels is warranted.

Reference Range

Sample size: 0.5-2 mL blood (red top tube) or 0.1-1 mL serum (separated)

Therapeutic levels:

Peak:

Life-threatening infections: 25-40 mcg/mL

Serious infections: 20-25 mcg/mL

Urinary tract infections: 15-20 mcg/mL

Trough: <8 mcg/mL

The American Thoracic Society (ATS) recommends trough levels of <4-5 mcg/mL for patients with hospital-acquired pneumonia.

Toxic concentration: Peak: >40 mcg/mL; Trough: >10 mcg/mL

Timing of serum samples: Draw peak 30 minutes after completion of 30-minute infusion or at 1 hour following initiation of infusion or I.M. injection; draw trough within 30 minutes prior to next dose

Test Interactions Some penicillin derivatives may accelerate the degradation of aminoglycosides *in vitro*, leading to a potential underestimation of aminoglycoside serum concentration.

Additional Information Aminoglycoside levels measured from blood taken from central venous catheters can sometimes give falsely high readings (draw levels from alternate lumen or peripheral stick, if possible).

Dosage Forms Excipient information presented when available (limited, particularly for generics); consult specific product labeling. [DSC] = Discontinued product

Injection, solution, as sulfate: 50 mg/mL (2 mL [DSC]); 250 mg/mL (2 mL, 4 mL)

◆ **Amikacin Sulfate** *see* Amikacin *on page 87*

◆ **Amikacin Sulfate Injection, USP (Can)** *see* Amikacin *on page 87*

◆ **Amikin® (Can)** *see* Amikacin *on page 87*

AMILoride (a MIL oh ride)

Brand Names: Canada Apo-Amiloride®; Midamor

Index Terms Amiloride Hydrochloride

Pharmacologic Category Diuretic, Potassium-Sparing

Use Counteracts potassium loss induced by other diuretics in the treatment of hypertension or edematous conditions including CHF, hepatic cirrhosis, and hypoaldosteronism; usually used in conjunction with more potent diuretics such as thiazides or loop diuretics

Unlabeled Use Cystic fibrosis; reduction of lithium-induced polyuria; pediatric hypertension

Pregnancy Risk Factor B

Dosage Oral:

Children 1-17 years: Hypertension (unlabeled use): 0.4-0.625 mg/kg/day (maximum: 20 mg/day)

Adults: 5-10 mg/day (up to 20 mg)

Hypertension (JNC 7): 5-10 mg/day in 1-2 divided doses

Elderly: Initial: 5 mg once daily or every other day

Dosing adjustment in renal impairment:

Cl_{cr} 10-50 mL/minute: Administer at 50% of normal dose.

Cl_{cr} <10 mL/minute: Avoid use.

Additional Information Complete prescribing information for this medication should be consulted for additional detail.

Dosage Forms Excipient information presented when available (limited, particularly for generics); consult specific product labeling.

Tablet, oral, as hydrochloride: 5 mg

◆ **Amiloride Hydrochloride** *see* AMILoride *on page 89*

◆ **2-Amino-6-Mercaptopurine** *see* Thioguanine *on page 1670*

◆ **2-Amino-6-Methoxypurine Arabinoside** *see* Nelarabine *on page 1184*

◆ **2-Amino-6-Trifluoromethoxy-benzothiazole** *see* Riluzole *on page 1491*

◆ **Aminobenzylpenicillin** *see* Ampicillin *on page 115*

Aminocaproic Acid (a mee noe ka PROE ik AS id)

Brand Names: U.S. Amicar®

Index Terms EACA; Epsilon Aminocaproic Acid

Pharmacologic Category Antifibrinolytic Agent; Antihemophilic Agent; Hemostatic Agent; Lysine Analog

Use To enhance hemostasis when fibrinolysis contributes to bleeding (causes may include cardiac surgery, hematologic disorders, neoplastic disorders, abruption placentae, hepatic cirrhosis, and urinary fibrinolysis)

Unlabeled Use Treatment of traumatic hyphema; control bleeding in thrombocytopenia; control oral bleeding in congenital and acquired coagulation disorders; topical treatment (mouth rinse) of bleeding associated with dental procedures in patients on oral anticoagulant therapy; prevention of perioperative bleeding associated with cardiac surgery; prevention of bleeding associated with extracorporeal membrane oxygenation (ECMO); prevention of perioperative bleeding associated with spinal surgery (eg, idiopathic scoliosis)

Pregnancy Risk Factor C

Dosage

Acute bleeding: Adults: Oral, I.V.: Loading dose: 4-5 g during the first hour, followed by 1 g/hour (or 1.25 g/hour using oral solution) for 8 hours or until bleeding controlled (maximum daily dose: 30 g)

Control of bleeding with severe thrombocytopenia (unlabeled use) (Bartholomew, 1989; Gardner, 1980): Adults:

Initial: I.V.: 100 mg/kg (maximum dose: 5 g) over 30-60 minutes

Maintenance: Oral, I.V.: 1-4 g every 4-8 hours or 1 g/hour (maximum daily dose: 24 g)

Control of oral bleeding in congenital and acquired coagulation disorder (unlabeled use): Adults: Oral: 50-60 mg/kg every 4 hours (Mannucci, 1998)

Prevention of dental procedure bleeding in patients on oral anticoagulant therapy (unlabeled use): Adults: Oral rinse: Hold 4 g/10 mL in mouth for 2 minutes then spit out. Repeat every 6 hours for 2 days after procedure (Souto, 1996). Concentration and frequency may vary by institution and product availability.

Prevention of perioperative bleeding associated with cardiac surgery (unlabeled use): I.V.:

Children: 100 mg/kg given over 20-30 minutes after induction and prior to incision, 100 mg/kg during cardiopulmonary bypass, and 100 mg/kg after heparin reversal over 3 hours (Chauhan, 2004)

Adults: Loading dose of 75-150 mg/kg (typically 5-10 g), followed by 10-15 mg/kg/hour (typically 1 g/hour); may add 2-2.5 g/L of cardiopulmonary bypass circuit priming solution (Gravlee, 2008)

or

Loading dose of 10 g followed by 2 g/hour during surgery; no medication added to the bypass circuit (Fergusson, 2008)

or

10 g over 20-30 minutes prior to skin incision, followed by 10 g after heparin administration then 10 g at discontinuation of cardiopulmonary bypass (Vander Salm, 1996)

Prevention of bleeding associated with extracorporeal membrane oxygenation (ECMO) (unlabeled use): Children: I.V.: 100 mg/kg prior to or immediately after cannulation, followed by 25-30 mg/kg/hour for up to 72 hours (Downard, 2003; Horwitz, 1998; Wilson, 1993)

Prevention of perioperative bleeding associated with spinal surgery (eg, idiopathic scoliosis) (unlabeled use): Children and Adolescents: I.V.: 100 mg/kg given over 15-20 minutes after induction, followed by 10 mg/kg/hour for the remainder of the surgery; discontinue at time of wound closure (Florentino-Pineda, 2001; Florentino-Pineda, 2004)

Traumatic hyphema (unlabeled use): Children and Adults: Oral: 50 mg/kg/dose every 4 hours (maximum daily dose: 30 g) for 5 days (Brandt, 2001; Crouch, 1999)

Dosing adjustment in renal impairment: May accumulate in patients with decreased renal function. When used during cardiopulmonary bypass in anephric patients, a normal or slightly reduced loading dose and a continuous infusion rate of 5 mg/kg/hour has been recommended (Gravlee, 2008).

Additional Information Complete prescribing information for this medication should be consulted for additional detail.

Dosage Forms Excipient information presented when available (limited, particularly for generics); consult specific product labeling.

Injection, solution: 250 mg/mL (20 mL)
Solution, oral: 1.25 g/5 mL (237 mL, 473 mL)
Syrup, oral:
Amicar®: 1.25 g/5 mL (473 mL) [raspberry flavor]
Tablet, oral: 500 mg
Amicar®: 500 mg, 1000 mg [scored]

Aminolevulinic Acid (a MEE noh lev yoo lin ik AS id)

Brand Names: U.S. Levulan® Kerastick®

Brand Names: Canada Levulan® Kerastick®

Index Terms 5-ALA; 5-Aminolevulinic Acid; ALA; Amino Levulinic Acid; Aminolevulinic Acid Hydrochloride

Pharmacologic Category Photosensitizing Agent, Topical; Topical Skin Product

Use Treatment of minimally to moderately thick actinic keratoses (grade 1 or 2) of the face or scalp; to be used in conjunction with blue light illumination

Unlabeled Use Photodynamic treatment of low-risk superficial basal cell skin cancer and low-risk squamous cell skin cancer *in situ* (Bowen's disease)

Pregnancy Risk Factor C

Dosage Adults: Topical: Apply to actinic keratoses (**not** perilesional skin) followed 14-18 hours later by blue light illumination. Application/treatment may be repeated at a treatment site (once) after 8 weeks.

Additional Information Complete prescribing information for this medication should be consulted for additional detail.

Dosage Forms Excipient information presented when available (limited, particularly for generics); consult specific product labeling.

Powder for solution, topical, as hydrochloride:
Levulan® Kerastick®: 20% (6s) [contains ethanol 48% (in diluent); supplied with diluent]

◆ **Amino Levulinic Acid** *see* Aminolevulinic Acid *on page 90*
◆ **5-Aminolevulinic Acid** *see* Aminolevulinic Acid *on page 90*
◆ **Aminolevulinic Acid Hydrochloride** *see* Aminolevulinic Acid *on page 90*
◆ **4-aminopyridine** *see* Dalfampridine *on page 440*
◆ **5-Aminosalicylic Acid** *see* Mesalamine *on page 1081*
◆ **Aminoxin® [OTC]** *see* Pyridoxine *on page 1437*

Amiodarone (a MEE oh da rone)

Brand Names: U.S. Cordarone®; Nexterone®; Pacerone®

Brand Names: Canada Amiodarone Hydrochloride Injection; Apo-Amiodarone®; Cordarone®; Dom-Amiodarone; Mylan-Amiodarone; Novo-Amiodarone; PHL-Amiodarone; PMS-Amiodarone; PRO-Amiodarone; ratio-Amiodarone; Riva-Amiodarone; Sandoz-Amiodarone; Teva-Amiodarone

Index Terms Amiodarone Hydrochloride

Pharmacologic Category Antiarrhythmic Agent, Class III

Additional Appendix Information

Beers Criteria – Potentially Inappropriate Medications for Geriatrics *on page 1973*

Use Management of life-threatening recurrent ventricular fibrillation (VF) or hemodynamically-unstable ventricular tachycardia (VT) refractory to other antiarrhythmic agents or in patients intolerant of other agents used for these conditions

Unlabeled Use

Atrial fibrillation (AF): Pharmacologic conversion of AF to and maintenance of normal sinus rhythm; treatment of AF in patients with heart failure [no accessory pathway] who require heart rate control (ACC/AHA/ESC Practice Guidelines) or in patients with hypertrophic cardiomyopathy (ACCF/AHA Practice Guidelines); prevention of postoperative AF associated with cardiothoracic surgery

Paroxysmal supraventricular tachycardia (SVT) (not initial drug of choice)

Ventricular tachyarrhythmias (ACLS/PALS guidelines): Cardiac arrest with persistent VT or VF if defibrillation, CPR, and vasopressor administration have failed; control of hemodynamically-stable monomorphic VT, polymorphic VT with a normal baseline QT interval, or wide-complex tachycardia of uncertain origin; control of rapid ventricular rate due to accessory pathway conduction in pre-excited atrial arrhythmias (ACLS guidelines) or stable narrow-complex tachycardia (ACLS guidelines)

Adjunct to ICD therapy to suppress symptomatic ventricular tachyarrhythmias in otherwise optimally-treated patients with heart failure (ACC/AHA/ESC Practice Guidelines)

Pregnancy Risk Factor D

Pregnancy Considerations May cause fetal harm when administered to a pregnant woman, leading to congenital goiter and hypo- or hyperthyroidism.

Lactation Enters breast milk/not recommended (AAP rates "of concern"; AAP 2001 update pending)

Medication Guide Available Yes

Contraindications Hypersensitivity to amiodarone, iodine, or any component of the formulation; severe sinus-node dysfunction; second- and third-degree heart block (except in patients with a functioning artificial pacemaker); bradycardia causing syncope (except in patients with a functioning artificial pacemaker); cardiogenic shock

Warnings/Precautions [U.S. Boxed Warning]: Only indicated for patients with life-threatening arrhythmias because of risk of toxicity. Alternative therapies should be tried first before using amiodarone. Patients should be hospitalized when amiodarone is initiated. Currently, the 2005 ACLS guidelines recommend I.V. amiodarone as the preferred antiarrhythmic for the treatment of pulseless VT/VF, both life-threatening arrhythmias. In patients with non-life-threatening arrhythmias (eg, atrial fibrillation), amiodarone should be used only if the use of other antiarrhythmics has proven ineffective or are contraindicated.

[U.S. Boxed Warning]: Lung damage (abnormal diffusion capacity) may occur without symptoms. Monitor for pulmonary toxicity. Evaluate new respiratory symptoms; pre-existing pulmonary disease does not increase risk of developing pulmonary toxicity, but if pulmonary toxicity develops then the prognosis is worse. The lowest effective dose should be used as appropriate for the acuity/severity of the arrhythmia being treated. **[U.S. Boxed Warning]: Liver toxicity is common, but usually mild with evidence of increased liver enzymes. Severe liver toxicity can occur and has been fatal in a few cases.**

[U.S. Boxed Warning]: Amiodarone can exacerbate arrhythmias, by making them more difficult to tolerate or reverse; other types of arrhythmias have occurred, including significant heart block, sinus bradycardia new ventricular fibrillation, incessant ventricular tachycardia, increased resistance to cardioversion, and polymorphic ventricular tachycardia associated with QT_c prolongation (torsade de pointes [TdP]). Risk may be increased with concomitant use of other antiarrhythmic agents or drugs that prolong the QT_c interval. Proarrhythmic effects may be prolonged.

Monitor pacing or defibrillation thresholds in patients with implantable cardiac devices (eg, pacemakers, defibrillators). Use very cautiously and with close monitoring in patients with thyroid or liver disease. May cause hyper- or hypothyroidism. Hyperthyroidism may result in thyrotoxicosis and may aggravate or cause breakthrough arrhythmias. If any new signs of arrhythmia appear, hyperthyroidism should be considered. Thyroid function should be monitored prior to treatment and periodically thereafter.

May cause optic neuropathy and/or optic neuritis, usually resulting in visual impairment. Corneal microdeposits occur in a majority of patients, and may cause visual disturbances in some patients (blurred vision, halos); these are not generally considered a reason to discontinue treatment. Corneal refractive laser surgery is generally contraindicated in amiodarone users. Avoid excessive exposure to sunlight; may cause photosensitivity.

Amiodarone is a potent inhibitor of CYP enzymes and transport proteins (including p-glycoprotein), which may lead to increased serum concentrations/toxicity of a number of medications. Particular caution must be used when a drug with QT_c-prolonging potential relies on metabolism via these enzymes, since the effect of elevated concentrations may be additive with the effect of amiodarone. Carefully assess risk:benefit of coadministration of other drugs which may prolong QT_c interval. Patients may still be at risk for amiodarone–related drug interactions after the drug has been discontinued. The pharmacokinetics are complex (due to prolonged duration of action and half-life) and difficult to predict. Correct electrolyte disturbances, especially hypokalemia or hypomagnesemia, prior to use and throughout therapy. Use caution when initiating amiodarone in patients on warfarin. Cases of increased INR with or without bleeding have occurred in patients treated with warfarin; monitor INR closely after initiating amiodarone in these patients.

May cause hypotension and bradycardia (infusion-rate related). Hypotension with rapid administration has been attributed to the emulsifier polysorbate 80. Commercially-prepared premixed solutions do not contain polysorbate 80 and may have a lower incidence of hypotension. Caution in surgical patients; may enhance hemodynamic effect of anesthetics; associated with increased risk of adult respiratory distress syndrome (ARDS) postoperatively. May be inappropriate in the elderly due to a risk of QT_c-interval prolongation, torsade de pointes, and lack of efficacy in the elderly (Beers Criteria). Vials for injection contain benzyl alcohol, which has been associated with "gasping syndrome" in neonates. Commercially-prepared premixed solutions do not contain benzyl alcohol. Commercially-prepared premixed infusion contains the excipient cyclodextrin (sulfobutyl ether beta-cyclodextrin), which may accumulate in patients with renal insufficiency.

Adverse Reactions In a recent meta-analysis, patients taking lower doses of amiodarone (152-330 mg daily for at least 12 months) were more likely to develop thyroid, neurologic, skin, ocular, and bradycardic abnormalities than those taking placebo (Vorperian, 1997). Pulmonary toxicity was similar in both the low-dose amiodarone group and in the placebo group, but there was a trend towards increased toxicity in the amiodarone group. Gastrointestinal and hepatic events were seen to a similar extent in both the low-dose amiodarone group and placebo group. As the frequency of adverse events varies considerably across studies as a function of route and dose, a consolidation of adverse event rates is provided by Goldschlager, 2000.

>10%:

Cardiovascular: Hypotension (I.V. 16%, refractory in rare cases)

Central nervous system (3% to 40%): Abnormal gait/ataxia, dizziness, fatigue, headache, malaise, impaired memory, involuntary movement, insomnia, poor coordination, peripheral neuropathy, sleep disturbances, tremor

Dermatologic: Photosensitivity (10% to 75%)

Endocrine & Metabolic: Hypothyroidism (1% to 22%)

Gastrointestinal: Nausea, vomiting, anorexia, and constipation (10% to 33%)

Hepatic: AST or ALT level >2x normal (15% to 50%)

Ocular: Corneal microdeposits (>90%; causes visual disturbance in <10%)

1% to 10%:

Cardiovascular: CHF (3%), bradycardia (3% to 5%), AV block (5%), conduction abnormalities, SA node dysfunction (1% to 3%), cardiac arrhythmia, flushing, edema. Additional effects associated with I.V. administration include asystole, atrial fibrillation, cardiac arrest, electromechanical dissociation, pulseless electrical activity (PEA), ventricular tachycardia, and cardiogenic shock.

Dermatologic: Slate blue skin discoloration (<10%)

Endocrine & metabolic: Hyperthyroidism (3% to 10%; more common in iodine-deficient regions of the world), libido decreased

Gastrointestinal: Abdominal pain, abnormal salivation, abnormal taste (oral), diarrhea, nausea (I.V.)

Hematologic: Coagulation abnormalities

Hepatic: Hepatitis and cirrhosis (<3%)

Local: Phlebitis (I.V., with concentrations >3 mg/mL)

Ocular: Visual disturbances (2% to 9%), halo vision (<5% occurring especially at night), optic neuritis (1%)

Respiratory: Pulmonary toxicity has been estimated to occur at a frequency between 2% and 7% of patients (some reports indicate a frequency as high as 17%). Toxicity may present as hypersensitivity pneumonitis; pulmonary fibrosis (cough, fever, malaise); pulmonary inflammation; interstitial pneumonitis; or alveolar pneumonitis. ARDS has been reported in up to 2% of patients receiving amiodarone, and postoperatively in patients receiving oral amiodarone.

Miscellaneous: Abnormal smell (oral)

<1% (Limited to important or life-threatening): Acute intracranial hypertension (I.V.), acute renal failure, acute respiratory distress syndrome, agranulocytosis, alopecia, anaphylactic shock, angioedema, aplastic anemia, bone marrow granuloma, bronchiolitis obliterans organizing pneumonia (BOOP), bronchospasm, cholestatic hepatitis, confusion, delirium, demyelinating polyneuropathy, disorientation, drug rash with eosinophilia and systemic symptoms (DRESS), dyspnea, encephalopathy, eczema, eosinophilic pneumonia, epididymitis (noninfectious), erectile dysfunction, erythema multiforme, exfoliative dermatitis, fever, granuloma, hallucination, hemolytic anemia, hemoptysis, hyperglycemia, hypertriglyceridemia, hypotension (oral), hypoxia, impotence, injection site reactions, leukocytoclastic vasculitis, muscle weakness, myopathy, neutropenia, optic neuropathy, pancreatitis, pancytopenia, parkinsonian symptoms, photophobia, pleural effusion, pleuritis, proarrhythmia, pruritus, pseudotumor cerebri, pulmonary alveolar hemorrhage, pulmonary edema, pulmonary infiltrates, pulmonary mass, QT interval increased, rash, renal impairment, renal insufficiency, respiratory failure, rhabdomyolysis, SIADH, sinus arrest, skin cancer, spontaneous ecchymosis, Stevens-Johnson syndrome, thrombocytopenia, thyroid nodules, thyroid cancer, thyrotoxicosis, torsade de pointes (rare), toxic epidermal necrolysis, urticaria, vasculitis, ventricular fibrillation, wheezing

Drug Interactions

Metabolism/Transport Effects Substrate of CYP1A2 (minor), CYP2C19 (minor), CYP2C8 (major), CYP2D6 (minor), CYP3A4 (major), P-glycoprotein; **Note:** Assignment of Major/Minor substrate status based on clinically relevant drug interaction potential; **Inhibits** CYP1A2 (weak), CYP2A6 (moderate), CYP2B6 (weak), CYP2C9 (moderate), CYP2D6 (moderate), CYP3A4 (moderate), P-glycoprotein

Avoid Concomitant Use

Avoid concomitant use of Amiodarone with any of the following: Agalsidase Alfa; Agalsidase Beta; Artemether; Conivaptan; Dronedarone; Grapefruit Juice; Lumefantrine; Nilotinib; Pimozide; Propafenone; Protease Inhibitors; QUEtiapine; QuiNINE; Silodosin; Tetrabenazine; Thioridazine; Topotecan; Toremifene; Vandetanib; Vemurafenib; Ziprasidone

Increased Effect/Toxicity

Amiodarone may increase the levels/effects of: Antiarrhythmic Agents (Class Ia); ARIPiprazole; Beta-Blockers; Budesonide (Systemic, Oral Inhalation); Cardiac Glycosides; Colchicine; CycloSPORINE; CycloSPORINE (Systemic); CYP2A6 Substrates; CYP2C9 Substrates; CYP2D6 Substrates; CYP3A4 Substrates; Dabigatran Etexilate; Dronedarone; Eplerenone; Everolimus; FentaNYL; Fesoterodine; Flecainide; Fosphenytoin; HMG-CoA Reductase Inhibitors; Lidocaine; Lidocaine (Systemic); Lidocaine (Topical); Loratadine; Lurasidone; P-glycoprotein/ABCB1 Substrates; Phenytoin; Pimecrolimus; Pimozide; Porfimer; Propafenone; QTc-Prolonging Agents; QuiNINE; Rivaroxaban; Salmeterol; Silodosin; Tetrabenazine; Thioridazine; Topotecan; Toremifene; Vandetanib; Vemurafenib; Vilazodone; Vitamin K Antagonists; Ziprasidone

The levels/effects of Amiodarone may be increased by: Alfuzosin; Artemether; Azithromycin; Azithromycin (Systemic); Boceprevir; Calcium Channel Blockers (Nondihydropyridine); Chloroquine; Cimetidine; Ciprofloxacin; Ciprofloxacin (Systemic); Conivaptan; CYP2C8 Inhibitors (Moderate); CYP2C8 Inhibitors (Strong); CYP3A4 Inhibitors (Moderate); CYP3A4 Inhibitors (Strong); Deferasirox; Eribulin; Fingolimod; Gadobutrol; Grapefruit Juice; Indacaterol; Lidocaine (Topical); Lumefantrine; Nilotinib; P-glycoprotein/ABCB1 Inhibitors; Protease Inhibitors; QUEtiapine; QuiNINE; Telaprevir

Decreased Effect

Amiodarone may decrease the levels/effects of: Agalsidase Alfa; Agalsidase Beta; Clopidogrel; Codeine; Sodium Iodide I 131; TraMADol

The levels/effects of Amiodarone may be decreased by: Bile Acid Sequestrants; CYP2C8 Inducers (Strong); CYP3A4 Inducers (Strong); Cyproterone; Deferasirox; Etravirine; Fosphenytoin; Grapefruit Juice; Orlistat; Peginterferon Alfa-2b; P-glycoprotein/ABCB1 Inducers; Phenytoin; Rifamycin Derivatives; Tocilizumab

Ethanol/Nutrition/Herb Interactions

Food: Increases the rate and extent of absorption of amiodarone. Grapefruit juice increases bioavailability of oral amiodarone by 50% and decreases the conversion of amiodarone to N-DEA (active metabolite); altered effects are possible; use should be avoided during therapy.

Herb/Nutraceutical: St John's wort may decrease amiodarone levels or enhance photosensitization. Avoid ephedra (may worsen arrhythmia). Avoid dong quai.

Stability Store undiluted vials and premixed solutions at 20°C to 25°C (68°F to 77°F). Protect from light.

Vials for injection: When admixed in D_5W to a final concentration of 1-6 mg/mL, the solution is stable at room temperature for 24 hours in polyolefin or glass, or for 2 hours in PVC. Infusions >2 hours must be administered in a non-PVC container (eg, glass or polyolefin). Do not use evacuated glass containers; buffer may cause precipitation.

Mechanism of Action Class III antiarrhythmic agent which inhibits adrenergic stimulation (alpha- and beta-blocking properties), affects sodium, potassium, and calcium channels, prolongs the action potential and refractory period in myocardial tissue; decreases AV conduction and sinus node function

Pharmacodynamics/Kinetics

Absorption: Slow and variable

Onset of action: Oral: 2 days to 3 weeks; I.V.: May be more rapid

Peak effect: 1 week to 5 months

Duration after discontinuing therapy: 7-50 days

Note: Mean onset of effect and duration after discontinuation may be shorter in children than adults

Distribution: V_d: 66 L/kg (range: 18-148 L/kg)

Protein binding: 96%

Metabolism: Hepatic via CYP2C8 and 3A4 to active N-desethylamiodarone metabolite; possible enterohepatic recirculation

Bioavailability: Oral: 35% to 65%

Half-life elimination: Terminal: 40-55 days (range: 26-107 days); shorter in children

Time to peak, serum: 3-7 hours

Excretion: Feces; urine (<1% as unchanged drug)

Dosage Note: Lower loading and maintenance doses are preferable in women and all patients with low body weight.

Oral:

Children: Arrhythmias (unlabeled use):

Loading dose: 10-20 mg/kg/day in 1-2 doses for 4-14 days or until adequate control of arrhythmia or prominent adverse effects occur; alternative loading dose in children <1 year: 600-800 mg/1.73 m^2/day in 1-2 divided doses/day

Maintenance dose: Dose may be reduced to 5 mg/kg/day for several weeks (or 200-400 mg/1.73 m^2/day given once daily); if no recurrence of arrhythmia, dose may be further reduced to 2.5 mg/kg/day; maintenance doses may be given 5-7 days/week

Adults:

Ventricular arrhythmias: 800-1600 mg/day in 1-2 doses for 1-3 weeks, then when adequate arrhythmia control is achieved, decrease to 600-800 mg/day in 1-2 doses for 1 month; maintenance: 400 mg/day. Lower doses are recommended for supraventricular arrhythmias.

Atrial fibrillation:

Pharmacologic cardioversion (unlabeled use): ACC/AHA/ESC Practice Guidelines: *Inpatient:* 1.2-1.8 g/day in divided doses until 10 g total, then 200-400 mg/day maintenance. *Outpatient:* 600-800 mg/day in divided doses until 10 g total, then 200-400 mg/day maintenance; although not supported by clinical evidence, a maintenance dose of 100 mg/day is commonly used especially for the elderly or patients with low body mass (Fuster, 2006; Zimetbaum, 2007). **Note:** Other regimens have been described and may be used clinically:

400 mg 3 times/day for 5-7 days, then 400 mg/day for 1 month, then 200 mg/day

or

10 mg/kg/day for 14 days, followed by 300 mg/day for 4 weeks, followed by maintenance dosage of 200 mg/day (Roy, 2000)

Prophylaxis following open heart surgery (unlabeled use): Starting in postop recovery: 400 mg twice daily for up to 7 days. Alternative regimen of amiodarone: 600 mg/day for 7 days prior to surgery, followed by 200 mg/day until hospital discharge, has also been shown to decrease the risk of postoperative atrial fibrillation. **Note:** A variety of regimens have been used in clinical trials.

I.V.:

Children:

Arrhythmias (unlabeled use, dosing based on limited data): Loading dose: 5 mg/kg over 30 minutes; may repeat up to 3 times if no response. Maintenance dose: Continuous infusion: 10-20 mg/kg/day followed by conversion to oral therapy as appropriate

Note: I.V. administration at low flow rates (potentially associated with use in pediatrics) may result in leaching of plasticizers (DEHP) from intravenous tubing. DEHP may adversely affect male reproductive tract development. Alternative means of dosing and administration (1 mg/kg aliquots) may need to be considered.

Pulseless VT or VF (PALS dosing): 5 mg/kg (maximum: 300 mg/dose) rapid I.V. bolus or I.O.; repeat up to a maximum daily dose of 15 mg/kg. (**Note:** Maximum recommended daily dose in adolescents is 2.2 g.)

Perfusing tachycardias (PALS dosing): Loading dose: 5 mg/kg (maximum: 300 mg/dose) I.V. over 20-60 minutes or I.O.; may repeat up to maximum dose of 15 mg/kg/day. (**Note:** Maximum recommended daily dose in adolescents is 2.2 g.)

Adults:

Atrial fibrillation:

Pharmacologic cardioversion (ACC/AHA/ESC Practice Guidelines) (unlabeled use): 5-7 mg/kg over 30-60 minutes, then 1.2-1.8 g/day continuous infusion until 10 g total. Maintenance: See oral dosing.

Prophylaxis following open heart surgery (unlabeled use): Starting at postop recovery, 1000 mg infused over 24 hours for 2 days has been shown to reduce the risk of postoperative atrial fibrillation. **Note:** A variety of regimens have been used in clinical trials.

Pulseless VT or VF (ACLS, 2010): I.V. push, I.O.: Initial: 300 mg; if pulseless VT or VF continues after subsequent defibrillation attempt or recurs, administer supplemental dose of 150 mg. **Note:** In this setting, administering **undiluted** is preferred (Dager, 2006; Skrifvars, 2004). *The Handbook of Emergency Cardiovascular Care* (Hazinski, 2010) and the 2010 ACLS guidelines, do not make any specific recommendations regarding dilution of amiodarone in this setting. Experience limited with I.O. administration of amiodarone (ACLS, 2010).

Upon return of spontaneous circulation, follow with an infusion of 1 mg/minute for 6 hours, then 0.5 mg/minute for 18 hours (mean daily doses >2.1 g/day have been associated with hypotension).

Stable VT or SVT (unlabeled use): First 24 hours: 1050 mg according to following regimen

Step 1: 150 mg (100 mL) over first 10 minutes (mix 3 mL in 100 mL D_5W)

Step 2: 360 mg (200 mL) over next 6 hours (mix 18 mL in 500 mL D_5W): 1 mg/minute

Step 3: 540 mg (300 mL) over next 18 hours: 0.5 mg/minute

Note: After the first 24 hours: 0.5 mg/minute utilizing concentration of 1-6 mg/mL

Breakthrough stable VT or SVT: 150 mg supplemental doses in 100 mL D_5W or NS over 10 minutes (mean daily doses >2.1 g/day have been associated with hypotension)

I.V. to oral therapy conversion: Use the following as a guide:

<1-week I.V. infusion: 800-1600 mg/day

1- to 3-week I.V. infusion: 600-800 mg/day

>3-week I.V. infusion: 400 mg/day

Note: Conversion from I.V. to oral therapy has not been formally evaluated. Some experts recommend a 1-2 day overlap when converting from I.V. to oral therapy especially when treating ventricular arrhythmias.

Recommendations for conversion to intravenous amiodarone after oral administration: During long-term amiodarone therapy (ie, ≥4 months), the mean plasma-elimination half-life of the active metabolite of amiodarone is 61 days. Replacement therapy may not be necessary in such patients if oral therapy is discontinued for a period <2 weeks, since any changes in serum amiodarone concentrations during this period may **not** be clinically significant.

Elderly: No specific guidelines available. Dose selection should be cautious, at low end of dosage range, and titration should be slower to evaluate response. Although not supported by clinical evidence, a maintenance dose of 100 mg/day is commonly used especially for the elderly or patients with low body mass (Fuster, 2006; Zimetbaum, 2007).

Dosing adjustment in renal impairment: No dosage adjustment necessary

Hemodialysis: Not dialyzable (0% to 5%); supplemental dose is not necessary.

Peritoneal dialysis: Not dialyzable (0% to 5%); supplemental dose is not necessary.

Dosing adjustment in hepatic impairment: Dosage adjustment is probably necessary in substantial hepatic impairment. No specific guidelines available. If hepatic enzymes exceed 3 times normal or double in a patient with an elevated baseline, consider decreasing the dose or discontinuing amiodarone.

Dietary Considerations Take consistently with regard to meals. Amiodarone is a potential source of large amounts of inorganic iodine; ~3 mg of inorganic iodine per 100 mg of amiodarone is released into the systemic circulation. Recommended daily allowance for iodine in adults is 150 mcg.

Grapefruit juice is not recommended.

Administration

Oral: Administer consistently with regard to meals. Take in divided doses with meals if GI upset occurs or if taking large daily dose. If GI intolerance occurs with single-dose therapy, use twice daily dosing.

I.V.: For infusions >1 hour, use concentrations ≤2 mg/mL unless a central venous catheter is used; commercially-prepared premixed solutions in concentrations of 1.5 mg/mL and 1.8 mg/mL are available. Use only volumetric infusion pump; use of drop counting may lead to underdosage. Administer through an I.V. line located as centrally as possible. For continuous infusions, an in-line filter has been recommended during administration to reduce the incidence of phlebitis. During pulseless VT/VF, administering **undiluted** is preferred (Dager, 2006; Skrifvars, 2004). *The Handbook of Emergency Cardiovascular Care* (Hazinski, 2010) and the 2010 ACLS guidelines do not make any specific recommendations regarding dilution of amiodarone in this setting.

Adjust administration rate to urgency (give more slowly when perfusing arrhythmia present). Slow the infusion rate if hypotension or bradycardia develops. Infusions >2 hours must be administered in a non-PVC container (eg, glass or polyolefin). PVC tubing is recommended for administration regardless of infusion duration. **Note:** I.V. administration at lower flow rates (potentially associated with use in pediatrics) and higher concentrations than recommended may result in leaching of plasticizers (DEHP) from intravenous tubing. DEHP may adversely affect male reproductive tract development. Alternative means of dosing and administration (1 mg/kg aliquots) may need to be considered.

Monitoring Parameters Blood pressure, heart rate (ECG) and rhythm throughout therapy; assess patient for signs of lethargy, edema of the hands or feet, weight loss, and pulmonary toxicity (baseline pulmonary function tests and chest X-ray; continue monitoring chest X-ray annually during therapy); liver function tests (semiannually); monitor serum electrolytes, especially potassium and magnesium. Assess thyroid function tests before initiation of treatment and then periodically thereafter (some experts suggest every 3-6 months). If signs or symptoms of thyroid disease or arrhythmia breakthrough/exacerbation occur then immediate re-evaluation is necessary. Amiodarone partially inhibits the peripheral conversion of thyroxine (T_4) to triiodothyronine (T_3); serum T_4 and reverse triiodothyronine (rT_3) concentrations may be increased and serum T_3 may be decreased; most patients remain clinically euthyroid, however, clinical hypothyroidism or hyperthyroidism may occur.

Perform regular ophthalmic exams.

Patients with implantable cardiac devices: Monitor pacing or defibrillation thresholds with initiation of amiodarone and during treatment.

Reference Range Therapeutic: 0.5-2.5 mg/L (SI: 1-4 micromole/L) (parent); desethyl metabolite is active and is present in equal concentration to parent drug

Dosage Forms Excipient information presented when available (limited, particularly for generics); consult specific product labeling.

Infusion, premixed iso-osmotic dextrose solution, as hydrochloride:
Nexterone®: 150 mg (100 mL); 360 mg (200 mL) [contains cyclodextrin]

Injection, solution, as hydrochloride: 50 mg/mL (3 mL, 9 mL, 18 mL)

Tablet, oral, as hydrochloride: 200 mg, 400 mg
Cordarone®: 200 mg [scored]
Pacerone®: 100 mg
Pacerone®: 200 mg, 400 mg [scored]

Extemporaneous Preparations A 5 mg/mL oral suspension may be made with tablets and either a 1:1 mixture of Ora-Sweet® and Ora-Plus® or a 1:1 mixture of Ora-Sweet® SF and Ora-Plus® adjusted to a pH between 6-7 using a sodium bicarbonate solution (5 g/100 mL of distilled water). Crush five 200 mg tablets in a mortar and reduce to a fine powder. Add small portions of the chosen vehicle and mix to a uniform paste; mix while adding the vehicle in incremental proportions to **almost** 200 mL; transfer to a calibrated bottle, rinse mortar with vehicle, and add quantity of vehicle sufficient to make 200 mL. Label "shake well" and "protect from light". Stable for 42 days at room temperature or 91 days refrigerated (preferred) (Nahata, 2004).

Nahata MC, Pai VB, and Hipple TF, *Pediatric Drug Formulations*, 5th ed, Cincinnati, OH: Harvey Whitney Books Co, 2004.

◆ **Amiodarone Hydrochloride** *see* Amiodarone *on page 90*

◆ **Amiodarone Hydrochloride Injection (Can)** *see* Amiodarone *on page 90*

◆ **Amitiza®** *see* Lubiprostone *on page 1040*

Amitriptyline (a mee TRIP ti leen)

Brand Names: Canada Apo-Amitriptyline®; Bio-Amitriptyline; Dom-Amitriptyline; Elavil; Levate®; Novo-Triptyn; PMS-Amitriptyline

Index Terms Amitriptyline Hydrochloride; Elavil

Pharmacologic Category Antidepressant, Tricyclic (Tertiary Amine)

Additional Appendix Information

Antidepressant Agents *on page 1874*

Beers Criteria – Potentially Inappropriate Medications for Geriatrics *on page 1973*

Use Relief of symptoms of depression

Unlabeled Use Analgesic for certain chronic and neuropathic pain (including diabetic neuropathy); prophylaxis against migraine headaches; treatment of depressive disorders in children; post-traumatic stress disorder (PTSD)

Pregnancy Risk Factor C

Pregnancy Considerations Teratogenic effects have been observed in animal studies. Amitriptyline crosses the human placenta; CNS effects, limb deformities and developmental delay have been noted in case reports.

Lactation Enters breast milk/not recommended (AAP rates "of concern"; AAP 2001 update pending)

Medication Guide Available Yes

Contraindications Hypersensitivity to amitriptyline or any component of the formulation (cross-sensitivity with other tricyclics may occur); use of MAO inhibitors within past 14 days; acute recovery phase following myocardial infarction; concurrent use of cisapride

Warnings/Precautions [U.S. Boxed Warning]: Antidepressants increase the risk of suicidal thinking and behavior in children, adolescents, and young adults (18-24 years of age) with major depressive disorder (MDD) and other psychiatric disorders; consider risk prior to prescribing. Short-term studies did not show an increased risk in patients >24 years of age and showed a decreased risk in patients ≥65 years. Closely monitor for clinical worsening, suicidality, or unusual changes in behavior; the patient's family or caregiver should be instructed to closely observe the patient and communicate condition with healthcare provider. Such observation would generally include at least weekly face-to-face contact with patients or their family members or caregivers during the first 4 weeks of treatment, then every other week visits for the next 4 weeks, then at 12 weeks, and as clinically indicated beyond 12 weeks. Additional contact by telephone may be appropriate between face-to-face visits. Adults treated with antidepressants should be observed similarly for clinical worsening and suicidality, especially during the initial few months of a course of drug therapy, or at times of dose changes, either increases or decreases. A medication guide should be dispensed with each prescription. **Amitriptyline is not FDA-approved for use in children <12 years of age.**

The possibility of a suicide attempt is inherent in major depression and may persist until remission occurs. Monitor for worsening of depression or suicidality, especially during initiation of therapy (generally first 1-2 months) or with dose increases or decreases. Worsening depression and severe abrupt suicidality that are not part of the presenting symptoms may require discontinuation or modification of drug therapy. The patient's family or caregiver should be alerted to monitor patients for the emergence of suicidality and associated behaviors (such as agitation, irritability, hostility, impulsivity, and hypomania) and notify healthcare provider.

May worsen psychosis in some patients or precipitate a shift to mania or hypomania in patients with bipolar disorder. Patients presenting with depressive symptoms should be screened for bipolar disorder. Monotherapy in patients with bipolar disorder should be avoided. **Amitriptyline is not FDA approved for bipolar depression.**

The degree of sedation, anticholinergic effects, orthostasis, and conduction abnormalities are high relative to other antidepressants. Amitriptyline often causes drowsiness/sedation, resulting in impaired performance of tasks requiring alertness (eg, operating machinery or driving). Sedative effects may be additive with other CNS depressants and/or ethanol. Use with caution in patients with a history of cardiovascular disease (including previous MI, stroke, tachycardia, or conduction abnormalities). Use with caution in patients with urinary retention, benign prostatic hyperplasia, narrow-angle glaucoma, xerostomia, visual problems, constipation, or a history of bowel obstruction.

TCAs may rarely cause bone marrow suppression; monitor for any signs of infection and obtain CBC if symptoms (eg, fever, sore throat) evident. May alter glucose control - use with caution in patients with diabetes. Consider discontinuing, when possible, prior to elective surgery. Therapy should not be abruptly discontinued in patients receiving high doses for prolonged periods. May lower seizure threshold - use caution in patients with a previous seizure disorder or condition predisposing to seizures such as brain damage, alcoholism, or concurrent therapy with other drugs which lower the seizure threshold. Hyperpyrexia has been observed with TCAs in combination with anticholinergics and/or neuroleptics, particularly during hot weather. May increase the risks associated with electroconvulsive therapy. Use with caution in hyperthyroid patients or those receiving thyroid supplementation. Use with caution in patients with hepatic or renal dysfunction. Use with caution in the elderly; may be inappropriate in this age group due to its potent anticholinergic and sedative properties (Beers Criteria).

Adverse Reactions Anticholinergic effects may be pronounced; moderate to marked sedation can occur (tolerance to these effects usually occurs).

Frequency not defined.

Cardiovascular: Orthostatic hypotension, tachycardia, ECG changes (nonspecific), AV conduction changes, cardiomyopathy (rare), MI, stroke, heart block, arrhythmia, syncope, hypertension, palpitation

Central nervous system: Restlessness, dizziness, insomnia, sedation, fatigue, anxiety, cognitive function impaired, seizure, extrapyramidal symptoms, coma, hallucinations, confusion, disorientation, coordination impaired, ataxia, headache, nightmares, hyperpyrexia

Dermatologic: Allergic rash, urticaria, photosensitivity, alopecia

Endocrine & metabolic: Syndrome of inappropriate ADH secretion

Gastrointestinal: Weight gain, xerostomia, constipation, paralytic ileus, nausea, vomiting, anorexia, stomatitis, peculiar taste, diarrhea, black tongue

Genitourinary: Urinary retention

Hematologic: Bone marrow depression, purpura, eosinophilia

Neuromuscular & skeletal: Numbness, paresthesia, peripheral neuropathy, tremor, weakness

Ocular: Blurred vision, mydriasis, ocular pressure increased

Otic: Tinnitus

Miscellaneous: Diaphoresis, withdrawal reactions (nausea, headache, malaise)

Postmarketing and/or case reports: Neuroleptic malignant syndrome (rare), serotonin syndrome (rare)

Drug Interactions

Metabolism/Transport Effects Substrate of CYP1A2 (minor), CYP2B6 (minor), CYP2C19 (minor), CYP2C9 (minor), CYP2D6 (major), CYP3A4 (minor); **Note:** Assignment of Major/Minor substrate status based on clinically relevant drug interaction potential; **Inhibits** CYP1A2 (weak), CYP2C19 (weak), CYP2C9 (weak), CYP2D6 (weak), CYP2E1 (weak)

Avoid Concomitant Use

Avoid concomitant use of Amitriptyline with any of the following: Artemether; Cisapride; Dronedarone; Iobenguane I 123; Lumefantrine; MAO Inhibitors; Methylene Blue; Nilotinib; Pimozide; QUEtiapine; QuiNINE; Tetrabenazine; Thioridazine; Toremifene; Vandetanib; Vemurafenib; Ziprasidone

Increased Effect/Toxicity

Amitriptyline may increase the levels/effects of: Alpha-/Beta-Agonists (Direct-Acting); Alpha1-Agonists; Amphetamines; Anticholinergics; Aspirin; Beta2-Agonists; Cisapride; Desmopressin; Dronedarone; Methylene Blue; Metoclopramide; NSAID (COX-2 Inhibitor); NSAID (Nonselective); Pimozide; QTc-Prolonging Agents; QuiNIDine; QuiNINE; Serotonin Modulators; Sodium Phosphates; Sulfonylureas; Tetrabenazine; Thioridazine; Toremifene; TraMADol; Vandetanib; Vemurafenib; Vitamin K Antagonists; Yohimbine; Ziprasidone

The levels/effects of Amitriptyline may be increased by: Abiraterone Acetate; Alfuzosin; Altretamine; Antipsychotics; Artemether; BuPROPion; Chloroquine; Cimetidine; Cinacalcet; Ciprofloxacin; Ciprofloxacin (Systemic); Conivaptan; CYP2D6 Inhibitors (Moderate); CYP2D6 Inhibitors (Strong); Dexmethylphenidate; Divalproex; DULoxetine; Gadobutrol; Indacaterol; Linezolid; Lithium; Lumefantrine; MAO Inhibitors; Methylphenidate; Metoclopramide; Nilotinib; Pramlintide; Protease Inhibitors; QUEtiapine; QuiNIDine; QuiNINE; Selective Serotonin Reuptake Inhibitors; Terbinafine; Terbinafine (Systemic); Valproic Acid

Decreased Effect

Amitriptyline may decrease the levels/effects of: Acetylcholinesterase Inhibitors (Central); Alpha2-Agonists; Iobenguane I 123

The levels/effects of Amitriptyline may be decreased by: Acetylcholinesterase Inhibitors (Central); Barbiturates; CarBAMazepine; Cyproterone; Peginterferon Alfa-2b; St Johns Wort; Tocilizumab

Ethanol/Nutrition/Herb Interactions

Ethanol: May increase CNS depression; monitor for increased effects with coadministration. Caution patients about effects.

Food: Grapefruit juice may inhibit the metabolism of some TCAs and clinical toxicity may result.

Herb/Nutraceutical: St John's wort may decrease amitriptyline levels. Avoid valerian, St John's wort, kava kava, gotu kola (may increase CNS depression).

Mechanism of Action Increases the synaptic concentration of serotonin and/or norepinephrine in the central nervous system by inhibition of their reuptake by the presynaptic neuronal membrane

Pharmacodynamics/Kinetics

Onset of action: Migraine prophylaxis: 6 weeks, higher dosage may be required in heavy smokers because of increased metabolism; Depression: 4-6 weeks, reduce dosage to lowest effective level

Distribution: Crosses placenta; enters breast milk

Metabolism: Hepatic to nortriptyline (active), hydroxy and conjugated derivatives; may be impaired in the elderly

Half-life elimination: Adults: 9-27 hours (average: 15 hours)

Time to peak, serum: ~4 hours

Excretion: Urine (18% as unchanged drug); feces (small amounts)

Dosage

Children:

Chronic pain management (unlabeled use): Oral: Initial: 0.1 mg/kg at bedtime, may advance as tolerated over 2-3 weeks to 0.5-2 mg/kg at bedtime

Depressive disorders (unlabeled use): Oral: Initial doses of 1 mg/kg/day given in 3 divided doses with increases to 1.5 mg/kg/day have been reported in a small number of children (n=9) 9-12 years of age; clinically, doses up to 3 mg/kg/day (5 mg/kg/day if monitored closely) have been proposed

Migraine prophylaxis (unlabeled use): Oral: Initial: 0.25 mg/kg/day, given at bedtime; increase dose by 0.25 mg/kg/day to maximum 1 mg/kg/day. Reported dosing ranges: 0.1-2 mg/kg/day; maximum suggested dose: 10 mg.

Adolescents: Depressive disorders: Oral: Initial: 25-50 mg/day; may administer in divided doses; increase gradually to 100 mg/day in divided doses

Adults:
Depression: Oral: 50-150 mg/day single dose at bedtime or in divided doses; dose may be gradually increased up to 300 mg/day
Chronic pain management (unlabeled use): Oral: Initial: 25 mg at bedtime; may increase as tolerated to 100 mg/day
Diabetic neuropathy (unlabeled use): Oral: 25-100 mg/day (Bril, 2011)
Migraine prophylaxis (unlabeled use): Oral: Initial: 10-25 mg at bedtime; usual dose: 150 mg; reported dosing ranges: 10-400 mg/day
Post-traumatic stress disorder (PTSD) (unlabeled use): Oral: 75-200 mg/day
Elderly: Depression: Oral: Initial: 10-25 mg at bedtime; dose should be increased in 10-25 mg increments every week if tolerated; dose range: 25-150 mg/day
Dosing interval in hepatic impairment: Use with caution and monitor plasma levels and patient response
Hemodialysis: Nondialyzable

Monitoring Parameters Monitor blood pressure and pulse rate prior to and during initial therapy; evaluate mental status, suicide ideation (especially at the beginning of therapy or when doses are increased or decreased); ECG in older adults and patients with cardiac disease

Reference Range Therapeutic: Amitriptyline and nortriptyline 100-250 ng/mL (SI: 360-900 nmol/L); nortriptyline 50-150 ng/mL (SI: 190-570 nmol/L); Toxic: >0.5 mcg/mL; plasma levels do not always correlate with clinical effectiveness

Test Interactions May cause false-positive reaction to EMIT immunoassay for imipramine

Dosage Forms Excipient information presented when available (limited, particularly for generics); consult specific product labeling.
Tablet, oral, as hydrochloride: 10 mg, 25 mg, 50 mg, 75 mg, 100 mg, 150 mg

Amitriptyline and Chlordiazepoxide

(a mee TRIP ti leen & klor dye az e POKS ide)

Index Terms Chlordiazepoxide and Amitriptyline Hydrochloride; Limbitrol

Pharmacologic Category Antidepressant, Tricyclic (Tertiary Amine); Benzodiazepine

Additional Appendix Information
Beers Criteria – Potentially Inappropriate Medications for Geriatrics *on page 1973*

Use Treatment of moderate-to-severe anxiety and/or agitation and depression

Pregnancy Risk Factor D

Medication Guide Available Yes

Dosage Initial: 3-4 tablets in divided doses; this may be increased to 6 tablets/day as required; some patients respond to smaller doses and can be maintained on 2 tablets

Additional Information Complete prescribing information for this medication should be consulted for additional detail.

Dosage Forms Excipient information presented when available (limited, particularly for generics); consult specific product labeling.
Tablet: 12.5/5: Amitriptyline hydrochloride 12.5 mg and chlordiazepoxide 5 mg; 25/10: Amitriptyline hydrochloride 25 mg and chlordiazepoxide 10 mg

Controlled Substance C-IV

Amitriptyline and Perphenazine

(a mee TRIP ti leen & per FEN a zeen)

Brand Names: Canada PMS-Levazine

Index Terms Perphenazine and Amitriptyline Hydrochloride

Pharmacologic Category Antidepressant, Tricyclic (Tertiary Amine); Antipsychotic Agent, Typical, Phenothiazine

Additional Appendix Information
Beers Criteria – Potentially Inappropriate Medications for Geriatrics *on page 1973*

Use Treatment of patients with moderate-to-severe anxiety and/or agitation and depression; schizophrenia with depressive symptoms

Medication Guide Available Yes

Dosage Oral: Adults:
Depression and anxiety:
Initial: One tablet (amitriptyline 25 mg/perphenazine 2 mg or amitriptyline 25 mg/perphenazine 4 mg) 3-4 times/day **or** 1 tablet (amitriptyline 50 mg/perphenazine 4 mg) 2 times/day; initial therapeutic response may be observed after several days or upwards of a few weeks or longer (maximum daily dose: amitriptyline 200 mg/perphenazine 16 mg)
Maintenance: Smallest dose necessary for symptom relief; usually 1 tablet (amitriptyline 25 mg/perphenazine 2 mg or amitriptyline 25 mg/perphenazine 4 mg) 2-4 times/day **or** 1 tablet (amitriptyline 50 mg/perphenazine 4 mg) 2 times/day
Schizophrenia and depression:
Initial: Two tablets (amitriptyline 25 mg/perphenazine 4 mg) 3 times/day; if necessary, a fourth dose may be given at bedtime; initial therapeutic response may be observed after several days or upwards of a few weeks or longer (maximum daily dose: amitriptyline 200 mg/perphenazine 16 mg) (maximum: 64 mg/day of perphenazine)
Maintenance: Smallest dose necessary for symptom relief; usually 1 tablet (amitriptyline 25 mg/perphenazine 2 mg or amitriptyline 25 mg/perphenazine 4 mg) 2-4 times/day **or** 1 tablet (amitriptyline 50 mg/perphenazine 4 mg) 2 times/day
Elderly: One tablet (amitriptyline 10 mg/perphenazine 4 mg) 3-4 times/day
Dosage adjustment in renal impairment: No dosage adjustment provided in manufacturer's labeling.
Dosage adjustment in hepatic impairment: Use caution; no dosage adjustment provided in manufacturer's labeling.

Additional Information Complete prescribing information for this medication should be consulted for additional detail.

Dosage Forms Excipient information presented when available (limited, particularly for generics); consult specific product labeling.
Tablet:
2-10: Amitriptyline hydrochloride 10 mg and perphenazine 2 mg
4-10: Amitriptyline hydrochloride 10 mg and perphenazine 4 mg
2-25: Amitriptyline hydrochloride 25 mg and perphenazine 2 mg
4-25: Amitriptyline hydrochloride 25 mg and perphenazine 4 mg
4-50: Amitriptyline hydrochloride 50 mg and perphenazine 4 mg

◆ **Amitriptyline Hydrochloride** *see* Amitriptyline *on page 94*

◆ **AMJ 9701** *see* Palifermin *on page 1276*

Amlexanox (am LEKS an oks)

Brand Names: U.S. Aphthasol®

Pharmacologic Category Anti-inflammatory, Locally Applied

Use Treatment of aphthous ulcers (ie, canker sores)

Unlabeled Use Allergic disorders

Pregnancy Risk Factor B

Dosage Topical: Administer ~1/4 inch (0.5 cm) directly on ulcers 4 times/day following oral hygiene, after meals, and at bedtime

Additional Information Complete prescribing information for this medication should be consulted for additional detail.

Dosage Forms Excipient information presented when available (limited, particularly for generics); consult specific product labeling.

Paste, oral:

Aphthasol®: 5% (3 g) [contains benzyl alcohol]

AmLODIPine (am LOE di peen)

Brand Names: U.S. Norvasc®

Brand Names: Canada Accel-Amlodipine; Apo-Amlodipine®; CO Amlodipine; Dom-Amlodipine; GD-Amlodipine; JAMP-Amlodipine; Mint-Amlodipine; Mylan-Amlodipine; Norvasc®; PHL-Amlodipine; PMS-Amlodipine; RAN™-Amlodipine; ratio-Amlodipine; Riva-Amlodipine; Sandoz Amlodipine; Septa-Amlodipine; Teva-Amlodipine; ZYM-Amlodipine

Index Terms Amlodipine Besylate

Pharmacologic Category Antianginal Agent; Calcium Channel Blocker; Calcium Channel Blocker, Dihydropyridine

Additional Appendix Information

Calcium Channel Blockers *on page 1887*

Use Treatment of hypertension; treatment of symptomatic chronic stable angina, vasospastic (Prinzmetal's) angina (confirmed or suspected); prevention of hospitalization due to angina with documented CAD (limited to patients without heart failure or ejection fraction <40%)

Pregnancy Risk Factor C

Pregnancy Considerations Embryotoxic effects have been demonstrated in animal studies. No well-controlled studies have been conducted in pregnant women. Use in pregnancy only when clearly needed and when the benefits outweigh the potential hazard to the fetus.

Lactation Excretion in breast milk unknown/not recommended

Contraindications Hypersensitivity to amlodipine or any component of the formulation

Warnings/Precautions Increased angina and/or MI has occurred with initiation or dosage titration of calcium channel blockers. Symptomatic hypotension with or without syncope can rarely occur; blood pressure must be lowered at a rate appropriate for the patient's clinical condition. Use caution in severe aortic stenosis and/or hypertrophic cardiomyopathy with outflow tract obstruction. Use caution in patients with hepatic impairment; may require lower starting dose; titrate slowly with severe hepatic impairment. The most common side effect is peripheral edema; occurs within 2-3 weeks of starting therapy. Reflex tachycardia may occur with use. Peak antihypertensive effect is delayed; dosage titration should occur after 7-14 days on a given dose. Initiate at a lower dose in the elderly.

Adverse Reactions

>10%: Cardiovascular: Peripheral edema (2% to 15% dose related; HF patients: 27% [Packer, 1996])

1% to 10%:

Cardiovascular: Flushing (1% to 5% dose related), palpitation (1% to 5% dose related)

Central nervous system: Dizziness (1% to 3% dose related), fatigue (5%), somnolence (1% to 2%)

Dermatologic: Rash (1% to 2%), pruritus (1% to 2%)

Endocrine & metabolic: Male sexual dysfunction (1% to 2%)

Gastrointestinal: Nausea (3%), abdominal pain (1% to 2%), dyspepsia (1% to 2%)

Neuromuscular & skeletal: Muscle cramps (1% to 2%), weakness (1% to 2%)

Respiratory: Dyspnea (1% to 2%), pulmonary edema (HF patients: 27% [Packer, 1996])

<1% (Limited to important or life-threatening): Abnormal dreams, abnormal vision, abnormal visual accommodation, acute interstitial nephritis, allergic reactions, agitation, alopecia, amnesia, angioedema, anorexia, anxiety, apathy, appetite increased, arrhythmia, arthralgia, arthrosis, ataxia, atrial fibrillation, back pain, bradycardia, cardiac failure, chest pain, cholestasis, cold and clammy skin, conjunctivitis, constipation, cough, depersonalization, depression, dermatitis, diaphoresis increased, diarrhea, diplopia, dysphagia, dysuria, epistaxis, erythema multiforme, exfoliative dermatitis, extrasystoles, eye pain, female sexual dysfunction, flatulence, gastritis, gingival hyperplasia, gynecomastia, hepatitis, hot flushes, hyperglycemia, hypertonia, hypoesthesia, hypotension, insomnia, jaundice, leukocytoclastic vasculitis, leukopenia, loose stools, malaise, micturition disorder, micturition frequency, migraine, muscle weakness, myalgia, nervousness, nocturia, nonthrombocytopenic purpura, pain, pancreatitis, paresthesia, parosmia, peripheral ischemia, peripheral neuropathy, phototoxicity, polyuria, postural dizziness, postural hypotension, pulse irregularity, purpura, rash erythematous, rash maculopapular, rhinitis, rigors, skin discoloration, skin dryness, Stevens-Johnson syndrome, syncope, tachycardia, taste perversion, thirst, thrombocytopenia, tinnitus, transaminases increased, tremor, twitching, urticaria, vasculitis, ventricular tachycardia, vertigo, vomiting, weight gain/loss, xerophthalmia, xerostomia

Drug Interactions

Metabolism/Transport Effects Substrate of CYP3A4 (major); **Note:** Assignment of Major/Minor substrate status based on clinically relevant drug interaction potential; **Inhibits** CYP1A2 (moderate), CYP2A6 (weak), CYP2B6 (weak), CYP2C8 (weak), CYP2C9 (weak), CYP2D6 (weak), CYP3A4 (weak)

Avoid Concomitant Use

Avoid concomitant use of AmLODIPine with any of the following: Conivaptan; Pimozide

Increased Effect/Toxicity

AmLODIPine may increase the levels/effects of: Amifostine; Antihypertensives; Beta-Blockers; Calcium Channel Blockers (Nondihydropyridine); CYP1A2 Substrates; Fosphenytoin; Hypotensive Agents; Magnesium Salts; Neuromuscular-Blocking Agents (Nondepolarizing); Nitroprusside; Phenytoin; Pimozide; QuiNIDine; RiTUXimab; Simvastatin; Tacrolimus; Tacrolimus (Systemic)

The levels/effects of AmLODIPine may be increased by: Alpha1-Blockers; Antifungal Agents (Azole Derivatives, Systemic); Calcium Channel Blockers (Nondihydropyridine); Conivaptan; CycloSPORINE; CycloSPORINE (Systemic); CYP3A4 Inhibitors (Moderate); CYP3A4 Inhibitors (Strong); Dasatinib; Diazoxide; Fluconazole; Grapefruit Juice; Herbs (Hypotensive Properties); Macrolide Antibiotics; Magnesium Salts; MAO Inhibitors; Pentoxifylline; Phosphodiesterase 5 Inhibitors; Prostacyclin Analogues; Protease Inhibitors; QuiNIDine

Decreased Effect

AmLODIPine may decrease the levels/effects of: Clopidogrel; QuiNIDine

The levels/effects of AmLODIPine may be decreased by: Barbiturates; Calcium Salts; CarBAMazepine; CYP3A4 Inducers (Strong); Deferasirox; Herbs (CYP3A4 Inducers); Herbs (Hypertensive Properties); Methylphenidate; Nafcillin; Rifamycin Derivatives; Tocilizumab; Yohimbine

Ethanol/Nutrition/Herb Interactions
Food: Grapefruit juice may modestly increase amlodipine levels.
Herb/Nutraceutical: St John's wort may decrease amlodipine levels. Avoid herbs with *hypertensive* properties (bayberry, blue cohosh, cayenne, ephedra, ginger, ginseng [American], kola, licorice). Avoid herbs with *hypotensive* properties (black cohosh, California poppy, coleus, garlic, goldenseal, hawthorn, mistletoe, periwinkle, quinine, shepherd's purse).

Stability Store at room temperature of 15°C to 30°C (59°F to 86°F).

Mechanism of Action Inhibits calcium ion from entering the "slow channels" or select voltage-sensitive areas of vascular smooth muscle and myocardium during depolarization, producing a relaxation of coronary vascular smooth muscle and coronary vasodilation; increases myocardial oxygen delivery in patients with vasospastic angina. Amlodipine directly acts on vascular smooth muscle to produce peripheral arterial vasodilation reducing peripheral vascular resistance and blood pressure.

Pharmacodynamics/Kinetics
Duration of antihypertensive effect: 24 hours
Absorption: Oral: Well absorbed
Distribution: V_d: 21 L/kg
Protein binding: 93% to 98%
Metabolism: Hepatic (>90%) to inactive metabolites
Bioavailability: 64% to 90%
Half-life elimination: Terminal: 30-50 hours; increased with hepatic dysfunction
Time to peak, plasma: 6-12 hours
Excretion: Urine (10% of total dose as unchanged drug, 60% of total dose as metabolites)

Dosage Oral:
Children 6-17 years: Hypertension: 2.5-5 mg once daily
Adults:
Hypertension: Initial dose: 5 mg once daily; maximum dose: 10 mg once daily. In general, titrate in 2.5 mg increments over 7-14 days. Usual dosage range (JNC 7): 2.5-10 mg once daily.
Angina: Usual dose: 5-10 mg; most patients require 10 mg for adequate effect
Elderly: Dosing should start at the lower end of dosing range and titrated to response due to possible increased incidence of hepatic, renal, or cardiac impairment. Elderly patients also show decreased clearance of amlodipine.
Hypertension: 2.5 mg once daily
Angina: 5 mg once daily

Dosage adjustment in renal impairment: Dialysis: Hemodialysis and peritoneal dialysis do not enhance elimination. Supplemental dose is not necessary.

Dosage adjustment in hepatic impairment:
Angina: Administer 5 mg once daily.
Hypertension: Administer 2.5 mg once daily.

Dietary Considerations May be taken without regard to meals.

Administration May be administered without regard to meals.

Monitoring Parameters Heart rate, blood pressure, peripheral edema

Dosage Forms Excipient information presented when available (limited, particularly for generics); consult specific product labeling.
Tablet, oral: 2.5 mg, 5 mg, 10 mg
Norvasc®: 2.5 mg, 5 mg, 10 mg

Extemporaneous Preparations A 1 mg/mL oral suspension may be made with tablets and either a 1:1 mixture of simple syrup and 1% methylcellulose or a 1:1 mixture of Ora-Plus® and Ora-Sweet®. Crush fifty 5 mg tablets in a mortar and reduce to a fine powder. Add small portions of the chosen vehicle and mix to a uniform paste; mix while adding the vehicle in incremental proportions to **almost** 250 mL; transfer to a calibrated bottle, rinse mortar with vehicle, and add quantity of vehicle sufficient to make 250 mL. Label "shake well" and "refrigerate". Stable for 56 days at room temperature or 91 days refrigerated.

Nahata MC, Morosco RS, and Hipple TF, "Stability of Amlodipine Besylate in Two Liquid Dosage Forms," *J Am Pharm Assoc (Wash)*, 1999, 39(3):375-7.

◆ **Amlodipine, Aliskiren, and Hydrochlorothiazide** *see* Aliskiren, Amlodipine, and Hydrochlorothiazide *on page 67*

Amlodipine and Atorvastatin

(am LOW di peen & a TORE va sta tin)

Brand Names: U.S. Caduet®
Brand Names: Canada Caduet®
Index Terms Atorvastatin and Amlodipine; Atorvastatin Calcium and Amlodipine Besylate
Pharmacologic Category Antianginal Agent; Antilipemic Agent, HMG-CoA Reductase Inhibitor; Calcium Channel Blocker; Calcium Channel Blocker, Dihydropyridine
Use For use when treatment with both amlodipine and atorvastatin is appropriate:
Amlodipine: Treatment of hypertension; treatment of chronic stable angina, vasospastic (Prinzmetal's) angina (confirmed or suspected); prevention of hospitalization or to decrease coronary revascularization procedure due to angina with documented CAD (limited to patients without heart failure or ejection fraction <40%)
Atorvastatin: Treatment of dyslipidemias or primary prevention of cardiovascular disease (atherosclerotic) as detailed here:
Primary prevention of cardiovascular disease (high-risk for CVD): To reduce the risk of MI or stroke in patients without evidence of coronary heart disease who have multiple CVD risk factors or type 2 diabetes; also reduces the risk for angina or revascularization procedures in patients with multiple CVD risk factors without evidence of coronary heart disease
Secondary prevention of cardiovascular disease: To reduce the risk of MI, stroke, revascularization procedures, angina, and hospitalization for heart failure
Treatment of dyslipidemias: To reduce elevations in total cholesterol, LDL-C, apolipoprotein B, and triglycerides in patients with elevations of one or more components, and/or to increase low HDL-C as present in heterozygous familial/nonfamilial hypercholesterolemia and mixed dyslipidemia (Fredrickson type IIa and IIb hyperlipidemias); treatment of primary dysbetalipoproteinemia (Fredrickson type III), elevated serum TG levels (Fredrickson type IV), and homozygous familial hypercholesterolemia
Treatment of heterozygous familial hypercholesterolemia (HeFH) in adolescent patients (10-17 years of age, females >1 year postmenarche) having LDL-C ≥190 mg/dL or LDL-C ≥160 mg/dL with positive family history of premature cardiovascular disease (CVD) or with two or more CVD risk factors.
Pregnancy Risk Factor X
Dosage Oral: **Note:** Dose is individualized; combination product may be used as initial therapy or substituted for individual components in patients currently maintained on both agents separately or in patients not adequately controlled with monotherapy (using one of the agents or an agent within same pharmacologic class).
Children 10-17 years (females >1 year postmenarche):
Hypertension and hyperlipidemia:
Initial therapy: Amlodipine 2.5 mg and atorvastatin 10 mg once daily; dose may be titrated after 1-2 weeks (amlodipine component) and after 2-4 weeks (atorvastatin component) to a maximum daily dose: Amlodipine 5 mg; atorvastatin 20 mg

Add-on therapy/replacement therapy: Amlodipine 2.5-5 mg and atorvastatin 10-20 mg once daily; dose may be titrated after 1-2 weeks (amlodipine component) and after 2-4 weeks (atorvastatin component) to a maximum daily dose: Amlodipine 5 mg; atorvastatin 20 mg

Adults: Hypertension, angina, and hyperlipidemia:

Initial therapy: Amlodipine 5 mg and atorvastatin 10-20 mg once daily; dose may be titrated after 1-2 weeks (amlodipine component) and after 2-4 weeks (atorvastatin component) to a maximum daily dose: Amlodipine 10 mg; atorvastatin 80 mg

Add-on therapy/replacement therapy: Amlodipine 5-10 mg and atorvastatin 10-80 mg once daily; dose may be titrated after 1-2 weeks (amlodipine component) and after 2-4 weeks (atorvastatin component) to a maximum daily dose: Amlodipine 10 mg; atorvastatin 80 mg

Elderly: Consider starting amlodipine at the lower end of dosing range due to increased incidence of hepatic, renal, or cardiac impairment. Elderly patients also show decreased clearance of amlodipine.

Dosage adjustment for atorvastatin with concomitant medications:

Cyclosporine: Atorvastatin dose should not exceed 10 mg/day

Clarithromycin, itraconazole, ritonavir plus saquinavir, or lopinavir plus ritonavir when atorvastatin dose >20 mg: Ensure that the lowest dose necessary of atorvastatin is used

Dosage adjustment in renal impairment: No dosage adjustment is necessary

Dosage adjustment in hepatic impairment: Contraindicated in patients with active liver disease

Additional Information Complete prescribing information for this medication should be consulted for additional detail.

Dosage Forms Excipient information presented when available (limited, particularly for generics); consult specific product labeling.

Tablet, oral: Amlodipine 2.5 mg and atorvastatin 10 mg; Amlodipine 2.5 mg and atorvastatin 20 mg; Amlodipine 2.5 mg and atorvastatin 40 mg; Amlodipine 5 mg and atorvastatin 10 mg; Amlodipine 5 mg and atorvastatin 20 mg; Amlodipine 5 mg and atorvastatin 40 mg; Amlodipine 5 mg and atorvastatin 80 mg; Amlodipine 10 mg and atorvastatin 10 mg; Amlodipine 10 mg and atorvastatin 20 mg; Amlodipine 10 mg and atorvastatin 40 mg; Amlodipine 10 mg and atorvastatin 80 mg

Caduet®:

2.5/10: Amlodipine 2.5 mg and atorvastatin 10 mg
2.5/20: Amlodipine 2.5 mg and atorvastatin 20 mg
2.5/40: Amlodipine 2.5 mg and atorvastatin 40 mg
5/10: Amlodipine 5 mg and atorvastatin 10 mg
5/20: Amlodipine 5 mg and atorvastatin 20 mg
5/40: Amlodipine 5 mg and atorvastatin 40 mg
5/80: Amlodipine 5 mg and atorvastatin 80 mg
10/10: Amlodipine 10 mg and atorvastatin 10 mg
10/20: Amlodipine 10 mg and atorvastatin 20 mg
10/40: Amlodipine 10 mg and atorvastatin 40 mg
10/80: Amlodipine 10 mg and atorvastatin 80 mg

Amlodipine and Benazepril

(am LOE di peen & ben AY ze pril)

Brand Names: U.S. Lotrel®

Index Terms Benazepril Hydrochloride and Amlodipine Besylate

Pharmacologic Category Angiotensin-Converting Enzyme (ACE) Inhibitor; Antianginal Agent; Calcium Channel Blocker; Calcium Channel Blocker, Dihydropyridine

Use Treatment of hypertension

Pregnancy Risk Factor D

Dosage Oral: **Note:** Dose is individualized; combination product may be substituted for individual components in patients currently maintained on both agents separately or in patients not adequately controlled with monotherapy (using one of the agents or an agent within same antihypertensive class).

Adults: 2.5-10 mg (amlodipine) and 10-40 mg (benazepril) once daily; maximum: Amlodipine: 10 mg/day; benazepril: 80 mg/day

Elderly: Initial dose: 2.5 mg based on amlodipine component

Dosage adjustment in renal impairment: Cl_{cr} ≤30 mL/minute: Use of combination product is not recommended.

Dosage adjustment in hepatic impairment: Initial dose: 2.5 mg based on amlodipine component

Additional Information Complete prescribing information for this medication should be consulted for additional detail.

Dosage Forms Excipient information presented when available (limited, particularly for generics); consult specific product labeling.

Capsule:

2.5/10: Amlodipine 2.5 mg and benazepril hydrochloride 10 mg
5/10: Amlodipine 5 mg and benazepril hydrochloride 10 mg
5/20: Amlodipine 5 mg and benazepril hydrochloride 20 mg
5/40: Amlodipine 5 mg and benazepril hydrochloride 40 mg
10/20: Amlodipine 10 mg and benazepril hydrochloride 20 mg
10/40: Amlodipine 10 mg and benazepril hydrochloride 40 mg
Lotrel® 2.5/10: Amlodipine 2.5 mg and benazepril hydrochloride 10 mg
Lotrel® 5/10: Amlodipine 5 mg and benazepril hydrochloride 10 mg
Lotrel® 5/20: Amlodipine 5 mg and benazepril hydrochloride 20 mg
Lotrel® 5/40: Amlodipine 5 mg and benazepril hydrochloride 40 mg
Lotrel® 10/20: Amlodipine 10 mg and benazepril hydrochloride 20 mg
Lotrel® 10/40: Amlodipine 10 mg and benazepril hydrochloride 40 mg

Amlodipine and Olmesartan

(am LOE di peen & olme SAR tan)

Brand Names: U.S. Azor™

Index Terms Amlodipine Besylate and Olmesartan Medoxomil; Olmesartan and Amlodipine

Pharmacologic Category Angiotensin II Receptor Blocker; Antianginal Agent; Calcium Channel Blocker; Calcium Channel Blocker, Dihydropyridine

Use Treatment of hypertension, including initial treatment in patients who will require multiple antihypertensives for adequate control

Pregnancy Risk Factor C/D (2nd and 3rd trimesters)

Dosage Oral: Dose is individualized; combination product may be substituted for individual components in patients currently maintained on both agents separately or in patients not adequately controlled with monotherapy (using one of the agents or an agent the within same antihypertensive class). May also be used as initial therapy in patients who are likely to need >1 antihypertensive to control blood pressure.

Adults: Hypertension:

Initial therapy (antihypertensive naive): Amlodipine 5 mg/olmesartan 20 mg once daily; dose may be increased after 1-2 weeks of therapy. Maximum recommended dose: Amlodipine 10 mg/day; olmesartan 40 mg/day.

Add-on/replacement therapy: Amlodipine 5-10 mg and olmesartan 20-40 mg once daily depending upon previous doses, current control, and goals of therapy; dose may be titrated after 2 weeks of therapy. Maximum recommended doses: Amlodipine 10 mg/day; olmesartan 40 mg/day.

Elderly: Initial therapy is not recommended in patients ≥75 years of age.

Dosing adjustment in renal impairment: No specific guidelines for dosage adjustment

Dosing adjustment in hepatic impairment: Initial therapy is not recommended

Additional Information Complete prescribing information for this medication should be consulted for additional detail.

Dosage Forms Excipient information presented when available (limited, particularly for generics); consult specific product labeling.

Tablet:

Azor™ 5/20: Amlodipine 5 mg and olmesartan medoxomil 20 mg

Azor™ 5/40: Amlodipine 5 mg and olmesartan medoxomil 40 mg

Azor™ 10/20: Amlodipine 10 mg and olmesartan medoxomil 20 mg

Azor™ 10/40: Amlodipine 10 mg and olmesartan medoxomil 40 mg

◆ **Amlodipine and Telmisartan** *see* Telmisartan and Amlodipine *on page 1637*

Amlodipine and Valsartan

(am LOE di peen & val SAR tan)

Brand Names: U.S. Exforge®

Index Terms Amlodipine Besylate and Valsartan; Valsartan and Amlodipine

Pharmacologic Category Angiotensin II Receptor Blocker; Antianginal Agent; Calcium Channel Blocker; Calcium Channel Blocker, Dihydropyridine

Use Treatment of hypertension

Pregnancy Risk Factor D

Dosage Oral: Dose is individualized; combination product may be used as initial therapy or substituted for individual components in patients currently maintained on both agents separately or in patients not adequately controlled with monotherapy (using one of the agents or an agent within same antihypertensive class).

Adults: Hypertension:

Initial therapy: Amlodipine 5 mg and valsartan 160 mg once daily, dose may be titrated after 1-2 weeks of therapy. Maximum recommended doses: Amlodipine 10 mg/day; valsartan 320 mg/day

Add-on/replacement therapy: Amlodipine 5-10 mg and valsartan 160-320 mg once daily; dose may be titrated after 3-4 weeks of therapy. Maximum recommended doses: Amlodipine 10 mg/day; valsartan 320 mg/day

Elderly: Initiate amlodipine at 2.5 mg/day due to decreased clearance

Dosing adjustment in renal impairment:

Cl_{cr} >10 mL/minute: No dosage adjustment necessary

Cl_{cr} ≤10 mL/minute: Use caution; titrate slowly

Dosing adjustment in hepatic impairment: Mild-to-moderate hepatic impairment: No initial dosage adjustment required, titrate slowly. Amlodipine and valsartan exposure increased in presence of hepatic impairment.

Amlodipine: Use caution in severe hepatic impairment; lower initial doses may be required

Valsartan: Mild-to-moderate hepatic impairment: No dosage adjustment required; however, patients with mild-to-moderate chronic disease have twice the exposure as healthy volunteers.

Additional Information Complete prescribing information for this medication should be consulted for additional detail.

Dosage Forms Excipient information presented when available (limited, particularly for generics); consult specific product labeling.

Tablet:

Exforge®:

5/160: Amlodipine 5 mg and valsartan 160 mg

5/320 mg: Amlodipine 5 mg and valsartan 320 mg

10/160: Amlodipine 10 mg and valsartan 160 mg

10/320: Amlodipine 10 mg and valsartan 320 mg

◆ **Amlodipine Besylate** *see* AmLODIPine *on page 97*

◆ **Amlodipine Besylate, Aliskiren Hemifumarate, and Hydrochlorothiazide** *see* Aliskiren, Amlodipine, and Hydrochlorothiazide *on page 67*

◆ **Amlodipine Besylate and Olmesartan Medoxomil** *see* Amlodipine and Olmesartan *on page 99*

◆ **Amlodipine Besylate and Telmisartan** *see* Telmisartan and Amlodipine *on page 1637*

◆ **Amlodipine Besylate and Valsartan** *see* Amlodipine and Valsartan *on page 100*

◆ **Amlodipine Besylate, Olmesartan Medoxomil, and Hydrochlorothiazide** *see* Olmesartan, Amlodipine, and Hydrochlorothiazide *on page 1238*

◆ **Amlodipine Besylate, Valsartan, and Hydrochlorothiazide** *see* Amlodipine, Valsartan, and Hydrochlorothiazide *on page 100*

◆ **Amlodipine, Hydrochlorothiazide, and Aliskiren** *see* Aliskiren, Amlodipine, and Hydrochlorothiazide *on page 67*

◆ **Amlodipine, Hydrochlorothiazide, and Olmesartan** *see* Olmesartan, Amlodipine, and Hydrochlorothiazide *on page 1238*

◆ **Amlodipine, Hydrochlorothiazide, and Valsartan** *see* Amlodipine, Valsartan, and Hydrochlorothiazide *on page 100*

Amlodipine, Valsartan, and Hydrochlorothiazide

(am LOE di peen, val SAR tan, & hye droe klor oh THYE a zide)

Brand Names: U.S. Exforge HCT®

Index Terms Amlodipine Besylate, Valsartan, and Hydrochlorothiazide; Amlodipine, Hydrochlorothiazide, and Valsartan; Hydrochlorothiazide, Amlodipine, and Valsartan; Valsartan, Hydrochlorothiazide, and Amlodipine

Pharmacologic Category Angiotensin II Receptor Blocker; Antianginal Agent; Calcium Channel Blocker; Calcium Channel Blocker, Dihydropyridine; Diuretic, Thiazide

Use Treatment of hypertension (not for initial therapy)

Pregnancy Risk Factor D

Dosage Oral: **Note:** Not for initial therapy. Dose is individualized; combination product may be substituted for individual components in patients currently maintained on all three agents separately or in patients not adequately controlled with any two of the following antihypertensive classes: Calcium channel blockers, angiotensin II receptor blockers, and diuretics.

Adults: Hypertension: Add-on/switch/replacement therapy: Amlodipine 5-10 mg and valsartan 160-320 mg and hydrochlorothiazide 12.5-25 mg once daily; dose may be titrated after 2 weeks of therapy. Maximum recommended daily dose: Amlodipine 10 mg/valsartan 320 mg/hydrochlorothiazide 25 mg

Dosage adjustment in renal impairment:
Cl_{cr} >30 mL/minute: No adjustment needed
Cl_{cr} ≤30 mL/minute: Use of combination not recommended; contraindicated in patients with anuria

Dosage adjustment in hepatic impairment: Use of combination is not recommended in severe hepatic impairment. Use with caution in mild-to-moderate hepatic impairment; monitor for worsening of hepatic or renal function and adverse reactions.

Additional Information Complete prescribing information for this medication should be consulted for additional detail.

Dosage Forms Excipient information presented when available (limited, particularly for generics); consult specific product labeling.

Tablet, oral:
Exforge HCT®:
Amlodipine 5 mg, valsartan 160 mg, and hydrochlorothiazide 12.5 mg
Amlodipine 5 mg, valsartan 160 mg, and hydrochlorothiazide 25 mg
Amlodipine 10 mg, valsartan 160 mg, and hydrochlorothiazide 12.5 mg
Amlodipine 10 mg, valsartan 160 mg, and hydrochlorothiazide 25 mg
Amlodipine 10 mg, valsartan 320 mg, and hydrochlorothiazide 25 mg

- ◆ **Ammens® Original Medicated [OTC]** *see* Zinc Oxide *on page 1817*
- ◆ **Ammens® Shower Fresh [OTC]** *see* Zinc Oxide *on page 1817*
- ◆ **Ammonapse** *see* Sodium Phenylbutyrate *on page 1573*

Ammonium Chloride (a MOE nee um KLOR ide)

Pharmacologic Category Electrolyte Supplement, Parenteral

Use Treatment of hypochloremic states or metabolic alkalosis

Pregnancy Risk Factor C

Dosage Metabolic alkalosis: The following equations represent different methods of correction utilizing either the serum HCO_3^-, the serum chloride, or the base excess

Dosing of mEq NH_4 Cl via the chloride-deficit method (hypochloremia):
Dose of mEq NH_4Cl = [0.2 L/kg x body weight (kg)] x [103 - observed serum chloride]; administer 50% of dose over 12 hours, then re-evaluate
Note: 0.2 L/kg is the estimated chloride volume of distribution and 103 is the average normal serum chloride concentration (mEq/L)

Dosing of mEq NH_4 Cl via the bicarbonate-excess method (refractory hypochloremic metabolic alkalosis):
Dose of NH_4Cl = [0.5 L/kg x body weight (kg)] x (observed serum HCO_3^- - 24); administer 50% of dose over 12 hours, then re-evaluate
Note: 0.5 L/kg is the estimated bicarbonate volume of distribution and 24 is the average normal serum bicarbonate concentration (mEq/L)

These equations will yield different requirements of ammonium chloride

Additional Information Complete prescribing information for this medication should be consulted for additional detail.

Dosage Forms Excipient information presented when available (limited, particularly for generics); consult specific product labeling.

Injection, solution: Ammonium 5 mEq/mL and chloride 5 mEq/mL (20 mL) [equivalent to ammonium chloride 267.5 mg/mL]

- ◆ **Ammonul®** *see* Sodium Phenylacetate and Sodium Benzoate *on page 1572*
- ◆ **AMN107** *see* Nilotinib *on page 1205*
- ◆ **Amnesteem®** *see* ISOtretinoin *on page 939*

Amobarbital (am oh BAR bi tal)

Brand Names: U.S. Amytal®

Brand Names: Canada Amytal®

Index Terms Amobarbital Sodium; Amylobarbitone

Pharmacologic Category Barbiturate; General Anesthetic; Hypnotic; Sedative

Use Hypnotic in short-term treatment of insomnia; reduce anxiety and provide sedation preoperatively

Unlabeled Use Therapeutic or diagnostic "Amytal® Interviewing"; Wada test

Pregnancy Risk Factor D

Dosage
Children:
Sedative: I.M., I.V.: 6-12 years: Manufacturer's dosing range: 65-500 mg
Hypnotic (unlabeled use): I.M.: 2-3 mg/kg (maximum: 500 mg)
Adults:
Hypnotic: I.M., I.V.: 65-200 mg at bedtime (maximum single dose: 1000 mg)
Sedative: I.M., I.V.: 30-50 mg 2-3 times/day (maximum single dose: 1000 mg)
"Amytal® interview" (unlabeled use): I.V.: 50-100 mg/minute for total dose of 200-1000 mg or until patient experiences drowsiness, impaired attention, slurred speech, or nystagmus
Wada test (unlabeled use): Intra-arterial: 100 mg over 4-5 seconds via percutaneous transfemoral catheter

Dosing adjustment in renal/hepatic impairment: Dosing should be reduced; specific recommendations not available.

Additional Information Complete prescribing information for this medication should be consulted for additional detail.

Dosage Forms Excipient information presented when available (limited, particularly for generics); consult specific product labeling.

Injection, powder for reconstitution, as sodium:
Amytal®: 0.5 g

Controlled Substance C-II

- ◆ **Amobarbital Sodium** *see* Amobarbital *on page 101*
- ◆ **Amoclan** *see* Amoxicillin and Clavulanate *on page 105*

Amoxapine (a MOKS a peen)

Index Terms Asendin [DSC]

Pharmacologic Category Antidepressant, Tricyclic (Secondary Amine)

Additional Appendix Information
Antidepressant Agents *on page 1874*

Use Treatment of depression (including endogenous, neurotic, psychotic, and reactive depression); treatment of depression accompanied by anxiety or agitation

Pregnancy Risk Factor C

Pregnancy Considerations Teratogenic effects were not observed in animal reproduction studies; however, fetotoxic and embryotoxic effects were seen in some studies.

Lactation Enters breast milk/use caution (AAP rates "of concern"; AAP 2001 update pending)

Medication Guide Available Yes

Contraindications Hypersensitivity to amoxapine or any component of the formulation; use with or within 14 days of MAO inhibitors; acute recovery phase following myocardial infarction

Warnings/Precautions [U.S. Boxed Warning]: Antidepressants increase the risk of suicidal thinking and behavior in children, adolescents, and young adults (18-24 years of age) with major depressive disorder (MDD) and other psychiatric disorders; consider risk prior to prescribing. Short-term studies did not show an increased risk in patients >24 years of age and showed a decreased risk in patients ≥65 years. Closely monitor for clinical worsening, suicidality, or unusual changes in behavior; the patient's family or caregiver should be instructed to closely observe the patient and communicate condition with healthcare provider. A medication guide should be dispensed with each prescription. **Amoxapine is not FDA approved for use in pediatric patients.**

The possibility of a suicide attempt is inherent in major depression and may persist until remission occurs. Monitor for worsening of depression or suicidality, especially during initiation of therapy (generally first 1-2 months) or with dose increases or decreases. Use caution in high-risk patients. Worsening depression and severe abrupt suicidality that are not part of the presenting symptoms may require discontinuation or modification of drug therapy. The patient's family or caregiver should be alerted to monitor patients for the emergence of suicidality and associated behaviors (such as agitation, irritability, hostility, impulsivity, and hypomania) and notify the healthcare provider.

May worsen psychosis in some patients or precipitate a shift to mania or hypomania in patients with bipolar disorder. Patients presenting with depressive symptoms should be screened for bipolar disorder. Monotherapy in patients with bipolar disorder should be avoided. **Amoxapine is not FDA approved for bipolar depression.** May cause extrapyramidal symptoms, including pseudoparkinsonism, acute dystonic reactions, akathisia, and tardive dyskinesia (risk of these reactions is low). The risk for tardive dyskinesia (may be irreversible) increases with long-term treatment and higher cumulative doses. Therapy should be discontinued in any patient if signs/symptoms of tardive dyskinesia appear. May be associated with neuroleptic malignant syndrome.

The degree of sedation, anticholinergic effects, orthostasis, and conduction abnormalities are moderate relative to other antidepressants. May cause drowsiness/sedation, resulting in impaired performance of tasks requiring alertness (eg, operating machinery or driving). Sedative effects may be additive with other CNS depressants and/or ethanol. Use with caution in patients with a history of cardiovascular disease (including previous MI, stroke, tachycardia, or conduction abnormalities). Use with caution in patients with urinary retention, benign prostatic hyperplasia, narrow-angle glaucoma, xerostomia, visual problems, constipation, or a history of bowel obstruction.

Consider discontinuing, when possible, prior to elective surgery. Therapy should not be abruptly discontinued in patients receiving high doses for prolonged periods. May lower seizure threshold - use caution in patients with a previous seizure disorder or condition predisposing to seizures such as brain damage, alcoholism, or concurrent therapy with other drugs which lower the seizure threshold. May increase the risks associated with electroconvulsive therapy. Use with caution in hyperthyroid patients or those receiving thyroid supplementation. Use with caution or avoid in the elderly; not the drug of choice for elderly patients; may have increased risk of adverse events, including tardive dyskinesia (particularly older women) and sedation.

Adverse Reactions

>10%:

- Central nervous system: Drowsiness (14%)
- Gastrointestinal: Xerostomia (14%), constipation (12%)

1% to 10%:

- Cardiovascular: Palpitations
- Central nervous system: Anxiety, ataxia, confusion, dizziness, EEG abnormalities, excitement, fatigue, headache, insomnia, nervousness, nightmares, restlessness
- Dermatologic: Edema, skin rash
- Endocrine: Prolactin levels increased
- Gastrointestinal: Appetite increased, nausea
- Neuromuscular & skeletal: Tremor, weakness
- Ocular: Blurred vision (7%)
- Miscellaneous: Diaphoresis

<1% (Limited to important or life-threatening): Agranulocytosis, allergic reactions, diarrhea, extrapyramidal symptoms, fever, galactorrhea, hepatitis, hypertension, hypomania. impotence, incoordination, intraocular pressure increased, leukopenia, menstrual irregularity, mydriasis, neuroleptic malignant syndrome, numbness, painful ejaculation, paresthesia, photosensitivity, seizure, SIADH, syncope, tardive dyskinesia, testicular edema, tinnitus, urinary retention, vasculitis, vomiting

Drug Interactions

Metabolism/Transport Effects Substrate of CYP2D6 (major); **Note:** Assignment of Major/Minor substrate status based on clinically relevant drug interaction potential

Avoid Concomitant Use

Avoid concomitant use of Amoxapine with any of the following: Artemether; Dronedarone; Iobenguane I 123; Lumefantrine; MAO Inhibitors; Methylene Blue; Nilotinib; Pimozide; QUEtiapine; QuiNINE; Tetrabenazine; Thioridazine; Toremifene; Vandetanib; Vemurafenib; Ziprasidone

Increased Effect/Toxicity

Amoxapine may increase the levels/effects of: Alpha-/Beta-Agonists (Direct-Acting); Alpha1-Agonists; Amphetamines; Anticholinergics; Beta2-Agonists; Desmopressin; Dronedarone; Methylene Blue; Metoclopramide; Pimozide; QTc-Prolonging Agents; QuiNIDine; QuiNINE; Serotonin Modulators; Sodium Phosphates; Sulfonylureas; Tetrabenazine; Thioridazine; Toremifene; TraMADol; Vandetanib; Vemurafenib; Vitamin K Antagonists; Yohimbine; Ziprasidone

The levels/effects of Amoxapine may be increased by: Abiraterone Acetate; Alfuzosin; Altretamine; Antipsychotics; Artemether; Chloroquine; Cimetidine; Cinacalcet; Ciprofloxacin; Ciprofloxacin (Systemic); CYP2D6 Inhibitors (Moderate); CYP2D6 Inhibitors (Strong); Dexmethylphenidate; Divalproex; DULoxetine; Gadobutrol; Indacaterol; Linezolid; Lithium; Lumefantrine; MAO Inhibitors; Methylphenidate; Metoclopramide; Nilotinib; Pramlintide; Protease Inhibitors; QUEtiapine; QuiNIDine; QuiNINE; Selective Serotonin Reuptake Inhibitors; Terbinafine; Terbinafine (Systemic); Valproic Acid

Decreased Effect

Amoxapine may decrease the levels/effects of: Acetylcholinesterase Inhibitors (Central); Alpha2-Agonists; Iobenguane I 123

The levels/effects of Amoxapine may be decreased by: Acetylcholinesterase Inhibitors (Central); Barbiturates; CarBAMazepine; Peginterferon Alfa-2b; St Johns Wort

Ethanol/Nutrition/Herb Interactions

Ethanol: May increase CNS depression; monitor for increased effects with coadministration. Caution patients about effects.

Food: Grapefruit juice may inhibit the metabolism of some TCAs and clinical toxicity may result.

Herb/Nutraceutical: Avoid valerian, St John's wort, SAMe, kava kava.

Stability Store at 20°C to 25°C (68°F to 77°F).

Mechanism of Action Reduces the reuptake of serotonin and norepinephrine. The metabolite, 7-OH-amoxapine has significant dopamine receptor blocking activity similar to haloperidol.

Pharmacodynamics/Kinetics

Onset of antidepressant effect: Usually occurs after 1-2 weeks, but may require 4-6 weeks

Absorption: Rapid and well absorbed

Distribution: V_d: 0.9-1.2 L/kg; enters breast milk

Protein binding: ~90%

Metabolism: Extensively metabolized; hepatic hydroxylation produces two active metabolites, 7-hydroxyamoxapine (7-OH-amoxapine) and 8-hydroxyamoxapine (8-OH-amoxapine); metabolites undergo conjugation to form glucuronides

Half-life elimination: 8 hours; 7-hydroxyamoxapine metabolite: 4-6 hours; 8-hydroxyamoxapine metabolite: 30 hours

Time to peak, serum: ~90 minutes

Excretion: Urine (as unchanged drug and metabolites)

Dosage Oral:

Adults:

Outpatients: Initial: 50 mg 2-3 times/day; dose may be increased to 100 mg 2-3 times/day by the end of the first week, if tolerated. Usual effective dose: 200-300 mg/day; if 300 mg daily has been reached and maintained for at least 2 weeks and no response is observed, may further increase to 400 mg/day. Once an effective dose is reached, doses ≤300 mg may be given once daily at bedtime and doses >300 mg/day should be divided.

Inpatients: Hospitalized patients refractory to antidepressant therapy (and no history of seizures) may be cautiously titrated to 600 mg/day in divided doses.

Maintenance: Outpatients and Inpatients: Once symptoms are controlled, gradually decrease to lowest dose that will maintain remission.

Elderly: Use caution or avoid in the elderly. Initial: 25 mg 2-3 times/day; dose may be increased to 50 mg 2-3 times/day by the end of the first week, if tolerated; usual effective dose: 100-150 mg/day; if dose is ineffective, may further increase cautiously to 300 mg/day; once an effective dose is reached, doses ≤300 mg may be given once daily at bedtime. Maintenance: Once symptoms are controlled, gradually decrease to the lowest dose that will maintain remission.

Monitoring Parameters Monitor blood pressure and pulse rate prior to and during initial therapy evaluate mental status, suicide ideation (especially at the beginning of therapy or when doses are increased or decreased); ECG in older adults and patients with cardiac disease

Test Interactions Increased glucose, liver function tests; decreased WBC

Additional Information Extrapyramidal reactions and tardive dyskinesia may occur.

Dosage Forms Excipient information presented when available (limited, particularly for generics); consult specific product labeling.

Tablet, oral: 25 mg, 50 mg, 100 mg, 150 mg

Amoxicillin (a moks i SIL in)

Brand Names: U.S. Moxatag™

Brand Names: Canada Apo-Amoxi®; Gen-Amoxicillin; Lin-Amox; Mylan-Amoxicillin; Novamoxin®; Nu-Amoxi; PHL-Amoxicillin; PMS-Amoxicillin

Index Terms *p*-Hydroxyampicillin; Amoxicillin Trihydrate; Amoxil; Amoxycillin

Pharmacologic Category Antibiotic, Penicillin

Additional Appendix Information

Prevention of Infective Endocarditis *on page 1952*

Use Treatment of otitis media, sinusitis, and infections caused by susceptible organisms involving the upper and lower respiratory tract, skin, and urinary tract; prophylaxis of infective endocarditis in patients undergoing surgical or dental procedures; as part of a multidrug regimen for *H. pylori* eradication

Unlabeled Use Postexposure prophylaxis for anthrax exposure with documented susceptible organisms

Pregnancy Risk Factor B

Pregnancy Considerations Adverse events have not been observed in animal studies; therefore, amoxicillin is classified as pregnancy category B. There is no documented increased risk of adverse pregnancy outcome or teratogenic effects caused by amoxicillin. It is the drug of choice for the treatment of chlamydial infections in pregnancy and for anthrax prophylaxis when penicillin susceptibility is documented.

Due to pregnancy-induced physiologic changes, amoxicillin clearance is increased during pregnancy resulting in lower concentrations and smaller AUCs. Oral ampicillin-class antibiotics are poorly-absorbed during labor.

Lactation Enters breast milk/use caution (AAP rates "compatible"; AAP 2001 update pending)

Contraindications Hypersensitivity to amoxicillin, penicillin, other beta-lactams, or any component of the formulation

Warnings/Precautions In patients with renal impairment, doses and/or frequency of administration should be modified in response to the degree of renal impairment; in addition, use of certain dosage forms (eg, extended release 775 mg tablet and immediate release 875 mg tablet) should be avoided in patients with Cl_{cr} <30 mL/minute or patients requiring hemodialysis. A high percentage of patients with infectious mononucleosis have developed rash during therapy with amoxicillin; ampicillin-class antibiotics not recommended in these patients. Serious and occasionally severe or fatal hypersensitivity (anaphylactoid) reactions have been reported in patients on penicillin therapy, especially with a history of beta-lactam hypersensitivity, history of sensitivity to multiple allergens, or previous IgE-mediated reactions (eg, anaphylaxis, angioedema, urticaria). Use with caution in asthmatic patients. Prolonged use may result in fungal or bacterial superinfection, including *C. difficile*-associated diarrhea (CDAD) and pseudomembranous colitis; CDAD has been observed >2 months postantibiotic treatment. Chewable tablets contain phenylalanine.

Adverse Reactions Frequency not defined.

Central nervous system: Agitation, anxiety, behavioral changes, confusion, dizziness, headache, hyperactivity (reversible), insomnia, seizure

Dermatologic: Acute exanthematous pustulosis, erythematous maculopapular rash, erythema multiforme, exfoliative dermatitis, hypersensitivity vasculitis, mucocutaneous candidiasis, Stevens-Johnson syndrome, toxic epidermal necrolysis, urticaria

Gastrointestinal: Black hairy tongue, diarrhea, hemorrhagic colitis, nausea, pseudomembranous colitis, tooth discoloration (brown, yellow, or gray; rare), vomiting

Hematologic: Agranulocytosis, anemia, eosinophilia, hemolytic anemia, leukopenia,thrombocytopenia, thrombocytopenia purpura

Hepatic: Acute cytolytic hepatitis, ALT increased, AST increased, cholestatic jaundice, hepatic cholestasis

Renal: Crystalluria

Miscellaneous: Anaphylaxis, serum sickness-like reaction

Drug Interactions

Metabolism/Transport Effects None known.

Avoid Concomitant Use

Avoid concomitant use of Amoxicillin with any of the following: BCG

Increased Effect/Toxicity

Amoxicillin may increase the levels/effects of: Methotrexate; Vitamin K Antagonists

The levels/effects of Amoxicillin may be increased by: Allopurinol; Probenecid

Decreased Effect

Amoxicillin may decrease the levels/effects of: BCG; Mycophenolate; Typhoid Vaccine

The levels/effects of Amoxicillin may be decreased by: Fusidic Acid; Tetracycline Derivatives

Stability

Amoxil®: Oral suspension remains stable for 14 days at room temperature or if refrigerated (refrigeration preferred). Unit-dose antibiotic oral syringes are stable at room temperature for at least 72 hours (Tu, 1988).

Moxatag™: Store at 25°C (77°F); excursions permitted to 15°C to 30°C (59°F to 86°F).

Mechanism of Action Inhibits bacterial cell wall synthesis by binding to one or more of the penicillin-binding proteins (PBPs) which in turn inhibits the final transpeptidation step of peptidoglycan synthesis in bacterial cell walls, thus inhibiting cell wall biosynthesis. Bacteria eventually lyse due to ongoing activity of cell wall autolytic enzymes (autolysins and murein hydrolases) while cell wall assembly is arrested.

Pharmacodynamics/Kinetics

Absorption: Oral: Rapid and nearly complete; food does not interfere

Extended-release tablet: Rate of absorption is slower compared to immediate-release formulations; food decreases the rate but not extent of absorption

Distribution: Widely to most body fluids and bone; poor penetration into cells, eyes, and across normal meninges

Pleural fluids, lungs, and peritoneal fluid; high urine concentrations are attained; also into synovial fluid, liver, prostate, muscle, and gallbladder; penetrates into middle ear effusions, maxillary sinus secretions, tonsils, sputum, and bronchial secretions

CSF:blood level ratio: Normal meninges: <1%; Inflamed meninges: 8% to 90%

Protein binding: 17% to 20%

Metabolism: Partially hepatic

Half-life elimination:

Neonates, full-term: 3.7 hours

Infants and Children: 1-2 hours

Adults: Normal renal function: 0.7-1.4 hours

Cl_{cr} <10 mL/minute: 7-21 hours

Time to peak: Capsule: 2 hours; Extended-release tablet: 3.1 hours; Suspension: 1 hour

Excretion: Urine (60% as unchanged drug); lower in neonates

Note: Extended-release tablets: In healthy volunteers, serum drug concentrations were below 0.25 mcg/mL and undetectable at 16 hours following dosing.

Dosage

Usual dosage range:

Children ≤3 months: Oral: 20-30 mg/kg/day divided every 12 hours

Children >3 months and <40 kg: Oral: 20-100 mg/kg/day in divided doses every 8-12 hours

Children >3 months and ≥40 kg: Refer to adult dosing

Children ≥12 years: Oral: Extended-release tablet: 775 mg once daily

Adults: Oral: 250-500 mg every 8 hours or 500-875 mg twice daily

Extended-release tablet: 775 mg once daily

Indication-specific dosing:

Children >3 months and <40 kg: Oral: **Note:** In general, children >3 months and ≥40 kg should be dosed according to the adult recommendations except where indicated.

Acute otitis media: 80-90 mg/kg/day divided every 12 hours

Community-acquired pneumonia (CAP) (IDSA/PIDS, 2011): Note: In children ≥5 years, a macrolide antibiotic should be added if atypical pneumonia cannot be ruled out.

Empiric treatment or *S. pneumoniae* (MICs to penicillin ≤2.0 mcg/mL) (preferred): 90 mg/kg/day in 2-3 divided doses (maximum: 4 g/day). **Note:** Dividing in 3 doses is recommended for MIC = 2 mcg/mL.

Group A *Streptococcus* (moderate-to-severe) (preferred): 50-75 mg/kg/day in 2 divided doses (maximum: 4 g/day)

H. influenzae (beta-lactamase negative) mild infection (preferred): 75-100 mg/kg/day in 3 divided doses (maximum: 4 g/day)

Ear, nose, throat, genitourinary tract, or skin/skin structure infections:

Mild-to-moderate: 25 mg/kg/day in divided doses every 12 hours **or** 20 mg/kg/day in divided doses every 8 hours

Severe: 45 mg/kg/day in divided doses every 12 hours **or** 40 mg/kg/day in divided doses every 8 hours

Tonsillitis and/or pharyngitis: Children ≥12 years: Extended-release tablet: 775 mg once daily

Lower respiratory tract infections: 45 mg/kg/day in divided doses every 12 hours **or** 40 mg/kg/day in divided doses every 8 hours

Lyme disease: 25-50 mg/kg/day divided every 8 hours (maximum: 500 mg)

Postexposure inhalational anthrax prophylaxis (ACIP recommendations): Children <40 kg: 45 mg/kg/day divided into 3 daily doses (maximum: 500 mg/dose) (ACIP, 2010). **Note:** The AAP recommends a higher dose (80 mg/kg/day divided into 3 daily doses [maximum: 500 mg/dose]) due to the lack of data on amoxicillin dosages for treating anthrax and the high mortality rate.

Note: Use **only** if isolates of the specific *B. anthracis* are sensitive to amoxicillin (MIC ≤0.125 mcg/mL). Duration of antibiotic postexposure prophylaxis (PEP) is ≥60 days in a previously-unvaccinated exposed person. Antimicrobial therapy should continue for 14 days after the third dose of PEP vaccine. Those who are partially or fully vaccinated should receive at least a 30-day course of antimicrobial PEP and continue with licensed vaccination regimen. Unvaccinated workers, even those wearing personal protective equipment with adequate respiratory protection, should receive antimicrobial PEP. Antimicrobial PEP is not required for fully-vaccinated people (five-dose I.M. vaccination series with a yearly booster) who enter an anthrax area clothed in personal protective equipment. If respiratory protection is disrupted, a 30-day course of antimicrobial therapy is recommended (ACIP, 2010).

Prophylaxis against infective endocarditis: 50 mg/kg 1 hour before procedure. **Note:** American Heart Association (AHA) guidelines now recommend prophylaxis only in patients undergoing invasive procedures and in whom underlying cardiac conditions may predispose to a higher risk of adverse outcomes should infection occur. As of April 2007, routine prophylaxis for GI/GU procedures is no longer recommended by the AHA.

Adults: Oral:

Chlamydial infection during pregnancy (unlabeled use): 500 mg 3 times/day for 7 days (CDC, 2010)

Ear, nose, throat, genitourinary tract, or skin/skin structure infections:
Mild-to-moderate: 500 mg every 12 hours **or** 250 mg every 8 hours
Severe: 875 mg every 12 hours **or** 500 mg every 8 hours
Tonsillitis and/or pharyngitis: Extended-release tablet: 775 mg once daily

***Helicobacter pylori* eradication:** 1000 mg twice daily; requires combination therapy with at least one other antibiotic and an acid-suppressing agent (proton pump inhibitor or H_2 blocker)

Lower respiratory tract infections: 875 mg every 12 hours **or** 500 mg every 8 hours

Lyme disease: 500 mg every 6-8 hours (depending on size of patient) for 21-30 days

Postexposure inhalational anthrax prophylaxis (ACIP recommendations): 500 mg every 8 hours. **Note:** Use **only** if isolates of the specific *B. anthracis* are sensitive to amoxicillin (MIC ≤0.125 mcg/mL); may be administered to pregnant and breast-feeding women. Duration of antibiotic postexposure prophylaxis (PEP) is ≥60 days in a previously unvaccinated exposed person. Antimicrobial therapy should continue for 14 days after the third dose of PEP vaccine. Those who are partially or fully vaccinated should receive at least a 30-day course of antimicrobial PEP and continue with licensed vaccination regimen. Unvaccinated workers, even those wearing personal protective equipment with adequate respiratory protection, should receive antimicrobial PEP. Antimicrobial PEP is not required for fully vaccinated people (five-dose I.M. vaccination series with a yearly booster) who enter an anthrax area clothed in personal protective equipment. If respiratory protection is disrupted, a 30-day course of antimicrobial therapy is recommended (ACIP, 2010).

Prophylaxis against infective endocarditis: 2 g 30-60 minutes before procedure. **Note:** American Heart Association (AHA) guidelines now recommend prophylaxis only in patients undergoing invasive procedures and in whom underlying cardiac conditions may predispose to a higher risk of adverse outcomes should infection occur. As of April 2007, routine prophylaxis for GI/GU procedures is no longer recommended by the AHA.

Prophylaxis in total joint replacement patients undergoing dental procedures which produce bacteremia: 2 g 1 hour prior to procedure

Dosing interval in renal impairment: Use of certain dosage forms (eg, extended-release 775 mg tablet and immediate-release 875 mg tablet) should be avoided in patients with Cl_{cr} <30 mL/minute or patients requiring hemodialysis.
Cl_{cr} 10-30 mL/minute: 250-500 mg every 12 hours
Cl_{cr} <10 mL/minute: 250-500 mg every 24 hours

Dialysis: Moderately dialyzable (20% to 50%) by hemo- or peritoneal dialysis; approximately 50 mg of amoxicillin per liter of filtrate is removed by continuous arteriovenous or venovenous hemofiltration; dose as per Cl_{cr} <10 mL/minute guidelines

Dietary Considerations May be taken with food.
Moxatag™: Take within 1 hour of finishing a meal.

Administration Administer around-the-clock to promote less variation in peak and trough serum levels. The appropriate amount of suspension may be mixed with formula, milk, fruit juice, water, ginger ale, or cold drinks; administer dose immediately after mixing.

Moxatag™ extended release tablet: Administer within 1 hour of finishing a meal.

Some penicillins (eg, carbenicillin, ticarcillin, and piperacillin) have been shown to inactivate aminoglycosides *in vitro*. This has been observed to a greater extent with tobramycin and gentamicin, while amikacin has shown greater stability against inactivation. Concurrent use of these agents may pose a risk of reduced antibacterial efficacy *in vivo*, particularly in the setting of profound renal impairment. However, definitive clinical evidence is lacking. If combination penicillin/aminoglycoside therapy is desired in a patient with renal dysfunction, separation of doses (if feasible), and routine monitoring of aminoglycoside levels, CBC, and clinical response should be considered.

Monitoring Parameters With prolonged therapy, monitor renal, hepatic, and hematologic function periodically; assess patient at beginning and throughout therapy for infection; monitor for signs of anaphylaxis during first dose

Test Interactions May interfere with urinary glucose tests using cupric sulfate (Benedict's solution, Clinitest®)
Some penicillin derivatives may accelerate the degradation of aminoglycosides *in vitro*, leading to a potential underestimation of aminoglycoside serum concentration.

Dosage Forms Excipient information presented when available (limited, particularly for generics); consult specific product labeling.
Capsule, oral: 250 mg, 500 mg
Powder for suspension, oral: 125 mg/5 mL (80 mL, 100 mL, 150 mL); 200 mg/5 mL (50 mL, 75 mL, 100 mL); 250 mg/5 mL (80 mL, 100 mL, 150 mL); 400 mg/5 mL (50 mL, 75 mL, 100 mL)
Tablet, oral: 500 mg, 875 mg
Tablet, chewable, oral: 125 mg, 200 mg, 250 mg, 400 mg
Tablet, extended release, oral:
Moxatag™: 775 mg

Amoxicillin and Clavulanate

(a moks i SIL in & klav yoo LAN ate)

Brand Names: U.S. Amoclan; Augmentin ES-600® [DSC]; Augmentin XR®; Augmentin®

Brand Names: Canada Amoxi-Clav; Apo-Amoxi-Clav®; Clavulin®; Novo-Clavamoxin; ratio-Aclavulanate

Index Terms Amoxicillin and Clavulanate Potassium; Amoxicillin and Clavulanic Acid; Clavulanic Acid and Amoxicillin

Pharmacologic Category Antibiotic, Penicillin

Use Treatment of otitis media, sinusitis, and infections caused by susceptible organisms involving the lower respiratory tract, skin and skin structure, and urinary tract; spectrum same as amoxicillin with additional coverage of beta-lactamase producing *B. catarrhalis*, *H. influenzae*, *N. gonorrhoeae*, and *S. aureus* (not MRSA). The expanded coverage of this combination makes it a useful alternative when amoxicillin resistance is present and patients cannot tolerate alternative treatments.

Pregnancy Risk Factor B

Pregnancy Considerations Adverse events have not been observed in animal studies; therefore, amoxicillin/clavulanate is classified as pregnancy category B. Both amoxicillin and clavulanic acid cross the placenta. There is no documented increased risk of teratogenic effects caused by amoxicillin/clavulanate. A potential increased risk of necrotizing enterocolitis in the newborn has been noted after maternal use of amoxicillin/clavulanate for preterm labor or premature prolonged rupture of membranes. When used during pregnancy, pharmacokinetic changes have been observed with amoxicillin alone (refer to the Amoxicillin monograph for details).

Lactation Enters breast milk/use caution

Contraindications Hypersensitivity to amoxicillin, clavulanic acid, penicillin, or any component of the formulation; history of cholestatic jaundice or hepatic dysfunction with amoxicillin/clavulanate potassium therapy; Augmentin XR™: severe renal impairment (Cl_{cr} <30 mL/minute) and hemodialysis patients

Warnings/Precautions Hypersensitivity reactions, including anaphylaxis (some fatal), have been reported. Prolonged use may result in fungal or bacterial superinfection, including *C. difficile*-associated diarrhea (CDAD) and pseudomembranous colitis; CDAD has been observed >2 months postantibiotic treatment. In patients with renal impairment, doses and/or frequency of administration should be modified in response to the degree of renal impairment. High percentage of patients with infectious mononucleosis have developed rash during therapy; ampicillin-class antibiotics not recommended in these patients. Incidence of diarrhea is higher than with amoxicillin alone. Due to differing content of clavulanic acid, not all formulations are interchangeable. Low incidence of cross-allergy with cephalosporins exists. Some products contain phenylalanine.

Adverse Reactions

>10%: Gastrointestinal: Diarrhea (3% to 34%; incidence varies upon dose and regimen used)

1% to 10%:

Dermatologic: Diaper rash, skin rash, urticaria

Gastrointestinal: Abdominal discomfort, loose stools, nausea, vomiting

Genitourinary: Vaginitis, vaginal mycosis

Miscellaneous: Moniliasis

<1% (Limited to important or life-threatening): Alkaline phosphatase increased, cholestatic jaundice, flatulence, headache, hepatic dysfunction, hepatitis, liver function tests increased, prothrombin time increased, thrombocytosis, vasculitis (hypersensitivity)

Additional adverse reactions seen with **ampicillin-class antibiotics:** Agitation, agranulocytosis, alkaline phosphatase increased, anaphylaxis, anemia, angioedema, anxiety, behavioral changes, bilirubin increased, black "hairy" tongue, confusion, convulsions, crystalluria, dizziness, enterocolitis, eosinophilia, erythema multiforme, exanthematous pustulosis, exfoliative dermatitis, gastritis, glossitis, hematuria, hemolytic anemia, hemorrhagic colitis, indigestion, insomnia, hyperactivity, interstitial nephritis, leukopenia, mucocutaneous candidiasis, pruritus, pseudomembranous colitis, serum sickness-like reaction, Stevens-Johnson syndrome, stomatitis, transaminases increased, thrombocytopenia, thrombocytopenic purpura, tooth discoloration, toxic epidermal necrolysis

Drug Interactions

Metabolism/Transport Effects None known.

Avoid Concomitant Use

Avoid concomitant use of Amoxicillin and Clavulanate with any of the following: BCG

Increased Effect/Toxicity

Amoxicillin and Clavulanate may increase the levels/effects of: Methotrexate; Vitamin K Antagonists

The levels/effects of Amoxicillin and Clavulanate may be increased by: Allopurinol; Probenecid

Decreased Effect

Amoxicillin and Clavulanate may decrease the levels/effects of: BCG; Mycophenolate; Typhoid Vaccine

The levels/effects of Amoxicillin and Clavulanate may be decreased by: Fusidic Acid; Tetracycline Derivatives

Stability

Powder for oral suspension: Store dry powder at room temperature of 25°C (77°F). Reconstitute powder for oral suspension with appropriate amount of water as specified on the bottle. Shake vigorously until suspended. Reconstituted oral suspension should be kept in refrigerator. Discard unused suspension after 10 days. Unit-dose antibiotic oral syringes are stable under refrigeration for 24 hours (Tu, 1988).

Tablet: Store at room temperature of 25°C (77°F).

Mechanism of Action Clavulanic acid binds and inhibits beta-lactamases that inactivate amoxicillin resulting in amoxicillin having an expanded spectrum of activity. Amoxicillin inhibits bacterial cell wall synthesis by binding to one or more of the penicillin-binding proteins (PBPs) which in turn inhibits the final transpeptidation step of peptidoglycan synthesis in bacterial cell walls, thus inhibiting cell wall biosynthesis. Bacteria eventually lyse due to ongoing activity of cell wall autolytic enzymes (autolysins and murein hydrolases) while cell wall assembly is arrested.

Pharmacodynamics/Kinetics Amoxicillin pharmacokinetics are not affected by clavulanic acid.

Amoxicillin: See Amoxicillin monograph.

Clavulanic acid:

Protein binding: ~25%

Metabolism: Hepatic

Half-life elimination: 1 hour

Time to peak: 1 hour

Excretion: Urine (30% to 40% as unchanged drug)

Dosage Note: Dose is based on the amoxicillin component; see "Augmentin® Product-Specific Considerations" table on next page.

Usual dosage range:

Infants <3 months: Oral: 30 mg/kg/day divided every 12 hours using the 125 mg/5 mL suspension

Children ≥3 months and <40 kg: Oral: 20-90 mg/kg/day divided every 8-12 hours

Children >40 kg and Adults: Oral: 250-500 mg every 8 hours or 875 mg every 12 hours

Indication-specific dosing:

Children ≥3 months and <40 kg: Oral:

Community-acquired pneumonia (CAP) (IDSA/PIDS, 2011): Infants >3 months and Children: **Note:** In children ≥5 years, a macrolide antibiotic should be added if atypical pneumonia cannot be ruled out.

Presumed bacterial (mild-to-moderate infection) (alternative to amoxicillin): 45 mg/kg/dose in 2 doses (maximum: 4 g/day)

H. influenzae (typable or nontypable; beta-lactamase producing), step-down therapy or mild infection (preferred): 15 mg/kg/dose in 3 doses **or** 45 mg/kg/dose in 2 doses

Lower respiratory tract infections, severe infections, sinusitis: 45 mg/kg/day divided every 12 hours **or** 40 mg/kg/day divided every 8 hours

Mild-to-moderate infections: 25 mg/kg/day divided every 12 hours or 20 mg/kg/day divided every 8 hours

Otitis media (Augmentin ES-600®): 90 mg/kg/day divided every 12 hours for 10 days in children with severe illness and when coverage for β-lactamase-positive *H. influenzae* and *M. catarrhalis* is needed.

Children ≥16 years and Adults: Oral:

Acute bacterial sinusitis: Extended release tablet: Two 1000 mg tablets every 12 hours for 10 days

Bite wounds (animal/human): 875 mg every 12 hours **or** 500 mg every 8 hours

Chronic obstructive pulmonary disease: 875 mg every 12 hours **or** 500 mg every 8 hours

Diabetic foot: Extended release tablet: Two 1000 mg tablets every 12 hours for 7-14 days

Diverticulitis, perirectal abscess: Extended release tablet: Two 1000 mg tablets every 12 hours for 7-10 days

Erysipelas: 875 mg every 12 hours **or** 500 mg every 8 hours

Febrile neutropenia: 875 mg every 12 hours

Pneumonia:
Aspiration: 875 mg every 12 hours
Community-acquired: Extended release tablet: Two 1000 mg tablets every 12 hours for 7-10 days
Pyelonephritis (acute, uncomplicated): 875 mg every 12 hours **or** 500 mg every 8 hours
Skin abscess: 875 mg every 12 hours

Dosing interval in renal impairment:
Cl_{cr} <30 mL/minute: Do not use 875 mg tablet or extended release tablets
Cl_{cr} 10-30 mL/minute: 250-500 mg every 12 hours
Cl_{cr} <10 mL/minute: 250-500 every 24 hours
Hemodialysis: Moderately dialyzable (20% to 50%)
250-500 mg every 24 hours; administer dose during and after dialysis. Do not use extended release tablets.
Peritoneal dialysis: Moderately dialyzable (20% to 50%)
Amoxicillin: Administer 250 mg every 12 hours
Clavulanic acid: Dose for Cl_{cr} <10 mL/minute
Continuous arteriovenous or venovenous hemofiltration effects:
Amoxicillin: ~50 mg of amoxicillin/L of filtrate is removed
Clavulanic acid: Dose for Cl_{cr} <10 mL/minute

Augmentin® Product-Specific Considerations

Strength	Form	Consideration
125 mg	S	q8h dosing
	S	For adults having difficulty swallowing tablets, 125 mg/5 mL suspension may be substituted for 500 mg tablet.
200 mg	CT, S	q12h dosing
	CT	Contains phenylalanine
	S	For adults having difficulty swallowing tablets, 200 mg/5 mL suspension may be substituted for 875 mg tablet.
250 mg	S, T	q8h dosing
	T	Not for use in patients <40 kg
	S	For adults having difficulty swallowing tablets, 250 mg/5 mL suspension may be substituted for 500 mg tablet.
400 mg	CT, S	q12h dosing
	CT	Contains phenylalanine
	S	For adults having difficulty swallowing tablets, 400 mg/5 mL suspension may be substituted for 875 mg tablet.
500 mg	T	q8h or q12h dosing
600 mg	S	q12h dosing
		Not for use in adults or children ≥40 kg
		600 mg/5 mL suspension is not equivalent to or interchangeable with 200 mg/5 mL or 400 mg/5 mL due to differences in clavulanic acid.
875 mg	T	q12h dosing; not for use in Cl_{cr} <30 mL/minute
1000 mg	XR	q12h dosing
		Not for use in children <16 years of age
		Not interchangeable with two 500 mg tablets
		Not for use if Cl_{cr} <30 mL/minute or hemodialysis

Legend: CT = chewable tablet, S = suspension, T = tablet, XR = extended release.

Dietary Considerations May be taken with meals or on an empty stomach; take with meals to increase absorption and decrease GI upset; may mix with milk, formula, or juice. Extended release tablets should be taken with food. Some products may contain sodium. Some products contain phenylalanine; if you have phenylketonuria or PKU, avoid use. All dosage forms contain potassium.

Administration Administer around-the-clock to promote less variation in peak and trough serum levels. Administer with food to increase absorption and decrease stomach upset; shake suspension well before use. Extended release tablets should be administered with food.

Some penicillins (eg, carbenicillin, ticarcillin, and piperacillin) have been shown to inactivate aminoglycosides *in vitro*. This has been observed to a greater extent with tobramycin and gentamicin, while amikacin has shown greater stability against inactivation. Concurrent use of these agents may pose a risk of reduced antibacterial efficacy *in vivo*, particularly in the setting of profound renal impairment. However, definitive clinical evidence is lacking. If combination penicillin/aminoglycoside therapy is desired in a patient with renal dysfunction, separation of doses (if feasible), and routine monitoring of aminoglycoside levels, CBC, and clinical response should be considered.

Monitoring Parameters Assess patient at beginning and throughout therapy for infection; with prolonged therapy, monitor renal, hepatic, and hematologic function periodically; monitor for signs of anaphylaxis during first dose

Test Interactions May interfere with urinary glucose tests using cupric sulfate (Benedict's solution, Clinitest®, Fehling's solution); may inactivate aminoglycosides *in vitro*. Some penicillin derivatives may accelerate the degradation of aminoglycosides *in vitro*, leading to a potential underestimation of aminoglycoside serum concentration.

Additional Information Two 250 mg tablets are not equivalent to a 500 mg tablet (both tablet sizes contain equivalent clavulanate). Two 500 mg tablets are not equivalent to a single 1000 mg extended release tablet.

Dosage Forms Excipient information presented when available (limited, particularly for generics); consult specific product labeling. [DSC] = Discontinued product

Powder for suspension, oral: 200: Amoxicillin 200 mg and clavulanate potassium 28.5 mg per 5 mL (50 mL, 75 mL, 100 mL); 250: Amoxicillin 250 mg and clavulanate potassium 62.5 mg per 5 mL (75 mL, 100 mL, 150 mL); 400: Amoxicillin 400 mg and clavulanate potassium 57 mg per 5 mL (50 mL, 75 mL, 100 mL); 600: Amoxicillin 600 mg and clavulanate potassium 42.9 mg per 5 mL (75 mL, 125 mL, 200 mL)

Amoclan:
200: Amoxicillin 200 mg and clavulanate potassium 28.5 mg per 5 mL (50 mL, 75 mL, 100 mL) [contains phenylalanine 7 mg/5 mL and potassium 0.14 mEq/5 mL; fruit flavor]
400: Amoxicillin 400 mg and clavulanate potassium 57 mg per 5 mL (50 mL, 75 mL, 100 mL) [contains phenylalanine 7 mg/5 mL and potassium 0.29 mEq/5 mL; fruit flavor]
600: Amoxicillin 600 mg and clavulanate potassium 42.9 mg per 5 mL (75 mL, 125 mL 200 mL) [contains phenylalanine 7 mg/5 mL, potassium 0.248 mEq/5 mL; orange flavor]

Augmentin®:
125: Amoxicillin 125 mg and clavulanate potassium 31.25 mg per 5 mL (75 mL, 100 mL, 150 mL) [contains potassium 0.16 mEq/5 mL; banana flavor]
200: Amoxicillin 200 mg and clavulanate potassium 28.5 mg per 5 mL (50 mL, 75 mL, 100 mL) [contains phenylalanine 7 mg/5 mL and potassium 0.14 mEq/5 mL; orange flavor] [DSC]
250: Amoxicillin 250 mg and clavulanate potassium 62.5 mg per 5 mL (75 mL, 100 mL, 150 mL) [contains potassium 0.32 mEq/5 mL; orange flavor]
400: Amoxicillin 400 mg and clavulanate potassium 57 mg per 5 mL (50 mL, 75 mL, 100 mL) [contains phenylalanine 7 mg/5 mL and potassium 0.29 mEq/5 mL; orange flavor] [DSC]

Augmentin ES-600®: Amoxicillin 600 mg and clavulanate potassium 42.9 mg per 5 mL (75 mL, 125 mL, 200 mL) [contains phenylalanine 7 mg/5 mL and potassium 0.23 mEq/5 mL; strawberry cream flavor] [DSC]

Tablet: 250: Amoxicillin 250 mg and clavulanate potassium 125 mg; 500: Amoxicillin 500 mg and clavulanate potassium 125 mg; 875: Amoxicillin 875 mg and clavulanate potassium 125 mg

Augmentin®:

250: Amoxicillin 250 mg and clavulanate potassium 125 mg [contains potassium 0.63 mEq/tablet] [DSC]

500: Amoxicillin 500 mg and clavulanate potassium 125 mg [contains potassium 0.63 mEq/tablet]

875: Amoxicillin 875 mg and clavulanate potassium 125 mg [contains potassium 0.63 mEq/tablet]

Tablet, chewable: 200: Amoxicillin 200 mg and clavulanate potassium 28.5 mg [contains phenylalanine]; 400: Amoxicillin 400 mg and clavulanate potassium 57 mg [contains phenylalanine]

Tablet, extended release: Amoxicillin 1000 mg and clavulanate acid 62.5 mg

Augmentin XR®: 1000: Amoxicillin 1000 mg and clavulanate acid 62.5 mg [contains potassium 12.6 mg (0.32 mEq) and sodium 29.3 mg (1.27 mEq) per tablet; packaged in either a 7-day or 10-day package]

◆ **Amoxicillin and Clavulanate Potassium** *see* Amoxicillin and Clavulanate *on page* 105

◆ **Amoxicillin and Clavulanic Acid** *see* Amoxicillin and Clavulanate *on page* 105

◆ **Amoxicillin, Clarithromycin, and Lansoprazole** *see* Lansoprazole, Amoxicillin, and Clarithromycin *on page* 975

◆ **Amoxicillin Trihydrate** *see* Amoxicillin *on page* 103

◆ **Amoxi-Clav (Can)** *see* Amoxicillin and Clavulanate *on page* 105

◆ **Amoxil** *see* Amoxicillin *on page* 103

◆ **Amoxycillin** *see* Amoxicillin *on page* 103

◆ **Amphetamine and Dextroamphetamine** *see* Dextroamphetamine and Amphetamine *on page* 488

◆ **Amphojel® (Can)** *see* Aluminum Hydroxide *on page* 79

◆ **Amphotec®** *see* Amphotericin B Cholesteryl Sulfate Complex *on page* 108

Amphotericin B Cholesteryl Sulfate Complex

(am foe TER i sin bee kole LES te ril SUL fate KOM plecks)

Brand Names: U.S. Amphotec®

Brand Names: Canada Amphotec®

Index Terms ABCD; Amphotericin B Colloidal Dispersion

Pharmacologic Category Antifungal Agent, Parenteral

Use Treatment of invasive aspergillosis in patients who have failed amphotericin B deoxycholate treatment, or who have renal impairment or experience unacceptable toxicity which precludes treatment with amphotericin B deoxycholate in effective doses.

Unlabeled Use Effective in patients with serious *Candida* species infections

Pregnancy Risk Factor B

Pregnancy Considerations Adverse events were not observed in animal reproduction studies. Amphotericin crosses the placenta and enters the fetal circulation. Amphotericin B is recommended for the treatment of serious systemic fungal diseases in pregnant women; refer to current guidelines (King, 1998).

Lactation Excretion in breast milk unknown/not recommended

Contraindications Hypersensitivity to amphotericin B or any component of the formulation

Warnings/Precautions Anaphylaxis has been reported with amphotericin B-containing drugs. If severe respiratory distress occurs, the infusion should be immediately discontinued. During the initial dosing, the drug should be administered under close clinical observation. Infusion reactions, sometimes severe, usually subside with continued therapy - manage with decreased rate of infusion and pretreatment with antihistamines/corticosteroids.

Adverse Reactions

>10%: Central nervous system: Chills, fever

1% to 10%:

Cardiovascular: Hypotension, tachycardia

Central nervous system: Headache

Dermatologic: Rash

Endocrine & metabolic: Hypokalemia, hypomagnesemia

Gastrointestinal: Nausea, diarrhea, abdominal pain

Hematologic: Thrombocytopenia

Hepatic: LFT change

Neuromuscular & skeletal: Rigors

Renal: Creatinine increased

Respiratory: Dyspnea

Note: Amphotericin B colloidal dispersion has an improved therapeutic index compared to conventional amphotericin B, and has been used safely in patients with amphotericin B-related nephrotoxicity; however, continued decline of renal function has occurred in some patients.

Drug Interactions

Metabolism/Transport Effects None known.

Avoid Concomitant Use

Avoid concomitant use of Amphotericin B Cholesteryl Sulfate Complex with any of the following: Gallium Nitrate

Increased Effect/Toxicity

Amphotericin B Cholesteryl Sulfate Complex may increase the levels/effects of: Aminoglycosides; Colistimethate; CycloSPORINE; CycloSPORINE (Systemic); Flucytosine; Gallium Nitrate

The levels/effects of Amphotericin B Cholesteryl Sulfate Complex may be increased by: Corticosteroids (Orally Inhaled); Corticosteroids (Systemic)

Decreased Effect

Amphotericin B Cholesteryl Sulfate Complex may decrease the levels/effects of: Saccharomyces boulardii

The levels/effects of Amphotericin B Cholesteryl Sulfate Complex may be decreased by: Antifungal Agents (Azole Derivatives, Systemic)

Stability Store intact vials under refrigeration. Reconstitute 50 mg and 100 mg vials with 10 mL and 20 mL of SWI, respectively. The reconstituted vials contain 5 mg/mL of amphotericin B. Shake the vial gently by hand until all solid particles have dissolved. After reconstitution, the solution should be refrigerated at 2°C to 8°C (36°F to 46°F) and used within 24 hours.

Further dilute amphotericin B colloidal dispersion with D_5W. Concentrations of 0.1-2 mg/mL in D_5W are stable for 14 days at 4°C and 23°C if protected from light, however, due to the occasional formation of subvisual particles, solutions should be used within 48 hours.

Mechanism of Action Binds to ergosterol altering cell membrane permeability in susceptible fungi and causing leakage of cell components with subsequent cell death. Proposed mechanism suggests that amphotericin causes an oxidation-dependent stimulation of macrophages (Lyman, 1992).

Pharmacodynamics/Kinetics

Distribution: V_d: Total volume increases with higher doses, reflects increasing uptake by tissues (with 4 mg/kg/day = 4 L/kg); predominantly distributed in the liver; concentrations in kidneys and other tissues are lower than observed with conventional amphotericin B

Half-life elimination: 28-29 hours; prolonged with higher doses

Dosage Children and Adults: I.V.:

Premedication: For patients who experience chills, fever, hypotension, nausea, or other nonanaphylactic infusion-related immediate reactions, premedicate with the following drugs 30-60 minutes prior to drug administration: A nonsteroidal (eg, ibuprofen, choline magnesium trisalicylate) with or without diphenhydramine **or** acetaminophen with diphenhydramine **or** hydrocortisone 50-100 mg. If the patient experiences rigors during the infusion, meperidine may be administered.

Range: 3-4 mg/kg/day (infusion of 1 mg/kg/hour); maximum: 7.5 mg/kg/day

A regimen of 6 mg/kg/day has been used for treatment of life-threatening invasive mold infections in immunocompromised patients; maximum: 7.5 mg/kg/day

Initially infuse at 1 mg/kg/hour. Rate of infusion may be increased with subsequent doses to 3 mg/kg/hour as patient tolerance allows. Treatment should continue as patient tolerance allows, until complete resolution of microbiologic and clinical evidence of fungal disease.

Administration Avoid injection faster than 1 mg/kg/hour. For a patient who experiences chills, fever, hypotension, nausea, or other nonanaphylactic infusion-related reactions, premedicate with the following drugs 30-60 minutes prior to drug administration: A nonsteroidal (eg, ibuprofen, choline magnesium trisalicylate) with or without diphenhydramine **or** acetaminophen with diphenhydramine **or** hydrocortisone 50-100 mg. If the patient experiences rigors during the infusion, meperidine may be administered. If severe respiratory distress occurs, the infusion should be immediately discontinued.

Monitoring Parameters Liver function tests, electrolytes, BUN, Cr, temperature, CBC, I/O, signs of hypokalemia (muscle weakness, cramping, drowsiness, ECG changes)

Additional Information Controlled trials which compare the original formulation of amphotericin B to the newer liposomal formulations (ie, Amphotec®) are lacking. Thus, comparative data discussing differences among the formulations should be interpreted cautiously. Although the risk of nephrotoxicity and infusion-related adverse effects may be less with Amphotec®, the efficacy profiles of Amphotec® and the original amphotericin formulation are comparable. Consequently, Amphotec® should be restricted to those patients who cannot tolerate or fail a standard amphotericin B formulation.

Dosage Forms Excipient information presented when available (limited, particularly for generics); consult specific product labeling.

Injection, powder for reconstitution:

Amphotec®: 50 mg [contains edetate disodium, lactose 950 mg]

Amphotec®: 100 mg [contains edetate disodium, lactose 1900 mg]

◆ **Amphotericin B Colloidal Dispersion** *see* Amphotericin B Cholesteryl Sulfate Complex *on page 108*

Amphotericin B (Conventional)

(am foe TER i sin bee con VEN sha nal)

Brand Names: Canada Fungizone®

Index Terms Amphotericin B Deoxycholate; Amphotericin B Desoxycholate; Conventional Amphotericin B

Pharmacologic Category Antifungal Agent, Parenteral

Additional Appendix Information

Antifungal Agents *on page 1876*

Use Treatment of severe systemic and central nervous system infections caused by susceptible fungi such as *Candida* species, *Histoplasma capsulatum*, *Cryptococcus neoformans*, *Aspergillus* species, *Blastomyces dermatitidis*, *Torulopsis glabrata*, and *Coccidioides immitis*; fungal peritonitis; irrigant for bladder fungal infections; used in fungal infection in patients with bone marrow transplantation, amebic meningoencephalitis, ocular aspergillosis (intraocular injection), candidal cystitis (bladder irrigation), chemoprophylaxis (low-dose I.V.), immunocompromised patients at risk of aspergillosis (intranasal/nebulized), refractory meningitis (intrathecal), coccidioidal arthritis (intra-articular/I.M.).

Low-dose amphotericin B has been administered after bone marrow transplantation to reduce the risk of invasive fungal disease.

Pregnancy Risk Factor B

Pregnancy Considerations Adverse events were not observed in animal reproduction studies. Amphotericin crosses the placenta and enters the fetal circulation. No teratogenic or undue systemic toxicity (electrolyte imbalance or renal dysfunction) has been reported in the mother or fetus. Toxic maternal effects are to be expected and must be monitored (Perfect, 2010). Amphotericin B is recommended for the treatment of serious systemic fungal diseases in pregnant women. Refer to current guidelines (King, 1998).

Lactation Excretion in breast milk unknown/not recommended

Contraindications Hypersensitivity to amphotericin or any component of the formulation

Warnings/Precautions Anaphylaxis has been reported with amphotericin B-containing drugs. During the initial dosing, the drug should be administered under close clinical observation. May cause nephrotoxicity; usual risk factors include underlying renal disease, concomitant nephrotoxic medications and daily and/or cumulative dose of amphotericin. Avoid use with other nephrotoxic drugs; drug-induced renal toxicity usually improves with interrupting therapy, decreasing dosage, or increasing dosing interval. However permanent impairment may occur, especially in patients receiving large cumulative dose (eg, >5 g) and in those also receiving other nephrotoxic drugs. Hydration and sodium repletion prior to administration may reduce the risk of developing nephrotoxicity. Frequent monitoring of renal function is recommended. Acute reactions (eg, fever, shaking chills, hypotension, anorexia, nausea, vomiting, headache, tachypnea) are most common 1-3 hours after starting the infusion and diminish with continued therapy. Avoid rapid infusion to prevent hypotension, hypokalemia, arrhythmias, and shock. If therapy is stopped for >7 days, restart at the lowest dose recommended and increase gradually. Leukoencephalopathy has been reported following administration of amphotericin. Total body irradiation has been reported to be a possible predisposition.

[U.S. Boxed Warning]: Should be used primarily for treatment of progressive, potentially life-threatening fungal infections, not noninvasive forms of infection. [U.S. Boxed warning]: Verify the product name and dosage if dose exceeds 1.5 mg/kg.

Adverse Reactions

Systemic:

>10%:

Cardiovascular: Hypotension, tachypnea

Central nervous system: Fever, chills, headache (less frequent with I.T.), malaise

Endocrine & metabolic: Hypokalemia, hypomagnesemia

Gastrointestinal: Anorexia, nausea (less frequent with I.T.), vomiting (less frequent with I.T.), diarrhea, heartburn, cramping epigastric pain

Hematologic: Normochromic-normocytic anemia

Local: Pain at injection site with or without phlebitis or thrombophlebitis (incidence may increase with peripheral infusion of admixtures)

Neuromuscular & skeletal: Generalized pain, including muscle and joint pains (less frequent with I.T.)

Renal: Decreased renal function and renal function abnormalities including azotemia, renal tubular acidosis, nephrocalcinosis (>0.1 mg/mL)

1% to 10%:

Cardiovascular: Hypertension, flushing

Central nervous system: Delirium, arachnoiditis, pain along lumbar nerves (especially I.T. therapy)

Genitourinary: Urinary retention

Hematologic: Leukocytosis

Neuromuscular & skeletal: Paresthesia (especially with I.T. therapy)

<1% (Limited to important or life-threatening): Acute liver failure, agranulocytosis, anuria, arrhythmias, bone marrow suppression, bronchospasm, cardiac arrest, cardiac failure, coagulation defects, convulsions, diplopia, dyspnea, eosinophilia, hearing loss, hemorrhagic gastroenteritis, hepatitis, hypersensitivity pneumonitis, increased liver function tests, jaundice, leukoencephalopathy, leukopenia, maculopapular rash, melena, nephrogenic diabetes insipidus, oliguria, peripheral neuropathy, pruritus, pulmonary edema, renal failure, renal tubular acidosis, shock, skin exfoliation, Stevens-Johnson syndrome, thrombocytopenia, tinnitus, toxic epidermal necrolysis, transient vertigo, ventricular fibrillation, vision changes, wheezing

Drug Interactions

Metabolism/Transport Effects None known.

Avoid Concomitant Use

Avoid concomitant use of Amphotericin B (Conventional) with any of the following: Gallium Nitrate

Increased Effect/Toxicity

Amphotericin B (Conventional) may increase the levels/effects of: Aminoglycosides; Colistimethate; CycloSPORINE; CycloSPORINE (Systemic); Flucytosine; Gallium Nitrate

The levels/effects of Amphotericin B (Conventional) may be increased by: Corticosteroids (Orally Inhaled); Corticosteroids (Systemic)

Decreased Effect

Amphotericin B (Conventional) may decrease the levels/effects of: Saccharomyces boulardii

The levels/effects of Amphotericin B (Conventional) may be decreased by: Antifungal Agents (Azole Derivatives, Systemic)

Stability Store intact vials under refrigeration. Protect from light. Add 10 mL of SWFI (without a bacteriostatic agent) to each vial of amphotericin B. Further dilute with 250-500 mL D_5W; final concentration should not exceed 0.1 mg/mL (peripheral infusion) or 0.25 mg/mL (central infusion).

Reconstituted vials are stable, protected from light, for 24 hours at room temperature and 1 week when refrigerated. Parenteral admixtures are stable, protected from light, for 24 hours at room temperature and 2 days under refrigeration. Short-term exposure (<24 hours) to light during I.V. infusion does **not** appreciably affect potency.

Mechanism of Action Binds to ergosterol altering cell membrane permeability in susceptible fungi and causing leakage of cell components with subsequent cell death. Proposed mechanism suggests that amphotericin causes an oxidation-dependent stimulation of macrophages (Lyman, 1992).

Pharmacodynamics/Kinetics

Distribution: Minimal amounts enter the aqueous humor, bile, CSF (inflamed or noninflamed meninges), pericardial fluid, pleural fluid, and synovial fluid

Protein binding, plasma: 90%

Half-life elimination: Biphasic: Initial: 15-48 hours; Terminal: 15 days

Time to peak: Within 1 hour following a 4- to 6-hour dose

Excretion: Urine (2% to 5% as biologically active form); ~40% eliminated over a 7-day period and may be detected in urine for at least 7 weeks after discontinued use

Dosage Premedication: For patients who experience infusion-related immediate reactions, premedicate with the following drugs 30-60 minutes prior to drug administration: NSAID ± diphenhydramine **or** acetaminophen with diphenhydramine **or** hydrocortisone. If the patient experiences rigors during the infusion, meperidine may be administered.

Usual dosage ranges:

Infants and Children:

Test dose: I.V.: 0.1 mg/kg/dose to a maximum of 1 mg; infuse over 30-60 minutes. Many clinicians believe a test dose is unnecessary.

Maintenance dose: 0.25-1 mg/kg/day given once daily; infuse over 2-6 hours. Once therapy has been established, amphotericin B can be administered on an every-other-day basis at 1-1.5 mg/kg/dose; cumulative dose: 1.5-2 g over 6-10 weeks.

Duration of therapy: Varies with nature of infection, usual duration is 4-12 weeks or cumulative dose of 1-4 g

Adults:

Test dose: 1 mg infused over 20-30 minutes. Many clinicians believe a test dose is unnecessary.

Maintenance dose: Usual: 0.3-1.5 mg/kg/day; 1-1.5 mg/kg over 4-6 hours every other day may be given once therapy is established; aspergillosis, rhinocerebral mucormycosis, often require 1-1.5 mg/kg/day; do not exceed 1.5 mg/kg/day

Indication-specific dosing:

Infants and Children:

Aspergillosis (HIV-exposed/-positive): I.V.: 1-1.5 mg/kg/day once daily (CDC, 2009)

Candidiasis (HIV-exposed/-positive):

Invasive: I.V.: 0.5-1.5 mg/kg/day once daily (CDC, 2009)

Esophageal: I.V.: 0.3-0.5 mg/kg/day once daily (CDC, 2009)

Oropharyngeal, refractory: I.V.: 0.3-0.5 mg/kg/day (CDC, 2009)

Coccidioidomycosis (HIV-exposed/-positive): I.V.: 0.5-1 mg/kg/day (CDC, 2009)

***Cryptococcus,* CNS disease (HIV-exposed/-positive):** I.V.: 0.7-1 mg/kg/day plus flucytosine; **Note:** Minimum 2 week induction followed by consolidation and chronic suppressive therapy; may increase amphotericin dose to 1.5 mg/kg/day if flucytosine is not tolerated.

***Cryptococcus,* disseminated (non-CNS disease) or severe pulmonary disease (HIV-exposed/-positive):** I.V.: 0.7-1 mg/kg/day once daily with or without flucytosine

Histoplasma, CNS or severe disseminated: I.V.: 1 mg/kg/day once daily (CDC, 2009)

Adults:

Aspergillosis, disseminated: I.V.: 0.6-0.7 mg/kg/day for 3-6 months

Bone marrow transplantation (prophylaxis): I.V.: Low-dose amphotericin B 0.1-0.25 mg/kg/day has been administered after bone marrow transplantation to reduce the risk of invasive fungal disease.

Candidemia (neutropenic or non-neutropenic): I.V.: 0.5-1 mg/kg/day until 14 days after first negative blood culture and resolution of signs and symptoms (Pappas, 2009)

Candidiasis, chronic, disseminated: I.V.: 0.5-0.7 mg/kg/day for 3-6 months and resolution of radiologic lesions (Pappas, 2009)

Dematiaceous fungi: I.V.: 0.7 mg/kg/day in combination with an azole

Endocarditis: I.V.: 0.6-1 mg/kg/day (with or without flucytosine) for 6 weeks after valve replacement; **Note:** If isolates susceptible and/or clearance demonstrated, guidelines recommend step-down to fluconazole; also for long-term suppression therapy if valve replacement is not possible (Pappas, 2009)

Endophthalmitis, fungal:

Intravitreal (unlabeled use): 10 mcg in 0.1 mL (in conjunction with systemic therapy)

I.V.: 0.7-1 mg/kg/day (with or without flucytosine) for at least 4-6 weeks (Pappas, 2009)

Esophageal candidiasis: I.V.: 0.3-0.7 mg/kg/day for 14-21 days after clinical improvement (Pappas, 2009)

Histoplasmosis: Chronic, severe pulmonary or disseminated: I.V.: 0.5-1 mg/kg/day for 7 days, then 0.8 mg/kg every other day (or 3 times/week) until total dose of 10-15 mg/kg; may continue itraconazole as suppressive therapy (lifelong for immunocompromised patients)

Meningitis:

Candidal: I.V.: 0.7-1 mg/kg/day (with or without flucytosine) for at least 4 weeks; **Note:** Liposomal amphotericin favored by IDSA guidelines based on decreased risk of nephrotoxicity and potentially better CNS penetration (Pappas, 2009)

Cryptococcal or Coccidioides: I.T.: Initial: 0.01-0.05 mg as single daily dose; may increase daily in increments of 0.025-0.1 mg as tolerated (maximum: 1.5 mg/day; most patients will tolerate a maximum dose of ~0.5 mg/treatment). Once titration to a maximum tolerated dose is achieved, that dose is administered daily. Once CSF improvement noted, may decrease frequency on a weekly basis (eg, 5 times/week, then 3 times/week, then 2 times/week, then once weekly, then once every other week, then once every 2 weeks, etc) until administration occurs once every 6 weeks. Typically, concurrent oral azole therapy is maintained (Stevens, 2001). **Note:** IDSA notes that the use of I.T. amphotericin for cryptococcal meningitis is generally discouraged and rarely necessary (Perfect, 2010).

Histoplasma: I.V.: 0.5-1 mg/kg/day for 7 days, then 0.8 mg/kg every other day (or 3 times/week) for 3 months total duration; follow with fluconazole suppressive therapy for up to 12 months

Meningoencephalitis, cryptococcal (Perfect, 2010): I.V.:

HIV positive: Induction: 0.7-1 mg/kg/day (plus flucytosine 100 mg/kg/day) for 2 weeks, then change to oral fluconazole for at least 8 weeks; alternatively, amphotericin (0.7-1 mg/kg/day) may be continued uninterrupted for 4-6 weeks; maintenance: amphotericin 1 mg/kg/week for ≥1 year may be considered, but inferior to use of azoles

HIV negative: Induction: 0.7-1 mg/kg/day (plus flucytosine 100 mg/kg/day) for 2 weeks (low-risk patients), ≥4 weeks (non-low-risk, but without neurologic complication, immunosuppression, underlying disease, and negative CSF culture at 2 weeks), >6 weeks (neurologic complication or patients intolerant of flucytosine) Follow with azole consolidation/maintenance treatment.

Oropharyngeal candidiasis: I.V.: 0.3 mg/kg/day for 7-14 days (Pappas, 2009)

Osteoarticular candidiasis: I.V.: 0.5-1 mg/kg/day for several weeks, followed by fluconazole for 6-12 months (osteomyelitis) or 6 weeks (septic arthritis) (Pappas, 2009)

Penicillium marneffei: I.V.: 0.6 mg/kg/day for 2 weeks

Pneumonia: Cryptococcal (mild-to-moderate): I.V.:

HIV positive: 0.5-1 mg/kg/day

HIV negative: 0.5-0.7 mg/kg/day (plus flucytosine) for 2 weeks

Sporotrichosis: Pulmonary, meningeal, osteoarticular, or disseminated: I.V.: Total dose of 1-2 g, then change to oral itraconazole or fluconazole for suppressive therapy

Urinary tract candidiasis (Pappas, 2009):

Fungus balls: I.V.: 0.5-0.7 mg/kg/day with or without flucytosine 25 mg/kg 4 times daily

Pyelonephritis: I.V.: 0.5-0.7 mg/kg/day with or without flucytosine 25 mg/kg 4 times daily for 2 weeks

Symptomatic cystitis: I.V.: 0.3-0.6 mg/kg/day for 1-7 days

Bladder irrigation: Irrigate with 50 mcg/mL solution instilled periodically or continuously for 5-10 days or until cultures are clear for fluconazole-resistant *Candida*

Dosing adjustment in renal impairment: If renal dysfunction is due to the drug, the daily total can be decreased by 50% or the dose can be given every other day; I.V. therapy may take several months

Renal replacement therapy: Poorly dialyzed; no supplemental dose or dosage adjustment necessary, including patients on intermittent hemodialysis or CRRT.

Peritoneal dialysis (PD): Administration in dialysate: 1-2 mg/L of peritoneal dialysis fluid either with or without low-dose I.V. amphotericin B (a total dose of 2-10 mg/kg given over 7-14 days). Precipitate may form in ionic dialysate solutions.

Administration May be infused over 4-6 hours. For a patient who experiences chills, fever, hypotension, nausea, or other nonanaphylactic infusion-related reactions, premedicate with the following drugs 30-60 minutes prior to drug administration: A nonsteroidal (eg, ibuprofen, choline magnesium trisalicylate) ± diphenhydramine **or** acetaminophen with diphenhydramine **or** hydrocortisone. If the patient experiences rigors during the infusion, meperidine may be administered. Bolus infusion of normal saline immediately preceding, or immediately preceding and following amphotericin B may reduce drug-induced nephrotoxicity. Risk of nephrotoxicity increases with amphotericin B doses >1 mg/kg/day. Infusion of admixtures more concentrated than 0.25 mg/mL should be limited to patients absolutely requiring volume contraction.

Monitoring Parameters Renal function (monitor frequently during therapy), electrolytes (especially potassium and magnesium), liver function tests, temperature, PT/PTT, CBC; monitor input and output; monitor for signs of hypokalemia (muscle weakness, cramping, drowsiness, ECG changes, etc)

Reference Range Therapeutic: 1-2 mcg/mL (SI: 1-2.2 micromole/L)

Test Interactions Increased BUN (S), serum creatinine, alkaline phosphate, bilirubin; decreased magnesium, potassium (S)

Additional Information Premedication with diphenhydramine and acetaminophen may reduce the severity of acute infusion-related reactions. Meperidine reduces the duration of amphotericin B-induced rigors and chilling. Hydrocortisone may be used in patients with severe or refractory infusion-related reactions. Bolus infusion of normal saline immediately preceding, or immediately preceding and following amphotericin B may reduce drug-induced nephrotoxicity. Risk of nephrotoxicity increases with amphotericin B doses >1 mg/kg/day. Infusion of admixtures more concentrated than 0.25 mg/mL should be limited to patients absolutely requiring volume restriction. Amphotericin B does not have a bacteriostatic constituent, subsequently admixture expiration is determined by sterility more than chemical stability.

Dosage Forms Excipient information presented when available (limited, particularly for generics); consult specific product labeling.

Injection, powder for reconstitution, as desoxycholate: 50 mg

- **Amphotericin B Deoxycholate** *see* Amphotericin B (Conventional) *on page 109*
- **Amphotericin B Desoxycholate** *see* Amphotericin B (Conventional) *on page 109*

Amphotericin B (Lipid Complex)

(am foe TER i sin bee LIP id KOM pleks)

Brand Names: U.S. Abelcet®

Brand Names: Canada Abelcet®

Index Terms ABLC

Pharmacologic Category Antifungal Agent, Parenteral

Use Treatment of aspergillosis or any type of progressive fungal infection in patients who are refractory to or intolerant of conventional amphotericin B therapy

Unlabeled Use Effective in patients with serious *Candida* species infections

Pregnancy Risk Factor B

Pregnancy Considerations Adverse events were not observed in animal reproduction studies. Amphotericin crosses the placenta and enters the fetal circulation. Amphotericin B is recommended for the treatment of serious, systemic fungal diseases in pregnant women, refer to current guidelines (King, 1998).

Lactation Enters breast milk/not recommended

Contraindications Hypersensitivity to amphotericin or any component of the formulation

Warnings/Precautions Anaphylaxis has been reported with amphotericin B-containing drugs. If severe respiratory distress occurs, the infusion should be immediately discontinued. During the initial dosing, the drug should be administered under close clinical observation. Acute reactions (including fever and chills) may occur 1-2 hours after starting an intravenous infusion. These reactions are usually more common with the first few doses and generally diminish with subsequent doses.

Adverse Reactions Nephrotoxicity and infusion-related hyperpyrexia, rigor, and chilling are reduced relative to amphotericin deoxycholate.

>10%:

Central nervous system: Chills, fever

Renal: Serum creatinine increased

Miscellaneous: Multiple organ failure

1% to 10%:

Cardiovascular: Hypotension, cardiac arrest

Central nervous system: Headache, pain

Dermatologic: Rash

Endocrine & metabolic: Bilirubinemia, hypokalemia, acidosis

Gastrointestinal: Nausea, vomiting, diarrhea, gastrointestinal hemorrhage, abdominal pain

Renal: Renal failure

Respiratory: Respiratory failure, dyspnea, pneumonia

Drug Interactions

Metabolism/Transport Effects None known.

Avoid Concomitant Use

Avoid concomitant use of Amphotericin B (Lipid Complex) with any of the following: Gallium Nitrate

Increased Effect/Toxicity

Amphotericin B (Lipid Complex) may increase the levels/effects of: Aminoglycosides; Colistimethate; CycloSPORINE; CycloSPORINE (Systemic); Flucytosine; Gallium Nitrate

The levels/effects of Amphotericin B (Lipid Complex) may be increased by: Corticosteroids (Orally Inhaled); Corticosteroids (Systemic)

Decreased Effect

Amphotericin B (Lipid Complex) may decrease the levels/effects of: Saccharomyces boulardii

The levels/effects of Amphotericin B (Lipid Complex) may be decreased by: Antifungal Agents (Azole Derivatives, Systemic)

Stability Intact vials should be stored at 2°C to 8°C (35°F to 46°F); do not freeze. Protect intact vials from exposure to light. Solutions for infusion are stable for 48 hours under refrigeration and for 6 hours at room temperature. Shake the vial gently until there is no evidence of any yellow sediment at the bottom. Dilute with D_5W to 1-2 mg/mL. Protect from light.

Do not dilute with saline solutions or mix with other drugs or electrolytes - compatibility has not been established

Do not use an in-line filter during administration.

Mechanism of Action Binds to ergosterol altering cell membrane permeability in susceptible fungi and causing leakage of cell components with subsequent cell death. Proposed mechanism suggests that amphotericin causes an oxidation-dependent stimulation of macrophages.

Pharmacodynamics/Kinetics

Distribution: V_d: Increases with higher doses; reflects increased uptake by tissues (131 L/kg with 5 mg/kg/day)

Half-life elimination: ~24 hours

Excretion: Clearance: Increases with higher doses (5 mg/kg/day): 400 mL/hour/kg

Dosage I.V.:

Note: Premedication: For patients who experience infusion-related immediate reactions, premedicate with the following drugs 30-60 minutes prior to drug administration: A nonsteroidal anti-inflammatory agent ± diphenhydramine **or** acetaminophen with diphenhydramine **or** hydrocortisone. If the patient experiences rigors during the infusion, meperidine may be administered.

Children:

Usual dosage range: 2.5-5 mg/kg/day as a single infusion

Aspergillosis, coccidioidomycosis (non-CNS), *Cryptococcus* (non-CNS), or invasive candidiasis (HIV-exposed/-positive): 5 mg/kg/dose once daily; may consider addition of flucytosine for severe candidal or cryptococcal disease (CDC, 2009)

Adults: Usual dosage range: 2.5-5 mg/kg/day as a single infusion

Dosing adjustment in renal impairment: None necessary; effects of renal impairment are not currently known

Hemodialysis: No supplemental dosage necessary

Peritoneal dialysis: No supplemental dosage necessary

Continuous renal replacement therapy (CRRT): No supplemental dosage necessary

Administration For patients who experience nonanaphylactic infusion-related reactions, premedicate 30-60 minutes prior to drug administration with a nonsteroidal anti-inflammatory agent ± diphenhydramine **or** acetaminophen with diphenhydramine **or** hydrocortisone. If the patient experiences rigors during the infusion, meperidine may be administered.

Administer at an infusion rate of 2.5 mg/kg/hour (over 2 hours). Invert infusion container several times prior to administration and every 2 hours during infusion if it exceeds 2 hours.

Monitoring Parameters Renal function (monitor frequently during therapy), electrolytes (especially potassium and magnesium), liver function tests, temperature, PT/PTT, CBC; monitor input and output; monitor for signs of hypokalemia (muscle weakness, cramping, drowsiness, ECG changes, etc)

Test Interactions Increased BUN (S), serum creatinine, alkaline phosphate, bilirubin; decreased magnesium, potassium (S)

Additional Information As a modification of dimyristoyl phosphatidylcholine:dimyristoyl phosphatidylglycerol 7:3 (DMPC:DMPG) liposome, amphotericin B lipid-complex has a higher drug to lipid ratio and the concentration of amphotericin B is 33 M. ABLC is a ribbon-like structure, not a liposome.

Controlled trials which compare the original formulation of amphotericin B to the newer liposomal formulations (ie, Abelcet®) are lacking. Thus, comparative data discussing differences among the formulations should be interpreted cautiously. Although the risk of nephrotoxicity and infusion-related adverse effects may be less with Abelcet®, the efficacy profiles of Abelcet® and the original amphotericin formulation are comparable. Consequently, Abelcet® should be restricted to those patients who cannot tolerate or fail a standard amphotericin B formulation.

Dosage Forms Excipient information presented when available (limited, particularly for generics); consult specific product labeling.

Injection, suspension [preservative free]:
- Abelcet®: 5 mg/mL (20 mL)

Amphotericin B (Liposomal)

(am foe TER i sin bee lye po SO mal)

Brand Names: U.S. AmBisome®

Brand Names: Canada AmBisome®

Index Terms L-AmB

Pharmacologic Category Antifungal Agent, Parenteral

Use Empirical therapy for presumed fungal infection in febrile, neutropenic patients; treatment of patients with *Aspergillus* species, *Candida* species, and/or *Cryptococcus* species infections refractory to amphotericin B desoxycholate (conventional amphotericin), or in patients where renal impairment or unacceptable toxicity precludes the use of amphotericin B desoxycholate; treatment of cryptococcal meningitis in HIV-infected patients; treatment of visceral leishmaniasis

Unlabeled Use Treatment of systemic *Histoplasmosis* infection

Pregnancy Risk Factor B

Pregnancy Considerations Adverse events were not observed in animal reproduction studies. Amphotericin crosses the placenta and enters the fetal circulation. Amphotericin B is recommended for the treatment of serious systemic fungal diseases in pregnant women; refer to current guidelines (King, 1998).

Lactation Excretion in breast milk unknown/not recommended

Contraindications Hypersensitivity to amphotericin B deoxycholate or any component of the formulation

Warnings/Precautions Patients should be under close clinical observation during initial dosing. As with other amphotericin B-containing products, anaphylaxis has been reported. Facilities for cardiopulmonary resuscitation should be available during administration. Acute infusion reactions (including fever and chills) may occur 1-2 hours after starting infusions; reactions are more common with the first few doses and generally diminish with subsequent doses. Immediately discontinue infusion if severe respiratory distress occurs; the patient should not receive further infusions. Concurrent use of amphotericin B with other nephrotoxic drugs may enhance the potential for drug-induced renal toxicity. Concurrent use with antineoplastic agents may enhance the potential for renal toxicity, bronchospasm or hypotension. Acute pulmonary toxicity has been reported in patients receiving simultaneous leukocyte transfusions and amphotericin B. Safety and efficacy have not been established in patients <1 month of age.

Adverse Reactions Percentage of adverse reactions is dependent upon population studied and may vary with respect to premedications and underlying illness. Incidence of decreased renal function and infusion-related events are lower than rates observed with amphotericin B deoxycholate.

>10%:

Cardiovascular: Peripheral edema (15%), edema (12% to 14%), tachycardia (9% to 19%), hypotension (7% to 14%), hypertension (8% to 20%), chest pain (8% to 12%), hypervolemia (8% to 12%)

Central nervous system: Chills (29% to 48%), insomnia (17% to 22%), headache (9% to 20%), anxiety (7% to 14%), pain (14%), confusion (9% to 13%)

Dermatologic: Rash (5% to 25%), pruritus (11%)

Endocrine & metabolic: Hypokalemia (31% to 51%), hypomagnesemia (15% to 50%), hyperglycemia (8% to 23%), hypocalcemia (5% to 18%), hyponatremia (9% to 12%)

Gastrointestinal: Nausea (16% to 40%), vomiting (11% to 32%), diarrhea (11% to 30%), abdominal pain (7% to 20%), constipation (15%), anorexia (10% to 14%)

Hematologic: Anemia (27% to 48%), blood transfusion reaction (9% to 18%), leukopenia (15% to 17%), thrombocytopenia (6% to 13%)

Hepatic: Alkaline phosphatase increased (7% to 22%), bilirubinemia (≤18%), ALT increased (15%), AST increased (13%), liver function tests abnormal (not specified) (4% to 13%)

Local: Phlebitis (9% to 11%)

Neuromuscular & skeletal: Weakness (6% to 13%), back pain (12%)

Renal: Nephrotoxicity (14% to 47%), creatinine increased (18% to 40%), BUN increased (7% to 21%), hematuria (14%)

Respiratory: Dyspnea (18% to 23%), lung disorder (14% to 18%), cough (2% to 18%), epistaxis (9% to 15%), pleural effusion (13%), rhinitis (11%)

Miscellaneous: Infusion reactions (4% to 21%), sepsis (7% to 14%), infection (11% to 13%)

2% to 10%:

Cardiovascular: Arrhythmia, atrial fibrillation, bradycardia, cardiac arrest, cardiomegaly, facial swelling, flushing, postural hypotension, valvular heart disease, vascular disorder, vasodilation

Central nervous system: Agitation, abnormal thinking, coma, depression, dysesthesia, dizziness (7% to 9%), hallucinations, malaise, nervousness, seizure, somnolence

Dermatologic: Alopecia, bruising, cellulitis, dry skin, maculopapular rash, petechia, purpura, skin discoloration, skin disorder, skin ulcer, urticaria, vesiculobullous rash

Endocrine & metabolic: Acidosis, fluid overload, hypernatremia (4%), hyperchloremia, hyperkalemia, hypermagnesemia, hyperphosphatemia, hypophosphatemia, hypoproteinemia, lactate dehydrogenase increased, nonprotein nitrogen increased

Gastrointestinal: Abdomen enlarged, amylase increased, dyspepsia, dysphagia, eructation, fecal incontinence, flatulence, gastrointestinal hemorrhage (10%), hematemesis, hemorrhoids, gum/oral hemorrhage, ileus, mucositis, rectal disorder, stomatitis, ulcerative stomatitis, xerostomia

Genitourinary: Vaginal hemorrhage

Hematologic: Coagulation disorder, hemorrhage, prothrombin decreased
Hepatic: Hepatocellular damage, hepatomegaly, veno-occlusive liver disease
Local: Injection site inflammation
Neuromuscular & skeletal: Arthralgia, bone pain, dystonia, myalgia, neck pain, paresthesia, rigors, tremor
Ocular: Conjunctivitis, dry eyes, eye hemorrhage
Renal: Abnormal renal function, acute renal failure, dysuria, renal failure, toxic nephropathy, urinary incontinence
Respiratory: Asthma, atelectasis, dry nose, hemoptysis, hyperventilation, pharyngitis, pneumonia, pulmonary edema, respiratory alkalosis, respiratory insufficiency, respiratory failure, sinusitis, hypoxia (6% to 8%)
Miscellaneous: Allergic reaction, cell-mediated immunological reaction, flu-like syndrome, graft-versus-host disease, herpes simplex, hiccup, procedural complication (8% to 10%), diaphoresis (7%)

Postmarketing and/or case reports: Agranulocytosis, angioedema, bronchospasm, cyanosis/hypoventilation, erythema, hemorrhagic cystitis

Drug Interactions

Metabolism/Transport Effects None known.

Avoid Concomitant Use

Avoid concomitant use of Amphotericin B (Liposomal) with any of the following: Gallium Nitrate

Increased Effect/Toxicity

Amphotericin B (Liposomal) may increase the levels/effects of: Aminoglycosides; Colistimethate; CycloSPORINE; CycloSPORINE (Systemic); Flucytosine; Gallium Nitrate

The levels/effects of Amphotericin B (Liposomal) may be increased by: Corticosteroids (Orally Inhaled); Corticosteroids (Systemic)

Decreased Effect

Amphotericin B (Liposomal) may decrease the levels/effects of: Saccharomyces boulardii

The levels/effects of Amphotericin B (Liposomal) may be decreased by: Antifungal Agents (Azole Derivatives, Systemic)

Stability Store intact vials at ≤25°C (≤77°F). Reconstituted vials are stable refrigerated at 2°C to 8°C (36°F to 46°F) for 24 hours. Do not freeze. Manufacturer's labeling states infusion should begin within 6 hours of dilution with D_5W; data on file with Astellas Pharma shows extended formulation stability when admixed in D_5W at 0.2-2 mg/mL (in polyolefin or PVC bags) for up to 11 days when stored refrigerated at 2°C to 8°C (36°F to 46°F).

Reconstitution: Reconstitute with 12 mL SWFI to a concentration of 4 mg/mL. The use of any solution other than those recommended, or the presence of a bacteriostatic agent in the solution, may cause precipitation. **Shake the vial vigorously** for 30 seconds, until dispersed into a translucent yellow suspension.

Filtration and dilution: The 5-micron filter should be on the syringe used to remove the reconstituted AmBisome®. Dilute to a final concentration of 1-2 mg/mL (0.2-0.5 mg/mL for infants and small children).

Mechanism of Action Binds to ergosterol altering cell membrane permeability in susceptible fungi and causing leakage of cell components with subsequent cell death. Proposed mechanism suggests that amphotericin causes an oxidation-dependent stimulation of macrophages (Lyman, 1992).

Pharmacodynamics/Kinetics

Distribution: V_d: 131 L/kg
Half-life elimination: Terminal: 174 hours

Dosage

Usual dosage range:

Children ≥1 month: I.V.: 3-6 mg/kg/day
Adults: I.V.: 3-6 mg/kg/day; **Note:** Higher doses (15 mg/kg/day) have been used clinically (Walsh, 2001)

Note: Premedication: For patients who experience non-anaphylactic infusion-related immediate reactions, premedicate with the following drugs 30-60 minutes prior to drug administration: A nonsteroidal anti-inflammatory agent ± diphenhydramine; **or** acetaminophen with diphenhydramine; **or** hydrocortisone. If the patient experiences rigors during the infusion, meperidine may be administered.

Indication-specific dosing:

Children ≥1 month: I.V.:

Empiric therapy: 3 mg/kg/day

Systemic fungal infections *(Aspergillus, Candida, Cryptococcus)*: 3-5 mg/kg/day

Systemic fungal infections (HIV-exposed/-positive [CDC, 2009; unlabeled use]):

Aspergillosis: 5 mg/kg/day once daily
Candida, invasive: 5 mg/kg/day once daily (may consider addition of oral flucytosine for severe disease)
Cryptococcal meningitis: 4-6 mg/kg/day once daily plus oral flucytosine
Cryptococcus, disseminated (non-CNS): 3-5 mg/kg/day (may consider addition of oral flucytosine)
Histoplasmosis: 3-5 mg/kg/day once daily

Visceral leishmaniasis:

Immunocompetent: 3 mg/kg/day on days 1-5, and 3 mg/kg/day on days 14 and 21; a repeat course may be given in patients who do not achieve parasitic clearance

Note: Alternate regimen of 10 mg/kg/day for 2 days has been reportedly effective.

Immunocompromised: 4 mg/kg/day on days 1-5, and 4 mg/kg/day on days 10, 17, 24, 31, and 38

Adults: I.V.:

Cryptococcal meningitis (HIV-positive): 6 mg/kg/day or 4-6 mg/kg/day in combination with addition of oral flucytosine 25 mg/kg 4 times daily (unlabeled combination; CDC, 2009)

Empiric candidiasis therapy: 3-5 mg/kg/day (Pappas, 2009)

Endocarditis: I.V.: 3-5 mg/kg/day (with or without flucytosine 25 mg/kg 4 times daily) for 6 weeks after valve replacement; **Note:** If isolates susceptible and/or clearance demonstrated, guidelines recommend step-down to fluconazole; also for long-term suppression therapy if valve replacement is not possible (Pappas, 2009)

Fungal sinusitis: Limited data in immunocompromised patients have shown efficacy with 3-10 mg/kg/day (Barron, 2005; Pagano, 2004; Rokicka, 2006). **Note:** An azole antifungal is recommended if causative organism is *Aspergillus* spp or *Pseudallescheria boydii* (*Scedosporium* sp).

Osteoarticular candidiasis: I.V.: 3-5 mg/kg/day for several weeks, followed by fluconazole for 6-12 months (osteomyelitis) or 6 weeks (septic arthritis) (Pappas, 2009)

Systemic fungal infections *(Aspergillus, Candida, Cryptococcus)* : 3-5 mg/kg/day

General invasive Candidal disease: 3-5 mg/kg/day with oral flucytosine 25 mg/kg 4 times daily (unlabeled combination; Pappas, 2009)
Candidal meningitis: 3-5 mg/kg/day with or without oral flucytosine 25 mg/kg 4 times daily (unlabeled combination; Pappas, 2009)
Histoplasmosis (unlabeled use): 3-5 mg/kg/day (CDC, 2009)

Visceral leishmaniasis:

Immunocompetent: 3 mg/kg/day on days 1-5, and 3 mg/kg/day on days 14 and 21; a repeat course may be given in patients who do not achieve parasitic clearance

Note: Alternate regimen of 2 mg/kg/day for 5 days has been reportedly effective.

Immunocompromised: 4 mg/kg/day on days 1-5, and 4 mg/kg/day on days 10, 17, 24, 31, and 38

Dosing adjustment in renal impairment: None necessary; effects of renal impairment are not currently known

Poorly dialyzed; no supplemental dose or dosage adjustment necessary, including patients on intermittent hemodialysis, peritoneal dialysis, or continuous renal replacement therapy (eg, CVVHD).

Administration Administer via intravenous infusion, over a period of approximately 2 hours. Infusion time may be reduced to approximately 1 hour in patients in whom the treatment is well-tolerated. If the patient experiences discomfort during infusion, the duration of infusion may be increased. Administer at a rate of 2.5 mg/kg/hour. Existing intravenous line should be flushed with D_5W prior to infusion (if not feasible, administer through a separate line). An in-line membrane filter (not less than 1 micron) may be used.

For a patient who experiences chills, fever, hypotension, nausea, or other nonanaphylactic infusion-related reactions, premedicate with the following drugs, 30-60 minutes prior to drug administration: A nonsteroidal (eg, ibuprofen, choline magnesium trisalicylate) ± diphenhydramine **or** acetaminophen with diphenhydramine **or** hydrocortisone. If the patient experiences rigors during the infusion, meperidine may be administered.

Monitoring Parameters Renal function (monitor frequently during therapy), electrolytes (especially potassium and magnesium), liver function tests, temperature, PT/PTT, CBC; monitor input and output; monitor for signs of hypokalemia (muscle weakness, cramping, drowsiness, ECG changes, etc); monitor cardiac function if used concurrently with corticosteroids

Additional Information Amphotericin B (liposomal) is a true single bilayer liposomal drug delivery system. Liposomes are closed, spherical vesicles created by mixing specific proportions of amphophilic substances such as phospholipids and cholesterol so that they arrange themselves into multiple concentric bilayer membranes when hydrated in aqueous solutions. Single bilayer liposomes are then formed by microemulsification of multilamellar vesicles using a homogenizer. Amphotericin B (liposomal) consists of these unilamellar bilayer liposomes with amphotericin B intercalated within the membrane. Due to the nature and quantity of amphophilic substances used, and the lipophilic moiety in the amphotericin B molecule, the drug is an integral part of the overall structure of the amphotericin B liposomal liposomes. Amphotericin B (liposomal) contains true liposomes that are <100 nm in diameter.

Dosage Forms Excipient information presented when available (limited, particularly for generics); consult specific product labeling.

Injection, powder for reconstitution:

AmBisome®: 50 mg [contains soy, sucrose 900 mg]

Ampicillin (am pi SIL in)

Brand Names: Canada Apo-Ampi®; Novo-Ampicillin; Nu-Ampi

Index Terms Aminobenzylpenicillin; Ampicillin Sodium; Ampicillin Trihydrate

Pharmacologic Category Antibiotic, Penicillin

Additional Appendix Information

Antibiotic Treatment of Adults With Infective Endocarditis *on page 1956*

Prevention of Infective Endocarditis *on page 1952*

Use Treatment of susceptible bacterial infections (nonbeta-lactamase-producing organisms); treatment or prophylaxis of infective endocarditis; susceptible bacterial infections caused by streptococci, pneumococci, nonpenicillinase-producing staphylococci, *Listeria*, meningococci; some strains of *H. influenzae*, *Salmonella*, *Shigella*, *E. coli*, *Enterobacter*, and *Klebsiella*

Pregnancy Risk Factor B

Pregnancy Considerations Adverse events have not been observed in animal studies; therefore, ampicillin is classified as pregnancy category B. Ampicillin crosses the human placenta, providing detectable concentrations in the cord serum and amniotic fluid. Most studies have not identified a teratogenic potential for ampicillin use during pregnancy. Two possible associations (congenital heart disease and cleft palate) have been noted; each of these was observed in a single study, was not substantiated by other studies, and may have been chance associations. Ampicillin is recommended for use in pregnant women for the management of premature rupture of membranes. Ampicillin is considered an acceptable alternative to penicillin for the prevention of early-onset Group B Streptococcal (GBS) disease in newborns.

The volume of distribution of ampicillin is increased during pregnancy and the half-life is decreased. As a result, serum concentrations in pregnant patients are approximately 50% of those in nonpregnant patients receiving the same dose. Higher doses may be needed during pregnancy. Although oral absorption is not altered during pregnancy, oral ampicillin is poorly-absorbed during labor.

Lactation Enters breast milk/use caution

Contraindications Hypersensitivity to ampicillin, any component of the formulation, or other penicillins

Warnings/Precautions Dosage adjustment may be necessary in patients with renal impairment. Serious and occasionally severe or fatal hypersensitivity (anaphylactoid) reactions have been reported in patients on penicillin therapy, especially with a history of beta-lactam hypersensitivity, history of sensitivity to multiple allergens, or previous IgE-mediated reactions (eg, anaphylaxis, angioedema, urticaria). Use with caution in asthmatic patients. High percentage of patients with infectious mononucleosis have developed rash during therapy with ampicillin; ampicillin-class antibiotics not recommended in these patients. Appearance of a rash should be carefully evaluated to differentiate a nonallergic ampicillin rash from a hypersensitivity reaction. Ampicillin rash occurs in 5% to 10% of children receiving ampicillin and is a generalized dull red, maculopapular rash, generally appearing 3-14 days after the start of therapy. It normally begins on the trunk and spreads over most of the body. It may be most intense at pressure areas, elbows, and knees. Prolonged use may result in fungal or bacterial superinfection, including *C. difficile*-associated diarrhea (CDAD) and pseudomembranous colitis; CDAD has been observed >2 months post-antibiotic treatment.

Adverse Reactions Frequency not defined.

Central nervous system: Fever, penicillin encephalopathy, seizure

Dermatologic: Erythema multiforme, exfoliative dermatitis, rash, urticaria

Note: Appearance of a rash should be carefully evaluated to differentiate (if possible) nonallergic ampicillin rash from hypersensitivity reaction. Incidence is higher in patients with viral infection, *Salmonella* infection, lymphocytic leukemia, or patients that have hyperuricemia.

Gastrointestinal: Black hairy tongue, diarrhea, enterocolitis, glossitis, nausea, pseudomembranous colitis, sore mouth or tongue, stomatitis, vomiting, oral candidiasis
Hematologic: Agranulocytosis, anemia, hemolytic anemia, eosinophilia, leukopenia, thrombocytopenia purpura
Hepatic: AST increased
Renal: Interstitial nephritis (rare)
Respiratory: Laryngeal stridor
Miscellaneous: Anaphylaxis, serum sickness-like reaction

Drug Interactions

Metabolism/Transport Effects None known.

Avoid Concomitant Use

Avoid concomitant use of Ampicillin with any of the following: BCG

Increased Effect/Toxicity

Ampicillin may increase the levels/effects of: Methotrexate; Vitamin K Antagonists

The levels/effects of Ampicillin may be increased by: Allopurinol; Probenecid

Decreased Effect

Ampicillin may decrease the levels/effects of: Atenolol; BCG; Mycophenolate; Typhoid Vaccine

The levels/effects of Ampicillin may be decreased by: Chloroquine; Fusidic Acid; Lanthanum; Tetracycline Derivatives

Ethanol/Nutrition/Herb Interactions Food: Food decreases ampicillin absorption rate; may decrease ampicillin serum concentration.

Stability

Oral: Oral suspension is stable for 7 days at room temperature or for 14 days under refrigeration.

I.V.:

I.V. minimum volume: Concentration should not exceed 30 mg/mL due to concentration-dependent stability restrictions. Solutions for I.M. or direct I.V. should be used within 1 hour. Solutions for I.V. infusion will be inactivated by dextrose at room temperature. If dextrose-containing solutions are to be used, the resultant solution will only be stable for 2 hours versus 8 hours in the 0.9% sodium chloride injection. D_5W has limited stability.

Stability of parenteral admixture in NS at room temperature (25°C) is 8 hours.

Stability of parenteral admixture in NS at refrigeration temperature (4°C) is 2 days.

Standard diluent: 500 mg/50 mL NS; 1 g/50 mL NS; 2 g/100 mL NS

Mechanism of Action Inhibits bacterial cell wall synthesis by binding to one or more of the penicillin-binding proteins (PBPs) which in turn inhibits the final transpeptidation step of peptidoglycan synthesis in bacterial cell walls, thus inhibiting cell wall biosynthesis. Bacteria eventually lyse due to ongoing activity of cell wall autolytic enzymes (autolysins and murein hydrolases) while cell wall assembly is arrested.

Pharmacodynamics/Kinetics

Absorption: Oral: 50%
Distribution: Bile, blister, and tissue fluids; penetration into CSF occurs with inflamed meninges only, good only with inflammation (exceeds usual MICs)
Normal meninges: Nil; Inflamed meninges: 5% to 10%
Protein binding: 15% to 25%
Half-life elimination:
Children and Adults: 1-1.8 hours
Anuria/end-stage renal disease: 7-20 hours
Time to peak: Oral: Within 1-2 hours
Excretion: Urine (~90% as unchanged drug) within 24 hours

Dosage

Usual dosage range:

Infants and Children:
Oral: 50-100 mg/kg/day in doses divided every 6 hours (maximum: 2-4 g/day)
I.M., I.V.: 100-400 mg/kg/day in divided doses every 6 hours (maximum: 12 g/day)
Adults: Oral, I.M., I.V.: 250-500 mg every 6 hours

Indication-specific dosing:

Infants and Children:

Community-acquired pneumonia (CAP) (IDSA/PIDS, 2011): Infants >3 months and Children: I.V.: **Note:** May consider addition of vancomycin or clindamycin to empiric therapy if community-acquired MRSA suspected. In children ≥ 5 years, a macrolide antibiotic should be added if atypical pneumonia cannot be ruled out.

Empiric treatment or *S. pneumoniae* (moderate-to-severe; MICs to penicillin ≤2.0 mcg/mL) or *H. influenzae* (beta-lactamase negative) (preferred): 150-200 mg/kg/day divided every 6 hours

Group A *Streptococcus* (moderate-to-severe) (preferred): 200 mg/kg/day every 6 hours

S. pneumoniae (moderate-to-severe; MICs to penicillin ≥4.0 mcg/mL) (alternative to ceftriaxone): 300-400 mg/kg/day divided every 6 hours

Prophylaxis against infective endocarditis:

Dental, oral, or respiratory tract procedures: I.M., I.V.: 50 mg/kg within 30-60 minutes prior to procedure in patients not allergic to penicillin and unable to take oral amoxicillin. Intramuscular injections should be avoided in patients who are receiving anticoagulant therapy. In these circumstances, orally administered regimens should be given whenever possible. Intravenously administered antibiotics should be used for patients who are unable to tolerate or absorb oral medications.

Note: American Heart Association (AHA) guidelines now recommend prophylaxis only in patients undergoing invasive procedures and in whom underlying cardiac conditions may predispose to a higher risk of adverse outcomes should infection occur.

Genitourinary and gastrointestinal tract procedures: I.M., I.V.:

High-risk patients: 50 mg/kg (maximum: 2 g) within 30 minutes prior to procedure, followed by ampicillin 25 mg/kg (or amoxicillin 25 mg/kg orally) 6 hours later; must be used in combination with gentamicin. **Note:** As of April 2007, routine prophylaxis for GI/GU procedures is no longer recommended by the AHA.

Moderate-risk patients: 50 mg/kg within 30 minutes prior to procedure

Mild-to-moderate infections:

Oral: 50-100 mg/kg/day in doses divided every 6 hours (maximum: 2-4 g/day)

I.M., I.V.: 100-150 mg/kg/day in divided doses every 6 hours (maximum: 2-4 g/day)

Severe infections, meningitis: I.M., I.V.: 200-400 mg/kg/day in divided doses every 6 hours (maximum: 6-12 g/day)

Adults:

Actinomycosis: I.V.: 50 mg/kg/day for 4-6 weeks then oral amoxicillin

Cholangitis (acute): I.V.: 2 g every 4 hours with gentamicin

Diverticulitis: I.M., I.V.: 2 g every 6 hours with metronidazole

Endocarditis:

Infective: I.V.: 12 g/day via continuous infusion or divided every 4 hours

Prophylaxis: Dental, oral, or respiratory tract: I.M., I.V.: 2 g within 30-60 minutes prior to procedure in patients not allergic to penicillin and unable to take oral amoxicillin. Intramuscular injections should be avoided in patients who are receiving anticoagulant therapy. In these circumstances, orally administered regimens should be given whenever possible. Intravenously administered antibiotics should be used for patients who are unable to tolerate or absorb oral medications.

Note: American Heart Association (AHA) guidelines now recommend prophylaxis only in patients undergoing invasive procedures and in whom underlying cardiac conditions may predispose to a higher risk of adverse outcomes should infection occur.

Prophylaxis in total joint replacement patient: I.M., I.V.: 2 g 1 hour prior to the procedure

Genitourinary and gastrointestinal tract procedures:

High-risk patients: I.M., I.V.: 2 g within 30 minutes prior to procedure, followed by ampicillin 1 g (or amoxicillin 1 g orally) 6 hours later; must be used in combination with gentamicin. **Note:** As of April 2007, routine prophylaxis for GI/GU procedures is no longer recommended by the AHA.

Moderate-risk patients: I.M., I.V.: 2 g within 30 minutes prior to procedure

Group B strep prophylaxis (intrapartum): I.V.: 2 g initial dose, then 1 g every 4 hours until delivery

***Listeria* infections:** I.V.: 2 g every 4 hours (consider addition of aminoglycoside)

Sepsis/meningitis: I.M., I.V.: 150-250 mg/kg/day divided every 3-4 hours (range: 6-12 g/day)

Urinary tract infections (*Enterococcus* suspected): I.V.: 1-2 g every 6 hours with gentamicin

Dosing interval in renal impairment:

Cl_{cr} >50 mL/minute: Administer every 6 hours

Cl_{cr} 10-50 mL/minute: Administer every 6-12 hours

Cl_{cr} <10 mL/minute: Administer every 12-24 hours

Intermittent hemodialysis (IHD) (administer after hemodialysis on dialysis days): Dialyzable (20% to 50%): I.V.: 1-2 g every 12-24 hours (Heintz, 2009). **Note:** Dosing dependent on the assumption of 3 times/week, complete IHD sessions.

Peritoneal dialysis (PD): 250 mg every 12 hours

Continuous renal replacement therapy (CRRT) (Heintz, 2009): Drug clearance is highly dependent on the method of renal replacement, filter type, and flow rate. Appropriate dosing requires close monitoring of pharmacologic response, signs of adverse reactions due to drug accumulation, as well as drug concentrations in relation to target trough (if appropriate). The following are general recommendations only (based on dialysate flow/ultrafiltration rates of 1-2 L/hour and minimal residual renal function) and should not supersede clinical judgment:

CVVH: Loading dose of 2 g followed by 1-2 g every 8-12 hours

CVVHD: Loading dose of 2 g followed by 1-2 g every 8 hours

CVVHDF: Loading dose of 2 g followed by 1-2 g every 6-8 hours

Dietary Considerations Take on an empty stomach 1 hour before or 2 hours after meals. Some products may contain sodium.

Administration Administer around-the-clock to promote less variation in peak and trough serum levels.

Oral: Administer on an empty stomach (ie, 1 hour prior to, or 2 hours after meals) to increase total absorption.

I.V.: Administer over 3-5 minutes (125-500 mg) or over 10-15 minutes (1-2 g). More rapid infusion may cause seizures. Ampicillin and gentamicin should not be mixed in the same I.V. tubing.

Some penicillins (eg, carbenicillin, ticarcillin, and piperacillin) have been shown to inactivate aminoglycosides *in vitro*. This has been observed to a greater extent with tobramycin and gentamicin, while amikacin has shown greater stability against inactivation. Concurrent use of these agents may pose a risk of reduced antibacterial efficacy *in vivo*, particularly in the setting of profound renal impairment. However, definitive clinical evidence is lacking. If combination penicillin/aminoglycoside therapy is desired in a patient with renal dysfunction, separation of doses (if feasible), and routine monitoring of aminoglycoside levels, CBC, and clinical response should be considered.

Monitoring Parameters With prolonged therapy, monitor renal, hepatic, and hematologic function periodically; observe signs and symptoms of anaphylaxis during first dose

Test Interactions May interfere with urinary glucose tests using cupric sulfate (Benedict's solution, Clinitest®)

Some penicillin derivatives may accelerate the degradation of aminoglycosides *in vitro*, leading to a potential underestimation of aminoglycoside serum concentration.

Dosage Forms Excipient information presented when available (limited, particularly for generics); consult specific product labeling.

Capsule, oral: 250 mg, 500 mg

Injection, powder for reconstitution, as sodium [strength expressed as base]: 125 mg, 250 mg, 500 mg, 1 g, 2 g, 10 g

Powder for suspension, oral: 125 mg/5 mL (100 mL, 200 mL); 250 mg/5 mL (100 mL, 200 mL)

Ampicillin and Sulbactam

(am pi SIL in & SUL bak tam)

Brand Names: U.S. Unasyn®

Brand Names: Canada Unasyn®

Index Terms Sulbactam and Ampicillin

Pharmacologic Category Antibiotic, Penicillin

Additional Appendix Information

Antibiotic Treatment of Adults With Infective Endocarditis *on page 1956*

Prevention of Wound Infection and Sepsis in Surgical Patients *on page 1954*

Use Treatment of susceptible bacterial infections involved with skin and skin structure, intra-abdominal infections, gynecological infections; spectrum is that of ampicillin plus organisms producing beta-lactamases such as *S. aureus*, *H. influenzae*, *E. coli*, *Klebsiella*, *Acinetobacter*, *Enterobacter*, and anaerobes

Pregnancy Risk Factor B

Pregnancy Considerations Adverse events have not been observed in animal studies; therefore, ampicillin/sulbactam is classified as pregnancy category B. Both ampicillin and sulbactam cross the placenta. When used during pregnancy, pharmacokinetic changes have been observed with ampicillin alone (refer to the Ampicillin monograph for details).

Lactation Enters breast milk/use caution

Contraindications Hypersensitivity to ampicillin, sulbactam, penicillins, or any component of the formulations

Warnings/Precautions Dosage adjustment may be necessary in patients with renal impairment. Serious and occasionally severe or fatal hypersensitivity (anaphylactoid) reactions have been reported in patients on penicillin therapy, especially with a history of beta-lactam hypersensitivity, history of sensitivity to multiple allergens, or previous IgE-mediated reactions (eg, anaphylaxis, angioedema, urticaria). Use with caution in asthmatic patients. High percentage of patients with infectious mononucleosis have developed rash during therapy with ampicillin; ampicillin-class antibiotics not recommended in these patients. Appearance of a rash should be carefully evaluated to differentiate a nonallergic ampicillin rash from a hypersensitivity reaction. Prolonged use may result in fungal or bacterial superinfection, including *C. difficile*-associated diarrhea (CDAD) and pseudomembranous colitis; CDAD has been observed >2 months postantibiotic treatment.

Adverse Reactions Also see Ampicillin.

>10%: Local: Pain at injection site (I.M.)

1% to 10%:

Dermatologic: Rash

Gastrointestinal: Diarrhea

Local: Pain at injection site (I.V.), thrombophlebitis

Miscellaneous: Allergic reaction (may include serum sickness, urticaria, bronchospasm, hypotension, etc)

<1% (Limited to important or life-threatening): Abdominal distension, candidiasis, chest pain, chills, dysuria, edema, epistaxis, erythema, facial swelling, fatigue, flatulence, glossitis, hairy tongue, headache, interstitial nephritis, itching, liver enzymes increased, malaise, mucosal bleeding, nausea, pseudomembranous colitis, seizure, substernal pain, throat tightness, thrombocytopenia, urine retention, vomiting

Drug Interactions

Metabolism/Transport Effects None known.

Avoid Concomitant Use

Avoid concomitant use of Ampicillin and Sulbactam with any of the following: BCG

Increased Effect/Toxicity

Ampicillin and Sulbactam may increase the levels/effects of: Methotrexate; Vitamin K Antagonists

The levels/effects of Ampicillin and Sulbactam may be increased by: Allopurinol; Probenecid

Decreased Effect

Ampicillin and Sulbactam may decrease the levels/effects of: Atenolol; BCG; Mycophenolate; Typhoid Vaccine

The levels/effects of Ampicillin and Sulbactam may be decreased by: Chloroquine; Fusidic Acid; Lanthanum; Tetracycline Derivatives

Stability Prior to reconstitution, store at ≤30°C (86°F).

I.M. and direct I.V. administration: Use within 1 hour after preparation. Reconstitute with sterile water for injection or 0.5% or 2% lidocaine hydrochloride injection (I.M.). Sodium chloride 0.9% (NS) is the diluent of choice for I.V. piggyback use. Solutions made in NS are stable up to 72 hours when refrigerated whereas dextrose solutions (same concentration) are stable for only 4 hours.

Mechanism of Action The addition of sulbactam, a beta-lactamase inhibitor, to ampicillin extends the spectrum of ampicillin to include some beta-lactamase-producing organisms; inhibits bacterial cell wall synthesis by binding to one or more of the penicillin-binding proteins (PBPs) which in turn inhibits the final transpeptidation step of peptidoglycan synthesis in bacterial cell walls, thus inhibiting cell wall biosynthesis. Bacteria eventually lyse due to ongoing activity of cell wall autolytic enzymes (autolysins and murein hydrolases) while cell wall assembly is arrested.

Pharmacodynamics/Kinetics

Ampicillin: See Ampicillin.

Sulbactam:

Distribution: Bile, blister, and tissue fluids

Protein binding: 38%

Half-life elimination: Normal renal function: 1-1.3 hours

Excretion: Urine (~75% to 85% as unchanged drug) within 8 hours

Dosage Note: Unasyn® (ampicillin/sulbactam) is a combination product. Dosage recommendations for Unasyn® are based on the ampicillin component.

Usual dosage range:

Children ≥1 year: I.V.: 100-400 mg ampicillin/kg/day divided every 6 hours (maximum: 8 g ampicillin/day, 12 g Unasyn®). **Note:** The American Academy of Pediatrics recommends a dose of up to 300 mg/kg/day for severe infection in infants >1 month of age.

Adults: I.M., I.V.: 1-2 g ampicillin (1.5-3 g Unasyn®) every 6 hours (maximum: 8 g ampicillin/day, 12 g Unasyn®)

Indication-specific dosing:

Children: ≥1 year:

Epiglottitis: I.V.: 100-200 mg ampicillin/kg/day divided in 4 doses

Mild-to-moderate infections: I.V.: 100-200 mg ampicillin/kg/day (150-300 mg Unasyn®) divided every 6 hours (maximum: 8 g ampicillin/day, 12 g Unasyn®)

Peritonsillar and retropharyngeal abscess: I.V.: 50 mg ampicillin/kg/dose every 6 hours

Severe infections: I.V.: 200-400 mg ampicillin/kg/day divided every 6 hours (maximum: 8 g ampicillin/day, 12 g Unasyn®)

Adults: Doses expressed as ampicillin/sulbactam combination:

Amnionitis, cholangitis, diverticulitis, endometritis, endophthalmitis, epididymitis/orchitis, liver abscess, osteomyelitis (diabetic foot), peritonitis: I.V.: 3 g every 6 hours; **Note:** Due to high rates of *E. coli* resistance, not recommended for the treatment of community-acquired intra-abdominal infections (Solomkin, 2010)

Endocarditis: I.V.: 3 g every 6 hours with gentamicin or vancomycin for 4-6 weeks

Orbital cellulitis: I.V.: 1.5 g every 6 hours

Parapharyngeal space infections: I.V.: 3 g every 6 hours

Pasteurella multocida **(human, canine/feline bites):** I.V.: 1.5-3 g every 6 hours

Pelvic inflammatory disease: I.V.: 3 g every 6 hours with doxycycline

Peritonitis associated with CAPD: Intraperitoneal:

Anuric, intermittent: 3 g every 12 hours (Li, 2010)

Anuric, continuous: Loading dose: 1.5 g per liter of dialysate; maintenance dose: 150 mg per liter of dialysate (Li, 2010)

Pneumonia:

Aspiration, community-acquired: I.V.: 1.5-3 g every 6 hours

Hospital-acquired: I.V.: 3 g every 6 hours

Urinary tract infections, pyelonephritis: I.V.: 3 g every 6 hours for 14 days

Dosing interval in renal impairment: Note: Estimation of renal function for the purpose of drug dosing should be done using the Cockcroft-Gault formula.

Cl_{cr} 15-29 mL/minute/1.73 m^2: 1.5-3 g every 12 hours

Cl_{cr} 5-14 mL/minute/1.73 m^2: 1.5-3 g every 24 hours

Intermittent hemodialysis (IHD) (administer after hemodialysis on dialysis days): 1.5-3 g every 12-24 hours (Heintz, 2009). **Note:** Dosing dependent on the assumption of 3 times/week, complete IHD sessions.

Peritoneal dialysis (PD): 3 g every 24 hours

Continuous renal replacement therapy (CRRT): Drug clearance is highly dependent on the method of renal replacement, filter type, and flow rate. Appropriate dosing requires close monitoring of pharmacologic response, signs of adverse reactions due to drug accumulation, as well as drug levels in relation to target trough (if appropriate). The following are general recommendations only (based on dialysate flow/ultrafiltration rates of 1-2 L/hour and minimal residual renal function) and should not supersede clinical judgment (Heintz, 2009; Trotman, 2005):

CVVH: Initial: 3 g; maintenance: 1.5-3 g every 8-12 hours

CVVHD: Initial: 3 g; maintenance: 1.5-3 g every 8 hours

CVVHDF: Initial: 3 g; maintenance: 1.5-3 g every 6-8 hours

Dietary Considerations Some products may contain sodium.

Administration Administer around-the-clock to promote less variation in peak and trough serum levels. Administer by slow injection over 10-15 minutes or I.V. over 15-30 minutes. Ampicillin and gentamicin should not be mixed in the same I.V. tubing.

Some penicillins (eg, carbenicillin, ticarcillin, and piperacillin) have been shown to inactivate aminoglycosides *in vitro*. This has been observed to a greater extent with tobramycin and gentamicin, while amikacin has shown greater stability against inactivation. Concurrent use of these agents may pose a risk of reduced antibacterial efficacy *in vivo*, particularly in the setting of profound renal impairment. However, definitive clinical evidence is lacking. If combination penicillin/aminoglycoside therapy is desired in a patient with renal dysfunction, separation of doses (if feasible), and routine monitoring of aminoglycoside levels, CBC, and clinical response should be considered.

Monitoring Parameters With prolonged therapy, monitor hematologic, renal, and hepatic function; monitor for signs of anaphylaxis during first dose

Test Interactions May interfere with urinary glucose tests using cupric sulfate (Benedict's solution, Clinitest®).

Some penicillin derivatives may accelerate the degradation of aminoglycosides *in vitro*, leading to a potential underestimation of aminoglycoside serum concentration.

Dosage Forms Excipient information presented when available (limited, particularly for generics); consult specific product labeling.

Injection, powder for reconstitution: 1.5 g: Ampicillin 1 g and sulbactam 0.5 g; 3 g: Ampicillin 2 g and sulbactam 1 g; 15 g: Ampicillin 10 g and sulbactam 5 g

Unasyn®:

1.5 g: Ampicillin 1 g and sulbactam 0.5 g [contains sodium 115 mg (5 mEq)/1.5 g)]

3 g: Ampicillin 2 g and sulbactam 1 g [contains sodium 115 mg (5 mEq)/1.5 g)]

15 g: Ampicillin 10 g and sulbactam 5 g [bulk package; contains sodium 115 mg (5 mEq)/1.5 g)]

- ◆ **Ampicillin Sodium** *see* Ampicillin *on page 115*
- ◆ **Ampicillin Trihydrate** *see* Ampicillin *on page 115*
- ◆ **AMPT** *see* Metyrosine *on page 1123*
- ◆ **Ampyra™** *see* Dalfampridine *on page 440*
- ◆ **Amrinone Lactate** *see* Inamrinone *on page 884*
- ◆ **Amrix®** *see* Cyclobenzaprine *on page 419*
- ◆ **Amturnide™** *see* Aliskiren, Amlodipine, and Hydrochlorothiazide *on page 67*
- ◆ **Amvisc®** *see* Hyaluronate and Derivatives *on page 831*
- ◆ **Amvisc® Plus** *see* Hyaluronate and Derivatives *on page 831*
- ◆ **Amylase, Lipase, and Protease** *see* Pancrelipase *on page 1285*

Amyl Nitrite (AM il NYE trite)

Index Terms Isoamyl Nitrite

Pharmacologic Category Antianginal Agent; Antidote; Vasodilator

Use Coronary vasodilator in angina pectoris

Note: Given the widespread use of newer nitrate compounds, the use of amyl nitrite for patients experiencing angina pectoris has fallen out of favor.

Unlabeled Use Adjunct treatment of cyanide toxicity; produce changes in the intensity of heart murmurs; provocation of latent left ventricular outflow tract (LVOT) gradient during echocardiography in patients with hypertrophic cardiomyopathy (HCM)

Pregnancy Risk Factor C

Dosage Nasal inhalation:

Angina: Adults: 2-6 inhalations from 1 crushed ampul; may repeat in 3-5 minutes

Cyanide toxicity (unlabeled use): Children and Adults: Inhale the vapor from 1 crushed ampul over a 30-60 second period; repeat every 30-60 seconds for ~5 minutes (Lavon, 2010). **Note:** Amyl nitrite is a temporary intervention that should only be used until I.V. sodium nitrite infusion is ready for administration.

Pharmacologic provocation of latent left ventricular outflow tract (LVOT) gradient in hypertrophic cardiomyopathy (HCM) (unlabeled use): Adults: 3-4 deep inhalations from 1 crushed ampul over a 10-15 second period (Nagueh, 2011; Reagan, 2005). **Note:** The use of more physiologic testing (eg, treadmill testing with Doppler echocardiography) may be preferred over amyl nitrite inhalation (Maron, 2003: Nagueh, 2011).

Additional Information Complete prescribing information for this medication should be consulted for additional detail.

Dosage Forms Excipient information presented when available (limited, particularly for generics); consult specific product labeling.

Liquid, for inhalation: USP: 85% to 103% (0.3 mL) [crushable covered glass capsule]

- ◆ **Amylobarbitone** *see* Amobarbital *on page 101*
- ◆ **Amytal®** *see* Amobarbital *on page 101*
- ◆ **AN100226** *see* Natalizumab *on page 1181*
- ◆ **Anacin® Advanced Headache Formula [OTC]** *see* Acetaminophen, Aspirin, and Caffeine *on page 32*
- ◆ **Anadrol®-50** *see* Oxymetholone *on page 1270*
- ◆ **Anafranil®** *see* ClomiPRAMINE *on page 388*

Anagrelide (an AG gre lide)

Brand Names: U.S. Agrylin®

Brand Names: Canada Agrylin®; Dom-Anagrelide; Mylan-Anagrelide; PMS-Anagrelide; Sandoz-Anagrelide

Index Terms Anagrelide Hydrochloride; BL4162A

Pharmacologic Category Phospholipase A_2 Inhibitor; Platelet Reducing Agent

Use Treatment of thrombocythemia associated with myeloproliferative disorders (eg, chronic myelogenous leukemia, essential thrombocythemia, polycythemia vera, myeloid metaplasia with myelofibrosis, or other myeloproliferative disorder) to reduce the risk of thrombosis and reduce associated symptoms (including thrombo-hemorrhagic events)

Pregnancy Risk Factor C

Dosage Note: Maintain initial dose for ≥1 week, then adjust to the lowest effective dose to reduce and maintain platelet count <600,000/mm³ ideally to the normal range; the dose must not be increased by >0.5 mg/day in any 1 week; maximum dose: 10 mg/day or 2.5 mg/dose

Oral: Thrombocythemia:

Children: Initial: 0.5 mg/day (range: 0.5 mg 1-4 times/day)

Adults: Initial: 0.5 mg 4 times/day or 1 mg twice daily (most patients will experience adequate response at dose ranges of 1.5-3 mg/day)

Elderly: There are no special requirements for dosing in the elderly

Dosage adjustment in renal impairment: No adjustment required in renal insufficiency; monitor closely

Dosage adjustment in hepatic impairment:

Moderate impairment: Initial: 0.5 mg once daily; maintain for at least 1 week with careful monitoring of cardiovascular status; the dose must not be increased by >0.5 mg/day in any 1 week.

Severe impairment: Use is contraindicated

Additional Information Complete prescribing information for this medication should be consulted for additional detail.

Dosage Forms Excipient information presented when available (limited, particularly for generics); consult specific product labeling.

Capsule, oral: 0.5 mg, 1 mg

Agrylin®: 0.5 mg

◆ **Anagrelide Hydrochloride** *see* Anagrelide *on page 119*

Anakinra (an a KIN ra)

Brand Names: U.S. Kineret®

Brand Names: Canada Kineret®

Index Terms IL-1Ra; Interleukin-1 Receptor Antagonist

Pharmacologic Category Antirheumatic, Disease Modifying; Interleukin-1 Receptor Antagonist

Use Treatment of moderately- to severely-active rheumatoid arthritis in adult patients who have failed one or more disease-modifying antirheumatic drugs (DMARDs); may be used alone or in combination with DMARDs (other than tumor necrosis factor-blocking agents)

Pregnancy Risk Factor B

Pregnancy Considerations Animal reproduction studies have not revealed any evidence of impaired fertility or harm to fetus. There are no adequate and well-controlled studies in pregnant women. Women exposed to anakinra during pregnancy may contact the Organization of Teratology Information Services (OTIS), Rheumatoid Arthritis and Pregnancy Study at 1-877-311-8972.

Lactation Excretion in breast milk unknown/use caution

Contraindications Hypersensitivity to *E. coli*-derived proteins, anakinra, or any component of the formulation

Warnings/Precautions Anakinra may affect defenses against infections and malignancies. Safety and efficacy in patients with immunosuppression or chronic infections have not been evaluated. Discontinue administration if patient develops a serious infection. Do not start drug administration in patients with an active infection. Patients with asthma may be at an increased risk of serious infections. Use is not recommended in combination with tumor necrosis factor antagonists. Impact on the development and course of malignancies is not fully defined. As compared to the general population, an increased risk of lymphoma has been noted in clinical trials; however, rheumatoid arthritis has been previously associated with an increased rate of lymphoma.

Use caution in patients with a history of significant hematologic abnormalities; has been associated with uncommon, but significant decreases in hematologic parameters (particularly neutrophil counts). Patients must be advised to seek medical attention if they develop signs and symptoms suggestive of blood dyscrasias. Discontinue if significant hematologic abnormalities are confirmed.

Use is not recommended in combination with tumor necrosis factor antagonists. Patients should be brought up to date with all immunizations before initiating therapy. Live vaccines should not be given concurrently. Patients with a significant exposure to varicella virus should temporarily discontinue anakinra. Hypersensitivity reactions may occur; discontinue use if severe hypersensitivity occurs. Impact on the development and course of malignancies is not fully defined. Use caution in patients with renal impairment; consider extended dosing intervals for severe renal dysfunction (Cl_{cr} <30 mL/minute). Use with caution in patients with asthma; may have increased risk of serious infection. Use caution in the elderly due to the potential for higher risk of infections. The packaging (needle cover) contains latex.

Adverse Reactions

>10%:

Central nervous system: Headache (12%)

Local: Injection site reaction (majority mild, typically lasting 14-28 days, characterized by erythema, ecchymosis, inflammation, and pain; up to 71%)

Miscellaneous: Infection (39% versus 37% in placebo; serious infection 2% to 3%)

1% to 10%:

Gastrointestinal: Nausea (8%), diarrhea (7%)

Hematologic: Neutropenia (8%; grades 3/4: 0.4%)

Respiratory: Sinusitis (7%)

<1% (Limited to important or life-threatening): Cellulitis, leukopenia, hypersensitivity reactions (including anaphylaxis, angioedema, pruritus, rash, urticaria), opportunistic infection, malignancies (including lymphoma, melanoma), pneumonia (bacterial), pulmonary fibrosis, thrombocytopenia

Drug Interactions

Metabolism/Transport Effects None known.

Avoid Concomitant Use

Avoid concomitant use of Anakinra with any of the following: Anti-TNF Agents; BCG; Canakinumab; Natalizumab; Pimecrolimus; Tacrolimus (Topical); Vaccines (Live)

Increased Effect/Toxicity

Anakinra may increase the levels/effects of: Canakinumab; Leflunomide; Natalizumab; Vaccines (Live)

The levels/effects of Anakinra may be increased by: Anti-TNF Agents; Denosumab; Pimecrolimus; Roflumilast; Tacrolimus (Topical); Trastuzumab

Decreased Effect

Anakinra may decrease the levels/effects of: BCG; Coccidioidin Skin Test; Sipuleucel-T; Vaccines (Inactivated); Vaccines (Live)

The levels/effects of Anakinra may be decreased by: Echinacea

Stability Store in refrigerator at 2°C to 8°C (36°F to 46°F); do not freeze. Do not shake. Protect from light.

Mechanism of Action Antagonist of the interleukin-1 (IL-1) receptor. Endogenous IL-1 is induced by inflammatory stimuli and mediates a variety of immunological responses, including degradation of cartilage (loss of proteoglycans) and stimulation of bone resorption.

Pharmacodynamics/Kinetics

Bioavailability: SubQ: 95%

Half-life elimination: Terminal: 4-6 hours; Severe renal impairment (Cl_{cr} <30 mL/minute): ~7 hours; ESRD: 9.7 hours (Yang, 2003)

Time to peak: SubQ: 3-7 hours

Dosage Adults: SubQ: Rheumatoid arthritis: 100 mg once daily (administer at approximately the same time each day)

Dosage adjustment in renal impairment: Cl_{cr} <30 mL/minute and/or end-stage renal disease: 100 mg every other day

Dosage adjustment in hepatic impairment: There are no dosage adjustments recommended in manufacturer's labeling.

Administration Rotate injection sites (thigh, abdomen, upper arm, buttocks); injection should be given at least 1 inch away from previous injection site. Allow solution to warm to room temperature prior to use (60-90 minutes). Do not shake. Provided in single-use, preservative free syringes with 27-gauge needles; discard any unused portion.

Monitoring Parameters CBC with differential (baseline, then monthly for 3 months, then every 3 months for a period up to 1 year); serum creatinine

Additional Information Anakinra is produced by recombinant DNA/*E. coli* technology.

Dosage Forms Excipient information presented when available (limited, particularly for generics); consult specific product labeling.

Injection, solution [preservative free]:

Kineret®: 100 mg/0.67 mL (0.67 mL) [contains edetate disodium, natural rubber/natural latex in packaging, polysorbate 80]

◆ **Analpram E™** *see* Pramoxine and Hydrocortisone *on page 1393*

◆ **Analpram HC®** *see* Pramoxine and Hydrocortisone *on page 1393*

◆ **Anandron® (Can)** *see* Nilutamide *on page 1205*

◆ **Anaprox®** *see* Naproxen *on page 1177*

◆ **Anaprox® DS** *see* Naproxen *on page 1177*

◆ **Anascorp®** *see* *Centruroides* Immune F(ab')$_2$ (Equine) *on page 326*

◆ **Anaspaz®** *see* Hyoscyamine *on page 854*

Anastrozole (an AS troe zole)

Brand Names: U.S. Arimidex®

Brand Names: Canada Arimidex®

Index Terms ICI-D1033; ZD1033

Pharmacologic Category Antineoplastic Agent, Aromatase Inhibitor

Use First-line treatment of locally-advanced or metastatic breast cancer (hormone receptor-positive or unknown) in postmenopausal women; treatment of advanced breast cancer in postmenopausal women with disease progression following tamoxifen therapy; adjuvant treatment of early hormone receptor-positive breast cancer in postmenopausal women

Unlabeled Use Treatment of recurrent or metastatic endometrial or uterine cancers, treatment of recurrent ovarian cancer

Pregnancy Risk Factor X

Pregnancy Considerations Fetotoxicity was observed in animal studies. Anastrozole is contraindicated in women who are or may become pregnant (may cause fetal harm if administered during pregnancy). Use in premenopausal women with breast cancer does not provide any clinical benefit.

Lactation Excretion in breast milk unknown/not recommended

Contraindications Hypersensitivity to anastrozole or any component of the formulation; use in women who are or may become pregnant

Warnings/Precautions Hazardous agent - use appropriate precautions for handling and disposal. Use is contraindicated in women who are or may become pregnant. Anastrozole offers no clinical benefit in premenopausal women with breast cancer. Patients with pre-existing ischemic cardiac disease have an increased risk for ischemic cardiovascular events.

Due to decreased circulating estrogen levels, anastrozole is associated with a reduction in bone mineral density (BMD); decreases (from baseline) in total hip and lumbar spine BMD have been reported. Patients with pre-existing osteopenia are at higher risk for developing osteoporosis (Eastell, 2008). When initiating anastrozole treatment, follow available guidelines for bone mineral density management in postmenopausal women with similar fracture risk; concurrent use of bisphosphonates may be useful in patients at risk for fractures.

Elevated total cholesterol levels (contributed to by LDL cholesterol increases) have been reported in patients receiving anastrozole; use with caution in patients with hyperlipidemias; cholesterol levels should be monitored/managed in accordance with current guidelines for patients with LDL elevations. Plasma concentrations in patients with stable hepatic cirrhosis were within the range of concentrations seen in normal subjects across all clinical trials; use has not been studied in patients with severe hepatic impairment. Safety and efficacy in children have not been established.

Adverse Reactions

>10%:

Cardiovascular: Vasodilatation (25% to 36%), ischemic cardiovascular disease (4%; 17% in patients with pre-existing ischemic heart disease), hypertension (2% to 13%), angina (2%; 12% in patients with pre-existing ischemic heart disease)

Central nervous system: Mood disturbance (19%), fatigue (19%), pain (11% to 17%), headache (9% to 13%), depression (5% to 13%)

Dermatologic: Rash (6% to 11%)

Endocrine & metabolic: Hot flashes (12% to 36%)

Gastrointestinal: Nausea (11% to 19%), vomiting (8% to 13%)

Neuromuscular & skeletal: Weakness (16% to 19%), arthritis (17%), arthralgia (2% to 15%), back pain (10% to 12%), bone pain (6% to 11%), osteoporosis (11%)

Respiratory: Pharyngitis (6% to 14%), cough increased (8% to 11%)

1% to 10%:

Cardiovascular: Peripheral edema (5% to 10%), chest pain (5% to 7%), edema (7%), venous thromboembolic events (2% to 4%), ischemic cerebrovascular events (2%), MI (1%)

Central nervous system: Insomnia (2% to 10%), dizziness (6% to 8%), anxiety (2% to 6%), fever (2% to 5%), malaise (2% to 5%), confusion (2% to 5%), nervousness (2% to 5%), somnolence (2% to 5%), lethargy (1%)

Dermatologic: Alopecia (2% to 5%), pruritus (2% to 5%)

Endocrine & metabolic: Hypercholesterolemia (9%), breast pain (2% to 8%)

Gastrointestinal: Diarrhea (8% to 9%), constipation (7% to 9%), abdominal pain (7% to 9%), weight gain (2% to 9%), anorexia (5% to 7%), xerostomia (6%), dyspepsia (7%), weight loss (2% to 5%)

Genitourinary: Urinary tract infection (2% to 8%), vulvovaginitis (6%), pelvic pain (5%), vaginal bleeding (1% to 5%), vaginitis (4%), vaginal discharge (4%), vaginal hemorrhage (2% to 4%), leukorrhea (2% to 3%), vaginal dryness (2% to 5%)

Hematologic: Anemia (2% to 5%), leukopenia (2% to 5%)

Hepatic: Liver function tests increased (1% to 10%), alkaline phosphatase increased (1% to 10%), gamma GT increased (≤5%)

Local: Thrombophlebitis (2% to 5%)

Neuromuscular & skeletal: Fracture (1% to 10%), arthrosis (7%), paresthesia (5% to 7%), joint disorder (6%), myalgia (2% to 6%), neck pain (2% to 5%), carpal tunnel syndrome (3%), hypertonia (3%)

Ocular: Cataracts (6%)
Respiratory: Dyspnea (8% to 10%), sinusitis (2% to 6%), bronchitis (2% to 5%), rhinitis (2% to 5%)
Miscellaneous: Lymphedema (10%), infection (2% to 9%), flu-like syndrome (2% to 7%), diaphoresis (2% to 5%), cyst (5%), neoplasm (5%), tumor flare (3%)
<1% (Limited to important or life-threatening): Anaphylaxis, angioedema, bilirubin increased, CVA, cerebral ischemia, cerebral infarct, cutaneous vasculitis (including Henoch-Schönlein purpura), endometrial cancer, erythema multiforme, hepatitis, jaundice, joint pain, joint stiffness, liver inflammation, liver pain, liver swelling, myocardial ischemia, pulmonary embolus, retinal vein thrombosis; skin reactions (eg, blisters, lesions, ulcers); Stevens-Johnson syndrome, trigger finger, urticaria

Drug Interactions

Metabolism/Transport Effects Inhibits CYP1A2 (weak), CYP2C8 (weak), CYP2C9 (weak), CYP3A4 (weak)

Avoid Concomitant Use

Avoid concomitant use of Anastrozole with any of the following: Estrogen Derivatives; Pimozide

Increased Effect/Toxicity

Anastrozole may increase the levels/effects of: Pimozide

Decreased Effect

The levels/effects of Anastrozole may be decreased by: Estrogen Derivatives; Tamoxifen

Stability Store at 20°C to 25°C (68°F to 77°F).

Mechanism of Action Potent and selective nonsteroidal aromatase inhibitor. By inhibiting aromatase, the conversion of androstenedione to estrone, and testosterone to estradiol, is prevented, thereby decreasing tumor mass or delaying progression in patients with tumors responsive to hormones. Anastrozole causes an 85% decrease in estrone sulfate levels.

Pharmacodynamics/Kinetics

Onset of estradiol reduction: 70% reduction after 24 hours; 80% after 2 weeks therapy
Duration of estradiol reduction: 6 days
Absorption: Well absorbed; extent of absorption not affected by food
Protein binding, plasma: 40%
Metabolism: Extensively hepatic (~85%) via N-dealkylation, hydroxylation, and glucuronidation; primary metabolite (triazole) inactive
Half-life elimination: ~50 hours
Time to peak, plasma: ~2 hours without food; 5 hours with food
Excretion: Feces; urine (urinary excretion accounts for ~10% of total elimination, mostly as metabolites)

Dosage Oral: Adults: Females: Postmenopausal:
Breast cancer, advanced: 1 mg once daily; continue until tumor progression
Breast cancer, early (adjuvant treatment): 1 mg once daily; optimal duration unknown, duration in clinical trial is 5 years

Dosage adjustment in renal impairment: Dosage adjustment not necessary

Dosage adjustment in hepatic impairment:
Mild-to-moderate impairment or stable hepatic cirrhosis: Dosage adjustment is not required
Severe hepatic impairment: Has not been studied in this population

Dietary Considerations May be taken with or without food.

Administration May be administered with or without food.

Monitoring Parameters Bone mineral density; total cholesterol and LDL

Additional Information Oncology Comment: The American Society of Clinical Oncology (ASCO) guidelines for adjuvant endocrine therapy in postmenopausal women with HR-positive breast cancer (Burstein, 2010) recommend considering aromatase inhibitor (AI) therapy at some point in the treatment course (primary, sequentially, or extended). Optimal duration at this time is not known; however, treatment with an AI should not exceed 5 years in primary and extended therapies, and 2-3 years if followed by tamoxifen in sequential therapy (total of 5 years). If initial therapy with AI has been discontinued before the 5 years, consideration should be taken to receive tamoxifen for a total of 5 years. The optimal time to switch to an AI is also not known, but data supports switching after 2-3 years of tamoxifen (sequential) or after 5 years of tamoxifen (extended). If patient becomes intolerant or has poor adherence, consideration should be made to switch to another AI or initiate tamoxifen.

Dosage Forms Excipient information presented when available (limited, particularly for generics); consult specific product labeling.
Tablet, oral: 1 mg
Arimidex®: 1 mg

- ◆ **A-Natural [OTC]** *see* Vitamin A *on page* 1795
- ◆ **A-Natural-25 [OTC]** *see* Vitamin A *on page* 1795
- ◆ **Anbesol® [OTC]** *see* Benzocaine *on page* 202
- ◆ **Anbesol® Baby [OTC]** *see* Benzocaine *on page* 202
- ◆ **Anbesol® Baby (Can)** *see* Benzocaine *on page* 202
- ◆ **Anbesol® Cold Sore Therapy [OTC]** *see* Benzocaine *on page* 202
- ◆ **Anbesol® Jr. [OTC]** *see* Benzocaine *on page* 202
- ◆ **Anbesol® Maximum Strength [OTC]** *see* Benzocaine *on page* 202
- ◆ **Ancef** *see* CeFAZolin *on page* 301
- ◆ **Ancobon®** *see* Flucytosine *on page* 720
- ◆ **Andriol® (Can)** *see* Testosterone *on page* 1654
- ◆ **Androderm®** *see* Testosterone *on page* 1654
- ◆ **AndroGel®** *see* Testosterone *on page* 1654
- ◆ **Android®** *see* MethylTESTOSTERone *on page* 1114
- ◆ **Andropository (Can)** *see* Testosterone *on page* 1654
- ◆ **Androxy™** *see* Fluoxymesterone *on page* 735
- ◆ **AneCream™ [OTC]** *see* Lidocaine (Topical) *on page* 1009
- ◆ **Anectine®** *see* Succinylcholine *on page* 1596
- ◆ **Anestafoam™ [OTC]** *see* Lidocaine (Topical) *on page* 1009
- ◆ **Aneurine Hydrochloride** *see* Thiamine *on page* 1669
- ◆ **Anexate® (Can)** *see* Flumazenil *on page* 725
- ◆ **Angiomax®** *see* Bivalirudin *on page* 222

Anidulafungin (ay nid yoo la FUN jin)

Brand Names: U.S. Eraxis™

Brand Names: Canada Eraxis™

Index Terms LY303366

Pharmacologic Category Antifungal Agent, Parenteral; Echinocandin

Additional Appendix Information

Antifungal Agents *on page* 1876

Use Treatment of candidemia and other forms of *Candida* infections (including those of intra-abdominal, peritoneal, and esophageal locus)

Unlabeled Use Treatment of infections due to *Aspergillus* spp.

Pregnancy Risk Factor C

Pregnancy Considerations Skeletal teratogenic effects were noted in animal studies. There are no adequate and well-controlled studies in pregnant women. Use only if benefit outweighs risk.

Lactation Excretion in breast milk unknown/use caution

Contraindications Hypersensitivity to anidulafungin, other echinocandins, or any component of the formulation

Warnings/Precautions Histamine-mediated reactions (eg, urticaria, flushing, hypotension) have been observed; these may be related to infusion rate. Elevated liver function tests, hepatitis, and worsening hepatic failure have been reported. Monitor for progressive hepatic impairment if increased transaminase enzymes noted. Safety and efficacy in pediatric patients, neutropenic patients, or other *Candida* infections (eg, endocarditis, osteomyelitis, meningitis) have not been established.

Adverse Reactions

2% to 10%:

Endocrine & metabolic: Hypokalemia (3%)

Gastrointestinal: Diarrhea (3%)

Hepatic: Transaminase increased (<1% to 2%)

<2% (Limited to important or life-threatening): Abdominal pain, alkaline phosphatase increased, amylase increased, angioneurotic edema, atrial fibrillation, back pain, bilirubin increased, bundle branch block (right), candidiasis, cholestasis, clostridial infection, coagulopathy, constipation, cough, CPK increased, creatinine increased, diaphoresis, diarrhea, dizziness, DVT, dyspepsia, ECG abnormality (including QT prolongation), erythema, eye pain, fecal incontinence, flushing, fungemia, GGT increased, headache, hepatic necrosis, hepatitis, hepatic dysfunction, hot flushes, hypercalcemia, hyperglycemia, hyperkalemia, hypernatremia, hyper-/hypotension, hypomagnesemia, infusion-related reaction, leukopenia (0.7%), lipase increased, nausea, neutropenia (1%), peripheral edema, phlebitis, platelet count increased, prothrombin time prolonged, pruritus, pyrexia, rash, rigors, seizure, sinus arrhythmia, thrombocytopenia, thrombophlebitis, urea increased, urticaria, ventricular extrasystoles, vision blurred, visual disturbance, vomiting

Drug Interactions

Metabolism/Transport Effects None known.

Avoid Concomitant Use There are no known interactions where it is recommended to avoid concomitant use.

Increased Effect/Toxicity There are no known significant interactions involving an increase in effect.

Decreased Effect

Anidulafungin may decrease the levels/effects of: Saccharomyces boulardii

Stability Store vials at 2°C to 8°C (36°F to 46°F); do not freeze. Aseptically add 15 mL (50 mg vial) or 30 mL (100 mg vial) of sterile water for injection to each vial. Swirl to dissolve; do not shake. The reconstituted solution can be stored for up to 1 hour at 2°C to 8°C (36°F to 46°F) prior to dilution into the infusion solution; do not freeze. Further dilute 50 mg, 100 mg, or 200 mg in 50 mL, 100 mL, or 200 mL, respectively, of D_5W or NS. If the infusion solution is not used immediately, it should be stored in a refrigerator at 2°C to 8°C (36°F to 46°F) and administered within 24 hours of preparation; do not freeze.

Mechanism of Action Noncompetitive inhibitor of 1,3-beta-D-glucan synthase resulting in reduced formation of 1,3-beta-D-glucan, an essential polysaccharide comprising 30% to 60% of *Candida* cell walls (absent in mammalian cells); decreased glucan content leads to osmotic instability and cellular lysis

Pharmacodynamics/Kinetics

Distribution: 30-50 L

Protein binding: 84%

Metabolism: No hepatic metabolism observed; undergoes slow chemical hydrolysis to open-ring peptide-lacking antifungal activity

Half-life elimination: 27 hours

Excretion: Feces (30%, 10% as unchanged drug); urine (<1%)

Dosage I.V.: Adults:

Candidemia, intra-abdominal or peritoneal candidiasis: 200 mg loading dose on day 1, followed by 100 mg daily for at least 14 days after last positive culture

Esophageal candidiasis: 100 mg loading dose on day 1, followed by 50 mg daily for at least 14 days and for at least 7 days after symptom resolution

Dosage adjustment in renal impairment: No adjustment necessary, including dialysis patients

Dosage adjustment in hepatic impairment: No adjustment necessary

Administration For intravenous use only; infusion rate should not exceed 1.1 mg/minute

Monitoring Parameters Liver function tests

Dosage Forms Excipient information presented when available (limited, particularly for generics); consult specific product labeling. [DSC] = Discontinued product

Injection, powder for reconstitution:

Eraxis™: 50 mg [contains polysorbate 80]

Eraxis™: 100 mg [DSC] [contains dehydrated ethanol (in diluent), polysorbate 80]

Eraxis™: 100 mg [contains polysorbate 80]

◆ **Anolor 300** *see* Butalbital, Acetaminophen, and Caffeine *on page 255*

◆ **Ansaid® (Can)** *see* Flurbiprofen (Systemic) *on page 737*

◆ **Ansamycin** *see* Rifabutin *on page 1483*

◆ **Antabuse®** *see* Disulfiram *on page 529*

◆ **Antagon** *see* Ganirelix *on page 779*

◆ **Antara®** *see* Fenofibrate *on page 693*

◆ **Anthraforte® (Can)** *see* Anthralin *on page 123*

Anthralin (AN thra lin)

Brand Names: U.S. Dritho-Creme®; Dritho-Scalp®; Zithranol®-RR

Brand Names: Canada Anthraforte®; Anthranol®; Anthrascalp®; Micanol®

Index Terms Dithranol

Pharmacologic Category Antipsoriatic Agent; Keratolytic Agent

Use Treatment of psoriasis (quiescent or chronic psoriasis)

Pregnancy Risk Factor C

Dosage Children (unlabeled) and Adults: Topical: Generally, apply once a day or as directed. The irritant potential of anthralin is directly related to the strength being used and each patient's individual tolerance. Always commence treatment using a short, daily contact time (5-10 minutes) for at least 1 week using the lowest strength possible. Contact time may be gradually increased (to 20-30 minutes) as tolerated.

Skin application: Apply sparingly only to psoriatic lesions and rub gently and carefully into the skin until absorbed. Avoid applying an excessive quantity which may cause unnecessary soiling and staining of the clothing or bed linen.

Scalp application: Comb hair to remove scalar debris, wet hair and, after suitably parting, rub cream well into the lesions, taking care to prevent the cream from spreading onto the forehead.

Remove by washing or showering; optimal period of contact will vary according to the strength used and the patient's response to treatment. Continue treatment until the skin is entirely clear (ie, when there is nothing to feel with the fingers and the texture is normal).

Additional Information Complete prescribing information for this medication should be consulted for additional detail.

Dosage Forms Excipient information presented when available (limited, particularly for generics); consult specific product labeling.

Cream, topical:

Dritho-Creme®: 1% (50 g)

Dritho-Scalp®: 0.5% (50 g)

Zithranol®-RR: 1.2% (45 g)

◆ **Anthranol® (Can)** *see* Anthralin *on page 123*

◆ **Anthrascalp® (Can)** *see* Anthralin *on page 123*

Anthrax Vaccine Adsorbed

(AN thraks vak SEEN ad SORBED)

Brand Names: U.S. BioThrax®

Index Terms AVA

Pharmacologic Category Vaccine, Inactivated (Bacterial)

Use Immunization against *Bacillus anthracis* in persons at high risk for exposure.

The Advisory Committee on Immunization Practices (ACIP) recommends routine vaccination (pre-exposure vaccination) for the following:

- Persons who work directly with the organism in the laboratory
- Persons who handle animals or animal products only when
  - potentially infected in research settings;
  - in areas of high incidence of enzootic anthrax; or
  - where standards and restrictions are not sufficient to prevent exposure
- Military personnel deployed to areas with high risk of exposure as recommended by the Department of Defense (DoD)
- Persons engaged in environmental investigations or remediation efforts

Routine immunization for the general population is not recommended. Routine vaccination may be offered to emergency and other responders (police and fire departments, the National Guard, etc) on a voluntary basis under the direction of a comprehensive occupational health and safety program.

The ACIP recommends postexposure prophylaxis for the following (in the absence of completing a pre-exposure, routine vaccination schedule):

- The general public, including pregnant and breast-feeding women
- Medical professionals
- Children ages 0-18 years as determined on an event-by-event basis
- Persons engaged in handling certain animals or animal products
- Persons who work directly with the organism in the laboratory (postexposure vaccination dependant upon pre-event vaccination status)
- Military personnel as recommended by the DoD
- Persons engaged in environmental investigations or remediation efforts (postexposure vaccination dependent upon pre-event vaccination status)
- Emergency and other responders (police and fire departments, the National Guard, etc)
- Persons working in postal facilities

Pregnancy Risk Factor D

Pregnancy Considerations Adverse events were not observed in animal developmental toxicity studies. Data from the Department of Defense suggest the vaccine may be linked with a slightly increased number of atrial septal defects when given during the first trimester of pregnancy; however, when premature infants are excluded from analysis, the association is not statistically significant. Current ACIP guidelines recommend deferring pre-exposure vaccination when possible; however, postexposure prophylaxis is recommended in pregnant women. Male fertility is not affected by vaccine administration.

Lactation Excretion in breast milk unknown/use caution

Prescribing and Access Restrictions Not commercially available in U.S.; presently, all anthrax vaccine lots are owned by the U.S. Department of Defense. The Center for Disease Control (CDC) does not currently recommend routine vaccination of the general public.

Contraindications Hypersensitivity to anthrax vaccine or any component of the formulation

Warnings/Precautions Immediate treatment for anaphylactic/anaphylactoid reaction should be available during vaccine use. May consider deferring administration in patients with moderate or severe acute illness (with or without fever) in pre-exposure vaccination programs; may administer to patients with mild acute illness (with or without fever). When used for postexposure prophylaxis, consider the benefits versus risks in patients with moderate or severe acute illness. Use with caution in severely immunocompromised patients (eg, patients receiving chemo/radiation therapy or other immunosuppressive therapy (including high dose corticosteroids)); may have a reduced response to vaccination. In general, household and close contacts of persons with altered immunocompetence may receive all age appropriate vaccines. Persons with a history of anthrax disease may have an increased risk for adverse reactions from the vaccine.

Use with caution in patients with a history of bleeding disorders (including thrombocytopenia) and/or patients on anticoagulant therapy; bleeding/hematoma may occur from I.M. administration. For patients at risk of hemorrhage following intramuscular injection, the vaccine can be administered SubQ. In order to maximize vaccination rates, the ACIP recommends simultaneous administration of all age-appropriate vaccines (live or inactivated) for which a person is eligible at a single clinic visit, unless contraindications exist. Packaging may contain natural latex rubber. Safety and efficacy in children <18 years of age or adults ≥65 years have not been established. Use in children <18 years is recommended by the ACIP as determined on an event-by-event basis.

Adverse Reactions All serious adverse reactions must be reported to the U.S. Department of Health and Human Services (DHHS) Vaccine Adverse Event Reporting System (VAERS) 1-800-822-7967 or online at https://vaers.hhs.gov/esub/index.

Note: Percentages reported with I.M. administration; the incidence of local reactions may be increased with SubQ administration.

>10%:

Central nervous system: Headache (4% to 64%), fatigue (5% to 62%)

Local: Tenderness (10% to 61%), erythema (8% to 31%), pain (4% to 23%), edema (1% to 16%), limitation of arm motion (1% to 16%), induration (3% to 14%), warmth (1% to 11%)

Neuromuscular & skeletal: Myalgia (2% to 72%)

Respiratory: Nasopharyngitis (12% to 15%), pharyngolaryngeal pain (12%)

1% to 10%:

Dermatologic: Pruritus (≤2%), rash (≤2%)

Endocrine & metabolic: Dysmenorrhea (7%)

Gastrointestinal: Diarrhea (6% to 8%), nausea (6%)

Local: Itching (≤9%), bruising (3% to 6%), nodule (1% to 6%)

Neuromuscular & skeletal: Back pain (7% to 9%), neck pain (3%), joint sprain (≤2%), rigors (1% to 2%)

Respiratory: Sinusitis (5% to 7%), upper respiratory tract infection (2% to 3%), sinus headache (1% to 3%)

Miscellaneous: Hypersensitivity (2% to 4%), lymphadenopathy (2% to 3%), flu-like illness (2%), tender/painful axillary adenopathy (≤1%)

Postmarketing and/or case reports: Allergic reactions, anaphylactoid reaction, erythema multiforme, rhabdomyolysis, Stevens-Johnson syndrome, syncope, tremor, ulnar nerve neuropathy

Drug Interactions

Metabolism/Transport Effects None known.

Avoid Concomitant Use There are no known interactions where it is recommended to avoid concomitant use.

Increased Effect/Toxicity There are no known significant interactions involving an increase in effect.

Decreased Effect

The levels/effects of Anthrax Vaccine Adsorbed may be decreased by: Belimumab; Fingolimod; Immunosuppressants

Stability Store under refrigeration at 2°C to 8°C (36°F to 46°F); do not freeze.

Mechanism of Action Active immunization against *Bacillus anthracis*. The vaccine is prepared from a cell-free filtrate of *B. anthracis*, but no dead or live bacteria. Completion of the entire vaccination series is required for full protection.

Dosage

Children <18 years: Safety and efficacy have not been established. **Note:** Use in children is recommended by the ACIP as determined on an event-by-event basis; refer to adult dosing for postexposure prophylaxis.

Adults:

I.M.:

Primary immunization: Five injections of 0.5 mL each given at day 0, week 4, then 6-, 12-, and 18 months

Subsequent booster injections: 0.5 mL at 1-year intervals are recommended for immunity to be maintained in persons who remain at risk

SubQ: Postexposure prophylaxis (ACIP recommendations): Three injections of 0.5 mL each given at day 0, week 2, and week 4. Administer with a 60-day course of antibiotics. (Vaccination should begin within 10 days of exposure. Refer to guidelines provided as part of emergency use authorization or IND at the time of the event). **Note:** Additional considerations for postexposure prophylaxis following occupational exposures:

Fully vaccinated: Personnel who have completed the 5-dose primary vaccination series and booster injections do not require postexposure prophylaxis if wearing protective equipment. If respiratory protection is disrupted, a 30-day course of antimicrobial therapy is recommended.

Previously unvaccinated: Workers should receive the vaccine as directed per postexposure prophylaxis along with the 60-day course of antimicrobial therapy (antimicrobial therapy should continue for 14 days after the third dose of PEP vaccine), then switch to the licensed regimen at the 6-month dose.

Partially vaccinated: Any person who started but did not complete the primary vaccination series should receive a 30-day course of antimicrobial therapy and continue with the primary vaccination schedule.

Elderly: Safety and efficacy have not been established for patients >65 years of age

Administration Shake well before use. Do not use if discolored or contains particulate matter. Do not use the same site for more than one injection. Do not mix with other injections.

Pre-exposure (routine vaccination): For I.M. administration; do not inject I.V. or intradermally. For patients at risk of hemorrhage following intramuscular injection, the vaccine can be administered SubQ.

Postexposure prophylaxis: Administer SubQ.

Simultaneous administration of vaccines helps ensure the patients will be fully vaccinated by the appropriate age. Simultaneous administration of vaccines is defined as administering >1 vaccine on the same day at different anatomic sites. Separate vaccines should not be combined in the same syringe unless indicated by product specific labeling. Separate needles and syringes should be used for each injection. The ACIP prefers each dose of a specific vaccine in a series come from the same manufacturer when possible. Adolescents and adults should be vaccinated while seated or lying down. In general, preterm infants should be vaccinated at the same chronological age as full-term infants (CDC, 2011).

Antipyretics have not been shown to prevent febrile seizures. Antipyretics may be used to treat fever or discomfort following vaccination (CDC, 2011). One study reported that routine prophylactic administration of acetaminophen to prevent fever prior to vaccination decreased the immune response of some vaccines; the clinical significance of this reduction in immune response has not been established (Prymula, 2009).

Monitoring Parameters Monitor for local reactions, chills, fever, anaphylaxis; syncope for ≥15 minutes following vaccination

Additional Information Not commercially available in the U.S.

Federal law requires that the name of medication, date of administration, the vaccine manufacturer, lot number of vaccine, and the administering person's name, title and address be entered into the patient's permanent medical record.

Dosage Forms Excipient information presented when available (limited, particularly for generics); consult specific product labeling.

Injection, suspension:

BioThrax®: *Bacillus anthracis* proteins (5 mL) [contains aluminum, natural rubber/natural latex in packaging]

◆ **Anti-4 Alpha Integrin** *see* Natalizumab *on page* 1181

◆ **131 I Anti-B1 Antibody** *see* Tositumomab and Iodine I 131 Tositumomab *on page* 1714

◆ **131 I-Anti-B1 Monoclonal Antibody** *see* Tositumomab and Iodine I 131 Tositumomab *on page* 1714

◆ **Antibody-Drug Conjugate SGN-35** *see* Brentuximab Vedotin *on page* 234

◆ **Anti-CD20 Monoclonal Antibody** *see* RiTUXimab *on page* 1503

◆ **Anti-CD20-Murine Monoclonal Antibody I-131** *see* Tositumomab and Iodine I 131 Tositumomab *on page* 1714

◆ **Anti-CD30 ADC SGN-35** *see* Brentuximab Vedotin *on page* 234

◆ **Anti-CD30 Antibody-Drug Conjugate SGN-35** *see* Brentuximab Vedotin *on page* 234

◆ **Anti-CD52 Monoclonal Antibody** *see* Alemtuzumab *on page* 58

◆ **anti-c-erB-2** *see* Trastuzumab *on page* 1722

◆ **Anti-Diarrheal [OTC]** *see* Loperamide *on page* 1026

◆ **Antidigoxin Fab Fragments, Ovine** *see* Digoxin Immune Fab *on page* 506

◆ **Antidiuretic Hormone** *see* Vasopressin *on page* 1775

◆ **anti-ERB-2** *see* Trastuzumab *on page* 1722

◆ **Anti-Fungal™ [OTC]** *see* Clotrimazole (Topical) *on page* 399

Antihemophilic Factor (Human)

(an tee hee moe FIL ik FAK tor HYU man)

Brand Names: U.S. Hemofil M; Koāte®-DVI; Monoclate-P®

Brand Names: Canada Hemofil M

Index Terms AHF (Human); Factor VIII (Human)

Pharmacologic Category Antihemophilic Agent; Blood Product Derivative

Use Prevention and treatment of hemorrhagic episodes in patients with hemophilia A (classic hemophilia); perioperative management of hemophilia A; can be of significant therapeutic value in patients with acquired factor VIII inhibitors not exceeding 10 Bethesda units/mL

Pregnancy Risk Factor C

Pregnancy Considerations Reproduction studies have not been conducted. Safety and efficacy in pregnant women have not been established. Use during pregnancy only if clearly needed. Parvovirus B19 or hepatitis A, which may be present in plasma-derived products, may affect a pregnant woman more seriously than nonpregnant women.

Lactation Excretion in breast milk unknown/use caution

Contraindications Hypersensitivity to any component of the formulation

Warnings/Precautions Risk of viral transmission is not totally eradicated. Because antihemophilic factor is prepared from pooled plasma, it may contain the causative agent of viral hepatitis and other viral diseases. Hepatitis B vaccination is recommended for all patients. Hepatitis A vaccination is also recommended for seronegative patients. Antihemophilic factor contains trace amounts of blood groups A and B isohemagglutinins and when large or frequently repeated doses are given to individuals with blood groups A, B, and AB, the patient should be monitored for signs of progressive anemia and the possibility of intravascular hemolysis should be considered. The dosage requirement will vary in patients with factor VIII inhibitors; optimal treatment should be determined by clinical response. Natural rubber latex is a component of Hemofil M packaging. Hemofil M and Monoclate-P® contain trace amounts of mouse protein. Products contain naturally-occurring von Willebrand factor for stabilization, however efficacy has not been established for the treatment of von Willebrand disease. Products vary by preparation method; final formulations contain human albumin.

Adverse Reactions <1% (Limited to important or life-threatening): Acute hemolytic anemia, AHF inhibitor development, allergic reactions (rare), anaphylaxis (rare), bleeding tendency increased, blurred vision, chest tightness, chills, fever, headache, hyperfibrinogenemia, jittery feeling, lethargy, nausea, somnolence, stinging at the infusion site, stomach discomfort, tingling, urticaria, vasomotor reactions with rapid infusion, vomiting

Drug Interactions

Metabolism/Transport Effects None known.

Avoid Concomitant Use There are no known interactions where it is recommended to avoid concomitant use.

Increased Effect/Toxicity There are no known significant interactions involving an increase in effect.

Decreased Effect There are no known significant interactions involving a decrease in effect.

Stability Store under refrigeration, 2°C to 8°C (36°F to 46°F); avoid freezing. If refrigerated, the dried concentrate and diluent should be warmed to room temperature before reconstitution. Gently swirl or rotate vial after adding diluent; do not shake vigorously. Use within 3 hours of reconstitution. Do not refrigerate after reconstitution, precipitation may occur.

Hemofil M: May also be stored at room temperature not to exceed 30°C (86°F).

Koāte®-DVI; Monoclate-P®: May also be stored at room temperature of 25°C (77°F) for ≤6 months.

Mechanism of Action Protein (factor VIII) in normal plasma which is necessary for clot formation and maintenance of hemostasis; activates factor X in conjunction with activated factor IX; activated factor X converts prothrombin to thrombin, which converts fibrinogen to fibrin, and with factor XIII forms a stable clot

Pharmacodynamics/Kinetics Half-life elimination: Mean: 8-27 hours

Dosage Children and Adults: I.V.: Individualize dosage based on coagulation studies performed prior to treatment and at regular intervals during treatment. In general, administration of factor VIII 1 int. unit/kg will increase circulating factor VIII levels by ~2 int. units/dL. (General guidelines presented; consult individual product labeling for specific dosing recommendations.)

Dosage based on desired factor VIII increase (%):

To calculate dosage needed based on desired factor VIII increase (%):

Body weight (kg) x 0.5 int. units/kg x desired factor VIII increase (%) = int. units factor VIII required

For example:

50 kg x 0.5 int. units/kg x 30 (% increase) = 750 int. units factor VIII

Dosage based on expected factor VIII increase (%):

It is also possible to calculate the **expected** % factor VIII increase:

(# int. units administered x 2%/int. units/kg) divided by body weight (kg) = expected % factor VIII increase

For example:

(1400 int. units x 2%/int. units/kg) divided by 70 kg = 40%

General guidelines:

Minor hemorrhage: 10-20 int. units/kg as a single dose to achieve FVIII plasma level ~20% to 40% of normal. Mild superficial or early hemorrhages may respond to a single dose; may repeat dose every 12-24 hours for 1-3 days until bleeding is resolved or healing achieved.

Moderate hemorrhage/minor surgery: 15-25 int. units/kg to achieve FVIII plasma level 30% to 50% of normal. If needed, may continue with a maintenance dose of 10-15 int. units/kg every 8-12 hours.

Major to life-threatening hemorrhage: Initial dose 40-50 int. units/kg, followed by a maintenance dose of 20-25 int. units/kg every 8-12 hours until threat is resolved, to achieve FVIII plasma level 80% to 100% of normal.

Major surgery: 50 int. units/kg given preoperatively to raise factor VIII level to 100% before surgery begins. May repeat as necessary after 6-12 hours initially and for a total of 10-14 days until healing is complete. Intensity of therapy may depend on type of surgery and postoperative regimen.

Bleeding prophylaxis: May be administered on a regular basis for bleeding prophylaxis. Doses of 24-40 int. units/kg 3 times/week have been reported in patients with severe hemophilia to prevent joint bleeding.

If bleeding is not controlled with adequate dose, test for presence of inhibitor. It may not be possible or practical to control bleeding if inhibitor titers are >10 Bethesda units/mL.

Elderly: Response in the elderly is not expected to differ from that of younger patients; dosage should be individualized

Administration Administer I.V. over 5-10 minutes (maximum: 10 mL/minute). Infuse Monoclate-P® at 2 mL/minute.

Monitoring Parameters Heart rate and blood pressure (before and during I.V. administration); AHF levels prior to and during treatment; in patients with circulating inhibitors, the inhibitor level should be monitored; hematocrit; monitor for signs and symptoms of intravascular hemolysis; bleeding

Reference Range Classification of hemophilia; normal is defined as 1 int. unit/mL of factor VIII

Severe: Factor level <1% of normal

Moderate: Factor level 1% to 5% of normal

Mild: Factor level >5% to <40% of normal

Dosage Forms Excipient information presented when available (limited, particularly for generics); consult specific product labeling. [DSC] = Discontinued product

Injection, powder for reconstitution:

Hemofil M: ~250 int. units, ~500 int. units, ~1000 int. units, ~1700 int. units [contains albumin (human); derived from mouse proteins; packaging may contain natural rubber latex]. Supplied with diluent.

Koāte®-DVI: ~250 int. units [DSC], ~500 int. units, ~1000 int. units [contains albumin (human), aluminum, polysorbate 80]. Supplied with diluent.

Monoclate-P®: ~250 int. units, ~500 int. units, ~1000 int. units, ~1500 int. units [contains albumin (human); derived from mouse proteins]. Supplied with diluent.

Antihemophilic Factor (Recombinant)

(an tee hee moe FIL ik FAK tor ree KOM be nant)

Brand Names: U.S. Advate; Helixate® FS; Kogenate® FS; Recombinate; Xyntha®; Xyntha® Solofuse™

Brand Names: Canada Advate; Helixate® FS; Kogenate® FS; Xyntha®

Index Terms AHF (Recombinant); Factor VIII (Recombinant); rAHF

Pharmacologic Category Antihemophilic Agent

Use Prevention and treatment of hemorrhagic episodes in patients with hemophilia A (classic hemophilia or congenital factor VIII deficiency); perioperative management of hemophilia A; routine prophylaxis in patients with hemophilia A to prevent bleeding episodes (Advate, Helixate® FS, Kogenate® FS)

Note: Helixate® FS and Kogenate® FS are also approved in children with hemophilia A with no pre-existing joint damage to reduce risk of joint damage. In addition, Recombinate can be of therapeutic value in patients with acquired factor VIII inhibitors ≤10 Bethesda units/mL.

Pregnancy Risk Factor C

Pregnancy Considerations Animal reproduction studies have not been conducted. Safety and efficacy in pregnant women has not been established. Use during pregnancy only if clearly needed.

Lactation Excretion in breast milk unknown/use caution

Contraindications Hypersensitivity to any component of the formulation

Warnings/Precautions Monitor for signs of formation of antibodies to factor VIII; may occur at anytime but more common in young children with severe hemophilia. The dosage requirement will vary in patients with factor VIII inhibitors; optimal treatment should be determined by clinical response. Allergic hypersensitivity reactions (including anaphylaxis) may occur; monitor. Products vary by preparation method. Recombinate is stabilized using human albumin. Helixate® FS and Kogenate® FS are stabilized with sucrose. Advate, Helixate® FS, Kogenate® FS, and Xyntha® may contain trace amounts of mouse or hamster protein. Recombinate may contain mouse, hamster or bovine protein. Some products may contain polysorbate 80. Products may contain von Willebrand factor for stabilization; however, efficacy has not been established for the treatment of von Willebrand's disease.

Adverse Reactions Actual frequency may vary by product.

>1%:

Central nervous system: Chills, dizziness, fever, headache, pain

Dermatologic: Pruritus, rash, urticaria

Gastrointestinal: Constipation, diarrhea, nausea, taste perversion, vomiting

Local: Injection/infusion site reactions

Neuromuscular & skeletal: Arthralgia, joint swelling, pain in extremity, weakness

Otic: Ear infection, ear pain

Respiratory: Cough, nasal congestion, nasopharyngitis, pharyngolaryngeal pain, rhinorrhea, sinusitis

Miscellaneous: Catheter thrombosis, catheter infection, factor VIII inhibitor formation, flu-like syndrome, influenza

≤1% (Limited to important or life-threatening): Abdominal pain, adenopathy, allergic reactions, anaphylaxis, anemia, angioedema, anorexia, arthralgia, AST increased, chest discomfort, chest pain, cyanosis, depersonalization, diaphoresis, dyspnea, edema, epistaxis, erythema, facial edema, facial flushing, factor VIII decreased, fatigue, GI hemorrhage, hematoma, hives, hot flashes, hyperhidrosis, hypersensitivity reaction, hyper-/hypotension (slight), infection, laryngeal edema, lethargy, malaise, pallor, paresthesia, restlessness, rhinitis, rigors, shortness of breath, somnolence, tachycardia, tremor, urinary tract infection, vasodilation, venous catheter access complications

Drug Interactions

Metabolism/Transport Effects None known.

Avoid Concomitant Use There are no known interactions where it is recommended to avoid concomitant use.

Increased Effect/Toxicity There are no known significant interactions involving an increase in effect.

Decreased Effect There are no known significant interactions involving a decrease in effect.

Stability Prior to reconstitution, store refrigerated at 2°C to 8°C (36°F to 46°F); avoid freezing. Use within 3 hours of reconstitution. Gently agitate or rotate vial after adding diluent, do not shake vigorously. Do not refrigerate after reconstitution.

Advate: May also be stored at room temperature for up to 6 months.

Helixate® FS: May also be stored at room temperature (not to exceed 25°C [77°F]) up to 3 months; do not return to refrigerator. Avoid prolonged exposure to light during storage.

Kogenate® FS: May also be stored at room temperature (not to exceed 25°C [77°F]) up to 12 months; do not return to refrigerator. Avoid prolonged exposure to light during storage.

Recombinate: May also be stored at room temperature, not to exceed 30°C (86°F).

Xyntha®: May also be stored at room temperature (not to exceed 25°C [77°F]) up to 3 months; after room temperature storage, product may be returned to the refrigerator until the expiration date; however, do not store at room temperature and return to refrigerator temperature more than once. Avoid prolonged exposure to light during storage.

Xyntha® Solofuse™: May also be stored at room temperature not to exceed 25°C [77°F]) up to 3 months; do not return to refrigerator; after 3 months at room temperature, must use immediately or discard.

If refrigerated, the dried concentrate and diluent should be warmed to room temperature before reconstitution.

Mechanism of Action Factor VIII replacement, necessary for clot formation and maintenance of hemostasis. It activates factor X in conjunction with activated factor IX; activated factor X converts prothrombin to thrombin, which converts fibrinogen to fibrin, and with factor XIII forms a stable clot.

Pharmacodynamics/Kinetics

Distribution: V_{ss}: ~0.4 dL/kg

Half-life elimination: Mean: ~11-15 hours

Dosage I.V.:

Hemophilia A: Children and Adults: Individualize dosage based on coagulation studies performed prior to treatment and at regular intervals during treatment. In general, administration of factor VIII 1 int. unit/kg will increase circulating factor VIII levels by ~2 int. units/dL. (General guidelines presented; consult individual product labeling for specific dosing recommendations.)

Dosage based on desired factor VIII increase (%):
To calculate dosage needed based on desired factor VIII increase (%):
[Body weight (kg) x desired factor VIII increase (%)] divided by 2%/int. units/kg = int. units factor VIII required
For example:
50 kg x 30 (% increase) divided by 2%/int. units/kg = 750 int. units factor VIII

Dosage based on expected factor VIII increase (%):
It is also possible to calculate the **expected** % factor VIII increase:
(# int. units administered x 2%/int. units/kg) divided by body weight (kg) = expected % factor VIII increase
For example:
(1400 int. units x 2%/int. units/kg) divided by 70 kg = 40%

General guidelines (consult individual product labeling for specific dosage recommendations): Note: Children <6 years may require more frequent administration.
Minor hemorrhage: 10-20 int. units/kg as a single dose to achieve FVIII plasma level ~20% to 40% of normal. Mild superficial or early hemorrhages may respond to a single dose; may repeat dose every 12-24 hours for 1-3 days until bleeding is resolved or healing achieved.
Moderate hemorrhage/minor surgery: 15-30 int. units/kg to achieve FVIII plasma level 30% to 60% of normal. May repeat 1 dose at 12-24 hours if needed. Some products suggest continuing for ≥3 days until pain and disability are resolved.
Major to life-threatening hemorrhage: Initial dose 30-50 int. units/kg followed by a maintenance dose of 20-50 int. units/kg every 8-24 hours until threat is resolved, to achieve FVIII plasma level 60% to 100% of normal.
Minor surgery (including tooth extraction): 15-50 int. units/kg to raise factor VIII level to ~30-100% before procedure/surgery. May repeat every 12-24 hours until bleeding is resolved.
Major surgery: 40-60 int. units/kg given preoperatively to raise factor VIII level to ~60% to 120% before surgery begins. May repeat as necessary after 6-24 hours until wound healing. Intensity of therapy may depend on type of surgery and postoperative regimen.
If bleeding is not controlled with adequate dose, test for presence of inhibitor. It may not be possible or practical to control bleeding if inhibitor titers >10 Bethesda units/mL.

Routine prophylaxis to prevent bleeding episodes and joint damage (Helixate® FS, Kogenate® FS): Children (without pre-existing joint damage): 25 int. units/kg every other day

Routine prophylaxis to prevent bleeding episodes (Advate): Children and Adults: 20-40 int. units/kg every other day (3-4 times weekly). Alternatively, an every-third-day dosing regimen may be used to target factor VIII trough levels of ≥1%.

Elderly: Response in the elderly is not expected to differ from that of younger patients; dosage should be individualized

Dietary Considerations Some products may contain sodium.

Administration Use administration sets/tubing provided by manufacturer (if provided).
Advate: Infuse over ≤5 minutes (maximum: 10 mL/minute)
Helixate® FS, Kogenate® FS: Infuse over 1-15 minutes; based on patient tolerability
Recombinate reconstituted with 5 mL of SWFI: Infuse at a rate of ≤5 mL/minute (maximum: 5 mL/minute)
Recombinate reconstituted with 10 mL of SWFI: Infuse at a rate of ≤10 mL/minute (maximum: 10 mL/minute)
Xyntha®, Xyntha® Solufuse™: Infuse over several minutes; adjust based on patient comfort. Do not admix or administer in same tubing as other medications.

Monitoring Parameters Heart rate and blood pressure (before and during I.V. administration); plasma factor VIII activity prior to and during treatment; development of factor VIII inhibitors; signs of bleeding; hemoglobin, hematocrit

Reference Range Classification of hemophilia; normal is defined as 1 int. unit/mL of factor VIII
Severe: Factor level <1% of normal
Moderate: Factor level 1% to 5% of normal
Mild: Factor level >5% to <40% of normal

Dosage Forms Excipient information presented when available (limited, particularly for generics); consult specific product labeling.
Injection, powder for reconstitution:
Recombinate: 2000 int. units [contains albumin (human), natural rubber/natural latex in packaging, polysorbate 80, sodium 180 mEq/L; derived from or manufactured using bovine, hamster or mouse protein]
Injection, powder for reconstitution [preservative free]:
Advate: 250 int. units, 500 int. units, 1000 int. units, 1500 int. units, 2000 int. units, 3000 int. units [plasma/albumin free; contains mannitol, polysorbate 80, sodium 108 mEq/L; derived from or manufactured using hamster or mouse protein]
Helixate® FS: 250 int. units, 500 int. units, 1000 int. units [contains polysorbate 80, sodium 27-36 mEq/L, sucrose 28 mg/vial; derived from or manufactured using hamster or mouse protein]
Helixate® FS: 2000 int. units, 3000 int. units [contains polysorbate 80, sodium 26-34 mEq/L, sucrose 52 mg/vial; derived from or manufactured using hamster or mouse protein]
Kogenate® FS: 250 int. units, 500 int. units, 1000 int. units [contains polysorbate 80, sodium 27-36 mEq/L, sucrose 28 mg/vial; derived from or manufactured using hamster or mouse protein]
Kogenate® FS: 2000 int. units, 3000 int. units [contains polysorbate 80, sodium 26-34 mEq/L, sucrose 52 mg/vial; derived from or manufactured using hamster or mouse protein]
Recombinate: 250 int. units, 500 int. units, 1000 int. units, 1500 int. units [contains albumin (human), natural rubber/natural latex in packaging, polysorbate 80, sodium 180 mEq/L; derived from or manufactured using bovine, hamster or mouse protein]
Xyntha®: 250 int. units, 500 int. units, 1000 int. units, 2000 int. units [albumin free; contains polysorbate 80, sucrose; derived from or manufactured using hamster protein; supplied with diluent]
Xyntha® Solofuse™: 1000 int. units, 2000 int. units, 3000 int. units [albumin free; contains polysorbate 80, sucrose; derived from or manufactured using hamster protein; dual-chamber syringe]

Antihemophilic Factor/von Willebrand Factor Complex (Human)

(an tee hee moe FIL ik FAK tor von WILL le brand FAK tor KOM plex HYU man)

Brand Names: U.S. Alphanate®; Humate-P®; Wilate®
Brand Names: Canada Humate-P®
Index Terms AHF (Human); Factor VIII (Human); Factor VIII Concentrate; FVIII/vWF; von Willebrand Factor/Factor VIII Complex; VWF/FVIII Concentrate; VWF:RCo; vWF:RCof
Pharmacologic Category Antihemophilic Agent; Blood Product Derivative

Use

Factor VIII deficiency: Alphanate®, Humate-P®: Prevention and treatment of hemorrhagic episodes in patients with hemophilia A (classical hemophilia) or acquired factor VIII deficiency (Alphanate® only); **Note:** Wilate® is not approved for use in patients with hemophilia A or acquired factor VIII deficiency

von Willebrand disease (VWD):

Alphanate®: Prophylaxis with surgical and/or invasive procedures in patients with VWD when desmopressin is either ineffective or contraindicated; **Note:** Not indicated for patients with severe VWD undergoing major surgery

Humate-P®: Treatment of spontaneous or trauma-induced bleeding, as well as prevention of excessive bleeding during and after surgery in patients with severe VWD, including mild or moderate disease where use of desmopressin is known or suspected to be inadequate; **Note:** Not indicated for the prophylaxis of spontaneous bleeding episodes

Wilate®: Treatment of spontaneous and trauma-induced bleeding in patients with severe VWD, including mild or moderate disease where use of desmopressin is known or suspected to be inadequate or contraindicated; **Note:** Not indicated for prophylaxis of spontaneous bleeding or prevention of excessive bleeding during and after surgery)

Pregnancy Risk Factor C

Dosage

Factor VIII deficiency: General guidelines (consult specific product labeling for Alphanate® or Humate-P®): Children and Adults: I.V.:

Individualize dosage based on coagulation studies performed prior to treatment and at regular intervals during treatment; in general, administration of factor VIII 1 int. unit/kg will increase circulating factor VIII levels by ~2 int. units/dL.

Minor hemorrhage: Loading dose: FVIII:C 15 int. units/kg to achieve FVIII:C plasma level ~30% of normal. If second infusion is needed, half the loading dose may be given once or twice daily for 1-2 days.

Moderate hemorrhage: Loading dose: FVIII:C 25 int. units/kg to achieve FVIII:C plasma level ~50% of normal; Maintenance: FVIII:C 15 int. units/kg every 8-12 hours for 1-2 days in order to maintain FVIII:C plasma levels at 30% of normal. Repeat the same dose once or twice daily for up to 7 days or until adequate wound healing.

Life-threatening hemorrhage/major surgery: Loading dose: FVIII:C 40-50 int. units/kg; Maintenance: FVIII:C 20-25 int. units/kg every 8-12 hours to maintain FVIII:C plasma levels at 80% to 100% of normal for 7 days. Continue same dose once or twice daily for another 7 days in order to maintain FVIII:C levels at 30% to 50% of normal.

von Willebrand disease (VWD): Treatment:

Humate-P®: Children and Adults: I.V.: Individualize dosage based on coagulation studies performed prior to treatment and at regular intervals during treatment; in general, administration of factor VIII 1 int. unit/kg would be expected to raise circulating VWF:RCo ~5 int. units/dL

Type 1, mild VWD: Minor hemorrhage (if desmopressin is not appropriate) or major hemorrhage:

Loading dose: VWF:RCo 40-60 int. units/kg

Maintenance dose: VWF:RCo 40-50 int. units/kg every 8-12 hours for 3 days, keeping VWF:RCo nadir >50%; follow with 40-50 int. units/kg daily for up to 7 days

Type 1, moderate or severe VWD:

Minor hemorrhage: VWF:RCo 40-50 int. units/kg for 1-2 doses

Major hemorrhage:

Loading dose: VWF:RCo 50-75 int. units/kg

Maintenance dose: VWF:RCo 40-60 int. units/kg every 8-12 hours for 3 days to keep the VWF:RCo nadir >50%, then 40-60 int. units/kg daily for a total of up to 7 days

Types 2 and 3 VWD:

Minor hemorrhage: VWF:RCo 40-50 int. units/kg for 1-2 doses

Major hemorrhage:

Loading dose: VWF:RCo 60-80 int. units/kg

Maintenance dose: VWF:RCo 40-60 int. units/kg every 8-12 hours for 3 days, keeping the VWF:RCo nadir >50%; follow with 40-60 int. units/kg daily for a total of up to 7 days

Wilate®: Children and Adults: I.V.:

Minor hemorrhage:

Loading dose: VWF:RCo: 20-40 int. units/kg

Maintenance dose: 20-30 int. units/kg every 12-24 hours for ≤3 days, keeping the VWF:RCo nadir >30%

Major hemorrhage:

Loading dose: VWF:RCo: 40-60 int. units/kg

Maintenance dose: 20-40 int. units/kg every 12-24 hours for 5-7 days, keeping the VWF:RCo nadir >50%

von Willebrand disease (VWD): Prophylaxis:

Alphanate®: Surgery/procedure prophylaxis (except patients with type 3 undergoing major surgery):

Children: I.V.:

Preoperative dose: VWF:RCo: 75 int. units/kg 1 hour prior to surgery

Maintenance dose: VWF:RCo: 50-75 int. units/kg every 8-12 hours as clinically needed. May reduce dose after third postoperative day; continue treatment until healing is complete.

Adults: I.V.:

Preoperative dose: VWF:RCo: 60 int. units/kg 1 hour prior to surgery

Maintenance dose: VWF:RCo: 40-60 int. units/kg every 8-12 hours as clinically needed. May reduce dose after third postoperative day; continue treatment until healing is complete. For minor procedures, maintain VWF of 40% to 50% during postoperative days 1-3; for major procedures maintain VWF of 40% to 50% for ≥3-7 days.

Humate-P®: Surgery/procedure prevention of bleeding: Children and Adults: I.V.:

Emergency surgery: Administer VWF:RCo 50-60 int. units/kg; monitor trough coagulation factor levels for subsequent doses

Surgical management (nonemergency):

Loading dose calculation based on baseline target VWF:RCo: (Target peak VWF:RCo - Baseline VWF:RCo) x weight (in kg) / IVR = int. units VWF:RCo required. Administer loading dose 1-2 hours prior to surgery. **Note:** If *in vivo* recovery (IVR) not available, assume 2 int. units/dL per int. units/kg of VWF:RCo product administered.

Target concentrations for VWF:RCo following loading dose:

Major surgery: 100 int. units/dL

Minor surgery: 50-60 int. units/dL

Maintenance dose: Initial: One-half loading dose, followed by subsequent dosing determined by target trough concentrations, generally every 8-12 hours. Patients with shorter half-lives may require dosing every 6 hours.

Target maintenance trough VWF:RCo concentrations:

Major surgery: >50 int. units/dL for up to 3 days, followed by >30 int. units/dL for a minimum total treatment of 72 hours

Minor surgery: ≥30 int. units/dL for a minimum duration of 48 hours

Oral surgery: ≥30 int. units/dL for a minimum duration of 8-12 hours

Elderly: Response in the elderly is not expected to differ from that of younger patients; dosage should be individualized

Additional Information Complete prescribing information for this medication should be consulted for additional detail.

Dosage Forms Excipient information presented when available (limited, particularly for generics); consult specific product labeling.

Injection, powder for reconstitution [human derived]:

Alphanate®:

250 int. units [Factor VIII and VWF:RCo ratio varies by lot; contains sodium ≥10 mEq/vial, albumin and polysorbate 80; packaged with diluent]

500 int. units [Factor VIII and VWF:RCo ratio varies by lot; contains sodium ≥10 mEq/vial, albumin and polysorbate 80; packaged with diluent]

1000 int. units [Factor VIII and VWF:RCo ratio varies by lot; contains sodium ≥10 mEq/vial, albumin and polysorbate 80; packaged with diluent]

1500 int. units [Factor VIII and VWF:RCo ratio varies by lot; contains sodium ≥10 mEq/vial, albumin and polysorbate 80; packaged with diluent]

Humate-P®:

FVIII 250 int. units and VWF:RCo 600 int. units [contains albumin; packaged with diluent]

FVIII 500 int. units and VWF:RCo 1200 int. units [contains albumin; packaged with diluent]

FVIII 1000 int. units and VWF:RCo 2400 int. units [contains albumin; packaged with diluent]

◆ **Anti-Hist [OTC]** *see* DiphenhydrAMINE (Systemic) *on page 516*

Anti-inhibitor Coagulant Complex

(an TEE in HI bi tor coe AG yoo lant KOM pleks)

Brand Names: U.S. Feiba NF; Feiba VH [DSC]

Brand Names: Canada Feiba NF

Index Terms AICC; aPCC; Coagulant Complex Inhibitor

Pharmacologic Category Activated Prothrombin Complex Concentrate (aPCC); Antihemophilic Agent; Blood Product Derivative

Use Hemophilia A & B patients with inhibitors who are to undergo surgery or those who are bleeding

Unlabeled Use Acquired hemophilia with factor VIII or factor IX inhibitor titers >5 Bethesda units (BU)

Pregnancy Risk Factor C

Dosage I.V.: Children and Adults: **Note:** Considered a first-line treatment when factor VIII inhibitor titer is >5 Bethesda units (BU) (antihemophilic factor may be preferred when titer <5 BU)

General dosing guidelines: 50-100 units/kg (maximum: 200 units/kg/day)

Joint hemorrhage: 50 units/kg every 12 hours; may increase to 100 units/kg every 12 hours; continue until signs of clinical improvement occur (maximum: 200 units/kg/day)

Mucous membrane bleeding: 50 units/kg every 6 hours; may increase to 100 units/kg every 6 hours up to 2 doses only (maximum: 200 units/kg/day)

Soft tissue hemorrhage (eg, retroperitoneal bleed): 100 units/kg every 12 hours (maximum: 200 units/kg/day)

Other severe hemorrhage (eg, intracranial hemorrhage): 100 units/kg every 12 hours; may be used every 6 hours if needed; continue until clinical improvement (maximum: 200 units/kg/day unless severity of hemorrhage justifies higher doses). **Note:** If total single dose exceeds 100 units/kg or total daily dose exceeds 200 units/kg/day, monitor closely for DIC and/or coronary ischemia.

Additional Information Complete prescribing information for this medication should be consulted for additional detail.

Dosage Forms Excipient information presented when available (limited, particularly for generics); consult specific product labeling. [DSC] = Discontinued product

Injection, powder for reconstitution:

Feiba NF: ~500 units, ~1000 units, ~2500 units [heparin free; contains natural rubber/natural latex in packaging; exact potency labeled on each vial]

Feiba VH: ~500 units, ~1000 units, ~2500 units [heparin free; contains natural rubber/natural latex in packaging; exact potency labeled on each vial] [DSC]

Antipyrine and Benzocaine

(an tee PYE reen & BEN zoe kane)

Brand Names: Canada Auralgan®

Index Terms Benzocaine and Antipyrine

Pharmacologic Category Otic Agent, Analgesic; Otic Agent, Cerumenolytic

Use Temporary relief of pain and reduction of swelling associated with acute congestive and serous otitis media; facilitates ear wax removal

Pregnancy Risk Factor C

Dosage Otic: Children and Adults:

Otitis media: Fill ear canal with solution; moisten cotton pledget with antipyrine and benzocaine solution, place in external ear, repeat every 1-2 hours until pain and congestion are relieved

Ear wax removal: Instill drops 3 times/day for 2-3 days; before and after ear wax removal, moisten cotton pledget with antipyrine and benzocaine solution and place in external ear after solution instillation.

Additional Information Complete prescribing information for this medication should be consulted for additional detail.

Dosage Forms Excipient information presented when available (limited, particularly for generics); consult specific product labeling.

Solution, otic [drops]: Antipyrine 5.4% and benzocaine 1.4% (10 mL, 15 mL)

Antithrombin (an tee THROM bin)

Brand Names: U.S. Atryn®; Thrombate III®

Brand Names: Canada Thrombate III®

Index Terms Antithrombin Alfa; Antithrombin III; AT; AT-III; hpAT; rhAT; rhATIII

Pharmacologic Category Anticoagulant; Blood Product Derivative

Use Prophylaxis (ATryn®, Thrombate III®) of thromboembolic events in patients with hereditary antithrombin (AT or AT-III) deficiency undergoing surgical or obstetrical procedures (eg, childbirth); treatment (Thrombate III®) of thromboembolism in patients with hereditary AT deficiency

Pregnancy Risk Factor B (Thrombate III®); C (ATryn®)

Dosage I.V.: Adults: Antithrombin deficiency:

Atryn®: Prophylaxis of thrombosis during surgical or obstetrical procedures:

Dosing is individualized based on pretherapy antithrombin (AT) activity levels. Therapy should begin before delivery or ~24 hours prior to surgery to obtain target AT activity levels. Dosing should be targeted to keep levels between 80% to 120% of normal. Loading dose should be given as a 15-minute infusion, followed by maintenance dose as a continuous infusion. Doses may be calculated based on the following formulas:

Surgical patients (nonpregnant):

Loading dose: [(100 - baseline AT activity level) **divided** by 2.3] x body weight (kg) = int. units of antithrombin required

Maintenance infusion: [(100 - baseline AT activity level) **divided** by 10.2] x body weight (kg) = int. units of antithrombin required/hour

Pregnant patients: **Note:** Pregnant women undergoing surgical procedures (other than a Cesarean section) should also be dosed according to the formula below.

Loading dose: [(100 - baseline AT activity level) **divided** by 1.3] x body weight (kg) = int. units of antithrombin required

Maintenance infusion: [(100 - baseline AT activity level) **divided** by 5.4] x body weight (kg) = int. units of antithrombin required/hour

Dosing adjustments: Adjustments should be made based on AT activity levels to maintain levels between 80% to 120% of normal. Surgery or delivery may rapidly decrease AT levels; check AT level just after surgery or delivery. The first AT level should be obtained 2 hours after initiation and adjusted as follows:

AT activity level <80%: Increase infusion rate by 30%; recheck AT level 2 hours after adjustment. Alternatively, an additional bolus dose (using loading dose formula) may be needed to rapidly restore AT levels. Calculate the additional bolus/loading dose using the last available AT activity result. After additional loading/bolus dose given, resume maintenance infusion at the same rate prior to bolus administration.

AT activity level 80% to 120%: No dosage adjustment needed; recheck AT level in 6 hours

AT activity level >120%: Decrease infusion rate by 30%; recheck AT level 2 hours after adjustment

Thrombate III®: Prophylaxis of thrombosis during surgical or obstetrical procedures or treatment of thromboembolism:

Initial loading dose: Dosing is individualized based on pretherapy antithrombin (AT) levels. The initial dose should raise AT levels to 120% and may be calculated based on the following formula:

[(desired AT level % - baseline AT level %) x body weight (kg)] **divided** by 1.4 = int. units of antithrombin required

For example, if a 70 kg adult patient had a baseline AT level of 57%, the initial dose would be

[(120% - 57%) x 70] divided by 1.4 = 3150 int. units

Maintenance dose: In general, subsequent dosing should be targeted to keep levels between 80% to 120% which may be achieved by administering 60% of the initial loading dose every 24 hours. Adjustments may be made by adjusting dose or interval. Maintain level within normal range for 2-8 days depending on type of procedure/situation.

Additional Information Complete prescribing information for this medication should be consulted for additional detail.

Dosage Forms Excipient information presented when available (limited, particularly for generics); consult specific product labeling.

Injection, powder for reconstitution [human, preservative free]:

Thrombate III®: ~500 int. units [contains heparin; exact potency labeled on each vial]

Injection, powder for reconstitution [recombinant, preservative free]:

Atryn®: ~1750 int. units [contains goat protein; exact potency labeled on each vial]

◆ **Antithrombin III** *see* Antithrombin *on page* 130

◆ **Antithrombin Alfa** *see* Antithrombin *on page* 130

Antithymocyte Globulin (Equine)

(an te THY moe site GLOB yu lin, E kwine)

Brand Names: U.S. Atgam®

Brand Names: Canada Atgam®

Index Terms Antithymocyte Immunoglobulin; ATG; Horse Antihuman Thymocyte Gamma Globulin; Lymphocyte Immune Globulin

Pharmacologic Category Immune Globulin; Immunosuppressant Agent; Polyclonal Antibody

Use Prevention and treatment of acute renal allograft rejection; treatment of moderate-to-severe aplastic anemia in patients not considered suitable candidates for bone marrow transplantation

Unlabeled Use Prevention and treatment of other solid organ allograft rejection; prevention or treatment of graft-versus-host disease (GVHD) following allogeneic stem cell transplantation; treatment of myelodysplastic syndrome (MDS)

Pregnancy Risk Factor C

Pregnancy Considerations Reproduction studies have not been conducted; use during pregnancy is not recommended. Use in pregnant women is not recommended and should be considered only in exceptional circumstances. Women exposed to Atgam® during pregnancy may be enrolled in the National Transplantation Pregnancy Registry (877-955-6877).

Lactation Excretion in breast milk unknown/use caution

Contraindications History of severe systemic reaction to prior administration of antithymocyte globulin or other equine gamma globulins

Warnings/Precautions For I.V. use only. Must be administered via central line due to chemical phlebitis. **[U.S. Boxed Warning]: Should only be used by physicians experienced in immunosuppressive therapy or management of solid organ or bone marrow transplant patients. Adequate laboratory and supportive medical resources must be readily available in the facility for patient management.** Hypersensitivity and anaphylactic reactions can occur; immediate treatment (including epinephrine 1:1000) should be available. Rash, dyspnea, hypotension, tachycardia, or anaphylaxis precludes further administration of the drug. Respiratory distress, hypotension, or pain (chest, flank or back) may indicate an anaphylactoid/anaphylactic reaction. Discontinue if severe and unremitting thrombocytopenia and/or leukopenia occur in transplant patients. Clinically significant hemolysis has been reported (rarely); severe and unremitting hemolysis may require treatment discontinuation; chest, flank or back pain may indicate hemolysis. Monitor closely for signs of infection; there may be an increased incidence of cytomegalovirus (CMV) infection. Dose must be administered over at least 4 hours. Patient may need to be pretreated with an antipyretic, antihistamine, and/or corticosteroid. Intradermal skin testing is recommended prior to first-dose administration. Product of equine and human plasma; may have a risk of transmitting disease, including a theoretical risk of Creutzfeldt-Jakob disease (CJD). Product potency and activity may vary from lot to lot.

Adverse Reactions

>10%:

Central nervous system: Chills, fever, headache

Dermatologic: Pruritus, rash, urticaria, wheal/flare

Hematologic: Leukopenia, thrombocytopenia

Neuromuscular & skeletal: Arthralgia

1% to 10%:

Cardiovascular: Bradycardia, cardiac irregularity, chest pain, edema, heart failure, hyper-/hypotension, myocarditis

Central nervous system: Agitation, encephalitis, lethargy, lightheadedness, listlessness, seizure, viral encephalopathy

Gastrointestinal: Diarrhea, nausea, stomatitis, vomiting
Hepatic: Hepatosplenomegaly, liver function tests abnormal
Local: Injection site reactions (pain, redness, swelling), phlebitis, thrombophlebitis, burning soles/palms
Neuromuscular & skeletal: Aches, back pain, joint stiffness, myalgia
Ocular: Periorbital edema
Renal: Proteinuria, renal function tests abnormal
Respiratory: Dyspnea, pleural effusion, respiratory distress
Miscellaneous: Anaphylactic reaction, diaphoresis, lymphadenopathy, night sweats, serum sickness, viral infection

<1% (Limited to important or life-threatening: Abdominal pain, acute renal failure, anaphylactoid reaction, anemia, aplasia, apnea, confusion, cough, deep vein thrombosis, disorientation, dizziness, eosinophilia, epigastric pain, epistaxis, erythema, faintness, flank pain, GI bleeding, GI perforation, granulocytopenia, hemolysis, hemolytic anemia, herpes simplex reactivation, hiccups, hyperglycemia, iliac vein obstruction, infection, involuntary movement, kidney enlarged/ruptured, laryngospasm, malaise, neutropenia, pancytopenia, paresthesia, pulmonary edema, renal artery thrombosis, rigidity, sore mouth/throat, tachycardia, toxic epidermal necrosis, tremor, vasculitis, viral hepatitis, weakness, wound dehiscence

Drug Interactions

Metabolism/Transport Effects None known.

Avoid Concomitant Use

Avoid concomitant use of Antithymocyte Globulin (Equine) with any of the following: BCG; Natalizumab; Pimecrolimus; Tacrolimus (Topical); Vaccines (Live)

Increased Effect/Toxicity

Antithymocyte Globulin (Equine) may increase the levels/effects of: Leflunomide; Natalizumab; Vaccines (Live)

The levels/effects of Antithymocyte Globulin (Equine) may be increased by: Denosumab; Pimecrolimus; Roflumilast; Tacrolimus (Topical); Trastuzumab

Decreased Effect

Antithymocyte Globulin (Equine) may decrease the levels/effects of: BCG; Coccidioidin Skin Test; Sipuleucel-T; Vaccines (Inactivated); Vaccines (Live)

The levels/effects of Antithymocyte Globulin (Equine) may be decreased by: Echinacea

Stability Refrigerate ampuls at 2°C to 8°C (36°F to 46°F); do not freeze. Dilute into inverted bottle of sterile vehicle to ensure that undiluted lymphocyte immune globulin does not contact air. Gently rotate or swirl to mix; do not shake. Final concentration should be 4 mg/mL. May be diluted in NS, $D_5$1/4NS, $D_5$1/2NS **(do not use D_5W; low salt concentrations may result in precipitation)**. Diluted solution is stable for 24 hours (including infusion time) at refrigeration. Allow infusion solution to reach room temperature prior to administration.

Mechanism of Action Immunosuppressant involved in the elimination of antigen-reactive T lymphocytes (killer cells) in peripheral blood or alteration in the function of T-lymphocytes, which are involved in humoral immunity and partly in cell-mediated immunity; induces complete or partial hematologic response in aplastic anemia

Pharmacodynamics/Kinetics

Distribution: Poorly into lymphoid tissues; binds to circulating lymphocytes, granulocytes, platelets, bone marrow cells

Half-life elimination, plasma: 1.5-12 days

Excretion: Urine (~1%)

Dosage An intradermal skin test is recommended prior to administration of the initial dose of ATG; use 0.1 mL of a fresh 1:1000 dilution of ATG in normal saline; observe every 15-20 minutes for 1 hour. A positive skin reaction consists of a wheal ≥10 mm in diameter. If a positive skin test occurs, the first infusion should be administered in a controlled environment with intensive life support immediately available. A systemic reaction precludes further administration of the drug. The absence of a reaction does **not** preclude the possibility of an immediate sensitivity reaction.

Premedication with diphenhydramine, hydrocortisone, and acetaminophen is recommended prior to first dose.

Children: I.V.:

Aplastic anemia protocol: 10-20 mg/kg/day for 8-14 days; then administer every other day for 7 more doses; additional doses may be given every other day for 21 total doses in 28 days **or**

Unlabeled dosing: Children >10 kg: 40 mg/kg/day for 4 days (Rosenfeld, 1995)

Renal allograft: 5-25 mg/kg/day

Acute GVHD treatment (unlabeled use): 30 mg/kg/dose every other day for 6 doses (MacMillan, 2007) **or** 15 mg/kg/dose twice daily for 10 doses (MacMillan, 2002)

Adults: I.V.:

Aplastic anemia protocol: 10-20 mg/kg/day for 8-14 days, then administer every other day for 7 more doses, for a total of 21 doses in 28 days **or**

Unlabeled dosing: 40 mg/kg/day for 4 days (Rosenfeld, 1995)

Renal allograft:

Rejection prophylaxis: 15 mg/kg/day for 14 days, then give every other day for 7 more doses for a total of 21 doses in 28 days; the initial dose should be administered within 24 hours before or after transplantation

Rejection treatment: 10-15 mg/kg/day for 14 days, then administer every other day for 7 more doses for a total of 21 doses in 28 days

Acute GVHD treatment (unlabeled use): 30 mg/kg/dose every other day for 6 doses (MacMillan, 2007) **or** 15 mg/kg/dose twice daily for 10 doses (MacMillan, 2002)

Myelodysplastic syndrome (unlabeled use): 40 mg/kg/dose once daily for 4 days; an intradermal test dose was administered prior to treatment (Molldrem, 2002)

Dosage adjustment for toxicity:

Anaphylaxis: Stop infusion immediately; administer epinephrine. May require corticosteroids, respiration assistance, and/or other resuscitative measures. Do not resume infusion.

Hemolysis (severe and unremitting): May require discontinuation of treatment.

Administration Infuse dose over at least 4 hours. Any severe systemic reaction to the skin test, such as generalized rash, tachycardia, dyspnea, hypotension, or anaphylaxis, should preclude further therapy. Epinephrine and resuscitative equipment should be nearby. Patient may need to be pretreated with an antipyretic, antihistamine, and/or corticosteroid. Mild itching and erythema can be treated with antihistamines. May cause vein irritation (chemical phlebitis) if administered peripherally. Infuse into a vascular shunt, arterial venous fistula, or high-flow central vein through a 0.2-1 micron in-line filter.

First dose: Premedicate with diphenhydramine orally 30 minutes prior to and hydrocortisone I.V. 15 minutes prior to infusion and acetaminophen 2 hours after start of infusion.

Monitoring Parameters Lymphocyte profile, CBC with differential and platelet count, vital signs during administration

Dosage Forms Excipient information presented when available (limited, particularly for generics); consult specific product labeling.

Injection, solution:

Atgam®: 50 mg/mL (5 mL)

Antithymocyte Globulin (Rabbit)

(an te THY moe site GLOB yu lin RAB bit)

Brand Names: U.S. Thymoglobulin®

Index Terms Antithymocyte Immunoglobulin; rATG

Pharmacologic Category Immune Globulin; Immunosuppressant Agent; Polyclonal Antibody

Use Treatment of acute rejection of renal transplant; used in conjunction with concomitant immunosuppression

Unlabeled Use Induction therapy in renal transplant; treatment of myelodysplastic syndrome (MDS)

Pregnancy Risk Factor C

Pregnancy Considerations Reproduction studies have not been conducted.

Lactation Excretion in breast milk unknown/use caution

Contraindications Hypersensitivity to antithymocyte globulin, rabbit proteins, or any component of the formulation; acute or chronic infection

Warnings/Precautions [U.S. Boxed Warning]: Should only be used by physicians experienced in immunosuppressive therapy for the treatment of renal transplant patients. Medical surveillance is required during the infusion. Initial dose must be administered over at least 6 hours into a high flow vein; patient may need pretreatment with an antipyretic, antihistamine, and/or corticosteroid. Hypersensitivity and fatal anaphylactic reactions can occur; immediate treatment (including epinephrine 1:1000) should be available. An increased incidence of lymphoma, post-transplant lymphoproliferative disease (PTLD), other malignancies, or severe infections may develop following concomitant use of immunosuppressants and prolonged use or overdose of antithymocyte globulin. Appropriate antiviral, antibacterial, antiprotozoal, and/or antifungal prophylaxis is recommended. Reversible neutropenia or thrombocytopenia may result from the development of cross-reactive antibodies.

Release of cytokines by activated monocytes and lymphocytes may cause fatal cytokine release syndrome (CRS) during administration of antithymocyte globulin. Rapid infusion rates of have been associated with CRS in case reports. Symptoms range from a mild, self-limiting "flu-like reaction" to severe, life-threatening reactions. Severe or life-threatening symptoms include hypotension, acute respiratory distress syndrome, pulmonary edema, myocardial infarction, and tachycardia. Patients should not be immunized with attenuated live viral vaccines during or shortly after treatment; safety of immunization following therapy has not been studied.

Adverse Reactions

>10%:

Cardiovascular: Hypertension, peripheral edema, tachycardia

Central nervous system: Chills, fever, headache, pain, malaise

Endocrine & metabolic: Hyperkalemia

Gastrointestinal: Abdominal pain, diarrhea, nausea

Genitourinary: Urinary tract infection

Hematologic: Leukopenia, thrombocytopenia

Neuromuscular & skeletal: Weakness

Respiratory: Dyspnea

Miscellaneous: Antirabbit antibody development, cytomegalovirus infection, sepsis, systemic infection

1% to 10%:

Central nervous system: Dizziness

Gastrointestinal: Gastritis, gastrointestinal moniliasis

Miscellaneous: Herpes simplex infection, oral moniliasis

Postmarketing and/or case reports: Anaphylaxis, cytokine release syndrome, PTLD, neutropenia, serum sickness (delayed)

Drug Interactions

Metabolism/Transport Effects None known.

Avoid Concomitant Use

Avoid concomitant use of Antithymocyte Globulin (Rabbit) with any of the following: BCG; Natalizumab; Pimecrolimus; Tacrolimus (Topical); Vaccines (Live)

Increased Effect/Toxicity

Antithymocyte Globulin (Rabbit) may increase the levels/effects of: Leflunomide; Natalizumab; Vaccines (Live)

The levels/effects of Antithymocyte Globulin (Rabbit) may be increased by: Denosumab; Pimecrolimus; Roflumilast; Tacrolimus (Topical); Trastuzumab

Decreased Effect

Antithymocyte Globulin (Rabbit) may decrease the levels/effects of: BCG; Coccidioidin Skin Test; Sipuleucel-T; Vaccines (Inactivated); Vaccines (Live)

The levels/effects of Antithymocyte Globulin (Rabbit) may be decreased by: Echinacea

Stability Store powder under refrigeration at 2°C to 8°C (36°F to 46°F); do not freeze. Protect from light. Allow vials to reach room temperature, then reconstitute each vial with SWFI 5 mL. Rotate vial gently until dissolved. Prior to administration, further dilute one vial in 50 mL saline or dextrose (total volume is usually 50-500 mL depending on total number of vials needed per dose). Mix by gently inverting infusion bag once or twice. Reconstituted product is stable for up to 24 hours at room temperature; however, since it contains no preservatives, it should be used immediately following reconstitution.

Mechanism of Action Polyclonal antibody which appears to cause immunosuppression by acting on T-cell surface antigens and depleting CD4 lymphocytes

Pharmacodynamics/Kinetics

Duration: Lymphopenia may persist ≥1 year

Half-life elimination, plasma: 2-3 days

Dosage I.V.: Children and Adults: Treatment of acute rejection: 1.5 mg/kg/day for 7-14 days

Dosage adjustment for toxicity:

WBC count 2000-3000 cells/mm^3 or platelet count 50,000-75,000 cells/mm^3: Reduce dose by 50%

WBC count <2000 cells/mm^3 or platelet count <50,000 cells/mm^3: Consider discontinuing treatment

Administration The first dose should be infused over at least 6 hours through a high-flow vein. Subsequent doses should be administered over at least 4 hours. Administer through an in-line 0.22 micron filter. Premedication with corticosteroids, acetaminophen, and/or an antihistamine may reduce infusion-related reactions.

Monitoring Parameters Lymphocyte profile, CBC with differential and platelet count; vital signs during administration; signs and symptoms of infection

Test Interactions Potential interference with rabbit antibody-based immunoassays

Dosage Forms Excipient information presented when available (limited, particularly for generics); consult specific product labeling.

Injection, powder for reconstitution:

Thymoglobulin®: 25 mg

- ◆ **Antithymocyte Immunoglobulin** *see* Antithymocyte Globulin (Equine) *on page 131*
- ◆ **Antithymocyte Immunoglobulin** *see* Antithymocyte Globulin (Rabbit) *on page 133*
- ◆ **Antitumor Necrosis Factor Alpha (Human)** *see* Adalimumab *on page 42*
- ◆ **Anti-VEGF Monoclonal Antibody** *see* Bevacizumab *on page 212*
- ◆ **Anti-VEGF rhuMAb** *see* Bevacizumab *on page 212*
- ◆ **Antivenin (*Centruroides*) Immune F(ab')$_2$ (Equine)** *see Centruroides* Immune F(ab')$_2$ (Equine) *on page 326*
- ◆ **Antivenin Scorpion** *see Centruroides* Immune F(ab')$_2$ (Equine) *on page 326*

- **Apo-Sulfatrim® DS (Can)** *see* Sulfamethoxazole and Trimethoprim *on page 1602*
- **Apo-Sulfatrim® Pediatric (Can)** *see* Sulfamethoxazole and Trimethoprim *on page 1602*
- **Apo-Sulin® (Can)** *see* Sulindac *on page 1608*
- **Apo-Sumatriptan® (Can)** *see* SUMAtriptan *on page 1609*
- **Apo-Tamox® (Can)** *see* Tamoxifen *on page 1624*
- **Apo-Temazepam® (Can)** *see* Temazepam *on page 1638*
- **Apo-Terazosin® (Can)** *see* Terazosin *on page 1647*
- **Apo-Terbinafine® (Can)** *see* Terbinafine (Systemic) *on page 1648*
- **Apo-Tetra® (Can)** *see* Tetracycline *on page 1661*
- **Apo-Theo LA® (Can)** *see* Theophylline *on page 1667*
- **Apo-Ticlopidine® (Can)** *see* Ticlopidine *on page 1682*
- **Apo-Timol® (Can)** *see* Timolol (Systemic) *on page 1686*
- **Apo-Timop® (Can)** *see* Timolol (Ophthalmic) *on page 1687*
- **Apo-Tizanidine® (Can)** *see* TiZANidine *on page 1695*
- **Apo-Tolbutamide® (Can)** *see* TOLBUTamide *on page 1702*
- **Apo-Topiramate® (Can)** *see* Topiramate *on page 1706*
- **Apo-Tramadol/Acet® (Can)** *see* Acetaminophen and Tramadol *on page 32*
- **Apo-Trazodone® (Can)** *see* TraZODone *on page 1725*
- **Apo-Trazodone D® (Can)** *see* TraZODone *on page 1725*
- **Apo-Triazide® (Can)** *see* Hydrochlorothiazide and Triamterene *on page 836*
- **Apo-Triazo® (Can)** *see* Triazolam *on page 1736*
- **Apo-Trifluoperazine® (Can)** *see* Trifluoperazine *on page 1736*
- **Apo-Trimethoprim® (Can)** *see* Trimethoprim *on page 1740*
- **Apo-Valacyclovir® (Can)** *see* ValACYclovir *on page 1753*
- **Apo-Valproic® (Can)** *see* Valproic Acid *on page 1757*
- **Apo-Verap® (Can)** *see* Verapamil *on page 1783*
- **Apo-Verap® SR (Can)** *see* Verapamil *on page 1783*
- **Apo-Warfarin® (Can)** *see* Warfarin *on page 1802*
- **Apo-Zidovudine® (Can)** *see* Zidovudine *on page 1814*
- **APPG** *see* Penicillin G Procaine *on page 1325*

Apraclonidine (a pra KLOE ni deen)

Brand Names: U.S. Iopidine®
Brand Names: Canada Iopidine®
Index Terms Aplonidine; Apraclonidine Hydrochloride; p-Aminoclonidine
Pharmacologic Category Alpha$_2$ Agonist, Ophthalmic
Use Prevention and treatment of postsurgical intraocular pressure (IOP) elevation; short-term, adjunctive therapy in patients who require additional reduction of IOP
Pregnancy Risk Factor C
Dosage Adults: Ophthalmic:
0.5%: Instill 1-2 drops in the affected eye(s) 3 times/day
1%: Instill 1 drop in operative eye 1 hour prior to anterior segment laser surgery, second drop in eye immediately upon completion of procedure

Dosing adjustment in renal impairment: Although the topical use of apraclonidine has not been studied in renal failure patients, structurally-related clonidine undergoes a significant increase in half-life in patients with severe renal impairment; close monitoring of cardiovascular parameters in patients with impaired renal function is advised.

Dosing adjustment in hepatic impairment: Close monitoring of cardiovascular parameters in patients with impaired liver function is advised because the systemic dosage form of clonidine is partially metabolized in the liver.

Additional Information Complete prescribing information for this medication should be consulted for additional detail.
Dosage Forms Excipient information presented when available (limited, particularly for generics); consult specific product labeling.
Solution, ophthalmic [drops]: 0.5% (5 mL, 10 mL)
Iopidine®: 0.5% (5 mL, 10 mL); 1% (0.1 mL) [contains benzalkonium chloride]

- **Apraclonidine Hydrochloride** *see* Apraclonidine *on page 137*

Aprepitant (ap RE pi tant)

Brand Names: U.S. Emend®
Brand Names: Canada Emend®
Index Terms L 754030; MK 869
Pharmacologic Category Antiemetic; Substance P/Neurokinin 1 Receptor Antagonist
Use Prevention of acute and delayed nausea and vomiting associated with moderately- and highly-emetogenic chemotherapy (in combination with other antiemetics); prevention of postoperative nausea and vomiting (PONV)
Pregnancy Risk Factor B
Pregnancy Considerations Teratogenic effects were not observed in animal studies. There are no adequate and well-controlled studies in pregnant women; use only if clearly needed. Efficacy of hormonal contraceptive may be reduced; alternative or additional methods of contraception should be used both during treatment with fosaprepitant or aprepitant and for at least 1 month following the last fosaprepitant/aprepitant dose.
Lactation Excretion in breast milk unknown/not recommended
Contraindications Hypersensitivity to aprepitant or any component of the formulation; concurrent use with cisapride or pimozide
Warnings/Precautions Use caution with agents primarily metabolized via CYP3A4; aprepitant is a 3A4 inhibitor. Effect on orally administered 3A4 substrates is greater than those administered intravenously. Chronic continuous use is not recommended; however, a single 40 mg aprepitant oral dose is not likely to alter plasma concentrations of CYP3A4 substrates. Use caution with severe hepatic impairment; has not been studied in patients with severe hepatic impairment (Child-Pugh class C). Not studied for treatment of existing nausea and vomiting. Chronic continuous administration is not recommended.
Adverse Reactions Note: Adverse reactions reported as part of a combination chemotherapy regimen or with general anesthesia.

>10%:
Central nervous system: Fatigue (≤18%)
Gastrointestinal: Nausea (6% to 13%), constipation (9% to 10%)
Neuromuscular & skeletal: Weakness (≤18%)
Miscellaneous: Hiccups (11%)

1% to 10%:
Cardiovascular: Hypotension (≤6%), bradycardia (≤4%)
Central nervous system: Dizziness (≤7%)
Endocrine & metabolic: Dehydration (≤6%)

Gastrointestinal: Diarrhea (≤10%), dyspepsia (≤6%), abdominal pain (≤5%), epigastric discomfort (4%), gastritis (4%), stomatitis (3%)

Hepatic: ALT increased (≤6%), AST increased (3%)

Renal: Proteinuria (7%), BUN increased (5%)

>0.5% (Limited to important or life-threatening): Acid reflux, acne, albumin decreased, alkaline phosphatase increased, anaphylactic reaction, anemia, angioedema, anxiety, appetite decreased, arthralgia, back pain, bilirubin increased, candidiasis, confusion, conjunctivitis, cough, deglutition disorder, depression, diabetes mellitus, diaphoresis, disorientation, duodenal ulcer (perforating), DVT, dysarthria, dysphagia, dyspnea, dysuria, edema, enterocolitis, eructation, erythrocyturia, febrile neutropenia, flatulence, flushing, glucosuria, herpes simplex, hyperglycemia, hypersensitivity reaction, hypertension, hypoesthesia, hypokalemia, hyponatremia, hypothermia, hypovolemia, hypoxia, leukocytes increased, leukocyturia, malaise, MI, miosis, muscular weakness, musculoskeletal pain, myalgia, nasal secretion, neutropenic sepsis, obstipation, pain, palpitation, pelvic pain, peripheral neuropathy, pharyngitis, pharyngolaryngeal pain, pneumonia, pneumonitis, pruritus, pulmonary embolism, rash, renal insufficiency, respiratory infection, respiratory insufficiency, rigors, salivation increased, sensory disturbance, sensory neuropathy, septic shock, Stevens-Johnson syndrome, syncope, tachycardia, taste disturbance, thrombocytopenia, tremor, urinary tract infection, urticaria, visual acuity decreased, vocal disturbance, weight loss, wheezing, xerostomia

Drug Interactions

Metabolism/Transport Effects Substrate of CYP1A2 (minor), CYP2C19 (minor), CYP3A4 (major); **Note:** Assignment of Major/Minor substrate status based on clinically relevant drug interaction potential; **Inhibits** CYP2C19 (weak), CYP2C9 (weak), CYP3A4 (moderate); **Induces** CYP2C9 (strong), CYP3A4 (weak/moderate)

Avoid Concomitant Use

Avoid concomitant use of Aprepitant with any of the following: Cisapride; Conivaptan; Pimozide; Tolvaptan

Increased Effect/Toxicity

Aprepitant may increase the levels/effects of: ARIPiprazole; Benzodiazepines (metabolized by oxidation); Budesonide (Systemic, Oral Inhalation); Cisapride; Colchicine; Corticosteroids (Systemic); CYP3A4 Substrates; Diltiazem; Eplerenone; Everolimus; FentaNYL; Halofantrine; Lurasidone; Pimecrolimus; Pimozide; Propafenone; Ranolazine; Salmeterol; Saxagliptin; Tolvaptan; Vilazodone; Zuclopenthixol

The levels/effects of Aprepitant may be increased by: Antifungal Agents (Azole Derivatives, Systemic); Conivaptan; CYP3A4 Inhibitors (Moderate); CYP3A4 Inhibitors (Strong); Dasatinib; Diltiazem

Decreased Effect

Aprepitant may decrease the levels/effects of: ARIPiprazole; Contraceptives (Estrogens); Contraceptives (Progestins); CYP2C9 Substrates; Diclofenac; PARoxetine; Saxagliptin; TOLBUTamide; Warfarin

The levels/effects of Aprepitant may be decreased by: CYP3A4 Inducers (Strong); Cyproterone; Deferasirox; Herbs (CYP3A4 Inducers); PARoxetine; Rifamycin Derivatives; Tocilizumab

Ethanol/Nutrition/Herb Interactions

Food: Aprepitant serum concentration may be increased when taken with grapefruit juice; avoid concurrent use.

Herb/Nutraceutical: Avoid St John's wort (may decrease aprepitant levels).

Stability Store at room temperature of 20°C to 25°C (68°F to 77°F).

Mechanism of Action Prevents acute and delayed vomiting by inhibiting the substance P/neurokinin 1 (NK_1) receptor; augments the antiemetic activity of 5-HT_3 receptor antagonists and corticosteroids to inhibit acute and delayed phases of chemotherapy-induced emesis.

Pharmacodynamics/Kinetics

Distribution: V_d: ~70 L; crosses the blood-brain barrier

Protein binding: >95%

Metabolism: Extensively hepatic via CYP3A4 (major); CYP1A2 and CYP2C19 (minor); forms 7 metabolites (weakly active)

Bioavailability: ~60% to 65%

Half-life elimination: Terminal: ~9-13 hours

Time to peak, plasma: ~3-4 hours

Dosage Oral: Adults:

Prevention of chemotherapy-induced nausea/vomiting: 125 mg 1 hour prior to chemotherapy on day 1, followed by 80 mg once daily on days 2 and 3 (in combination with a corticosteroid and 5-HT_3 antagonist antiemetic)

Prevention of PONV: 40 mg within 3 hours prior to induction

Dosage adjustment in renal impairment: No dose adjustment necessary in patients with renal disease or end-stage renal disease maintained on hemodialysis.

Dosage adjustment in hepatic impairment:

Mild-to-moderate impairment (Child-Pugh classes A and B): No adjustment necessary

Severe impairment (Child-Pugh class C): Use caution; no data available

Dietary Considerations May be taken with or without food.

Administration

Chemotherapy induced nausea/vomiting: Administer with or without food. First dose should be given 1 hour prior to antineoplastic therapy; subsequent doses should be given in the morning.

PONV: Administer within 3 hours prior to induction; follow healthcare providers instructions about food/drink restrictions prior to surgery.

Additional Information Oncology Comment: Aprepitant is recommended in the American Society of Clinical Oncology (ASCO) oncology antiemetic guidelines for use in combination with a serotonin receptor antagonist and dexamethasone for chemotherapy with high emetic risk and for chemotherapy regimens of moderate emetic risk which contain an anthracycline and cyclophosphamide (Kris, 2006). The National Comprehensive Cancer Network® (NCCN) Clinical Practice Guidelines in Oncology for Antiemesis (version 1.2011) recommend the same use of aprepitant as is in the ASCO recommendation. In addition to the moderately emetogenic chemotherapy listed above, the NCCN guidelines suggest that aprepitant may also be used for select moderately emetogenic regimens containing carboplatin, cisplatin, doxorubicin, epirubicin, ifosfamide, irinotecan and methotrexate. Either fosaprepitant 115 mg or aprepitant (125 mg orally) are administered on day 1; for day 2 and 3, patients should receive aprepitant 80 mg orally.

Dosage Forms Excipient information presented when available (limited, particularly for generics); consult specific product labeling.

Capsule, oral:

Emend®: 40 mg, 80 mg, 125 mg

Combination package, oral [each package contains]:

Emend®: Capsule: 80 mg (2s) and Capsule: 125 mg (1s)

Extemporaneous Preparations A 20 mg/mL oral aprepitant suspension may be prepared with capsules and a 1:1 combination of Ora-Sweet® and Ora-Plus® (or Ora-Blend®). Empty the contents of four 125 mg capsules into a mortar and reduce to a fine powder (process will take 10-15 minutes). Add small portions of vehicle and mix to a uniform paste. Add sufficient vehicle to form a liquid;

transfer to a graduated cylinder, rinse mortar with vehicle, and add quantity of vehicle sufficient to make 25 mL. Label "shake well" and "refrigerate". Stable for 90 days refrigerated.

Dupuis LL, Lingertat-Walsh K, and Walker SE, "Stability of an Extemporaneous Oral Liquid Aprepitant Formulation," *Support Care Cancer*, 2009, 17(6):701-6.

- **Aprepitant Injection** *see* Fosaprepitant *on page 759*
- **Apresoline [DSC]** *see* HydrALAZINE *on page 833*
- **Apresoline® (Can)** *see* HydrALAZINE *on page 833*
- **Apri®** *see* Ethinyl Estradiol and Desogestrel *on page 653*
- **Apriso™** *see* Mesalamine *on page 1081*
- **Aprodine [OTC]** *see* Triprolidine and Pseudoephedrine *on page 1741*

Aprotinin (a proe TYE nin)

Brand Names: Canada Trasylol®

Pharmacologic Category Blood Product Derivative; Hemostatic Agent

Use Prevention of perioperative blood loss in patients who are at increased risk for blood loss and blood transfusions in association with cardiopulmonary bypass in coronary artery bypass graft (CABG) surgery

Note: Aprotinin has been withdrawn from the worldwide market due to evidence demonstrating an increased risk of renal dysfunction, myocardial infarction, and mortality in patients undergoing cardiac surgery (Canada has lifted this suspension); use limited to investigational use in the U.S. only according to a special treatment protocol allowing for treatment in select patients at increased risk of blood loss and transfusion during CABG surgery when alternative therapies are unacceptable.

Pregnancy Risk Factor B

Prescribing and Access Restrictions Available in U.S. under an investigational new drug (IND) process. The program will provide aprotinin for the treatment of adult patients undergoing coronary artery bypass graft (CABG) surgery requiring cardiopulmonary bypass (CPB) who are at increased risk of bleeding and transfusion during CABG surgery with no acceptable therapeutic alternative. Healthcare providers using aprotinin for this situation must also ensure that the benefits outweigh the risks for their patient. Healthcare providers with patients who may qualify can access information and forms for enrollment at http://www.trasylol.com/main.htm or contact Bayer Medical Communications at (888) 842-2937.

Dosage Adults: Test dose: **All** patients should receive a 1 mL (1.4 mg) I.V. test dose at least 10 minutes prior to the loading dose to assess the potential for allergic reactions.

Note:

The loading dose should be given after induction of anesthesia but prior to sternotomy. In patients with previous exposure to aprotinin, administer loading dose just prior to cannulation. A constant infusion is continued until surgery is complete.

To avoid physical incompatibility with heparin when adding to pump-prime solution, each agent should be added during recirculation to assure adequate dilution.

Regimen A (standard dose):

2 million KIU (280 mg; 200 mL) loading dose I.V. over 20-30 minutes

2 million KIU (280 mg; 200 mL) into pump prime volume

500,000 KIU/hour (70 mg/hour; 50 mL/hour) I.V. during operation

Regimen B (low dose):

1 million KIU (140 mg; 100 mL) loading dose I.V. over 20-30 minutes

1 million KIU (140 mg; 100 mL) into pump prime volume

250,000 KIU/hour (35 mg/hour; 25 mL/hour) I.V. during operation

Dosage adjustment in renal impairment: No adjustment required, but increased risk of worsening renal dysfunction with use; monitor closely

Dosage adjustment in hepatic impairment: No information available

Additional Information Complete prescribing information for this medication should be consulted for additional detail.

Dosage Forms Excipient information presented when available (limited, particularly for generics); consult specific product labeling.

Injection, solution:

Trasylol®: 1.4 mg/mL [10,000 KIU/mL] (100 mL, 200 mL) [bovine derived]

- **Aptivus®** *see* Tipranavir *on page 1691*
- **Aqua-Ban® Maximum Strength [OTC]** *see* Pamabrom *on page 1282*
- **Aqua Care® [OTC]** *see* Urea *on page 1749*
- **Aquacort® (Can)** *see* Hydrocortisone (Topical) *on page 841*
- **Aqua Gem-E™ [OTC]** *see* Vitamin E *on page 1796*
- **AquaMEPHYTON® (Can)** *see* Phytonadione *on page 1351*
- **Aquanil HC® [OTC]** *see* Hydrocortisone (Topical) *on page 841*
- **Aquaphilic® with Carbamide [OTC]** *see* Urea *on page 1749*
- **Aquasol A®** *see* Vitamin A *on page 1795*
- **Aquasol E® [OTC]** *see* Vitamin E *on page 1796*
- **Aquavan** *see* Fospropofol *on page 767*
- **Aqueous Procaine Penicillin G** *see* Penicillin G Procaine *on page 1325*
- **Ara-C** *see* Cytarabine (Conventional) *on page 428*
- **Arabinosylcytosine** *see* Cytarabine (Conventional) *on page 428*
- **Aralen®** *see* Chloroquine *on page 343*
- **Aranelle®** *see* Ethinyl Estradiol and Norethindrone *on page 660*
- **Aranesp®** *see* Darbepoetin Alfa *on page 447*
- **Aranesp® SingleJect®** *see* Darbepoetin Alfa *on page 447*
- **Arava®** *see* Leflunomide *on page 978*
- **Arbinoxa™** *see* Carbinoxamine *on page 287*
- **Arcalyst™** *see* Rilonacept *on page 1489*
- **Arcapta™ Neohaler™** *see* Indacaterol *on page 885*
- **Aredia®** *see* Pamidronate *on page 1282*
- **Arestin Microspheres (Can)** *see* Minocycline *on page 1137*

Arformoterol (ar for MOE ter ol)

Brand Names: U.S. Brovana®

Index Terms (R,R)-Formoterol L-Tartrate; Arformoterol Tartrate

Pharmacologic Category $Beta_2$-Adrenergic Agonist; $Beta_2$-Adrenergic Agonist, Long-Acting

Additional Appendix Information
Bronchodilators *on page 1886*

Use Long-term maintenance treatment of bronchoconstriction in chronic obstructive pulmonary disease (COPD), including chronic bronchitis and emphysema

Pregnancy Risk Factor C

Medication Guide Available Yes

Dosage Nebulization: Adults: COPD: 15 mcg twice daily; maximum: 30 mcg/day

Dosage adjustment in renal impairment: No adjustment required

Dosage adjustment in hepatic impairment: No dosage adjustment required, but use caution; systemic drug exposure prolonged (1.3- to 2.4-fold)

Additional Information Complete prescribing information for this medication should be consulted for additional detail.

Dosage Forms Excipient information presented when available (limited, particularly for generics); consult specific product labeling.

Solution, for nebulization:

Brovana®: 15 mcg/2 mL (30s, 60s)

◆ **Arformoterol Tartrate** *see* Arformoterol *on page 139*

Argatroban (ar GA troh ban)

Pharmacologic Category Anticoagulant, Thrombin Inhibitor

Use Prophylaxis or treatment of thrombosis in patients with heparin-induced thrombocytopenia (HIT); adjunct to percutaneous coronary intervention (PCI) in patients who have or are at risk of thrombosis associated with HIT

Unlabeled Use To maintain extracorporeal circuit patency (prefilter administration) of continuous renal replacement therapy (CRRT) in critically-ill patients with HIT

Pregnancy Risk Factor B

Pregnancy Considerations Adverse events were not observed in animal studies. There are no adequate and well-controlled studies in pregnant women. Argatroban should be used in pregnant women only if clearly needed.

Lactation Excretion in breast milk unknown/not recommended

Contraindications Hypersensitivity to argatroban or any component of the formulation; overt major bleeding

Warnings/Precautions Hemorrhage can occur at any site in the body. Extreme caution should be used when there is an increased danger of hemorrhage, such as severe hypertension, immediately following lumbar puncture, spinal anesthesia, major surgery (including brain, spinal cord, or eye surgery), congenital or acquired bleeding disorders, and gastrointestinal ulcers. Use caution in critically-ill patients; reduced clearance may require dosage reduction. Use caution with hepatic dysfunction. Argatroban prolongs the PT/INR. Concomitant use with warfarin will cause increased prolongation of the PT and INR greater than that of warfarin alone. If warfarin is initiated concurrently with argatroban, initial PT/INR goals while on argatroban may require modification; alternative guidelines for monitoring therapy should be followed. Safety and efficacy for use with other thrombolytic agents has not been established. Discontinue all parenteral anticoagulants prior to starting therapy. Allow reversal of heparin's effects before initiation. Patients with hepatic dysfunction may require >4 hours to achieve full reversal of argatroban's anticoagulant effect following treatment. Avoid use during PCI in patients with elevations of ALT/AST (≥3 times ULN); the use of argatroban in these patients has not been evaluated. Limited pharmacokinetic and dosing information is available from use in critically-ill children with heparin-induced thrombocytopenia.

Adverse Reactions As with all anticoagulants, bleeding is the major adverse effect of argatroban. Hemorrhage may occur at virtually any site. Risk is dependent on multiple variables, including the intensity of anticoagulation and patient susceptibility.

>10%:

Cardiovascular: Chest pain (PCI related: <1% to 15%), hypotension (7% to 11%)

Gastrointestinal: Gastrointestinal bleed (major: <1% to 3%; minor: 3% to 14%)

Genitourinary: Genitourinary bleed and hematuria (major: <1%; minor: 2% to 12%)

1% to 10%:

Cardiovascular: Vasodilation (1% to 10%), cardiac arrest (6%), ventricular tachycardia (5%), bradycardia (5%), myocardial infarction (PCI: 4%), atrial fibrillation (3%), angina (2%), CABG-related bleeding (minor, 2%), myocardial ischemia (2%), cerebrovascular disorder (<1% to 2%), thrombosis (<1% to 2%)

Central nervous system: Fever (<1% to 7%), headache (5%), pain (5%), intracranial bleeding (1% to 4%)

Dermatologic: Skin reactions (bullous eruption, rash; 1% to <10%)

Gastrointestinal: Nausea (5% to 7%), diarrhea (6%), vomiting (4% to 6%), abdominal pain (3% to 4%)

Genitourinary: Urinary tract infection (5%)

Hematologic: Hemoglobin decreased (<2 g/dL), hematocrit decreased (minor: 2% to 10%; major: <1%)

Local: Bleeding at injection or access site (minor: 2% to 5%)

Neuromuscular & skeletal: Back pain (PCI related: 8%)

Renal: Abnormal renal function (3%)

Respiratory: Dyspnea (8% to 10%), cough (3% to 10%), hemoptysis (minor: <1% to 3%), pneumonia (3%)

Miscellaneous: Sepsis (6%), infection (4%)

<1% (Limited to important or life-threatening): Allergic reactions, GERD, limb and below-the-knee stump bleed, multisystem hemorrhage and DIC, pulmonary edema, retroperitoneal bleeding

Drug Interactions

Metabolism/Transport Effects None known.

Avoid Concomitant Use

Avoid concomitant use of Argatroban with any of the following: Rivaroxaban

Increased Effect/Toxicity

Argatroban may increase the levels/effects of: Anticoagulants; Collagenase (Systemic); Deferasirox; Ibritumomab; Rivaroxaban; Tositumomab and Iodine I 131 Tositumomab

The levels/effects of Argatroban may be increased by: Antiplatelet Agents; Dasatinib; Herbs (Anticoagulant/Antiplatelet Properties); Nonsteroidal Anti-Inflammatory Agents; Pentosan Polysulfate Sodium; Prostacyclin Analogues; Salicylates; Thrombolytic Agents

Decreased Effect There are no known significant interactions involving a decrease in effect.

Stability

Vials for injection, 2.5 mL (100 mg/mL) concentrate: Prior to use, store at 15°C to 30°C (59°F to 86°F). Protect from light. May be mixed with 0.9% sodium chloride injection, 5% dextrose injection, or lactated Ringer's injection. Do not mix with other medications. To prepare solution for I.V. administration, each vial must be diluted to a final concentration of 1 mg/mL; dilute each 250 mg vial with 250 mL of diluent or dilute 500 mg per 500 mL of diluent. Mix by repeated inversion for 1 minute. A slight but brief haziness may occur prior to mixing. The diluted, prepared solution is stable for 24 hours at 15°C to 30°C (59°F to 86°F) in ambient indoor light. Do not expose to direct sunlight. Prepared solutions that are protected from light and kept at controlled room temperature of 20°C to 25°C (68°F to 77°F) or under refrigeration at 2°C to 8°C (36°F to 46°F) are stable for up to 96 hours.

Premixed vials for infusion, 50 mL or 125 mL (1 mg/mL): Store at controlled room temperature of 20°C to 25°C (68°F to 77°F). Keep in original container to protect from light. No further dilution is required.

Mechanism of Action A direct, highly-selective thrombin inhibitor. Reversibly binds to the active thrombin site of free and clot-associated thrombin. Inhibits fibrin formation; activation of coagulation factors V, VIII, and XIII; activation of protein C; and platelet aggregation.

Pharmacodynamics/Kinetics

Onset of action: Immediate

Distribution: 174 mL/kg

Protein binding: Albumin: 20%; α_1-acid glycoprotein: 35%

Metabolism: Hepatic via hydroxylation and aromatization. Metabolism via CYP3A4/5 to four known metabolites plays a minor role. Unchanged argatroban is the major plasma component. Plasma concentration of metabolite M1 is 0% to 20% of the parent drug and is three- to fivefold weaker.

Half-life elimination: 39-51 minutes; Hepatic impairment: ≤181 minutes

Time to peak: Steady-state: 1-3 hours

Excretion: Feces (65%); urine (22%); low quantities of metabolites M2-4 in urine

Clearance is decreased in critically-ill pediatric patients

Dosage I.V.:

Children: **Heparin-induced thrombocytopenia** (dosing based on limited data from critically-ill patients):

Initial dose: 0.75 mcg/kg/minute

Maintenance dose: Patient may not be at steady-state but measure aPTT after 2 hours; adjust dose until the steady-state aPTT is 1.5-3 times the initial baseline value, not exceeding 100 seconds; dosage may be adjusted in increments of 0.1-0.25 mcg/kg/minute. **Note:** Frequent dosage adjustments may be required to maintain desired anticoagulant activity.

Adults:

Heparin-induced thrombocytopenia:

Initial dose: 2 mcg/kg/minute; **Note:** Pharmacokinetics and pharmacodynamics have not been evaluated prospectively in obese patients; however, retrospective data suggests using actual body weight to dose and that adjustment of initial dose is unnecessary in obesity (BMI up to 51 kg/m^2) (Rice, 2007); weight range included in phase II and III clinical trials: 33-204 kg (actual body weight).

Maintenance dose: Patient may not be at steady-state but measure aPTT after 2 hours; adjust dose until the steady-state aPTT is 1.5-3 times the initial baseline value, not exceeding 100 seconds; dosage should not exceed 10 mcg/kg/minute

Note: Critically-ill patients with normal hepatic function have become excessively anticoagulated with FDA-approved or lower starting doses of argatroban. Doses between 0.15-1.3 mcg/kg/minute were required to maintain aPTTs in the target range (Reichert, 2003). In a prospective observational study of critically-ill patients with multiple organ dysfunction (MODS) and suspected or proven HIT, an initial infusion dose of 0.2 mcg/kg/minute was found to be sufficient and safe in this population (Beiderlinden, 2007). Consider reducing starting dose to 0.2 mcg/kg/minute in critically-ill patients with MODS defined as a minimum number of two organ failures. Another report of a cardiac patient with anasarca secondary to acute renal failure had a reduction in argatroban clearance similar to patients with hepatic dysfunction. Reduced clearance may have been due to reduced liver perfusion (de Denus, 2003). The American College of Chest Physicians has recommended an initial infusion rate of 0.5-1.2 mcg/kg/minute for patients with heart failure, MODS, severe anasarca, or postcardiac surgery (Hirsh, 2008).

Conversion to oral anticoagulant: Because there may be a combined effect on the INR when argatroban is combined with warfarin, loading doses of warfarin should not be used. Warfarin therapy should be started at the expected daily dose.

Patients receiving ≤2 mcg/kg/minute of argatroban: Argatroban therapy can be stopped when the combined INR on warfarin and argatroban is >4; repeat INR measurement in 4-6 hours; if INR is below therapeutic level, argatroban therapy may be restarted. Repeat procedure daily until desired INR on warfarin alone is obtained.

Patients receiving >2 mcg/kg/minute of argatroban: In order to predict the INR on warfarin alone, reduce dose of argatroban to 2 mcg/kg/minute; measure INR for argatroban and warfarin 4-6 hours after dose reduction; argatroban therapy can be stopped when the combined INR on warfarin and argatroban is >4. Repeat INR measurement in 4-6 hours; if INR is below therapeutic level, argatroban therapy may be restarted. Repeat procedure daily until desired INR on warfarin alone is obtained.

Note: The American College of Chest Physicians recommends monitoring chromogenic factor X assay when transitioning from argatroban to warfarin (Hirsh, 2008). Factor X levels <45% have been associated with INR values >2 after the effects of argatroban have been eliminated (Arpino, 2005).

Prefilter administration for continuous renal replacement therapy (CRRT) in critically-ill patients with HIT (unlabeled use; Link, 2009): 0.1-1.5 mcg/kg/minute. **Note:** Loading dose of 100 mcg/kg was administered during clinical trial; however, this may be unnecessary.

Percutaneous coronary intervention (PCI):

Initial: Begin infusion of 25 mcg/kg/minute and administer bolus dose of 350 mcg/kg (over 3-5 minutes). ACT should be checked 5-10 minutes after bolus infusion; proceed with procedure if ACT >300 seconds. **Note:** Pharmacokinetics and pharmacodynamics have not been evaluated prospectively in obese patients; however, retrospective data suggests using actual body weight to dose and that adjustment of initial dose is unnecessary in obesity (BMI up to 51 kg/m^2) (Hursting, 2008); weight range included in phase II and III clinical trials: 49-141 kg (actual body weight).

Following initial bolus:

ACT <300 seconds: Give an additional 150 mcg/kg bolus, and increase infusion rate to 30 mcg/kg/minute (recheck ACT in 5-10 minutes)

ACT >450 seconds: Decrease infusion rate to 15 mcg/kg/minute (recheck ACT in 5-10 minutes)

Once a therapeutic ACT (300-450 seconds) is achieved, infusion should be continued at this dose for the duration of the procedure.

If dissection, impending abrupt closure, thrombus formation during PCI, or inability to achieve ACT >300 seconds: An additional bolus of 150 mcg/kg, followed by an increase in infusion rate to 40 mcg/kg/minute may be administered.

Note: Post-PCI anticoagulation, if required, may be achieved by continuing infusion at a reduced dose of 2-10 mcg/kg/minute, with close monitoring of aPTT.

Elderly: No adjustment is necessary for patients with normal liver function

Dosage adjustment in renal impairment: Removal during hemodialysis and continuous venovenous hemofiltration is clinically insignificant. No dosage adjustment required.

Dosage adjustment in hepatic impairment: Decreased clearance and increased elimination half-life are seen with hepatic impairment; dose should be reduced.

Children: Initial dose: 0.2 mcg/kg/minute; adjust dose in increments of ≤0.05 mcg/kg/minute

Adults: Initial dose for moderate hepatic impairment is 0.5 mcg/kg/minute. **Note:** During PCI, avoid use in patients with elevations of ALT/AST (≥3 times ULN); the use of argatroban in these patients has not been evaluated.

Administration The 2.5 mL (100 mg/mL) **concentrated** vial **must be diluted to 1 mg/mL** prior to administration. The premixed 50 mL or 125 mL (1 mg/mL) vial requires no further dilution. The premixed 1 mg/mL vial may be inverted for use with an infusion set.

Monitoring Parameters Obtain baseline aPTT prior to start of therapy. Patient may not be at steady-state but check aPTT 2 hours after start of therapy to adjust dose, keeping the steady-state aPTT 1.5-3 times the initial baseline value (not exceeding 100 seconds). Monitor hemoglobin, hematocrit, signs and symptoms of bleeding.

PCI: Monitor ACT before dosing, 5-10 minutes after bolus dosing, and after any change in infusion rate and at the end of the procedure. Additional ACT assessments should be made every 20-30 minutes during extended PCI procedures.

Test Interactions Argatroban may elevate PT/INR levels in the absence of warfarin. If warfarin is started, initial PT/INR goals while on argatroban may require modification. The American College of Chest Physicians recommends monitoring chromogenic factor X assay when transitioning from argatroban to warfarin (Hirsh, 2008). Factor Xa levels <45% have been associated with INR values >2 after the effects of argatroban have been eliminated (Arpino, 2005).

Additional Information Platelet counts recovered by day 3 in 53% of patients with heparin-induced thrombocytopenia and in 58% of patients with heparin-induced thrombocytopenia with thrombosis syndrome.

Dosage Forms Excipient information presented when available (limited, particularly for generics); consult specific product labeling.

Infusion, premixed in NS: 125 mg (125 mL)

Infusion, premixed in water for injection: 50 mg (50 mL)

Injection, solution: 100 mg/mL (2.5 mL)

Arginine (AR ji neen)

Brand Names: U.S. R-Gene® 10

Index Terms Arginine HCl; Arginine Hydrochloride; L-Arginine; L-Arginine Hydrochloride

Pharmacologic Category Diagnostic Agent

Use Pituitary function test (growth hormone)

Unlabeled Use Management of severe, uncompensated, metabolic alkalosis (pH ≥7.55) **after** optimizing therapy with sodium and potassium supplements

Pregnancy Risk Factor B

Dosage I.V.: Pituitary function test:

Children: 0.5 g/kg/dose administered over 30 minutes

Adults: 30 g (300 mL) administered over 30 minutes

Additional Information Complete prescribing information for this medication should be consulted for additional detail.

Dosage Forms Excipient information presented when available (limited, particularly for generics); consult specific product labeling.

Injection, solution, as hydrochloride:

R-Gene® 10: 10% [100 mg/mL] (300 mL) [contains chloride 0.475 mEq/mL; 950 mOsm/L]

◆ **Arginine HCl** *see* Arginine *on page 142*
◆ **Arginine Hydrochloride** *see* Arginine *on page 142*
◆ **8-Arginine Vasopressin** *see* Vasopressin *on page 1775*
◆ **Aricept®** *see* Donepezil *on page 543*
◆ **Aricept® ODT** *see* Donepezil *on page 543*
◆ **Aricept® RDT (Can)** *see* Donepezil *on page 543*
◆ **Aridol™** *see* Mannitol *on page 1049*
◆ **Arimidex®** *see* Anastrozole *on page 121*

ARIPiprazole (ay ri PIP ray zole)

Brand Names: U.S. Abilify Discmelt®; Abilify®

Brand Names: Canada Abilify®

Index Terms BMS 337039; OPC-14597

Pharmacologic Category Antipsychotic Agent, Atypical

Additional Appendix Information

Antipsychotic Agents *on page 1880*

Use

Oral: Acute and maintenance treatment of schizophrenia; acute (manic and mixed episodes) and maintenance treatment of bipolar I disorder as monotherapy or as an adjunct to lithium or valproic acid; adjunctive treatment of major depressive disorder; treatment of irritability associated with autistic disorder

Injection: Agitation associated with schizophrenia or bipolar I disorder

Unlabeled Use Depression with psychotic features; aggression (children); conduct disorder (children); Tourette syndrome (children); psychosis/agitation related to Alzheimer's dementia

Pregnancy Risk Factor C

Pregnancy Considerations Aripiprazole demonstrated developmental toxicity and teratogenic effects in animal models. Antipsychotic use during the third trimester of pregnancy has a risk for abnormal muscle movements (extrapyramidal symptoms [EPS]) and withdrawal symptoms in newborns following delivery. Symptoms in the newborn may include agitation, feeding disorder, hypertonia, hypotonia, respiratory distress, somnolence, and tremor; these effects may be self-limiting or require hospitalization. Information specific to the use of aripiprazole in pregnancy is limited. Treatment algorithms have been developed by the ACOG and the APA for the management of depression in women prior to conception and during pregnancy (Yonkers, 2009). Healthcare providers are encouraged to enroll women 18-45 years of age exposed to aripiprazole during pregnancy in the Atypical Antipsychotics Pregnancy Registry (866-961-2388).

Lactation Excretion in breast milk unknown/not recommended

Medication Guide Available Yes

Contraindications Hypersensitivity to aripiprazole or any component of the formulation

Warnings/Precautions [U.S. Boxed Warning]: Elderly patients with dementia-related psychosis treated with antipsychotics are at an increased risk of death compared to placebo. Most deaths appeared to be either cardiovascular (eg, heart failure, sudden death) or infectious (eg, pneumonia) in nature. In addition, an increased incidence of cerebrovascular effects (eg, transient ischemic attack, cerebrovascular accidents) has been reported in studies of placebo-controlled trials of aripiprazole in elderly patients with dementia-related psychosis. Aripiprazole is not approved for the treatment of dementia-related psychosis.

[U.S. Boxed Warning]: Antidepressants increase the risk of suicidal thinking and behavior in children, adolescents, and young adults (18-24 years of age) with major depressive disorder (MDD) and other psychiatric disorders; consider risk prior to prescribing. The possibility of a suicide attempt is inherent in major depression and may persist until remission occurs. Patients treated with antidepressants should be observed for clinical worsening and suicidality, especially during the initial few months of a course of drug therapy, or at times of dose changes, either increases or decreases. Prescriptions should be written for the smallest quantity consistent with good patient care. The patient's family or caregiver should be alerted to monitor patients for the emergence of suicidality and associated behaviors; patients should be instructed to notify their healthcare provider if any of these symptoms or worsening depression or psychosis occur.

Leukopenia, neutropenia, and agranulocytosis (sometimes fatal) have been reported in clinical trials and postmarketing reports with antipsychotic use; presence of risk factors (eg, pre-existing low WBC or history of drug-induced leuko-/neutropenia) should prompt periodic blood count assessment. Discontinue therapy at first signs of blood dyscrasias or if absolute neutrophil count <1000/mm^3.

A medication guide concerning the use of antidepressants should be dispensed with each prescription. **Aripiprazole is not FDA approved for adjunctive treatment of depression in children.**

May cause extrapyramidal symptoms (EPS), including pseudoparkinsonism, acute dystonic reactions, akathisia, and tardive dyskinesia (risk of these reactions is very low relative to typical/conventional antipsychotics, frequencies reported are similar to placebo). Risk of dystonia (and probably other EPS) may be greater with increased doses, use of conventional antipsychotics, males, and younger patients. May be associated with neuroleptic malignant syndrome (NMS).

May be sedating, use with caution in disorders where CNS depression is a feature. May cause orthostatic hypotension (although reported rates are similar to placebo); use caution in patients at risk of this effect or those who would not tolerate transient hypotensive episodes (cerebrovascular disease, cardiovascular disease, or other medications which may predispose).

Use caution in patients with Parkinson's disease; predisposition to seizures; and severe cardiac disease. May alter cardiac conduction; life-threatening arrhythmias have occurred with therapeutic doses of antipsychotics. Esophageal dysmotility and aspiration have been associated with antipsychotic use; use caution in patients at risk of pneumonia (eg, Alzheimer's disease). May alter temperature regulation. Significant weight gain has been observed with antipsychotic therapy; incidence varies with product. Monitor waist circumference and BMI.

Atypical antipsychotics have been associated with development of hyperglycemia; in some cases, may be extreme and associated with ketoacidosis, hyperosmolar coma, or death. Reports of hyperglycemia with aripiprazole therapy have been few and specific risk associated with this agent is not known. Use caution in patients with diabetes or other disorders of glucose regulation; monitor for worsening of glucose control.

Tablets contain lactose; avoid use in patients with galactose intolerance or glucose-galactose malabsorption.

Abilify Discmelt®: Use caution in phenylketonuria; contains phenylalanine.

Adverse Reactions Unless otherwise noted, frequency of adverse reactions is shown as reported for adult patients receiving oral administration. Spectrum and incidence of adverse effects similar in children; exceptions noted when incidence much higher in children.

>10%:

Central nervous system: Headache (27%; injection 12%), agitation (19%), insomnia (18%), anxiety (17%), EPS (dose related; 5% to 16%; children 6% to 26%), akathisia (dose related; 8% to 13%; injection 2%), sedation (dose related; 5% to 11%; children 8% to 24%; injection 3% to 9%)

Gastrointestinal: Weight gain (2% to 30%; highest frequency in patients with baseline BMI <23 and prolonged use), nausea (15%; injection 9%), constipation (11%), vomiting (11%; children 9% to 14%; injection 3%), dyspepsia (9%)

1% to 10%:

Cardiovascular: Orthostatic hypotension (1% to 4%; injection 1% to 3%), tachycardia (injection 2%), chest pain, hypertension, peripheral edema

Central nervous system: Dizziness (10%; injection 8%), pyrexia (children 5% to 9%), restlessness (5% to 6%), fatigue (dose related; 6%; children 8% to 17%; injection 2%), lethargy (children 2% to 5%), lightheadedness (4%), pain (3%), dystonia (children 1%), hypersomnia (1%), irritability (children 1%), coordination impaired, suicidal ideation

Dermatologic: Rash (children 2%), hyperhidrosis

Endocrine & metabolic: Dysmenorrhea (children 2%)

Gastrointestinal: Salivation increased (dose related; children 4% to 9%), appetite decreased (children 4% to 7%), appetite increased (children 7%), xerostomia (5%), toothache (4%), abdominal discomfort (3%), diarrhea (children 5%), weight loss

Local: Injection site reaction (injection)

Neuromuscular & skeletal: Tremor (dose related; 5% to 6%; children 6% to 10%), extremity pain (4%), stiffness (4%), myalgia (2%), spasm (2%), arthralgia (children 1%), dyskinesia (children 1%), CPK increased, weakness

Ocular: Blurred vision (3%; children 3% to 8%)

Respiratory: Nasopharyngitis (children 6%), pharyngolaryngeal pain (3%), cough (3%), rhinorrhea (children 2%), aspiration pneumonia, dyspnea, nasal congestion

Miscellaneous: Thirst (children 1%)

<1% (Limited to important or life-threatening): Aggression, agranulocytosis, alopecia, akinesia, amenorrhea, anaphylactic reaction, anger, angina pectoris, angioedema, anorexia, anorgasmia, atrial fibrillation, atrial flutter, atrioventricular block, bilirubin increased, bradycardia, bradykinesia, breast pain, cardiopulmonary failure, cardiorespiratory arrest, catatonia, cerebrovascular accident, choreoathetosis, cogwheel rigidity, creatinine increased, delirium, diplopia, diabetes mellitus, DKA, dysphagia, edema (facial), erectile dysfunction, esophagitis, extrasystoles, GGT increased, glycosylated hemoglobin increased, gynecomastia, heat stroke, hepatic enzyme increased, hepatitis, homicidal ideation, hostility, hyper-/hypoglycemia, hyper-/hypotonia, hyperlipidemia, hypersensitivity, hypokalemia, hypokinesia, hyponatremia, hypotension, hypothermia, intentional self injury, jaundice, lactate dehydrogenase increased, leukopenia, libido changes, memory impairment, menstrual irregularities, MI, muscle rigidity, myocardial ischemia, myoclonus, neutropenia, nocturia, oropharyngeal spasm, palpitation, pancreatitis, parkinsonism, photophobia, polydypsia, polyuria, priapism, prolactin increased, pruritus, QT_c prolonged, rhabdomyolysis, seizure (grand mal), speech disorder, suicide, suicide attempt, supraventricular tachycardia, swollen tongue, syncope, tardive dyskinesia, thrombocytopenia, tic, urea increased, urinary retention, urticaria, ventricular tachycardia

Drug Interactions

Metabolism/Transport Effects Substrate of CYP2D6 (major), CYP3A4 (major); **Note:** Assignment of Major/Minor substrate status based on clinically relevant drug interaction potential

Avoid Concomitant Use

Avoid concomitant use of ARIPiprazole with any of the following: Conivaptan; Metoclopramide

Increased Effect/Toxicity

ARIPiprazole may increase the levels/effects of: Alcohol (Ethyl); CNS Depressants; Methotrimeprazine; Methylphenidate; Serotonin Modulators

The levels/effects of ARIPiprazole may be increased by: Abiraterone Acetate; Acetylcholinesterase Inhibitors (Central); Conivaptan; CYP2D6 Inhibitors (Moderate); CYP2D6 Inhibitors (Strong); CYP3A4 Inhibitors; CYP3A4 Inhibitors (Strong); Darunavir; Dasatinib; Droperidol; HydrOXYzine; Lithium formulations; Methotrimeprazine; Methylphenidate; Metoclopramide; Tetrabenazine

Decreased Effect

ARIPiprazole may decrease the levels/effects of: Amphetamines; Anti-Parkinson's Agents (Dopamine Agonist); Quinagolide

The levels/effects of ARIPiprazole may be decreased by: CYP3A4 Inducers; Deferasirox; Lithium formulations; Peginterferon Alfa-2b; Tocilizumab

Ethanol/Nutrition/Herb Interactions

Ethanol: May increase CNS depression; monitor for increased effects with coadministration. Caution patients about effects.

Food: Ingestion with a high-fat meal delays time to peak plasma level.

Herb/Nutraceutical: St John's wort may decrease aripiprazole levels. Avoid kava kava, gotu kola, valerian, St John's wort (may increase CNS depression).

Stability

Injection solution: Store at controlled room temperature of 25°C (77°F); excursions permitted to 15°C to 30°C (59°F to 86°F). Protect from light.

Oral solution: Store at controlled room temperature of 25°C (77°F); excursions permitted to 15°C to 30°C (59°F to 86°F). Use within 6 months after opening.

Tablet: Store at controlled room temperature of 25°C (77°F); excursions permitted to 15°C to 30°C (59°F to 86°F).

Mechanism of Action Aripiprazole is a quinolinone antipsychotic which exhibits high affinity for D_2, D_3, 5-HT_{1A}, and 5-HT_{2A} receptors; moderate affinity for D_4, 5-HT_{2C}, 5-HT_7, $alpha_1$ adrenergic, and H_1 receptors. It also possesses moderate affinity for the serotonin reuptake transporter; has no affinity for muscarinic (cholinergic) receptors. Aripiprazole functions as a partial agonist at the D_2 and 5-HT_{1A} receptors, and as an antagonist at the 5-HT_{2A} receptor.

Pharmacodynamics/Kinetics

Onset of action: Initial: 1-3 weeks

Absorption: Well absorbed

Distribution: V_d: 4.9 L/kg

Protein binding: ≥99%, primarily to albumin

Metabolism: Hepatic, via CYP2D6, CYP3A4 (dehydro-aripiprazole metabolite has affinity for D_2 receptors similar to the parent drug and represents 40% of the parent drug exposure in plasma)

Bioavailability: I.M.: 100%; Tablet: 87%

Half-life elimination: Aripiprazole: 75 hours; dehydro-aripiprazole: 94 hours

CYP2D6 poor metabolizers: Aripiprazole: 146 hours

Time to peak, plasma: I.M.: 1-3 hours; Tablet: 3-5 hours

With high-fat meal: Aripiprazole: Delayed by 3 hours; dehydro-aripiprazole: Delayed by 12 hours

Excretion: Feces (55%, ~18% of the total dose as unchanged drug); urine (25%, <1% of the total dose as unchanged drug)

Dosage Note: Oral solution may be substituted for the oral tablet on a mg-per-mg basis, up to 25 mg. Patients receiving 30 mg tablets should be given 25 mg oral solution. Orally disintegrating tablets (Abilify Discmelt®) are bioequivalent to the immediate release tablets (Abilify®).

Children: Oral: Aggression, conduct disorder, Tourette syndrome (unlabeled uses): 5-20 mg/day

Children ≥6 years: Oral: Irritability associated with autistic disorder: Initial: 2 mg daily for 7 days, followed by an increase to target dose of 5 mg daily; subsequent dose increases may be made in 5 mg increments at intervals of ≥1 week as needed, up to a maximum of 15 mg/day

Children ≥10 years: Oral: Bipolar I disorder (acute manic or mixed episodes): Initial: 2 mg daily for 2 days, followed by 5 mg daily for 2 days with a further increase to target dose of 10 mg daily as monotherapy or as adjunct to lithium or valproic acid; subsequent dose increases may be made in 5 mg increments, up to a maximum of 30 mg/day

Adolescents ≥13 years (U.S. labeling) or ≥15 years (Canadian labeling): Oral: Schizophrenia: Initial: 2 mg daily for 2 days, followed by 5 mg daily for 2 days with a further increase to target dose of 10 mg daily; subsequent dose increases may be made in 5 mg increments up to a maximum of 30 mg/day (30 mg/day not shown to be more efficacious than 10 mg/day)

Adults:

Acute agitation (schizophrenia/bipolar mania): I.M.: 9.75 mg as a single dose (range: 5.25-15 mg); repeated doses may be given at ≥2-hour intervals to a maximum of 30 mg/day. **Note:** If ongoing therapy with aripiprazole is necessary, transition to oral therapy as soon as possible.

Bipolar I disorder (acute manic or mixed episodes): Oral:

Stabilization:

Monotherapy: Initial: 15 mg once daily. May increase to 30 mg once daily if clinically indicated; safety of doses >30 mg/day has not been evaluated

Adjunct to lithium or valproic acid: Initial: 10-15 mg once daily. May increase to 30 mg once daily if clinically indicated; safety of doses >30 mg/day has not been evaluated.

Maintenance: Continue stabilization dose for up to 6 weeks; efficacy of continued treatment >6 weeks has not been established

Depression (adjunctive with antidepressants): Oral: Initial: 2-5 mg/day (range: 2-15 mg/day); dose adjustments of up to 5 mg/day may be made in intervals of ≥1 week. **Note:** Dosing based on patients already receiving antidepressant therapy.

Schizophrenia: Oral: 10-15 mg once daily; may be increased to a maximum of 30 mg once daily (efficacy at dosages above 10-15 mg has not been shown to be increased). Dosage titration should not be more frequent than every 2 weeks.

Dosage adjustment with concurrent CYP450 inducer or inhibitor therapy: Oral:

CYP3A4 inducers (eg, carbamazepine): Aripiprazole dose should be doubled (20-30 mg/day); dose should be subsequently reduced (10-15 mg/day) if concurrent inducer agent discontinued.

CYP3A4 inhibitors (eg, ketoconazole): Aripiprazole dose should be reduced to 1/2 of the usual dose, and proportionally increased upon discontinuation of the inhibitor agent.

CYP2D6 inhibitors (eg, fluoxetine, paroxetine): Aripiprazole dose should be reduced to 1/2 of the usual dose, and proportionally increased upon discontinuation of the inhibitor agent.

Dosage adjustment in renal impairment: No dosage adjustment required

Dosage adjustment in hepatic impairment: No dosage adjustment required

Dietary Considerations May be taken with or without food. Some products may contain phenylalanine.

Administration

Injection: For I.M. use only; do not administer SubQ or I.V.; inject slowly into deep muscle mass

Oral: May be administered with or without food. Tablet and oral solution may be interchanged on a mg-per-mg basis, up to 25 mg. Doses using 30 mg tablets should be exchanged for 25 mg oral solution. Orally disintegrating tablets (Abilify Discmelt®) are bioequivalent to the immediate release tablets (Abilify®).

Orally-disintegrating tablet: Remove from foil blister by peeling back (do not push tablet through the foil). Place tablet in mouth immediately upon removal. Tablet dissolves rapidly in saliva and may be swallowed without liquid. If needed, can be taken with liquid. Do not split tablet.

Monitoring Parameters Vital signs; fasting lipid profile and fasting blood glucose/Hb A_{1c} (prior to treatment, at 3 months, then annually); CBC frequently during first few months of therapy in patients with pre-existing low WBC or a history of drug-induced leukopenia/neutropenia; BMI, personal/family history of diabetes, waist circumference, blood pressure, mental status, abnormal involuntary movement scale (AIMS), extrapyramidal symptoms (EPS). Weight should be assessed prior to treatment, at 4 weeks, 8 weeks, 12 weeks, and then at quarterly intervals. Consider titrating to a different antipsychotic agent for a weight gain ≥5% of the initial weight.

Dosage Forms Excipient information presented when available (limited, particularly for generics); consult specific product labeling.

Injection, solution:

Abilify®: 7.5 mg/mL (1.3 mL)

Solution, oral:

Abilify®: 1 mg/mL (150 mL) [contains fructose 200 mg/mL, propylene glycol, sucrose 400 mg/mL; orange cream flavor]

Tablet, oral:

Abilify®: 2 mg, 5 mg, 10 mg, 15 mg, 20 mg, 30 mg

Tablet, orally disintegrating, oral:

Abilify Discmelt®: 10 mg [contains phenylalanine 1.12 mg/tablet; creme de vanilla flavor]

Abilify Discmelt®: 15 mg [contains phenylalanine 1.68 mg/tablet; creme de vanilla flavor]

◆ **Aristospan®** *see* Triamcinolone (Systemic) *on page 1732*

◆ **Arixtra®** *see* Fondaparinux *on page 752*

Armodafinil (ar moe DAF i nil)

Brand Names: U.S. Nuvigil®

Index Terms R-modafinil

Pharmacologic Category Stimulant

Use Improve wakefulness in patients with excessive daytime sleepiness associated with narcolepsy and shift work sleep disorder (SWSD); adjunctive therapy for obstructive sleep apnea/hypopnea syndrome (OSAHS)

Pregnancy Risk Factor C

Pregnancy Considerations There are no well-controlled studies of armodafinil in pregnant women. There have been reports of intrauterine growth retardation and spontaneous abortions in women using the both armodafinil and modafinil, but relationship to the drug is unknown.

Adverse events have been observed in animal studies. Armodafinil and modafinil have been studied in both rats and rabbits. Developmental toxicity (including visceral and skeletal abnormalities and decreased fetal weight) in rats (armodafinil and modafinil) and rabbits (modafinil) has been observed at doses correlating to those used clinically. Efficacy of steroidal contraceptives may be decreased; alternate means of contraception should be considered during therapy and for 1 month after modafinil is discontinued.

Lactation Excretion in breast milk unknown/use caution

Medication Guide Available Yes

Contraindications Hypersensitivity to armodafinil, modafinil, or any component of the formulation

Warnings/Precautions For use following complete evaluation of sleepiness and in conjunction with other standard treatments (eg, CPAP). The degree of sleepiness should be reassessed frequently; some patients may not return to a normal level of wakefulness. Use is not recommended with a history of angina, cardiac ischemia, recent history of myocardial infarction, left ventricular hypertrophy, or patients with mitral valve prolapse who have developed mitral valve prolapse syndrome with previous CNS stimulant use. Blood pressure monitoring may be required in patients on armodafinil. New or additional antihypertensive therapy may be needed.

Serious and life-threatening rashes including Stevens-Johnson syndrome, toxic epidermal necrolysis, and drug rash with eosinophilia and systemic symptoms have been reported with modafinil, the racemate of armodafinil. In clinical trials of modafinil, these rashes were more likely to occur in children; however, in the postmarketing period, serious reactions have occurred in both adults and children. Most cases have been reported within the first 5 weeks of initiating therapy; however, rare cases have occurred after prolonged therapy.

Caution should be exercised when modafinil is given to patients with a history of psychosis; may impair the ability to engage in potentially hazardous activities. Stimulants may unmask tics in individuals with coexisting Tourette's syndrome. Use caution with renal or hepatic impairment (dosage adjustment in hepatic dysfunction is recommended). Use reduced doses in elderly patients. Safety and efficacy in children <17 years of age have not been established.

Adverse Reactions

>10%: Central nervous system: Headache (14% to 23%; dose-related)

1% to 10%:

Cardiovascular: Palpitation (2%), increased heart rate (1%)

Central nervous system: Dizziness (5%), insomnia (4% to 6%; dose related), anxiety (4%), depression (1% to 3%; dose related), fatigue (2%), agitation (1%), attention disturbance (1%), depressed mood (1%), migraine (1%), nervousness (1%), pain (1%), pyrexia (1%), tremor (1%)

Dermatologic: Rash (1% to 4%; dose related), contact dermatitis (1%), hyperhidrosis (1%)

Gastrointestinal: Nausea (6% to 9%; dose related), xerostomia (2% to 7%; dose related), diarrhea (4%), abdominal pain (2%), dyspepsia (2%), anorexia (1%), appetite decreased (1%), constipation (1%), loose stools (1%), vomiting (1%)

Genitourinary: Polyuria (1%)

Hepatic: GGT increased (1%)

Neuromuscular & skeletal: Paresthesia (1%)

Respiratory: Dyspnea (1%)

Miscellaneous: Flu-like syndrome (1%), thirst (1%)

Postmarketing and/or case reports: Anaphylactoid reaction, angioedema, hypersensitivity, liver enzymes increased, pancytopenia, systolic blood pressure increased

Drug Interactions

Metabolism/Transport Effects **Substrate** of CYP3A4 (major); **Note:** Assignment of Major/Minor substrate status based on clinically relevant drug interaction potential; **Inhibits** CYP2C19 (moderate); **Induces** CYP3A4 (weak/moderate)

Avoid Concomitant Use

Avoid concomitant use of Armodafinil with any of the following: Clopidogrel; Conivaptan; Iobenguane I 123

Increased Effect/Toxicity

Armodafinil may increase the levels/effects of: Citalopram; CYP2C19 Substrates; Sympathomimetics

The levels/effects of Armodafinil may be increased by: Atomoxetine; Cannabinoids; Conivaptan; CYP3A4 Inhibitors (Moderate); CYP3A4 Inhibitors (Strong); Dasatinib; Linezolid

Decreased Effect

Armodafinil may decrease the levels/effects of: ARIPiprazole; Clopidogrel; Contraceptives (Estrogens); CycloSPORINE; CycloSPORINE (Systemic); Iobenguane I 123; Saxagliptin

The levels/effects of Armodafinil may be decreased by: CYP3A4 Inducers (Strong); Deferasirox; Herbs (CYP3A4 Inducers); Tocilizumab

Ethanol/Nutrition/Herb Interactions

Ethanol: Avoid or limit ethanol.

Food: Delays absorption, but minimal effects on bioavailability. Food may affect the onset and time course of armodafinil.

Stability Store at 20°C to 25°C (68°F to 77°F).

Mechanism of Action The exact mechanism of action of armodafinil is unknown. It is the R-enantiomer of modafinil. Armodafinil binds to the dopamine transporter and inhibits dopamine reuptake, which may result in increased extracellular dopamine levels in the brain. However, it does not appear to be a dopamine receptor agonist and also does not appear to bind to or inhibit the most common receptors or enzymes that are relevant for sleep/wake regulation.

Pharmacodynamics/Kinetics

Absorption: Readily absorbed

Distribution: V_d: 42 L

Protein binding: ~60% (based on modafinil; primarily albumin)

Metabolism: Hepatic, multiple pathways, including CYP3A4/5; metabolites include R-modafinil acid and modafinil sulfone

Clearance: 33 mL/minute, mainly via hepatic metabolism

Half-life elimination: 15 hours; Steady state: ~7 days

Time to peak, plasma: 2 hours (fasted)

Excretion: Urine (80% predominantly as metabolites; <10% as unchanged drug)

Dosage Oral:

Adults:

Narcolepsy: 150-250 mg once daily in the morning

Obstructive sleep apnea/hypopnea syndrome (OSAHS): 150-250 mg once daily in the morning; 250 mg was not shown to have any increased benefit over 150 mg

Shift work sleep disorder (SWSD): 150 mg given once daily ~1 hour prior to work shift

Elderly: Consider lower initial dosage. Concentrations were almost doubled in clinical trials (based on modafinil)

Dosage adjustment in renal impairment: Inadequate data to determine safety and efficacy in severe renal impairment.

Dosage adjustment in hepatic impairment: Severe hepatic impairment (Child-Pugh classes B and C): Based on modafinil, dose should be reduced by half

Dietary Considerations Take with or without meals.

Administration May be administered without regard to food.

Monitoring Parameters Signs of hypersensitivity, rash, psychiatric symptoms, levels of sleepiness, blood pressure, and drug abuse

Dosage Forms Excipient information presented when available (limited, particularly for generics); consult specific product labeling.

Tablet, oral:

Nuvigil®: 50 mg, 150 mg, 250 mg

Controlled Substance C-IV

- **Armour® Thyroid** *see* Thyroid, Desiccated *on page 1676*
- **Aromasin®** *see* Exemestane *on page 677*
- **Arranon®** *see* Nelarabine *on page 1184*

Arsenic Trioxide (AR se nik tri OKS id)

Brand Names: U.S. Trisenox®

Index Terms As_2O_3

Pharmacologic Category Antineoplastic Agent, Miscellaneous

Use Remission induction and consolidation in patients with relapsed or refractory acute promyelocytic leukemia (APL) characterized by t(15;17) translocation or PML/RAR-alpha gene expression

Unlabeled Use Initial treatment of APL, treatment of myelodysplastic syndrome (MDS)

Pregnancy Risk Factor D

Pregnancy Considerations Increased resorptions, neural-tube defects, and ophthalmic abnormalities have been observed in animal studies. Arsenic crosses the human placenta. In studies of women exposed to high levels of arsenic from drinking water, cord blood levels were similar to maternal serum levels. Dimethylarsinic acid (DMA) was the form of arsenic found in the fetus. An increased risk of low birth weight and still births were observed in women who ingested high levels of dietary arsenic. Women of childbearing potential should avoid pregnancy.

Lactation Enters breast milk/not recommended

Contraindications Hypersensitivity to arsenic or any component of the formulation

Warnings/Precautions Hazardous agent - use appropriate precautions for handling and disposal. **[U.S. Boxed Warnings]: May prolong the QT interval. May lead to torsade de pointes or complete AV block.** Risk factors for torsade de pointes include extent of prolongation, HF, a history of torsade de pointes, pre-existing QT interval prolongation, patients taking medications know to prolong the QT interval or potassium-wasting diuretics, and conditions which cause hypokalemia or hypomagnesemia. If possible, discontinue all medications known to prolong the QT interval. **[U.S. Boxed Warning]: A baseline 12-lead ECG, serum electrolytes (potassium, calcium, magnesium), and creatinine should be obtained prior to treatment.** Correct electrolyte abnormalities prior to treatment and monitor potassium and magnesium levels during therapy (maintain potassium >4 mEq/dL and magnesium >1.8 mg/dL). If baseline QT_c >500 msec, correct prior to treatment. If QT_c >500 msec during treatment, reassess, correct contributing factors, and consider temporarily withholding treatment. If syncope or irregular heartbeat develop during therapy, hospitalize patient and do not reinitiate until QT_c <460 msec, electrolyte abnormalities are corrected and syncope/irregular heartbeat has resolved. Monitor ECG weekly; more frequently if clinically indicated.

[U.S. Boxed Warning]: May cause APL differentiation syndrome (formerly called retinoic-acid-APL [RA-APL] syndrome) in patients with APL, which is characterized by dyspnea, fever, weight gain, pulmonary infiltrates, and pleural or pericardial effusions. May be fatal. High-dose steroids (dexamethasone 10 mg I.V. twice daily for ≥3 days; begin at initial presentation) have been used for treatment; in general, most patients may continue arsenic trioxide during treatment of APL differentiation syndrome. May lead to the development of hyperleukocytosis (leukocytes ≥10,000/mm^3); did not correlate with baseline WBC counts and generally was not as high during consolidation as observed during induction treatment. Use with caution in patients with hepatic impairment; in patients with severe hepatic impairment, monitor closely for toxicity. Use with caution in patients with severe renal impairment; systemic exposure to metabolites may be higher; has not been studied in dialysis patients. Monitor electrolytes, CBC with differential, and coagulation parameters at least twice a week during induction and weekly during consolidation; more frequently if clinically indicated. **[U.S. Boxed Warning]: Should be administered under the supervision of a physician experienced in acute leukemia management.**

Adverse Reactions

>10%:

Cardiovascular: Tachycardia (55%), edema (40%), QT interval >500 msec (40%), chest pain (25%; grades 3/4: 5%), hypotension (25%; grades 3/4: 5%)

Central nervous system: Fatigue (63%), fever (63%), headache (60%), insomnia (43%), anxiety (30%), dizziness (23%), depression (20%), pain (15%)

Dermatologic: Dermatitis (43%), pruritus (33%), bruising (20%), dry skin (15%), erythema (13%)

Endocrine & metabolic: Hypokalemia (50%; grades 3/4: 13%), hyperglycemia (45%; grades 3/4: 13%), hypomagnesemia (45%; grades 3/4: 13%), hyperkalemia (18%; grades 3/4: 5%)

Gastrointestinal: Nausea (75%), abdominal pain (58%), vomiting (58%), diarrhea (53%), sore throat (35%), constipation (28%), anorexia (23%), appetite decreased (15%), weight gain (13%)

Genitourinary: Vaginal hemorrhage (13%)

Hematologic: Leukocytosis (50%; grades 3/4: 3%), APL differentiation syndrome (23%; grades 3/4: 8%), anemia (20%; grades 3/4: 5%), thrombocytopenia (18%; grades 3/4: 13%), febrile neutropenia (13%; grades 3/4: 8%)

Hepatic: ALT increased (20%; grades 3/4: 5%), AST increased (13%; grades 3/4: 3%)

Local: Injection site: Pain (20%), erythema (13%)

Neuromuscular & skeletal: Rigors (38%), arthralgia (33%), paresthesia (33%), myalgia (25%), bone pain (23%), back pain (18%), limb pain (13%), neck pain (13%), tremor (13%)

Respiratory: Cough (65%), dyspnea (53%; grades 3/4: 10%), epistaxis (25%), hypoxia (23%), pleural effusion (20%), sinusitis (20%), postnasal drip (13%), upper respiratory tract infection (13%), wheezing (13%)

Miscellaneous: Herpes simplex (13%), diaphoresis (13%)

1% to 10%:

Cardiovascular: Hypertension (10%), flushing (10%), pallor (10%), palpitation (10%), facial edema (8%), abnormal ECG (not QT prolongation) (8%), atrial dysrhythmia (5%), torsade de pointes (3%)

Central nervous system: Seizure (8%; grades 3/4: 5%), somnolence (8%), agitation (5%), coma (5%), confusion (5%)

Dermatologic: Hyperpigmentation (8%), petechia (8%), skin lesions (8%), urticaria (8%), local exfoliation (5%)

Endocrine & metabolic: Hypocalcemia (10%), hypoglycemia (8%), intermenstrual bleeding (8%), acidosis (5%)

Gastrointestinal: Dyspepsia (10%), loose stools (10%), abdominal distension (8%), abdominal tenderness (8%), caecitis (children: 8%), fecal incontinence (8%), gastrointestinal hemorrhage (8%), hemorrhagic diarrhea (8%), oral blistering (8%), weight loss (8%), xerostomia (8%), oral candidiasis (5%)

Genitourinary: Incontinence (5%)

Hematologic: Neutropenia (10%; grades 3/4: 10%), DIC (8%), hemorrhage (8%)

Local: Injection site edema (10%)

Neuromuscular & skeletal: Weakness (10%)

Ocular: Blurred vision (10%), eye irritation (10%), dry eye (8%), eyelid edema (5%), painful red eye (5%)

Otic: Earache (8%), tinnitus (5%)

Renal: Renal failure (8%; grades 3/4: 3%), renal impairment (8%), oliguria (5%)

Respiratory: Breath sounds decreased (10%), crepitations (10%), rales (10%), hemoptysis (8%), pulmonary edema (children: 8%), rhonchi (8%), tachypnea (8%), nasopharyngitis (5%)

Miscellaneous: Bacterial infection (8%), herpes zoster (8%), lymphadenopathy (8%), night sweats (8%), hypersensitivity (5%), sepsis (5%; grades 3/4: 5%)

<1% (Limited to important or life-threatening): Acute respiratory distress syndrome, AV block, capillary leak syndrome, CHF, heart block, hypoalbuminemia, hyponatremia, hypophosphatemia, lipase increased, pancytopenia, peripheral neuropathy, pneumonitis, pulmonary infiltrate, respiratory distress, stomatitis, ventricular extrasystoles, ventricular tachycardia

Drug Interactions

Metabolism/Transport Effects None known.

Avoid Concomitant Use

Avoid concomitant use of Arsenic Trioxide with any of the following: Artemether; CloZAPine; Dronedarone; Lumefantrine; Nilotinib; Pimozide; QUEtiapine; QuiNINE; Tetrabenazine; Thioridazine; Toremifene; Vandetanib; Vemurafenib; Ziprasidone

Increased Effect/Toxicity

Arsenic Trioxide may increase the levels/effects of: CloZAPine; Dronedarone; Hypoglycemic Agents; Pimozide; QTc-Prolonging Agents; QuiNINE; Tetrabenazine; Thioridazine; Toremifene; Vandetanib; Vemurafenib; Ziprasidone

The levels/effects of Arsenic Trioxide may be increased by: Alfuzosin; Artemether; Chloroquine; Ciprofloxacin; Ciprofloxacin (Systemic); Gadobutrol; Herbs (Hypoglycemic Properties); Indacaterol; Lumefantrine; Nilotinib; QUEtiapine; QuiNINE

Decreased Effect There are no known significant interactions involving a decrease in effect.

Ethanol/Nutrition/Herb Interactions Herb/Nutraceutical: Avoid homeopathic products (arsenic is present in some homeopathic medications). Avoid hypoglycemic herbs, including alfalfa, aloe, bilberry, bitter melon, burdock, celery, damiana, fenugreek, garcinia, garlic, ginger, ginseng, gymnema, marshmallow, and stinging nettle (may enhance the hypoglycemic effect of arsenic trioxide).

Stability Store at 25°C (77°F); excursions permitted to 15°C to 30°C (59°F to 86°F); do not freeze. Following dilution, stable for 24 hours at room temperature or 48 hours when refrigerated. Dilute in 100-250 mL D_5W or 0.9% NaCl. Discard unused portion of ampul. Use appropriate precautions for handling and disposal.

Mechanism of Action Induces apoptosis in APL cells via morphological changes and DNA fragmentation; also damages or degrades the fusion protein PML-RAR alpha

Pharmacodynamics/Kinetics

Distribution: V_{dss}: As^{III}: 562 L; widely distributed throughout body tissues; orally administered arsenic trioxide distributes into the CNS

Metabolism: Arsenic trioxide is immediately hydrolyzed to the active form, arsenious acid (As^{III}) which is methylated (hepatically) to the less active pentavalent metabolites, monomethylarsonic acid (MMA^V) and dimethylarsinic acid (DMA^V) by methyltransferases; As^{III} is also oxidized to the minor metabolite, arsenic acid (As^V)

Half-life elimination: AS^{III}: 10-14 hours; MMA^V: ~32 hours; DMA^V: ~72 hours

Time to peak: As^{III}: At the end of infusion; MMA^V and DMA^V; ~10-24 hours

Excretion: Urine (MMA^V, DMA^V, and 15% of a dose as unchanged As^{III})

Dosage I.V.:

APL, relapsed or refractory: Children ≥4 years and Adults:

Induction: 0.15 mg/kg/day; administer daily until bone marrow remission; maximum induction: 60 doses

Consolidation: 0.15 mg/kg/day starting 3-6 weeks after completion of induction therapy; maximum consolidation: 25 doses over a period of up to 5 weeks

APL initial treatment (unlabeled use):

Children: Induction, consolidation, and maintenance (Mathews, 2006):

Induction: 0.15 mg/kg/day (maximum dose: 10 mg); administer daily until bone marrow remission; maximum induction: 60 doses

Consolidation: 0.15 mg/kg/day (maximum dose: 10 mg) for 4 weeks, starting 4 weeks after completion of induction therapy

Maintenance: 0.15 mg/kg/dose (maximum dose: 10 mg) administered 10 days per month for 6 months, starting 4 weeks after completion of consolidation therapy

Adults:

Induction, consolidation, and maintenance (Mathews, 2006):

Induction: 10 mg/day; administer daily until bone marrow remission; maximum induction: 60 doses

Consolidation: 10 mg/day for 4 weeks, starting 4 weeks after completion of induction therapy

Maintenance: 10 mg/dose administered 10 days per month for 6 months, starting 4 weeks after completion of consolidation therapy

Consolidation therapy after remission induction with tretinoin, daunorubicin and cytarabine (Powell, 2007; Powell, 2010): Two consolidation courses (2 weeks apart): 0.15 mg/kg/day 5 days/week for 5 weeks

In combination with tretinoin (Estey, 2006; Ravandi, 2009):

Induction (beginning 10 days after initiation of tretinoin): 0.15 mg/kg/day until bone marrow remission; maximum induction: 75 doses

Consolidation: 0.15 mg/kg/day Monday through Friday for 4 weeks every 8 weeks for 4 cycles (weeks 1 to 4, 9 to 12, 17 to 20, and 25 to 28)

MDS (unlabeled uses): Adults: 0.25 mg/kg/day 5 consecutive days/week for 2 weeks, followed by a 2-week rest period (Schiller, 2006)

Dosage adjustment in renal impairment:

Severe renal impairment (Cl_{cr} <30 mL/minute): Use with caution (systemic exposure to metabolites may be higher); may require dosage reduction; monitor closely for toxicity

Dialysis patients: Has not been studied

Dosage adjustment in hepatic impairment:

Hepatic impairment: Use with caution

Severe hepatic impairment (Child-Pugh class C): Monitor closely for toxicity

Administration Administer as I.V. infusion over 1-2 hours. If acute vasomotor reactions occur, infuse over a maximum of 4 hours. Does not require administration via a central venous catheter.

Monitoring Parameters Baseline then weekly 12-lead ECG; monitor electrolytes, CBC with differential, and coagulation at baseline then at least twice weekly during induction and at least weekly during consolidation; more frequent monitoring may be necessary in unstable patients

Dosage Forms Excipient information presented when available (limited, particularly for generics); consult specific product labeling.

Injection, solution [preservative free]:

Trisenox®: 1 mg/mL (10 mL)

◆ **Artane** *see* Trihexyphenidyl *on page 1738*

◆ **Artemether and Benflumetol** *see* Artemether and Lumefantrine *on page 148*

Artemether and Lumefantrine

(ar TEM e ther & loo me FAN treen)

Brand Names: U.S. Coartem®

Index Terms Artemether and Benflumetol; Benflumetol and Artemether; Lumefantrine and Artemether

Pharmacologic Category Antimalarial Agent

Use Treatment of acute, uncomplicated malaria infections due to *Plasmodium falciparum*, including geographical regions where chloroquine resistance has been reported

Pregnancy Risk Factor C

Dosage Oral: Three-day schedule for the treatment of uncomplicated malaria (chloroquine-resistant uncomplicated *P. falciparum*):

Children 2 months to ≤16 years:

5 to <15 kg: One tablet at hour 0 and hour 8 on the first day, then 1 tablet twice daily on day 2 and day 3 (total of 6 tablets per treatment course)

15 to <25 kg: Two tablets at hour 0 and hour 8 on the first day, then 2 tablets twice daily on day 2 and day 3 (total of 12 tablets per treatment course)

25 to <35 kg: Three tablets at hour 0 and hour 8 on the first day, then 3 tablets twice daily on day 2 and day 3 (total of 18 tablets per treatment course)

≥35 kg: Four tablets at hour 0 and hour 8 on the first day, then 4 tablets twice daily on day 2 and day 3 (total of 24 tablets per treatment course)

Children >16 years and Adults:

25 to <35 kg: Three tablets at hour 0 and hour 8 on the first day, then 3 tablets twice daily on day 2 and day 3 (total of 18 tablets per treatment course)

≥35 kg: Four tablets at hour 0 and hour 8 on the first day, then 4 tablets twice daily on day 2 and day 3 (total of 24 tablets per treatment course)

Dosage adjustment in renal impairment: Not adequately studied in renal impairment; however, no specific dosage adjustments are recommended in mild or moderate impairment. Use caution in severe renal impairment.

Dosage adjustment in hepatic impairment: Not adequately studied in hepatic impairment; however, no specific dosage adjustments are recommended in mild or moderate impairment. Use caution in severe impairment.

Additional Information Complete prescribing information for this medication should be consulted for additional detail.

Dosage Forms Excipient information presented when available (limited, particularly for generics); consult specific product labeling.

Tablet:

Coartem®: Artemether 20 mg and lumefantrine 120 mg

◆ **Artemisinin Derivative** *see* Artesunate *on page 148*

Artesunate (ar TES oo nate)

Index Terms Artemisinin Derivative; Artesunic Acid; Dihydroartemisinin Hemisuccinate Sodium; Dihydroqinghaosu Hemisuccinate Sodium; Nuartez™; P01BE03; Qinghao Derivative; Qinghaosu Derivative; Sodium Artesunate

Pharmacologic Category Antimalarial Agent; Artemisinin Derivative

Unlabeled Use Treatment of severe malaria

Pregnancy Considerations Teratogenic effects have been observed in animal reproduction studies. Limited studies in pregnant women have not revealed an increased risk of congenital abnormalities in newborns (McGready, 1998; McGready, 2008). Malaria infection in pregnant women may be more severe than in nonpregnant women. Because *P. falciparum* malaria can cause maternal death, congenital malaria, and fetal loss, pregnant women traveling to malaria-endemic areas must use personal protection against mosquito bites.

Prescribing and Access Restrictions Investigational agent – not approved for use in the U.S.

Artesunate is available in the U.S. for I.V. use in patients with malaria through an Investigational New Drug (IND) protocol. To obtain artesunate via the IND protocol, clinicians must contact the Centers for Disease Control (CDC) Malaria Hotline at 770-488-7788 (business hours) or 770-488-7100 (nonbusiness hours) and request to speak with a CDC Malaria Branch clinician.

Eligibility criteria under the IND protocol include (Hess, 2010):

- **Patients must have malaria:** Diagnosis by microscopy or strong clinical suspicion of *Plasmodium falciparum* or other *Plasmodium* spp. infection
- **Patients must require parenteral therapy:** Unable to take oral medications, high-density parasitemia (eg, >5%), or diagnosis of severe malaria
- **I.V. artesunate must be the preferred treatment:** I.V. artesunate is at least as readily available as I.V. quinidine or the patient has experienced quinidine failure (eg, parasitemia >10% baseline after 48 hours of quinidine therapy), quinidine intolerance, or contraindications to quinidine

For medical access to I.V. artesunate in Canada, please refer to special access information on the Public Health Agency of Canada website, http://www.phac-aspc.gc.ca/tmp-pmv/quinine/.

Contraindications Hypersensitivity to artesunate or any component of the formulation (Hess, 2010)

Warnings/Precautions Severe allergic reactions have been reported with oral administration of artesunate (Leonardi, 2001); monitor for signs of hypersensitivity and discontinue treatment in patients who develop severe hypersensitivity reactions (eg, angioedema, dyspnea, erythema, anaphylaxis). QT prolongation has been reported with other artemisinin derivatives (eg, artemether); however, one report suggests that the mean QT_c interval was unaffected by artesunate (Maude, 2010).

Adverse Reactions Frequency not defined.

Cardiovascular: Hypotension

Central nervous system: Anxiety, dizziness, headache, restlessness, slurred speech

Dermatologic: Angioedema, erythema, pruritus, rash, urticaria

Endocrine & metabolic: Hypoglycemia

Gastrointestinal: Anorexia, diarrhea, metallic taste, nausea, vomiting

Hematologic: Anemia, hemolysis, neutropenia, reticulocytopenia

Hepatic: ALT increased

Neuromuscular & skeletal: Ataxia, hyperreflexia, tremor

Renal: BUN increased

Respiratory: Dyspnea

Miscellaneous: Hypersensitivity reaction

Stability Reconstitute vial with 11 mL of phosphate buffer diluent to a final concentration of 10 mg/mL; gently swirl for 5-6 minutes to mix. Resulting solution is stable for 1 hour after reconstitution.

Mechanism of Action

Artesunate, a semisynthetic derivative of artemisinin, is a prodrug which is converted to dihydroartemisinin (DHA). DHA is an antimalarial agent active against all of the erythrocytic stages of the parasite including gametocytes; inhibits parasite metabolism and enhances the clearance of infected erythrocytes.

Antiparasitic activity is hypothesized to involve cleavage of the $Fe^{2+}$of endoperoxide bridge, thereby producing free radicals and damaging parasite proteins. DHA may also inhibit calcium adenosine triphosphatase (cATP) of the sarcoplasmic endoplasmic reticulum and impair parasite protein folding.

Pharmacodynamics/Kinetics

Distribution: V_{dss}: Adults infected with severe malaria: Artesunate: 15.2 L/kg (range: 2.2-39 L/kg); Dihydroartemisinin (DHA): 1.9 L/kg (range: 0.8-11.5 L/kg) (Newton, 2006)

Protein binding: Dihydroartemisinin (DHA): 47% to 76%

Metabolism: Artesunate (prodrug) is rapidly hydrolyzed to an active metabolite, dihydroartemisinin (DHA). DHA undergoes hepatic metabolism via CYP2B6, CYP2C19, and CYP3A4 to inactive metabolites (Hess, 2010).

Half-life elimination: Artesunate: Adults infected with severe malaria: 0.22 hours (range: 0.08-0.61 hours); Dihydroartesiminin (DHA): 0.34 hours (range: 0.14-0.87 hours) (Newton, 2006)

Time to peak: Dihyrdoartemisinin (DHA): Adults infected with severe malaria: Within 15 minutes (Newton, 2006)

Dosage I.V.: Children and Adults: 2.4 mg/kg/dose initially, followed by 2.4 mg/kg/dose at 12 hours, 24 hours, and 48 hours after the initial dose for a total of 4 doses over a period of 3 days; longer treatment duration (eg, an additional 4 days [Hess, 2010]) may be required in severely-ill patients or in patients unable to transition to oral therapy (Hess, 2010; Rosenthal, 2008). **Note:** Because of the short half-life of artesunate and a high risk of recrudescence, oral antimalarial therapy must begin ≤4 hours after the last I.V. artesunate infusion. Appropriate oral therapies include atovaquone-proguanil, doxycycline (in patients >8 years of age and nonpregnant adults), clindamycin, **or** mefloquine (CDC, 2009, Hess, 2010; Rosenthal, 2008).

Dosage adjustment in renal impairment: No dosage adjustment necessary (Rosenthal, 2008).

Dosage adjustment in hepatic impairment: No dosage adjustment necessary (Rosenthal, 2008).

Administration I.V.: Administer via I.V. bolus over 1–2 minutes through a 0.8-micron hydrophilic polyethersulfone filter (Hess, 2010)

- ◆ **Artesunic Acid** *see* Artesunate *on page 148*
- ◆ **Arthrotec®** *see* Diclofenac and Misoprostol *on page 498*
- ◆ **Arzerra™** *see* Ofatumumab *on page 1229*
- ◆ **As_2O_3** *see* Arsenic Trioxide *on page 146*
- ◆ **ASA** *see* Aspirin *on page 154*
- ◆ **5-ASA** *see* Mesalamine *on page 1081*
- ◆ **ASA and Diphenhydramine** *see* Aspirin and Diphenhydramine *on page 157*
- ◆ **Asacol®** *see* Mesalamine *on page 1081*
- ◆ **Asacol® 800 (Can)** *see* Mesalamine *on page 1081*
- ◆ **Asacol® HD** *see* Mesalamine *on page 1081*
- ◆ **Asaphen (Can)** *see* Aspirin *on page 154*
- ◆ **Asaphen E.C. (Can)** *see* Aspirin *on page 154*
- ◆ **Asclera™** *see* Polidocanol *on page 1370*
- ◆ **Asco-Caps-500 [OTC]** *see* Ascorbic Acid *on page 149*
- ◆ **Asco-Caps-1000 [OTC]** *see* Ascorbic Acid *on page 149*
- ◆ **Ascocid® [OTC]** *see* Ascorbic Acid *on page 149*
- ◆ **Ascocid®-500 [OTC]** *see* Ascorbic Acid *on page 149*
- ◆ **Ascor L 500® [DSC]** *see* Ascorbic Acid *on page 149*
- ◆ **Ascor L NC® [DSC]** *see* Ascorbic Acid *on page 149*

Ascorbic Acid (a SKOR bik AS id)

Brand Names: U.S. Acerola [OTC]; Asco-Caps-1000 [OTC]; Asco-Caps-500 [OTC]; Asco-Tabs-1000 [OTC];

Ascocid® [OTC]; Ascocid®-500 [OTC]; Ascor L 500® [DSC]; Ascor L NC® [DSC]; C-Gel [OTC]; C-Gram [OTC]; C-Time [OTC]; Cemill 1000 [OTC]; Cemill 500 [OTC]; Chew-C [OTC]; Dull-C® [OTC]; Mild-C® [OTC]; One Gram C [OTC]; Time-C® [OTC]; Vicks® Vitamin C [OTC]; Vita-C® [OTC]

Brand Names: Canada Proflavanol C™; Revitalose C-1000®

Index Terms Vitamin C

Pharmacologic Category Vitamin, Water Soluble

Use Prevention and treatment of scurvy; acidify the urine

Unlabeled Use In large doses, to decrease the severity of "colds"; dietary supplementation; a 20-year study was recently completed involving 730 individuals which indicates a possible decreased risk of death by stroke when ascorbic acid at doses ≥45 mg/day was administered

Pregnancy Risk Factor A/C (dose exceeding RDA recommendation)

Dosage Oral, I.M., I.V., SubQ:

Recommended adequate intake (AI):

0-6 months: 40 mg

6-12 months: 50 mg

Recommended daily allowance (RDA):

1-3 years: 15 mg; upper limit of intake should not exceed 400 mg/day

4-8 years: 25 mg; upper limit of intake should not exceed 650 mg/day

9-13 years: 45 mg; upper limit of intake should not exceed 1200 mg/day

14-18 years: Upper limit of intake should not exceed 1800 mg/day

Males: 75 mg

Females: 65 mg

Adults: Upper limit of intake should not exceed 2000 mg/day

Males: 90 mg

Females: 75 mg

Pregnant females:

≤18 years: 80 mg; upper limit of intake should not exceed 1800 mg/day

19-50 years: 85 mg; upper limit of intake should not exceed 2000 mg/day

Lactating females:

≤18 years: 115 mg; upper limit of intake should not exceed 1800 mg/day

19-50 years: 120 mg; upper limit of intake should not exceed 2000 mg/day

Adult smoker: Add an additional 35 mg/day

Children:

Scurvy: 100-300 mg/day in divided doses for at least 2 weeks

Urinary acidification: 500 mg every 6-8 hours

Dietary supplement: 35-100 mg/day

Adults:

Scurvy: 100-250 mg 1-2 times/day for at least 2 weeks

Urinary acidification: 4-12 g/day in 3-4 divided doses

Prevention and treatment of colds: 1-3 g/day

Dietary supplement: 50-200 mg/day

Additional Information Complete prescribing information for this medication should be consulted for additional detail.

Dosage Forms Excipient information presented when available (limited, particularly for generics); consult specific product labeling. [DSC] = Discontinued product

Caplet, oral: 1000 mg

Caplet, timed release, oral: 500 mg, 1000 mg

Capsule, oral:

Mild-C®: 500 mg

Capsule, softgel, oral:

C-Gel: 1000 mg

Capsule, sustained release, oral:

C-Time: 500 mg

Capsule, timed release, oral: 500 mg

Asco-Caps-500: 500 mg

Asco-Caps-1000: 1000 mg [sugar free]

Time-C®: 500 mg

Crystals for solution, oral: (170 g, 1000 g)

Mild-C®: (170 g, 1000 g)

Vita-C®: (113 g, 454 g) [dye free, gluten free, sugar free]

Injection, solution: 500 mg/mL (50 mL)

Ascor L 500®: 500 mg/mL (50 mL [DSC]) [contains edetate disodium]

Injection, solution [preservative free]: 500 mg/mL (50 mL)

Ascor L NC®: 500 mg/mL (50 mL [DSC]) [contains edetate disodium]

Liquid, oral: 500 mg/5 mL (118 mL, 473 mL)

Lozenge, oral:

Vicks® Vitamin C: 25 mg (20s) [contains sodium 5 mg/lozenge; orange flavor]

Powder for solution, oral:

Ascocid®: (227 g, 454 g)

Dull-C®: (113 g, 454 g) [dye free, gluten free, sugar free]

Tablet, oral: 100 mg, 250 mg, 500 mg, 1000 mg

Asco-Tabs-1000: 1000 mg [sugar free]

Ascocid®-500: 500 mg [sugar free]

C-Gram: 1000 mg [dye free, gluten free, sugar free]

One Gram C: 1000 mg

Tablet, chewable, oral: 250 mg, 500 mg

Acerola: 500 mg [cherry flavor]

Mild-C®: 250 mg [orange-tangerine flavor]

Tablet, chewable, oral [buffered]:

Chew-C: 500 mg [orange flavor]

Tablet, timed release, oral: 500 mg, 1000 mg

Cemill 500: 500 mg

Cemill 1000: 1000 mg

Mild-C®: 1000 mg

◆ **Asco-Tabs-1000 [OTC]** *see* Ascorbic Acid *on page 149*

◆ **Ascriptin® Maximum Strength [OTC]** *see* Aspirin *on page 154*

◆ **Ascriptin® Regular Strength [OTC]** *see* Aspirin *on page 154*

Asenapine (a SEN a peen)

Brand Names: U.S. Saphris®

Pharmacologic Category Antimanic Agent; Antipsychotic Agent, Atypical

Additional Appendix Information

Antipsychotic Agents *on page 1880*

Use Acute and maintenance treatment of schizophrenia; treatment of acute mania or mixed episodes associated with bipolar I disorder (as monotherapy or in combination with lithium or valproate)

Pregnancy Risk Factor C

Dosage Sublingual: Adults: **Note:** Safety of doses >20 mg/day has not been evaluated:

Schizophrenia:

Acute treatment: Initial: 5 mg twice daily. Daily doses >20 mg/day in clinical trials did not appear to offer any additional benefits and increased risk of adverse effects.

Maintenance treatment: Initial: 5 mg twice daily; may increase to 10 mg twice daily after 1 week based on tolerability

Bipolar disorder:

Monotherapy: Initial: 10 mg twice daily; decrease to 5 mg twice daily if dose not tolerated

Combination therapy (with lithium or valproate): 5 mg twice daily; may increase to 10 mg twice daily based on tolerability

Dosing adjustment in renal impairment: No dosage adjustment is necessary

Dosing adjustment in hepatic impairment:
Mild-to-moderate hepatic impairment (Child-Pugh class A or B): No dosage adjustment is necessary
Severe hepatic impairment (Child-Pugh class C): Use is not recommended

Additional Information Complete prescribing information for this medication should be consulted for additional detail.

Dosage Forms Excipient information presented when available (limited, particularly for generics); consult specific product labeling.

Tablet, sublingual:
Saphris®: 5 mg [unflavored]
Saphris®: 5 mg [black cherry flavor]
Saphris®: 10 mg [unflavored]
Saphris®: 10 mg [black cherry flavor]

◆ **Asendin [DSC]** *see* Amoxapine *on page 101*
◆ **Asmanex® Twisthaler®** *see* Mometasone (Oral Inhalation) *on page 1149*
◆ **Asparaginase** *see* Asparaginase (*E. coli*) *on page 151*

Asparaginase (*E. coli*) (a SPEAR a ji nase e ko lye)

Brand Names: U.S. Elspar®
Brand Names: Canada Kidrolase®
Index Terms *E. coli* Asparaginase; Asparaginase; L-asparaginase (*E. coli*)
Pharmacologic Category Antineoplastic Agent, Miscellaneous; Enzyme
Use Treatment (in combination with other chemotherapy) of acute lymphoblastic leukemia (ALL)
Unlabeled Use Treatment of lymphoblastic lymphoma
Pregnancy Risk Factor C
Pregnancy Considerations Decreased weight gain, resorptions, gross abnormalities, and skeletal abnormalities were observed in animal studies. There are no adequate and well-controlled studies in pregnant women. Use during pregnancy only if clearly needed.
Lactation Excretion in breast milk unknown/not recommended
Contraindications History of serious allergic reaction to asparaginase or any *E. coli*-derived L-asparaginase; history of serious thrombosis, pancreatitis, or serious hemorrhagic events with prior L-asparaginase treatment
Warnings/Precautions Hazardous agent - use appropriate precautions for handling and disposal. Monitor for severe allergic reactions; immediate treatment for hypersensitivity reactions should be available during administration. May alter hepatic function; use caution with preexisting liver impairment. Serious thrombosis, including sagittal sinus thrombosis may occur; discontinue with serious thrombotic events. Increased prothrombin time, partial thromboplastin time and hypofibrinogenemia may occur; cerebrovascular hemorrhage has been reported; monitor coagulation parameters; use cautiously in patients with an underlying coagulopathy. Monitor blood glucose; may cause hyperglycemia/glucose intolerance (possibly irreversible). May cause serious and possibly fatal pancreatitis; promptly evaluate patients with abdominal pain; discontinue permanently if pancreatitis develops. Appropriate measures must be taken to prevent tumor lysis syndrome and subsequent hyperuricemia and uric acid nephropathy; monitor, consider allopurinol, hydration and urinary alkalization.

Severe allergic reactions may occur; monitor; immediate treatment for hypersensitivity reactions should be available during administration. Risk factors for allergic reactions include: I.V. administration, doses >6000-12,000 units/m^2, patients who have received previous cycles of asparaginase, and intervals of even a few days between doses. Up to 33% of patients who have an allergic reaction to *E. coli* asparaginase will also react to the *Erwinia* form or pegaspargase. A test dose may be administered prior to the first dose of asparaginase, or prior to restarting therapy after a hiatus of several days. **False-negative rates of up to 80% to test doses of 2-50 units are reported.** Desensitization may be performed in patients found to be hypersensitive by the intradermal test dose or who have received previous courses of therapy with the drug.

Adverse Reactions Note: Immediate effects: Fever, chills, nausea, and vomiting occur in 50% to 60% of patients.

>10%:
Central nervous system: Fatigue, fever, chills, depression, agitation, seizure (10% to 60%), somnolence, stupor, confusion, coma (25%)
Endocrine & metabolic: Hyperglycemia/glucose intolerance (10%)
Gastrointestinal: Nausea, vomiting (50% to 60%), anorexia, abdominal cramps (70%), acute pancreatitis (15%, may be severe in some patients)
Hematologic: Hypofibrinogenemia and depression of clotting factors V and VIII, variable decrease in factors VII and IX, severe protein C deficiency and decrease in antithrombin III (may be dose limiting or fatal)
Hepatic: Transaminases, bilirubin, and alkaline phosphatase increased (transient)
Hypersensitivity: Acute allergic reactions (fever, rash, urticaria, arthralgia, hypotension, angioedema, bronchospasm, anaphylaxis (15% to 35%); may be dose limiting in some patients, may be fatal)
Renal: Azotemia (66%)

1% to 10%:
Endocrine & metabolic: Hyperuricemia
Gastrointestinal: Stomatitis
Miscellaneous: Allergic reaction (including anaphylaxis), antibody formation/immunogenicity (~25%)

<1% (Limited to important or life-threatening) and/or frequency not defined: Acute renal failure, albumin decreased, cerebrovascular hemorrhage, cerebrovascular thrombosis, disorientation, fatty liver, fibrinogen decreased, glucosuria, hallucinations, headache, hemorrhagic pancreatitis, hyper-/hypolipidemia, hyperthermia, hypocholesterolemia, hypotension, insulin-dependent diabetes, intracranial hemorrhage, irritability, ketoacidosis, laryngospasm, malabsorption syndrome, myelosuppression (mild–to-moderate anemia, leukopenia, and thrombocytopenia; onset: 7 days; nadir: 14 days; recovery: 21 days), pancreatic pseudocyst, Parkinsonian symptoms (including tremor and increased muscle tone), partial thromboplastin time increased, peripheral edema, polyuria, proteinuria, prothrombin time increased, pruritus, rash, renal insufficiency, serum ammonia increased, serum cholesterol decreased, sagittal sinus thrombosis, stroke (hemorrhagic and thrombotic), thrombosis, urticaria, venous thrombosis

Drug Interactions
Metabolism/Transport Effects None known.
Avoid Concomitant Use There are no known interactions where it is recommended to avoid concomitant use.
Increased Effect/Toxicity
Asparaginase (E. coli) may increase the levels/effects of: Dexamethasone; Dexamethasone (Systemic)
Decreased Effect There are no known significant interactions involving a decrease in effect.

Stability Intact vials of powder should be refrigerated at 2°C to 8°C (36°F to 48°F). For I.V. administration, reconstitute lyophilized powder with 5 mL sterile water for injection or NS. For I.M. administration, the manufacturer recommends reconstitution of the lyophilized powder with 2 mL NS to a concentration of 5000 units/mL; however, some institutions reconstitute with 1 mL NS for I.M use, resulting in a concentration of 10,000 units/mL. Shake well, but not too vigorously. A 5 micron filter may be used to remove fiber-like particles in the solution (do not use a 0.2 micron filter; has been associated with loss of potency). Reconstituted solutions are stable 1 week refrigerated at 8°C (Stecher, 1999), although the manufacturer recommends use within 8 hours.

Standard I.M. dilution: 5000 units/mL (10,000 units/mL has been used by some institutions)

Standard I.V. dilution: Dilute in NS or D_5W; solutions for I.V. infusion are stable for 8 hours at room temperature or under refrigeration

Mechanism of Action Asparaginase inhibits protein synthesis by hydrolyzing asparagine to aspartic acid and ammonia. Leukemia cells, especially lymphoblasts, require exogenous asparagine; normal cells can synthesize asparagine. Asparaginase is cycle-specific for the G_1 phase.

Pharmacodynamics/Kinetics

Absorption: I.M.: Produces peak blood levels 50% lower than those from I.V. administration

Distribution: V_d: 4-5 L/kg; 70% to 80% of plasma volume; <1% CSF penetration

Metabolism: Systemically degraded

Half-life elimination: I.M.: 39-49 hours; I.V.: 8-30 hours

Time to peak, plasma: I.M.: 14-24 hours

Dosage Refer to individual protocols. **Note:** Dose, frequency, number of doses, and start date may vary by protocol and treatment phase.

Children:

I.V.:

6000 units/m²/dose 3 times/week for ~6-9 doses **or** 1000 units/kg/day for 10 days **or**

High-dose therapy (unlabeled dose): 10,000 units/m²/dose every ~3 days for ~4-8 doses

I.M.:

6000 units/m²/dose 3 times/week **or** 6000 units/m²/dose every ~3 days for ~6-9 doses

High-dose therapy (unlabeled dose): 10,000 units/m²/dose every ~3 days for ~4-8 doses **or** 25,000 units/m²/dose weekly for ~9 doses (generally used in high-risk continuation therapy)

Adults:

I.V.:

6000 units/m²/dose 3 times/week for ~6-9 doses **or** 1000 units/kg/day for 10 days **or**

High-dose therapy (unlabeled dose): 10,000 units/m²/day for ~3-12 doses

Single agent therapy (rare): 200 units/kg/day for 28 days

I.M.:

6000 units/m²/dose 3 times/week for ~6-9 doses **or** 6000 units/m²/dose every ~3 days for ~6-9 doses

High-dose therapy (unlabeled dose): 10,000 units/m²/day for ~3-12 doses

Test dose: A test dose is often recommended prior to the first dose of asparaginase, or prior to restarting therapy after a hiatus of several days. Most commonly, 0.1 mL of a 20 units/mL (2 units) asparaginase dilution is injected intradermally, and the patient observed for at least 1 hour. False-negative rates of up to 80% to test doses of 2-50 units are reported.

Some practitioners recommend an asparaginase desensitization regimen for patients who react to a test dose, or are being retreated following a break in therapy. Doses are doubled and given every 10 minutes until the total daily dose for that day has been administered. One schedule begins with a total of 1 unit given I.V. and doubles the dose every 10 minutes until the total amount given is the planned dose for that day. For example, if a patient was to receive a total dose of 4000 units, he/she would receive injections 1 through 12 during the desensitization. See table.

Asparaginase Desensitization

Injection No.	Elspar Dose (int. units)	Accumulated Total Dose
1	1	1
2	2	3
3	4	7
4	8	15
5	16	31
6	32	63
7	64	127
8	128	255
9	256	511
10	512	1023
11	1024	2047
12	2048	4095
13	4096	8191
14	8192	16,383
15	16,384	32,767
16	32,768	65,535
17	65,536	131,071
18	131,072	262,143

Administration May be administered I.M., I.V., or intradermal (skin test only); has been administered SubQ in specific protocols

I.M.: Doses should be given as a deep intramuscular injection into a large muscle; volumes >2 mL should be divided and administered in 2 separate sites

Note: I.V. administration greatly increases the risk of allergic reactions and should be avoided if possible.

I.V.: I.V. infusion in 50-250 mL of D_5W or NS over at least 30-60 minutes. The manufacturer recommends a test dose (0.1 mL of a dilute 20 unit/mL solution) prior to initial administration and when given after an interval of 7 days or more. Institutional policies vary. The skin test site should be observed for at least 1 hour for a wheal or erythema. Note that a negative skin test does not preclude the possibility of an allergic reaction. Desensitization may be performed in patients who have been found to be hypersensitive by the intradermal skin test or who have received previous courses of therapy with the drug. Have epinephrine, diphenhydramine, and hydrocortisone at the bedside. Have a running I.V. in place. A physician should be readily accessible.

Gelatinous fiber-like particles may develop on standing. Filtration through a 5-micron filter during administration will remove the particles with no loss of potency.

Monitoring Parameters Vital signs during administration; CBC with differential, urinalysis, amylase, liver enzymes, coagulation parameters (baseline and periodic), renal function tests, urine dipstick for glucose, blood glucose, uric acid. Monitor for allergic reaction, be prepared to treat anaphylaxis at each administration; monitor for onset of abdominal pain and mental status changes.

Test Interactions Decreased thyroxine and thyroxine-binding globulin

Additional Information Some institutions recommended the following precautions for asparaginase administration: Parenteral epinephrine, diphenhydramine, and hydrocortisone available at bedside; freely running I.V. in place; physician readily accessible; monitor the patient closely for 30-60 minutes; avoid administering at night.

The *E. coli* and the *Erwinia* strains of asparaginase differ slightly in their gene sequencing, and have slight differences in their enzyme characteristics. Both are highly specific for asparagine and have <10% activity for the D-isomer.

Dosage Forms Excipient information presented when available (limited, particularly for generics); consult specific product labeling.

Injection, powder for reconstitution:

Elspar®: 10,000 int. units

◆ **Asparaginase *Erwinia chrysanthemi*** *see* Asparaginase (*Erwinia*) *on page 153*

Asparaginase (*Erwinia*)

(a SPEAR a ji nase er WIN i ah)

Brand Names: U.S. Erwinaze™

Brand Names: Canada Erwinase®

Index Terms *Erwinia chrysanthemi*; Asparaginase *Erwinia chrysanthemi*; L-asparaginase (*Erwinia*)

Pharmacologic Category Antineoplastic Agent, Miscellaneous; Enzyme

Use Treatment (in combination with other chemotherapy) of acute lymphoblastic leukemia (ALL) in patients with hypersensitivity to *E. coli*-derived asparaginase

Pregnancy Risk Factor C

Pregnancy Considerations Animal reproduction studies have not been conducted. The effects on human pregnancy are unknown.

Lactation Excretion in breast milk unknown/not recommended

Prescribing and Access Restrictions Erwinaze™ is distributed through Accredo Health Group, Inc. (1-877-900-9223).

Contraindications History of serious hypersensitivity reactions, including anaphylaxis to asparaginase (*Erwinia*) or any component of the formulation; history of serious pancreatitis, serious thrombosis, or serious hemorrhagic event with prior asparaginase treatment

Canadian labeling: Additional contraindications (not in the U.S. labeling): Women who are or may become pregnant

Warnings/Precautions Hazardous agent - use appropriate precautions for handling and disposal.

Serious hypersensitivity reactions, including anaphylaxis, have occurred in 5% of patients in clinical trials. Immediate treatment for hypersensitivity reactions should be available during treatment; discontinue for serious hypersensitivity (and administer appropriate treatment for reaction).

Pancreatitis has been reported in 4% of patients in clinical trials; promptly evaluate with symptoms suggestive of pancreatitis. For mild pancreatitis, withhold treatment until signs and symptoms subside and amylase returns to normal; may resume after resolution. Discontinue for severe or hemorrhagic pancreatitis characterized by abdominal pain >72 hours and amylase ≥2 x ULN. Further use is contraindicated if severe pancreatitis is diagnosed.

Serious thrombotic events, including sagittal sinus thrombosis, have been reported with asparaginase formulations. Decreases in fibrinogen, protein C activity, protein S activity, and antithrombin III have been noted following a 2-week treatment course. Discontinue for hemorrhagic or thrombotic events; may resume treatment after resolution (contraindicated with history of serious thrombosis or hemorrhagic event with prior asparaginase treatment).

In clinical trials, 2% of patients experienced glucose intolerance; may be irreversible; monitor glucose levels (baseline and periodic) during treatment; may require insulin administration.

Adverse Reactions

>10%: Miscellaneous: Allergic reaction/hypersensitivity (17%; grades 3/4: 5% to 9%; includes anaphylaxis, urticaria)

1% to 10%:

Cardiovascular: Thrombosis (2%; grades 3/4: ≤1%)

Central nervous system: Fever (3%), headache (1%), seizure (1%)

Endocrine & metabolic: Glucose intolerance (2%), hyperglycemia (2%; grades 3/4: 2%), hyperammonemia (1%)

Gastrointestinal: Pancreatitis (4%; grades 3/4: ≤1%), nausea (2%), vomiting (2%), abdominal pain (1%), diarrhea (1%)

Hematologic: Coagulation abnormalities (3%; grades 3/4: ≤1%), hemorrhage (1%; grades 3/4: <1%)

Hepatic: Transaminases increased (3%; grades 3/4: ≤2%), hyperbilirubinemia (1%)

<1% (Limited to important or life-threatening): Acute renal failure, albumin decreased, alkaline phosphatase increased, anorexia, azotemia, bone marrow depression (rare), chills, cholesterol decreased, disseminated intravascular coagulation (DIC), hepatomegaly, injection site reactions, irritability, lipids (total) decreased/increased, malabsorption syndrome, proteinuria, transient ischemic event, weight loss

Drug Interactions

Metabolism/Transport Effects None known.

Avoid Concomitant Use There are no known interactions where it is recommended to avoid concomitant use.

Increased Effect/Toxicity

Asparaginase (Erwinia) may increase the levels/effects of: Dexamethasone; Dexamethasone (Systemic)

Decreased Effect There are no known significant interactions involving a decrease in effect.

Stability Store intact vials refrigerated at 2°C to 8°C (36°F to 48°F). Protect from light. Hazardous agent; use appropriate precautions for handling and disposal. Reconstitute each vial with 1 mL of preservative free sodium chloride 0.9% (NS) to obtain a concentration of 10,000 units/mL, or with 2 mL preservative free NS to obtain a concentration of 5000 units/mL. Gently direct the NS down the wall of the vial (do not inject forcefully into or onto the powder). Dissolve by gently swirling or mixing; do not shake or invert the vial. Resulting reconstituted solution should be clear and colorless and free of visible particles or protein aggregates. Within 15 minutes of reconstitution, withdraw appropriate volume for dose into a polypropylene syringe. Do not freeze or refrigerate reconstituted solution; discard if not administered within 4 hours.

Mechanism of Action Asparaginase catalyzes the deamidation of asparagine to aspartic acid and ammonia, reducing circulating levels of asparagine. Leukemia cells lack asparagine synthetase and are unable to synthesize asparagine. Asparaginase reduces the exogenous asparagine source for the leukemic cells, resulting in cytotoxicity specific to leukemic cells.

Pharmacodynamics/Kinetics Half-life elimination: I.M.: ~16 hours (Asselin, 1993; Avramis, 2005)

Dosage

I.M.: Children and Adults: Acute lymphoblastic leukemia (ALL):

As a substitute for pegaspargase: 25,000 units/m^2 3 times/week (Mon, Wed, Fri) for 6 doses for each planned pegaspargase dose

As a substitute for asparaginase (E. coli): 25,000 units/m^2 for each planned asparaginase (*E. coli*) dose

Canadian labeling (not in the U.S. labeling): ALL induction:

Children <14 years: I.M.: 6000 units/m^2 3 times/week for 9 doses beginning day 4 of week 1 (in combination with vincristine, prednisone, methotrexate, and daunorubicin)

Children >14 years and Adults: SubQ: 10,000 units/m^2 days 1, 3, and 5 of week 4 and day 1 of week 5 (in combination with prednisolone, vincristine, mercaptopurine, and methotrexate) **or** 10,000 units/m^2 3 times/week (starting week 4) for 4 weeks (in combination with prednisolone, vincristine, and daunorubicin)

Dosage adjustment for toxicity:

Hemorrhagic or thrombotic event: Discontinue treatment; may resume treatment upon symptom resolution

Pancreatitis:

Mild pancreatitis: Withhold treatment until signs and symptoms subside and amylase returns to normal; may resume after resolution

Severe or hemorrhagic pancreatitis (abdominal pain >72 hours and amylase ≥2 x ULN): Discontinue treatment; further use is contraindicated.

Serious hypersensitivity: Discontinue treatment

Dosage adjustment in renal impairment: No dosage adjustment provided in the manufacturer's labeling.

Dosage adjustment in hepatic impairment: No dosage adjustment provided in the manufacturer's labeling.

Administration

Administer I.M.; volume of each single injection site should be limited to 2 mL; use multiple injections for volumes >2 mL

Canadian labeling (additional administration routes not in the U.S. labeling): May also be administered SubQ and I.V., although I.M. and SubQ are preferred

Monitoring Parameters CBC with differential, amylase, liver enzymes, blood glucose, coagulation parameters, symptoms of hypersensitivity, symptoms of pancreatitis, thrombosis, or hemorrhage

Dosage Forms Excipient information presented when available (limited, particularly for generics); consult specific product labeling.

Injection, powder for reconstitution:

Erwinaze™: 10,000 int. units [contains glucose 5 mg/vial]

◆ **Aspart Insulin** *see* Insulin Aspart *on page 903*

◆ **Aspercin [OTC]** *see* Aspirin *on page 154*

◆ ***Aspergillus niger*** *see* Alpha-Galactosidase *on page 71*

◆ **Aspergum® [OTC]** *see* Aspirin *on page 154*

Aspirin (AS pir in)

Brand Names: U.S. Ascriptin® Maximum Strength [OTC]; Ascriptin® Regular Strength [OTC]; Aspercin [OTC]; Aspergum® [OTC]; Aspir-low [OTC]; Aspirtab [OTC]; Bayer® Aspirin Extra Strength [OTC]; Bayer® Aspirin Regimen Adult Low Strength [OTC]; Bayer® Aspirin Regimen Children's [OTC]; Bayer® Aspirin Regimen Regular Strength [OTC]; Bayer® Genuine Aspirin [OTC]; Bayer® Plus Extra Strength [OTC]; Bayer® Women's Low Dose Aspirin [OTC]; Buffasal [OTC]; Bufferin® Extra Strength [OTC]; Bufferin® [OTC]; Buffinol [OTC]; Ecotrin® Arthritis Strength [OTC]; Ecotrin® Low Strength [OTC]; Ecotrin® [OTC]; Halfprin® [OTC]; St Joseph® Adult Aspirin [OTC]; Tri-Buffered Aspirin [OTC]

Brand Names: Canada Asaphen; Asaphen E.C.; Entrophen®; Novasen; Praxis ASA EC 81 Mg Daily Dose

Index Terms Acetylsalicylic Acid; ASA; Baby Aspirin

Pharmacologic Category Antiplatelet Agent; Salicylate

Use Treatment of mild-to-moderate pain, inflammation, and fever; prevention and treatment of myocardial infarction (MI), acute ischemic stroke, and transient ischemic episodes; management of rheumatoid arthritis, rheumatic fever, osteoarthritis; adjunctive therapy in revascularization procedures (coronary artery bypass graft [CABG], percutaneous transluminal coronary angioplasty [PTCA], carotid endarterectomy), stent implantation

Unlabeled Use Low doses have been used in the prevention of pre-eclampsia, complications associated with autoimmune disorders such as lupus or antiphospholipid syndrome; colorectal cancer; Kawasaki disease; alternative therapy for prevention of thromboembolism associated with atrial fibrillation in patients not candidates for warfarin; pericarditis associated with MI; prosthetic valve thromboprophylaxis; peripheral arterial occlusive disease

Pregnancy Considerations Salicylates have been noted to cross the placenta and enter fetal circulation. Adverse effects reported in the fetus include mortality, intrauterine growth retardation, salicylate intoxication, bleeding abnormalities, and neonatal acidosis. Use of aspirin close to delivery may cause premature closure of the ductus arteriosus. Adverse effects reported in the mother include anemia, hemorrhage, prolonged gestation, and prolonged labor. Aspirin has been used for the prevention of pre-eclampsia; however, the ACOG currently recommends that it not be used in low-risk women. Low-dose aspirin is used to treat complications resulting from antiphospholipid syndrome in pregnancy (either primary or secondary to SLE). In general, low doses during pregnancy needed for the treatment of certain medical conditions have not been shown to cause fetal harm, however, discontinuing therapy prior to delivery is recommended. Use of safer agents for routine management of pain or headache should be considered.

Lactation Enters breast milk (AAP recommends use "with caution"; AAP 2001 update pending)

Contraindications Hypersensitivity to salicylates, other NSAIDs, or any component of the formulation; asthma; rhinitis; nasal polyps; inherited or acquired bleeding disorders (including factor VII and factor IX deficiency); do not use in children (<16 years of age) for viral infections (chickenpox or flu symptoms), with or without fever, due to a potential association with Reye's syndrome; pregnancy (3rd trimester especially)

Warnings/Precautions Use with caution in patients with platelet and bleeding disorders, renal dysfunction, dehydration, erosive gastritis, or peptic ulcer disease. Heavy ethanol use (>3 drinks/day) can increase bleeding risks. Avoid use in severe renal failure or in severe hepatic failure. Low-dose aspirin for cardioprotective effects is associated with a two- to fourfold increase in UGI events (eg, symptomatic or complicated ulcers); risks of these events increase with increasing aspirin dose; during the chronic phase of aspirin dosing, doses >81 mg are not recommended unless indicated (Bhatt, 2008).

Discontinue use if tinnitus or impaired hearing occurs. Caution in mild-to-moderate renal failure (only at high dosages). Patients with sensitivity to tartrazine dyes, nasal polyps, and asthma may have an increased risk of salicylate sensitivity. In the treatment of acute ischemic stroke, avoid aspirin for 24 hours following administration of alteplase; administration within 24 hours increases the risk of hemorrhagic transformation. Concurrent use of aspirin and clopidogrel is not recommended for secondary prevention of ischemic stroke or TIA in patients unable to take oral anticoagulants due to hemorrhagic risk (Furie, 2011). Surgical patients should avoid ASA if possible, for 1-2 weeks prior to surgery, to reduce the risk of excessive bleeding (except in patients with cardiac stents that have not completed their full course of dual antiplatelet therapy [aspirin, clopidogrel]; patient-specific situations need to be discussed with cardiologist; AHA/ACC/SCAI/ACS/ADA Science Advisory provides recommendations). When used concomitantly with ≤325 mg of aspirin, NSAIDs (including selective COX-2 inhibitors) substantially increase the risk of gastrointestinal complications (eg, ulcer); concomitant gastroprotective therapy (eg, proton pump inhibitors) is recommended (Bhatt, 2008).

When used for self-medication (OTC labeling): Children and teenagers who have or are recovering from chickenpox or flu-like symptoms should not use this product. Changes in behavior (along with nausea and vomiting) may be an early sign of Reye's syndrome; patients should be instructed to contact their healthcare provider if these occur.

Adverse Reactions As with all drugs which may affect hemostasis, bleeding is associated with aspirin. Hemorrhage may occur at virtually any site. Risk is dependent on multiple variables including dosage, concurrent use of multiple agents which alter hemostasis, and patient susceptibility. Many adverse effects of aspirin are dose related, and are extremely rare at low dosages. Other serious reactions are idiosyncratic, related to allergy or individual sensitivity. Accurate estimation of frequencies is not possible.

Cardiovascular: Hypotension, tachycardia, dysrhythmias, edema

Central nervous system: Fatigue, insomnia, nervousness, agitation, confusion, dizziness, headache, lethargy, cerebral edema, hyperthermia, coma

Dermatologic: Rash, angioedema, urticaria

Endocrine & metabolic: Acidosis, hyperkalemia, dehydration, hypoglycemia (children), hyperglycemia, hypernatremia (buffered forms)

Gastrointestinal: Nausea, vomiting, dyspepsia, epigastric discomfort, heartburn, stomach pain, gastrointestinal ulceration (6% to 31%), gastric erosions, gastric erythema, duodenal ulcers

Hematologic: Anemia, disseminated intravascular coagulation (DIC), prothrombin times prolonged, coagulopathy, thrombocytopenia, hemolytic anemia, bleeding, iron-deficiency anemia

Hepatic: Hepatotoxicity, transaminases increased, hepatitis (reversible)

Neuromuscular & skeletal: Rhabdomyolysis, weakness, acetabular bone destruction (OA)

Otic: Hearing loss, tinnitus

Renal: Interstitial nephritis, papillary necrosis, proteinuria, renal failure (including cases caused by rhabdomyolysis), BUN increased, serum creatinine increased

Respiratory: Asthma, bronchospasm, dyspnea, laryngeal edema, hyperpnea, tachypnea, respiratory alkalosis, noncardiogenic pulmonary edema

Miscellaneous: Anaphylaxis, prolonged pregnancy and labor, stillbirths, low birth weight, peripartum bleeding, Reye's syndrome

Postmarketing and/or case reports: Colonic ulceration, esophageal stricture, esophagitis with esophageal ulcer, esophageal hematoma, oral mucosal ulcers (aspirin-containing chewing gum), coronary artery spasm, conduction defect and atrial fibrillation (toxicity), delirium, ischemic brain infarction, colitis, rectal stenosis (suppository), cholestatic jaundice, periorbital edema, rhinosinusitis

Drug Interactions

Metabolism/Transport Effects Substrate of CYP2C9 (minor); **Note:** Assignment of Major/Minor substrate status based on clinically relevant drug interaction potential

Avoid Concomitant Use

Avoid concomitant use of Aspirin with any of the following: Floctafenine; Influenza Virus Vaccine (Live/Attenuated); Ketorolac; Ketorolac (Nasal); Ketorolac (Systemic)

Increased Effect/Toxicity

Aspirin may increase the levels/effects of: Alendronate; Anticoagulants; Carbonic Anhydrase Inhibitors; Collagenase (Systemic); Corticosteroids (Systemic); Divalproex; Drotrecogin Alfa (Activated); Heparin; Ibritumomab; Methotrexate; PRALAtrexate; Rivaroxaban; Salicylates; Sulfonylureas; Thrombolytic Agents; Ticagrelor; Tositumomab and Iodine I 131 Tositumomab; Valproic Acid; Varicella Virus-Containing Vaccines; Vitamin K Antagonists

The levels/effects of Aspirin may be increased by: Ammonium Chloride; Antidepressants (Tricyclic, Tertiary Amine); Antiplatelet Agents; Calcium Channel Blockers (Nondihydropyridine); Dasatinib; Floctafenine; Ginkgo Biloba; Glucosamine; Herbs (Anticoagulant/Antiplatelet Properties); Influenza Virus Vaccine (Live/Attenuated); Ketorolac; Ketorolac (Nasal); Ketorolac (Systemic); Loop Diuretics; Nonsteroidal Anti-Inflammatory Agents; NSAID (Nonselective); Omega-3-Acid Ethyl Esters; Pentosan Polysulfate Sodium; Pentoxifylline; Potassium Acid Phosphate; Prostacyclin Analogues; Selective Serotonin Reuptake Inhibitors; Serotonin/Norepinephrine Reuptake Inhibitors; Treprostinil; Vitamin E

Decreased Effect

Aspirin may decrease the levels/effects of: ACE Inhibitors; Loop Diuretics; NSAID (Nonselective); Probenecid; Ticagrelor; Tiludronate

The levels/effects of Aspirin may be decreased by: Corticosteroids (Systemic); Nonsteroidal Anti-Inflammatory Agents; NSAID (Nonselective)

Ethanol/Nutrition/Herb Interactions

Ethanol: Avoid ethanol (may enhance gastric mucosal damage).

Food: Food may decrease the rate but not the extent of oral absorption.

Folic acid: Hyperexcretion of folate; folic acid deficiency may result, leading to macrocytic anemia.

Iron: With chronic aspirin use and at doses of 3-4 g/day, iron-deficiency anemia may result.

Sodium: Hypernatremia resulting from buffered aspirin solutions or sodium salicylate containing high sodium content. Avoid or use with caution in CHF or any condition where hypernatremia would be detrimental.

Benedictine liqueur, prunes, raisins, tea, and gherkins: Potential salicylate accumulation.

Fresh fruits containing vitamin C: Displace drug from binding sites, resulting in increased urinary excretion of aspirin.

Herb/Nutraceutical: Avoid cat's claw, dong quai, evening primrose, feverfew, garlic, ginger, ginkgo, red clover, horse chestnut, green tea, ginseng (all have additional antiplatelet activity). Limit curry powder, paprika, licorice; may cause salicylate accumulation. These foods contain 6 mg salicylate/100 g. An ordinary American diet contains 10-200 mg/day of salicylate.

Stability Keep suppositories in refrigerator; do not freeze. Hydrolysis of aspirin occurs upon exposure to water or moist air, resulting in salicylate and acetate, which possess a vinegar-like odor. Do not use if a strong odor is present.

Mechanism of Action Irreversibly inhibits cyclooxygenase-1 and 2 (COX-1 and 2) enzymes, via acetylation, which results in decreased formation of prostaglandin precursors; irreversibly inhibits formation of prostaglandin derivative, thromboxane A_2, via acetylation of platelet cyclooxygenase, thus inhibiting platelet aggregation; has antipyretic, analgesic, and anti-inflammatory properties

Pharmacodynamics/Kinetics

Duration: 4-6 hours

Absorption: Rapid

Distribution: V_d: 10 L; readily into most body fluids and tissues

Metabolism: Hydrolyzed to salicylate (active) by esterases in GI mucosa, red blood cells, synovial fluid, and blood; metabolism of salicylate occurs primarily by hepatic conjugation; metabolic pathways are saturable

Bioavailability: 50% to 75% reaches systemic circulation

Half-life elimination: Parent drug: 15-20 minutes; Salicylates (dose dependent): 3 hours at lower doses (300-600 mg), 5-6 hours (after 1 g), 10 hours with higher doses

Time to peak, serum: ~1-2 hours

Excretion: Urine (75% as salicyluric acid, 10% as salicylic acid)

Dosage

Children:

Analgesic and antipyretic: Oral, rectal: 10-15 mg/kg/dose every 4-6 hours, up to a total of 4 g/day

Anti-inflammatory: Oral: Initial: 60-90 mg/kg/day in divided doses; usual maintenance: 80-100 mg/kg/day divided every 6-8 hours; monitor serum concentrations

Antiplatelet effects: Adequate pediatric studies have not been performed; pediatric dosage is derived from adult studies and clinical experience and is not well established; suggested doses have ranged from 3-5 mg/kg/day to 5-10 mg/kg/day given as a single daily dose. Doses are rounded to a convenient amount (eg, 1/2 of 81 mg tablet).

Mechanical prosthetic heart valves: 6-20 mg/kg/day given as a single daily dose (used in combination with an oral anticoagulant in children who have systemic embolism despite adequate oral anticoagulation therapy (INR 2.5-3.5) and used in combination with low-dose anticoagulation (INR 2-3) and dipyridamole when full-dose oral anticoagulation is contraindicated)

Blalock-Taussig shunts (unlabeled use): 1-5 mg/kg/day given as a single daily dose (Monagle, 2008)

Cerebrovascular accident (non-sickle cell-related ischemic stroke) (unlabeled use): 1-5 mg/kg/day for at least 2 years (Monagle, 2008)

Kawasaki disease (unlabeled use): Oral: 80-100 mg/kg/day divided every 6 hours; monitor serum concentrations; after fever resolves: 1-5 mg/kg/day once daily; in patients without coronary artery abnormalities, give lower dose for at least 6-8 weeks or until ESR and platelet count are normal; in patients with coronary artery abnormalities, low-dose aspirin should be continued indefinitely (Monagle, 2008)

Adults:

Analgesic and antipyretic:

Oral: 325-650 mg every 4-6 hours up to 4 g/day

Rectal: 300-600 mg every 4-6 hours up to 4 g/day

Anti-inflammatory: Oral: Initial: 2.4-3.6 g/day in divided doses; usual maintenance: 3.6-5.4 g/day; monitor serum concentrations

Atrial fibrillation (in patients not candidates for warfarin or at low risk of ischemic stroke): Oral: 75-325 mg once daily (Fuster, 2006; Singer, 2008) **or** 75-100 mg once daily (Furie, 2011)

CABG: Oral: 100-325 mg once daily initiated either preoperatively or within 6 hours postoperatively; continue indefinitely (Hillis, 2011)

Carotid artery stenting: Oral: 81-325 mg once daily beginning at least 24 hours (preferably 4 days) prior to procedure with concomitant clopidogrel (Bates, 2007)

Carotid endarterectomy: Oral: 50-100 mg once daily preoperatively and daily thereafter; usual dose: 81 mg once daily (Albers, 2008)

Heart valve (bioprosthetic, mechanical): Oral: 50-100 mg once daily (in addition to warfarin) (Furie, 2011); usual dose: 81 mg once daily (Salem, 2008)

Mechanical heart valve (history of thromboembolism while receiving oral anticoagulants): Oral: 75-100 mg once daily (in addition to warfarin) (Furie, 2011); usual dose: 81 mg once daily

Mitral valve (prolapse, annular calcification) (with documented stroke or TIA): Oral: 50-100 mg once daily; usual dose: 81 mg once daily (Salem, 2008)

Myocardial infarction (primary prevention): Oral: 75-162 mg once daily (Antman, 2004) **or** 75-100 mg (usual dose: 81 mg) once daily (Hirsh, 2008)

Myocardial infarction (ST-segment elevation myocardial infarction [STEMI], non-ST-segment elevation myocardial infarction [NSTEMI]): Oral: Initial: 162-325 mg given on presentation (patient should chew nonenteric-coated aspirin especially if not taking before presentation); for patients unable to take oral, may use rectal suppository (300 mg). Maintenance (secondary prevention): 75-162 mg once daily indefinitely (Anderson, 2007; Antman, 2004).

PCI: Oral: Preprocedure: 81-325 mg (325 mg [nonenteric coated] in aspirin-naive patients) starting at least 2 hours (preferably 24 hours) before procedure; postprocedure: 81 mg once daily continued indefinitely (Levine, 2011).

Pericarditis associated with myocardial infarction: Oral: 162-325 mg once daily; doses as high as 650 mg every 4-6 hours may be required; enteric-coated recommended (Antman, 2004)

Peripheral arterial disease: Oral: 75-100 mg once daily; usual dose: 81 mg once daily (Sobel, 2008) **or** 75-325 mg once daily; may use in conjunction with clopidogrel in those who are not at an increased risk of bleeding but are of high cardiovascular risk (Class IIb recommendation). **Note:** These recommendations also pertain to those with intermittent claudication or critical limb ischemia, prior lower extremity revascularization, or prior amputation for lower extremity ischemia (Rooke, 2011).

Pre-eclampsia prevention: Oral: 60-81 mg once daily (usual dose: 81 mg) during gestational weeks 13-26 (patient selection criteria not established) (Bates, 2008; CLASP, 1994)

Stroke (acute ischemic): Oral: Initial: 150-325 mg within 48 hours of stroke onset (in patients who are not candidates for thrombolytic therapy), followed by 50-100 mg once daily (Albers, 2008)

Stroke (cardioembolic, anticoagulation contraindicated): Oral: 75-325 mg once daily (Albers, 2008)

Stroke/TIA (noncardioembolic, secondary prevention): Oral: 50-325 mg once daily (Adams, 2007; Smith, 2011) **or** 50-100 mg once daily; usual dose: 81 mg once daily (Hirsh, 2008). **Note:** Combination aspirin 25 mg and extended release dipyridamole 200 mg twice daily is preferred over aspirin alone (Albers, 2008)

Stroke (women at high risk for CVA, primary prevention): Oral: 81 mg once daily **or** 100 mg every other day (Goldstein, 2010)

Dosing adjustment in renal impairment: Cl_{cr} <10 mL/minute: Avoid use.

Hemodialysis: Dialyzable (50% to 100%)

Dosing adjustment in hepatic disease: Avoid use in severe liver disease.

Dietary Considerations Take with food or large volume of water or milk to minimize GI upset.

Administration Do not crush enteric coated tablet. Administer with food or a full glass of water to minimize GI distress. For acute myocardial infarction, have patient chew tablet.

Reference Range Timing of serum samples: Peak levels usually occur 2 hours after ingestion. Salicylate serum concentrations correlate with the pharmacological actions and adverse effects observed. The serum salicylate concentration (mcg/mL) and the corresponding clinical correlations are as follows: See table.

Serum Salicylate: Clinical Correlations

Serum Salicylate Concentration (mcg/mL)	Desired Effects	Adverse Effects / Intoxication
~100	Antiplatelet Antipyresis Analgesia	GI intolerance and bleeding, hypersensitivity, hemostatic defects
150-300	Anti-inflammatory	Mild salicylism
250-400	Treatment of rheumatic fever	Nausea/vomiting, hyperventilation, salicylism, flushing, sweating, thirst, headache, diarrhea, and tachycardia
>400-500		Respiratory alkalosis, hemorrhage, excitement, confusion, asterixis, pulmonary edema, convulsions, tetany, metabolic acidosis, fever, coma, cardiovascular collapse, renal and respiratory failure

Test Interactions False-negative results for glucose oxidase urinary glucose tests (Clinistix®); false-positives using the cupric sulfate method (Clinitest®); also, interferes with Gerhardt test, VMA determination; 5-HIAA, xylose tolerance test and T_3 and T_4

Dosage Forms Excipient information presented when available (limited, particularly for generics); consult specific product labeling.

Caplet, oral: 500 mg
  Bayer® Aspirin Extra Strength: 500 mg
  Bayer® Genuine Aspirin: 325 mg
  Bayer® Women's Low Dose Aspirin: 81 mg [contains elemental calcium 300 mg]
Caplet, oral [buffered]:
  Ascriptin® Maximum Strength: 500 mg [contains aluminum hydroxide, calcium carbonate, magnesium hydroxide]
  Bayer® Plus Extra Strength: 500 mg [contains calcium carbonate]
Caplet, enteric coated, oral:
  Bayer® Aspirin Regimen Regular Strength: 325 mg
Gum, chewing, oral:
  Aspergum®: 227 mg (12s) [cherry flavor]
  Aspergum®: 227 mg (12s) [orange flavor]
Suppository, rectal: 300 mg (12s); 600 mg (12s)
Tablet, oral: 325 mg
  Aspercin: 325 mg
  Aspirtab: 325 mg
  Bayer® Genuine Aspirin: 325 mg
Tablet, oral [buffered]: 325 mg
  Ascriptin® Regular Strength: 325 mg [contains aluminum hydroxide, calcium carbonate, magnesium hydroxide]
  Buffasal: 325 mg [contains magnesium oxide]
  Bufferin®: 325 mg [contains calcium carbonate, magnesium carbonate, magnesium oxide]
  Bufferin® Extra Strength: 500 mg [contains calcium carbonate, magnesium carbonate, magnesium oxide]
  Buffinol: 324 mg [sugar free; contains magnesium oxide]
  Tri-Buffered Aspirin: 325 mg [contains calcium carbonate, magnesium carbonate, magnesium hydroxide]
  Tri-Buffered Aspirin: 325 mg [contains calcium carbonate, magnesium oxide]
Tablet, chewable, oral: 81 mg
  Bayer® Aspirin Regimen Children's: 81 mg [cherry flavor]
  Bayer® Aspirin Regimen Children's: 81 mg [orange flavor]
  St Joseph® Adult Aspirin: 81 mg
Tablet, enteric coated, oral: 81 mg, 325 mg, 650 mg
  Aspir-low: 81 mg
  Bayer® Aspirin Regimen Adult Low Strength: 81 mg
  Ecotrin®: 325 mg
  Ecotrin® Arthritis Strength: 500 mg
  Ecotrin® Low Strength: 81 mg
  Halfprin®: 81 mg, 162 mg
  St Joseph® Adult Aspirin: 81 mg

◆ **Aspirin, Acetaminophen, and Caffeine** *see* Acetaminophen, Aspirin, and Caffeine *on page* 32

◆ **Aspirin and Carisoprodol** *see* Carisoprodol and Aspirin *on page* 292

Aspirin and Diphenhydramine
(AS pir in & dye fen HYE dra meen)

Brand Names: U.S. Bayer® PM [OTC]

Index Terms ASA and Diphenhydramine; Aspirin and Diphenhydramine Citrate; Diphenhydramine and ASA; Diphenhydramine and Aspirin; Diphenhydramine Citrate and Aspirin

Pharmacologic Category Analgesic, Miscellaneous

Use Aid in the relief of insomnia accompanied by minor pain or headache

Dosage Oral: Children ≥12 years and Adults: Pain-associated insomnia: Two caplets (1000 mg aspirin/77 mg diphenhydramine citrate) at bedtime if needed or as directed by physician; do not exceed recommended dosage; not for use in children <12 years of age

Additional Information Complete prescribing information for this medication should be consulted for additional detail.

Dosage Forms Excipient information presented when available (limited, particularly for generics); consult specific product labeling.

Caplet, oral:
  Bayer® PM: Aspirin 500 mg and diphenhydramine citrate 38.3 mg

◆ **Aspirin and Diphenhydramine Citrate** *see* Aspirin and Diphenhydramine *on page* 157

Aspirin and Dipyridamole
(AS pir in & dye peer ID a mole)

Brand Names: U.S. Aggrenox®

Brand Names: Canada Aggrenox®

Index Terms Aspirin and Extended-Release Dipyridamole; Dipyridamole and Aspirin

Pharmacologic Category Antiplatelet Agent

Use Reduction in the risk of stroke in patients who have had transient ischemia of the brain or ischemic stroke due to thrombosis

Unlabeled Use Hemodialysis graft patency

Pregnancy Risk Factor D

Dosage Oral: Adults:

Stroke prevention: One capsule (dipyridamole 200 mg, aspirin 25 mg) twice daily

Alternative regimen for patients with intolerable headache: One capsule at bedtime and low-dose aspirin in the morning. Return to usual dose (1 capsule twice daily) as soon as tolerance to headache develops (usually within a week).

Hemodialysis graft patency (unlabeled use): One capsule (dipyridamole 200 mg, aspirin 25 mg) twice daily

Dosage adjustment in renal impairment: Avoid use in patients with severe renal dysfunction (Cl_{cr} <10 mL/minute). Studies have not been done in patients with renal impairment.

Dosage adjustment in hepatic impairment: Avoid use in patients with severe hepatic impairment. Studies have not been done in patients with varying degrees of hepatic impairment.

Elderly: Plasma concentrations were 40% higher, but specific dosage adjustments have not been recommended.

Additional Information Complete prescribing information for this medication should be consulted for additional detail.

Dosage Forms Excipient information presented when available (limited, particularly for generics); consult specific product labeling.

Capsule, variable release:

Aggrenox®: Aspirin 25 mg [immediate release] and dipyridamole 200 mg [extended release] [contains lactose, sucrose]

- **Aspirin and Extended-Release Dipyridamole** *see* Aspirin and Dipyridamole *on page* 157
- **Aspirin and Oxycodone** *see* Oxycodone and Aspirin *on page* 1269
- **Aspirin, Caffeine and Acetaminophen** *see* Acetaminophen, Aspirin, and Caffeine *on page* 32
- **Aspirin, Caffeine, and Butalbital** *see* Butalbital, Aspirin, and Caffeine *on page* 255
- **Aspirin, Caffeine, and Orphenadrine** *see* Orphenadrine, Aspirin, and Caffeine *on page* 1252
- **Aspirin, Carisoprodol, and Codeine** *see* Carisoprodol, Aspirin, and Codeine *on page* 292
- **Aspirin Free Anacin® Extra Strength [OTC]** *see* Acetaminophen *on page* 27
- **Aspirin, Orphenadrine, and Caffeine** *see* Orphenadrine, Aspirin, and Caffeine *on page* 1252
- **Aspir-low [OTC]** *see* Aspirin *on page* 154
- **Aspirtab [OTC]** *see* Aspirin *on page* 154
- **Astelin®** *see* Azelastine (Nasal) *on page* 179
- **Astepro®** *see* Azelastine (Nasal) *on page* 179
- **Astramorph®/PF** *see* Morphine (Systemic) *on page* 1153
- **AT** *see* Antithrombin *on page* 130
- **AT-III** *see* Antithrombin *on page* 130
- **Atacand®** *see* Candesartan *on page* 273
- **Atacand HCT®** *see* Candesartan and Hydrochlorothiazide *on page* 274
- **Atacand® Plus (Can)** *see* Candesartan and Hydrochlorothiazide *on page* 274
- **Atarax® (Can)** *see* HydrOXYzine *on page* 853
- **Atasol® (Can)** *see* Acetaminophen *on page* 27

Atazanavir (at a za NA veer)

Brand Names: U.S. Reyataz®

Brand Names: Canada Reyataz®

Index Terms Atazanavir Sulfate; ATV; BMS-232632

Pharmacologic Category Antiretroviral Agent, Protease Inhibitor

Additional Appendix Information

Management of Healthcare Worker Exposures to HBV, HCV, and HIV *on page* 1935

Perinatal HIV Guidelines *on page* 1946

Use Treatment of HIV-1 infections in combination with at least two other antiretroviral agents

Pregnancy Risk Factor B

Pregnancy Considerations Teratogenic effects have not been observed in animal reproduction studies. Atazanavir crosses the placenta with cord blood concentrations reported as 10% to 21% of maternal serum concentrations at delivery. An increased risk of teratogenic effects has not been observed based on information collected by the antiretroviral pregnancy registry. A small increased risk of preterm birth has been associated with maternal use of protease inhibitor-based combination antiretroviral (ARV) therapy during pregnancy; however, the benefits of use generally outweigh this risk and protease inhibitors (PIs) should not be withheld if otherwise recommended. Hyperglycemia, new onset of diabetes mellitus, or diabetic ketoacidosis have been reported with PIs; it is not clear if pregnancy increases this risk. Hyperbilirubinemia or hypoglycemia may occur in neonates following *in utero* exposure to atazanavir, although data is conflicting.

The DHHS Perinatal HIV Guidelines recommend atazanavir as an alternate PI when combined with low-dose ritonavir boosting. Pharmacokinetic studies suggest that standard dosing during pregnancy may provide decreased plasma concentrations. However, dose adjustment is not required unless using concomitant H_2-receptor blockers or tenofovir. May give as once-daily dosing.

Regardless of CD4 count or HIV RNA copy number, all HIV-infected pregnant women should receive a combination antepartum ARV drug regimen; this includes women who require therapy for their own health, as well as women who do not yet require therapy for their own health. ARV therapy should be started as soon as possible if required for the woman's health or immediately after the first trimester if not needed for the mothers health (although earlier initiation may be considered). Long-term follow-up is recommended for all infants exposed to ARV medications.

Healthcare providers are encouraged to enroll pregnant women exposed to antiretroviral medications in the Antiretroviral Pregnancy Registry (1-800-258-4263 or www.APRegistry.com). Healthcare providers caring for HIV-infected women and their infants may contact the National Perinatal HIV Hotline (888-448-8765) for clinical consultation (DHHS [perinatal], 2011).

Lactation Enters breast milk/contraindicated

Contraindications Hypersensitivity (eg, Stevens-Johnson syndrome, erythema multiforme, or toxic skin eruptions) to atazanavir or any component of the formulation; concurrent therapy with alfuzosin, cisapride, ergot derivatives (dihydroergotamine, ergonovine, ergotamine, methylergonovine), etravirine, indinavir, irinotecan, lovastatin, midazolam (oral), pimozide, rifampin, sildenafil (when used for pulmonary artery hypertension [eg, Revatio®]), simvastatin, St John's wort, or triazolam

Warnings/Precautions Use with caution in patients taking strong CYP3A4 inhibitors, moderate or strong CYP3A4 inducers, and major CYP2C8 substrates; consider alternative agents that avoid or lessen the potential for CYP- or glucuronidation-mediated interactions. Contraindicated with drugs that are major CYP3A4 or UGT1A1 substrates (see Drug Interactions). Do not coadminister colchicine in patient with renal or hepatic impairment; avoid concurrent use with salmeterol.

Atazanavir may prolong PR interval, use with caution in patients with pre-existing conduction abnormalities or with medications which prolong AV conduction (dosage adjustment required with some agents); rare cases of second-degree AV block have been reported. May exacerbate pre-existing hepatic dysfunction; use caution in patients with hepatitis B or C or in patients with elevated transaminases. Asymptomatic elevations in bilirubin (unconjugated) occur commonly during therapy with atazanavir; consider alternative therapy if bilirubin is >5 times ULN. Evaluate alternative etiologies if transaminase elevations also occur.

Cases of nephrolithiasis have been reported in postmarketing surveillance; temporary or permanent discontinuation of therapy should be considered if symptoms develop.

Protease inhibitors have been associated with a variety of hypersensitivity events (some severe), including rash, anaphylaxis (rare), angioedema, bronchospasm, erythema multiforme, and/or Stevens-Johnson syndrome (rare). It is generally recommended to discontinue treatment if severe rash or moderate symptoms accompanied by other systemic symptoms occur.

Use with caution in patients with hemophilia A or B; increased bleeding during protease inhibitor therapy has been reported. Changes in glucose tolerance, hyperglycemia, exacerbation of diabetes, DKA, and new-onset diabetes mellitus have been reported in patients receiving protease inhibitors. May be associated with fat redistribution (buffalo hump, increased abdominal girth, breast engorgement, facial atrophy). Immune reconstitution syndrome may develop resulting in the occurrence of an inflammatory response to an indolent or residual opportunistic infection; further evaluation and treatment may be required. Do not use in children <3 months of age due to potential for kernicterus.

Adverse Reactions Includes data from both treatment-naive and treatment-experienced patients. Percentages listed for adults unless otherwise specified.

>10%:
- Dermatologic: Rash (3% to 21%; median onset 7 weeks)
- Endocrine & metabolic: Cholesterol increased (≥240 mg/dL: 6% to 25%)
- Gastrointestinal: Nausea (3% to 14%), amylase increased (≤14%)
- Hepatic: Bilirubin increased (≥2.6 times ULN: 35% to 49%)
- Neuromuscular & skeletal: CPK increased (6% to 11%)
- Respiratory: Cough (children 21%)

2% to 10%:
- Cardiovascular: AV block (first degree: 6%; second degree [children] 2%)
- Central nervous system: Headache (1% to 6%; children 7%), peripheral neuropathy (<1% to 4%), insomnia (<1% to 3%), depression (2%), fever (2%; children 19%), dizziness (<1% to 2%)
- Endocrine & metabolic: Triglycerides increased (<1% to 8%), hyperglycemia (≥251 mg/dL: 5%)
- Gastrointestinal: Lipase increased (<1% to 5%), abdominal pain (4%), vomiting (3% to 4%; children 8%), diarrhea (1% to 3%; children 8%)
- Hematologic: Neutropenia (3% to 7%), hemoglobin decreased (<1% to 5%), thrombocytopenia (2%)
- Hepatic: Jaundice (5% to 9%; children 13%), ALT increased (>5 times ULN: 3% to 9%; 10% to 25% in patients seropositive for hepatitis B and/or C), AST increased (>5 times ULN: 2% to 7%; 9% to 10% in patients seropositive for hepatitis B and/or C)
- Neuromuscular & skeletal: Myalgia (4%)
- Respiratory: Rhinorrhea (children 6%)

<2%, postmarketing, and/or case reports: Alopecia, arthralgia, AV block (second- and third-degree, rare), cholecystitis, cholelithiasis, cholestasis, diabetes mellitus, edema, erythema multiforme, immune reconstitution syndrome, left bundle branch block, macropapular rash, nephrolithiasis, pancreatitis, PR prolongation, pruritus, QT_c prolongation, Stevens-Johnson syndrome, torsade de pointes

Drug Interactions

Metabolism/Transport Effects Substrate of CYP3A4 (major); **Note:** Assignment of Major/Minor substrate status based on clinically relevant drug interaction potential; **Inhibits** CYP1A2 (weak), CYP2C8 (weak), CYP2C9 (weak), CYP3A4 (strong), UGT1A1

Avoid Concomitant Use

Avoid concomitant use of Atazanavir with any of the following: Alfuzosin; Amiodarone; Buprenorphine; Cisapride; Conivaptan; Crizotinib; Dronedarone; Eplerenone; Ergot Derivatives; Etravirine; Everolimus; Fluticasone (Oral Inhalation); Halofantrine; Indinavir; Irinotecan; Lapatinib; Lovastatin; Lurasidone; Midazolam; Nevirapine; Nilotinib; Nisoldipine; Pimozide; QuiNIDine; Ranolazine; Rifampin; Rivaroxaban; RomiDEPsin; Salmeterol; Silodosin; Simvastatin; St Johns Wort; Tamsulosin; Ticagrelor; Tolvaptan; Toremifene; Triazolam

Increased Effect/Toxicity

Atazanavir may increase the levels/effects of: Alfuzosin; Almotriptan; Alosetron; ALPRAZolam; Amiodarone; Antifungal Agents (Azole Derivatives, Systemic); ARIPiprazole; Bortezomib; Brentuximab Vedotin; Brinzolamide; Budesonide (Nasal); Budesonide (Systemic, Oral Inhalation); Buprenorphine; Calcium Channel Blockers (Dihydropyridine); Calcium Channel Blockers (Nondihydropyridine); CarBAMazepine; Ciclesonide; Cisapride; Clarithromycin; Colchicine; Conivaptan; Corticosteroids (Orally Inhaled); Crizotinib; CycloSPORINE; CycloSPORINE (Systemic); CYP3A4 Substrates; Dienogest; Digoxin; Dronedarone; Dutasteride; Enfuvirtide; Eplerenone; Ergot Derivatives; Etravirine; Everolimus; FentaNYL; Fesoterodine; Fluticasone (Nasal); Fluticasone (Oral Inhalation); Fusidic Acid; GuanFACINE; Halofantrine; HMG-CoA Reductase Inhibitors; Iloperidone; Indinavir; Irinotecan; Ixabepilone; Lapatinib; Lovastatin; Lumefantrine; Lurasidone; Maraviroc; Meperidine; MethylPREDNISolone; Midazolam; Nefazodone; Nevirapine; Nilotinib; Nisoldipine; Paricalcitol; Pazopanib; Pimecrolimus; Pimozide; Pitavastatin; Propafenone; Protease Inhibitors; QuiNIDine; Ranolazine; Rifabutin; Rivaroxaban; RomiDEPsin; Ruxolitinib; Salmeterol; Saxagliptin; Sildenafil; Silodosin; Simvastatin; Sirolimus; SORAfenib; Tacrolimus; Tacrolimus (Systemic); Tacrolimus (Topical); Tadalafil; Tamsulosin; Temsirolimus; Tenofovir; Ticagrelor; Tolterodine; Tolvaptan; Toremifene; TraZODone; Triazolam; Tricyclic Antidepressants; Vardenafil; Vemurafenib; Vilazodone; Warfarin; Zuclopenthixol

The levels/effects of Atazanavir may be increased by: Antifungal Agents (Azole Derivatives, Systemic); Clarithromycin; CycloSPORINE; CycloSPORINE (Systemic); CYP3A4 Inhibitors (Moderate); CYP3A4 Inhibitors (Strong); Dasatinib; Delavirdine; Efavirenz; Enfuvirtide; Fusidic Acid; Indinavir; Telaprevir

Decreased Effect

Atazanavir may decrease the levels/effects of: Abacavir; Clarithromycin; Contraceptives (Estrogens); Delavirdine; Didanosine; Divalproex; Meperidine; Prasugrel; Telaprevir; Theophylline Derivatives; Ticagrelor; Valproic Acid; Zidovudine

The levels/effects of Atazanavir may be decreased by: Antacids; Buprenorphine; CarBAMazepine; CYP3A4 Inducers (Strong); Deferasirox; Didanosine; Efavirenz; Etravirine; Garlic; H2-Antagonists; Minocycline; Nevirapine; Proton Pump Inhibitors; Rifampin; St Johns Wort; Tenofovir; Tocilizumab

Ethanol/Nutrition/Herb Interactions

Food: Bioavailability of atazanavir increased when taken with food.

Herb/Nutraceutical: St John's wort (*Hypericum perforatum*) decreases serum concentrations of protease inhibitors and may lead to treatment failures; concurrent use is contraindicated.

Stability Store at 25°C (77°F); excursions permitted to 15°C to 30°C (59°F to 86°F).

Mechanism of Action Binds to the site of HIV-1 protease activity and inhibits cleavage of viral Gag-Pol polyprotein precursors into individual functional proteins required for infectious HIV. This results in the formation of immature, noninfectious viral particles.

Pharmacodynamics/Kinetics

Absorption: Rapid; enhanced with food

Protein binding: 86%

Metabolism: Hepatic, via multiple pathways including CYP3A4; forms two metabolites (inactive)

Half-life elimination: Unboosted therapy: 7-8 hours; Boosted therapy (with ritonavir): 9-18 hours

Time to peak, plasma: 2-3 hours

Excretion: Feces (79%, 20% of total dose as unchanged drug); urine (13%, 7% of total dose as unchanged drug)

Dosage Oral:

Children 6-17 years:

Antiretroviral-naive patients:

15-24 kg: Atazanavir 150 mg once daily **plus** ritonavir 80 mg once daily

25-31 kg: Atazanavir 200 mg once daily **plus** ritonavir 100 mg once daily

32-38 kg: Atazanavir 250 mg once daily **plus** ritonavir 100 mg once daily

≥39 kg: Atazanavir 300 mg once daily **plus** 100 mg ritonavir once daily. **Note:** Treatment-naive patients ≥39 kg and ≥13 years of age who are unable to tolerate ritonavir, refer to adult dosing.

or

15-19 kg: Atazanavir 8.5 mg/kg/dose once daily (rounded to available capsule strengths) **plus** ritonavir 4 mg/kg/dose once daily

≥20 kg: Atazanavir 7 mg/kg/dose once daily (round to available capsule strengths) (maximum: 300 mg/day) **plus** ritonavir 4 mg/kg/dose once daily (maximum: 100 mg/day)

Antiretroviral-experienced patients: **Note:** Atazanavir without ritonavir is not recommended in antiretroviral-experienced patients with prior virologic failure:

25-31 kg: Atazanavir 200 mg once daily **plus** ritonavir 100 mg once daily

32-38 kg: Atazanavir 250 mg once daily **plus** ritonavir 100 mg once daily

≥39 kg: Atazanavir 300 mg once daily **plus** 100 mg ritonavir once daily

Adults:

Antiretroviral-naive patients: Atazanavir 300 mg once daily **plus** ritonavir 100 mg once daily **or** 400 mg once daily in patients unable to tolerate ritonavir. **Note:** Recommended (with ritonavir) as a first-line therapy with tenofovir/emtricitabine in nonpregnant antiretroviral-naive patients (DHHS, 2011). If using without ritonavir, consider also using two nucleoside reverse transcriptase inhibitors (other than didanosine/emtricitabine or didanosine/lamivudine) (DHHS, 2011).

Antiretroviral-experienced patients: Atazanavir 300 mg once daily **plus** ritonavir 100 mg once daily. **Note:** Atazanavir without ritonavir is not recommended in antiretroviral-experienced patients with prior virologic failure.

Pregnant patients (antiretroviral-naive): Atazanavir 300 mg once daily **plus** ritonavir 100 mg once daily. **Note:** Postpartum dosage adjustment not needed. Observe patient for adverse events, especially within 2 months after delivery. Dose adjustments required for concomitant tenofovir *or* H_2 antagonist use (insufficient information for dose adjustment if *both* tenofovir and an H_2 antagonist are used).

Dosage adjustments for concomitant therapy: Adults:

Coadministration with bosentan:

Coadministration of bosentan in patients currently receiving atazanavir/ritonavir: For patients receiving ritonavir for at least 10 days, begin with bosentan 62.5 mg once daily or every other day based on tolerability

Coadministration of atazanavir/ritonavir in patients currently receiving bosentan: Discontinue bosentan 36 hours prior to the initiation of ritonavir. After at least 10 days of ritonavir; resume bosentan 62.5 mg once daily or every other day based on tolerability.

Coadministration with colchicine:

Familial Mediterranean fever (FMF): Maximum colchicine dose: 0.6 mg/day (0.3 mg twice daily)

Gout prophylaxis:

If original colchicine dose is 0.6 mg twice daily, adjust dose to 0.3 mg once daily

If original colchicine dose is 0.6 mg once daily, adjust dose to 0.3 mg every other day

Gout flare treatment: Initial: Colchicine 0.6 mg, followed in 1 hour by a single dose of 0.3 mg; do not repeat for at least 3 days

Coadministration with efavirenz:

Antiretroviral-naive patients: Atazanavir 400 mg plus ritonavir 100 mg given with efavirenz 600 mg (all once daily but administered at different times; atazanavir and ritonavir with food and efavirenz on an empty stomach). This combination/dose may be used after the first trimester in pregnant women when other alternatives are not available (DHHS [perinatal], 2011).

Antiretroviral-experienced patients: Concurrent use not recommended due to decreased atazanavir exposure.

Coadministration with didanosine buffered or enteric-coated formulations: Administer atazanavir 2 hours before or 1 hour after didanosine buffered or enteric coated formulations

Coadministration with H_2 antagonists:

Antiretroviral-naive patients: Atazanavir 300 mg plus ritonavir 100 mg given simultaneously with, or at least 10 hours after an H_2 antagonist equivalent dose of ≤80 mg famotidine/day

Patients unable to tolerate ritonavir: Atazanavir 400 mg once daily given at least 2 hours before or at least 10 hours after an H_2 antagonist equivalent daily dose of ≤40 mg famotidine (single dose ≤20 mg)

Antiretroviral-experienced patients: Atazanavir 300 mg plus ritonavir 100 mg given simultaneously with, or at least 10 hours after an H_2 antagonist equivalent dose of ≤40 mg famotidine/day

Antiretroviral-experienced pregnant patients in the second or third trimester: Atazanavir 400 mg plus ritonavir 100 mg simultaneously with, or at least 10 hours after an H_2 antagonist. **Note:** Insufficient information for dose adjustment if tenofovir **and** an H_2 antagonist are used.

Coadministration with maraviroc: Atazanavir 300 mg plus ritonavir 100 mg once daily plus maraviroc 150 mg twice daily

Coadministration with phosphodiesterase-5 enzyme (PDE-5) inhibitor:

Pulmonary arterial hypertension: Atazanavir coadministered with tadalafil:

Patient receiving atazanavir with or without ritonavir for at least 1 week: Initiate tadalafil at 20 mg once daily; increase to 40 mg once daily based on individual tolerability

Patient receiving tadalafil when initiating atazanavir with or without ritonavir: Stop tadalafil at least 24 hours prior to starting atazanavir (with or without ritonavir). After at least 1 week following the initiation of atazanavir (with or without ritonavir), resume tadalafil at 20 mg once daily; increase to 40 mg once daily based on individual tolerability.

Erectile dysfunction: Atazanavir coadministered with:

Sildenafil (Viagra®): Maximum sildenafil dose: 25 mg in a 48-hour period

Tadalafil (Cialis®): Maximum tadalafil dose: 10 mg in a 72-hour period

Vardenafil: Maximum vardenafil dose: 2.5 mg in a 24-hour period

Ritonavir and vardenafil: Maximum vardenafil dose: 2.5 mg in a 72-hour period

Coadministration with proton pump inhibitors:

Antiretroviral-naive patients: Atazanavir 300 mg plus ritonavir 100 mg given 12 hours after a proton pump inhibitor equivalent dose of ≤20 mg omeprazole/day

Antiretroviral-experienced patients: Concurrent use not recommended. (**Note:** One study noted adequate serum concentrations when atazanavir 400 mg plus ritonavir 100 mg was given at the same time or 12 hours after omeprazole 20 mg.)

Coadministration with tenofovir:

Antiretroviral-naive patients: Atazanavir 300 mg plus ritonavir 100 mg given with tenofovir 300 mg (all as a single daily dose); if H_2 antagonist coadministered, administer atazanavir simultaneously with, or at least 10 hours after, an H_2 antagonist equivalent dose of ≤40 mg famotidine once daily

Antiretroviral-experienced patients: Atazanavir 300 mg plus ritonavir 100 mg given with tenofovir 300 mg (all as a single daily dose); if H_2 antagonist coadministered (not to exceed equivalent daily dose of ≤40 mg famotidine), increase atazanavir to 400 mg (plus ritonavir 100 mg) once daily

Antiretroviral-experienced pregnant patients in the second or third trimester: Atazanavir 400 mg plus ritonavir 100 mg. **Note:** Insufficient information for dose adjustment if tenofovir **and** an H_2 antagonist are used

Dosage adjustment in renal impairment:

Not on hemodialysis: No adjustment necessary

Hemodialysis:

Antiretroviral-naive patients: Use boosted therapy of atazanavir 300 mg with ritonavir 100 mg once daily

Antiretroviral-experienced patients: Not recommended

Dosage adjustment in hepatic impairment:

Atazanavir:

Mild-to-moderate hepatic insufficiency: Use with caution; if moderate insufficiency (Child-Pugh class B) and no prior virologic failure, reduce dose to 300 mg once daily.

Severe hepatic insufficiency (Child-Pugh class C): Not recommended

Note: Patients with underlying hepatitis B or C may be at increased risk of hepatic decompensation.

Atazanavir/ritonavir: Use not recommended in hepatic impairment.

Dietary Considerations Must be taken with food; enhances absorption.

Administration Administer with food.

Monitoring Parameters Viral load, CD4, serum glucose; liver function tests, bilirubin, drug levels (with certain concomitant medications), ECG monitoring in patients with prolonged PR interval or with concurrent AV nodal blocking drugs

Additional Information A listing of medications that should not be used concurrently is available with each bottle and patients should be provided with this information.

Dosage Forms Excipient information presented when available (limited, particularly for generics); consult specific product labeling.

Capsule, oral, as sulfate:

Reyataz®: 100 mg, 150 mg, 200 mg, 300 mg

◆ **Atazanavir Sulfate** *see* Atazanavir *on page 158*

◆ **Atelvia™** *see* Risedronate *on page 1494*

Atenolol (a TEN oh lole)

Brand Names: U.S. Tenormin®

Brand Names: Canada Apo-Atenol®; CO Atenolol; Dom-Atenolol; JAMP-Atenolol; Mint-Atenolol; Mylan-Atenolol; Nu-Atenol; PHL-Atenolol; PMS-Atenolol; RAN™-Atenolol; ratio-Atenolol; Riva-Atenolol; Sandoz-Atenolol; Septa-Atenolol; Tenormin®; Teva-Atenolol

Pharmacologic Category Antianginal Agent; Beta Blocker, Beta-1 Selective

Additional Appendix Information

Beta-Blockers *on page 1884*

Use Treatment of hypertension, alone or in combination with other agents; management of angina pectoris; secondary prevention postmyocardial infarction

Unlabeled Use Acute ethanol withdrawal (in combination with a benzodiazepine), supraventricular and ventricular arrhythmias, and migraine headache prophylaxis

Pregnancy Risk Factor D

Pregnancy Considerations Studies in pregnant women have demonstrated a risk to the fetus; therefore, the manufacturer classifies atenolol as pregnancy category D. Atenolol crosses the placenta and is found in cord blood. In a cohort study, an increased risk of cardiovascular defects was observed following maternal use of beta-blockers during pregnancy. Intrauterine growth restriction (IUGR), small placentas, as well as fetal/neonatal bradycardia, hypoglycemia, and/or respiratory depression have been observed following *in utero* exposure to beta-blockers as a class. Adequate facilities for monitoring infants at birth should be available. Untreated chronic maternal hypertension and pre-eclampsia are also associated with adverse events in the fetus, infant, and mother. The maternal pharmacokinetic parameters of atenolol during the second and third trimesters are within the ranges reported in nonpregnant patients. Although atenolol has shown efficacy in the treatment of hypertension in pregnancy, it is not the drug of choice due to potential IUGR in the infant.

Lactation Enters breast milk/use caution (AAP recommends "use with caution"; AAP 2001 update pending)

Contraindications Hypersensitivity to atenolol or any component of the formulation; sinus bradycardia; sinus node dysfunction; heart block greater than first-degree (except in patients with a functioning artificial pacemaker); cardiogenic shock; uncompensated cardiac failure; pulmonary edema; pregnancy

Warnings/Precautions Consider pre-existing conditions such as sick sinus syndrome before initiating. Administer cautiously in compensated heart failure and monitor for a worsening of the condition (efficacy of atenolol in heart failure has not been established). **[U.S. Boxed Warning]: Beta-blocker therapy should not be withdrawn abruptly (particularly in patients with CAD), but gradually tapered to avoid acute tachycardia, hypertension, and/or ischemia.** Chronic beta-blocker therapy should not be routinely withdrawn prior to major surgery. Beta-blockers should be avoided in patients with bronchospastic disease (asthma). Atenolol, with B_1 selectivity, has been used cautiously in bronchospastic disease with close monitoring. May precipitate or aggravate symptoms of arterial insufficiency in patients with PVD and Raynaud's disease; use with caution and monitor for progression of arterial obstruction. Use cautiously in patients with diabetes - may mask hypoglycemic symptoms. May mask signs of hyperthyroidism (eg, tachycardia); use caution if hyperthyroidism is suspected, abrupt withdrawal may precipitate thyroid storm. Alterations in thyroid function tests may be observed. Use cautiously in the renally impaired (dosage adjustment required). Caution in myasthenia gravis or psychiatric disease (may cause CNS depression). Bradycardia may be observed more frequently in elderly patients (>65 years of age); dosage reductions may be necessary. Adequate alpha-blockade is required prior to use of any beta-blocker for patients with untreated pheochromocytoma. May induce or exacerbate psoriasis. Use caution with history of severe anaphylaxis to allergens; patients taking beta-blockers may become more sensitive to repeated challenges. Treatment of anaphylaxis (eg, epinephrine) in patients taking beta-blockers may be ineffective or promote undesirable effects. Use with caution in patients on concurrent digoxin, verapamil, or diltiazem; bradycardia or heart block can occur. Use with caution in patients receiving inhaled anesthetic agents known to depress myocardial contractility.

Adverse Reactions

1% to 10%:

Cardiovascular: Persistent bradycardia, hypotension, chest pain, edema, heart failure, second- or third-degree AV block, Raynaud's phenomenon

Central nervous system: Dizziness, fatigue, insomnia, lethargy, confusion, mental impairment, depression, headache, nightmares

Gastrointestinal: Constipation, diarrhea, nausea

Genitourinary: Impotence

Miscellaneous: Cold extremities

<1% (Limited to important or life-threatening): Alopecia, dyspnea (especially with large doses), hallucinations, impotence, liver enzymes increased, lupus syndrome, Peyronie's disease, positive ANA, psoriasiform rash, psychosis, thrombocytopenia, wheezing

Drug Interactions

Metabolism/Transport Effects None known.

Avoid Concomitant Use

Avoid concomitant use of Atenolol with any of the following: Floctafenine; Methacholine

Increased Effect/Toxicity

Atenolol may increase the levels/effects of: Alpha-/Beta-Agonists (Direct-Acting); Alpha1-Blockers; Alpha2-Agonists; Amifostine; Antihypertensives; Bupivacaine; Cardiac Glycosides; Cholinergic Agonists; Fingolimod; Hypotensive Agents; Insulin; Lidocaine; Lidocaine (Systemic); Lidocaine (Topical); Mepivacaine; Methacholine; Midodrine; RiTUXimab; Sulfonylureas

The levels/effects of Atenolol may be increased by: Acetylcholinesterase Inhibitors; Amiodarone; Anilidopiperidine Opioids; Calcium Channel Blockers (Dihydropyridine); Calcium Channel Blockers (Nondihydropyridine); Diazoxide; Dipyridamole; Disopyramide; Dronedarone; Floctafenine; Glycopyrrolate; Herbs (Hypotensive Properties); MAO Inhibitors; Pentoxifylline; Phosphodiesterase 5 Inhibitors; Prostacyclin Analogues; Reserpine

Decreased Effect

Atenolol may decrease the levels/effects of: Beta2-Agonists; Theophylline Derivatives

The levels/effects of Atenolol may be decreased by: Ampicillin; Herbs (Hypertensive Properties); Methylphenidate; Nonsteroidal Anti-Inflammatory Agents; Yohimbine

Ethanol/Nutrition/Herb Interactions

Food: Atenolol serum concentrations may be decreased if taken with food.

Herb/Nutraceutical: Avoid dong quai if using for hypertension (has estrogenic activity). Avoid ephedra, yohimbe, ginseng (may worsen hypertension). Avoid garlic (may have increased antihypertensive effect).

Stability Protect from light.

Mechanism of Action Competitively blocks response to beta-adrenergic stimulation, selectively blocks $beta_1$-receptors with little or no effect on $beta_2$-receptors except at high doses

Pharmacodynamics/Kinetics

Onset of action: Peak effect: Oral: 2-4 hours

Duration: Normal renal function: 12-24 hours

Absorption: Oral: Rapid, incomplete (~50%)

Distribution: Low lipophilicity; does not cross blood-brain barrier

Protein binding: 6% to 16%

Metabolism: Limited hepatic

Half-life elimination: Beta:

Neonates: ≤35 hours; Mean: 16 hours

Children: 4.6 hours; children >10 years may have longer half-life (>5 hours) compared to children 5-10 years (<5 hours)

Adults: Normal renal function: 6-7 hours, prolonged with renal impairment; End-stage renal disease: 15-35 hours

Time to peak, plasma: Oral: 2-4 hours

Excretion: Feces (50%); urine (40% as unchanged drug)

Dosage Oral:

Children: Hypertension: 0.5-1 mg/kg/dose given daily; range of 0.5-1.5 mg/kg/day; maximum dose: 2 mg/kg/day up to 100 mg/day

Adults:

Hypertension: 25-50 mg once daily, may increase to 100 mg/day. Doses >100 mg are unlikely to produce any further benefit.

Angina pectoris: 50 mg once daily, may increase to 100 mg/day. Some patients may require 200 mg/day.

Postmyocardial infarction: 100 mg/day or 50 mg twice daily for 6-9 days postmyocardial infarction.

Thyrotoxicosis (unlabeled use): 25-100 mg once or twice daily (Bahn, 2011)

Elderly: Hypertension: Consider lower initial doses and titrate to response (Aronow, 2011).

Dosing interval for oral atenolol in renal impairment:

Cl_{cr} 15-35 mL/minute: Administer 50 mg/day maximum.

Cl_{cr} <15 mL/minute: Administer 50 mg every other day maximum.

Hemodialysis: Moderately dialyzable (20% to 50%) via hemodialysis; administer dose postdialysis or administer 25-50 mg supplemental dose.

Peritoneal dialysis: Elimination is not enhanced; supplemental dose is not necessary.

Dietary Considerations May be taken without regard to meals.

Administration When administered acutely for cardiac treatment, monitor ECG and blood pressure. May be administered without regard to meals.

Monitoring Parameters Acute cardiac treatment: Monitor ECG and blood pressure

Test Interactions Increased glucose; decreased HDL

Dosage Forms Excipient information presented when available (limited, particularly for generics); consult specific product labeling.

Tablet, oral: 25 mg, 50 mg, 100 mg

Tenormin®: 25 mg

Tenormin®: 50 mg [scored]

Tenormin®: 100 mg

Extemporaneous Preparations A 2 mg/mL oral suspension may be made with tablets. Crush four 50 mg tablets in a mortar and reduce to a fine powder. Add a small amount of glycerin and mix to a uniform paste. Mix while adding Ora-Sweet® SF vehicle in incremental proportions to **almost** 100 mL; transfer to a calibrated bottle, rinse mortar with vehicle, and add quantity of vehicle sufficient to make 100 mL. Label "shake well" and "refrigerate". Stable for 90 days.

Nahata MC, Pai VB, and Hipple TF, *Pediatric Drug Formulations*, 5th ed, Cincinnati, OH: Harvey Whitney Books Co, 2004.

◆ **ATG** *see* Antithymocyte Globulin (Equine) *on page 131*

◆ **Atgam®** *see* Antithymocyte Globulin (Equine) *on page 131*

◆ **Ativan®** *see* LORazepam *on page 1032*
◆ **Atlizumab** *see* Tocilizumab *on page 1700*
◆ **ATNAA** *see* Atropine and Pralidoxime *on page 172*

Atomoxetine (AT oh mox e teen)

Brand Names: U.S. Strattera®

Brand Names: Canada Strattera®

Index Terms Atomoxetine Hydrochloride; LY139603; Methylphenoxy-Benzene Propanamine; Tomoxetine

Pharmacologic Category Norepinephrine Reuptake Inhibitor, Selective

Use Treatment of attention deficit/hyperactivity disorder (ADHD)

Pregnancy Risk Factor C

Pregnancy Considerations Decreased pup weight and survival were observed in animal studies. There are no adequate and well-controlled studies in pregnant women. Use only if potential benefit to the mother outweighs possible risk to fetus.

Lactation Excretion in breast milk unknown/use caution

Medication Guide Available Yes

Contraindications Hypersensitivity to atomoxetine or any component of the formulation; use with or within 14 days of MAO inhibitors; narrow-angle glaucoma; current or past history of pheochromocytoma; severe cardiovascular disorders in which the condition would be expected to deteriorate with clinically relevant blood pressure or heart rate increases

Canadian labeling: Additional contraindications (not in U.S. labeling): Symptomatic cardiovascular diseases, moderate-to-severe hypertension; advanced arteriosclerosis; uncontrolled hyperthyroidism

Warnings/Precautions [U.S. Boxed Warning]: Use caution in pediatric patients; may be an increased risk of suicidal ideation. Closely monitor for clinical worsening, suicidality, or unusual changes in behavior; especially during the initial few months of a course of drug therapy, or at times of dose changes, either increases or decreases. The child's family or caregiver should be instructed to closely observe the patient and communicate condition with healthcare provider. New or worsening symptoms of hostility or aggressive behaviors have been associated with atomoxetine, particularly with the initiation of therapy. Use caution in patients with a history of psychotic illness or bipolar disorder; therapy may induce mixed/manic disorder or psychotic symptoms. Atomoxetine is not approved for major depressive disorder. Patients presenting with depressive symptoms should be screened for bipolar disorder. Recommended to be used as part of a comprehensive treatment program for attention deficit disorders. Atomoxetine does not worsen anxiety in patients with existing anxiety disorders or tics related to Tourette's disorder.

Use caution with hepatic disease (dosage adjustments necessary in hepatic impairment). Use may be associated with rare but severe hepatotoxicity; discontinue and do not restart if signs or symptoms of hepatotoxic reaction (eg, jaundice, pruritus, flu-like symptoms) or laboratory evidence of liver disease are noted. Use caution in patients who are poor metabolizers of CYP2D6 metabolized drugs ("poor metabolizers"), bioavailability increases.

Orthostasis can occur; use caution in patients predisposed to hypotension or those with abrupt changes in heart rate or blood pressure. CNS stimulant use has been associated with serious cardiovascular events including sudden death in patients with pre-existing structural cardiac abnormalities or other serious heart problems (sudden death in children and adolescents; sudden death, stroke, and MI in adults). These products should be avoided in patients with known serious structural cardiac abnormalities, cardiomyopathy, serious heart rhythm abnormalities, or other serious cardiac problems that could increase the risk of sudden death that these conditions alone carry. Patients should be carefully evaluated for cardiac disease prior to initiation of therapy. May cause increased heart rate or blood pressure; use caution with hypertension or other cardiovascular disease. Use caution with renal impairment. May cause urinary retention/hesitancy; use caution in patients with history of urinary retention or bladder outlet obstruction. Priapism has been associated with use (rarely). Allergic reactions (including angioneurotic edema, urticaria, and rash) may occur (rare).

Growth should be monitored during treatment. Height and weight gain may be reduced during the first 9-12 months of treatment, but should recover by 3 years of therapy. Safety and efficacy have not been evaluated in pediatric patients <6 years of age.

Adverse Reactions Percentages as reported in children and adults; some adverse reactions may be increased in "poor metabolizers" (CYP2D6).

>10%:

Central nervous system: Headache (2% to 19%), insomnia (2% to 15%), somnolence (4% to 11%)

Gastrointestinal: Xerostomia (21%), nausea (7% to 21%), abdominal pain (7% to 18%), appetite decreased (11% to 16%), vomiting (3% to 11%)

1% to 10%:

Cardiovascular: Systolic blood pressure increased (4% to 5%), diastolic pressure increased (≤4%), palpitation (3%), flushing (≥2%), tachycardia (≤2%), orthostatic hypotension (<2%)

Central nervous system: Fatigue/lethargy (6% to 9%), dizziness (5% to 6%), irritability (≤6%), chills (3%), sleep disturbance (3%), mood swings (1% to 2%)

Dermatologic: Hyperhidrosis (4%), rash (2%)

Endocrine & metabolic: Hot flashes (8%), dysmenorrhea (6%), libido decreased (4%), menstruation disturbance (2%), orgasm abnormal (2%)

Gastrointestinal: Constipation (1% to 9%), dyspepsia (4%), anorexia (<3%), weight loss (2% to 3%)

Genitourinary: Erectile disturbance (9%), urinary hesitation/retention (7%), dysuria (3%), ejaculatory disturbance (3%), prostatitis (2%)

Neuromuscular & skeletal: Paresthesia (3% adults; postmarketing observation in children), tremor (2%)

Ocular: Mydriasis (≥2%)

Respiratory: Sinus headache (3%)

Miscellaneous: Jittery feeling (2%)

Postmarketing and/or case reports: Aggressiveness, agitation, akathisia, allergic reactions, allergy, anaphylaxis, angioedema, anxiety, delusional thinking, depression, growth suppression (children), hallucinations, hepatotoxicity, hostility, hyperhidrosis, hypoesthesia, hypomania, impulsiveness, jaundice, mania, MI, panic attacks, paresthesia, pelvic pain, peripheral vascular instability, priapism, pruritus, QT prolongation, Raynaud's phenomenon, seizure (including patients with no prior history or known risk factors for seizure), stroke, suicidal ideation, syncope, tics, urticaria

Drug Interactions

Metabolism/Transport Effects Substrate of CYP2C19 (minor), CYP2D6 (major); **Note:** Assignment of Major/Minor substrate status based on clinically relevant drug interaction potential; **Inhibits** CYP2D6 (weak), CYP3A4 (weak)

Avoid Concomitant Use

Avoid concomitant use of Atomoxetine with any of the following: Iobenguane I 123; MAO Inhibitors; Pimozide

Increased Effect/Toxicity

Atomoxetine may increase the levels/effects of: Beta2-Agonists; Pimozide; Sympathomimetics

The levels/effects of Atomoxetine may be increased by: Abiraterone Acetate; CYP2D6 Inhibitors (Moderate); CYP2D6 Inhibitors (Strong); Darunavir; MAO Inhibitors

Decreased Effect

Atomoxetine may decrease the levels/effects of: Iobenguane I 123

The levels/effects of Atomoxetine may be decreased by: Peginterferon Alfa-2b

Ethanol/Nutrition/Herb Interactions Ethanol: May increase CNS depression; monitor for increased effects with coadministration. Caution patients about effects.

Stability Store at room temperature of 25°C (77°F).

Mechanism of Action Selectively inhibits the reuptake of norepinephrine (Ki 4.5nM) with little to no activity at the other neuronal reuptake pumps or receptor sites.

Pharmacodynamics/Kinetics

Absorption: Rapid

Distribution: V_d: I.V.: 0.85 L/kg

Protein binding: 98%, primarily albumin

Metabolism: Hepatic, via CYP2D6 and CYP2C19; forms metabolites (4-hydroxyatomoxetine, active, equipotent to atomoxetine; N-desmethylatomoxetine in poor metabolizers, limited activity)

Bioavailability: 63% in extensive metabolizers; 94% in poor metabolizers

Half-life elimination: Atomoxetine: 5 hours (up to 24 hours in poor metabolizers); Active metabolites: 4-hydroxyatomoxetine: 6-8 hours; N-desmethylatomoxetine: 6-8 hours (34-40 hours in poor metabolizers)

Time to peak, plasma: 1-2 hours

Excretion: Urine (80%, as conjugated 4-hydroxy metabolite); feces (17%)

Dosage Oral: **Note:** Atomoxetine may be discontinued without the need for tapering dose.

ADHD:

U.S. labeling:

Children ≥6 years and ≤70 kg:

Initial: 0.5 mg/kg/day, increase after minimum of 3 days to ~1.2 mg/kg/day; may administer as either a single daily dose or 2 evenly divided doses in morning and late afternoon/early evening. Maximum daily dose: 1.4 mg/kg or 100 mg, whichever is less.

Dosage adjustment in patients receiving strong CYP2D6 inhibitors (eg, paroxetine, fluoxetine, quinidine) or patients known to be CYP2D6 poor metabolizers: Initial: 0.5 mg/kg/day; if tolerating therapy but inadequate response, may increase after minimum of 4 weeks to 1.2 mg/kg/day. Maximum daily dose: 1.2 mg/kg/day.

Children ≥6 years and >70 kg and Adults:

Initial: 40 mg/day, increased after minimum of 3 days to ~80 mg/day; may administer as either a single daily dose or two evenly divided doses in morning and late afternoon/early evening. May increase to 100 mg/day in 2-4 additional weeks to achieve optimal response. Maximum daily dose: 100 mg/day.

Dosage adjustment in patients receiving strong CYP2D6 inhibitors (eg, paroxetine, fluoxetine, quinidine) or patients known to be CYP2D6 poor metabolizers: Initial: 40 mg/day; if tolerating therapy but inadequate response, may increase after minimum of 4 weeks to 80 mg/day. Maximum daily dose: 80 mg/day.

Canadian labeling:

Children ≥6 years and ≤70 kg:

Initial: ~0.5 mg/kg/day for 7-14 days (Step 1); if tolerated, may increase to ~0.8 mg/kg/day for 7-14 days (Step 2), then to ~1.2 mg/kg/day (Step 3); re-evaluate after ≥30 days and adjust for response if necessary. Maximum daily dose: 1.4 mg/kg or 100 mg, whichever is less. **Note:** Children should weigh at least 20 kg at the time of initiation as 10 mg is the lowest available capsule strength and capsules are to be swallowed whole.

Dosing recommendations according to weight:

Initial (Step 1):

20-29 kg: 10 mg/day
30-44 kg: 18 mg/day
45-64 kg: 25 mg/day
65-70 kg: 40 mg/day

First titration (Step 2):

20-29 kg: 18 mg/day
30-44 kg: 25 mg/day
45-64 kg: 40 mg/day
65-70 kg: 60 mg/day

Second titration (Step 3):

20-29 kg: 25 mg/day
30-44 kg: 40 mg/day
45-64 kg: 60 mg/day
65-70 kg: 80 mg/day

Dosage adjustment in patients receiving strong CYP2D6 inhibitors: Initial: 0.5 mg/kg/day; may increase to next dosage level after 14 days if previous dose is well tolerated but response is inadequate. **Note:** Canadian labeling does not include specific dosing recommendations in regards to patients who are poor CYP2D6 metabolizers although similar dose reductions would appear necessary.

Children ≥6 years and >70 kg and Adults:

Initial: 40 mg/day for 7-14 days (Step 1); if tolerated, may increase dose at 7-14 day intervals to 60 mg/day (Step 2) then to 80 mg/day (Step 3). If optimal response is not obtained after 2-4 additional weeks, may increase to a maximum dose of 100 mg/day.

Dosage adjustment in patients receiving strong CYP2D6 inhibitors: Initial: 40 mg/day; may increase to next dosage level after 14 days if previous dose is well tolerated but response is inadequate. **Note:** Canadian labeling does not include specific dosing recommendations in regards to patients who are poor CYP2D6 metabolizers although similar dose reductions would appear necessary.

Elderly: Use has not been evaluated in the elderly

Dosage adjustment in renal impairment: No dosage adjustment necessary

Dosage adjustment in hepatic impairment:

Mild impairment (Child-Pugh class A): No dosage adjustment provided in manufacturer's labeling.

Moderate impairment (Child-Pugh class B): All doses should be reduced to 50% of normal.

Severe impairment (Child-Pugh class C): All doses should be reduced to 25% of normal.

Dietary Considerations May be taken with or without food.

Administration May be administered with or without food as a single daily dose in the morning or as two evenly divided doses in morning and late afternoon/early evening. Swallow capsules whole; do not open capsules. If opened accidentally, do not touch eyes; wash hands immediately (product is an ocular irritant).

Monitoring Parameters Patient growth (weight/height gain in children); attention, hyperactivity, anxiety, worsening of aggressive behavior or hostility; blood pressure and pulse (baseline and following dose increases and periodically during treatment)

Family members and caregivers need to monitor patient daily for emergence of irritability, agitation, unusual changes in behavior, and suicide ideation. Pediatric patients should be monitored closely for suicidality, clinical worsening, or unusual changes in behavior, especially during the initial for months of therapy or at times of dose changes. Appearance of symptoms needs to be immediately reported to healthcare provider.

When used for the treatment of ADHD, thoroughly evaluate for cardiovascular risk. Monitor heart rate, blood pressure, and consider obtaining ECG prior to initiation (Vetter, 2008)

Dosage Forms Excipient information presented when available (limited, particularly for generics); consult specific product labeling.

Capsule, oral:

Strattera®: 10 mg, 18 mg, 25 mg, 40 mg, 60 mg, 80 mg, 100 mg

◆ **Atomoxetine Hydrochloride** *see* Atomoxetine *on page 163*

Atorvastatin (a TORE va sta tin)

Brand Names: U.S. Lipitor®

Brand Names: Canada Apo-Atorvastatin®; CO Atorvastatin; GD-Atorvastatin; Lipitor®; Novo-Atorvastatin; PMS-Atorvastatin; RAN™-Atorvastatin; ratio-Atorvastatin; Sandoz-Atorvastatin

Index Terms Atorvastatin Calcium

Pharmacologic Category Antilipemic Agent, HMG-CoA Reductase Inhibitor

Additional Appendix Information

Hyperlipidemia Management *on page 1996*

Use Treatment of dyslipidemias or primary prevention of cardiovascular disease (atherosclerotic) as detailed below:

Primary prevention of cardiovascular disease (high-risk for CVD): To reduce the risk of MI or stroke in patients without evidence of heart disease who have multiple CVD risk factors or type 2 diabetes. Treatment reduces the risk for angina or revascularization procedures in patients with multiple risk factors.

Secondary prevention of cardiovascular disease: To reduce the risk of nonfatal MI, nonfatal stroke, revascularization procedures, hospitalization for heart failure, and angina in patients with evidence of coronary heart disease.

Treatment of dyslipidemias: To reduce elevations in total cholesterol (C), LDL-C, apolipoprotein B, and triglycerides in patients with elevations of one or more components, and/or to increase low HDL-C as present in Fredrickson type IIa, IIb, III, and IV hyperlipidemias, heterozygous familial and nonfamilial hypercholesterolemia, and homozygous familial hypercholesterolemia

Treatment of heterozygous familial hypercholesterolemia (HeFH) in adolescent patients (10-17 years of age, females >1 year postmenarche) having LDL-C ≥190 mg/dL or LDL-C ≥160 mg/dL with positive family history of premature cardiovascular disease (CVD) or with two or more CVD risk factors.

Unlabeled Use Secondary prevention in patients who have experienced a noncardioembolic stroke/TIA or following an ACS event regardless of baseline LDL-C using intensive lipid-lowering therapy

Pregnancy Risk Factor X

Pregnancy Considerations Cholesterol biosynthesis may be important in fetal development. Contraindicated in pregnancy. Administer to women of childbearing potential only when conception is highly unlikely and patients have been informed of potential hazards.

Lactation Excretion in breast milk unknown/contraindicated

Contraindications Hypersensitivity to atorvastatin or any component of the formulation; active liver disease; unexplained persistent elevations of serum transaminases; pregnancy; breast-feeding

Warnings/Precautions Secondary causes of hyperlipidemia should be ruled out prior to therapy. Atorvastatin has not been studied when the primary lipid abnormality is chylomicron elevation (Fredrickson types I and V). Liver function must be monitored by periodic laboratory assessment. May cause hepatic dysfunction. Use with caution in patients who consume large amounts of ethanol or have a history of liver disease; use is contraindicated in patients with active liver disease or unexplained persistent elevations of serum transaminases. Monitoring is recommended. Patients with a history of hemorrhagic stroke may be at increased risk for another hemorrhagic stroke with use.

Rhabdomyolysis with acute renal failure has occurred. Risk is dose related and is increased with concurrent use of lipid-lowering agents which may cause rhabdomyolysis (fibric acid derivatives or niacin at doses ≥1 g/day) or during concurrent use with potent CYP3A4 inhibitors (including amiodarone, clarithromycin, cyclosporine, erythromycin, itraconazole, ketoconazole, nefazodone, grapefruit juice in large quantities, verapamil, or protease inhibitors such as indinavir, nelfinavir, or ritonavir). Ensure patient is on the lowest effective atorvastatin dose. If concurrent use of clarithromycin or combination protease inhibitors (eg, lopinavir/ritonavir or ritonavir/saquinavir) is warranted consider dose adjustment of atorvastatin. Monitor closely if used with other drugs associated with myopathy. Weigh the risk versus benefit when combining any of these drugs with atorvastatin. The manufacturer recommends temporary discontinuation for elective major surgery, acute medical or surgical conditions, or in any patient experiencing an acute or serious condition predisposing to renal failure (eg, sepsis, hypotension, trauma, uncontrolled seizures). However, based upon current evidence, HMG-CoA reductase inhibitor therapy should be continued in the perioperative period unless risk outweighs cardioprotective benefit. Use with caution in patients with advanced age, these patients are predisposed to myopathy. Safety and efficacy have not been established in patients <10 years of age or in premenarcheal girls.

Adverse Reactions

>10%:

- Gastrointestinal: Diarrhea (5% to 14%)
- Neuromuscular & skeletal: Arthralgia (4% to 12%)
- Respiratory: Nasopharyngitis (4% to 13%)

2% to 10%:

- Central nervous system: Insomnia (1% to 5%)
- Gastrointestinal: Nausea (4% to 7%), dyspepsia (3% to 6%)
- Genitourinary: Urinary tract infection (4% to 8%)
- Hepatic: Transaminases increased (2% to 3% with 80 mg/day dosing)
- Neuromuscular & skeletal: Limb pain (3% to 9%), myalgia (3% to 8%), muscle spasms (2% to 5%), musculoskeletal pain (2% to 5%)
- Respiratory: Pharyngolaryngeal pain (1% to 4%)

<2% (Limited to important or life-threatening): Alkaline phosphatase increased, alopecia, anaphylaxis, anemia, angioneurotic edema, anorexia, biliary pain, blurred vision, bullous rash, bullous rash, bursitis, cholestasis, cholestatic jaundice, colitis, CPK increased, depression, dizziness, duodenal ulcer, dysphagia, ecchymosis, emotional lability, epistaxis, eructation, erythema multiforme, esophagitis, fatigue, flatulence, gastritis, gastroenteritis, gingival hemorrhage, glossitis, hematuria, hepatic failure, hepatitis, hyper-/hypoglycemia, incoordination, jaundice, joint swelling, leg cramps, malaise, melena, memory impairment, metrorrhagia, migraine, muscle fatigue,

myasthenia, myopathy, myositis, neck pain, neck rigidity, nephritis, nightmare, pancreatitis, paresthesia, parosmia, peripheral neuropathy, petechiae, photosensitivity, pruritus, rectal hemorrhage, rhabdomyolysis, Stevens-Johnson syndrome, stomatitis, syncope, taste loss, taste perversion, tendinous contracture, tendon rupture, tenesmus, thrombocytopenia, tinnitus, torticollis, toxic epidermal necrolysis, urticaria, vaginal hemorrhage, vomiting

Additional class-related events or case reports (not necessarily reported with atorvastatin therapy): Cataracts, cirrhosis, dermatomyositis, eosinophilia, erectile dysfunction, extraocular muscle movement impaired, fulminant hepatic necrosis, gynecomastia, hemolytic anemia, interstitial lung disease, ophthalmoplegia, peripheral nerve palsy, polymyalgia rheumatica, positive ANA, renal failure (secondary to rhabdomyolysis), systemic lupus erythematosus-like syndrome, thyroid dysfunction, tremor, vasculitis, vertigo

Drug Interactions

Metabolism/Transport Effects Substrate of CYP3A4 (major), P-glycoprotein, SLCO1B1; **Note:** Assignment of Major/Minor substrate status based on clinically relevant drug interaction potential; **Inhibits** CYP3A4 (weak), P-glycoprotein

Avoid Concomitant Use

Avoid concomitant use of Atorvastatin with any of the following: Conivaptan; Pimozide; Red Yeast Rice; Silodosin; Telaprevir; Topotecan

Increased Effect/Toxicity

Atorvastatin may increase the levels/effects of: Aliskiren; Colchicine; Dabigatran Etexilate; DAPTOmycin; Digoxin; Diltiazem; Everolimus; Midazolam; P-glycoprotein/ABCB1 Substrates; Pimozide; Rivaroxaban; Silodosin; Topotecan; Trabectedin; Verapamil

The levels/effects of Atorvastatin may be increased by: Amiodarone; Antifungal Agents (Azole Derivatives, Systemic); Boceprevir; Colchicine; Conivaptan; CycloSPORINE; CycloSPORINE (Systemic); CYP3A4 Inhibitors (Moderate); CYP3A4 Inhibitors (Strong); Cyproterone; Danazol; Dasatinib; Diltiazem; Dronedarone; Eltrombopag; Fenofibrate; Fenofibric Acid; Fluconazole; Fusidic Acid; Gemfibrozil; Grapefruit Juice; Macrolide Antibiotics; Niacin; Niacinamide; P-glycoprotein/ABCB1 Inhibitors; Protease Inhibitors; QuiNINE; Red Yeast Rice; Sildenafil; Telaprevir; Verapamil

Decreased Effect

Atorvastatin may decrease the levels/effects of: Dabigatran Etexilate; Lanthanum

The levels/effects of Atorvastatin may be decreased by: Antacids; Bexarotene; Bexarotene (Systemic); Bosentan; CYP3A4 Inducers (Strong); Deferasirox; Efavirenz; Etravirine; Fosphenytoin; P-glycoprotein/ABCB1 Inducers; Phenytoin; Rifamycin Derivatives; St Johns Wort; Tocilizumab

Ethanol/Nutrition/Herb Interactions

Ethanol: Avoid excessive ethanol consumption (due to potential hepatic effects).

Food: Atorvastatin serum concentrations may be increased by grapefruit juice; avoid concurrent intake of large quantities (>1 quart/day). Red yeast rice contains an estimated 2.4 mg lovastatin per 600 mg rice.

Herb/Nutraceutical: St John's wort may decrease atorvastatin levels.

Stability Store at controlled room temperature of 20°C to 25°C (68°F to 77°F).

Mechanism of Action Inhibitor of 3-hydroxy-3-methylglutaryl coenzyme A (HMG-CoA) reductase, the rate-limiting enzyme in cholesterol synthesis (reduces the production of mevalonic acid from HMG-CoA); this then results in a compensatory increase in the expression of LDL receptors on hepatocyte membranes and a stimulation of LDL catabolism

Pharmacodynamics/Kinetics

Onset of action: Initial changes: 3-5 days; Maximal reduction in plasma cholesterol and triglycerides: 2 weeks

Absorption: Rapid

Distribution: V_d: ~381 L

Protein binding: ≥98%

Metabolism: Hepatic; forms active ortho- and parahydroxylated derivates and an inactive beta-oxidation product

Bioavailability: ~14% (parent drug); ~30% (parent drug and equipotent metabolites)

Half-life elimination: Parent drug: 14 hours; Equipotent metabolites: 20-30 hours

Time to peak, serum: 1-2 hours

Excretion: Bile; urine (<2% as unchanged drug)

Dosage Oral:

Primary prevention: Note: Doses should be individualized according to the baseline LDL-cholesterol concentrations, the recommended goal of therapy, and patient response; adjustments should be made at intervals of 2-4 weeks (4 weeks for children)

Children 10-17 years (females >1 year postmenarche): HeFH: 10 mg once daily (maximum: 20 mg/day)

Adults:

Hypercholesterolemia (heterozygous familial and nonfamilial) and mixed hyperlipidemia (Fredrickson types IIa and IIb): Initial: 10-20 mg once daily; patients requiring >45% reduction in LDL-C may be started at 40 mg once daily; range: 10-80 mg once daily

Homozygous familial hypercholesterolemia: 10-80 mg once daily

Secondary prevention:

Clinically-evident coronary heart disease: Initial: 80 mg once daily; adjust based on patient tolerability and recommended goal LDL-C (LaRosa, 2005)

Intensive lipid-lowering after an ACS event regardless of baseline LDL (unlabeled use): Initial: 80 mg once daily; adjust based on patient tolerability and recommended goal LDL-C (Cannon, 2004; Pederson, 2005; Schwartz, 2001). **Note:** Currently, the ACC/AHA guidelines for UA/NSTEMI do not specify which statin to use (Anderson, 2007).

Noncardioembolic stroke/TIA (unlabeled use): Initial: 80 mg once daily; adjust based on patient tolerability and recommended goal LDL-C (Adams, 2008; Amarenco, 2006)

Dosage adjustment for atorvastatin with concomitant medications:

Cyclosporine: Atorvastatin dose should not exceed 10 mg/day

Clarithromycin, itraconazole, ritonavir plus saquinavir, or lopinavir plus ritonavir when atorvastatin dose >20 mg: Ensure that the lowest dose necessary of atorvastatin is used.

Dosing adjustment in renal impairment: No dosage adjustment is necessary.

Dosing adjustment in hepatic impairment: Contraindicated in active liver disease or in patients with unexplained persistent elevations of serum transaminases.

Dietary Considerations May take with food if desired; may take without regard to time of day. Before initiation of therapy, patients should be placed on a standard cholesterol-lowering diet for 3-6 months and the diet should be continued during drug therapy. Red yeast rice contains an estimated 2.4 mg lovastatin per 600 mg rice. Atorvastatin serum concentration may be increased when taken with grapefruit juice; avoid concurrent intake of large quantities (>1 quart/day).

Administration May be administered with food if desired; may take without regard to time of day.

Monitoring Parameters Lipid levels after 2-4 weeks; LFTs; baseline CPK (recheck CPK in any patient with symptoms suggestive of myopathy)

It is recommended that liver function tests (LFTs) be performed prior to and at 12 weeks following both the initiation of therapy and any elevation in dose, and periodically (eg, semiannually) thereafter. Monitor LDL-C at intervals no less than 4 weeks.

Dosage Forms Excipient information presented when available (limited, particularly for generics); consult specific product labeling.

Tablet, oral: 10 mg, 20 mg, 40 mg, 80 mg

Lipitor®: 10 mg, 20 mg, 40 mg, 80 mg

- **Atorvastatin and Amlodipine** *see* Amlodipine and Atorvastatin *on page 98*
- **Atorvastatin Calcium** *see* Atorvastatin *on page 165*
- **Atorvastatin Calcium and Amlodipine Besylate** *see* Amlodipine and Atorvastatin *on page 98*

Atovaquone (a TOE va kwone)

Brand Names: U.S. Mepron®
Brand Names: Canada Mepron®
Pharmacologic Category Antiprotozoal

Use Acute oral treatment of mild-to-moderate *Pneumocystis jirovecii* pneumonia (PCP) in patients who are intolerant to co-trimoxazole; prophylaxis of PCP in patients who are intolerant to co-trimoxazole

Unlabeled Use Treatment of babesiosis; treatment/suppression of *Toxoplasma gondii* encephalitis; primary prophylaxis of HIV-infected persons at high risk for developing *Toxoplasma gondii* encephalitis

Pregnancy Risk Factor C

Pregnancy Considerations There are no adequate and well-controlled studies of atovaquone in pregnant women. Use in pregnant women only if the potential benefit outweighs the possible risk to the fetus.

Lactation Excretion in breast milk unknown/use caution

Contraindications Life-threatening allergic reaction to atovaquone or any component of the formulation

Warnings/Precautions When used for treatment, has only been indicated in mild-to-moderate *Pneumocystis jirovecii* pneumonia (PCP); not studied for use in severe PCP. Use with caution in elderly patients due to potentially impaired renal, hepatic, and cardiac function. Absorption may be decreased in patients who have diarrhea or vomiting; monitor closely and consider use of an antiemetic. If severe, consider use of an alternative antimalarial. Use with caution in patients with severe hepatic impairment; rare cases of hepatitis, elevated liver function tests, and liver failure have been reported.

Adverse Reactions Note: Adverse reaction statistics have been compiled from studies including patients with advanced HIV disease. Consequently, it is difficult to distinguish reactions attributed to atovaquone from those caused by the underlying disease or a combination thereof.

>10%:

Central nervous system: Fever (14% to 40%), headache (16% to 31%), insomnia (10% to 19%), depression, pain

Dermatologic: Rash (22% to 46%), pruritus (5% to ≥10%)

Gastrointestinal: Diarrhea (19% to 42%), nausea (21% to 32%), vomiting (14% to 22%), abdominal pain (4% to 21%)

Neuromuscular & skeletal: Weakness (8% to 31%), myalgia

Respiratory: Cough (14% to 25%), rhinitis (5% to 24%), dyspnea (15% to 21%), sinusitis (7% to ≥10%)

Miscellaneous: Infection (18% to 22%), diaphoresis, flu-like syndrome

1% to 10%:

Cardiovascular: Hypotension (≤1%)

Central nervous system: Dizziness (3% to 8%), anxiety (≤7%)

Endocrine & metabolic: Hyponatremia (7% to 10%), hyperglycemia (≤9%), hypoglycemia (≤1%)

Gastrointestinal: Amylase increased (7% to 8%), anorexia (≤7%), dyspepsia (≤5%), constipation (≤3%), taste perversion (≤3%)

Hematologic: Anemia (4% to 6%), neutropenia (3% to 5%)

Hepatic: Liver enzymes increased (4% to 8%)

Renal: BUN increased (≤1%), creatinine increased (≤1%)

Respiratory: Bronchospasm (2% to 4%)

Miscellaneous: Oral moniliasis (5% to 10%)

Postmarketing and/or case reports: Acute renal failure, allergic reaction, angioedema, erythema multiforme, hepatitis (rare), hypersensitivity reactions, liver failure (rare), methemoglobinemia, pancreatitis, skin desquamation, Stevens-Johnson syndrome, throat tightness, thrombocytopenia, urticaria, vortex keratopathy

Drug Interactions

Metabolism/Transport Effects None known.

Avoid Concomitant Use There are no known interactions where it is recommended to avoid concomitant use.

Increased Effect/Toxicity

Atovaquone may increase the levels/effects of: Etoposide; Hypoglycemic Agents

The levels/effects of Atovaquone may be increased by: Herbs (Hypoglycemic Properties)

Decreased Effect

Atovaquone may decrease the levels/effects of: Indinavir

The levels/effects of Atovaquone may be decreased by: Rifamycin Derivatives; Ritonavir; Tetracycline

Ethanol/Nutrition/Herb Interactions

Food: Ingestion with a fatty meal increases absorption.

Herb/Nutraceutical: Herbs with hypoglycemic properties may enhance the hypoglycemic effect of atovaquone. This includes alfalfa, aloe, bilberry, bitter melon, burdock, celery, damiana, fenugreek, garcinia, garlic, ginger, ginseng (American), gymnema, marshmallow, stinging nettle.

Stability Store at 15°C to 25°C (59°F to 77°F). Do not freeze.

Mechanism of Action Inhibits electron transport in mitochondria resulting in the inhibition of key metabolic enzymes responsible for the synthesis of nucleic acids and ATP

Pharmacodynamics/Kinetics

Absorption: Significantly increased with a high-fat meal

Distribution: V_{dss}: 0.6 ± 0.17 L/kg

Protein binding: >99%

Metabolism: Undergoes enterohepatic recirculation

Bioavailability: 32% to 62%

Half-life elimination: 1.5-4 days

Excretion: Feces (>94% as unchanged drug); urine (<1%)

Dosage Oral:

Children <13 years (unlabeled uses):

Prevention of PCP (CDC, 2009):

1-3 months: 30 mg/kg once daily with food

4-24 months: 45 mg/kg once daily with food

>24 months: 30 mg/kg once daily with food

Treatment of mild-to-moderate PCP (CDC, 2009):

Birth to 3 months: 30-40 mg/kg/day in 2 divided doses with food (maximum: 1500 mg/day)

3-24 months: 45 mg/kg/day in 2 divided doses with food (maximum: 1500 mg/day)

≥24 months: 30-40 mg/kg/day in 2 divided doses with food (maximum: 1500 mg/day)

Toxoplasma gondii prophylaxis (CDC, 2009):
1-3 months: 30 mg/kg once daily with food
4-24 months: 45 mg/kg once daily with food
>24 months: 30 mg/kg once daily with food
Babesiosis: 40 mg/kg/day in 2 divided doses with food for 7-10 days
Adolescents 13-16 years and Adults:
Prevention of PCP: 1500 mg once daily with food
Treatment of mild-to-moderate PCP: 750 mg twice daily with food for 21 days
Toxoplasma gondii encephalitis (unlabeled use; AIDS*info* guidelines):
Prophylaxis: 1500 mg once daily with food
Treatment: 750 mg 4 times daily or 1500 mg twice daily with food for at least 6 weeks after resolution of signs and symptoms
Suppression after treatment: 750 mg 2-4 times/day with food
Babesiosis (unlabeled use): 750 mg twice daily with azithromycin for 7-10 days

Dietary Considerations Must be taken with meals.

Administration Must be administered with meals. Shake suspension gently before use. Once opened, the foil pouch can be emptied on a dosing spoon, in a cup, or directly into the mouth.

Dosage Forms Excipient information presented when available (limited, particularly for generics); consult specific product labeling.
Suspension, oral:
Mepron®: 750 mg/5 mL (5 mL, 210 mL) [contains benzyl alcohol; citrus flavor]

Atovaquone and Proguanil

(a TOE va kwone & pro GWA nil)

Brand Names: U.S. Malarone®

Brand Names: Canada Malarone®; Malarone® Pediatric

Index Terms Atovaquone and Proguanil Hydrochloride; Proguanil and Atovaquone; Proguanil Hydrochloride and Atovaquone

Pharmacologic Category Antimalarial Agent

Use Prevention or treatment of acute, uncomplicated *P. falciparum* malaria

Pregnancy Risk Factor C

Pregnancy Considerations Teratogenic effects were not observed with the combination of atovaquone/proguanil in animal reproduction studies using concentrations similar to the estimated human exposure. The pharmacokinetics of atovaquone and proguanil are changed during pregnancy. Malaria infection in pregnant women may be more severe than in nonpregnant women. Because *P. falciparum* malaria can cause maternal death and fetal loss, pregnant women traveling to malaria-endemic areas must use personal protection against mosquito bites. Atovaquone/proguanil may be used as an alternative treatment of malaria in pregnant women; consult current CDC guidelines.

Lactation
Atovaquone: Excretion in breast milk unknown/use caution
Proguanil: Enters breast milk/use caution

Contraindications Hypersensitivity to atovaquone, proguanil, or any component of the formulation; prophylactic use in severe renal impairment (Cl_{cr} <30 mL/minute)

Warnings/Precautions Not indicated for severe or complicated malaria. Absorption of atovaquone may be decreased in patients who have diarrhea or vomiting; monitor closely and consider use of an antiemetic. If severe, consider use of an alternative antimalarial. Increased transaminase levels and hepatitis (rare) have been reported with prophylactic use; single case report of hepatic failure requiring transplantation documented. Monitor closely and use caution in patients with existing hepatic impairment. Data from clinical trials indicates that elevations in AST/ALT may persist for up to 4 weeks following treatment. Administer with caution to patients with pre-existing renal disease. May use for 3-day treatment in patients with severe renal impairment if benefit outweighs risk. Contraindicated for prophylactic use in severe renal impairment (Cl_{cr} <30 mL/minute). Not for use in patients <5 kg. Treatment failures have been reported in patients >100 kg (case reports); follow-up monitoring is recommended. Delayed cases of *P. falciparum* malaria may occur after stopping prophylaxis. Recrudescent infections or infections following prophylaxis with this agent should be treated with an alternative agent(s).

Adverse Reactions The following adverse reactions were reported in patients being treated for malaria. When used for prophylaxis, reactions are similar to those seen with placebo.

>10%:
Gastrointestinal: Abdominal pain (17%), nausea (12%), vomiting (children 10% to 13%, adults 12%)
Hepatic: Transaminase increases (ALT 27%, AST 17%; increased LFT values typically normalized after ~4 weeks)

1% to 10%:
Central nervous system: Headache (10%), dizziness (5%)
Dermatologic: Pruritus (children 6%)
Gastrointestinal: Diarrhea (children 6%, adults 8%), anorexia (5%)
Neuromuscular & skeletal: Weakness (8%)

Postmarketing and/or case reports: Anaphylaxis (rare), anemia (rare), angioedema, cholestasis, erythema multiforme (rare), hallucinations, hepatitis (rare), hepatic failure (case report), neutropenia, pancytopenia (with severe renal impairment), photosensitivity, psychotic episodes (rare), rash, seizure (rare), Stevens-Johnson syndrome (rare), stomatitis, urticaria, vasculitis (rare)

Drug Interactions

Metabolism/Transport Effects None known.

Avoid Concomitant Use

Avoid concomitant use of Atovaquone and Proguanil with any of the following: Artemether; Lumefantrine

Increased Effect/Toxicity

Atovaquone and Proguanil may increase the levels/effects of: Antipsychotic Agents (Phenothiazines); Dapsone; Dapsone (Systemic); Dapsone (Topical); Etoposide; Hypoglycemic Agents; Lumefantrine

The levels/effects of Atovaquone and Proguanil may be increased by: Artemether; Dapsone; Dapsone (Systemic); Herbs (Hypoglycemic Properties)

Decreased Effect

Atovaquone and Proguanil may decrease the levels/effects of: Indinavir

The levels/effects of Atovaquone and Proguanil may be decreased by: Rifamycin Derivatives; Ritonavir; Tetracycline

Ethanol/Nutrition/Herb Interactions
Food: Atovaquone taken with dietary fat significantly increases the rate and extent of absorption.
Herb/Nutraceutical: Herbs with hypoglycemic properties may enhance the hypoglycemic effect of atovaquone. This includes alfalfa, aloe, bilberry, bitter melon, burdock, celery, damiana, fenugreek, garcinia, garlic, ginger, ginseng (American), gymnema, marshmallow, stinging nettle.

Stability Store 25°C (77°F); excursions permitted to 15°C to 30°C (59°F to 86°F).

Mechanism of Action
Atovaquone: Selectively inhibits parasite mitochondrial electron transport.
Proguanil: The metabolite cycloguanil inhibits dihydrofolate reductase, disrupting deoxythymidylate synthesis.

Together, atovaquone/cycloguanil affect the erythrocytic and exoerythrocytic stages of development.

Pharmacodynamics/Kinetics

Atovaquone: See Atovaquone.

Proguanil:

Absorption: Extensive

Distribution: V_d: Adults and Children >15 years of age and 31-110 kg: 1617-2502 L; Pediatric patients ≤15 years and 11-56 kg: 62-966 L; concentrated in erythrocytes

Protein binding: 75%

Metabolism: Hepatic to active metabolites, cycloguanil (via CYP2C19) and 4-chlorophenylbiguanide

Bioavailability: ≤60%

Half-life elimination: 12-21 hours

Time to peak, plasma: 2-4 hours

Excretion: Urine (40% to 60%)

Dosage Oral:

Children (dosage based on body weight):

Prevention of malaria: Start 1-2 days prior to entering a malaria-endemic area, continue throughout the stay and for 7 days after returning. Take as a single dose, once daily.

5-8 kg (unlabeled dosing): Atovaquone/proguanil 31.25 mg/12.5 mg (Boggild, 2007)

9-10 kg (unlabeled dosing): Atovaquone/proguanil 46.8 mg/18.75 mg (Boggild, 2007)

11-20 kg: Atovaquone/proguanil 62.5 mg/25 mg

21-30 kg: Atovaquone/proguanil 125 mg/50 mg

31-40 kg: Atovaquone/proguanil 187.5 mg/75 mg

>40 kg: Atovaquone/proguanil 250 mg/100 mg

Treatment of acute malaria: Take as a single dose, once daily for 3 consecutive days.

5-8 kg: Atovaquone/proguanil 125 mg/50 mg

9-10 kg: Atovaquone/proguanil 187.5 mg/75 mg

11-20 kg: Atovaquone/proguanil 250 mg/100 mg

21-30 kg: Atovaquone/proguanil 500 mg/200 mg

31-40 kg: Atovaquone/proguanil 750 mg/300 mg

>40 kg: Atovaquone/proguanil 1 g/400 mg

Adults:

Prevention of malaria: Atovaquone/proguanil 250 mg/100 mg once daily; start 1-2 days prior to entering a malaria-endemic area, continue throughout the stay and for 7 days after returning

Treatment of acute malaria: Atovaquone/proguanil 1 g/400 mg as a single dose, once daily for 3 consecutive days

Elderly: Use with caution due to possible decrease in renal and hepatic function, as well as possible decreases in cardiac function, concomitant diseases, or other drug therapy.

Dosage adjustment in renal impairment: No dosage adjustment required in mild-to-moderate renal impairment. Contraindicated as prophylaxis in severe renal impairment (Cl_{cr} <30 mL/minute). May use for 3-day treatment in patients with severe renal impairment if benefit outweighs risk.

Dosage adjustment in hepatic impairment: No dosage adjustment required in mild-to-moderate hepatic impairment. No data available for use in severe hepatic impairment.

Dietary Considerations Must be taken with food or milk-based drink.

Administration Administer with food or milk-based drink at the same time each day. If vomiting occurs within 1 hour of administration, repeat the dose. For children who have difficulty swallowing tablets, tablets may be crushed and mixed with condensed milk just prior to administration.

Monitoring Parameters Liver and renal function; closely monitor response to treatment in patients >100 kg

Dosage Forms Excipient information presented when available (limited, particularly for generics); consult specific product labeling.

Tablet, oral:

Malarone®: Atovaquone 250 mg and proguanil hydrochloride 100 mg

Tablet, oral [pediatric]:

Malarone®: Atovaquone 62.5 mg and proguanil hydrochloride 25 mg

◆ **Atovaquone and Proguanil Hydrochloride** *see* Atovaquone and Proguanil *on page 168*

◆ **ATRA** *see* Tretinoin (Systemic) *on page 1729*

Atracurium (a tra KYOO ree um)

Brand Names: Canada Atracurium Besylate Injection

Index Terms Atracurium Besylate

Pharmacologic Category Neuromuscular Blocker Agent, Nondepolarizing

Use Adjunct to general anesthesia to facilitate endotracheal intubation and to relax skeletal muscles during surgery; to facilitate mechanical ventilation in ICU patients; does not relieve pain or produce sedation

Pregnancy Risk Factor C

Pregnancy Considerations Adverse events were observed in animal reproduction studies. Small amounts of atracurium have been shown to cross the placenta when given to women during cesarean section.

Lactation Excretion in breast milk unknown/use caution

Contraindications Hypersensitivity to atracurium besylate or any component of the formulation

Warnings/Precautions Reduce initial dosage and inject slowly (over 1-2 minutes) in patients in whom substantial histamine release would be potentially hazardous (eg, patients with clinically-important cardiovascular disease). Maintenance of an adequate airway and respiratory support is critical. Certain clinical conditions may result in potentiation or antagonism of neuromuscular blockade:

Potentiation: Electrolyte abnormalities, severe hyponatremia, severe hypocalcemia, severe hypokalemia, hypermagnesemia, neuromuscular diseases, acidosis, acute intermittent porphyria, renal failure, hepatic failure

Antagonism: Alkalosis, hypercalcemia, demyelinating lesions, peripheral neuropathies, diabetes mellitus

Increased sensitivity in patients with myasthenia gravis, Eaton-Lambert syndrome; resistance in burn patients (>30% of body) for period of 5-70 days postinjury; resistance in patients with muscle trauma, denervation, immobilization, infection, chronic treatment with atracurium. Cross-sensitivity with other neuromuscular-blocking agents may occur; use extreme caution in patients with previous anaphylactic reactions. Use caution in the elderly. Bradycardia may be more common with atracurium than with other neuromuscular-blocking agents since it has no clinically-significant effects on heart rate to counteract the bradycardia produced by anesthetics. Should be administered by adequately trained individuals familiar with its use. Some dosage forms may contain benzyl alcohol which has been associated with "gasping syndrome" in neonates.

Adverse Reactions Mild, rare, and generally suggestive of histamine release

1% to 10%: Cardiovascular: Flushing

<1%: Bronchial secretions, erythema, hives, itching, wheezing

Postmarketing and/or case reports: Allergic reaction, bradycardia, bronchospasm, dyspnea, hypotension, injection site reaction, seizure, acute quadriplegic myopathy syndrome (prolonged use), laryngospasm, myositis ossificans (prolonged use), tachycardia, urticaria

Causes of prolonged neuromuscular blockade: Excessive drug administration; cumulative drug effect, metabolism/excretion decreased (hepatic and/or renal impairment); accumulation of active metabolites; electrolyte imbalance (hypokalemia, hypocalcemia, hypermagnesemia, hypernatremia); hypothermia

Drug Interactions

Metabolism/Transport Effects None known.

Avoid Concomitant Use

Avoid concomitant use of Atracurium with any of the following: QuiNINE

Increased Effect/Toxicity

Atracurium may increase the levels/effects of: Cardiac Glycosides; Corticosteroids (Systemic); OnabotulinumtoxinA; RimabotulinumtoxinB

The levels/effects of Atracurium may be increased by: AbobotulinumtoxinA; Aminoglycosides; Calcium Channel Blockers; Capreomycin; Colistimethate; Inhalational Anesthetics; Ketorolac; Ketorolac (Nasal); Ketorolac (Systemic); Lincosamide Antibiotics; Lithium; Loop Diuretics; Magnesium Salts; Polymyxin B; Procainamide; QuiNIDine; QuiNINE; Spironolactone; Tetracycline Derivatives; Vancomycin

Decreased Effect

The levels/effects of Atracurium may be decreased by: Acetylcholinesterase Inhibitors; Loop Diuretics

Stability Refrigerate intact vials at 2°C to 8°C (36°F to 46°F); protect from freezing. Use vials within 14 days upon removal from the refrigerator to room temperature of 25°C (77°F). Dilutions of 0.2 mg/mL or 0.5 mg/mL in 0.9% sodium chloride, dextrose 5% in water, or 5% dextrose in sodium chloride 0.9% are stable for up to 24 hours at room temperature or under refrigeration. Atracurium should not be mixed with alkaline solutions.

Mechanism of Action Blocks neural transmission at the myoneural junction by binding with cholinergic receptor sites

Pharmacodynamics/Kinetics

Onset of action (dose dependent): 2-3 minutes

Duration: Recovery begins in 20-35 minutes following initial dose of 0.4-0.5 mg/kg under balanced anesthesia; recovery to 95% of control takes 60-70 minutes

Metabolism: Undergoes ester hydrolysis and Hofmann elimination (nonbiologic process independent of renal, hepatic, or enzymatic function); metabolites have no neuromuscular blocking properties; laudanosine, a product of Hofmann elimination, is a CNS stimulant and can accumulate with prolonged use. Laudanosine is hepatically metabolized.

Half-life elimination: Biphasic: Adults: Initial (distribution): 2 minutes; Terminal: 20 minutes

Excretion: Urine (<5%)

Dosage I.V. (not to be used I.M.): Dose to effect; doses must be individualized due to interpatient variability; use ideal body weight for obese patients

Children 1 month to 2 years: Initial: 0.3-0.4 mg/kg followed by maintenance doses as needed to maintain neuromuscular blockade

Children >2 years to Adults: 0.4-0.5 mg/kg, then 0.08-0.1 mg/kg 20-45 minutes after initial dose to maintain neuromuscular block; repeat dose at 15- to 25-minute intervals

Initial dose after succinylcholine for intubation (balanced anesthesia): Adults: 0.2-0.4 mg/kg

Pretreatment/priming: 10% of intubating dose given 3-5 minutes before initial dose

Continuous infusion:

Surgery: Initial: 9-10 mcg/kg/minute at initial signs of recovery from bolus dose; block usually maintained by a rate of 5-9 mcg/kg/minute under balanced anesthesia

ICU: Block usually maintained by rate of 11-13 mcg/kg/minute (rates for pediatric patients may be higher)

Dosage adjustment for hepatic or renal impairment is not necessary

Administration May be given undiluted as a bolus injection; not for I.M. injection due to tissue irritation; administration via infusion requires the use of an infusion pump; use infusion solutions within 24 hours of preparation

Monitoring Parameters Vital signs (heart rate, blood pressure, respiratory rate); degree of muscle relaxation (via peripheral nerve stimulator and presence of spontaneous movement); renal function (serum creatinine, BUN) and liver function when in ICU

In the ICU setting, prolonged paralysis and generalized myopathy, following discontinuation of agent, may be minimized by appropriately monitoring degree of blockade.

Additional Information Atracurium is classified as an intermediate-duration neuromuscular-blocking agent. It does not appear to have a cumulative effect on the duration of blockade. It does not relieve pain or produce sedation.

Dosage Forms Excipient information presented when available (limited, particularly for generics); consult specific product labeling.

Injection, solution, as besylate: 10 mg/mL (10 mL)

Injection, solution, as besylate [preservative free]: 10 mg/mL (5 mL)

- **Atracurium Besylate** *see* Atracurium *on page 169*
- **Atracurium Besylate Injection (Can)** *see* Atracurium *on page 169*
- **Atralin™** *see* Tretinoin (Topical) *on page 1731*
- **Atriance™ (Can)** *see* Nelarabine *on page 1184*
- **Atripla®** *see* Efavirenz, Emtricitabine, and Tenofovir *on page 577*
- **AtroPen®** *see* Atropine *on page 170*

Atropine (A troe peen)

Brand Names: U.S. AtroPen®; Atropine Care™; Isopto® Atropine

Brand Names: Canada Dioptic's Atropine Solution; Isopto® Atropine

Index Terms Atropine Sulfate

Pharmacologic Category Anticholinergic Agent; Anticholinergic Agent, Ophthalmic; Antidote; Antispasmodic Agent, Gastrointestinal; Ophthalmic Agent, Mydriatic

Use

Injection: Preoperative medication to inhibit salivation and secretions; treatment of symptomatic sinus bradycardia, AV block (nodal level); antidote for acetylcholinesterase inhibitor poisoning (carbamate insecticides, nerve agents, organophosphate insecticides); adjuvant use with anticholinesterases (eg, edrophonium, neostigmine) to decrease their side effects during reversal of neuromuscular blockade

Note: Use is no longer recommended in the management of asystole or pulseless electrical activity (PEA) (ACLS, 2010).

Ophthalmic: Produce mydriasis and cycloplegia for examination of the retina and optic disc and accurate measurement of refractive errors; uveitis

Oral: Inhibit salivation and secretions

Pregnancy Risk Factor B/C (manufacturer specific)

Pregnancy Considerations Animal reproduction studies have not been conducted. Atropine has been found to cross the human placenta.

Lactation Enters breast milk/use caution (AAP rates "compatible"; AAP 2001 update pending)

Prescribing and Access Restrictions The AtroPen® formulation is available for use primarily by the Department of Defense.

Contraindications Hypersensitivity to atropine or any component of the formulation; narrow-angle glaucoma; adhesions between the iris and lens; tachycardia; obstructive GI disease; paralytic ileus; intestinal atony of the elderly or debilitated patient; severe ulcerative colitis; toxic megacolon complicating ulcerative colitis; hepatic disease; obstructive uropathy; renal disease; myasthenia gravis (unless used to treat side effects of acetylcholinesterase inhibitor); asthma; thyrotoxicosis; Mobitz type II block

Warnings/Precautions Use with caution in children with spastic paralysis; use with caution in elderly patients. Low doses cause a paradoxical decrease in heart rates. Heat prostration may occur in hot weather. Use with caution in patients with autonomic neuropathy, prostatic hyperplasia, hyperthyroidism, HF, cardiac arrhythmias, chronic lung disease, biliary tract disease; anticholinergic agents are generally not well tolerated in the elderly and their use should be avoided when possible. Atropine is rarely used except as a preoperative agent or in the acute treatment of bradyarrhythmias. In heart transplant recipients, atropine will likely be ineffective in treatment of bradycardia due to lack of vagal innervation of the transplanted heart; cholinergic reinnervation may occur over time (years), so atropine may be used cautiously; however, some may experience paradoxical slowing of the heart rate and high-degree AV block upon administration (ACLS, 2010: Bernheim, 2004).

Avoid relying on atropine for effective treatment of type II second-degree or third-degree AV block (with or without a new wide QRS complex). Asystole or bradycardic pulseless electrical activity (PEA): Although no evidence exists for significant detrimental effects, routine use is unlikely to have a therapeutic benefit and is no longer recommended (ACLS, 2010).

AtroPen®: There are no absolute contraindications for the use of atropine in severe organophosphate poisonings, however in mild poisonings, use caution in those patients where the use of atropine would be otherwise contraindicated. Formulation for use by trained personnel only.

Adverse Reactions Severity and frequency of adverse reactions are dose related and vary greatly; listed reactions are limited to significant and/or life-threatening.

Cardiovascular: Arrhythmia, flushing, hypotension, palpitation, tachycardia

Central nervous system: Ataxia, coma, delirium, disorientation, dizziness, drowsiness, excitement, fever, hallucinations, headache, insomnia, nervousness

Dermatologic: Anhidrosis, urticaria, rash, scarlatiniform rash

Gastrointestinal: Bloating, constipation, delayed gastric emptying, loss of taste, nausea, paralytic ileus, vomiting, xerostomia, dry throat, nasal dryness

Genitourinary: Urinary hesitancy, urinary retention

Neuromuscular & skeletal: Weakness

Ocular: Angle-closure glaucoma, blurred vision, cycloplegia, dry eyes, mydriasis, ocular tension increased

Respiratory: Dyspnea, laryngospasm, pulmonary edema

Miscellaneous: Anaphylaxis

Drug Interactions

Metabolism/Transport Effects None known.

Avoid Concomitant Use There are no known interactions where it is recommended to avoid concomitant use.

Increased Effect/Toxicity

Atropine may increase the levels/effects of: AbobotulinumtoxinA; Anticholinergics; Cannabinoids; OnabotulinumtoxinA; Potassium Chloride; RimabotulinumtoxinB

The levels/effects of Atropine may be increased by: Pramlintide

Decreased Effect

Atropine may decrease the levels/effects of: Acetylcholinesterase Inhibitors (Central); Secretin

The levels/effects of Atropine may be decreased by: Acetylcholinesterase Inhibitors (Central)

Stability Store injection at controlled room temperature of 15°C to 30°C (59°F to 86°F); avoid freezing. In addition, AtroPen® should be protected from light.

Mechanism of Action Blocks the action of acetylcholine at parasympathetic sites in smooth muscle, secretory glands, and the CNS; increases cardiac output, dries secretions. Atropine reverses the muscarinic effects of cholinergic poisoning. The primary goal in cholinergic poisonings is reversal of bronchorrhea and bronchoconstriction. Atropine has no effect on the nicotinic receptors responsible for muscle weakness, fasciculations, and paralysis.

Pharmacodynamics/Kinetics

Onset of action: I.V.: Rapid

Absorption: Complete

Distribution: Widely throughout the body; crosses placenta; trace amounts enter breast milk; crosses blood-brain barrier

Metabolism: Hepatic

Half-life elimination: 2-3 hours

Excretion: Urine (30% to 50% as unchanged drug and metabolites)

Dosage

Infants and Children: Doses <0.1 mg have been associated with paradoxical bradycardia.

Inhibit salivation and secretions (preanesthesia): Oral, I.M., I.V., SubQ:

<5 kg: 0.02 mg/kg/dose 30-60 minutes preop then every 4-6 hours as needed. Use of a minimum dosage of 0.1 mg in neonates <5 kg will result in dosages >0.02 mg/kg. There is no documented minimum dosage in this age group.

>5 kg: 0.01-0.02 mg/kg/dose to a maximum 0.4 mg/dose 30-60 minutes preop; minimum dose: 0.1 mg

Alternate dosing:

3-7 kg (7-16 lb): 0.1 mg

8-11 kg (17-24 lb): 0.15 mg

11-18 kg (24-40 lb): 0.2 mg

18-29 kg (40-65 lb): 0.3 mg

>30 kg (>65 lb): 0.4 mg

Bradycardia:

I.V., I.O.: 0.02 mg/kg, minimum dose 0.1 mg, maximum single dose: 0.5 mg; may repeat once in 3-5 minutes to a maximum total dose of 0.04 mg/kg or 1 mg (PALS, 2010). When treating bradycardia in neonates, reserve use for those patients unresponsive to improved oxygenation and epinephrine.

Intratracheal: 0.04-0.06 mg/kg; may repeat once if needed (PALS, 2010)

Infants and Children: Nerve agent toxicity management: See **"Note"** under adult dosing.

Prehospital ("in the field"): I.M.:

Birth to <2 years: Mild-to-moderate symptoms: 0.05 mg/kg; severe symptoms: 0.1 mg/kg

2-10 years: Mild-to-moderate symptoms: 1 mg; severe symptoms: 2 mg

>10 years: Mild-to-moderate symptoms: 2 mg; severe symptoms: 4 mg

Hospital/emergency department: I.M.:

Birth to <2 years: Mild-to-moderate symptoms: 0.05 mg/kg I.M. **or** 0.02 mg/kg I.V.; severe symptoms: 0.1 mg/kg I.M. **or** 0.02 mg/kg I.V.

2-10 years: Mild-to-moderate symptoms: 1 mg; severe symptoms: 2 mg

>10 years: Mild-to-moderate symptoms: 2 mg; severe symptoms: 4 mg

Note: Pralidoxime is a component of the management of nerve agent toxicity; consult Pralidoxime for specific route and dose. For prehospital ("in the field") management, repeat atropine I.M. (children: 0.05-0.1 mg/kg) at 5-10 minute intervals until secretions have diminished and breathing is comfortable or airway resistance has returned to near normal. For hospital management, repeat atropine I.M. (infants 1 mg; all others: 2 mg) at 5-10 minute intervals until secretions have diminished and breathing is comfortable or airway resistance has returned to near normal.

Children: Organophosphate or carbamate poisoning:

I.V.: 0.03-0.05 mg/kg every 10-20 minutes until atropine effect, then every 1-4 hours for at least 24 hours

I.M. (AtroPen®): Mild symptoms: Administer dose listed below as soon as exposure is known or suspected. If severe symptoms develop after first dose, 2 additional doses should be repeated in 10 minutes; do not administer more than 3 doses. Severe symptoms: Immediately administer 3 doses as follows:

<6.8 kg (15 lb): Use of **AtroPen® formulation not recommended;** administer atropine 0.05 mg/kg

6.8-18 kg (15-40 lb): 0.5 mg/dose

18-41 kg (40-90 lb): 1 mg/dose

>41 kg (>90 lb): 2 mg/dose

Adults (doses <0.5 mg have been associated with paradoxical bradycardia):

Inhibit salivation and secretions (preanesthesia):

I.M., I.V., SubQ: 0.4-0.6 mg 30-60 minutes preop and repeat every 4-6 hours as needed

Oral: 0.4 mg; may repeat in 4 hours if necessary; 0.4 mg initial dose may be exceeded in certain cases and may repeat in 4 hours if necessary

Bradycardia: **Note:** Atropine may be ineffective in heart transplant recipients: I.V.: 0.5 mg every 3-5 minutes, not to exceed a total of 3 mg or 0.04 mg/kg (ACLS, 2010)

Neuromuscular blockade reversal: I.V.: 25-30 mcg/kg 30-60 seconds before neostigmine or 7-10 mcg/kg 30-60 seconds before edrophonium

Organophosphate or carbamate poisoning: **Note:** The dose of atropine required varies considerably with the severity of poisoning. Total amount of atropine used in carbamate poisoning is usually less. Severely poisoned patients may exhibit significant tolerance to atropine; ≥2 times the suggested doses may be needed. Titrate to pulmonary status (decreased bronchial secretions). Once patient is stable for a period of time, the dose/dosing frequency may be decreased. If atropinization occurs after 1-2 mg of atropine then re-evaluate working diagnosis.

I.V.: Initial: 1-5 mg; doses should be doubled every 5 minutes until signs of muscarinic excess abate (clearing of bronchial secretions, bronchospasm, and adequate oxygenation). Overly aggressive dosing may cause anticholinergic toxicity (eg, delirium, hyperthermia, and muscle twitching).

I.V. Infusion: 0.5-1 mg/hour or 10% to 20% of loading dose/hour

I.M. (AtroPen®): Mild symptoms: Administer 2 mg as soon as exposure is known or suspected. If severe symptoms develop after first dose, 2 additional doses should be repeated in 10 minutes; do not administer more than 3 doses. Severe symptoms: Immediately administer three 2 mg doses.

Nerve agent toxicity management: I.M.: See **"Note"**. Prehospital ("in the field") or hospital/emergency department: Mild-to-moderate symptoms: 2-4 mg; severe symptoms: 6 mg

Note: Pralidoxime is a component of the management of nerve agent toxicity; consult Pralidoxime for specific route and dose. For prehospital ("in the field") management, repeat atropine I.M. (2 mg) at 5-10 minute intervals until secretions have diminished and breathing is comfortable or airway resistance has returned to near normal. For hospital management, repeat atropine I.M. (2 mg) at 5-10 minute intervals until secretions have diminished and breathing is comfortable or airway resistance has returned to near normal.

Mydriasis, cycloplegia (preprocedure): Ophthalmic (1% solution): Instill 1-2 drops 1 hour before procedure.

Uveitis: Ophthalmic:

1% solution: Instill 1-2 drops 4 times/day

Ointment: Apply a small amount in the conjunctival sac up to 3 times/day; compress the lacrimal sac by digital pressure for 1-3 minutes after instillation

Elderly, frail patients: Nerve agent toxicity management (unlabeled use): I.M.: See **"Note"** under adult dosing.

Prehospital ("in the field"): Mild-to-moderate symptoms: 1 mg; severe symptoms: 2-4 mg

Hospital/emergency department: Mild-to-moderate symptoms: 1 mg; severe symptoms: 2 mg

Administration

I.M.: AtroPen®: Administer to outer thigh. May be given through clothing as long as pockets at the injection site are empty. Hold autoinjector in place for 10 seconds following injection; massage the injection site.

I.V.: Administer undiluted by rapid I.V. injection; slow injection may result in paradoxical bradycardia. In bradycardia, atropine administration should not delay treatment with external pacing.

Intratracheal: Dilute in NS or sterile water (absorption may be greater with sterile water). Spray drug quickly down tube. Follow immediately with several quick insufflations.

Monitoring Parameters Heart rate, blood pressure, pulse, mental status; intravenous administration requires a cardiac monitor

Dosage Forms Excipient information presented when available (limited, particularly for generics); consult specific product labeling. [DSC] = Discontinued product

Injection, solution, as sulfate: 0.05 mg/mL (5 mL); 0.1 mg/mL (5 mL, 10 mL); 0.4 mg/mL (1 mL [DSC], 20 mL [DSC]); 1 mg/mL (1 mL [DSC])

AtroPen®: 0.25 mg/0.3 mL (0.3 mL); 0.5 mg/0.7 mL (0.7 mL); 1 mg/0.7 mL (0.7 mL); 2 mg/0.7 mL (0.7 mL)

Injection, solution, as sulfate [preservative free]: 0.4 mg/0.5 mL (0.5 mL); 0.4 mg/mL (1 mL); 1 mg/mL (1 mL)

Ointment, ophthalmic, as sulfate: 1% (3.5 g)

Solution, ophthalmic, as sulfate [drops]: 1% (2 mL, 5 mL, 15 mL)

Atropine Care™: 1% (2 mL, 5 mL, 15 mL) [contains benzalkonium chloride]

Isopto® Atropine: 1% (5 mL, 15 mL) [contains benzalkonium chloride]

◆ **Atropine and Diphenoxylate** *see* Diphenoxylate and Atropine *on page 519*

Atropine and Pralidoxime

(A troe peen & pra li DOKS eem)

Brand Names: U.S. ATNAA; Duodote™

Index Terms Atropine and Pralidoxime Chloride; Mark 1™; NAAK; Nerve Agent Antidote Kit; Pralidoxime and Atropine

Pharmacologic Category Anticholinergic Agent; Antidote

Use

ATNAA: Treatment of poisoning by susceptible organophosphorous nerve agents having acetylcholinesterase-inhibiting activity for self or buddy-administration by military personnel

Duodote™: Treatment of poisoning by organophosphorous nerve agents (eg, tabun, sarin, soman) or organophosphorous insecticide for use by trained emergency medical services personnel

Pregnancy Risk Factor C

Prescribing and Access Restrictions
ATNAA (**A**ntidote **T**reatment-**N**erve **A**gent **A**uto-Injector) is only available for use by U.S. Armed Forces military personnel. Information on distribution is available at Defense Services Supply Center-Philadelphia at https://dmmonline.dscp.dla.mil/pharm/nerve.asp.
Duodote™ is only available for use by trained emergency medical services personnel to treat civilians. Distribution is limited to directly from manufacturer (Meridian Medical Technologies, Inc) to emergency medical service organizations or their suppliers.

Dosage I.M.: Adults: Organophosphorous poisoning: **Note:** If suspected, antidotal therapy should be given immediately as soon as symptoms appear (critical to administer immediately in case of soman exposure). Definitive medical care should be sought after any injection given. One injection only may be given as self-aid. If repeat injections needed, administration must be done by another trained individual. Emergency medical personnel who have self-administered a dose must determine capacity to continue to provide care.

ATNAA:
Mild symptoms (some or all mild symptoms): Self-Aid or Buddy-Aid: 1 injection (wait 10-15 minutes for effect); if patient is able to ambulate, and knows who and where they are, then no more injections are needed. If symptoms still present: Buddy-Aid: May repeat 1-2 more injections
Severe symptoms (if most or all): Buddy-Aid: If no self-aid given, 3 injections in rapid succession; if 1 self-aid injection given, 2 injections in rapid succession
Maximum cumulative dose: 3 injections
Symptoms provided by manufacturer in ATNAA product labeling to guide therapy:
Mild symptoms: Breathing difficulties, chest tightness, coughing, difficulty in seeing, drooling, headache, localized sweating and muscular twitching, miosis, nausea (with or without vomiting), runny nose, stomach cramps, tachycardia (followed by bradycardia), wheezing
Severe symptoms: Bradycardia, confused/strange behavior, convulsions, increased wheezing and breathing difficulties, involuntary urination/defecation, miosis (severe), muscular twitching/generalized weakness (severe), red/teary eyes, respiratory failure, unconsciousness, vomiting

Duodote™:
Mild symptoms (≥2 mild symptoms): 1 injection (wait 10-15 minutes for effect); if after 10-15 minutes no severe symptoms emerge, no further injections are indicated; if any severe symptoms emerge at any point following initial injection, repeat dose by giving 2 additional injections in rapid succession. Transport to medical care facility.
Severe symptoms (≥1 severe symptom): 3 injections in rapid succession. Transport to medical care facility.
Maximum cumulative dose: 3 injections unless medical care support (eg, hospital, respiratory support) is available
Symptoms provided by manufacturer in Duodote™ product labeling to guide therapy:
Mild symptoms: Airway secretions increased, blurred vision, bradycardia, breathing difficulties, chest tightness, drooling miosis, nausea, vomiting, runny nose, salivation, stomach cramps (acute onset), tachycardia, teary eyes, tremors/muscular twitching, wheezing/coughing
Severe symptoms: Breathing difficulties (severe), confused/strange behavior, convulsions, copious secretions from lung or airway, involuntary urination/defecation, muscular twitching/generalized weakness (severe)

Dosage adjustment in renal impairment: Use caution in renal impairment; pralidoxime is renally eliminated

Additional Information Complete prescribing information for this medication should be consulted for additional detail.

Dosage Forms Excipient information presented when available (limited, particularly for generics); consult specific product labeling.
Injection, solution:
ATNAA, Duodote™: Atropine 2.1 mg/0.7 mL and pralidoxime chloride 600 mg/2 mL [contains benzyl alcohol; prefilled autoinjector]

- ◆ **Atropine and Pralidoxime Chloride** *see* Atropine and Pralidoxime *on page* *172*
- ◆ **Atropine Care™** *see* Atropine *on page* *170*
- ◆ **Atropine, Hyoscyamine, Phenobarbital, and Scopolamine** *see* Hyoscyamine, Atropine, Scopolamine, and Phenobarbital *on page* *855*
- ◆ **Atropine Sulfate** *see* Atropine *on page* *170*
- ◆ **Atropine Sulfate and Edrophonium Chloride** *see* Edrophonium and Atropine *on page* *574*
- ◆ **Atrovent®** *see* Ipratropium (Nasal) *on page* *924*
- ◆ **Atrovent® HFA** *see* Ipratropium (Systemic) *on page* *923*
- ◆ **Atryn®** *see* Antithrombin *on page* *130*
- ◆ **ATV** *see* Atazanavir *on page* *158*
- ◆ **Augmentin®** *see* Amoxicillin and Clavulanate *on page* *105*
- ◆ **Augmentin ES-600® [DSC]** *see* Amoxicillin and Clavulanate *on page* *105*
- ◆ **Augmentin XR®** *see* Amoxicillin and Clavulanate *on page* *105*
- ◆ **Auralgan® (Can)** *see* Antipyrine and Benzocaine *on page* *130*

Auranofin (au RANE oh fin)

Brand Names: U.S. Ridaura®
Brand Names: Canada Ridaura®
Pharmacologic Category Gold Compound
Use Management of active stage classic or definite rheumatoid arthritis in patients who do not respond to or tolerate other agents
Pregnancy Risk Factor C
Dosage Oral: Adults: 6 mg/day in 1-2 divided doses; after 6 months may be increased to 9 mg/day in 3 divided doses; discontinue therapy if no response after 3 months at 9 mg/day
Note: Signs of clinical improvement may not be evident until after 3 months of therapy.
Dosing adjustment in renal impairment: There are no dosage adjustments provided in the manufacturer's labeling. The following guidelines have been used by some clinicians (Aronoff, 2007):
Cl_{cr} 50-80 mL/minute: Reduce dose to 50%
Cl_{cr} <50 mL/minute: Avoid use

Additional Information Complete prescribing information for this medication should be consulted for additional detail.

Dosage Forms Excipient information presented when available (limited, particularly for generics); consult specific product labeling.
Capsule, oral:
Ridaura®: 3 mg [gold 29%]

- ◆ **Auraphene B® [OTC]** *see* Carbamide Peroxide *on page* *283*
- ◆ **Auro® [OTC]** *see* Carbamide Peroxide *on page* *283*
- ◆ **Auro-Nevirapine (Can)** *see* Nevirapine *on page* *1193*

◆ **Auro-Terbinafine (Can)** *see* Terbinafine (Systemic) *on page 1648*

◆ **AVA** *see* Anthrax Vaccine Adsorbed *on page 124*

◆ **Ava-Azithromycin (Can)** *see* Azithromycin (Systemic) *on page 180*

◆ **Ava-Bupropion SR (Can)** *see* BuPROPion *on page 247*

◆ **Ava-Clarithromycin (Can)** *see* Clarithromycin *on page 374*

◆ **Ava-Diltiazem (Can)** *see* Diltiazem *on page 510*

◆ **Ava-Famciclovir (Can)** *see* Famciclovir *on page 687*

◆ **Avagard™ [OTC]** *see* Chlorhexidine Gluconate *on page 341*

◆ **Avage®** *see* Tazarotene *on page 1630*

◆ **Avakine** *see* InFLIXimab *on page 893*

◆ **Ava-Levetiracetam (Can)** *see* LevETIRAcetam *on page 994*

◆ **Avalide®** *see* Irbesartan and Hydrochlorothiazide *on page 926*

◆ **Avamys® (Can)** *see* Fluticasone (Nasal) *on page 741*

◆ **Avandamet®** *see* Rosiglitazone and Metformin *on page 1523*

◆ **Avandaryl®** *see* Rosiglitazone and Glimepiride *on page 1523*

◆ **Avandia®** *see* Rosiglitazone *on page 1521*

◆ **Ava-Pantoprazole (Can)** *see* Pantoprazole *on page 1289*

◆ **Ava-Pioglitazone (Can)** *see* Pioglitazone *on page 1355*

◆ **Ava-Pramipexole (Can)** *see* Pramipexole *on page 1389*

◆ **Avapro®** *see* Irbesartan *on page 925*

◆ **Avapro® HCT** *see* Irbesartan and Hydrochlorothiazide *on page 926*

◆ **AVAR™** *see* Sulfur and Sulfacetamide *on page 1607*

◆ **Ava-Ramipril (Can)** *see* Ramipril *on page 1459*

◆ **AVAR™-e** *see* Sulfur and Sulfacetamide *on page 1607*

◆ **AVAR™-e Green [DSC]** *see* Sulfur and Sulfacetamide *on page 1607*

◆ **AVAR™-e LS** *see* Sulfur and Sulfacetamide *on page 1607*

◆ **Ava-Risperidone (Can)** *see* RisperiDONE *on page 1496*

◆ **AVAR™ LS** *see* Sulfur and Sulfacetamide *on page 1607*

◆ **Avastin®** *see* Bevacizumab *on page 212*

◆ **Ava-Sumatriptan (Can)** *see* SUMAtriptan *on page 1609*

◆ **Ava-Tamsulosin CR (Can)** *see* Tamsulosin *on page 1626*

◆ **Avaxim® (Can)** *see* Hepatitis A Vaccine *on page 824*

◆ **Avaxim®-Pediatric (Can)** *see* Hepatitis A Vaccine *on page 824*

◆ **AVC™** *see* Sulfanilamide *on page 1605*

◆ **AVE 0005** *see* Aflibercept *on page 48*

◆ **Avelox®** *see* Moxifloxacin (Systemic) *on page 1159*

◆ **Avelox® ABC Pack** *see* Moxifloxacin (Systemic) *on page 1159*

◆ **Avelox® I.V.** *see* Moxifloxacin (Systemic) *on page 1159*

◆ **Aventyl® (Can)** *see* Nortriptyline *on page 1220*

◆ **Aviane™** *see* Ethinyl Estradiol and Levonorgestrel *on page 656*

◆ **Aviane® (Can)** *see* Ethinyl Estradiol and Levonorgestrel *on page 656*

◆ **Avian Influenza Virus Vaccine** *see* Influenza Virus Vaccine (H5N1) *on page 896*

◆ **AVINza®** *see* Morphine (Systemic) *on page 1153*

◆ **Avita®** *see* Tretinoin (Topical) *on page 1731*

◆ **Avodart®** *see* Dutasteride *on page 568*

◆ **Avonex®** *see* Interferon Beta-1a *on page 916*

◆ **AVP** *see* Vasopressin *on page 1775*

◆ **Axert®** *see* Almotriptan *on page 70*

◆ **Axid®** *see* Nizatidine *on page 1215*

◆ **Axiron®** *see* Testosterone *on page 1654*

◆ **Axiron®** *see* Testosterone *on page 1654*

◆ **AY-25650** *see* Triptorelin *on page 1742*

◆ **Aygestin®** *see* Norethindrone *on page 1217*

◆ **Ayr® Allergy Sinus [OTC]** *see* Sodium Chloride *on page 1567*

◆ **Ayr® Baby Saline [OTC]** *see* Sodium Chloride *on page 1567*

◆ **Ayr® Saline [OTC]** *see* Sodium Chloride *on page 1567*

◆ **Ayr® Saline No-Drip [OTC]** *see* Sodium Chloride *on page 1567*

◆ **5-Aza-2'-deoxycytidine** *see* Decitabine *on page 460*

AzaCITIDine (ay za SYE ti deen)

Brand Names: U.S. Vidaza®

Index Terms 5-Azacytidine; 5-AZC; AZA-CR; Azacytidine; Ladakamycin

Pharmacologic Category Antineoplastic Agent, DNA Methylation Inhibitor

Use Treatment of myelodysplastic syndrome (MDS)

Unlabeled Use Treatment of acute myelogenous leukemia (AML)

Pregnancy Risk Factor D

Pregnancy Considerations Embryotoxicity, fetal death, and fetal abnormalities were observed in animal studies. There are no adequate and well-controlled studies in pregnant women. Women of childbearing potential should be advised to avoid pregnancy during treatment. In addition, males should be advised to avoid fathering a child while on azacitidine therapy.

Lactation Excretion in breast milk unknown/not recommended

Contraindications Hypersensitivity to azacitidine, mannitol, or any component of the formulation; advanced malignant hepatic tumors

Warnings/Precautions Hazardous agent - use appropriate precautions for handling and disposal. Azacitidine may be hepatotoxic, use caution with hepatic impairment; use is contraindicated in patients with advanced malignant hepatic tumors. Progressive hepatic coma leading to death has been reported (rare) in patients with extensive tumor burden, especially those with a baseline albumin <30 g/L. Use caution with renal impairment; dose adjustment may be required. Serum creatinine elevations, renal tubular acidosis, and renal failure have been reported with combination chemotherapy; decrease or withhold dose for unexplained elevations in BUN or serum creatinine or reductions in serum bicarbonate to <20 mEq/L. Patients with renal and hepatic impairment were excluded from clinical studies. Neutropenia, thrombocytopenia, and anemia are common; may cause therapy delays and/or dosage reductions. Not FDA approved for use in children.

Adverse Reactions

>10%:

Cardiovascular: Peripheral edema (7% to 19%), chest pain (16%), pallor (16%), pitting edema (15%)

Central nervous system: Fever (30% to 52%), fatigue (13% to 36%), headache (22%), dizziness (19%), anxiety (5% to 13%), depression (12%), insomnia (9% to 11%), malaise (11%), pain (11%)

Dermatologic: Bruising (19% to 31%), petechiae (11% to 24%), erythema (7% to 17%), skin lesion (15%), rash (10% to 14%), pruritus (12%)
Endocrine & metabolic: Hypokalemia (6% to 13%)
Gastrointestinal: Nausea (48% to 71%), vomiting (27% to 54%), diarrhea (36%), constipation (34% to 50%), anorexia (13% to 21%), weight loss (16%), abdominal pain (11% to 16%), abdominal tenderness (12%)
Hematologic: Thrombocytopenia (66% to 70%; grades 3/4: 58%), anemia (51% to 70%; grades 3/4: 14%), neutropenia (32% to 66%; grades 3/4: 61%), leukopenia (18% to 48%; grades 3/4: 15%), febrile neutropenia (14% to 16%; grades 3/4: 13%), myelosuppression (nadir: days 10-17; recovery: days 28-31)
Local: Injection site reactions (14% to 29%): Erythema (35% to 43%; more common with I.V. administration), pain (19% to 23%; more common with I.V. administration), bruising (5% to 14%)
Neuromuscular & skeletal: Weakness (29%), rigors (26%), arthralgia (22%), limb pain (20%), back pain (19%), myalgia (16%)
Respiratory: Cough (11% to 30%), dyspnea (5% to 29%), pharyngitis (20%), epistaxis (16%), nasopharyngitis (15%), upper respiratory tract infection (9% to 13%), pneumonia (11%), crackles (11%)
Miscellaneous: Diaphoresis (11%)

5% to 10%:
Cardiovascular: Cardiac murmur (10%), hypertension (≤9%), tachycardia (9%), hypotension (7%), syncope (6%), chest wall pain (5%)
Central nervous system: Lethargy (7% to 8%), hypoesthesia (5%), postprocedural pain (5%)
Dermatologic: Cellulitis (8%), urticaria (6%), dry skin (5%), skin nodule (5%)
Gastrointestinal: Gingival bleeding (10%), oral mucosal petechiae (8%), stomatitis (8%), weight loss (≤8%), dyspepsia (6% to 7%), hemorrhoids (7%), abdominal distension (6%), loose stools (6%), dysphagia (5%), oral hemorrhage (5%), tongue ulceration (5%)
Genitourinary: Dysuria (8%), urinary tract infection (8% to 9%)
Hematologic: Hematoma (9%), postprocedural hemorrhage (6%)
Local: Injection site reactions: Pruritus (7%), hematoma (6%), rash (6%), granuloma (5%), induration (5%), pigmentation change (5%), swelling (5%)
Neuromuscular & skeletal: Muscle cramps (6%)
Renal: Hematuria (≤6%)
Respiratory: Rhinorrhea (10%), rales (9%), wheezing (9%), breath sounds decreased (8%), pharyngolaryngeal pain (6%), pleural effusion (6%), postnasal drip (6%), rhinitis (6%), rhonchi (6%), nasal congestion (6%), atelectasis (5%), sinusitis (5%)
Miscellaneous: Lymphadenopathy (10%), herpes simplex (9%), night sweats (9%), transfusion reaction (7%), mouth hemorrhage (5%)

<5% (Limited to important or life-threatening): Abscess (limb), acute febrile neutrophilic dermatosis (Sweet's syndrome), agranulocytosis, anaphylactic shock, atrial fibrillation, azotemia, blastomycosis, bone marrow depression/failure, bone pain aggravated, cardiac failure, cardiorespiratory arrest, catheter site hemorrhage, cellulitis, cerebral hemorrhage, CHF, cholecystectomy, cholecystitis, congestive cardiomyopathy, dehydration, diverticulitis, eye hemorrhage, fibrosis (interstitial and alveolar), gastrointestinal hemorrhage, glycosuria, hemoptysis, hepatic coma, hypersensitivity reaction, hypophosphatemia, infection (bacterial), injection site infection, intracranial hemorrhage, leukemia cutis, lung infiltration, melena, neutropenic sepsis, orthostatic hypotension, pancytopenia, pneumonitis, polyuria, pyoderma gangrenosum, renal failure, renal tubular acidosis, seizure, respiratory distress, sepsis, septic shock, serum bicarbonate levels decreased, serum creatinine increased, splenomegaly, systemic inflammatory response syndrome, toxoplasmosis

Drug Interactions

Metabolism/Transport Effects None known.

Avoid Concomitant Use

Avoid concomitant use of AzaCITIDine with any of the following: BCG; CloZAPine; Natalizumab; Pimecrolimus; Tacrolimus (Topical); Vaccines (Live)

Increased Effect/Toxicity

AzaCITIDine may increase the levels/effects of: CloZAPine; Leflunomide; Natalizumab; Vaccines (Live)

The levels/effects of AzaCITIDine may be increased by: Denosumab; Pimecrolimus; Roflumilast; Tacrolimus (Topical); Trastuzumab

Decreased Effect

AzaCITIDine may decrease the levels/effects of: BCG; Coccidioidin Skin Test; Sipuleucel-T; Vaccines (Inactivated); Vaccines (Live)

The levels/effects of AzaCITIDine may be decreased by: Echinacea

Stability Prior to reconstitution, store powder at room temperature of 25°C (77°F); excursions permitted to 15°C to 30°C (59°F to 86°F). Use appropriate precautions for handling and disposal.

SubQ: To prepare a 25 mg/mL suspension, slowly add 4 mL SWFI to each vial. Vigorously shake or roll vial until a suspension is formed (suspension will be cloudy). Following reconstitution, suspension may be stored at room temperature for up to 1 hour, or immediately refrigerated at 2°C to 8°C (36°F to 46°F) and stored for up to 8 hours.

I.V.: **Solutions for I.V. administration have very limited stability and must be prepared immediately prior to each dose.** Reconstitute vial with 10 mL SWFI to form a 10 mg/mL solution; vigorously shake until solution is dissolved and clear. Mix in 50-100 mL of NS or lactated Ringer's injection for infusion. Administration must be completed within 1 hour of (vial) reconstitution.

Mechanism of Action Antineoplastic effects may be a result of azacitidine's ability to promote hypomethylation of DNA leading to direct toxicity of abnormal hematopoietic cells in the bone marrow.

Pharmacodynamics/Kinetics

Absorption: SubQ: Rapid and complete
Distribution: V_d: I.V.: 76 ± 26 L; does not cross blood-brain barrier
Metabolism: Hepatic; hydrolysis to several metabolites
Bioavailability: SubQ: ~89%
Half-life elimination: I.V., SubQ: ~4 hours
Time to peak, plasma: SubQ: 30 minutes
Excretion: Urine (50% to 85%); feces (minor)

Dosage

Children: I.V.: Refractory AML (unlabeled use): 250 mg/m²/dose days 4 and 5 every 4 weeks (Steuber, 1996) **or** 300 mg/m²/dose days 4 and 5 every 4 weeks (Hurwitz, 1995)

Adults:

MDS: I.V., SubQ: 75 mg/m²/day for 7 days repeated every 4 weeks. Dose may be increased to 100 mg/m²/day if no benefit is observed after 2 cycles and no toxicity other than nausea and vomiting have occurred. Treatment is recommended for at least 4 cycles; treatment may be continued as long as patient continues to benefit.

Note: Alternate (unlabeled) schedules (which have produced hematologic response) have been used for convenience in community oncology centers (Lyons, 2009):

75 mg/m^2/day for 5 days (Mon-Fri), 2 days rest (Sat, Sun), then 75 mg/m^2/day for 2 days (Mon, Tues); repeat cycle every 28 days **or**

50 mg/m^2/day for 5 days (Mon-Fri), 2 days rest (Sat, Sun), then 50 mg/m^2/day for 5 days (Mon-Fri); repeat cycle every 28 days **or**

75 mg/m^2/day for 5 days (Mon-Fri), repeat cycle every 28 days

AML (unlabeled use): SubQ: 75 mg/m^2/day for 7 days repeated every 4 weeks (Sudan, 2006)

Elderly: Refer to adult dosing; due to the potential for decreased renal function in the elderly, select dose carefully and closely monitor renal function

Dosage adjustment based on hematology: Adults: MDS: I.V., SubQ:

For baseline WBC ≥3.0 x 10^9/L, ANC ≥1.5 x 10^9/L, and platelets ≥75 x 10^9/L:

Nadir count: ANC <0.5 x 10^9/L or platelets <25 x 10^9/L: Administer 50% of dose during next treatment course

Nadir count: ANC 0.5-1.5 x 10^9/L or platelets 25-50 x 10^9/L: Administer 67% of dose during next treatment course

Nadir count: ANC >1.5 x 10^9/L or platelets >50 x 10^9/L: Administer 100% of dose during next treatment course

For baseline WBC <3 x 10^9/L, ANC <1.5 x 10^9/L, or platelets <75 x 10^9/L: Adjust dose as follows based on nadir counts and bone marrow biopsy cellularity at the time of nadir, unless clear improvement in differentiation at the time of the next cycle:

WBC or platelet nadir decreased 50% to 75% from baseline and bone marrow biopsy cellularity at time of nadir 30% to 60%: Administer 100% of dose during next treatment course

WBC or platelet nadir decreased 50% to 75% from baseline and bone marrow biopsy cellularity at time of nadir 15% to 30%: Administer 50% of dose during next treatment course

WBC or platelet nadir decreased 50% to 75% from baseline and bone marrow biopsy cellularity at time of nadir <15%: Administer 33% of dose during next treatment course

WBC or platelet nadir decreased >75% from baseline and bone marrow biopsy cellularity at time of nadir 30% to 60%: Administer 75% of dose during next treatment course

WBC or platelet nadir decreased >75% from baseline and bone marrow biopsy cellularity at time of nadir 15% to 30%: Administer 50% of dose during next treatment course

WBC or platelet nadir decreased >75% from baseline and bone marrow biopsy cellularity at time of nadir <15%: Administer 33% of dose during next treatment course

Note: If a nadir defined above occurs, administer the next treatment course 28 days after the start of the preceding course as long as WBC and platelet counts are >25% above the nadir and rising. If a >25% increase above the nadir is not seen by day 28, reassess counts every 7 days. If a 25% increase is not seen by day 42, administer 50% of the scheduled dose.

Dosage adjustment based on serum electrolytes: The manufacturer recommends that if serum bicarbonate falls to <20 mEq/L (unexplained decrease): Reduce dose by 50% for next treatment course

Dosage adjustment based on renal toxicity: If increases in BUN or serum creatinine (unexplained) occur, delay next cycle until values reach baseline or normal, then reduce dose by 50% for next treatment course.

Dosage adjustment in renal impairment: Not studied in patients with renal impairment; select dose carefully (excretion is primarily renal; consider dose reduction); monitor closely for toxicity

Dosage adjustment in hepatic impairment: Not studied in patients with hepatic impairment; use caution. Contraindicated in patients with advanced malignant hepatic tumors.

Administration

SubQ: Premedication for nausea and vomiting is recommended. The manufacturer recommends equally dividing volumes >4 mL into 2 syringes and injecting into 2 separate sites; however, policies for maximum SubQ administration volume may vary by institution; interpatient variations may also apply. Administer subsequent injections at least 1 inch from previous injection sites. Allow refrigerated suspensions to come to room temperature (up to 30 minutes) prior to administration. Resuspend by inverting the syringe 2-3 times and then rolling the syringe between the palms for 30 seconds. If azacitidine suspension comes in contact with the skin, immediately wash with soap and water.

I.V.: Premedication for nausea and vomiting is recommended. Infuse over 10-40 minutes; infusion must be completed within 1 hour of (vial) reconstitution.

Monitoring Parameters Liver function tests, electrolytes, CBC with differential and platelets, renal function tests (BUN and serum creatinine) should be obtained prior to initiation of therapy. Electrolytes, renal function (BUN and creatinine), CBC should be monitored prior to each cycle and periodically as needed to monitor response and toxicity.

Additional Information Oncology Comment: Azacitidine treatment for MDS is associated with an improvement in quality of life (including a reduction in transfusion requirements), a decrease in transformation to AML, and improved survival, when compared to best supportive care. Treatment should be continued for a minimum of 4-6 cycles (NCCN MDS guidelines v.2.2009).

Dosage Forms Excipient information presented when available (limited, particularly for generics); consult specific product labeling.

Injection, powder for suspension:

Vidaza®: 100 mg [contains mannitol]

- **AZA-CR** *see* AzaCITIDine *on page* *174*
- **Azactam®** *see* Aztreonam *on page* *184*
- **Azacytidine** *see* AzaCITIDine *on page* *174*
- **5-Azacytidine** *see* AzaCITIDine *on page* *174*
- **5-Aza-dCyd** *see* Decitabine *on page* *460*
- **Azaepothilone B** *see* Ixabepilone *on page* *945*
- **Azasan®** *see* AzaTHIOprine *on page* *176*
- **AzaSite®** *see* Azithromycin (Ophthalmic) *on page* *183*

AzaTHIOprine (ay za THYE oh preen)

Brand Names: U.S. Azasan®; Imuran®

Brand Names: Canada Apo-Azathioprine®; Imuran®; Mylan-Azathioprine; Teva-Azathioprine

Index Terms Azathioprine Sodium

Pharmacologic Category Immunosuppressant Agent

Use Adjunctive therapy in prevention of rejection of kidney transplants; management of active rheumatoid arthritis (RA)

Unlabeled Use Adjunct in prevention of rejection of solid organ (nonrenal) transplants; remission maintenance or reduction of steroid use in Crohn's disease (CD) and in ulcerative colitis (UC); dermatomyositis/polymyositis; erythema multiforme; pemphigus vulgaris, lupus nephritis, chronic refractory immune (idiopathic) thrombocytopenic purpura, relapsed/remitting multiple sclerosis

Pregnancy Risk Factor D

Pregnancy Considerations Azathioprine was found to be teratogenic in animal studies; temporary depression in spermatogenesis and reduction in sperm viability and sperm count were also reported in mice. Azathioprine crosses the placenta in humans; congenital anomalies, immunosuppression, hematologic toxicities (lymphopenia, pancytopenia), and intrauterine growth retardation have been reported. There are no adequate and well-controlled studies in pregnant women. Azathioprine should not be used to treat rheumatoid arthritis during pregnancy. The potential benefit to the mother versus possible risk to the fetus should be considered when treating other disease states. Women of childbearing potential should avoid becoming pregnant during treatment.

The National Transplantation Pregnancy Registry (NTPR, Temple University) is a registry for pregnant women taking immunosuppressants following any solid organ transplant. The NTPR encourages reporting of all immunosuppressant exposures during pregnancy in transplant recipients at 877-955-6877.

Lactation Enters breast milk/not recommended

Contraindications Hypersensitivity to azathioprine or any component of the formulation; pregnancy (in patients with rheumatoid arthritis); patients with rheumatoid arthritis and a history of treatment with alkylating agents (eg, cyclophosphamide, chlorambucil, melphalan) may have a prohibitive risk of neoplasia with azathioprine treatment

Warnings/Precautions [U.S. Boxed Warning]: Immunosuppressive agents, including azathioprine, are associated with the development of lymphoma and other malignancies, especially of the skin. Hepatosplenic T-Cell Lymphoma (HSTCL), a rare white blood cell cancer that is usually fatal, has predominantly occurred in adolescents and young adults treated for Crohn's disease or ulcerative colitis and receiving TNF blockers (eg, adalimumab, certolizumab pegol, etanercept, golimumab), azathioprine, and/or mercaptopurine. Most cases have occurred in patients treated with a combination of immunosuppressant agents, although there have been reports of HSTCL in patients receiving azathioprine or mercaptopurine monotherapy. Renal transplant patients are also at increased risk for malignancy (eg, skin cancer, lymphoma); limit sun and ultraviolet light exposure and use appropriate sun protection. Dose-related hematologic toxicities (leukopenia, thrombocytopenia, and anemias, including macrocytic anemia, or pancytopenia) may occur; delayed toxicities may also occur. May be more severe with renal transplants undergoing rejection; dosage modification for hematologic toxicity may be necessary. Chronic immunosuppression increases the risk of serious infections; may require dosage reduction. Use with caution in patients with liver disease or renal impairment; monitor hematologic function closely. Azathioprine is metabolized to mercaptopurine; concomitant use may result in profound myelosuppression and should be avoided. Patients with genetic deficiency of thiopurine methyltransferase (TPMT) or concurrent therapy with drugs which may inhibit TPMT may be sensitive to myelosuppressive effects. Patients with intermediate TPMT activity may be at risk for increased myelosuppression; those with low or absent TPMT activity are at risk for developing severe myelotoxicity. TPMT genotyping or phenotyping may assist in identifying patients at risk for developing toxicity. Consider TPMT testing in patients with abnormally low CBC unresponsive to dose reduction. TPMT testing does not substitute for CBC monitoring. Xanthine oxidase inhibitors may increase risk for hematologic toxicity; reduce azathioprine dose when used concurrently with allopurinol; patients with low or absent TPMT activity may require further dose reductions or discontinuation.

Hepatotoxicity (transaminase, bilirubin, and alkaline phosphatase elevations) may occur, usually in renal transplant patients and generally within 6 months of transplant; normally reversible with discontinuation; monitor liver function periodically. Rarely, hepatic sinusoidal obstruction syndrome (SOS; formerly called veno-occlusive disease) has been reported; discontinue if hepatic SOS is suspected. Severe nausea, vomiting, diarrhea, rash, fever, malaise, myalgia, hypotension, and liver enzyme abnormalities may occur within the first several weeks of treatment and are generally reversible upon discontinuation. **[U.S. Boxed Warning]: Should be prescribed by physicians familiar with the risks, including hematologic toxicities and mutagenic potential.** Immune response to vaccines may be diminished. Hazardous agent - use appropriate precautions for handling and disposal.

Adverse Reactions Frequency not always defined; dependent upon dose, duration, indication, and concomitant therapy.

Central nervous system: Fever, malaise

Gastrointestinal: Nausea/vomiting (RA 12%), diarrhea

Hematologic: Leukopenia (renal transplant >50%; RA 28%), thrombocytopenia

Hepatic: Alkaline phosphatase increased, bilirubin increased, hepatotoxicity, transaminases increased

Neuromuscular & skeletal: Myalgia

Miscellaneous: Infection (renal transplant 20%; RA <1%; includes bacterial, fungal, protozoal, viral), neoplasia (renal transplant 3% [other than lymphoma], 0.5% [lymphoma])

Postmarketing and/or case reports: Abdominal pain, alopecia, anemia, arthralgia, bleeding, bone marrow suppression, fever, hepatic sinusoidal obstruction syndrome (SOS; veno-occlusive disease), hepatosplenic T-cell lymphoma, hypersensitivity, hypotension, interstitial pneumonitis, lymphoma, macrocytic anemia, negative nitrogen balance, pancreatitis, pancytopenia, rash, skin cancer, steatorrhea, Sweet's syndrome (acute febrile neutrophilic dermatosis)

Drug Interactions

Metabolism/Transport Effects None known.

Avoid Concomitant Use

Avoid concomitant use of AzaTHIOprine with any of the following: BCG; Febuxostat; Mercaptopurine; Natalizumab; Pimecrolimus; Tacrolimus (Topical)

Increased Effect/Toxicity

AzaTHIOprine may increase the levels/effects of: Leflunomide; Mercaptopurine; Natalizumab; Vaccines (Live)

The levels/effects of AzaTHIOprine may be increased by: 5-ASA Derivatives; ACE Inhibitors; Allopurinol; Denosumab; Febuxostat; Pimecrolimus; Ribavirin; Roflumilast; Sulfamethoxazole; Tacrolimus (Topical); Trastuzumab; Trimethoprim

Decreased Effect

AzaTHIOprine may decrease the levels/effects of: BCG; Coccidioidin Skin Test; Sipuleucel-T; Vaccines (Inactivated); Vitamin K Antagonists

The levels/effects of AzaTHIOprine may be decreased by: Echinacea

Ethanol/Nutrition/Herb Interactions Herb/Nutraceutical: Avoid cat's claw, echinacea (have immunostimulant properties).

Stability

Tablet: Store at room temperature of 15°C to 25°C (59°F to 77°F). Protect from light and moisture.

Powder for injection: Store intact vials at room temperature of 15°C to 25°C (59°F to 77°F). Protect from light. Reconstitute each vial with 10 mL sterile water for injection; may further dilute for infusion (in D_5W, 1/2NS, or NS). Reconstituted solution should be used within 24 hours; solutions diluted in D_5W, 1/2NS, or NS for infusion are stable at room temperature or refrigerated for up to 16 days (Johnson, 1981); however, the manufacturer recommends use within 24 hours of reconstitution. Use appropriate precautions for handling and disposal.

Mechanism of Action Azathioprine is an imidazolyl derivative of mercaptopurine; antagonizes purine metabolism and may inhibit synthesis of DNA, RNA, and proteins; may also interfere with cellular metabolism and inhibit mitosis. The 6-thioguanine nucleotides appear to mediate the majority of azathioprine's immunosuppressive and toxic effects.

Pharmacodynamics/Kinetics

Absorption: Oral: Well absorbed

Distribution: Crosses placenta

Protein binding: ~30%

Metabolism: Hepatic, to 6-mercaptopurine, possibly by glutathione S-transferase (GST). Further metabolism of 6-mercaptopurine (in the liver and GI tract), via three major pathways: Hypoxanthine guanine phosphoribosyltransferase (to 6-thioguanine-nucleotides, or 6-TGN), xanthine oxidase (to 6-thiouric acid), and thiopurine methyltransferase (TPMT), which forms 6-methylmercaptopurine (6-MMP).

Half-life elimination: Parent drug: 12 minutes; mercaptopurine: 0.7-3 hours; End-stage renal disease: Slightly prolonged

Time to peak, plasma: Oral: 1-2 hours (including metabolites)

Excretion: Urine (primarily as metabolites)

Dosage Note: Patients with intermediate TPMT activity may be at risk for increased myelosuppression; those with low or absent TPMT activity receiving conventional azathioprine doses are at risk for developing severe, life-threatening myelotoxicity. Dosage reductions are recommended for patients with reduced TPMT activity.

I.V. dose is equivalent to oral dose (dosing should be transitioned from I.V. to oral as soon as tolerated):

Children:

Crohn's disease (unlabeled use): Oral: 3 mg/kg once daily (**Note:** Prior to initiating oral therapy, may administer I.V. [same dosage] for initial 5 days) (Fuentes, 2003)

Immune (idiopathic) thrombocytopenic purpura, chronic refractory (unlabeled use): Oral: Maintenance: 2-2.5 mg/kg/day, rounded to the nearest 50 mg (Boruchov, 2006)

Renal transplantation (unlabeled use): Oral: 1-2 mg/kg/day (Grenda, 2006; Webb, 2009)

Ulcerative colitis, maintenance (unlabeled use): Oral: 1.5-2.5 mg/kg/day (Hyams, 2011; Timmer, 2008)

Adults:

Renal transplantation (treatment usually started the day of transplant, however, has been initiated [rarely] 1-3 days prior to transplant): Oral, I.V.: Initial: 3-5 mg/kg/day usually given as a single daily dose, then 1-3 mg/kg/day maintenance

Rheumatoid arthritis: Oral:

Initial: 1 mg/kg/day (50-100 mg) given once daily or divided twice daily for 6-8 weeks; may increase by 0.5 mg/kg every 4 weeks until response or up to 2.5 mg/kg/day; an adequate trial should be a minimum of 12 weeks

Maintenance dose: Reduce dose by 0.5 mg/kg (~25 mg daily) every 4 weeks until lowest effective dose is reached; optimum duration of therapy not specified; may be discontinued abruptly

Crohn's disease, remission maintenance or reduction of steroid use (unlabeled use): Oral: 2-3 mg/kg/day (Lichtenstein, 2009)

Dermatomyositis/polymyositis, adjunctive management (unlabeled use): Oral: 50 mg/day in conjunction with prednisone; increase by 50 mg/week to total dose of 2-3 mg/kg/day (Briemberg, 2003); **Note:** Onset of beneficial effects may take 3-6 months; however, may be preferred over methotrexate in patients with pulmonary or hepatic toxicity.

Immune (idiopathic) thrombocytopenic purpura, chronic refractory (unlabeled use): Oral: Maintenance: 100-200 mg/day (Boruchov, 2007)

Lupus nephritis (unlabeled use): Oral: Initial: 2 mg/kg/day; may reduce to 1.5 mg/kg/day after 1 month (if proteinuria <1 g/day and serum creatinine stable) (Moroni, 2006) **or** target dose: 2 mg/kg/day (Houssiau, 2010)

Ulcerative colitis, remission maintenance or reduction of steroid use (unlabeled use): Oral: 1.5-2.5 mg/kg/day (Kornbluth, 2010)

Dosage adjustment for concomitant use with allopurinol: Reduce azathioprine dose to one-third or one-fourth the usual dose when used concurrently with allopurinol. Patients with low or absent TPMT activity may require further dose reductions or discontinuation.

Dosage adjustment for toxicity:

Rapid WBC count decrease, persistently low WBC count, or serious infection: Reduce dose or temporarily withhold treatment

Severe toxicity in renal transplantation: May require discontinuation

Hepatic sinusoidal obstruction syndrome (SOS; veno-occlusive disease): Permanently discontinue

Dosing adjustment in renal impairment: Although dosage reductions are recommended, specific guidelines are not available in the FDA-approved labeling; the following guidelines have been used by some clinicians (Aronoff, 2007):

Cl_{cr} >50 mL/minute: No adjustment recommended

Cl_{cr} 10-50 mL/minute: Administer 75% of normal dose

Cl_{cr} <10 mL/minute: Administer 50% of normal dose

Hemodialysis (dialyzable; ~45% removed in 8 hours): Children: Administer 50% of normal dose; Adults: Administer 50% of normal dose; supplement: 0.25 mg/kg

CAPD: Children: Administer 50% of normal dose; Adults: Unknown

CRRT: Children and Adults: Administer 75% of normal dose

Dietary Considerations May be taken with food.

Administration

I.V.: Azathioprine can be administered IVP over 5 minutes at a concentration not to exceed 10 mg/mL **or** azathioprine can be further diluted with normal saline, 1/2NS, or D_5W and administered by intermittent infusion usually over 30-60 minutes or by an extended infusion up to 8 hours.

Oral: Administering tablets after meals or in divided doses may decrease adverse GI events.

Monitoring Parameters CBC with differential and platelets (weekly during first month, twice monthly for months 2 and 3, then monthly; monitor more frequently with dosage modifications), total bilirubin, liver function tests, creatinine clearance, TPMT genotyping or phenotyping (consider TPMT testing in patients with abnormally low CBC unresponsive to dose reduction); monitor for symptoms of infection

For use as immunomodulatory therapy in CD or UC, monitor CBC with differential weekly for 1 month, then biweekly for 1 month, followed by monitoring every 1-2 months throughout the course of therapy; monitor more frequently if symptomatic. LFTs should be assessed every 3 months

Test Interactions TPMT phenotyping results will not be accurate following recent blood transfusions.

Dosage Forms Excipient information presented when available (limited, particularly for generics); consult specific product labeling.

Injection, powder for reconstitution: 100 mg

Tablet, oral: 50 mg

Azasan®: 75 mg, 100 mg [scored]

Imuran®: 50 mg [scored]

Extemporaneous Preparations Hazardous agent: Use appropriate precautions for handling and disposal.

A 50 mg/mL oral suspension may be prepared with tablets. Crush one-hundred-twenty 50 mg tablets in a mortar and reduce to a fine powder. Add 40 mL of either cherry syrup (diluted 1:4 with Simple Syrup, USP); a 1:1 mixture of Ora-Sweet® and Ora-Plus®; or a 1:1 mixture of Ora-Sweet® SF and Ora-Plus®, and mix to a uniform paste. Mix while adding the vehicle in incremental proportions to **almost** 120 mL; transfer to a calibrated bottle, rinse mortar with vehicle, and add quantity of vehicle sufficient to make 120 mL. Label "shake well", "refrigerate", and "protect from light". Stable for 60 days refrigerated.

Allen LV Jr and Erickson MA 3rd, "Stability of Acetazolamide, Allopurinol, Azathioprine, Clonazepam, and Flucytosine in Extemporaneously Compounded Oral Liquids," *Am J Health Syst Pharm*, 1996, 53(16):1944-9.

- **Azathioprine Sodium** *see* AzaTHIOprine *on page 176*
- **5-AZC** *see* AzaCITIDine *on page 174*
- **AZD6140** *see* Ticagrelor *on page 1679*
- **AZD6474** *see* Vandetanib *on page 1767*

Azelaic Acid (a zeh LAY ik AS id)

Brand Names: U.S. Azelex®; Finacea®; Finacea® Plus™

Brand Names: Canada Finacea®

Pharmacologic Category Topical Skin Product, Acne

Use

Azelex®: Treatment of mild-to-moderate inflammatory acne vulgaris

Finacea®: Treatment of inflammatory papules and pustules of mild-to-moderate rosacea

Pregnancy Risk Factor B

Dosage Topical:

Adolescents ≥12 years and Adults: Acne vulgaris: Cream 20%: Apply a thin film to the affected area(s) twice daily, in the morning and evening; may reduce to once daily if persistent skin irritation occurs. Improvement in condition is usually seen within 4 weeks.

Adults: Rosacea: Gel 15%: Apply a thin layer to the affected area(s) of the face twice daily, in the morning and evening; reassess if no improvement after 12 weeks of therapy.

Additional Information Complete prescribing information for this medication should be consulted for additional detail.

Dosage Forms Excipient information presented when available (limited, particularly for generics); consult specific product labeling.

Cream, topical:

Azelex®: 20% (30 g, 50 g) [contains benzoic acid]

Gel, topical:

Finacea®: 15% (50 g) [contains benzoic acid]

Finacea® Plus™: 15% (50 g) [contains benzoic acid; packaged with cleanser and lotion]

Azelastine (Nasal) (a ZEL as teen)

Brand Names: U.S. Astelin®; Astepro®

Brand Names: Canada Astelin®

Index Terms Azelastine Hydrochloride

Pharmacologic Category Histamine H_1 Antagonist; Histamine H_1 Antagonist, Second Generation

Use Treatment of the symptoms of seasonal allergic rhinitis such as rhinorrhea, sneezing, and nasal pruritus; treatment of the symptoms of vasomotor rhinitis

Pregnancy Risk Factor C

Dosage Intranasal:

Seasonal allergic rhinitis:

Children 5-11 years (Astelin®): 1 spray in each nostril twice daily

Children ≥12 years and Adults (Astelin®, Astepro®): 1-2 sprays in each nostril twice daily

Vasomotor rhinitis: Children ≥12 years and Adults (Astelin®): 2 sprays in each nostril twice daily

Additional Information Complete prescribing information for this medication should be consulted for additional detail.

Dosage Forms Excipient information presented when available (limited, particularly for generics); consult specific product labeling.

Solution, intranasal, as hydrochloride [spray]: 0.1% [137 mcg/spray] (30 mL)

Astelin®: 0.1% [137 mcg/spray] (30 mL) [contains benzalkonium chloride; 200 metered sprays]

Astepro®: 0.15% [205.5 mcg/spray] (30 mL) [contains benzalkonium chloride; 200 metered sprays]

Azelastine (Ophthalmic) (a ZEL as teen)

Brand Names: U.S. Optivar®

Index Terms Azelastine Hydrochloride

Pharmacologic Category Histamine H_1 Antagonist; Histamine H_1 Antagonist, Second Generation

Use Treatment of itching of the eye associated with seasonal allergic conjunctivitis

Pregnancy Risk Factor C

Dosage Ophthalmic: Children ≥3 years and Adults: Instill 1 drop into affected eye(s) twice daily.

Additional Information Complete prescribing information for this medication should be consulted for additional detail.

Dosage Forms Excipient information presented when available (limited, particularly for generics); consult specific product labeling.

Solution, ophthalmic, as hydrochloride [drops]: 0.05% (6 mL)

Optivar®: 0.05% (6 mL) [contains benzalkonium chloride]

- **Azelastine Hydrochloride** *see* Azelastine (Nasal) *on page 179*
- **Azelastine Hydrochloride** *see* Azelastine (Ophthalmic) *on page 179*
- **Azelex®** *see* Azelaic Acid *on page 179*
- **Azidothymidine** *see* Zidovudine *on page 1814*
- **Azidothymidine, Abacavir, and Lamivudine** *see* Abacavir, Lamivudine, and Zidovudine *on page 20*
- **Azilect®** *see* Rasagiline *on page 1466*

Azilsartan (ay zil SAR tan)

Brand Names: U.S. Edarbi™

Index Terms Azilsartan Medoxomil; AZL-M

Pharmacologic Category Angiotensin II Receptor Blocker

Additional Appendix Information

Angiotensin Agents *on page 1869*

Use Treatment of hypertension; may be used alone or in combination with other antihypertensives

Pregnancy Risk Factor D

Pregnancy Considerations Medications which act on the renin-angiotensin system are reported to have the following fetal/neonatal effects: Hypotension, neonatal skull hypoplasia, anuria, renal failure, and death; oligohydramnios is also reported. These effects are reported to occur with exposure during the second and third trimesters. **[U.S. Boxed Warning]: Based on human data, drugs that act on the renin-angiotensin system can cause injury and death to the developing fetus. Angiotensin receptor blockers should be discontinued as soon as possible once pregnancy is detected.**

Lactation Excretion in breast milk unknown/not recommended

Contraindications There are no contraindications listed in manufacturer's labeling.

Warnings/Precautions [U.S. Boxed Warning]: Based on human data, drugs that act on the renin-angiotensin system can cause injury and death to the developing fetus. Angiotensin receptor blockers should be discontinued as soon as possible once pregnancy is detected. Angiotensin II receptor blockers may cause hyperkalemia; avoid potassium supplementation unless specifically required by healthcare provider. Avoid use or use a smaller dose in patients who are volume depleted; correct depletion first. May be associated with deterioration of renal function and/or increases in serum creatinine, particularly in patients with low renal blood flow (eg, renal artery stenosis, heart failure, volume depletion) whose glomerular filtration rate (GFR) is dependent on efferent arteriolar vasoconstriction by angiotensin II. Use with caution in unstented unilateral/bilateral renal artery stenosis. When unstented bilateral renal artery stenosis is present, use is generally avoided due to the elevated risk of deterioration in renal function unless possible benefits outweigh risks. Use with caution in pre-existing renal insufficiency; significant aortic/mitral stenosis. Concurrent use with ACE inhibitors may increase the risk of clinically-significant adverse events (eg, renal dysfunction, hyperkalemia).

Adverse Reactions

Cardiovascular: Hypotension, orthostatic hypotension
Central nervous system: Dizziness, fatigue
Gastrointestinal: Diarrhea (2%), nausea
Hematologic: Hemoglobin decreased, hematocrit decreased, leukopenia (rare), RBC decreased, thrombocytopenia (rare)
Neuromuscular & skeletal: Muscle spasm, weakness
Renal: Serum creatinine increased
Respiratory: Cough

Drug Interactions

Metabolism/Transport Effects Substrate of CYP2C9 (minor); **Note:** Assignment of Major/Minor substrate status based on clinically relevant drug interaction potential

Avoid Concomitant Use There are no known interactions where it is recommended to avoid concomitant use.

Increased Effect/Toxicity

Azilsartan may increase the levels/effects of: ACE Inhibitors; Amifostine; Antihypertensives; Hypotensive Agents; Lithium; Nonsteroidal Anti-Inflammatory Agents; Potassium-Sparing Diuretics; RiTUXimab; Sodium Phosphates

The levels/effects of Azilsartan may be increased by: Alfuzosin; Diazoxide; Eplerenone; Herbs (Hypotensive Properties); MAO Inhibitors; Pentoxifylline; Phosphodiesterase 5 Inhibitors; Potassium Salts; Prostacyclin Analogues; Tolvaptan; Trimethoprim

Decreased Effect

The levels/effects of Azilsartan may be decreased by: Herbs (Hypertensive Properties); Methylphenidate; Nonsteroidal Anti-Inflammatory Agents; Rifamycin Derivatives; Yohimbine

Ethanol/Nutrition/Herb Interactions Herb/Nutraceutical: Avoid ephedra, yohimbe, ginseng (may worsen hypertension). Avoid garlic (may have increased antihypertensive effect).

Stability Store at 25°C (77°F); excursions permitted to 15°C to 30°C (59°F to 86°F). Protect from moisture and light. Dispense and store in original container.

Mechanism of Action Angiotensin II (which is formed by enzymatic conversion from angiotensin I) is the primary pressor agent of the renin-angiotensin system. Effects of angiotensin II include vasoconstriction, stimulation of aldosterone synthesis/release, cardiac stimulation, and renal sodium reabsorption. Azilsartan inhibits angiotensin II's vasoconstrictor and aldosterone-secreting effects by selectively blocking the binding of angiotensin II to the AT_1 receptor in vascular smooth muscle and adrenal gland tissues (azilsartan has a stronger affinity for the AT_1 receptor than the AT_2 receptor). The action is independent of the angiotensin II synthesis pathways. Azilsartan does not inhibit ACE (kininase II), therefore it does not affect the response to bradykinin (the clinical relevance of this is unknown) and does not bind to or inhibit other receptors or ion channels of importance in cardiovascular regulation.

Pharmacodynamics/Kinetics

Distribution: V_d: ~16 L
Protein binding: >99%; primarily to serum albumin
Metabolism: Gut: prodrug hydrolyzed to active metabolite; Hepatic: primarily via CYP2C9 to inactive metabolites
Bioavailability: ~60%
Half-life elimination: ~11 hours
Time to peak, serum: 1.5-3 hours
Excretion: Feces (~55%); urine (~42%, 15% as unchanged drug)
Clearance: 2.3 mL/minute

Dosage Oral: Adults: 80 mg once daily; consider initial dose of 40 mg once daily in patients with volume depletion (eg, patients receiving high-dose diuretics)

Dosage adjustment in renal impairment: No starting dosage adjustment is necessary; however, carefully monitor the patient.

Dosage adjustment in hepatic impairment: No starting dosage adjustment is necessary in patients with mild-to-moderate impairment; however, carefully monitor the patient. Not studied in patients with severe impairment.

Dietary Considerations May be taken with or without food.

Administration Administer without regard to food.

Monitoring Parameters Electrolytes, serum creatinine, BUN; blood pressure

Dosage Forms Excipient information presented when available (limited, particularly for generics); consult specific product labeling.

Tablet, oral, as medoxomil:
Edarbi™: 40 mg, 80 mg

◆ **Azilsartan Medoxomil** *see* Azilsartan *on page 179*

Azithromycin (Systemic) (az ith roe MYE sin)

Brand Names: U.S. Zithromax®; Zithromax® TRI-PAK™; Zithromax® Z-PAK®; Zmax®

Brand Names: Canada Apo-Azithromycin®; Ava-Azithromycin; Azithromycin for Injection; CO Azithromycin; Dom-Azithromycin; GD-Azithromycin; Mylan-Azithromycin; Novo-Azithromycin; PHL-Azithromycin; PMS-Azithromycin; PRO-Azithromycin; ratio-Azithromycin; Riva-Azithromycin; Sandoz-Azithromycin; Zithromax®; Zmax SR™

Index Terms Azithromycin Dihydrate; Azithromycin Hydrogencitrate; Azithromycin Monohydrate; Z-Pak; Zithromax TRI-PAK™; Zithromax Z-PAK®

Pharmacologic Category Antibiotic, Macrolide

Additional Appendix Information

Prevention of Infective Endocarditis *on page 1952*

Use Oral, I.V.: Treatment of acute otitis media due to *H. influenzae*, *M. catarrhalis*, or *S. pneumoniae*; pharyngitis/tonsillitis due to *S. pyogenes*; treatment of mild-to-moderate upper and lower respiratory tract infections, infections of the skin and skin structure, community-acquired pneumonia, pelvic inflammatory disease (PID), sexually-transmitted diseases (urethritis/cervicitis), and genital ulcer disease (chancroid) due to susceptible strains of *Chlamydophila pneumoniae, C. trachomatis, M. catarrhalis, H. influenzae, S. aureus, S. pneumoniae, Mycoplasma genitalium, Mycoplasma pneumoniae*, and *C. psittaci*; acute bacterial exacerbations of chronic obstructive pulmonary disease (COPD) due to *H. influenzae, M. catarrhalis,* or *S. pneumoniae*; acute bacterial sinusitis; prevention, alone or in combination with rifabutin, of MAC in patients with advanced HIV infection; treatment, in combination with ethambutol, of disseminated MAC in patients with advanced HIV infection

Unlabeled Use Prophylaxis of infective endocarditis in patients who are allergic to penicillin and undergoing surgical or dental procedures; pertussis

Pregnancy Risk Factor B

Pregnancy Considerations Adverse events were not observed in animal studies; therefore, azithromycin is classified as pregnancy category B. Azithromycin crosses the placenta. Fetal malformations have not been observed following maternal use of azithromycin. The maternal serum half-life of azithromycin is unchanged in early pregnancy and decreased at term; however, high concentrations of azithromycin are sustained in the myometrium and adipose tissue. Azithromycin is recommended for the treatment of several infections, including chlamydia and *Mycobacterium avium* complex (MAC) in pregnant patients.

Lactation Enters breast milk/use caution

Contraindications Hypersensitivity to azithromycin, other macrolide (eg, azalide or ketolide) antibiotics, or any component of the formulation; history of cholestatic jaundice/hepatic dysfunction associated with prior azithromycin use

Warnings/Precautions Use with caution in patients with pre-existing liver disease; hepatocellular and/or cholestatic hepatitis, with or without jaundice, hepatic necrosis, failure and death have occurred. Discontinue immediately if symptoms of hepatitis occur (malaise, nausea, vomiting, abdominal colic, fever). Allergic reactions have been reported (rare); reappearance of allergic reaction may occur shortly after discontinuation without further azithromycin exposure. May mask or delay symptoms of incubating gonorrhea or syphilis, so appropriate culture and susceptibility tests should be performed prior to initiating azithromycin. Prolonged use may result in fungal or bacterial superinfection, including *C. difficile*-associated diarrhea (CDAD); CDAD has been observed >2 months postantibiotic treatment. Use caution with renal dysfunction. Prolongation of the QT_c interval has been reported with macrolide antibiotics; use caution in patients at risk of prolonged cardiac repolarization. Use with caution in patients with myasthenia gravis.

Oral suspensions (immediate release and extended release) are not interchangeable.

Adverse Reactions

>10%: Gastrointestinal: Diarrhea (4% to 9%; high single-dose regimens 12% to 14%), nausea (≤7%; high single-dose regimens 18%)

2% to 10%:

Dermatologic: Pruritus, rash

Gastrointestinal: Abdominal pain, anorexia, cramping, vomiting (especially with high single-dose regimens)

Genitourinary: Vaginitis

Local: (with I.V. administration): Injection site pain, inflammation

≤1% (Limited to important or life-threatening): Acute renal failure, aggressive behavior agitation, allergic reaction, anaphylaxis, anemia, angioedema, anxiety, arrhythmia (including ventricular tachycardia), arthralgia, bronchospasm, candidiasis, chest pain, cholestatic jaundice, conjunctivitis (pediatric patients), constipation, cough increased, deafness, dehydration, dermatitis (fungal), diaphoresis, dizziness, dyspepsia, eczema, edema, enteritis, erythema multiforme (rare), facial edema, fatigue fever, flatulence, fungal infection, gastritis, headache, hearing disturbance, hearing loss, hepatic failure, hepatic necrosis, hepatitis, hyperactivity, hyperkinesia, hypotension, insomnia, interstitial nephritis, jaundice, leukopenia, LFTs increased, loss of smell, loss of taste, malaise, melena, mucositis, nephritis, nervousness, neutropenia (mild), oral candidiasis, oral moniliasis, pain, palpitation, pancreatitis, paresthesia, pharyngitis, photosensitivity, pleural effusion, pseudomembranous colitis, pyloric stenosis, QT_c prolongation (rare), rhinitis, seizure, smell perversion, somnolence, somnolence, Stevens-Johnson syndrome (rare), syncope, taste perversion, thrombocytopenia, tinnitus, tongue discoloration (rare), torsade de pointes (rare), toxic epidermal necrolysis (rare), urticaria, vertigo, vesiculobullous rash, weakness

Drug Interactions

Metabolism/Transport Effects **Substrate** of CYP3A4 (minor); **Note:** Assignment of Major/Minor substrate status based on clinically relevant drug interaction potential; **Inhibits** CYP1A2 (weak)

Avoid Concomitant Use

Avoid concomitant use of Azithromycin (Systemic) with any of the following: Artemether; BCG; Dronedarone; Lumefantrine; Nilotinib; Pimozide; QUEtiapine; QuiNINE; Terfenadine; Tetrabenazine; Thioridazine; Toremifene; Vandetanib; Vemurafenib; Ziprasidone

Increased Effect/Toxicity

Azithromycin (Systemic) may increase the levels/effects of: Amiodarone; Cardiac Glycosides; CycloSPORINE; CycloSPORINE (Systemic); Dronedarone; Pimozide; QTc-Prolonging Agents; QuiNINE; Tacrolimus; Tacrolimus (Systemic); Tacrolimus (Topical); Terfenadine; Tetrabenazine; Thioridazine; Toremifene; Vandetanib; Vemurafenib; Vitamin K Antagonists; Ziprasidone

The levels/effects of Azithromycin (Systemic) may be increased by: Alfuzosin; Artemether; Chloroquine; Ciprofloxacin; Ciprofloxacin (Systemic); Conivaptan; Gadobutrol; Indacaterol; Lumefantrine; Nelfinavir; Nilotinib; QUEtiapine; QuiNINE

Decreased Effect

Azithromycin (Systemic) may decrease the levels/effects of: BCG; Typhoid Vaccine

The levels/effects of Azithromycin (Systemic) may be decreased by: Tocilizumab

Ethanol/Nutrition/Herb Interactions Food: Rate and extent of GI absorption may be altered depending upon the formulation. Azithromycin suspension, not tablet form, has significantly increased absorption (46%) with food.

Stability

Injection (Zithromax®): Store intact vials of injection at room temperature. Reconstitute the 500 mg vial with 4.8 mL of sterile water for injection and shake until all of the drug is dissolved. Each mL contains 100 mg azithromycin. Reconstituted solution is stable for 24 hours when stored below 30°C (86°F). Use of a standard syringe is recommended due to the vacuum in the vial (which may draw additional solution through an automated syringe).

The initial solution should be further diluted to a concentration of 1 mg/mL (500 mL) to 2 mg/mL (250 mL) in 0.9% sodium chloride, 5% dextrose in water, or lactated Ringer's. The diluted solution is stable for 24 hours at or below room temperature (30°C or 86°F) and for 7 days if stored under refrigeration (5°C or 41°F).

Suspension, immediate release (Zithromax®): Store dry powder below 30°C (86°F). Following reconstitution, store at 5°C to 30°C (41°F to 86°F).

Suspension, extended release (Zmax®): Store dry powder ≤30°C (86°F). Following reconstitution, store at 25°C (77°F); excursions permitted to 15°C to 30°C (59°F to 86°F); do not refrigerate or freeze. Should be consumed within 12 hours following reconstitution.

Tablet (Zithromax®): Store between 15°C to 30°C (59°F to 86°F).

Mechanism of Action Inhibits RNA-dependent protein synthesis at the chain elongation step; binds to the 50S ribosomal subunit resulting in blockage of transpeptidation

Pharmacodynamics/Kinetics

Absorption: Oral: Rapid

Distribution: Extensive tissue; distributes well into skin, lungs, sputum, tonsils, and cervix; penetration into CSF is poor; I.V.: 33.3 L/kg; Oral: 31.1 L/kg

Protein binding (concentration dependent): Oral, I.V.: 7% to 51%

Metabolism: Hepatic

Bioavailability: Oral: 38%, decreased by 17% with extended release suspension; variable effect with food (increased with immediate or delayed release oral suspension, unchanged with tablet)

Half-life elimination: Oral, I.V.: Terminal: Immediate release: 68-72 hours; Extended release: 59 hours

Time to peak, serum: Oral: Immediate release: 2-3 hours; Extended release: 5 hours

Excretion: Oral, I.V.: Biliary (major route); urine (6%)

Dosage Note: Extended release suspension (Zmax®) is not interchangeable with immediate release formulations. Use should be limited to approved indications. All doses are expressed as immediate release azithromycin unless otherwise specified.

Usual dosage range:

Children ≥6 months: Oral: 5-12 mg/kg given once daily (maximum: 500 mg/day) **or** 30 mg/kg as a single dose (maximum: 1500 mg)

Extended release suspension (Zmax®): 60 mg/kg as a single dose; **Note:** Extended release suspension (Zmax®): Dose in mL is equal to the weight in lbs for patients <75 lbs (34 kg). Pediatric patients ≥75 lbs should receive the adult dose.

Adolescents ≥16 years and Adults:

Oral: 250-600 mg once daily **or** 1-2 g as a single dose

Extended release suspension (Zmax®): 2 g as a single dose

I.V.: 250-500 mg once daily

Indication-specific dosing:

Children:

Bacterial sinusitis: Oral: 10 mg/kg once daily for 3 days (maximum: 500 mg/day)

Cat scratch disease (unlabeled use): Oral: <45.5 kg: 10 mg/kg as a single dose, then 5 mg/kg once daily for 4 days

Community-acquired pneumonia (CAP) (IDSA/PIDS, 2011): Infants >3 months and Children: **Note:** A beta-lactam antibiotic should be added if typical bacterial pneumonia cannot be ruled out

Presumed mild infection or step-down therapy, atypical *(M. pneumoniae, C. pneumoniae, C. trachomatis)* (preferred): Oral: 10 mg/kg (maximum dose: 500 mg) as a single dose on the first day, followed by 5 mg/kg/day (maximum dose: 250 mg) on days 2 through 5.

Presumed moderate-to-severe infection, atypical *(M. pneumoniae, C. pneumoniae, C. trachomatis)*: I.V.: 10 mg/kg/day on days 1 and 2, then switch to oral azithromycin therapy if possible to finish the 5-day course

Alternative regimens for community-acquired pneumonia: Oral: 10 mg/kg (maximum dose: 500 mg) once daily for 3 days (Kogan, 2003)

Extended release suspension (Zmax®):

<75 lbs (34 kg): 60 mg/kg as a single dose

≥75 lbs (34 kg): Refer to adult dosing

Disseminated *M. avium* complex disease in patients with advanced HIV infection (unlabeled use; CDC, 2009):

Treatment: 10-12 mg/kg/day (maximum: 500 mg) in combination with ethambutol; patients with severe disease should also receive rifabutin

Primary prophylaxis: 20 mg/kg (maximum: 1200 mg) once weekly (preferred) or alternatively, 5 mg/kg/day once daily (maximum: 250 mg/day)

Secondary prophylaxis: 5 mg/kg/day once daily (maximum: 250 mg/day) in combination with ethambutol, with or without rifabutin

Otitis media: Oral:

1-day regimen: 30 mg/kg as a single dose (maximum: 1500 mg)

3-day regimen: 10 mg/kg once daily for 3 days (maximum: 500 mg/day)

5-day regimen: 10 mg/kg on day 1 (maximum: 500 mg/day) followed by 5 mg/kg/day once daily on days 2-5 (maximum: 250 mg/day)

Pertussis (CDC, 2005):

Children <6 months: 10 mg/kg/day for 5 days

Children ≥6 months: 10 mg/kg on day 1 (maximum: 500 mg/day) followed by 5 mg/kg/day once daily on days 2-5 (maximum: 250 mg/day)

Pharyngitis, tonsillitis: Children ≥2 years: 12 mg/kg/day once daily for 5 days (maximum: 500 mg/day)

Prophylaxis against infective endocarditis (unlabeled use): 15 mg/kg 30-60 minutes before procedure (maximum: 500 mg). **Note:** American Heart Association (AHA) guidelines now recommend prophylaxis only in patients undergoing invasive procedures and in whom underlying cardiac conditions may predispose to a higher risk of adverse outcomes should infection occur. As of April 2007, routine prophylaxis for GI/GU procedures is no longer recommended by the AHA.

Uncomplicated chlamydial urethritis or cervicitis (unlabeled use): Children ≥45 kg: 1 g as a single dose (CDC, 2010)

Adolescents ≥16 years and Adults:

Bacterial sinusitis: Oral: 500 mg/day for a total of 3 days

Extended release suspension (Zmax®): 2 g as a single dose

Cat scratch disease (unlabeled use): Oral: >45.5 kg: 500 mg as a single dose, then 250 mg once daily for 4 days

Chancroid due to *H. ducreyi*: Oral: 1 g as a single dose (CDC, 2010)

Community-acquired pneumonia:

Oral: 500 mg on day 1 followed by 250 mg once daily on days 2-5

Extended release suspension (Zmax®): 2 g as a single dose

I.V.: 500 mg as a single dose for at least 2 days, follow I.V. therapy by the oral route with a single daily dose of 500 mg to complete a 7- to 10-day course of therapy.

Disseminated *M. avium* complex disease in patients with advanced HIV infection: Oral:

Treatment: 600 mg/day in combination with ethambutol

Primary prophylaxis: 1200 mg once weekly (preferred), with or without rifabutin **or** alternatively, 600 mg twice weekly (CDC, 2009)

Secondary prophylaxis: 500-600 mg/day in combination with ethambutol (CDC, 2009)

Gonococcal infection, uncomplicated (cervix, pharynx, rectum, urethra): Oral: 1 g as a single dose (in combination with a cephalosporin) (CDC, 2010)

Note: Monotherapy with azithromycin (1 g and 2 g) have been associated with resistance and/or treatment failure; use in combination with a cephalosporin (CDC, 2010). However, a single 2 g azithromycin dose is still an FDA-approved dose for gonococcal urethritis and cervicitis and also may be appropriate for treatment of a gonococcal infection in pregnant women who cannot tolerate a cephalosporin (CDC, 2010).

Granuloma inguinale (donovanosis): Oral: 1 g once a week for at least 3 weeks (and until lesions have healed) (CDC, 2010)

Mild-to-moderate respiratory tract, skin, and soft tissue infections: Oral: 500 mg in a single loading dose on day 1 followed by 250 mg/day as a single dose on days 2-5

Alternative regimen: Bacterial exacerbation of COPD: 500 mg/day for a total of 3 days

Pelvic inflammatory disease (PID): I.V.: 500 mg as a single dose for 1-2 days, follow I.V. therapy by the oral route with a single daily dose of 250 mg to complete a 7-day course of therapy

Pertussis (CDC, 2005): Oral: 500 mg on day 1 followed by 250 mg/day on days 2-5 (maximum: 500 mg/day)

Prophylaxis against infective endocarditis (unlabeled use): Oral: 500 mg 30-60 minutes prior to the procedure. **Note:** American Heart Association (AHA) guidelines now recommend prophylaxis only in patients undergoing invasive procedures and in whom underlying cardiac conditions may predispose to a higher risk of adverse outcomes should infection occur. As of April 2007, routine prophylaxis for GI/GU procedures is no longer recommended by the AHA.

Prophylaxis against sexually-transmitted diseases following sexual assault: Oral: 1 g as a single dose (in combination with a cephalosporin and metronidazole) (CDC, 2010)

Urethritis/cervicitis: Oral: *Due to C. trachomatis or M. genitalium*: 1 g as a single dose

Dosage adjustment in renal impairment: Use caution in patients with GFR <10 mL/minute

Poorly dialyzed; no supplemental dose or dosage adjustment necessary, including patients on intermittent hemodialysis, peritoneal dialysis, or continuous renal replacement therapy (eg, CVVHD).

Dosage adjustment in hepatic impairment: Use with caution due to potential for hepatotoxicity (rare). Specific guidelines for dosing in hepatic impairment have not been established.

Dietary Considerations

Some products may contain sodium and/or sucrose.

Oral suspension, immediate release, may be administered with or without food.

Oral suspension, extended release, should be taken on an empty stomach (at least 1 hour before or 2 hours following a meal).

Tablet may be administered with food to decrease GI effects.

Administration

I.V.: Infusate concentration and rate of infusion for azithromycin for injection should be either 1 mg/mL over 3 hours or 2 mg/mL over 1 hour. Other medications should not be infused simultaneously through the same I.V. line.

Oral: Immediate release suspension and tablet may be taken without regard to food; extended release suspension should be taken on an empty stomach (at least 1 hour before or 2 hours following a meal), within 12 hours of reconstitution.

Monitoring Parameters Liver function tests, CBC with differential

Additional Information Zithromax® tablets and immediate release suspension may be interchanged (eg, two Zithromax® 250 mg tablets may be substituted for one Zithromax® 500 mg tablet or the tablets may be substituted with the immediate release suspension); however, the extended release suspension (Zmax®) is not bioequivalent with Zithromax® and therefore should not be interchanged.

Dosage Forms Excipient information presented when available (limited, particularly for generics); consult specific product labeling. [DSC] = Discontinued product

Injection, powder for reconstitution, as dihydrate [strength expressed as base]: 500 mg

Zithromax®: 500 mg [contains sodium 114 mg (4.96 mEq)/vial]

Injection, powder for reconstitution, as hydrogencitrate [strength expressed as base]: 500 mg [DSC]

Injection, powder for reconstitution, as monohydrate [strength expressed as base]: 500 mg

Microspheres for suspension, extended release, oral, as dihydrate [strength expressed as base]:

Zmax®: 2 g/bottle (60 mL) [contains sodium 148 mg/bottle, sucrose 19 g/bottle; cherry-banana flavor; product contains azithromycin 27 mg/mL after constitution]

Powder for suspension, oral, as dihydrate [strength expressed as base]: 100 mg/5 mL (15 mL); 200 mg/5 mL (15 mL, 22.5 mL, 30 mL); 1 g/packet (3s)

Zithromax®: 100 mg/5 mL (15 mL) [contains sodium 3.7 mg/5 mL; cherry-crème de vanilla-banana flavor]

Zithromax®: 200 mg/5 mL (15 mL, 22.5 mL, 30 mL) [contains sodium 7.4 mg/5 mL; cherry-crème de vanilla-banana flavor]

Zithromax®: 1 g/packet (3s, 10s) [contains sodium 37 mg/packet; banana-cherry flavor]

Powder for suspension, oral, as monohydrate [strength expressed as base]: 100 mg/5 mL (15 mL); 200 mg/5 mL (15 mL, 22.5 mL, 30 mL)

Tablet, oral, as anhydrous: 250 mg, 500 mg, 600 mg

Tablet, oral, as dihydrate [strength expressed as base]: 250 mg, 500 mg, 600 mg

Zithromax®: 250 mg [contains sodium 0.9 mg/tablet]

Zithromax®: 500 mg [contains sodium 1.8 mg/tablet]

Zithromax®: 600 mg [contains sodium 2.1 mg/tablet]

Zithromax® TRI-PAK™: 500 mg [contains sodium 1.8 mg/tablet]

Zithromax® Z-PAK®: 250 mg [contains sodium 0.9 mg/tablet]

Tablet, oral, as monohydrate [strength expressed as base]: 250 mg, 500 mg, 600 mg

Azithromycin (Ophthalmic) (az ith roe MYE sin)

Brand Names: U.S. AzaSite®

Pharmacologic Category Antibiotic, Macrolide; Antibiotic, Ophthalmic

Use Bacterial conjunctivitis

Pregnancy Risk Factor B

Dosage Ophthalmic: **Usual dosage range:** Bacterial conjunctivitis: Children ≥1 year and Adults: Instill 1 drop into affected eye(s) twice daily (8-12 hours apart) for 2 days, then 1 drop once daily for 5 days

Additional Information Complete prescribing information for this medication should be consulted for additional detail.

Dosage Forms Excipient information presented when available (limited, particularly for generics); consult specific product labeling.

Solution, ophthalmic [drops]:

AzaSite®: 1% (2.5 mL) [contains benzalkonium chloride]

- **Azithromycin Dihydrate** *see* Azithromycin (Systemic) *on page 180*
- **Azithromycin for Injection (Can)** *see* Azithromycin (Systemic) *on page 180*
- **Azithromycin Hydrogencitrate** *see* Azithromycin (Systemic) *on page 180*
- **Azithromycin Monohydrate** *see* Azithromycin (Systemic) *on page 180*
- **AZL-M** *see* Azilsartan *on page 179*
- **Azo-Gesic™ [OTC]** *see* Phenazopyridine *on page 1337*
- **Azopt®** *see* Brinzolamide *on page 236*
- **Azor™** *see* Amlodipine and Olmesartan *on page 99*
- **AZO Standard® [OTC]** *see* Phenazopyridine *on page 1337*
- **AZO Standard® Maximum Strength [OTC]** *see* Phenazopyridine *on page 1337*
- **AZT™ (Can)** *see* Zidovudine *on page 1814*
- **AZT + 3TC (error-prone abbreviation)** *see* Lamivudine and Zidovudine *on page 967*
- **AZT, Abacavir, and Lamivudine** *see* Abacavir, Lamivudine, and Zidovudine *on page 20*
- **AZT (error-prone abbreviation)** *see* Zidovudine *on page 1814*
- **Azthreonam** *see* Aztreonam *on page 184*

Aztreonam (AZ tree oh nam)

Brand Names: U.S. Azactam®; Cayston®

Index Terms Azthreonam

Pharmacologic Category Antibiotic, Miscellaneous

Use

Injection: Treatment of patients with urinary tract infections, lower respiratory tract infections, septicemia, skin/skin structure infections, intra-abdominal infections, and gynecological infections caused by susceptible gram-negative bacilli

Inhalation: Improve respiratory symptoms in cystic fibrosis (CF) patients with *Pseudomonas aeruginosa*

Pregnancy Risk Factor B

Pregnancy Considerations Adverse events have not been observed in animal reproduction studies; therefore, the manufacturer classifies aztreonam as pregnancy category B. Aztreonam crosses the placenta and enters cord blood during middle and late pregnancy. Distribution to the fetus is minimal in early pregnancy. The amount of aztreonam available systemically following inhalation is significantly less in comparison to doses given by injection.

Lactation Enters breast milk/not recommended (AAP rates "compatible"; AAP 2001 update pending)

Prescribing and Access Restrictions Cayston® (aztreonam inhalation solution) is only available through a select group of specialty pharmacies and cannot be obtained through a retail pharmacy. Because Cayston® may only be used with the Altera® Nebulizer System, it can only be obtained from the following specialty pharmacies: Cystic Fibrosis Services, Inc; IV Solutions; Foundation Care; and Pharmaceutical Specialties, Inc. This network of specialty pharmacies ensures proper access to both the drug and device. To obtain the medication and proper nebulizer, contact the Cayston Access Program at 1-877-7CAYSTON (1-877-722-9786) or at www.cayston.com.

Contraindications Hypersensitivity to aztreonam or any component of the formulation

Warnings/Precautions Rare cross-allergenicity to penicillins and cephalosporins has been reported. Use caution in renal impairment; dosing adjustment required for the injectable formulation. Prolonged use may result in fungal or bacterial superinfection, including *C. difficile*-associated diarrhea (CDAD) and pseudomembranous colitis; CDAD has been observed >2 months postantibiotic treatment. Patients colonized with *Burkholderia cepacia* have not been studied. Safety and efficacy has not been established in patients with FEV_1 <25% or >75% predicted. To reduce the development of resistant bacteria and maintain efficacy reserve use for CF patients with known *Pseudomonas aeruginosa*. Bronchospasm may occur occur following nebulization; administer a bronchodilator prior to treatment.

Adverse Reactions

Injection: Adults:

1% to 10%:

Dermatologic: Rash

Gastrointestinal: Diarrhea, nausea, vomiting

Local: Thrombophlebitis, pain at injection site

<1% (Limited to important or life-threatening): Abdominal cramps, abnormal taste, anaphylaxis, anemia, angioedema, aphthous ulcer, breast tenderness, bronchospasm, *C. difficile*-associated diarrhea, chest pain, confusion, diaphoresis, diplopia, dizziness, dyspnea, eosinophilia, erythema multiforme, exfoliative dermatitis, fever, flushing, halitosis, headache, hepatitis, hypotension, insomnia, jaundice, leukopenia, liver enzymes increased, muscular aches myalgia, neutropenia, numb tongue, pancytopenia, paresthesia, petechiae, pruritus, pseudomembranous colitis, purpura, seizure, sneezing, thrombocytopenia, tinnitus, toxic epidermal necrolysis, urticaria, vaginitis, vertigo, weakness, wheezing

Inhalation:

>10%:

Central nervous system: Pyrexia (13%; more often observed in children)

Respiratory: Cough (54%), nasal congestion (16%), pharyngeal pain (12%), wheezing (16%)

1% to 10%:

Cardiovascular: Chest discomfort (8%)

Dermatologic: Rash (2%)

Gastrointestinal: Abdominal pain (7%), vomiting (6%)

Respiratory: Bronchospasm (3%)

<1% (Limited to important or life-threatening): Facial edema, hypersensitivity reaction, throat tightness

Drug Interactions

Metabolism/Transport Effects None known.

Avoid Concomitant Use

Avoid concomitant use of Aztreonam with any of the following: BCG

Increased Effect/Toxicity There are no known significant interactions involving an increase in effect.

Decreased Effect

Aztreonam may decrease the levels/effects of: BCG; Typhoid Vaccine

Stability

Inhalation: Prior to reconstitution, store at 2°C to 8°C (36°F to 46°F). Once removed from refrigeration, aztreonam and the diluent may be stored at room temperature (up to 25°C/77°F) for ≤28 days. Protect from light. Reconstitute immediately prior to use. Squeeze diluent into opened glass vial. Replace rubber stopper and gently swirl vial until contents have completely dissolved. Use immediately after reconstitution.

Injection: Prior to reconstitution, store at room temperature; avoid excessive heat. Reconstituted solutions are colorless to light yellow straw and may turn pink upon standing without affecting potency. Use reconstituted solutions and I.V. solutions (in NS and D_5W) within 48 hours if kept at room temperature (25°C) or 7 days under refrigeration (4°C).

I.M.: Reconstitute with at least 3 mL SWFI, sterile bacteriostatic water for injection, NS, or bacteriostatic sodium chloride.

I.V.:

Bolus injection: Reconstitute with 6-10 mL SWFI.

Infusion: Reconstitute to a final concentration ≤2%; the final concentration should not exceed 20 mg/mL. Solution for infusion may be frozen at less than -2°C (less than -4°F) for up to 3 months. Thawed solution should be used within 24 hours if thawed at room temperature or within 72 hours if thawed under refrigeration. **Do not refreeze.**

Mechanism of Action Inhibits bacterial cell wall synthesis by binding to one or more of the penicillin-binding proteins (PBPs) which in turn inhibits the final transpeptidation step of peptidoglycan synthesis in bacterial cell walls, thus inhibiting cell wall biosynthesis. Bacteria eventually lyse due to ongoing activity of cell wall autolytic enzymes (autolysins and murein hydrolases) while cell wall assembly is arrested. Monobactam structure makes cross-allergenicity with beta-lactams unlikely.

Pharmacodynamics/Kinetics

Absorption: I.M.: Well absorbed; I.M. and I.V. doses produce comparable serum concentrations; Inhalation: Low systemic absorption

Distribution: Injection: Widely to most body fluids and tissues

V_d: Children: 0.2-0.29 L/kg; Adults: 0.2 L/kg

Relative diffusion of antimicrobial agents from blood into CSF: Good only with inflammation (exceeds usual MICs)

CSF:blood level ratio: Meninges: Inflamed: 8% to 40%; Normal: ~1%

Protein binding: 56%

Metabolism: Injection: Hepatic (minor %)

Half-life elimination: Injection:

Children 2 months to 12 years: 1.7 hours

Adults: Normal renal function: 1.7-2.9 hours

End-stage renal disease: 6-8 hours

Time to peak: I.M., I.V. push: Within 60 minutes; I.V. infusion: 1.5 hours

Excretion: Injection: Urine (60% to 70% as unchanged drug); feces (~13% to 15%)

Dosage

Children >1 month: I.M., I.V.:

Mild-to-moderate infections: I.M., I.V.: 30 mg/kg every 8 hours

Moderate-to-severe infections: I.M., I.V.: 30 mg/kg every 6-8 hours; maximum: 120 mg/kg/day (8 g/day)

Cystic fibrosis: I.V.: 50 mg/kg/dose every 6-8 hours (ie, up to 200 mg/kg/day); maximum: 8 g/day

Children ≥7 years and Adults: Inhalation (nebulizer): Cystic fibrosis: 75 mg 3 times daily (at least 4 hours apart) for 28 days; do not repeat for 28 days after completion

Adults:

Urinary tract infection: I.M., I.V.: 500 mg to 1 g every 8-12 hours

Moderately-severe systemic infections: 1 g I.V. or I.M. or 2 g I.V. every 8-12 hours

Severe systemic or life-threatening infections (especially caused by *Pseudomonas aeruginosa*): I.V.: 2 g every 6-8 hours; maximum: 8 g/day

Meningitis (gram-negative): I.V.: 2 g every 6-8 hours

Dosing adjustment in renal impairment:

Oral inhalation: Dosage adjustment not required for mild, moderate, or severe renal impairment

I.M., I.V.: Adults: Following initial dose, maintenance doses should be given as follows:

Cl_{cr} 10-30 mL/minute: 50% of usual dose at the usual interval

Cl_{cr} <10 mL/minute: 25% of usual dosage at the usual interval

Intermittent hemodialysis (IHD): Dialyzable (20% to 50%): Loading dose of 500 mg, 1 g, or 2 g, followed by 25% of initial dose at usual interval; for serious/life-threatening infections, administer one-eighth (1/8) of initial dose after each hemodialysis session (given in addition to the maintenance doses). Alternatively, may administer 500 mg every 12 hours (Heintz, 2009). **Note:** Dosing dependent on the assumption of 3 times/week, complete IHD sessions.

Peritoneal dialysis (PD): Administer as for Cl_{cr} <10 mL/minute

Continuous renal replacement therapy (CRRT) (Heintz, 2009; Trotman, 2005): Drug clearance is highly dependent on the method of renal replacement, filter type, and flow rate. Appropriate dosing requires close monitoring of pharmacologic response, signs of adverse reactions due to drug accumulation, as well as drug concentrations in relation to target trough (if appropriate). The following are general recommendations only (based on dialysate flow/ultrafiltration rates of 1-2 L/hour and minimal residual renal function) and should not supersede clinical judgment:

CVVH: Loading dose of 2 g followed by 1-2 g every 12 hours

CVVHD/CVVHDF: Loading dose of 2 g followed by either 1 g every 8 hours **or** 2 g every 12 hours (Heintz, 2009)

Administration

Inhalation: Administer using only an Altera® nebulizer system; **administer alone; do not mix with other nebulizer medications**. Administer a bronchodilator before administration of aztreonam (short-acting: 15 minutes to 4 hours before; long-acting: 30 minutes to 12 hours before). For patients on multiple inhaled therapies, administer bronchodilator first, then mucolytic, and lastly, aztreonam.

To administer Cayston®, pour reconstituted solution into the handset of the nebulizer system, turn unit on. Place the mouthpiece in the patient's mouth and encourage to breath normally through the mouth. Administration time is usually 2-3 minutes. Administer doses ≥4 hours apart.

Injection: Doses >1 g should be administered I.V.

I.M.: Administer by deep injection into large muscle mass, such as upper outer quadrant of gluteus maximus or the lateral part of the thigh

I.V.: Administer by slow I.V. push over 3-5 minutes or by intermittent infusion over 20-60 minutes.

Monitoring Parameters

Injection: Periodic liver function test; monitor for signs of anaphylaxis during first dose

Inhalation: Consider measuring FEV_1 prior to initiation of therapy

Test Interactions May interfere with urine glucose tests containing cupric sulfate (Benedict's solution, Clinitest®); positive Coombs' test

Additional Information Although marketed as an agent similar to aminoglycosides, aztreonam is a monobactam antimicrobial with almost pure gram-negative aerobic activity. It cannot be used for gram-positive infections.

Dosage Forms Excipient information presented when available (limited, particularly for generics); consult specific product labeling.

Infusion, premixed iso-osmotic solution:

Azactam®: 1 g (50 mL); 2 g (50 mL)

Injection, powder for reconstitution: 1 g, 2 g
Azactam®: 1 g, 2 g
Powder for reconstitution, for oral inhalation [preservative free]:
Cayston®: 75 mg [supplied with diluent]

Bacitracin (bas i TRAY sin)

Brand Names: U.S. Baciguent® [OTC]; BACiiM™

Brand Names: Canada Baciguent®; Baciject®

Pharmacologic Category Antibiotic, Miscellaneous; Antibiotic, Ophthalmic; Antibiotic, Topical

Use Treatment of susceptible bacterial infections mainly (has activity against gram-positive bacilli); due to toxicity risks, systemic and irrigant uses of bacitracin should be limited to situations where less toxic alternatives would not be effective

Unlabeled Use Oral administration: Treatment of *Clostridium difficile*-associated diarrhea; has been used for enteric eradication of vancomycin-resistant enterococci (VRE)

Dosage Do not administer I.V.:
Infants: I.M.:
≤2.5 kg: 900 units/kg/day in 2-3 divided doses
>2.5 kg: 1000 units/kg/day in 2-3 divided doses
Adults: Oral:
Clostridium difficile-associated diarrhea (unlabeled use): 25,000 units 4 times/day for 7-10 days (Dudley 1986; Young, 1985). **Note:** May be considered when other more established regimens (eg, metronidazole or vancomycin) fail; not routinely used (Cohen, 2010).
Enteric VRE eradication (unlabeled use): 25,000 units 4 times/day for 7-10 days (Chia, 1995; O'Donovan, 1994)
Children and Adults:
Topical: Apply 1-3 times/day
Ophthalmic, ointment: Instill 1/4" to 1/2" ribbon every 3-4 hours into conjunctival sac for acute infections, or 2-3 times/day for mild-to-moderate infections for 7-10 days

Additional Information Complete prescribing information for this medication should be consulted for additional detail.

Dosage Forms Excipient information presented when available (limited, particularly for generics); consult specific product labeling.
Injection, powder for reconstitution: 50,000 units
BACiiM™: 50,000 units
Ointment, ophthalmic: 500 units/g (3.5 g)
Ointment, topical, as zinc [strength expressed as base]: 500 units/g (0.9 g, 15 g, 30 g, 120 g, 454 g)
Baciguent®: 500 units/g (30 g)

Bacitracin and Polymyxin B
(bas i TRAY sin & pol i MIKS in bee)

Brand Names: U.S. AK-Poly-Bac™; Polycin™; Polysporin® [OTC]

Brand Names: Canada LID-Pack®; Optimyxin®

Index Terms Polymyxin B and Bacitracin

Pharmacologic Category Antibiotic, Ophthalmic; Antibiotic, Topical

Use Treatment of superficial infections caused by susceptible organisms

Pregnancy Risk Factor C

Dosage Children and Adults:
Ophthalmic ointment: Instill 1/2" ribbon in the affected eye(s) every 3-4 hours for acute infections or 2-3 times/day for mild-to-moderate infections for 7-10 days
Topical ointment/powder: Apply to affected area 1-4 times/day; may cover with sterile bandage if needed

Additional Information Complete prescribing information for this medication should be consulted for additional detail.

Dosage Forms Excipient information presented when available (limited, particularly for generics); consult specific product labeling.
Ointment, ophthalmic: Bacitracin 500 units and polymyxin B 10,000 units per g (3.5 g)
AK-Poly-Bac™: Bacitracin 500 units and polymyxin B 10,000 units per g (3.5 g)
Polycin™: Bacitracin 500 units and polymyxin B 10,000 units per g (3.5 g)
Ointment, topical: Bacitracin 500 units and polymyxin B 10,000 units per g in white petrolatum (15 g, 30 g)
Polysporin®: Bacitracin 500 units and polymyxin B 10,000 units per g (0.9 g, 15 g, 30 g)
Powder, topical:
Polysporin®: Bacitracin 500 units and polymyxin B 10,000 units per g (10 g)

Bacitracin, Neomycin, and Polymyxin B
(bas i TRAY sin, nee oh MYE sin, & pol i MIKS in bee)

Brand Names: U.S. Neo-Polycin™; Neosporin® Neo To Go® [OTC]; Neosporin® Topical [OTC]

Index Terms Neomycin, Bacitracin, and Polymyxin B; Polymyxin B, Bacitracin, and Neomycin; Triple Antibiotic

Pharmacologic Category Antibiotic, Ophthalmic; Antibiotic, Topical

Use Helps prevent infection in minor cuts, scrapes, and burns; short-term treatment of superficial external ocular infections caused by susceptible organisms

Pregnancy Risk Factor C

Dosage Children and Adults:
Ophthalmic: Ointment: Instill 1/2" into the conjunctival sac every 3-4 hours for 7-10 days for acute infections
Topical: Apply 1-3 times/day to infected area; may cover with sterile bandage as needed

Additional Information Complete prescribing information for this medication should be consulted for additional detail.

Dosage Forms Excipient information presented when available (limited, particularly for generics); consult specific product labeling.
Ointment, ophthalmic: Bacitracin 400 units, neomycin 3.5 mg, and polymyxin B 10,000 units per g (3.5 g)
Neo-Polycin™: Bacitracin 400 units, neomycin 3.5 mg, and polymyxin B 10,000 units per g (3.5 g)

Ointment, topical: Bacitracin 400 units, neomycin 3.5 mg, and polymyxin B 5000 units per g (0.9 g, 15 g, 30 g, 454 g)

Neosporin®: Bacitracin 400 units, neomycin 3.5 mg, and polymyxin B 5000 units per g (15 g, 30 g)

Neosporin® Neo To Go®: Bacitracin 400 units, neomycin 3.5 mg, and polymyxin B 5000 units per g (0.9 g)

Bacitracin, Neomycin, Polymyxin B, and Hydrocortisone

(bas i TRAY sin, nee oh MYE sin, pol i MIKS in bee, & hye droe KOR ti sone)

Brand Names: U.S. Cortisporin® Ointment; Neo-Polycin™ HC

Brand Names: Canada Cortisporin® Topical Ointment

Index Terms Hydrocortisone, Bacitracin, Neomycin, and Polymyxin B; Neomycin, Bacitracin, Polymyxin B, and Hydrocortisone; Polymyxin B, Bacitracin, Neomycin, and Hydrocortisone

Pharmacologic Category Antibiotic, Ophthalmic; Antibiotic, Topical; Corticosteroid, Ophthalmic; Corticosteroid, Topical

Use Prevention and treatment of susceptible inflammatory conditions where bacterial infection (or risk of infection) is present

Pregnancy Risk Factor C

Dosage Children and Adults:

Ophthalmic: Ointment: Instill 1/2 inch ribbon to inside of lower lid every 3-4 hours until improvement occurs

Topical: Apply sparingly 2-4 times/day. Therapy should be discontinued when control is achieved; if no improvement is seen, reassessment of diagnosis may be necessary.

Additional Information Complete prescribing information for this medication should be consulted for additional detail.

Dosage Forms Excipient information presented when available (limited, particularly for generics); consult specific product labeling.

Ointment, ophthalmic: Bacitracin 400 units, neomycin 3.5 mg, polymyxin B 10,000 units, and hydrocortisone 10 mg per g (3.5 g)

Neo-Polycin™ HC: Bacitracin 400 units, neomycin 3.5 mg, polymyxin B 10,000 units, and hydrocortisone 10 mg per g (3.5 g)

Ointment, topical:

Cortisporin®: Bacitracin 400 units, neomycin 3.5 mg, polymyxin B 5000 units, and hydrocortisone 10 mg per g (15 g)

Baclofen (BAK loe fen)

Brand Names: U.S. Gablofen®; Lioresal®

Brand Names: Canada Apo-Baclofen®; Dom-Baclofen; Lioresal®; Liotec; Med-Baclofen; Mylan-Baclofen; Novo-Baclofen; Nu-Baclo; PHL-Baclofen; PMS-Baclofen; ratio-Baclofen; Riva-Baclofen

Pharmacologic Category Skeletal Muscle Relaxant

Use Treatment of reversible spasticity associated with multiple sclerosis or spinal cord lesions

Orphan drug: Intrathecal: Treatment of intractable spasticity caused by spinal cord injury, multiple sclerosis, and other spinal disease (spinal ischemia or tumor, transverse myelitis, cervical spondylosis, degenerative myelopathy)

Unlabeled Use Intractable hiccups, intractable pain relief, bladder spasticity, trigeminal neuralgia, cerebral palsy, short-term treatment of spasticity in children with cerebral palsy, Huntington's chorea

Pregnancy Risk Factor C

Pregnancy Considerations Adverse events were observed in animal reproduction studies. Withdrawal symptoms in the neonate were noted in a case report following the maternal use of oral baclofen 20 mg 4 times/day throughout pregnancy (Ratnayaka, 2001). Plasma concentrations following administration of intrathecal baclofen are significantly less than those with oral doses; exposure to the fetus is expected to be limited (Morton, 2009).

Lactation Enters breast milk/not recommended

Contraindications Hypersensitivity to baclofen or any component of the formulation

Warnings/Precautions Use with caution in patients with seizure disorder or impaired renal function. **[U.S. Boxed Warning]: Avoid abrupt withdrawal of the drug; abrupt withdrawal of intrathecal baclofen has resulted in severe sequelae (hyperpyrexia, obtundation, rebound/exaggerated spasticity, muscle rigidity, and rhabdomyolysis), leading to organ failure and some fatalities.** Risk may be higher in patients with injuries at T-6 or above, history of baclofen withdrawal, or limited ability to communicate. May cause CNS depression, which may impair physical or mental abilities; patients must be cautioned about performing tasks which require mental alertness (eg, operating machinery or driving). Elderly are more sensitive to the effects of baclofen and are more likely to experience adverse CNS effects at higher doses.

Cases (most from pharmacy compounded preparations) of intrathecal mass formation at the implanted catheter tip have been reported; may lead to loss of clinical response, pain or new/worsening neurological effects. Neurosurgical evaluation and/or an appropriate imaging study should be considered if a mass is suspected.

Adverse Reactions

>10%:

Central nervous system: Drowsiness, vertigo, dizziness, psychiatric disturbances, insomnia, slurred speech, ataxia, hypotonia

Neuromuscular & skeletal: Weakness

1% to 10%:

Cardiovascular: Hypotension

Central nervous system: Fatigue, confusion, headache

Dermatologic: Rash

Gastrointestinal: Nausea, constipation

Genitourinary: Polyuria

<1% (Limited to important or life-threatening): Chest pain, dyspnea, dysuria, enuresis, hematuria, impotence, inability to ejaculate, nocturia, palpitation, syncope, urinary retention; withdrawal reactions have occurred with abrupt discontinuation (particularly severe with intrathecal use).

Drug Interactions

Metabolism/Transport Effects None known.

Avoid Concomitant Use There are no known interactions where it is recommended to avoid concomitant use.

Increased Effect/Toxicity

Baclofen may increase the levels/effects of: Alcohol (Ethyl); CNS Depressants; Methotrimeprazine; Selective Serotonin Reuptake Inhibitors

The levels/effects of Baclofen may be increased by: Droperidol; HydrOXYzine; Methotrimeprazine

Decreased Effect There are no known significant interactions involving a decrease in effect.

Ethanol/Nutrition/Herb Interactions

Ethanol: May increase CNS depression; monitor for increased effects with coadministration. Caution patients about effects.

Herb/Nutraceutical: Avoid valerian, St John's wort, kava kava, gotu kola.

Mechanism of Action Inhibits the transmission of both monosynaptic and polysynaptic reflexes at the spinal cord level, possibly by hyperpolarization of primary afferent fiber terminals, with resultant relief of muscle spasticity

Pharmacodynamics/Kinetics

Onset of action: 3-4 days

Peak effect: 5-10 days

Absorption (dose dependent): Oral: Rapid

Protein binding: 30%

Metabolism: Hepatic (15% of dose)

Half-life elimination: 3.5 hours

Time to peak, serum: Oral: Within 2-3 hours

Excretion: Urine and feces (85% as unchanged drug)

Dosage

Oral (avoid abrupt withdrawal of drug):

Children (unlabeled use):

Spasticity: Caution: Pediatric dosing expressed as a daily amount, and **NOT** in mg/kg. Limited published data in children; the following is a compilation of small prospective studies (Albright, 1996; Milla, 1977; Scheinberg, 2006) and one large retrospective study (Lubsch, 2006):

<2 years: 10-20 mg daily divided every 8 hours; titrate dose every 3 days in increments of 5-15mg/day to a maximum of 40 mg daily

2-7 years: Initial: 20-30 mg daily divided every 8 hours; titrate dose every 3 days in increments of 5-15 mg/day to a maximum of 60 mg daily

≥8 years: 30-40 mg daily divided every 8 hours; titrate dose every 3 days in increments of 5-15 mg/day to a maximum of 120 mg daily

Note: Baclofen dose may need to be increased over time. One retrospective analysis (Lubsch, 2006) suggested that increased doses were needed as the time increased from spasticity onset, as age increased, and as the number of concomitant anti-spasticity medications increased. A small number of patients required daily doses exceeding 200 mg.

Spasticity in cerebral palsy (unlabeled use): Initial: 5-10 mg/day in 3 divided doses (Delgado, 2010)

Adults: 5 mg 3 times/day, may increase 5 mg/dose every 3 days to a maximum of 80 mg/day

Hiccups (unlabeled use): Usual effective dose: 10-20 mg 2-3 times/day

Intrathecal: Children and Adults:

Test dose: 50-100 mcg, doses >50 mcg should be given in 25 mcg increments, separated by 24 hours. A screening dose of 25 mcg may be considered in very small patients. Patients not responding to screening dose of 100 mcg should not be considered for chronic infusion/implanted pump.

Maintenance: After positive response to test dose, a maintenance intrathecal infusion can be administered via an implanted intrathecal pump. Initial dose via pump: Infusion at a 24-hour rate dosed at twice the test dose. Avoid abrupt discontinuation.

Elderly: Oral (the lowest effective dose is recommended): Initial: 5 mg 2-3 times/day, increasing gradually as needed; if benefits are not seen, withdraw the drug slowly.

Dosing adjustment in renal impairment: May be necessary to reduce dosage in renal impairment, but there are no specific guidelines available

Hemodialysis: Poor water solubility allows for accumulation during chronic hemodialysis. Low-dose therapy is recommended. There have been several case reports of accumulation of baclofen resulting in toxicity symptoms (organic brain syndrome, myoclonia, deceleration and steep potentials in EEG) in patients with renal failure who have received normal doses of baclofen.

Administration Intrathecal: For screening dosages, dilute with preservative-free sodium chloride to a final concentration of 50 mcg/mL for bolus injection into the subarachnoid space. For maintenance infusions, concentrations of 500-2000 mcg/mL may be used.

Test Interactions Increased alkaline phosphatase, AST, glucose, ammonia (B); decreased bilirubin (S)

Dosage Forms Excipient information presented when available (limited, particularly for generics); consult specific product labeling.

Injection, solution, intrathecal [preservative free]:

Gablofen®: 50 mcg/mL (1 mL); 500 mcg/mL (20 mL); 2000 mcg/mL (20 mL)

Lioresal®: 500 mcg/mL (20 mL); 2000 mcg/mL (5 mL, 20 mL)

Injection, solution, intrathecal [for screening, preservative free]:

Lioresal®: 50 mcg/mL (1 mL)

Tablet, oral: 10 mg, 20 mg

Extemporaneous Preparations A 5 mg/mL oral suspension may be made with tablets. Crush thirty 20 mg tablets in a mortar and reduce to a fine powder. Add a small amount of glycerin and mix to a uniform paste. Mix while adding Simple Syrup, NF in incremental proportions to **almost** 120 mL; transfer to a calibrated bottle, rinse mortar with vehicle, and add a sufficient quantity of vehicle to make 120 mL. Label "shake well" and "refrigerate". Stable for 35 days (Johnson, 1993).

A 10 mg/mL oral suspension may be made with tablets. Crush one-hundred-twenty 10 mg tablets in a mortar and reduce to a fine powder. Add small portions (60 mL) of a 1:1 mixture of Ora-Sweet® and Ora-Plus® and mix to a uniform paste; mix while adding the vehicle in incremental proportions to **almost** 120 mL; transfer to a calibrated bottle, rinse mortar with vehicle, and add quantity of vehicle sufficient to make 120 mL. Label "shake well" and "refrigerate". Stable for 60 days (Allen, 1996).

Allen LV Jr and Erickson MA 3rd, "Stability of Baclofen, Captopril, Diltiazem Hydrochloride, Dipyridamole, and Flecainide Acetate in Extemporaneously Compounded Oral Liquids," *Am J Health Syst Pharm*, 1996, 53(18):2179-84.

Johnson CE and Hart SM, "Stability of an Extemporaneously Compounded Baclofen Oral Liquid," *Am J Hosp Pharm*, 1993, 50 (11):2353-5.

◆ **Bactoshield® CHG [OTC]** *see* Chlorhexidine Gluconate *on page 341*

◆ **Bactrim™** *see* Sulfamethoxazole and Trimethoprim *on page 1602*

◆ **Bactrim™ DS** *see* Sulfamethoxazole and Trimethoprim *on page 1602*

◆ **Bactroban®** *see* Mupirocin *on page 1161*

◆ **Bactroban Cream®** *see* Mupirocin *on page 1161*

◆ **Bactroban Nasal®** *see* Mupirocin *on page 1161*

◆ **Baking Soda** *see* Sodium Bicarbonate *on page 1566*

◆ **BAL** *see* Dimercaprol *on page 513*

◆ **BAL in Oil®** *see* Dimercaprol *on page 513*

◆ **Balmex® [OTC]** *see* Zinc Oxide *on page 1817*

◆ **Balminil Decongestant (Can)** *see* Pseudoephedrine *on page 1430*

◆ **Balminil DM D (Can)** *see* Pseudoephedrine and Dextromethorphan *on page 1431*

◆ **Balminil DM + Decongestant + Expectorant (Can)** *see* Guaifenesin, Pseudoephedrine, and Dextromethorphan *on page 814*

◆ **Balminil DM E (Can)** *see* Guaifenesin and Dextromethorphan *on page 810*

◆ **Balminil Expectorant (Can)** *see* GuaiFENesin *on page 809*

Balsalazide (bal SAL a zide)

Brand Names: U.S. Colazal®

Index Terms Balsalazide Disodium

Pharmacologic Category 5-Aminosalicylic Acid Derivative; Anti-inflammatory Agent

Use Treatment of mildly- to moderately-active ulcerative colitis

Pregnancy Risk Factor B

Pregnancy Considerations Teratogenic effects were not observed in animal reproduction studies. Mesalamine (5-aminosalicylic acid) is the active metabolite of balsalazide; mesalamine is known to cross the placenta.

Lactation Excretion in breast milk unknown/use caution

Contraindications Hypersensitivity to balsalazide or its metabolites, salicylates, or any component of the formulation

Warnings/Precautions Pyloric stenosis may prolong gastric retention of balsalazide capsules. Renal toxicity and hepatic failure have been observed with other mesalamine (5-aminosalicylic acid) products; use with caution in patients with known renal or hepatic disease. Symptomatic worsening of ulcerative colitis may occur following initiation of treatment. May cause staining of teeth or tongue if capsule is opened and sprinkled on food. Safety and efficacy of use beyond 12 weeks in adults or 8 weeks in children has not been established.

Adverse Reactions

>10%:

Central nervous system: Headache (children 15%; adults 8%)

Gastrointestinal: Abdominal pain (children 12% to 13%; adults 6%)

1% to 10%:

Central nervous system: Insomnia (adults 2%), fatigue (children 4%; adults 2%), fever (children 6%; adults 2%)

Endocrine & metabolic: Dysmenorrhea (children 3%)

Gastrointestinal: Diarrhea (children 9%; adults 5%), ulcerative colitis exacerbation (children 6%; adults 1%), nausea (children 4%; adults 5%), vomiting (children 10%; adults 4%), hematochezia (children 4%), stomatitis (children 3%), anorexia (adults 2%), dyspepsia (adults 2%), flatulence (adults 2%), cramps (adults 1%), constipation (adults 1%), xerostomia (adults 1%)

Genitourinary: Urinary tract infection (adults 1%)

Neuromuscular & skeletal: Arthralgia (adults 4%), myalgia (adults 1%)

Respiratory: Respiratory infection (adults 4%), cough (children 3%; adults 2%), pharyngitis (children 6%; adults 2%), pharyngolaryngeal pain (children 3%), rhinitis (adults 2%)

Miscellaneous: Flu-like syndrome (children 4%; adults 1%)

<1% (Limited to important or life-threatening): Alopecia, alveolitis, cholestatic jaundice, cirrhosis, hepatocellular damage, hepatotoxicity, hypersensitivity, interstitial nephritis, jaundice, Kawasaki-like syndrome, liver failure, liver necrosis, liver function tests increased, myocarditis, pancreatitis, pericarditis, pleural effusion, pneumonia (with and without eosinophilia), pruritus, renal failure, vasculitis

Drug Interactions

Metabolism/Transport Effects None known.

Avoid Concomitant Use There are no known interactions where it is recommended to avoid concomitant use.

Increased Effect/Toxicity

Balsalazide may increase the levels/effects of: Heparin; Heparin (Low Molecular Weight); Thiopurine Analogs; Varicella Virus-Containing Vaccines

Decreased Effect

Balsalazide may decrease the levels/effects of: Cardiac Glycosides

Stability Store at controlled room temperature of 20°C to 25°C (68°F to 77°F); excursions permitted to 15°C to 30°C (59°F to 86°F).

Mechanism of Action Balsalazide is a prodrug, converted by bacterial azoreduction to 5-aminosalicylic acid (mesalamine, active), 4-aminobenzoyl-β-alanine (inert), and their metabolites. 5-aminosalicylic acid may decrease inflammation by blocking the production of arachidonic acid metabolites topically in the colon mucosa.

Pharmacodynamics/Kinetics

Onset of action: Delayed; may require several days to weeks

Absorption: Very low and variable

Protein binding: Balsalazide: ≥99%

Metabolism: Azoreduced in the colon to 5-aminosalicylic acid (active), 4-aminobenzoyl-β-alanine (inert), and N-acetylated metabolites

Half-life elimination: Primary effect is topical (colonic mucosa); systemic half-life not determined

Time to peak: Balsalazide: 1-2 hours

Excretion: Feces (65% as 5-aminosalicylic acid, 4-aminobenzoyl-β-alanine, and N-acetylated metabolites); urine (<16% as N-acetylated metabolites); Parent drug: Urine or feces (<1%)

Dosage Oral:

Children 5-17 years: 750 mg 3 times/day for up to 8 weeks **or** 2.25 g (three 750 mg capsules) 3 times/day for up to 8 weeks

Adults: 2.25 g (three 750 mg capsules) 3 times/day for up to 8-12 weeks

Elderly: Refer to adult dosing.

Dosage adjustment in renal impairment: No dosage adjustment provided in manufacturer's labeling. Renal toxicity has been observed with other 5-aminosalicylic acid products; use with caution.

Dosage adjustment in hepatic impairment: No dosage adjustment provided in manufacturer's labeling.

Dietary Considerations Some products may contain sodium.

Administration Capsules should be swallowed whole or may be opened and sprinkled on applesauce. Applesauce mixture may be chewed; swallow immediately, do not store mixture for later use. When sprinkled on food, may cause staining of teeth or tongue.

Monitoring Parameters Improvement or worsening of symptoms

Additional Information Balsalazide 750 mg is equivalent to mesalamine 267 mg

Dosage Forms Excipient information presented when available (limited, particularly for generics); consult specific product labeling.

Capsule, oral, as disodium: 750 mg

Colazal®: 750 mg [contains sodium ~86 mg/capsule]

- ◆ **Balsalazide Disodium** *see* Balsalazide *on page* 189
- ◆ **Balsam Peru, Castor Oil, and Trypsin** *see* Trypsin, Balsam Peru, and Castor Oil *on page* 1744
- ◆ **Balziva™** *see* Ethinyl Estradiol and Norethindrone *on page* 660
- ◆ **Band-Aid® Hurt Free™ Antiseptic Wash [OTC]** *see* Lidocaine (Topical) *on page* 1009
- ◆ **Banophen™ [OTC]** *see* DiphenhydrAMINE (Systemic) *on page* 516
- ◆ **Banzel®** *see* Rufinamide *on page* 1528
- ◆ **Banzel™ (Can)** *see* Rufinamide *on page* 1528
- ◆ **Baraclude®** *see* Entecavir *on page* 592
- ◆ **Baridium [OTC]** *see* Phenazopyridine *on page* 1337
- ◆ **Basaljel® (Can)** *see* Aluminum Hydroxide *on page* 79
- ◆ **Base Ointment** *see* Zinc Oxide *on page* 1817

Basiliximab (ba si LIK si mab)

Brand Names: U.S. Simulect®

Brand Names: Canada Simulect®

Pharmacologic Category Immunosuppressant Agent; Monoclonal Antibody

Use Prophylaxis of acute organ rejection in renal transplantation (in combination with cyclosporine and corticosteroids)

Unlabeled Use Treatment of refractory acute graft-versus-host disease (GVHD); prevention of liver or cardiac transplant rejection

Pregnancy Risk Factor B

Pregnancy Considerations Teratogenic effects were not observed in animal studies. IL-2 receptors play an important role in the development of the immune system. Use in pregnant women only when benefit exceeds potential risk to the fetus. Women of childbearing potential should use effective contraceptive measures before beginning treatment and for 4 months after completion of therapy with this agent. The National Transplantation Pregnancy Registry (NTPR, Temple University) is a registry for pregnant women taking immunosuppressants following any solid organ transplant. The NTPR encourages reporting of all immunosuppressant exposures during pregnancy in transplant recipients at 877-955-6877.

Lactation Excretion in breast milk unknown/not recommended

Contraindications Hypersensitivity to basiliximab or any component of the formulation

Warnings/Precautions To be used as a component of an immunosuppressive regimen which includes cyclosporine and corticosteroids. The incidence of lymphoproliferative disorders and/or opportunistic infections may be increased by immunosuppressive therapy. Severe hypersensitivity reactions, occurring within 24 hours, have been reported. Reactions, including anaphylaxis, have occurred both with the initial exposure and/or following re-exposure after several months. Use caution during re-exposure to a subsequent course of therapy in a patient who has previously received basiliximab; patients in whom concomitant immunosuppression was prematurely discontinued due to abandoned transplantation or early graft loss are at increased risk for developing a severe hypersensitivity reaction upon re-exposure. Discontinue permanently if a severe reaction occurs. Medications for the treatment of hypersensitivity reactions should be available for immediate use. Treatment may result in the development of human antimurine antibodies (HAMA); however, limited evidence suggesting the use of muromonab-CD3 or other murine products is not precluded. **[U.S. Boxed Warning]: Should be administered under the supervision of a physician experienced in immunosuppression therapy and organ transplant management.** In renal transplant patients receiving basiliximab plus prednisone, cyclosporine, and mycophenolate, new-onset diabetes, glucose intolerance, and impaired fasting glucose were observed at rates significantly higher than observed in patients receiving prednisone, cyclosporine, and mycophenolate without basiliximab (Aasebo, 2010).

Adverse Reactions Administration of basiliximab did not appear to increase the incidence or severity of adverse effects in clinical trials. Adverse events were reported in 96% of both the placebo and basiliximab groups.

>10%:

- Cardiovascular: Hypertension, peripheral edema
- Central nervous system: Fever, headache, insomnia, pain
- Dermatologic: Acne, wound complications
- Endocrine & metabolic: Hypercholesterolemia, hyperglycemia, hyper-/hypokalemia, hyperuricemia, hypophosphatemia
- Gastrointestinal: Abdominal pain, constipation, diarrhea, dyspepsia, nausea, vomiting
- Genitourinary: Urinary tract infection
- Hematologic: Anemia
- Neuromuscular & skeletal: Tremor
- Respiratory: Dyspnea, infection (upper respiratory)
- Miscellaneous: Viral infection

3% to 10%:

- Cardiovascular: Abnormal heart sounds, angina, arrhythmia, atrial fibrillation, chest pain, generalized edema, heart failure, hypotension, tachycardia
- Central nervous system: Agitation, anxiety, depression, dizziness, fatigue, hypoesthesia, malaise
- Dermatologic: Cyst, hypertrichosis, pruritus, rash, skin disorder, skin ulceration
- Endocrine & metabolic: Acidosis, dehydration, diabetes mellitus, fluid overload, glucocorticoids increased, hyper-/hypocalcemia, hyperlipemia, hypertriglyceridemia, hypoglycemia, hypomagnesemia, hyponatremia, hypoproteinemia
- Gastrointestinal: Abdomen enlarged, esophagitis, flatulence, gastroenteritis, GI hemorrhage, gingival hyperplasia, melena, moniliasis, stomatitis (including ulcerative), weight gain
- Genitourinary: Bladder disorder, dysuria, genital edema (male), impotence, ureteral disorder, urinary frequency, urinary retention
- Hematologic: Hematoma, hemorrhage, leukopenia, polycythemia, purpura, thrombocytopenia, thrombosis
- Neuromuscular & skeletal: Arthralgia, arthropathy, back pain, cramps, fracture, hernia, leg pain, myalgia, neuropathy, paresthesia, rigors, weakness
- Ocular: Abnormal vision, cataract, conjunctivitis
- Renal: Albuminuria, hematuria, nonprotein nitrogen increased, oliguria, renal function abnormal, renal tubular necrosis
- Respiratory: Bronchitis, bronchospasm, cough, pharyngitis, pneumonia, pulmonary edema, rhinitis, sinusitis
- Miscellaneous: Accidental trauma, cytomegalovirus (CMV) infection, herpes infection (simplex and zoster), infection, sepsis

Postmarketing and/or case reports: Anaphylaxis, capillary leak syndrome, cytokine release syndrome, diabetes (new onset), fasting glucose impaired, glucose intolerance, hypersensitivity reaction (including heart failure, hypotension, tachycardia, bronchospasm, dyspnea, pulmonary edema, respiratory failure, sneezing, pruritus, rash, urticaria), lymphoproliferative disease

Drug Interactions

Metabolism/Transport Effects None known.

Avoid Concomitant Use

Avoid concomitant use of Basiliximab with any of the following: BCG; Belimumab; Natalizumab; Pimecrolimus; Tacrolimus (Topical); Vaccines (Live)

Increased Effect/Toxicity

Basiliximab may increase the levels/effects of: Belimumab; Hypoglycemic Agents; Leflunomide; Natalizumab; Vaccines (Live)

The levels/effects of Basiliximab may be increased by: Abciximab; Denosumab; Herbs (Hypoglycemic Properties); Pimecrolimus; Roflumilast; Tacrolimus (Topical); Trastuzumab

Decreased Effect

Basiliximab may decrease the levels/effects of: BCG; Coccidioidin Skin Test; Sipuleucel-T; Vaccines (Inactivated); Vaccines (Live)

The levels/effects of Basiliximab may be decreased by: Echinacea

Ethanol/Nutrition/Herb Interactions Herb/Nutraceutical: Echinacea may diminish the therapeutic effect of basiliximab. Avoid hypoglycemic herbs, including alfalfa, bilberry, bitter melon, burdock, celery, damiana, fenugreek, garcinia, garlic, ginger, ginseng, gymnema, marshmallow, and stinging nettle (may enhance the hypoglycemic effect of basiliximab).

Stability Store intact vials refrigerated at 2°C to 8°C (36°F to 46°F). Reconstitute with preservative-free sterile water for injection (reconstitute 10 mg vial with 2.5 mL, 20 mg vial with 5 mL). Shake gently to dissolve. Should be used immediately after reconstitution; however, if not used immediately, reconstituted solution may be stored at 2°C to 8°C for up to 24 hours or at room temperature for up to 4 hours. Discard the reconstituted solution if not used within 24 hours. May further dilute reconstituted solution with 25 mL (10 mg) or 50 mL (20 mg) 0.9% sodium chloride or dextrose 5% in water. When mixing the solution, gently invert the bag to avoid foaming. Do not shake solutions diluted for infusion.

Mechanism of Action Chimeric (murine/human) immunosuppressant monoclonal antibody which blocks the alpha-chain of the interleukin-2 (IL-2) receptor complex; this receptor is expressed on activated T lymphocytes and is a critical pathway for activating cell-mediated allograft rejection

Pharmacodynamics/Kinetics

Duration: Mean: 36 days (determined by IL-2R alpha saturation)

Distribution: Mean: V_d: Children 1-11 years: 4.8 ± 2.1 L; Adolescents 12-16 years: 7.8 ± 5.1 L; Adults: 8.6 ± 4.1 L

Half-life elimination: Children 1-11 years: 9.5 days; Adolescents 12-16 years: 9.1 days; Adults: Mean: 7.2 days

Dosage Note: Patients previously administered basiliximab should only be re-exposed to a subsequent course of therapy with extreme caution.

I.V.:

Children <35 kg: Acute renal transplant rejection prophylaxis: 10 mg within 2 hours prior to transplant surgery, followed by a second 10 mg dose 4 days after transplantation; the second dose should be withheld if complications occur (including severe hypersensitivity reactions or graft loss)

Children ≥35 kg and Adults: Acute renal transplant rejection prophylaxis: 20 mg within 2 hours prior to transplant surgery, followed by a second 20 mg dose 4 days after transplantation; the second dose should be withheld if complications occur (including severe hypersensitivity reactions or graft loss)

Adults:

Acute cardiac transplant rejection prophylaxis (unlabeled use): 20 mg on the day of transplant, followed by a second dose 4 days after transplantation (Mehra, 2005); usually given within the first hour postoperatively

Acute liver transplant rejection prophylaxis (unlabeled use): 20 mg within 6 hours of organ reperfusion, followed by a second 20 mg dose 4 days after transplantation (Neuhaus, 2002)

Treatment of refractory acute GVHD (unlabeled use): 20 mg on days 1 and 4; may repeat for recurrent acute GVHD (Schmidt-Hieber, 2005)

Administration For intravenous administration only. Infuse as a bolus or I.V. infusion over 20-30 minutes. (Bolus dosing is associated with nausea, vomiting, and local pain at the injection site.) Administer only after assurance that patient will receive renal graft and immunosuppression. For the treatment of acute GVHD (unlabeled use), the dose was diluted in 250 mL NS and administered over 30 minutes (Schmidt-Hieber, 2005).

Monitoring Parameters Signs and symptoms of acute rejection; hypersensitivity, infection

Dosage Forms Excipient information presented when available (limited, particularly for generics); consult specific product labeling.

Injection, powder for reconstitution:

Simulect®: 10 mg [contains sucrose 10 mg/vial]

Simulect®: 20 mg [contains sucrose 20 mg/vial]

◆ **BAY 43-9006** *see* SORAfenib *on page 1584*

◆ **BAY 59-7939** *see* Rivaroxaban *on page 1507*

◆ **Baycadron™** *see* Dexamethasone (Systemic) *on page 480*

◆ **Bayer® Aspirin Extra Strength [OTC]** *see* Aspirin *on page 154*

◆ **Bayer® Aspirin Regimen Adult Low Strength [OTC]** *see* Aspirin *on page 154*

◆ **Bayer® Aspirin Regimen Children's [OTC]** *see* Aspirin *on page 154*

◆ **Bayer® Aspirin Regimen Regular Strength [OTC]** *see* Aspirin *on page 154*

◆ **Bayer® Genuine Aspirin [OTC]** *see* Aspirin *on page 154*

◆ **Bayer® Plus Extra Strength [OTC]** *see* Aspirin *on page 154*

◆ **Bayer® PM [OTC]** *see* Aspirin and Diphenhydramine *on page 157*

◆ **Bayer® Women's Low Dose Aspirin [OTC]** *see* Aspirin *on page 154*

◆ **BayGam® (Can)** *see* Immune Globulin *on page 880*

◆ **Baza® Antifungal [OTC]** *see* Miconazole (Topical) *on page 1126*

◆ **Baza® Clear [OTC]** *see* Vitamin A and Vitamin D *on page 1796*

◆ **β,β-Dimethylcysteine** *see* PenicillAMINE *on page 1319*

◆ **B-Caro-T™ [OTC]** *see* Beta-Carotene *on page 207*

BCG (bee see jee)

Brand Names: U.S. BCG Vaccine; TheraCys®; TICE® BCG

Brand Names: Canada ImmuCyst®; Oncotice™; Pacis™

Index Terms Bacillus Calmette-Guérin (BCG) Live; BCG Vaccine U.S.P. *(percutaneous use product)*; BCG, Live

Pharmacologic Category Biological Response Modulator; Vaccine, Live (Bacterial)

Use

BCG intravesical: Treatment and prophylaxis of carcinoma *in situ* of the bladder; prophylaxis of primary or recurrent superficial papillary tumors following transurethral resection

BCG vaccine: Immunization against *Mycobacterium tuberculosis* in persons not previously infected and who are at high risk for exposure

BCG vaccine is not routinely administered for the prevention of *M. tuberculosis* in the United States. The Advisory Committee on Immunization Practices (ACIP) recommends vaccination be considered for the following:

- Children with a negative tuberculin skin test who are continually exposed to (and cannot be separated from) adults who are untreated or ineffectively treated for TB disease when the child cannot be given long-term treatment for infection **or** if the adult has TB caused by strains resistant to isoniazid and rifampin.

- Healthcare workers with a high percentage of patients with *M. tuberculosis* strains resistant to both isoniazid and rifampin, if there is ongoing transmission of the resistant strains and subsequent infection is likely, or if comprehensive infection-control precautions have not been successful. In addition, healthcare workers should be counseled on the risks and benefits of vaccination and treatment of latent TB infection

Pregnancy Risk Factor C

Dosage

Immunization against tuberculosis: Percutaneous: **Note:** Initial lesion usually appears after 10-14 days consisting of small, red papule at injection site and reaches maximum diameter of 3 mm in 4-6 weeks.

Children <1 month: 0.2-0.3 mL (half-strength dilution). Administer tuberculin test (5 TU) after 2-3 months; repeat vaccination after 1 year of age for negative tuberculin test if indications persist.

Children >1 month and Adults: 0.2-0.3 mL (full strength dilution); conduct postvaccinal tuberculin test (5 TU of PPD) in 2-3 months; if test is negative, repeat vaccination.

Immunotherapy for bladder cancer: Intravesicular: Adults: **Note:** Treatment should begin 7-14 days after biopsy or TUR.

TheraCys®: One dose instilled into bladder (for 2 hours) once weekly for 6 weeks followed by 1 treatment at 3, 6, 12, 18, and 24 months after initial treatment

TICE® BCG: One dose instilled into the bladder (for 2 hours) once weekly for 6 weeks (may repeat cycle 1 time) followed by once monthly for 6-12 months

Additional Information Complete prescribing information for this medication should be consulted for additional detail.

Dosage Forms Excipient information presented when available (limited, particularly for generics); consult specific product labeling.

Injection, powder for reconstitution, intravesical:
TICE® BCG: 50 mg

Injection, powder for reconstitution, intravesical [preservative free]:
TheraCys®: 81 mg [contains natural rubber/natural latex in packaging, polysorbate 80 (in diluent); supplied with diluent]

Injection, powder for reconstitution, percutaneous:
BCG Vaccine: 50 mg

◆ **BCG, Live** *see* BCG *on page 191*

◆ **BCG Vaccine** *see* BCG *on page 191*

◆ **BCG Vaccine U.S.P.** ***(percutaneous use product)*** *see* BCG *on page 191*

◆ **BCNU** *see* Carmustine *on page 293*

◆ **beano® [OTC]** *see* Alpha-Galactosidase *on page 71*

◆ **beano® Meltaways [OTC]** *see* Alpha-Galactosidase *on page 71*

◆ **Bebulin® VH** *see* Factor IX Complex (Human) *on page 684*

Becaplermin (be KAP ler min)

Brand Names: U.S. Regranex®

Brand Names: Canada Regranex®

Index Terms Recombinant Human Platelet-Derived Growth Factor B; rPDGF-BB

Pharmacologic Category Growth Factor, Platelet-Derived; Topical Skin Product

Use Adjunctive treatment of diabetic neuropathic ulcers occurring on the lower limbs and feet that extend into subcutaneous tissue (or beyond) and have adequate blood supply

Pregnancy Risk Factor C

Dosage Topical: Adults: Diabetic ulcers: Apply appropriate amount of gel once daily with a cotton swab or similar tool, as a coating over the ulcer. The amount of becaplermin to be applied will vary depending on the size of the ulcer area.

Note: If the ulcer does not decrease in size by ~30% after 10 weeks of treatment or complete healing has not occurred in 20 weeks, continued treatment with becaplermin gel should be reassessed.

To calculate the length of gel applied to the ulcer, measure the greatest length of the ulcer by the greatest width of the ulcer. Tube size and unit of measure will determine the formula used in the calculation. Recalculate amount of gel needed every 1-2 weeks, depending on the rate of change in ulcer area.

Centimeters:

15 g tube: [ulcer length (cm) x width (cm)] divided by 4 = length of gel (cm)

2 g tube: [ulcer length (cm) x width (cm)] divided by 2 = length of gel (cm)

Inches:

15 g tube: [length (in) x width (in)] x 0.6 = length of gel (in)

2 g tube: [length (in) x width (in)] x 1.3 = length of gel (in)

Additional Information Complete prescribing information for this medication should be consulted for additional detail.

Dosage Forms Excipient information presented when available (limited, particularly for generics); consult specific product labeling. [DSC] = Discontinued product

Gel, topical:
Regranex®: 0.01% (2 g [DSC], 15 g)

Beclomethasone (Systemic)
(be kloe METH a sone)

Brand Names: U.S. QVAR®

Brand Names: Canada QVAR®; Vanceril® AEM

Index Terms Vancenase

Pharmacologic Category Corticosteroid, Inhalant (Oral)

Additional Appendix Information

Asthma *on page 1967*

Use Oral inhalation: Maintenance and prophylactic treatment of asthma; includes those who require corticosteroids and those who may benefit from a dose reduction/elimination of systemically-administered corticosteroids. Not for relief of acute bronchospasm.

Pregnancy Risk Factor C

Pregnancy Considerations Teratogenic effects were observed in animal studies. No human data on beclomethasone crossing the placenta or effects on the fetus. A decrease in fetal growth has not been observed with inhaled corticosteroid use during pregnancy. Inhaled corticosteroids are recommended for the treatment of asthma (most information available using budesonide) and allergic rhinitis during pregnancy.

Lactation Excretion in breast milk unknown/use caution

Contraindications Hypersensitivity to beclomethasone or any component of the formulation; status asthmaticus

Warnings/Precautions May cause hypercorticism or suppression of hypothalamic-pituitary-adrenal (HPA) axis, particularly in younger children or in patients receiving high doses for prolonged periods. HPA axis suppression may lead to adrenal crisis. Withdrawal and discontinuation of a corticosteroid should be done slowly and carefully. Particular care is required when patients are transferred from systemic corticosteroids to inhaled products due to possible adrenal insufficiency or withdrawal from steroids, including an increase in allergic symptoms. Patients receiving >20 mg per day of prednisone (or equivalent) may be most susceptible. Fatalities have occurred due to adrenal insufficiency in asthmatic patients during and after transfer from systemic corticosteroids to aerosol steroids; aerosol steroids do **not** provide the systemic steroid needed to treat patients having trauma, surgery, or infections.

Bronchospasm may occur with wheezing after inhalation; if this occurs, stop steroid and treat with a fast-acting bronchodilator. Supplemental steroids (oral or parenteral) may be needed during stress or severe asthma attacks. Not to be used in status asthmaticus or for the relief of acute bronchospasm. Corticosteroid use may cause psychiatric disturbances, including depression, euphoria, insomnia, mood swings, and personality changes. Pre-existing psychiatric conditions may be exacerbated by corticosteroid use. Prolonged use of corticosteroids may also increase the incidence of secondary infection, mask acute infection (including fungal infections), prolong or exacerbate viral infections, or limit response to vaccines. Exposure to chickenpox should be avoided; corticosteroids should not be used to treat ocular herpes simplex. Corticosteroids should not be used for cerebral malaria. Close observation is required in patients with latent tuberculosis and/or TB reactivity; restrict use in active TB (only in conjunction with antituberculosis treatment). Prolonged treatment with corticosteroids has been associated with the development of Kaposi's sarcoma (case reports); if noted, discontinuation of therapy should be considered.

Use with caution in patients with thyroid disease, hepatic impairment, renal impairment, cardiovascular disease, diabetes, glaucoma, cataracts, myasthenia gravis, patients at risk for osteoporosis, patients at risk for seizures, or GI diseases (diverticulitis, peptic ulcer, ulcerative colitis) due to perforation risk. Use caution following acute MI (corticosteroids have been associated with myocardial rupture). Because of the risk of adverse effects, systemic corticosteroids should be used cautiously in the elderly in the smallest possible effective dose for the shortest duration.

Orally-inhaled corticosteroids may cause a reduction in growth velocity in pediatric patients (~1 centimeter per year [range: 0.3-1.8 cm per year] and related to dose and duration of exposure). To minimize the systemic effects of orally-inhaled corticosteroids, each patient should be titrated to the lowest effective dose. Growth should be routinely monitored in pediatric patients. Safety and efficacy have not been established in children <5 years of age. There have been reports of systemic corticosteroid withdrawal symptoms (eg, joint/muscle pain, lassitude, depression) when withdrawing oral inhalation therapy.

Adverse Reactions Frequency not defined.

Central nervous system: Agitation, depression, dizziness, dysphonia, headache, lightheadedness, mental disturbances

Dermatologic: Acneiform lesions, angioedema, atrophy, bruising, pruritus, purpura, striae, rash, urticaria

Endocrine & metabolic: Cushingoid features, growth velocity reduction in children and adolescents, HPA function suppression

Gastrointestinal: Dry/irritated nose, throat and mouth, hoarseness, localized *Candida* or *Aspergillus* infection, loss of smell, loss of taste, nausea, unpleasant smell, unpleasant taste, vomiting, weight gain

Ocular: Cataracts, glaucoma, intraocular pressure increased

Respiratory: Cough, paradoxical bronchospasm, pharyngitis, sinusitis, wheezing

Miscellaneous: Anaphylactic/anaphylactoid reactions, death (due to adrenal insufficiency, reported during and after transfer from systemic corticosteroids to aerosol in asthmatic patients), immediate and delayed hypersensitivity reactions

Drug Interactions

Metabolism/Transport Effects None known.

Avoid Concomitant Use

Avoid concomitant use of Beclomethasone (Oral Inhalation) with any of the following: Aldesleukin; BCG; Natalizumab; Pimecrolimus; Tacrolimus (Topical)

Increased Effect/Toxicity

Beclomethasone (Oral Inhalation) may increase the levels/effects of: Amphotericin B; Deferasirox; Leflunomide; Loop Diuretics; Natalizumab; Thiazide Diuretics

The levels/effects of Beclomethasone (Oral Inhalation) may be increased by: Denosumab; Pimecrolimus; Tacrolimus (Topical); Telaprevir; Trastuzumab

Decreased Effect

Beclomethasone (Oral Inhalation) may decrease the levels/effects of: Aldesleukin; Antidiabetic Agents; BCG; Coccidioidin Skin Test; Corticorelin; Sipuleucel-T; Telaprevir; Vaccines (Inactivated)

The levels/effects of Beclomethasone (Oral Inhalation) may be decreased by: Echinacea

Stability Do not store near heat or open flame. Do not puncture canisters. Store at 25°C (77°F); excursions permitted between 15°C to 30°C (59°F to 86°F). Rest QVAR® on concave end of canister with actuator on top.

Mechanism of Action Controls the rate of protein synthesis; depresses the migration of polymorphonuclear leukocytes, fibroblasts; reverses capillary permeability and lysosomal stabilization at the cellular level to prevent or control inflammation

Pharmacodynamics/Kinetics

Onset of action: Therapeutic effect: 1-4 weeks

Absorption: Readily; quickly hydrolyzed by pulmonary esterases to active metabolite (beclomethasone-17-monoproprionate [17-BMP]) prior to absorption

Distribution: Beclomethasone dipropionate (BDP): 20 L; 17-BMP: 424 L

Protein binding: 17-BMP: 94% to 96%

Metabolism: Pro-drug; undergoes rapid conversion to 17-BMP during absorption; followed by additional metabolism via CYP3A4 to other, less active metabolites (beclomethasone-21-monopropionate [21-BMP] and beclomethasone [BOH])

Half-life elimination: BDP: 0.5 hours; 17-BMP: 3 hours

Time to peak, plasma: Oral inhalation: BDP: 0.5 hours; 17-BMP: 0.7 hours

Excretion: Feces (60%); urine (<10% to 12%)

Dosage Nasal inhalation and oral inhalation dosage forms are not to be used interchangeably.

Inhalation, oral: Asthma (doses should be titrated to the lowest effective dose once asthma is controlled) (QVAR®):

Children 5-11 years: Initial: 40 mcg twice daily; maximum dose: 80 mcg twice daily

Children ≥12 years and Adults:

Patients previously on bronchodilators only: Initial dose 40-80 mcg twice daily; maximum dose: 320 mcg twice day

Patients previously on inhaled corticosteroids: Initial dose 40-160 mcg twice daily; maximum dose: 320 mcg twice daily

NIH Asthma Guidelines (NIH, 2007): HFA formulation (eg, QVAR®): Administer in divided doses:

Children 5-11 years:

"Low" dose: 80-160 mcg/day

"Medium" dose: >160-320 mcg/day

"High" dose: >320 mcg/day

Children ≥12 years and Adults:

"Low" dose: 80-240 mcg/day

"Medium" dose: >240-480 mcg/day

"High" dose: >480 mcg/day

Administration QVAR®: Rinse mouth and throat after use to prevent *Candida* infection. Do not wash or put inhaler in water; mouth piece may be cleaned with a dry tissue or cloth. Prime canister before using.

Additional Information Effects of inhaled steroids on growth have been observed in the absence of laboratory evidence of HPA axis suppression, suggesting that growth velocity is a more sensitive indicator of systemic corticosteroid exposure in pediatric patients than some commonly used tests of HPA axis function. The long-term effects of this reduction in growth velocity associated with orally-inhaled corticosteroids, including the impact on final adult height, are unknown. The potential for "catch up" growth following discontinuation of treatment with inhaled corticosteroids has not been adequately studied.

Dosage Forms Excipient information presented when available (limited, particularly for generics); consult specific product labeling. [DSC] = Discontinued product

Aerosol, for oral inhalation, as dipropionate:

QVAR®: 40 mcg/inhalation (7.3 g [DSC]) [chlorofluorocarbon free; contains ethanol; 100 metered actuations]

QVAR®: 40 mcg/inhalation (8.7 g) [chlorofluorocarbon free; contains ethanol; 120 metered actuations]

QVAR®: 80 mcg/inhalation (7.3 g [DSC]) [chlorofluorocarbon free; contains ethanol; 100 metered actuations]

QVAR®: 80 mcg/inhalation (8.7 g) [chlorofluorocarbon free; contains ethanol; 120 metered actuations]

Beclomethasone (Nasal) (be kloe METH a sone)

Brand Names: U.S. Beconase AQ®

Brand Names: Canada Apo-Beclomethasone®; Gen-Beclo; Nu-Beclomethasone; Rivanase AQ

Index Terms Beclomethasone Dipropionate

Pharmacologic Category Corticosteroid, Nasal

Use Symptomatic treatment of seasonal or perennial rhinitis; prevent recurrence of nasal polyps following surgery.

Pregnancy Risk Factor C

Dosage Nasal inhalation and oral inhalation dosage forms are not to be used interchangeably.

Inhalation, nasal: Rhinitis, nasal polyps (Beconase® AQ): Children ≥6 years and Adults: 1-2 inhalations each nostril twice daily; total dose 168-336 mcg/day

Additional Information Complete prescribing information for this medication should be consulted for additional detail.

Dosage Forms Excipient information presented when available (limited, particularly for generics); consult specific product labeling.

Suspension, intranasal, as dipropionate [spray]:

Beconase AQ®: 42 mcg/inhalation (25 g) [contains benzalkonium chloride, ethanol 0.25%; 180 metered actuations]

◆ **Beclomethasone Dipropionate** *see* Beclomethasone (Nasal) *on page 194*

◆ **Beconase AQ®** *see* Beclomethasone (Nasal) *on page 194*

◆ **Behenyl Alcohol** *see* Docosanol *on page 537*

Belatacept (bel AT a sept)

Brand Names: U.S. Nulojix®

Index Terms BMS-224818; LEA29Y

Pharmacologic Category Selective T-Cell Costimulation Blocker

Use Prophylaxis of organ rejection concomitantly with basiliximab, mycophenolate, and corticosteroids in Epstein-Barr virus (EBV) seropositive kidney transplant recipients

Pregnancy Risk Factor C

Pregnancy Considerations Teratogenic effects were not observed in animal studies. There are no adequate and well-controlled studies in pregnant women. Due to the potential risk for development of autoimmune disease in the fetus, use during pregnancy only if clearly needed. A pregnancy registry has been established to monitor outcomes of women exposed to belatacept during pregnancy (1-877-955-6877).

Lactation Excretion in breast milk unknown/not recommended

Medication Guide Available Yes

Contraindications Transplant patients who are Epstein-Barr virus (EBV) seronegative or with unknown EBV status

Warnings/Precautions [U.S. Boxed Warning]: Risk of post-transplant lymphoproliferative disorder (PTLD) is increased, primarily involving the CNS, in patients receiving belatacept compared to patients receiving cyclosporine-based regimens. Degree of immunosuppression is a risk factor for PTLD developing; do not exceed recommended dosing. Patients who are Epstein-Barr virus seronegative (EBV) are at an even higher risk; use is contraindicated in patients without evidence of immunity to EBV. Therapy is only appropriate in patients who are EBV seropositive via evidence of acquired immunity, such as presence of IgG antibodies to viral capsid antigen [VCA] and EBV nuclear antigen [EBNA]. Cytomegalovirus (CMV) infection also increases the risk for PTLD; CMV prophylaxis is recommended for a minimum of 3 months following transplantation. Although CMV disease is a risk for PTLD and CMV seronegative patients are at an increased risk for CMV disease, the clinical role, if any, of determining CMV serology to determine risk of PTLD development has not been determined.

[U.S. Boxed Warning]: Risk for infection is increased. Immunosuppressive therapy may lead to opportunistic infections, sepsis, and/or fatal infections. Tuberculosis (TB) is increased; test patients for latent TB prior to initiation, and treat latent TB infection prior to use. Patients receiving immunosuppressive therapy are at an increased risk of activation of latent viral infections, including John Cunningham virus (JCV) and BK virus infection. Activation of JCV may result in progressive multifocal leukoencephalopathy (PML), a rare and potentially fatal condition affecting the CNS. Symptoms of PML include apathy, ataxia, cognitive deficiencies, confusion, and hemiparesis. Polyoma virus-associated nephropathy (PVAN), primarily from activation of BK virus, may also occur and lead to the deterioration of renal function and/or renal graft loss. Risk factors for the development of PML and PVAN include immunosuppression and treatment with immunosuppressant therapy. The onset of PML or PVAN may warrant a reduction in immunosuppressive therapy; however, in transplant recipients, the risk of reduced immunosuppression and graft rejection should be considered.

[U.S. Boxed Warning]: Risk for malignancy is increased. Malignancy, including skin malignancy and post-transplant lymphoproliferative disease, is associated with the use of immunosuppressants, including belatacept; higher than recommended doses or more frequent dosing is not recommended; patients should be advised to limit their exposure to sunlight/UV light.

[U.S. Boxed Warning]: Therapy is not recommended in liver transplant patients due to increased risk of graft loss and death. [U.S. Boxed Warning]: Should be administered under the supervision of a physician experienced in immunosuppressive therapy. Patients should not be immunized with attenuated or live viral vaccines during or shortly after treatment; safety of immunization following therapy has not been studied. The ENLiST registry has been created to further determine the safety of belatacept, particularly the incidence of PTLD and PML, in EBV seropositive kidney transplant patients. Transplant centers are encouraged to participate (1-800-321-1335).

Adverse Reactions Incidences reported occurred during clinical trials using belatacept compared to a cyclosporine control regimen. All patients also received basiliximab induction, mycophenolate mofetil, and corticosteroids, and were followed up to 3 years.

>10%:

Cardiovascular: Peripheral edema (34%), hypertension (32%), hypotension (18%)

Central nervous system: Fever (28%), headache (21%), insomnia (15%)

Endocrine & metabolic: Hypokalemia (21%), hyperkalemia (20%), hypophosphatemia (19%), dyslipidemia (19%), hyperglycemia (16%), hypocalcemia (13%), hypercholesterolemia (11%)

Gastrointestinal: Diarrhea (39%), constipation (33%), nausea (24%), vomiting (22%), abdominal pain (19%)

Genitourinary: Urinary tract infection (37%), dysuria (11%)

Hematologic: Anemia (45%), leukopenia (20%)

Neuromuscular & skeletal: Arthralgia (17%), back pain (13%)

Renal: Proteinuria (16%; up to 33% 2+ proteinuria at 1 month post-transplant), renal graft dysfunction (25%), hematuria (16%), serum creatinine increased (15%)

Respiratory: Cough (24%), upper respiratory infection (15%), nasopharyngitis (13%), dyspnea (12%)

Miscellaneous: Infection (72% to 82%; serious infection: 24% to 36%), herpes (7% to 14%), CMV (11% to 13%), influenza (11%)

1% to 10%:

Cardiovascular: Arteriovenous fistula thrombosis (<10%), atrial fibrillation (<10%)

Central nervous system: Anxiety (10%), dizziness (9%)

Dermatologic: Alopecia (<10%), hyperhidrosis (<10%), acne (8%)

Endocrine & metabolic: New-onset diabetes (5% to 8%), hypomagnesemia (7%), hyperuricemia (5%)

Gastrointestinal: Stomatitis (<10%), upper abdominal pain (9%)

Genitourinary: Urinary incontinence (<10%)

Hematologic: Hematoma (<10%), neutropenia (<10%)

Neuromuscular & skeletal: Musculoskeletal pain (<10%), tremor (8%)

Renal: Chronic allograft nephropathy (<10%), hydronephrosis (<10%), renal impairment (<10%), renal artery stenosis (<10%), renal tubular necrosis (9%)

Respiratory: Bronchitis (10%)

Miscellaneous: Guillain-Barré syndrome (<10%), lymphocele (<10%), infusion reactions (5%), malignancy (4%), polyoma virus (3% to 4%), antibelatacept antibody development (2%), nonmelanoma skin cancer (2%), tuberculosis (1% to 2%), BK virus-associated nephropathy (1%)

<1% (Limited to important or life-threatening): Cerebral aspergillosis (higher dosing regimen), Chagas encephalitis (higher dosing regimen), cryptococcal meningitis, post-transplant lymphoproliferative disorder (incidence is 9-fold higher in non-EBV seropositive patients), progressive multifocal leukoencephalopathy (higher dosing regimen), West Nile encephalitis (higher dosing regimen)

Drug Interactions

Metabolism/Transport Effects None known.

Avoid Concomitant Use

Avoid concomitant use of Belatacept with any of the following: BCG; Belimumab; Natalizumab; Pimecrolimus; Tacrolimus (Topical); Vaccines (Live)

Increased Effect/Toxicity

Belatacept may increase the levels/effects of: Belimumab; Leflunomide; Mycophenolate; Natalizumab; Vaccines (Live)

The levels/effects of Belatacept may be increased by: Denosumab; Pimecrolimus; Roflumilast; Tacrolimus (Topical); Trastuzumab

Decreased Effect

Belatacept may decrease the levels/effects of: BCG; Coccidioidin Skin Test; Sipuleucel-T; Vaccines (Inactivated); Vaccines (Live)

The levels/effects of Belatacept may be decreased by: Echinacea

Stability Prior to use, store refrigerated at 2°C to 8°C (36°F to 46°F). Protect from light. After dilution, the infusion solution (reconstituted solution must be further diluted immediately) may be stored refrigerated for up to 24 hours, with a maximum of 4 hours of the 24 hours at room temperature, 20°C to 25°C (68°F to 77°F), and room light. Infusion must be completed within 24 hours of reconstitution.

Reconstitute each vial with 10.5 mL of diluent (SWFI, NS, or D_5W) using the provided silicone-free disposable syringe, and an 18- to 21-gauge needle. Reconstituted using **only** the silicone-free syringe provided (discard if powder is inadvertently mixed using a siliconized syringe, translucent particles may develop). Inject the diluent down the side of the vial to avoid foaming. Rotate the vial and invert with gentle swirling until completely dissolved; do **not** shake vial. The reconstituted solution should be clear to slightly opalescent and colorless to pale yellow. Immediately transfer the reconstituted solution using the same silicone-free syringe to an infusion bag or bottle with NS or D_5W (if NS or D_5W were used to reconstitute, the same fluid should be used to further dilute). The final concentration should range from 2 mg/mL and 10 mg/mL (typical infusion volume is 100 mL). Prior to adding belatacept to the infusion solution, the manufacturer recommends withdrawing a volume equal to the amount of belatacept to be added. Mix gently; do not shake.

Mechanism of Action Fusion protein which acts as a selective T-cell (lymphocyte) costimulation blocker by binding to CD80 and CD86 receptors on antigen presenting cells (APC), blocking the required CD28 mediated interaction between APCs and T cells needed to activate T lymphocytes. T-cell stimulation results in cytokine production and proliferation, mediators in immunologic rejection associated with kidney transplantation.

Pharmacodynamics/Kinetics

Distribution: V_{ss}: 0.11 L/kg (transplant patients)

Half-life elimination: ~10 days (healthy patients and kidney transplant patients)

Dosage Note: Dosing is based on actual body weight at the time of transplantation; do not modify weight-based dosing during course of therapy unless the change in body weight is >10%. The prescribed dose must be evenly divisible by 12.5 mg to allow accurate preparation of the reconstituted solution using the provided required disposable syringe for preparation. For example, the calculated dose for a 64 kg patient: 64 kg x 10 mg per kg = 640 mg. The nearest doses to 640 mg that are evenly divisible by 12.5 mg would be 637.5 mg or 650 mg; the closest dose to the calculated dose is 637.5 mg, therefore, 637.5 should be the actual prescribed dose for the patient.

I.V.: Adults: Kidney transplant, prophylaxis of organ rejection:

Initial phase: 10 mg/kg/dose on Day 1 (day of transplant, prior to implantation) and on day 5 (~96 hours after Day 1 dose), followed by 10 mg/kg/dose given at the end of Week 2, Week 4, Week 8, and Week 12 following transplantation

Maintenance phase: 5 mg/kg/dose every 4 weeks (plus or minus 3 days) beginning at Week 16 following transplantation

Dosing adjustment in renal impairment: There are no dosage adjustments provided in manufacturer's labeling. Pharmacokinetic studies in kidney transplant patients indicated that renal function did not affect the clearance of belatacept.

Dosing adjustment in hepatic impairment: There are no dosage adjustments provided in manufacturer's labeling. Pharmacokinetic studies in kidney transplant patients indicated that hepatic function did not affect the clearance of belatacept.

Dietary Considerations Some products may contain sucrose.

Administration Administer as an I.V. infusion over 30 minutes using an infusion set with a 0.2-1.2 micron low protein-binding filter. Prior to administration, inspect visually and do not use if solution is discolored or contains particulate matter.

Monitoring Parameters New-onset or worsening neurological, cognitive, or behavioral signs/symptoms; signs/symptoms of infection; TB screening prior to therapy initiation; EBV seropositive verification prior to therapy initiation

Additional Information If additional silicone-free disposable syringes are needed, contact Bristol-Myers Squibb at 1-888-NULOJIX.

Dosage Forms Excipient information presented when available (limited, particularly for generics); consult specific product labeling.

Injection, powder for reconstitution:

Nulojix®: 250 mg [contains sucrose 500 mg/vial]

Belimumab (be LIM yoo mab)

Brand Names: U.S. Benlysta®

Brand Names: Canada Benlysta™

Pharmacologic Category Monoclonal Antibody

Use Treatment of autoantibody-positive (antinuclear antibody [ANA] and/or anti-double-stranded DNA [anti-ds-DNA]) systemic lupus erythematosus (SLE) in addition to standard therapy

Pregnancy Risk Factor C

Pregnancy Considerations Animal studies have not demonstrated teratogenic effects on the fetus but increased fetal and infant deaths have been observed. Reversible reductions in IgM were noted in infant monkeys. IgG molecules are known to cross the placenta (belimumab is an engineered IgG molecule). B-Cell lymphocytopenia lasting <3 months occurred in exposed infant animals. Effective contraception should be used during and for at least 4 months following treatment. Healthcare providers are encouraged to enroll women exposed to belimumab during pregnancy in a pregnancy registry (877-681-6296).

Lactation Excretion in breast milk unknown/not recommended

Medication Guide Available Yes

Contraindications Hypersensitivity to belimumab or any component of the formulation

Warnings/Precautions Hazardous agent - use appropriate precautions for handling and disposal. Deaths due to infection, cardiovascular disease, and suicide were higher in belimumab patients compared to placebo during clinical trials. Use is not recommended if severe active infection is present; consider discontinuing in patients who develop infections and initiate appropriate anti-infective treatment. Hypersensitivity and infusion reactions have been associated with use; discontinue for severe reactions (anaphylaxis, angioedema); infusion may be slowed or temporarily interrupted for minor reactions (headache, nausea, skin reactions). May increase risk of malignancy. May cause psychiatric adverse effects, including anxiety, insomnia, or new/worsening depression. Combined use with other immune modifying therapy or intravenous cyclophosphamide is not recommended. Live vaccines should not be given within 30 days or concurrently with belimumab. African-American patients may have a lower response rate. Has not been studied in patients with severe active lupus nephritis or CNS lupus; use not recommended.

Adverse Reactions

>10%: Gastrointestinal: Nausea (15%), diarrhea (12%)

≥3% to 10%:

Central nervous system: Fever (10%), insomnia (7%), migraine (5%), depression (5%), anxiety (4%)

Gastrointestinal: Viral gastroenteritis (3%)

Genitourinary: Cystitis (4%)

Hematologic: Leukopenia (4%)

Neuromuscular & skeletal: Pain in extremity (6%)

Respiratory: Bronchitis (9%), nasopharyngitis (9%), pharyngitis (5%)

<3% (Limited to important or life-threatening): Angioedema, antibody formation, bradycardia, cellulitis, dyspnea, eyelid edema, headache, hypersensitivity reactions, hypotension, influenza, myalgia, pneumonia, pruritus, upper respiratory infection, rash, sinusitis, urinary tract infection, urticaria

Drug Interactions

Metabolism/Transport Effects None known.

Avoid Concomitant Use

Avoid concomitant use of Belimumab with any of the following: Abatacept; Alefacept; BCG; Belatacept; Cyclophosphamide; Denileukin Diftitox; Etanercept; Monoclonal Antibodies; Natalizumab; Pimecrolimus; Tacrolimus (Topical); Vaccines (Live)

Increased Effect/Toxicity

Belimumab may increase the levels/effects of: Cyclophosphamide; Leflunomide; Natalizumab; Vaccines (Live)

The levels/effects of Belimumab may be increased by: Abatacept; Abciximab; Alefacept; Belatacept; Denileukin Diftitox; Denosumab; Etanercept; Monoclonal Antibodies; Pimecrolimus; Roflumilast; Tacrolimus (Topical); Trastuzumab

Decreased Effect

Belimumab may decrease the levels/effects of: BCG; Coccidioidin Skin Test; Sipuleucel-T; Vaccines (Inactivated); Vaccines (Live)

The levels/effects of Belimumab may be decreased by: Echinacea

Stability Prior to reconstitution, store unused vials between 2°C to 8°C (36°F to 46°F); do not freeze. Protect from light. To reconstitute, allow vial to reach room temperature. Reconstitute 120 mg vial with 1.5 mL of SWFI. Reconstitute 400 mg vial with 4.8 mL of SWFI. Gently swirl for 60 seconds every 5 minutes until powder has dissolved (usual reconstitution time is 10-15 minutes, but may take up to 30 minutes); do not shake. Further dilute reconstituted solution in 250 mL of 0.9% sodium chloride by first removing and discarding the volume equivalent to the volume of the reconstituted solution to be added to prepare the appropriate dose; add the appropriate volume of the reconstituted solution to the infusion container and invert to mix solution. Protect from light. Solution may be stored refrigerated or at room temperature. Storage time, including infusion to the patient, must be completed within 8 hours of reconstitution.

Mechanism of Action Belimumab is an IgG1-lambda monoclonal antibody that prevents the survival of B lymphocytes by blocking the binding of soluble human B lymphocyte stimulator protein (BLyS) to receptors on B lymphocytes. This reduces the activity of B-cell mediated immunity and the autoimmune response.

Pharmacodynamics/Kinetics

Onset of action: B cells: 8 weeks; Clinical improvement (SLE Responder Index and flare reduction): 16 weeks (Navarra, 2011)

Distribution: V_d: 5.29 L

Half-life elimination: 19.4 days

Dosage I.V.: Adults: Initial: 10 mg/kg every 2 weeks for 3 doses; Maintenance: 10 mg/kg every 4 weeks

Dosing adjustment in renal impairment: No dosage adjustment necessary for Cl_{cr} ≥15 mL/minute; has not been studied in Cl_{cr}<15 mL/minute

Dosing adjustment in hepatic impairment: Has not been studied

Administration Administer intravenously over 1 hour through a dedicated I.V. line. Do not give as an I.V. push or bolus. Discontinue infusion for severe hypersensitivity reaction (eg, anaphylaxis, angioedema). The infusion may be slowed or temporarily interrupted for minor reactions. Consider premedicating for prophylaxis against infusion reactions.

Monitoring Parameters Monitor for infusion reactions; worsening of depression, mood changes, or suicidal thoughts

Dosage Forms Excipient information presented when available (limited, particularly for generics); consult specific product labeling.

Injection, powder for reconstitution:

Benlysta®: 120 mg, 400 mg [contains polysorbate 80, sucrose 80 mg/mL]

◆ **Belladonna Alkaloids With Phenobarbital** *see* Hyoscyamine, Atropine, Scopolamine, and Phenobarbital *on page 855*

Belladonna and Opium (bel a DON a & OH pee um)

Index Terms B&O; Opium and Belladonna

Pharmacologic Category Analgesic Combination (Opioid); Antispasmodic Agent, Urinary

Use Relief of moderate-to-severe pain associated with ureteral spasms not responsive to nonopioid analgesics and to space intervals between injections of opiates

Pregnancy Risk Factor C

Dosage Rectal: Children >12 years and Adults: 1 suppository 1-2 times/day, up to 4 doses/day

Additional Information Complete prescribing information for this medication should be consulted for additional detail.

Dosage Forms Excipient information presented when available (limited, particularly for generics); consult specific product labeling.

Suppository: Belladonna extract 16.2 mg and opium 30 mg; belladonna extract 16.2 mg and opium 60 mg

Controlled Substance C-II

◆ **Benadryl® (Can)** *see* DiphenhydrAMINE (Systemic) *on page 516*

◆ **Benadryl-D® Allergy & Sinus [OTC]** *see* Diphenhydramine and Phenylephrine *on page 518*

◆ **Benadryl-D® Children's Allergy & Sinus [OTC]** *see* Diphenhydramine and Phenylephrine *on page 518*

◆ **Benadryl® Allergy [OTC]** *see* DiphenhydrAMINE (Systemic) *on page 516*

◆ **Benadryl® Allergy Quick Dissolve [OTC]** *see* DiphenhydrAMINE (Systemic) *on page 516*

◆ **Benadryl® Children's Allergy [OTC]** *see* DiphenhydrAMINE (Systemic) *on page 516*

◆ **Benadryl® Children's Allergy FastMelt® [OTC]** *see* DiphenhydrAMINE (Systemic) *on page 516*

◆ **Benadryl® Children's Allergy Perfect Measure™ [OTC]** *see* DiphenhydrAMINE (Systemic) *on page 516*

◆ **Benadryl® Children's Dye Free Allergy [OTC]** *see* DiphenhydrAMINE (Systemic) *on page 516*

◆ **Benadryl® Dye-Free Allergy [OTC]** *see* DiphenhydrAMINE (Systemic) *on page 516*

Benazepril (ben AY ze pril)

Brand Names: U.S. Lotensin®

Brand Names: Canada Lotensin®

Index Terms Benazepril Hydrochloride

Pharmacologic Category Angiotensin-Converting Enzyme (ACE) Inhibitor

Additional Appendix Information

Angiotensin Agents *on page 1869*

Use Treatment of hypertension, either alone or in combination with other antihypertensive agents

Pregnancy Risk Factor D

Pregnancy Considerations Due to adverse events observed in humans, benazepril is considered pregnancy category D. Benazepril crosses the placenta. First trimester exposure to ACE inhibitors may cause major congenital malformations. An increased risk of cardiovascular and/or central nervous system malformations was observed in one study; however, an increased risk of teratogenic events was not observed in other studies. Second and third trimester use of an ACE inhibitor is associated with oligohydramnios. Oligohydramnios due to decreased fetal renal function may lead to fetal limb contractures, craniofacial deformation, and hypoplastic lung development. The use of ACE inhibitors during the second and third trimesters is also associated with anuria, hypotension, renal failure (reversible or irreversible), skull hypoplasia, and death in the fetus/neonate. Chronic maternal hypertension itself is also associated with adverse events in the fetus/infant. ACE inhibitors are not recommended during pregnancy to treat maternal hypertension or heart failure. Those who are planning a pregnancy should be considered for other medication options if an ACE inhibitor is currently prescribed or the ACE inhibitor should be discontinued as soon as possible once pregnancy is detected. The exposed fetus should be monitored for fetal growth, amniotic fluid volume, and organ formation. Infants exposed to an ACE inhibitor *in utero*, especially during the second and third trimester, should be monitored for hyperkalemia, hypotension, and oliguria.

[U.S. Boxed Warning]: Based on human data, ACE inhibitors can cause injury and death to the developing fetus. ACE inhibitors should be discontinued as soon as possible once pregnancy is detected.

Lactation Enters breast milk

Contraindications Hypersensitivity to benazepril or any component of the formulation; patients with a history of angioedema (with or without prior ACE inhibitor therapy)

Warnings/Precautions Anaphylactic reactions may occur rarely with ACE inhibitors. At any time during treatment (especially following first dose) angioedema may occur rarely with ACE inhibitors. It may involve the head and neck (potentially compromising airway) or the intestine (presenting with abdominal pain). African-Americans and patients with idiopathic or hereditary angioedema may be at an increased risk. Prolonged frequent monitoring may be required especially if tongue, glottis, or larynx are involved as they are associated with airway obstruction. Patients with a history of airway surgery may have a higher risk of airway obstruction. Aggressive early and appropriate management is critical. Contraindicated in patients with history of angioedema with or without prior ACE inhibitor therapy. Hypersensitivity reactions may be seen during hemodialysis (eg, CVVHD) with high-flux dialysis membranes (eg, AN69), and rarely, during low density lipoprotein apheresis with dextran sulfate cellulose. Rare cases of anaphylactoid reactions have been reported in patients undergoing sensitization treatment with hymenoptera (bee, wasp) venom while receiving ACE inhibitors.

Symptomatic hypotension with or without syncope can occur with ACE inhibitors (usually with the first several doses); effects are most often observed in volume depleted patients; close monitoring of patient is required especially with initial dosing and dosing increases; blood pressure must be lowered at a rate appropriate for the patient's clinical condition. Initiation of therapy in patients with ischemic heart disease or cerebrovascular disease warrants close observation due to the potential consequences posed by falling blood pressure (eg, MI, stroke). **[U.S. Boxed Warning]: Based on human data, ACEIs can cause injury and death to the developing fetus when used in the second and third trimesters. ACEIs should be discontinued as soon as possible once pregnancy is detected.** Use with caution in hypertrophic cardiomyopathy with outflow tract obstruction, severe aortic stenosis, or before, during, or immediately after major surgery.

Hyperkalemia may occur with ACE inhibitors; risk factors include renal dysfunction, diabetes mellitus, concomitant use of potassium-sparing diuretics, potassium supplements and/or potassium containing salts. Use cautiously, if at all, with these agents and monitor potassium closely. Cough may occur with ACE inhibitors. Other causes of cough should be considered (eg, pulmonary congestion in patients with heart failure) and excluded prior to discontinuation. Use with caution in patients with diabetes receiving insulin or oral antidiabetic agents; may be at increased risk for episodes of hypoglycemia.

May be associated with deterioration of renal function and/or increases in serum creatinine, particularly in patients with low renal blood flow (eg, renal artery stenosis, heart failure) whose glomerular filtration rate (GFR) is dependent on efferent arteriolar vasoconstriction by angiotensin II; deterioration may result in oliguria, acute renal failure, and progressive azotemia. Small increases in serum creatinine may occur following initiation; consider discontinuation only in patients with progressive and/or significant deterioration in renal function. Use with caution in patients with unstented unilateral/bilateral renal artery stenosis. When unstented bilateral renal artery stenosis is present, use is generally avoided due to the elevated risk of deterioration in renal function unless possible benefits outweigh risks. Concurrent use of angiotensin receptor blockers may increase the risk of clinically-significant adverse events (eg, renal dysfunction, hyperkalemia).

Rare toxicities associated with ACE inhibitors include cholestatic jaundice (which may progress to fulminant hepatic necrosis), agranulocytosis, neutropenia, or leukopenia with myeloid hypoplasia. Patients with collagen vascular diseases (especially with concomitant renal impairment) or renal impairment alone may be at increased risk for hematologic toxicity; periodically monitor CBC with differential in these patients.

Adverse Reactions

1% to 10%:

Cardiovascular: Postural dizziness (2%)

Central nervous system: Headache (6%), dizziness (4%), somnolence (2%)

Renal: Serum creatinine increased (2%), worsening of renal function may occur in patients with bilateral renal artery stenosis or hypovolemia

Respiratory: Cough (1% to 10%)

<1% (Limited to important or life-threatening): Agranulocytosis, alopecia, anaphylactoid reaction, angina, angioedema (includes head, neck and intestinal angioedema), arthralgia, arthritis, asthma, BUN increased (transient), dermatitis, dyspnea, ECG changes, eosinophilia, flushing, gastritis, hemolytic anemia, hyperbilirubinemia, hyperglycemia, hyperkalemia, hypersensitivity, hypertonia, hyponatremia, hypotension, impotence, insomnia, leukopenia, myalgia, neutropenia, palpitations, pancreatitis, paresthesia, pemphigus, peripheral edema, photosensitivity, postural hypotension, proteinuria, pruritus, rash, shock, Stevens-Johnson syndrome, syncope, thrombocytopenia, transaminases increased, uric acid increased, vomiting

Eosinophilic pneumonitis, anaphylaxis, renal insufficiency, and renal failure have been reported with other ACE inhibitors. In addition, a syndrome including fever, myalgia, arthralgia, interstitial nephritis, vasculitis, rash, eosinophilia, and elevated ESR has been reported to be associated with ACE inhibitors.

Drug Interactions

Metabolism/Transport Effects None known.

Avoid Concomitant Use There are no known interactions where it is recommended to avoid concomitant use.

Increased Effect/Toxicity

Benazepril may increase the levels/effects of: Allopurinol; Amifostine; Antihypertensives; AzaTHIOprine; CycloSPORINE; CycloSPORINE (Systemic); Ferric Gluconate; Gold Sodium Thiomalate; Hypotensive Agents; Iron Dextran Complex; Lithium; Nonsteroidal Anti-Inflammatory Agents; RiTUXimab; Sodium Phosphates

The levels/effects of Benazepril may be increased by: Alfuzosin; Angiotensin II Receptor Blockers; Diazoxide; DPP-IV Inhibitors; Eplerenone; Everolimus; Herbs (Hypotensive Properties); Loop Diuretics; MAO Inhibitors; Pentoxifylline; Phosphodiesterase 5 Inhibitors; Potassium Salts; Potassium-Sparing Diuretics; Prostacyclin Analogues; Sirolimus; Temsirolimus; Thiazide Diuretics; TiZANidine; Tolvaptan; Trimethoprim

Decreased Effect

The levels/effects of Benazepril may be decreased by: Antacids; Aprotinin; Herbs (Hypertensive Properties); Icatibant; Lanthanum; Methylphenidate; Nonsteroidal Anti-Inflammatory Agents; Salicylates; Yohimbine

Ethanol/Nutrition/Herb Interactions Herb/Nutraceutical: Avoid bayberry, blue cohosh, cayenne, ephedra, ginger, ginseng (American), kola, licorice (may worsen hypertension). Avoid black cohosh, California poppy, coleus, golden seal, hawthorn, mistletoe, periwinkle, quinine, shepherd's purse (may have increased antihypertensive effect).

Stability Store at ≤30°C (86°F). Protect from moisture.

Mechanism of Action Competitive inhibition of angiotensin I being converted to angiotensin II, a potent vasoconstrictor, through the angiotensin I-converting enzyme (ACE) activity, with resultant lower levels of angiotensin II which causes an increase in plasma renin activity and a reduction in aldosterone secretion

Pharmacodynamics/Kinetics

Reduction in plasma angiotensin-converting enzyme (ACE) activity:

Onset of action: Peak effect: 1-2 hours after 2-20 mg dose

Duration: >90% inhibition for 24 hours after 5-20 mg dose

Reduction in blood pressure:

Peak effect: Single dose: 2-4 hours; Continuous therapy: 2 weeks

Absorption: Rapid (37%); food does not alter significantly; metabolite (benazeprilat) itself unsuitable for oral administration due to poor absorption
Distribution: V_d: ~8.7 L
Protein binding:
Benazepril: ~97%
Benazeprilat: ~95%
Metabolism: Rapidly and extensively hepatic to its active metabolite, benazeprilat, via enzymatic hydrolysis; extensive first-pass effect
Half-life elimination: Benazeprilat: Effective: 10-11 hours; Terminal: Children: 5 hours, Adults: 22 hours
Time to peak: Parent drug: 0.5-1 hour
Excretion:
Urine (trace amounts as benazepril; 20% as benazeprilat; 12% as other metabolites)
Clearance: Nonrenal clearance (ie, biliary, metabolic) appears to contribute to the elimination of benazeprilat (11% to 12%), particularly patients with severe renal impairment; hepatic clearance is the main elimination route of unchanged benazepril
Dialysis: ~6% of metabolite removed within 4 hours of dialysis following 10 mg of benazepril administered 2 hours prior to procedure; parent compound not found in dialysate

Dosage Oral: Hypertension:
Children ≥6 years: Initial: 0.2 mg/kg/day (up to 10 mg/day) as monotherapy; dosing range: 0.1-0.6 mg/kg/day (maximum dose: 40 mg/day)
Adults: Initial: 10 mg/day in patients not receiving a diuretic; 20-80 mg/day as a single dose or 2 divided doses; the need for twice-daily dosing should be assessed by monitoring peak (2-6 hours after dosing) and trough responses.
Note: Patients taking diuretics should have them discontinued 2-3 days prior to starting benazepril. If they cannot be discontinued, then initial dose should be 5 mg; restart after blood pressure is stabilized if needed.
Elderly: Oral: Initial: 5-10 mg/day in single or divided doses; usual range: 20-40 mg/day; adjust for renal function; also see **"Note"** in adult dosing.
Dosing interval in renal impairment: Cl_{cr} <30 mL/minute:
Children: Use is not recommended.
Adults: Administer 5 mg/day initially; maximum daily dose: 40 mg.
Hemodialysis: Moderately dialyzable (20% to 50%); administer dose postdialysis or administer 25% to 35% supplemental dose.
Peritoneal dialysis: Supplemental dose is not necessary.

Monitoring Parameters Blood pressure; serum creatinine and potassium; if patient has collagen vascular disease and/or renal impairment, periodically monitor CBC with differential

Dosage Forms Excipient information presented when available (limited, particularly for generics); consult specific product labeling. [DSC] = Discontinued product
Tablet, oral: 10 mg, 20 mg, 40 mg
Tablet, oral, as hydrochloride: 5 mg, 10 mg, 20 mg, 40 mg
Lotensin®: 5 mg [DSC], 10 mg, 20 mg, 40 mg

Extemporaneous Preparations A 2 mg/mL oral suspension may be made with tablets. Mix fifteen benazepril 20 mg tablets in an amber polyethylene terephthalate bottle with Ora-Plus® 75 mL. Shake for 2 minutes, allow suspension to stand for ≥1 hour, then shake again for at least 1 additional minute. Add Ora-Sweet® 75 mL to suspension and shake to disperse. Will make 150 mL of a 2 mg/mL suspension. Label "shake well" and "refrigerate". Stable for 30 days.

Lotensin® prescribing information, Novartis Pharmaceuticals Corporation, Suffern, NY, 2009.

Benazepril and Hydrochlorothiazide
(ben AY ze pril & hye droe klor oh THYE a zide)

Brand Names: U.S. Lotensin HCT®
Index Terms Benazepril Hydrochloride and Hydrochlorothiazide; Hydrochlorothiazide and Benazepril
Pharmacologic Category Angiotensin-Converting Enzyme (ACE) Inhibitor; Diuretic, Thiazide
Use Treatment of hypertension
Pregnancy Risk Factor D
Dosage Note: Not for initial therapy; dose should be individualized.
Oral: Range: Benazepril: 5-20 mg; Hydrochlorothiazide: 6.25-25 mg/day
Add-on therapy:
Patients not adequately controlled on benazepril monotherapy: Initiate benazepril 10-20 mg/hydrochlorothiazide 12.5 mg; titrate to effect at 2- to 3-week intervals
Patients controlled on hydrochlorothiazide 25 mg/day but experience significant potassium loss with this regimen: Initiate benazepril 5 mg/hydrochlorothiazide 6.25 mg
Replacement therapy: Substitute for the individually titrated components

Dosage adjustment in renal impairment: Cl_{cr} ≤30 mL/minute: Not recommended; loop diuretics are preferred.
Additional Information Complete prescribing information for this medication should be consulted for additional detail.
Dosage Forms Excipient information presented when available (limited, particularly for generics); consult specific product labeling.
Tablet: 5/6.25: Benazepril hydrochloride 5 mg and hydrochlorothiazide 6.25 mg; 10/12.5: Benazepril hydrochloride 10 mg and hydrochlorothiazide 12.5 mg; 20/12.5: Benazepril hydrochloride 20 mg and hydrochlorothiazide 12.5 mg; 20/25: Benazepril hydrochloride 20 mg and hydrochlorothiazide 25 mg
Lotensin HCT® 10/12.5: Benazepril hydrochloride 10 mg and hydrochlorothiazide 12.5 mg
Lotensin HCT® 20/12.5: Benazepril hydrochloride 20 mg and hydrochlorothiazide 12.5 mg
Lotensin HCT® 20/25: Benazepril hydrochloride 20 mg and hydrochlorothiazide 25 mg

◆ **Benazepril Hydrochloride** *see* Benazepril *on page 197*
◆ **Benazepril Hydrochloride and Amlodipine Besylate** *see* Amlodipine and Benazepril *on page 99*
◆ **Benazepril Hydrochloride and Hydrochlorothiazide** *see* Benazepril and Hydrochlorothiazide *on page 199*

Bendamustine (ben da MUS teen)

Brand Names: U.S. Treanda®
Index Terms Bendamustine Hydrochloride; Cytostasan; SDX-105
Pharmacologic Category Antineoplastic Agent; Antineoplastic Agent, Alkylating Agent; Antineoplastic Agent, Alkylating Agent (Nitrogen Mustard)
Use Treatment of chronic lymphocytic leukemia (CLL); treatment of progressed indolent B-cell non-Hodgkin's lymphoma (NHL)
Unlabeled Use Treatment of mantle cell lymphoma; salvage therapy for relapsed multiple myeloma; first-line therapy for follicular lymphoma; treatment of Waldenstrom's macroglobulinemia
Pregnancy Risk Factor D
Pregnancy Considerations Teratogenic and nonteratogenic events were observed in animal studies following intraperitoneal dosing. There are no adequate and well-controlled studies in pregnant women. May cause fetal

harm if administered during pregnancy. Effective contraception is recommended during and for 3 months after treatment for women and men of reproductive potential.

Lactation Excretion in breast milk unknown/not recommended

Contraindications Hypersensitivity to bendamustine, mannitol, or any component of the formulation

Warnings/Precautions Hazardous agent - use appropriate precautions for handling and disposal. Myelosuppression (neutropenia, thrombocytopenia, and anemia) is a common toxicity; may require therapy delay and/or dose reduction; monitor. Complications due to febrile neutropenia and severe thrombocytopenia have been reported. ANC should recover to ≥1000/mm^3 and platelets to ≥75,000/mm^3 prior to therapy/cycle initiation. Infections, including pneumonia and sepsis have been reported with use; may require hospitalization; septic shock and fatalities have occurred. Patients with myelosuppression are more susceptible to infection; monitor closely.

Infusion reactions, including chills, fever, pruritus, and rash are common; rarely, anaphylactic and anaphylactoid reactions have occurred, particularly with the second or subsequent cycle(s). In general, patients who experienced grade 3 or 4 allergic reactions were not rechallenged in CLL clinical trials. Consider premedication with antihistamines, antipyretics and/or corticosteroids for patients with a history of grade 1 or 2 infusion reaction. Discontinue for severe allergic reaction; consider discontinuation with grade 3 or 4 infusion reaction. Rash, toxic skin reactions and bullous exanthema have been reported with monotherapy and in combination with other antineoplastics; may be progressive or worsen with continued treatment; discontinue bendamustine treatment for severe or progressive skin reaction; monitor closely; discontinue bendamustine treatment for severe or progressive skin reaction. The risk for severe skin toxicity is increased with concurrent use of allopurinol and other medications known to cause skin toxicity; Stevens-Johnson syndrome and toxic epidermal necrolysis (TEN) have been reported. TEN has also been reported when used in combination with rituximab. Erythema, marked swelling, and pain have been reported with extravasation; monitor infusion site; avoid extravasation.

Tumor lysis syndrome may occur as a consequence of leukemia treatment, including treatment with bendamustine, usually occurring in the first treatment cycle. May lead to life threatening acute renal failure; adequate hydration and prophylactic allopurinol should be instituted prior to treatment in high-risk patients; monitor closely.

Use is not recommended in patients with moderate (AST or ALT 2.5-10 times ULN and total bilirubin 1.5-3 times ULN) or severe (total bilirubin >3 times ULN) hepatic impairment; use with caution in patients with mild hepatic impairment. Use is not recommended in patient with Cl_{cr} <40 mL/minute; use with caution in patients with mild-to-moderate renal impairment. Malignancies (including myelodysplastic syndrome, myeloproliferative disorders, acute myeloid leukemia and bronchial cancer) and premalignant diseases have been reported in patients who have received bendamustine. Safety and efficacy have not been established in children.

Adverse Reactions

>10%:

Cardiovascular: Peripheral edema (≤13%)

Central nervous system: Fatigue (9% to 57%), fever (24% to 34%), headache (≤21%), chills (6% to 14%), dizziness (≤14%), insomnia (≤13%)

Dermatologic: Rash (8% to 16%; grades 3/4: ≤3%)

Endocrine & metabolic: Dehydration (≤14%)

Gastrointestinal: Nausea (20% to 75%), vomiting (16% to 40%), diarrhea (9% to 37%), constipation (≤29%), anorexia (≤23%), weight loss (7% to 18%), stomatitis (≤15%), abdominal pain (5% to 13%), appetite loss (≤13%), dyspepsia (≤11%)

Hematologic: Myelosuppression (nadir: in week 3), lymphopenia (68% to 99%; grades 3/4: 47% to 94%), leukopenia (61% to 94%; grades 3/4: 28% to 56%), anemia (88% to 89%; grades 3/4: 11% to 13%), thrombocytopenia (77% to 86%; grades 3/4: 11% to 25%), neutropenia (75% to 86%; grades 3/4: 43% to 60%)

Hepatic: Bilirubin increased (≤34%; grades 3/4: 3%)

Neuromuscular & skeletal: Back pain (≤14%), weakness (8% to 11%)

Respiratory: Cough (4% to 22%), dyspnea (≤16%)

1% to 10%:

Cardiovascular: Tachycardia (≤7%), hypotension (≤6%), chest pain (≤6%), hypertension aggravated (≤3%)

Central nervous system: Anxiety (≤8%), depression (≤6%), pain (≤6%)

Dermatologic: Pruritus (5% to 6%), dry skin (≤5%)

Endocrine & metabolic: Hypokalemia (≤9%), hyperuricemia (≤7%; grades 3/4: 2%), hyperglycemia (grades 3/4: ≤3%), hypocalcemia (grades 3/4: ≤2%), hyponatremia (grades 3/4: ≤2%)

Gastrointestinal: Gastroesophageal reflux disease (≤10%), xerostomia (9%), taste alteration (≤7%), oral candidiasis (≤6%), abdominal distention (≤5%)

Genitourinary: Urinary tract infection (≤10%)

Hematologic: Febrile neutropenia (3% to 6%)

Hepatic: ALT increased (grades 3/4: ≤3%), AST increased (grades 3/4: ≤1%)

Local: Infusion site pain (≤6%), catheter site pain (≤5%)

Neuromuscular & skeletal: Arthralgia (≤6%), bone pain (≤5%), limb pain (≤5%)

Renal: Creatinine increased (grades 3/4: ≤2%)

Respiratory: Upper respiratory infection (10%), sinusitis (≤9%), pharyngolaryngeal pain (≤8%), pneumonia (≤8%), nasopharyngitis (6% to 7%), wheezing (≤5%), nasal congestion (≤5%)

Miscellaneous: Herpes infection (3% to 10%), infection (≤6%; grades 3/4: 2%), hypersensitivity (≤5%; grades 3/4: 1%), diaphoresis (≤5%), night sweats (≤5%)

<1% (Limited to important or life-threatening): Acute myeloid leukemia, acute renal failure, alopecia, anaphylaxis, bronchial carcinoma, bullous exanthema, cardiac failure, dermatitis, erythema, hemolysis, infusion reaction, injection/infusion site reaction (erythema, irritation, pain, phlebitis, pruritus, swelling), malaise, mucosal inflammation, myelodysplastic syndrome, myeloproliferative disorders, pulmonary fibrosis, sepsis, septic shock, skin necrosis, somnolence, Stevens-Johnson syndrome, toxic epidermal necrolysis, toxic skin reactions, tumor lysis syndrome

Drug Interactions

Metabolism/Transport Effects Substrate of BCRP, CYP1A2 (minor), P-glycoprotein; **Note:** Assignment of Major/Minor substrate status based on clinically relevant drug interaction potential

Avoid Concomitant Use

Avoid concomitant use of Bendamustine with any of the following: CloZAPine

Increased Effect/Toxicity

Bendamustine may increase the levels/effects of: CloZAPine

The levels/effects of Bendamustine may be increased by: CYP1A2 Inhibitors (Strong)

Decreased Effect

The levels/effects of Bendamustine may be decreased by: CYP1A2 Inducers (Strong); Cyproterone

Stability Prior to reconstitution, store intact vials up to 25°C (77°F); excursions permitted up to 30°C (86°F). Protect from light. Use appropriate precautions for handling and disposal. Reconstitute 25 mg vial with 5 mL and 100 mg vial with 20 mL of sterile water for injection to a concentration of 5 mg/mL; powder usually dissolves within 5 minutes. Prior to administration, dilute appropriate dose in 500 mL NS (or $D_{2.5}$1/2NS) to a final concentration of 0.2-0.6 mg/mL; mix thoroughly. The solution in the vial (reconstituted with SWFI) is stable for 30 minutes (transfer to 500 mL infusion bag within that 30 minutes). The solution diluted in 500 mL for infusion is stable for 24 hours refrigerated or 3 hours at room temperature and room light. Infusion must be completed within these time frames.

Mechanism of Action Bendamustine is an alkylating agent (nitrogen mustard derivative) with a benzimidazole ring (purine analog) which demonstrates only partial cross-resistance (*in vitro*) with other alkylating agents. It leads to cell death via single and double strand DNA cross-linking. Bendamustine is active against quiescent and dividing cells. The primary cytotoxic activity is due to bendamustine (as compared to metabolites).

Pharmacodynamics/Kinetics

Distribution: V_{ss}: ~25 L

Protein binding: 94% to 96%

Metabolism: Hepatic, via CYP1A2 to active (minor) metabolites gamma-hydroxy bendamustine (M3) and N-desmethyl-bendamustine (M4)

Half-life elimination: Bendamustine: ~40 minutes; M3: ~3 hours; M4: ~30 minutes

Time to peak, serum: At end of infusion

Excretion: Feces (~90%); urine (1% to 10%)

Dosage I.V.: Adults:

CLL: 100 mg/m^2 on days 1 and 2 of a 28-day treatment cycle for up to 6 cycles

NHL, refractory: 120 mg/m^2 on days 1 and 2 of a 21-day treatment cycle for up to 8 cycles

Follicular lymphoma, first-line (unlabeled use): 90 mg/m^2 days 1 and 2 of a 28-day treatment cycle in combination with rituximab for up to 6 cycles (Rummel, 2009)

Mantle cell lymphoma (unlabeled use): 90 mg/m^2 days 2 and 3 of a 28-day treatment cycle in combination with rituximab for up to 4 cycles (Rummel, 2005)

Multiple myeloma (unlabeled use): 90-100 mg/m^2 on days 1 and 2 of a 28-day treatment cycle for at least 2 cycles (Knop, 2005)

Dosage adjustment for toxicity:

Infusion reactions:

Grade 1 or 2: Consider premedication with antihistamines, antipyretics, and corticosteroids in subsequent cycles

Grade 3 or 4: Consider discontinuing treatment

Treatment delay:

Hematologic toxicity ≥grade 4: Delay treatment until resolves (ANC ≥1000/mm^3, platelets ≥75,000/mm^3)

Nonhematologic toxicity ≥grade 2 (clinically significant): Delay treatment until resolves to ≤grade 1

Dose modification in CLL:

Hematologic toxicity ≥grade 3: Reduce dose to 50 mg/m^2 on days 1 and 2 of each treatment cycle. For recurrent hematologic toxicity (≥grade 3), further reduce dose to 25 mg/m^2 on days 1 and 2 of the treatment cycle. May cautiously re-escalate dose in subsequent cycles.

Nonhematologic toxicity ≥grade 3 (clinically significant): Reduce dose to 50 mg/m^2 on days 1 and 2 of the treatment cycle with discretion. May cautiously re-escalate dose in subsequent cycles.

Dose modification in NHL:

Hematologic toxicity grade 4: Reduce dose to 90 mg/m^2 on days 1 and 2 of each treatment cycle. For recurrent hematologic toxicity (grade 4), further reduce dose to 60 mg/m^2 on days 1 and 2 of each treatment cycle.

Nonhematologic toxicity ≥grade 3: Reduce dose to 90 mg/m^2 on days 1 and 2 of the treatment cycle with discretion. For recurrent toxicity ≥grade 3, further reduce dose to 60 mg/m^2 on days 1 and 2 of each treatment cycle.

Dosage adjustment in renal impairment:

Mild-to-moderate renal impairment: Use with caution

Cl_{cr} <40 mL/minute: Use is not recommended

Dosage adjustment in hepatic impairment:

Mild hepatic impairment: Use with caution

Moderate hepatic impairment (AST or ALT 2.5-10 times ULN and total bilirubin 1.5-3 times ULN): Use is not recommended

Severe hepatic impairment (total bilirubin >3 times ULN): Use is not recommended

Administration Infuse over 30 minutes for the treatment of CLL and over 60 minutes for NHL. Prophylactic treatment with allopurinol may be needed in patients at risk for tumor lysis syndrome. Consider premedication with antihistamines, antipyretics, and/or corticosteroids for patients with a previous grade 1 or 2 infusion reaction to bendamustine. Avoid extravasation; monitor I.V. site for redness, swelling, or pain.

Monitoring Parameters CBC with differential (monitored weekly [initially] in clinical trials); serum creatinine (pretreatment); ALT, AST, and total bilirubin (pretreatment); monitor potassium and uric acid levels in patients at risk for tumor lysis syndrome; monitor for infusion reactions anaphylaxis, infection and dermatologic toxicity; monitor I.V. site during and after infusion

Dosage Forms Excipient information presented when available (limited, particularly for generics); consult specific product labeling.

Injection, powder for reconstitution:

Treanda®: 25 mg, 100 mg [contains mannitol]

- **Bendamustine Hydrochloride** *see* Bendamustine *on page 199*
- **Benefiber® [OTC]** *see* Wheat Dextrin *on page 1805*
- **Benefiber® Plus Calcium [OTC]** *see* Wheat Dextrin *on page 1805*
- **BeneFix®** *see* Factor IX *on page 683*
- **Benemid [DSC]** *see* Probenecid *on page 1407*
- **Benflumetol and Artemether** *see* Artemether and Lumefantrine *on page 148*
- **BenGay® [OTC]** *see* Methyl Salicylate and Menthol *on page 1113*
- **Benicar®** *see* Olmesartan *on page 1236*
- **Benicar HCT®** *see* Olmesartan and Hydrochlorothiazide *on page 1238*
- **Benlysta®** *see* Belimumab *on page 196*
- **Benlysta™ (Can)** *see* Belimumab *on page 196*
- **Benoxinate Hydrochloride and Fluorescein Sodium** *see* Fluorescein and Benoxinate *on page 728*

Bentoquatam (BEN toe kwa tam)

Brand Names: U.S. Ivy Block® [OTC]

Index Terms Quaternium-18 Bentonite

Pharmacologic Category Topical Skin Product

Use Skin protectant for the prevention of allergic contact dermatitis to poison oak, ivy, and sumac

Dosage Children >6 years and Adults: Topical: Apply to skin 15 minutes prior to potential exposure to poison ivy, poison oak, or poison sumac, and reapply every 4 hours

Additional Information Complete prescribing information for this medication should be consulted for additional detail.

Dosage Forms Excipient information presented when available (limited, particularly for generics); consult specific product labeling.

Lotion, topical:

Ivy Block®: 5% (120 mL) [contains benzyl alcohol, ethanol 25%]

- ◆ **Bentyl®** *see* Dicyclomine *on page 499*
- ◆ **Bentylol® (Can)** *see* Dicyclomine *on page 499*
- ◆ **Benuryl™ (Can)** *see* Probenecid *on page 1407*
- ◆ **Benylin® 3.3 mg-D-E (Can)** *see* Guaifenesin, Pseudoephedrine, and Codeine *on page 813*
- ◆ **Benylin® D for Infants (Can)** *see* Pseudoephedrine *on page 1430*
- ◆ **Benylin® DM-D (Can)** *see* Pseudoephedrine and Dextromethorphan *on page 1431*
- ◆ **Benylin® DM-D-E (Can)** *see* Guaifenesin, Pseudoephedrine, and Dextromethorphan *on page 814*
- ◆ **Benylin® DM-E (Can)** *see* Guaifenesin and Dextromethorphan *on page 810*
- ◆ **Benylin® E Extra Strength (Can)** *see* GuaiFENesin *on page 809*
- ◆ **Benzamycin®** *see* Erythromycin and Benzoyl Peroxide *on page 620*
- ◆ **Benzamycin® Pak** *see* Erythromycin and Benzoyl Peroxide *on page 620*
- ◆ **Benzathine Benzylpenicillin** *see* Penicillin G Benzathine *on page 1321*
- ◆ **Benzathine Penicillin G** *see* Penicillin G Benzathine *on page 1321*
- ◆ **Benzene Hexachloride** *see* Lindane *on page 1013*
- ◆ **Benzhexol Hydrochloride** *see* Trihexyphenidyl *on page 1738*
- ◆ **Benzmethyzin** *see* Procarbazine *on page 1410*

Benzocaine (BEN zoe kane)

Brand Names: U.S. Americaine® Hemorrhoidal [OTC]; Anbesol® Baby [OTC]; Anbesol® Cold Sore Therapy [OTC]; Anbesol® Jr. [OTC]; Anbesol® Maximum Strength [OTC]; Anbesol® [OTC]; Benzodent® [OTC]; Bi-Zets [OTC]; Boil-Ease® Pain Relieving [OTC]; Cepacol® Fizzlers™ [OTC]; Cepacol® Sore Throat & Coating [OTC]; Cepacol® Sore Throat Pain Relief [OTC] [DSC]; Cepacol® Sore Throat Plus Coating Relief [OTC]; Cepacol® Sore Throat [OTC]; Cepacol® Ultra Sore Throat [OTC]; Chiggerex® Plus [OTC]; ChiggerTox® [OTC]; Dent's Extra Strength Toothache Gum [OTC]; Dentapaine [OTC]; Dermoplast® Antibacterial [OTC]; Dermoplast® Pain Relieving [OTC]; Detane® [OTC]; Foille® [OTC]; HDA® Toothache [OTC]; Hurricaine® [OTC]; Ivy-Rid® [OTC]; Kank-A® Soft Brush [OTC]; Lanacane® Maximum Strength [OTC]; Lanacane® [OTC]; Little Teethers® [OTC]; Medicone® Hemorrhoidal [OTC]; Mycinettes® [OTC]; Orabase® with Benzocaine [OTC]; Orajel® Baby Daytime and Nighttime [OTC]; Orajel® Baby Teething Nighttime [OTC]; Orajel® Baby Teething [OTC]; Orajel® Cold Sore [OTC]; Orajel® Denture Plus [OTC]; Orajel® Maximum Strength [OTC]; Orajel® Medicated Mouth Sore [OTC]; Orajel® Medicated Toothache [OTC]; Orajel® Mouth Sore [OTC]; Orajel® Multi-Action Cold Sore [OTC]; Orajel® PM Maximum Strength [OTC]; Orajel® Ultra Mouth Sore [OTC]; Orajel® [OTC]; Outgro® [OTC]; Red Cross™ Canker Sore [OTC]; Rid-A-Pain Dental [OTC]; Sepasoothe® [OTC]; Skeeter Stik® [OTC]; Sore Throat Relief [OTC]; Sting-Kill® [OTC]; Tanac® [OTC]; Thorets [OTC]; Trocaine® [OTC]; Zilactin® Tooth & Gum Pain [OTC]; Zilactin®-B [OTC]

Brand Names: Canada Anbesol® Baby; Zilactin Baby®; Zilactin-B®

Index Terms Ethyl Aminobenzoate

Pharmacologic Category Local Anesthetic

Use Temporary relief of pain associated with pruritic dermatosis, pruritus, minor burns, acute congestive, bee stings, and insect bites; mouth and gum irritations (toothache, minor sore throat pain, canker sores, dentures, orthodontia, teething, mucositis, stomatitis); sunburn; hemorrhoids; anesthetic lubricant for passage of catheters and endoscopic tubes

Pregnancy Risk Factor C

Pregnancy Considerations Reproduction studies have not been conducted.

Lactation Excretion in breast milk unknown/use caution

Contraindications Hypersensitivity to benzocaine, other ester-type local anesthetics, or any component of the formulation; secondary bacterial infection of area; ophthalmic use

Warnings/Precautions Methemoglobinemia has been reported following topical use, particularly with higher concentration (14% to 20%) spray formulations applied to the mouth or mucous membranes. When applied as a spray to the mouth or throat, multiple sprays (or sprays of longer than indicated duration) are not recommended. Use caution with breathing problems (asthma, bronchitis, emphysema, in smokers), inflamed/damaged mucosa, heart disease, and hemoglobin or enzyme abnormalities (glucose-6-phosphate dehydrogenase deficiency, hemoglobin-M disease, NADH-methemoglobin reductase deficiency, pyruvate-kinase deficiency). Alternatives to benzocaine sprays, such as topical lidocaine preparations, should be considered for patients at higher risk of this reaction. Due to the heightened risk of methemoglobinemia, not recommended for use in patients <2 years of age unless under the advice and supervision by a healthcare professional.

The classical clinical finding of methemoglobinemia is chocolate brown-colored arterial blood. However, suspected cases should be confirmed by co-oximetry, which yields a direct and accurate measure of methemoglobin levels. Standard pulse oximetry readings or arterial blood gas values are not reliable. Clinically significant methemoglobinemia requires immediate treatment.

When topical anesthetics are used prior to cosmetic or medical procedures, the lowest amount of anesthetic necessary for pain relief should be applied. High systemic levels and toxic effects (eg, methemoglobinemia, irregular heart beats, respiratory depression, seizures, death) have been reported in patients who (without supervision of a trained professional) have applied topical anesthetics in large amounts (or to large areas of the skin), left these products on for prolonged periods of time, or have used wraps/dressings to cover the skin following application.

When used for self-medication (OTC), notify healthcare provider if condition worsens or does not improve within the timeframe noted on the product labeling or if accompanied by additional symptoms (eg, swelling, rash, headache, nausea, vomiting, or fever). Do not use topical products on open wounds; avoid contact with the eyes.

Adverse Reactions Frequency not defined.

Hematologic: Methemoglobinemia

Local: Burning, contact dermatitis, edema, erythema, pruritus, rash, stinging, tenderness, urticaria

Miscellaneous: Hypersensitivity

Drug Interactions

Metabolism/Transport Effects None known.

Avoid Concomitant Use There are no known interactions where it is recommended to avoid concomitant use.

Increased Effect/Toxicity
Benzocaine may increase the levels/effects of: Prilocaine

Decreased Effect There are no known significant interactions involving a decrease in effect.

Mechanism of Action Ester local anesthetic blocks both the initiation and conduction of nerve impulses by decreasing the neuronal membrane's permeability to sodium ions, which results in inhibition of depolarization with resultant blockade of conduction

Pharmacodynamics/Kinetics
Absorption: Topical: Poor to intact skin; well absorbed from mucous membranes and traumatized skin
Metabolism: Hepatic (to a lesser extent) and plasma via hydrolysis by cholinesterase
Excretion: Urine (as metabolites)

Dosage Note: These are general dosing guidelines; refer to specific product labeling for dosing instructions.

Children ≥4 months: Topical (oral): Teething pain: 7.5% to 10%: Apply to affected gum area up to 4 times daily
Children ≥2 years and Adults:
Topical:
Bee stings, insect bites, minor burns, sunburn: 5% to 20%: Apply to affected area 3-4 times daily as needed. In cases of bee stings, remove stinger before treatment.
Boils: 20%: Apply to affected area up to 2 times daily (maximum: 2 times/day)
Lubricant for passage of catheters and instruments: 20%: Apply evenly to exterior of instrument prior to use.
Topical (oral): Mouth and gum irritation: 10% to 20%: Apply thin layer to affected area up to 4 times daily
Children ≥5 years and Adults: Oral: Sore throat: Allow 1 lozenge (10-15 mg) to dissolve slowly in mouth; may repeat every 2 hours as needed
Children ≥6 years and Adults: Topical (oral) spray: 5%: Sore throat or mouth: One spray to affected area, then wait ≥1 minute and spit; may repeat up to 4 times daily. **Note:** Children 6-11 years should only use under adult supervision.
Children ≥12 years and Adults: Rectal: Hemorrhoids: 5% to 20%: Apply externally to affected area up to 6 times daily

Dietary Considerations Some products may contain sodium.

Administration Avoid application to large areas of broken skin, especially in children. When possible, apply to clean, dry area. When administering a spray formulation, the number of sprays administered and the length of each spray should be monitored and recorded.

Monitoring Parameters Monitor patients for signs and symptoms of methemoglobinemia such as pallor, cyanosis, nausea, muscle weakness, dizziness, confusion, agitation, dyspnea and tachycardia. The classical clinical finding of methemoglobinemia is chocolate brown-colored arterial blood. However, suspected cases should be confirmed by co-oximetry, which yields a direct and accurate measure of methemoglobin levels. Standard pulse oximetry readings or arterial blood gas values are not reliable. Clinically significant methemoglobinemia requires immediate treatment.

Dosage Forms Excipient information presented when available (limited, particularly for generics); consult specific product labeling. [DSC] = Discontinued product
Aerosol, spray, oral:
Hurricaine®: 20% (60 mL) [dye free; wild cherry flavor]
Aerosol, spray, topical:
Dermoplast® Antibacterial: 20% (82.5 mL) [contains aloe, benzethonium chloride, menthol]
Dermoplast® Pain Relieving: 20% (60 mL, 82.5 mL) [contains menthol]
Ivy-Rid®: 2% (85 g)
Lanacane® Maximum Strength: 20% (120 mL) [contains ethanol 36%]
Combination package, oral:
Orajel® Baby Daytime and Nighttime: gel, oral (Daytime Regular formula): benzocaine 7.5% (5.3 g) [1 tube] and gel, oral (Nighttime formula): benzocaine 10% (5.3 g) [1 tube]
Cream, oral:
Benzodent®: 20% (7.5 g, 30 g)
Orajel® PM Maximum Strength: 20% (5.3 g, 7 g) [contains menthol]
Cream, topical:
Lanacane®: 6% (28 g, 60 g)
Lanacane® Maximum Strength: 20% (28 g)
Gel, oral: 20% (15 g)
Anbesol®: 10% (7.1 g) [contains benzyl alcohol; cool mint flavor]
Anbesol® Baby: 7.5% (7.1 g) [contains benzoic acid; grape flavor]
Anbesol® Jr.: 10% (7.1 g) [contains benzyl alcohol; bubblegum flavor]
Anbesol® Maximum Strength: 20% (7.1 g, 10 g) [contains benzyl alcohol]
Dentapaine: 20% (11 g) [contains clove oil]
HDA® Toothache: 6.5% (15 mL) [contains benzyl alcohol]
Hurricaine®: 20% (30 g) [dye free; fresh mint flavor]
Hurricaine®: 20% (30 g) [dye free; pina colada flavor]
Hurricaine®: 20% (30 g) [dye free; watermelon flavor]
Hurricaine®: 20% (5.25 g, 30 g) [dye free; wild cherry flavor]
Kank-A® Soft Brush: 20% (2 g)
Little Teethers®: 7.5% (9.4 g) [cherry flavor]
Orabase® with Benzocaine: 20% (7 g) [contains ethanol 48%; fresh mint flavor]
Orajel®: 10% (5.3 g, 7 g, 9.4 g)
Orajel® Baby Teething: 7.5% (11.9 g); 7.5% (9.4 g) [cherry flavor]
Orajel® Baby Teething Nighttime: 10% (5.3 g)
Orajel® Denture Plus: 15% (9 g) [contains ethanol 66.7%, menthol]
Orajel® Maximum Strength: 20% (5.4 g, 7 g, 9.4 g, 11.9 g)
Orajel® Mouth Sore: 20% (5.3 g, 9.4 g, 11.9 g) [contains allantoin, benzalkonium chloride, zinc chloride]
Orajel® Multi-Action Cold Sore: 20% (9.4 g) [contains allantoin, camphor, dimethicone]
Orajel® Ultra Mouth Sore: 15% (9.4 g) [contains ethanol 66.7%, menthol]
Zilactin®-B: 10% (7.5 g)
Gel, topical:
Detane®: 7.5% (15 g)
Liquid, oral: 20% (15 mL)
Anbesol®: 10% (9.3 mL) [contains benzyl alcohol; cool mint flavor]
Anbesol® Maximum Strength: 20% (9.3 mL) [contains benzyl alcohol]
Hurricaine®: 20% (30 mL) [dye free; pina colada flavor]
Orajel® Baby Teething: 7.5% (13.3 mL) [very berry flavor]
Orajel® Maximum Strength: 20% (13.5 mL) [contains ethanol 44.2%, tartrazine]
Tanac®: 10% (13 mL) [contains benzalkonium chloride]
Liquid, oral [drops]:
Rid-A-Pain Dental: 6.3% (30 mL) [contains ethanol 70%]
Liquid, oral [spray]:
Cepacol® Ultra Sore Throat: 5% (22.2 mL) [sugar free; cherry flavor]
Liquid, topical:
ChiggerTox®: 2% (30 mL)
Outgro®: 20% (9.3 mL)
Skeeter Stik®: 5% (14 mL) [contains isopropyl alcohol, menthol]

Lozenge, oral: 6 mg (18s)
 Bi-Zets: 15 mg (10s)
 Cepacol® Sore Throat: 15 mg (16s) [contains cetylpyridinium, menthol; cherry flavor]
 Cepacol® Sore Throat: 15 mg (16s) [contains cetylpyridinium, menthol; honey-lemon flavor]
 Cepacol® Sore Throat: 15 mg (16s) [sugar free; contains cetylpyridinium, menthol; cherry flavor]
 Cepacol® Sore Throat & Coating: 15 mg (16s) [sugar free; contains cetylpyridinium, pectin; lemon-lime flavor]
 Cepacol® Sore Throat Pain Relief: 15 mg (18s [DSC]) [contains cetylpyridinium, menthol; cherry flavor]
 Cepacol® Sore Throat Pain Relief: 15 mg (18s [DSC]) [contains cetylpyridinium, menthol; citrus flavor]
 Cepacol® Sore Throat Pain Relief: 15 mg (18s [DSC]) [contains cetylpyridinium, menthol; honey-lemon flavor]
 Cepacol® Sore Throat Pain Relief: 15 mg (18s [DSC]) [contains cetylpyridinium, menthol; menthol flavor]
 Cepacol® Sore Throat Pain Relief: 15 mg (16s [DSC]) [sugar free; contains cetylpyridinium, menthol; cherry flavor]
 Cepacol® Sore Throat Plus Coating Relief: 15 mg (18s) [sugar free; contains cetylpyridinium, pectin; lemon-lime flavor]
 Mycinettes®: 15 mg (12s) [sugar free; contains sodium 9 mg/lozenge; cherry flavor]
 Mycinettes®: 15 mg (12s) [sugar free; contains sodium 9 mg/lozenge; regular flavor]
 Sepasoothe®: 10 mg (6s, 24s, 100s, 250s, 500s) [sugar free; contains cetylpyridinium 0.5 mg/lozenge; wild cherry flavor]
 Sore Throat Relief: 10 mg (100s, 250s, 500s) [sugar free]
 Thorets: 18 mg (300s) [sugar free]
 Trocaine®: 10 mg (50s, 300s) [cherry-menthol flavor]
Ointment, oral:
 Anbesol® Cold Sore Therapy: 20% (7.1 g) [contains allantoin, aloe, benzyl alcohol, camphor, menthol, vitamin E]
 Red Cross™ Canker Sore: 20% (7.5 g) [contains coconut oil]
Ointment, rectal:
 Americaine® Hemorrhoidal: 20% (30 g)
 Medicone® Hemorrhoidal: 20% (28.4 g)
Ointment, topical:
 Boil-Ease® Pain Relieving: 20% (30 g)
 Chiggerex® Plus: 6% (50 g) [contains aloe]
 Foille®: 5% (3.5 g, 14 g, 28 g) [contains benzyl alcohol, chloroxylenol, corn oil]
Pad, topical:
 Sting-Kill®: 20% (8s) [contains menthol, tartrazine]
Paste, oral:
 Orabase® with Benzocaine: 20% (6 g)
Solution, oral:
 Hurricaine®: 20% (30 mL) [dye free; wild cherry flavor]
Swab, oral:
 Hurricaine®: 20% (8s, 72s) [dye free; wild cherry flavor]
 Orajel® Baby Teething: 7.5% (12s) [berry flavor]
 Orajel® Cold Sore: 20% (12s) [contains tartrazine]
 Orajel® Medicated Mouth Sore: 20% (8s, 12s) [contains tartrazine]
 Orajel® Medicated Toothache: 20% (8s, 12s) [contains tartrazine]
 Zilactin® Tooth & Gum Pain: 20% (8s) [grape flavor]
Swab, topical:
 Boil-Ease® Pain Relieving: 20% (12s) [contains tartrazine]
 Sting-Kill®: 20% (5s) [contains menthol, tartrazine]
Tablet, orally dissolving, oral:
 Cepacol® Fizzlers™: 6 mg (12s) [grape flavor]
Wax, oral:
 Dent's Extra Strength Toothache Gum: 20% (1 g)

◆ **Benzocaine and Antipyrine** *see* Antipyrine and Benzocaine *on page* 130

Benzocaine, Butamben, and Tetracaine

(BEN zoe kane, byoo TAM ben, & TET ra kane)

Brand Names: U.S. Cetacaine®; Exactacain®

Index Terms Benzocaine, Butamben, and Tetracaine Hydrochloride; Benzocaine, Butyl Aminobenzoate, and Tetracaine; Butamben, Tetracaine, and Benzocaine; Tetracaine, Benzocaine, and Butamben

Pharmacologic Category Local Anesthetic

Use Topical anesthetic to control pain in surgical or endoscopic procedures; anesthetic for accessible mucous membranes except for the eyes

Dosage Topical anesthetic: **Note:** Decrease dose in the acutely-ill patient.

Children: Dose has not been established; dose reduction is suggested

Adults:
 Cetacaine®:
  Aerosol: Apply for ≤1 second; use of sprays >2 seconds is contraindicated
  Gel: Apply ~1/2 inch (13 mm) x 3/16 inch (5 mm); application of >1 inch (26 cm) x 3/16 inch (5 mm) is contraindicated
  Liquid: Apply 6-7 drops (0.2 mL); application of >12-14 drops (0.4 mL) is contraindicated
 Exactacain™: 3 metered sprays (use of >6 metered sprays is contraindicated)

Elderly: Dose reduction is suggested

Additional Information Complete prescribing information for this medication should be consulted for additional detail.

Dosage Forms Excipient information presented when available (limited, particularly for generics); consult specific product labeling.

Aerosol, spray, topical [kit]:
 Cetacaine®: Benzocaine 14%, butamben 2%, and tetracaine hydrochloride 2% (56 g) [delivers benzocaine 28 mg, butamben 4 mg, and tetracaine hydrochloride 4 mg per second; contains benzalkonium chloride, chlorofluorocarbon; packaged with cannula assortment]
Aerosol, spray, topical:
 Cetacaine®: Benzocaine 14%, butamben 2%, and tetracaine hydrochloride 2% (56 g) [delivers benzocaine 28 mg, butamben 4 mg, and tetracaine hydrochloride 4 mg per second; contains benzalkonium chloride, chlorofluorocarbon; packaged with cannula]
 Exactacain®: Benzocaine 14%, butamben 2%, and tetracaine hydrochloride 2% (60 g) [chlorofluorocarbon free; delivers benzocaine 9.3 mg, butamben 1.3 mg, and tetracaine hydrochloride 1.3 mg per metered spray; contains benzalkonium chloride; cherry flavor; packaged with 100 disposable applicators]
Gel, topical:
 Cetacaine®: Benzocaine 14%, butamben 2%, and tetracaine hydrochloride 2% (29 g [DSC]) [provides benzocaine 28 mg, butamben 4 mg and tetracaine hydrochloride 4 mg per 0.5 inch (13 mm) x 3/16 inch (5 mm) application; contains benzalkonium chloride]
 Cetacaine®: Benzocaine 14%, butamben 2%, and tetracaine hydrochloride 2% (32 g) [delivers benzocaine 28 mg, butamben 4 mg and tetracaine hydrochloride 4 mg per pump actuation ~0.25 inch (6.5 mm) x 0.5 inch (13 mm) long application; contains benzalkonium chloride]
Liquid, topical [kit]:
 Cetacaine®: Benzocaine 14%, butamben 2%, and tetracaine hydrochloride 2% (14 g) [provides benzocaine 28 mg, butamben 4 mg, and tetracaine hydrochloride 4 mg per 6-7 drops (0.2 mL); contains benzalkonium chloride; packaged with syringes and applicator tips]

Liquid, topical:

Cetacaine®: Benzocaine 14%, butamben 2%, and tetracaine hydrochloride 2% (14 g, 30 g) [provides benzocaine 28 mg, butamben 4 mg, and tetracaine hydrochloride 4 mg per 6-7 drops (0.2 mL); contains benzalkonium chloride]

- **Benzocaine, Butamben, and Tetracaine Hydrochloride** *see* Benzocaine, Butamben, and Tetracaine *on page 204*
- **Benzocaine, Butyl Aminobenzoate, and Tetracaine** *see* Benzocaine, Butamben, and Tetracaine *on page 204*
- **Benzodent® [OTC]** *see* Benzocaine *on page 202*
- **Benzoic Acid, Hyoscyamine, Methenamine, Methylene Blue, and Phenyl Salicylate** *see* Methenamine, Phenyl Salicylate, Methylene Blue, Benzoic Acid, and Hyoscyamine *on page 1094*
- **Benzoic Acid, Methenamine, Methylene Blue, Phenyl Salicylate, and Hyoscyamine** *see* Methenamine, Phenyl Salicylate, Methylene Blue, Benzoic Acid, and Hyoscyamine *on page 1094*

Benzonatate (ben ZOE na tate)

Brand Names: U.S. Tessalon®; Zonatuss™

Index Terms Tessalon Perles

Pharmacologic Category Antitussive

Use Symptomatic relief of nonproductive cough

Pregnancy Risk Factor C

Dosage Children >10 years and Adults: Oral: 100-200 mg 3 times/day as needed for cough; maximum dose: 600 mg/day

Additional Information Complete prescribing information for this medication should be consulted for additional detail.

Dosage Forms Excipient information presented when available (limited, particularly for generics); consult specific product labeling.

Capsule, oral:

Zonatuss™: 150 mg

Capsule, softgel, oral: 100 mg, 200 mg

Tessalon®: 100 mg, 200 mg

- **Benzoyl Peroxide and Adapalene** *see* Adapalene and Benzoyl Peroxide *on page 44*
- **Benzoyl Peroxide and Erythromycin** *see* Erythromycin and Benzoyl Peroxide *on page 620*

Benzoyl Peroxide and Hydrocortisone

(BEN zoe il peer OKS ide & hye droe KOR ti sone)

Brand Names: U.S. Vanoxide-HC®

Brand Names: Canada Vanoxide-HC®

Index Terms Hydrocortisone and Benzoyl Peroxide

Pharmacologic Category Acne Products; Topical Skin Product; Topical Skin Product, Acne

Use Treatment of acne vulgaris and oily skin

Pregnancy Risk Factor C

Dosage Adolescents ≥12 years and Adults: Topical: Apply thin film 1-3 times/day

Additional Information Complete prescribing information for this medication should be consulted for additional detail.

Dosage Forms Excipient information presented when available (limited, particularly for generics); consult specific product labeling.

Lotion, topical:

Vanoxide-HC®: Benzoyl peroxide 5% and hydrocortisone 0.5% (25 g)

Lotion, topical [kit]:

Vanoxide-HC®: Benzoyl peroxide 5% and hydrocortisone 0.5% (25 g) packaged with cleanser

Benztropine (BENZ troe peen)

Brand Names: U.S. Cogentin®

Brand Names: Canada Apo-Benztropine®

Index Terms Benztropine Mesylate

Pharmacologic Category Anti-Parkinson's Agent, Anticholinergic; Anticholinergic Agent

Additional Appendix Information

Antiparkinsonian Agents *on page 1879*

Use Adjunctive treatment of Parkinson's disease; treatment of drug-induced extrapyramidal symptoms (except tardive dyskinesia)

Pregnancy Risk Factor C

Pregnancy Considerations Animal reproduction studies have not been conducted. Paralytic ileus (which resolved rapidly) was reported in two newborns exposed to a combination of benztropine and chlorpromazine during the second and third trimesters and the last 6 weeks of pregnancy, respectively (Falterman, 1980).

Lactation Excretion in breast milk unknown/use caution

Contraindications Hypersensitivity to benztropine or any component of the formulation; pyloric or duodenal obstruction, stenosing peptic ulcers; bladder neck obstructions; achalasia; myasthenia gravis; children <3 years of age

Warnings/Precautions Use with caution in older children (dose has not been established). Use with caution in hot weather or during exercise. May cause anhydrosis and hyperthermia, which may be severe. The risk is increased in hot environments, particularly in the elderly, alcoholics, patients with CNS disease, and those with prolonged outdoor exposure.

Elderly patients frequently develop increased sensitivity and require strict dosage regulation - side effects may be more severe in elderly patients with atherosclerotic changes. Use with caution in patients with tachycardia, cardiac arrhythmias, hypertension, hypotension, glaucoma, prostatic hyperplasia (especially in the elderly), any tendency toward urinary retention, liver or kidney disorders, and obstructive disease of the GI or GU tract. When given in large doses or to susceptible patients, may cause weakness and inability to move particular muscle groups.

May be associated with confusion or hallucinations (generally at higher dosages). Intensification of symptoms or toxic psychosis may occur in patients with mental disorders. May cause CNS depression, which may impair physical or mental abilities; patients must be cautioned about performing tasks which require mental alertness (eg, operating machinery or driving). Benztropine does not relieve symptoms of tardive dyskinesia.

Adverse Reactions Frequency not defined.

Cardiovascular: Tachycardia

Central nervous system: Confusion, disorientation, memory impairment, toxic psychosis, visual hallucinations

Dermatologic: Rash

Endocrine & metabolic: Heat stroke, hyperthermia

Gastrointestinal: Constipation, dry throat, ileus, nasal dryness, nausea, vomiting, xerostomia

Genitourinary: Urinary retention, dysuria

Ocular: Blurred vision, mydriasis

Miscellaneous: Fever

Drug Interactions

Metabolism/Transport Effects Substrate of CYP2D6 (minor); **Note:** Assignment of Major/Minor substrate status based on clinically relevant drug interaction potential

Avoid Concomitant Use There are no known interactions where it is recommended to avoid concomitant use.

Increased Effect/Toxicity
Benztropine may increase the levels/effects of: AbobotulinumtoxinA; Anticholinergics; Cannabinoids; OnabotulinumtoxinA; Potassium Chloride; RimabotulinumtoxinB

The levels/effects of Benztropine may be increased by: Pramlintide

Decreased Effect
Benztropine may decrease the levels/effects of: Acetylcholinesterase Inhibitors (Central); Ioflupane I 123; Secretin

The levels/effects of Benztropine may be decreased by: Acetylcholinesterase Inhibitors (Central); Peginterferon Alfa-2b

Ethanol/Nutrition/Herb Interactions Ethanol: Avoid ethanol (may increase CNS depression).

Mechanism of Action Possesses both anticholinergic and antihistaminic effects. *In vitro* anticholinergic activity approximates that of atropine; *in vivo* it is only about half as active as atropine. Animal data suggest its antihistaminic activity and duration of action approach that of pyrilamine maleate. May also inhibit the reuptake and storage of dopamine, thereby prolonging the action of dopamine.

Pharmacodynamics/Kinetics
Onset of action: Oral: Within 1 hour; Parenteral: Within 15 minutes
Duration: 6-48 hours
Metabolism: Hepatic (N-oxidation, N-dealkylation, and ring hydroxylation)
Bioavailability: 29%

Dosage
Drug-induced extrapyramidal symptom: Oral, I.M., I.V.:
Children >3 years (unlabeled dose): 0.02-0.05 mg/kg/dose 1-2 times/day
Adults: 1-4 mg 1-2 times/day or 1-2 mg 2-3 times/day for reactions developing soon after initiation of antipsychotic medication; usually provides relief within 1-2 days, but may continue for up to 1-2 weeks; withdraw after 1-2 weeks to reassess continued need for therapy
Acute dystonia: Adults: I.M., I.V.: 1-2 mg
Parkinsonism, idiopathic or postencephalitic: Adults: Oral, I.M., I.V.: Usual dose: 1-2 mg/day; range: 0.5-6 mg/day in a single dose at bedtime or divided in 2-4 doses; titrate dose in 0.5 mg increments at 5- to 6-day intervals up to a maximum of 6 mg.
Elderly: Use caution or avoid; anticholinergics generally not tolerated in older adults.

Dietary Considerations Tablet may be taken with or without food.

Administration
Oral: May be given with or without food.
Injectable: May administer I.M or I.V. if oral route is unacceptable. Manufacturer's labeling states there is no difference in onset of effect after I.V. or I.M. injection and therefore there is usually no need to use the I.V. route. No specific instructions on administering benztropine I.V. are provided in the labeling. The I.V. route has been reported in the literature (slow I.V. push when reported), although specific instructions are lacking (Duncan, 2001; Lydon, 1998; Sachdev, 1993; Schramm, 2002).

Monitoring Parameters Symptoms of EPS or Parkinson's, pulse, anticholinergic effects

Dosage Forms Excipient information presented when available (limited, particularly for generics); consult specific product labeling.
Injection, solution, as mesylate: 1 mg/mL
Cogentin®: 1 mg/mL
Tablet, oral, as mesylate: 0.5 mg, 1 mg, 2 mg

◆ **Benztropine Mesylate** *see* Benztropine *on page 205*

Benzyl Alcohol (BEN zill AL koe hol)

Brand Names: U.S. Ulesfia®; Zilactin®-L [OTC]

Pharmacologic Category Analgesic, Topical; Antiparasitic Agent, Topical; Pediculocide; Topical Skin Product

Use
Liquid (Zilactin®-L): Temporary relief of pain from cold sores/fever blisters
Lotion (Ulesfia™): Treatment of head lice infestation

Pregnancy Risk Factor B

Dosage Topical:
Lotion: Head lice: Children ≥6 months and Adults: Apply appropriate volume for hair length to dry hair and completely saturate the scalp; leave on for 10 minutes; rinse thoroughly with water; repeat in 7 days
Hair length 0-2 inches: 4-6 ounces
Hair length 2-4 inches: 6-8 ounces
Hair length 4-8 inches: 8-12 ounces
Hair length 8-16 inches: 12-24 ounces
Hair length 16-22 inches: 24-32 ounces
Hair length >22 inches: 32-48 ounces
Liquid (topical): Cold sores/fever blisters: Children ≥2 years and Adults: Apply to affected area up to 4 times/day

Additional Information Complete prescribing information for this medication should be consulted for additional detail.

Dosage Forms Excipient information presented when available (limited, particularly for generics); consult specific product labeling.
Liquid, topical:
Zilactin®-L: 10% (5.9 mL) [contains ethanol 80%]
Lotion, topical:
Ulesfia®: 5% (227 g)

◆ **Benzylpenicillin Benzathine** *see* Penicillin G Benzathine *on page 1321*

◆ **Benzylpenicillin Potassium** *see* Penicillin G (Parenteral/Aqueous) *on page 1323*

◆ **Benzylpenicillin Sodium** *see* Penicillin G (Parenteral/Aqueous) *on page 1323*

Bepotastine (be poe TAS teen)

Brand Names: U.S. Bepreve®

Index Terms Bepotastine Besilate

Pharmacologic Category Histamine H_1 Antagonist; Histamine H_1 Antagonist, Second Generation; Mast Cell Stabilizer

Use Treatment of itching associated with allergic conjunctivitis

Pregnancy Risk Factor C

Dosage Ophthalmic: Children ≥2 years and Adults: Allergic conjunctivitis: Instill 1 drop into the affected eye(s) twice daily

Additional Information Complete prescribing information for this medication should be consulted for additional detail.

Dosage Forms Excipient information presented when available (limited, particularly for generics); consult specific product labeling.
Solution, ophthalmic, as besilate [drops]:
Bepreve®: 1.5% (5 mL, 10 mL) [contains benzalkonium chloride]

◆ **Bepotastine Besilate** *see* Bepotastine *on page 206*

◆ **Bepreve®** *see* Bepotastine *on page 206*

Beractant (ber AKT ant)

Brand Names: U.S. Survanta®

Brand Names: Canada Survanta®

Index Terms Bovine Lung Surfactant; Natural Lung Surfactant

Pharmacologic Category Lung Surfactant

Use Prevention and treatment of respiratory distress syndrome (RDS) in premature infants

Prophylactic therapy: Body weight <1250 g in infants at risk for developing, or with evidence of, surfactant deficiency (administer within 15 minutes of birth)

Rescue therapy: Treatment of infants with RDS confirmed by x-ray and requiring mechanical ventilation (administer as soon as possible - within 8 hours of age)

Contraindications There are no contraindications listed within the FDA-approved labeling

Warnings/Precautions For endotracheal administration only. Rapidly affects oxygenation and lung compliance; restrict use to a highly-supervised clinical setting with immediate availability of clinicians experienced in intubation and ventilatory management of premature infants. Transient episodes of bradycardia and decreased oxygen saturation occur. Discontinue dosing procedure and initiate measures to alleviate the condition; may reinstitute after the patient is stable. Produces rapid improvements in lung oxygenation and compliance that may require frequent adjustments to oxygen delivery and ventilator settings.

Adverse Reactions During the dosing procedure:

>10%: Cardiovascular: Transient bradycardia

1% to 10%: Respiratory: Oxygen desaturation

<1% (Limited to important or life-threatening): Apnea, endotracheal tube blockage, hypercarbia, hyper-/hypotension, post-treatment nosocomial sepsis probability increased, pulmonary air leaks, pulmonary interstitial emphysema, vasoconstriction

Drug Interactions

Metabolism/Transport Effects None known.

Avoid Concomitant Use There are no known interactions where it is recommended to avoid concomitant use.

Increased Effect/Toxicity There are no known significant interactions involving an increase in effect.

Decreased Effect There are no known significant interactions involving a decrease in effect.

Stability Refrigerate; protect from light. Prior to administration, warm by standing at room temperature for 20 minutes or held in hand for 8 minutes. **Artificial warming methods should not be used.** Unused, unopened vials warmed to room temperature may be returned to the refrigerator within 24 hours of warming only once.

Mechanism of Action Replaces deficient or ineffective endogenous lung surfactant in neonates with respiratory distress syndrome (RDS) or in neonates at risk of developing RDS. Surfactant prevents the alveoli from collapsing during expiration by lowering surface tension between air and alveolar surfaces.

Pharmacodynamics/Kinetics Excretion: Clearance: Alveolar clearance is rapid

Dosage

Endotracheal: Premature infants:

Prophylactic treatment: Administer 4 mL/kg (100 mg phospholipids/kg) as soon as possible; as many as 4 doses may be administered during the first 48 hours of life, no more frequently than 6 hours apart. The need for additional doses is determined by evidence of continuing respiratory distress; if the infant is still intubated and requiring at least 30% inspired oxygen to maintain a PaO_2 ≤80 torr.

Rescue treatment: Administer 4 mL/kg (100 mg phospholipids/kg) as soon as the diagnosis of RDS is made; may repeat if needed, no more frequently than every 6 hours to a maximum of 4 doses

Administration For endotracheal administration only

Suction infant prior to administration. Inspect solution to verify complete mixing of the suspension (may swirl gently, but DO NOT SHAKE). Do not filter dose and avoid shaking.

Administer endotracheally by instillation through a 5-French end-hole catheter inserted into the infant's endotracheal tube.

Administer the dose in four 1 mL/kg aliquots. Each quarter-dose is instilled over 2-3 seconds followed by at least 30 seconds of manual ventilation or until stable; each quarter-dose is administered with the infant in a different position. Slightly downward inclination with head turned to the right, then repeat with head turned to the left; then slightly upward inclination with head turned to the right, then repeat with head turned to the left. Following administration of one full dose, withhold suctioning for 1 hour unless signs of significant airway obstruction.

Monitoring Parameters Continuous ECG and transcutaneous O_2 saturation should be monitored during administration; frequent arterial blood gases are necessary to prevent postdosing hyperoxia and hypocarbia

Additional Information Each mL contains 25 mg phospholipids suspended in 0.9% sodium chloride solution. Contents of 1 mL: 0.5-1.75 mg triglycerides, 1.4-3.5 mg free fatty acids, and <1 mg protein.

Dosage Forms Excipient information presented when available (limited, particularly for generics); consult specific product labeling.

Suspension, intratracheal [bovine derived, preservative free]:

Survanta®: Phospholipids 25 mg/mL (4 mL, 8 mL)

◆ **Berinert®** *see* C1 Inhibitor (Human) *on page 257*

Besifloxacin (be si FLOX a sin)

Brand Names: U.S. Besivance™

Index Terms Besifloxacin Hydrochloride; BOL-303224-A; SS734

Pharmacologic Category Antibiotic, Ophthalmic; Antibiotic, Quinolone

Use Treatment of bacterial conjunctivitis

Pregnancy Risk Factor C

Dosage Ophthalmic: Children ≥1 year and Adults: Bacterial conjunctivitis: Instill 1 drop into affected eye(s) 3 times/day (4-12 hours apart) for 7 days

Additional Information Complete prescribing information for this medication should be consulted for additional detail.

Dosage Forms Excipient information presented when available (limited, particularly for generics); consult specific product labeling.

Suspension, ophthalmic [drops]:

Besivance™: 0.6% (5 mL) [contains benzalkonium chloride]

◆ **Besifloxacin Hydrochloride** *see* Besifloxacin *on page 207*

◆ **Besivance™** *see* Besifloxacin *on page 207*

◆ **9-Beta-D-Ribofuranosyladenine** *see* Adenosine *on page 46*

◆ **Betacaine® (Can)** *see* Lidocaine (Topical) *on page 1009*

Beta-Carotene (BAY ta KARE oh teen)

Brand Names: U.S. A-Caro-25 [OTC]; B-Caro-T™ [OTC]; Lumitene™ [OTC]

Pharmacologic Category Vitamin, Fat Soluble

Unlabeled Use Prophylaxis and treatment of polymorphous light eruption; prophylaxis against photosensitivity reactions in erythropoietic protoporphyria

Pregnancy Risk Factor C

Dosage Oral:

Children <14 years: 30-150 mg/day

Adults: 30-300 mg/day

Additional Information Complete prescribing information for this medication should be consulted for additional detail.

Dosage Forms Excipient information presented when available (limited, particularly for generics); consult specific product labeling.

Capsule, oral:

Lumitene™: 50,000 int. units [30 mg]

Capsule, softgel, oral: 10,000 int. units [6 mg], 25,000 int. units [15 mg]

A-Caro-25: 25,000 int. units [contains soy; 15 mg]

B-Caro-T™: 25,000 int. units [contains soybean lecithin, soybean oil; 15 mg]

Tablet, oral: 10,000 int. units [6 mg]

- **Betaderm (Can)** *see* Betamethasone *on page 208*
- **Betagan®** *see* Levobunolol *on page 995*
- **Beta-HC® [OTC]** *see* Hydrocortisone (Topical) *on page 841*

Betaine (BAY ta een)

Brand Names: U.S. Cystadane®

Brand Names: Canada Cystadane®

Index Terms Betaine Anhydrous

Pharmacologic Category Homocystinuria, Treatment Agent

Use Treatment of homocystinuria (eg, deficiencies or defects in cystathionine beta-synthase [CBS], 5,10-methylene tetrahydrofolate reductase [MTHFR], and cobalamin cofactor metabolism [CBL])

Pregnancy Risk Factor C

Prescribing and Access Restrictions Cystadane® may be obtained by contacting Accredo Health Group Inc at 1-888-454-8860.

Dosage Oral:

Children <3 years: Initial dose: 100 mg/kg/day administered in 2 divided doses; increase weekly by 50 mg/kg increments, as needed

Children ≥3 years and Adults: Usual dose: 6 g/day administered in divided doses of 3 g twice daily; dosages of up to 20 g/day have been necessary to control homocysteine levels in some patients

Note: Dosage in all patients can be gradually increased until plasma total homocysteine is undetectable or present only in small amounts. One study in six patients with CBS deficiency, ranging from 6-17 years of age, showed minimal benefit from exceeding a twice daily dosing schedule and a 150 mg/kg/day dosage.

Additional Information Complete prescribing information for this medication should be consulted for additional detail.

Dosage Forms Excipient information presented when available (limited, particularly for generics); consult specific product labeling.

Powder for solution, oral, as anhydrous:

Cystadane®: 1 g/scoop (180 g) [1 scoop = 1.7 mL]

- **Betaine Anhydrous** *see* Betaine *on page 208*
- **Betaject™ (Can)** *see* Betamethasone *on page 208*
- **Betaloc® (Can)** *see* Metoprolol *on page 1117*

Betamethasone (bay ta METH a sone)

Brand Names: U.S. Celestone®; Celestone® Soluspan®; Diprolene®; Diprolene® AF; Luxiq®

Brand Names: Canada Betaderm; Betaject™; Betnesol®; Betnovate®; Celestone® Soluspan®; Diprolene®; Diprolene® Glycol; Diprosone®; Ectosone; Prevex® B; ratio-Ectosone; ratio-Topilene; ratio-Topisone; Rivasone; Rolene; Rosone; Taro-Sone; Topilene®; Topisone®; Valisone® Scalp Lotion

Index Terms Betamethasone Dipropionate; Betamethasone Dipropionate, Augmented; Betamethasone Sodium Phosphate; Betamethasone Valerate; Flubenisolone

Pharmacologic Category Corticosteroid, Systemic; Corticosteroid, Topical

Additional Appendix Information

Corticosteroids *on page 1888*

Use Inflammatory dermatoses such as seborrheic or atopic dermatitis, neurodermatitis, anogenital pruritus, psoriasis, inflammatory phase of xerosis

Unlabeled Use Accelerate fetal lung maturation in patients with preterm labor

Pregnancy Risk Factor C

Pregnancy Considerations Adverse events have been observed with corticosteroids in animal reproduction studies. Betamethasone crosses the placenta; approximately 25% is metabolized by placental enzymes to an inactive metabolite. Due to its positive effect on stimulating fetal lung maturation, the injection is often used in patients with premature labor (24-34 weeks gestation). Topical products are not recommended for extensive use, in large quantities, or for long periods of time in pregnant women. Some studies have shown an association between first trimester systemic corticosteroid use and oral clefts; adverse events in the fetus/neonate have been noted in case reports following large doses of systemic corticosteroids during pregnancy. Women exposed to betamethasone during pregnancy for the treatment of an autoimmune disease may contact the OTIS Autoimmune Diseases Study at 877-311-8972.

Lactation Excretion in breast milk unknown/use caution

Contraindications Hypersensitivity to betamethasone, other corticosteroids, or any component of the formulation; systemic fungal infections; I.M. administration contraindicated in idiopathic thrombocytopenia purpura

Warnings/Precautions Very high potency topical products are not for treatment of rosacea, perioral dermatitis; not for use on face, groin, or axillae; not for use in a diapered area. Avoid concurrent use of other corticosteroids.

May cause hypercorticism or suppression of hypothalamic-pituitary-adrenal (HPA) axis, particularly in younger children or in patients receiving high doses for prolonged periods. HPA axis suppression may lead to adrenal crisis. Withdrawal and discontinuation of a corticosteroid should be done slowly and carefully. Particular care is required when patients are transferred from systemic corticosteroids to inhaled products due to possible adrenal insufficiency or withdrawal from steroids, including an increase in allergic symptoms. Patients receiving >20 mg per day of prednisone (or equivalent) may be most susceptible. Fatalities have occurred due to adrenal insufficiency in asthmatic patients during and after transfer from systemic corticosteroids to aerosol steroids; aerosol steroids do not provide the systemic steroid needed to treat patients having trauma, surgery, or infections. In stressful situations, HPA axis-suppressed patients should receive adequate supplementation with natural glucocorticoids (hydrocortisone or cortisone) rather than betamethasone (due to lack of mineralocorticoid activity).

Topical corticosteroids may be absorbed percutaneously. Absorption of topical corticosteroids may cause manifestations of Cushing's syndrome, hyperglycemia, or glycosuria. Absorption is increased by the use of occlusive dressings, application to denuded skin, or application to large surface areas.

Acute myopathy has been reported with high dose corticosteroids, usually in patients with neuromuscular transmission disorders; may involve ocular and/or respiratory muscles; monitor creatine kinase; recovery may be delayed. Corticosteroid use may cause psychiatric disturbances, including depression, euphoria, insomnia, mood swings, and personality changes. Pre-existing psychiatric conditions may be exacerbated by corticosteroid use. Prolonged use of corticosteroids may also increase the incidence of secondary infection, mask acute infection (including fungal infections), prolong or exacerbate viral infections, or limit response to vaccines. Exposure to chickenpox should be avoided; corticosteroids should not be used to treat ocular herpes simplex. Corticosteroids should not be used for cerebral malaria or viral hepatitis. Close observation is required in patients with latent tuberculosis and/or TB reactivity; restrict use in active TB (only in conjunction with antituberculosis treatment). Prolonged treatment with corticosteroids has been associated with the development of Kaposi's sarcoma (case reports); if noted, discontinuation of therapy should be considered. High-dose corticosteroids should not be used to manage acute head injury.

Use with caution in patients with thyroid disease, hepatic impairment, renal impairment, cardiovascular disease, diabetes, glaucoma, cataracts, myasthenia gravis, patients at risk for osteoporosis, patients at risk for seizures, or GI diseases (diverticulitis, peptic ulcer, ulcerative colitis) due to perforation risk. Use caution following acute MI (corticosteroids have been associated with myocardial rupture). Because of the risk of adverse effects, systemic corticosteroids should be used cautiously in the elderly in the smallest possible effective dose for the shortest duration. Discontinue if skin irritation or contact dermatitis should occur; do not use in patients with decreased skin circulation. Withdraw therapy with gradual tapering of dose.

Topical use in patients ≤12 years of age is not recommended. Children may absorb proportionally larger amounts after topical application and may be more prone to systemic effects. HPA axis suppression, intracranial hypertension, and Cushing's syndrome have been reported in children receiving topical corticosteroids. Prolonged use may affect growth velocity; growth should be routinely monitored in pediatric patients.

Adverse Reactions

Systemic:

Cardiovascular: Congestive heart failure, edema, hyper-/hypotension

Central nervous system: Dizziness, headache, insomnia, intracranial pressure increased, lightheadedness, nervousness, pseudotumor cerebri, seizure, vertigo

Dermatologic: Ecchymoses, facial erythema, fragile skin, hirsutism, hyper-/hypopigmentation, perioral dermatitis (oral), petechiae, striae, wound healing impaired

Endocrine & metabolic: Amenorrhea, Cushing's syndrome, diabetes mellitus, growth suppression, hyperglycemia, hypokalemia, menstrual irregularities, pituitary-adrenal axis suppression, protein catabolism, sodium retention, water retention

Gastrointestinal: Abdominal distention, appetite increased, hiccups, indigestion, peptic ulcer, pancreatitis, ulcerative esophagitis

Local: Injection site reactions (intra-articular use), sterile abscess

Neuromuscular & skeletal: Arthralgia, muscle atrophy, fractures, muscle weakness, myopathy, osteoporosis, necrosis (femoral and humeral heads)

Ocular: Cataracts, glaucoma, intraocular pressure increased

Miscellaneous: Anaphylactoid reaction, diaphoresis, hypersensitivity, secondary infection

Topical:

Dermatologic: Acneiform eruptions, allergic dermatitis, burning, dry skin, erythema, folliculitis, hypertrichosis, irritation, miliaria, pruritus, skin atrophy, striae, vesiculation

Endocrine and metabolic effects have occasionally been reported with topical use.

Drug Interactions

Metabolism/Transport Effects None known.

Avoid Concomitant Use

Avoid concomitant use of Betamethasone with any of the following: Aldesleukin; BCG; Natalizumab; Pimecrolimus; Tacrolimus (Topical)

Increased Effect/Toxicity

Betamethasone may increase the levels/effects of: Acetylcholinesterase Inhibitors; Amphotericin B; Deferasirox; Leflunomide; Loop Diuretics; Natalizumab; NSAID (COX-2 Inhibitor); NSAID (Nonselective); Thiazide Diuretics; Vaccines (Live); Warfarin

The levels/effects of Betamethasone may be increased by: Antifungal Agents (Azole Derivatives, Systemic); Aprepitant; Calcium Channel Blockers (Nondihydropyridine); Denosumab; Estrogen Derivatives; Fluconazole; Fosaprepitant; Indacaterol; Macrolide Antibiotics; Neuromuscular-Blocking Agents (Nondepolarizing); Pimecrolimus; Quinolone Antibiotics; Roflumilast; Salicylates; Tacrolimus (Topical); Telaprevir; Trastuzumab

Decreased Effect

Betamethasone may decrease the levels/effects of: Aldesleukin; Antidiabetic Agents; BCG; Calcitriol; Coccidioidin Skin Test; Corticorelin; Isoniazid; Salicylates; Sipuleucel-T; Telaprevir; Vaccines (Inactivated)

The levels/effects of Betamethasone may be decreased by: Aminoglutethimide; Antacids; Barbiturates; Bile Acid Sequestrants; Echinacea; Mitotane; Primidone; Rifamycin Derivatives

Ethanol/Nutrition/Herb Interactions

Ethanol: Avoid ethanol (may enhance gastric mucosal irritation).

Food: Betamethasone interferes with calcium absorption.

Herb/Nutraceutical: Avoid cat's claw, echinacea (have immunostimulant properties).

Mechanism of Action Controls the rate of protein synthesis; depresses the migration of polymorphonuclear leukocytes, fibroblasts; reverses capillary permeability and lysosomal stabilization at the cellular level to prevent or control inflammation

Pharmacodynamics/Kinetics

Protein binding: 64%

Metabolism: Hepatic

Half-life elimination: 6.5 hours

Time to peak, serum: I.V.: 10-36 minutes

Excretion: Urine (<5% as unchanged drug)

Dosage Base dosage on severity of disease and patient response

Children: Use lowest dose listed as initial dose for adrenocortical insufficiency (physiologic replacement)

I.M.: ≤12 years: 0.0175-0.125 mg base/kg/day divided every 6-12 hours **or** 0.5-7.5 mg base/m^2/day divided every 6-12 hours

Oral: ≤12 years: 0.0175-0.25 mg/kg/day divided every 6-8 hours **or** 0.5-7.5 mg/m^2/day divided every 6-8 hours ▶

Topical:
≤12 years: Use is not recommended.
≥13 years: Use minimal amount for shortest period of time to avoid HPA axis suppression
Gel, augmented formulation: Apply once or twice daily; rub in gently. **Note:** Do not exceed 2 weeks of treatment or 50 g/week.
Lotion: Apply a few drops twice daily
Augmented formulation: Apply a few drops once or twice daily; rub in gently. **Note:** Do not exceed 2 weeks of treatment or 50 mL/week.
Cream/ointment: Apply once or twice daily.
Augmented formulation: Apply once or twice daily. **Note:** Do not exceed 2 weeks of treatment or 45 g/week.
Adolescents and Adults:
Oral: 2.4-4.8 mg/day in 2-4 doses; range: 0.6-7.2 mg/day
I.M.: Betamethasone sodium phosphate and betamethasone acetate: 0.6-9 mg/day (generally, 1/3 to 1/2 of oral dose) divided every 12-24 hours
Adults:
Intrabursal, intra-articular, intradermal: 0.25-2 mL
Intralesional: Rheumatoid arthritis/osteoarthritis:
Very large joints: 1-2 mL
Large joints: 1 mL
Medium joints: 0.5-1 mL
Small joints: 0.25-0.5 mL
Topical:
Foam: Apply to the scalp twice daily, once in the morning and once at night
Gel, augmented formulation: Apply once or twice daily; rub in gently. **Note:** Do not exceed 2 weeks of treatment or 50 g/week.
Lotion: Apply a few drops twice daily
Augmented formulation: Apply a few drops once or twice daily; rub in gently. **Note:** Do not exceed 2 weeks of treatment or 50 mL/week.
Cream/ointment: Apply once or twice daily
Augmented formulation: Apply once or twice daily. **Note:** Do not exceed 2 weeks of treatment or 45 g/week.

Dosing adjustment in hepatic impairment: Adjustments may be necessary in patients with liver failure because betamethasone is extensively metabolized in the liver

Dietary Considerations May be taken with food to decrease GI distress.

Administration
Oral: Not for alternate day therapy; once daily doses should be given in the morning. May be administered with food to decrease GI distress.
I.M.: Do **not** give injectable sodium phosphate/acetate suspension I.V.
Topical: Apply topical sparingly to areas. Not for use on broken skin or in areas of infection. Do not apply to wet skin unless directed; do not cover with occlusive dressing. Do not apply very high potency agents to face, groin, axillae, or diaper area.
Foam: Invert can and dispense a small amount onto a saucer or other cool surface. Do not dispense directly into hands. Pick up small amounts of foam and gently massage into affected areas until foam disappears. Repeat until entire affected scalp area is treated.

Monitoring Parameters Growth in children

Test Interactions May suppress the wheal and flare reactions to skin test antigens

Additional Information
Very high potency: Augmented betamethasone dipropionate ointment, lotion
High potency: Augmented betamethasone dipropionate cream, betamethasone dipropionate cream and ointment
Intermediate potency: Betamethasone dipropionate lotion, betamethasone valerate cream

Dosage Forms Excipient information presented when available (limited, particularly for generics); consult specific product labeling. [DSC] = Discontinued product
Aerosol, foam, topical, as valerate:
Luxiq®: 0.12% (50 g, 100 g) [contains ethanol 60.4%]
Cream, topical, as dipropionate [strength expressed as base]: 0.05% (15 g, 45 g, 50 g)
Cream, topical, as dipropionate [strength expressed as base, augmented]: 0.05% (15 g, 50 g)
Diprolene® AF: 0.05% (15 g, 50 g)
Cream, topical, as valerate [strength expressed as base]: 0.1% (15 g, 45 g)
Gel, topical, as dipropionate [strength expressed as base, augmented]: 0.05% (15 g, 50 g)
Injection, suspension: Betamethasone sodium phosphate 3 mg and betamethasone acetate 3 mg per 1 mL (5 mL)
Celestone® Soluspan®: Betamethasone sodium phosphate 3 mg and betamethasone acetate 3 mg per 1 mL (5 mL) [contains benzalkonium chloride, edetate disodium; total of 6 mg/mL]
Lotion, topical, as dipropionate [strength expressed as base]: 0.05% (60 mL)
Lotion, topical, as dipropionate [strength expressed as base, augmented]: 0.05% (30 mL, 60 mL)
Diprolene®: 0.05% (30 mL, 60 mL) [contains isopropyl alcohol 30%]
Lotion, topical, as valerate [strength expressed as base]: 0.1% (60 mL)
Ointment, topical, as dipropionate [strength expressed as base]: 0.05% (15 g, 45 g)
Ointment, topical, as dipropionate [strength expressed as base, augmented]: 0.05% (15 g, 45 g, 50 g [DSC])
Diprolene®: 0.05% (15 g, 50 g)
Ointment, topical, as valerate [strength expressed as base]: 0.1% (15 g, 45 g)
Solution, oral, as base:
Celestone®: 0.6 mg/5 mL (118 mL) [contains ethanol <1%, propylene glycol, sodium benzoate]

Betamethasone and Clotrimazole

(bay ta METH a sone & kloe TRIM a zole)

Brand Names: U.S. Lotrisone®

Brand Names: Canada Lotriderm®

Index Terms Clotrimazole and Betamethasone

Pharmacologic Category Antifungal Agent, Topical; Corticosteroid, Topical

Use Topical treatment of various dermal fungal infections (including tinea pedis, cruris, and corpora in patients ≥17 years of age)

Pregnancy Risk Factor C

Dosage
Children <17 years: Do not use
Children ≥17 years and Adults:
Allergic or inflammatory diseases: Topical: Apply to affected area twice daily, morning and evening
Tinea corporis, tinea cruris: Topical: Massage into affected area twice daily, morning and evening; do not use for longer than 2 weeks; re-evaluate after 1 week if no clinical improvement; do not exceed 45 g cream/week or 45 mL lotion/week
Tinea pedis: Topical: Massage into affected area twice daily, morning and evening; do not use for longer than 4 weeks; re-evaluate after 2 weeks if no clinical improvement; do not exceed 45 g cream/week or 45 mL lotion/week
Elderly: Use with caution; skin atrophy and skin ulceration (rare) have been reported in patients with thinning skin; do not use for diaper dermatitis or under occlusive dressings

Additional Information Complete prescribing information for this medication should be consulted for additional detail.

Dosage Forms Excipient information presented when available (limited, particularly for generics); consult specific product labeling.

Cream: Betamethasone dipropionate 0.05% (base) and clotrimazole 1% (15 g, 45 g)

Lotrisone®: Betamethasone dipropionate 0.05% (base) and clotrimazole 1% (15 g, 45 g) [contains benzyl alcohol]

Lotion: Betamethasone dipropionate 0.05% (base) and clotrimazole 1% (30 mL)

Lotrisone®: Betamethasone dipropionate 0.05% (base) and clotrimazole 1% (30 mL) [contains benzyl alcohol]

◆ **Betamethasone Dipropionate** *see* Betamethasone *on page 208*

◆ **Betamethasone Dipropionate and Calcipotriene Hydrate** *see* Calcipotriene and Betamethasone *on page 261*

◆ **Betamethasone Dipropionate, Augmented** *see* Betamethasone *on page 208*

◆ **Betamethasone Sodium Phosphate** *see* Betamethasone *on page 208*

◆ **Betamethasone Valerate** *see* Betamethasone *on page 208*

◆ **Betapace®** *see* Sotalol *on page 1586*

◆ **Betapace AF®** *see* Sotalol *on page 1586*

◆ **Betasept® [OTC]** *see* Chlorhexidine Gluconate *on page 341*

◆ **Betaseron®** *see* Interferon Beta-1b *on page 918*

◆ **Betaxin® (Can)** *see* Thiamine *on page 1669*

Betaxolol (Systemic) (be TAKS oh lol)

Brand Names: U.S. Kerlone®

Brand Names: Canada Sandoz-Betaxolol

Index Terms Betaxolol Hydrochloride

Pharmacologic Category Beta Blocker, Beta-1 Selective

Additional Appendix Information

Beta-Blockers *on page 1884*

Use Management of hypertension

Unlabeled Use Treatment of coronary artery disease

Pregnancy Risk Factor C

Dosage Oral:

Adults: 5-10 mg/day; may increase dose to 20 mg/day after 7-14 days if desired response is not achieved.

Elderly: Refer to adult dosing; initial dose: 5 mg/day

Dosage adjustment in renal impairment: Severe impairment: Initial dose: 5 mg/day; may increase every 2 weeks up to a maximum of 20 mg/day

Hemodialysis: Initial dose: 5 mg/day; may increase every 2 weeks up to a maximum of 20 mg/day. Supplemental dose not required.

Additional Information Complete prescribing information for this medication should be consulted for additional detail.

Dosage Forms Excipient information presented when available (limited, particularly for generics); consult specific product labeling.

Tablet, oral, as hydrochloride: 10 mg, 20 mg

Kerlone®: 10 mg [scored]

Kerlone®: 20 mg

Betaxolol (Ophthalmic) (be TAKS oh lol)

Brand Names: U.S. Betoptic S®

Brand Names: Canada Betoptic® S

Index Terms Betaxolol Hydrochloride

Pharmacologic Category Ophthalmic Agent, Antiglaucoma

Use Treatment of chronic open-angle glaucoma or ocular hypertension

Pregnancy Risk Factor C

Dosage

Children and Adults: Ophthalmic suspension (Betoptic® S): Instill 1 drop into affected eye(s) twice daily.

Adults: Ophthalmic solution: Instill 1-2 drops into affected eye(s) twice daily.

Elderly: Ophthalmic: Refer to adult dosing.

Additional Information Complete prescribing information for this medication should be consulted for additional detail.

Dosage Forms Excipient information presented when available (limited, particularly for generics); consult specific product labeling.

Solution, ophthalmic [drops]: 0.5% (5 mL, 10 mL, 15 mL) [contains benzalkonium chloride]

Suspension, ophthalmic [drops]:

Betoptic S®: 0.25% (10 mL, 15 mL) [contains benzalkonium chloride]

◆ **Betaxolol Hydrochloride** *see* Betaxolol (Ophthalmic) *on page 211*

◆ **Betaxolol Hydrochloride** *see* Betaxolol (Systemic) *on page 211*

Bethanechol (be THAN e kole)

Brand Names: U.S. Urecholine®

Brand Names: Canada Duvoid®; PMS-Bethanechol

Index Terms Bethanechol Chloride

Pharmacologic Category Cholinergic Agonist

Use Treatment of acute postoperative and postpartum nonobstructive (functional) urinary retention; treatment of neurogenic atony of the urinary bladder with retention

Unlabeled Use Gastroesophageal reflux

Pregnancy Risk Factor C

Pregnancy Considerations Reproduction studies have not been conducted.

Lactation Excretion in breast milk unknown/not recommended

Contraindications Hypersensitivity to bethanechol or any component of the formulation; mechanical obstruction of the GI or GU tract or when the strength or integrity of the GI or bladder wall is in question; hyperthyroidism, peptic ulcer disease, epilepsy, asthma, bradycardia, vasomotor instability, coronary artery disease, hypotension, or parkinsonism

Warnings/Precautions Potential for reflux infection if the sphincter fails to relax as bethanechol contracts the bladder.

Adverse Reactions Frequency not defined.

Cardiovascular: Hypotension, tachycardia, flushed skin

Central nervous system: Headache, malaise, seizure

Gastrointestinal: Abdominal cramps, belching, borborygmi, colicky pain, diarrhea, nausea, vomiting, salivation

Genitourinary: Urinary urgency

Ocular: Lacrimation, miosis

Respiratory: Asthmatic attacks, bronchial constriction

Miscellaneous: Diaphoresis

Drug Interactions

Metabolism/Transport Effects None known.

Avoid Concomitant Use There are no known interactions where it is recommended to avoid concomitant use.

Increased Effect/Toxicity

The levels/effects of Bethanechol may be increased by: Acetylcholinesterase Inhibitors; Beta-Blockers

Decreased Effect There are no known significant interactions involving a decrease in effect.

Stability Store at room temperature of 15°C to 30°C (59°F to 86°F).

Mechanism of Action Due to stimulation of the parasympathetic nervous system, bethanechol increases bladder muscle tone causing contractions which initiate urination. Bethanechol also stimulates gastric motility, increases gastric tone and may restore peristalsis.

Pharmacodynamics/Kinetics
Onset of action: 30-90 minutes
Duration: Up to 6 hours
Absorption: Variable

Dosage Oral:
Children:
Urinary retention (unlabeled use): 0.3-0.6 mg/kg/day in 3-4 divided doses
Gastroesophageal reflux (unlabeled use): 0.3-0.6 mg/kg/day in 3-4 divided doses
Adults:
Urinary retention, neurogenic bladder: Initial: 10-50 mg 3-4 times/day (some patients may require dosages of 50-100 mg 4 times/day). To determine effective dose, may initiate at a dose of 5-10 mg, with additional doses of 5-10 mg hourly until an effective cumulative dose is reached. Cholinergic effects at higher oral dosages may be cumulative.
Gastroesophageal reflux (unlabeled): 25 mg 4 times/day
Elderly: Use the lowest effective dose

Dietary Considerations Should be taken 1 hour before meals or 2 hours after meals.

Administration Should be administered 1 hour before meals or 2 hours after meals.

Monitoring Parameters Observe closely for side effects.

Test Interactions Increased lipase, amylase (S), bilirubin, aminotransferase [ALT/AST] (S)

Dosage Forms Excipient information presented when available (limited, particularly for generics); consult specific product labeling.
Tablet, oral, as chloride: 5 mg, 10 mg, 25 mg, 50 mg
Urecholine®: 5 mg, 10 mg, 25 mg, 50 mg [scored]

Dosage Forms: Canada Excipient information presented when available (limited, particularly for generics); consult specific product labeling.
Tablet, as chloride:
Duvoid®: 10 mg, 25 mg, 50 mg

Extemporaneous Preparations A 1 mg/mL solution may be made with tablets. Crush twelve 10 mg tablets in a mortar and reduce to a fine powder. Add small portions of sterile water and mix to a uniform paste; mix while adding sterile water in incremental proportions to **almost** 120 mL; transfer to a calibrated bottle, rinse mortar with sterile water, and add quantity of sterile water sufficient to make 120 mL. Label "shake well" and "refrigerate". Stable for 30 days (Schlatter, 1997).

A 5 mg/mL suspension may be made with tablets and either a 1:1 mixture of Ora-Plus® and Ora-Sweet® or Ora-Plus® and Ora-Sweet® SF or 1:4 concentrated cherry syrup and simple syrup, NF mixture. Crush twelve 50 mg tablets in a mortar and reduce to a fine powder. Add small portions of chosen vehicle and mix to a uniform paste; mix while adding the vehicle in incremental proportions to **almost** 120 mL; transfer to a calibrated bottle, rinse mortar with vehicle, and add quantity of vehicle sufficient to make 120 mL. Label "shake well" and "refrigerate". Stable for 60 days refrigerated (preferred) or at room temperature (Allen, 1998; Nahata, 2004).

Allen LV Jr and Erickson MA, "Stability of Bethanechol Chloride, Pyrazinamide, Quinidine Sulfate, Rifampin, and Tetracycline Hydrochloride in Extemporaneously Compounded Oral Liquids," *Am J Health Syst Pharm*, 1998, 55(17):1804-9.
Nahata MC, Pai VB, and Hipple TF, *Pediatric Drug Formulations*, 5th ed, Cincinnati, OH: Harvey Whitney Books Co, 2004.
Schlatter JL and Saulnier JL, "Bethanechol Chloride Oral Solutions: Stability and Use in Infants," *Ann Pharmacother*, 1997, 31(3):294-6.

◆ **Bethanechol Chloride** *see* Bethanechol *on page 211*
◆ **Betimol®** *see* Timolol (Ophthalmic) *on page 1687*
◆ **Betnesol® (Can)** *see* Betamethasone *on page 208*
◆ **Betnovate® (Can)** *see* Betamethasone *on page 208*
◆ **Betoptic S®** *see* Betaxolol (Ophthalmic) *on page 211*
◆ **Betoptic® S (Can)** *see* Betaxolol (Ophthalmic) *on page 211*

Bevacizumab (be vuh SIZ uh mab)

Brand Names: U.S. Avastin®

Brand Names: Canada Avastin®

Index Terms Anti-VEGF Monoclonal Antibody; Anti-VEGF rhuMAb; rhuMAb-VEGF

Pharmacologic Category Antineoplastic Agent, Monoclonal Antibody; Vascular Endothelial Growth Factor (VEGF) Inhibitor

Use Treatment of metastatic colorectal cancer; treatment of unresectable, locally advanced, recurrent or metastatic nonsquamous, nonsmall cell lung cancer; treatment of progressive glioblastoma; treatment of metastatic renal cell cancer (not an approved use in Canada)

Note: For the treatment of glioblastoma, effectiveness is based on improvement in objective response rate.

Unlabeled Use Treatment of metastatic breast cancer, recurrent cervical cancer, recurrent ovarian cancer, soft tissue sarcomas (angiosarcoma or hemangiopericytoma/solitary fibrous tumor), age-related macular degeneration (AMD)

Pregnancy Risk Factor C

Pregnancy Considerations Teratogenic effects have been observed in animal reproduction studies. Angiogenesis is of critical importance to human fetal development, and bevacizumab inhibits angiogenesis. Adequate contraception during therapy is recommended (and for ≥6 months following last dose of bevacizumab). Patients should also be counseled regarding prolonged exposure following discontinuation of therapy due to the long half-life of bevacizumab.

Based on animal studies, bevacizumab may disrupt normal menstrual cycles and impair fertility by several effects, including reduced endometrial proliferation and follicular developmental arrest. Some parameters do not recover completely, or recover very slowly following discontinuation.

Lactation Excretion in breast milk unknown/not recommended

Contraindications There are no contraindications listed in the FDA-approved manufacturer's labeling.

Canadian labeling: Hypersensitivity to bevacizumab, any component of the formulation, Chinese hamster ovary cell products or other recombinant human or humanized antibodies; untreated CNS metastases

Warnings/Precautions [U.S. Boxed Warning]: Gastrointestinal (GI) perforation (sometimes fatal) has occurred in 0.3 to 2.4% of clinical study patients receiving bevacizumab; discontinue if GI perforation occurs. Most cases occur within 50 days of treatment initiation; monitor patients for signs/symptoms (eg, fever, abdominal pain with constipation and/or nausea/vomiting). GI fistula (including enterocutaneous, esophageal, duodenal, and rectal fistulas), and intra-abdominal abscess have been reported in patients receiving bevacizumab for colorectal cancer and other cancers (not related to treatment duration). Non-GI fistula formation (including tracheoesophageal, bronchopleural, biliary, vaginal, renal, and bladder fistulas) has been observed, most commonly within the first 6 months of treatment; permanently discontinue in patients who develop internal organ fistulas. **[U.S. Boxed**

Warning]: The incidence of wound healing and surgical complications is increased in patients who have received bevacizumab; discontinue with wound dehiscence. Although the appropriate interval between withholding bevacizumab and elective surgery has not been defined, bevacizumab should be discontinued at least 28 days prior to surgery and should not be reinitiated for at least 28 days after surgery and until wound is fully healed. In a retrospective review of central venous access device placements, a greater risk of wound dehiscence was observed when port placement and bevacizumab administration were separated by <14 days (Erinjeri, 2011).

Bevacizumab is associated with an increased risk for arterial thromboembolic events (ATE), including cerebral infarction, stroke, MI, TIA, angina, and other ATEs, when used in combination with chemotherapy. History of ATE or ≥65 years of age may present an even greater risk; permanently discontinue with serious ATE; the safety of treatment reinitiation after ATE has not been studied. Although patients with cancer are at risk for venous thromboembolism (VTE), a meta-analysis of 15 controlled trials has demonstrated an increased risk for VTE in patients who received bevacizumab (Nalluri, 2008). Discontinue therapy in patients with severe arteriothrombotic event or life-threatening pulmonary embolism.

Use with caution in patients with cardiovascular disease. Among all approved indications, the incidence of heart failure (HF) and/or left ventricular dysfunction, is higher in patients receiving bevacizumab plus chemotherapy when compared to chemotherapy alone. Bevacizumab may potentiate the cardiotoxic effects of anthracyclines. HF is more common with prior anthracycline exposure and/or left chest wall irradiation. The safety of therapy resumption or continuation in patients with cardiac dysfunction has not been studied. In studies of patients with metastatic breast cancer (an unlabeled use), the incidence of grades 3 or 4 HF was increased in patients receiving bevacizumab plus paclitaxel, compared to the control arm. Patients with metastatic breast cancer who had received prior anthracycline therapy had a higher rate of HF compared to those receiving paclitaxel alone (3.8% vs 0.6% respectively). A meta-analysis of 5 studies which enrolled patients with metastatic breast cancer who received bevacizumab suggested an association with an increased risk of heart failure; all trials included in the analysis enrolled patients who either received prior or were receiving concurrent anthracycline therapy (Choueiri, 2011).

Bevacizumab may cause and/or worsen hypertension; use caution in patients with pre-existing hypertension and monitor BP closely in all patients. Permanent discontinuation is recommended in patients who experience a hypertensive crisis or encephalopathy. Temporarily discontinue in patients who develop uncontrolled hypertension. Cases of reversible posterior leukoencephalopathy syndrome (RPLS) have been reported. Symptoms (which include headache, seizure, confusion, lethargy, blindness and/or other vision, or neurologic disturbances) may occur from 16 hours to 1 year after treatment initiation. Resolution of symptoms usually occurs within days after discontinuation; however, neurologic sequelae may remain. RPLS may be associated with hypertension; discontinue bevacizumab and begin management of hypertension, if present.

[U.S. Boxed Warning]: Severe or fatal hemorrhage, including hemoptysis, gastrointestinal bleeding, central nervous system hemorrhage, epistaxis, and vaginal bleeding have been reported (up to 5 times more frequently if receiving bevacizumab). Avoid use in patients with serious hemorrhage or recent hemoptysis (≥2.5 mL blood). Serious pulmonary hemorrhage has been reported in patients receiving bevacizumab (primarily in patients with nonsmall cell lung cancer with squamous cell histology [not an FDA-approved indication]). Intracranial hemorrhage, including cases of grade 3 or 4 hemorrhage, has occurred in patients with previously treated glioblastoma. Treatment discontinuation is recommended in all patients with intracranial or other serious hemorrhage. Use with caution in patients with CNS metastases; once case of CNS hemorrhage was observed in an ongoing study of NSCLC patients with CNS metastases. Use in patients with untreated CNS metastases is contraindicated in the Canadian labeling. Use with caution in patients at risk for thrombocytopenia.

Infusion reactions (eg, hypertension, hypertensive crisis, wheezing, oxygen desaturation, hypersensitivity [including anaphylactic/anaphylactoid reactions], chest pain, rigors, headache, diaphoresis) may occur with the first infusion (uncommon); interrupt therapy in patients experiencing severe infusion reactions; there are no data to address routine premedication use or reinstitution of therapy in patients who experience severe infusion reactions. Proteinuria and/or nephrotic syndrome have been associated with bevacizumab; risk may be increased in patients with a history of hypertension; thrombotic microangiopathy has been associated with bevacizumab-induced proteinuria. Withhold treatment for ≥2 g proteinuria/24 hours and resume when proteinuria is <2 g/24 hours; discontinue in patients with nephrotic syndrome. Elderly patients (≥65 years of age) are at higher risk for adverse events, including thromboembolic events and proteinuria; serious adverse events occurring more frequently in the elderly also include deep thrombophlebitis, sepsis, hyper-/hypotension, MI, CHF, leukopenia, anemia, dehydration, hypokalemia, and hyponatremia. Microangiopathic hemolytic anemia (MAHA) has been reported when bevacizumab has been used in combination with sunitinib. Concurrent therapy with sunitinib and bevacizumab is also associated with dose-limiting hypertension in patients with metastatic renal cell cancer. The incidence of hand-foot syndrome is increased in patients treated with bevacizumab plus sorafenib in comparison to those treated with sorafenib monotherapy. When used in combination with myelosuppressive chemotherapy, increased rates of severe or febrile neutropenia and neutropenic infection were reported. Bevacizumab, in combination with chemotherapy (or biologic therapy), is associated with an increased risk of treatment-related mortality; a higher risk of fatal adverse events was identified in a meta-analysis of 16 trials in which bevacizumab was used for the treatment of various cancers (breast cancer, colorectal cancer, non small cell lung cancer, pancreatic cancer, prostate cancer, and renal cell cancer) and compared to chemotherapy alone (Ranpura, 2011). When bevacizumab is used in combination with myelosuppressive chemotherapy, increased rates of severe or febrile neutropenia and neutropenic infection have been reported. In premenopausal women receiving bevacizumab in combination with mFOLFOX (fluorouracil/oxaliplatin based chemotherapy) the incidence of ovarian failure (amenorrhea ≥3 months) was higher (34%) compared to women who received mFOLFOX alone (2%); ovarian function recovered in some patients after treatment was discontinued; premenopausal women should be informed of the potential risk of ovarian failure.

Adverse Reactions Percentages reported as monotherapy and as part of combination chemotherapy regimens. Some studies only reported hematologic toxicities grades ≥4 and nonhematologic toxicities grades ≥3.

>10%:

Cardiovascular: Hypertension (12% to 34%; grades 3/4: 5% to 18%), thromboembolic event (≤21%; grades 3/4: 15%; venous thrombus/embolus: 8%; grades 3/4: 5% to 7%; arterial thrombosis 6%; grades 3/4: 3%), hypotension (7% to 15%)

Central nervous system: Pain (8% to 62%), headache (24% to 37%; grades 3/4: 2% to 4%), dizziness (19% to 26%), fatigue (≤45%; grades 3/4: 4% to 19%), sensory neuropathy (grades 3/4: 1% to 17%; in combination with paclitaxel: 24%)

Dermatologic: Alopecia (6% to 32%), dry skin (7% to 20%), exfoliative dermatitis (3% to 19%), skin discoloration (2% to 16%)

Gastrointestinal: Abdominal pain (8% to 61%; grades 3/4: 8%), vomiting (47% to 52%; grades 3/4: ≤11%), anorexia (35% to 43%), constipation (4% to 40%), diarrhea (grades 3/4: 1% to 34%), stomatitis (30% to 32%), gastrointestinal hemorrhage (19% to 24%), dyspepsia (17% to 24%), taste disorder (14% to 21%), weight loss (15% to 20%), flatulence (11% to 19%), nausea (grades 3/4: ≤12%)

Hematologic: Hemorrhage (≤40%; grades 3/4: 1% to 5%), leukopenia (grades 3/4: 37%), neutropenia (grade 4: 21% to 27%)

Neuromuscular & skeletal: Myalgia (8% to 19%), back pain (≤12%)

Renal: Proteinuria (4% to 36%; grades 3/4: ≤7%; median onset: 5.6 months; median time to resolution: 6.1 months)

Respiratory: Upper respiratory infection (40% to 47%), epistaxis (19% to 35%), dyspnea (25% to 26%), rhinitis

Miscellaneous: Infection (≤55%; serious: 7% to 14%; pneumonia, catheter, or wound infections)

1% to 10%:

Cardiovascular: DVT (6% to 9%; grades 3/4: 9%), HF (grades 3/4: 1% to 4%), syncope (grades 3/4: 3%), intra-abdominal venous thrombosis (grades 3/4: 3%), cardio-/cerebrovascular arterial thrombotic event (2% to 4%), left ventricular dysfunction (grades 3/4: 1%)

Central nervous system: CNS hemorrhage (1% to 5%; grades 3/4: 1%), dysphonia (≤5%)

Dermatologic: Skin ulcer (≤6%), wound dehiscence (1% to 6%), acne (≤1%)

Endocrine & metabolic: Dehydration (grades 3/4: ≤10%), hyponatremia (grades 3/4: 4%)

Gastrointestinal: Xerostomia (4% to 7%), colitis (1% to 6%), ileus (grades 3/4: 4% to 5%), gingival bleeding (2% to 4%), fistula (1%), gastrointestinal perforation (≤4%), gastroesophageal reflux (≤2%), gingivitis (≤2%), mouth ulceration (≤2%), tooth abscess (≤2%), intra-abdominal abscess (1%), gastritis (≤1%), gingival pain (≤1%)

Genitourinary: Vaginal hemorrhage (4%)

Hematologic: Neutropenic fever/infection (5%; grades 3 and/or 4: 4% to 5%), thrombocytopenia (5%)

Neuromuscular & skeletal: Weakness (10%), neuropathy (other than sensory: grades 3/4: 1% to 5%)

Ocular: Blurred vision (≤2%)

Otic: Tinnitus (≤2%), deafness (≤1%)

Respiratory: Voice alteration (5% to 9%), pneumonitis/pulmonary infiltrates (grades 3/4: 5%), hemoptysis (nonsquamous histology 2%), pulmonary embolism (≤1%)

Miscellaneous: Infusion reactions (<3%)

<1% (Limited to important or life-threatening): Anaphylaxis, anastomotic ulceration, angina, bladder perforation, cerebral infarction; fistula (biliary, bladder, bronchopleural, duodenal, enterocutaneous, esophageal, gastrointestinal, rectal, renal, tracheoesophageal [TE] and vaginal); gastrointestinal ulcer, hemorrhagic stroke, hypersensitivity, hypertensive crises, hypertensive encephalopathy, intestinal necrosis, intestinal obstruction, mesenteric venous occlusion, microangiopathic hemolytic anemia (when used in combination with sunitinib), MI, nasal septum perforation, nephrotic syndrome, osteonecrosis (jaw), ovarian failure, pancytopenia, polyserositis, pulmonary hemorrhage, pulmonary hypertension, renal failure, renal thrombotic microangiopathy, reversible posterior leukoencephalopathy syndrome (RPLS), sepsis, subarachnoid hemorrhage, toxic anterior segment syndrome (TASS), transient ischemic attack, ureteral stricture wound healing complications

Reported from unlabeled use: Eye disorders: Endophthalmitis (infectious and sterile), hemorrhage (conjunctival, retinal or vitreous), intraocular inflammation (iritis, vitritis), intraocular pressure increased, ocular hyperemia, ocular pain/discomfort, permanent vision loss, retinal detachment, visual disturbance, vitreous floaters

Drug Interactions

Metabolism/Transport Effects None known.

Avoid Concomitant Use

Avoid concomitant use of Bevacizumab with any of the following: CloZAPine; SUNItinib

Increased Effect/Toxicity

Bevacizumab may increase the levels/effects of: Antineoplastic Agents (Anthracycline, Systemic); CloZAPine; Irinotecan; SORAfenib; SUNItinib

The levels/effects of Bevacizumab may be increased by: SUNItinib

Decreased Effect There are no known significant interactions involving a decrease in effect.

Stability Store vials at 2°C to 8°C (36°F to 46°F); do not freeze. Protect from light; do not shake. Prior to I.V. infusion, dilute prescribed dose of bevacizumab in a total volume of 100 mL NS. Do not mix with dextrose-containing solutions. Diluted solutions are stable for up to 8 hours under refrigeration. Discard unused portion of vial.

Mechanism of Action Bevacizumab is a recombinant, humanized monoclonal antibody which binds to, and neutralizes, vascular endothelial growth factor (VEGF), preventing its association with endothelial receptors, Flt-1 and KDR. VEGF binding initiates angiogenesis (endothelial proliferation and the formation of new blood vessels). The inhibition of microvascular growth is believed to retard the growth of all tissues (including metastatic tissue).

Pharmacodynamics/Kinetics

Distribution: V_d: 46 mL/kg

Half-life elimination: ~20 days (range: 11-50 days)

Excretion: Clearance: 2.75-5 mL/kg/day

Dosage Adults: Details concerning dosing in combination regimens should also be consulted.

I.V.:

Colorectal cancer, metastatic: 5 or 10 mg/kg every 2 weeks (in combination with fluorouracil-based chemotherapy)

Canadian labeling: 5 mg/kg every 2 weeks (in combination with fluorouracil-based chemotherapy)

Glioblastoma: 10 mg/kg every 2 weeks as monotherapy **or** (unlabeled) 10 mg/kg every 2 weeks (in combination with irinotecan) (Vredenburgh, 2007)

Nonsmall cell lung cancer (nonsquamous cell histology): 15 mg/kg every 3 weeks (in combination with carboplatin and paclitaxel) for 4-6 cycles followed by maintenance treatment (unlabeled use) of bevacizumab 15 mg/kg every 3 weeks as monotherapy until disease progression or unacceptable toxicity (Sandler, 2006)

Renal cell cancer, metastatic: 10 mg/kg every 2 weeks (in combination with interferon alfa) **or** (unlabeled) 10 mg/kg every 2 weeks as monotherapy (Yang, 2003)

Breast cancer, metastatic (unlabeled use): 10 mg/kg every 2 weeks (in combination with paclitaxel) (Miller, 2007)

Ovarian cancer (unlabeled use): 15 mg/kg every 3 weeks (Burger, 2007; Cannistra, 2007)

Intravitreal: Age-related macular degeneration (unlabeled use): 1.25 mg (0.05 mL) monthly until improvement/resolution, usually ~1-3 injections (Avery, 2006) **or** 2.5 mg (0.1 mL) every 4 weeks for 3 doses (Bashshur, 2006)

Dosage adjustment for toxicity: I.V. administration (systemic): There are no recommended dosage reductions.

Temporary suspension is recommended for severe infusion reactions, at least 4 weeks prior to (and after) elective surgery, in moderate-to-severe proteinuria (in most studies, treatment was withheld for ≥2 g proteinuria/24 hours), or in patients with severe hypertension which is not controlled with medical management. Permanent discontinuation is recommended (by the manufacturer) in patients who develop wound dehiscence and wound healing complications requiring intervention, fistula (gastrointestinal and nongastrointestinal), gastrointestinal perforation, intra-abdominal abscess, hypertensive crisis, hypertensive encephalopathy, serious bleeding/hemorrhage, severe arterial thromboembolic event, nephrotic syndrome, or RPLS.

Dosage adjustment in renal impairment: There are no dosage adjustments provided in manufacturer's labeling

Dosage adjustment in hepatic impairment: There are no dosage adjustments provided in manufacturer's labeling

Administration

I.V. infusion, usually after the other antineoplastic agents. Infuse the initial dose over 90 minutes. The second infusion may be shortened to 60 minutes if the initial infusion is well tolerated. The third and subsequent infusions may be shortened to 30 minutes if the 60-minute infusion is well tolerated. Monitor closely during the infusion for signs/symptoms of an infusion reaction. Some institutions use a 10-minute infusion (0.5 mg/kg/minute) for bevacizumab dosed at 5 mg/kg (after tolerance at the 90-, 60-, and 30-minute infusion rates has been established; Reidy, 2007). Do not administer I.V. push.

Intravitreal injection (unlabeled use): Adequate local anesthesia and a topical broad-spectrum antimicrobial agent should be administered prior to the procedure; administer topical ophthalmic antibiotics for 3 days after procedure (Avery, 2006; Bashshur, 2006).

Monitoring Parameters Monitor closely during the infusion for signs/symptoms of an infusion reaction. Monitor CBC with differential; signs/symptoms of gastrointestinal perforation, fistula, or abscess (including abdominal pain, constipation, vomiting, and fever); signs/symptoms of bleeding, including hemoptysis, gastrointestinal, and/or CNS bleeding, and/or epistaxis. Monitor blood pressure every 2-3 weeks; more frequently if hypertension develops during therapy. Continue to monitor blood pressure after discontinuing due to bevacizumab-induced hypertension. Monitor for proteinuria/nephrotic syndrome with urine dipstick; collect 24 hour urine in patients with ≥2+ reading.

AMD: Monitor intraocular pressure and retinal artery perfusion

Dosage Forms Excipient information presented when available (limited, particularly for generics); consult specific product labeling.

Injection, solution [preservative free]:

Avastin®: 25 mg/mL (4 mL, 16 mL) [derived from or manufactured using Chinese hamster ovary cells]

Bexarotene (Systemic) (beks AIR oh teen)

Brand Names: U.S. Targretin®

Brand Names: Canada Targretin®

Pharmacologic Category Antineoplastic Agent, Miscellaneous

Use Treatment of cutaneous manifestations of cutaneous T-cell lymphoma in patients who are refractory to at least one prior systemic therapy

Pregnancy Risk Factor X

Pregnancy Considerations **[U.S. Boxed Warning]: Bexarotene is a retinoid, a drug class associated with birth defects in humans; do not administer during pregnancy.** Bexarotene caused birth defects when administered orally to pregnant rats. It must not be given to a pregnant woman or a woman who intends to become pregnant. If a woman becomes pregnant while taking the drug, it must be stopped immediately and appropriate counseling be given. In women of childbearing potential, therapy should be started on the second or third day of a normal menstrual period. Either abstinence or two forms of reliable contraception (one should be nonhormonal) must be used for at least 1 month before initiating therapy, during therapy, and for 1 month following discontinuation of bexarotene. A negative pregnancy test (sensitivity of at least 50 mIU/mL) within 1 week prior to beginning therapy, and monthly thereafter is required for women of childbearing potential. Male patients must use a condom during any sexual contact with women of childbearing age during therapy, and for 1 month following discontinuation of bexarotene.

Lactation Excretion in breast milk unknown/not recommended

Contraindications Hypersensitivity to bexarotene or any component of the formulation; pregnancy

Warnings/Precautions Hazardous agent - use appropriate precautions for handling and disposal. **[U.S. Boxed Warning]: Bexarotene is a retinoid, a drug class associated with birth defects in humans; do not administer during pregnancy.** Pregnancy test needed 1 week before initiation and every month thereafter. Effective contraception must be in place 1 month before initiation, during therapy, and for at least 1 month after discontinuation. Male patients with sexual partners who are pregnant, possibly pregnant, or who could become pregnant, must use condoms during sexual intercourse during treatment and for 1 month after last dose. Induces significant lipid abnormalities in a majority of patients (triglyceride, total cholesterol, and HDL); reversible on discontinuation. Use extreme caution in patients with underlying hypertriglyceridemia. Pancreatitis secondary to hypertriglyceridemia has been reported. Patients with risk factors for pancreatitis (eg, prior pancreatitis, uncontrolled hyperlipidemia, excess ethanol consumption, uncontrolled diabetes, biliary tract disease) should generally not receive bexarotene (oral). Monitor for liver function test abnormalities and discontinue drug if tests are three times the upper limit of normal values for AST, ALT, or bilirubin. Hypothyroidism occurs in about a third of patients. Monitor for signs and symptoms of infection about 4-8 weeks after initiation (leukopenia may occur). Any new visual abnormalities experienced by the patient should be evaluated by an ophthalmologist (cataracts can form, or worsen, especially in the geriatric population). May cause photosensitization. Safety and efficacy are not established in the pediatric population. Use only with extreme caution in patients with hepatic impairment. Limit additional vitamin A intake to <15,000 int. units/day. Use caution with diabetic patients.

Adverse Reactions First percentage is at a dose of 300 mg/m^2/day; the second percentage is at a dose >300 mg/m^2/day.

>10%:

Cardiovascular: Peripheral edema (13% to 11%)

Central nervous system: Headache (30% to 42%), chills (10% to 13%)

Dermatologic: Rash (17% to 23%), exfoliative dermatitis (10% to 28%)

Endocrine & metabolic: Hyperlipidemia (about 79% in both dosing ranges), hypercholesteremia (32% to 62%), hypothyroidism (29% to 53%)

Hematologic: Leukopenia (17% to 47%)

Neuromuscular & skeletal: Weakness (20% to 45%)

Miscellaneous: Infection (13% to 23%)

<10% (Limited to important or life-threatening):
Cardiovascular: Hemorrhage, hypertension, angina pectoris, right heart failure, tachycardia, cerebrovascular accident, syncope
Central nervous system: Fever (5% to 17%), insomnia (5% to 11%), subdural hematoma, depression, agitation, ataxia
Dermatologic: Dry skin (about 10% for both dosing ranges), alopecia (4% to 11%), skin ulceration, maculopapular rash, vesicular bullous rash, cheilitis
Endocrine & metabolic: Hypoproteinemia, hyperglycemia
Gastrointestinal: Abdominal pain (11% to 4%), nausea (16% to 8%), diarrhea (7% to 42%), vomiting (4% to 13%), anorexia (2% to 23%), colitis, gastroenteritis, gingivitis, melena, pancreatitis
Genitourinary: Albuminuria, hematuria, dysuria
Hematologic: Hypochromic anemia (4% to 13%), anemia (6% to 25%), eosinophilia, thrombocythemia, coagulation time increased, lymphocytosis, thrombocytopenia
Hepatic: LDH increased (7% to 13%), hepatic failure
Neuromuscular & skeletal: Back pain (2% to 11%), arthralgia, myalgia, myasthenia, neuropathy
Ocular: Conjunctivitis, blepharitis, corneal lesion, visual field defects, keratitis
Otic: Ear pain, otitis externa
Renal: Renal dysfunction
Respiratory: Pharyngitis, rhinitis, dyspnea, pleural effusion, bronchitis, cough increased, lung edema, hemoptysis, hypoxia
Miscellaneous: Flu-like syndrome (4% to 13%), infection (1% to 13%)

Drug Interactions

Metabolism/Transport Effects Substrate of CYP3A4 (minor); **Note:** Assignment of Major/Minor substrate status based on clinically relevant drug interaction potential; **Induces** CYP3A4 (weak/moderate)

Avoid Concomitant Use

Avoid concomitant use of Bexarotene (Systemic) with any of the following: Gemfibrozil; Tetracycline Derivatives; Vitamin A

Increased Effect/Toxicity

Bexarotene (Systemic) may increase the levels/effects of: Porfimer; Vitamin A

The levels/effects of Bexarotene (Systemic) may be increased by: CARBOplatin; Conivaptan; Gemfibrozil; PACLitaxel; Tetracycline Derivatives

Decreased Effect

Bexarotene (Systemic) may decrease the levels/effects of: ARIPiprazole; Atorvastatin; Contraceptives (Estrogens); Contraceptives (Progestins); PACLitaxel; Saxagliptin

The levels/effects of Bexarotene (Systemic) may be decreased by: Tocilizumab

Ethanol/Nutrition/Herb Interactions

Food: Bioavailability is increased when administered with a fat-containing meal. Bexarotene serum levels may be increased by grapefruit juice; avoid concurrent use.

Herb/Nutraceutical: Avoid dong quai, St John's wort (may also cause photosensitization). St John's wort may decrease bexarotene levels. Additional vitamin A supplements may lead to vitamin A toxicity (dry skin, irritation, arthralgias, myalgias, abdominal pain, hepatic changes).

Stability Store at 2°C to 25°C (36°F to 77°F). Protect from light.

Mechanism of Action The exact mechanism is unknown. Binds and activates retinoid X receptor subtypes. Once activated, these receptors function as transcription factors that regulate the expression of genes which control cellular differentiation and proliferation. Bexarotene inhibits the growth *in vitro* of some tumor cell lines of hematopoietic and squamous cell origin.

Pharmacodynamics/Kinetics

Absorption: Significantly improved by a fat-containing meal
Protein binding: >99%
Metabolism: Hepatic via CYP3A4 isoenzyme; four metabolites identified; further metabolized by glucuronidation
Half-life elimination: ~7 hours
Time to peak: ~2 hours
Excretion: Primarily feces; urine (<1% as unchanged drug and metabolites)

Dosage Oral: Adults: 300-400 mg/m^2/day taken as a single daily dose.

Dosing adjustment in renal impairment: No studies have been conducted; however, renal insufficiency may result in significant protein binding changes and alter pharmacokinetics of bexarotene

Dosing adjustment in hepatic impairment: No studies have been conducted; however, hepatic impairment would be expected to result in decreased clearance of bexarotene due to the extensive hepatic contribution to elimination

Dietary Considerations It is preferable to take the oral capsule following a fat-containing meal. Avoid grapefruit juice.

Administration Administer capsule following a fat-containing meal.

Monitoring Parameters If female, pregnancy test 1 week before initiation then monthly while on bexarotene; lipid panel before initiation, then weekly until lipid response established and then at 8-week intervals thereafter; baseline LFTs, repeat at 1, 2, and 4 weeks after initiation then at 8-week intervals thereafter if stable; baseline and periodic thyroid function tests; baseline CBC with periodic monitoring

Dosage Forms Excipient information presented when available (limited, particularly for generics); consult specific product labeling.

Capsule, oral:
Targretin®: 75 mg

Extemporaneous Preparations Hazardous agent: Use appropriate precautions for handling and disposal.

A 1 mg/mL oral suspension may be prepared with capsules. Cut one 75 mg capsule in half, rinse the interior contents of the capsule, and suspend with 75 mL sterile water. Administer immediately after preparation. To ensure administration of full dose, rinse empty glass with half a glass of water and administer residue.

Targretin® data on file, Eisai Inc.

Bexarotene (Topical) (beks AIR oh teen)

Brand Names: U.S. Targretin®

Brand Names: Canada Targretin®

Pharmacologic Category Antineoplastic Agent, Miscellaneous

Use Treatment of cutaneous lesions in patients with refractory cutaneous T-cell lymphoma (stage 1A and 1B) or who have not tolerated other therapies

Pregnancy Risk Factor X

Pregnancy Considerations Bexarotene is a retinoid, a drug class associated with birth defects in humans; do not administer during pregnancy. Bexarotene caused birth defects when administered orally to pregnant rats. It must not be given to a pregnant woman or a woman who intends to become pregnant. If a woman becomes pregnant while using the gel, it must be stopped immediately and appropriate counseling be given. In women of childbearing potential, therapy should be started on the second or third day of a normal menstrual period. Either abstinence or two forms of reliable contraception (one should be nonhormonal) must be used for at least 1 month before initiating therapy, during therapy, and for 1 month following discontinuation of bexarotene. A negative pregnancy test (sensitivity of at least 50 mIU/mL) within 1 week prior to beginning therapy, and monthly thereafter is required for women of childbearing potential. Males patients must use a condom during any sexual contact with women of childbearing age during therapy, and for 1 month following discontinuation of bexarotene

Lactation Excretion in breast milk unknown/not recommended

Contraindications Hypersensitivity to bexarotene or any component of the formulation; pregnancy

Warnings/Precautions Hazardous agent - use appropriate precautions for handling and disposal. **Bexarotene is a retinoid, a drug class associated with birth defects in humans; do not administer during pregnancy.** Pregnancy test needed 1 week before initiation and every month thereafter. Effective contraception must be in place 1 month before initiation, during therapy, and for at least 1 month after discontinuation. Male patients with sexual partners who are pregnant, possibly pregnant, or who could become pregnant, must use condoms during sexual intercourse during treatment and for 1 month after last dose. May induce lipid abnormalities; reversible on discontinuation. Use extreme caution in patients with underlying hypertriglyceridemia. Monitor for signs and symptoms of infection about 4-8 weeks after initiation (leukopenia may occur). May cause photosensitization. Safety and efficacy are not established in the pediatric population. Use only with extreme caution in patients with hepatic impairment. Limit additional vitamin A intake to <15,000 int. units/day.

Adverse Reactions

Cardiovascular: Edema (10%)

Central nervous system: Headache (14%), weakness (6%), pain (30%)

Dermatologic: Rash (14% to 72%), pruritus (6% to 40%), contact dermatitis (14%), exfoliative dermatitis (6%)

Endocrine & metabolic: Hyperlipidemia (10%)

Hematologic: Leukopenia (6%), lymphadenopathy (6%)

Neuromuscular & skeletal: Paresthesia (6%)

Respiratory: Cough (6%), pharyngitis (6%)

Miscellaneous: Diaphoresis (6%), infection (18%)

Drug Interactions

Metabolism/Transport Effects Substrate of CYP3A4 (minor); **Note:** Assignment of Major/Minor substrate status based on clinically relevant drug interaction potential; **Induces** CYP3A4 (weak/moderate)

Avoid Concomitant Use

Avoid concomitant use of Bexarotene (Topical) with any of the following: Tetracycline Derivatives; Vitamin A

Increased Effect/Toxicity

Bexarotene (Topical) may increase the levels/effects of: Porfimer; Vitamin A

The levels/effects of Bexarotene (Topical) may be increased by: Conivaptan; Tetracycline Derivatives

Decreased Effect

Bexarotene (Topical) may decrease the levels/effects of: ARIPiprazole; Contraceptives (Estrogens); Contraceptives (Progestins); Saxagliptin

The levels/effects of Bexarotene (Topical) may be decreased by: Tocilizumab

Stability Store at 2°C to 25°C (36°F to 77°F). Protect from light.

Mechanism of Action The exact mechanism is unknown. Binds and activates retinoid X receptor subtypes. Once activated, these receptors function as transcription factors that regulate the expression of genes which control cellular differentiation and proliferation.

Pharmacodynamics/Kinetics Absorption: Systemically absorbed following topical application (1% gel: <55 ng/mL)

Dosage Topical: Adults: Apply once every other day for first week, then increase on a weekly basis to once daily, 2 times/day, 3 times/day, and finally 4 times/day, according to tolerance

Dosing adjustment in renal impairment: No studies have been conducted; however, renal insufficiency may result in significant protein binding changes and alter pharmacokinetics of bexarotene

Dosing adjustment in hepatic impairment: No studies have been conducted; however, hepatic impairment would be expected to result in decreased clearance of bexarotene due to the extensive hepatic contribution to elimination

Administration Allow gel to dry before covering with clothing. Avoid application to normal skin. Use of occlusive dressings is not recommended.

Monitoring Parameters If female, pregnancy test 1 week before initiation then monthly while on bexarotene; lipid panel before initiation, then weekly until lipid response established and then at 8-week intervals thereafter; baseline LFTs, repeat at 1, 2, and 4 weeks after initiation then at 8-week intervals thereafter if stable; baseline and periodic thyroid function tests; baseline CBC with periodic monitoring

Dosage Forms Excipient information presented when available (limited, particularly for generics); consult specific product labeling.

Gel, topical:

Targretin®: 1% (60 g) [contains dehydrated ethanol]

- ◆ **Bexxar®** *see* Tositumomab and Iodine I 131 Tositumomab *on page 1714*
- ◆ **Beyaz™** *see* Ethinyl Estradiol, Drospirenone, and Levomefolate *on page 664*
- ◆ **BG 9273** *see* Alefacept *on page 57*
- ◆ **BI-1356** *see* Linagliptin *on page 1012*
- ◆ **Biaxin®** *see* Clarithromycin *on page 374*
- ◆ **Biaxin® XL** *see* Clarithromycin *on page 374*

Bicalutamide (bye ka LOO ta mide)

Brand Names: U.S. Casodex®

Brand Names: Canada Apo-Bicalutamide®; Casodex®; CO Bicalutamide; Dom-Bicalutamide; JAMP-Bicalutamide; Mylan-Bicalutamide; Novo-Bicalutamide; PHL-Bicalutamide; PMS-Bicalutamide; PRO-Bicalutamide; ratio-Bicalutamide; Sandoz-Bicalutamide

Index Terms CDX; ICI-176334

Pharmacologic Category Antineoplastic Agent, Antiandrogen

Use Treatment of metastatic prostate cancer (in combination with an LHRH agonist)

Unlabeled Use Monotherapy for locally-advanced prostate cancer

Pregnancy Risk Factor X

Pregnancy Considerations Animal studies have demonstrated teratogenicity. Bicalutamide use is contraindicated in women. Androgen receptor inhibition during pregnancy may affect fetal development.

Lactation Excretion in breast milk unknown/contraindicated

Contraindications Hypersensitivity to bicalutamide or any component of the formulation; use in women, especially women who are or may become pregnant

Warnings/Precautions Hazardous agent - use appropriate precautions for handling and disposal. Rare cases of death or hospitalization due to hepatitis have been reported postmarketing. Use with caution in moderate-to-severe hepatic dysfunction. Hepatotoxicity generally occurs within the first 3-4 months of use; patients should ▶

be monitored for signs and symptoms of liver dysfunction. Bicalutamide should be discontinued if patients have jaundice or ALT is >2 times the upper limit of normal. Androgen-deprivation therapy may increase the risk for cardiovascular disease (Levine, 2010). May cause gynecomastia, breast pain, or lead to spermatogenesis inhibition. When used in combination with LHRH agonists, a loss of glycemic control and decrease in glucose tolerance has been reported in patients with diabetes; monitor. May cause gynecomastia or breast pain (at higher, unlabeled doses), or lead to spermatogenesis inhibition.

Adverse Reactions Adverse reaction percentages reported as part of combination regimen with an LHRH analogue unless otherwise noted.

>10%:

Cardiovascular: Peripheral edema (13%)

Central nervous system: Pain (35%)

Endocrine & metabolic: Hot flashes (53%), breast pain (6%; monotherapy [150 mg]: 39% to 85%), gynecomastia (9%; monotherapy [150 mg]: 38% to 73%)

Gastrointestinal: Constipation (22%), nausea (15%), diarrhea (12%), abdominal pain (11%)

Genitourinary: Pelvic pain (21%), hematuria (12%), nocturia (12%)

Hematologic: Anemia (11%)

Neuromuscular & skeletal: Back pain (25%), weakness (22%)

Respiratory: Dyspnea (13%)

Miscellaneous: Infection (18%)

≥2% to 10%:

Cardiovascular: Chest pain (8%), hypertension (8%), angina pectoris (2% to <5%), cardiac arrest (2% to <5%), CHF (2% to <5%), edema (2% to <5%), MI (2% to <5%), coronary artery disorder (2% to <5%), syncope (2% to <5%)

Central nervous system: Dizziness (10%), headache (7%), insomnia (7%), anxiety (5%), depression (4%), chills (2% to <5%), confusion (2% to <5%), fever (2% to <5%), nervousness (2% to <5%), somnolence (2% to <5%)

Dermatologic: Rash (9%), alopecia (2% to <5%), dry skin (2% to <5%), pruritus (2% to <5%), skin carcinoma (2% to <5%)

Endocrine & metabolic: Hyperglycemia (6%), dehydration (2% to <5%), gout (2% to <5%), hypercholesterolemia (2% to <5%), libido decreased (2% to <5%)

Gastrointestinal: Dyspepsia (7%), weight loss (7%), anorexia (6%), flatulence (6%), vomiting (6%), weight gain (5%), dysphagia (2% to <5%), gastrointestinal carcinoma (2% to <5%), melena (2% to <5%), periodontal abscess (2% to <5%), rectal hemorrhage (2% to <5%), xerostomia (2% to <5%)

Genitourinary: Urinary tract infection (9%), impotence (7%), polyuria (6%), urinary retention (5%), urinary impairment (5%), urinary incontinence (4%), dysuria (2% to <5%), urinary urgency (2% to <5%)

Hepatic: LFTs increased (7%), alkaline phosphatase increased (5%)

Neuromuscular & skeletal: Bone pain (9%), paresthesia (8%), myasthenia (7%), arthritis (5%), pathological fracture (4%), hypertonia (2% to <5%), leg cramps (2% to <5%), myalgia (2% to <5%), neck pain (2% to <5%), neuropathy (2% to <5%)

Ocular: Cataract (2% to <5%)

Renal: BUN increased (2% to <5%), creatinine increased (2% to <5%), hydronephrosis (2% to <5%)

Respiratory: Cough (8%), pharyngitis (8%), bronchitis (6%), pneumonia (4%), rhinitis (4%), asthma (2% to <5%), epistaxis (2% to <5%), sinusitis (2% to <5%)

Miscellaneous: Flu-like syndrome (7%), diaphoresis (6%), cyst (2% to <5%), hernia (2% to <5%), herpes zoster (2% to <5%), sepsis (2% to <5%)

Postmarketing and/or case reports: Bilirubin increased, glucose tolerance decreased, hemoglobin decreased, hepatitis, hepatotoxicity, hypersensitivity reactions (including angioneurotic edema and urticaria), interstitial pneumonitis, pulmonary fibrosis, WBC decreased

Drug Interactions

Metabolism/Transport Effects **Inhibits** CYP3A4 (moderate)

Avoid Concomitant Use

Avoid concomitant use of Bicalutamide with any of the following: Pimozide; Tolvaptan

Increased Effect/Toxicity

Bicalutamide may increase the levels/effects of: ARIPiprazole; Budesonide (Systemic, Oral Inhalation); Colchicine; CYP3A4 Substrates; Eplerenone; Everolimus; FentaNYL; Halofantrine; Lurasidone; Pimecrolimus; Pimozide; Propafenone; Ranolazine; Salmeterol; Saxagliptin; Tolvaptan; Vilazodone; Vitamin K Antagonists; Zuclopenthixol

Decreased Effect There are no known significant interactions involving a decrease in effect.

Stability Store at room temperature of 20°C to 25°C (68°F to 77°F).

Mechanism of Action Androgen receptor inhibitor; pure nonsteroidal antiandrogen that binds to androgen receptors; specifically a competitive inhibitor for the binding of dihydrotestosterone and testosterone; prevents testosterone stimulation of cell growth in prostate cancer

Pharmacodynamics/Kinetics

Absorption: Rapid and complete; unaffected by food

Protein binding: 96%

Metabolism: Extensively hepatic; glucuronidation and oxidation of the R (active) enantiomer to inactive metabolites; the S enantiomer is inactive

Half-life elimination: Active enantiomer: ~6 days, ~10 days in severe liver disease

Time to peak, plasma: Active enantiomer: ~31 hours

Excretion: Urine (36%, as inactive metabolites); feces (42%, as unchanged drug and inactive metabolites)

Dosage Oral: Adults:

Prostate cancer, metastatic: 50 mg once daily (in combination with an LHRH analogue)

Prostate cancer, locally-advanced (unlabeled use): 150 mg once daily (as monotherapy) (McLeod, 2006)

Dosage adjustment in renal impairment: No adjustment required

Dosage adjustment in hepatic impairment: No adjustment required for mild, moderate, or severe hepatic impairment; use caution with moderate-to-severe impairment. Discontinue if ALT >2 times ULN or patient develops jaundice.

Dietary Considerations May be taken with or without food.

Administration Dose should be taken at the same time each day with or without food. Treatment for metastatic cancer should be started concomitantly with an LHRH analogue.

Monitoring Parameters Periodically monitor CBC, ECG, echocardiograms, serum testosterone, luteinizing hormone, and prostate specific antigen (PSA). Liver function tests should be obtained at baseline and repeated regularly during the first 4 months of treatment, and periodically thereafter; monitor for signs and symptoms of liver dysfunction (discontinue if jaundice is noted or ALT is >2 times the upper limit of normal). Monitor blood glucose in patients with diabetes. If initiating bicalutamide in patients who are on warfarin, closely monitor prothrombin time.

Dosage Forms Excipient information presented when available (limited, particularly for generics); consult specific product labeling.
Tablet, oral: 50 mg
Casodex®: 50 mg

◆ **Bicillin® L-A** *see* Penicillin G Benzathine *on page 1321*
◆ **Bicillin® C-R** *see* Penicillin G Benzathine and Penicillin G Procaine *on page 1322*
◆ **Bicillin® C-R 900/300** *see* Penicillin G Benzathine and Penicillin G Procaine *on page 1322*
◆ **Bicitra** *see* Sodium Citrate and Citric Acid *on page 1570*
◆ **BiCNU®** *see* Carmustine *on page 293*
◆ **Bidex®-400 [OTC]** *see* GuaiFENesin *on page 809*
◆ **BiDil®** *see* Isosorbide Dinitrate and Hydralazine *on page 938*
◆ **BIG-IV** *see* Botulism Immune Globulin (Intravenous-Human) *on page 232*
◆ **Biltricide®** *see* Praziquantel *on page 1395*

Bimatoprost (bi MAT oh prost)

Brand Names: U.S. Latisse®; Lumigan®
Brand Names: Canada Lumigan®; Lumigan® RC
Pharmacologic Category Ophthalmic Agent, Antiglaucoma; Ophthalmic Agent, Miscellaneous; Prostaglandin, Ophthalmic
Use Reduction of intraocular pressure (IOP) in patients with open-angle glaucoma or ocular hypertension; hypotrichosis treatment of the eyelashes
Pregnancy Risk Factor C
Dosage Adults:
Ophthalmic: Open-angle glaucoma or ocular hypertension: Instill 1 drop into affected eye(s) once daily in the evening; do not exceed once-daily dosing (may decrease IOP-lowering effect). If used with other topical ophthalmic agents, separate administration by at least 5 minutes.
Ophthalmic, topical: Hypotrichosis of the eyelashes: Place one drop on applicator and apply evenly along the skin of the upper eyelid at base of eyelashes once daily at bedtime; repeat procedure for second eye (use a clean applicator)
Additional Information Complete prescribing information for this medication should be consulted for additional detail.
Dosage Forms Excipient information presented when available (limited, particularly for generics); consult specific product labeling.
Solution, ophthalmic [drops]:
Latisse®: 0.03% (3 mL) [contains benzalkonium chloride]
Lumigan®: 0.01% (2.5 mL, 5 mL, 7.5 mL); 0.03% (2.5 mL, 5 mL, 7.5 mL) [contains benzalkonium chloride]

◆ **Bio-Amitriptyline (Can)** *see* Amitriptyline *on page 94*
◆ **Bio-Furosemide (Can)** *see* Furosemide *on page 771*
◆ **BioGlo™** *see* Fluorescein *on page 727*
◆ **Bio-Hydrochlorothiazide (Can)** *see* Hydrochlorothiazide *on page 835*
◆ **Bionect®** *see* Hyaluronate and Derivatives *on page 831*
◆ **Bioniche Promethazine (Can)** *see* Promethazine *on page 1416*
◆ **Bio-Oxazepam (Can)** *see* Oxazepam *on page 1261*
◆ **BioQuin® Durules™ (Can)** *see* QuiNIDine *on page 1446*
◆ **BioThrax®** *see* Anthrax Vaccine Adsorbed *on page 124*
◆ **Biphentin® (Can)** *see* Methylphenidate *on page 1107*
◆ **Bird Flu Vaccine** *see* Influenza Virus Vaccine (H5N1) *on page 896*
◆ **Bisac-Evac™ [OTC]** *see* Bisacodyl *on page 219*

Bisacodyl (bis a KOE dil)

Brand Names: U.S. Alophen® [OTC]; Bisac-Evac™ [OTC]; Biscolax™ [OTC]; Correctol® Tablets [OTC]; Dacodyl™ [OTC]; Doxidan® [OTC]; Dulcolax® [OTC]; ex-lax® Ultra [OTC]; Femilax™ [OTC]; Fleet® Bisacodyl [OTC]; Fleet® Stimulant Laxative [OTC]; Veracolate® [OTC]
Brand Names: Canada Apo-Bisacodyl®; Carter's Little Pills®; Dulcolax®; Gentlax®
Pharmacologic Category Laxative, Stimulant
Additional Appendix Information
Beers Criteria – Potentially Inappropriate Medications for Geriatrics *on page 1973*
Laxatives, Classification and Properties *on page 1893*
Use Treatment of constipation; colonic evacuation prior to procedures or examination
Pregnancy Risk Factor C
Dosage
Children:
Oral: >6 years: 5-10 mg (0.3 mg/kg) at bedtime or before breakfast
Rectal suppository:
<2 years: 5 mg as a single dose
>2 years: 10 mg
Adults:
Oral: 5-15 mg as single dose (up to 30 mg when complete evacuation of bowel is required)
Rectal suppository: 10 mg as single dose
Additional Information Complete prescribing information for this medication should be consulted for additional detail.
Dosage Forms Excipient information presented when available (limited, particularly for generics); consult specific product labeling.
Solution, rectal [enema]:
Fleet® Bisacodyl: 10 mg/30 mL (37 mL)
Suppository, rectal: 10 mg (12s, 50s, 100s)
Bisac-Evac™: 10 mg (8s, 12s, 50s, 100s, 500s, 1000s)
Biscolax™: 10 mg (12s, 100s)
Dulcolax®: 10 mg (4s, 8s, 16s, 28s, 50s)
Tablet, oral: 5 mg, 10 mg
Tablet, delayed release, oral: 5 mg
Doxidan®: 5 mg
Fleet® Stimulant Laxative: 5 mg
Tablet, enteric coated, oral: 5 mg
Alophen®: 5 mg
Bisac-Evac™: 5 mg
Correctol® Tablets: 5 mg
Dacodyl™: 5 mg
Dulcolax®: 5 mg
ex-lax® Ultra: 5 mg [contains sodium 0.1 mg/tablet]
Femilax™: 5 mg
Veracolate®: 5 mg

◆ **bis(chloroethyl) nitrosourea** *see* Carmustine *on page 293*
◆ **bis-chloronitrosourea** *see* Carmustine *on page 293*
◆ **Biscolax™ [OTC]** *see* Bisacodyl *on page 219*
◆ **Bismatrol** *see* Bismuth *on page 220*
◆ **Bismatrol [OTC]** *see* Bismuth *on page 220*

◆ **Bismatrol Maximum Strength [OTC]** *see* Bismuth *on page 220*

Bismuth (BIZ muth)

Brand Names: U.S. Bismatrol Maximum Strength [OTC]; Bismatrol [OTC]; Diotame [OTC]; Kao-Tin [OTC]; Kaopectate® Extra Strength [OTC]; Kaopectate® [OTC]; Peptic Relief [OTC]; Pepto Relief [OTC]; Pepto-Bismol® Maximum Strength [OTC]; Pepto-Bismol® [OTC]

Index Terms Bismatrol; Bismuth Subsalicylate; Pink Bismuth

Pharmacologic Category Antidiarrheal

Use Subsalicylate formulation: Symptomatic treatment of mild, nonspecific diarrhea; control of traveler's diarrhea (enterotoxigenic *Escherichia coli*); as part of a multidrug regimen for *H. pylori* eradication to reduce the risk of duodenal ulcer recurrence

Pregnancy Risk Factor C/D (3rd trimester)

Dosage Oral:

Treatment of nonspecific diarrhea, control/relieve traveler's diarrhea: Subsalicylate: Children >12 years and Adults: 524 mg every 30 minutes to 1 hour as needed up to 8 doses/24 hours

Helicobacter pylori eradication: Subsalicylate: Adults: 524 mg 4 times/day with meals and at bedtime; requires combination therapy

Dosing adjustment in renal impairment: Bismuth has been associated with nephrotoxicity in overdose (Leussink, 2002); although there are no specific recommendations by the manufacturer, consider using with caution in patients with renal impairment.

Additional Information Complete prescribing information for this medication should be consulted for additional detail.

Dosage Forms Excipient information presented when available (limited, particularly for generics); consult specific product labeling.

Caplet, oral, as subsalicylate:
- Pepto-Bismol®: 262 mg [sugar free; contains sodium 2 mg/caplet]

Liquid, oral, as subsalicylate: 262 mg/15 mL (120 mL, 240 mL, 360 mL, 480 mL); 525 mg/15 mL (240 mL, 360 mL)
- Bismatrol: 262 mg/15 mL (240 mL)
- Bismatrol Maximum Strength: 525 mg/15 mL (240 mL)
- Diotame: 262 mg/15 mL (30 mL) [sugar free]
- Kao-Tin: 262 mg/15 mL (240 mL, 473 mL) [contains sodium benzoate]
- Kaopectate®: 262 mg/15 mL (236 mL) [contains potassium 5 mg/15 mL, sodium 5 mg/15 mL; peppermint flavor]
- Kaopectate®: 262 mg/15 mL (177 mL) [contains sodium 4 mg/15 mL; cherry flavor]
- Kaopectate®: 262 mg/15 mL (236 mL, 354 mL) [contains sodium 4 mg/15 mL; vanilla flavor]
- Kaopectate® Extra Strength: 525 mg/15 mL (236 mL) [contains potassium 5 mg/15 mL, sodium 5 mg/15 mL; peppermint flavor]
- Peptic Relief: 262 mg/15 mL (237 mL) [sugar free; mint flavor]
- Pepto-Bismol®: 262 mg/15 mL (240 mL, 360 mL, 480 mL) [sugar free; contains benzoic acid, sodium 6 mg/15 mL; cherry flavor]
- Pepto-Bismol®: 262 mg/15 mL (120 mL, 240 mL, 360 mL, 480 mL) [sugar free; contains benzoic acid, sodium 6 mg/15 mL; wintergreen flavor]
- Pepto-Bismol® Maximum Strength: 525 mg/15 mL (120 mL, 240 mL, 360 mL) [sugar free; contains benzoic acid, sodium 6 mg/15 mL; wintergreen flavor]

Suspension, oral, as subsalicylate: 262 mg/15 mL (30 mL)

Tablet, chewable, oral, as subsalicylate: 262 mg
- Bismatrol: 262 mg
- Diotame: 262 mg [sugar free]
- Peptic Relief: 262 mg
- Pepto Relief: 262 mg
- Pepto-Bismol®: 262 mg [sugar free; contains sodium <1 mg/tablet; cherry flavor]
- Pepto-Bismol®: 262 mg [sugar free; contains sodium <1 mg/tablet; wintergreen flavor]

◆ **Bismuth Subsalicylate** *see* Bismuth *on page 220*

Bisoprolol (bis OH proe lol)

Brand Names: U.S. Zebeta®

Brand Names: Canada Apo-Bisoprolol®; Novo-Bisoprolol; PHL-Bisoprolol; PMS-Bisoprolol; PRO-Bisoprolol; Sandoz-Bisoprolol; ZYM-Bisoprolol

Index Terms Bisoprolol Fumarate

Pharmacologic Category Beta Blocker, Beta-1 Selective

Additional Appendix Information

Beta-Blockers *on page 1884*

Heart Failure (Systolic) *on page 1991*

Use Treatment of hypertension, alone or in combination with other agents

Unlabeled Use Chronic stable angina, supraventricular arrhythmias, PVCs, heart failure (HF)

Pregnancy Risk Factor C

Pregnancy Considerations Adverse events were observed in animal reproduction studies; therefore, the manufacturer classifies bisoprolol as pregnancy category C. In a cohort study, an increased risk of cardiovascular defects was observed following maternal use of beta-blockers during pregnancy. Intrauterine growth restriction (IUGR), small placentas, as well as fetal/neonatal bradycardia, hypoglycemia, and/or respiratory depression have been observed following *in utero* exposure to beta-blockers as a class. Adequate facilities for monitoring infants at birth should be available. Untreated chronic maternal hypertension and pre-eclampsia are also associated with adverse events in the fetus, infant, and mother. Limited information is available related to the use of bisoprolol for the treatment of hypertension in pregnancy; other agents may be more appropriate for use.

Lactation Excretion unknown/use caution

Contraindications Cardiogenic shock; overt cardiac failure; marked sinus bradycardia or heart block greater than first-degree (except in patients with a functioning artificial pacemaker)

Warnings/Precautions Consider pre-existing conditions such as sick sinus syndrome before initiating. Use caution in patients with heart failure; use gradual and careful titration; monitor for symptoms of congestive heart failure. Use with caution in patients with myasthenia gravis, psychiatric disease (may cause CNS depression), bronchospastic disease, undergoing anesthesia; and in those with impaired hepatic function. Bradycardia may be observed more frequently in elderly patients (>65 years of age); dosage reductions may be necessary. Beta-blocker therapy should not be withdrawn abruptly (particularly in patients with CAD), but gradually tapered to avoid acute tachycardia, hypertension, and/or ischemia. Chronic beta-blocker therapy should not be routinely withdrawn prior to major surgery. Can precipitate or aggravate symptoms of arterial insufficiency in patients with PVD and Raynaud's disease; use with caution and monitor for progression of arterial obstruction. Use caution with concurrent use of digoxin, verapamil, or diltiazem; bradycardia or heart block may occur. Use with caution in patients receiving inhaled anesthetic agents known to depress myocardial contractility. Bisoprolol, with $beta_1$-selectivity, may be used cautiously in bronchospastic disease with close monitoring.

Use cautiously in patients with diabetes because it can mask prominent hypoglycemic symptoms. May mask signs of hyperthyroidism (eg, tachycardia); use caution if hyperthyroidism is suspected, abrupt withdrawal may precipitate thyroid storm. Dosage adjustment is required in patients with significant hepatic or renal dysfunction. Adequate alpha-blockade is required prior to use of any beta-blocker for patients with untreated pheochromocytoma. May induce or exacerbate psoriasis. Use caution with history of severe anaphylaxis to allergens; patients taking beta-blockers may become more sensitive to repeated challenges. Treatment of anaphylaxis (eg, epinephrine) in patients taking beta-blockers may be ineffective or promote undesirable effects.

Adverse Reactions

1% to 10%:

Cardiovascular: Chest pain (1% to 2%)

Central nervous system: Fatigue (dose related; 6% to 8%), insomnia (2% to 3%), hypoesthesia (1% to 2%)

Gastrointestinal: Diarrhea (dose related; 3% to 4%), nausea (2%), vomiting (1% to 2%)

Neuromuscular & skeletal: Arthralgia (2% to 3%), weakness (dose related; ≤2%)

Respiratory: Upper respiratory infection (5%), rhinitis (3% to 4%), sinusitis (dose related; 2%), dyspnea (1% to 2%)

<1% (Limited to important or life-threatening): Abdominal pain, acne, alopecia, angioedema, anxiety, arrhythmia, asthma, back/neck pain, bradycardia (dose related), bronchitis, bronchospasm, BUN/creatinine increased, claudication, cold extremities, confusion (especially in the elderly), congestive heart failure, constipation, coughing, cutaneous vasculitis, cystitis, depression, dermatitis, dizziness, dyspepsia, dyspnea on exertion, eczema, edema, exfoliative dermatitis, flushing, gastritis, gout, hallucinations, headache, hearing decreased, hyperesthesia, hyperglycemia, hyperkalemia, hyperphosphatemia, hypertriglyceridemia, hypotension, impotence, lacrimation (abnormal), leukopenia, libido decreased, malaise, memory loss, muscle cramps, muscle/joint pain, nervousness, ocular pain/pressure, orthostatic hypotension, palpitations, paresthesia, peptic ulcer, Peyronie's disease, pharyngitis, polyuria, positive ANA titers, pruritus, psoriasis, psoriasiform eruption, purpura, rash, renal colic, restlessness, rhythm disturbances, sleep disturbances, somnolence, syncope, taste abnormality, thrombocytopenia, tinnitus, transaminases increased, tremor, twitching, uric acid increased, vasculitis, vertigo, visual disturbances, weight gain, xerostomia

Drug Interactions

Metabolism/Transport Effects Substrate of CYP2D6 (minor), CYP3A4 (major); **Note:** Assignment of Major/Minor substrate status based on clinically relevant drug interaction potential

Avoid Concomitant Use

Avoid concomitant use of Bisoprolol with any of the following: Conivaptan; Floctafenine; Methacholine

Increased Effect/Toxicity

Bisoprolol may increase the levels/effects of: Alpha-/Beta-Agonists (Direct-Acting); Alpha1-Blockers; Alpha2-Agonists; Amifostine; Antihypertensives; Antipsychotic Agents (Phenothiazines); Bupivacaine; Cardiac Glycosides; Cholinergic Agonists; Fingolimod; Hypotensive Agents; Insulin; Lidocaine; Lidocaine (Systemic); Lidocaine (Topical); Mepivacaine; Methacholine; Midodrine; RiTUXimab; Sulfonylureas

The levels/effects of Bisoprolol may be increased by: Acetylcholinesterase Inhibitors; Aminoquinolines (Antimalarial); Amiodarone; Anilidopiperidine Opioids; Antipsychotic Agents (Phenothiazines); Calcium Channel Blockers (Dihydropyridine); Calcium Channel Blockers (Nondihydropyridine); Conivaptan; CYP3A4 Inhibitors (Moderate); CYP3A4 Inhibitors (Strong); Dasatinib; Diazoxide; Dipyridamole; Disopyramide; Dronedarone; Floctafenine; Herbs (Hypotensive Properties); MAO Inhibitors; Pentoxifylline; Phosphodiesterase 5 Inhibitors; Propafenone; Prostacyclin Analogues; QuiNIDine; Reserpine

Decreased Effect

Bisoprolol may decrease the levels/effects of: Beta2-Agonists; Theophylline Derivatives

The levels/effects of Bisoprolol may be decreased by: Barbiturates; CYP3A4 Inducers (Strong); Deferasirox; Herbs (CYP3A4 Inducers); Herbs (Hypertensive Properties); Methylphenidate; Nonsteroidal Anti-Inflammatory Agents; Peginterferon Alfa-2b; Rifamycin Derivatives; Tocilizumab; Yohimbine

Ethanol/Nutrition/Herb Interactions Herb/Nutraceutical: Avoid dong quai if using for hypertension (has estrogenic activity). Avoid ephedra, yohimbe, ginseng (may worsen hypertension). Avoid garlic (may have increased antihypertensive effect).

Stability Store at controlled room temperature 20°C to 25°C (68°F to 77°F). Protect from moisture.

Mechanism of Action Selective inhibitor of $beta_1$-adrenergic receptors; competitively blocks $beta_1$-receptors, with little or no effect on $beta_2$-receptors at doses ≤20 mg

Pharmacodynamics/Kinetics

Onset of action: 1-2 hours

Absorption: Rapid and almost complete

Distribution: Widely; highest concentrations in heart, liver, lungs, and saliva; crosses blood-brain barrier

Protein binding: ~30%

Metabolism: Extensively hepatic; significant first-pass effect (~20%)

Bioavailability: ~80%

Half-life elimination: Normal renal function: 9-12 hours; Cl_{cr} <40 mL/minute: 27-36 hours; Hepatic cirrhosis: 8-22 hours

Time to peak: 2-4 hours

Excretion: Urine (50% as unchanged drug, remainder as inactive metabolites); feces (<2%)

Dosage Oral:

Adults:

Hypertension: Initial: 2.5-5 mg once daily; may be increased to 10 mg and then up to 20 mg once daily, if necessary; usual dose range (JNC 7): 2.5-10 mg once daily

Heart failure (unlabeled use): Initial: 1.25 mg once daily; maximum recommended dose: 10 mg once daily. **Note:** Increase dose gradually and monitor for signs and symptoms of CHF (Hunt, 2009; Lindenfeld, 2010)

Elderly: Refer to adult dosing.

Dosing adjustment in renal impairment: Cl_{cr} <40 mL/minute: Initial: 2.5 mg/day; increase cautiously.

Hemodialysis: Not dialyzable

Dietary Considerations May be taken without regard to meals.

Administration May be administered without regard to meals.

Monitoring Parameters Blood pressure, heart rate, ECG; serum glucose regularly (in patients with diabetes)

Dosage Forms Excipient information presented when available (limited, particularly for generics); consult specific product labeling.

Tablet, oral, as fumarate: 5 mg, 10 mg

Zebeta®: 5 mg [scored]

Zebeta®: 10 mg

Bisoprolol and Hydrochlorothiazide

(bis OH proe lol & hye droe klor oh THYE a zide)

Brand Names: U.S. Ziac®

Brand Names: Canada Ziac®

Index Terms Bisoprolol Fumarate and Hydrochlorothiazide; Hydrochlorothiazide and Bisoprolol

Pharmacologic Category Beta Blocker, Beta-1 Selective; Diuretic, Thiazide

Use Treatment of hypertension

Unlabeled Use Treatment of hypertension in the pediatric patient

Pregnancy Risk Factor C

Dosage Oral: Hypertension:

Children (unlabeled use): Initial: Bisoprolol 2.5 mg/hydrochlorothiazide 6.25 mg once daily; up to a maximum of bisoprolol 10 mg/hydrochlorothiazide 6.25 mg daily

Adults: Initial: Bisoprolol 2.5 mg and hydrochlorothiazide 6.25 mg once daily; dose may be titrated at ≥2-week intervals. Maximum dose (manufacturer recommended): Bisoprolol 20 mg/hydrochlorothiazide 12.5 mg once daily

Add-on/replacement therapy: Bisoprolol 2.5-20 mg and hydrochlorothiazide 6.25-12.5 mg once daily

Dosage adjustment in renal impairment: Caution should be used in dosing/titrating patients with renal impairment. Discontinue use with progressive renal impairment; use is contraindicated in patients with anuria.

Dosage adjustment in hepatic impairment: Caution should be used in dosing/titrating patients. Dosage adjustment necessary with severe impairment. Specific dosing recommendations are not provided in manufacturer labeling.

Additional Information Complete prescribing information for this medication should be consulted for additional detail.

Dosage Forms Excipient information presented when available (limited, particularly for generics); consult specific product labeling.

Tablet, oral: 2.5/6.25: Bisoprolol fumarate 2.5 mg and hydrochlorothiazide 6.25 mg; 5/6.25: Bisoprolol fumarate 5 mg and hydrochlorothiazide 6.25 mg; 10/6.25: Bisoprolol fumarate 10 mg and hydrochlorothiazide 6.25 mg

Ziac®: 2.5/6.25: Bisoprolol fumarate 2.5 mg and hydrochlorothiazide 6.25 mg

Ziac®: 5/6.25: Bisoprolol fumarate 5 mg and hydrochlorothiazide 6.25 mg

Ziac®: 10/6.25: Bisoprolol fumarate 10 mg and hydrochlorothiazide 6.25 mg

◆ **Bisoprolol Fumarate** *see* Bisoprolol *on page 220*

◆ **Bisoprolol Fumarate and Hydrochlorothiazide** *see* Bisoprolol and Hydrochlorothiazide *on page 221*

◆ **Bis-POM PMEA** *see* Adefovir *on page 44*

◆ **Bistropamide** *see* Tropicamide *on page 1743*

◆ **Bivalent Human Papillomavirus Vaccine** *see* Papillomavirus (Types 16, 18) Vaccine (Human, Recombinant) *on page 1292*

Bivalirudin (bye VAL i roo din)

Brand Names: U.S. Angiomax®

Brand Names: Canada Angiomax®

Index Terms Hirulog

Pharmacologic Category Anticoagulant, Thrombin Inhibitor

Use Anticoagulant used in conjunction with aspirin for patients with unstable angina undergoing percutaneous transluminal coronary angioplasty (PTCA) or percutaneous coronary intervention (PCI) with provisional glycoprotein IIb/IIIa inhibitor; anticoagulant used in conjunction with aspirin for patients undergoing PCI with (or at risk of) heparin-induced thrombocytopenia (HIT) / thrombosis syndrome (HITTS)

Unlabeled Use Heparin-induced thrombocytopenia (HIT); ST-elevation myocardial infarction (STEMI) undergoing primary PCI

Pregnancy Risk Factor B

Pregnancy Considerations Although animal studies have not shown harm to the fetus, safety and efficacy for use in pregnant women have not been established. Bivalirudin is used in conjunction with aspirin, which may lead to maternal or fetal adverse effects, especially during the third trimester. Use during pregnancy only if clearly needed.

Lactation Excretion in breast milk unknown/use caution

Contraindications Hypersensitivity to bivalirudin or any component of the formulation; active major bleeding

Warnings/Precautions Not for intramuscular use. Safety and efficacy have not been established in patients with unstable angina or acute coronary syndromes who are not undergoing PTCA or PCI. Increased risk of thrombus formation (some fatal) has been reported with bivalirudin use in gamma brachytherapy. As with all anticoagulants, bleeding may occur at any site and should be considered following an unexplained fall in blood pressure or hematocrit, or any unexplained symptom. Use with caution in patients with disease states associated with increased risk of bleeding. Use with caution in patients with renal impairment; dosage reduction required.

Adverse Reactions As with all anticoagulants, bleeding is the major adverse effect of bivalirudin. Hemorrhage may occur at virtually any site. Risk is dependent on multiple variables, including the intensity of anticoagulation, concurrent use of a glycoprotein IIb/IIIa inhibitor, and patient susceptibility. Additional adverse effects are often related to idiosyncratic reactions, and the frequency is difficult to estimate. Adverse reactions reported were generally less than those seen with heparin.

>10%:

Cardiovascular: Hypotension (≤12%)

Central nervous system: Pain (≤15%), headache (≤12%)

Gastrointestinal: Nausea (≤15%)

Hematologic: Minor hemorrhage (REPLACE-2 study: Protocol defined: 14%, compared to 26% with heparin; TIMI defined: 1%, compared to 3% with heparin)

Neuromuscular & skeletal: Back pain (9% to 42%)

1% to 10%:

Cardiovascular: Hypertension (6%), bradycardia (5%), angina (≤5%)

Central nervous system: Insomnia (7%), anxiety (6%), fever (5%), nervousness (5%)

Gastrointestinal: Vomiting (≤6%), dyspepsia (5%), abdominal pain (5%)

Genitourinary: Urinary retention (4%)

Hematologic: Major hemorrhage (Protocol defined: 2% to 4%, compared to 4% to 9% with heparin; REPLACE-2 Study: TIMI defined: 0.6%, compared to 0.9% with heparin), transfusion required (1% to 2%, compared to 2% to 6% with heparin)

Local: Injection site pain (≤8%)

Neuromuscular & skeletal: Pelvic pain (6%)

<1% (Limited to important or life-threatening): Allergic reaction (including anaphylaxis), cerebral ischemia, confusion, facial paralysis, fatal bleeding, infection, intracranial bleeding, pulmonary edema, renal failure, retroperitoneal bleeding, syncope, thrombocytopenia, thrombus formation (during PCI, including intracoronary brachytherapy), ventricular fibrillation

Drug Interactions

Metabolism/Transport Effects None known.

Avoid Concomitant Use

Avoid concomitant use of Bivalirudin with any of the following: Rivaroxaban

Increased Effect/Toxicity

Bivalirudin may increase the levels/effects of: Anticoagulants; Collagenase (Systemic); Deferasirox; Ibritumomab; Rivaroxaban; Tositumomab and Iodine I 131 Tositumomab

The levels/effects of Bivalirudin may be increased by: Antiplatelet Agents; Dasatinib; Herbs (Anticoagulant/Antiplatelet Properties); Nonsteroidal Anti-Inflammatory Agents; Pentosan Polysulfate Sodium; Prostacyclin Analogues; Salicylates; Thrombolytic Agents

Decreased Effect There are no known significant interactions involving a decrease in effect.

Stability Store unopened vials at 20°C to 25°C (68°F to 77°F); excursions permitted between 15°C to 30°C. Reconstitute each 250 mg with 5 mL SWFI. Gently swirl to dissolve. Further dilution in D_5W or NS (50 mL to make 5 mg/mL solution **or** 500 mL to make 0.5 mg/mL solution) is required prior to infusion. Following reconstitution, vials should be stored at 2°C to 8°C for up to 24 hours. Do not freeze. Final dilutions of 0.5 mg/mL or 5 mg/mL are stable at room temperature for up to 24 hours.

Mechanism of Action Bivalirudin acts as a specific and reversible direct thrombin inhibitor; it binds to the catalytic and anionic exosite of both circulating and clot-bound thrombin. Catalytic binding site occupation functionally inhibits coagulant effects by preventing thrombin-mediated cleavage of fibrinogen to fibrin monomers, and activation of factors V, VIII, and XIII. Shows linear dose- and concentration-dependent prolongation of ACT, aPTT, PT, and TT.

Pharmacodynamics/Kinetics

Onset of action: Immediate

Duration: Coagulation times return to baseline ~1 hour following discontinuation of infusion

Distribution: 0.2 L/kg

Protein binding, plasma: Does not bind other than thrombin

Metabolism: Blood proteases

Half-life elimination: Normal renal function (Cl_{cr} ≥90 mL/minute): 25 minutes; Severe renal impairment (Cl_{cr} 10-29 mL/minute): 57 minutes; Dialysis-dependent patients (off dialysis): 3.5 hours

Excretion: Urine (20%), proteolytic cleavage

Dosage I.V.: Adults: **Note:** If clinically indicated, a glycoprotein IIb/IIIa inhibitor may be concomitantly administered during percutaneous coronary intervention (PCI). In addition to aspirin, concomitant administration of clopidogrel or prasugrel is also recommended for patients undergoing PCI (King, 2005; Kushner, 2009).

PTCA/PCI with or without HIT/HITTS: Initial: 0.75 mg/kg bolus immediately prior to procedure, followed by 1.75 mg/kg/hour for the duration of procedure and up to 4 hours postprocedure if needed; determine ACT 5 minutes after bolus dose; may administer additional bolus of 0.3 mg/kg if necessary. If continued anticoagulation is needed after the initial 4-hour postprocedure infusion, the infusion may be continued at 0.2 mg/kg/hour for up to an additional 20 hours.

If patient received prior unfractionated heparin: Discontinue heparin, wait 30 minutes, then initiate bivalirudin (Levine, 2011).

Unstable angina/non-ST-elevation myocardial infarction (UA/NSTEMI) (moderate-high risk) undergoing early invasive strategy (unlabeled dose): Initial: 0.1 mg/kg bolus, followed by 0.25 mg/kg/hour. Once PCI is determined to be necessary, give an additional bolus of 0.5 mg/kg and increase infusion rate to 1.75 mg/kg/hour; may discontinue at end of procedure or continue for up to 4 hours postprocedure if necessary. If cardiac surgery is deemed necessary, discontinue bivalirudin 3 hours prior to surgery and dose with unfractionated heparin per institutional practice (Anderson, 2007; Stone, 2006).

STEMI undergoing primary PCI (unlabeled use): Initial: 0.75 mg/kg bolus, followed by 1.75 mg/kg/hour for the duration of procedure; may continue postprocedure at a reduced dose if clinically indicated. **Note:** For patients who received unfractionated heparin (UFH) prior to procedure, wait 30 minutes before administering bivalirudin bolus dose (Kushner, 2009; Stone, 2008).

Cardiac surgery in patients with acute or subacute (if surgery cannot be delayed) heparin-induced thrombocytopenia (unlabeled use; Warkentin, 2008):

Off-pump: Initial bolus: 0.75 mg/kg, followed by continuous infusion 1.75 mg/kg/hour to maintain ACT >300 seconds

On-pump: Initial bolus: 1 mg/kg, followed by continuous infusion 2.5 mg/kg/hour; 50 mg bolus added to priming solution of cardiopulmonary bypass (CPB) circuit. Additional boluses of 0.1-0.5 mg/kg may be given to maintain ACT >2.5 times baseline ACT. **Note:** Special maneuvers needed to prevent stasis and consequent clotting within CPB circuit during or after surgery.

Heparin-induced thrombocytopenia (HIT) (unlabeled use): Initial dose: 0.15-0.2 mg/kg/hour; adjust to aPTT 1.5-2.5 times baseline value (Warkentin, 2008)

Elderly: No dosage adjustment is needed in elderly patients with normal renal function. Puncture site hemorrhage and catheterization site hemorrhage were seen more often in patients ≥65 years of age.

Dosage adjustment in renal impairment: Infusion dose should be reduced based on degree of renal impairment; initial bolus dose remains unchanged; monitor activated coagulation time (ACT) or aPTT depending on indication.

For use in PCI:

Cl_{cr} ≥30 mL/minute: No adjustment required

Cl_{cr} 10-29 mL/minute: Decrease infusion rate to 1 mg/kg/hour

Dialysis-dependent patients (off dialysis during administration): Decrease infusion rate to 0.25 mg/kg/hour

Hemodialysis: Approximately 25% removed during hemodialysis

For use in HIT: No dosage adjustment provided in manufacturer's labeling for this population; however, the following dose ranges have been observed in small retrospective observational studies (Kiser 2006; Kiser, 2008; Tsu, 2011). Of note, critically-ill patients comprised a significant proportion of patients in these observational studies. The following dose recommendations are based on the mean dose achieving aPTT goal within these studies; overlaps may exist; **Note:** The Cockcroft-Gault equation was used in all studies to define creatinine clearance:

Cl_{cr} >60 mL/minute: 0.13 mg/kg/hour

Cl_{cr} 30-60 mL/minute: 0.08-0.1 mg/kg/hour

Cl_{cr} <30 mL/minute: 0.04-0.05 mg/kg/hour

Intermittent hemodialysis (IHD): 0.07 mg/kg/hour (Tsu, 2011)

CRRT (eg, CVVH or CVVHDF): 0.03-0.07 mg/kg/hour (Kiser, 2006; Tsu, 2011)

Sustained low-efficiency daily diafiltration (SLEDD): 0.09 mg/kg/hour (Tsu, 2011)

Dosage adjustment in hepatic impairment: No dosage adjustment is needed

Administration For I.V. administration only.

Monitoring Parameters Depends upon indication for use of bivalirudin: ACT or aPTT

Test Interactions PT/INR levels may become elevated in the absence of warfarin. If warfarin is initiated, initial PT/INR goals while on bivalirudin may require modification.

Dosage Forms Excipient information presented when available (limited, particularly for generics); consult specific product labeling.

Injection, powder for reconstitution:

Angiomax®: 250 mg [contains sodium 12.5 mg/vial]

- ◆ **Bi-Zets [OTC]** *see* Benzocaine *on page 202*
- ◆ **BL4162A** *see* Anagrelide *on page 119*
- ◆ **Blenoxane** *see* Bleomycin *on page 224*
- ◆ **Blenoxane® (Can)** *see* Bleomycin *on page 224*
- ◆ **Bleo** *see* Bleomycin *on page 224*

Bleomycin (blee oh MYE sin)

Brand Names: Canada Blenoxane®; Bleomycin Injection, USP

Index Terms Blenoxane; Bleo; Bleomycin Sulfate; BLM

Pharmacologic Category Antineoplastic Agent, Antibiotic

Use Treatment of squamous cell carcinomas of the head and neck, penis, cervix, or vulva, testicular carcinoma, Hodgkin's lymphoma, and non-Hodgkin's lymphoma; sclerosing agent for malignant pleural effusion

Unlabeled Use Treatment of ovarian germ cell tumors

Pregnancy Risk Factor D

Pregnancy Considerations Animal studies have demonstrated teratogenic and abortifacient effects. There are no adequate and well-controlled studies in pregnant women. Women of childbearing potential should avoid becoming pregnant during treatment.

Lactation Excretion in breast milk unknown/not recommended

Contraindications Hypersensitivity to bleomycin or any component of the formulation

Warnings/Precautions Hazardous agent - use appropriate precautions for handling and disposal. **[U.S. Boxed Warning]: Occurrence of pulmonary fibrosis (commonly presenting as pneumonitis; occasionally progressing to pulmonary fibrosis) is the most severe toxicity. Risk is higher in elderly patients or patients receiving >400 units total lifetime dose;** other possible risk factors include smoking and patients with prior radiation therapy or receiving concurrent oxygen. **A severe idiosyncratic reaction consisting of hypotension, mental confusion, fever, chills, and wheezing (similar to anaphylaxis) has been reported in 1% of lymphoma patients treated with bleomycin.** Since these reactions usually occur after the first or second dose, careful monitoring is essential after these doses. Use caution when administering O_2 during surgery to patients who have received bleomycin; the risk of bleomycin-related pulmonary toxicity is increased. Use caution with renal impairment (Cl_{cr} <50 mL/minute), may require dose adjustment. May cause renal or hepatic toxicity. **[U.S. Boxed Warning]: Should be administered under the supervision of an experienced cancer chemotherapy physician.**

Adverse Reactions

>10%:

Dermatologic: Pain at the tumor site, phlebitis. About 50% of patients develop erythema, rash, striae, induration, hyperkeratosis, vesiculation, and peeling of the skin, particularly on the palmar and plantar surfaces of the hands and feet. Hyperpigmentation (50%), alopecia, nailbed changes may also occur. These effects appear dose related and reversible with discontinuation.

Gastrointestinal: Stomatitis and mucositis (30%), anorexia, weight loss

Respiratory: Tachypnea, rales, acute or chronic interstitial pneumonitis, and pulmonary fibrosis (5% to 10%); hypoxia and death (1%). Symptoms include cough, dyspnea, and bilateral pulmonary infiltrates. The pathogenesis is not certain, but may be due to damage of pulmonary, vascular, or connective tissue. Response to steroid therapy is variable and somewhat controversial.

Miscellaneous: Acute febrile reactions (25% to 50%)

1% to 10%:

Dermatologic: Skin thickening, diffuse scleroderma, onycholysis, pruritus

Miscellaneous: Anaphylactoid-like reactions (characterized by hypotension, confusion, fever, chills, and wheezing; onset may be immediate or delayed for several hours); idiosyncratic reactions (1% in lymphoma patients)

<1% (Limited to important or life-threatening): Angioedema, cerebrovascular accident, cerebral arteritis, chest pain, coronary artery disease, flagellate hyperpigmentation, hepatotoxicity, malaise, MI, myelosuppression (rare), myocardial ischemia, nausea, pericarditis, Raynaud's phenomenon, renal toxicity, scleroderma-like skin changes, Stevens-Johnson syndrome, thrombotic microangiopathy, toxic epidermal necrolysis, vomiting

Drug Interactions

Metabolism/Transport Effects None known.

Avoid Concomitant Use

Avoid concomitant use of Bleomycin with any of the following: BCG; Brentuximab Vedotin; Natalizumab; Pimecrolimus; Tacrolimus (Topical); Vaccines (Live)

Increased Effect/Toxicity

Bleomycin may increase the levels/effects of: Leflunomide; Natalizumab; Vaccines (Live)

The levels/effects of Bleomycin may be increased by: Brentuximab Vedotin; Denosumab; Filgrastim; Gemcitabine; Pimecrolimus; Roflumilast; Sargramostim; Tacrolimus (Topical); Trastuzumab

Decreased Effect

Bleomycin may decrease the levels/effects of: BCG; Cardiac Glycosides; Coccidioidin Skin Test; Sipuleucel-T; Vaccines (Inactivated); Vaccines (Live)

The levels/effects of Bleomycin may be decreased by: Echinacea

Stability

Refrigerate intact vials of powder. Intact vials are stable for up to 4 weeks at room temperature. Solutions for infusion are stable for 96 hours at room temperature and 14 days under refrigeration.

For I.V. use, reconstitute 15-unit vial with 5 mL NS and the 30-unit vial with 10 mL NS; for I.M. or SubQ use, reconstitute 15-unit vial with 1-5 mL of SWFI, BWFI, or NS and the 30-unit vial with 2-10 mL of SWFI, BWFI, or NS. Use appropriate precautions for handling and disposal. Solutions reconstituted in NS for are stable for up to 28 days refrigerated and 14 days at room temperature; however, the manufacturer recommends stability of 24 hours in NS at room temperature.

For intrapleural use, mix in 50-100 mL of NS.

Mechanism of Action Inhibits synthesis of DNA; binds to DNA leading to single- and double-strand breaks; also inhibits (to a lesser degree) RNA and protein synthesis

Pharmacodynamics/Kinetics

Absorption: I.M. and intrapleural administration: 30% to 50% of I.V. serum concentrations; intraperitoneal and SubQ routes produce serum concentrations equal to those of I.V.

Distribution: V_d: 22 L/m^2; highest concentrations in skin, kidney, lung, heart tissues; lowest in testes and GI tract; does not cross blood-brain barrier

Protein binding: 1%

Metabolism: Via several tissues including hepatic, GI tract, skin, pulmonary, renal, and serum

Half-life elimination: Biphasic (renal function dependent):

Normal renal function: Initial: 1.3 hours; Terminal: 9 hours

End-stage renal disease: Initial: 2 hours; Terminal: 30 hours

Time to peak, serum: I.M.: Within 30 minutes

Excretion: Urine (50% to 70% as active drug)

Dosage The risk for pulmonary toxicity increases with age >70 years and cumulative lifetime dose of >400 units; 1 unit = 1 mg; details concerning dosage in combination regimens should also be consulted.

Children and Adults: Test dose for lymphoma patients: I.M., I.V., SubQ: Because of the possibility of an anaphylactoid reaction, the manufacturer recommends administering 1-2 units of bleomycin before the first 1-2 doses; monitor vital signs every 15 minutes; wait a minimum of 1 hour before administering remainder of dose; if no acute reaction occurs, then the regular dosage schedule may be followed. **Note:** Test doses may not be predictive of a reaction (Lam, 2005) and/or may produce false-negative results.

I.V.:

Children: Hodgkin's lymphoma (unlabeled dosing; combination regimen): ABVD: 10 units/m^2 days 1 and 15 of a 28-day treatment cycle (Hutchinson, 1998)

Adults:

Hodgkin's lymphoma (unlabeled dosing; combination regimens):

ABVD: 10 units/m^2 days 1 and 15 of a 28-day treatment cycle (Straus, 2004)

BEACOPP: 10 units/m^2 day 8 of a 21-day treatment cycle (Dann, 2007; Diehl, 2003)

Stanford V: 5 units/m^2/dose in weeks 2, 4, 6, 8, 10 and 12 (Horning, 2000; Horning, 2002)

Testicular cancer (unlabeled dosing; combination therapy): 30 units/dose days 1, 8, and 15 of a 21-day treatment cycle for 4 cycles (Culine, 2008; Nichols, 1998)

Ovarian germ cell cancer (unlabeled use; combination therapy): 30 units/dose days 1, 8, and 15 of a 21-day treatment cycle for 3 cycles (Williams, 1994) **or** 15 units/m^2 day 1 of a 21-day treatment cycle for 4 cycles (Cushing, 2004)

Intrapleural: Adults: Malignant pleural effusion: 60 units as a single instillation; mix in 50-100 mL of NS

Dosing adjustment in renal impairment:

The FDA-approved labeling recommends the following adjustments:

Cl_{cr} >50 mL/minute: No adjustment required

Cl_{cr} 40-50 mL/minute: Administer 70% of normal dose

Cl_{cr} 30-40 mL/minute: Administer 60% of normal dose

Cl_{cr} 20-30 mL/minute: Administer 55% of normal dose

Cl_{cr} 10-20 mL/minute: Administer 45% of normal dose

Cl_{cr} 5-10 mL/minute: Administer 40% of normal dose

The following guidelines have been used by some clinicians:

Aronoff, 2007: Adults: Continuous renal replacement therapy (CRRT): Administer 75% of dose

Kintzel, 1995:

Cl_{cr} 46-60 mL/minute: Administer 70% of dose

Cl_{cr} 31-45 mL/minute: Administer 60% of dose

Cl_{cr} <30 mL/minute: Consider use of alternative drug

Dosing adjustment in hepatic impairment: Not studied in patients with hepatic impairment; adjustment for hepatic impairment may be needed.

Administration

I.V. doses should be administered slowly over 10 minutes.

I.M. or SubQ: May cause pain at injection site

Intrapleural: 60 units in 50-100 mL NS; use of topical anesthetics or narcotic analgesia is usually not necessary

Monitoring Parameters Pulmonary function tests (total lung volume, forced vital capacity, carbon monoxide diffusion), renal function, liver function, chest x-ray, temperature initially; check body weight at regular intervals

Dosage Forms Excipient information presented when available (limited, particularly for generics); consult specific product labeling.

Injection, powder for reconstitution: 15 units, 30 units

- ◆ **Bleomycin Injection, USP (Can)** *see* Bleomycin *on page 224*
- ◆ **Bleomycin Sulfate** *see* Bleomycin *on page 224*
- ◆ **Bleph®-10** *see* Sulfacetamide (Ophthalmic) *on page 1599*
- ◆ **Bleph 10 DPS (Can)** *see* Sulfacetamide (Ophthalmic) *on page 1599*
- ◆ **Blephamide®** *see* Sulfacetamide and Prednisolone *on page 1600*
- ◆ **Blis-To-Sol® [OTC]** *see* Tolnaftate *on page 1704*
- ◆ **BLM** *see* Bleomycin *on page 224*
- ◆ **BMS-188667** *see* Abatacept *on page 20*
- ◆ **BMS-224818** *see* Belatacept *on page 194*
- ◆ **BMS-232632** *see* Atazanavir *on page 158*
- ◆ **BMS-247550** *see* Ixabepilone *on page 945*
- ◆ **BMS 337039** *see* ARIPiprazole *on page 142*
- ◆ **BMS-354825** *see* Dasatinib *on page 454*
- ◆ **BMS-477118** *see* Saxagliptin *on page 1540*
- ◆ **B&O** *see* Belladonna and Opium *on page 197*

Boceprevir (boe SE pre vir)

Brand Names: U.S. Victrelis™

Brand Names: Canada Victrelis™

Index Terms SCH503034

Pharmacologic Category Antiviral Agent; Protease Inhibitor

Use Treatment of chronic hepatitis C (CHC) genotype 1 (in combination with peginterferon alfa and ribavirin) in adult patients with compensated liver disease (including cirrhosis) who were previously untreated or have failed prior therapy with peginterferon alfa and ribavirin therapy

Pregnancy Risk Factor B / X (in combination with ribavirin)

Pregnancy Considerations Adverse events were not observed in boceprevir animal developmental studies; however, boceprevir must not be used as monotherapy (must be used in combination with peginterferon alfa and ribavirin). Significant ribavirin teratogenic effects have been observed in all animal studies at ~0.01 times the maximum recommended daily human dose. Use of ribavirin is contraindicated in pregnancy. In addition, animal studies with interferons have demonstrated abortifacient effects. Negative pregnancy test is required before initiation and monthly thereafter. Avoid pregnancy in female patients and female partners of male patients during therapy by using two effective forms of contraception; continue contraceptive measures for at least 6 months after completion of therapy. If patient or female partner becomes pregnant during treatment, she should be counseled about potential risks of exposure. If pregnancy occurs during use or within 6 months after treatment, report to the ribavirin pregnancy registry (800-593-2214).

Lactation Excretion in breast milk unknown/not recommended

Medication Guide Available Yes

Contraindications Hypersensitivity to boceprevir or any component of the formulation; pregnancy; male partners of pregnant women

Coadministration with CYP 3A4/5 highly-dependent substrates (alfuzosin, cisapride, drospirenone, ergot derivatives, lovastatin, midazolam [oral], pimozide, sildenafil/tadalafil [when used for treatment of pulmonary arterial hypertension], simvastatin, triazolam) or strong CYP 3A4/5 inducers (carbamazepine, phenobarbital, phenytoin, rifampin, St John's wort)

Refer to Peginterferon Alfa and Ribavirin monographs for individual product contraindications.

Canadian labeling: Additional contraindications (not in U.S. labeling): Autoimmune hepatitis, hepatic decompensation (Child-Pugh class B or C)

Warnings/Precautions Avoid pregnancy in female patients and female partners of male patients, during therapy, and for at least 6 months after treatment; two forms of contraception should be used. Safety and efficacy have not been established in patients who have uncompensated cirrhosis, received organ transplants, or been coinfected with hepatitis B or HIV. Monotherapy is not effective for chronic hepatitis C infection. Safety and efficacy have not been established in patients documented to have less than a 2-$\log_{10}$ HCV-RNA decline by treatment week 12 with prior peginterferon alfa and ribavirin therapy. Patients who have less than 0.5-$\log_{10}$ HCV-RNA decline at treatment week 4 with peginterferon alfa and ribavirin when **initiating** boceprevir therapy are predicted to have less than a 2-$\log_{10}$ HCV-RNA decline by treatment week 12. Those poor responders treated with boceprevir will likely not have a sustained virologic response and have a predisposition to viral resistance at treatment failure.

Anemia has been reported with peginterferon alfa and ribavirin; addition of boceprevir is associated with further hemoglobin decreases. With anemia management, average hemoglobin decrease in clinical trials was ~1 g/dL. The addition of boceprevir to peginterferon alfa and ribavirin therapy is also associated with a higher incidence of neutropenia. Dose modifications of peginterferon alfa and ribavirin were needed more often in patients also taking boceprevir. Complete blood counts should be obtained pretreatment and at weeks 4, 8, and 12, as well as other times during treatment. May be severe or life-threatening (rare); discontinuation of therapy may be necessary.

Adverse Reactions

>10%:

- Central nervous system: Fatigue (55% to 58%), chills (33% to 34%), insomnia (30% to 34%), irritability (21% to 22%), dizziness (16% to 19%), headache
- Dermatologic: Alopecia (22% to 27%), dry skin (18% to 22%), rash (16% to 17%)
- Gastrointestinal: Nausea (43% to 46%), abnormal taste (35% to 44%), appetite decreased (25% to 26%), diarrhea (24% to 25%), vomiting (15% to 20%), xerostomia (11% to 15%)
- Hematologic: Anemia (45% to 50%), neutropenia (14% to 31%)
- Neuromuscular & skeletal: Arthralgia (19% to 23%), weakness (15% to 21%)
- Respiratory: Dyspnea (8% to 11%)

1% to 10%: Hematologic: Thrombocytopenia

<1% (Limited to important or life-threatening): Thromboembolic events

Drug Interactions

Metabolism/Transport Effects **Substrate** of CYP3A4 (major), P-glycoprotein; **Note:** Assignment of Major/Minor substrate status based on clinically relevant drug interaction potential; **Inhibits** CYP3A4 (strong), P-glycoprotein

Avoid Concomitant Use

Avoid concomitant use of Boceprevir with any of the following: Alfuzosin; CarBAMazepine; Cisapride; Conivaptan; Crizotinib; Dihydroergotamine; Dronedarone; Drospirenone; Efavirenz; Eplerenone; Ergotamine; Everolimus; Fluticasone (Oral Inhalation); Fosphenytoin; Halofantrine; Lapatinib; Lovastatin; Lurasidone; Methylergonovine; Midazolam; Nilotinib; Nisoldipine; PHENobarbital; Phenytoin; Pimozide; Primidone; Ranolazine; Rifabutin; Rifampin; Rivaroxaban; RomiDEPsin; Salmeterol; Sildenafil; Silodosin; Simvastatin; St Johns Wort; Tadalafil; Tamsulosin; Ticagrelor; Tolvaptan; Toremifene; Triazolam

Increased Effect/Toxicity

Boceprevir may increase the levels/effects of: Alfuzosin; Almotriptan; Alosetron; ALPRAZolam; Amiodarone; ARIPiprazole; Atorvastatin; Bepridil [Off Market]; Bortezomib; Brentuximab Vedotin; Brinzolamide; Budesonide (Nasal); Budesonide (Systemic, Oral Inhalation); Buprenorphine; Ciclesonide; Cisapride; Colchicine; Conivaptan; Contraceptives (Progestins); Corticosteroids (Orally Inhaled); Crizotinib; CYP3A4 Substrates; Desipramine; Dienogest; Digoxin; Dihydroergotamine; Dronedarone; Drospirenone; Dutasteride; Efavirenz; Eplerenone; Ergotamine; Everolimus; FentaNYL; Fesoterodine; Flecainide; Fluticasone (Nasal); Fluticasone (Oral Inhalation); GuanFACINE; Halofantrine; Iloperidone; Itraconazole; Ixabepilone; Ketoconazole; Ketoconazole (Systemic); Lapatinib; Lovastatin; Lumefantrine; Lurasidone; Maraviroc; Methadone; Methylergonovine; MethylPREDNISolone; Midazolam; Nilotinib; Nisoldipine; Paricalcitol; Pazopanib; Pimecrolimus; Pimozide; Posaconazole; Propafenone; QuiNIDine; Ranolazine; Rifabutin; Rivaroxaban; RomiDEPsin; Ruxolitinib; Salmeterol; Saxagliptin; Sildenafil; Silodosin; Simvastatin; SORAfenib; Tadalafil; Tamsulosin; Ticagrelor; Tolterodine; Tolvaptan; Toremifene; Triazolam; Vardenafil; Vemurafenib; Vilazodone; Voriconazole; Warfarin; Zuclopenthixol

The levels/effects of Boceprevir may be increased by: Itraconazole; Ketoconazole; Ketoconazole (Systemic); Posaconazole; Voriconazole

Decreased Effect

Boceprevir may decrease the levels/effects of: Buprenorphine; Contraceptives (Estrogens); Methadone; Prasugrel; Ticagrelor; Warfarin

The levels/effects of Boceprevir may be decreased by: CarBAMazepine; CYP3A4 Inducers (Strong); Deferasirox; Efavirenz; Fosphenytoin; PHENobarbital; Phenytoin; Primidone; Rifabutin; Rifampin; St Johns Wort; Tocilizumab

Stability Store refrigerated at 2°C to 8°C (36°F to 46°F). After dispensing, may be stored at room temperature of up to 25°C (77°F) for 3 months; keep container closed tightly; avoid excessive heat.

Mechanism of Action Binds reversibly to nonstructural protein 3 (NS 3) serine protease and inhibits replication of the hepatitis C virus. Considered a direct-acting antiviral treatment for HCV, also called a specifically targeted antiviral therapy for HCV (STAT-C).

Pharmacodynamics/Kinetics

Absorption: Food (type or timing is not important) enhances absorption by up to 65%

Distribution: V_d: ~772 L

Protein binding: ~75%

Metabolism: Primarily hepatic via aldo-ketoreductase pathway to inactive metabolites. Also some oxidative CYP 3A4/5 metabolism.

Half-life elimination: Plasma: Adults: ~3 hours

Time to peak, serum: 2 hours

Excretion: Feces (79%); urine (9%)

Dosage Oral: Adults: 800 mg 3 times/day (in combination with peginterferon alfa and ribavirin)

Treatment-naive patients (interferon-responsive at week 4):

Weeks 1-4: Peginterferon alfa with concomitant ribavirin only

Weeks 5-8: Boceprevir 800 mg 3 times/day with continued peginterferon alfa and ribavirin

Weeks 9-24 (based on HCV-RNA results at week 8):

HCV-RNA **undetectable** or **detectable** at a level of <100 int. units/mL: Boceprevir 800 mg 3 times/day with continued peginterferon alfa and ribavirin

HCV-RNA ≥100 int. units/mL (treatment futility): Recheck HCV-RNA at week 12. If HCV-RNA ≥100 int. units/mL at week 12, discontinue treatment (boceprevir, peginterferon alfa, and ribavirin)

Weeks ≥24:

HCV-RNA **undetectable** at week 8 and week 24: Boceprevir 800 mg 3 times/day with continued peginterferon alfa and ribavirin for 4 additional weeks (through week 28)

HCV-RNA **detectable** at Week 8 and **undetectable** at week 24:

U.S. labeling: Boceprevir 800 mg 3 times/day with continued peginterferon alfa and ribavirin for 12 additional weeks (through week 36), followed by peginterferon alfa and ribavirin for additional 12 weeks (through week 48)

Canadian labeling: Boceprevir 800 mg 3 times/day with continued peginterferon alfa and ribavirin for 4 additional weeks (through week 28), followed by peginterferon alfa and ribavirin for additional 20 weeks (through week 48)

HCV-RNA **detectable** at week 24: Discontinue treatment (boceprevir, peginterferon alfa, and ribavirin)

Treatment-naive patients (interferon nonresponsive [<0.5-log_{10} HCV-RNA decline in viral load] at week 4):

Weeks 1-4: Peginterferon alfa with concomitant ribavirin only

Weeks 5-48: Boceprevir 800 mg 3 times/day with continued peginterferon alfa and ribavirin

Previously-treated patients (partial response, relapsed):

Note: Previously treated does not include prior treatment with boceprevir. "Partial response" includes patients with a >2-log_{10} HCV-RNA decrease by week 12, but a nonsustained virologic response thereafter. "Relapsed" includes patients with an undetectable HCV-RNA upon completion of previous treatment, but with detectable HCV-RNA during the follow-up period.

Weeks 1-4: Peginterferon alfa with concomitant ribavirin only

Weeks 5-8: Boceprevir 800 mg 3 times/day with continued peginterferon alfa and ribavirin

Weeks 9-24 (based on HCV-RNA results at week 8):

HCV-RNA **undetectable** or <100 int. units/mL: Boceprevir 800 mg 3 times/day with continued peginterferon alfa and ribavirin

HCV-RNA ≥100 int. units/mL: Recheck HCV-RNA at week 12. If HCV-RNA ≥100 int. units/mL at week 12, discontinue treatment (boceprevir, peginterferon alfa, and ribavirin)

Weeks ≥24:

HCV-RNA **undetectable** at week 8 and week 24: Boceprevir 800 mg 3 times/day with continued peginterferon alfa and ribavirin for 12 additional weeks (through week 36)

HCV-RNA **detectable** at Week 8 and **undetectable** at week 24: Boceprevir 800 mg 3 times/day with continued peginterferon alfa and ribavirin for 12 additional weeks (through week 36), followed by peginterferon alfa and ribavirin for additional 12 weeks (through week 48)

HCV-RNA **detectable** at week 24: Discontinue treatment (boceprevir, peginterferon alfa, and ribavirin)

Previously treated patients with <2-log_{10} HCV-RNA decline at week 12 (null responders):

Weeks 1-4: Peginterferon alfa with concomitant ribavirin only

Weeks 5-48: Boceprevir 800 mg 3 times/day with continued peginterferon alfa and ribavirin

Cirrhosis, compensated:

Weeks 1-4: Peginterferon alfa with concomitant ribavirin only

Weeks 5-48: Boceprevir 800 mg 3 times/day with continued peginterferon alfa and ribavirin

Dosage adjustment in renal impairment: No dosage adjustments are recommended. Not removed by hemodialysis.

Dosage adjustment in hepatic impairment:

Mild, moderate, or severe impairment: No dosage adjustments are recommended.

Decompensated cirrhosis: Has not been studied; also refer to Peginterferon Alfa and Ribavirin individual monographs.

Dietary Considerations Take with food. The type or timing of a meal is not important as long as dose is taken with food.

Administration Administer with food. Doses should be taken approximately every 7-9 hours. Administer concurrently with peginterferon alfa and ribavirin.

Monitoring Parameters

CBC with differential at baseline and weeks 4, 8 and 12, then periodically (and when clinically indicated)

Serum HCV RNA at baseline, weeks 4, 8, 12 and 24, end of treatment, during treatment follow up, and when clinically indicated

Pretreatment and monthly pregnancy test up to 6 months following discontinuation of therapy for women of childbearing age

Reference Range

Treatment futility: HCV-RNA ≥100 int. units/mL at treatment week 12 or confirmed, detectable HCV-RNA at treatment week 24

Rapid virological response (RVR): Absence of detectable HCV RNA after 4 weeks of treatment

Early viral response (EVR): ≥2-log decrease in HCV RNA after 8-12 weeks of treatment

End of treatment response (ETR): Absence of detectable HCV RNA at end of the recommended treatment period

Sustained treatment response (STR): Absence of HCV RNA in the serum 6 months following completion of full treatment course

Additional Information In clinical studies of treatment-naive patients, a sustained virologic response (SVR) with peginterferon alfa, ribavirin, and boceprevir was achieved in ~68% of non-African-American patients versus 40% of controls (peginterferon alfa and ribavirin only). African-American patients had a lower rate of SVR compared to controls (42% to 53% dependent upon treatment duration versus 23% of controls). Rapid virologic response (RVR) at week 4 of lead-in treatment with peginterferon alfa and ribavirin can predict patient success after the addition of boceprevir and guide treatment duration. Patients who have marginal response during the lead-in treatment phase have a lower SVR after the addition of boceprevir; these patients may need close monitoring for regimen adherence and resistance development.

Dosage Forms Excipient information presented when available (limited, particularly for generics); consult specific product labeling.

Capsule, oral:

Victrelis™: 200 mg

- **Boil-Ease® Pain Relieving [OTC]** *see* Benzocaine *on page 202*
- **BOL-303224-A** *see* Besifloxacin *on page 207*
- **Bonamine™ (Can)** *see* Meclizine *on page 1057*
- **Bonine® [OTC]** *see* Meclizine *on page 1057*
- **Bonine® (Can)** *see* Meclizine *on page 1057*
- **Boniva®** *see* Ibandronate *on page 856*
- **Boostrix®** *see* Diphtheria and Tetanus Toxoids, and Acellular Pertussis Vaccine *on page 523*

Bortezomib (bore TEZ oh mib)

Brand Names: U.S. Velcade®

Brand Names: Canada Velcade®

Index Terms LDP-341; MLN341; PS-341

Pharmacologic Category Antineoplastic Agent; Proteasome Inhibitor

Use Treatment of multiple myeloma; treatment of relapsed or refractory mantle cell lymphoma

Unlabeled Use Treatment of Waldenström's macroglobulinemia, peripheral T-cell lymphoma, cutaneous T-Cell lymphomas (mycosis fungoides), systemic light-chain amyloidosis

Pregnancy Risk Factor D

Pregnancy Considerations Adverse effects (fetal loss and decreased fetal weight) were observed in animal studies. There are no adequate and well-controlled studies in pregnant women. Effective contraception is recommended for women of childbearing potential.

Lactation Excretion in breast milk unknown/not recommended

Contraindications Hypersensitivity to bortezomib, boron, mannitol, or any component of the formulation

Warnings/Precautions Hazardous agent - use appropriate precautions for handling and disposal. May cause peripheral neuropathy (usually sensory but may be mixed sensorimotor); risk may be increased with previous use of neurotoxic agents or pre-existing peripheral neuropathy; adjustment of dose and schedule may be required; the majority of patients with ≥grade 2 peripheral neuropathy have improvement in or resolution of symptoms with dose adjustments or discontinuation; in a study of elderly patients receiving weekly bortezomib with combination chemotherapy, the incidence of peripheral neuropathy was significantly reduced without an effect on outcome (Boccadoro, 2010; Palumbo, 2009). May cause hypotension (including postural and orthostatic); use caution with dehydration, history of syncope, or medications associated with hypotension (may require adjustment of antihypertensive medication, hydration, and mineralocorticoids and/or sympathomimetics). Has been associated with the development or exacerbation of heart failure (HF) and decreased left ventricular ejection fraction; monitor closely in patients with risk factors for HF or existing heart disease. Has also been associated with QT_c prolongation.

Pulmonary disorders (some fatal) including pneumonitis, interstitial pneumonia, lung infiltrates, and acute respiratory distress syndrome (ARDS) have been reported. Pulmonary hypertension (without left heart failure or significant pulmonary disease has been reported rarely). May cause tumor lysis syndrome; risk is increased in patients with high tumor burden prior to treatment. Reversible posterior leukoencephalopathy syndrome (RPLS) has been reported (rarely). Promptly evaluate with new or worsening cardiopulmonary symptoms. Symptoms of RPLS include confusion, headache, hypertension, lethargy, seizure, blindness and/or other vision, or neurologic disturbances; discontinue bortezomib if RPLS occurs. MRI is recommended for RPLS diagnosis. The safety of reinitiating bortezomib in patients previously experiencing RPLS is unknown. Herpes (zoster and simplex) reactivation has been reported with bortezomib; consider antiviral prophylaxis during therapy. Hematologic toxicity, including neutropenia and severe thrombocytopenia, may occur; risk is increased in patients with pretreatment platelet counts <75,000/µL; frequent monitoring is required throughout treatment; may require dosage adjustments; withhold treatment for platelets <30,000/µL. Hemorrhage (gastrointestinal and intracerebral) due to low platelet count has been observed. Acute liver failure has been reported (rarely) in patients receiving multiple concomitant medications and with serious underlying conditions. Hepatitis, transaminase increases, and hyperbilirubinemia have also been reported; may be reversible when discontinued. Use caution in patients with hepatic dysfunction; reduced initial doses are recommended for moderate and severe hepatic impairment (exposure is increased); closely monitor for toxicities. Hyper- and hypoglycemia may occur in diabetic patients receiving oral hypoglycemics; may require adjustment of diabetes medications. Nausea, vomiting, diarrhea or constipation may occur; may require antiemetics or antidiarrheals; ileus may occur; administer fluid and electrolytes to prevent dehydration.

Adverse Reactions

>10%:

Cardiovascular: Edema (11% to 23%), cardiac disorder (treatment emergent; 15%), hypotension (13%; grades 3/4: 3%)

Central nervous system: Psychiatric disturbance (≤35%), fever (34%), dysesthesia (22% to 27%), headache (22%), insomnia (20%), dizziness (17%; excludes vertigo)

Dermatologic: Rash (18%)

Gastrointestinal: Nausea (55%), diarrhea (52%), constipation (41%), anorexia (36%), vomiting (33%), abdominal pain (15%), abnormal taste, dyspepsia

Hematologic: Thrombocytopenia (36%; grade 4: 5%; nadir: day 11; recovery: by day 21), anemia (29%; grade 4: <1%), neutropenia (17%; grade 4: 3%; nadir: day 11; recovery: by day 21)

Neuromuscular & skeletal: Weakness (64%; grades 3/4: 16%), peripheral neuropathy (39%; grade 3: 11%; grade 4: <1%), paresthesia (22%), arthralgia (17%), limb pain (15%), bone pain (14%), back pain (13%), myalgia (12%), muscle cramps (11%), rigors (≤11%)

Respiratory: Dyspnea (21%), cough (20%), respiratory tract infection (12% to 15%), nasopharyngitis (12%), pneumonia (12%)

Miscellaneous: Herpesvirus infections (2% to 12%)

1% to 10%:

Cardiovascular: Heart failure (5%; includes acute pulmonary edema, cardiac failure, congestive cardiac failure, cardiogenic shock, pulmonary edema)

Central nervous system: Anxiety (10%)

Endocrine & metabolic: Dehydration (10%), hypercalcemia (grade 4: 2%)

Hematologic: Bleeding events (≥grade 3: 4%)

Local: Injection site irritation (5%)

Frequency not defined (including postmarketing and/or case reports; limited to important or life-threatening): Acute diffuse infiltrative pulmonary disease, acute respiratory distress syndrome, alkaline phosphatase increased, amyloidosis, anaphylaxis, angina, angioedema, ascites, aspergillosis, atelectasis, atrial fibrillation, atrial flutter, AV block, bacteremia, bradycardia, cardiac amyloidosis, blurred vision, cardiac arrest, cardiac tamponade, cardiopulmonary arrest, cerebral hemorrhage, cerebrovascular accident, cholestasis, coma, conjunctival infection/irritation, cranial palsy, deep venous thrombosis, diplopia, disseminated intravascular coagulation (DIC), duodenitis (hemorrhagic), DVT, dysautonomia, dysphagia, encephalopathy, embolism, epistaxis, fecal impaction, gastritis (hemorrhagic), gastroenteritis, GGT increased, glomerular nephritis, hearing impairment, hematemesis, hematuria, hemoptysis, hemorrhagic cystitis, hepatic failure, hepatic hemorrhage, hepatitis, hepatocellular damage, herpes meningoencephalitis, hyperbilirubinemia, hyper-/hypoglycemia, hyper-/hypokalemia, hyper-/hyponatremia, hypersensitivity, hyperuricemia, hypocalcemia, hypoxia, ileus, immune complex hypersensitivity, inappropriate ADH secretion, injection site reaction, interstitial pneumonia, intestinal obstruction, intestinal perforation, intracerebral hemorrhage, ischemic colitis, ischemic stroke, laryngeal edema, left ventricular ejection fraction decreased, leukocytoclastic vasculitis, leukopenia, listeriosis, lymphopenia, melena, MI, myocardial ischemia, neuralgia, neutropenic fever, ophthalmic herpes, oral candidiasis, pancreatitis, paralytic ileus, pericardial effusion, pericarditis, peritonitis, pleural effusion, pneumonitis, portal vein thrombosis, proliferative glomerular nephritis, pruritus, psychosis, pulmonary embolism, pulmonary hypertension, pulmonary infiltrate, QT_c prolongation, renal failure, respiratory failure, respiratory insufficiency, reversible posterior leukoencephalopathy syndrome (RPLS), seizure, septic shock, sepsis, sinus arrest, spinal cord compression, Stevens-Johnson syndrome, stomatitis, stroke (hemorrhagic), subarachnoid hemorrhage, subdural hematoma, suicidal ideation, Sweet's syndrome (acute febrile neutrophilic dermatosis), syncope, tachycardia, torsade de pointes, toxic epidermal necrolysis, toxoplasmosis, transaminases increased, transient ischemic attack, tumor lysis syndrome, urticaria, ventricular tachycardia

Drug Interactions

Metabolism/Transport Effects Substrate of CYP1A2 (minor), CYP2C19 (major), CYP2C9 (minor), CYP2D6 (minor), CYP3A4 (major); **Note:** Assignment of Major/Minor substrate status based on clinically relevant drug interaction potential; **Inhibits** CYP1A2 (weak), CYP2C19 (moderate), CYP2C9 (weak), CYP2D6 (weak), CYP3A4 (weak)

Avoid Concomitant Use

Avoid concomitant use of Bortezomib with any of the following: Clopidogrel; CloZAPine; CYP3A4 Inducers (Strong); Green Tea; Pimozide; St Johns Wort

Increased Effect/Toxicity

Bortezomib may increase the levels/effects of: Citalopram; CloZAPine; CYP2C19 Substrates; Pimozide

The levels/effects of Bortezomib may be increased by: CYP3A4 Inhibitors (Moderate); CYP3A4 Inhibitors (Strong); Dasatinib

Decreased Effect

Bortezomib may decrease the levels/effects of: Clopidogrel

The levels/effects of Bortezomib may be decreased by: Ascorbic Acid; CYP3A4 Inducers (Strong); Cyproterone; Deferasirox; Green Tea; Peginterferon Alfa-2b; St Johns Wort; Tocilizumab

Ethanol/Nutrition/Herb Interactions

Food: Avoid grapefruit juice (may increase bortezomib levels).

Herb/Nutraceutical: Avoid St John's wort (may decrease bortezomib levels). Avoid green tea and green tea extracts (may diminish the therapeutic effect of bortezomib) (Golden, 2009). Avoid ascorbic acid supplements, including multivitamins containing ascorbic acid (may diminish bortezomib activity) during treatment, especially 12 hours before and after bortezomib treatment (Perrone, 2009).

Stability Prior to reconstitution, store at room temperature of 25°C (77°F); excursions permitted between 15°C to 30°C (59°F to 86°F). Protect from light. Use appropriate precautions for handling and disposal.

I.V.: Dilute each 3.5 mg vial with 3.5 mL NS to a final concentration of 1 mg/mL. Once reconstituted, although the manufacturer recommends use within 8 hours, solution may be stored at room temperature for up to 3 days, or under refrigeration for up to 5 days, in vial or syringe (Andre, 2005).

SubQ (unlabeled route): Reconstitute each 3.5 mg vial with 1.4 mL NS to a concentration of 2.5 mg/mL (Moreau, 2011).

Mechanism of Action Bortezomib inhibits proteasomes, enzyme complexes which regulate protein homeostasis within the cell. Specifically, it reversibly inhibits chymotrypsin-like activity at the 26S proteasome, leading to activation of signaling cascades, cell-cycle arrest, and apoptosis.

Pharmacodynamics/Kinetics

Distribution: 498-1884 L/m^2; distributes widely to peripheral tissues

Protein binding: ~83%

Metabolism: Hepatic primarily via CYP2C19 and 3A4 and to a lesser extent CYP1A2; forms metabolites (inactive) via deboronization followed by hydroxylation

Half-life elimination: Single dose: 9-15 hours; multiple dosing: 1 mg/m^2: 40-193 hours; 1.3 mg/m^2: 76-108 hours

Dosage Details concerning dosing in combination regimens should also be consulted. **Note:** Consecutive doses should be separated by at least 72 hours. I.V.: Adults:

Multiple myeloma (first-line therapy; in combination with melphalan and prednisone): 1.3 mg/m^2 days 1, 4, 8, 11, 22, 25, 29, and 32 of a 42-day treatment cycle for 4 cycles, followed by 1.3 mg/m^2 days 1, 8, 22, and 29 of a 42-day treatment cycle for 5 cycles.

Alternative first-line therapy (studied in patients ≥65 years of age; unlabeled dosing): 1.3 mg/m^2/dose days 1, 8, 15, and 22 of a 5-week treatment cycle, in combination with **either** melphalan and prednisone or melphalan, prednisone, and thalidomide (Boccadoro, 2010; Bringhen, 2010; Palumbo, 2009)

Relapsed multiple myeloma and mantle cell lymphoma: 1.3 mg/m^2 twice weekly for 2 weeks on days 1, 4, 8, and 11 of a 21-day treatment cycle. Therapy extending beyond 8 cycles may be administered by the standard schedule or may be given once weekly for 4 weeks (days 1, 8, 15, and 22), followed by a 13-day rest (days 23 through 35).

Cutaneous and peripheral T-cell lymphoma (unlabeled use): 1.3 mg/m^2 twice weekly for 2 weeks on days 1, 4, 8, and 11 of a 21-day treatment cycle (Zinzani, 2007)

Systemic light-chain amyloidosis (unlabeled use): 1.3 mg/m^2 days 1, 4, 8, and 11 of a 21-day treatment cycle (with or without dexamethasone) (Kastritis, 2010)

Waldenström's macroglobulinemia (unlabeled use): 1.3 mg/m^2 days 1, 4, 8, and 11 of a 21-day treatment cycle (Chen, 2007) **or** 1.3 mg/m^2 days 1, 4, 8, and 11 of a 21-day treatment cycle (in combination with dexamethasone and rituximab) (Treon, 2009) **or** 1.6 mg/m^2 days 1, 8, and 15 of a 28-day treatment cycle (in combination with rituximab) (Ghobrial, 2010)

Dosage adjustment in renal impairment: Dosage adjustment not necessary. **Note:** Dialysis may reduce bortezomib concentrations; administer postdialysis.

Dosage adjustment in hepatic impairment:

Mild impairment (bilirubin ≤1 times ULN and AST >UNL or bilirubin >1-1.5 times ULN): No initial dose adjustment required

Moderate (bilirubin >1.5-3 times ULN) and severe impairment (bilirubin >3 times ULN): Reduce initial dose to 0.7 mg/m^2 in the first cycle; based on patient tolerance, may consider dose escalation to 1 mg/m^2 or further dose reduction to 0.5 mg/m^2 in subsequent cycles

Dosage adjustment for toxicity:

Myeloma (first-line therapy):

Platelets should be ≥70,000/mm^3, ANC should be ≥1000/mm^3, and nonhematologic toxicities should resolve to grade 1 or baseline prior to therapy initiation.

Platelets ≤30,000/mm^3 or ANC ≤750/mm^3 on bortezomib day(s) (except day 1): Withhold bortezomib; if several bortezomib doses in consecutive cycles are withheld, reduce dose 1 level (1.3 mg/m^2/dose reduced to 1 mg/m^2/dose; 1 mg/m^2/dose reduced to 0.7 mg/m^2/dose)

Grade ≥3 nonhematological toxicity (other than neuropathy): Withhold bortezomib until toxicity resolves to grade 1 or baseline. May reinitiate bortezomib at 1 dose level reduction (1.3 mg/m²/dose reduced to 1 mg/m²/dose; 1 mg/m²/dose reduced to 0.7 mg/m²/dose).

Neuropathic pain and/or peripheral sensory or motor neuropathy: See "Neuropathic pain and/or peripheral sensory or motor neuropathy" toxicity adjustment guidelines.

Relapsed multiple myeloma and mantle cell lymphoma:

Grade 3 nonhematological (excluding neuropathy) or Grade 4 hematological toxicity: Withhold until toxicity resolved; may reinitiate with a 25% dose reduction (1.3 mg/m²/dose reduced to 1 mg/m²/dose; 1 mg/m²/dose reduced to 0.7 mg/m²/dose)

Neuropathic pain and/or peripheral sensory or motor neuropathy:

Grade 1 without pain or loss of function: No action needed

Grade 1 with pain or Grade 2 interfering with function but not activities of daily living: Reduce dose to 1 mg/m²

Grade 2 with pain or Grade 3 interfering with activities of daily living: Withhold until toxicity resolved, may reinitiate at 0.7 mg/m² once weekly

Grade 4: Discontinue therapy

Dietary Considerations Green tea and green tea extracts may diminish the therapeutic effect of bortezomib and should be avoided (Golden, 2009). Avoid grapefruit juice. Avoid additional, nondietary sources of ascorbic acid supplements, including multivitamins containing ascorbic acid (may diminish bortezomib activity) during treatment, especially 12 hours before and after bortezomib treatment (Perrone, 2009).

Administration

I.V.: Administer via rapid I.V. push (3-5 seconds)

SubQ (unlabeled route): Subcutaneous administration of bortezomib 1.3 mg/m² days 1, 4, 8, and 11 of a 21-day treatment cycle has been studied in a limited number of patients with relapsed multiple myeloma; doses were administered subcutaneously (concentration of 2.5 mg/mL) into the thigh or abdomen, rotating the injection site with each dose; injections at the same site within a single cycle were avoided (Moreau, 2010; Moreau, 2011). Response rates were similar to I.V. administration; decreased incidence of grade 3 or higher adverse events were observed with SubQ administration.

Monitoring Parameters Signs/symptoms of peripheral neuropathy, dehydration, hypotension, or RPLS; CBC with differential and platelets (monitor frequently throughout therapy); renal function, pulmonary function (with new or worsening pulmonary symptoms), liver function tests (in patients with existing hepatic impairment)

Dosage Forms Excipient information presented when available (limited, particularly for generics); consult specific product labeling.

Injection, powder for reconstitution:

Velcade®: 3.5 mg [contains mannitol]

Bosentan (boe SEN tan)

Brand Names: U.S. Tracleer®

Brand Names: Canada Tracleer®

Pharmacologic Category Endothelin Antagonist; Vasodilator

Use Treatment of pulmonary artery hypertension (PAH) (WHO Group I) in patients with NYHA Class II, III, or IV symptoms to improve exercise capacity and decrease the rate of clinical deterioration

Pregnancy Risk Factor X

Pregnancy Considerations [U.S. Boxed Warning]: Use in pregnancy is contraindicated; may cause birth defects. Exclude pregnancy prior to initiation of therapy, monthly during therapy and one month after stopping bosentan. Two reliable methods of contraception must be used during therapy and for one month after stopping treatment except in patients with tubal ligation or an implanted IUD (Copper T 380A or LNg 20). No other contraceptive measures are required for these patients. Women of childbearing potential should avoid exposure to dust generated from broken or split tablets, especially if repeated exposure is expected (tablet splitting is currently outside of product labeling). Sperm counts may be reduced in men during treatment. No changes in sperm function or hormone levels have been noted.

Lactation Excretion in breast milk unknown/not recommended

Prescribing and Access Restrictions As a requirement of the REMS program, access to this medication is restricted. Bosentan (Tracleer®) is only available through Tracleer® Access Program (T.A.P.). Only prescribers and pharmacies registered with T.A.P. may prescribe and dispense bosentan. Further information may be obtained from the manufacturer, Actelion Pharmaceuticals (1-866-228-3546).

Medication Guide Available Yes

Contraindications Hypersensitivity to bosentan or any component of the formulation; concurrent use of cyclosporine or glyburide; pregnancy

Canadian labeling: Additional contraindications (not in U.S. labeling): Moderate-to-severe hepatic impairment and/or baseline ALT or AST >3 times the upper limit of normal (ULN), particularly when total bilirubin >2 times ULN

Warnings/Precautions Hazardous agent - use appropriate precautions for handling and disposal. **[U.S. Boxed Warning]: Avoid use in moderate-to-severe hepatic impairment.** Has been associated with a high incidence (~11%) of significant transaminase elevations, and rare cases of unexplained hepatic cirrhosis have occurred, including after long-term therapy. Transaminase elevations are dose dependent, generally asymptomatic, occur both early and late in therapy, progress slowly, and are usually reversible after treatment interruption or discontinuation. Avoid use in patients with elevated serum transaminases (>3 times upper limit of normal [ULN]) at baseline. Monitor hepatic function closely (at least monthly) for the duration of treatment. Treatment should be stopped in patients who develop elevated transaminases (ALT or AST) in combination with symptoms of hepatic injury (unusual fatigue, jaundice, nausea, vomiting, abdominal pain, and/or fever) or elevated serum bilirubin ≥2 times ULN. Safety of reintroduction is unknown.

[U.S. Boxed Warning]: Use in pregnancy is contraindicated; may cause birth defects. Exclude pregnancy prior to initiation of therapy, monthly during therapy and 1 month after stopping bosentan. Two reliable methods of contraception must be used during therapy and for one month after stopping treatment except in patients with tubal ligation or an implanted IUD (Copper T 380A or LNg 20). No other contraceptive measures are required for these patients. A missed menses should be reported to healthcare provider and prompt immediate pregnancy testing. Women of childbearing potential should avoid exposure to dust generated from broken or split tablets, especially if repeated exposure is expected (tablet splitting is currently outside of product labeling). Sperm counts may be reduced in men during treatment. No changes in sperm function or hormone levels have been noted.

[U.S. Boxed Warning]: Because of the risks of hepatic impairment and the high likelihood of teratogenic effects, bosentan is only available through the T.A.P. restricted distribution program. Patients, prescribers, and pharmacies must be registered with and meet conditions of T.A.P. Call 1-866-228-3546 for more information.

A reduction in hematocrit/hemoglobin may be observed within the first few weeks of therapy with subsequent stabilization of levels. Hemoglobin reductions >15% have been observed in some patients. Measure hemoglobin prior to initiating therapy, at 1 and 3 months, and every 3 months thereafter. Significant decreases in hemoglobin in the absence of other causes may warrant the discontinuation of therapy.

Development of peripheral edema due to treatment and/or disease state (pulmonary arterial hypertension) may occur. There have also been postmarketing reports of fluid retention requiring treatment (eg, diuretics, fluid management, hospitalization). Further evaluation may be necessary to determine cause and appropriate treatment or discontinuation of therapy. Bosentan should be discontinued in any patient with pulmonary edema suggestive of pulmonary veno-occlusive disease (PVOD). Bosentan may interact with many medications, resulting in potentially serious and/or life-threatening adverse events (see Drug Interactions).

Adverse Reactions

>10%:

Cardiovascular: Edema (11%)

Central nervous system: Headache (15%)

Endocrine & metabolic: Spermatogenesis inhibition (25%)

Hematologic: Hemoglobin decreased (≥1 g/dL in up to 57%; <11 g/dL: 3% to 6%; typically in first 6 weeks of therapy)

Hepatic: Transaminases increased (≥3 times ULN; up to 12%; dose-related)

Respiratory: Respiratory tract infection (22%)

1% to 10%:

Cardiovascular: Chest pain (5%), syncope (5%), flushing (4%), hypotension (4%), palpitation (4%)

Dermatologic: Pruritus (2%)

Hematologic: Anemia (3%)

Hepatic: Abnormal hepatic function (4%)

Neuromuscular & skeletal: Arthralgia (4%)

Respiratory: Sinusitis (4%)

<1% (Limited to important or life-threatening): Anaphylaxis, angioneurotic edema, heart failure (exacerbation), cirrhosis (prolonged therapy), hyperbilirubinemia, hypersensitivity, jaundice, leukocytoclastic vasculitis, leukopenia, liver failure (rare), neutropenia, peripheral edema, rash, thrombocytopenia, weight gain

Drug Interactions

Metabolism/Transport Effects Substrate of CYP2C9 (major), CYP3A4 (major), SLCO1B1; **Note:** Assignment of Major/Minor substrate status based on clinically relevant drug interaction potential; **Induces** CYP2C9 (strong), CYP3A4 (strong)

Avoid Concomitant Use

Avoid concomitant use of Bosentan with any of the following: Bortezomib; Conivaptan; Crizotinib; CycloSPORINE; CycloSPORINE (Systemic); Dronedarone; Everolimus; GlyBURIDE; Lapatinib; Lurasidone; Nilotinib; Nisoldipine; Pazopanib; Praziquantel; Ranolazine; Rivaroxaban; Roflumilast; RomiDEPsin; SORAfenib; Ticagrelor; Tolvaptan; Toremifene; Vandetanib

Increased Effect/Toxicity

Bosentan may increase the levels/effects of: Clarithromycin

The levels/effects of Bosentan may be increased by: Antifungal Agents (Azole Derivatives, Systemic); Clarithromycin; Conivaptan; CycloSPORINE; CycloSPORINE (Systemic); CYP2C9 Inhibitors (Moderate); CYP2C9 Inhibitors (Strong); CYP3A4 Inhibitors (Moderate); CYP3A4 Inhibitors (Strong); Dasatinib; Eltrombopag; GlyBURIDE; Indinavir; Nelfinavir; Phosphodiesterase 5 Inhibitors; Ritonavir; Telaprevir

Decreased Effect

Bosentan may decrease the levels/effects of: ARIPiprazole; Boceprevir; Bortezomib; Brentuximab Vedotin; Clarithromycin; Contraceptives (Estrogens); Contraceptives (Progestins); Crizotinib; CycloSPORINE; CycloSPORINE (Systemic); CYP2C9 Substrates; CYP3A4 Substrates; Dasatinib; Diclofenac; Dronedarone; Everolimus; Exemestane; Gefitinib; GlyBURIDE; GuanFACINE; HMG-CoA Reductase Inhibitors; Imatinib; Indinavir; Ixabepilone; Lapatinib; Linagliptin; Lurasidone; Maraviroc; Nelfinavir; NIFEdipine; Nilotinib; Nisoldipine; Pazopanib; Phosphodiesterase 5 Inhibitors; Praziquantel; Ranolazine; Rivaroxaban; Roflumilast; RomiDEPsin; Saxagliptin; SORAfenib; SUNItinib; Telaprevir; Ticagrelor; Tolvaptan; Toremifene; Ulipristal; Vandetanib; Vemurafenib; Vitamin K Antagonists; Zuclopenthixol

The levels/effects of Bosentan may be decreased by: CYP2C9 Inducers (Strong); CYP3A4 Inducers (Strong); Deferasirox; GlyBURIDE; Herbs (CYP3A4 Inducers); Peginterferon Alfa-2b; Tocilizumab

Ethanol/Nutrition/Herb Interactions

Food: Bioavailability of bosentan is not affected by food. Bosentan serum concentrations may be increased by grapefruit juice.

Herb/Nutraceutical: Avoid St John's wort (may decrease serum concentrations of bosentan).

Stability Store at 20°C to 25°C (68°F to 77°F); excursions permitted to 15°C to 30°C (59°F to 86°F).

Mechanism of Action Blocks endothelin receptors on vascular endothelium and smooth muscle. Stimulation of these receptors is associated with vasoconstriction. Although bosentan blocks both ET_A and ET_B receptors, the affinity is higher for the A subtype.

Pharmacodynamics/Kinetics

Distribution: V_d: ~18 L

Protein binding, plasma: >98% primarily to albumin

Metabolism: Hepatic via CYP2C9 and 3A4 to three primary metabolites (one contributing ~10% to 20% pharmacologic activity); autoinduction may occur with chronic dosing

Bioavailability: ~50%

Half-life elimination: 5 hours; prolonged with heart failure, possibly in PAH

Time to peak, plasma: 3-5 hours

Excretion: Feces (as metabolites); urine (<3% as unchanged drug)

Dosage Oral:

Adolescents >12 years and Adults: Pulmonary artery hypertension:

<40 kg: Initial and maintenance: 62.5 mg twice daily

≥40 kg: Initial: 62.5 mg twice daily for 4 weeks; increase to maintenance dose of 125 mg twice daily. Doses >125 mg twice daily do not appear to confer additional clinical benefit, but may increase risk of liver toxicity.

Note: When discontinuing treatment, consider a reduction in dosage to 62.5 mg twice daily for 3-7 days (to avoid clinical deterioration).

Canadian labeling (not in U.S. labeling): Children 3-18 years:

10-20 kg: Initial: 31.25 mg once daily for 4 weeks; increase to maintenance dose of 31.25 mg twice daily

>20-40 kg: Initial: 31.25 mg twice daily for 4 weeks; increase to maintenance dose of 62.5 mg twice daily

>40 kg: Initial: 62.5 mg twice daily for 4 weeks; increase to maintenance dose of 125 mg twice daily

Coadministration with protease inhibitor regimen:

Dosage adjustment for concurrent use with atazanavir/ritonavir, darunavir/ritonavir, fosamprenavir, lopinavir/ritonavir, ritonavir, saquinavir/ritonavir, tipranavir/ritonavir: Coadministration of bosentan in patients currently receiving one of these protease inhibitor regimens for at least

10 days: Begin with bosentan 62.5 mg once daily or every other day based on tolerability

Coadministration of one of these protease inhibitor regimens in patients currently receiving bosentan: Discontinue bosentan 36 hours prior to the initiation of an above regimen. After at least 10 days of the protease inhibitor regimen, resume bosentan 62.5 mg once daily or every other day based on tolerability.

Dosage adjustment for concurrent use with indinavir or nelfinavir:

Coadministration of bosentan in patients currently receiving indinavir or nelfinavir: Begin with bosentan 62.5 mg once daily or every other day based on tolerability

Coadministration of indinavir or nelfinavir in patients currently receiving bosentan: Adjust bosentan to 62.5 mg once daily or every other day based on tolerability

Dosage adjustment in renal impairment: No dosage adjustment required.

Dosage adjustment in hepatic impairment: Avoid use in patients with **pretreatment** moderate-to-severe hepatic insufficiency and/or transaminase increases >3 times ULN

Modification based on transaminase elevation:

If any elevation, regardless of degree, is accompanied by clinical symptoms of hepatic injury (unusual fatigue, nausea, vomiting, abdominal pain, fever, or jaundice) or a serum bilirubin ≥2 times ULN, treatment should be stopped.

AST/ALT >3 times but ≤5 times ULN: Confirm with additional test; if confirmed, reduce dose or interrupt treatment. Monitor transaminase levels at least every 2 weeks. May continue or reintroduce treatment, as appropriate, following return to pretreatment values. When reintroducing treatment, begin with starting dose and recheck transaminases within 3 days and at least every 2 weeks thereafter.

AST/ALT >5 times but ≤8 times ULN: Confirm with additional test; if confirmed, stop treatment. Monitor transaminase levels at least every 2 weeks. May reintroduce treatment, as appropriate, at starting dose, following return to pretreatment values. Recheck within 3 days and at least every 2 weeks thereafter following reinitiation.

AST/ALT >8 times ULN: Stop treatment and do not reintroduce.

Dietary Considerations May be taken with or without food. Avoid grapefruit and grapefruit juice.

Administration May be administered with or without food, once in the morning and once in the evening. Women of childbearing potential should avoid excessive handling of broken tablets.

Monitoring Parameters Serum transaminase (AST and ALT) and bilirubin should be determined prior to the initiation of therapy and at monthly intervals thereafter. Monitor for clinical signs and symptoms of liver injury (eg, abdominal pain, fatigue, fever, jaundice, nausea, vomiting).

A woman of childbearing potential must have a negative pregnancy test prior to the initiation of therapy and monthly thereafter (prior to shipment of monthly refill). Hemoglobin and hematocrit should be measured at baseline, at 1 month and 3 months of treatment, and every 3 months thereafter (generally stabilizes after 4-12 weeks of treatment).

Dosage Forms Excipient information presented when available (limited, particularly for generics); consult specific product labeling.

Tablet, oral:

Tracleer®: 62.5 mg, 125 mg

Extemporaneous Preparations Hazardous agent: Use appropriate precautions for handling and disposal.

Note: Tablets are not scored; a commercial pill cutter should be used to prepare a 31.25 mg dose from the 62.5 mg tablet; the half-cut 62.5 mg tablets are stable for up to 4 weeks when stored at room temperature in the high-density polyethylene plastic bottle provided by the manufacturer. Since bosentan is classified as a teratogen (Pregnancy Risk Factor X), individuals should avoid exposure to bosentan powder (dust) by taking appropriate measures (eg, using gloves and mask); women of childbearing potential should avoid exposure to dust generated from broken or split tablets.

Crushing of the tablets is not recommended; bosentan tablets will disintegrate rapidly (within 5 minutes) in 5-25 mL of water to create a suspension. An appropriate aliquot of the suspension can be used to deliver the prescribed dose. Any remaining suspension should be discarded. Bosentan should not be mixed or dissolved in liquids with a low (acidic) pH (eg, fruit juices) due to poor solubility; the drug is most soluble in solutions with a pH >8.5.

- **Botox®** *see* OnabotulinumtoxinA *on page 1244*
- **Botox® Cosmetic** *see* OnabotulinumtoxinA *on page 1244*

Botulinum Pentavalent (ABCDE) Toxoid

(BOT yoo lin num pen ta VAY lent [aye, bee, cee, dee, ee] TOKS oyd)

Index Terms Botulinum Toxoid, Pentavalent Vaccine (Against Types A / B / C / D / E Strains of *C. botulinum*)

Pharmacologic Category Toxoid

Unlabeled Use Prophylaxis for *C. botulinum* exposure (high-risk research laboratory personnel actively working with, or expect to work with, known cultures and purified botulinum toxin)

Dosage Do not inject intracutaneously or into superficial structures.

Initial vaccination series: 0.5 mL deep SubQ at 0-, 2-, and 12 weeks

First booster: 0.5 mL deep SubQ 12 months after first injection of the initial series

Subsequent boosters: 0.5 mL deep SubQ at 2-year intervals based on antitoxin titers as checked by CDC

Additional Information Complete prescribing information for this medication should be consulted for additional detail.

Dosage Forms Excipient information presented when available (limited, particularly for generics); consult specific product labeling.

- **Botulinum Toxin Type A** *see* AbobotulinumtoxinA *on page 25*
- **Botulinum Toxin Type A** *see* IncobotulinumtoxinA *on page 884*
- **Botulinum Toxin Type A** *see* OnabotulinumtoxinA *on page 1244*
- **Botulinum Toxin Type B** *see* RimabotulinumtoxinB *on page 1492*
- **Botulinum Toxoid, Pentavalent Vaccine (Against Types A / B / C / D / E Strains of *C. botulinum*)** *see* Botulinum Pentavalent (ABCDE) Toxoid *on page 232*

Botulism Immune Globulin (Intravenous-Human)

(BOT yoo lism i MYUN GLOB you lin, in tra VEE nus, YU man)

Brand Names: U.S. BabyBIG®

Index Terms BIG-IV

Pharmacologic Category Blood Product Derivative; Immune Globulin

Use Treatment of infant botulism caused by toxin type A or B

Pregnancy Considerations Reproduction studies have not been conducted.

Prescribing and Access Restrictions Access to botulism immune globulin is restricted through the Infant Botulism Treatment and Prevention Program (IBTPP). Healthcare providers must contact the IBTPP on-call physician at (510) 231-7600 to review treatment indications and to obtain the medication. For more information, refer to http://www.infantbotulism.org or contact IBTPP@infantbotulism.org.

Contraindications Hypersensitivity to human immune globulin preparations or any component of the formulation; selective immunoglobulin A deficiency

Warnings/Precautions Hypersensitivity and anaphylactic reactions can occur; immediate treatment (including epinephrine 1:1000) should be available. Aseptic meningitis syndrome (AMS) has been reported with intravenous immune globulin administration (rare); may occur with high doses (≥2 g/kg). Immune globulin intravenous (IGIV) has been associated with antiglobulin hemolysis; monitor for signs of hemolytic anemia. Hyperproteinemia, increased serum viscosity, and hyponatremia may occur following administration of IGIV products; distinguish hyponatremia from pseudohyponatremia to prevent volume depletion, a further increase in serum viscosity, and a higher risk of thrombotic events. These adverse events have not reported with botulism immune globulin. Thrombotic events have been reported with administration of IGIV; use with caution in patients with a history of atherosclerosis or cardiovascular and/or thrombotic risk factors or patients with known/suspected hyperviscosity. Consider a baseline assessment of blood viscosity in patients at risk for hyperviscosity. Infuse at lowest practical rate in patients at risk for thrombotic events. Monitor for transfusion-related acute lung injury (TRALI); noncardiogenic pulmonary edema has been reported with IGIV use. TRALI is characterized by severe respiratory distress, pulmonary edema, hypoxemia, and fever in the presence of normal left ventricular function. Usually occurs within 1-6 hours after infusion.

Acute renal dysfunction (increased serum creatinine, oliguria, acute renal failure) can rarely occur; usually within 7 days of use (more likely with products stabilized with sucrose). Use with caution in the elderly, patients with renal disease, diabetes mellitus, volume depletion, sepsis, paraproteinemia, and nephrotoxic medications due to risk of renal dysfunction. In patients at risk of renal dysfunction, the rate of infusion and concentration of solution should be minimized. discontinue if renal function deteriorates. Patients should not be volume depleted prior to therapy. Product of human plasma; may potentially contain infectious agents which could transmit disease. Screening of donors, as well as testing and/or inactivation or removal of certain viruses, reduces the risk. Infections thought to be transmitted by this product should be reported to the manufacturer. For I.V. infusion only; do not exceed recommended rate of administration. Not indicated for use in adults. Safety and efficacy established for infants <1 year of age; not indicated for children ≥1 year of age.

Adverse Reactions Percentages reported in open-label study except where otherwise noted; may reflect pathophysiology of infant botulism.

>10%:

Cardiovascular: Blood pressure increased (transient, 75%), pallor (28%), edema (18%); blood pressure decreased (transient, 16%), cardiac murmur (15%)

Central nervous system: Irritability (41%), pyrexia (17%), body temperature decreased (16%)

Dermatologic: Contact dermatitis (24%), erythematous rash (22%, reported as 14% vs 8% in placebo-controlled study)

Gastrointestinal: Dysphagia (65%), loose stools (25%), vomiting (20%), abdominal distension (11%)

Otic: Otitis media (11%, reported in placebo-controlled study)

Respiratory: Atelectasis (39%), rhonchi (34%), nasal congestion (18%), oxygen saturation decreased (17%), cough (13%), rales (13%)

1% to 10%:

Cardiovascular: Tachycardia (7%), peripheral coldness (7%)

Central nervous system: Agitation (10%)

Endocrine & metabolic: Dehydration (10%), hyponatremia (6%), metabolic acidosis (5%)

Hematologic: Hemoglobin decreased (9%), anemia (5%)

Local: Injection site reaction (7%), injection site erythema (5%)

Renal: Neurogenic bladder

Respiratory: Breath sounds decreased (10%), stridor (9%), lower respiratory tract infection (8%), dyspnea (6%), tachypnea (5%)

Miscellaneous: Oral candidiasis (8%), intubation (5%), infusion rate reactions (<5%, includes chills, back pain, fever, muscle cramps, nausea, vomiting, wheezing)

Drug Interactions

Metabolism/Transport Effects None known.

Avoid Concomitant Use There are no known interactions where it is recommended to avoid concomitant use.

Increased Effect/Toxicity There are no known significant interactions involving an increase in effect.

Decreased Effect

Botulism Immune Globulin (Intravenous-Human) may decrease the levels/effects of: Vaccines (Live)

Stability Prior to reconstitution, store between 2°C to 8°C (35.6°F to 46.4°F). Infusion should begin within 2 hours of reconstitution and be completed within 4 hours of reconstitution. Reconstitute with SWFI 2 mL. Swirl gently to wet powder; do not shake. Powder should dissolve in ~30 minutes.

Mechanism of Action BIG-IV is purified immunoglobulin derived from the plasma of adults immunized with botulinum toxoid types A and B. BIG-IV provides antibodies to neutralize circulating toxins.

Pharmacodynamics/Kinetics

Duration: Protective neutralizing antibody levels: 6 months

Half-life elimination: 28 days

Dosage I.V.: Children <1 year: Infant botulism: 100 mg/kg as a single dose; infuse at 25 mg/kg/hour for the first 15 minutes; if well tolerated, may increase to 50 mg/kg/hour

Administration For I.V. infusion only. Do not administer if solution is turbid. Epinephrine should be available for the treatment of acute allergic reaction. Administer using low volume tubing and infusion pump with an in-line or syringe tip 18 μm filter. Infuse at 25 mg/kg/hour (0.5 mL/kg/hour) for the first 15 minutes; if well tolerated, may increase to 50 mg/kg/hour (1 mL/kg/hour). Infusion should take 127.5 minutes at the recommended rates and should be concluded within 4 hours of reconstitution. Infusion should be slowed or temporarily interrupted for minor side effects; discontinue in case of hypotension or anaphylaxis.

Monitoring Parameters Renal function (BUN, serum creatinine, urinary output); vital signs (continuously during infusion); aseptic meningitis syndrome (may occur hours to days following IGIV therapy); signs of relapse (may occur up to 1 month following recovery)

Dosage Forms Excipient information presented when available (limited, particularly for generics); consult specific product labeling.

Injection, powder for reconstitution [preservative free]:

BabyBIG®: ~100 mg [contains albumin (human), sucrose; supplied with diluent]

◆ **Boudreaux's® Butt Paste [OTC]** *see* Zinc Oxide *on page 1817*

◆ **Bovine Lung Surfactant** *see* Beractant *on page 206*
◆ **BP10-1** *see* Sulfur and Sulfacetamide *on page 1607*
◆ **BP 50%** *see* Urea *on page 1749*
◆ **BP Cleansing Wash** *see* Sulfur and Sulfacetamide *on page 1607*
◆ **BRAF(V600E) Kinase Inhibitor RO5185426** *see* Vemurafenib *on page 1778*
◆ **Bravelle®** *see* Urofollitropin *on page 1750*
◆ **Breathe Free® [OTC]** *see* Sodium Chloride *on page 1567*
◆ **Brentuximab** *see* Brentuximab Vedotin *on page 234*

Brentuximab Vedotin (bren TUX i mab ve DOE tin)

Brand Names: U.S. Adcetris™

Index Terms Anti-CD30 ADC SGN-35; Anti-CD30 Antibody-Drug Conjugate SGN-35; Antibody-Drug Conjugate SGN-35; Brentuximab; SGN-35

Pharmacologic Category Antineoplastic Agent, Monoclonal Antibody

Use Treatment of Hodgkin lymphoma after failure of at least 2 prior chemotherapy regimens (in patients ineligible for transplant) or after stem cell transplant failure; treatment of systemic anaplastic large cell lymphoma (sALCL) after failure of at least 1 prior chemotherapy regimen

Pregnancy Risk Factor D

Pregnancy Considerations Embryo-fetal toxicities and fetal malformations were noted in animal reproduction studies. Based on the mechanism of action, may cause fetal harm if administered to a pregnant woman.

Lactation Excretion in breast milk unknown/not recommended

Contraindications Concurrent use with bleomycin

Warnings/Precautions Hazardous agent - use appropriate precautions for handling and disposal.

[U.S. Boxed Warning]: Cases of PML and death due to JC virus infection have been reported. Immunosuppression due to prior chemotherapy treatments or underlying disease may also contribute to PML development. New-onset signs/symptoms of central nervous system abnormalities (eg, changes in mood, memory, cognition, motor incoordination and/or weakness, speech and/or visual disturbances) should receive prompt evaluation with neurology consultation, brain MRI, and lumbar puncture or brain biopsy. Withhold treatment with new-onset symptoms suggestive of PML; discontinue if diagnosis of PML is confirmed.

Peripheral neuropathy is common and is generally cumulative; usually sensory neuropathy, although motor neuropathy has also been observed; neuropathy completely resolved in nearly half of patients; almost one-third had partial improvement. Monitor for symptoms of neuropathy; dose interruption, reduction or discontinuation may be recommended.

Neutropenia, thrombocytopenia and anemia may occur; neutropenia may be prolonged (≥1 week); monitor blood counts; may require dose interruption, reduction or discontinuation. Infusion reactions, including anaphylaxis have been reported; monitor during infusion. For anaphylaxis, immediately and permanently discontinue and administer appropriate medical intervention. For infusion-related reaction, interrupt infusion and administer appropriate medical intervention; premedicate for subsequent infusions (with acetaminophen, an antihistamine, and/or a corticosteroid).

Due to the risk for pulmonary injury, concurrent use with bleomycin is contraindicated. In a study comparing brentuximab combined with ABVD (doxorubicin, bleomycin, vinblastine, and dacarbazine) to brentuximab combined with AVD (doxorubicin, vinblastine, and dacarbazine), the occurrence of pulmonary toxicity was 40% in the brentuximab/ABVD group compared to a literature-based frequency of ≤25% for other bleomycin-containing regimens. There were no cases of pulmonary toxicity documented with brentuximab in combination with AVD. Pulmonary symptoms/toxicities reported with brentuximab in combination with ABVD consisted of cough, dyspnea, and interstitial infiltration/inflammation; most patients responded to corticosteroids.

Stevens-Johnson syndrome has been observed; discontinue and administer appropriate medical intervention. Tumor lysis syndrome (TLS) may occur; risk of TLS is higher in patients with a high tumor burden or with rapid tumor proliferation; monitor closely. A component of brentuximab vedotin, the microtubule-disrupting agent MMAE is excreted renally and hepatically; the impact of renal or hepatic impairment on MMAE pharmacokinetics is undetermined.

Adverse Reactions

>10%:

Cardiovascular: Peripheral edema (4% to 16%)

Central nervous system: Fatigue (41% to 49%), fever (29% to 38%), pain (7% to 28%), headache (16% to 19%), insomnia (14% to 16%), dizziness (11% to 16%), chills (12% to 13%), anxiety (7% to 11%)

Dermatologic: Rash (27% to 31%), pruritus (17% to 19%), alopecia (13% to 14%)

Gastrointestinal: Nausea (38% to 42%), diarrhea (29% to 36%), abdominal pain (9% to 25%), vomiting (17% to 22%), constipation (16% to 19%), appetite decreased (11% to 16%), weight loss (6% to 12%)

Hematologic: Neutropenia (54% to 55%; grade 4: 6% to 9%); anemia (33% to 52%; grade 4: ≤2%), thrombocytopenia (16% to 28%; grade 4: 2% to 5%)

Neuromuscular & skeletal: Peripheral sensory neuropathy (52% to 53%; grade 3: 8% to 10%), arthralgia (9% to 19%), myalgia (16% to 17%), peripheral motor neuropathy (7% to 16%; grade 3: 3% to 4%), back pain (10% to 14%)

Respiratory: Upper respiratory tract infection (12% to 47%), cough (17% to 25%), dyspnea (13% to 19%), oropharyngeal pain (9% to 11%)

Miscellaneous: Infusion reactions (grades 1/2: 12%), night sweats (9% to 12%), lymphadenopathy (10% to 11%)

1% to 10%:

Cardiovascular: Supraventricular arrhythmia

Dermatologic: Dry skin

Genitourinary: Urinary tract infection

Neuromuscular & skeletal: Limb pain, muscle spasms

Renal: Pyelonephritis

Respiratory: Pneumonitis, pneumothorax, pulmonary embolism

Miscellaneous: Antibrentuximab antibody formation, septic shock

<1% (Limited to important or life-threatening): Anaphylaxis, progressive multifocal leukoencephalopathy (PML), Stevens-Johnson syndrome, tachycardia, tumor lysis syndrome

Drug Interactions

Metabolism/Transport Effects Substrate of CYP3A4 (major); **Note:** Assignment of Major/Minor substrate status based on clinically relevant drug interaction potential

Avoid Concomitant Use

Avoid concomitant use of Brentuximab Vedotin with any of the following: BCG; Bleomycin; Natalizumab; Pimecrolimus; Tacrolimus (Topical); Vaccines (Live)

Increased Effect/Toxicity

Brentuximab Vedotin may increase the levels/effects of: Bleomycin; Leflunomide; Natalizumab; Vaccines (Live); Vitamin K Antagonists

The levels/effects of Brentuximab Vedotin may be increased by: CYP3A4 Inhibitors (Strong); Denosumab; Pimecrolimus; Roflumilast; Tacrolimus (Topical); Trastuzumab

Decreased Effect

Brentuximab Vedotin may decrease the levels/effects of: BCG; Cardiac Glycosides; Coccidioidin Skin Test; Sipuleucel-T; Vaccines (Inactivated); Vaccines (Live); Vitamin K Antagonists

The levels/effects of Brentuximab Vedotin may be decreased by: CYP3A4 Inducers (Strong); Deferasirox; Echinacea; Herbs (CYP3A4 Inducers); Tocilizumab

Stability Store intact vials refrigerated at 2°C to 8°C (36°F to 46°F) in the original carton. Protect from light. Use appropriate precautions for handling and disposal. Reconstitute each 50 mg vial with 10.5 mL sterile water for injection (SWFI), resulting in a concentration of 5 mg/mL. Direct SWFI toward the vial wall; do not direct toward the cake or powder. Swirl gently to dissolve, do not shake. Reconstituted solution should be clear to slightly opalescent without visible particles. Reconstituted solution may be stored refrigerated for up to 24 hours; do not freeze. Further dilute in at least 100 mL of either NS, D_5W, or lactated Ringer's to a final concentration of 0.4 to 1.8 mg/mL; gently invert bag to mix. Solutions diluted for infusion may be stored for 24 hours refrigerated (do not freeze); use within 24 hours of initial reconstitution. Do not mix with other medications.

Mechanism of Action Brentuximab vedotin is an antibody drug conjugate (ADC) directed at CD30 consisting of 3 components: 1) a CD30-specific chimeric IgG1 antibody cAC10; 2) a microtubule-disrupting agent, monomethylauristatin E (MMAE); and 3) a protease cleavable dipeptide linker (which covalently conjugates MMAE to cAC10). The conjugate binds to cells which express CD30, and forms a complex which is internalized within the cell and releases MMAE. MMAE binds to the tubules and disrupts the cellular microtubule network, inducing cell cycle arrest (G2/M phase) and apoptosis.

Pharmacodynamics/Kinetics

Distribution: V_{dss}: ADC: 6-10 L

Metabolism: MMAE: Minimal, primarily via oxidation by CYP3A4/5

Half-life elimination: Terminal: ADC: ~4-6 days

Time to peak: ADC: At end of infusion; MMAE: ~1-3 days

Excretion: MMAE: Feces (~72%, primarily unchanged); urine

Dosage I.V.: Adults: **Note:** For patients weighing >100 kg, dose should be calculated using a weight of 100 kg.

Hodgkin lymphoma, refractory: 1.8 mg/kg (maximum dose: 180 mg) every 3 weeks, continue until disease progression, unacceptable toxicities, or a maximum of 16 cycles

Systemic anaplastic large cell lymphoma (sALCL), refractory: 1.8 mg/kg (maximum dose: 180 mg) every 3 weeks, continue until disease progression, unacceptable toxicities, or a maximum of 16 cycles

Dosage adjustment for toxicity:

Hematologic toxicity:

Grade 3 or 4 neutropenia: Withhold treatment until resolves to baseline or ≤grade 2, consider growth factor support in subsequent cycles.

Recurrent grade 4 neutropenia (despite the use of growth factor support): Consider reducing the dose to 1.2 mg/kg or discontinuing treatment

Nonhematologic toxicities:

Anaphylaxis: Discontinue immediately and permanently

Infusion reaction: Interrupt infusion and administer appropriate medical intervention. Premedicate subsequent infusions with acetaminophen, an antihistamine, and/or a corticosteroid.

Peripheral neuropathy, new or worsening grade 2 or 3: Withhold treatment until improves or returns to grade 1 or baseline; then resume with dose reduced to 1.2 mg/kg

Peripheral neuropathy, grade 4: Discontinue treatment

Progressive multifocal leukoencephalopathy (PML): Withhold treatment with new-onset symptoms suggestive of PML; discontinue if PML diagnosis confirmed

Stevens-Johnson syndrome: Discontinue and administer appropriate medical intervention

Dosage adjustment in renal impairment: No dosage adjustment provided in the manufacturer's labeling; active drug (MMAE) pharmacokinetics have not been determined in renal impairment.

Dosage adjustment in hepatic impairment: No dosage adjustment provided in the manufacturer's labeling; active drug (MMAE) pharmacokinetics have not been determined in hepatic impairment.

Administration Infuse over 30 minutes. Do not administer as I.V. push or bolus.

Monitoring Parameters CBC with differential prior to each dose (more frequently if clinically indicated). Monitor for infusion reaction, tumor lysis syndrome, and for signs of neuropathy (hyperesthesia, paresthesia, discomfort, burning sensation, or neuropathic pain or weakness).

Dosage Forms Excipient information presented when available (limited, particularly for generics); consult specific product labeling.

Injection, powder for reconstitution:

Adcetris™: 50 mg [contains polysorbate 80; derived from or manufactured using hamster or mouse protein]

◆ **Brethaire [DSC]** *see* Terbutaline *on page* 1650

◆ **Brethine** *see* Terbutaline *on page* 1650

◆ **Brevibloc** *see* Esmolol *on page* 622

◆ **Brevibloc® (Can)** *see* Esmolol *on page* 622

◆ **Brevicon®** *see* Ethinyl Estradiol and Norethindrone *on page* 660

◆ **Brevicon® 0.5/35 (Can)** *see* Ethinyl Estradiol and Norethindrone *on page* 660

◆ **Brevicon® 1/35 (Can)** *see* Ethinyl Estradiol and Norethindrone *on page* 660

◆ **Brevital® (Can)** *see* Methohexital *on page* 1097

◆ **Brevital® Sodium** *see* Methohexital *on page* 1097

◆ **Bricanyl [DSC]** *see* Terbutaline *on page* 1650

◆ **Bricanyl® (Can)** *see* Terbutaline *on page* 1650

◆ **Brilinta™** *see* Ticagrelor *on page* 1679

Brimonidine (bri MOE ni deen)

Brand Names: U.S. Alphagan® P

Brand Names: Canada Alphagan®; Apo-Brimonidine P®; Apo-Brimonidine®; PMS-Brimonidine Tartrate; ratio-Brimonidine; Sandoz-Brimonidine

Index Terms Brimonidine Tartrate

Pharmacologic Category $Alpha_2$ Agonist, Ophthalmic; Ophthalmic Agent, Antiglaucoma

Use Lowering of intraocular pressure (IOP) in patients with open-angle glaucoma or ocular hypertension

Pregnancy Risk Factor B

Dosage Ophthalmic: Children ≥2 years and Adults: Glaucoma, ocular hypertension: Instill 1 drop in affected eye(s) 3 times/day (approximately every 8 hours)

Additional Information Complete prescribing information for this medication should be consulted for additional detail.

Dosage Forms Excipient information presented when available (limited, particularly for generics); consult specific product labeling.

Solution, ophthalmic, as tartrate [drops]: 0.15% (5 mL, 10 mL, 15 mL); 0.2% (5 mL, 10 mL, 15 mL)

Alphagan® P: 0.1% (5 mL, 10 mL, 15 mL); 0.15% (5 mL, 10 mL, 15 mL) [contains Purite®]

Brimonidine and Timolol (bri MOE ni deen & TIM oh lol)

Brand Names: U.S. Combigan®

Brand Names: Canada Combigan®

Index Terms Brimonidine Tartrate and Timolol Maleate; Timolol and Brimonidine

Pharmacologic Category $Alpha_2$ Agonist, Ophthalmic; Beta Blocker, Nonselective; Ophthalmic Agent, Antiglaucoma

Use Reduction of intraocular pressure (IOP) in patients with glaucoma or ocular hypertension

Pregnancy Risk Factor C

Dosage Ophthalmic: Children ≥2 years and Adults: Instill 1 drop into affected eye(s) twice daily

Note: In the Canadian labeling, use in children (at any age) is not recommended

Additional Information Complete prescribing information for this medication should be consulted for additional detail.

Dosage Forms Excipient information presented when available (limited, particularly for generics); consult specific product labeling.

Solution, ophthalmic [drops]:

Combigan®: Brimonidine tartrate 0.2% and timolol 0.5% (5 mL,10 mL) [contains benzalkonium chloride]

Dosage Forms: Canada Excipient information presented when available (limited, particularly for generics); consult specific product labeling.

Solution, ophthalmic [drops]:

Combigan®: Brimonidine tartrate 0.2% and timolol maleate 0.5% (2.5 mL, 5 mL,10 mL) [contains benzalkonium chloride]

◆ **Brimonidine Tartrate** *see* Brimonidine *on page* 235

◆ **Brimonidine Tartrate and Timolol Maleate** *see* Brimonidine and Timolol *on page* 236

Brinzolamide (brin ZOH la mide)

Brand Names: U.S. Azopt®

Brand Names: Canada Azopt®

Pharmacologic Category Carbonic Anhydrase Inhibitor; Ophthalmic Agent, Antiglaucoma

Use Treatment of elevated intraocular pressure in patients with ocular hypertension or open-angle glaucoma

Pregnancy Risk Factor C

Dosage Ophthalmic: Adults: Ocular hypertension or open-angle glaucoma: Instill 1 drop in affected eye(s) 3 times/day

Dosage adjustment in renal impairment: Severe renal impairment (Cl_{cr} <30 mL/minute): Use is not recommended (has not been studied; brinzolamide and metabolite are excreted predominately by the kidney).

Additional Information Complete prescribing information for this medication should be consulted for additional detail.

Dosage Forms Excipient information presented when available (limited, particularly for generics); consult specific product labeling.

Suspension, ophthalmic [drops]:

Azopt®: 1% (10 mL, 15 mL) [contains benzalkonium chloride]

◆ **Brioschi® [OTC]** *see* Sodium Bicarbonate *on page* 1566

◆ **British Anti-Lewisite** *see* Dimercaprol *on page* 513

◆ **BRL 43694** *see* Granisetron *on page* 807

◆ **Bromax [DSC]** *see* Brompheniramine *on page* 237

◆ **Bromday™** *see* Bromfenac *on page* 236

Bromfenac (BROME fen ak)

Brand Names: U.S. Bromday™; Xibrom® [DSC]

Index Terms Bromfenac Sodium

Pharmacologic Category Nonsteroidal Anti-inflammatory Drug (NSAID), Ophthalmic

Use Treatment of postoperative inflammation and reduction in ocular pain following cataract removal

Pregnancy Risk Factor C

Dosage Ophthalmic: Adults:

Bromday™: Instill 1 drop into affected eye(s) once daily beginning 1 day prior to surgery and continuing on the day of surgery and for 2 weeks postoperatively

Xibrom®: Instill 1 drop into affected eye(s) twice daily beginning 24 hours after surgery and continuing for 2 weeks postoperatively

Additional Information Complete prescribing information for this medication should be consulted for additional detail.

Dosage Forms Excipient information presented when available (limited, particularly for generics); consult specific product labeling. [DSC] = Discontinued product

Solution, ophthalmic [drops]: 0.09% (2.5 mL)

Bromday™: 0.09% (1.7 mL) [contains benzalkonium chloride, sodium sulfite]

Xibrom®: 0.09% (2.5 mL [DSC], 5 mL [DSC]) [contains benzalkonium chloride, sodium sulfite]

◆ **Bromfenac Sodium** *see* Bromfenac *on page* 236

Bromocriptine (broe moe KRIP teen)

Brand Names: U.S. Cycloset®; Parlodel®; Parlodel® SnapTabs®

Brand Names: Canada Apo-Bromocriptine®; Dom-Bromocriptine; PMS-Bromocriptine

Index Terms Bromocriptine Mesylate; Cycloset®

Pharmacologic Category Anti-Parkinson's Agent, Dopamine Agonist; Antidiabetic Agent, Dopamine Agonist; Ergot Derivative

Additional Appendix Information

Antiparkinsonian Agents *on page* 1879

Use Treatment of hyperprolactinemia associated with amenorrhea with or without galactorrhea, infertility, or hypogonadism; treatment of prolactin-secreting adenomas; treatment of acromegaly; treatment of Parkinson's disease

Cycloset®: Management of type 2 diabetes mellitus (noninsulin dependent, NIDDM) as an adjunct to diet and exercise

Unlabeled Use Neuroleptic malignant syndrome

Pregnancy Risk Factor B

Dosage Oral:

Children: Hyperprolactinemia:

11-15 years (based on limited information): Initial: 1.25-2.5 mg daily; dosage may be increased as tolerated to achieve a therapeutic response (range: 2.5-10 mg daily).

≥16 years: Refer to adult dosing

Adults:

Acromegaly: Initial: 1.25-2.5 mg daily increasing by 1.25-2.5 mg daily as necessary every 3-7 days; usual dose: 20-30 mg/day (maximum: 100 mg/day)

Hyperprolactinemia: Initial: 1.25-2.5 mg/day; may be increased by 2.5 mg/day as tolerated every 2-7 days until optimal response (range: 2.5-15 mg/day)

Parkinsonism: 1.25 mg twice daily, increased by 2.5 mg/day in 2- to 4-week intervals as needed (maximum: 100 mg/day)

Type 2 diabetes (Cycloset®): Initial: 0.8 mg once daily; may increase at weekly intervals in 0.8 mg increments as tolerated; usual dose: 1.6-4.8 mg/day (maximum: 4.8 mg/day)

Neuroleptic malignant syndrome (unlabeled use): 2.5 mg (orally or via gastric tube) every 8-12 hours, increased to a maximum of 45 mg/day, if needed; continue therapy until NMS is controlled, then taper slowly (Gortney, 2009; Strawn, 2007)

Dosing adjustment in hepatic impairment: No guidelines are available; however, adjustment may be necessary due to extensive hepatic metabolism.

Additional Information Complete prescribing information for this medication should be consulted for additional detail.

Dosage Forms Excipient information presented when available (limited, particularly for generics); consult specific product labeling.

Capsule, oral: 5 mg

Parlodel®: 5 mg

Tablet, oral: 2.5 mg

Cycloset®: 0.8 mg

Parlodel® SnapTabs®: 2.5 mg [scored]

◆ **Bromocriptine Mesylate** *see* Bromocriptine *on page 236*

Brompheniramine (brome fen IR a meen)

Brand Names: U.S. Bromax [DSC]; Lodrane® 24 [DSC]; LoHist-12 [DSC]; Respa®-BR [DSC]; TanaCof-XR [DSC]

Index Terms Brompheniramine Maleate; Brompheniramine Tannate

Pharmacologic Category Alkylamine Derivative; Histamine H_1 Antagonist; Histamine H_1 Antagonist, First Generation

Use Symptomatic relief of perennial and seasonal allergic rhinitis, vasomotor rhinitis, and other respiratory allergies

Pregnancy Risk Factor C

Dosage Oral: Allergic rhinitis, allergic symptoms, vasomotor rhinitis:

Children 6-12 years:

Lodrane® 24: One capsule once daily

LoHist-12: One tablet every 12 hours (maximum: 2 tablets/day)

Children >12 years (Bromax, Lodrane® 24, LoHist-12, Respa®-BR): Refer to adult dosing

Adults:

Bromax, Respa®-BR: One tablet twice daily

Lodrane® 24: 1-2 capsules once daily

LoHist-12: 1-2 tablets every 12 hours (maximum: 4 tablets/day)

Additional Information Complete prescribing information for this medication should be consulted for additional detail.

Dosage Forms Excipient information presented when available (limited, particularly for generics); consult specific product labeling. [DSC] = Discontinued product

Capsule, extended release, oral, as maleate:

Lodrane® 24: 12 mg [DSC] [dye free]

Suspension, oral, as tannate:

TanaCof-XR: 8 mg/5 mL (480 mL [DSC]) [ethanol free, sugar free; contains phenylalanine; strawberry cream flavor]

Tablet, chewable, oral, as tannate: 12 mg [DSC]

Tablet, extended release, oral, as maleate:

Bromax: 11 mg [DSC] [dye free]

LoHist-12: 6 mg [DSC] [scored; dye free]

Tablet, prolonged release, oral, as maleate:

Respa®-BR: 11 mg [DSC] [dye free]

Tablet, timed release, oral, as maleate: 6 mg [DSC]

◆ **Brompheniramine Maleate** *see* Brompheniramine *on page 237*

◆ **Brompheniramine Tannate** *see* Brompheniramine *on page 237*

◆ **Brovana®** *see* Arformoterol *on page 139*

◆ **BSF208075** *see* Ambrisentan *on page 84*

◆ **BTX-A** *see* OnabotulinumtoxinA *on page 1244*

◆ **B-type Natriuretic Peptide (Human)** *see* Nesiritide *on page 1191*

◆ **Budeprion XL®** *see* BuPROPion *on page 247*

◆ **Budeprion SR®** *see* BuPROPion *on page 247*

Budesonide (Systemic) (byoo DES oh nide)

Brand Names: U.S. Entocort® EC; Pulmicort Flexhaler®; Pulmicort Respules®

Brand Names: Canada Entocort®; Pulmicort®

Pharmacologic Category Corticosteroid, Inhalant (Oral); Corticosteroid, Systemic

Additional Appendix Information

Asthma *on page 1967*

Use

Nebulization: Maintenance and prophylactic treatment of asthma

Oral capsule: Treatment of active Crohn's disease (mild-to-moderate) involving the ileum and/or ascending colon; maintenance of remission (for up to 3 months) of Crohn's disease (mild-to-moderate) involving the ileum and/or ascending colon

Oral inhalation: Maintenance and prophylactic treatment of asthma; includes patients who require oral corticosteroids and those who may benefit from systemic dose reduction/elimination

Pregnancy Risk Factor C (capsule)/B (inhalation)

Pregnancy Considerations Adverse events have been observed with corticosteroids in animal reproduction studies. Studies of pregnant women using inhaled budesonide have not demonstrated an increased risk of abnormalities. Some studies have shown an association between first trimester systemic corticosteroid use and oral clefts; adverse events in the fetus/neonate have been noted in case reports following large doses of systemic corticosteroids during pregnancy. Budesonide is the preferred inhaled corticosteroid for the treatment of asthma in pregnant women.

Lactation Enters breast milk/use caution

Contraindications Hypersensitivity to budesonide or any component of the formulation; primary treatment of status asthmaticus, acute episodes of asthma; not for relief of acute bronchospasm

Canadian labeling: Additional contraindications (not in U.S. labeling): Moderate-to-severe bronchiectasis, pulmonary tuberculosis (active or quiescent), untreated respiratory infection (bacterial, fungal, or viral)

Warnings/Precautions May cause hypercorticism or suppression of hypothalamic-pituitary-adrenal (HPA) axis, particularly in younger children or in patients receiving high doses for prolonged periods. HPA axis suppression may ▶

lead to adrenal crisis. Withdrawal and discontinuation of a corticosteroid should be done slowly and carefully. Particular care is required when patients are transferred from systemic corticosteroids to inhaled products due to possible adrenal insufficiency or withdrawal from steroids, including an increase in allergic symptoms. Patients receiving >20 mg per day of prednisone (or equivalent) may be most susceptible. Fatalities have occurred due to adrenal insufficiency in asthmatic patients during and after transfer from systemic corticosteroids to aerosol steroids; aerosol steroids do not provide the systemic steroid needed to treat patients having trauma, surgery, or infections. Do not use this product to transfer patients directly from oral corticosteroid therapy.

Bronchospasm may occur with wheezing after inhalation; if this occurs stop steroid and treat with a fast-acting bronchodilator (eg, albuterol). Supplemental steroids (oral or parenteral) may be needed during stress or severe asthma attacks. Not to be used in status asthmaticus or for the relief of acute bronchospasm. Acute myopathy has been reported with high-dose corticosteroids, usually in patients with neuromuscular transmission disorders; may involve ocular and/or respiratory muscles; monitor creatine kinase; recovery may be delayed. Corticosteroid use may cause psychiatric disturbances, including depression, euphoria, insomnia, mood swings, and personality changes. Preexisting psychiatric conditions may be exacerbated by corticosteroid use. Prolonged use of corticosteroids may also increase the incidence of secondary infection, mask acute infection (including fungal infections), prolong or exacerbate viral infections, or limit response to vaccines. Exposure to chickenpox should be avoided; corticosteroids should not be used to treat ocular herpes simplex. Corticosteroids should not be used for cerebral malaria or viral hepatitis. Close observation is required in patients with latent tuberculosis and/or TB reactivity; restrict use in active TB (only in conjunction with antituberculosis treatment). *Candida albicans* infections may occur in the mouth and pharynx; rinsing (and spitting) with water after inhaler use may decrease risk. Prolonged treatment with corticosteroids has been associated with the development of Kaposi's sarcoma (case reports); if noted, discontinuation of therapy should be considered.

Use with caution in patients with thyroid disease, hepatic impairment, renal impairment, cardiovascular disease, diabetes, glaucoma, cataracts, myasthenia gravis, patients at risk for osteoporosis, patients at risk for seizures, or GI diseases (diverticulitis, peptic ulcer, ulcerative colitis) due to perforation risk. Use caution following acute MI (corticosteroids have been associated with myocardial rupture). Because of the risk of adverse effects, systemic corticosteroids should be used cautiously in the elderly in the smallest possible effective dose for the shortest duration.

Orally-inhaled corticosteroids may cause a reduction in growth velocity in pediatric patients (~1 centimeter per year [range: 0.3-1.8 cm per year] and related to dose and duration of exposure). To minimize the systemic effects of orally-inhaled corticosteroids, each patient should be titrated to the lowest effective dose. Growth should be routinely monitored in pediatric patients. Withdraw systemic therapy with gradual tapering of dose. There have been reports of systemic corticosteroid withdrawal symptoms (eg, joint/muscle pain, lassitude, depression) when withdrawing oral inhalation therapy. Pulmicort Flexhaler™ contains lactose; very rare anaphylactic reactions have been reported in patients with severe milk protein allergy.

Adverse Reactions Reaction severity varies by dose and duration; not all adverse reactions have been reported with each dosage form.

>10%:

Central nervous system: Headache (≤21%)

Gastrointestinal: Nausea (≤11%)

Respiratory: Respiratory infection, rhinitis

Miscellaneous: Symptoms of HPA axis suppression and/or hypercorticism may occur in >10% of patients following administration of dosage forms which result in higher systemic exposure (ie, oral capsule), but may be less frequent than rates observed with comparator drugs (prednisolone). These symptoms may be rare (<1%) following administration via methods which result in lower exposures (topical).

1% to 10%:

Cardiovascular: Chest pain, edema, flushing, hypertension, palpitation, syncope, tachycardia

Central nervous system: Amnesia, dizziness, dysphonia, emotional lability, fatigue, fever, insomnia, malaise, migraine, nervousness, pain, sleep disorder, somnolence, vertigo

Dermatologic: Acne, alopecia, bruising, contact dermatitis, eczema, hirsutism, pruritus, pustular rash, rash, striae

Endocrine & metabolic: Adrenal insufficiency, hypokalemia, menstrual disorder

Gastrointestinal: Abdominal pain, anorexia, diarrhea, dyspepsia, flatulence, gastroenteritis (including viral), glossitis, intestinal obstruction, oral candidiasis, taste perversion, tongue edema, vomiting, weight gain, xerostomia

Genitourinary: Dysuria, hematuria, nocturia, pyuria

Hematologic: Cervical lymphadenopathy, leukocytosis, purpura

Hepatic: Alkaline phosphatase increased

Neuromuscular & skeletal: Arthralgia, back pain, fracture, hyperkinesis, hypertonia, myalgia, neck pain, paresthesia, weakness

Ocular: Conjunctivitis, eye infection

Otic: Earache, ear infection, external ear infection

Respiratory: Bronchitis, bronchospasm, cough, epistaxis, hoarseness, nasal congestion, nasal irritation, pharyngitis, sinusitis, stridor, throat irritation

Miscellaneous: Abscess, allergic reaction, C-reactive protein increased, erythrocyte sedimentation rate increased, fat distribution (moon face, buffalo hump); flu-like syndrome, herpes simplex, infection, moniliasis, viral infection, voice alteration

<1% (Limited to important or life-threatening): Aggressive reactions, alopecia, angioedema, anxiety, avascular necrosis of the femoral head, benign intracranial hypertension, bone mineral density decreased, cataracts, depression, dyspnea, glaucoma, growth suppression, hypersensitivity reactions (immediate and delayed [includes rash, contact dermatitis, angioedema, bronchospasm]), hypocorticism, intermenstrual bleeding, irritability, nasal septum perforation, osteoporosis, psychosis, somnolence, urticaria, wheezing (patients with severe milk allergy)

Drug Interactions

Metabolism/Transport Effects Substrate of CYP3A4 (major); **Note:** Assignment of Major/Minor substrate status based on clinically relevant drug interaction potential

Avoid Concomitant Use

Avoid concomitant use of Budesonide (Systemic, Oral Inhalation) with any of the following: Aldesleukin; BCG; Grapefruit Juice; Natalizumab; Pimecrolimus; Tacrolimus (Topical)

Increased Effect/Toxicity

Budesonide (Systemic, Oral Inhalation) may increase the levels/effects of: Amphotericin B; Deferasirox; Leflunomide; Loop Diuretics; Natalizumab; Thiazide Diuretics

The levels/effects of Budesonide (Systemic, Oral Inhalation) may be increased by: CYP3A4 Inhibitors (Moderate); CYP3A4 Inhibitors (Strong); Dasatinib; Denosumab; Grapefruit Juice; Pimecrolimus; Tacrolimus (Topical); Telaprevir; Trastuzumab

Decreased Effect

Budesonide (Systemic, Oral Inhalation) may decrease the levels/effects of: Aldesleukin; Antidiabetic Agents; BCG; Coccidioidin Skin Test; Corticorelin; Sipuleucel-T; Telaprevir; Vaccines (Inactivated)

The levels/effects of Budesonide (Systemic, Oral Inhalation) may be decreased by: Antacids; Bile Acid Sequestrants; Echinacea; Tocilizumab

Ethanol/Nutrition/Herb Interactions Food: Grapefruit juice may double systemic exposure of orally-administered budesonide. Administration of capsules with a high-fat meal delays peak concentration, but does not alter the extent of absorption.

Stability

Suspension for nebulization: Store upright at 20°C to 25°C (68°F to 77°F). Protect from light. Do not refrigerate or freeze. Once aluminum package is opened, solution should be used within 2 weeks. Continue to protect from light.

Oral inhaler (Pulmicort Flexhaler™): Store at controlled room temperature of 20°C to 25°C (68°F to 77°F). Protect from moisture.

Mechanism of Action Controls the rate of protein synthesis; depresses the migration of polymorphonuclear leukocytes, fibroblasts; reverses capillary permeability and lysosomal stabilization at the cellular level to prevent or control inflammation. Has potent glucocorticoid activity and weak mineralocorticoid activity.

Pharmacodynamics/Kinetics

Onset of action: Pulmicort Respules®: 2-8 days; Inhalation: 24 hours

Peak effect: Pulmicort Respules®: 4-6 weeks; Inhalation: 1-2 weeks

Distribution: 2.2-3.9 L/kg

Protein binding: 85% to 90%

Metabolism: Hepatic via CYP3A4 to two metabolites: 16 alpha-hydroxyprednisolone and 6 beta-hydroxybudesonide; minor activity

Bioavailability: Limited by high first-pass effect; Capsule: 9% to 21%; Pulmicort Respules®: 6%; Inhalation: 6% to 13%

Half-life elimination: 2-3.6 hours

Time to peak: Capsule: 0.5-10 hours (variable in Crohn's disease); Pulmicort Respules®: 10-30 minutes; Inhalation: 1-2 hours

Excretion: Urine (60%) and feces as metabolites

Dosage

Nebulization: Children 12 months to 8 years: Asthma: Pulmicort Respules®: Titrate to lowest effective dose once patient is stable; start at 0.25 mg/day or use as follows:

Previous therapy of bronchodilators alone: 0.5 mg/day administered as a single dose or divided twice daily (maximum daily dose: 0.5 mg)

Previous therapy of inhaled corticosteroids: 0.5 mg/day administered as a single dose or divided twice daily (maximum daily dose: 1 mg)

Previous therapy of oral corticosteroids: 1 mg/day administered as a single dose or divided twice daily (maximum daily dose: 1 mg)

NIH Asthma Guidelines (NIH, 2007):

Children 0-4 years:

"Low" dose: 0.25-0.5 mg/day

"Medium" dose: >0.5-1 mg/day

"High" dose: >1 mg/day

Children 5-11 years:

"Low" dose: 0.5 mg/day

"Medium" dose: 1 mg/day

"High" dose: 2 mg/day

Oral inhalation: Asthma:

Children ≥6 years:

Pulmicort Flexhaler™: Initial: 180 mcg twice daily (some patients may be initiated at 360 mcg twice daily); maximum: 360 mcg twice daily

NIH Asthma Guidelines (NIH, 2007) (administer in divided doses twice daily):

Children 5-11 years:

"Low" dose: 180-400 mcg/day

"Medium" dose: >400-800 mcg/day

"High" dose: >800 mcg/day

Children ≥12 years: Refer to adult dosing.

Pulmicort® Turbuhaler®: [CAN, not available in the U.S.]: Initial (during periods of severe asthma or when switching from oral corticosteroid therapy): 200-400 mcg daily in 2 divided doses; Maintenance: Individualized, lowest effective dose.

Adults:

Pulmicort Flexhaler™: Initial: 360 mcg twice daily (selected patients may be initiated at 180 mcg twice daily); maximum: 720 mcg twice daily

NIH Asthma Guidelines (NIH, 2007) (administer in divided doses twice daily):

"Low" dose: 180-600 mcg/day

"Medium" dose: >600-1200 mcg/day

"High" dose: >1200 mcg/day

Pulmicort® Turbuhaler® [CAN, not available in the U.S.]: Initial (during periods of severe asthma or when switching from oral corticosteroid therapy): 400-2400 mcg daily in 2-4 divided doses; Maintenance: 200-400 mcg twice daily (higher doses may be needed for short periods of time). **Note:** Patients taking 400 mcg/day may take as a single daily dose

Oral: Crohn's disease (active): Adults: 9 mg once daily in the morning for up to 8 weeks; recurring episodes may be treated with a repeat 8-week course of treatment

Note: Patients receiving CYP3A4 inhibitors should be monitored closely for signs and symptoms of hypercorticism; dosage reduction may be required. If switching from oral prednisolone, prednisolone dosage should be tapered while budesonide (Entocort™ EC) treatment is initiated.

Maintenance of remission: Following treatment of active disease (control of symptoms with CDAI <150), treatment may be continued at a dosage of 6 mg once daily for up to 3 months. If symptom control is maintained for 3 months, tapering of the dosage to complete cessation is recommended. Continued dosing beyond 3 months has not been demonstrated to result in substantial benefit.

Dosage adjustment in hepatic impairment: Monitor closely for signs and symptoms of hypercorticism; dosage reduction may be required.

Dietary Considerations Avoid grapefruit juice when using oral capsules.

Administration

Oral capsule: Capsule should be swallowed whole; do not crush or chew.

Powder for inhalation:

Pulmicort Flexhaler™: Hold inhaler in upright position (mouthpiece up) to load dose. Do not shake prior to use. Unit should be primed prior to first use only. It will not need primed again, even if not used for a long time. Place mouthpiece between lips and inhale forcefully and deeply. Do not exhale through inhaler; do not use a spacer. Dose indicator does not move with every dose, usually only after 5 doses. Discard when dose indicator reads "0". Rinse mouth with water after each use to reduce incidence of candidiasis.

Pulmicort Turbuhaler® [CAN, not available in the U.S.]: Hold inhaler in upright position (mouthpiece up) to load dose. Do not shake inhaler after dose is loaded. Unit should be primed prior to first use. Place mouthpiece between lips and inhale forcefully and deeply; mouthpiece should face up. Do not exhale through inhaler; do not use a spacer. When a red mark appears in the dose indicator window, 20 doses are left. When the red mark reaches the bottom of the window, the inhaler should be discarded. Rinse mouth with water after use to reduce incidence of candidiasis.

Suspension for nebulization: Shake well before using. Use Pulmicort Respules® with jet nebulizer connected to an air compressor; administer with mouthpiece or facemask. Do not use ultrasonic nebulizer. Do not mix with other medications in nebulizer. Rinse mouth following treatments to decrease risk of oral candidiasis (wash face if using face mask).

Monitoring Parameters Monitor growth in pediatric patients; blood pressure, serum glucose, weight with high-dose or long-term oral use

Asthma: FEV_1, peak flow, and/or other pulmonary function tests

Additional Information Effects of inhaled steroids on growth have been observed in the absence of laboratory evidence of HPA axis suppression, suggesting that growth velocity is a more sensitive indicator of systemic corticosteroid exposure in pediatric patients than some commonly used tests of HPA axis function. The long-term effects of this reduction in growth velocity associated with orally-inhaled corticosteroids, including the impact on final adult height, are unknown. The potential for "catch up" growth following discontinuation of treatment with inhaled corticosteroids has not been adequately studied.

Dosage Forms Excipient information presented when available (limited, particularly for generics); consult specific product labeling.

Capsule, enteric coated, oral: 3 mg

Entocort® EC: 3 mg

Powder, for oral inhalation:

Pulmicort Flexhaler®: 90 mcg/inhalation (165 mg) [contains lactose; delivers ~80 mcg/inhalation; 60 actuations]

Pulmicort Flexhaler®: 180 mcg/inhalation (225 mg) [contains lactose; delivers ~160 mcg/inhalation; 120 actuations]

Suspension, for nebulization: 0.25 mg/2 mL (30s); 0.5 mg/2 mL (30s)

Pulmicort Respules®: 0.25 mg/2 mL (30s); 0.5 mg/2 mL (30s); 1 mg/2 mL (30s)

Dosage Forms: Canada Excipient information presented when available (limited, particularly for generics); consult specific product labeling.

Powder for oral inhalation:

Pulmicort Turbuhaler®: 100 mcg/inhalation [delivers 200 metered actuations]; 200 mcg/inhalation [delivers 200 metered actuations]; 400 mcg/inhalation [delivers 200 metered actuations]

Budesonide (Nasal) (byoo DES oh nide)

Brand Names: U.S. Rhinocort Aqua®

Brand Names: Canada Gen-Budesonide AQ; Mylan-Budesonide AQ; Rhinocort® Aqua™; Rhinocort® Turbuhaler®

Pharmacologic Category Corticosteroid, Nasal

Use Management of symptoms of seasonal or perennial rhinitis

Canadian labeling: Additional use (not in U.S. labeling): Prevention and treatment of nasal polyps

Pregnancy Risk Factor B

Dosage Nasal inhalation:

U.S. labeling (Rhinocort® Aqua®): Rhinitis: Children ≥6 years and Adults: 64 mcg/day as a single 32 mcg spray in each nostril. Some patients who do not achieve adequate control may benefit from increased dosage. A reduced dosage may be effective after initial control is achieved.

Maximum dose: Children <12 years: 128 mcg/day; Adults: 256 mcg/day

Canadian labeling:

Rhinocort® Aqua®: Children ≥6 years and Adults:

Nasal polyps: 256 mcg/day administered as a single 64 mcg spray in each nostril twice daily

Rhinitis: Initial: 256 mcg/day administered as two 64 mcg sprays in each nostril once daily or a single 64 mcg spray in each nostril twice daily; Maintenance: Individualize, lowest effective dose

Maximum dose: 256 mcg/day

Rhinocort® Turbuhaler®: Children ≥6 years and Adults:

Nasal polyps: 100 mcg into each nostril twice daily (maximum: 400 mcg/day)

Rhinitis: Initial: 200 mcg into each nostril once daily; Maintenance: Individualize, lowest effective dose (maximum: 400 mcg/day)

Additional Information Complete prescribing information for this medication should be consulted for additional detail.

Dosage Forms Excipient information presented when available (limited, particularly for generics); consult specific product labeling.

Suspension, intranasal [spray]:

Rhinocort Aqua®: 32 mcg/inhalation (8.6 g) [120 metered actuations]

Dosage Forms: Canada Excipient information presented when available (limited, particularly for generics); consult specific product labeling.

Powder for nasal inhalation:

Rhinocort® Turbuhaler®: 100 mcg/inhalation [delivers 200 metered actuations]

Suspension, intranasal [spray]:

Rhinocort® Aqua®: 64 mcg/inhalation [120 metered actuations]

◆ **Budesonide and Eformoterol** *see* Budesonide and Formoterol *on page 240*

Budesonide and Formoterol

(byoo DES oh nide & for MOH te rol)

Brand Names: U.S. Symbicort®

Brand Names: Canada Symbicort®

Index Terms Budesonide and Eformoterol; Eformoterol and Budesonide; Formoterol and Budesonide; Formoterol Fumarate Dihydrate and Budesonide

Pharmacologic Category $Beta_2$-Adrenergic Agonist; $Beta_2$-Adrenergic Agonist, Long-Acting; Corticosteroid, Inhalant (Oral)

Use Treatment of asthma in patients ≥12 years of age where combination therapy is indicated; maintenance treatment of airflow obstruction associated with chronic obstructive pulmonary disease (COPD; including chronic bronchitis and emphysema)

Unlabeled Use Treatment of asthma in children 5-11 years of age where combination therapy is indicated

Pregnancy Risk Factor C

Medication Guide Available Yes

Dosage Oral inhalation:

Asthma:

Children 5-11 years (NIH Guidelines): Symbicort® 80/4.5: Two inhalations twice daily. Do not exceed 4 inhalations per day.

Children ≥12 years and Adults:

U.S. labeling: Symbicort® 80/4.5, Symbicort® 160/4.5: Two inhalations twice daily (maximum: 4 inhalations/day). Recommended starting dose combination is determined according to asthma severity. In patients not adequately controlled on the lower combination dose following 1-2 weeks of therapy, consider the higher dose combination.

Canadian labeling:

Symbicort® 100 Turbuhaler® [CAN; not available in U.S.], Symbicort® 200 Turbuhaler® [CAN; not available in U.S.]:

Initial: 1-2 inhalations twice daily until symptom control, then titrate to lowest effective dosage to maintain control

Maintenance: 1-2 inhalations once or twice daily (maximum: 8 inhalations/day as temporary treatment in periods of worsening asthma)

Symbicort® Maintenance and Reliever Therapy (Symbicort® SMART): **Note:** Not approved in the U.S.:

Maintenance: Symbicort® 100 Turbuhaler® [CAN] **or** Symbicort® 200 Turbuhaler® [CAN]: 1-2 inhalations twice daily **or** 2 inhalations once daily

Reliever therapy: Symbicort® 100 Turbuhaler [CAN] **or** Symbicort® 200 Turbuhaler® [CAN]: One additional inhalation as needed, may repeat if no relief for up to 6 inhalations total (maximum: 8 inhalations/day)

COPD: Adults:

U.S. labeling: Symbicort® 160/4.5: Two inhalations twice daily (maximum: 4 inhalations/day)

Canadian labeling: Symbicort® 200 Turbuhaler® [CAN; not available in U.S.]: Two inhalations twice daily (maximum: 4 inhalations/day)

Dosing adjustment in hepatic impairment: Use of this combination has not been studied in patients with hepatic impairment; however, the manufacturer recommends close monitoring of patients with hepatic disease.

Additional Information Complete prescribing information for this medication should be consulted for additional detail.

Dosage Forms Excipient information presented when available (limited, particularly for generics); consult specific product labeling.

Aerosol for oral inhalation:

Symbicort® 80/4.5: Budesonide 80 mcg and formoterol fumarate dihydrate 4.5 mcg per actuation (6.9 g) [60 metered inhalations]; budesonide 80 mcg and formoterol fumarate dihydrate 4.5 mcg per actuation (10.2 g) [120 metered inhalations]

Symbicort® 160/4.5: Budesonide 160 mcg and formoterol fumarate dihydrate 4.5 mcg per actuation (6 g) [60 metered inhalations]; budesonide 160 mcg and formoterol fumarate dihydrate 4.5 mcg per actuation (10.2 g) [120 metered inhalations]

Dosage Forms: Canada Excipient information presented when available (limited, particularly for generics); consult specific product labeling.

Powder for oral inhalation:

Symbicort® 100 Turbuhaler®: Budesonide 100 mcg and formoterol dihydrate 6 mcg per inhalation (available in 60 or 120 metered doses) [delivers ~80 mcg budesonide and 4.5 mcg formoterol per inhalation; contains lactose]

Symbicort® 200 Turbuhaler®: Budesonide 200 mcg and formoterol dihydrate 6 mcg per inhalation (available in 60 or 120 metered doses) [delivers ~160 mcg budesonide and 4.5 mcg formoterol per inhalation; contains lactose]

◆ **Buffasal [OTC]** *see* Aspirin *on page 154*

◆ **Bufferin® [OTC]** *see* Aspirin *on page 154*

◆ **Bufferin® Extra Strength [OTC]** *see* Aspirin *on page 154*

◆ **Buffinol [OTC]** *see* Aspirin *on page 154*

◆ **Bulk-K [OTC]** *see* Psyllium *on page 1432*

Bumetanide (byoo MET a nide)

Brand Names: Canada Burinex®

Index Terms Bumex

Pharmacologic Category Diuretic, Loop

Additional Appendix Information

Heart Failure (Systolic) *on page 1991*

Use Management of edema secondary to heart failure or hepatic or renal disease (including nephrotic syndrome)

Unlabeled Use Treatment of hypertension

Pregnancy Risk Factor C

Pregnancy Considerations Adverse events have been observed in some animal studies.

Lactation Excretion in breast milk unknown/not recommended

Contraindications Hypersensitivity to bumetanide or any component of the formulation; anuria; patients with hepatic coma or in states of severe electrolyte depletion until the condition improves or is corrected

Warnings/Precautions [U.S. Boxed Warning]: Excessive amounts can lead to profound diuresis with fluid and electrolyte loss; close medical supervision and dose evaluation are required. Potassium supplementation and/or use of potassium-sparing diuretics may be necessary to prevent hypokalemia. In cirrhosis, initiate bumetanide therapy with conservative dosing and close monitoring of electrolytes; avoid sudden changes in fluid and electrolyte balance and acid/base status which may lead to hepatic encephalopathy. *In vitro* studies using pooled sera from critically-ill neonates have shown bumetanide to be a potent displacer of bilirubin; avoid use in neonates at risk for kernicterus. Coadministration of antihypertensives may increase the risk of hypotension.

Monitor fluid status and renal function in an attempt to prevent oliguria, azotemia, and reversible increases in BUN and creatinine; close medical supervision of aggressive diuresis required. Bumetanide-induced ototoxicity (usually transient) may occur with rapid I.V. administration, renal impairment, excessive doses, and concurrent use of other ototoxins (eg, aminoglycosides). Asymptomatic hyperuricemia has been reported with use.

Chemical similarities are present among sulfonamides, sulfonylureas, carbonic anhydrase inhibitors, thiazides, and loop diuretics (except ethacrynic acid); the manufacturer's labeling states that bumetanide may be used in patients allergic to furosemide. Use in patients with sulfonylurea allergy is not specifically contraindicated in product labeling; however, a risk of cross-reaction exists in patients with allergy to any of these compounds; avoid use when previous reaction has been severe. Discontinue if signs of hypersensitivity are noted.

Adverse Reactions

>10%:

Endocrine & metabolic: Hyperuricemia (18%), hypochloremia (15%), hypokalemia (15%)

Renal: Azotemia (11%)

1% to 10%:

Central nervous system: Dizziness (1%)

Endocrine & metabolic: Hyponatremia (9%), hyperglycemia (7%), phosphorus altered (5%), CO_2 content altered (4%), bicarbonate altered (3%), calcium altered (2%)

Neuromuscular & skeletal: Muscle cramps (1%)

Renal: Serum creatinine increased (7%)

Miscellaneous: LDH altered (1%)

<1% (Limited to important or life-threatening): Abdominal pain, alkaline phosphatase altered, arthritic pain, asterixis, bilirubin altered, chest pain, cholesterol altered, creatinine clearance altered, dehydration, diaphoresis, diarrhea, ear discomfort, ECG changes, encephalopathy (in patients with pre-existing liver disease), erectile dysfunction, fatigue, headache, hearing impaired, hemoglobin/hematocrit altered, hives, hypernatremia, hyperventilation, hypotension, musculoskeletal pain, nausea, nipple tenderness, orthostatic hypotension, ototoxicity, premature ejaculation, prothrombin time altered, pruritus, rash, renal failure, Stevens-Johnson syndrome, thrombocytopenia, toxic epidermal necrolysis, transaminase altered, upset stomach, urine glucose increased, urine protein increased, vertigo, vomiting, WBC altered, weakness, xerostomia

Drug Interactions

Metabolism/Transport Effects None known.

Avoid Concomitant Use There are no known interactions where it is recommended to avoid concomitant use.

Increased Effect/Toxicity

Bumetanide may increase the levels/effects of: ACE Inhibitors; Allopurinol; Amifostine; Aminoglycosides; Antihypertensives; Cardiac Glycosides; CISplatin; Dofetilide; Hypotensive Agents; Lithium; Methotrexate; Neuromuscular-Blocking Agents; RisperiDONE; RiTUXimab; Salicylates; Sodium Phosphates

The levels/effects of Bumetanide may be increased by: Alfuzosin; Beta2-Agonists; Corticosteroids (Orally Inhaled); Corticosteroids (Systemic); CycloSPORINE (Systemic); Diazoxide; Herbs (Hypotensive Properties); Licorice; MAO Inhibitors; Methotrexate; Pentoxifylline; Phosphodiesterase 5 Inhibitors; Probenecid; Prostacyclin Analogues

Decreased Effect

Bumetanide may decrease the levels/effects of: Lithium; Neuromuscular-Blocking Agents

The levels/effects of Bumetanide may be decreased by: Bile Acid Sequestrants; Fosphenytoin; Herbs (Hypertensive Properties); Methotrexate; Methylphenidate; Nonsteroidal Anti-Inflammatory Agents; Phenytoin; Probenecid; Salicylates; Yohimbine

Ethanol/Nutrition/Herb Interactions

Food: Bumetanide serum levels may be decreased if taken with food. It has been recommended that bumetanide be administered without food (Bard, 2004).

Herb/Nutraceutical: Avoid ephedra, yohimbe, ginseng (may worsen hypertension). Avoid dong quai if using for hypertension (has estrogenic activity). Avoid garlic (may have increased antihypertensive effect).

Stability

I.V.: Store vials at 15°C to 30°C (59°F to 86°F). Infusion solutions should be used within 24 hours after preparation. Light sensitive; discoloration may occur when exposed to light.

Tablet: Store at 15°C to 30°C (59°F to 86°F).

Mechanism of Action Inhibits reabsorption of sodium and chloride in the ascending loop of Henle and proximal renal tubule, interfering with the chloride-binding cotransport system, thus causing increased excretion of water, sodium, chloride, magnesium, phosphate, and calcium; it does not appear to act on the distal tubule

Pharmacodynamics/Kinetics

Onset of action: Oral, I.M.: 0.5-1 hour; I.V.: 2-3 minutes

Peak effect: Oral: 1-2 hours; I.V.: 15-30 minutes

Duration: 4-6 hours

Distribution: V_d: Neonates and Infants: 0.26-0.39 L/kg; Adults: 9-25 L

Protein binding: 94% to 96%

Metabolism: Partially hepatic

Bioavailability: 59% to 89% (median: 80%)

Half-life elimination: Neonates: ~6 hours; Infants (1 month): ~2.4 hours; Adults: 1-1.5 hours

Excretion: Urine (81% of total dose; 45% of which is unchanged drug); feces (2% of total dose)

Dosage

Infants and Children: Oral, I.M., I.V.: 0.015-0.1 mg/kg/dose every 6-24 hours (maximum dose: 10 mg/day)

Adults:

Edema:

Oral: 0.5-2 mg/dose 1-2 times/day; if diuretic response to initial dose is not adequate, may repeat in 4-5 hours for up to 2 doses (maximum dose: 10 mg/day)

I.M., I.V.: 0.5-1 mg/dose; if diuretic response to initial dose is not adequate, may repeat in 2-3 hours for up to 2 doses (maximum dose: 10 mg/day)

Continuous I.V. infusion (unlabeled dose): Initial: 1 mg I.V. load then 0.5-2 mg/hour (Hunt, 2009)

Hypertension (unlabeled use): Oral: 0.5 mg daily (maximum dose: 5 mg/day); usual dosage range (JNC 7): 0.5-2 mg/day in 2 divided doses (Chobanian, 2003)

Dietary Considerations Administration with food slows the rate and reduces the extent of absorption and may reduce diuretic efficacy (Bard, 2004). May require increased intake of potassium-rich foods.

Administration

I.V.: Administer slowly, over 1-2 minutes.

Oral: An alternate-day schedule or a 3-4 daily dosing regimen with rest periods of 1-2 days in between may be the most tolerable and effective regimen for the continued control of edema.

Monitoring Parameters Blood pressure; serum electrolytes, renal function; fluid status (weight and I & O), blood pressure

Dosage Forms Excipient information presented when available (limited, particularly for generics); consult specific product labeling.

Injection, solution: 0.25 mg/mL (2 mL, 4 mL, 10 mL)

Tablet, oral: 0.5 mg, 1 mg, 2 mg

◆ **Bumex** *see* Bumetanide *on page 241*

◆ **Buminate** *see* Albumin *on page 51*

◆ **Bupap** *see* Butalbital and Acetaminophen *on page 255*

◆ **Buphenyl®** *see* Sodium Phenylbutyrate *on page 1573*

Bupivacaine (byoo PIV a kane)

Brand Names: U.S. Bupivacaine Spinal; Marcaine®; Marcaine® Spinal; Sensorcaine®; Sensorcaine®-MPF; Sensorcaine®-MPF Spinal

Brand Names: Canada Marcaine®; Sensorcaine®

Index Terms Bupivacaine Hydrochloride

Pharmacologic Category Local Anesthetic

Use Local or regional anesthesia; spinal anesthesia; diagnostic and therapeutic procedures; obstetrical procedures (only 0.25% and 0.5% concentrations)

0.25%: Local infiltration, peripheral nerve block, sympathetic block, caudal or epidural block

0.5%: Peripheral nerve block, caudal and epidural block

0.75% **(not for obstetrical anesthesia)**: Retrobulbar block, epidural block. **Note:** Reserve for surgical procedures where a high degree of muscle relaxation and prolonged effect are necessary

Pregnancy Risk Factor C

Pregnancy Considerations Decreased pup survival and embryocidal effects were observed in animal studies. Bupivacaine is approved for use at term in obstetrical anesthesia or analgesia. **[U.S. Boxed Warning]: The 0.75% is not recommended for obstetrical anesthesia.** Bupivacaine 0.75% solutions have been associated with cardiac arrest following epidural anesthesia in obstetrical patients and use of this concentration is not recommended for this purpose. Use in obstetrical paracervical block anesthesia is contraindicated.

Lactation Enters breast milk/not recommended

Contraindications Hypersensitivity to bupivacaine hydrochloride, amide-type local anesthetics, or any component of the formulation; obstetrical paracervical block anesthesia

Note: Use as intravenous regional anesthesia (Bier block) is considered contraindicated per accepted clinical practice.

Warnings/Precautions **Do not use solutions containing preservatives for caudal or epidural block.** Use with caution in patients with hepatic impairment. Local anesthetics have been associated with rare occurrences of sudden respiratory arrest; convulsions due to systemic toxicity leading to cardiac arrest have also been reported, presumably following unintentional intravascular injection. Intravenous regional anesthesia (Bier block) is **not** recommended; cardiac arrest and death have occurred with this method of administration. **[U.S. Boxed Warning]: The 0.75% concentration is not recommended for obstetrical epidural anesthesia; cardiac arrest with difficult resuscitation or death has occurred.** A test dose is recommended prior to epidural administration (prior to initial dose) and all reinforcing doses with continuous catheter technique. Use caution with cardiovascular dysfunction including patients with hypotension or heart block. Use caution in debilitated, elderly, or acutely ill patients; dose reduction may be required. Resuscitative equipment, oxygen, and other resuscitative drugs should be available for immediate use. Continuous intra-articular infusion of local anesthetics after arthroscopic or other surgical procedures is **not** an approved use; chondrolysis (primarily shoulder joint) has occurred following infusion, with some requiring arthroplasty or shoulder replacement.

Adverse Reactions Note: Incidence of adverse reactions is difficult to define. Most effects are dose related, and are often due to accelerated absorption from the injection site, unintentional intravascular injection, or slow metabolic degradation. The development of any central nervous system symptoms may be an early indication of more significant toxicity (seizure).

Cardiovascular: Hypotension, bradycardia, palpitation, heart block, ventricular arrhythmia, cardiac arrest

Central nervous system: Restlessness, anxiety, dizziness, seizure (0.1%); rare symptoms (usually associated with unintentional subarachnoid injection during high spinal anesthesia) include persistent anesthesia, paresthesia, paralysis, headache, septic meningitis, and cranial nerve palsies

Gastrointestinal: Nausea, vomiting; rare symptoms (usually associated with unintentional subarachnoid injection during high spinal anesthesia) include fecal incontinence and loss of sphincter control

Genitourinary: Rare symptoms (usually associated with unintentional subarachnoid injection during high spinal anesthesia) include urinary incontinence, loss of perineal sensation, and loss of sexual function

Neuromuscular & skeletal: Chondrolysis (continuous intra-articular administration), weakness

Ocular: Blurred vision, pupillary constriction

Otic: Tinnitus

Respiratory: Apnea, hypoventilation (usually associated with unintentional subarachnoid injection during high spinal anesthesia)

Miscellaneous: Allergic reactions (urticaria, pruritus, angioedema), anaphylactoid reactions

Drug Interactions

Metabolism/Transport Effects **Substrate** of CYP1A2 (minor), CYP2C19 (minor), CYP2D6 (minor), CYP3A4 (minor); **Note:** Assignment of Major/Minor substrate status based on clinically relevant drug interaction potential

Avoid Concomitant Use There are no known interactions where it is recommended to avoid concomitant use.

Increased Effect/Toxicity

The levels/effects of Bupivacaine may be increased by: Beta-Blockers; Conivaptan

Decreased Effect

The levels/effects of Bupivacaine may be decreased by: Cyproterone; Peginterferon Alfa-2b; Tocilizumab

Stability Store at controlled room temperature of 20°C to 25°C (68°F to 77°F).

Mechanism of Action Blocks both the initiation and conduction of nerve impulses by decreasing the neuronal membrane's permeability to sodium ions, which results in inhibition of depolarization with resultant blockade of conduction

Pharmacodynamics/Kinetics

Onset of action: Anesthesia (route and dose dependent): 1-17 minutes

Duration (route and dose dependent): 2-9 hours

Protein binding: ~95%

Metabolism: Hepatic; forms metabolite (pipecoloxylidine [PPX])

Half-life elimination (age dependent): Neonates: 8.1 hours; Adults: 2.7 hours

Time to peak, plasma: Caudal, epidural, or peripheral nerve block: 30-45 minutes

Excretion: Urine (~6% unchanged)

Dosage Dose varies with procedure, depth of anesthesia, vascularity of tissues, duration of anesthesia, and condition of patient. Do not use solutions containing preservatives for caudal or epidural block.

Children >12 years and Adults:

Local anesthesia: Infiltration: 0.25% infiltrated locally; maximum: 175 mg

Caudal block (preservative free): 15-30 mL of 0.25% or 0.5%

Epidural block (other than caudal block; preservative free): Administer in 3-5 mL increments, allowing sufficient time to detect toxic manifestations of inadvertent I.V. or I.T. administration: 10-20 mL of 0.25% or 0.5%

Surgical procedures requiring a high degree of muscle relaxation and prolonged effects **only**: 10-20 mL of 0.75% (**Note:** Not to be used in obstetrical cases)

Peripheral nerve block: 5 mL of 0.25% or 0.5%; maximum: 400 mg/day

Sympathetic nerve block: 20-50 mL of 0.25%

Retrobulbar anesthesia: 2-4 mL of 0.75%

Adults: Spinal anesthesia: Preservative free solution of 0.75% bupivacaine in 8.25% dextrose:

Lower extremity and perineal procedures: 1 mL

Lower abdominal procedures: 1.6 mL

Normal vaginal delivery: 0.8 mL (higher doses may be required in some patients)

Cesarean section: 1-1.4 mL

Administration Solutions containing preservatives should not be used for epidural or caudal blocks.

Monitoring Parameters Vital signs, state of consciousness; signs of CNS toxicity

Dosage Forms Excipient information presented when available (limited, particularly for generics); consult specific product labeling.

Injection, solution, as hydrochloride: 0.25% [2.5 mg/mL] (20 mL, 50 mL); 0.5% [5 mg/mL] (20 mL, 50 mL)

Marcaine®: 0.5% [5 mg/mL] (50 mL) [contains methylparaben]

Sensorcaine®: 0.25% [2.5 mg/mL] (50 mL); 0.5% [5 mg/mL] (50 mL) [contains methylparaben]

Injection, solution, as hydrochloride [preservative free]: 0.25% [2.5 mg/mL] (10 mL, 20 mL, 30 mL); 0.5% [5 mg/mL] (10 mL, 20 mL, 30 mL); 0.75% [7.5 mg/mL] (10 mL, 30 mL)
Marcaine®: 0.25% [2.5 mg/mL] (10 mL, 30 mL, 50 mL); 0.5% [5 mg/mL] (10 mL, 30 mL); 0.75% [7.5 mg/mL] (10 mL, 30 mL)
Sensorcaine®-MPF: 0.25% [2.5 mg/mL] (10 mL, 30 mL); 0.5% [5 mg/mL] (10 mL, 30 mL); 0.75% [7.5 mg/mL] (10 mL, 30 mL)
Injection, solution, premixed in $D_{8.25}W$, as hydrochloride [preservative free]:
Bupivacaine Spinal: 0.75% [7.5 mg/mL] (2 mL)
Marcaine® Spinal: 0.75% [7.5 mg/mL] (2 mL)
Sensorcaine®-MPF Spinal: 0.75% [7.5 mg/mL] (2 mL)

◆ **Bupivacaine Hydrochloride** *see* Bupivacaine *on page 242*
◆ **Bupivacaine Spinal** *see* Bupivacaine *on page 242*
◆ **Buprenex®** *see* Buprenorphine *on page 244*

Buprenorphine (byoo pre NOR feen)

Brand Names: U.S. Buprenex®; Butrans®; Subutex® [DSC]
Brand Names: Canada Buprenex®; Subutex®
Index Terms Buprenorphine Hydrochloride
Pharmacologic Category Analgesic, Opioid; Analgesic, Opioid Partial Agonist
Additional Appendix Information
Opioid Analgesics *on page 1896*
Use
Injection: Management of moderate-to-severe pain
Sublingual tablet: Treatment of opioid dependence
Transdermal patch: Management of moderate-to-severe chronic pain in patients requiring an around-the-clock opioid analgesic for an extended period of time
Unlabeled Use Injection: Management of opioid withdrawal in heroin-dependent hospitalized patients
Pregnancy Risk Factor C
Pregnancy Considerations Adverse effects have been observed in animal reproduction studies following buprenorphine subcutaneous and transdermal administration. In humans, withdrawal has been reported in infants of women receiving buprenorphine during pregnancy. Onset of symptoms ranged from day 1 to day 8 of life, most occurring on day 1.
Lactation Enters breast milk/not recommended
Prescribing and Access Restrictions Prescribing of tablets for opioid dependence is limited to physicians who have met the qualification criteria and have received a DEA number specific to prescribing this product. Tablets will be available through pharmacies and wholesalers which normally provide controlled substances.
Medication Guide Available Yes
Contraindications Hypersensitivity to buprenorphine or any component of the formulation

Transdermal patch: Additional contraindications: Significant respiratory depression; severe asthma; known or suspected paralytic ileus; management of mild, acute, or intermittent pain; management of pain requiring short-term opioid analgesia; management of postoperative pain

Warnings/Precautions An opioid-containing analgesic regimen should be tailored to each patient's needs and based upon the type of pain being treated (acute versus chronic), the route of administration, degree of tolerance for opioids (naive versus chronic user), age, weight, and medical condition. The optimal analgesic dose varies widely among patients. Doses should be titrated to pain relief/prevention.

May cause CNS depression, which may impair physical or mental abilities. Effects with other sedative drugs or ethanol may be potentiated. Elderly may be more sensitive to CNS depressant and constipating effects. May cause respiratory depression - use caution in patients with respiratory disease or pre-existing respiratory depression. Hypersensitivity reactions, including bronchospasm, angioneurotic edema, and anaphylactic shock, have also been reported. Potential for drug dependency exists, abrupt cessation may precipitate withdrawal. Use caution in elderly, debilitated, pediatric patients, depression or suicidal tendencies. Tolerance, psychological and physical dependence may occur with prolonged use. Partial antagonist activity may precipitate acute narcotic withdrawal in opioid-dependent individuals.

Hepatitis has been reported with buprenorphine use; hepatic events ranged from transient, asymptomatic transaminase elevations to hepatic failure; in many cases, patients had preexisting hepatic dysfunction. Monitor liver function tests in patients at increased risk for hepatotoxicity (eg, history of alcohol abuse, pre-existing hepatic dysfunction, I.V. drug abusers) prior to and during therapy. Use with caution in patients with hepatic impairment; dosage adjustments are recommended in hepatic impairment.

Use with caution in patients with pulmonary or renal function impairment. Also use caution in patients with head injury or increased ICP, biliary tract dysfunction, patients with history of hyperthyroidism, morbid obesity, adrenal insufficiency, prostatic hyperplasia, urinary stricture, CNS depression, toxic psychosis, pancreatitis, alcoholism, delirium tremens, or kyphoscoliosis. May cause hypotension; use with caution in patients with hypovolemia, cardiovascular disease (including acute MI), or drugs which may exaggerate hypotensive effects (including phenothiazines or general anesthetics). May obscure diagnosis or clinical course of patients with acute abdominal conditions. Opioid therapy may lower seizure threshold; use caution in patients with a history of seizure disorders.

Transdermal patch: **[U.S. Boxed Warning]: Do not exceed one 20 mcg/hour transdermal patch due to the risk of QT_c-interval prolongation.** Avoid using in patients with history of long QT syndrome or in patients with predisposing factors increasing the risk of QT abnormalities (eg, concurrent medications such as antiarrhythmics, hypokalemia, unstable heart failure, unstable atrial fibrillation). **[U.S. Boxed Warning]: Healthcare provider should be alert to problems of abuse, misuse, and diversion.**

Sublingual tablets, which are used for induction treatment of opioid dependence, should not be started until effects of withdrawal are evident.

Adverse Reactions
Injection:
>10%: Central nervous system: Sedation
1% to 10%:
Cardiovascular: Hypotension
Central nervous system: Respiratory depression, dizziness, headache
Gastrointestinal: Vomiting, nausea
Ocular: Miosis
Otic: Vertigo
Miscellaneous: Diaphoresis
<1%: Agitation, allergic reaction, apnea, appetite decreased, blurred vision, bradycardia, confusion, constipation, convulsion, coma, cyanosis, depersonalization, depression, diplopia, dyspnea, dysphoria, euphoria, fatigue, flatulence, flushing, hallucinations, hypertension, injection site reaction, malaise, nervousness, pallor, paresthesia, pruritus, psychosis, rash, slurred speech, tachycardia, tinnitus, tremor, urinary retention, urticaria, weakness, Wenckebach block, xerostomia

Tablet:

>10%:

Central nervous system: Headache (30%), pain (24%), insomnia (21% to 25%), anxiety (12%), depression (11%)

Gastrointestinal: Nausea (10% to 14%), abdominal pain (12%), constipation (8% to 11%)

Neuromuscular & skeletal: Back pain (14%), weakness (14%)

Respiratory: Rhinitis (11%)

Miscellaneous: Withdrawal syndrome (19%; placebo 37%), infection (12% to 20%), diaphoresis (12% to 13%)

1% to 10%:

Central nervous system: Chills (6%), nervousness (6%), somnolence (5%), dizziness (4%), fever (3%)

Gastrointestinal: Vomiting (5% to 8%), diarrhea (5%), dyspepsia (3%)

Ocular: Lacrimation (5%)

Respiratory: Cough (4%), pharyngitis (4%)

Miscellaneous: Flu-like syndrome (6%)

Transdermal patch:

>10%:

Central nervous system: Headache (16%), dizziness (16%), somnolence (14%),

Gastrointestinal: Nausea (23%), constipation (14%), vomiting (11%)

Local: Application site pruritus (15%)

1% to 10%:

Cardiovascular: Peripheral edema (7%), chest pain, hypertension

Central nervous system: Fatigue (5%), insomnia (3%), hypoesthesia (2%), anxiety, depression, fever, migraine

Dermatologic: Pruritus (4%), rash (2%)

Gastrointestinal: Xerostomia (7%), diarrhea (3%), abdominal discomfort (2%), anorexia (2%), upper abdominal pain

Genitourinary: Urinary tract infection (3%)

Local: Application site erythema (7%); application site rash (6%), application site irritation

Neuromuscular & skeletal: Pain in extremity (3%), back pain (3%), joint swelling (3%), paresthesia (2%), tremor (2%), muscles spasms, musculoskeletal pain, myalgia, neck pain, weakness

Respiratory: Dyspnea (3%), bronchitis, cough, nasopharyngitis, pharyngolaryngeal pain, sinusitis, upper respiratory tract infection

Miscellaneous: Hyperhydrosis (4%), fall (4%), flu-like syndrome

<1% (Limited to important or life-threatening): ALT increased, angina, angioedema, application site dermatitis, contact dermatitis, hypersensitivity, facial edema, hallucination, hypotension, ileus, loss of consciousness, mental status changes, miosis (dose-related), orthostatic hypotension, respiratory depression, respiratory distress, respiratory failure, syncope, tachycardia, urinary incontinence, urinary retention, visual disturbances, withdrawal syndrome

Drug Interactions

Metabolism/Transport Effects Substrate of CYP3A4 (major); **Note:** Assignment of Major/Minor substrate status based on clinically relevant drug interaction potential; **Inhibits** CYP1A2 (weak), CYP2A6 (weak), CYP2C19 (weak), CYP2D6 (weak)

Avoid Concomitant Use

Avoid concomitant use of Buprenorphine with any of the following: Atazanavir; Conivaptan; MAO Inhibitors

Increased Effect/Toxicity

Buprenorphine may increase the levels/effects of: Alcohol (Ethyl); Alvimopan; CNS Depressants; Desmopressin; MAO Inhibitors; Selective Serotonin Reuptake Inhibitors; Thiazide Diuretics

The levels/effects of Buprenorphine may be increased by: Amphetamines; Antipsychotic Agents (Phenothiazines); Atazanavir; Boceprevir; Conivaptan; CYP3A4 Inhibitors (Moderate); CYP3A4 Inhibitors (Strong); Dasatinib; Droperidol; HydrOXYzine; Succinylcholine

Decreased Effect

Buprenorphine may decrease the levels/effects of: Analgesics (Opioid); Atazanavir; Pegvisomant

The levels/effects of Buprenorphine may be decreased by: Ammonium Chloride; Boceprevir; CYP3A4 Inducers (Strong); Deferasirox; Efavirenz; Etravirine; Herbs (CYP3A4 Inducers); Mixed Agonist / Antagonist Opioids; Tocilizumab

Ethanol/Nutrition/Herb Interactions

Ethanol: May increase CNS depression; monitor for increased effects with coadministration. Caution patients about effect.

Herb/Nutraceutical: Avoid valerian, St John's wort, kava kava, gotu kola (may increase CNS depression).

Stability

Injection: Protect from excessive heat >40°C (>104°F). Protect from light.

Patch, tablet: Store at room temperature of 25°C (77°F).

Mechanism of Action Buprenorphine exerts its analgesic effect via high affinity binding to μ opiate receptors in the CNS; displays partial mu agonist and weak kappa antagonist activity

Pharmacodynamics/Kinetics

Onset of action: Analgesic: I.M: Within 15 minutes

Peak effect: I.M.: ~1 hour; Transdermal patch: Steady state achieved by day 3

Duration: I.M.: ≥6 hours

Absorption: I.M., SubQ: 30% to 40%

Distribution: V_d: 97-187 L/kg

Protein binding: High (~96%, primarily to alpha- and beta globulin)

Metabolism: Primarily hepatic via N-dealkylation by CYP3A4 to norbuprenorphine (active metabolite), and to a lesser extent via glucuronidation by UGT1A1 and 2B7 to buprenorphine 3-O-glucuronide; the major metabolite, norbuprenorphine, also undergoes glucuronidation via UGT1A3; extensive first-pass effect

Bioavailability (relative to I.V. administration): I.M.: 70%; Sublingual tablet: 29%; Transdermal patch: ~15%

Half-life elimination: I.V.: 2.2-3 hours; Apparent terminal half-life: Sublingual tablet: ~37 hours; Transdermal patch: ~26 hours. **Note:** Extended elimination half-life for sublingual administration may be due to depot effect (Kuhlman, 1996).

Time to peak, plasma: Sublingual: 30 minutes to 1 hour (Kuhlman, 1996)

Excretion: Feces (~70%); urine (27% to 30%)

Dosage

I.M., I.V.: Acute pain (moderate-to-severe): **Note: Long-term use is not recommended.** The following recommendations are guidelines and do not represent the maximum doses that may be required in all patients. Doses should be titrated to pain relief/prevention. In high-risk patients (eg, elderly, debilitated, presence of respiratory disease) and/or concurrent CNS depressant use, reduce dose by one-half. Buprenorphine has an analgesic ceiling.

Children 2-12 years: I.M., slow I.V.: 2-6 mcg/kg every 4-6 hours

Children ≥13 years and Adults:

I.M.: Initial: Opiate-naive: 0.3 mg every 6-8 hours as needed; initial dose (up to 0.3 mg) may be repeated once in 30-60 minutes after the initial dose if needed; usual dosage range: 0.15-0.6 mg every 4-8 hours as needed

Slow I.V.: Initial: Opiate-naive: 0.3 mg every 6-8 hours as needed; initial dose (up to 0.3 mg) may be repeated once in 30-60 minutes after the initial dose if needed

Adults: I.V. infusion: Opiate withdrawal in heroin-dependent hospitalized patients (unlabeled): 0.3-0.9 mg (diluted in 50-100 mL of NS) over 20-30 minutes every 6-12 hours (Welsh, 2002)

Sublingual tablet: Children ≥16 years and Adults: Opioid dependence: **Note:** The combination product, buprenorphine and naloxone, is preferred therapy over buprenorphine monotherapy for induction treatment (and stabilization/maintenance treatment) for short-acting opioid dependence (U.S. Department of Health and Human Services, 2005).

Manufacturer's labeling:

Induction: Day 1: 8 mg; Day 2 and subsequent induction days: 16 mg; usual induction dosage range: 12-16 mg/day (induction usually accomplished over 3-4 days). Treatment should begin at least 4 hours after last use of heroin or other short-acting opioids, preferably when first signs of withdrawal appear. Titrating dose to clinical effectiveness should be done as rapidly as possible to prevent undue withdrawal symptoms and patient drop-out during the induction period. There is little controlled experience with induction in patients on methadone or other long-acting opioids; consult expert physician experienced with this procedure.

Maintenance: Target dose: 16 mg/day; in some patients 12 mg/day may be effective; patients should be switched to the buprenorphine/naloxone combination product for maintenance and unsupervised therapy

Transdermal patch: Adults: Chronic pain (moderate-to-severe):

Opioid-naive patients: Initial: 5 mcg/hour applied once every 7 days

Opioid-experienced patients (conversion from other opioids to buprenorphine): Taper the current around-the-clock opioid for up to 7 days to ≤30 mg/day of oral morphine or equivalent before initiating therapy. Short-acting analgesics as needed may be continued until analgesia with transdermal buprenorphine is attained. There is a potential for buprenorphine to precipitate withdrawal in patients already receiving opioids.

Patients who were receiving daily dose of <30 mg of oral morphine equivalents: Initial: 5 mcg/hour applied once every 7 days

Patients who were receiving daily dose of 30-80 mg of oral morphine equivalents: Initial: 10 mcg/hour applied once every 7 days

Dose titration (opioid-naive or opioid-experienced patients): May increase dose, based on patient's supplemental short-acting analgesic requirements, with a minimum titration interval of 72 hours (maximum dose: 20 mcg/hour applied once every 7 days; risk for QT_c prolongation increases with doses ≥20 mcg/hour patch).

Discontinuation of therapy: Taper dose gradually to prevent withdrawal; consider initiating immediate-release opioids, if needed.

Elderly:

I.M., slow I.V.: 0.15 mg every 6 hours; elderly patients are more likely to suffer from confusion and drowsiness compared to younger patients

Transdermal patch: Chronic pain (moderate-to-severe): No specific dosage adjustments required; use caution due to potential for increased risk of adverse events. Refer to adult dosing.

Dosage adjustment in hepatic impairment:

Injection, sublingual tablet: Use caution due to extensive hepatic metabolism; dosage adjustments recommended although no specific recommendations are provided by the manufacturer.

Transdermal patch:

Mild-to-moderate impairment: Initial: 5 mcg/hour applied once every 7 days

Severe impairment: Not studied; consider alternative therapy with more flexibility for dosing adjustments

Administration

I.M.: Administer via deep I.M. injection

I.V.: Administer slowly, over at least 2 minutes. Administration over 20-30 minutes preferred when managing opioid withdrawal in heroin-dependent hospitalized patients (Welsh, 2002).

Oral: Sublingual tablet: Tablet should be placed under the tongue until dissolved; should not be swallowed. If two or more tablets are needed per dose, all may be placed under the tongue at once, or two at a time. To ensure consistent bioavailability, subsequent doses should always be taken the same way.

Transdermal patch: Apply to patch to intact, nonirritated skin only. Apply to a hairless or nearly hairless skin site. If hairless site is not available, do not shave skin; hair at application site should be clipped. Prior to application, if the site must be cleaned, clean with clear water and allow to dry completely; do not use soaps, alcohol, lotions or abrasives due to potential for increased skin absorption. Do not use any patch that has been damaged, cut or manipulated in any way. Remove patch from protective pouch immediately before application. Remove the protective backing, and apply the sticky side of the patch to one of eight possible application sites (upper outer arm, upper chest, upper back or the side of the chest [on either side of the body]). Firmly press patch in place and hold for ~15 seconds. Change patch every 7 days. Rotate patch application sites; wait ≥21 days before reapplying another patch to the same skin site. Avoid exposing application site to external heat sources (eg, heating pad, electric blanket, heat lamp, hot tub). If there is difficulty with patch adhesion, the edges of the system may be taped in place with first-aid tape. If the patch falls off during the 7-day dosing interval, dispose of the patch and apply a new patch to a different skin site.

Monitoring Parameters Pain relief, respiratory and mental status, CNS depression, blood pressure; LFTs (prior to initiation and during therapy); symptoms of withdrawal; application site reactions (transdermal patch)

Dosage Forms Excipient information presented when available (limited, particularly for generics); consult specific product labeling. [DSC] = Discontinued product

Injection, solution: 0.3 mg/mL (1 mL)

Buprenex®: 0.3 mg/mL (1 mL)

Injection, solution [preservative free]: 0.3 mg/mL (1 mL)

Patch, transdermal:

Butrans®: 5 mcg/hr (4s) [total buprenorphine 5 mg]

Butrans®: 10 mcg/hr (4s) [total buprenorphine 10 mg]

Butrans®: 20 mcg/hr (4s) [total buprenorphine 20 mg]

Tablet, sublingual: 2 mg, 8 mg

Subutex®: 2 mg [DSC], 8 mg [DSC]

Controlled Substance C-III

Buprenorphine and Naloxone

(byoo pre NOR feen & nal OKS one)

Brand Names: U.S. Suboxone®

Brand Names: Canada Suboxone®

Index Terms Buprenorphine Hydrochloride and Naloxone Hydrochloride Dihydrate; Naloxone and Buprenorphine; Naloxone Hydrochloride Dihydrate and Buprenorphine Hydrochloride

Pharmacologic Category Analgesic, Opioid; Analgesic, Opioid Partial Agonist

Use Maintenance treatment for opioid dependence

Pregnancy Risk Factor C

Prescribing and Access Restrictions Prescribing of tablets for opioid dependence is limited to physicians who have met the qualification criteria and have received a DEA number specific to prescribing this product. Tablets will be available through pharmacies and wholesalers which normally provide controlled substances.

Medication Guide Available Yes

Dosage Sublingual: Opioid dependence: **Note:** Buprenorphine and naloxone combination product is not recommended for use during the induction period for long-acting opioids (eg, methadone); initial treatment should begin using buprenorphine oral sublingual tablets under supervision. Patients should be switched to the combination product for maintenance and unsupervised therapy. Doses provided based on buprenorphine content.

Children ≥16 years (sublingual tablet) and Adults (sublingual tablet or sublingual film):

Manufacturer's labeling: Maintenance: Target dose: 16 mg/day as a single daily dose; dosage should be adjusted in increments of 2 mg or 4 mg to a level which maintains treatment and suppresses opioid withdrawal symptoms; usual range: 4-24 mg/day

Unlabeled dosing recommendations (U.S. Department of Health and Human Services, 2005):

Induction (only administer combination product for induction in patients who are dependent on **short-acting** opioids and whose last dose of opioids was >12-24 hours prior to induction):

Day 1 induction dose: Initial: 4 mg; may repeat dose after >2 hours if withdrawal symptoms not relieved; maximum daily dose on day 1: 8 mg/day

Day 2 induction dose: Previous dose from day 1 if no withdrawal symptoms present; if symptoms of withdrawal present, increase day 1 dose by 4 mg. If withdrawal symptoms not relieved after >2 hours, may administer 4 mg; maximum daily dose on day 2: 16 mg/day

Subsequent induction days: If withdrawal symptoms are not present, daily dose is established. If withdrawal symptoms are present, increase dose in increments of 2 mg or 4 mg each day as needed for symptom relief. Target daily dose by the end of the first week: 12 mg or 16 mg/day; maximum daily dose: 32 mg/day

Stabilization: Usual dose: 16-24 mg/day; maximum dose: 32 mg/day

Switching between sublingual tablets and sublingual film: Same dosage should be used as the previous administered product. **Note:** Potential for greater bioavailability with the sublingual film compared to the sublingual tablet; monitor closely for either over- or underdosing when switching patients from one formulation to another.

Dosing adjustment in hepatic impairment: Moderate-to-severe impairment: Dosage adjustments recommended; however, no specific dosage adjustment recommendations provided by manufacturer.

Additional Information Complete prescribing information for this medication should be consulted for additional detail.

Dosage Forms Excipient information presented when available (limited, particularly for generics); consult specific product labeling.

Film, sublingual:

Suboxone®: Buprenorphine 2 mg and naloxone 0.5 mg; buprenorphine 8 mg and naloxone 2 mg [lime flavor]

Tablet, sublingual:

Suboxone®:Buprenorphine 2 mg and naloxone 0.5 mg; buprenorphine 8 mg and naloxone 2 mg [lemon-lime flavor]

Controlled Substance C-III

◆ **Buprenorphine Hydrochloride** *see* Buprenorphine *on page 244*

◆ **Buprenorphine Hydrochloride and Naloxone Hydrochloride Dihydrate** *see* Buprenorphine and Naloxone *on page 246*

◆ **Buproban®** *see* BuPROPion *on page 247*

BuPROPion (byoo PROE pee on)

Brand Names: U.S. Aplenzin™; Budeprion SR®; Budeprion XL®; Buproban®; Wellbutrin SR®; Wellbutrin XL®; Wellbutrin®; Zyban®

Brand Names: Canada Ava-Bupropion SR; Bupropion SR®; Novo-Bupropion SR; PMS-Bupropion SR; ratio-Bupropion SR; Sandoz-Bupropion SR; Wellbutrin® SR; Wellbutrin® XL; Zyban®

Index Terms Bupropion Hydrobromide; Bupropion Hydrochloride

Pharmacologic Category Antidepressant, Dopamine-Reuptake Inhibitor; Smoking Cessation Aid

Additional Appendix Information

Antidepressant Agents *on page 1874*

Use Treatment of major depressive disorder, including seasonal affective disorder (SAD); adjunct in smoking cessation

Unlabeled Use Attention-deficit/hyperactivity disorder (ADHD); depression associated with bipolar disorder

Pregnancy Risk Factor C

Pregnancy Considerations Due to adverse events observed in some animal studies, bupropion is classified as pregnancy category C. A significant increase in major teratogenic effects has not been observed following exposure to bupropion during pregnancy; however, the risk of spontaneous abortions may be increased (additional studies are needed to confirm). The long-term effects on development and behavior have not been studied.

Pregnancy itself does not provide protection against depression. The ACOG recommends that therapy with antidepressants during pregnancy be individualized and should incorporate the clinical expertise of the mental health clinician, obstetrician, primary care provider, and pediatrician. If treatment is needed, consider gradually stopping antidepressants 10-14 days before the expected date of delivery to prevent potential withdrawal symptoms in the infant. If this is done and the woman is considered to be at risk of relapse from her major depressive disorder, the medication can be restarted following delivery, although the dose should be readjusted to that required before pregnancy. Bupropion has also been evaluated for smoking cessation during pregnancy; current recommendations suggest that pharmacologic treatments be considered only after other therapies have failed. Treatment algorithms have been developed by the ACOG and the APA for the management of depression in women prior to conception and during pregnancy (Yonkers, 2009).

Lactation Enters breast milk/not recommended (AAP rates "of concern"; AAP 2001 update pending)

Medication Guide Available Yes

Contraindications Hypersensitivity to bupropion or any component of the formulation; seizure disorder; history of anorexia/bulimia; use of MAO inhibitors within 14 days; patients undergoing abrupt discontinuation of ethanol or sedatives (including benzodiazepines); patients receiving other dosage forms of bupropion

Warnings/Precautions [U.S. Boxed Warning]: Use in treating psychiatric disorders: Antidepressants increase the risk of suicidal thinking and behavior in children, adolescents, and young adults (18-24 years of age) with major depressive disorder (MDD) and other psychiatric disorders; consider risk prior to prescribing. Short-term studies did not show an increased risk in patients >24 years of age and showed a decreased risk in patients ≥65 years. All patients must be closely monitored for clinical worsening, suicidality, or unusual changes in behavior, especially during the initiation of therapy (generally first 1-2 months) or following an increase or decrease in dosage. The patient's family or caregiver should be instructed to closely observe the patient and communicate condition with healthcare provider. A medication guide should be dispensed with each prescription. **Bupropion is not FDA approved for use in children.**

[U.S. Boxed Warning]: Use in smoking cessation: Serious neuropsychiatric events, including depression, suicidal thoughts, and suicide, have been reported with use; some cases may have been complicated by symptoms of nicotine withdrawal following smoking cessation. Smoking cessation (with or without treatment) is associated with nicotine withdrawal symptoms and the exacerbation of underlying psychiatric illness; however, some of the behavioral disturbances were reported in treated patients who continued to smoke. These neuropsychiatric symptoms (eg, mood disturbances, psychosis, hostility) have occurred in patients with and without pre-existing psychiatric disease; many cases resolved following therapy discontinuation although in some cases, symptoms persisted. Monitor all patients for behavioral changes and psychiatric symptoms (eg, agitation, depression, suicidal behavior, suicidal ideation); inform patients to discontinue treatment and contact their healthcare provider immediately if they experience any behavioral and/or mood changes.

The possibility of a suicide attempt is inherent in major depression and may persist until remission occurs. Use caution in high-risk patients. Worsening depression and severe abrupt suicidality that are not part of the presenting symptoms may require discontinuation or modification of drug therapy. The patient's family or caregiver should be alerted to monitor patients for the emergence of suicidality and associated behaviors (such as agitation, irritability, hostility, impulsivity, and hypomania) and notify the healthcare provider.

May worsen psychosis in some patients or precipitate a shift to mania or hypomania in patients with bipolar disorder. Patients presenting with depressive symptoms should be screened for bipolar disorder. Monotherapy in patients with bipolar disorder should be avoided. **Bupropion is not FDA approved for bipolar depression.**

The risk of seizures is dose-dependent and increased in patients with a history of seizures, anorexia/bulimia, head trauma, CNS tumor, severe hepatic cirrhosis, abrupt discontinuation of sedative-hypnotics or ethanol, medications which lower seizure threshold (antipsychotics, antidepressants, theophyllines, systemic steroids), stimulants, or hypoglycemic agents. Risk of seizures may also be increased by chewing, crushing, or dividing long-acting products. Risk may be reduced by limiting the daily dose to bupropion hydrochloride ≤450 mg or bupropion hydrobromide 522 mg. Gradually increase dose incrementally to reduce risk. Discontinue and do not restart in patients experiencing a seizure.

May cause CNS stimulation (restlessness, anxiety, insomnia) or anorexia. May increase the risks associated with electroconvulsive therapy. Consider discontinuing, when possible, prior to elective surgery. May cause weight loss; use caution in patients where weight loss is not desirable. The incidence of sexual dysfunction with bupropion is generally lower than with SSRIs.

Use caution in patients with cardiovascular disease, history of hypertension, or coronary artery disease; treatment-emergent hypertension (including some severe cases) has been reported, both with bupropion alone and in combination with nicotine transdermal systems. All children diagnosed with ADHD who may be candidates for stimulant medications should have a thorough cardiovascular assessment to identify risk factors for sudden cardiac death prior to initiation of drug therapy. Use with caution in patients with hepatic or renal dysfunction and in elderly patients; reduced dose and/or frequency may be recommended. Elderly patients may be at greater risk of accumulation during chronic dosing. May cause motor or cognitive impairment in some patients; use with caution if tasks requiring alertness such as operating machinery or driving are undertaken. Arthralgia, myalgia, and fever with rash and other symptoms suggestive of delayed hypersensitivity resembling serum sickness have been reported.

Extended release tablet: Insoluble tablet shell may remain intact and be visible in the stool.

Adverse Reactions Frequencies, when reported, reflect highest incidence reported with sustained release product.

>10%:
- Cardiovascular: Tachycardia (11%)
- Central nervous system: Headache (25% to 34%), insomnia (11% to 20%), dizziness (6% to 11%)
- Gastrointestinal: Xerostomia (17% to 26%), weight loss (14% to 23%), nausea (1% to 18%)
- Respiratory: Pharyngitis (3% to 13%)

1% to 10%:
- Cardiovascular: Palpitation (2% to 6%), arrhythmias (5%), chest pain (3% to 4%), hypertension (2% to 4%; may be severe), flushing (1% to 4%), hypotension (3%)
- Central nervous system: Agitation (2% to 9%), confusion (8%), anxiety (5% to 7%), hostility (6%), nervousness (3% to 5%), sleep disturbance (4%), sensory disturbance (4%), migraine (1% to 4%), abnormal dreams (3%), irritability (2% to 3%), somnolence (2% to 3%), pain (2% to 3%), memory decreased (≤3%), fever (1% to 2%), CNS stimulation (1% to 2%), depression
- Dermatologic: Rash (1% to 5%), pruritus (2% to 4%), urticaria (1% to 2%)
- Endocrine & metabolic: Menstrual complaints (2% to 5%), hot flashes (1% to 3%), libido decreased (3%)
- Gastrointestinal: Constipation (5% to 10%), abdominal pain (2% to 9%), diarrhea (5% to 7%), flatulence (6%), anorexia (3% to 5%), appetite increased (4%), taste perversion (2% to 4%), vomiting (2% to 4%), dyspepsia (3%), dysphagia (≤2%)
- Genitourinary: Polyuria (2% to 5%), urinary urgency (≤2%), vaginal hemorrhage (≤2%), UTI (≤1%)
- Neuromuscular & skeletal: Tremor (3% to 6%), myalgia (2% to 6%), weakness (2% to 4%), arthralgia (1% to 4%), arthritis (2%), akathisia (≤2%), paresthesia (1% to 2%), twitching (1% to 2%), neck pain
- Ocular: Blurred vision (2% to 3%), amblyopia (2%)
- Otic: Tinnitus (3% to 6%), auditory disturbance (5%)
- Respiratory: Upper respiratory infection (9%), cough increased (1% to 4%), sinusitis (1% to 5%)
- Miscellaneous: Infection (8% to 9%), diaphoresis (5% to 6%), allergic reaction (including anaphylaxis, pruritus, urticaria)

<1% (Limited to important or life-threatening): Accommodation abnormality, aggression, akinesia, alopecia, amnesia, anaphylactic shock, anemia, angioedema, aphasia, ataxia, atrioventricular block, bronchospasm, bruxism, colitis, coma, coordination abnormal, cystitis, deafness, delayed hypersensitivity, delirium, delusions,

depersonalization, derealization, diplopia, dysarthria, dyskinesia, dyspareunia, dysphoria, dystonia, dysuria, edema, EEG abnormality, emotional lability, erythema multiforme, esophagitis, euphoria, exfoliative dermatitis, extrapyramidal syndrome, extrasystoles, facial edema, gastric reflux, gastrointestinal hemorrhage, glossitis, glycosuria, gum hemorrhage, gynecomastia, hallucinations, hepatic damage, hepatitis, hirsutism, hyper-/hypoglycemia, hyper-/hypokinesia, hypertonia, hypoesthesia, hypomania, impotence, intestinal perforation, intraocular pressure increased, jaundice, leukocytosis, leukopenia, libido increased, liver function abnormal, lymphadenopathy, manic reaction, MI, muscle weakness, musculoskeletal chest pain, mydriasis, myoclonus, neuralgia, neuropathy, painful erection, pancreatitis, pancytopenia, paranoia, pneumonia, photosensitivity, postural hypotension, pulmonary embolism, rhabdomyolysis, salpingitis, sciatica, seizures (dose-related), SIADH, stomach ulcer, Stevens-Johnson syndrome, stomatitis, stroke, suicidal ideation, syncope, tardive dyskinesia, thrombocytopenia, tongue edema, urinary incontinence, urinary retention, vasodilation

Drug Interactions

Metabolism/Transport Effects Substrate of CYP1A2 (minor), CYP2A6 (minor), CYP2B6 (major), CYP2C9 (minor), CYP2D6 (minor), CYP2E1 (minor), CYP3A4 (minor); **Note:** Assignment of Major/Minor substrate status based on clinically relevant drug interaction potential; **Inhibits** CYP2D6 (strong)

Avoid Concomitant Use

Avoid concomitant use of BuPROPion with any of the following: MAO Inhibitors; Methylene Blue; Pimozide; Tamoxifen; Thioridazine

Increased Effect/Toxicity

BuPROPion may increase the levels/effects of: Alcohol (Ethyl); Atomoxetine; CYP2D6 Substrates; Fesoterodine; Iloperidone; Methylene Blue; Nebivolol; Pimozide; Propafenone; Tamoxifen; Tetrabenazine; Thioridazine; Tricyclic Antidepressants

The levels/effects of BuPROPion may be increased by: Alcohol (Ethyl); Conivaptan; CYP2B6 Inhibitors (Moderate); CYP2B6 Inhibitors (Strong); MAO Inhibitors; Quazepam

Decreased Effect

BuPROPion may decrease the levels/effects of: Codeine; Iloperidone; Ioflupane I 123; TraMADol

The levels/effects of BuPROPion may be decreased by: CYP2B6 Inducers (Strong); Cyproterone; Efavirenz; Lopinavir; Peginterferon Alfa-2b; Ritonavir; Tocilizumab

Ethanol/Nutrition/Herb Interactions

Ethanol: May increase CNS depression; monitor for increased effects with coadministration. Caution patients about effects.

Herb/Nutraceutical: Avoid valerian, St John's wort, SAMe, gotu kola, kava kava (may increase CNS depression).

Stability Store at controlled room temperature of 20°C to 25°C (68°F to 77°F).

Aplenzin™, Wellbutrin XL®: Store at 15°C to 30°C (59°F to 86°F).

Mechanism of Action Aminoketone antidepressant structurally different from all other marketed antidepressants; like other antidepressants the mechanism of bupropion's activity is not fully understood. Bupropion is a relatively weak inhibitor of the neuronal uptake of norepinephrine and dopamine, and does not inhibit monoamine oxidase or the reuptake of serotonin. Metabolite inhibits the reuptake of norepinephrine. The primary mechanism of action is thought to be dopaminergic and/or noradrenergic.

Pharmacodynamics/Kinetics

Absorption: Rapid

Distribution: V_d: ~20-47 L/kg (Laizure, 1985)

Protein binding: 84%

Metabolism: Extensively hepatic via CYP2B6 to hydroxybupropion; non-CYP-mediated metabolism to erythrohydrobupropion and threohydrobupropion. Metabolite activity ranges from 20% to 50% potency of bupropion.

Half-life:

Distribution: 3-4 hours

Elimination: 21 ± 9 hours; Metabolites: Hydroxybupropion: 20 ± 5 hours; Erythrohydrobupropion: 33 ± 10 hours; Threohydrobupropion: 37 ± 13 hours

Extended release (Aplenzin™): 21 ± 7 hours; Metabolites: Hydroxybupropion: 24 ± 5 hours; Erythrohydrobupropion: 31 ± 8 hours; Threohydrobupropion: 51 ± 9 hours

Time to peak, serum:

Bupropion: Immediate release: Within 2 hours; Sustained release: Within 3 hours; Extended release: ~5 hours

Metabolite: Hydroxybupropion: Immediate release: ~3 hours; Extended release, sustained release: ~6-7 hours

Excretion: Urine (87%, primarily as metabolites); feces (10%, primarily as metabolites)

Dosage Oral:

Children and Adolescents: ADHD (unlabeled use): Hydrochloride salt: 1.4-6 mg/kg/day

Adults:

Depression:

Immediate release hydrochloride salt: 100 mg 3 times/day; begin at 100 mg twice daily; may increase to a maximum dose of 450 mg/day

Sustained release hydrochloride salt: Initial: 150 mg/day in the morning; may increase to 150 mg twice daily by day 4 if tolerated; target dose: 300 mg/day given as 150 mg twice daily; maximum dose: 400 mg/day given as 200 mg twice daily

Extended release:

Hydrochloride salt: Initial: 150 mg/day in the morning; may increase as early as day 4 of dosing to 300 mg/day; maximum dose: 450 mg/day

Hydrobromide salt (Aplenzin™): Target dose: 348 mg/day in the morning. Patients not previously on bupropion: Initial: 174 mg/day in the morning; may increase as early as day 4 of dosing to 348 mg/day; maximum dose: 522 mg/day. **Note:** 174 mg strength currently not available; 348 mg tablet cannot be split.

Switching from hydrochloride salt formulation (eg, Wellbutrin® immediate release, SR®, XL®) to hydrobromide salt formulation (Aplenzin™): **Note:** Patients being treated twice daily with bupropion hydrochloride would be switched to the equivalent once daily dose of bupropion hydrobromide.

Bupropion hydrochloride 150 mg is equivalent to bupropion hydrobromide 174 mg

Bupropion hydrochloride 300 mg is equivalent to bupropion hydrobromide 348 mg

Bupropion hydrochloride 450 mg is equivalent to bupropion hydrobromide 522 mg

SAD (Wellbutrin XL®): Initial: 150 mg/day in the morning; if tolerated, may increase after 1 week to 300 mg/day

Note: Prophylactic treatment should be reserved for those patients with frequent depressive episodes and/or significant impairment. Initiate treatment in the Autumn prior to symptom onset, and discontinue in early Spring with dose tapering to 150 mg/day for 2 weeks

Smoking cessation (Zyban®): Initiate with 150 mg once daily for 3 days; increase to 150 mg twice daily; treatment should continue for 7-12 weeks

Note: Therapy should begin at least 1 week before target quit date. Target quit dates are generally in the second week of treatment. If patient successfully quits smoking after 7-12 weeks, may consider ongoing maintenance therapy based on individual patient risk: benefit. Efficacy of maintenance therapy (300 mg/day) has been demonstrated for up to 6 months. Conversely, if significant progress has not been made by the seventh week of therapy, success is unlikely and treatment discontinuation should be considered.

Elderly: Depression: Hydrochloride salt: 50-100 mg/day, increase by 50-100 mg every 3-4 days as tolerated; there is evidence that the elderly respond at 150 mg/day in divided doses, but some may require a higher dose. **Note:** Patients with Alzheimer's dementia-related depression may require a lower starting dosage of 37.5 mg once or twice daily (100 mg/day sustained release), increased as needed up to 300 mg/day in divided doses (300 mg/day for sustained release)

Dosing conversion between hydrochloride salt (eg, Wellbutrin®) immediate, sustained, and extended release products: Convert using same total daily dose (up to the maximum recommended dose for a given dosage form), but adjust frequency as indicated for sustained (twice daily) or extended (once daily) release products.

Dosing adjustment/comments in renal impairment: Use with caution and consider a reduction in dosing frequency; limited pharmacokinetic information suggests elimination of bupropion and/or the active metabolites may be reduced.

Moderate-to-severe renal impairment: Bupropion exposure was approximately twofold higher compared to normal subjects following a 150 mg single dose administration.

End-stage renal failure: Per the manufacturer, the elimination of hydroxybupropion and threohydrobupropion are reduced in patients with end-stage renal failure.

Dosing adjustment in hepatic impairment:

Note: The mean AUC increased by ~1.5-fold for hydroxybupropion and ~2.5-fold for erythro/threohydrobupropion; median T_{max} was observed 19 hours later for hydroxybupropion, 31 hours later for erythro/threohydrobupropion; mean half-life for hydroxybupropion increased fivefold, and increased twofold for erythro/threohydrobupropion in patients with severe hepatic cirrhosis compared to healthy volunteers.

Mild-to-moderate hepatic impairment: Use with caution and/or reduced dose/frequency

Severe hepatic cirrhosis: Use with extreme caution; maximum dose:
- Aplenzin™: 174 mg every other day
- Wellbutrin®: 75 mg/day
- Wellbutrin SR®: 100 mg/day or 150 mg every other day
- Wellbutrin XL®: 150 mg every other day
- Zyban®: 150 mg every other day

Administration May be taken without regard to meals. Zyban® and extended release tablets (hydrochloride and hydrobromide salt formulations) should be swallowed whole; do not crush, chew, or divide. The insoluble shell of the extended-release tablet may remain intact during GI transit and is eliminated in the feces.

Monitoring Parameters Body weight; mental status for depression, suicidal ideation (especially at the beginning of therapy or when doses are increased or decreased), anxiety, social functioning, mania, panic attacks

When used for the treatment of ADHD, thoroughly evaluate for cardiovascular risk. Monitor heart rate, blood pressure, and consider obtaining ECG prior to initiation (Vetter, 2008).

Reference Range Therapeutic levels (trough, 12 hours after last dose): 50-100 ng/mL

Test Interactions May interfere with urine detection of amphetamine/methamphetamine (false-positive). Decreased prolactin levels.

Additional Information Risk of seizures: When using bupropion hydrochloride immediate release tablets, seizure risk is increased at total daily dosage >450 mg, individual dosages >150 mg, or by sudden, large increments in dose. Data for the immediate-release formulation of bupropion revealed a seizure incidence of 0.4% in patients treated at doses in the 300-450 mg/day range. The estimated seizure incidence increases almost 10-fold between 450 mg and 600 mg per day. Data for the sustained release dosage form revealed a seizure incidence of 0.1% in patients treated at a dosage range of 100-300 mg/day, and increases to ~0.4% at the maximum recommended dose of 400 mg/day.

Dosage Forms Excipient information presented when available (limited, particularly for generics); consult specific product labeling.

Tablet, oral, as hydrochloride: 75 mg [generic for Wellbutrin®], 100 mg [generic for Wellbutrin®]
- Wellbutrin®: 75 mg, 100 mg

Tablet, extended release, oral, as hydrobromide:
- Aplenzin™: 174 mg, 348 mg, 522 mg

Tablet, extended release, oral, as hydrochloride: 100 mg [generic for Wellbutrin SR®], 150 mg [generic for Wellbutrin SR®], 150 mg [generic for Wellbutrin XL®], 150 mg [generic for Zyban®], 200 mg [generic for Wellbutrin SR®], 300 mg [generic for Wellbutrin XL®]
- Budeprion SR®: 100 mg [contains tartrazine; generic for Wellbutrin SR®]
- Budeprion SR®: 150 mg [generic for Wellbutrin SR®]
- Budeprion XL®: 150 mg [generic for Wellbutrin XL®]
- Budeprion XL®: 300 mg [contains tartrazine; generic for Wellbutrin XL®]
- Buproban®: 150 mg [generic for Zyban®]
- Wellbutrin XL®: 150 mg, 300 mg

Tablet, sustained release, oral, as hydrochloride:
- Wellbutrin SR®: 100 mg, 150 mg, 200 mg
- Zyban®: 150 mg

- ◆ **Bupropion Hydrobromide** *see* BuPROPion *on page 247*
- ◆ **Bupropion Hydrochloride** *see* BuPROPion *on page 247*
- ◆ **Bupropion SR® (Can)** *see* BuPROPion *on page 247*
- ◆ **Burinex® (Can)** *see* Bumetanide *on page 241*
- ◆ **Burn Jel® [OTC]** *see* Lidocaine (Topical) *on page 1009*
- ◆ **Burn Jel Plus [OTC]** *see* Lidocaine (Topical) *on page 1009*
- ◆ **Buscopan® (Can)** *see* Scopolamine (Systemic) *on page 1542*
- ◆ **BuSpar** *see* BusPIRone *on page 250*
- ◆ **BuSpar® (Can)** *see* BusPIRone *on page 250*
- ◆ **Buspirex (Can)** *see* BusPIRone *on page 250*

BusPIRone (byoo SPYE rone)

Brand Names: Canada Apo-Buspirone®; BuSpar®; Buspirex; Bustab®; CO Buspirone; Dom-Buspirone; Gen-Buspirone; Lin-Buspirone; Mylan-Buspirone; Novo-Buspirone; Nu-Buspirone; PMS-Buspirone; ratio-Buspirone; Riva-Buspirone

Index Terms BuSpar; Buspirone Hydrochloride

Pharmacologic Category Antianxiety Agent, Miscellaneous

Use Management of generalized anxiety disorder (GAD)

Unlabeled Use Management of aggression in mental retardation and secondary mental disorders; major depression; potential augmenting agent for antidepressants; premenstrual syndrome

Pregnancy Risk Factor B

Pregnancy Considerations No impairment of fertility or fetotoxic effects were noted in animal studies with doses 30 times maximum recommended human dose. There are no adequate and well-controlled studies in pregnant women.

Lactation Excretion in breast milk unknown/not recommended

Contraindications Hypersensitivity to buspirone or any component of the formulation

Warnings/Precautions Use in severe hepatic or renal impairment is not recommended; does not prevent or treat withdrawal from benzodiazepines. Low potential for cognitive or motor impairment. Use with MAO inhibitors may result in hypertensive reactions. Restlessness syndrome has been reported in small number of patients; monitor for signs of any dopamine-related movement disorders. Buspirone does not exhibit cross-tolerance with benzodiazepines or other sedative/hypnotic agents. If substituting buspirone for any of these agents, gradually withdraw the drug(s) prior to initiating buspirone. Safety and efficacy of buspirone have not been established in children <6 years of age; no long-term safety/efficacy data available in children.

Adverse Reactions

>10%: Central nervous system: Dizziness (12%)

1% to 10%:

Cardiovascular: Chest pain (≥1%)

Central nervous system: Drowsiness (10%), headache (6%), nervousness (5%), lightheadedness (3%), anger/hostility (2%), confusion (2%), excitement (2%), dream disturbance (≥1%)

Dermatologic: Rash (1%)

Gastrointestinal: Nausea (8%), diarrhea (2%)

Neuromuscular & skeletal: Numbness (2%), weakness (2%), musculoskeletal pain (1%), paresthesia (1%), incoordination (1%), tremor (1%)

Ocular: Blurred vision (2%)

Otic: Tinnitus (≥1%)

Respiratory: Nasal congestion (≥1%), sore throat (≥1%)

Miscellaneous: Diaphoresis (1%)

<1% (Limited to important or life-threatening): Akathisia, allergic reaction, angioedema, anorexia, bradycardia, bruising, cardiomyopathy, cogwheel rigidity, conjunctivitis, CVA, dyskinesia, dyspnea, dystonia, edema, enuresis, eosinophilia, epistaxis, EPS, galactorrhea, hallucination, heart failure, hyper-/hypotension, hyperventilation, irritable colon, leukopenia, menstrual irregularity, MI, muscle spasms, parkinsonism, personality disorders, PID, psychosis, rectal bleeding, restless leg syndrome, seizure, serotonin syndrome, suicidal ideation, syncope, thrombocytopenia, thyroid abnormality, transaminase increases, visual disturbances (tunnel vision)

Drug Interactions

Metabolism/Transport Effects **Substrate** of CYP2D6 (minor), CYP3A4 (major); **Note:** Assignment of Major/Minor substrate status based on clinically relevant drug interaction potential

Avoid Concomitant Use

Avoid concomitant use of BusPIRone with any of the following: Conivaptan; MAO Inhibitors; Methylene Blue

Increased Effect/Toxicity

BusPIRone may increase the levels/effects of: Alcohol (Ethyl); Antidepressants (Serotonin Reuptake Inhibitor/Antagonist); CNS Depressants; MAO Inhibitors; Methylene Blue; Metoclopramide; Selective Serotonin Reuptake Inhibitors; Serotonin Modulators

The levels/effects of BusPIRone may be increased by: Antifungal Agents (Azole Derivatives, Systemic); Antipsychotics; Calcium Channel Blockers (Nondihydropyridine); Conivaptan; CYP3A4 Inhibitors (Moderate); CYP3A4 Inhibitors (Strong); Dasatinib; Grapefruit Juice; HydrOXYzine; Macrolide Antibiotics; Selective Serotonin Reuptake Inhibitors

Decreased Effect

BusPIRone may decrease the levels/effects of: Ioflupane I 123

The levels/effects of BusPIRone may be decreased by: CYP3A4 Inducers (Strong); Deferasirox; Peginterferon Alfa-2b; Rifamycin Derivatives; Tocilizumab; Yohimbine

Ethanol/Nutrition/Herb Interactions

Ethanol: May increase CNS depression; monitor for increased effects with coadministration. Caution patients about effects.

Food: Food may decrease the absorption of buspirone, but it may also decrease the first-pass metabolism, thereby increasing the bioavailability of buspirone. Grapefruit juice may cause increased buspirone concentrations; avoid intake of large quantities of grapefruit juice.

Herb/Nutraceutical: St John's wort may decrease buspirone levels or increase CNS depression. Avoid valerian, gotu kola, kava kava (may increase CNS depression).

Stability Store at USP controlled room temperature of 25°C (77°F). Protect from light.

Mechanism of Action The mechanism of action of buspirone is unknown. Buspirone has a high affinity for serotonin 5-HT_{1A} and 5-HT_2 receptors, without affecting benzodiazepine-GABA receptors. Buspirone has moderate affinity for dopamine D_2 receptors.

Pharmacodynamics/Kinetics

Absorption: Rapid

Distribution: V_d: 5.3 L/kg

Protein binding: 86% to 95%

Metabolism: Hepatic oxidation, primarily via CYP3A4; extensive first-pass effect

Bioavailability: ~4%

Half-life elimination: 2-3 hours

Time to peak, serum: 40-90 minutes

Excretion: Urine: 29% to 63% (<0.1% dose excreted unchanged); feces: 18% to 38%

Dosage Oral:

Generalized anxiety disorder:

Children ≥6 years and Adolescents: Initial: 5 mg daily; increase in increments of 5 mg/day at weekly intervals as needed, to a maximum dose of 60 mg/day divided into 2-3 doses

Adults: 15 mg/day (7.5 mg twice daily); may increase in increments of 5 mg/day every 2-3 days to a maximum of 60 mg/day; target dose for most people is 20-30 mg/day (10-15 mg twice daily)

Elderly: Initial: 5 mg twice daily, increase by 5 mg/day every 2-3 days as needed up to 20-30 mg/day; maximum daily dose: 60 mg/day.

Dosing adjustment in renal impairment: Patients with impaired renal function demonstrated increased plasma levels and a prolonged half-life of buspirone. Use in patients with severe renal impairment not recommended.

Dosing adjustment in hepatic impairment: Patients with impaired hepatic function demonstrated increased plasma levels and a prolonged half-life of buspirone. Use in patients with severe hepatic impairment not recommended.

Dietary Considerations Avoid large quantities of grapefruit juice.

Monitoring Parameters Mental status, symptoms of anxiety

Additional Information Has shown little potential for abuse; needs continuous use. Because of slow onset, not appropriate for "as needed" (prn) use or for brief, situational anxiety. Ineffective for treatment of benzodiazepine or ethanol withdrawal.

Dosage Forms Excipient information presented when available (limited, particularly for generics); consult specific product labeling.

Tablet, oral, as hydrochloride: 5 mg, 7.5 mg, 10 mg, 15 mg, 30 mg

◆ **Buspirone Hydrochloride** *see* BusPIRone *on page 250*

◆ **Bussulfam** *see* Busulfan *on page 252*

◆ **Bustab® (Can)** *see* BusPIRone *on page 250*

Busulfan (byoo SUL fan)

Brand Names: U.S. Busulfex®; Myleran®

Brand Names: Canada Busulfex®; Myleran®

Index Terms Bussulfam; Busulfanum; Busulphan

Pharmacologic Category Antineoplastic Agent, Alkylating Agent

Use Palliative treatment of chronic myelogenous leukemia (CML) (oral); conditioning regimen prior to allogeneic hematopoietic progenitor cell transplantation (I.V.) for CML

Unlabeled Use Conditioning regimen prior to hematopoietic stem cell transplant (HSCT) (oral); treatment of polycythemia vera and essential thrombocytosis

Pregnancy Risk Factor D

Pregnancy Considerations Animal studies have demonstrated teratogenic effects. There are no adequate and well-controlled studies in pregnant women. May cause fetal harm if administered during pregnancy. The solvent in I.V. busulfan, DMA, is also associated with teratogenic effects and may impair fertility. Women of childbearing potential should avoid pregnancy while receiving busulfan treatment.

Lactation Excretion in breast milk unknown/not recommended

Contraindications Hypersensitivity to busulfan or any component of the formulation; oral busulfan is contraindicated in patients without a definitive diagnosis of CML

Warnings/Precautions Hazardous agent - use appropriate precautions for handling and disposal. **[U.S. Boxed Warning]: Severe bone marrow suppression is common; reduce dose or discontinue oral busulfan for unusual suppression; may require bone marrow biopsy.** May result in severe neutropenia, thrombocytopenia, anemia, bone marrow failure, and/or pancytopenia; pancytopenia may be prolonged (1 month up to 2 years) and may be reversible. Use with caution in patients with compromised bone marrow reserve (due to prior treatment or radiation therapy). Monitor closely for signs of infection (due to neutropenia) or bleeding (due to thrombocytopenia) Seizures have been reported with use; use caution in patients predisposed to seizures, history of seizures or head trauma; when using as a conditioning regimen for transplant, initiate prophylactic anticonvulsant therapy (eg, phenytoin) prior to treatment. Phenytoin increases busulfan clearance by ≥15%; busulfan kinetics and dosing recommendations for high-dose HSCT conditioning were studied with concomitant phenytoin. If alternate anticonvulsants are used, busulfan clearance may be decreased and dosing should be monitored accordingly.

Bronchopulmonary dysplasia with pulmonary fibrosis ("busulfan lung") is associated with busulfan; onset is delayed with symptoms occurring at an average of 4 years (range: 4 months to 10 years) after treatment; may be fatal. Symptoms generally include a slow onset of cough, dyspnea, and fever (low-grade), although acute symptomatic onset may also occur. Diminished diffusion capacity and decreased pulmonary compliance have been noted with pulmonary function testing. Differential diagnosis should rule out opportunistic pulmonary infection or leukemic pulmonary infiltrates; may require lung biopsy. Discontinue busulfan if toxicity develops. Pulmonary toxicity may be additive if administered with other cytotoxic agents also associated with pulmonary toxicity. Cardiac tamponade as been reported in children with thalassemia treated with high-dose oral busulfan in combination with cyclophosphamide. Busulfan has been causally related to the development of secondary malignancies (tumors and acute leukemias); chromosomal alterations may also occur. Busulfan has been associated with ovarian failure (including failure to achieve puberty).

High busulfan area under the concentration versus time curve (AUC) values (>1500 micromolar•minute) are associated with increased risk of hepatic sinusoidal obstruction syndrome (SOS; formerly called veno-occlusive disease [VOD]) due to conditioning for allogenic HSCT; patients with a history of radiation therapy, prior chemotherapy (≥3 cycles), or prior stem cell transplantation are at increased risk; monitor liver function tests periodically. Oral busulfan doses above 16 mg/kg (based on IBW) and concurrent use with alkylating agents may also increase the risk for hepatic SOS. The solvent in I.V. busulfan, DMA, may impair fertility. DMA may also be associated with hepatotoxicity, hallucinations, somnolence, lethargy, and confusion. **[U.S. Boxed Warning]: Should be administered under the supervision of an experienced cancer chemotherapy physician; for the I.V. formulation, should be experienced in management of HSCT and management of patients with severe pancytopenia; according to the manufacturer, oral busulfan should not be used until CML diagnosis has been established.** Cellular dysplasia in many organs has been observed (in addition to lung dysplasia); giant hyperchromatic nuclei have been noted in adrenal glands, liver, lymph nodes, pancreas, thyroid, and bone marrow. May obscure routine diagnostic cytologic exams (eg, cervical smear).

Adverse Reactions

I.V.:

>10%:

Cardiovascular: Tachycardia (44%), hypertension (36%; grades 3/4: 7%), edema (28% to 79%), thrombosis (33%), chest pain (26%), vasodilation (25%), hypotension (11%; grades 3/4: 3%)

Central nervous system: Insomnia (84%), fever (80%), anxiety (72% to 75%), headache (69%), chills (46%), pain (44%), dizziness (30%), depression (23%), confusion (11%)

Dermatologic: Rash (57%), pruritus (28%), alopecia (17%)

Endocrine & metabolic: Hypomagnesemia (77%), hyperglycemia (66% to 67%; grades 3/4: 15%), hypokalemia (64%), hypocalcemia (49%), hypophosphatemia (17%)

Gastrointestinal: Vomiting (43% to 100%), nausea (83% to 98%), mucositis/stomatitis (79% to 97%; grades 3/4: 26%), anorexia (85%), diarrhea (84%; grades 3/4: 5%), abdominal pain (72%), dyspepsia (44%), constipation (38%), xerostomia (26%), rectal disorder (25%), abdominal fullness (23%)

Hematologic: Myelosuppression (≤100%), neutropenia (100%; onset: 4 days; median recovery: 13 days [with G-CSF support]), thrombocytopenia (98%; median onset: 5-6 days), lymphopenia (children: 79%), anemia (69%)

Hepatic: Hyperbilirubinemia (49%; grades 3/4: 30%), ALT increased (31%; grades 3/4: 7%), hepatic sinusoidal obstruction syndrome (SOS; veno-occlusive disease) (adults: 8% to 12%; children: 21%), alkaline phosphatase increased (15%), jaundice (12%)

Local: Injection site inflammation (25%), injection site pain (15%)

Neuromuscular & skeletal: Weakness (51%), back pain (23%), myalgia (16%), arthralgia (13%)

Renal: Creatinine increased (21%), oliguria (15%)

Respiratory: Rhinitis (44%), lung disorder (34%), cough (28%), epistaxis (25%), dyspnea (25%), pneumonia (children: 21%), hiccup (18%), pharyngitis (18%)
Miscellaneous: Infection (51%; includes severe bacterial, viral [CMV], and fungal infections), allergic reaction (26%)

1% to 10%:
Cardiovascular: Arrhythmia (5%), cardiomegaly (5%), atrial fibrillation (2%), ECG abnormal (2%), heart block (2%), heart failure (grade 3/4: 2%), pericardial effusion (2%), tamponade (children with thalassemia: 2%), ventricular extrasystoles (2%), hypervolemia
Central nervous system: Lethargy (7%), hallucination (5%), agitation (2%), delirium (2%), encephalopathy (2%), seizure (2%), somnolence (2%), cerebral hemorrhage (1%)
Dermatologic: Vesicular rash (10%), vesiculobullous rash (10%), skin discoloration (8%), maculopapular rash (8%), acne (7%), exfoliative dermatitis (5%), erythema nodosum (2%)
Endocrine & metabolic: Hyponatremia (2%)
Gastrointestinal: Ileus (8%), weight gain (8%), esophagitis (grade 3: 2%), hematemesis (2%), pancreatitis (2%)
Hematologic: Prothrombin time increased (2%)
Hepatic: Hepatomegaly (6%)
Renal: Hematuria (8%), dysuria (7%), hemorrhagic cystitis (grade 3/4: 7%), BUN increased (3%; grades 3/4: 2%)
Respiratory: Asthma (8%), alveolar hemorrhage (5%), hyperventilation (5%), hemoptysis (3%), pleural effusion (3%), sinusitis (3%), atelectasis (2%), hypoxia (2%)

Oral: Frequency not defined:
Dermatologic: Hyperpigmentation of skin (5% to 10%), rash
Endocrine & metabolic: Amenorrhea, ovarian suppression
Gastrointestinal: Xerostomia
Hematologic: Myelosuppression (anemia, leukopenia, thrombocytopenia)

I.V. and/or Oral: Infrequent, postmarketing, and/or case reports: Acute leukemias, adrenal insufficiency, alopecia (permanent), aplastic anemia (may be irreversible), azoospermia, bronchopulmonary dysplasia, capillary leak syndrome, cataracts (rare), cheilosis, cholestatic jaundice, corneal thinning, dry skin, endocardial fibrosis, erythema multiforme, esophageal varices, gynecomastia, hepatic dysfunction, hepatocellular atrophy, hyperuricemia, hyperuricosuria, interstitial pulmonary fibrosis, malignant tumors, myasthenia gravis, neutropenic fever, ocular (lens) changes, ovarian failure, pancytopenia, porphyria cutanea tarda, pulmonary fibrosis, radiation myelopathy, radiation recall (skin rash), sepsis, sterility, testicular atrophy, thrombotic microangiopathy (TMA), tumor lysis syndrome, urticaria

Drug Interactions

Metabolism/Transport Effects **Substrate** of CYP3A4 (major); **Note:** Assignment of Major/Minor substrate status based on clinically relevant drug interaction potential

Avoid Concomitant Use

Avoid concomitant use of Busulfan with any of the following: BCG; CloZAPine; Conivaptan; Natalizumab; Pimecrolimus; Tacrolimus (Topical); Vaccines (Live)

Increased Effect/Toxicity

Busulfan may increase the levels/effects of: CloZAPine; Leflunomide; Natalizumab; Vaccines (Live); Vitamin K Antagonists

The levels/effects of Busulfan may be increased by: Acetaminophen; Antifungal Agents (Azole Derivatives, Systemic); Conivaptan; CYP3A4 Inhibitors (Moderate); CYP3A4 Inhibitors (Strong); Dasatinib; Denosumab; MetroNIDAZOLE; MetroNIDAZOLE (Systemic); Pimecrolimus; Roflumilast; Tacrolimus (Topical); Trastuzumab

Decreased Effect

Busulfan may decrease the levels/effects of: BCG; Coccidioidin Skin Test; Sipuleucel-T; Vaccines (Inactivated); Vaccines (Live); Vitamin K Antagonists

The levels/effects of Busulfan may be decreased by: CYP3A4 Inducers (Strong); Deferasirox; Echinacea; Fosphenytoin; Herbs (CYP3A4 Inducers); Phenytoin; Tocilizumab

Ethanol/Nutrition/Herb Interactions

Ethanol: Avoid ethanol due to GI irritation.
Food: No clear or firm data on the effect of food on busulfan bioavailability.
Herb/Nutraceutical: Avoid St John's wort (may decrease busulfan levels).

Stability

Injection: Store intact vials under refrigeration at 2°C to 8°C (36°F to 46°F). Dilute in 0.9% sodium chloride (NS) injection or dextrose 5% in water (D_5W). The dilution volume should be ten times the volume of busulfan injection, ensuring that the final concentration of busulfan is 0.5 mg/mL. Always add busulfan to the diluent, and not the diluent to the busulfan. Mix with several inversions. Solutions diluted in NS or D_5W for infusion are stable for up to 8 hours at room temperature (25°C [77°F]); the infusion must also be completed within that 8-hour timeframe. Dilution of busulfan injection in NS is stable for up to 12 hours at refrigeration (2°C to 8°C); the infusion must be completed within that 12-hour timeframe. Do not use polycarbonate syringes or filters for preparation or administration.
Tablet: Store at 25°C (77°F); excursions permitted to 15°C to 30°C (59°F to 86°F).

Mechanism of Action Busulfan is an alkylating agent which reacts with the N-7 position of guanosine and interferes with DNA replication and transcription of RNA. Busulfan has a more marked effect on myeloid cells than on lymphoid cells and is also very toxic to hematopoietic stem cells. Busulfan exhibits little immunosuppressive activity. Interferes with the normal function of DNA by alkylation and cross-linking the strands of DNA.

Pharmacodynamics/Kinetics

Absorption: Rapid and complete
Distribution: V_d: ~1 L/kg; distributes into CSF with levels equal to plasma
Protein binding: 32% to plasma proteins and 47% to red blood cells
Metabolism: Extensively hepatic (may increase with multiple doses); glutathione conjugation followed by oxidation
Bioavailability: Oral: Children ≥13 years and adults: 80% ± 20%; Children 1.5-6 years: 68% ± 31%
Half-life elimination: 2-3 hours
Time to peak, serum: Oral: ~1 hour; I.V.: Within 5 minutes
Excretion: Urine (25% to 60% predominantly as metabolites; <2% as unchanged drug)

Dosage Note: Premedicate with prophylactic anticonvulsant therapy (eg, phenytoin) prior to high-dose busulfan treatment. Prophylactic antiemetics may be necessary for high-dose (HSCT) regimens.

Children:
CML, palliation (manufacturer's labeling): Oral:
Remission induction: 60 mcg/kg/day or 1.8 mg/m²/day; titrate dose (or withhold) to maintain leukocyte counts ≥15,000/mm³ (doses >4 mg/day should be reserved for patients with the most compelling symptoms)
Maintenance: When leukocyte count ≥50,000/mm³: Resume induction dose **or** (if remission <3 months) 1-3 mg/day (to control hematologic status and prevent relapse)

HSCT conditioning regimen:
I.V.:
≤12 kg: 1.1 mg/kg/dose (actual body weight) every 6 hours for 16 doses
>12 kg: 0.8 mg/kg/dose (actual body weight) every 6 hours for 16 doses
Adjust dose to desired AUC (1125 micromolar•minute) using the following formula:
Adjusted dose (mg) = Actual dose (mg) x [target AUC (micromolar•minute) / actual AUC (micromolar•minute)]
Reduced intensity conditioning regimen (unlabeled dosing): 0.8 mg/kg/dose for 1 dose 7-10 days prior to transplant, followed by ~0.8 mg/kg/dose (busulfan kinetics calculated after initial dose) every 6 hours for 7 doses beginning 3-6 days prior to transplant (in combination with fludarabine and antithymocyte globulin) (Pulsipher, 2009)
Oral (unlabeled use): 1 mg/kg/dose every 6 hours for 16 doses beginning 9 days prior to transplant (in combination with cyclophosphamide) (Cassileth, 1998)
Adults:
CML, palliation (manufacturer's labeling): Oral:
Remission induction: 60 mcg/kg/day or 1.8 mg/m^2/day; usual range: 4-8 mg/day; titrate dose (or withhold) to maintain leukocyte counts ≥15,000/mm^3 (doses >4 mg/day should be reserved for patients with the most compelling symptoms)
Maintenance: When leukocyte count ≥50,000/mm^3: Resume induction dose **or** (if remission <3 months) 1-3 mg/day (to control hematologic status and prevent relapse)
HSCT conditioning regimen:
I.V.:
0.8 mg/kg every 6 hours for 4 days (a total of 16 doses); **Note:** Use ideal body weight or actual body weight, (whichever is lower) for dosing. For obese or severely-obese patients, use of an adjusted body weight [IBW + 0.25 x (actual – IBW)] is recommended.
Reduced intensity conditioning regimen (unlabeled dosing): 0.8 mg/kg/day for 4 days starting 5 days prior to transplant (in combinations with fludarabine) (Ho, 2009)
Oral (unlabeled use): 1 mg/kg/dose every 6 hours for 16 doses (in combination with cyclophosphamide) (Socié, 2001) **or** 1 mg/kg/dose every 6 hours for 16 doses beginning 9 days prior to transplant (in combination with cyclophosphamide) (Cassileth, 1993) **or** 0.44 mg/kg/dose every 6 hours for 16 doses (in combination with cyclophosphamide) (Anderson, 1996) **or** 1 mg/kg/dose every 6 hours for 16 doses beginning 6 days prior to transplant (in combination with melphalan) (Fermand, 2005)
Polycythemia vera and essential thrombocythemia (unlabeled uses): Oral: 2-4 mg/day (Fabris, 2009; Tefferi, 2011)

Dosing adjustment in renal impairment:
I.V.: No dosage adjustment provided in the manufacturer's labeling (has not been studied).
Oral: No dosage adjustment provided in the manufacturer's labeling (elimination appears to be independent of renal function); however, some clinicians suggest adjustment is not necessary (Aronoff, 2007).

Dosing adjustment in hepatic impairment:
I.V.: No dosage adjustment provided in the manufacturer's labeling (has not been studied).
Oral: No dosage adjustment provided in the manufacturer's labeling.

Administration Intravenous busulfan should be infused over 2 hours via central line. Flush line before and after each infusion with 5 mL D_5W or NS. Do not use polycarbonate syringes or filters for preparation or administration

HSCT only: To facilitate ingestion of high oral doses, may insert multiple tablets into gelatin capsules.

Monitoring Parameters CBC with differential and platelet count (weekly for palliative treatment; daily until engraftment for HSCT); liver function tests (evaluate transaminases, alkaline phosphatase, and bilirubin daily for at least 28 days post transplant). If conducting therapeutic drug monitoring for AUC calculations in HSCT, monitor blood samples at appropriate collections times (record collection times).

Dosage Forms Excipient information presented when available (limited, particularly for generics); consult specific product labeling.
Injection, solution:
Busulfex®: 6 mg/mL (10 mL) [contains N,N-dimethylacetamide (DMA), polyethylene glycol 400]
Tablet, oral:
Myleran®: 2 mg [scored]

Extemporaneous Preparations Hazardous agent: Use appropriate precautions for handling and disposal.

A 2 mg/mL oral suspension can be prepared in a vertical flow hood with tablets and simple syrup. Crush one-hundred-twenty 2 mg tablets in a mortar and reduce to a fine powder. Add small portions of simple syrup and mix to a uniform paste; mix while adding the simple syrup in incremental proportions to **almost** 120 mL; transfer to a graduated cylinder, rinse mortar and pestle with simple syrup, and add quantity of vehicle sufficient to make 120 mL. Transfer contents of the graduated cylinder into an amber prescription bottle. Label "shake well", "refrigerate", and "caution chemotherapy". Stable for 30 days.

Allen LV, "Busulfan Oral Suspension," *US Pharm*, 1990, 15:94-5.

◆ **Busulfanum** *see* Busulfan *on page* 252
◆ **Busulfex®** *see* Busulfan *on page* 252
◆ **Busulphan** *see* Busulfan *on page* 252

Butabarbital (byoo ta BAR bi tal)

Brand Names: U.S. Butisol Sodium®
Pharmacologic Category Barbiturate
Use Sedative; hypnotic
Pregnancy Risk Factor D
Dosage Oral:
Children: Preoperative sedation: 2-6 mg/kg/dose (maximum: 100 mg)
Adults:
Sedative: 15-30 mg 3-4 times/day
Hypnotic: 50-100 mg at bedtime. When used for insomnia, treatment should be limited since barbiturates lose effectiveness for sleep induction and maintenance after 2 weeks.
Preop: 50-100 mg 1-1½ hours before surgery
Elderly: Use with caution; reduce dose if use is needed

Dosage adjustment in renal impairment: Reduce dose if use is needed

Dosage adjustment in hepatic impairment: Reduce dose if use is needed

Additional Information Complete prescribing information for this medication should be consulted for additional detail.

Dosage Forms Excipient information presented when available (limited, particularly for generics); consult specific product labeling.

Elixir, oral, as sodium:

Butisol Sodium®: 30 mg/5 mL (480 mL) [contains ethanol 7%, propylene glycol, sodium benzoate, tartrazine]

Tablet, oral, as sodium:

Butisol Sodium®: 30 mg, 50 mg [scored; contains tartrazine]

Controlled Substance C-III

Butalbital, Acetaminophen, and Caffeine

(byoo TAL bi tal, a seet a MIN oh fen, & KAF een)

Brand Names: U.S. Alagesic LQ; Anolor 300; Dolgic® Plus; Esgic-Plus™; Esgic®; Fioricet®; Margesic; Orbivan™; Repan®; Zebutal®

Index Terms Acetaminophen, Butalbital, and Caffeine

Pharmacologic Category Barbiturate

Use Relief of the symptomatic complex of tension or muscle contraction headache

Pregnancy Risk Factor C

Dosage

Adults: Oral: 1-2 tablets or capsules (or 15-30 mL solution) every 4 hours; not to exceed 6 tablets or capsules (or 180 mL solution) daily

Elderly: Not recommended for use in the elderly

Dosing interval in renal or hepatic impairment: Should be reduced

Additional Information Complete prescribing information for this medication should be consulted for additional detail.

Dosage Forms Excipient information presented when available (limited, particularly for generics); consult specific product labeling.

Capsule, oral:

Anolor 300, Esgic®, Margesic: Butalbital 50 mg, acetaminophen 325 mg, and caffeine 40 mg

Esgic-Plus™, Zebutal®: Butalbital 50 mg, acetaminophen 500 mg, and caffeine 40 mg

Orbivan™: Butalbital 50 mg, acetaminophen 300 mg, and caffeine 40 mg

Liquid, oral:

Alagesic LQ: Butalbital 50 mg, acetaminophen 325 mg, and caffeine 40 mg per 15 mL (480 mL) [contains ethanol 7%; propylene glycol]

Tablet, oral: Butalbital 50 mg, acetaminophen 325 mg, and caffeine 40 mg; butalbital 50 mg, acetaminophen 500 mg, and caffeine 40 mg

Dolgic® Plus: Butalbital 50 mg, acetaminophen 750 mg, and caffeine 40 mg

Esgic®, Fioricet®, Repan®: Butalbital 50 mg, acetaminophen 325 mg, and caffeine 40 mg

Esgic-Plus™: Butalbital 50 mg, acetaminophen 500 mg, and caffeine 40 mg

Butalbital and Acetaminophen

(byoo TAL bi tal & a seet a MIN oh fen)

Brand Names: U.S. Bupap; Cephadyn; Phrenilin®; Phrenilin® Forte; Promacet; Sedapap®

Index Terms Acetaminophen and Butalbital

Pharmacologic Category Analgesic, Miscellaneous; Barbiturate

Use Relief of the symptomatic complex of tension or muscle contraction headache

Pregnancy Risk Factor C

Dosage Oral: Adults: One tablet/capsule every 4 hours as needed (maximum dose: 6 tablets/day)

Phrenilin®: 1-2 tablets every 4 hours as needed (maximum: 6 tablets in 24 hours)

Elderly: Use with caution; see adult dosing

Dosage adjustment in renal impairment: Mild-to-moderate: Should decrease dose; in severe impairment, use with caution

Dosage adjustment in hepatic impairment: Mild-to-moderate: Should decrease dose; in severe impairment, use with caution

Additional Information Complete prescribing information for this medication should be consulted for additional detail.

Dosage Forms Excipient information presented when available (limited, particularly for generics); consult specific product labeling.

Tablet:

Phrenilin®: Butalbital 50 mg and acetaminophen 325 mg

Bupap, Cephadyn, Promacet, Sedapap®: Butalbital 50 mg and acetaminophen 650 mg

Capsule:

Phrenilin® Forte: Butalbital 50 mg and acetaminophen 650 mg [may contain benzyl alcohol]

Butalbital, Aspirin, and Caffeine

(byoo TAL bi tal, AS pir in, & KAF een)

Brand Names: U.S. Fiorinal®

Brand Names: Canada Fiorinal®

Index Terms Aspirin, Caffeine, and Butalbital; Butalbital Compound

Pharmacologic Category Barbiturate

Use Relief of the symptomatic complex of tension or muscle contraction headache

Pregnancy Risk Factor C/D (prolonged use or high doses at term)

Dosage

Oral: Adults: 1-2 tablets or capsules every 4 hours; not to exceed 6 tablets or capsules/day

Elderly: Not recommended for use in the elderly

Dosing adjustment in renal/hepatic impairment: Dosage should be reduced

Additional Information Complete prescribing information for this medication should be consulted for additional detail.

Dosage Forms Excipient information presented when available (limited, particularly for generics); consult specific product labeling.

Capsule: Butalbital 50 mg, aspirin 325 mg, and caffeine 40 mg

Fiorinal®: Butalbital 50 mg, aspirin 325 mg, and caffeine 40 mg

Tablet: Butalbital 50 mg, aspirin 325 mg, and caffeine 40 mg

Controlled Substance C-III

◆ **Butalbital Compound** *see* Butalbital, Aspirin, and Caffeine *on page* 255

◆ **Butamben, Tetracaine, and Benzocaine** *see* Benzocaine, Butamben, and Tetracaine *on page* 204

Butenafine (byoo TEN a feen)

Brand Names: U.S. Lotrimin® ultra™ [OTC]; Mentax®

Index Terms Butenafine Hydrochloride

Pharmacologic Category Antifungal Agent, Topical

Use Topical treatment of tinea pedis (athlete's foot), tinea cruris (jock itch), tinea corporis (ringworm), and tinea versicolor

Pregnancy Risk Factor C

Dosage Children >12 years and Adults: Topical:

Tinea corporis, tinea cruris (Lotrimin® Ultra™): Apply once daily for 2 weeks to affected area and surrounding skin

Tinea versicolor (Mentax®): Apply once daily for 2 weeks to affected area and surrounding skin

Tinea pedis (Lotrimin® Ultra™): Apply to affected skin between and around the toes, twice daily for 1 week, or once daily for 4 weeks

Additional Information Complete prescribing information for this medication should be consulted for additional detail.

Dosage Forms Excipient information presented when available (limited, particularly for generics); consult specific product labeling.

Cream, topical, as hydrochloride:

Lotrimin® ultra™: 1% (12 g, 24 g) [contains benzyl alcohol, sodium benzoate; for athlete's foot]

Lotrimin® ultra™: 1% (12 g) [contains benzyl alcohol, sodium benzoate; for jock itch]

Mentax®: 1% (15 g, 30 g) [contains benzyl alcohol, sodium benzoate]

◆ **Butenafine Hydrochloride** *see* Butenafine *on page 255*

◆ **Butisol Sodium®** *see* Butabarbital *on page 254*

Butoconazole (byoo toe KOE na zole)

Brand Names: U.S. Gynazole-1® [DSC]

Brand Names: Canada Femstat® One; Gynazole-1®

Index Terms Butoconazole Nitrate

Pharmacologic Category Antifungal Agent, Vaginal

Use Local treatment of vulvovaginal candidiasis

Pregnancy Risk Factor C (use only in 2nd or 3rd trimester)

Dosage Adults: Females: Gynazole-1®: Insert 1 applicatorful (~5 g) intravaginally as a single dose; treatment may need to be extended for up to 6 days in pregnant women (use in pregnancy during 2nd or 3rd trimester only)

Additional Information Complete prescribing information for this medication should be consulted for additional detail.

Dosage Forms Excipient information presented when available (limited, particularly for generics); consult specific product labeling. [DSC] = Discontinued product

Cream, vaginal, as nitrate:

Gynazole-1®: 2% (5 g [DSC])

◆ **Butoconazole Nitrate** *see* Butoconazole *on page 256*

Butorphanol (byoo TOR fa nole)

Brand Names: Canada Apo-Butorphanol®; PMS-Butorphanol

Index Terms Butorphanol Tartrate; Stadol

Pharmacologic Category Analgesic, Opioid; Analgesic, Opioid Partial Agonist

Additional Appendix Information

Opioid Analgesics *on page 1896*

Use

Parenteral: Management of moderate-to-severe pain; preoperative medication; supplement to balanced anesthesia; management of pain during labor

Nasal spray: Management of moderate-to-severe pain, including migraine headache pain

Pregnancy Risk Factor C

Dosage Note: These are guidelines and do not represent the maximum doses that may be required in all patients. Doses should be titrated to pain relief/prevention. Butorphanol has an analgesic ceiling.

Adults:

Parenteral:

Acute pain (moderate-to-severe):

I.M.: Initial: 2 mg, may repeat every 3-4 hours as needed; usual range: 1-4 mg every 3-4 hours as needed

I.V.: Initial: 1 mg, may repeat every 3-4 hours as needed; usual range: 0.5-2 mg every 3-4 hours as needed

Preoperative medication: I.M.: 2 mg 60-90 minutes before surgery

Supplement to balanced anesthesia: I.V.: 2 mg shortly before induction and/or an incremental dose of 0.5-1 mg (up to 0.06 mg/kg), depending on previously administered sedative, analgesic, and hypnotic medications

Pain during labor (fetus >37 weeks gestation and no signs of fetal distress):

I.M., I.V.: 1-2 mg; may repeat in 4 hours

Note: Alternative analgesia should be used for pain associated with delivery or if delivery is anticipated within 4 hours

Nasal spray:

Moderate-to-severe pain (including migraine headache pain): Initial: 1 spray (~1 mg per spray) in 1 nostril; if adequate pain relief is not achieved within 60-90 minutes, an additional 1 spray in 1 nostril may be given; may repeat initial dose sequence in 3-4 hours after the last dose as needed

Alternatively, an initial dose of 2 mg (1 spray in each nostril) may be used in patients who will be able to remain recumbent (in the event drowsiness or dizziness occurs); additional 2 mg doses should not be given for 3-4 hours

Note: In some clinical trials, an initial dose of 2 mg (as 2 doses 1 hour apart or 2 mg initially - 1 spray in each nostril) has been used, followed by 1 mg in 1 hour; side effects were greater at these dosages

Elderly:

I.M., I.V.: Initial dosage should generally be 1/2 of the recommended dose; repeated dosing must be based on initial response rather than fixed intervals, but generally should be at least 6 hours apart

Nasal spray: Initial dose should not exceed 1 mg; a second dose may be given after 90-120 minutes

Dosage adjustment in renal impairment:

I.M., I.V.: Initial dosage should generally be 1/2 of the recommended dose; repeated dosing must be based on initial response rather than fixed intervals, but generally should be at least 6 hours apart

Nasal spray: Initial dose should not exceed 1 mg; a second dose may be given after 90-120 minutes

Dosage adjustment in hepatic impairment:

I.M., I.V.: Initial dosage should generally be 1/2 of the recommended dose; repeated dosing must be based on initial response rather than fixed intervals, but generally should be at least 6 hours apart

Nasal spray: Initial dose should not exceed 1 mg; a second dose may be given after 90-120 minutes

Additional Information Complete prescribing information for this medication should be consulted for additional detail.

Dosage Forms Excipient information presented when available (limited, particularly for generics); consult specific product labeling.

Injection, solution, as tartrate: 1 mg/mL (1 mL); 2 mg/mL (1 mL, 2 mL, 10 mL)

Injection, solution, as tartrate [preservative free]: 1 mg/mL (1 mL); 2 mg/mL (1 mL, 2 mL)

Solution, intranasal, as tartrate [spray]: 10 mg/mL (2.5 mL)

Controlled Substance C-IV

◆ **Butorphanol Tartrate** *see* Butorphanol *on page 256*

◆ **Butrans®** *see* Buprenorphine *on page 244*

◆ **BW-430C** *see* LamoTRIgine *on page 967*

◆ **BW524W91** *see* Emtricitabine *on page 581*

- ◆ **Byetta®** *see* Exenatide *on page 678*
- ◆ **Bystolic®** *see* Nebivolol *on page 1183*
- ◆ **C1 Esterase Inhibitor** *see* C1 Inhibitor (Human) *on page 257*
- ◆ **C1-INH** *see* C1 Inhibitor (Human) *on page 257*
- ◆ **C1-Inhibitor** *see* C1 Inhibitor (Human) *on page 257*
- ◆ **C1INHRP** *see* C1 Inhibitor (Human) *on page 257*
- ◆ **C2B8 Monoclonal Antibody** *see* RiTUXimab *on page 1503*
- ◆ **C7E3** *see* Abciximab *on page 22*
- ◆ **311C90** *see* ZOLMitriptan *on page 1824*
- ◆ **C225** *see* Cetuximab *on page 332*

C1 Inhibitor (Human) (cee won in HIB i ter HYU man)

Brand Names: U.S. Berinert®; Cinryze™
Brand Names: Canada Berinert®
Index Terms C1 Esterase Inhibitor; C1-INH; C1-Inhibitor; C1INHRP; Human C1 Inhibitor
Pharmacologic Category Blood Product Derivative
Use

Berinert®: Treatment of acute abdominal or facial attacks of hereditary angioedema (HAE)

Cinryze™: Routine prophylaxis against angioedema attacks in patients with HAE or inherited C1 inhibitor deficiency

Pregnancy Risk Factor C

Prescribing and Access Restrictions Assistance with procurement and reimbursement of Cinryze™ is available for healthcare providers and patients through the CINRYZE*Solutions*® program (telephone: 1-877-945-1000) or at http://www.cinryze.com/Cinryze_Solutions/Default.aspx

Dosage I.V.: Adolescents and Adults:

Routine prophylaxis against HAE attacks (Cinryze™): 1000 units every 3-4 days

Treatment of abdominal or facial HAE attacks (Berinert®): 20 units/kg

Additional Information Complete prescribing information for this medication should be consulted for additional detail.

Dosage Forms Excipient information presented when available (limited, particularly for generics); consult specific product labeling.

Injection, powder for reconstitution:

Berinert®: 500 units [supplied with SWFI diluent]

Cinryze™: 500 units [contains sucrose 21 mg/mL]

Cabazitaxel (ca baz i TAKS el)

Brand Names: U.S. Jevtana®
Brand Names: Canada Jevtana®
Index Terms RPR-116258A; XRP6258
Pharmacologic Category Antineoplastic Agent, Antimicrotubular; Antineoplastic Agent, Taxane Derivative

Use Treatment of hormone-refractory metastatic prostate cancer (in patients previously treated with a docetaxel-containing regimen)

Pregnancy Risk Factor D

Pregnancy Considerations Animal studies have demonstrated adverse effects (embryotoxicity, fetotoxicity and fetal loss) at doses significantly lower than human doses. There are no adequate and well-controlled studies in pregnant women. May cause fetal harm if administered during pregnancy. Pregnant women should avoid exposure to cabazitaxel.

Lactation Excretion in breast milk unknown/not recommended

Contraindications Hypersensitivity to cabazitaxel, polysorbate 80, or any component of the formulation; neutrophil count ≤1500/mm^3

Warnings/Precautions Hazardous agent - use appropriate precautions for handling and disposal. **[U.S. Boxed Warning]: Severe hypersensitivity reactions, including generalized rash, erythema, hypotension, and bronchospasm may occur; may require immediate discontinuation if hypersensitivity is severe. Premedicate with an I.V. antihistamine, corticosteroid and H2 antagonist prior to infusion. Use in patients with history of severe hypersensitivity to cabazitaxel or polysorbate 80 is contraindicated.** Observe closely during infusion, especially during the first and second infusions; reaction may occur within minutes. Do not rechallenge after severe hypersensitivity reactions.

[U.S. Boxed Warning]: Deaths due to neutropenia have been reported. Do not administer in patients with neutrophil count ≤1500/mm$_3$; monitor blood counts frequently. Dose reductions are recommended following neutropenic fever or prolonged neutropenia. Administration of WBC growth factors may reduce the risk of complications due to neutropenia; consider primary WBC growth factor prophylaxis in high-risk patients (eg, >65 years of age, poor performance status, history of neutropenic fever, extensive prior radiation, poor nutrition status, or other serious comorbidities); secondary prophylaxis and therapeutic WBC growth factors should be considered in all patients with increased risk for neutropenic complications. Patients ≥65 years of age are more likely to experience certain adverse reactions, including neutropenia and neutropenic fever.

Use is not recommended in patients with hepatic impairment (total bilirubin ≥ULN or AST and/or ALT ≥1.5 times ULN). Due to extensive hepatic metabolism, cabazitaxel exposure is increased in patients with hepatic impairment. Renal failure has been reported from clinical trials; generally associated with dehydration, sepsis, or obstructive uropathy; use with caution in patients with severe renal impairment (Cl_{cr} <30 mL/minute) and end-stage renal disease. Nausea, vomiting and diarrhea may occur. Diarrhea may be severe and may result in dehydration and electrolyte imbalance. Antiemetics, antidiarrhea medication, and fluid and electrolyte replacement may be necessary. Diarrhea ≥ grade 3 may require treatment delay and or dosage reduction.

Avoid concomitant use of strong CYP3A4 inducers or inhibitors; use with moderate CYP3A4 inhibitors with caution. Strong CYP3A4 inducers (eg, carbamazepine, phenobarbital, phenytoin, rifabutin rifampin, rifapentine) may decrease the levels/effects of cabazitaxel. Strong CYP3A4 inhibitors (eg, atazanavir, clarithromycin, indinavir, itraconazole, ketoconazole, nefazodone, nelfinavir, ritonavir, saquinavir, telithromycin, voriconazole) may increase the levels/effects of cabazitaxel.

Adverse Reactions Note: Adverse reactions reported for combination therapy with prednisone.

>10%:

Central nervous system: Fatigue (37%), fever (12%)

Gastrointestinal: Diarrhea (47%; grades 3/4: 6%), nausea (34%), vomiting (22%), constipation (20%), abdominal pain (17%), anorexia (16%), taste alteration (11%)

Hematologic: Anemia (98%; grades 3/4: 11%), leukopenia (96%; grades 3/4: 69%), neutropenia (94%; grades 3/4: 82%; nadir: 12 days [range: 4-17 days]), thrombocytopenia (48%; grades 3/4: 4%)

Neuromuscular & skeletal: Weakness (20%), back pain (16%), peripheral neuropathy (13%; grades 3/4: <1%), arthralgia (11%)

Renal: Hematuria (17%)

Respiratory: Dyspnea (12%), cough (11%)

1% to 10%:
- Cardiovascular: Peripheral edema (9%), arrhythmia (5%), hypotension (5%)
- Central nervous system: Dizziness (8%), headache (8%), pain (5%)
- Dermatologic: Alopecia (10%)
- Endocrine & metabolic: Dehydration (5%)
- Gastrointestinal: Dyspepsia (10%), weight loss (9%), mucosal inflammation (6%)
- Genitourinary: Urinary tract infection (8%), dysuria (7%)
- Hematologic: Neutropenic fever (grades 3/4: 7%)
- Hepatic: ALT increased (grades 3/4: ≤1%), AST increased (grades 3/4: ≤1%), bilirubin increased (grades 3/4: ≤1%)
- Neuromuscular & skeletal: Muscle spasm (7%)

<1% (Limited to important or life-threatening): Hypersensitivity (eg, rash, erythema, hypotension, bronchospasm), electrolyte imbalance, renal failure, sepsis, septic shock

Drug Interactions

Metabolism/Transport Effects Substrate of CYP2C8 (minor), CYP3A4 (major); **Note:** Assignment of Major/Minor substrate status based on clinically relevant drug interaction potential

Avoid Concomitant Use

Avoid concomitant use of Cabazitaxel with any of the following: BCG; CloZAPine; Conivaptan; Natalizumab; Pimecrolimus; Tacrolimus (Topical); Vaccines (Live)

Increased Effect/Toxicity

Cabazitaxel may increase the levels/effects of: Antineoplastic Agents (Anthracycline, Systemic); CloZAPine; DOXOrubicin; Leflunomide; Natalizumab; Vaccines (Live); Vitamin K Antagonists

The levels/effects of Cabazitaxel may be increased by: Conivaptan; CYP3A4 Inhibitors (Moderate); CYP3A4 Inhibitors (Strong); Dasatinib; Denosumab; Pimecrolimus; Platinum Derivatives; Roflumilast; Tacrolimus (Topical); Trastuzumab

Decreased Effect

Cabazitaxel may decrease the levels/effects of: BCG; Cardiac Glycosides; Coccidioidin Skin Test; Sipuleucel-T; Vaccines (Inactivated); Vaccines (Live); Vitamin K Antagonists

The levels/effects of Cabazitaxel may be decreased by: CYP3A4 Inducers (Strong); Deferasirox; Echinacea; Herbs (CYP3A4 Inducers); Tocilizumab

Ethanol/Nutrition/Herb Interactions

Food: Avoid grapefruit juice (may increase the levels/effects of cabazitaxel).

Herb/Nutraceutical: Avoid St John's wort (may increase metabolism and decrease cabazitaxel concentrations).

Stability Store intact vials at 25°C (77°F); excursions permitted between 15°C and 30°C (59°F and 86°F). Do not refrigerate. Use appropriate precautions for handling and disposal. Do not prepare in PVC-containing infusion containers. Cabazitaxel and diluent vials contain overfill.

Preparation requires 2 steps. Slowly inject the entire contents of the provided diluent into the 60 mg/1.5 mL cabazitaxel vial, directing the diluent down the vial wall. Mix gently by inverting the vial for at least 45 seconds; do not shake. Allow vial to sit so that foam dissipates and solution appears homogeneous. This results in an intermediate reconstituted concentration of 10 mg/mL, which is stable for 30 minutes in the vial. Further dilute into a 250 mL D_5W or NS non-PVC infusion container to final concentration of 0.1-0.26 mg/mL (total doses >65 mg will require a larger infusion volume; final concentration should not exceed 0.26 mg/mL). Gently invert to mix. Solutions for infusion are stable for 8 hours at room temperature or 24 hours refrigerated. Infusion should be completed within 8 hours if stored at room temperature or 24 hours if refrigerated. Do not use infusion solutions if crystals or precipitate appear; discard.

Mechanism of Action Cabazitaxel is a taxane derivative which is a microtubule inhibitor; it binds to tubulin promoting assembly into microtubules and inhibiting disassembly which stabilizes microtubules. This inhibits microtubule depolymerization and cell division, arresting the cell cycle and inhibiting tumor proliferation. Unlike other taxanes, cabazitaxel has a poor affinity for multidrug resistance (MDR) proteins, therefore conferring activity in resistant tumors.

Pharmacodynamics/Kinetics

Distribution: V_{dss}: 4864 L; has greater CNS penetration than other taxanes

Protein binding: 89% to 92%; primarily to serum albumin and lipoproteins

Metabolism: Extensively hepatic; primarily via CYP3A4 and 3A5; also via CYP2C8 (minor)

Half-life elimination: Terminal: 95 hours

Excretion: Feces (76% as metabolites); Urine (~4%)

Dosage Note: Premedicate at least 30 minutes prior to each dose of cabazitaxel with an antihistamine (eg, diphenhydramine I.V. 25 mg or equivalent), a corticosteroid (eg, dexamethasone 8 mg I.V. or equivalent), and an H_2 antagonist (eg, ranitidine 50 mg I.V. or equivalent). Antiemetic prophylaxis is also recommended. Details concerning dosing in combination regimens should also be consulted.

I.V.: Adults: Prostate cancer: 25 mg/m²/dose once every 3 weeks (in combination with prednisone)

Dosage adjustment for toxicity:

Hematologic toxicity:

Neutropenia ≥grade 3 for >1 week despite WBC growth factors: Delay treatment until ANC >1500/mm³ and then reduce dose to 20 mg/m² with continued WBC growth factor secondary prophylaxis

Neutropenic fever: Delay treatment until improvement/resolution and ANC >1500/mm³ and then reduce dose to 20 mg/m² with continued WBC growth factor secondary prophylaxis

Persistent hematologic toxicity (despite dosage reduction): Discontinue treatment

Nonhematologic toxicity:

Severe hypersensitivity: Discontinue immediately

Diarrhea ≥grade 3 or persistent despite appropriate medication, fluids, and electrolyte replacement: Delay treatment until improves or resolves and then reduce dose to 20 mg/m²

Persistent diarrhea (despite dosage reduction): Discontinue treatment

Dosage adjustment in renal impairment: Severe renal impairment (Cl_{cr} <30 mL/minute) or end-stage renal disease: Use with caution

Dosage adjustment in hepatic impairment: Hepatic impairment (total bilirubin ≥ULN or AST and/or ALT ≥1.5 times ULN): Use is not recommended

Dietary Considerations Avoid grapefruit juice.

Administration I.V.: Infuse over 1 hour using a 0.22 micron inline filter. Do not use polyurethane-containing infusion sets for administration. Allow to reach room temperature prior to infusion. Premedicate with an antihistamine, a corticosteroid, and an H_2 antagonist at least 30 minutes prior to infusion. Observe closely during infusion (for hypersensitivity). Antiemetic prophylaxis (oral or I.V.) is also recommended.

Monitoring Parameters CBC with differential and platelets (weekly during first cycle, then prior to each treatment cycle); monitor for hypersensitivity

Dosage Forms Excipient information presented when available (limited, particularly for generics); consult specific product labeling.

Injection, solution:

Jevtana®: 40 mg/mL (1.5 mL) [contains ethanol 13% (in diluent), polysorbate 80; supplied with diluent]

Cabergoline (ca BER goe leen)

Brand Names: Canada CO Cabergoline; Dostinex®

Pharmacologic Category Ergot Derivative

Additional Appendix Information

Antiparkinsonian Agents *on page 1879*

Use Treatment of hyperprolactinemic disorders, either idiopathic or due to pituitary adenomas

Canadian labeling: Additional use (not in U.S. labeling): Prevention of the onset of physiological lactation in the puerperium when clinically indicated (eg, still born baby or neonatal death, conditions that interfere with suckling, severe acute or chronic mental illness). Note: Not indicated for suppression of established postpartum lactation.

Pregnancy Risk Factor B

Dosage Oral: Adults:

Hyperprolactinemia:

U.S. labeling: Initial dose: 0.25 mg twice weekly; the dose may be increased by 0.25 mg twice weekly up to a maximum of 1 mg twice weekly according to the patient's serum prolactin level. Dosage increases should not occur more rapidly than every 4 weeks. Once a normal serum prolactin level is maintained for 6 months, the dose may be discontinued and prolactin levels monitored to determine if cabergoline is still required. The durability of efficacy beyond 24 months of therapy has not been established.

Canadian labeling: Initial dose: 0.5 mg once weekly or 0.25 mg twice weekly; weekly dose may be increased by 0.5 mg per week at 4 week intervals until optimal therapeutic response. Therapeutic dose: Usual: 1 mg/week (range: 0.25-2 mg/week). **Note:** May divide weekly dose into 2 or more divided doses per week (recommended for doses >1 mg/week) based on tolerability.

Lactation inhibition (Canadian labeling; not in U.S. labeling): 1 mg single dose on first day postpartum

Elderly: No dosage recommendations suggested; however, start at the low end of the dosage range

Dosage adjustment in renal impairment: No dosage adjustment required; pharmacokinetics not altered with moderate-severe renal impairment.

Dosage adjustment in hepatic impairment:

Mild-to-moderate dysfunction (Child-Pugh classes A and B): No dosage adjustment required; no effect on C_{max} or AUC.

Severe dysfunction (Child-Pugh class C): There are no dosage adjustments provided in manufacturer's labeling; use caution; significant increase in AUC.

Additional Information Complete prescribing information for this medication should be consulted for additional detail.

Dosage Forms Excipient information presented when available (limited, particularly for generics); consult specific product labeling.

Tablet, oral: 0.5 mg

◆ **Caduet®** *see* Amlodipine and Atorvastatin *on page 98*

◆ **CaEDTA** *see* Edetate CALCIUM Disodium *on page 572*

◆ **Caelyx® (Can)** *see* DOXOrubicin (Liposomal) *on page 555*

◆ **Cafcit®** *see* Caffeine *on page 259*

◆ **CAFdA** *see* Clofarabine *on page 385*

Caffeine (KAF een)

Brand Names: U.S. Cafcit®; Enerjets [OTC]; No Doz® Maximum Strength [OTC]; Vivarin® [OTC]

Index Terms Caffeine and Sodium Benzoate; Caffeine Citrate; Caffeine Sodium Benzoate; Sodium Benzoate and Caffeine

Pharmacologic Category Stimulant

Use

Caffeine citrate: Treatment of idiopathic apnea of prematurity

Caffeine and sodium benzoate: Treatment of acute respiratory depression (not a preferred agent)

Caffeine [OTC labeling]: Restore mental alertness or wakefulness when experiencing fatigue

Unlabeled Use Caffeine and sodium benzoate: Treatment of spinal puncture headache; CNS stimulant; diuretic; augmentation of seizure induction during electroconvulsive therapy (ECT)

Pregnancy Risk Factor C

Pregnancy Considerations Caffeine crosses the placenta; serum levels in the fetus are similar to those in the mother. When large bolus doses are administered to animals, teratogenic effects have been reported. Similar doses are not probable following normal caffeine consumption and moderate consumption is not associated with congenital malformations, spontaneous abortions, preterm birth or low birth weight. According to one source, pregnant women who do not smoke or drink alcohol could consume ≤5 mg/kg of caffeine over the course of a day without reproductive risk. Other sources recommend limiting caffeine intake to <150-200 mg/day. The half-life of caffeine is prolonged during the second and third trimesters of pregnancy.

Lactation Enters breast milk/use caution (AAP rates "compatible"; AAP 2001 update pending)

Contraindications Hypersensitivity to caffeine or any component of the formulation; sodium benzoate is not for use in neonates

Warnings/Precautions Use with caution in patients with a history of peptic ulcer, gastroesophageal reflux, impaired renal or hepatic function, seizure disorders, or cardiovascular disease. Avoid use in patients with symptomatic cardiac arrhythmias, agitation, anxiety, or tremor. Over-the-counter [OTC] products contain an amount of caffeine similar to one cup of coffee; limit the use of other caffeine-containing beverages or foods.

Caffeine citrate should not be interchanged with caffeine and sodium benzoate. Avoid use of products containing sodium benzoate in neonates; has been associated with a potentially fatal toxicity ("gasping syndrome"). Neonates receiving caffeine citrate should be closely monitored for the development of necrotizing enterocolitis. Caffeine serum levels should be closely monitored to optimize therapy and prevent serious toxicity.

Adverse Reactions Frequency not specified; primarily serum-concentration related.

Cardiovascular: Angina, arrhythmia (ventricular), chest pain, flushing, palpitation, sinus tachycardia, tachycardia (supraventricular), vasodilation

Central nervous system: Agitation, delirium, dizziness, hallucinations, headache, insomnia, irritability, psychosis, restlessness

Dermatologic: Urticaria

Gastrointestinal: Esophageal sphincter tone decreased, gastritis

Neuromuscular & skeletal: Fasciculations

Ocular: Intraocular pressure increased (>180 mg caffeine), miosis

Renal: Diuresis

Drug Interactions

Metabolism/Transport Effects Substrate of CYP1A2 (major), CYP2C9 (minor), CYP2D6 (minor), CYP2E1 (minor), CYP3A4 (minor); **Note:** Assignment of Major/Minor substrate status based on clinically relevant drug interaction potential; **Inhibits** CYP1A2 (weak)

Avoid Concomitant Use

Avoid concomitant use of Caffeine with any of the following: Iobenguane I 123

Increased Effect/Toxicity

Caffeine may increase the levels/effects of: Formoterol; Indacaterol; Sympathomimetics

The levels/effects of Caffeine may be increased by: Abiraterone Acetate; Atomoxetine; Cannabinoids; Conivaptan; CYP1A2 Inhibitors (Moderate); CYP1A2 Inhibitors (Strong); Deferasirox; Linezolid; Quinolone Antibiotics

Decreased Effect

Caffeine may decrease the levels/effects of: Adenosine; Iobenguane I 123; Regadenoson

The levels/effects of Caffeine may be decreased by: Cyproterone; Peginterferon Alfa-2b; Tocilizumab

Stability Store at 20°C to 25°C (68°F to 77°F).

Caffeine citrate: Injection and oral solution contain no preservatives; injection is chemically stable for at least 24 hours at room temperature when diluted to 10 mg/mL (as caffeine citrate) with D_5W, $D_{50}W$, Intralipid® 20%, and Aminosyn® 8.5%; also compatible with dopamine (600 mcg/mL), calcium gluconate 10%, heparin (1 unit/mL), and fentanyl (10 mcg/mL) at room temperature for 24 hours.

Mechanism of Action Increases levels of 3'5' cyclic AMP by inhibiting phosphodiesterase; CNS stimulant which increases medullary respiratory center sensitivity to carbon dioxide, stimulates central inspiratory drive, and improves skeletal muscle contraction (diaphragmatic contractility); prevention of apnea may occur by competitive inhibition of adenosine

Pharmacodynamics/Kinetics

Distribution: V_d:

Neonates: 0.8-0.9 L/kg

Children >9 months to Adults: 0.6 L/kg

Protein binding: 17% (children) to 36% (adults)

Metabolism: Hepatic, via demethylation by CYP1A2. **Note:** In neonates, interconversion between caffeine and theophylline has been reported (caffeine levels are ~25% of measured theophylline after theophylline administration and ~3% to 8% of caffeine would be expected to be converted to theophylline)

Half-life elimination:

Neonates: 72-96 hours (range: 40-230 hours)

Children >9 months and Adults: 5 hours

Time to peak, serum: Oral: Within 30 minutes to 2 hours

Excretion:

Neonates ≤1 month: 86% excreted unchanged in urine

Infants >1 month and Adults: In urine, as metabolites

Dosage

Note: Caffeine citrate should not be interchanged with the caffeine sodium benzoate formulation.

Caffeine citrate: Neonates: Apnea of prematurity: Oral, I.V.:

Loading dose: 10-20 mg/kg as caffeine citrate (5-10 mg/kg as caffeine base). If theophylline has been administered to the patient within the previous 3 days, a full or modified loading dose (50% to 75% of a loading dose) may be given.

Maintenance dose: 5 mg/kg/day as caffeine citrate (2.5 mg/kg/day as caffeine base) once daily starting 24 hours after the loading dose. Maintenance dose is adjusted based on patient's response and serum caffeine concentrations.

Caffeine and sodium benzoate:

Children: Stimulant: I.M., I.V., SubQ: 8 mg/kg every 4 hours as needed

Children ≥12 years and Adults: OTC labeling (stimulant): Oral: 100-200 mg every 3-4 hours as needed

Adults:

Electroconvulsive therapy: I.V.: 300-2000 mg

Respiratory depression: I.M., I.V.: 250 mg as a single dose; may repeat as needed. Maximum single dose should be limited to 500 mg; maximum amount in any 24-hour period should generally be limited to 2500 mg.

Spinal puncture headache (unlabeled use):

I.V.: 500 mg in 1000 mL NS infused over 1 hour, followed by 1000 mL NS infused over 1 hour; a second course of caffeine can be given for unrelieved headache pain in 4 hours.

Oral: 300 mg as a single dose

Stimulant/diuretic (unlabeled use): I.M., I.V.: 500 mg, maximum single dose: 1 g

Dosage adjustment in renal impairment: No dosage adjustment required.

Dietary Considerations Oral formulations may be taken without regard to feedings or meals.

Administration

Oral: May be administered without regard to feedings or meals. May administer injectable formulation (caffeine citrate) orally.

Parenteral:

Caffeine citrate: Infuse loading dose over at least 30 minutes; maintenance dose may be infused over at least 10 minutes. May administer without dilution or diluted with D_5W to 10 mg caffeine citrate/mL.

Caffeine and sodium benzoate: I.V. as slow direct injection. For spinal headaches, dilute in 1000 mL NS and infuse over 1 hour. Follow with 1000 mL NS; infuse over 1 hour. May administer I.M. undiluted.

Reference Range

Therapeutic: Apnea of prematurity: 8-20 mcg/mL

Potentially toxic: >20 mcg/mL

Toxic: >50 mcg/mL

Dosage Forms Excipient information presented when available (limited, particularly for generics); consult specific product labeling. [DSC] = Discontinued product

Caplet:

NoDoz® Maximum Strength, Vivarin®: 200 mg

Injection, solution, as citrate [preservative free]: 20 mg/mL (3 mL) [equivalent to 10 mg/mL caffeine base]

Cafcit®: 20 mg/mL (3 mL) [equivalent to 10 mg/mL caffeine base]

Injection, solution [with sodium benzoate]: Caffeine 125 mg/mL and sodium benzoate 125 mg/mL (2 mL); caffeine 121 mg/mL and sodium benzoate 129 mg/mL (2 mL) [DSC]

Lozenge:

Enerjets®: 75 mg (12s) [classic coffee, hazelnut cream, or mochamint flavor]

Solution, oral, as citrate [preservative free]: 20 mg/mL (3 mL) [equivalent to 10 mg/mL caffeine base]

Cafcit®: 20 mg/mL (3 mL) [equivalent to 10 mg/mL caffeine base]

Tablet: 200 mg

Vivarin®: 200 mg

Extemporaneous Preparations A 10 mg/mL oral solution of caffeine (as citrate) may be prepared from 10 g caffeine (anhydrous) combined with 10 g citric acid USP and dissolved in 1000 mL sterile water. Label "shake well" and "refrigerate". Stable for 3 months (Nahata, 2004).

A 20 mg/mL oral solution of caffeine (as citrate) may be made from 5 g caffeine (anhydrous) combined with 5 g citric acid USP and dissolved in 250 mL sterile water. Stir solution until completely clear, then add a 2:1 mixture of simple syrup and cherry syrup in sufficient quantity to make 500 mL. Label "shake well" and "refrigerate". Stable for 90 days (Eisenberg, 1984).

Eisenberg MG and Kang N, "Stability of Citrated Caffeine Solutions for Injectable and Enteral Use," *Am J Hosp Pharm*, 1984, 41(11):2405-6.
Nahata MC, Pai VB, and Hipple TF, *Pediatric Drug Formulations*, 5th ed, Cincinnati, OH: Harvey Whitney Books Co, 2004.

◆ **Caffeine, Acetaminophen, and Aspirin** *see* Acetaminophen, Aspirin, and Caffeine *on page 32*
◆ **Caffeine and Sodium Benzoate** *see* Caffeine *on page 259*
◆ **Caffeine, Aspirin, and Acetaminophen** *see* Acetaminophen, Aspirin, and Caffeine *on page 32*
◆ **Caffeine Citrate** *see* Caffeine *on page 259*
◆ **Caffeine, Orphenadrine, and Aspirin** *see* Orphenadrine, Aspirin, and Caffeine *on page 1252*
◆ **Caffeine Sodium Benzoate** *see* Caffeine *on page 259*
◆ **Cal-C-Caps [OTC]** *see* Calcium Citrate *on page 269*

Calamine (KAL a meen)

Index Terms Calamine Lotion
Pharmacologic Category Topical Skin Product
Use Employed primarily as an astringent, protectant, and soothing agent for conditions such as poison ivy, poison oak, poison sumac, sunburn, insect bites, or minor skin irritations
Dosage Topical: Children and Adults: Apply to affected area as often as needed
Additional Information Complete prescribing information for this medication should be consulted for additional detail.
Dosage Forms Excipient information presented when available (limited, particularly for generics); consult specific product labeling.
Suspension, topical: 8% (118 mL, 177 mL, 240 mL)

◆ **Calamine Lotion** *see* Calamine *on page 261*
◆ **Calan®** *see* Verapamil *on page 1783*
◆ **Calan® SR** *see* Verapamil *on page 1783*
◆ **Calcarb 600 [OTC] [DSC]** *see* Calcium Carbonate *on page 266*
◆ **Cal-Cee [OTC]** *see* Calcium Citrate *on page 269*
◆ **Calci-Chew® [OTC]** *see* Calcium Carbonate *on page 266*
◆ **Calciferol™ [OTC]** *see* Ergocalciferol *on page 610*
◆ **Calcijex®** *see* Calcitriol *on page 263*
◆ **Calcimar® (Can)** *see* Calcitonin *on page 262*
◆ **Calci-Mix® [OTC]** *see* Calcium Carbonate *on page 266*
◆ **Calcionate [OTC]** *see* Calcium Glubionate *on page 269*

Calcipotriene (kal si POE try een)

Brand Names: U.S. Calcitrene™; Dovonex®
Brand Names: Canada Dovonex®
Pharmacologic Category Topical Skin Product; Vitamin D Analog
Use Treatment of plaque psoriasis; chronic, moderate-to-severe psoriasis of the scalp
Unlabeled Use Vitiligo
Pregnancy Risk Factor C
Dosage Topical: Adults:
Cream: Apply a thin film to the affected skin twice daily for up to 8 weeks
Ointment: Apply a thin film to the affected skin once or twice daily
Solution: Apply to the affected scalp twice daily for up to 8 weeks
Additional Information Complete prescribing information for this medication should be consulted for additional detail.
Dosage Forms Excipient information presented when available (limited, particularly for generics); consult specific product labeling.
Cream, topical:
Dovonex®: 0.005% (60 g, 120 g)
Ointment, topical:
Calcitrene™: 0.005% (60 g)
Solution, topical: 0.005% (60 mL)
Dovonex®: 0.005% (60 mL) [contains isopropyl alcohol 51% v/v]

Calcipotriene and Betamethasone
(kal si POE try een & bay ta METH a sone)

Brand Names: U.S. Taclonex Scalp®; Taclonex®
Brand Names: Canada Dovobet®; Xamiol®
Index Terms Betamethasone Dipropionate and Calcipotriene Hydrate; Calcipotriol and Betamethasone Dipropionate
Pharmacologic Category Corticosteroid, Topical; Vitamin D Analog
Use Treatment of psoriasis vulgaris
Unlabeled Use Treatment of corticosteroid-responsive dermatoses
Pregnancy Risk Factor C
Dosage Topical: Adults: Psoriasis vulgaris:
Gel (Xamiol® [CAN]): Apply to affected areas of scalp once daily for up to 4 weeks (maximum recommended dose: 15 g/day or 100 g/week). Application to >30% of body surface area is not recommended
Ointment: Apply to affected area once daily for up to 4 weeks (maximum recommended dose: 100 g/week). Application to >30% of body surface area is not recommended.
Suspension: Apply to affected area of the scalp once daily for 2 weeks or until clear; may continue for up to 8 weeks (maximum recommended dose: 100 g/week)

Dosing adjustment in renal impairment: Safety and efficacy have not been established with severe renal impairment.

Dosing adjustment in hepatic impairment: Safety and efficacy have not been established with severe hepatic impairment.

Additional Information Complete prescribing information for this medication should be consulted for additional detail.
Dosage Forms Excipient information presented when available (limited, particularly for generics); consult specific product labeling.
Ointment, topical:
Taclonex®: Calcipotriene 0.005% and betamethasone dipropionate 0.064% (60 g, 100 g)
Suspension, topical:
Taclonex Scalp®: Calcipotriene 0.005% and betamethasone dipropionate 0.064% (60 mL) [contains castor oil]
Dosage Forms: Canada Excipient information presented when available (limited, particularly for generics); consult specific product labeling.
Gel, topical:
Xamiol®: Calcipotriol 50 mcg/g and betamethasone dipropionate 0.5 mg/g (30 g, 60 g, 2 x 60 g)
Ointment, topical:
Dovobet®: Calcipotriol 50 mcg/g and betamethasone 0.5 mg/g (30 g, 60 g, 120 g)

◆ **Calcipotriol and Betamethasone Dipropionate** *see* Calcipotriene and Betamethasone *on page 261*
◆ **Calcite-500 (Can)** *see* Calcium Carbonate *on page 266*

Calcitonin (kal si TOE nin)

Brand Names: U.S. Fortical®; Miacalcin®

Brand Names: Canada Apo-Calcitonin®; Calcimar®; Caltine®; Miacalcin® NS; PRO-Calcitonin; Sandoz-Calcitonin

Index Terms Calcitonin (Salmon)

Pharmacologic Category Antidote; Hormone

Use Treatment of Paget's disease of bone (osteitis deformans); adjunctive therapy for hypercalcemia; treatment of osteoporosis in women >5 years postmenopause

Pregnancy Risk Factor C

Pregnancy Considerations Decreased birth weight was observed in animal studies. Calcitonin does not cross the placenta.

Lactation Excretion in breast milk unknown/not recommended

Contraindications Hypersensitivity to calcitonin salmon or any component of the formulation

Warnings/Precautions A skin test should be performed prior to initiating therapy of calcitonin salmon in patients with suspected sensitivity; have epinephrine immediately available for a possible hypersensitivity reaction. A detailed skin testing protocol is available from the manufacturers. Temporarily withdraw use of nasal spray if ulceration of nasal mucosa occurs. Discontinue for ulcerations >1.5 mm or those that penetrate below the mucosa. Patients >65 years of age may experience a higher incidence of nasal adverse events with calcitonin nasal spray.

Adverse Reactions Unless otherwise noted, frequencies reported are with nasal spray.

>10%: Respiratory: Rhinitis (≤12%, including ulcerative)

1% to 10%:

Cardiovascular: Flushing (nasal spray: <1%; injection: 2% to 5%), angina (1% to 3%), hypertension (1% to 3%)

Central nervous system: Depression (1% to 3%), dizziness (1% to 3%), fatigue (1% to 3%)

Dermatologic: Erythematous rash (1% to 3%)

Gastrointestinal: Nausea (injection: 10%; nasal spray: 2%), abdominal pain (1% to 3%), constipation (1% to 3%), diarrhea (1% to 3%), dyspepsia (1% to 3%)

Genitourinary: Cystitis (1% to 3%)

Local: Injection site reactions (injection: 10%)

Neuromuscular & skeletal: Back pain (5%), arthrosis (1% to 3%), myalgia (1% to 3%), paresthesia (1% to 3%)

Ocular: Conjunctivitis (1% to 3%), lacrimation abnormality (1% to 3%)

Respiratory: Nasal ulcerations (3%), bronchospasm (1% to 3%), sinusitis (1% to 3%), upper respiratory tract infection (1% to 3%)

Miscellaneous: Flu-like syndrome (1% to 3%), infection (1% to 3%), lymphadenopathy (1% to 3%)

<1% (Limited to important or life-threatening): Agitation, allergic reactions, allergic rhinitis, alopecia, anaphylactoid reaction, anaphylaxis/anaphylactic shock, anemia, anorexia, anxiety, appetite increased, arthralgia, arthritis, blurred vision, bronchitis, bundle branch block, cerebrovascular accident, cholelithiasis, cough, diaphoresis, dyspnea, earache, eczema, edema, eye pain, fever, flatulence, gastritis, goiter, hearing loss, hematuria, hepatitis, hypersensitivity, hyperthyroidism, insomnia, migraine, mucosal excoriation, myocardial infarction, nasal congestion, nasal odor, neuralgia, nocturia, palpitation, parosmia, periorbital edema, pharyngitis, pneumonia, polymyalgia rheumatica, polyuria, pruritus, pyelonephritis, rash, renal calculus, skin ulceration, sneezing, stiffness, tachycardia, taste perversion, thirst, thrombophlebitis, tinnitus, urine sediment abnormality, vertigo, visual disturbances, vitreous floater, vomiting, weight gain, xerostomia

Drug Interactions

Metabolism/Transport Effects None known.

Avoid Concomitant Use There are no known interactions where it is recommended to avoid concomitant use.

Increased Effect/Toxicity There are no known significant interactions involving an increase in effect.

Decreased Effect

Calcitonin may decrease the levels/effects of: Lithium

Ethanol/Nutrition/Herb Interactions Ethanol: Avoid ethanol (may increase risk of osteoporosis).

Stability

Injection: Store under refrigeration at 2°C to 8°C (36°F to 46°F); protect from freezing. NS has been recommended for the dilution to prepare a skin test in patients with suspected sensitivity. The following stability information has also been reported: May be stored at room temperature for up to 14 days (Cohen, 2007).

Nasal: Store unopened bottle under refrigeration at 2°C to 8°C (36°F to 46°F); do not freeze.

Fortical®: After opening, store for up to 30 days at 20°C to 25°C (68°F to 77°F); excursions permitted to 15°C to 30°C (59°F to 86°F). Store in upright position.

Miacalcin®: After opening, store for up to 35 days at room temperature of 15°C to 30°C (59°F to 86°F). Store in upright position.

Mechanism of Action Peptide sequence similar to human calcitonin; functionally antagonizes the effects of parathyroid hormone. Directly inhibits osteoclastic bone resorption; promotes the renal excretion of calcium, phosphate, sodium, magnesium, and potassium by decreasing tubular reabsorption; increases the jejunal secretion of water, sodium, potassium, and chloride

Pharmacodynamics/Kinetics

Onset of action:

Hypercalcemia: I.M., SubQ: ~2 hours

Paget's disease: Within a few months; may take up to 1 year for neurologic symptom improvement

Duration: Hypercalcemia: I.M., SubQ: 6-8 hours

Distribution: V_d: 0.15-0.3 L/kg

Metabolism: Metabolized in kidneys, blood and peripheral tissue

Bioavailability: I.M.: 66%; SubQ: 71%; Nasal: ~3% to 5% (relative to I.M.)

Half-life elimination (terminal): I.M. 58 minutes; SubQ 59-64 minutes; Nasal: ~18 minutes

Time to peak, plasma: SubQ ~23 minutes; Nasal: ~13 minutes

Excretion: Urine (as inactive metabolites)

Dosage

Children: Dosage not established

Adults:

Paget's disease (Miacalcin®): I.M., SubQ: Initial: 100 units/day; maintenance: 50 units/day or 50-100 units every 1-3 days

Hypercalcemia (Miacalcin®): Initial: I.M., SubQ: 4 units/kg every 12 hours; may increase up to 8 units/kg every 12 hours; if the response remains unsatisfactory, a further increase up to a maximum of 8 units/kg every 6 hours may be considered

Postmenopausal osteoporosis:

I.M., SubQ: Miacalcin®: 100 units/every other day

Intranasal: Fortical®, Miacalcin®: 200 units (1 spray) in one nostril daily

Dietary Considerations Recommended amounts of vitamin D and calcium intake is essential for preventing/treating osteoporosis. Patients with Paget's disease and hypercalcemia should follow a low calcium diet as prescribed.

Administration

Injection solution: May be administered I.M. or SubQ. I.M route is preferred if the injection volume is >2 mL. SubQ route is preferred for outpatient self-administration unless the injection volume is >2 mL.

Nasal spray: Before first use, allow bottle to reach room temperature, then prime pump by releasing at least 5 sprays until full spray is produced. To administer, place nozzle into nostril with head in upright position. Alternate nostrils daily. Do not prime pump before each daily use. Discard after 30 doses.

Monitoring Parameters Serum electrolytes and calcium; alkaline phosphatase and 24-hour urine collection for hydroxyproline excretion (Paget's disease), urinalysis (urine sediment); bone mineral density

Nasal formulation: Visualization of nasal mucosa, turbinate, septum, and mucosal blood vessels (at baseline and with nasal complaints)

Dosage Forms Excipient information presented when available (limited, particularly for generics); consult specific product labeling.

Injection, solution [calcitonin-salmon]:

Miacalcin®: 200 int. units/mL (2 mL)

Solution, intranasal [calcitonin-salmon/rDNA origin/spray]:

Fortical®: 200 int. units/actuation (3.7 mL) [contains benzyl alcohol; delivers 30 doses]

Solution, intranasal [calcitonin-salmon/spray]: 200 int. units/actuation (3.7 mL)

Miacalcin®: 200 int. units/actuation (3.7 mL) [contains benzalkonium chloride; delivers 30 doses]

◆ **Calcitonin (Salmon)** *see* Calcitonin *on page 262*

◆ **Calcitrate [OTC]** *see* Calcium Citrate *on page 269*

◆ **Cal-Citrate™ 225 [OTC]** *see* Calcium Citrate *on page 269*

◆ **Calcitrene™** *see* Calcipotriene *on page 261*

Calcitriol (kal si TRYE ole)

Brand Names: U.S. Calcijex®; Rocaltrol®; Vectical™

Brand Names: Canada Calcijex®; Rocaltrol®

Index Terms 1,25 Dihydroxycholecalciferol

Pharmacologic Category Vitamin D Analog

Use

Oral, injection: Management of hypocalcemia in patients on chronic renal dialysis; management of secondary hyperparathyroidism in patients with chronic kidney disease (CKD); management of hypocalcemia in hypoparathyroidism and pseudohypoparathyroidism

Topical: Management of mild-to-moderate plaque psoriasis

Unlabeled Use Decrease severity of psoriatic lesions in psoriatic vulgaris; vitamin D-dependent rickets

Pregnancy Risk Factor C

Pregnancy Considerations Teratogenic effects have been observed in animal studies. Mild hypercalcemia has been reported in a newborn following maternal use of calcitriol during pregnancy. If calcitriol is used for the management of hypoparathyroidism in pregnancy, dose adjustments may be needed as pregnancy progresses and again following delivery. Vitamin D and calcium levels should be monitored closely and kept in the lower normal range.

Lactation Enters breast milk/not recommended

Contraindications Hypersensitivity to calcitriol or any component of the formulation; hypercalcemia, vitamin D toxicity

Topical: There are no contraindications listed in the manufacturer's labeling.

Warnings/Precautions

Oral, injection: Adequate dietary (supplemental) calcium is necessary for clinical response to vitamin D. Excessive vitamin D may cause severe hypercalcemia, hypercalciuria, and hyperphosphatemia; calcium-phosphate product (serum calcium times phosphorus) must not exceed 70 mg^2/dL^2. Other forms of vitamin D should be withheld during therapy. Immobilization may increase risk of hypercalcemia and/or hypercalciuria. Maintain adequate hydration. Use caution in patients with malabsorption syndromes (efficacy may be limited and/or response may be unpredictable). Use of calcitriol for the treatment of secondary hyperparathyroidism associated with CKD is not recommended in patients with rapidly worsening kidney function or in noncompliant patients. Increased serum phosphate levels in patients with renal failure may lead to calcification; the use of an aluminum-containing phosphate binder is recommended along with a low phosphate diet in these patients. Use with caution in patients taking cardiac glycosides; digitalis toxicity is potentiated by hypocalcemia. Products may contain coconut (capsule) or palm seed oil (oral solution). Some products may contain tartrazine.

Topical: May cause hypercalcemia; if alterations in calcium occur, discontinue treatment until levels return to normal. For external use only; not for ophthalmic, oral, or intravaginal use. Do not apply to facial skin, eyes, or lips. Absorption may be increased with occlusive dressings. Avoid or limit excessive exposure to natural or artificial sunlight, or phototherapy. The safety and effectiveness has not been evaluated in patients with erythrodermic, exfoliative, or pustular psoriasis.

Adverse Reactions

Oral, I.V.: Frequency not defined.

Cardiovascular: Cardiac arrhythmia, hypertension

Central nervous system: Apathy, headache, hypothermia, psychosis, sensory disturbances, somnolence

Dermatologic: Erythema multiforme, pruritus

Endocrine & metabolic: Dehydration, growth suppression, hypercalcemia, hypercholesterolemia, hypermagnesemia, hyperphosphatemia, libido decreased, polydipsia

Gastrointestinal: Abdominal pain, anorexia, constipation, metallic taste, nausea, pancreatitis, stomach ache, vomiting, weight loss, xerostomia

Genitourinary: Nocturia, urinary tract infection

Hepatic: ALT increased, AST increased

Local: Injection site pain (mild)

Neuromuscular & skeletal: Bone pain, myalgia, dystrophy, soft tissue calcification, weakness

Ocular: Conjunctivitis, photophobia

Renal: Albuminuria, BUN increased, creatinine increased, hypercalciuria, nephrocalcinosis, polyuria

Respiratory: Rhinorrhea

Miscellaneous: Allergic reaction

Topical:

>10%: Endocrine: Hypercalcemia (≤24%)

1% to 10%:

Dermatologic: Skin discomfort (3%), pruritus (1% to 3%)

Genitourinary: Urine abnormality (4%)

Renal: Hypercalciuria (3%)

Postmarketing and/or case reports: Dermatitis (acute; blistering), erythema, hypercalcemia, kidney stones, skin burning

Drug Interactions

Metabolism/Transport Effects Substrate of CYP3A4 (major); **Note:** Assignment of Major/Minor substrate status based on clinically relevant drug interaction potential; **Induces** CYP3A4 (weak/moderate)

Avoid Concomitant Use

Avoid concomitant use of Calcitriol with any of the following: Aluminum Hydroxide; Conivaptan; Sucralfate; Vitamin D Analogs

Increased Effect/Toxicity

Calcitriol may increase the levels/effects of: Aluminum Hydroxide; Cardiac Glycosides; Magnesium Salts; Sucralfate; Vitamin D Analogs

The levels/effects of Calcitriol may be increased by: Calcium Salts; Conivaptan; CYP3A4 Inhibitors (Moderate); CYP3A4 Inhibitors (Strong); Danazol; Dasatinib; Thiazide Diuretics

Decreased Effect

Calcitriol may decrease the levels/effects of: ARIPiprazole; Saxagliptin

The levels/effects of Calcitriol may be decreased by: Bile Acid Sequestrants; Corticosteroids (Systemic); CYP3A4 Inducers (Strong); Deferasirox; Herbs (CYP3A4 Inducers); Mineral Oil; Orlistat; Sevelamer; Tocilizumab

Stability

Injection: Store at room temperature of 15°C to 30°C (59°F to 86°F). Protect from light.

Oral capsule, solution: Store at room temperature of 20°C to 25°C (68°F to 77°F). Protect from light.

Topical: Store at room temperature of 25°C (77°F); excursions permitted to 15°C to 30°C (59°F to 86°F); do not refrigerate; do not freeze.

Mechanism of Action Calcitriol is a potent active metabolite of vitamin D. Vitamin D promotes absorption of calcium in the intestines and retention at the kidneys thereby increasing calcium levels in the serum; decreases excessive serum phosphatase levels, parathyroid hormone levels, and decreases bone resorption; increases renal tubule phosphate resorption

The mechanism by which calcitriol is beneficial in the treatment of psoriasis has not been established.

Pharmacodynamics/Kinetics

Onset of action: Oral: ~2-6 hours

Duration: Oral, I.V.: 3-5 days

Absorption: Oral: Rapid

Protein binding: 99.9%

Metabolism: Primarily to 1,24,25-trihydroxycholecalciferol and 1,24,25-trihydroxy ergocalciferol

Half-life elimination: Children ~27 hours; Normal adults: 5-8 hours; Hemodialysis: 16-22 hours

Time to peak, serum: Oral: 3-6 hours; Hemodialysis: 8-12 hours

Excretion: Primarily feces; urine

Dosage

Hypocalcemia in patients on chronic renal dialysis (manufacturer labeling): *Adults:*

Oral: 0.25 mcg/day or every other day (may require 0.5-1 mcg/day); increases should be made at 4- to 8-week intervals

I.V.: Initial: 1-2 mcg 3 times/week (0.02 mcg/kg) approximately every other day. Adjust dose at 2-4 week intervals; dosing range: 0.5-4 mcg 3 times/week

Hypocalcemia in hypoparathyroidism/pseudohypoparathyroidism (manufacturers labeling): Oral (evaluate dosage at 2- to 4-week intervals):

Children <1 year (unlabeled use): 0.04-0.08 mcg/kg once daily

Children 1-5 years: 0.25-0.75 mcg once daily

Children ≥6 years and Adults: Initial: 0.25 mcg/day, range: 0.5-2 mcg once daily

Secondary hyperparathyroidism associated with moderate-to-severe CKD in patients not on dialysis (manufacturer labeling): Oral:

Children <3 years: Initial dose: 0.01-0.015 mcg/kg/day

Children ≥3 years and Adults: 0.25 mcg/day; may increase to 0.5 mcg/day

K/DOQI guidelines for vitamin D therapy in CKD:

Children:

CKD stage 2, 3: Oral:

<10 kg: 0.05 mcg every other day

10-20 kg: 0.1-0.15 mcg/day

>20 kg: 0.25 mcg/day

Note: Treatment should only be started with serum 25 (OH) D >30 ng/mL, serum iPTH >70 pg/mL, serum calcium <10 mg/dL and serum phosphorus less than or equal to the age appropriate level.

CKD stage 4: Oral:

<10 kg: 0.05 mcg every other day

10-20 kg: 0.1-0.15 mcg/day

>20 kg: 0.25 mcg/day

Note: Treatment should only be started with serum 25 (OH) D >30 ng/mL, serum iPTH >110 pg/mL, serum calcium <10 mg/dL and serum phosphorus less than or equal to the age appropriate level.

CKD stage 5: Oral, I.V.: **Note:** The following initial doses are based on plasma PTH and serum calcium levels for patients with serum phosphorus <5.5 mg/dL in adolescents or <6.5 in infants and children, and Ca-P product <55 in adolescents or <65 in infants and children <12 years. Adjust dose based on serum phosphate, calcium and PTH levels. Administer dose with each dialysis session (3 times/week). Intermittent I.V./oral administration is more effective than daily oral dosing.

Plasma PTH 300-500 pg/mL and serum Ca <10 mg/dL: 0.0075 mcg/kg (maximum: 0.25 mcg/day)

Plasma PTH >500-1000 pg/mL and serum Ca <10 mg/dL: 0.015 mcg/kg (maximum: 0.5 mcg/day)

Plasma PTH >1000 pg/mL and serum Ca <10.5 mg/dL: 0.025 mcg/kg (maximum: 1 mcg/day)

Adults:

CKD stage 3: Oral: 0.25 mcg/day. Treatment should only be started with serum 25(OH) D >30 ng/mL, serum iPTH >70 pg/mL, serum calcium <9.5 mg/dL and serum phosphorus <4.6 mg/dL

CKD stage 4: Oral: 0.25 mcg/day. Treatment should only be started with serum 25(OH) D >30 ng/mL, serum iPTH >110 pg/mL, serum calcium <9.5 mg/dL and serum phosphorus <4.6 mg/dL

CKD stage 5:

Peritoneal dialysis: Oral: Initial: 0.5-1 mcg 2-3 times/week or 0.25 mcg/day

Hemodialysis: **Note:** The following initial doses are based on plasma PTH and serum calcium levels for patients with serum phosphorus <5.5 mg/dL and Ca-P product <55. Adjust dose based on serum phosphate, calcium, and PTH levels. Intermittent I.V. administration may be more effective than daily oral dosing.

Plasma PTH 300-600 pg/mL and serum Ca <9.5 mg/dL: Oral, I.V.: 0.5-1.5 mcg

Plasma PTH 600-1000 pg/mL and serum Ca <9.5 mg/dL:

Oral: 1-4 mcg

I.V.: 1-3 mcg

Plasma PTH >1000 pg/mL and serum Ca <10 mg/dL:

Oral: 3-7 mcg

I.V.: 3-5 mcg

Psoriasis: Adults: Topical: Apply twice daily to affected areas (maximum: 200 g/week)

Vitamin D-dependent rickets (unlabeled use): Children and Adults: Oral: 1 mcg once daily

Elderly: No dosage recommendations, but start at the lower end of the dosage range

Dosage adjustment for toxicity: K/DOQI guidelines: Children and Adults: CKD stage 3 and 4:

iPTH below target: Hold calcitriol until levels rise then resume treatment at half the previous dose. If the lowest dose was being used, switch to alternate day therapy.

Corrected total calcium >9.5 mg/dL (adults) or 10.2 mg/dL (children): Hold calcitriol until serum calcium returns to <9.5 mg/dL (adults) or <9.8 mg/dL (children) then resume treatment at half the previous dose. If the lowest dose was being used, switch to alternate day therapy.

Serum phosphorus >4.6 mg/dL (adults) or greater than the age appropriate limits in children: Hold calcitriol (or add/increase dose of phosphate binder) until levels of phosphorous decrease, then resume at half the prior dose.

Dietary Considerations May be taken without regard to food. Give with meals to reduce GI problems. Adequate calcium intake should be maintained during therapy; dietary phosphorous may need to be restricted.

Administration

I.V.: May be administered as a bolus dose I.V. through the catheter at the end of hemodialysis.

Oral: May be administered without regard to food. Administer with meals to reduce GI problems.

Topical: Apply externally; not for ophthalmic, oral, or intravaginal use. Do not apply to eyes, lips, or facial skins. Rub in gently so that no medication remains visible. Limit application to only the areas of skin affected by psoriasis.

Monitoring Parameters

Serum calcium and phosphorus: Frequency of measurement may be dependent upon the presence and magnitude of abnormalities, the rate of progression of CKD, and the use of treatments for CKD-mineral and bone disorders (KDIGO, 2009):

CKD stage 3: Every 6-12 months

CKD stage 4: Every 3-6 months

CKD stage 5 and 5D: Every 1-3 months

Periodic 24-hour urinary calcium and phosphorus; magnesium; alkaline phosphatase every 12 months or more frequently in the presence of elevated PTH; creatinine, BUN, albumin; intact parathyroid hormone (iPTH) every 3-12 months depending on CKD severity

Reference Range

Corrected total serum calcium (K/DOQI, 2003): CKD stages 3 and 4: 8.4-10.2 mg/dL (2.1-2.6 mmol/L); CKD stage 5: 8.4-9.5 mg/dL (2.1-2.37 mmol/L); KDIGO guidelines recommend maintaining normal ranges for all stages of CKD (3-5D) (KDIGO, 2009)

Phosphorus (K/DOQI, 2003):

CKD stages 3 and 4: 2.7-4.6 mg/dL (0.87-1.48 mmol/L) (adults); maintain within age-appropriate limits (children)

CKD stage 5 (including those treated with dialysis): 3.5-5.5 mg/dL (1.13-1.78 mmol/L) (children >12 years and adults); 4-6 mg/dL (1.29-1.94 mmol/L) (children 1-12 years)

KDIGO guidelines recommend maintaining normal ranges for CKD stages 3-5 and lowering elevated phosphorus levels toward the normal range for CKD stage 5D (KDIGO, 2009)

Serum calcium-phosphorus product (K/DOQI, 2003): CKD stage 3-5: <55 mg^2/dL^2 (children >12 years and adults); <65 mg^2/dL^2 (children ≤12 years)

PTH: Whole molecule, immunochemiluminometric assay (ICMA): 1.0-5.2 pmol/L; whole molecule, radioimmunoassay (RIA): 10.0-65.0 pg/mL; whole molecule, immunoradiometric, double antibody (IRMA): 1.0-6.0 pmol/L

Target ranges by stage of chronic kidney disease (KDIGO, 2009): CKD stage 3-5: Optimal iPTH is unknown; maintain normal range (assay-dependent); CKD stage 5D: Maintain iPTH within 2-9 times the upper limit of normal for the assay used

Dosage Forms Excipient information presented when available (limited, particularly for generics); consult specific product labeling.

Capsule, softgel, oral: 0.25 mcg, 0.5 mcg

Rocaltrol®: 0.25 mcg, 0.5 mcg [contains coconut oil]

Injection, solution: 1 mcg/mL (1 mL)

Calcijex®: 1 mcg/mL (1 mL) [contains aluminum]

Ointment, topical:

Vectical™: 3 mcg/g (100 g)

Solution, oral: 1 mcg/mL (15 mL)

Rocaltrol®: 1 mcg/mL (15 mL) [contains palm oil]

Calcium Acetate (KAL see um AS e tate)

Brand Names: U.S. Eliphos™; PhosLo®; Phoslyra™

Brand Names: Canada PhosLo®

Pharmacologic Category Antidote; Calcium Salt; Phosphate Binder

Use Control of hyperphosphatemia in end-stage renal failure; does not promote aluminum absorption

Pregnancy Risk Factor C

Dosage Oral: Adults, on dialysis: Initial: 1334 mg with each meal, can be increased gradually (ie, every 2-3 weeks) to bring the serum phosphate value to <6 mg/dL as long as hypercalcemia does not develop (usual dose: 2001-2668 mg calcium acetate with each meal); do not give additional calcium supplements

Additional Information Complete prescribing information for this medication should be consulted for additional detail.

Dosage Forms Excipient information presented when available (limited, particularly for generics); consult specific product labeling.

Gelcap, oral: 667 mg [equivalent to elemental calcium 169 mg (8.45 mEq)]

PhosLo®: 667 mg [equivalent to elemental calcium 169 mg (8.45 mEq)]

Solution, oral:

Phoslyra™: 667 mg/5 mL (473 mL) [contains maltitol (1 g/5 mL), propylene glycol; black cherry-menthol flavor; equivalent to elemental calcium 169 mg (8.45 mEq)/5 mL]

Tablet, oral:

Eliphos™: 667 mg [equivalent to elemental calcium 169 mg (8.45 mEq)]

◆ **Calcium Acetate and Aluminum Sulfate** *see* Aluminum Sulfate and Calcium Acetate *on page 81*

◆ **Calcium Acetylhomotaurinate** *see* Acamprosate *on page 25*

Calcium and Vitamin D

(KAL see um & VYE ta min dee)

Brand Names: U.S. Cal-CYUM [OTC]; Caltrate® 600+D [OTC]; Caltrate® 600+Soy™ [OTC]; Caltrate® Colon-Health™ [OTC]; Chew-Cal [OTC]; Citracal® Maximum [OTC]; Citracal® Petites [OTC]; Citracal® Regular [OTC]; Liqua-Cal [OTC]; Os-Cal® 500+D [OTC]; Oysco 500+D [OTC]; Oysco D [OTC]; Oyst-Cal-D 500 [OTC]; Oyst-Cal-D [OTC]

Index Terms Vitamin D and Calcium Carbonate

Pharmacologic Category Calcium Salt; Electrolyte Supplement, Oral; Vitamin, Fat Soluble

Use Dietary supplement, antacid

Dosage Oral: Adults: Refer to individual monographs for dietary reference intake.

Dosage adjustment in renal impairment: Use caution in severe renal impairment

Additional Information Complete prescribing information for this medication should be consulted for additional detail.

Dosage Forms Excipient information presented when available (limited, particularly for generics); consult specific product labeling.

Caplet, oral:

Citracal® Maximum: Calcium 315 mg and vitamin D 250 int. units [gluten free]

Capsule, softgel, oral: Calcium 500 mg and vitamin D 500 int. units; calcium 600 mg and vitamin D 100 int. units; calcium 600 mg and vitamin D 200 int. units

Liqua-Cal: Calcium 600 mg and vitamin D 200 int. units [contains beeswax, lecithin, and soybean oil]

Tablet, oral: Calcium 250 mg and vitamin D 125 int. units; calcium 500 mg and vitamin D 125 int. units; calcium 500 mg and vitamin D 200 int. units; calcium 600 mg and vitamin D 125 int. units; calcium 600 mg and vitamin D 200 int. units

Caltrate® 600+D: Calcium 600 mg and vitamin D 200 int. units [contains soybean oil]

Caltrate® 600+Soy™: Calcium 600 mg and vitamin D 200 int. units [contains soy isoflavones 25 mg]

Caltrate® ColonHealth™: Calcium 600 mg and vitamin D 200 int. units [contains soybean oil]

Citracal® Petites: Calcium 200 mg and vitamin D 250 int. units [gluten free]

Citracal® Regular: Calcium 250 mg and vitamin D 200 int. units [gluten free]

Oysco D: Calcium 250 mg and vitamin D 125 int. units

Oysco 500+D: Calcium 500 mg and vitamin D 200 int. units [contains tartrazine]

Oyst-Cal-D: Calcium 250 mg and vitamin D 125 int. units [sodium free, sugar free; contains tartrazine]

Oyst-Cal-D 500: Calcium 500 mg and vitamin D 200 int. units [sodium free, sugar free; contains tartrazine]

Tablet, chewable: Calcium 500 mg and vitamin D 100 int. units; Calcium 600 mg and vitamin D 400 int. units

Os-Cal® 500+D: Calcium 500 mg and vitamin D 400 int. units [sugar free; contains phenylalanine; light lemon flavor]

Wafer, chewable:

Cal-CYUM: Calcium 519 mg and vitamin D 150 int. units (50s) [dye free; vanilla flavor]

Chew-Cal: Calcium 333 mg and vitamin D 40 int. units (100s, 250s)

Calcium Carbonate (KAL see um KAR bun ate)

Brand Names: U.S. Alcalak [OTC]; Alka-Mints® [OTC]; Cal-Gest [OTC]; Cal-Mint [OTC]; Calcarb 600 [OTC] [DSC]; Calci-Chew® [OTC]; Calci-Mix® [OTC]; Caltrate® 600 [OTC]; Children's Pepto [OTC]; Chooz® [OTC]; Florical® [OTC]; Maalox® Children's [OTC]; Maalox® Regular Strength [OTC]; Nephro-Calci® [OTC]; Nutralox® [OTC]; Oysco 500 [OTC]; Oystercal™ 500 [OTC]; Rolaids® Extra Strength [OTC]; Super Calcium 600 [OTC]; Titralac™ [OTC]; Tums® E-X [OTC]; Tums® Extra Strength Sugar Free [OTC]; Tums® Quickpak [OTC]; Tums® Smoothies™ [OTC]; Tums® Ultra [OTC]; Tums® [OTC]

Brand Names: Canada Apo-Cal®; Calcite-500; Caltrate®; Caltrate® Select; Os-Cal®; Tums Extra Strength; Tums Smoothies; Tums® Chews Extra Strength; Tums® Regular Strength; Tums® Ultra Strength

Index Terms Oscal

Pharmacologic Category Antacid; Antidote; Calcium Salt; Electrolyte Supplement, Oral

Use As an antacid; treatment and prevention of calcium deficiency or hyperphosphatemia (eg, osteoporosis, osteomalacia, mild/moderate renal insufficiency, hypoparathyroidism, postmenopausal osteoporosis, rickets); has been used to bind phosphate

Dosage Oral (dosage is in terms of **elemental** calcium):

Dietary Reference Intake for Calcium:

1-6 months: Adequate intake: 200 mg/day
7-12 months: Adequate intake: 260 mg/day
1-3 years: RDA: 700 mg/day
4-8 years: RDA: 1000 mg/day
9-18 years: RDA:1300 mg/day
Adults, Females/Males: RDA:
19-50 years: 1000 mg/day
≥51 years, females: 1200 mg/day
51-70 years, males: 1000 mg/day
>70 years, males: 1200 mg/day
Females: Pregnancy/Lactating: RDA: Requirements are the same as in nonpregnant or nonlactating females

Hypocalcemia (dose depends on clinical condition and serum calcium level): Dose expressed in mg of **elemental calcium**

Children: 45-65 mg/kg/day in 4 divided doses
Adults: 1-2 g or more/day in 3-4 divided doses

Antacid:

Children 2-5 years (24-47 lb): Elemental calcium 161 mg as needed; maximum 483 mg per 24 hours

Children 6-11 years (48-95 lb): Elemental calcium 322 mg as needed; maximum: 966 mg per 24 hours

Adults: Dosage based on acid-neutralizing capacity of specific product; generally, 1-2 tablets or 5-10 mL every 2 hours; maximum: 7000 mg calcium carbonate per 24 hours; specific product labeling should be consulted

Dietary supplementation: Adults: 500 mg to 2 g divided 2-4 times/day

Osteoporosis: Adults >51 years: 1200 mg/day

Dosing adjustment in renal impairment: Cl_{cr} <25 mL/minute: Dosage adjustments may be necessary depending on the serum calcium levels

Additional Information Complete prescribing information for this medication should be consulted for additional detail.

Dosage Forms Excipient information presented when available (limited, particularly for generics); consult specific product labeling. [DSC] = Discontinued product

Capsule, oral:

Calci-Mix®: 1250 mg [equivalent to elemental calcium 500 mg]

Florical®: 364 mg [equivalent to elemental calcium 145 mg; contains fluoride]

Gum, chewing, oral:

Chooz®: 500 mg (12s) [sugar free; contains phenylalanine 1.4 mg/tablet; mint flavor; equivalent to elemental calcium 200 mg]

Powder, oral: (480 g)

Tums® Quickpak: 1000 mg/packet (24s) [contains sodium <5 mg/packet; berry fusion flavor; equivalent to elemental calcium 400 mg]

Suspension, oral: 1250 mg/5 mL (5 mL, 500 mL, 16 oz) [equivalent to elemental calcium 500 mg/5 mL]

Tablet, oral: 648 mg [equivalent to elemental calcium 260 mg], 650 mg [equivalent to elemental calcium 260 mg], 1250 mg [equivalent to elemental calcium 500 mg], 1500 mg [equivalent to elemental calcium 600 mg]

Calcarb 600: 1500 mg [DSC] [scored; sugar free; equivalent to elemental calcium 600 mg]

Caltrate® 600: 1500 mg [scored; equivalent to elemental calcium 600 mg]

Florical®: 364 mg [equivalent to elemental calcium 145 mg; contains fluoride]

Nephro-Calci®: 1500 mg [equivalent to elemental calcium 600 mg]

Oysco 500: 1250 mg [equivalent to elemental calcium 500 mg]

Oystercal™ 500: 1250 mg [equivalent to elemental calcium 500 mg]

Super Calcium 600: 1500 mg [gluten free, sugar free; equivalent to elemental calcium 600 mg]
Super Calcium 600: 1500 mg [sugar free; equivalent to elemental calcium 600 mg]
Tablet, chewable, oral: 420 mg [equivalent to elemental calcium 168 mg], 500 mg [equivalent to elemental calcium 200 mg], 500 mg, 600 mg [equivalent to elemental calcium 222 mg], 650 mg [equivalent to elemental calcium 260 mg], 750 mg [equivalent to elemental calcium 300 mg], 1250 mg [equivalent to elemental calcium 500 mg]
Alcalak: 420 mg [aluminum free; mint flavor; equivalent to elemental calcium 168 mg]
Alka-Mints®: 850 mg [spearmint flavor; equivalent to elemental calcium 340 mg]
Cal-Gest: 500 mg [equivalent to elemental calcium 200 mg]
Cal-Mint: 650 mg [aluminum free, dye free, gluten free, sugar free; mint flavor; equivalent to elemental calcium 260 mg]
Calci-Chew®: 1250 mg [cherry flavor; equivalent to elemental calcium 500 mg]
Children's Pepto: 400 mg [bubblegum flavor; equivalent to elemental calcium 161 mg]
Children's Pepto: 400 mg [watermelon flavor; equivalent to elemental calcium 161 mg]
Maalox® Children's: 400 mg [contains phenylalanine 0.3 mg/tablet; wildberry flavor; equivalent to elemental calcium 160 mg]
Maalox® Regular Strength: 600 mg [contains phenylalanine 0.5 mg/tablet; wildberry flavor; equivalent to elemental calcium 240 mg]
Nutralox®: 420 mg [sugar free; mint flavor; equivalent to elemental calcium 168 mg]
Titralac™: 420 mg [sugar free; contains sodium 1.1 mg/tablet; spearmint flavor; equivalent to elemental calcium 168 mg]
Tums®: 500 mg [contains tartrazine; assorted fruit flavor; equivalent to elemental calcium 200 mg]
Tums®: 500 mg [contains tartrazine; peppermint flavor; equivalent to elemental calcium 200 mg]
Tums® E-X: 750 mg [tropical fruit flavor; equivalent to elemental calcium 300 mg]
Tums® E-X: 750 mg [wintergreen flavor; equivalent to elemental calcium 300 mg]
Tums® E-X: 750 mg [contains tartrazine; assorted berries flavor; equivalent to elemental calcium 300 mg]
Tums® E-X: 750 mg [contains tartrazine; assorted fruit flavor; equivalent to elemental calcium 300 mg]
Tums® E-X: 750 mg [contains tartrazine; cool relief mint flavor; equivalent to elemental calcium 300 mg]
Tums® E-X: 750 mg [contains tartrazine; fresh blend flavor; equivalent to elemental calcium 300 mg]
Tums® E-X: 750 mg [contains tartrazine; tropical fruit flavor; equivalent to elemental calcium 300 mg]
Tums® Extra Strength Sugar Free: 750 mg [sugar free; contains phenylalanine <1 mg/tablet; orange cream flavor; equivalent to elemental calcium 300 mg]
Tums® Smoothies™: 750 mg [contains tartrazine; assorted fruit flavor; equivalent to elemental calcium 300 mg]
Tums® Smoothies™: 750 mg [contains tartrazine; peppermint flavor; equivalent to elemental calcium 300 mg]
Tums® Smoothies™: 750 mg [contains tartrazine; tropical assorted fruits flavor; equivalent to elemental calcium 300 mg]
Tums® Ultra: 1000 mg [contains tartrazine; assorted berries flavor; equivalent to elemental calcium 400 mg]
Tums® Ultra: 1000 mg [contains tartrazine; assorted fruit flavor; equivalent to elemental calcium 400 mg]
Tums® Ultra: 1000 mg [contains tartrazine; peppermint flavor; equivalent to elemental calcium 400 mg]
Tums® Ultra: 1000 mg [contains tartrazine; spearmint flavor; equivalent to elemental calcium 400 mg]
Tums® Ultra: 1000 mg [contains tartrazine; tropical assorted fruits flavor; equivalent to elemental calcium 400 mg]
Tablet, softchew, oral:
Rolaids® Extra Strength: 1177 mg [contains coconut oil, soya lecithin; vanilla crème flavor; equivalent to elemental calcium 471 mg]
Rolaids® Extra Strength: 1177 mg [contains coconut oil, soya lecithin; wild cherry flavor; equivalent to elemental calcium 471 mg]

Calcium Carbonate and Magnesium Hydroxide

(KAL see um KAR bun ate & mag NEE zhum hye DROKS ide)

Brand Names: U.S. Mi-Acid™ Double Strength [OTC]; Mylanta® Gelcaps® [OTC]; Mylanta® Supreme [OTC]; Mylanta® Ultra [OTC]; Rolaids® Extra Strength [OTC]; Rolaids® [OTC]

Index Terms Magnesium Hydroxide and Calcium Carbonate

Pharmacologic Category Antacid

Use Hyperacidity

Dosage Adults: Oral: 2-4 tablets between meals, at bedtime, or as directed by healthcare provider

Additional Information Complete prescribing information for this medication should be consulted for additional detail.

Dosage Forms Excipient information presented when available (limited, particularly for generics); consult specific product labeling.

Gelcap (Mylanta® Gelcaps®): Calcium carbonate 550 mg and magnesium hydroxide 125 mg
Liquid (Mylanta® Supreme): Calcium carbonate 400 mg and magnesium hydroxide 135 mg per 5 mL (360 mL, 720 mL) [cherry flavor]
Tablet, chewable:
Mi-Acid™ Double Strength: Calcium carbonate 700 mg and magnesium hydroxide 300 mg
Mylanta® Ultra: Calcium carbonate 700 mg and magnesium hydroxide 300 mg [cherry créme and cool mint flavors]
Rolaids®: Calcium carbonate 550 mg and magnesium hydroxide 110 mg [sodium free; contains elemental calcium 220 mg and elemental magnesium 45 mg; original (peppermint), cherry, and spearmint flavors]
Rolaids® Extra Strength: Calcium carbonate 675 mg and magnesium hydroxide 135 mg [sodium free; contains elemental calcium 271 mg and elemental magnesium 56 mg, fruit flavor contains tartrazine; cool strawberry, fresh mint, fruit, and tropical fruit punch flavors]

Calcium Chloride (KAL see um KLOR ide)

Pharmacologic Category Calcium Salt; Electrolyte Supplement, Parenteral

Use Treatment of acute symptomatic hypocalcemia; cardiac disturbances of hyperkalemia or hypocalcemia; emergent treatment of hypocalcemic tetany; treatment of severe hypermagnesemia

Unlabeled Use Calcium channel blocker overdose; beta-blocker overdose; severe hyperkalemia (K+ >6.5 mEq/L with toxic ECG changes) [ACLS guidelines]; malignant arrhythmias (including cardiac arrest) associated with hypermagnesemia [ACLS guidelines]

Pregnancy Risk Factor C

Pregnancy Considerations Animal reproduction studies have not been conducted. Calcium crosses the placenta. The amount of calcium reaching the fetus is determined by maternal physiological changes. Calcium requirements are ▶

the same in pregnant and nonpregnant females (IOM, 2011). Information related to use as an antidote in pregnancy is limited. In general, medications used as antidotes should take into consideration the health and prognosis of the mother (Bailey, 2003).

Contraindications Hypercalcemia, known or suspected digoxin toxicity; not recommended as routine treatment in cardiac arrest (includes asystole, ventricular fibrillation, pulseless ventricular tachycardia, or pulseless electrical activity)

Warnings/Precautions For I.V. use only; do not inject SubQ or I.M.; avoid rapid I.V. administration (<100 mg/minute) unless being given emergently. Avoid extravasation. Use with caution in patients with hyperphosphatemia, respiratory acidosis, renal impairment, or respiratory failure; acidifying effect of calcium chloride may potentiate acidosis. Use with caution in patients with chronic renal failure to avoid hypercalcemia; frequent monitoring of serum calcium and phosphorus is necessary. Use with caution in hypokalemic or digitalized patients since acute rises in serum calcium levels may precipitate cardiac arrhythmias. Solutions may contain aluminum; toxic levels may occur following prolonged administration in premature neonates or patients with renal impairment. Avoid metabolic acidosis (ie, administer only 2-3 days then change to another calcium salt).

Adverse Reactions Frequency not defined. I.V.:

Cardiovascular: Arrhythmia, bradycardia, cardiac arrest, hypotension, syncope, vasodilation

Endocrine & metabolic: Hypercalcemia

Gastrointestinal: Irritation, chalky taste

Hepatic: Serum amylase increased

Neuromuscular & skeletal: Tingling sensation

Renal: Renal calculi

Miscellaneous: Hot flashes

Postmarketing and/or case reports: Calcinosis cutis

Drug Interactions

Metabolism/Transport Effects None known.

Avoid Concomitant Use

Avoid concomitant use of Calcium Chloride with any of the following: Calcium Acetate

Increased Effect/Toxicity

Calcium Chloride may increase the levels/effects of: Calcium Acetate; CefTRIAXone; Vitamin D Analogs

The levels/effects of Calcium Chloride may be increased by: Thiazide Diuretics

Decreased Effect

Calcium Chloride may decrease the levels/effects of: Bisphosphonate Derivatives; Calcium Channel Blockers; Deferiprone; DOBUTamine; Eltrombopag; Phosphate Supplements; Tetracycline Derivatives; Thyroid Products; Trientine

The levels/effects of Calcium Chloride may be decreased by: Trientine

Stability Do not refrigerate solutions; IVPB solutions/I.V. infusion solutions are stable for 24 hours at room temperature.

Although calcium chloride is not routinely used in the preparation of parenteral nutrition, it is important to note that phosphate salts may precipitate when mixed with calcium salts. Solubility is improved in amino acid parenteral nutrition solutions. Check with a pharmacist to determine compatibility.

Mechanism of Action Moderates nerve and muscle performance via action potential excitation threshold regulation

Pharmacodynamics/Kinetics Excretion: Primarily feces (80% as insoluble calcium); urine (20%)

Dosage Note: One gram of calcium chloride is equal to 270 mg of elemental calcium.

Dosages are expressed in terms of the calcium chloride salt based on a solution concentration of 100 mg/mL (10%) containing 1.4 mEq (27.3 mg)/mL elemental calcium.

Acute, symptomatic ionized hypocalcemia, hyperkalemia, or hypermagnesemia: **Note:** Routine use in cardiac arrest is not recommended due to the lack of improved survival (PALS, 2010): I.V.:

Infants and Children: 20 mg/kg (maximum: 2000 mg/dose); may repeat as necessary (PALS, 2010)

Adults: 500-1000 mg; may repeat as necessary (ACLS, 2010)

Beta-blocker overdose, refractory to glucagon and high-dose vasopressors (unlabeled use): Adults: I.V.: 1000 mg bolus via central line reported to quickly increase blood pressure (O'Grady, 2001).

Calcium channel blocker overdose (unlabeled use):

Infants and Children (PALS, 2010):

I.V., I.O.: 20 mg/kg (maximum: 2000 mg/dose) over 5-10 minutes; if favorable response obtained, consider I.V. infusion

I.V. infusion: 20-50 mg/kg/hour

Adults:

I.V.: 1000 mg every 10-20 minutes (total of 4 doses) **or** 1000 mg every 2-3 minutes until clinical effect is achieved; if favorable response obtained, consider I.V. infusion (ACLS, 2010)

I.V. infusion: 20-50 mg/kg/hour

Hypocalcemia secondary to citrated blood transfusion: I.V.: **Note:** Routine administration of calcium, in the absence of signs/symptoms of hypocalcemia, is generally not recommended. A number of recommendations have been published seeking to address potential hypocalcemia during massive transfusion of citrated blood; however, many practitioners recommend replacement only as guided by clinical evidence of hypocalcemia and/or serial monitoring of ionized calcium. In adults, clinically-significant hypocalcemia usually dose not occur until >5 units of packed red blood cells have been administered.

Infants and Children: Give 32 mg (0.45 mEq elemental calcium) for each 100 mL citrated blood infused

Adults: 200-500 mg per 500 mL of citrated blood (infused into another vein)

Hypocalcemic tetany: I.V.:

Infants and Children: 10 mg/kg over 5-10 minutes; may repeat after 6-8 hours or follow with an infusion with a maximum dose of 200 mg/kg/day; alternatively, higher doses of 35-50 mg/kg/dose repeated every 6-8 hours have been used

Adults: 1000 mg over 10-30 minutes; may repeat after 6 hours

Dosing adjustment in renal impairment: Cl_{cr} <25 mL/minute: Dosage adjustments may be necessary depending on the serum calcium concentration

Administration For I.V. administration only; avoid extravasation. Avoid rapid administration (do not exceed 100 mg/minute except in emergency situations). May be given over 2-5 minutes if rapid increase in serum calcium concentration is required. For I.V. infusion, dilute to a maximum concentration of 20 mg/mL and infuse over 1 hour or no greater than 45-90 mg/kg/hour (0.6-1.2 mEq/kg/hour); administration via a central or deep vein is preferred; do not use scalp, small hand or foot veins for I.V. administration since severe necrosis and sloughing may occur. Monitor ECG if calcium is infused faster than 2.5 mEq/minute; **stop the infusion if the patient complains of pain or discomfort.** Warm to body temperature. **Do not infuse calcium chloride in the same I.V. line as phosphate-containing solutions.**

Monitoring Parameters Monitor infusion site, ECG when appropriate; serum calcium and ionized calcium (normal: 8.5-10.2 mg/dL [total]; 4.5-5.0 mg/dL [ionized]), albumin, serum phosphate

Calcium channel blocker overdose, beta-blocker overdose: Hemodynamic response, serum ionized calcium levels

Reference Range

Serum total calcium: 8.4-10.2 mg/dL. **Note:** Due to a poor correlation between the serum ionized calcium (free) and total serum calcium, particularly in states of low albumin or acid/base imbalances, direct measurement of ionized calcium is recommended.

In low albumin states, the corrected **total** serum calcium may be estimated by the following equation (assuming a normal albumin of 4 g/dL).

Corrected total calcium = total serum calcium + 0.8 (4.0 - measured serum albumin)

or

Corrected calcium = measured calcium - measured albumin + 4.0

Serum/plasma chloride: 95-108 mEq/L

Test Interactions Increased calcium

Additional Information 14 mEq calcium/g (10 mL); 270 mg elemental calcium/g calcium chloride (27% elemental calcium)

Dosage Forms Excipient information presented when available (limited, particularly for generics); consult specific product labeling.

Injection, solution: 10% (10 mL) [equivalent to elemental calcium 27.2 mg (1.36 mEq)/mL]

Injection, solution [preservative free]: 10% (10 mL) [equivalent to elemental calcium 27.2 mg (1.36 mEq)/mL]

Calcium Citrate (KAL see um SIT rate)

Brand Names: U.S. Cal-C-Caps [OTC]; Cal-Cee [OTC]; Cal-Citrate™ 225 [OTC]; Calcitrate [OTC]

Brand Names: Canada Osteocit®

Pharmacologic Category Calcium Salt

Use Dietary supplement

Dosage Oral: Dosage is in terms of **elemental** calcium

Dietary Reference Intake for Calcium:

1-6 months: Adequate intake: 200 mg/day
7-12 months: Adequate intake: 260 mg/day
1-3 years: RDA: 700 mg/day
4-8 years: RDA: 1000 mg/day
9-18 years: RDA: 1300 mg/day
Adults, Females/Males: RDA:
19-50 years: 1000 mg/day
≥51 years, females: 1200 mg/day
51-70 years, males: 1000 mg/day
>70 years, males: 1200 mg/day

Female: Pregnancy/Lactating: RDA: Requirements are the same as in nonpregnant or nonlactating females

Additional Information Complete prescribing information for this medication should be consulted for additional detail.

Dosage Forms Excipient information presented when available (limited, particularly for generics); consult specific product labeling. [DSC] = Discontinued product

Capsule, oral:
Cal-C-Caps: Elemental calcium 180 mg
Cal-Citrate™ 225: Elemental calcium 225 mg

Granules, oral: (480 g)

Tablet, oral: Elemental calcium 200 mg [DSC], Elemental calcium 250 mg
Cal-Cee: Elemental calcium 250 mg
Calcitrate: Elemental calcium 200 mg

◆ **Calcium Disodium Edetate** *see* Edetate CALCIUM Disodium *on page 572*

◆ **Calcium Disodium Versenate®** *see* Edetate CALCIUM Disodium *on page 572*

◆ **Calcium Folinate** *see* Leucovorin Calcium *on page 987*

Calcium Glubionate (KAL see um gloo BYE oh nate)

Brand Names: U.S. Calcionate [OTC]

Pharmacologic Category Calcium Salt

Use Dietary supplement

Dosage Dosage is in terms of **elemental** calcium

Dietary Reference Intake for Calcium: Oral:

1-6 months: Adequate intake: 200 mg/day
7-12 months: Adequate intake: 260 mg/day
1-3 years: RDA: 700 mg/day
4-8 years: RDA: 1000 mg/day
9-18 years: RDA: 1300 mg/day
Adults, Females/Males: RDA:
19-50 years: 1000 mg/day
≥51 years, females: 1200 mg/day
51-70 years, males: 1000 mg/day
>70 years, males: 1200 mg/day

Females: Pregnancy/Lactating: RDA: Requirements are the same as in nonpregnant or nonlactating females

Dietary supplement: Oral:

Infants <12 months: 5 mL 5 times/day; may mix with juice or formula
Children <4 years: 10 mL 3 times/day
Children ≥4 years and Adults: 15 mL 3 times/day

Additional Information Complete prescribing information for this medication should be consulted for additional detail.

Dosage Forms Excipient information presented when available (limited, particularly for generics); consult specific product labeling.

Syrup, oral:
Calcionate: 1.8 g/5 mL (473 mL) [contains benzoic acid; caramel-orange flavor; equivalent to elemental calcium 115 mg/5 mL]

Calcium Gluconate (KAL see um GLOO koe nate)

Brand Names: U.S. Cal-G [OTC]; Cal-GLU™ [OTC]

Pharmacologic Category Calcium Salt; Electrolyte Supplement, Oral; Electrolyte Supplement, Parenteral

Use Treatment and prevention of hypocalcemia; treatment of tetany, cardiac disturbances of hyperkalemia, cardiac resuscitation when epinephrine fails to improve myocardial contractions, hypocalcemia; calcium supplementation; hydrofluoric acid (HF) burns

Unlabeled Use Calcium channel blocker overdose

Pregnancy Risk Factor C

Pregnancy Considerations Animal reproduction studies have not been conducted. Calcium crosses the placenta. The amount of calcium reaching the fetus is determined by maternal physiological changes. Calcium requirements are the same in pregnant and nonpregnant females (IOM, 2011). Information related to use as an antidote in pregnancy is limited. In general, medications used as antidotes should take into consideration the health and prognosis of the mother (Bailey, 2003).

Lactation Enters breast milk

Contraindications Hypersensitivity to calcium gluconate or any component of the formulation; ventricular fibrillation during cardiac resuscitation; digitalis toxicity or suspected digoxin toxicity; hypercalcemia

Warnings/Precautions Injection solution is for I.V. use only; do not inject SubQ or I.M. Avoid too rapid I.V. administration and avoid extravasation. Use with caution in digitalized patients, severe hyperphosphatemia, respiratory failure, or acidosis. May produce cardiac arrest. Hypercalcemia may occur in patients with renal failure; ▶

frequent determination of serum calcium is necessary. Use caution with renal disease. Use caution when administering calcium supplements to patients with a history of kidney stones. Solutions may contain aluminum; toxic levels may occur following prolonged administration in premature neonates or patients with renal dysfunction. Oral: Constipation, bloating, and gas are common with oral calcium supplements (especially carbonate salt). Taking calcium (≤500 mg) with food improves absorption. Calcium administration interferes with absorption of some minerals and drugs; use with caution. It is recommended to concomitantly administer vitamin D for optimal calcium absorption.

Adverse Reactions Frequency not defined.

I.V.:

Cardiovascular: Arrhythmia, bradycardia, cardiac arrest, hypotension, vasodilation, and syncope may occur following rapid I.V. injection

Central nervous system: Sense of oppression

Gastrointestinal: Chalky taste

Local: Abscess and necrosis following I.M. administration

Neuromuscular & skeletal: Tingling sensation

Miscellaneous: Heat waves

Postmarketing and/or case reports: Calcinosis cutis

Oral: Gastrointestinal: Constipation

Drug Interactions

Metabolism/Transport Effects None known.

Avoid Concomitant Use

Avoid concomitant use of Calcium Gluconate with any of the following: Calcium Acetate

Increased Effect/Toxicity

Calcium Gluconate may increase the levels/effects of: Calcium Acetate; CefTRIAXone; Vitamin D Analogs

The levels/effects of Calcium Gluconate may be increased by: Thiazide Diuretics

Decreased Effect

Calcium Gluconate may decrease the levels/effects of: Bisphosphonate Derivatives; Calcium Channel Blockers; Deferiprone; DOBUTamine; Eltrombopag; Estramustine; Phosphate Supplements; Quinolone Antibiotics; Tetracycline Derivatives; Thyroid Products; Trientine

The levels/effects of Calcium Gluconate may be decreased by: Trientine

Stability

Do not refrigerate solutions. IVPB solutions/I.V. infusion solutions are stable for 24 hours at room temperature.

Standard diluent: 1 g/100 mL D_5W or NS; 2 g/100 mL D_5W or NS.

Maximum concentration in parenteral nutrition solutions is variable depending upon concentration and solubility (consult detailed reference).

Mechanism of Action As dietary supplement, used to prevent or treat negative calcium balance; in osteoporosis, it helps to prevent or decrease the rate of bone loss. The calcium in calcium salts moderates nerve and muscle performance and allows normal cardiac function.

Pharmacodynamics/Kinetics

Absorption: Requires vitamin D; calcium is absorbed in soluble, ionized form; solubility of calcium is increased in an acid environment

Protein binding: Primarily albumin

Excretion: Primarily feces (as unabsorbed calcium); urine (20%)

Dosage

Dietary Reference Intake for Calcium:

1-6 months: Adequate intake: 200 mg/day

7-12 months: Adequate intake: 260 mg/day

1-3 years: RDA: 700 mg/day

4-8 years: RDA: 1000 mg/day

9-18 years: RDA: 1300 mg/day

Adults, Females/Males: RDA:

19-50 years: 1000 mg/day

≥51 years, females: 1200 mg/day

51-70 years, males: 1000 mg/day

>70 years, males: 1200 mg/day

Females: Pregnancy/Lactating: RDA: Requirements are the same as in nonpregnant or nonlactating females

Dosage note: Calcium chloride has 3 times more elemental calcium than calcium gluconate. Calcium chloride is 27% elemental calcium; calcium gluconate is 9% elemental calcium. One gram of calcium chloride is equal to 270 mg of elemental calcium; 1 gram of calcium gluconate is equal to 90 mg of elemental calcium. The following dosages are expressed in terms of the calcium gluconate salt based on a solution concentration of 100 mg/mL (10%) containing 0.465 mEq (9.3 mg)/mL elemental calcium:

Hypocalcemia: I.V.:

Infants and Children: 200-500 mg/kg/day as a continuous infusion or in 4 divided doses (maximum: 2-3 g/dose)

Adults: 2-15 g/24 hours as a continuous infusion or in divided doses

Hypocalcemia: Oral:

Children: 200-500 mg/kg/day divided every 6 hours

Adults: 500 mg to 2 g 2-4 times/day

Hypocalcemia secondary to citrated blood infusion: I.V.: **Note:** Routine administration of calcium, in the absence of signs/symptoms of hypocalcemia, is generally not recommended. A number of recommendations have been published seeking to address potential hypocalcemia during massive transfusion of citrated blood; however, many practitioners recommend replacement only as guided by clinical evidence of hypocalcemia and/or serial monitoring of ionized calcium.

Infants and Children: Give 98 mg (0.45 mEq **elemental** calcium) for each 100 mL citrated blood infused

Adults: 500 mg to 1 g per 500 mL of citrated blood (infused into another vein). Single doses up to 2 g have also been recommended.

Hypocalcemic tetany: I.V.:

Infants and Children: 100-200 mg/kg/dose over 5-10 minutes; may repeat every 6-8 hours **or** follow with an infusion of 500 mg/kg/day

Adults: 1-3 g may be administered until therapeutic response occurs

Magnesium intoxication, cardiac arrest in the presence of hyperkalemia or hypocalcemia: I.V.:

Infants and Children: 60-100 mg/kg/dose (maximum: 3 g/dose)

Adults: 500-800 mg/dose (maximum: 3 g/dose)

Maintenance electrolyte requirements for total parenteral nutrition: I.V.: Daily requirements: Adults: 1.7-3.4 g/1000 kcal/24 hours

Calcium channel blocker overdose (unlabeled use): Adults: I.V. infusion: 10% solution: 0.6-1.2 mL/kg/hour or I.V. 0.2-0.5 ml/kg every 15-20 minutes for 4 doses (maximum: 2-3 g/dose). In life-threatening situations, 1 g has been given every 1-10 minutes until clinical effect is achieved (case reports of resistant hypotension reported use of 12-18 g total).

Dosing adjustment in renal impairment: Cl_{cr} <25 mL/minute: Dosage adjustments may be necessary depending on the serum calcium levels

Administration Not for I.M. or SubQ administration. For I.V. administration only; administer slowly (~1.5 mL calcium gluconate 10% per minute) through a small needle into a large vein in order to avoid too rapid increased in serum calcium and extravasation.

Extravasation treatment example: Hyaluronidase: Add 1 mL NS to 150 unit vial to make 150 units/mL of concentration; mix 0.1 mL of above with 0.9 mL NS in 1 mL syringe to make final concentration = 15 units/mL

Reference Range

Serum calcium: 8.5-10.5 mg/dL. Monitor plasma calcium levels if using calcium salts as electrolyte supplements for deficiency.

Due to a poor correlation between the serum ionized calcium (free) and total serum calcium, particularly in states of low albumin or acid/base imbalances, direct measurement of ionized calcium is recommended

In low albumin states, the corrected **total** serum calcium may be estimated by:

Corrected total calcium = total serum calcium + 0.8 (4.0 - measured serum albumin)

Test Interactions Increased calcium (S); decreased magnesium

Additional Information A topical 2.5% to 5% calcium gel for the treatment of hydrofluoric acid (HF) burns can be prepared by adding calcium gluconate to a surgical lubricant (water soluble such as K-Y® Jelly). Calcium chloride should not be used for this purpose. Use of injectable calcium gluconate (I.V., SubQ) has also been reported in the literature for the treatment of HF burns not amenable to topical treatment.

Dosage Forms Excipient information presented when available (limited, particularly for generics); consult specific product labeling.

Capsule, oral:

Cal-G: 700 mg [gluten free; equivalent to elemental calcium 65 mg]

Cal-GLU™: 515 mg [dye free, sugar free; equivalent to elemental calcium 50 mg]

Injection, solution [preservative free]: 10% (10 mL, 50 mL, 100 mL) [equivalent to elemental calcium 9.3 mg (0.465 mEq)/mL]

Powder, oral: (480 g)

Tablet, oral: 500 mg [equivalent to elemental calcium 45 mg], 648 mg [equivalent to elemental calcium 60 mg]

Extemporaneous Preparations A calcium gluconate gel may be made with tablets or solution for injection. Crush seven 500 mg calcium gluconate tablets in a mortar and reduce to a fine powder and add 5 oz tube of water-soluble surgical lubricant (eg, K-Y® Jelly) **or** add 3.5 g calcium gluconate injection solution to 5 oz of water-soluble surgical lubricant. Calcium carbonate may be substituted; do not use calcium chloride due to potential for irritation.

◆ **Calcium Leucovorin** *see* Leucovorin Calcium *on page 987*

◆ **Calcium Levoleucovorin** *see* LEVOleucovorin *on page 1000*

◆ **Cal-CYUM [OTC]** *see* Calcium and Vitamin D *on page 265*

◆ **Caldecort® [OTC]** *see* Hydrocortisone (Topical) *on page 841*

◆ **Caldolor™** *see* Ibuprofen *on page 860*

Calfactant (kaf AKT ant)

Brand Names: U.S. Infasurf®

Pharmacologic Category Lung Surfactant

Use Prevention of respiratory distress syndrome (RDS) in premature infants at high risk for RDS and for the treatment ("rescue") of premature infants who develop RDS

Prophylaxis: Therapy at birth with calfactant is indicated for premature infants <29 weeks of gestational age at significant risk for RDS. Should be administered as soon as possible, preferably within 30 minutes after birth.

Treatment: For infants ≤72 hours of age with RDS (confirmed by clinical and radiologic findings) and requiring endotracheal intubation.

Warnings/Precautions For intratracheal administration only. Rapidly affects oxygenation and lung compliance; restrict use to a highly-supervised clinical setting with immediate availability of clinicians experienced in intubation and ventilatory management of premature infants. Transient episodes of bradycardia, decreased oxygen saturation, endotracheal tube blockage or reflux of calfactant into endotracheal tube may occur. Discontinue dosing procedure and initiate measures to alleviate the condition; may reinstitute after the patient is stable. Produces rapid improvements in lung oxygenation and compliance that may require frequent adjustments to oxygen delivery and ventilator settings.

Adverse Reactions

Cardiovascular: Bradycardia (34%), cyanosis (65%)

Respiratory: Airway obstruction (39%), reflux (21%), requirement for manual ventilation (16%), reintubation (1% to 10%)

Drug Interactions

Metabolism/Transport Effects None known.

Avoid Concomitant Use There are no known interactions where it is recommended to avoid concomitant use.

Increased Effect/Toxicity There are no known significant interactions involving an increase in effect.

Decreased Effect There are no known significant interactions involving a decrease in effect.

Stability Gentle swirling or agitation of the vial of suspension is often necessary for redispersion. **Do not shake**. Visible flecks of the suspension and foaming under the surface are normal. Calfactant should be stored at refrigeration (2°C to 8°C/36°F to 46°F). Warming before administration is not necessary. Unopened and unused vials of calfactant that have been warmed to room temperature can be returned to the refrigeration storage within 24 hours for future use. Repeated warming to room temperature should be avoided. Each single-use vial should be entered only once and the vial with any unused material should be discarded after the initial entry.

Mechanism of Action Endogenous lung surfactant is essential for effective ventilation because it modifies alveolar surface tension, thereby stabilizing the alveoli. Lung surfactant deficiency is the cause of respiratory distress syndrome (RDS) in premature infants and lung surfactant restores surface activity to the lungs of these infants.

Pharmacodynamics/Kinetics No human studies of absorption, biotransformation, or excretion have been performed

Dosage Intratracheal administration **only**: Each dose is 3 mL/kg body weight at birth; should be administered every 12 hours for a total of up to 3 doses

Administration Gentle swirling or agitation of the vial is often necessary for redispersion as suspension settles during storage; do **not** shake; visible flecks in the suspension and foaming at the surface are normal; does not require reconstitution; do not dilute or sonicate.

Should be administered intratracheally through an endotracheal tube. Dose is drawn into a syringe from the single-use vial using a 20-gauge or larger needle with care taken to avoid excessive foaming. Should be administered in two aliquots of 1.5 mL/kg each. After each aliquot is instilled, the infant should be positioned with either the right or the left side dependent. Administration is made while ventilation is continued over 20-30 breaths for each aliquot, with small bursts timed only during the inspiratory cycles. A pause followed by evaluation of the respiratory status and repositioning should separate the two aliquots.

Monitoring Parameters Following administration, patients should be carefully monitored so that oxygen therapy and ventilatory support can be modified in response to changes in respiratory status.

Additional Information Each mL = 35 mg total phospholipids (including 26 mg phosphatidylcholine, of which 16 mg is disaturated phosphatidylcholine) and 0.7 mg proteins (including 0.26 mg SP-B)

Dosage Forms Excipient information presented when available (limited, particularly for generics); consult specific product labeling.

Suspension, intratracheal [preservative free]:

Infasurf®: 35 mg phospholipids and 0.7 mg protein per mL (3 mL, 6 mL) [production involves products derived from bovine sources]

- ◆ **Cal-G [OTC]** *see* Calcium Gluconate *on page 269*
- ◆ **Cal-Gest [OTC]** *see* Calcium Carbonate *on page 266*
- ◆ **Cal-GLU™ [OTC]** *see* Calcium Gluconate *on page 269*
- ◆ **Cal-Mint [OTC]** *see* Calcium Carbonate *on page 266*
- ◆ **Calmylin with Codeine (Can)** *see* Guaifenesin, Pseudoephedrine, and Codeine *on page 813*
- ◆ **CaloMist™ [DSC]** *see* Cyanocobalamin *on page 418*
- ◆ **Caltine® (Can)** *see* Calcitonin *on page 262*
- ◆ **Caltrate® (Can)** *see* Calcium Carbonate *on page 266*
- ◆ **Caltrate® 600 [OTC]** *see* Calcium Carbonate *on page 266*
- ◆ **Caltrate® 600+D [OTC]** *see* Calcium and Vitamin D *on page 265*
- ◆ **Caltrate® 600+Soy™ [OTC]** *see* Calcium and Vitamin D *on page 265*
- ◆ **Caltrate® ColonHealth™ [OTC]** *see* Calcium and Vitamin D *on page 265*
- ◆ **Caltrate® Select (Can)** *see* Calcium Carbonate *on page 266*
- ◆ **Cambia™** *see* Diclofenac (Systemic) *on page 495*
- ◆ **Camila®** *see* Norethindrone *on page 1217*
- ◆ **Campath®** *see* Alemtuzumab *on page 58*
- ◆ **Campath-1H** *see* Alemtuzumab *on page 58*
- ◆ **Camphorated Tincture of Opium (error-prone synonym)** *see* Paregoric *on page 1296*
- ◆ **Campral®** *see* Acamprosate *on page 25*
- ◆ **Camptosar®** *see* Irinotecan *on page 926*
- ◆ **Camptothecin-11** *see* Irinotecan *on page 926*
- ◆ **camrese™** *see* Ethinyl Estradiol and Levonorgestrel *on page 656*

Canakinumab (can a KIN ue mab)

Brand Names: U.S. Ilaris®

Index Terms ACZ885

Pharmacologic Category Interleukin-1 Beta Inhibitor; Interleukin-1 Inhibitor; Monoclonal Antibody

Use Treatment of cryopyrin-associated periodic syndromes (CAPS), including familial cold autoinflammatory syndrome (FCAS) and Muckle-Wells syndrome (MWS)

Pregnancy Risk Factor C

Pregnancy Considerations Animal studies have demonstrated fetal skeletal development delays. There are no adequate and well-controlled studies in pregnant women. Use during pregnancy only if potential benefit to the mother outweighs potential risk to the fetus.

Lactation Excretion in breast milk unknown/use caution

Contraindications There are no contraindications listed in the manufacturer's labeling.

Warnings/Precautions Caution should be exercised when considering use in patients with a history of new/recurrent infections, with conditions that predispose them to infections, or with latent or localized infections. Therapy should not be initiated in patients with active or chronic infections. Patients should be evaluated for latent tuberculosis infection with a tuberculin skin test prior to starting therapy. Treat latent TB infections prior to initiating canakinumab therapy. During and following treatment, monitor for signs/symptoms of active TB. Use may impair defenses against malignancies; impact on the development and course of malignancies is not fully defined. Tumor necrosis factor (TNF)-blocking agents should not be used in combination with canakinumab; risk of serious infection is increased. Immunizations should be up to date including pneumococcal and influenza vaccines before initiating therapy. Live vaccines should not be given concurrently. Administration of inactivated (killed) vaccines while on therapy may not be effective. Use with caution in the elderly due to the potential higher risk for infections. Safety and efficacy has not been established in patients <4 years of age.

Adverse Reactions

>10%:

Central nervous system: Headache (14%), vertigo (9% to 14%)

Gastrointestinal: Diarrhea (20%), nausea (14%), gastroenteritis (11%), weight gain (11%)

Neuromuscular and skeletal: Musculoskeletal pain (11%)

Respiratory: Nasopharyngitis (34%), rhinitis (17%), bronchitis (11%), pharyngitis (11%)

Miscellaneous: Influenza (17%)

1% to 10%: Local: Injection site reactions (7% to 9%)

Drug Interactions

Metabolism/Transport Effects None known.

Avoid Concomitant Use

Avoid concomitant use of Canakinumab with any of the following: Anti-TNF Agents; BCG; Interleukin-1 Inhibitors; Interleukin-1 Receptor Antagonist; Natalizumab; Pimecrolimus; Tacrolimus (Topical); Vaccines (Live)

Increased Effect/Toxicity

Canakinumab may increase the levels/effects of: Leflunomide; Natalizumab; Vaccines (Live)

The levels/effects of Canakinumab may be increased by: Anti-TNF Agents; Denosumab; Interleukin-1 Inhibitors; Interleukin-1 Receptor Antagonist; Pimecrolimus; Roflumilast; Tacrolimus (Topical); Trastuzumab

Decreased Effect

Canakinumab may decrease the levels/effects of: BCG; Coccidioidin Skin Test; Sipuleucel-T; Vaccines (Inactivated); Vaccines (Live)

The levels/effects of Canakinumab may be decreased by: Echinacea

Stability Store powder in refrigerator at 2°C to 8°C (36°F to 46°F); do not freeze. Protect from light. Reconstitute vial with 1 mL of SWFI; do not use bacteriostatic water containing benzyl alcohol or parabens. After reconstituting with SWFI, swirl the vial at an angle for ~1 minute, then allow solution to sit for 5 minutes. Gently turn vial (without touching rubber stopper) upside down and back 10 times. Allow to sit at room temperature for ~15 minutes until solution is clear. Do not shake. Solution may have a slight brownish-yellow tint; do not use if distinctly brown in color. Each reconstituted vial results in a final concentration of 150 mg/mL. After reconstitution, vials may be stored at controlled room temperature for up to 1 hour or in a refrigerator for up to 4 hours.

Mechanism of Action Canakinumab reduces inflammation by binding to interleukin-1 beta (IL-1β) (no binding to IL-1 alpha or IL-1 receptor antagonist) and preventing interaction with cell surface receptors. Cryopyrin-associated periodic syndromes (CAPS) refers to rare genetic syndromes caused by mutations in the nucleotide-binding domain, leucine rich family (NLR), pyrin domain containing 3 (NLRP-3) gene or the cold-induced autoinflammatory syndrome-1 (CIAS1) gene. Cryopyrin, a protein encoded by this gene, regulates IL-1β activation. Deficiency of cryopyrin results in excessive inflammation.

Pharmacodynamics/Kinetics
Distribution: V_d: 6 L
Bioavailability: Subcutaneous: 70%
Half-life elimination: 26 days
Time to peak, serum: Children: 2-7 days; Adults: ~7 days

Dosage SubQ: Cryopyrin-associated periodic syndromes:
Children ≥4 years:
15-40 kg: 2 mg/kg every 8 weeks; may increase to 3 mg/kg if response inadequate
>40 kg: 150 mg every 8 weeks
Adults >40 kg: 150 mg every 8 weeks

Administration SubQ: Do not inject into scar tissue.

Monitoring Parameters CBC with differential, C-reactive protein (CRP), serum amyloid A; signs of infection; latent TB screening (prior to initiating therapy)

Dosage Forms Excipient information presented when available (limited, particularly for generics); consult specific product labeling.
Injection, powder for reconstitution:
Ilaris®: 180 mg [contains polysorbate 80, sucrose]

◆ **Canasa®** *see* Mesalamine *on page* 1081

◆ **Cancidas®** *see* Caspofungin *on page* 298

Candesartan (kan de SAR tan)

Brand Names: U.S. Atacand®

Brand Names: Canada Apo-Candesartan; Atacand®; CO Candesartan; Sandoz-Candesartan

Index Terms Candesartan Cilexetil

Pharmacologic Category Angiotensin II Receptor Blocker; Antihypertensive Agent

Additional Appendix Information
Angiotensin Agents *on page* 1869
Heart Failure (Systolic) *on page* 1991

Use Alone or in combination with other antihypertensive agents in treating hypertension; treatment of heart failure (NYHA class II-IV)

Pregnancy Risk Factor C (1st trimester); D (2nd and 3rd trimesters)

Pregnancy Considerations Medications which act on the renin-angiotensin system are reported to have the following fetal/neonatal effects: Hypotension, neonatal skull hypoplasia, anuria, renal failure, and death; oligohydramnios is also reported. These effects are reported to occur with exposure during the second and third trimesters. There are no adequate and well-controlled studies in pregnant women. **[U.S. Boxed Warning]: Based on human data, drugs that act on the angiotensin system can cause injury and death to the developing fetus when used in the second and third trimesters. Angiotensin receptor blockers should be discontinued as soon as possible once pregnancy is detected.**

Lactation Enters breast milk/contraindicated

Contraindications Hypersensitivity to candesartan or any component of the formulation

Warnings/Precautions [U.S. Boxed Warning]: Based on human data, drugs that act on the angiotensin system can cause injury and death to the developing fetus when used in the second and third trimesters. Angiotensin receptor blockers should be discontinued as soon as possible once pregnancy is detected. May cause hyperkalemia; avoid potassium supplementation unless specifically required by healthcare provider. Avoid use or use a smaller dose in patients who are volume depleted; correct depletion first. May be associated with deterioration of renal function and/or increases in serum creatinine, particularly in patients with low renal blood flow (eg, renal artery stenosis, heart failure) whose glomerular filtration rate (GFR) is dependent on efferent arteriolar vasoconstriction by angiotensin II. Use with caution in unstented unilateral/bilateral renal artery stenosis, preexisting renal insufficiency, or significant aortic/mitral stenosis. Use with caution in patients with moderate hepatic impairment. Contraindicated with severe hepatic impairment and/or cholestasis. Use caution when initiating in heart failure; may need to adjust dose, and/or concurrent diuretic therapy, because of candesartan-induced hypotension. Hypotension may occur during major surgery and anesthesia; use cautiously before, during, and immediately after such interventions. Although concurrent therapy with an ACE inhibitor may be rational in select patients, concurrent use of ACE inhibitors may increase the risk of clinically-significant adverse events (eg, renal dysfunction, hyperkalemia). Pediatric patients with a GFR <30 mL/minute/1.73m^2 or children <1 year of age should not receive candesartan; has not been evaluated.

Adverse Reactions
Cardiovascular: Angina, hypotension (heart failure 19%), MI, palpitation, tachycardia
Central nervous system: Anxiety, depression, dizziness, drowsiness, fever, headache, lightheadedness, somnolence, vertigo
Dermatologic: Angioedema, rash
Endocrine & metabolic: Hyperglycemia, hyperkalemia (heart failure <1% to 6%), hypertriglyceridemia, hyperuricemia
Gastrointestinal: Dyspepsia, gastroenteritis
Neuromuscular & skeletal: Back pain, CPK increased, myalgia, paresthesia, weakness
Renal: Serum creatinine increased (up to 13% in patients with heart failure with drug discontinuation required in 6%), hematuria
Respiratory: Dyspnea, epistaxis, pharyngitis, rhinitis, upper respiratory tract infection
Miscellaneous: Diaphoresis increased
<1%, postmarketing, and/or case reports: Abnormal hepatic function, agranulocytosis, anemia, hepatitis, hyponatremia, leukopenia, neutropenia, pruritus, renal failure, renal impairment, rhinitis, sinusitis, thrombocytopenia, urticaria; rhabdomyolysis has been reported (rarely) with angiotensin-receptor antagonists

Drug Interactions

Metabolism/Transport Effects Substrate of CYP2C9 (minor); **Note:** Assignment of Major/Minor substrate status based on clinically relevant drug interaction potential; **Inhibits** CYP2C8 (weak), CYP2C9 (weak)

Avoid Concomitant Use There are no known interactions where it is recommended to avoid concomitant use.

Increased Effect/Toxicity

Candesartan may increase the levels/effects of: ACE Inhibitors; Amifostine; Antihypertensives; Hypotensive Agents; Lithium; Nonsteroidal Anti-Inflammatory Agents; Potassium-Sparing Diuretics; RiTUXimab; Sodium Phosphates

The levels/effects of Candesartan may be increased by: Alfuzosin; Diazoxide; Eplerenone; Herbs (Hypotensive Properties); MAO Inhibitors; Pentoxifylline; Phosphodiesterase 5 Inhibitors; Potassium Salts; Prostacyclin Analogues; Tolvaptan; Trimethoprim

Decreased Effect

The levels/effects of Candesartan may be decreased by: Herbs (Hypertensive Properties); Methylphenidate; Nonsteroidal Anti-Inflammatory Agents; Yohimbine

Ethanol/Nutrition/Herb Interactions Herb/Nutraceutical: Avoid dong quai if using for hypertension (has estrogenic activity). Avoid ephedra, yohimbe, ginseng (may worsen hypertension). Avoid garlic (may have increased antihypertensive effect).

Stability Store at 25°C (77°F); excursions permitted to 15°C to 30°C (59°F to 86°F).

Mechanism of Action Candesartan is an angiotensin receptor antagonist. Angiotensin II acts as a vasoconstrictor. In addition to causing direct vasoconstriction, angiotensin II also stimulates the release of aldosterone. Once aldosterone is released, sodium as well as water are reabsorbed. The end result is an elevation in blood pressure. Candesartan binds to the AT1 angiotensin II receptor. This binding prevents angiotensin II from binding to the receptor thereby blocking the vasoconstriction and the aldosterone secreting effects of angiotensin II.

Pharmacodynamics/Kinetics

Onset of action: 2-3 hours

Peak effect: 6-8 hours

Duration: >24 hours

Distribution: V_d: 0.13 L/kg

Protein binding: >99%

Metabolism: Parent compound bioactivated during absorption via ester hydrolysis within intestinal wall to candesartan

Bioavailability: 15%

Half-life elimination (dose dependent): 5-9 hours

Time to peak: 3-4 hours

Excretion: Urine (26%)

Dosage Oral:

Hypertension:

Children 1 to <6 years: Initial: 0.2 mg/kg/day in 1-2 divided doses; titrate to response (within 2 weeks, antihypertensive effect usually observed); usual range: 0.05 to 0.4 mg/kg/day; maximum daily dose: 0.4 mg/kg/day

Children 6 to <17 years:

<50 kg: Initial: 4-8 mg/day in 1-2 divided doses; titrate to response (within 2 weeks, antihypertensive effect usually observed); usual range: 2-16 mg/day; maximum daily dose: 32 mg/day

>50 kg: Initial: 8-16 mg/day in 1-2 divided doses; titrate to response (within 2 weeks, antihypertensive effect usually observed); usual range: 4-32 mg/day; maximum daily dose: 32 mg/day

Adults: Dosage must be individualized. Initial: 16 mg once daily; titrate to response (within 2 weeks, antihypertensive effect usually observed); usual range: 8-32 mg/day in 1-2 divided doses; maximum daily dose: 32 mg/day.

Heart failure: Adults: Initial: 4 mg once daily; double the dose at 2-week intervals, as tolerated; target dose: 32 mg once daily

Note: In selected cases, concurrent therapy with an ACE inhibitor may provide additional benefit.

Elderly: No initial dosage adjustment is necessary for elderly patients (although higher concentrations (C_{max}) and AUC were observed in these populations), for patients with mildly impaired renal function, or for patients with mildly impaired hepatic function.

Dosage adjustment in renal impairment:

Children 1 to <17 years: No dosage adjustment provided in manufacturer's labeling (has not been studied). Children with GFR <30 mL/minute/1.73 m^2 should not receive candesartan.

Adults: No initial dosage adjustment necessary; however, in patients with severe renal impairment (Cl_{cr} <30 mL/minute/1.73 m^2) AUC and C_{max} were approximately doubled after repeated dosing.

Dosage adjustment in hepatic impairment:

Mild impairment: No initial dosage adjustment necessary.

Moderate impairment: Consider initiation at lower dosages (AUC increased by 145%).

Severe impairment: No dosage adjustment provided in manufacturer's labeling (has not been studied).

Administration Administer without regard to meals.

Monitoring Parameters Supine blood pressure, electrolytes, serum creatinine, BUN, urinalysis, symptomatic hypotension, and tachycardia; in heart failure, serum potassium during dose escalation and periodically thereafter

Additional Information May have an advantage over losartan due to minimal metabolism requirements and consequent use in mild-to-moderate hepatic impairment

Dosage Forms Excipient information presented when available (limited, particularly for generics); consult specific product labeling.

Tablet, oral, as cilexetil:

Atacand®: 4 mg, 8 mg, 16 mg, 32 mg [scored]

Extemporaneous Preparations Oral suspension may be made in concentrations ranging from 0.1-2 mg/mL; typically 1 mg/mL oral suspension suitable for majority of prescribed doses; any strength tablet may be used. A 1 mg/mL (total volume: 160 mL) oral suspension may be made with tablets and a 1:1 mixture of Ora-Plus® and Ora-Sweet SF®. Prepare the vehicle by adding 80 mL of Ora-Plus® and 80 mL of Ora-Sweet SF® or, alternatively, use 160 mL of Ora-Blend SF®. Add a small amount of vehicle to five 32 mg tablets and grind into a smooth paste using a mortar and pestle. Transfer the paste to a calibrated amber PET bottle, rinse the mortar and pestle clean using the vehicle, add this to the bottle, and then add a quantity of vehicle sufficient to make 160 mL. The suspension is stable at room temperature for 100 days unopened or 30 days after the first opening; do not freeze (Atacand® prescribing information, 2011).

Atacand® prescribing information, AstraZeneca LP, Wilmington, DE, 2011.

Candesartan and Hydrochlorothiazide

(kan de SAR tan & hye droe klor oh THYE a zide)

Brand Names: U.S. Atacand HCT®

Brand Names: Canada Atacand® Plus

Index Terms Candesartan Cilexetil and Hydrochlorothiazide; Hydrochlorothiazide and Candesartan

Pharmacologic Category Angiotensin II Receptor Blocker; Diuretic, Thiazide

Use Treatment of hypertension; combination product should not be used for initial therapy

Pregnancy Risk Factor C/D (2nd and 3rd trimesters)

Dosage Oral: Adults: Replacement therapy: Combination product can be substituted for individual agents; maximum therapeutic effect would be expected within 4 weeks

Usual dosage range:

Candesartan: 16-32 mg/day, given once daily or twice daily in divided doses

Hydrochlorothiazide: 12.5-25 mg once daily

Elderly: No initial dosage adjustment is recommended in patients with normal renal and hepatic function; some patients may have increased sensitivity.

Dosage adjustment in renal impairment: Serum levels of candesartan are increased and the half-life of hydrochlorothiazide is prolonged in patients with renal impairment.

Cl_{cr} <30 mL/minute: Contraindicated

Dosage adjustment in hepatic impairment: Use with caution with moderate hepatic impairment.

Severe hepatic impairment and/or cholestasis: Use is contraindicated.

Additional Information Complete prescribing information for this medication should be consulted for additional detail.

Dosage Forms Excipient information presented when available (limited, particularly for generics); consult specific product labeling.

Tablet:

Atacand HCT®:

16/12.5: Candesartan cilexetil 16 mg and hydrochlorothiazide 12.5 mg

32/12.5: Candesartan cilexetil 32 mg and hydrochlorothiazide 12.5 mg

32/25: Candesartan cilexetil 32 mg and hydrochlorothiazide 25 mg

◆ **Candesartan Cilexetil** *see* Candesartan *on page 273*

◆ **Candesartan Cilexetil and Hydrochlorothiazide** *see* Candesartan and Hydrochlorothiazide *on page 274*

◆ **Candistatin® (Can)** *see* Nystatin (Topical) *on page 1225*

◆ **CanesOral® (Can)** *see* Fluconazole *on page 718*

◆ **Canesten® Topical (Can)** *see* Clotrimazole (Topical) *on page 399*

◆ **Canesten® Vaginal (Can)** *see* Clotrimazole (Topical) *on page 399*

◆ **Cankaid® [OTC]** *see* Carbamide Peroxide *on page 283*

◆ **CAPE** *see* Capecitabine *on page 275*

Capecitabine (ka pe SITE a been)

Brand Names: U.S. Xeloda®

Brand Names: Canada Xeloda®

Index Terms CAPE

Pharmacologic Category Antineoplastic Agent, Antimetabolite; Antineoplastic Agent, Antimetabolite (Pyrimidine Analog)

Use Treatment of metastatic colorectal cancer; adjuvant therapy of Dukes' C colon cancer; treatment of metastatic breast cancer

Unlabeled Use Treatment of gastric cancer, pancreatic cancer, esophageal cancer, ovarian cancer, metastatic renal cell cancer, neuroendocrine tumors, metastatic CNS lesions

Pregnancy Risk Factor D

Pregnancy Considerations Animal studies have demonstrated teratogenicity and fetal loss. There are no adequate and well-controlled studies in pregnant women; however, fetal harm may occur. Women of childbearing potential should avoid pregnancy.

Lactation Excretion in breast milk unknown/not recommended

Contraindications Hypersensitivity to capecitabine, fluorouracil, or any component of the formulation; known deficiency of dihydropyrimidine dehydrogenase (DPD); severe renal impairment (Cl_{cr} <30 mL/minute)

Warnings/Precautions Hazardous agent - use appropriate precautions for handling and disposal. Use with caution in patients ≥80 years of age, or with renal or hepatic dysfunction. Patients with baseline moderate renal impairment require dose reduction. Patients with mild-to-moderate renal impairment require careful monitoring and subsequent dose reduction with any grade 2 or higher adverse event. Bone marrow suppression may occur, hematologic toxicity is more common when used in combination therapy; use with caution; dosage adjustments may be required. Canadian labeling recommends that patients with baseline platelets <100,000/mm^3 and/or neutrophils <1500/mm^3 not receive capecitabine therapy and also to withhold for grade 3 or 4 hematologic toxicity during treatment. Use with caution in patients who have received extensive pelvic radiation or alkylating therapy. Use cautiously with warfarin. Rare and unexpected severe toxicity may be attributed to dihydropyrimidine dehydrogenase (DPD) deficiency. Necrotizing enterocolitis (typhlitis) has been reported.

Capecitabine can cause severe diarrhea; median time to first occurrence is 34 days. Subsequent doses should be reduced after grade 3 or 4 diarrhea or recurrence of grade 2 diarrhea. Dehydration may occur rapidly in patients with diarrhea, nausea, vomiting, anorexia, and/or weakness; adequately hydrate prior to treatment initiation. Elderly patients may be a higher risk for dehydration. **Note:** the Canadian labeling recommends treatment interruption for dehydration requiring I.V. hydration lasting <24 hours and dosage reduction if I.V hydration required for ≥24 hours; correct precipitating factors and ensure rehydration prior to resuming therapy.

Hand-and-foot syndrome is characterized by numbness, dysesthesia/paresthesia, tingling, painless or painful swelling, erythema, desquamation, blistering, and severe pain. If grade 2 or 3 hand-and-foot syndrome occurs, interrupt administration of capecitabine until decreases to grade 1. Following grade 3 hand-and-foot syndrome, decrease subsequent doses of capecitabine. In patients with colorectal cancer, treatment with capecitabine immediately following 6 weeks of fluorouracil/leucovorin (FU/LV) therapy has been associated with an increased incidence of grade ≥3 toxicity, when compared to patients receiving the reverse sequence, capecitabine (two 3-week courses) followed by FU/LV (Hennig, 2008).

There has been cardiotoxicity associated with fluorinated pyrimidine therapy. May be more common in patients with a history of coronary artery disease. **[U.S. Boxed Warning]: Capecitabine may increase the anticoagulant effects of warfarin; monitor closely.**

Safety and efficacy in children <18 years of age have not been established.

Adverse Reactions Frequency listed derived from monotherapy trials.

>10%:

Cardiovascular: Edema (9% to 15%)

Central nervous system: Fatigue (16% to 42%), fever (7% to 18%), pain (12%)

Dermatologic: Palmar-plantar erythrodysesthesia (hand-and-foot syndrome) (54% to 60%; grade 3: 11% to 17%; may be dose limiting), dermatitis (27% to 37%)

Gastrointestinal: Diarrhea (47% to 57%; may be dose limiting; grade 3: 12% to 13%; grade 4: 2% to 3%), nausea (34% to 53%), vomiting (15% to 37%), abdominal pain (7% to 35%), stomatitis (22% to 25%), appetite decreased (26%), anorexia (9% to 23%), constipation (9% to 15%)

Hematologic: Lymphopenia (94%; grade 4: 14%), anemia (72% to 80%; grade 4: <1% to 1%), neutropenia (2% to 26%; grade 4: 2%), thrombocytopenia (24%; grade 4: 1%)
Hepatic: Bilirubin increased (22% to 48%; grades 3/4: 11% to 23%)
Neuromuscular & skeletal: Paresthesia (21%)
Ocular: Eye irritation (13% to 15%)
Respiratory: Dyspnea (14%)

5% to 10%:
Cardiovascular: Venous thrombosis (8%), chest pain (6%)
Central nervous system: Headache (5% to 10%), lethargy (10%), dizziness (6% to 8%), insomnia (7% to 8%), mood alteration (5%), depression (5%)
Dermatologic: Nail disorder (7%), rash (7%), skin discoloration (7%), alopecia (6%), erythema (6%)
Endocrine & metabolic: Dehydration (7%)
Gastrointestinal: Motility disorder (10%), oral discomfort (10%), dyspepsia (6% to 8%), upper GI inflammatory disorders (colorectal cancer: 8%), hemorrhage (6%), ileus (6%), taste perversion (colorectal cancer: 6%)
Neuromuscular & skeletal: Back pain (10%), weakness (10%), neuropathy (10%), myalgia (9%), arthralgia (8%), limb pain (6%)
Ocular: Abnormal vision (colorectal cancer: 5%), conjunctivitis (5%)
Respiratory: Cough (7%)
Miscellaneous: Viral infection (colorectal cancer: 5%)

<5% (Limited to important or life-threatening): Angina, ascites, asthma, atrial fibrillation, bradycardia, bronchitis, bronchopneumonia, bronchospasm, cachexia, cardiac arrest, cardiac failure, cardiomyopathy, cerebral vascular accident, cholestatic hepatitis, coagulation disorder, colitis, confusion, deep vein thrombosis, diaphoresis, duodenitis, dysarthria, dysphagia, dysrhythmia, ecchymoses, ECG changes, encephalopathy, epistaxis, esophagitis, fibrosis, fingerprint distortion (secondary to hand-and-foot syndrome), fungal infection, gastric ulcer, gastritis, gastroenteritis, gastrointestinal perforation, hematemesis, hemoptysis, hepatic failure, hepatic fibrosis, hepatitis, hypokalemia, hypomagnesemia, hyper-/hypotension, hypersensitivity, hypertriglyceridemia, idiopathic thrombocytopenia purpura, ileus, infection, intestinal obstruction (~1%), keratoconjunctivitis, lacrimal duct stenosis, leukopenia, loss of consciousness, lymphedema, MI, multifocal leukoencephalopathy, myocardial ischemia, myocarditis, necrotizing enterocolitis (typhlitis), oral candidiasis, pericardial effusion, thrombocytopenic purpura, pancytopenia, photosensitivity reaction, pneumonia, pruritus, pulmonary embolism, radiation recall syndrome, renal impairment, respiratory distress, sedation, sepsis, skin ulceration, Stevens-Johnson syndrome, tachycardia, thrombophlebitis, toxic epidermal necrolysis, toxic megacolon, tremor, ventricular extrasystoles

Drug Interactions

Metabolism/Transport Effects Inhibits CYP2C9 (strong)

Avoid Concomitant Use

Avoid concomitant use of Capecitabine with any of the following: BCG; CloZAPine; Natalizumab; Pimecrolimus; Tacrolimus (Topical); Vaccines (Live)

Increased Effect/Toxicity

Capecitabine may increase the levels/effects of: Carvedilol; CloZAPine; CYP2C9 Substrates; Diclofenac; Fosphenytoin; Leflunomide; Natalizumab; Phenytoin; Vaccines (Live); Vitamin K Antagonists

The levels/effects of Capecitabine may be increased by: Denosumab; Leucovorin Calcium-Levoleucovorin; Pimecrolimus; Roflumilast; Tacrolimus (Topical); Trastuzumab

Decreased Effect

Capecitabine may decrease the levels/effects of: BCG; Coccidioidin Skin Test; Sipuleucel-T; Vaccines (Inactivated); Vaccines (Live)

The levels/effects of Capecitabine may be decreased by: Echinacea

Ethanol/Nutrition/Herb Interactions Food: Food reduced the rate and extent of absorption of capecitabine.

Stability Store at room temperature of 25°C (77°F); excursions permitted between 15°C and 30°C (59°F and 86°F).

Mechanism of Action Capecitabine is a prodrug of fluorouracil. It undergoes hydrolysis in the liver and tissues to form fluorouracil which is the active moiety. Fluorouracil is a fluorinated pyrimidine antimetabolite that inhibits thymidylate synthetase, blocking the methylation of deoxyuridylic acid to thymidylic acid, interfering with DNA, and to a lesser degree, RNA synthesis. Fluorouracil appears to be phase specific for the G_1 and S phases of the cell cycle.

Pharmacodynamics/Kinetics

Absorption: Rapid and extensive
Protein binding: <60%; ~35% to albumin
Metabolism:
Hepatic: Inactive metabolites: 5'-deoxy-5-fluorocytidine, 5'-deoxy-5-fluorouridine
Tissue: Active metabolite: Fluorouracil
Half-life elimination: 0.5-1 hour
Time to peak: 1.5 hours; Fluorouracil: 2 hours
Excretion: Urine (96%, 57% as α-fluoro-β-alanine); feces (<3%)

Dosage Oral:

Adults: **Note:** Details concerning dosing in combination regimens should also be consulted. Capecitabine toxicities, particularly hand-foot syndrome, may be higher in North American populations (for the treatment of colorectal cancer); therapy initiation at doses of 1000 mg/m^2 twice daily (for 2 weeks every 21 days) may be considered (Haller, 2008; NCCN Colon Cancer Guidelines)

Metastatic breast cancer, metastatic colorectal cancer: 1250 mg/m^2 twice daily (morning and evening) for 2 weeks, every 21 days

Adjuvant therapy of Dukes' C colon cancer: Recommended for a total of 24 weeks (8 cycles of 2 weeks of drug administration and 1 week rest period).

Pancreatic cancer (unlabeled use): 1000 mg/m^2 twice daily for 2 weeks, every 21 days (NCCN Pancreatic Cancer Guidelines v.1.2009) **or** 1250 mg/m^2 twice daily for 2 weeks, every 21 days (Cartwright, 2002)

Elderly: The elderly may be more sensitive to the toxic effects of fluorouracil. Insufficient data are available to provide dosage modifications.

Dosing adjustment in renal impairment:
Cl_{cr} 51-80 mL/minute: No adjustment of initial dose
Cl_{cr} 30-50 mL/minute: Administer 75% of normal dose
Cl_{cr} <30 mL/minute: Use is contraindicated

Dosing adjustment in hepatic impairment:
Mild-to-moderate impairment: No starting dose adjustment is necessary; however, carefully monitor patients
Severe hepatic impairment: Patients have not been studied

Dosage modification guidelines: See table.

Refer to package labeling for modifications when administered in combination with docetaxel.

Recommended Dose Modifications

Toxicity NCI Grades	During a Course of Therapy (Monotherapy)	Dose Adjustment for Next Cycle (% of starting dose)
Grade 1	Maintain dose level	Maintain dose level
Grade 2		
1st appearance	Interrupt until resolved to grade 0-1	100%
2nd appearance	Interrupt until resolved to grade 0-1	75%
3rd appearance	Interrupt until resolved to grade 0-1	50%
4th appearance	Discontinue treatment permanently	
Grade 3		
1st appearance	Interrupt until resolved to grade 0-1	75%
2nd appearance	Interrupt until resolved to grade 0-1	50%
3rd appearance	Discontinue treatment permanently	
Grade 4		
1st appearance	Discontinue permanently **or** If physician deems it to be in the patient's best interest to continue, interrupt until resolved to grade 0-1	50%

Dosage adjustments for hematologic toxicity in combination therapy with ixabepilone:

Neutrophils $<500/mm^3$ for ≥7 days or neutropenic fever: Hold for concurrent diarrhea or stomatitis until neutrophils recover to $>1000/mm^3$, then continue at same dose

Platelets $<25,000/mm^3$ (or $<50,000/mm^3$ with bleeding): Hold for concurrent diarrhea or stomatitis until platelets recover to $>50,000/mm^3$, then continue at same dose

Dietary Considerations Because current safety and efficacy data are based upon administration with food, it is recommended that capecitabine be administered with food. In all clinical trials, patients were instructed to take with water within 30 minutes after a meal.

Administration Usually administered in 2 divided doses taken 12 hours apart. Doses should be taken with water within 30 minutes after a meal.

Monitoring Parameters Renal function should be estimated at baseline to determine initial dose. During therapy, CBC with differential, hepatic function, and renal function should be monitored.

Additional Information Oncology Comment: An investigational uridine prodrug, uridine triacetate (formerly called vistonuridine), has been studied in a limited number of cases of fluorouracil overdose. Of 17 patients receiving uridine triacetate beginning within 8-96 hours after fluorouracil overdose, all patients fully recovered (von Borstel, 2009). Updated data has described a total of 28 patients treated with uridine triacetate for fluorouracil overdose (including overdoses related to continuous infusions delivering fluorouracil at rates faster than prescribed), all of whom recovered fully (Bamat, 2010). Refer to Uridine Triacetate monograph.

Dosage Forms Excipient information presented when available (limited, particularly for generics); consult specific product labeling.

Tablet, oral:

Xeloda®: 150 mg, 500 mg

Extemporaneous Preparations Hazardous agent: Use appropriate precautions for handling and disposal.

A 10 mg/mL oral solution may be made with tablets. Crush four 500 mg tablets in a mortar and reduce to a fine powder; add to 200 mL water. Capecitabine tablets are water soluble (data on file from Roche). Administer immediately after preparation, 30 minutes after a meal.

Judson IR, Beale PJ, Trigo JM, et al, "A Human Capecitabine Excretion Balance and Pharmacokinetic Study After Administration of a Single Oral Dose of ^{14}C-Labelled Drug," *Invest New Drugs*, 1999, 17 (1):49-56.

- **Capex®** *see* Fluocinolone (Topical) *on page 726*
- **Capital® and Codeine** *see* Acetaminophen and Codeine *on page 30*
- **Capoten® (Can)** *see* Captopril *on page 277*
- **Caprelsa®** *see* Vandetanib *on page 1767*

Captopril (KAP toe pril)

Brand Names: Canada Apo-Capto®; Capoten®; Dom-Captopril; Mylan-Captopril; Nu-Capto; PMS-Captopril; Teva-Captopril

Index Terms ACE

Pharmacologic Category Angiotensin-Converting Enzyme (ACE) Inhibitor

Additional Appendix Information

Angiotensin Agents *on page 1869*

Heart Failure (Systolic) *on page 1991*

Hypertension *on page 2001*

Use Management of hypertension; treatment of heart failure, left ventricular dysfunction after myocardial infarction, diabetic nephropathy

Unlabeled Use To delay the progression of nephropathy and reduce risks of cardiovascular events in hypertensive patients with type 1 or 2 diabetes mellitus; treatment of hypertensive crisis, rheumatoid arthritis; diagnosis of anatomic renal artery stenosis, hypertension secondary to scleroderma renal crisis; diagnosis of aldosteronism, idiopathic edema, Bartter's syndrome, postmyocardial infarction for prevention of ventricular failure; increase circulation in Raynaud's phenomenon, hypertension secondary to Takayasu's disease

Pregnancy Risk Factor C (1st trimester); D (2nd and 3rd trimesters)

Pregnancy Considerations Due to adverse events observed in some animal studies, captopril is considered pregnancy category C during the first trimester. Based on human data, captopril is considered pregnancy category D if used during the second and third trimesters (per the manufacturer; however, one study suggests that fetal injury may occur at anytime during pregnancy). Captopril crosses the placenta and may affect ACE activity in the fetus. First trimester exposure to ACE inhibitors may cause major congenital malformations. An increased risk of cardiovascular and/or central nervous system malformations was observed in one study; however, an increased risk of teratogenic events was not observed in other studies. Second and third trimester use of an ACE inhibitor is associated with oligohydramnios. Oligohydramnios due to decreased fetal renal function may lead to fetal limb contractures, craniofacial deformation, and hypoplastic lung development. The use of ACE inhibitors during the second and third trimesters is also associated with anuria, hypotension, renal failure (reversible or irreversible), skull hypoplasia, and death in the fetus/neonate. Chronic maternal hypertension itself is also associated with adverse events in the fetus/infant. ACE inhibitors are not recommended during pregnancy to treat maternal hypertension or heart failure. Those who are planning a pregnancy should be considered for other medication options if an ACE inhibitor is currently prescribed or the ACE inhibitor should be discontinued as soon as possible once pregnancy is detected. The exposed fetus should be monitored for fetal growth, amniotic fluid volume, and organ formation. Infants exposed to an ACE inhibitor *in utero*, especially during the second and third trimester, should be monitored for hyperkalemia, hypotension, and oliguria.

[U.S. Boxed Warning]: Based on human data, ACE inhibitors can cause injury and death to the developing fetus when used in the second and third trimesters. ACE inhibitors should be discontinued as soon as possible once pregnancy is detected.

Lactation Enters breast milk/not recommended (AAP rates "compatible"; AAP 2001 update pending)

Contraindications Hypersensitivity to captopril, any other ACE inhibitor, or any component of the formulation; angioedema related to previous treatment with an ACE inhibitor

Warnings/Precautions Anaphylactic reactions may occur rarely with ACE inhibitors. At any time during treatment (especially following first dose) angioedema may occur rarely with ACE inhibitors; may involve the head and neck (potentially compromising airway) or the intestine (presenting with abdominal pain). African-Americans and patients with idiopathic or hereditary angioedema may be at an increased risk. Prolonged frequent monitoring may be required especially if tongue, glottis, or larynx are involved as they are associated with airway obstruction. Patients with a history of airway surgery may have a higher risk of airway obstruction. Aggressive early and appropriate management is critical. Use in patients with previous angioedema associated with ACE inhibitor therapy is contraindicated. Severe anaphylactoid reactions may be seen during hemodialysis (eg, CVVHD) with high-flux dialysis membranes (eg, AN69), and rarely, during low density lipoprotein apheresis with dextran sulfate cellulose. Rare cases of anaphylactoid reactions have been reported in patients undergoing sensitization treatment with hymenoptera (bee, wasp) venom while receiving ACE inhibitors.

Symptomatic hypotension with or without syncope can occur with ACE inhibitors (usually with the first several doses); effects are most often observed in volume depleted patients; close monitoring of patient is required especially with initial dosing and dosing increases; blood pressure must be lowered at a rate appropriate for the patient's clinical condition. Initiation of therapy in patients with ischemic heart disease or cerebrovascular disease warrants close observation due to the potential consequences posed by falling blood pressure (eg, MI, stroke). Use with caution in hypertrophic cardiomyopathy with outflow tract obstruction, severe aortic stenosis, or before, during, or immediately after major surgery. **[U.S. Boxed Warning]: Based on human data, ACEIs can cause injury and death to the developing fetus when used in the second and third trimesters. ACEIs should be discontinued as soon as possible once pregnancy is detected.**

Hyperkalemia may occur with ACE inhibitors; risk factors include renal dysfunction, diabetes mellitus, concomitant use of potassium-sparing diuretics, potassium supplements and/or potassium containing salts. Use cautiously, if at all, with these agents and monitor potassium closely. Cough may occur with ACE inhibitors. Other causes of cough should be considered (eg, pulmonary congestion in patients with heart failure) and excluded prior to discontinuation.

May be associated with deterioration of renal function and/or increases in serum creatinine, particularly in patients with low renal blood flow (eg, renal artery stenosis, heart failure) whose glomerular filtration rate (GFR) is dependent on efferent arteriolar vasoconstriction by angiotensin II; deterioration may result in oliguria, acute renal failure, and progressive azotemia. Small increases in serum creatinine may occur following initiation; consider discontinuation only in patients with progressive and/or significant deterioration in renal function. Use with caution in patients with unstented unilateral/bilateral renal artery stenosis. When unstented bilateral renal artery stenosis is present, use is generally avoided due to the elevated risk of deterioration in renal function unless possible benefits outweigh risks. Concurrent use of angiotensin receptor blockers may increase the risk of clinically-significant adverse events (eg, renal dysfunction, hyperkalemia).

Rare toxicities associated with ACE inhibitors include cholestatic jaundice (which may progress to fulminant hepatic necrosis), agranulocytosis, neutropenia, or leukopenia with myeloid hypoplasia. Patients with collagen vascular diseases (especially with concomitant renal impairment) or renal impairment alone may be at increased risk for hematologic toxicity; closely monitor CBC with differential for the first 3 months of therapy and periodically thereafter in these patients.

Adverse Reactions

Frequency not defined:

Cardiovascular: Angioedema, cardiac arrest, cerebrovascular insufficiency, rhythm disturbances, orthostatic hypotension, syncope, flushing, pallor, angina, MI, Raynaud's syndrome, CHF

Central nervous system: Ataxia, confusion, depression, nervousness, somnolence

Dermatologic: Bullous pemphigus, erythema multiforme, Stevens-Johnson syndrome, exfoliative dermatitis

Endocrine & metabolic: Alkaline phosphatase increased, bilirubin increased, gynecomastia

Gastrointestinal: Pancreatitis, glossitis, dyspepsia

Genitourinary: Urinary frequency, impotence

Hematologic: Anemia, thrombocytopenia, pancytopenia, agranulocytosis, anemia

Hepatic: Jaundice, hepatitis, hepatic necrosis (rare), cholestasis, hyponatremia (symptomatic), transaminases increased

Neuromuscular & skeletal: Asthenia, myalgia, myasthenia

Ocular: Blurred vision

Renal: Renal insufficiency, renal failure, nephrotic syndrome, polyuria, oliguria

Respiratory: Bronchospasm, eosinophilic pneumonitis, rhinitis

Miscellaneous: Anaphylactoid reactions

1% to 10%:

Cardiovascular: Hypotension (1% to 3%), tachycardia (1%), chest pain (1%), palpitation (1%)

Dermatologic: Rash (maculopapular or urticarial) (4% to 7%), pruritus (2%); in patients with rash, a positive ANA and/or eosinophilia has been noted in 7% to 10%.

Endocrine & metabolic: Hyperkalemia (1% to 11%)

Hematologic: Neutropenia may occur in up to 4% of patients with renal insufficiency or collagen-vascular disease.

Renal: Proteinuria (1%), serum creatinine increased, worsening of renal function (may occur in patients with bilateral renal artery stenosis or hypovolemia)

Respiratory: Cough (<1% to 2%)

Miscellaneous: Hypersensitivity reactions (rash, pruritus, fever, arthralgia, and eosinophilia) have occurred in 4% to 7% of patients (depending on dose and renal function); dysgeusia - loss of taste or diminished perception (2% to 4%)

Postmarketing and/or case reports: Aplastic anemia, hemolytic anemia, bronchospasm, alopecia, systemic lupus erythematosus, Kaposi's sarcoma, pericarditis, exacerbations of Huntington's disease, Guillain-Barré syndrome, seizure (in premature infants). A syndrome which may include fever, myalgia, arthralgia, interstitial nephritis, vasculitis, rash, eosinophilia, and elevated ESR has been reported for captopril and other ACE inhibitors.

Drug Interactions

Metabolism/Transport Effects Substrate of CYP2D6 (major); **Note:** Assignment of Major/Minor substrate status based on clinically relevant drug interaction potential

Avoid Concomitant Use There are no known interactions where it is recommended to avoid concomitant use.

Increased Effect/Toxicity

Captopril may increase the levels/effects of: Allopurinol; Amifostine; Antihypertensives; AzaTHIOprine; CycloSPORINE; CycloSPORINE (Systemic); Ferric Gluconate; Gold Sodium Thiomalate; Hypotensive Agents; Iron Dextran Complex; Lithium; Nonsteroidal Anti-Inflammatory Agents; RiTUXimab; Sodium Phosphates

The levels/effects of Captopril may be increased by: Abiraterone Acetate; Alfuzosin; Angiotensin II Receptor Blockers; CYP2D6 Inhibitors (Moderate); CYP2D6 Inhibitors (Strong); Darunavir; Diazoxide; DPP-IV Inhibitors; Eplerenone; Everolimus; Herbs (Hypotensive Properties); Loop Diuretics; MAO Inhibitors; Pentoxifylline; Phosphodiesterase 5 Inhibitors; Potassium Salts; Potassium-Sparing Diuretics; Prostacyclin Analogues; Sirolimus; Temsirolimus; Thiazide Diuretics; TiZANidine; Tolvaptan; Trimethoprim

Decreased Effect

The levels/effects of Captopril may be decreased by: Antacids; Aprotinin; Herbs (Hypertensive Properties); Icatibant; Lanthanum; Methylphenidate; Nonsteroidal Anti-Inflammatory Agents; Peginterferon Alfa-2b; Salicylates; Yohimbine

Ethanol/Nutrition/Herb Interactions

Food: Captopril serum concentrations may be decreased if taken with food. Long-term use of captopril may result in a zinc deficiency which can result in a decrease in taste perception.

Herb/Nutraceutical: Avoid bayberry, blue cohosh, cayenne, ephedra, ginger, ginseng (American), kola, licorice (may worsen hypertension). Avoid black cohosh, california poppy, coleus, golden seal, hawthorn, mistletoe, periwinkle, quinine, shepherd's purse (may have increased antihypertensive effect).

Mechanism of Action Competitive inhibitor of angiotensin-converting enzyme (ACE); prevents conversion of angiotensin I to angiotensin II, a potent vasoconstrictor; results in lower levels of angiotensin II which causes an increase in plasma renin activity and a reduction in aldosterone secretion

Pharmacodynamics/Kinetics

Onset of action: Peak effect: Blood pressure reduction: 1-1.5 hours after dose

Duration: Dose related, may require several weeks of therapy before full hypotensive effect

Absorption: 60% to 75%; reduced 30% to 40% by food

Protein binding: 25% to 30%

Metabolism: 50%

Half-life elimination (renal and cardiac function dependent):

Adults, healthy volunteers: 1.9 hours; Heart failure: 2.06 hours; Anuria: 20-40 hours

Time to peak: 1 hour

Excretion: Urine (>95%) within 24 hours (40% to 50% as unchanged drug)

Dosage Note: Titrate dose according to patient's response; use lowest effective dose. Oral:

Infants: Initial: 0.15-0.3 mg/kg/dose; titrate dose upward to maximum of 6 mg/kg/day in 1-4 divided doses; usual required dose: 2.5-6 mg/kg/day

Children: Initial: 0.5 mg/kg/dose; titrate upward to maximum of 6 mg/kg/day in 2-4 divided doses

Older Children: Initial: 6.25-12.5 mg/dose every 12-24 hours; titrate upward to maximum of 6 mg/kg/day

Adolescents: Initial: 12.5-25 mg/dose given every 8-12 hours; increase by 25 mg/dose to maximum of 450 mg/day

Adults:

Acute hypertension (urgency/emergency): 12.5-25 mg, may repeat as needed (may be given sublingually, but no therapeutic advantage demonstrated)

Heart failure:

Initial dose: 6.25-12.5 mg 3 times/day in conjunction with cardiac glycoside and diuretic therapy; initial dose depends upon patient's fluid/electrolyte status

Target dose: 50 mg 3 times/day

Hypertension:

Initial dose: 12.5-25 mg 2-3 times/day; may increase by 12.5-25 mg/dose at 1- to 2-week intervals up to 50 mg 3 times/day; maximum dose: 150 mg 3 times/day; add diuretic before further dosage increases

Usual dose range (JNC 7): 25-100 mg/day in 2 divided doses

LV dysfunction after MI: Initial dose: 6.25 mg followed by 12.5 mg 3 times/day; then increase to 25 mg 3 times/day during next several days and then gradually increase over next several weeks to target dose of 50 mg 3 times/day (some dose schedules are more aggressive to achieve an increased goal dose within the first few days of initiation.)

Diabetic nephropathy: 25 mg 3 times/day; other antihypertensives often given concurrently

Elderly: Hypertension: Consider lower initial doses and titrate to response (Aronow, 2011)

Dosing adjustment in renal impairment:

Cl_{cr} 10-50 mL/minute: Administer at 75% of normal dose.

Cl_{cr} <10 mL/minute: Administer at 50% of normal dose.

Note: Smaller dosages given every 8-12 hours are indicated in patients with renal dysfunction; renal function and leukocyte count should be carefully monitored during therapy.

Hemodialysis: Moderately dialyzable (20% to 50%); administer dose postdialysis or administer 25% to 35% supplemental dose.

Peritoneal dialysis: Supplemental dose is not necessary.

Dietary Considerations Should be taken at least 1 hour before or 2 hours after eating.

Administration Unstable in aqueous solutions; to prepare solution for oral administration, mix prior to administration and use within 10 minutes.

Monitoring Parameters BUN, electrolytes, serum creatinine; blood pressure. In patients with renal impairment and/or collagen vascular disease, closely monitor CBC with differential for the first 3 months of therapy and periodically thereafter.

Test Interactions Positive Coombs' [direct]; may cause false-positive results in urine acetone determinations using sodium nitroprusside reagent

Dosage Forms Excipient information presented when available (limited, particularly for generics); consult specific product labeling.

Tablet, oral: 12.5 mg, 25 mg, 50 mg, 100 mg

Extemporaneous Preparations A 1 mg/mL oral solution may be made by allowing two 50 mg tablets to dissolve in 50 mL of distilled water. Add the contents of one 500 mg sodium ascorbate injection ampul or one 500 mg ascorbic acid tablet and allow to dissolve. Add quantity of distilled water sufficient to make 100 mL. Label "shake well" and "refrigerate". Stable for 56 days refrigerated.

Nahata MC, Pai VB, and Hipple TF, *Pediatric Drug Formulations*, 5th ed, Cincinnati, OH: Harvey Whitney Books Co, 2004.

Captopril and Hydrochlorothiazide

(KAP toe pril & hye droe klor oh THYE a zide)

Index Terms Hydrochlorothiazide and Captopril

Pharmacologic Category Angiotensin-Converting Enzyme (ACE) Inhibitor; Diuretic, Thiazide

Use Management of hypertension

Pregnancy Risk Factor C/D (2nd and 3rd trimesters)

Dosage Oral: Adults: Hypertension, CHF: May be substituted for previously titrated dosages of the individual components; alternatively, may initiate as follows:

Initial: Single tablet (captopril 25 mg/hydrochlorothiazide 15 mg) taken once daily; daily dose of captopril should not exceed 150 mg; daily dose of hydrochlorothiazide should not exceed 50 mg

Dosing adjustment/comments in renal impairment: May respond to smaller or less frequent doses.

Additional Information Complete prescribing information for this medication should be consulted for additional detail.

Dosage Forms Excipient information presented when available (limited, particularly for generics); consult specific product labeling.

Tablet: 25/15: Captopril 25 mg and hydrochlorothiazide 15 mg; 25/25: Captopril 25 mg and hydrochlorothiazide 25 mg; 50/15: Captopril 50 mg and hydrochlorothiazide 15 mg; 50/25: Captopril 50 mg and hydrochlorothiazide 25 mg

- **Carac®** *see* Fluorouracil (Topical) *on page 731*
- **Carafate®** *see* Sucralfate *on page 1598*
- **Carapres® (Can)** *see* CloNIDine *on page 392*

Carbachol (KAR ba kole)

Brand Names: U.S. Isopto® Carbachol; Miostat®

Brand Names: Canada Isopto® Carbachol; Miostat®

Index Terms Carbacholine; Carbamylcholine Chloride

Pharmacologic Category Cholinergic Agonist; Ophthalmic Agent, Antiglaucoma; Ophthalmic Agent, Miotic

Use Lowers intraocular pressure in the treatment of glaucoma; cause miosis during surgery

Pregnancy Risk Factor C

Dosage Adults:

Ophthalmic: Instill 1-2 drops up to 3 times/day

Intraocular: 0.5 mL instilled into anterior chamber before or after securing sutures

Additional Information Complete prescribing information for this medication should be consulted for additional detail.

Dosage Forms Excipient information presented when available (limited, particularly for generics); consult specific product labeling.

Solution, intraocular:

Miostat®: 0.01% (1.5 mL)

Solution, ophthalmic:

Isopto® Carbachol: 1.5% (15 mL); 3% (15 mL) [contains benzalkonium chloride]

- **Carbacholine** *see* Carbachol *on page 280*
- **Carbaglu®** *see* Carglumic Acid *on page 291*

CarBAMazepine (kar ba MAZ e peen)

Brand Names: U.S. Carbatrol®; Epitol®; Equetro®; TEGretol®; TEGretol®-XR

Brand Names: Canada Apo-Carbamazepine®; Dom-Carbamazepine; Mapezine®; Mylan-Carbamazepine CR; Nu-Carbamazepine; PMS-Carbamazepine; Sandoz-Carbamazepine; Taro-Carbamazepine Chewable; Tegretol®; Teva-Carbamazepine

Index Terms CBZ; SPD417

Pharmacologic Category Anticonvulsant, Miscellaneous

Additional Appendix Information

Anticonvulsant Drugs of Choice *on page 1873*

Use

Carbatrol®, Tegretol®, Tegretol®-XR: Partial seizures with complex symptomatology (psychomotor, temporal lobe), generalized tonic-clonic seizures (grand mal), mixed seizure patterns, trigeminal neuralgia

Equetro®: Acute manic and mixed episodes associated with bipolar 1 disorder

Unlabeled Use Treatment of restless leg syndrome and post-traumatic stress disorders

Pregnancy Risk Factor D

Pregnancy Considerations Studies in pregnant women have demonstrated a risk to the fetus; therefore, the manufacturer classifies carbamazepine as pregnancy category D. Carbamazepine and its metabolites can be found in the fetus. Carbamazepine may be associated with teratogenic effects, including spina bifida, craniofacial defects, cardiovascular malformations, and hypospadias. The risk of teratogenic effects is higher with anticonvulsant polytherapy than monotherapy.

Developmental delays have also been observed following *in utero* exposure to carbamazepine (per manufacturer); however, socioeconomic factors, maternal and paternal IQ, and polytherapy may contribute to these findings. Pregnancy may cause small decreases of carbamazepine plasma concentrations in the second and third trimesters; monitoring should be considered. When used for the treatment of bipolar disorder, use of carbamazepine should be avoided during the first trimester of pregnancy if possible. The use of a single medication for the treatment of bipolar disorder or epilepsy in pregnancy is preferred. Carbamazepine may decrease plasma concentrations of hormonal contraceptives; breakthrough bleeding or unintended pregnancy may occur and alternate or back-up methods of contraception should be considered.

Patients exposed to carbamazepine during pregnancy are encouraged to enroll themselves into the AED Pregnancy Registry by calling 1-888-233-2334. Additional information is available at www.aedpregnancyregistry.org.

Lactation Enters breast milk/not recommended (AAP rates "compatible"; AAP 2001 update pending)

Medication Guide Available Yes

Contraindications Hypersensitivity to carbamazepine, tricyclic antidepressants, or any component of the formulation; bone marrow depression; with or within 14 days of MAO inhibitor use; concurrent use of nefazodone

Warnings/Precautions **[U.S. Boxed Warning]: Potentially fatal blood cell abnormalities have been reported.** Patients with a previous history of adverse hematologic reaction to any drug may be at increased risk.

Antiepileptics are associated with an increased risk of suicidal behavior/thoughts with use (regardless of indication); patients should be monitored for signs/symptoms of depression, suicidal tendencies, and other unusual behavior changes during therapy and instructed to inform their healthcare provider immediately if symptoms occur.

Administer carbamazepine with caution to patients with history of cardiac damage, ECG abnormalities (or at risk for ECG abnormalities), hepatic or renal disease. When used to treat bipolar disorder, the smallest effective dose is suggested to reduce the risk for overdose/suicide; high-risk patients should be monitored for suicidal ideations. Prescription should be written for the smallest quantity consistent with good patient care. May activate latent psychosis and/or cause confusion or agitation; elderly patients may be at an increased risk for psychiatric effects. Potentially serious, sometimes fatal multiorgan hypersensitivity reactions have been reported with some antiepileptic drugs; monitor for signs and symptoms of possible disparate manifestations associated with lymphatic, hepatic, renal, and/or hematologic organ systems; gradual discontinuation and conversion to alternate therapy may be required.

Carbamazepine is not effective in absence, myoclonic, or akinetic seizures; exacerbation of certain seizure types have been seen after initiation of carbamazepine therapy in children with mixed seizure disorders. Abrupt discontinuation is not recommended in patients being treated for seizures. Dizziness or drowsiness may occur; caution should be used when performing tasks which require alertness until the effects are known. Effects with other sedative drugs or ethanol may be potentiated. Carbamazepine has a high potential for drug interactions; use caution in patients taking strong CYP3A4 inducers or inhibitors or medications significantly metabolized via CYP1A2, 2B6, 2C9, 2C19, and 3A4. Coadministration of carbamazepine and nefazodone may lead to insufficient plasma levels of nefazodone; combination is contraindicated. Carbamazepine has mild anticholinergic activity; use with caution in patients with increased intraocular pressure, or sensitivity to anticholinergic effects. Severe dermatologic reactions, including toxic epidermal necrolysis and Stevens-Johnson syndrome, although rarely reported, have resulted in fatalities. **[U.S. Boxed Warning]: Use caution and screen for the genetic susceptibility genotype (*HLA-B*1502* allele) in Asian patients. Patients with a positive result should not be started on carbamazepine.** Discontinue if there are any signs of hypersensitivity. Elderly patients may have an increased risk of SIADH-like syndrome.

Administration of the suspension will yield higher peak and lower trough serum levels than an equal dose of the tablet form; consider a lower starting dose given more frequently (same total daily dose) when using the suspension.

Adverse Reactions Frequency not defined, unless otherwise specified.

Cardiovascular: Arrhythmias, AV block, bradycardia, chest pain (bipolar use), CHF, edema, hyper-/hypotension, lymphadenopathy, syncope, thromboembolism, thrombophlebitis

Central nervous system: Amnesia (bipolar use), anxiety (bipolar use), aseptic meningitis (case report), ataxia (bipolar use 15%), confusion, depression (bipolar use), dizziness (bipolar use 44%), fatigue, headache (bipolar use 22%), sedation, slurred speech, somnolence (bipolar use 32%)

Dermatologic: Alopecia, alterations in skin pigmentation, erythema multiforme, exfoliative dermatitis, photosensitivity reaction, pruritus (bipolar use 8%), purpura, rash, Stevens-Johnson syndrome, toxic epidermal necrolysis, urticaria

Endocrine & metabolic: Chills, fever, hyponatremia, syndrome of inappropriate ADH secretion (SIADH)

Gastrointestinal: Abdominal pain, anorexia, constipation, diarrhea, dyspepsia (bipolar use), gastric distress, nausea (bipolar use 29%), pancreatitis, vomiting (bipolar use 18%), xerostomia (bipolar use)

Genitourinary: Azotemia, impotence, renal failure, urinary frequency, urinary retention

Hematologic: Acute intermittent porphyria, agranulocytosis, aplastic anemia, bone marrow suppression, eosinophilia, leukocytosis, leukopenia, pancytopenia, thrombocytopenia

Hepatic: Abnormal liver function tests, hepatic failure, hepatitis, jaundice

Neuromuscular & skeletal: Back pain, pain (bipolar use 12%), peripheral neuritis, weakness

Ocular: Blurred vision, conjunctivitis, lens opacities, nystagmus

Otic: Hyperacusis, tinnitus

Miscellaneous: Diaphoresis, hypersensitivity (including multiorgan reactions, may include disorders mimicking lymphoma, eosinophilia, hepatosplenomegaly, vasculitis); infection (bipolar use 12%)

Postmarketing and/or case reports: Suicidal ideation

Drug Interactions

Metabolism/Transport Effects Substrate of CYP2C8 (minor), CYP3A4 (major); **Note:** Assignment of Major/Minor substrate status based on clinically relevant drug interaction potential; **Induces** CYP1A2 (strong), CYP2B6 (strong), CYP2C19 (strong), CYP2C8 (strong), CYP2C9 (strong), CYP3A4 (strong), P-glycoprotein

Avoid Concomitant Use

Avoid concomitant use of CarBAMazepine with any of the following: Boceprevir; Bortezomib; CloZAPine; Conivaptan; Dabigatran Etexilate; Dronedarone; Etravirine; Lurasidone; MAO Inhibitors; Nefazodone; Nilotinib; Praziquantel; Rilpivirine; Roflumilast; SORAfenib; Telaprevir; Ticagrelor; Toremifene; Vandetanib; Voriconazole

Increased Effect/Toxicity

CarBAMazepine may increase the levels/effects of: Adenosine; Alcohol (Ethyl); ClomiPRAMINE; CloZAPine; CNS Depressants; Desmopressin; Fosphenytoin; Lithium; MAO Inhibitors; Methotrimeprazine; Phenytoin

The levels/effects of CarBAMazepine may be increased by: Allopurinol; Antifungal Agents (Azole Derivatives, Systemic); Calcium Channel Blockers (Nondihydropyridine); Carbonic Anhydrase Inhibitors; Cimetidine; Conivaptan; CYP3A4 Inhibitors (Moderate); CYP3A4 Inhibitors (Strong); Danazol; Darunavir; Dasatinib; Droperidol; Fluconazole; Grapefruit Juice; HydrOXYzine; Isoniazid; LamoTRIgine; Macrolide Antibiotics; Methotrimeprazine; Nefazodone; Protease Inhibitors; QuiNINE; Selective Serotonin Reuptake Inhibitors; Telaprevir; Thiazide Diuretics; Zolpidem

Decreased Effect

CarBAMazepine may decrease the levels/effects of: Acetaminophen; ARIPiprazole; Bendamustine; Benzodiazepines (metabolized by oxidation); Boceprevir; Bortezomib; Brentuximab Vedotin; Calcium Channel Blockers (Dihydropyridine); Calcium Channel Blockers (Nondihydropyridine); Caspofungin; CloZAPine; Contraceptives (Estrogens); Contraceptives (Progestins); CycloSPORINE; CycloSPORINE (Systemic); CYP1A2 Substrates; CYP2B6 Substrates; CYP2C19 Substrates; CYP2C8 Substrates; CYP2C9 Substrates; CYP3A4 Substrates; Dabigatran Etexilate; Dasatinib; Diclofenac; Divalproex; Doxycycline; Dronedarone; Etravirine; Exemestane; Felbamate; Flunarizine; Fosphenytoin; Gefitinib; GuanFACINE; Haloperidol; Irinotecan; Ixabepilone; Lacosamide; LamoTRIgine; Linagliptin; Lopinavir; Lurasidone; Maraviroc; Mebendazole; Methadone; Nefazodone; Nilotinib; Paliperidone; P-glycoprotein/ABCB1 Substrates; Phenytoin; Praziquantel; Protease Inhibitors; QuiNINE; Rilpivirine; RisperiDONE; Roflumilast; Rufinamide; Selective Serotonin Reuptake Inhibitors; SORAfenib; SUNItinib; Tadalafil; Telaprevir; Temsirolimus; Theophylline Derivatives; Thyroid Products; Ticagrelor; Topiramate; Toremifene; Treprostinil; Tricyclic

Antidepressants; Ulipristal; Valproic Acid; Vandetanib; Vecuronium; Vitamin K Antagonists; Voriconazole; Ziprasidone; Zolpidem; Zuclopenthixol

The levels/effects of CarBAMazepine may be decreased by: CYP3A4 Inducers (Strong); Deferasirox; Divalproex; Felbamate; Fosphenytoin; Herbs (CYP3A4 Inducers); Ketorolac; Ketorolac (Nasal); Ketorolac (Systemic); Mefloquine; Methylfolate; Phenytoin; Rufinamide; Theophylline Derivatives; Tocilizumab; Valproic Acid

Ethanol/Nutrition/Herb Interactions

Ethanol: May increase CNS depression; monitor for increased effects with coadministration. Caution patients about effects.

Food: Carbamazepine serum levels may be increased if taken with food. Carbamazepine serum concentration may be increased if taken with grapefruit juice; avoid concurrent use.

Herb/Nutraceutical: Avoid evening primrose (seizure threshold decreased). Avoid valerian, St John's wort, kava kava, gotu kola (may increase CNS depression).

Mechanism of Action In addition to anticonvulsant effects, carbamazepine has anticholinergic, antineuralgic, antidiuretic, muscle relaxant, antimanic, antidepressive, and antiarrhythmic properties; may depress activity in the nucleus ventralis of the thalamus or decrease synaptic transmission or decrease summation of temporal stimulation leading to neural discharge by limiting influx of sodium ions across cell membrane or other unknown mechanisms; stimulates the release of ADH and potentiates its action in promoting reabsorption of water; chemically related to tricyclic antidepressants

Pharmacodynamics/Kinetics

Absorption: Slow

Distribution: V_d: Neonates: 1.5 L/kg; Children: 1.9 L/kg; Adults: 0.59-2 L/kg

Protein binding: Carbamazepine: 75% to 90%, may be decreased in newborns; Epoxide metabolite: 50%

Metabolism: Hepatic via CYP3A4 to active epoxide metabolite; induces hepatic enzymes to increase metabolism

Bioavailability: 85%

Half-life elimination: **Note:** Half-life is variable because of autoinduction which is usually complete 3-5 weeks after initiation of a fixed carbamazepine regimen.

Carbamazepine: Initial: 25-65 hours; Extended release: 35-40 hours; Multiple doses: Children: 8-14 hours; Adults: 12-17 hours

Epoxide metabolite: Initial: 25-43 hours

Time to peak, serum: Unpredictable:

Immediate release: Suspension: 1.5 hour; tablet: 4-5 hours

Extended release: Carbatrol®, Equetro®: 12-26 hours (single dose), 4-8 hours (multiple doses); Tegretol®-XR: 3-12 hours

Excretion: Urine 72% (1% to 3% as unchanged drug); feces (28%)

Dosage Dosage must be adjusted according to patient's response and serum concentrations. Administer tablets (chewable or conventional) in 2-3 divided doses daily and suspension in 4 divided doses daily. Oral:

Epilepsy:

Children:

<6 years: Initial: 10-20 mg/kg/day divided twice or 3 times daily as tablets or 4 times/day as suspension; increase dose every week until optimal response and therapeutic levels are achieved

Maintenance dose: Divide into 3-4 doses daily (tablets or suspension); maximum recommended dose: 35 mg/kg/day

6-12 years: Initial: 200 mg/day in 2 divided doses (tablets or extended release tablets) or 4 divided doses (oral suspension); increase by up to 100 mg/day at weekly intervals using a twice daily regimen of extended release tablets or 3-4 times daily regimen of other formulations until optimal response and therapeutic levels are achieved

Maintenance: Usual: 400-800 mg/day; maximum recommended dose: 1000 mg/day

Note: Children <12 years who receive ≥400 mg/day of carbamazepine may be converted to extended release capsules (Carbatrol®) using the same total daily dosage divided twice daily

Children >12 years and Adults: Initial: 400 mg/day in 2 divided doses (tablets or extended release tablets) or 4 divided doses (oral suspension); increase by up to 200 mg/day at weekly intervals using a twice daily regimen of extended release tablets or capsules, or a 3-4 times/day regimen of other formulations until optimal response and therapeutic levels are achieved; usual dose: 800-1200 mg/day

Maximum recommended doses:

Children 12-15 years: 1000 mg/day

Children >15 years: 1200 mg/day

Adults: 1600 mg/day; however, some patients have required up to 1.6-2.4 g/day

Trigeminal or glossopharyngeal neuralgia: Adults: Initial: 200 mg/day in 2 divided doses (tablets, extended release tablets, or extended release capsules) or 4 divided doses (oral suspension) with food, gradually increasing in increments of 200 mg/day as needed

Maintenance: Usual: 400-800 mg daily in 2 divided doses (tablets, extended release tablets, or extended release capsules) or 4 divided doses (oral suspension); maximum dose: 1200 mg/day

Bipolar disorder: Adults: Initial: 400 mg/day in 2 divided doses (tablets, extended release tablets, or extended release capsules) or 4 divided doses (oral suspension), may adjust by 200 mg/day increments; maximum dose: 1600 mg/day.

Note: Equetro® is the only formulation specifically approved by the FDA for the management of bipolar disorder.

Dosing adjustment in renal impairment: Dosage adjustments are not required or recommended in the manufacturer's labeling; however, the following guidelines have been used by some clinicians (Aronoff, 2007):

Children and Adults:

GFR <10 mL/minute: Administer 75% of dose

Hemodialysis, peritoneal dialysis: Administer 75% of dose

Continuous renal replacement therapy (CRRT):

Children: Administer 75% of dose

Adults: No dosage adjustment recommended

Dosing adjustment in hepatic impairment: Use with caution in hepatic impairment; metabolized primarily in the liver

Dietary Considerations Drug may cause GI upset, take with large amount of water or food to decrease GI upset. May need to split doses to avoid GI upset.

Administration

Suspension: Must be given on a 3-4 times/day schedule versus tablets which can be given 2-4 times/day. Since a given dose of suspension will produce higher peak and lower trough levels than the same dose given as the tablet form, patients given the suspension should be started on lower doses given more frequently (same total daily dose) and increased slowly to avoid unwanted side effects. When carbamazepine suspension has been combined with chlorpromazine or thioridazine solutions, a precipitate forms which may result in loss of effect. Therefore, it is recommended that the carbamazepine suspension dosage form not be administered at the same time with other liquid medicinal agents or diluents. Should be administered with meals.

Extended release capsule (Carbatrol®, Equetro®): Consists of three different types of beads: Immediate release, extended-release, and enteric release. The bead types are combined in a ratio to allow twice daily dosing. May be opened and contents sprinkled over food such as a teaspoon of applesauce; may be administered with or without food; do not crush or chew.

Extended release tablet: Should be inspected for damage. Damaged extended release tablets (without release portal) should not be administered. Should be administered with meals; swallow whole, do not crush or chew.

Monitoring Parameters CBC with platelet count, reticulocytes, serum iron, lipid panel, liver function tests, urinalysis, BUN, serum carbamazepine levels, thyroid function tests, serum sodium; pregnancy test; ophthalmic exams (pupillary reflexes); observe patient for excessive sedation, especially when instituting or increasing therapy; signs of rash; *HLA-B*1502* genotype screening prior to therapy initiation in patients of Asian descent; suicidality (eg, suicidal thoughts, depression, behavioral changes)

Reference Range

Timing of serum samples: Absorption is slow, peak levels occur 6-8 hours after ingestion of the first dose; the half-life ranges from 8-60 hours, therefore, steady-state is achieved in 2-5 days

Therapeutic levels: 4-12 mcg/mL (SI: 17-51 micromole/L)

Toxic concentration: >15 mcg/mL; patients who require higher levels of 8-12 mcg/mL (SI: 34-51 micromole/L) should be watched closely. Side effects including CNS effects occur commonly at higher dosage levels. If other anticonvulsants are given therapeutic range is 4-8 mcg/mL.

Test Interactions May cause false-positive serum TCA screen; may interact with some pregnancy tests

Dosage Forms Excipient information presented when available (limited, particularly for generics); consult specific product labeling.

Capsule, extended release, oral:
- Carbatrol®: 100 mg, 200 mg, 300 mg
- Equetro®: 100 mg, 200 mg, 300 mg

Suspension, oral: 100 mg/5 mL (5 mL, 10 mL, 450 mL)
- TEGretol®: 100 mg/5 mL (450 mL) [contains propylene glycol; citrus-vanilla flavor]

Tablet, oral: 200 mg
- Epitol®: 200 mg [scored]
- TEGretol®: 200 mg [scored]

Tablet, chewable, oral: 100 mg
- TEGretol®: 100 mg [scored]

Tablet, extended release, oral: 200 mg, 400 mg
- TEGretol®-XR: 100 mg, 200 mg, 400 mg

Extemporaneous Preparations Note: Commercial oral suspension is available (20 mg/mL)

A 40 mg/mL oral suspension may be made with tablets. Crush twenty 200 mg tablets in a mortar and reduce to a fine powder. Add small portions of Simple Syrup, NF and mix to a uniform paste; mix while adding the vehicle in incremental proportions to **almost** 100 mL; transfer to a calibrated bottle, rinse mortar with vehicle, and add sufficient quantity of vehicle to make 100 mL. Label "shake well" and "refrigerate". Stable for 90 days.

Nahata MC, Pai VB, and Hipple TF, *Pediatric Drug Formulations*, 5th ed, Cincinnati, OH: Harvey Whitney Books Co, 2004.

◆ **Carbamide** *see* Urea *on page 1749*

Carbamide Peroxide (KAR ba mide per OKS ide)

Brand Names: U.S. Auraphene B® [OTC]; Auro® [OTC]; Cankaid® [OTC]; Debrox® [OTC]; E-R-O® [OTC]; Gly-Oxide® [OTC]; Murine® Ear Wax Removal Kit [OTC]; Murine® Ear [OTC]; Otix® [OTC]; Wax Away [OTC]

Index Terms Urea Peroxide

Pharmacologic Category Anti-inflammatory, Locally Applied; Otic Agent, Cerumenolytic

Use Relief of minor inflammation of gums, oral mucosal surfaces, and lips including canker sores and dental irritation; emulsify and disperse ear wax

Dosage Children and Adults:

Oral: Inflammation/dental irritation: Solution (should not be used for >7 days): Oral preparation should not be used in children <2 years of age; apply several drops undiluted on affected area 4 times/day after meals and at bedtime; expectorate after 2-3 minutes **or** place 10 drops onto tongue, mix with saliva, swish for several minutes, expectorate

Otic:

Children <12 years: Tilt head sideways and individualize the dose according to patient size; 3 drops (range: 1-5 drops) twice daily for up to 4 days, tip of applicator should not enter ear canal; keep drops in ear for several minutes by keeping head tilted and placing cotton in ear

Children ≥12 years and Adults: Tilt head sideways and instill 5-10 drops twice daily up to 4 days, tip of applicator should not enter ear canal; keep drops in ear for several minutes by keeping head tilted and placing cotton in ear

Additional Information Complete prescribing information for this medication should be consulted for additional detail.

Dosage Forms Excipient information presented when available (limited, particularly for generics); consult specific product labeling.

Liquid, oral: 10% (60 mL)
- Cankaid®: 10% (15 mL)
- Gly-Oxide®: 10% (15 mL, 60 mL)

Solution, otic [drops]: 6.5% (15 mL)
- Auraphene B®: 6.5% (15 mL)
- Auro®: 6.5% (22.2 mL)
- Debrox®: 6.5% (15 mL, 30 mL)
- E-R-O®: 6.5% (15 mL) [ethanol free]
- Murine® Ear: 6.5% (15 mL) [contains ethanol 6.3%]
- Murine® Ear Wax Removal Kit: 6.5% (15 mL) [contains ethanol 6.3%]
- Otix®: 6.5% (15 mL)
- Wax Away: 6.5% (15 mL)

◆ **Carbamylcholine Chloride** *see* Carbachol *on page 280*
◆ **Carbatrol®** *see* CarBAMazepine *on page 280*

Carbetapentane and Pseudoephedrine
(kar bay ta PEN tane & soo doe e FED rin)

Brand Names: U.S. Corzall™ Liquid [DSC]

Index Terms Carbetapentane Tannate and Pseudoephedrine Tannate; Pseudoephedrine and Carbetapentane

Pharmacologic Category Antitussive/Decongestant

Use Relief of cough and congestion due to the common cold, influenza, sinusitis, or bronchitis

Pregnancy Risk Factor C

Dosage Relief of cough and congestion: Oral:

Children: 6-12 years: 2.5-5 mL every 4-6 hours (maximum: 30 mL/24 hours)

Children >12 years and Adults: 5-10 mL every 4-6 hours (maximum: 60 mL/24 hours)

Additional Information Complete prescribing information for this medication should be consulted for additional detail.

Dosage Forms Excipient information presented when available (limited, particularly for generics); consult specific product labeling. [DSC] = Discontinued product

Liquid, oral:

Corzall™: Carbetapentane citrate 20 mg and pseudoephedrine hydrochloride 30 mg per 5 mL (473 mL) [dye free, ethanol free, sugar free; contains propylene glycol; grape flavor] [DSC]

◆ **Carbetapentane Tannate and Pseudoephedrine Tannate** *see* Carbetapentane and Pseudoephedrine *on page 283*

Carbidopa (kar bi DOE pa)

Brand Names: U.S. Lodosyn®

Pharmacologic Category Anti-Parkinson's Agent, Decarboxylase Inhibitor

Use Given with carbidopa-levodopa in the treatment of parkinsonism to enable a lower dosage of levodopa to be used and a more rapid response to be obtained and to decrease side effects; use with carbidopa-levodopa in patients requiring additional carbidopa; has no effect without levodopa

Pregnancy Risk Factor C

Dosage Oral: Adults: **Note:** Optimal daily dosage determined by careful titration; generally if carbidopa is ≥70 mg/day, a 1:10 proportion of carbidopa:levodopa provides the most patient response.

Carbidopa augmentation in patients receiving carbidopa-levodopa:

Patients receiving Sinemet® 10/100: 25 mg carbidopa daily with first daily dose of Sinemet® 10/100; if necessary, 12.5-25 mg carbidopa may be given with each subsequent dose of Sinemet® 10/100; maximum: 200 mg carbidopa/day (including carbidopa from Sinemet®)

Patients receiving Sinemet® 25/250 or Sinemet® 25/100: 25 mg carbidopa with any dose of Sinemet® 25/250 or Sinemet® 25/100 throughout the day; maximum: 200 mg carbidopa/day (including carbidopa from Sinemet®)

Individual titration of carbidopa and levodopa: Initial: 25 mg carbidopa 3-4 times/day; administer at the same time as levodopa, initial dose of levodopa should be 20% to 25% of the previous levodopa dose in carbidopa-naive patients; first dose of carbidopa should be taken ≥12 hours after the last dose of levodopa in carbidopa-naive patients; increase or decrease dose by 1/2 or 1 tablet/day

Additional Information Complete prescribing information for this medication should be consulted for additional detail.

Dosage Forms Excipient information presented when available (limited, particularly for generics); consult specific product labeling.

Tablet, oral:

Lodosyn®: 25 mg [scored]

Carbidopa and Levodopa
(kar bi DOE pa & lee voe DOE pa)

Brand Names: U.S. Parcopa®; Sinemet®; Sinemet® CR

Brand Names: Canada Apo-Levocarb®; Apo-Levocarb® CR; Dom-Levo-Carbidopa; Duodopa™; Endo®-Levodopa/Carbidopa; Levocarb CR; Novo-Levocarbidopa; Nu-Levocarb; PRO-Levocarb; Sinemet®; Sinemet® CR

Index Terms Levodopa and Carbidopa

Pharmacologic Category Anti-Parkinson's Agent, Decarboxylase Inhibitor; Anti-Parkinson's Agent, Dopamine Precursor

Additional Appendix Information

Antiparkinsonian Agents *on page 1879*

Use Idiopathic Parkinson's disease; postencephalitic parkinsonism; symptomatic parkinsonism

Duodopa™ intestinal gel: Canadian labeling (not available in U.S.): Treatment of advanced levodopa-responsive Parkinson's disease in which severe motor symptoms are not controlled by other Parkinson's agents

Unlabeled Use Restless leg syndrome

Pregnancy Risk Factor C

Pregnancy Considerations Teratogenic effects were observed with levodopa and carbidopa in animal studies. There are case reports of levodopa crossing the placenta in humans.

Lactation Excretion in breast milk unknown/use caution

Prescribing and Access Restrictions Duodopa™ intestinal gel (Canadian labeling; product not available in U.S.): In Canada, the Duodopa™ Education Program is a risk mitigation program established to provide safe and effective use of Duodopa™ in advanced Parkinson's patients. The program involves:

- Education of prescribing neurologists and other healthcare providers on suitable candidates for treatment, surgical procedures (PEG tube placement), and follow-up care including infusion device education.
- Distribution of educational materials to patients and caregivers describing Duodopa™ intestinal gel and its proper use, PEG tube placement, and complications associated with the mode of administration and/or PEG tube placement.

Contraindications Hypersensitivity to levodopa, carbidopa, or any component of the formulation; narrow-angle glaucoma; use of MAO inhibitors within prior 14 days (however, may be administered concomitantly with the manufacturer's recommended dose of an MAO inhibitor with selectivity for MAO type B); history of melanoma or undiagnosed skin lesions

Canadian labeling: Additional contraindications: Clinical or laboratory evidence of uncompensated cardiovascular, cerebrovascular, endocrine, renal, hepatic, hematologic or pulmonary disease; when administration of a sympathomimetic amine (eg, epinephrine, norepinephrine or isoproterenol) is contraindicated; intestinal gel therapy in patients with any condition preventing the required placement of a PEG tube for administration.

Warnings/Precautions Use with caution in patients with history of cardiovascular disease (including myocardial infarction and arrhythmias), pulmonary diseases (such as asthma), psychosis, wide-angle glaucoma, peptic ulcer disease, seizure disorder or prone to seizures, and in severe renal and hepatic dysfunction. Use with caution when interpreting plasma/urine catecholamine levels; falsely diagnosed pheochromocytoma has been rarely reported. Severe cases or rhabdomyolysis have been reported. Sudden discontinuation of levodopa may cause a worsening of Parkinson's disease. Elderly may be more sensitive to CNS effects of levodopa. May cause or exacerbate dyskinesias. Patients have reported falling asleep while engaging in activities of daily living; this has been reported to occur without significant warning signs. May cause orthostatic hypotension; Parkinson's disease patients appear to have an impaired capacity to respond to a postural challenge; use with caution in patients at risk of hypotension (such as those receiving antihypertensive drugs) or where transient hypotensive episodes would be poorly tolerated (cardiovascular disease or cerebrovascular disease). Observe patients closely for development of depression with concomitant suicidal tendencies.

Dopamine agonists have been associated with compulsive behaviors and/or loss of impulse control, which has manifested as pathological gambling, libido increases (hypersexuality), and/or binge eating. Causality has not been established, and controversy exists as to whether this phenomenon is related to the underlying disease, prior behaviors/addictions and/or drug therapy. Dose reduction or discontinuation of therapy has been reported to reverse these behaviors in some, but not all cases. Risk for melanoma development is increased in Parkinson's disease patients; drug causation or factors contributing to risk have not been established. Patients should be monitored closely and periodic skin examinations should be performed. Dopaminergic agents have been associated with a syndrome resembling neuroleptic malignant syndrome on abrupt withdrawal or significant dosage reduction after long-term use. Protein in the diet should be distributed throughout the day to avoid fluctuations in levodopa absorption.

Intestinal gel (available in Canada, not available in U.S.): Product should be prescribed only by neurologists experienced in the treatment of Parkinson's disease and who have completed the Duodopa™ Education Program. Response to levodopa/carbidopa intestinal gel therapy should be assessed with a test period (~3 days) of administration via a temporary nasoduodenal tube prior to placement of a percutaneous endoscopic gastrostomy (PEG) tube for permanent access and administration. Sudden deterioration in therapy response with recurring motor symptoms may indicate PEG tube complications (eg, displacement) or obstruction of the infusion device. Tube or infusion device complications may require initiation of oral levodopa/carbidopa therapy until complications are resolved. Discontinue therapy 2-3 hours prior to surgical procedures requiring general anesthesia, if possible. May resume therapy postoperatively when oral fluid intake is permitted.

Adverse Reactions Frequency not defined.

Cardiovascular: Arrhythmia, chest pain, edema, flushing, hypotension, hypertension, MI, orthostatic hypotension, palpitation, phlebitis, syncope

Central nervous system: Agitation, anxiety, ataxia, confusion, delusions, dementia, depression (with or without suicidal tendencies), disorientation, dizziness, dreams abnormal, EPS, euphoria, faintness, falling, fatigue, gait abnormalities, headache, hallucinations, impulse control symptoms, insomnia, malaise, memory impairment, mental acuity decreased, nervousness, neuroleptic malignant syndrome, nightmares, on-off phenomena, paranoid ideation, pathological gambling, psychosis, seizure (causal relationship not established), somnolence

Dermatologic: Alopecia, malignant melanoma, rash

Endocrine & metabolic: Hot flashes, hyperglycemia, hypokalemia, libido increased (including hypersexuality), uric acid increased

Gastrointestinal: Abdominal pain, abdominal distress, anorexia, bruxism, constipation, diarrhea, discoloration of saliva, duodenal ulcer, dyspepsia, dysphagia, flatulence, GI bleeding, heartburn, nausea, sialorrhea, taste alterations, tongue burning sensation, weight gain/loss, vomiting, xerostomia

Genitourinary: Discoloration of urine, glycosuria, urinary frequency, priapism, proteinuria, urinary incontinence, urinary retention, urinary tract infection

Hematologic: Agranulocytosis, anemia, Coombs' test abnormal, hematocrit decreased, hemoglobin decreased, hemolytic anemia, leukopenia

Hepatic: Alkaline phosphatase abnormal, ALT abnormal, AST abnormal, bilirubin abnormal, LDH abnormal

Neuromuscular & skeletal: Back pain, dyskinesias (including choreiform, dystonic and other involuntary movements), leg pain, muscle cramps, muscle twitching, numbness, paresthesia, peripheral neuropathy, shoulder pain, tremor increased, trismus, weakness

Ocular: Blepharospasm, blurred vision, diplopia, Horner's syndrome reactivation, mydriasis, oculogyric crises (may be associated with acute dystonic reactions)

Renal: Difficult urination

Respiratory: Cough, dyspnea, hoarseness, pharyngeal pain, upper respiratory infection

Miscellaneous: Discoloration of sweat, diaphoresis increased, hiccups, hypersensitivity reactions (angioedema, pruritus, urticaria, bullous lesions [including pemphigus-like reactions], Henoch-Schönlein purpura)

Drug Interactions

Metabolism/Transport Effects None known.

Avoid Concomitant Use There are no known interactions where it is recommended to avoid concomitant use.

Increased Effect/Toxicity

Carbidopa and Levodopa may increase the levels/effects of: MAO Inhibitors

The levels/effects of Carbidopa and Levodopa may be increased by: Antipsychotics (Typical); MAO Inhibitors; Methylphenidate; Sapropterin

Decreased Effect

Carbidopa and Levodopa may decrease the levels/effects of: Antipsychotics (Typical)

The levels/effects of Carbidopa and Levodopa may be decreased by: Antipsychotics (Atypical); Fosphenytoin; Glycopyrrolate; Iron Salts; Methionine; Metoclopramide; Phenytoin; Pyridoxine

Ethanol/Nutrition/Herb Interactions

Ethanol: Avoid ethanol (due to CNS depression).

Food: Avoid high protein diets due to potential for impaired levodopa absorption; levodopa competes with certain amino acids for transport across the gut wall or across the blood-brain barrier.

Herb/Nutraceutical: Avoid kava kava (may decrease effects). Pyridoxine (vitamin B_6) in doses >10-25 mg (for levodopa alone) may decrease efficacy. Iron supplements or iron-containing multivitamins may reduce absorption of levodopa.

Stability

Tablet: Store at 20°C to 25°C (68°F to 77°F); excursions permitted between 15°C to 30°C (59°F to 86°F). Protect from light and moisture.

Intestinal gel (Canadian labeling; not available in U.S.): Store in refrigerator at 2°C to 8°C (36°F to 46°F). Keep in outer carton to protect from light. Cassettes are for single use only and should be discarded daily following infusion (up to 16 hours).

Mechanism of Action Parkinson's symptoms are due to a lack of striatal dopamine; levodopa circulates in the plasma to the blood-brain-barrier (BBB), where it crosses, to be converted by striatal enzymes to dopamine; carbidopa inhibits the peripheral plasma breakdown of levodopa by inhibiting its decarboxylation, and thereby increases available levodopa at the BBB

Pharmacodynamics/Kinetics

Distribution: Levodopa: 0.9-1.6 L/kg (in presence of carbidopa), crosses the blood-brain barrier;Carbidopa: Does not cross the blood-brain barrier

Metabolism: Levodopa: Two major pathways (decarboxylation and O-methylation) and two minor pathways (transamination and oxidation) of metabolism; Carbidopa inhibits the decarboxylation of levodopa to dopamine in the peripheral tissue to allow greater levodopa distribution into the CNS

Bioavailability:

Controlled release: Levodopa: Bioavailability is 70% to 75% relative to availability from immediate release formulation; Carbidopa: Bioavailability is ~58% relative to availability from immediate release formulation

Intestinal gel: Levodopa: Similar bioavailability relative to oral administration of tablet formulations (81% to 98%)

Half-life elimination: Immediate release: Levodopa (in presence of carbidopa): 1.5 hours; Half-life may be prolonged with controlled release formulations due to continuous absorption

Time to peak: Immediate release: 0.5 hours; Controlled release: 2 hours; Intestinal gel: therapeutic plasma levels reached 10-30 minutes following morning bolus dose

Excretion: Levodopa: Urine (as metabolites); Carbidopa: Urine (~50% of an oral dose)

Dosage

Adults:

Parkinson's disease:

Oral:

Immediate release tablet, orally-disintegrating tablet:

Initial: Carbidopa 25 mg/levodopa 100 mg 3 times/day

Dosage adjustment: Alternate tablet strengths may be substituted according to individual carbidopa/levodopa requirements. Increase by 1 tablet every 1-2 days as necessary, except when using the carbidopa 25 mg/ levodopa 250 mg tablets where increases should be made using 1/2-1 tablet every 1-2 days. Use of more than 1 dosage strength or dosing 4 times/day may be required (maximum: 8 tablets of any strength/day or 200 mg of carbidopa and 2000 mg of levodopa)

Controlled release tablet:

Patients not currently receiving levodopa: Initial: Carbidopa 50 mg/levodopa 200 mg 2 times/day, at intervals not <6 hours

Patients converting from immediate release formulation to controlled release: Initial: Dosage should be substituted at an amount that provides ~10% more of levodopa/day; total calculated dosage is administered in divided doses 2-3 times/day (or ≥3 times/day for patients maintained on levodopa ≥700 mg). Intervals between doses should be 4-8 hours while awake; when divided doses are not equal, smaller doses should be given toward the end of the day. Depending on clinical response, dosage may need to be increased to provide up to 30% more levodopa/day.

Dosage adjustment: May adjust every 3 days; intervals should be between 4-8 hours during the waking day (maximum dose: 8 tablets/day)

Intestinal infusion via PEG tube: Intestinal gel (Canadian labeling; not available in U.S.): **Note:** Conversion to/from oral levodopa tablet formulations and the intestinal gel formulation can be done on a 1:1 ratio. Total daily dose (expressed in terms of levodopa) consists of a morning bolus dose, a continuous maintenance dose, and additional bolus doses when necessary. Nighttime dosing may be necessary in certain rare situations (eg, nocturnal akinesia). Dosage adjustments should be carried out over a period of a few weeks.

Morning bolus dose (based on previous morning levodopa intake and volume to fill intestinal tubing): Usual: Levodopa 100-200 mg (5-10 mL); Maximum: Levodopa 300 mg (15 mL)

Continuous maintenance dose: Adjustable in increments of 2 mg/hour (0.1 mL/hour) and based on previous daily intake of levodopa: Usual: Levodopa 40-120 mg/hour (2-6 mL/hour) infused up to 16 hours; Range: Levodopa 20-200 mg/hour (1-10 mL/hour)

Additional bolus doses: Usual: Levodopa: 10-40 mg (0.5-2 mL), if needed for daytime hypokinesia; in patients requiring >5 additional boluses/day, the maintenance dose should be increased

Restless leg syndrome (RLS) (unlabeled use; Silber, 2004): Oral:

Immediate release tablet: Carbidopa 25 mg/levodopa 100 mg (0.5-1 tablet) given in the evening, at bedtime, or upon waking during the night with RLS symptoms

Controlled release tablet: Carbidopa 25 mg/levodopa 100 mg (1 tablet) before bedtime for RLS symptoms that awaken patient during the night

Elderly: Refer to adult dosing

Dosage adjustment in renal impairment: Use with caution; manufacturer labeling makes no specific dosing recommendations

Dosage adjustment in hepatic impairment: Use with caution; manufacturer labeling makes no specific dosing recommendations

Dietary Considerations Avoid high protein diets (>2 g/kg) which may decrease the efficacy of levodopa via competition with amino acids in crossing the blood-brain barrier. Some products may contain phenylalanine.

Administration

Oral tablet formulations: Space doses evenly over the waking hours. Give with meals to decrease GI upset. Controlled release product should not be chewed or crushed. Orally-disintegrating tablets do not require water; the tablet should disintegrate on the tongue's surface before swallowing.

Intestinal gel (Canadian labeling; not available in U.S.): Gel is administered directly to the duodenum via a portable infusion pump (CADD-legacy Duodopa™ pump). Administer through a temporary nasoduodenal tube for at least 3 days to evaluate patient response and for dose optimization. Long-term administration requires placement of PEG tube for intestinal infusion. Continuous maintenance dose is infused throughout the day for up to 16 hours.

Monitoring Parameters Periodic hepatic function tests, BUN, creatinine, and CBC; periodic skin examinations; blood pressure, standing and sitting/supine; symptoms of parkinsonism, dyskinesias, mental status

Test Interactions False-positive reaction for urinary glucose with Clinitest®; false-negative reaction using Clinistix®; false-positive urine ketones with Acetest®, Ketostix®, Labstix®

Additional Information To block the peripheral conversion of levodopa to dopamine, ≥70 mg/day of carbidopa is needed. "On-off" (a clinical syndrome characterized by sudden periods of drug activity/inactivity), can be managed by giving smaller, more frequent doses of Sinemet® or adding a dopamine agonist or selegiline; when adding a new agent, doses of Sinemet® can usually be decreased. Protein in the diet should be distributed throughout the day to avoid fluctuations in levodopa absorption. Levodopa is the drug of choice when rigidity is the predominant presenting symptom.

Conversion from levodopa to carbidopa/levodopa: **Note:** Levodopa must be discontinued at least 12 hours prior to initiation of levodopa/carbidopa:

Initial dose: Levodopa portion of carbidopa/levodopa should be at least 25% of previous levodopa therapy.

Levodopa <1500 mg/day: Sinemet® or Parcopa™ (levodopa 25 mg/carbidopa 100 mg) 3-4 times/day

Levodopa ≥1500 mg/day: Sinemet® or Parcopa™ (levodopa 25 mg/carbidopa 250 mg) 3-4 times/day

Conversion from immediate release carbidopa/levodopa (Sinemet® or Parcopa™) to Sinemet® CR (50/200):

Sinemet® or Parcopa™ [total daily dose of levodopa]/ Sinemet® CR:

Sinemet® or Parcopa™ (levodopa 300-400 mg/day): Sinemet® CR (50/200) 1 tablet twice daily

Sinemet® or Parcopa™ (levodopa 500-600 mg/day): Sinemet® CR (50/200) 1 1/2 tablets twice daily or 1 tablet 3 times/day

Sinemet® or Parcopa™ (levodopa 700-800 mg/day): Sinemet® CR (50/200) 4 tablets in 3 or more divided doses
Sinemet® or Parcopa™ (levodopa 900-1000 mg/day): Sinemet® CR (50/200) 5 tablets in 3 or more divided doses
Intervals between doses of Sinemet® CR should be 4-8 hours while awake; when divided doses are not equal, smaller doses should be given toward the end of the day

Dosage Forms Excipient information presented when available (limited, particularly for generics); consult specific product labeling.
Tablet: 10/100: Carbidopa 10 mg and levodopa 100 mg; 25/100: Carbidopa 25 mg and levodopa 100 mg; 25/250: Carbidopa 25 mg and levodopa 250 mg
Sinemet®:
10/100: Carbidopa 10 mg and levodopa 100 mg
25/100: Carbidopa 25 mg and levodopa 100 mg
25/250: Carbidopa 25 mg and levodopa 250 mg
Tablet, extended release: 25/100: Carbidopa 25 mg and levodopa 100 mg; 50/200: Carbidopa 50 mg and levodopa 200 mg
Tablet, orally disintegrating: 10/100: Carbidopa 10 mg and levodopa 100 mg; 25/100: Carbidopa 25 mg and levodopa 100 mg; 25/250: Carbidopa 25 mg and levodopa 250 mg
Parcopa®:
10/100: Carbidopa 10 mg and levodopa 100 mg [contains phenylalanine 3.4 mg/tablet; mint flavor]
25/100: Carbidopa 25 mg and levodopa 100 mg [contains phenylalanine 3.4 mg/tablet; mint flavor]
25/250: Carbidopa 25 mg and levodopa 250 mg [contains phenylalanine 8.4 mg/tablet; mint flavor]
Tablet, sustained release: 25/100: Carbidopa 25 mg and levodopa 100 mg; 50/200: Carbidopa 50 mg and levodopa 200 mg
Sinemet® CR:
25/100: Carbidopa 25 mg and levodopa 100 mg
50/200: Carbidopa 50 mg and levodopa 200 mg

Dosage Forms: Canada Excipient information presented when available (limited, particularly for generics); consult specific product labeling.
Intestinal gel:
Duodopa™: Carbidopa 5 mg and levodopa 20 mg/1 mL (100 mL)

Extemporaneous Preparations An oral suspension containing carbidopa 1.25 mg and levodopa 5 mg per mL may be made with tablets. Crush ten tablets each containing carbidopa 25 mg and levodopa 100 mg and reduce to a fine powder. Add small portions of a 1:1 mixture of Ora-Sweet® and Ora-Plus® and mix to a uniform paste; mix while adding the vehicle in equal proportions to **almost** 200 mL; transfer to a calibrated bottle, rinse mortar with vehicle, and add sufficient quantity of vehicle to make 200 mL. Label "shake well" and "refrigerate". Stable 42 days under refrigeration. Also stable 28 days at room temperature.

Nahata MC, Morosco RS, and Leguire LE, "Development of Two Stable Oral Suspensions of Levodopa-Carbidopa for Children With Amblyopia," *J Pediatr Ophthalmol Strabismus*, 2000, 37(6):333-7.

◆ **Carbidopa, Entacapone, and Levodopa** *see* Levodopa, Carbidopa, and Entacapone *on page 996*
◆ **Carbidopa, Levodopa, and Entacapone** *see* Levodopa, Carbidopa, and Entacapone *on page 996*

Carbinoxamine (kar bi NOKS a meen)

Brand Names: U.S. Arbinoxa™; Palgic®
Index Terms Carbinoxamine Maleate
Pharmacologic Category Ethanolamine Derivative; Histamine H_1 Antagonist; Histamine H_1 Antagonist, First Generation
Use Seasonal and perennial allergic rhinitis; vasomotor rhinitis; allergic conjunctivitis; mild manifestations of urticaria and angioedema; dermatographism; adjunct therapy for anaphylactic reactions (after acute manifestations controlled)
Pregnancy Risk Factor C
Dosage Oral:
Children:
2-5 years: 0.2-0.4 mg/kg/day divided into 3-4 doses (weight-based dosing preferred) **or** 1-2 mg 3-4 times/day
6-11 years: 2-4 mg 3-4 times/day
Adults: 4-8 mg 3-4 times/day

Additional Information Complete prescribing information for this medication should be consulted for additional detail.

Dosage Forms Excipient information presented when available (limited, particularly for generics); consult specific product labeling.
Solution, oral, as maleate: 4 mg/5 mL (118 mL, 473 mL)
Arbinoxa™: 4 mg/5 mL (480 mL) [contains propylene glycol; bubblegum flavor]
Palgic®: 4 mg/5 mL (480 mL) [contains propylene glycol; bubblegum flavor]
Tablet, oral, as maleate: 4 mg
Arbinoxa™: 4 mg [scored]
Palgic®: 4 mg [scored]

◆ **Carbinoxamine Maleate** *see* Carbinoxamine *on page 287*
◆ **Carbocaine®** *see* Mepivacaine *on page 1076*
◆ **Carbolith™ (Can)** *see* Lithium *on page 1023*

CARBOplatin (KAR boe pla tin)

Brand Names: Canada Carboplatin Injection; Paraplatin-AQ
Index Terms CBDCA; Paraplatin
Pharmacologic Category Antineoplastic Agent, Alkylating Agent; Antineoplastic Agent, Platinum Analog
Use Treatment of advanced ovarian cancer
Unlabeled Use Treatment of bladder cancer, breast cancer (metastatic), central nervous system tumors, cervical cancer (recurrent or metastatic), endometrial cancer, esophageal cancer, head and neck cancer, Hodgkin's lymphoma (relapsed or refractory), malignant pleural mesothelioma, melanoma (advanced or metastatic), merkel cell carcinoma, neuroendocrine tumors (adrenal gland and carcinoid tumors), non-Hodgkin's lymphomas (relapsed or refractory), nonsmall cell lung cancer, prostate cancer, sarcomas (Ewing's sarcoma and osteosarcoma), small-cell lung cancer, testicular cancer, thymic malignancies, unknown primary adenocarcinoma, and as a conditioning regimen prior to hematopoietic stem cell transplantation
Pregnancy Risk Factor D
Pregnancy Considerations Embryotoxicity and teratogenicity have been observed in animal studies. There are no adequate and well-controlled studies in pregnant women. May cause fetal harm if administered during pregnancy. Women of childbearing potential should avoid becoming pregnant during treatment.
Lactation Excretion in breast milk unknown/not recommended
Contraindications History of severe allergic reaction to cisplatin, carboplatin, other platinum-containing formulations, mannitol, or any component of the formulation; should not be used in patients with severe bone marrow depression or significant bleeding
Warnings/Precautions Hazardous agent - use appropriate precautions for handling and disposal. High doses have resulted in severe abnormalities of liver function ▶

tests. **[U.S. Boxed Warning]: Bone marrow suppression, which may be severe, is dose related;** reduce dosage in patients with bone marrow suppression; cycles should be delayed until WBC and platelet counts have recovered. Patients who have received prior myelosuppressive therapy and patients with renal dysfunction are at increased risk for bone marrow suppression. Anemia is cumulative.

When calculating the carboplatin dose using the Calvert formula and an estimated glomerular filtration rate (GFR), the laboratory method used to measure serum creatinine may impact dosing. Compared to other methods, standardized isotope dilution mass spectrometry (IDMS) may underestimate serum creatinine values in patients with low creatinine values (eg, ≤0.7 mg/dL) and may overestimate GFR in patients with normal renal function. This may result in higher calculated carboplatin doses and increased toxicities. If using IDMS, the Food and Drug Administration (FDA) recommends that clinicians consider capping estimated GFR at a maximum of 125 mL/minute to avoid potential toxicity.

[U.S. Boxed Warning]: Anaphylactic-like reactions have been reported with carboplatin; may occur within minutes of administration. Epinephrine, corticosteroids and antihistamines have been used to treat symptoms. The risk of allergic reactions (including anaphylaxis) is increased in patients previously exposed to platinum therapy. Skin testing and desensitization protocols have been reported (Confina-Cohen, 2005; Lee, 2004; Markman, 2003). When administered as sequential infusions, taxane derivatives (docetaxel, paclitaxel) should be administered before the platinum derivatives (carboplatin, cisplatin) to limit myelosuppression and to enhance efficacy. Clinically significant hearing loss has been reported to occur in pediatric patients when carboplatin was administered at higher than recommended doses in combination with other ototoxic agents (eg, aminoglycosides). Loss of vision (reversible) has been reported with higher than recommended doses. Peripheral neuropathy occurs infrequently, the incidence of peripheral neuropathy is increased patients >65 years of age and those who have previously received cisplatin treatment. Patients >65 years of age are more likely to develop severe thrombocytopenia. **[U.S. Boxed Warning]: Vomiting may occur;** may be severe in patients who have received prior emetogenic therapy. **[U.S. Boxed Warning]: Should be administered under the supervision of an experienced cancer chemotherapy physician.**

Adverse Reactions Percentages reported with single-agent therapy.

>10%:
- Central nervous system: Pain (23%)
- Endocrine & metabolic: Hyponatremia (29% to 47%), hypomagnesemia (29% to 43%), hypocalcemia (22% to 31%), hypokalemia (20% to 28%)
- Gastrointestinal: Vomiting (65% to 81%), abdominal pain (17%), nausea (without vomiting: 10% to 15%)
- Hematologic: Myelosuppression (dose related and dose limiting; nadir at ~21 days; recovery by ~28 days), anemia (71% to 90%; grades 3/4: 21%), leukopenia (85%; grades 3/4: 15% to 26%), neutropenia (67%; grades 3/4: 16% to 21%), thrombocytopenia (62%; grades 3/4: 25% to 35%)
- Hepatic: Alkaline phosphatase increased (24% to 37%), AST increased (15% to 19%)
- Neuromuscular & skeletal: Weakness (11%)
- Renal: Creatinine clearance decreased (27%), BUN increased (14% to 22%)
- Miscellaneous: Hypersensitivity/allergic reaction (2% to 16%)

1% to 10%:
- Central nervous system: Neurotoxicity (5%)
- Dermatologic: Alopecia (2% to 3%)
- Gastrointestinal: Constipation (6%), diarrhea (6%), stomatitis/mucositis (1%), taste dysgeusia (1%)
- Hematologic: Bleeding (5%), hemorrhagic complications (5%)
- Hepatic: Bilirubin increased (5%)
- Neuromuscular & skeletal: Peripheral neuropathy (4% to 6%)
- Ocular: Visual disturbance (1%)
- Otic: Ototoxicity (1%)
- Renal: Creatinine increased (6% to 10%)
- Miscellaneous: Infection (5%)

<1% (Limited to important or life-threatening): Anaphylactic reaction, bronchospasm, cardiac failure, cerebrovascular accident, dehydration, embolism, erythema, hemolytic anemia (acute), hemolytic uremic syndrome (HUS), hyper-/hypotension, injection site reactions (pain, redness, swelling), limb ischemia (acute), necrosis (associated with extravasation), neutropenic fever, pruritus, rash, secondary malignancies, urticaria, vision loss

Drug Interactions

Metabolism/Transport Effects None known.

Avoid Concomitant Use

Avoid concomitant use of CARBOplatin with any of the following: BCG; CloZAPine; Natalizumab; Pimecrolimus; SORAfenib; Tacrolimus (Topical); Vaccines (Live)

Increased Effect/Toxicity

CARBOplatin may increase the levels/effects of: Bexarotene; Bexarotene (Systemic); CloZAPine; Leflunomide; Natalizumab; Taxane Derivatives; Topotecan; Vaccines (Live)

The levels/effects of CARBOplatin may be increased by: Aminoglycosides; Denosumab; Pimecrolimus; Roflumilast; SORAfenib; Tacrolimus (Topical); Trastuzumab

Decreased Effect

CARBOplatin may decrease the levels/effects of: BCG; Coccidioidin Skin Test; Sipuleucel-T; Vaccines (Inactivated); Vaccines (Live)

The levels/effects of CARBOplatin may be decreased by: Echinacea

Ethanol/Nutrition/Herb Interactions Herb/Nutraceutical: Avoid black cohosh, dong quai in estrogen-dependent tumors.

Stability Store intact vials at room temperature of 25°C (77°F); excursions permitted to 15°C to 30°C (59°F to 86°F). Protect from light. Further dilution to a concentration as low as 0.5 mg/mL is stable at room temperature (25°C) for 8 hours in NS; stable at room temperature or under refrigeration for at least 9 days in D_5W, although the manufacturer states to use within 8 hours due to lack of preservative. Use appropriate precautions for handling and disposal.

Powder for reconstitution: Reconstitute powder to yield a final concentration of 10 mg/mL which is stable for 5 days at room temperature (25°C). Reconstituted carboplatin 10 mg/mL should be further diluted to a final concentration of 0.5-2 mg/mL with D_5W or NS for administration.

Solution for injection: Multidose vials are stable for up to 14 days after opening when stored at room temperature.

Mechanism of Action Carboplatin is a platinum compound alkylating agent which covalently binds to DNA; interferes with the function of DNA by producing interstrand DNA cross-links

Pharmacodynamics/Kinetics

Distribution: V_d: 16 L (based on a dose of 300-500 mg/m^2); into liver, kidney, skin, and tumor tissue

Protein binding: Carboplatin: 0%; Platinum (from carboplatin): Irreversibly binds to plasma proteins

Metabolism: Minimally hepatic to aquated and hydroxylated compounds
Half-life elimination: Cl_{cr} >60 mL/minute: Carboplatin: 2.6-5.9 hours (based on a dose of 300-500 mg/m^2); Platinum (from carboplatin): ≥5 days
Excretion: Urine (~70% as carboplatin within 24 hours; 3% to 5% as platinum within 1-4 days)

Dosage Details concerning dosing in combination regimens should also be consulted. **Note:** Doses for adults are commonly calculated by the target AUC using the Calvert formula, where **Total dose (mg) = Target AUC x (GFR + 25)**. If estimating glomerular filtration rate (GFR) instead of a measured GFR, the Food and Drug Administration (FDA) recommends that clinicians consider capping estimated GFR at a maximum of 125 mL/minute to avoid potential toxicity.

Children: I.V.:
Glioma (unlabeled use): 175 mg/m^2 weekly for 4 weeks every 6 weeks, with a 2-week recovery period between courses (in combination with vincristine) (Packer, 1997)
Sarcomas: Ewing's sarcoma, osteosarcoma (unlabeled uses): 400 mg/m^2/day for 2 days every 21 days (in combination with ifosfamide and etoposide) (van Winkle, 2005)

Adults: I.V.:
Ovarian cancer, advanced: 360 mg/m^2 every 4 weeks (as a single agent) **or** 300 mg/m^2 every 4 weeks (in combination with cyclophosphamide) **or** Target AUC 4-6 (single agent; in previously-treated patients)
Unlabeled dosing: Target AUC 5-7.5 every 3 weeks (in combination with paclitaxel) (Ozols, 2003; Parmar, 2003)
Bladder cancer (unlabeled use): Target AUC 5 every 3 weeks (in combination with gemcitabine and paclitaxel) (Hainsworth, 2005) **or** Target AUC 5 every 3 weeks (in combination with gemcitabine) (Bamias, 2006) **or** Target AUC 6 every 3 weeks (in combination with paclitaxel) (Vaughn, 2002)
Breast cancer, metastatic (unlabeled use): Target AUC 6 every 3 weeks (in combination with trastuzumab and paclitaxel) (Robert, 2006) **or** Target AUC 6 every 3 weeks (in combination with trastuzumab and docetaxel) (Pegram, 2004)
Cervical cancer, recurrent or metastatic (unlabeled use): Target AUC 5 every 3 weeks (in combination with paclitaxel) (Pectasides, 2009) **or** Target AUC 5-6 every 4 weeks (in combination with paclitaxel) (Tinker, 2005) **or** 400 mg/m^2 every 28 days (as a single agent) (Weiss, 1990)
Endometrial cancer (unlabeled use): Target AUC 5 every 3 weeks (in combination with paclitaxel) (Pectasides, 2008) **or** Target AUC 2 on days 1, 8, and 15 every 28 days (in combination with paclitaxel) (Secord, 2007)
Esophageal cancer (unlabeled use): Target AUC 2 on days 1, 8, 15, 22, and 29 for 1 cycle (in combination with paclitaxel) (van Meerten, 2006) **or** Target AUC 5 every 3 weeks (in combination with paclitaxel) (El-Rayes, 2004)
Head and neck cancer (unlabeled use): Target AUC 5 every 3 weeks (in combination with cetuximab) (Chan, 2005) **or** Target AUC 5 every 3 weeks (in combination with cetuximab and fluorouracil) (Vermorken, 2008) **or** 300 mg/m^2 every 4 weeks (in combination with fluorouracil) (Forastiere, 1992) **or** Target AUC 6 every 3 weeks (in combination with paclitaxel) (Clark, 2001)
Hodgkin's lymphoma, relapsed or refractory (unlabeled use): Target AUC 5 (maximum dose 800 mg) for 2 cycles (in combination with ifosfamide and etoposide) (Moskowitz, 2001)
Malignant pleural mesothelioma (unlabeled use): Target AUC 5 every 3 weeks (in combination with pemetrexed) (Castagneto, 2008; Ceresoli, 2006)
Melanoma, advanced or metastatic (unlabeled use): Target AUC 2 on days 1, 8, and 15 every 4 weeks (in combination with paclitaxel) (Rao, 2006)
Non-Hodgkin's lymphomas, relapsed or refractory (unlabeled use): Target AUC 5 (maximum dose 800 mg) per cycle for 3 cycles (in combination with rituximab, ifosfamide and etoposide) (Kewalramani, 2004)
Nonsmall cell lung cancer (unlabeled use): Target AUC 6 every 3 weeks (in combination with paclitaxel) (Schiller, 2002; Strauss, 2008) **or** Target AUC 6 every 3 weeks (in combination with bevacizumab and paclitaxel) (Sandler, 2006) **or** in combination with radiation therapy and paclitaxel (Belani, 2005):
Target AUC 6 every 3 weeks for 2 cycles **or**
Target AUC 6 every 3 weeks for 2 cycles; then target AUC 2 weekly for 7 weeks **or**
Target AUC 2 every week for 7 weeks; then target AUC 6 every 3 weeks for 2 cycles
Sarcomas: Ewing's sarcoma, osteosarcoma (unlabeled uses): 400 mg/m^2/day for 2 days every 21 days (in combination with ifosfamide and etoposide) (van Winkle, 2005)
Small cell lung cancer (unlabeled use): Target AUC 6 every 3 weeks (in combination with etoposide) (Skarlos, 2001) **or** Target AUC 5 every 3 weeks (in combination with irinotecan) (Hermes, 2008) **or** Target AUC 5 every 28 days (in combination with irinotecan) (Schmittel, 2006)
Thymic malignancies (unlabeled use): Target AUC 5 every 3 weeks (in combination with paclitaxel) (Lemma, 2008)
Unknown primary adenocarcinoma (unlabeled use): Target AUC 6 every 3 weeks (in combination with paclitaxel) (Briasoulis, 2000) **or** Target AUC 6 every 3 weeks (in combination with docetaxel) (Greco, 2000) **or** Target AUC 6 every 3 weeks (in combination with paclitaxel and etoposide) (Hainsworth, 2006) **or** Target AUC 5 every 3 weeks (in combination with paclitaxel and gemcitabine) (Greco, 2002)

Elderly: The Calvert formula should be used to calculate dosing for elderly patients.

Dosage adjustment for toxicity: Platelets <50,000 cells/mm^3 or ANC <500 cells/mm^3: Administer 75% of dose

Dosing adjustment in renal impairment: Note: Dose determination with Calvert formula uses GFR and, therefore, inherently adjusts for renal dysfunction.
The FDA-approved labeling recommends the following dosage adjustment guidelines for single-agent therapy:
Baseline Cl_{cr} 41-59 mL/minute: Initiate at 250 mg/m^2 and adjust subsequent doses based on bone marrow toxicity
Baseline Cl_{cr} 16-40 mL/minute: Initiate at 200 mg/m^2 and adjust subsequent doses based on bone marrow toxicity
Baseline Cl_{cr} ≤15 mL/minute: No guidelines are available.
The following dosage adjustments have been used by some clinicians (Aronoff, 2007): Adults (for dosing based on mg/m^2):
Hemodialysis: Administer 50% of dose
Continuous ambulatory peritoneal dialysis (CAPD): Administer 25% of dose
Continuous renal replacement therapy (CRRT): 200 mg/m^2

Dosing adjustment in hepatic impairment: Minimal hepatic metabolism; dosage adjustment may not be needed. No specific dosage adjustment guidelines are available.

Administration Usually infused over 15-60 minutes, although some protocols may require infusions up to 24 hours. When administered as sequential infusions, taxane derivatives (docetaxel, paclitaxel) should be administered before platinum derivatives to limit myelosuppression and to enhance efficacy.

Monitoring Parameters CBC (with differential and platelet count), serum electrolytes, serum creatinine and BUN, creatinine clearance, liver function tests

Dosage Forms Excipient information presented when available (limited, particularly for generics); consult specific product labeling. [DSC] = Discontinued product

Injection, powder for reconstitution: 50 mg [DSC], 150 mg [DSC], 450 mg [DSC]

Injection, solution: 10 mg/mL (5 mL, 15 mL, 45 mL, 60 mL)

Injection, solution [preservative free]: 10 mg/mL (5 mL, 15 mL, 45 mL, 60 mL)

◆ **Carboplatin Injection (Can)** *see* CARBOplatin *on page 287*

◆ **Carboprost** *see* Carboprost Tromethamine *on page 290*

Carboprost Tromethamine

(KAR boe prost tro METH a meen)

Brand Names: U.S. Hemabate®

Brand Names: Canada Hemabate®

Index Terms Carboprost; Prostaglandin F_2

Pharmacologic Category Abortifacient; Prostaglandin

Use Termination of pregnancy; treatment of refractory postpartum uterine bleeding

Unlabeled Use Hemorrhagic cystitis

Pregnancy Risk Factor C

Pregnancy Considerations Teratogenic effects were not observed in animal studies. Carboprost tromethamine is not considered feticidal, but is used to terminate pregnancy due to its ability to stimulate uterine contractions. Use is not indicated if the fetus has reached a stage of viability *in utero*. Complete abortion may not be induced in ~20% of cases.

Lactation Excretion in breast milk unknown

Contraindications Hypersensitivity to carboprost tromethamine or any component of the formulation; acute pelvic inflammatory disease; active cardiac, pulmonary, renal, or hepatic dysfunction

Warnings/Precautions [U.S. Boxed Warning] Potent oxytocic agent; use with strict adherence to recommended dosing. Immediate intensive care and acute surgical facilities must be available. Transient pyrexia and increased blood pressure may be observed with treatment. Use caution with history of asthma; hypotension or hypertension; cardiovascular, adrenal, renal, or hepatic disease; anemia; jaundice; diabetes; epilepsy; or compromised uteri. Concomitant use of antiemetic and antidiarrheal agents is recommended to decrease incidence of GI side effects. Safety and efficacy have not been established in pediatric patients.

Adverse Reactions Frequency not defined. Effects due to increased smooth muscle contractility are most common.

Cardiovascular: Chest pain, flushing, hypertension, syncope, palpitation, tachycardia, tightness of chest

Central nervous system: Anxiety, chills/shivering, dizziness, drowsiness, dystonia, faintness, headache, lethargy, lightheadedness, nervousness, sleep disturbance, temperature elevation (may be drug induced or due to postabortion endometritis), vasovagal syndrome, vertigo

Dermatologic: Rash

Endocrine & metabolic: Breast tenderness, dysmenorrhea-like pain, endometritis, hot flashes, thyroid storm

Gastrointestinal: Choking sensation, diarrhea (~2/3 patients), dry throat, epigastric pain, gagging/retching, hematemesis, nausea (~1/3 patients), taste alteration, thirst, throat fullness, vomiting (~2/3 patients), xerostomia

Genitourinary: Perforated uterus, posterior cervical perforation, urinary tract infection, uterine bleeding (excessive), uterine rupture, uterine sacculation

Local: Injection site pain

Neuromuscular & skeletal: Backache, leg cramps, muscular pain, paresthesia, torticollis, weakness

Ocular: Blurred vision, eye pain, eyelid twitching

Otic: Tinnitus

Respiratory: Asthma, cough, bronchospasm, dyspnea, epistaxis, hyperventilation, pulmonary edema, respiratory distress, upper respiratory tract infection, wheezing

Miscellaneous: Diaphoresis, hiccups, retained placental fragment, septic shock

Drug Interactions

Metabolism/Transport Effects None known.

Avoid Concomitant Use There are no known interactions where it is recommended to avoid concomitant use.

Increased Effect/Toxicity There are no known significant interactions involving an increase in effect.

Decreased Effect There are no known significant interactions involving a decrease in effect.

Stability Store under refrigeration at 2°C to 8°C (36°F to 46°F).

Bladder irrigation: Dilute immediately prior to administration in NS; stability unknown.

Mechanism of Action Carboprost tromethamine is a prostaglandin similar to prostaglandin F_2 alpha (dinoprost) except for the addition of a methyl group at the C-15 position. This substitution produces longer duration of activity than dinoprost; carboprost stimulates uterine contractility which usually results in expulsion of the products of conception and is used to induce abortion between 13-20 weeks of pregnancy. Hemostasis at the placentation site is achieved through the myometrial contractions produced by carboprost.

Pharmacodynamics/Kinetics Excretion: Urine

Dosage I.M.: Adults:

Abortion: Initial: 250 mcg, then 250 mcg at 1.5- to 3.5-hour intervals, depending on uterine response; a 500 mcg dose may be given if uterine response is not adequate after several 250 mcg doses; do not exceed 12 mg total dose or continuous administration for >2 days

Refractory postpartum uterine bleeding: Initial: 250 mcg; if needed, may repeat at 15- to 90-minute intervals; maximum total dose: 2 mg (8 doses)

Bladder irrigation for hemorrhagic cystitis (unlabeled use): [0.1-1.0 mg/dL as solution] 50 mL instilled into bladder 4 times/day for 1 hour

Administration Do not inject I.V.; may result in bronchospasm, hypertension, vomiting, or anaphylaxis. Administer deep I.M.; rotate site if repeat injections are required.

Dosage Forms Excipient information presented when available (limited, particularly for generics); consult specific product labeling.

Injection, solution [strength expressed as base]:

Hemabate®: 250 mcg/mL (1 mL) [contains benzyl alcohol]

◆ **Carboxypeptidase-G2** *see* Glucarpidase *on page 798*

◆ **Cardene® I.V.** *see* NiCARdipine *on page 1198*

◆ **Cardene® SR** *see* NiCARdipine *on page 1198*

◆ **Cardizem®** *see* Diltiazem *on page 510*

◆ **Cardizem® CD** *see* Diltiazem *on page 510*

◆ **Cardizem® LA** *see* Diltiazem *on page 510*

◆ **Cardura®** *see* Doxazosin *on page 548*

◆ **Cardura-1™ (Can)** *see* Doxazosin *on page 548*

◆ **Cardura-2™ (Can)** *see* Doxazosin *on page 548*

◆ **Cardura-4™ (Can)** *see* Doxazosin *on page 548*
◆ **Cardura® XL** *see* Doxazosin *on page 548*

Carglumic Acid (kar GLU mik AS id)

Brand Names: U.S. Carbaglu®

Index Terms N-Carbamoyl-L-Glutamic Acid; N-Carbamyl-glutamate

Pharmacologic Category Antidote; Metabolic Alkalosis Agent; Urea Cycle Disorder (UCD) Treatment Agent

Use Adjunctive treatment of acute hyperammonemia and maintenance therapy of chronic hyperammonemia due to the deficiency of the hepatic enzyme N-acetylglutamate synthase (NAGS)

Pregnancy Risk Factor C

Pregnancy Considerations Teratogenic effects were reported in some animal reproductive studies. There are no adequate and well-controlled studies in pregnant women. However, due to the potential for irreversible fetal neurologic damage for untreated NAGS deficiency, women with this condition should remain on treatment throughout pregnancy.

Lactation Excretion in breast milk is unknown/not recommended

Prescribing and Access Restrictions Carbaglu® is not available through pharmaceutical wholesalers or retail pharmacies, but only through direct shipping from the Accredo specialty pharmacy. Prescribers must contact Accredo Health Group at 888-454-8860 or refer to www.accredo.com to initiate patients on this product.

Contraindications There are no contraindications listed in the manufacturers labeling.

Warnings/Precautions With acute episodes of hyperammonemia, protein restriction and a hypercaloric diet are recommended until normalization of plasma ammonia concentrations.

Adverse Reactions

>10%:

- Central nervous system: Fever (17%), headache (13%)
- Gastrointestinal: Vomiting (26%), abdominal pain (17%), diarrhea (13%)
- Hematologic: Anemia (13%)
- Otic: Ear infection (13%)
- Respiratory: Tonsillitis (17%), nasopharyngitis (13%)
- Miscellaneous: Infections (13%)

1% to 10%:

- Central nervous system: Somnolence (9%)
- Dermatologic: Hyperhidrosis (9%), rash (9%)
- Gastrointestinal: Anorexia (9%), dysgeusia (9%), weight loss (9%)
- Neuromuscular & skeletal: Weakness (9%)
- Respiratory: Pneumonia (9%)
- Miscellaneous: Influenza (9%)

Drug Interactions

Metabolism/Transport Effects None known.

Avoid Concomitant Use There are no known interactions where it is recommended to avoid concomitant use.

Increased Effect/Toxicity There are no known significant interactions involving an increase in effect.

Decreased Effect There are no known significant interactions involving a decrease in effect.

Stability Store at 2°C to 8°C (36°F to 46°F). After opening, do not refrigerate or store above 30°C (86°F). Discard 1 month after opening.

Mechanism of Action N-acetylglutamate synthase (NAGS) is a mitochondrial enzyme which produces N-acetylglutamate (NAG). NAG is a required allosteric activator of the hepatic mitochondrial enzyme, carbamoyl phosphate synthetase 1 (CPS 1), which converts ammonia into urea in the first step of the urea cycle. In NAGS-deficient patients, carglumic acid serves as a structural analogue to NAG.

Pharmacodynamics/Kinetics

Distribution: V_d: ~2657 L
Metabolism: Via intestinal flora to carbon dioxide
Half-life: elimination: 5.6 hours
Time to peak: 3 hours
Excretion: Feces (60% as unchanged drug); urine (9% as unchanged drug)

Dosage Oral: Infants, Children, and Adults:

Acute hyperammonemia: 100-250 mg/kg/day given in 2 or 4 divided doses; titrate to age-appropriate plasma ammonia levels. Concomitant adjunctive ammonia-lowering therapy recommended.

Chronic hyperammonemia: Usual dose: <100 mg/kg/day given in 2 or 4 divided doses; titrate to age-appropriate plasma ammonia levels

Dietary Considerations Take immediately prior to meals.

Administration Administer immediately prior to meals.

Oral: Carglumic acid tablets should not be crushed or swallowed whole. Each 200 mg tablet should be dispersed in at least 2.5 mL of water (no other foods/liquids) and taken immediately. Tablets do not dissolve completely, and some particles may remain; container should be rinsed with water and swallowed immediately.

Nasogastric tube: Disperse each 200 mg tablet in 2.5 mL of water and shake gently. Immediately administer through a nasogastric tube, followed by flush with additional water to clear the tube. Carglumic acid tablets should not be mixed with any other foods or liquids other than water.

Oral syringe: Disperse each 200 mg tablet in 2.5 mL of water to yield a concentration of 80 mg/mL (shake gently in container). Appropriate volume of dispersion should be drawn up in an oral syringe and administered immediately (discard unused dispersion). Oral syringe should be refilled with a minimum of 1-2 mL of water and administered immediately.

Monitoring Parameters Blood ammonia; monitor for physical signs/symptoms of hyperammonemia (eg, lethargy, ataxia, confusion, vomiting, seizures, and memory impairment)

Dosage Forms Excipient information presented when available (limited, particularly for generics); consult specific product labeling.

Tablet for solution, oral:
Carbaglu®: 200 mg [scored]

◆ **Carimune® NF** *see* Immune Globulin *on page 880*
◆ **Carisoprodate** *see* Carisoprodol *on page 291*

Carisoprodol (kar eye soe PROE dole)

Brand Names: U.S. Soma®

Index Terms Carisoprodate; Isobamate

Pharmacologic Category Skeletal Muscle Relaxant

Additional Appendix Information

Beers Criteria – Potentially Inappropriate Medications for Geriatrics *on page 1973*

Use Short-term (2-3 weeks) treatment of acute musculoskeletal pain

Pregnancy Risk Factor C

Pregnancy Considerations Animal data suggests that carisoprodol crosses placenta and adverse events have been observed in animal studies. Limited postmarketing data with meprobamate (the active metabolite) demonstrate a possible risk for congenital malformations. Use only if benefit outweighs the risk.

Lactation Enters breast milk/use caution

Contraindications Hypersensitivity to carisoprodol, meprobamate, or any component of the formulation; acute intermittent porphyria

Warnings/Precautions Can cause CNS depression, which may impair physical or mental abilities. Patients must be cautioned about performing tasks which require mental alertness (eg, operating machinery or driving); postmarketing reports of motor vehicle accidents have been associated with use. Effects with other CNS-depressant drugs or ethanol may be potentiated. Use with caution in patients with hepatic/renal dysfunction. Tolerance or drug dependence may result from extended use. Limit use to 2-3 weeks; use caution in patients who may be prone to addiction. May precipitate withdrawal after abrupt cessation of prolonged use.

Idiosyncratic reactions and/or severe allergic reactions may occur. Idiosyncratic reactions occur following the initial dose and may include severe weakness, transient quadriplegia, euphoria, or vision loss (temporary). Has been associated (rarely) with seizures in patients with and without seizure history. Carisoprodol should be used with caution in patients who are poor CYP2C19 metabolizers; poor metabolizers have been shown to have a fourfold increase in exposure to carisoprodol and a 50% reduced exposure to the metabolite meprobamate compared to normal metabolizers. This class of medication is poorly tolerated by the elderly due to anticholinergic effects, sedation, and weakness. Efficacy is questionable at dosages tolerated by elderly patients (Beers Criteria).

Adverse Reactions

>10%: Central nervous system: Drowsiness (13% to 17%)

1% to 10%: Central nervous system: Dizziness (7% to 8%), headache (3% to 5%)

Postmarketing and/or case reports: Agitation, anaphylaxis, angioedema, asthma exacerbation, ataxia, burning eyes, depression, dependence, dermatitis (allergic), dyspnea, epigastric pain, eosinophilia, erythema multiforme, fixed drug eruption, flushing of face, headache, hiccups, hypersensitivity reactions, hypotension (postural), idiosyncratic reaction (symptoms may include agitation, ataxia, confusion, diplopia, disorientation, dysarthria, euphoria, extreme weakness, mydriasis, temporary vision loss, and/or transient quadriplegia); insomnia, irritability, leukopenia, nausea, pancytopenia, paradoxical CNS stimulation, pruritus, rash, seizure, syncope, tachycardia, tremor, urticaria, vertigo, vomiting, weakness, withdrawal syndrome (abdominal cramps, headache, insomnia, nausea, seizure)

Drug Interactions

Metabolism/Transport Effects Substrate of CYP2C19 (major); **Note:** Assignment of Major/Minor substrate status based on clinically relevant drug interaction potential

Avoid Concomitant Use There are no known interactions where it is recommended to avoid concomitant use.

Increased Effect/Toxicity

Carisoprodol may increase the levels/effects of: Alcohol (Ethyl); CNS Depressants; Methotrimeprazine; Selective Serotonin Reuptake Inhibitors

The levels/effects of Carisoprodol may be increased by: CYP2C19 Inhibitors (Moderate); CYP2C19 Inhibitors (Strong); Droperidol; HydrOXYzine; Methotrimeprazine

Decreased Effect

The levels/effects of Carisoprodol may be decreased by: CYP2C19 Inducers (Strong)

Ethanol/Nutrition/Herb Interactions Ethanol: May increase CNS depression; monitor for increased effects with coadministration. Caution patients about effects.

Stability Store at controlled room temperature of 20°C to 25°C (68°F to 77°F).

Mechanism of Action Precise mechanism is not yet clear, but many effects have been ascribed to its central depressant actions. In animals, carisoprodol blocks interneuronal activity and depresses polysynaptic neuron transmission in the spinal cord and reticular formation of the brain. It is also metabolized to meprobamate, which has anxiolytic and sedative effects.

Pharmacodynamics/Kinetics

Onset of action: ~30 minutes

Duration: 4-6 hours

Metabolism: Hepatic, via CYP2C19 to active metabolite (meprobamate)

Half-life elimination: ~2 hours; Meprobamate: 10 hours

Time to peak, plasma: 1.5-2 hours

Excretion: Urine, as metabolite

Dosage Note: Carisoprodol should only be used for short periods (2-3 weeks) due to lack of evidence of effectiveness with prolonged use.

Oral: Children ≥16 years and Adults: 250-350 mg 3 times/day and at bedtime

Dosing adjustment in renal impairment: Use in renal impairment has not been studied; use with caution

Dialysis: Removed by hemo- and peritoneal dialysis

Dosing adjustment in hepatic impairment: Use in hepatic impairment has not been studied; use with caution

Dietary Considerations May be taken with or without food.

Administration Administer with or without food.

Monitoring Parameters CNS effects (eg, mental status, excessive drowsiness); relief of pain and/or muscle spasm; signs of drug abuse in addiction-prone individuals

Dosage Forms Excipient information presented when available (limited, particularly for generics); consult specific product labeling.

Tablet, oral: 350 mg

Soma®: 250 mg, 350 mg

Controlled Substance C-IV

Carisoprodol and Aspirin

(kar eye soe PROE dole & AS pir in)

Brand Names: U.S. Soma® Compound

Index Terms Aspirin and Carisoprodol

Pharmacologic Category Skeletal Muscle Relaxant

Use Relief of discomfort associated with acute, painful skeletal muscle conditions

Pregnancy Risk Factor D

Dosage Oral:

Children ≥16 years and Adults: Acute skeletal muscle pain: 1-2 tablets 4 times/day for 2-3 weeks (maximum: 8 tablets/24 hours)

Elderly: Avoid use in the elderly due to risk of orthostatic hypotension and CNS depression

Dosing adjustment in renal impairment: Use in renal impairment has not been studied; use with caution

Dosing adjustment in hepatic impairment: Use in hepatic impairment has not been studied; use with caution

Additional Information Complete prescribing information for this medication should be consulted for additional detail.

Dosage Forms Excipient information presented when available (limited, particularly for generics); consult specific product labeling.

Tablet: Carisoprodol 200 mg and aspirin 325 mg

Soma® Compound: Carisoprodol 200 mg and aspirin 325 mg

Controlled Substance C-IV

Carisoprodol, Aspirin, and Codeine

(kar eye soe PROE dole, AS pir in, and KOE deen)

Index Terms Aspirin, Carisoprodol, and Codeine; Codeine, Aspirin, and Carisoprodol; Soma Compound w/Codeine

Pharmacologic Category Skeletal Muscle Relaxant

Use Skeletal muscle relaxant

Pregnancy Risk Factor D

Dosage Oral:

Adults: 1 or 2 tablets 4 times/day (maximum: 8 tablets/day); treatment should be temporary (2-3 weeks)

Elderly: Avoid or use with caution in the elderly (>65 years of age); adverse effects (eg, orthostatic hypotension and CNS depression) may be potentiated.

Additional Information Complete prescribing information for this medication should be consulted for additional detail.

Dosage Forms Excipient information presented when available (limited, particularly for generics); consult specific product labeling. [DSC] = Discontinued product

Tablet: Carisoprodol 200 mg, aspirin 325 mg, and codeine phosphate 16 mg

Controlled Substance C-III

- ◆ **Carmol® 10 [OTC]** *see* Urea *on page 1749*
- ◆ **Carmol® 20 [OTC]** *see* Urea *on page 1749*
- ◆ **Carmol® 40** *see* Urea *on page 1749*
- ◆ **Carmol® Deep Cleansing [OTC]** *see* Urea *on page 1749*
- ◆ **Carmol-HC®** *see* Urea and Hydrocortisone *on page 1750*
- ◆ **Carmol® Scalp Treatment** *see* Sulfacetamide (Topical) *on page 1599*

Carmustine (kar MUS teen)

Brand Names: U.S. BiCNU®; Gliadel®

Brand Names: Canada BiCNU®; Gliadel Wafer®

Index Terms BCNU; bis(chloroethyl) nitrosourea; bis-chloronitrosourea; Carmustine Polymer Wafer; Carmustinum; WR-139021

Pharmacologic Category Antineoplastic Agent; Antineoplastic Agent, Alkylating Agent; Antineoplastic Agent, Alkylating Agent (Nitrosourea)

Use

Injection: Treatment of brain tumors (glioblastoma, brainstem glioma, medulloblastoma, astrocytoma, ependymoma, and metastatic brain tumors), multiple myeloma, Hodgkin's lymphoma (relapsed or refractory), non-Hodgkin's lymphomas (relapsed or refractory)

Wafer (implant): Adjunct to surgery in patients with recurrent glioblastoma multiforme; adjunct to surgery and radiation in patients with newly-diagnosed high-grade malignant glioma

Unlabeled Use Treatment of mycosis fungoides (topical)

Pregnancy Risk Factor D

Pregnancy Considerations Teratogenicity and embryotoxicity have been demonstrated in animal studies. Carmustine can cause fetal harm if administered to a pregnant woman. There are no adequate and well-controlled studies in pregnant women. Women of childbearing potential should avoid becoming pregnant while on treatment.

Lactation Excretion in breast milk unknown/not recommended

Contraindications Hypersensitivity to carmustine or any component of the formulation

Warnings/Precautions Hazardous agent - use appropriate precautions for handling and disposal.

[U.S. Boxed Warning]: Injection: Bone marrow suppression (primarily thrombocytopenia and leukopenia) is the major carmustine toxicity; generally is delayed. Monitor blood counts weekly for at least 6 weeks after administration. Myelosuppression is cumulative. When given at the FDA-approved doses, treatment should not be administered less than 6 weeks apart. Consider nadir blood counts from prior dose for dosage adjustment. May cause bleeding (due to thrombocytopenia) or infections (due to neutropenia); monitor closely. Patients must have platelet counts >100,000/mm^3 and leukocytes >4000/mm^3 for a repeat dose. Anemia may occur (less common and less severe than leukopenia or thrombocytopenia). Long-term use is associated with the development of secondary malignancies (acute leukemias and bone marrow dysplasias).

[U.S. Boxed Warnings]: Injection: Dose-related pulmonary toxicity may occur; patients receiving cumulative doses >1400 mg/m^2 are at higher risk. Delayed onset of pulmonary fibrosis (may be fatal) has occurred in children up to 17 years after treatment; this occurred in ages 1-16 for the treatment of intracranial tumors; cumulative doses ranged from 770-1800 mg/m^2 (in combination with cranial radiotherapy). Pulmonary toxicity is characterized by pulmonary infiltrates and/or fibrosis and has been reported from 9 days to 43 months after nitrosourea treatment (including carmustine). Although pulmonary toxicity generally occurs in patients who have received prolonged treatment, pulmonary fibrosis has been reported with cumulative doses <1400 mg/m^2. In addition to high cumulative doses, other risk factors for pulmonary toxicity include history of lung disease and baseline predicted forced vital capacity (FVC) or carbon monoxide diffusing capacity (DL_{CO}) <70%. Baseline and periodic pulmonary function tests are recommended. For high-dose treatment (transplant; unlabeled dose), acute lung injury may occur ~1-3 months post transplant; advise patients to contact their transplant physician for dyspnea, cough, or fever; interstitial pneumonia may be managed with a course of corticosteroids. Children are at higher risk for delayed pulmonary toxicity.

Injection site burning and local tissue reactions, including swelling, pain, erythema, and necrosis have been reported. Monitor infusion site closely for infiltration or injection site reactions. Reversible increases in transaminases, bilirubin and alkaline phosphatase have been reported (rare); monitor liver function tests periodically during treatment. Renal failure, progressive azotemia, and decreased kidney size have been reported in patients who have received large cumulative doses or prolonged treatment (renal toxicity has also been reported in patients who have received lower cumulative doses); monitor renal function tests periodically during treatment. Unlabeled administration (intraarterial intracarotid route) has been associated with ocular toxicity. Consider initiating treatment at the lower end of the dose range in the elderly. Diluent contains ethanol. With wafer implantation, monitor closely for known craniotomy-related complications (seizure, intracranial infection, abnormal wound healing, brain edema); intracerebral mass effect (unresponsive to corticosteroids) has been reported; may lead to brain herniation; avoid communication between the resection cavity and the ventricular system to prevent wafer migration; communications larger than the wafer should be closed prior to implantation; wafer migration may cause obstructive hydrocephalus. **[U.S. Boxed Warning]: Injection: Should be administered under the supervision of an experienced cancer chemotherapy physician.**

Adverse Reactions

I.V.: Frequency not defined:

Cardiovascular: Arrhythmia (with high doses), chest pain, flushing (with rapid infusion), hypotension, tachycardia

Central nervous system: Ataxia, dizziness

Central nervous system: Ethanol intoxication (with high doses), headache

Dermatologic: Hyperpigmentation/skin burning (after skin contact)

Gastrointestinal: Nausea (common; dose related), vomiting (common; dose related), mucositis (with high doses), toxic enterocolitis (with high doses)

Hematologic: Leukopenia (common; onset: 5-6 weeks; recovery: after 1-2 weeks), thrombocytopenia (common: onset:~4 weeks; recovery: after 1-2 weeks), anemia, neutropenic fever, secondary malignancies (acute leukemia, bone marrow dysplasias)

Hepatic: Alkaline phosphatase increased, bilirubin increased, hepatic sinusoidal obstruction syndrome (SOS; veno-occlusive disease; with high doses), transaminases increased

Local: Injection site reactions (burning, erythema, necrosis, pain, swelling)

Ocular: Conjunctival suffusion (with rapid infusion), neuroretinitis

Renal: Kidney size decreased, progressive azotemia, renal failure

Respiratory: Interstitial pneumonitis (with high doses), pulmonary fibrosis, pulmonary hypoplasia, pulmonary infiltrates

Miscellaneous: Allergic reaction, infection (with high doses)

Wafer:

≥4% (percentages reported only where incidence was greater compared to placebo):

Cardiovascular: Deep thrombophlebitis (10%), facial edema (6%), chest pain (5%)

Central nervous system: Brain edema (4% to 23%), confusion (10% to 23%), depression (16%), headache (15%), somnolence (14%), fever (12%), speech disorder (11%), intracranial hypertension (9%), anxiety (7%), facial paralysis (7%), pain (7%), ataxia (6%), hypesthesia (6%), hallucination (5%), seizure (grand mal 5%), meningitis (4%)

Dermatologic: Abnormal wound healing (14% to 16%), rash (5% to 12%)

Endocrine: Diabetes (5%)

Gastrointestinal: Nausea (8% to 22%), vomiting (8% to 21%), constipation (19%), abdominal pain (8%), diarrhea (5%)

Genitourinary: Urinary tract infection (21%)

Hematologic: Hemorrhage (7%)

Local: Abscess (4% to 8%)

Neuromuscular & skeletal: Weakness (22%), back pain (7%)

<4% (Limited to important or life-threatening): Abnormal thinking, allergic reaction, amnesia, aspiration pneumonia, cerebral hemorrhage, cerebral infarction, coma, cyst formation, diplopia, dizziness, dysphagia, eye pain, fecal incontinence, gastrointestinal hemorrhage, hydrocephalus, hyperglycemia, hyper-/hypotension, hypokalemia, hyponatremia, insomnia, leukocytosis, monoplegia, neck pain, paranoia, peripheral edema, sepsis, thrombocytopenia, urinary incontinence, visual field defect

Drug Interactions

Metabolism/Transport Effects None known.

Avoid Concomitant Use

Avoid concomitant use of Carmustine with any of the following: BCG; CloZAPine; Natalizumab; Pimecrolimus; Tacrolimus (Topical); Vaccines (Live)

Increased Effect/Toxicity

Carmustine may increase the levels/effects of: CloZAPine; Leflunomide; Natalizumab; Vaccines (Live)

The levels/effects of Carmustine may be increased by: Cimetidine; Denosumab; Melphalan; Pimecrolimus; Roflumilast; Tacrolimus (Topical); Trastuzumab

Decreased Effect

Carmustine may decrease the levels/effects of: BCG; Cardiac Glycosides; Coccidioidin Skin Test; Sipuleucel-T; Vaccines (Inactivated); Vaccines (Live)

The levels/effects of Carmustine may be decreased by: Echinacea

Stability

Injection: Store intact vials under refrigeration at 2°C to 8°C (36°F to 46°F); provided diluent may be stored in refrigerator or at room temperature; intact vials are stable for 7 days at room temperature. Reconstitute initially with 3 mL of supplied diluent (dehydrated alcohol injection, USP); then further dilute with SWFI (27 mL), this provides a concentration of 3.3 mg/mL in ethanol 10%; protect from light; further dilute for infusion with D_5W using a non-PVC container. Reconstituted solutions are stable for 24 hours refrigerated (2°C to 8°C) and protected from light. Solutions diluted to a concentration of 0.2 mg/mL in D_5W are stable for 8 hours at room temperature (25°C) in glass or polyolefin containers and protected from light.

Wafer: Store at or below -20°C (-4°F). Unopened foil pouches may be kept at room temperature for up to 6 hours.

Mechanism of Action Interferes with the normal function of DNA and RNA by alkylation and cross-linking the strands of DNA and RNA, and by possible protein modification; may also inhibit enzyme processes by carbamylation of amino acids in protein

Pharmacodynamics/Kinetics

Distribution: 3.3 L/kg; readily crosses blood-brain barrier producing CSF levels >50% of blood plasma levels; highly lipid soluble

Metabolism: Rapidly hepatic; forms active metabolites

Half-life elimination: Biphasic: Initial: 1.4 minutes; Secondary: 20 minutes (active metabolites: plasma half-life of 67 hours)

Excretion: Urine (~60% to 70%) within 96 hours; lungs (6% to 10% as CO_2)

Dosage

I.V.: Adults: Brain tumors, Hodgkin's lymphoma, multiple myeloma, non-Hodgkin's lymphoma (per manufacturer labeling): 150-200 mg/m^2 every 6 weeks or 75-100 mg/m^2/day for 2 days every 6 weeks

Indication-specific dosing: I.V.:

Brain tumor, primary (unlabeled doses):

80 mg/m^2/day for 3 days every 8 weeks for 6 cycles (Brandes, 2004)

200 mg/m^2 every 8 weeks [maximum cumulative dose: 1500 mg/m^2] (Selker, 2002)

Hodgkin's lymphoma, relapsed or refractory (unlabeled dose): Mini-BEAM regimen: 60 mg/m^2 day 1 every 4-6 weeks (in combination with etoposide, cytarabine, and melphalan) (Colwill, 1995; Martin, 2001)

Multiple myeloma, relapsed, refractory (unlabeled dose): VBMCP regimen: 20 mg/m^2 day 1 every 35 days (in combination with vincristine, melphalan, cyclophosphamide, and prednisone) (Kyle, 2006; Oken, 1997)

Stem cell or bone marrow transplant, autologous (unlabeled use):

BEAM regimen: 300 mg/m^2 six days prior to transplant (in combination with etoposide, cytarabine, and melphalan) (Chopra, 1993; Linch, 2010)

CBV regimen: 600 mg/m^2 three days prior to transplant (in combination with cyclophosphamide and etoposide) (Reece, 1991)

Implantation (wafer): Adults: Recurrent glioblastoma multiforme, newly-diagnosed high-grade malignant glioma: 8 wafers placed in the resection cavity (total dose 61.6 mg); should the size and shape not accommodate 8 wafers, the maximum number of wafers allowed (up to 8) should be placed

Topical: Mycosis fungoides, early stage (unlabeled use; Zackheim, 2003):

Ointment (10 mg/100 grams petrolatum): Apply (with gloves) once daily to affected areas

Solution (0.2% solution in alcohol; dilute 5 mL in 60 mL water): Apply (with gloves) once daily to affected areas

Dosing adjustments for hematologic toxicity: Based on nadir counts with previous dose (manufacturer's labeling). I.V.:

If leukocytes >3000/mm^3 and platelets >75,000/mm^3: Administer 100% of dose

If leukocytes 2000-2999/mm^3 or platelets 25,000-74,999/mm^3: Administer 70% of dose

If leukocytes <2000/mm^3 or platelets <25,000/mm^3: Administer 50% of dose

Dosing adjustment in renal impairment: I.V.: The FDA-approved labeling does not contain renal dosing adjustment guidelines. The following dosage adjustments have been used by some clinicians (Kintzel, 1995):

Cl_{cr} 46-60 mL/minute: Administer 80% of dose

Cl_{cr} 31-45 mL/minute: Administer 75% of dose

Cl_{cr} ≤30 mL/minute: Consider use of alternative drug

Dosing adjustment in hepatic impairment: Dosage adjustment may be necessary; however, no specific guidelines are available.

Administration

Injection: Hazardous agent; use appropriate precautions for handling and disposal. Irritant (alcohol-based diluent). Significant absorption to PVC containers; should be prepared in either glass or polyolefin containers. Infuse over 2 hours (infusions <2 hours may lead to injection site pain or burning); infuse through a free-flowing saline or dextrose infusion, or administer through a central catheter to alleviate venous pain/irritation.

High-dose carmustine (transplant dose; unlabeled use): Infuse over a least 2 hours to avoid excessive flushing, agitation, and hypotension; was infused over 1 hour in some trials (Chopra, 1993). **High-dose carmustine may be fatal if not followed by stem cell rescue.** Monitor vital signs frequently during infusion; patients should be supine during infusion and may require the Trendelenburg position, fluid support, and vasopressor support.

Implant: Hazardous agent; use appropriate precautions for handling and disposal; double glove before handling; outer gloves should be discarded as chemotherapy waste after handling wafers. Any wafer or remnant that is removed upon repeat surgery should be discarded as chemotherapy waste. The outer surface of the external foil pouch is not sterile. Open pouch gently; avoid pressure on the wafers to prevent breakage. Wafer that are broken in half may be used, however, wafers broken into more than 2 pieces should be discarded in a biohazard container. Oxidized regenerated cellulose (Surgicel®) may be placed over the wafer to secure; irrigate cavity prior to closure.

Topical (unlabeled use): Hazardous agent; use appropriate precautions for handling and disposal. Apply solution with brush or gauze pads; ointment and solution should be applied while wearing gloves to involved areas only; avoid contact with eyes or mouth (Zackheim, 2003).

Monitoring Parameters CBC with differential and platelet count (weekly for at least 6 weeks after a dose), pulmonary function tests (FVC, DL_{CO}; at baseline and frequently during treatment), liver function (periodically), renal function tests (periodically); monitor blood pressure and vital signs during administration, monitor infusion site for possible infiltration

Wafer: Complications of craniotomy (seizures, intracranial infection, brain edema)

Dosage Forms Excipient information presented when available (limited, particularly for generics); consult specific product labeling.

Injection, powder for reconstitution:

BiCNU®: 100 mg [supplied with diluent]

Wafer, for implantation:

Gliadel®: 7.7 mg (8s)

◆ **Carmustine Polymer Wafer***see* Carmustine *on page 293*

◆ **Carmustinum***see* Carmustine *on page 293*

◆ **Carrington® Antifungal [OTC]***see* Miconazole (Topical) *on page 1126*

◆ **Carter's Little Pills® (Can)***see* Bisacodyl *on page 219*

◆ **Cartia XT®***see* Diltiazem *on page 510*

Carvedilol (KAR ve dil ole)

Brand Names: U.S. Coreg CR®; Coreg®

Brand Names: Canada Apo-Carvedilol®; Coreg®; Dom-Carvedilol; JAMP-Carvedilol; Mylan-Carvedilol; Novo-Carvedilol; PHL-Carvedilol; PMS-Carvedilol; RAN™-Carvedilol; ratio-Carvedilol; ZYM-Carvedilol

Pharmacologic Category Beta Blocker With Alpha-Blocking Activity

Additional Appendix Information

Beta-Blockers *on page 1884*

Heart Failure (Systolic) *on page 1991*

Use Mild-to-severe heart failure of ischemic or cardiomyopathic origin (usually in addition to standard therapy); left ventricular dysfunction following myocardial infarction (MI) (clinically stable with LVEF ≤40%); management of hypertension

Unlabeled Use Angina pectoris

Pregnancy Risk Factor C

Pregnancy Considerations Because adverse events were not observed in animal reproduction studies, carvedilol is classified as pregnancy category C. In a cohort study, an increased risk of cardiovascular defects was observed following maternal use of beta-blockers during pregnancy. Intrauterine growth restriction (IUGR), small placentas, as well as fetal/neonatal bradycardia, hypoglycemia, and/or respiratory depression have been observed following *in utero* exposure to beta-blockers as a class. Adequate facilities for monitoring infants at birth should be available. Untreated chronic maternal hypertension and pre-eclampsia are also associated with adverse events in the fetus, infant, and mother. Carvedilol is not currently recommended for the initial treatment of maternal hypertension during pregnancy.

Lactation Excretion in breast milk unknown/not recommended

Contraindications Serious hypersensitivity to carvedilol or any component of the formulation; decompensated cardiac failure requiring intravenous inotropic therapy; bronchial asthma or related bronchospastic conditions; second- or third-degree AV block, sick sinus syndrome, and severe bradycardia (except in patients with a functioning artificial pacemaker); cardiogenic shock; severe hepatic impairment

Warnings/Precautions Consider pre-existing conditions such as sick sinus syndrome before initiating. Heart failure patients may experience a worsening of renal function (rare); risk factors include ischemic heart disease, diffuse vascular disease, underlying renal dysfunction, and systolic BP <100 mm Hg. Initiate cautiously and monitor for possible deterioration in patient status (eg, symptoms of HF). Worsening heart failure or fluid retention may occur during upward titration; dose reduction or temporary discontinuation may be necessary. Adjustment of other medications (ACE inhibitors and/or diuretics) may also be required. Bradycardia may be observed more frequently in elderly patients (>65 years of age); dosage reductions may be necessary.

Symptomatic hypotension with or without syncope may occur with carvedilol (usually within the first 30 days of therapy); close monitoring of patient is required especially with initial dosing and dosing increases; blood pressure must be lowered at a rate appropriate for the patient's clinical condition. Initiation with a low dose, gradual up-titration, and administration with food may help to decrease the occurrence of hypotension or syncope. Patients should be advised to avoid driving or other hazardous tasks during initiation of therapy due to the risk of syncope. Beta-blocker therapy should not be withdrawn abruptly (particularly in patients with CAD), but gradually tapered to avoid acute tachycardia, hypertension, and/or ischemia. Chronic beta-blocker therapy should not be routinely withdrawn prior to major surgery.

In general, patients with bronchospastic disease should not receive beta-blockers; if used at all, should be used cautiously with close monitoring. May precipitate or aggravate symptoms of arterial insufficiency in patients with PVD and Raynaud's disease; use with caution and monitor for progression of arterial obstruction. Use caution with concurrent use of digoxin, verapamil or diltiazem; bradycardia or heart block can occur. Use with caution in patients receiving inhaled anesthetic agents known to depress myocardial contractility. Use cautiously in patients with diabetes because it can mask prominent hypoglycemic symptoms. In patients with heart failure and diabetes, use of carvedilol may worsen hyperglycemia; may require adjustment of antidiabetic agents. May mask signs of hyperthyroidism (eg, tachycardia); if hyperthyroidism is suspected, carefully manage and monitor; abrupt withdrawal may exacerbate symptoms of hyperthyroidism or precipitate thyroid storm. May induce or exacerbate psoriasis. Use with caution in patients with myasthenia gravis or psychiatric disease (may cause CNS depression). Use with caution in patients with mild-to-moderate hepatic impairment; use is contraindicated in patients with severe impairment. Manufacturer recommends discontinuation of therapy if liver injury occurs (confirmed by laboratory testing). Adequate alpha-blockade is required prior to use of any beta-blocker for patients with untreated pheochromocytoma. Use caution with history of severe anaphylaxis to allergens; patients taking beta-blockers may become more sensitive to repeated challenges. Treatment of anaphylaxis (eg, epinephrine) in patients taking beta-blockers may be ineffective or promote undesirable effects.

Intraoperative floppy iris syndrome has been observed in cataract surgery patients who were on or were previously treated with alpha$_1$-blockers; causality has not been established and there appears to be no benefit in discontinuing alpha-blocker therapy prior to surgery. Instruct patients to inform ophthalmologist of carvedilol use when considering eye surgery.

Adverse Reactions Note: Frequency ranges include data from hypertension and heart failure trials. Higher rates of adverse reactions have generally been noted in patients with heart failure. However, the frequency of adverse effects associated with placebo is also increased in this population.

>10%:

Cardiovascular: Hypotension (9% to 20%)

Central nervous system: Dizziness (2% to 32%), fatigue (4% to 24%)

Endocrine & metabolic: Hyperglycemia (5% to 12%)

Gastrointestinal: Diarrhea (1% to 12%), weight gain (10% to 12%)

Neuromuscular & skeletal: Weakness (7% to 11%)

1% to 10%:

Cardiovascular: Bradycardia (2% to 10%), syncope (3% to 8%), peripheral edema (1% to 7%), generalized edema (5% to 6%), angina (1% to 6%), dependent edema (≤4%), AV block, cerebrovascular accident, hypertension, hyper-/hypovolemia, postural hypotension, palpitation

Central nervous system: Headache (5% to 8%), depression, fever, hypoesthesia, hypotonia, insomnia, malaise, somnolence, vertigo

Endocrine & metabolic: Hypercholesterolemia (1% to 4%), hypertriglyceridemia (1%), diabetes mellitus, gout, hyperkalemia, hyperuricemia, hypoglycemia, hyponatremia

Gastrointestinal: Nausea (2% to 9%), vomiting (1% to 6%), abdominal pain, melena, periodontitis, weight loss

Genitourinary: Impotence

Hematologic: Anemia, prothrombin decreased, purpura, thrombocytopenia

Hepatic: Alkaline phosphatase increased (1% to 3%), GGT increased, transaminases increased

Neuromuscular & skeletal: Back pain (2% to 7%), arthralgia (1% to 6%), arthritis, muscle cramps, paresthesia

Ocular: Blurred vision (1% to 5%)

Renal: BUN increased (≤6%), nonprotein nitrogen increased (6%), albuminuria, creatinine increased, glycosuria, hematuria, renal insufficiency

Respiratory: Cough (5% to 8%), nasopharyngitis (4%), rales (4%), dyspnea (>3%), pulmonary edema (>3%), rhinitis (2%), nasal congestion (1%), sinus congestion (1%)

Miscellaneous: Injury (3% to 6%), allergy, flu-like syndrome, sudden death

<1% (Limited to important or life-threatening): Anaphylactoid reaction, alopecia, angioedema, aplastic anemia, amnesia, asthma, bronchospasm, bundle branch block, cholestatic jaundice, concentration decreased, diaphoresis, erythema multiforme, exfoliative dermatitis, GI hemorrhage, HDL decreased, hearing decreased, hyperbilirubinemia, hypersensitivity reaction, hypokalemia, hypokinesia, interstitial pneumonitis, leukopenia, libido decreased, migraine, myocardial ischemia, nervousness, neuralgia, nightmares, pancytopenia, paresis, peripheral ischemia, photosensitivity, pruritus, rash (erythematous, maculopapular, and psoriaform), respiratory alkalosis, seizure, Stevens-Johnson syndrome, tachycardia, tinnitus, toxic epidermal necrolysis, urinary incontinence, urticaria, xerostomia

Drug Interactions

Metabolism/Transport Effects Substrate of CYP1A2 (minor), CYP2C9 (minor), CYP2D6 (major), CYP2E1 (minor), CYP3A4 (minor), P-glycoprotein; **Note:** Assignment of Major/Minor substrate status based on clinically relevant drug interaction potential; **Inhibits** P-glycoprotein

Avoid Concomitant Use

Avoid concomitant use of Carvedilol with any of the following: Beta2-Agonists; Floctafenine; Methacholine; Silodosin; Topotecan

Increased Effect/Toxicity

Carvedilol may increase the levels/effects of: Alpha-/Beta-Agonists (Direct-Acting); Alpha1-Blockers; Alpha2-Agonists; Amifostine; Antihypertensives; Antipsychotic Agents (Phenothiazines); Bupivacaine; Cardiac Glycosides; Cholinergic Agonists; Colchicine; CycloSPORINE; CycloSPORINE (Systemic); Dabigatran Etexilate; Digoxin; Everolimus; Fingolimod; Hypotensive Agents; Insulin; Lidocaine; Lidocaine (Systemic); Lidocaine (Topical); Mepivacaine; Methacholine; Midodrine; P-glycoprotein/ABCB1 Substrates; RiTUXimab; Rivaroxaban; Silodosin; Sulfonylureas; Topotecan

The levels/effects of Carvedilol may be increased by: Acetylcholinesterase Inhibitors; Aminoquinolines (Antimalarial); Amiodarone; Anilidopiperidine Opioids; Antipsychotic Agents (Phenothiazines); Calcium Channel Blockers (Dihydropyridine); Calcium Channel Blockers (Nondihydropyridine); Cimetidine; Conivaptan; CYP2C9 Inhibitors (Moderate); CYP2C9 Inhibitors (Strong); CYP2D6 Inhibitors (Moderate); CYP2D6 Inhibitors (Strong); Diazoxide; Dipyridamole; Disopyramide; Dronedarone; Floctafenine; Herbs (Hypotensive Properties); MAO Inhibitors; Pentoxifylline; P-glycoprotein/ABCB1 Inhibitors; Phosphodiesterase 5 Inhibitors; Propafenone; Prostacyclin Analogues; QuiNIDine; Reserpine; Selective Serotonin Reuptake Inhibitors

Decreased Effect

Carvedilol may decrease the levels/effects of: Beta2-Agonists; Theophylline Derivatives

The levels/effects of Carvedilol may be decreased by: Barbiturates; Cyproterone; Herbs (Hypertensive Properties); Methylphenidate; Nonsteroidal Anti-Inflammatory Agents; Peginterferon Alfa-2b; P-glycoprotein/ABCB1 Inducers; Rifamycin Derivatives; Tocilizumab; Yohimbine

Ethanol/Nutrition/Herb Interactions

Food: Food decreases rate but not extent of absorption. Administration with food minimizes risks of orthostatic hypotension.

Herb/Nutraceutical: Avoid herbs with hypertensive properties (bayberry, blue cohosh, cayenne, ephedra, ginger, ginseng [American], kola, licorice); may diminish the antihypertensive effect of carvedilol. Avoid herbs with hypotensive properties (black cohosh, California poppy, coleus, golden seal, hawthorn, mistletoe, periwinkle, quinine, shepherd's purse); may enhance the hypotensive effect of carvedilol.

Stability

Coreg®: Store at <30°C (<86°F). Protect from moisture.

Coreg CR®: Store at 25°C (77°F); excursions permitted to 15°C to 30°C (59°F to 86°F).

Mechanism of Action As a racemic mixture, carvedilol has nonselective beta-adrenoreceptor and alpha-adrenergic blocking activity. No intrinsic sympathomimetic activity has been documented. Associated effects in hypertensive patients include reduction of cardiac output, exercise- or beta-agonist-induced tachycardia, reduction of reflex orthostatic tachycardia, vasodilation, decreased peripheral vascular resistance (especially in standing position), decreased renal vascular resistance, reduced plasma renin activity, and increased levels of atrial natriuretic peptide. In CHF, associated effects include decreased pulmonary capillary wedge pressure, decreased pulmonary artery pressure, decreased heart rate, decreased systemic vascular resistance, increased stroke volume index, and decreased right arterial pressure (RAP).

Pharmacodynamics/Kinetics

Onset of action: 1-2 hours

Peak antihypertensive effect: ~1-2 hours

Absorption: Rapid and extensive

Distribution: V_d: 115 L

Protein binding: >98%, primarily to albumin

Metabolism: Extensively hepatic, via CYP2C9, 2D6, 3A4, and 2C19 (2% excreted unchanged); three active metabolites (4-hydroxyphenyl metabolite is 13 times more potent than parent drug for beta-blockade); first-pass effect; plasma concentrations in the elderly and those with cirrhotic liver disease are 50% and 4-7 times higher, respectively

Bioavailability: Immediate release: 25% to 35% (due to significant first-pass metabolism); Extended release: 85% of immediate release

Half-life elimination: 7-10 hours

Time to peak, plasma: Extended release: 5 hours

Excretion: Primarily feces

Dosage Oral: Adults: Reduce dosage if heart rate drops to <55 beats/minute.

Hypertension:

Immediate release: 6.25 mg twice daily; if tolerated, dose should be maintained for 1-2 weeks, then increased to 12.5 mg twice daily. If necessary, dosage may be increased to a maximum of 25 mg twice daily after 1-2 weeks.

Extended release: Initial: 20 mg once daily, if tolerated, dose should be maintained for 1-2 weeks then increased to 40 mg once daily if necessary; maximum dose: 80 mg once daily

Heart failure:

Immediate release: 3.125 mg twice daily for 2 weeks; if this dose is tolerated, may increase to 6.25 mg twice daily. Double the dose every 2 weeks to the highest dose tolerated by patient. (Prior to initiating therapy, other heart failure medications should be stabilized and fluid retention minimized.)

Maximum recommended dose:

Mild-to-moderate heart failure:

<85 kg: 25 mg twice daily

>85 kg: 50 mg twice daily

Severe heart failure: 25 mg twice daily

Extended release: Initial: 10 mg once daily for 2 weeks; if the dose is tolerated, increase dose to 20 mg, 40 mg, and 80 mg over successive intervals of at least 2 weeks. Maintain on lower dose if higher dose is not tolerated.

Left ventricular dysfunction following MI: **Note**: Should be initiated only after patient is hemodynamically stable and fluid retention has been minimized.

Immediate release: Initial 3.125-6.25 mg twice daily; increase dosage incrementally (ie, from 6.25-12.5 mg twice daily) at intervals of 3-10 days, based on tolerance, to a target dose of 25 mg twice daily.

Extended release: Initial: 10-20 mg once daily; increase dosage incrementally at intervals of 3-10 days, based on tolerance, to a target dose of 80 mg once daily.

Angina pectoris (unlabeled use): Immediate release: 25-50 mg twice daily

Elderly: Hypertension: Consider lower initial dose and titrate to response (Aronow, 2011)

Conversion from immediate release to extended release (Coreg CR®):

Current dose immediate release tablets 3.125 mg twice daily: Convert to extended release capsules 10 mg once daily

Current dose immediate release tablets 6.25 mg twice daily: Convert to extended release capsules 20 mg once daily

Current dose immediate release tablets 12.5 mg twice daily: Convert to extended release capsules 40 mg once daily

Current dose immediate release tablets 25 mg twice daily: Convert to extended release capsules 80 mg once daily

Dosing adjustment in renal impairment: None necessary

Dosing adjustment in hepatic impairment: Use is contraindicated in severe liver dysfunction.

Dietary Considerations Should be taken with food to minimize the risk of orthostatic hypotension.

Administration Administer with food to minimize the risk of orthostatic hypotension. Extended release capsules should not be crushed or chewed. Capsules may be opened and sprinkled on applesauce for immediate use.

Monitoring Parameters Heart rate, blood pressure (base need for dosage increase on trough blood pressure measurements and for tolerance on standing systolic pressure 1 hour after dosing); renal studies, BUN, liver function; in patient with increase risk for developing renal dysfunction, monitor during dosage titration.

Additional Information Fluid retention during therapy should be treated with an increase in diuretic dosage.

Dosage Forms Excipient information presented when available (limited, particularly for generics); consult specific product labeling.

Capsule, extended release, oral, as phosphate:
Coreg CR®: 10 mg, 20 mg, 40 mg, 80 mg
Tablet, oral: 3.125 mg, 6.25 mg, 12.5 mg, 25 mg
Coreg®: 3.125 mg, 6.25 mg, 12.5 mg, 25 mg

Extemporaneous Preparations A 1.25 mg/mL carvedilol oral suspension may be made with tablets and one of two different vehicles (Ora-Blend™ or 1:1 mixture of Ora-Sweet® and Ora-Plus®). Crush five 25 mg tablets in a mortar and reduce to a fine powder; add 15 mL of purified water and mix to a uniform paste. Mix while adding chosen vehicle in incremental proportions to almost 100 mL; transfer to a calibrated amber bottle, rinse mortar with vehicle, and add quantity of vehicle sufficient to make 100 mL. Label "shake well". Stable for 84 days when stored in amber prescription bottles at room temperature (Loyd, 2006).

Carvedilol oral liquid suspensions (0.1 mg/mL and 1.67 mg/mL) made from tablets, water, Ora-Plus®, and Ora-Sweet® were stable for 12 weeks when stored in glass amber bottles at room temperature (25°C). Use one 3.125 mg tablet for the 0.1 mg/mL suspension or two 25 mg tablets for the 1.67 mg/mL suspension; grind the tablet(s) and compound a mixture with 5 mL of water, 15 mL Ora-Plus®, and 10 mL Ora-Sweet®. Final volume of each suspension: 30 mL; label "shake well" (data on file, GlaxoSmithKline, Philadelphia, PA: DOF #132 [**Note:** Manufacturer no longer disseminates this document]).

Loyd A Jr, "Carvedilol 1.25 mg/mL Oral Suspension," *Int J Pharm Compounding*, 2006, 10(3):220.

◆ **Casodex®** *see* Bicalutamide *on page 217*

Caspofungin (kas poe FUN jin)

Brand Names: U.S. Cancidas®

Brand Names: Canada Cancidas®

Index Terms Caspofungin Acetate

Pharmacologic Category Antifungal Agent, Parenteral; Echinocandin

Additional Appendix Information

Antifungal Agents *on page 1876*

Use Treatment of invasive *Aspergillus* infections in patients who are refractory or intolerant of other therapy; treatment of candidemia and other *Candida* infections (intra-abdominal abscesses, esophageal, peritonitis, pleural space); empirical treatment for presumed fungal infections in febrile neutropenic patient

Pregnancy Risk Factor C

Pregnancy Considerations Adverse events have been observed in animal studies. There are no adequate and well-controlled studies in pregnant women. Should be used during pregnancy only if potential benefit justifies the potential risk to the fetus.

Lactation Excretion in breast milk unknown/use caution

Contraindications Hypersensitivity to caspofungin or any component of the formulation

Warnings/Precautions Concurrent use of cyclosporine should be limited to patients for whom benefit outweighs risk, due to a high frequency of hepatic transaminase elevations observed during concurrent use. Use caution in hepatic impairment; increased transaminases and rare cases of liver impairment have been reported in pediatric and adult patients. Dosage reduction required in adults with moderate hepatic impairment; safety and efficacy have not been established in children with any degree of hepatic impairment and adults with severe hepatic impairment.

Adverse Reactions

>10%:

Cardiovascular: Hypotension (3% to 20%), peripheral edema (6% to 11%), tachycardia (4% to 11%)
Central nervous system: Fever (6% to 30%), chills (9% to 23%), headache (5% to 15%)
Dermatologic: Rash (4% to 23%)
Endocrine & metabolic: Hypokalemia (5% to 23%)
Gastrointestinal: Diarrhea (6% to 27%), vomiting (6% to 17%), nausea (4% to 15%)
Hematologic: Hemoglobin decreased (18% to 21%), hematocrit decreased (13% to 18%), WBC decreased (12%), anemia (2% to 11%)
Hepatic: Serum alkaline phosphatase increased (9% to 22%), transaminases increased (2% to 18%), bilirubin increased (5% to 13%)
Local: Phlebitis/thrombophlebitis (18%)
Renal: Serum creatinine increased (3% to 11%)
Respiratory: Respiratory failure (2% to 20%), cough (6% to 11%), pneumonia (4% to 11%)
Miscellaneous: Infusion reactions (20% to 35%), septic shock (11% to 14%)

5% to 10%:

Cardiovascular: Hypertension (5% to 6%; children 9% to 10%)
Dermatologic: Erythema (4% to 9%), pruritus (6% to 7%)
Endocrine & metabolic: Hypomagnesemia (7%), hyperglycemia (6%)
Gastrointestinal: Mucosal inflammation (4% to 10%), abdominal pain (4% to 9%)
Hepatic: Albumin decreased (7%)
Local: Infection (1% to 9%, central line)
Renal: Hematuria (10%), blood urea nitrogen increased (4% to 9%)
Respiratory: Dyspnea (9%), pleural effusion (9%), respiratory distress (≤8%), rales (7%)
Miscellaneous: Sepsis (5% to 7%)

<5% (Limited to important or life-threatening): Abdominal distention, anaphylaxis, anorexia, anxiety, appetite decrease, arrhythmia, arthralgia, atrial fibrillation, back pain, bacteremia, bradycardia, cardiac arrest, coagulopathy, confusion, constipation, depression, dizziness, dyspepsia, dystonia, edema, epistaxis, erythema multiforme, fatigue, febrile neutropenia, fluid overload, flushing, hematuria, hepatic necrosis, hepatomegaly, hepatotoxicity, hypercalcemia, hyperkalemia, hypoxia, infusion site reactions (pain/pruritus/swelling), insomnia, jaundice, liver failure, MI, nephrotoxicity (serum creatinine ≥2 x baseline value or ≥1 mg/dL in patients with serum creatinine above ULN range), pain (extremities), pancreatitis, petechiae, pulmonary edema, renal failure/insufficiency, seizure, skin exfoliation, skin lesion, somnolence, stridor, Stevens-Johnson syndrome, tachypnea, thrombocytopenia, tremor, urinary tract infection, urticaria, weakness; histamine-mediated reactions (including facial swelling, bronchospasm, sensation of warmth) have been reported

Drug Interactions

Metabolism/Transport Effects None known.

Avoid Concomitant Use There are no known interactions where it is recommended to avoid concomitant use.

Increased Effect/Toxicity

The levels/effects of Caspofungin may be increased by: CycloSPORINE; CycloSPORINE (Systemic)

Decreased Effect

Caspofungin may decrease the levels/effects of: Saccharomyces boulardii; Tacrolimus; Tacrolimus (Systemic)

The levels/effects of Caspofungin may be decreased by: Inducers of Drug Clearance; Rifampin

Stability Store vials at 2°C to 8°C (36°F to 46°F). Reconstituted solution may be stored at ≤25°C (≤77°F) for 1 hour prior to preparation of infusion solution. Infusion solutions may be stored at ≤25°C (≤77°F) and should be used within 24 hours; up to 48 hours if stored at 2°C to 8°C (36°F to 46°F).

Bring refrigerated vial to room temperature. Reconstitute vials using 0.9% sodium chloride for injection, SWFI, or bacteriostatic water for injection. Mix gently until clear solution is formed; do not use if cloudy or contains particles. Solution should be further diluted with 0.9%, 0.45%, or 0.225% sodium chloride or LR (do not exceed final concentration of 0.5 mg/mL).

Mechanism of Action Inhibits synthesis of β(1,3)-D-glucan, an essential component of the cell wall of susceptible fungi. Highest activity in regions of active cell growth. Mammalian cells do not require β(1,3)-D-glucan, limiting potential toxicity.

Pharmacodynamics/Kinetics

Protein binding: ~97% to albumin

Metabolism: Slowly, via hydrolysis and *N*-acetylation as well as by spontaneous degradation, with subsequent metabolism to component amino acids. Overall metabolism is extensive.

Half-life elimination: Beta (distribution): 9-11 hours; Terminal: 40-50 hours

Excretion: Urine (41%; primarily as metabolites, ~1% of total dose as unchanged drug); feces (35%; primarily as metabolites)

Dosage I.V.:

Children: 3 months to 17 years: Initial dose: 70 mg/m^2 on day 1, subsequent dosing: 50 mg/m^2 once daily, if clinical response inadequate, may increase to 70 mg/m^2 once daily if tolerated, but increased efficacy not demonstrated (maximum dose: 70 mg/day)

Adults: **Note:** Duration of caspofungin treatment should be determined by patient status and clinical response. Empiric therapy should be given until neutropenia resolves. In patients with positive cultures, treatment should continue until 14 days after last positive culture. In neutropenic patients, treatment should be given at least 7 days after both signs and symptoms of infection **and** neutropenia resolve.

Aspergillosis, invasive: Initial dose: 70 mg on day 1; subsequent dosing: 50 mg/day. If clinical response inadequate, may increase up to 70 mg/day if tolerated, but increased efficacy not demonstrated. **Note:** Duration of therapy should be a minimum of 6-12 weeks or throughout period of immunosuppression.

Candidiasis: Initial dose: 70 mg on day 1; subsequent dosing: 50 mg/day; higher doses (150 mg once daily infused over ~2 hours) compared to the standard adult dosing regimen (50 mg once daily) have not demonstrated additional benefit or toxicity in patients with invasive candidiasis (Betts, 2009)

Esophageal: 50 mg/day; **Note:** The majority of patients studied for this indication also had oropharyngeal involvement.

Empiric therapy: Initial dose: 70 mg on day 1; subsequent dosing: 50 mg/day; if clinical response inadequate, may increase up to 70 mg/day if tolerated, but increased efficacy not demonstrated

Concomitant use of an enzyme inducer:

Children: Patients receiving carbamazepine, dexamethasone, efavirenz, nevirapine, phenytoin, or rifampin (and possibly other enzyme inducers): Consider 70 mg/m^2 once daily (maximum: 70 mg/day)

Adults:

Patients receiving rifampin: 70 mg caspofungin daily

Patients receiving carbamazepine, dexamethasone, efavirenz, nevirapine, **or** phenytoin (and possibly other enzyme inducers) may require an increased daily dose of caspofungin (70 mg/day).

Elderly: The number of patients >65 years of age in clinical studies was not sufficient to establish whether a difference in response may be anticipated.

Dosage adjustment in renal impairment: No dosage adjustment required in renal impairment.

Poorly dialyzed; no supplemental dose or dosage adjustment necessary, including patients on intermittent hemodialysis, peritoneal dialysis, or continuous renal replacement therapy (eg, CVVHD).

Dosage adjustment in hepatic impairment:

Children: Mild-to-severe hepatic insufficiency: No clinical experience

Adults:

Mild hepatic insufficiency (Child-Pugh score 5-6): No adjustment necessary

Moderate hepatic insufficiency (Child-Pugh score 7-9): 70 mg on day 1 (where recommended), followed by 35 mg once daily

Severe hepatic insufficiency (Child-Pugh score >9): No clinical experience

Administration Infuse slowly, over 1 hour; monitor during infusion. Isolated cases of possible histamine-related reactions have occurred during clinical trials (rash, flushing, pruritus, facial edema).

Monitoring Parameters Liver function

Dosage Forms Excipient information presented when available (limited, particularly for generics); consult specific product labeling.

Injection, powder for reconstitution, as acetate:

Cancidas®: 50 mg [contains sucrose 39 mg]

Cancidas®: 70 mg [contains sucrose 54 mg]

- ◆ **Caspofungin Acetate** *see* Caspofungin *on page* 298
- ◆ **Castor Oil, Trypsin, and Balsam Peru** *see* Trypsin, Balsam Peru, and Castor Oil *on page* 1744
- ◆ **Cataflam®** *see* Diclofenac (Systemic) *on page* 495
- ◆ **Catapres®** *see* CloNIDine *on page* 392
- ◆ **Catapres-TTS®-1** *see* CloNIDine *on page* 392
- ◆ **Catapres-TTS®-2** *see* CloNIDine *on page* 392
- ◆ **Catapres-TTS®-3** *see* CloNIDine *on page* 392
- ◆ **Cathflo® Activase®** *see* Alteplase *on page* 76
- ◆ **Caverject®** *see* Alprostadil *on page* 74
- ◆ **Caverject Impulse®** *see* Alprostadil *on page* 74
- ◆ **CaviRinse™** *see* Fluoride *on page* 728
- ◆ **Cayston®** *see* Aztreonam *on page* 184
- ◆ **Caziant®** *see* Ethinyl Estradiol and Desogestrel *on page* 653
- ◆ **CB-1348** *see* Chlorambucil *on page* 337
- ◆ **CB7630** *see* Abiraterone Acetate *on page* 23
- ◆ **CBDCA** *see* CARBOplatin *on page* 287
- ◆ **CBZ** *see* CarBAMazepine *on page* 280
- ◆ **CC-5013** *see* Lenalidomide *on page* 981
- ◆ **CCI-779** *see* Temsirolimus *on page* 1641
- ◆ **CCNU** *see* Lomustine *on page* 1025
- ◆ **2-CdA** *see* Cladribine *on page* 372
- ◆ **CDB-2914** *see* Ulipristal *on page* 1748
- ◆ **CDCA** *see* Chenodiol *on page* 336
- ◆ **CDDP** *see* CISplatin *on page* 368
- ◆ **CDP870** *see* Certolizumab Pegol *on page* 328
- ◆ **CDX** *see* Bicalutamide *on page* 217

Cefaclor (SEF a klor)

Brand Names: Canada Apo-Cefaclor®; Ceclor®; Novo-Cefaclor; Nu-Cefaclor; PMS-Cefaclor

Pharmacologic Category Antibiotic, Cephalosporin (Second Generation)

Use Treatment of susceptible bacterial infections including otitis media, lower respiratory tract infections, acute exacerbations of chronic bronchitis, pharyngitis and tonsillitis, urinary tract infections, skin and skin structure infections

Pregnancy Risk Factor B

Pregnancy Considerations Adverse events were not observed in animal reproduction studies; therefore, cefaclor is classified as pregnancy category B. It is not known if cefaclor crosses the placenta; other cephalosporins cross the placenta and are considered safe for use during pregnancy. An increased risk of teratogenic effects has not been observed following maternal use of cefaclor.

Lactation Enters breast milk/use caution

Contraindications Hypersensitivity to cefaclor, any component of the formulation, or other cephalosporins

Warnings/Precautions Modify dosage in patients with severe renal impairment. Prolonged use may result in fungal or bacterial superinfection, including *C. difficile*-associated diarrhea (CDAD) and pseudomembranous colitis; CDAD has been observed >2 months postantibiotic treatment. Use with caution in patients with a history of penicillin allergy, especially IgE-mediated reactions (eg, anaphylaxis, urticaria). Beta-lactamase-negative, ampicillin-resistant (BLNAR) strains of *H. influenzae* should be considered resistant to cefaclor. Extended release tablets are not approved for use in children <16 years of age.

Adverse Reactions

1% to 10%:

Dermatologic: Rash (maculopapular, erythematous, or morbilliform) (1% to 2%)

Gastrointestinal: Diarrhea (3%)

Genitourinary: Vaginitis (2%)

Hematologic: Eosinophilia (2%)

Hepatic: Transaminases increased (3%)

Miscellaneous: Moniliasis (2%)

<1% (Limited to important or life-threatening): Agitation, agranulocytosis, anaphylaxis, angioedema, aplastic anemia, arthralgia, cholestatic jaundice, CNS irritability, confusion, dizziness, hallucinations, hemolytic anemia, hepatitis, hyperactivity, insomnia, interstitial nephritis, nausea, nervousness, neutropenia, paresthesia, PT prolonged, pruritus, pseudomembranous colitis, seizure, serum-sickness, somnolence, Stevens-Johnson syndrome, thrombocytopenia, toxic epidermal necrolysis, urticaria, vomiting

Reactions reported with other cephalosporins: Abdominal pain, cholestasis, fever, hemorrhage, renal dysfunction, superinfection, toxic nephropathy

Drug Interactions

Metabolism/Transport Effects None known.

Avoid Concomitant Use

Avoid concomitant use of Cefaclor with any of the following: BCG

Increased Effect/Toxicity

Cefaclor may increase the levels/effects of: Aminoglycosides

The levels/effects of Cefaclor may be increased by: Probenecid

Decreased Effect

Cefaclor may decrease the levels/effects of: BCG; Typhoid Vaccine

Ethanol/Nutrition/Herb Interactions Food: Cefaclor serum levels may be decreased slightly if taken with food. The bioavailability of cefaclor extended release tablets is decreased 23% and the maximum concentration is decreased 67% when taken on an empty stomach.

Stability Store at controlled room temperature. Refrigerate suspension after reconstitution. Discard after 14 days. Do not freeze.

Mechanism of Action Inhibits bacterial cell wall synthesis by binding to one or more of the penicillin-binding proteins (PBPs) which in turn inhibits the final transpeptidation step of peptidoglycan synthesis in bacterial cell walls, thus inhibiting cell wall biosynthesis. Bacteria eventually lyse due to ongoing activity of cell wall autolytic enzymes (autolysins and murein hydrolases) while cell wall assembly is arrested.

Pharmacodynamics/Kinetics

Absorption: Well absorbed, acid stable

Distribution: Widely throughout the body and reaches therapeutic concentration in most tissues and body fluids, including synovial, pericardial, pleural, peritoneal fluids; bile, sputum, and urine; bone, myocardium, gallbladder, skin and soft tissue

Protein binding: 25%

Metabolism: Partially hepatic

Half-life elimination: 0.5-1 hour; prolonged with renal impairment

Time to peak: Capsule: 60 minutes; Suspension: 45 minutes

Excretion: Urine (80% as unchanged drug)

Dosage

Usual dosage range:

Children >1 month: Oral: 20-40 mg/kg/day divided every 8-12 hours (maximum dose: 1 g/day)

Adults: Oral: 250-500 mg every 8 hours

Indication-specific dosing:

Children: Oral:

Otitis media: 40 mg/kg/day divided every 12 hours

Pharyngitis: 20 mg/kg/day divided every 12 hours

Dosing adjustment in renal impairment:

Cl_{cr} 10-50 mL/minute: Administer 50% to 100% of dose

Cl_{cr} <10 mL/minute: Administer 50% of dose

Hemodialysis: Moderately dialyzable (20% to 50%)

Dietary Considerations Capsule and suspension may be taken with or without food.

Administration Administer around-the-clock to promote less variation in peak and trough serum levels.

Oral suspension: Shake well before using.

Monitoring Parameters Assess patient at beginning and throughout therapy for infection; monitor for signs of anaphylaxis during first dose

Test Interactions Positive direct Coombs', false-positive urinary glucose test using cupric sulfate (Benedict's solution, Clinitest®, Fehling's solution), false-positive serum or urine creatinine with Jaffé reaction

Dosage Forms Excipient information presented when available (limited, particularly for generics); consult specific product labeling.

Capsule, oral: 250 mg, 500 mg

Powder for suspension, oral: 125 mg/5 mL (75 mL, 150 mL); 250 mg/5 mL (75 mL, 150 mL); 375 mg/5 mL (50 mL, 100 mL)

Tablet, extended release, oral: 500 mg

Cefadroxil (sef a DROKS il)

Brand Names: Canada Apo-Cefadroxil®; Novo-Cefadroxil; PRO-Cefadroxil

Index Terms Cefadroxil Monohydrate; Duricef

Pharmacologic Category Antibiotic, Cephalosporin (First Generation)

Use Treatment of susceptible bacterial infections, including those caused by group A beta-hemolytic *Streptococcus*

Pregnancy Risk Factor B

Pregnancy Considerations Adverse events were not observed in animal reproduction studies; therefore, cefadroxil is classified as pregnancy category B. Cefadroxil crosses the placenta. Limited data is available concerning the use of cefadroxil in pregnancy; however, adverse fetal effects were not noted in a small clinical trial. Adequate and well-controlled studies have been not completed in pregnant women.

Lactation Enters breast milk (small amounts)/use caution (AAP rates "compatible"; AAP 2001 update pending)

Contraindications Hypersensitivity to cefadroxil, any component of the formulation, or other cephalosporins

Warnings/Precautions Modify dosage in patients with severe renal impairment. Use with caution in patients with a history of penicillin allergy, especially IgE-mediated reactions (eg, anaphylaxis, angioedema, urticaria). Prolonged use may result in fungal or bacterial superinfection, including *C. difficile*-associated diarrhea (CDAD) and pseudomembranous colitis; CDAD has been observed >2 months postantibiotic treatment.

Adverse Reactions

1% to 10%: Gastrointestinal: Diarrhea

<1% (Limited to important or life-threatening): Abdominal pain, agranulocytosis, anaphylaxis, angioedema, arthralgia, cholestasis, dyspepsia, erythema multiforme, fever, nausea, neutropenia, pruritus, pseudomembranous colitis, rash (maculopapular and erythematous), serum sickness, Stevens-Johnson syndrome, thrombocytopenia, transaminases increased, urticaria, vaginitis, vomiting

Reactions reported with other cephalosporins: Abdominal pain, aplastic anemia, BUN increased, creatinine increased, eosinophilia, hemolytic anemia, hemorrhage, pancytopenia, prothrombin time prolonged, renal dysfunction, seizure, superinfection, toxic epidermal necrolysis, toxic nephropathy

Drug Interactions

Metabolism/Transport Effects None known.

Avoid Concomitant Use

Avoid concomitant use of Cefadroxil with any of the following: BCG

Increased Effect/Toxicity

The levels/effects of Cefadroxil may be increased by: Probenecid

Decreased Effect

Cefadroxil may decrease the levels/effects of: BCG; Typhoid Vaccine

Ethanol/Nutrition/Herb Interactions Food: Concomitant administration with food, infant formula, or cow's milk does **not** significantly affect absorption.

Stability Refrigerate suspension after reconstitution; discard after 14 days.

Mechanism of Action Inhibits bacterial cell wall synthesis by binding to one or more of the penicillin-binding proteins (PBPs) which in turn inhibits the final transpeptidation step of peptidoglycan synthesis in bacterial cell walls, thus inhibiting cell wall biosynthesis. Bacteria eventually lyse due to ongoing activity of cell wall autolytic enzymes (autolysins and murein hydrolases) while cell wall assembly is arrested.

Pharmacodynamics/Kinetics

Absorption: Rapid and well absorbed

Distribution: Widely throughout the body and reaches therapeutic concentrations in most tissues and body fluids, including synovial, pericardial, pleural, and peritoneal fluids; bile, sputum, and urine; bone, myocardium, gallbladder, skin, and soft tissue

Protein binding: 20%

Half-life elimination: 1-2 hours; Renal failure: 20-24 hours

Time to peak, serum: 70-90 minutes

Excretion: Urine (>90% as unchanged drug)

Dosage

Usual dosage range: Oral:

Children: 30 mg/kg/day divided twice daily up to a maximum of 2 g/day

Adults: 1-2 g/day in 2 divided doses

Indication-specific dosing: Orofacial infections: Adults: 250-500 mg every 8 hours

Dosing interval in renal impairment:

Cl_{cr} 10-25 mL/minute: Administer every 24 hours

Cl_{cr} <10 mL/minute: Administer every 36 hours

Administration Administer around-the-clock to promote less variation in peak and trough serum levels.

Monitoring Parameters Observe for signs and symptoms of anaphylaxis during first dose.

Test Interactions Positive direct Coombs', false-positive urinary glucose test using cupric sulfate (Benedict's solution, Clinitest®, Fehling's solution), false-positive serum or urine creatinine with Jaffé reaction

Dosage Forms Excipient information presented when available (limited, particularly for generics); consult specific product labeling.

Capsule, oral, as hemihydrate [strength expressed as base]: 500 mg

Capsule, oral, as monohydrate [strength expressed as base]: 500 mg

Powder for suspension, oral, as monohydrate [strength expressed as base]: 250 mg/5 mL (50 mL, 100 mL); 500 mg/5 mL (75 mL, 100 mL)

Tablet, oral, as hemihydrate [strength expressed as base]: 1 g

Tablet, oral, as monohydrate [strength expressed as base]: 1 g

◆ **Cefadroxil Monohydrate** *see* Cefadroxil *on page 301*

CeFAZolin (sef A zoe lin)

Index Terms Ancef; Cefazolin Sodium

Pharmacologic Category Antibiotic, Cephalosporin (First Generation)

Additional Appendix Information

Antibiotic Treatment of Adults With Infective Endocarditis *on page 1956*

Prevention of Infective Endocarditis *on page 1952*

Prevention of Wound Infection and Sepsis in Surgical Patients *on page 1954*

Use Treatment of respiratory tract, skin, genital, urinary tract, biliary tract, bone and joint infections, and septicemia due to susceptible gram-positive cocci (except *Enterococcus*); some gram-negative bacilli including *E. coli*, *Proteus*, and *Klebsiella* may be susceptible; surgical prophylaxis

Unlabeled Use Prophylaxis against infective endocarditis

Pregnancy Risk Factor B

Pregnancy Considerations Adverse effects were not observed in animal reproduction studies; therefore, cefazolin is classified as pregnancy category B. Cefazolin crosses the placenta. Adverse events have not been reported in the fetus following administration of cefazolin prior to caesarean section. Cefazolin is recommended for group B streptococcus prophylaxis in pregnant patients with a nonanaphylactic penicillin allergy.

Due to pregnancy-induced physiologic changes, the pharmacokinetics of cefazolin are altered. The half-life is shorter and the AUC is smaller. The volume of distribution is unchanged.

Lactation Enters breast milk (small amounts)/use caution (AAP rates "compatible"; AAP 2001 update pending)

Contraindications Hypersensitivity to cefazolin sodium, any component of the formulation, or other cephalosporins

Warnings/Precautions Modify dosage in patients with severe renal impairment. Use with caution in patients with a history of penicillin allergy, especially IgE-mediated reactions (eg, anaphylaxis, angioedema, urticaria). Prolonged use may result in fungal or bacterial superinfection, including *C. difficile*-associated diarrhea (CDAD) and pseudomembranous colitis; CDAD has been observed >2 months postantibiotic treatment. May be associated with increased INR, especially in nutritionally-deficient patients, prolonged treatment, hepatic or renal disease. Use with caution in patients with a history of seizure disorder; high levels, particularly in the presence of renal impairment, may increase risk of seizures.

Adverse Reactions Frequency not defined.

Central nervous system: Fever, seizure

Dermatologic: Rash, pruritus, Stevens-Johnson syndrome

Gastrointestinal: Diarrhea, nausea, vomiting, abdominal cramps, anorexia, pseudomembranous colitis, oral candidiasis

Genitourinary: Vaginitis

Hepatic: Transaminases increased, hepatitis

Hematologic: Eosinophilia, neutropenia, leukopenia, thrombocytopenia, thrombocytosis

Local: Pain at injection site, phlebitis

Renal: BUN increased, serum creatinine increased, renal failure

Miscellaneous: Anaphylaxis

Reactions reported with other cephalosporins: Toxic epidermal necrolysis, abdominal pain, cholestasis, superinfection, toxic nephropathy, aplastic anemia, hemolytic anemia, hemorrhage, prothrombin time prolonged, pancytopenia

Drug Interactions

Metabolism/Transport Effects None known.

Avoid Concomitant Use

Avoid concomitant use of CeFAZolin with any of the following: BCG

Increased Effect/Toxicity

CeFAZolin may increase the levels/effects of: Fosphenytoin; Phenytoin; Vitamin K Antagonists

The levels/effects of CeFAZolin may be increased by: Probenecid

Decreased Effect

CeFAZolin may decrease the levels/effects of: BCG; Typhoid Vaccine

Stability Store intact vials at room temperature and protect from temperatures exceeding 40°C. Dilute large vial with 2.5 mL SWFI; 10 g vial may be diluted with 45 mL to yield 1 g/5 mL or 96 mL to yield 1 g/10 mL. May be injected or further dilution for I.V. administration in 50-100 mL compatible solution. Standard diluent is 1 g/50 mL D_5W or 2 g/50 mL D_5W.

Reconstituted solutions of cefazolin are light yellow to yellow. Protection from light is recommended for the powder and for the reconstituted solutions. Reconstituted solutions are stable for 24 hours at room temperature and for 10 days under refrigeration. Stability of parenteral admixture at room temperature (25°C) is 48 hours. Stability of parenteral admixture at refrigeration temperature (4°C) is 14 days.

DUPLEX™: Store at 20°C to 25°C (68°F to 77°F); excursions permitted to 15°C to 30°C (59°F to 86°F) prior to activation. Following activation, stable for 24 hours at room temperature and for 7 days under refrigeration.

Mechanism of Action Inhibits bacterial cell wall synthesis by binding to one or more of the penicillin-binding proteins (PBPs) which in turn inhibits the final transpeptidation step of peptidoglycan synthesis in bacterial cell walls, thus inhibiting cell wall biosynthesis. Bacteria eventually lyse due to ongoing activity of cell wall autolytic enzymes (autolysins and murein hydrolases) while cell wall assembly is arrested.

Pharmacodynamics/Kinetics

Distribution: Widely into most body tissues and fluids including gallbladder, liver, kidneys, bone, sputum, bile, pleural, and synovial; CSF penetration is poor

Protein binding: 74% to 86%

Metabolism: Minimally hepatic

Half-life elimination: 90-150 minutes; prolonged with renal impairment

Time to peak, serum: I.M.: 0.5-2 hours

Excretion: Urine (80% to 100% as unchanged drug)

Dosage

Usual dosage range: I.M., I.V.:

Children >1 month: 25-100 mg/kg/day divided every 6-8 hours; maximum: 6 g/day

Adults: 250 mg to 1.5 g every 6-12 (usually 8) hours, depending on severity of infection; maximum dose: 12 g/day

Indication-specific dosing:

Infants and Children: I.M., I.V.:

Community-acquired pneumonia (CAP) (IDSA/PIDS, 2011), moderate-to-severe infection, *S. aureus* (methicillin-susceptible) (preferred): Infants >3 months and Children: 150 mg/kg/day divided every 8 hours

Prophylaxis against infective endocarditis (unlabeled use): 50 mg/kg 30-60 minutes before procedure; maximum dose: 1 g. Intramuscular injections should be avoided in patients who are receiving anticoagulant therapy. In these circumstances, orally administered regimens should be given whenever possible. Intravenously administered antibiotics should be used for patients who are unable to tolerate or absorb oral medications.

Note: American Heart Association (AHA) guidelines now recommend prophylaxis only in patients undergoing invasive procedures and in whom underlying cardiac conditions may predispose to a higher risk of adverse outcomes should infection occur. As of April 2007, routine prophylaxis for GI/GU procedures is no longer recommended by the AHA.

Adults: I.M., I.V.:

Cholecystitis, mild-to-moderate: I.V.: 1-2 g every 8 hours for 4-7 days (provided source controlled)

Endocarditis due to MSSA (without prosthesis) (unlabeled use): I.V.: 2 g every 8 hours; **Note:** Recommended for penicillin-allergic (nonanaphylactoid) patients (Baddour, 2005)

Intra-abdominal infection, complicated, community-acquired, mild-to-moderate (in combination with metronidazole): I.V.: 1-2 g every 8 hours for 4-7 days (provided source controlled)

Prophylaxis against infective endocarditis (unlabeled use): 1 g 30-60 minutes before procedure. Intramuscular injections should be avoided in patients who are receiving anticoagulant therapy. In these circumstances, orally administered regimens should be given whenever possible. Intravenously administered antibiotics should be used for patients who are unable to tolerate or absorb oral medications.

Note: American Heart Association (AHA) guidelines now recommend prophylaxis only in patients undergoing invasive procedures and in whom underlying cardiac conditions may predispose to a higher risk of adverse outcomes should infection occur. As of April 2007, routine prophylaxis for GI/GU procedures is no longer recommended by the AHA.

Moderate-to-severe infections: 500 mg to 1 g every 6-8 hours

Mild infection with gram-positive cocci: 250-500 mg every 8 hours

Perioperative prophylaxis: 1-2 g within 60 minutes prior to surgery (may repeat in 2-5 hours intraoperatively); followed by 500 mg to 1 g every 6-8 hours for 24 hours postoperatively

Cardiothoracic surgery: 1 g within 60 minutes prior to incision, followed by 1 g at sternotomy and 1 g after cardiopulmonary bypass; may continue 1 g every 6 hours for 24-48 hours postoperatively (Eagle, 2004)

Cholecystectomy: 1-2 g every 8 hours, discontinue within 24 hours unless infection outside gallbladder suspected

Total joint replacement: 1 g 1 hour prior to the procedure

Pneumococcal pneumonia: 500 mg every 12 hours

Severe infection: 1-1.5 g every 6 hours

UTI (uncomplicated): 1 g every 12 hours

Dosing adjustment in renal impairment:

Cl_{cr} 35-54 mL/minute: Administer full dose in intervals of ≥8 hours

Cl_{cr} 11-34 mL/minute: Administer 50% of usual dose every 12 hours

Cl_{cr} ≤10 mL/minute: Administer 50% of usual dose every 18-24 hours

Intermittent hemodialysis (IHD) (administer after hemodialysis on dialysis days): Dialyzable (20% to 50%): 0.5-1 g every 24 hours **or** use 1-2 g every 48-72 hours (Heintz, 2009); **Note:** Dosing dependent on the assumption of 3 times/week, complete IHD sessions. Alternatively, may administer 15-20 mg/kg (maximum dose: 2 g) after dialysis without regularly scheduled dosing (Ahern, 2003; Sowinski, 2001).

Peritoneal dialysis (PD): 0.5 g every 12 hours

Continuous renal replacement therapy (CRRT) (Heintz, 2009; Trotman, 2005): Drug clearance is highly dependent on the method of renal replacement, filter type, and flow rate. Appropriate dosing requires close monitoring of pharmacologic response, signs of adverse reactions due to drug accumulation, as well as drug concentrations in relation to target trough (if appropriate). The following are general recommendations only (based on dialysate flow/ultrafiltration rates of 1-2 L/hour and minimal residual renal function) and should not supersede clinical judgment:

CVVH: Loading dose of 2 g followed by 1-2 g every 12 hours

CVVHD/CVVHDF: Loading dose of 2 g followed by either 1 g every 8 hours **or** 2 g every 12 hours. **Note:** Dosage of 1 g every 8 hours results in similar steady-state concentrations as 2 g every 12 hours and is more cost effective (Heintz, 2009).

Dietary Considerations Some products may contain sodium.

Administration

I.M.: Inject deep I.M. into large muscle mass.

I.V.: Inject direct I.V. over 5 minutes. Infuse intermittent infusion over 30-60 minutes.

Some penicillins (eg, carbenicillin, ticarcillin and piperacillin) have been shown to inactivate aminoglycosides *in vitro*. This has been observed to a greater extent with tobramycin and gentamicin, while amikacin has shown greater stability against inactivation. Concurrent use of these agents may pose a risk of reduced antibacterial efficacy *in vivo*, particularly in the setting of profound renal impairment. However, definitive clinical evidence is lacking. If combination penicillin/aminoglycoside therapy is desired in a patient with renal dysfunction, separation of doses (if feasible), and routine monitoring of aminoglycoside levels, CBC, and clinical response should be considered.

Monitoring Parameters Renal function periodically when used in combination with other nephrotoxic drugs, hepatic function tests, CBC; monitor for signs of anaphylaxis during first dose

Test Interactions Positive direct Coombs', false-positive urinary glucose test using cupric sulfate (Benedict's solution, Clinitest®, Fehling's solution), false-positive serum or urine creatinine with Jaffé reaction.

Some penicillin derivatives may accelerate the degradation of aminoglycosides *in vitro*, leading to a potential underestimation of aminoglycoside serum concentration.

Dosage Forms Excipient information presented when available (limited, particularly for generics); consult specific product labeling.

Infusion, premixed iso-osmotic dextrose solution: 1 g (50 mL) [contains sodium 46 mg/g]

Injection, powder for reconstitution: 500 mg [contains sodium 48 mg (2 mEq)/g], 1 g [contains sodium 48 mg (2 mEq)/g], 10 g [contains sodium 48 mg (2 mEq)/g], 20 g [contains sodium 48 mg (2 mEq)/g], 100 g [contains sodium 48 mg (2 mEq)/g], 300 g [contains sodium 48 mg (2 mEq)/g]

◆ **Cefazolin Sodium** *see* CeFAZolin *on page 301*

Cefdinir (SEF di ner)

Brand Names: U.S. Omnicef®

Brand Names: Canada Omnicef®

Index Terms CFDN

Pharmacologic Category Antibiotic, Cephalosporin (Third Generation)

Use Treatment of community-acquired pneumonia, acute exacerbations of chronic bronchitis, acute bacterial otitis media, acute maxillary sinusitis, pharyngitis/tonsillitis, and uncomplicated skin and skin structure infections.

Pregnancy Risk Factor B

Pregnancy Considerations Teratogenic events have not been observed in animal studies; therefore, cefdinir is classified as pregnancy category B. It is not known if cefdinir crosses the human placenta.

Lactation Excretion in breast milk unknown

Contraindications Hypersensitivity to cefdinir, any component of the formulation, other cephalosporins, or related antibiotics

Warnings/Precautions Administer cautiously to penicillin-sensitive patients, especially IgE-mediated reactions (eg, anaphylaxis, urticaria). Prolonged use may result in fungal or bacterial superinfection, including *C. difficile*-associated diarrhea (CDAD) and pseudomembranous colitis; CDAD has been observed >2 months postantibiotic treatment. Use caution with renal dysfunction (Cl_{cr} <30 mL/minute); dose adjustment may be required.

Adverse Reactions

>10%: Gastrointestinal: Diarrhea (8% to 15%)

1% to 10%:

Central nervous system: Headache (2%)

Dermatologic: Rash (≤3%)

Endocrine & metabolic: Bicarbonate decreased (≤1%), hyperglycemia (≤1%), hyperphosphatemia (≤1%)

Gastrointestinal: Nausea (≤3%), abdominal pain (≤1%), vomiting (≤1%)

Genitourinary: Vaginal moniliasis (≤4%), urine leukocytes increased (≤2%), urine pH increased (≤1%), urine specific gravity increased (≤1%), vaginitis (≤1%)

Hematologic: Lymphocytes increased (≤2%), eosinophils increased (1%), lymphocytes decreased (1%), platelets increased (≤1%), PMN changes (≤1%), WBC decreased/increased (≤1%)

Hepatic: Alkaline phosphatase increased (≤1%), ALT increased (≤1%)

Renal: Proteinuria (1% to 2%), microhematuria (≤1%), glycosuria (≤1%)

Miscellaneous: GGT increased (≤1%), lactate dehydrogenase increased (≤1%)

<1%, postmarketing, and/or case reports: Allergic vasculitis, amylase increased, anaphylaxis, anorexia, asthma, AST increased, bilirubin increased, bleeding tendency, bloody diarrhea, BUN increased, cardiac failure, chest pain, cholestasis, coagulation disorder, conjunctivitis, constipation, cutaneous moniliasis, disseminated intravascular coagulation (DIC), dizziness, dyspepsia, enterocolitis (acute), eosinophilic pneumonia, erythema multiforme, erythema nodosum, exfoliative dermatitis, facial edema, fever, flatulence, fulminant hepatitis, granulocytopenia, hemoglobin decreased, hemolytic anemia, hemorrhagic colitis, hepatic failure, hepatitis (acute), hyperkalemia, hyperkinesia, hypertension, hypocalcemia, hypophosphatemia, idiopathic thrombocytopenia purpura, ileus, insomnia, interstitial pneumonia (idiopathic), involuntary movement, jaundice, laryngeal edema, leukopenia, leukorrhea, loss of consciousness, maculopapular rash, melena, moniliasis, monocytes increased, myocardial infarction, nephropathy, pancytopenia, peptic ulcer, pneumonia (drug-induced), pruritus, pseudomembranous colitis, renal failure (acute), respiratory failure (acute), rhabdomyolysis, serum sickness, shock, somnolence, Stevens-Johnson syndrome, stomatitis, stools abnormal, thrombocytopenia, toxic epidermal necrolysis, upper GI bleed, urine specific gravity decreased, weakness, xerostomia

Additional reactions reported with other cephalosporins: Agranulocytosis, angioedema, aplastic anemia, asterixis, encephalopathy, hemorrhage, interstitial nephritis, neuromuscular excitability, PT prolonged, seizure, superinfection, and toxic nephropathy

Drug Interactions

Metabolism/Transport Effects None known.

Avoid Concomitant Use

Avoid concomitant use of Cefdinir with any of the following: BCG

Increased Effect/Toxicity

Cefdinir may increase the levels/effects of: Aminoglycosides

The levels/effects of Cefdinir may be increased by: Probenecid

Decreased Effect

Cefdinir may decrease the levels/effects of: BCG; Typhoid Vaccine

The levels/effects of Cefdinir may be decreased by: Iron Salts

Stability Capsules and unmixed powder should be stored at 25°C (77°F); excursions permitted to 15°C to 30°C (59°F to 86°F). Oral suspension should be mixed with 38 mL water for the 60 mL bottle and 63 mL of water for the 100 mL bottle. After mixing, the suspension can be stored at room temperature of 25°C (77°F) for 10 days.

Mechanism of Action Inhibits bacterial cell wall synthesis by binding to one or more of the penicillin-binding proteins (PBPs) which in turn inhibits the final transpeptidation step of peptidoglycan synthesis in bacterial cell walls, thus inhibiting cell wall biosynthesis. Bacteria eventually lyse due to ongoing activity of cell wall autolytic enzymes (autolysins and murein hydrolases) while cell wall assembly is arrested.

Pharmacodynamics/Kinetics

Distribution: V_d:

Children 6 months to 12 years: 0.29-1.05 L/kg

Adults: 0.06-0.64 L/kg

Protein binding: 60% to 70%

Metabolism: Minimal

Bioavailability: Capsule: 16% to 21%; suspension 25%

Half-life elimination: ~100 minutes

Time to peak, plasma: 3 hours

Excretion: Primarily urine (7% to 25% as unchanged drug)

Dosage

Usual dosage range:

Children 6 months to 12 years: Oral: 7 mg/kg/dose twice daily or 14 mg/kg/dose once daily (maximum: 600 mg/day)

Adolescents and Adults: Oral: 300 mg twice daily or 600 mg once daily

Indication-specific dosing:

Children 6 months to 12 years: Oral:

Acute bacterial otitis media, pharyngitis/tonsillitis: 7 mg/kg/dose twice daily for 5-10 days **or** 14 mg/kg/dose once daily for 10 days (maximum: 600 mg/day)

Acute maxillary sinusitis: 7 mg/kg/dose twice daily **or** 14 mg/kg/dose once daily for 10 days (maximum: 600 mg/day)

Uncomplicated skin and skin structure infections: 7 mg/kg/dose twice daily for 10 days (maximum: 600 mg/day)

Adolescents and Adults:

Acute exacerbations of chronic bronchitis, pharyngitis/tonsillitis: 300 mg twice daily for 5-10 days **or** 600 mg once daily for 10 days

Acute maxillary sinusitis: 300 mg twice daily **or** 600 mg once daily for 10 days

Community-acquired pneumonia, uncomplicated skin and skin structure infections: 300 mg twice daily for 10 days

Dosing adjustment in renal impairment: Cl_{cr} <30 mL/minute:

Children: 7 mg/kg once daily (maximum: 300 mg/day)

Adults: 300 mg once daily

Hemodialysis removes cefdinir; recommended initial dose: 300 mg (or 7 mg/kg/dose) every other day. At the conclusion of each hemodialysis session, 300 mg (or 7 mg/kg/dose) should be given. Subsequent doses (300 mg or 7 mg/kg/dose) should be administered every other day.

Dosing adjustment in hepatic impairment: No adjustment necessary.

Administration Twice daily doses should be given every 12 hours. May be administered with or without food. Manufacturer recommends administering at least 2 hours before or after antacids or iron supplements. Shake suspension well before use.

Monitoring Parameters Observe for signs and symptoms of anaphylaxis during first dose.

Test Interactions False-positive reaction for urinary ketones may occur with nitroprusside- but not nitroferricyanide-based tests. False-positive urine glucose results may occur when using Clinitest®, Benedict's solution, or Fehling's solution; glucose-oxidase-based reaction systems (eg, Clinistix®, Tes-Tape®) are recommended. May cause positive direct Coombs' test.

Dosage Forms Excipient information presented when available (limited, particularly for generics); consult specific product labeling.

Capsule, oral: 300 mg

Omnicef®: 300 mg

Powder for suspension, oral: 125 mg/5 mL (60 mL, 100 mL); 250 mg/5 mL (60 mL, 100 mL)

Omnicef®: 125 mg/5 mL (60 mL, 100 mL); 250 mg/5 mL (60 mL, 100 mL) [contains sodium benzoate, sucrose 2.86 g/5 mL; strawberry flavor]

Cefditoren (sef de TOR en)

Brand Names: U.S. Spectracef®

Index Terms Cefditoren Pivoxil

Pharmacologic Category Antibiotic, Cephalosporin (Third Generation)

Use Treatment of acute bacterial exacerbation of chronic bronchitis or community-acquired pneumonia (due to susceptible organisms including *Haemophilus influenzae*, *Haemophilus parainfluenzae*, *Streptococcus pneumoniae*-penicillin susceptible only, *Moraxella catarrhalis*); pharyngitis or tonsillitis (*Streptococcus pyogenes*); and uncomplicated skin and skin-structure infections (*Staphylococcus aureus* - not MRSA, *Streptococcus pyogenes*)

Pregnancy Risk Factor B

Pregnancy Considerations Adverse events have not been observed in animal reproduction studies; therefore, the manufacturer classifies cefditoren as pregnancy category B. Other cephalosporins cross the placenta and are considered safe in pregnancy.

Lactation Excretion in breast milk unknown/use caution

Contraindications Hypersensitivity to cefditoren, any component of the formulation, other cephalosporins, or milk protein; carnitine deficiency

Warnings/Precautions Use with caution in patients with a history of penicillin allergy, especially IgE-mediated reactions (eg, anaphylaxis, urticaria). Prolonged use may result in fungal or bacterial superinfection, including *C. difficile*-associated diarrhea (CDAD) and pseudomembranous colitis; CDAD has been observed >2 months postantibiotic treatment. Caution in individuals with seizure disorders; high levels, particularly in the presence of renal impairment, may increase risk of seizures. Use caution in patients with renal or hepatic impairment; modify dosage in patients with severe renal impairment. Cefditoren causes renal excretion of carnitine; do not use in patients with carnitine deficiency; not for long-term therapy due to the possible development of carnitine deficiency over time. May prolong prothrombin time; use with caution in patients with a history of bleeding disorder. Cefditoren tablets contain sodium caseinate, which may cause hypersensitivity reactions in patients with milk protein hypersensitivity; this does not affect patients with lactose intolerance.

Adverse Reactions

>10%: Gastrointestinal: Diarrhea (11% to 15%)

1% to 10%:

- Central nervous system: Headache (2% to 3%)
- Endocrine & metabolic: Glucose increased (1% to 2%)
- Gastrointestinal: Nausea (4% to 6%), abdominal pain (2%), dyspepsia (1% to 2%), vomiting (1%)
- Genitourinary: Vaginal moniliasis (3% to 6%)
- Hematologic: Hematocrit decreased (2%)
- Renal: Hematuria (3%), urinary white blood cells increased (2%)

<1% (Limited to important or life-threatening): Acute renal failure, albumin decreased, allergic reaction, arthralgia, asthma, BUN increased, calcium decreased, eosinophilic pneumonia, coagulation time increased, erythema multiforme, fungal infection, hyperglycemia, interstitial pneumonia, leukopenia, leukorrhea, positive direct Coombs' test, potassium increased, pseudomembranous colitis, rash, sodium decreased, Stevens-Johnson syndrome, thrombocythemia, thrombocytopenia, toxic epidermal necrolysis, white blood cells increased/decreased

Reactions reported with other cephalosporins: Anaphylaxis, aplastic anemia, cholestasis, hemorrhage, hemolytic anemia, renal dysfunction, reversible hyperactivity, serum sickness-like reaction, toxic nephropathy

Drug Interactions

Metabolism/Transport Effects None known.

Avoid Concomitant Use There are no known interactions where it is recommended to avoid concomitant use.

Increased Effect/Toxicity

The levels/effects of Cefditoren may be increased by: Probenecid

Decreased Effect

The levels/effects of Cefditoren may be decreased by: Antacids; H2-Antagonists; Proton Pump Inhibitors

Ethanol/Nutrition/Herb Interactions Food: Moderate- to high-fat meals increase bioavailability and maximum plasma concentration.

Stability Store at controlled room temperature of 15°C to 30°C (59°F to 86°F). Protect from light and moisture.

Mechanism of Action Inhibits bacterial cell wall synthesis by binding to one or more of the penicillin-binding proteins (PBPs) which in turn inhibits the final transpeptidation step of peptidoglycan synthesis in bacterial cell walls, thus inhibiting cell wall biosynthesis. Bacteria eventually lyse due to ongoing activity of cell wall autolytic enzymes (autolysins and murein hydrolases) while cell wall assembly is arrested.

Pharmacodynamics/Kinetics

Distribution: 9.3 ± 1.6 L

Protein binding: 88% (*in vitro*), primarily to albumin

Metabolism: Cefditoren pivoxil is hydrolyzed to cefditoren (active) and pivalate

Bioavailability: ~14% to 16%, increased by moderate- to high-fat meal

Half-life elimination: 1.6 ± 0.4 hours

Time to peak: 1.5-3 hours

Excretion: Urine (as cefditoren and pivaloylcarnitine)

Dosage

Usual dosage range:

Children ≥12 years and Adults: Oral: 200-400 mg twice daily

Indication-specific dosing:

Children ≥12 years and Adults: Oral:

Acute bacterial exacerbation of chronic bronchitis: 400 mg twice daily for 10 days

Dental infections (unlabeled use): 400 mg twice daily for 10 days

Community-acquired pneumonia: 400 mg twice daily for 14 days

Pharyngitis, tonsillitis, uncomplicated skin and skin structure infections: 200 mg twice daily for 10 days

Dosage adjustment in renal impairment:

Cl_{cr} 30-49 mL/minute/1.73 m^2: Maximum dose: 200 mg twice daily

Cl_{cr} <30 mL/minute/1.73 m^2: Maximum dose: 200 mg once daily

End-stage renal disease: Appropriate dosing not established

Dosage adjustment in hepatic impairment:

Mild-to-moderate impairment: Adjustment not required

Severe impairment (Child-Pugh Class C): Specific guidelines not available

Dietary Considerations Cefditoren should be taken with meals. Plasma carnitine levels are decreased during therapy (39% with 200 mg dosing, 63% with 400 mg dosing); normal concentrations return within 7-10 days after treatment is discontinued.

Administration Administer with meals.

Monitoring Parameters Assess patient at beginning and throughout therapy for infection; monitor for signs of anaphylaxis during first dose.

Test Interactions May induce a positive direct Coomb's test. May cause a false-negative ferricyanide test. Glucose oxidase or hexokinase methods recommended for blood/plasma glucose determinations. False-positive urine glucose test when using copper reduction based assays (eg, Clinitest®).

Dosage Forms Excipient information presented when available (limited, particularly for generics); consult specific product labeling.

Tablet, oral: 200 mg, 400 mg

Spectracef®: 200 mg, 400 mg [contains sodium caseinate]

◆ **Cefditoren Pivoxil** *see* Cefditoren *on page 305*

Cefepime (SEF e pim)

Brand Names: U.S. Maxipime®

Brand Names: Canada Maxipime®

Index Terms Cefepime Hydrochloride

Pharmacologic Category Antibiotic, Cephalosporin (Fourth Generation)

Use Treatment of uncomplicated and complicated urinary tract infections, including pyelonephritis caused by *Escherichia coli, Klebsiella pneumoniae*, or *Proteus mirabilis*; monotherapy for febrile neutropenia; uncomplicated skin and skin structure infections caused by *Streptococcus pyogenes* or methicillin-susceptible staphylococci; moderate-to-severe pneumonia caused by *Streptococcus pneumoniae, Pseudomonas aeruginosa, Klebsiella pneumoniae*, or *Enterobacter* species; complicated intra-abdominal infections (in combination with metronidazole) caused by *E. coli, P. aeruginosa, K. pneumoniae, Enterobacter* species, or *Bacteroides fragilis* against methicillin-susceptible staphylococci, *Enterobacter* sp, and many other gram-negative bacilli.

Children 2 months to 16 years: Empiric therapy of febrile neutropenia patients, uncomplicated skin/soft tissue infections, pneumonia, and uncomplicated/complicated urinary tract infections, including pyelonephritis.

Unlabeled Use Brain abscess (postneurosurgical prevention); malignant otitis externa; septic lateral/cavernous sinus thrombosis

Pregnancy Risk Factor B

Pregnancy Considerations Teratogenic effects were not observed in animal studies; therefore, cefepime is classified as pregnancy category B. It is not known if cefepime crosses the human placenta.

Lactation Enters breast milk/use caution

Contraindications Hypersensitivity to cefepime, other cephalosporins, penicillins, other beta-lactam antibiotics, or any component of the formulation

Warnings/Precautions Modify dosage in patients with renal impairment (Cl_{cr} ≤60 mL/minute); may increase risk of encephalopathy, myoclonus, and seizures. Use with caution in patients with a history of penicillin or cephalosporin allergy, especially IgE-mediated reactions (eg, anaphylaxis, urticaria). Prolonged use may result in fungal or bacterial superinfection, including *C. difficile*-associated diarrhea (CDAD) and pseudomembranous colitis; CDAD has been observed >2 months postantibiotic treatment. Use with caution in patients with a history of gastrointestinal disease, especially colitis. May be associated with increased INR, especially in nutritionally-deficient patients, prolonged treatment, hepatic or renal disease. Use with caution in patients with a history of seizure disorder; high levels, particularly in the presence of renal impairment, may increase risk of seizures.

Adverse Reactions

>10%: Hematologic: Positive Coombs' test without hemolysis (16%)

1% to 10%:

Central nervous system: Fever (1%), headache (1%)

Dermatologic: Rash (1% to 4%), pruritus (1%)

Endocrine & metabolic: Hypophosphatemia (3%)

Gastrointestinal: Diarrhea (≤3%), nausea (≤2%), vomiting (≤1%)

Hematologic: Eosinophils (2%)

Hepatic: ALT increased (3%), AST increased (2%), PTT abnormal (2%), PT abnormal (1%)

Local: Inflammation, phlebitis, and pain (1%)

<1% (Limited to important or life-threatening): Agranulocytosis, alkaline phosphatase increased, anaphylactic shock, anaphylaxis, bilirubin increased, BUN increased, colitis, coma, confusion, creatinine increased, encephalopathy, hallucinations, hematocrit decreased, hypercalcemia, hyperkalemia, hyperphosphatemia, hypocalcemia, leucopenia, myoclonus, neutropenia, oral moniliasis, pseudomembranous colitis, seizure, stupor, thrombocytopenia, urticaria, vaginitis

Reactions reported with other cephalosporins: Aplastic anemia, erythema multiforme, hemolytic anemia, hemorrhage, pancytopenia, PT prolonged, renal dysfunction, Stevens-Johnson syndrome, superinfection, toxic epidermal necrolysis, toxic nephropathy, vaginitis

Drug Interactions

Metabolism/Transport Effects None known.

Avoid Concomitant Use

Avoid concomitant use of Cefepime with any of the following: BCG

Increased Effect/Toxicity

Cefepime may increase the levels/effects of: Aminoglycosides

The levels/effects of Cefepime may be increased by: Probenecid

Decreased Effect

Cefepime may decrease the levels/effects of: BCG; Typhoid Vaccine

Stability

Vials: Store at 20°C to 25°C (68°F to 77°F). Protect from light. After reconstitution, stable in normal saline, D_5W, and a variety of other solutions for 24 hours at room temperature and 7 days refrigerated.

Premixed solution: Store frozen at -20°C (-4°F). Thawed solution is stable for 24 hours at room temperature or 7 days under refrigeration; do not refreeze.

Mechanism of Action Inhibits bacterial cell wall synthesis by binding to one or more of the penicillin-binding proteins (PBPs) which in turn inhibits the final transpeptidation step of peptidoglycan synthesis in bacterial cell walls, thus inhibiting cell wall biosynthesis. Bacteria eventually lyse due to ongoing activity of cell wall autolytic enzymes (autolysis and murein hydrolases) while cell wall assembly is arrested.

Pharmacodynamics/Kinetics

Absorption: I.M.: Rapid and complete

Distribution: V_d: Adults: 16-20 L; penetrates into inflammatory fluid at concentrations ~80% of serum levels and into bronchial mucosa at levels ~60% of those reached in the plasma; crosses blood-brain barrier

Protein binding, plasma: ~20%

Metabolism: Minimally hepatic

Half-life elimination: 2 hours

Time to peak: I.M.: 1-2 hours; I.V.: 0.5 hours

Excretion: Urine (85% as unchanged drug)

Dosage

Usual dosage range:

Children: I.M., I.V.: 50 mg/kg/dose every 8-12 hours (not to exceed maximum adult dosing)

Adults: I.V.: 1-2 g every 8-12 hours; I.M.: 0.5-1 g every 12 hours

Indication-specific dosing:

Children ≥2 months to 16 years (<40 kg):

Febrile neutropenia: I.V.: 50 mg/kg/dose every 8 hours for 7 days or until neutropenia resolves

Skin and skin structure infections (uncomplicated) and pneumonia: I.V.: 50 mg/kg/dose every 12 hours for 10 days

Urinary tract infections, complicated and uncomplicated: I.M., I.V.: 50 mg/kg/dose every 12 hours for 7-10 days; **Note:** I.M. may be considered for mild-to-moderate infection only

Adults:

Brain abscess, postneurosurgical prevention (unlabeled use): I.V.: 2 g every 8 hours with vancomycin

Febrile neutropenia, monotherapy: I.V: 2 g every 8 hours for 7 days or until the neutropenia resolves

Intra-abdominal infections, complicated, severe (in combination with metronidazole): I.V.: 2 g every 12 hours for 7-10 days. **Note:** 2010 IDSA guidelines recommend 2 g every 8-12 hours for 4-7 days (provided source controlled). Not recommended for hospital-acquired intra-abdominal infections (IAI) associated with multidrug-resistant gram negative organisms or in mild-to-moderate community-acquired IAIs due to risk of toxicity and the development of resistant organisms (Solomkin, 2010).

Otitis externa, malignant (unlabeled use): I.V.: 2 g every 12 hours

Pneumonia: I.V.:

Nosocomial (HAP/VAP): 1-2 g every 8-12 hours; **Note:** Duration of therapy may vary considerably (7-21 days); usually longer courses are required if *Pseudomonas*. In absence of *Pseudomonas*, and if appropriate empiric treatment used and patient responsive, it may be clinically appropriate to reduce duration of therapy to 7-10 days (American Thoracic Society Guidelines, 2005).

Community-acquired (including pseudomonal): 1-2 g every 12 hours for 10 days

Septic lateral/cavernous sinus thrombosis (unlabeled use): I.V.: 2 g every 8-12 hours; with metronidazole for lateral

Skin and skin structure, uncomplicated: I.V.: 2 g every 12 hours for 10 days

Urinary tract infections, complicated and uncomplicated:

Mild-to-moderate: I.M., I.V.: 0.5-1 g every 12 hours for 7-10 days

Severe: I.V.: 2 g every 12 hours for 10 days

Dosing adjustment in renal impairment: Adults: Recommended maintenance schedule based on creatinine clearance (mL/minute), compared to normal dosing schedule: See table.

Cefepime Hydrochloride

Creatinine Clearance (mL/minute)	Recommended Maintenance Schedule			
>60 (normal recommended dosing schedule)	500 mg every 12 hours	1 g every 12 hours	2 g every 12 hours	2 g every 8 hours
30-60	500 mg every 24 hours	1 g every 24 hours	2 g every 24 hours	2 g every 12 hours
11-29	500 mg every 24 hours	500 mg every 24 hours	1 g every 24 hours	2 g every 24 hours
<11	250 mg every 24 hours	250 mg every 24 hours	500 mg every 24 hours	1 g every 24 hours

Intermittent hemodialysis (IHD) (administer after hemodialysis on dialysis days): I.V.: Initial: 1 g (single dose) on day 1. Maintenance: 0.5-1 g every 24 hours **or** 1-2 g every 48-72 hours (Heintz, 2009). **Note:** Dosing dependent on the assumption of 3 times/week, complete IHD sessions.

Peritoneal dialysis (PD): Removed to a lesser extent than hemodialysis; administer normal recommended dose every 48 hours

Continuous renal replacement therapy (CRRT) (Heintz, 2009; Trotman, 2005): Drug clearance is highly dependent on the method of renal replacement, filter type, and flow rate. Appropriate dosing requires close monitoring of pharmacologic response, signs of adverse reactions due to drug accumulation, as well as drug concentrations in relation to target trough (if appropriate). The following are general recommendations only (based on dialysate flow/ultrafiltration rates of 1-2 L/hour and minimal residual renal function) and should not supersede clinical judgment:

CVVH: Loading dose of 2 g followed by 1-2 g every 12 hours

CVVHD/CVVHDF: Loading dose of 2 g followed by either 1 g every 8 hours **or** 2 g every 12 hours. **Note:** Dosage of 1 g every 8 hours results in similar steady-state concentrations as 2 g every 12 hours and is more cost effective (Heintz, 2009).

Note: Consider higher dosage of 4 g/day if treating *Pseudomonas* or life-threatening infections in order to maximize time above MIC (Trotman, 2005). Dosage of 2 g every 8 hours may be needed for gram-negative rods with MIC ≥4 mg/L (Heintz, 2009).

Administration May be administered either I.M. or I.V. Inject deep I.M. into large muscle mass. Inject direct I.V. over 5 minutes. Infuse intermittent infusion over 30 minutes.

Monitoring Parameters Obtain specimen for culture and susceptibility prior to the first dose. Monitor for signs of anaphylaxis during first dose.

Test Interactions Positive direct Coombs', false-positive urinary glucose test using cupric sulfate (Benedict's solution, Clinitest®, Fehling's solution), false-positive serum or urine creatinine with Jaffé reaction, false-positive urinary proteins and steroids

Dosage Forms Excipient information presented when available (limited, particularly for generics); consult specific product labeling.

Infusion, premixed iso-osmotic dextrose solution, as hydrochloride: 1 g (50 mL); 2 g (100 mL)

Injection, powder for reconstitution, as hydrochloride: 500 mg, 1 g, 2 g

Maxipime®: 500 mg, 1 g, 2 g

◆ **Cefepime Hydrochloride** *see* Cefepime *on page 306*

Cefixime (sef IKS eem)

Brand Names: U.S. Suprax®

Brand Names: Canada Suprax®

Index Terms Cefixime Trihydrate

Pharmacologic Category Antibiotic, Cephalosporin (Third Generation)

Use Treatment of urinary tract infections, otitis media, respiratory infections due to susceptible organisms including *S. pneumoniae* and *S. pyogenes*, *H. influenzae*, and many Enterobacteriaceae; uncomplicated cervical/urethral gonorrhea due to *N. gonorrhoeae*

Pregnancy Risk Factor B

Pregnancy Considerations Teratogenic effects were not observed in animal studies; therefore cefixime is classified as pregnancy category B. It is not known if cefixime crosses the human placenta; other cephalosporins cross the placenta and are considered safe in pregnancy. Congenital anomalies have not been associated with cefixime use during pregnancy (limited data). Cefixime is recommended for use in pregnant women for the treatment of gonococcal infections.

Lactation Excretion in breast milk unknown

Contraindications Hypersensitivity to cefixime, any component of the formulation, or other cephalosporins

Warnings/Precautions Prolonged use may result in fungal or bacterial superinfection, including *C. difficile*-associated diarrhea (CDAD) and pseudomembranous colitis; CDAD has been observed >2 months postantibiotic treatment. Modify dosage in patients with renal impairment. Use with caution in patients with a history of penicillin allergy, especially IgE-mediated reactions (eg, anaphylaxis, urticaria).

Adverse Reactions

>10%: Gastrointestinal: Diarrhea (16%)

2% to 10%: Gastrointestinal: Abdominal pain, nausea, dyspepsia, flatulence, loose stools

<2% (Limited to important or life-threatening): Acute renal failure, anaphylactic/anaphylactoid reactions, angioedema, BUN increased, candidiasis, creatinine increased, dizziness, drug fever, eosinophilia, erythema multiforme, facial edema, fever, headache, hepatitis, hyperbilirubinemia, jaundice, leukopenia, neutropenia, pruritus, pseudomembranous colitis, PT prolonged, rash, seizure, serum sickness-like reaction, Stevens-Johnson syndrome, thrombocytopenia, toxic epidermal necrolysis, transaminases increased, urticaria, vaginitis, vomiting

Reactions reported with other cephalosporins: Agranulocytosis, aplastic anemia, colitis, hemolytic anemia, hemorrhage, interstitial nephritis, pancytopenia, superinfection

Drug Interactions

Metabolism/Transport Effects None known.

Avoid Concomitant Use

Avoid concomitant use of Cefixime with any of the following: BCG

Increased Effect/Toxicity

Cefixime may increase the levels/effects of: Aminoglycosides

The levels/effects of Cefixime may be increased by: Probenecid

Decreased Effect

Cefixime may decrease the levels/effects of: BCG; Typhoid Vaccine

Ethanol/Nutrition/Herb Interactions Food: Delays cefixime absorption.

Stability After reconstitution, suspension may be stored for 14 days at room temperature or under refrigeration.

Mechanism of Action Inhibits bacterial cell wall synthesis by binding to one or more of the penicillin-binding proteins (PBPs); which in turn inhibits the final transpeptidation step of peptidoglycan synthesis in bacterial cell walls, thus inhibiting cell wall biosynthesis. Bacteria eventually lyse due to ongoing activity of cell wall autolytic enzymes (autolysins and murein hydrolases) while cell wall assembly is arrested.

Pharmacodynamics/Kinetics

Absorption: 40% to 50%

Distribution: Widely throughout the body and reaches therapeutic concentration in most tissues and body fluids, including synovial, pericardial, pleural, peritoneal; bile, sputum, and urine; bone, myocardium, gallbladder, and skin and soft tissue

Protein binding: 65%

Half-life elimination: Normal renal function: 3-4 hours; Renal failure: Up to 11.5 hours

Time to peak, serum: 2-6 hours; delayed with food

Excretion: Urine (50% of absorbed dose as active drug); feces (10%)

Dosage

Usual dosage range:

Children ≥6 months: Oral: 8 mg/kg/day divided every 12-24 hours (maximum: 400 mg/day)

Children >50 kg or >12 years and Adults: Oral: 400 mg/day divided every 12-24 hours

Indication-specific dosing:

Children: Oral:

S. pyogenes **infections:** Treat for 10 days

Typhoid fever (unlabeled use): 20 mg/kg/day for 10-14 days; maximum 400 mg/day

Uncomplicated gonococcal infection: Note: Due to increased antimicrobial resistance, the Public Health Agency of Canada recommends 800 mg as a single dose (unlabeled dose) for treatment of uncomplicated gonococcal infections in children ≥9 years of age.

Adults: Oral:

S. pyogenes **infections:** Treat for 10 days

Typhoid fever (unlabeled use): 20-30 mg/kg/day in 2 divided doses for 7-14 days after I.V. therapy

Uncomplicated cervical/urethral gonorrhea due to ***N. gonorrhoeae:*** 400 mg as a single dose

Note: Due to increased antimicrobial resistance, the Public Health Agency of Canada recommends 800 mg as a single dose (unlabeled dose) for treatment of uncomplicated gonococcal infections.

Dosing adjustment in renal impairment:

Cl_{cr} 21-60 mL/minute or with renal hemodialysis: Administer 75% of the standard dose

Cl_{cr} <20 mL/minute or with CAPD: Administer 50% of the standard dose

Moderately dialyzable (10%)

Dietary Considerations May be taken with food to decrease GI distress.

Administration May be administered with or without food; administer with food to decrease GI distress. Shake oral suspension well before use.

Monitoring Parameters With prolonged therapy, monitor renal and hepatic function periodically. Observe for signs and symptoms of anaphylaxis during first dose.

Test Interactions Positive direct Coombs', false-positive urinary glucose test using cupric sulfate (Benedict's solution, Clinitest®, Fehling's solution), false-positive serum or urine creatinine with Jaffé reaction; false-positive urine ketones using tests with nitroprusside

Dosage Forms Excipient information presented when available (limited, particularly for generics); consult specific product labeling.

Powder for suspension, oral, as trihydrate:

Suprax®: 100 mg/5 mL (50 mL, 100 mL); 200 mg/5 mL (50 mL, 75 mL) [contains sodium benzoate; strawberry flavor]

Tablet, oral, as trihydrate:

Suprax®: 400 mg [scored]

◆ **Cefixime Trihydrate** *see* Cefixime *on page 307*

◆ **Cefotan** *see* CefoTEtan *on page 310*

Cefotaxime (sef oh TAKS eem)

Brand Names: U.S. Claforan®

Brand Names: Canada Claforan®

Index Terms Cefotaxime Sodium

Pharmacologic Category Antibiotic, Cephalosporin (Third Generation)

Additional Appendix Information

Antibiotic Treatment of Adults With Infective Endocarditis *on page 1956*

Use Treatment of susceptible infection in respiratory tract, skin and skin structure, bone and joint, urinary tract, gynecologic as well as septicemia, and documented or suspected meningitis. Active against most gram-negative bacilli (not *Pseudomonas*) and gram-positive cocci (not enterococcus). Active against many penicillin-resistant pneumococci.

Pregnancy Risk Factor B

Pregnancy Considerations Teratogenic effects were not observed in animal studies; therefore, cefotaxime is classified as pregnancy category B. Cefotaxime crosses the placenta and can be found in fetal tissue. An increased risk of teratogenic effects has not been observed following maternal use. During pregnancy, peak cefotaxime serum concentrations are decreased and the serum half-life is shorter.

Lactation Enters breast milk/use caution (AAP rates "compatible"; AAP 2001 update pending)

Contraindications Hypersensitivity to cefotaxime, any component of the formulation, or other cephalosporins

Warnings/Precautions Modify dosage in patients with severe renal impairment. Prolonged use may result in superinfection. A potentially life-threatening arrhythmia has been reported in patients who received a rapid bolus injection via central line. Granulocytopenia and more rarely agranulocytosis may develop during prolonged treatment (>10 days). Minimize tissue inflammation by changing infusion sites when needed. Use with caution in patients with a history of penicillin allergy, especially IgE-mediated reactions (eg, anaphylaxis, urticaria). Prolonged use may result in fungal or bacterial superinfection, including *C. difficile*-associated diarrhea (CDAD) and pseudomembranous colitis; CDAD has been observed >2 months postantibiotic treatment.

Adverse Reactions

1% to 10%:

Dermatologic: Rash, pruritus

Gastrointestinal: Diarrhea, nausea, vomiting, colitis

Local: Pain at injection site

<1% (Limited to important or life-threatening): Anaphylaxis, arrhythmia (after rapid I.V. injection via central catheter), BUN increased, candidiasis, creatinine increased, eosinophilia, erythema multiforme, fever, headache, interstitial nephritis, neutropenia, phlebitis, pseudomembranous colitis, Stevens-Johnson syndrome, thrombocytopenia, transaminases increased, toxic epidermal necrolysis, urticaria, vaginitis

Reactions reported with other cephalosporins: Agranulocytosis, aplastic anemia, cholestasis, hemolytic anemia, hemorrhage, pancytopenia, renal dysfunction, seizure, superinfection, toxic nephropathy.

Drug Interactions

Metabolism/Transport Effects None known.

Avoid Concomitant Use

Avoid concomitant use of Cefotaxime with any of the following: BCG

Increased Effect/Toxicity

Cefotaxime may increase the levels/effects of: Aminoglycosides

The levels/effects of Cefotaxime may be increased by: Probenecid

Decreased Effect

Cefotaxime may decrease the levels/effects of: BCG; Typhoid Vaccine

Stability Reconstituted solution is stable for 12-24 hours at room temperature and 7-10 days when refrigerated and for 13 weeks when frozen. For I.V. infusion in NS or D_5W, solution is stable for 24 hours at room temperature, 5 days when refrigerated, or 13 weeks when frozen in Viaflex® plastic containers. Thawed solutions previously of frozen premixed bags are stable for 24 hours at room temperature or 10 days when refrigerated.

Mechanism of Action Inhibits bacterial cell wall synthesis by binding to one or more of the penicillin-binding proteins (PBPs) which in turn inhibits the final transpeptidation step of peptidoglycan synthesis in bacterial cell walls, thus inhibiting cell wall biosynthesis. Bacteria eventually lyse due to ongoing activity of cell wall autolytic enzymes (autolysins and murein hydrolases) while cell wall assembly is arrested.

Pharmacodynamics/Kinetics

Distribution: Widely to body tissues and fluids including aqueous humor, ascitic and prostatic fluids, bone; penetrates CSF best when meninges are inflamed

Metabolism: Partially hepatic to active metabolite, desacetylcefotaxime

Half-life elimination:

Cefotaxime: Premature neonates <1 week: 5-6 hours; Full-term neonates <1 week: 2-3.4 hours; Adults: 1-1.5 hours; prolonged with renal and/or hepatic impairment

Desacetylcefotaxime: 1.5-1.9 hours; prolonged with renal impairment

Time to peak, serum: I.M.: Within 30 minutes

Excretion: Urine (as unchanged drug and metabolites)

Dosage

Usual dosage range:

Infants and Children 1 month to 12 years <50 kg: I.M., I.V.: 50-200 mg/kg/day in divided doses every 6-8 hours

Children >12 years and Adults: I.M., I.V.: 1-2 g every 4-12 hours

Indication-specific dosing:

Infants >3 months and Children:

Community-acquired pneumonia (CAP) (IDSA/PIDS, 2011): I.V.: **Note:** May consider addition of vancomycin or clindamycin to empiric therapy if community-acquired MRSA suspected. In children ≥5 years, a macrolide antibiotic should be added if atypical pneumonia cannot be ruled out.

Empiric treatment, *Haemophilus influenzae*, group A *Streptococcus*, or *S. pneumoniae* (MICs to penicillin ≤2.0 mcg/mL), patient fully immunized for *H. influenzae* type b and *S. pneumoniae*, or minimal local resistance to penicillin in invasive pneumococcal strains (alternative to ampicillin or penicillin): 50 mg/kg/dose every 8 hours

Moderate-to-severe infection, patient not fully immunized for *H. influenzae* type b and *S. pneumoniae*, or significant local resistance to penicillin in invasive pneumococcal strains (preferred): 50 mg/kg/dose every 8 hours

Moderate-to-severe infection, *H. influenzae* (beta-lactamase producing) (preferred): 50 mg/kg/dose every 8 hours

Infants and Children ≤12 years:

Epiglottitis: I.M., I.V.: 150-200 mg/kg/day in 4 divided doses with clindamycin for 7-10 days

Meningitis: I.M., I.V.: 200 mg/kg/day in divided doses every 6 hours

Sepsis: I.V.: 150 mg/kg/day divided every 8 hours

Typhoid fever: I.M., I.V.: 150-200 mg/kg/day in 3-4 divided doses (maximum: 12 g/day); fluoroquinolone resistant: 80 mg/kg/day in 3-4 divided doses (maximum: 12 g/day)

Children >12 years and Adults:

Arthritis (septic): I.V.: 1 g every 8 hours

Brain abscess, meningitis: I.V.: 2 g every 4-6 hours

Caesarean section: I.M., I.V.: 1 g as soon as the umbilical cord is clamped, then 1 g at 6- and 12-hour intervals

Epiglottitis: I.V.: 2 g every 4-8 hours

Gonorrhea: I.M.: 1 g as a single dose

Disseminated: I.V.: 1 g every 8 hours

Life-threatening infections: I.V.: 2 g every 4 hours

Liver abscess: I.V.: 1-2 g every 6 hours

Lyme disease:

Cardiac manifestations: I.V.: 2 g every 4 hours

CNS manifestations: I.V.: 2 g every 8 hours for 14-28 days

Moderate-to-severe infections: I.M., I.V.: 1-2 g every 8 hours

Orbital cellulitis: I.V.: 2 g every 4 hours

Peritonitis (spontaneous): I.V.: 2 g every 8 hours, unless life-threatening then 2 g every 4 hours

Septicemia: I.V.: 2 g every 6-8 hours

Skin and soft tissue:

Mixed, necrotizing: I.V.: 2 g every 6 hours, with metronidazole or clindamycin

Bite wounds (animal): I.V.: 2 g every 6 hours

Surgical prophylaxis: I.M., I.V.: 1 g 30-90 minutes before surgery

Uncomplicated infections: I.M., I.V.: 1 g every 12 hours

Adults:

Intra-abdominal infection, complicated, community-acquired, mild-to-moderate (in combination with metronidazole): I.V.: 1-2 g every 6 -8 hours for 4-7 days (provided source controlled)

Dosing interval in renal impairment:

Manufacturer's labeling: **Note:** Renal function may be estimated using Cockcroft-Gault formula for dosage adjustment purposes.

Cl_{cr} <20 mL/minute/1.73 m^2: Dose should be decreased by 50%.

Alternate recommendations:

Children: **Note:** Glomerular filtration rate (GFR) should be estimated using an acceptable pediatric method (eg, Schwartz equation, Traub-Johnson equation, or a height/weight nomogram):

The following dosage adjustments have been used by some clinicians (Aronoff, 2007):

GFR 30-50 mL/minute/1.73 m^2: 35-70 mg/kg/dose every 8-12 hours

GFR 10-29 mL/minute/1.73 m^2: 35-70 mg/kg/dose every 12 hours

GFR <10 mL/minute/1.73 m^2: 35-70 mg/kg/dose every 24 hours

Intermittent hemodialysis (IHD): 35-70 mg/kg/dose every 24 hours

Peritoneal dialysis: 35-70 mg/kg/dose every 24 hours

Continuous renal replacement therapy (CRRT): 35-70 mg/kg/dose every 12 hours

Adults: The following dosage adjustments have been used by some clinicians (Aronoff, 2007; Heintz, 2009; Trotman, 2005):

GFR >50 mL/minute: Administer every 6 hours (Aronoff, 2007)

GFR 10-50 mL/minute: Administer every 6-12 hours (Aronoff, 2007)

GFR <10 mL/minute: Administer every 24 hours **or** decrease the dose by 50% (and administer at usual intervals) (Aronoff, 2007)

Intermittent hemodialysis (IHD): Administer 1-2 g every 24 hours (on dialysis days, administer after hemodialysis). **Note:** Dosing dependent on the assumption of 3 times/week, complete IHD sessions (Heintz, 2009).

Peritoneal dialysis (PD): 1 g every 24 hours (Aronoff, 2007)

Continuous renal replacement therapy (CRRT) (Heintz, 2009; Trotman, 2005): Drug clearance is highly dependent on the method of renal replacement, filter type, and flow rate. Appropriate dosing requires close monitoring of pharmacologic response, signs of adverse reactions due to drug accumulation, as well as drug concentrations in relation to target trough (if appropriate). The following are general recommendations only (based on dialysate flow/ultrafiltration rates of 1-2 L/hour and minimal residual renal function) and should not supersede clinical judgment:

CVVH: 1-2 g every 8-12 hours

CVVHD: 1-2 g every 8 hours

CVVHDF: 1-2 g every 6-8 hours

Dosing adjustment in hepatic impairment: Dosage reduction generally not necessary unless concurrent severe renal impairment. Consider dose reduction to 0.5 g every 12 hours in patients with Cl_{cr} <5 mL/minute (Wise, 1985).

Dietary Considerations Some products may contain sodium.

Administration Can be administered IVP over 3-5 minutes or I.V. intermittent infusion over 15-30 minutes.

Monitoring Parameters Observe for signs and symptoms of anaphylaxis during first dose; CBC with differential (especially with long courses)

Test Interactions Positive direct Coombs', false-positive urinary glucose test using cupric sulfate (Benedict's solution, Clinitest®, Fehling's solution), false-positive serum or urine creatinine with Jaffé reaction

Dosage Forms Excipient information presented when available (limited, particularly for generics); consult specific product labeling. [DSC] = Discontinued product

Infusion, premixed iso-osmotic solution:

Claforan®: 1 g (50 mL); 2 g (50 mL) [contains sodium ~50.5 mg (2.2 mEq) per cefotaxime 1 g]

Injection, powder for reconstitution: 500 mg, 1 g, 2 g, 10 g, 20 g [DSC]

Claforan®: 500 mg, 1 g, 2 g, 10 g [contains sodium ~50.5 mg (2.2 mEq) per cefotaxime 1 g]

◆ **Cefotaxime Sodium** *see* Cefotaxime *on page* 308

CefoTEtan (SEF oh tee tan)

Index Terms Cefotan; Cefotetan Disodium

Pharmacologic Category Antibiotic, Cephalosporin (Second Generation)

Additional Appendix Information

Prevention of Wound Infection and Sepsis in Surgical Patients *on page* 1954

Use Surgical prophylaxis; intra-abdominal infections and other mixed infections; respiratory tract, skin and skin structure, bone and joint, urinary tract and gynecologic as well as septicemia; active against gram-negative enteric bacilli including *E. coli*, *Klebsiella*, and *Proteus*; less active against staphylococci and streptococci than first generation cephalosporins, but active against anaerobes including *Bacteroides fragilis*

Pregnancy Risk Factor B

Pregnancy Considerations Adverse events have not been observed in animal reproduction studies; therefore, the manufacturer classifies cefotetan as pregnancy category B. Cefotetan crosses the placenta and produces therapeutic concentrations in the amniotic fluid and cord serum.

Lactation Enters breast milk (small amounts)/use caution

Contraindications Hypersensitivity to cefotetan, any component of the formulation, or other cephalosporins; previous cephalosporin-associated hemolytic anemia

Warnings/Precautions Modify dosage in patients with severe renal impairment. Although cefotetan contains the methyltetrazolethiol side chain, bleeding has not been a significant problem. Use with caution in patients with a history of penicillin allergy, especially IgE-mediated reactions (eg, anaphylaxis, urticaria). Cefotetan has been associated with a higher risk of hemolytic anemia relative to other cephalosporins (approximately threefold); monitor carefully during use and consider cephalosporin-associated immune anemia in patients who have received cefotetan within 2-3 weeks (either as treatment or prophylaxis). Prolonged use may result in fungal or bacterial superinfection, including *C. difficile*-associated diarrhea (CDAD) and pseudomembranous colitis; CDAD has been observed >2 months postantibiotic treatment. May be associated with increased INR, especially in nutritionally-deficient patients, prolonged treatment, hepatic or renal disease.

Adverse Reactions

1% to 10%:

Gastrointestinal: Diarrhea (1%)

Hepatic: Transaminases increased (1%)

Miscellaneous: Hypersensitivity reactions (1%)

<1%: Anaphylaxis, urticaria, rash, pruritus, pseudomembranous colitis, nausea, vomiting, eosinophilia, thrombocytosis, agranulocytosis, hemolytic anemia, leukopenia, thrombocytopenia, prolonged PT, bleeding, BUN increased, creatinine increased, nephrotoxicity, phlebitis, fever

Reactions reported with other cephalosporins: Seizure, Stevens-Johnson syndrome, toxic epidermal necrolysis, renal dysfunction, toxic nephropathy, cholestasis, aplastic anemia, hemolytic anemia, hemorrhage, pancytopenia, agranulocytosis, colitis, superinfection

Drug Interactions

Metabolism/Transport Effects None known.

Avoid Concomitant Use

Avoid concomitant use of CefoTEtan with any of the following: BCG

Increased Effect/Toxicity

CefoTEtan may increase the levels/effects of: Alcohol (Ethyl); Aminoglycosides; Vitamin K Antagonists

The levels/effects of CefoTEtan may be increased by: Probenecid

Decreased Effect

CefoTEtan may decrease the levels/effects of: BCG; Typhoid Vaccine

Ethanol/Nutrition/Herb Interactions Ethanol: Avoid ethanol (may cause a disulfiram-like reaction).

Stability Reconstituted solution is stable for 24 hours at room temperature and 96 hours when refrigerated. For I.V. infusion in NS or D_5W solution and after freezing, thawed solution is stable for 24 hours at room temperature or 96 hours when refrigerated. Frozen solution is stable for 12 weeks.

Mechanism of Action Inhibits bacterial cell wall synthesis by binding to one or more of the penicillin-binding proteins (PBPs) which in turn inhibits the final transpeptidation step of peptidoglycan synthesis in bacterial cell walls, thus inhibiting cell wall biosynthesis. Bacteria eventually lyse due to ongoing activity of cell wall autolytic enzymes (autolysins and murein hydrolases) while cell wall assembly is arrested.

Pharmacodynamics/Kinetics

Distribution: Widely to body tissues and fluids including bile, sputum, prostatic, peritoneal; low concentrations enter CSF

Protein binding: 76% to 90%

Half-life elimination: 3-5 hours

Time to peak, serum: I.M.: 1.5-3 hours

Excretion: Primarily urine (as unchanged drug); feces (20%)

Dosage

Usual dosage range:

Children (unlabeled use): I.M., I.V.: 20-40 mg/kg/dose every 12 hours (maximum: 6 g/day)

Adults: I.M., I.V.: 1-6 g/day in divided doses every 12 hours

Indication-specific dosing:

Children (unlabeled use):

Preoperative prophylaxis: I.M., I.V.: 40 mg/kg 30-60 minutes prior to surgery

Adolescents and Adults:

Pelvic inflammatory disease: I.V.: 2 g every 12 hours; used in combination with doxycycline

Adults:

Orbital cellulitis, odontogenic infections: I.V.: 2 g every 12 hours

Preoperative prophylaxis: I.M., I.V.: 1-2 g 30-60 minutes prior to surgery; when used for cesarean section, dose should be given as soon as umbilical cord is clamped

Susceptible infections: I.M., I.V.: 1-6 g/day in divided doses every 12 hours; usual dose: 1-2 g every 12 hours for 5-10 days; 1-2 g may be given every 24 hours for urinary tract infection; **Note:** Due to high rates of *B. fragilis* group resistance, not recommended for the treatment of community-acquired intra-abdominal infections (Solomkin, 2010)

Urinary tract infection: I.M., I.V.: 1-2 g may be given every 24 hours

Dosing interval in renal impairment:

Cl_{cr} 10-30 mL/minute: Administer every 24 hours

Cl_{cr} <10 mL/minute: Administer every 48 hours

Hemodialysis: Dialyzable (5% to 20%); administer 1/4 the usual dose every 24 hours on days between dialysis; administer 1/2 the usual dose on the day of dialysis.

Continuous arteriovenous or venovenous hemodiafiltration effects: Administer 750 mg every 12 hours

Dietary Considerations Some products may contain sodium.

Administration

I.M.: Inject deep I.M. into large muscle mass.

I.V.: Inject direct I.V. over 3-5 minutes. Infuse intermittent infusion over 30 minutes.

Monitoring Parameters Observe for signs and symptoms of anaphylaxis during first dose; monitor for signs and symptoms of hemolytic anemia, including hematologic parameters where appropriate.

Test Interactions Positive direct Coombs', false-positive urinary glucose test using cupric sulfate (Benedict's solution, Clinitest®, Fehling's solution), false-positive serum or urine creatinine with Jaffé reaction

Dosage Forms Excipient information presented when available (limited, particularly for generics); consult specific product labeling.

Injection, powder for reconstitution: 1 g [contains sodium 80 mg (3.5 mEq)/g], 2 g [contains sodium 80 mg (3.5 mEq)/g], 10 g [contains sodium 80 mg (3.5 mEq)/g]

◆ **Cefotetan Disodium** *see* CefoTEtan *on page 310*

CefOXitin (se FOKS i tin)

Brand Names: U.S. Mefoxin®

Brand Names: Canada Apo-Cefoxitin®

Index Terms Cefoxitin Sodium

Pharmacologic Category Antibiotic, Cephalosporin (Second Generation)

Additional Appendix Information

Prevention of Wound Infection and Sepsis in Surgical Patients *on page 1954*

Use Less active against staphylococci and streptococci than first generation cephalosporins, but active against anaerobes including *Bacteroides fragilis*; active against gram-negative enteric bacilli including *E. coli*, *Klebsiella*, and *Proteus*; used predominantly for respiratory tract, skin, bone and joint, urinary tract and gynecologic as well as septicemia; surgical prophylaxis; intra-abdominal infections and other mixed infections; indicated for bacterial *Eikenella corrodens* infections

Pregnancy Risk Factor B

Pregnancy Considerations Adverse events have not been observed in animal reproduction studies; therefore, cefoxitin is classified as pregnancy category B. Cefoxitin crosses the placenta and reaches the cord serum and amniotic fluid. Adequate well-controlled studies are not available in pregnant women.

Peak serum concentrations of cefoxitin during pregnancy may be similar to or decreased compared to nonpregnant values. Maternal half-life may be shorter at term. Pregnancy-induced hypertension increases trough concentrations in the immediate postpartum period.

Lactation Enters breast milk/use caution (AAP rates "compatible"; AAP 2001 update pending)

Contraindications Hypersensitivity to cefoxitin, any component of the formulation, or other cephalosporins

Warnings/Precautions Modify dosage in patients with severe renal impairment. Prolonged use may result in superinfection. Use with caution in patients with a history of penicillin allergy, especially IgE-mediated reactions (eg, anaphylaxis, urticaria). Prolonged use may result in fungal or bacterial superinfection, including *C. difficile*-associated diarrhea (CDAD) and pseudomembranous colitis; CDAD has been observed >2 months postantibiotic treatment.

Adverse Reactions

1% to 10%: Gastrointestinal: Diarrhea

<1% (Limited to important or life-threatening): Anaphylaxis, angioedema, bone marrow suppression, BUN increased, creatinine increased, dyspnea, eosinophilia, exacerbation of myasthenia gravis, exfoliative dermatitis, fever, hemolytic anemia, hypotension, interstitial nephritis, jaundice, leukopenia, nausea, nephrotoxicity (with aminoglycosides), phlebitis, prolonged PT, pruritus, pseudomembranous colitis, rash, thrombocytopenia, thrombophlebitis, toxic epidermal necrolysis, transaminases increased, urticaria, vomiting

Reactions reported with other cephalosporins: Agranulocytosis, aplastic anemia, cholestasis, colitis, erythema multiforme, hemolytic anemia, hemorrhage, pancytopenia, renal dysfunction, seizure, serum-sickness reactions, Stevens-Johnson syndrome, superinfection, toxic nephropathy, vaginitis

Drug Interactions

Metabolism/Transport Effects None known.

Avoid Concomitant Use

Avoid concomitant use of CefOXitin with any of the following: BCG

Increased Effect/Toxicity

CefOXitin may increase the levels/effects of: Aminoglycosides; Vitamin K Antagonists

The levels/effects of CefOXitin may be increased by: Probenecid

Decreased Effect

CefOXitin may decrease the levels/effects of: BCG; Typhoid Vaccine

Stability Reconstitute vials with SWFI, bacteriostatic water for injection, NS, or D_5W. For I.V. infusion, solutions may be further diluted in NS, $D_5$1/4NS, $D_5$1/2NS, D_5NS, D_5W, $D_{10}W$, LR, D_5LR, mannitol 10%, or sodium bicarbonate 5%. Reconstituted solution is stable for 6 hours at room temperature or 7 days when refrigerated; I.V. infusion in NS or D_5W solution is stable for 18 hours at room temperature or 48 hours when refrigerated. Premixed frozen solution, when thawed, is stable for 24 hours at room temperature or 21 days when refrigerated.

Mechanism of Action Inhibits bacterial cell wall synthesis by binding to one or more of the penicillin-binding proteins (PBPs) which in turn inhibits the final transpeptidation step of peptidoglycan synthesis in bacterial cell walls, thus inhibiting cell wall biosynthesis. Bacteria eventually lyse due to ongoing activity of cell wall autolytic enzymes (autolysins and murein hydrolases) while cell wall assembly is arrested.

Pharmacodynamics/Kinetics

Distribution: Widely to body tissues and fluids including pleural, synovial, ascitic, bile; poorly penetrates into CSF even with inflammation of the meninges

Protein binding: 65% to 79%

Half-life elimination: 45-60 minutes; significantly prolonged with renal impairment

Time to peak, serum: I.M.: 20-30 minutes

Excretion: Urine (85% as unchanged drug)

Dosage

Usual dosage range:

Infants >3 months and Children: I.M., I.V.: 80-160 mg/kg/day in divided doses every 4-6 hours (maximum dose: 12 g/day)

Adults: I.M., I.V.: 1-2 g every 6-8 hours (maximum dose: 12 g/day)

Note: I.M. injection is painful

Indication-specific dosing:

Infants >3 months and Children:

Mild-to-moderate infection: I.M., I.V.: 80-100 mg/kg/day in divided doses every 4-6 hours

Perioperative prophylaxis: I.V.: 30-40 mg/kg 30-60 minutes prior to surgery followed by 30-40 mg/kg/dose every 6 hours for no more than 24 hours after surgery depending on the procedure

Severe infection: I.M., I.V.: 100-160 mg/kg/day in divided doses every 4-6 hours

Adolescents and Adults:

Perioperative prophylaxis: I.M., I.V.: 1-2 g 30-60 minutes prior to surgery (may repeat in 2-5 hours intraoperatively) followed by 1-2 g every 6-8 hours for no more than 24 hours after surgery depending on the procedure

Adults:

Amnionitis, endomyometritis: I.M., I.V.: 2 g every 6-8 hours

Aspiration pneumonia, empyema, orbital cellulitis, parapharyngeal space, human bites: I.M., I.V.: 2 g every 8 hours

Intra-abdominal infection, complicated, community acquired, mild-to-moderate: I.V.: 2 g every 6 hours for 4-7 days (provided source controlled)

Liver abscess: I.V.: 1 g every 4 hours

Mycobacterium species, not MTB or MAI: I.V.: 12 g/day with amikacin

Pelvic inflammatory disease:

Inpatients: I.V.: 2 g every 6 hours **plus** doxycycline 100 mg I.V. or 100 mg orally every 12 hours until improved, followed by doxycycline 100 mg orally twice daily to complete 14 days

Outpatients: I.M.: 2 g **plus** probenecid 1 g orally as a single dose, followed by doxycycline 100 mg orally twice daily for 14 days

Dosing interval in renal impairment:

Cl_{cr} 30-50 mL/minute: Administer 1-2 g every 8-12 hours

Cl_{cr} 10-29 mL/minute: Administer 1-2 g every 12-24 hours

Cl_{cr} 5-9 mL/minute: Administer 0.5-1 g every 12-24 hours

Cl_{cr} <5 mL/minute: Administer 0.5-1 g every 24-48 hours

Hemodialysis: Moderately dialyzable (20% to 50%); administer a loading dose of 1-2 g after each hemodialysis; maintenance dose as noted above based on Cl_{cr}

Continuous arteriovenous or venovenous hemodiafiltration effects: Dose as for Cl_{cr} 10-50 mL/minute

Dietary Considerations Some products may contain sodium.

Administration

I.M.: Inject deep I.M. into large muscle mass.

I.V.: Can be administered IVP over 3-5 minutes at a maximum concentration of 100 mg/mL or I.V. intermittent infusion over 10-60 minutes at a final concentration for I.V. administration not to exceed 40 mg/mL

Monitoring Parameters Monitor renal function periodically when used in combination with other nephrotoxic drugs; observe for signs and symptoms of anaphylaxis during first dose

Test Interactions Positive direct Coombs', false-positive urinary glucose test using cupric sulfate (Benedict's solution, Clinitest®, Fehling's solution), false-positive serum or urine creatinine with Jaffé reaction

Dosage Forms Excipient information presented when available (limited, particularly for generics); consult specific product labeling.

Infusion, premixed iso-osmotic dextrose solution:
Mefoxin®: 1 g (50 mL); 2 g (50 mL) [contains sodium 53.8 mg (2.3 mEq)/g]

Injection, powder for reconstitution: 1 g, 2 g, 10 g

◆ **Cefoxitin Sodium** *see* CefOXitin *on page 311*

Cefpodoxime (sef pode OKS eem)

Index Terms Cefpodoxime Proxetil; Vantin

Pharmacologic Category Antibiotic, Cephalosporin (Third Generation)

Use Treatment of susceptible acute, community-acquired pneumonia caused by *S. pneumoniae* or nonbeta-lactamase producing *H. influenzae*; acute uncomplicated gonorrhea caused by *N. gonorrhoeae*; uncomplicated skin and skin structure infections caused by *S. aureus* or *S. pyogenes*; acute otitis media caused by *S. pneumoniae*, *H. influenzae*, or *M. catarrhalis*; pharyngitis or tonsillitis; and uncomplicated urinary tract infections caused by *E. coli*, *Klebsiella*, and *Proteus*

Pregnancy Risk Factor B

Pregnancy Considerations Teratogenic events were not observed in animal studies; therefore, cefpodoxime is classified as pregnancy category B. It is not known if cefpodoxime crosses the human placenta. Other cephalosporins cross the placenta and are considered safe in pregnancy.

Lactation Enters breast milk (small amounts)/not recommended

Contraindications Hypersensitivity to cefpodoxime, any component of the formulation, or other cephalosporins

Warnings/Precautions Modify dosage in patients with severe renal impairment. Prolonged use may result in fungal or bacterial superinfection, including *C. difficile*-associated diarrhea (CDAD) and pseudomembranous colitis; CDAD has been observed >2 months postantibiotic treatment. Use with caution in patients with a history of penicillin allergy, especially IgE-mediated reactions (eg, anaphylaxis, urticaria).

Adverse Reactions

>10%:
- Dermatologic: Diaper rash (12.1%)
- Gastrointestinal: Diarrhea in infants and toddlers (15.4%)

1% to 10%:
- Central nervous system: Headache (1.1%)
- Dermatologic: Rash (1.4%)
- Gastrointestinal: Diarrhea (7.2%), nausea (3.8%), abdominal pain (1.6%), vomiting (1.1% to 2.1%)
- Genitourinary: Vaginal infection (3.1%)

<1% (Limited to important or life-threatening): Anaphylaxis, anxiety, appetite decreased, chest pain, cough, dizziness, epistaxis, eye itching, fatigue, fever, flatulence, flushing, fungal skin infection, hypotension, insomnia, malaise, nightmares, pruritus, pseudomembranous colitis, purpuric nephritis, salivation decreased, taste alteration, tinnitus, vaginal candidiasis, weakness

Reactions reported with other cephalosporins: Agranulocytosis, aplastic anemia, cholestasis, colitis, erythema multiforme, hemolytic anemia, hemorrhage, interstitial nephritis, toxic nephropathy, pancytopenia, renal dysfunction, seizure, serum-sickness reactions, Stevens-Johnson syndrome, superinfection, toxic epidermal necrolysis, urticaria, vaginitis

Drug Interactions

Metabolism/Transport Effects None known.

Avoid Concomitant Use

Avoid concomitant use of Cefpodoxime with any of the following: BCG

Increased Effect/Toxicity

Cefpodoxime may increase the levels/effects of: Aminoglycosides

The levels/effects of Cefpodoxime may be increased by: Probenecid

Decreased Effect

Cefpodoxime may decrease the levels/effects of: BCG; Typhoid Vaccine

The levels/effects of Cefpodoxime may be decreased by: Antacids; H2-Antagonists

Ethanol/Nutrition/Herb Interactions Food: Food delays absorption; cefpodoxime serum levels may be increased if taken with food.

Stability Shake well before using. After mixing, keep suspension in refrigerator. Discard unused portion after 14 days.

Mechanism of Action Inhibits bacterial cell wall synthesis by binding to one or more of the penicillin-binding proteins (PBPs) which in turn inhibits the final transpeptidation step of peptidoglycan synthesis in bacterial cell walls, thus inhibiting cell wall biosynthesis. Bacteria eventually lyse due to ongoing activity of cell wall autolytic enzymes (autolysins and murein hydrolases) while cell wall assembly is arrested.

Pharmacodynamics/Kinetics

Absorption: Rapid and well absorbed (50%), acid stable; enhanced in the presence of food or low gastric pH

Distribution: Good tissue penetration, including lung and tonsils; penetrates into pleural fluid

Protein binding: 18% to 23%

Metabolism: De-esterified in GI tract to active metabolite, cefpodoxime

Half-life elimination: 2.2 hours; prolonged with renal impairment

Time to peak: Within 1 hour

Excretion: Urine (80% as unchanged drug) in 24 hours

Dosage

Usual dosage range:

Children 2 months to 12 years: Oral: 10 mg/kg/day divided every 12 hours (maximum dose: 400 mg/day)

Children ≥12 years and Adults: Oral: 100-400 mg every 12 hours

Indication-specific dosing:

Children 2 months to 12 years: Oral:

Acute maxillary sinusitis: 10 mg/kg/day divided every 12 hours for 10 days (maximum: 200 mg/dose)

Acute otitis media: 10 mg/kg/day divided every 12 hours (400 mg/day) for 5 days (maximum: 200 mg/dose)

Pharyngitis/tonsillitis: 10 mg/kg/day in 2 divided doses for 5-10 days (maximum: 100 mg/dose)

Children ≥12 years and Adults: Oral:

Acute community-acquired pneumonia and bacterial exacerbations of chronic bronchitis: 200 mg every 12 hours for 14 days and 10 days, respectively

Acute maxillary sinusitis: 200 mg every 12 hours for 10 days

Pharyngitis/tonsillitis: 100 mg every 12 hours for 5-10 days

Skin and skin structure: 400 mg every 12 hours for 7-14 days

Uncomplicated gonorrhea (male and female) and rectal gonococcal infections (female): 200 mg as a single dose

Uncomplicated urinary tract infection: 100 mg every 12 hours for 7 days

Dosing adjustment in renal impairment: Cl_{cr} <30 mL/minute: Administer every 24 hours

Hemodialysis: Administer dose 3 times/week following hemodialysis

Dietary Considerations May be taken with food.

Administration Administer around-the-clock to promote less variation in peak and trough serum levels.

Monitoring Parameters Observe for signs and symptoms of anaphylaxis during first dose

Test Interactions Positive direct Coombs', false-positive urinary glucose test using cupric sulfate (Benedict's solution, Clinitest®, Fehling's solution), false-positive serum or urine creatinine with Jaffé reaction

Dosage Forms Excipient information presented when available (limited, particularly for generics); consult specific product labeling.

Granules for suspension, oral: 50 mg/5 mL (50 mL, 100 mL); 100 mg/5 mL (50 mL, 100 mL)

Tablet, oral: 100 mg, 200 mg

◆ **Cefpodoxime Proxetil** *see* Cefpodoxime *on page 313*

Cefprozil (sef PROE zil)

Brand Names: Canada Apo-Cefprozil®; Cefzil®; Mint-Cefprozil; RAN™-Cefprozil; Sandoz-Cefprozil

Index Terms Cefzil

Pharmacologic Category Antibiotic, Cephalosporin (Second Generation)

Use Treatment of otitis media and infections involving the respiratory tract and skin and skin structure; active against methicillin-sensitive staphylococci, many streptococci, and various gram-negative bacilli including *E. coli*, some *Klebsiella*, *P. mirabilis*, *H. influenzae*, and *Moraxella*.

Pregnancy Risk Factor B

Pregnancy Considerations Adverse events were not observed in animal reproduction studies; therefore, cefprozil is classified as pregnancy category B. It is not known if cefprozil crosses the human placenta. Other cephalosporins cross the placenta and are considered safe for use during pregnancy.

Lactation Enters breast milk/use caution (AAP rates "compatible"; AAP 2001 update pending)

Contraindications Hypersensitivity to cefprozil, any component of the formulation, or other cephalosporins

Warnings/Precautions Modify dosage in patients with severe renal impairment. Use with caution in patients with a history of penicillin allergy, especially IgE-mediated reactions (eg, anaphylaxis, urticaria). Prolonged use may result in fungal or bacterial superinfection, including *C. difficile*-associated diarrhea (CDAD) and pseudomembranous colitis; CDAD has been observed >2 months post-antibiotic treatment. Some products may contain phenylalanine.

Adverse Reactions

1% to 10%:

Central nervous system: Dizziness (1%)

Dermatologic: Diaper rash (1.5%)

Gastrointestinal: Diarrhea (2.9%), nausea (3.5%), vomiting (1%), abdominal pain (1%)

Genitourinary: Vaginitis, genital pruritus (1.6%)

Hepatic: Transaminases increased (2%)

Miscellaneous: Superinfection

<1% (Limited to important or life-threatening): Anaphylaxis, angioedema, arthralgia, BUN increased, cholestatic jaundice, confusion, creatinine increased, eosinophilia, erythema multiforme, fever, headache, hyperactivity, insomnia, leukopenia, pseudomembranous colitis, rash, serum sickness, somnolence, Stevens-Johnson syndrome, thrombocytopenia, urticaria

Reactions reported with other cephalosporins: Agranulocytosis, aplastic anemia, colitis, hemolytic anemia, hemorrhage, interstitial nephritis, pancytopenia, renal dysfunction, seizure, superinfection, toxic epidermal necrolysis, toxic nephropathy, vaginitis

Drug Interactions

Metabolism/Transport Effects None known.

Avoid Concomitant Use

Avoid concomitant use of Cefprozil with any of the following: BCG

Increased Effect/Toxicity

Cefprozil may increase the levels/effects of: Aminoglycosides

The levels/effects of Cefprozil may be increased by: Probenecid

Decreased Effect

Cefprozil may decrease the levels/effects of: BCG; Typhoid Vaccine

Ethanol/Nutrition/Herb Interactions Food: Food delays cefprozil absorption.

Mechanism of Action Inhibits bacterial cell wall synthesis by binding to one or more of the penicillin-binding proteins (PBPs) which in turn inhibits the final transpeptidation step of peptidoglycan synthesis in bacterial cell walls, thus inhibiting cell wall biosynthesis. Bacteria eventually lyse due to ongoing activity of cell wall autolytic enzymes (autolysins and murein hydrolases) while cell wall assembly is arrested.

Pharmacodynamics/Kinetics

Absorption: Well absorbed (94%)

Protein binding: 35% to 45%

Half-life elimination: Normal renal function: 1.3 hours

Time to peak, serum: Fasting: 1.5 hours

Excretion: Urine (61% as unchanged drug)

Dosage

Usual dosage range:

Infants and Children >6 months to 12 years: Oral: 7.5-15 mg/kg/day divided every 12 hours

Children >12 years and Adults: Oral: 250-500 mg every 12 hours or 500 mg every 24 hours

Indication-specific dosing:

Infants and Children >6 months to 12 years: Oral:

Otitis media: 15 mg/kg every 12 hours for 10 days

Children 2-12 years: Oral:

Pharyngitis/tonsillitis: 7.5-15 mg/kg/day divided every 12 hours for 10 days (administer for >10 days if due to *S. pyogenes*); maximum: 1 g/day

Uncomplicated skin and skin structure infections: 20 mg/kg every 24 hours for 10 days; maximum: 1 g/day

Children >12 years and Adults: Oral:

Pharyngitis/tonsillitis: 500 mg every 24 hours for 10 days

Secondary bacterial infection of acute bronchitis or acute bacterial exacerbation of chronic bronchitis: 500 mg every 12 hours for 10 days

Uncomplicated skin and skin structure infections: 250 mg every 12 hours or 500 mg every 12-24 hours for 10 days

Dosing adjustment in renal impairment: Cl_{cr} <30 mL/minute: Reduce dose by 50%

Hemodialysis: Reduced by hemodialysis; administer dose after the completion of hemodialysis

Dietary Considerations May be taken with food. Oral suspension may contain phenylalanine; consult product labeling.

Administration Administer around-the-clock to promote less variation in peak and trough serum levels. Chilling the reconstituted oral suspension improves flavor (do not freeze).

Monitoring Parameters Assess patient at beginning and throughout therapy for infection; monitor for signs of anaphylaxis during first dose

Test Interactions Positive direct Coombs', false-positive urinary glucose test using cupric sulfate (Benedict's solution, Clinitest®, Fehling's solution), false-positive serum or urine creatinine with Jaffé reaction

Dosage Forms Excipient information presented when available (limited, particularly for generics); consult specific product labeling.

Powder for suspension, oral: 125 mg/5 mL (50 mL, 75 mL, 100 mL); 250 mg/5 mL (50 mL, 75 mL, 100 mL)

Tablet, oral: 250 mg, 500 mg

Ceftaroline Fosamil (sef TAR oh leen FOS a mil)

Brand Names: U.S. Teflaro™

Index Terms PPI-0903; PPI-0903M; T-91825; TAK-599

Pharmacologic Category Antibiotic, Cephalosporin (Fifth Generation)

Use Treatment of acute bacterial skin and skin structure infections (ABSSSI) caused by susceptible isolates of *Staphylococcus aureus* (including methicillin-susceptible and –resistant isolates), *Streptococcus pyogenes, Streptococcus agalactiae, Escherichia coli, Klebsiella pneumoniae*, and *Klebsiella oxytoca*, and community-acquired pneumonia (CAP) caused by *Streptococcus pneumoniae* (including cases with concurrent bacteremia), *Staphylococcus aureus* (methicillin-susceptible isolates only), *Haemophilus influenzae, Klebsiella pneumoniae, Klebsiella oxytoca*, and *Escherichia coli*

Pregnancy Risk Factor B

Pregnancy Considerations Skeletal abnormalities have been observed in some but not all animal studies using maternally toxic doses. There are no adequate and well-controlled studies in pregnant women.

Lactation Excretion in breast milk unknown/use caution

Contraindications Hypersensitivity to ceftaroline, other cephalosporins, or any component of the formulation

Warnings/Precautions Use with caution in patients with a history of penicillin allergy, especially IgE-mediated reactions (eg, anaphylaxis, angioedema, urticaria). Prolonged use may result in fungal or bacterial superinfection, including *C. difficile*-associated diarrhea (CDAD) and pseudomembranous colitis; CDAD has been observed >2 months postantibiotic treatment. Use with caution in patients with renal impairment (Cl_{cr} ≤50 mL/minute); dosage adjustments recommended.

Adverse Reactions

>10%: Hematologic: Positive Coombs' test without hemolysis (~11%)

2% to 10%:

Central nervous system: Headache (3% to 5%), insomnia (3% to 4%)

Dermatologic: Pruritus (3% to 4%), rash (3%)

Endocrine & metabolic: Hypokalemia (2%)

Gastrointestinal: Diarrhea (5%), nausea (4%), constipation (2%), vomiting (2%)

Hepatic: Transaminases increased (2%)

Local: Phlebitis (2%)

<2% (Limited to important or life-threatening): Abdominal pain, anaphylaxis, anemia, bradycardia, dizziness, *C. difficile*-associated diarrhea (CDAD), eosinophilia, fever, hepatitis, hyperglycemia, hyperkalemia, hypersensitivity, neutropenia, palpitation, seizures, renal failure, thrombocytopenia, urticaria

Drug Interactions

Metabolism/Transport Effects None known.

Avoid Concomitant Use

Avoid concomitant use of Ceftaroline Fosamil with any of the following: BCG

Increased Effect/Toxicity

The levels/effects of Ceftaroline Fosamil may be increased by: Probenecid

Decreased Effect

Ceftaroline Fosamil may decrease the levels/effects of: BCG; Typhoid Vaccine

Stability Store unused vials at 2°C to 8°C (36°F to 46°F); unused vials may be stored at room temperature, up to 25°C (77°F), for ≤7 days. Reconstitute 400 mg or 600 mg vial with 20 mL SWFI; mix gently; reconstituted solution should be further diluted for I.V. administration in >250 mL of a compatible solution (eg, D_5W, NS); use within 6 hours at room temperature or within 24 hours if refrigerated; color of infusion solutions ranges from clear and light to dark yellow depending on concentration and storage conditions.

Mechanism of Action Inhibits bacterial cell wall synthesis by binding to penicillin-binding proteins (PBPs) 1 through 3. This action blocks the final transpeptidation step of peptidoglycan synthesis in bacterial cell walls and inhibits cell wall biosynthesis.Bacteria eventually lyse due to ongoing activity of cell wall autolytic enzymes (autolysis and murein hydrolases) while cell wall assembly is arrested. Ceftaroline has a strong affinity for PBP2a, a modified PBP in MRSA, and PBP2x in *S. pneumoniae*, contributing to its spectrum of activity against these bacteria.

Pharmacodynamics/Kinetics

Distribution: V_d: 18.3-21.6 L

Protein binding: ~20%

Metabolism: Ceftaroline fosamil (inactive prodrug) undergoes rapid conversion to bioactive ceftaroline in plasma by phosphatase enzyme; ceftaroline is hydrolyzed to form inactive ceftaroline M-1 metabolite

Half-life elimination: Normal renal function: 2.4 hours; Moderate renal impairment (Cl_{cr} 30-50 ml/minute): 4.5 hours

Time to peak: 1 hour

Excretion: Urine (~88%); feces (~6%)

Dosage I.V.: Adults:

Usual dosage range: 600 mg every 12 hours

Indication-specific dosage:

Pneumonia, community-acquired: 600 mg every 12 hours for 5-7 days

Skin and skin structure, complicated: 600 mg every 12 hours for 5-14 days

Dosage adjustment in renal impairment:

Cl_{cr} 31-50 mL/minute: Administer 400 mg every 12 hours

Cl_{cr} 15-30 mL/minute: Administer 300 mg every 12 hours

Cl_{cr} <15mL/minute and ESRD patients receiving hemodialysis: Administer 200 mg every 12 hours; should be given after hemodialysis, if applicable

Administration Administer by slow I.V. infusion over 60 minutes.

Monitoring Parameters Obtain specimen for culture and susceptibility prior to the first dose. Monitor for signs of anaphylaxis during first dose. Monitor renal function.

Additional Information Considered to be ineffective against *Pseudomonas aeruginosa*, *Enterococcus* species (including vancomycin-susceptible and –resistant isolates), extended-spectrum beta-lactamase (ESBL) producing or AmpC overexpressing Enterobacteriaceae.

Dosage Forms Excipient information presented when available (limited, particularly for generics); consult specific product labeling.

Injection, powder for reconstitution:

Teflaro™: 600 mg

CefTAZidime (SEF tay zi deem)

Brand Names: U.S. Fortaz®; Tazicef®

Brand Names: Canada Fortaz®

Pharmacologic Category Antibiotic, Cephalosporin (Third Generation)

Use Treatment of documented susceptible *Pseudomonas aeruginosa* infection and infections due to other susceptible aerobic gram-negative organisms; empiric therapy of a febrile, granulocytopenic patient

Unlabeled Use Bacterial endophthalmitis

Pregnancy Risk Factor B

Pregnancy Considerations Teratogenic effects were not observed in animal studies; therefore, ceftazidime is classified as pregnancy category B. Ceftazidime crosses the placenta and reaches the cord serum and amniotic fluid. Maternal peak serum concentration is unchanged in the first trimester. After the first trimester, serum concentrations decrease by approximately 50% of those in nonpregnant patients. Renal clearance is increased during pregnancy.

Lactation Enters breast milk/use caution (AAP rates "compatible"; AAP 2001 update pending)

Contraindications Hypersensitivity to ceftazidime, any component of the formulation, or other cephalosporins

Warnings/Precautions Modify dosage in patients with severe renal impairment. Use with caution in patients with a history of penicillin allergy, especially IgE-mediated reactions (eg, anaphylaxis, urticaria). Prolonged use may result in fungal or bacterial superinfection, including *C. difficile*-associated diarrhea (CDAD) and pseudomembranous colitis; CDAD has been observed >2 months postantibiotic treatment. May be associated with increased INR, especially in nutritionally-deficient patients, prolonged treatment, hepatic or renal disease. Use with caution in patients with a history of seizure disorder; high levels, particularly in the presence of renal impairment, may increase risk of seizures.

Adverse Reactions

1% to 10%:

Gastrointestinal: Diarrhea (1%)

Local: Pain at injection site (1%)

Miscellaneous: Hypersensitivity reactions (2%)

<1% (Limited to important or life-threatening): Anaphylaxis, angioedema, asterixis, BUN increased, candidiasis, creatinine increased, dizziness, encephalopathy, eosinophilia, erythema multiforme, fever, headache, hemolytic anemia, hyperbilirubinemia, jaundice, leukopenia, myoclonus, nausea, neuromuscular excitability, paresthesia, phlebitis, pruritus, pseudomembranous colitis, rash, Stevens-Johnson syndrome, thrombocytosis, toxic epidermal necrolysis, transaminases increased, vaginitis, vomiting

Reactions reported with other cephalosporins: Agranulocytosis, aplastic anemia, cholestasis, colitis, hemolytic anemia, hemorrhage, interstitial nephritis, pancytopenia, prolonged PT, renal dysfunction, seizure, serum-sickness reactions, superinfection, toxic nephropathy, urticaria

Drug Interactions

Metabolism/Transport Effects None known.

Avoid Concomitant Use

Avoid concomitant use of CefTAZidime with any of the following: BCG

Increased Effect/Toxicity

CefTAZidime may increase the levels/effects of: Aminoglycosides

The levels/effects of CefTAZidime may be increased by: Probenecid

Decreased Effect

CefTAZidime may decrease the levels/effects of: BCG; Typhoid Vaccine

Stability

Fortaz®: Store dry vials at 15°C to 30°C (59°F to 86°F). Protect from light. Reconstituted solution and solution further diluted for I.V. infusion are stable for 12 hours at room temperature, for 3 days when refrigerated, or for 12 weeks when frozen at -20°C (-4°F). After freezing, thawed solution in SWFI for I.M. administration is stable for 3 hours at room temperature or for 3 days when refrigerated; thawed solution in NS in a Viaflex® small volume container for I.V. administration is stable for 12 hours at room temperature or for 3 days when refrigerated; and thawed solution in SWFI in the original container is stable for 8 hours at room temperature or for 3 days when refrigerated.

Premixed frozen solution: Store frozen at -20°C (-4°F). Thawed solution is stable for 8 hours at room temperature or for 3 days under refrigeration; do not refreeze.

Fortaz®, Tazicef®: ADD-Vantage® vials: Diluted in 50 or 100 mL of D_5W, NS, or 0.45% sodium chloride in an ADD-Vantage® flexible diluent container only, may be stored for up to 12 hours at room temperature or for 3 days under refrigeration. Freezing solutions in the ADD-Vantage® system is not recommended. Joined vials that have not been activated may be used within 14 days.

Tazicef® vials: Store dry vials at 20°C to 25°C (68°F to 77°F). Protect from light. Reconstituted vials and solution further diluted for I.V. infusion are stable for 24 hours at room temperature, for 7 days when refrigerated, or for 12 weeks when frozen at -20°C (-4°F). When thawed, solution is stable for 8 hours at room temperature and 4 days when refrigerated.

Reconstitution:

I.M.: Using SWFI, bacteriostatic water, lidocaine 0.5%, or lidocaine 1%, reconstitute the 500 mg vials with 1.5 mL or the 1 g vials with 3 mL; final concentration of *~280 mg/mL*

I.V.: Using SWFI, reconstitute as follows (**Note:** After reconstitution, may dilute further with a compatible solution to administer via I.V. infusion):

Fortaz®:

~100 mg/mL solution:

500 mg vial: 5.3 mL SWFI (withdraw 5 mL from the reconstituted vial to obtain a 500 mg dose)

1 g vial: 10 mL SWFI (withdraw 10 mL from the reconstituted vial to obtain a 1 g dose)

6 g vial: 56 mL SWFI (withdraw 10 mL from the reconstituted vial to obtain a 1 g dose)

~170 mg/mL solution: 2 g vial: 10 mL SWFI (withdraw 11.5 mL from the reconstituted vial to obtain a 2 g dose)

~200 mg/mL solution: 6 g vial: 26 mL SWFI (withdraw 5 mL from the reconstituted vial to obtain a 1 g dose)

Tazicef®:

~95 mg/mL solution: 1 g vial: 10 mL SWFI (withdraw 10.6 mL from the reconstituted vial to obtain a 1 g dose)

~180 mg/mL solution: 2 g vial: 10 mL SWFI (withdraw 11.2 mL from the reconstituted vial to obtain a 2 g dose)

Fortaz®, Tazicef®: ADD-Vantage® vials: Dilute in 50 or 100 mL of D_5W, NS, or 0.45% sodium chloride in an ADD-Vantage® flexible diluent container only.

Mechanism of Action Inhibits bacterial cell wall synthesis by binding to one or more of the penicillin-binding proteins (PBPs) which in turn inhibits the final transpeptidation step of peptidoglycan synthesis in bacterial cell walls, thus inhibiting cell wall biosynthesis. Bacteria eventually lyse due to ongoing activity of cell wall autolytic enzymes (autolysins and murein hydrolases) while cell wall assembly is arrested.

Pharmacodynamics/Kinetics

Distribution: Widely throughout the body including bone, bile, skin, CSF (higher concentrations achieved when meninges are inflamed), endometrium, heart, pleural and lymphatic fluids

Protein binding: 17%

Half-life elimination: 1-2 hours, prolonged with renal impairment; Neonates <23 days: 2.2-4.7 hours

Time to peak, serum: I.M.: ~1 hour

Excretion: Urine (80% to 90% as unchanged drug)

Dosage

Usual dosage range:

Infants and Children 1 month to 12 years: I.V.: 30-50 mg/kg/dose every 8 hours (maximum dose: 6 g/day)

Adults: I.M., I.V.: 500 mg to 2 g every 8-12 hours

Indication-specific dosing:

Bacterial arthritis (gram-negative bacilli): I.V.: 1-2 g every 8 hours

Cystic fibrosis: I.V.: 30-50 mg/kg/dose every 8 hours (maximum: 6 g/day)

Endophthalmitis, bacterial (unlabeled use): Intravitreal: 2.25 mg/0.1 mL NS in combination with vancomycin

Intra-abdominal infection, severe (in combination with metronidazole): I.V.: 2 g every 8 hours for 4-7 days (provided source controlled). Not recommended for hospital-acquired intra-abdominal infections (IAI) associated with multidrug-resistant gram negative organisms or in mild-to-moderate community-acquired IAIs due to risk of toxicity and the development of resistant organisms (Solomkin, 2010).

Melioidosis: I.V.: 40 mg/kg/dose every 8 hours for 10 days, followed by oral therapy with doxycycline or TMP/SMX

Otitis externa: I.V.: 2 g every 8 hours

Peritonitis (CAPD):

Anuric, intermittent: 1000-1500 mg/day

Anuric, continuous (per liter exchange): Loading dose: 250 mg; maintenance dose: 125 mg

Severe infections, including meningitis, complicated pneumonia, endophthalmitis, CNS infection, osteomyelitis, gynecological, skin and soft tissue: I.V.: 2 g every 8 hours

Dosing interval in renal impairment:

Cl_{cr} 30-50 mL/minute: Administer every 12 hours

Cl_{cr} 10-30 mL/minute: Administer every 24 hours

Cl_{cr} <10 mL/minute: Administer every 48-72 hours

Intermittent hemodialysis (IHD) (administer after hemodialysis on dialysis days): Dialyzable (50% to 100%): 0.5-1 g every 24 hours **or** 1-2 g every 48-72 hours (Heintz, 2009). **Note:** Dosing dependent on the assumption of 3 times/week, complete IHD sessions.

Peritoneal dialysis (PD): Loading dose of 1 g, followed by 500 mg every 24 hours

Continuous renal replacement therapy (CRRT) (Heintz, 2009; Trotman, 2005): Drug clearance is highly dependent on the method of renal replacement, filter type, and flow rate. Appropriate dosing requires close monitoring of pharmacologic response, signs of adverse reactions due to drug accumulation, as well as drug concentrations in relation to target trough (if appropriate). The following are general recommendations only (based on dialysate flow/ultrafiltration rates of 1-2 L/hour and minimal residual renal function) and should not supersede clinical judgment:

CVVH: Loading dose of 2 g followed by 1-2 g every 12 hours

CVVHD/CVVHDF: Loading dose of 2 g followed by either 1 g every 8 hours **or** 2 g every 12 hours. **Note:** Dosage of 1 g every 8 hours results in similar steady-state concentrations as 2 g every 12 hours and is more cost effective. Dosage of 2 g every 8 hours may be needed for gram-negative rods with MIC ≥4 mg/L (Heintz, 2009).

Note: For patients receiving CVVHDF, some recommend giving a loading dose of 2 g followed by 3 g over 24 hours as a continuous I.V. infusion to maintain concentrations ≥4 times the MIC for susceptible pathogens (Heintz, 2009).

Dietary Considerations Some products may contain sodium.

Administration Any carbon dioxide bubbles that may be present in the withdrawn solution should be expelled prior to injection. Administer around-the-clock to promote less variation in peak and trough serum levels. Ceftazidime can be administered deep I.M. into large mass muscle, IVP over 3-5 minutes, or I.V. intermittent infusion over 15-30 minutes. Do not admix with aminoglycosides in same bottle/bag. Final concentration for I.V. administration should not exceed 100 mg/mL.

Monitoring Parameters Observe for signs and symptoms of anaphylaxis during first dose

Test Interactions Positive direct Coombs', false-positive urinary glucose test using cupric sulfate (Benedict's solution, Clinitest®, Fehling's solution), false-positive serum or urine creatinine with Jaffé reaction

Additional Information With some organisms, resistance may develop during treatment (including *Enterobacter* spp and *Serratia* spp). Consider combination therapy or periodic susceptibility testing for organisms with inducible resistance.

Dosage Forms Excipient information presented when available (limited, particularly for generics); consult specific product labeling. [DSC] = Discontinued product

Infusion, premixed iso-osmotic solution, as sodium [strength expressed as base]:

Fortaz®: 1 g (50 mL); 2 g (50 mL) [contains sodium ~54 mg (2.3 mEq)/g]

Injection, powder for reconstitution: 500 mg [DSC], 1 g, 2 g, 6 g

Fortaz®: 500 mg, 1 g, 2 g, 6 g [contains sodium ~54 mg (2.3 mEq)/g]

Tazicef®: 1 g, 2 g, 6 g [contains sodium ~54 mg (2.3 mEq)/g]

Ceftibuten (sef TYE byoo ten)

Brand Names: U.S. Cedax®

Pharmacologic Category Antibiotic, Cephalosporin (Third Generation)

Use Treatment of acute exacerbations of chronic bronchitis, acute bacterial otitis media, and pharyngitis/tonsillitis

Pregnancy Risk Factor B

Pregnancy Considerations Teratogenic effects were not observed in animal studies; therefore, ceftibuten is classified as pregnancy category B. It is not know if ceftibuten crosses the placenta; other cephalosporins cross the placenta and are considered safe for use during pregnancy. Adequate and well-controlled studies have not been completed in pregnant women.

Lactation Excretion in breast milk unknown/use caution

Contraindications Hypersensitivity to ceftibuten, any component of the formulation, or other cephalosporins

Warnings/Precautions Modify dosage in patients with moderate-to-severe renal impairment. Prolonged use may result in fungal or bacterial superinfection, including *C. difficile*-associated diarrhea (CDAD) and pseudomembranous colitis; CDAD has been observed >2 months postantibiotic treatment. Use with caution in patients with a history of colitis and other gastrointestinal diseases. Use with caution in patients with a history of penicillin allergy, especially IgE-mediated reactions (eg, anaphylaxis, urticaria). Oral suspension formulation contains sucrose.

Adverse Reactions

1% to 10%:

Central nervous system: Headache (≤3%), dizziness (≤1%)

Gastrointestinal: Nausea (≤4%), diarrhea (3% to 4%), dyspepsia (≤2%), loose stools (≤2%), abdominal pain (1% to 2%), vomiting (1% to 2%)

Hematologic: Eosinophils increased (3%), hemoglobin decreased (1% to 2%), platelets increased (≤1%)

Hepatic: ALT increased (≤1%), bilirubin increased (≤1%)

Renal: BUN increased (2% to 4%)

<1% (Limited to important or life-threatening): Agitation, alkaline phosphatase increased, anorexia, aphasia, AST increased, constipation, creatinine increased, dehydration, diaper rash, dyspnea, dysuria, eructation, fatigue, fever, flatulence, hematuria, hyperkinesia, insomnia, irritability, jaundice, leukopenia, melena, moniliasis, nasal congestion, paresthesia, platelets increased, pruritus, pseudomembranous colitis, psychosis, rash, rigors, serum-sickness reactions, somnolence, Stevens-Johnson syndrome, stridor, taste perversion, thrombocytopenia, toxic epidermal necrolysis, urticaria, vaginitis, xerostomia

Additional reactions reported with other cephalosporins: Allergic reaction, agranulocytosis, angioedema, aplastic anemia, anaphylaxis, asterixis, cholestasis, drug fever, encephalopathy, erythema multiforme, hemolytic anemia, hemorrhage, interstitial nephritis, neuromuscular excitability, neutropenia, pancytopenia, prolonged PT, renal dysfunction, seizure, superinfection, toxic nephropathy

Drug Interactions

Metabolism/Transport Effects None known.

Avoid Concomitant Use

Avoid concomitant use of Ceftibuten with any of the following: BCG

Increased Effect/Toxicity

Ceftibuten may increase the levels/effects of: Aminoglycosides

The levels/effects of Ceftibuten may be increased by: Probenecid

Decreased Effect

Ceftibuten may decrease the levels/effects of: BCG; Typhoid Vaccine

Stability Store capsules and powder for suspension at 2°C to 25°C (36°F to 77°F). Reconstituted suspension is stable for 14 days when refrigerated at 2°C to 8°C (36°F to 46°F).

Mechanism of Action Inhibits bacterial cell wall synthesis by binding to one or more of the penicillin-binding proteins (PBPs) which in turn inhibits the final transpeptidation step of peptidoglycan synthesis in bacterial cell walls, thus inhibiting cell wall biosynthesis. Bacteria eventually lyse due to ongoing activity of cell wall autolytic enzymes (autolysins and murein hydrolases) while cell wall assembly is arrested.

Pharmacodynamics/Kinetics

Absorption: Rapid; food decreases peak concentrations, delays T_{max}, and lowers AUC

Distribution: V_d: Children: 0.5 L/kg; Adults: 0.21 L/kg

Protein binding: 65%

Half-life elimination: 2 hours; Cl_{cr} 30-49 mL/minute: 7 hours; Cl_{cr} 5-29 mL/minute: 13 hours; Cl_{cr} <5 mL/minute: 22 hours

Time to peak: 2-3 hours

Excretion: Urine (~56%); feces (39%)

Dosage

Usual dosage range:

Children 6 months to <12 years: Oral: 9 mg/kg/day for 10 days (maximum dose: 400 mg/day)

Children ≥12 years and Adults: Oral: 400 mg once daily for 10 days

Dosage adjustment in renal impairment:

Cl_{cr} ≥50 mL//minute: No adjustment needed

Cl_{cr} 30-49 mL//minute: Administer 4.5 mg/kg or 200 mg every 24 hours

Cl_{cr} 5-29 mL/minute: Administer 2.25 mg/kg or 100 mg every 24 hours.

Hemodialysis: Administer 400 mg or 9 mg/kg (maximum: 400 mg) after each hemodialysis session

Dietary Considerations

Capsule: Take without regard to food.

Suspension: Take 2 hours before or 1 hour after meals.

Administration

Capsule: Administer without regard to food.

Suspension: Administer 2 hours before or 1 hour after meals. Shake well before use.

Monitoring Parameters Observe for signs and symptoms of anaphylaxis during first dose; with prolonged therapy, monitor renal, hepatic, and hematologic function periodically

Test Interactions Positive direct Coombs', false-positive urinary glucose test using cupric sulfate (Benedict's solution, Clinitest®, Fehling's solution), false-positive serum or urine creatinine with Jaffé reaction

Dosage Forms Excipient information presented when available (limited, particularly for generics); consult specific product labeling.

Capsule, oral:

Cedax®: 400 mg

Powder for suspension, oral:

Cedax®: 90 mg/5 mL (60 mL, 90 mL, 120 mL); 180 mg/5 mL (60 mL) [contains sodium benzoate, sucrose ~1 g/5 mL; cherry flavor]

◆ Ceftin® *see* Cefuroxime *on page 322*

CefTRIAXone (sef trye AKS one)

Brand Names: U.S. Rocephin®

Brand Names: Canada Ceftriaxone for Injection; Ceftriaxone Sodium for Injection BP; Rocephin®

Index Terms Ceftriaxone Sodium

Pharmacologic Category Antibiotic, Cephalosporin (Third Generation)

Additional Appendix Information

Antibiotic Treatment of Adults With Infective Endocarditis *on page 1956*

Prevention of Infective Endocarditis *on page 1952*

Use Treatment of lower respiratory tract infections, acute bacterial otitis media, skin and skin structure infections, bone and joint infections, intra-abdominal and urinary tract infections, pelvic inflammatory disease (PID), uncomplicated gonorrhea, bacterial septicemia, and meningitis; used in surgical prophylaxis

Unlabeled Use Treatment of chancroid, epididymitis, complicated gonococcal infections; sexually-transmitted diseases (STD); periorbital or buccal cellulitis; salmonellosis or shigellosis; atypical community-acquired pneumonia; epiglottitis, Lyme disease; used in chemoprophylaxis for high-risk contacts (close exposure to patients with invasive meningococcal disease); sexual assault; typhoid fever, Whipple's disease

Pregnancy Risk Factor B

Pregnancy Considerations Teratogenic effects have not been observed in animal studies; therefore, ceftriaxone is classified as pregnancy category B. The pharmacokinetics of ceftriaxone in the third trimester are similar to those of nonpregnant patients, with the possible exception of lower peak concentrations during labor. Ceftriaxone crosses the placenta and distributes to amniotic fluid. Ceftriaxone is recommended for use in pregnant women for the treatment of gonococcal infections.

Lactation Enters breast milk/use caution (AAP rates "compatible"; AAP 2001 update pending)

Contraindications Hypersensitivity to ceftriaxone sodium, any component of the formulation, or other cephalosporins; **do not use in hyperbilirubinemic neonates**, particularly those who are premature since ceftriaxone is reported to displace bilirubin from albumin binding sites; concomitant use with intravenous calcium-containing solutions/products in neonates (≤28 days)

Warnings/Precautions Use with caution in patients with a history of penicillin allergy, especially IgE-mediated reactions (eg, anaphylaxis, urticaria). Abnormal gallbladder sonograms have been reported, possibly due to cetriaxone-calcium precipitates; discontinue in patients who develop signs and symptoms of gallbladder disease. Secondary to biliary obstruction, pancreatitis has been reported rarely. Use with caution in patients with a history of GI disease, especially colitis. Severe cases (including some fatalities) of immune-related hemolytic anemia have been reported in patients receiving cephalosporins, including ceftriaxone. Prolonged use may result in fungal or bacterial superinfection, including *C. difficile*-associated diarrhea (CDAD) and pseudomembranous colitis; CDAD has been observed >2 months postantibiotic treatment.

May be associated with increased INR (rarely), especially in nutritionally-deficient patients, prolonged treatment, hepatic or renal disease. No adjustment is generally necessary in patients with renal impairment; use with caution in patients with concurrent hepatic dysfunction and significant renal disease, dosage should not exceed 2 g/day. Ceftriaxone may complex with calcium causing precipitation. Fatal lung and kidney damage associated with calcium-ceftriaxone precipitates has been observed in premature and term neonates. Do not reconstitute, admix, or coadminister with calcium-containing solutions, even via separate infusion lines/sites or at different times in any neonatal patient. Ceftriaxone should not be diluted or administered simultaneously with any calcium-containing solution via a Y-site in any patient. However, ceftriaxone and calcium-containing solution may be administered sequentially of one another for use in patients **other than neonates** if infusion lines are thoroughly flushed, with a compatible fluid, between infusions

Adverse Reactions

>10%: Local: Induration (I.M. 5% to 17%), warmth (I.M.), tightness (I.M.)

1% to 10%:

Dermatologic: Rash (2%)

Gastrointestinal: Diarrhea (3%)

Hematologic: Eosinophilia (6%), thrombocytosis (5%), leukopenia (2%)

Hepatic: Transaminases increased (3%)

Local: Tenderness at injection site (I.V. 1%), pain

Renal: BUN increased (1%)

<1% (Limited to important or life-threatening): Abdominal pain, agranulocytosis, alkaline phosphatase increased, allergic dermatitis, allergic pneumonitis, anaphylaxis, anemia, basophilia, biliary lithiasis, bilirubin increased, bronchospasm, chills, colitis, creatinine increased, diaphoresis, dizziness, dysgeusia, dyspepsia, edema, epistaxis, erythema multiforme, exanthema, fever, flatulence, flushing, gallbladder sludge, gallstones, glossitis, glycosuria, headache, hematuria, hemolytic anemia, jaundice, leukocytosis, Lyell's syndrome, lymphocytosis, lymphopenia, moniliasis, monocytosis, nausea, nephrolithiasis, neutropenia, oliguria, palpitation, pancreatitis, phlebitis, prolonged or decreased PT, pruritus, pseudomembranous colitis, renal and pulmonary ceftriaxone-calcium precipitations (neonates including some fatalities), seizure, serum sickness Stevens-Johnson syndrome, stomatitis, thrombocytopenia, toxic epidermal necrolysis, urinary casts, urticaria, vaginitis, vomiting

Reactions reported with other cephalosporins: Angioedema, allergic reaction, aplastic anemia, asterixis, cholestasis, encephalopathy, hemorrhage, hepatic dysfunction, hyperactivity (reversible), hypertonia, interstitial nephritis, LDH increased, neuromuscular excitability, pancytopenia, paresthesia, renal dysfunction, superinfection, toxic nephropathy

Drug Interactions

Metabolism/Transport Effects None known.

Avoid Concomitant Use

Avoid concomitant use of CefTRIAXone with any of the following: BCG

Increased Effect/Toxicity

CefTRIAXone may increase the levels/effects of: Aminoglycosides; Vitamin K Antagonists

The levels/effects of CefTRIAXone may be increased by: Calcium Salts (Intravenous); Probenecid; Ringer's Injection (Lactated)

Decreased Effect

CefTRIAXone may decrease the levels/effects of: BCG; Typhoid Vaccine

Stability

Powder for injection: Prior to reconstitution, store at room temperature ≤25°C (≤77°F). Protect from light.

Premixed solution (manufacturer premixed): Store at -20°C. Once thawed, solutions are stable for 3 days at room temperature of 25°C (77°F) or for 21 days refrigerated at 5°C (41°F). Do not refreeze.

Stability of reconstituted solutions:

10-40 mg/mL: Reconstituted in D_5W, $D_{10}W$, NS, or SWFI: Stable for 2 days at room temperature of 25°C (77°F) or for 10 days when refrigerated at 4°C (39°F). Stable for 26 weeks when frozen at -20°C when reconstituted with D_5W or NS. Once thawed (at room temperature), solutions are stable for 2 days at room temperature of 25°C (77°F) or for 10 days when refrigerated at 4°C (39°F); does not apply to manufacturer's premixed bags. Do not refreeze.

100 mg/mL:

Reconstituted in D_5W, SWFI, or NS: Stable for 2 days at room temperature of 25°C (77°F) or for 10 days when refrigerated at 4°C (39°F).

Reconstituted in lidocaine 1% solution or bacteriostatic water: Stable for 24 hours at room temperature of 25°C (77°F) or for 10 days when refrigerated at 4°C (39°F).

250-350 mg/mL: Reconstituted in D_5W, NS, lidocaine 1% solution, bacteriostatic water, or SWFI: Stable for 24 hours at room temperature of 25°C (77°F) or for 3 days when refrigerated at 4°C (39°F).

Reconstitution:

I.M. injection: Vials should be reconstituted with appropriate volume of diluent (including D_5W, NS, SWFI, bacteriostatic water, or 1% lidocaine) to make a final concentration of 250 mg/mL or 350 mg/mL.

Volume to add to create a **250 mg/mL** solution:

250 mg vial: 0.9 mL

500 mg vial: 1.8 mL

1 g vial: 3.6 mL

2 g vial: 7.2 mL

Volume to add to create a **350 mg/mL** solution:

500 mg vial: 1.0 mL

1 g vial: 2.1 mL

2 g vial: 4.2 mL

I.V. infusion: Infusion is prepared in two stages: Initial reconstitution of powder, followed by dilution to final infusion solution.

Vials: Reconstitute powder with appropriate I.V. diluent (including SWFI, D_5W, $D_{10}W$, NS) to create an initial solution of ~100 mg/mL. Recommended volume to add:

250 mg vial: 2.4 mL

500 mg vial: 4.8 mL

1 g vial: 9.6 mL

2 g vial: 19.2 mL

Note: After reconstitution of powder, further dilution into a volume of compatible solution (eg, 50-100 mL of D_5W or NS) is recommended.

Piggyback bottle: Reconstitute powder with appropriate I.V. diluent (D_5W or NS) to create a resulting solution of ~100 mg/mL. Recommended initial volume to add:

1 g bottle:10 mL

2 g bottle: 20 mL

Note: After reconstitution, to prepare the final infusion solution, further dilution to 50 mL or 100 mL volumes with the appropriate I.V. diluent (including D_5W or NS) is recommended.

Mechanism of Action Inhibits bacterial cell wall synthesis by binding to one or more of the penicillin-binding proteins (PBPs) which in turn inhibits the final transpeptidation step of peptidoglycan synthesis in bacterial cell walls, thus inhibiting cell wall biosynthesis. Bacteria eventually lyse due to ongoing activity of cell wall autolytic enzymes (autolysins and murein hydrolases) while cell wall assembly is arrested.

Pharmacodynamics/Kinetics

Absorption: I.M.: Well absorbed

Distribution: V_d: 6-14 L; widely throughout the body including gallbladder, lungs, bone, bile, CSF (higher concentrations achieved when meninges are inflamed)

Protein binding: 85% to 95%

Half-life elimination: Normal renal and hepatic function: 5-9 hours; Renal impairment (mild-to-severe): 12-16 hours

Time to peak, serum: I.M.: 2-3 hours

Excretion: Urine (33% to 67% as unchanged drug); feces (as inactive drug)

Dosage

Usual dosage range:

Infants and Children: I.M., I.V.: 50-100 mg/kg/day in 1-2 divided doses (maximum: 4 g/day [meningitis]; 2 g/day [nonmeningeal infections])

Adults: I.M., I.V.: 1-2 g every 12-24 hours

Indication-specific dosing:

Infants and Children:

Community-acquired pneumonia (CAP) (IDSA/PIDS, 2011): Infants >3 months and Children: I.V.: 50-100 mg/kg/day once daily or divided every 12 hours. **Note:** May consider addition of vancomycin or clindamycin to empiric therapy if community-acquired MRSA suspected. Use the higher end of the range for penicillin-resistant *S. pneumoniae*; in children ≥5 years, a macrolide antibiotic should be added if atypical pneumonia cannot be ruled out; preferred in patients not fully immunized for *H. influenzae* type b and *S. pneumoniae*, or significant local resistance to penicillin in invasive pneumococcal strains

Epiglottitis (unlabeled use): I.M., I.V.: 50-100 mg/kg once daily; reported duration of treatment ranged from 2-14 days

Gonococcal infections:

Conjunctivitis, complicated (unlabeled use): I.M.:

<45 kg: 50 mg/kg in a single dose (maximum: 1 g)

≥45 kg: 1 g in a single dose

Disseminated (unlabeled use): I.M., I.V.:

Infants: 25-50 mg/kg/day as single daily dose for 7 days (10-14 days for meningitis) (CDC, 2010); **Note**: Use contraindicated in hyperbilirubinemic neonates.

Children <45 kg: 25-50 mg/kg once daily (maximum: 1 g)

Children ≥45 kg: 1 g once daily for 7 days

Endocarditis (unlabeled use):

<45 kg: I.M., I.V.: 50 mg/kg/day every 12 hours (maximum: 2 g/day) for at least 28 days

≥45 kg: I.V.: 1-2 g every 12 hours, for at least 28 days

Prophylaxis (due to maternal gonococcal infection): I.M., I.V.: 25-50 mg/kg as a single dose (maximum: 125 mg) (CDC, 2010)

Uncomplicated cervicitis, pharyngitis, proctitis, urethritis, vulvovaginitis (unlabeled use) (CDC, 2010):

≤45 kg: I.M.: 125 mg as a single dose

>45 kg: Refer to adult dosing

Infective endocarditis: I.M., I.V.:

Native valve: 100 mg/kg once daily for 2-4 weeks; **Note:** If using 2-week regimen, concurrent gentamicin is recommended

Prosthetic valve: 100 mg/kg once daily for 6 weeks (with or without 2 weeks of gentamicin [dependent on penicillin MIC]); **Note:** For HACEK organisms, duration of therapy is 4 weeks

Enterococcus faecalis (resistant to penicillin, aminoglycoside, and vancomycin), native or prosthetic valve: 100 mg/kg once daily for ≥8 weeks administered concurrently with ampicillin

Prophylaxis: 50 mg/kg 30-60 minutes before procedure; maximum dose: 1 g. Intramuscular injections should be avoided in patients who are receiving anticoagulant therapy. In these circumstances, orally administered regimens should be given whenever possible. Intravenously administered antibiotics should be used for patients who are unable to tolerate or absorb oral medications.

Note: American Heart Association (AHA) guidelines now recommend prophylaxis only in patients undergoing invasive procedures and in whom underlying cardiac conditions may predispose to a higher risk of adverse outcomes should infection occur. As of April 2007, routine prophylaxis for GI/GU procedures is no longer recommended by the AHA.

Lyme disease, persistent arthritis (unlabeled use): I.M., I.V.: 75-100 mg/kg (maximum: 2 g) for 2-4 weeks

Mild-to-moderate infections: I.M., I.V.: 50-75 mg/kg/day in 1-2 divided doses every 12-24 hours (maximum: 2 g/day); continue until at least 2 days after signs and symptoms of infection have resolved

Meningitis:

Gonococcal, complicated:

≤45 kg: I.V.: 50 mg/kg/day given every 12 hours (maximum: 2 g/day); usual duration of treatment is 10-14 days

>45 kg: I.V.: 1-2 g every 12 hours; usual duration of treatment is 10-14 days

Uncomplicated: I.M., I.V.: Loading dose of 100 mg/kg (maximum: 4 g), followed by 100 mg/kg/day divided every 12-24 hours (maximum: 4 g/day); usual duration of treatment is 7-14 days

Otitis media:

Acute: I.M.: 50 mg/kg in a single dose (maximum: 1 g)

Persistent or relapsing (unlabeled use): I.M., I.V.: 50 mg/kg once daily for 3 days

Pneumonia: I.V.: 50-75 mg/kg once daily

Prophylaxis against sexually-transmitted diseases following sexual assault (unlabeled use):

≤45 kg: I.M.: 125 mg in a single dose (in combination with azithromycin and metronidazole) (CDC, 2010)

>45 kg: Refer to adult dosing

Serious infections: I.V.: 80-100 mg/kg/day in 1-2 divided doses (maximum: 4 g/day)

Skin/skin structure infections: I.M., I.V.: 50-75 mg/kg/day in 1-2 divided doses (maximum: 2 g/day)

Typhoid fever (unlabeled use): I.V.: 75-80 mg/kg once daily for 5-14 days

Children >8 years (≥45 kg) and Adolescents:

Epididymitis, acute (unlabeled use): I.M.: 125 mg in a single dose

Children <15 years:

Chemoprophylaxis for high-risk contacts (close exposure to patients with invasive meningococcal disease) (unlabeled use): I.M.: 125 mg in a single dose. Children ≥15 years: Refer to adult dosing.

Adults:

Arthritis, septic (unlabeled use): I.V.: 1-2 g once daily

Brain abscess (unlabeled use): I.V.: 2 g every 12 hours with metronidazole

Cavernous sinus thrombosis (unlabeled use): I.V.: 2 g once daily with vancomycin or linezolid

Chancroid (unlabeled use): I.M.: 250 mg as single dose (CDC, 2010)

Chemoprophylaxis for high-risk contacts (close exposure to patients with invasive meningococcal disease) (unlabeled use): I.M.: 250 mg in a single dose

Cholecystitis, mild-to-moderate: 1-2 g every 12-24 hours for 4-7 days (provided source controlled)

Gonococcal infections (CDC, 2010):

Conjunctivitis, complicated (unlabeled use): I.M.: 1 g in a single dose

Disseminated (unlabeled use): I.M., I.V.: 1 g once daily for 24-48 hours may switch to cefixime (after improvement noted) to complete a total of 7 days of therapy

Endocarditis (unlabeled use): I.M., I.V.: 1-2 g every 12 hours for at least 28 days

Epididymitis, acute (unlabeled use): I.M.: 250 mg in a single dose with doxycycline

Meningitis: I.M., I.V.: 1-2 g every 12 hours for 10-14 days

Proctitis (unlabeled use): I.M.: 250 mg in a single dose with doxycycline

Prostatitis (unlabeled use): I.M.: 125-250 mg in a single dose with doxycycline

Uncomplicated cervicitis, pharyngitis, urethritis (unlabeled use): I.M.: 250 mg in a single dose with doxycycline or azithromycin

Infective endocarditis: I.M., I.V.:

Native valve: 2 g once daily for 2-4 weeks; **Note:** If using 2-week regimen, concurrent gentamicin is recommended

Prosthetic valve: I.M., I.V.: 2 g once daily for 6 weeks (with or without 2 weeks of gentamicin [dependent on penicillin MIC]); **Note:** For HACEK organisms, duration of therapy is 4 weeks

Enterococcus faecalis (resistant to penicillin, aminoglycoside, and vancomycin), native or prosthetic valve: 2 g twice daily for ≥8 weeks administered concurrently with ampicillin

Prophylaxis: I.M., I.V.: 1 g 30-60 minutes before procedure. Intramuscular injections should be avoided in patients who are receiving anticoagulant therapy. In these circumstances, orally administered regimens should be given whenever possible. Intravenously administered antibiotics should be used for patients who are unable to tolerate or absorb oral medications.

Note: American Heart Association (AHA) guidelines now recommend prophylaxis only in patients undergoing invasive procedures and in whom underlying cardiac conditions may predispose to a higher risk of adverse outcomes should infection occur. As of April 2007, routine prophylaxis for GI/GU procedures is no longer recommended by the AHA.

Intra-abdominal infection, complicated, community-acquired, mild-to-moderate (in combination with metronidazole): 1-2 g every 12-24 hours for 4-7 days (provided source controlled)

Lyme disease (unlabeled use): I.V.: 2 g once daily for 14-28 days

Mastoiditis (hospitalized; unlabeled use): I.V.: 2 g once daily; >60 years old: 1 g once daily

Meningitis: I.V.: 2 g every 12 hours for 7-14 days (longer courses may be necessary for selected organisms)

Orbital cellulitis (unlabeled use) and endophthalmitis: I.V.: 2 g once daily

Pelvic inflammatory disease: I.M.: 250 mg in a single dose plus doxycycline (with or without metronidazole) (CDC, 2010)

Pneumonia, community-acquired: I.V.: 1 g once daily, usually in combination with a macrolide; consider 2 g/day for patients at risk for more severe infection and/or resistant organisms (ICU status, age >65 years, disseminated infection)

Prophylaxis against sexually-transmitted diseases following sexual assault: I.M.: 250 mg as a single dose (in combination with azithromycin and metronidazole) (CDC, 2010)

Pyelonephritis (acute, uncomplicated): Females: I.V.: 1-2 g once daily (Stamm, 1993). Many physicians administer a single parenteral dose before initiating oral therapy (Warren, 1999).

Septic/toxic shock/necrotizing fasciitis (unlabeled use): I.V.: 2 g once daily; with clindamycin for toxic shock

Surgical prophylaxis: I.V.: 1 g 30 minutes to 2 hours before surgery

Cholecystectomy: 1-2 g every 12-24 hours, discontinue within 24 hours unless infection outside gallbladder suspected

Syphilis (unlabeled use): I.M., I.V.: 1 g once daily for 10-14 days; **Note:** Alternative treatment for early syphilis, optimal dose, and duration have not been defined (CDC, 2010)

Typhoid fever (unlabeled use): I.V.: 2 g once daily for 14 days

Whipple's disease (unlabeled use): Initial: 2 g once daily for 10-14 days, then oral therapy for ~1 year.

Dosage adjustment in renal impairment: No dosage adjustment is generally necessary in renal impairment; **Note:** Concurrent renal and hepatic dysfunction: Maximum dose: ≤2 g/day

Poorly dialyzed; no supplemental dose or dosage adjustment necessary, including patients on intermittent hemodialysis, peritoneal dialysis, or continuous renal replacement therapy (eg, CVVHD).

Dosage adjustment in hepatic impairment: No adjustment necessary unless there is concurrent renal dysfunction (see dosage adjustment in renal impairment).

Dietary Considerations Some products may contain sodium.

Administration Do not admix with aminoglycosides in same bottle/bag. Do not reconstitute, admix, or coadminister with calcium-containing solutions. Infuse intermittent infusion over 30 minutes.

I.M.: Inject deep I.M. into large muscle mass; a concentration of 250 mg/mL or 350 mg/mL is recommended for all vial sizes except the 250 mg size (250 mg/mL is suggested); can be diluted with 1:1 water and 1% lidocaine for I.M. administration.

I.V.: Infuse intermittent infusion over 30 minutes.

Monitoring Parameters Observe for signs and symptoms of anaphylaxis

Test Interactions Positive direct Coombs', false-positive urinary glucose test using cupric sulfate (Benedict's solution, Clinitest®, Fehling's solution), false-positive serum or urine creatinine with Jaffé reaction

Dosage Forms Excipient information presented when available (limited, particularly for generics); consult specific product labeling.

Infusion, premixed in D_5W: 1 g (50 mL); 2 g (50 mL)

Injection, powder for reconstitution: 250 mg, 500 mg, 1 g, 2 g, 10 g

Rocephin®: 500 mg, 1 g [contains sodium ~83 mg (3.6 mEq) per ceftriaxone 1 g]

◆ **Ceftriaxone for Injection (Can)** *see* CefTRIAXone *on page 318*

◆ **Ceftriaxone Sodium** *see* CefTRIAXone *on page 318*

◆ **Ceftriaxone Sodium for Injection BP (Can)** *see* CefTRIAXone *on page 318*

Cefuroxime (se fyoor OKS eem)

Brand Names: U.S. Ceftin®; Zinacef®

Brand Names: Canada Apo-Cefuroxime®; Ceftin®; Cefuroxime For Injection; PRO-Cefuroxime; ratio-Cefuroxime

Index Terms Cefuroxime Axetil; Cefuroxime Sodium

Pharmacologic Category Antibiotic, Cephalosporin (Second Generation)

Additional Appendix Information

Prevention of Wound Infection and Sepsis in Surgical Patients *on page 1954*

Use Treatment of infections caused by staphylococci, group B streptococci, *H. influenzae* (type A and B), *E. coli*, *Enterobacter*, *Salmonella*, and *Klebsiella*; treatment of susceptible infections of the upper and lower respiratory tract, otitis media, urinary tract, uncomplicated skin and soft tissue, bone and joint, sepsis, uncomplicated gonorrhea, and early Lyme disease; surgical prophylaxis

Pregnancy Risk Factor B

Pregnancy Considerations Adverse events were not observed in animal studies; therefore, cefuroxime is classified as pregnancy category B. Cefuroxime crosses the placenta and reaches the cord serum and amniotic fluid. Placental transfer is decreased in the presence of oligohydramnios. Several studies have failed to identify a teratogenic risk to the fetus from maternal cefuroxime use.

During pregnancy, mean plasma concentrations of cefuroxime are 50% lower, the AUC is 25% lower, and the plasma half-life is shorter than nonpregnant values. At term, plasma half-life is similar to nonpregnant values and peak maternal concentrations after I.M. administration are slightly decreased. Pregnancy does not alter the volume of distribution.

Lactation Enters breast milk/use caution

Contraindications Hypersensitivity to cefuroxime, any component of the formulation, or other cephalosporins

Warnings/Precautions Modify dosage in patients with severe renal impairment. Use with caution in patients with a history of penicillin allergy, especially IgE-mediated reactions (eg, anaphylaxis, urticaria). Prolonged use may result in fungal or bacterial superinfection, including *C. difficile*-associated diarrhea (CDAD) and pseudomembranous colitis; CDAD has been observed >2 months postantibiotic treatment. May be associated with increased INR, especially in nutritionally-deficient patients, prolonged treatment, hepatic or renal disease. Tablets and oral suspension are not bioequivalent (do not substitute on a mg-per-mg basis). Some products may contain phenylalanine.

Adverse Reactions

>10%: Gastrointestinal: Diarrhea (4% to 11%, duration-dependent)

1% to 10%:

Dermatologic: Diaper rash (3%)

Endocrine & metabolic: Alkaline phosphatase increased (2%), lactate dehydrogenase increased (1%)

Gastrointestinal: Nausea/vomiting (3% to 7%)

Genitourinary: Vaginitis (≤5%)

Hematologic: Eosinophilia (7%), hemoglobin and hematocrit decreased (10%)

Hepatic: Transaminases increased (2% to 4%)

Local: Thrombophlebitis (2%)

<1% (Limited to important or life-threatening): Anaphylaxis, angioedema, BUN increased, chest pain, cholestasis, colitis, creatinine increased, dyspnea, erythema multiforme, fever, GI bleeding, hemolytic anemia, hepatitis, hives, hyperbilirubinemia, hypersensitivity, interstitial nephritis, jaundice, leukopenia, neutropenia, pain at injection site, pancytopenia, positive Coombs test, prolonged PT/INR, pseudomembranous colitis, rash, renal dysfunction, seizure, Stevens-Johnson syndrome, stomach cramps, tachycardia, thrombocytopenia (rare), tongue swelling, toxic epidermal necrolysis, urticaria

Reactions reported with other cephalosporins: Agranulocytosis, aplastic anemia, asterixis, colitis, encephalopathy, hemorrhage, neuromuscular excitability, serum-sickness reactions, superinfection, toxic nephropathy

Drug Interactions

Metabolism/Transport Effects None known.

Avoid Concomitant Use

Avoid concomitant use of Cefuroxime with any of the following: BCG

Increased Effect/Toxicity

Cefuroxime may increase the levels/effects of: Aminoglycosides

The levels/effects of Cefuroxime may be increased by: Probenecid

Decreased Effect

Cefuroxime may decrease the levels/effects of: BCG; Typhoid Vaccine

The levels/effects of Cefuroxime may be decreased by: Antacids; H2-Antagonists

Ethanol/Nutrition/Herb Interactions Food: Bioavailability is increased with food; cefuroxime serum levels may be increased if taken with food or dairy products.

Stability

Injection: Reconstituted solution is stable for 24 hours at room temperature and 48 hours when refrigerated. I.V. infusion in NS or D_5W solution is stable for 24 hours at room temperature, 7 days when refrigerated, or 26 weeks when frozen. After freezing, thawed solution is stable for 24 hours at room temperature or 21 days when refrigerated.

Oral suspension: Prior to reconstitution, store at 2°C to 30°C (36°F to 86°F). Reconstituted suspension is stable for 10 days at 2°C to 8°C (36°F to 46°F).

Tablet: Store at 15°C to 30°C (59°F to 86°F).

Mechanism of Action Inhibits bacterial cell wall synthesis by binding to one or more of the penicillin-binding proteins (PBPs) which in turn inhibits the final transpeptidation step of peptidoglycan synthesis in bacterial cell walls, thus inhibiting cell wall biosynthesis. Bacteria eventually lyse due to ongoing activity of cell wall autolytic enzymes (autolysins and murein hydrolases) while cell wall assembly is arrested.

Pharmacodynamics/Kinetics

Absorption: Oral (cefuroxime axetil): Increases with food

Distribution: Widely to body tissues and fluids; crosses blood-brain barrier; therapeutic concentrations achieved in CSF even when meninges are not inflamed

Protein binding: 33% to 50%

Bioavailability: Tablet: Fasting: 37%; Following food: 52%

Half-life elimination: Children 1-2 hours; Adults: 1-2 hours; prolonged with renal impairment

Time to peak, serum: I.M.: ~15-60 minutes; I.V.: 2-3 minutes; Oral: Children: 3-4 hours; Adults: 2-3 hours

Excretion: Urine (66% to 100% as unchanged drug)

Dosage Note: Cefuroxime axetil film-coated tablets and oral suspension are not bioequivalent and are not substitutable on a mg/mg basis

Usual dosage range:

Children 3 months to 12 years:

Oral: 20-30 mg/kg/day in 2 divided doses

I.M., I.V.: 75-150 mg/kg/day divided every 8 hours (maximum dose: 6 g/day)

Children ≥13 years and Adults:
Oral: 250-500 mg twice daily
I.M., I.V.: 750 mg to 1.5 g every 6-8 hours or 100-150 mg/kg/day in divided doses every 6-8 hours (maximum: 6 g/day)

Indication-specific dosing:

Children ≥3 months to 12 years:

Acute bacterial maxillary sinusitis, acute otitis media, and impetigo:
Oral: Suspension: 30 mg/kg/day in 2 divided doses for 10 days (maximum dose: 1 g/day); tablet: 250 mg twice daily for 10 days
I.M., I.V.: 75-150 mg/kg/day divided every 8 hours (maximum dose: 6 g/day)

Epiglottitis: Oral: 150 mg/kg/day in 3 divided doses for 7-10 days

Pharyngitis/tonsillitis:
Oral: Suspension: 20 mg/kg/day (maximum: 500 mg/day) in 2 divided doses for 10 days; tablet: 125 mg every 12 hours for 10 days
I.M., I.V.: 75-150 mg/kg day divided every 8 hours (maximum: 6 g/day)

Children ≥13 years and Adults (all oral doses listed are for tablet formulation):

Bronchitis (acute and exacerbations of chronic bronchitis):
Oral: 250-500 mg every 12 hours for 10 days
I.V.: 500-750 mg every 8 hours (complete therapy with oral dosing)

Cellulitis, orbital: I.V.: 1.5 g every 8 hours

Gonorrhea:
Disseminated: I.M., I.V.: 750 mg every 8 hours
Uncomplicated:
Oral: 1 g as a single dose
I.M.: 1.5 g as single dose (administer in 2 different sites with probenecid)

Lyme disease (early): Oral: 500 mg twice daily for 20 days

Pharyngitis/tonsillitis and sinusitis: Oral: 250 mg twice daily for 10 days

Pneumonia (uncomplicated): I.V.: 750 mg every 8 hours

Severe or complicated infections: I.M., I.V.: 1.5 g every 8 hours (up to 1.5 g every 6 hours in life-threatening infections)

Skin/skin structure infection (uncomplicated):
Oral: 250-500 mg every 12 hours for 10 days
I.M., I.V.: 750 mg every 8 hours

Surgical prophylaxis: I.V.: 1.5 g 30 minutes to 1 hour prior to procedure (if procedure is prolonged can give 750 mg every 8 hours I.M.)
Open heart: I.V.: 1.5 g every 12 hours to a total of 6 g

Urinary tract infection (uncomplicated):
Oral: 125-250 mg every 12 hours for 7-10 days
I.M., I.V.: 750 mg every 8 hours

Adults:

Cholecystitis, mild-to-moderate: I.V.: 1.5 g every 8 hours for 4-7 days (provided source controlled)

Intra-abdominal infection, complicated, community-acquired, mild-to-moderate (in combination with metronidazole): I.V.: 1.5 g every 8 hours for 4-7 days (provided source controlled)

Surgical prophylaxis:
Cholecystectomy: I.V.: 1.5 g every 8 hours, discontinue within 24 hours unless infection outside gallbladder suspected

Dosing adjustment in renal impairment:
Cl_{cr} 10-20 mL/minute: Administer every 12 hours
Cl_{cr} <10 mL/minute: Administer every 24 hours
Hemodialysis: Dialyzable (25%)
Peritoneal dialysis: Dose every 24 hours
Continuous renal replacement therapy (CRRT): 1 g every 12 hours

Dietary Considerations Some products may contain phenylalanine and/or sodium.
Oral suspension: May be taken with food.

Administration
Oral suspension: Administer with food. Shake well before use.
I.M.: Inject deep I.M. into large muscle mass.
I.V.: Inject direct I.V. over 3-5 minutes. Infuse intermittent infusion over 15-30 minutes.

Monitoring Parameters Observe for signs and symptoms of anaphylaxis during first dose; with prolonged therapy, monitor renal, hepatic, and hematologic function periodically; monitor prothrombin time in patients at risk of prolongation during cephalosporin therapy (nutritionally-deficient, prolonged treatment, renal or hepatic disease)

Test Interactions Positive direct Coombs', false-positive urinary glucose test using cupric sulfate (Benedict's solution, Clinitest®, Fehling's solution); false-negative may occur with ferricyanide test. Glucose oxidase or hexokinase-based methods should be used.

Dosage Forms Excipient information presented when available (limited, particularly for generics); consult specific product labeling.
Infusion, premixed iso-osmotic solution, as sodium [strength expressed as base]:
Zinacef®: 750 mg (50 mL); 1.5 g (50 mL) [contains sodium 4.8 mEq (111 mg) per 750 mg]
Injection, powder for reconstitution, as sodium [strength expressed as base]: 750 mg, 1.5 g, 7.5 g, 75 g
Zinacef®: 750 mg, 1.5 g, 7.5 g [contains sodium ~1.8 mEq (41 mg) per 750 mg]
Powder for suspension, oral, as axetil [strength expressed as base]: 125 mg/5 mL (100 mL); 250 mg/5 mL (50 mL, 100 mL)
Ceftin®: 125 mg/5 mL (100 mL) [contains phenylalanine 11.8 mg/5 mL; tutti frutti flavor]
Ceftin®: 250 mg/5 mL (50 mL, 100 mL) [contains phenylalanine 25.2 mg/5 mL; tutti frutti flavor]
Tablet, oral, as axetil [strength expressed as base]: 250 mg, 500 mg
Ceftin®: 250 mg, 500 mg

◆ **Cefuroxime Axetil** *see* Cefuroxime *on page 322*
◆ **Cefuroxime For Injection (Can)** *see* Cefuroxime *on page 322*
◆ **Cefuroxime Sodium** *see* Cefuroxime *on page 322*
◆ **Cefzil** *see* Cefprozil *on page 314*
◆ **Cefzil® (Can)** *see* Cefprozil *on page 314*
◆ **CeleBREX®** *see* Celecoxib *on page 323*
◆ **Celebrex® (Can)** *see* Celecoxib *on page 323*

Celecoxib (se le KOKS ib)

Brand Names: U.S. CeleBREX®
Brand Names: Canada Celebrex®

Pharmacologic Category Nonsteroidal Anti-inflammatory Drug (NSAID), COX-2 Selective

Use Relief of the signs and symptoms of osteoarthritis, ankylosing spondylitis, juvenile idiopathic arthritis (JIA), and rheumatoid arthritis; management of acute pain; treatment of primary dysmenorrhea

Pregnancy Risk Factor C (prior to 30 weeks gestation)/D (≥30 weeks gestation)

Pregnancy Considerations Teratogenic effects have been observed in some animal studies; therefore, celecoxib is classified as pregnancy category C. Celecoxib is a NSAID that primarily inhibits COX-2 whereas other currently available NSAIDs are nonselective for COX-1 and COX-2. The effects of this selective inhibition to the fetus have not been well studied and limited information is available specific to celecoxib. NSAID exposure during the first trimester is not strongly associated with congenital malformations; however, cardiovascular anomalies and cleft palate have been observed following NSAID exposure in some studies. The use of a NSAID close to conception may be associated with an increased risk of miscarriage. Nonteratogenic effects have been observed following NSAID administration during the third trimester including: Myocardial degenerative changes, prenatal constriction of the ductus arteriosus, fetal tricuspid regurgitation, failure of the ductus arteriosus to close postnatally; renal dysfunction or failure, oligohydramnios; gastrointestinal bleeding or perforation, increased risk of necrotizing enterocolitis; intracranial bleeding (including intraventricular hemorrhage), platelet dysfunction with resultant bleeding; pulmonary hypertension. Because it may cause premature closure of the ductus arteriosus, the use of celecoxib is not recommended ≥30 weeks gestation. The chronic use of NSAIDs in women of reproductive age may be associated with infertility that is reversible upon discontinuation of the medication. A registry is available for pregnant women exposed to autoimmune medications including celecoxib. For additional information contact the Organization of Teratology Information Specialists, OTIS Autoimmune Diseases Study, at 877-311-8972.

Lactation Enters breast milk/use caution

Medication Guide Available Yes

Contraindications Hypersensitivity to celecoxib, sulfonamides, aspirin, other NSAIDs, or any component of the formulation; perioperative pain in the setting of coronary artery bypass graft (CABG) surgery

Canadian labeling: Additional contraindications (not in U.S. labeling): Pregnancy (third trimester); women who are breast-feeding; severe, uncontrolled heart failure; active gastrointestinal ulcer (gastric, duodenal, peptic) or bleeding; inflammatory bowel disease; cerebrovascular bleeding; severe liver impairment or active hepatic disease; severe renal impairment (Cl_{cr} <30 mL/minute) or deteriorating renal disease; known hyperkalemia; use in children

Warnings/Precautions [U.S. Boxed Warning]: NSAIDs are associated with an increased risk of serious (and potentially fatal) adverse cardiovascular thrombotic events, including MI and stroke. Risk may be increased with duration of use or pre-existing cardiovascular risk factors or disease. Carefully evaluate individual cardiovascular risk profiles prior to prescribing. New-onset or exacerbation of hypertension may occur (NSAIDS may impair response to thiazide or loop diuretics); may contribute to cardiovascular events; monitor blood pressure; use with caution in patients with hypertension. May cause sodium and fluid retention; use with caution in patients with edema, cerebrovascular disease, or ischemic heart disease. Avoid use in heart failure. Long-term cardiovascular risk in children has not been evaluated.

[U.S. Boxed Warning]: Celecoxib is contraindicated for treatment of perioperative pain in the setting of coronary artery bypass graft (CABG) surgery. Risk of MI and stroke may be increased with use following CABG surgery.

[U.S. Boxed Warning]: NSAIDs may increase risk of serious gastrointestinal ulceration, bleeding, and perforation (may be fatal). These events may occur at any time during therapy and without warning. Use caution with a history of GI disease (bleeding or ulcers), concurrent therapy with aspirin, anticoagulants and/or corticosteroids, smoking, use of alcohol, the elderly or debilitated patients. When used concomitantly with ≤325 mg of aspirin, a substantial increase in the risk of gastrointestinal complications (eg, ulcer) occurs; concomitant gastroprotective therapy (eg, proton pump inhibitors) is recommended (Bhatt, 2008).

Use the lowest effective dose for the shortest duration of time, consistent with individual patient goals, to reduce risk of cardiovascular or GI adverse events. Alternate therapies should be considered for patients at high risk.

NSAIDs may cause serious skin adverse events including exfoliative dermatitis, Stevens-Johnson syndrome (SJS), and toxic epidermal necrolysis (TEN); may occur without warning and in patients without prior known sulfa allergy. Anaphylactoid reactions may occur, even without prior exposure; patients with "aspirin triad" (bronchial asthma, aspirin intolerance, rhinitis) may be at increased risk. Do not use in patients who experience bronchospasm, asthma, rhinitis, or urticaria with NSAID or aspirin therapy. Use with caution in other forms of asthma.

Use with caution in patients with decreased hepatic (dosage adjustments are recommended for moderate hepatic impairment; not recommended for patients with severe hepatic impairment) or renal function. Transaminase elevations have been reported with use; closely monitor patients with any abnormal LFT. Severe hepatic reactions (eg, fulminant hepatitis, liver failure) have occurred with NSAID use, rarely; discontinue if signs or symptoms of liver disease develop, if systemic manifestations occur, or with persistent or worsening abnormal hepatic function tests. NSAID use may compromise existing renal function; dose-dependent decreases in prostaglandin synthesis may result from NSAID use, causing a reduction in renal blood flow which may cause renal decompensation (usually reversible). Patients with impaired renal function, dehydration, heart failure, liver dysfunction, those taking diuretics, ACE inhibitors, angiotensin II receptor blockers, and the elderly are at greater risk for renal toxicity. Rehydrate patient before starting therapy; monitor renal function closely. Not recommended for use in patients with advanced renal disease or severe renal insufficiency; discontinue use with persistent or worsening abnormal renal function tests. Long-term NSAID use may result in renal papillary necrosis. Should not be considered a treatment or replacement of corticosteroid-dependent diseases.

Anaphylactoid reactions may occur, even with no prior exposure to celecoxib. Use with caution in patients with known or suspected deficiency of cytochrome P450 isoenzyme 2C9; poor metabolizers may have higher plasma levels due to reduced metabolism; consider reduced initial doses. Alternate therapies should be considered in patients with JIA who are poor metabolizers of CYP2C9.

Anemia may occur with use; monitor hemoglobin or hematocrit in patients on long-term treatment. Celecoxib does not affect PT, PTT or platelet counts; does not inhibit platelet aggregation at approved doses.

When used for juvenile idiopathic arthritis (JIA), celecoxib is not FDA-approved in children <2 years of age or in children <10 kg. Use caution with systemic onset JIA (may be at risk for disseminated intravascular coagulation). Safety and efficacy have not been established for use in children for indications other than JIA.

Adverse Reactions

≥2%

- Cardiovascular: Peripheral edema
- Central nervous system: Dizziness, fever, headache, insomnia
- Dermatologic: Rash
- Gastrointestinal: Abdominal pain, diarrhea, dyspepsia, flatulence, nausea, vomiting
- Neuromuscular & skeletal: Arthralgia, back pain
- Respiratory: Cough, nasopharyngitis, pharyngitis, rhinitis, sinusitis, upper respiratory tract infection

0.1% to 1.9%:

Cardiovascular: Angina, aortic valve incompetence, chest pain, coronary artery disorder, edema, facial edema, hypertension (aggravated), MI, palpitation, sinus bradycardia, tachycardia, ventricular hypertrophy

Central nervous system: Anxiety, depression, fatigue, hypoesthesia, migraine, nervousness, pain, somnolence, vertigo

Dermatologic: Alopecia, bruising, cellulitis, dermatitis, dry skin, photosensitivity, pruritus, rash (erythematous), rash (maculopapular), urticaria

Endocrine & metabolic: Hot flashes, hypercholesterolemia, hyperglycemia, hypokalemia, ovarian cyst, testosterone decreased

Gastrointestinal: Anorexia, appetite increased, constipation, diverticulitis, dysphagia, eructation, esophagitis, gastritis, gastroenteritis, gastroesophageal reflux, gastrointestinal ulcer, hemorrhoids, hiatal hernia, melena, stomatitis, tenesmus, weight gain, xerostomia

Genitourinary: Cystitis, dysuria, urinary frequency

Hematologic: Anemia, thrombocythemia

Hepatic: Alkaline phosphatase increased, transaminases increased

Neuromuscular & skeletal: Arthrosis, CPK increased, hypertonia, leg cramps, myalgia, paresthesia, synovitis, tendonitis

Ocular: Conjunctival hemorrhage, vitreous floaters

Otic: Deafness, labyrinthitis, tinnitus

Renal: Albuminuria, BUN increased, creatinine increased, hematuria, nonprotein nitrogen increased, renal calculi

Respiratory: Bronchitis, bronchospasm, dyspnea, epistaxis, laryngitis, pneumonia

Miscellaneous: Allergic reactions, allergy aggravated, cyst, diaphoresis, flu-like syndrome

<0.1% (Limited to important or life-threatening): Acute renal failure, agranulocytosis, anaphylactoid reactions, angioedema, anosmia, aplastic anemia, aseptic meningitis, cerebrovascular accident, CHF, cholelithiasis, colitis, DVT, erythema multiforme, esophageal perforation, exfoliative dermatitis, gangrene, gastrointestinal bleeding, hepatic failure, hepatic necrosis, hepatitis (including fulminant), hypoglycemia, hyponatremia, ileus, interstitial nephritis, intestinal obstruction, intestinal perforation, intracranial hemorrhage, jaundice, leukopenia, pancreatitis, pancytopenia, pulmonary embolism, renal papillary necrosis, sepsis, Stevens-Johnson syndrome, sudden death, suicide, syncope, thrombocytopenia, thrombophlebitis, toxic epidermal necrolysis, vasculitis, ventricular fibrillation

Drug Interactions

Metabolism/Transport Effects Substrate of CYP2C9 (major), CYP3A4 (minor); **Note:** Assignment of Major/Minor substrate status based on clinically relevant drug interaction potential; **Inhibits** CYP2C8 (moderate), CYP2D6 (moderate)

Avoid Concomitant Use

Avoid concomitant use of Celecoxib with any of the following: Floctafenine; Ketorolac; Ketorolac (Nasal); Ketorolac (Systemic); Thioridazine

Increased Effect/Toxicity

Celecoxib may increase the levels/effects of: Aminoglycosides; Anticoagulants; Antiplatelet Agents; Bisphosphonate Derivatives; CycloSPORINE; CycloSPORINE (Systemic); CYP2C8 Substrates; CYP2D6 Substrates; Deferasirox; Desmopressin; Digoxin; Eplerenone; Fesoterodine; Haloperidol; Lithium; Methotrexate; Nebivolol; Nonsteroidal Anti-Inflammatory Agents; Porfimer; Potassium-Sparing Diuretics; PRALAtrexate; Prilocaine; Quinolone Antibiotics; Tamoxifen; Thioridazine; Thrombolytic Agents; Vancomycin; Vitamin K Antagonists

The levels/effects of Celecoxib may be increased by: ACE Inhibitors; Angiotensin II Receptor Blockers; Antidepressants (Tricyclic, Tertiary Amine); Conivaptan; Corticosteroids (Systemic); CycloSPORINE; CycloSPORINE (Systemic); CYP2C9 Inhibitors (Moderate); CYP2C9 Inhibitors (Strong); Floctafenine; Herbs (Anticoagulant/Antiplatelet Properties); Ketorolac; Ketorolac (Nasal); Ketorolac (Systemic); Probenecid; Propafenone; Selective Serotonin Reuptake Inhibitors; Sodium Phosphates; Treprostinil

Decreased Effect

Celecoxib may decrease the levels/effects of: ACE Inhibitors; Angiotensin II Receptor Blockers; Antiplatelet Agents; Beta-Blockers; Codeine; Eplerenone; HydrALAZINE; Loop Diuretics; Potassium-Sparing Diuretics; Thiazide Diuretics; TraMADol

The levels/effects of Celecoxib may be decreased by: Bile Acid Sequestrants; CYP2C9 Inducers (Strong); Peginterferon Alfa-2b; Tocilizumab

Ethanol/Nutrition/Herb Interactions

Ethanol: Avoid ethanol (increased GI irritation).

Food: Peak concentrations are delayed and AUC is increased by 10% to 20% when taken with a high-fat meal.

Herb/Nutraceutical: Avoid concomitant use with herbs possessing anticoagulation/antiplatelet properties, including alfalfa, anise, bilberry, bladderwrack, bromelain, cat's claw, celery, chamomile, coleus, cordyceps, dong quai, evening primrose, fenugreek, feverfew, garlic, ginger, ginkgo biloba, ginseng (American, Panax, Siberian), grapeseed, green tea, guggul, horse chestnuts, horseradish, licorice, prickly ash, red clover, reishi, SAMe (S-adenosylmethionine), sweet clover, turmeric, white willow.

Stability Store at 25°C (77°F); excursions permitted to 15°C to 30°C (59°F to 86°F).

Mechanism of Action Inhibits prostaglandin synthesis by decreasing the activity of the enzyme, cyclooxygenase-2 (COX-2), which results in decreased formation of prostaglandin precursors; has antipyretic, analgesic, and anti-inflammatory properties. Celecoxib does not inhibit cyclooxygenase-1 (COX-1) at therapeutic concentrations.

Pharmacodynamics/Kinetics

Distribution: V_d (apparent): ~400 L

Protein binding: ~97% primarily to albumin

Metabolism: Hepatic via CYP2C9; forms inactive metabolites

Bioavailability: Absolute: Unknown

Half-life elimination: ~11 hours (fasted)

Time to peak: ~3 hours

Excretion: Feces (~57% as metabolites, <3% as unchanged drug); urine (27% as metabolites, <3% as unchanged drug)

Dosage Note: Use the lowest effective dose for the shortest duration of time, consistent with individual patient treatment goals. Oral:

Children ≥2 years: Juvenile idiopathic arthritis (JIA):

≥10 kg to ≤25 kg: 50 mg twice daily

>25 kg: 100 mg twice daily

Adults:

Acute pain or primary dysmenorrhea: Initial dose: 400 mg, followed by an additional 200 mg if needed on day 1; maintenance dose: 200 mg twice daily as needed.

Canadian labeling: Recommended maximum dose for treatment of acute pain: 400 mg/day up to 7 days

Ankylosing spondylitis: 200 mg/day as a single dose or in divided doses twice daily; if no effect after 6 weeks, may increase to 400 mg/day. If no response following 6 weeks of treatment with 400 mg/day, consider discontinuation and alternative treatment.

Canadian labeling: Recommended maximum dose: 200 mg/day

Osteoarthritis: 200 mg/day as a single dose or in divided doses twice daily

Rheumatoid arthritis: 100-200 mg twice daily

Elderly: No specific adjustment based on age is recommended. However, the AUC in elderly patients may be increased by 50% as compared to younger subjects. Initiate at the lowest recommended dose in patients weighing <50 kg.

*Dosing adjustment in poor CYP2C9 metabolizers (eg, CYP2C9*3/*3):* Consider reducing initial dose by 50%; consider alternative treatment in patients with JIA who are poor CYP2C9 metabolizers.

Canadian labeling: Recommended maximum dose: 100 mg/day

Dosing adjustment in renal impairment:

Advanced renal disease: Use is not recommended; however, if celecoxib treatment cannot be avoided, monitor renal function closely

Severe renal insufficiency: Use is not recommended.

Canadian labeling: Cl_{cr} <30 mL/minute: Use is contraindicated.

Abnormal renal function tests (persistent or worsening): Discontinue use

Dosing adjustment in hepatic impairment:

Moderate hepatic impairment (Child-Pugh class B): Reduce dose by 50%

Severe hepatic impairment (Child-Pugh class C): Use is not recommended

Canadian labeling: Use is contraindicated.

Abnormal liver function tests (persistent or worsening): Discontinue use

Dietary Considerations May be taken without regard to meals.

Administration May be administered without regard to meals. Capsules may be swallowed whole or the entire contents emptied onto a teaspoon of cool or room temperature applesauce. The contents of the capsules sprinkled onto applesauce may be stored under refrigeration for up to 6 hours.

Monitoring Parameters CBC; blood chemistry profile; occult blood loss and periodic liver function tests; monitor renal function (urine output, serum BUN and creatinine; monitor response (pain, range of motion, grip strength, mobility, ADL function), inflammation; blood pressure (baseline and during treatment); observe for weight gain, edema; observe for bleeding, bruising; evaluate gastrointestinal effects (abdominal pain, bleeding, dyspepsia)

JIA: Monitor for development of abnormal coagulation tests with systemic onset JIA

Dosage Forms Excipient information presented when available (limited, particularly for generics); consult specific product labeling.

Capsule, oral:

CeleBREX®: 50 mg, 100 mg, 200 mg, 400 mg

◆ **Celestone®***see* Betamethasone *on page 208*

◆ **Celestone® Soluspan®***see* Betamethasone *on page 208*

◆ **CeleXA®***see* Citalopram *on page 370*

◆ **Celexa® (Can)***see* Citalopram *on page 370*

◆ **CellCept®***see* Mycophenolate *on page 1162*

◆ **Celontin®***see* Methsuximide *on page 1103*

◆ **Celsentri™ (Can)***see* Maraviroc *on page 1052*

◆ **Cemill 500 [OTC]***see* Ascorbic Acid *on page 149*

◆ **Cemill 1000 [OTC]***see* Ascorbic Acid *on page 149*

◆ **Cenestin®***see* Estrogens (Conjugated A/Synthetic) *on page 637*

◆ **Cenestin (Can)***see* Estrogens (Conjugated A/Synthetic) *on page 637*

◆ **Centany®***see* Mupirocin *on page 1161*

◆ **Centany® AT***see* Mupirocin *on page 1161*

◆ ***Centruroides* Immune FAB2 (Equine)***see Centruroides* Immune F(ab')$_2$ (Equine) *on page 326*

Centruroides Immune F(ab')$_2$ (Equine)

(sen tra ROY dez i MYUN fab too E kwine)

Brand Names: U.S. Anascorp®

Index Terms *Centruroides* Immune FAB2 (Equine); Antivenin (*Centruroides*) Immune F(ab')$_2$ (Equine); Antivenin Scorpion; Antivenom (*Centruroides*) Immune F(ab')$_2$ (Equine); Antivenom Scorpion; Scorpion Antivenin; Scorpion Antivenom

Pharmacologic Category Antivenin

Use Treatment of scorpion envenomation

Pregnancy Risk Factor C

Pregnancy Considerations Animal reproduction studies have not been conducted.

Lactation Excretion in breast milk unknown/use caution

Contraindications There are no contraindications listed within the manufacturer's labeling.

Warnings/Precautions Derived from equine (horse) immune globulin F(ab')$_2$ fragments; anaphylaxis and anaphylactoid reactions are possible, especially in patients with known allergies to horse protein. Patients who have had previous treatment with *Centruroides* immune F(ab')$_2$ or other equine-derived antivenom/antitoxin may be at a higher risk for acute hypersensitivity reactions. In patients who develop an anaphylactic reaction, discontinue the infusion and administer emergency care. Immediate treatment (eg, epinephrine 1:1000, corticosteroids, diphenhydramine) should be available. In addition, delayed serum sickness may occur, usually within 2 weeks; monitor patients with follow-up visits for signs and symptoms (eg, arthralgia, fever, myalgia, rash).

Product of equine (horse) plasma; may potentially contain infectious agents (eg, viruses) which could transmit disease. May contain small amounts of cresol resulting from the manufacturing process; local reactions and myalgias may occur.

Adverse Reactions

1% to 10%:

Central nervous system: Fever (4%), fatigue (2%), headache (2%), lethargy (1%)

Dermatologic: Rash (3%), pruritus (2%)

Gastrointestinal: Vomiting (5%), nausea (2%), diarrhea (1%)

Neuromuscular & skeletal: Myalgia (2%)

Respiratory: Rhinorrhea (2%), cough (1%)

<1% (Limited to important or life-threatening): Aspiration, ataxia, chest tightness, eye edema, hypersensitivity, hypoxia, palpitation, pneumonia, respiratory distress, serum sickness (delayed)

Drug Interactions

Metabolism/Transport Effects None known.

Avoid Concomitant Use There are no known interactions where it is recommended to avoid concomitant use.

Increased Effect/Toxicity There are no known significant interactions involving an increase in effect.

Decreased Effect There are no known significant interactions involving a decrease in effect.

Stability Store unused vials at room temperature of 25°C (77°F); excursions permitted up to 40°C (104°F); do not freeze. Reconstitute each vial with 5 mL NS; gently swirl to mix. Dilute dose (eg, 1-3 vials) with NS to a total volume of 50 mL. Inspect diluted solution; do not use if it contains particulate matter or is discolored or turbid; discard partially used vials.

Mechanism of Action Contains venom-specific $F(ab')_2$ fragments of IgG which bind and neutralize venom toxins; thereby helping to remove the toxin from the target tissue and eliminate it from the body.

Pharmacodynamics/Kinetics

Onset: Time to resolution of symptoms: Adults: 1.91 ± 1.4 hours; Children: 1.28 ± 0.8 hours; >95% of all patients will experience resolution of symptoms within 4 hours

Distribution: V_{dss}: 13.6 L ± 5.4 L

Half-life, elimination: 159 ± 57 hours

Dosage I.V.: Children and Adults: **Note:** Initiate therapy as soon as possible after scorpion sting. Initial: 3 vials; may administer additional vials in 1-vial increments every 30-60 minutes as needed.

Dosing adjustment in renal impairment: There are no dosage adjustments provided in manufacturer's labeling.

Dosing adjustment in hepatic impairment: There are no dosage adjustments provided in manufacturer's labeling.

Administration I.V.: Administer over 10 minutes; monitor for return of symptoms of envenomation and repeat as needed. Medications (eg, epinephrine, corticosteroids, diphenhydramine) and equipment for resuscitation should be readily available in case of hypersensitivity reactions. Avoid I.M. since the time to peak blood concentration may be prolonged with this route of administration (Vasquez, 2010; Turri, 2011).

Monitoring Parameters Signs and symptoms of envenomation (eg, opsoclonus, involuntary muscle movement, slurred speech, paresthesias, respiratory distress, salivation, frothy sputum, vomiting); signs and symptoms of hypersensitivity reactions; follow-up visits for signs and symptoms of serum sickness (eg, arthralgia, fever, myalgia, rash)

Additional Information Each vial of *Centruroides* immune $F(ab')_2$ (equine) contains ≤120 mg total protein and ≥150 LD50 (mouse) neutralizing units.

Dosage Forms Excipient information presented when available (limited, particularly for generics); consult specific product labeling.

Injection, powder for reconstitution:

Anascorp®: ≤120 mg total protein [contains cresol, sucrose 4.3-38.3 mg/vial; derived from Centruroides limpidus limpidus, C. l. tecomanus, C. noxius, and C. suffusus suffusus venom; equine origin]

◆ **Cepacol® Fizzlers™ [OTC]***see* Benzocaine *on page 202*

◆ **Cepacol® Sore Throat [OTC]***see* Benzocaine *on page 202*

◆ **Cepacol® Sore Throat & Coating [OTC]** *see* Benzocaine *on page 202*

◆ **Cepacol® Sore Throat Pain Relief [OTC] [DSC]** *see* Benzocaine *on page 202*

◆ **Cepacol® Sore Throat Plus Coating Relief [OTC]***see* Benzocaine *on page 202*

◆ **Cepacol® Ultra Sore Throat [OTC]***see* Benzocaine *on page 202*

◆ **Cephadyn***see* Butalbital and Acetaminophen *on page 255*

Cephalexin (sef a LEKS in)

Brand Names: U.S. Keflex®

Brand Names: Canada Apo-Cephalex®; Dom-Cephalexin; Keflex®; Keftab®; Novo-Lexin; Nu-Cephalex; PMS-Cephalexin

Index Terms Cephalexin Monohydrate

Pharmacologic Category Antibiotic, Cephalosporin (First Generation)

Additional Appendix Information

Prevention of Infective Endocarditis *on page 1952*

Use Treatment of susceptible bacterial infections including respiratory tract infections, otitis media, skin and skin structure infections, bone infections, and genitourinary tract infections, including acute prostatitis; alternative therapy for acute infective endocarditis prophylaxis

Pregnancy Risk Factor B

Pregnancy Considerations Adverse events were not observed in animal reproduction studies; therefore, cephalexin is classified as pregnancy category B. Cephalexin crosses the placenta and produces therapeutic concentrations in the fetal circulation and amniotic fluid. An increased risk of teratogenic effects has not been observed following maternal use of cephalexin; however, adequate and well-controlled studies have not been completed in pregnant women. Peak concentrations in pregnant patients are similar to those in nonpregnant patients. Prolonged labor may decrease oral absorption.

Lactation Enters breast milk (small amounts)/use caution

Contraindications Hypersensitivity to cephalexin, any component of the formulation, or other cephalosporins

Warnings/Precautions Modify dosage in patients with severe renal impairment. Use with caution in patients with a history of penicillin allergy, especially IgE-mediated reactions (eg, anaphylaxis, urticaria). Prolonged use may result in fungal or bacterial superinfection, including *C. difficile*-associated diarrhea (CDAD) and pseudomembranous colitis; CDAD has been observed >2 months postantibiotic treatment. May be associated with increased INR, especially in nutritionally-deficient patients, prolonged treatment, hepatic or renal disease.

Adverse Reactions Frequency not defined.

Central nervous system: Agitation, confusion, dizziness, fatigue, hallucinations, headache

Dermatologic: Angioedema, erythema multiforme (rare), rash, Stevens-Johnson syndrome (rare), toxic epidermal necrolysis (rare), urticaria

Gastrointestinal: Abdominal pain, diarrhea, dyspepsia, gastritis, nausea (rare), pseudomembranous colitis, vomiting (rare)

Genitourinary: Genital pruritus, genital moniliasis, vaginitis, vaginal discharge

Hematologic: Eosinophilia, hemolytic anemia, neutropenia, thrombocytopenia

Hepatic: ALT increased, AST increased, cholestatic jaundice (rare), transient hepatitis (rare)

Neuromuscular & skeletal: Arthralgia, arthritis, joint disorder

Renal: Interstitial nephritis (rare)

Miscellaneous: Allergic reactions, anaphylaxis

Drug Interactions

Metabolism/Transport Effects None known.

Avoid Concomitant Use

Avoid concomitant use of Cephalexin with any of the following: BCG

Increased Effect/Toxicity

Cephalexin may increase the levels/effects of: MetFORMIN

The levels/effects of Cephalexin may be increased by: Probenecid

Decreased Effect

Cephalexin may decrease the levels/effects of: BCG; Typhoid Vaccine

The levels/effects of Cephalexin may be decreased by: Zinc Salts

Ethanol/Nutrition/Herb Interactions Food: Peak antibiotic serum concentration is lowered and delayed, but total drug absorbed is not affected. Cephalexin serum levels may be decreased if taken with food.

Stability
Capsule: Store at 15°C to 30°C (59°F to 86°F).
Powder for oral suspension: Refrigerate suspension after reconstitution; discard after 14 days.

Mechanism of Action Inhibits bacterial cell wall synthesis by binding to one or more of the penicillin-binding proteins (PBPs) which in turn inhibits the final transpeptidation step of peptidoglycan synthesis in bacterial cell walls, thus inhibiting cell wall biosynthesis. Bacteria eventually lyse due to ongoing activity of cell wall autolytic enzymes (autolysins and murein hydrolases) while cell wall assembly is arrested.

Pharmacodynamics/Kinetics
Absorption: Rapid (90%); delayed in young children
Distribution: Widely into most body tissues and fluids, including gallbladder, liver, kidneys, bone, sputum, bile, and pleural and synovial fluids; CSF penetration is poor
Protein binding: 6% to 15%
Half-life elimination: Adults: 0.5-1.2 hours; prolonged with renal impairment
Time to peak, serum: ~1 hour
Excretion: Urine (80% to 100% as unchanged drug) within 8 hours

Dosage
Usual dosage range:
Children >1 year: Oral: 25-100 mg/kg/day every 6-8 hours (maximum: 4 g/day)
Adults: Oral: 250-1000 mg every 6 hours; maximum: 4 g/day
Indication-specific dosing:
Infants >3 months and Children: Oral:
Community-acquired pneumonia (CAP) (IDSA/PIDS, 2011), *S. aureus* (methicillin-susceptible), mild infection or step-down therapy (preferred): 75-100 mg/kg/day in 3-4 divided doses
Children: Oral:
Furunculosis: 25-50 mg/kg/day in 4 divided doses
Impetigo: 25 mg/kg/day in 4 divided doses
Otitis media: 75-100 mg/kg/day in 4 divided doses
Prophylaxis against infective endocarditis (dental, oral, or respiratory tract procedures): 50 mg/kg 30-60 minutes prior to procedure (maximum: 2 g). **Note:** American Heart Association (AHA) guidelines now recommend prophylaxis only in patients undergoing invasive procedures and in whom underlying cardiac conditions may predispose to a higher risk of adverse outcomes should infection occur.
Severe infections: 50-100 mg/kg/day in divided doses every 6-8 hours
Skin abscess: 50 mg/kg/day in 4 divided doses (maximum: 4 g)
Streptococcal pharyngitis, skin and skin structure infections: Children >1 year: 25-50 mg/kg/day divided every 12 hours
Adolescents >15 years and Adults: Oral:
Cellulitis and mastitis: 500 mg every 6 hours
Furunculosis/skin abscess: 250 mg 4 times/day
Prophylaxis against infective endocarditis (dental, oral, or respiratory tract procedures): 2 g 30-60 minutes prior to procedure. **Note:** American Heart Association (AHA) guidelines now recommend prophylaxis only in patients undergoing invasive procedures and in whom underlying cardiac conditions may predispose to a higher risk of adverse outcomes should infection occur.
Prophylaxis in total joint replacement patients undergoing dental procedures which produce bacteremia: 2 g 1 hour prior to procedure
Streptococcal pharyngitis, skin and skin structure infections: 500 mg every 12 hours
Uncomplicated cystitis: 500 mg every 12 hours for 7-14 days

Dosing adjustment in renal impairment: Adults:
Cl_{cr} 10-50 mL/minute: 500 mg every 8-12 hours
Cl_{cr} <10: 250-500 mg every 12-24 hours
Hemodialysis: 250 mg every 12-24 hours; moderately dialyzable (20% to 50%); give dose after dialysis session

Dietary Considerations Take without regard to food. If GI distress, take with food.

Administration Take without regard to food. If GI distress, take with food. Give around-the-clock to promote less variation in peak and trough serum levels.

Monitoring Parameters With prolonged therapy monitor renal, hepatic, and hematologic function periodically; monitor for signs of anaphylaxis during first dose

Test Interactions Positive direct Coombs', false-positive urinary glucose test using cupric sulfate (Benedict's solution, Clinitest®, Fehling's solution), false-positive serum or urine creatinine with Jaffé reaction, false-positive urinary proteins and steroids

Dosage Forms Excipient information presented when available (limited, particularly for generics); consult specific product labeling.
Capsule, oral: 250 mg, 500 mg
Keflex®: 250 mg, 500 mg, 750 mg
Powder for suspension, oral: 125 mg/5 mL (100 mL, 200 mL); 250 mg/5 mL (100 mL, 200 mL)
Tablet, oral: 250 mg, 500 mg

◆ **Cephalexin Monohydrate** *see* Cephalexin *on page 327*

◆ **Ceprotin** *see* Protein C Concentrate (Human) *on page 1429*

◆ **Cerebyx®** *see* Fosphenytoin *on page 765*

◆ **Ceredase®** *see* Alglucerase *on page 65*

◆ **Cerefolin® NAC** *see* Methylfolate, Methylcobalamin, and Acetylcysteine *on page 1106*

◆ **Cerezyme®** *see* Imiglucerase *on page 874*

◆ **Ceron [DSC]** *see* Chlorpheniramine and Phenylephrine *on page 345*

◆ **Ceron-DM [DSC]** *see* Chlorpheniramine, Phenylephrine, and Dextromethorphan *on page 346*

Certolizumab Pegol (cer to LIZ u mab PEG ol)

Brand Names: U.S. Cimzia®

Brand Names: Canada Cimzia®

Index Terms CDP870

Pharmacologic Category Antirheumatic, Disease Modifying; Gastrointestinal Agent, Miscellaneous; Tumor Necrosis Factor (TNF) Blocking Agent

Use Treatment of moderately- to severely-active Crohn's disease in patients who have inadequate response to conventional therapy; moderately- to severely-active rheumatoid arthritis (as monotherapy or in combination with nonbiological disease-modifying antirheumatic drugs [DMARDS])

Pregnancy Risk Factor B

Pregnancy Considerations Adverse effects were not observed in animal studies. There are no adequate and well-controlled studies in pregnant women.

Lactation Excretion in breast milk unknown/not recommended

Medication Guide Available Yes

Contraindications There are no contraindications listed within the manufacturer's labeling.

Warnings/Precautions [U.S. Boxed Warning]: Patients receiving certolizumab are at increased risk for serious infections which may result in hospitalization and/or fatality; infections usually developed in patients receiving concomitant immunosuppressive agents (eg, methotrexate or corticosteroids) and may present as disseminated (rather than local) disease. Active

tuberculosis (or reactivation of latent tuberculosis), invasive fungal (including aspergillosis, blastomycosis, candidiasis, coccidioidomycosis, histoplasmosis, and pneumocystosis) and bacterial, viral or other opportunistic infections (including legionellosis and listeriosis) have been reported in patients receiving TNF-blocking agents, including certolizumab. Monitor closely for signs/symptoms of infection. Discontinue for serious infection or sepsis. Consider risks versus benefits prior to use in patients with a history of chronic or recurrent infection. Consider empiric antifungal therapy in patients who are at risk for invasive fungal infection and develop severe systemic illness. Caution should be exercised when considering use in the elderly or in patients with conditions that predispose them to infections (eg, diabetes) or residence/travel from areas of endemic mycoses (blastomycosis, coccidioidomycosis, histoplasmosis), or with latent or localized infections. Do not initiate certolizumab therapy with clinically important active infection. Patients who develop a new infection while undergoing treatment should be monitored closely. **[U.S. Boxed Warning]: Lymphoma and other malignancies have been reported in children and adolescent patients receiving other TNF-blocking agents.** Use of TNF blockers may affect defenses against malignancies; impact on the development and course of malignancies is not fully defined. Lymphoma has been noted in clinical trials. Chronic immunosuppressant therapy use may be a predisposing factor for malignancy development; rheumatoid arthritis alone has been previously associated with an increased rate of lymphoma.

Tuberculosis has been reported with certolizumab treatment. **[U.S. Boxed Warnings]: Patients should be evaluated for tuberculosis risk factors and for latent tuberculosis infection (with a tuberculin skin test) prior to therapy. Treatment of latent tuberculosis should be initiated before use. Patients with initial negative tuberculin skin tests should receive continued monitoring for tuberculosis throughout treatment;** active tuberculosis has developed in this population during treatment. Use with caution in patients who have resided in regions where tuberculosis is endemic. If appropriate, antituberculosis therapy should be considered (prior to certolizumab treatment) in patients with several or with highly significant risk factors for tuberculosis development.

Rare reactivation of hepatitis B virus (HBV) has occurred in chronic virus carriers; use with caution; evaluate prior to initiation and during treatment.

Hypersensitivity reactions, including angioedema, dyspnea, rash, serum sickness and urticaria have been reported (rarely) with treatment; discontinue and do not resume therapy if hypersensitivity occurs. Use with caution in patients who have experienced hypersensitivity with other TNF blockers. Use with caution in heart failure patients; worsening heart failure and new onset heart failure have been reported with TNF blockers, including certolizumab pegol; monitor closely. Rare cases of pancytopenia and other significant cytopenias, including aplastic anemia and have been reported with TNF-blocking agents. Leukopenia and thrombocytopenia have occurred with certolizumab; use with caution in patients with underlying hematologic disorders; consider discontinuing therapy with significant hematologic abnormalities. Autoantibody formation may develop; rarely resulting in autoimmune disorder, including lupus-like syndrome; monitor and discontinue if symptoms develop. A small number of patients (8%) develop antibodies to certolizumab during therapy. Antibody-positive patients may have an increased incidence of adverse events (including injection site pain/erythema, abdominal pain and erythema nodosum). Use with caution in patients with pre-existing or recent-onset CNS demyelinating disorders; rare cases of optic neuritis, seizure, peripheral neuropathy, and demyelinating disease (new onset or exacerbation) have been reported.

The manufacturer does not recommend concurrent use with anakinra or other tumor necrosis factor (TNF) blocking agents due to the risk of serious infections. Do not use in combination with biologic DMARDS. Patients should be up to date with all immunizations before initiating therapy; live vaccines should not be given concurrently. There is no data available concerning the effects of therapy on vaccination or secondary transmission of live vaccines in patients receiving therapy. Use has not been studied in patients with renal impairment; however, the pharmacokinetics of the pegylated (polyethylene glycol) component may be dependent on renal function. Use with caution in the elderly, may be at higher risk for infections.

Adverse Reactions

>10%:
- Central nervous system: Headache (5% to 18%)
- Gastrointestinal: Nausea (≤11%)
- Respiratory: Upper respiratory infection (6% to 20%), nasopharyngitis (4% to 13%)
- Miscellaneous: Infection (14% to 38%; serious: 3%)

1% to 10%:
- Cardiovascular: Hypertension (≤5%)
- Central nervous system: Dizziness (≤6%), fever (≤5%), fatigue (≤3%)
- Dermatologic: Rash (9%)
- Gastrointestinal: Abdominal pain (≤6%), vomiting (5%)
- Genitourinary: Urinary tract infection (≤8%)
- Local: Injection site reactions (includes bleeding, burning, erythema, inflammation, pain, rash: ≤7%; incidence higher with placebo)
- Neuromuscular & skeletal: Arthralgia (6% to 7%), back pain (≤4%)
- Respiratory: Cough (≤6%), bronchitis (≤3%), pharyngitis (≤3%)
- Miscellaneous: Antibody formation (7% to 8%), positive ANA (≤4%)

<1% (Limited to important or life-threatening): Abdominal mass, abscess, alopecia, anemia, angina, anxiety, aphthous stomatitis, aplastic anemia, arrhythmia, atrial fibrillation, bacterial arthritis, bipolar disorder, blurred vision, cytopenia, demyelinating disorder exacerbation, dermatitis, diarrhea, erysipelas, erythema nodosum, gastroenteritis, heart failure (new or worsening), hepatitis, hepatitis B reactivation; hypersensitivity reaction (eg, allergic dermatitis, angioedema, dizziness [postural], dyspnea, hot flush, hypotension, malaise, serum sickness, syncope); intestinal obstruction, leukemias, leukopenia, limb pain, lupus erythematosus rash, lupus-like syndrome, lymphadenopathy, lymphomas, malignancy, mastitis, menstrual disorder, MI, myocardial ischemia, nephrotic syndrome, opportunistic infection (rare), optic neuritis, pancytopenia, paralytic ileus, pericardial effusion, pericarditis, peripheral edema, peripheral neuropathy, pneumonia, psoriasis (including new onset, palmoplantar, pustular, or exacerbation), pyelonephritis, rectal hemorrhage, renal failure, retinal hemorrhage, seizure, stroke, suicide attempt, thrombocytopenia, thrombophilia, thrombophlebitis, tooth abscess, transaminases increased, transient ischemic attack, tuberculosis (peritoneal, pulmonary and disseminated), urosepsis, urticaria, uveitis, vasculitis, viral infection, visual acuity decreased, wound infection

Drug Interactions

Metabolism/Transport Effects None known.

Avoid Concomitant Use

Avoid concomitant use of Certolizumab Pegol with any of the following: Abatacept; Anakinra; Anti-TNF Agents; BCG; Canakinumab; Natalizumab; Pimecrolimus; Rilonacept; RiTUXimab; Tacrolimus (Topical); Vaccines (Live)

Increased Effect/Toxicity

Certolizumab Pegol may increase the levels/effects of: Abatacept; Anakinra; Canakinumab; Leflunomide; Natalizumab; Rilonacept; Vaccines (Live)

The levels/effects of Certolizumab Pegol may be increased by: Anti-TNF Agents; Denosumab; Pimecrolimus; RiTUXimab; Roflumilast; Tacrolimus (Topical); Trastuzumab

Decreased Effect

Certolizumab Pegol may decrease the levels/effects of: BCG; Coccidioidin Skin Test; Sipuleucel-T; Vaccines (Inactivated); Vaccines (Live)

The levels/effects of Certolizumab Pegol may be decreased by: Echinacea; Pegloticase

Ethanol/Nutrition/Herb Interactions Herb/Nutraceutical: Echinacea may decrease the therapeutic effects of certolizumab; avoid concurrent use.

Stability Prior to reconstitution, store refrigerated at 2°C to 8°C (36°F to 46°F); do not freeze. Bring to room temperature prior to administration.

Prefilled syringe: Protect from light.

Vials: Allow to reach room temperature prior to reconstitution. Using aseptic technique, reconstitute each vial with 1 mL sterile water for injection (provided) to a concentration of ~200 mg/mL; the manufacturer recommends using a 20-gauge needle (provided). Gently swirl to facilitate wetting of powder; do not shake. Allow vials to set undisturbed (may take up to 30 minutes) until fully reconstituted. Reconstituted solutions should not contain visible particles or gels in the solution. Reconstituted vials may be retained at room temperature for ≤2 hours or refrigerated (do not freeze) for ≤24 hours prior to administration.

Mechanism of Action Certolizumab pegol is a pegylated humanized antibody Fab' fragment of tumor necrosis factor alpha (TNF-alpha) monoclonal antibody. Certolizumab pegol binds to and selectively neutralizes human TNF-alpha activity. (Elevated levels of TNF-alpha have a role in the inflammatory process associated with Crohn's disease and in joint destruction associated with rheumatoid arthritis.) Since it is not a complete antibody (lacks Fc region), it does not induce complement activation, antibody-dependent cell-mediated cytotoxicity, or apoptosis. Pegylation of certolizumab allows for delayed elimination and therefore an extended half-life.

Pharmacodynamics/Kinetics

Distribution: V_{ss}: 6-8 L

Bioavailability: SubQ: ~80% (range: 76% to 88%)

Half-life elimination: ~14 days

Time to peak, plasma: 54-171 hours

Dosage Note: Each 400 mg dose should be administered as 2 injections of 200 mg each

SubQ: Adults:

Crohn's disease: Initial: 400 mg, repeat dose 2 and 4 weeks after initial dose; Maintenance: 400 mg every 4 weeks

Rheumatoid arthritis: Initial: 400 mg, repeat dose 2 and 4 weeks after initial dose; Maintenance: 200 mg every other week. May consider maintenance dose of 400 mg every 4 weeks.

Dosing adjustment in renal impairment: Moderate-to-severe renal impairment: The pharmacokinetics of the pegylated (polyethylene glycol) component may be dependent on renal function; however, data is insufficient to provide a dosing recommendation.

Administration SubQ: Bring to room temperature prior to administration. Total dose requires 2 vials **or** 2 prefilled syringes. After reconstitution (of vials), draw each vial into separate syringes (using 20-gauge needles).

Administer each syringe subcutaneously (using provided 23-gauge needle) to separate sites on abdomen or thigh. Rotate injections sites; do not administer to areas where skin is tender, bruised, red, or hard.

Monitoring Parameters Monitor improvement of symptoms and physical function assessments. Latent TB screening prior to initiating and during therapy; signs/symptoms of infection (prior to, during, and following therapy); CBC with differential; signs/symptoms/worsening of heart failure; HBV screening prior to initiating (all patients), HBV carriers (during and for several months following therapy); signs and symptoms of hypersensitivity reaction; symptoms of lupus-like syndrome.

Test Interactions Tests for latent tuberculosis may be falsely negative while on certolizumab pegol treatment. Falsely elevated aPTT assays have been reported with PTT-Lupus Anticoagulant (LA) and Standard Target Activated Partial Thromboplastin time (STA-PTT) tests from Diagnostica Stago, and with HemosiL APTT-SP liquid and HemosiL lyophilized silica tests from Instrumentation Laboratories.

Dosage Forms Excipient information presented when available (limited, particularly for generics); consult specific product labeling.

Injection, powder for reconstitution [preservative free]:

Cimzia®: 200 mg [contains sucrose 100 mg]

Injection, solution [preservative free]:

Cimzia®: 200 mg/mL (1 mL)

◆ **Cerubidine®** *see* DAUNOrubicin (Conventional) *on page 457*

◆ **Cervarix®** *see* Papillomavirus (Types 16, 18) Vaccine (Human, Recombinant) *on page 1292*

◆ **Cervidil®** *see* Dinoprostone *on page 514*

◆ **C.E.S.** *see* Estrogens (Conjugated/Equine, Systemic) *on page 641*

◆ **C.E.S.** *see* Estrogens (Conjugated/Equine, Topical) *on page 643*

◆ **C.E.S.® (Can)** *see* Estrogens (Conjugated/Equine, Systemic) *on page 641*

◆ **Cesia® [DSC]** *see* Ethinyl Estradiol and Desogestrel *on page 653*

◆ **Cetacaine®** *see* Benzocaine, Butamben, and Tetracaine *on page 204*

◆ **Cetafen® [OTC]** *see* Acetaminophen *on page 27*

◆ **Cetafen® Extra [OTC]** *see* Acetaminophen *on page 27*

Cetirizine (se TI ra zeen)

Brand Names: U.S. All Day Allergy [OTC]; ZyrTEC® Allergy [OTC]; ZyrTEC® Children's Allergy [OTC]; ZyrTEC® Children's Hives Relief [OTC]

Brand Names: Canada Apo-Cetirizine®; PMS-Cetirizine; Reactine™

Index Terms Cetirizine Hydrochloride; P-071; UCB-P071

Pharmacologic Category Histamine H_1 Antagonist; Histamine H_1 Antagonist, Second Generation; Piperazine Derivative

Use Perennial and seasonal allergic rhinitis and other allergic symptoms including urticaria; chronic idiopathic urticaria

Pregnancy Considerations Maternal use of cetirizine has not been associated with an increased risk of major malformations. The use of antihistamines for the treatment of rhinitis during pregnancy is generally considered to be safe at recommended doses. Although safety data is limited, cetirizine may be a preferred second generation antihistamine for the treatment of rhinitis during pregnancy.

Contraindications Hypersensitivity to cetirizine, hydroxyzine, or any component of the formulation

Warnings/Precautions Cetirizine should be used cautiously in patients with hepatic or renal dysfunction; dosage adjustment recommended. Use with caution in the elderly; may be more sensitive to adverse effects. May cause drowsiness; use caution performing tasks which require alertness (eg, operating machinery or driving). Effects may be potentiated when used with other sedative drugs or ethanol.

Adverse Reactions

>10%: Central nervous system: Headache (children 11% to 14%, placebo 12%), somnolence (adults 14%, children 2% to 4%)

2% to 10%:

Central nervous system: Insomnia (children 9%, adults <2%), fatigue (adults 6%), malaise (4%), dizziness (adults 2%)

Gastrointestinal: Abdominal pain (children 4% to 6%), dry mouth (adults 5%), diarrhea (children 2% to 3%), nausea (children 2% to 3%, placebo 2%), vomiting (children 2% to 3%)

Respiratory: Epistaxis (children 2% to 4%, placebo 3%), pharyngitis (children 3% to 6%, placebo 3%), bronchospasm (children 2% to 3%, placebo 2%)

<2% (Limited to important or life-threatening; as reported in adults and/or children): Aggressive reaction, anaphylaxis, angioedema, ataxia, chest pain, confusion, convulsions, depersonalization, depression, edema, fussiness, hallucinations, hemolytic anemia, hepatitis, hypertension, hypotension (severe), irritability, liver function abnormal, nervousness, ototoxicity, palpitation, paralysis, paresthesia, photosensitivity, rash, suicidal ideation, suicide, taste perversion, tongue discoloration, tongue edema, tremor, visual field defect, weakness

Drug Interactions

Metabolism/Transport Effects Substrate of CYP3A4 (minor), P-glycoprotein; **Note:** Assignment of Major/Minor substrate status based on clinically relevant drug interaction potential

Avoid Concomitant Use There are no known interactions where it is recommended to avoid concomitant use.

Increased Effect/Toxicity

Cetirizine may increase the levels/effects of: Alcohol (Ethyl); Anticholinergics; CNS Depressants; Methotrimeprazine; Selective Serotonin Reuptake Inhibitors

The levels/effects of Cetirizine may be increased by: Conivaptan; Droperidol; HydrOXYzine; Methotrimeprazine; P-glycoprotein/ABCB1 Inhibitors; Pramlintide

Decreased Effect

Cetirizine may decrease the levels/effects of: Acetylcholinesterase Inhibitors (Central); Benzylpenicilloyl Polylysine; Betahistine

The levels/effects of Cetirizine may be decreased by: Acetylcholinesterase Inhibitors (Central); Amphetamines; P-glycoprotein/ABCB1 Inducers; Tocilizumab

Ethanol/Nutrition/Herb Interactions Ethanol: May increase CNS depression; monitor for increased effects with coadministration. Caution patients about effects.

Stability Store at room temperature.

Syrup: Store at room temperature of 15°C to 30°C (59°F to 86°F), or under refrigeration at 2°C to 8°C (36°F to 46°F).

Mechanism of Action Competes with histamine for H_1-receptor sites on effector cells in the gastrointestinal tract, blood vessels, and respiratory tract

Pharmacodynamics/Kinetics

Onset of action: Suppression of skin wheal and flare: 0.7 hours (Simons, 1999)

Duration of action: Suppression of skin wheal and flare: ≥24 hours (Simons, 1999)

Absorption: Rapid

Distribution: 0.56 L/kg (Simons, 1999)

Protein binding, plasma: Mean: 93%

Metabolism: Limited hepatic

Half-life elimination: 8 hours

Time to peak, serum: 1 hour

Excretion: Urine (70%); feces (10%)

Dosage Oral:

Children:

6-12 months: Chronic urticaria, perennial allergic rhinitis: 2.5 mg once daily

12 months to <2 years: Chronic urticaria, perennial allergic rhinitis: 2.5 mg once daily; may increase to 2.5 mg every 12 hours if needed

2-5 years: Chronic urticaria, perennial or seasonal allergic rhinitis: Initial: 2.5 mg once daily; may be increased to 2.5 mg every 12 hours **or** 5 mg once daily

Children ≥6 years and Adults: Chronic urticaria, perennial or seasonal allergic rhinitis: 5-10 mg once daily, depending upon symptom severity

Elderly: Initial: 5 mg once daily; may increase to 10 mg/day. **Note:** Manufacturer recommends 5 mg/day in patients ≥77 years of age.

Dosage adjustment in renal/hepatic impairment:

Children <6 years: Cetirizine use not recommended

Children 6-11 years: <2.5 mg once daily

Children ≥12 and Adults:

Cl_{cr} 11-31 mL/minute, hemodialysis, or hepatic impairment: Administer 5 mg once daily

Cl_{cr} <11 mL/minute, not on dialysis: Cetirizine use not recommended

Dietary Considerations May be taken with or without food.

Administration May be administered with or without food.

Monitoring Parameters Relief of symptoms, sedation and anticholinergic effects

Test Interactions May cause false-positive serum TCA screen.

Dosage Forms Excipient information presented when available (limited, particularly for generics); consult specific product labeling.

Capsule, liquid gel, oral, as hydrochloride:

ZyrTEC® Allergy: 10 mg

Solution, oral, as hydrochloride: 5 mg/5 mL (5 mL)

Syrup, oral, as hydrochloride: 5 mg/5 mL (5 mL, 118 mL, 120 mL, 473 mL, 480 mL, 480s)

ZyrTEC® Children's Allergy: 5 mg/5 mL (118 mL) [contains propylene glycol; grape flavor]

ZyrTEC® Children's Allergy: 5 mg/5 mL (118 mL) [dye free, sugar free; contains propylene glycol, sodium benzoate; bubblegum flavor]

ZyrTEC® Children's Hives Relief: 5 mg/5 mL (118 mL) [contains propylene glycol; grape flavor]

Tablet, oral, as hydrochloride: 5 mg, 10 mg

All Day Allergy: 10 mg

ZyrTEC® Allergy: 10 mg

Tablet, chewable, oral, as hydrochloride: 5 mg, 10 mg

All Day Allergy: 5 mg [fruit flavor]

ZyrTEC® Children's Allergy: 5 mg, 10 mg [grape flavor]

◆ **Cetirizine Hydrochloride** *see* Cetirizine *on page* 330

◆ **Cetraxal®** *see* Ciprofloxacin (Otic) *on page* 366

Cetrorelix (set roe REL iks)

Brand Names: U.S. Cetrotide®

Brand Names: Canada Cetrotide®

Index Terms Cetrorelix Acetate

Pharmacologic Category Gonadotropin Releasing Hormone Antagonist

Use Inhibits premature luteinizing hormone (LH) surges in women undergoing controlled ovarian stimulation

Pregnancy Risk Factor X

Pregnancy Considerations Adverse effects, including fetal resorption and implantation loss, have been observed in animal reproduction studies. Resorption resulting in fetal loss would be expected if used in a pregnant woman; use is contraindicated during pregnancy.

Lactation Excretion in breast milk unknown/contraindicated

Contraindications Hypersensitivity to cetrorelix or any component of the formulation; extrinsic peptide hormones, mannitol, gonadotropin releasing hormone (GnRH) or GnRH analogs; severe renal impairment; pregnancy; breast-feeding

Warnings/Precautions Should only be prescribed by fertility specialists. Monitor carefully after first injection for possible hypersensitivity reactions. Use caution in women with active allergic conditions or a history of allergies; use in women with severe allergic conditions is not recommended. Pregnancy should be excluded before treatment is begun.

Adverse Reactions

1% to 10%:

Central nervous system: Headache (1%)

Endocrine & metabolic: Ovarian hyperstimulation syndrome, WHO grade II or III (4%)

Gastrointestinal: Nausea (1%)

Hepatic: ALT, AST, GGT, and alkaline phosphatase increased (1% to 2%)

Postmarketing and/or case reports: Anaphylactic reactions (cough, hypotension, rash); local injection site reactions (bruising, erythema, itching, pruritus, redness, swelling)

Drug Interactions

Metabolism/Transport Effects None known.

Avoid Concomitant Use There are no known interactions where it is recommended to avoid concomitant use.

Increased Effect/Toxicity There are no known significant interactions involving an increase in effect.

Decreased Effect There are no known significant interactions involving a decrease in effect.

Stability Store in outer carton. Once mixed, solution should be used immediately.

0.25 mg vials: Store under refrigeration at 2°C to 8°C (36°F to 46°F).

3 mg vials: Store at controlled room temperature at 25°C (77°F); excursions permitted to 15°C to 30°C (59°F to 86°F).

Mechanism of Action Competes with naturally-occurring GnRH for binding on receptors of the pituitary. This delays luteinizing hormone surge, preventing ovulation until the follicles are of adequate size.

Pharmacodynamics/Kinetics

Onset of action: 0.25 mg dose: 2 hours; 3 mg dose: 1 hour

Duration: 3 mg dose (single dose): 4 days

Absorption: Rapid

Distribution: V_d: ~1 L/kg

Protein binding: 86%

Metabolism: Transformed by peptidases; cetrorelix and peptides (1-9), (1-7), (1-6), and (1-4) are found in the bile; peptide (1-4) is the predominant metabolite

Bioavailability: 85%

Half-life elimination: 0.25 mg dose: 5 hours; 0.25 mg multiple doses: 20.6 hours; 3 mg dose: 62.8 hours

Time to peak: 0.25 mg dose: 1 hour; 3 mg dose: 1.5 hours

Excretion: Feces (5% to 10% as unchanged drug and metabolites); urine (2% to 4% as unchanged drug); within 24 hours

Dosage

Adults: Females: SubQ: Used in conjunction with controlled ovarian stimulation therapy using gonadotropins (FSH, hMG):

Single-dose regimen: 3 mg given when serum estradiol levels show appropriate stimulation response, usually stimulation day 7 (range: days 5-9). If hCG is not administered within 4 days, continue cetrorelix at 0.25 mg/day until hCG is administered.

Multiple-dose regimen: 0.25 mg morning or evening of stimulation day 5, or morning of stimulation day 6; continue until hCG is administered.

Elderly: Not intended for use in women ≥65 years of age (Phase 2 and Phase 3 studies included women 19-40 years of age)

Dosing adjustment in renal impairment:

Severe impairment: Use is contraindicated

Mild-to-moderate impairment: No dosage adjustment provided in manufacturer's labeling.

Dosing adjustment in hepatic impairment: No dosage adjustment provided in manufacturer's labeling.

Administration Cetrorelix is administered by SubQ injection following proper aseptic technique procedures. Injections should be to the lower abdomen, preferably around the navel (but staying at least 1 inch from the navel). The injection site should be rotated daily. The needle should be inserted completely into the skin at a 45-degree angle.

Monitoring Parameters Ultrasound to assess follicle size

Dosage Forms Excipient information presented when available (limited, particularly for generics); consult specific product labeling.

Injection, powder for reconstitution:

Cetrotide®: 0.25 mg, 3 mg [contains mannitol; supplied with diluent]

◆ **Cetrorelix Acetate** *see* Cetrorelix *on page* 331

◆ **Cetrotide®** *see* Cetrorelix *on page* 331

Cetuximab (se TUK see mab)

Brand Names: U.S. Erbitux®

Brand Names: Canada Erbitux®

Index Terms C225; IMC-C225; MOAB C225

Pharmacologic Category Antineoplastic Agent, Monoclonal Antibody; Epidermal Growth Factor Receptor (EGFR) Inhibitor

Use Treatment of EGFR-expressing metastatic colorectal cancer (as a single agent or in combination with irinotecan); treatment of squamous cell cancer of the head and neck (as a single agent for recurrent or metastatic disease after platinum-based chemotherapy failure; in combination with radiation therapy as initial treatment of locally or regionally advanced disease; in combination with platinum and fluorouracil-based chemotherapy as first-line treatment of locoregional or metastatic disease)

Note: Subset analyses (retrospective) in metastatic colorectal cancer trials have not shown a benefit with EGFR inhibitor treatment in patients whose tumors have codon 12 or 13 *KRAS* mutations; use is not recommended in these patients.

Unlabeled Use Treatment of EGFR-expressing advanced nonsmall cell lung cancer (NSCLC)

Pregnancy Risk Factor C

Pregnancy Considerations In pregnant cynomolgus monkeys, cetuximab was detected in the amniotic fluid and in the serum of embryos. Although teratogenic effects were not observed in animal studies, increases in embryolethality and fetal loss were noted. It is not known whether cetuximab can cause fetal harm or affect reproductive capacity. Because cetuximab inhibits epidermal growth factor (EGF), a component of fetal development, adverse effects on pregnancy would be expected. Cetuximab should only be given to a pregnant woman if the potential benefit justifies the potential risk to the fetus.

Lactation Excretion in breast milk is unknown/not recommended

Contraindications There are no contraindications listed in the manufacturer's labeling

Warnings/Precautions [U.S. Boxed Warning]: Serious infusion reactions have been reported in ~3% of patients; fatal outcome has been reported rarely; interrupt infusion promptly and permanently discontinue for serious infusion reactions. Reactions have included airway obstruction (bronchospasm, stridor, hoarseness), hypotension, loss of consciousness, shock, MI, and/or cardiac arrest. Approximately 90% of reactions occur with the first infusion despite the use of prophylactic antihistamines. Immediate treatment for anaphylactic/anaphylactoid reactions should be available during administration. The manufacturer recommends monitoring patients for at least 1 hour following completion of infusion, or longer if a reaction occurs. Mild-to-moderate infusion reactions are managed by slowing the infusion rate (by 50%) and administering antihistamines. Patients with pre-existing IgE antibody against cetuximab (specific for galactose-α-1,3-galactose) are reported to have a higher incidence of severe hypersensitivity reaction. Severe hypersensitivity reaction has been reported more frequently in patients living in the middle south area of the United States, including North Carolina and Tennessee (Chung, 2008; O'Neil, 2007).

[U.S. Boxed Warning]: In patients with squamous cell head and neck cancer, cardiopulmonary arrest and/or sudden death has occurred in 2% of patients receiving radiation therapy in combination with cetuximab and in 3% of patients receiving combination chemotherapy (platinum and fluorouracil-based) with cetuximab. Closely monitor serum electrolytes (magnesium, potassium, calcium) during and after cetuximab treatment (monitor for at least 8 weeks after treatment). Use caution with history of coronary artery disease, HF, and arrhythmias; fatalities have been reported. Interstitial lung disease (ILD) has been reported; use caution with pre-existing lung disease; interrupt treatment for acute onset or worsening of pulmonary symptoms; permanently discontinue with confirmed ILD.

Acneiform rash has been reported in 76% to 88% of patients (severe in 1% to 17%), usually developing within the first 2 weeks of therapy; may require dose modification; generally resolved after discontinuation in most patients, although persisted beyond 28 days in some patients; monitor for dermatologic toxicity and corresponding infections. Acneiform rash should be treated with topical and/or oral antibiotics; topical corticosteroids are not recommended. Other dermatologic toxicities, including dry skin, fissures, hypertrichosis, paronychial inflammation, and skin infections have been reported; related ocular toxicities (blepharitis, conjunctivitis, keratitis) may also occur. Sunlight may exacerbate skin reactions (limit sun exposure). Hypomagnesemia is common (may be severe); the onset of electrolyte disturbance may occur within days to months after initiation of treatment; monitor magnesium, calcium, and potassium during treatment and for at least 8 weeks after completion; may require electrolyte replacement. Non-neutralizing anticetuximab antibodies were detected in 5% of evaluable patients. Safety has not been established when used in combination with radiation therapy **and** cisplatin; fatalities and serious cardiotoxicity, pneumonia or other adverse events have been observed. Patients with colorectal cancer with tumors with a codon 12 or 13 *KRAS* mutation are unlikely to benefit from EGFR inhibitor therapy and should not receive cetuximab treatment. In trials for colorectal cancer, evidence of EGFR expression was required, although the response rate did not correlate with either the percentage of cells positive for EGFR or the intensity of expression. EGFR expression has been detected in nearly all patients with head and neck cancer, therefore laboratory evidence of EGFR expression is not necessary for head and neck cancers.

Adverse Reactions Except where noted, percentages reported for studies with cetuximab monotherapy.

>10%:

Central nervous system: Fatigue (89%), pain (51%), headache (33%), fever (30%), insomnia (30%), confusion (15%), anxiety (14%), chills/rigors (13%), depression (13%)

Dermatologic: Acneiform rash (all studies: 76% to 88%; grades 3/4: 1% to 17%; onset: ≤14 days), rash (89%), dry skin (49%), pruritus (40%), nail changes (21%)

Endocrine & metabolic: Hypomagnesemia (all studies: 55%; grades 3/4: 6% to 17%)

Gastrointestinal: Abdominal pain (59%), constipation (46%), diarrhea (39%), vomiting (37%), stomatitis (25%), xerostomia (11%)

Neuromuscular & skeletal: Bone pain (15%)

Respiratory: Dyspnea (48%), cough (29%)

Miscellaneous: Infection (all studies: 13% to 35%), infusion reaction (all studies: 15% to 21%; grades 3/4: 2% to 5%; 90% of severe reactions occurred with first infusion)

1% to 10%:

Cardiovascular: Cardiopulmonary arrest (2%; with radiation therapy; 3% with platinum/fluorouracil-based chemotherapy)

Renal: Renal failure (all studies: 1%)

Miscellaneous: Sepsis (all studies: 1% to 4%)

<1% (Limited to important or life-threatening; all studies): Abscess formation, arrhythmia, aseptic meningitis, blepharitis, bronchospasm, cardiac arrest, cellulitis, cheilitis, conjunctivitis, electrolyte abnormality, hoarseness, hypertrichosis, hypotension, interstitial lung disease (occurred between the fourth and eleventh doses), keratitis, leukopenia, loss of consciousness, MI, paronychial inflammation, pulmonary embolism, radiation dermatitis, shock, skin fissure, skin infection, stridor

Drug Interactions

Metabolism/Transport Effects None known.

Avoid Concomitant Use There are no known interactions where it is recommended to avoid concomitant use.

Increased Effect/Toxicity There are no known significant interactions involving an increase in effect.

Decreased Effect There are no known significant interactions involving a decrease in effect.

Stability Store unopened vials refrigerated at 2°C to 8°C (36°F to 46°F); do not freeze. Reconstitution is not required. Appropriate dose should be added to empty sterile container; do not shake or dilute. Preparations in infusion containers are stable for up to 12 hours refrigerated at 2°C to 8°C (36°F to 46°F) and up to 8 hours at room temperature of 20°C to 25°C (68°F to 77°F).

Mechanism of Action Recombinant human/mouse chimeric monoclonal antibody which binds specifically to the epidermal growth factor receptor (EGFR, HER1, c-ErbB-1) and competitively inhibits the binding of epidermal growth factor (EGF) and other ligands. Binding to the EGFR blocks phosphorylation and activation of receptor-associated kinases, resulting in inhibition of cell growth, induction of apoptosis, and decreased matrix metalloproteinase and vascular endothelial growth factor production. EGFR signal transduction results in *KRAS* wild-type activation; cells with *KRAS* mutations appear to be unaffected by EGFR inhibition.

Pharmacodynamics/Kinetics

Distribution: V_d: ~2-3 L/m^2

Half-life elimination: ~112 hours (range: 63-230 hours)

Dosage I.V.: Adults: **Note:** Premedicate with an H_1 antagonist (eg, diphenhydramine 50 mg) I.V. 30-60 minutes prior to the first dose; premedication for subsequent doses is based on clinical judgement.

Colorectal cancer:

Initial loading dose: 400 mg/m² infused over 120 minutes

Maintenance dose: 250 mg/m² infused over 60 minutes weekly until disease progression or unacceptable toxicity

Biweekly administration (unlabeled dosing): 500 mg/m² every 2 weeks (initial dose infused over 120 minutes, subsequent doses infused over 60 minutes) (Pfeiffer, 2007)

Head and neck cancer (squamous cell):

Initial loading dose: 400 mg/m² infused over 120 minutes

Maintenance dose: 250 mg/m² infused over 60 minutes weekly

Note: If given in combination with radiation therapy, administer loading dose 1 week prior to initiation of radiation course; weekly maintenance dose should be completed 1 hour prior to radiation for the duration of radiation therapy (6-7 weeks). If given in combination with chemotherapy, administer loading dose on the day of initiation of platinum and fluorouracil-based chemotherapy, cetuximab infusion should be completed 1 hour prior to initiation of chemotherapy; weekly maintenance dose should be completed 1 hour prior to chemotherapy; continue until disease progression or unacceptable toxicity. Monotherapy weekly doses should be continued until disease progression or unacceptable toxicity.

NSCLC (unlabeled use): Initial loading dose: 400 mg/m², followed by maintenance dose: 250 mg/m² weekly (Pirker, 2009)

Dosage adjustment for toxicity:

Infusion reactions, grade 1 or 2 and nonserious grades 3 or 4: Reduce the infusion rate by 50% and continue to use prophylactic antihistamines

Infusion reactions, severe: Immediately and permanently discontinue treatment

Pulmonary toxicity:

Acute onset or worsening pulmonary symptoms: Hold treatment

Interstitial lung disease: Permanently discontinue

Skin toxicity, mild-to-moderate: No dosage modification required

Acneiform rash, severe (grade 3 or 4):

First occurrence: Delay cetuximab infusion 1-2 weeks

If improvement, continue at 250 mg/m²

If no improvement, discontinue therapy

Second occurrence: Delay cetuximab infusion 1-2 weeks

If improvement, continue at reduced dose of 200 mg/m²

If no improvement, discontinue therapy

Third occurrence: Delay cetuximab infusion 1-2 weeks

If improvement, continue at reduced dose of 150 mg/m²

If no improvement, discontinue therapy

Fourth occurrence: Discontinue therapy

Note: Dose adjustments are not recommended for severe **radiation** dermatitis.

Administration Administer via I.V. infusion; loading dose over 2 hours, weekly maintenance dose over 1 hour. Do not administer as I.V. push or bolus. Do not shake or dilute. Administer via infusion pump or syringe pump. Following the infusion, an observation period (1 hour) is recommended; longer observation time (following an infusion reaction) may be required. Premedication with an H_1 antagonist prior to the initial dose is recommended. The maximum infusion rate is 10 mg/minute. Administer through a low protein-binding 0.22 micrometer in-line filter. Use 0.9% NaCl to flush line at the end of infusion.

For biweekly administration (unlabeled frequency and dose), the initial dose was infused over 120 minutes and subsequent doses infused over 60 minutes (Pfeiffer, 2007).

Monitoring Parameters Vital signs during infusion and observe for at least 1 hour postinfusion. Patients developing dermatologic toxicities should be monitored for the development of complications. Periodic monitoring of serum magnesium, calcium, and potassium are recommended to continue over an interval consistent with the half-life (8 weeks); monitor closely (during and after treatment) for cetuximab plus radiation therapy. *KRAS* genotyping of tumor tissue in patients with colorectal cancer.

Additional Information Oncology Comment: The National Comprehensive Cancer Network® (NCCN) guidelines for colon cancer (v.2.2012) and the American Society of Clinical Oncology (ASCO) provisional clinical opinion (Allegra, 2009) recommend genotyping tumor tissue for *KRAS* mutation in all patients with metastatic colorectal cancer (genotyping may be done on archived specimens). Patients with known codon 12 or 13 *KRAS* gene mutations are unlikely to respond to EGFR inhibitors and should not receive cetuximab. Favorable progression-free survival and overall survival has been demonstrated with cetuximab in patients with *KRAS* wild-type (Karapetis, 2008; Van Cutsem, 2008). Because EGFR testing in colorectal tumors does not correlate with response, the NCCN guidelines do not recommend routine EGFR testing in colorectal cancer. Dermatologic toxicity with cetuximab is predictive for response; the presence of acneiform rash correlates with treatment response and prolonged survival (Cunningham, 2004).

Dosage Forms Excipient information presented when available (limited, particularly for generics); consult specific product labeling.

Injection, solution [preservative free]:

Erbitux®: 2 mg/mL (50 mL, 100 mL)

Cevimeline (se vi ME leen)

Brand Names: U.S. Evoxac®

Brand Names: Canada Evoxac®

Index Terms Cevimeline Hydrochloride

Pharmacologic Category Cholinergic Agonist

Use Treatment of symptoms of dry mouth in patients with Sjögren's syndrome

Pregnancy Risk Factor C

Dosage Oral:

Adults: 30 mg 3 times/day

Elderly: No specific dosage adjustment is recommended; however, use caution when initiating due to potential for increased sensitivity

Dosage adjustment in renal impairment: No dosage adjustment provided in the manufacturer's labeling.

Dosage adjustment in hepatic impairment: No dosage adjustment provided in the manufacturer's labeling.

Additional Information Complete prescribing information for this medication should be consulted for additional detail.

Dosage Forms Excipient information presented when available (limited, particularly for generics); consult specific product labeling.

Capsule, oral, as hydrochloride:

Evoxac®: 30 mg

- **Cevimeline Hydrochloride** *see* Cevimeline *on page 334*
- **CFDN** *see* Cefdinir *on page 303*
- **CG** *see* Chorionic Gonadotropin (Human) *on page 352*
- **CG5503** *see* Tapentadol *on page 1628*
- **C-Gel [OTC]** *see* Ascorbic Acid *on page 149*
- **CGP 33101** *see* Rufinamide *on page 1528*
- **CGP-39393** *see* Desirudin *on page 475*
- **CGP-42446** *see* Zoledronic Acid *on page 1821*
- **CGP-57148B** *see* Imatinib *on page 870*

- ◆ **C-Gram [OTC]** *see* Ascorbic Acid *on page 149*
- ◆ **CGS-20267** *see* Letrozole *on page 986*
- ◆ **Champix® (Can)** *see* Varenicline *on page 1771*
- ◆ **Chantix®** *see* Varenicline *on page 1771*
- ◆ **Charcadole® (Can)** *see* Charcoal, Activated *on page 335*
- ◆ **Charcadole®, Aqueous (Can)** *see* Charcoal, Activated *on page 335*
- ◆ **Charcadole® TFS (Can)** *see* Charcoal, Activated *on page 335*

Charcoal, Activated (CHAR kole AK tiv ay ted)

Brand Names: U.S. Actidose® with Sorbitol [OTC]; Actidose®-Aqua [OTC]; Charcoal Plus® DS [OTC]; CharcoCaps® [OTC]; EZ-Char® [OTC]; Kerr Insta-Char® in Aqueous Base [OTC]; Kerr Insta-Char® in Sorbitol Base [OTC]; Requa® Activated Charcoal [OTC]

Brand Names: Canada Charcadole®; Charcadole® TFS; Charcadole®, Aqueous

Index Terms Activated Carbon; Activated Charcoal; Adsorbent Charcoal; Liquid Antidote; Medicinal Carbon; Medicinal Charcoal

Pharmacologic Category Antidote

Use

Suspension: Activated charcoal is a nonabsorbable adsorbent that may be considered in the management of poisonings when gastrointestinal decontamination of drugs or chemicals is indicated (eg, presentation to a treatment facility within 1 hour of ingestion). Activated charcoal is generally an effective adsorbent of drugs and chemicals with a molecular weight range of 100-1000 daltons. Multidose activated charcoal may be considered if a patient has ingested a life-threatening amount of carbamazepine, dapsone, phenobarbital, quinine, or theophylline (Vale, 1999).

Capsules, tablets: Digestive aid

Pregnancy Considerations Activated charcoal is not absorbed systemically following oral administration. Systemic absorption would be required in order for activated charcoal to cross the placenta and reach the fetus. In general, medications used as antidotes should take into consideration the health and prognosis of the mother (Bailey, 2003).

Lactation Use with caution

Contraindications There are no absolute contraindications listed within the manufacturer's labeling.

Note: The American Academy of Clinical Toxicology (AACT) and European Association of Poisons Centres and Clinical Toxicologists (EAPCCT) consider the following to be contraindications to the use of charcoal (Chyka, 2005; Vale, 1999): Presence of intestinal obstruction or GI tract not anatomically intact; patients at risk of GI hemorrhage or perforation; patients with an unprotected airway (eg, CNS depression without intubation); if use would increase the risk and severity of aspiration

Warnings/Precautions Charcoal may cause vomiting; the risk appears to be greater when charcoal is administered with sorbitol (Chyka, 2005). I.V. antiemetics may be required to reduce the risk of vomiting or to control vomiting to facilitate administration (Vale, 1999). Due to the risk of vomiting, avoid the use of charcoal in hydrocarbon and caustic ingestions. Use caution with decreased peristalsis. Some products may contain sorbitol. Coadministration of a cathartic is **not** recommended; cathartics (eg, sorbitol, mannitol, magnesium sulfate) have not been demonstrated to change patient outcome and have no role in the management of the poisoned patient. Cathartics subject the patient to the risk of developing significant fluid and electrolyte abnormalities (AACT, 2004a). Do not use products containing sorbitol in persons with a genetic intolerance to fructose or in patients who are dehydrated; may cause excessive diarrhea. Ipecac should not be administered routinely in the management of poisoned patients (AACT, 2004b).

Not effective in the treatment of poisonings due to the ingestion of low molecular weight compounds such as cyanide, iron, ethanol, methanol, or lithium. Most effective when administered within 30-60 minutes of ingestion. Based on experimental and clinical studies, multidose activated charcoal, in most acute poisonings, has not been shown to reduce morbidity or mortality (Vale, 1999). It may be considered if a patient has ingested a life-threatening amount of carbamazepine, dapsone, phenobarbital, quinine, or theophylline, although no controlled studies have demonstrated clinical benefit.

Commercial charcoal products may contain propylene glycol. Capsules and tablets should not be used for the treatment of poisoning.

Adverse Reactions Frequency not defined.

Gastrointestinal: Abdominal distention, appendicitis, bowel obstruction, constipation, vomiting

Ocular: Corneal abrasion (with direct contact)

Respiratory: Aspiration, respiratory failure

Miscellaneous: Fecal discoloration (black)

Drug Interactions

Metabolism/Transport Effects None known.

Avoid Concomitant Use There are no known interactions where it is recommended to avoid concomitant use.

Increased Effect/Toxicity There are no known significant interactions involving an increase in effect.

Decreased Effect

Charcoal, Activated may decrease the levels/effects of: Leflunomide

Ethanol/Nutrition/Herb Interactions Food: The addition of some flavoring agents (eg, milk, ice cream, sherbet, marmalade) are known to reduce the adsorptive capacity, and therefore the efficacy, of activated charcoal and should be avoided in preference to activated charcoal-water slurries; nevertheless, these flavoring agents do not completely compromise the effectiveness of activated charcoal and may be necessary in some circumstances (eg, administration in pediatric patients) to enhance compliance (Cooney, 1995; Dagnone, 2002).

Stability Adsorbs gases from air, store in a closed container. Dilute powder with at least 8 mL of water per 1 g of charcoal, or mix in a charcoal to water ratio of 1:4 to 1:8; mix to form a slurry (eg, mix 25 g with sufficient tap water to create a 4-ounce slurry or mix 50 g with sufficient tap water to create an 8-ounce slurry).

Mechanism of Action Adsorbs toxic substances, thus inhibiting GI absorption

Pharmacodynamics/Kinetics Excretion: Feces (as charcoal)

Dosage Oral, NG: **Note:** Some products may contain sorbitol; coadministration of a cathartic, including sorbitol, is **not** recommended. Some clinicians still recommend dosing activated charcoal in a 10:1 (charcoal:poison) ratio for optimal efficacy (Gude, 2009); however, the amount of poison ingested is commonly unknown, which makes this approach challenging and often impractical (Chyka, 2005).

Single dose (Chyka, 2005):

Infants <1 year: 10-25 g; **Note:** Although dosing by body weight is reported in children (0.5-1 g/kg) and published in many resources, there are no data or scientific rationale to support this recommendation.

Children 1-12 years: 25-50 g

Children >12 years and Adults: 25-100 g

Multidose:
Children: Initial dose: 25-50 g followed by multiple doses of 10-25 g every 4 hours
Adults: Initial dose: 50-100 g followed by 25-50 g every 4 hours

Administration Flavoring agents (eg, chocolate, concentrated fruit juice) or thickening agents (eg, bentonite, carboxymethylcellulose) can enhance charcoal's palatability. Check for presence of bowel sounds before administration. I.V. antiemetics may be required to reduce the risk of vomiting. The activated charcoal container should be agitated thoroughly before administration. The container should be rinsed with a small quantity of water to insure that the patient has received all of the activated charcoal (Krenzelok, 1991).

Capsules and tablets should not be used for the treatment of poisoning.

Dosage Forms Excipient information presented when available (limited, particularly for generics); consult specific product labeling.
Capsule, oral:
CharcoCaps®: 260 mg [dietary supplement]
Pellets for suspension, oral:
EZ-Char®: 25 g/bottle (1s)
Powder for suspension, oral: USP: 100% (30 g, 240 g)
Suspension, oral:
Actidose®-Aqua: 15 g (72 mL); 25 g (120 mL); 50 g (240 mL)
Kerr Insta-Char® in Aqueous Base: 25 g (120 mL); 50 g (240 mL) [contains propylene glycol (in flavoring packet), sodium benzoate]
Kerr Insta-Char® in Aqueous Base: 50 g (240 mL) [contains sodium benzoate]
Suspension, oral [with sorbitol]:
Actidose® with Sorbitol: 25 g (120 mL); 50 g (240 mL) [contains sorbitol]
Kerr Insta-Char® in Sorbitol Base: 25 g (120 mL); 50 g (240 mL) [contains propylene glycol (in flavoring packet), sodium benzoate, sorbitol]
Tablet, oral:
Requa® Activated Charcoal: 250 mg
Tablet, enteric coated, oral:
Charcoal Plus® DS: 250 mg

- **Charcoal Plus® DS [OTC]** *see* Charcoal, Activated *on page 335*
- **CharcoCaps® [OTC]** *see* Charcoal, Activated *on page 335*
- **Chemet®** *see* Succimer *on page 1595*
- **Chenodal™** *see* Chenodiol *on page 336*
- **Chenodeoxycholic Acid** *see* Chenodiol *on page 336*

Chenodiol (kee noe DYE ole)

Brand Names: U.S. Chenodal™
Index Terms CDCA; Chenodeoxycholic Acid
Pharmacologic Category Bile Acid
Use Oral dissolution of radiolucent cholesterol gallstones in selected patients as an alternative to surgery
Unlabeled Use Cerebrotendinous xanthomatosis (CTX)
Pregnancy Risk Factor X
Dosage Oral:
Cerebrotendinous xanthomatosis (unlabeled use):
Children: 15 mg/kg/day in 3 divided doses (van Heijst, 1998)
Adults: 750 mg/day in 3 divided doses (Beringer, 1984)
Gallstone dissolution (monotherapy): Adults: Initial: 250 mg twice daily for the first 2 weeks and increasing by 250 mg/day each week thereafter until the recommended or maximum tolerated dose is achieved; maintenance: 13-16 mg/kg/day in 2 divided doses. **Note:** Dosages <10 mg/kg are usually ineffective and may increase the risk of cholecystectomy.
Gallstone dissolution (combination therapy; unlabeled dose): Adults: 5-7.5 mg/kg/day once daily at bedtime, in combination with ursodeoxycholic acid, with or without adjuvant lithotripsy (Jazrawi, 1992; Pereira, 1997; Petroni, 2001)

Dosing comments in hepatic impairment: Use extreme caution; contraindicated for use in presence of known hepatocyte dysfunction or bile ductal abnormalities

Additional Information Complete prescribing information for this medication should be consulted for additional detail.

Dosage Forms Excipient information presented when available (limited, particularly for generics); consult specific product labeling.
Tablet, oral:
Chenodal™: 250 mg

- **Cheracol® D [OTC]** *see* Guaifenesin and Dextromethorphan *on page 810*
- **Cheracol® Plus [OTC]** *see* Guaifenesin and Dextromethorphan *on page 810*
- **Cheratussin** *see* GuaiFENesin *on page 809*
- **Chew-C [OTC]** *see* Ascorbic Acid *on page 149*
- **Chew-Cal [OTC]** *see* Calcium and Vitamin D *on page 265*
- **CHG** *see* Chlorhexidine Gluconate *on page 341*
- **Chickenpox Vaccine** *see* Varicella Virus Vaccine *on page 1773*
- **Chiggerex® Plus [OTC]** *see* Benzocaine *on page 202*
- **ChiggerTox® [OTC]** *see* Benzocaine *on page 202*
- **Children's Advil® Cold (Can)** *see* Pseudoephedrine and Ibuprofen *on page 1432*
- **Children's Nasal Decongestant [OTC]** *see* Pseudoephedrine *on page 1430*
- **Children's Pepto [OTC]** *see* Calcium Carbonate *on page 266*
- **Children's Motion Sickness Liquid (Can)** *see* DimenhyDRINATE *on page 513*
- **Chloditan** *see* Mitotane *on page 1144*
- **Chlodithane** *see* Mitotane *on page 1144*
- **Chloral** *see* Chloral Hydrate *on page 336*

Chloral Hydrate (KLOR al HYE drate)

Brand Names: U.S. Somnote®
Brand Names: Canada PMS-Chloral Hydrate
Index Terms Chloral; Hydrated Chloral; Trichloroacetaldehyde Monohydrate
Pharmacologic Category Hypnotic, Nonbenzodiazepine
Use Short-term sedative and hypnotic (<2 weeks); sedative/hypnotic for diagnostic procedures; sedative prior to EEG evaluations
Pregnancy Risk Factor C
Dosage
Children:
Sedation or anxiety: Oral, rectal: 5-15 mg/kg/dose every 8 hours (maximum: 500 mg/dose)
Prior to EEG: Oral, rectal: 20-25 mg/kg/dose, 30-60 minutes prior to EEG; may repeat in 30 minutes to maximum of 100 mg/kg or 2 g total

Hypnotic: Oral, rectal: 20-40 mg/kg/dose up to a maximum of 50 mg/kg/24 hours or 1 g/dose or 2 g/24 hours
Conscious sedation: Oral: 50-75 mg/kg/dose 30-60 minutes prior to procedure; may repeat 30 minutes after initial dose if needed, to a total maximum dose of 120 mg/kg or 1 g total

Adults: Oral:
Sedation, anxiety: 250 mg 3 times/day
Hypnotic: 500-1000 mg at bedtime or 30 minutes prior to procedure, not to exceed 2 g/24 hours

Discontinuation: Withdraw gradually over 2 weeks if patient has been maintained on high doses for prolonged period of time. Do not stop drug abruptly; sudden withdrawal may result in delirium.

Dosing adjustment/comments in renal impairment: Cl_{cr} <50 mL/minute: Avoid use

Hemodialysis: Dialyzable (50% to 100%); supplemental dose is not necessary

Dosing adjustment/comments in hepatic impairment: Avoid use in patients with severe hepatic impairment

Additional Information Complete prescribing information for this medication should be consulted for additional detail.

Dosage Forms Excipient information presented when available (limited, particularly for generics); consult specific product labeling.

Capsule, oral:
Somnote®: 500 mg

Syrup, oral: 500 mg/5 mL (5 mL, 473 mL)

Controlled Substance C-IV

Chlorambucil (klor AM byoo sil)

Brand Names: U.S. Leukeran®

Brand Names: Canada Leukeran®

Index Terms CB-1348; Chlorambucilum; Chloraminophene; Chlorbutinum; WR-139013

Pharmacologic Category Antineoplastic Agent, Alkylating Agent

Use Management of chronic lymphocytic leukemia (CLL), Hodgkin lymphoma, non-Hodgkin's lymphomas (NHL)

Unlabeled Use Treatment of nephrotic syndrome (steroid sensitive) in children, treatment of Waldenström's macroglobulinemia

Pregnancy Risk Factor D

Pregnancy Considerations Animal studies have demonstrated teratogenicity. Chlorambucil crosses the human placenta. Following exposure during the first trimester, case reports have noted adverse renal effects (unilateral agenesis). Women of childbearing potential should avoid becoming pregnant while receiving treatment. **[U.S. Boxed Warning]: Affects human fertility; probably mutagenic and teratogenic as well**; chromosomal damage has been documented. Reversible and irreversible sterility (when administered to prepubertal and pubertal males), azoospermia (in adult males) and amenorrhea (in females) have been observed. Fibrosis, vasculitis and depletion of primordial follicles have been noted on autopsy of the ovaries.

Lactation Excretion in breast milk unknown/not recommended

Contraindications Hypersensitivity to chlorambucil or any component of the formulation; hypersensitivity to other alkylating agents (may have cross-hypersensitivity); prior (demonstrated) resistance to chlorambucil

Warnings/Precautions Hazardous agent - use appropriate precautions for handling and disposal. Seizures have been observed; use with caution in patients with seizure disorder or head trauma; history of nephrotic syndrome and high pulse doses are at higher risk of seizures. **[U.S. Boxed Warning]: May cause severe bone marrow suppression;** neutropenia may be severe. Reduce initial dosage if patient has received myelosuppressive or radiation therapy within the previous 4 weeks, or has a depressed baseline leukocyte or platelet count. Irreversible bone marrow damage may occur with total doses approaching 6.5 mg/kg. Progressive lymphopenia may develop (recovery is generally rapid after discontinuation). Avoid administration of live vaccines to immunocompromised patients. Rare instances of severe skin reactions (eg, erythema multiforme, Stevens-Johnson syndrome) have been reported; discontinue promptly if skin reaction occurs.

Chlorambucil is primarily metabolized in the liver. Dosage reductions should be considered in patients with hepatic impairment. **[U.S. Boxed Warning]: Affects human fertility; carcinogenic in humans and probably mutagenic and teratogenic as well;** chromosomal damage has been documented. Reversible and irreversible sterility (when administered to prepubertal and pubertal males), azoospermia (in adult males) and amenorrhea (in females) have been observed. **[U.S. Boxed Warning]: Carcinogenic;** acute myelocytic leukemia and secondary malignancies may be associated with chronic therapy. Duration of treatment and higher cumulative doses are associated with a higher risk for development of leukemia.

Adverse Reactions Frequency not always defined.

Central nervous system: Agitation (rare), ataxia (rare), confusion (rare), drug fever, fever, focal/generalized seizure (rare), hallucinations (rare)
Dermatologic: Angioneurotic edema, erythema multiforme (rare), rash, skin hypersensitivity, Stevens-Johnson syndrome (rare), toxic epidermal necrolysis (rare), urticaria
Endocrine & metabolic: Amenorrhea, infertility, SIADH (rare)
Gastrointestinal: Diarrhea (infrequent), nausea (infrequent), oral ulceration (infrequent), vomiting (infrequent)
Genitourinary: Azoospermia, cystitis (sterile)
Hematologic: Neutropenia (onset: 3 weeks; recovery: 10 days after last dose), bone marrow failure (irreversible), bone marrow suppression, anemia, leukemia (secondary), leukopenia, lymphopenia, pancytopenia, thrombocytopenia
Hepatic: Hepatotoxicity, jaundice
Neuromuscular & skeletal: Flaccid paresis (rare), muscular twitching (rare), myoclonia (rare), peripheral neuropathy, tremor (rare)
Respiratory: Interstitial pneumonia, pulmonary fibrosis
Miscellaneous: Allergic reactions, malignancies (secondary)

Drug Interactions

Metabolism/Transport Effects None known.

Avoid Concomitant Use

Avoid concomitant use of Chlorambucil with any of the following: BCG; CloZAPine; Natalizumab; Pimecrolimus; Tacrolimus (Topical); Vaccines (Live)

Increased Effect/Toxicity

Chlorambucil may increase the levels/effects of: CloZAPine; Leflunomide; Natalizumab; Vaccines (Live)

The levels/effects of Chlorambucil may be increased by: Denosumab; Pimecrolimus; Roflumilast; Tacrolimus (Topical); Trastuzumab

Decreased Effect

Chlorambucil may decrease the levels/effects of: BCG; Coccidioidin Skin Test; Sipuleucel-T; Vaccines (Inactivated); Vaccines (Live)

The levels/effects of Chlorambucil may be decreased by: Echinacea

Ethanol/Nutrition/Herb Interactions Food: Absorption is decreased when administered with food.

Stability Store in refrigerator at 2°C to 8°C (36°F to 46°F). Protect from light.

Mechanism of Action Alkylating agent; interferes with DNA replication and RNA transcription by alkylation and cross-linking the strands of DNA

Pharmacodynamics/Kinetics

Absorption: Rapid and complete (>70%); reduced with food

Distribution: V_d: ~0.3 L/kg

Protein binding: ~99%; primarily to albumin

Metabolism: Hepatic (extensively); primarily to active metabolite, phenylacetic acid mustard

Half-life elimination: ~1.5 hours; Phenylacetic acid mustard: ~1.8 hours

Time to peak, plasma: Within 1 hour; Phenylacetic acid mustard: 1.2-2.6 hours

Excretion: Urine (~20% to 60%, primarily as inactive metabolites, <1% as unchanged drug or phenylacetic acid mustard)

Dosage Oral:

Children: Nephrotic syndrome, steroid sensitive (unlabeled use): 0.2 mg/kg once daily for 8 weeks (Hodson, 2010)

Adults: **Note:** With bone marrow lymphocytic infiltration involvement (in CLL, Hodgkin lymphoma, or NHL), the maximum dose is 0.1 mg/kg/day. While short treatment courses are preferred, if maintenance therapy is required, the maximum dose is 0.1 mg/kg/day.

Chronic lymphocytic leukemia (CLL):

Labeled dosing: 0.1 mg/kg/day for 3-6 weeks **or** 0.4 mg/kg pulsed doses administered intermittently, biweekly, or monthly (increased by 0.1 mg/kg/dose until response/toxicity observed)

Unlabeled dosing: 30 mg/m^2 day 1 every 2 weeks (in combination with prednisone) (Raphael, 1991) **or** 0.4 mg/kg day 1 every 2 weeks; if tolerated may increase by 0.1 mg/kg with each treatment course to a maximum dose of 0.8 mg/kg and maximum of 24 cycles (Eichhorst, 2009) **or** 40 mg/m^2 day 1 every 4 weeks for up to 12 cycles or until disease progression or complete remission or response plateau (Rai, 2000)

Hodgkin lymphoma: 0.2 mg/kg/day for 3-6 weeks

Non-Hodgkin's lymphomas (NHL): 0.1 mg/kg/day for 3-6 weeks

Waldenström's macroglobulinemia (unlabeled use): 0.1 mg/kg/day (continuously) for at least 6 months **or** 0.3 mg/kg/day for 7 days every 6 weeks for at least 6 months (Kyle, 2000)

Elderly: Refer to adult dosing; begin at the lower end of dosing range(s)

Dosage adjustment for toxicity:

Skin reactions: Discontinue treatment

Hematologic:

WBC or platelets below normal: Reduce dose

Severely depressed WBC or platelet counts: Discontinue

Persistently low neutrophil or platelet counts or peripheral lymphocytosis: May be suggestive of bone marrow infiltration; if infiltration confirmed, do not exceed 0.1 mg/kg/day.

Concurrent or within 4 weeks (before or after) of chemotherapy/radiotherapy: Initiate treatment cautiously; reduce dose; monitor closely.

Dosing adjustment in renal impairment: No dosage adjustment provided in manufacturer's labeling; however, renal elimination of unchanged chlorambucil and active metabolite (phenylacetic acid mustard) is minimal and renal impairment is not likely to affect elimination. The following recommendations have been used by some clinicians: Adults:

Aronoff, 2007:

Cl_{cr} >50 mL/minute: No adjustment necessary

Cl_{cr} 10-50 mL/minute: Administer 75% of dose

Cl_{cr} <10 mL/minute: Administer 50% of dose

Peritoneal dialysis (PD): Administer 50% of dose

Kintzel, 1995: Based on the pharmacokinetics, dosage adjustment is not indicated

Dosing adjustment in hepatic impairment: Chlorambucil undergoes extensive hepatic metabolism. Although dosage reduction should be considered in patients with hepatic impairment, no dosage adjustment is provided in the manufacturer's labeling (data is insufficient).

Administration Usually administered as a single dose; preferably on an empty stomach.

Monitoring Parameters Liver function tests, CBC with differential (weekly, with WBC monitored twice weekly during the first 3-6 weeks of treatment), serum uric acid

Dosage Forms Excipient information presented when available (limited, particularly for generics); consult specific product labeling.

Tablet, oral:

Leukeran®: 2 mg

Extemporaneous Preparations Hazardous agent: Use appropriate precautions for handling and disposal.

A 2 mg/mL oral suspension may be made with tablets. Crush sixty 2 mg tablets in a mortar and reduce to a fine powder. Add small portions of methylcellulose 1% and mix to a uniform paste (total methylcellulose: 30 mL); mix while adding simple syrup in incremental proportions to **almost** 60 mL; transfer to a graduated cylinder, rinse mortar and pestle with simple syrup, and add quantity of vehicle sufficient to make 60 mL. Transfer contents of graduated cylinder to an amber prescription bottle. Label "shake well", "refrigerate", and "protect from light". Stable for 7 days refrigerated.

Dressman JB and Poust RI, "Stability of Allopurinol and of Five Antineoplastics in Suspension," *Am J Hosp Pharm*, 1983, 40(4):616-8.

Nahata MC, Pai VB, and Hipple TF, *Pediatric Drug Formulations*, 5th ed, Cincinnati, OH: Harvey Whitney Books Co, 2004.

◆ **Chlorambucilum** *see* Chlorambucil *on page* 337

◆ **Chloraminophene** *see* Chlorambucil *on page* 337

Chloramphenicol (klor am FEN i kole)

Brand Names: Canada Chloromycetin®; Chloromycetin® Succinate; Diochloram®; Pentamycetin®

Pharmacologic Category Antibiotic, Miscellaneous

Use Treatment of serious infections due to organisms resistant to other less toxic antibiotics or when its penetrability into the site of infection is clinically superior to other antibiotics to which the organism is sensitive; useful in infections caused by *Bacteroides*, *H. influenzae*, *Neisseria meningitidis*, *Salmonella*, and *Rickettsia*; active against many vancomycin-resistant enterococci

Pregnancy Considerations Chloramphenicol crosses the placenta producing cord concentrations approaching maternal serum concentrations. An increased risk of teratogenic effects has not been identified for chloramphenicol and there have been no reports of fetal harm related to use of chloramphenicol in pregnancy. "Gray Syndrome" has occurred in premature infants and newborns receiving chloramphenicol. In most cases, chloramphenicol was started during the first 48 hours of life, but it has also occurred in older patients after high doses. Symptoms began after 3-4 days of therapy, starting with abdominal distention and continuing to progressive pallid cyanosis, vasomotor collapse, irregular respiration, and death within a few hours of symptom onset. Stopping therapy can reverse the process and allow complete recovery. There is one case report of an infant with gray baby syndrome after *in utero* exposure to a single maternal dose during labor, followed by a 10-fold overdose of chloramphenicol in the first day of life. The extent of the contribution of the single dose given during labor is unknown. The manufacturer recommends caution if used in a pregnant patient near term or during labor.

Lactation Enters breast milk/use with caution (AAP rates "of concern"; AAP 2001 update pending)

Contraindications Hypersensitivity to chloramphenicol or any component of the formulation; treatment of trivial or viral infections; bacterial prophylaxis

Warnings/Precautions Hazardous agent - use appropriate precautions for handling and disposal. Gray syndrome characterized by circulatory collapse, cyanosis, acidosis, abdominal distention, myocardial depression, coma, and death has occurred. Use with caution in patients with impaired renal or hepatic function and in neonates. Reduce dose with impaired liver function. Use with care in patients with glucose 6-phosphate dehydrogenase deficiency. **[U.S. Boxed Warning]: Serious and fatal blood dyscrasias (aplastic anemia, hypoplastic anemia, thrombocytopenia, and granulocytopenia) have occurred after both short-term and prolonged therapy. Monitor CBC frequently in all patients;** discontinue if evidence of myelosuppression. Irreversible bone marrow suppression may occur weeks or months after therapy. Avoid repeated courses of treatment. Should not be used for minor infections or when less potentially toxic agents are effective. Prolonged use may result in fungal or bacterial superinfection, including *C. difficile*-associated diarrhea (CDAD) and pseudomembranous colitis; CDAD has been observed >2 months postantibiotic treatment.

Adverse Reactions Frequency not defined.

Central nervous system: Confusion, delirium, depression, fever, headache

Dermatologic: Angioedema, rash, urticaria

Gastrointestinal: Diarrhea, enterocolitis, glossitis, nausea, stomatitis, vomiting

Hematologic: Aplastic anemia, bone marrow suppression, granulocytopenia, hypoplastic anemia, pancytopenia, thrombocytopenia

Ocular: Optic neuritis

Miscellaneous: Anaphylaxis, hypersensitivity reactions, Gray syndrome

Drug Interactions

Metabolism/Transport Effects Inhibits CYP2C19 (strong), CYP2C9 (weak), CYP3A4 (strong)

Avoid Concomitant Use

Avoid concomitant use of Chloramphenicol with any of the following: Alfuzosin; BCG; Clopidogrel; CloZAPine; Conivaptan; Crizotinib; Dronedarone; Eplerenone; Everolimus; Fluticasone (Oral Inhalation); Halofantrine; Lapatinib; Lovastatin; Lurasidone; Nilotinib; Nisoldipine; Pimozide; Ranolazine; Rivaroxaban; RomiDEPsin; Salmeterol; Silodosin; Simvastatin; Tamsulosin; Ticagrelor; Tolvaptan; Toremifene

Increased Effect/Toxicity

Chloramphenicol may increase the levels/effects of: Alfuzosin; Almotriptan; Alosetron; Anticonvulsants (Hydantoin); ARIPiprazole; Barbiturates; Bortezomib; Brentuximab Vedotin; Brinzolamide; Budesonide (Nasal); Budesonide (Systemic, Oral Inhalation); Ciclesonide; Citalopram; CloZAPine; Colchicine; Conivaptan; Corticosteroids (Orally Inhaled); Crizotinib; CycloSPORINE; CycloSPORINE (Systemic); CYP2C19 Substrates; CYP3A4 Substrates; Dienogest; Dronedarone; Dutasteride; Eplerenone; Everolimus; FentaNYL; Fesoterodine; Fluticasone (Nasal); Fluticasone (Oral Inhalation); GuanFACINE; Halofantrine; Iloperidone; Ixabepilone; Lapatinib; Lovastatin; Lumefantrine; Lurasidone; Maraviroc; MethylPREDNISolone; Nilotinib; Nisoldipine; Paricalcitol; Pazopanib; Pimecrolimus; Pimozide; Propafenone; Ranolazine; Rivaroxaban; RomiDEPsin; Ruxolitinib; Salmeterol; Saxagliptin; Sildenafil; Silodosin; Simvastatin; SORAfenib; Sulfonylureas; Tacrolimus; Tacrolimus (Systemic); Tadalafil; Tamsulosin; Ticagrelor; Tolterodine; Tolvaptan; Toremifene; Vardenafil; Vemurafenib; Vilazodone; Vitamin K Antagonists; Voriconazole; Zuclopenthixol

Decreased Effect

Chloramphenicol may decrease the levels/effects of: BCG; Clopidogrel; Cyanocobalamin; Prasugrel; Ticagrelor; Typhoid Vaccine

The levels/effects of Chloramphenicol may be decreased by: Anticonvulsants (Hydantoin); Barbiturates; Rifampin

Ethanol/Nutrition/Herb Interactions Food: May decrease intestinal absorption of vitamin B_{12} may have increased dietary need for riboflavin, pyridoxine, and vitamin B_{12}.

Stability Store at room temperature prior to reconstitution. Reconstituted solutions remain stable for 30 days. Use only clear solutions. Frozen solutions remain stable for 6 months.

Mechanism of Action Reversibly binds to 50S ribosomal subunits of susceptible organisms preventing amino acids from being transferred to growing peptide chains thus inhibiting protein synthesis

Pharmacodynamics/Kinetics

Distribution: To most tissues and body fluids
- Chloramphenicol: V_d: 0.5-1 L/kg
- Chloramphenicol succinate: V_d: 0.2-3.1 L/kg; decreased with hepatic or renal dysfunction

Protein binding: Chloramphenicol: ~60%; decreased with hepatic or renal dysfunction and in newborn infants

Metabolism:
- Chloramphenicol: Hepatic to metabolites (inactive)
- Chloramphenicol succinate: Hydrolyzed in the liver, kidney and lungs to chloramphenicol (active)

Bioavailability:
- Chloramphenicol: Oral: ~80%
- Chloramphenicol succinate: I.V.: ~70%; highly variable, dependent upon rate and extent of metabolism to chloramphenicol

Half-life elimination:
- Normal renal function:
  - Chloramphenicol: Adults: ~4 hours; Children 4-6 hours; Infants: Significantly prolonged
  - Chloramphenicol succinate: Adults: ~3 hours
- End-stage renal disease: Chloramphenicol: 3-7 hours
- Hepatic disease: Prolonged

Excretion: Urine (~30% as unchanged chloramphenicol succinate in adults, 6% to 80% in children; 5% to 15% as chloramphenicol)

Dosage

Children: Usual dosing range: I.V.: 50-100 mg/kg/day in divided doses every 6 hours; maximum daily dose: 4 g/day
- Meningitis: I.V.: Infants >30 days and Children: 75-100 mg/kg/day divided every 6 hours

Adults: 50-100 mg/kg/day in divided doses every 6 hours; maximum daily dose: 4 g/day

Dosing adjustment in renal impairment: Use with caution; monitor serum concentrations

Dosing adjustment/comments in hepatic impairment: Use with caution; monitor serum concentrations

Dietary Considerations May have increased dietary need for riboflavin, pyridoxine, and vitamin B_{12}. Some products may contain sodium.

Administration Do not administer I.M.; can be administered IVP over at least 1 minute at a concentration of 100 mg/mL, or I.V. intermittent infusion over 15-30 minutes at a final concentration for administration of ≤20 mg/mL.

Monitoring Parameters CBC with differential (baseline and every 2 days during therapy), periodic liver and renal function tests, serum drug concentration

Reference Range

Therapeutic levels:
- Meningitis:
  - Peak: 15-25 mcg/mL; toxic concentration: >40 mcg/mL
  - Trough: 5-15 mcg/mL

Other infections:
Peak: 10-20 mcg/mL
Trough: 5-10 mcg/mL
Timing of serum samples: Draw levels 0.5-1.5 hours after completion of I.V. dose

Test Interactions May cause false-positive results in urine glucose tests when using cupric sulfate (Benedict's solution, Clinitest®).

Dosage Forms Excipient information presented when available (limited, particularly for generics); consult specific product labeling.

Injection, powder for reconstitution: 1 g [contains sodium [~52 mg (2.25 mEq)/g]]

◆ **ChloraPrep® [OTC]** *see* Chlorhexidine Gluconate *on page 341*

◆ **ChloraPrep® Frepp® [OTC]** *see* Chlorhexidine Gluconate *on page 341*

◆ **ChloraPrep® Sepp® [OTC]** *see* Chlorhexidine Gluconate *on page 341*

◆ **Chlorascrub™ [OTC]** *see* Chlorhexidine Gluconate *on page 341*

◆ **Chlorascrub™ Maxi [OTC]** *see* Chlorhexidine Gluconate *on page 341*

◆ **Chlorbutinum** *see* Chlorambucil *on page 337*

ChlordiazePOXIDE (klor dye az e POKS ide)

Brand Names: Canada Apo-Chlordiazepoxide®

Index Terms Librium; Methaminodiazepoxide Hydrochloride

Pharmacologic Category Benzodiazepine

Additional Appendix Information

Beers Criteria - Potentially Inappropriate Medications for Geriatrics *on page 1973*

Benzodiazepines *on page 1882*

Use Management of anxiety disorder or for the short-term relief of symptoms of anxiety; withdrawal symptoms of acute alcoholism; preoperative apprehension and anxiety

Pregnancy Considerations Adverse events were observed in some animal reproduction studies. Chlordiazepoxide crosses the human placenta and fetal serum concentrations are similar to those in the mother. Teratogenic effects have been observed with some benzodiazepines (including chlordiazepoxide); however, additional studies are needed. The incidence of premature birth and low birth weights may be increased following maternal use of benzodiazepines; hypoglycemia and respiratory problems in the neonate may occur following exposure late in pregnancy. Neonatal withdrawal symptoms may occur within days to weeks after birth and "floppy infant syndrome" (which also includes withdrawal symptoms) has been reported with some benzodiazepines.

Lactation Enters breast milk

Contraindications Hypersensitivity to chlordiazepoxide or any component of the formulation (cross-sensitivity with other benzodiazepines may also exist)

Warnings/Precautions Active metabolites with extended half-lives may lead to delayed accumulation and adverse effects. Use with caution in elderly or debilitated patients, pediatric patients, patients with hepatic disease (including alcoholics) or renal impairment, patients with respiratory disease or impaired gag reflex, patients with porphyria.

Causes CNS depression (dose related) resulting in sedation, dizziness, confusion, or ataxia which may impair physical and mental capabilities. Patients must be cautioned about performing tasks which require mental alertness (eg, operating machinery or driving). Use with caution in patients receiving other CNS depressants or psychoactive agents (lithium, phenothiazines). Effects with other sedative drugs or ethanol may be potentiated. Benzodiazepines have been associated with falls and traumatic injury and should be used with extreme caution in patients who are at risk of these events (especially the elderly). Benzodiazepines with long half-lives may produce prolonged sedation and increase the risk of falls and fracture. Short- or intermediate-acting benzodiazepines are preferred in elderly patients (Beers Criteria).

Use caution in patients with depression, particularly if suicidal risk may be present. Use with caution in patients with a history of drug dependence. Benzodiazepines have been associated with dependence and acute withdrawal symptoms on discontinuation or reduction in dose. Acute withdrawal, including seizures, may be precipitated in patients after administration of flumazenil to patients receiving long-term benzodiazepine therapy.

Benzodiazepines have been associated with anterograde amnesia. Paradoxical reactions, including hyperactive or aggressive behavior have been reported with benzodiazepines, particularly in adolescent/pediatric or psychiatric patients. Does not have analgesic, antidepressant, or antipsychotic properties.

Adverse Reactions

>10%:

Central nervous system: Drowsiness, fatigue, ataxia, lightheadedness, memory impairment, dysarthria, irritability
Dermatologic: Rash
Endocrine & metabolic: Libido decreased, menstrual disorders
Gastrointestinal: Xerostomia, salivation decreased, appetite increased or decreased, weight gain/loss
Genitourinary: Micturition difficulties

1% to 10%:

Cardiovascular: Hypotension
Central nervous system: Confusion, dizziness, disinhibition, akathisia
Dermatologic: Dermatitis
Endocrine & metabolic: Libido increased
Gastrointestinal: Salivation increased
Genitourinary: Sexual dysfunction, incontinence
Neuromuscular & skeletal: Rigidity, tremor, muscle cramps
Otic: Tinnitus
Respiratory: Nasal congestion

<1% (Limited to important or life-threatening): Photosensitivity

Drug Interactions

Metabolism/Transport Effects Substrate of CYP3A4 (major); **Note:** Assignment of Major/Minor substrate status based on clinically relevant drug interaction potential

Avoid Concomitant Use

Avoid concomitant use of ChlordiazePOXIDE with any of the following: Conivaptan; OLANZapine

Increased Effect/Toxicity

ChlordiazePOXIDE may increase the levels/effects of: Alcohol (Ethyl); CloZAPine; CNS Depressants; Fosphenytoin; Methotrimeprazine; Phenytoin; Selective Serotonin Reuptake Inhibitors

The levels/effects of ChlordiazePOXIDE may be increased by: Antifungal Agents (Azole Derivatives, Systemic); Aprepitant; Calcium Channel Blockers (Nondihydropyridine); Cimetidine; Conivaptan; Contraceptives (Estrogens); Contraceptives (Progestins); CYP3A4 Inhibitors (Moderate); CYP3A4 Inhibitors (Strong); Dasatinib; Disulfiram; Droperidol; Fluconazole; Fosaprepitant; Grapefruit Juice; HydrOXYzine; Isoniazid; Macrolide Antibiotics; MAO Inhibitors; Methotrimeprazine; Nefazodone; OLANZapine; Proton Pump Inhibitors; Selective Serotonin Reuptake Inhibitors

Decreased Effect

The levels/effects of ChlordiazePOXIDE may be decreased by: CarBAMazepine; CYP3A4 Inducers (Strong); Deferasirox; Rifamycin Derivatives; St Johns Wort; Theophylline Derivatives; Tocilizumab; Yohimbine

Ethanol/Nutrition/Herb Interactions

Ethanol: May increase CNS depression; monitor for increased effects with coadministration. Caution patients about effects.

Food: Serum concentrations/effects may be increased with grapefruit juice, but unlikely because of high oral bioavailability of chlordiazepoxide.

Herb/Nutraceutical: Avoid valerian, St John's wort, kava kava, gotu kola (may increase CNS depression).

Stability Store at controlled room temperature. Protect from light and moisture.

Mechanism of Action Binds to stereospecific benzodiazepine receptors on the postsynaptic GABA neuron at several sites within the central nervous system, including the limbic system, reticular formation. Enhancement of the inhibitory effect of GABA on neuronal excitability results by increased neuronal membrane permeability to chloride ions. This shift in chloride ions results in hyperpolarization (a less excitable state) and stabilization.

Pharmacodynamics/Kinetics

Distribution: V_d: 3.3 L/kg

Protein binding: 90% to 98%

Metabolism: Extensively hepatic to desmethyldiazepam (active and long-acting)

Half-life elimination: 6.6-25 hours; End-stage renal disease: 5-30 hours; Cirrhosis: 30-63 hours

Time to peak, serum: Within 2 hours

Excretion: Urine (minimal as unchanged drug)

Dosage Oral:

Children:

<6 years: Not recommended

≥6 years: Anxiety: Usual daily dose: 5 mg 2-4 times/day. Dose may be increased to 10 mg 2-3 times/day in some patients, if necessary.

Adults:

Anxiety:

Mild-moderate anxiety: Usual daily dose: 5-10 mg 3-4 times/day

Severe anxiety: Usual daily dose: 20-25 mg 3-4 times/day

Preoperative anxiety: 5-10 mg 3-4 times/day on the days preceding surgery

Ethanol withdrawal symptoms: 50-100 mg to start; dose may be repeated in 2-4 hours as necessary to a maximum of 300 mg/24 hours. **Note:** Frequency of repeat doses is often based on institution-specific protocols.

Elderly or debilitated patients: Usual daily dose: 5 mg 2-4 times/day. Avoid use if possible due to long-acting metabolite.

Dosing adjustment in renal impairment: Dosage adjustments are not provided in the manufacturer's labeling; however, the following guidelines have been used by some clinicians (Aronoff, 2007): Adults: Cl_{cr} <10 mL/minute: Administer 50% of dose

Peritoneal dialysis: Administer 50% of the dose

Dosing adjustment/comments in hepatic impairment: There are no specific hepatic dosage adjustments provided in the manufacturer's labeling. Use with caution or avoid use in hepatic impairment; hepatic metabolism occurs.

Administration Administer orally in divided doses.

Monitoring Parameters Respiratory and cardiovascular status, mental status, check for orthostasis

Reference Range Therapeutic: 0.1-3 mcg/mL (SI: 0-10 micromole/L); Toxic: >23 mcg/mL (SI: >77 micromole/L)

Additional Information The parenteral formulation of chlordiazepoxide is no longer commercially available in the U.S. or Canada.

Dosage Forms Excipient information presented when available (limited, particularly for generics); consult specific product labeling.

Capsule, oral, as hydrochloride: 5 mg, 10 mg, 25 mg

Controlled Substance C-IV

◆ **Chlordiazepoxide and Amitriptyline Hydrochloride** *see* Amitriptyline and Chlordiazepoxide *on page 96*

◆ **Chlordiazepoxide and Clidinium** *see* Clidinium and Chlordiazepoxide *on page 378*

◆ **Chlorethazine** *see* Mechlorethamine *on page 1056*

◆ **Chlorethazine Mustard** *see* Mechlorethamine *on page 1056*

Chlorhexidine Gluconate

(klor HEKS i deen GLOO koe nate)

Brand Names: U.S. Avagard™ [OTC]; Bactoshield® CHG [OTC]; Betasept® [OTC]; ChloraPrep® Frepp® [OTC]; ChloraPrep® Sepp® [OTC]; ChloraPrep® [OTC]; Chlorascrub™ Maxi [OTC]; Chlorascrub™ [OTC]; Dyna-Hex® [OTC]; Hibiclens® [OTC]; Hibistat® [OTC]; Operand® Chlorhexidine Gluconate [OTC]; Peridex®; periochip®; PerioGard® [OTC]

Brand Names: Canada Hibidil® 1:2000; ORO-Clense; Peridex® Oral Rinse

Index Terms 3M™ Avagard™ [OTC]; CHG

Pharmacologic Category Antibiotic, Oral Rinse; Antibiotic, Topical

Use Skin cleanser for line placement, skin wounds, preoperative skin preparation; germicidal hand rinse; antibacterial dental rinse. Chlorhexidine is active against gram-positive and gram-negative organisms, facultative anaerobes, aerobes, and yeast. Chip, for periodontal pocket insertion: Reduces pocket depth in patients with adult periodontitis

Orphan drug: Peridex®: Oral mucositis with cytoreductive therapy when used for patients undergoing bone marrow transplant

Pregnancy Risk Factor B/C (manufacturer specific)

Dosage Adults:

Oral rinse (Peridex®, PerioGard®):

Floss and brush teeth, completely rinse toothpaste from mouth and swish 15 mL (one capful) undiluted oral rinse around in mouth for 30 seconds, then expectorate. Caution patient not to swallow the medicine and instruct not to eat for 2-3 hours after treatment (cap on bottle measures 15 mL).

Treatment of gingivitis: Oral prophylaxis: Swish for 30 seconds with 15 mL chlorhexidine, then expectorate; repeat twice daily (morning and evening). Patient should have a re-evaluation followed by a dental prophylaxis every 6 months.

Periodontal chip: One chip is inserted into a periodontal pocket with a probing pocket depth ≥5 mm. Up to 8 chips may be inserted in a single visit. Treatment is recommended every 3 months in pockets with a remaining depth ≥5 mm. If dislodgment occurs 7 days or more after placement, the subject is considered to have had the full course of treatment. If dislodgment occurs within 48 hours, a new chip should be inserted. The chip biodegrades completely and does not need to be removed. Patients should avoid dental floss at the site of periochip® insertion for 10 days after placement because flossing might dislodge the chip.

Insertion of periodontal chip: Pocket should be isolated and surrounding area dried prior to chip insertion. The chip should be grasped using forceps with the rounded edges away from the forceps. The chip should be ▶

inserted into the periodontal pocket to its maximum depth. It may be maneuvered into position using the tips of the forceps or a flat instrument.

Cleanser:

Surgical scrub: Scrub 3 minutes and rinse thoroughly, wash for an additional 3 minutes

Hand sanitizer (Avagard™): Dispense 1 pumpful in palm of one hand; dip fingertips of opposite hand into solution and work it under nails. Spread remainder evenly over hand and just above elbow, covering all surfaces. Repeat on other hand. Dispense another pumpful in each hand and reapply to each hand up to the wrist. Allow to dry before gloving.

Hand wash: Wash for 15 seconds and rinse

Hand rinse: Rub 15 seconds and rinse

Additional Information Complete prescribing information for this medication should be consulted for additional detail.

Dosage Forms Excipient information presented when available (limited, particularly for generics); consult specific product labeling. [DSC] = Discontinued product

Chip, for periodontal pocket insertion:
- periochip®: 2.5 mg (20s)

Liquid, oral [rinse]: 0.12% (15 mL, 473 mL, 480 mL)
- Peridex®: 0.12% (118 mL, 473 mL, 1893 mL, 1920 mL [DSC]) [contains ethanol 11.6%; mint flavor]
- PerioGard®: 0.12% (480 mL) [contains ethanol 11.6%; mint flavor]

Liquid, topical [surgical scrub]:
- Betasept®: 4% (118 mL, 237 mL, 473 mL, 946 mL, 3840 mL) [contains isopropyl alcohol 4%]
- Dyna-Hex®: 2% (120 mL, 480 mL, 960 mL, 3840 mL); 4% (120 mL, 240 mL, 480 mL, 960 mL, 3840 mL) [contains isopropyl alcohol]
- Hibiclens®: 4% (15 mL, 118 mL, 236 mL, 473 mL, 946 mL, 3840 mL) [contains isopropyl alcohol 4%]
- Operand® Chlorhexidine Gluconate: 2% (118 mL); 4% (118 mL, 237 mL, 472 mL, 946 mL, 3785 mL) [contains isopropyl alcohol 4%]

Lotion, topical [surgical scrub]:
- Avagard™: 1% (500 mL) [contains ethanol 61%, moisturizers]

Solution, topical [surgical scrub]:
- Bactoshield® CHG: 2% (120 mL, 480 mL, 750 mL, 960 mL, 3840 mL); 4% (120 mL, 473 mL, 960 mL, 3840 mL) [contains isopropyl alcohol]

Sponge, topical [surgical scrub]:
- ChloraPrep®: 2% (25s) [contains isopropyl alcohol 70%; 3 mL; clear]
- ChloraPrep®: 2% (25s) [contains isopropyl alcohol 70%; 3 mL; Hi-Lite Orange™ tint]
- ChloraPrep®: 2% (25s) [contains isopropyl alcohol 70%; 10.5 mL; clear]
- ChloraPrep®: 2% (25s) [contains isopropyl alcohol 70%; 10.5 mL; Hi-Lite Orange™ tint]
- ChloraPrep®: 2% (25s) [contains isopropyl alcohol 70%; 10.5 mL; Scrub Teal™ tint]
- ChloraPrep®: 2% (25s) [contains isopropyl alcohol 70%; 26 mL; clear]
- ChloraPrep®: 2% (25s) [contains isopropyl alcohol 70%; 26 mL; Hi-Lite Orange™ tint]
- ChloraPrep®: 2% (25s) [contains isopropyl alcohol 70%; 26 mL; Scrub Teal™ tint]
- ChloraPrep® Frepp®: 2% (20s) [contains isopropyl alcohol 70%; 1.5 mL]
- ChloraPrep® Sepp®: 2% (200s) [contains isopropyl alcohol 70%; 0.67 mL]

Sponge/Brush, topical [surgical scrub]:
- Bactoshield® CHG: 4% (300s) [contains isopropyl alcohol 4%; 25 mL]

Swab, topical [prep pads]:
- Chlorascrub™: 3.15% (100s) [contains isopropyl alcohol 70%; 1 mL]

Swabsticks, topical [surgical scrub]:
- ChloraPrep®: 2% (48s) [contains isopropyl alcohol 70%; 1.75 mL]
- ChloraPrep®: 2% (120s) [contains isopropyl alcohol 70%; 5.25 mL]
- Chlorascrub™: 3.15% (50s) [contains isopropyl alcohol 70%; 1.6 mL]
- Chlorascrub™ Maxi: 3.15% (30s) [contains isopropyl alcohol 70%; 5.1 mL]

Wipe, topical [towelette]:
- Hibistat®: 0.5% (50s) [contains isopropyl alcohol 70%; 5 mL]

◆ **Chlormeprazine** *see* Prochlorperazine *on page 1412*

◆ **2-Chlorodeoxyadenosine** *see* Cladribine *on page 372*

◆ **Chloromag®** *see* Magnesium Chloride *on page 1044*

◆ **Chloromycetin® (Can)** *see* Chloramphenicol *on page 338*

◆ **Chloromycetin® Succinate (Can)** *see* Chloramphenicol *on page 338*

Chloroprocaine (klor oh PROE kane)

Brand Names: U.S. Nesacaine®; Nesacaine®-MPF

Brand Names: Canada Nesacaine®-CE

Index Terms Chloroprocaine Hydrochloride

Pharmacologic Category Local Anesthetic

Use Infiltration anesthesia, peripheral nerve block, epidural anesthesia

Pregnancy Risk Factor C

Dosage Dosage varies with anesthetic procedure, the area to be anesthetized, the vascularity of the tissues, depth of anesthesia required, degree of muscle relaxation required, and duration of anesthesia; range.

Children >3 years (normally developed): Maximum dose (without epinephrine): 11 mg/kg; for infiltration, concentrations of 0.5% to 1% are recommended; for nerve block, concentrations of 1% to 1.5% are recommended

Adults:
- Maximum single dose (without epinephrine): 11 mg/kg; maximum dose: 800 mg
- Maximum single dose (with epinephrine): 14 mg/kg; maximum dose: 1000 mg
- Infiltration and peripheral nerve block:
  - Mandibular: 2%: 2-3 mL; total dose 40-60 mg
  - Infraorbital: 2%: 0.5-1 mL; total dose 10-20 mg
  - Brachial plexus: 2%; 30-40 mL; total dose 600-800 mg
  - Digital (without epinephrine): 1%; 3-4 mL; total dose: 30-40 mg
  - Pudendal: 2%; 10 mL each side; total dose: 400 mg
  - Paracervical: 1%; 3 mL per each of four sites
- Caudal block: Preservative-free: 2% or 3%: 15-25 mL; may repeat at 40-60 minute intervals
- Lumbar epidural block: Preservative-free: 2% or 3%: 2-2.5 mL per segment; usual total volume: 15-25 mL; may repeat with doses that are 2-6 mL less than initial dose every 40-50 minutes.

Additional Information Complete prescribing information for this medication should be consulted for additional detail.

Dosage Forms Excipient information presented when available (limited, particularly for generics); consult specific product labeling.

Injection, solution, as hydrochloride: 2% [20 mg/mL] (30 mL); 3% [30 mg/mL] (30 mL)
- Nesacaine®: 1% [10 mg/mL] (30 mL); 2% [20 mg/mL] (30 mL) [contains edetate disodium, methylparaben]

Injection, solution, as hydrochloride [preservative free]: 2% [20 mg/mL] (20 mL); 3% [30 mg/mL] (20 mL)
- Nesacaine®-MPF: 2% [20 mg/mL] (20 mL); 3% [30 mg/mL] (20 mL)

◆ **Chloroprocaine Hydrochloride** *see* Chloroprocaine *on page 342*

Chloroquine (KLOR oh kwin)

Brand Names: U.S. Aralen®
Brand Names: Canada Aralen®; Novo-Chloroquine
Index Terms Chloroquine Phosphate
Pharmacologic Category Aminoquinoline (Antimalarial)
Use Suppression/chemoprophylaxis or treatment of acute malaria due to susceptible *Plasmodium malariae, P. vivax, P. ovale, P. falciparum*; extraintestinal amebiasis
Unlabeled Use Rheumatoid arthritis; discoid lupus erythematosus
Pregnancy Considerations There are no adequate and well-controlled studies using chloroquine during pregnancy. However, based on clinical experience and because malaria infection in pregnant women may be more severe than in nonpregnant women, chloroquine prophylaxis may be considered in areas of chloroquine-sensitive *P. falciparum* malaria. Pregnant women should be advised not to travel to areas of *P. falciparum* resistance to chloroquine. Consult current CDC guidelines for the treatment of malaria during pregnancy.
Lactation Enters breast milk/not recommended (AAP considers "compatible"; AAP 2001 update pending)
Contraindications Hypersensitivity to 4-aminoquinoline compounds (eg, chloroquine, hydroxychloroquine) or any component of the formulation; retinal or visual field changes
Warnings/Precautions [U.S. Boxed Warning]: Physicians should be familiar with chloroquine before prescribing. Use with caution in patients with liver disease, alcoholism or in conjunction with hepatotoxic drugs. May exacerbate psoriasis or porphyria. Use caution in patients with seizure disorders. Use caution in G6PD deficiency; 4-aminoquinolines such as chloroquine has been associated with hemolysis and renal impairment. Use with caution in patients with pre-existing auditory damage; discontinue immediately if hearing defects are noted. Retinopathy (irreversible) and neuropathy/myopathy have occurred with long or high-dose therapy; discontinue drug if any abnormality in the visual field or if muscular weakness develops during treatment. Chloroquine has been associated with ECG changes, AV block, and cardiomyopathy. May cause QT prolongation and subsequent torsade de pointes; avoid use in patients with diagnosed or suspected congenital long QT syndrome. Avoid concurrent use with other drugs known to prolong QT_c interval. Aminoquinolones have been associated with rare hematologic reactions including agranulocytosis, aplastic anemia, and thrombocytopenia; monitoring (CBC) is recommended in prolonged therapy. Also consult current CDC guidelines for treatment recommendations.
Adverse Reactions Frequency not defined.
Cardiovascular: Cardiomyopathy, ECG changes (rare; including prolonged QRS and QT_c intervals), hypotension (rare), torsade de pointes (rare)
Central nervous system: Agitation, anxiety, confusion, delirium, depression, hallucinations, headache, insomnia, personality changes, polyneuritis, psychosis,
Dermatologic: Alopecia, erythema multiforme (rare), exfoliative dermatitis (rare), hair bleaching, lichen planus eruptions, photosensitivity, pleomorphic skin eruptions, pruritus, skin/mucosal pigmentary changes (blue-black), Stevens-Johnson syndrome (rare), toxic epidermal necrolysis (rare), urticaria
Gastrointestinal: Abdominal cramps, anorexia, diarrhea, nausea, vomiting
Hematologic: Rare cases of agranulocytosis (reversible), aplastic anemia, neutropenia, pancytopenia, thrombocytopenia
Hepatic: Hepatitis, liver enzymes increased
Neuromuscular & skeletal: Depression of deep tendon reflexes, myopathy, neuromyopathy, proximal muscle atrophy
Ocular: Accommodation disturbances, blurred vision, corneal opacities (reversible), nyctalopia, retinopathy (including irreversible changes in some patients long-term or high-dose therapy), visual field defects
Otic: Hearing reduced (risk increased in patients with pre-existing auditory damage), nerve deafness, tinnitus
Miscellaneous: Anaphylaxis, angioedema
Drug Interactions
Metabolism/Transport Effects Substrate of CYP2D6 (major), CYP3A4 (major); **Note:** Assignment of Major/Minor substrate status based on clinically relevant drug interaction potential; **Inhibits** CYP2D6 (moderate)
Avoid Concomitant Use
Avoid concomitant use of Chloroquine with any of the following: Agalsidase Alfa; Agalsidase Beta; Artemether; Conivaptan; Lumefantrine; Mefloquine
Increased Effect/Toxicity
Chloroquine may increase the levels/effects of: Antipsychotic Agents (Phenothiazines); Beta-Blockers; Cardiac Glycosides; CYP2D6 Substrates; Dapsone; Dapsone (Systemic); Dapsone (Topical); Fesoterodine; Lumefantrine; Mefloquine; Prilocaine; QTc-Prolonging Agents; Tamoxifen

The levels/effects of Chloroquine may be increased by: Abiraterone Acetate; Artemether; Conivaptan; CYP2D6 Inhibitors (Moderate); CYP2D6 Inhibitors (Strong); CYP3A4 Inhibitors (Moderate); CYP3A4 Inhibitors (Strong); Dapsone; Dapsone (Systemic); Darunavir; Mefloquine
Decreased Effect
Chloroquine may decrease the levels/effects of: Agalsidase Alfa; Agalsidase Beta; Ampicillin; Anthelmintics; Codeine; Rabies Vaccine; TraMADol

The levels/effects of Chloroquine may be decreased by: Antacids; CYP3A4 Inducers (Strong); Deferasirox; Herbs (CYP3A4 Inducers); Kaolin; Lanthanum; Peginterferon Alfa-2b; Tocilizumab
Ethanol/Nutrition/Herb Interactions Ethanol: Avoid ethanol (may increase GI irritation).
Stability Store tablets at 25°C (77°F); excursions permitted to 15°C to 30°C (59°F to 86°F).
Mechanism of Action Binds to and inhibits DNA and RNA polymerase; interferes with metabolism and hemoglobin utilization by parasites; inhibits prostaglandin effects; chloroquine concentrates within parasite acid vesicles and raises internal pH resulting in inhibition of parasite growth; may involve aggregates of ferriprotoporphyrin IX acting as chloroquine receptors causing membrane damage; may also interfere with nucleoprotein synthesis
Pharmacodynamics/Kinetics
Duration: Small amounts may be present in urine months following discontinuation of therapy
Absorption: Oral: Rapid (~89%)
Distribution: Widely in body tissues (eg, brain, eyes, heart, kidneys, leukocytes, liver, lungs, spleen) where retention prolonged
Protein binding: 55%
Metabolism: Partially hepatic
Half-life elimination: 3-5 days
Time to peak, serum: 1-2 hours
Excretion: Urine (~70% as unchanged drug); acidification of urine increases elimination

Dosage Oral:
Malaria chemoprophylaxis:
Children: Administer 8.3 mg/kg/week (5 mg/kg base) on the same day each week (not to exceed 500 mg/dose [300 mg base/dose]); begin 1-2 weeks prior to exposure; continue while in endemic area and for 4 weeks after leaving endemic area (CDC, 2010)
Adults: 500 mg/week (300 mg base) on the same day each week; begin 1-2 weeks prior to exposure; continue while in endemic area and for 4 weeks after leaving endemic area (CDC, 2010)
Malaria treatment:
Children: 16.6 mg/kg (10 mg/kg base) on day 1 (maximum: 1000 mg [600 mg base]), followed by 8.3 mg/kg (5 mg/kg base) (maximum: 500 mg [300 mg base]) 6-, 24-, and 48 hours after first dose (CDC, 2009)
Adults: 1 g (600 mg base) on day 1, followed by 500 mg (300 mg base) 6-8 hours later, followed by 500 mg (300 mg base) 6-, 24-, and 48 hours after first dose (CDC, 2009)
Extraintestinal amebiasis: Adults: 1 g/day (600 mg base) for 2 days followed by 500 mg/day (300 mg base) for at least 2-3 weeks
Rheumatoid arthritis, lupus erythematosus (unlabeled uses): Adults: 250 mg (150 mg base) once daily; reduce dosage following maximal response (taper to discontinue after response in lupus); generally requires 3-6 weeks
Note: Not considered first-line agent.

Dosing adjustment in renal impairment: The FDA-approved labeling does not contain renal dosing adjustment guidelines; the following guidelines have been used by some clinicians (Arnoff, 2007):
Cl_{cr} ≥10 mL/minute: No dosage adjustment needed
Cl_{cr} <10 mL/minute: Administer 50% of dose
Hemodialysis effects: Minimally removed by hemodialysis
Hemodialysis, peritoneal dialysis: Administer 50% of dose
Continuous renal replacement therapy (CRRT): Administer 100% of normal dose

Dietary Considerations May be taken with meals to decrease GI upset.

Administration May be taken with meals to decrease GI upset. Chloroquine phosphate tablets have also been mixed with chocolate syrup or enclosed in gelatin capsules to mask the bitter taste.

Monitoring Parameters Ophthalmic exams at baseline and every 3 months during prolonged therapy. Visual acuity, slit-lamp, fundoscopic and visual field examination are recommended. Evaluate neuromuscular function during prolonged therapy. Periodic CBC in patients receiving prolonged therapy

Dosage Forms Excipient information presented when available (limited, particularly for generics); consult specific product labeling.
Tablet, oral, as phosphate: 250 mg [equivalent to chloroquine base 150 mg], 500 mg [equivalent to chloroquine base 300 mg]
Aralen®: 500 mg [equivalent to chloroquine base 300 mg]

Extemporaneous Preparations A 15 mg chloroquine phosphate/mL oral suspension (equivalent to 9 mg chloroquine base/mL) may be made from tablets and a 1:1 mixture of Ora-Sweet® and Ora-Plus®. Crush three 500 mg chloroquine phosphate tablets (equivalent to 300 mg base/tablet) in a mortar and reduce to a fine powder. Add 15 mL of the vehicle and mix to a uniform paste; mix while adding the vehicle in incremental proportions to **almost** 100 mL; transfer to a calibrated bottle, rinse mortar with vehicle, and add quantity of vehicle sufficient to make 100 mL. Label "shake well before using" and "protect from light". Stable for up to 60 days when stored in the dark at room temperature or refrigerated (preferred).

Allen LV Jr and Erickson MA 3rd, "Stability of Alprazolam, Chloroquine Phosphate, Cisapride, Enalapril Maleate, and Hydralazine Hydrochloride in Extemporaneously Compounded Oral Liquids," *Am J Health Syst Pharm*, 1998, 55(18):1915-20.

◆ **Chloroquine Phosphate** *see* Chloroquine *on page 343*

Chlorothiazide (klor oh THYE a zide)

Brand Names: U.S. Diuril®; Sodium Diuril®
Brand Names: Canada Diuril®
Pharmacologic Category Diuretic, Thiazide
Use Management of mild-to-moderate hypertension; adjunctive treatment of edema
Pregnancy Risk Factor C
Dosage Note: The manufacturer states that I.V. and oral dosing are equivalent. Some clinicians may use lower I.V. doses; however, because of chlorothiazide's poor oral absorption. I.V. dosing in infants and children has not been well established.
Infants <6 months:
Oral: 10-30 mg/kg/day in 2 divided doses (maximum dose: 375 mg/day); anecdotal reports have used up to 40 mg/kg/day (unlabeled).
I.V. (unlabeled): 2-8 mg/kg/day in 2 divided doses; anecdotal reports have used up to 20 mg/kg/day
Infants >6 months and Children:
Oral: 10-20 mg/kg/day in 1-2 divided doses (maximum dose: 375 mg/day in children <2 years or 1 g/day in children 2-12 years)
I.V. (unlabeled route): 4 mg/kg/day in 1-2 divided doses; anecdotal reports have used up to 20 mg/kg/day
Adults:
Hypertension: Oral: 500-2000 mg/day divided in 1-2 doses (manufacturer labeling); doses of 125-500 mg/day have also been recommended (JNC 7)
Edema: Oral, I.V.: 500-1000 mg once or twice daily; intermittent treatment (eg, therapy on alternative days) may be appropriate for some patients
ACC/AHA 2009 Heart Failure guidelines:
Oral: 250-500 mg once or twice daily (maximum daily dose: 1000 mg)
I.V.: 500-1000 mg once or twice daily plus a loop diuretic

Dosage adjustment in renal impairment: Cl_{cr} <10 mL/minute: Avoid use. Ineffective with Cl_{cr} <30 mL/minute unless in combination with a loop diuretic (Aronoff, 2007)
Note: ACC/AHA 2009 Heart Failure guidelines suggest that thiazides lose their efficacy when Cl_{cr} <40 mL/minute

Additional Information Complete prescribing information for this medication should be consulted for additional detail.

Dosage Forms Excipient information presented when available (limited, particularly for generics); consult specific product labeling.
Injection, powder for reconstitution, as sodium [strength expressed as base]: 500 mg
Sodium Diuril®: 0.5 g
Suspension, oral:
Diuril®: 250 mg/5 mL (237 mL) [contains benzoic acid, ethanol 0.5%]
Tablet, oral: 250 mg, 500 mg

Chlorpheniramine and Acetaminophen
(klor fen IR a meen & a seet a MIN oh fen)

Brand Names: U.S. Coricidin HBP® Cold and Flu [OTC]
Index Terms Acetaminophen and Chlorpheniramine

Pharmacologic Category Alkylamine Derivative; Analgesic, Miscellaneous; Histamine H_1 Antagonist; Histamine H_1 Antagonist, First Generation

Use Symptomatic relief of congestion, headache, aches and pains of colds and flu

Dosage Adults: Oral: 2 tablets every 4 hours

Additional Information Complete prescribing information for this medication should be consulted for additional detail.

Dosage Forms Excipient information presented when available (limited, particularly for generics); consult specific product labeling.

Tablet: Chlorpheniramine maleate 2 mg and acetaminophen 325 mg

◆ **Chlorpheniramine and Dextromethorphan** *see* Dextromethorphan and Chlorpheniramine *on page 489*

Chlorpheniramine and Phenylephrine

(klor fen IR a meen & fen il EF rin)

Brand Names: U.S. Actifed® Cold & Allergy [OTC] *[reformulation]*; C-Phen [DSC]; Ceron [DSC]; Dallergy Drops [DSC]; Dallergy®-JR [DSC]; Dec-Chlorphen [DSC]; Ed A-Hist™ [DSC]; Ed ChlorPed D; LoHist [OTC]; NoHist LQ [OTC]; NoHist [DSC]; PD-Hist-D; Phenabid® [DSC]; R-Tanna; R-Tanna Pediatric; Rynatan® Pediatric [DSC]; Rynatan® [DSC]; Sildec PE [DSC]; Sudafed PE® Sinus + Allergy [OTC]; Triaminic® Cold and Allergy [OTC]

Index Terms Chlorpheniramine Maleate and Phenylephrine Hydrochloride; Chlorpheniramine Tannate and Phenylephrine Tannate; Phenylephrine and Chlorpheniramine

Pharmacologic Category Alkylamine Derivative; Alpha-Adrenergic Agonist; Decongestant; Histamine H_1 Antagonist; Histamine H_1 Antagonist, First Generation

Use Temporary relief of upper respiratory conditions such as nasal congestion, runny nose, and sneezing due to the common cold, hay fever, or allergic or vasomotor rhinitis

Pregnancy Risk Factor C

Dosage Antihistamine/decongestant: Oral:

Children:

2-6 years:

Dallergy®-JR suspension: 2.5 mL every 12 hours

Rynatan® suspension: 2.5 -5 mL every 12 hours

6-12 years:

Dallergy®-JR: One capsule every 12 hours; maximum: 2 capsules/24 hours

Dallergy®-JR suspension: 5 mL every 12 hours

Ed A-Hist™: One-half caplet every 12 hours

Rynatan® suspension: 5-10 mL every 12 hours

≥12 years: Refer to adult dosing.

Adults:

Dallergy®-JR: Two capsules every 12 hours; maximum: 4 capsules/24 hours

Dallergy®-JR suspension: 10 mL every 12 hours

Ed A-Hist™: One caplet every 12 hours

R-Tanna: 1-2 tablets every 12 hours

Rynatan® tablet: 1-2 tablets every 12 hours

Additional Information Complete prescribing information for this medication should be consulted for additional detail.

Dosage Forms Excipient information presented when available (limited, particularly for generics); consult specific product labeling. [DSC] = Discontinued product

Caplet, prolonged release:

Ed A-Hist™ [DSC], NoHist [DSC]: Chlorpheniramine maleate 8 mg and phenylephrine hydrochloride 20 mg

Capsule, extended release:

Dallergy®-JR [DSC]: Chlorpheniramine maleate 4 mg and phenylephrine hydrochloride 20 mg

Liquid:

Ed A-Hist™: Chlorpheniramine maleate 4 mg and phenylephrine hydrochloride 10 mg per 5 mL (480 mL) [sugar free; contains alcohol 5%; grape flavor] [DSC]

Triaminic® Cold and Allergy: Chlorpheniramine maleate 1 mg and phenylephrine hydrochloride 2.5 mg per 5 mL (120 mL) [contains sodium 5 mg/5 mL and benzoic acid; orange flavor]

Liquid, oral [drops]:

Dallergy: Chlorpheniramine maleate 1 mg and phenylephrine hydrochloride 2 mg per 1 mL (30 mL) [ethanol free, sugar free; contains propylene glycol; peach flavor] [DSC]

LoHist: Chlorpheniramine maleate 1 mg and phenylephrine hydrochloride 2.5 mg per 1 mL (30 mL) [dye free, ethanol free, sugar free; contains propylene glycol; cherry flavor]

NoHist LQ: Chlorpheniramine maleate 4 mg and phenylephrine hydrochloride 10 mg per 5 mL (473 mL) [ethanol free, sugar free; contains propylene glycol; bubblegum flavor]

Solution, oral [drops]:

C-Phen [DSC], PD-Hist-D: Chlorpheniramine maleate 1 mg and phenylephrine hydrochloride 3.5 mg per mL (30 mL) [ethanol free, sugar free; bubblegum flavor]

Ceron: Chlorpheniramine maleate 1 mg and phenylephrine hydrochloride 3.5 mg per mL (30 mL) [raspberry flavor] [DSC]

Dec-Chlorphen: Chlorpheniramine maleate 1 mg and phenylephrine hydrochloride 3.5 mg per mL (30 mL) [ethanol free, dye free, sugar free; grape flavor] [DSC]

Suspension, oral:

Dallergy®-JR: Chlorpheniramine tannate 4 mg and phenylephrine tannate 20 mg per 5 mL (480 mL) [contains sodium benzoate; peaches and cream flavor]

R-Tanna Pediatric: Chlorpheniramine tannate 4.5 mg and phenylephrine tannate 5 mg per 5 mL (480 mL) [contains benzoic acid and tartrazine]

Rynatan® Pediatric: Chlorpheniramine tannate 4.5 mg and phenylephrine tannate 5 mg per 5 mL (480 mL) [contains benzoic acid and tartrazine; strawberry-currant flavor] [DSC]

Suspension, oral [drops]:

Ed ChlorPed D: Chlorpheniramine tannate 2 mg and phenylephrine tannate 6 mg per 1 mL (60 mL) [apple sauce flavor]

Syrup:

C-Phen: Chlorpheniramine maleate 4 mg and phenylephrine hydrochloride 12.5 mg per 5 mL (120 mL, 480 mL) [ethanol free, sugar free; contains sodium benzoate; bubble gum flavor] [DSC]

Ceron [DSC], Sildec PE [DSC]: Chlorpheniramine maleate 4 mg and phenylephrine hydrochloride 12.5 mg per 5 mL (480 mL) [raspberry flavor]

PD-Hist-D: Chlorpheniramine maleate 4 mg and phenylephrine hydrochloride 12.5 mg per 5 mL (480 mL) [ethanol free, sugar free; bubblegum flavor]

Tablet:

Actifed® Cold & Allergy, Sudafed PE® Sinus + Allergy: Chlorpheniramine maleate 4 mg and phenylephrine hydrochloride 10 mg

R-Tanna, Rynatan® [DSC]: Chlorpheniramine tannate 9 mg and phenylephrine tannate 25 mg

Tablet, chewable:

Rynatan® [DSC]: Chlorpheniramine tannate 4.5 mg and phenylephrine tannate 5 mg [grape flavor]

Tablet, timed release:

Phenabid®: Chlorpheniramine maleate 8 mg and phenylephrine hydrochloride 20 mg [dye free, sugar free] [DSC]

Chlorpheniramine and Pseudoephedrine

(klor fen IR a meen & soo doe e FED rin)

Brand Names: U.S. Dicel® Chewable [OTC]; Dicel® Suspension; LoHist-D; Neutrahist Pediatric [OTC] [DSC]; Suclor™ [DSC]; SudaHist® [DSC]

Brand Names: Canada Triaminic® Cold & Allergy

Index Terms Allerest; Chlorpheniramine Maleate and Pseudoephedrine Hydrochloride; Chlorpheniramine Tannate and Pseudoephedrine Tannate; Pseudoephedrine and Chlorpheniramine

Pharmacologic Category Alkylamine Derivative; Alpha/Beta Agonist; Decongestant; Histamine H_1 Antagonist; Histamine H_1 Antagonist, First Generation

Use Relief of nasal congestion associated with the common cold, hay fever, and other allergies, sinusitis, eustachian tube blockage, and vasomotor and allergic rhinitis

Pregnancy Risk Factor C

Dosage General dosing guidelines; consult specific product labeling. Rhinitis/decongestant: Oral:

Children:

2-6 years:

Chlorpheniramine maleate 1 mg and pseudoephedrine hydrochloride 15 mg every 4-6 hours

Chlorpheniramine tannate 4.5 mg and pseudoephedrine tannate 75 mg: 2.5-5 mL every 12 hours (maximum: 10 mL/24 hours)

6-12 years: Chlorpheniramine maleate 2 mg and pseudoephedrine hydrochloride 30 mg every 4-6 hours (immediate release products)

Children ≥12 years and Adults:

Chlorpheniramine maleate 4 mg and pseudoephedrine hydrochloride 60 mg every 4-6 hours (immediate release products)

Chlorpheniramine tannate 4.5 mg and pseudoephedrine tannate 75 mg: 10-20 mL every 12 hours (maximum: 40 mL/24 hours)

Deconamine® SR: Chlorpheniramine maleate 8 mg and pseudoephedrine hydrochloride 120 mg every 12 hours

Additional Information Complete prescribing information for this medication should be consulted for additional detail.

Dosage Forms Excipient information presented when available (limited, particularly for generics); consult specific product labeling. [DSC] = Discontinued product

Capsule, extended release, oral:

Suclor™: Chlorpheniramine maleate 8 mg and pseudoephedrine hydrochloride 120 mg [DSC]

Liquid, oral:

LoHist-D: Chlorpheniramine maleate 2 mg and pseudoephedrine hydrochloride 30 mg per 5 mL (480 mL) [alcohol free, dye free; peach flavor]

Liquid, oral [drops]:

Neutrahist Pediatric: Chlorpheniramine maleate 0.8 mg and pseudoephedrine sulfate 9 mg per 1 mL (30 mL) [contains propylene glycol; cherry flavor] [DSC]

Suspension, oral:

Dicel®: Chlorpheniramine tannate 5 mg and pseudoephedrine tannate 75 mg per 5 mL (480 mL) [contains sodium benzoate; strawberry banana flavor]

Syrup, oral: Chlorpheniramine maleate 2 mg and pseudoephedrine hydrochloride 30 mg per 5 mL (480 mL) [DSC]

Tablet, oral: Chlorpheniramine maleate 4 mg and pseudoephedrine hydrochloride 60 mg

Tablet, chewable, oral:

Dicel®: Chlorpheniramine maleate 2 mg and pseudoephedrine hydrochloride 30 mg [contains sodium 17 mg/tablet, soy lecithin; strawberry-banana cream flavor]

Tablet, sustained release, oral:

SudaHist: Chlorpheniramine maleate 12 mg and pseudoephedrine hydrochloride 120 mg [DSC]

◆ **Chlorpheniramine, Dextromethorphan, and Pseudoephedrine** *see* Chlorpheniramine, Pseudoephedrine, and Dextromethorphan *on page 347*

◆ **Chlorpheniramine Maleate and Dextromethorphan Hydrobromide** *see* Dextromethorphan and Chlorpheniramine *on page 489*

◆ **Chlorpheniramine Maleate and Hydrocodone Bitartrate** *see* Hydrocodone and Chlorpheniramine *on page 838*

◆ **Chlorpheniramine Maleate and Phenylephrine Hydrochloride** *see* Chlorpheniramine and Phenylephrine *on page 345*

◆ **Chlorpheniramine Maleate and Pseudoephedrine Hydrochloride** *see* Chlorpheniramine and Pseudoephedrine *on page 346*

◆ **Chlorpheniramine Maleate, Dihydrocodeine Bitartrate, and Phenylephrine Hydrochloride** *see* Dihydrocodeine, Chlorpheniramine, and Phenylephrine *on page 508*

◆ **Chlorpheniramine Maleate, Pseudoephedrine Hydrochloride, and Dextromethorphan Hydrobromide** *see* Chlorpheniramine, Pseudoephedrine, and Dextromethorphan *on page 347*

Chlorpheniramine, Phenylephrine, and Dextromethorphan

(klor fen IR a meen, fen il EF rin, & deks troe meth OR fan)

Brand Names: U.S. Ceron-DM [DSC]; Corfen DM [DSC]; De-Chlor DM [DSC]; De-Chlor DR [DSC]; Ed A-Hist DM [DSC]; EndoCof [OTC]; Father John's® Plus [OTC]; Neo DM; NoHist DM [OTC]; NoHist-DMX [DSC]; PD-Cof [DSC]; PE-Hist-DM [OTC]; Sildec PE-DM [DSC]

Index Terms Dextromethorphan, Chlorpheniramine, and Phenylephrine; Phenylephrine, Chlorpheniramine, and Dextromethorphan

Pharmacologic Category Alkylamine Derivative; Alpha-Adrenergic Agonist; Antitussive; Decongestant; Histamine H_1 Antagonist; Histamine H_1 Antagonist, First Generation

Use Temporary relief of cough and upper respiratory symptoms associated with allergies or the common cold

Pregnancy Risk Factor C

Dosage Oral: Relief of cough and cold symptoms:

Children: 6-12 years (Ceron-DM syrup): 2.5 mL every 6 hours (maximum: 10 mL/24 hours)

Children ≥12 years and Adults (Ceron-DM syrup): 5 mL every 6 hours (maximum: 20 mL/24 hours)

Additional Information Complete prescribing information for this medication should be consulted for additional detail.

Dosage Forms Excipient information presented when available (limited, particularly for generics); consult specific product labeling. [DSC] = Discontinued product

Liquid, oral:

Corfen DM: Chlorpheniramine maleate 4 mg, phenylephrine hydrochloride 10 mg, and dextromethorphan hydrobromide 15 mg per 5 mL (480 mL) [grape flavor] [DSC]

De-Chlor DM: Chlorpheniramine maleate 2 mg, phenylephrine hydrochloride 10 mg, and dextromethorphan hydrobromide 15 mg per 5 mL (480 mL) [strawberry flavor] [DSC]

De-Chlor DR: Chlorpheniramine maleate 2 mg, phenylephrine hydrochloride 6 mg, and dextromethorphan hydrobromide 15 mg per 5 mL (480 mL) [strawberry flavor] [DSC]

Father John's® Plus: Chlorpheniramine maleate 2 mg, phenylephrine hydrochloride 5 mg, and dextromethorphan hydrobromide 5 mg per 15 mL (118 mL) [ethanol free]

NoHist DM: Chlorpheniramine maleate 4 mg, phenylephrine hydrochloride 10 mg, and dextromethorphan hydrobromide 15 mg per 5 mL (473 mL) [dye free, ethanol free, sugar free; contains propylene glycol; grape flavor]

PE-Hist-DM: Chlorpheniramine maleate 2 mg, phenylephrine hydrochloride 5 mg, and dextromethorphan hydrobromide 15 mg per 5 mL (480 mL) [dye free, ethanol free, sugar free; contains propylene glycol; grape flavor]

Liquid, oral [drops]:

EndaCof: Chlorpheniramine maleate 1 mg, phenylephrine hydrochloride 2.5 mg, and dextromethorphan hydrobromide 2.5 mg per 1 mL (30 mL) [dye free, ethanol free, sugar free; contains propylene glycol; grape flavor]

Neo DM: Chlorpheniramine maleate 0.75 mg, phenylephrine hydrochloride 1.75 mg, and dextromethorphan hydrobromide 2.75 mg per 1 mL (30 mL) [ethanol free, sugar free; contains propylene glycol; black cherry flavor]

Syrup, oral:

Ceron-DM: Chlorpheniramine maleate 4 mg, phenylephrine hydrochloride 12.5 mg, and dextromethorphan hydrobromide 15 mg per 5 mL (118 mL, 480 mL) [ethanol free, sugar free; contains sodium benzoate; grape flavor] [DSC]

Ed A-Hist DM: Chlorpheniramine maleate 4 mg, phenylephrine hydrochloride 10 mg, and dextromethorphan hydrobromide 15 mg per 5 mL (480 mL) [ethanol free, sugar free; contains propylene glycol; banana flavor] [DSC]

Sildec PE-DM: Chlorpheniramine maleate 4 mg, phenylephrine hydrochloride 12.5 mg, and dextromethorphan hydrobromide 15 mg per 5 mL (480 mL) [grape flavor] [DSC]

Tablet, sustained release, oral:

NoHist-DMX: Chlorpheniramine maleate 8 mg, phenylephrine hydrochloride 20 mg, and dextromethorphan hydrobromide 30 mg [DSC]

◆ **Chlorpheniramine, Phenylephrine, and Pyrilamine** *see* Chlorpheniramine, Pyrilamine, and Phenylephrine *on page 348*

Chlorpheniramine, Pseudoephedrine, and Dextromethorphan

(klor fen IR a meen, soo doe e FED rin, & deks troe meth OR fan)

Brand Names: U.S. Dicel® DM Chewable [OTC]; Dicel® DM Suspension; Entre-S; Kidkare Children's Cough/Cold [OTC]; Neutrahist PDX; Pedia Relief™ Cough-Cold [OTC]; Rescon DM [OTC]; Tanafed DMX™

Index Terms Chlorpheniramine Maleate, Pseudoephedrine Hydrochloride, and Dextromethorphan Hydrobromide; Chlorpheniramine Tannate, Pseudoephedrine Tannate, and Dextromethorphan Tannate; Chlorpheniramine, Dextromethorphan, and Pseudoephedrine; Dexchlorpheniramine Tannate, Pseudoephedrine Tannate, and Dextromethorphan Tannate; Dextromethorphan, Chlorpheniramine, and Pseudoephedrine; Pseudoephedrine, Chlorpheniramine, and Dextromethorphan

Pharmacologic Category Alkylamine Derivative; Alpha/Beta Agonist; Antitussive; Decongestant; Histamine H_1 Antagonist; Histamine H_1 Antagonist, First Generation

Use Temporarily relieves nasal congestion, runny nose, cough, and sneezing due to the common cold, hay fever, or allergic rhinitis

Pregnancy Risk Factor C

Dosage General dosing guidelines; consult specific product labeling. Relief of cold symptoms: Oral:

Children:

2-6 years: Dexchlorpheniramine tannate 2.5 mg, pseudoephedrine tannate 75 mg, and dextromethorphan tannate 25 mg (Tanafed DMX™): 2.5-5 mL every 12 hours (maximum: 10 mL/24 hours)

6-12 years:

Chlorpheniramine maleate 1 mg, pseudoephedrine 15 mg, and dextromethorphan hydrobromide 5 mg per tablet or 5 mL: 2 tablets or 10 mL every 4-6 hours (maximum: 4 doses/24 hours)

Chlorpheniramine maleate 2 mg, pseudoephedrine 30 mg, and dextromethorphan hydrobromide 10 mg per tablet or 5 mL (Rescon DM): 5 mL every 4-6 hours (maximum: 4 doses/24 hours)

Dexchlorpheniramine tannate 2.5 mg, pseudoephedrine tannate 75 mg, and dextromethorphan tannate 25 mg (Tanafed DMX™): 5-10 mL every 12 hours (maximum: 20 mL/24 hours)

>12 years: Refer to adult dosing

Adults:

Chlorpheniramine maleate 2 mg, pseudoephedrine 30 mg, and dextromethorphan hydrobromide 10 mg per tablet or 5 mL (Rescon DM): 10 mL every 4-6 hours (maximum: 4 doses/24 hours)

Dexchlorpheniramine tannate 2.5 mg, pseudoephedrine tannate 75 mg, and dextromethorphan tannate 25 mg (Tanafed DMX™): 10-20 mL every 12 hours (maximum: 40 mL/24 hours)

Additional Information Complete prescribing information for this medication should be consulted for additional detail.

Dosage Forms Excipient information presented when available (limited, particularly for generics); consult specific product labeling.

Liquid, oral: Chlorpheniramine maleate 1 mg, pseudoephedrine hydrochloride 15 mg, and dextromethorphan hydrobromide 5 mg per 5 mL (120 mL)

Kidkare Children's Cough/Cold: Chlorpheniramine maleate 1 mg, pseudoephedrine hydrochloride 15 mg, and dextromethorphan hydrobromide 5 mg per 5 mL (118 mL) [ethanol free; contains propylene glycol and sodium benzoate; cherry flavor]

Pedia Relief™ Cough-Cold: Chlorpheniramine maleate 1 mg, pseudoephedrine hydrochloride 15 mg, and dextromethorphan hydrobromide 5 mg per 5 mL (120 mL) [ethanol free; contains propylene glycol and sodium benzoate; cherry flavor]

Rescon DM: Chlorpheniramine maleate 2 mg, pseudoephedrine hydrochloride 30 mg, and dextromethorphan hydrobromide 10 mg per 5 mL (120 mL, 480 mL) [dye free; contains propylene glycol; cherry flavor]

Liquid, oral [drops]:

Neutrahist PDX: Chlorpheniramine maleate 0.8 mg, pseudoephedrine hydrochloride 9 mg, and dextromethorphan hydrobromide 3 mg per 1 mL (30 mL) [ethanol free, sugar free; contains propylene glycol; grape flavor]

Suspension, oral:

Dicel® DM: Chlorpheniramine tannate 5 mg, pseudoephedrine tannate 75 mg, and dextromethorphan tannate 25 mg per 5 mL (480 mL) [contains sodium benzoate; cotton candy flavor]

Entre-S: Chlorpheniramine maleate 4 mg, pseudoephedrine hydrochloride 30 mg, and dextromethorphan hydrobromide 30 mg per 5 mL (120 mL, 480 mL)

Tanafed DMX™: Dexchlorpheniramine tannate 2.5 mg, pseudoephedrine tannate 75 mg, and dextromethorphan tannate 25 mg per 5 mL (120 mL, 480 mL) [contains sodium benzoate; cotton candy flavor]

Tablet, chewable, oral:
Dicel® DM: Chlorpheniramine maleate 2 mg, pseudoephedrine hydrochloride 30 mg, and dextromethorphan hydrobromide 10 mg [contains sodium 19 mg/tablet, soy lecithin; cotton candy flavor]

Chlorpheniramine, Pyrilamine, and Phenylephrine

(klor fen IR a meen, pye RIL a meen, & fen il EF rin)

Brand Names: U.S. MyHist-PD; Nalex A 12; Pyrichlor PE™; Ru-Hist Forte [DSC]; Triplex™ AD [DSC]

Index Terms Chlorpheniramine, Phenylephrine, and Pyrilamine; Phenylephrine, Chlorpheniramine, and Pyrilamine; Pyrilamine, Chlorpheniramine, and Phenylephrine

Pharmacologic Category Alkylamine Derivative; Alpha-Adrenergic Agonist; Decongestant; Ethylenediamine Derivative; Histamine H_1 Antagonist; Histamine H_1 Antagonist, First Generation

Use Symptomatic relief of rhinitis and nasal congestion due to colds or allergy

Pregnancy Risk Factor C

Dosage Oral:
Tablet (Ru-Hist Forte):
Children <6 years: Dosage not established.
Children 6-12 years: 1/2 tablet 2-3 times/day
Children >12 years and Adults: 1 tablet 2-3 times/day
Liquid (MyHist-PD):
Children 2-6 years: 2.5 mL every 4-6 hours (maximum: 10 mL/day)
Children 6-12 years: 5 mL every 4-6 hours (maximum: 20 mL/day)
Children >12 years and Adults: 5-10 mL every 4-6 hours (maximum: 40 mL/day)
Liquid (Triplex™ AD):
Children <6 years: Dosage not established
Children 6-12 years: 5 mL every 4-6 hours (maximum: 20 mL/day)
Children >12 and Adults: 5-10 mL every 4-6 hours (maximum: 40 mL/day)

Additional Information Complete prescribing information for this medication should be consulted for additional detail.

Dosage Forms Excipient information presented when available (limited, particularly for generics); consult specific product labeling. [DSC] = Discontinued product
Liquid, oral:
MyHist-PD: Chlorpheniramine maleate 2 mg, pyrilamine maleate 12.5 mg, and phenylephrine hydrochloride 7.5 mg per 5 mL (473 mL) [dye free, ethanol free, sugar free; bubblegum flavor]
Pyrichlor PE™: Chlorpheniramine maleate 2 mg, pyrilamine maleate 10 mg, and phenylephrine hydrochloride 10 mg per 5 mL (480 mL) [dye free, ethanol free, sugar free; contains sodium benzoate; grape flavor]
Triplex™ AD: Chlorpheniramine maleate 2 mg, pyrilamine maleate 12.5 mg, and phenylephrine hydrochloride 7.5 mg per 5 mL (473 mL) [dye free, ethanol free, sugar free; contains sodium benzoate; bubblegum flavor] [DSC]
Suspension, oral:
Nalex A 12: Chlorpheniramine tannate 2 mg, pyrilamine tannate 12.5 mg, and phenylephrine tannate 5 mg per 5 mL (120 mL) [contains benzoic acid; raspberry flavor]
Tablet, time-released, oral: Chlorpheniramine maleate 4 mg, pyrilamine maleate 25 mg, and phenylephrine hydrochloride 10 mg
Ru-Hist Forte: Chlorpheniramine maleate 4 mg, pyrilamine maleate 25 mg, and phenylephrine hydrochloride 10 mg [DSC]

◆ **Chlorpheniramine Tannate and Phenylephrine Tannate** *see* Chlorpheniramine and Phenylephrine *on page 345*

◆ **Chlorpheniramine Tannate and Pseudoephedrine Tannate** *see* Chlorpheniramine and Pseudoephedrine *on page 346*

◆ **Chlorpheniramine Tannate, Pseudoephedrine Tannate, and Dextromethorphan Tannate** *see* Chlorpheniramine, Pseudoephedrine, and Dextromethorphan *on page 347*

ChlorproMAZINE (klor PROE ma zeen)

Brand Names: Canada Largactil®; Novo-Chlorpromazine

Index Terms Chlorpromazine Hydrochloride; CPZ; Thorazine

Pharmacologic Category Antimanic Agent; Antipsychotic Agent, Typical, Phenothiazine

Additional Appendix Information
Antipsychotic Agents *on page 1880*

Use Management of psychotic disorders (control of mania, treatment of schizophrenia); control of nausea and vomiting; relief of restlessness and apprehension before surgery; acute intermittent porphyria; adjunct in the treatment of tetanus; intractable hiccups; combativeness and/or explosive hyperexcitable behavior in children 1-12 years of age and in short-term treatment of hyperactive children

Unlabeled Use Behavioral symptoms associated with dementia (elderly); psychosis/agitation related to Alzheimer's dementia

Pregnancy Considerations Embryotoxicity was observed in animal reproduction studies. Jaundice or hyper-/hyporeflexia have been reported in newborn infants following maternal use of phenothiazines. Antipsychotic use during the third trimester of pregnancy has a risk for abnormal muscle movements (extrapyramidal symptoms [EPS]) and withdrawal symptoms in newborns following delivery. Symptoms in the newborn may include agitation, feeding disorder, hypertonia, hypotonia, respiratory distress, somnolence, and tremor; these effects may be self-limiting or require hospitalization.

Lactation Enters breast milk/not recommended (AAP rates "of concern"; AAP 2001 update pending)

Contraindications Hypersensitivity to chlorpromazine or any component of the formulation (cross-reactivity between phenothiazines may occur); severe CNS depression; coma

Warnings/Precautions [U.S. Boxed Warning]: Elderly patients with dementia-related psychosis treated with antipsychotics are at an increased risk of death compared to placebo. Most deaths appeared to be either cardiovascular (eg, heart failure, sudden death) or infectious (eg, pneumonia) in nature. Chlorpromazine is not approved for the treatment of dementia-related psychosis. Highly sedating, use with caution in disorders where CNS depression is a feature and in patients with Parkinson's disease. Use with caution in patients with hemodynamic instability, predisposition to seizures, subcortical brain damage, severe cardiac, hepatic, or renal disease. Use caution in respiratory disease (eg, severe asthma, emphysema) due to potential for CNS effects.

Leukopenia, neutropenia, and agranulocytosis (sometimes fatal) have been reported in clinical trials and postmarketing reports with antipsychotic use; presence of risk factors (eg, pre-existing low WBC or history of drug-induced leuko/neutropenia) should prompt periodic blood count assessment. Discontinue therapy at first signs of blood dyscrasias or if absolute neutrophil count $<1000/mm^3$.

Esophageal dysmotility and aspiration have been associated with antipsychotic use; use with caution in patients at risk of aspiration pneumonia (ie, Alzheimer's disease). Use associated with increased prolactin levels; clinical significance of hyperprolactinemia in patients with breast cancer or other prolactin-dependent tumors is unknown. May alter temperature regulation or mask toxicity of other drugs due to antiemetic effects. May alter cardiac conduction; life-threatening arrhythmias have occurred with therapeutic doses of neuroleptics. May cause QT prolongation and subsequent torsade de pointes; avoid use in patients with diagnosed or suspected congenital long QT syndrome. Avoid concurrent use with other drugs known to prolong QT_c interval.

Use with caution in patients at risk of hypotension (orthostasis is common) or those who would tolerate transient hypotensive episodes (cerebrovascular disease, cardiovascular disease, or other medications which may predispose). Significant hypotension may occur, particularly with parenteral administration. Injection contains sulfites.

Use with caution in patients with decreased gastrointestinal motility, urinary retention, BPH, xerostomia, or visual problems (ie, narrow-angle glaucoma), and myasthenia gravis. Relative to other neuroleptics, chlorpromazine has a moderate potency of cholinergic blockade. May cause pigmentary retinopathy, and lenticular and corneal deposits, particularly with prolonged therapy.

May cause extrapyramidal symptoms (EPS), including pseudoparkinsonism, acute dystonic reactions, akathisia, and tardive dyskinesia. Risk of dystonia (and possibly other EPS) may be greater with increased doses, use of conventional antipsychotics, males, and younger patients. May cause neuroleptic malignant syndrome (NMS). Use with caution in the elderly.

Adverse Reactions Frequency not defined.

Cardiovascular: Postural hypotension, tachycardia, dizziness, nonspecific QT changes

Central nervous system: Drowsiness, dystonias, akathisia, pseudoparkinsonism, tardive dyskinesia, neuroleptic malignant syndrome, seizure

Dermatologic: Photosensitivity, dermatitis, skin pigmentation (slate gray)

Endocrine & metabolic: Lactation, breast engorgement, false-positive pregnancy test, amenorrhea, gynecomastia, hyper- or hypoglycemia

Gastrointestinal: Xerostomia, constipation, nausea

Genitourinary: Urinary retention, ejaculatory disorder, impotence

Hematologic: Agranulocytosis, eosinophilia, leukopenia, hemolytic anemia, aplastic anemia, thrombocytopenic purpura

Hepatic: Jaundice

Ocular: Blurred vision, corneal and lenticular changes, epithelial keratopathy, pigmentary retinopathy

Drug Interactions

Metabolism/Transport Effects **Substrate** of CYP1A2 (minor), CYP2D6 (major), CYP3A4 (minor); **Note:** Assignment of Major/Minor substrate status based on clinically relevant drug interaction potential; **Inhibits** CYP2D6 (moderate), CYP2E1 (weak)

Avoid Concomitant Use

Avoid concomitant use of ChlorproMAZINE with any of the following: Artemether; Dronedarone; Lumefantrine; Metoclopramide; Nilotinib; Pimozide; QUEtiapine; QuiNINE; Tetrabenazine; Thioridazine; Toremifene; Vandetanib; Vemurafenib; Ziprasidone

Increased Effect/Toxicity

ChlorproMAZINE may increase the levels/effects of: Alcohol (Ethyl); Analgesics (Opioid); Anticholinergics; Antidepressants (Serotonin Reuptake Inhibitor/Antagonist); Anti-Parkinson's Agents (Dopamine Agonist); Beta-Blockers; CNS Depressants; CYP2D6 Substrates; Desmopressin; Divalproex; Dronedarone; Fesoterodine; Haloperidol; Methylphenidate; Pimozide; Porfimer; QTc-Prolonging Agents; QuiNINE; Serotonin Modulators; Tamoxifen; Tetrabenazine; Thioridazine; Toremifene; Valproic Acid; Vandetanib; Vemurafenib; Ziprasidone

The levels/effects of ChlorproMAZINE may be increased by: Abiraterone Acetate; Acetylcholinesterase Inhibitors (Central); Alfuzosin; Antidepressants (Serotonin Reuptake Inhibitor/Antagonist); Antimalarial Agents; Artemether; Beta-Blockers; Chloroquine; Ciprofloxacin; Ciprofloxacin (Systemic); Conivaptan; CYP2D6 Inhibitors (Moderate); CYP2D6 Inhibitors (Strong); Darunavir; Gadobutrol; Haloperidol; HydrOXYzine; Indacaterol; Lithium formulations; Lumefantrine; Methylphenidate; Metoclopramide; Nilotinib; Pramlintide; QUEtiapine; QuiNINE; Tetrabenazine

Decreased Effect

ChlorproMAZINE may decrease the levels/effects of: Amphetamines; Quinagolide

The levels/effects of ChlorproMAZINE may be decreased by: Antacids; Anti-Parkinson's Agents (Dopamine Agonist); Cyproterone; Lithium formulations; Peginterferon Alfa-2b; Tocilizumab

Ethanol/Nutrition/Herb Interactions

Ethanol: May increase CNS depression; monitor for increased effects with coadministration. Caution patients about effects.

Herb/Nutraceutical: Avoid St John's wort (may decrease chlorpromazine levels, increase photosensitization, or enhance sedative effect). Avoid dong quai (may enhance photosensitization). Avoid kava kava, gotu kola, valerian (may increase CNS depression).

Stability Injection: Protect from light. A slightly yellowed solution does not indicate potency loss, but a markedly discolored solution should be discarded. Diluted injection (1 mg/mL) with NS and stored in 5 mL vials remains stable for 30 days.

Mechanism of Action Chlorpromazine is an aliphatic phenothiazine antipsychotic which blocks postsynaptic mesolimbic dopaminergic receptors in the brain; exhibits a strong alpha-adrenergic blocking effect and depresses the release of hypothalamic and hypophyseal hormones; believed to depress the reticular activating system, thus affecting basal metabolism, body temperature, wakefulness, vasomotor tone, and emesis

Pharmacodynamics/Kinetics

Onset of action: I.M.: 15 minutes; Oral: 30-60 minutes

Absorption: Rapid

Distribution: V_d: 20 L/kg

Protein binding: 92% to 97%

Metabolism: Extensively hepatic to active and inactive metabolites

Bioavailability: 20%

Half-life, biphasic: Initial: 2 hours; Terminal: 30 hours

Excretion: Urine (<1% as unchanged drug) within 24 hours

Dosage

Children ≥6 months:

- Schizophrenia/psychoses:
  - Oral: 0.5-1 mg/kg/dose every 4-6 hours; older children may require 200 mg/day or higher
  - I.M., I.V.: 0.5-1 mg/kg/dose every 6-8 hours
    - <5 years (<22.7 kg): Maximum: 40 mg/day
    - 5-12 years (22.7-45.5 kg): Maximum: 75 mg/day
- Nausea and vomiting:
  - Oral: 0.5-1 mg/kg/dose every 4-6 hours as needed
  - I.M., I.V.: 0.5-1 mg/kg/dose every 6-8 hours
    - <5 years (<22.7 kg): Maximum: 40 mg/day
    - 5-12 years (22.7-45.5 kg): Maximum: 75 mg/day

Adults:

Schizophrenia/psychoses:

Oral: Range: 30-800 mg/day in 1-4 divided doses, initiate at lower doses and titrate as needed; usual dose: 200-600 mg/day; some patients may require 1-2 g/day

I.M., I.V.: Initial: 25 mg, may repeat (25-50 mg) in 1-4 hours, gradually increase to a maximum of 400 mg/dose every 4-6 hours until patient is controlled; usual dose: 300-800 mg/day

Intractable hiccups:

Oral, I.M.: 25-50 mg 3-4 times/day

I.V. (refractory to oral or I.M. treatment): 25-50 mg via slow I.V. infusion

Nausea and vomiting:

Oral: 10-25 mg every 4-6 hours

I.M., I.V.: 25-50 mg every 4-6 hours

Elderly: Behavioral symptoms associated with dementia (unlabeled use): Initial: 10-25 mg 1-2 times/day; increase at 4- to 7-day intervals by 10-25 mg/day. Increase dose intervals (bid, tid, etc) as necessary to control behavior response or side effects; maximum daily dose: 800 mg; gradual increases (titration) may prevent some side effects or decrease their severity.

Dosing comments in renal impairment: Hemodialysis: Not dialyzable (0% to 5%)

Dosing adjustment/comments in hepatic impairment: Avoid use in severe hepatic dysfunction

Administration Do not administer SubQ (tissue damage and irritation may occur); for direct I.V. injection: Dilute with normal saline to a maximum concentration of 1 mg/mL, administer slow I.V. at a rate not to exceed 0.5 mg/minute in children and 1 mg/minute in adults. For treatment of intractable hiccups the manufacturer recommends diluting 25-50 mg of chlorpromazine in 500-1000 ml of normal saline. To reduce the risk of hypotension, patients receiving I.V. chlorpromazine must remain lying down during and for 30 minutes after the injection. **Note:** Avoid skin contact with solution; may cause contact dermatitis.

Monitoring Parameters Vital signs (especially with parenteral use); lipid profile, fasting blood glucose/Hgb A_{1c}; BMI; mental status; abnormal involuntary movement scale (AIMS); extrapyramidal symptoms (EPS); CBC in patients with risk factors for leukopenia/neutropenia

Reference Range

Therapeutic: 50-300 ng/mL (SI: 157-942 nmol/L)

Toxic: >750 ng/mL (SI: >2355 nmol/L); serum concentrations poorly correlate with expected response

Test Interactions False-positives for phenylketonuria, amylase, uroporphyrins, urobilinogen. May cause false-positive pregnancy test. May interfere with urine detection of amphetamine/methamphetamine and methadone (false-positives).

Dosage Forms Excipient information presented when available (limited, particularly for generics); consult specific product labeling.

Injection, solution, as hydrochloride: 25 mg/mL (1 mL, 2 mL)

Tablet, oral, as hydrochloride: 10 mg, 25 mg, 50 mg, 100 mg, 200 mg

◆ **Chlorpromazine Hydrochloride** *see* ChlorproMAZINE *on page 348*

ChlorproPAMIDE (klor PROE pa mide)

Brand Names: Canada Apo-Chlorpropamide®

Pharmacologic Category Antidiabetic Agent, Sulfonylurea

Additional Appendix Information

Beers Criteria – Potentially Inappropriate Medications for Geriatrics *on page 1973*

Diabetes Mellitus Management, Adults *on page 1983*

Use Management of blood sugar in type 2 diabetes mellitus (noninsulin dependent, NIDDM)

Unlabeled Use Neurogenic diabetes insipidus

Pregnancy Risk Factor C

Dosage Oral: The dosage of chlorpropamide is variable and should be individualized based upon the patient's response

Initial dose:

Adults: 250 mg/day in mild-to-moderate diabetes in middle-aged, stable diabetic

Elderly: 100-125 mg/day in older patients

Subsequent dosages may be increased or decreased by 50-125 mg/day at 3- to 5-day intervals

Maintenance dose: 100-250 mg/day; severe diabetics may require 500 mg/day; avoid doses >750 mg/day

Dosing adjustment/comments in renal impairment: Cl_{cr} <50 mL/minute: Avoid use

Hemodialysis: Removed with hemoperfusion

Peritoneal dialysis: Supplemental dose is not necessary

Dosing adjustment in hepatic impairment: Dosage reduction is recommended. Conservative initial and maintenance doses are recommended in patients with liver impairment because chlorpropamide undergoes extensive hepatic metabolism.

Additional Information Complete prescribing information for this medication should be consulted for additional detail.

Dosage Forms Excipient information presented when available (limited, particularly for generics); consult specific product labeling.

Tablet, oral: 100 mg, 250 mg

Chlorthalidone (klor THAL i done)

Brand Names: U.S. Thalitone®

Brand Names: Canada Apo-Chlorthalidone®

Index Terms Hygroton

Pharmacologic Category Diuretic, Thiazide

Use Management of mild-to-moderate hypertension when used alone or in combination with other agents; treatment of edema associated with heart failure or nephrotic syndrome. Recent studies have found chlorthalidone effective in the treatment of isolated systolic hypertension in the elderly.

Unlabeled Use Pediatric hypertension

Pregnancy Risk Factor B

Dosage Oral:

Children (nonapproved): 2 mg/kg/dose 3 times/week or 1-2 mg/kg/day

Hypertension (unlabeled use): Initial: 0.3 mg/kg once daily, up to 2 mg/kg/day; maximum: 50 mg/day

Adults:

Hypertension: 25-100 mg/day or 100 mg 3 times/week; usual dosage range (JNC 7): 12.5-25 mg/day

Edema: Initial: 50-100 mg/day or 100 mg on alternate days; maximum dose: 200 mg/day

Heart failure-associated edema: 12.5-25 mg once daily; maximum daily dose: 100 mg (ACC/AHA 2009 Heart Failure Guidelines)

Elderly: Initial: 12.5-25 mg/day or every other day; there is little advantage to using doses >25 mg/day

Dosage adjustment in renal impairment: Cl_{cr} <10 mL/minute: Avoid use. Ineffective with low GFR (Aronoff, 2002)

Note: ACC/AHA 2009 Heart Failure Guidelines suggest that thiazides lose their efficacy when Cl_{cr} <40 mL/minute

Additional Information Complete prescribing information for this medication should be consulted for additional detail.

Dosage Forms Excipient information presented when available (limited, particularly for generics); consult specific product labeling. [DSC] = Discontinued product

Tablet, oral: 25 mg, 50 mg, 100 mg [DSC]

Thalitone®: 15 mg

◆ **Chlor-Tripolon ND® (Can)** *see* Loratadine and Pseudoephedrine *on page 1032*

Chlorzoxazone (klor ZOKS a zone)

Brand Names: U.S. Lorzone™; Parafon Forte® DSC

Brand Names: Canada Parafon Forte®; Strifon Forte®

Pharmacologic Category Skeletal Muscle Relaxant

Additional Appendix Information

Beers Criteria – Potentially Inappropriate Medications for Geriatrics *on page 1973*

Use Symptomatic treatment of muscle spasm and pain associated with acute musculoskeletal conditions

Dosage Oral:

Children: 20 mg/kg/day or 600 mg/m²/day in 3-4 divided doses

Adults: 250-500 mg 3-4 times/day up to 750 mg 3-4 times/day

Additional Information Complete prescribing information for this medication should be consulted for additional detail.

Dosage Forms Excipient information presented when available (limited, particularly for generics); consult specific product labeling.

Caplet, oral:

Parafon Forte® DSC: 500 mg [scored]

Tablet, oral: 500 mg

Lorzone™: 375 mg

Lorzone™: 750 mg [scored]

◆ **Cholecalciferol and Alendronate** *see* Alendronate and Cholecalciferol *on page 62*

Cholestyramine Resin (koe LES teer a meen REZ in)

Brand Names: U.S. Prevalite®; Questran®; Questran® Light

Brand Names: Canada Novo-Cholamine; Novo-Cholamine Light; Olestyr; PMS-Cholestyramine; Questran®; Questran® Light Sugar Free; ZYM-Cholestyramine-Light; ZYM-Cholestyramine-Regular

Pharmacologic Category Antilipemic Agent, Bile Acid Sequestrant

Additional Appendix Information

Hyperlipidemia Management *on page 1996*

Use Adjunct in the management of primary hypercholesterolemia; pruritus associated with elevated levels of bile acids; regression of arteriolosclerosis

Unlabeled Use Diarrhea associated with excess fecal bile acids (Westergaard, 2007); may be used to enhance elimination of digoxin when non-life-threatening toxicity occurs (Henderson, 1988)

Pregnancy Risk Factor C

Dosage Oral (dosages are expressed in terms of anhydrous resin):

Children (unlabeled use): 240 mg/kg/day in 2-3 divided doses; need to titrate dose depending on indication, response and tolerance; maximum: 8 g/day

Adults: Initial: 4 g 1-2 times/day; increase gradually over ≥1-month intervals; maintenance: 8-16 g/day divided in 2 doses; maximum: 24 g/day

Dosage adjustment in renal impairment: No dosage adjustment provided in manufacturer's labeling; however, use with caution in renal impairment; may cause hyperchloremic acidosis.

Dosage adjustment in hepatic impairment: No dosage adjustment necessary; not absorbed from the gastrointestinal tract.

Additional Information Complete prescribing information for this medication should be consulted for additional detail.

Dosage Forms Excipient information presented when available (limited, particularly for generics); consult specific product labeling.

Powder for suspension, oral: Cholestyramine resin 4 g/5 g of powder (210 g); Cholestyramine resin 4 g/5.7 g of powder (239.4 g); Cholestyramine resin 4 g/9 g of powder (378 g); Cholestyramine resin 4 g/5 g packet (60s); Cholestyramine resin 4 g/5.7 g packet (60s); Cholestyramine resin 4 g/9 g packet (60s)

Prevalite®: Cholestyramine resin 4 g/5.5 g of powder (231 g); Cholestyramine resin 4 g/5.5 g packet (42s, 60s) [contains phenylalanine 14.1 mg/5.5 g; orange flavor]

Questran®: Cholestyramine resin 4 g/9 g of powder (378 g); Cholestyramine resin 4 g/9 g packet (60s) [orange flavor]

Questran® Light: Cholestyramine resin 4 g/5 g of powder (210 g); Cholestyramine resin 4 g/5 g packet (60s) [contains phenylalanine 14 mg/5 g; orange flavor]

◆ **Choline Fenofibrate** *see* Fenofibric Acid *on page 695*

Choline Magnesium Trisalicylate
(KOE leen mag NEE zhum trye sa LIS i late)

Index Terms Tricosal; Trilisate

Pharmacologic Category Salicylate

Use Management of osteoarthritis, rheumatoid arthritis, and other arthritis; acute painful shoulder

Pregnancy Risk Factor C/D (3rd trimester)

Pregnancy Considerations Animal reproduction studies have not been conducted. Due to the known effects of other salicylates (closure of ductus arteriosus), use during late pregnancy should be avoided.

Lactation Enters breast milk/use caution

Contraindications Hypersensitivity to salicylates, other nonacetylated salicylates, other NSAIDs, or any component of the formulation; bleeding disorders; pregnancy (3rd trimester)

Warnings/Precautions Salicylate salts may not inhibit platelet aggregation and, therefore, should not be substituted for aspirin in the prophylaxis of thrombosis. Use with caution in patients with impaired hepatic or renal function, dehydration, erosive gastritis, asthma, or peptic ulcer. Children and teenagers who have or are recovering from chickenpox or flu-like symptoms should not use this product. Changes in behavior (along with nausea and vomiting) may be an early sign of Reye's syndrome; patients should be instructed to contact their healthcare provider if these occur.

Elderly are a high-risk population for adverse effects from NSAIDs. As many as 60% of elderly can develop peptic ulceration and/or hemorrhage asymptomatically. Use lowest effective dose for shortest period possible. Tinnitus or impaired hearing may indicate toxicity. Tinnitus may be a difficult and unreliable indication of toxicity due to age-related hearing loss or eighth cranial nerve damage. CNS adverse effects may be observed in the elderly at lower doses than younger adults.

Adverse Reactions
<20%:
Gastrointestinal: Nausea, vomiting, diarrhea, heartburn, dyspepsia, epigastric pain, constipation
Otic: Tinnitus
<2%:
Central nervous system: Headache, lightheadedness, dizziness, drowsiness, lethargy
Otic: Hearing impairment
<1%: Anorexia, asthma, BUN and creatinine increased, bruising, confusion, duodenal ulceration, dysgeusia, edema, epistaxis, erythema multiforme, esophagitis, hallucinations, hearing loss (irreversible), hepatic enzymes increased, gastric ulceration, occult bleeding, pruritus, rash, weight gain

Drug Interactions

Metabolism/Transport Effects None known.

Avoid Concomitant Use

Avoid concomitant use of Choline Magnesium Trisalicylate with any of the following: Influenza Virus Vaccine (Live/Attenuated)

Increased Effect/Toxicity

Choline Magnesium Trisalicylate may increase the levels/effects of: Anticoagulants; Carbonic Anhydrase Inhibitors; Corticosteroids (Systemic); Divalproex; Drotrecogin Alfa (Activated); Methotrexate; PRALAtrexate; Salicylates; Sulfonylureas; Thrombolytic Agents; Valproic Acid; Varicella Virus-Containing Vaccines; Vitamin K Antagonists

The levels/effects of Choline Magnesium Trisalicylate may be increased by: Ammonium Chloride; Antiplatelet Agents; Calcium Channel Blockers (Nondihydropyridine); Ginkgo Biloba; Herbs (Anticoagulant/Antiplatelet Properties); Influenza Virus Vaccine (Live/Attenuated); Loop Diuretics; Potassium Acid Phosphate; Treprostinil

Decreased Effect

Choline Magnesium Trisalicylate may decrease the levels/effects of: ACE Inhibitors; Loop Diuretics; Probenecid

The levels/effects of Choline Magnesium Trisalicylate may be decreased by: Corticosteroids (Systemic)

Ethanol/Nutrition/Herb Interactions
Ethanol: Avoid ethanol (may enhance gastric mucosal irritation).
Food: May decrease the rate but not the extent of oral absorption.
Herb/Nutraceutical: Avoid cat's claw, dong quai, evening primrose, feverfew, garlic, ginger, ginkgo, red clover, horse chestnut, green tea, ginseng (all have additional antiplatelet activity). Limit curry powder, paprika, licorice, Benedictine liqueur, prunes, raisins, tea, and gherkins; may cause salicylate accumulation. These foods contain 6 mg salicylate/100 g.

Stability Store at controlled room temperature of 15°C to 30°C (59°F to 86°F).

Mechanism of Action Weakly inhibits cyclooxygenase enzymes, which results in decreased formation of prostaglandin precursors; antipyretic, analgesic, and anti-inflammatory properties.

Other proposed mechanisms not fully elucidated (and possibly contributing to the anti-inflammatory effect to varying degrees) include inhibiting chemotaxis, altering lymphocyte activity, inhibiting neutrophil aggregation/activation, and decreasing proinflammatory cytokine levels.

Pharmacodynamics/Kinetics
Onset of action: Peak effect: ~2 hours
Absorption: Stomach and small intestines
Distribution: Readily into most body fluids and tissues; crosses placenta; enters breast milk
Half-life elimination (dose dependent): Low dose: 2-3 hours; High dose: 30 hours
Time to peak, serum: ~2 hours

Dosage Oral (based on total salicylate content):
Children <37 kg: 50 mg/kg/day given in 2 divided doses; 2250 mg/day for heavier children
Adults: 500 mg to 1.5 g 2-3 times/day **or** 3 g at bedtime; usual maintenance dose: 1-4.5 g/day
Elderly: 750 mg 3 times/day
Dosing adjustment/comments in renal impairment: Avoid use in severe renal impairment

Dietary Considerations Take with food or large volume of water or milk to minimize GI upset. Liquid may be mixed with fruit juice just before drinking. Hypermagnesemia resulting from magnesium salicylate; avoid or use with caution in renal insufficiency.

Administration Liquid may be mixed with fruit juice just before drinking. Do not administer with antacids. Take with a full glass of water and remain in an upright position for 15-30 minutes after administration.

Monitoring Parameters Serum magnesium with high dose therapy or in patients with impaired renal function; serum salicylate levels, renal function, hearing changes or tinnitus, abnormal bruising, weight gain and response (ie, pain)

Reference Range Salicylate blood levels for anti-inflammatory effect: 150-300 mcg/mL; analgesia and antipyretic effect: 30-50 mcg/mL

Test Interactions False-negative results for glucose oxidase urinary glucose tests (Clinistix®); false-positives using the cupric sulfate method (Clinitest®); also, interferes with Gerhardt test (urinary ketone analysis), VMA determination; 5-HIAA, xylose tolerance test, and T_3 and T_4; increased PBI

Dosage Forms Excipient information presented when available (limited, particularly for generics); consult specific product labeling. [DSC] = Discontinued product
Liquid, oral: 500 mg/5 mL (240 mL) [choline salicylate 293 mg and magnesium salicylate 362 mg per 5 mL]
Tablet, oral: 500 mg [DSC] [choline salicylate 293 mg and magnesium salicylate 362 mg], 750 mg [DSC] [choline salicylate 440 mg and magnesium salicylate 544 mg], 1000 mg [DSC] [choline salicylate 587 mg and magnesium salicylate 725 mg]

◆ **Chondroitin Sulfate and Sodium Hyaluronate** *see* Sodium Chondroitin Sulfate and Sodium Hyaluronate *on page 1570*
◆ **Chooz® [OTC]** *see* Calcium Carbonate *on page 266*
◆ **Choriogonadotropin Alfa** *see* Chorionic Gonadotropin (Recombinant) *on page 353*
◆ **Chorionic Gonadotropin for Injection (Can)** *see* Chorionic Gonadotropin (Human) *on page 352*

Chorionic Gonadotropin (Human)
(kor ee ON ik goe NAD oh troe pin, HYU man)

Brand Names: U.S. Novarel®; Pregnyl®

Brand Names: Canada Chorionic Gonadotropin for Injection; Pregnyl®

Index Terms CG; hCG

Pharmacologic Category Gonadotropin; Ovulation Stimulator

Use Induces ovulation and pregnancy in anovulatory, infertile females; treatment of hypogonadotropic hypogonadism, prepubertal cryptorchidism; spermatogenesis induction with follitropin alfa

Pregnancy Risk Factor X

Pregnancy Considerations Teratogenic effects (forelimb, CNS) have been noted in animal studies at doses intended to induce superovulation (used in combination with gonadotropin). Testicular tumors in otherwise healthy men have been reported when treating secondary infertility.

Lactation Excretion in breast milk unknown/use caution

Contraindications Hypersensitivity to chorionic gonadotropin or any component of the formulation; precocious puberty; prostatic carcinoma or similar neoplasms; pregnancy

Warnings/Precautions Use with caution in asthma, seizure disorders, migraine, cardiac or renal disease. **Not** effective in the treatment of obesity. Safety and efficacy in children <4 years of age have not been established.

Cryptorchidism: May induce precocious puberty in children being treated for cryptorchidism; discontinue if signs of precocious puberty occur.

Ovulation induction: These medications should only be used by physicians who are thoroughly familiar with infertility problems and their management. May cause ovarian hyperstimulation syndrome (OHSS); characterized by severe ovarian enlargement, abdominal pain/distention, nausea, vomiting, diarrhea, dyspnea, and oliguria, and may be accompanied by ascites, pleural effusion, hypovolemia, electrolyte imbalance, hemoperitoneum, and thromboembolic events. If severe hyperstimulation occurs, stop treatment and hospitalize patient. This syndrome develops rapidly with 24 hours to several days and generally occurs during the 7-10 days immediately following treatment. Ovarian enlargement may be accompanied by abdominal distention or abdominal pain and generally regresses without treatment within 2-3 weeks. If ovaries are abnormally enlarged on the last day of treatment, withhold hCG to reduce the risk of OHSS. In association with and separate from OHSS, thromboembolic events have been reported. May result from the use of these medications; advise patients of the potential risk of multiple births before starting the treatment.

Adverse Reactions Frequency not always defined.

Cardiovascular: Edema

Central nervous system: Depression, fatigue, headache, irritability, restlessness

Endocrine & metabolic: Gynecomastia, precocious puberty

Local: Injection site reaction, pain at injection site

Miscellaneous: Hypersensitivity reaction (local or systemic)

<1% (Limited to important or life-threatening): Arterial thrombus, ovarian cyst rupture, ovarian hyperstimulation syndrome

Drug Interactions

Metabolism/Transport Effects None known.

Avoid Concomitant Use There are no known interactions where it is recommended to avoid concomitant use.

Increased Effect/Toxicity There are no known significant interactions involving an increase in effect.

Decreased Effect There are no known significant interactions involving a decrease in effect.

Stability Following reconstitution with the provided diluent, solutions are stable for 30-60 days, depending on the specific preparation, when stored at 2°C to 15°C.

Mechanism of Action Luteinizing hormone obtained from the urine of pregnant women. Stimulates production of gonadal steroid hormones by causing production of androgen by the testes; as a substitute for luteinizing hormone (LH) to stimulate ovulation

Pharmacodynamics/Kinetics

Half-life elimination: Biphasic: Initial: 11 hours; Terminal: 23 hours

Excretion: Urine

Dosage I.M.:

Children: Various regimens:

Prepubertal cryptorchidism:

4000 units 3 times/week for 3 weeks **or**

5000 units every second day for 4 injections **or**

500 units 3 times/week for 4-6 weeks **or**

15 injections of 500-1000 units given over 6 weeks

Hypogonadotropic hypogonadism: Males:

500-1000 units 3 times/week for 3 weeks, followed by the same dose twice weekly for 3 weeks **or**

4000 units 3 times/week for 6-9 months, then reduce dosage to 2000 units 3 times/week for additional 3 months

Adults:

Induction of ovulation: Females: 5000-10,000 units one day following last dose of menotropins

Spermatogenesis induction associated with hypogonadotropic hypogonadism: Males: Treatment regimens vary (range: 1000-2000 units 2-3 times a week). Administer hCG until serum testosterone levels are normal (may require 2-3 months of therapy), then may add follitropin alfa or menopausal gonadotropin if needed to induce spermatogenesis; continue hCG at the dose required to maintain testosterone levels.

Administration I.M. administration only

Monitoring Parameters

Male: Serum testosterone levels, semen analysis

Female: Ultrasound and/or estradiol levels to assess follicle development; ultrasound to assess number and size of follicles; ovulation (basal body temperature, serum progestin level, menstruation, sonography)

Reference Range Depends on application and methodology; <3 mIU/mL (SI: <3 units/L) usually normal (nonpregnant)

Test Interactions Cross-reacts with radioimmunoassay of gonadotropins, especially LH

Dosage Forms Excipient information presented when available (limited, particularly for generics); consult specific product labeling.

Injection, powder for reconstitution: 10,000 units

Novarel®: 10,000 units [contains benzyl alcohol (in diluent)]

Pregnyl®: 10,000 units [contains benzyl alcohol (in diluent)]

Chorionic Gonadotropin (Recombinant)

(kor ee ON ik goe NAD oh troe pin ree KOM be nant)

Brand Names: U.S. Ovidrel®

Brand Names: Canada Ovidrel®

Index Terms Choriogonadotropin Alfa; r-hCG

Pharmacologic Category Gonadotropin; Ovulation Stimulator

Use As part of an assisted reproductive technology (ART) program, induces ovulation in infertile females who have been pretreated with follicle stimulating hormones (FSH); induces ovulation and pregnancy in infertile females when the cause of infertility is functional

Pregnancy Risk Factor X

Pregnancy Considerations Intrauterine death and impaired birth were observed in animal studies. Ectopic pregnancy, premature labor, postpartum fever, and spontaneous abortion have been reported in clinical trials. Congenital abnormalities have also been observed, however, the incidence is similar during natural conception.

Lactation Excretion in breast milk unknown/use caution

Contraindications Hypersensitivity to hCG preparations or any component of the formulation; primary ovarian failure; uncontrolled thyroid or adrenal dysfunction; uncontrolled organic intracranial lesion (ie, pituitary tumor); abnormal uterine bleeding, ovarian cyst or enlargement of undetermined origin; sex hormone dependent tumors; pregnancy

Warnings/Precautions Ovarian enlargement may occur; may be accompanied by abdominal distention or abdominal pain and generally regresses without treatment within 2-3 weeks. If ovaries are abnormally enlarged on the last day of treatment, withhold hCG to reduce the risk of ovarian hyperstimulation syndrome (OHSS). OHSS is characterized by severe ovarian enlargement, abdominal pain/distention, nausea, vomiting, diarrhea, dyspnea, and oliguria, and may be accompanied by ascites, pleural effusion, hypovolemia, electrolyte imbalance, hemoperitoneum, and thromboembolic events. If severe hyperstimulation occurs, stop treatment and hospitalize patient. This syndrome develops rapidly with 24 hours to several days and generally occurs during the 7-10 days immediately following treatment.

Arterial thromboembolic events have been reported in association with and separate from OHSS. These medications should only be used by healthcare providers who are thoroughly familiar with infertility problems and their management. Multiple births may result from the use of these medications; advise patients of the potential risk of multiple births before starting the treatment. Safety and efficacy have not been established in the elderly or in children.

Adverse Reactions
2% to 10%:
Endocrine & metabolic: Ovarian cyst (3%), ovarian hyperstimulation (<2% to 3%)
Gastrointestinal: Abdominal pain (3% to 4%), nausea (3%), vomiting (3%)
Local: Injection site: Pain (8%), bruising (3% to 5%), reaction (<2% to 3%), inflammation (<2% to 2%)
Miscellaneous: Postoperative pain (5%)
<2% (Limited to important or life-threatening): Abdominal enlargement, albuminuria, allergic reaction, back pain, breast pain, cardiac arrhythmia, cervical carcinoma, cervical lesion, cough, diarrhea, dizziness, dysuria, ectopic pregnancy, emotional lability, fever, flatulence, genital herpes, genital moniliasis, headache, heart murmur, hiccups, hot flashes, hyperglycemia, insomnia, intermenstrual bleeding, leukocytosis, leukorrhea, malaise, paresthesia, pharyngitis, pruritus, rash, upper respiratory tract infection, urinary incontinence, urinary tract infection, vaginal discomfort, vaginal hemorrhage, vaginitis
In addition, the following have been reported with menotropin therapy: Adnexal torsion, hemoperitoneum, mild-to-moderate ovarian enlargement, pulmonary and vascular complications. Ovarian neoplasms have also been reported (rare) with multiple drug regimens used for ovarian induction (relationship not established).

Drug Interactions
Metabolism/Transport Effects None known.
Avoid Concomitant Use There are no known interactions where it is recommended to avoid concomitant use.
Increased Effect/Toxicity There are no known significant interactions involving an increase in effect.
Decreased Effect There are no known significant interactions involving a decrease in effect.

Stability Prefilled syringe: Prior to dispensing, store at 2°C to 8°C (36°F to 46°F). Patient may store at 25°C (77°F) for up to 30 days. Protect from light.

Mechanism of Action Luteinizing hormone analogue produced by recombinant DNA techniques; stimulates late follicular maturation and intitates rupture of the ovarian follicle once follicular development has occurred

Pharmacodynamics/Kinetics
Distribution: V_d: 21.4L
Bioavailability: 40%
Half-life elimination: Initial: 4 hours; Terminal: 29 hours
Time to peak: 12-24 hours
Excretion: Urine (10% of dose)

Dosage SubQ:
Adults: Females:
Assisted reproductive technologies (ART) and ovulation induction: 250 mcg given 1 day following the last dose of follicle stimulating agent. Use only after adequate follicular development has been determined. Hold treatment when there is an excessive ovarian response.
Elderly: Safety and efficacy have not been established
Dosage adjustment in renal impairment: Safety and efficacy have not been established
Dosage adjustment in hepatic impairment: Safety and efficacy have not been established

Administration For SubQ use only; inject into stomach area.

Monitoring Parameters Ultrasound and/or estradiol levels to assess follicle development; ultrasound to assess number and size of follicles; ovulation (basal body temperature, serum progestin level, menstruation, sonography)

Test Interactions May interfere with interpretation of pregnancy tests; may cross-react with radioimmunoassay of luteinizing hormone and other gonadotropins

Additional Information Clinical studies have shown r-hCG to be clinically and statistically equivalent to urinary-derived hCG products.

Dosage Forms Excipient information presented when available (limited, particularly for generics); consult specific product labeling.
Injection, solution:
Ovidrel®: 257.5 mcg/0.515 mL (0.515 mL) [delivers 250 mcg r-hCG/0.5 mL; derived from Chinese Hamster Ovary cells]

Chromic Phosphate P 32
(KROME ik FOS fate pe THUR tee too)

Brand Names: U.S. Phosphocol® P 32
Index Terms P32; Phosphorus p32
Pharmacologic Category Radiopharmaceutical
Use Treatment of peritoneal or pleural effusions caused by metastatic disease by intracavitary instillation; may be injected interstitially for the treatment of cancer
Dosage Adults: **Note:** Consult manufacturer potency tables when applicable. All doses should be individualized.
General dosing ranges (based on 70 kg patient):
Intraperitoneal instillation: 370-740 megabecquerels (10-20 millicuries)
Intrapleural instillation: 222-444 megabecquerels (6-12 millicuries)
Interstitial use: ~3.7-18.5 megabecquerels/g of tumor weight (0.1-0.5 millicuries/g)
Additional Information Complete prescribing information for this medication should be consulted for additional detail.
Dosage Forms Excipient information presented when available (limited, particularly for generics); consult specific product labeling.
Injection, suspension:
Phosphocol® P 32: 185 MBq (5mCi) per mL

◆ **CI-1008** *see* Pregabalin *on page* 1402
◆ **Cialis®** *see* Tadalafil *on page* 1621

Ciclesonide (Systemic) (sye KLES oh nide)

Brand Names: U.S. Alvesco®
Brand Names: Canada Alvesco®
Pharmacologic Category Corticosteroid, Inhalant (Oral)
Use Prophylactic management of bronchial asthma
Pregnancy Risk Factor C
Pregnancy Considerations Teratogenic effects were reported in some, but not all animal studies. There are no adequate and well-controlled studies in pregnant women. The extent of intranasal absorption of ciclesonide systemically is low but variable; use during pregnancy with caution. Hypoadrenalism may occur in infants born to mothers receiving corticosteroids during pregnancy.
Lactation Excretion in breast milk unknown/use caution

Contraindications Hypersensitivity to ciclesonide or any component of the formulation; primary treatment of acute asthma or status asthmaticus; moderate-to-severe bronchiectasis

Canadian labeling: Additional contraindications (not in U.S. labeling): Untreated fungal, bacterial, or tuberculosis infections of the respiratory tract; moderate-to-severe bronchiectasis

Warnings/Precautions May cause hypercorticism or suppression of hypothalamic-pituitary-adrenal (HPA) axis, particularly in younger children or in patients receiving high doses for prolonged periods. HPA axis suppression may lead to adrenal crisis. Withdrawal and discontinuation of a corticosteroid should be done slowly and carefully. Particular care is required when patients are transferred from systemic corticosteroids to inhaled products due to possible adrenal insufficiency or withdrawal from steroids, including an increase in allergic symptoms. Patients receiving >20 mg per day of prednisone (or equivalent) may be most susceptible. Fatalities have occurred due to adrenal insufficiency in asthmatic patients during and after transfer from systemic corticosteroids to aerosol steroids; aerosol steroids do **not** provide the systemic steroid needed to treat patients having trauma, surgery, or infections.

Bronchospasm may occur with wheezing after inhalation; if this occurs stop steroid and treat with a fast-acting bronchodilator. Supplemental steroids (oral or parenteral) may be needed during stress or severe asthma attacks. Not to be used in status asthmaticus or for the relief of acute bronchospasm. Oropharyngeal thrush due to candida albicans infection may occur with use. Prolonged use of corticosteroids may also increase the incidence of secondary infection, mask acute infection (including fungal infections), prolong or exacerbate viral infections, or limit response to vaccines. Exposure to chickenpox and measles should be avoided; corticosteroids should not be used to treat ocular herpes simplex. Close observation is required in patients with latent tuberculosis and/or TB reactivity; restrict use in active TB (only in conjunction with antituberculosis treatment). Use in patients with TB is contraindicated in the Canadian labeling. Prolonged treatment with corticosteroids has been associated with the development of Kaposi's sarcoma (case reports); if noted, discontinuation of therapy should be considered.

Use with caution in patients with thyroid disease, severe hepatic impairment, glaucoma, cataracts, patients at risk for osteoporosis, and patients at risk for seizures.

Orally inhaled corticosteroids may cause a reduction in growth velocity in pediatric patients (~1 cm per year [range: 0.3-1.8 cm per year] and related to dose and duration of exposure). To minimize the systemic effects of orally inhaled corticosteroids, each patient should be titrated to the lowest effective dose. Growth should be routinely monitored in pediatric patients.

Adverse Reactions

>10%:
- Central nervous system: Headache (≤11%)
- Respiratory: Nasopharyngitis (≤11%)

1% to 10%:
- Cardiovascular: Facial edema (≥3%)
- Central nervous system: Dizziness (≥3%), fatigue (≥3%), dysphonia (1%)
- Dermatologic: Urticaria (≥3%)
- Gastrointestinal: Gastroenteritis (≥3%), oral candidiasis (≥3%)
- Neuromuscular & skeletal: Arthralgia (≤4%), musculoskeletal chest pain (≥3%), back pain (≥3%), extremity pain (≥3%)
- Ocular: Conjunctivitis (≥3%)
- Otic: Ear pain (2%)
- Respiratory: Upper respiratory infection (≤9%), epistaxis (≤8%), nasal congestion (≤6%), sinusitis (≤6%), pharyngolaryngeal pain (≤ 5%), hoarseness (≥3%), pneumonia (≥3%), paradoxical bronchospasm (2%)
- Miscellaneous: Influenza (≥3%)

<1% (Limited to important or life-threatening): ALT increased, angioedema (with swelling of lip/pharynx/tongue), bruising, candidiasis (nasal/pharyngeal/systemic), cataract, chest discomfort, cough, dry throat, dysgeusia, dyspepsia, GGT increased, intraocular pressure increased, nausea, nasal septum disorder, palpitation, pharyngitis, rash, rhinorrhea, throat irritation, WBC increased, weight gain, xerostomia

Drug Interactions

Metabolism/Transport Effects Substrate of CYP3A4 (major); **Note:** Assignment of Major/Minor substrate status based on clinically relevant drug interaction potential

Avoid Concomitant Use

Avoid concomitant use of Ciclesonide (Oral Inhalation) with any of the following: Aldesleukin

Increased Effect/Toxicity

Ciclesonide (Oral Inhalation) may increase the levels/effects of: Deferasirox

The levels/effects of Ciclesonide (Oral Inhalation) may be increased by: CYP3A4 Inhibitors (Moderate); Dasatinib; Telaprevir

Decreased Effect

Ciclesonide (Oral Inhalation) may decrease the levels/effects of: Aldesleukin; Corticorelin; Telaprevir

The levels/effects of Ciclesonide (Oral Inhalation) may be decreased by: Tocilizumab

Stability Store at 15°C to 30°C (59°F to 86°F); do not freeze.

Mechanism of Action Ciclesonide is a nonhalogenated, glucocorticoid prodrug that is hydrolyzed to the pharmacologically active metabolite des-ciclesonide following administration. Des-ciclesonide has a high affinity for the glucocorticoid receptor and exhibits anti-inflammatory activity. The mechanism of action for corticosteroids is believed to be a combination of three important properties – anti-inflammatory activity, immunosuppressive properties, and antiproliferative actions.

Pharmacodynamics/Kinetics

- Absorption: 52% (lung deposition)
- Protein binding: ≥99%
- Metabolism: Ciclesonide hydrolyzed to active metabolite, des-ciclesonide via esterases in nasal mucosa and lungs; further metabolism via hepatic CYP3A4 and 2D6
- Bioavailability: >50% (active metabolite)
- Half-life elimination: ~5-7 hours
- Time to peak: ~1 hour (active metabolite)
- Excretion: Feces (78%)

Dosage Oral inhalation (Alvesco®):

Asthma: **Note:** Titrate to the lowest effective dose once asthma stability is achieved:

U.S. labeling: Children ≥12 years and Adults:
- Prior therapy with bronchodilators alone: Initial: 80 mcg twice daily (maximum dose: 320 mcg/day)
- Prior therapy with inhaled corticosteroids: Initial: 80 mcg twice daily (maximum dose: 640 mcg/day)
- Prior therapy with oral corticosteroids: Initial: 320 mcg twice daily (maximum dose: 640 mcg/day)

Canadian labeling:
- Children 6-11 years: Initial: 100-200 mcg once daily; maintenance: 100-200 mcg/day (1-2 puffs once daily)
- Children ≥12 years and Adults: Initial: 400 mcg once daily; maintenance: 100-800 mcg/day (1-2 puffs once or twice daily)

Conversion from oral to inhaled steroid: Initiation of oral inhalation therapy should begin in patients who have previously been stabilized on oral corticosteroids (OCS). A gradual dose reduction of OCS should begin ~7-10 days after starting inhaled therapy. U.S. labeling recommends reducing prednisone dose no more rapidly than ≤2.5 mg/day on a weekly basis. The Canadian labeling recommends decreasing the daily dose of prednisone by 1 mg (or equivalent of other OCS) every 7 days in closely monitored patients, and every 10 days in patients whom close monitoring is not possible. In the presence of withdrawal symptoms, resume previous OCS dose for 1 week before attempting further dose reductions.

Administration Remove mouthpiece cover, place inhaler in mouth, close lips around mouthpiece, and inhale slowly and deeply. Press down on top of inhaler after slow inhalation has begun. Remove inhaler while holding breath for approximately 10 seconds. Breathe out slowly and replace mouthpiece on inhaler. Do not wash or place inhaler in water. Clean mouthpiece using a dry cloth or tissue once weekly. Discard after the "discard by" date or after labeled number of doses has been used, even if container is not completely empty.

Shaking is not necessary since drug is formulated as a solution aerosol. Prime inhaler prior to initial use or if not in use for ≥1 week by releasing 3 puffs into the air.

Monitoring Parameters Growth (adolescents) and signs/symptoms of HPA axis suppression/adrenal insufficiency; ocular effects (eg, cataracts, increased intraocular pressure, glaucoma)

Additional Information The incidence of oral candidiasis, as well as other localized oropharyngeal effects, observed with ciclesonide use has been reported to be approximately one-half of that seen with other commonly inhaled corticosteroids such as budesonide and fluticasone. Small particle size, minimal activation, and deposition in the oropharynx may explain this decreased incidence.

Dosage Forms Excipient information presented when available (limited, particularly for generics); consult specific product labeling.

Aerosol, for oral inhalation:

Alvesco®: 80 mcg/inhalation (6.1 g); 160 mcg/inhalation (6.1 g) [60 metered actuations]

Dosage Forms: Canada Excipient information presented when available (limited, particularly for generics); consult specific product labeling.

Aerosol for oral inhalation:

Alvesco®: 50 mcg/inhalation [30-, 60-, and 120 metered actuations]; 100 mcg/inhalation [30-, 60-, and 120 metered actuations]; 200 mcg/inhalation [30-, 60-, and 120 metered actuations]

Ciclesonide (Nasal) (sye KLES oh nide)

Brand Names: U.S. Omnaris™

Brand Names: Canada Omnaris™

Pharmacologic Category Corticosteroid, Nasal

Use Management of seasonal and perennial allergic rhinitis

Pregnancy Risk Factor C

Dosage Intranasal (Omnaris™):

Seasonal allergic rhinitis:

U.S. labeling: Children ≥6 years and Adults: 2 sprays (50 mcg/spray) per nostril once daily; maximum: 200 mcg/day

Canadian labeling: Children ≥12 years and Adults: 2 sprays (50 mcg/spray) per nostril once daily; maximum: 200 mcg/day

Perennial allergic rhinitis: Children ≥12 years and Adults: 2 sprays (50 mcg/spray) per nostril once daily; maximum: 200 mcg/day

Additional Information Complete prescribing information for this medication should be consulted for additional detail.

Dosage Forms Excipient information presented when available (limited, particularly for generics); consult specific product labeling.

Suspension, intranasal [spray]:

Omnaris™: 50 mcg/inhalation (12.5 g) [120 metered actuations]

◆ **Ciclodan™** *see* Ciclopirox *on page* 356

◆ **Ciclodan™ Kit** *see* Ciclopirox *on page* 356

Ciclopirox (sye kloe PEER oks)

Brand Names: U.S. Ciclodan™; Ciclodan™ Kit; Loprox®; Penlac®

Brand Names: Canada Loprox®; Penlac®; Stieprox®

Index Terms Ciclopirox Olamine

Pharmacologic Category Antifungal Agent, Topical

Use

Cream/suspension: Treatment of tinea pedis (athlete's foot), tinea cruris (jock itch), tinea corporis (ringworm), cutaneous candidiasis, and tinea versicolor (pityriasis)

Gel: Treatment of tinea pedis (athlete's foot), tinea corporis (ringworm); seborrheic dermatitis of the scalp

Lacquer (solution): Topical treatment of mild-to-moderate onychomycosis of the fingernails and toenails due to *Trichophyton rubrum* (not involving the lunula) and the immediately-adjacent skin

Shampoo: Treatment of seborrheic dermatitis of the scalp

Pregnancy Risk Factor B

Dosage Topical:

Children >10 years and Adults: Tinea pedis, tinea cruris, tinea corporis, cutaneous candidiasis, and tinea versicolor: Cream/suspension: Apply twice daily, gently massage into affected areas; if no improvement after 4 weeks of treatment, re-evaluate the diagnosis.

Children ≥12 years and Adults: Onychomycosis of the fingernails and toenails: Lacquer (solution): Apply to adjacent skin and affected nails daily (as a part of a comprehensive management program for onychomycosis). Remove with alcohol every 7 days.

Children >16 years and Adults:

Tinea pedis, tinea corporis: Gel: Apply twice daily, gently massage into affected areas and surrounding skin; if no improvement after 4 weeks of treatment, re-evaluate diagnosis

Seborrheic dermatitis of the scalp:

Gel: Apply twice daily, gently massage into affected areas and surrounding skin; if no improvement after 4 weeks of treatment, re-evaluate diagnosis.

Shampoo: Apply ~5 mL to wet hair; lather, and leave in place ~3 minutes; rinse. May use up to 10 mL for longer hair. Repeat twice weekly for 4 weeks; allow a minimum of 3 days between applications.

Additional Information Complete prescribing information for this medication should be consulted for additional detail.

Dosage Forms Excipient information presented when available (limited, particularly for generics); consult specific product labeling.

Cream, topical, as olamine: 0.77% (15 g, 30 g, 90 g)

Gel, topical: 0.77% (30 g, 45 g, 100 g)

Loprox®: 0.77% (30 g, 45 g, 100 g) [contains isopropyl alcohol]

Shampoo, topical: 1% (120 mL)

Loprox®: 1% (120 mL)

Solution, topical [nail lacquer]: 8% (6.6 mL)
Ciclodan™: 8% (6.6 mL) [contains isopropyl alcohol]
Ciclodan™ Kit: 8% (6.6 mL) [contains isopropyl alcohol; packaged with Toetal Fresh™]
Penlac®: 8% (6.6 mL) [contains isopropyl alcohol]
Suspension, topical, as olamine: 0.77% (30 mL, 60 mL)

◆ **Ciclopirox Olamine** *see* Ciclopirox *on page 356*
◆ **Cidecin** *see* DAPTOmycin *on page 446*

Cidofovir (si DOF o veer)

Brand Names: U.S. Vistide®
Pharmacologic Category Antiviral Agent
Use Treatment of cytomegalovirus (CMV) retinitis in patients with acquired immunodeficiency syndrome (AIDS). **Note:** Should be administered with probenecid.
Pregnancy Risk Factor C
Pregnancy Considerations [U.S. Boxed Warning]: Possibly carcinogenic and teratogenic based on animal data. May cause hypospermia. Cidofovir was shown to be teratogenic and embryotoxic in animal studies, some at doses which also produced maternal toxicity. Reduced testes weight and hypospermia were also noted in animal studies. There are no adequate and well-controlled studies in pregnant women; use during pregnancy only if the potential benefit to the mother outweighs the possible risk to the fetus. Women of childbearing potential should use effective contraception during therapy and for 1 month following treatment. Males should use a barrier contraceptive during therapy and for 3 months following treatment.
Lactation Excretion in breast milk unknown/contraindicated
Contraindications Hypersensitivity to cidofovir; history of clinically-severe hypersensitivity to probenecid or other sulfa-containing medications; serum creatinine >1.5 mg/dL; Cl_{cr} <55 mL/minute; urine protein ≥100 mg/dL (≥2+ proteinuria); use with or within 7 days of nephrotoxic agents; direct intraocular injection
Warnings/Precautions Hazardous agent - use appropriate precautions for handling and disposal. **[U.S. Boxed Warning]: Dose-dependent nephrotoxicity requires dose adjustment or discontinuation if changes in renal function occur during therapy (eg, proteinuria, glycosuria, decreased serum phosphate, uric acid or bicarbonate, and elevated creatinine). Neutropenia has been reported;** monitor counts during therapy. Cases of ocular hypotony have also occurred; monitor intraocular pressure. Monitor for signs of metabolic acidosis. Safety and efficacy have not been established in children or the elderly. Administration must be accompanied by oral probenecid and intravenous saline prehydration. **[U.S. Boxed Warning]: Indicated only for CMV retinitis treatment in HIV patients; possibly carcinogenic and teratogenic based on animal data. May cause hypospermia.**
Adverse Reactions
>10%:
Central nervous system: Chills, fever, headache, pain
Dermatologic: Alopecia, rash
Gastrointestinal: Nausea, vomiting, diarrhea, anorexia
Hematologic: Anemia, neutropenia
Neuromuscular & skeletal: Weakness
Ocular: Intraocular pressure decreased, iritis, ocular hypotony, uveitis
Renal: Creatinine increased, proteinuria, renal toxicity
Respiratory: Cough, dyspnea
Miscellaneous: Infection, oral moniliasis, serum bicarbonate decreased
1% to 10%:
Renal: Fanconi syndrome
Respiratory: Pneumonia
<1%: Hepatic failure, metabolic acidosis, pancreatitis
Frequency not defined (limited to important or life-threatening reactions):
Cardiovascular: Cardiomyopathy, cardiovascular disorder, CHF, edema, postural hypotension, shock, syncope, tachycardia
Central nervous system: Agitation, amnesia, anxiety, confusion, convulsion, dizziness, hallucinations, insomnia, malaise, vertigo
Dermatologic: Photosensitivity reaction, skin discoloration, urticaria
Endocrine & metabolic: Adrenal cortex insufficiency
Gastrointestinal: Abdominal pain, aphthous stomatitis, colitis, constipation, dysphagia, fecal incontinence, gastritis, GI hemorrhage, gingivitis, melena, proctitis, splenomegaly, stomatitis, tongue discoloration
Genitourinary: Urinary incontinence
Hematologic: Hypochromic anemia, leukocytosis, leukopenia, lymphadenopathy, lymphoma-like reaction, pancytopenia, thrombocytopenia, thrombocytopenic purpura
Hepatic: Hepatomegaly, hepatosplenomegaly, jaundice, liver function tests abnormal, liver damage, liver necrosis
Local: Injection site reaction
Neuromuscular & skeletal: Tremor
Ocular: Amblyopia, blindness, cataract, conjunctivitis, corneal lesion, diplopia, vision abnormal
Otic: Hearing loss
Miscellaneous: Allergic reaction, sepsis
Drug Interactions
Metabolism/Transport Effects None known.
Avoid Concomitant Use There are no known interactions where it is recommended to avoid concomitant use.
Increased Effect/Toxicity There are no known significant interactions involving an increase in effect.
Decreased Effect There are no known significant interactions involving a decrease in effect.
Stability Store at controlled room temperature 20°C to 25°C (68°F to 77°F). Dilute dose in NS 100 mL prior to infusion. Store admixtures under refrigeration for ≤24 hours. Cidofovir infusion admixture should be administered within 24 hours of preparation at room temperature or refrigerated. Admixtures should be allowed to equilibrate to room temperature prior to use.
Mechanism of Action Cidofovir is converted to cidofovir diphosphate which is the active intracellular metabolite; cidofovir diphosphate suppresses CMV replication by selective inhibition of viral DNA synthesis. Incorporation of cidofovir into growing viral DNA chain results in reductions in the rate of viral DNA synthesis.
Pharmacodynamics/Kinetics The following pharmacokinetic data is based on a combination of cidofovir administered with probenecid:
Distribution: V_d: 0.54 L/kg; does not cross significantly into CSF
Protein binding: <6%
Metabolism: Minimal; phosphorylation occurs intracellularly
Half-life elimination, plasma: ~2.6 hours
Excretion: Urine
Dosage Adults:
Induction: 5 mg/kg I.V. over 1 hour once weekly for 2 consecutive weeks
Maintenance: 5 mg/kg over 1 hour once every other week
Note: Administer with probenecid 2 g orally 3 hours prior to each cidofovir dose and 1 g at 2 hours and 8 hours after completion of the infusion (total: 4 g)

Hydrate with at least 1 L of 0.9% NS I.V. prior to each cidofovir infusion; infuse saline over a 1- to 2-hour period immediately prior to cidofovir infusion. A second liter may be administered over a 1- to 3-hour period at the start of cidofovir infusion or immediately following infusion, if tolerated

Dosing adjustment in renal impairment:

Changes in renal function during therapy: If the creatinine increases by 0.3-0.4 mg/dL, reduce the cidofovir dose to 3 mg/kg; discontinue therapy for increases ≥0.5 mg/dL or development of ≥3+ proteinuria

Pre-existing renal impairment: Use is contraindicated with serum creatinine >1.5 mg/dL, Cl_{cr} <55 mL/minute, or urine protein ≥100 mg/dL (≥2+ proteinuria)

Administration For I.V. infusion only. Infuse over 1 hour. Hydrate with 1 L of 0.9% NS I.V. prior to cidofovir infusion. A second liter may be administered over a 1- to 3-hour period immediately following infusion, if tolerated.

Monitoring Parameters Renal function (Cr, BUN, UAs) within 48 hours of each dose, LFTs, WBCs; intraocular pressure and visual acuity, signs and symptoms of uveitis/iritis

Dosage Forms Excipient information presented when available (limited, particularly for generics); consult specific product labeling.

Injection, solution [preservative free]:

Vistide®: 75 mg/mL (5 mL)

Cilostazol (sil OH sta zol)

Brand Names: U.S. Pletal®

Index Terms OPC-13013

Pharmacologic Category Antiplatelet Agent; Phosphodiesterase Enzyme Inhibitor

Use Symptomatic management of peripheral vascular disease, primarily intermittent claudication

Unlabeled Use Adjunct with aspirin and clopidogrel for prevention of stent thrombosis and restenosis after coronary stent placement

Pregnancy Risk Factor C

Pregnancy Considerations In animal studies, abnormalities of the skeletal, renal and cardiovascular system were increased. In addition, the incidence of stillbirth and decreased birth weights were increased.

Lactation Excretion in breast milk unknown/not recommended

Contraindications Hypersensitivity to cilostazol or any component of the formulation; heart failure (HF) of any severity; hemostatic disorders or active bleeding

Warnings/Precautions [U.S. Boxed Warning]: The use of this drug is contraindicated in patients with heart failure. Use with caution in severe underlying heart disease. Use with caution in patients receiving other platelet aggregation inhibitors or in patients with thrombocytopenia. Discontinue therapy if thrombocytopenia or leukopenia occur; progression to agranulocytosis (reversible) has been reported when cilostazol was not immediately stopped. When cilostazol and clopidogrel are used concurrently, manufacturer recommends checking bleeding times. Withhold for at least 4-6 half-lives prior to elective surgical procedures. Use with caution in patients receiving CYP3A4 inhibitors (eg, ketoconazole or erythromycin) or CYP2C19 inhibitors (eg, omeprazole). If concurrent use is warranted, consider dosage adjustment of cilostazol. Use caution in moderate-to-severe hepatic impairment. Use cautiously in severe renal impairment (Cl_{cr} <25 mL/minute).

Adverse Reactions

>10%:

Central nervous system: Headache (27% to 34%)

Gastrointestinal: Abnormal stools (12% to 15%), diarrhea (12% to 19%)

Respiratory: Rhinitis (7% to 12%)

Miscellaneous: Infection (10% to 14%)

2% to 10%:

Cardiovascular: Peripheral edema (7% to 9%), palpitation (5% to 10%), tachycardia (4%)

Central nervous system: Dizziness (9% to 10%), vertigo (up to 3%)

Gastrointestinal: Dyspepsia (6%), nausea (6% to 7%), abdominal pain (4% to 5%), flatulence (2% to 3%)

Neuromuscular & skeletal: Back pain (6% to 7%), myalgia (2% to 3%)

Respiratory: Pharyngitis (7% to 10%), cough (3% to 4%)

<2% (Limited to important or life-threatening): Agranulocytosis, anemia, aplastic anemia, asthma, atrial fibrillation, atrial flutter, blindness, blood pressure increased, bursitis, cardiac arrest, cerebral infarction/ischemia, cerebrovascular accident, chest pain, CHF, cholelithiasis, colitis, coronary stent thrombosis, cystitis, diabetes mellitus, duodenal ulcer, duodenitis, esophageal hemorrhage, esophagitis, extradural hematoma, gastrointestinal hemorrhage, gout, granulocytopenia, hemorrhage, hepatic dysfunction, hot flashes, hyperglycemia, hypotension, interstitial pneumonia, intracranial hemorrhage, jaundice, leukopenia, myocardial infarction/ischemia, neuralgia, nodal arrhythmia, pain, periodontal abscess, peptic ulcer, pneumonia, polycythemia, postural hypotension, pulmonary hemorrhage, pruritus, QT_c prolongation, rectal hemorrhage, retinal hemorrhage, retroperitoneal hemorrhage, Stevens-Johnson syndrome, subcutaneous hemorrhage, subdural hematoma, supraventricular tachycardia, syncope, thrombocytopenia, thrombosis, torsade de pointes, uric acid increased, ventricular tachycardia

Drug Interactions

Metabolism/Transport Effects Substrate of CYP1A2 (minor), CYP2C19 (major), CYP2D6 (minor), CYP3A4 (major); **Note:** Assignment of Major/Minor substrate status based on clinically relevant drug interaction potential

Avoid Concomitant Use

Avoid concomitant use of Cilostazol with any of the following: Conivaptan

Increased Effect/Toxicity

Cilostazol may increase the levels/effects of: Anticoagulants; Antiplatelet Agents; Collagenase (Systemic); Drotrecogin Alfa (Activated); Ibritumomab; Rivaroxaban; Salicylates; Thrombolytic Agents; Tositumomab and Iodine I 131 Tositumomab

The levels/effects of Cilostazol may be increased by: Antifungal Agents (Azole Derivatives, Systemic); Conivaptan; CYP2C19 Inhibitors (Moderate); CYP2C19 Inhibitors (Strong); CYP3A4 Inhibitors (Moderate); CYP3A4 Inhibitors (Strong); Dasatinib; Esomeprazole; Glucosamine; Herbs (Anticoagulant/Antiplatelet Properties); Macrolide Antibiotics; Nonsteroidal Anti-Inflammatory Agents; Omega-3-Acid Ethyl Esters; Omeprazole; Pentosan Polysulfate Sodium; Pentoxifylline; Prostacyclin Analogues; Vitamin E

Decreased Effect

The levels/effects of Cilostazol may be decreased by: CYP3A4 Inducers (Strong); Cyproterone; Deferasirox; Herbs (CYP3A4 Inducers); Nonsteroidal Anti-Inflammatory Agents; Peginterferon Alfa-2b; Tocilizumab

Ethanol/Nutrition/Herb Interactions

Food: Taking cilostazol with a high-fat meal may increase peak concentration by 90%. Avoid concurrent ingestion of grapefruit juice due to the potential to inhibit CYP3A4.

Herb/Nutraceutical: St John's wort may decrease the levels/effects of cilostazol. Avoid alfalfa, anise, bilberry, bladderwrack, bromelain, cat's claw, chamomile, coleus, cordyceps, dong quai, evening primrose oil, fenugreek, feverfew, garlic, ginger, ginkgo biloba, ginseng (American), ginseng (Panax), ginseng (Siberian), grape seed, green tea, guggul, horse chestnut seed, horseradish, licorice, prickly ash, red clover, reishi, SAMe (S-adenosylmethionine), sweet clover, turmeric, white willow (all have additional antiplatelet activity).

Stability Store at 25°C (77°F); excursions permitted to 15°C to 30°C (59°F to 86°F).

Mechanism of Action Cilostazol and its metabolites are inhibitors of phosphodiesterase III. As a result, cyclic AMP is increased leading to reversible inhibition of platelet aggregation, vasodilation, and inhibition of vascular smooth muscle cell proliferation.

Pharmacodynamics/Kinetics

Onset of action: 2-4 weeks; may require up to 12 weeks

Protein binding: Cilostazol 95% to 98%; active metabolites 66% to 97%

Metabolism: Hepatic via CYP3A4 (primarily), 1A2, 2C19, and 2D6; at least one metabolite has significant activity

Half-life elimination: 11-13 hours

Excretion: Urine (74%) and feces (20%) as metabolites

Dosage Adults: Oral: 100 mg twice daily

Dosage adjustment for cilostazol with concomitant medications:

CYP2C19 inhibitors (see Drug Interactions): Dosage of cilostazol should be reduced to 50 mg twice daily

CYP3A4 inhibitors (see Drug Interactions): Dosage of cilostazol should be reduced to 50 mg twice daily

Dietary Considerations It is best to take cilostazol 30 minutes before or 2 hours after meals.

Administration Administer cilostazol 30 minutes before or 2 hours after meals.

Dosage Forms Excipient information presented when available (limited, particularly for generics); consult specific product labeling.

Tablet, oral: 50 mg, 100 mg

Pletal®: 50 mg, 100 mg

◆ **Ciloxan®** *see* Ciprofloxacin (Ophthalmic) *on page 366*

Cimetidine (sye MET i deen)

Brand Names: U.S. Tagamet HB 200® [OTC]

Brand Names: Canada Apo-Cimetidine®; Dom-Cimetidine; Mylan-Cimetidine; Novo-Cimetidine; Nu-Cimet; PMS-Cimetidine; Tagamet® HB

Pharmacologic Category Histamine H_2 Antagonist

Additional Appendix Information

Beers Criteria – Potentially Inappropriate Medications for Geriatrics *on page 1973*

Use Short-term treatment of active duodenal ulcers and benign gastric ulcers; maintenance therapy of duodenal ulcer; treatment of gastric hypersecretory states; treatment of gastroesophageal reflux disease (GERD)

OTC labeling: Prevention or relief of heartburn, acid indigestion, or sour stomach

Unlabeled Use Part of a multidrug regimen for *H. pylori* eradication to reduce the risk of duodenal ulcer recurrence

Pregnancy Risk Factor B

Pregnancy Considerations Teratogenic effects were not observed in animal reproduction studies; therefore, cimetidine is classified as pregnancy category B. Cimetidine crosses the placenta. An increased risk of congenital malformations or adverse events in the newborn has generally not been observed following maternal use of cimetidine during pregnancy. Histamine H_2 antagonists have been evaluated for the treatment of gastroesophageal reflux disease (GERD), as well as gastric and duodenal ulcers during pregnancy. Although if needed, cimetidine is not the agent of choice. Histamine H_2 antagonists may be used for aspiration prophylaxis prior to cesarean delivery.

Lactation Enters breast milk/not recommended (AAP rates "compatible"; AAP 2001 update pending)

Contraindications Hypersensitivity to cimetidine, any component of the formulation, or other H_2 antagonists

Warnings/Precautions Reversible confusional states, usually clearing within 3-4 days after discontinuation, have been linked to use. Increased age (>50 years) and renal or hepatic impairment are thought to be associated. May be inappropriate for use in the elderly due to risk of confusion and other CNS effects (Beers Criteria). Dosage should be adjusted in renal/hepatic impairment or in patients receiving drugs metabolized through the P450 system.

Over the counter (OTC) cimetidine should not be taken by individuals experiencing painful swallowing, vomiting with blood, or bloody or black stools; medical attention should be sought. A physician should be consulted prior to use when pain in the stomach, shoulder, arms or neck is present; if heartburn has occurred for >3 months; or if unexplained weight loss, or nausea and vomiting occur. Frequent wheezing, shortness of breath, lightheadedness, or sweating, especially with chest pain or heartburn, should also be reported. Consultation of a healthcare provider should occur by patients if also taking theophylline, phenytoin, or warfarin; if heartburn or stomach pain continues or worsens; or if use is required for >14 days. Symptoms of GI distress may be associated with a variety of conditions; symptomatic response to H_2 antagonists does not rule out the potential for significant pathology (eg, malignancy). OTC cimetidine is not approved for use in patients <12 years of age.

Adverse Reactions

1% to 10%:

Central nervous system: Headache (2% to 4%), dizziness (1%), somnolence (1%), agitation

Endocrine & metabolic: Gynecomastia (<1% to 4%)

Gastrointestinal: Diarrhea (1%)

Frequency not defined:

Cardiovascular: AV block, bradycardia, hypotension, tachycardia, vasculitis

Central nervous system: Confusion, fever

Dermatologic: Alopecia, erythema multiforme, exfoliative dermatitis, Stevens-Johnson syndrome, toxic epidermal necrolysis, rash

Endocrine & metabolic: Edema of the breasts, sexual ability decreased

Gastrointestinal: Nausea, pancreatitis, vomiting

Hematologic: Agranulocytosis, aplastic anemia, hemolytic anemia (immune-based), neutropenia, pancytopenia, thrombocytopenia

Hepatic: ALT increased, AST increased, hepatic fibrosis (case report)

Neuromuscular & skeletal: Arthralgia, myalgia, polymyositis

Renal: Creatinine increased, interstitial nephritis

Miscellaneous: Anaphylaxis, pneumonia (causal relationship not established)

Drug Interactions

Metabolism/Transport Effects **Substrate** of P-glycoprotein; **Inhibits** CYP1A2 (moderate), CYP2C19 (moderate), CYP2C9 (weak), CYP2D6 (moderate), CYP2E1 (weak), CYP3A4 (moderate)

Avoid Concomitant Use

Avoid concomitant use of Cimetidine with any of the following: Clopidogrel; Delavirdine; Dofetilide; Epirubicin; Pimozide; Thioridazine; Tolvaptan

Increased Effect/Toxicity

Cimetidine may increase the levels/effects of: Alfentanil; Amiodarone; Anticonvulsants (Hydantoin); ARIPiprazole; Benzodiazepines (metabolized by oxidation); Bromazepam; Budesonide (Systemic, Oral Inhalation); Calcium Channel Blockers; CarBAMazepine; Carmustine; Carvedilol; Cisapride; CloZAPine; Colchicine; CYP1A2 Substrates; CYP2C19 Substrates; CYP2D6 Substrates; CYP3A4 Substrates; Dexmethylphenidate; Dofetilide; ▶

Epirubicin; Eplerenone; Everolimus; Fesoterodine; Halofantrine; Lurasidone; MetFORMIN; Methylphenidate; Moclobemide; Nebivolol; Nicotine; Pentoxifylline; Pimecrolimus; Pimozide; Pramipexole; Praziquantel; Procainamide; Propafenone; QuiNIDine; QuiNINE; Roflumilast; Salmeterol; Saquinavir; Saxagliptin; Selective Serotonin Reuptake Inhibitors; Sulfonylureas; Theophylline Derivatives; Thioridazine; Tolvaptan; Tricyclic Antidepressants; Varenicline; Vitamin K Antagonists; Zaleplon; ZOLMitriptan; Zuclopenthixol

The levels/effects of Cimetidine may be increased by: P-glycoprotein/ABCB1 Inhibitors

Decreased Effect

Cimetidine may decrease the levels/effects of: Atazanavir; Cefditoren; Cefpodoxime; Cefuroxime; Clopidogrel; Dasatinib; Delavirdine; Erlotinib; Fosamprenavir; Gefitinib; Indinavir; Iron Salts; Itraconazole; Ketoconazole; Ketoconazole (Systemic); Mesalamine; Nelfinavir; Posaconazole; Rilpivirine

The levels/effects of Cimetidine may be decreased by: P-glycoprotein/ABCB1 Inducers

Ethanol/Nutrition/Herb Interactions

Ethanol: Avoid ethanol (may enhance gastric mucosal irritation).

Food: Cimetidine may increase serum caffeine levels if taken with caffeine. Cimetidine peak serum levels may be decreased if taken with food.

Herb/Nutraceutical: St John's wort may decrease cimetidine levels.

Stability Tablet: Store between 15°C and 30°C (59°F to 86°F). Protect from light.

Mechanism of Action Competitive inhibition of histamine at H_2 receptors of the gastric parietal cells resulting in reduced gastric acid secretion, gastric volume and hydrogen ion concentration reduced

Pharmacodynamics/Kinetics

Onset of action: 1 hour

Duration: 80% reduction in gastric acid secretion for 4-5 hours after 300 mg dose

Absorption: Rapid

Distribution: 1.3 L/kg

Protein binding: 20%

Metabolism: Partially hepatic, forms metabolites

Bioavailability: 60% to 70%

Half-life elimination: Neonates: 3.6 hours; Children: 1.4 hours; Adults: 2 hours

Time to peak, serum: Oral: 1-2 hours

Excretion: Primarily urine (48% as unchanged drug); feces (some)

Dosage Oral:

Children: 20-40 mg/kg/day in divided doses every 6 hours

Children ≥12 years and Adults: Heartburn, acid indigestion, sour stomach (OTC labeling): 200 mg up to twice daily; may take 30 minutes prior to eating foods or beverages expected to cause heartburn or indigestion

Adults:

Short-term treatment of active ulcers: 300 mg 4 times/day or 800 mg at bedtime or 400 mg twice daily for up to 8 weeks

Note: Higher doses of 1600 mg at bedtime for 4 weeks may be beneficial for a subpopulation of patients with larger duodenal ulcers (>1 cm defined endoscopically) who are also heavy smokers (≥1 pack/day).

Duodenal ulcer prophylaxis: 400 mg at bedtime

Gastric hypersecretory conditions: 300-600 mg every 6 hours; dosage not to exceed 2.4 g/day

Gastroesophageal reflux disease: 400 mg 4 times/day or 800 mg twice daily for 12 weeks

Helicobacter pylori eradication (unlabeled use): 400 mg twice daily; requires combination therapy with antibiotics

Dosing adjustment/interval in renal impairment: Children and Adults:

Cl_{cr} 10-50 mL/minute: Administer 50% of normal dose

Cl_{cr} <10 mL/minute: Administer 25% of normal dose

Hemodialysis: Slightly dialyzable (5% to 20%); administer after dialysis

Dosing adjustment/comments in hepatic impairment: Usual dose is safe in mild liver disease but use with caution and in reduced dosage in severe liver disease; increased risk of CNS toxicity in cirrhosis suggested by enhanced penetration of CNS

Administration Administer with meals so that the drug's peak effect occurs at the proper time (peak inhibition of gastric acid secretion occurs at 1 and 3 hours after dosing in fasting subjects and approximately 2 hours in nonfasting subjects; this correlates well with the time food is no longer in the stomach offering a buffering effect)

Monitoring Parameters CBC, gastric pH, occult blood with GI bleeding; monitor renal function to correct dose.

Dosage Forms Excipient information presented when available (limited, particularly for generics); consult specific product labeling.

Solution, oral, as hydrochloride [strength expressed as base]: 300 mg/5 mL (237 mL, 473 mL)

Tablet, oral: 200 mg, 300 mg, 400 mg, 800 mg

Tagamet HB 200®: 200 mg

Extemporaneous Preparations Note: Commercial oral solution is available (strength expressed as base: 60 mg/mL)

A 60 mg/mL oral suspension may be made with tablets. Place twenty-four 300 mg tablets in 5 mL of sterile water for ~3-5 minutes to dissolve film coating. Crush tablets in a mortar and reduce to a fine powder. Add 10 mL of glycerin and mix to a uniform paste; mix while adding Simple Syrup, NF in incremental proportions to **almost** 120 mL; transfer to a calibrated bottle, rinse mortar with vehicle, and add quantity of vehicle sufficient to make 120 mL. Label "shake well" and "refrigerate". Stable for 17 days.

Nahata MC, Pai VB, and Hipple TF, *Pediatric Drug Formulations*, 5th ed, Cincinnati, OH: Harvey Whitney Books Co, 2004.

◆ **Cimzia®** *see* Certolizumab Pegol *on page* 328

Cinacalcet (sin a KAL cet)

Brand Names: U.S. Sensipar®

Brand Names: Canada Sensipar®

Index Terms AMG 073; Cinacalcet Hydrochloride

Pharmacologic Category Calcimimetic

Use Treatment of secondary hyperparathyroidism in patients with chronic kidney disease (CKD) on dialysis; treatment of hypercalcemia in patients with parathyroid carcinoma; treatment of severe hypercalcemia in patients with primary hyperparathyroidism who are unable to undergo parathyroidectomy

Pregnancy Risk Factor C

Pregnancy Considerations In animal studies, there were no teratogenic effects observed, although decreased pup weights were noted. There are no adequate or well-controlled studies in pregnant women. Use in pregnancy only if potential benefit to mother justifies risk to the fetus. Women who become pregnant during cinacalcet treatment are encouraged to enroll in Amgen's Pregnancy Surveillance Program (1-800-772-6436).

Lactation Excretion in breast milk unknown/not recommended

Contraindications Hypocalcemia (serum calcium lower than the lower limit of normal range)

Canadian labeling: Additional contraindications (not in U.S. labeling): Hypersensitivity to any component of the formulation

Warnings/Precautions Use is contraindicated in hypocalcemia. Monitor serum calcium and for symptoms of hypocalcemia (eg, cramps, myalgia, paresthesia, seizure, tetany); may require treatment interruption, dose reduction, or initiation (or dose increases) of calcium-based phosphate binder or vitamin D to raise serum calcium depending on calcium levels or symptoms of hypocalcemia. Use with caution in patients with a seizure disorder (seizure threshold is lowered by significant serum calcium reductions); monitor calcium levels closely. Adynamic bone disease may develop if intact parathyroid hormone (iPTH) levels are suppressed (<100 pg/mL).

Use caution in patients with moderate-to-severe hepatic impairment (Child-Pugh classes B and C); monitor serum calcium, serum phosphorus and iPTH closely. In the U.S., the long-term safety and efficacy of cinacalcet has not been evaluated in chronic kidney disease (CKD) patients with hyperparathyroidism not requiring dialysis. Not indicated for CKD patients not receiving dialysis. Although possibly related to lower baseline calcium levels, clinical studies have shown an increased incidence of hypocalcemia (<8.4 mg/dL) in patients not requiring dialysis. Monitor serum calcium and iPTH concentrations closely in patients on concurrent CYP3A4 inhibitors; dosage adjustment may be required. Cinacalcet is a strong inhibitor of CYP2D6; if on concurrent therapy with a CYP2D6 substrate, dosage adjustment of the CYP2D6 substrate may be necessary. May cause a decrease in testosterone levels (free and total); although below normal testosterone levels may occur in patients with end-stage renal disease, the clinical significance has not been determined. Use with caution in patients with cardiovascular disease; idiosyncratic hypotension, worsening of heart failure, and/or arrhythmia have been reported in patients with impaired cardiovascular function; may correlate with decreased serum calcium.

Adverse Reactions

>10%:

Central nervous system: Fatigue (12% to 21%), headache (≤21%), depression (10% to 18%)

Endocrine & metabolic: Hypocalcemia (≤66%), dehydration (≤24%), hypercalcemia (12% to 21%)

Gastrointestinal: Nausea (31% to 66%), vomiting (27% to 52%), diarrhea (≤21%), anorexia (6% to 21%), constipation (10% to 18%)

Hematologic: Anemia (6% to 17%)

Neuromuscular & skeletal: Parasthesia (14% to 29%), fracture (12% to 21%), weakness (7% to 17%), arthralgia (6% to 17%), myalgia (≤15%), limb pain (10% to 12%)

Respiratory: Upper respiratory infection (10% to 12%)

1% to 10%:

Cardiovascular: Hypertension (≤7%)

Central nervous system: Dizziness (≤10%), seizure (1%)

Endocrine & metabolic: Testosterone decreased

Neuromuscular & skeletal: Chest pain (noncardiac; ≤6%)

Postmarketing and/or case reports: Adynamic bone disease, angioedema, arrhythmia, heart failure, hypersensitivity reactions, hypotension (idiosyncratic), rash, urticaria

Drug Interactions

Metabolism/Transport Effects Substrate of CYP1A2 (minor), CYP2D6 (minor), CYP3A4 (major); **Note:** Assignment of Major/Minor substrate status based on clinically relevant drug interaction potential; **Inhibits** CYP2D6 (strong)

Avoid Concomitant Use

Avoid concomitant use of Cinacalcet with any of the following: Conivaptan; Pimozide; Tamoxifen; Thioridazine

Increased Effect/Toxicity

Cinacalcet may increase the levels/effects of: Atomoxetine; CYP2D6 Substrates; Fesoterodine; Iloperidone; Nebivolol; Pimozide; Propafenone; Tamoxifen; Tetrabenazine; Thioridazine; Tricyclic Antidepressants

The levels/effects of Cinacalcet may be increased by: Antifungal Agents (Azole Derivatives, Systemic); Conivaptan; CYP3A4 Inhibitors (Moderate); CYP3A4 Inhibitors (Strong); Dasatinib

Decreased Effect

Cinacalcet may decrease the levels/effects of: Codeine; Iloperidone; Tacrolimus; Tacrolimus (Systemic); TraMADol

The levels/effects of Cinacalcet may be decreased by: Cyproterone; Peginterferon Alfa-2b; Tocilizumab

Ethanol/Nutrition/Herb Interactions Food: Food increases bioavailability.

Stability Store at 25°C (77°F); excursions permitted to 15°C to 30°C (59°F to 86°F).

Mechanism of Action Increases the sensitivity of the calcium-sensing receptor on the parathyroid gland thereby, concomitantly lowering parathyroid hormone (PTH), serum calcium, and serum phosphorus levels, preventing progressive bone disease and adverse events associated with mineral metabolism disorders.

Pharmacodynamics/Kinetics

Distribution: V_d: ~1000 L

Protein binding: ~93% to 97%

Metabolism: Hepatic (extensive) via CYP3A4, 2D6, 1A2; forms inactive metabolites

Half-life elimination: Terminal: 30-40 hours; moderate hepatic impairment: 65 hours; severe hepatic impairment: 84 hours

Time to peak, plasma: ~2-6 hours

Excretion: Urine ~80% (as metabolites); feces ~15%

Dosage Oral: Adults: **Do not titrate dose more frequently than every 2-4 weeks.** Dosage adjustment may be required in patients on concurrent CYP3A4 inhibitors.

Secondary hyperparathyroidism: Initial: 30 mg once daily (maximum daily dose: 180 mg); increase dose incrementally (60 mg, 90 mg, 120 mg, 180 mg once daily) as necessary to maintain iPTH level between 150-300 pg/mL.

Parathyroid carcinoma, primary hyperparathyroidism: Initial: 30 mg twice daily (maximum daily dose: 360 mg daily as 90 mg 4 times/day); increase dose incrementally (60 mg twice daily, 90 mg twice daily, 90 mg 3-4 times/day) as necessary to normalize serum calcium levels.

Elderly: No adjustment required; refer to adult dosing

Dosage adjustment for hypocalcemia:

If serum calcium >7.5 mg/dL but <8.4 mg/dL **or** if hypocalcemia symptoms occur: Use calcium-containing phosphate binders and/or vitamin D to raise calcium levels.

If serum calcium <7.5 mg/dL **or** if hypocalcemia symptoms persist and the dose of vitamin D cannot be increased: Withhold cinacalcet until serum calcium ≥8 mg/dL and/or symptoms of hypocalcemia resolve. Reinitiate cinacalcet at the next lowest dose.

If iPTH <150-300 pg/mL: Reduce dose or discontinue cinacalcet and/or vitamin D.

Dosage adjustment in renal impairment: No adjustment required.

Dosage adjustment in hepatic impairment: Patients with moderate-to-severe dysfunction (Child-Pugh classes B and C) have an increased exposure to cinacalcet and increased half-life. Dosage adjustments may be necessary based on serum calcium, serum phosphorus and/or iPTH.

Dietary Considerations Take with food or shortly after a meal. May be taken with vitamin D and/or phosphate binders.

Administration Administer with food or shortly after a meal. Do not break or divide tablet; should be taken whole.

Monitoring Parameters

Secondary hyperparathyroidism: Serum calcium and phosphorus levels prior to initiation and within a week of initiation or dosage adjustment; iPTH should be measured 1-4 weeks after initiation or dosage adjustment. After the maintenance dose is established, monthly calcium and phosphorus levels and iPTH every 1-3 months are required. Wait at least 12 hours after dose before drawing iPTH levels.

Parathyroid carcinoma and primary hyperparathyroidism: Serum calcium levels prior to initiation and within a week of initiation or dosage adjustment; once maintenance dose is established, obtain serum calcium every 2 months.

Reference Range

CKD K/DOQI guidelines definition of stages; chronic disease is kidney damage or GFR <60 mL/minute/1.73 m^2 for ≥3 months:

Stage 2: GFR 60-89 mL/minute/1.73 m^2 (kidney damage with mild decrease GFR)

Stage 3: GFR 30-59 mL/minute/1.73 m^2 (moderate decrease GFR)

Stage 4: GFR 15-29 mL/minute/1.73 m^2 (severe decrease GFR)

Stage 5: GFR <15 mL/minute/1.73 m^2 or dialysis (kidney failure)

Target range for iPTH: Adults:

Stage 3 CKD: 35-70 pg/mL

Stage 4 CKD: 70-110 pg/mL

Stage 5 CKD: 150-300 pg/mL

Serum phosphorus: Adults:

Stage 3 and 4 CKD: ≥2.7 to <4.6 mg/dL

Stage 5 CKD: 3.5-5.5 mg/dL

Serum calcium-phosphorus product: Adults: Stage 3-5 CKD: <55 mg^2/dL^2

Dosage Forms Excipient information presented when available (limited, particularly for generics); consult specific product labeling.

Tablet, oral:

Sensipar®: 30 mg, 60 mg, 90 mg

- **Cinacalcet Hydrochloride** *see* Cinacalcet *on page 360*
- **Cinryze™** *see* C1 Inhibitor (Human) *on page 257*
- **Cipralex® (Can)** *see* Escitalopram *on page 620*
- **Cipro®** *see* Ciprofloxacin (Systemic) *on page 362*
- **Cipro® XL (Can)** *see* Ciprofloxacin (Systemic) *on page 362*
- **Ciprodex®** *see* Ciprofloxacin and Dexamethasone *on page 366*

Ciprofloxacin (Systemic) (sip roe FLOKS a sin)

Brand Names: U.S. Cipro®; Cipro® I.V.; Cipro® XR

Brand Names: Canada Apo-Ciproflox®; Cipro®; Cipro® XL; CO Ciprofloxacin; Dom-Ciprofloxacin; Mint-Ciprofloxacin; Mylan-Ciprofloxacin; Novo-Ciprofloxacin; PHL-Ciprofloxacin; PMS-Ciprofloxacin; PRO-Ciprofloxacin; RAN™-Ciprofloxacin; ratio-Ciprofloxacin; Riva-Ciprofloxacin; Sandoz-Ciprofloxacin; Taro-Ciprofloxacin

Index Terms Ciprofloxacin Hydrochloride

Pharmacologic Category Antibiotic, Quinolone

Additional Appendix Information

Antibiotic Treatment of Adults With Infective Endocarditis *on page 1956*

Prevention of Wound Infection and Sepsis in Surgical Patients *on page 1954*

Use

Children: Complicated urinary tract infections and pyelonephritis due to *E. coli*. **Note:** Although effective, ciprofloxacin is not the drug of first choice in children.

Children and Adults: To reduce incidence or progression of disease following exposure to aerolized *Bacillus anthracis*.

Adults: Treatment of the following infections when caused by susceptible bacteria: Urinary tract infections; acute uncomplicated cystitis in females; chronic bacterial prostatitis; lower respiratory tract infections (including acute exacerbations of chronic bronchitis); acute sinusitis; skin and skin structure infections; bone and joint infections; complicated intra-abdominal infections (in combination with metronidazole); infectious diarrhea; typhoid fever due to *Salmonella typhi* (eradication of chronic typhoid carrier state has not been proven); uncomplicated cervical and urethra gonorrhea (due to *N. gonorrhoeae*); nosocomial pneumonia; empirical therapy for febrile neutropenic patients (in combination with piperacillin)

Note: As of April 2007, the CDC no longer recommends the use of fluoroquinolones for the treatment of gonococcal disease.

Unlabeled Use Acute pulmonary exacerbations in cystic fibrosis (children); cutaneous/gastrointestinal/oropharyngeal anthrax (treatment, children and adults); disseminated gonococcal infection (adults); chancroid (adults); prophylaxis to *Neisseria meningitidis* following close contact with an infected person; empirical therapy (oral) for febrile neutropenia in low-risk cancer patients; HACEK group endocarditis; infectious diarrhea (children); periodontitis

Pregnancy Risk Factor C

Pregnancy Considerations Adverse events have been observed in some animal studies; therefore, the manufacturer classifies ciprofloxacin as pregnancy category C. Ciprofloxacin crosses the placenta and produces measurable concentrations in the amniotic fluid and cord serum. An increased risk of teratogenic effects has not been observed in animals or humans following ciprofloxacin use during pregnancy; however, because of concerns of cartilage damage in immature animals, ciprofloxacin should only be used during pregnancy if a safer option is not available. Ciprofloxacin is recommended for prophylaxis and treatment of pregnant women exposed to anthrax. Serum concentrations of ciprofloxacin may be lower during pregnancy than in nonpregnant patients.

Lactation Enters breast milk/not recommended (AAP rates "compatible"; AAP 2001 update pending)

Medication Guide Available Yes

Contraindications Hypersensitivity to ciprofloxacin, any component of the formulation, or other quinolones; concurrent administration of tizanidine

Warnings/Precautions **[U.S. Boxed Warning]: There have been reports of tendon inflammation and/or rupture with quinolone antibiotics; risk may be increased with concurrent corticosteroids, organ transplant recipients, and in patients >60 years of age.** Rupture of the Achilles tendon sometimes requiring surgical repair has been reported most frequently; but other tendon sites (eg, rotator cuff, biceps) have also been reported. Strenuous physical activity, rheumatoid arthritis, and renal impairment may be an independent risk factor for tendonitis. Discontinue at first sign of tendon inflammation or pain. May occur even after discontinuation of therapy. Use with caution in patients with rheumatoid arthritis; may increase risk of tendon rupture. CNS stimulation may occur (tremor, restlessness, confusion, and very rarely hallucinations or seizures). Use with caution in patients with known or suspected CNS disorder. Potential for seizures, although very rare, may be increased with concomitant NSAID therapy. Use with caution in individuals at risk of seizures. Fluoroquinolones may prolong QT_c interval; avoid use in patients with a history of QT_c prolongation, uncorrected hypokalemia, hypomagnesemia, or concurrent administration of other medications known to prolong the QT interval (including Class Ia and Class III antiarrhythmics, cisapride, erythromycin, antipsychotics, and tricyclic antidepressants). Prolonged use may result in fungal or bacterial superinfection, including *C. difficile*-associated diarrhea (CDAD) and pseudomembranous colitis; CDAD has been observed >2 months postantibiotic treatment. Rarely crystalluria has occurred; urine alkalinity may increase the risk. Ensure adequate hydration during therapy. Adverse effects, including those related to joints and/or surrounding tissues, are increased in pediatric patients and therefore, ciprofloxacin should not be considered as drug of choice in children (exception is anthrax treatment). Rare cases of peripheral neuropathy may occur.

Fluoroquinolones have been associated with the development of serious, and sometimes fatal, hypoglycemia, most often in elderly diabetics but also in patients without diabetes. This occurred most frequently with gatifloxacin (no longer available systemically), but may occur at a lower frequency with other quinolones.

Severe hypersensitivity reactions, including anaphylaxis, have occurred with quinolone therapy. Reactions may present as typical allergic symptoms after a single dose, or may manifest as severe idiosyncratic dermatologic, vascular, pulmonary, renal, hepatic, and/or hematologic events, usually after multiple doses. Prompt discontinuation of drug should occur if skin rash or other symptoms arise. **[U.S. Boxed Warning]: Quinolones may exacerbate myasthenia gravis; avoid use (rare, potentially life-threatening weakness of respiratory muscles may occur).** Use caution in renal impairment. Avoid excessive sunlight and take precautions to limit exposure (eg, loose fitting clothing, sunscreen); may cause moderate-to-severe phototoxicity reactions. Discontinue use if photosensitivity occurs. Since ciprofloxacin is ineffective in the treatment of syphilis and may mask symptoms, all patients should be tested for syphilis at the time of gonorrheal diagnosis and 3 months later. Hemolytic reactions may (rarely) occur with quinolone use in patients with latent or actual G6PD deficiency.

Ciprofloxacin is a potent inhibitor of CYP1A2. Coadministration of drugs which depend on this pathway may lead to substantial increases in serum concentrations and adverse effects.

Adverse Reactions

1% to 10%:

Central nervous system: Neurologic events (children 2%, includes dizziness, insomnia, nervousness, somnolence); fever (children 2%); headache (I.V. administration); restlessness (I.V. administration)

Dermatologic: Rash (children 2%, adults 1%)

Gastrointestinal: Nausea (3%); diarrhea (children 5%, adults 2%); vomiting (children 5%, adults 1%); abdominal pain (children 3%, adults <1%); dyspepsia (children 3%)

Hepatic: ALT increased, AST increased (adults 1%)

Local: Injection site reactions (I.V. administration)

Respiratory: Rhinitis (children 3%)

<1% (Limited to important or life-threatening): Abnormal gait, acute renal failure, agitation, agranulocytosis, albuminuria, allergic reactions, anaphylactic shock, anaphylaxis, anemia, angina pectoris, angioedema, anorexia, anosmia, arthralgia, ataxia, atrial flutter, bone marrow depression (life-threatening), breast pain, bronchospasm, candidiasis, candiduria, cardiopulmonary arrest, cerebral thrombosis, chills, cholestatic jaundice, chromatopsia, confusion, constipation, crystalluria (particularly in alkaline urine), cylindruria, delirium, depersonalization, depression, dizziness, drowsiness, dyspepsia (adults), dysphagia, dyspnea, edema, eosinophilia, erythema multiforme, erythema nodosum, exfoliative dermatitis, fever (adults), fixed eruption, flatulence, gastrointestinal bleeding, hallucinations, headache (oral), hematuria, hemolytic anemia, hepatic failure (some fatal), hepatic necrosis, hyperesthesia, hyperglycemia, hyperpigmentation, hyper-/hypotension, hypertonia, insomnia, interstitial nephritis, intestinal perforation, irritability, jaundice, joint pain, laryngeal edema, lightheadedness, lymphadenopathy, malaise, manic reaction, methemoglobinemia, MI, migraine, moniliasis, myalgia, myasthenia gravis exacerbation, myoclonus, nephritis, nightmares, nystagmus, orthostatic hypotension, palpitation, pancreatitis, pancytopenia (life-threatening or fatal), paranoia, paresthesia, peripheral neuropathy, petechia, photosensitivity, pneumonitis, prolongation of PT/INR, pseudomembranous colitis, psychosis, pulmonary edema, renal calculi, seizure; serum cholesterol, glucose, triglycerides increased; serum sickness-like reactions, Stevens-Johnson syndrome, syncope, tachycardia, taste loss, tendon rupture, tendonitis, thrombophlebitis, tinnitus, torsade de pointes, toxic epidermal necrolysis (Lyell's syndrome), tremor, twitching, urethral bleeding, vaginal candidiasis, vaginitis, vasculitis, ventricular ectopy, visual disturbance, weakness

Drug Interactions

Metabolism/Transport Effects Substrate of P-glycoprotein; **Inhibits** CYP1A2 (strong), CYP3A4 (weak)

Avoid Concomitant Use

Avoid concomitant use of Ciprofloxacin (Systemic) with any of the following: BCG; TiZANidine

Increased Effect/Toxicity

Ciprofloxacin (Systemic) may increase the levels/effects of: Bendamustine; Caffeine; Corticosteroids (Systemic); CYP1A2 Substrates; Erlotinib; Methotrexate; Pentoxifylline; Porfimer; QTc-Prolonging Agents; ROPINIRole; Ropivacaine; Sulfonylureas; Theophylline Derivatives; TiZANidine; Varenicline; Vitamin K Antagonists

The levels/effects of Ciprofloxacin (Systemic) may be increased by: Insulin; Nonsteroidal Anti-Inflammatory Agents; P-glycoprotein/ABCB1 Inhibitors; Probenecid

Decreased Effect

Ciprofloxacin (Systemic) may decrease the levels/effects of: BCG; Fosphenytoin; Mycophenolate; Phenytoin; Sulfonylureas; Typhoid Vaccine

The levels/effects of Ciprofloxacin (Systemic) may be decreased by: Antacids; Calcium Salts; Didanosine; Iron Salts; Lanthanum; Magnesium Salts; P-glycoprotein/ABCB1 Inducers; Quinapril; Sevelamer; Sucralfate; Zinc Salts

Ethanol/Nutrition/Herb Interactions

Food: Food decreases rate, but not extent, of absorption. Ciprofloxacin serum levels may be decreased if taken with dairy products or calcium-fortified juices. Ciprofloxacin may increase serum caffeine levels if taken with caffeine.

Enteral feedings may decrease plasma concentrations of ciprofloxacin probably by >30% inhibition of absorption. Ciprofloxacin should not be administered with enteral feedings. The feeding would need to be discontinued for 1-2 hours prior to and after ciprofloxacin administration. Nasogastric administration produces a greater loss of ciprofloxacin bioavailability than does nasoduodenal administration.

Herb/Nutraceutical: Avoid dong quai, St John's wort (may also cause photosensitization).

Stability

Injection:

Premixed infusion: Store between 5°C to 25°C (41°F to 77°F); avoid freezing. Protect from light.

Vial: Store between 5°C to 30°C (41°F to 86°F); avoid freezing. Protect from light. May be diluted with NS, D_5W, SWFI, $D_{10}W$, $D_5{}^1\!/\!_4NS$, $D_5{}^1\!/\!_2NS$, LR. Diluted solutions of 0.5-2 mg/mL are stable for up to 14 days refrigerated or at room temperature.

Microcapsules for oral suspension: Prior to reconstitution, store below 25°C (77°F); protect from freezing. Following reconstitution, store below 30°C (86°F) for up to 14 days; protect from freezing.

Tablet:

Immediate release: Store below 30°C (86°F).

Extended release: Store at room temperature of 15°C to 30°C (59°F to 86°F).

Mechanism of Action Inhibits DNA-gyrase in susceptible organisms; inhibits relaxation of supercoiled DNA and promotes breakage of double-stranded DNA

Pharmacodynamics/Kinetics

Absorption: Oral: Immediate release tablet: Rapid (~50% to 85%)

Distribution: V_d: 2.1-2.7 L/kg; tissue concentrations often exceed serum concentrations especially in kidneys, gallbladder, liver, lungs, gynecological tissue, and prostatic tissue; CSF concentrations: 10% of serum concentrations (noninflamed meninges), 14% to 37% (inflamed meninges)

Protein binding: 20% to 40%

Metabolism: Partially hepatic; forms 4 metabolites (limited activity)

Half-life elimination: Children: 2.5 hours; Adults: Normal renal function: 3-5 hours

Time to peak: Oral:

Immediate release tablet: 0.5-2 hours

Extended release tablet: Cipro® XR: 1-2.5 hours

Excretion: Urine (30% to 50% as unchanged drug); feces (15% to 43%)

Dosage Note: Extended release tablets and immediate release formulations are not interchangeable. Unless otherwise specified, oral dosing reflects the use of immediate release formulations.

Usual dosage ranges:

Children (see Warnings/Precautions):

Oral: 20-30 mg/kg/day in 2 divided doses; maximum dose: 1.5 g/day

I.V.: 20-30 mg/kg/day divided every 12 hours; maximum dose: 800 mg/day

Adults:

Oral: 250-750 mg every 12 hours

I.V.: 200-400 mg every 12 hours

Indication-specific dosing:

Infants >3 months and Children:

Community-acquired pneumonia (CAP) (IDSA/PIDS, 2011): *H. influenzae,* moderate-to-severe infection (alternative to ampicillin, ceftriaxone, or cefotaxime): I.V.: 30 mg/kg/day divided every 12 hours

Children:

Anthrax:

Inhalational (postexposure prophylaxis):

Oral: 15 mg/kg/dose every 12 hours for 60 days; maximum: 500 mg/dose

I.V.: 10 mg/kg/dose every 12 hours for 60 days; do **not** exceed 400 mg/dose (800 mg/day)

Cutaneous (treatment, CDC guidelines): Oral: 10-15 mg/kg every 12 hours for 60 days (maximum: 1 g/day); amoxicillin 80 mg/kg/day divided every 8 hours is an option for completion of treatment after clinical improvement. **Note:** In the presence of systemic involvement, extensive edema, lesions on head/neck, refer to I.V. dosing for treatment of inhalational/gastrointestinal/oropharyngeal anthrax.

Inhalational/gastrointestinal/oropharyngeal (treatment, CDC guidelines): I.V.: Initial: 10-15 mg/kg every 12 hours for 60 days (maximum: 500 mg/dose); switch to oral therapy when clinically appropriate; refer to adult dosing for notes on combined therapy and duration

Cystic fibrosis (unlabeled use):

Oral: 40 mg/kg/day divided every 12 hours administered following 1 week of I.V. therapy has been reported in a clinical trial; total duration of therapy: 10-21 days

I.V.: 30 mg/kg/day divided every 8 hours for 1 week, followed by oral therapy, has been reported in a clinical trial

Urinary tract infection (complicated) or pyelonephritis:

Oral: 20-30 mg/kg/day in 2 divided doses (every 12 hours) for 10-21 days; maximum: 1.5 g/day

I.V.: 6-10 mg/kg every 8 hours for 10-21 days (maximum: 400 mg/dose)

Adults:

Anthrax:

Inhalational (postexposure prophylaxis):

Oral: 500 mg every 12 hours for 60 days

I.V.: 400 mg every 12 hours for 60 days

Cutaneous (treatment, CDC guidelines): Oral: Immediate release formulation: 500 mg every 12 hours for 60 days. **Note:** In the presence of systemic involvement, extensive edema, lesions on head/neck, refer to I.V. dosing for treatment of inhalational/gastrointestinal/oropharyngeal anthrax

Inhalational/gastrointestinal/oropharyngeal (treatment, CDC guidelines): I.V.: 400 mg every 12 hours. **Note:** Initial treatment should include two or more agents predicted to be effective (per CDC recommendations). Continue combined therapy for 60 days.

Bone/joint infections:

Oral: 500-750 mg twice daily for 4-6 weeks

I.V.: Mild-to-moderate: 400 mg every 12 hours for 4-6 weeks; Severe/complicated: 400 mg every 8 hours for 4-6 weeks

Chancroid (unlabeled use): Oral: 500 mg twice daily for 3 days (CDC, 2010)

Endocarditis due to HACEK organisms (AHA guidelines, unlabeled use): Note: Not first-line option; use only if intolerant of beta-lactam therapy:

Oral: 500 mg every 12 hours for 4 weeks

I.V.: 400 mg every 12 hours for 4 weeks

Febrile neutropenia: I.V.: 400 mg every 8 hours for 7-14 days (combination therapy generally recommended)

Gonococcal infections:

Urethral/cervical gonococcal infections: Oral: 250-500 mg as a single dose (CDC recommends concomitant doxycycline or azithromycin due to possible coinfection with *Chlamydia*; **Note:** As of April 2007, the CDC no longer recommends the use of fluoroquinolones for the treatment of uncomplicated gonococcal disease.

Disseminated gonococcal infection (CDC guidelines): Oral: 500 mg twice daily to complete 7 days of therapy (initial treatment with ceftriaxone 1 g I.M./I.V. daily for 24-48 hours after improvement begins); **Note:** As of April 2007, the CDC no longer recommends the use of fluoroquinolones for the treatment of more serious gonococcal disease, unless no other options exist and susceptibility can be confirmed via culture.

Granuloma inguinale (donovanosis) (unlabeled use): Oral: 750 mg twice daily for at least 3 weeks (and until lesions have healed) (CDC, 2010)

Infectious diarrhea: Oral:

Salmonella: 500 mg twice daily for 5-7 days

Shigella: 500 mg twice daily for 3 days

Traveler's diarrhea: Mild: 750 mg for one dose; Severe: 500 mg twice daily for 3 days

Vibrio cholerae: 1 g for one dose

Intra-abdominal, complicated, community-acquired (in combination with metronidazole): Note: Avoid using in settings where *E. coli* susceptibility to fluoroquinolones is <90%:
Oral: 500 mg every 12 hours for 7-14 days
I.V.: 400 mg every 12 hours for 7-14 days; **Note:** 2010 IDSA guidelines recommend treatment duration of 4-7 days (provided source controlled)

Lower respiratory tract, skin/skin structure infections:
Oral: 500-750 mg twice daily for 7-14 days
I.V.: Mild-to-moderate: 400 mg every 12 hours for 7-14 days; Severe/complicated: 400 mg every 8 hours for 7-14 days

Nosocomial pneumonia: I.V.: 400 mg every 8 hours for 10-14 days

Periodontitis (unlabeled use): Oral: 500 mg every 12 hours for 8-10 days

Prostatitis (chronic, bacterial): Oral: 500 mg every 12 hours for 28 days

Sinusitis (acute): Oral: 500 mg every 12 hours for 10 days

Typhoid fever: Oral: 500 mg every 12 hours for 10 days

Urinary tract infection:
Acute uncomplicated, cystitis:
Oral:
Immediate release formulation: 250 mg every 12 hours for 3 days
Extended release formulation (Cipro® XR): 500 mg every 24 hours for 3 days
I.V.: 200 mg every 12 hours for 7-14 days
Complicated (including pyelonephritis):
Oral:
Immediate release formulation: 500 mg every 12 hours for 7-14 days
Extended release formulation (Cipro® XR): 1000 mg every 24 hours for 7-14 days
I.V.: 400 mg every 12 hours for 7-14 days

Elderly: No adjustment needed in patients with normal renal function

Dosing adjustment in renal impairment: Adults:
Cl_{cr} 30-50 mL/minute: Oral: 250-500 mg every 12 hours
Cl_{cr} <30 mL/minute: Acute uncomplicated pyelonephritis or complicated UTI: Oral: Extended release formulation: 500 mg every 24 hours
Cl_{cr} 5-29 mL/minute:
Oral: 250-500 mg every 18 hours
I.V.: 200-400 mg every 18-24 hours

Intermittent hemodialysis (IHD) (administer after hemodialysis on dialysis days): Minimally dialyzable (<10%): Oral: 250-500 mg every 24 hours **or** I.V.: 200-400 mg every 24 hours (Heintz, 2009). **Note:** Dosing dependent on the assumption of 3 times/week, complete IHD sessions.

Continuous renal replacement therapy (CRRT) (Heintz, 2009; Trotman, 2005): Drug clearance is highly dependent on the method of renal replacement, filter type, and flow rate. Appropriate dosing requires close monitoring of pharmacologic response, signs of adverse reactions due to drug accumulation, as well as drug concentrations in relation to target trough (if appropriate). The following are general recommendations only (based on dialysate flow/ultrafiltration rates of 1-2 L/hour and minimal residual renal function) and should not supersede clinical judgment:
CVVH/CVVHD/CVVHDF: I.V.: 200-400 mg every 12-24 hours

Dietary Considerations Food: Drug may cause GI upset; take without regard to meals (manufacturer prefers that immediate release tablet is taken 2 hours after meals). Extended release tablet may be taken with meals that contain dairy products (calcium content <800 mg), but not with dairy products alone.

Dairy products, calcium-fortified juices, oral multivitamins, and mineral supplements: Absorption of ciprofloxacin is decreased by divalent and trivalent cations. The manufacturer states that the usual dietary intake of calcium (including meals which include dairy products) has not been shown to interfere with ciprofloxacin absorption. Immediate release ciprofloxacin and Cipro® XR may be taken 2 hours before or 6 hours after any of these products.

Caffeine: Patients consuming regular large quantities of caffeinated beverages may need to restrict caffeine intake if excessive cardiac or CNS stimulation occurs.

Administration
Oral: May administer with food to minimize GI upset; avoid antacid use; maintain proper hydration and urine output. Administer immediate release ciprofloxacin and Cipro® XR at least 2 hours before or 6 hours after antacids or other products containing calcium, iron, or zinc (including dairy products or calcium-fortified juices). Separate oral administration from drugs which may impair absorption (see Drug Interactions).
Oral suspension: Should not be administered through feeding tubes (suspension is oil-based and adheres to the feeding tube). Patients should avoid chewing on the microcapsules.
Nasogastric/orogastric tube: Crush immediate-release tablet and mix with water. Flush feeding tube before and after administration. Hold tube feedings at least 1 hour before and 2 hours after administration.
Tablet, extended release: Do not crush, split, or chew. May be administered with meals containing dairy products (calcium content <800 mg), but not with dairy products alone.
Parenteral: Administer by slow I.V. infusion over 60 minutes to reduce the risk of venous irritation (burning, pain, erythema, and swelling); final concentration for administration should not exceed 2 mg/mL.

Monitoring Parameters CBC, renal and hepatic function during prolonged therapy

Reference Range Therapeutic: 2.6-3 mcg/mL; Toxic: >5 mcg/mL

Test Interactions Some quinolones may produce a false-positive urine screening result for opiates using commercially-available immunoassay kits. This has been demonstrated most consistently for levofloxacin and ofloxacin, but other quinolones have shown cross-reactivity in certain assay kits. Confirmation of positive opiate screens by more specific methods should be considered.

Additional Information Although the systemic use of ciprofloxacin is only FDA-approved in children for the treatment of complicated UTI and postexposure treatment of inhalation anthrax, use of the fluoroquinolones in pediatric patients is increasing. Current recommendations by the American Academy of Pediatrics note that the systemic use of these agents in children should be restricted to infections caused by multidrug resistant pathogens with no safe or effective alternative, and when parenteral therapy is not feasible or other oral agents are not available.

Dosage Forms Excipient information presented when available (limited, particularly for generics); consult specific product labeling. [DSC] = Discontinued product
Infusion, premixed in D_5W: 200 mg (100 mL); 400 mg (200 mL)
Cipro® I.V.: 200 mg (100 mL); 400 mg (200 mL)
Infusion, premixed in D_5W [preservative free]: 200 mg (100 mL); 400 mg (200 mL)
Injection, solution: 10 mg/mL (20 mL, 40 mL)
Injection, solution [preservative free]: 10 mg/mL (20 mL, 40 mL [DSC])

Microcapsules for suspension, oral:
Cipro®: 250 mg/5 mL (100 mL); 500 mg/5 mL (100 mL) [strawberry flavor]
Tablet, oral, as hydrochloride [strength expressed as base]: 100 mg, 250 mg, 500 mg, 750 mg
Cipro®: 250 mg, 500 mg
Tablet, extended release, oral, as base and hydrochloride [strength expressed as base]: 500 mg, 1000 mg
Cipro® XR: 500 mg, 1000 mg

Extemporaneous Preparations A 50 mg/mL oral suspension may be made using 2 different vehicles (a 1:1 mixture of Ora-Sweet® and Ora-Plus® or a 1:1 mixture of Methylcellulose 1% and Simple Syrup, NF). Crush twenty 500 mg tablets and reduce to a fine powder. Add a small amount of vehicle and mix to a uniform paste; mix while adding the vehicle in geometric proportions to **almost** 200 mL; transfer to a calibrated bottle, rinse mortar with vehicle, and add quantity of vehicle sufficient to make 200 mL. Label "shake well" and "refrigerate". Stable 91 days refrigerated and 70 days at room temperature. **Note:** Microcapsules for oral suspension available (50 mg/mL; 100 mg/mL); not for use in feeding tubes.

Nahata MC, Pai VB, and Hipple TF, *Pediatric Drug Formulations*, 5th ed, Cincinnati, OH: Harvey Whitney Books Co, 2004.

Ciprofloxacin (Ophthalmic) (sip roe FLOKS a sin)

Brand Names: U.S. Ciloxan®
Brand Names: Canada Ciloxan®
Index Terms Ciprofloxacin Hydrochloride
Pharmacologic Category Antibiotic, Ophthalmic; Antibiotic, Quinolone
Use Treatment of superficial ocular infections (corneal ulcers, conjunctivitis) due to susceptible strains
Pregnancy Risk Factor C
Dosage Ophthalmic:
Bacterial conjunctivitis:
Ophthalmic solution: Children >1 year and Adults: Instill 1-2 drops in eye(s) every 2 hours while awake for 2 days and 1-2 drops every 4 hours while awake for the next 5 days
Ophthalmic ointment: Children >2 years and Adults: Apply a 1/2" ribbon into the conjunctival sac 3 times/day for the first 2 days, followed by a 1/2" ribbon applied twice daily for the next 5 days
Corneal ulcer: Ophthalmic solution: Children >1 year and Adults: Instill 2 drops into affected eye every 15 minutes for the first 6 hours, then 2 drops into the affected eye every 30 minutes for the remainder of the first day. On day 2, instill 2 drops into the affected eye hourly. On days 3-14, instill 2 drops into affected eye every 4 hours. Treatment may continue after day 14 if re-epithelialization has not occurred.

Additional Information Complete prescribing information for this medication should be consulted for additional detail.

Dosage Forms Excipient information presented when available (limited, particularly for generics); consult specific product labeling.
Ointment, ophthalmic, as hydrochloride:
Ciloxan®: 3.33 mg/g (3.5 g) [equivalent to ciprofloxacin base 0.3%]
Solution, ophthalmic, as hydrochloride [drops]: 3.5 mg/mL (2.5 mL, 5 mL, 10 mL) [equivalent to ciprofloxacin base 0.3%]
Ciloxan®: 3.5 mg/mL (5 mL) [contains benzalkonium chloride; equivalent to ciprofloxacin base 0.3%]

Ciprofloxacin (Otic) (sip roe FLOKS a sin)

Brand Names: U.S. Cetraxal®
Index Terms Ciprofloxacin Hydrochloride
Pharmacologic Category Antibiotic, Otic; Antibiotic, Quinolone
Use Treatment of acute otitis externa due to susceptible strains of *Pseudomonas aeruginosa* or *Staphylococcus aureus*
Pregnancy Risk Factor C
Dosage Otic: Children ≥1 year and Adults: Acute otitis externa: Instill 0.25 mL solution (contents of 1 single-dose container) into affected ear twice daily for 7 days

Additional Information Complete prescribing information for this medication should be consulted for additional detail.

Dosage Forms Excipient information presented when available (limited, particularly for generics); consult specific product labeling.
Solution, otic, as hydrochloride [preservative free]:
Cetraxal®: 0.5 mg/0.25 mL (14s) [equivalent to ciprofloxacin base 0.2%]

Ciprofloxacin and Dexamethasone
(sip roe FLOKS a sin & deks a METH a sone)

Brand Names: U.S. Ciprodex®
Brand Names: Canada Ciprodex®
Index Terms Ciprofloxacin Hydrochloride and Dexamethasone; Dexamethasone and Ciprofloxacin
Pharmacologic Category Antibiotic, Otic; Antibiotic/Corticosteroid, Otic; Corticosteroid, Otic
Use Treatment of acute otitis media in pediatric patients with tympanostomy tubes or acute otitis externa in children and adults
Pregnancy Risk Factor C
Dosage Otic:
Children: Acute otitis media in patients with tympanostomy tubes or acute otitis externa: Instill 4 drops into affected ear(s) twice daily for 7 days
Adults: Acute otitis externa: Instill 4 drops into affected ear(s) twice daily for 7 days

Additional Information Complete prescribing information for this medication should be consulted for additional detail.

Dosage Forms Excipient information presented when available (limited, particularly for generics); consult specific product labeling.
Suspension, otic:
Ciprodex®: Ciprofloxacin 0.3% and dexamethasone 0.1% (7.5 mL) [contains benzalkonium chloride]

Ciprofloxacin and Hydrocortisone
(sip roe FLOKS a sin & hye droe KOR ti sone)

Brand Names: U.S. Cipro® HC
Brand Names: Canada Cipro® HC
Index Terms Ciprofloxacin Hydrochloride and Hydrocortisone; Hydrocortisone and Ciprofloxacin
Pharmacologic Category Antibiotic/Corticosteroid, Otic
Use Treatment of acute otitis externa, sometimes known as "swimmer's ear"
Pregnancy Risk Factor C
Dosage Children >1 year of age and Adults: Otic: The recommended dosage for all patients is three drops of the suspension in the affected ear twice daily for 7 days; twice-daily dosing schedule is more convenient for patients than that of existing treatments with hydrocortisone, which are typically administered 3 or 4 times a day; a twice-daily dosage schedule may be especially helpful for parents and caregivers of young children

Additional Information Complete prescribing information for this medication should be consulted for additional detail.

Dosage Forms Excipient information presented when available (limited, particularly for generics); consult specific product labeling.

Suspension, otic:

Cipro® HC: Ciprofloxacin hydrochloride 0.2% and hydrocortisone 1% (10 mL) [contains benzyl alcohol]

◆ **Ciprofloxacin Hydrochloride** *see* Ciprofloxacin (Ophthalmic) *on page 366*

◆ **Ciprofloxacin Hydrochloride** *see* Ciprofloxacin (Otic) *on page 366*

◆ **Ciprofloxacin Hydrochloride** *see* Ciprofloxacin (Systemic) *on page 362*

◆ **Ciprofloxacin Hydrochloride and Dexamethasone** *see* Ciprofloxacin and Dexamethasone *on page 366*

◆ **Ciprofloxacin Hydrochloride and Hydrocortisone** *see* Ciprofloxacin and Hydrocortisone *on page 366*

◆ **Cipro® HC** *see* Ciprofloxacin and Hydrocortisone *on page 366*

◆ **Cipro® I.V.** *see* Ciprofloxacin (Systemic) *on page 362*

◆ **Cipro® XR** *see* Ciprofloxacin (Systemic) *on page 362*

Cisatracurium (sis a tra KYOO ree um)

Brand Names: U.S. Nimbex®

Brand Names: Canada Nimbex®

Index Terms Cisatracurium Besylate

Pharmacologic Category Neuromuscular Blocker Agent, Nondepolarizing

Use Adjunct to general anesthesia to facilitate endotracheal intubation and to relax skeletal muscles during surgery; to facilitate mechanical ventilation in ICU patients; does not relieve pain or produce sedation

Pregnancy Risk Factor B

Pregnancy Considerations Adverse events have not been observed in animal reproduction studies.

Lactation Excretion in breast milk unknown/use caution

Contraindications Hypersensitivity to cisatracurium besylate or any component of the formulation

Warnings/Precautions Maintenance of an adequate airway and respiratory support is critical; certain clinical conditions may result in potentiation or antagonism of neuromuscular blockade:

Potentiation: Electrolyte abnormalities, severe hyponatremia, severe hypocalcemia, severe hypokalemia, hypermagnesemia, neuromuscular diseases, acidosis, acute intermittent porphyria, renal failure, hepatic failure

Antagonism: Alkalosis, hypercalcemia, demyelinating lesions, peripheral neuropathies, diabetes mellitus

Increased sensitivity in patients with myasthenia gravis, Eaton-Lambert syndrome; resistance in burn patients (>30% of body) for period of 5-70 days postinjury; resistance in patients with muscle trauma, denervation, immobilization, infection. Cross-sensitivity with other neuromuscular-blocking agents may occur; use extreme caution in patients with previous anaphylactic reactions. Bradycardia may be more common with cisatracurium than with other neuromuscular blocking agents since it has no clinically significant effects on heart rate to counteract the bradycardia produced by anesthetics. Use caution in the elderly. Should be administered by adequately trained individuals familiar with its use. Some dosage forms may contain benzyl alcohol which has been associated with "gasping syndrome" in neonates.

Adverse Reactions <1%: Effects are minimal and transient, bradycardia and hypotension, flushing, pruritus, rash, bronchospasm, acute quadriplegic myopathy syndrome (prolonged use), myositis ossificans (prolonged use)

Drug Interactions

Metabolism/Transport Effects None known.

Avoid Concomitant Use

Avoid concomitant use of Cisatracurium with any of the following: QuiNINE

Increased Effect/Toxicity

Cisatracurium may increase the levels/effects of: Cardiac Glycosides; Corticosteroids (Systemic); OnabotulinumtoxinA; RimabotulinumtoxinB

The levels/effects of Cisatracurium may be increased by: AbobotulinumtoxinA; Aminoglycosides; Calcium Channel Blockers; Capreomycin; Colistimethate; Inhalational Anesthetics; Ketorolac; Ketorolac (Nasal); Ketorolac (Systemic); Lincosamide Antibiotics; Lithium; Loop Diuretics; Magnesium Salts; Polymyxin B; Procainamide; QuiNIDine; QuiNINE; Spironolactone; Tetracycline Derivatives; Vancomycin

Decreased Effect

The levels/effects of Cisatracurium may be decreased by: Acetylcholinesterase Inhibitors; Loop Diuretics

Stability Refrigerate intact vials at 2°C to 8°C (36°F to 46°F). Use vials within 21 days upon removal from the refrigerator to room temperature (25°C to 77°F). Per the manufacturer, dilutions of 0.1-0.2 mg/mL in 0.9% sodium chloride (NS) or dextrose 5% in water (D_5W) are stable for up to 24 hours at room temperature or under refrigeration and in D_5LR for up to 24 hours in the refrigerator. *Additional stability data:* Dilutions of 0.1, 2, and 5 mg/mL in D_5W or NS are stable in the refrigerator for up to 30 days; at room temperature (23°C), dilutions of 0.1 and 2 mg/mL began exhibiting substantial drug loss between 7-14 days; dilutions of 5 mg/mL in D_5W or NS are stable for up to 30 days at room temperature (23°C) (Xu, 1998). Usual concentration: 0.1-0.4 mg/mL.

Mechanism of Action Blocks neural transmission at the myoneural junction by binding with cholinergic receptor sites

Pharmacodynamics/Kinetics

Onset of action: I.V.: 2-3 minutes

Peak effect: 3-5 minutes

Duration: Recovery begins in 20-35 minutes when anesthesia is balanced; recovery is attained in 90% of patients in 25-93 minutes

Metabolism: Undergoes rapid nonenzymatic degradation in the bloodstream (Hofmann elimination) to laudanosine and inactive metabolites; laudanosine may cause CNS stimulation (association not established in humans) and has less accumulation with prolonged use than atracurium due to lower requirements for clinical effect

Half-life elimination: 22-29 minutes

Dosage I.V. (not to be used I.M.):

Operating room administration:

Infants 1-23 months: Intubating dose: 0.15 mg/kg over 5-10 seconds

Children 2-12 years: Intubating dose: 0.1-0.15 mg/kg over 5-15 seconds. (**Note:** When given during stable opioid/nitrous oxide/oxygen anesthesia, 0.1 mg/kg produces maximum neuromuscular block in an average of 2.8 minutes and clinically effective block for 28 minutes.)

Adults: Intubating dose: 0.15-0.2 mg/kg as component of propofol/nitrous oxide/oxygen induction-intubation technique. (**Note:** May produce generally good or excellent conditions for tracheal intubation in 1.5-2 minutes with clinically effective duration of action during propofol anesthesia of 55-61 minutes.) Initial dose after succinylcholine for intubation: 0.1 mg/kg; maintenance dose: 0.03 mg/kg 40-60 minutes after initial dose, then at ~20-minute intervals based on clinical criteria

Children ≥2 years and Adults: Continuous infusion: After an initial bolus, a diluted solution can be given by continuous infusion for maintenance of neuromuscular blockade during extended surgery; adjust the rate of administration according to the patient's response as determined by peripheral nerve stimulation. An initial infusion rate of 3 mcg/kg/minute may be required to rapidly counteract the spontaneous recovery of neuromuscular function; thereafter, a rate of 1-2 mcg/kg/minute should be adequate to maintain continuous neuromuscular block in the 89% to 99% range in most pediatric and adult patients. Consider reduction of the infusion rate by 30% to 40% when administering during stable isoflurane, enflurane, sevoflurane, or desflurane anesthesia. Spontaneous recovery from neuromuscular blockade following discontinuation of infusion of cisatracurium may be expected to proceed at a rate comparable to that following single bolus administration.

Intensive care unit administration: Follow the principles for infusion in the operating room. At initial signs of recovery from bolus dose, begin the infusion at a dose of 3 mcg/kg/minute and adjust rates accordingly; dosage ranges of 0.5-10 mcg/kg/minute have been reported. If patient is allowed to recover from neuromuscular blockade, readministration of a bolus dose may be necessary to quickly re-establish neuromuscular block prior to reinstituting the infusion.

Dosing adjustment in renal impairment: Because slower times to onset of complete neuromuscular block were observed in renal dysfunction patients, extending the interval between the administration of cisatracurium and intubation attempt may be required to achieve adequate intubation conditions.

Administration Administer I.V. only; the use of a peripheral nerve stimulator will permit the most advantageous use of cisatracurium, minimize the possibility of overdosage or underdosage and assist in the evaluation of recovery

Give undiluted as a bolus injection; not for I.M. injection, too much tissue irritation; continuous administration requires the use of an infusion pump

Monitoring Parameters Vital signs (heart rate, blood pressure, respiratory rate)

Additional Information Cisatracurium is classified as an intermediate-duration neuromuscular-blocking agent. It does not appear to have a cumulative effect on the duration of blockade. Neuromuscular-blocking potency is 3 times that of atracurium; maximum block is up to 2 minutes longer than for equipotent doses of atracurium.

Dosage Forms Excipient information presented when available (limited, particularly for generics); consult specific product labeling.

Injection, solution:

Nimbex®: 2 mg/mL (5 mL)

Nimbex®: 2 mg/mL (10 mL) [contains benzyl alcohol]

Nimbex®: 10 mg/mL (20 mL)

◆ **Cisatracurium Besylate** *see* Cisatracurium *on page 367*

CISplatin (SIS pla tin)

Index Terms CDDP; Platinol; Platinol-AQ

Pharmacologic Category Antineoplastic Agent, Alkylating Agent; Antineoplastic Agent, Platinum Analog

Use Treatment of advanced bladder cancer, metastatic testicular cancer, and metastatic ovarian cancer

Unlabeled Use Treatment of head and neck cancer, breast cancer, gastric cancer, esophageal cancer, cervical cancer, prostate cancer, nonsmall cell lung cancer, small cell lung cancer; Hodgkin's and non-Hodgkin's lymphoma; neuroblastoma; sarcomas, myeloma, melanoma, mesothelioma, hepatoblastoma, and osteosarcoma

Pregnancy Risk Factor D

Pregnancy Considerations Animal studies have demonstrated teratogenicity and embryotoxicity. There are no adequate and well-controlled studies in pregnant women. Women of childbearing potential should be advised to avoid pregnancy. If used in pregnancy, or if patient becomes pregnant during treatment, the patient should be apprised of potential hazard to the fetus.

Lactation Enters breast milk/not recommended

Contraindications Hypersensitivity to cisplatin, other platinum-containing compounds, or any component of the formulation (anaphylactic-like reactions have been reported); pre-existing renal impairment; myelosuppression; hearing impairment

Warnings/Precautions Hazardous agent - use appropriate precautions for handling and disposal. **[U.S. Boxed Warning]: Doses >100 mg/m^2 once every 3-4 weeks are rarely used and should be verified with the prescriber.** Patients should receive adequate hydration, with or without diuretics, prior to and for 24 hours after cisplatin administration. Reduce dosage in renal impairment. **[U.S. Boxed Warning]: Cumulative renal toxicity may be severe.** Elderly patients may be more susceptible to nephrotoxicity and peripheral neuropathy; select dose cautiously and monitor closely. **[U.S. Boxed Warnings]: Dose-related toxicities include myelosuppression, nausea, and vomiting. Ototoxicity, especially pronounced in children, is manifested by tinnitus or loss of high frequency hearing and occasionally, deafness.** Severe and possibly irreversible neuropathies may occur with higher than recommended doses or more frequent regimen. Serum electrolytes, particularly magnesium and potassium, should be monitored and replaced as needed during and after cisplatin therapy. When administered as sequential infusions, taxane derivatives (docetaxel, paclitaxel) should be administered before platinum derivatives (carboplatin, cisplatin). **[U.S. Boxed Warnings]: Anaphylactic-like reactions have been reported; may be managed with epinephrine, corticosteroids, and/or antihistamines. Should be administered under the supervision of an experienced cancer chemotherapy physician.**

Adverse Reactions

>10%:

Central nervous system: Neurotoxicity: Peripheral neuropathy is dose- and duration-dependent.

Gastrointestinal: Nausea and vomiting (76% to 100%)

Hematologic: Myelosuppression (25% to 30%; nadir: day 18-23; recovery: by day 39; mild with moderate doses, mild-to-moderate with high-dose therapy)

Hepatic: Liver enzymes increased

Renal: Nephrotoxicity (acute renal failure and chronic renal insufficiency)

Otic: Ototoxicity (10% to 30%; manifested as high frequency hearing loss; ototoxicity is especially pronounced in children)

1% to 10%: Local: Tissue irritation

<1% (Limited to important or life-threatening): Alopecia (mild), anaphylactic reaction, arrhythmias, arterial vasospasm (acute), blurred vision, bradycardia, diarrhea, heart block, heart failure, hemolytic anemia (acute), hemolytic uremic syndrome, hypercholesterolemia, hypocalcemia, hypokalemia, hypomagnesemia, hyponatremia, hypophosphatemia, limb ischemia (acute), mesenteric ischemia (acute), MI, myocardial ischemia, mouth sores, neutropenic typhlitis, optic neuritis, orthostatic hypotension, pancreatitis, papilledema, phlebitis,

reversible posterior leukoencephalopathy syndrome (RPLS), SIADH, stroke, thrombophlebitis, thrombotic thrombocytopenic purpura

Drug Interactions

Metabolism/Transport Effects None known.

Avoid Concomitant Use

Avoid concomitant use of CISplatin with any of the following: BCG; CloZAPine; Natalizumab; Pimecrolimus; Tacrolimus (Topical); Vaccines (Live)

Increased Effect/Toxicity

CISplatin may increase the levels/effects of: Aminoglycosides; CloZAPine; Leflunomide; Natalizumab; Taxane Derivatives; Topotecan; Vaccines (Live); Vinorelbine

The levels/effects of CISplatin may be increased by: Denosumab; Loop Diuretics; Pimecrolimus; Roflumilast; Tacrolimus (Topical); Trastuzumab

Decreased Effect

CISplatin may decrease the levels/effects of: BCG; Coccidioidin Skin Test; Fosphenytoin; Phenytoin; Sipuleucel-T; Vaccines (Inactivated); Vaccines (Live)

The levels/effects of CISplatin may be decreased by: Echinacea

Ethanol/Nutrition/Herb Interactions Herb/Nutraceutical: Avoid black cohosh, dong quai in estrogen-dependent tumors.

Stability

Store intact vials at room temperature of 15°C to 25°C (59°F to 77°F). Protect from light. Do not refrigerate solution, a precipitate may form. Further dilution **stability is dependent on the chloride ion concentration** and should be mixed in solutions of NS (at least 0.3% NaCl). Further dilutions in NS, D_5/0.45% NaCl or D_5/NS to a concentration of 0.05-2 mg/mL are stable for 72 hours at 4°C to 25°C. The infusion solution should have a final sodium chloride concentration ≥0.2%.

After initial entry into the vial, solution is stable for 28 days protected from light or for at least 7 days under fluorescent room light at room temperature.

Standard I.V. dilution: Dose/250-1000 mL NS, D_5/NS, or D_5/0.45% NaCl

Mechanism of Action Inhibits DNA synthesis by the formation of DNA cross-links; denatures the double helix; covalently binds to DNA bases and disrupts DNA function; may also bind to proteins; the *cis*-isomer is 14 times more cytotoxic than the *trans*-isomer; both forms cross-link DNA but cis-platinum is less easily recognized by cell enzymes and, therefore, not repaired. Cisplatin can also bind two adjacent guanines on the same strand of DNA producing intrastrand cross-linking and breakage.

Pharmacodynamics/Kinetics

Distribution: I.V.: Rapidly into tissue; high concentrations in kidneys, liver, ovaries, uterus, and lungs

Protein binding: >90%

Metabolism: Nonenzymatic; inactivated (in both cell and bloodstream) by sulfhydryl groups; covalently binds to glutathione and thiosulfate

Half-life elimination: Initial: 20-30 minutes; Beta: 60 minutes; Terminal: ~24 hours; Secondary half-life: 44-73 hours

Excretion: Urine (>90%); feces (10%)

Dosage VERIFY ANY CISPLATIN DOSE EXCEEDING 100 mg/m² PER COURSE. Pretreatment hydration with 1-2 L of I.V. fluid is recommended. Details concerning dosing in combination regimens should also be consulted.

Children: I.V.:

Hepatoblastoma (unlabeled use; combination chemotherapy): 80 mg/m² continuous infusion over 24 hours on day 1 of a 21-day treatment cycle (Pritchard, 2000)

Medulloblastoma (unlabeled use; combination chemotherapy): 75 mg/m² on either day 0 or day 1 of each chemotherapy cycle (Packer, 2006)

Osteosarcoma (unlabeled use; combination chemotherapy): 60 mg/m²/day for 2 days weeks 2, 7, 25, and 28 (neoadjuvant) or weeks 5, 10, 25, and 28 (adjuvant) (Goorin, 2003)

Bone marrow/stem cell transplant (unlabeled use): Continuous infusion: High dose: 55 mg/m²/day for 72 hours; total dose = 165 mg/m²

Adults: I.V.:

Advanced bladder cancer: 50-70 mg/m² every 3-4 weeks

Metastatic ovarian cancer: 75-100 mg/m² every 4 weeks (combination therapy) or 100 mg/m² every 4 weeks (as a single agent)

Metastatic testicular cancer: 10-20 mg/m²/day for 5 days repeated every 3 weeks (Saxman, 1998)

Head and neck cancer (unlabeled use): 100 mg/m² every 3 weeks for 3 doses (as a single agent) (Bernier, 2004; Cooper, 2004)

Malignant pleural mesothelioma (unlabeled use): 75 mg/m² on day 1 of each 21-day cycle (in combination with pemetrexed) (Vogelzang, 2003) **or** 100 mg/m² on day 1 of a 28-day cycle (in combination with gemcitabine) (Nowak, 2002) **or** 80 mg/m² on day 1 of a 21-day cycle (in combination with gemcitabine) (van Haarst, 2002)

Adults: Intraperitoneal: Ovarian cancer (unlabeled use): 100 mg/m² on day 2 of a 21-day treatment cycle (Armstrong, 2006)

Elderly: Select dose cautiously and monitor closely in the elderly; may be more susceptible to nephrotoxicity and peripheral neuropathy.

Dosing adjustment in renal impairment: Note: The manufacturer(s) recommend that repeat courses of cisplatin should not be given until serum creatinine is <1.5 mg/dL and/or BUN is <25 mg/dL. The FDA-approved labeling does not contain renal dosing adjustment guidelines. The following guidelines have been used by some clinicians:

Aronoff, 2007:

Cl_{cr} 10-50 mL/minute: Administer 75% of dose

Cl_{cr} <10 mL/minute: Administer 50% of dose

Hemodialysis: Partially cleared by hemodialysis

Administer 50% of dose posthemodialysis

Continuous ambulatory peritoneal dialysis (CAPD): Administer 50% of dose

Continuous renal replacement therapy (CRRT): Administer 75% of dose

Kintzel, 1995:

Cl_{cr} 46-60 mL/minute: Administer 75% of dose

Cl_{cr} 31-45 mL/minute: Administer 50% of dose

Cl_{cr} <30 mL/minute: Consider use of alternative drug

Dietary Considerations Some products may contain sodium.

Administration Pretreatment hydration with 1-2 L of fluid is recommended prior to cisplatin administration; adequate hydration and urinary output (>100 mL/hour) should be maintained for 24 hours after administration.

I.V.: Rate of administration has varied from a 15- to 120-minute infusion, 1 mg/minute infusion, 6- to 8-hour infusion, 24-hour infusion, or per protocol.

Monitoring Parameters Renal function (serum creatinine, BUN, Cl_{cr}); electrolytes (particularly magnesium, calcium, potassium) before and within 48 hours after cisplatin therapy; audiography (baseline and prior to each subsequent dose), neurologic exam (with high dose); liver function tests periodically, CBC with differential and platelet count; urine output, urinalysis

Dosage Forms Excipient information presented when available (limited, particularly for generics); consult specific product labeling.

Injection, solution [preservative free]: 1 mg/mL (50 mL, 100 mL, 200 mL)

◆ **13-*cis*-Retinoic Acid** *see* ISOtretinoin *on page 939*

Citalopram (sye TAL oh pram)

Brand Names: U.S. CeleXA®

Brand Names: Canada Apo-Citalopram®; Celexa®; Citalopram-Odan; CO Citalopram; CTP 30; Dom-Citalopram; JAMP-Citalopram; Mint-Citalopram; Mylan-Citalopram; NG-Citalopram; Novo-Citalopram; PHL-Citalopram; PMS-Citalopram; RAN™-Citalo; ratio-Citalopram; Riva-Citalopram; Sandoz-Citalopram; Septa-Citalopram; Teva-Citalopram

Index Terms Citalopram Hydrobromide; Nitalapram

Pharmacologic Category Antidepressant, Selective Serotonin Reuptake Inhibitor

Additional Appendix Information

Antidepressant Agents *on page 1874*

Selective Serotonin Reuptake Inhibitors (SSRIs) Pharmacokinetics *on page 1897*

Use Treatment of depression

Unlabeled Use Smoking cessation; ethanol abuse; obsessive-compulsive disorder (OCD) in children; diabetic neuropathy

Pregnancy Risk Factor C

Pregnancy Considerations Due to adverse effects observed in animal studies, citalopram is classified as pregnancy category C. Citalopram and its metabolites cross the human placenta. Nonteratogenic effects in the newborn following SSRI exposure late in the third trimester include respiratory distress, cyanosis, apnea, seizures, temperature instability, feeding difficulty, vomiting, hypoglycemia, hypo- or hypertonia, hyper-reflexia, jitteriness, irritability, constant crying, and tremor. An increased risk of low birth weight and lower Apgar scores have also been reported. Exposure to SSRIs after the twentieth week of gestation has been associated with persistent pulmonary hypertension of the newborn (PPHN). Adverse effects may be due to toxic effects of the SSRI or drug withdrawal without a taper. The long-term effects of *in utero* SSRI exposure on infant development and behavior are not known.

Due to pregnancy-induced physiologic changes, women who are pregnant may require increased doses of citalopram to achieve euthymia. Women treated for major depression and who are euthymic prior to pregnancy are more likely to experience a relapse when medication is discontinued as compared to pregnant women who continue taking antidepressant medications. The ACOG recommends that therapy with SSRIs or SNRIs during pregnancy be individualized; treatment of depression during pregnancy should incorporate the clinical expertise of the mental health clinician, obstetrician, primary healthcare provider, and pediatrician. If treatment during pregnancy is required, consider tapering therapy during the third trimester in order to prevent withdrawal symptoms in the infant. If this is done and the woman is considered to be at risk of relapse from her major depressive disorder, the medication can be restarted following delivery, although the dose should be readjusted to that required before pregnancy. Treatment algorithms have been developed by the ACOG and the APA for the management of depression in women prior to conception and during pregnancy (Yonkers, 2009).

Lactation Enters breast milk/consider risk:benefit

Medication Guide Available Yes

Contraindications Hypersensitivity to citalopram or any component of the formulation; concomitant use with MAO inhibitors or within 2 weeks of discontinuing MAO inhibitors; concomitant use with pimozide; patients with congenital long QT syndrome

Warnings/Precautions [U.S. Boxed Warning]: Antidepressants increase the risk of suicidal thinking and behavior in children, adolescents, and young adults (18-24 years of age) with major depressive disorder (MDD) and other psychiatric disorders; consider risk prior to prescribing. Short-term studies did not show an increased risk in patients >24 years of age and showed a decreased risk in patients ≥65 years. Closely monitor patients for clinical worsening, suicidality, or unusual changes in behavior, particularly during the initial 1-2 months of therapy or during periods of dosage adjustments (increases or decreases); the patient's family or caregiver should be instructed to closely observe the patient and communicate condition with healthcare provider. A medication guide concerning the use of antidepressants should be dispensed with each prescription. **Citalopram is not FDA approved for use in children.**

The possibility of a suicide attempt is inherent in major depression and may persist until remission occurs. Use caution in high-risk patients. Worsening depression and severe abrupt suicidality that are not part of the presenting symptoms may require discontinuation or modification of drug therapy. The patient's family or caregiver should be alerted to monitor patients for the emergence of suicidality and associated behaviors (such as agitation, irritability, hostility, impulsivity, and hypomania) and call healthcare provider.

May worsen psychosis in some patients or precipitate a shift to mania or hypomania in patients with bipolar disorder. Patients presenting with depressive symptoms should be screened for bipolar disorder. Monotherapy in patients with bipolar disorder should be avoided. **Citalopram is not FDA approved for the treatment of bipolar depression.**

Serotonin syndrome and neuroleptic malignant syndrome (NMS)-like reactions have occurred with serotonin/norepinephrine reuptake inhibitors (SNRIs) and selective serotonin reuptake inhibitors (SSRIs) when used alone, and particularly when used in combination with serotonergic agents (eg, triptans) or antidopaminergic agents (eg, antipsychotics). Concurrent use with MAO inhibitors is contraindicated. May increase the risks associated with electroconvulsive therapy. Has a low potential to impair cognitive or motor performance; caution operating hazardous machinery or driving.

May result in QT_c prolongation. Risk may be increased by conditions or concomitant medications which cause bradycardia, heart failure, hypokalemia, and/or hypomagnesemia; ECG monitoring is recommended. Avoid doses >40 mg/day. Use is contraindicated in patients with congenital long QT syndrome. Use with caution in patients with hepatic or renal dysfunction, in elderly patients, concomitant CNS depressants, and pregnancy (high doses of citalopram have been associated with teratogenicity in animals). Use with caution in patients with a previous seizure disorder or condition predisposing to seizures such as brain damage or alcoholism. Use caution with concomitant use of aspirin, NSAIDs, warfarin, or other drugs that affect coagulation; the risk of bleeding may be potentiated. May cause hyponatremia/SIADH (elderly at increased risk); volume depletion and diuretics may increase risk. May cause or exacerbate sexual dysfunction. Upon discontinuation of citalopram therapy, gradually taper dose. If intolerable symptoms occur following a decrease in dosage or upon discontinuation of therapy, then resuming the previous dose with a more gradual taper should be considered.

Adverse Reactions

>10%:

Central nervous system: Somnolence (18%; dose related), insomnia (15%; dose related)

Gastrointestinal: Nausea (21%), xerostomia (20%)

Miscellaneous: Diaphoresis (11%; dose related)

1% to 10%:

Cardiovascular: Postural hypotension, tachycardia

Central nervous system: Fatigue (5%; dose related), anorexia (4%), anxiety (4%), agitation (3%), fever (2%), yawning (2%; dose related), amnesia, apathy, concentration impaired, confusion, depression, migraine, suicide attempt
Dermatologic: Rash, pruritus
Endocrine & metabolic: Libido decreased (1% to 4%), dysmenorrhea (3%), amenorrhea, sexual dysfunction
Gastrointestinal: Diarrhea (8%), dyspepsia (5%), vomiting (4%), abdominal pain (3%), flatulence, salivation increased, taste perversion, weight gain/loss
Genitourinary: Ejaculation disorder (6%), impotence (3%; dose related), polyuria
Neuromuscular & skeletal: Tremor (8%), arthralgia (2%), myalgia (2%), paresthesia
Ocular: Abnormal accommodation
Respiratory: Rhinitis (5%), upper respiratory tract infection (5%), sinusitis (3%), cough

<1% (Limited to important or life threatening): Acute renal failure, aggressiveness, akathisia, alkaline phosphatase increased, allergic reaction, alopecia, anaphylaxis, anemia, angina pectoris, angioedema, ataxia, bradycardia, cardiac failure, cerebrovascular accident, choreoathetosis, delirium, dyskinesia, dyspnea, dystonia, ecchymosis, eczema, edema (extremities), epidermal necrolysis, epistaxis, erythema multiforme, extrapyramidal symptoms, extrasystoles, gastrointestinal hemorrhage, glaucoma, grand mal seizure, hallucinations, hemolytic anemia, hepatic necrosis, hypertension, hyponatremia, leukocytosis, leukopenia, liver enzymes increased, lymphadenopathy, muscle weakness, myocardial infarction, myoclonus, neuralgia, neuroleptic malignant syndrome, nystagmus, pancreatitis, photosensitivity, priapism, prolactinemia, prothrombin decreased, purpura, QT prolonged, rhabdomyolysis, rigors, serotonin syndrome, SIADH, spontaneous abortion, thrombocytopenia, thrombosis, tinnitus, torsade de pointes, urinary incontinence, urinary retention, urticaria, ventricular arrhythmia, withdrawal syndrome

Drug Interactions

Metabolism/Transport Effects Substrate of CYP2C19 (major), CYP2D6 (minor), CYP3A4 (major); **Note:** Assignment of Major/Minor substrate status based on clinically relevant drug interaction potential; **Inhibits** CYP1A2 (weak), CYP2B6 (weak), CYP2C19 (weak), CYP2D6 (weak)

Avoid Concomitant Use

Avoid concomitant use of Citalopram with any of the following: Artemether; Conivaptan; Dronedarone; Iobenguane I 123; Lumefantrine; MAO Inhibitors; Methylene Blue; Nilotinib; Pimozide; QUEtiapine; QuiNINE; Tetrabenazine; Thioridazine; Toremifene; Tryptophan; Vandetanib; Vemurafenib; Ziprasidone

Increased Effect/Toxicity

Citalopram may increase the levels/effects of: Alpha-/Beta-Blockers; Anticoagulants; Antidepressants (Serotonin Reuptake Inhibitor/Antagonist); Antiplatelet Agents; Aspirin; BusPIRone; CarBAMazepine; CloZAPine; Collagenase (Systemic); Desmopressin; Dextromethorphan; Dronedarone; Drotrecogin Alfa (Activated); Ibritumomab; Lithium; Methadone; Methylene Blue; Metoclopramide; Mexiletine; NSAID (COX-2 Inhibitor); NSAID (Nonselective); Pimozide; QTc-Prolonging Agents; QuiNINE; RisperiDONE; Rivaroxaban; Salicylates; Serotonin Modulators; Tetrabenazine; Thioridazine; Thrombolytic Agents; Toremifene; Tositumomab and Iodine I 131 Tositumomab; TraMADol; Tricyclic Antidepressants; Vandetanib; Vemurafenib; Vitamin K Antagonists; Ziprasidone

The levels/effects of Citalopram may be increased by: Alcohol (Ethyl); Alfuzosin; Analgesics (Opioid); Antipsychotics; Artemether; BusPIRone; Chloroquine; Cimetidine; Ciprofloxacin; Ciprofloxacin (Systemic); CNS Depressants; Conivaptan; CYP2C19 Inhibitors (Moderate); CYP2C19 Inhibitors (Strong); CYP3A4 Inhibitors (Moderate); CYP3A4 Inhibitors (Strong); Fluconazole; Gadobutrol; Glucosamine; Herbs (Anticoagulant/Antiplatelet Properties); Indacaterol; Linezolid; Lumefantrine; Macrolide Antibiotics; MAO Inhibitors; Metoclopramide; Nilotinib; Omega-3-Acid Ethyl Esters; Pentosan Polysulfate Sodium; Pentoxifylline; Prostacyclin Analogues; QUEtiapine; QuiNINE; TraMADol; Tryptophan; Vitamin E

Decreased Effect

Citalopram may decrease the levels/effects of: Iobenguane I 123; Ioflupane I 123

The levels/effects of Citalopram may be decreased by: CarBAMazepine; CYP2C19 Inducers (Strong); CYP3A4 Inducers (Strong); Cyproheptadine; Deferasirox; NSAID (Nonselective); Peginterferon Alfa-2b; Tocilizumab

Ethanol/Nutrition/Herb Interactions

Ethanol: May increase CNS depression; monitor for increased effects with coadministration. Caution patients about effects.
Herb/Nutraceutical: Avoid valerian, St John's wort, SAMe, kava kava, and gotu kola (may increase CNS depression).

Stability Store at 20°C to 25°C (68°F to 77°F); excursions permitted to 15°C to 30°C (59°F to 86°F). Protect from light.

Mechanism of Action A racemic bicyclic phthalane derivative, citalopram selectively inhibits serotonin reuptake in the presynaptic neurons and has minimal effects on norepinephrine or dopamine. Uptake inhibition of serotonin is primarily due to the *S*-enantiomer of citalopram. Displays little to no affinity for serotonin, dopamine, adrenergic, histamine, GABA, or muscarinic receptor subtypes.

Pharmacodynamics/Kinetics

Onset of action: Depression: The onset of action is within a week; however, individual response varies greatly and full response may not be seen until 8-12 weeks after initiation of treatment.
Distribution: V_d: 12 L/kg
Protein binding, plasma: ~80%
Metabolism: Extensively hepatic, via CYP3A4 and 2C19 (major pathways), and 2D6 (minor pathway); forms metabolites, N-demethylcitalopram (DCT) and didemethylcitalopram (DDCT) which are at least eight times less potent than citalopram
Bioavailability: 80%
Half-life elimination: 24-48 hours (average: 35 hours); doubled with hepatic impairment
Time to peak, serum: 1-6 hours, average within 4 hours
Excretion: Urine (Citalopram 10% and DCT 5%)

Note: Clearance was decreased, while AUC and half-life were significantly increased in elderly patients and in patients with hepatic impairment. Mild-to-moderate renal impairment may reduce clearance (17%) and prolong half-life of citalopram. No pharmacokinetic information is available concerning patients with severe renal impairment.

Dosage Oral:

Children and Adolescents: Obsessive-compulsive disorder (unlabeled use): 10-40 mg/day (Mukaddes, 2003; Thomsen, 1997; Thomsen, 2001)
Adults: Depression: Initial: 20 mg once daily; may increase the dose in 20 mg increments at intervals of ≥1 week; maximum dose in adults <60 years: 40 mg/day; maximum recommended dose in adults ≥60 years: 20 mg/day, although up to 40 mg/day may be considered in nonresponders

Poor metabolizers of CYP2C19 or concurrent use of moderate-to-strong CYP2C19 inhibitors (eg, cimetidine): Maximum dose: 20 mg/day

Elderly: Refer to adult dosing. **Note:** Due to increased serum concentrations in patients ≥60 years and the risk of QT prolongation, the maximum recommended dose in elderly patients is 20 mg/day, although up to 40 mg/day may be considered in nonresponders.

Dosage adjustment in renal impairment:
Mild-to-moderate impairment: No dosage adjustment needed
Severe impairment: Cl_{cr} <20 mL/minute: Use with caution

Dosage adjustment in hepatic impairment: 20 mg once daily; maximum recommended dose: 20 mg/day due to increased serum concentrations and the risk of QT prolongation; although up to 40 mg/day may be considered in nonresponders

Dietary Considerations May be taken without regard to food.

Administration May be administered without regard to food.

Monitoring Parameters ECG; liver function tests and CBC with continued therapy; monitor patient periodically for symptom resolution; mental status for depression, suicidal ideation (especially at the beginning of therapy or when doses are increased or decreased), anxiety, social functioning, mania, panic attacks; akathisia

Dosage Forms Excipient information presented when available (limited, particularly for generics); consult specific product labeling.
Solution, oral: 10 mg/5 mL (240 mL)
Tablet, oral: 10 mg, 20 mg, 40 mg
CeleXA®: 10 mg
CeleXA®: 20 mg, 40 mg [scored]

◆ **Citalopram Hydrobromide** *see* Citalopram *on page 370*

◆ **Citalopram-Odan (Can)** *see* Citalopram *on page 370*

◆ **Citracal® Maximum [OTC]** *see* Calcium and Vitamin D *on page 265*

◆ **Citracal® Petites [OTC]** *see* Calcium and Vitamin D *on page 265*

◆ **Citracal® Regular [OTC]** *see* Calcium and Vitamin D *on page 265*

◆ **Citrate of Magnesia** *see* Magnesium Citrate *on page 1044*

◆ **Citric Acid and Potassium Citrate** *see* Potassium Citrate and Citric Acid *on page 1382*

◆ **Citric Acid and Sodium Citrate** *see* Sodium Citrate and Citric Acid *on page 1570*

Citric Acid, Sodium Citrate, and Potassium Citrate

(SIT rik AS id, SOW dee um SIT rate, & poe TASS ee um SIT rate)

Brand Names: U.S. Cytra-3; Tricitrates

Index Terms Polycitra; Potassium Citrate, Citric Acid, and Sodium Citrate; Sodium Citrate, Citric Acid, and Potassium Citrate

Pharmacologic Category Alkalinizing Agent, Oral

Use Conditions where long-term maintenance of an alkaline urine is desirable as in control and dissolution of uric acid and cystine calculi of the urinary tract

Pregnancy Risk Factor Not established

Dosage Oral:
Children: 5-15 mL diluted in water after meals and at bedtime
Adults: 15-30 mL diluted in water after meals and at bedtime

Additional Information Complete prescribing information for this medication should be consulted for additional detail.

Dosage Forms Excipient information presented when available (limited, particularly for generics); consult specific product labeling. [DSC] = Discontinued product
Solution, oral:
Cytra-3: Citric acid 334 mg, sodium citrate 500 mg, and potassium citrate 550 mg per 5 mL (480 mL) [equivalent to potassium 1 mEq, sodium 1 mEq, and bicarbonate 2 mEq per 1 mL; alcohol free, sugar free; contains sodium benzoate and propylene glycol; raspberry flavor]
Tricitrates: Citric acid 334 mg, sodium citrate 500 mg, and potassium citrate 550 mg per 5 mL (480 mL) [equivalent to potassium 1 mEq, sodium 1 mEq, and bicarbonate 2 mEq per 1 mL; alcohol free; contains sodium benzoate; raspberry flavor]
Tricitrates: Citric acid 334 mg, sodium citrate 500 mg, and potassium citrate 550 mg per 5 mL (15 mL [DSC]; 30 mL [DSC]; 480 mL) [equivalent to potassium 1 mEq, sodium 1 mEq, and bicarbonate 2 mEq per 1 mL; alcohol free, sugar free; contains sodiuim benzoate and propylene glycol; raspberry flavor]

◆ **Citroma® [OTC]** *see* Magnesium Citrate *on page 1044*

◆ **Citro-Mag® (Can)** *see* Magnesium Citrate *on page 1044*

◆ **Citrovorum Factor** *see* Leucovorin Calcium *on page 987*

◆ **CL-118,532** *see* Triptorelin *on page 1742*

◆ **Cl-719** *see* Gemfibrozil *on page 785*

◆ **CL-184116** *see* Porfimer *on page 1376*

◆ **CL-232315** *see* MitoXANtrone *on page 1145*

Cladribine (KLA dri been)

Brand Names: U.S. Leustatin®

Brand Names: Canada Leustatin®

Index Terms 2-CdA; 2-Chlorodeoxyadenosine

Pharmacologic Category Antineoplastic Agent, Antimetabolite; Antineoplastic Agent, Antimetabolite (Purine Analog)

Use Treatment of hairy cell leukemia

Unlabeled Use Treatment of acute myeloid leukemia (AML), chronic lymphocytic leukemia (CLL), non-Hodgkin's lymphomas (mantle cell), Waldenström's macroglobulinemia, refractory Langerhans cell histiocytosis

Pregnancy Risk Factor D

Pregnancy Considerations Teratogenic effects and fetal mortality were observed in animal studies. There are no adequate and well-controlled studies in pregnant women. Do not administer during pregnancy. Women of childbearing potential should avoid becoming pregnant during treatment.

Lactation Excretion in breast milk unknown/not recommended

Contraindications Hypersensitivity to cladribine or any component of the formulation

Warnings/Precautions Hazardous agent - use appropriate precautions for handling and disposal. **[U.S. Boxed Warning]: Dose-dependent, reversible myelosuppression (neutropenia, anemia, and thrombocytopenia) is common and generally reversible;** use with caution in patients with pre-existing hematologic or immunologic abnormalities; monitor blood counts, especially during the first 4-8 weeks after treatment. **[U.S. Boxed Warning]: Serious, delayed (~1-3 months) neurologic toxicity, including irreversible paresis, has been reported, usually with continuous infusions of higher doses (4-9 times the FDA-approved dose); may occur at approved doses (rare);** diagnostics with electromyography and nerve conduction studies were consistent with demyelinating disease. **[U.S. Boxed Warning]: Acute nephrotoxicity (eg, acidosis, anuria, increased serum creatinine), possibly requiring dialysis, has been reported with high doses (4-9 times the FDA-approved dose); use**

caution when administering with other nephrotoxic agents. Use with caution in patients with renal or hepatic impairment. Fever (>100°F) may occur, with or without neutropenia, observed more commonly in the first month of treatment. Infections (bacterial, viral, and fungal) were reported more commonly in the first month after treatment (generally mild or moderate in severity); the incidence is reduced in the second month; due to neutropenia and T-cell depletion, risk versus benefit of treatment should be evaluated in patients with active infections. Use caution in patients with high tumor burden; tumor lysis syndrome may occur (rare). **[U.S. Boxed Warning]: Should be administered under the supervision of an experienced cancer chemotherapy physician.**

Adverse Reactions

>10%:

Central nervous system: Fever (69%; ≥100°F: 67%; ≥104°F: 11%), fatigue (11% to 45%), headache (7% to 22%)

Dermatologic: Rash (10% to 27%)

Gastrointestinal: Nausea (28%), appetite decreased (17%), vomiting (13%)

Hematologic: Neutropenia (grade 4: 70%; recovery: by week 5); anemia (grade 4: 37%; recovery: by week 8); bone marrow hypocellularity (34%; prolonged), neutropenic fever (47%; severe: 32%), thrombocytopenia (grade 4: 12%; recovery: by day 12), CD4 lymphocytopenia (nadir: 4-6 months)

Local: Injection site reactions (9% to 19%)

Respiratory: Abnormal breath sounds (11%)

Miscellaneous: Infection (month 1: 28% [serious: 6%]; month 2: 6%)

1% to 10%:

Cardiovascular: Edema (6%), tachycardia (6%), thrombosis (2%)

Central nervous system: Dizziness (9%), chills (9%), insomnia (7%), malaise (5% to 7%), pain (6%)

Dermatologic: Purpura (10%), petechiae (8%), pruritus (6%), erythema (6%)

Gastrointestinal: Diarrhea (10%), constipation (9%), abdominal pain (6%)

Local: Phlebitis (2%)

Neuromuscular & skeletal: Weakness (9%), myalgia (7%), arthralgia (5%)

Respiratory: Cough (7% to 10%), abnormal chest sounds (9%), dyspnea (7%), epistaxis (5%)

Miscellaneous: Diaphoresis (9%)

<1% (Limited to important or life-threatening): Aplastic anemia, bilirubin increased, hemolytic anemia, hypereosinophilia, myelodysplastic syndrome, neurologic toxicity, opportunistic infections (cytomegalovirus, fungal infections, herpes virus infections, listeriosis, *Pneumocystis jirovecii*), pancytopenia (prolonged), paraparesis, pneumonia, polyneuropathy (with high doses), progressive multifocal leukoencephalopathy (PML), pulmonary interstitial infiltrates, quadriplegia (reported at high doses); renal dysfunction (with high doses), Stevens-Johnson syndrome, stroke, toxic epidermal necrolysis, transaminases increased, tuberculosis reactivation, tumor lysis syndrome, urticaria

Drug Interactions

Metabolism/Transport Effects None known.

Avoid Concomitant Use

Avoid concomitant use of Cladribine with any of the following: BCG; CloZAPine; Natalizumab; Pimecrolimus; Tacrolimus (Topical); Vaccines (Live)

Increased Effect/Toxicity

Cladribine may increase the levels/effects of: CloZAPine; Leflunomide; Natalizumab; Vaccines (Live)

The levels/effects of Cladribine may be increased by: Denosumab; Pimecrolimus; Roflumilast; Tacrolimus (Topical); Trastuzumab

Decreased Effect

Cladribine may decrease the levels/effects of: BCG; Coccidioidin Skin Test; Sipuleucel-T; Vaccines (Inactivated); Vaccines (Live)

The levels/effects of Cladribine may be decreased by: Echinacea

Ethanol/Nutrition/Herb Interactions Ethanol: Avoid ethanol (due to GI irritation).

Stability Store intact vials under refrigeration 2°C to 8°C (36°F to 46°F). Protect from light. Use appropriate precautions for handling and disposal. To prepare a 24-hour continuous infusion, dilute in 500 mL NS; to prepare a 7-day continuous infusion, dilute to a total volume of 100 mL in a CADD® medication cassette reservoir using bacteriostatic NS. The manufacturer recommends filtering with a 0.22 micron filter when preparing 7-day infusions. Dilutions for infusion should be used promptly; if not used promptly, both the 24-hour and 7-day infusion may be stored refrigerated for up to 8 hours prior to administration. Stability has been demonstrated for 7 days (when diluted in bacteriostatic NS) in a CADD® medication cassette reservoir.

Mechanism of Action A purine nucleoside analogue; prodrug which is activated via phosphorylation by deoxycytidine kinase to a 5'-triphosphate derivative. This active form incorporates into DNA to result in the breakage of DNA strand and shutdown of DNA synthesis and repair. This also results in a depletion of nicotinamide adenine dinucleotide and adenosine triphosphate (ATP). Cladribine is cell-cycle nonspecific.

Pharmacodynamics/Kinetics

Distribution: V_d: ~9 L/kg; penetrates CSF (CSF concentrations are ~25% of plasma concentrations)

Protein binding: ~20%

Half-life elimination: After a 2-hour infusion (with normal renal function): 5.4 hours

Excretion: Urine (18%)

Dosage

Children: I.V.:

Acute myeloid leukemia (unlabeled use): 8.9 mg/m²/day continuous infusion for 5 days for 1 or 2 courses (Krance, 2001) **or** 9 mg/m²/day over 30 minutes for 5 days for 1 course (in combination with cytarabine) (Crews, 2002; Rubnitz, 2009)

Langerhans cell histiocytosis, refractory (unlabeled use): 5 mg/m²/day over 2 hours for 5 days every 21 days for up to 6 cycles (Weitzman, 2009)

Adults: Details concerning dosing in combination regimens should also be consulted.

Hairy cell leukemia: I.V.: 0.09 mg/kg/day continuous infusion for 7 days for 1 cycle **or** (unlabeled dosing) 0.1 mg/kg/day continuous infusion for 7 days for 1 cycle (Goodman, 2003; Saven, 1998)

Acute myeloid leukemia, induction (unlabeled use): I.V.: CLAG or CLAG-M regimen: 5 mg/m²/day over 2 hours for 5 days; a second induction may be administered if needed (Robak, 2000; Wierzbowska, 2008; Wrzesień-Kuś, 2003)

Chronic lymphocytic leukemia (unlabeled use): I.V.: 0.1 mg/kg/day continuous infusion for 7 days every 4-5 weeks (Saven, 1995) **or** 0.14 mg/kg/day over 2 hours for 5 days every 28 days for 3-6 cycles (Byrd, 2003)

Mantle cell lymphoma (unlabeled use): I.V.: 5 mg/m²/day over 2 hours for 5 days every 4 weeks for 2-6 cycles (Inwards, 2008; Rummel, 1999) **or** 5 mg/m²/day over 2 hours for 5 days every 4 weeks for 2-6 cycles (in combination with rituximab) (Inwards, 2008)

Waldenström's macroglobulinemia (unlabeled use):
I.V.: 0.1 mg/kg/day continuous infusion for 7 days every 4 weeks for 2 cycles (Dimopoulos, 1994)
SubQ: 0.1 mg/kg/day for 5 consecutive days every month for 4 cycles (in combination with rituximab) (Laszlo, 2010)

Dosing adjustment in renal impairment: The FDA-approved labeling recommends that caution should be used in patients with renal impairment; however, no specific dosage adjustment guidelines are available due to lack of data. The following guidelines have been used by some clinicians (Aronoff, 2007):
Children:
Cl_{cr} 10-50 mL/minute: Administer 50% of dose
Cl_{cr} <10 mL/minute: Administer 30% of dose
Hemodialysis: Administer 30% of dose
Continuous renal replacement therapy (CRRT): Administer 50% of dose
Adults:
Cl_{cr} 10-50 mL/minute: Administer 75% of dose
Cl_{cr} <10 mL/minute: Administer 50% of dose
Continuous ambulatory peritoneal dialysis (CAPD): Administer 50% of dose

Dosing adjustment in hepatic impairment: The FDA-approved labeling recommends that caution should be used in patients with hepatic impairment; however, no specific dosage adjustment guidelines are available due to lack of data.

Administration
I.V.: Administer as a continuous infusion. May also be administered over 30 minutes or over 2 hours (unlabeled administration rates) depending on indication and/or protocol.
SubQ (unlabeled route): May also be administered SubQ (Laszlo, 2010)

Monitoring Parameters CBC with differential (particularly during the first 4-8 weeks post-treatment), renal and hepatic function; monitor for fever

Dosage Forms Excipient information presented when available (limited, particularly for generics); consult specific product labeling.
Injection, solution [preservative free]: 1 mg/mL (10 mL)
Leustatin®: 1 mg/mL (10 mL)

- **Claforan®** *see* Cefotaxime *on page 308*
- **Claravis™** *see* ISOtretinoin *on page 939*
- **Clarifoam™ EF** *see* Sulfur and Sulfacetamide *on page 1607*
- **Clarinex®** *see* Desloratadine *on page 475*
- **Clarinex-D® 12 Hour** *see* Desloratadine and Pseudoephedrine *on page 476*
- **Clarinex-D® 24 Hour** *see* Desloratadine and Pseudoephedrine *on page 476*

Clarithromycin (kla RITH roe mye sin)

Brand Names: U.S. Biaxin®; Biaxin® XL

Brand Names: Canada Apo-Clarithromycin®; Ava-Clarithromycin; Biaxin®; Biaxin® XL; Dom-Clarithromycin; Mylan-Clarithromycin; PMS-Clarithromycin; RAN™-Clarithromycin; ratio-Clarithromycin; Riva-Clarithromycin; Sandoz-Clarithromycin

Pharmacologic Category Antibiotic, Macrolide

Additional Appendix Information
Prevention of Infective Endocarditis *on page 1952*

Use
Children:
Acute otitis media (*H. influenzae, M. catarrhalis*, or *S. pneumoniae*)
Community-acquired pneumonia due to susceptible *Mycoplasma pneumoniae, S. pneumoniae*, or *Chlamydia pneumoniae* (TWAR)
Pharyngitis/tonsillitis due to susceptible *S. pyogenes*, acute maxillary sinusitis due to susceptible *H. influenzae, S. pneumoniae*, or *Moraxella catarrhalis*, uncomplicated skin/skin structure infections due to susceptible *S. aureus, S. pyogenes*, and mycobacterial infections
Prevention of disseminated mycobacterial infections due to MAC disease in patients with advanced HIV infection
Adults:
Pharyngitis/tonsillitis due to susceptible *S. pyogenes*
Acute maxillary sinusitis due to susceptible *H. influenzae, M. catarrhalis*, or *S. pneumoniae*
Acute exacerbation of chronic bronchitis due to susceptible *H. influenzae, H. parainfluenzae, M. catarrhalis*, or *S. pneumoniae*
Community-acquired pneumonia due to susceptible *H. influenzae, H. parainfluenzae, Mycoplasma pneumoniae, S. pneumoniae*, or *Chlamydia pneumoniae* (TWAR), *Moraxella catarrhalis*
Uncomplicated skin/skin structure infections due to susceptible *S. aureus, S. pyogenes*
Disseminated mycobacterial infections due to *M. avium* or *M. intracellulare*
Prevention of disseminated mycobacterial infections due to *M. avium* complex (MAC) disease (eg, patients with advanced HIV infection)
Duodenal ulcer disease due to *H. pylori* in regimens with other drugs including amoxicillin and lansoprazole or omeprazole, ranitidine bismuth citrate, bismuth subsalicylate, tetracycline, and/or an H_2 antagonist

Unlabeled Use Pertussis (CDC guidelines); alternate antibiotic for prophylaxis of infective endocarditis in patients who are allergic to penicillin and undergoing surgical or dental procedures (ACC/AHA guidelines)

Pregnancy Risk Factor C

Pregnancy Considerations Adverse fetal effects have been documented in some animal studies; therefore, clarithromycin is classified as pregnancy category C. Clarithromycin crosses the placenta. The manufacturer recommends that clarithromycin not be used in a pregnant woman unless there are no alternative therapies. An increased risk of teratogenic events has not been observed following maternal use of clarithromycin.

Lactation Excretion in breast milk unknown/use caution

Contraindications Hypersensitivity to clarithromycin, erythromycin, or any macrolide antibiotic; use with ergot derivatives, pimozide, cisapride, astemizole, terfenadine, colchicine (if patient has concomitant renal or hepatic impairment); history of cholestatic jaundice or hepatic dysfunction with prior clarithromycin use

Warnings/Precautions Dosage adjustment required with severe renal impairment; decreased dosage or prolonged dosing interval may be appropriate. May cause hepatotoxicity (elevated liver function tests, hepatitis, jaundice, hepatic failure); use caution with preexisting hepatic disease or hepatotoxic medications. Use with caution in patients with myasthenia gravis. Colchicine toxicity (including fatalities) has been reported with concomitant use; concomitant use is contraindicated in patients with renal or hepatic impairment. Prolonged use may result in fungal or bacterial superinfection, including *C. difficile*-associated diarrhea (CDAD) and pseudomembranous colitis; CDAD has been observed >2 months postantibiotic treatment. Macrolides (including clarithromycin) have been associated with rare QT prolongation and ventricular arrhythmias, including torsade de pointes. Use caution in patients with coronary artery disease. Avoid use of extended release tablets (Biaxin® XL) in patients with known stricture/narrowing of the GI tract.

Adverse Reactions

1% to 10%:

Central nervous system: Headache (adults and children 2%)

Dermatologic: Rash (children 3%)

Gastrointestinal: Abnormal taste (adults 3% to 7%), diarrhea (adults 3% to 6%; children 6%), vomiting (children 6%), nausea (adults 3%), abdominal pain (adults 2%; children 3%), dyspepsia (adults 2%)

Hepatic: Prothrombin time increased (adults 1%)

Renal: BUN increased (4%)

<1% (Limited to important or life-threatening): Alkaline phosphatase increased, ALT increased, anaphylaxis, anorexia, anxiety, AST increased, behavioral changes, bilirubin increased, cholestatic hepatitis, *Clostridium difficile* colitis, confusion, depersonalization, depression, disorientation, dizziness, GGT increased, glossitis, hallucinations, hearing loss (reversible), hepatic dysfunction, hepatic failure, hepatitis, hypoglycemia, insomnia, interstitial nephritis, jaundice, leukopenia, LDH increased, manic behavior, neutropenia, nightmares, oral moniliasis, pancreatitis, psychosis, QT prolongation, seizure, serum creatinine increased, smell loss, Stevens-Johnson syndrome, stomatitis, thrombocytopenia, tinnitus, tongue discoloration, tooth discoloration (reversible), torsade de pointes, toxic epidermal necrolysis, tremor, urticaria, ventricular tachycardia, ventricular arrhythmia, vertigo, white blood cell count decreased

Drug Interactions

Metabolism/Transport Effects Substrate of CYP3A4 (major); **Note:** Assignment of Major/Minor substrate status based on clinically relevant drug interaction potential; **Inhibits** CYP1A2 (weak), CYP3A4 (strong), P-glycoprotein

Avoid Concomitant Use

Avoid concomitant use of Clarithromycin with any of the following: Alfuzosin; Artemether; BCG; Cisapride; Conivaptan; Crizotinib; Dihydroergotamine; Disopyramide; Dronedarone; Eplerenone; Ergotamine; Everolimus; Fluticasone (Oral Inhalation); Halofantrine; Lapatinib; Lovastatin; Lumefantrine; Lurasidone; Nilotinib; Nisoldipine; Pimozide; QUEtiapine; QuiNINE; Ranolazine; Rivaroxaban; RomiDEPsin; Salmeterol; Silodosin; Simvastatin; Tamsulosin; Terfenadine; Tetrabenazine; Thioridazine; Ticagrelor; Tolvaptan; Topotecan; Toremifene; Vandetanib; Vemurafenib; Ziprasidone

Increased Effect/Toxicity

Clarithromycin may increase the levels/effects of: Alfentanil; Alfuzosin; Almotriptan; Alosetron; Antifungal Agents (Azole Derivatives, Systemic); Antineoplastic Agents (Vinca Alkaloids); ARIPiprazole; Benzodiazepines (metabolized by oxidation); Bortezomib; Brentuximab Vedotin; Brinzolamide; Budesonide (Nasal); Budesonide (Systemic, Oral Inhalation); BusPIRone; Calcium Channel Blockers; CarBAMazepine; Cardiac Glycosides; Ciclesonide; Cilostazol; Cisapride; CloZAPine; Colchicine; Conivaptan; Corticosteroids (Orally Inhaled); Corticosteroids (Systemic); Crizotinib; CycloSPORINE; CycloSPORINE (Systemic); CYP3A4 Inducers (Strong); CYP3A4 Substrates; Dabigatran Etexilate; Dienogest; Dihydroergotamine; Disopyramide; Dronedarone; Dutasteride; Eletriptan; Eplerenone; Ergot Derivatives; Ergotamine; Everolimus; FentaNYL; Fesoterodine; Fluticasone (Nasal); Fluticasone (Oral Inhalation); GlipiZIDE; GlyBURIDE; GuanFACINE; Halofantrine; HMG-CoA Reductase Inhibitors; Iloperidone; Ixabepilone; Lapatinib; Lovastatin; Lumefantrine; Lurasidone; Maraviroc; MethylPREDNISolone; Nilotinib; Nisoldipine; Paricalcitol; Pazopanib; P-glycoprotein/ABCB1 Substrates; Pimecrolimus; Pimozide; Propafenone; Protease Inhibitors; QTc-Prolonging Agents; QuiNIDine; QuiNINE; Ranolazine; Repaglinide; Rifamycin Derivatives; Rivaroxaban; RomiDEPsin; Ruxolitinib; Salmeterol; Saxagliptin; Selective Serotonin Reuptake Inhibitors; Sildenafil; Silodosin; Simvastatin; Sirolimus; SORAfenib; Tacrolimus; Tacrolimus (Systemic); Tacrolimus (Topical); Tadalafil; Tamsulosin; Telaprevir; Temsirolimus; Terfenadine; Tetrabenazine; Theophylline Derivatives; Thioridazine; Ticagrelor; Tolterodine; Tolvaptan; Topotecan; Toremifene; Vandetanib; Vardenafil; Vemurafenib; Vilazodone; Vitamin K Antagonists; Zidovudine; Ziprasidone; Zopiclone; Zuclopenthixol

The levels/effects of Clarithromycin may be increased by: Alfuzosin; Antifungal Agents (Azole Derivatives, Systemic); Artemether; Chloroquine; Ciprofloxacin; Ciprofloxacin (Systemic); CYP3A4 Inducers (Strong); CYP3A4 Inhibitors (Moderate); CYP3A4 Inhibitors (Strong); Gadobutrol; Indacaterol; Lumefantrine; Nilotinib; Protease Inhibitors; QUEtiapine; QuiNINE; Telaprevir

Decreased Effect

Clarithromycin may decrease the levels/effects of: BCG; Clopidogrel; Prasugrel; Ticagrelor; Typhoid Vaccine; Zidovudine

The levels/effects of Clarithromycin may be decreased by: CYP3A4 Inducers (Strong); Deferasirox; Etravirine; Herbs (CYP3A4 Inducers); Protease Inhibitors; Tocilizumab

Ethanol/Nutrition/Herb Interactions

Food: Immediate release: Food delays rate, but not extent of absorption; Extended release: Food increases clarithromycin AUC by ~30% relative to fasting conditions.

Herb/Nutraceutical: St John's wort may decrease clarithromycin levels.

Stability

Immediate release 250 mg tablets and granules for oral suspension: Store at controlled room temperature of 15°C to 30°C (59°F to 86°F). Reconstituted oral suspension should not be refrigerated because it might gel; microencapsulated particles of clarithromycin in suspension are stable for 14 days when stored at room temperature. Protect tablets from light.

Immediate release 500 mg tablets and Biaxin® XL: Store at controlled room temperature of 20°C to 25°C (68°F to 77°F); excursions permitted to 15°C to 30°C (59°F to 86°F).

Mechanism of Action Exerts its antibacterial action by binding to 50S ribosomal subunit resulting in inhibition of protein synthesis. The 14-OH metabolite of clarithromycin is twice as active as the parent compound against certain organisms.

Pharmacodynamics/Kinetics

Absorption: Immediate release: Rapid; food delays rate, but not extent of absorption

Distribution: Widely into most body tissues except CNS

Protein binding: 42% to 50%

Metabolism: Partially hepatic via CYP3A4; converted to 14-OH clarithromycin (active metabolite)

Bioavailability: ~50%

Half-life elimination: Immediate release: Clarithromycin: 3-7 hours; 14-OH-clarithromycin: 5-9 hours

Time to peak: Immediate release: 2-3 hours

Excretion: Primarily urine (20% to 40% as unchanged drug; additional 10% to 15% as metabolite)

Clearance: Approximates normal GFR

Dosage

Usual dosage range:

Children ≥6 months: Oral: 7.5 mg/kg every 12 hours (maximum: 500 mg/dose) for 10 days

Adults: Oral: 250-500 mg every 12 hours **or** 1000 mg (two 500 mg extended release tablets) once daily for 7-14 days

Indication-specific dosing:

Children: Oral:

Community-acquired pneumonia (CAP) (IDSA/PIDS, 2011): Infants >3 months and Children: **Note:** A beta-lactam antibiotic should be added if typical bacterial pneumonia cannot be ruled out.

Presumed atypical *(M. pneumoniae, C. pneumoniae, C. trachomatis)* infection, mild-to-severe atypical infection or step-down therapy (alternative to azithromycin): 7.5 mg/kg/dose (maximum: 1 g) every 12 hours

Mycobacterial infection (prevention and treatment): Manufacturer's recommendation: 7.5 mg/kg/dose (maximum: 500 mg/dose) twice daily. **Note:** Safety of clarithromycin for MAC not studied in children <20 months.

HIV-exposed/-positive (unlabeled use; CDC, 2009):

Primary prophylaxis: 7.5 mg/kg/dose (maximum: 500 mg/dose) twice daily

Secondary prophylaxis: 7.5 mg/kg/dose (maximum: 500 mg/dose) twice daily, plus ethambutol, with or without rifabutin

Treatment: 7.5-15 mg/kg/dose (maximum: 500 mg/dose) twice daily plus ethambutol, plus rifabutin (for severe disease)

Pertussis (unlabeled use; CDC, 2005):

Children 1-5 months: 7.5 mg/kg/dose every 12 hours for 7 days

Children ≥6 months: 7.5 mg/kg/dose every 12 hours for 7 days (maximum: 1 g/day)

Prophylaxis against infective endocarditis (unlabeled use): 15 mg/kg 30-60 minutes before procedure. **Note:** American Heart Association (AHA) guidelines now recommend prophylaxis only in patients undergoing invasive procedures and in whom underlying cardiac conditions may predispose to a higher risk of adverse outcomes should infection occur. As of April 2007, routine prophylaxis for GI/GU procedures is no longer recommended by the AHA.

Sinusitis, bronchitis, skin infections: 7.5 mg/kg/dose every 12 hours for 10 days

Adults: Oral:

Acute exacerbation of chronic bronchitis:

M. catarrhalis and *S. pneumoniae*: 250 mg every 12 hours for 7-14 days **or** 1000 mg (two 500 mg extended release tablets) once daily for 7 days

H. influenzae: 500 mg every 12 hours for 7-14 days **or** 1000 mg (two 500 mg extended release tablets) once daily for 7 days

H. parainfluenzae: 500 mg every 12 hours for 7 days **or** 1000 mg (two 500 mg extended release tablets) once daily for 7 days

Acute maxillary sinusitis: 500 mg every 12 hours **or** 1000 mg (two 500 mg extended release tablets) once daily for 14 days

Mycobacterial infection (prevention and treatment): 500 mg twice daily (use with other antimycobacterial drugs, eg, ethambutol or rifampin)

Peptic ulcer disease: Eradication of *Helicobacter pylori*: Dual or triple combination regimens with bismuth subsalicylate, amoxicillin, an H_2-receptor antagonist, or proton-pump inhibitor: 500 mg every 8-12 hours for 10-14 days

Pertussis (unlabeled use; CDC, 2005): 500 mg twice daily for 7 days

Pharyngitis, tonsillitis: 250 mg every 12 hours for 10 days

Pneumonia:

C. pneumoniae, M. pneumoniae, and *S. pneumoniae*: 250 mg every 12 hours for 7-14 days **or** 1000 mg (two 500 mg extended release tablets) once daily for 7 days

H. influenzae: 250 mg every 12 hours for 7 days **or** 1000 mg (two 500 mg extended release tablets) once daily for 7 days

H. parainfluenzae and *M. catarrhalis*: 1000 mg (two 500 mg extended release tablets) once daily for 7 days

Prophylaxis against infective endocarditis (unlabeled use): 500 mg 30-60 minutes prior to procedure. **Note:** American Heart Association (AHA) guidelines now recommend prophylaxis only in patients undergoing invasive procedures and in whom underlying cardiac conditions may predispose to a higher risk of adverse outcomes should infection occur. As of April 2007, routine prophylaxis for GI/GU procedures is no longer recommended by the AHA.

Skin and skin structure infection, uncomplicated: 250 mg every 12 hours for 7-14 days

Elderly: Pharmacokinetics are similar to those in younger adults; may have age-related reductions in renal function; monitor and adjust dose if necessary

Dosing adjustment in renal impairment:

Cl_{cr} <30 mL/minute: Decrease clarithromycin dose by 50%

Hemodialysis: Administer after HD session is completed (Aronoff, 2007).

In combination with atazanavir or ritonavir:

Cl_{cr} 30-60 mL/minute: Decrease clarithromycin dose by 50%

Cl_{cr} <30 mL/minute: Decrease clarithromycin dose by 75%

Dosing adjustment in hepatic impairment: No dosing adjustment is needed as long as renal function is normal

Dietary Considerations Clarithromycin immediate release tablets and oral suspension may be given with or without meals, and may be taken with milk. Extended release tablets should be taken with food.

Administration Clarithromycin immediate release tablets and oral suspension may be administered with or without meals. Give every 12 hours rather than twice daily to avoid peak and trough variation. Shake suspension well before each use.

Extended release tablets: Should be given with food. Do not crush or chew extended release tablet.

Monitoring Parameters CBC with differential, BUN, creatinine; perform culture and sensitivity studies prior to initiating drug therapy

Dosage Forms Excipient information presented when available (limited, particularly for generics); consult specific product labeling.

Granules for suspension, oral: 125 mg/5 mL (50 mL, 100 mL); 250 mg/5 mL (50 mL, 100 mL)

Biaxin®: 125 mg/5 mL (50 mL, 100 mL); 250 mg/5 mL (50 mL, 100 mL) [fruit-punch flavor]

Tablet, oral: 250 mg, 500 mg

Biaxin®: 250 mg, 500 mg

Tablet, extended release, oral: 500 mg

Biaxin® XL: 500 mg

◆ **Clarithromycin, Lansoprazole, and Amoxicillin** *see* Lansoprazole, Amoxicillin, and Clarithromycin *on page 975*

◆ **Claritin® (Can)** *see* Loratadine *on page 1031*

◆ **Claritin® 24 Hour Allergy [OTC]** *see* Loratadine *on page 1031*

◆ **Claritin-D® 12 Hour Allergy & Congestion [OTC]** *see* Loratadine and Pseudoephedrine *on page 1032*

◆ **Claritin-D® 24 Hour Allergy & Congestion [OTC]** *see* Loratadine and Pseudoephedrine *on page 1032*

◆ **Claritin® Children's Allergy [OTC]** *see* Loratadine *on page 1031*

◆ **Claritin® Extra (Can)** *see* Loratadine and Pseudoephedrine *on page 1032*

◆ **Claritin™ Eye [OTC]** *see* Ketotifen (Ophthalmic) *on page 959*

◆ **Claritin® Kids (Can)** *see* Loratadine *on page 1031*

◆ **Claritin® Liberator (Can)** *see* Loratadine and Pseudoephedrine *on page 1032*

◆ **Claritin® Liqui-Gels® 24 Hour Allergy [OTC]** *see* Loratadine *on page 1031*

◆ **Claritin® RediTabs® 24 Hour Allergy [OTC]** *see* Loratadine *on page 1031*

◆ **Clarus™ (Can)** *see* ISOtretinoin *on page 939*

◆ **Clavulanic Acid and Amoxicillin** *see* Amoxicillin and Clavulanate *on page 105*

◆ **Clavulin® (Can)** *see* Amoxicillin and Clavulanate *on page 105*

◆ **Clear eyes® for Dry Eyes Plus ACR Relief [OTC]** *see* Naphazoline (Ophthalmic) *on page 1176*

◆ **Clear eyes® for Dry Eyes plus Redness Relief [OTC]** *see* Naphazoline (Ophthalmic) *on page 1176*

◆ **Clear eyes® Redness Relief [OTC]** *see* Naphazoline (Ophthalmic) *on page 1176*

◆ **Clear eyes® Seasonal Relief [OTC]** *see* Naphazoline (Ophthalmic) *on page 1176*

Clemastine (KLEM as teen)

Brand Names: U.S. Tavist® Allergy [OTC]

Index Terms Clemastine Fumarate

Pharmacologic Category Ethanolamine Derivative; Histamine H_1 Antagonist; Histamine H_1 Antagonist, First Generation

Use Perennial and seasonal allergic rhinitis and other allergic symptoms including urticaria

Pregnancy Risk Factor B

Dosage Oral:

Infants and Children <6 years: 0.05 mg/kg/day as **clemastine base** or 0.335-0.67 mg/day clemastine fumarate (0.25-0.5 mg base/day) divided into 2 or 3 doses; maximum daily dosage: 1.34 mg (1 mg base)

Children 6-12 years: 0.67-1.34 mg clemastine fumarate (0.5-1 mg base) twice daily; do not exceed 4.02 mg/day (3 mg/day base)

Children ≥12 years and Adults:

1.34 mg clemastine fumarate (1 mg base) twice daily to 2.68 mg (2 mg base) 3 times/day; do not exceed 8.04 mg/day (6 mg base)

OTC labeling: 1.34 mg clemastine fumarate (1 mg base) twice daily; do not exceed 2 mg base/24 hours

Elderly: Lower doses should be considered in patients >60 years

Additional Information Complete prescribing information for this medication should be consulted for additional detail.

Dosage Forms Excipient information presented when available (limited, particularly for generics); consult specific product labeling.

Syrup, oral, as fumarate: 0.67 mg/5 mL (120 mL) [equivalent to clemastine base 0.5 mg/5 mL; prescription formulation]

Tablet, oral, as fumarate: 1.34 mg [equivalent to clemastine base 1 mg; OTC], 2.68 mg [equivalent to clemastine base 2 mg; prescription formulation]

Tavist® Allergy: 1.34 mg [scored; equivalent to clemastine base 1 mg]

◆ **Clemastine Fumarate** *see* Clemastine *on page 377*

◆ **Clenia™** *see* Sulfur and Sulfacetamide *on page 1607*

◆ **Cleocin®** *see* Clindamycin (Topical) *on page 381*

◆ **Cleocin HCl®** *see* Clindamycin (Systemic) *on page 378*

◆ **Cleocin Pediatric®** *see* Clindamycin (Systemic) *on page 378*

◆ **Cleocin Phosphate®** *see* Clindamycin (Systemic) *on page 378*

◆ **Cleocin T®** *see* Clindamycin (Topical) *on page 381*

◆ **Cleocin® Vaginal Ovule** *see* Clindamycin (Topical) *on page 381*

Clevidipine (klev ID i peen)

Brand Names: U.S. Cleviprex®

Index Terms Clevidipine Butyrate

Pharmacologic Category Calcium Channel Blocker; Calcium Channel Blocker, Dihydropyridine

Additional Appendix Information

Calcium Channel Blockers *on page 1887*

Hypertension *on page 2001*

Use Management of hypertension

Pregnancy Risk Factor C

Pregnancy Considerations Adverse events were observed in animal reproduction studies. There are no adequate and well-controlled studies in pregnant women. Use only if potential benefit justifies potential risks.

Lactation Excretion in breast milk unknown/not recommended

Contraindications Hypersensitivity to clevidipine or any component of the formulation (soybeans, soy products, eggs, egg products); hypertriglyceridemia or complications of hypertriglyceridemia (eg, acute pancreatitis); lipoid nephrosis; severe aortic stenosis

Warnings/Precautions Symptomatic hypotension with or without syncope and reflex tachycardia may rarely occur. Blood pressure must be lowered at a rate appropriate for the patient's clinical condition; dosage reductions may be necessary. Treatment of clevidipine-induced tachycardia with beta-blockers is **not** recommended. After prolonged use, discontinuation may cause rebound hypertension; monitor closely for ≥8 hours after discontinuation. Use with caution in patients with heart failure (may worsen symptoms). Clevidipine is formulated within a 20% fat emulsion (0.2 g/mL); hypertriglyceridemia is an expected side effect with high-dose or extended treatment periods; median infusion duration in clinical trials was approximately 6.5 hours (Aronson, 2008). Patients who develop hypertriglyceridemia (eg, >500 mg/dL) are at risk of developing pancreatitis. A reduction in the quantity of concurrently administered lipids may be necessary. Use is contraindicated in patients with hypertriglyceridemia or complications associated with hypertriglyceridemia (eg, acute pancreatitis) and lipoid nephrosis. Withdrawal from concomitant beta-blocker therapy should be done gradually. Initiate therapy at the low end of the dosage range in the elderly, with careful upward titration if needed. Use within 12 hours of puncturing vial; maintain aseptic technique while handling.

Adverse Reactions

>10%:

Central nervous system: Fever (19%), insomnia (12%)

Gastrointestinal: Nausea (5% to 21%)

1% to 10%:

Central nervous system: Headache (6%)

Gastrointestinal: Vomiting (3%)

Hematologic: Postprocedural hemorrhage (3%)

Renal: Acute renal failure (9%)

Respiratory: Pneumonia (3%), respiratory failure (3%)

<1% (Limited to important or life-threatening): Cardiac arrest, dyspnea, MI, syncope, thrombophlebitis

Drug Interactions

Metabolism/Transport Effects None known.

Avoid Concomitant Use There are no known interactions where it is recommended to avoid concomitant use.

Increased Effect/Toxicity

Clevidipine may increase the levels/effects of: Amifostine; Antihypertensives; Beta-Blockers; Calcium Channel Blockers (Nondihydropyridine); Hypotensive Agents; Magnesium Salts; Neuromuscular-Blocking Agents (Nondepolarizing); Nitroprusside; QuiNIDine; RiTUXimab

The levels/effects of Clevidipine may be increased by: Alpha1-Blockers; Calcium Channel Blockers (Nondihydropyridine); Diazoxide; Herbs (Hypotensive Properties); Magnesium Salts; MAO Inhibitors; Pentoxifylline; Phosphodiesterase 5 Inhibitors; Prostacyclin Analogues; QuiNIDine

Decreased Effect

Clevidipine may decrease the levels/effects of: QuiNIDine

The levels/effects of Clevidipine may be decreased by: Calcium Salts; Herbs (Hypertensive Properties); Methylphenidate; Yohimbine

Ethanol/Nutrition/Herb Interactions Herb/Nutraceutical: Avoid bayberry, blue cohosh, cayenne, ephedra, ginger, ginseng (American), kola, licorice (may worsen hypertension). Avoid black cohosh, California poppy, coleus, golden seal, hawthorn, mistletoe, periwinkle, quinine, shepherd's purse (may have increased antihypertensive effect).

Stability Store in refrigerator at 2°C to 8°C (36°F to 46°F). Unopened vials are stable for 2 months at room temperature. Vials are stable for 12 hours once opened. Protect from light during storage. Do not freeze.

Mechanism of Action Dihydropyridine calcium channel blocker with potent arterial vasodilating activity. Inhibits calcium ion influx through the L-type calcium channels during depolarization in arterial smooth muscle, producing a decrease in mean arterial pressure (MAP) by reducing systemic vascular resistance.

Pharmacodynamics/Kinetics

Onset of action: 2-4 minutes after start of infusion

Duration: I.V.: 5-15 minutes

Distribution: V_{dss}: 0.17 L/kg

Protein binding: >99.5%

Metabolism: Rapid hydrolysis primarily by esterases in blood and extravascular tissues to an inactive carboxylic acid metabolite and formaldehyde

Half-life elimination: Biphasic: Initial: 1 minute (predominant); Terminal: 15 minutes

Excretion: Urine (63% to 74% as metabolites); feces (7% to 22% as metabolites)

Dosage I.V.:

Adults: Initial: 1-2 mg/hour

Titration: Initial: dose may be doubled at 90-second intervals toward blood pressure goal. As blood pressure approaches goal, dose may be increased by less than double every 5-10 minutes. **Note:** For every 1-2 mg/hour increase in dose, an approximate reduction of 2-4 mm Hg in systolic blood pressure may occur.

Usual maintenance: 4-6 mg/hour; maximum: 21 mg/hour (1000 mL within a 24-hour period due to lipid load restriction). There is limited short-term experience with doses up to 32 mg/hour. Data is limited beyond 72 hours.

Elderly: Initiate at the low end of the dosage range.

Dosing adjustment in renal impairment: No adjustment required with initial infusion rate

Dosing adjustment in hepatic impairment: No adjustment required with initial infusion rate

Dietary Considerations Clevidipine is formulated in an oil-in-water emulsion containing 200 mg/mL of lipid (2 kcal/mL). If on parenteral nutrition, may need to adjust the amount of lipid infused. Emulsion contains soybean oil, egg yolk phospholipids, and glycerin.

Administration I.V.: Maintain aseptic technique. Do not use if contamination is suspected. Do not dilute. Invert vial gently several times to ensure uniformity of emulsion prior to administration. Administer as a slow continuous infusion via central or peripheral line, using infusion device allowing for calibrated infusion rates. Use within 12 hours of puncturing vial; discard any tubing and unused portion, including that currently being infused.

Monitoring Parameters Blood pressure, heart rate; patients who receive prolonged infusions of clevidipine and are not transitioned to other antihypertensive therapy should be monitored for at least 8 hours after discontinuation

Dosage Forms Excipient information presented when available (limited, particularly for generics); consult specific product labeling. [DSC] = Discontinued product

Injection, emulsion:

Cleviprex®: 0.5 mg/mL (50 mL, 100 mL) [contains edetate disodium, egg yolk phospholipid, soybean oil]

Cleviprex®: 0.5 mg/mL (50 mL [DSC], 100 mL [DSC]) [contains egg yolk phospholipid, soybean oil]

- **Clevidipine Butyrate** *see* Clevidipine *on page 377*
- **Cleviprex®** *see* Clevidipine *on page 377*

Clidinium and Chlordiazepoxide

(kli DI nee um & klor dye az e POKS ide)

Brand Names: U.S. Librax®

Brand Names: Canada Apo-Chlorax®; Librax®

Index Terms Chlordiazepoxide and Clidinium

Pharmacologic Category Antispasmodic Agent, Gastrointestinal; Benzodiazepine

Additional Appendix Information

Beers Criteria – Potentially Inappropriate Medications for Geriatrics *on page 1973*

Use Adjunct treatment of peptic ulcer; treatment of irritable bowel syndrome

Pregnancy Risk Factor D

Dosage Oral: 1-2 capsules 3-4 times/day, before meals or food and at bedtime

Caution: Do not abruptly discontinue after prolonged use; taper dose gradually.

Additional Information Complete prescribing information for this medication should be consulted for additional detail.

Dosage Forms Excipient information presented when available (limited, particularly for generics); consult specific product labeling.

Capsule: Clidinium bromide 2.5 mg and chlordiazepoxide hydrochloride 5 mg

Librax®: Clidinium bromide 2.5 mg and chlordiazepoxide hydrochloride 5 mg

- **Climara®** *see* Estradiol (Systemic) *on page 627*
- **ClimaraPro®** *see* Estradiol and Levonorgestrel *on page 635*
- **Clindagel®** *see* Clindamycin (Topical) *on page 381*
- **ClindaMax®** *see* Clindamycin (Topical) *on page 381*

Clindamycin (Systemic) (klin da MYE sin)

Brand Names: U.S. Cleocin HCl®; Cleocin Pediatric®; Cleocin Phosphate®

Brand Names: Canada Alti-Clindamycin; Apo-Clindamycin®; Clindamycin Injection, USP; Clindamycine; Gen-Clindamycin; Mylan-Clindamycin; Novo-Clindamycin; NV-Clindamycin; PMS-Clindamycin; ratio-Clindamycin; Riva-Clindamycin; Teva-Clindamycin

Index Terms Clindamycin Hydrochloride; Clindamycin Palmitate

Pharmacologic Category Antibiotic, Lincosamide

Additional Appendix Information

Prevention of Infective Endocarditis *on page 1952*
Prevention of Wound Infection and Sepsis in Surgical Patients *on page 1954*

Use Treatment of susceptible bacterial infections, mainly those caused by anaerobes, streptococci, pneumococci, and staphylococci; pelvic inflammatory disease (I.V.)

Unlabeled Use May be useful in PCP; alternate treatment for toxoplasmosis; bacterial vaginosis (oral); alternate treatment for MRSA infections; alternate antibiotic for prophylaxis of infective endocarditis in patients who are allergic to penicillin and undergoing surgical or dental procedures (ACC/AHA guidelines); treatment of severe or uncomplicated malaria; treatment of babesiosis

Pregnancy Risk Factor B

Pregnancy Considerations Adverse events were not observed in animal reproduction studies. Clindamycin crosses the placenta throughout pregnancy and at term, but use during pregnancy has not been shown to cause adverse fetal effects. Clindamycin pharmacokinetics are not affected by pregnancy. Clindamycin therapy is recommended in certain pregnant patients for prophylaxis of group B streptococcal disease in newborns, prophylaxis and treatment of *Toxoplasma gondii* encephalitis, or for the treatment of *Pneumocystis* pneumonia (PCP), bacterial vaginosis, or malaria.

Lactation Enters breast milk/not recommended (AAP rates "compatible"; AAP 2001 update pending)

Contraindications Hypersensitivity to clindamycin, lincomycin, or any component of the formulation

Warnings/Precautions Dosage adjustment may be necessary in patients with severe hepatic dysfunction. **[U.S. Boxed Warning]: Can cause severe and possibly fatal colitis.** Prolonged use may result in fungal or bacterial superinfection, including *C. difficile*-associated diarrhea (CDAD) and pseudomembranous colitis; CDAD has been observed >2 months postantibiotic treatment. Use with caution in patients with a history of gastrointestinal disease. Discontinue drug if significant diarrhea, abdominal cramps, or passage of blood and mucus occurs. Some dosage forms contain benzyl alcohol or tartrazine. Use caution in atopic patients. Not appropriate for use in the treatment of meningitis due to inadequate penetration into the CSF.

Adverse Reactions Frequency not defined.

Cardiovascular: Cardiac arrest (rare; I.V. administration), hypotension (rare; I.V. administration)

Dermatologic: Erythema multiforme (rare), exfoliative dermatitis (rare), pruritus, rash, Stevens-Johnson syndrome (rare), urticaria

Gastrointestinal: Abdominal pain, diarrhea, esophagitis, nausea, pseudomembranous colitis, vomiting

Genitourinary: Vaginitis

Hematologic: Agranulocytosis, eosinophilia (transient), neutropenia (transient), thrombocytopenia

Hepatic: Jaundice, liver function test abnormalities

Local: Induration/pain/sterile abscess (I.M.), thrombophlebitis (I.V.)

Neuromuscular & skeletal: Polyarthritis (rare)

Renal: Renal dysfunction (rare)

Miscellaneous: Anaphylactoid reactions (rare)

Drug Interactions

Metabolism/Transport Effects None known.

Avoid Concomitant Use

Avoid concomitant use of Clindamycin (Systemic) with any of the following: BCG; Erythromycin; Erythromycin (Systemic)

Increased Effect/Toxicity

Clindamycin (Systemic) may increase the levels/effects of: Neuromuscular-Blocking Agents

Decreased Effect

Clindamycin (Systemic) may decrease the levels/effects of: BCG; Erythromycin (Systemic); Typhoid Vaccine

The levels/effects of Clindamycin (Systemic) may be decreased by: Erythromycin; Kaolin

Ethanol/Nutrition/Herb Interactions

Food: Peak concentrations may be delayed with food.

Herb/Nutraceutical: St John's wort may decrease clindamycin levels.

Stability

Capsule: Store at room temperature of 20°C to 25°C (68°F to 77°F).

I.V.: Infusion solution in NS or D_5W solution is stable for 16 days at room temperature, 32 days refrigerated, or 8 weeks frozen. Prior to use, store vials and premixed bags at controlled room temperature 20°C to 25°C (68°F to 77°F). After initial use, discard any unused portion of vial after 24 hours.

Oral solution: Do not refrigerate reconstituted oral solution (it will thicken); following reconstitution, oral solution is stable for 2 weeks at room temperature of 20°C to 25°C (68°F to 77°F).

Mechanism of Action Reversibly binds to 50S ribosomal subunits preventing peptide bond formation thus inhibiting bacterial protein synthesis; bacteriostatic or bactericidal depending on drug concentration, infection site, and organism

Pharmacodynamics/Kinetics

Absorption: Oral, hydrochloride: Rapid (90%)

Distribution: High concentrations in bone and urine; no significant levels in CSF, even with inflamed meninges

V_d: ~2 L/kg

Metabolism: Hepatic; forms metabolites (variable activity); Clindamycin phosphate is converted to clindamycin HCl (active)

Half-life elimination: Neonates: Premature: 8.7 hours; Full-term: 3.6 hours; Children: ~2 hours; Adults: ~2-3 hours; Elderly 4 hours (range 3.4-5.1 hours)

Time to peak, serum: Oral: Within 60 minutes; I.M.: 1-3 hours

Excretion: Urine (10%) and feces (~4%) as active drug and metabolites

Dosage

Usual dosage ranges:

Infants and Children:

Oral: 8-40 mg/kg/day in 3-4 divided doses; Manufacturer's labeling: 8-20 mg/kg/day (as hydrochloride) or 8-25 mg/kg/day (as palmitate) in 3-4 divided doses; minimum dose of palmitate: 37.5 mg 3 times/day

I.M., I.V.: Manufacturer's labeling: 20-40 mg/kg/day in 3-4 divided doses

Adults:

Oral: 150-450 mg/dose every 6-8 hours; maximum dose: 1.8 g/day

I.M., I.V.: 1.2-2.7 g/day in 2-4 divided doses; maximum dose: 4.8 g/day

Indication-specific dosing:

Infants >3 months and Children:

Community-acquired pneumonia (CAP) (IDSA/PIDS, 2011): Note: In children ≥5 years, a macrolide antibiotic should be added if atypical pneumonia cannot be ruled out.

Group A *Streptococcus:*

Moderate-to-severe infection (alternative to ampicillin/penicillin): I.V.: 40 mg/kg/day divided every 6-8 hours

Mild infection, step-down therapy (alternative to amoxicillin/penicillin): Oral: 40 mg/kg/day divided every 8 hours

Presumed bacterial (in addition to recommended antibiotic therapy), *S. pneumoniae* moderate-to-severe (MICs to penicillin ≤2.0 mcg/mL) (alternative to ampicillin/penicillin): I.V.: 40 mg/kg/day divided every 6-8 hours

S. pneumoniae:

Moderate-to-severe infection (MICs to penicillin ≥4.0 mcg/mL) (alternative to ceftriaxone): I.V.: 40 mg/kg/day divided every 6-8 hours

Mild infection, step-down therapy (MICs to penicillin ≥4.0 mcg/mL) (alternative to levofloxacin or linezolid): Oral: 30-40 mg/kg/day divided every 8 hours

S. aureus (methicillin-susceptible):

Moderate-to-severe infection (alternative to cefazolin or oxacillin): I.V.: 40 mg/kg/day divided every 6-8 hours

Mild infection, step-down therapy (alternative to cephalexin): Oral: 30-40 mg/kg/day divided every 6-8 hours

S. aureus (methicillin-resistant/clindamycin-susceptible):

Moderate-to-severe infection (preferred): I.V.: 40 mg/kg/day divided every 6-8 hours; recommended duration: 7-21 days (Liu, 2011)

Mild infection, step-down therapy (preferred): Oral: 30-40 mg/kg/day divided every 6-8 hours; recommended duration: 7-21 days (Liu, 2011)

Children:

Anthrax (unlabeled use): I.V.: 30 mg/kg/day divided every 6 hours

Babesiosis (unlabeled use): Oral: 20-40 mg/kg/day divided every 8 hours for 7-10 days *plus* quinine (*Medical Letter*, 2007)

Cellulitis due to MRSA (unlabeled use): Oral: 10-13 mg/kg/dose every 6-8 hours for 5-10 days (maximum: 40 mg/kg/day) (Liu, 2011)

Complicated skin/soft tissue infection due to MRSA (unlabeled use): Oral, I.V.: 10-13 mg/kg/dose every 6-8 hours for 7-14 days (maximum: 40 mg/kg/day) (Liu, 2011)

Healthcare-associated pneumonia (HAP) (methicillin-resistant/clindamycin-susceptible): Oral, I.V.: 30-40 mg/kg/day divided every 6-8 hours for 7-21 days (Liu, 2011)

Malaria, severe (unlabeled use): I.V.: Load: 10 mg/kg followed by 15 mg/kg/day divided every 8 hours *plus* I.V. quinidine gluconate; switch to oral therapy (clindamycin *plus* quinine) when able for total clindamycin treatment duration of 7 days (**Note:** Quinine duration is region specific, consult CDC for current recommendations) (CDC, 2009)

Malaria, uncomplicated treatment (unlabeled use): Oral: 20 mg/kg/day divided every 8 hours for 7 days *plus* quinine (CDC, 2009)

Osteomyelitis due to MRSA (unlabeled use): Oral, I.V.: 10-13 mg/kg/dose every 6-8 hours for a minimum of 4-6 weeks (maximum: 40 mg/kg/day) (Liu, 2011)

Prophylaxis against infective endocarditis (unlabeled use):

Oral: 20 mg/kg 30-60 minutes before procedure (Wilson, 2007)

I.M., I.V.: 20 mg/kg 30-60 minutes before procedure. Intramuscular injections should be avoided in patients who are receiving anticoagulant therapy. In these circumstances, orally administered regimens should be given whenever possible. Intravenously administered antibiotics should be used for patients who are unable to tolerate or absorb oral medications. (Wilson, 2007)

Note: American Heart Association (AHA) guidelines now recommend prophylaxis only in patients undergoing invasive procedures and in whom underlying cardiac conditions may predispose to a higher risk of adverse outcomes should infection occur. As of April 2007, routine prophylaxis for GI/GU procedures is no longer recommended by the AHA.

Septic arthritis due to MRSA (unlabeled use): Oral, I.V.: 10-13 mg/kg/dose every 6-8 hours for minimum of 3-4 weeks (maximum: 40 mg/kg/day) (Liu, 2011)

Toxoplasmosis (HIV-exposed/-positive; secondary prevention [unlabeled use]): Oral: 20-30 mg/kg/day divided every 6-8 hours (*plus* pyrimethamine and leucovorin calcium) (CDC, 2009)

Adults:

Amnionitis: I.V.: 450-900 mg every 8 hours

Anthrax (unlabeled use): I.V.: 900 mg every 8 hours with ciprofloxacin or doxycycline

Babesiosis (unlabeled use):

Oral: 600 mg 3 times/day for 7-10 days with quinine (*Medical Letter*, 2007)

I.V.: 1.2 g twice daily for 7-10 days with quinine (*Medical Letter*, 2007)

Bacterial vaginosis (unlabeled use): Oral: 300 mg twice daily for 7 days (CDC, 2010)

Bite wounds (canine): Oral: 300 mg 4 times/day with a fluoroquinolone

Cellulitis due to MRSA (unlabeled use): Oral: 300-450 mg 3 times/day for 5-10 days (Liu, 2011)

Complicated skin/soft tissue infection due to MRSA (unlabeled use): I.V., Oral: 600 mg 3 times/day for 7-14 days (Liu, 2011)

Gangrenous pyomyositis: I.V.: 900 mg every 8 hours with penicillin G

Group B streptococcus (neonatal prophylaxis): I.V.: 900 mg every 8 hours until delivery

Malaria, severe (unlabeled use): I.V.: Load: 10 mg/kg followed by 15 mg/kg/day divided every 8 hours *plus* I.V. quinidine gluconate; switch to oral therapy (clindamycin *plus* quinine) when able for total clindamycin treatment duration of 7 days (**Note:** Quinine duration is region specific, consult CDC for current recommendations) (CDC, 2009)

Malaria, uncomplicated treatment (unlabeled use): Oral: 20 mg/kg/day divided every 8 hours for 7 days *plus* quinine (CDC, 2009)

Orofacial/parapharyngeal space infections:

Oral: 150-450 mg every 6 hours for 7 days, maximum 1.8 g/day

I.V.: 600-900 mg every 8 hours

Osteomyelitis due to MRSA (unlabeled use): I.V., Oral: 600 mg 3 times/day for a minimum of 8 weeks (some experts combine with rifampin) (Liu, 2011)

Pelvic inflammatory disease: I.V.: 900 mg every 8 hours with gentamicin (conventional or single daily dosing); 24 hours after clinical improvement may convert to oral doxycycline 100 mg twice daily **or** clindamycin 450 mg 4 times/day to complete 14 days of total therapy. Avoid doxycycline if tubo-ovarian abscess is present (CDC, 2010).

***Pneumocystis jirovecii* pneumonia (unlabeled use):**

I.V.: 600-900 mg every 6-8 hours with primaquine for 21 days (CDC, 2009)

Oral: 300-450 mg every 6-8 hours with primaquine for 21 days (CDC, 2009)

Pneumonia due to MRSA (unlabeled use): I.V., Oral: 600 mg 3 times/day for 7-21 days (Liu, 2011)

Prophylaxis against infective endocarditis (unlabeled use):

Oral: 600 mg 30-60 minutes before procedure (Wilson, 2007)

I.M., I.V.: 600 mg 30-60 minutes before procedure. Intramuscular injections should be avoided in patients who are receiving anticoagulant therapy. In these circumstances, orally administered regimens should be given whenever possible. Intravenously administered antibiotics should be used for patients who are unable to tolerate or absorb oral medications. (Wilson, 2007)

Note: American Heart Association (AHA) guidelines now recommend prophylaxis only in patients undergoing invasive procedures and in whom underlying cardiac conditions may predispose to a higher risk of adverse outcomes should infection occur. As of April 2007, routine prophylaxis for GI/GU procedures is no longer recommended by the AHA.

Prophylaxis in total joint replacement patients undergoing dental procedures which produce bacteremia (unlabeled use):

Oral: 600 mg 1 hour prior to procedure (ADA, 2003)

I.V.: 600 mg 1 hour prior to procedure (for patients unable to take oral medication) (ADA, 2003)

Septic arthritis due to MRSA (unlabeled use): I.V., Oral: 600 mg 3 times/day for 3-4 weeks (Liu, 2011)

Toxic shock syndrome: I.V.: 900 mg every 8 hours with penicillin G or ceftriaxone

Toxoplasmosis (HIV-exposed/positive; secondary prevention [unlabeled use]): Oral: 600 mg every 8 hours (with pyrimethamine and leucovorin calcium) (CDC, 2009)

Dosing adjustment in renal impairment: No dosage adjustment required in renal impairment.

Poorly dialyzed; no supplemental dose or dosage adjustment necessary, including patients on intermittent hemodialysis, peritoneal dialysis, or continuous renal replacement therapy (eg, CVVHD).

Dosing adjustment in hepatic impairment: No adjustment required. Use caution with severe hepatic impairment.

Dietary Considerations May be taken with food.

Administration

I.M.: Deep I.M. sites, rotate sites; do not exceed 600 mg in a single injection.

I.V.: **Never administer as bolus**; administer by I.V. intermittent infusion over at least 10-60 minutes, at a rate **not** to exceed 30 mg/minute (do not exceed 1200 mg/hour); final concentration for administration should not exceed 18 mg/mL.

Oral: Administer with a full glass of water to minimize esophageal ulceration; give around-the-clock to promote less variation in peak and trough serum levels.

Monitoring Parameters Observe for changes in bowel frequency. Monitor for colitis and resolution of symptoms. During prolonged therapy monitor CBC, liver and renal function tests periodically.

Additional Information *In vitro* susceptibility rates to clindamycin are higher in community acquired versus hospital acquired MRSA, although this may vary by geographic region. The D-zone test is recommended for detection of inducible resistance to clindamycin in erythromycin-resistant but clindamycin-susceptible isolates (Liu, 2011).

Dosage Forms Excipient information presented when available (limited, particularly for generics); consult specific product labeling.

Capsule, oral, as hydrochloride [strength expressed as base]: 75 mg, 150 mg, 300 mg

Cleocin HCl®: 75 mg, 150 mg [contains tartrazine]

Cleocin HCl®: 300 mg

Granules for solution, oral, as palmitate hydrochloride [strength expressed as base]: 75 mg/5 mL (100 mL)

Cleocin Pediatric®: 75 mg/5 mL (100 mL) [cherry flavor]

Infusion, premixed in D_5W, as phosphate [strength expressed as base]:

Cleocin Phosphate®: 300 mg (50 mL); 600 mg (50 mL); 900 mg (50 mL) [contains edetate disodium]

Injection, solution, as phosphate [strength expressed as base]: 150 mg/mL (2 mL, 4 mL, 6 mL, 60 mL)

Cleocin Phosphate®: 150 mg/mL (2 mL, 4 mL, 6 mL, 60 mL) [contains benzyl alcohol, edetate disodium]

Clindamycin (Topical) (klin da MYE sin)

Brand Names: U.S. Cleocin T®; Cleocin®; Cleocin® Vaginal Ovule; Clindagel®; ClindaMax®; ClindaReach®; Clindesse®; Evoclin®

Brand Names: Canada Clinda-T; Clindasol™; Clindets; Dalacin® C; Dalacin® T; Dalacin® Vaginal; Taro-Clindamycin

Index Terms Clindamycin Phosphate

Pharmacologic Category Antibiotic, Lincosamide; Topical Skin Product, Acne

Use Treatment of bacterial vaginosis (vaginal cream, vaginal suppository); topically in treatment of severe acne

Pregnancy Risk Factor B

Dosage Indication-specific dosing:

Children ≥12 years and Adults: **Acne vulgaris:** Topical:

Gel, pledget, lotion, solution: Apply a thin film twice daily

Foam (Evoclin®): Apply once daily

Adults: **Bacterial vaginosis:** Intravaginal:

Suppositories: Insert one ovule (100 mg clindamycin) daily into vagina at bedtime for 3 days

Cream:

Cleocin®: One full applicator inserted intravaginally once daily before bedtime for 3 or 7 consecutive days in nonpregnant patients or for 7 consecutive days in pregnant patients

Clindesse®: One full applicator inserted intravaginally as a single dose at anytime during the day in nonpregnant patients

Additional Information Complete prescribing information for this medication should be consulted for additional detail.

Dosage Forms Excipient information presented when available (limited, particularly for generics); consult specific product labeling. [DSC] = Discontinued product

Aerosol, foam, topical, as phosphate [strength expressed as base]: 1% (50 g, 100 g)

Evoclin®: 1% (50 g, 100 g) [contains ethanol 58%]

Cream, vaginal, as phosphate [strength expressed as base]: 2% (40 g)

Cleocin®: 2% (40 g) [contains benzyl alcohol, mineral oil]

Clindesse®: 2% (5 g) [contains mineral oil]

Gel, topical, as phosphate [strength expressed as base]: 1% (30 g, 60 g)

Cleocin T®: 1% (30 g, 60 g)

Clindagel®: 1% (40 mL, 75 mL)

ClindaMax®: 1% (30 g, 60 g)

Lotion, topical, as phosphate [strength expressed as base]: 1% (60 mL)

Cleocin T®: 1% (60 mL)

ClindaMax®: 1% (60 mL)

Pledget, topical, as phosphate [strength expressed as base]: 1% (60s, 69s [DSC])

Cleocin T®: 1% (60s) [contains isopropyl alcohol 50%]

ClindaReach®: 1% (120s) [contains isopropyl alcohol 50%]

Solution, topical, as phosphate [strength expressed as base]: 1% (30 mL, 60 mL)

Cleocin T®: 1% (30 mL, 60 mL) [contains isopropyl alcohol 50%]

Suppository, vaginal, as phosphate [strength expressed as base]:
Cleocin® Vaginal Ovule: 100 mg (3s) [contains oleaginous base]

Clindamycin and Tretinoin

(klin da MYE sin & TRET i noyn)

Brand Names: U.S. Veltin™; Ziana®

Index Terms Clindamycin Phosphate and Tretinoin; Tretinoin and Clindamycin; Veltin™

Pharmacologic Category Acne Products; Retinoic Acid Derivative; Topical Skin Product; Topical Skin Product, Acne

Use Treatment of acne vulgaris

Pregnancy Risk Factor C

Dosage Topical: Children ≥12 years and Adults: Apply once daily

Additional Information Complete prescribing information for this medication should be consulted for additional detail.

Dosage Forms Excipient information presented when available (limited, particularly for generics); consult specific product labeling.

Gel, topical:
Veltin™: Clindamycin phosphate 1.2% and tretinoin 0.025% (30 g, 60 g)
Ziana®: Clindamycin phosphate 1.2% and tretinoin 0.025% (30 g, 60 g)

◆ **Clindamycine (Can)** *see* Clindamycin (Systemic) *on page 378*
◆ **Clindamycin Hydrochloride** *see* Clindamycin (Systemic) *on page 378*
◆ **Clindamycin Injection, USP (Can)** *see* Clindamycin (Systemic) *on page 378*
◆ **Clindamycin Palmitate** *see* Clindamycin (Systemic) *on page 378*
◆ **Clindamycin Phosphate** *see* Clindamycin (Topical) *on page 381*
◆ **Clindamycin Phosphate and Tretinoin** *see* Clindamycin and Tretinoin *on page 382*
◆ **ClindaReach®** *see* Clindamycin (Topical) *on page 381*
◆ **Clindasol™ (Can)** *see* Clindamycin (Topical) *on page 381*
◆ **Clinda-T (Can)** *see* Clindamycin (Topical) *on page 381*
◆ **Clindesse®** *see* Clindamycin (Topical) *on page 381*
◆ **Clindets (Can)** *see* Clindamycin (Topical) *on page 381*
◆ **Clinoril®** *see* Sulindac *on page 1608*
◆ **Clinpro™ 5000** *see* Fluoride *on page 728*

Clobazam (KLOE ba zam)

Brand Names: U.S. Onfi™

Brand Names: Canada Apo-Clobazam®; Clobazam-10; Dom-Clobazam; Frisium®; Novo-Clobazam; PMS-Clobazam

Pharmacologic Category Benzodiazepine

Use Adjunctive treatment of seizures associated with Lennox-Gastaut syndrome

Canadian labeling: Adjunctive treatment of epilepsy

Unlabeled Use Catamenial epilepsy; epilepsy (monotherapy)

Pregnancy Considerations Clobazam was shown to be teratogenic in some animal studies. Clobazam crosses the placenta. Teratogenic effects have been observed with some benzodiazepines; however, additional studies are needed. Epilepsy itself, the number of medications, genetic factors, or a combination of these probably influence the teratogenicity of anticonvulsant therapy. The incidence of premature birth and low birth weights may be increased following maternal use of benzodiazepines; hypoglycemia and respiratory problems in the neonate may occur following exposure late in pregnancy. Neonatal withdrawal symptoms may occur within days to weeks after birth and "floppy infant syndrome" (which also includes withdrawal symptoms) has been reported with some benzodiazepines. An increased risk of fetal malformations may be associated with first trimester exposure. The Canadian labeling contraindicates use in the first trimester.

Patients exposed to clobazam during pregnancy are encouraged to enroll themselves into the AED Pregnancy Registry by calling 1-888-233-2334. Additional information is available at www.aedpregnancyregistry.org.

Lactation Enters breast milk/not recommended

Medication Guide Available Yes

Contraindications There are no contraindications in the manufacturer's labeling.

Canadian labeling (not in U.S. labeling): Hypersensitivity to clobazam or any component of the formulation (cross sensitivity with other benzodiazepines may exist); myasthenia gravis; narrow-angle glaucoma; severe hepatic or respiratory disease; sleep apnea; history of substance abuse; use in the first trimester of pregnancy; breastfeeding

Warnings/Precautions Rebound or withdrawal symptoms may occur following abrupt discontinuation or large decreases in dose (more common with prolonged treatment). Cautiously taper dose if drug discontinuation is required. Use with caution in elderly or debilitated patients, patients with mild-to-moderate hepatic impairment or with pre-existing muscle weakness or ataxia (may cause muscle weakness).

Causes CNS depression (dose related) resulting in sedation, dizziness, confusion, or ataxia which may impair physical and mental capabilities. Patients must be cautioned about performing tasks which require mental alertness (eg, operating machinery or driving). Use with caution in patients receiving other CNS depressants or psychoactive agents. Effects with other sedative drugs or ethanol may be potentiated. Use with caution in patients with an impaired gag reflex or respiratory disease.

Tolerance, psychological and physical dependence may occur with prolonged use. Where possible, avoid use in patients with drug abuse, alcoholism, or psychiatric disease (eg, depression, psychosis). May increase risk of suicidal thoughts/behavior.

Acute withdrawal, including seizures, may be precipitated in patients after administration of flumazenil to patients receiving long-term benzodiazepine therapy.

Benzodiazepines have been associated with anterograde amnesia. Paradoxical reactions, including hyperactive or aggressive behavior, have been reported with benzodiazepines, particularly in adolescent/pediatric or psychiatric patients. Does not have analgesic, antidepressant, or antipsychotic properties.

Adverse Reactions

Central nervous system: Drowsiness (17%), ataxia (4%), dizziness (2%), nervousness (2%), behavior disorder (1%), hostility (1%), anterograde amnesia, confusion, disorientation, headache, lethargy, sedation, slurred speech; paradoxical reactions (including aggression, agitation, anxiety, delusions, difficulty falling asleep, excitation, hallucinations, irritability, nightmares, rage, restlessness, psychosis, and suicidal tendencies)

Dermatologic: Rash, Stevens-Johnson syndrome, toxic epidermal necrolysis, urticaria

Endocrine: Libido decreased

Gastrointestinal: Weight gain (2%), constipation, nausea, xerostomia

Hematologic: Decreased WBCs and other hematologic abnormalities have been rarely associated with benzodiazepines

Neuromuscular & skeletal: Gait instability, muscle spasm, muscle weakness, tremor

Ocular: Blurred vision (1%), double vision, nystagmus

Drug Interactions

Metabolism/Transport Effects Substrate of CYP2B6 (minor), CYP2C19 (major), CYP3A4 (minor), P-glycoprotein; **Note:** Assignment of Major/Minor substrate status based on clinically relevant drug interaction potential; **Inhibits** CYP2C9 (weak), CYP2D6 (moderate), UGT1A4, UGT1A6, UGT2B4; **Induces** CYP3A4 (weak/moderate)

Avoid Concomitant Use

Avoid concomitant use of Clobazam with any of the following: OLANZapine; Thioridazine

Increased Effect/Toxicity

Clobazam may increase the levels/effects of: CloZAPine; CNS Depressants; CYP2D6 Substrates; Deferiprone; Fesoterodine; Fosphenytoin; Methotrimeprazine; Nebivolol; Phenytoin; Selective Serotonin Reuptake Inhibitors; Tamoxifen; Thioridazine

The levels/effects of Clobazam may be increased by: Alcohol (Ethyl); Antifungal Agents (Azole Derivatives, Systemic); Aprepitant; Calcium Channel Blockers (Nondihydropyridine); Cimetidine; Conivaptan; Contraceptives (Estrogens); Contraceptives (Progestins); CYP2C19 Inhibitors (Moderate); CYP2C19 Inhibitors (Strong); Droperidol; Fluconazole; Fosaprepitant; Grapefruit Juice; HydrOXYzine; Isoniazid; Macrolide Antibiotics; Methotrimeprazine; Nefazodone; OLANZapine; Propafenone; Proton Pump Inhibitors; Selective Serotonin Reuptake Inhibitors

Decreased Effect

Clobazam may decrease the levels/effects of: ARIPiprazole; Codeine; Contraceptives (Estrogens); Contraceptives (Progestins); Saxagliptin; TraMADol

The levels/effects of Clobazam may be decreased by: CarBAMazepine; CYP2C19 Inducers (Strong); Rifamycin Derivatives; St Johns Wort; Theophylline Derivatives; Tocilizumab; Yohimbine

Ethanol/Nutrition/Herb Interactions

Ethanol: Concomitant administration may increase bioavailability of clobazam by 50%. Ethanol may also increase CNS depression; monitor for increased effects with coadministration. Caution patients about effects.

Food: Serum concentrations may be increased by grapefruit juice.

Herb/Nutraceutical: St John's wort may decrease benzodiazepine levels. Avoid valerian, St John's wort, kava kava, gotu kola (may increase CNS depression).

Stability Store at 20°C to 25°C (68°F to 77°F).

Mechanism of Action Clobazam is a 1,5 benzodiazepine which binds to stereospecific benzodiazepine receptors on the postsynaptic GABA neuron at several sites within the central nervous system, including the limbic system, reticular formation. Enhancement of the inhibitory effect of GABA on neuronal excitability results by increased neuronal membrane permeability to chloride ions. This shift in chloride ions results in hyperpolarization (a less excitable state) and stabilization.

Pharmacodynamics/Kinetics

Absorption: Rapid; ~87%

Protein binding: 80% to 90%

Metabolism: Hepatic via CYP3A4 and to a lesser extent via CYP2C19 and 2B6 (N-demethylation to active metabolite [N-desmethyl] with ~20% activity of clobazam). CYP2C19 primarily mediates subsequent hydroxylation of the N-desmethyl metabolite.

Half-life elimination: 36-42 hours; N-desmethyl (active): 71-82 hours

Time to peak: 30 minutes to 4 hours

Excretion: Urine (~94%), as metabolites

Dosage Oral:

Children:

Lennox-Gastaut (adjunctive): U.S. labeling: ≥2 years: Refer to adult dosing.

Epilepsy (adjunctive): Canadian labeling (not in U.S. labeling):

<2 years: Initial 0.5-1 mg/kg/day

2-16 years: Initial: 5 mg/day; may be increased (no more frequently than every 5 days) to a maximum of 40 mg/day

Epilepsy (monotherapy) (unlabeled use): 2-16 years: Initial: Titrate slowly over 1-3 weeks to target dose of ~0.5 mg/kg/day in 2 divided doses (Canadian Study Group, 1998)

Adults:

Lennox-Gastaut (adjunctive): U.S. labeling: **Note:** Dose should be titrated according to patient tolerability and response.

≤30 kg: Initial: 5 mg once daily for ≥1 week, then increase to 5 mg twice daily for ≥1 week, then increase to 10 mg twice daily thereafter

>30 kg: Initial: 5 mg twice daily for ≥1 week, then increase to 10 mg twice daily for ≥1 week, then increase to 20 mg twice daily thereafter

CYP2C19 poor metabolizers:

≤30 kg: Initial: 5 mg once daily for ≥2 weeks, then increase to 5 mg twice daily; after ≥1 week may increase to 10 mg twice daily

>30 kg: Initial: 5 mg once daily for ≥1 week, then increase to 5 mg twice daily for ≥1 week, then increase to 10 mg twice daily; after ≥1 week may increase to 20 mg twice daily

Epilepsy (adjunctive): Canadian labeling (not in U.S. labeling): Initial: 5-15 mg/day; dosage may be gradually adjusted (based on tolerance and seizure control) to a maximum of 80 mg/day. **Note:** Daily doses of up to 30 mg may be taken as a single dose at bedtime; higher doses should be divided.

Catamenial epilepsy (unlabeled use): 20-30 mg daily for 10 days during the perimenstrual period (Feely, 1984)

Elderly: Lennox-Gastaut (adjunctive):

≤30 kg: Initial: 5 mg once daily for ≥2 weeks, then increase to 5 mg twice daily; after ≥1 week may increase to 10 mg twice daily based on patient tolerability and response

>30 kg: Initial: 5 mg once daily for ≥1 week, then increase to 5 mg twice daily for ≥1 week, then increase to 10 mg twice daily; after ≥1 week may increase to 20 mg twice daily based on patient tolerability and response

Dosage adjustment in renal impairment:

U.S. labeling:

Cl_{cr} ≥30 mL/minute: No dosage adjustment necessary.

Cl_{cr} <30 mL/minute: No dosage adjustment provided in manufacturer's labeling (has not been studied); use with caution.

Canadian labeling: No dosage adjustment provided in manufacturer's labeling; however, a reduced dosage is recommended.

Dosage adjustment in hepatic impairment:

U.S. labeling:

Mild-to-moderate impairment:

≤30 kg: Initial: 5 mg once daily for ≥2 weeks, then increase to 5 mg twice daily; after ≥1 week may increase to 10 mg twice daily based on patient tolerability and response

>30 kg: Initial: 5 mg once daily for ≥1 week, then increase to 5 mg twice daily for ≥1 week, then increase to 10 mg twice daily; after ≥1 week may increase to 20 mg twice daily based on patient tolerability and response

Severe impairment: No dosage adjustment provided in manufacturer's labeling (has not been studied). Use with caution; undergoes extensive hepatic metabolism.

Canadian labeling:

Mild-to-moderate impairment: No dosage adjustment provided in manufacturer's labeling; however, a reduced dosage is recommended.

Severe impairment: Use is contraindicated.

Dietary Considerations May be taken with or without food.

Administration May be administered with or without food. Tablets can be crushed and mixed in applesauce.

Monitoring Parameters Respiratory and mental status/suicidality (eg, suicidal thoughts, depression, behavioral changes). The Canadian labeling recommends periodic CBC, liver function, renal function and thyroid function tests.

Dosage Forms Excipient information presented when available (limited, particularly for generics); consult specific product labeling.

Tablet, oral:

Onfi™: 5 mg, 10 mg, 20 mg

Dosage Forms: Canada Excipient information presented when available (limited, particularly for generics); consult specific product labeling.

Tablet:

Alti-Clobazam, Apo-Clobazam®, Clobazam-10, Dom-Clobazam, Frisium®, Novo-Clobazam, PMS-Clobazam, ratio-Clobazam: 10 mg

Controlled Substance C-IV

◆ **Clobazam-10 (Can)** *see* Clobazam *on page 382*

Clobetasol (kloe BAY ta sol)

Brand Names: U.S. Clobex®; Cormax®; Olux-E™; Olux®; Olux®/Olux-E™ CP [DSC]; Temovate E®; Temovate®

Brand Names: Canada Clobex®; Dermovate®; Gen-Clobetasol; Mylan-Clobetasol Cream; Mylan-Clobetasol Ointment; Mylan-Clobetasol Scalp Application; Novo-Clobetasol; PMS-Clobetasol; ratio-Clobetasol; Taro-Clobetasol

Index Terms Clobetasol Propionate

Pharmacologic Category Corticosteroid, Topical

Additional Appendix Information

Corticosteroids *on page 1888*

Use Short-term relief of inflammation of moderate-to-severe corticosteroid-responsive dermatoses (very high potency topical corticosteroid)

Pregnancy Risk Factor C

Dosage Topical: Discontinue when control achieved; if improvement not seen within 2 weeks, reassessment of diagnosis may be necessary.

Children <12 years: Use is not recommended

Children ≥12 years and Adults:

Oral mucosal inflammation, dental (unlabeled use): Cream: Apply twice daily for up to 2 weeks (maximum dose: 50 g/week); discontinue application when control is achieved; if no improvement is seen, reassessment of diagnosis may be necessary

Steroid-responsive dermatoses:

Cream, emollient cream, gel, ointment: Apply twice daily for up to 2 weeks (maximum dose: 50 g/week)

Foam (Olux-E™): Apply to affected area twice daily for up to 2 weeks (maximum dose: 50 g/week); do not apply to face or intertriginous areas

Steroid-responsive dermatoses: Foam (Olux®), solution: Apply to affected scalp twice daily for up to 2 weeks (maximum dose: 50 g/week or 50 mL/week)

Mild-to-moderate plaque-type psoriasis of nonscalp areas: Foam (Olux®): Apply to affected area twice daily for up to 2 weeks (maximum dose: 50 g/week); do not apply to face or intertriginous areas

Children ≥16 years and Adults: Moderate-to-severe plaque-type psoriasis: Emollient cream, lotion: Apply twice daily for up to 2 weeks, has been used for up to 4 weeks when application is <10% of body surface area; use with caution (maximum dose: 50 g/week)

Children ≥18 years and Adults:

Moderate-to-severe plaque-type psoriasis: Spray: Apply by spraying directly onto affected area twice daily; should be gently rubbed into skin. Should be used for not longer than 4 weeks; treatment beyond 2 weeks should be limited to localized lesions which have not improved sufficiently. Total dose should not exceed 50 g/week or 59 mL/week.

Scalp psoriasis: Shampoo: Apply thin film to dry scalp once daily; leave in place for 15 minutes, then add water, lather; rinse thoroughly

Steroid-responsive dermatoses: Lotion: Apply twice daily for up to 2 weeks (maximum dose: 50 g/week)

Additional Information Complete prescribing information for this medication should be consulted for additional detail.

Dosage Forms Excipient information presented when available (limited, particularly for generics); consult specific product labeling. [DSC] = Discontinued product

Aerosol, foam, topical, as propionate: 0.05% (50 g, 100 g)

Olux-E™: 0.05% (50 g, 100 g) [chlorofluorocarbon free, ethanol free]

Olux®: 0.05% (50 g, 100 g) [chlorofluorocarbon free; contains ethanol 60%; for scalp application]

Aerosol, foam, topical, as propionate [combination package]:

Olux®/Olux-E™ CP: Olux-E™: 0.05% (50 g) and Olux® 0.05% (50 g) [contains ethanol 60%] (1s [DSC]); Olux-E™: 0.05% (10 g) and Olux® 0.05% (100 g) [contains ethanol 60%] (1s [DSC])

Cream, topical, as propionate: 0.05% (15 g, 30 g, 45 g, 60 g)

Temovate®: 0.05% (30 g, 60 g)

Cream, topical, as propionate [emollient-based]: 0.05% (15 g, 30 g, 60 g)

Temovate E®: 0.05% (60 g)

Gel, topical, as propionate: 0.05% (15 g, 30 g, 60 g)

Temovate®: 0.05% (60 g)

Lotion, topical, as propionate: 0.05% (59 mL, 118 mL)

Clobex®: 0.05% (30 mL, 59 mL, 118 mL)

Ointment, topical, as propionate: 0.05% (15 g, 30 g, 45 g, 60 g)

Cormax®: 0.05% (15 g, 45 g)

Temovate®: 0.05% (15 g, 30 g)

Shampoo, topical, as propionate: 0.05% (118 mL)

Clobex®: 0.05% (118 mL) [contains ethanol]

Solution, topical, as propionate [for scalp application]: 0.05% (25 mL, 50 mL)

Cormax®: 0.05% (25 mL, 50 mL) [contains isopropyl alcohol 40%]

Temovate®: 0.05% (50 mL) [contains isopropyl alcohol 39.3%]

Solution, topical, as propionate [spray]:

Clobex®: 0.05% (59 mL, 125 mL) [contains ethanol]

◆ **Clobetasol Propionate** *see* Clobetasol *on page 384*

◆ **Clobex®** *see* Clobetasol *on page 384*

Clocortolone (kloe KOR toe lone)

Brand Names: U.S. Cloderm®
Brand Names: Canada Cloderm®
Index Terms Clocortolone Pivalate
Pharmacologic Category Corticosteroid, Topical
Additional Appendix Information
Corticosteroids *on page 1888*
Use Inflammation of corticosteroid-responsive dermatoses (intermediate-potency topical corticosteroid)
Pregnancy Risk Factor C
Dosage Adults: Apply sparingly and gently; rub into affected area from 1-4 times/day. Therapy should be discontinued when control is achieved; if no improvement is seen, reassessment of diagnosis may be necessary.
Additional Information Complete prescribing information for this medication should be consulted for additional detail.
Dosage Forms Excipient information presented when available (limited, particularly for generics); consult specific product labeling.
Cream, topical, as pivalate:
Cloderm®: 0.1% (30 g, 45 g, 75 g, 90 g)

◆ **Clocortolone Pivalate** *see* Clocortolone *on page 385*
◆ **Cloderm®** *see* Clocortolone *on page 385*

Clofarabine (klo FARE a been)

Brand Names: U.S. Clolar®
Index Terms CAFdA; Clofarex
Pharmacologic Category Antineoplastic Agent, Antimetabolite (Purine Analog)
Use Treatment of relapsed or refractory acute lymphoblastic leukemia (ALL) in children (ages 1-21 years)
Unlabeled Use Treatment of acute myeloid leukemia (AML) in adults ≥60 years of age
Pregnancy Risk Factor D
Pregnancy Considerations Teratogenic effects and resorptions were observed in animal studies. May cause fetal harm if administered to a pregnant woman. Women of childbearing potential should be advised to use effective contraception and avoid becoming pregnant during therapy.
Lactation Excretion in breast milk unknown/not recommended
Contraindications There are no contraindications listed within the manufacturer's labeling.
Warnings/Precautions Hazardous agent - use appropriate precautions for handling and disposal. Cytokine release may develop into capillary leak syndrome, systemic inflammatory response syndrome (SIRS), and organ dysfunction; discontinue with signs/symptoms of SIRS or capillary leak syndrome and consider diuretics, corticosteroids, and albumin. Prophylactic corticosteroids may prevent the signs/symptoms of cytokine release. Monitor blood pressure during 5 days of treatment; discontinue if hypotension develops. Monitor if on concurrent medications known to affect blood pressure. Dose-dependent, reversible myelosuppression (neutropenia, thrombocytopenia, and anemia) is common; may be severe. Monitor blood counts. May be at increased risk for infection due to neutropenia; opportunistic infection is increased due to prolonged neutropenia and immunocompromised state; monitor for signs and symptoms of infection and treat promptly if infection develops.

Has not been studied in patients with hepatic or renal impairment; use with caution (per manufacturer's labeling); however, a pharmacokinetic study demonstrated that systemic exposure increases as creatinine clearance decreases (Cl_{cr} <60 mL/minute) (Bonate, 2011). Avoid the use of drugs that may cause hepatic or renal toxicity during the 5-day treatment period. Tumor lysis syndrome/hyperuricemia may occur as a consequence of leukemia treatment, including treatment with clofarabine, usually occurring in the first treatment cycle. May lead to life-threatening acute renal failure; adequate hydration and prophylactic allopurinol throughout treatment will reduce the risk/effects of tumor lysis syndrome; monitor closely. Transaminases and bilirubin may be increased during treatment; may require dosage modification. Transaminase elevations generally occur within 10 days of administration, with a duration of ≤15 days. The risk for hepatotoxicity, including hepatic sinusoidal obstruction syndrome (SOS; formerly called veno-occlusive disease), is increased in patients who have previously undergone a hematopoietic stem cell transplant.

Adverse Reactions
>10%:
Cardiovascular: Tachycardia (35%), hypotension (29%; grades 3/4: 19%), flushing (19%), hypertension (13%), edema (12%)
Central nervous system: Headache (43%), fever (39%), chills (34%), fatigue (34%), anxiety (21%), pain (15%)
Dermatologic: Pruritus (43%), rash (38%), petechiae (26%), palmar-plantar erythrodysesthesia syndrome (16%), erythema (11%)
Gastrointestinal: Vomiting (78%; grades 3/4: 9%), nausea (73%; grades 3/4: 15%), diarrhea (56%), abdominal pain (8% to 35%), anorexia (30%), mucosal inflammation (16%), gingival bleeding (14%), oral candidiasis (11%)
Hematologic: Leukopenia (grades 3/4: 88%), anemia (83%; grades 3/4: 75%), lymphopenia (grades 3/4: 82%), thrombocytopenia (81%; grades 3/4: 80%), neutropenia (grades 3/4: 10% to 64%), febrile neutropenia (55%; grade 4: 3%)
Hepatic: ALT increased (81%; grades 3/4: 43% to 44%), AST increased (74%; grades 3/4: 36%), bilirubin increased (45%; grades 3/4: 13%)
Neuromuscular & skeletal: Limb pain (30%), myalgia (14%)
Renal: Creatinine increased (50%; grades 3/4: 8%), hematuria (13%)
Respiratory: Epistaxis (27%), dyspnea (13%), pleural effusion (12%)
Miscellaneous: Infection (83%; includes bacterial, fungal, and viral), catheter-related infection (12%)
1% to 10%:
Cardiovascular: Pericardial effusion (8%)
Central nervous system: Irritability (10%), lethargy (10%), somnolence (10%), agitation (5%), mental status change (1% to 4%)
Dermatologic: Cellulitis (8%), pruritic rash (8%)
Gastrointestinal: Proctalgia (8%), clostridium colitis (7%), stomatitis (7%), mouth hemorrhage (5%), oral mucosal petechiae (5%), cecitis (1% to 4%), pancreatitis (1% to 4%)
Hepatic: Jaundice (8%)
Neuromuscular & skeletal: Back pain (10%), bone pain (10%), weakness (10%), arthralgia (9%)
Respiratory: Pneumonia (10%), respiratory distress (10%), tachypnea (9%), upper respiratory tract infection (5%), pulmonary edema (1% to 4%)
Miscellaneous: Herpes simplex (10%), sepsis (10%), bacteremia (9%), candidiasis (7%), herpes zoster (7%), septic shock (7%), staphylococcus bacteremia (6%), tumor lysis syndrome (grade 3: 6%), capillary leak syndrome (4%), hypersensitivity (1% to 4%), SIRS (2%) ▶

<1% (Limited to important or life-threatening): Bone marrow failure, dermatitis, hallucination, hepatic sinusoidal obstruction syndrome (SOS; veno-occlusive disease), hepatomegaly, hypokalemia, hypophosphatemia, left ventricular systolic function decreased, right ventricular pressure increased, Stevens-Johnson syndrome, toxic epidermal necrolysis

Drug Interactions

Metabolism/Transport Effects None known.

Avoid Concomitant Use

Avoid concomitant use of Clofarabine with any of the following: BCG; CloZAPine; Natalizumab; Pimecrolimus; Tacrolimus (Topical); Vaccines (Live)

Increased Effect/Toxicity

Clofarabine may increase the levels/effects of: CloZAPine; Leflunomide; Natalizumab; Vaccines (Live); Vitamin K Antagonists

The levels/effects of Clofarabine may be increased by: Denosumab; Pimecrolimus; Roflumilast; Tacrolimus (Topical); Trastuzumab

Decreased Effect

Clofarabine may decrease the levels/effects of: BCG; Cardiac Glycosides; Coccidioidin Skin Test; Sipuleucel-T; Vaccines (Inactivated); Vaccines (Live); Vitamin K Antagonists

The levels/effects of Clofarabine may be decreased by: Echinacea

Stability Store intact vials at room temperature of 25°C (77°F); excursions permitted to 15°C to 30°C (59°F to 86°F). The manufacturer recommends the product be filtered through a 0.2 micron filter prior to dilution. Clofarabine should be diluted with NS or D_5W to a final concentration of 0.15-0.4 mg/mL. Solutions diluted for infusion in D_5W or NS are stable for 24 hours at room temperature. Use appropriate precautions for handling and disposal.

Mechanism of Action Clofarabine, a purine (deoxyadenosine) nucleoside analog, is metabolized to clofarabine 5'-triphosphate. Clofarabine 5'-triphosphate decreases cell replication and repair as well as causing cell death. To decrease cell replication and repair, clofarabine 5'-triphosphate competes with deoxyadenosine triphosphate for the enzymes ribonucleotide reductase and DNA polymerase. Cell replication is decreased when clofarabine 5'-triphosphate inhibits ribonucleotide reductase from reacting with deoxyadenosine triphosphate to produce deoxynucleotide triphosphate which is needed for DNA synthesis. Cell replication is also decreased when clofarabine 5'-triphosphate competes with DNA polymerase for incorporation into the DNA chain; when done during the repair process, cell repair is affected. To cause cell death, clofarabine 5'-triphosphate alters the mitochondrial membrane by releasing proteins, an inducing factor and cytochrome C.

Pharmacodynamics/Kinetics

Distribution: V_d: Children: 172 L/m^2 or 5.8 L/kg (Bonate, 2011); Elderly: 268 L/kg (Bonate, 2011)

Protein binding: 47%, primarily to albumin

Metabolism: Intracellulary by deoxycytidine kinase and mono- and diphosphokinases to active metabolite clofarabine 5′-triphosphate; limited hepatic metabolism (0.2%)

Half-life elimination: Children: ~5 hours; Children and Adults: 7 hours (Bonate, 2011); half-life may be increased in elderly and in patients with renal impairment (Bonate, 2011)

Excretion: Urine (49% to 60%, as unchanged drug)

Dosage Consider prophylactic corticosteroids (hydrocortisone 100 mg/m^2 on days 1-3) to prevent signs/symptoms of capillary leak syndrome or systemic inflammatory response syndrome (SIRS), hydration and allopurinol (to reduce the risk of tumor lysis syndrome/hyperuricemia), and prophylactic antiemetics.

Children ≥1 year and Adults ≤21 years: Acute lymphoblastic leukemia (ALL): I.V.: 52 mg/m^2/day days 1 through 5; repeat every 2-6 weeks; subsequent cycles should begin no sooner than 14 days from day 1 of the previous cycle (subsequent cycles may be administered when ANC ≥750/mm^3)

Adults ≥60 years (unlabeled use): Acute myelocytic leukemia (AML): I.V.:

Monotherapy (Kantarjian, 2010):

Induction: 30 mg/m^2/day for 5 days; may repeat one time after day 28 (if needed) with 20 mg/m^2/day for 5 days

Consolidation: 20 mg/m^2/day for 5 days for up to a maximum total 6 cycles, including induction cycles

Combination therapy with cytarabine (Faderl, 2008):

Induction: 30 mg/m^2/day for 5 days; may repeat one time if needed

Consolidation: 30 mg/m^2/day for 3 days every 4-7 weeks for up to a total of 12 consolidation cycles

Dosage adjustment for toxicity:

Hematologic toxicity: ANC <500/mm^3 lasting ≥4 weeks: Reduce clofarabine dose by 25% for next cycle

Nonhematologic toxicity:

Clinically significant infection: Withhold treatment until infection is under control, then restart clofarabine at full dose

Grade 3 toxicity (excluding infection, nausea and vomiting, and transient elevations in transaminases and bilirubin): Withhold treatment; may reinitiate clofarabine with a 25% dose-reduction with resolution or return to baseline

Grade ≥3 increase in creatinine or bilirubin: Discontinue clofarabine; may reinitiate with 25% dosage reduction when creatinine or bilirubin return to baseline and patient is stable; administer allopurinol for hyperuricemia

Grade 4 toxicity (noninfectious): Discontinue clofarabine treatment

Capillary leak or SIRS early signs/symptoms (eg, hypotension, tachycardia, tachypnea, pulmonary edema): Discontinue clofarabine; institute supportive measures

Dosage adjustment in renal impairment: No dosage adjustment provided in manufacturer's labeling; use with caution (has not been studied). Clofarabine undergoes renal elimination and exposure is increased as creatinine clearance decreases (Bonate, 2011)

NCCN AML guidelines (v.2.2011): Adults >60 years with creatinine clearance <60 mL/minute: Use is not recommended

Dosage adjustment in hepatic impairment: No dosage adjustment provided in manufacturer's labeling; use with caution (has not been studied)

Administration

Acute lymphoblastic leukemia (ALL): I.V. infusion: Over 2 hours. Continuous I.V. fluids are encouraged to decrease adverse events and tumor lysis effects. Hypotension may be a sign of capillary leak syndrome or systemic inflammatory response syndrome (SIRS). Discontinue if the patient becomes hypotensive during administration. Retreatment should only be considered if the hypotension is not related to capillary leak syndrome or SIRS.

Acute myelocytic leukemia (AML): Was infused over 1 hour in AML studies (Faderl, 2008; Kantarjian, 2010)

Monitoring Parameters Blood pressure, cardiac function, and respiratory status during infusion; CBC with differential (periodic; increase frequency in patients who develop cytopenias); liver and kidney function (during 5 days of clofarabine administration); signs and symptoms of tumor lysis syndrome and cytokine release syndrome (tachypnea, tachycardia, hypotension, pulmonary edema); hydration status

Dosage Forms Excipient information presented when available (limited, particularly for generics); consult specific product labeling.

Injection, solution [preservative free]:

Clolar®: 1 mg/mL (20 mL)

◆ **Clofarex** *see* Clofarabine *on page 385*

◆ **Clolar®** *see* Clofarabine *on page 385*

◆ **Clomid®** *see* ClomiPHENE *on page 387*

ClomiPHENE (KLOE mi feen)

Brand Names: U.S. Clomid®; Serophene®

Brand Names: Canada Clomid®; Milophene®; Serophene®

Index Terms Clomiphene Citrate

Pharmacologic Category Ovulation Stimulator; Selective Estrogen Receptor Modulator (SERM)

Use Treatment of ovulatory failure in patients desiring pregnancy

Pregnancy Risk Factor X

Pregnancy Considerations Embryotoxic effects were observed in animal studies. The incidence of adverse fetal effects following maternal use of clomiphene for ovulation induction is similar to those seen in the general population. Clomiphene is not indicated for use in women who are already pregnant.

Lactation Excretion in breast milk unknown/use caution

Contraindications Hypersensitivity to clomiphene citrate or any of its components; liver disease; abnormal uterine bleeding; enlargement or development of ovarian cyst (not due to polycystic ovarian syndrome); uncontrolled thyroid or adrenal dysfunction; presence of an organic intracranial lesion such as pituitary tumor; pregnancy

Warnings/Precautions Ovarian enlargement may occur with use; may be accompanied by abdominal distention or abdominal pain and generally regresses without treatment within 2-3 weeks. Do not continue dosing until ovaries are of normal size. Ovarian hyperstimulation syndrome (OHSS) is characterized by severe ovarian enlargement, abdominal pain/distention, nausea, vomiting, diarrhea, dyspnea, and oliguria, and may be accompanied by ascites, pleural effusion, hypovolemia, electrolyte imbalance, hemoperitoneum, and thromboembolic events. If severe hyperstimulation occurs, stop treatment and hospitalize patient. This syndrome develops rapidly within 24 hours to several days and generally occurs during the 7-10 days immediately following treatment. Use with caution in patients unusually sensitive to pituitary gonadotropins (eg, PCOS). To minimize risks, use only at the lowest effective dose. Blurring or other visual symptoms can occur; patients with visual disturbances should discontinue therapy and have an eye exam. Multiple births may result from the use of these medications; advise patient of the potential risk of multiple births before starting the treatment.

Adverse Reactions

>10%: Endocrine & metabolic: Ovarian enlargement (14%)

1% to 10%:

Central nervous system: Headache (1%)

Endocrine & metabolic: Hot flashes (10%), breast discomfort (2%), abnormal uterine bleeding (1%)

Gastrointestinal: Distention/bloating/discomfort (6%), nausea (2%), vomiting (2%)

Ocular: Visual symptoms (2%, includes blurring of vision, diplopia, floaters, lights, phosphenes, photophobia, scotomata, waves)

<1% (Limited to important or life-threatening): Abnormal accommodation, acne, acute abdomen, allergic reaction, appetite increased, arrhythmia, chest pain, constipation, depression, dermatitis, diarrhea, dizziness, dry hair, edema, endometriosis, erythema multiforme, erythema nodosum, eye pain, fatigue, fever, hypertension, hypertrichosis, insomnia, lightheadedness, macular edema, migraine, mood changes, neoplasms, nervousness, optic neuritis, ovarian cyst, ovarian hemorrhage, palpitation, PE, pruritus, rash, retinal hemorrhage, retinal thrombosis, seizure, stroke, syncope, tachycardia, temporary loss of vision, thrombophlebitis, thyroid disorder, tinnitus, transaminase increased, tubal pregnancy, urinary frequency/volume increased, uterine hemorrhage, vaginal dryness, vertigo, weight gain/loss

Drug Interactions

Metabolism/Transport Effects None known.

Avoid Concomitant Use There are no known interactions where it is recommended to avoid concomitant use.

Increased Effect/Toxicity There are no known significant interactions involving an increase in effect.

Decreased Effect There are no known significant interactions involving a decrease in effect.

Stability Store at room temperature of 15°C to 30°C (59°F to 86°F). Protect from light, heat, and excessive humidity.

Mechanism of Action Clomiphene is a racemic mixture consisting of zuclomiphene (~38%) and enclomiphene (~62%), each with distinct pharmacologic properties. Enclomiphene is much less potent in inducing ovulation; however, it is more rapidly absorbed and metabolized, allowing the more potent activity of zuclomiphene to predominate. Zuclomiphene acts at the level of the hypothalamus, occupying cell surface and intracellular estrogen receptors (ERs) for longer durations than estrogen. This interferes with receptor recycling, effectively depleting hypothalamic ERs and inhibiting normal estrogenic negative feedback. Impairment of the feedback signal results in increased pulsatile GnRH secretion from the hypothalamus and subsequent pituitary gonadotropin (FSH, LH) release, causing growth of the ovarian follicle, followed by follicular rupture.

Pharmacodynamics/Kinetics

Onset of action: Ovulation: 5-10 days following course of treatment

Duration: Effects are cumulative; ovulation may occur in the cycle following the last treatment

Metabolism: Hepatic; undergoes enterohepatic recirculation

Half-life elimination: 5-7 days

Time to peak, plasma: ~6 hours

Excretion: Primarily feces; urine (small amounts)

Dosage Oral: Adults: Ovulation induction: Females:

Initial course: 50 mg once daily for 5 days. Begin on or about the fifth day of cycle if progestin-induced bleeding is scheduled or spontaneous uterine bleeding occurs prior to therapy.

Dose adjustment: Subsequent doses may be increased to 100 mg once daily for 5 days only if ovulation does not occur at the initial dose. A low dose or duration of course is recommended in patients where unusual sensitivity to pituitary gonadotropin is suspected (eg, PCOS).

Repeat courses: If needed, the 5-day cycle may be repeated as early as 30 days after the previous one. Exclude the presence of pregnancy.

Maximum dose: 100 mg once daily for 5 days for 6 cycles. Discontinue if ovulation does not occur after 3 courses of treatment; or if 3 ovulatory responses occur but pregnancy is not achieved. Re-evaluate if menses does not occur following ovulatory response. Doses larger than 150 mg have been reported, however, pregnancy rates are low.

Administration The total daily dose should be taken at one time to maximize effectiveness.

Monitoring Parameters Basal body temperature, serum progesterone, urinary luteinizing hormone; follicular growth and endometrial thickness may be useful in some cases; pregnancy test prior to repeat courses

Reference Range Serum progesterone: Ovulation generally occurs with levels ≥3 ng/mL; best results with levels >10 ng/mL

Test Interactions Clomiphene may increase levels of serum thyroxine and thyroxine-binding globulin (TBG)

Dosage Forms Excipient information presented when available (limited, particularly for generics); consult specific product labeling.

Tablet, oral, as citrate: 50 mg
  Clomid®: 50 mg [scored]
  Serophene®: 50 mg [scored]

◆ **Clomiphene Citrate** *see* ClomiPHENE *on page 387*

ClomiPRAMINE (kloe MI pra meen)

Brand Names: U.S. Anafranil®

Brand Names: Canada Anafranil®; Apo-Clomipramine®; CO Clomipramine; Gen-Clomipramine

Index Terms Clomipramine Hydrochloride

Pharmacologic Category Antidepressant, Tricyclic (Tertiary Amine)

Additional Appendix Information

Antidepressant Agents *on page 1874*

Use Treatment of obsessive-compulsive disorder (OCD)

Unlabeled Use Depression, panic attacks, chronic pain

Pregnancy Risk Factor C

Pregnancy Considerations Adverse events were observed in some animal reproduction studies. Withdrawal symptoms (including jitteriness, tremor, and seizures) have been observed in neonates whose mothers took clomipramine up to delivery.

Lactation Enters breast milk/not recommended (AAP rates "of concern"; AAP 2001 update pending)

Medication Guide Available Yes

Contraindications Hypersensitivity to clomipramine, other tricyclic agents, or any component of the formulation; use of MAO inhibitors within 14 days; use in a patient during the acute recovery phase of MI

Warnings/Precautions [U.S. Boxed Warning]: Antidepressants increase the risk of suicidal thinking and behavior in children, adolescents, and young adults (18-24 years of age) with major depressive disorder (MDD) and other psychiatric disorders; consider risk prior to prescribing. Short-term studies did not show an increased risk in patients >24 years of age and showed a decreased risk in patients ≥65 years. Closely monitor for clinical worsening, suicidality, or unusual changes in behavior; the patient's family or caregiver should be instructed to closely observe the patient and communicate condition with healthcare provider. A medication guide should be dispensed with each prescription. **Clomipramine is FDA approved for the treatment of OCD in children ≥10 years of age.**

The possibility of a suicide attempt is inherent in major depression and may persist until remission occurs. Monitor for worsening of depression or suicidality, especially during initiation of therapy (generally first 1-2 months) or with dose increases or decreases. Use caution in high-risk patients. Worsening depression and severe abrupt suicidality that are not part of the presenting symptoms may require discontinuation or modification of drug therapy. The patient's family or caregiver should be alerted to monitor patients for the emergence of suicidality and associated behaviors (such as agitation, irritability, hostility, impulsivity, and hypomania) and notify the healthcare provider.

May worsen psychosis in some patients or precipitate a shift to mania or hypomania in patients with bipolar disorder. Patients presenting with depressive symptoms should be screened for bipolar disorder. Monotherapy in patients with bipolar disorder should be avoided. **Clomipramine is not FDA approved for bipolar depression.**

TCAs may rarely cause bone marrow suppression; monitor for any signs of infection and obtain CBC if symptoms (eg, fever, sore throat) evident. May cause seizures (relationship to dose and/or duration of therapy) - do not exceed maximum doses. Use caution in patients with a previous seizure disorder or condition predisposing to seizures such as brain damage, alcoholism, or concurrent therapy with other drugs which lower the seizure threshold. May increase the risks associated with electroconvulsive therapy. Has been associated with a high incidence of sexual dysfunction. Weight gain may occur. Hyperpyrexia has been observed with TCAs in combination with anticholinergics and/or neuroleptics, particularly during hot weather.

The degree of sedation, anticholinergic effects, and conduction abnormalities are high relative to other antidepressants. Clomipramine often causes drowsiness/sedation, resulting in impaired performance of tasks requiring alertness (eg, operating machinery or driving). Sedative effects may be additive with other CNS depressants and/or ethanol. The risk of orthostasis is moderate to high relative to other antidepressants. Use with caution in patients with a history of cardiovascular disease (including previous MI, stroke, tachycardia, or conduction abnormalities). Use with caution in patients with urinary retention, benign prostatic hyperplasia, narrow-angle glaucoma, xerostomia, visual problems, constipation, or a history of bowel obstruction.

Consider discontinuing, when possible, prior to elective surgery. Therapy should not be abruptly discontinued in patients receiving high doses for prolonged periods. Use with caution in hyperthyroid patients or those receiving thyroid supplementation. Use with caution in patients with hepatic or renal dysfunction and in elderly patients.

Adverse Reactions Data shown for children reflects both children and adolescents studied in clinical trials.

>10%:
  Central nervous system: Dizziness (54%), somnolence (54%), drowsiness, headache (52%; children 28%), fatigue (39%), insomnia (25%; children 11%), malaise, nervousness (18%; children 4%)
  Endocrine & metabolic: Libido changes (21%), hot flushes (5%)
  Gastrointestinal: Xerostomia (84%, children 63%) constipation (47%; children 22%), nausea (33%; children 9%), dyspepsia (22%; children 13%), weight gain (18%; children 2%), diarrhea (13%; children 7%), anorexia (12%; children 22%), abdominal pain (11%), appetite increased (11%)
  Genitourinary: Ejaculation failure (42%), impotence (20%), micturition disorder (14%; children 4%)
  Neuromuscular & skeletal: Tremor (54%), myoclonus (13%; children 2%), myalgia (13%)
  Ocular: Abnormal vision (18%; children 7%)
  Respiratory: Pharyngitis (14%), rhinitis (12%)
  Miscellaneous: Diaphoresis increased (29%; children 9%)

1% to 10%:
  Cardiovascular: Flushing (8%), postural hypotension (6%), palpitation (4%), tachycardia (4%; children 2%), chest pain (4%), edema (2%)
  Central nervous system: Anxiety (9%), memory impairment (9%), twitching (7%), depression (5%), concentration impaired (5%), fever (4%), hypertonia (4%), abnormal dreaming (3%), agitation (3%), confusion (3%), migraine (3%), pain (3%), psychosomatic disorder (3%), speech disorder (3%), yawning (3%), aggressiveness (children 2%), chills (2%), depersonalization (2%), emotional lability (2%), irritability (2%), panic reaction (1%)

Dermatologic: Rash (8%), pruritus (6%), purpura (3%), dermatitis (2%), acne (2%), dry skin (2%), urticaria (1%)

Endocrine & metabolic: Amenorrhea (1%), breast enlargement (2%), breast pain (1%), hot flashes (5%), lactation (nonpuerperal) (4%)

Gastrointestinal: Taste disturbance (8%), vomiting (7%), flatulence (6%), dental caries and teeth grinding (5%), dysphagia (2%), esophagitis (1%)

Genitourinary: UTI (2% to 6%), micturition frequency (5%), dysuria (2%), leucorrhea (2%), vaginitis (2%), urinary retention (2%)

Neuromuscular & skeletal: Paresthesia (9%), back pain (6%), arthralgia (3%), paresis (children 2%), weakness (1%)

Ocular: Lacrimation abnormal (3%), mydriasis (2%), conjunctivitis (1%)

Otic: Tinnitus (6%)

Respiratory: Sinusitis (6%), coughing (6%), bronchospasm (2%; children 7%), epistaxis (2%)

<1% (Limited to important or life-threatening): Accommodation abnormal, albuminuria, aneurysm, anticholinergic syndrome, aphasia, apraxia, arrhythmia, ataxia, atrial flutter, blepharitis, blood in stool, bradycardia, breast fibroadenosis, bronchitis, bundle branch block, cardiac arrest, cardiac failure, catalepsy, cellulitis, cerebral hemorrhage, cervical dysplasia, cheilitis, cholinergic syndrome, choreoathetosis, chromatopsia, chronic enteritis, coma, conjunctival hemorrhage, cyanosis, deafness, dehydration, delirium, delusion, diabetes mellitus, diplopia, dyskinesia, dysphonia, dystonia, EEG abnormal, encephalopathy, endometrial hyperplasia, endometriosis, epididymitis, erythematous rash, exophthalmos, extrapyramidal disorder, extrasystoles, gastric ulcer, generalized spasm, glaucoma, glycosuria, goiter, gynecomastia, hallucinations, heart block, hematuria, hemiparesis, hemoptysis, hepatitis, hostility, hyperacusis, hypercholesterolemia, hyper-/hypoesthesia, hyperglycemia, hyper-/hypokinesia, hyper-reflexia, hyper-/hypothyroidism, hyperuricemia, hyper-/hypoventilation, hypnagogic hallucination, hypokalemia, ideation, intestinal obstruction, irritable bowel syndrome, keratitis, laryngismus, leukemoid reaction, lupus erythematosus rash, lymphadenopathy, lymphoma-like disorder, maculopapular rash, manic reaction, marrow depression, myocardial infarction, myocardial ischemia, myopathy, myositis, neuralgia, neuropathy, oculogyric crisis, oculomotor nerve paralysis, oral/pharyngeal edema, ovarian cyst, paralytic ileus, paranoia, parosmia, peptic ulcer, peripheral ischemia, phobic disorder, photophobia, photosensitivity reaction, pneumonia, polyarteritis nodosa, premature ejaculation, psychosis, pyelonephritis, pyuria, rectal hemorrhage, renal calculus, renal cyst, schizophrenic reaction, scleritis, seizure, sensory disturbance, skin ulceration, strabismus, stupor, suicidal ideation, suicide, suicide attempt, thrombophlebitis, tongue ulceration, torticollis, urinary incontinence, uterine hemorrhage, uterine inflammation, vaginal hemorrhage, vasospasm, ventricular tachycardia, visual field defect, withdrawal syndrome

Drug Interactions

Metabolism/Transport Effects Substrate of CYP1A2 (major), CYP2C19 (major), CYP2D6 (major), CYP3A4 (minor); **Note:** Assignment of Major/Minor substrate status based on clinically relevant drug interaction potential; **Inhibits** CYP2D6 (moderate)

Avoid Concomitant Use

Avoid concomitant use of ClomiPRAMINE with any of the following: Artemether; Dronedarone; Iobenguane I 123; Lumefantrine; MAO Inhibitors; Methylene Blue; Nilotinib; Pimozide; QUEtiapine; QuiNINE; Tetrabenazine; Thioridazine; Toremifene; Vandetanib; Vemurafenib; Ziprasidone

Increased Effect/Toxicity

ClomiPRAMINE may increase the levels/effects of: Alpha-/Beta-Agonists (Direct-Acting); Alpha1-Agonists; Amphetamines; Anticholinergics; Aspirin; Beta2-Agonists; CYP2D6 Substrates; Desmopressin; Dronedarone; Fesoterodine; Methylene Blue; Metoclopramide; Milnacipran; Nebivolol; NSAID (COX-2 Inhibitor); NSAID (Nonselective); Pimozide; QTc-Prolonging Agents; QuiNIDine; QuiNINE; Serotonin Modulators; Sodium Phosphates; Sulfonylureas; Tamoxifen; Tetrabenazine; Thioridazine; Toremifene; TraMADol; Vandetanib; Vemurafenib; Vitamin K Antagonists; Yohimbine; Ziprasidone

The levels/effects of ClomiPRAMINE may be increased by: Abiraterone Acetate; Alfuzosin; Altretamine; Antipsychotics; Artemether; BuPROPion; CarBAMazepine; Chloroquine; Cimetidine; Cinacalcet; Ciprofloxacin; Ciprofloxacin (Systemic); Conivaptan; CYP1A2 Inhibitors (Moderate); CYP1A2 Inhibitors (Strong); CYP2C19 Inhibitors (Moderate); CYP2C19 Inhibitors (Strong); CYP2D6 Inhibitors (Moderate); CYP2D6 Inhibitors (Strong); Deferasirox; Dexmethylphenidate; Divalproex; DULoxetine; Gadobutrol; Grapefruit Juice; Indacaterol; Linezolid; Lithium; Lumefantrine; MAO Inhibitors; Methylphenidate; Metoclopramide; Nilotinib; Pramlintide; Protease Inhibitors; QUEtiapine; QuiNIDine; QuiNINE; Selective Serotonin Reuptake Inhibitors; Terbinafine; Terbinafine (Systemic); Valproic Acid

Decreased Effect

ClomiPRAMINE may decrease the levels/effects of: Acetylcholinesterase Inhibitors (Central); Alpha2-Agonists; Codeine; Iobenguane I 123

The levels/effects of ClomiPRAMINE may be decreased by: Acetylcholinesterase Inhibitors (Central); Barbiturates; CYP1A2 Inducers (Strong); CYP2C19 Inducers (Strong); Cyproterone; Peginterferon Alfa-2b; St Johns Wort; Tocilizumab

Ethanol/Nutrition/Herb Interactions

Ethanol: May increase CNS depression; monitor for increased effects with coadministration. Caution patients about effects.

Food: Serum concentrations/toxicity may be increased by grapefruit juice.

Herb/Nutraceutical: Avoid valerian, St John's wort, SAMe, kava kava.

Mechanism of Action Clomipramine appears to affect serotonin uptake while its active metabolite, desmethylclomipramine, affects norepinephrine uptake

Pharmacodynamics/Kinetics

Absorption: Rapid

Protein binding: 97%, primarily to albumin

Metabolism: Hepatic to desmethylclomipramine (DMI; active); extensive first-pass effect

Half-life elimination: Clomipramine: mean 32 hours (19-37 hours); DMI: mean 69 hours (range 54-77 hours)

Time to peak, plasma: 2-6 hours

Excretion: Urine and feces

Dosage Oral:

Children:

<10 years: Safety and efficacy have not been established.

≥10 years: OCD:

Initial: 25 mg/day; may gradually increase as tolerated over the first 2 weeks to 3 mg/kg/day or 100 mg/day (whichever is less) in divided doses

Maintenance: May further increase to recommended maximum of 3 mg/kg/day or 200 mg/day (whichever is less); may give as a single daily dose at bedtime once tolerated

Adults: OCD:

Initial: 25 mg/day; may gradually increase as tolerated over the first 2 weeks to 100 mg/day in divided doses

Maintenance: May further increase to recommended maximum of 250 mg/day; may give as a single daily dose at bedtime once tolerated

Administration During titration, may divide doses and administer with meals to decrease gastrointestinal side effects. After titration, may administer total daily dose at bedtime to decrease daytime sedation.

Monitoring Parameters Pulse rate and blood pressure prior to and during therapy; ECG/cardiac status in older adults and patients with cardiac disease; suicidal ideation (especially at the beginning of therapy, after initiation, or when doses are increased or decreased)

Test Interactions Increased glucose; may interfere with urine detection of methadone (false-positive)

Dosage Forms Excipient information presented when available (limited, particularly for generics); consult specific product labeling.

Capsule, oral, as hydrochloride: 25 mg, 50 mg, 75 mg

Anafranil®: 25 mg, 50 mg, 75 mg

◆ **Clomipramine Hydrochloride** *see* ClomiPRAMINE *on page 388*

◆ **Clonapam (Can)** *see* ClonazePAM *on page 390*

ClonazePAM (kloe NA ze pam)

Brand Names: U.S. KlonoPIN®

Brand Names: Canada Alti-Clonazepam; Apo-Clonazepam®; Clonapam; CO Clonazepam; Gen-Clonazepam; Klonopin®; Mylan-Clonazepam; Novo-Clonazepam; Nu-Clonazepam; PMS-Clonazepam; PRO-Clonazepam; Rho®-Clonazepam; Rivotril®; Sandoz-Clonazepam; ZYM-Clonazepam

Pharmacologic Category Benzodiazepine

Additional Appendix Information

Anticonvulsant Drugs of Choice *on page 1873*

Benzodiazepines *on page 1882*

Use Alone or as an adjunct in the treatment of petit mal variant (Lennox-Gastaut), akinetic, and myoclonic seizures; petit mal (absence) seizures unresponsive to succimides; panic disorder with or without agoraphobia

Unlabeled Use Restless legs syndrome; neuralgia; multifocal tic disorder; parkinsonian dysarthria; bipolar disorder; adjunct therapy for schizophrenia; burning mouth syndrome

Pregnancy Risk Factor D

Pregnancy Considerations Clonazepam was shown to be teratogenic in some animal studies. Clonazepam crosses the placenta. Teratogenic effects have been observed with some benzodiazepines; however, additional studies are needed. Epilepsy itself, the number of medications, genetic factors, or a combination of these probably influence the teratogenicity of anticonvulsant therapy. The incidence of premature birth and low birth weights may be increased following maternal use of benzodiazepines; hypoglycemia and respiratory problems in the neonate may occur following exposure late in pregnancy. Neonatal withdrawal symptoms may occur within days to weeks after birth and "floppy infant syndrome" (which also includes withdrawal symptoms) has been reported with some benzodiazepines, including clonazepam.

Patients exposed to clonazepam during pregnancy are encouraged to enroll themselves into the AED Pregnancy Registry by calling 1-888-233-2334. Additional information is available at www.aedpregnancyregistry.org.

Lactation Enters breast milk/not recommended

Medication Guide Available Yes

Contraindications Hypersensitivity to clonazepam or any component of the formulation (cross-sensitivity with other benzodiazepines may exist); significant liver disease; narrow-angle glaucoma; pregnancy

Warnings/Precautions Antiepileptics are associated with an increased risk of suicidal behavior/thoughts with use (regardless of indication); patients should be monitored for signs/symptoms of depression, suicidal tendencies, and other unusual behavior changes during therapy and instructed to inform their healthcare provider immediately if symptoms occur.

Use with caution in elderly or debilitated patients, patients with hepatic disease (including alcoholics), or renal impairment. Use with caution in patients with respiratory disease or impaired gag reflex or ability to protect the airway from secretions (salivation may be increased). Worsening of seizures may occur when added to patients with multiple seizure types. Concurrent use with valproic acid may result in absence status. Monitoring of CBC and liver function tests has been recommended during prolonged therapy.

Causes CNS depression (dose related) resulting in sedation, dizziness, confusion, or ataxia which may impair physical and mental capabilities. Patients must be cautioned about performing tasks which require mental alertness (eg, operating machinery or driving). Use with caution in patients receiving other CNS depressants or psychoactive agents. Effects with other sedative drugs or ethanol may be potentiated. Benzodiazepines have been associated with falls and traumatic injury and should be used with extreme caution in patients who are at risk of these events (especially the elderly).

Use caution in patients with depression, particularly if suicidal risk may be present. Use with caution in patients with a history of drug dependence. Benzodiazepines have been associated with dependence and acute withdrawal symptoms, including seizures, on discontinuation or reduction in dose. Acute withdrawal, including seizures, may be precipitated in patients after administration of flumazenil to patients receiving long-term benzodiazepine therapy.

Benzodiazepines have been associated with anterograde amnesia. Paradoxical reactions, including hyperactive or aggressive behavior, have been reported with benzodiazepines, particularly in adolescent/pediatric or psychiatric patients. Does not have analgesic, antidepressant, or antipsychotic properties.

Adverse Reactions Reactions reported in patients with seizure and/or panic disorder. Frequency not always defined.

Cardiovascular: Edema (ankle or facial), palpitation

Central nervous system: Amnesia, ataxia (seizure disorder ~30%; panic disorder 5%), behavior problems (seizure disorder ~25%), coma, confusion, depression, dizziness, drowsiness (seizure disorder ~50%), emotional lability, fatigue, fever, hallucinations, headache, hypotonia, hysteria, insomnia, intellectual ability reduced, memory disturbance, nervousness; paradoxical reactions (including aggressive behavior, agitation, anxiety, excitability, hostility, irritability, nervousness, nightmares, sleep disturbance, vivid dreams); psychosis, slurred speech, somnolence (panic disorder 37%), suicidal attempt, suicide ideation, vertigo

Dermatologic: Hair loss, hirsutism, skin rash

Endocrine & metabolic: Dysmenorrhea, libido increased/decreased

Gastrointestinal: Abdominal pain, anorexia, appetite increased/decreased, coated tongue, constipation, dehydration, diarrhea, gastritis, gum soreness, nausea, weight changes (loss/gain), xerostomia

Genitourinary: Colpitis, dysuria, ejaculation delayed, enuresis, impotence, micturition frequency, nocturia, urinary retention, urinary tract infection

Hematologic: Anemia, eosinophilia, leukopenia, thrombocytopenia

Hepatic: Alkaline phosphatase increased (transient), hepatomegaly, transaminases increased (transient)

Neuromuscular & skeletal: Choreiform movements, coordination abnormal, dysarthria, muscle pain, muscle weakness, myalgia, tremor

Ocular: Blurred vision, eye movements abnormal, diplopia, nystagmus

Respiratory: Chest congestion, cough, bronchitis, hypersecretions, pharyngitis, respiratory depression, respiratory tract infection, rhinitis, rhinorrhea, shortness of breath, sinusitis

Miscellaneous: Allergic reaction, aphonia, dysdiadochokinesis, encopresis, "glassy-eyed" appearance, hemiparesis, lymphadenopathy

Drug Interactions

Metabolism/Transport Effects **Substrate** of CYP3A4 (major); **Note:** Assignment of Major/Minor substrate status based on clinically relevant drug interaction potential

Avoid Concomitant Use

Avoid concomitant use of ClonazePAM with any of the following: Conivaptan; OLANZapine

Increased Effect/Toxicity

ClonazePAM may increase the levels/effects of: Alcohol (Ethyl); CloZAPine; CNS Depressants; Fosphenytoin; Methotrimeprazine; Phenytoin; Selective Serotonin Reuptake Inhibitors

The levels/effects of ClonazePAM may be increased by: Antifungal Agents (Azole Derivatives, Systemic); Aprepitant; Calcium Channel Blockers (Nondihydropyridine); Cimetidine; Conivaptan; Contraceptives (Estrogens); Contraceptives (Progestins); CYP3A4 Inhibitors (Moderate); CYP3A4 Inhibitors (Strong); Dasatinib; Droperidol; Fluconazole; Fosaprepitant; Grapefruit Juice; HydrOXYzine; Isoniazid; Macrolide Antibiotics; Methotrimeprazine; Nefazodone; OLANZapine; Proton Pump Inhibitors; Selective Serotonin Reuptake Inhibitors

Decreased Effect

The levels/effects of ClonazePAM may be decreased by: CarBAMazepine; CYP3A4 Inducers (Strong); Deferasirox; Rifamycin Derivatives; St Johns Wort; Theophylline Derivatives; Tocilizumab; Yohimbine

Ethanol/Nutrition/Herb Interactions

Ethanol: May increase CNS depression; monitor for increased effects with coadministration. Caution patients about effects.

Food: Clonazepam serum concentration is unlikely to be increased by grapefruit juice because of clonazepam's high oral bioavailability.

Herb/Nutraceutical: St John's wort may decrease clonazepam levels. Avoid valerian, St John's wort, kava kava, gotu kola (may increase CNS depression).

Mechanism of Action The exact mechanism is unknown, but believed to be related to its ability to enhance the activity of GABA; suppresses the spike-and-wave discharge in absence seizures by depressing nerve transmission in the motor cortex

Pharmacodynamics/Kinetics

Onset of action: 20-60 minutes

Duration: Infants and young children: 6-8 hours; Adults: ≤12 hours

Absorption: Well absorbed

Distribution: Adults: V_d: 1.5-4.4 L/kg

Protein binding: 85%

Metabolism: Extensively hepatic via glucuronide and sulfate conjugation

Half-life elimination: Children: 22-33 hours; Adults: 19-50 hours

Time to peak, serum: 1-3 hours; Steady-state: 5-7 days

Excretion: Urine (<2% as unchanged drug); metabolites excreted as glucuronide or sulfate conjugates

Dosage Oral:

Children <10 years or 30 kg: Seizure disorders:

Initial daily dose: 0.01-0.03 mg/kg/day (maximum: 0.05 mg/kg/day) given in 2-3 divided doses; increase by no more than 0.5 mg every third day until seizures are controlled or adverse effects seen

Usual maintenance dose: 0.1-0.2 mg/kg/day divided 3 times/day, not to exceed 0.2 mg/kg/day

Adults:

Burning mouth syndrome (unlabeled use): 0.25-3 mg/day in 2 divided doses, in morning and evening

Seizure disorders:

Initial daily dose not to exceed 1.5 mg given in 3 divided doses; may increase by 0.5-1 mg every third day until seizures are controlled or adverse effects seen (maximum: 20 mg/day)

Usual maintenance dose: 0.05-0.2 mg/kg; do not exceed 20 mg/day

Panic disorder: 0.25 mg twice daily; increase in increments of 0.125-0.25 mg twice daily every 3 days; target dose: 1 mg/day (maximum: 4 mg/day)

Discontinuation of treatment: To discontinue, treatment should be withdrawn gradually. Decrease dose by 0.125 mg twice daily every 3 days until medication is completely withdrawn.

Elderly: Initiate with low doses and observe closely

Hemodialysis: Supplemental dose is not necessary

Administration Orally-disintegrating tablet: Open pouch and peel back foil on the blister; do not push tablet through foil. Use dry hands to remove tablet and place in mouth. May be swallowed with or without water. Use immediately after removing from package.

Monitoring Parameters CBC, liver function tests; observe patient for excess sedation, respiratory depression; suicidality (eg, suicidal thoughts, depression, behavioral changes)

Reference Range Relationship between serum concentration and seizure control is not well established

Timing of serum samples: Peak serum levels occur 1-3 hours after oral ingestion; the half-life is 20-40 hours; therefore, steady-state occurs in 5-7 days

Therapeutic levels: 20-80 ng/mL; Toxic concentration: >80 ng/mL

Additional Information Ethosuximide or valproic acid may be preferred for treatment of absence (petit mal) seizures. Clonazepam-induced behavioral disturbances may be more frequent in mentally handicapped patients. Abrupt discontinuation after sustained use (generally >10 days) may cause withdrawal symptoms. Flumazenil, a competitive benzodiazepine antagonist at the CNS receptor site, reverses benzodiazepine-induced CNS depression.

Dosage Forms Excipient information presented when available (limited, particularly for generics); consult specific product labeling.

Tablet, oral: 0.5 mg, 1 mg, 2 mg

KlonoPIN®: 0.5 mg [scored]

KlonoPIN®: 1 mg, 2 mg

Tablet, orally disintegrating, oral: 0.125 mg, 0.25 mg, 0.5 mg, 1 mg, 2 mg

Controlled Substance C-IV

Extemporaneous Preparations A 0.1 mg/mL oral suspension may be made with tablets and one of three different vehicles (cherry syrup; a 1:1 mixture of Ora-Sweet® and Ora-Plus®; or a 1:1 mixture of Ora-Sweet® SF and Ora-Plus®). Crush six 2 mg tablets in a mortar and reduce to a fine powder. Add 10 mL of the chosen vehicle and mix to a uniform paste; mix while adding the vehicle in incremental proportions to **almost** 120 mL; transfer to a calibrated bottle, rinse mortar with vehicle, and add quantity of vehicle sufficient to make 120 mL. Label "shake well" and "protect from light". Stable for 60 days when stored in amber prescription bottles in the dark at room temperature or refrigerated.

Allen LV Jr and Erickson MA 3rd, "Stability of Acetazolamide, Allopurinol, Azathioprine, Clonazepam, and Flucytosine in Extemporaneously Compounded Oral Liquids," Am *J Health Syst Pharm*, 1996, 53(16):1944-9.

CloNIDine (KLON i deen)

Brand Names: U.S. Catapres-TTS®-1; Catapres-TTS®-2; Catapres-TTS®-3; Catapres®; Duraclon®; Kapvay™; Nexiclon™ XR

Brand Names: Canada Apo-Clonidine®; Carapres®; Dixarit®; Dom-Clonidine; Novo-Clonidine; Nu-Clonidine

Index Terms Clonidine Hydrochloride

Pharmacologic Category Alpha$_2$-Adrenergic Agonist

Additional Appendix Information

Beers Criteria – Potentially Inappropriate Medications for Geriatrics *on page 1973*

Hypertension *on page 2001*

Use

Oral:

Immediate release: Management of hypertension (monotherapy or as adjunctive therapy)

Extended release:

Kapvay™: Treatment of attention-deficit/hyperactivity disorder (ADHD) (monotherapy or as adjunctive therapy)

Nexiclon™ XR: Management of hypertension (monotherapy or as adjunctive therapy)

Epidural (Duraclon®): For continuous epidural administration as adjunctive therapy with opioids for treatment of severe cancer pain in patients tolerant to or unresponsive to opioids alone; epidural clonidine is generally more effective for neuropathic pain and less effective (or possibly ineffective) for somatic or visceral pain

Transdermal patch: Management of hypertension (monotherapy or as adjunctive therapy)

Unlabeled Use Heroin or nicotine withdrawal; severe pain; dysmenorrhea; vasomotor symptoms associated with menopause; ethanol dependence; prophylaxis of migraines; glaucoma; diabetes-associated diarrhea; impulse control disorder, clozapine-induced sialorrhea; aid in the diagnosis of growth hormone deficiency; attention-deficit/hyperactivity disorder (ADHD) and associated insomnia in children; Tourette's syndrome in children; aggression associated with conduct disorder

Pregnancy Risk Factor C

Pregnancy Considerations Adverse events have been observed in some animal reproduction studies. Clonidine crosses the placenta; concentrations in the umbilical cord plasma are similar to those in the maternal serum and concentrations in the amniotic fluid may be 4 times those in the maternal serum. **[U.S. Boxed Warning]: Epidural clonidine is not recommended for obstetrical or postpartum pain** due to risk of hemodynamic instability.

Lactation Enters breast milk/not recommended

Contraindications Hypersensitivity to clonidine hydrochloride or any component of the formulation

Epidural administration: Injection site infection; concurrent anticoagulant therapy; bleeding diathesis; administration above the C4 dermatome

Warnings/Precautions May cause CNS depression, which may impair physical or mental abilities; patients must be cautioned about performing tasks which require mental alertness (eg, operating machinery or driving). Sedating effects may be potentiated when used with other CNS-depressant drugs or ethanol. Use with caution in patients with severe coronary insufficiency; conduction disturbances; recent MI, CVA, or chronic renal insufficiency. May cause dose dependent reductions in heart rate; use with caution in patients with preexisting bradycardia or those predisposed to developing bradycardia. Caution in sinus node dysfunction. Use with caution in patients concurrently receiving agents known to reduce SA node function and/or AV nodal conduction (eg, digoxin, diltiazem, metoprolol, verapamil). May cause significant xerostomia. Clonidine may cause eye dryness in patients who wear contact lenses.

[U.S. Boxed Warning]: Must dilute concentrated epidural injectable (500 mcg/mL) solution prior to use. Epidural clonidine is not recommended for perioperative, obstetrical, or postpartum pain due to risk of hemodynamic instability. Clonidine injection should be administered via a continuous epidural infusion device. Monitor closely for catheter-related infection such as meningitis or epidural abscess. Epidural clonidine is not recommended for use in patients with severe cardiovascular disease or hemodynamic instability; may lead to cardiovascular instability (hypotension, bradycardia). Symptomatic hypotension may occur with use; in all patients, use epidural clonidine with caution due to the potential for severe hypotension especially in women and those of low body weight. Most hypotensive episodes occur within the first 4 days of initiation; however, episodes may occur throughout the duration of therapy.

Gradual withdrawal is needed (taper oral immediate release or epidural dose gradually over 2-4 days to avoid rebound hypertension) if drug needs to be stopped. Patients should be instructed about abrupt discontinuation (causes rapid increase in BP and symptoms of sympathetic overactivity). In patients on both a beta-blocker and clonidine where withdrawal of clonidine is necessary, withdraw the beta-blocker first and several days before clonidine withdrawal, then slowly decrease clonidine. In children and adolescents, extended release formulation (Kapvay™) should be tapered in decrements of no more than 0.1 mg every 3-7 days. Discontinue oral immediate release formulations within 4 hours of surgery then restart as soon as possible afterwards. Discontinue oral extended release formulations up to 28 hours prior to surgery, then restart the following day.

Oral formulations of clonidine (immediate release versus extended release) are not interchangeable on a mg:mg basis due to different pharmacokinetic profiles. This includes commercially available oral suspension (Nexiclon™ XR) which is an extended release preparation and should not be used interchangeably with any extemporaneously prepared clonidine oral suspension.

Transdermal patch may contain conducting metal (eg, aluminum); remove patch prior to MRI. Due to the potential for altered electrical conductivity, remove transdermal patch before cardioversion or defibrillation. Localized contact sensitization to the transdermal system has been reported; in these patients, allergic reactions (eg, generalized rash, urticaria, angioedema) have also occurred following subsequent substitution of oral therapy.

Clonidine may be inappropriate for use in the elderly due to CNS adverse events and orthostatic hypotension (Beers Criteria). In pediatric patients, epidural clonidine should be reserved for cancer patients with severe intractable pain, unresponsive to other analgesics or epidural or spinal opioids. Use oral formulations with caution in pediatric patients since children commonly have gastrointestinal illnesses with vomiting and are susceptible to hypertensive episodes due to abrupt inability to take oral medication.

Adverse Reactions Frequency not always defined.

Oral, Transdermal: Incidence of adverse events may be less with transdermal compared to oral due to the lower peak/trough ratio.

Cardiovascular: Bradycardia (≤4%), palpitation (1%), tachycardia (1%), arrhythmia, atrioventricular block, chest pain, CHF, ECG abnormalities, flushing, orthostatic hypotension, pallor, Raynaud's phenomenon, syncope

Central nervous system: Drowsiness (12% to 38%), headache (1% to 29%), fatigue (4% to 16%), dizziness (2% to 16%), sedation (3% to 10%), insomnia (≤6%), lethargy (3%), nervousness (1% to 3%), mental depression (1%), aggression, agitation, anxiety, behavioral changes, CVA, delirium, delusional perception, fever, hallucinations (visual and auditory), irritability, malaise, nightmares, restlessness, vivid dreams

Dermatologic: Transient localized skin reactions characterized by pruritus and erythema (transdermal 15% to 50%), contact dermatitis (transdermal 8% to 34%), vesiculation (transdermal 7%), allergic contact sensitization (transdermal 5%), hyperpigmentation (transdermal 5%), burning (transdermal 3%), edema (3%), excoriation (transdermal 3%) blanching (transdermal 1%), generalized macular rash (1%), papules (transdermal 1%), throbbing (transdermal 1%), alopecia, angioedema, hives, localized hypopigmentation (transdermal), rash, urticaria

Endocrine & metabolic: Sexual dysfunction (3%), gynecomastia (1%), creatine phosphokinase increased (transient; oral), hyperglycemia (transient; oral), libido decreased

Gastrointestinal: Xerostomia (≤40%), constipation (2% to 10%), anorexia (1%), taste perversion (1%), weight gain (<1%), abdominal pain (oral), diarrhea, nausea, parotid gland pain (oral), parotitis (oral), pseudo-obstruction (oral), throat pain, vomiting

Genitourinary: Erectile dysfunction (2% to 3%), nocturia (1%), dysuria, enuresis, urinary retention

Hematologic: Thrombocytopenia (oral)

Hepatic: Liver function test (mild transient abnormalities; ≤1%), hepatitis

Neuromuscular & skeletal: Weakness (10%), arthralgia (1%), myalgia (1%), leg cramps (<1%), numbness (localized, transdermal), pain in extremities, paresthesia, tremor

Ocular: Accommodation disorder, blurred vision, burning eyes, dry eyes, lacrimation decreased, lacrimation increased

Otic: Ear pain, otitis media

Renal: Pollakiuria

Respiratory: Asthma, epistaxis, nasal congestion, nasal dryness, nasopharyngitis, respiratory tract infection, rhinorrhea

Miscellaneous: Withdrawal syndrome (1%), flu-like syndrome, thirst

Epidural: Note: The following adverse events occurred more often than placebo in cancer patients with intractable pain being treated with concurrent epidural morphine.

>10%:

Cardiovascular: Hypotension (45%), postural hypotension (32%)

Central nervous system: Confusion (13%), dizziness (13%)

Gastrointestinal: Xerostomia (13%)

1% to 10%:

Cardiovascular: Chest pain (5%)

Central nervous system: Hallucinations (5%)

Gastrointestinal: Nausea/vomiting (8%)

Otic: Tinnitus (5%)

Miscellaneous: Diaphoresis (5%)

Drug Interactions

Metabolism/Transport Effects None known.

Avoid Concomitant Use

Avoid concomitant use of CloNIDine with any of the following: Iobenguane I 123

Increased Effect/Toxicity

CloNIDine may increase the levels/effects of: Amifostine; Antihypertensives; Hypotensive Agents; RiTUXimab

The levels/effects of CloNIDine may be increased by: Alfuzosin; Beta-Blockers; Diazoxide; Herbs (Hypotensive Properties); MAO Inhibitors; Methylphenidate; Pentoxifylline; Phosphodiesterase 5 Inhibitors; Prostacyclin Analogues

Decreased Effect

CloNIDine may decrease the levels/effects of: Iobenguane I 123

The levels/effects of CloNIDine may be decreased by: Antidepressants (Alpha2-Antagonist); Herbs (Hypertensive Properties); Serotonin/Norepinephrine Reuptake Inhibitors; Tricyclic Antidepressants; Yohimbine

Ethanol/Nutrition/Herb Interactions

Ethanol: Avoid ethanol (may increase CNS depression). *In vitro* studies have shown high concentrations of alcohol may increase the rate of release of Nexiclon™ XR.

Herb/Nutraceutical: Avoid dong quai if using for hypertension (has estrogenic activity). Avoid ephedra, yohimbe, ginseng (may worsen hypertension). Avoid valerian, St John's wort, kava kava, gotu kola (may increase CNS depression).

Stability

Epidural formulation: Store at 25°C (77°F); excursions permitted to 15°C to 30°C (59°F to 86°F). **Preservative free;** discard unused portion. Prior to administration, the 500 mcg/mL concentration must be diluted in 0.9% sodium chloride for injection (preservative-free) to a final concentration of 100 mcg/mL.

Oral suspension, tablets: Store at 25°C (77°F); excursions permitted to 15°C to 30°C (59°F to 86°F). Protect from light.

Transdermal patches: Store below 30°C (86°F).

Mechanism of Action Stimulates alpha$_2$-adrenoceptors in the brain stem, thus activating an inhibitory neuron, resulting in reduced sympathetic outflow from the CNS, producing a decrease in peripheral resistance, renal vascular resistance, heart rate, and blood pressure; epidural clonidine may produce pain relief at spinal presynaptic and postjunctional alpha$_2$-adrenoceptors by preventing pain signal transmission; pain relief occurs only for the body regions innervated by the spinal segments where analgesic concentrations of clonidine exist. For the treatment of ADHD, the mechanism of action is unknown; it has been proposed that postsynaptic alpha$_2$-agonist stimulation regulates subcortical activity in the prefrontal cortex, the area of the brain responsible for emotions, attentions, and behaviors and causes reduced hyperactivity, impulsiveness, and distractibility.

Pharmacodynamics/Kinetics

Onset of action: Oral: 0.5-1 hour; Transdermal: Initial application: 2-3 days

Duration: 6-10 hours

Absorption: Oral: Extended release tablets (Kapvay™) are not bioequivalent with immediate release formulations; peak plasma concentrations are 50% lower compared to immediate release formulations

Distribution: V_d: Adults: 2.1 L/kg; highly lipid soluble; distributes readily into extravascular sites

Note: Epidurally administered clonidine readily distributes into plasma via the epidural veins and attains clinically significant systemic concentrations.

Protein binding: 20% to 40%

Metabolism: Extensively hepatic to inactive metabolites; undergoes enterohepatic recirculation

Bioavailability: Oral: Immediate release: 75% to 85%; Extended release (Kapvay™): 89% (relative to immediate release formulation)

Half-life elimination: Adults: Normal renal function: 12-16 hours; Renal impairment: Up to 41 hours

Epidural administration: CSF half-life elimination: 0.8-1.8 hours

Time to peak: Oral: Immediate release: 3-5 hours; Extended release: 7-8 hours

Excretion: Urine (40% to 60%as unchanged drug)

Dosage Note: Dosing is expressed as the salt (clonidine hydrochloride) unless otherwise noted. Formulations of clonidine (immediate release versus extended release) are not interchangeable on a mg:mg basis due to different pharmacokinetic profiles. This includes commercially available oral suspension (Nexiclon™ XR) which is an extended release preparation and should not be used interchangeably with any extemporaneously prepared clonidine oral suspension.

Children:

Oral:

Hypertension (unlabeled use): Children ≥12 years: Immediate release: Initial: 0.2 mg/day in 2 divided doses; increase gradually, if needed, in 0.1 mg/day increments at weekly intervals; maximum: 2.4 mg/day (rarely required) (NHBPEP, Fourth Report)

Severe hypertension (unlabeled use): Children: Immediate release: 0.05-0.1 mg/dose; may repeat up to a maximum total dose of 0.8 mg (NHBPEP, Fourth Report)

Clonidine tolerance test (test of growth hormone release from pituitary) (unlabeled use):

0.15 mg/m^2 as a single dose (Lanes, 1982)

or

5 mcg/kg as a single dose; maximum dose: 250 mcg (Richmond, 2008)

ADHD: **Note:** May be used alone or as an adjunct to stimulants.

Immediate release (unlabeled indication; Pliszka, 2007):

Children ≤45 kg: Initial: 0.05 mg at bedtime; sequentially increase every 3-7 days by 0.05 mg increments as twice daily, then 3 times daily, then 4 times daily; maximum daily dose: 0.2 mg/day for patients weighing 27-40.5 kg; 0.3 mg/day for patients weighing 40.5-45 kg. When discontinuing therapy, taper gradually over 1-2 weeks.

Children >45 kg: Initial: 0.1 mg at bedtime; sequentially increase every 3-7 days by 0.1 mg increments as twice daily, then 3 times daily, then 4 times daily; maximum daily dose: 0.4 mg/day. When discontinuing therapy, taper gradually over 1-2 weeks.

Extended release (Kapvay™): Children ≥6 years: Initial: 0.1 mg at bedtime; increase in 0.1 mg/day increments every 7 days until desired response, doses should be administered twice daily (either split equally or with the higher split dosage given at bedtime); maximum: 0.4 mg/day. **Note:** Maintenance treatment for >5 weeks has not been evaluated. When discontinuing therapy, taper daily dose by ≤0.1 mg every 3-7 days.

Epidural infusion: Pain management: Reserved for cancer patients with severe intractable pain, unresponsive to other opioid analgesics: Initial: 0.5 mcg/kg/**hour**; adjust with caution, based on clinical effect

Adults:

Oral:

Hypertension:

Immediate release: Initial dose: 0.1 mg twice daily (maximum recommended dose: 2.4 mg/day); usual dose range (JNC 7): 0.1-0.8 mg/day in 2 divided doses

Extended release (Nexiclon™ XR): Initial: 0.17 mg clonidine base once daily at bedtime; may increase increments of 0.09 mg/day every 7 days; maintenance: usual dose range: 0.17-0.52 mg clonidine base once daily; maximum: 0.52 mg/day clonidine base

Conversion between immediate release clonidine hydrochloride and extended release (Nexiclon™ XR) clonidine base:

Current dose immediate release tablets 0.05 mg twice daily: Convert to extended release tablet of 0.09 mg clonidine base once daily

Current dose immediate release tablets 0.1 mg twice daily: Convert to extended release tablet of 0.17 mg clonidine base once daily

Current dose immediate release tablets 0.2 mg twice daily: Convert to extended release tablet of 0.34 mg clonidine base once daily

Current dose immediate release tablets 0.3 mg twice daily: convert to extended release tablets of 0.52 mg clonidine base once daily

Acute hypertension (urgency) (unlabeled use): Initial 0.1-0.2 mg; may be followed by additional doses of 0.1 mg every hour, if necessary, to a maximum total dose of 0.7 mg (Atkin, 1992; Jaker, 1989)

Unlabeled route of administration: Sublingual: Initial: 0.1-0.2 mg; followed by 0.05-0.1 mg every hour until blood pressure controlled or a cumulative dose of 0.7 mg is reached (Cunningham, 1994; Matuschka, 1999)

Nicotine withdrawal symptoms (unlabeled use): Initial: 0.1 mg twice daily; titrate by 0.1 mg/day every 7 days if needed; dosage range used in clinical trials: 0.15-0.75 mg/day; duration of therapy ranged from 3-10 weeks in clinical trials (Fiore, 2008)

Transdermal:

Hypertension: Initial: 0.1 mg/24 hour patch applied once every 7 days and increase by 0.1 mg at 1- to 2-week intervals (dosages >0.6 mg/24 hours do not improve efficacy); usual dose range (JNC 7): 0.1-0.3 mg/24 hour patch applied once every 7 days

Nicotine withdrawal symptoms (unlabeled use): Initial: 0.1 mg/24 hour patch applied once every 7 days and increase by 0.1 mg at 1-week intervals if necessary; dosage range used in clinical trials: 0.1-0.2 mg/24 hour patch applied once every 7 days; duration of therapy ranged from 3-10 weeks in clinical trials (Fiore, 2008)

Epidural infusion: Pain management: Reserved for cancer patients with severe intractable pain, unresponsive to other opioid analgesics: Starting dose: 30 mcg/hour; titrate as required for relief of pain or presence of side effects; experience with doses >40 mcg/hour is limited; should be considered an adjunct to opioid therapy

Conversion from oral to transdermal: **Note:** If transitioning from oral to transdermal therapy, overlap oral regimen for 1-2 days; transdermal route takes 2-3 days to achieve therapeutic effects. An example transition is below:

Day 1: Place Catapres-TTS® 1; administer 100% of oral dose.

Day 2: Administer 50% of oral dose.

Day 3: Administer 25% of oral dose.

Day 4: Patch remains, no further oral supplement necessary.

Conversion from transdermal to oral: After transdermal patch removal, therapeutic clonidine levels persist for ~8 hours and then slowly decrease over several days. Consider starting oral clonidine no sooner than 8 hours after patch removal.

Elderly: Oral: Hypertension:

Immediate release: Initial: 0.1 mg once daily at bedtime, increase gradually as needed

Extended release (Nexiclon™ XR): No specific recommendations are provided by the manufacturer although a lower initial dose is recommended.

Dosing adjustment in renal impairment: Bradycardia, sedation, and hypotension may be more likely to occur in patients with renal failure; may consider using doses at the lower end of the dosing range and monitor closely

Not dialyzable (0% to 5%) via hemodialysis; supplemental dose is not necessary; unclear how much is removed via peritoneal dialysis. Oral antihypertensive drugs given preferentially at night may reduce the nocturnal surge of blood pressure and minimize the intradialytic hypotension that may occur when taken the morning before a dialysis session (K/DOQI, 2005).

Oral: Extended release (Nexiclon™ XR):

Moderate-to-severe impairment (not on dialysis): No dosage adjustment recommended; titrate slowly

End-stage kidney disease (on maintenance dialysis): Initial: 0.09 mg clonidine base/day; titrate slowly

Administration

Epidural: Specialized techniques are required for continuous epidural administration; administration via this route should only be performed by qualified individuals familiar with the techniques of epidural administration and patient management problems associated with this route. Familiarization of the epidural infusion device is essential. Do not discontinue clonidine abruptly; if needed, gradually reduce dose over 2-4 days to avoid withdrawal symptoms.

Oral: May be taken with or without food. Do not discontinue clonidine abruptly. If needed, gradually reduce dose over 2-4 days to avoid rebound hypertension.

Extended release products:

Kapvay™: Swallow whole; do not crush, split, or chew.

Nexiclon™ XR: Tablets may be split. Shake suspension well before use.

Transdermal patch: Patches should be applied weekly at a consistent time to a clean, hairless area of the upper outer arm or chest. Rotate patch sites weekly. Redness under patch may be reduced if a topical corticosteroid spray is applied to the area before placement of the patch.

Monitoring Parameters Blood pressure, standing and sitting/supine, mental status, heart rate

When used for the treatment of ADHD, thoroughly evaluate for cardiovascular risk. Monitor heart rate, blood pressure (when started and weaned), and consider obtaining ECG prior to initiation (Vetter, 2008).

Clonidine tolerance test: In addition to growth hormone concentrations, monitor blood pressure and blood glucose (Huang, 2001).

Epidural: Carefully monitor infusion pump; inspect catheter tubing for obstruction or dislodgement to reduce risk of inadvertent abrupt withdrawal of infusion. Monitor closely for catheter-related infection (eg, meningitis or epidural abscess).

Test Interactions Positive Coombs' test

Additional Information Each 0.1 mg of clonidine hydrochloride (salt form) is equivalent to 0.087 mg of the free base.

Transdermal clonidine should only be used in patients unable to take oral medication. The transdermal product is much more expensive than oral clonidine and produces no better therapeutic effects.

When used for ADHD treatment, clonidine is recommended to be used as part of a comprehensive treatment program (eg, psychological, educational, and social) for attention-deficit disorder.

Dosage Forms Excipient information presented when available (limited, particularly for generics); consult specific product labeling.

Injection, solution, as hydrochloride [epidural, preservative free]: 100 mcg/mL (10 mL); 500 mcg/mL (10 mL)

Duraclon®: 100 mcg/mL (10 mL); 500 mcg/mL (10 mL)

Patch, transdermal: 0.1 mg/24 hours (4s); 0.2 mg/24 hours (4s); 0.3 mg/24 hours (4s)

Catapres-TTS®-1: 0.1 mg/24 hours (4s) [contains metal]

Catapres-TTS®-2: 0.2 mg/24 hours (4s) [contains metal]

Catapres-TTS®-3: 0.3 mg/24 hours (4s) [contains metal]

Suspension, extended release, oral, as base:

Nexiclon™ XR: 0.09 mg/mL (118 mL)

Tablet, oral, as hydrochloride: 0.1 mg, 0.2 mg, 0.3 mg

Catapres®: 0.1 mg, 0.2 mg, 0.3 mg [scored]

Tablet, extended release, oral, as base:

Nexiclon™ XR: 0.17 mg [scored]

Tablet, extended release, oral, as hydrochloride:

Kapvay™: 0.1 mg

Extemporaneous Preparations Note: Extended-release oral suspension commercially available (0.09 mg/mL as clonidine base). The commercially available oral suspension (Nexiclon™ XR) is an extended-release preparation and should not be in used interchangeably with any extemporaneously prepared clonidine oral suspension.

A 0.1 mg/mL oral suspension may be made from tablets. Crush thirty 0.2 mg tablets in a glass mortar and reduce to a fine powder. Slowly add 2 mL Purified Water USP and mix to a uniform paste. Slowly add Simple Syrup, NF in 15 mL increments; transfer to a calibrated bottle, rinse mortar with vehicle, and add quantity of vehicle sufficient to make 60 mL. Label "shake well" and "refrigerate". Stable for 28 days when stored in amber glass bottles and refrigerated.

Levinson ML and Johnson CE, "Stability of an Extemporaneously Compounded Clonidine Hydrochloride Oral Liquid," Am J Hosp Pharm, 1992, 49(1):122-5.

◆ **Clonidine Hydrochloride** *see* CloNIDine *on page* 392

Clopidogrel (kloh PID oh grel)

Brand Names: U.S. Plavix®

Brand Names: Canada Plavix®

Index Terms Clopidogrel Bisulfate

Pharmacologic Category Antiplatelet Agent; Antiplatelet Agent, Thienopyridine

Use Reduces rate of atherothrombotic events (myocardial infarction, stroke, vascular deaths) in patients with recent MI or stroke, or established peripheral arterial disease; reduces rate of atherothrombotic events in patients with unstable angina (UA) or non-ST-segment elevation (NSTEMI) managed medically or with percutaneous coronary intervention (PCI) (with or without stent) or CABG; reduces rate of death and atherothrombotic events in patients with ST-segment elevation MI (STEMI) managed medically

Canadian labeling: Additional use (not in U.S. labeling): Prevention of atherothrombotic and thromboembolic events, including stroke, in patients with atrial fibrillation with at least 1 risk factor for vascular events who are not suitable for treatment with an anticoagulant and are at a low risk for bleeding.

Unlabeled Use In patients with allergy or major gastrointestinal intolerance to aspirin, initial treatment of acute coronary syndromes (ACS) or prevention of coronary artery bypass graft closure (saphenous vein); stable coronary artery disease (in combination with aspirin)

Pregnancy Risk Factor B

Pregnancy Considerations Teratogenic effects were not observed in animal studies. Use during pregnancy only if clearly needed.

Lactation Excretion in breast milk unknown/not recommended

Medication Guide Available Yes

Contraindications Hypersensitivity to clopidogrel or any component of the formulation; active pathological bleeding such as peptic ulcer or intracranial hemorrhage

Canadian labeling: Additional contraindications (not in U.S. labeling): Significant liver impairment or cholestatic jaundice

Warnings/Precautions [U.S. Boxed Warning]: Patients with one or more copies of the variant *CYP2C19*2* and/or *CYP2C19*3* alleles (and potentially other reduced-function variants) may have reduced conversion of clopidogrel to its active thiol metabolite. Lower active metabolite exposure may result in reduced platelet inhibition and, thus, a higher rate of cardiovascular events following MI or stent thrombosis following PCI. Although evidence is insufficient to recommend routine genetic testing, tests are available to determine CYP2C19 genotype and may be used to determine therapeutic strategy; alternative treatment or treatment strategies may be considered if patient is identified as a CYP2C19 poor metabolizer. Genetic testing may be considered prior to initiating clopidogrel in patients at moderate or high risk for poor outcomes (eg, PCI in patients with extensive and/or very complex disease). The optimal dose for CYP2C19 poor metabolizers has yet to be determined. After initiation of clopidogrel, functional testing (eg, VerifyNow® P2Y12 assay) may also be done to determine clopidogrel responsiveness (Holmes, 2010).

Use with caution in patients who may be at risk of increased bleeding, including patients with PUD, trauma, or surgery. In patients with coronary stents, premature interruption of therapy may result in stent thrombosis with subsequent fatal and nonfatal MI. Duration of therapy, in general, is determined by the type of stent placed (bare metal or drug eluting) and whether an ACS event was ongoing at the time of placement. Consider discontinuing 5 days before elective surgery (except in patients with cardiac stents that have not completed their full course of dual antiplatelet therapy; patient-specific situations need to be discussed with cardiologist; AHA/ACC/SCAI/ACS/ADA Science Advisory provides recommendations). Discontinue at least 5 days before elective CABG; when urgent CABG is necessary, the ACCF/AHA CABG guidelines recommend discontinuation for at least 24 hours prior to surgery (Hillis, 2011).

Because of structural similarities, cross-reactivity is possible among the thienopyridines (clopidogrel, prasugrel, and ticlopidine); use with caution or avoid in patients with previous thienopyridine hypersensitivity. Use of clopidogrel is contraindicated in patients with hypersensitivity to clopidogrel, although desensitization may be considered for mild-to-moderate hypersensitivity.

Use caution in concurrent treatment with anticoagulants (eg, heparin, warfarin) or other antiplatelet drugs; bleeding risk is increased. Concurrent use with drugs known to inhibit CYP2C19 (eg, proton pump inhibitors) may reduce levels of active metabolite and subsequently reduce clinical efficacy and increase the risk of cardiovascular events; if possible, avoid concurrent use of moderate-to-strong CYP2C19 inhibitors. In patients requiring antacid therapy, consider use of an acid-reducing agent lacking (eg, ranitidine) or with less CYP2C19 inhibition. According to the manufacturer, if a PPI is necessary, the use of pantoprazole, a weak CYP2C19 inhibitor, is recommended since it has been shown to have less of an effect on the pharmacologic activity of clopidogrel; lansoprazole exhibits the most potent CYP2C19 inhibition (Li, 2004). Others have recommended the continued use of PPIs, regardless of the degree of inhibition, in patients with multiple risk factors for GI bleeding who are also receiving clopidogrel since no evidence has established clinically meaningful differences in outcome; however, a clinically-significant interaction cannot be excluded in those who are poor metabolizers of clopidogrel. Staggering PPIs with clopidogrel is not recommended until further evidence is available (Abraham, 2010). Concurrent use of aspirin and clopidogrel is not recommended for secondary prevention of ischemic stroke or TIA in patients unable to take oral anticoagulants due to hemorrhagic risk (Furie, 2011).

Use with caution in patients with severe liver or renal disease (experience is limited). Cases of TTP (usually occurring within the first 2 weeks of therapy), resulting in some fatalities, have been reported; urgent plasmapheresis is required. Use in patients with severe hepatic impairment or cholestatic jaundice is contraindicated in the Canadian labeling. Cases of TTP (usually occurring within the first 2 weeks of therapy), resulting in some fatalities, have been reported; urgent plasmapheresis is required.

Assess bleeding risk carefully prior to initiating therapy in patients with atrial fibrillation (Canadian labeling; not an approved use in U.S. labeling); in clinical trials, a significant increase in major bleeding events (including intracranial hemorrhage and fatal bleeding events) were observed in patients receiving clopidogrel plus aspirin versus aspirin alone. Vitamin K antagonist (VKA) therapy (in suitable patients) has demonstrated a greater benefit in stroke reduction than aspirin (with or without clopidogrel).

Adverse Reactions As with all drugs which may affect hemostasis, bleeding is associated with clopidogrel. Hemorrhage may occur at virtually any site. Risk is dependent on multiple variables, including the concurrent use of multiple agents which alter hemostasis and patient susceptibility.

3% to 10%:

- Dermatologic: Rash (4%), pruritus (3%)
- Hematologic: Bleeding (major 4%; minor 5%), purpura/bruising (5%), epistaxis (3%)

1% to 3%:

- Gastrointestinal: GI hemorrhage (2%)
- Hematologic: Hematoma

<1% (Limited to important or life-threatening): Acute liver failure, agranulocytosis, anaphylactoid reaction, angioedema, aplastic anemia, arthralgia, arthritis, bronchospasm, bullous eruption, colitis (including ulcerative or lymphocytic), confusion, creatinine increased, eczema, erythema multiforme, fever, glomerulopathy, hallucination, hemorrhagic stroke (≤0.2%), hepatitis, hypersensitivity reaction, hypotension, interstitial pneumonitis, intracranial hemorrhage (≤0.4%), lichen planus, liver function tests (abnormal), musculoskeletal bleeding, myalgia, ocular bleeding (including conjunctival and retinal), pancreatitis, pancytopenia, pulmonary hemorrhage, rash (erythematous or maculopapular), retroperitoneal hemorrhage, serum sickness, Stevens-Johnson syndrome, stomatitis, taste disorder, thrombotic thrombocytopenic purpura (TTP), toxic epidermal necrolysis, vasculitis, wound hemorrhage

Drug Interactions

Metabolism/Transport Effects Substrate of CYP2C19 (major), CYP3A4 (minor); **Note:** Assignment of Major/Minor substrate status based on clinically relevant drug interaction potential; **Inhibits** CYP2B6 (moderate), CYP2C9 (weak)

Avoid Concomitant Use

Avoid concomitant use of Clopidogrel with any of the following: CYP2C19 Inhibitors (Moderate); CYP2C19 Inhibitors (Strong); Omeprazole

Increased Effect/Toxicity

Clopidogrel may increase the levels/effects of: Anticoagulants; Antiplatelet Agents; Collagenase (Systemic); CYP2B6 Substrates; Drotrecogin Alfa (Activated); Ibritumomab; Rivaroxaban; Salicylates; Thrombolytic Agents; Tositumomab and Iodine I 131 Tositumomab; Warfarin

The levels/effects of Clopidogrel may be increased by: Conivaptan; Dasatinib; Glucosamine; Herbs (Anticoagulant/Antiplatelet Properties); Nonsteroidal Anti-Inflammatory Agents; Omega-3-Acid Ethyl Esters; Pentosan Polysulfate Sodium; Pentoxifylline; Prostacyclin Analogues; Rifamycin Derivatives; Vitamin E

Decreased Effect

The levels/effects of Clopidogrel may be decreased by: Amiodarone; Calcium Channel Blockers; CYP2C19 Inhibitors (Moderate); CYP2C19 Inhibitors (Strong); Dexlansoprazole; Esomeprazole; Lansoprazole; Macrolide Antibiotics; Nonsteroidal Anti-Inflammatory Agents; Omeprazole; Pantoprazole; RABEprazole; Tocilizumab

Ethanol/Nutrition/Herb Interactions Herb/Nutraceutical: Avoid alfalfa, anise, bilberry, bladderwrack, bromelain, cat's claw, chamomile, coleus, cordyceps, dong quai, evening primrose oil, fenugreek, feverfew, garlic, ginger, ginkgo biloba, ginseng (American), ginseng (Panax), ginseng (Siberian), grape seed, green tea, guggul, horse chestnut seed, horseradish, licorice, prickly ash, red clover, reishi, SAMe (S-adenosylmethionine), sweet clover, turmeric, white willow (all have additional antiplatelet activity).

Stability Store at 25°C (77°F); excursions permitted to 15°C to 30°C (59°F to 86°F).

Mechanism of Action Clopidogrel requires *in vivo* biotransformation to an active thiol metabolite. The active metabolite irreversibly blocks the $P2Y_{12}$ component of ADP receptors on the platelet surface, which prevents activation of the GPIIb/IIIa receptor complex, thereby reducing platelet aggregation. Platelets blocked by clopidogrel are affected for the remainder of their lifespan (~7-10 days).

Pharmacodynamics/Kinetics

Onset of action: Inhibition of platelet aggregation (IPA): Dose-dependent:

300-600 mg loading dose: Detected within 2 hours

50-100 mg/day: Detected by the second day of treatment

Peak effect: Time to maximal IPA: Dose-dependent: **Note:** Degree of IPA based on adenosine diphosphate (ADP) concentration used during light aggregometry:

300-600 mg loading dose:

ADP 5 micromole/L: 20% to 30% IPA at 6 hours post administration (Montelescot, 2006)

ADP 20 micromole/L: 30% to 37% IPA at 6 hours post administration (Montelescot, 2006)

50-100 mg/day: ADP 5 micromole/L: 50% to 60% IPA at 5-7 days (Herbert, 1993)

Absorption: Well absorbed

Protein binding: Parent drug: 98%; Inactive metabolite: 94%

Metabolism: Extensively hepatic via esterase-mediated hydrolysis to a carboxylic acid derivative (inactive) and via CYP450-mediated (CYP2C19 primarily) oxidation to a thiol metabolite (active)

Half-life elimination: Parent drug: ~6 hours; Active metabolite: ~30 minutes

Time to peak, serum: ~0.75 hours

Excretion: Urine (50%); feces (46%)

Dosage Oral: Adults:

Recent MI, recent stroke, or established peripheral arterial disease (PAD): 75 mg once daily. **Note:** The ACCF/AHA guidelines for PAD recommend clopidogrel as an alternative to aspirin (Class Ib recommendation) or in conjunction with aspirin for those who are not at an increased risk of bleeding but are of high cardiovascular risk (Class IIb recommendation). These recommendations also pertain to those with intermittent claudication or critical limb ischemia, prior lower extremity revascularization, or prior amputation for lower extremity ischemia (Rooke, 2011).

Acute coronary syndrome (ACS):

Unstable angina, non-ST-segment elevation myocardial infarction (UA/NSTEMI): Initial: 300 mg loading dose, followed by 75 mg once daily for at least 1 month and ideally up to 12 months (in combination with aspirin 75-162 mg once daily indefinitely) (Wright, 2011).

ST-segment elevation myocardial infarction (STEMI): 75 mg once daily (in combination with aspirin 162-325 mg initially followed by 81-162 mg/day). **Note:** CLARITY-TIMI 28 used a 300 mg loading dose (with thrombolysis) demonstrating an improvement in patency rate of the infarct related artery and reduction in ischemic complications. The duration of therapy was <28 days (usually until hospital discharge) unless non-primary percutaneous coronary intervention (PCI) was performed (Sabatine, 2005).

The American College of Chest Physicians (Goodman, 2008) recommends:

Patients ≤75 years: Initial: 300 mg loading dose, followed by 75 mg once daily for up to 28 days (in combination with aspirin)

Patients >75 years: 75 mg once daily for up to 28 days (with or without thrombolysis)

Percutaneous coronary intervention (PCI) for acute coronary syndrome (eg, UA/NSTEMI or STEMI): Loading dose: 600 mg given as early as possible before or at the time of PCI, followed by 75 mg once daily. **Note:** If fibrinolytic administered within the previous 24 hours, administer 300 mg loading dose instead (Levine, 2011).

Higher versus standard maintenance dosing: May consider a maintenance dose of 150 mg once daily for 6 days, then 75 mg once daily thereafter in patients not at high risk for bleeding (CURRENT-OASIS 7 Investigators, 2010; Wright, 2011); however, in another study, in patients with high on-treatment platelet reactivity, the use of 150 mg once daily for 6 months did not demonstrate a difference in 6-month incidence of death from cardiovascular causes, nonfatal MI, or stent thrombosis compared to standard dose therapy (Price, 2011).

Duration of clopidogrel (in combination with aspirin) after stent placement: **Premature interruption of therapy may result in stent thrombosis with subsequent fatal and nonfatal MI.** At least 12 months of clopidogrel is recommended for those with ACS receiving either stent type (bare metal [BMS] or drug eluting stent [DES]) or those receiving a DES for a non-ACS indication. Those receiving a BMS for a non-ACS indication should be given at least 1 month and ideally up to 12 months; if patient is at increased risk of bleeding, give for a minimum of 2 weeks (Levine, 2011). A duration >12 months, regardless of indication, may be considered in patients with DES placement (Levine, 2011; Wright, 2011).

CYP2C19 poor metabolizers (ie, *CYP2C19*2* or **3* carriers): Although routine genetic testing is not recommended in patients treated with clopidogrel undergoing PCI, testing may be considered to identify poor metabolizers who would be at risk for poor outcomes while receiving clopidogrel; if identified, these patients may be considered for an alternative $P2Y_{12}$ inhibitor (Levine, 2011). An appropriate regimen for this patient population has not been established in clinical outcome trials. Although the manufacturer suggests a 600 mg loading dose, followed by 150 mg once daily, it does not appear that this dosing strategy improves outcomes for this patient population (Price, 2011).

Atrial fibrillation (in patients not candidates for warfarin and at a low risk of bleeding) (Canadian labeling; ACTIVE Investigators, 2009; unlabeled use in U.S.): 75 mg once daily (in combination with aspirin 75-100 mg once daily)

Prevention of coronary artery bypass graft closure (saphenous vein) [*Chest* guidelines, 2008]: Aspirin-allergic patients (unlabeled use): Loading dose: 300 mg administered 6 hours following procedure; maintenance: 75 mg once daily

Dosing adjustment in renal impairment and elderly: None necessary

Dosing adjustment in hepatic impairment: Use with caution; experience is limited. **Note:** Inhibition of ADP-induced platelet aggregation and mean bleeding time prolongation were similar in patients with severe hepatic impairment compared to healthy subjects after repeated doses of 75 mg once daily for 10 days.

Dietary Considerations May be taken without regard to meals.

Administration May be administered without regard to meals.

Monitoring Parameters Signs of bleeding; hemoglobin and hematocrit periodically. Consider platelet function testing to determine platelet inhibitory response if results of testing may alter management (Wright, 2011).

Dosage Forms Excipient information presented when available (limited, particularly for generics); consult specific product labeling.

Tablet, oral:

Plavix®: 75 mg, 300 mg

Extemporaneous Preparations A 5 mg/mL oral suspension may be made using tablets. Crush four 75 mg tablets and reduce to a fine powder. Add a small amount of a 1:1 mixture of Ora-Sweet® and Ora-Plus® and mix to a uniform paste; mix while adding the vehicle in geometric proportions to **almost** 60 mL; transfer to a calibrated bottle, rinse mortar with vehicle, and add quantity of vehicle sufficient to make 60 mL. Label "shake well". Stable 60 days at room temperature or under refrigeration.

Skillman KL, Caruthers RL, and Johnson CE, "Stability of an Extemporaneously Prepared Clopidogrel Oral Suspension," *Am J Health Syst Pharm*, 2010, 67(7):559-61.

◆ **Clopidogrel Bisulfate** *see* Clopidogrel *on page 395*

Clorazepate (klor AZ e pate)

Brand Names: U.S. Tranxene® T-Tab®

Brand Names: Canada Apo-Clorazepate®; Novo-Clopate

Index Terms Clorazepate Dipotassium; Tranxene T-Tab

Pharmacologic Category Benzodiazepine

Additional Appendix Information

Benzodiazepines *on page 1882*

Use Treatment of generalized anxiety disorder; management of ethanol withdrawal; adjunct anticonvulsant in management of partial seizures

Pregnancy Considerations Nordiazepam, the active metabolite of clorazepate, crosses the placenta and is measurable in cord blood and amniotic fluid. Teratogenic effects have been observed with some benzodiazepines (including clorazepate); however, additional studies are needed. The incidence of premature birth and low birth weights may be increased following maternal use of benzodiazepines; hypoglycemia and respiratory problems in the neonate may occur following exposure late in pregnancy. Neonatal withdrawal symptoms may occur within days to weeks after birth and "floppy infant syndrome" (which also includes withdrawal symptoms) has been reported with some benzodiazepines.

Patients exposed to clorazepate during pregnancy are encouraged to enroll themselves into the AED Pregnancy Registry by calling 1-888-233-2334. Additional information is available at www.aedpregnancyregistry.org.

Lactation Enters breast milk/not recommended

Medication Guide Available Yes

Contraindications Hypersensitivity to clorazepate or any component of the formulation (cross-sensitivity with other benzodiazepines may exist); narrow-angle glaucoma

Warnings/Precautions Antiepileptics are associated with an increased risk of suicidal behavior/thoughts with use (regardless of indication); patients should be monitored for signs/symptoms of depression, suicidal tendencies, and other unusual behavior changes during therapy and instructed to inform their healthcare provider immediately if symptoms occur.

Not recommended for use in patients <9 years of age or patients with depressive or psychotic disorders. Use with caution in elderly or debilitated patients, patients with hepatic disease (including alcoholics), or renal impairment. Active metabolites with extended half-lives may lead to delayed accumulation and adverse effects. Use with caution in patients with respiratory disease or impaired gag reflex. Avoid use in patients with sleep apnea.

Causes CNS depression (dose related) resulting in sedation, dizziness, confusion, or ataxia which may impair physical and mental capabilities. Patients must be cautioned about performing tasks which require mental alertness (eg, operating machinery or driving). Use with caution in patients receiving other CNS depressants or psychoactive agents. Effects with other sedative drugs or ethanol may be potentiated. Benzodiazepines have been associated with falls and traumatic injury and should be used with extreme caution in patients who are at risk of these events. Benzodiazepines with long half-lives may produce prolonged sedation and increase the risk of falls and fracture; short- or intermediate-acting benzodiazepines are preferred in elderly patients (Beers Criteria).

Use caution in patients with depression, particularly if suicidal risk may be present. Use with caution in patients with a history of drug dependence. Benzodiazepines have been associated with dependence and acute withdrawal symptoms on discontinuation or reduction in dose. Acute withdrawal, including seizures, may be precipitated in patients after administration of flumazenil to patients receiving long-term benzodiazepine therapy.

Benzodiazepines have been associated with anterograde amnesia. Paradoxical reactions, including hyperactive or aggressive behavior, have been reported with benzodiazepines, particularly in adolescent/pediatric or psychiatric patients. Does not have analgesic, antidepressant, or antipsychotic properties.

Adverse Reactions Frequency not defined.

Cardiovascular: Hypotension

Central nervous system: Drowsiness, fatigue, ataxia, lightheadedness, memory impairment, insomnia, anxiety, headache, depression, slurred speech, confusion, nervousness, dizziness, irritability

Dermatologic: Rash

Endocrine & metabolic: Libido decreased

Gastrointestinal: Xerostomia, constipation, diarrhea, salivation decreased, nausea, vomiting, appetite increased or decreased

Hepatic: Jaundice, transaminase increased

Neuromuscular & skeletal: Dysarthria, tremor

Ocular: Blurred vision, diplopia

Drug Interactions

Metabolism/Transport Effects Substrate of CYP3A4 (major); **Note:** Assignment of Major/Minor substrate status based on clinically relevant drug interaction potential

Avoid Concomitant Use

Avoid concomitant use of Clorazepate with any of the following: Conivaptan; OLANZapine

Increased Effect/Toxicity

Clorazepate may increase the levels/effects of: Alcohol (Ethyl); CloZAPine; CNS Depressants; Fosphenytoin; Methotrimeprazine; Phenytoin; Selective Serotonin Reuptake Inhibitors

The levels/effects of Clorazepate may be increased by: Antifungal Agents (Azole Derivatives, Systemic); Aprepitant; Calcium Channel Blockers (Nondihydropyridine); Cimetidine; Conivaptan; Contraceptives (Estrogens); Contraceptives (Progestins); CYP3A4 Inhibitors (Moderate); CYP3A4 Inhibitors (Strong); Dasatinib; Droperidol; Fluconazole; Fosamprenavir; Fosaprepitant; Grapefruit Juice; HydrOXYzine; Isoniazid; Macrolide Antibiotics; MAO Inhibitors; Methotrimeprazine; Nefazodone; OLANZapine; Proton Pump Inhibitors; Ritonavir; Saquinavir; Selective Serotonin Reuptake Inhibitors

Decreased Effect

The levels/effects of Clorazepate may be decreased by: CarBAMazepine; CYP3A4 Inducers (Strong); Deferasirox; Rifamycin Derivatives; St Johns Wort; Theophylline Derivatives; Tocilizumab; Yohimbine

Ethanol/Nutrition/Herb Interactions

Ethanol: May increase CNS depression; monitor for increased effects with coadministration. Caution patients about effects.

Food: Serum concentrations/toxicity may be increased by grapefruit juice.

Herb/Nutraceutical: Avoid valerian, St John's wort, kava kava, gotu kola (may increase CNS depression).

Stability Store at controlled room temperature at 20° to 25°C (68° to 77°F). Protect from moisture; keep bottle tightly closed; dispense in tightly closed, light-resistant container.

Mechanism of Action Binds to stereospecific benzodiazepine receptors on the postsynaptic GABA neuron at several sites within the central nervous system, including the limbic system, reticular formation. Enhancement of the inhibitory effect of GABA on neuronal excitability results by increased neuronal membrane permeability to chloride ions. This shift in chloride ions results in hyperpolarization (a less excitable state) and stabilization.

Pharmacodynamics/Kinetics

Onset of action: 1-2 hours

Duration: Variable, 8-24 hours

Distribution: Appears in urine

Protein binding: Nordiazepam 97% to 98%

Metabolism: Rapidly decarboxylated to nordiazepam (active) in acidic stomach prior to absorption; hepatically to oxazepam (active)

Half-life elimination: Adults: Nordiazepam: 40-50 hours; Oxazepam: 6-8 hours

Time to peak, serum: ~1 hour

Excretion: Primarily urine

Dosage Oral:

Children 9-12 years: Anticonvulsant: Initial: 3.75-7.5 mg/dose twice daily; increase dose by 3.75 mg at weekly intervals, not to exceed 60 mg/day in 2-3 divided doses

Children >12 years and Adults: Anticonvulsant: Initial: Up to 7.5 mg/dose 2-3 times/day; increase dose by 7.5 mg at weekly intervals, not to exceed 90 mg/day

Adults:

Anxiety: 7.5-15 mg 2-4 times/day

Ethanol withdrawal: Initial: 30 mg, then 15 mg 2-4 times/day on first day; maximum daily dose: 90 mg; gradually decrease dose over subsequent days

Monitoring Parameters Respiratory and cardiovascular status, excess CNS depression; suicidality (eg, suicidal thoughts, depression, behavioral changes)

Reference Range Therapeutic: 0.12-1 mcg/mL (SI: 0.36-3.01 micromole/L)

Test Interactions Decreased hematocrit; abnormal liver and renal function tests

Additional Information Abrupt discontinuation after sustained use (generally >10 days) may cause withdrawal symptoms.

Dosage Forms Excipient information presented when available (limited, particularly for generics); consult specific product labeling.

Tablet, oral, as dipotassium: 3.75 mg, 7.5 mg, 15 mg

Tranxene® T-Tab®: 3.75 mg, 7.5 mg, 15 mg [scored]

Controlled Substance C-IV

◆ **Clorazepate Dipotassium** *see* Clorazepate *on page 398*

◆ **Clotrimaderm (Can)** *see* Clotrimazole (Topical) *on page 399*

Clotrimazole (Oral) (kloe TRIM a zole)

Index Terms Mycelex

Pharmacologic Category Antifungal Agent, Oral Nonabsorbed

Use Treatment of susceptible fungal infections, including oropharyngeal candidiasis; limited data suggest that clotrimazole troches may be effective for prophylaxis against oropharyngeal candidiasis in neutropenic patients

Pregnancy Risk Factor C

Dosage Oral: Children >3 years and Adults:

Prophylaxis: 10 mg troche dissolved 3 times/day for the duration of chemotherapy or until steroids are reduced to maintenance levels

Treatment: 10 mg troche dissolved slowly 5 times/day for 14 consecutive days

Additional Information Complete prescribing information for this medication should be consulted for additional detail.

Dosage Forms Excipient information presented when available (limited, particularly for generics); consult specific product labeling.

Troche, oral: 10 mg

Clotrimazole (Topical) (kloe TRIM a zole)

Brand Names: U.S. Anti-Fungal™ [OTC]; Cruex® [OTC]; Gyne-Lotrimin® 3 [OTC]; Gyne-Lotrimin® 7 [OTC]; Lotrimin® AF Athlete's Foot [OTC]; Lotrimin® AF for Her [OTC]; Lotrimin® AF Jock Itch [OTC]

Brand Names: Canada Canesten® Topical; Canesten® Vaginal; Clotrimaderm; Trivagizole-3®

Pharmacologic Category Antifungal Agent, Topical; Antifungal Agent, Vaginal

Use Treatment of susceptible fungal infections, including dermatophytoses, superficial mycoses, and cutaneous candidiasis, as well as vulvovaginal candidiasis

Pregnancy Risk Factor B

Dosage

Children >3 years and Adults: Topical (cream, solution): Apply twice daily; if no improvement occurs after 4 weeks of therapy, re-evaluate diagnosis

Children >12 years and Adults:

Vaginal: Cream:

1%: Insert 1 applicatorful vaginal cream daily (preferably at bedtime) for 7 consecutive days

2%: Insert 1 applicatorful vaginal cream daily (preferably at bedtime) for 3 consecutive days

Topical (cream, solution): Apply to affected area twice daily (morning and evening) for 7 consecutive days

Additional Information Complete prescribing information for this medication should be consulted for additional detail.

Dosage Forms Excipient information presented when available (limited, particularly for generics); consult specific product labeling.

Cream, topical: 1% (15 g, 30 g, 45 g)

Anti-Fungal™: 1% (113 g)

Cruex®: 1% (15 g) [contains benzyl alcohol]

Lotrimin® AF Athlete's Foot: 1% (12 g) [contains benzyl alcohol]

Lotrimin® AF for Her: 1% (24 g) [contains benzyl alcohol]
Lotrimin® AF Jock Itch: 1% (12 g) [contains benzyl alcohol]
Cream, vaginal: 1% (45 g); 2% (21 g)
Gyne-Lotrimin® 7: 1% (45 g) [contains benzyl alcohol]
Gyne-Lotrimin® 3: 2% (21 g) [contains benzyl alcohol]
Solution, topical: 1% (10 mL, 30 mL)

◆ **Clotrimazole and Betamethasone** *see* Betamethasone and Clotrimazole *on page 210*

CloZAPine (KLOE za peen)

Brand Names: U.S. Clozaril®; FazaClo®

Brand Names: Canada Apo-Clozapine®; Clozaril®; Gen-Clozapine

Pharmacologic Category Antipsychotic Agent, Atypical

Additional Appendix Information
Antipsychotic Agents *on page 1880*

Use Treatment-refractory schizophrenia; to reduce risk of recurrent suicidal behavior in schizophrenia or schizoaffective disorder

Unlabeled Use Schizoaffective disorder, bipolar disorder, childhood psychosis, severe obsessive-compulsive disorder; psychosis/agitation related to Alzheimer's dementia

Pregnancy Risk Factor B

Pregnancy Considerations Teratogenic effects were not seen in animal studies. Clozapine crosses the placenta and can be detected in the fetal blood and amniotic fluid. Antipsychotic use during the third trimester of pregnancy has a risk for abnormal muscle movements (extrapyramidal symptoms [EPS]) and withdrawal symptoms in newborns following delivery. Symptoms in the newborn may include agitation, feeding disorder, hypertonia, hypotonia, respiratory distress, somnolence, and tremor; these effects may be self-limiting or require hospitalization. Healthcare providers are encouraged to enroll women 18-45 years of age exposed to clozapine during pregnancy in the Atypical Antipsychotics Pregnancy Registry (1-866-961-2388). Women with amenorrhea associated with use of other antipsychotic agents may return to normal menstruation when switching to clozapine therapy. Reliable contraceptive measures should be employed by women of childbearing potential switching to clozapine therapy.

Lactation Enters breast milk/not recommended (AAP rates "of concern"; AAP 2001 update pending)

Prescribing and Access Restrictions

U.S.: Clozaril® is deemed to have an approved REMS program. As a requirement of the REMS program, access to this medication is restricted. Patient-specific registration is required to dispense clozapine. Monitoring systems for individual clozapine manufacturers are independent. If a patient is switched from one brand/manufacturer of clozapine to another, the patient must be entered into a new registry (must be completed by the prescriber and delivered to the dispensing pharmacy). Healthcare providers, including pharmacists dispensing clozapine, should verify the patient's hematological status and qualification to receive clozapine with all existing registries. The manufacturer of Clozaril® requests that healthcare providers submit all WBC/ANC values following discontinuation of therapy to the Clozaril National Registry for all nonrechallengable patients until WBC is ≥3500/mm^3 and ANC is ≥2000/mm^3.

Canada: Distribution of clozapine is available only through the Clozaril Support and Assistance Network (CSAN). Details regarding CSAN are available to Canadian practitioners at (800-267-2726).

Contraindications Hypersensitivity to clozapine or any component of the formulation; history of agranulocytosis or severe granulocytopenia with clozapine; uncontrolled epilepsy, severe central nervous system depression or comatose state; paralytic ileus; myeloproliferative disorders or use with other agents which have a well-known risk of agranulocytosis or bone marrow suppression

Canadian labeling: Additional contraindications (not in U.S. labeling): Active hepatic disease associated with nausea, anorexia, or jaundice; progressive hepatic disease or hepatic failure; severe renal impairment; severe cardiac disease (eg, myocarditis); patients unable to undergo blood testing

Warnings/Precautions [U.S. Boxed Warning]: Elderly patients with dementia-related psychosis treated with antipsychotics are at an increased risk of death compared to placebo. Most deaths appeared to be either cardiovascular (eg, heart failure, sudden death) or infectious (eg, pneumonia) in nature. Clozapine is not approved for the treatment of dementia-related psychosis.

[U.S. Boxed Warning]: Significant risk of agranulocytosis, potentially life-threatening. Therapy should not be initiated in patients with WBC <3500 cells/mm^3 or ANC <2000 cells/mm^3 or history of myeloproliferative disorder. WBC testing should occur periodically on an on-going basis (see prescribing information for monitoring details) to ensure that acceptable WBC/ANC counts are maintained. Initial episodes of moderate leukopenia or granulopoietic suppression confer up to a 12-fold increased risk for subsequent episodes of agranulocytosis. WBCs must be monitored weekly for at least 4 weeks after therapy discontinuation or until WBC is ≥3500/mm^3 and ANC is ≥2000/mm^3. Use with caution in patients receiving other marrow suppressive agents. Eosinophilia has been reported to occur with clozapine. Interrupt therapy for eosinophil count >4000/mm^3. May resume therapy when eosinophil count <3000/mm^3. (**Note:** The Canadian labeling recommends discontinuing therapy for eosinophil count >3000/mm^3; may resume therapy when eosinophil count <1000/mm^3). Due to the significant risk of agranulocytosis, it is strongly recommended that a patient must fail at least two trials of other primary medications for the treatment of schizophrenia (of adequate dose and duration) before initiating therapy with clozapine.

Cognitive and/or motor impairment (sedation) is common with clozapine, resulting in impaired performance of tasks requiring alertness (eg, operating machinery or driving); use caution in patients receiving general anesthesia. **[U.S. Boxed Warning]: Seizures have been associated with clozapine use in a dose-dependent manner;** use with caution in patients at risk of seizures, including those with a history of seizures, head trauma, brain damage, alcoholism, or concurrent therapy with medications which may lower seizure threshold. Benign transient temperature elevation (>100.4°F) may occur; peaking within the first 3 weeks of treatment. Rule out infection, agranulocytosis, and neuroleptic malignant syndrome (NMS) in patients presenting with fever. However, clozapine may also be associated with severe febrile reactions, including neuroleptic malignant syndrome (NMS). Clozapine's potential for extrapyramidal symptoms (including tardive dyskinesia) appears to be extremely low. Risk of dystonia (and probably other EPS) may be greater with increased doses, use of conventional antipsychotics, males, and younger patients.

Deep vein thrombosis, myocarditis, pericarditis, pericardial effusion, cardiomyopathy, and HF have also been associated with clozapine. **[U.S. Boxed Warning]: Fatalities due to myocarditis have been reported; highest risk in the first month of therapy, however, later cases also reported.** Myocarditis or cardiomyopathy should be considered in patients who present with signs/symptoms of heart failure (dyspnea, fatigue, orthopnea, paroxysmal nocturnal dyspnea, peripheral edema), chest pain, palpitations, new electrocardiographic abnormalities (arrhythmias, ST-T wave abnormalities), or unexplained fever. Patients with tachycardia during the first month of therapy should be closely monitored for other signs of myocarditis. Discontinue clozapine if myocarditis is suspected; do not rechallenge in patients with clozapine-related myocarditis. The reported rate of myocarditis in clozapine-treated patients appears to be 17-322 times greater than in the general population. Clozapine should be discontinued in patients with confirmed cardiomyopathy unless benefit clearly outweighs risk. Rare cases of thromboembolism, including pulmonary embolism and stroke resulting in fatalities, have been associated with clozapine.

An increased incidence of cerebrovascular effects (eg, transient ischemic attack, stroke), including fatalities, has been reported in placebo-controlled trials of atypical antipsychotics in elderly patients with dementia-related psychosis.

May cause anticholinergic effects; use with caution in patients with urinary retention, benign prostatic hyperplasia, narrow-angle glaucoma, xerostomia, visual problems, constipation, or history of bowel obstruction. May cause hyperglycemia; in some cases may be extreme and associated with ketoacidosis, hyperosmolar coma, or death. Use with caution in patients with diabetes or other disorders of glucose regulation; monitor for worsening of glucose control. Antipsychotic use has been associated with esophageal dysmotility and aspiration; use with caution in patients at risk of pneumonia (eg, Alzheimer's disease). Use with caution in patients with hepatic disease or impairment; monitor hepatic function regularly. Hepatitis has been reported as a consequence of therapy. Discontinuation of therapy may be necessary with significant elevations in liver function tests; may reinitiate with close monitoring and if values return to normal. Use with caution in patients with renal disease.

Use caution with cardiovascular or pulmonary disease; gradually increase dose. **[U.S. Boxed Warning]: May cause orthostatic hypotension (with or without syncope);** generally occurs more frequently with initial titration and in association with rapid dose increases; use with caution in patients at risk of hypotension or in patients where transient hypotensive episodes would be poorly tolerated (cardiovascular disease or cerebrovascular disease). Concurrent use with benzodiazepines may increase the risk of severe cardiopulmonary reactions. May cause tachycardia (including sustained); sustained tachycardia is not limited to a reflex response to orthostatic hypotension, and is present in all positions.

The possibility of a suicide attempt is inherent in psychotic illness or bipolar disorder; use caution in high-risk patients during initiation of therapy. Prescriptions should be written for the smallest quantity consistent with good patient care.

Medication should not be stopped abruptly; taper off over 1-2 weeks. If conditions warrant abrupt discontinuation (leukopenia, myocarditis, cardiomyopathy), monitor patient for psychosis and cholinergic rebound (headache, nausea, vomiting, diarrhea). Significant weight gain has been observed with antipsychotic therapy; incidence varies with product. Monitor waist circumference and BMI. Elderly patients are more susceptible to adverse effects (including agranulocytosis, cardiovascular, anticholinergic, and tardive dyskinesia). Clozapine levels may be lower in patients who smoke. Smoking cessation may cause toxicity in a patient stabilized on clozapine. Monitor change in smoking. FazaClo® oral disintegrating tablets contain phenylalanine.

Adverse Reactions

>10%:

Cardiovascular: Tachycardia (25%)

Central nervous system: Drowsiness (39% to 46%), dizziness (19% to 27%), insomnia (2% to 20%)

Gastrointestinal: Sialorrhea (31% to 48%), weight gain (4% to 31%), constipation (14% to 25%), nausea/vomiting (3% to 17%)

1% to 10%:

Cardiovascular: Hypotension (9%), syncope (6%), hypertension (4%), angina (1%), ECG changes (1%)

Central nervous system: Headache (7%), fever (5%), agitation (4%), akinesia (4%), nightmares (4%), restlessness (4%), akathisia (3%), confusion (3%), seizure (3%), anxiety (1%), ataxia (1%), depression (1%), lethargy (1%), myoclonic jerks (1%), slurred speech (1%)

Dermatologic: Rash (2%)

Gastrointestinal: Abdominal discomfort/heartburn (4% to 14%), xerostomia (6%), diarrhea (2%), anorexia (1%), throat discomfort (1%)

Genitourinary: Urinary abnormalities (eg, abnormal ejaculation, retention, urgency, incontinence; 1% to 2%)

Hematologic: Agranulocytosis (1%), eosinophilia (1%), leukocytosis, leukopenia

Hepatic: Liver function tests abnormal (1%)

Neuromuscular & skeletal: Tremor (6%), hypokinesia (4%), rigidity (3%), hyperkinesia (1%), weakness (1%), pain (1%), spasm (1%)

Ocular: Visual disturbances (5%)

Respiratory: Dyspnea (1%), nasal congestion (1%)

Miscellaneous: Diaphoresis (6%), tongue numbness (1%)

<1%, postmarketing, and/or case reports (limited to important or life-threatening): Amentia, amnesia, anemia, arrhythmia (atrial or ventricular), aspiration, blurred vision, bradycardia, bronchitis, cardiomyopathy (usually dilated), cataplexy, CHF, cholestasis, CPK increased, cyanosis, delirium, delusions, dermatitis, diabetes mellitus, difficult urination, DVT, dysphagia, eczema, edema, EEG abnormal, erythema multiforme, ESR increased, fecal impaction, gastric ulcer, gastroenteritis, granulocytopenia, hallucinations, hematemesis, hepatitis, hypercholesterolemia (rare), hyperglycemia, hypersensitivity reaction, hypertriglyceridemia (rare), hyperuricemia, hyponatremia, hyperosmolar coma, hypothermia, impotence, interstitial nephritis (acute), intestinal obstruction, jaundice, ketoacidosis, loss of speech, MI, mitral valve insufficiency, myasthenia syndrome, mydriasis, myocarditis, narrow-angle glaucoma, neuroleptic malignant syndrome, obsessive compulsive symptoms, palpitations, pancreatitis (acute), paralytic ileus, paresthesia, Parkinsonism, pericardial effusion, pericarditis, periorbital edema, phlebitis, photosensitivity, pleural effusion, pneumonia, priapism, pruritus, psychosis exacerbated, pulmonary embolism, rectal bleeding, respiratory arrest, rhabdomyolysis, salivary gland swelling, sepsis, status epilepticus, stroke, Stevens-Johnson syndrome, tardive dyskinesia, thrombocytopenia, thrombocytosis, thromboembolism, thrombophlebitis, urticaria, vasculitis, weight loss, wheezing

Drug Interactions

Metabolism/Transport Effects **Substrate** of CYP1A2 (major), CYP2A6 (minor), CYP2C19 (minor), CYP2C9 (minor), CYP2D6 (minor), CYP3A4 (minor); **Note:** Assignment of Major/Minor substrate status based on clinically relevant drug interaction potential; **Inhibits** CYP1A2 (weak), CYP2C19 (weak), CYP2C9 (weak), CYP2D6 (moderate), CYP2E1 (weak), CYP3A4 (weak)

Avoid Concomitant Use

Avoid concomitant use of CloZAPine with any of the following: Artemether; Dronedarone; Lumefantrine; Metoclopramide; Myelosuppressive Agents; Nilotinib; Pimozide; QUEtiapine; QuiNINE; Tetrabenazine; Thioridazine; Toremifene; Vandetanib; Vemurafenib; Ziprasidone

Increased Effect/Toxicity

CloZAPine may increase the levels/effects of: Alcohol (Ethyl); Anticholinergics; CNS Depressants; CYP2D6 Substrates; Dronedarone; Fesoterodine; Methylphenidate; Nebivolol; Pimozide; QTc-Prolonging Agents; QuiNINE; Serotonin Modulators; Tamoxifen; Tetrabenazine; Thioridazine; Toremifene; Vandetanib; Vemurafenib; Ziprasidone

The levels/effects of CloZAPine may be increased by: Abiraterone Acetate; Acetylcholinesterase Inhibitors (Central); Alfuzosin; Artemether; Benzodiazepines; Chloroquine; Cimetidine; Ciprofloxacin; Ciprofloxacin (Systemic); Conivaptan; CYP1A2 Inhibitors (Moderate); CYP1A2 Inhibitors (Strong); Deferasirox; Gadobutrol; HydrOXYzine; Indacaterol; Lithium formulations; Lumefantrine; Macrolide Antibiotics; MAO Inhibitors; Methylphenidate; Metoclopramide; Myelosuppressive Agents; Nefazodone; Nilotinib; Omeprazole; Pramlintide; QUEtiapine; QuiNINE; Selective Serotonin Reuptake Inhibitors; Tetrabenazine

Decreased Effect

CloZAPine may decrease the levels/effects of: Amphetamines; Anti-Parkinson's Agents (Dopamine Agonist); Codeine; Quinagolide

The levels/effects of CloZAPine may be decreased by: CarBAMazepine; CYP1A2 Inducers (Strong); Cyproterone; Fosphenytoin; Lithium formulations; Omeprazole; Phenytoin; Tocilizumab

Ethanol/Nutrition/Herb Interactions

Ethanol: May increase CNS depression; monitor for increased effects with coadministration. Caution patients about effects.

Herb/Nutraceutical: St John's wort may decrease clozapine levels. Avoid kava kava, gotu kola, valerian, St John's wort (may increase CNS depression).

Stability Store at ≤30°C (86°F).

FazaClo®: Store at 25°C (77°F); excursions permitted to 15°C to 30°C (59°F to 86°F). Protect from moisture; do not remove from package until ready to use.

Mechanism of Action Clozapine (dibenzodiazepine antipsychotic) exhibits weak antagonism of D_1, D_2, D_3, and D_5 dopamine receptor subtypes, but shows high affinity for D_4; in addition, it blocks the serotonin ($5HT_2$), alpha-adrenergic, histamine H_1, and cholinergic receptors

Pharmacodynamics/Kinetics

Protein binding: 97% to serum proteins

Metabolism: Extensively hepatic; forms metabolites with limited or no activity

Bioavailability: 50% to 60% (not affected by food)

Half-life elimination: Steady state: 12 hours (range: 4-66 hours)

Time to peak: 2.5 hours (range: 1-6 hours)

Excretion: Urine (~50%) and feces (30%) with trace amounts of unchanged drug

Dosage Oral:

Children and Adolescents: Childhood psychosis (unlabeled use): Initial: 12.5-25 mg/day; increase to a target dose of 25-400 mg/day (Kumra, 2008; Turetz, 1997)

Adults:

Schizophrenia: Initial: 12.5 mg once or twice daily; increased, as tolerated, in increments of 25-50 mg/day to a target dose of 300-450 mg/day after 2 weeks; may further titrate in increments not exceeding 100 mg and no more frequently than once or twice weekly. May require doses as high as 600-900 mg/day (maximum dose: 900 mg/day). **Note:** In some efficacy studies, total daily dosage was administered in 3 divided doses.

Suicidal behavior in schizophrenia or schizoaffective disorder: Initial: 12.5 mg once or twice daily; increased, as tolerated, in increments of 25-50 mg/day to a target dose of 300-450 mg/day after 2 weeks; mean dose is ~300 mg/day (range: 12.5-900 mg); treatment duration 2 years then reassess need. **Note:** If no longer a suicide risk, may resume prior antipsychotic therapy after gradually tapering off clozapine over 1-2 weeks.

Elderly:

Schizophrenia: Experience in the elderly is limited; initial dose should be 12.5-25 mg/day; increase as tolerated by 25 mg/day to desired response. Elderly may require slower titration and daily increases may not be tolerated.

Psychosis/agitation related to Alzheimer's dementia (unlabeled use): Initial: 12.5 mg/day; if necessary, gradually increase as tolerated not to exceed 75-100 mg/day (Rabins, 2007)

Termination of therapy: If dosing is interrupted for ≥48 hours, therapy must be reinitiated at 12.5-25 mg/day; may be increased more rapidly than with initial titration, unless cardiopulmonary arrest occurred during initial titration.

In the event of planned termination of clozapine, gradual reduction in dose over a 1- to 2-week period is recommended. If conditions warrant abrupt discontinuation (leukopenia), monitor patient for psychosis and cholinergic rebound (headache, nausea, vomiting, diarrhea).

Dosage adjustment for toxicity:

Eosinophilia:

U.S. labeling: Interrupt therapy for eosinophil count >4000/mm^3; may resume therapy when eosinophil count <3000/mm^3

Canadian labeling: Interrupt therapy for eosinophil count >3000/mm^3; may resume therapy when eosinophil count <1000/ mm^3

Moderate leukopenia or granulocytopenia (WBC <3000/mm^3 and/or ANC <1500/mm^3): Discontinue therapy; may rechallenge patient when WBC is >3500/mm^3 and ANC is >2000/mm^3. **Note:** Patient is at greater risk for developing agranulocytosis.

Severe leukopenia or granulocytopenia (WBC <2000/mm^3 and/or ANC <1000/mm^3 [U.S. labeling] or ANC <1500/mm^3 [Canadian labeling]): Discontinue therapy and do not rechallenge patient.

Platelets <50,000/mm^3: Canadian labeling recommends discontinuing therapy

Dietary Considerations May be taken without regard to food. Some products may contain phenylalanine.

Administration May be taken without regard to food. Total daily dose may be divided into uneven doses with larger dose administered at bedtime.

Canadian labeling: Maintenance dosing ≤200 mg/day may be administered as single dose in the evening.

Orally-disintegrating tablet: Should be removed from foil blister by peeling apart (do not push tablet through the foil). Remove immediately prior to use. Place tablet in mouth and allow to dissolve; swallow with saliva. If dosing requires splitting tablet, throw unused portion away.

Monitoring Parameters Note: The Canadian labeling recommends initiating treatment in an inpatient setting or an outpatient setting with medical supervision and monitoring of vital signs for at least 6-8 hours after the first few doses.

Mental status, ECG, WBC (see below), vital signs, fasting lipid profile and fasting blood glucose/Hgb A_{1c} (prior to treatment, at 3 months, then annually; liver function tests; BMI, personal/family history of obesity; waist circumference (weight should be assessed prior to treatment, at 4 weeks, 8 weeks, 12 weeks, and then at quarterly intervals. Consider titrating to a different antipsychotic agent for a weight gain ≥5% of the initial weight); blood pressure; abnormal involuntary movement scale (AIMS).

WBC and ANC should be obtained at baseline and at least weekly for the first 6 months (26 weeks) of continuous treatment. If counts remain acceptable (WBC ≥3500/mm^3, ANC ≥2000/mm^3) during this time period, then they may be monitored every other week for the next 6 months (26 weeks). If WBC/ANC continue to remain within these acceptable limits after the second 6 months (26 weeks) of therapy, monitoring can be decreased to every 4 weeks. If clozapine is discontinued, a weekly WBC should be conducted for an additional 4 weeks or until WBC is ≥3500/mm^3 and ANC is ≥2000/mm^3. If clozapine therapy is interrupted due to moderate leukopenia, weekly WBC/ANC monitoring is required for 12 months in patients restarted on clozapine treatment. (**Note:** When therapy is interrupted for >3 days, the Canadian labeling recommends weekly hematologic testing for an additional 6 weeks). If therapy is interrupted for reasons other than leukopenia/granulocytopenia, the 6-month time period for initiation of biweekly WBCs may need to be reset. **This determination depends upon the treatment duration, the length of the break in therapy, and whether or not an abnormal blood event occurred.**

Consult manufacturer prescribing information for determination of appropriate WBC/ANC monitoring interval.

Dosage Forms Excipient information presented when available (limited, particularly for generics); consult specific product labeling.

Tablet, oral: 25 mg, 50 mg, 100 mg, 200 mg
  Clozaril®: 25 mg, 100 mg [scored]
Tablet, orally disintegrating, oral:
  FazaClo®: 12.5 mg [contains phenylalanine 0.87 mg/tablet; mint flavor]
  FazaClo®: 25 mg [contains phenylalanine 1.74 mg/tablet; mint flavor]
  FazaClo®: 100 mg [contains phenylalanine 6.96 mg/tablet; mint flavor]
  FazaClo®: 150 mg [contains phenylalanine 10.44 mg/tablet; mint flavor]
  FazaClo®: 200 mg [contains phenylalanine 13.92 mg/tablet; mint flavor]

- ◆ **Clozaril®** *see* CloZAPine *on page 400*
- ◆ **CMA-676** *see* Gemtuzumab Ozogamicin *on page 788*
- ◆ **C-Met/Hepatocyte Growth Factor Receptor Tyrosine Kinase Inhibitor PF-02341066** *see* Crizotinib *on page 416*
- ◆ **C-Met/HGFR Tyrosine Kinase Inhibitor PF-02341066** *see* Crizotinib *on page 416*
- ◆ **CMV-IGIV** *see* Cytomegalovirus Immune Globulin (Intravenous-Human) *on page 434*
- ◆ **CNJ-016®** *see* Vaccinia Immune Globulin (Intravenous) *on page 1752*
- ◆ **CNTO-148** *see* Golimumab *on page 803*
- ◆ **CNTO 1275** *see* Ustekinumab *on page 1751*
- ◆ **Coagulant Complex Inhibitor** *see* Anti-inhibitor Coagulant Complex *on page 130*
- ◆ **Coagulation Factor I** *see* Fibrinogen Concentrate (Human) *on page 710*
- ◆ **Coagulation Factor VIIa** *see* Factor VIIa (Recombinant) *on page 681*
- ◆ **CO Alendronate (Can)** *see* Alendronate *on page 61*
- ◆ **CO Amlodipine (Can)** *see* AmLODIPine *on page 97*
- ◆ **Coartem®** *see* Artemether and Lumefantrine *on page 148*
- ◆ **CO Atenolol (Can)** *see* Atenolol *on page 161*
- ◆ **CO Atorvastatin (Can)** *see* Atorvastatin *on page 165*
- ◆ **CO Azithromycin (Can)** *see* Azithromycin (Systemic) *on page 180*
- ◆ **CO Bicalutamide (Can)** *see* Bicalutamide *on page 217*
- ◆ **CO Buspirone (Can)** *see* BusPIRone *on page 250*
- ◆ **CO Cabergoline (Can)** *see* Cabergoline *on page 259*

Cocaine (koe KANE)

Index Terms Cocaine Hydrochloride

Pharmacologic Category Local Anesthetic

Use Topical anesthesia for mucous membranes

Pregnancy Risk Factor C/X (nonmedicinal use)

Dosage Topical application (ear, nose, throat, bronchoscopy): Dosage depends on the area to be anesthetized, tissue vascularity, technique of anesthesia, and individual patient tolerance; the lowest dose necessary to produce adequate anesthesia should be used; concentrations of 1% to 10% are used (not to exceed 1 mg/kg). Lasts for 30 minutes or longer depending on concentration and vascularity of anesthetized tissue. Use reduced dosages for children, elderly, or debilitated patients.

Additional Information Complete prescribing information for this medication should be consulted for additional detail.

Dosage Forms Excipient information presented when available (limited, particularly for generics); consult specific product labeling. [DSC] = Discontinued product

Powder, for prescription compounding, as hydrochloride: USP: 100% (5 g, 25 g)

Solution, topical, as hydrochloride: 4% (4 mL, 10 mL); 10% (4 mL, 10 mL [DSC])

Controlled Substance C-II

- ◆ **Cocaine Hydrochloride** *see* Cocaine *on page 403*
- ◆ **CO Candesartan (Can)** *see* Candesartan *on page 273*
- ◆ **CO Ciprofloxacin (Can)** *see* Ciprofloxacin (Systemic) *on page 362*
- ◆ **CO Citalopram (Can)** *see* Citalopram *on page 370*
- ◆ **CO Clomipramine (Can)** *see* ClomiPRAMINE *on page 388*
- ◆ **CO Clonazepam (Can)** *see* ClonazePAM *on page 390*
- ◆ **Codar® GF** *see* Guaifenesin and Codeine *on page 810*

Codeine (KOE deen)

Brand Names: Canada Codeine Contin®; PMS-Codeine; ratio-Codeine

Index Terms Codeine Phosphate; Codeine Sulfate; Methylmorphine

Pharmacologic Category Analgesic, Opioid; Antitussive

Use Treatment of mild-to-moderate pain

Unlabeled Use Short-term relief of coughing in select patients

Pregnancy Risk Factor C

Pregnancy Considerations Adverse events have been observed in animal reproduction studies. Neonatal abstinence syndrome (NAS) has been observed in the newborn following maternal use of codeine during pregnancy. Symptoms of opioid withdrawal may include excessive crying, diarrhea, fever, hyper-reflexia, irritability, tremors, or vomiting. Perinatal stroke has also been reported.

Lactation Enters breast milk/use caution (AAP rates "compatible"; AAP 2001 update pending)

Contraindications Hypersensitivity to codeine or any component of the formulation; respiratory depression in the absence of resuscitative equipment; acute or severe bronchial asthma or hypercarbia; presence or suspicion of paralytic ileus

Canadian labeling: Additional contraindications (not in U.S. labeling): Hypersensitivity to other opioid analgesics; cor pulmonale; acute alcoholism; delirium tremens; severe

CNS depression; convulsive disorders; increased cerebrospinal or intracranial pressure; head injury; suspected surgical abdomen; use with or within 14 days of MAO inhibitors.

Warnings/Precautions May cause dose-related respiratory depression. The risk is increased in elderly patients, debilitated patients, and patients with conditions associated with hypoxia, hypercapnia, or upper airway obstruction. Use with caution in patients with pre-existing respiratory compromise (hypoxia and/or hypercapnia), COPD or other obstructive pulmonary disease, and kyphoscoliosis or other skeletal disorder which may alter respiratory function; critical respiratory depression may occur, even at therapeutic dosages.

Use may cause or aggravate constipation; chronic use may result in obstructive bowel disease, particularly in those with underlying intestinal motility disorders. Avoid use in patients with gastrointestinal obstruction, particularly paralytic ileus. May cause hypotension; use with caution in patients with hypovolemia, cardiovascular disease (including acute MI), or drugs which may exaggerate hypotensive effects (including phenothiazines or general anesthetics). May cause CNS depression, which may impair physical or mental abilities; patients must be cautioned about performing tasks which require mental alertness (eg, operating machinery or driving).

Use with extreme caution in patients with head injury, intracranial lesions, or elevated intracranial pressure; exaggerated elevation of ICP may occur. Use with caution in patients with hypersensitivity reactions to other phenanthrene-derivative opioid agonists (hydrocodone, hydromorphone, levorphanol, oxycodone, oxymorphone), adrenal insufficiency (including Addison's disease), biliary tract dysfunction, CNS depression or coma, thyroid dysfunction, morbid obesity, prostatic hyperplasia and/or urinary stricture, or severe hepatic or renal impairment. Use may obscure diagnosis or clinical course of patients with acute abdominal conditions. May induce or aggravate seizures; use with caution in patients with seizure disorders.

Use with caution in patients with a history of drug abuse or acute alcoholism; potential for drug dependency exists. Tolerance, psychological and physical dependence may occur with prolonged use. Effects may be potentiated when used with other sedative drugs or ethanol. Concurrent use of agonist/antagonist analgesics may precipitate withdrawal symptoms and/or reduced analgesic efficacy in patients following prolonged therapy with mu opioid agonists. Abrupt discontinuation following prolonged use may also lead to withdrawal symptoms.

Use caution in patients with two or more copies of the variant CYP2D6*2 allele; may have extensive conversion to morphine and thus increased opioid-mediated effects.

Some preparations contain sulfites which may cause allergic reactions.

Adverse Reactions Frequency not defined.

Cardiovascular: Bradycardia, cardiac arrest, circulatory depression, flushing, hyper-/hypotension, palpitation, shock, syncope, tachycardia

Central nervous system: Abnormal dreams, agitation, anxiety, apprehension, chills, coordination impaired, depression, disorientation, dizziness, drowsiness, dysphoria, euphoria, faintness, fatigue, hallucinations, headache, insomnia, intracranial pressure increased, lightheadedness, nervousness, sedation, shakiness, somnolence, vertigo

Dermatologic: Pruritus, rash, urticaria

Gastrointestinal: Abdominal cramps/pain, anorexia, biliary tract spasm, constipation, diarrhea, nausea, pancreatitis, taste disturbance, vomiting, xerostomia

Genitourinary: Urinary hesitancy/retention

Neuromuscular & skeletal: Paresthesia, rigidity, tremor, weakness

Ocular: Blurred vision, diplopia, miosis, nystagmus, visual disturbances

Respiratory: Bronchospasm, dyspnea, laryngospasm, respiratory arrest, respiratory depression

Miscellaneous: Allergic reaction, diaphoresis

Drug Interactions

Metabolism/Transport Effects Substrate of CYP2D6 (major); **Note:** Assignment of Major/Minor substrate status based on clinically relevant drug interaction potential

Avoid Concomitant Use There are no known interactions where it is recommended to avoid concomitant use.

Increased Effect/Toxicity

Codeine may increase the levels/effects of: Alcohol (Ethyl); Alvimopan; CNS Depressants; Desmopressin; Selective Serotonin Reuptake Inhibitors; Thiazide Diuretics

The levels/effects of Codeine may be increased by: Amphetamines; Antipsychotic Agents (Phenothiazines); Droperidol; HydrOXYzine; Somatostatin Analogs; Succinylcholine

Decreased Effect

Codeine may decrease the levels/effects of: Pegvisomant

The levels/effects of Codeine may be decreased by: Ammonium Chloride; CYP2D6 Inhibitors (Moderate); CYP2D6 Inhibitors (Strong); Mixed Agonist / Antagonist Opioids

Ethanol/Nutrition/Herb Interactions

Ethanol: May increase CNS depression; monitor for increased effects with coadministration. Caution patients about effects.

Herb/Nutraceutical: St John's wort may decrease codeine levels. Avoid valerian, St John's wort, kava kava, gotu kola (may increase CNS depression).

Stability Store at 15°C to 30°C (59°F to 86°F). Protect from light.

Mechanism of Action Binds to opioid receptors in the CNS, causing inhibition of ascending pain pathways, altering the perception of and response to pain; causes cough suppression by direct central action in the medulla; produces generalized CNS depression

Pharmacodynamics/Kinetics

Onset of action: Oral: Immediate release: 0.5-1 hour

Peak effect: Oral: Immediate release: 1-1.5 hours

Duration: Immediate release: 4-6 hours

Distribution: ~3-6 L/kg

Protein binding: ~7% to 25%

Metabolism: Hepatic via UGT2B7 and UGT2B4 to codeine-6-glucuronide, via CYP2D6 to morphine (active), and via CYP3A4 to norcodeine. Morphine is further metabolized via glucuronidation to morphine-3-glucuronide and morphine-6-glucuronide (active).

Bioavailability: 53%

Half-life elimination: ~3 hours

Time to peak, plasma: Immediate release: 1 hour; Controlled release (Canadian availability; not available in the U.S.): 3.3 hours

Excretion: Urine (~90%, ~10% of the total dose as unchanged drug); feces

Dosage Oral:

Pain management (analgesic): **Note:** These are guidelines and do not represent the maximum doses that may be required in all patients. Doses should be titrated to pain relief/prevention.

Children (unlabeled use): Initial: 0.5-1 mg/kg/dose every 4 hours as needed; maximum: 60 mg/dose (American Pain Society, 2008)

Adults:

Immediate release: Initial: 15-60 mg every 4 hours as needed; maximum total daily dose: 360 mg/day; patients with prior opioid exposure may require higher initial doses. **Note:** The American Pain Society recommends an initial dose of 30-60 mg for adults with moderate pain (American Pain Society, 2008).

Controlled release: Codeine Contin® (Canadian availability; not available in U.S.): **Note:** Titrate at intervals of ≥48 hours until adequate analgesia has been achieved. Daily doses >600 mg/day should not be used; patients requiring higher doses should be switched to an opioid approved for use in severe pain. In patients who receive both Codeine Contin® and an immediate release or combination codeine phosphate product for breakthrough pain, the rescue dose of codeine base should be ≤12.5% of the total daily Codeine Contin® dose.

Opioid-naive patients: Initial: 50 mg every 12 hours

Conversion from immediate release codeine phosphate preparations: Codeine phosphate preparations contain ~75% codeine base. Therefore, patients who are switching from immediate release codeine phosphate preparations may be transferred to a ~25% lower total daily dose of Codeine Contin®, equally divided into 2 daily doses.

*Conversion from a combination codeine product (eg, codeine with acetaminophen **or** aspirin):* See table:

Number of 30 mg Codeine Combination Tablets Daily	Initial Dose of Codeine Contin®	Maintenance Dose of Codeine Contin®
≤6	50 mg every 12 h	100 mg every 12 h
7-9	100 mg every 12 h	150 mg every 12 h
10-12	150 mg every 12 h	200 mg every 12 h
>12	200 mg every 12 h	200-300 every 12 h (maximum: 300 mg every 12 h)

Conversion from another opioid analgesic: Using the patient's current opioid dose, calculate an equivalent daily dose of codeine phosphate. A ~25% lower dose of Codeine Contin® should then be initiated, equally divided into 2 daily doses.

Discontinuation of therapy: **Note:** Gradual dose reduction is recommended if clinically appropriate. Initially reduce the total daily dose by 50% and administer equally divided into 2 daily doses for 2 days followed by a 25% reduction every 2 days thereafter.

Treatment of cough (unlabeled use): Adults: Reported doses vary; range: 7.5-120 mg/day as a single dose or in divided doses (Bolser, 2006; Smith, 2010); **Note:** The American College of Chest Physicians does not recommend the routine use of codeine as an antitussive in patients with upper respiratory infections (Bolser, 2006).

Dosing adjustment in renal impairment:

Manufacturer's recommendations: Clearance may be reduced; active metabolites may accumulate. Initiate at lower doses or longer dosing intervals followed by careful titration.

Alternate recommendations: The following guidelines have been used by some clinicians (Aronoff, 2007):

Cl_{cr} 10-50 mL/minute: Administer 75% of dose

Cl_{cr} <10 mL/minute: Administer 50% of dose

Dosing adjustment in hepatic impairment: No dosage adjustment provided in manufacturer's labeling (has not been studied); however, initial lower doses or longer dosing intervals followed by careful titration are recommended.

Administration May administer without regard to meals. Take with food or milk to decrease adverse GI effects.

Controlled release tablets: Codeine Contin® (Canadian availability; not available in U.S.): Tablets should be swallowed whole; do not chew, dissolve, or crush. All strengths may be halved, **except** the 50 mg tablets; half tablets should also be swallowed intact.

Monitoring Parameters Pain relief, respiratory and mental status, blood pressure, heart rate

Reference Range Therapeutic: Not established; Toxic: >1.1 mcg/mL

Test Interactions Some quinolones may produce a false-positive urine screening result for opioids using commercially-available immunoassay kits. This has been demonstrated most consistently for levofloxacin and ofloxacin, but other quinolones have shown cross-reactivity in certain assay kits. Confirmation of positive opioid screens by more specific methods should be considered.

Dosage Forms Excipient information presented when available (limited, particularly for generics); consult specific product labeling. [DSC] = Discontinued product

Powder, for prescription compounding, as phosphate: USP: 100% (10 g, 25 g)

Tablet, oral, as phosphate: 30 mg [DSC], 60 mg [DSC]

Tablet, oral, as sulfate: 15 mg, 30 mg, 60 mg

Dosage Forms: Canada Excipient information presented when available (limited, particularly for generics); consult specific product labeling.

Tablet, controlled release:

Codeine Contin®: 50 mg, 100 mg, 150 mg, 200 mg

Controlled Substance C-II

Extemporaneous Preparations A 3 mg/mL oral suspension may be made with codeine phosphate powder, USP. Add 600 mg of powder to a 400 mL beaker. Add 2.5 mL of Sterile Water for Irrigation, USP, and stir to dissolve the powder. Mix for 10 minutes while adding Ora-Sweet® to make 200 mL; transfer to a calibrated bottle. Stable 98 days at room temperature.

Dentinger PJ and Swenson CF, "Stability of Codeine Phosphate in an Extemporaneously Compounded Syrup," *Am J Health Syst Pharm*, 2007, 64(24):2569-73.

◆ **Codeine and Acetaminophen** *see* Acetaminophen and Codeine *on page* 30
◆ **Codeine and Guaifenesin** *see* Guaifenesin and Codeine *on page* 810
◆ **Codeine and Promethazine** *see* Promethazine and Codeine *on page* 1418
◆ **Codeine, Aspirin, and Carisoprodol** *see* Carisoprodol, Aspirin, and Codeine *on page* 292
◆ **Codeine Contin® (Can)** *see* Codeine *on page* 403
◆ **Codeine, Guaifenesin, and Pseudoephedrine** *see* Guaifenesin, Pseudoephedrine, and Codeine *on page* 813
◆ **Codeine Phosphate** *see* Codeine *on page* 403
◆ **Codeine Sulfate** *see* Codeine *on page* 403
◆ **CO Diltiazem CD (Can)** *see* Diltiazem *on page* 510
◆ **CO Diltiazem T (Can)** *see* Diltiazem *on page* 510
◆ **Cod Liver Oil** *see* Vitamin A and Vitamin D *on page* 1796
◆ **CO Enalapril (Can)** *see* Enalapril *on page* 584
◆ **Co-Etidronate (Can)** *see* Etidronate *on page* 666
◆ **CO Famciclovir (Can)** *see* Famciclovir *on page* 687
◆ **CO Finasteride (Can)** *see* Finasteride *on page* 713
◆ **CO Fluconazole (Can)** *see* Fluconazole *on page* 718
◆ **CO Fluoxetine (Can)** *see* FLUoxetine *on page* 731
◆ **CO Gabapentin (Can)** *see* Gabapentin *on page* 773
◆ **Cogentin®** *see* Benztropine *on page* 205
◆ **CO Glimepiride (Can)** *see* Glimepiride *on page* 793

- ◆ **CO Ipra-Sal (Can)** *see* Ipratropium and Albuterol *on page 924*
- ◆ **CO Irbesartan (Can)** *see* Irbesartan *on page 925*
- ◆ **CO Irbesartan HCT (Can)** *see* Irbesartan and Hydrochlorothiazide *on page 926*
- ◆ **Colace® [OTC]** *see* Docusate *on page 537*
- ◆ **Colace® (Can)** *see* Docusate *on page 537*
- ◆ **CO Latanoprost (Can)** *see* Latanoprost *on page 978*
- ◆ **Colax-C® (Can)** *see* Docusate *on page 537*
- ◆ **Colazal®** *see* Balsalazide *on page 189*
- ◆ **ColBenemid** *see* Colchicine and Probenecid *on page 408*

Colchicine (KOL chi seen)

Brand Names: U.S. Colcrys®

Pharmacologic Category Antigout Agent

Use Prevention and treatment of acute gout flares; treatment of familial Mediterranean fever (FMF)

Unlabeled Use Primary biliary cirrhosis; pericarditis

Pregnancy Risk Factor C

Pregnancy Considerations Adverse events were observed in animal reproduction studies. Colchicine crosses the human placenta. Use during pregnancy in the treatment of familial Mediterranean fever has not shown an increase in miscarriage, stillbirth, or teratogenic effects (limited data).

Lactation Enters breast milk/use caution (AAP rates "compatible"; AAP 2001 update pending)

Medication Guide Available Yes

Contraindications Concomitant use of a P-glycoprotein (P-gp) or strong CYP3A4 inhibitor in presence of renal or hepatic impairment

Warnings/Precautions Hazardous agent - use appropriate precautions for handling and disposal. Myelosuppression (eg, thrombocytopenia, leukopenia, granulocytopenia, pancytopenia) and aplastic anemia have been reported in patients receiving therapeutic doses. Neuromuscular toxicity (including rhabdomyolysis) has been reported in patients receiving therapeutic doses; patients with renal dysfunction and elderly patients are at increased risk. Concomitant use of cyclosporine, diltiazem, verapamil, fibrates, and statins may increase the risk of myopathy. Clearance is decreased in renal or hepatic impairment; monitor closely for adverse effects/toxicity. Dosage adjustments may be required depending on degree of impairment or indication, and may be affected by the use of concurrent medication (CYP3A4 or P-gp inhibitors). Concurrent use of P-gp or strong CYP3A4 inhibitors is contraindicated in renal impairment; fatal toxicity has been reported. Colchicine does not have analgesic activity and should not be used to treat pain from other causes. Colchicine requires dosage adjustment when used concurrently with protease inhibitor regimens. Colchicine does not have analgesic activity and should not be used to treat pain from other causes.

Adverse Reactions

>10%: Gastrointestinal: Gastrointestinal disorders including abdominal pain, cramping, nausea, vomiting (up to 26%), diarrhea (up to 23%)

1% to 10%: Respiratory: Pharyngolaryngeal pain (3%)

<1% (Limited to important or life-threatening): Alopecia, ALT increased, aplastic anemia, AST increased, azoospermia, bone marrow suppression, CPK increased, dermatosis, granulocytopenia, hepatotoxicity, hypersensitivity reaction, lactose intolerance, leukopenia, maculopapular rash, muscle weakness, myalgia, myopathy, myotonia, neuropathy, oligospermia, pancytopenia, peripheral neuritis, purpura, rash, rhabdomyolysis, thrombocytopenia

Drug Interactions

Metabolism/Transport Effects Substrate of CYP3A4 (major), P-glycoprotein; **Note:** Assignment of Major/Minor substrate status based on clinically relevant drug interaction potential; **Induces** CYP2C9 (weak/moderate), CYP2E1 (weak/moderate), CYP3A4 (weak/moderate)

Avoid Concomitant Use There are no known interactions where it is recommended to avoid concomitant use.

Increased Effect/Toxicity

Colchicine may increase the levels/effects of: HMG-CoA Reductase Inhibitors

The levels/effects of Colchicine may be increased by: CYP3A4 Inhibitors (Moderate); CYP3A4 Inhibitors (Strong); Dasatinib; Digoxin; Fibric Acid Derivatives; P-glycoprotein/ABCB1 Inhibitors; Telaprevir

Decreased Effect

Colchicine may decrease the levels/effects of: ARIPiprazole; Cyanocobalamin; Saxagliptin

The levels/effects of Colchicine may be decreased by: P-glycoprotein/ABCB1 Inducers; Tocilizumab

Ethanol/Nutrition/Herb Interactions

Ethanol: Avoid ethanol.

Food: Cyanocobalamin (vitamin B_{12}): Malabsorption of the substrate. May result in macrocytic anemia or neurologic dysfunction. Grapefruit juice may increase colchicine serum concentrations.

Herb/Nutraceutical: Vitamin B_{12} absorption may be decreased by colchicine.

Stability Store at 20°C to 25°C (68°F to 77°F). Protect from light.

Mechanism of Action Disrupts cytoskeletal functions by inhibiting β-tubulin polymerization into microtubules, preventing activation, degranulation, and migration of neutrophils associated with mediating some gout symptoms. In familial Mediterranean fever, may interfere with intracellular assembly of the inflammasome complex present in neutrophils and monocytes that mediate activation of interleukin-1β.

Pharmacodynamics/Kinetics

Onset of action: Oral: Pain relief: ~18-24 hours

Distribution: Concentrates in leukocytes, kidney, spleen, and liver; does not distribute in heart, skeletal muscle, and brain

V_d: 5-8 L/kg

Protein binding: ~39%

Metabolism: Hepatic via CYP3A4; 3 metabolites (2 primary, 1 minor)

Bioavailability: ~45%

Half-life elimination: 27-31 hours (multiple oral doses; young, healthy volunteers)

Time to peak, serum: Oral: 0.5-3 hours

Excretion: Urine (40% to 65% as unchanged drug); enterohepatic recirculation and biliary excretion also possible

Dosage Oral:

Familial Mediterranean fever (FMF):

Children:

4-6 years: 0.3-1.8 mg/day in 1-2 divided doses

6-12 years: 0.9-1.8 mg/day in 1-2 divided doses

Children >12 years and Adults: 1.2-2.4 mg/day in 1-2 divided doses. Titration: Increase or decrease dose in 0.3 mg/day increments based on efficacy or adverse effects; maximum: 2.4 mg/day

Gout: Children >16 years and Adults:

Flare treatment: Initial: 1.2 mg at the first sign of flare, followed in 1 hour with a single dose of 0.6 mg (maximum: 1.8 mg within 1 hour). Patients receiving prophylaxis therapy may receive treatment dosing; wait 12 hours before resuming prophylaxis dose. **Note:** Current FDA-approved dose for gout flare is substantially lower than what has been historically used clinically. Doses larger than the currently recommended dosage for gout flare have not been proven to be more effective.

Prophylaxis: 0.6 mg once or twice daily; maximum: 1.2 mg/day

Pericarditis post-STEMI (unlabeled use): Adults: 0.6 mg twice daily (Antman, 2004)

Recurrent pericarditis due to previous autoimmune or idiopathic cause (unlabeled use; Imazio, 2011): **Note:** Dosage strength not available in the U.S.: Oral: 0.5-1 mg every 12 hours for 1 day, followed by 0.25-0.5 mg every 12 hours for 6 months (in combination with high-dose aspirin or ibuprofen)

Patients <70 kg or unable to tolerate higher dosing regimen: 0.5 mg every 12 hours for 1 day followed by 0.5 mg once daily.

Primary biliary cirrhosis (unlabeled use): Adults: 0.6 mg twice daily (Kaplan, 2005); **Note:** Use reserved for patients refractory to ursodiol.

Elderly: Use caution; reduce prophylactic daily dose by 50% in individuals >70 years (Terkeltaub, 2009)

Dosage adjustment for concomitant therapy with CYP3A4 or P-glycoprotein (P-gp) inhibitors: *Dosage adjustment also required in patients receiving CYP3A4 or P-gp inhibitors up to 14 days prior to initiation of colchicine.* **Note:** Treatment of gout flare with colchicine is not recommended in patients receiving prophylactic colchicine and CYP3A4 inhibitors.

Coadministration of **strong** CYP3A4 inhibitor (eg, atazanavir, clarithromycin, darunavir, indinavir, itraconazole, ketoconazole, lopinavir/ritonavir, nefazodone, nelfinavir, ritonavir, saquinavir, telithromycin, tipranavir):

FMF: Maximum dose: 0.6 mg/day (0.3 mg twice daily)

Gout prophylaxis:

If original dose is 0.6 mg twice daily, adjust dose to 0.3 mg once daily

If original dose is 0.6 mg once daily, adjust dose to 0.3 mg every other day

Gout flare treatment: Initial: 0.6 mg, followed in 1 hour by a single dose of 0.3 mg; do not repeat for at least 3 days

Coadministration of **moderate** CYP3A4 inhibitor (eg, aprepitant, diltiazem, erythromycin, fluconazole, fosamprenavir, grapefruit juice, verapamil):

FMF: Maximum dose: 1.2 mg/day (0.6 mg twice daily)

Gout prophylaxis:

If original dose is 0.6 mg twice daily, adjust dose to 0.3 mg twice daily **or** 0.6 mg once daily

If original dose is 0.6 mg once daily, adjust dose to 0.3 mg once daily

Gout flare treatment: 1.2 mg as a single dose; do not repeat for at least 3 days

Coadministration of P-gp inhibitor (eg, cyclosporine, ranolazine):

FMF: Maximum dose: 0.6 mg/day (0.3 mg twice daily)

Gout prophylaxis:

If original dose is 0.6 mg twice daily, adjust dose to 0.3 mg once daily

If original dose is 0.6 mg once daily, adjust dose to 0.3 mg every other day

Gout flare treatment: Initial: 0.6 mg as a single dose; do not repeat for at least 3 days

Dosing adjustment in renal impairment: Concurrent use of colchicine and P-gp or strong CYP3A4 inhibitors is **contraindicated** in renal impairment. Fatal toxicity has been reported. Treatment of gout flares is not recommended in patients with renal impairment receiving prophylactic colchicine.

FMF:

Cl_{cr} 30-80 mL/minute: Monitor closely for adverse effects; dose reduction may be necessary

Cl_{cr} <30 mL/minute: Initial dose: 0.3 mg/day; use caution if dose titrated; monitor for adverse effects

Dialysis: 0.3 mg as a single dose; use caution if dose titrated; dosing can be increased with close monitoring; monitor for adverse effects. Not removed by dialysis.

Gout prophylaxis:

Cl_{cr} 30-80 mL/minute: Dosage adjustment not required; monitor closely for adverse effects

Cl_{cr} <30 mL/minute: Initial dose: 0.3 mg/day; use caution if dose titrated; monitor for adverse effects

Dialysis: 0.3 mg twice weekly; monitor closely for adverse effects

Gout flare treatment:

Cl_{cr} 30-80 mL/minute: Dosage adjustment not required; monitor closely for adverse effects

Cl_{cr} <30 mL/minute: Dosage reduction not required but may be considered; treatment course should not be repeated more frequently than every 14 days

Dialysis: 0.6 mg as a single dose; treatment course should not be repeated more frequently than every 14 days. Not removed by dialysis.

Hemodialysis: Avoid chronic use of colchicine.

Dosage adjustment in hepatic impairment: Concurrent use of colchicine and P-gp or strong CYP3A4 inhibitors is **contraindicated** in hepatic impairment. Fatal toxicity has been reported. Treatment of gout flare with colchicine is not recommended in patients with hepatic impairment receiving prophylactic colchicine.

FMF:

Mild-to-moderate impairment: Use caution; monitor closely for adverse effects

Severe impairment: Consider dosage reduction

Gout prophylaxis:

Mild-to-moderate impairment: Dosage adjustment not required; monitor closely for adverse effects

Severe impairment: Dosage adjustment should be considered

Gout flare treatment:

Mild-to-moderate impairment: Dosage adjustment not required; monitor closely for adverse effects

Severe impairment: Dosage reduction not required but may be considered; treatment course should not be repeated more frequently than every 14 days

Dietary Considerations May be taken without regard to meals. May need to supplement with vitamin B_{12}. Avoid grapefruit juice.

Administration Administer orally with water and maintain adequate fluid intake. May be administered without regard to meals.

Monitoring Parameters CBC, renal and hepatic function tests

Test Interactions May cause false-positive results in urine tests for erythrocytes or hemoglobin

Additional Information Oral colchicine had been available as an unapproved medication without FDA-approved prescribing information. In August 2009, the FDA approved prescribing information for a brand name colchicine product. The currently approved prescribing information recommends a lower than historically used dosage for the treatment of acute gout. This recommendation is based on data from the AGREE trial. In this trial, low-dose colchicine (1.8 mg total) had similar efficacy to high dose colchicine (4.8 mg total). Additionally, the low dosage regimen was associated with a lower incidence (26% vs 77%) of GI adverse events. Parenteral formulation of colchicine is no longer available in the U.S.; serious life-threatening complications (eg, neutropenia, acute renal failure, thrombocytopenia, heart failure) associated with intravenous colchicine have occurred prior to market withdrawal. The risks associated with oral colchicine are believed to be lower compared to intravenous use.

Dosage Forms Excipient information presented when available (limited, particularly for generics); consult specific product labeling.

Tablet, oral: 0.6 mg

Colcrys®: 0.6 mg [scored]

Dosage Forms: Canada Excipient information presented when available (limited, particularly for generics); consult specific product labeling.

Tablet, oral: 1 mg [scored]

Colchicine and Probenecid

(KOL chi seen & proe BEN e sid)

Index Terms ColBenemid; Probenecid and Colchicine

Pharmacologic Category Anti-inflammatory Agent; Antigout Agent; Uricosuric Agent

Use Treatment of chronic gouty arthritis when complicated by frequent, recurrent acute attacks of gout

Dosage Oral: Adults: One tablet daily for 1 week, then 1 tablet twice daily thereafter

Note: Current prescribing information states a maximum dose of 4 tablets per day; however this exceeds the usual maximum dose of colchicine for gout prophylaxis (1.2 mg per day).

Dosage adjustment in renal impairment: See individual agents.

Additional Information Complete prescribing information for this medication should be consulted for additional detail.

Dosage Forms Excipient information presented when available (limited, particularly for generics); consult specific product labeling.

Tablet: Colchicine 0.5 mg and probenecid 0.5 g

◆ **Colcrys®** *see* Colchicine *on page 406*

◆ **Coldcough PD** *see* Dihydrocodeine, Chlorpheniramine, and Phenylephrine *on page 508*

Colesevelam (koh le SEV a lam)

Brand Names: U.S. Welchol®

Brand Names: Canada Welchol®

Pharmacologic Category Antilipemic Agent, Bile Acid Sequestrant

Additional Appendix Information

Diabetes Mellitus Management, Adults *on page 1983*

Hyperlipidemia Management *on page 1996*

Use Management of elevated LDL in primary hypercholesterolemia (Fredrickson type IIa) when used alone or in combination with an HMG-CoA reductase inhibitor; management of heterozygous familial hypercholesterolemia (heFH) in adolescent patients (males and postmenarcheal females 10-17 years of age) when used alone or in combination with an HMG-CoA reductase inhibitor, in patients who after an adequate trial of dietary therapy have LDL-C ≥190 mg/dL or LDL-C ≥160 mg/dL with positive family history of premature cardiovascular disease (CVD) or with two or more CVD risk factors; improve glycemic control in type 2 diabetes mellitus (noninsulin dependent, NIDDM) in conjunction with diet, exercise, and insulin or oral antidiabetic agents

Pregnancy Risk Factor B

Dosage Oral:

Children 10-17 years (males and postmenarchal females): Dyslipidemia (heterozygous familial hypercholesterolemia):

Once-daily dosing: 3.75 g (oral suspension or 6 tablets)

Twice-daily dosing: 1.875 g (3 tablets)

Note: Due to large tablet size, oral suspension is recommended in pediatric patients.

Adults: Dyslipidemia, type 2 diabetes (combination therapy with insulin or oral antidiabetic agents):

Once-daily dosing: 3.75 g (oral suspension or 6 tablets)

Twice-daily dosing: 1.875 g (3 tablets)

Elderly: Refer to adult dosing.

Dosage adjustment in renal impairment: No dosage adjustment necessary; not absorbed from the gastrointestinal tract.

Dosage adjustment in hepatic impairment: No dosage adjustment necessary; not absorbed from the gastrointestinal tract.

Additional Information Complete prescribing information for this medication should be consulted for additional detail.

Dosage Forms Excipient information presented when available (limited, particularly for generics); consult specific product labeling.

Granules for suspension, oral, as hydrochloride:

Welchol®: 3.75 g/packet (30s) [contains phenylalanine 48 mg/packet; citrus flavor]

Tablet, oral, as hydrochloride:

Welchol®: 625 mg

◆ **Colestid®** *see* Colestipol *on page 408*

◆ **Colestid® Flavored** *see* Colestipol *on page 408*

Colestipol (koe LES ti pole)

Brand Names: U.S. Colestid®; Colestid® Flavored

Brand Names: Canada Colestid®

Index Terms Colestipol Hydrochloride

Pharmacologic Category Antilipemic Agent, Bile Acid Sequestrant

Additional Appendix Information

Hyperlipidemia Management *on page 1996*

Use Adjunct in management of primary hypercholesterolemia

Unlabeled Use Diarrhea associated with excess fecal bile acids (Westergaard, 2007); relief of pruritus associated with elevated levels of bile acids (Datta, 1963; Scaldaferri, 2011)

Dosage Adults: Oral:

Granules: Initial: 5 g 1-2 times/day; maintenance: 5-30 g/day given once or in divided doses; increase by 5 g/day at 1- to 2-month intervals

Tablets: Initial: 2 g 1-2 times/day; maintenance: 2-16 g/day given once or in divided doses; increase by 2 g once or twice daily at 1- to 2-month intervals

Dosage adjustment in renal impairment: No dosage adjustment necessary; not absorbed from the gastrointestinal tract.

Dosage adjustment in hepatic impairment: No dosage adjustment necessary; not absorbed from the gastrointestinal tract.

Additional Information Complete prescribing information for this medication should be consulted for additional detail.

Dosage Forms Excipient information presented when available (limited, particularly for generics); consult specific product labeling.

Granules for suspension, oral, as hydrochloride: 5 g/scoop (500 g); 5 g/packet (30s, 90s)

Colestid®: 5 g/scoop (300 g, 500 g); 5 g/packet (30s, 90s) [unflavored]

Colestid® Flavored: 5 g/scoop (450 g) [contains phenylalanine 18.2 mg/scoop; orange flavor]

Colestid® Flavored: 5 g/packet (60s) [contains phenylalanine 18.2 mg/packet; orange flavor]

Tablet, oral, as hydrochloride: 1 g

Tablet, oral, as hydrochloride [micronized]: 1 g

Colestid®: 1 g

◆ **Colestipol Hydrochloride** *see* Colestipol *on page 408*

◆ **CO Levetiracetam (Can)** *see* LevETIRAcetam *on page 994*

◆ **CO Lisinopril (Can)** *see* Lisinopril *on page 1020*

Colistimethate (koe lis ti METH ate)

Brand Names: U.S. Coly-Mycin® M

Brand Names: Canada Coly-Mycin® M

Index Terms Colistimethate Sodium; Colistin Methanesulfonate; Colistin Sulfomethate; Pentasodium Colistin Methanesulfonate

Pharmacologic Category Antibiotic, Miscellaneous

Use Treatment of infections due to sensitive strains of certain gram-negative bacilli which are resistant to other antibacterials or in patients allergic to other antibacterials

Unlabeled Use Used as nebulized inhalation in the prevention of *Pseudomonas aeruginosa* respiratory tract infections in immunocompromised patients, and used as nebulized inhalation adjunct agent for the treatment of *P. aeruginosa* infections in patients with cystic fibrosis and other seriously ill or chronically ill patients

Pregnancy Risk Factor C

Pregnancy Considerations Adverse events have been observed in animal reproduction studies; therefore, the manufacturer classifies colistimethate as pregnancy category C. Colistimethate crosses the placenta in humans. There are no adequate and well-controlled studies in pregnant women.

Lactation Excretion in breast milk unknown/use caution

Contraindications Hypersensitivity to colistimethate, colistin, or any component of the formulation

Warnings/Precautions Nephrotoxicity has been reported; use with caution in patients with pre-existing renal disease; dosage adjustments may be required. Respiratory arrest has been reported with use; impaired renal function may increase the risk for neuromuscular blockade and apnea. Transient, reversible neurological disturbances (eg, dizziness, numbness, paresthesia, tingling, vertigo) may occur. Prolonged use may result in fungal or bacterial superinfection, including *C. difficile*-associated diarrhea (CDAD) and pseudomembranous colitis; CDAD has been observed >2 months postantibiotic treatment.

Adverse Reactions Frequency not defined.

Central nervous system: Dizziness, fever, headache, slurred speech, vertigo

Dermatologic: Pruritus, rash, urticaria

Gastrointestinal: GI upset

Neuromuscular & skeletal: Paresthesia (extremities, oral); weakness (lower limb)

Renal: BUN increased, creatinine increased, nephrotoxicity, proteinuria, urine output decreased

Respiratory: Apnea, respiratory arrest

Postmarketing, and/or case reports: Lung toxicity (bronchoconstriction, bronchospasm, chest tightness, respiratory distress, acute respiratory failure following inhalation)

Drug Interactions

Metabolism/Transport Effects None known.

Avoid Concomitant Use

Avoid concomitant use of Colistimethate with any of the following: BCG

Increased Effect/Toxicity

Colistimethate may increase the levels/effects of: Neuromuscular-Blocking Agents

The levels/effects of Colistimethate may be increased by: Aminoglycosides; Amphotericin B; Capreomycin; Polymyxin B; Vancomycin

Decreased Effect

Colistimethate may decrease the levels/effects of: BCG; Typhoid Vaccine

Stability Store intact vials (prior to reconstitution) at 20°C to 25°C (68°F to 77°F); reconstituted vials may be refrigerated at 2°C to 8°C (36°F to 46°F) or stored at 20°C to 25°C (68°F to 77°F) for up to 24 hours. Solutions for infusion should be freshly prepared; do not use beyond 24 hours.

For I.V. use, reconstitute each vial with 2 mL of SWFI; swirl gently to avoid foaming. May further dilute in D_5W or NS for I.V. infusion.

For nebulized inhalation (unlabeled use), reconstitute with NS; should be used promptly after preparation; do not use after 24 hours.

For intrathecal/intraventricular use (unlabeled route), reconstitute with preservative-free diluent (SWFI or NS) only; use promptly after preparation; discard unused portion of vial.

Mechanism of Action Hydrolyzed to colistin, which acts as a cationic detergent which damages the bacterial cytoplasmic membrane causing leaking of intracellular substances and cell death

Pharmacodynamics/Kinetics

Distribution: Widely, except for CNS, synovial, pleural, and pericardial fluids

Metabolism: Colistimethate is hydrolyzed to colistin

Half-life elimination: I.M., I.V.: 2-3 hours; Anuria: ≤2-3 days

Time to peak: I.V.: 10 minutes

Excretion: Primarily urine (as unchanged drug)

Dosage Note: Doses should be based on ideal body weight in obese patients; dosage expressed in terms of colistin.

Children and Adults:

Susceptible infections:

I.M., I.V.: 2.5-5 mg/kg/day in 2-4 divided doses

Inhalation (unlabeled use): 50-75 mg in NS (3-4 mL total) via nebulizer 2-3 times/day

Cystic fibrosis (unlabeled use): I.V.:

Children: 3-8 mg/kg/day in 3 divided doses (maximum dose: 70 mg)

Adults: 3-8 mg/kg/day in 3 divided doses **or** 60-70 mg every 8 hours, if tolerated, may increase to 80-100 mg every 8 hours

Adults: Meningitis (susceptible gram-negative organisms): Intrathecal/Intraventricular (unlabeled route): 10 mg/day (IDSA, 2004); **Note:** Dosage in clinical reports has ranged from 1.6-20 mg/day in 1 or 2 divided doses (maximum single dose: 10 mg) (administered with concomitant systemic antimicrobial therapy) (Guardado, 2008; Kasiakou, 2005; Katragkou, 2005)

Dosing interval in renal impairment: Adults:

S_{cr} 1.3-1.5 mg/dL: 75-115 mg twice daily (approximately 2.5-3.8 mg/kg/day)

S_{cr} 1.6-2.5 mg/dL: 66-150 mg once or twice daily (approximately 2.5 mg/kg/day)

S_{cr} 2.6-4 mg/dL: 100-150 mg every 36 hours (approximately 1.5 mg/kg/day)

Intermittent hemodialysis (IHD) (administer after hemodialysis on dialysis days): 1.5 mg/kg every 24-48 hours (Heintz, 2009). **Note:** Dosing dependent on the assumption of 3 times/week, complete IHD sessions.

Continuous renal replacement therapy (CRRT) (Heintz, 2009; Trotman, 2005): Drug clearance is highly dependent on the method of renal replacement, filter type, and flow rate. Appropriate dosing requires close monitoring of pharmacologic response, signs of adverse reactions due to drug accumulation, as well as drug concentrations in relation to target trough (if appropriate). The following are general recommendations only (based on dialysate flow/ultrafiltration rates of 1-2 L/hour and minimal residual renal function) and should not supersede clinical judgment:

CVVH/CVVHD/CVVHDF: 2.5 mg/kg every 24-48 hours (frequency dependent upon site or severity of infection or susceptibility of pathogen)

Note: A single case report has demonstrated that the use of 2.5 mg/kg every 48 hours with a dialysate flow rate of 1 L/hour may be inadequate and that dosing every 24 hours was well-tolerated. Based on pharmacokinetic analysis, the authors recommend dosing as frequent as every 12 hours in patients receiving CVVHDF (Li, 2005).

Administration

Parenteral: Reconstitute vial with 2 mL SWFI resulting in a concentration of 75 mg colistin/mL; swirl gently to avoid frothing. Administer by I.M., direct I.V. injection over 3-10 minutes, intermittent infusion over 30 minutes, or by continuous I.V. infusion. For continuous I.V. infusion, one-half of the total daily dose is administered by direct I.V. injection over 3-10 minutes followed 1-2 hours later by the remaining one-half of the total daily dose diluted in a compatible I.V. solution infused over 22-23 hours. The final concentration for administration should be based on the patient's fluid needs.

Inhalation (unlabeled): Reconstitute vial with 2 mL SWFI resulting in a concentration of 75 mg colistin/mL; further dilute dose to a total volume of 3-4 mL in NS and administer via nebulizer. If patient is on a ventilator, place medicine in a T-piece at the midinspiratory circuit of the ventilator. Administer solution promptly following preparation to decrease possibility of high concentrations of colistin from forming which may lead to potentially life-threatening lung toxicity.

Intrathecal/intraventricular (unlabeled route): Administer only preservative-free solutions via intrathecal/intraventricular routes. Administer promptly after preparation. Discard unused portion of vial.

Monitoring Parameters Serum creatinine, BUN; urine output; signs of neurotoxicity

Dosage Forms Excipient information presented when available (limited, particularly for generics); consult specific product labeling.

Injection, powder for reconstitution [strength expressed as base]: colistin 150 mg

Coly-Mycin® M: colistin 150 mg

◆ **Colistimethate Sodium** *see* Colistimethate *on page 409*

◆ **Colistin, Hydrocortisone, Neomycin, and Thonzonium** *see* Neomycin, Colistin, Hydrocortisone, and Thonzonium *on page 1189*

◆ **Colistin Methanesulfonate** *see* Colistimethate *on page 409*

◆ **Colistin Sulfomethate** *see* Colistimethate *on page 409*

Collagenase (Systemic) (KOL la je nase)

Brand Names: U.S. Xiaflex®

Index Terms Collagenase Clostridium Histolyticum

Pharmacologic Category Enzyme

Use Treatment of Dupuytren's contracture with a palpable cord

Pregnancy Risk Factor B

Medication Guide Available Yes

Dosage Intralesional: Adults: Dupuytren's contracture: Inject 0.58 mg per cord affecting a metacarpophalangeal (MP) joint or a proximal interphalangeal (PIP) joint. If contracture persists, finger extension procedure should be performed 24 hours following injection to facilitate cord disruption. If MP or PIP contracture remains, may reinject cord 4 weeks following initial injection; injections and finger extension procedures may be administered up to 3 times per cord separated by ~4 week intervals. **Note:** Only one cord should be injected at a time; if other palpable cords exist, inject in a sequential order.

Dosage adjustment in renal impairment: No adjustment necessary

Dosage adjustment in hepatic impairment: No adjustment necessary

Additional Information Complete prescribing information for this medication should be consulted for additional detail.

Dosage Forms Excipient information presented when available (limited, particularly for generics); consult specific product labeling.

Injection, powder for reconstitution:

Xiaflex®: 0.9 mg [contains sucrose 18.5 mg/vial; supplied with diluent]

Collagenase (Topical) (KOL la je nase)

Brand Names: U.S. Santyl®

Brand Names: Canada Santyl®

Pharmacologic Category Enzyme, Topical Debridement

Use Promotes debridement of necrotic tissue in dermal ulcers and severe burns

Pregnancy Risk Factor C

Dosage Topical: Apply once daily (or more frequently if the dressing becomes soiled)

Additional Information Complete prescribing information for this medication should be consulted for additional detail.

Dosage Forms Excipient information presented when available (limited, particularly for generics); consult specific product labeling.

Ointment, topical:

Santyl®: 250 units/g (30 g)

◆ **Collagenase Clostridium Histolyticum** *see* Collagenase (Systemic) *on page 410*

◆ **Colocort®** *see* Hydrocortisone (Topical) *on page 841*

◆ **CO Lovastatin (Can)** *see* Lovastatin *on page 1038*

◆ **Coly-Mycin® M** *see* Colistimethate *on page 409*

◆ **Coly-Mycin® S** *see* Neomycin, Colistin, Hydrocortisone, and Thonzonium *on page 1189*

◆ **Colyte®** *see* Polyethylene Glycol-Electrolyte Solution *on page 1372*

◆ **Colyte™ (Can)** *see* Polyethylene Glycol-Electrolyte Solution *on page 1372*

◆ **Combantrin™ (Can)** *see* Pyrantel Pamoate *on page 1434*

◆ **Combigan®** *see* Brimonidine and Timolol *on page 236*

◆ **CombiPatch®** *see* Estradiol and Norethindrone *on page 635*

◆ **Combivent®** *see* Ipratropium and Albuterol *on page 924*

◆ **Combivent UDV (Can)** *see* Ipratropium and Albuterol *on page 924*

◆ **Combivir®** *see* Lamivudine and Zidovudine *on page 967*

◆ **CO Meloxicam (Can)** *see* Meloxicam *on page 1063*

◆ **CO Memantine (Can)** *see* Memantine *on page 1068*

◆ **CO Metformin (Can)** *see* MetFORMIN *on page 1086*

◆ **CO Mirtazapine (Can)** *see* Mirtazapine *on page 1140*

◆ **Commit® [OTC]** *see* Nicotine *on page 1200*

◆ **Compazine** *see* Prochlorperazine *on page 1412*

◆ **Complera™** *see* Emtricitabine, Rilpivirine, and Tenofovir *on page 583*

◆ **Compound E** *see* Cortisone *on page 413*

◆ **Compound F** *see* Hydrocortisone (Systemic) *on page 839*

◆ **Compound F** *see* Hydrocortisone (Topical) *on page 841*

◆ **Compound S** *see* Zidovudine *on page 1814*

◆ **Compound S, Abacavir, and Lamivudine** *see* Abacavir, Lamivudine, and Zidovudine *on page 20*

◆ **Compoz® [OTC]** *see* DiphenhydrAMINE (Systemic) *on page* 516
◆ **Compro®** *see* Prochlorperazine *on page* 1412
◆ **Comtan®** *see* Entacapone *on page* 591
◆ **Comvax®** *see* *Haemophilus* b Conjugate and Hepatitis B Vaccine *on page* 815
◆ **Conceptrol® [OTC]** *see* Nonoxynol 9 *on page* 1216
◆ **Concerta®** *see* Methylphenidate *on page* 1107
◆ **Congest (Can)** *see* Estrogens (Conjugated/Equine, Systemic) *on page* 641
◆ **Congestac® [OTC]** *see* Guaifenesin and Pseudoephedrine *on page* 813

Conivaptan (koe NYE vap tan)

Brand Names: U.S. Vaprisol®

Index Terms Conivaptan Hydrochloride; YM087

Pharmacologic Category Vasopressin Antagonist

Use Treatment of euvolemic and hypervolemic hyponatremia in hospitalized patients

Pregnancy Risk Factor C

Pregnancy Considerations Animal studies indicate that conivaptan accumulates in the placenta (2.2-fold relative to maternal plasma); systemic exposure to fetus is likely. No teratogenic effects have been observed in animal studies; however, these studies have shown decreased neonatal viability and delayed growth and development at doses lower than those required for therapeutic efficacy. There are no adequate and well-controlled studies in pregnant women. Use only if benefit outweighs risk.

Lactation Excretion in breast milk unknown/not recommended

Contraindications Hypersensitivity to conivaptan, corn or corn products, or any component of the formulation; use in hypovolemic hyponatremia; concurrent use with strong CYP3A4 inhibitors (eg, ketoconazole, itraconazole, ritonavir, indinavir, and clarithromycin); anuria

Warnings/Precautions Monitor closely for rate of serum sodium increase and neurological status; overly rapid serum sodium correction (>12 mEq/L/24 hours) can lead to seizures, permanent neurological damage, coma, or death. Discontinue use if rate of serum sodium increase is undesirable; may reinitiate infusion (at reduced dose) if hyponatremia persists in the absence of neurological symptoms typically associated with rapid sodium rise. Of note, raising serum sodium concentrations with conivaptan has not demonstrated symptomatic benefit. Discontinue if hypovolemia or hypotension occurs. Safety and efficacy in heart failure patients have not been established. Use in small numbers of hypervolemic, hyponatremic heart failure patients led to increased adverse events. In other heart failure studies, conivaptan did not show significant improvements in outcomes over placebo. Coadministration with digoxin may increase digoxin concentrations; monitor digoxin concentrations. Use with caution in patients with hepatic and renal impairment; dosage adjustment required. Do not use in patients with severe renal impairment (Cl_{cr} <30 mL/minute). Contraindicated in patients with anuria. May cause injection-site reactions.

Adverse Reactions

>10%:

Cardiovascular: Orthostatic hypotension (6% to 14%)
Central nervous system: Fever (5% to 11%)
Endocrine & metabolic: Hypokalemia (10% to 22%)
Local: Injection site reactions including pain, erythema, phlebitis, swelling (63% to 73%)

1% to 10%:

Cardiovascular: Hypertension (6% to 8%), hypotension (5% to 8%), peripheral edema (3% to 8%), phlebitis (5%), atrial fibrillation (2% to 5%), ECG abnormality (≤5%)
Central nervous system: Headache (8% to 10%), insomnia (4% to 5%), confusion (≤5%), pain (2%)
Dermatologic: Pruritus (1% to 5%), erythema (3%)
Endocrine & metabolic: Hyponatremia (6% to 8%), hypomagnesemia (2% to 5%), hyper-/hypoglycemia (3%)
Gastrointestinal: Constipation (6% to 8%), vomiting (5% to 7%), diarrhea (≤7%), nausea (3% to 5%), dry mouth (4%), dehydration (2%), oral candidiasis (2%)
Genitourinary: Urinary tract infection (4% to 5%)
Hematologic: Anemia (5% to 6%)
Renal: Polyuria (5% to 6%), hematuria (2%)
Respiratory: Pneumonia (2% to 5%), pharyngolaryngeal pain (1% to 5%)
Miscellaneous: Thirst (3% to 6%)

<1%, postmarketing, and/or case reports (limited to important or life-threatening): Atrial arrhythmias, sepsis

Drug Interactions

Metabolism/Transport Effects Substrate of CYP3A4 (major); **Note:** Assignment of Major/Minor substrate status based on clinically relevant drug interaction potential; **Inhibits** CYP3A4 (strong)

Avoid Concomitant Use

Avoid concomitant use of Conivaptan with any of the following: Alfuzosin; Antifungal Agents (Azole Derivatives, Systemic); Crizotinib; CYP3A4 Inhibitors (Strong); CYP3A4 Substrates; Dronedarone; Eplerenone; Everolimus; Fluticasone (Oral Inhalation); Halofantrine; Lapatinib; Lovastatin; Lurasidone; Nilotinib; Nisoldipine; Pimozide; Ranolazine; Rivaroxaban; RomiDEPsin; Salmeterol; Silodosin; Simvastatin; Tamsulosin; Ticagrelor; Tolvaptan; Toremifene

Increased Effect/Toxicity

Conivaptan may increase the levels/effects of: Alfuzosin; Almotriptan; Alosetron; ARIPiprazole; Bortezomib; Brentuximab Vedotin; Brinzolamide; Budesonide (Nasal); Budesonide (Systemic, Oral Inhalation); Ciclesonide; Colchicine; Corticosteroids (Orally Inhaled); Crizotinib; CYP3A4 Substrates; CYP3A4 Substrates (Low risk); Dienogest; Digoxin; Dronedarone; Dutasteride; Eplerenone; Everolimus; FentaNYL; Fesoterodine; Fluticasone (Nasal); Fluticasone (Oral Inhalation); GuanFACINE; Halofantrine; Iloperidone; Ixabepilone; Lapatinib; Lovastatin; Lumefantrine; Lurasidone; Maraviroc; MethylPREDNISolone; Nilotinib; Nisoldipine; Paricalcitol; Pazopanib; Pimecrolimus; Pimozide; Propafenone; Ranolazine; Rivaroxaban; RomiDEPsin; Ruxolitinib; Salmeterol; Saxagliptin; Sildenafil; Silodosin; Simvastatin; SORAfenib; Tadalafil; Tamsulosin; Ticagrelor; Tolterodine; Tolvaptan; Toremifene; Vardenafil; Vemurafenib; Vilazodone; Zuclopenthixol

The levels/effects of Conivaptan may be increased by: Antifungal Agents (Azole Derivatives, Systemic); CYP3A4 Inhibitors (Moderate); CYP3A4 Inhibitors (Strong); Dasatinib

Decreased Effect

Conivaptan may decrease the levels/effects of: Prasugrel; Ticagrelor

The levels/effects of Conivaptan may be decreased by: CYP3A4 Inducers (Strong); Deferasirox; Herbs (CYP3A4 Inducers); Tocilizumab

Ethanol/Nutrition/Herb Interactions Herb/Nutraceutical: St John's wort may decrease the levels/effects of conivaptan.

Stability Store at 25°C (77°F); brief excursions permitted up to 40°C (104°F). Protect from light and freezing. Do not remove protective overwrap until ready for use.

Mechanism of Action Conivaptan is an arginine vasopressin (AVP) receptor antagonist with affinity for AVP receptor subtypes V_{1A} and V_2. The antidiuretic action of AVP is mediated through activation of the V_2 receptor, which functions to regulate water and electrolyte balance at the level of the collecting ducts in the kidney. Serum levels of AVP are commonly elevated in euvolemic or hypervolemic hyponatremia, which results in the dilution of serum sodium and the relative hyponatremic state. Antagonism of the V_2 receptor by conivaptan promotes the excretion of free water (without loss of serum electrolytes) resulting in net fluid loss, increased urine output, decreased urine osmolality, and subsequent restoration of normal serum sodium concentrations.

Pharmacodynamics/Kinetics

Protein binding: 99%

Metabolism: Hepatic via CYP3A4 to four minimally-active metabolites

Half-life elimination: ~5-8 hours

Excretion: Feces (83%); urine (12%, primarily as metabolites)

Dosage I.V.: Adults: 20 mg infused over 30 minutes as a loading dose, followed by a continuous infusion of 20 mg over 24 hours (0.83 mg/hour); may increase to a maximum dose of 40 mg over 24 hours (1.7 mg/hour) if serum sodium not rising sufficiently; total duration of therapy not to exceed 4 days. **Note:** If patient requires 40 mg/24 hours, may administer two consecutive 20 mg/100 mL premixed solutions over 24 hours (ie, 20 mg over 12 hours followed by 20 mg over 12 hours).

Dosing adjustment in renal impairment:

Cl_{cr} >60 mL/minute: Dose adjustment is not necessary.

Moderate renal impairment (Cl_{cr} 30-60 mL/minute): 10 mg infused over 30 minutes as a loading dose, followed by a continuous infusion of 10 mg over 24 hours; may increase to a maximum dose of 20 mg over 24 hours if serum sodium not rising sufficiently; total duration of therapy not to exceed 4 days.

Severe renal impairment (Cl_{cr} <30 mL/minute): Use is not recommended.

Dosing adjustment in hepatic impairment: Child-Pugh classes A-C: 10 mg infused over 30 minutes as a loading dose, followed by a continuous infusion of 10 mg over 24 hours; may increase to a maximum dose of 20 mg over 24 hours if serum sodium not rising sufficiently; total duration of therapy not to exceed 4 days.

Administration For intravenous use only; infuse into large veins and change infusion site every 24 hours to minimize vascular irritation. Do not administer with any other product in the same intravenous line or container.

Monitoring Parameters Rate of serum sodium increase, blood pressure, volume status, urine output

Dosage Forms Excipient information presented when available (limited, particularly for generics); consult specific product labeling.

Infusion, premixed in D_5W, as hydrochloride:

Vaprisol®: 20 mg (100 mL)

- **Conivaptan Hydrochloride** *see* Conivaptan *on page 411*
- **Conjugated Estrogen** *see* Estrogens (Conjugated/ Equine, Systemic) *on page 641*
- **Conjugated Estrogen** *see* Estrogens (Conjugated/ Equine, Topical) *on page 643*
- **CO Norfloxacin (Can)** *see* Norfloxacin *on page 1219*
- **Constulose** *see* Lactulose *on page 964*
- **Contac® Cold 12 Hour Relief Non Drowsy (Can)** *see* Pseudoephedrine *on page 1430*
- **Contac® Cold and Sore Throat, Non Drowsy, Extra Strength (Can)** *see* Acetaminophen and Pseudoephedrine *on page 31*
- **Contac® Cold-Chest Congestion, Non Drowsy, Regular Strength (Can)** *see* Guaifenesin and Pseudoephedrine *on page 813*
- **Contac® Cold + Flu Maximum Strength Non-Drowsy [OTC]** *see* Pseudoephedrine *on page 1430*
- **Continuous Renal Replacement Therapy** *see* Electrolyte Solution, Renal Replacement *on page 578*
- **ControlRx™** *see* Fluoride *on page 728*
- **ControlRx™ Multi** *see* Fluoride *on page 728*
- **Conventional Amphotericin B** *see* Amphotericin B (Conventional) *on page 109*
- **Conventional Cytarabine** *see* Cytarabine (Conventional) *on page 428*
- **Conventional Daunomycin** *see* DAUNOrubicin (Conventional) *on page 457*
- **Conventional Doxorubicin** *see* DOXOrubicin *on page 552*
- **Conventional Paclitaxel** *see* PACLitaxel *on page 1273*
- **ConZip™** *see* TraMADol *on page 1715*
- **CO Olanzapine (Can)** *see* OLANZapine *on page 1233*
- **CO Olanzapine ODT (Can)** *see* OLANZapine *on page 1233*
- **CO Ondansetron (Can)** *see* Ondansetron *on page 1246*
- **CO Pantoprazole (Can)** *see* Pantoprazole *on page 1289*
- **CO Paroxetine (Can)** *see* PARoxetine *on page 1299*
- **Copaxone®** *see* Glatiramer Acetate *on page 792*
- **COPD [DSC]** *see* Dyphylline and Guaifenesin *on page 568*
- **Copegus®** *see* Ribavirin *on page 1479*
- **CO Pioglitazone (Can)** *see* Pioglitazone *on page 1355*
- **Copolymer-1** *see* Glatiramer Acetate *on page 792*

Copper (KOP er)

Index Terms Cupric Chloride; Cupric Chloride Dihydrate

Pharmacologic Category Trace Element, Parenteral

Use Supplement to intravenous solutions given for total parenteral nutrition (TPN) to maintain copper serum levels and to prevent depletion of endogenous stores and subsequent deficiency symptoms

Pregnancy Risk Factor C

Dosage I.V. (incorporated into parenteral nutrition):

Infants and Children: 20 mcg/kg/day

Adults: 0.3-0.5 mg/day (ASPEN, 2002); 0.5-1.5 mg/day (manufacturer's product labeling)

High output intestinal fistula: Some clinicians may use twice the recommended daily allowance (ASPEN, 2002)

Elderly: Use caution. Start at the low end of dosing range.

Dosage adjustment in renal impairment: Use caution; contains aluminum

Dosage adjustment in hepatic impairment: Use caution; dosage reduction may be required

Additional Information Complete prescribing information for this medication should be consulted for additional detail.

Dosage Forms Excipient information presented when available (limited, particularly for generics); consult specific product labeling.

Injection, solution [preservative free]: 0.4 mg/mL (10 mL)

- **CO Pramipexole (Can)** *see* Pramipexole *on page 1389*
- **CO Pravastatin (Can)** *see* Pravastatin *on page 1394*
- **CO Quetiapine (Can)** *see* QUEtiapine *on page 1440*
- **CO Ramipril (Can)** *see* Ramipril *on page 1459*

Corticorelin (kor ti koe REL in)

Brand Names: U.S. Acthrel®

Index Terms Corticorelin Ovine Triflutate; Human Corticotrophin-Releasing Hormone, Analogue; Ovine Corticotrophin-Releasing Hormone

Pharmacologic Category Diagnostic Agent, ACTH-Dependent Hypercortisolism

Use Diagnostic test used in adrenocorticotropic hormone (ACTH)-dependent Cushing's syndrome to differentiate between pituitary and ectopic production of ACTH

Pregnancy Risk Factor C

Dosage I.V.: Adults: Testing pituitary corticotrophin function: 1 mcg/kg; dosages >100 mcg have been associated with an increase in adverse effects

Note: Venous blood samples should be drawn 15 minutes before and immediately prior to corticorelin administration to determine baseline ACTH and cortisol. At 15-, 30-, and 60 minutes after administration, venous blood samples should be drawn again to determine response. **Basal and peak responses differ depending on AM or PM administration; therefore, any repeat evaluations are recommended to be done at the same time of day as initial testing.**

Additional Information Complete prescribing information for this medication should be consulted for additional detail.

Dosage Forms Excipient information presented when available (limited, particularly for generics); consult specific product labeling.

Injection, powder for reconstitution, as trifluoroacetate [ovine derived]:

Acthrel®: 100 mcg [contains lactose 10 mg]

Cortisone (KOR ti sone)

Index Terms Compound E; Cortisone Acetate

Pharmacologic Category Corticosteroid, Systemic

Additional Appendix Information

Corticosteroids *on page 1888*

Use Management of adrenocortical insufficiency

Pregnancy Considerations Adverse events have been observed with corticosteroids in animal reproduction studies. Cortisone is found in cord blood; endogenous maternal cortisol (active) is metabolized by placental enzymes to cortisone (inactive), regulating the amount of maternal glucocorticoids reaching the fetus. Some studies have shown an association between first trimester systemic corticosteroid use and oral clefts; adverse events in the fetus/neonate have been noted in case reports following large doses of systemic corticosteroids during pregnancy. Women exposed to cortisone during pregnancy for the treatment of an autoimmune disease may contact the OTIS Autoimmune Diseases Study at 877-311-8972.

Lactation Excretion in breast milk unknown/use caution

Contraindications Hypersensitivity to cortisone acetate or any component of the formulation; serious infections, except septic shock or tuberculous meningitis; administration of live virus vaccines

Warnings/Precautions Use with caution in patients with thyroid disease, hepatic impairment, renal impairment, cardiovascular disease, diabetes, glaucoma, cataracts, myasthenia gravis, patients at risk for osteoporosis, patients at risk for seizures, or GI diseases (diverticulitis, peptic ulcer, ulcerative colitis) due to perforation risk. Use caution following acute MI (corticosteroids have been associated with myocardial rupture). Because of the risk of adverse effects, systemic corticosteroids should be used cautiously in the elderly in the smallest possible effective dose for the shortest duration. May affect growth velocity; growth should be routinely monitored in pediatric patients. Withdraw therapy with gradual tapering of dose.

May cause hypercorticism or suppression of hypothalamic-pituitary-adrenal (HPA) axis, particularly in younger children or in patients receiving high doses for prolonged periods. HPA axis suppression may lead to adrenal crisis. Withdrawal and discontinuation of a corticosteroid should be done slowly and carefully. Particular care is required when patients are transferred from systemic corticosteroids to inhaled products due to possible adrenal insufficiency or withdrawal from steroids, including an increase in allergic symptoms. Patients receiving >20 mg per day of prednisone (or equivalent) may be most susceptible. Fatalities have occurred due to adrenal insufficiency in asthmatic patients during and after transfer from systemic corticosteroids to aerosol steroids; aerosol steroids do not provide the systemic steroid needed to treat patients having trauma, surgery, or infections.

Acute myopathy has been reported with high dose corticosteroids, usually in patients with neuromuscular transmission disorders; may involve ocular and/or respiratory muscles; monitor creatine kinase; recovery may be delayed. Corticosteroid use may cause psychiatric disturbances, including depression, euphoria, insomnia, mood swings, and personality changes. Pre-existing psychiatric conditions may be exacerbated by corticosteroid use. Prolonged use of corticosteroids may also increase the incidence of secondary infection, mask acute infection (including fungal infections), prolong or exacerbate viral infections, or limit response to vaccines. Exposure to chickenpox should be avoided; corticosteroids should not be used to treat ocular herpes simplex. Corticosteroids should not be used for cerebral malaria or viral hepatitis. Close observation is required in patients with latent tuberculosis and/or TB reactivity; restrict use in active TB (only in conjunction with antituberculosis treatment). Prolonged treatment with corticosteroids has been associated with the development of Kaposi's sarcoma (case reports); if noted, discontinuation of therapy should be considered.

Adverse Reactions

>10%:

Central nervous system: Insomnia, nervousness

Gastrointestinal: Increased appetite, indigestion

1% to 10%:

Dermatologic: Hirsutism

Endocrine & metabolic: Diabetes mellitus

Neuromuscular & skeletal: Arthralgia

Ocular: Cataracts, glaucoma

Respiratory: Epistaxis

<1% (Limited to important or life-threatening): Alkalosis, Cushing's syndrome, delirium, edema, euphoria, fractures, hallucinations, hypersensitivity reactions, hypertension, hypokalemia, muscle wasting, myalgia, osteoporosis, pancreatitis, peptic ulcer, pituitary-adrenal axis suppression, pseudotumor cerebri, psychoses, seizure, skin atrophy, ulcerative esophagitis

Drug Interactions

Metabolism/Transport Effects None known.

Avoid Concomitant Use

Avoid concomitant use of Cortisone with any of the following: Aldesleukin; BCG; Natalizumab; Pimecrolimus; Tacrolimus (Topical)

Increased Effect/Toxicity

Cortisone may increase the levels/effects of: Acetylcholinesterase Inhibitors; Amphotericin B; Deferasirox; Leflunomide; Loop Diuretics; Natalizumab; NSAID (COX-2 Inhibitor); NSAID (Nonselective); Thiazide Diuretics; Vaccines (Live); Warfarin

The levels/effects of Cortisone may be increased by: Antifungal Agents (Azole Derivatives, Systemic); Aprepitant; Calcium Channel Blockers (Nondihydropyridine); Denosumab; Estrogen Derivatives; Fluconazole; Fosaprepitant; Indacaterol; Macrolide Antibiotics; Neuromuscular-Blocking Agents (Nondepolarizing); Pimecrolimus; Quinolone Antibiotics; Roflumilast; Salicylates; Tacrolimus (Topical); Telaprevir; Trastuzumab

Decreased Effect

Cortisone may decrease the levels/effects of: Aldesleukin; Antidiabetic Agents; BCG; Calcitriol; Coccidioidin Skin Test; Corticorelin; Isoniazid; Salicylates; Sipuleucel-T; Telaprevir; Vaccines (Inactivated)

The levels/effects of Cortisone may be decreased by: Aminoglutethimide; Antacids; Barbiturates; Bile Acid Sequestrants; Echinacea; Mitotane; Primidone; Rifamycin Derivatives; Somatropin; Tesamorelin

Ethanol/Nutrition/Herb Interactions Food: Limit caffeine intake.

Mechanism of Action Decreases inflammation by suppression of migration of polymorphonuclear leukocytes and reversal of increased capillary permeability

Pharmacodynamics/Kinetics

Onset of action: Peak effect: Oral: ~2 hours; I.M.: 20-48 hours

Duration: 30-36 hours

Absorption: Slow

Distribution: Muscles, liver, skin, intestines, and kidneys; crosses placenta; enters breast milk

Metabolism: Hepatic to inactive metabolites

Half-life elimination: 0.5-2 hours; End-stage renal disease: 3.5 hours

Excretion: Urine and feces

Dosage If possible, administer glucocorticoids before 9 AM to minimize adrenocortical suppression; dosing depends upon the condition being treated and the response of the patient. **Note:** Supplemental doses may be warranted during times of stress in the course of withdrawing therapy.

Children:

Anti-inflammatory or immunosuppressive: Oral: 2.5-10 mg/kg/day **or** 20-300 mg/m^2/day in divided doses every 6-8 hours

Physiologic replacement: Oral: 0.5-0.75 mg/kg/day **or** 20-25 mg/m^2/day in divided doses every 8 hours

Adults:

Anti-inflammatory or immunosuppressive: Oral: 25-300 mg/day in divided doses every 12-24 hours

Physiologic replacement: Oral: 25-35 mg/day

Hemodialysis: Supplemental dose is not necessary

Peritoneal dialysis: Supplemental dose is not necessary

Dietary Considerations May need diet with increased potassium, pyridoxine, vitamin C, vitamin D, folate, calcium, and phosphorus and decreased sodium; may be taken with food to decrease GI distress.

Administration Insoluble in water.

Test Interactions May suppress the wheal and flare reactions to skin test antigens

Dosage Forms Excipient information presented when available (limited, particularly for generics); consult specific product labeling.

Tablet, oral, as acetate: 25 mg

◆ **Cortisone Acetate** *see* Cortisone *on page 413*

◆ **Cortisporin®** *see* Neomycin, Polymyxin B, and Hydrocortisone *on page 1190*

◆ **Cortisporin® Ointment** *see* Bacitracin, Neomycin, Polymyxin B, and Hydrocortisone *on page 187*

◆ **Cortisporin® Otic (Can)** *see* Neomycin, Polymyxin B, and Hydrocortisone *on page 1190*

◆ **Cortisporin®-TC** *see* Neomycin, Colistin, Hydrocortisone, and Thonzonium *on page 1189*

◆ **Cortisporin® Topical Ointment (Can)** *see* Bacitracin, Neomycin, Polymyxin B, and Hydrocortisone *on page 187*

◆ **Cortizone-10® Hydratensive Healing [OTC]** *see* Hydrocortisone (Topical) *on page 841*

◆ **Cortizone-10® Hydratensive Soothing [OTC]** *see* Hydrocortisone (Topical) *on page 841*

◆ **Cortizone-10® Intensive Healing Eczema [OTC]** *see* Hydrocortisone (Topical) *on page 841*

◆ **Cortizone-10® Maximum Strength [OTC]** *see* Hydrocortisone (Topical) *on page 841*

◆ **Cortizone-10® Maximum Strength Cooling Relief [OTC]** *see* Hydrocortisone (Topical) *on page 841*

◆ **Cortizone-10® Maximum Strength Easy Relief [OTC]** *see* Hydrocortisone (Topical) *on page 841*

◆ **Cortizone-10® Maximum Strength Intensive Healing Formula [OTC]** *see* Hydrocortisone (Topical) *on page 841*

◆ **Cortizone-10® Plus Maximum Strength [OTC]** *see* Hydrocortisone (Topical) *on page 841*

Cosyntropin (koe sin TROE pin)

Brand Names: U.S. Cortrosyn®
Brand Names: Canada Cortrosyn®
Index Terms Synacthen; Tetracosactide
Pharmacologic Category Diagnostic Agent
Use Diagnostic test to differentiate primary adrenal from secondary (pituitary) adrenocortical insufficiency
Pregnancy Risk Factor C
Pregnancy Considerations Animal reproduction studies have not been conducted.
Lactation Excretion in breast milk unknown/use caution
Contraindications Hypersensitivity to cosyntropin or any component of the formulation
Warnings/Precautions Use with caution in patients with pre-existing allergic disease or a history of allergic reactions to corticotropin.
Adverse Reactions Frequency not defined.
Cardiovascular: Bradycardia, hypertension, peripheral edema, tachycardia
Dermatologic: Rash
Local: Whealing with redness at the injection site
Miscellaneous: Anaphylaxis, hypersensitivity reaction
Drug Interactions
Metabolism/Transport Effects None known.
Avoid Concomitant Use There are no known interactions where it is recommended to avoid concomitant use.
Increased Effect/Toxicity There are no known significant interactions involving an increase in effect.
Decreased Effect There are no known significant interactions involving a decrease in effect.
Stability
Powder for injection: Store at controlled room temperature of 15°C to 30°C (59°F to 86°F).
Solution for injection: Store refrigerated between 2°C to 8°C (36°F to 46°F). Protect from light and freezing.
I.M.: Reconstitute cosyntropin 0.25 mg with NS 1 mL.
I.V. push: Reconstitute cosyntropin 0.25 mg with NS 2-5 mL.
I.V. infusion: Mix in NS or D_5W. Stable for 12 hours at room temperature; stable for 21 days under refrigeration.
Mechanism of Action Stimulates the adrenal cortex to secrete adrenal steroids (including hydrocortisone, cortisone), androgenic substances, and a small amount of aldosterone
Pharmacodynamics/Kinetics Time to peak, serum: I.M., IVP: ~1 hour; plasma cortisol levels rise in healthy individuals within 5 minutes
Dosage Diagnosis of adrenocortical insufficiency: I.M., I.V.:
Note: Cosyntropin injection **solution** is not recommended for I.M. administration (manufacturer recommendation).
Children ≤2 years: 0.125 mg
Children >2 years and Adults:
Conventional dose: 0.25 mg
Note: Doses in the range of 0.25-0.75 mg have been used in clinical studies; however, maximal response is seen with 0.25 mg dose. When greater cortisol stimulation is needed, an I.V. infusion may be used: 0.25 mg administered at 0.04 mg/hour over 6 hours
Low–dose protocol (unlabeled dose): 1 mcg (Abdu, 1999)
Note: The use of the low-dose protocol has been advocated by some clinicians, particularly in mild or secondary adrenal insufficiency. The low-dose protocol is not recommended in critically-ill patients (Marik, 2008).
Administration
I.V.: May administer by I.V. injection over 2 minutes or as an I.V. infusion over 4-8 hours.
I.M.: May administer I.M. (reconstituted powder for injection only); cosyntropin injection **solution** is not recommended for I.M. administration (manufacturer recommendation).
Reference Range Normal baseline cortisol >5 mcg/dL; normal response 30 minutes after cosyntropin injection: increase in serum cortisol concentration of >7 mcg/dL or peak response >18 mcg/dL; plasma cortisol concentrations should be measured immediately before and exactly 30 minutes after a dose. If increase in plasma cortisol levels at 30 minutes is equivocal, consider repeat cortisol sampling at 60 and/or 90 minutes.
Test Interactions Concurrent or recent use of spironolactone, hydrocortisone, cortisone, etomidate, estrogens
Additional Information Each 0.25 mg of cosyntropin is equivalent to 25 units of corticotropin.

Patient should not receive corticosteroids or spironolactone the day of the test.
Dosage Forms Excipient information presented when available (limited, particularly for generics); consult specific product labeling.
Injection, powder for reconstitution: 0.25 mg
Cortrosyn®: 0.25 mg
Injection, solution [preservative free]: 0.25 mg/mL (1 mL)

◆ **Crestor®** *see* Rosuvastatin *on page 1524*

◆ **Crinone®** *see* Progesterone *on page 1414*

◆ **Critic-Aid® Clear AF [OTC]** *see* Miconazole (Topical) *on page 1126*

◆ **Critic-Aid Skin Care® [OTC]** *see* Zinc Oxide *on page 1817*

◆ **Crixivan®** *see* Indinavir *on page 888*

Crizotinib (kriz OH ti nib)

Brand Names: U.S. Xalkori®

Index Terms C-Met/Hepatocyte Growth Factor Receptor Tyrosine Kinase Inhibitor PF-02341066; C-Met/HGFR Tyrosine Kinase Inhibitor PF-02341066; MET Tyrosine Kinase Inhibitor PF-02341066; PF-02341066

Pharmacologic Category Antineoplastic Agent, Anaplastic Lymphoma Kinase Inhibitor; Antineoplastic Agent, Tyrosine Kinase Inhibitor

Use Treatment of locally advanced or metastatic nonsmall cell lung cancer (NSCLC) that is anaplastic lymphoma kinase positive (as detected by an FDA-approved test)

Pregnancy Risk Factor D

Pregnancy Considerations Embryotoxicity and fetal toxicity were observed in animal studies. There are no adequate and well-controlled studies in pregnant women. Based on the mechanism of action, crizotinib may cause fetal harm if administered during pregnancy. Women of childbearing potential and men of reproductive potential should use adequate contraception methods during and for at least 90 days after treatment.

Lactation Excretion in breast milk unknown/not recommended

Prescribing and Access Restrictions Available through specialty pharmacies. Further information may be obtained from the manufacturer, Pfizer, at 1-877-744-5675, or at http://www.pfizerpro.com/resources/minisites/xalkori_home/aval/docs/pharmacy_financial_info.pdf

Contraindications There are no contraindications listed within the manufacturer's labeling.

Warnings/Precautions Approved for use only in patients with locally advanced or metastatic nonsmall cell lung cancer (NSCLC) who test positive for the abnormal anaplastic lymphoma kinase (ALK) gene. The Vysis ALK break-apart FISH probe kit is approved to test for the gene abnormality.

Grade 3 or 4 ALT increases (usually asymptomatic and reversible) have been observed in clinical trials. May require dosage interruption and/or reduction; permanent discontinuation was necessary in some cases; concurrent ALT elevations >3 x ULN and total bilirubin elevations >2 x ULN (without alkaline phosphatase elevations) were observed rarely. Monitor liver function tests, including ALT and total bilirubin. Use with caution in patients with hepatic impairment (has not been studied); crizotinib is extensively metabolized in the liver and liver impairment is likely to increase crizotinib levels.

Severe, life-threatening, and potentially fatal pneumonitis has been associated with crizotinib. Onset was generally within 2 months of treatment initiation. Monitor for pulmonary symptoms which may indicate pneumonitis; exclude other potential causes (eg, disease progression, infection, other pulmonary disease, or radiation therapy). Permanently discontinue if treatment-related pneumonitis is confirmed.

QT_c prolongation has been observed; consider periodic monitoring of ECG and electrolytes in patients with heart failure, bradyarrhythmias, electrolyte abnormalities, or who are taking medications known to prolong the QT interval. May require treatment interruption, dosage reduction, or discontinuation. Avoid use in patients with congenital long QT syndrome.

Ocular toxicities (eg, blurred vision, diplopia, photophobia, photopsia, visual acuity decreased, visual brightness, visual field defect, visual impairment, and/or vitreous floaters) commonly occur. Onset is generally within 2 weeks of treatment initiation; consider ophthalmology exam, especially if photopsia or vitreous floaters occur. Severe or worsening vitreous floaters or photopsia could be a sign of retinal hole or impending detachment. Use with caution in patients with severe renal impairment; only one patient with severe renal impairment was studied in clinical trials and end stage renal disease was not studied. CYP3A4 inhibitors may increase crizotinib levels; avoid concomitant use with strong CYP3A4 inhibitors and use moderate CYP3A4 inhibitors with caution. CYP3A4 inducers may decrease crizotinib levels; avoid concomitant use with strong CYP3A4 inducers. Avoid concomitant use with CYP3A4 substrates.

Adverse Reactions

>10%:

Cardiovascular: Edema (28%)

Central nervous system: Fatigue (20%), dizziness (16%)

Gastrointestinal: Nausea (53%), diarrhea (43%), vomiting (40%), constipation (27%), appetite decreased (19%), taste alteration (12%), esophageal disorder (11%; includes dyspepsia, dysphagia, epigastric burning/discomfort/pain, esophageal obstruction/pain/spasm/ulcer, esophagitis, gastroesophageal reflux, odynophagia, reflux esophagitis)

Hematologic: Lymphopenia (grades 3/4: 11%)

Hepatic: ALT increased (13%; grades 3/4: 5%)

Neuromuscular & skeletal: Neuropathy (13%; grades 3/4: <1%)

Ocular: Vision disorder (62%; onset: <2 weeks; includes blurred vision, diplopia, photophobia, photopsia, visual acuity decreased, visual brightness, visual field defect, visual impairment, vitreous floaters)

1% to 10%:

Cardiovascular: Bradycardia (5%), chest pain (1%)

Central nervous system: Headache (4%), insomnia (3%)

Dermatologic: Rash (10%)

Gastrointestinal: Abdominal pain (8%), stomatitis (6%)

Hematologic: Neutropenia (grades 3/4: 5%)

Hepatic: AST increased (9%; grades 3/4: 2%)

Neuromuscular & skeletal: Arthralgia (2%)

Renal: Renal cysts (1%)

Respiratory: Cough (4%), dyspnea (2%), pneumonitis (2%), upper respiratory infection (2%)

<1% (Limited to important or life-threatening): Back pain, fever, QT_c prolongation, thrombocytopenia

Drug Interactions

Metabolism/Transport Effects Substrate of CYP3A4 (major), P-glycoprotein; **Note:** Assignment of Major/Minor substrate status based on clinically relevant drug interaction potential; **Inhibits** CYP3A4 (moderate), P-glycoprotein

Avoid Concomitant Use

Avoid concomitant use of Crizotinib with any of the following: Alfentanil; Artemether; CycloSPORINE; CycloSPORINE (Systemic); CYP3A4 Inducers (Strong); CYP3A4 Inhibitors (Strong); Dihydroergotamine; Dronedarone; Ergotamine; FentaNYL; Grapefruit Juice; Lumefantrine; Nilotinib; Pimozide; QUEtiapine; QuiNIDine; QuiNINE; Silodosin; Sirolimus; St Johns Wort; Tacrolimus; Tacrolimus (Systemic); Tetrabenazine; Thioridazine; Topotecan; Toremifene; Vandetanib; Vemurafenib; Ziprasidone

Increased Effect/Toxicity

Crizotinib may increase the levels/effects of: Alfentanil; ARIPiprazole; Budesonide (Systemic, Oral Inhalation);

Colchicine; CycloSPORINE; CycloSPORINE (Systemic); CYP3A4 Substrates; Dabigatran Etexilate; Dihydroergotamine; Dronedarone; Eplerenone; Ergotamine; Everolimus; FentaNYL; Lurasidone; P-glycoprotein/ABCB1 Substrates; Pimecrolimus; Pimozide; QTc-Prolonging Agents; QuiNIDine; QuiNINE; Rivaroxaban; Salmeterol; Silodosin; Sirolimus; Tacrolimus; Tacrolimus (Systemic); Tetrabenazine; Thioridazine; Topotecan; Toremifene; Vandetanib; Vemurafenib; Vilazodone; Vitamin K Antagonists; Ziprasidone

The levels/effects of Crizotinib may be increased by: Alfuzosin; Artemether; Chloroquine; Ciprofloxacin; Ciprofloxacin (Systemic); CYP3A4 Inhibitors (Moderate); CYP3A4 Inhibitors (Strong); Gadobutrol; Grapefruit Juice; Indacaterol; Lumefantrine; Nilotinib; P-glycoprotein/ABCB1 Inhibitors; QUEtiapine; QuiNINE

Decreased Effect

Crizotinib may decrease the levels/effects of: Cardiac Glycosides; Vitamin K Antagonists

The levels/effects of Crizotinib may be decreased by: CYP3A4 Inducers (Strong); Deferasirox; P-glycoprotein/ABCB1 Inducers; St Johns Wort; Tocilizumab

Ethanol/Nutrition/Herb Interactions Food: Avoid grapefruit and grapefruit juice (may increase crizotinib levels). Although may be administered with or without food, bioavailability is reduced 14% with a high-fat meal.

Stability Store at room temperature of 20°C to 25°C (68°F to 77°F); excursions permitted to 15°C and 30°C (59°F and 86°F).

Mechanism of Action Tyrosine kinase receptor inhibitor, which inhibits anaplastic lymphoma kinase (ALK), Hepatocyte Growth Factor Receptor (HGFR, c-MET), and Recepteur d'Origine Nantais (RON). ALK gene abnormalities due to mutations or translocations may result in expression of oncogenic fusion proteins (eg, ALK fusion protein) which alter signaling and expression and result in increased cellular proliferation and survival in tumors which express these fusion proteins. Approximately 2% to 7% of patients with NSCLC have the abnormal echinoderm microtubule-associated protein-like 4, or EML4-ALK gene (which has a higher prevalence in never smokers or light smokers and in patients with adenocarcinoma). Crizotinib selectively inhibits ALK tyrosine kinase, which reduces proliferation of cells expressing the genetic alteration.

Pharmacodynamics/Kinetics

Distribution: V_{ss}: 1772 L

Protein binding: 91%

Metabolism: Hepatic, via CYP3A4/5

Bioavailability: 43% (range: 32% to 66%); bioavailability is reduced 14% with a high-fat meal

Half-life elimination: Terminal: 42 hours

Time to peak: 4-6 hours

Excretion: Feces (63%; 53% as unchanged drug); urine (22%; 2% as unchanged drug)

Dosage Oral: Adults: Nonsmall cell lung cancer, locally advanced or metastatic (ALK-positive): 250 mg twice a day, continue treatment as long as clinically benefiting

Dosage adjustment for toxicity: Note: If dose reduction is necessary, reduce dose to 200 mg orally twice a day, if necessary, further reduce to 250 mg once daily.

Hematologic toxicity (except lymphopenia, unless lymphopenia is associated with clinical events such as opportunistic infection):

Grade 3 toxicity (WBC 1000-2000/mm^3, ANC 500-1000/mm^3, platelets 25,000-50,000/mm^3, hemoglobin 6.5-8 g/dL): Withhold treatment until recovers to ≤grade 2, then resume at the same dose and schedule

Grade 4 toxicity (WBC <1000/mm^3, ANC <500/mm^3, platelets <25,000/mm^3, hemoglobin <6.5 g/dL): Withhold treatment until recovers to ≤grade 2, then resume at 200 mg twice a day

Recurrent grade 4 toxicity on 200 mg twice a day: Withhold treatment until recovers to ≤grade 2, then resume at 250 mg once daily

Recurrent grade 4 toxicity on 250 mg once daily: Permanently discontinue

Nonhematologic toxicities:

Grade 3 or 4 ALT or AST elevation (ALT or AST >5 x ULN) with ≤grade 1 total bilirubin elevation (total bilirubin ≤1.5 x ULN): Withhold treatment until recovers to ≤grade 1 (<2.5 X ULN) or baseline, then resume at 200 mg twice a day

Recurrent grade 3 or 4 ALT or AST elevation with ≤grade 1 total bilirubin elevation: Withhold treatment until recovers to ≤grade 1, then resume at 250 mg once daily

Recurrent grade 3 or 4 ALT or AST elevation on 250 mg once daily: Permanently discontinue

Grade 2, 3, or 4 ALT or AST elevation (ALT or AST >2.5 x ULN) with concurrent grade 2, 3, or 4 total bilirubin elevation (>1.5 x ULN) in the absence of cholestasis or hemolysis: Permanently discontinue

Pneumonitis (any grade; not attributable to disease progression, infection, other pulmonary disease or radiation therapy): Permanently discontinue

Grade 3 QT_c prolongation (QT_c >500 msec without life-threatening signs or symptoms): Withhold treatment until recovers to ≤grade 1 (QT_c ≤470 msec), then resume at 200 mg twice daily

Recurrent grade 3 QT_c prolongation at 200 mg twice a day: Withhold treatment until recovers to ≤grade 1, then resume at 250 mg once daily

Recurrent grade 3 QT_c prolongation at 250 mg once daily: Permanently discontinue

Grade 4 QT_c prolongation (QT_c >500 msec with life-threatening signs or symptoms or torsade de pointes): Permanently discontinue.

Dosage adjustment in renal impairment:

Mild (Cl_{cr} 30-60 mL/minute) to moderate impairment (Cl_{cr} 60-90 mL/minute): No adjustment required

Severe impairment (Cl_{cr} <30 mL/minute): Data are insufficient to determine if dosage adjustment necessary; use with caution

End-stage renal disease (ESRD): Was not studied in patients with ESRD; use with caution

Dosage adjustment in hepatic impairment: Data are insufficient to determine if dosage adjustment necessary; use with caution

Dietary Considerations May be taken with or without food. Avoid grapefruit and grapefruit juice.

Administration Swallow capsules whole (do not crush, dissolve, or open capsules). May be administered with or without food. If a dose is missed, take as soon as remembered unless it is <6 hours prior to the next scheduled dose (skip the dose if <6 hours before the next dose); do not take 2 doses at the same time to make up for a missed dose.

Monitoring Parameters CBC with differential monthly and as clinically appropriate (monitor more frequently if grades 3 or 4 abnormalities observed or with fever or infection), liver function tests monthly and as clinically appropriate (monitor more frequently if grades 2, 3 or 4 abnormalities observed). Consider monitoring ECG and electrolytes in patients with heart failure, bradyarrhythmias, electrolyte abnormalities, or who are taking medications known to prolong the QT interval. Consider ophthalmic evaluation, especially if photopsia or vitreous floaters occur.

Dosage Forms Excipient information presented when available (limited, particularly for generics); consult specific product labeling.

Capsule, oral:

Xalkori®: 200 mg, 250 mg

◆ **Cromoglycic Acid** *see* Cromolyn (Nasal) *on page 418*

◆ **Cromoglycic Acid** *see* Cromolyn (Ophthalmic) *on page 418*

Cromolyn (Nasal) (KROE moe lin)

Brand Names: U.S. NasalCrom® [OTC]

Brand Names: Canada Rhinaris-CS Anti-Allergic Nasal Mist

Index Terms Cromoglycic Acid; Cromolyn Sodium; Disodium Cromoglycate; DSCG

Pharmacologic Category Mast Cell Stabilizer

Use Prevention and treatment of seasonal and perennial allergic rhinitis

Dosage Intranasal: Allergic rhinitis (treatment and prophylaxis): Children ≥2 years and Adults: 1 spray into each nostril 3-4 times/day; may be increased to 6 times/day (symptomatic relief may require 2-4 weeks)

Additional Information Complete prescribing information for this medication should be consulted for additional detail.

Dosage Forms Excipient information presented when available (limited, particularly for generics); consult specific product labeling.

Solution, intranasal, as sodium [spray]: 40 mg/mL (26 mL)
NasalCrom®: 40 mg/mL (13 mL) [contains benzalkonium chloride; 5.2 mg/inhalation]

Cromolyn (Ophthalmic) (KROE moe lin)

Brand Names: Canada Opticrom®

Index Terms Cromoglycic Acid; Cromolyn Sodium; Disodium Cromoglycate; DSCG

Pharmacologic Category Mast Cell Stabilizer

Use Treatment of vernal keratoconjunctivitis, vernal conjunctivitis, and vernal keratitis

Pregnancy Risk Factor B

Dosage Ophthalmic: Children >4 years and Adults: 1-2 drops in each eye 4-6 times/day

Additional Information Complete prescribing information for this medication should be consulted for additional detail.

Dosage Forms Excipient information presented when available (limited, particularly for generics); consult specific product labeling.

Solution, ophthalmic, as sodium [drops]: 4% (10 mL)

◆ **Cromolyn Sodium** *see* Cromolyn (Nasal) *on page 418*

◆ **Cromolyn Sodium** *see* Cromolyn (Ophthalmic) *on page 418*

Crotamiton (kroe TAM i tonn)

Brand Names: U.S. Eurax®

Pharmacologic Category Scabicidal Agent

Use Treatment of scabies (*Sarcoptes scabiei*) and symptomatic treatment of pruritus

Pregnancy Risk Factor C

Dosage Topical:

Scabicide: Children and Adults: Wash thoroughly and scrub away loose scales, then towel dry; apply a thin layer and massage drug onto skin of the entire body from the neck to the toes (with special attention to skin folds, creases, and interdigital spaces). Repeat application in 24 hours. Take a cleansing bath 48 hours after the final application. Treatment may be repeated after 7-10 days if live mites are still present.

Pruritus: Massage into affected areas until medication is completely absorbed; repeat as necessary

Additional Information Complete prescribing information for this medication should be consulted for additional detail.

Dosage Forms Excipient information presented when available (limited, particularly for generics); consult specific product labeling.

Cream, topical:
Eurax®: 10% (60 g)

Lotion, topical:
Eurax®: 10% (60 mL, 480 mL)

◆ **CRRT** *see* Electrolyte Solution, Renal Replacement *on page 578*

◆ **Cruex® [OTC]** *see* Clotrimazole (Topical) *on page 399*

◆ **Cryselle® 28** *see* Ethinyl Estradiol and Norgestrel *on page 664*

◆ **Crystalline Penicillin** *see* Penicillin G (Parenteral/Aqueous) *on page 1323*

◆ **Crystal Violet** *see* Gentian Violet *on page 792*

◆ **Crystapen® (Can)** *see* Penicillin G (Parenteral/Aqueous) *on page 1323*

◆ **CS-747** *see* Prasugrel *on page 1393*

◆ **CsA** *see* CycloSPORINE (Ophthalmic) *on page 427*

◆ **CsA** *see* CycloSPORINE (Systemic) *on page 422*

◆ **C-Time [OTC]** *see* Ascorbic Acid *on page 149*

◆ **CTLA-4Ig** *see* Abatacept *on page 20*

◆ **CTP 30 (Can)** *see* Citalopram *on page 370*

◆ **CTX** *see* Cyclophosphamide *on page 421*

◆ **Cubicin®** *see* DAPTOmycin *on page 446*

◆ **Cupric Chloride** *see* Copper *on page 412*

◆ **Cupric Chloride Dihydrate** *see* Copper *on page 412*

◆ **Cuprimine®** *see* PenicillAMINE *on page 1319*

◆ **Cutivate®** *see* Fluticasone (Topical) *on page 741*

◆ **Cutivate™ (Can)** *see* Fluticasone (Topical) *on page 741*

◆ **Cuvposa™** *see* Glycopyrrolate *on page 802*

◆ **CyA** *see* CycloSPORINE (Ophthalmic) *on page 427*

◆ **CyA** *see* CycloSPORINE (Systemic) *on page 422*

Cyanocobalamin (sye an oh koe BAL a min)

Brand Names: U.S. CaloMist™ [DSC]; Ener-B® [OTC]; Nascobal®; Twelve Resin-K [OTC]

Index Terms Vitamin B_{12}

Pharmacologic Category Vitamin, Water Soluble

Use Treatment of pernicious anemia; vitamin B_{12} deficiency due to dietary deficiencies or malabsorption diseases, inadequate secretion of intrinsic factor, and inadequate utilization of B_{12} (eg, during neoplastic treatment); increased B_{12} requirements due to pregnancy, thyrotoxicosis, hemorrhage, malignancy, liver or kidney disease

CaloMist™: Maintenance of vitamin B_{12} concentrations after initial correction in patients with B_{12} deficiency without CNS involvement

Pregnancy Risk Factor A/C (dose exceeding RDA recommendation); C (intranasal)

Dosage

Adequate intake:

Children:
0-6 months: 0.4 mcg/day
7-12 months: 0.5 mcg/day

Recommended intake:

Children:
1-3 years: 0.9 mcg/day
4-8 years: 1.2 mcg/day
9-13 years: 1.8 mcg/day

Children >14 years and Adults: 2.4 mcg/day
Pregnancy: 2.6 mcg/day
Lactation: 2.8 mcg/day

Vitamin B_{12} deficiency:
I.M., deep SubQ:
Children (dosage not well established): 0.2 mcg/kg for 2 days, followed by 1000 mcg/day for 2-7 days, followed by 100 mcg/week for one month; for malabsorptive causes of B_{12} deficiency, monthly maintenance doses of 100 mcg have been recommended **or** as an alternative 100 mcg/day for 10-15 days, then once or twice weekly for several months
Adults: Initial: 30 mcg/day for 5-10 days; maintenance: 100-200 mcg/month
Intranasal: Adults:
Nascobal®: 500 mcg in one nostril once weekly
CaloMist™: Maintenance therapy (following correction of vitamin B_{12} deficiency): 25 mcg in each nostril daily (50 mcg/day). If inadequate response, 25 mcg in each nostril twice daily (100 mcg/day).
Oral: Adults: 250 mcg/day
Pernicious anemia: I.M., deep SubQ (administer concomitantly with folic acid if needed, 1 mg/day for 1 month):
Children: 30-50 mcg/day for 2 or more weeks (to a total dose of 1000-5000 mcg), then follow with 100 mcg/month as maintenance dosage
Adults: 100 mcg/day for 6-7 days; if improvement, administer same dose on alternate days for 7 doses, then every 3-4 days for 2-3 weeks; once hematologic values have returned to normal, maintenance dosage: 100 mcg/month. **Note:** Alternative dosing of 1000 mcg/day for 5 days (followed by 500-1000 mcg/month) has been used.
Hematologic remission (without evidence of nervous system involvement): Adults:
Intranasal (Nascobal®): 500 mcg in one nostril once weekly
Oral: 1000-2000 mcg/day
I.M., SubQ: 100-1000 mcg/month
Schilling test: Adults: I.M.: 1000 mcg

Additional Information Complete prescribing information for this medication should be consulted for additional detail.

Dosage Forms Excipient information presented when available (limited, particularly for generics); consult specific product labeling. [DSC] = Discontinued product
Injection, solution: 1000 mcg/mL (1 mL, 10 mL, 30 mL)
Lozenge, oral: 50 mcg (100s); 100 mcg (100s); 250 mcg (100s, 250s); 500 mcg (100s, 250s)
Lozenge, sublingual: 500 mcg (100s)
Solution, intranasal [spray]:
CaloMist™: 25 mcg/spray (10.7 mL [DSC]) [contains benzalkonium chloride, benzyl alcohol; 60 metered sprays]
Nascobal®: 500 mcg/spray (2.3 mL) [contains benzalkonium chloride; delivers 8 doses]
Tablet, for buccal application/oral/sublingual:
Twelve Resin-K: 1000 mcg [gluten free]
Tablet, oral: 50 mcg, 100 mcg, 250 mcg, 500 mcg, 1000 mcg
Ener-B®: 100 mcg, 500 mcg, 1000 mcg
Tablet, sublingual: 1000 mcg, 2500 mcg, 5000 mcg
Tablet, timed release, oral: 1000 mcg
Ener-B®: 1500 mcg

◆ **Cyanocobalamin, Folic Acid, and Pyridoxine** *see* Folic Acid, Cyanocobalamin, and Pyridoxine *on page 749*

◆ **Cyanokit®** *see* Hydroxocobalamin *on page 847*

◆ **Cyclafem™ 1/35** *see* Ethinyl Estradiol and Norethindrone *on page 660*

◆ **Cyclafem™ 7/7/7** *see* Ethinyl Estradiol and Norethindrone *on page 660*

◆ **Cyclen® (Can)** *see* Ethinyl Estradiol and Norgestimate *on page 663*

◆ **Cyclessa®** *see* Ethinyl Estradiol and Desogestrel *on page 653*

Cyclobenzaprine (sye kloe BEN za preen)

Brand Names: U.S. Amrix®; Fexmid®; Flexeril®

Brand Names: Canada Apo-Cyclobenzaprine®; Dom-Cyclobenzaprine; Flexeril®; Flexitec; Gen-Cyclobenzaprine; Mylan-Cyclobenzaprine; Novo-Cycloprine; Nu-Cyclobenzaprine; PHL-Cyclobenzaprine; PMS-Cyclobenzaprine; ratio-Cyclobenzaprine; Riva-Cycloprine

Index Terms Cyclobenzaprine Hydrochloride

Pharmacologic Category Skeletal Muscle Relaxant

Additional Appendix Information
Beers Criteria – Potentially Inappropriate Medications for Geriatrics *on page 1973*

Use Treatment of muscle spasm associated with acute, painful musculoskeletal conditions

Unlabeled Use Treatment of muscle spasm associated with acute temporomandibular joint pain (TMJ)

Pregnancy Risk Factor B

Pregnancy Considerations Teratogenic effects were not observed in animal studies. There are no adequate and well-controlled studies in pregnant women. Use during pregnancy only if clearly needed.

Lactation Excretion in breast milk unknown/use caution

Contraindications Hypersensitivity to cyclobenzaprine or any component of the formulation; during or within 14 days of MAO inhibitors; hyperthyroidism; congestive heart failure; arrhythmias; heart block or conduction disturbances; acute recovery phase of MI

Warnings/Precautions May cause CNS depression, which may impair physical or mental abilities; patients must be cautioned about performing tasks which require mental alertness (eg, operating machinery or driving). Cyclobenzaprine shares the toxic potentials of the tricyclic antidepressants (including arrhythmias, tachycardia, and conduction time prolongation) and the usual precautions of tricyclic antidepressant therapy should be observed; use with caution in patients with urinary hesitancy or retention, angle-closure glaucoma or increased intraocular pressure, hepatic impairment, or in the elderly. This class of medication is poorly tolerated by the elderly due to anticholinergic effects, sedation, and weakness; efficacy is questionable at dosages tolerated by elderly patients (Beers Criteria). Extended release capsules not recommended for use in mild-to-severe hepatic impairment or in the elderly. Do not use concomitantly or within 14 days after MAO inhibitors; combination may cause hypertensive crisis, severe convulsions. Effects may be potentiated when used with other CNS depressants or ethanol.

Adverse Reactions
>10%:
Central nervous system: Drowsiness (29% to 39%), dizziness (1% to 11%)
Gastrointestinal: Xerostomia (21% to 32%)
1% to 10%:
Central nervous system: Fatigue (1% to 6%), headache (1% to 5%), confusion (1% to 3%), irritability (1% to 3%), mental acuity decreased (1% to 3%), nervousness (1% to 3%), somnolence (1% to 2%)
Gastrointestinal: Dyspepsia (≤4%), abdominal pain (1% to 3%), constipation (1% to 3%), diarrhea (1% to 3%), gastric regurgitation (1% to 3%), nausea (1% to 3%), unpleasant taste (1% to 3%)
Neuromuscular & skeletal: Weakness (1% to 3%)
Ocular: Blurred vision (1% to 3%)
Respiratory: Pharyngitis (1% to 3%), upper respiratory infection (1% to 3%)

<1% (Limited to important or life-threatening): Anaphylaxis, angioedema, arrhythmia, ataxia, dysarthria, hepatitis (rare), hypertonia, hypotension, paresthesia, psychosis, rash, seizures, syncope, tachycardia, tremor

Drug Interactions

Metabolism/Transport Effects Substrate of CYP1A2 (major), CYP2D6 (minor), CYP3A4 (minor); **Note:** Assignment of Major/Minor substrate status based on clinically relevant drug interaction potential

Avoid Concomitant Use

Avoid concomitant use of Cyclobenzaprine with any of the following: MAO Inhibitors

Increased Effect/Toxicity

Cyclobenzaprine may increase the levels/effects of: Alcohol (Ethyl); Anticholinergics; CNS Depressants; MAO Inhibitors; Metoclopramide; Serotonin Modulators

The levels/effects of Cyclobenzaprine may be increased by: Abiraterone Acetate; Antipsychotics; Conivaptan; CYP1A2 Inhibitors (Moderate); CYP1A2 Inhibitors (Strong); Deferasirox; HydrOXYzine; Pramlintide

Decreased Effect

Cyclobenzaprine may decrease the levels/effects of: Acetylcholinesterase Inhibitors (Central)

The levels/effects of Cyclobenzaprine may be decreased by: Acetylcholinesterase Inhibitors (Central); Cyproterone; Peginterferon Alfa-2b; Tocilizumab

Ethanol/Nutrition/Herb Interactions

Ethanol: May increase CNS depression; monitor for increased effects with coadministration. Caution patients about effects.

Food: Food increases bioavailability (peak plasma concentrations increased by 35% and area under the curve by 20%) of the extended release capsule.

Herb/Nutraceutical: Avoid valerian, kava kava, gotu kola (may increase CNS depression).

Stability

Amrix®, Flexeril®: Store at 25°C (77°F); excursions permitted to 15°C to 30°C (59°F to 86°F).

Fexmid®: Store at 20°C to 25°C (68°F to 77°F).

Mechanism of Action Centrally-acting skeletal muscle relaxant pharmacologically related to tricyclic antidepressants; reduces tonic somatic motor activity influencing both alpha and gamma motor neurons

Pharmacodynamics/Kinetics

Metabolism: Hepatic via CYP3A4, 1A2, and 2D6; may undergo enterohepatic recirculation

Bioavailability: 33% to 55%

Half-life elimination: Range: 8-37 hours; Immediate release tablet: 18 hours; Extended release capsule: 32-33 hours

Time to peak, serum: Extended release capsule: 7-8 hours

Excretion: Urine (as inactive metabolites); feces (as unchanged drug)

Dosage Oral: Muscle spasm: **Note:** Do not use longer than 2-3 weeks

Capsule, extended release:

Adults: Usual: 15 mg once daily; some patients may require up to 30 mg once daily

Elderly: Use not recommended

Tablet, immediate release:

Children ≥15 years and Adults: Initial: 5 mg 3 times/day; may increase up to 10 mg 3 times/day if needed

Elderly: Initial: 5 mg; titrate dose slowly and consider less frequent dosing

Dosage adjustment in hepatic impairment:

Capsule, extended release: Mild-to-severe impairment: Use not recommended.

Tablet, immediate release:

Mild impairment: Initial: 5 mg; use with caution; titrate slowly and consider less frequent dosing

Moderate-to-severe impairment: Use not recommended

Administration Oral: Extended release capsules: Administer at the same time each day. Do not crush or chew.

Test Interactions May cause false-positive serum TCA screen.

Dosage Forms Excipient information presented when available (limited, particularly for generics); consult specific product labeling.

Capsule, extended release, oral, as hydrochloride: 15 mg, 30 mg

Amrix®: 15 mg, 30 mg

Tablet, oral, as hydrochloride: 5 mg, 10 mg

Fexmid®: 7.5 mg

Flexeril®: 5 mg, 10 mg

◆ **Cyclobenzaprine Hydrochloride** *see* Cyclobenzaprine *on page 419*

◆ **Cyclogyl®** *see* Cyclopentolate *on page 420*

◆ **Cyclomen® (Can)** *see* Danazol *on page 443*

◆ **Cyclomydril®** *see* Cyclopentolate and Phenylephrine *on page 420*

Cyclopentolate (sye kloe PEN toe late)

Brand Names: U.S. AK-Pentolate™; Cyclogyl®; Cylate™

Brand Names: Canada Cyclogyl®; Diopentolate®

Index Terms Cyclopentolate Hydrochloride

Pharmacologic Category Anticholinergic Agent, Ophthalmic

Use Diagnostic procedures requiring mydriasis and cycloplegia

Pregnancy Risk Factor C

Dosage Ophthalmic:

Infants: **Note:** Cyclopentolate and phenylephrine combination formulation is the preferred agent for use in infants due to lower cyclopentolate concentration and reduced risk for systemic reactions

Children: Instill 1 drop of 0.5%, 1%, or 2% in eye followed by 1 drop of 0.5% or 1% in 5 minutes, if necessary

Adults: Instill 1 drop of 1% followed by another drop in 5 minutes; 2% solution in heavily pigmented iris

Additional Information Complete prescribing information for this medication should be consulted for additional detail.

Dosage Forms Excipient information presented when available (limited, particularly for generics); consult specific product labeling.

Solution, ophthalmic, as hydrochloride [drops]: 1% (2 mL, 15 mL)

AK-Pentolate™: 1% (2 mL, 15 mL) [contains benzalkonium chloride]

Cyclogyl®: 0.5% (15 mL); 1% (2 mL, 5 mL, 15 mL); 2% (2 mL, 5 mL, 15 mL) [contains benzalkonium chloride]

Cylate™: 1% (2 mL, 15 mL) [contains benzalkonium chloride]

Cyclopentolate and Phenylephrine
(sye kloe PEN toe late & fen il EF rin)

Brand Names: U.S. Cyclomydril®

Index Terms Phenylephrine and Cyclopentolate

Pharmacologic Category Ophthalmic Agent, Antiglaucoma

Use Induce mydriasis greater than that produced with cyclopentolate HCl alone

Pregnancy Risk Factor C

Dosage Ophthalmic: Infants, Children, and Adults: Instill 1 drop into the eye every 5-10 minutes, for up to 3 doses, approximately 40-50 minutes before the examination

Additional Information Complete prescribing information for this medication should be consulted for additional detail.

Dosage Forms Excipient information presented when available (limited, particularly for generics); consult specific product labeling.

Solution, ophthalmic:

Cyclomydril®: Cyclopentolate hydrochloride 0.2% and phenylephrine hydrochloride 1% (2 mL, 5 mL) [contains benzalkonium chloride]

◆ **Cyclopentolate Hydrochloride** *see* Cyclopentolate *on page 420*

Cyclophosphamide (sye kloe FOS fa mide)

Brand Names: Canada Procytox®

Index Terms CPM; CTX; CYT; Cytoxan; Neosar

Pharmacologic Category Antineoplastic Agent, Alkylating Agent

Use

Oncology-related uses: Treatment of Hodgkin's lymphoma, non-Hodgkin's lymphoma (including Burkitt's lymphoma), chronic lymphocytic leukemia (CLL), chronic myelocytic leukemia (CML), acute myelocytic leukemia (AML), acute lymphocytic leukemia (ALL), mycosis fungoides, multiple myeloma, neuroblastoma, retinoblastoma; breast cancer; ovarian adenocarcinoma

Nononcology uses: Treatment of refractory nephrotic syndrome in children

Unlabeled Use

Oncology-related uses: Ewing's sarcoma, rhabdomyosarcoma, Wilms tumor, ovarian germ cell tumors, small cell lung cancer, testicular cancer, pheochromocytoma, bone marrow transplantation conditioning regimen

Nononcology uses: Severe rheumatoid disorders, Wegener's granulomatosis, myasthenia gravis, multiple sclerosis, systemic lupus erythematosus, lupus nephritis, autoimmune hemolytic anemia, idiopathic thrombocytic purpura (ITP), and antibody-induced pure red cell aplasia; juvenile idiopathic arthritis (JIA)

Pregnancy Risk Factor D

Pregnancy Considerations Studies in pregnant women have demonstrated a risk to the fetus. Women of childbearing potential should avoid pregnancy while receiving cyclophosphamide treatment. Cyclophosphamide may also cause sterility in males and females (reversible in some cases).

Lactation Enters breast milk/not recommended

Contraindications Hypersensitivity to cyclophosphamide or any component of the formulation; severely depressed bone marrow function

Warnings/Precautions Hazardous agent - use appropriate precautions for handling and disposal. Dosage adjustment may be needed for renal or hepatic failure. Hemorrhagic cystitis may occur; increased hydration and frequent voiding is recommended. Immunosuppression may occur; monitor for infections. May cause cardiotoxicity (HF, usually with higher doses); may potentiate the cardiotoxicity of anthracyclines. May impair fertility; interferes with oogenesis and spermatogenesis. Secondary malignancies (usually delayed) have been reported

Adverse Reactions

>10%:

Dermatologic: Alopecia (40% to 60%) but hair will usually regrow although it may be a different color and/or texture. Hair loss usually begins 3-6 weeks after the start of therapy.

Endocrine & metabolic: Fertility: May cause sterility; interferes with oogenesis and spermatogenesis; may be irreversible in some patients; gonadal suppression (amenorrhea)

Gastrointestinal: Nausea and vomiting (usually beginning 6-10 hours after administration; severe with high-dose therapy); anorexia, diarrhea, mucositis, and stomatitis are also seen

Genitourinary: Severe, potentially fatal, acute hemorrhagic cystitis or urinary fibrosis (7% to 40%)

Hematologic: Anemia, leukopenia (dose-related; recovery: 7-10 days after cessation), thrombocytopenia

1% to 10%:

Cardiovascular: Facial flushing

Central nervous system: Headache

Dermatologic: Skin rash

Respiratory: Nasal congestion occurs when I.V. doses are administered too rapidly; patients experience runny eyes, rhinorrhea, sinus congestion, and sneezing during or immediately after the infusion.

<1% (Limited to important or life-threatening): Acute respiratory distress syndrome, anaphylactic reactions, arrhythmias (with high-dose [HSCT] therapy), cardiac tamponade (with high-dose [HSCT] therapy), CHF (with high-dose [HSCT] therapy), dyspnea, heart block, hemorrhagic colitis, hemorrhagic myocarditis (with high-dose [HSCT] therapy), hemorrhagic ureteritis, hepatotoxicity, hyperuricemia, hypokalemia, hyponatremia, interstitial pneumonitis, interstitial pulmonary fibrosis (with high doses), jaundice, mesenteric ischemia (acute), methemoglobinemia (with high-dose [HSCT] therapy), myocardial necrosis (with high-dose [HSCT] therapy), neutrophilic eccrine hidradenitis, pulmonary infiltrates, radiation recall, renal tubular necrosis, reversible posterior leukoencephalopathy syndrome (RPLS), secondary malignancy, SIADH, Stevens-Johnson syndrome, thrombocytopenia (immune mediated), toxic epidermal necrolysis, toxic megacolon, veno-occlusive liver disease

Drug Interactions

Metabolism/Transport Effects Substrate of CYP2A6 (minor), CYP2B6 (major), CYP2C19 (minor), CYP2C9 (minor), CYP3A4 (minor); **Note:** Assignment of Major/Minor substrate status based on clinically relevant drug interaction potential; **Inhibits** CYP3A4 (weak); **Induces** CYP2B6 (weak/moderate), CYP2C9 (weak/moderate)

Avoid Concomitant Use

Avoid concomitant use of Cyclophosphamide with any of the following: BCG; Belimumab; CloZAPine; Etanercept; Natalizumab; Pimecrolimus; Pimozide; Tacrolimus (Topical); Vaccines (Live)

Increased Effect/Toxicity

Cyclophosphamide may increase the levels/effects of: CloZAPine; Leflunomide; Natalizumab; Pimozide; Succinylcholine; Vaccines (Live); Vitamin K Antagonists

The levels/effects of Cyclophosphamide may be increased by: Allopurinol; Belimumab; Conivaptan; CYP2B6 Inhibitors (Moderate); CYP2B6 Inhibitors (Strong); Denosumab; Etanercept; Pentostatin; Pimecrolimus; Quazepam; Roflumilast; Tacrolimus (Topical); Trastuzumab

Decreased Effect

Cyclophosphamide may decrease the levels/effects of: BCG; Cardiac Glycosides; Coccidioidin Skin Test; Sipuleucel-T; Vaccines (Inactivated); Vaccines (Live); Vitamin K Antagonists

The levels/effects of Cyclophosphamide may be decreased by: CYP2B6 Inducers (Strong); Echinacea; Tocilizumab

Ethanol/Nutrition/Herb Interactions Herb/Nutraceutical: Avoid black cohosh, dong quai in estrogen-dependent tumors.

Stability Store intact vials of powder at room temperature of 15°C to 30°C (59°F to 86°F). Reconstitute vials with sterile water, normal saline, or 5% dextrose to a concentration of 20 mg/mL. Reconstituted solutions are stable for 24 hours at room temperature and 6 days under refrigeration at 2°C to 8°C (36°F to 46°F). Further dilutions in D_5W or NS are stable for 24 hours at room temperature and 6 days at refrigeration.

Mechanism of Action Cyclophosphamide is an alkylating agent that prevents cell division by cross-linking DNA strands and decreasing DNA synthesis. It is a cell cycle phase nonspecific agent. Cyclophosphamide also possesses potent immunosuppressive activity. Cyclophosphamide is a prodrug that must be metabolized to active metabolites in the liver.

Pharmacodynamics/Kinetics

Absorption: Oral: Well absorbed

Distribution: V_d: 0.48-0.71 L/kg; crosses into CSF (not in high enough concentrations to treat meningeal leukemia)

Protein binding: 10% to 60%

Metabolism: Hepatic to active metabolites acrolein, 4-aldophosphamide, 4-hydroperoxycyclophosphamide, and nor-nitrogen mustard

Bioavailability: >75%

Half-life elimination: 3-12 hours

Time to peak, serum: Oral: ~1 hour

Excretion: Urine (<30% as unchanged drug, 85% to 90% as metabolites)

Dosage Details concerns dosing in combination regimens should also be consulted.

Children: Oral:

Malignancy: Usual range (in the manufacturer's labeling): 1-5 mg/kg/day (initial and maintenance dosing)

Nephrotic syndrome: 2.5-3 mg/kg/day every day for 60-90 days (when refractory or intolerant to corticosteroid treatment)

Children and Adults: I.V.:

Single doses: 400-1800 mg/m^2 (30-50 mg/kg) per treatment course (1-5 days) which can be repeated at 2-4 week intervals

Continuous daily doses: 60-120 mg/m^2 (1-2.5 mg/kg) per day

Autologous BMT (unlabeled use): IVPB: 50 mg/kg/dose x 4 days **or** 60 mg/kg/dose for 2 days; total dose is usually divided over 2-4 days

JIA/vasculitis (unlabeled use): 10 mg/kg every 2 weeks

SLE (unlabeled use): 500 mg/m^2 every month; may increase up to a maximum dose of 1 g/m^2 every month (Austin, 1986)

Adults: Oral:

Malignancy: Usual range (in the manufacturer's labeling): 1-5 mg/kg/day (initial and maintenance dosing)

Breast cancer (unlabeled dosing; combination chemotherapy):

CEF: 75 mg/m^2/day days 1-14 every 28 days (Levine, 1998)

CMF: 100 mg/m^2/day days 1-14 every 28 days (Bonadonna, 1995; Levine, 1998)

Nephrotic syndrome (refractory; unlabeled use): 2.5-3 mg/kg/day every day for 60-90 days (when refractory or intolerant to corticosteroid treatment)

Dosing adjustment in renal impairment: The FDA-approved labeling states there is insufficient evidence to recommend dosage adjustment and therefore, does not contain renal dosing adjustment guidelines. The following guidelines have been used by some clinicians (Aronoff, 2007): Children and Adults:

Cl_{cr} <10 mL/minute: Administer 75% of normal dose

Hemodialysis effects: Moderately dialyzable (20% to 50%) Administer 50% of dose posthemodialysis

Continuous ambulatory peritoneal dialysis (CAPD): Administer 75% of normal dose

Continuous renal replacement therapy (CRRT): Administer 100% of normal dose

Dosing adjustment in hepatic impairment: The pharmacokinetics of cyclophosphamide are not significantly altered in the presence of hepatic insufficiency. The FDA-approved labeling does not contain hepatic dosing adjustment guidelines. The following guidelines have been used by some clinicians (Floyd, 2006):

Serum bilirubin 3.1-5 mg/dL or transaminases >3 times ULN: Administer 75% of dose

Serum bilirubin >5 mg/mL: Avoid use

Dietary Considerations Tablets should be administered during or after meals.

Administration

Injection: Administer IVPB or continuous I.V. infusion; may also be administered slow IVP in doses ≤1 g.

I.V. infusions may be administered over 1-24 hours

Doses >500 mg to approximately 2 g may be administered over 20-30 minutes

To minimize bladder toxicity, increase normal fluid intake during and for 1-2 days after cyclophosphamide dose. Most adult patients will require a fluid intake of at least 2 L/day. High-dose regimens should be accompanied by vigorous hydration with or without mesna therapy.

Oral: Tablets are not scored and should not be cut or crushed. To minimize the risk of bladder irritation, do not administer tablets at bedtime.

Monitoring Parameters CBC with differential and platelet count, BUN, UA, serum electrolytes, serum creatinine

Additional Information In patients with CYP2B6 G516T variant allele, cyclophosphamide metabolism is markedly increased; metabolism is not influenced by CYP2C9 and CYP2C19 isotypes.

Dosage Forms Excipient information presented when available (limited, particularly for generics); consult specific product labeling.

Injection, powder for reconstitution: 500 mg, 1 g, 2 g

Tablet, oral: 25 mg, 50 mg

Extemporaneous Preparations Hazardous agent: Use appropriate precautions for handling and disposal.

A 10 mg/mL oral suspension may be prepared by reconstituting one 2 g vial for injection with 100 mL of NaCl 0.9%, providing an initial concentration of 20 mg/mL. Mix this solution in a 1:1 ratio with either Simple Syrup, NF or Ora-Plus® to obtain a final concentration of 10 mg/mL. Label "shake well" and "refrigerate". Stable for 56 days refrigerated.

Kennedy R, Groepper D, Tagen M, et al, "Stability of Cyclophosphamide in Extemporaneous Oral Suspensions," *Ann Pharmacother*, 2010, 44(2):295-301.

◆ **Cycloset®** *see* Bromocriptine *on page 236*

◆ **Cycloset®** *see* Bromocriptine *on page 236*

◆ **Cyclosporin A** *see* CycloSPORINE (Ophthalmic) *on page 427*

◆ **Cyclosporin A** *see* CycloSPORINE (Systemic) *on page 422*

CycloSPORINE (Systemic) (SYE kloe spor een)

Brand Names: U.S. Gengraf®; Neoral®; SandIMMUNE®

Brand Names: Canada Apo-Cyclosporine®; Neoral®; Rhoxal-cyclosporine; Sandimmune® I.V.; Sandoz-Cyclosporine

Index Terms CsA; CyA; Cyclosporin A

Pharmacologic Category Calcineurin Inhibitor; Immunosuppressant Agent

Use Prophylaxis of organ rejection in kidney, liver, and heart transplants, has been used with azathioprine and/or corticosteroids; severe, active rheumatoid arthritis (RA) not responsive to methotrexate alone; severe, recalcitrant plaque psoriasis in nonimmunocompromised adults unresponsive to or unable to tolerate other systemic therapy

Unlabeled Use Allogenic stem cell transplants for prevention and treatment of graft-versus-host disease; also used in some cases of severe autoimmune disease (eg, SLE) that are resistant to corticosteroids and other therapy; focal segmental glomerulosclerosis; severe ulcerative colitis

Pregnancy Risk Factor C

Pregnancy Considerations Adverse events were not observed following the use of oral cyclosporine in animal reproduction studies (using doses that were not maternally toxic). In humans, cyclosporine crosses the placenta; maternal concentrations do not correlate with those found in the umbilical cord. Cyclosporine may be detected in the serum of newborns for several days after birth. Based on clinical use, premature births and low birth weight were consistently observed in pregnant transplant patients (additional pregnancy complications also present).

A pregnancy registry has been established for pregnant women taking immunosuppressants following any solid organ transplant (National Transplantation Pregnancy Registry, Temple University, 877-955-6877).

A pregnancy registry has also been established for pregnant women taking Neoral® for psoriasis or rheumatoid arthritis (Neoral® Pregnancy Registry for Psoriasis and Rheumatoid Arthritis, Thomas Jefferson University, 888-522-5581).

Lactation Enters breast milk/not recommended

Contraindications Hypersensitivity to cyclosporine or any component of the formulation. I.V. cyclosporine is contraindicated in hypersensitivity to polyoxyethylated castor oil (Cremophor® EL).

Rheumatoid arthritis and psoriasis: Abnormal renal function, uncontrolled hypertension, malignancies. Concomitant treatment with PUVA or UVB therapy, methotrexate, other immunosuppressive agents, coal tar, or radiation therapy are also contraindications for use in patients with psoriasis.

Warnings/Precautions Hazardous agent - use appropriate precautions for handling and disposal. **[U.S. Boxed Warning]: Renal impairment, including structural kidney damage has occurred (when used at high doses); monitor renal function closely.** Elevations in serum creatinine and BUN generally respond to dosage reductions. Use caution with other potentially nephrotoxic drugs (eg, acyclovir, aminoglycoside antibiotics, amphotericin B, ciprofloxacin). **[U.S. Boxed Warning]: Increased risk of lymphomas and other malignancies, particularly those of the skin;** risk is related to intensity/duration of therapy and the use of >1 immunosuppressive agent; all patients should avoid excessive sun/UV light exposure. **[U.S. Boxed Warning]: Increased risk of infection; fatal infections have been reported.** Latent viral infections may be activated (including BK virus which is associated with nephropathy) and result in serious adverse effects. **[U.S. Boxed Warning]: May cause hypertension.** Use caution when changing dosage forms. **[U.S. Boxed Warning]: Cyclosporine (modified) has increased bioavailability as compared to cyclosporine (non-modified) and cannot be used interchangeably without close monitoring.** Monitor cyclosporine concentrations closely following the addition, modification, or deletion of other medications; live, attenuated vaccines may be less effective; use should be avoided. Increased hepatic enzymes and bilirubin have occurred (when used at high doses); improvement usually seen with dosage reduction.

Transplant patients: To be used initially with corticosteroids. May cause significant hyperkalemia and hyperuricemia, seizures (particularly if used with high dose corticosteroids), and encephalopathy. Other neurotoxic events (eg, optic disc edema including papilledema and visual impairment) have been reported rarely. Make dose adjustments based on cyclosporine blood concentrations. **[U.S. Boxed Warning]: Adjustment of dose should only be made under the direct supervision of an experienced physician.** Anaphylaxis has been reported with I.V. use; reserve for patients who cannot take oral form. **[U.S. Boxed Warning]: Risk of skin cancer may be increased in transplant patients.** Due to the increased risk for nephrotoxicity in renal transplantation, avoid using standard doses of cyclosporine in combination with everolimus; reduced cyclosporine doses are recommended; monitor cyclosporine concentrations closely. Cyclosporine and everolimus combination therapy may increase the risk for proteinuria. Cyclosporine combined with either everolimus or sirolimus may increase the risk for thrombotic microangiopathy/thrombotic thrombocytopenic purpura/hemolytic uremic syndrome (TMA/TTP/HUS).

Psoriasis: Patients should avoid excessive sun exposure; safety and efficacy in children <18 years of age have not been established. **[U.S. Boxed Warning]: Risk of skin cancer may be increased with a history of PUVA and possibly methotrexate or other immunosuppressants, UVB, coal tar, or radiation.**

Rheumatoid arthritis: Safety and efficacy for use in juvenile idiopathic arthritis (JIA) have not been established. If receiving other immunosuppressive agents, radiation or UV therapy, concurrent use of cyclosporine is not recommended.

Products may contain corn oil, ethanol, or propylene glycol; injection also contains Cremophor® EL (polyoxyethylated castor oil), which has been associated with rare anaphylactic reactions.

Adverse Reactions Adverse reactions reported with systemic use, including rheumatoid arthritis, psoriasis, and transplantation (kidney, liver, and heart). Percentages noted include the highest frequency regardless of indication/dosage. Frequencies may vary for specific conditions or formulation.

>10%:
- Cardiovascular: Hypertension (8% to 53%), edema (5% to 14%)
- Central nervous system: Headache (2% to 25%)
- Dermatologic: Hirsutism (21% to 45%), hypertrichosis (5% to 19%)
- Endocrine & metabolic: Triglycerides increased (15%), female reproductive disorder (9% to 11%)
- Gastrointestinal: Nausea (23%), diarrhea (3% to 13%), gum hyperplasia (2% to 16%), abdominal discomfort (<1% to 15%), dyspepsia (2% to 12%)
- Neuromuscular & skeletal: Tremor (7% to 55%), paresthesia (1% to 11%), leg cramps/muscle contractions (2% to 12%)
- Renal: Renal dysfunction/nephropathy (10% to 38%), creatinine increased (16% to ≥50%)
- Respiratory: Upper respiratory infection (1% to 14%)
- Miscellaneous: Infection (3% to 25%)

1% to 10%:
- Cardiovascular: Chest pain (4% to 6%), arrhythmia (2% to 5%), abnormal heart sounds, cardiac failure, flushes (<1% to 5%), MI, peripheral ischemia
- Central nervous system: Dizziness (8%), pain (6%), convulsions (1% to 5%), insomnia (4%), psychiatric events (4% to 5%), pain (3% to 4%), depression (1% to 6%), migraine (2% to 3%), anxiety, confusion, fever, hypoesthesia, emotional lability, impaired concentration, lethargy, malaise, nervousness, paranoia, somnolence, vertigo
- Dermatologic: Purpura (3% to 4%), acne (1% to 6%), brittle fingernails, hair breaking, abnormal pigmentation, angioedema, cellulitis, dermatitis, dry skin, eczema, folliculitis, keratosis, pruritus, rash, skin disorder, skin malignancies, urticaria

Endocrine & metabolic: Gynecomastia (<1% to 4%), menstrual disorder (1% to 3%), breast fibroadenosis, breast pain, hyper-/hypoglycemia, diabetes mellitus, goiter, hot flashes, hyperkalemia, hyperuricemia, libido increased/decreased

Gastrointestinal: Vomiting (2% to 10%), flatulence (5%), gingivitis (up to 4%), cramps (up to 4%), anorexia, constipation, dry mouth, dysphagia, enanthema, eructation, esophagitis, gastric ulcer, gastritis, gastroenteritis, gastrointestinal bleeding (upper), gingival bleeding, glossitis, mouth sores, peptic ulcer, pancreatitis, swallowing difficulty, salivary gland enlargement, taste perversion, tongue disorder, gum hyperplasia, weight loss/gain

Genitourinary: Leukorrhea (1%), abnormal urine, micturition increased, micturition urgency, nocturia, polyuria, pyelonephritis, urinary incontinence, uterine hemorrhage

Hematologic: Leukopenia (<1% to 6%), anemia, bleeding disorder, clotting disorder, platelet disorder, red blood cell disorder, thrombocytopenia

Hepatic: Hepatotoxicity (<1% to 7%), hyperbilirubinemia

Neuromuscular & skeletal: Arthralgia (1% to 6%), bone fracture, joint dislocation, joint pain, muscle pain, myalgia, neuropathy, stiffness, synovial cyst, tendon disorder, tingling, weakness

Ocular: Abnormal vision, cataract, conjunctivitis, eye pain, visual disturbance

Otic: Deafness, hearing loss, tinnitus, vestibular disorder

Renal: BUN increased, hematuria, renal abscess

Respiratory: Sinusitis (<1% to 7%), bronchospasm (up to 5%), cough (3% to 5%), pharyngitis (3% to 5%), dyspnea (1% to 5%), rhinitis (up to 5%), abnormal chest sounds, epistaxis, respiratory infection, pneumonia (up to 1%)

Miscellaneous: Flu-like syndrome (8% to 10%), lymphoma (<1% to 6% reported in transplant), abscess, allergic reactions, bacterial infection, carcinoma, diaphoresis increased, fungal infection, herpes simplex, herpes zoster, hiccups, lymphadenopathy, moniliasis, night sweats, tonsillitis, viral infection

Postmarketing and/or case reports (any indication): Anaphylaxis/anaphylactoid reaction (possibly associated with Cremophor® EL vehicle in injection formulation), benign intracranial hypertension, BK virus-associated nephropathy, cholesterol increased, death (due to renal deterioration), encephalopathy, gout, hyperbilirubinemia, hyperkalemia, hypomagnesemia (mild), impaired consciousness, neurotoxicity, papilloedema, pulmonary edema (noncardiogenic), reversible posterior leukoencephalopathy syndrome (RPLS), uric acid increased

Drug Interactions

Metabolism/Transport Effects Substrate of CYP3A4 (major), P-glycoprotein; **Note:** Assignment of Major/Minor substrate status based on clinically relevant drug interaction potential; **Inhibits** CYP2C9 (weak), CYP3A4 (moderate), P-glycoprotein

Avoid Concomitant Use

Avoid concomitant use of CycloSPORINE (Systemic) with any of the following: Aliskiren; BCG; Bosentan; Conivaptan; Crizotinib; Dronedarone; Eplerenone; Natalizumab; Pimecrolimus; Pimozide; Pitavastatin; Potassium-Sparing Diuretics; Silodosin; Sitaxentan; Tacrolimus; Tacrolimus (Systemic); Tacrolimus (Topical); Topotecan; Vaccines (Live)

Increased Effect/Toxicity

CycloSPORINE (Systemic) may increase the levels/effects of: Aliskiren; Ambrisentan; ARIPiprazole; Bosentan; Budesonide (Systemic, Oral Inhalation); Calcium Channel Blockers (Dihydropyridine); Calcium Channel Blockers (Nondihydropyridine); Cardiac Glycosides; Caspofungin; Colchicine; CYP3A4 Substrates; Dabigatran Etexilate; Dexamethasone; Dexamethasone (Systemic); DOXOrubicin; Dronedarone; Etoposide; Etoposide Phosphate; Everolimus; Ezetimibe; FentaNYL; Fibric Acid Derivatives; Halofantrine; HMG-CoA Reductase Inhibitors; Imipenem; Leflunomide; Loop Diuretics; Lurasidone; Methotrexate; MethylPREDNISolone; Minoxidil; Minoxidil (Systemic); Minoxidil (Topical); Natalizumab; Nonsteroidal Anti-Inflammatory Agents; P-glycoprotein/ABCB1 Substrates; Pimozide; Pitavastatin; PrednisoLONE; PrednisoLONE (Systemic); PredniSONE; Propafenone; Protease Inhibitors; Repaglinide; Rivaroxaban; Salmeterol; Silodosin; Sirolimus; Sitaxentan; Tacrolimus; Tacrolimus (Systemic); Tacrolimus (Topical); Topotecan; Vaccines (Live); Vilazodone; Zuclopenthixol

The levels/effects of CycloSPORINE (Systemic) may be increased by: ACE Inhibitors; AcetaZOLAMIDE; Aminoglycosides; Amiodarone; Amphotericin B; Androgens; Antifungal Agents (Azole Derivatives, Systemic); Bromocriptine; Calcium Channel Blockers (Nondihydropyridine); Carvedilol; Chloramphenicol; Conivaptan; Crizotinib; CYP3A4 Inhibitors (Moderate); CYP3A4 Inhibitors (Strong); Dasatinib; Denosumab; Dexamethasone; Dexamethasone (Systemic); Eplerenone; Ezetimibe; Fluconazole; GlyBURIDE; Grapefruit Juice; Imatinib; Imipenem; Macrolide Antibiotics; Melphalan; Methotrexate; MethylPREDNISolone; Metoclopramide; MetroNIDAZOLE; MetroNIDAZOLE (Systemic); Nonsteroidal Anti-Inflammatory Agents; Norfloxacin; Omeprazole; P-glycoprotein/ABCB1 Inhibitors; Pimecrolimus; Potassium-Sparing Diuretics; PrednisoLONE; PrednisoLONE (Systemic); PredniSONE; Protease Inhibitors; Pyrazinamide; Quinupristin; Roflumilast; Sirolimus; Sulfonamide Derivatives; Tacrolimus; Tacrolimus (Systemic); Tacrolimus (Topical); Telaprevir; Temsirolimus; Trastuzumab

Decreased Effect

CycloSPORINE (Systemic) may decrease the levels/effects of: BCG; Coccidioidin Skin Test; GlyBURIDE; Mycophenolate; Sipuleucel-T; Vaccines (Inactivated); Vaccines (Live)

The levels/effects of CycloSPORINE (Systemic) may be decreased by: Armodafinil; Ascorbic Acid; Barbiturates; Bosentan; CarBAMazepine; Colesevelam; CYP3A4 Inducers (Strong); Deferasirox; Dexamethasone; Dexamethasone (Systemic); Echinacea; Efavirenz; Fibric Acid Derivatives; Fosphenytoin; Griseofulvin; Imipenem; MethylPREDNISolone; Modafinil; Nafcillin; Orlistat; P-glycoprotein/ABCB1 Inducers; Phenytoin; PrednisoLONE; PrednisoLONE (Systemic); PredniSONE; Rifamycin Derivatives; Somatostatin Analogs; St Johns Wort; Sulfinpyrazone [Off Market]; Sulfonamide Derivatives; Terbinafine; Tocilizumab; Vitamin E

Ethanol/Nutrition/Herb Interactions

Food: Grapefruit juice increases cyclosporine serum concentrations.

Herb/Nutraceutical: Avoid St John's wort; as an enzyme inducer, it may increase the metabolism of and decrease plasma levels of cyclosporine; organ rejection and graft loss have been reported. Avoid cat's claw, echinacea (have immunostimulant properties).

Stability

Capsule: Store at controlled room temperature.

Injection: Store at controlled room temperature; do not refrigerate. Ampuls and vials should be protected from light. Stability of injection of parenteral admixture at room temperature (25°C) is 6 hours in PVC; 12-24 hours in Excel®, PAB® containers, or glass. To minimize leaching of DEHP, non-PVC containers and sets should be used for preparation and administration.

Sandimmune® injection: Injection should be further diluted [1 mL (50 mg) of concentrate in 20-100 mL of D_5W or NS] for administration by intravenous infusion.

Oral solution: Store at controlled room temperature; do not refrigerate. Use within 2 months after opening; should be mixed in glass containers.

Neoral® oral solution: Orange juice, apple juice; avoid changing diluents frequently; mix thoroughly and drink at once.

Sandimmune® oral solution: Milk, chocolate milk, orange juice; avoid changing diluents frequently; mix thoroughly and drink at once.

Mechanism of Action Inhibition of production and release of interleukin II and inhibits interleukin II-induced activation of resting T-lymphocytes.

Pharmacodynamics/Kinetics

Absorption: Oral:

Cyclosporine (non-modified): Erratic and incomplete; dependent on presence of food, bile acids, and GI motility; larger oral doses are needed in pediatrics due to shorter bowel length and limited intestinal absorption

Cyclosporine (modified): Erratic and incomplete; increased absorption, up to 30% when compared to cyclosporine (non-modified); less dependent on food, bile acids, or GI motility when compared to cyclosporine (non-modified)

Distribution: Widely in tissues and body fluids including the liver, pancreas, and lungs

V_{dss}: 4-6 L/kg in renal, liver, and marrow transplant recipients (slightly lower values in cardiac transplant patients; children <10 years have higher values)

Protein binding: 90% to 98% to lipoproteins

Metabolism: Extensively hepatic via CYP3A4; forms at least 25 metabolites; extensive first-pass effect following oral administration

Bioavailability: Oral:

Cyclosporine (non-modified): Dependent on patient population and transplant type (<10% in adult liver transplant patients and as high as 89% in renal transplant patients); bioavailability of Sandimmune® capsules and oral solution are equivalent; bioavailability of oral solution is ~30% of the I.V. solution

Children: 28% (range: 17% to 42%); gut dysfunction common in BMT patients and oral bioavailability is further reduced

Cyclosporine (modified): Bioavailability of Neoral® capsules and oral solution are equivalent:

Children: 43% (range: 30% to 68%)

Adults: 23% greater than with cyclosporine (non-modified) in renal transplant patients; 50% greater in liver transplant patients

Half-life elimination: Oral: May be prolonged in patients with hepatic impairment and shorter in pediatric patients due to the higher metabolism rate

Cyclosporine (non-modified): Biphasic: Alpha: 1.4 hours; Terminal: 19 hours (range: 10-27 hours)

Cyclosporine (modified): Biphasic: Terminal: 8.4 hours (range: 5-18 hours)

Time to peak, serum: Oral:

Cyclosporine (non-modified): 2-6 hours; some patients have a second peak at 5-6 hours

Cyclosporine (modified): Renal transplant: 1.5-2 hours

Excretion: Primarily feces; urine (6%, 0.1% as unchanged drug and metabolites)

Dosage Neoral®/Gengraf® and Sandimmune® are not bioequivalent and cannot be used interchangeably.

Children: Transplant: Refer to adult dosing; children may require, and are able to tolerate, larger doses than adults.

Adults:

Newly-transplanted patients: Adjunct therapy with corticosteroids is recommended. Initial dose should be given 4-12 hours prior to transplant or may be given postoperatively; adjust initial dose to achieve desired plasma concentration

Oral: Dose is dependent upon type of transplant and formulation:

Cyclosporine (modified):

Renal: 9 ± 3 mg/kg/day, divided twice daily

Liver: 8 ± 4 mg/kg/day, divided twice daily

Heart: 7 ± 3 mg/kg/day, divided twice daily

Cyclosporine (non-modified): Initial doses of 10-14 mg/kg/day have been used for renal transplants (the manufacturer's labeling includes dosing from initial clinical trials of 15 mg/kg/day [range: 14-18 mg/kg/day]; however, this higher dosing level is rarely used any longer). Continue initial dose daily for 1-2 weeks; taper by 5% per week to a maintenance dose of 5-10 mg/kg/day; some renal transplant patients may be dosed as low as 3 mg/kg/day

Note: When using the non-modified formulation, cyclosporine levels may increase in liver transplant patients when the T-tube is closed; dose may need decreased

I.V.: Cyclosporine (non-modified): Manufacturer's labeling: Initial dose: 5-6 mg/kg/day or one-third of the oral dose as a single dose, infused over 2-6 hours; use should be limited to patients unable to take capsules or oral solution; patients should be switched to an oral dosage form as soon as possible

Note: Many transplant centers administer cyclosporine as "divided dose" infusions (in 2-3 doses/day) or as a continuous (24-hour) infusion; dosages range from 3-7.5 mg/kg/day. Specific institutional protocols should be consulted.

Conversion to cyclosporine (modified) from cyclosporine (non-modified): Start with daily dose previously used and adjust to obtain preconversion cyclosporine trough concentration. Plasma concentrations should be monitored every 4-7 days and dose adjusted as necessary, until desired trough level is obtained. When transferring patients with previously poor absorption of cyclosporine (non-modified), monitor trough levels at least twice weekly (especially if initial dose exceeds 10 mg/kg/day); high plasma levels are likely to occur.

Rheumatoid arthritis: Oral: Cyclosporine (modified): Initial dose: 2.5 mg/kg/day, divided twice daily; salicylates, NSAIDs, and oral glucocorticoids may be continued (refer to Drug Interactions); dose may be increased by 0.5-0.75 mg/kg/day if insufficient response is seen after 8 weeks of treatment; additional dosage increases may be made again at 12 weeks (maximum dose: 4 mg/kg/day). Discontinue if no benefit is seen by 16 weeks of therapy.

Note: Increase the frequency of blood pressure monitoring after each alteration in dosage of cyclosporine. Cyclosporine dosage should be decreased by 25% to 50% in patients with no history of hypertension who develop sustained hypertension during therapy and, if hypertension persists, treatment with cyclosporine should be discontinued.

Psoriasis: Oral: Cyclosporine (modified): Initial dose: 2.5 mg/kg/day, divided twice daily; dose may be increased by 0.5 mg/kg/day if insufficient response is seen after 4 weeks of treatment. Additional dosage increases may be made every 2 weeks if needed (maximum dose: 4 mg/kg/day). Discontinue if no benefit is seen by 6 weeks of therapy. Once patients are adequately controlled, the dose should be decreased to the lowest effective dose. Doses lower than 2.5 mg/kg/day may be effective. Treatment longer than 1 year is not recommended.

Note: Increase the frequency of blood pressure monitoring after each alteration in dosage of cyclosporine. Cyclosporine dosage should be decreased by 25% to 50% in patients with no history of hypertension who develop sustained hypertension during therapy and, if hypertension persists, treatment with cyclosporine should be discontinued.

Focal segmental glomerulosclerosis (unlabeled use): Oral: Initial: 3.5-5 mg/kg/day divided every 12 hours (in combination with oral prednisone) (Braun, 2008; Cattran, 1999)

Lupus nephritis (unlabeled use): Oral: Initial: 4 mg/kg/day for 1 month (reduce dose if trough concentrations >200 ng/mL); reduce dose by 0.5 mg/kg every 2 weeks to a maintenance dose of 2.5-3 mg/kg/day (Moroni, 2006)

Severe ulcerative colitis (steroid-refractory) (unlabeled use):

I.V.: Cyclosporine (non-modified): 2-4 mg/kg/day, infused continuously over 24 hours. (Lichtiger, 1994; Van Assche, 2003). **Note:** Some studies suggest no therapeutic difference between low-dose (2 mg/kg) and high-dose (4 mg/kg) cyclosporine regimens (Van Assche, 2003).

Oral: Cyclosporine (modified): 2.3-3 mg/kg every 12 hours (De Saussure 2005; Weber 2006)

Note: Patients responsive to I.V. therapy should be switched to oral therapy when possible.

Dosage adjustment in renal impairment: For severe psoriasis:

Serum creatinine levels ≥25% above pretreatment levels: Take another sample within 2 weeks; if the level remains ≥25% above pretreatment levels, decrease dosage of cyclosporine (modified) by 25% to 50%. If two dosage adjustments do not reverse the increase in serum creatinine levels, treatment should be discontinued.

Serum creatinine levels ≥50% above pretreatment levels: Decrease cyclosporine dosage by 25% to 50%. If two dosage adjustments do not reverse the increase in serum creatinine levels, treatment should be discontinued.

Hemodialysis: Supplemental dose is not necessary.

Peritoneal dialysis: Supplemental dose is not necessary.

Dosage adjustment in hepatic impairment: Probably necessary; monitor levels closely

Dietary Considerations Administer this medication consistently with relation to time of day and meals. Avoid grapefruit juice with oral cyclosporine use.

Administration

Oral solution: Do not administer liquid from plastic or styrofoam cup. May dilute Neoral® oral solution with orange juice or apple juice. May dilute Sandimmune® oral solution with milk, chocolate milk, or orange juice. Avoid changing diluents frequently. Mix thoroughly and drink at once. Use syringe provided to measure dose. Mix in a glass container and rinse container with more diluent to ensure total dose is taken. Do not rinse syringe before or after use (may cause dose variation).

Combination therapy with renal transplantation:

Everolimus: Administer cyclosporine at the same time as everolimus

Sirolimus: Administer cyclosporine 4 hours prior to sirolimus

I.V.: The manufacturer recommends that following dilution, intravenous admixture be administered over 2-6 hours. However, many transplant centers administer as divided doses (2-3 doses/day) or as a 24-hour continuous infusion. Discard solution after 24 hours. Anaphylaxis has been reported with I.V. use; reserve for patients who cannot take oral form. Patients should be under continuous observation for at least the first 30 minutes of the infusion, and should be monitored frequently thereafter. Maintain patent airway; other supportive measures and agents for treating anaphylaxis should be present when I.V. drug is given. To minimize leaching of DEHP, non-PVC sets should be used for administration.

Monitoring Parameters Monitor blood pressure and serum creatinine after any cyclosporine dosage changes or addition, modification, or deletion of other medications. Monitor plasma concentrations periodically.

Transplant patients: Cyclosporine trough levels, serum electrolytes, renal function, hepatic function, blood pressure, lipid profile

Psoriasis therapy: Baseline blood pressure, serum creatinine (2 levels each), BUN, CBC, serum magnesium, potassium, uric acid, lipid profile. Biweekly monitoring of blood pressure, complete blood count, and levels of BUN, uric acid, potassium, lipids, and magnesium during the first 3 months of treatment for psoriasis. Monthly monitoring is recommended after this initial period. Also evaluate any atypical skin lesions prior to therapy. Increase the frequency of blood pressure monitoring after each alteration in dosage of cyclosporine. Cyclosporine dosage should be decreased by 25% to 50% in patients with no history of hypertension who develop sustained hypertension during therapy and, if hypertension persists, treatment with cyclosporine should be discontinued.

Rheumatoid arthritis: Baseline blood pressure, and serum creatinine (2 levels each); serum creatinine every 2 weeks for first 3 months, then monthly if patient is stable. Increase the frequency of blood pressure monitoring after each alteration in dosage of cyclosporine. Cyclosporine dosage should be decreased by 25% to 50% in patients with no history of hypertension who develop sustained hypertension during therapy and, if hypertension persists, treatment with cyclosporine should be discontinued.

Reference Range Reference ranges are method dependent and specimen dependent; use the same analytical method consistently

Method-dependent and specimen-dependent: Trough levels should be obtained:

Oral: 12-18 hours after dose (chronic usage)

I.V.: 12 hours after dose **or** immediately prior to next dose

Therapeutic range: Not absolutely defined, dependent on organ transplanted, time after transplant, organ function and CsA toxicity:

General range of 100-400 ng/mL

Toxic level: Not well defined, nephrotoxicity may occur at any level

Recommend cyclosporine therapeutic ranges when administered in combination with everolimus for renal transplant (Zortress® product labeling, 2010):

Month 1 post-transplant: 100-200 ng/mL

Months 2 and 3 post-transplant: 75-150 ng/mL

Months 4 and 5 post-transplant: 50-100 ng/mL

Months 6-12 post-transplant: 25-50 ng/mL

Test Interactions Specific whole blood assay for cyclosporine may be falsely elevated if sample is drawn from the same central venous line through which dose was administered (even if flush has been administered and/or dose was given hours before); cyclosporine metabolites cross-react with radioimmunoassay and fluorescence polarization immunoassay

Additional Information Cyclosporine (modified): Refers to the capsule dosage formulation of cyclosporine in an aqueous dispersion (previously referred to as "microemulsion"). Cyclosporine (modified) has increased bioavailability as compared to cyclosporine (non-modified) and cannot be used interchangeably without close monitoring.

Dosage Forms Excipient information presented when available (limited, particularly for generics); consult specific product labeling. [DSC] = Discontinued product

Capsule, oral [modified]:

Gengraf®: 25 mg, 100 mg [contains ethanol 12.8%]

Capsule, oral [non-modified]: 25 mg [DSC], 100 mg

Capsule, softgel, oral [modified]: 25 mg, 50 mg, 100 mg

Neoral®: 25 mg, 100 mg [contains corn oil, dehydrated ethanol 11.9%]

Capsule, softgel, oral [non-modified]:
SandIMMUNE®: 25 mg, 100 mg [contains corn oil, dehydrated ethanol 12.7%]
Injection, solution [non-modified]: 50 mg/mL (5 mL)
SandIMMUNE®: 50 mg/mL (5 mL) [contains ethanol 32.9%, polyoxyethylated castor oil]
Solution, oral [modified]: 100 mg/mL (50 mL)
Gengraf®: 100 mg/mL (50 mL) [contains propylene glycol]
Neoral®: 100 mg/mL (50 mL) [contains corn oil, dehydrated ethanol 11.9%, propylene glycol]
Solution, oral [non-modified]: 100 mg/mL (50 mL [DSC])
SandIMMUNE®: 100 mg/mL (50 mL) [contains ethanol 12.5%]

CycloSPORINE (Ophthalmic)

(SYE kloe spor een)

Brand Names: U.S. Restasis®

Index Terms CsA; CyA; Cyclosporin A

Pharmacologic Category Immunosuppressant Agent

Use Increase tear production when suppressed tear production is presumed to be due to keratoconjunctivitis sicca-associated ocular inflammation (in patients not already using topical anti-inflammatory drugs or punctal plugs)

Pregnancy Risk Factor C

Dosage Ophthalmic (Restasis®): Children ≥16 years and Adults: Keratoconjunctivitis sicca: Instill 1 drop in each eye every 12 hours

Additional Information Complete prescribing information for this medication should be consulted for additional detail.

Dosage Forms Excipient information presented when available (limited, particularly for generics); consult specific product labeling.

Emulsion, ophthalmic [drops, preservative free]:
Restasis®: 0.05% (0.4 mL) [contains castor oil]

◆ **Cyklokapron®** *see* Tranexamic Acid *on page 1719*

◆ **Cylate™** *see* Cyclopentolate *on page 420*

◆ **Cymbalta®** *see* DULoxetine *on page 565*

Cyproheptadine (si proe HEP ta deen)

Index Terms Cyproheptadine Hydrochloride; Periactin

Pharmacologic Category Histamine H_1 Antagonist; Histamine H_1 Antagonist, First Generation; Piperidine Derivative

Additional Appendix Information

Beers Criteria - Potentially Inappropriate Medications for Geriatrics *on page 1973*

Use Perennial and seasonal allergic rhinitis and other allergic symptoms including urticaria

Unlabeled Use Migraine headache prophylaxis, pruritus, spasticity associated with spinal cord damage

Pregnancy Risk Factor B

Lactation Excretion in breast milk unknown/contraindicated

Contraindications Hypersensitivity to cyproheptadine or any component of the formulation; narrow-angle glaucoma; bladder neck obstruction; pyloroduodenal obstruction; symptomatic prostatic hyperplasia; stenosing peptic ulcer; concurrent use of MAO inhibitors; use in debilitated elderly patients; use in premature and term newborns due to potential association with SIDS; breast-feeding

Warnings/Precautions May cause CNS depression, which may impair physical or mental abilities; patients must be cautioned about performing tasks which require mental alertness (eg, operating machinery or driving). Effects may be potentiated when used with other sedative drugs or ethanol. Use with caution in patients with cardiovascular disease; increased intraocular pressure; respiratory disease; or thyroid dysfunction. May be inappropriate for use in the elderly due to potent anticholinergic effects (Beers Criteria). Antihistamines may cause excitation in young children.

Adverse Reactions Frequency not defined.

Cardiovascular: Extrasystoles, hypotension, palpitation, tachycardia

Central nervous system: Confusion, coordination disturbed, dizziness, excitation, euphoria, faintness, hallucinations, headache, hysteria, insomnia, irritability, nervousness, neuritis, restlessness, sedation, seizure, sleepiness, tremor, vertigo

Dermatologic: Angioedema, photosensitivity, rash, urticaria

Gastrointestinal: Abdominal pain, anorexia, appetite increased, constipation, diarrhea, nausea, vomiting, xerostomia

Genitourinary: Difficult urination, urinary frequency, urinary retention

Hematologic: Agranulocytosis, hemolytic anemia, leukopenia, thrombocytopenia

Hepatic: Cholestasis, hepatic failure, hepatitis, jaundice

Neuromuscular & skeletal: Paresthesia

Ocular: Blurred vision, diplopia

Otic: Labyrinthitis (acute), tinnitus

Respiratory: Bronchial secretions (thickening), nasal congestion, pharyngitis

Miscellaneous: Allergic reactions, anaphylactic shock, chills, diaphoresis, fatigue

Drug Interactions

Metabolism/Transport Effects None known.

Avoid Concomitant Use There are no known interactions where it is recommended to avoid concomitant use.

Increased Effect/Toxicity

Cyproheptadine may increase the levels/effects of: Alcohol (Ethyl); Anticholinergics; CNS Depressants; Methotrimeprazine

The levels/effects of Cyproheptadine may be increased by: Droperidol; HydrOXYzine; Methotrimeprazine; Pramlintide

Decreased Effect

Cyproheptadine may decrease the levels/effects of: Acetylcholinesterase Inhibitors (Central); Benzylpenicilloyl Polylysine; Betahistine; Selective Serotonin Reuptake Inhibitors

The levels/effects of Cyproheptadine may be decreased by: Acetylcholinesterase Inhibitors (Central); Amphetamines

Ethanol/Nutrition/Herb Interactions Ethanol: May increase CNS depression; monitor for increased effects with coadministration. Caution patients about effects.

Mechanism of Action A potent antihistamine and serotonin antagonist, competes with histamine for H_1-receptor sites on effector cells in the gastrointestinal tract, blood vessels, and respiratory tract

Pharmacodynamics/Kinetics

Absorption: Completely

Metabolism: Almost completely hepatic

Time to peak, plasma: 6-9 hours (Hintze, 1975)

Excretion: Urine (~40% primarily as metabolites); feces (2% to 20%)

Dosage Oral:

Children:

Allergic conditions: 0.25 mg/kg/day or 8 mg/m²/day in 2-3 divided doses **or**

2-6 years: 2 mg every 8-12 hours (not to exceed 12 mg/day)

7-14 years: 4 mg every 8-12 hours (not to exceed 16 mg/day)

▶

Migraine headache prophylaxis (unlabeled use): 4 mg every 8-12 hours
Adults:
Allergic conditions: 4-20 mg/day divided every 8 hours (not to exceed 0.5 mg/kg/day); some patients may require up to 32 mg/day for adequate control of symptoms
Spasticity associated with spinal cord damage (unlabeled use): Initial: 2-4 mg every 8 hours; maximum: 8 mg every 8 hours (Barbeau, 1982; Wainberg, 1990)
Elderly: Initiate therapy at the lower end of the dosage range

Test Interactions Diagnostic antigen skin test results may be suppressed; false positive serum TCA screen

Dosage Forms Excipient information presented when available (limited, particularly for generics); consult specific product labeling.
Syrup, oral, as hydrochloride: 2 mg/5 mL (473 mL, 480 mL)
Tablet, oral, as hydrochloride: 4 mg

◆ **Cyproheptadine Hydrochloride** *see* Cyproheptadine *on page 427*
◆ **Cystadane®** *see* Betaine *on page 208*
◆ **Cystagon®** *see* Cysteamine *on page 428*

Cysteamine (sis TEE a meen)

Brand Names: U.S. Cystagon®
Index Terms Cysteamine Bitartrate
Pharmacologic Category Anticystine Agent; Urinary Tract Product
Use Treatment of nephropathic cystinosis
Pregnancy Risk Factor C
Dosage Oral: Initiate therapy with 1/4 to 1/6 of maintenance dose; titrate slowly upward over 4-6 weeks. **Note:** Dosage may be increased if cystine levels are <1 nmol/1/2 cystine/mg protein, although intolerance and incidence of adverse events may be increased.

Children <12 years: Maintenance: 1.3 g/m²/day or 60 mg/kg/day divided into 4 doses (maximum dose: 1.95 g/m²/day or 90 mg/kg/day)
Children >12 years and Adults (>110 lb): 2 g/day in 4 divided doses; maximum dose: 1.95 g/m²/day or 90 mg/kg/day

Additional Information Complete prescribing information for this medication should be consulted for additional detail.

Dosage Forms Excipient information presented when available (limited, particularly for generics); consult specific product labeling.
Capsule, oral:
Cystagon®: 50 mg, 150 mg

◆ **Cysteamine Bitartrate** *see* Cysteamine *on page 428*
◆ **Cystistat® (Can)** *see* Hyaluronate and Derivatives *on page 831*
◆ **CYT** *see* Cyclophosphamide *on page 421*
◆ **Cytarabine** *see* Cytarabine (Conventional) *on page 428*

Cytarabine (Conventional)
(sye TARE a been con VEN sha nal)

Brand Names: Canada Cytosar®
Index Terms Ara-C; Arabinosylcytosine; Conventional Cytarabine; Cytarabine; Cytarabine Hydrochloride; Cytosar-U; Cytosine Arabinosine Hydrochloride
Pharmacologic Category Antineoplastic Agent, Antimetabolite; Antineoplastic Agent, Antimetabolite (Pyrimidine Analog)
Use Remission induction in acute myeloid leukemia (AML), treatment of acute lymphocytic leukemia (ALL) and chronic myelocytic leukemia (CML; blast phase); prophylaxis and treatment of meningeal leukemia
Unlabeled Use AML consolidation treatment, AML salvage treatment; acute promyelocytic leukemia (APL) consolidation treatment; treatment of primary central nervous system (CNS) lymphoma; treatment of chronic lymphocytic leukemia (CLL); treatment of relapsed or refractory Hodgkin lymphoma; treatment of non-Hodgkin's lymphomas (NHL)
Pregnancy Risk Factor D
Pregnancy Considerations Teratogenic effects were demonstrated in animal studies; limb and ear defects have been noted in case reports of cytarabine exposure during the first trimester of pregnancy. The following have also been noted in the neonate: Pancytopenia, WBC depression, electrolyte abnormalities, prematurity, low birth weight, decreased hematocrit or platelets. Risk to the fetus is decreased if treatment can be avoided during the first trimester; however, women of childbearing potential should be advised of the potential risks.
Lactation Excretion in breast milk unknown/not recommended
Contraindications Hypersensitivity to cytarabine or any component of the formulation
Warnings/Precautions Hazardous agent - use appropriate precautions for handling and disposal. **[U.S. Boxed Warning]: Myelosuppression (leukopenia, thrombocytopenia and anemia) is the major toxicity of cytarabine.** Use with caution in patients with prior drug-induced bone marrow suppression. Monitor blood counts frequently; once blasts are no longer apparent in the peripheral blood, bone marrow should be monitored frequently. Monitor for signs of infection or neutropenic fever due to neutropenia or bleeding due to thrombocytopenia.

High-dose regimens are associated with CNS, gastrointestinal, ocular (reversible corneal toxicity and hemorrhagic conjunctivitis; prophylaxis with ophthalmic corticosteroid drops is recommended), pulmonary toxicities and cardiomyopathy. Neurotoxicity associated with high-dose treatment may present as acute cerebellar toxicity (with or without cerebral impairment), personality changes, or may be severe with seizure and/or coma; may be delayed, occurring up to 3-8 days after treatment has begun. Risk factors for neurotoxicity include cumulative cytarabine dose, prior CNS disease and renal impairment; high-dose therapy (>18 g/m² per cycle) and age >50 years also increase the risk for cerebellar toxicity (Herzig, 1987). Tumor lysis syndrome and subsequent hyperuricemia may occur with high dose cytarabine; monitor, consider allopurinol and hydrate accordingly. There have been case reports of fatal cardiomyopathy when high dose cytarabine was used in combination with cyclophosphamide as a preparation regimen for transplantation.

Use with caution in patients with impaired renal and hepatic function; may be at higher risk for CNS toxicities; dosage adjustments may be necessary. A sudden respiratory arrest syndrome is characterized by fever, myalgia, bone pain, chest pain, maculopapular rash, conjunctivitis, and malaise, and may occur 6-12 hours following administration; may be managed with corticosteroids. Anaphylaxis resulting in acute cardiopulmonary arrest has been reported (rare). There have been reports of acute pancreatitis in patients receiving continuous infusion and in patients previously treated with L-asparaginase. **[U.S. Boxed Warning]: Should be administered under the supervision of an experienced cancer chemotherapy physician. Due to the potential toxicities, induction treatment with cytarabine should be in a facility with sufficient laboratory and supportive resources.** Some products may contain benzyl alcohol; do not use products containing benzyl alcohol or products reconstituted with bacteriostatic diluent intrathecally or for high-dose cytarabine regimens. When used for intrathecal administration, should not be prepared during the preparation of any other agents; after preparation, store intrathecal medications in an isolated location or container clearly marked with a label identifying as "intrathecal" use only; delivery of intrathecal medications to the patient should only be with other medications also intended for administration into the central nervous system (Jacobson, 2009).

Adverse Reactions

Frequent:

Central nervous system: Fever
Dermatologic: Rash
Gastrointestinal: Anal inflammation, anal ulceration, anorexia, diarrhea, mucositis, nausea, vomiting
Hematologic: Myelosuppression, neutropenia (onset: 1-7 days; nadir [biphasic]: 7-9 days and at 15-24 days; recovery [biphasic]: 9-12 days and at 24-34 days), thrombocytopenia (onset: 5 days; nadir: 12-15 days; recovery 15-25 days), anemia, bleeding, leukopenia, megaloblastosis, reticulocytes decreased
Hepatic: Hepatic dysfunction, transaminases increased (acute)
Local: Thrombophlebitis

Less frequent:

Cardiovascular: Chest pain, pericarditis
Central nervous system: Dizziness, headache, neural toxicity, neuritis
Dermatologic: Alopecia, pruritus, skin freckling, skin ulceration, urticaria
Gastrointestinal: Abdominal pain, bowel necrosis, esophageal ulceration, esophagitis, pancreatitis, sore throat
Genitourinary: Urinary retention
Hepatic: Jaundice
Local: Injection site cellulitis
Ocular: Conjunctivitis
Renal: Renal dysfunction
Respiratory: Dyspnea
Miscellaneous: Allergic edema, anaphylaxis, sepsis

Infrequent and/or case reports: Acute respiratory distress syndrome, amylase increased, angina, aseptic meningitis, cardiopulmonary arrest (acute), cerebral dysfunction, cytarabine syndrome (bone pain, chest pain, conjunctivitis, fever, maculopapular rash, malaise, myalgia); exanthematous pustulosis, hepatic sinusoidal obstruction syndrome (SOS; veno-occlussive disease), hyperuricemia, injection site inflammation (SubQ injection), injection site pain (SubQ injection), interstitial pneumonitis, lipase increased, paralysis (intrathecal and I.V. combination therapy), reversible posterior leukoencephalopathy syndrome (RPLS), rhabdomyolysis, toxic megacolon

Adverse events associated with high-dose cytarabine (CNS, gastrointestinal, ocular, and pulmonary toxicities are more common with high-dose regimens):

Cardiovascular: Cardiomegaly, cardiomyopathy (in combination with cyclophosphamide)
Central nervous system: Cerebellar toxicity, coma, neurotoxicity (up to 55% in patients with renal impairment), personality change, somnolence
Dermatologic: Alopecia (complete), desquamation, rash (severe)
Gastrointestinal: Gastrointestinal ulcer, pancreatitis, peritonitis, pneumatosis cystoides intestinalis
Hepatic: Hyperbilirubinemia, liver abscess, liver damage, necrotizing colitis
Neuromuscular & skeletal: Peripheral neuropathy (motor and sensory)
Ocular: Corneal toxicity, hemorrhagic conjunctivitis
Respiratory: Pulmonary edema, syndrome of sudden respiratory distress
Miscellaneous: Sepsis

Adverse events associated with intrathecal cytarabine administration:

Central nervous system: Accessory nerve paralysis, fever, necrotizing leukoencephalopathy (with concurrent cranial irradiation, I.T. methotrexate, and I.T. hydrocortisone), neurotoxicity, paraplegia
Gastrointestinal: Dysphagia, nausea, vomiting
Ocular: Blindness (with concurrent systemic chemotherapy and cranial irradiation), diplopia
Respiratory: Cough, hoarseness
Miscellaneous: Aphonia

Drug Interactions

Metabolism/Transport Effects None known.

Avoid Concomitant Use

Avoid concomitant use of Cytarabine (Conventional) with any of the following: BCG; CloZAPine; Natalizumab; Pimecrolimus; Tacrolimus (Topical); Vaccines (Live)

Increased Effect/Toxicity

Cytarabine (Conventional) may increase the levels/effects of: CloZAPine; Leflunomide; Natalizumab; Vaccines (Live)

The levels/effects of Cytarabine (Conventional) may be increased by: Denosumab; Pimecrolimus; Roflumilast; Tacrolimus (Topical); Trastuzumab

Decreased Effect

Cytarabine (Conventional) may decrease the levels/effects of: BCG; Cardiac Glycosides; Coccidioidin Skin Test; Flucytosine; Sipuleucel-T; Vaccines (Inactivated); Vaccines (Live)

The levels/effects of Cytarabine (Conventional) may be decreased by: Echinacea

Stability Use appropriate precautions for handling and disposal. Store intact vials of powder for injection at room temperature of 20°C to 25°C (68°F to 77°F); store intact vials of solution at room temperature of 15°C to 30°C (59°F to 86°F). **Note:** Solutions containing bacteriostatic agents may be used for SubQ and standard-dose (100-200 mg/m^2) I.V. cytarabine preparations, but should not be used for the preparation of either intrathecal doses or high-dose I.V. therapies.

I.V.:

Powder for reconstitution: Reconstitute with bacteriostatic water for injection (for standard-dose). Reconstituted solutions should be stored at room temperature and used within 48 hours.

For I.V. infusion: Further dilute in 250-1000 mL 0.9% NaCl or D_5W. Solutions for I.V. infusion diluted in D_5W or NS are stable for 7 days at room temperature, although the manufacturer recommends administration as soon as possible after preparation.

Intrathecal: Powder for reconstitution: Reconstitute with preservative free sodium chloride 0.9%; may further dilute to preferred final volume (volume generally based on institution or practitioner preference; may be up to 12 mL) with Elliott's B solution, sodium chloride 0.9% or lactated Ringer's. Administer as soon as possible after preparation. Intrathecal medications should not be prepared during the preparation of any other agents. After preparation, store intrathecal medications in an isolated location or container clearly marked with a label identifying as "intrathecal" use only.

Triple intrathecal therapy (TIT): Cytarabine 30-50 mg with hydrocortisone sodium succinate 15-25 mg and methotrexate 12 mg; compatible together for up to 24 hours in a syringe; however, should be administered administer as soon as possible after preparation because intrathecal preparations are preservative-free

Mechanism of Action Inhibits DNA synthesis. Cytosine gains entry into cells by a carrier process, and then must be converted to its active compound, aracytidine triphosphate. Cytosine is a pyrimidine analog and is incorporated into DNA; however, the primary action is inhibition of DNA polymerase resulting in decreased DNA synthesis and repair. The degree of cytotoxicity correlates linearly with incorporation into DNA; therefore, incorporation into the DNA is responsible for drug activity and toxicity. Cytarabine is specific for the S phase of the cell cycle (blocks progression from the G_1 to the S phase).

Pharmacodynamics/Kinetics

Distribution: V_d: Total body water; widely and rapidly since it enters the cells readily; crosses blood-brain barrier with CSF levels of 40% to 50% of plasma level

Metabolism: Primarily hepatic; metabolized by deoxycytidine kinase and other nucleotide kinases to aracytidine triphosphate (active); about 86% to 96% of dose is metabolized to inactive uracil arabinoside (ARA-U); intrathecal administration results in little conversion to ARA-U due to the low levels of deaminase in the cerebral spinal fluid

Half-life elimination: I.V.: Initial: 7-20 minutes; Terminal: 1-3 hours; I.T.: 2-6 hours

Time to peak, plasma: SubQ: 20-60 minutes

Excretion: Urine (~80%; 90% as metabolite ARA-U) within 24 hours

Dosage Details concerning dosing in combination regimens should also be consulted.

Acute myeloid leukemia (AML) remission induction: I.V.: Children and Adults: Standard-dose (provided in the FDA-approved labeling): 100 mg/m²/day continuous infusion for 7 days **or** 200 mg/m²/day continuous infusion (as 100 mg/m² over 12 hours every 12 hours) for 7 days

Pediatric indication-specific dosing:

AML induction: *7 + 3 regimen:* I.V.:

Children <3 years (unlabeled dosing): 3.3 mg/kg/day continuous infusion for 7 days; minimum of 2 courses (in combination with daunorubicin) (Woods, 1990)

Children ≥3 years: 100 mg/m²/day continuous infusion for 7 days; minimum of 2 courses (in combination with daunorubicin) (Woods, 1990)

AML consolidation (unlabeled use): *5 + 2 + 5 regimen:* I.V.: Children ≥15 years: 100 mg/m²/day continuous infusion for 5 days for 2 consolidation courses (in combination with daunorubicin and etoposide) (Bishop, 1996)

AML salvage treatment (unlabeled use):

FLAG regimen: I.V.: Children ≥11 years: 2000 mg/m²/day over 4 hours for 5 days (in combination with fludarabine and G-CSF); may repeat once if needed (Montillo, 1998)

MEC regimen: I.V.: Children ≥5 years: 1000 mg/m²/day over 6 hours for 6 days (in combination with etoposide and mitoxantrone) (Amadori, 1991)

Acute lymphocytic leukemia (ALL; unlabeled dosing): *POG 8602/PVA regimen, intensification phase:* I.V.: Children ≥1 year: 1000 mg/m² continuous infusion over 24 hours day 1 (beginning 12 hours after start of methotrexate) every 3 weeks or every 12 weeks for 6 cycles (Land, 1994)

Chronic myeloid leukemia (CML; unlabeled dosing): SubQ: Children ≥7 years: 20 mg/m² once daily days 15-24 every month (in combination with interferon alfa-2b) (Guilhot, 1997)

Non-Hodgkin's lymphomas (unlabeled use): *CODOX-M/IVAC regimen:* I.V.: Children ≥3 years: Cycles 2 and 4 (IVAC): 2000 mg/m² every 12 hours days 1 and 2 (total of 4 doses/cycle) (IVAC is combination with ifosfamide, mesna and etoposide; IVAC alternates with CODOX-M) (Magrath, 1996)

Adult indication-specific dosing:

AML induction: I.V.:

7 + 3 regimens (a second induction may be administered if needed; refer to specific references): 100 mg/m²/day continuous infusion for 7 days (in combination with daunorubicin **or** idarubicin **or** mitoxantrone) (Arlin, 1990; Dillman, 1991; Fernandez, 2009; Wiernick, 1992) **or** (Adults <60 years) 200 mg/m²/day continuous infusion for 7 days (in combination with daunorubicin) (Dillman, 1991)

Low intensity therapy (unlabeled dosing): Adults ≥65 years: SubQ: 20 mg/m²/day for 14 days out of every 28-day cycle for at least 4 cycles (Fenaux, 2010) **or** 10 mg/m² every 12 hours for 21 days; if complete response not achieved, may repeat a second course after 15 days (Tilly, 1990)

AML consolidation (unlabeled use): I.V.:

5 + 2 regimens: 100 mg/m²/day continuous infusion for 5 days (in combination with daunorubicin **or** idarubicin **or** mitoxantrone) (Arlin, 1990; Wiernick, 1992)

5 + 2 + 5 regimen: 100 mg/m²/day continuous infusion for 5 days (in combination with daunorubicin **and** etoposide) (Bishop, 1996)

Single-agent: Adults ≤60 years: 3000 mg/m² over 3 hours every 12 hours on days 1, 3, and 5 (total of 6 doses); repeat every 28-35 days for 4 courses (Mayer, 1994)

AML salvage treatment (unlabeled use): I.V.:

ADE regimen: Course 1: 100 mg/m² I.V push every 12 hours for 10 days (in combination with daunorubicin and etoposide) followed by Course 2: 100 mg/m² I.V push every 12 hours for 8 days (Milligan, 2006)

CLAG regimen: 2000 mg/m²/day over 4 hours for 5 days (in combination with cladribine and G-CSF); may repeat once if needed (Wrzesień -Kuś, 2003)

CLAG-M regimen: 2000 mg/m²/day over 4 hours for 5 days (in combination with cladribine, G-CSF, and mitoxantrone); may repeat once if needed (Wierzbowska, 2008)

FLAG regimen: 2000 mg/m²/day over 4 hours for 5 days (in combination with fludarabine and G-CSF); may repeat once if needed (Montillo, 1998)

HiDAC (high-dose cytarabine) ± an anthracycline: 3000 mg/m² over 1 hour every 12 hours for 12 doses (Herzig, 1985)

MEC regimen: 1000 mg/m²/day over 6 hours for 6 days (in combination with mitoxantrone and etoposide) (Amadori, 1991) **or**

Adults <60 years: 500 mg/m²/day continuous infusion days 1, 2, and 3 and days 8, 9, and 10 (in combination with mitoxantrone and etoposide); may administer a second course if needed (Archimbaud, 1991; Archimbaud, 1995)

Acute promyelocytic leukemia (APL) induction (unlabeled dosing): I.V.: 200 mg/m²/day continuous infusion for 7 days beginning on day 3 of treatment (in combination with tretinoin and daunorubicin) (Ades, 2006; Powell, 2010)

APL consolidation (unlabeled use): I.V.:

In combination with idarubicin and tretinoin: High-risk patients (WBC ≥10,000/mm³) (Sanz, 2010): Adults ≤60 years:

First consolidation course: 1000 mg/m²/day for 4 days

Third consolidation course: 150 mg/m² every 8 hours for 4 days

In combination with idarubicin, tretinoin, and thioguanine: High-risk patients (WBC >10,000/mm³) (Lo Coco, 2010): Adults ≤61 years:

First consolidation course: 1000 mg/m²/day for 4 days

Third consolidation course: 150 mg/m² every 8 hours for 5 days

In combination with daunorubicin (Ades, 2006; Ades, 2008):
First consolidation course: 200 mg/m^2/day for 7 days
Second consolidation course:
Age ≤60 years and low risk (WBC <10,000/mm^3): 1000 mg/m^2 every 12 hours for 4 days (8 doses)
Age <50 years and high risk (WBC ≥10,000/mm^3): 2000 mg/m^2 every 12 hours for 5 days (10 doses)
Age 50-60 years and high risk (WBC ≥10,000/mm^3): 1500 mg/m^2 every 12 hours for 5 days (10 doses) (Ades, 2008)
Age >60 years and high risk (WBC ≥10,000/mm^3): 1000 mg/m^2 every 12 hours for 4 days (8 doses)

Acute lymphocytic leukemia (ALL; unlabeled dosing):
Induction regimen, relapsed or refractory: I.V.: 3000 mg/m^2 over 3 hours daily for 5 days (in combination with idarubicin [day 3]) (Weiss, 2002)
Dose-intensive regimen: I.V.: 3000 mg/m^2 over 2 hours every 12 hours days 2 and 3 (4 doses/cycle) of even numbered cycles (in combination with methotrexate; alternates with Hyper-CVAD) (Kantarjian, 2000)
Larson regimen (Larson, 1995): SubQ
Early intensification phase: 75 mg/m^2/dose days 1-4 and 8-11 (4-week cycle; repeat once)
Late intensification phase: 75 mg/m^2/dose days 29-32 and 36-39
Linker protocol: I.V.: 300 mg/m^2/day days 1, 4, 8, and 11 of even numbered consolidation cycles (in combination with teniposide) (Linker, 1991)

Chronic lymphocytic leukemia (CLL; unlabeled use):
OFAR regimen: I.V.: 1000 mg/m^2/dose over 2 hours days 2 and 3 every 4 weeks for up to 6 cycles (in combination with oxaliplatin, fludarabine, and rituximab) (Tsimberidou, 2008)

Chronic myeloid leukemia (CML; unlabeled dosing): SubQ: 20 mg/m^2 once daily days 15-24 every month (in combination with interferon alfa-2b) (Guilhot, 1997)

CNS lymphoma, primary (unlabeled use): I.V.: 2000 mg/m^2 over 1 hour every 12 hours days 2 and 3 (total of 4 doses) every 3 weeks (in combination with methotrexate and followed by whole brain irradiation) for a total of 4 courses (Ferreri, 2009)

Hodgkin lymphoma, relapsed or refractory (unlabeled use): I.V.:
DHAP regimen: 2000 mg/m^2 over 3 hours every 12 hours day 2 (total of 2 doses/cycle) for 2 cycles (in combination with dexamethasone and cisplatin) (Josting, 2002)
ESHAP regimen: 2000 mg/m^2 day 5 (in combination with etoposide, methylprednisolone, and cisplatin) every 3-4 weeks for 3 or 6 cycles (Aparicio, 1999)
Mini-BEAM regimen: 100 mg/m^2 every 12 hours days 2-5 (total of 8 doses) every 4-6 weeks (in combination with carmustine, etoposide, and melphalan) (Colwill, 1995; Martin, 2001)
BEAM regimen (transplant preparative regimen): 200 mg/m^2 twice daily for 4 days beginning 5 days prior to transplant (in combination with carmustine, etoposide, and melphalan) (Chopra, 1993)

Non-Hodgkin's lymphomas (unlabeled use): I.V.:
CALGB 9251 regimen: Cycles 2, 4, and 6: 150 mg/m^2/day continuous infusion days 4 and 5 (Lee, 2001; Rizzieri, 2004)
CODOX-M/IVAC regimen:
Adults ≤60 years: Cycles 2 and 4 (IVAC): 2000 mg/m^2 every 12 hours days 1 and 2 (total of 4 doses/cycle) (IVAC is combination with ifosfamide, mesna, and etoposide; IVAC alternates with CODOX-M) (Magrath, 1996)
Adults ≤65 years: Cycles 2 and 4 (IVAC): 2000 mg/m^2 over 3 hours every 12 hours days 1 and 2 (total of 4 doses/cycle) (IVAC is combination with ifosfamide, mesna, and etoposide; IVAC alternates with CODOX-M) (Mead, 2008)
Adults >65 years: Cycles 2 and 4 (IVAC): 1000 mg/m^2 over 3 hours every 12 hours days 1 and 2 (total of 4 doses/cycle) (IVAC is combination with ifosfamide, mesna, and etoposide; IVAC alternates with CODOX-M) (Mead, 2008)
DHAP regimen:
Adults ≤70 years: 2000 mg/m^2 over 3 hours every 12 hours day 2 (total of 2 doses/cycle) every 3-4 weeks for 6-10 cycles (in combination with dexamethasone and cisplatin) (Velasquez, 1988)
Adults >70 years: 1000 mg/m^2 over 3 hours every 12 hours day 2 (total of 2 doses/cycle) every 3-4 weeks for 6-10 cycles (in combination with dexamethasone and cisplatin) (Velasquez, 1988)
ESHAP regimen: 2000 mg/m^2 over 2 hours day 5 every 3-4 weeks for 6-8 cycles (in combination with etoposide, methylprednisolone, and cisplatin) (Velasquez, 1994)
BEAM regimen (transplant preparative regimen): 200 mg/m^2 twice daily for 3 days beginning 4 days prior to transplant (in combination with carmustine, etoposide, and melphalan) (Linch 2010) **or** 100 mg/m^2 over 1 hour every 12 hours for 4 days beginning 5 days prior to transplant (in combination with carmustine, etoposide, and melphalan) (van Imhoff, 2005)

Intrathecal (I.T.):

Meningeal leukemia: Note: Optimal intrathecal chemotherapy dosing should be based on age rather than on body surface area (BSA); CSF volume correlates with age and not to BSA (Bleyer, 1983; Kerr, 2001). Dosing provided in the FDA-approved labeling is BSA-based (usual dose 30 mg/m^2 every 4 days; range: 5-75 mg/m^2 once daily for 4 days or once every 4 days until CNS findings normalize, followed by 1 additional treatment).

Children: Age-based intrathecal dosing (unlabeled):
CNS prophylaxis:
<1 year: 20 mg per dose
1 to 1.99 years: 30 mg per dose
2 to 2.99 years: 50 mg per dose
≥3 years: 70 mg per dose
ALL CNS prophylaxis, age-specific doses from literature:
Administer on day 0 of induction therapy (Gaynon, 1993):
1 to <2 years: 30 mg per dose
2 to <3 years: 50 mg per dose
≥3 years: 70 mg per dose
Administer as part of triple intrathecal therapy (TIT) on days 1 and 15 of induction therapy; days 1, 15, 50, and 64 (standard risk patients) or days 1, 15, 29, and 43 (high-risk patients) during consolidation therapy; day 1 of reinduction therapy, and during maintenance therapy (very high-risk patients receive on days 1, 22, 45, and 59 of induction, days 8, 22, 36, and 50 of consolidation therapy, days 8 and 38 of reinduction therapy, and during maintenance) (Lin, 2007):
<1 year: 18 mg per dose
1-2 years: 24 mg per dose
2-3 years: 30 mg per dose
≥3 years: 36 mg per dose
Administer on day 0 of induction therapy, then as part of TIT on days 7, 14, and 21 during consolidation therapy; as part of TIT on days 0, 28, and 35 for 2 cycles of delayed intensification therapy, and then maintenance treatment as part of TIT on day 0 every 12 weeks for 38 months (boys) or 26 months (girls) from initial induction treatment (Matloub, 2006):
1 to <2 years: 16 mg per dose
2 to <3 years: 20 mg per dose
≥3 years: 24-30 mg per dose

Administer on day 15 of induction therapy, days 1 and 15 of reinduction phase; and day 1 of cycle 2 of maintenance 1A phase (Pieters, 2007):
<1 year: 15 mg per dose
≥1 year: 20 mg per dose

Treatment, CNS leukemia (ALL): Children: Administer as part of TIT weekly until CSF remission, then every 4 weeks throughout continuation treatment (Lin, 2007):
<1 year: 18 mg per dose
1-2 years: 24 mg per dose
2-3 years: 30 mg per dose
≥3 years: 36 mg per dose

Adult unlabeled uses or doses for intrathecal therapy:
CNS prophylaxis (ALL): 100 mg weekly for 8 doses, then every 2 weeks for 8 doses, then monthly for 6 doses (high-risk patients) **or** 100 mg on day 7 or 8 with each chemotherapy cycle for 4 doses (low risk patients) **or** 16 doses (high-risk patients) (Cortes, 1995)
or as part of TIT: 40 mg days 0 and 14 during induction, days 1, 4, 8, and 11 during CNS therapy phase, every 18 weeks during intensification and maintenance phases (Storring, 2009)
CNS prophylaxis (APL, as part of TIT): 50 mg per dose; administer 1 dose prior to consolidation and 2 doses during each of 2 consolidation phases (total of 5 doses) (Ades, 2006; Ades, 2008)
CNS leukemia treatment (ALL, as part of TIT): 40 mg twice weekly until CSF cleared (Storring, 2009)
CNS lymphoma treatment: 50 mg twice a week for 4 weeks, then weekly for 4-8 weeks, then every other week for 4 weeks, then every 4 weeks for 4 doses (Glantz, 1999)
Leptomeningeal metastases treatment: 50 mg twice a week for 4 weeks, then weekly for 4 weeks then monthly for 4 doses (NCCN CNS cancer guidelines v.1.2010) **or** 40-60 mg per dose (DeAngelis, 2005)

Dosage adjustment in renal impairment: The FDA-approved labeling does not contain renal dosing adjustment guidelines; the following guidelines have been used by some clinicians:
Aronoff, 2007 (Cytarabine 100-200 mg/m^2): Children and Adults: No adjustment necessary
Kintzel, 1995 (High-dose cytarabine 1-3 g/m^2):
Cl_{cr} 46-60 mL/minute: Administer 60% of dose
Cl_{cr} 31-45 mL/minute: Administer 50% of dose
Cl_{cr} <30 mL/minute: Consider use of alternative drug
Smith, 1997 (High-dose cytarabine; ≥2 g/m^2/dose):
Serum creatinine 1.5-1.9 mg/dL or increase (from baseline) of 0.5-1.2 mg/dL: Reduce dose to 1 g/m^2/dose
Serum creatinine ≥2 mg/dL or increase (from baseline) of >1.2 mg/dL: Reduce dose to 0.1 g/m^2/day as a continuous infusion
Hemodialysis: In 4 hour dialysis sessions (with high flow polysulfone membrane) 6 hours after cytarabine 1 g/m^2 over 2 hours, 63% of the metabolite ARA-U was extracted from plasma (based on a single adult case report) (based on a single adult case report) (Radeski, 2011)

Dosage adjustment in hepatic impairment: Dose may need to be adjusted in patients with liver failure since cytarabine is partially detoxified in the liver. The FDA-approved labeling does not contain hepatic dosing adjustment guidelines; the following guideline has been used by some clinicians:
Floyd, 2006: Transaminases (any elevation): Administer 50% of dose; may increase subsequent doses in the absence of toxicities
Koren, 1992 (dose level not specified): Bilirubin >2 mg/dL: Administer 50% of dose; may increase subsequent doses in the absence of toxicities

Administration
I.V.: Infuse standard dose therapy for AML (100-200 mg/m^2/day) as a continuous infusion. Infuse high-dose therapy (unlabeled) over 1-3 hours (usually). Other rates have been used, refer to specific reference.
I.T.: Intrathecal doses should be administered as soon as possible after preparation.
May also be administered SubQ.

Monitoring Parameters Liver function tests, CBC with differential and platelet count, serum creatinine, BUN, serum uric acid

Additional Information I.V. doses ≥1.5 g/m^2 may produce conjunctivitis which can be ameliorated with prophylactic use of corticosteroid (0.1% dexamethasone) eye drops. Dexamethasone eye drops should be administered at 1-2 drops every 6 hours during and for 2-7 days after completion of cytarabine.

Dosage Forms Excipient information presented when available (limited, particularly for generics); consult specific product labeling.
Injection, powder for reconstitution: 100 mg [contains benzyl alcohol (in diluent)], 500 mg [contains benzyl alcohol (in diluent)], 1 g [contains benzyl alcohol (in diluent)], 2 g [contains benzyl alcohol (in diluent)]
Injection, solution: 20 mg/mL (25 mL) [contains benzyl alcohol]; 100 mg/mL (20 mL)
Injection, solution [preservative free]: 20 mg/mL (5 mL, 50 mL); 100 mg/mL (20 mL)

◆ **Cytarabine Hydrochloride** *see* Cytarabine (Conventional) *on page 428*

◆ **Cytarabine Lipid Complex** *see* Cytarabine (Liposomal) *on page 432*

Cytarabine (Liposomal)

(sye TARE a been lye po SO mal)

Brand Names: U.S. DepoCyt®
Brand Names: Canada DepoCyt®
Index Terms Cytarabine Lipid Complex; Cytarabine Liposome; DepoFoam-Encapsulated Cytarabine; DTC 101; Liposomal Cytarabine
Pharmacologic Category Antineoplastic Agent, Antimetabolite (Pyrimidine Antagonist)
Use Treatment of lymphomatous meningitis
Pregnancy Risk Factor D
Pregnancy Considerations Reproductive studies have not been conducted with cytarabine liposomal. Cytarabine, the active component, has been associated with fetal malformations when given as a component of systemic combination chemotherapy during the first trimester. Systemic exposure following intrathecal administration of cytarabine liposomal is negligible; however, women of childbearing potential should avoid becoming pregnant during treatment.
Lactation Excretion in breast milk unknown/not recommended
Contraindications Hypersensitivity to cytarabine or any component of the formulation; active meningeal infection
Warnings/Precautions Hazardous agent - use appropriate precautions for handling and disposal. **[U.S. Boxed Warning]: Chemical arachnoiditis (nausea, vomiting, headache, fever) occurs commonly; may be fatal if untreated. The incidence and severity of chemical arachnoiditis is reduced by coadministration with dexamethasone; dexamethasone should be administered concomitantly with cytarabine (liposomal) to diminish chemical arachnoid symptoms.** Hydrocephalus has been reported and may be precipitated by chemical arachnoiditis. May cause neurotoxicity (including myelopathy), which may lead to permanent neurologic deficit (rare); monitor for neurotoxicity; reduce subsequent doses;

discontinue with persistent neurotoxicity. The risk of neurotoxicity is increased with concurrent radiation therapy or systemic chemotherapy. The risk for neurotoxicity is increased when administered with other antineoplastic agents or with cranial/spinal irradiation. Persistent (extreme) somnolence, hemiplegia, visual disturbances (including blindness; may be permanent), deafness, cranial nerve palsies, peripheral neuropathy, and even combined neurologic features (cauda equina syndrome) have been reported. CSF flow blockage may lead to increased free cytarabine concentrations in the CSF and increase the risk for neurotoxicity; assess CSF flow prior to administration. Infectious meningitis may be associated with intrathecal administration. **[U.S. Boxed Warning]: Should be administered under the supervision of an experienced cancer chemotherapy physician; facilities appropriate for diagnosis and management of complications should be readily available.** For intrathecal use only. Intrathecal medications should not be prepared during the preparation of any other agents; after preparation, store intrathecal medications in an isolated location or container clearly marked with a label identifying as "intrathecal" use only; delivery of intrathecal medications to the patient should only be with other medications intended for administration into the central nervous system (Jacobson, 2009).

Adverse Reactions

>10%:

Cardiovascular: Peripheral edema (11%)

Central nervous system: Chemical arachnoiditis (without dexamethasone premedication: 100%; with dexamethasone premedication: 33% to 42%; grade 4: 19% to 30%; onset: ≤5 days); headache (56%), confusion (33%), fever (32%), fatigue (25%), seizure (20% to 22%), dizziness (18%), lethargy (16%), insomnia (14%), memory impairment (14%), pain (14%)

Endocrine & metabolic: Dehydration (13%)

Gastrointestinal: Nausea (46%), vomiting (44%), constipation (25%), diarrhea (12%), appetite decreased (11%)

Genitourinary: Urinary tract infection (14%)

Hematologic: Anemia (12%), thrombocytopenia (3% to 11%)

Neuromuscular & skeletal: Weakness (40%), back pain (24%), abnormal gait (23%), limb pain (15%), neck pain (14%), arthralgia (11%), neck stiffness (11%)

Ocular: Blurred vision (11%)

1% to 10%:

Cardiovascular: Tachycardia (9%), hypotension (8%), hypertension (6%), syncope (3%), edema (2%)

Central nervous system: Agitation (10%), hypoesthesia (10%), depression (8%), anxiety (7%), sensory neuropathy (3%)

Dermatologic: Pruritus (2%)

Endocrine & metabolic: Hypokalemia (7%), hyponatremia (7%), hyperglycemia (6%)

Gastrointestinal: Abdominal pain (9%), dysphagia (8%), anorexia (5%), hemorrhoids (3%), mucosal inflammation (3%)

Genitourinary: Incontinence (7%), urinary retention (5%)

Hematologic: Neutropenia (10%), contusion (2%)

Neuromuscular & skeletal: Muscle weakness (10%), tremor (9%), peripheral neuropathy (3% to 4%), abnormal reflexes (3%)

Otic: Hypoacusis (6%)

Respiratory: Dyspnea (10%), cough (7%), pneumonia (6%)

Miscellaneous: Diaphoresis (2%)

1% (Limited to important or life-threatening): Anaphylaxis, bladder control impaired, blindness, bowel control impaired, cauda equine syndrome, cranial nerve palsies, CSF protein increased, CSF WBC increased, deafness, encephalopathy, hemiplegia, hydrocephalus, infectious meningitis, intracranial pressure increased, myelopathy, neurologic deficit, numbness, papilledema, somnolence, visual disturbance

Drug Interactions

Metabolism/Transport Effects None known.

Avoid Concomitant Use There are no known interactions where it is recommended to avoid concomitant use.

Increased Effect/Toxicity There are no known significant interactions involving an increase in effect.

Decreased Effect There are no known significant interactions involving a decrease in effect.

Stability Store under refrigeration at 2°C to 8°C (36°F to 46°F); protect from freezing. Use appropriate precautions for handling and disposal. Avoid aggressive agitation. Allow vial to warm to room temperature prior to withdrawal from vial. Particles may settle in diluent over time, and may be resuspended with gentle agitation or inversion immediately prior to withdrawing from the vial. Withdraw from the vial immediately prior to administration. Solutions should be used within 4 hours of withdrawal from the vial. Do not further dilute or mix with any other medications.

Intrathecal medications should not be prepared during the preparation of any other agents. After preparation, store intrathecal medications in an isolated location or container clearly marked with a label identifying as "intrathecal" use only.

Mechanism of Action Cytarabine liposomal is a sustained-release formulation of the active ingredient cytarabine, an antimetabolite which acts through inhibition of DNA synthesis and is cell cycle-specific for the S phase of cell division. Cytarabine is converted intracellularly to its active metabolite cytarabine-5'-triphosphate (ara-CTP). Ara-CTP also appears to be incorporated into DNA and RNA; however, the primary action is inhibition of DNA polymerase, resulting in decreased DNA synthesis and repair. The liposomal formulation allows for gradual release, resulting in prolonged exposure.

Pharmacodynamics/Kinetics

Absorption: Systemic exposure following intrathecal administration is negligible since transfer rate from CSF to plasma is slow

Half-life elimination, CSF: 6-82 hours

Time to peak, CSF: Intrathecal: <1 hour

Dosage Note: Initiate dexamethasone 4 mg twice daily (oral or I.V.) for 5 days, beginning on the day of cytarabine liposomal administration.

Intrathecal: Adults:

Induction: 50 mg every 14 days for a total of 2 doses (weeks 1 and 3)

Consolidation: 50 mg every 14 days for 3 doses (weeks 5, 7, and 9), followed by an additional dose at week 13

Maintenance: 50 mg every 28 days for 4 doses (weeks 17, 21, 25, and 29)

Dosage reduction for toxicity: If drug-related neurotoxicity develops, reduce dose to 25 mg. If toxicity persists, discontinue treatment.

Administration For intrathecal use only. Dose should be removed from vial immediately before administration (must be administered within 4 hours of removal). An in-line filter should **NOT** be used. Administer directly into the CSF via an intraventricular reservoir or by direct injection into the lumbar sac. Injection should be made slowly (over 1-5 minutes). Patients should lie flat for 1 hour after lumbar puncture.

Monitoring Parameters Monitor closely for signs of an immediate reaction; neurotoxicity

Test Interactions Since cytarabine liposomes are similar in appearance to WBCs, care must be taken in interpreting CSF examinations in patients receiving cytarabine liposomal.

Dosage Forms Excipient information presented when available (limited, particularly for generics); consult specific product labeling.

Injection, suspension, intrathecal [preservative free]:
DepoCyt®: 10 mg/mL (5 mL)

- ◆ **Cytarabine Liposome** *see* Cytarabine (Liposomal) *on page 432*
- ◆ **CytoGam®** *see* Cytomegalovirus Immune Globulin (Intravenous-Human) *on page 434*

Cytomegalovirus Immune Globulin (Intravenous-Human)

(sye toe meg a low VYE rus i MYUN GLOB yoo lin in tra VEE nus HYU man)

Brand Names: U.S. CytoGam®
Brand Names: Canada CytoGam®
Index Terms CMV-IGIV
Pharmacologic Category Blood Product Derivative; Immune Globulin
Use Prophylaxis of cytomegalovirus (CMV) disease associated with kidney, lung, liver, pancreas, and heart transplants; concomitant use with ganciclovir should be considered in organ transplants (other than kidney) from CMV seropositive donors to CMV seronegative recipients
Unlabeled Use Adjunct therapy in the treatment of CMV disease in immunocompromised patients
Pregnancy Risk Factor C
Pregnancy Considerations Reproduction studies have not been conducted.
Lactation Excretion in breast milk unknown
Contraindications Hypersensitivity to CMV-IGIV, other immunoglobulins, or any component of the formulation; immunoglobulin A deficiency
Warnings/Precautions Hypersensitivity and anaphylactic reactions can occur; immediate treatment (including epinephrine 1:1000) should be available. Aseptic meningitis syndrome (AMS) has been reported with intravenous immune globulin administration (rare); may occur with high doses (≥2 g/kg). Intravenous immune globulin has been associated with antiglobulin hemolysis; monitor for signs of hemolytic anemia. Monitor for transfusion-related acute lung injury (TRALI); noncardiogenic pulmonary edema has been reported with intravenous immune globulin use. Acute renal dysfunction (increased serum creatinine, oliguria, acute renal failure) can rarely occur; usually within 7 days of use (more likely with products stabilized with sucrose). Use with caution in the elderly, patients with renal disease, diabetes mellitus, volume depletion, sepsis, paraproteinemia, and nephrotoxic medications due to risk of renal dysfunction. In patients at risk of renal dysfunction, the rate of infusion and concentration of solution should be minimized. discontinue if renal function deteriorates. Patients should not be volume depleted prior to therapy. Thrombotic events have been reported with administration of intravenous immune globulin; use with caution in patients with cardiovascular risk factors. Use with caution in patients >65 years of age. Product is stabilized with albumin. Product of human plasma; may potentially contain infectious agents which could transmit disease. Screening of donors, as well as testing and/or inactivation or removal of certain viruses, reduces the risk. Infections thought to be transmitted by this product should be reported to the manufacturer. Product is stabilized with sucrose.

Adverse Reactions
<6%:
Cardiovascular: Flushing
Central nervous system: Chills, fever
Gastrointestinal: Nausea, vomiting
Neuromuscular & skeletal: Arthralgia, back pain, muscle cramps
Respiratory: Wheezing
<1% (Limited to important or life-threatening): Acute renal failure, acute tubular necrosis, AMS, anaphylactic shock, angioneurotic edema, anuria, blood presure decreased, BUN increase, oliguria, osmotic nephrosis, proximal tubular nephropathy, serum creatinine increased

Drug Interactions
Metabolism/Transport Effects None known.
Avoid Concomitant Use There are no known interactions where it is recommended to avoid concomitant use.
Increased Effect/Toxicity There are no known significant interactions involving an increase in effect.
Decreased Effect
Cytomegalovirus Immune Globulin (Intravenous-Human) may decrease the levels/effects of: Vaccines (Live)

Stability Store between 2°C and 8°C (35.6°F and 46.4°F). Use reconstituted product within 6 hours; do not admix with other medications; do not use if turbid. Do not shake vials. Dilution is not recommended. Infusion with other products is not recommended.
Mechanism of Action CMV-IGIV is a preparation of immunoglobulin G derived from pooled healthy blood donors with a high titer of CMV antibodies; administration provides a passive source of antibodies against cytomegalovirus
Dosage I.V.: Adults:
Kidney transplant:
Initial dose (within 72 hours of transplant): 150 mg/kg/dose
2-, 4-, 6-, and 8 weeks after transplant: 100 mg/kg/dose
12 and 16 weeks after transplant: 50 mg/kg/dose
Liver, lung, pancreas, or heart transplant:
Initial dose (within 72 hours of transplant): 150 mg/kg/dose
2-, 4-, 6-, and 8 weeks after transplant: 150 mg/kg/dose
12 and 16 weeks after transplant: 100 mg/kg/dose
Severe CMV pneumonia (unlabeled): Various regimens have been used, including 400 mg/kg CMV-IGIV in combination with ganciclovir on days 1, 2, 7, or 8, followed by 200 mg/kg CMV-IGIV on days 14 and 21
Elderly: Use with caution in patients >65 years of age, may be at increased risk of renal insufficiency
Dosage adjustment in renal impairment: Use with caution; specific dosing adjustments are not available. Infusion rate should be the minimum practical; do not exceed 180 mg/kg/hour
Dietary Considerations Some products may contain sodium.
Administration Administer through an I.V. line containing an in-line filter (pore size 15 micron) using an infusion pump. Do not mix with other infusions; do not use if turbid. Begin infusion within 6 hours of entering vial, complete infusion within 12 hours.

Infuse at 15 mg/kg/hour. If no adverse reactions occur within 30 minutes, may increase rate to 30 mg/kg/hour. If no adverse reactions occur within the second 30 minutes, may increase rate to 60 mg/kg/hour; maximum rate of infusion: 75 mL/hour. When infusing subsequent doses, may decrease titration interval from 30 minutes to 15 minutes. If patient develops nausea, back pain, or flushing during infusion, slow the rate or temporarily stop the infusion. Discontinue if blood pressure drops or in case of anaphylactic reaction.
Monitoring Parameters Vital signs (throughout infusion), flushing, chills, muscle cramps, back pain, fever, nausea, vomiting, wheezing, decreased blood pressure, or anaphylaxis; renal function and urine output

Dosage Forms Excipient information presented when available (limited, particularly for generics); consult specific product labeling.

Injection, solution [preservative free]:

CytoGam®: 50 mg (± 10 mg)/mL (50 mL) [contains sodium 20-30 mEq/L, human albumin, and sucrose 50 mg/mL]

Dabigatran Etexilate (da BIG a tran ett EX ill ate)

Brand Names: U.S. Pradaxa®

Brand Names: Canada Pradax™

Index Terms Dabigatran Etexilate Mesylate

Pharmacologic Category Anticoagulant, Thrombin Inhibitor

Use Prevention of stroke and systemic embolism in patients with nonvalvular atrial fibrillation

2011 ACCF/AHA/HRS atrial fibrillation guidelines: Not recommended for patients with coexisting prosthetic heart valve or hemodynamically significant valve disease, severe renal failure (Cl_{cr} <15 mL/minute), or advanced liver disease (impaired baseline clotting function)

Canadian labeling: Additional uses (not in U.S. labeling): Postoperative thromboprophylaxis in patients who have undergone total hip or knee replacement procedures

Pregnancy Risk Factor C

Pregnancy Considerations Adverse events were observed in some animal reproductive studies. There are no adequate and well-controlled studies in pregnant women. Dabigatran etexilate should be used in pregnant women only if clinical benefit outweighs risks of therapy.

Lactation Excretion in breast milk unknown/use caution

Medication Guide Available Yes

Contraindications

Serious hypersensitivity (eg, anaphylaxis) to dabigatran or any component of the formulation; active pathological bleeding

Canadian labeling: Additional contraindications (not in U.S. labeling): Severe renal impairment (Cl_{cr} <30 mL/minute); bleeding diathesis or patients with spontaneous or pharmacological hemostatic impairment; lesions at risk of clinically significant bleeding (eg, hemorrhagic or ischemic cerebral infarction) within previous 6 months; concomitant therapy with oral ketoconazole

Warnings/Precautions The most common complication is bleeding, and sometimes fatal bleeding. Risk factors for bleeding include concurrent use of drugs that increase the risk of bleeding (eg, antiplatelet agents, heparin) and labor and delivery. Monitor for signs and symptoms of bleeding; discontinue in patients with active pathological bleeding; **no specific antidote exists for dabigatran reversal.** Therapy for severe hemorrhage may include transfusions of fresh frozen plasma, packed red blood cells, or surgical intervention when appropriate (Wann, 2011). The use of a PCC (Cofact ®, not available in the U.S.) has been shown **not** to be effective for dabigatran reversal (Eerenberg, 2011). Use in patients with moderate hepatic impairment (Child-Pugh class B) demonstrated large inter-subject variability; however no consistent change in exposure or pharmacodynamics was seen. Use in patients with advanced liver disease (impaired baseline clotting function) is not recommended (Wann, 2011). Use in patients with a coexisting prosthetic heart valve or hemodynamically significant valve disease is not recommended (Wann, 2011).

Due to an increased risk of bleeding, avoid use with other direct thrombin inhibitors (eg, bivalirudin), unfractionated heparin or heparin derivatives, low molecular weight heparins (eg, enoxaparin), fondaparinux, thienopyridines (eg, clopidogrel, ticlodipine), GPIIb/IIIa antagonists (eg, eptifibatide), aspirin, coumarin derivatives, and sulfinpyrazone. NSAIDs should be used cautiously. Appropriate doses of unfractionated heparin may be used to maintain catheter patency. The concomitant use of P-gp inducers (eg, rifampin) may reduce dabigatran bioavailability and should be avoided. Concurrent use of certain P-gp inhibitors ((ie, verapamil, amiodarone, quinidine, and clarithromycin) does not require dosage adjustment if Cl_{cr} ≥30 mL/minute; however, this should not be extrapolated to other P-gp inhibitors. A dabigatran dose reduction should be considered with concurrent use of dronedarone or oral ketoconazole in patients with Cl_{cr} 30-50 mL/minute. Concurrent use of oral ketoconazole is contraindicated in the Canadian labeling. Use of any P-gp inhibitor should be avoided for Cl_{cr}<30 mL/minute.

Evaluate renal function prior to and during therapy; dabigatran exposure may increase in any degree of renal impairment. In moderate impairment, serum concentrations may increase 3 times higher than normal compared to concentrations in patients with normal renal function. However, U.S. labeling only requires dosage reduction in patients with severe renal impairment (Cl_{cr}15-30 mL/minute) and recommends avoiding use in patients with Cl_{cr} <15 mL/minute due to insufficient evidence. The Canadian labeling contraindicates use in severe renal impairment (Cl_{cr} <30 mL/minute) and recommends indication-specific dose reductions in patients with moderate impairment (Cl_{cr} 30-50 mL/minute). Discontinue therapy in any patient who develops acute renal failure.

In the elderly, use with extreme caution or consider other treatment options. No dosage adjustment is recommended in the U.S. labeling based on age alone (unless renal impairment coexists); however, numerous case reports of hemorrhage, including hemorrhagic stroke, have been reported in elderly patients (median age: 80 years), with a quarter of these reports occurring in patients ≥84 years of age. Some reports have resulted in fatality, particularly in those with low body weight and mild-to-moderate renal impairment; the risk is expected to be higher in patients receiving interacting drugs (eg, amiodarone) (Legrand, 2011). The RE-LY trial, although not powered to assess safety in the elderly, employed 110 mg and 150 mg twice daily regiments. The 110 mg twice daily regimen was not approved for use in the U.S. The Canadian labeling recommends a dose reduction for patients ≥80 years of age with atrial fibrillation and suggests that dose reductions may be considered in patients >75 years receiving postoperative thromboprophylaxis.

If possible, discontinue dabigatran 1-2 days (Cl_{cr} ≥50 mL/minute) or 3-5 days (Cl_{cr} <50 mL/minute) before invasive or surgical procedures due to the risk of bleeding; consider longer times for patients undergoing major surgery, spinal puncture, or insertion of a spinal or epidural catheter or port. If surgery cannot be delayed, the risk of bleeding is elevated; weigh risk of bleeding with urgency of procedure. Bleeding risk can be assessed by the ecarin clotting time (ECT) if available; if ECT is not available, use of aPTT may provide an approximation of dabigatran's anticoagulant activity. When temporarily discontinuing anticoagulants, including dabigatran, for active bleeding, elective surgery, or invasive procedures, the risk of stroke may increase (dependent on amount of elapsed time); avoid lapses in therapy and reinitiate therapy as soon as possible if discontinuation is warranted.

Adverse Reactions Adverse reactions listed below are reflective of both the U.S. and Canadian product information. **Important:** No specific antidote exists for dabigatran reversal. Therapy for severe hemorrhage may include transfusions of fresh frozen plasma, packed red blood cells, or surgical intervention when appropriate (Wann, 2011). The use of a prothrombin complex concentrate (PCC) (Cofact®, not available in the U.S.) has been shown to be **ineffective** for dabigatran reversal (Eerenberg, 2011).

>10%:
- Gastrointestinal: Dyspepsia (11%; includes abdominal discomfort/pain, epigastric discomfort)
- Hematologic: Bleeding (8% to 33%; major: ≤6%)

1% to 10%:
- Gastrointestinal: GI hemorrhage (≤6%), gastritis-like symptoms (eg, GERD, esophagitis, erosive gastritis, GI ulcer)
- Hematologic: Anemia (1% to 4%), hematoma (1% to 2%), hemoglobin decreased (1% to 2%), hemorrhage (post-procedural or wound: 1% to 2%)
- Hepatic: ALT increased (≥3 x ULN: 2% to 3%)
- Renal: Hematuria (1%)
- Miscellaneous: Wound secretion (5%), postprocedural discharge (1%)

<1% (Limited to important or life-threatening): Allergic edema, anaphylactic shock, anaphylaxis, AST increased, bloody discharge, ecchymosis, epistaxis, hemarthrosis, hematocrit decreased, hemorrhage (catheter site, hemorrhoidal, incision site, rectal), hepatic function abnormal, occult blood positive, pruritus, rash, thrombocytopenia, urticaria

Drug Interactions

Metabolism/Transport Effects None known.

Avoid Concomitant Use

Avoid concomitant use of Dabigatran Etexilate with any of the following: P-glycoprotein/ABCB1 Inducers; Rivaroxaban

Increased Effect/Toxicity

Dabigatran Etexilate may increase the levels/effects of: Anticoagulants; Collagenase (Systemic); Deferasirox; Ibritumomab; Rivaroxaban; Tositumomab and Iodine I 131 Tositumomab

The levels/effects of Dabigatran Etexilate may be increased by: Amiodarone; Antiplatelet Agents; Dasatinib; Dronedarone; Herbs (Anticoagulant/Antiplatelet Properties); Ketoconazole; Ketoconazole (Systemic); Nonsteroidal Anti-Inflammatory Agents; Pentosan Polysulfate Sodium; P-glycoprotein/ABCB1 Inhibitors; Prostacyclin Analogues; QuiNIDine; Salicylates; Thrombolytic Agents; Verapamil

Decreased Effect

The levels/effects of Dabigatran Etexilate may be decreased by: Antacids; Atorvastatin; P-glycoprotein/ABCB1 Inducers; Proton Pump Inhibitors

Ethanol/Nutrition/Herb Interactions

Food: Food has no affect on the bioavailability of dabigatran, but delays the time to peak plasma concentrations by 2 hours.

Herb/Nutraceutical: St John's wort may decrease levels/effects of dabigatran (concomitant use is not recommended). Concomitant use of dabigatran with herbs possessing anticoagulant/antiplatelet properties may increase the risk for bleeding.

Stability

Blister: Store at 25°C (77°F); excursions permitted between 15°C to 30°C (59°F to 86°F). Protect from moisture.

Bottle: Store at 25°C (77°F); excursions permitted between 15°C to 30°C (59°F to 86°F). Dispense and store in original manufacturer's bottle to protect from moisture; discard 4 months after opening original container.

Mechanism of Action Prodrug lacking anticoagulant activity that is converted *in vivo* to the active dabigatran, a specific, reversible, direct thrombin inhibitor that inhibits both free and fibrin-bound thrombin. Inhibits coagulation by preventing thrombin-mediated effects, including cleavage of fibrinogen to fibrin monomers, activation of factors V, VIII, XI, and XIII, and inhibition of thrombin-induced platelet aggregation.

Pharmacodynamics/Kinetics

Absorption: Rapid; initially slow postoperatively

Distribution: V_d: 50-70 L

Protein binding: 35%

Metabolism: Hepatic; dabigatran etexilate is rapidly and completely hydrolyzed to dabigatran (active form) by plasma and hepatic esterases; dabigatran undergoes hepatic glucuronidation to active acylglucuronide isomers (similar activity to parent compound; accounts for <10% of total dabigatran in plasma)

Bioavailability: 3% to 7%

Half-life elimination: 12-17 hours; Elderly: 14-17 hours; Mild-to-moderate renal impairment: 15-18 hours; Severe renal impairment: 28 hours (Stangier, 2010)

Time to peak, plasma: Dabigatran: 1 hour; delayed 2 hours by food (no effect on bioavailability)

Excretion: Urine (80%)

Dosage Oral:

Adults:

Nonvalvular atrial fibrillation (to prevent stroke and systemic embolism): 150 mg twice daily

Conversion from a parenteral anticoagulant: Initiate dabigatran ≤2 hours prior to the time of the next scheduled dose of the parenteral anticoagulant (eg, enoxaparin) or at the time of discontinuation for a continuously administered parenteral drug (eg, I.V. heparin); discontinue parenteral anticoagulant at the time of dabigatran initiation.

Conversion to a parenteral anticoagulant: Wait 12 hours (Cl_{cr} ≥30 mL/minute) or 24 hours (Cl_{cr} <30 mL/minute) after the last dose of dabigatran before initiating a parenteral anticoagulant.

Conversion from warfarin: Discontinue warfarin and initiate dabigatran when INR <2.0

Conversion to warfarin: Start time must be adjusted based on Cl_{cr}:

Cl_{cr} >50 mL/minute: Initiate warfarin 3 days before discontinuation of dabigatran

Cl_{cr} 31-50 mL/minute: Initiate warfarin 2 days before discontinuation of dabigatran

Cl_{cr} 15-30 mL/minute: Initiate warfarin 1 day before discontinuation of dabigatran

Cl_{cr} <15 mL/minute: No recommendations provided

Note: Since dabigatran contributes to INR elevation, warfarin's effect on the INR will be better reflected after dabigatran has been stopped for ≥2 days

Dosing adjustment with concomitant medications:

Dronedarone with Cl_{cr} 30-50 mL/minute: Consider dabigatran dose reduction to 75 mg twice daily

Ketoconazole (oral) with Cl_{cr} 30-50 mL/minute: Consider dabigatran dose reduction to 75 mg twice daily

Postoperative thromboprophylaxis (Canadian labeling): **Note:** Therapy should not be initiated until hemostasis has been established. When transitioning from parenteral anticoagulation therapy, initiate oral dabigatran therapy ≤2 hours prior to the time of next regularly scheduled dose of intermittent parenteral anticoagulant or at the time of discontinuation for continuously administered parenteral anticoagulation therapy. When transitioning from dabigatran to I.V. anticoagulation therapy, allow 24 hours after the last dabigatran dose before initiating I.V. anticoagulation therapy.

Knee replacement: Initial: 110 mg given 1-4 hours after completion of surgery and establishment of hemostasis **OR** 220 mg as 1 dose in postoperative patients in whom therapy is not initiated on day of surgery regardless of reason; maintenance: 220 mg once daily (total duration of therapy: 10 days)

Hip replacement: Initial: 110 mg given 1-4 hours after completion of surgery and establishment of hemostasis **OR** 220 mg as 1 dose in postoperative patients in whom therapy is not initiated on day of surgery regardless of reason; maintenance: 220 mg once daily (total duration of therapy: 28-35 days)

Elderly:

Nonvalvular atrial fibrillation (to prevent stroke and systemic embolism):

U.S. labeling:

Patients >65 years: Refer to adult dosing. No dosage adjustment required unless renal impairment exists; however, increased risk of bleeding has been observed, particularly in elderly patients with low body weight and/or concomitant renal impairment.

Patients ≥80 years: **Use with extreme caution or consider other treatment options;** no dosage adjustment provided in manufacturer's labeling; however, numerous cases of hemorrhage, including hemorrhagic stroke, have been reported postmarketing, particularly in this age group of octogenarians. Due to a lack of available dosing options available in the U.S., consider avoiding use of dabigatran in this population.

Canadian labeling:

Patients <80 years: 150 mg twice daily; **Note:** The manufacturer labeling suggests that a dose reduction to 110 mg twice daily may be considered in patients >75 years with at least one other risk factor for bleeding, however, efficacy in stroke prevention may be lessened with this dose reduction.

Patients ≥80 years: 110 mg twice daily

Postoperative thromboprophylaxis (Canadian labeling): Patients >75 years: 220 mg/day. Manufacturer labeling suggests that a dose reduction to 150 mg/day may be considered.

Dosing adjustment in renal impairment:

Nonvalvular atrial fibrillation (to prevent stroke and systemic embolism):

U.S. labeling:

Cl_{cr} >30 mL/minute: No dosage adjustment provided in manufacturer's labeling (unless patient receiving certain concomitant medications); however, use with caution in mild-to-moderate renal impairment due to risk for increased dabigatran exposure (concentrations may be increased 3 times higher than normal concentrations in moderate impairment), particularly if patient is also of advanced age.

Cl_{cr} 30-50 mL/minute and patient receiving concomitant dronedarone or oral ketoconazole: Consider dose reduction to 75 mg twice daily.

Cl_{cr} 15-30 mL/minute: 75 mg twice daily; if concomitant administration with any P-gp inhibitor (including dronedarone or oral ketoconazole), avoid concurrent use. **Note:** Patients with Cl_{cr} <30 mL/minute were excluded from the RE-LY trial (Connolly, 2009)

Cl_{cr} <15 mL/minute: Use not recommended (has not been studied)

ESRD requiring hemodialysis: Use not recommended (has not been studied); **Note:** Hemodialysis removes ~60% over 2-3 hours

Canadian labeling:

Cl_{cr} ≥30 mL/minute: No dosage adjustment recommended

Severe renal impairment (Cl_{cr} <30 mL/minute): Use is contraindicated

Postoperative thromboprophylaxis (Canadian labeling):

Moderate renal impairment (Cl_{cr} 30-50 mL/minute): Initial: 75 mg given 1-4 hours after completion of surgery and establishment of hemostasis; Maintenance: 150 mg/day

Severe renal impairment (Cl_{cr} < 30 mL/minute): Use is contraindicated

Dosing adjustment in hepatic impairment: Nonvalvular atrial fibrillation (to prevent stroke and systemic embolism): No dosage adjustment required

Dietary Considerations May be taken without regard to meals.

Administration Do not break, chew, or open capsules, as this will lead to 75% increase in absorption and potentially serious adverse reactions. Administer with water. May be taken without regard to meals.

Monitoring Parameters Activated partial thromboplastin time (aPTT) (values >2.5 x control may indicate overanticoagulation), ecarin clotting test (ECT) if available, thrombin time (TT), CBC with differential, renal function (at least annually if Cl_{cr} <50 mL/minute or age >75 years)

Reference Range

At therapeutic dabigatran doses, aPTT, ECT (ecarin clotting time), and TT (thrombin time) are prolonged. A median peak aPTT of ~2 x control and a median trough aPTT of 1.5 x control were observed in subjects taking dabigatran 150 mg twice daily in the RE-LY trail

A therapeutic range has not been established for aPTT or for other tests of anticoagulant activity

Dosage Forms Excipient information presented when available (limited, particularly for generics); consult specific product labeling.

Capsule, oral:

Pradaxa®: 75 mg, 150 mg

Dosage Forms: Canada Excipient information presented when available (limited, particularly for generics); consult specific product labeling.

Capsule, oral:

Pradax™: 75 mg, 110 mg, 150 mg

◆ **Dabigatran Etexilate Mesylate** *see* Dabigatran Etexilate *on page 435*

◆ **DABIL2** *see* Denileukin Diftitox *on page 469*

Dacarbazine (da KAR ba zeen)

Brand Names: Canada Dacarbazine for Injection

Index Terms DIC; Dimethyl Triazeno Imidazole Carboxamide; DTIC; DTIC-Dome; Imidazole Carboxamide; Imidazole Carboxamide Dimethyltriazene; WR-139007

Pharmacologic Category Antineoplastic Agent, Alkylating Agent (Triazene)

Use Treatment of malignant melanoma, Hodgkin's disease

Unlabeled Use Treatment of soft-tissue sarcomas, islet cell tumors, pheochromocytoma, medullary carcinoma of the thyroid

Pregnancy Risk Factor C

Pregnancy Considerations [U.S. Boxed Warning]: This agent is carcinogenic and/or teratogenic when used in animals; adverse effects have been observed in animal studies. There are no adequate and well-controlled trials in pregnant women; use in pregnancy only if the potential benefit outweighs the potential risk to the fetus.

Lactation Excretion in breast milk unknown/not recommended

Contraindications Hypersensitivity to dacarbazine or any component of the formulation

Warnings/Precautions Hazardous agent - use appropriate precautions for handling and disposal. **[U.S. Boxed Warnings]: Bone marrow suppression is a common toxicity;** leukopenia and thrombocytopenia may be severe; may result in treatment delays or discontinuation; monitor closely. **Hepatotoxicity with hepatocellular necrosis and hepatic vein thrombosis has been reported (rare),** usually with combination chemotherapy, but may occur with dacarbazine alone. The half-life is increased in patients with renal and/or hepatic impairment; use caution, monitor for toxicity and consider dosage reduction. Anaphylaxis may occur following dacarbazine administration. Extravasation may result in tissue damage and severe pain. **[U.S. Boxed Warnings]: May be carcinogenic and/or teratogenic. Should be administered under the supervision of an experienced cancer chemotherapy physician.** Carefully evaluate the potential benefits of therapy against the risk for toxicity.

Adverse Reactions Frequency not always defined.

Dermatologic: Alopecia

Gastrointestinal: Nausea and vomiting (>90%), anorexia

Hematologic: Myelosuppression (onset: 5-7 days; nadir: 7-10 days; recovery: 21-28 days), leukopenia, thrombocytopenia

Local: Pain on infusion

Infrequent, postmarketing, and/or case reports: Anaphylactic reactions, anemia, diarrhea, eosinophilia, erythema, facial flushing, facial paresthesia, flu-like syndrome (fever, myalgia, malaise), hepatic necrosis, hepatic vein occlusion, liver enzymes increased (transient), paresthesia, photosensitivity, rash, renal functions test abnormalities, taste alteration, urticaria

Drug Interactions

Metabolism/Transport Effects Substrate of CYP1A2 (major), CYP2E1 (major); **Note:** Assignment of Major/Minor substrate status based on clinically relevant drug interaction potential

Avoid Concomitant Use

Avoid concomitant use of Dacarbazine with any of the following: BCG; CloZAPine; Natalizumab; Pimecrolimus; Tacrolimus (Topical); Vaccines (Live)

Increased Effect/Toxicity

Dacarbazine may increase the levels/effects of: CloZAPine; Leflunomide; Natalizumab; Vaccines (Live)

The levels/effects of Dacarbazine may be increased by: Abiraterone Acetate; CYP1A2 Inhibitors (Moderate); CYP1A2 Inhibitors (Strong); CYP2E1 Inhibitors (Moderate); CYP2E1 Inhibitors (Strong); Deferasirox; Denosumab; MAO Inhibitors; Pimecrolimus; Roflumilast; Tacrolimus (Topical); Trastuzumab

Decreased Effect

Dacarbazine may decrease the levels/effects of: BCG; Coccidioidin Skin Test; Sipuleucel-T; Vaccines (Inactivated); Vaccines (Live)

The levels/effects of Dacarbazine may be decreased by: CYP1A2 Inducers (Strong); Cyproterone; Echinacea; SORAfenib

Ethanol/Nutrition/Herb Interactions

Ethanol: Avoid ethanol (due to GI irritation).

Herb/Nutraceutical: Avoid dong quai, St John's wort (may also cause photosensitization).

Stability Store intact vials under refrigeration (2°C to 8°C). Protect from light. The following stability information has also been reported: Intact vials are stable for 3 months at room temperature (Cohen, 2007). Reconstituted solution is stable for 24 hours at room temperature (20°C) and 96 hours under refrigeration (4°C) when protected from light, although the manufacturer recommends use within 72 hours if refrigerated and 8 hours at room temperature. Solutions for infusion (in D_5W or NS) are stable for 24 hours at room temperature if protected from light. Decomposed drug turns pink.

The manufacturer recommends reconstituting 100 mg and 200 mg vials with 9.9 mL and 19.7 mL SWFI, respectively, to a concentration of 10 mg/mL; some institutions use different standard dilutions (eg, 20 mg/mL). Use appropriate precautions for handling and disposal.

Standard I.V. dilution: Dilute in 250-1000 mL D_5W or NS.

Mechanism of Action Dacarbazine is an alkylating agent. It is converted to the active alkylating metabolite MTIC [(methyl-triazene-1-yl)-imidazole-4-carboxamide]. The cytotoxic effects of MTIC are manifested through alkylation of DNA at the O^6, N^7 guanine positions which appears to attack cross-links strands of DNA resulting in the inhibition of DNA, RNA, and protein synthesis.

Pharmacodynamics/Kinetics

Distribution: V_d: 0.6 L/kg, exceeding total body water; suggesting binding to some tissue (probably liver)

Protein binding: ~5%

Metabolism: Extensively hepatic to the active metabolite MTIC [(methyl-triazene-1-yl)-imidazole-4-carboxamide]

Half-life elimination: Biphasic: Initial: 20-40 minutes, Terminal: 5 hours; Patients with renal and hepatic dysfunction: Initial: 55 minutes, Terminal: 7.2 hours

Excretion: Urine (~40% as unchanged drug)

Dosage Details concerning dosing in combination regimens should also be consulted. I.V.:

Children: Hodgkin's disease (combination chemotherapy): 375 mg/m^2/dose days 1 and 15 every 4 weeks (ABVD regimen; Hutchinson, 1998)

Adults:

Hodgkin's disease (combination chemotherapy): 375 mg/m^2/dose days 1 and 15 every 4 weeks (ABVD regimen)

Metastatic melanoma: 250 mg/m^2/dose days 1-5 every 3 weeks

Metastatic melanoma (unlabeled dosing; in combination with cisplatin and vinblastine): 800 mg/m^2 on day 1 every 3 weeks (Atkins, 2008; Eton, 2002)

Soft tissue sarcoma (unlabeled use; MAID regimen): 250 mg/m^2/day continuous infusion for 4 days every 3 weeks (total of 1000 mg/m^2/cycle) (Antman, 1993; Antman, 1998)

Dosage adjustment in renal impairment: The FDA-approved labeling does not contain dosage adjustment guidelines. The following guidelines have been used by some clinicians (Kintzel, 1995):
Cl_{cr} 46-60 mL/minute: Administer 80% of dose
Cl_{cr} 31-45 mL/minute: Administer 75% of dose
Cl_{cr} <30 mL/minute: Administer 70% of dose

Dosage adjustment in hepatic impairment: The FDA-approved labeling does not contain adjustment guidelines. May cause hepatotoxicity; monitor closely for signs of toxicity.

Administration Infuse over 30-60 minutes; rapid infusion may cause severe venous irritation. May also be administered as a continuous infusion (unlabeled administration rate) depending on the protocol.

Extravasation management: Local pain, burning sensation, and irritation at the injection site may be relieved by local application of hot packs. If extravasation occurs, apply cold packs. Protect exposed tissue from light following extravasation.

Monitoring Parameters CBC with differential, liver function

Dosage Forms Excipient information presented when available (limited, particularly for generics); consult specific product labeling.
Injection, powder for reconstitution: 100 mg, 200 mg

◆ **Dacarbazine for Injection (Can)** *see* Dacarbazine *on page 438*
◆ **Dacodyl™ [OTC]** *see* Bisacodyl *on page 219*
◆ **Dacogen®** *see* Decitabine *on page 460*
◆ **DACT** *see* DACTINomycin *on page 439*

DACTINomycin (dak ti noe MYE sin)

Brand Names: U.S. Cosmegen®
Brand Names: Canada Cosmegen®
Index Terms ACT-D; Actinomycin; Actinomycin Cl; Actinomycin D; DACT
Pharmacologic Category Antineoplastic Agent, Antibiotic
Use Treatment of Wilms' tumor, childhood rhabdomyosarcoma, Ewing's sarcoma, metastatic testicular tumors (nonseminomatous), gestational trophoblastic neoplasm; regional perfusion (palliative or adjunctive) of locally recurrent or locoregional solid tumors (sarcomas, carcinomas and adenocarcinomas)
Unlabeled Use Treatment of ovarian cancer (germ cell or stromal tumors), osteosarcoma, soft tissue sarcoma (other than rhabdomyosarcoma)
Pregnancy Risk Factor D
Pregnancy Considerations Animal studies have demonstrated teratogenic effects and fetal loss. There are no adequate and well-controlled studies in pregnant women. Women of childbearing potential are advised not to become pregnant. Use only when potential benefit justifies potential risk to the fetus. **[U.S. Boxed Warning]: Avoid exposure during pregnancy.**
Lactation Excretion in breast milk unknown/not recommended
Contraindications Hypersensitivity to dactinomycin or any component of the formulation; patients with concurrent or recent chickenpox or herpes zoster
Warnings/Precautions [U.S. Boxed Warnings]: Hazardous agent - use appropriate precautions for handling and disposal. Dactinomycin is extremely irritating to tissues; if extravasation occurs during I.V. use, severe damage to soft tissues will occur; has led to contracture of the arm (rare). Avoid inhalation of vapors or contact with skin, mucous membrane, or eyes; avoid exposure during pregnancy. Recommended for I.V. administration only. The manufacturer recommends intermittent ice (15 minutes 4 times/day) for suspected extravasation.

May cause hepatic sinusoidal obstruction syndrome (SOS; formerly called veno-occlusive liver disease); use with caution in hepatobiliary dysfunction. Monitor for signs or symptoms of hepatic SOS, including bilirubin >1.4 mg/dL, unexplained weight gain, ascites, hepatomegaly, or unexplained right upper quadrant pain (Arndt, 2004). The risk of fatal SOS is increased in children <4 years of age.

Dactinomycin potentiates the effects of radiation therapy; use with caution in patients who have received radiation therapy; reduce dosages in patients who are receiving dactinomycin and radiation therapy simultaneously; combination with radiation therapy may result in increased GI toxicity and myelosuppression. Avoid dactinomycin use within 2 months of radiation treatment for right-sided Wilms' tumor, may increase the risk of hepatotoxicity.

Toxic effects may be delayed in onset (2-4 days following a course of treatment) and may require 1-2 weeks to reach maximum severity. Long-term observation of cancer survivors is recommended due to the increased risk of second primary tumors following treatment with radiation and antineoplastic agents. Regional perfusion therapy may result in local limb edema, soft tissue damage, and possible venous thrombosis; leakage of dactinomycin into systemic circulation may result in hematologic toxicity, infection, impaired wound healing, and mucositis. Dosage is usually expressed in **MICRO**grams and should be calculated on the basis of body surface area (BSA) in obese or edematous adult patients (to relate dose to lean body mass). Avoid administration of live vaccines during dactinomycin treatment. Avoid use in infants <6 months of age (toxic effects may occur more frequently). May be associated with an increased risk of myelosuppression in the elderly; use with caution. **[U.S. Boxed Warning]: Should be administered under the supervision of an experienced cancer chemotherapy physician.**

Adverse Reactions Frequency not defined.
Central nervous system: Fatigue, fever, lethargy, malaise
Dermatologic: Acne, alopecia (reversible), cheilitis; increased pigmentation, sloughing, or erythema of previously irradiated skin; skin eruptions
Endocrine & metabolic: Growth retardation, hyperuricemia, hypocalcemia
Gastrointestinal: Abdominal pain, anorexia, diarrhea, dysphagia, esophagitis, GI ulceration, mucositis, nausea, pharyngitis, proctitis, stomatitis, vomiting
Hematologic: Agranulocytosis, anemia, aplastic anemia, febrile neutropenia, leukopenia, myelosuppression (onset: 7 days, nadir: 14-21 days, recovery: 21-28 days), neutropenia, pancytopenia, reticulocytopenia, thrombocytopenia, thrombocytopenia (immune mediated)
Hepatic: Ascites, bilirubin increased, hepatic failure, hepatitis, hepatomegaly, hepatopathy thrombocytopenia syndrome, hepatotoxicity, liver function test abnormality, hepatic sinusoidal obstruction syndrome (SOS; veno-occlusive liver disease)
Local: Erythema, edema, epidermolysis, pain, tissue necrosis, and ulceration (following extravasation)
Neuromuscular & skeletal: Myalgia
Renal: Renal function abnormality
Respiratory: Pneumonitis
Miscellaneous: Anaphylactoid reaction, infection

Drug Interactions
Metabolism/Transport Effects None known.
Avoid Concomitant Use
Avoid concomitant use of DACTINomycin with any of the following: BCG; CloZAPine; Natalizumab; Pimecrolimus; Tacrolimus (Topical); Vaccines (Live)

Increased Effect/Toxicity
DACTINomycin may increase the levels/effects of: CloZAPine; Leflunomide; Natalizumab; Vaccines (Live)

The levels/effects of DACTINomycin may be increased by: Denosumab; Pimecrolimus; Roflumilast; Tacrolimus (Topical); Trastuzumab

Decreased Effect
DACTINomycin may decrease the levels/effects of: BCG; Coccidioidin Skin Test; Sipuleucel-T; Vaccines (Inactivated); Vaccines (Live)

The levels/effects of DACTINomycin may be decreased by: Echinacea

Stability Store at controlled room temperature of 15°C to 30°C (59°F to 86°F). Protect from light and humidity. Use appropriate precautions for handling and disposal. Dilute with 1.1 mL of preservative-free SWFI to yield a final concentration of 500 mcg/mL (diluent containing preservatives will cause precipitation). Reconstituted solutions retain potency for 24 hours at room temperature or refrigerated. May further dilute in D_5W or NS. Solutions in 50 mL D_5W are stable for 24 hours at room temperature. Cellulose ester membrane filters may partially remove dactinomycin from solution and should not be used during preparation or administration.

Mechanism of Action Binds to the guanine portion of DNA intercalating between guanine and cytosine base pairs inhibiting DNA and RNA synthesis and protein synthesis

Pharmacodynamics/Kinetics
Distribution: Children: Extensive extravascular distribution (59-714 L); does not penetrate blood-brain barrier
Metabolism: Minimal
Half-life elimination: ~36 hours; Children: Range: 14-43 hours
Excretion: Urine and feces

Dosage Details concerning dosing in combination regimens should also be consulted.

Note: Medication orders for dactinomycin are commonly written in MICROgrams (eg, 150 mcg) although many regimens list the dose in MILLIgrams (eg, mg/kg or mg/m²). One-time doses for >1000 mcg, or multiple-day doses for >500 mcg/day are not common. The dose intensity per 2-week cycle for adults and children should not exceed 15 mcg/kg/day for 5 days or 400-600 mcg/m²/day for 5 days. Some practitioners recommend calculation of the dosage for obese or edematous adult patients on the basis of body surface area in an effort to relate dosage to lean body mass.

I.V.:
Children >6 months:
Usual dose: 15 mcg/kg/day for 5 days every 3-6 weeks **or** 400-600 mcg/m²/day for 5 days every 3-6 weeks
Wilms' tumor, rhabdomyosarcoma, Ewing's sarcoma: 15 mcg/kg/day for 5 days (in various combination regimens and schedules)
Osteosarcoma (unlabeled use): 600 mcg/m²/dose days 1, 2, and 3 as part of a combination chemotherapy regimen (Goorin, 2003)

Adults:
Usual doses: 15 mcg/kg/day for 5 days every 3-6 weeks **or** 400-600 mcg/m²/day for 5 days every 3-6 weeks **or** 1000 mcg/m² on day 1 **or** 12 mcg/kg/day for 5 days (monotherapy) **or** 500 mcg/dose days 1 and 2 (as part of a combination chemotherapy regimen)
Testicular cancer: 1000 mcg/m² on day 1 (as part of a combination chemotherapy regimen)
Gestational trophoblastic neoplasm: 12 mcg/kg/day for 5 days (monotherapy) **or** 500 mcg/dose days 1 and 2 (as part of a combination chemotherapy regimen)
Wilms' tumor, Ewing's sarcoma, rhabdomyosarcoma: 15 mcg/kg/day for 5 days (in various combination regimens and schedules)
Osteosarcoma (unlabeled use): 600 mcg/m²/dose days 1, 2, and 3 as part of a combination chemotherapy regimen (Goorin, 2003)
Ovarian (germ cell) tumor (unlabeled use): 500 mcg/day for 5 days every 4 weeks (Gershenson, 1985) **or** 300 mcg/m²/day for 5 days every 4 weeks (Slayton,1985)

Regional perfusion: Adults (dosages and techniques may vary by institution; obese patients and patients with prior chemotherapy or radiation therapy may require lower doses): Lower extremity or pelvis: 50 mcg/kg; Upper extremity: 35 mcg/kg

Elderly: Elderly patients are at increased risk of myelosuppression; dosing should begin at the low end of the dosing range.

Dosage adjustment in renal impairment: No adjustment required

Administration I.V.: Administer by slow I.V. push or infuse over 10-15 minutes. Avoid extravasation. Do not filter with cellulose ester membrane filters. Do not administer I.M. or SubQ.

Monitoring Parameters CBC with differential and platelet count, liver function tests, and renal function tests; monitor for signs/symptoms of hepatic SOS, including unexplained weight gain, ascites, hepatomegaly, or unexplained right upper quadrant pain (Arndt, 2004)

Test Interactions May interfere with bioassays of antibacterial drug levels

Dosage Forms Excipient information presented when available (limited, particularly for generics); consult specific product labeling.
Injection, powder for reconstitution: 0.5 mg
Cosmegen®: 0.5 mg [contains mannitol]

◆ **Dakin's Solution** *see* Sodium Hypochlorite Solution *on page 1570*

◆ **Dalacin® C (Can)** *see* Clindamycin (Topical) *on page 381*

◆ **Dalacin® T (Can)** *see* Clindamycin (Topical) *on page 381*

◆ **Dalacin® Vaginal (Can)** *see* Clindamycin (Topical) *on page 381*

Dalfampridine (dal FAM pri deen)

Brand Names: U.S. Ampyra™

Index Terms 4-aminopyridine; 4-AP; EL-970; Fampridine-SR

Pharmacologic Category Potassium Channel Blocker

Use Treatment to improve walking in multiple sclerosis (MS) patients

Pregnancy Risk Factor C

Medication Guide Available Yes

Dosage Oral: Adults: Multiple sclerosis: 10 mg every 12 hours (maximum daily dose: 20 mg); no additional benefit seen with doses >20 mg/day

Dosing adjustment in renal impairment:
Mild renal impairment (Cl_{cr} 51-80 mL/minute): No specific adjustment recommended by the manufacturer; however, risk of seizure may be increased secondary to reduced clearance.
Moderate-to-severe renal impairment (Cl_{cr} ≤50 mL/minute): Contraindicated

Additional Information Complete prescribing information for this medication should be consulted for additional detail.

Dosage Forms Excipient information presented when available (limited, particularly for generics); consult specific product labeling.

Tablet, extended release, oral:

Ampyra™: 10 mg

- ◆ **Dalfopristin and Quinupristin** *see* Quinupristin and Dalfopristin *on page 1450*
- ◆ **Daliresp®** *see* Roflumilast *on page 1514*
- ◆ **Dallergy Drops [DSC]** *see* Chlorpheniramine and Phenylephrine *on page 345*
- ◆ **Dallergy®-JR [DSC]** *see* Chlorpheniramine and Phenylephrine *on page 345*
- ◆ **Dalmane® (Can)** *see* Flurazepam *on page 737*
- ◆ **d-Alpha Gems™ [OTC]** *see* Vitamin E *on page 1796*
- ◆ ***d*-Alpha Tocopherol** *see* Vitamin E *on page 1796*

Dalteparin (dal TE pa rin)

Brand Names: U.S. Fragmin®
Brand Names: Canada Fragmin®
Index Terms Dalteparin Sodium
Pharmacologic Category Low Molecular Weight Heparin
Use Prevention of deep vein thrombosis (DVT) which may lead to pulmonary embolism, in patients requiring abdominal surgery who are at risk for thromboembolism complications (eg, patients >40 years of age, obesity, patients with malignancy, history of DVT or pulmonary embolism, and surgical procedures requiring general anesthesia and lasting >30 minutes); prevention of DVT in patients undergoing hip-replacement surgery; patients immobile during an acute illness; prevention of ischemic complications in patients with unstable angina or non-Q-wave myocardial infarction on concurrent aspirin therapy; in patients with cancer, extended treatment (6 months) of acute symptomatic venous thromboembolism (DVT and/or PE) to reduce the recurrence of venous thromboembolism
Unlabeled Use Active treatment of deep vein thrombosis (noncancer patients)
Pregnancy Risk Factor B
Pregnancy Considerations Multiple-dose vials contain benzyl alcohol (avoid in pregnant women due to association with gasping syndrome in premature infants). Adverse effects were not observed in animal studies. There are no adequate and well-controlled studies in pregnant women. Use during pregnancy only if clearly needed.
Lactation Enters breast milk/use caution
Contraindications Hypersensitivity to dalteparin or any component of the formulation; history of heparin-induced thrombocytopenia (HIT) or HIT with thrombosis; hypersensitivity to heparin or pork products; patients with active major bleeding; patients with unstable angina, non-Q-wave MI, or acute venous thromboembolism undergoing epidural/neuraxial anesthesia
Warnings/Precautions [U.S. Boxed Warning]: Spinal or epidural hematomas, including subsequent paralysis, may occur with recent or anticipated neuraxial anesthesia (epidural or spinal) or spinal puncture in patients anticoagulated with LMWH or heparinoids. Consider risk versus benefit prior to spinal procedures; risk is increased by the use of concomitant agents which may alter hemostasis, the use of indwelling epidural catheters for analgesia, a history of spinal deformity or spinal surgery, as well as traumatic or repeated epidural or spinal punctures. Use of dalteparin is contraindicated in patients undergoing epidural/neuraxial anesthesia. Patient should be observed closely for bleeding if enoxaparin is administered during or immediately following diagnostic lumbar puncture, epidural anesthesia, or spinal anesthesia.

Use with caution in patients with pre-existing thrombocytopenia, recent childbirth, subacute bacterial endocarditis, peptic ulcer disease, pericarditis or pericardial effusion, liver or renal function impairment, recent lumbar puncture, vasculitis, concurrent use of aspirin (increased bleeding risk), previous hypersensitivity to heparin, heparin-associated thrombocytopenia. Monitor platelet count closely. Rare cases of thrombocytopenia (some with thrombosis) have occurred. Consider discontinuation of dalteparin in any patient developing significant thrombocytopenia related to initiation of dalteparin especially when associated with a positive *in vitro* test for antiplatelet antibodies. Use caution in patients with congenital or drug-induced thrombocytopenia or platelet defects. Cancer patients with thrombocytopenia may require dose adjustments for treatment of acute venous thromboembolism. In patients with a history of heparin-induced thrombocytopenia (HIT) or HIT with thrombosis, dalteparin is contraindicated.

Monitor patient closely for signs or symptoms of bleeding. Certain patients are at increased risk of bleeding. Risk factors include bacterial endocarditis; congenital or acquired bleeding disorders; active ulcerative or angiodysplastic GI diseases; severe uncontrolled hypertension; hemorrhagic stroke; or use shortly after brain, spinal, or ophthalmology surgery; in patients treated concomitantly with platelet inhibitors; recent GI bleeding; thrombocytopenia or platelet defects; severe liver disease; hypertensive or diabetic retinopathy; or in patients undergoing invasive procedures.

Use with caution in patients with severe renal impairment; accumulation may occur with repeated dosing increasing the risk for bleeding. Multidose vials contain benzyl alcohol and should not be used in pregnant women. In neonates, large amounts of benzyl alcohol (>100 mg/kg/day) have been associated with fatal toxicity (gasping syndrome). Heparin can cause hyperkalemia by affecting aldosterone. Similar reactions could occur with dalteparin. Monitor for hyperkalemia. Do **not** administer intramuscularly. Not to be used interchangeably (unit for unit) with heparin or any other low molecular weight heparins.

There is no consensus for adjusting/correcting the weight-based dosage of LMWH for patients who are morbidly obese (BMI ≥40 kg/m^2). For patients undergoing inpatient bariatric surgery, the American College of Chest Physicians Practice Guidelines suggest using a higher thromboprophylaxis dose of LMWH for obese patients (Geerts, 2008).

Adverse Reactions Note: As with all anticoagulants, bleeding is the major adverse effect of dalteparin. Hemorrhage may occur at virtually any site. Risk is dependent on multiple variables.

>10%: Hematologic: Bleeding (3% to 14%), thrombocytopenia (including heparin-induced thrombocytopenia), <1%; cancer clinical trials: ~11%)

1% to 10%:

Hematologic: Major bleeding (up to 6%), wound hematoma (up to 3%)

Hepatic: AST >3 times upper limit of normal (5% to 9%), ALT >3 times upper limit of normal (4% to 10%)

Local: Pain at injection site (up to 12%), injection site hematoma (up to 7%)

<1% (Limited to important or life-threatening): Allergic reaction (fever, pruritus, rash, injections site reaction, bullous eruption), alopecia, anaphylactoid reaction, gastrointestinal bleeding, hemoptysis, operative site bleeding, skin necrosis, subdural hematoma, thrombosis (associated with heparin-induced thrombocytopenia). Spinal or epidural hematomas can occur following neuraxial anesthesia or spinal puncture, resulting in paralysis.

Drug Interactions

Metabolism/Transport Effects None known.

Avoid Concomitant Use

Avoid concomitant use of Dalteparin with any of the following: Rivaroxaban

Increased Effect/Toxicity

Dalteparin may increase the levels/effects of: Anticoagulants; Collagenase (Systemic); Deferasirox; Drotrecogin Alfa (Activated); Ibritumomab; Rivaroxaban; Tositumomab and Iodine I 131 Tositumomab

The levels/effects of Dalteparin may be increased by: 5-ASA Derivatives; Antiplatelet Agents; Dasatinib; Herbs (Anticoagulant/Antiplatelet Properties); Nonsteroidal Anti-Inflammatory Agents; Pentosan Polysulfate Sodium; Pentoxifylline; Prostacyclin Analogues; Salicylates; Thrombolytic Agents

Decreased Effect There are no known significant interactions involving a decrease in effect.

Ethanol/Nutrition/Herb Interactions Herb/Nutraceutical: Alfalfa, anise, bilberry, bladderwrack, bromelain, cat's claw, celery, chamomile, coleus, cordyceps, dong quai, evening primrose oil, fenugreek, feverfew, garlic, ginger, ginkgo biloba, ginseng (American), ginseng (panax), ginseng (Siberian), grapeseed, green tea, guggul, horse chestnut seed, horseradish, licorice, prickly ash, red clover, reishi, SAMe (s-adenosylmethionine), sweet clover, turmeric, white willow (all have additional antiplatelet/anticoagulant activity)

Stability Store at temperatures of 20°C to 25°C (68°F to 77°F). Multidose vials may be stored for up to 2 weeks at room temperature after entering.

Mechanism of Action Low molecular weight heparin analog with a molecular weight of 4000-6000 daltons; the commercial product contains 3% to 15% heparin with a molecular weight <3000 daltons, 65% to 78% with a molecular weight of 3000-8000 daltons and 14% to 26% with a molecular weight >8000 daltons; while dalteparin has been shown to inhibit both factor Xa and factor IIa (thrombin), the antithrombotic effect of dalteparin is characterized by a higher ratio of antifactor Xa to antifactor IIa activity (ratio = 4)

Pharmacodynamics/Kinetics

Onset of action: Anti-Xa activity: Within 1-2 hours

Duration: >12 hours

Distribution: V_d: 40-60 mL/kg

Protein binding: Low affinity for plasma proteins (Hirsh, 2008)

Bioavailability: SubQ: 81% to 93%

Half-life elimination (route dependent): Anti-Xa activity: 2-5 hours; prolonged in chronic renal insufficiency: 3.7-7.7 hours (following a single 5000 int. unit dose)

Time to peak, serum: Anti-Xa activity: ~4 hours

Excretion: Primarily renal (Hirsh, 2008)

Dosage Adults: SubQ: **Note:** Each 2500 int. units of anti-Xa activity is equal to 16 mg of dalteparin.

DVT prophylaxis: **Note:** In morbidly obese patients (BMI ≥40 kg/m^2), increasing the prophylactic dose by 30% may be appropriate (Nutescu, 2009):

Abdominal surgery:

Low-to-moderate DVT risk: 2500 int. units 1-2 hours prior to surgery, then once daily for 5-10 days postoperatively

High DVT risk: 5000 int. units the evening prior to surgery and then once daily for 5-10 days postoperatively. Alternatively in patients with malignancy: 2500 int. units 1-2 hours prior to surgery, 2500 int. units 12 hours later, then 5000 int. units once daily for 5-10 days postoperatively.

Total hip replacement surgery: **Note:** Three treatment options are currently available. Dose is given for 5-10 days, although up to 14 days of treatment have been tolerated in clinical trials:

Postoperative regimen:

Initial: 2500 int. units 4-8 hours* after surgery

Maintenance: 5000 int. units once daily; start at least 6 hours after postsurgical dose

Preoperative regimen (starting day of surgery):

Initial: 2500 int. units within 2 hours before surgery

Adjustment: 2500 int. units 4-8 hours* after surgery

Maintenance: 5000 int. units once daily; start at least 6 hours after postsurgical dose

Preoperative regimen (starting evening prior to surgery):

Initial: 5000 int. units 10-14 hours before surgery

Adjustment: 5000 int. units 4-8 hours* after surgery

Maintenance: 5000 int. units once daily, allowing 24 hours between doses.

***Dose may be delayed if hemostasis is not yet achieved.**

Immobility during acute illness: 5000 int. units once daily

Unstable angina or non-Q-wave myocardial infarction: 120 int. units/kg body weight (maximum dose: 10,000 int. units) every 12 hours for up to 8 days with concurrent aspirin therapy. Discontinue dalteparin once patient is clinically stable.

Obesity: Use actual body weight to calculate dose; dose capping at 10,000 int. units recommended (Nutescu, 2009)

Venous thromboembolism, extended treatment in cancer patients:

Initial (month 1): 200 int. units/kg (maximum dose: 18,000 int. units) once daily for 30 days

Maintenance (months 2-6): ~150 int. units/kg (maximum dose: 18,000 int. units) once daily. If platelet count between 50,000-100,000/mm^3, reduce dose by 2,500 int. units until platelet count recovers to ≥100,000/mm^3. If platelet count <50,000/mm^3, discontinue dalteparin until platelet count recover to >50,000/mm^3.

Obesity: Use actual body weight to calculate dose; dose capping is not recommended (Nutescu, 2009). However, the manufacturer recommends a maximum dose of 18,000 units per day for the treatment of VTE in cancer patients.

DVT (with or without PE) treatment in noncancer patients (unlabeled use): SubQ: 200 int. units/kg once daily (Feissinger, 1996; Jaff, 2011; Wells, 2005) or 100 int. units/kg twice daily (Jaff, 2011)

Obesity: Use actual body weight to calculate dose; dose capping is not recommended (Nutescu, 2009). One study demonstrated similar anti-Xa levels after 3 days of therapy in obese patients (>40% above IBW; range: 82-190 kg) compared to those ≤20% above IBW or between 20% to 40% above IBW (Wilson, 2001).

Dosing adjustment in renal impairment: Half-life is increased in patients with chronic renal failure, use with caution, accumulation can be expected; specific dosage adjustments have not been recommended. Accumulation was not observed in critically ill patients with severe renal insufficiency (Cl_{cr} <30 mL/minute) receiving prophylactic doses (5000 int. units) for a median of 7 days (Douketis, 2008). In cancer patients, receiving treatment for venous thromboembolism, if Cl_{cr} <30 mL/minute, manufacturer recommends monitoring anti-Xa levels to determine appropriate dose.

Dosing adjustment in hepatic impairment: Use with caution in patients with hepatic insufficiency; specific dosage adjustments have not been recommended

Administration For deep SubQ injection **only**. May be injected in a U-shape to the area surrounding the navel, the upper outer side of the thigh, or the upper outer quadrangle of the buttock. Use thumb and forefinger to lift a fold of skin when injecting dalteparin to the navel area or thigh. Insert needle at a 45- to 90-degree angle. The entire length of needle should be inserted. Do not expel air bubble from fixed-dose syringe prior to injection. Air bubble (and extra solution, if applicable) may be expelled from graduated syringes. In order to minimize bruising, do not rub injection site.

To convert from I.V. unfractionated heparin (UFH) infusion to SubQ dalteparin (Nutescu, 2007): Calculate specific dose for dalteparin based on indication, discontinue UFH and begin dalteparin within 1 hour

To convert from SubQ dalteparin to I.V. UFH infusion (Nutescu, 2007): Discontinue dalteparin; calculate specific dose for I.V. UFH infusion based on indication; omit heparin bolus/loading dose

Converting from SubQ dalteparin dosed every 12 hours: Start I.V. UFH infusion 10-11 hours after last dose of dalteparin

Converting from SubQ dalteparin dosed every 24 hours: Start I.V. UFH infusion 22-23 hours after last dose of dalteparin

Monitoring Parameters Periodic CBC including platelet count; stool occult blood tests; monitoring of PT and PTT is not necessary. Once patient has received 3-4 doses, anti-Xa levels, drawn 4-6 hours after dalteparin administration, may be used to monitor effect in patients with severe renal dysfunction or if abnormal coagulation parameters or bleeding should occur. For patients >190 kg, if anti-Xa monitoring is available, adjusting dose based on anti-Xa levels is recommended; if anti-Xa monitoring is unavailable, reduce dose if bleeding occurs (Nutescu, 2009).

Reference Range Treatment: Venous thromboembolism: Target anti-Xa range: 0.5-1.5 int. units/mL

Dosage Forms Excipient information presented when available (limited, particularly for generics); consult specific product labeling. [DSC] = Discontinued product

Injection, solution:

Fragmin®: 10,000 anti-Xa int. units/mL (9.5 mL [DSC]); 25,000 anti-Xa int. units/mL (3.8 mL) [contains benzyl alcohol]

Injection, solution [preservative free]:

Fragmin®: 10,000 anti-Xa int. units/mL (1 mL); 2500 anti-Xa int. units/0.2 mL (0.2 mL); 5000 anti-Xa int. units/0.2 mL (0.2 mL); 7500 anti-Xa int. units/0.3 mL (0.3 mL); 12,500 anti-Xa int. units/0.5 mL (0.5 mL); 15,000 anti-Xa int. units/0.6 mL (0.6 mL); 18,000 anti-Xa int. units/0.72 mL (0.72 mL)

◆ **Dalteparin Sodium** *see* Dalteparin *on page 441*

Danazol (DA na zole)

Brand Names: Canada Cyclomen®

Index Terms Danocrine

Pharmacologic Category Androgen

Use Treatment of endometriosis, fibrocystic breast disease, and hereditary angioedema

Pregnancy Risk Factor X

Dosage Adults: Oral:

Females: Endometriosis: Initial: 200-400 mg/day in 2 divided doses for mild disease; individualize dosage. Usual maintenance dose: 800 mg/day in 2 divided doses to achieve amenorrhea and rapid response to painful symptoms. Continue therapy uninterrupted for 3-6 months (up to 9 months).

Females: Fibrocystic breast disease: Range: 100-400 mg/day in 2 divided doses

Males/Females: Hereditary angioedema: Initial: 200 mg 2-3 times/day; after favorable response, decrease the dosage by 50% or less at intervals of 1-3 months or longer if the frequency of attacks dictates. If an attack occurs, increase the dosage by up to 200 mg/day.

Additional Information Complete prescribing information for this medication should be consulted for additional detail.

Dosage Forms Excipient information presented when available (limited, particularly for generics); consult specific product labeling.

Capsule, oral: 50 mg, 100 mg, 200 mg

◆ **Dandrex** *see* Selenium Sulfide *on page 1547*

◆ **Danocrine** *see* Danazol *on page 443*

◆ **Dantrium®** *see* Dantrolene *on page 443*

Dantrolene (DAN troe leen)

Brand Names: U.S. Dantrium®; Revonto™

Brand Names: Canada Dantrium®

Index Terms Dantrolene Sodium

Pharmacologic Category Skeletal Muscle Relaxant

Use Treatment of spasticity associated with upper motor neuron disorders (eg, spinal cord injury, stroke, cerebral palsy, or multiple sclerosis); management of malignant hyperthermia; prevention of malignant hyperthermia in susceptible individuals (preoperative/postoperative administration)

Unlabeled Use Neuroleptic malignant syndrome (NMS)

Pregnancy Risk Factor C

Pregnancy Considerations Animal studies indicate an increased risk in fetal mortality. Dantrolene crosses the human placenta; cord blood concentrations are similar to those in the maternal plasma at term. There are no adequate and well-controlled studies in pregnant women.

Lactation Enters breast milk/not recommended

Contraindications

I.V.: There are no contraindications listed within the manufacturers labeling.

Oral: Active hepatic disease; should not be used when spasticity is used to maintain posture/balance during locomotion or to obtain/maintain increased function

Warnings/Precautions [U.S. Boxed Warning]: Has potential for hepatotoxicity. Overt hepatitis has been most frequently observed between the third and twelfth month of therapy. Hepatic injury appears to be greater in females and in patients >35 years of age. Idiosyncratic and hypersensitivity reactions (sometimes fatal) of the liver have also occurred. Discontinue therapy if benefits not observed within 45 days when utilized for chronic spasticity.

Use oral therapy with caution in patients with impaired cardiac, hepatic, or pulmonary function (particularly in obstructive pulmonary disease). May cause photosensitivity. Patients should be cautioned about performing tasks which require mental alertness (eg, operating machinery or driving). The combination of I.V. dantrolene and calcium channel blockers is not recommended. Injection contains 3 g mannitol/vial; caution if additional mannitol required. Alkaline solution may cause tissue necrosis if extravasated. In addition to I.V. dantrolene, supportive measures must also be utilized for management of malignant hyperthermia. Long-term use in patients <5 years of age has not been established.

Adverse Reactions Frequency not defined.

Cardiovascular: Blood pressure (altered), heart failure, tachycardia

Central nervous system: Chills, confusion, dizziness, drowsiness, fatigue, fever, headache, insomnia, lightheadedness, malaise, mental depression, nervousness, seizure, speech disturbance

Dermatologic: Eczematoid eruption, hair growth (abnormal), pruritus, rash, urticaria

Gastrointestinal: Abdominal cramps, anorexia, constipation, diarrhea, dysphagia, gastric irritation, gastrointestinal hemorrhage, nausea, taste change, vomiting

Genitourinary: Crystalluria, difficult erection, difficult urination, nocturia, polyuria, urinary frequency, urinary incontinence, urinary retention

Hematologic: Anemia (aplastic), leukopenia, thrombocytopenia

Hepatic: Hepatitis

Local: Injection site reaction (pain, erythema, swelling), thrombophlebitis, tissue necrosis

Neuromuscular & skeletal: Back pain, muscle weakness, myalgia

Ocular: Blurred vision, diplopia, tearing (excessive)

Renal: Hematuria

Respiratory: Feeling of suffocation, pleural effusion (associated with pericarditis), pulmonary edema, respiratory depression

Miscellaneous: Anaphylaxis, diaphoresis, lymphocytic lymphoma, sialorrhea

Drug Interactions

Metabolism/Transport Effects Substrate of CYP3A4 (major); **Note:** Assignment of Major/Minor substrate status based on clinically relevant drug interaction potential

Avoid Concomitant Use

Avoid concomitant use of Dantrolene with any of the following: Conivaptan

Increased Effect/Toxicity

Dantrolene may increase the levels/effects of: Alcohol (Ethyl); CNS Depressants; Methotrimeprazine; Selective Serotonin Reuptake Inhibitors

The levels/effects of Dantrolene may be increased by: Conivaptan; CYP3A4 Inhibitors (Moderate); CYP3A4 Inhibitors (Strong); Dasatinib; Droperidol; HydrOXYzine; Methotrimeprazine

Decreased Effect

The levels/effects of Dantrolene may be decreased by: CYP3A4 Inducers (Strong); Deferasirox; Herbs (CYP3A4 Inducers); Tocilizumab

Ethanol/Nutrition/Herb Interactions

Ethanol: May increase CNS depression; monitor for increased effects with coadministration. Caution patients about effects.

Herb/Nutraceutical: Avoid valerian, St John's wort, kava kava, gotu kola (may increase CNS depression).

Stability Reconstitute vial by adding 60 mL of sterile water for injection USP (**not bacteriostatic water for injection**); incompatible with D_5W, NS, and other acidic solutions. Protect from light. Use reconstituted solution within 6 hours; avoid glass bottles for I.V. infusion due to potential for precipitate formation.

Dantrium®: Store unreconstituted vials and reconstituted solutions at controlled room temperature of 15°C to 30°C (59°F to 86°F).

Revonto™: Dissolution time reduced; shake vial for ~20 seconds or until solution is clear. Store unreconstituted vials and reconstituted solutions at controlled room temperature of 20°C to 25°C (68°F to 77°F).

Mechanism of Action Acts directly on skeletal muscle by interfering with release of calcium ion from the sarcoplasmic reticulum; prevents or reduces the increase in myoplasmic calcium ion concentration that activates the acute catabolic processes associated with malignant hyperthermia

Pharmacodynamics/Kinetics

Absorption: Oral: Slow and incomplete

Metabolism: Hepatic

Half-life elimination: 4-8 hours

Excretion: Feces (45% to 50%); urine (25% as unchanged drug and metabolites)

Dosage

Spasticity: Oral:

Children: Children: Initial: 0.5 mg/kg/dose once daily for 7 days; increase to 0.5 mg/kg/dose 3 times/day for 7 days, increase to 1 mg/kg/dose 3 times/day for 7 days, and then increase to 2 mg/kg/dose 3 times/day; not to exceed 400 mg/day

Adults: Initial: 25 mg once daily for 7 days; increase to 25 mg 3 times/day for 7 days, increase to 50 mg 3 times/day for 7 days, and then increase to 100 mg 3 times/day; not to exceed 400 mg/day

Malignant hyperthermia: Children and Adults:

Preoperative prophylaxis:

Oral: 4-8 mg/kg/day in 4 divided doses, begin 1-2 days prior to surgery with last dose 3-4 hours prior to surgery

I.V.: 2.5 mg/kg ~1¼ hours prior to anesthesia and infused over 1 hour with additional doses as needed and individualized

Crisis: I.V.: 2.5 mg/kg; continuously repeat dose until symptoms subside or a cumulative dose of 10 mg/kg is reached; if physiologic and metabolic abnormalities reappear, repeat regimen (**Note:** Manufacturer's labeling suggests an initial dose of 1 mg/kg; however, guidelines recommend 2.5 mg/kg initially [www.mhaus.org]).

Postcrisis follow-up: Oral: 4-8 mg/kg/day in 4 divided doses for 1-3 days; I.V. dantrolene may be used when oral therapy is not practical; individualize dosage beginning with 1 mg/kg or more as the clinical situation dictates

Neuroleptic malignant syndrome (unlabeled use): I.V.: 1-2.5 mg/kg, may repeat dose up to maximum cumulative dose of 10 mg/kg/day, then switch to oral dosage (Strawn, 2007; Susman, 2001)

Administration I.V.: Therapeutic or emergency dose can be administered with rapid continuous I.V. push. Follow-up doses should be administered over 2-3 minutes.

Monitoring Parameters Motor performance should be monitored for therapeutic outcomes; nausea, vomiting, and liver function tests should be monitored for potential hepatotoxicity; intravenous administration requires cardiac monitor and blood pressure monitor

Dosage Forms Excipient information presented when available (limited, particularly for generics); consult specific product labeling.

Capsule, oral, as sodium: 25 mg, 50 mg, 100 mg

Dantrium®: 25 mg, 50 mg, 100 mg

Injection, powder for reconstitution, as sodium:

Dantrium®: 20 mg [contains mannitol 3 g]

Revonto™: 20 mg [contains mannitol 3 g]

Extemporaneous Preparations A 5 mg/mL oral suspension may be made with dantrolene capsules, a citric acid solution, and either simple syrup or syrup BP (containing 0.15% w/v methylhydroxybenzoate). Add the contents of five 100 mg dantrolene capsules to a citric acid solution (150 mg citric acid powder in 10 mL water); mix while adding the chosen vehicle in incremental proportions to **almost** 100 mL. Transfer to a calibrated bottle and add quantity of vehicle sufficient to make 100 mL. Label "shake well" and "refrigerate". Simple syrup suspension is stable for 2 days refrigerated; syrup BP suspension is stable for 30 days refrigerated.

Nahata MC, Pai VB, and Hipple TF, *Pediatric Drug Formulations*, 5th ed, Cincinnati, OH: Harvey Whitney Books Co, 2004.

◆ **Dantrolene Sodium** *see* Dantrolene *on page 443*

◆ **Dapcin** *see* DAPTOmycin *on page 446*

Dapsone (Systemic) (DAP sone)

Index Terms Diaminodiphenylsulfone

Pharmacologic Category Antibiotic, Miscellaneous

Use Treatment of leprosy and dermatitis herpetiformis (infections caused by *Mycobacterium leprae*)

Unlabeled Use Prophylaxis of toxoplasmosis in severely-immunocompromised patients; alternative agent for *Pneumocystis jirovecii* pneumonia (PCP) prophylaxis (monotherapy) and treatment (in combination with trimethoprim); pemphigus vulgaris (oral), aphthous ulcers (severe), bullous systemic lupus erythematosus; all in consultation with patient's physician as significant monitoring required

Pregnancy Risk Factor C

Pregnancy Considerations Because of adverse events observed in some animal studies, dapsone is classified as pregnancy category C. Per the manufacturer, dapsone has not shown an increased risk of congenital anomalies when given during all trimesters of pregnancy. Several reports have described adverse effects in the newborn after *in utero* exposure to dapsone, including neonatal hemolytic disease, methemoglobinemia, and hyperbilirubinemia. Dapsone is an alternative for prophylaxis and treatment of *Pneumocystis jirovecii* pneumonia (PCP) in pregnant, HIV-infected patients. Dapsone is also recommended for pregnant women requiring maintenance therapy of either leprosy or dermatitis herpetiformis

Lactation Enters breast milk/not recommended (AAP rates "compatible"; AAP 2001 update pending)

Contraindications Hypersensitivity to dapsone or any component of the formulation

Warnings/Precautions Use with caution in patients with severe anemia, G6PD, methemoglobin reductase deficiency or hemoglobin M deficiency; hypersensitivity to other sulfonamides; aplastic anemia, agranulocytosis and other severe blood dyscrasias have resulted in death; monitor carefully; serious dermatologic reactions (including toxic epidermal necrolysis) are rare but potential occurrences; sulfone reactions may also occur as potentially fatal hypersensitivity reactions; these, but not leprosy reactional states, require drug discontinuation. Motor loss and muscle weakness have been reported with use. Prolonged use may result in fungal or bacterial superinfection, including *C. difficile*-associated diarrhea and pseudomembranous colitis.

Adverse Reactions Frequency not always defined.

>10%: Hematologic: Reticulocyte increase (2% to 12%), hemolysis (>10%; dose related; seen in patients with and without G6PD deficiency), hemoglobin decrease (>10%; 1-2 g/dL; almost all patients), methemoglobinemia (>10%), red cell life span shortened (>10%), Agranulocytosis, anemia, leukopenia, pure red cell aplasia (case report)

Cardiovascular: Tachycardia

Central nervous system: Fever, headache, insomnia, psychosis, vertigo

Dermatologic: Bullous and exfoliative dermatitis, erythema nodosum, exfoliative dermatitis, morbilliform and scarlatiniform reactions, phototoxicity, Stevens-Johnson syndrome, toxic epidural necrolysis, urticaria

Endocrine & metabolic: Hypoalbuminemia (without proteinuria), male infertility

Gastrointestinal: Abdominal pain, nausea, pancreatitis, vomiting

Hepatic: Cholestatic jaundice, hepatitis

Neuromuscular & skeletal: Drug-induced lupus erythematosus, lower motor neuron toxicity (prolonged therapy), peripheral neuropathy (rare, nonleprosy patients)

Ocular: Blurred vision

Otic: Tinnitus

Renal: Albuminuria, nephrotic syndrome, renal papillary necrosis

Respiratory: Interstitial pneumonitis, pulmonary eosinophilia

Miscellaneous: Infectious mononucleosis-like syndrome (rash, fever, lymphadenopathy, hepatic dysfunction)

Drug Interactions

Metabolism/Transport Effects Substrate of CYP2C19 (minor), CYP2C8 (minor), CYP2C9 (major), CYP2E1 (minor), CYP3A4 (major); **Note:** Assignment of Major/Minor substrate status based on clinically relevant drug interaction potential

Avoid Concomitant Use

Avoid concomitant use of Dapsone (Systemic) with any of the following: BCG; Conivaptan

Increased Effect/Toxicity

Dapsone (Systemic) may increase the levels/effects of: Antimalarial Agents; Trimethoprim

The levels/effects of Dapsone (Systemic) may be increased by: Antimalarial Agents; Conivaptan; CYP2C9 Inhibitors (Moderate); CYP2C9 Inhibitors (Strong); CYP3A4 Inhibitors (Moderate); CYP3A4 Inhibitors (Strong); Dasatinib; Probenecid; Trimethoprim

Decreased Effect

Dapsone (Systemic) may decrease the levels/effects of: BCG; Typhoid Vaccine

The levels/effects of Dapsone (Systemic) may be decreased by: CYP2C9 Inducers (Strong); CYP3A4 Inducers (Strong); Cyproterone; Deferasirox; Herbs (CYP3A4 Inducers); Peginterferon Alfa-2b; Rifamycin Derivatives; Tocilizumab

Ethanol/Nutrition/Herb Interactions Herb/Nutraceutical: St John's wort may decrease dapsone levels.

Stability Store at 20°C to 25°C (68°F to 76°F). Protect from light.

Mechanism of Action Competitive antagonist of para-aminobenzoic acid (PABA) and prevents normal bacterial utilization of PABA for the synthesis of folic acid

Pharmacodynamics/Kinetics

Absorption: Well-absorbed

Protein binding: Dapsone: 70% to 90%; Metabolite: ~99%

Distribution: V_d: 1.5 L/kg; throughout total body water and present in all tissues, especially liver and kidney

Metabolism: Hepatic (acetylation and hydroxylation); forms multiple metabolites

Half-life elimination: 30 hours (range: 10-50 hours)

Excretion: Urine (~85%)

Dosage Oral:

Aphthous ulcers, severe (unlabeled use): Adults: 50 mg once daily

Bullous systemic lupus erythematosus (unlabeled use): Adults: 100 mg once daily

Leprosy:

- Children: 1-2 mg/kg/24 hours, up to a maximum of 100 mg/day, in combination with other antileprosy agents; duration of therapy is variable
- Adults: 100 mg/day, in combination with other antileprosy agents; duration of therapy is variable

Dermatitis herpetiformis: Adults: Start at 50 mg/day, increase to 300 mg/day, or higher to achieve full control, reduce dosage to minimum level as soon as possible

Pneumocystis jirovecii pneumonia, alternative therapy (unlabeled use):

Prophylaxis (primary or secondary):

- Infants and Children: 2 mg/kg/day once daily (maximum dose: 100 mg/day) or 4 mg/kg/dose once weekly (maximum dose: 200 mg) (CDC, 2009)
- Adolescents and Adults: 100 mg/day once daily or divided in 2 doses as monotherapy **or** 50 mg daily in combination with weekly pyrimethamine and leucovorin (CDC, 2009)

Treatment:

Infants and Children: 2 mg/kg/day once daily (maximum dose: 100 mg/day) in combination with trimethoprim for 21 days

Adolescents and Adults: 100 mg/day once daily in combination with trimethoprim for 21 days

Dosing adjustment in renal impairment: No specific guidelines are available

Dietary Considerations Do not give with antacids, alkaline foods, or drugs.

Administration May administer with meals if GI upset occurs.

Monitoring Parameters Check G6PD levels prior to initiation. Monitor patients for signs of jaundice and hemolysis; CBC weekly for first month, monthly for 6 months and semiannually thereafter.

Dosage Forms Excipient information presented when available (limited, particularly for generics); consult specific product labeling.

Tablet, oral: 25 mg, 100 mg

Extemporaneous Preparations A 2 mg/mL oral suspension may be made with tablets and a 1:1 mixture of Ora-Sweet® and Ora-Plus®. Crush eight 25 mg tablets in a mortar and reduce to a fine powder. Add small portions of vehicle and mix to a uniform paste; mix while adding the vehicle in incremental proportions to **almost** 100 mL; transfer to a calibrated bottle, rinse mortar with vehicle, and add quantity of vehicle sufficient to make 100 mL. Label "shake well". Stable for 90 days at room temperature or refrigerated.

Jacobus Pharmaceutical Company makes a 2 mg/mL proprietary liquid formulation available under an IND for the prophylaxis of *Pneumocystis jirovecii* pneumonia.

Nahata MC, Morosco RS, and Trowbridge JM, "Stability of Dapsone in Two Oral Liquid Dosage Forms," *Ann Pharmacother*, 2000, 34 (7-8):848-50.

◆ **Daptacel®** *see* Diphtheria and Tetanus Toxoids, and Acellular Pertussis Vaccine *on page* 523

DAPTOmycin (DAP toe mye sin)

Brand Names: U.S. Cubicin®

Brand Names: Canada Cubicin®

Index Terms Cidecin; Dapcin; LY146032

Pharmacologic Category Antibiotic, Cyclic Lipopeptide

Use Treatment of complicated skin and skin structure infections caused by susceptible aerobic gram-positive organisms; *Staphylococcus aureus* bacteremia, including right-sided native valve infective endocarditis caused by MSSA or MRSA

Unlabeled Use Treatment of severe infections caused by MRSA or VRE

Pregnancy Risk Factor B

Pregnancy Considerations Because adverse events were not observed in animal reproduction studies, daptomycin is classified as pregnancy category B. Successful use of daptomycin during the second and third trimesters of pregnancy has been described; however, only limited information is available from case reports.

Lactation Excreted in breast milk/use caution

Contraindications Hypersensitivity to daptomycin or any component of the formulation

Warnings/Precautions May be associated with an increased incidence of myopathy; discontinue in patients with signs and symptoms of myopathy in conjunction with an increase in CPK (>5 times ULN or 1000 units/L) or in asymptomatic patients with a CPK ≥10 times ULN. Myopathy may occur more frequently at dose and/or frequency in excess of recommended dosages. Use caution in patients receiving other drugs associated with myopathy (eg, HMG-CoA reductase inhibitors). Not indicated for the treatment of pneumonia (inactivation by pulmonary surfactant). Use caution in renal impairment (dosage adjustment required severe renal impairment [Cl_{cr} <30 mL/minute]). Limited data (eg, subgroup analysis) from cSSSI and endocarditis trials suggest possibly reduced clinical efficacy (relative to comparators) in patients with baseline moderate renal impairment (<50 mL/minute). Symptoms suggestive of peripheral neuropathy have been observed with treatment; monitor for new-onset or worsening neuropathy. Prolonged use may result in fungal or bacterial superinfection, including *C. difficile*-associated diarrhea and pseudomembranous colitis. Hypersensitivity reactions and anaphylaxis have been reported with use; discontinue use immediately with signs/symptoms of hypersensitivity and initiate appropriate treatment. Use has been associated with eosinophilic pneumonia; generally develops 2-4 weeks after therapy initiation. Monitor for signs/symptoms of eosinophilic pneumonia, including new onset or worsening fever, dyspnea, difficulty breathing, new infiltrates on chest imaging studies, and/or >25% eosinophils present in bronchoalveolar lavage. Discontinue use immediately with signs/symptoms of eosinophilic pneumonia and initiate appropriate treatment (ie, corticosteroids). May reoccur with re-exposure.

Adverse Reactions

>10%:

Gastrointestinal: Diarrhea (5% to 12%), vomiting (3% to 12%), constipation (6% to 11%)

Hematologic: Anemia (2% to 13%)

1% to 10%:

Cardiovascular: Peripheral edema (7%), chest pain (7%), hypertension (1% to 6%), hypotension (2% to 5%)

Central nervous system: Insomnia (5% to 9%), headache (5% to7%), fever (2% to 7%), dizziness (2% to 6%), anxiety (5%)

Dermatologic: Rash (4% to 7%), pruritus (3% to 6%), erythema (5%)

Endocrine & metabolic: Hypokalemia (9%), hyperkalemia (5%), hyperphosphatemia (3%)

Gastrointestinal: Nausea (6% to 10%), abdominal pain (6%), dyspepsia (1% to 4%), loose stool (4%), GI hemorrhage (2%)

Genitourinary: Urinary tract infection (2% to 7%)

Hematologic: INR increased (2%), eosinophilia (2%)

Hepatic: Transaminases increased (2% to 3%), alkaline phosphatase increased (2%)

Local: Injection site reaction (3% to 6%)

Neuromuscular & skeletal: CPK increased (3% to 9%), limb pain (2% to 9%), back pain (7%), weakness (5%), arthralgia (1% to 3%)

Renal: Renal failure (2% to 3%)

Respiratory: Pharyngolaryngeal pain (8%), pleural effusion (6%), cough (3%), pneumonia (3%), dyspnea (2% to 3%)

Miscellaneous: Osteomyelitis (6%), bacteremia (5%), diaphoresis (5%), sepsis (5%), infection (fungal, 2% to 3%)

<1% (Limited to important or life-threatening): Anaphylaxis, appetite decreased, arthralgia, atrial fibrillation, atrial flutter, cardiac arrest, coma (post anaesthesia/surgery), dyskinesia, dysphagia, eczema, electrolyte disturbance, eosinophilia, eosinophilic pneumonia, erythema (truncal), eye irritation, fatigue, flatulence, flushing, GI discomfort, gingival pain, hallucination, hives, hypomagnesemia, hypersensitivity, hypoesthesia, jaundice, jitteriness, LDH increased, leukocytosis, lymphadenopathy, mental status change, muscle cramps, muscle weakness, myalgia, myoglobin increased, osteomyelitis, paresthesia, peripheral neuropathy, proteinuria, prothrombin time prolonged, pulmonary eosinophilia, rhabdomyolysis, rigors, serum bicarbonate increased, shortness of breath, stomatitis, supraventricular arrhythmia, taste disturbance,

thrombocytopenia, thrombocythemia, tinnitus, vertigo, vesiculobullous rash, vision blurred, xerostomia

Drug Interactions

Metabolism/Transport Effects None known.

Avoid Concomitant Use There are no known interactions where it is recommended to avoid concomitant use.

Increased Effect/Toxicity

The levels/effects of DAPTOmycin may be increased by: HMG-CoA Reductase Inhibitors

Decreased Effect There are no known significant interactions involving a decrease in effect.

Stability Store under refrigeration at 2°C to 8°C (36°F to 46°F). Intact vials may be stored at room temperature for up to 12 months (data on file [Cubist Pharmaceuticals, 2011]). However, the manufacturer recommends storage under refrigeration. Room temperature stability information should only be utilized in situations where the drug has been inadvertently exposed to prolonged room temperature.

Reconstitute vial with 10 mL NS. Add NS to vial and rotate gently to wet powder. Allow to stand for 10 minutes, then gently swirl to obtain completely reconstituted solution. Do not shake or agitate vial vigorously. If administering via IVPB, further dilute following reconstitution in an appropriate volume of NS. Reconstituted solution (either in vial or in infusion bag) is stable for a cumulative time of 12 hours at room temperature and 48 hours if refrigerated (2°C to 8°C). Incompatible with ReadyMED® elastomeric infusion pumps (Cardinal Health, Inc) due to an impurity (2-mercaptobenzothiazole) leaching from the pump system into the daptomycin solution.

Mechanism of Action Daptomycin binds to components of the cell membrane of susceptible organisms and causes rapid depolarization, inhibiting intracellular synthesis of DNA, RNA, and protein. Daptomycin is bactericidal in a concentration-dependent manner.

Pharmacodynamics/Kinetics

Distribution: V_{ss}: 0.1 L/kg; Critically-ill patients: V_{ss}: 0.23 ± 0.14 L/kg (Vilay, 2010)

Protein binding: 90% to 93%; 84% to 88% in patients with Cl_{cr}<30 mL/minute

Half-life elimination: 8-9 hours (up to 28 hours in renal impairment)

Excretion: Urine (78%; primarily as unchanged drug); feces (6%)

Dosage I.V.: Adults:

Skin and soft tissue: 4 mg/kg once daily for 7-14 days

Bacteremia, right-sided native valve endocarditis caused by MSSA or MRSA: 6 mg/kg once daily for 2-6 weeks (some experts recommend 8-10 mg/kg once daily for complicated bacteremia or infective endocarditis [Liu, 2011])

Osteomyelitis (unlabeled use): 6 mg/kg once daily for a minimum of 8 weeks (some experts combine with rifampin) (Liu, 2011)

Septic arthritis (unlabeled use): 6 mg/kg once daily for 3-4 weeks (Liu, 2011)

Dosage adjustment in renal impairment: Cl_{cr} <30 mL/minute:

Skin and soft tissue infections: 4 mg/kg every 48 hours

Staphylococcal bacteremia: 6 mg/kg every 48 hours

Intermittent hemodialysis or peritoneal dialysis (PD): Dose as in Cl_{cr} <30 mL/minute (administer after hemodialysis on dialysis days) or (unlabeled dosing) may administer 6 mg/kg after hemodialysis 3 times weekly (Salama, 2010)

Note: High permeability intermittent hemodialysis removes ~50% during a 4-hour session (Salama, 2010).

Continuous renal replacement therapy (CRRT) (Heintz, 2009; Trotman, 2005): Drug clearance is highly dependent on the method of renal replacement, filter type, and flow rate. Appropriate dosing requires close monitoring of pharmacologic response, signs of adverse reactions due to drug accumulation, as well as drug concentrations in relation to target trough (if appropriate). The following are general recommendations only (based on dialysate flow/ultrafiltration rates of 1-2 L/hour and minimal residual renal function) and should not supersede clinical judgment:

Continuous veno-venous hemodialysis (CVVHD): 8 mg/kg every 48 hours (Vilay, 2010)

Note: For other forms of CRRT (eg, CVVH or CVVHDF), dosing as with Cl_{cr}<30 mL/minute may result in low C_{max}. May consider 4-6 mg/kg every 24 hours (or 8 mg/kg every 48 hours) depending on site or severity of infection or if not responding to standard dosing; therapeutic drug monitoring and/or more frequent serum CPK levels may be necessary (Heintz, 2009).

Slow extended daily dialysis (or extended dialysis): 6 mg/kg every 24 hours (Kielstein, 2010); **Note:** Dialysis should be initiated within 8 hours of administering daptomycin dose to avoid dose accumulation.

Dosage adjustment in hepatic impairment: No adjustment required for mild-to-moderate impairment (Child-Pugh class A or B); not evaluated in severe hepatic impairment (Child-Pugh class C)

Administration May administer I.V. push over 2 minutes or infuse IVPB over 30 minutes. Do not use in conjunction with ReadyMED® elastomeric infusion pumps (Cardinal Health, Inc) due to an impurity (2-mercaptobenzothiazole) leaching from the pump system into the daptomycin solution.

Monitoring Parameters Monitor signs and symptoms of infection. CPK should be monitored at least weekly during therapy; more frequent monitoring if current or prior statin therapy, unexplained CPK increases, and/or renal impairment. Monitor for muscle pain or weakness, especially if noted in distal extremities. Canadian labeling recommends CPK monitoring every 48 hours with unexplained muscle pain, tenderness, weakness or cramps. Monitor for signs/symptoms of eosinophilic pneumonia.

Reference Range

Trough concentrations at steady-state:

4 mg/kg once daily: 5.9 ± 1.6 mcg/mL

6 mg/kg once daily: 6.7 ± 1.6 mcg/mL

Note: Trough concentrations are not predictive of efficacy/toxicity. Drug exhibits concentration-dependent bactericidal activity, so C_{max}:MIC ratios may be a more useful parameter.

Test Interactions Daptomycin may cause false prolongation of the PT and increase of INR with certain reagents. This appears to be a dose-dependent phenomenon. Therefore, it is recommended to obtain blood samples immediately prior to next daptomycin dose (eg, trough). If PT/INR elevated, clinicians should repeat PT/INR and evaluate for other causes of hypocoagulation.

Dosage Forms Excipient information presented when available (limited, particularly for generics); consult specific product labeling.

Injection, powder for reconstitution:

Cubicin®: 500 mg

◆ **Daraprim®** *see* Pyrimethamine *on page 1438*

Darbepoetin Alfa (dar be POE e tin AL fa)

Brand Names: U.S. Aranesp®; Aranesp® SingleJect®

Brand Names: Canada Aranesp®

Index Terms Erythropoiesis-Stimulating Agent (ESA); Erythropoiesis-Stimulating Protein; NESP; Novel Erythropoiesis-Stimulating Protein

Pharmacologic Category Colony Stimulating Factor; Growth Factor; Recombinant Human Erythropoietin

Use Treatment of anemia due to concurrent myelosuppressive chemotherapy in patients with cancer (nonmyeloid malignancies) receiving chemotherapy (palliative intent) for a planned minimum of 2 additional months of chemotherapy; treatment of anemia due to chronic kidney disease (including patients on dialysis and not on dialysis)

Note: Darbepoetin is **not** indicated for use under the following conditions:

- Cancer patients receiving hormonal therapy, therapeutic biologic products, or radiation therapy unless also receiving concurrent myelosuppressive chemotherapy
- Cancer patients receiving myelosuppressive chemotherapy when the expected outcome is curative
- As a substitute for RBC transfusion in patients requiring immediate correction of anemia

Note: In clinical trials, darbepoetin has not demonstrated improved quality of life, fatigue, or well-being.

Unlabeled Use Treatment of symptomatic anemia in myelodysplastic syndrome (MDS)

Pregnancy Risk Factor C

Pregnancy Considerations Darbepoetin has been shown to have adverse effects (reduced weights, early postimplantation loss) in animal studies. There are no adequate and well-controlled studies in pregnant women. Darbepoetin alfa should be used in a pregnant woman only if potential benefit justifies the potential risk to the fetus. Women who become pregnant during treatment with darbepoetin are encouraged to enroll in Amgen's Pregnancy Surveillance Program (1-800-772-6436).

Lactation Excretion in breast milk unknown/use caution

Prescribing and Access Restrictions As a requirement of the REMS program, access to this medication is restricted. Healthcare providers and hospitals must be enrolled in the ESA APPRISE (Assisting Providers and Cancer Patients with Risk Information for the Safe use of ESAs) Oncology Program (866-284-8089; http://www.esa-apprise.com) to prescribe or dispense ESAs (ie, darbepoetin alfa, epoetin alfa) to patients with cancer.

Medication Guide Available Yes

Contraindications Hypersensitivity to darbepoetin or any component of the formulation; uncontrolled hypertension; pure red cell aplasia (due to darbepoetin or other erythropoietin protein drugs)

Warnings/Precautions **[U.S. Boxed Warning]: Erythropoiesis-stimulating agents (ESAs) increased the risk of serious cardiovascular events, thromboembolic events, stroke, and/or tumor progression in clinical studies when administered to target hemoglobin levels >11 g/dL** (and provide no additional benefit); a rapid rise in hemoglobin (>1 g/dL over 2 weeks) may also contribute to these risks. **[U.S. Boxed Warning]: A shortened overall survival and/or increased risk of tumor progression or recurrence has been reported in studies with breast, cervical, head and neck, lymphoid, and nonsmall cell lung cancer patients.** It is of note that in these studies, patients received ESAs to a target hemoglobin of ≥12 g/dL; although risk has not been excluded when dosed to achieve a target hemoglobin of <12 g/dL. **[U.S. Boxed Warnings]: To decrease these risks, and risk of cardio- and thrombovascular events, use ESAs in cancer patients only for the treatment of anemia related to concurrent myelosuppressive chemotherapy and use the lowest dose needed to avoid red blood cell transfusions. Discontinue ESA following completion of the chemotherapy course. ESAs are not indicated for patients receiving myelosuppressive therapy when the anticipated outcome is curative.** A dosage modification is appropriate if hemoglobin levels rise >1 g/dL per 2-week time period during treatment (Rizzo, 2010). Use of ESAs has been associated with an increased risk of venous thromboembolism (VTE) without a reduction in transfusions in patients >65 years of age with cancer (Hershman, 2009). Improved anemia symptoms, quality of life, fatigue, or well-being have not been demonstrated in controlled clinical trials. **[U.S. Boxed Warning]: Because of the risks of decreased survival and increased risk of tumor growth or progression, all healthcare providers and hospitals are required to enroll and comply with the ESA APPRISE (Assisting Providers and Cancer Patients with Risk Information for the Safe use of ESAs) Oncology Program prior to prescribing or dispensing ESAs to cancer patients.** Prescribers and patients will have to provide written documentation of discussed risks prior to each course.

[U.S. Boxed Warning]: An increased risk of death, serious cardiovascular events, and stroke was reported in patients with chronic kidney disease (CKD) administered ESAs to target hemoglobin levels ≥11 g/dL; use the lowest dose sufficient to reduce the need for RBC transfusions. An optimal target hemoglobin level, dose or dosing strategy to reduce these risks has not been identified in clinical trials. Hemoglobin rising >1 g/dL in a 2-week period may contribute to the risk (dosage reduction recommended). CKD patients who exhibit an inadequate hemoglobin response to ESA therapy may be at a higher risk for cardiovascular events and mortality compared to other patients. ESA therapy may reduce dialysis efficacy (due to increase in red blood cells and decrease in plasma volume); adjustments in dialysis parameters may be needed. Patients treated with epoetin may require increased heparinization during dialysis to prevent clotting of the extracorporeal circuit. CKD patients not requiring dialysis may have a better response to darbepoetin and may require lower doses. An increased risk of DVT has been observed in patients treated with epoetin undergoing surgical orthopedic procedures. Darbepoetin is **not** approved for reduction in allogeneic red blood cell transfusions in patients scheduled for surgical procedures. The risk for seizures is increased with darbepoetin use in patients with CKD; use with caution in patients with a history of seizures. Monitor closely for neurologic symptoms during the first several months of therapy. Use with caution in patients with hypertension; hypertensive encephalopathy has been reported. Use is contraindicated in patients with uncontrolled hypertension. If hypertension is difficult to control, reduce or hold darbepoetin alfa. Due to the delayed onset of erythropoiesis, darbepoetin alfa is **not** recommended for acute correction of severe anemia or as a substitute for emergency transfusion. Consider discontinuing in patients who receive a renal transplant.

Prior to treatment, correct or exclude deficiencies of iron, vitamin B_{12}, and/or folate, as well as other factors which may impair erythropoiesis (inflammatory conditions, infections, bleeding). Prior to and during therapy, iron stores must be evaluated. Supplemental iron is recommended if serum ferritin <100 mcg/L or serum transferrin saturation <20%; most patients with CKD will require iron supplementation. Poor response should prompt evaluation of these potential factors, as well as possible malignant processes and hematologic disease (thalassemia, refractory anemia, myelodysplastic disorder), occult blood loss, hemolysis, osteitis fibrosa cystic, and/or bone marrow fibrosis. Severe anemia and pure red cell aplasia (PRCA) with associated neutralizing antibodies to erythropoietin has been reported, predominantly in patients with CKD receiving SubQ darbepoetin (the I.V. route is preferred for hemodialysis patients). Cases have also been reported in patients with hepatitis C who were receiving ESAs, interferon, and ribavirin. Patients with a sudden loss of response to darbepoetin (with severe anemia and a low reticulocyte count) should be evaluated for PRCA with associated neutralizing antibodies to erythropoietin; discontinue treatment (permanently) in patients with PRCA secondary to neutralizing antibodies to erythropoietin. Antibodies may cross-react; do not switch to another ESA in patients who develop antibody-mediated anemia.

Potentially serious allergic reactions have been reported (rarely). Discontinue immediately (and permanently) in patients who experience serious allergic/anaphylactic reactions. Some products may contain albumin and the packaging of some formulations may contain latex.

Adverse Reactions

>10%:

Cardiovascular: Hypertension (31%), peripheral edema (17%), edema (6% to 13%)

Gastrointestinal: Abdominal pain (10% to 13%)

Respiratory: Dyspnea (17%), cough (12%)

1% to 10%:

Cardiovascular: Angina, fluid overload, hypotension, MI, thromboembolic events

Central nervous system: Cerebrovascular disorder

Dermatologic: Rash/erythema

Local: AV graft thrombosis, vascular access complications

Respiratory: Pulmonary embolism

<1% (Limited to important or life-threatening): Allergic reaction, anaphylactic reactions, anemia associated with neutralizing antibodies (severe; with or without other cytopenias), angioedema, bronchospasm, hypertensive encephalopathy, pure red cell aplasia (PRCA), seizure, stroke, tumor progression/recurrence (cancer patients), urticaria

Drug Interactions

Metabolism/Transport Effects None known.

Avoid Concomitant Use There are no known interactions where it is recommended to avoid concomitant use.

Increased Effect/Toxicity There are no known significant interactions involving an increase in effect.

Decreased Effect There are no known significant interactions involving a decrease in effect.

Ethanol/Nutrition/Herb Interactions Ethanol: Should be avoided due to adverse effects on erythropoiesis.

Stability Store at 2°C to 8°C (36°F to 46°F); do not freeze. Do not shake. Protect from light. Store in original carton until use. The following stability information has also been reported: May be stored at room temperature for up to 7 days (Cohen, 2007). Do not dilute or administer with other solutions.

Mechanism of Action Induces erythropoiesis by stimulating the division and differentiation of committed erythroid progenitor cells; induces the release of reticulocytes from the bone marrow into the bloodstream, where they mature to erythrocytes. There is a dose response relationship with this effect. This results in an increase in reticulocyte counts followed by a rise in hematocrit and hemoglobin levels. When administered SubQ or I.V., darbepoetin's half-life is ~3 times that of epoetin alfa concentrations.

Pharmacodynamics/Kinetics

Onset of action: Increased hemoglobin levels not generally observed until 2-6 weeks after initiating treatment

Absorption: SubQ: Slow

Distribution: V_d: 0.06 L/kg

Bioavailability: CKD: SubQ: Adults: ~37% (range: 30% to 50%); Children: 54% (range: 32% to 70%)

Half-life elimination:

CKD: Adults:

I.V.: 21 hours

SubQ: Nondialysis patients: 70 hours (range: 35-139 hours); Dialysis patients: 46 hours (range: 12-89 hours)

Cancer: Adults: SubQ: 74 hours (range: 24-144 hours); Children: 49 hours

Note: Darbepoetin half-life is approximately threefold longer than epoetin alfa following I.V. administration

Time to peak: SubQ:

CKD: Adults: 48 hours (range: 12-72 hours; independent of dialysis); Children: 36 hours (range: 10-58 hours)

Cancer: Adults: 71-90 hours (range: 28-123 hours); Children: 71 hours (range: 21-143 hours)

Dosage

Anemia associated with chronic kidney disease: Individualize dosing and use the lowest dose necessary to reduce the need for RBC transfusions.

*Chronic kidney disease patients **ON dialysis*** (I.V. route is preferred for hemodialysis patients; initiate treatment when hemoglobin is <10 g/dL; reduce dose or interrupt treatment if hemoglobin approaches or exceeds 11 g/dL):

Children ≥1 year: Conversion from epoetin alfa: I.V., SubQ: Initial dose: Epoetin alfa doses of 1500 to ≥90,000 units per week may be converted to doses ranging from 6.25-200 mcg darbepoetin alfa per week (see pediatric column in conversion table on next page).

Adults: I.V., SubQ: Initial: 0.45 mcg/kg once weekly **or** 0.75 mcg/kg once every 2 weeks **or** epoetin alfa doses of <1500 to ≥90,000 units per week may be converted to doses ranging from 6.25-200 mcg darbepoetin alfa per week (see adult column in conversion table on next page).

*Chronic kidney disease patients **NOT on dialysis*** (consider initiating treatment when hemoglobin is <10 g/dL; use only if rate of hemoglobin decline would likely result in RBC transfusion and desire is to reduce risk of alloimmunization or other RBC transfusion-related risks; reduce dose or interrupt treatment if hemoglobin exceeds 10 g/dL):

Adults: I.V., SubQ: Initial: 0.45 mcg/kg once every 4 weeks

Dosage adjustments for chronic kidney disease patients (either on dialysis or not on dialysis): Do not increase dose more frequently than every 4 weeks (dose decreases may occur more frequently).

If hemoglobin increases >1 g/dL in any 2-week period: Decrease dose by ≥25%

If hemoglobin does not increase by >1 g/dL after 4 weeks: Increase dose by 25%

Inadequate or lack of response: If adequate response is not achieved over 12 weeks, further increases are unlikely to be of benefit and may increase the risk for adverse events; use the minimum effective dose that will maintain a hemoglobin level sufficient to avoid red blood cell transfusions **and** evaluate patient for other causes of anemia; discontinue treatment if responsiveness does not improve

Anemia due to chemotherapy in cancer patients: Initiate treatment only if hemoglobin <10 g/dL and anticipated duration of myelosuppressive chemotherapy is ≥2 months. Titrate dosage to use the minimum effective dose that will maintain a hemoglobin level sufficient to avoid red blood cell transfusions. Discontinue darbepoetin following completion of chemotherapy. SubQ:

Adults: Initial: 2.25 mcg/kg once weekly **or** 500 mcg once every 3 weeks until completion of chemotherapy

Dosage adjustments:

Increase dose: If hemoglobin does not increase by 1 g/dL **and** remains below 10 g/dL after initial 6 weeks (for patients receiving weekly therapy only), increase dose to 4.5 mcg/kg once weekly (no dosage adjustment if using every 3 week dosing).

Reduce dose by 40% if hemoglobin increases >1g/dL in any 2-week period **or** hemoglobin reaches a level sufficient to avoid red blood cell transfusion.

Withhold dose if hemoglobin exceeds a level needed to avoid red blood cell transfusion. Resume treatment with a 40% dose reduction when hemoglobin approaches a level where transfusions may be required.

Discontinue: On completion of chemotherapy or if after 8 weeks of therapy there is no hemoglobin response or RBC transfusions still required

Symptomatic anemia associated with MDS (unlabeled use): Adults: SubQ: 150-300 mcg once weekly (NCCN MDS guidelines v.2.2011)

Conversion from epoetin alfa to darbepoetin alfa: See table.

Conversion From Epoetin Alfa to Darbepoetin Alfa (Initial Dose)

Previous Dosage of Epoetin Alfa (units/week)	Children Darbepoetin Alfa Dosage (mcg/week)	Adults Darbepoetin Alfa Dosage (mcg/week)
<1500	Not established	6.25
1500-2499	6.25	6.25
2500-4999	10	12.5
5000-10,999	20	25
11,000-17,999	40	40
18,000-33,999	60	60
34,000-89,999	100	100
≥90,000	200	200

Note: In patients receiving epoetin alfa 2-3 times per week, darbepoetin alfa is administered once weekly. In patients receiving epoetin alfa once weekly, darbepoetin alfa is administered once every 2 weeks. The darbepoetin dose to be administered every 2 weeks is derived by adding together 2 weekly epoetin alfa doses and then converting to the appropriate darbepoetin dose. Titrate dose to hemoglobin response thereafter (see dosage adjustment in renal impairment).

Dietary Considerations Supplemental iron intake may be required in patients with low iron stores.

Administration May be administered by SubQ or I.V. injection. The I.V. route is recommended in hemodialysis patients. Do not shake; vigorous shaking may denature darbepoetin alfa, rendering it biologically inactive. Do not dilute or administer in conjunction with other drug solutions. Discard any unused portion of the vial; do not pool unused portions.

Monitoring Parameters Hemoglobin (at least once per week until maintenance dose established and after dosage changes; monitor less frequently once hemoglobin is stabilized); CKD patients should be also be monitored at least monthly following hemoglobin stability); iron stores (transferrin saturation and ferritin) prior to and during therapy; serum chemistry (CKD patients); blood pressure; fluid balance (CKD patients); seizures (CKD patients following initiation for first few months, includes new-onset or change in seizure frequency or premonitory symptoms)

Cancer patients: Examinations recommended by the ASCO/ASH guidelines (Rizzo, 2010) prior to treatment include peripheral blood smear (in some situations a bone marrow exam may be necessary), assessment for iron, folate, or vitamin B_{12} deficiency, reticulocyte count, renal function status, and occult blood loss; during ESA treatment, assess baseline and periodic iron, total iron-binding capacity, and transferrin saturation or ferritin levels.

Additional Information Oncology Comment: The American Society of Clinical Oncology (ASCO) and American Society of Hematology (ASH) 2010 updates to the clinical practice guidelines for the use of erythropoiesis-stimulating agents (ESAs) in patients with cancer indicate that ESAs are appropriate when used according to the parameters identified within the Food and Drug Administration (FDA) approved labeling for epoetin and darbepoetin (Rizzo, 2010). ESAs are an option for chemotherapy associated anemia when the hemoglobin has fallen to <10 g/dL to decrease the need for RBC transfusions. ESAs should only be used in conjunction with concurrent chemotherapy. Although the FDA label now limits ESA use to the palliative setting, the ASCO/ASH guidelines suggest using clinical judgment in weighing risks versus benefits as formal outcomes studies of ESA use defined by intent of chemotherapy treatment have not been conducted.

The ASCO/ASH guidelines continue to recommend following the FDA approved dosing (and dosing adjustment) guidelines as alternate dosing and schedules have not demonstrated consistent differences in effectiveness with regard to hemoglobin response. In patients who do not have a response within 6-8 weeks (hemoglobin rise <1-2 g/dL or no reduction in transfusions) ESA therapy should be discontinued.

Prior to the initiation of ESAs, other sources of anemia (in addition to chemotherapy or underlying hematologic malignancy) should be investigated. Examinations recommended prior to treatment include peripheral blood smear (in some situations a bone marrow exam may be necessary), assessment for iron, folate, or vitamin B_{12} deficiency, reticulocyte count, renal function status, and occult blood loss. During ESA treatment, assess baseline and periodic iron, total iron-binding capacity, and transferrin saturation or ferritin levels. Iron supplementation may be necessary.

The guidelines note that patients with an increased risk of thromboembolism (generally includes previous history of thrombosis, surgery, and/or prolonged periods of immobilization) and patients receiving concomitant medications that may increase thromboembolic risk, should begin ESA therapy only after careful consideration. With the exception of low-risk myelodysplasia-associated anemia (which has evidence supporting the use of ESAs without concurrent chemotherapy), the guidelines do not support the use of ESAs in the absence of concurrent chemotherapy.

Dosage Forms Excipient information presented when available (limited, particularly for generics); consult specific product labeling.

Injection, solution [preservative free]:

Aranesp®: 25 mcg/mL (1 mL); 40 mcg/mL (1 mL); 60 mcg/mL (1 mL); 100 mcg/mL (1 mL); 150 mcg/0.75 mL (0.75 mL); 200 mcg/mL (1 mL); 300 mcg/mL (1 mL) [contains polysorbate 80]

Aranesp® SingleJect®: 25 mcg/0.42 mL (0.42 mL); 40 mcg/0.4 mL (0.4 mL); 60 mcg/0.3 mL (0.3 mL); 100 mcg/0.5 mL (0.5 mL); 150 mcg/0.3 mL (0.3 mL); 200 mcg/0.4 mL (0.4 mL); 300 mcg/0.6 mL (0.6 mL); 500 mcg/mL (1 mL) [contains natural rubber/natural latex in packaging, polysorbate 80]

Darifenacin (dar i FEN a sin)

Brand Names: U.S. Enablex®

Brand Names: Canada Enablex®

Index Terms Darifenacin Hydrobromide; UK-88,525

Pharmacologic Category Anticholinergic Agent

Use Management of symptoms of bladder overactivity (urge incontinence, urgency, and frequency)

Pregnancy Risk Factor C

Pregnancy Considerations Teratogenic effects and developmental delay were observed in some animal studies. There are no adequate and well-controlled studies in pregnant women; should be used only if potential benefit outweighs possible risk to the fetus.

Lactation Excretion in breast milk unknown/use caution

Contraindications Hypersensitivity to darifenacin or any component of the formulation; uncontrolled narrow-angle glaucoma; urinary retention, paralytic ileus, GI or GU obstruction

Warnings/Precautions May cause drowsiness and/or blurred vision, which may impair physical or mental abilities; patients must be cautioned about performing tasks which require mental alertness (eg, operating machinery or driving). May occur in the presence of increased environmental temperature; use caution in hot weather and/or exercise. Use with caution with hepatic impairment; dosage limitation is required in moderate hepatic impairment (Child-Pugh class B). Not recommended for use in severe hepatic impairment (Child-Pugh class C). Use with caution in patients with clinically-significant bladder outlet obstruction or prostatic hyperplasia (nonobstructive). Use caution in patients with decreased GI motility, constipation, hiatal hernia, reflux esophagitis, and ulcerative colitis. Use caution in patients with myasthenia gravis. In patients with controlled narrow-angle glaucoma, darifenacin should be used with extreme caution and only when the potential benefit outweighs risks of treatment. Use with caution in patients taking strong CYP3A4 inhibitors (see Drug Interactions); dosage limitation of darifenacin is required.

Adverse Reactions

>10%: Gastrointestinal: Xerostomia (19% to 35%), constipation (15% to 21%)

1% to 10%:

Cardiovascular: Hypertension (≥1%), peripheral edema (≥1%)

Central nervous system: Headache (7%), dizziness (<2%), pain (≥1%)

Dermatological: Dry skin (≥1%), pruritus (≥1%), rash (≥1%)

Gastrointestinal: Dyspepsia (3% to 8%), abdominal pain (2% to 4%), nausea (2% to 4%), vomiting (≥1%), weight gain (≥1%)

Genitourinary: Urinary tract infection (4% to 5%), vaginitis (≥1%), urinary retention (acute)

Neuromuscular & skeletal: Weakness (<3%), arthralgia (≥1%), back pain (≥1%)

Ocular: Dry eyes (2%), abnormal vision (≥1%)

Respiratory: Bronchitis (≥1%), pharyngitis (≥1%), rhinitis (≥1%), sinusitis (≥1%)

Miscellaneous: Flu-like syndrome (1% to 3%)

Postmarketing and/or case reports: Angioedema, confusion, hallucinations, hypersensitivity reactions, palpitation

Drug Interactions

Metabolism/Transport Effects Substrate of CYP2D6 (minor), CYP3A4 (major); **Note:** Assignment of Major/Minor substrate status based on clinically relevant drug interaction potential; **Inhibits** CYP2D6 (moderate), CYP3A4 (weak)

Avoid Concomitant Use

Avoid concomitant use of Darifenacin with any of the following: Conivaptan; Pimozide; Thioridazine

Increased Effect/Toxicity

Darifenacin may increase the levels/effects of: AbobotulinumtoxinA; Anticholinergics; Cannabinoids; CYP2D6 Substrates; Fesoterodine; Nebivolol; OnabotulinumtoxinA; Pimozide; Potassium Chloride; RimabotulinumtoxinB; Tamoxifen; Thioridazine

The levels/effects of Darifenacin may be increased by: Conivaptan; CYP3A4 Inhibitors (Moderate); CYP3A4 Inhibitors (Strong); Dasatinib; Pramlintide; Propafenone

Decreased Effect

Darifenacin may decrease the levels/effects of: Acetylcholinesterase Inhibitors (Central); Codeine; Secretin; TraMADol

The levels/effects of Darifenacin may be decreased by: Acetylcholinesterase Inhibitors (Central); CYP3A4 Inducers (Strong); Deferasirox; Herbs (CYP3A4 Inducers); Peginterferon Alfa-2b; Tocilizumab

Ethanol/Nutrition/Herb Interactions Herb/Nutraceutical: Darifenacin serum concentration may be decreased by St John's wort (avoid concurrent use.)

Stability Store at 25°C (77°F); excursions permitted to 15°C to 30°C (59°F to 86°F). Protect from light.

Mechanism of Action Selective antagonist of the M3 muscarinic (cholinergic) receptor subtype. Blockade of the receptor limits bladder contractions, reducing the symptoms of bladder irritability/overactivity (urge incontinence, urgency and frequency).

Pharmacodynamics/Kinetics

Distribution: V_{dss}: ~163 L

Protein binding: ~98% (primarily alpha$_1$-acid glycoprotein)

Metabolism: Hepatic, via CYP3A4 (major) and CYP2D6 (minor)

Bioavailability: 15% to 19%

Half-life elimination: ~13-19 hours

Time to peak, plasma: ~7 hours

Excretion: As metabolites (inactive); urine (60%), feces (40%)

Dosage Oral: Adults: Initial: 7.5 mg once daily. If response is not adequate after a minimum of 2 weeks, dosage may be increased to 15 mg once daily.

Dosage adjustment with concomitant potent CYP3A4 inhibitors (eg, azole antifungals, erythromycin, isoniazid, protease inhibitors): Daily dosage should not exceed 7.5 mg/day

Dosage adjustment in renal impairment: No adjustment required.

Dosage adjustment in hepatic impairment:

Moderate impairment (Child-Pugh class B): Daily dosage should not exceed 7.5 mg/day

Severe impairment (Child-Pugh class C): Has not been evaluated; use is not recommended

Dietary Considerations May be taken without regard to meals, with or without food.

Administration Tablet should be taken with liquid and swallowed whole; do not chew, crush, or split tablet. May be taken without regard to food.

Dosage Forms Excipient information presented when available (limited, particularly for generics); consult specific product labeling.

Tablet, extended release, oral:

Enablex®: 7.5 mg, 15 mg

◆ **Darifenacin Hydrobromide** *see* Darifenacin *on page 450*

Darunavir (dar OO na veer)

Brand Names: U.S. Prezista®

Brand Names: Canada Prezista®

Index Terms Darunavir Ethanolate; TMC-114

Pharmacologic Category Antiretroviral Agent, Protease Inhibitor

Additional Appendix Information

Perinatal HIV Guidelines *on page 1946*

Use Treatment of HIV-1 infections in combination with ritonavir and other antiretroviral agents

Pregnancy Risk Factor C

Pregnancy Considerations Teratogenic effects have not been observed in animal reproduction studies. Darunavir crosses the placenta (concentrations vary by report). The DHHS Perinatal HIV Guidelines note there is insufficient data to recommend use during pregnancy; however, if used, darunavir must be given with low-dose ritonavir boosting. A small increased risk of preterm birth has been associated with maternal use of protease inhibitor-based combination antiretroviral (ARV) therapy during pregnancy; however, the benefits of use generally outweigh this risk and protease inhibitors (PIs) should not be withheld if otherwise recommended. Hyperglycemia, new onset of diabetes mellitus, or diabetic ketoacidosis have been reported with PIs; it is not clear if pregnancy increases this risk.

Regardless of CD4 count or HIV RNA copy number, all HIV-infected pregnant women should receive a combination antepartum ARV drug regimen; this includes women who require therapy for their own health, as well as women who do not yet require therapy for their own health. ARV therapy should be started as soon as possible if required for the woman's health or immediately after the first trimester if not needed for the mothers health (although earlier initiation may be considered). Long-term follow-up is recommended for all infants exposed to ARV medications.

Healthcare providers are encouraged to enroll pregnant women exposed to antiretroviral medications in the Antiretroviral Pregnancy Registry (1-800-258-4263 or www.-APRegistry.com). Healthcare providers caring for HIV-infected women and their infants may contact the National Perinatal HIV Hotline (888-448-8765) for clinical consultation (DHHS [perinatal], 2011).

Lactation Excretion in breast milk unknown/not recommended

Contraindications Coadministration with medications highly dependent upon CYP3A4 for clearance and for which increased levels are associated with serious and/or life-threatening events (includes alfuzosin, cisapride, ergot alkaloids [eg, dihydroergotamine, ergonovine, ergotamine, methylergonovine], lovastatin, midazolam [oral], pimozide, rifampin, sildenafil (when used for pulmonary artery hypertension [eg, Revatio®]), simvastatin, St John's wort, triazolam

Canadian labeling: Additional contraindications: Hypersensitivity to darunavir or any component of the formulation; coadministration with amiodarone, lidocaine (systemic), quinidine; severe (Child-Pugh class C) hepatic impairment

Warnings/Precautions Coadministration with ritonavir is required (DHHS, 2011). Use with caution in patients taking strong CYP3A4 inhibitors, moderate or strong CYP3A4 inducers and major CYP3A4 substrates (see Drug Interactions); consider alternative agents that avoid or lessen the potential for CYP-mediated interactions. Do not coadminister colchicine in patient with renal or hepatic impairment; avoid concurrent use with salmeterol.

Use with caution in patients with hepatic impairment, including active chronic hepatitis; consider interruption or discontinuation with worsening hepatic function. Not recommended in severe hepatic impairment (contraindicated in Canadian labeling). Infrequent cases of drug-induced hepatitis (including acute and cytolytic) have been reported. Liver injury has been reported with use (including some fatalities), though generally in patients on multiple medications, with advanced HIV disease, hepatitis B/C coinfection, and/or immune reconstitution syndrome. Monitor patients closely; consider interrupting or discontinuing therapy if signs/symptoms of liver impairment occur.

May cause fat redistribution (buffalo hump, increased abdominal girth, breast engorgement, facial atrophy). Immune reconstitution syndrome, including inflammatory responses to indolent infections, has been associated with antiretroviral therapy; additional evaluation and treatment may be required. May increase cholesterol and/or triglycerides. Pancreatitis has been observed with use. Risk for pancreatitis may be increased in patients with elevated triglycerides, advanced HIV disease, or history of pancreatitis. Protease inhibitors have been associated with glucose dysregulation; use caution in patients with diabetes. Use with caution in patients with sulfonamide allergy (contains sulfa moiety) or hemophilia. Protease inhibitors have been associated with a variety of hypersensitivity events (some severe), including rash, anaphylaxis (rare), angioedema, bronchospasm, erythema multiforme, Stevens-Johnson syndrome (rare), and/or toxic epidermal necrolysis. Discontinue treatment if severe skin reactions develop. Severe skin reactions may be accompanied by fever, malaise, fatigue, arthralgias, hepatitis, oral lesion, blisters, conjunctivitis, and/or eosinophilia. Mild-to-moderate rash may occur early in treatment and resolve with continued therapy. Treatment history and resistance data should guide use of darunavir with ritonavir.

Adverse Reactions As a class, protease inhibitors potentially cause dyslipidemias which includes elevated cholesterol and triglycerides and a redistribution of body fat centrally to cause increased abdominal girth, buffalo hump, facial atrophy, and breast enlargement. These agents also cause hyperglycemia. Frequency of adverse events is reported for darunavir/ritonavir. See also Ritonavir monograph.

>10%:

Endocrine & metabolic: Hypercholesterolemia (grade 2: 16% to 25%; grade 3: 1% to 10%), LDL increased (grade 2: 14%; grade 3: 5% to 8%)

Gastrointestinal: Vomiting (children 13%; adults 2% to 5%), diarrhea (8% to 14%)

2% to 10%:

Central nervous system: Headache (children 9%; adults 3% to 6%), fatigue (children 3%; adults ≤2%)

Dermatologic: Rash (5% to 10%)

Endocrine & metabolic: Hyperglycemia (grade 2: 7% to 10%; grade 3: ≤1%; grade 4: <1%), triglycerides increased (grade 2: 3% to 10%; grade 3: 1% to 7%; grade 4: ≤3%), diabetes mellitus (2%)

Gastrointestinal: Abdominal pain (children 10%; adults 5% to 6%), nausea (3% to 7%), amylase increased (grade 2: 5% to 6%; grade 3: 3% to 7%), lipase increased (grade 2: 2% to 3%; grade 3: ≤2%; grade 4: <1%), abdominal distention (2%), anorexia (2%), dyspepsia (2%)

Hepatic: ALT increased (grade 2: 7%, grade 3: 2% to 3%; grade 4: ≤1%), AST increased (grade 2: 6%; grade 3: 2% to 4%; grade 4: <1%), alkaline phosphatase (grade 2: ≤2%; grade 3: <1%)

Neuromuscular & skeletal: Weakness (≤3%)

<2% (Limited to important or life-threatening): Acute renal failure, acute respiratory distress syndrome, allergic dermatitis, alopecia, anemia, angioedema, appetite decreased, arthralgia, bile duct obstruction, bradycardia, cerebrovascular accident, dermatitis medicamentosa, dyspnea, erythema multiforme, extremity pain, facial edema, fat redistribution (eg, buffalo hump, increased abdominal girth, breast engorgement, facial atrophy), fever, folliculitis, gynecomastia, hematuria, hepatic cirrhosis, hepatic failure, hepatic neoplasm (malignant), hepatitis (acute and cytolytic), hepatotoxicity, hiccups, hyperbilirubinemia, hyperhidrosis, hyperkalemia, hyperlipidemia, hypersensitivity, hypertension, hyperthermia, hypoesthesia, immune reconstitution syndrome, infection (including clostridium, cryptosporidiosis, cytomegalovirus encephalitis, hepatitis B, esophageal candidiasis), jaundice, large B-cell neoplasm (diffuse), lipoatrophy, lymphoma, maculopapular rash, metabolic acidosis, MI, myalgia, myocarditis, myositis, nephrolithiasis, neuromyopathy, night sweats, nightmare, obesity, osteonecrosis, osteopenia, osteoporosis, pancreatitis, pancytopenia, paresthesia, peripheral edema, peripheral neuropathy, pharyngeal lesion, pneumothorax, polydipsia, polyuria, progressive multifocal leukoencephalopathy, pruritus, rectal hemorrhage, renal insufficiency, renal tubular

necrosis, rhabdomyolysis (coadministration with HMG-CoA reductase inhibitors), respiratory failure, rigors, seizure, sepsis, skin inflammation, somnolence, Stevens-Johnson syndrome, suicide (completed), tachycardia, toxic skin eruption, toxic epidermal necrolysis, transient ischemic attack, urticaria, vertigo, xerostomia

Drug Interactions

Metabolism/Transport Effects **Substrate** of CYP3A4 (major); **Note:** Assignment of Major/Minor substrate status based on clinically relevant drug interaction potential; **Inhibits** CYP2D6 (weak), CYP3A4 (strong), P-glycoprotein

Avoid Concomitant Use

Avoid concomitant use of Darunavir with any of the following: Alfuzosin; Amiodarone; Cisapride; Conivaptan; Crizotinib; Dronedarone; Eplerenone; Ergot Derivatives; Everolimus; Fluticasone (Oral Inhalation); Fosphenytoin; Halofantrine; Lapatinib; Lopinavir; Lovastatin; Lurasidone; Midazolam; Nilotinib; Nisoldipine; PHENobarbital; Phenytoin; Pimozide; QuiNIDine; Ranolazine; Rifampin; Rivaroxaban; RomiDEPsin; Salmeterol; Saquinavir; Silodosin; Simvastatin; St Johns Wort; Tamsulosin; Telaprevir; Ticagrelor; Tolvaptan; Topotecan; Toremifene; Triazolam; Voriconazole

Increased Effect/Toxicity

Darunavir may increase the levels/effects of: Alfuzosin; Almotriptan; Alosetron; ALPRAZolam; Amiodarone; Antifungal Agents (Azole Derivatives, Systemic); ARIPiprazole; Bortezomib; Brentuximab Vedotin; Brinzolamide; Budesonide (Nasal); Budesonide (Systemic, Oral Inhalation); Calcium Channel Blockers (Dihydropyridine); Calcium Channel Blockers (Nondihydropyridine); CarBAMazepine; Ciclesonide; Cisapride; Clarithromycin; Colchicine; Conivaptan; Corticosteroids (Orally Inhaled); Crizotinib; CycloSPORINE; CycloSPORINE (Systemic); CYP2D6 Substrates; CYP3A4 Substrates; Dabigatran Etexilate; Dienogest; Digoxin; Dronedarone; Dutasteride; Efavirenz; Enfuvirtide; Eplerenone; Ergot Derivatives; Everolimus; FentaNYL; Fesoterodine; Fluticasone (Nasal); Fluticasone (Oral Inhalation); Fusidic Acid; GuanFACINE; Halofantrine; HMG-CoA Reductase Inhibitors; Iloperidone; Ixabepilone; Lapatinib; Lidocaine; Lidocaine (Systemic); Lidocaine (Topical); Lovastatin; Lumefantrine; Lurasidone; Maraviroc; Meperidine; MethylPREDNISolone; Midazolam; Nefazodone; Nilotinib; Nisoldipine; Paricalcitol; Pazopanib; P-glycoprotein/ABCB1 Substrates; Pimecrolimus; Pimozide; Propafenone; Protease Inhibitors; QuiNIDine; Ranolazine; Rifabutin; Rilpivirine; Rivaroxaban; RomiDEPsin; Ruxolitinib; Salmeterol; Saxagliptin; Sildenafil; Silodosin; Simvastatin; Sirolimus; SORAfenib; Tacrolimus; Tacrolimus (Systemic); Tacrolimus (Topical); Tadalafil; Tamsulosin; Temsirolimus; Tenofovir; Ticagrelor; Tolterodine; Tolvaptan; Topotecan; Toremifene; TraZODone; Triazolam; Tricyclic Antidepressants; Vardenafil; Vemurafenib; Vilazodone; Zuclopenthixol

The levels/effects of Darunavir may be increased by: Antifungal Agents (Azole Derivatives, Systemic); Clarithromycin; CycloSPORINE; CycloSPORINE (Systemic); CYP3A4 Inhibitors (Moderate); CYP3A4 Inhibitors (Strong); Dasatinib; Delavirdine; Efavirenz; Enfuvirtide; Etravirine; Fusidic Acid; Rifabutin

Decreased Effect

Darunavir may decrease the levels/effects of: Abacavir; Clarithromycin; Contraceptives (Estrogens); Delavirdine; Didanosine; Divalproex; Etravirine; Meperidine; Methadone; Norethindrone; PARoxetine; Prasugrel; Sertraline; Telaprevir; Theophylline Derivatives; Ticagrelor; Valproic Acid; Voriconazole; Warfarin; Zidovudine

The levels/effects of Darunavir may be decreased by: CarBAMazepine; CYP3A4 Inducers (Strong); Deferasirox; Efavirenz; Fosphenytoin; Garlic; Lopinavir; PHENobarbital; Phenytoin; Rifampin; Saquinavir; St Johns Wort; Telaprevir; Tenofovir; Tocilizumab

Ethanol/Nutrition/Herb Interactions

Food: Bioavailability is increased when administered with food.

Herb/nutraceutical: St John's wort may decrease the plasma levels of darunavir; concomitant use is contraindicated.

Stability Store at 25°C (77°F); excursions permitted to 15°C to 30°C (59°F to 86°F).

Mechanism of Action Binds to the site of HIV-1 protease activity and inhibits cleavage of viral Gag-Pol polyprotein precursors into individual functional proteins required for infectious HIV. This results in the formation of immature, noninfectious viral particles.

Pharmacodynamics/Kinetics All kinetic parameters derived in the presence of ritonavir coadministration.

Absorption: Increased 30% with food

Protein binding: ~95%; primarily to alpha$_1$ acid glycoprotein (AAG)

Metabolism: Hepatic, via CYP3A4 to minimally-active metabolites

Bioavailability: 82%

Half-life elimination: ~15 hours

Time to peak, plasma: 2.5-4 hours

Excretion: Feces (~80%, 41% as unchanged drug); urine (~14%, 8% as unchanged drug)

Dosage Oral:

Children ≥6 years: **Note:** Do not use once daily dosing in pediatric patients; maximum dose: 600 mg darunavir/100 mg ritonavir twice daily

≥20 kg to <30 kg: 375 mg twice daily; coadministration with ritonavir 50 mg twice daily is required

≥30 kg to <40 kg: 450 mg twice daily; coadministration with ritonavir 60 mg twice daily is required

≥40 kg: 600 mg twice daily; coadministration with ritonavir 100 mg twice daily is required

Adults:

Therapy-naive: 800 mg once daily; coadministration with ritonavir 100 mg once daily is required. **Note:** Recommended (with ritonavir) as a first-line therapy with tenofovir/emtricitabine in antiretroviral naïve patients (DHHS, 2011).

Therapy-experienced: **Note:** If genotypic testing is not possible, 600 mg twice daily, coadministered with ritonavir 100 mg twice daily, is recommended.

With no resistance-associated substitutions: 800 mg once daily; coadministration with ritonavir 100 mg once daily is required

With ≥1 resistance-associated substitution: 600 mg twice daily; coadministration with ritonavir 100 mg twice daily is required

Dosage adjustment for toxicity:

Severe rash: Discontinue treatment

New or worsening liver dysfunction: Consider interrupting or discontinuing treatment

Dosage adjustments for concomitant therapy:

Coadministration with bosentan:

Coadministration of bosentan in patients currently receiving darunavir/ritonavir: For patients receiving ritonavir for at least 10 days, begin with bosentan 62.5 mg once daily or every other day based on tolerability

Coadministration of darunavir/ritonavir in patients currently receiving bosentan: Discontinue bosentan 36 hours prior to the initiation of ritonavir. After at least 10 days of ritonavir, resume bosentan 62.5 mg once daily or every other day based on tolerability.

Coadministration with colchicine:

Familial Mediterranean fever (FMF): Maximum colchicine dose: 0.6 mg/day (0.3 mg twice daily)

Gout prophylaxis:
If original colchicine dose is 0.6 mg twice daily, adjust dose to 0.3 mg once daily
If original colchicine dose is 0.6 mg once daily, adjust dose to 0.3 mg every other day
Gout flare treatment: Initial: Colchicine 0.6 mg, followed in 1 hour by a single dose of 0.3 mg; do not repeat for at least 3 days

Coadministration with phosphodiesterase-5 enzyme (PDE-5) inhibitor:
Pulmonary arterial hypertension: Darunavir/ritonavir coadministered with tadalafil:
Patient receiving darunavir with ritonavir for at least 1 week: Initiate tadalafil at 20 mg once daily; increase to 40 mg once daily based on individual tolerability
Patient receiving tadalafil when initiating darunavir/ritonavir: Discontinue tadalafil at least 24 hours prior to starting darunavir/ritonavir. After at least 1 week following the initiation of ritonavir, resume tadalafil at 20 mg once daily; increase to 40 mg once daily based on individual tolerability.
Erectile dysfunction: Darunavir/ritonavir coadministered with:
Sildenafil (Viagra®): Maximum sildenafil dose: 25 mg in a 48-hour period
Tadalafil (Cialis®): Maximum tadalafil dose: 10 mg in a 72-hour period
Vardenafil: Maximum vardenafil dose: 2.5 mg in a 72-hour period

Dosage adjustment in renal impairment: No adjustment required for mild-to-moderate impairment. No data available for use in severe renal failure or end-stage renal disease.

Dosage adjustment in hepatic impairment: No adjustment for mild-to-moderate impairment (Child-Pugh classes A and B). Not recommended for patients with severe impairment (contraindicated in Canadian labeling).

Dietary Considerations Absorption increased with food. Take with meals.

Administration Coadministration with ritonavir and food is required (bioavailability is increased).

Monitoring Parameters Viral load, CD4, serum glucose; transaminase levels prior to and during therapy (increase monitoring in patients at risk for liver impairment), cholesterol, triglycerides

Product Availability Prezista® 100 mg/mL oral suspension: FDA approved December 2011; availability expected in the second quarter of 2012

Dosage Forms Excipient information presented when available (limited, particularly for generics); consult specific product labeling.
Tablet, oral:
Prezista®: 75 mg, 150 mg, 400 mg, 600 mg

Dosage Forms: Canada Excipient information presented when available (limited, particularly for generics); consult specific product labeling.
Tablet:
Prezista®: 300 mg, 400 mg, 600 mg

◆ **Darunavir Ethanolate** *see* Darunavir *on page 451*

Dasatinib (da SA ti nib)

Brand Names: U.S. Sprycel®
Brand Names: Canada Sprycel®
Index Terms BMS-354825
Pharmacologic Category Antineoplastic Agent, Tyrosine Kinase Inhibitor

Use Treatment of chronic myelogenous leukemia (CML) in chronic, accelerated or blast (myeloid or lymphoid) phase resistant or intolerant to prior therapy (including imatinib); treatment of newly-diagnosed Philadelphia chromosome-positive (Ph+) CML in chronic phase; treatment of Philadelphia chromosome-positive (Ph+) acute lymphoblastic leukemia (ALL) resistant or intolerant to prior therapy

Unlabeled Use Post-stem cell transplant (allogeneic) follow-up treatment of CML; treatment of gastrointestinal stromal tumor (GIST)

Pregnancy Risk Factor D

Pregnancy Considerations Animal studies have demonstrated fetal abnormalities (skeletal malformations, reduced ossification, edema, microhepatia) and fetal death. There are no adequate and well-controlled studies in pregnant women. May cause fetal harm if administered to a pregnant woman. Not recommended for use during pregnancy or if contemplating pregnancy. Effective contraception is recommended for men and women of child-bearing potential. Pregnant women are advised to avoid contact with crushed or broken tablets.

Lactation Excretion in breast milk unknown/not recommended

Contraindications There are no contraindications listed within the FDA-approved manufacturer's labeling.

Canadian labeling: Hypersensitivity to dasatinib or any other component of the formulation

Warnings/Precautions Hazardous agent - use appropriate precautions for handling and disposal. Severe dose-related bone marrow suppression (thrombocytopenia, neutropenia, anemia) is associated with treatment; dosage adjustment or temporary interruption may be required for severe myelosuppression; the incidence of myelosuppression is higher in patients with advanced CML and Ph+ ALL. Fatal intracranial hemorrhage has been reported in association with dasatinib use; monitor blood counts. Severe hemorrhage (including CNS, GI) may occur due to thrombocytopenia; in addition to thrombocytopenia, dasatinib may also cause platelet dysfunction. Use caution with patients taking anticoagulants or medications interfering with platelet function; not studied in clinical trials. Avoid concomitant use with CYP3A4 inducers and inhibitors; if concomitant use cannot be avoided, consider dasatinib dosage adjustments.

Cardiomyopathy, diastolic dysfunction, heart failure (congestive), left ventricular dysfunction, and MI have been reported; monitor for signs and symptoms of cardiac dysfunction. Fluid retention, including pleural and pericardial effusions, severe ascites, severe pulmonary edema, and generalized edema were reported; may be dose-related. A chest x-ray is recommended for symptoms suggestive of effusion (dyspnea or dry cough). Utilizing once-daily dosing is associated with a decreased frequency of fluid retention. The risk for pleural effusion is increased in patients with hypertension, prior cardiac history and a twice a day administration schedule; interrupt treatment for grade ≥2 effusion; may consider reinitiating at a reduced dose after resolution (Quintás-Cardama, 2007). Use caution in patients where fluid accumulation may be poorly tolerated, such as in cardiovascular disease (HF or hypertension) and pulmonary disease. Elderly may be more likely to experience dyspnea and fluid retention. Pulmonary arterial hypertension (PAH) has been reported with use, sometimes after >12 months of therapy. Evaluate for underlying cardiopulmonary disease prior to therapy initiation and during therapy; evaluate and rule out alternative etiologies in patients with symptoms suggestive of PAH (eg, dyspnea, fatigue) and interrupt therapy if symptoms are severe. Discontinue permanently with confirmed PAH diagnosis.

May prolong QT interval; use caution in patients at risk for QT prolongation, including patients with long QT syndrome; patients taking antiarrhythmic medications or other medications that lead to QT prolongation or potassium-wasting diuretics; patients with cumulative high-dose anthracycline therapy, and conditions which cause hypokalemia or hypomagnesemia. Correct hypokalemia and hypomagnesemia prior to initiation of therapy. Use caution with hepatic impairment due to extensive hepatic metabolism; patients with ALT or AST >2.5 times the upper limit of normal (ULN) or total bilirubin >2 times the ULN were excluded from clinical trials.

Adverse Reactions

≥10%:

Cardiovascular: Fluid retention (21% to 35%; grades 3/4: 1% to 8%), superficial edema (3% to 19%; grades 3/4: ≤1%)

Central nervous system: Headache (12% to 33%), fatigue (8% to 24%), fever (5% to 18%)

Dermatologic: Rash (11% to 21%; includes drug eruption, erythema, erythema multiforme, erythematous rash, erythrosis, exfoliative rash, follicular rash, heat rash, macular rash, maculopapular rash, milia, papular rash, pruritic rash, pustular rash, skin exfoliation, skin irritation, urticaria vesiculosa, vesicular rash)

Endocrine & metabolic: Hypophosphatemia (grades 3/4: 5% to 18%), hypokalemia (grades 3/4: ≤15%), hypocalcemia (grades 3/4: <1% to 12%)

Gastrointestinal: Diarrhea (18% to 31%; grades 3/4: ≤5%), nausea (9% to 24%), vomiting (5% to 16%), abdominal pain (3% to 12%)

Hematologic: Thrombocytopenia (grades 3/4: 19% to 85%), neutropenia (grades 3/4: 22% to 79%), anemia (grades 3/4: 11% to 74%), hemorrhage (6% to 26%; grades 3/4: 1% to 9%), neutropenic fever (grades 3/4: 1% to 12%)

Neuromuscular & skeletal: Musculoskeletal pain (≤19%), myalgia (3% to 13%), arthralgia (≤12%)

Respiratory: Pleural effusion (12% to 24%; grades 3/4: ≤11%), dyspnea (3% to 20%; grades 3/4: 2% to 3%)

Miscellaneous: Infection (9% to 12%, includes bacterial, fungal, viral)

1% to <10%:

Cardiovascular: Generalized edema (≤1%), pericardial effusion (≤3%; grades 3/4: ≤1%), CHF/cardiac dysfunction (≤4%; includes cardiac failure, cardiomyopathy, diastolic dysfunction, ejection fraction decreased, left ventricular dysfunction, ventricular failure); arrhythmia, chest pain, flushing, hypertension, palpitation

Central nervous system: CNS bleeding (≤3%; grades 3/4: ≤3%), chills, depression, dizziness, insomnia, pain, somnolence

Dermatologic: Acne, alopecia, dermatitis, dry skin, eczema, hyperhydrosis, pruritus, urticaria

Gastrointestinal: Gastrointestinal bleeding (2% to 9%; grades 3/4: 1% to 7%), abdominal distention, anorexia, colitis (including neutropenic colitis), constipation, dyspepsia, enterocolitis, gastritis, mucositis/stomatitis, oral soft tissue disorder, taste alteration, weight loss/gain

Hematologic: Contusion, pancytopenia

Hepatic: Bilirubin increased (grades 3/4: ≤6%), ALT increased (grades 3/4: ≤5%), AST increased (grades 3/4: ≤4%)

Neuromuscular & skeletal: Muscle inflammation (4%), muscle weakness, neuropathy, peripheral neuropathy, weakness

Ocular: Visual disorder (blurred vision, acuity reduced, visual disturbance), xerophthalmia

Otic: Tinnitus

Renal: Serum creatinine increased (grades 3/4: ≤8%)

Respiratory: Pulmonary edema (≤4%; grades 3/4: ≤3%), cough, lung infiltration, pneumonia (bacterial, viral or fungal), pneumonitis, pulmonary hypertension, upper respiratory tract infection/inflammation

Miscellaneous: Herpes virus infection

<1% (Limited to important or life-threatening): Acute coronary syndrome, acute febrile neutrophilic dermatosis, acute respiratory distress syndrome, amnesia, anal fissure, angina, anxiety, ascites, asthma, atrial fibrillation, atrial flutter, bronchospasm, bullous conditions, cardiomegaly, cerebrovascular accident, cholecystitis, cholestasis, conjunctivitis, cor pulmonale, creatine phosphokinase increased, dysphagia, embolism, erythema nodosum, esophagitis, gynecomastia, hand-foot syndrome (palmar-plantar erythrodysesthesia syndrome), hematoma, hematuria, hepatitis, hypersensitivity, hyperuricemia, hypoalbuminemia, hypotension, interstitial lung disease, libido decreased, livedo reticularis, malaise, menstrual irregularities, MI, myocarditis, neutropenic colitis, optic neuritis, pancreatitis, panniculitis, pericarditis, petechiae, photosensitivity, pigmentation disorder, platelet aggregation abnormal, polyuria, proteinuria, pulmonary arterial hypertension, pure red cell aplasia, QT_c prolongation, renal failure, rhabdomyolysis, seizure, sepsis, skin ulcer, syncope, temperature intolerance, tendonitis, thrombophlebitis, thrombosis, TIA, tremor, tumor lysis syndrome, upper gastrointestinal ulcer, ventricular arrhythmia, ventricular tachycardia

Drug Interactions

Metabolism/Transport Effects Substrate of CYP3A4 (major); **Note:** Assignment of Major/Minor substrate status based on clinically relevant drug interaction potential; **Inhibits** CYP3A4 (weak)

Avoid Concomitant Use

Avoid concomitant use of Dasatinib with any of the following: Artemether; BCG; CloZAPine; Conivaptan; Dronedarone; Lumefantrine; Natalizumab; Nilotinib; Pimecrolimus; Pimozide; QUEtiapine; QuiNINE; St Johns Wort; Tacrolimus (Topical); Tetrabenazine; Thioridazine; Toremifene; Vaccines (Live); Vandetanib; Vemurafenib; Ziprasidone

Increased Effect/Toxicity

Dasatinib may increase the levels/effects of: Acetaminophen; Anticoagulants; Antiplatelet Agents; CloZAPine; CYP3A4 Substrates; Dronedarone; Leflunomide; Natalizumab; Pimozide; QTc-Prolonging Agents; QuiNINE; Tetrabenazine; Thioridazine; Toremifene; Vaccines (Live); Vandetanib; Vemurafenib; Vitamin K Antagonists; Ziprasidone

The levels/effects of Dasatinib may be increased by: Acetaminophen; Alfuzosin; Artemether; Chloroquine; Ciprofloxacin; Ciprofloxacin (Systemic); Conivaptan; CYP3A4 Inhibitors (Moderate); CYP3A4 Inhibitors (Strong); Denosumab; Gadobutrol; Indacaterol; Lumefantrine; Nilotinib; Pimecrolimus; QUEtiapine; QuiNINE; Roflumilast; Tacrolimus (Topical); Trastuzumab

Decreased Effect

Dasatinib may decrease the levels/effects of: BCG; Cardiac Glycosides; Coccidioidin Skin Test; Sipuleucel-T; Vaccines (Inactivated); Vaccines (Live); Vitamin K Antagonists

The levels/effects of Dasatinib may be decreased by: Antacids; CYP3A4 Inducers (Strong); Deferasirox; Echinacea; H2-Antagonists; Proton Pump Inhibitors; St Johns Wort; Tocilizumab

Ethanol/Nutrition/Herb Interactions Herb/Nutraceutical: Avoid St John's wort (may increase metabolism and decrease dasatinib plasma concentration).

Stability Store at 25°C (77°F); excursions permitted to 15°C to 30°C (59°F to 86°F).

Mechanism of Action BCR-ABL tyrosine kinase inhibitor; targets most imatinib-resistant BCR-ABL mutations (except the T315I and F317V mutants) by distinctly binding to active and inactive ABL-kinase. Kinase inhibition halts proliferation of leukemia cells. Also inhibits SRC family (including SRC, LKC, YES, FYN); c-KIT, EPHA2 and platelet derived growth factor receptor (PDGFRβ)

Pharmacodynamics/Kinetics

Distribution: 2505 L

Protein binding: Dasatinib: 96%; metabolite (active): 93%

Metabolism: Hepatic (extensive); metabolized by CYP3A4 (primarily), flavin-containing mono-oxygenase-3 (FOM-3) and uridine diphosphate-glucuronosyltransferase (UGT) to an active metabolite and other inactive metabolites (the active metabolite plays only a minor role in the pharmacology of dasatinib)

Half-life elimination: Terminal: 3-5 hours

Time to peak, plasma: 0.5-6 hours

Excretion: Feces (85%, 19% as unchanged drug); urine (4%, 0.1% as unchanged drug)

Dosage Oral: Adults: **Note:** In clinical trials, dasatinib was continued until disease progression or until unacceptable toxicity; the effect of discontinuation after complete cytogenetic remission is achieved has not been studied.

CML, newly-diagnosed Ph+ in chronic phase: 100 mg once daily, a dose escalation to 140 mg once daily was allowed in patients not achieving cytogenetic response at recommended initial dosage.

CML, resistant or intolerant:

Chronic phase: 100 mg once daily. In clinical studies, a dose escalation to 140 mg once daily was allowed in patients not achieving cytogenetic response at recommended initial dosage.

Accelerated or blast phase: 140 mg once daily. In clinical studies, a dose escalation to 180 mg once daily was allowed in patients not achieving cytogenetic response at recommended initial dosage.

Ph+ ALL: 140 mg once daily. In clinical studies, a dose escalation to 180 mg once daily was allowed in patients not achieving cytogenetic response at recommended initial dosage.

Dosage adjustment for concomitant CYP3A4 inhibitors: Avoid concomitant administration with strong CYP3A4 inhibitors (eg, clarithromycin, itraconazole, ketoconazole, nefazodone, protease inhibitors, telithromycin, voriconazole, grapefruit juice); if concomitant administration with a strong CYP3A4 inhibitor cannot be avoided, consider reducing dasatinib from 100 mg once daily to 20 mg once daily **or** from 140 mg once daily to 40 mg once daily, with careful monitoring. If reduced dose is not tolerated, the strong CYP3A4 inhibitor must be discontinued or dasatinib therapy temporarily held until concomitant inhibitor use has ceased. When a strong CYP3A4 inhibitor is discontinued, allow a washout period (~1 week) prior to adjusting dasatinib dose upward.

Dosage adjustment for concomitant CYP3A4 inducers: Avoid concomitant administration with strong CYP3A4 inducers (eg, carbamazepine, dexamethasone, phenobarbital, phenytoin, rifampin, St John's wort); if concomitant administration with a strong CYP3A4 inducer cannot be avoided, consider increasing the dasatinib dose with careful monitoring.

Dosage adjustment for toxicity:

Hematologic toxicity:

Chronic phase CML (100 mg daily starting dose): For ANC <500/mm^3 or platelets <50,000/mm^3, withhold treatment until ANC ≥1000/mm^3 and platelets ≥50,000/mm^3; then resume treatment at the original starting dose if recovery occurs in ≤7 days. If platelets <25,000/mm^3 or recurrence of ANC <500/mm^3 for >7 days, withhold treatment until ANC ≥1000/mm^3 and platelets ≥50,000/mm^3; then resume treatment at 80 mg once daily (second episode). For third episode, further reduce dose to 50 mg once daily (for newly-diagnosed patients) or discontinue (for patients resistant or intolerant to prior therapy)

Accelerated or blast phase CML and Ph+ ALL (140 mg once daily starting dose): For ANC <500/mm^3 or platelets <10,000/mm^3, if cytopenia unrelated to leukemia, withhold treatment until ANC ≥1000/mm^3 and platelets ≥20,000/mm^3; then resume treatment at the original starting dose. If cytopenia recurs, withhold treatment until ANC ≥1000/mm^3 and platelets ≥20,000/mm^3; then resume treatment at 100 mg once daily (second episode) or 80 mg once daily (third episode). For cytopenias related to leukemia (confirm with marrow aspirate or biopsy), consider dose escalation to 180 mg once daily.

Nonhematologic toxicity: Withhold treatment until toxicity improvement or resolution; if appropriate, resume treatment at a reduced dose based on the event severity. Fluid retention is managed with diuretics and supportive care. Effusions may require diuretics and/or dose interruption. Corticosteroids (eg, prednisone 20 mg/day for 3 days) may be considered for pleural or pericardial effusion with significant symptoms (hold dasatinib and reinitiate at a decreased dose when effusion resolves). Rash may be managed with steroids (topical or systemic), treatment interruption, dose reduction, or discontinuation (NCCN CML guidelines v.2.2011).

Dosage adjustment for hepatic impairment: No adjustment required; use with caution

Dietary Considerations May be taken without regard to food. Avoid grapefruit juice.

Administration Administer once daily (morning or evening). May be taken without regard to food. Swallow whole; do not break, crush, or chew tablets. Take with a meal or with a large glass of water if GI upset occurs.

Monitoring Parameters CBC with differential (weekly for 2 months, then monthly or as clinically necessary); bone marrow biopsy; liver function tests, electrolytes including calcium, phosphorus, magnesium; monitor for fluid retention; ECG monitoring if at risk for QT_c prolongation; chest x-ray is recommended for symptoms suggestive of pleural effusion (eg, cough, dyspnea)

Additional Information Oncology Comment: In a dose finding study in chronic-phase CML, dasatinib 100 mg once daily provided comparable efficacy to the original FDA-approved dose of 70 mg twice daily. The 100 mg once daily dose was better tolerated (lower rates of pleural effusion and grades 3/4 thrombocytopenia), required fewer dose reductions, and fewer dosing interruptions or discontinuations (Shah, 2008).

Dosage Forms Excipient information presented when available (limited, particularly for generics); consult specific product labeling.

Tablet, oral:

Sprycel®: 20 mg, 50 mg, 70 mg, 100 mg

Extemporaneous Preparations Hazardous agent: Use appropriate precautions for handling and disposal.

An oral suspension may be prepared by dissolving dasatinib tablet(s) for one dose in 30 mL chilled orange or apple juice (without preservatives). After 5 minutes, swirl the contents for 3 seconds and repeat the process every 5 minutes for a total of 20 minutes following addition of tablet(s). Minimize time between end of 20 minutes and administration since suspension will taste more bitter if allowed to stand longer. Swirl contents of container one last time, then administer immediately. To ensure the full dose is administered, rinse container with 15 mL juice and administer residue. May be administered orally (or by nasogastric tube). Discard any unused portion after 60 minutes.

Sprycel® data on file, Bristol-Myers Squibb

◆ **DaTSCAN** *see* Ioflupane I 123 *on page 921*

◆ **DaTscan™** *see* Ioflupane I 123 *on page 921*

◆ **Daunomycin** *see* DAUNOrubicin (Conventional) *on page 457*

◆ **DAUNOrubicin Citrate** *see* DAUNOrubicin (Liposomal) *on page 458*

◆ **DAUNOrubicin Citrate (Liposomal)** *see* DAUNOrubicin (Liposomal) *on page 458*

◆ **DAUNOrubicin Citrate Liposome** *see* DAUNOrubicin (Liposomal) *on page 458*

DAUNOrubicin (Conventional)

(daw noe ROO bi sin con VEN sha nal)

Brand Names: U.S. Cerubidine®

Brand Names: Canada Cerubidine®

Index Terms Conventional Daunomycin; Daunomycin; DAUNOrubicin Hydrochloride; Rubidomycin Hydrochloride

Pharmacologic Category Antineoplastic Agent, Anthracycline

Use Treatment of acute lymphocytic leukemia (ALL) and acute myeloid leukemia (AML)

Pregnancy Risk Factor D

Pregnancy Considerations May cause fetal harm when administered to a pregnant woman. Animal studies have shown an increased incidence of fetal abnormalities.

Lactation Excretion in breast milk unknown/not recommended

Contraindications Hypersensitivity to daunorubicin or any component of the formulation

Warnings/Precautions Hazardous agent - use appropriate precautions for handling and disposal. Use with caution in patients who have received radiation therapy; reduce dosage in patients who are receiving radiation therapy simultaneously. **[U.S. Boxed Warnings]: Use caution with renal impairment or in the presence of hepatic dysfunction; dosage reduction is recommended. Potent vesicant; if extravasation occurs, severe local tissue damage leading to ulceration and necrosis, and pain may occur. For I.V. administration only. Severe bone marrow suppression may occur.**

[U.S. Boxed Warning]: May cause cumulative, dose-related myocardial toxicity (concurrent or delayed). Total cumulative dose should take into account previous or concomitant treatment with cardiotoxic agents or irradiation of chest. The incidence of irreversible myocardial toxicity increases as the total cumulative (lifetime) dosages approach:

- 550 mg/m² in adults
- 400 mg/m² in adults receiving chest radiation
- 300 mg/m² in children >2 years of age
- 10 mg/kg in children <2 years of age

Although the risk increases with cumulative dose, irreversible cardiotoxicity may occur at any dose level. Patients with pre-existing heart disease, hypertension, concurrent administration of other antineoplastic agents, prior or concurrent chest irradiation, advanced age; and infants and children are at increased risk. Monitor left ventricular (LV) function (baseline and periodic) with ECHO or MUGA scan; monitor ECG.

Secondary leukemias may occur when used with combination chemotherapy or radiation therapy. **[U.S. Boxed Warning]: Should be administered under the supervision of an experienced cancer chemotherapy physician.**

Adverse Reactions

>10%:

Cardiovascular: Transient ECG abnormalities (supraventricular tachycardia, S-T wave changes, atrial or ventricular extrasystoles); generally asymptomatic and self-limiting. CHF, dose related, may be delayed for 7-8 years after treatment.

Dermatologic: Alopecia (reversible), radiation recall

Gastrointestinal: Mild nausea or vomiting, stomatitis

Genitourinary: Discoloration of urine (red)

Hematologic: Myelosuppression (onset: 7 days; nadir: 10-14 days; recovery: 21-28 days), primarily leukopenia; thrombocytopenia and anemia

1% to 10%:

Dermatologic: Skin "flare" at injection site; discoloration of saliva, sweat, or tears

Endocrine & metabolic: Hyperuricemia

Gastrointestinal: Abdominal pain, GI ulceration, diarrhea

<1% (Limited to important or life-threatening): Anaphylactoid reaction, arrhythmia, bilirubin increased, cardiomyopathy, hepatitis, infertility; local (cellulitis, pain, thrombophlebitis at injection site); MI, myocarditis, neutropenic typhlitis, pericarditis, secondary leukemia, skin rash, sterility, systemic hypersensitivity (including urticaria, pruritus, angioedema, dysphagia, dyspnea); transaminases increased

Drug Interactions

Metabolism/Transport Effects Substrate of P-glycoprotein

Avoid Concomitant Use

Avoid concomitant use of DAUNOrubicin (Conventional) with any of the following: BCG; CloZAPine; Natalizumab; Pimecrolimus; Tacrolimus (Topical); Vaccines (Live)

Increased Effect/Toxicity

DAUNOrubicin (Conventional) may increase the levels/effects of: CloZAPine; Leflunomide; Natalizumab; Vaccines (Live)

The levels/effects of DAUNOrubicin (Conventional) may be increased by: Bevacizumab; Denosumab; P-glycoprotein/ABCB1 Inhibitors; Pimecrolimus; Roflumilast; Tacrolimus (Topical); Taxane Derivatives; Trastuzumab

Decreased Effect

DAUNOrubicin (Conventional) may decrease the levels/effects of: BCG; Cardiac Glycosides; Coccidioidin Skin Test; Sipuleucel-T; Vaccines (Inactivated); Vaccines (Live)

The levels/effects of DAUNOrubicin (Conventional) may be decreased by: Cardiac Glycosides; Echinacea; P-glycoprotein/ABCB1 Inducers

Ethanol/Nutrition/Herb Interactions Ethanol: Avoid ethanol (due to GI irritation).

Stability Store intact vials of powder for injection at room temperature of 15°C to 30°C (59°F to 86°F); intact vials of solution for injection should be refrigerated at 2°C to 8°C (36°F to 46°F). Protect from light. Dilute vials of powder for injection with 4 mL SWFI for a final concentration of 5 mg/mL. May further dilute in 100 mL D_5W or NS. Reconstituted solution is stable for 4 days at 15°C to 25°C. Further dilution in D_5W, LR, or NS is stable at room temperature (25°C) for up to 4 weeks if protected from light.

Mechanism of Action Inhibition of DNA and RNA synthesis by intercalation between DNA base pairs and by steric obstruction. Daunomycin intercalates at points of local uncoiling of the double helix. Although the exact mechanism is unclear, it appears that direct binding to DNA (intercalation) and inhibition of DNA repair (topoisomerase II inhibition) result in blockade of DNA and RNA synthesis and fragmentation of DNA.

Pharmacodynamics/Kinetics

Distribution: Many body tissues, particularly the liver, kidneys, lung, spleen, and heart; not into CNS; crosses placenta; V_d: 40 L/kg

Metabolism: Primarily hepatic to daunorubicinol (active), then to inactive aglycones, conjugated sulfates, and glucuronides

Half-life elimination: Distribution: 2 minutes; Elimination: 14-20 hours; Terminal: 18.5 hours; Daunorubicinol plasma half-life: 24-48 hours

Excretion: Feces (40%); urine (~25% as unchanged drug and metabolites)

Dosage I.V. (refer to individual protocols):

Children: **Note:** Cumulative dose should not exceed 300 mg/m^2 in children >2 years or 10 mg/kg in children <2 years of age; maximum cumulative doses for younger children are unknown.

Children <2 years or BSA <0.5 m^2: ALL combination therapy: 1 mg/kg/dose per protocol, with frequency dependent on regimen employed

Children ≥2 years and BSA ≥0.5 m^2:

ALL combination therapy: Remission induction: 25 mg/m^2 on day 1 every week for up to 4-6 cycles

AML combination therapy: Induction: I.V. continuous infusion: 30-60 mg/m^2/day on days 1-3 of cycle

Adults: **Note:** Cumulative dose should not exceed 550 mg/m^2 in adults without risk factors for cardiotoxicity and should not exceed 400 mg/m^2 in adults receiving chest irradiation.

Range: 30-60 mg/m^2/day for 3 days, repeat dose in 3-4 weeks

ALL combination therapy: 45 mg/m^2/day for 3 days

AML combination therapy:

Adults <60 years: Induction: 45 mg/m^2/day for 3 days of the first course of induction therapy; subsequent courses: 45 mg/m^2/day for 2 days

Adults ≥60 years: Induction: 30 mg/m^2/day for 3 days of the first course of induction therapy; subsequent courses: 30 mg/m^2/day for 2 days

Dosing adjustment in renal impairment:

The FDA-approved labeling recommends the following adjustment: S_{cr} >3 mg/dL: Administer 50% of normal dose

The following guidelines have been used by some clinicians (Aronoff, 2007):

Children:

Cl_{cr} <30 mL/minute: Administer 50% of dose

Hemodialysis/continuous ambulatory peritoneal dialysis (CAPD): Administer 50% of dose

Adults: No adjustment recommended

Dosing adjustment in hepatic impairment:

The FDA-approved labeling recommends the following adjustments:

Serum bilirubin 1.2-3 mg/dL: Administer 75% of dose

Serum bilirubin >3 mg/dL: Administer 50% of dose

The following guidelines have been used by some clinicians (Floyd, 2006):

Serum bilirubin 1.2-3 mg/dL: Administer 75% of dose

Serum bilirubin 3.1-5 mg/dL: Administer 50% of dose

Serum bilirubin >5 mg/dL: Avoid use

Administration Not for I.M. or SubQ administration. Administer as slow I.V. push over 1-5 minutes into the tubing of a rapidly infusing I.V. solution of D_5W or NS or dilute in 100 mL of D_5W or NS and infuse over 15-30 minutes.

Monitoring Parameters CBC with differential and platelet count, liver function test, ECG, left ventricular ejection function (echocardiography [ECHO] or multigated radionuclide angiography [MUGA] scan), renal function test

Dosage Forms Excipient information presented when available (limited, particularly for generics); consult specific product labeling.

Injection, powder for reconstitution [strength expressed as base]: 20 mg

Cerubidine®: 20 mg [contains mannitol]

Injection, solution [strength expressed as base, preservative free]: 5 mg/mL (4 mL, 10 mL)

◆ **DAUNOrubicin Hydrochloride** *see* DAUNOrubicin (Conventional) *on page 457*

DAUNOrubicin (Liposomal)

(daw noe ROO bi sin lye po SO mal)

Brand Names: U.S. DaunoXome®

Index Terms DAUNOrubicin Citrate; DAUNOrubicin Citrate (Liposomal); DAUNOrubicin Citrate Liposome; Liposomal DAUNOrubicin; NSC-697732

Pharmacologic Category Antineoplastic Agent, Anthracycline

Use First-line treatment of advanced HIV-associated Kaposi's sarcoma (KS)

Pregnancy Risk Factor D

Pregnancy Considerations Teratogenic effects and embryotoxicity were noted in animal studies. There are no adequate and well-controlled studies in pregnant women. Women of childbearing potential should avoid becoming pregnant while receiving treatment.

Lactation Excretion in breast milk unknown/not recommended

Contraindications Hypersensitivity to daunorubicin citrate (liposomal), daunorubicin, or any component of the formulation

Warnings/Precautions Hazardous agent - use appropriate precautions for handling and disposal. **[U.S. Boxed Warning]: Monitor cardiac function regularly; especially in patients with previous therapy with high cumulative doses of anthracyclines, cyclophosphamide, or thoracic radiation, or who have pre-existing cardiac disease.** Although the risk increases with cumulative dose, irreversible cardiotoxicity may occur with anthracycline treatment at any dose level. Patients with pre-existing heart disease, hypertension, concurrent administration of other antineoplastic agents, prior or concurrent chest irradiation, and advanced age are at increased risk. Evaluate left ventricular ejection fraction (LVEF) prior to treatment and periodically during treatment.

[U.S. Boxed Warning]: May cause bone marrow suppression, particularly neutropenia; monitor closely for infections. **[U.S. Boxed Warning]: Use caution with hepatic impairment;** dosage reduction is recommended. Use caution with renal impairment; may require dose adjustment. **[U.S. Boxed Warning]: The lipid component is associated with infusion-related reactions (back pain, flushing, chest tightness) usually within the first 5 minutes of infusion;** monitor, interrupt infusion, and resume at reduced infusion rate. Safety and efficacy in children and the elderly have not been established. **[U.S. Boxed Warning]: Should be administered under the supervision of an experienced cancer chemotherapy physician.**

Adverse Reactions

>10%:

Cardiovascular: Edema (11%)

Central nervous system: Fatigue (49%), fever (47%), headache (25%), neutropenic fever (17%)

Gastrointestinal: Nausea (54%), diarrhea (38%), abdominal pain (23%), anorexia (23%), vomiting (23%)

Hematologic: Myelosuppression (onset: 7 days; nadir: 14 days; recovery 21 days), neutropenia (up to 55%; grade 4: 15%), anemia (up to 55%; grade 4: 2%), thrombocytopenia (up to 12%; grade 4: 1%)

Neuromuscular & skeletal: Rigors (19%), back pain (16%), neuropathy (13%)

Respiratory: Cough (28%), dyspnea (26%), rhinitis (12%)
Miscellaneous: Opportunistic infections (40%), allergic reactions (24%), diaphoresis (14%), infusion-related reactions (14%; includes back pain, flushing, chest tightness)

1% to 10%:
Cardiovascular: Chest pain (10%), hypertension (≤5%), palpitation (≤5%), syncope (≤5%), tachycardia (≤5%), LVEF decreased (3%), CHF/cardiomyopathy
Central nervous system: Depression (10%), malaise (10%), dizziness (8%), insomnia (6%), abnormal thinking (≤5%), amnesia (≤5%), anxiety (≤5%), ataxia (≤5%), confusion (≤5%), emotional lability (≤5%), hallucination (≤5%), meningitis (≤5%), seizure (≤5%), somnolence (≤5%)
Dermatologic: Alopecia (8%), pruritus (7%), dry skin (≤5%), folliculitis (≤5%), seborrhea (≤5%)
Endocrine & metabolic: Dehydration (≤5%), hot flashes (≤5%)
Gastrointestinal: Stomatitis (10%), constipation (7%), tenesmus (5%), appetite increased (≤5%), dental caries (≤5%), dysphagia (≤5%), gastrointestinal hemorrhage (≤5%), gastritis (≤5%), gingival bleeding (≤5%), hemorrhoids (≤5%), melena (≤5%), splenomegaly (≤5%), taste perversion (≤5%), xerostomia (≤5%)
Genitourinary: Dysuria (≤5%), nocturia (≤5%), polyuria (≤5%)
Hepatic: Hepatomegaly (≤5%)
Local: Injection site inflammation (≤5%)
Neuromuscular & skeletal: Arthralgia (7%), myalgia (7%), gait abnormal (≤5%), hyperkinesia (≤5%), hypertonia (≤5%), tremor (≤5%)
Ocular: Abnormal vision (5%) conjunctivitis (≤5%), eye pain (≤5%)
Otic: Deafness (≤5%), earache (≤5%), tinnitus (≤5%)
Respiratory: Sinusitis (8%), hemoptysis (≤5%), pulmonary infiltrate (≤5%), sputum increased (≤5%)
Miscellaneous: Flu-like syndrome (5%), hiccups (≤5%), lymphadenopathy (≤5%), thirst (≤5%)

Postmarketing and/or case reports: Angina, atrial fibrillation, cardiac arrest, MI, pericardial effusion, pericardial tamponade, pulmonary hypertension, supraventricular tachycardia, ventricular extrasystoles

Drug Interactions

Metabolism/Transport Effects **Substrate** of P-glycoprotein

Avoid Concomitant Use

Avoid concomitant use of DAUNOrubicin (Liposomal) with any of the following: BCG; CloZAPine; Natalizumab; Pimecrolimus; Tacrolimus (Topical); Vaccines (Live)

Increased Effect/Toxicity

DAUNOrubicin (Liposomal) may increase the levels/effects of: CloZAPine; Leflunomide; Natalizumab; Vaccines (Live)

The levels/effects of DAUNOrubicin (Liposomal) may be increased by: Bevacizumab; Denosumab; P-glycoprotein/ABCB1 Inhibitors; Pimecrolimus; Roflumilast; Tacrolimus (Topical); Taxane Derivatives; Trastuzumab

Decreased Effect

DAUNOrubicin (Liposomal) may decrease the levels/effects of: BCG; Cardiac Glycosides; Coccidioidin Skin Test; Sipuleucel-T; Vaccines (Inactivated); Vaccines (Live)

The levels/effects of DAUNOrubicin (Liposomal) may be decreased by: Cardiac Glycosides; Echinacea; P-glycoprotein/ABCB1 Inducers

Stability Store intact vials of solution under refrigeration at 2°C to 8°C (36°F to 46°F); do not freeze. Protect from light. Only fluid which may be mixed with DaunoXome® is D_5W. Dilute to a 1:1 solution (1 mg daunorubicin liposomal/mL D_5W). Must **not** be mixed with saline, bacteriostatic agents (such as benzyl alcohol), or any other solution. Diluted daunorubicin liposomal for infusion may be refrigerated at 2°C to 8°C (36°F to 46°F) for a maximum of 6 hours. Do not use with in-line filters.

Mechanism of Action Liposomes have been shown to penetrate solid tumors more effectively, possibly because of their small size and longer circulation time. Once in tissues, daunorubicin is released. Daunorubicin inhibits DNA and RNA synthesis by intercalation between DNA base pairs and by steric obstruction; and intercalates at points of local uncoiling of the double helix. Although the exact mechanism is unclear, it appears that direct binding to DNA (intercalation) and inhibition of DNA repair (topoisomerase II inhibition) result in blockade of DNA and RNA synthesis and fragmentation of DNA.

Pharmacodynamics/Kinetics

Distribution: V_d: 5-8 L
Metabolism: Similar to daunorubicin, but metabolite plasma levels are low
Half-life elimination: Distribution: 4.4 hours; Terminal: 3-5 hours
Excretion: Primarily feces; some urine
Clearance, plasma: 17.3 mL/minute

Dosage Refer to individual protocols. I.V.:
Adults: HIV-associated KS: 40 mg/m^2 every 2 weeks
Elderly: Use with caution.
Dosage adjustment for toxicity: Withhold treatment for ANC <750/mm^3
Elderly: Use with caution.
Dosing adjustment in renal impairment: Serum creatinine >3 mg/dL: Administer 50% of normal dose
Dosing adjustment in hepatic impairment:
Bilirubin 1.2-3 mg/dL: Administer 75% of normal dose
Bilirubin >3 mg/dL: Administer 50% of normal dose

Administration Infuse over 1 hour; do not mix with other drugs. Avoid extravasation.

Monitoring Parameters CBC with differential and platelets (prior to each dose), liver function tests, renal function tests; evaluate cardiac function (baseline left ventricular ejection fraction [LVEF] prior to treatment initiation; repeat LVEF at total cumulative doses of 320 mg/m^2, and every 160 mg/m^2 thereafter; patients with pre-existing cardiac disease, history of prior chest irradiation, or history of prior anthracycline treatment should have baseline LVEF and every 160 mg/m^2 thereafter); signs and symptoms of infection or disease progression; monitor closely for infusion reactions

Dosage Forms Excipient information presented when available (limited, particularly for generics); consult specific product labeling.
Injection, solution [strength expressed as base, preservative free]:
DaunoXome®: 2 mg/mL (25 mL) [contains sucrose 2125 mg/25 mL]

- ◆ **DaunoXome®** *see* DAUNOrubicin (Liposomal) *on page 458*
- ◆ **Daxas™ (Can)** *see* Roflumilast *on page 1514*
- ◆ **Daypro®** *see* Oxaprozin *on page 1260*
- ◆ **Daytrana®** *see* Methylphenidate *on page 1107*
- ◆ **dCF** *see* Pentostatin *on page 1331*
- ◆ **DDAVP®** *see* Desmopressin *on page 476*
- ◆ **DDAVP® Melt (Can)** *see* Desmopressin *on page 476*
- ◆ **ddI** *see* Didanosine *on page 499*
- ◆ **1-Deamino-8-D-Arginine Vasopressin** *see* Desmopressin *on page 476*
- ◆ **Debrox® [OTC]** *see* Carbamide Peroxide *on page 283*
- ◆ **Decadron** *see* Dexamethasone (Systemic) *on page 480*
- ◆ **Decavac®** *see* Diphtheria and Tetanus Toxoid *on page 520*

◆ **Dec-Chlorphen [DSC]** *see* Chlorpheniramine and Phenylephrine *on page 345*

◆ **De-Chlor DM [DSC]** *see* Chlorpheniramine, Phenylephrine, and Dextromethorphan *on page 346*

◆ **De-Chlor DR [DSC]** *see* Chlorpheniramine, Phenylephrine, and Dextromethorphan *on page 346*

Decitabine (de SYE ta been)

Brand Names: U.S. Dacogen®

Index Terms 5-Aza-2'-deoxycytidine; 5-Aza-dCyd; Deoxyazacytidine; Dezocitidine

Pharmacologic Category Antineoplastic Agent, DNA Methylation Inhibitor

Use Treatment of myelodysplastic syndrome (MDS)

Unlabeled Use Treatment of acute myelogenous leukemia (AML), sickle cell anemia

Pregnancy Risk Factor D

Pregnancy Considerations Teratogenic effects, decreased fetal weight, and increased fetal deaths were observed in animal studies. There are no adequate and well-controlled studies in pregnant women. Women of childbearing potential should be advised to avoid pregnancy during treatment and for 1 month after treatment. In addition, males should be advised to avoid fathering a child while on decitabine therapy and for 2 months after treatment.

Lactation Excretion in breast milk unknown/not recommended

Contraindications There are no contraindications listed within the manufacturer's labeling.

Warnings/Precautions Hazardous agent - use appropriate precautions for handling and disposal. The dose-limiting toxicity is bone marrow suppression; worsening neutropenia is common in first two treatment cycles and may not correlate with progression of underlying MDS; may require dosage adjustment (after the first cycle), growth factor support and/or antimicrobial agents; monitor for infection. Not studied in hepatic and renal disease; use caution.

Adverse Reactions

>10%:

Cardiovascular: Peripheral edema (25% to 27%), pallor (23%), edema (5% to 18%), cardiac murmur (16%), hypotension (6% to 11%)

Central nervous system: Fever (6% to 53%), fatigue (46%), headache (23% to 28%), insomnia (14% to 28%), dizziness (18% to 21%), chills (16%), pain (5% to 13%), confusion (8% to 12%), lethargy (12%), anxiety (9% to 11%), hypoesthesia (11%)

Dermatologic: Petechiae (12% to 39%), bruising (9% to 22%), rash (11% to 19%), erythema (5% to 14%), cellulitis (9% to 12%), lesions (5% to 11%), pruritus (9% to 11%)

Endocrine & metabolic: Hyperglycemia (6% to 33%), hypoalbuminemia (7% to 24%), hypomagnesemia (5% to 24%), hypokalemia (12% to 22%), hyperkalemia (13%), hyponatremia (19%)

Gastrointestinal: Nausea (40% to 42%), constipation (30% to 35%), diarrhea (28% to 34%), vomiting (16% to 25%), anorexia/appetite decreased (8% to 23%), abdominal pain (5% to 14%), oral mucosal petechiae (13%), stomatitis (11% to 12%), dyspepsia (10% to 12%)

Hematologic: Neutropenia (38% to 90%; grades 3/4: 37% to 87%; recovery 28-50 days), thrombocytopenia (27% to 89%; grades 3/4: 24% to 85%), anemia (31% to 82%; grades 3/4: 22%), febrile neutropenia (20% to 29%; grades 3/4: 23%), leukopenia (6% to 28%; grades 3/4: 22%), lymphadenopathy (12%)

Hepatic: Hyperbilirubinemia (6% to 14%), alkaline phosphatase increased (11%)

Local: Tenderness (11%)

Neuromuscular & skeletal: Rigors (22%), arthralgia (17% to 20%), limb pain (18% to 19%), back pain (17% to 18%), weakness (15%)

Respiratory: Cough (27% to 40%), dyspnea (29%), pneumonia (20% to 22%), pharyngitis (16%), lung crackles (14%), epistaxis (13%)

5% to 10%:

Cardiovascular: Tachycardia (8%), chest pain/discomfort (6% to 7%), facial edema (6%), hypertension (6%), heart failure (5%)

Central nervous system: Depression (9%), malaise (5%)

Dermatologic: Alopecia (8%), dry skin (8%), urticaria (6%)

Endocrine & metabolic: Hyperuricemia (10%), LDH increased (8%), bicarbonate increased (6%), dehydration (6% to 8%), hypochloremia (6%), bicarbonate decreased (5%), hypoproteinemia (5%)

Gastrointestinal: Mucosal inflammation (9%), weight loss (9%), gingival bleeding (8%), hemorrhoids (8%), loose stools (7%), tongue ulceration (7%), dysphagia (5% to 6%), oral candidiasis (6%), toothache (6%), abdominal distension (5%), gastroesophageal reflux (5%), glossodynia (5%), lip ulceration (5%), oral pain (5%), tooth abscess (5%)

Genitourinary: Urinary tract infection (7%), dysuria (6%), polyuria (5%)

Hematologic: Bacteremia (5% to 8%), hematoma (5%), pancytopenia (5%), thrombocythemia (5%)

Hepatic: Ascites (10%), AST increased (10%), hypobilirubinemia (5%)

Local: Catheter infection (8%), catheter site erythema (5%), catheter site pain (5%), injection site swelling (5%)

Neuromuscular & skeletal: Myalgia (5% to 9%), falling (8%), chest wall pain (7%), muscle spasm (7%), bone pain (6%), musculoskeletal pain/discomfort (5% to 6%), crepitation (5%)

Ocular: Blurred vision (6%)

Otic: Ear pain (6%)

Respiratory: Breath sounds abnormal (5% to 10%), hypoxia (10%), upper respiratory tract infection (10%), pharyngolaryngeal pain (8%), rales (8%), pulmonary edema (6%), sinusitis (5% to 6%), pleural effusion (5%), postnasal drip (5%), sinus congestion (5%)

Miscellaneous: Candidal infection (10%), staphylococcal infection (7%), transfusion reaction (7%), night sweats (5%)

<5% (Limited to important or life-threatening): Anaphylactic reaction, atrial fibrillation, bronchopulmonary aspergillosis, cardiomyopathy, cardiorespiratory arrest/failure, catheter site hemorrhage, cholecystitis, fungal infection, gastrointestinal hemorrhage, gingival pain, hemoptysis, hypersensitivity, intracranial hemorrhage, mental status change, MI, mycobacterium avium complex infection, peridiverticular abscess, pseudomonal lung infection, pulmonary embolism, pulmonary infiltrates, pulmonary mass, renal failure, respiratory arrest, sepsis, splenomegaly, supraventricular tachycardia, Sweet's syndrome (acute febrile neutrophilic dermatosis), urethral hemorrhage

Drug Interactions

Metabolism/Transport Effects None known.

Avoid Concomitant Use

Avoid concomitant use of Decitabine with any of the following: CloZAPine

Increased Effect/Toxicity

Decitabine may increase the levels/effects of: CloZAPine

Decreased Effect There are no known significant interactions involving a decrease in effect.

Stability Store vials at 25°C (77°F); excursions permitted to 15°C to 30°C (59°F to 86°F). Vials should be reconstituted with 10 mL SWFI to a concentration of 5 mg/mL.

Immediately further dilute with 50-250 mL NS, D_5W, or lactated Ringer's to a final concentration of 0.1-1 mg/mL. Use appropriate precautions for handling and disposal. Solutions not administered within 15 minutes of preparation should be prepared with cold (2°C to 8°C [36°F to 46°F]) infusion solutions. Solutions diluted for infusion may be stored for up to 7 hours under refrigeration at 2°C to 8°C (36°F to 46°F) if prepared with cold infusion fluids.

Mechanism of Action After phosphorylation, decitabine is incorporated into DNA and inhibits DNA methyltransferase causing hypomethylation and subsequent cell death (within the S-phase of the cell cycle).

Pharmacodynamics/Kinetics

Distribution: 63-89 L/m^2

Protein binding: <1%

Metabolism: Possibly via deamination by cytidine deaminase

Half-life elimination: ~30-35 minutes

Time to peak: At end of infusion

Dosage I.V.: Adults:

MDS:

15 mg/m^2 over 3 hours every 8 hours (45 mg/m^2/day) for 3 days (135 mg/m^2/cycle) every 6 weeks (treatment is recommended for at least 4 cycles and may continue until the patient no longer continues to benefit)

Adjustment for prolonged hematologic toxicity (ANC <1000/mm^3 and platelets <50,000/mm^3):

>6 weeks but <8 weeks: Delay dose for up to 2 weeks and temporarily reduce dose to 11 mg/m^2 every 8 hours (33 mg/m^2/day) for 3 days

>8 weeks but <10 weeks: Assess for disease progression; if no disease progression, delay dose for up to 2 weeks and reduce dose to 11 mg/m^2 every 8 hours (33 mg/m^2/day) for 3 days; maintain or increase dose with subsequent cycles if clinically indicated

or

20 mg/m^2 over 1 hour daily for 5 days every 28 days (delay subsequent treatment cycles until hematologic recovery (ANC ≥1000/mm^3 and platelets ≥50,000/mm^3)

AML (unlabeled use): 20 mg/m^2 over 1 hour daily for 5 days every 28 days (Cashen, 2010)

Dosage adjustment for toxicity:

Hematologic toxicity (ANC <1000/mm^3 and platelets <50,000/mm^3): Delay and/or reduce dose; see recommendations specific to each MDS dosing regimen

Nonhematologic toxicity: Temporarily hold treatment until resolution for any of the following toxicities:

Serum creatinine ≥2 mg/dL

ALT, bilirubin ≥2 times ULN

Active or uncontrolled infection

Administration Infuse over 1-3 hours. Premedication with antiemetics is recommended.

Monitoring Parameters CBC with differential and platelets with each cycle, more frequently if needed; liver enzymes; serum creatinine

Dosage Forms Excipient information presented when available (limited, particularly for generics); consult specific product labeling.

Injection, powder for reconstitution:

Dacogen®: 50 mg

◆ **Declomycin** *see* Demeclocycline *on page 468*

◆ **Deep Sea [OTC]** *see* Sodium Chloride *on page 1567*

Deferasirox (de FER a sir ox)

Brand Names: U.S. Exjade®

Brand Names: Canada Exjade®

Index Terms ICL670

Pharmacologic Category Chelating Agent

Use Treatment of chronic iron overload due to blood transfusions (transfusional hemosiderosis)

Pregnancy Risk Factor C

Pregnancy Considerations Teratogenic effects were observed in animal studies. There are no adequate and well-controlled studies in pregnant women. Use during pregnancy only if the potential benefit justifies the potential risk to the fetus.

Lactation Excretion in breast milk unknown/not recommended

Prescribing and Access Restrictions Deferasirox (Exjade®) is only available through a restricted distribution program called EPASS™ Complete Care. Prescribers must enroll patients in this program in order to obtain the medication. For patient enrollment, contact 1-888-90EPASS (1-888-903-7277).

Contraindications Hypersensitivity to deferasirox or any component of the formulation; platelet counts <50,000/mm^3; poor performance status and high-risk myelodysplastic syndromes or advanced malignancies; creatinine clearance <40 mL/minute or serum creatinine >2 x age-appropriate ULN

Canadian labeling: Additional contraindications (not in U.S. labeling): Cl_{cr} <60 mL/minute

Warnings/Precautions [U.S. Boxed Warning]: Renal impairment and renal failure (some fatal) have been reported; observed more frequently in elderly patients, high-risk myelodysplastic syndromes (MDS), underlying renal dysfunction, and/or other comorbidities. Monitor serum creatinine and/or creatinine clearance at baseline and monthly thereafter; in patients with underlying renal dysfunction or at risk for renal dysfunction, monitor weekly during the first month. Dose reduction, interruption, or discontinuation should be considered for serum creatinine elevations; interrupt for progressive increases beyond the upper limit of normal; may reinitiate with dose reduction once serum creatinine returns to age-appropriate normal range. Monitor closely if creatinine clearance is between 40-<60 mL/minute. Acute renal failure (some have required dialysis) has been reported; generally occurs in patients with multiple comorbidities. May cause proteinuria; closely monitor. Renal tubulopathy has also been reported, primarily in pediatric patients with β-thalassemia and serum ferritin levels <1500 mcg/L.

[U.S. Boxed Warning]: Hepatic dysfunction or failure (including fatalities) have occurred; observed more frequently in elderly patients, high-risk myelodysplastic syndromes (MDS), underlying hepatic dysfunction, and/or other comorbidities. Monitor transaminases and bilirubin at baseline, every 2 weeks for 1 month, then monthly thereafter. Hepatitis and elevated transaminases have also been reported. Avoid use in severe hepatic impairment, reduce dose for moderate impairment, and monitor closely in mild or moderate impairment. **[U.S. Boxed Warning]: Gastrointestinal (GI) hemorrhage, including fatalities, has occurred with use; observed more frequently in elderly patients with high-risk myelodysplastic syndromes (MDS) and/or low platelet counts (<50,000/mm^3).** Other GI effects including irritation and ulceration have been reported. Use caution with concurrent medications that may increase risk of adverse GI effects (eg, NSAIDs, corticosteroids, anticoagulants, oral bisphosphonates). Monitor patients closely for signs/symptoms of GI ulceration/bleeding.

May cause skin rash (dose-related), including erythema multiforme; mild-to-moderate rashes may resolve without treatment interruption; for severe rash, interrupt and consider restarting at a lower dose with dose escalation and oral steroids. Hypersensitivity reactions, including severe reactions (anaphylaxis and angioedema) have been reported, onset is usually within the first month of treatment; discontinue if severe. Auditory (decreased hearing and high frequency hearing loss) or ocular disturbances (lens opacities, cataracts, intraocular pressure elevation, and retinal disorders) have been reported (rare); monitor and consider dose reduction or treatment interruption. Cytopenias (including agranulocytosis, neutropenia, and thrombocytopenia) have been reported, predominately in patients with preexisting hematologic disorders; monitor blood counts regularly; interrupt treatment for unexplained cytopenias (may reinitiate once cause of cytopenia has been excluded). Potent UGT inducers (eg, rifampin) or cholestyramine may decrease the efficacy of deferasirox; avoid concomitant use. If coadministration necessary, dosage modifications may be needed; monitor serum ferritin and clinical response. Not approved for use in combination with other iron chelation therapies; safety of combinations has not been established. Treatment should be initiated with evidence of chronic iron overload (eg, transfusion of ~100 mL/kg of packed RBCs [~20 units for a 40 kg individual] and serum ferritin consistently >1000 mcg/L). Prior to use, consider risk versus anticipated benefit with respect to individual patient's life expectancy and prognosis. Use with caution in the elderly due to the higher incidence of hepatic, renal and cardiac dysfunction in the elderly.

Adverse Reactions

>10%:

- Central nervous system: Fever (19%), headache (16%)
- Dermatologic: Rash (dose related; 8% to 11%)
- Gastrointestinal: Abdominal pain (dose related; 21% to 28%), diarrhea (dose related; 12% to 20%), nausea (dose related; 11% to 23%), vomiting (dose related; 10% to 21%)
- Renal: Serum creatinine increased (dose related; 7% to 38%), proteinuria (19%)
- Respiratory: Cough (14%), nasopharyngitis (13%), pharyngolaryngeal pain (11%)
- Miscellaneous: Influenza (11%)

1% to 10%:

- Central nervous system: Fatigue (6%)
- Dermatologic: Urticaria (4%)
- Hepatic: ALT increased (2% to 8%), transaminitis (4%)
- Neuromuscular & skeletal: Arthralgia (7%), back pain (6%)
- Otic: Ear infection (5%)
- Respiratory: Respiratory tract infection (10%), bronchitis (9%), pharyngitis (8%), acute tonsillitis (6%), rhinitis (6%)

<1% (Limited to important or life-threatening): Acute renal failure, agranulocytosis, anaphylaxis, angioedema, ascites, bilirubin increased, cataract, cholecystitis, cholelithiasis, constipation, cytopenias, dizziness, drug fever, duodenal ulcer, edema, erythema multiforme, esophagitis, gastric ulcer, gastritis, gastrointestinal bleeding, gastrointestinal hemorrhage, glomerulonephritis, glucosuria, hearing loss (including high frequency), hematuria, Henoch-Schönlein purpura, hepatic dysfunction, hepatic encephalopathy, hepatic failure, hepatic transaminases increased, hepatitis, hyperactivity, hypersensitivity reaction, hypocalcemia, interstitial nephritis, intraocular pressure increased, jaundice, lens opacities, leukocytoclastic vasculitis, maculopathy, neutropenia, optic neuritis, pigment disorder, purpura, renal tubular necrosis, renal tubulopathy, retinal disorder, thrombocytopenia, visual disturbance

Drug Interactions

Metabolism/Transport Effects **Substrate** of UGT1A1; **Inhibits** CYP1A2 (moderate), CYP2C8 (moderate); **Induces** CYP3A4 (weak/moderate)

Avoid Concomitant Use

Avoid concomitant use of Deferasirox with any of the following: Aluminum Hydroxide; Theophylline

Increased Effect/Toxicity

Deferasirox may increase the levels/effects of: CYP1A2 Substrates; CYP2C8 Substrates; Theophylline

The levels/effects of Deferasirox may be increased by: Anticoagulants; Bisphosphonate Derivatives; Corticosteroids; Corticosteroids (Systemic); Nonsteroidal Anti-Inflammatory Agents

Decreased Effect

Deferasirox may decrease the levels/effects of: ARIPiprazole; CYP3A4 Substrates; Saxagliptin

The levels/effects of Deferasirox may be decreased by: Aluminum Hydroxide; Cholestyramine Resin; Fosphenytoin; PHENobarbital; Phenytoin; Rifampin; Ritonavir

Stability Store at room temperature of 25°C (77°F); excursions permitted to 15°C and 30°C (59°F and 86°F). Protect from moisture.

Mechanism of Action Selectively binds iron, forming a complex which is excreted primarily through the feces.

Pharmacodynamics/Kinetics

Distribution: Adults: 14.4 ± 2.7L

Protein binding: ~99% to serum albumin

Metabolism: Hepatic via glucuronidation by UGT1A1(primarily) and UGT1A3; minor oxidation by CYP450; undergoes enterohepatic recirculation

Bioavailability: 70%

Half-life elimination: 8-16 hours

Time to peak, plasma: ~1.5-4 hours

Excretion: Feces (84%); urine (8%)

Dosage Oral: Children ≥2 years and Adults: **Note:** Baseline serum ferritin and iron levels should be obtained prior to therapy; toxicity may be increased in patients with low iron burden or with only slightly elevated serum ferritin.

Initial: 20 mg/kg daily (calculate dose to nearest whole tablet); administer as a suspension (see **Administration**)

Maintenance: Adjust dose every 3-6 months based on serum ferritin trends; adjust by 5 or 10 mg/kg/day (calculate dose to nearest whole tablet); titrate to individual response and treatment goals. Usual range: 20-30 mg/kg/day; doses up to 40 mg/kg/day may be considered for serum ferritin levels persistently >2500 mcg/L (doses above 40 mg/kg/day are not recommended). **Note:** Consider interrupting therapy for serum ferritin <500 mcg/L and dose reduction or interruption for hearing loss or visual disturbances.

Dosage adjustment with concomitant cholestyramine or potent UGT inducers (eg, rifampin, phenytoin, phenobarbital, ritonavir): Avoid concomitant use; if coadministration necessary, consider increasing the initial dose of deferasirox dose to 30 mg/kg; monitor serum ferritin and clinical response. Doses above 40 mg/kg are not recommended.

Dosage adjustment for toxicity:

Cytopenias: Consider treatment interruption (may reinitiate once cause of cytopenia has been determined)

Hearing loss or visual disturbance: Consider dose reduction or treatment interruption

Severe rash: Interrupt treatment; may reintroduce at a lower dose (with future dose escalation) and short-term oral corticosteroids

Dosage adjustment in renal impairment:

Cl_{cr} ≥60 mL/minute: No initial adjustment necessary. Monitor renal function; increases in serum creatinine may require alteration or discontinuation of therapy.

Cl_{cr} ≥40 to <60 mL/minute: No initial adjustment necessary. Use caution; monitor renal function closely, particularly in patients at increased risk for further renal impairment (eg, concomitant nephrotoxic therapy, dehydration, severe infection); increases in serum creatinine may require alteration or discontinuation of therapy.

Cl_{cr} <40 mL/minute or serum creatinine >2 times age-appropriate ULN: Use is contraindicated

Increase in serum creatinine: Consider dose reduction, interruption, or discontinuation.

Progressive increase in serum creatinine above the age-appropriate ULN: Interrupt treatment; once serum creatinine recovers to within the normal range, reinitiate treatment at a reduced dose; gradually escalate the dose if the clinical benefit outweighs potential risk.

Children: For increase in serum creatinine above the age-appropriate ULN for 2 consecutive levels, reduce daily dose by 10 mg/kg; use in children with baseline serum creatinine >ULN has not been studied.

Adults: For increase in serum creatinine >33% above the average pretreatment level for 2 consecutive levels (and cannot be attributed to other causes), reduce daily dose by 10 mg/kg

Dosage adjustment in hepatic impairment:

Mild hepatic impairment (Child-Pugh class A): No adjustment necessary. Monitor closely for efficacy and for adverse reactions requiring dosage reduction

Moderate hepatic impairment (Child-Pugh class B): Reduce dose by 50%; monitor closely for efficacy and for adverse reactions requiring dosage reduction

Severe hepatic impairment (Child-Pugh class C): Avoid use

Dietary Considerations Bioavailability increased variably when taken with food; take on empty stomach 30 minutes before a meal.

Administration Oral: **Do not chew or swallow whole tablets.** Completely disperse tablets in water, orange juice, or apple juice (use 3.5 ounces for total doses <1 g; 7 ounces for doses ≥1 g); stir to form a fine suspension and drink entire contents. Rinse remaining residue with more fluid; drink. Administer at same time each day on an empty stomach, 30 minutes before food. Do not take simultaneously with aluminum-containing antacids.

Monitoring Parameters Serum ferritin (baseline, monthly thereafter), iron levels (baseline), CBC with differential, serum creatinine and/or creatinine clearance (2 baseline assessments then monthly thereafter; in patients who are at increased risk of complications [eg, pre-existing renal conditions, elderly, comorbid conditions, or receiving other potentially nephrotoxic medications]: weekly for the first month then monthly thereafter); urine protein (monthly); serum transaminases and bilirubin (baseline, every 2 weeks for the first month, then monthly); baseline and annual auditory and ophthalmic function (including slit lamp examinations and dilated fundoscopy); performance status (in patients with hematologic malignancies); signs and symptoms of GI ulcers or hemorrhage; number of RBC units received

Additional Information Deferasirox has a low affinity for binding with zinc and copper, may cause variable decreases in the serum concentration of these trace minerals.

Oncology Comment: The National Comprehensive Cancer Network (NCCN) guidelines for myelodysplastic syndromes (MDS) recommend considering iron chelation therapy in low- or intermediate-risk MDS patients to decrease iron overload due to multiple transfusions (v.2.2011). Treatment is generally recommended in MDS patients who have received >20-30 RBC transfusions and for those with serum ferritin levels >2500 mcg/L, with a goal to decrease ferritin levels to <1000 mcg/L.

Dosage Forms Excipient information presented when available (limited, particularly for generics); consult specific product labeling.

Tablet for suspension, oral:

Exjade®: 125 mg, 250 mg, 500 mg

Deferiprone (de FER i prone)

Brand Names: U.S. Ferriprox®

Index Terms APO-066; Ferriprox®

Pharmacologic Category Chelating Agent

Use Treatment of transfusional iron overload due to thalassemia syndromes with inadequate response to other chelation therapy

Pregnancy Risk Factor D

Dosage Oral: **Note:** Round dose to the nearest 250 mg (or 1/2 tablet). If serum ferritin falls consistently below 500 mcg/L, consider temporary treatment interruption.

Adults: Transfusional iron overload: Initial: 25 mg/kg 3 times/day (75 mg/kg/day); individualize dose based on response and therapeutic goal; maximum dose: 33 mg/kg 3 times/day (99 mg/kg/day)

Elderly: Begin at the low end of dosing range

Dosage adjustment for toxicity:

ANC <1500/mm^3: Interrupt treatment

ANC <500/mm^3: In addition to treatment interruption, consider hospitalization (and other clinically-appropriate management); do not resume or rechallenge unless the potential benefits outweigh potential risks

Infection: Interrupt treatment; monitor ANC more frequently

Dosage adjustment in renal impairment: No dosage adjustments are provided in the manufacturer's labeling (has not been studied).

Dosage adjustment in hepatic impairment: No dosage adjustments are provided in the manufacturer's labeling (has not been studied).

Additional Information Complete prescribing information for this medication should be consulted for additional detail.

Dosage Forms Excipient information presented when available (limited, particularly for generics); consult specific product labeling.

Tablet, oral:

Ferriprox®: 500 mg [scored]

Deferoxamine (de fer OKS a meen)

Brand Names: U.S. Desferal®

Brand Names: Canada Desferal®; PMS-Deferoxamine

Index Terms Deferoxamine Mesylate; Desferrioxamine

Pharmacologic Category Antidote; Chelating Agent

Use Adjunct in the treatment of acute iron intoxication; treatment of chronic iron overload secondary to multiple transfusions

Canadian labeling (unlabeled use in the U.S.): Diagnosis of aluminum overload; treatment of chronic aluminum overload in patients with end-stage renal failure undergoing maintenance dialysis

Unlabeled Use Diagnosis or treatment of aluminum induced toxicity associated with chronic kidney disease (CKD)

Pregnancy Risk Factor C

Pregnancy Considerations Skeletal anomalies and delayed ossification were observed in some but not all animal studies. Toxic amounts of iron or deferoxamine have not been noted to cross the placenta. In case of acute toxicity, treatment during pregnancy should not be withheld.

Lactation Excretion in breast milk unknown/use caution

Contraindications Hypersensitivity to deferoxamine or any component of the formulation; patients with severe renal disease or anuria

Note: Canadian labeling does not list severe renal disease or anuria within the contraindications.

Warnings/Precautions Flushing of the skin, hypotension, urticaria and shock are associated with rapid I.V. infusion; administer I.M., by slow subcutaneous or slow I.V. infusion only. Auditory disturbances (tinnitus and high frequency hearing loss) have been reported following prolonged administration, at high doses, or in patients with low ferritin levels; generally reversible with early detection and immediate discontinuation. Elderly patients are at increased risk for hearing loss. Audiology exams are recommended with long-term treatment. Ocular disturbances (blurred vision, cataracts, corneal opacities, decreased visual acuity, impaired peripheral, color, and night vision, optic neuritis, retinal pigment abnormalities, scotoma, visual loss/defect) have been reported following prolonged administration, at high doses, or in patients with low ferritin levels; generally reversible with early detection and immediate discontinuation. Elderly patients are at increased risk for ocular disorders. Periodic ophthalmic exams are recommended with long-term treatment.

Deferoxamine has been associated with acute respiratory distress syndrome following excessively high-dose I.V. treatment of acute intoxication or thalassemia (has been reported in children and adults). High deferoxamine doses and concurrent low ferritin levels are also associated with growth retardation. Growth velocity may partially resume to pretreatment velocity rates after deferoxamine dose reduction. Patients with iron overload are at increased susceptibility to infection with *Yersinia enterocolitica* and *Yersinia pseudotuberculosis*; treatment with deferoxamine may enhance this risk; if infection develops, discontinue therapy until resolved. Rare and serious cases of mucormycosis have been reported with use; withhold treatment with signs and symptoms of mucormycosis.

Increases in serum creatinine, acute renal failure and renal tubular disorders have been reported. When iron is chelated with deferoxamine, the chelate is excreted renally. Deferoxamine is readily dialyzable. Treatment with deferoxamine in patients with aluminum toxicity may cause hypocalcemia and aggravate hyperparathyroidism. Deferoxamine may cause neurological symptoms (including seizure) in patients with aluminum-related encephalopathy receiving dialysis and may precipitate dialysis dementia onset.

Deferoxamine is not indicated for the treatment of primary hemochromatosis (treatment of choice is phlebotomy). Patients should be informed that urine may have a reddish color. Combination treatment with ascorbic acid (>500 mg/day in adults) and deferoxamine may impair cardiac function (rare), reversible upon discontinuation of ascorbic acid. If combination treatment is warranted, initiate ascorbic acid after one month of deferoxamine treatment, do not exceed ascorbic acid dose of 200 mg/day for adults (in divided doses), 50 mg/day in children <10 years of age, or 100 mg/day in children ≥10 years of age; monitor cardiac function. Do not administer deferoxamine in combination with ascorbic acid in patients with pre-existing cardiac failure.

Adverse Reactions Frequency not defined.

Cardiovascular: Flushing, hypotension, shock, tachycardia
Central nervous system: Dizziness, encephalopathy (aluminum toxicity/dialysis-related), fever, headache, seizure
Dermatologic: Angioedema, rash, urticaria
Endocrine & metabolic: Growth retardation (children), hyperparathyroidism (aggravated), hypocalcemia
Gastrointestinal: Abdominal discomfort, abdominal pain, diarrhea, nausea, vomiting
Genitourinary: Dysuria, urine discoloration (reddish color)
Hematologic: Leukopenia, thrombocytopenia
Hepatic: Hepatic dysfunction, transaminases increased
Local: Injection site: Burning, crust, edema, erythema, eschar, induration, infiltration, irritation, pain, pruritus, swelling, vesicles, wheal formation
Neuromuscular & skeletal: Arthralgia, metaphyseal dysplasia (children <3 years; dose related), muscle spasms, myalgia, neuropathy (peripheral, sensory, motor, or mixed), paresthesia
Ocular: Blurred vision, cataract, corneal opacities, dyschromatopsia, loss of vision, night blindness, optic neuritis, peripheral vision impaired, retinal pigment abnormalities, scotoma, visual acuity decreased, visual field defects
Otic: Hearing loss, tinnitus
Renal: Acute renal failure, renal tubular disorders, serum creatinine increased
Respiratory: Acute respiratory distress syndrome (dyspnea, cyanosis, and/or interstitial infiltrates), asthma
Miscellaneous: Anaphylaxis (with or without shock), hypersensitivity reaction, infections (*Yersinia*, mucormycosis)

Drug Interactions

Metabolism/Transport Effects None known.

Avoid Concomitant Use There are no known interactions where it is recommended to avoid concomitant use.

Increased Effect/Toxicity

Deferoxamine may increase the levels/effects of: Prochlorperazine

The levels/effects of Deferoxamine may be increased by: Ascorbic Acid

Decreased Effect There are no known significant interactions involving a decrease in effect.

Stability Prior to reconstitution, store at ≤25°C (≤77°F). Following reconstitution, may be stored at room temperature for 24 hours, although the manufacturer recommends use begin within 3 hours of reconstitution. Do not refrigerate reconstituted solution. When stored at 30°C in polypropylene infusion pump syringes, deferoxamine 250 mg/mL in sterile water for injection retained 95% of initial concentration for 14 days (Stiles, 1996).

Reconstitution:

I.M.: Reconstitute with sterile water for injection (500 mg vial with 2 mL; 2000 mg vial with 8 mL) to a final concentration of 213 mg/mL

I.V.: Reconstitute with sterile water for injection (500 mg vial with 5 mL; 2000 mg vial with 20 mL) to a final concentration of 95 mg/mL; further dilute for infusion in sodium chloride 0.9%, sodium chloride 0.45%, D_5W, or LR.

SubQ: Reconstitute with sterile water for injection (500 mg vial with 5 mL; 2000 mg vial with 20 mL) to a final concentration of 95 mg/mL

Mechanism of Action Complexes with trivalent ions (ferric ions) to form ferrioxamine, which are removed by the kidneys, slows accumulation of hepatic iron and retards or eliminates progression of hepatic fibrosis. Also known to inhibit DNA synthesis *in vitro*.

Pharmacodynamics/Kinetics

Absorption: I.M., SubQ: Well absorbed
Distribution: Distributed throughout body fluids
Protein binding: <10%
Metabolism: Plasma enzymes; binds with iron to form ferrioxamine (iron complex)
Half-life elimination: 14 hours (plasma half-life: 20-30 minutes)
Excretion: Primarily urine (as unchanged drug and ferrioxamine); feces (via bile)

Dosage

Acute iron toxicity: **Note:** The I.V. route should be used for patients in a state of cardiovascular collapse.

Children ≥3 years:

I.M.: 90 mg/kg/dose every 8 hours (maximum: 6 g/24 hours)

I.V.: 15 mg/kg/hour (maximum: 6 g/24 hours)

Canadian labeling:
I.M.: Initial: 90 mg/kg/dose (maximum/dose: 1 g) followed by 45 mg/kg every 4-12 hours as needed (maximum: 6 g/24 hours)
I.V.: 15 mg/kg/hour up to a maximum of 80 mg/kg/dose or maximum of 6 g/24 hours
Adults: I.M., I.V.: Initial: 1000 mg, may be followed by 500 mg every 4 hours for 2 doses; subsequent doses of 500 mg have been administered every 4-12 hours based on clinical response (maximum recommended dose: 6 g/day [per manufacturer])
Canadian labeling:
I.M.: Initial: 90 mg/kg/dose (maximum/dose: 2 g) followed by 45 mg/kg every 4-12 hours as needed (maximum: 6 g/24 hours)
I.V.: 15 mg/kg/hour up to a maximum of 80 mg/kg/dose or maximum of 6 g/24 hours
Chronic iron overload:
Children ≥3 years:
I.V.: 15 mg/kg/hour (maximum: 6 g/24 hours)
SubQ: 20-40 mg/kg/day over 8-12 hours (maximum: 1000-2000 mg/day)
Unlabeled dosing: I.V., SubQ: 25-30 mg/kg over 8-10 hours 5-7 days/week (Brittenham, 2011)
Adults:
I.M., I.V.: Initial: I.M.: 500-1000 mg/day; in addition, 2000 mg should be given I.V. with each unit of blood transfused (administer separately from blood); maximum: 1 g/day in absence of transfusions; 6 g/day if patient received transfusions
SubQ: 1-2 g every day or 20-40 mg/kg/day over 8-24 hours
Unlabeled dosing: I.V., SubQ: 25-50 mg/kg over 8-10 hours 5-7 days/week (Brittenham, 2011)
Canadian labeling: I.V., SubQ: 1-4 g (20-60 mg/kg) over ~12 hours (may further increase iron excretion with infusion over 24 hours)
Diagnosis of aluminum-induced toxicity with CKD (unlabeled use; K/DOQI guidelines, 2003): Children and Adults: I.V.: Test dose: 5 mg/kg during the last hour of dialysis if serum aluminum levels are 60-200 mcg/L, or clinical signs/symptoms of toxicity, or aluminum exposure prior to parathyroid surgery. Measure aluminum just prior to deferoxamine; remeasure 2 days later (test is positive if serum aluminum is ≥50 mcg/L). Do not use if aluminum serum levels are >200 mcg/L.
Canadian labeling: **Note:** Measure serum aluminum levels prior to and after administration of deferoxamine.
Adults: I.V.: Test dose: 5 mg/kg/dose (infusion rate not to exceed 15 mg/kg/hour) following hemodialysis (preferred) or during the last hour of dialysis if serum aluminum levels are >60 mcg/L in association with serum ferritin levels >100 mcg/L; continuous rise in serum aluminum over the next 24-48 hours suggests overload. Remeasure serum aluminum levels prior to next hemodialysis, test is considered positive if serum aluminum levels increase >150 mcg/L above baseline.
Treatment of aluminum toxicity with CKD (unlabeled use; K/DOQI guidelines, 2003): Children and Adults: I.V.:
Administer after diagnostic deferoxamine test dose. **Note:** The risk for deferoxamine-associated neurotoxicity is increased if aluminum serum levels are >200 mcg/L; withhold deferoxamine and administer intensive dialysis until <200 mcg/L.
Aluminum rise ≥300 mcg/L: 5 mg/kg once a week 5 hours before dialysis for 4 months
Aluminum rise <300 mcg/L: 5 mg/kg once a week during the last hour of dialysis for 2 months
Canadian labeling: Adults: Treatment should be considered for symptomatic patients with serum aluminum levels >60 mcg/L and a positive deferoxamine test dose.
Hemodialysis: I.V.: 5 mg/kg/dose (infusion rate not to exceed 15 mg/kg/hour) once weekly for 3 months following hemodialysis (preferred) or during the last hour of dialysis administered. Withhold treatment for 1 month then perform deferoxamine test. Further treatment is not recommended if 2 consecutive tests (performed 1 month apart) yield an increase in serum aluminum levels <75 mcg/mL.
Continuous ambulatory or cyclic peritoneal dialysis: Intraperitoneal (preferred), I.M., SubQ infusion (slow), or I.V. infusion (slow): 5 mg/kg/dose once weekly prior to final daily exchange

Dosing adjustment in renal impairment: Severe renal disease or anuria: Use is contraindicated in the FDA-approved labeling.
The following adjustments have been used by some clinicians (Aronoff, 2007): Adults:
Cl_{cr} >50 mL/minute: No adjustment required
Cl_{cr} 10-50 mL/minute, CRRT: Administer 25% to 50% of normal dose
Cl_{cr}<10 mL/minute, hemodialysis, peritoneal dialysis: Avoid use

Dietary Considerations Vitamin C supplements may need to be limited. The manufacturer recommends a maximum ascorbic acid dose of 200 mg/day in adults (given in divided doses), 50 mg/day in children <10 years of age, or 100 mg/day in children ≥10 years of age. Avoid concurrent use with ascorbic acid in patients with heart failure.

Administration
I.V.: Urticaria, flushing of the skin, hypotension, and shock have occurred following rapid I.V. administration; limiting infusion rate to 15mg/kg/hour may help avoid infusion-related adverse effects.
Acute iron toxicity: The manufacturer states that the I.M. route is preferred; however, the I.V. route is generally preferred in patients with severe toxicity (ie, patients in shock). For the first 1000 mg, infuse at 15 mg/kg/hour. Subsequent doses may be given over 4-12 hours at a rate not to exceed 125 mg/hour.
Chronic iron overload: Longer infusion times (24 hours) and I.V. administration may be required in patients with severe cardiac iron deposition (Brittenham, 2011).
Diagnosis or treatment of aluminum-induced toxicity with CKD: Administer dose over 1 hour, during the last hour of dialysis (K/DOQI guidelines, 2003).
SubQ: When administered for chronic iron overload, daily dose is usually given over 8-12 hours using portable infusion pump. Topical anesthetic or glucocorticoid creams may be used for induration or erythema (Brittenham, 2011).

Monitoring Parameters Serum iron, ferritin, total iron-binding capacity, CBC with differential, serum creatinine, liver function tests, serum chemistries; ophthalmologic exam (visual acuity tests, fundoscopy, slit-lamp exam) and audiometry with long-term treatment; growth and body weight in children (every 3 months)
Dialysis patients: Serum aluminum (yearly; every 3 months in patients on aluminum-containing medications)
Aluminum-induced bone disease: Serum aluminum 2 days following test dose; test is considered positive if serum aluminum increases ≥50 mcg/L

Reference Range
Iron, serum: Normal: 50-150 mcg/dL; levels >500 mcg/dL associated with toxicity. Consider treatment with symptomatic patients with levels ≥350 mcg/dL; toxicity cannot be excluded with serum iron levels <350 mcg/dL
Aluminum, serum: <20 mcg/L recommended baseline level in dialysis patients (K/DOQI, 2003)

Test Interactions TIBC may be falsely elevated with high serum iron concentrations or deferoxamine therapy. Imaging results may be distorted due to rapid urinary excretion of deferoxamine-bound gallium-67; discontinue deferoxamine 48 hours prior to scintigraphy.

Additional Information Oncology Comment: The National Comprehensive Cancer Network (NCCN) guidelines for myelodysplastic syndromes (MDS) recommend considering iron chelation therapy in low- or intermediate-risk MDS patients to decrease iron overload due to multiple transfusions (v.2.2011). Treatment is generally recommended in MDS patients who have received ≥20 units of RBC transfusions and for those with serum ferritin levels >2500 mcg/L, with a goal to decrease ferritin levels to <1000 mcg/L.

Dosage Forms Excipient information presented when available (limited, particularly for generics); consult specific product labeling.

Injection, powder for reconstitution, as mesylate: 500 mg, 2 g

Desferal®: 500 mg, 2 g

◆ **Deferoxamine Mesylate** *see* Deferoxamine *on page 463*

Degarelix (deg a REL ix)

Brand Names: U.S. Firmagon®

Brand Names: Canada Firmagon®

Index Terms Degarelix Acetate; FE200486

Pharmacologic Category Antineoplastic Agent, Gonadotropin-Releasing Hormone Antagonist; Gonadotropin Releasing Hormone Antagonist

Use Treatment of advanced prostate cancer

Pregnancy Risk Factor X

Pregnancy Considerations Animal studies have demonstrated embryo and fetal loss. Use is contraindicated in women who are or may become pregnant.

Lactation Excretion in breast milk unknown/not recommended

Contraindications Hypersensitivity to degarelix or any component of the formulation; pregnancy (or potential to become pregnant)

Warnings/Precautions Hazardous agent - use appropriate precautions for handling and disposal. Long-term androgen deprivation therapy may prolong the QT interval; use with caution in patients with a known history of QT prolongation or other risk factors for QT prolongation (eg, concomitant use of medications known to prolong QT interval, heart failure, and/or electrolyte abnormalities). Androgen-deprivation therapy may increase the risk for cardiovascular disease (Levine, 2010) and decreased bone mineral density. Androgen deprivation therapy may cause obesity and insulin resistance; the risk for diabetes is increased.

Degarelix exposure is decreased in patients with hepatic impairment, dosage adjustment is not recommended in patients with mild-to-moderate hepatic impairment, although testosterone levels should be monitored. Has not been studied in patients with severe hepatic impairment; use with caution. Data for use in patients with moderate-to-severe renal impairment (Cl_{cr} <50 mL/minute) is limited; use with caution.

Adverse Reactions

>10%:

Endocrine & metabolic: Hot flashes (26%)

Local: Injections site reactions (35%, grade 3: ≤2%; pain 28%, erythema 17%, swelling 6%, induration 4%, nodule 3%)

1% to 10%:

Cardiovascular: Hypertension (6%)

Central nervous system: Chills (5%), dizziness (1% to 5%), fever (1% to 5%), headache (1% to 5%), insomnia (1% to 5%), fatigue (3%)

Dermatologic: Hyperhydrosis

Endocrine & metabolic: Hypercholesterolemia (3%), gynecomastia, testicular atrophy

Gastrointestinal: Weight gain (9%), constipation (5%), nausea (1% to 5%), diarrhea

Genitourinary: Urinary tract infection (5%), erectile dysfunction

Hepatic: ALT increased (10%; grade 3: <1%), AST increased (5%; grade 3: <1%), GGT increased

Neuromuscular & skeletal: Back pain (6%), arthralgia (5%), weakness (1% to 5%)

Miscellaneous: Antidegarelix antibody formation (10%), night sweats (1% to 5%)

<1% (Limited to important or life-threatening): Bone metastases worsening, cerebral stroke, depression, injection site pruritus, injection site soreness, lymphoma (malignant), mental status changes, MI, osteoarthritis, QT interval prolongation, squamous cell cancer, unstable angina

Drug Interactions

Metabolism/Transport Effects None known.

Avoid Concomitant Use

Avoid concomitant use of Degarelix with any of the following: Artemether; Dronedarone; Lumefantrine; Nilotinib; Pimozide; QUEtiapine; QuiNINE; Tetrabenazine; Thioridazine; Toremifene; Vandetanib; Vemurafenib; Ziprasidone

Increased Effect/Toxicity

Degarelix may increase the levels/effects of: Dronedarone; Pimozide; QTc-Prolonging Agents; QuiNINE; Tetrabenazine; Thioridazine; Toremifene; Vandetanib; Vemurafenib; Ziprasidone

The levels/effects of Degarelix may be increased by: Alfuzosin; Artemether; Chloroquine; Ciprofloxacin; Ciprofloxacin (Systemic); Gadobutrol; Indacaterol; Lumefantrine; Nilotinib; QUEtiapine; QuiNINE

Decreased Effect There are no known significant interactions involving a decrease in effect.

Stability Store at 25°C (77°F); excursions permitted to 15°C to 30°C (59°F to 86°F). Use appropriate precautions (wear gloves for preparation and administration) for handling and disposal. Reconstitute with preservative free sterile water for injection (reconstitute each 120 mg vial with 3 mL; reconstitute the 80 mg vial with 4.2 mL). Swirl gently; do not shake (to prevent foaming). Dissolution may take up to 15 minutes. Keep vial upright at all times. Tilt vial slightly, keeping needle in lowest section of vial to withdraw for administration. Administer within 1 hour of reconstitution.

Mechanism of Action Gonadotropin-releasing hormone (GnRH) antagonist which reversibly binds to GnRH receptors in the anterior pituitary gland, blocking the receptor and decreasing secretion of luteinizing hormone (LH) and follicle stimulation hormone (FSH), resulting in rapid androgen deprivation by decreasing testosterone production, thereby decreasing testosterone levels. Testosterone levels do not exhibit an initial surge, or flare, as is typical with GnRH agonists.

Pharmacodynamics/Kinetics

Onset of action: Rapid; ~96% of patients had testosterone levels ≤50 ng/dL within 3 days (Klotz, 2008)

Distribution: V_d: >1000 L

Protein binding: ~90%

Metabolism: Hepatobiliary, via peptide hydrolysis

Bioavailability: Biphasic release: Rapid release initially, then slow release from depot formed after subcutaneous injection administration (Tornoe, 2007)

Half-life elimination: Loading dose: SubQ: ~53 days

Time to peak, plasma: Loading dose: SubQ: Within 2 days

Excretion: Feces (~70% to 80%, primarily as peptide fragments); urine (~20% to 30%)

Dosage SubQ: Adults: Prostate cancer:

Loading dose: 240 mg administered as two 120 mg (3 mL) injections

Maintenance dose: 80 mg every 28 days (beginning 28 days after initial loading dose)

Dosage adjustment in renal impairment: Cl_{cr} <50 mL/minute: Use with caution

Dosage adjustment in hepatic impairment:

Mild-to-moderate hepatic impairment: No adjustment required; monitor serum testosterone levels

Severe hepatic impairment: Has not been studied; use with caution

Dietary Considerations Supplementation with 500 mg calcium and 400 int. units of vitamin D is recommended (due to the increased risk for osteoporosis with androgen deprivation therapy).

Administration Not for I.V. use. Administer SubQ in the abdominal area by grasping skin and elevating SubQ tissue; insert the needle deeply at an angle not ≤45 degrees. Avoid pressure exposed areas (eg, waistband, belt, or near ribs); rotate injection site. Inject loading dose as two 3 mL injections (40 mg/mL); maintenance dose should be administered as a single 4 mL injection (20 mg/mL); begin maintenance dose 28 days after initial loading dose.

Monitoring Parameters Prostate-specific antigen (PSA) periodically, serum testosterone levels (if PSA increases; in patients with hepatic impairment: monitor testosterone levels monthly until achieve castration levels, then consider monitoring every other month), liver function tests (at baseline), serum electrolytes (calcium, magnesium, potassium, sodium); bone mineral density

Screen for diabetes and cardiovascular risk prior to initiating treatment.

Test Interactions Suppression of pituitary-gonadal function may affect diagnostic tests of pituitary gonadotropic and gonadal functions.

Dosage Forms Excipient information presented when available (limited, particularly for generics); consult specific product labeling.

Injection, powder for reconstitution, as acetate:

Firmagon®: 80 mg, 120 mg

◆ **Degarelix Acetate** *see* Degarelix *on page 466*
◆ **Dehydral® (Can)** *see* Methenamine *on page 1093*
◆ **Dehydrobenzperidol** *see* Droperidol *on page 562*
◆ **Delatestryl®** *see* Testosterone *on page 1654*

Delavirdine (de la VIR deen)

Brand Names: U.S. Rescriptor®

Brand Names: Canada Rescriptor®

Index Terms DLV; U-90152S

Pharmacologic Category Antiretroviral Agent, Reverse Transcriptase Inhibitor (Non-nucleoside)

Additional Appendix Information

Management of Healthcare Worker Exposures to HBV, HCV, and HIV *on page 1935*

Perinatal HIV Guidelines *on page 1946*

Use Treatment of HIV-1 infection in combination with at least two additional antiretroviral agents

Pregnancy Risk Factor C

Pregnancy Considerations Adverse events were observed in some animal reproduction studies. Hypersensitivity reactions (including hepatic toxicity and rash) are more common in women on NNRTI therapy; it is not known if pregnancy increases this risk.

Regardless of CD4 count or HIV RNA copy number, all HIV-infected pregnant women should receive a combination antepartum antiretroviral (ARV) drug regimen; this includes women who require therapy for their own health, as well as women who do not yet require therapy for their own health. ARV therapy should be started as soon as possible if required for the woman's health or immediately after the first trimester if not needed for the mother's health (although earlier initiation may be considered). Long-term follow-up is recommended for all infants exposed to ARV medications.

Healthcare providers are encouraged to enroll pregnant women exposed to antiretroviral medications in the Antiretroviral Pregnancy Registry (1-800-258-4263 or www.-APRegistry.com). Healthcare providers caring for HIV-infected women and their infants may contact the National Perinatal HIV Hotline (888-448-8765) for clinical consultation (DHHS [perinatal], 2011).

Lactation Excretion in breast milk unknown/contraindicated

Contraindications Hypersensitivity to delavirdine or any component of the formulation; concurrent use of alprazolam, astemizole, cisapride, ergot alkaloids, midazolam, pimozide, rifampin, terfenadine, or triazolam

Warnings/Precautions Use with caution in patients with hepatic or renal dysfunction; due to rapid emergence of resistance, delavirdine should not be used as monotherapy or as a component of an initial antiretroviral regimen; cross-resistance may be conferred to other non-nucleoside reverse transcriptase inhibitors, although potential for cross-resistance with protease inhibitors is low. Long-term effects of delavirdine are not known. May cause redistribution of fat (eg, buffalo hump, peripheral wasting with increased abdominal girth, cushingoid appearance). Immune reconstitution syndrome may develop resulting in the occurrence of an inflammatory response to an indolent or residual opportunistic infection; further evaluation and treatment may be required. Safety and efficacy have not been established in children. Rash, which occurs frequently, may require discontinuation of therapy; usually occurs within 1-3 weeks and lasts <2 weeks. Most patients may resume therapy following a treatment interruption. Use with caution in patients taking strong CYP3A4 inhibitors, moderate or strong CYP3A4 inducers and major CYP3A4 substrates (see Drug Interactions); consider alternative agents that avoid or lessen the potential for CYP-mediated interactions.

Adverse Reactions

Frequency of adverse reactions reported from occurrence in clinical trials with delavirdine when used as part of combination antiretroviral therapy.

>10%:

Central nervous system: Headache (19% to 20%), depressive symptoms (10% to 15%), fever (4% to 12%)

Dermatologic: Rash (16% to 32%)

Gastrointestinal: Nausea (20% to 25%), vomiting (3% to 11%)

1% to 10%:

Central nervous system: Anxiety (6% to 8%)

Endocrine & metabolic: Transaminases increased (2% to 5%), amylase increased (3%), bilirubin increased (2%)

Gastrointestinal: Diarrhea, vomiting, abdominal pain (4% to 6%)

Hematologic: Prothrombin time increased (2%), hemoglobin decreased (1% to 3%)

Respiratory: Bronchitis (6% to 8%)

Frequency not defined (limited to important or life threatening): Abscess, adenopathy, alkaline phosphatase increased, allergic reaction, angioedema, anorexia, arrhythmia, bloody stool, bone pain, bruising, cardiac insufficiency, cardiac rate abnormal, cardiomyopathy, chest congestion, cognitive impairment, colitis, confusion, conjunctivitis, dermal leukocytoclastic vasculitis, desquamation, diverticulitis, dyspnea, emotional lability, eosinophilia, erythema multiforme, fecal incontinence, fungal dermatitis, gamma glutamyl transpeptidase increased, gastroenteritis, gastrointestinal bleeding, granulocytosis, gum hemorrhage, hallucination, hematuria, hepatomegaly, hyperglycemia, hyperkalemia, hypertension, hypertriglyceridemia, hyperuricemia, hypocalcemia, hyponatremia, hypophosphatemia, infection, jaundice, kidney pain, leukopenia, lipase increased, menstrual irregularities, moniliasis (oral/vaginal), pancreatitis, pancytopenia, paralysis, peripheral vascular disorder, pneumonia, postural hypotension, purpura, redistribution of body fat, renal calculi, serum creatinine increased, spleen disorder, Stevens-Johnson syndrome, tetany, thrombocytopenia, urinary tract infection, vertigo

Postmarketing and/or case reports: Acute renal failure, hemolytic anemia, hepatic failure, immune reconstitution syndrome, rhabdomyolysis

Drug Interactions

Metabolism/Transport Effects Substrate of CYP2D6 (minor), CYP3A4 (major); **Note:** Assignment of Major/Minor substrate status based on clinically relevant drug interaction potential; **Inhibits** CYP1A2 (weak), CYP2C19 (strong), CYP2C9 (strong), CYP2D6 (strong), CYP3A4 (strong)

Avoid Concomitant Use

Avoid concomitant use of Delavirdine with any of the following: Alfuzosin; Astemizole; Clopidogrel; Conivaptan; Crizotinib; Dronedarone; Eplerenone; Etravirine; Everolimus; Fluticasone (Oral Inhalation); Fosamprenavir; Fosphenytoin; H2-Antagonists; Halofantrine; Lapatinib; Lovastatin; Lurasidone; Nilotinib; Nisoldipine; Phenytoin; Pimozide; Proton Pump Inhibitors; Ranolazine; Rilpivirine; Rivaroxaban; RomiDEPsin; Salmeterol; Silodosin; Simvastatin; St Johns Wort; Tamoxifen; Tamsulosin; Terfenadine; Thioridazine; Ticagrelor; Tolvaptan; Toremifene

Increased Effect/Toxicity

Delavirdine may increase the levels/effects of: Alfuzosin; Almotriptan; Alosetron; ARIPiprazole; Astemizole; Atomoxetine; Bortezomib; Brentuximab Vedotin; Brinzolamide; Budesonide (Nasal); Budesonide (Systemic, Oral Inhalation); Carvedilol; Ciclesonide; Citalopram; Colchicine; Conivaptan; Corticosteroids (Orally Inhaled); Crizotinib; CYP2C19 Substrates; CYP2C9 Substrates; CYP2D6 Substrates; CYP3A4 Substrates; Diclofenac; Dienogest; Dronedarone; Dutasteride; Eplerenone; Etravirine; Everolimus; FentaNYL; Fesoterodine; Fluticasone (Nasal); Fluticasone (Oral Inhalation); Fosamprenavir; Fosphenytoin; GuanFACINE; Halofantrine; Iloperidone; Ixabepilone; Lapatinib; Lovastatin; Lumefantrine; Lurasidone; Maraviroc; MethylPREDNISolone; Nebivolol; Nilotinib; Nisoldipine; PACLitaxel; Paricalcitol; Pazopanib; Phenytoin; Pimecrolimus; Pimozide; Propafenone; Protease Inhibitors; Ranolazine; Rifamycin Derivatives; Rilpivirine; Rivaroxaban; RomiDEPsin; Ruxolitinib; Salmeterol; Saxagliptin; Sildenafil; Silodosin; Simvastatin; SORAfenib; Tadalafil; Tamoxifen; Tamsulosin; Terfenadine; Tetrabenazine; Thioridazine; Ticagrelor; Tolterodine; Tolvaptan; Toremifene; Vardenafil; Vemurafenib; Vilazodone; Zuclopenthixol

Decreased Effect

Delavirdine may decrease the levels/effects of: Clopidogrel; Codeine; Etravirine; Prasugrel; Rilpivirine; Ticagrelor; TraMADol

The levels/effects of Delavirdine may be decreased by: Antacids; CYP3A4 Inducers (Strong); Deferasirox; Fosamprenavir; Fosphenytoin; H2-Antagonists; Peginterferon Alfa-2b; Phenytoin; Protease Inhibitors; Proton Pump Inhibitors; Rifamycin Derivatives; St Johns Wort; Tocilizumab

Ethanol/Nutrition/Herb Interactions Herb/Nutraceutical: Delavirdine serum concentration may be decreased by St John's wort; avoid concurrent use.

Stability Store at 20°C to 25°C (68°F to 77°F). Protect from humidity.

Mechanism of Action Delavirdine binds directly to reverse transcriptase, blocking RNA-dependent and DNA-dependent DNA polymerase activities

Pharmacodynamics/Kinetics

Absorption: Rapid

Distribution: Low concentration in saliva and semen; CSF 0.4% concurrent plasma concentration

Protein binding: ~98%, primarily albumin

Metabolism: Hepatic via CYP3A4 and 2D6 (**Note:** May reduce CYP3A activity and inhibit its own metabolism.)

Bioavailability: Tablet: 85% as tablet; ~100% as oral slurry

Half-life elimination: 5.8 hours (range: 2-11 hours)

Time to peak, plasma: 1 hour

Excretion: Urine (51%, <5% as unchanged drug); feces (44%); nonlinear kinetics exhibited

Dosage Adolescents ≥16 years and Adults: Oral: 400 mg 3 times/day

Note: Only a single delavirdine mutation causes resistance; use is not recommended in initial antiretroviral regimens (DHHS, 2011).

Dietary Considerations May be taken without regard to meals.

Administration Patients with achlorhydria should take the drug with an acidic beverage; antacids and delavirdine should be separated by 1 hour. A dispersion of delavirdine may be prepared by adding four 100 mg tablets to at least 3 oz of water. Allow to stand for a few minutes and stir until uniform dispersion. Drink immediately. Rinse glass and mouth, then swallow the rinse to ensure total dose administered. The 200 mg tablets should be taken intact.

Monitoring Parameters Liver function tests if administered with saquinavir

Additional Information Potential compliance problems, frequency of administration, and adverse effects should be discussed with patients before initiating therapy to help prevent the emergence of resistance.

Dosage Forms Excipient information presented when available (limited, particularly for generics); consult specific product labeling.

Tablet, oral, as mesylate:

Rescriptor®: 100 mg, 200 mg

Extemporaneous Preparations A dispersion of delavirdine may be made with tablets. Add four 100 mg tablets to at least 3 oz of water; allow to stand for a few minutes and stir until uniform dispersion. Administer immediately. To ensure full dose is administered, rinse glass and drink liquid; also rinse mouth and swallow following ingestion.

- **Delestrogen®** *see* Estradiol (Systemic) *on page 627*
- **Delfen® [OTC]** *see* Nonoxynol 9 *on page 1216*
- **Delta-9-tetrahydro-cannabinol** *see* Dronabinol *on page 561*
- **Delta-9 THC** *see* Dronabinol *on page 561*
- **Deltacortisone** *see* PredniSONE *on page 1399*
- **Deltadehydrocortisone** *see* PredniSONE *on page 1399*
- **Demadex®** *see* Torsemide *on page 1712*

Demeclocycline (dem e kloe SYE kleen)

Index Terms Declomycin; Demeclocycline Hydrochloride; Demethylchlortetracycline

Pharmacologic Category Antibiotic, Tetracycline Derivative

Use Treatment of susceptible bacterial infections (acne, gonorrhea, pertussis, and urinary tract infections) caused by both gram-negative and gram-positive organisms

Unlabeled Use Treatment of chronic syndrome of inappropriate secretion of antidiuretic hormone (SIADH)

Pregnancy Risk Factor D

Pregnancy Considerations Demeclocycline has been shown to cross the placenta in rats and other tetracyclines cross the placenta in humans causing permanent discoloration of teeth if used during the second or third trimester. Because use during pregnancy may cause fetal harm, demeclocyline is classified as pregnancy category D.

Lactation Enters breast milk/not recommended

Contraindications Hypersensitivity to demeclocycline, tetracyclines, or any component of the formulation; children <8 years of age; concomitant use with methoxyflurane

Warnings/Precautions Photosensitivity reactions occur frequently with this drug; avoid prolonged exposure to sunlight and do not use tanning equipment. Use caution in patients with renal or hepatic impairment (eg, elderly); dosage modification required in patients with renal impairment. May act as an antianabolic agent and increase BUN. Pseudotumor cerebri has been reported with tetracycline use (usually resolves with discontinuation). Outdated drug can cause nephropathy. Prolonged use may result in fungal or bacterial superinfection, including *C. difficile*-associated diarrhea (CDAD) and pseudomembranous colitis; CDAD has been observed >2 months postantibiotic treatment. May cause tissue hyperpigmentation, enamel hypoplasia, or permanent tooth discoloration; use of tetracyclines should be avoided during tooth development (children <8 years of age) unless other drugs are not likely to be effective or are contraindicated. Do not use during pregnancy. In addition to affecting tooth development, tetracycline use has been associated with retardation of skeletal development and reduced bone growth.

Adverse Reactions Frequency not defined.

Cardiovascular: Pericarditis

Central nervous system: Bulging fontanels (infants), dizziness, headache, pseudotumor cerebri (adults)

Dermatologic: Angioneurotic edema, erythema multiforme, erythematous rash, maculopapular rash, photosensitivity, pigmentation of skin, Stevens-Johnson syndrome (rare), urticaria

Endocrine & metabolic: Discoloration of thyroid gland (brown/black), nephrogenic diabetes insipidus

Gastrointestinal: Anorexia, diarrhea, dysphagia, enterocolitis, esophageal ulcerations, glossitis, nausea, pancreatitis, vomiting

Genitourinary: Balanitis

Hematologic: Eosinophilia, neutropenia, hemolytic anemia, thrombocytopenia

Hepatic: Hepatitis (rare), hepatotoxicity (rare), liver enzymes increased, liver failure (rare)

Neuromuscular & skeletal: Myasthenic syndrome, polyarthralgia, tooth discoloration (children <8 years, rarely in adults)

Ocular: Visual disturbances

Otic: Tinnitus

Renal: Acute renal failure

Respiratory: Pulmonary infiltrates

Miscellaneous: Anaphylaxis, anaphylactoid purpura, lupus-like syndrome, systemic lupus erythematosus exacerbation

Drug Interactions

Metabolism/Transport Effects None known.

Avoid Concomitant Use

Avoid concomitant use of Demeclocycline with any of the following: BCG; Retinoic Acid Derivatives

Increased Effect/Toxicity

Demeclocycline may increase the levels/effects of: Neuromuscular-Blocking Agents; Porfimer; Retinoic Acid Derivatives; Vitamin K Antagonists

Decreased Effect

Demeclocycline may decrease the levels/effects of: BCG; Desmopressin; Penicillins; Typhoid Vaccine

The levels/effects of Demeclocycline may be decreased by: Antacids; Bile Acid Sequestrants; Bismuth; Bismuth Subsalicylate; Calcium Salts; Iron Salts; Lanthanum; Magnesium Salts; Quinapril; Sucralfate; Zinc Salts

Ethanol/Nutrition/Herb Interactions

Food: Demeclocycline serum levels may be decreased if taken with food.

Herb/Nutraceutical: Avoid dong quai, St John's wort (may also cause photosensitization).

Stability Tetracyclines form toxic products when outdated or when exposed to light, heat, or humidity (Fanconi-like syndrome).

Mechanism of Action Inhibits protein synthesis by binding with the 30S and possibly the 50S ribosomal subunit(s) of susceptible bacteria; may also cause alterations in the cytoplasmic membrane; inhibits the action of ADH in patients with chronic SIADH

Pharmacodynamics/Kinetics

Onset of action: SIADH: Several days

Absorption: ~50% to 80%; reduced by food and dairy products

Protein binding: 41% to 50%

Metabolism: Hepatic (small amounts) to inactive metabolites; undergoes enterohepatic recirculation

Half-life elimination: 10-17 hours

Time to peak, serum: 3-6 hours

Excretion: Urine (42% to 50% as unchanged drug)

Dosage Oral:

Children ≥8 years: 8-12 mg/kg/day divided every 6-12 hours

Adults: 150 mg 4 times/day or 300 mg twice daily

SIADH (unlabeled use): 900-1200 mg/day or 13-15 mg/kg/day divided every 6-8 hours initially, then decrease to 600-900 mg/day

Dosing adjustment/comments in renal/hepatic impairment: Should be avoided in patients with renal/hepatic dysfunction

Dietary Considerations Should be taken 1 hour before or 2 hours after food or milk with plenty of fluid.

Administration Administer 1 hour before or 2 hours after food or milk with plenty of fluid.

Monitoring Parameters CBC, renal and hepatic function

Test Interactions May interfere with tests for urinary glucose (false-negative urine glucose using Clinistix®, Tes-Tape®)

Dosage Forms Excipient information presented when available (limited, particularly for generics); consult specific product labeling.

Tablet, oral, as hydrochloride: 150 mg, 300 mg

- **Demeclocycline Hydrochloride** *see* Demeclocycline *on page 468*
- **Demerol®** *see* Meperidine *on page 1074*
- **4-Demethoxydaunorubicin** *see* IDArubicin *on page 865*
- **Demethylchlortetracycline** *see* Demeclocycline *on page 468*
- **Demser®** *see* Metyrosine *on page 1123*
- **Demulen® 30 (Can)** *see* Ethinyl Estradiol and Ethynodiol Diacetate *on page 655*
- **Denavir®** *see* Penciclovir *on page 1319*

Denileukin Diftitox (de ni LOO kin DIF ti toks)

Brand Names: U.S. ONTAK®

Index Terms DAB389 Interleukin-2; DAB_{389}IL-2; DABIL2

Pharmacologic Category Antineoplastic Agent, Miscellaneous

Use Treatment of persistent or recurrent cutaneous T-cell lymphoma (CTCL) whose malignant cells express the CD25 component of the IL-2 receptor

Unlabeled Use Treatment of CTCL types mycosis fungoides (MF) and Sézary syndrome (SS); peripheral T-cell lymphoma (second-line treatment)

Pregnancy Considerations Animal reproduction studies have not been conducted. There are no adequate and well-controlled studies in pregnant women. Should be given to a pregnant woman only if clearly needed

Lactation Excretion in breast milk unknown/not recommended

Contraindications There are no contraindications listed within the manufacturer's labeling.

Warnings/Precautions Hazardous agent - use appropriate precautions for handling and disposal. **[U.S. Boxed Warning]: Has been associated with a potentially severe, including life-threatening, capillary leak syndrome; monitor weight, edema, blood pressure, and serum albumin prior to and during treatment.** Symptoms of capillary leak syndrome (hypotension, edema, hypoalbuminemia) may be delayed, occurring up to 2 weeks post infusion; symptoms may persist or worsen after cessation of denileukin diftitox. Withhold treatment if serum albumin <3 g/dL; pre-existing low serum albumin levels may correlate with capillary leak syndrome. **[U.S. Boxed Warning]: Serious and fatal infusion reactions have occurred. Administer in a facility appropriate for cardiopulmonary resuscitation. Discontinue immediately and permanently with serious infusion reaction.** Infusion reaction symptoms usually occur within 24 hours of infusion and resolve within 48 hours of last infusion of cycle. Incidence of infusion reaction has been reported to be lower in cycles 3 and 4 (compared to cycles 1 and 2). The manufacturer recommends premedicating with an antihistamine and acetaminophen; corticosteroid (eg, dexamethasone) premedication may help to reduce the incidence of hypersensitivity and edema (Foss, 2001). **[U.S. Boxed Warning]: Loss of visual acuity, usually associated with loss of color vision (with or without retinal pigment mottling) has been reported;** most patients have persistent visual impairment.

Confirm CD25 expression on malignant cells prior to treatment. May develop immunogenicity; patients with antibodies have a two- to threefold increase in clearance; the presence of antibodies does not correlate with risk for hypersensitivity/infusion related reactions. Monitor closely for infection; may impair immune function. Use with caution in patients >65 years of age; adverse events (anemia, anorexia, confusion, hypotension, rash, nausea/vomiting) may occur more frequently. Safety and efficacy in children have not been established. Should be administered under the supervision of an experienced cancer chemotherapy physician.

Adverse Reactions

>10%:

Cardiovascular: Capillary leak syndrome (33%; serious: 11%), peripheral edema (20% to 26%), vasodilation (22%), hypotension (7% to 16%), chest pain (4% to 13%), tachycardia (12%), thrombosis-related events (7% to 11%)

Central nervous system: Fever (49% to 64%), fatigue (44% to 47%), headache (26% to 29%), dizziness (11% to 13%), pain (11% to 13%)

Dermatologic: Rash (20% to 24%), pruritus (16% to 18%)

Endocrine & metabolic: Hypoalbuminemia (14% to 17%)

Gastrointestinal: Nausea (47% to 60%), vomiting (13% to 35%), diarrhea (22%), anorexia (9% to 20%), taste disturbance (11% to 13%)

Hematologic: Lymphopenia (70%; 24% had lymphopenia at baseline)

Hepatic: ALT increased (84%), AST increased (84%)

Neuromuscular & skeletal: Rigors (42% to 47%), myalgia (18% to 20%), weakness (18%), back pain (16% to 18%), arthralgia (13% to 16%)

Respiratory: Cough (18% to 20%), upper respiratory infection (13%), dyspnea (11% to 13%)

Miscellaneous: Antibody formation (76% to 100%) neutralizing antibodies (45% to 97%), flu-like syndrome (≤85%), infusion reaction (71%; serious: 8%), infection (48%)

1% to 10%:

Cardiovascular: Arrhythmia (6%), hypertension (6%)

Hematologic: Leukopenia (grades 3/4: 3% to 6%), neutropenia (grades 3/4: 3%), thrombocytopenia (grades 3/4: 3%)

Local: Injection site reaction (8%)

Ocular: Visual changes (serious: 4%; includes loss of visual acuity)

Renal: Serum creatinine increased (3% to 10%), proteinuria/casts/hematuria (6%)

Postmarketing and/or case reports: Acute renal insufficiency, hyper-/hypothyroidism, oral ulcer, pancreatitis, thyroiditis, thyrotoxicosis, toxic epidermal necrolysis

Drug Interactions

Metabolism/Transport Effects None known.

Avoid Concomitant Use

Avoid concomitant use of Denileukin Diftitox with any of the following: BCG; Belimumab; Natalizumab; Pimecrolimus; Tacrolimus (Topical); Vaccines (Live)

Increased Effect/Toxicity

Denileukin Diftitox may increase the levels/effects of: Belimumab; Leflunomide; Natalizumab; Vaccines (Live)

The levels/effects of Denileukin Diftitox may be increased by: Denosumab; Pimecrolimus; Roflumilast; Tacrolimus (Topical); Trastuzumab

Decreased Effect

Denileukin Diftitox may decrease the levels/effects of: BCG; Coccidioidin Skin Test; Sipuleucel-T; Vaccines (Inactivated); Vaccines (Live)

The levels/effects of Denileukin Diftitox may be decreased by: Echinacea

Stability Store intact vials frozen at or below -10°C (14°F). Must be brought to room temperature (25°C or 77°F) before preparing the dose. Do not refreeze after thawing. Do **not** heat vials. Thaw in refrigerator for not >24 hours or at room temperature for 1-2 hours. Solution may be mixed by gentle swirling; avoid vigorous agitation. Dilute with NS to a concentration of ≥15 mcg/mL; the concentration must be ≥15 mcg/mL during all steps of preparation. This solution should be used within 6 hours. Add drug to the empty sterile I.V. bag first, then add NS. Do not prepare with glass syringes or in glass containers.

Mechanism of Action Denileukin diftitox is a fusion protein (a combination of amino acid sequences from diphtheria toxin and interleukin-2) which selectively delivers the cytotoxic activity of diphtheria toxin to targeted cells. It interacts with the high-affinity IL-2 receptor on the surface of malignant cells to inhibit intracellular protein synthesis, rapidly leading to cell death.

Pharmacodynamics/Kinetics

Distribution: V_d: 0.06-0.09 L/kg

Metabolism: Hepatic via proteolytic degradation (animal studies)

Half-life elimination: Distribution: 2-5 minutes; Terminal: 70-80 minutes

Dosage Note: Premedicate with an antihistamine and acetaminophen prior to each infusion; corticosteroid premedication (eg, dexamethasone) may reduce the incidence of hypersensitivity and edema (Foss, 2001). Withhold treatment if serum albumin <3 g/dL.

I.V.: Adults: CTCL: 9 or 18 mcg/kg/day days 1 through 5 every 21 days for 8 cycles

Dosage adjustment for toxicity:

Serum albumin <3 g/dL: Withhold treatment

Severe infusion reaction: Permanently discontinue treatment

Administration For I.V. use only. Infuse over 30-60 minutes. Should **not** be given as a rapid I.V. bolus. Discontinue or reduce infusion rate for infusion related reactions; discontinue for severe infusion reaction. Do not administer through an in-line filter. Premedicate with an antihistamine and acetaminophen; consider corticosteroid premedication.

Monitoring Parameters Baseline CD25 expression (on malignant cells); serum albumin level (prior to each treatment), CBC, blood chemistry panel, renal and hepatic function tests (prior to initiation of therapy and weekly during therapy). During the infusion, the patient should be monitored for symptoms of an infusion reaction. After infusion, the patient should be monitored for the development of a delayed capillary leak syndrome (usually in the first 2 weeks), including careful monitoring of weight, blood pressure, and serum albumin.

Information on assay for malignant cell CD25 expression is available at 1-877-873-4724.

Additional Information Oncology Comment: The National Comprehensive Cancer Network® (NCCN) Non-Hodgkin's Lymphoma Guidelines (v.2.2009) list denileukin diftitox as a second-line treatment option for systemic therapy of peripheral (cutaneous) T-cell lymphoma in patients who are not candidates for high dose therapy or autologous stem cell rescue. In mycosis fungoides (MF) and Sézary syndrome (SS), denileukin diftitox is a therapy option, either as monotherapy or in combination with bexarotene (Foss, 2005). Participation in a clinical trial is encouraged for this patient population.

Corticosteroids may be considered for prevention of hypersensitivity reaction. In a small study (Foss, 2001) reviewing denileukin diftitox and premedication with either prednisone 20 mg orally or dexamethasone 8 mg I.V. on day 1 followed by dexamethasone 8 mg I.V. on days 2-5, a reduction in adverse events was observed when compared to a previous (Olsen, 2001) phase III study. A statistically significant reduction in the incidence of edema was demonstrated. Improved response rates (compared to the phase III study) were noted, likely due to in increase in tolerability due to corticosteroid premedication. While some studies did not allow premedication with corticosteroids (Kuzel, 2007; Olsen, 2001) as part of the trial design, dexamethasone premedication has been utilized in other studies and case reports (Foss, 2005; Frankel, 2006; Gerena-Lewis, 2009; Talpur, 2002) with denileukin diftitox use for cutaneous T-cell lymphoma as well as other (unlabeled) uses.

Dosage Forms Excipient information presented when available (limited, particularly for generics); consult specific product labeling.

Injection, solution:

ONTAK®: 150 mcg/mL (2 mL) [contains edetate disodium]

Denosumab (den OH sue mab)

Brand Names: U.S. Prolia®; Xgeva™

Brand Names: Canada Prolia®; Xgeva™

Index Terms AMG-162

Pharmacologic Category Bone-Modifying Agent; Monoclonal Antibody

Use Treatment of osteoporosis in postmenopausal women at high risk for fracture; treatment of bone loss in men receiving androgen deprivation therapy (ADT) for nonmetastatic prostate cancer; treatment of bone loss in women receiving aromatase inhibitor (AI) therapy for breast cancer; prevention of skeletal-related events (eg, fracture, spinal cord compression, bone pain requiring surgery/radiation therapy) in patients with bone metastases from solid tumors

Unlabeled Use Treatment of bone destruction caused by rheumatoid arthritis

Pregnancy Risk Factor C

Pregnancy Considerations Adverse fetal events were observed in studies of genetically engineered mice developed to be missing RANKL (the target of denosumab). In studies of monkeys where denosumab was administered during the period of organogenesis, adverse fetal events were not observed (not studied beyond organogenesis). However, fetal exposure to monoclonal antibodies is expected to increase as pregnancy progresses. There are no adequate and well controlled trials in pregnant women. Use only if the potential benefit outweighs the potential risk to the fetus. If a pregnant woman is exposed, patients or their prescribers may contact the Amgen Pregnancy Surveillance Program (800-772-6436).

Lactation Excretion unknown/not recommended

Medication Guide Available Yes

Contraindications

Prolia®: Pre-existing hypocalcemia

Xgeva™: There are no contraindications listed in the manufacturer's labeling.

Warnings/Precautions Denosumab may cause or exacerbate hypocalcemia. Monitor calcium levels; correct pre-existing hypocalcemia prior to therapy. Use caution in patients with a history of hypoparathyroidism, thyroid surgery, parathyroid surgery, malabsorption syndromes, excision of small intestine, severe renal impairment/dialysis or other conditions which would predispose the patient to hypocalcemia; monitor calcium, phosphorus, and magnesium closely during therapy. Ensure adequate calcium and vitamin D intake; supplement with calcium and vitamin D; magnesium supplementation may also be necessary. Incidence of infections may be increased, including serious skin infections, abdominal, urinary, ear, or periodontal infections. Endocarditis has also been reported following use. Patients should be advised to contact healthcare provider if signs or symptoms of severe infection or cellulitis develop. Use with caution in patients with impaired immune systems or using concomitant immunosuppressive therapy; may be at increased risk for serious infections. Evaluate the need for continued treatment with serious infection. Osteonecrosis of the jaw (ONJ) has been reported in patients receiving denosumab. ONJ may manifest as jaw pain, osteomyelitis, osteitis, bone erosion, tooth/periodontal infection, toothache, gingival ulceration/ erosion. Risk factors include invasive dental procedures (eg, tooth extraction, dental implants, boney surgery); a diagnosis of cancer, concomitant chemotherapy or corticosteroids, poor oral hygiene, ill-fitting dentures; and comorbid disorders (anemia, coagulopathy, infection, pre-existing dental disease). Patients should maintain good oral hygiene during treatment. A dental exam and preventative dentistry should be performed prior to therapy. The benefit/risk must be assessed by the treating physician and/or dentist/surgeon prior to any invasive dental procedure; avoid invasive procedures in patients with bone metastases receiving therapy for prevention of skeletal-related events. Patients developing ONJ while on denosumab therapy should receive care by a dentist or oral surgeon; extensive dental surgery to treat ONJ may exacerbate ONJ; evaluate individually and consider discontinuing if extensive dental surgery is necessary.

Postmenopausal osteoporosis: For use in women at high risk for fracture which is defined as a history of osteoporotic fracture or multiple risk factors for fracture. May also be used in women who failed or did not tolerate other therapies.

Bone metastases: Denosumab is not indicated for the prevention of skeletal-related events in patients with multiple myeloma. In trials of with multiple myeloma patients, denosumab was noninferior to zoledronic acid in delaying time to first skeletal-related event and mortality was increased in a subset of the denosumab-treated group.

Denosumab therapy results in significant suppression of bone turnover; the long term effects of treatment are not known but may contribute to adverse outcomes such as ONJ, atypical fractures, or delayed fracture healing; monitor. Use with caution in patients with renal impairment (Cl_{cr} <30 mL/minute) or patients on dialysis; risk of hypocalcemia is increased. Dose adjustment is not needed. Dermatitis, eczema, and rash (which are not necessarily specific to the injection site) have been reported; consider discontinuing if severe symptoms occur. Packaging may contain natural latex rubber. May impair bone growth in children with open growth plates or inhibit eruption of dentition. Do not administer Prolia® and Xgeva™ to the same patient for different indications.

Adverse Reactions A postmarketing safety program for Prolia® is available to collect information on adverse events; more information is available at http://www.-proliasafety.com. To report adverse events for either Prolia® or Xgeva™, prescribers may also call Amgen at 800-772-6436 or FDA at 800-332-1088.

>10%:

Central nervous system: Fatigue (Xgeva™: 45%), headache (Xgeva™: 13%)

Dermatologic: Dermatitis (11%), eczema (11%), rash (3% to 11%)

Endocrine & metabolic: Hypophosphatemia (Xgeva™: 32%; grade 3: 15%), hypocalcemia (2%; Xgeva™: 18%; grade 3: 3%)

Gastrointestinal: Nausea (Xgeva™: 31%), diarrhea (Xgeva™: 20%)

Neuromuscular & skeletal: Weakness (Xgeva™: 45%), arthralgia (14%), limb pain (10% to 12%), back pain (12%)

Respiratory: Dyspnea (Xgeva™: 21%), cough (Xgeva™: 15%)

1% to 10%:

Cardiovascular: Peripheral edema (5%), angina (3%)

Endocrine & metabolic: Hypercholesterolemia (7%)

Gastrointestinal: Flatulence (2%)

Neuromuscular & skeletal: Musculoskeletal pain (6%), sciatica (5%), bone pain (4%), myalgia (3%), osteonecrosis of the jaw (ONJ; ≤2%)

Ocular: Cataracts (≤5%)

Respiratory: Upper respiratory tract infection (5%)

Miscellaneous: New malignancies (5%), infections (non-fatal, serious; 4%)

<1% (Limited to important or life-threatening): Antibody formation, constipation, cystitis, endocarditis, GERD, hypertension, influenza, pancreatitis

Drug Interactions

Metabolism/Transport Effects None known.

Avoid Concomitant Use There are no known interactions where it is recommended to avoid concomitant use.

Increased Effect/Toxicity

Denosumab may increase the levels/effects of: Immunosuppressants

Decreased Effect There are no known significant interactions involving a decrease in effect.

Ethanol/Nutrition/Herb Interactions Ethanol: Avoid ethanol (may increase risk of osteoporosis).

Stability Prior to use, store in original carton under refrigeration, 2°C to 8°C (36°F to 46°F). Do not freeze. Prior to use, bring to room temperature of 25°C (77°F) in original container (usually takes 15-30 minutes); do not use any other methods for warming. Use within 14 days once at room temperature. Protect from direct heat and light; do not expose to temperatures >25°C (77°F). Avoid vigorous shaking.

Mechanism of Action Denosumab is a monoclonal antibody with affinity for nuclear factor-kappa ligand (RANKL). Osteoblasts secrete RANKL; RANKL activates osteoclast precursors and subsequent osteolysis which promotes release of bone-derived growth factors, such as insulin-like growth factor-1 (IGF1) and transforming growth factor-beta (TGF-beta), and increases serum calcium levels. Denosumab binds to RANKL, blocks the interaction between RANKL and RANK (a receptor located on osteoclast surfaces), and prevents osteoclast formation, leading to decreased bone resorption and increased bone mass in osteoporosis. In solid tumors with bony metastases, RANKL inhibition decreases osteoclastic activity leading to decreased skeletal related events and tumor-induced bone destruction.

Pharmacodynamics/Kinetics

Onset of action: Decreases markers of bone resorption by ~85% within 3 days; maximal reductions observed within 1 month

Duration: Markers of bone resorption return to baseline within 12 months of discontinuing therapy

Bioavailability: SubQ: 62%

Half-life elimination: ~25-28 days

Time to peak, serum: 10 days (range: 3-21 days)

Dosage SubQ: Adults:

Prevention of skeletal-related events in bone metastases from solid tumors (Xgeva™): 120 mg every 4 weeks

Treatment of androgen deprivation-induced bone loss in men with prostate cancer (Prolia®): 60 mg as a single dose, once every 6 months (Smith, 2009)

Treatment of aromatase inhibitor-induced bone loss in women with breast cancer (Prolia®): 60 mg as a single dose, once every 6 months (Ellis, 2008)

Treatment of osteoporosis in postmenopausal females (Prolia®): 60 mg as a single dose, once every 6 months

Dosage adjustment in renal impairment: Dose adjustment is not needed; monitor patients with severe impairment (Cl_{cr} <30 mL/minute or on dialysis) due to increased risk of hypocalcemia.

Dietary Considerations Ensure adequate calcium and vitamin D intake to prevent or treat hypocalcemia. Calcium 1000 mg/day and vitamin D ≥400 units/day is recommended in product labeling (Prolia®).

Women and men >50 years of age should consume elemental calcium 1200-1500 mg/day and vitamin D 800-1000 int. units/day (National Osteoporosis Foundation Guidelines, 2010).

Administration SubQ: Prior to administration, bring to room temperature in original container (allow to stand ~15-30 minutes); do not warm by any other method. Solution may contain trace amounts of translucent to white protein particles; do not use if cloudy, discolored (normal solution should be clear and colorless to pale yellow), or contains excessive particles or foreign matter. Avoid vigorous shaking. Administer via SubQ injection in the upper arm, upper thigh, or abdomen.

Prolia®: If a dose is missed, administer as soon as possible, then continue dosing every 6 months from the date of the last injection.

Monitoring Parameters Recommend monitoring of serum creatinine, serum calcium, phosphorus and magnesium, signs and symptoms of hypocalcemia, especially in patients predisposed to hypocalcemia (severe renal impairment, thyroid/parathyroid surgery, malabsorption syndromes, hypoparathyroidism); infection, or dermatologic reactions; routine oral exam (prior to treatment); dental exam if risk factors for ONJ

Osteoporosis: Bone mineral density as measured by central dual-energy x-ray absorptiometry (DXA) of the hip or spine (prior to initiation of therapy and at least every 2 years; annual measurements of height and weight, assessment of chronic back pain; serum calcium and 25(OH)D; may consider monitoring biochemical markers of bone turnover (National Osteoporosis Foundation Guidelines, 2010)

Additional Information Oncology Comment: Metastatic breast cancer: The American Society of Clinical Oncology (ASCO) updated guidelines on the role of bone-modifying agents (BMAs) in the prevention and treatment of skeletal-related events for metastatic breast cancer patients (Van Poznak, 2011). The guidelines recommend initiating a BMA (denosumab, pamidronate, zoledronic acid) in patients with metastatic breast cancer to the bone. There is currently no literature indicating the superiority of one particular BMA. Optimal duration is not defined; however, the guidelines recommend continuing therapy until substantial decline in patient's performance status. In patients with normal creatinine clearance (Cl_{cr} >60 mL/minute), no dosage/interval/infusion rate changes for pamidronate or zoledronic acid are necessary. For patients with Cl_{cr} <30 mL/minute, pamidronate and zoledronic acid are not recommended. While no renal dose adjustments are recommended for denosumab, close monitoring is advised for risk of hypocalcemia in patients with Cl_{cr} <30 mL/minute or on dialysis. The ASCO guidelines are in alignment with package insert guidelines for dosing, renal dose adjustments, infusion times, prevention and management of osteonecrosis of the jaw, and monitoring of laboratory parameter recommendations. BMAs are not the first-line therapy for pain. BMAs are to be used as adjunctive therapy for cancer-related bone pain associated with bone metastasis, demonstrating a modest pain control benefit. BMAs should be used in conjunction with agents such as NSAIDs, opioid and nonopioid analgesics, corticosteroids, radiation/surgery, and interventional procedures.

Dosage Forms Excipient information presented when available (limited, particularly for generics); consult specific product labeling.

Injection, solution [preservative free]:
 Prolia®: 60 mg/mL (1 mL) [contains natural rubber/natural latex in packaging]
 Xgeva™: 70 mg/mL (1.7 mL)

- **Denta 5000 Plus™** *see* Fluoride *on page* 728
- **DentaGel™** *see* Fluoride *on page* 728
- **Dentapaine [OTC]** *see* Benzocaine *on page* 202
- **Dent's Extra Strength Toothache Gum [OTC]** *see* Benzocaine *on page* 202
- **Deodorized Tincture of Opium (error-prone synonym)** *see* Opium Tincture *on page* 1249
- **Deoxyazacytidine** *see* Decitabine *on page* 460
- **Deoxycoformycin** *see* Pentostatin *on page* 1331
- **2'-Deoxycoformycin** *see* Pentostatin *on page* 1331
- **Depacon®** *see* Valproic Acid *on page* 1757
- **Depakene®** *see* Valproic Acid *on page* 1757
- **Depakote®** *see* Divalproex *on page* 530
- **Depakote® ER** *see* Divalproex *on page* 530
- **Depakote® Sprinkle** *see* Divalproex *on page* 530
- **Depen®** *see* PenicillAMINE *on page* 1319
- **DepoCyt®** *see* Cytarabine (Liposomal) *on page* 432
- **DepoDur®** *see* Morphine (Liposomal) *on page* 1157
- **Depo®-Estradiol** *see* Estradiol (Systemic) *on page* 627
- **DepoFoam-Encapsulated Cytarabine** *see* Cytarabine (Liposomal) *on page* 432
- **Depo-Medrol®** *see* MethylPREDNISolone *on page* 1110
- **Depo-Prevera® (Can)** *see* MedroxyPROGESTERone *on page* 1058
- **Depo-Provera®** *see* MedroxyPROGESTERone *on page* 1058
- **Depo-Provera® Contraceptive** *see* MedroxyPROGESTERone *on page* 1058
- **depo-subQ provera 104®** *see* MedroxyPROGESTERone *on page* 1058
- **Depotest® 100 (Can)** *see* Testosterone *on page* 1654
- **Depo®-Testosterone** *see* Testosterone *on page* 1654
- **Deprenyl** *see* Selegiline *on page* 1544
- **Depsipeptide** *see* RomiDEPsin *on page* 1515
- **DermaFungal [OTC]** *see* Miconazole (Topical) *on page* 1126
- **Dermagran® [OTC]** *see* Aluminum Hydroxide *on page* 79
- **Dermagran® AF [OTC]** *see* Miconazole (Topical) *on page* 1126
- **Dermarest® Eczema Medicated [OTC]** *see* Hydrocortisone (Topical) *on page* 841
- **Derma-Smoothe/FS®** *see* Fluocinolone (Topical) *on page* 726
- **Dermatop®** *see* Prednicarbate *on page* 1396
- **Dermazene®** *see* Iodoquinol and Hydrocortisone *on page* 921
- **Dermazole (Can)** *see* Miconazole (Topical) *on page* 1126
- **Dermoplast® Antibacterial [OTC]** *see* Benzocaine *on page* 202
- **Dermoplast® Pain Relieving [OTC]** *see* Benzocaine *on page* 202
- **Dermovate® (Can)** *see* Clobetasol *on page* 384
- **Desferal®** *see* Deferoxamine *on page* 463
- **Desferrioxamine** *see* Deferoxamine *on page* 463
- **Desiccated Thyroid** *see* Thyroid, Desiccated *on page* 1676

Desipramine (des IP ra meen)

Brand Names: U.S. Norpramin®

Brand Names: Canada Alti-Desipramine; Apo-Desipramine®; Norpramin®; Nu-Desipramine; PMS-Desipramine

Index Terms Desipramine Hydrochloride; Desmethylimipramine Hydrochloride

Pharmacologic Category Antidepressant, Tricyclic (Secondary Amine)

Additional Appendix Information

Antidepressant Agents *on page* 1874

Use Treatment of depression

Unlabeled Use Analgesic adjunct in chronic pain; peripheral neuropathies (including diabetic neuropathy); attention-deficit/hyperactivity disorder (ADHD); depression in children ≤12 years of age

Pregnancy Considerations Animal reproduction studies are inconclusive.

Lactation Enters breast milk (AAP rates "of concern"; AAP 2001 update pending)

Medication Guide Available Yes

Contraindications Hypersensitivity to desipramine, drugs of similar chemical class, or any component of the formulation; use of MAO inhibitors with or within 14 days; use in a patient during the acute recovery phase of MI

Warnings/Precautions [U.S. Boxed Warning]: Antidepressants increase the risk of suicidal thinking and behavior in children, adolescents, and young adults (18-24 years of age) with major depressive disorder (MDD) and other psychiatric disorders; consider risk prior to prescribing. Short-term studies did not show an increased risk in patients >24 years of age and showed a decreased risk in patients ≥65 years. Closely monitor for clinical worsening, suicidality, or unusual changes in behavior; the patient's family or caregiver should be instructed to closely observe the patient and communicate condition with healthcare provider. A medication guide should be dispensed with each prescription. **Desipramine is FDA approved for the treatment of depression in adolescents.**

The possibility of a suicide attempt is inherent in major depression and may persist until remission occurs. Monitor for worsening of depression or suicidality, especially during initiation of therapy (generally first 1-2 months) or with dose increases or decreases. Use caution in high-risk patients. Worsening depression and severe abrupt suicidality that are not part of the presenting symptoms may require discontinuation or modification of drug therapy. The patient's family or caregiver should be alerted to monitor patients for the emergence of suicidality and associated behaviors (such as agitation, irritability, hostility, impulsivity, and hypomania) and notify healthcare provider.

May worsen psychosis in some patients or precipitate a shift to mania or hypomania in patients with bipolar disorder. Patients presenting with depressive symptoms should be screened for bipolar disorder. Monotherapy in patients with bipolar disorder should be avoided. **Desipramine is not FDA approved for the treatment of bipolar depression.**

TCAs may rarely cause bone marrow suppression; monitor for any signs of infection and obtain CBC if symptoms (eg, fever, sore throat) evident. The degree of anticholinergic blockade produced by this agent is low relative to other cyclic antidepressants - however, extreme caution should be used in patients with urinary retention, benign prostatic hyperplasia, narrow-angle glaucoma, xerostomia, visual problems, constipation, or a history of bowel obstruction. The degree of sedation with desipramine are low relative to other antidepressants. However, desipramine may cause drowsiness/sedation, resulting in impaired performance of tasks requiring alertness (eg, operating machinery or driving). Sedative effects may be additive with other CNS depressants and/or ethanol. The risk of orthostasis is moderate relative to other antidepressants. Due to risk of conduction abnormalities, use with extreme caution in patients with a history of cardiovascular disease (including previous MI, stroke, tachycardia, or conduction abnormalities) or in patients with a family history of sudden death, dysrhythmias, or conduction abnormalities. Use with caution in patients with diabetes mellitus; may alter glucose regulation.

Consider discontinuing, when possible, prior to elective surgery. Therapy should not be abruptly discontinued. May lower seizure threshold - use extreme caution in patients with a previous seizure disorder or condition predisposing to seizures such as brain damage, alcoholism, or concurrent therapy with other drugs which lower the seizure threshold. In some patients, seizures may precede cardiac dysrhythmias and death. May increase the risks associated with electroconvulsive therapy. Use with extreme caution in hyperthyroid patients or those receiving thyroid supplementation. Use with caution in patients with glaucoma, hepatic or renal dysfunction and in elderly patients.

Adverse Reactions Frequency not defined.

Cardiovascular: Arrhythmias, edema, flushing, heart block, hyper-/hypotension, MI, palpitation, stroke, tachycardia

Central nervous system: Agitation, anxiety, ataxia, confusion, delusions, disorientation, dizziness, drowsiness, EEG alterations, exacerbation of psychosis, extrapyramidal symptoms, fatigue, fever, hallucinations, headache, hypomania, incoordination, insomnia, neuroleptic malignant syndrome, nightmares, restlessness, seizure, suicidal thinking and behavior

Dermatologic: Alopecia, itching, petechiae, photosensitivity, skin rash, urticaria

Endocrine & metabolic: Breast enlargement, galactorrhea, gynecomastia, hyper-/hypoglycemia, impotence, libido changes, SIADH

Gastrointestinal: Abdominal cramps, anorexia, black tongue, constipation, diarrhea, epigastric distress, nausea, parotid edema, paralytic ileus, stomatitis, sublingual adenitis, unpleasant taste, vomiting, weight gain/loss, xerostomia

Genitourinary: Micturition delayed, nocturia, painful ejaculation, polyuria, testicular edema, urinary retention

Hematologic: Agranulocytosis, eosinophilia, purpura, thrombocytopenia

Hepatic: Alkaline phosphatase increased, cholestatic jaundice, hepatitis, liver enzymes increased

Neuromuscular & skeletal: Falling, numbness, paresthesia of extremities, peripheral neuropathy, tingling, tremor, weakness

Ocular: Blurred vision, disturbances of accommodation, intraocular pressure increased, mydriasis

Otic: Tinnitus

Miscellaneous: Allergic reaction, diaphoresis (excessive), withdrawal symptoms

Drug Interactions

Metabolism/Transport Effects Substrate of CYP1A2 (minor), CYP2D6 (major); **Note:** Assignment of Major/Minor substrate status based on clinically relevant drug interaction potential; **Inhibits** CYP2A6 (moderate), CYP2B6 (moderate), CYP2D6 (moderate), CYP2E1 (weak), CYP3A4 (moderate)

Avoid Concomitant Use

Avoid concomitant use of Desipramine with any of the following: Artemether; Dronedarone; Iobenguane I 123; Lumefantrine; MAO Inhibitors; Methylene Blue; Nilotinib; Pimozide; QUEtiapine; QuiNINE; Tetrabenazine; Thioridazine; Tolvaptan; Toremifene; Vandetanib; Vemurafenib; Ziprasidone

Increased Effect/Toxicity

Desipramine may increase the levels/effects of: Alpha-/Beta-Agonists (Direct-Acting); Alpha1-Agonists; Amphetamines; Anticholinergics; Beta2-Agonists; Budesonide (Systemic, Oral Inhalation); Colchicine; CYP2A6 Substrates; CYP2B6 Substrates; CYP2D6 Substrates; CYP3A4 Substrates; Desmopressin; Dronedarone; Eplerenone; Everolimus; FentaNYL; Fesoterodine; Methylene Blue; Metoclopramide; Nebivolol; Pimecrolimus; Pimozide; QTc-Prolonging Agents; QuiNIDine; QuiNINE; Saxagliptin; Serotonin Modulators; Sodium Phosphates; Sulfonylureas; Tamoxifen; Tetrabenazine; Thioridazine; Tolvaptan; Toremifene; TraMADol; Vandetanib; Vemurafenib; Vitamin K Antagonists; Yohimbine; Ziprasidone

The levels/effects of Desipramine may be increased by: Abiraterone Acetate; Alfuzosin; Altretamine; Antipsychotics; Artemether; Boceprevir; BuPROPion; Chloroquine; Cimetidine; Cinacalcet; Ciprofloxacin; Ciprofloxacin (Systemic); CYP2D6 Inhibitors (Moderate); CYP2D6 Inhibitors (Strong); Dexmethylphenidate; Divalproex; DULoxetine; Gadobutrol; Indacaterol; Linezolid; Lithium; Lumefantrine; MAO Inhibitors; Methylphenidate; Metoclopramide; Nilotinib; Pramlintide; Protease Inhibitors; QUEtiapine; QuiNIDine; QuiNINE; Selective Serotonin Reuptake Inhibitors; Telaprevir; Terbinafine; Terbinafine (Systemic); Valproic Acid

Decreased Effect

Desipramine may decrease the levels/effects of: Acetylcholinesterase Inhibitors (Central); Alpha2-Agonists; Codeine; Iobenguane I 123

The levels/effects of Desipramine may be decreased by: Acetylcholinesterase Inhibitors (Central); Barbiturates; CarBAMazepine; Cyproterone; Peginterferon Alfa-2b; St Johns Wort

Ethanol/Nutrition/Herb Interactions
Ethanol: May increase CNS depression; monitor for increased effects with coadministration. Caution patients about effects.
Food: Grapefruit juice may inhibit the metabolism of some TCAs and clinical toxicity may result.
Herb/Nutraceutical: Avoid valerian, St John's wort, SAMe, kava kava (may increase risk of serotonin syndrome and/or excessive sedation).

Stability Store at 20°C to 25°C (68°F to 77°F).

Mechanism of Action Traditionally believed to increase the synaptic concentration of norepinephrine (and to a lesser extent, serotonin) in the central nervous system by inhibition of its reuptake by the presynaptic neuronal membrane. However, additional receptor effects have been found including desensitization of adenyl cyclase, down regulation of beta-adrenergic receptors, and down regulation of serotonin receptors.

Pharmacodynamics/Kinetics
Onset of action: Earliest therapeutic effects: 2-5 days; Maximum antidepressant effect: >2 weeks
Metabolism: Hepatic
Half-life elimination: Adults: 15-24 hours (Weiner, 1981)
Time to peak, plasma: ~6 hours (Weiner, 1981)
Excretion: Urine (~70%)

Dosage Note: Not FDA approved for use in pediatric patients; controlled clinical trials have not shown tricyclic antidepressants to be superior to placebo for the treatment of depression in children and adolescents (Dopheide, 2006; Wagner, 2005).
Oral:
Children 6-12 years: Depression (unlabeled use): 1-3 mg/kg/day in divided doses; monitor carefully with doses >3 mg/kg/day; maximum dose: 5 mg/kg/day.
Adolescents: Depression: Initial dose: Start at the lower range and increase based on tolerance and response to 100 mg/day in divided or single dose; usual maintenance dose: 25-100 mg/day, but doses up to 150 mg/day may be necessary in severely depressed patients
Adults:
Depression: Initial dose: Start at the lower range and increase based on tolerance and response; usual maintenance dose: 100-200 mg/day, but doses up to 300 mg/day may be necessary in severely depressed patients
Neuropathic pain (unlabeled use): Initial: 10-25 mg/day; increase dose every 3 days as necessary until the desired effect is obtained; usual effective dose: 50-150 mg/day (maximum dose: 150 mg/day)
Elderly: Depression: Initial dose: Start at the lower range and increase based on tolerance and response to 100 mg/day in as single or divided doses; usual maintenance dose: 25-100 mg/day, but doses up to 150 mg/day may be necessary in severely depressed patients
Hemodialysis/peritoneal dialysis: Supplemental dose is not necessary

Monitoring Parameters Monitor blood pressure and pulse rate prior to and during initial therapy; evaluate mental status, suicide ideation (especially at the beginning of therapy or when doses are increased or decreased); monitor weight; ECG in older adults and those patients with cardiac disease

When used for the treatment of ADHD, thoroughly evaluate for cardiovascular risk. Monitor heart rate, blood pressure, and consider obtaining ECG prior to initiation (Vetter, 2008); ensure PR interval ≤200 ms, QRS duration ≤120 ms, and QT_c ≤460 ms.

Test Interactions Increased glucose; decreased glucose has also been reported. May interfere with urine detection of amphetamines/methamphetamines (false-positive).

Dosage Forms Excipient information presented when available (limited, particularly for generics); consult specific product labeling.
Tablet, oral, as hydrochloride: 10 mg, 25 mg, 50 mg, 75 mg, 100 mg, 150 mg
Norpramin®: 10 mg, 25 mg, 50 mg, 75 mg, 100 mg, 150 mg [contains soybean oil]

- **Desipramine Hydrochloride** *see* Desipramine *on page 473*

Desirudin (des i ROO din)

Brand Names: U.S. Iprivask®
Index Terms CGP-39393; Desulfato-Hirudin; Desulfatohirudin; Desulphatohirudin; r-Hirudin; Recombinant Desulfatohirudin; Recombinant Hirudin
Pharmacologic Category Anticoagulant, Thrombin Inhibitor
Use Prophylaxis of deep vein thrombosis (DVT) in patients undergoing surgery for hip replacement
Pregnancy Risk Factor C
Dosage SubQ: Adults: DVT prophylaxis: 15 mg every 12 hours; initial dose may be given up to 5-15 minutes prior to surgery (after induction of regional anesthesia, if used); has been administered for up to 12 days (average: 9-12 days) in clinical trials

Dosage adjustment in renal impairment:
Moderate renal impairment (Cl_{cr} ≥31-60 mL/minute/1.73 m^2): 5 mg every 12 hours
Severe renal impairment (Cl_{cr} <31 mL/minute/1.73 m^2): 1.7 mg every 12 hours; **Note:** The American College of Chest Physicians recommends against the use of desirudin in patients with Cl_{cr} <30 mL/minute (Hirsh, 2008).

Additional Information Complete prescribing information for this medication should be consulted for additional detail.
Dosage Forms Excipient information presented when available (limited, particularly for generics); consult specific product labeling.
Injection, powder for reconstitution [preservative free]:
Iprivask®: 15 mg [supplied with prefilled diluent syringe]

- **Desitin® [OTC]** *see* Zinc Oxide *on page 1817*
- **Desitin® Creamy [OTC]** *see* Zinc Oxide *on page 1817*

Desloratadine (des lor AT a deen)

Brand Names: U.S. Clarinex®
Brand Names: Canada Aerius®; Aerius® Kids
Pharmacologic Category Histamine H_1 Antagonist; Histamine H_1 Antagonist, Second Generation; Piperidine Derivative
Use Relief of nasal and non-nasal symptoms of seasonal allergic rhinitis (SAR) and perennial allergic rhinitis (PAR); treatment of chronic idiopathic urticaria (CIU)
Pregnancy Risk Factor C
Dosage Oral:
Children:
6-11 months: 1 mg once daily
12 months to 5 years: 1.25 mg once daily
6-11 years: 2.5 mg once daily
Children ≥12 years and Adults: 5 mg once daily
Dosage adjustment in renal/hepatic impairment:
Children: Not established
Adults: 5 mg every other day
Additional Information Complete prescribing information for this medication should be consulted for additional detail.

Dosage Forms Excipient information presented when available (limited, particularly for generics); consult specific product labeling.

Syrup, oral:

Clarinex®: 0.5 mg/mL (480 mL) [contains propylene glycol, sodium benzoate; bubblegum flavor]

Tablet, oral:

Clarinex®: 5 mg

Tablet, orally disintegrating, oral:

Clarinex®: 2.5 mg [contains phenylalanine 1.4 mg/tablet; tutti frutti flavor]

Clarinex®: 5 mg [contains phenylalanine 2.9 mg/tablet; tutti frutti flavor]

Desloratadine and Pseudoephedrine

(des lor AT a deen & soo doe e FED rin)

Brand Names: U.S. Clarinex-D® 12 Hour; Clarinex-D® 24 Hour

Index Terms Pseudoephedrine and Desloratadine

Pharmacologic Category Alpha/Beta Agonist; Decongestant; Histamine H_1 Antagonist; Histamine H_1 Antagonist, Second Generation; Piperidine Derivative

Use Relief of symptoms of seasonal allergic rhinitis, in children ≥12 years of age and adults

Pregnancy Risk Factor C

Dosage Oral: Children ≥12 years and Adults:

Clarinex-D® 12 Hour: One tablet twice daily

Clarinex-D® 24 Hour: One tablet daily

Dosage adjustment in renal impairment:

Clarinex-D® 12 Hour: Not recommended

Clarinex-D® 24 Hour: One tablet every other day

Dosage adjustment in hepatic impairment: Not recommended

Additional Information Complete prescribing information for this medication should be consulted for additional detail.

Dosage Forms Excipient information presented when available (limited, particularly for generics); consult specific product labeling.

Tablet, variable release:

Clarinex-D® 12 Hour: Desloratadine 2.5 mg [immediate release] and pseudoephedrine 120 mg [extended release]

Clarinex-D® 24 Hour: Desloratadine 5 mg [immediate release] and pseudoephedrine 240 mg [extended release]

◆ **Desmethylimipramine Hydrochloride** *see* Desipramine *on page 473*

Desmopressin (des moe PRES in)

Brand Names: U.S. DDAVP®; Stimate®

Brand Names: Canada Apo-Desmopressin®; DDAVP®; DDAVP® Melt; Minirin®; Novo-Desmopressin; Octostim®; PMS-Desmopressin

Index Terms 1-Deamino-8-D-Arginine Vasopressin; Desmopressin Acetate

Pharmacologic Category Antihemophilic Agent; Hemostatic Agent; Vasopressin Analog, Synthetic

Use

Injection: Treatment of diabetes insipidus; maintenance of hemostasis and control of bleeding in hemophilia A with factor VIII coagulant activity levels >5% and mild-to-moderate classic von Willebrand's disease (type 1) with factor VIII coagulant activity levels >5%

Nasal solutions (DDAVP® Nasal Spray and DDAVP® Rhinal Tube): Treatment of central diabetes insipidus

Nasal spray (Stimate®): Maintenance of hemostasis and control of bleeding in hemophilia A with factor VIII coagulant activity levels >5% and mild-to-moderate classic von Willebrand's disease (type 1) with factor VIII coagulant activity levels >5%

Tablet: Treatment of central diabetes insipidus, temporary polyuria and polydipsia following pituitary surgery or head trauma, primary nocturnal enuresis

Unlabeled Use Uremic bleeding associated with acute or chronic renal failure; prevention of surgical bleeding in patients with uremia

Pregnancy Risk Factor B

Pregnancy Considerations Adverse events were not observed in animal reproductive studies. There are no adequate and well-controlled studies in pregnant women. Anecdotal reports suggest congenital anomalies and low birth weight. However, causal relationship has not been established. Desmopressin has been used safely during pregnancy.

Lactation Excretion in breast milk unknown/use caution

Contraindications Hypersensitivity to desmopressin or any component of the formulation; hyponatremia or a history of hyponatremia; moderate-to-severe renal impairment (Cl_{cr}<50 mL/minute)

Canadian labeling: Additional contraindications (not in U.S. labeling): Type 2B or platelet-type (pseudo) von Willebrand's disease (injection, intranasal, oral, sublingual); known hyponatremia, habitual or psychogenic polydipsia, cardiac insufficiency or other conditions requiring diuretic therapy (intranasal, sublingual); nephrosis, severe hepatic dysfunction (sublingual); primary nocturnal enuresis (intranasal)

Warnings/Precautions Allergic reactions and anaphylaxis have been reported rarely with both the I.V. and intranasal formulations. Fluid intake should be adjusted downward in the elderly and very young patients to decrease the possibility of water intoxication and hyponatremia. Use may rarely lead to extreme decreases in plasma osmolality, resulting in seizures, coma, and death. Use caution with cystic fibrosis, heart failure, renal dysfunction, polydipsia (habitual or psychogenic [contraindicated in Canadian labeling]), or other conditions associated with fluid and electrolyte imbalance due to potential hyponatremia. Use caution with coronary artery insufficiency or hypertensive cardiovascular disease; may increase or decrease blood pressure leading to changes in heart rate. Consider switching from nasal to intravenous solution if changes in the nasal mucosa (scarring, edema) occur leading to unreliable absorption. Use caution in patients predisposed to thrombus formation; thrombotic events (acute cerebrovascular thrombosis, acute myocardial infarction) have occurred (rare).

Desmopressin (intranasal and I.V.), when used for hemostasis in hemophilia, is not for use in hemophilia B, type 2B von Willebrand disease, severe classic von Willebrand disease (type 1), or in patients with factor VIII antibodies. In general, desmopressin is also not recommended for use in patients with ≤5% factor VIII activity level, although it may be considered in selected patients with activity levels between 2% and 5%.

Consider switching from nasal to intravenous administration if changes in the nasal mucosa (scarring, edema) occur leading to unreliable absorption. Consider alternative rout of administration (I.V. or intranasal) with inadequate therapeutic response at maximum recommended oral doses. Therapy should be interrupted if patient experiences an acute illness (eg, fever, recurrent vomiting or diarrhea), vigorous exercise, or any condition associated with an increase in water consumption. Some patients may demonstrate a change in response after long-term therapy (>6 months) characterized as decreased response or a shorter duration of response.

Adverse Reactions Frequency may not be defined (may be dose or route related).

Cardiovascular: Blood pressure increased/decreased (I.V.), facial flushing
Central nervous system: Headache (2% to 5%), dizziness (intranasal; ≤3%), chills (intranasal; 2%)
Dermatologic: Rash
Endocrine & metabolic: Hyponatremia, water intoxication
Gastrointestinal: Abdominal pain (intranasal; 2%), gastrointestinal disorder (intranasal; ≤2%), nausea (intranasal; ≤2%), abdominal cramps, sore throat
Hepatic: Transient increases in liver transaminases (associated primarily with tablets)
Local: Injection: Burning pain, erythema, and swelling at the injection site
Neuromuscular & Skeletal: Weakness (intranasal; ≤2%)
Ocular: Conjunctivitis (intranasal; ≤2%), eye edema (intranasal; ≤2%), lacrimation disorder (intranasal; ≤2%)
Respiratory: Rhinitis (intranasal; 3% to 8%), epistaxis (intranasal; ≤3%), nostril pain (intranasal; ≤2%), cough, nasal congestion, upper respiratory infection
<1% (Limited to important or life-threatening): Acute cerebrovascular thrombosis (I.V.), acute MI (I.V.), agitation, allergic reactions (rare), anaphylaxis (rare), balanitis, chest pain, coma, diarrhea, dyspepsia, edema, insomnia, itching eyes, light-sensitive eyes, pain, palpitation, seizure, somnolence, tachycardia, thinking abnormal, vomiting, vulval pain, warmth

Drug Interactions

Metabolism/Transport Effects None known.

Avoid Concomitant Use There are no known interactions where it is recommended to avoid concomitant use.

Increased Effect/Toxicity

Desmopressin may increase the levels/effects of: Lithium

The levels/effects of Desmopressin may be increased by: Analgesics (Opioid); CarBAMazepine; ChlorproMAZINE; LamoTRIgine; Nonsteroidal Anti-Inflammatory Agents; Selective Serotonin Reuptake Inhibitors; Tricyclic Antidepressants

Decreased Effect

The levels/effects of Desmopressin may be decreased by: Demeclocycline; Lithium

Ethanol/Nutrition/Herb Interactions Ethanol: Avoid ethanol (may decrease antidiuretic effect).

Stability

DDAVP®:
Nasal spray: Store at controlled room temperature of 20°C to 25°C (68°F to 77°F). Keep nasal spray in upright position.
Rhinal Tube solution: Store refrigerated at 2°C to 8°C (36°F to 46°F). May store at controlled room temperature of 20°C to 25°C (68°F to 77°F) for up to 3 weeks.
Solution for injection: Store refrigerated at 2°C to 8°C (36°F to 46°F). Dilute solution for injection in 10-50 mL NS for I.V. infusion (10 mL for children ≤10 kg: 50 mL for adults and children >10 kg).
Tablet: Store at controlled room temperature of 20°C to 25°C (68°F to 77°F).
DDAVP® Melt (CAN; not available in U.S.): Store at 15°C to 25°C (59°F to 77°F) in original container. Protect from moisture.
Stimate® nasal spray: Store refrigerated at 2°C to 8°C (36°F to 46°F). May store at controlled room temperature of 22°C (72°F) for up to 3 weeks.

Mechanism of Action In a dose dependent manner, desmopressin increases cyclic adenosine monophosphate (cAMP) in renal tubular cells which increases water permeability resulting in decreased urine volume and increased urine osmolality; increases plasma levels of von Willebrand factor, factor VIII, and t-PA contributing to a shortened activated partial thromboplastin time (aPTT) and bleeding time.

Pharmacodynamics/Kinetics

Onset of action:
Intranasal: Antidiuretic: 15-30 minutes; Increased factor VIII and von Willebrand factor (vWF) activity (dose related): 30 minutes
Peak effect: Antidiuretic: 1 hour; Increased factor VIII and vWF activity: 1.5 hours
I.V. infusion: Increased factor VIII and vWF activity: 30 minutes (dose related)
Peak effect: 1.5-2 hours
Oral tablet: Antidiuretic: ~1 hour
Peak effect: 4-7 hours
Duration: Intranasal, I.V. infusion, Oral tablet: ~6-14 hours
Absorption: Sublingual: Rapid
Bioavailability: Intranasal: ~3.5%; Oral tablet: 5% compared to intranasal, 0.16% compared to I.V.
Half-life elimination: Intranasal: ~3.5 hours; I.V. infusion: 3 hours; Oral tablet: 2-3 hours
Renal impairment: ≤9 hours
Excretion: Urine

Dosage

Children:
Diabetes insipidus:
I.M., I.V., SubQ: Canadian labeling (not in U.S. labeling): Infants and Children ≥3 months: 0.4 mcg (0.1 mL) once daily or one-tenth (1/10) of the maintenance intranasal dose. Fluid restriction should be observed.
I.V., SubQ: Children <12 years: No definitive dosing available. Adult dosing should **not** be used in this age group; adverse events such as hyponatremia-induced seizures may occur. Dose should be reduced. Some have suggested an initial dosage range of 0.1-1 mcg in 1 or 2 divided doses (Cheetham, 2002). Initiate at low dose and increase as necessary. Closely monitor serum sodium levels and urine output; fluid restriction is recommended.
Intranasal (using 100 mcg/mL nasal solution): Infants and Children 3 months to 12 years: Initial: 5 mcg/day (0.05 mL/day) divided 1-2 times/day; range: 5-30 mcg/day (0.05-0.3 mL/day) divided 1-2 times/day; adjust morning and evening doses separately for an adequate diurnal rhythm of water turnover. **Note:** The nasal spray pump can only deliver doses of 10 mcg (0.1 mL) or multiples of 10 mcg (0.1 mL); if doses other than this are needed, the rhinal tube delivery system is preferred. Fluid restriction should be observed.
Oral:
U.S. labeling: Children ≥4 years: Initial: 0.05 mg twice daily; total daily dose should be increased or decreased as needed to obtain adequate antidiuresis (range: 0.1-1.2 mg divided 2-3 times/day). Fluid restriction should be observed.
Canadian labeling (not in U.S. labeling): Children ≥5 years: Initial: 0.1 mg 3 times/day; total daily dose should be increased or decreased as needed to obtain adequate antidiuresis (range: 0.3-1.2 mg divided 3 times/day). Divide daily doses so that the evening dose is 2 times higher than the morning or afternoon dose to ensure adequate antidiuresis during the night. Fluid restriction should be observed.
Sublingual formulation: Canadian labeling (not in U.S. labeling): Infants and Children ≥3 months: Initial: 60 mcg 3 times/day; total daily dose should be increased or decreased as needed to obtain adequate antidiuresis. Usual maintenance: 60-120 mcg 3 times/day (range: 120-720 mcg divided 2-3 times/day); divide daily doses so that the evening dose is 2 times higher than the morning or afternoon dose to ensure adequate antidiuresis during the night. Fluid restriction should be observed.

Hemophilia A and von Willebrand disease (type 1):
I.V.: Infants and Children ≥3 months: 0.3 mcg/kg by slow infusion; may repeat dose if needed; if used preoperatively, administer 30 minutes before procedure
Canadian labeling (not in U.S. labeling): Maximum I.V. dose: 20 mcg
Note: Adverse events such as hyponatremia-induced seizures have been reported especially in young children using this dosing regimen (Das, 2005; Molnar, 2005; Smith, 1989; Thumfart, 2005; Weinstein, 1989). Fluid restriction and careful monitoring of serum sodium levels and urine output are necessary.
Intranasal (using high concentration spray [1.5 mg/mL]): Infants and Children ≥11 months: Refer to adult dosing.
Nocturnal enuresis:
Oral: Children ≥6 years: 0.2 mg at bedtime; dose may be titrated up to 0.6 mg to achieve desired response. Fluid intake should be limited 1 hour prior to dose until the next morning, or at least 8 hours after administration. **Note:** In the Canadian labeling, use is approved for patients ≥5 years.
Sublingual formulation: Canadian labeling (not in U.S. labeling): Children ≥5 years: Initial: 120 mcg at bedtime; dose may be titrated up to 360 mcg to achieve desired response. Fluid intake should be limited 1 hour prior to dose until the next morning, or at least 8 hours after administration.
Children ≥12 years and Adults:
Diabetes insipidus:
I.V., SubQ: 2-4 mcg/day (0.5-1 mL) in 2 divided doses or one-tenth (1/10) of the maintenance intranasal dose. Fluid restriction should be observed.
Intranasal (using 100 mcg/mL nasal solution): 10-40 mcg/day (0.1-0.4 mL) divided 1-3 times/day; adjust morning and evening doses separately for an adequate diurnal rhythm of water turnover. **Note:** The nasal spray pump can only deliver doses of 10 mcg (0.1 mL) or multiples of 10 mcg (0.1 mL); if doses other than this are needed, the rhinal tube delivery system is preferred. Fluid restriction should be observed.
Oral:
U.S. labeling: Initial: 0.05 mg twice daily; total daily dose should be increased or decreased as needed to obtain adequate antidiuresis (range: 0.1-1.2 mg divided 2-3 times/day). Fluid restriction should be observed.
Canadian labeling (not in U.S. labeling): Initial: 0.1 mg 3 times/day; total daily dose should be increased or decreased as needed to obtain adequate antidiuresis (range: 0.3-1.2 mg divided 3 times/day). Fluid restriction should be observed.
Sublingual formulation: Canadian labeling (not in U.S. labeling): Initial: 60 mcg 3 times/day; total daily dose should be increased or decreased as needed to obtain adequate antidiuresis. Usual maintenance: 60-120 mcg 3 times/day (range: 120-720 mcg divided 2-3 times/day). Fluid restriction should be observed.
Hemophilia A and mild-to-moderate von Willebrand disease (type 1):
I.V.: 0.3 mcg/kg by slow infusion; if used preoperatively, administer 30 minutes before procedure
Canadian labeling (not in U.S. labeling): Maximum I.V. dose: 20 mcg
Intranasal (using high concentration spray [1.5 mg/mL]): <50 kg: 150 mcg (1 spray); >50 kg: 300 mcg (1 spray each nostril); repeat use is determined by the patient's clinical condition and laboratory work; if using preoperatively, administer 2 hours before surgery

Adults:
Diabetes insipidus: I.M., I.V., SubQ: Canadian labeling (not in U.S. labeling): 1-4 mcg (0.25-1 mL) once daily or one-tenth (1/10) of the maintenance intranasal dose. Fluid restriction should be observed.
Uremic bleeding associated with acute or chronic renal failure (unlabeled use) (Watson, 1984): I.V.: 0.4 mcg/kg over 10 minutes
Prevention of surgical bleeding in patients with uremia (unlabeled use) (Mannucci, 1983): I.V.: 0.3 mcg/kg over 30 minutes

Dosage adjustment in renal impairment: Cl_{cr} <50 mL/minute: Use is contraindicated according to the manufacturer; however, has been used in acute and chronic renal failure patients experiencing uremic bleeding or for prevention of surgical bleeding (unlabeled uses) (Mannucci, 1983; Watson, 1984)

Administration
I.M., I.V. push, SubQ injection: Central diabetes insipidus: Withdraw dose from ampul into appropriate syringe size (eg, insulin syringe). Further dilution is not required. Administer as direct injection.
I.V. infusion:
Hemophilia A, von Willebrand disease (type 1), and prevention of surgical bleeding in patients with uremia (unlabeled) (Mannucci, 1983): Infuse over 15-30 minutes
Acute uremic bleeding (unlabeled) (Watson, 1984): May infuse over 10 minutes
Intranasal:
DDAVP®: Nasal pump spray: Delivers 0.1 mL (10 mcg); for doses <10 mcg or for other doses which are not multiples, use rhinal tube. DDAVP® Nasal spray delivers fifty 10 mcg doses. For 10 mcg dose, administer in one nostril. Any solution remaining after 50 doses should be discarded. Pump must be primed prior to first use.
DDAVP® Rhinal tube: Insert top of dropper into tube (arrow marked end) in downward position. Squeeze dropper until solution reaches desired calibration mark. Disconnect dropper. Grasp the tube 3/4 inch from the end and insert tube into nostril until the fingertips reach the nostril. Place opposite end of tube into the mouth (holding breath). Tilt head back and blow with a strong, short puff into the nostril (for very young patients, an adult should blow solution into the child's nose). Reseal dropper after use.

Monitoring Parameters Blood pressure and pulse should be monitored during I.V. infusion

Note: For all indications, fluid intake, urine volume, and signs and symptoms of hyponatremia should be closely monitored especially in high-risk patient subgroups (eg, young children, elderly, patients with heart failure).
Diabetes insipidus: Urine specific gravity, plasma and urine osmolality, serum electrolytes
Hemophilia A: Factor VIII coagulant activity, factor VIII ristocetin cofactor activity, and factor VIII antigen levels, aPTT
von Willebrand disease: Factor VIII coagulant activity, factor VIII ristocetin cofactor activity, and factor VIII von Willebrand antigen levels, bleeding time
Nocturnal enuresis: Serum electrolytes if used for >7 days

Additional Information 10 mcg of desmopressin acetate is equivalent to 40 int. units

Dosage Forms Excipient information presented when available (limited, particularly for generics); consult specific product labeling.
Injection, solution, as acetate: 4 mcg/mL (1 mL, 10 mL)
DDAVP®: 4 mcg/mL (1 mL)
DDAVP®: 4 mcg/mL (10 mL) [contains chlorobutanol]

Solution, intranasal, as acetate: 0.1 mg/mL (2.5 mL)
DDAVP®: 0.1 mg/mL (2.5 mL) [contains chlorobutanol; with rhinal tube]
Solution, intranasal, as acetate [spray]: 0.1 mg/mL (5 mL)
DDAVP®: 0.1 mg/mL (5 mL) [contains benzalkonium chloride; delivers 10 mcg/spray]
Stimate®: 1.5 mg/mL (2.5 mL) [contains benzalkonium chloride; delivers 150 mcg/spray]
Tablet, oral, as acetate: 0.1 mg, 0.2 mg
DDAVP®: 0.1 mg, 0.2 mg [scored]

Dosage Forms: Canada Excipient information presented when available (limited, particularly for generics); consult specific product labeling.
Tablet, as acetate, sublingual:
DDAVP® Melt: 60 mcg, 120 mcg, 240 mcg

- ◆ **Desmopressin Acetate** *see* Desmopressin *on page 476*
- ◆ **Desocort® (Can)** *see* Desonide *on page 479*
- ◆ **Desogen®** *see* Ethinyl Estradiol and Desogestrel *on page 653*
- ◆ **Desogestrel and Ethinyl Estradiol** *see* Ethinyl Estradiol and Desogestrel *on page 653*
- ◆ **Desonate®** *see* Desonide *on page 479*

Desonide (DES oh nide)

Brand Names: U.S. Desonate®; DesOwen®; LoKara™; Verdeso®
Brand Names: Canada Desocort®; PMS-Desonide
Pharmacologic Category Corticosteroid, Topical
Additional Appendix Information
Corticosteroids *on page 1888*
Use Treatment of inflammatory and pruritic manifestations of corticosteroid responsive dermatosis (low-to-medium potency corticosteroid); mild-to-moderate atopic dermatitis
Pregnancy Risk Factor C
Dosage Topical:
Corticosteroid responsive dermatoses: Adults: Cream, ointment, lotion: Apply 2-3 times/day sparingly. Therapy should be discontinued when control is achieved. If no improvement is seen within 2 weeks, reassessment of diagnosis may be necessary.
Atopic dermatitis: Children ≥3 months and Adults: Foam, gel: Apply 2 times/day sparingly. Therapy should be discontinued when control is achieved. If no improvement is seen within 4 weeks, reassessment of diagnosis may be necessary.
Additional Information Complete prescribing information for this medication should be consulted for additional detail.
Dosage Forms Excipient information presented when available (limited, particularly for generics); consult specific product labeling. [DSC] = Discontinued product
Aerosol, foam, topical:
Verdeso®: 0.05% (50 g, 100 g)
Cream, topical: 0.05% (15 g, 60 g)
DesOwen®: 0.05% (60 g)
Gel, topical [aqueous]:
Desonate®: 0.05% (60 g)
Lotion, topical: 0.05% (59 mL, 60 mL, 118 mL)
DesOwen®: 0.05% (60 mL, 120 mL)
LoKara™: 0.05% (59 mL, 118 mL)
Ointment, topical: 0.05% (15 g, 60 g)
DesOwen®: 0.05% (60 g [DSC])

- ◆ **DesOwen®** *see* Desonide *on page 479*

Desoximetasone (des oks i MET a sone)

Brand Names: U.S. Topicort®; Topicort® LP
Brand Names: Canada Taro-Desoximetasone; Topicort®
Pharmacologic Category Corticosteroid, Topical
Additional Appendix Information
Corticosteroids *on page 1888*
Use Relieves inflammation and pruritic symptoms of corticosteroid-responsive dermatosis (intermediate- to high-potency topical corticosteroid)
Pregnancy Risk Factor C
Dosage Desoximetasone is a potent fluorinated topical corticosteroid. Therapy should be discontinued when control is achieved; if no improvement is seen, reassessment of diagnosis may be necessary.

Cream, gel: Children and Adults: Apply a thin film to affected area twice daily
Ointment: Children ≥10 years and Adults: Apply a thin film to affected area twice daily
Additional Information Complete prescribing information for this medication should be consulted for additional detail.
Dosage Forms Excipient information presented when available (limited, particularly for generics); consult specific product labeling.
Cream, topical: 0.05% (15 g, 60 g); 0.25% (15 g, 60 g, 100 g)
Topicort®: 0.25% (15 g, 60 g)
Topicort® LP: 0.05% (15 g, 60 g)
Gel, topical: 0.05% (15 g, 60 g)
Topicort®: 0.05% (15 g, 60 g) [contains ethanol]
Ointment, topical: 0.25% (15 g, 60 g)
Topicort®: 0.25% (15 g, 60 g) [contains coconut oil]

- ◆ **Desoxyephedrine Hydrochloride** *see* Methamphetamine *on page 1092*
- ◆ **Desoxyn®** *see* Methamphetamine *on page 1092*
- ◆ **Desoxyphenobarbital** *see* Primidone *on page 1405*
- ◆ **Desulfato-Hirudin** *see* Desirudin *on page 475*
- ◆ **Desulphatohirudin** *see* Desirudin *on page 475*

Desvenlafaxine (des ven la FAX een)

Brand Names: U.S. Pristiq®
Brand Names: Canada Pristiq®
Index Terms O-desmethylvenlafaxine; ODV
Pharmacologic Category Antidepressant, Serotonin/Norepinephrine Reuptake Inhibitor
Additional Appendix Information
Antidepressant Agents *on page 1874*
Use Treatment of major depressive disorder
Pregnancy Risk Factor C
Medication Guide Available Yes
Dosage Oral: Adults: Depression: 50 mg once daily; doses up to 400 mg once daily have been studied; however, the manufacturer states there is no evidence that doses >50 mg/day confer any additional benefit. A flat dose response curve for efficacy between 50-400 mg/day has been noted as well as an increase in adverse events.
Note: Gradually taper dose (by increasing dosing interval) if discontinuing.

Dosing adjustment in renal impairment:
Cl_{cr} >50 mL/minute: No dosage adjustment required
Cl_{cr} 30-50 mL/minute: 50 mg once daily (maximum)
Cl_{cr} <30 mL/minute: 50 mg every other day (maximum)
Hemodialysis: 50 mg every other day (maximum). Supplemental doses not required after HD.
Dosing adjustment in hepatic impairment: 50 mg once daily; maximum dose: 100 mg/day
Additional Information Complete prescribing information for this medication should be consulted for additional detail.

Dosage Forms Excipient information presented when available (limited, particularly for generics); consult specific product labeling.
Tablet, extended release, oral:
Pristiq®: 50 mg, 100 mg

- **Desyrel** *see* TraZODone *on page 1725*
- **Detane® [OTC]** *see* Benzocaine *on page 202*
- **Detemir Insulin** *see* Insulin Detemir *on page 904*
- **Detrol®** *see* Tolterodine *on page 1705*
- **Detrol® LA** *see* Tolterodine *on page 1705*
- **Detryptoreline** *see* Triptorelin *on page 1742*

Dexamethasone (Systemic)

(deks a METH a sone)

Brand Names: U.S. Baycadron™; Dexamethasone Intensol™; DexPak® 10 Day TaperPak®; DexPak® 13 Day TaperPak®; DexPak® 6 Day TaperPak®

Brand Names: Canada Apo-Dexamethasone®; Dexasone®

Index Terms Decadron; Dexamethasone Sodium Phosphate

Pharmacologic Category Anti-inflammatory Agent; Antiemetic; Corticosteroid, Systemic

Additional Appendix Information
Corticosteroids *on page 1888*

Use Primarily as an anti-inflammatory or immunosuppressant agent in the treatment of a variety of diseases including those of allergic, dermatologic, endocrine, hematologic, inflammatory, neoplastic, nervous system, renal, respiratory, rheumatic, and autoimmune origin; may be used in management of cerebral edema, chronic swelling, as a diagnostic agent, diagnosis of Cushing's syndrome, antiemetic

Unlabeled Use Dexamethasone suppression test as an indicator of depression and/or risk of suicide; prevention and treatment of acute mountain sickness and high altitude cerebral edema; accelerate fetal lung maturation in patients with preterm labor

Pregnancy Risk Factor C

Pregnancy Considerations Adverse events have been observed with corticosteroids in animal reproduction studies. Dexamethasone crosses the placenta; and is partially metabolized to an inactive metabolite by placental enzymes. Due to its positive effect on stimulating fetal lung maturation, the injection is often used in patients with premature labor (24-34 weeks gestation). Some studies have shown an association between first trimester systemic corticosteroid use and oral clefts; adverse events in the fetus/neonate have been noted in case reports following large doses of systemic corticosteroids during pregnancy. Women exposed to dexamethasone during pregnancy for the treatment of an autoimmune disease may contact the OTIS Autoimmune Diseases Study at 877-311-8972.

Lactation Excretion in breast milk unknown/use caution

Contraindications Hypersensitivity to dexamethasone or any component of the formulation; systemic fungal infections, cerebral malaria

Warnings/Precautions Use with caution in patients with thyroid disease, hepatic impairment, renal impairment, cardiovascular disease, diabetes, glaucoma, cataracts, myasthenia gravis, patients at risk for osteoporosis, patients at risk for seizures, or GI diseases (diverticulitis, peptic ulcer, ulcerative colitis) due to perforation risk. Use caution following acute MI (corticosteroids have been associated with myocardial rupture). Because of the risk of adverse effects, systemic corticosteroids should be used cautiously in the elderly in the smallest possible effective dose for the shortest duration. May affect growth velocity; growth should be routinely monitored in pediatric patients. Withdraw therapy with gradual tapering of dose.

May cause hypercorticism or suppression of hypothalamic-pituitary-adrenal (HPA) axis, particularly in younger children or in patients receiving high doses for prolonged periods. HPA axis suppression may lead to adrenal crisis. Withdrawal and discontinuation of a corticosteroid should be done slowly and carefully. Particular care is required when patients are transferred from systemic corticosteroids to inhaled products due to possible adrenal insufficiency or withdrawal from steroids, including an increase in allergic symptoms. Patients receiving >20 mg per day of prednisone (or equivalent) may be most susceptible. Fatalities have occurred due to adrenal insufficiency in asthmatic patients during and after transfer from systemic corticosteroids to aerosol steroids; aerosol steroids do not provide the systemic steroid needed to treat patients having trauma, surgery, or infections. Dexamethasone does not provide adequate mineralocorticoid activity in adrenal insufficiency (may be employed as a single dose while cortisol assays are performed). The lowest possible dose should be used during treatment; discontinuation and/or dose reductions should be gradual.

Acute myopathy has been reported with high dose corticosteroids, usually in patients with neuromuscular transmission disorders; may involve ocular and/or respiratory muscles; monitor creatine kinase; recovery may be delayed. Corticosteroid use may cause psychiatric disturbances, including depression, euphoria, insomnia, mood swings, and personality changes. Pre-existing psychiatric conditions may be exacerbated by corticosteroid use. Prolonged use of corticosteroids may also increase the incidence of secondary infection, mask acute infection (including fungal infections), prolong or exacerbate viral infections, or limit response to vaccines. Exposure to chickenpox should be avoided; corticosteroids should not be used to treat ocular herpes simplex. Corticosteroids should not be used for cerebral malaria or viral hepatitis. Close observation is required in patients with latent tuberculosis and/or TB reactivity; restrict use in active TB (only in conjunction with antituberculosis treatment). Prolonged treatment with corticosteroids has been associated with the development of Kaposi's sarcoma (case reports); if noted, discontinuation of therapy should be considered. High-dose corticosteroids should not be used to manage acute head injury.

Adverse Reactions Frequency not defined.

Cardiovascular: Arrhythmia, bradycardia, cardiac arrest, cardiomyopathy, CHF, circulatory collapse, edema, hypertension, myocardial rupture (post-MI), syncope, thromboembolism, vasculitis

Central nervous system: Depression, emotional instability, euphoria, headache, intracranial pressure increased, insomnia, malaise, mood swings, neuritis, personality changes, pseudotumor cerebri (usually following discontinuation), psychic disorders, seizure, vertigo

Dermatologic: Acne, allergic dermatitis, alopecia, angioedema, bruising, dry skin, erythema, fragile skin, hirsutism, hyper-/hypopigmentation, hypertrichosis, perianal pruritus (following I.V. injection), petechiae, rash, skin atrophy, skin test reaction impaired, striae, urticaria, wound healing impaired

Endocrine & metabolic: Adrenal suppression, carbohydrate tolerance decreased, Cushing's syndrome, diabetes mellitus, glucose intolerance decreased, growth suppression (children), hyperglycemia, hypokalemic alkalosis, menstrual irregularities, negative nitrogen balance, pituitary-adrenal axis suppression, protein catabolism, sodium retention

Gastrointestinal: Abdominal distention, appetite increased, gastrointestinal hemorrhage, gastrointestinal perforation, nausea, pancreatitis, peptic ulcer, ulcerative esophagitis, weight gain

Genitourinary: Altered (increased or decreased) spermatogenesis

Hepatic: Hepatomegaly, transaminases increased

Local: Postinjection flare (intra-articular use), thrombophlebitis

Neuromuscular & skeletal: Arthropathy, aseptic necrosis (femoral and humoral heads), fractures, muscle mass loss, myopathy (particularly in conjunction with neuromuscular disease or neuromuscular-blocking agents), neuropathy, osteoporosis, parasthesia, tendon rupture, vertebral compression fractures, weakness

Ocular: Cataracts, exophthalmos, glaucoma, intraocular pressure increased

Renal: Glucosuria

Respiratory: Pulmonary edema

Miscellaneous: Abnormal fat deposition, anaphylactoid reaction, anaphylaxis, avascular necrosis, diaphoresis, hiccups, hypersensitivity, impaired wound healing, infections, Kaposi's sarcoma, moon face, secondary malignancy

Drug Interactions

Metabolism/Transport Effects Substrate of CYP3A4 (major), P-glycoprotein; **Note:** Assignment of Major/Minor substrate status based on clinically relevant drug interaction potential; **Inhibits** P-glycoprotein; **Induces** CYP2A6 (weak/moderate), CYP2B6 (weak/moderate), CYP2C9 (weak/moderate), CYP3A4 (strong), P-glycoprotein

Avoid Concomitant Use

Avoid concomitant use of Dexamethasone (Systemic) with any of the following: Aldesleukin; BCG; Conivaptan; Dabigatran Etexilate; Lurasidone; Natalizumab; Nisoldipine; Pimecrolimus; Praziquantel; Rilpivirine; SORAfenib; Tacrolimus (Topical); Ticagrelor; Toremifene

Increased Effect/Toxicity

Dexamethasone (Systemic) may increase the levels/effects of: Acetylcholinesterase Inhibitors; Amphotericin B; CycloSPORINE; CycloSPORINE (Systemic); Deferasirox; Leflunomide; Lenalidomide; Loop Diuretics; Natalizumab; NSAID (COX-2 Inhibitor); NSAID (Nonselective); Thalidomide; Thiazide Diuretics; Vaccines (Live); Warfarin

The levels/effects of Dexamethasone (Systemic) may be increased by: Antifungal Agents (Azole Derivatives, Systemic); Aprepitant; Asparaginase (E. coli); Asparaginase (Erwinia); Calcium Channel Blockers (Nondihydropyridine); Conivaptan; CycloSPORINE; CycloSPORINE (Systemic); CYP3A4 Inhibitors (Moderate); CYP3A4 Inhibitors (Strong); Dasatinib; Denosumab; Estrogen Derivatives; Fluconazole; Fosaprepitant; Indacaterol; Macrolide Antibiotics; Neuromuscular-Blocking Agents (Nondepolarizing); P-glycoprotein/ABCB1 Inhibitors; Pimecrolimus; Quinolone Antibiotics; Roflumilast; Salicylates; Tacrolimus (Topical); Telaprevir; Trastuzumab

Decreased Effect

Dexamethasone (Systemic) may decrease the levels/effects of: Aldesleukin; Antidiabetic Agents; ARIPiprazole; BCG; Boceprevir; Brentuximab Vedotin; Calcitriol; Caspofungin; Coccidioidin Skin Test; Corticorelin; CycloSPORINE; CycloSPORINE (Systemic); CYP3A4 Substrates; Dabigatran Etexilate; Dasatinib; Exemestane; Gefitinib; GuanFACINE; Isoniazid; Ixabepilone; Linagliptin; Lurasidone; Maraviroc; NIFEdipine; Nisoldipine; P-glycoprotein/ABCB1 Substrates; Praziquantel; Rilpivirine; Salicylates; Sipuleucel-T; SORAfenib; Tadalafil; Telaprevir; Ticagrelor; Toremifene; Ulipristal; Vaccines (Inactivated); Zuclopenthixol

The levels/effects of Dexamethasone (Systemic) may be decreased by: Aminoglutethimide; Antacids; Barbiturates; Bile Acid Sequestrants; CYP3A4 Inducers (Strong); Echinacea; Mitotane; P-glycoprotein/ABCB1 Inducers; Primidone; Rifamycin Derivatives; Tocilizumab

Ethanol/Nutrition/Herb Interactions

Ethanol: Avoid ethanol (may enhance gastric mucosal irritation).

Food: Dexamethasone interferes with calcium absorption. Limit caffeine.

Herb/Nutraceutical: Avoid cat's claw, echinacea (have immunostimulant properties).

Stability Injection solution: Store at room temperature; protect from light and freezing.

Stability of injection of parenteral admixture at room temperature (25°C): 24 hours

Stability of injection of parenteral admixture at refrigeration temperature (4°C): 2 days; protect from light and freezing.

Injection should be diluted in 50-100 mL NS or D_5W.

Mechanism of Action Decreases inflammation by suppression of neutrophil migration, decreased production of inflammatory mediators, and reversal of increased capillary permeability; suppresses normal immune response. Dexamethasone's mechanism of antiemetic activity is unknown.

Pharmacodynamics/Kinetics

Onset of action: Acetate: Prompt

Duration of metabolic effect: 72 hours; acetate is a long-acting repository preparation

Metabolism: Hepatic

Half-life elimination: Normal renal function: 1.8-3.5 hours; Biological half-life: 36-54 hours

Time to peak, serum: Oral: 1-2 hours; I.M.: ~8 hours

Excretion: Urine and feces

Dosage Refer to individual protocols.

Children:

Antiemetic (prior to chemotherapy): Refer to individual protocols and emetogenic potential: I.V.: 10 mg/m^2/dose every 12-24 hours on days of chemotherapy for severely emetogenic chemotherapy courses

Anti-inflammatory immunosuppressant: Oral, I.M., I.V.: 0.08-0.3 mg/kg/day **or** 2.5-10 mg/m^2/day in divided doses every 6-12 hours

Extubation or airway edema: Oral, I.M., I.V.: 0.5-2 mg/kg/day in divided doses every 6 hours beginning 24 hours prior to extubation and continuing for 4-6 doses afterwards

Cerebral edema: I.V.: Loading dose: 1-2 mg/kg/dose as a single dose; maintenance: 1-1.5 mg/kg/day (maximum: 16 mg/day) in divided doses every 4-6 hours, taper off over 1-6 weeks

Croup (laryngotracheobronchitis): Oral, I.M., I.V.: 0.6 mg/kg once; usual maximum dose: 16 mg (doses as high as 20 mg have been used) (Bjornson, 2004; Hegenbarth, 2008; Rittichier, 2000); a single oral dose of 0.15 mg/kg has been shown effective in children with mild-to-moderate croup (Russell, 2004; Sparrow, 2006)

Bacterial meningitis: Infants and Children >6 weeks: I.V.: 0.15 mg/kg/dose every 6 hours for the first 2-4 days of antibiotic treatment; start dexamethasone 10-20 minutes before or with the first dose of antibiotic

Physiologic replacement: Oral, I.M., I.V.: 0.03-0.15 mg/kg/day **or** 0.6-0.75 mg/m^2/day in divided doses every 6-12 hours

Acute mountain sickness (AMS)/high altitude cerebral edema (HACE) (unlabeled use): Oral, I.M., I.V.: 0.15 mg/kg/dose every 6 hours; consider using for high altitude pulmonary edema because of associated HACE with this condition (Luks, 2010; Pollard, 2001)

Adults:
Antiemetic:
Prophylaxis: Oral, I.V.: 10-20 mg 15-30 minutes before treatment on each treatment day
Continuous infusion regimen: Oral or I.V.: 10 mg every 12 hours on each treatment day
Mildly emetogenic therapy: Oral, I.M., I.V.: 4 mg every 4-6 hours
Delayed nausea/vomiting: Oral: 4-10 mg 1-2 times/day for 2-4 days **or**
8 mg every 12 hours for 2 days; then
4 mg every 12 hours for 2 days **or**
20 mg 1 hour before chemotherapy; then
10 mg 12 hours after chemotherapy; then
8 mg every 12 hours for 4 doses; then
4 mg every 12 hours for 4 doses
Anti-inflammatory:
Oral, I.M., I.V. (injections should be given as sodium phosphate): 0.75-9 mg/day in divided doses every 6-12 hours
Intra-articular, intralesional, or soft tissue (as sodium phosphate): 0.4-6 mg/day
Multiple myeloma: Oral, I.V.: 40 mg/day, days 1 to 4, 9 to 12, and 17 to 20, repeated every 4 weeks (alone or as part of a regimen)
Cerebral edema: I.V. 10 mg stat, 4 mg I.M./I.V. every 6 hours until response is maximized, then switch to oral regimen, then taper off if appropriate; dosage may be reduced after 2-4 days and gradually discontinued over 5-7 days
Extubation or airway edema: Oral, I.M., I.V. (injections should be given as sodium phosphate): 0.5-2 mg/kg/day in divided doses every 6 hours beginning 24 hours prior to extubation and continuing for 4-6 doses afterwards
Dexamethasone suppression test (depression/suicide indicator) (unlabeled use): Oral: 1 mg at 11 PM, draw blood at 8 AM the following day for plasma cortisol determination
Cushing's syndrome, diagnostic: Oral: 1 mg at 11 PM, draw blood at 8 AM; greater accuracy for Cushing's syndrome may be achieved by the following:
Dexamethasone 0.5 mg by mouth every 6 hours for 48 hours (with 24-hour urine collection for 17-hydroxycorticosteroid excretion)
Differentiation of Cushing's syndrome due to ACTH excess from Cushing's due to other causes: Oral: Dexamethasone 2 mg every 6 hours for 48 hours (with 24-hour urine collection for 17-hydroxycorticosteroid excretion)
Multiple sclerosis (acute exacerbation): 30 mg/day for 1 week, followed by 4-12 mg/day for 1 month
Physiological replacement: Oral, I.M., I.V. (should be given as sodium phosphate): 0.03-0.15 mg/kg/day **or** 0.6-0.75 mg/m^2/day in divided doses every 6-12 hours
Treatment of shock:
Addisonian crisis/shock (ie, adrenal insufficiency/responsive to steroid therapy): I.V. (given as sodium phosphate): 4-10 mg as a single dose, which may be repeated if necessary
Unresponsive shock (ie, unresponsive to steroid therapy): I.V. (given as sodium phosphate): 1-6 mg/kg as a single I.V. dose or up to 40 mg initially followed by repeat doses every 2-6 hours while shock persists
Acute mountain sickness (AMS)/high altitude cerebral edema (HACE) (unlabeled use):
Prevention: Oral: 2 mg every 6 hours **or** 4 mg every 12 hours starting on the day of ascent; may be discontinued after staying at the same elevation for 2-3 days or if descent is initiated; do not exceed a 10 day duration (Luks, 2010). **Note:** In situations of rapid ascent to altitudes >3500 meters (such as rescue or military operations), 4 mg every 6 hours may be considered (Luks, 2010).
Treatment: Oral, I.M., I.V.:
AMS: 4 mg every 6 hours (Luks, 2010)
HACE: Initial: 8 mg as a single dose; Maintenance: 4 mg every 6 hours until symptoms resolve (Luks, 2010)

Dosing adjustment in renal impairment:
Hemodialysis: Supplemental dose is not necessary
Peritoneal dialysis: Supplemental dose is not necessary

Dietary Considerations May be taken with meals to decrease GI upset. May need diet with increased potassium, pyridoxine, vitamin C, vitamin D, folate, calcium, and phosphorus.

Administration
Oral: Administer with meals to decrease GI upset. **Note:** Oral administration of dexamethasone for croup may be prepared using a parenteral dexamethasone formulation and mixing it with an oral flavored syrup. (Bjornson, 2004)
I.V.: Administer as a 5-10 minute bolus; rapid injection is associated with a high incidence of perineal discomfort.

Monitoring Parameters Hemoglobin, occult blood loss, serum potassium, glucose, growth in children

Reference Range Dexamethasone suppression test, overnight: 8 AM cortisol <6 mcg/100 mL (dexamethasone 1 mg); plasma cortisol determination should be made on the day after giving dose

Test Interactions May suppress the wheal and flare reactions to skin test antigens

Additional Information Effects of inhaled/intranasal steroids on growth have been observed in the absence of laboratory evidence of HPA axis suppression, suggesting that growth velocity is a more sensitive indicator of systemic corticosteroid exposure in pediatric patients than some commonly used tests of HPA axis function. The long-term effects of this reduction in growth velocity associated with orally-inhaled and intranasal corticosteroids, including the impact on final adult height, are unknown. The potential for "catch up" growth following discontinuation of treatment with inhaled corticosteroids has not been adequately studied.

Withdrawal/tapering of therapy: Corticosteroid tapering following short-term use is limited primarily by the need to control the underlying disease state; tapering may be accomplished over a period of days. Following longer-term use, tapering over weeks to months may be necessary to avoid signs and symptoms of adrenal insufficiency and to allow recovery of the HPA axis. Testing of HPA axis responsiveness may be of value in selected patients. Subtle deficits in HPA response may persist for months after discontinuation of therapy, and may require supplemental dosing during periods of acute illness or surgical stress.

Dosage Forms Excipient information presented when available (limited, particularly for generics); consult specific product labeling.
Elixir, oral: 0.5 mg/5 mL (237 mL)
Baycadron™: 0.5 mg/5 mL (237 mL) [contains benzoic acid, ethanol 5.1%, propylene glycol; raspberry flavor]
Injection, solution, as sodium phosphate: 4 mg/mL (1 mL, 5 mL, 30 mL); 10 mg/mL (1 mL, 10 mL)
Injection, solution, as sodium phosphate [preservative free]: 10 mg/mL (1 mL)
Solution, oral: 0.5 mg/5 mL (240 mL, 500 mL)
Solution, oral [concentrate]:
Dexamethasone Intensol™: 1 mg/mL (30 mL) [dye free, sugar free; contains benzoic acid, ethanol 30%, propylene glycol]

Tablet, oral: 0.5 mg, 0.75 mg, 1 mg, 1.5 mg, 2 mg, 4 mg, 6 mg
DexPak® 6 Day TaperPak®: 1.5 mg [scored; 21 tablets on taper dose card]
DexPak® 10 Day TaperPak®: 1.5 mg [scored; 35 tablets on taper dose card]
DexPak® 13 Day TaperPak®: 1.5 mg [scored; 51 tablets on taper dose card]

Dexamethasone (Ophthalmic)

(deks a METH a sone)

Brand Names: U.S. Maxidex®; Ozurdex®
Brand Names: Canada Diodex®; Maxidex®
Index Terms Dexamethasone Sodium Phosphate
Pharmacologic Category Anti-inflammatory Agent, Ophthalmic; Corticosteroid, Ophthalmic
Use Management of steroid responsive inflammatory conditions such as allergic conjunctivitis, iritis, or cyclitis; symptomatic treatment of corneal injury from chemical, radiation, or thermal burns, or penetration of foreign bodies
Ophthalmic intravitreal implant (Ozurdex®): Treatment of macular edema following branch retinal vein occlusion (BRVO) or central retinal vein occlusion (CRVO); treatment of noninfective uveitis
Pregnancy Risk Factor C
Dosage Ophthalmic:
Children: Anti-inflammatory: Solution, suspension: Instill 1-2 drops every hour during the day and every other hour during the night; gradually reduce dose to every 3-4 hours, then to 3-4 times/day; others have used 2-4 times/day dosing (Cassidy, 2001)
Adults:
Anti-inflammatory:
Solution: Instill 1-2 drops into conjunctival sac every hour during the day and every other hour during the night; gradually reduce dose to every 3-4 hours, then to 3-4 times/day
Suspension: Instill 1-2 drops into conjunctival sac up to 4-6 times/day; may use hourly in severe disease; taper prior to discontinuation
Macular edema (following BRVO or CRVO): Ocular implant (Ozurdex®): Intravitreal injection: 0.7 mg implant injected in affected eye
Noninfective uveitis: Ocular implant (Ozurdex®): Intravitreal injection: 0.7 mg implant injected in affected eye
Additional Information Complete prescribing information for this medication should be consulted for additional detail.
Dosage Forms Excipient information presented when available (limited, particularly for generics); consult specific product labeling.
Implant, intravitreal:
Ozurdex®: 0.7 mg (1s)
Solution, ophthalmic, as phosphate [drops]: 0.1% (5 mL)
Suspension, ophthalmic [drops]:
Maxidex®: 0.1% (5 mL) [contains benzalkonium chloride]

- **Dexamethasone and Ciprofloxacin** *see* Ciprofloxacin and Dexamethasone *on page 366*
- **Dexamethasone and Tobramycin** *see* Tobramycin and Dexamethasone *on page 1700*
- **Dexamethasone Intensol™** *see* Dexamethasone (Systemic) *on page 480*
- **Dexamethasone, Neomycin, and Polymyxin B** *see* Neomycin, Polymyxin B, and Dexamethasone *on page 1189*
- **Dexamethasone Sodium Phosphate** *see* Dexamethasone (Ophthalmic) *on page 483*
- **Dexamethasone Sodium Phosphate** *see* Dexamethasone (Systemic) *on page 480*
- **Dexasone® (Can)** *see* Dexamethasone (Systemic) *on page 480*

Dexchlorpheniramine (deks klor fen EER a meen)

Index Terms Dexchlorpheniramine Maleate
Pharmacologic Category Alkylamine Derivative; Histamine H_1 Antagonist; Histamine H_1 Antagonist, First Generation
Additional Appendix Information
Beers Criteria – Potentially Inappropriate Medications for Geriatrics *on page 1973*
Use Perennial and seasonal allergic rhinitis and other allergic symptoms including urticaria
Pregnancy Risk Factor B
Dosage Oral:
Children:
2-5 years: 0.5 mg every 4-6 hours (do not use timed release)
6-11 years: 1 mg every 4-6 hours or 4 mg timed release at bedtime
Adults: 2 mg every 4-6 hours or 4-6 mg timed release at bedtime or every 8-10 hours
Additional Information Complete prescribing information for this medication should be consulted for additional detail.
Dosage Forms Excipient information presented when available (limited, particularly for generics); consult specific product labeling.
Syrup, oral, as maleate: 2 mg/5 mL (473 mL)

- **Dexchlorpheniramine Maleate** *see* Dexchlorpheniramine *on page 483*
- **Dexchlorpheniramine Tannate, Pseudoephedrine Tannate, and Dextromethorphan Tannate** *see* Chlorpheniramine, Pseudoephedrine, and Dextromethorphan *on page 347*
- **Dexedrine® (Can)** *see* Dextroamphetamine *on page 487*
- **Dexedrine® Spansule®** *see* Dextroamphetamine *on page 487*
- **Dexferrum®** *see* Iron Dextran Complex *on page 930*
- **Dexilant™** *see* Dexlansoprazole *on page 483*
- **Dexiron™ (Can)** *see* Iron Dextran Complex *on page 930*

Dexlansoprazole (deks lan SOE pra zole)

Brand Names: U.S. Dexilant™
Brand Names: Canada Dexilant™
Index Terms Kapidex; TAK-390MR
Pharmacologic Category Proton Pump Inhibitor; Substituted Benzimidazole
Use Short-term (4 weeks) treatment of heartburn associated with nonerosive GERD; short-term (up to 8 weeks) treatment of all grades of erosive esophagitis; to maintain healing of erosive esophagitis for up to 6 months
Pregnancy Risk Factor B
Dosage Oral: Adults:
Erosive esophagitis: Short-term treatment: 60 mg once daily for up to 8 weeks; maintenance therapy: 30 mg once daily for up to 6 months
Symptomatic GERD: Short-term treatment: 30 mg once daily for 4 weeks

Dosage adjustment in renal impairment: No dosage adjustment is needed
Dosage adjustment in hepatic impairment:
Mild hepatic impairment (Child-Pugh class A): No dosage adjustment is needed
Moderate hepatic impairment (Child-Pugh class B): Consider a maximum dose of 30 mg/day

Severe hepatic impairment (Child-Pugh class C): Use has not been studied in patients with severe hepatic impairment

Additional Information Complete prescribing information for this medication should be consulted for additional detail.

Dosage Forms Excipient information presented when available (limited, particularly for generics); consult specific product labeling.

Capsule, delayed release, oral:

Dexilant™: 30 mg, 60 mg

Dexmedetomidine (deks MED e toe mi deen)

Brand Names: U.S. Precedex®

Brand Names: Canada Precedex®

Index Terms Dexmedetomidine Hydrochloride

Pharmacologic Category $Alpha_2$-Adrenergic Agonist; Sedative

Use Sedation of initially intubated and mechanically ventilated patients during treatment in an intensive care setting; sedation prior to and/or during surgical or other procedures of nonintubated patients

Unlabeled Use Unlabeled uses include premedication prior to anesthesia induction with thiopental; relief of pain and reduction of opioid dose following laparoscopic tubal ligation; as an adjunct anesthetic in ophthalmic surgery; treatment of shivering; premedication to attenuate the cardiostimulatory and postanesthetic delirium of ketamine; use in children

Pregnancy Risk Factor C

Pregnancy Considerations Teratogenic effects were not observed in animal studies. There are no adequate and well-controlled studies in pregnant women.

Lactation Excretion in breast milk unknown/use caution

Contraindications There are no contraindications listed in the manufacturer's labeling.

Warnings/Precautions Should be administered only by persons skilled in management of patients in intensive care setting or operating room. Patients should be continuously monitored. Episodes of bradycardia, hypotension, and sinus arrest have been associated with dexmedetomidine. Use caution in patients with heart block, severe ventricular dysfunction, hypovolemia, diabetes, chronic hypertension, and elderly. Use with caution in patients with hepatic impairment; dosage reductions recommended. Use with caution in patients receiving vasodilators or drugs which decrease heart rate. If medical intervention is required, treatment may include stopping or decreasing the infusion; increasing the rate of I.V. fluid administration, use of pressor agents, and elevation of the lower extremities. Transient hypertension has been primarily observed during the loading dose administration and is associated with the initial peripheral vasoconstrictive effects of dexmedetomidine. Treatment of this is generally unnecessary; however, reduction of infusion rate may be required. Patients may be arousable and alert when stimulated. This alone should not be considered as lack of efficacy in the absence of other clinical signs/symptoms. When withdrawn abruptly in patients who have received >24 hours, withdrawal symptoms similar to clonidine withdrawal may result (eg, hypertension, nervousness, agitation, headaches). Use for >24 hours is not recommended by the manufacturer.

Adverse Reactions

>10%:

Cardiovascular: Hypotension (24% to 54%), bradycardia (5% to 14%)

Respiratory: Respiratory depression (37%; placebo 32%)

1% to 10%:

Cardiovascular: Atrial fibrillation (4% to 5%), hypovolemia (3%)

Endocrine & metabolic: Hypocalcemia (1%)

Gastrointestinal: Nausea (3% to 9%), xerostomia (3% to 4%)

Renal: Urine output decreased (1%)

Respiratory: Pleural effusion (2%), wheezing (≤1%)

Postmarketing and/or case reports: Abdominal pain, abnormal vision, acidosis, agitation, alkaline phosphatase increased, ALT increased, anemia, apnea, arrhythmia, AST increased, atrioventricular block, BUN increased, bronchospasm, cardiac arrest, confusion, delirium, diaphoresis, diarrhea, dizziness, dyspnea, extrasystoles, fever, GGT increased, hallucination, headache, heart block, hemorrhage, hepatic impairment, hyperbilirubinemia, hypercapnia, hyperkalemia, hypertension, hypoglycemia, hypoventilation, hypoxia, illusion, MI, neuralgia, neuritis, oliguria, pain, photopsia, pulmonary congestion, respiratory acidosis, rigors, seizure, speech disorder, supraventricular tachycardia, tachycardia, thirst, T-wave inversion, ventricular arrhythmia, ventricular tachycardia, vomiting

Drug Interactions

Metabolism/Transport Effects Substrate of CYP2A6 (major); **Note:** Assignment of Major/Minor substrate status based on clinically relevant drug interaction potential; **Inhibits** CYP1A2 (weak), CYP2C9 (weak), CYP3A4 (weak)

Avoid Concomitant Use

Avoid concomitant use of Dexmedetomidine with any of the following: Iobenguane I 123; Pimozide

Increased Effect/Toxicity

Dexmedetomidine may increase the levels/effects of: Hypotensive Agents; Pimozide

The levels/effects of Dexmedetomidine may be increased by: Beta-Blockers; CYP2A6 Inhibitors (Moderate); CYP2A6 Inhibitors (Strong); MAO Inhibitors

Decreased Effect

Dexmedetomidine may decrease the levels/effects of: Iobenguane I 123

The levels/effects of Dexmedetomidine may be decreased by: Antidepressants (Alpha2-Antagonist); Serotonin/Norepinephrine Reuptake Inhibitors; Tricyclic Antidepressants

Stability Store at controlled room temperature of 25°C (77°F); excursions permitted to 15°C to 30°C (59°F to 86°F). Add 2 mL (200 mcg) of dexmedetomidine to 48 mL of 0.9% sodium chloride for a total volume of 50 mL (4 mcg/mL). Shake gently to mix.

Mechanism of Action Selective $alpha_2$-adrenoceptor agonist with anesthetic and sedative properties thought to be due to activation of G-proteins by $apha_{2a}$-adrenoceptors in the brainstem resulting in inhibition of norepinephrine release; peripheral $alpha_{2b}$-adrenoceptors are activated at high doses or with rapid I.V. administration resulting in vasoconstriction.

Pharmacodynamics/Kinetics

Onset of action: I.V. Bolus: 5-10 minutes

Peak effect: 15-30 minutes

Duration (dose dependent): 60-120 minutes

Distribution: V_{ss}: ~118 L; rapid

Protein binding: ~94%

Metabolism: Hepatic via N-glucuronidation, N-methylation, and CYP2A6

Half-life elimination: ~6 minutes; Terminal: ~2 hours

Excretion: Urine (95%); feces (4%)

Dosage Note: Errors have occurred due to misinterpretation of dosing information. Maintenance dose expressed as mcg/kg/**hour**.

Individualized and titrated to desired clinical effect. Manufacturer recommends duration of infusion should not exceed 24 hours; however, randomized clinical trials have demonstrated efficacy and safety comparable to lorazepam and midazolam with longer-term infusions of up to approximately 5 days. (Pandharipande, 2007; Riker, 2009).

ICU sedation:

Adults: I.V.: Initial: Loading infusion (optional; see **"Note"** below) of 1 mcg/kg over 10 minutes, followed by a maintenance infusion of 0.2-0.7 mcg/kg/**hour**; adjust rate to desired level of sedation; titration no more frequently than every 30 minutes may reduce the incidence of hypotension (Gerlach, 2009)

Note: *Loading infusion:* Administration of a loading infusion may increase the risk of hemodynamic compromise. For this indication, the loading dose may be omitted. *Maintenance infusion:* Dosing ranges between 0.2-1.4 mcg/kg/**hour** have been reported during randomized controlled clinical trials (Pandharipande, 2007; Riker, 2009). Although infusion rates as high as 2.5 mcg/kg/**hour** have been used, it is thought that doses >1.5 mcg/kg/**hour** do not add to clinical efficacy (Venn, 2003).

Elderly (>65 years of age): Dosage reduction may need to be considered. No specific guidelines available. Dose selections should be cautious, at the low end of dosage range; titration should be slower, allowing adequate time to evaluate response.

Procedural sedation:

Adults: I.V.: Initial: Loading infusion of 1 mcg/kg (or 0.5 mcg/kg for less invasive procedures [eg, ophthalmic]) over 10 minutes, followed by a maintenance infusion of 0.6 mcg/kg/**hour**, titrate to desired effect; usual range: 0.2-1 mcg/kg/**hour**

Elderly (>65 years of age): Initial: Loading infusion of 0.5 mcg/kg over 10 minutes; Maintenance infusion: Dosage reduction should be considered

Fiberoptic intubation (awake): I.V. Initial: Loading infusion of 1 mcg/kg over 10 minutes, followed by a maintenance infusion of 0.7 mcg/kg/**hour** until endotracheal tube is secured.

Dosage adjustment in renal impairment: Dosage reduction may need to be considered. No specific guidelines available.

Dosage adjustment in hepatic impairment: Dosage reduction may need to be considered. No specific guidelines available.

Administration Administer using a controlled infusion device. Must be diluted in 0.9% sodium chloride solution to achieve the required concentration (4 mcg/mL) prior to administration. Advisable to use administration components made with synthetic or coated natural rubber gaskets. Parenteral products should be inspected visually for particulate matter and discoloration prior to administration. If loading dose used, administer over 10 minutes; may extend to 20 minutes to further reduce vasoconstrictive effects. Titration no more frequently than every 30 minutes may reduce the incidence of hypotension when used for ICU sedation (Gerlach, 2009).

Monitoring Parameters Level of sedation; heart rate, respiration, rhythm, blood pressure; pain control

Dosage Forms Excipient information presented when available (limited, particularly for generics); consult specific product labeling.

Injection, solution [preservative free]:

Precedex®: 100 mcg/mL (2 mL)

◆ **Dexmedetomidine Hydrochloride** *see* Dexmedetomidine *on page* 484

Dexmethylphenidate (dex meth il FEN i date)

Brand Names: U.S. Focalin XR®; Focalin®

Index Terms Dexmethylphenidate Hydrochloride

Pharmacologic Category Central Nervous System Stimulant

Use Treatment of attention-deficit/hyperactivity disorder (ADHD)

Pregnancy Risk Factor C

Medication Guide Available Yes

Dosage Treatment of ADHD: Oral:

Children ≥6 years: Patients not currently taking methylphenidate:

Immediate release: Initial: 2.5 mg twice daily; dosage may be adjusted in increments of 2.5-5 mg at weekly intervals (maximum dose: 20 mg/day); doses should be taken at least 4 hours apart

Extended release: Initial: 5 mg once daily; dosage may be adjusted in increments of 5 mg/day at weekly intervals (maximum dose: 30 mg/day)

Conversion to dexmethylphenidate from methylphenidate:

Immediate release: Initial: Half the total daily dose of racemic methylphenidate (maximum dexmethylphenidate dose: 20 mg/day)

Extended release: Initial: Half the total daily dose of racemic methylphenidate (maximum dexmethylphenidate dose: 30 mg/day)

Conversion from dexmethylphenidate immediate release to dexmethylphenidate extended release: When changing from Focalin® tablets to Focalin® XR capsules, patients may be switched to the same daily dose using Focalin® XR (maximum dose: 30 mg/day)

Adults: Patients not currently taking methylphenidate:

Immediate release: Initial: 2.5 mg twice daily; dosage may be adjusted in increments of 2.5-5 mg at weekly intervals (maximum dose: 20 mg/day); doses should be taken at least 4 hours apart

Extended release: Initial: 10 mg once daily; dosage may be adjusted in increments of 10 mg/day at weekly intervals (maximum dose: 40 mg/day)

Conversion to dexmethylphenidate from methylphenidate:

Immediate release: Initial: Half the total daily dose of racemic methylphenidate (maximum dexmethylphenidate dose: 20 mg/day)

Extended release: Initial: Half the total daily dose of racemic methylphenidate (maximum dexmethylphenidate dose: 40 mg/day)

Conversion from dexmethylphenidate immediate release to dexmethylphenidate extended release: When changing from Focalin® tablets to Focalin® XR capsules, patients may be switched to the same daily dose using Focalin® XR (maximum dose: 40 mg/day)

Dose reductions and discontinuation: Children ≥6 years and Adults: Reduce dose or discontinue in patients with paradoxical aggravation of symptoms. Discontinue if no improvement is seen after one month of treatment.

Dosage adjustment in renal impairment: No data available. However, considering extensive metabolism to inactive compounds, renal insufficiency expected to have minimal effect on kinetics of dexmethylphenidate.

Dosage adjustment in hepatic impairment: No data available.

Additional Information Complete prescribing information for this medication should be consulted for additional detail.

Dosage Forms Excipient information presented when available (limited, particularly for generics); consult specific product labeling.

Capsule, extended release, oral, as hydrochloride:

Focalin XR®: 5 mg, 10 mg, 15 mg, 20 mg, 25 mg, 30 mg, 35 mg, 40 mg [bimodal release]

Tablet, oral, as hydrochloride: 2.5 mg, 5 mg, 10 mg
Focalin®: 2.5 mg, 5 mg
Focalin®: 10 mg [dye free]

Controlled Substance C-II

◆ **Dexmethylphenidate Hydrochloride** *see* Dexmethylphenidate *on page 485*

◆ **DexPak® 6 Day TaperPak®** *see* Dexamethasone (Systemic) *on page 480*

◆ **DexPak® 10 Day TaperPak®** *see* Dexamethasone (Systemic) *on page 480*

◆ **DexPak® 13 Day TaperPak®** *see* Dexamethasone (Systemic) *on page 480*

Dexpanthenol (deks PAN the nole)

Index Terms Pantothenyl Alcohol

Pharmacologic Category Gastrointestinal Agent, Stimulant; Topical Skin Product

Use Prophylactic use to minimize paralytic ileus; treatment of postoperative distention; topical to relieve itching and to aid healing of minor dermatoses

Pregnancy Risk Factor C

Dosage I.M.: Adults:

Prevention of postoperative ileus: 250-500 mg stat, repeat in 2 hours, followed by doses every 6 hours until danger passes

Paralytic ileus: 500 mg stat, repeat in 2 hours, followed by doses every 6 hours, if needed

Additional Information Complete prescribing information for this medication should be consulted for additional detail.

Dosage Forms Excipient information presented when available (limited, particularly for generics); consult specific product labeling.

Injection, solution [preservative free]: 250 mg/mL (2 mL)

Dexrazoxane (deks ray ZOKS ane)

Brand Names: U.S. Totect®; Zinecard®

Brand Names: Canada Zinecard®

Index Terms ICRF-187

Pharmacologic Category Antidote; Cardioprotectant

Use

Zinecard®: Reduction of the incidence and severity of cardiomyopathy associated with doxorubicin administration in women with metastatic breast cancer who have received a cumulative doxorubicin dose of 300 mg/m^2 and who would benefit from continuing therapy with doxorubicin. (Not recommended for use with initial doxorubicin therapy.)

Totect®: Treatment of anthracycline-induced extravasation.

Unlabeled Use Reduction of the incidence and severity of cardiomyopathy associated with doxorubicin administration (cumulative doses >300 mg/m^2) in patients with malignancies other than metastatic breast cancer who would benefit from continuing therapy with doxorubicin; reduction of the incidence and severity of cardiomyopathy associated with continued epirubicin administration for advanced breast cancer

Pregnancy Risk Factor C (Zinecard®) / D (Totect®)

Dosage I.V.:

Children: Prevention of doxorubicin cardiomyopathy (unlabeled use): A 10:1 ratio of dexrazoxane:doxorubicin (eg, 300 mg/m^2 dexrazoxane: 30 mg/m^2 doxorubicin) was used in patients with high-risk acute lymphoblastic leukemia (Moghrabi, 2007)

Adults:

Prevention of doxorubicin cardiomyopathy: A 10:1 ratio of dexrazoxane:doxorubicin (500 mg/m^2 dexrazoxane: 50 mg/m^2 doxorubicin). **Note:** Cardiac monitoring should continue during dexrazoxane therapy; doxorubicin/dexrazoxane should be discontinued in patients who develop a decline in LVEF or clinical CHF.

Treatment of anthracycline extravasation: 1000 mg/m^2 on days 1 and 2 (maximum dose: 2000 mg), followed by 500 mg/m^2 on day 3 (maximum dose: 1000 mg); begin treatment as soon as possible, within 6 hours of extravasation

Dosage adjustment in renal impairment: Moderate-to-severe (Cl_{cr}<40 mL/minute):

Prevention of cardiomyopathy: Reduce dose by 50%, using a 5:1 dexrazoxane:doxorubicin ratio (250 mg/m^2 dexrazoxane: 50 mg/m^2 doxorubicin)

Anthracycline-induced extravasation: Reduce dose by 50%

Dosage adjustment in hepatic impairment:

Prevention of cardiomyopathy: Since doxorubicin dosage is reduced in hyperbilirubinemia, a proportional reduction in dexrazoxane dosage is recommended (maintain a 10:1 ratio of dexrazoxane:doxorubicin)

Anthracycline-induced extravasation: Use has not been evaluated in patients with hepatic dysfunction

Additional Information Complete prescribing information for this medication should be consulted for additional detail.

Dosage Forms Excipient information presented when available (limited, particularly for generics); consult specific product labeling.

Injection, powder for reconstitution: 250 mg, 500 mg
Totect®: 500 mg
Zinecard®: 250 mg, 500 mg

Dextran (DEKS tran)

Brand Names: U.S. LMD®

Index Terms 10% LMD; Dextran 40; Dextran, Low Molecular Weight

Pharmacologic Category Plasma Volume Expander, Colloid

Use Blood volume expander used in treatment of shock or impending shock when blood or blood products are not available; also used as a priming fluid in pump oxygenators during cardiopulmonary bypass and for prophylaxis of venous thrombosis and pulmonary embolism in surgical procedures associated with a high risk of thromboembolic complications

Pregnancy Risk Factor C

Dosage I.V.: Dose and infusion rate are dependent upon the patient's fluid status and must be individualized:

Volume expansion/shock:

Children (Dextran 40): Infuse 10 mL/kg as rapidly as possible (maximum: 20 mL/kg/day for the first 24 hours; 10 mL/kg/day thereafter); therapy should not be continued beyond 5 days

Adults (Dextran 40): Infuse 500-1000 mL (~10 mL/kg) as rapidly as possible (maximum: 20 mL/kg/day for first 24 hours; 10 mL/kg/day thereafter); therapy should not be continued beyond 5 days

Pump prime (Dextran 40): Varies with the volume of the pump oxygenator; generally, the solution is added in a dose of 10-20 mL/kg (or 1-2 g/kg); usual maximum total dose: 20 mL/kg (or 2 g/kg)

Postoperative prophylaxis of venous thrombosis/pulmonary embolism (Dextran 40): Begin during surgical procedure and give 500-1000 mL (~10 mL/kg); an additional 50 g (500 mL) should be administered every 2-3 days during the period of risk (up to 2 weeks postoperatively); usual maximum infusion rate for nonemergency use: 4 mL/minute

Dosing in renal and/or hepatic impairment: Use with extreme caution

Additional Information Complete prescribing information for this medication should be consulted for additional detail.

Dosage Forms Excipient information presented when available (limited, particularly for generics); consult specific product labeling.

Infusion, premixed in D_5W [low molecular weight]:
LMD®: 10% Dextran 40 (500 mL)

Infusion, premixed in NS [low molecular weight]:
LMD®: 10% Dextran 40 (500 mL)

◆ **Dextran 40** *see* Dextran *on page 486*

◆ **Dextran, Low Molecular Weight** *see* Dextran *on page 486*

◆ **Dextrin** *see* Wheat Dextrin *on page 1805*

Dextroamphetamine (deks troe am FET a meen)

Brand Names: U.S. Dexedrine® Spansule®; ProCentra®

Brand Names: Canada Dexedrine®

Index Terms Dextroamphetamine Sulfate

Pharmacologic Category Stimulant

Use Narcolepsy; attention-deficit/hyperactivity disorder (ADHD)

Unlabeled Use Depression

Pregnancy Risk Factor C

Pregnancy Considerations Teratogenic and embryocidal effects have been observed in animal studies. There are no adequate and well-controlled studies in pregnant women. Use only if potential benefit justifies the potential risk to the fetus.

Lactation Enters breast milk/not recommended

Medication Guide Available Yes

Contraindications Hypersensitivity or idiosyncrasy to dextroamphetamine, other sympathomimetic amines, or any component of the formulation; advanced arteriosclerosis, symptomatic cardiovascular disease, moderate-to-severe hypertension; hyperthyroidism; glaucoma; agitated states; patients with a history of drug abuse; during or within 14 days following MAO inhibitor therapy

Warnings/Precautions [U.S. Boxed Warning]: Use has been associated with serious cardiovascular events including sudden death in patients with pre-existing structural cardiac abnormalities or other serious heart problems (sudden death in children and adolescents; sudden death, stroke and MI in adults. These products should be avoided in the patients with known serious structural cardiac abnormalities, cardiomyopathy, serious heart rhythm abnormalities, or other serious cardiac problems that could increase the risk of sudden death that these conditions alone carry. Patients should be carefully evaluated for cardiac disease prior to initiation of therapy. Use with caution in patients with hypertension and other cardiovascular conditions that might be exacerbated by increases in blood pressure or heart rate. Amphetamines may impair the ability to engage in potentially hazardous activities. May cause visual disturbances.

Use with caution in patients with psychiatric or seizure disorders. May exacerbate symptoms of behavior and thought disorder in psychotic patients. Stimulants may unmask tics in individuals with coexisting Tourette's syndrome. **[U.S. Boxed Warning]: Potential for drug dependency exists; prolonged use may lead to drug dependency.** Use is contraindicated in patients with history of ethanol or drug abuse. Prescriptions should be written for the smallest quantity consistent with good patient care to minimize possibility of overdose. Abrupt discontinuation following high doses or for prolonged periods may result in symptoms for withdrawal.

May be inappropriate for use in the elderly due to CNS stimulant adverse effects (Beers Criteria). Appetite suppression may occur; monitor weight during therapy, particularly in children. Use of stimulants has been associated with suppression of growth; monitor growth rate during treatment.

Adverse Reactions Frequency not defined.

Cardiovascular: Cardiomyopathy, hypertension, palpitation, tachycardia

Central nervous system: Aggression, dizziness, dyskinesia, dysphoria, euphoria, exacerbation of motor and phonic tics, headache, insomnia, mania, overstimulation, psychosis, restlessness, Tourette's syndrome

Dermatologic: Urticaria

Endocrine & metabolic: Libido changes

Gastrointestinal: Anorexia, constipation, diarrhea, unpleasant taste, weight loss, xerostomia

Genitourinary: Impotence

Neuromuscular & skeletal: Tremor

Ocular: Accommodation abnormalities, blurred vision

Drug Interactions

Metabolism/Transport Effects Substrate of CYP2D6 (minor); **Note:** Assignment of Major/Minor substrate status based on clinically relevant drug interaction potential

Avoid Concomitant Use

Avoid concomitant use of Dextroamphetamine with any of the following: Iobenguane I 123; MAO Inhibitors

Increased Effect/Toxicity

Dextroamphetamine may increase the levels/effects of: Analgesics (Opioid); Sympathomimetics

The levels/effects of Dextroamphetamine may be increased by: Alkalinizing Agents; Antacids; Atomoxetine; Cannabinoids; Carbonic Anhydrase Inhibitors; MAO Inhibitors; Proton Pump Inhibitors; Tricyclic Antidepressants

Decreased Effect

Dextroamphetamine may decrease the levels/effects of: Antihistamines; Ethosuximide; Iobenguane I 123; Ioflupane I 123; PHENobarbital; Phenytoin

The levels/effects of Dextroamphetamine may be decreased by: Ammonium Chloride; Antipsychotics; Gastrointestinal Acidifying Agents; Lithium; Methenamine; Peginterferon Alfa-2b

Ethanol/Nutrition/Herb Interactions

Ethanol: Avoid ethanol (may increase CNS depression).

Food: Dextroamphetamine serum levels may be altered if taken with acidic food, juices, or vitamin C.

Herb/Nutraceutical: Avoid ephedra (may cause hypertension or arrhythmias).

Stability Store at controlled room temperature of 20°C to 25°C (68°F to 77°F). Protect from light.

Mechanism of Action Amphetamines are noncatecholamine, sympathomimetic amines that promote release of catecholamines (primarily dopamine and norepinephrine) from their storage sites in the presynaptic nerve terminals. A less significant mechanism may include their ability to block the reuptake of catecholamines by competitive inhibition.

Pharmacodynamics/Kinetics

Onset of action: 1-1.5 hours

Distribution: V_d: Adults: 3.5-4.6 L/kg; distributes into CNS; mean CSF concentrations are 80% of plasma; enters breast milk

Metabolism: Hepatic via CYP monooxygenase and glucuronidation

Half-life elimination: Adults: 10-13 hours

Time to peak, serum: Immediate release: ~3 hours; sustained release: ~8 hours

Excretion: Urine (as unchanged drug and inactive metabolites)

Dosage Oral:

Children:

Narcolepsy: 6-12 years: Initial: 5 mg/day; may increase at 5 mg/day increments in weekly intervals until side effects appear (maximum dose: 60 mg/day)

ADHD:

3-5 years: Immediate release tablets or oral solution: Initial: 2.5 mg/day; may increase at 2.5 mg/day increments in weekly intervals until optimal response is obtained; usual range: 0.1-0.5 mg/kg/dose (maximum dose: 40 mg/day)

≥6 years: Initial: 5 mg once or twice daily; may increase at 5 mg/day increments in weekly intervals until optimal response is obtained; usual range: 0.1-0.5 mg/kg/dose (5-20 mg/day) (maximum dose: 40 mg/day)

Children >12 years and Adults: Narcolepsy: 10 mg/day, may increase at 10 mg/day increments in weekly intervals until side effects appear (maximum dose: 60 mg/day)

Administration Administer initial dose upon awakening; do not administer doses late in the evening due to potential for insomnia.

Immediate release tablets and oral solution: If needed, 1-2 additional doses may be administered at intervals of 4-6 hours.

Extended release or sustained release capsules: Do not crush sustained release drug products. Formulations may be used for once-daily administration, if appropriate.

Monitoring Parameters Cardiac evaluation should be completed on any patient who develops chest pain, unexplained syncope, and any symptom of cardiac disease during treatment with stimulants; growth in children and CNS activity in all

When used for the treatment of ADHD, thoroughly evaluate for cardiovascular risk. Monitor heart rate, blood pressure, and consider obtaining ECG prior to initiation (Vetter, 2008).

Test Interactions Amphetamines may elevate plasma corticosteroid levels; may interfere with urinary steroid determinations.

Dosage Forms Excipient information presented when available (limited, particularly for generics); consult specific product labeling.

Capsule, extended release, oral, as sulfate: 5 mg, 10 mg, 15 mg

Capsule, sustained release, oral, as sulfate:

Dexedrine® Spansule®: 5 mg, 10 mg, 15 mg

Solution, oral, as sulfate:

ProCentra®: 5 mg/5 mL (480 mL) [contains benzoic acid; bubblegum flavor]

Tablet, oral, as sulfate: 5 mg, 10 mg

Controlled Substance C-II

Dextroamphetamine and Amphetamine

(deks troe am FET a meen & am FET a meen)

Brand Names: U.S. Adderall XR®; Adderall® [DSC]

Brand Names: Canada Adderall XR®

Index Terms Amphetamine and Dextroamphetamine

Pharmacologic Category Stimulant

Use Attention-deficit/hyperactivity disorder (ADHD); narcolepsy

Pregnancy Risk Factor C

Medication Guide Available Yes

Dosage Oral: **Note:** Use lowest effective individualized dose; administer first dose as soon as awake

ADHD:

Children: <3 years: Not recommended

Children: 3-5 years (Adderall®): Initial 2.5 mg/day given every morning; increase daily dose in 2.5 mg increments at weekly intervals until optimal response is obtained (maximum dose: 40 mg/day given in 1-3 divided doses); use intervals of 4-6 hours between additional doses

Children: ≥6 years:

Adderall®: Initial: 5 mg 1-2 times/day; increase daily dose in 5 mg increments at weekly intervals until optimal response is obtained (usual maximum dose: 40 mg/day given in 1-3 divided doses); use intervals of 4-6 hours between additional doses

Adderall XR®: 5-10 mg once daily in the morning; if needed, may increase daily dose in 5-10 mg increments at weekly intervals (maximum dose: 30 mg/day)

Adolescents 13-17 years (Adderall XR®): 10 mg once daily in the morning; maybe increased to 20 mg/day after 1 week if symptoms are not controlled; higher doses (up to 60 mg/day) have been evaluated; however, there is not adequate evidence that higher doses afford additional benefit.

Adults (Adderall XR®): Initial: 20 mg once daily in the morning; higher doses (up to 60 mg once daily) have been evaluated; however, there is not adequate evidence that higher doses afforded additional benefit

Narcolepsy (Adderall®):

Children: 6-12 years: Initial: 5 mg/day; increase daily dose in 5 mg at weekly intervals until optimal response is obtained (maximum dose: 60 mg/day given in 1-3 divided doses with intervals of 4-6 hours between doses)

Children >12 years and Adults: Initial: 10 mg/day; increase daily dose in 10 mg increments at weekly intervals until optimal response is obtained (maximum dose: 60 mg/day given in 1-3 divided doses with intervals of 4-6 hours between doses)

Additional Information Complete prescribing information for this medication should be consulted for additional detail.

Dosage Forms Excipient information presented when available (limited, particularly for generics); consult specific product labeling. [DSC] = Discontinued product

Capsule, extended release:

5 mg [dextroamphetamine sulfate 1.25 mg, dextroamphetamine saccharate 1.25 mg, amphetamine aspartate monohydrate 1.25 mg, amphetamine sulfate 1.25 mg (equivalent to amphetamine base 3.1 mg)]

10 mg [dextroamphetamine sulfate 2.5 mg, dextroamphetamine saccharate 2.5 mg, amphetamine aspartate monohydrate 2.5 mg, amphetamine sulfate 2.5 mg (equivalent to amphetamine base 6.3 mg)]

15 mg [dextroamphetamine sulfate 3.75 mg, dextroamphetamine saccharate 3.75 mg, amphetamine aspartate monohydrate 3.75 mg, amphetamine sulfate 3.75 mg (equivalent to amphetamine base 9.4 mg)]

20 mg [dextroamphetamine sulfate 5 mg, dextroamphetamine saccharate 5 mg, amphetamine aspartate monohydrate 5 mg, amphetamine sulfate 5 mg (equivalent to amphetamine base 12.5 mg)]

25 mg [dextroamphetamine sulfate 6.25 mg, dextroamphetamine saccharate 6.25 mg, amphetamine aspartate monohydrate 6.25 mg, amphetamine sulfate 6.25 mg (equivalent to amphetamine base 15.6 mg)]

30 mg [dextroamphetamine sulfate 7.5 mg, dextroamphetamine saccharate 7.5 mg, amphetamine aspartate monohydrate 7.5 mg, amphetamine sulfate 7.5 mg (equivalent to amphetamine base 18.8 mg)]

Adderall XR®:

5 mg [dextroamphetamine sulfate 1.25 mg, dextroamphetamine saccharate 1.25 mg, amphetamine aspartate monohydrate 1.25 mg, amphetamine sulfate 1.25 mg (equivalent to amphetamine base 3.1 mg)]

10 mg [dextroamphetamine sulfate 2.5 mg, dextroamphetamine saccharate 2.5 mg, amphetamine aspartate monohydrate 2.5 mg, amphetamine sulfate 2.5 mg (equivalent to amphetamine base 6.3 mg)]
15 mg [dextroamphetamine sulfate 3.75 mg, dextroamphetamine saccharate 3.75 mg, amphetamine aspartate monohydrate 3.75 mg, amphetamine sulfate 3.75 mg (equivalent to amphetamine base 9.4 mg)]
20 mg [dextroamphetamine sulfate 5 mg, dextroamphetamine saccharate 5 mg, amphetamine aspartate monohydrate 5 mg, amphetamine sulfate 5 mg (equivalent to amphetamine base 12.5 mg)]
25 mg [dextroamphetamine sulfate 6.25 mg, dextroamphetamine saccharate 6.25 mg, amphetamine aspartate monohydrate 6.25 mg, amphetamine sulfate 6.25 mg (equivalent to amphetamine base 15.6 mg)]
30 mg [dextroamphetamine sulfate 7.5 mg, dextroamphetamine saccharate 7.5 mg, amphetamine aspartate monohydrate 7.5 mg, amphetamine sulfate 7.5 mg (equivalent to amphetamine base 18.8 mg)]

Tablet:
5 mg [dextroamphetamine sulfate 1.25 mg, dextroamphetamine saccharate 1.25 mg, amphetamine aspartate monohydrate 1.25 mg, amphetamine sulfate 1.25 mg (equivalent to amphetamine base 3.13 mg)]
7.5 mg [dextroamphetamine 1.875 mg, dextroamphetamine saccharate 1.875 mg, amphetamine aspartate monohydrate 1.875 mg, amphetamine sulfate 1.875 mg (equivalent to amphetamine base 4.7 mg)]
10 mg [dextroamphetamine sulfate 2.5 mg, dextroamphetamine saccharate 2.5 mg, amphetamine aspartate monohydrate 2.5 mg, amphetamine sulfate 2.5 mg (equivalent to amphetamine base 6.3 mg)]
12.5 mg [dextroamphetamine sulfate 3.125 mg, dextroamphetamine saccharate 3.125 mg, amphetamine aspartate monohydrate 3.125 mg, amphetamine sulfate 3.125 mg (equivalent to amphetamine base 7.8 mg)]
15 mg [dextroamphetamine sulfate 3.75 mg, dextroamphetamine saccharate 3.75 mg, amphetamine aspartate monohydrate 3.75 mg, amphetamine sulfate 3.75 mg (equivalent to amphetamine base 9.4 mg)]
20 mg [dextroamphetamine sulfate 5 mg, dextroamphetamine saccharate 5 mg, amphetamine aspartate monohydrate 5 mg, amphetamine sulfate 5 mg (equivalent to amphetamine base 12.6 mg)]
30 mg [dextroamphetamine sulfate 7.5 mg, dextroamphetamine saccharate 7.5 mg, amphetamine aspartate monohydrate 7.5 mg, amphetamine sulfate 7.5 mg (equivalent to amphetamine base 18.8 mg)]

Adderall® [DSC]:
5 mg [dextroamphetamine sulfate 1.25 mg, dextroamphetamine saccharate 1.25 mg, amphetamine aspartate monohydrate 1.25 mg, amphetamine sulfate 1.25 mg (equivalent to amphetamine base 3.13 mg)]
7.5 mg [dextroamphetamine sulfate 1.875 mg, dextroamphetamine saccharate 1.875 mg, amphetamine aspartate monohydrate 1.875 mg, amphetamine sulfate 1.875 mg (equivalent to amphetamine base 4.7 mg)]
10 mg [dextroamphetamine sulfate 2.5 mg, dextroamphetamine saccharate 2.5 mg, amphetamine aspartate monohydrate 2.5 mg, amphetamine sulfate 2.5 mg (equivalent to amphetamine base 6.3 mg)]
12.5 mg [dextroamphetamine sulfate 3.125 mg, dextroamphetamine saccharate 3.125 mg, amphetamine aspartate monohydrate 3.125 mg, amphetamine sulfate 3.125 mg (equivalent to amphetamine base 7.8 mg)]
15 mg [dextroamphetamine sulfate 3.75 mg, dextroamphetamine saccharate 3.75 mg, amphetamine aspartate monohydrate 3.75 mg, amphetamine sulfate 3.75 mg (equivalent to amphetamine base 9.4 mg)]
20 mg [dextroamphetamine sulfate 5 mg, dextroamphetamine saccharate 5 mg, amphetamine aspartate monohydrate 5 mg, amphetamine sulfate 5 mg (equivalent to amphetamine base 12.6 mg)]
30 mg [dextroamphetamine sulfate 7.5 mg, dextroamphetamine saccharate 7.5 mg, amphetamine aspartate monohydrate 7.5 mg, amphetamine sulfate 7.5 mg (equivalent to amphetamine base 18.8 mg)]

Controlled Substance C-II

◆ **Dextroamphetamine Sulfate** *see* Dextroamphetamine *on page 487*

Dextromethorphan and Chlorpheniramine

(deks troe meth OR fan & klor fen IR a meen)

Brand Names: U.S. Coricidin® HBP Cough & Cold [OTC]; Dimetapp® Children's Long Acting Cough Plus Cold [OTC]; Robitussin® Children's Cough & Cold Long-Acting [OTC]; Robitussin® Cough & Cold Long-Acting [OTC] [DSC]; Scot-Tussin® DM Maximum Strength [OTC]; Triaminic® Children's Softchews® Cough & Runny Nose [OTC]

Index Terms Chlorpheniramine and Dextromethorphan; Chlorpheniramine Maleate and Dextromethorphan Hydrobromide; Dextromethorphan Hydrobromide and Chlorpheniramine Maleate

Pharmacologic Category Alkylamine Derivative; Antitussive; Histamine H_1 Antagonist; Histamine H_1 Antagonist, First Generation

Use Symptomatic relief of runny nose, sneezing, itchy/watery eyes, cough, and other upper respiratory symptoms associated with hay fever, common cold, or upper respiratory allergies

Dosage General dosing guidelines; consult specific product labeling.

Antitussive/antihistamine: Oral:
Children: 6-11 years:
Liquid: Dextromethorphan 15 mg and chlorpheniramine 2 mg every 6 hours as needed (maximum: 60 mg dextromethorphan and 8 mg chlorpheniramine/24 hours)
Chewable tablet: Dextromethorphan 10 mg and chlorpheniramine 2 mg every 4-6 hours as needed (maximum: 50 mg dextromethorphan and 10 mg chlorpheniramine/24 hours)
Children ≥12 years and Adults: Dextromethorphan 30 mg and chlorpheniramine 4 mg every 6 hours as needed (maximum: 120 mg dextromethorphan and 16 mg chlorpheniramine/24 hours)

Additional Information Complete prescribing information for this medication should be consulted for additional detail.

Dosage Forms Excipient information presented when available (limited, particularly for generics); consult specific product labeling. [DSC] = Discontinued product

Syrup:
Dimetapp® Children's Long Acting Cough Plus Cold: Dextromethorphan hydrobromide 7.5 mg and chlorpheniramine maleate 1 mg per 5 mL (118 mL) [ethanol free, sugar free; contains sodium 3 mg/5 mL, sodium benzoate, propylene glycol; grape flavor]
Robitussin® Children's Cough and Cold Long-Acting: Dextromethorphan hydrobromide 15 mg and chlorpheniramine maleate 2 mg per 5 mL (118 mL) [ethanol free; contains sodium 3 mg/5 mL, sodium benzoate, propylene glycol; fruit punch flavor]
Robitussin® Cough and Cold Long-Acting: Dextromethorphan hydrobromide 7.5 mg and chlorpheniramine maleate 1 mg per 5 mL (118 mL) [ethanol free; contains sodium benzoate, propylene glycol] [DSC]

Scot-Tussin® DM Maximum Strength: Dextromethorphan hydrobromide 15 mg and chlorpheniramine maleate 2 mg per 5 mL (118 mL) [ethanol free, dye free, sugar free; cherry-strawberry flavor]

Tablet:

Coricidin® HBP Cough and Cold: Dextromethorphan hydrobromide 30 mg and chlorpheniramine maleate 4 mg

Tablet, softchew:

Triaminic® Children's Softchews® Cough & Runny Nose: Dextromethorphan hydrobromide 5 mg and chlorpheniramine maleate 1 mg [contains coconut oil, phenylalanine 17.6 mg/softchew, sodium 5 mg/softchew; cherry flavor]

◆ **Dextromethorphan and Guaifenesin** *see* Guaifenesin and Dextromethorphan *on page 810*

Dextromethorphan and Phenylephrine

(deks troe meth OR fan & fen il EF rin)

Brand Names: U.S. PediaCare® Children's Multi-Symptom Cold [OTC]; Safetussin® CD [OTC]; Sudafed PE® Children's Cold & Cough [OTC]; Triaminic Thin Strips® Children's Day Time Cold & Cough [OTC]; Triaminic® Day Time Cold & Cough [OTC]

Index Terms Dextromethorphan Hydrobromide and Phenylephrine Hydrochloride; Phenylephrine and Dextromethorphan

Pharmacologic Category Antitussive; Decongestant

Use Temporary relief of symptoms of hay fever, the common cold, and upper respiratory allergies including sinus/nasal congestion, minor bronchial/throat irritation, and cough

Dosage Oral: Relief of nasal/sinus congestion and cough:

Children:

4-6 years:

PediaCare® Children's Multi-Symptom Cold, Sudafed PE® Children's Cold & Cough, Triaminic® Day Time Cold & Cough: 5 mL every 4 hours as needed (maximum: 30 mL/24 hours)

Triaminic Thin Strips® Children's Day Time Cold & Cough: Allow 1 strip to dissolve on tongue every 4 hours as needed (maximum: 6 strips/24 hours)

6-12 years:

PediaCare® Children's Multi-Symptom Cold, Sudafed PE® Children's Cold & Cough, Triaminic® Day Time Cold & Cough: 10 mL every 4 hours as needed (maximum: 60 mL/24 hours)

Safetussin® CD: 5 mL every 6 hours as needed (maximum: 20 mL/24 hours)

Triaminic Thin Strips® Children's Day Time Cold & Cough: Allow 2 strips to dissolve on tongue every 4 hours as needed (maximum: 12 strips/24 hours)

Children ≥12 years and Adults: Safetussin® CD: 10 mL every 6 hours as needed (maximum: 40 mL/24 hours)

Additional Information Complete prescribing information for this medication should be consulted for additional detail.

Dosage Forms Excipient information presented when available (limited, particularly for generics); consult specific product labeling.

Liquid, oral:

Sudafed PE® Children's Cold & Cough: Dextromethorphan hydrobromide 5 mg and phenylephrine hydrochloride 2.5 mg per 5 mL (118 mL) [ethanol free, sugar free; contains sodium 15 mg/5 mL, sodium benzoate; grape flavor]

Strip, orally disintegrating:

Triaminic Thin Strips® Children's Day Time Cold & Cough: Dextromethorphan hydrobromide 5 mg [equivalent to dextromethorphan 3.67 mg] and phenylephrine hydrochloride 2.5 mg (14s, 16s, 48s) [contains ethanol <0.5%; wild berry flavor]

Syrup:

PediaCare® Children's Multi-Symptom Cold: Dextromethorphan hydrobromide 5 mg and phenylephrine hydrochloride 2.5 mg per 5 mL (118 mL) [contains sodium 15 mg/5 mL; sodium benzoate; grape flavor]

Safetussin® CD: Dextromethorphan hydrobromide 15 mg and phenylephrine hydrochloride 2.5 mg per 5 mL (120 mL), [alcohol free; sugar free; contains menthol, propylene glycol; orange flavor]

Triaminic® Day Time Cold & Cough: Dextromethorphan hydrobromide 5 mg and phenylephrine hydrochloride 2.5 mg per 5 mL (120 mL, 240 mL) [contains benzoic acid; sodium 2 mg/5 mL; propylene glycol; cherry flavor]

◆ **Dextromethorphan and Promethazine** *see* Promethazine and Dextromethorphan *on page 1418*

◆ **Dextromethorphan and Pseudoephedrine** *see* Pseudoephedrine and Dextromethorphan *on page 1431*

Dextromethorphan and Quinidine

(deks troe meth OR fan & KWIN i deen)

Brand Names: U.S. Nuedexta™

Brand Names: Canada Nuedexta™

Index Terms Dextromethorphan Hydrobromide and Quinidine Sulfate; Quinidine and Dextromethorphan

Pharmacologic Category N-Methyl-D-Aspartate Receptor Antagonist

Use Treatment of pseudobulbar affect (PBA)

Pregnancy Risk Factor C

Pregnancy Considerations Adverse events were observed in animal reproduction studies using this combination.

Lactation Use caution

Contraindications Hypersensitivity to dextromethorphan, quinidine, quinine, mefloquine, or any component of the formulation; concomitant use with quinidine or other medications containing quinidine, quinine, or mefloquine; history of quinine-, mefloquine-, or quinidine-induced thrombocytopenia; hepatitis; bone marrow depression; or lupus-like syndrome; concurrent administration with or within 2 weeks of discontinuing an MAO inhibitor; patients with prolonged QT interval, congenital QT syndrome, or history of torsade de pointes; patients with heart failure; concurrent use of drugs that prolong the QT interval and are metabolized by CYP2D6 (eg, pimozide, thioridazine); patients with complete AV block without an implanted pacemaker or patients at high risk of complete AV block

Warnings/Precautions Immune-mediated thrombocytopenia (severe or fatal) may be associated with quinidine use. Unless clearly not drug related, discontinue immediately; continued use may be associated with an increase in fatal hemorrhage. Thrombocytopenia generally resolves within a few days of discontinuation. Therapy should not be restarted in sensitized patients. Agranulocytosis, angioedema, bronchospasm, lupus-like syndrome, rash or other hypersensitivity reactions may be associated with use. Quinidine has also been associated with severe hepatotoxic reactions including granulomatous hepatitis. Use is contraindicated in patients with prior history of immune-mediated thrombocytopenia associated with structurally related drugs (eg, quinine, mefloquine) and in patients with quinidine-, quinine-, or mefloquine-induced lupus-like syndrome.

Concomitant use of moderate or strong CYP3A4 inhibitors may increase quinidine levels and prolong the QT_c interval.

Quinidine inhibits CYP2D6; concomitant use with CYP2D6 substrates may cause an accumulation of concomitantly administered drug and/or reduce active metabolite formation, decreasing their safety and/or efficacy. Use with caution in patients who are poor metabolizers of CYP2D6 metabolized drugs. Quinidine in this combination product is used to inhibit CYP2D6 in order to increase plasma concentrations of dextromethorphan. In patients who are poor metabolizers, this effect would not be significant; however, adverse events related to quinidine may still be observed. Genotyping should be considered in patients considered to be at risk of quinidine toxicity prior to therapy. Symptoms associated with serotonin syndrome such as agitation, confusion, hallucinations, hyper-reflexia, myoclonus, shivering, and tachycardia may occur with concomitant proserotonergic drugs (ie, SSRIs/SNRIs or triptans); especially with higher dextromethorphan doses.

Use caution in patients with left ventricular hypertrophy or left ventricular dysfunction which are more common in patients with chronic hypertension, coronary artery disease or history of stroke; risk of QT_c prolongation may be increased. Use is contraindicated in patients with prolonged QT interval, congenital QT syndrome, or history of torsade de pointes, patients with heart failure, complete AV block without an implanted pacemaker or patients at high risk of complete AV block. Correct hypokalemia or hypomagnesemia prior to therapy. Use caution with medications which may further prolong the QT interval or cause cardiac arrhythmias. Dose dependent QT_c prolongation may occur. Monitor patients at risk following the first dose. Discontinue if arrhythmia occurs.

May cause anticholinergic effects; use caution in patients with myasthenia gravis or other conditions which may be affected. May cause dizziness; use caution in patients with motor impairment or history of falls. Safety and efficacy have not been established with severe hepatic or renal impairment; increased serum concentrations may occur. Has not shown to be safe or effective in other types of commonly occurring emotional labilities (eg, Alzheimer's disease and other dementias). Patients with a history of drug abuse should be monitored closely for signs of abuse/misuse of Nuedexta™ (eg, development of tolerance, increase in dose, or drug-seeking behavior). Abuse of dextromethorphan may cause brain damage, cardiac arrhythmia, loss of consciousness, or death. Periodically reassess the need for treatment; spontaneous improvement of PBA may occur.

Adverse Reactions Also refer to individual agents.

>10%: Gastrointestinal: Diarrhea (13%)

1% to 10%:

- Cardiovascular: Peripheral edema (5%)
- Central nervous system: Dizziness (10%)
- Gastrointestinal: Vomiting (5%), flatulence (3%)
- Genitourinary: Urinary tract infection (4%)
- Hepatic: GGT increased (3%)
- Neuromuscular & skeletal: Weakness (5%)
- Respiratory: Cough (5%)
- Miscellaneous: Influenza (4%)

Drug Interactions

Metabolism/Transport Effects Refer to individual components.

Avoid Concomitant Use

Avoid concomitant use of Dextromethorphan and Quinidine with any of the following: Antifungal Agents (Azole Derivatives, Systemic); Artemether; Conivaptan; Crizotinib; Dronedarone; Lumefantrine; MAO Inhibitors; Mefloquine; Nilotinib; Pimozide; Propafenone; Protease Inhibitors; QUEtiapine; QuiNINE; Silodosin; Tetrabenazine; Thioridazine; Topotecan; Toremifene; Vandetanib; Vemurafenib; Ziprasidone

Increased Effect/Toxicity

Dextromethorphan and Quinidine may increase the levels/effects of: Atomoxetine; Beta-Blockers; Calcium Channel Blockers (Dihydropyridine); Cardiac Glycosides; Colchicine; CYP2D6 Substrates; Dabigatran Etexilate; Dextromethorphan; Dronedarone; Everolimus; Fesoterodine; Haloperidol; Mefloquine; Metoclopramide; Neuromuscular-Blocking Agents; P-glycoprotein/ABCB1 Substrates; Pimozide; Propafenone; QTc-Prolonging Agents; QuiNINE; Rivaroxaban; Serotonin Modulators; Silodosin; Tetrabenazine; Thioridazine; Topotecan; Toremifene; Tricyclic Antidepressants; Vandetanib; Vemurafenib; Verapamil; Vitamin K Antagonists; Ziprasidone

The levels/effects of Dextromethorphan and Quinidine may be increased by: Alfuzosin; Amiodarone; Antacids; Antifungal Agents (Azole Derivatives, Systemic); Antipsychotics; Artemether; Barbiturates; Boceprevir; Calcium Channel Blockers (Dihydropyridine); Carbonic Anhydrase Inhibitors; Chloroquine; Cimetidine; Ciprofloxacin; Ciprofloxacin (Systemic); Conivaptan; Crizotinib; CYP2D6 Inhibitors (Moderate); CYP2D6 Inhibitors (Strong); CYP3A4 Inhibitors (Moderate); CYP3A4 Inhibitors (Strong); Diltiazem; Eribulin; Fingolimod; Fluconazole; Gadobutrol; Haloperidol; Indacaterol; Lumefantrine; Lurasidone; Macrolide Antibiotics; MAO Inhibitors; Nilotinib; P-glycoprotein/ABCB1 Inhibitors; Protease Inhibitors; QUEtiapine; QuiNIDine; QuiNINE; Reserpine; Selective Serotonin Reuptake Inhibitors; Telaprevir; Tricyclic Antidepressants; Verapamil

Decreased Effect

Dextromethorphan and Quinidine may decrease the levels/effects of: Codeine; Dihydrocodeine; Hydrocodone

The levels/effects of Dextromethorphan and Quinidine may be decreased by: Barbiturates; Calcium Channel Blockers (Dihydropyridine); CYP3A4 Inducers (Strong); Cyproterone; Deferasirox; Etravirine; Fosphenytoin; Kaolin; Peginterferon Alfa-2b; P-glycoprotein/ABCB1 Inducers; Phenytoin; Potassium-Sparing Diuretics; Primidone; Rifamycin Derivatives; Sucralfate; Tocilizumab

Ethanol/Nutrition/Herb Interactions

Ethanol: Use caution with ethanol as CNS effects may be enhanced.

Food: Avoid grapefruit juice (may increase levels of quinidine). Avoid tonic water (contains quinine).

Stability Store at controlled room temperature at 25°C (77°F); excursions permitted to 15°C to 30°C (59°F to 86°F).

Mechanism of Action Dextromethorphan may relieve the symptoms of PBA by binding to sigma-1 receptors in the brain which may be involved in behavior, however the exact mechanism of action is not known. Quinidine is used to block the rapid metabolism of dextromethorphan, thereby increasing serum concentrations. The dose of quinidine in this combination product provides serum concentrations 1% to 3% of those needed to treat cardiac arrhythmias.

Pharmacodynamics/Kinetics

Absorption: Bioavailability of dextromethorphan increased ~20-fold when administered with quinidine.

Protein binding: Dextromethorphan: 60% to 70%; Quinidine: 80% to 89%

Metabolism: Dextromethorphan: Hepatic via CYP2D6 to dextrorphan (active); Quinidine: Hepatic via CYP3A4 to 3-hydroxyquinidine (active) and other metabolites

Half-life elimination: Dextromethorphan: 13 hours in extensive metabolizers; Quinidine: 7 hours in extensive metabolizers

Time to peak: Dextromethorphan: 3-4 hours; Quinidine: 1-2 hours

Excretion: Urine

Dosage Oral: Adults: Pseudobulbar affect: One capsule once daily for 7 days, then increase to 1 capsule twice daily; reassess patient periodically to determine if continued use is necessary

Dosage adjustment in renal impairment: Dose adjustment not required for mild or moderate renal impairment; not studied with severe impairment

Dosage adjustment in hepatic impairment: Dose adjustment not required for mild or moderate hepatic impairment; however, an increase in adverse reactions is observed with moderate hepatic dysfunction; not studied with severe impairment

Dietary Considerations May be taken with or without food. Avoid grapefruit juice.

Administration May be administered with or without food. Administer twice-daily doses every 12 hours.

Monitoring Parameters QT interval 3-4 hours after the first dose in patients at risk for QTc prolongation; potassium and magnesium prior to and during therapy; CBC, liver and renal function tests; periodically assess risk factors for arrhythmias during treatment; periodically reassess the need for treatment (spontaneous improvement of PBA may occur)

Dosage Forms Excipient information presented when available (limited, particularly for generics); consult specific product labeling.

Capsule, oral:

Nuedexta™: Dextromethorphan hydrobromide 20 mg and quinidine sulfate 10 mg

◆ **Dextromethorphan, Chlorpheniramine, and Phenylephrine** *see* Chlorpheniramine, Phenylephrine, and Dextromethorphan *on page* 346

◆ **Dextromethorphan, Chlorpheniramine, and Pseudoephedrine** *see* Chlorpheniramine, Pseudoephedrine, and Dextromethorphan *on page* 347

◆ **Dextromethorphan, Guaifenesin, and Pseudoephedrine** *see* Guaifenesin, Pseudoephedrine, and Dextromethorphan *on page* 814

◆ **Dextromethorphan Hydrobromide and Chlorpheniramine Maleate** *see* Dextromethorphan and Chlorpheniramine *on page* 489

◆ **Dextromethorphan Hydrobromide and Phenylephrine Hydrochloride** *see* Dextromethorphan and Phenylephrine *on page* 490

◆ **Dextromethorphan Hydrobromide and Quinidine Sulfate** *see* Dextromethorphan and Quinidine *on page* 490

◆ **Dex-Tuss** *see* Guaifenesin and Codeine *on page* 810

◆ **Dezocitidine** *see* Decitabine *on page* 460

◆ **dFdC** *see* Gemcitabine *on page* 782

◆ **dFdCyd** *see* Gemcitabine *on page* 782

◆ **DFMO** *see* Eflornithine *on page* 577

◆ **DHAD** *see* MitoXANtrone *on page* 1145

◆ **DHAQ** *see* MitoXANtrone *on page* 1145

◆ **DHE** *see* Dihydroergotamine *on page* 508

◆ **D.H.E. 45®** *see* Dihydroergotamine *on page* 508

◆ **DHPG Sodium** *see* Ganciclovir (Systemic) *on page* 778

◆ **Diabeta** *see* GlyBURIDE *on page* 799

◆ **DiaBeta®** *see* GlyBURIDE *on page* 799

◆ **DiabetAid® Antifungal Foot Bath [OTC]** *see* Miconazole (Topical) *on page* 1126

◆ **Diabetic Siltussin DAS-Na [OTC]** *see* GuaiFENesin *on page* 809

◆ **Diabetic Siltussin-DM DAS-Na [OTC]** *see* Guaifenesin and Dextromethorphan *on page* 810

◆ **Diabetic Siltussin-DM DAS-Na Maximum Strength [OTC]** *see* Guaifenesin and Dextromethorphan *on page* 810

◆ **Diabetic Tussin® DM [OTC]** *see* Guaifenesin and Dextromethorphan *on page* 810

◆ **Diabetic Tussin® DM Maximum Strength [OTC]** *see* Guaifenesin and Dextromethorphan *on page* 810

◆ **Diabetic Tussin® EX [OTC]** *see* GuaiFENesin *on page* 809

◆ **Diaminocyclohexane Oxalatoplatinum** *see* Oxaliplatin *on page* 1257

◆ **Diaminodiphenylsulfone** *see* Dapsone (Systemic) *on page* 445

◆ **Diamode [OTC]** *see* Loperamide *on page* 1026

◆ **Diamox® (Can)** *see* AcetaZOLAMIDE *on page* 32

◆ **Diamox® Sequels®** *see* AcetaZOLAMIDE *on page* 32

◆ **Diarr-Eze (Can)** *see* Loperamide *on page* 1026

◆ **Diastat®** *see* Diazepam *on page* 492

◆ **Diastat® AcuDial™** *see* Diazepam *on page* 492

◆ **Diastat® Rectal Delivery System (Can)** *see* Diazepam *on page* 492

◆ **Diazemuls® (Can)** *see* Diazepam *on page* 492

Diazepam (dye AZ e pam)

Brand Names: U.S. Diastat®; Diastat® AcuDial™; Diazepam Intensol™; Valium®

Brand Names: Canada Apo-Diazepam®; Diastat®; Diastat® Rectal Delivery System; Diazemuls®; Novo-Dipam; Valium®

Pharmacologic Category Benzodiazepine

Additional Appendix Information

Beers Criteria – Potentially Inappropriate Medications for Geriatrics *on page* 1973

Benzodiazepines *on page* 1882

Patient Information for Disposal of Unused Medications *on page* 2026

Status Epilepticus *on page* 2010

Use Management of anxiety disorders, ethanol withdrawal symptoms; skeletal muscle relaxant; treatment of convulsive disorders; preoperative or preprocedural sedation and amnesia

Rectal gel: Management of selected, refractory epilepsy patients on stable regimens of antiepileptic drugs requiring intermittent use of diazepam to control episodes of increased seizure activity

Unlabeled Use Panic disorders; short-term treatment of spasticity in children with cerebral palsy; sedation for mechanically-ventilated patients in the intensive care unit

Pregnancy Risk Factor D

Pregnancy Considerations Teratogenic effects have been reported in animal studies. In humans, diazepam and its metabolites (N-desmethyldiazepam, temazepam, and oxazepam) cross the placenta. Teratogenic effects have been observed with diazepam; however, additional studies are needed. The incidence of premature birth and low birth weights may be increased following maternal use of benzodiazepines; hypoglycemia and respiratory problems in the neonate may occur following exposure late in pregnancy. Neonatal withdrawal symptoms may occur within days to weeks after birth and "floppy infant syndrome" (which also includes withdrawal symptoms) has been reported with some benzodiazepines (including diazepam).

Lactation Enters breast milk/not recommended (AAP rates "of concern"; AAP 2001 update pending)

Contraindications Hypersensitivity to diazepam or any component of the formulation (cross-sensitivity with other benzodiazepines may exist); myasthenia gravis; severe respiratory insufficiency; severe hepatic insufficiency; sleep apnea syndrome; acute narrow-angle glaucoma; not for use in children <6 months of age (oral)

Warnings/Precautions Withdrawal has also been associated with an increase in the seizure frequency. Use with caution with drugs which may decrease diazepam metabolism. Use with caution in debilitated patients, obese patients, patients with hepatic disease (including alcoholics), or renal impairment. Active metabolites with extended half-lives may lead to delayed accumulation and adverse effects. Use with caution in patients with respiratory disease or impaired gag reflex.

Acute hypotension, muscle weakness, apnea, and cardiac arrest have occurred with parenteral administration. Acute effects may be more prevalent in patients receiving concurrent barbiturates, narcotics, or ethanol. Appropriate resuscitative equipment and qualified personnel should be available during administration and monitoring. Avoid use of the injection in patients with shock, coma, or acute ethanol intoxication. Intra-arterial injection or extravasation of the parenteral formulation should be avoided. Parenteral formulation contains propylene glycol, which has been associated with toxicity when administered in high dosages. Administration of rectal gel should only be performed by individuals trained to recognize characteristic seizure activity and monitor response.

Causes CNS depression (dose-related) resulting in sedation, dizziness, confusion, or ataxia which may impair physical and mental capabilities. Patients must be cautioned about performing tasks which require mental alertness (eg, operating machinery or driving). Use with caution in patients receiving other CNS depressants or psychoactive agents. Effects with other sedative drugs or ethanol may be potentiated. The dosage of narcotics should be reduced by approximately 1/3 when diazepam is added. Benzodiazepines have been associated with falls and traumatic injury and should be used with extreme caution in patients who are at risk of these events (especially the elderly). Benzodiazepines with long half-lives may produce prolonged sedation and increase the risk of falls and fracture. Short- or intermediate-acting benzodiazepines are preferred in elderly patients (Beers Criteria).

Use with caution in patients taking strong CYP3A4 inhibitors, moderate or strong CYP3A4 and CYP2C19 inducers and major CYP3A4 substrates.

Use caution in patients with depression or anxiety associated with depression, particularly if suicidal risk may be present. Use with caution in patients with a history of drug dependence. Benzodiazepines have been associated with dependence and acute withdrawal symptoms on discontinuation or reduction in dose. Acute withdrawal, including seizures, may be precipitated in patients after administration of flumazenil to patients receiving long-term benzodiazepine therapy.

Diazepam has been associated with anterograde amnesia. Psychiatric and paradoxical reactions, including hyperactive or aggressive behavior, have been reported with benzodiazepines, particularly in adolescent/pediatric or elderly patients. Does not have analgesic, antidepressant, or antipsychotic properties.

Rectal gel: Safety and efficacy have not been established in children <2 years of age.

Oral: Safety and efficacy have not been established in children <6 months of age.

Injection: Safety and efficacy have not been established in children <30 days of age. Solution for injection may contain sodium benzoate, benzyl alcohol, or benzoic acid. Large amounts have been associated with "gasping syndrome" in neonates.

Adverse Reactions Frequency not defined. Adverse reactions may vary by route of administration.

Cardiovascular: Hypotension, vasodilatation

Central nervous system: Amnesia, ataxia, confusion, depression, drowsiness, fatigue, headache, slurred speech, paradoxical reactions (eg, aggressiveness, agitation, anxiety, delusions, hallucinations, inappropriate behavior, increased muscle spasms, insomnia, irritability, psychoses, rage, restlessness, sleep disturbances, stimulation), vertigo

Dermatologic: Rash

Endocrine & metabolic: Libido changes

Gastrointestinal: Constipation, diarrhea, nausea, salivation changes (dry mouth or hypersalivation)

Genitourinary: Incontinence, urinary retention

Hepatic: Jaundice

Local: Phlebitis, pain with injection

Neuromuscular & skeletal: Dysarthria, tremor, weakness

Ocular: Blurred vision, diplopia

Respiratory: Apnea, asthma, respiratory rate decreased

Drug Interactions

Metabolism/Transport Effects **Substrate** of CYP1A2 (minor), CYP2B6 (minor), CYP2C19 (major), CYP2C9 (minor), CYP3A4 (major); **Note:** Assignment of Major/Minor substrate status based on clinically relevant drug interaction potential; **Inhibits** CYP2C19 (weak), CYP3A4 (weak)

Avoid Concomitant Use

Avoid concomitant use of Diazepam with any of the following: Conivaptan; OLANZapine; Pimozide

Increased Effect/Toxicity

Diazepam may increase the levels/effects of: Alcohol (Ethyl); CloZAPine; CNS Depressants; Fosphenytoin; Methotrimeprazine; Phenytoin; Pimozide; Selective Serotonin Reuptake Inhibitors

The levels/effects of Diazepam may be increased by: Antifungal Agents (Azole Derivatives, Systemic); Aprepitant; Calcium Channel Blockers (Nondihydropyridine); Cimetidine; Conivaptan; Contraceptives (Estrogens); Contraceptives (Progestins); CYP2C19 Inhibitors (Moderate); CYP2C19 Inhibitors (Strong); CYP3A4 Inhibitors (Moderate); CYP3A4 Inhibitors (Strong); Dasatinib; Disulfiram; Droperidol; Fluconazole; Fosamprenavir; Fosaprepitant; Grapefruit Juice; HydrOXYzine; Isoniazid; Macrolide Antibiotics; Methotrimeprazine; Nefazodone; OLANZapine; Proton Pump Inhibitors; Ritonavir; Saquinavir; Selective Serotonin Reuptake Inhibitors

Decreased Effect

The levels/effects of Diazepam may be decreased by: CarBAMazepine; CYP2C19 Inducers (Strong); CYP3A4 Inducers (Strong); Cyproterone; Deferasirox; Rifamycin Derivatives; St Johns Wort; Theophylline Derivatives; Tocilizumab; Yohimbine

Ethanol/Nutrition/Herb Interactions

Ethanol: May increase CNS depression; monitor for increased effects with coadministration. Caution patients about effects.

Food: Diazepam serum concentrations may be increased if taken with food. Grapefruit juice may increase diazepam serum concentrations; avoid concurrent use.

Herb/Nutraceutical: St John's wort may decrease diazepam levels. Avoid valerian, St John's wort, kava kava, gotu kola (may increase CNS depression).

Stability

Injection: Store at 20° to 25°C (68° to 77°F); excursions permitted to 15°C to 30°C (59°F to 86°F). Protect from light. Potency is retained for up to 3 months when kept at room temperature. Most stable at pH 4-8; hydrolysis occurs at pH <3. Per manufacturer, do not mix I.V. product with other medications.

Rectal gel: Store at 25°C (77°F); excursion permitted to 15°C to 30°C (59°F to 86°F).

Tablet: Store at 15°C to 30°C (59°F to 86°F).

Mechanism of Action Binds to stereospecific benzodiazepine receptors on the postsynaptic GABA neuron at several sites within the central nervous system, including the limbic system, reticular formation. Enhancement of the inhibitory effect of GABA on neuronal excitability results by increased neuronal membrane permeability to chloride ions. This shift in chloride ions results in hyperpolarization (a less excitable state) and stabilization.

Pharmacodynamics/Kinetics

I.V.: Status epilepticus:
- Onset of action: Almost immediate
- Duration: 20-30 minutes

Absorption: Oral: 85% to 100%, more reliable than I.M.

Protein binding: 98%

Metabolism: Hepatic

Half-life elimination: Parent drug: Adults: 20-50 hours; increased half-life in neonates, elderly, and those with severe hepatic disorders; Active major metabolite (desmethyldiazepam): 50-100 hours; may be prolonged in neonates

Dosage Oral absorption is more reliable than I.M.

Children:

Conscious sedation for procedures: Oral: 0.2-0.3 mg/kg (maximum: 10 mg) 45-60 minutes prior to procedure

Muscle spasm associated with tetanus: I.V., I.M.:
- Infants >30 days and Children <5 years: 1-2 mg/dose every 3-4 hours as needed
- Children ≥5 years: 5-10 mg/dose every 3-4 hours as needed

Sedation/muscle relaxant/anxiety:
- Oral: 0.12-0.8 mg/kg/day in divided doses every 6-8 hours
- I.M., I.V.: 0.04-0.3 mg/kg/dose every 2-4 hours to a maximum of 0.6 mg/kg within an 8-hour period if needed

Spasticity in cerebral palsy (unlabeled use): Oral: Dose should be individualized:
- Children ≤5 years: <8.5 kg: 0.5-1 mg at bedtime; 8.5-15 kg: 1-2 mg at bedtime (Mathew, 2005)
- Children 5-16 years: 1.25 mg 3 times daily to 5 mg 4 times daily (Engle, 1966)

Status epilepticus:
- I.V.: Infants >30 days and Children: 0.1-0.3 mg/kg (maximum dose: 10 mg) given over ≤5 mg/minute; may repeat dose after 5-10 minutes (Hegenbarth, 2008)
  - Manufacturer's recommendations:
    - Infants >30 days and Children <5 years: 0.2-0.5 mg given slowly every 2-5 minutes (maximum total dose: 5 mg); repeat in 2-4 hours if needed
    - Children ≥5 years: 1 mg given slowly every 2-5 minutes (maximum total dose: 10 mg); repeat in 2-4 hours if needed
- Rectal gel: 0.5 mg/kg, then 0.25 mg/kg in 10 minutes if needed (maximum dose: 20 mg) (Hegenbarth, 2008).

Anticonvulsant (acute treatment): Rectal gel:
- Children <2 years: Safety and efficacy have not been studied
- Children 2-5 years: 0.5 mg/kg (maximum dose: 20 mg)
- Children 6-11 years: 0.3 mg/kg (maximum dose: 20 mg)
- Children ≥12 years: 0.2 mg/kg (maximum dose: 20 mg)
- **Note:** Dosage should be rounded upward to the next available dose, 2.5, 5, 7.5, 10, 12.5, 15, 17.5, and 20 mg/dose; dose may be repeated in 4-12 hours if needed; do not use for more than 5 episodes per month or more than one episode every 5 days

Adolescents: Conscious sedation for procedures:
- Oral: 10 mg
- I.V.: 5 mg, may repeat with 1/2 dose if needed

Adults:

Acute ethanol withdrawal: Oral: 10 mg 3-4 times during first 24 hours, then decrease to 5 mg 3-4 times/day as needed

Anticonvulsant (acute treatment): Rectal gel: 0.2 mg/kg
- **Note:** Dosage should be rounded upward to the next available dose, 2.5, 5, 7.5, 10, 12.5, 15, 17.5, and 20 mg/dose; dose may be repeated in 4-12 hours if needed; do not use for more than 5 episodes per month or more than one episode every 5 days.

Anxiety (symptoms/disorders): Oral, I.M, I.V.: 2-10 mg 2-4 times/day if needed

Muscle spasm: I.V., I.M.: Initial: 5-10 mg; then 5-10 mg in 3-4 hours, if necessary. Larger doses may be required if associated with tetanus.

Sedation in the ICU patient: I.V.: 0.03-0.1 mg/kg every 30 minutes to 6 hours (Jacobi, 2002)

Skeletal muscle relaxant (adjunct therapy): Oral: 2-10 mg 3-4 times/day

Status epilepticus:
- I.V.: 5-10 mg every 5-10 minutes given over ≤5 mg/minute; maximum dose: 30 mg
- Rectal gel: Premonitory/Out-of-hospital treatment: 10 mg once; may repeat once if necessary (Kälviäinen, 2007)

Rapid tranquilization of agitated patient (administer every 30-60 minutes): Oral: 5-10 mg; average total dose for tranquilization: 20-60 mg

Elderly/debilitated patients:
- Oral: 2-2.5 mg 1-2 times/day initially; increase gradually as needed and tolerated
- Rectal gel: Due to the increased half-life in elderly and debilitated patients, consider reducing dose.

Dosing adjustment in renal impairment: No dose adjustment recommended; decrease dose if administered for prolonged periods.
- I.V.: Risk of propylene glycol toxicity; monitor closely if using for prolonged periods or at high doses
- Hemodialysis: Not dialyzable (0% to 5%); supplemental dose is not necessary

Dosing adjustment in hepatic impairment: Decrease maintenance dose by 50%; half-life significantly prolonged.

Administration Intensol™ should be diluted before use.

Continuous infusion is not recommended because of precipitation in I.V. fluids and absorption of drug into infusion bags and tubing. In children, do not exceed 1-2 mg/minute IVP; adults 5 mg/minute.

Rectal gel: Prior to administration, confirm that prescribed dose is visible and correct, and that the green "ready" band is visible. Patient should be positioned on side (facing person responsible for monitoring), with top leg bent forward. Insert rectal tip (lubricated) into rectum and push in plunger gently over 3 seconds. Remove tip of rectal syringe after 3 additional seconds. Buttocks should be held together for 3 seconds after removal. Dispose of syringe appropriately.

Monitoring Parameters Respiratory, cardiovascular, and mental status; check for orthostasis

Reference Range Therapeutic: Diazepam: 0.2-1.5 mcg/mL (SI: 0.7-5.3 micromole/L); N-desmethyldiazepam (nordiazepam): 0.1-0.5 mcg/mL (SI: 0.35-1.8 micromole/L)

Test Interactions False-negative urinary glucose determinations when using Clinistix® or Diastix®

Additional Information Diazepam does not have any analgesic effects.

Diastat® AcuDial™: When dispensing, consult package information for directions on setting patient's dose; confirm green "ready" band is visible prior to dispensing product.

Dosage Forms Excipient information presented when available (limited, particularly for generics); consult specific product labeling.

Gel, rectal [adult rectal tip (6 cm)]: 20 mg (4 mL) [delivers set doses of 12.5 mg, 15 mg, 17.5 mg, 20 mg]

Diastat® AcuDial™: 20 mg (4 mL) [contains benzoic acid, benzyl alcohol, ethanol 10%, propylene glycol, sodium benzoate; 5 mg/mL (delivers set doses of 12.5 mg, 15 mg, 17.5 mg, and 20 mg)]

Gel, rectal [pediatric rectal tip (4.4 cm)]: 5 mg/mL (0.5 mL)

Diastat®: 5 mg/mL (0.5 mL) [contains benzoic acid, benzyl alcohol, ethanol 10%, propylene glycol, sodium benzoate]

Gel, rectal [pediatric/adult rectal tip (4.4 cm)]: 10 mg (2 mL) [delivers set doses of 5 mg, 7.5 mg, 10 mg]

Diastat® AcuDial™: 10 mg (2 mL) [contains benzoic acid, benzyl alcohol, ethanol 10%, propylene glycol, sodium benzoate; 5 mg/mL (delivers set doses of 5 mg, 7.5 mg, and 10 mg)]

Injection, solution: 5 mg/mL (2 mL, 10 mL)

Solution, oral: 5 mg/5 mL (5 mL, 500 mL)

Solution, oral [concentrate]:

Diazepam Intensol™: 5 mg/mL (30 mL) [contains ethanol 19%, propylene glycol]

Tablet, oral: 2 mg, 5 mg, 10 mg

Valium®: 5 mg, 10 mg [scored]

Valium®: 2 mg [scored; dye free]

Controlled Substance C-IV

◆ **Diazepam Intensol™** *see* Diazepam *on page 492*

Diazoxide (dye az OKS ide)

Brand Names: U.S. Proglycem®

Brand Names: Canada Proglycem®

Pharmacologic Category Antihypoglycemic Agent; Vasodilator, Direct-Acting

Use Hypoglycemia related to islet cell adenoma, carcinoma, hyperplasia, or adenomatosis; nesidioblastosis; leucine sensitivity; extrapancreatic malignancy

Pregnancy Risk Factor C

Dosage Oral: Hyperinsulinemic hypoglycemia:

Newborns and Infants: Initial dose: 10 mg/kg/day; dosing range: 8-15 mg/kg/day in divided doses every 8-12 hours

Children and Adults: Initial dose: 3 mg/kg/day; dosing range: 3-8 mg/kg/day in divided doses every 8-12 hours. **Note:** In certain instances, patients with refractory hypoglycemia may require higher doses.

Dosing adjustment in renal impairment: Half-life may be prolonged with renal impairment; a reduced dose should be considered.

Additional Information Complete prescribing information for this medication should be consulted for additional detail.

Dosage Forms Excipient information presented when available (limited, particularly for generics); consult specific product labeling.

Suspension, oral:

Proglycem®: 50 mg/mL (30 mL) [contains ethanol ~7.25%, propylene glycol, sodium benzoate; chocolate-mint flavor]

Dosage Forms: Canada Excipient information presented when available (limited, particularly for generics); consult specific product labeling.

Capsule, oral:

Proglycem®: 50 mg

◆ **Dibenzyline®** *see* Phenoxybenzamine *on page 1341*

◆ **DIC** *see* Dacarbazine *on page 438*

◆ **Dicel® Chewable [OTC]** *see* Chlorpheniramine and Pseudoephedrine *on page 346*

◆ **Dicel® DM Chewable [OTC]** *see* Chlorpheniramine, Pseudoephedrine, and Dextromethorphan *on page 347*

◆ **Dicel® DM Suspension** *see* Chlorpheniramine, Pseudoephedrine, and Dextromethorphan *on page 347*

◆ **Dicel® Suspension** *see* Chlorpheniramine and Pseudoephedrine *on page 346*

Diclofenac (Systemic) (dye KLOE fen ak)

Brand Names: U.S. Cambia™; Cataflam®; Voltaren®-XR; Zipsor™

Brand Names: Canada Apo-Diclo Rapide®; Apo-Diclo®; Apo-Diclo® SR®; Cataflam®; Diclofenac ECT; Diclofenac Sodium; Diclofenac Sodium SR; Diclofenac SR; Dom-Diclofenac; Dom-Diclofenac SR; Novo-Difenac ECT; Novo-Difenac K; Novo-Difenac Suppositories; Novo-Difenac-SR; Nu-Diclo; Nu-Diclo-SR; PMS-Diclofenac; PMS-Diclofenac SR; PMS-Diclofenac-K; PRO-Diclo-Rapide; Sandoz-Diclofenac; Sandoz-Diclofenac Rapide; Sandoz-Diclofenac SR; Voltaren Rapide®; Voltaren SR®; Voltaren®

Index Terms Diclofenac Potassium; Diclofenac Sodium; Voltaren

Pharmacologic Category Nonsteroidal Anti-inflammatory Drug (NSAID); Nonsteroidal Anti-inflammatory Drug (NSAID), Oral

Use

Capsule: Relief of mild-to-moderate acute pain

Immediate-release tablet: Relief of mild-to-moderate pain; primary dysmenorrhea; acute and chronic treatment of rheumatoid arthritis, osteoarthritis

Delayed-release tablet: Acute and chronic treatment of rheumatoid arthritis, osteoarthritis, ankylosing spondylitis

Extended-release tablet: Chronic treatment of osteoarthritis, rheumatoid arthritis

Oral solution: Treatment of acute migraine with or without aura

Suppository (CAN; not available in U.S.): Symptomatic treatment of rheumatoid arthritis and osteoarthritis (including degenerative joint disease of hip)

Unlabeled Use Juvenile idiopathic arthritis (JIA)

Pregnancy Risk Factor C (oral)/D (≥30 weeks gestation [oral])

Pregnancy Considerations Adverse events were not observed in the initial animal reproduction studies; therefore, manufacturers classify most dosage forms of diclofenac as pregnancy category C (oral: category D ≥30 weeks gestation). Diclofenac crosses the placenta and can be detected in fetal tissue and amniotic fluid. NSAID exposure during the first trimester is not strongly associated with congenital malformations; however, cardiovascular anomalies and cleft palate have been observed following NSAID exposure in some studies. The use of a NSAID close to conception may be associated with an increased risk of miscarriage. Nonteratogenic effects have been observed following NSAID administration during the third trimester including: Myocardial degenerative changes, prenatal constriction of the ductus arteriosus, fetal tricuspid regurgitation, failure of the ductus arteriosus to close postnatally; renal dysfunction or failure, oligohydramnios; gastrointestinal bleeding or perforation, increased risk of necrotizing enterocolitis; intracranial bleeding (including intraventricular hemorrhage), platelet dysfunction with resultant bleeding; pulmonary hypertension. Because they may cause premature closure of the ductus arteriosus, use of NSAIDs late in pregnancy should be avoided (use after 31 or 32 weeks gestation is not recommended by some clinicians). Product labeling for Zipsor™ specifically notes that use at ≥30 weeks gestation should be avoided and, therefore, classifies diclofenac as pregnancy category D at this time. Use in the third trimester is contraindicated in the Canadian labeling. The chronic use of NSAIDs in women of reproductive age may be associated with infertility that is reversible upon discontinuation of the medication. A registry is available for pregnant women exposed to autoimmune medications including diclofenac. For additional information contact the Organization of Teratology Information Specialists, OTIS Autoimmune Diseases Study, at 877-311-8972

Lactation Excreted in breast milk/not recommended

Medication Guide Available Yes

Contraindications Hypersensitivity to diclofenac or any component of the formulation; hypersensitivity to bovine protein (capsule formulation only); patients who exhibit asthma, urticaria, or other allergic-type reactions after taking aspirin or other NSAIDs; perioperative pain in the setting of coronary artery bypass graft (CABG) surgery

Canadian labeling: Additional contraindications (not in U.S. labeling): Uncontrolled heart failure, active gastric/duodenal/peptic ulcer; active GI bleed or perforation; regional ulcer, gastritis, or ulcerative colitis; cerebrovascular bleeding or other bleeding disorders; inflammatory bowel disease; severe hepatic impairment; active hepatic disease; severe renal impairment (Cl_{cr} <30 mL/minute) or deteriorating renal disease; known hyperkalemia; patients <16 years of age; breast-feeding; pregnancy (third trimester); use of diclofenac suppository if recent history of bleeding or inflammatory lesions of rectum/anus

Warnings/Precautions [U.S. Boxed Warning]: NSAIDs are associated with an increased risk of adverse cardiovascular thrombotic events, including MI and stroke. Risk may be increased with duration of use or pre-existing cardiovascular risk factors or disease. Carefully evaluate individual cardiovascular risk profiles prior to prescribing. May cause new-onset hypertension or worsening of existing hypertension. Monitor blood pressure closely. Use caution with fluid retention. Avoid use in heart failure. Concurrent administration of ibuprofen, and potentially other nonselective NSAIDs, may interfere with aspirin's cardioprotective effect. **[U.S. Boxed Warning]: Use is contraindicated for treatment of perioperative pain in the setting of coronary artery bypass graft (CABG) surgery.** Risk of MI and stroke may be increased with use following CABG surgery.

NSAID use may compromise existing renal function; dose-dependent decreases in prostaglandin synthesis may result from NSAID use, reducing renal blood flow which may cause renal decompensation. NSAID use may increase the risk for hyperkalemia. Patients with impaired renal function, dehydration, heart failure, liver dysfunction, those taking diuretics and ACEI, and the elderly are at greater risk of renal toxicity and hyperkalemia. Rehydrate patient before starting therapy; monitor renal function closely. Not recommended for use in patients with advanced renal disease. Long-term NSAID use may result in renal papillary necrosis while persistent urinary symptoms (eg, dysuria, bladder pain), cystitis, or hematuria may occur anytime after initiating NSAID therapy. Discontinue therapy with symptom onset and evaluate for origin.

[U.S. Boxed Warning]: NSAIDs may increase risk of gastrointestinal irritation, inflammation, ulceration, bleeding, and perforation. These events may occur at any time during therapy and without warning. Use caution with a history of GI disease (bleeding or ulcers), concurrent therapy with aspirin, anticoagulants and/or corticosteroids, smoking, use of alcohol, the elderly or debilitated patients. When used concomitantly with ≤325 mg of aspirin, a substantial increase in the risk of gastrointestinal complications (eg, ulcer) occurs; concomitant gastroprotective therapy (eg, proton pump inhibitors) is recommended (Bhatt, 2008).

Use the lowest effective dose for the shortest duration of time, consistent with individual patient goals, to reduce risk of cardiovascular or GI adverse events. Alternate therapies should be considered for patients at high risk.

NSAIDs may cause photosensitivity or serious skin adverse events including exfoliative dermatitis, Stevens-Johnson syndrome (SJS), and toxic epidermal necrolysis (TEN); discontinue use at first sign of skin rash or hypersensitivity. Anaphylactoid reactions may occur, even without prior exposure; patients with "aspirin triad" (bronchial asthma, aspirin intolerance, rhinitis) may be at increased risk. Do not use in patients who experience bronchospasm, asthma, rhinitis, or urticaria with NSAID or aspirin therapy. Use caution in other forms of asthma. Platelet adhesion and aggregation may be decreased; may prolong bleeding time; patients with coagulation disorders or who are receiving anticoagulants should be monitored closely. Anemia may occur; patients on long-term NSAID therapy should be monitored for anemia. Rarely, NSAID use may cause severe blood dyscrasias (eg, agranulocytosis, aplastic anemia, thrombocytopenia).

Use with caution in patients with impaired hepatic function. Closely monitor patients with any abnormal LFT. Diclofenac can cause transaminase elevations; initiate monitoring 4-8 weeks into therapy. Rarely, severe hepatic reactions (eg, fulminant hepatitis, liver failure) have occurred; discontinue all formulations if signs or symptoms of liver disease develop, or if systemic manifestations occur. Use with caution in hepatic porphyria (may trigger attack).

NSAIDS may cause drowsiness, dizziness, blurred vision, and other neurologic effects which may impair physical or mental abilities; patients must be cautioned about performing tasks which require mental alertness (eg, operating machinery or driving). Discontinue use with blurred or diminished vision and perform ophthalmologic exam. Monitor vision with long-term therapy. The elderly are at increased risk for adverse effects (especially peptic ulceration, CNS effects, and renal toxicity) from NSAIDs even at low doses. May increase the risk of aseptic meningitis, especially in patients with systemic lupus erythematosus (SLE) and mixed connective tissue disorders.

Withhold for at least 4-6 half-lives prior to surgical or dental procedures. Safety and efficacy have not been established in children.

Capsule: Contains gelatin; use is contraindicated in patients with history of hypersensitivity to bovine protein.

Oral solution: Only indicated for the acute treatment of migraine; not indicated for migraine prophylaxis or cluster headache. Not bioequivalent to other forms of diclofenac (even same dose); do not interchange products. Contains phenylalanine.

Adverse Reactions

Oral:

1% to 10%:

Cardiovascular: Edema
Central nervous system: Dizziness, headache
Dermatologic: Pruritus, rash
Endocrine & metabolic: Fluid retention
Gastrointestinal: Abdominal distension, abdominal pain, constipation, diarrhea, dyspepsia, flatulence, GI perforation, heartburn, nausea, peptic ulcer/GI bleed, vomiting
Hematologic: Anemia, bleeding time increased
Hepatic: Liver enzyme abnormalities (>3 x ULN; ≤4%)
Otic: Tinnitus
Renal: Renal function abnormal

Miscellaneous: Diaphoresis increased

<1% (Limited to important or life-threatening): Agranulocytosis, alopecia, anaphylactoid reactions, anaphylaxis, angioedema, aplastic anemia, anxiety, appetite changes, arrhythmia, aseptic meningitis, asthma, azotemia, blurred vision, chest pain, CHF, colitis, coma, confusion, conjunctivitis, cystitis, depression, diplopia, disorientation, dreams abnormal, drowsiness, dyspnea, dysuria, ecchymosis, eosinophilia, eructation, erythema multiforme, esophageal lesions, esophagitis, exfoliative dermatitis, fever, fulminant hepatitis, gastritis, glossitis,hallucination, hearing impairment, hearing loss, hematemesis, hematuria, hemoglobin decreased, hemolytic anemia, hepatic failure, hepatic necrosis, hepatitis, hepatotoxicity, hyper-/hypotension, hyper-/hypoglycemia, infection, insomnia, interstitial nephritis, intestinal perforation, jaundice, laryngeal edema, leukopenia, lymphadenopathy, malaise, melena, memory disturbance, meningitis, MI, nephrotic syndrome, nervousness, oliguria, palpitation, pancreatitis, pancytopenia, paresthesia, pharynx edema, photosensitivity, pneumonia, polyuria, proteinuria, psychotic reactions, purpura, rectal bleeding, renal failure, renal papillary necrosis, respiratory depression, seizure, sepsis, somnolence, Stevens-Johnson syndrome, stomatitis, stroke, swelling of lips and tongue, syncope, tachycardia, taste disorder, thrombocytopenia, toxic epidermal necrolysis, tremor, urticaria, vasculitis, vertigo, weight change, weakness, xerostomia

Rectal suppository (CAN; not available in U.S.):

Also refer to adverse reactions associated with oral formulations.

<1%, postmarketing, and/or case reports: Local: Bleeding, hemorrhoid exacerbation, proctitis, rectal irritation

Drug Interactions

Metabolism/Transport Effects **Substrate** of CYP1A2 (minor), CYP2B6 (minor), CYP2C19 (minor), CYP2C8 (minor), CYP2C9 (minor), CYP2D6 (minor), CYP3A4 (minor); **Note:** Assignment of Major/Minor substrate status based on clinically relevant drug interaction potential; **Inhibits** CYP1A2 (moderate), CYP2C9 (weak), CYP2E1 (weak), CYP3A4 (weak)

Avoid Concomitant Use

Avoid concomitant use of Diclofenac (Systemic) with any of the following: Floctafenine; Ketorolac; Ketorolac (Nasal); Ketorolac (Systemic); Pimozide

Increased Effect/Toxicity

Diclofenac (Systemic) may increase the levels/effects of: Aminoglycosides; Anticoagulants; Antiplatelet Agents; Bisphosphonate Derivatives; Collagenase (Systemic); CycloSPORINE; CycloSPORINE (Systemic); CYP1A2 Substrates; Deferasirox; Desmopressin; Digoxin; Drotrecogin Alfa (Activated); Eplerenone; Haloperidol; Ibritumomab; Lithium; Methotrexate; Nonsteroidal Anti-Inflammatory Agents; PEMEtrexed; Pimozide; Porfimer; Potassium-Sparing Diuretics; PRALAtrexate; Quinolone Antibiotics; Rivaroxaban; Salicylates; Thrombolytic Agents; Tositumomab and Iodine I 131 Tositumomab; Vancomycin; Vitamin K Antagonists

The levels/effects of Diclofenac (Systemic) may be increased by: ACE Inhibitors; Angiotensin II Receptor Blockers; Antidepressants (Tricyclic, Tertiary Amine); Conivaptan; Corticosteroids (Systemic); CycloSPORINE; CycloSPORINE (Systemic); Dasatinib; Floctafenine; Glucosamine; Herbs (Anticoagulant/Antiplatelet Properties); Ketorolac; Ketorolac (Nasal); Ketorolac (Systemic); Nonsteroidal Anti-Inflammatory Agents; Omega-3-Acid Ethyl Esters; Pentosan Polysulfate Sodium; Pentoxifylline; Probenecid; Prostacyclin Analogues; Selective Serotonin Reuptake Inhibitors; Serotonin/Norepinephrine Reuptake Inhibitors; Sodium Phosphates; Treprostinil; Vitamin E; Voriconazole

Decreased Effect

Diclofenac (Systemic) may decrease the levels/effects of: ACE Inhibitors; Angiotensin II Receptor Blockers; Antiplatelet Agents; Beta-Blockers; Eplerenone; HydrALAZINE; Loop Diuretics; Potassium-Sparing Diuretics; Salicylates; Selective Serotonin Reuptake Inhibitors; Thiazide Diuretics

The levels/effects of Diclofenac (Systemic) may be decreased by: Bile Acid Sequestrants; Cyproterone; Nonsteroidal Anti-Inflammatory Agents; Peginterferon Alfa-2b; Salicylates; Tocilizumab

Ethanol/Nutrition/Herb Interactions

Ethanol: Avoid ethanol (may enhance gastric mucosal irritation).

Herb/Nutraceutical: Avoid alfalfa, anise, bilberry, bladderwrack, bromelain, cat's claw, celery, chamomile, coleus, cordyceps, dong quai, evening primrose, fenugreek, feverfew, garlic, ginger, ginkgo biloba, grapeseed, green tea, ginseng (Siberian), guggul, horse chestnut, horseradish, licorice, prickly ash, red clover, reishi, SAMe (s-adenosylmethionine), sweet clover, turmeric, white willow (all have additional antiplatelet activity).

Stability

Capsule, oral solution: Store at 25°C (77°F); excursions permitted to 15°C to 30°C (59°F to 86°F). Protect from moisture.

Suppository (CAN; not available in U.S.): Store at 15°C to 30°C (59°F to 86°F); protect from heat.

Tablet: Store below 30°C (86°F). Protect from moisture; store in tight container.

Mechanism of Action Reversibly inhibits cyclooxygenase-1 and 2 (COX-1 and 2) enzymes, which results in decreased formation of prostaglandin precursors; has antipyretic, analgesic, and anti-inflammatory properties

Other proposed mechanisms not fully elucidated (and possibly contributing to the anti-inflammatory effect to varying degrees), include inhibiting chemotaxis, altering lymphocyte activity, inhibiting neutrophil aggregation/activation, and decreasing proinflammatory cytokine levels.

Pharmacodynamics/Kinetics

Onset of action:

Cataflam® (potassium salt) is more rapid than the sodium salt because it dissolves in the stomach instead of the duodenum

Suppository: More rapid onset, but slower rate of absorption when compared to enteric coated tablet

Distribution: ~1.4 L/kg

Protein binding: >99%, primarily to albumin

Metabolism: Hepatic; undergoes first-pass metabolism; forms several metabolites (1 with weak activity)

Bioavailability: 55%

Half-life elimination: ~2 hours

Time to peak, serum:

Cambia™: ~0.25 hours

Cataflam®: ~1 hour

Voltaren® XR ~5 hours

Zipsor™: ~0.5 hour

Suppository: ≤1 hour; **Note:** Suppository: C_{max}: Approximately two-thirds of that observed with enteric coated tablet (equivalent 50 mg dose)

Tablet, delayed release (diclofenac sodium): ~2 hours

Excretion: Urine (~65%); feces (~35%)

Dosage Adults:

Oral:

Analgesia:

Immediate release tablet: Starting dose: 50 mg 3 times/day (maximum dose: 150 mg/day); may administer 100 mg loading dose, followed by 50 mg every 8 hours (maximum dose day 1: 200 mg/day; maximum dose day 2 and thereafter: 150 mg/day)

Canadian labeling: Maximum loading dose day 1: 200 mg/day; maximum dose day 2 and up to 7 days: 150 mg/day (50 mg every 6-8 hours)

Immediate release capsule: 25 mg 4 times/day

Primary dysmenorrhea: Immediate release tablet: Starting dose: 50 mg 3 times/day (maximum dose: 150 mg/day); may administer 100 mg loading dose, followed by 50 mg every 8 hours (maximum dose day 1: 200 mg/day; maximum dose day 2 and thereafter: 150 mg/day)

Canadian labeling: Maximum loading dose day 1: 200 mg/day; maximum dose day 2 and up to 7 days: 150 mg/day (50 mg every 6-8 hours)

Rheumatoid arthritis: Immediate release tablet: 150-200 mg/day in 3-4 divided doses; Delayed release tablet: 150-200 mg/day in 2-4 divided doses; Extended release tablet: 100 mg/day (may increase dose to 200 mg/day in 2 divided doses)

Canadian labeling: 150 mg/day in 3 divided doses (75-150 mg/day of slow release tablet)

Osteoarthritis: Immediate or delayed release tablet: 100-150 mg/day in 2-3 divided doses; Extended release tablet: 100 mg/day

Canadian labeling: 150 mg/day in 3 divided doses (75-150 mg/day of slow release tablet)

Ankylosing spondylitis: Delayed release tablet: 100-125 mg/day in 4-5 divided doses

Migraine: Oral solution: 50 mg (one packet) as a single dose at the time of migraine onset; safety and efficacy of a second dose have not been established

Rectal suppository (not available in U.S.):

Osteoarthritis: *Canadian labeling:* Insert 50 mg or 100 mg suppository rectally as single dose to substitute for final (third) oral daily dose; maximum combined dose (rectal and oral): 150 mg/day

Rheumatoid arthritis: *Canadian labeling:* Insert 50 mg or 100 mg suppository rectally as single dose to substitute for final (third) oral daily dose (maximum combined dose [rectal and oral]: 150 mg/day

Dosage adjustment in renal impairment: Not recommended in patients with advanced renal disease or significant renal impairment

Dosage adjustment in hepatic impairment: May require dosage adjustment; use oral solution only if benefits outweigh risks

Elderly: No specific dosing recommendations; elderly may demonstrate adverse effects at lower doses than younger adults, and >60% may develop asymptomatic peptic ulceration with or without hemorrhage; monitor renal function

Dietary Considerations Oral formulations may be taken with food to decrease GI distress. Food may reduce effectiveness of oral solution. Some products may contain phenylalanine.

Diclofenac potassium = Cataflam®; potassium content: 5.8 mg (0.15 mEq) per 50 mg tablet

Administration

Oral: Do not crush delayed or extended release tablets. Administer with food or milk to avoid gastric distress. Take with full glass of water to enhance absorption.

Oral solution: Empty contents of packet into 1-2 ounces (30-60 mL) of water (do not use other liquids), mix well and administer immediately; food may reduce effectiveness.

Rectal suppository: Remove entire plastic wrapping prior to inserting rectally.

Monitoring Parameters Monitor CBC, liver enzymes (periodically during chronic therapy starting 4-8 weeks after initiation), BUN/serum creatinine; monitor urine output; occult blood loss

Dosage Forms Excipient information presented when available (limited, particularly for generics); consult specific product labeling.

Capsule, liquid filled, oral, as potassium:

Zipsor™: 25 mg [contains gelatin]

Powder for solution, oral, as potassium:

Cambia™: 50 mg/packet (1s) [contains phenylalanine 25 mg/packet; anise-mint flavor]

Tablet, oral, as potassium: 50 mg

Cataflam®: 50 mg

Tablet, delayed release, enteric coated, oral, as sodium: 25 mg, 50 mg, 75 mg

Tablet, extended release, oral, as sodium: 100 mg

Voltaren®-XR: 100 mg

Dosage Forms: Canada Excipient information presented when available (limited, particularly for generics); consult specific product labeling.

Suppository:

Voltaren®: 50 mg, 100mg

Diclofenac (Ophthalmic) (dye KLOE fen ak)

Brand Names: U.S. Voltaren Ophthalmic®

Brand Names: Canada Voltaren Ophtha®

Index Terms Diclofenac Sodium

Pharmacologic Category Nonsteroidal Anti-inflammatory Drug (NSAID); Nonsteroidal Anti-inflammatory Drug (NSAID), Ophthalmic

Use Treatment of postoperative inflammation following cataract extraction; temporary relief of pain and photophobia in patients undergoing corneal refractive surgery

Pregnancy Risk Factor C

Dosage Ophthalmic: Adults:

Cataract surgery: Instill 1 drop into affected eye 4 times/day beginning 24 hours after cataract surgery and continuing for 2 weeks

Corneal refractive surgery: Instill 1-2 drops into affected eye within the hour prior to surgery, within 15 minutes following surgery, and then continue for 4 times/day, up to 3 days

Additional Information Complete prescribing information for this medication should be consulted for additional detail.

Dosage Forms Excipient information presented when available (limited, particularly for generics); consult specific product labeling.

Solution, ophthalmic, as sodium [drops]: 0.1% (2.5 mL, 5 mL)

Voltaren Ophthalmic®: 0.1% (2.5 mL, 5 mL) [contains sorbic acid]

Diclofenac and Misoprostol

(dye KLOE fen ak & mye soe PROST ole)

Brand Names: U.S. Arthrotec®

Brand Names: Canada Arthrotec®

Index Terms Misoprostol and Diclofenac

Pharmacologic Category Nonsteroidal Anti-inflammatory Drug (NSAID), Oral; Prostaglandin

Use Treatment of osteoarthritis and rheumatoid arthritis in patients at high risk for NSAID-induced gastric and duodenal ulceration

Pregnancy Risk Factor X

Medication Guide Available Yes

Dosage Oral:

Adults:

Osteoarthritis: Arthotec® 50: 1 tablet 3 times/day

Rheumatoid arthritis: Arthotec® 50: 1 tablet 3 or 4 times/day

Note: For both indications, may administer Arthrotec® 50 or Arthrotec® 75 one tablet twice daily if recommended dose is not tolerated; however, these options are less effective in preventing GI ulceration. May adjust dose using individual agents in combination with Arthrotec®. The maximum daily dose of misoprostal is 800 mcg and the maximum single dose of misoprostal is 200 mcg. The maximum daily dose of diclofenac is 150 mg/day (osteoarthritis) or 225 mg/day (rheumatoid arthritis).

Elderly: No specific dosage adjustment is recommended; may require reduced dosage due to lower body weight; monitor renal function

Dosage adjustment in renal impairment: Not recommended in patients with advanced renal disease. In renal insufficiency, diclofenac should be used with caution due to potential detrimental effects on renal function, and misoprostol dosage reduction may be required if adverse effects occur (misoprostol is renally eliminated).

Dosage adjustment in hepatic impairment: May require dosage adjustment.

Additional Information Complete prescribing information for this medication should be consulted for additional detail.

Dosage Forms Excipient information presented when available (limited, particularly for generics); consult specific product labeling.

Tablet:

Arthrotec® 50: Diclofenac sodium 50 mg and misoprostol 200 mcg

Arthrotec® 75: Diclofenac sodium 75 mg and misoprostol 200 mcg

◆ **Diclofenac ECT (Can)** *see* Diclofenac (Systemic) *on page 495*

◆ **Diclofenac Potassium** *see* Diclofenac (Systemic) *on page 495*

◆ **Diclofenac Sodium** *see* Diclofenac (Ophthalmic) *on page 498*

◆ **Diclofenac Sodium** *see* Diclofenac (Systemic) *on page 495*

◆ **Diclofenac Sodium SR (Can)** *see* Diclofenac (Systemic) *on page 495*

◆ **Diclofenac SR (Can)** *see* Diclofenac (Systemic) *on page 495*

Dicloxacillin (dye kloks a SIL in)

Brand Names: Canada Dycill®; Pathocil®

Index Terms Dicloxacillin Sodium

Pharmacologic Category Antibiotic, Penicillin

Use Treatment of systemic infections such as pneumonia, skin and soft tissue infections, and osteomyelitis caused by penicillinase-producing staphylococci

Pregnancy Risk Factor B

Dosage

Usual dosage range:

Newborns: Use not recommended

Children <40 kg: Oral: 12.5-100 mg/kg/day divided every 6 hours

Children >40 kg: Oral: 125-250 mg every 6 hours

Adults: Oral: 125-1000 mg every 6 hours

Indication-specific dosing:

Children: Oral:

Furunculosis: 25-50 mg/kg/day divided every 6 hours

Osteomyelitis: 50-100 mg/kg/day in divided doses every 6 hours

Adults: Oral:

Erysipelas, furunculosis, mastitis, otitis externa, septic bursitis, skin abscess: 500 mg every 6 hours

Impetigo: 250 mg every 6 hours

Prosthetic joint (long-term suppression therapy): 250 mg twice daily

***Staphylococcus aureus*, methicillin susceptible infection if no I.V. access:** 500-1000 mg every 6-8 hours

Dosage adjustment in renal impairment: Not necessary

Hemodialysis: Not dialyzable (0% to 5%); supplemental dosage not necessary

Peritoneal dialysis: Supplemental dosage not necessary

Continuous arteriovenous or venovenous hemofiltration: Supplemental dosage not necessary

Additional Information Complete prescribing information for this medication should be consulted for additional detail.

Dosage Forms Excipient information presented when available (limited, particularly for generics); consult specific product labeling.

Capsule, oral: 250 mg, 500 mg

◆ **Dicloxacillin Sodium** *see* Dicloxacillin *on page 499*

Dicyclomine (dye SYE kloe meen)

Brand Names: U.S. Bentyl®

Brand Names: Canada Bentylol®; Formulex®; Lomine; Riva-Dicyclomine

Index Terms Dicyclomine Hydrochloride; Dicycloverine Hydrochloride

Pharmacologic Category Anticholinergic Agent

Additional Appendix Information

Beers Criteria – Potentially Inappropriate Medications for Geriatrics *on page 1973*

Use Treatment of functional bowel/irritable bowel syndrome

Unlabeled Use Urinary incontinence

Pregnancy Risk Factor B

Dosage Adults:

Oral: Initiate with 80 mg/day in 4 equally divided doses, then increase up to 160 mg/day. Duration: Safety data not available for duration >2 weeks.

I.M. **(should not be used I.V.)**: 80 mg/day in 4 divided doses (20 mg/dose)

Additional Information Complete prescribing information for this medication should be consulted for additional detail.

Dosage Forms Excipient information presented when available (limited, particularly for generics); consult specific product labeling.

Capsule, oral, as hydrochloride: 10 mg

Bentyl®: 10 mg

Injection, solution, as hydrochloride: 10 mg/mL (2 mL)

Bentyl®: 10 mg/mL (2 mL)

Syrup, oral, as hydrochloride:

Bentyl®: 10 mg/5 mL (480 mL) [contains propylene glycol]

Tablet, oral, as hydrochloride: 20 mg

Bentyl®: 20 mg

◆ **Dicyclomine Hydrochloride** *see* Dicyclomine *on page 499*

◆ **Dicycloverine Hydrochloride** *see* Dicyclomine *on page 499*

◆ **Di-Dak-Sol** *see* Sodium Hypochlorite Solution *on page 1570*

Didanosine (dye DAN oh seen)

Brand Names: U.S. Videx®; Videx® EC

Brand Names: Canada Videx®; Videx® EC

Index Terms ddI; Dideoxyinosine

Pharmacologic Category Antiretroviral Agent, Reverse Transcriptase Inhibitor (Nucleoside)

Additional Appendix Information

Management of Healthcare Worker Exposures to HBV, HCV, and HIV *on page 1935*

Perinatal HIV Guidelines *on page 1946*

Use Treatment of HIV infection; always to be used in combination with at least two other antiretroviral agents

Pregnancy Risk Factor B

Pregnancy Considerations Adverse events have not been observed in animal reproduction studies. Didanosine has been shown to cross the placenta. Based on data from the Antiretroviral Pregnancy Registry, birth defects have been observed in 4.7% of offspring with first trimester exposure (in comparison to 2.7% observed in U.S. population); no pattern of defects has been observed. Cases of lactic acidosis/hepatic steatosis syndrome related to mitochondrial toxicity have been reported in pregnant women with prolonged use of nucleoside analogues. It is not known if pregnancy itself potentiates this known side effect; however, women may be at increased risk of lactic acidosis and liver damage. In addition, these adverse events are similar to other rare but life-threatening syndromes which occur during pregnancy (eg, HELLP syndrome). Hepatic enzymes and electrolytes should be monitored in women receiving nucleoside analogues and clinicians should watch for early signs of the syndrome. In addition, mitochondrial dysfunction may develop in infants following *in utero* exposure. Due to the reports of lactic acidosis, maternal, and neonatal mortality, didanosine and stavudine should **not** be used in combination during pregnancy. Pharmacokinetics are not significantly altered during pregnancy; dose adjustments are not needed. The DHHS Perinatal HIV Guidelines consider didanosine to be an alternative NRTI in dual nucleoside combination regimens; use with stavudine only if no other alternatives are available.

Regardless of CD4 count or HIV RNA copy number, all HIV-infected pregnant women should receive a combination antepartum antiretroviral (ARV) drug regimen; this includes women who require therapy for their own health, as well as women who do not yet require therapy for their own health. ARV therapy should be started as soon as possible if required for the woman's health or immediately after the first trimester if not needed for the mother's health (although earlier initiation may be considered). Long-term follow-up is recommended for all infants exposed to ARV medications.

Healthcare providers are encouraged to enroll pregnant women exposed to antiretroviral medications in the Antiretroviral Pregnancy Registry (1-800-258-4263 or www.APRegistry.com). Healthcare providers caring for HIV-infected women and their infants may contact the National Perinatal HIV Hotline (888-448-8765) for clinical consultation (DHHS [perinatal], 2011).

Lactation Excretion in breast milk unknown/contraindicated

Medication Guide Available Yes

Contraindications Concurrent administration with allopurinol or ribavirin

Warnings/Precautions [U.S. Boxed Warning]: Pancreatitis (sometimes fatal) has been reported; incidence is dose related. Risk factors for developing pancreatitis may include a previous history of the condition, concurrent cytomegalovirus or *Mycobacterium avium-intracellulare* infection, renal impairment, advanced age, and concomitant use of stavudine, pentamidine, or hydroxyurea. Discontinue didanosine if clinical signs of pancreatitis occur. **[U.S. Boxed Warning]: Lactic acidosis, symptomatic hyperlactatemia, and severe hepatomegaly with steatosis (sometimes fatal) have occurred with antiretroviral nucleoside analogues, including didanosine.** Hepatotoxicity may occur even in the absence of marked transaminase elevations; suspend therapy in any patient developing clinical/laboratory findings which suggest hepatotoxicity. Hepatotoxicity and hepatic failure (including fatal cases) have been reported in HIV patients receiving combination drug therapy with didanosine and stavudine or hydroxyurea, or didanosine, stavudine, and hydroxyurea; avoid these combinations. Not currently recommended in combination with tenofovir due to failure and resistance. Noncirrhotic portal hypertension may develop within months to years of starting didanosine therapy. Signs may include elevated liver enzymes, esophageal varices, hematemesis, ascites, and splenomegaly. Noncirrhotic portal hypertension may lead to liver failure and/or death. Discontinue use in patients with evidence of this condition. Pregnant women may be at increased risk of lactic acidosis and liver damage. Use with caution in patients with hepatic impairment; safety and efficacy have not been established in patients with significant hepatic disease. Patients on combination antiretroviral therapy with hepatic impairment may be at increased risk of potentially severe and fatal hepatic toxicity; consider interruption or discontinuation of therapy if hepatic impairment worsens.

Peripheral neuropathy occurs in ~20% of patients receiving the drug. If symptomatic, discontinue therapy; after resolution of symptoms, reinitiation of therapy at a reduced dose may be tolerated. Permanently discontinue if neuropathy recurs. Retinal changes (including retinal depigmentation) and optic neuritis have been reported in adults and children using didanosine. Patients should undergo retinal examination every 6-12 months. Use caution in renal impairment; dose reduction recommended for Cl_{cr} <60 mL/minute. May cause redistribution of fat (eg, buffalo hump, peripheral wasting with increased abdominal girth, cushingoid appearance). Patients may develop immune reconstitution syndrome resulting in the occurrence of an inflammatory response to an indolent or residual opportunistic infection; further evaluation and treatment may be required. Didanosine delayed release capsules are indicated for once-daily use.

Adverse Reactions As reported in monotherapy studies; risk of toxicity may increase when combined with other agents.

>10%:

- Gastrointestinal: Diarrhea (19% to 28%), amylase increased (15% to 17%), abdominal pain (7% to 13%)
- Neuromuscular & skeletal: Peripheral neuropathy (17% to 20%)

1% to 10%:

- Dermatologic: Rash/pruritus (7% to 9%)
- Endocrine & metabolic: Uric acid increased (2% to 3%)
- Gastrointestinal: Pancreatitis (1% to 7% dose dependent); patients >65 years of age had a higher frequency of pancreatitis than younger patients patients (10% vs 5% in younger patients)
- Hepatic: AST increased (7% to 9%), ALT increased (6% to 9%), alkaline phosphatase increased (1% to 4%)

Postmarketing and/or case reports: Acute renal impairment, alopecia, anaphylactoid reaction, anemia, anorexia, arthralgia, chills/fever, diabetes mellitus, dry eyes, dyspepsia, flatulence, granulocytopenia, hepatic steatosis, hepatitis, hyper-/hypoglycemia, hyperlactatemia (symptomatic), hypersensitivity, immune reconstitution syndrome, lactic acidosis/hepatomegaly, leukopenia, lipodystrophy, liver failure, myalgia, myopathy, optic neuritis, pain, parotid gland enlargement, portal hypertension (noncirrhotic), retinal depigmentation, rhabdomyolysis, sialoadenitis, Stevens-Johnson syndrome, thrombocytopenia, weakness, xerostomia

Drug Interactions

Metabolism/Transport Effects None known.

Avoid Concomitant Use

Avoid concomitant use of Didanosine with any of the following: Alcohol (Ethyl); Allopurinol; Febuxostat; Hydroxyurea; Ribavirin; Tenofovir

Increased Effect/Toxicity

Didanosine may increase the levels/effects of: Hydroxyurea

The levels/effects of Didanosine may be increased by: Alcohol (Ethyl); Allopurinol; Febuxostat; Ganciclovir-Valganciclovir; Hydroxyurea; Ribavirin; Stavudine; Tenofovir

Decreased Effect

Didanosine may decrease the levels/effects of: Antifungal Agents (Azole Derivatives, Systemic); Atazanavir; Indinavir; Quinolone Antibiotics; Rilpivirine

The levels/effects of Didanosine may be decreased by: Atazanavir; Darunavir; Lopinavir; Methadone; Rilpivirine; Tenofovir; Tipranavir

Ethanol/Nutrition/Herb Interactions

Ethanol: Avoid ethanol (increases risk of pancreatitis).

Food: Decreases AUC and C_{max}. Didanosine serum levels may be decreased by 55% if taken with food.

Stability Delayed release capsules should be stored in tightly closed bottles at controlled room temperature of 25°C (77°F). Unreconstituted powder should be stored at 15°C to 30°C (59°F to 86°F). Reconstituted pediatric solution is stable for 30 days if refrigerated.

Videx® pediatric powder: Add 100 mL or 200 mL purified water, USP to the 2 g or 4 g container, respectively, to achieve a 20 mg/mL solution. Immediately mix the resulting solution with an equal volume of Mylanta® Maximum Strength (or equivalent) to achieve a final concentration of 10 mg/mL.

Mechanism of Action Didanosine, a purine nucleoside (adenosine) analog and the deamination product of dideoxyadenosine (ddA), inhibits HIV replication *in vitro* in both T cells and monocytes. Didanosine is converted within the cell to the mono-, di-, and triphosphates of ddA. These ddA triphosphates act as substrate and inhibitor of HIV reverse transcriptase substrate and inhibitor of HIV reverse transcriptase thereby blocking viral DNA synthesis and suppressing HIV replication.

Pharmacodynamics/Kinetics

Absorption: Subject to degradation by acidic pH of stomach; some formulations are buffered to resist acidic pH; ≤55% reduction in peak plasma concentration is observed in presence of food. Delayed release capsules contain enteric-coated beadlets which dissolve in the small intestine.

Distribution: V_d: Children: 28 L/m²; Adults: 1.08 L/kg

Protein binding: <5%

Metabolism: Has not been evaluated in humans; studies conducted in dogs show extensive metabolism with allantoin, hypoxanthine, xanthine, and uric acid being the major metabolites found in urine

Bioavailability: Children: 25%; Adults: 42%

Half-life elimination:

Children and Adolescents: 0.8 hour

Adults: Normal renal function: 1.5 hours; active metabolite, ddATP, has an intracellular half-life >12 hours *in vitro*; Renal impairment: 2.5-5 hours

Time to peak: Delayed release capsules: 2 hours; Powder for suspension: 0.25-1.5 hours

Excretion: Urine (~55% as unchanged drug)

Clearance: Total body: Averages 800 mL/minute

Dosage Oral: Treatment of HIV infection:

Pediatric powder for oral solution (Videx®): **Note:** Once-daily dosing of the oral solution is not FDA approved in children.

Infants: 2 weeks to 8 months: 100 mg/m² twice daily is recommended by the manufacturer; 50 mg/m² may be considered in infants 2 weeks to <3 months (AIDS*info* guidelines)

Infants and Children >8 months: 120 mg/m² twice daily, not to exceed adult dose, is recommended by the manufacturer. **Note:** AIDS*info* guidelines suggest a range of 90-150 mg/m² twice daily

Children 3-21 years (unlabeled dose): Treatment-naive: 240 mg/m²/dose once daily (maximum: 400 mg/dose) (AIDS*info* guidelines)

Adolescents and Adults: Dosing based on patient weight:

<60 kg: 125 mg twice daily (preferred) or 250 mg once daily

≥60 kg: 200 mg twice daily (preferred) or 400 mg once daily

Delayed release capsule (Videx® EC):

Children ≥6 years and Adults:

20 kg to <25 kg: 200 mg once daily

25 kg to <60 kg: 250 mg once daily

≥60 kg: 400 mg once daily

Children 3-21 years (unlabeled dose): Treatment-naive: 240 mg/m²/dose once daily (maximum: 400 mg/dose) (AIDS*info* guidelines)

Elderly: Higher frequency of pancreatitis (10% versus 5% in younger patients); monitor renal function and dose accordingly

When taken with tenofovir: Adults:

<60 kg and Cl_{cr} ≥60 mL/minute: 200 mg once daily

≥60 kg and Cl_{cr} ≥60 mL/minute: 250 mg once daily

Note: Combined use of tenofovir with didanosine is no longer recommended (DHHS, 2011).

Dosage adjustment in renal impairment:

Children: No specific guidelines available; consider dosage reduction using adjustments for adults.

Adults: Dosing based on patient weight, creatinine clearance, and dosage form: See table.

Recommended Dose (mg) of Didanosine by Body Weight – Adults

Creatinine Clearance (mL/min)	≥60 kg		<60 kg	
	Powder for Oral Solution	Delayed Release Capsule	Powder for Oral Solution	Delayed Release Capsule
≥60	400 mg daily or 200 mg twice daily	400 mg daily	250 mg daily or 125 mg twice daily	250 mg daily
30-59	200 mg daily or 100 mg twice daily	200 mg daily	150 mg daily or 75 mg twice daily	125 mg daily
10-29	150 mg daily	125 mg daily	100 mg daily	125 mg daily
<10	100 mg daily	125 mg daily	75 mg daily	See Note.

Note: Per manufacturer, not suitable for use in patients <60 kg with Cl_{cr} <10 mL/minute; use alternate formulation.

Patients requiring hemodialysis or CAPD: Dose per Cl_{cr} <10 mL/minute. Didanosine is not removed via CAPD and minimal amount of dose (≤7%) is removed by hemodialysis; no supplemental dosing necessary.

Dosing adjustment in hepatic impairment: No dosage adjustment needed

Dietary Considerations Take on an empty stomach; administer at least 30 minutes before or 2 hours after eating

Administration Pediatric powder for oral solution: Administer on an empty stomach at least 30 minutes before or 2 hours after eating. Prior to dispensing, the powder should be mixed with purified water USP to an initial concentration of 20 mg/mL and then further diluted with an appropriate antacid suspension to a final mixture of 10 mg/mL. Shake well prior to use.

Videx® EC: Administer on an empty stomach at least 1 hour before or 2 hours after eating; swallow capsule whole.

Monitoring Parameters Serum potassium, uric acid, creatinine; hemoglobin, CBC with neutrophil and platelet count, CD4 cells; viral load; liver function tests, serum bilirubin, albumin, INR, amylase; weight gain; perform dilated retinal exam every 6 months, ultrasonography (if portal hypertension suspected)

Additional Information A high rate of early virologic nonresponse was observed when the combination of didanosine, lamivudine, and tenofovir or the triple NRTI combination of didanosine, tenofovir and emtricitabine were used as the initial regimen in treatment-naive patients. Use of either of these combinations is not recommended; patients currently on these regimens should be closely monitored for modification of therapy. Early virologic failure and increased toxicity was also observed with tenofovir and didanosine delayed release capsules, plus either efavirenz or nevirapine; use is not recommended. In addition, preliminary data show inferior virologic response with the combination of atazanavir, didanosine and emtricitabine; use should be avoided (DHHS, 2011).

Dosage Forms Excipient information presented when available (limited, particularly for generics); consult specific product labeling.

Capsule, delayed release, enteric coated beadlets, oral: 125 mg, 200 mg, 250 mg, 400 mg

Videx® EC: 125 mg, 200 mg, 250 mg, 400 mg

Capsule, delayed release, enteric coated pellets, oral: 200 mg, 250 mg, 400 mg

Powder for solution, oral [pediatric]:

Videx®: 2 g/bottle, 4 g/bottle

◆ **Dideoxyinosine** *see* Didanosine *on page 499*

◆ **Didronel®** *see* Etidronate *on page 666*

◆ **Dienogest and Estradiol** *see* Estradiol and Dienogest *on page 634*

Diethylpropion (dye eth il PROE pee on)

Brand Names: Canada Tenuate®; Tenuate® Dospan®

Index Terms Amfepramone; Diethylpropion Hydrochloride

Pharmacologic Category Anorexiant; Sympathomimetic

Use Short-term (few weeks) adjunct in the management of exogenous obesity

Pharmacotherapy for weight loss is recommended only for obese patients with a body mass index ≥30 kg/m^2, or ≥27 kg/m^2 in the presence of other risk factors such as hypertension, diabetes, and/or dyslipidemia or a high waist circumference; therapy should be used in conjunction with a comprehensive weight management program.

Pregnancy Risk Factor B

Dosage Children >16 years and Adults: Oral:

Tablet: 25 mg 3 times/day before meals or food

Tablet, controlled release: 75 mg at midmorning

Additional Information Complete prescribing information for this medication should be consulted for additional detail.

Dosage Forms Excipient information presented when available (limited, particularly for generics); consult specific product labeling.

Tablet, oral, as hydrochloride: 25 mg

Tablet, controlled release, oral, as hydrochloride: 75 mg

Controlled Substance C-IV

◆ **Diethylpropion Hydrochloride** *see* Diethylpropion *on page 502*

◆ **Differin®** *see* Adapalene *on page 44*

◆ **Differin® XP (Can)** *see* Adapalene *on page 44*

◆ **Dificid™** *see* Fidaxomicin *on page 710*

◆ **Difil-G [DSC]** *see* Dyphylline and Guaifenesin *on page 568*

◆ **Difil-G® 400** *see* Dyphylline and Guaifenesin *on page 568*

◆ **Difil®-G Forte [DSC]** *see* Dyphylline and Guaifenesin *on page 568*

◆ **Difimicin** *see* Fidaxomicin *on page 710*

Diflorasone (dye FLOR a sone)

Brand Names: U.S. ApexiCon® E; ApexiCon™

Index Terms Diflorasone Diacetate

Pharmacologic Category Corticosteroid, Topical

Additional Appendix Information

Corticosteroids *on page 1888*

Use Relieves inflammation and pruritic symptoms of corticosteroid-responsive dermatosis (high to very high potency topical corticosteroid)

Pregnancy Risk Factor C

Dosage Topical: Apply ointment sparingly 1-3 times/day; apply cream sparingly 2-4 times/day. Therapy should be discontinued when control is achieved; if no improvement is seen, reassessment of diagnosis may be necessary.

Additional Information Complete prescribing information for this medication should be consulted for additional detail.

Dosage Forms Excipient information presented when available (limited, particularly for generics); consult specific product labeling.

Cream, topical, as diacetate: 0.05% (15 g, 30 g, 60 g)

ApexiCon® E: 0.05% (30 g, 60 g)

Ointment, topical, as diacetate: 0.05% (15 g, 30 g, 60 g)

ApexiCon™: 0.05% (30 g, 60 g)

◆ **Diflorasone Diacetate** *see* Diflorasone *on page 502*

◆ **Diflucan®** *see* Fluconazole *on page 718*

Diflunisal (dye FLOO ni sal)

Brand Names: Canada Apo-Diflunisal®; Novo-Diflunisal; Nu-Diflunisal

Index Terms Dolobid

Pharmacologic Category Nonsteroidal Anti-inflammatory Drug (NSAID), Oral

Use Management of inflammatory disorders usually including rheumatoid arthritis and osteoarthritis; can be used as an analgesic for treatment of mild-to-moderate pain

Pregnancy Risk Factor C

Medication Guide Available Yes

Dosage Adults: Oral:

Mild-to-moderate pain: Initial: 500-1000 mg followed by 250-500 mg every 8-12 hours; maximum daily dose: 1.5 g

Arthritis: 500-1000 mg/day in 2 divided doses; maximum daily dose: 1.5 g

Dosing adjustment in renal impairment: Use with caution; Cl_{cr} <50 mL/minute: Administer 50% of normal dose (Aronoff, 1998)

Hemodialysis: No supplement required

CAPD: No supplement require

CAVH: Dose for GFR 10-50

Additional Information Complete prescribing information for this medication should be consulted for additional detail.

Dosage Forms Excipient information presented when available (limited, particularly for generics); consult specific product labeling.

Tablet, oral: 500 mg

◆ **Difluorodeoxycytidine Hydrochlorothiazide** *see* Gemcitabine *on page 782*

Difluprednate (dye floo PRED nate)

Brand Names: U.S. Durezol®

Pharmacologic Category Corticosteroid, Ophthalmic

Use Treatment of inflammation and pain following ocular surgery

Pregnancy Risk Factor C

Dosage Ophthalmic: Adults: Instill 1 drop in conjunctival sac of the affected eye(s) 4 times/day beginning 24 hours after surgery, continue for 2 weeks, then decrease to 2 times/day for 1 week, then taper based on response

Additional Information Complete prescribing information for this medication should be consulted for additional detail.

Dosage Forms Excipient information presented when available (limited, particularly for generics); consult specific product labeling.

Emulsion, ophthalmic [drops]:

Durezol®: 0.05% (5 mL) [contains sorbic acid]

◆ **Digibind® [DSC]** *see* Digoxin Immune Fab *on page 506*

◆ **Digibind® (Can)** *see* Digoxin Immune Fab *on page 506*

◆ **DigiFab®** *see* Digoxin Immune Fab *on page 506*

◆ **Digitalis** *see* Digoxin *on page 503*

Digoxin (di JOKS in)

Brand Names: U.S. Lanoxin®

Brand Names: Canada Apo-Digoxin®; Digoxin CSD; Lanoxin®; Pediatric Digoxin CSD; PMS-Digoxin; Toloxin®

Index Terms Digitalis

Pharmacologic Category Antiarrhythmic Agent, Miscellaneous; Cardiac Glycoside

Additional Appendix Information

Beers Criteria – Potentially Inappropriate Medications for Geriatrics *on page 1973*

Heart Failure (Systolic) *on page 1991*

Use Treatment of mild-to-moderate (or stage C as recommended by the ACCF/AHA) heart failure (HF); atrial fibrillation (rate-control)

Note: In treatment of atrial fibrillation (AF), use is not considered first-line unless AF coexistent with heart failure or in sedentary patients (Fuster, 2006).

Unlabeled Use Fetal tachycardia with or without hydrops; to slow ventricular rate in supraventricular tachyarrhythmias such as supraventricular tachycardia (SVT) excluding atrioventricular reciprocating tachycardia (AVRT)

Pregnancy Risk Factor C

Pregnancy Considerations Animal reproduction studies have not been conducted. Digoxin crosses the placenta and can be detected in the fetus. Digoxin is recommended as first-line in the treatment of fetal tachycardia determined to be SVT. In pregnant women with atrial fibrillation or SVT, use of digoxin is recommended (Class I recommendation; Blomström-Lundqvist, 2003; Fuster, 2006).

Lactation Enters breast milk/use caution (AAP rates "compatible"; AAP 2001 update pending)

Contraindications Hypersensitivity to digoxin (rare) or other forms of digitalis, or any component of the formulation; ventricular fibrillation

Warnings/Precautions Watch for proarrhythmic effects (especially with digoxin toxicity). Withdrawal in clinically stable patients with HF may lead to recurrence of HF symptoms. During an episode of atrial fibrillation or flutter in patients with an accessory bypass tract (eg, Wolff-Parkinson-White syndrome), use has been associated with increased anterograde conduction down the accessory pathway leading to ventricular fibrillation; avoid use in such patients. Avoid use in patients with second- or third-degree heart block (except in patients with a functioning artificial pacemaker); incomplete AV block (eg, Stokes-Adams attack) may progress to complete block with digoxin administration. HF patients with preserved left ventricular function including patients with restrictive cardiomyopathy, constrictive pericarditis, and amyloid heart disease may be susceptible to digoxin toxicity; avoid use unless used to control ventricular response with atrial fibrillation. Digoxin should not be used in patients with low EF, sinus rhythm, and no HF symptoms since the risk of harm may be greater than clinical benefit. Avoid use in patients with hypertrophic cardiomyopathy (HCM) and outflow tract obstruction unless used to control ventricular response with atrial fibrillation; outflow obstruction may worsen due to the positive inotropic effects of digoxin.

Use with caution in patients with hyperthyroidism, hypothyroidism, recent acute MI (within 6 months), sinus nodal disease (eg, sick sinus syndrome). Reduce dose with renal impairment and when amiodarone, propafenone, quinidine, or verapamil are added to a patient on digoxin; use with caution in patients taking strong inducers or inhibitors of P-glycoprotein (eg, cyclosporine). Avoid rapid I.V. administration of calcium in digitalized patients; may produce serious arrhythmias.

Atrial arrhythmias associated with hypermetabolic states are very difficult to treat; treat underlying condition first; if digoxin is used, ensure digoxin toxicity does not occur. Patients with beri beri heart disease may fail to adequately respond to digoxin therapy; treat underlying thiamine deficiency concomitantly. Correct electrolyte disturbances, especially hypokalemia or hypomagnesemia, prior to use and throughout therapy; toxicity may occur despite therapeutic digoxin concentrations. Hypercalcemia may increase the risk of digoxin toxicity; maintain normocalcemia. It is not necessary to routinely reduce or hold digoxin therapy prior to elective electrical cardioversion for atrial fibrillation; however, exclusion of digoxin toxicity (eg, clinical and ECG signs) is necessary prior to cardioversion. If signs of digoxin excess exist, withhold digoxin and delay cardioversion until toxicity subsides; usually >24 hours. Use with caution in the elderly; may develop exaggerated serum/tissue concentrations due to age-related alterations in clearance and pharmacodynamics differences; dosage reduction may be necessary; in general, avoid doses >0.125 mg/day (Beers Criteria).

Adverse Reactions Incidence not always reported.

Cardiovascular: Accelerated junctional rhythm, asystole, atrial tachycardia with or without block, AV dissociation, first-, second- (Wenckebach), or third-degree heart block, facial edema, PR prolongation, PVCs (especially bigeminy or trigeminy), ST segment depression, ventricular tachycardia or ventricular fibrillation

Central nervous system: Dizziness (6%), mental disturbances (5%), headache (4%), apathy, anxiety, confusion, delirium, depression, fever, hallucinations

Dermatologic: Rash (erythematous, maculopapular [most common], papular, scarlatiniform, vesicular or bullous), pruritus, urticaria, angioneurotic edema

Gastrointestinal: Nausea (4%), vomiting (2%), diarrhea (4%), abdominal pain, anorexia

Neuromuscular & skeletal: Weakness

Ocular: Visual disturbances (blurred or yellow vision)

Respiratory: Laryngeal edema

<1% (Limited to important or life-threatening): Asymmetric chorea, gynecomastia, thrombocytopenia, palpitation, intestinal ischemia, hemorrhagic necrosis of the intestines, vaginal cornification, eosinophilia, sexual dysfunction, diaphoresis

Children are more likely to experience cardiac arrhythmia as a sign of excessive dosing. The most common are conduction disturbances or tachyarrhythmia (atrial tachycardia with or without block) and junctional tachycardia. Ventricular tachyarrhythmias are less common. In infants, sinus bradycardia may be a sign of digoxin toxicity. Any arrhythmia seen in a child on digoxin should be considered as digoxin toxicity. The gastrointestinal and central nervous system symptoms are not frequently seen in children.

Drug Interactions

Metabolism/Transport Effects Substrate of CYP3A4 (minor), P-glycoprotein; **Note:** Assignment of Major/Minor substrate status based on clinically relevant drug interaction potential

Avoid Concomitant Use There are no known interactions where it is recommended to avoid concomitant use.

Increased Effect/Toxicity

Digoxin may increase the levels/effects of: Adenosine; Colchicine; Dronedarone; Midodrine

The levels/effects of Digoxin may be increased by: Aminoquinolines (Antimalarial); Amiodarone; Antithyroid Agents; Atorvastatin; Beta-Blockers; Boceprevir; Calcium Channel Blockers (Nondihydropyridine); Calcium Polystyrene Sulfonate; Carvedilol; Conivaptan; CycloSPORINE; CycloSPORINE (Systemic); Dronedarone; Etravirine; Glycopyrrolate; Itraconazole; Loop Diuretics; Macrolide Antibiotics; Milnacipran; Nefazodone; Neuromuscular-Blocking Agents; NIFEdipine; Nonsteroidal Anti-Inflammatory Agents; Paricalcitol; P-glycoprotein/ABCB1 Inhibitors; Posaconazole; Potassium-Sparing Diuretics; Propafenone; Protease Inhibitors; QuiNIDine; QuiNINE; Ranolazine; Reserpine; SitaGLIPtin; Sodium Polystyrene Sulfonate; Spironolactone; Telaprevir; Telmisartan; Ticagrelor; Tolvaptan; Vitamin D Analogs

Decreased Effect

Digoxin may decrease the levels/effects of: Antineoplastic Agents (Anthracycline, Systemic)

The levels/effects of Digoxin may be decreased by: 5-ASA Derivatives; Acarbose; Aminoglycosides; Antineoplastic Agents; Antineoplastic Agents (Anthracycline, Systemic); Bile Acid Sequestrants; Kaolin; PenicillAMINE; P-glycoprotein/ABCB1 Inducers; Potassium-Sparing Diuretics; St Johns Wort; Sucralfate; Tocilizumab

Ethanol/Nutrition/Herb Interactions

Food: Digoxin peak serum concentrations may be decreased if taken with food. Meals containing increased fiber (bran) or foods high in pectin may decrease oral absorption of digoxin.

Herb/Nutraceutical: Avoid ephedra (risk of cardiac stimulation). Avoid natural licorice (causes sodium and water retention and increases potassium loss).

Stability Store at 25°C (77°F); excursions permitted to 15°C to 30°C (59°F to 86°F). Protect elixir, injection, and tablets from light.

Mechanism of Action

Heart failure: Inhibition of the sodium/potassium ATPase pump in myocardial cells results in a transient increase of intracellular sodium, which in turn promotes calcium influx via the sodium-calcium exchange pump leading to increased contractility.

Supraventricular arrhythmias: Direct suppression of the AV node conduction to increase effective refractory period and decrease conduction velocity - positive inotropic effect, enhanced vagal tone, and decreased ventricular rate to fast atrial arrhythmias. Atrial fibrillation may decrease sensitivity and increase tolerance to higher serum digoxin concentrations.

Pharmacodynamics/Kinetics

Onset of action: Heart rate control: Oral: 1-2 hours; I.V.: 5-60 minutes

Peak effect: Heart rate control: Oral: 2-8 hours; I.V.: 1-6 hours; **Note:** In patients with atrial fibrillation, median time to ventricular rate control in one study was 6 hours (range: 3-15 hours) (Siu, 2009)

Duration: Adults: 3-4 days

Absorption: By passive nonsaturable diffusion in the upper small intestine; food may delay, but does not affect extent of absorption

Distribution:

Normal renal function: 6-7 L/kg

V_d: Extensive to peripheral tissues, with a distinct distribution phase which lasts 6-8 hours; concentrates in heart, liver, kidney, skeletal muscle, and intestines. Heart/serum concentration is 70:1. Pharmacologic effects are delayed and do not correlate well with serum concentrations during distribution phase.

Hyperthyroidism: Increased V_d

Hyperkalemia, hyponatremia: Decreased digoxin distribution to heart and muscle

Hypokalemia: Increased digoxin distribution to heart and muscles

Concomitant quinidine therapy: Decreased V_d

Chronic renal failure: 4-6 L/kg

Decreased sodium/potassium ATPase activity - decreased tissue binding

Neonates, full-term: 7.5-10 L/kg

Children: 16 L/kg

Adults: 7 L/kg, decreased with renal disease

Protein binding: ~25%; in uremic patients, digoxin is displaced from plasma protein binding sites

Metabolism: Via sequential sugar hydrolysis in the stomach or by reduction of lactone ring by intestinal bacteria (in ~10% of population, gut bacteria may metabolize up to 40% of digoxin dose); once absorbed, only ~16% is metabolized to 3-beta-digoxigenin, 3-keto-digoxigenin, and glucuronide and sulfate conjugates; metabolites may contribute to therapeutic and toxic effects of digoxin; metabolism is reduced with decompensated HF

Bioavailability: Oral (formulation dependent): Elixir: 70% to 85%; Tablet: 60% to 80%

Half-life elimination (age, renal and cardiac function dependent):

Neonates: Premature: 61-170 hours; Full-term: 35-45 hours

Infants: 18-25 hours

Children: 18-36 hours

Adults: 36-48 hours

Adults, anephric: 3.5-5 days

Half-life elimination: Parent drug: 38 hours; Metabolites: Digoxigenin: 4 hours; Monodigitoxoside: 3-12 hours

Time to peak, serum: Oral: 1-3 hours

Excretion: Urine (50% to 70% as unchanged drug)

Dosage

Children: When changing from oral (tablets or liquid) or I.M. to I.V. therapy, dosage should be reduced by 20% to 25%. Refer to the following: See table.

Dosage Recommendations for Digoxin[1]

Age	Total Digitalizing Dose[2,3] (mcg/kg)		Daily Maintenance Dose[3,4] (mcg/kg)	
	Oral	I.V. or I.M.[5]	Oral	I.V. or I.M.[5]
Preterm infant	20-30	15-25	5-7.5	4-6
Full-term infant	25-35	20-30	6-10	5-8
1 mo - 2 y	35-60	30-50	10-15	7.5-12
2-5 y	30-40	25-35	7.5-10	6-9
5-10 y	20-35	15-30	5-10	4-8
>10 y	10-15	8-12	2.5-5	2-3

[1]**Heart failure:** A lower serum digoxin concentration may be adequate to treat heart failure (compared to cardiac arrhythmias); consider doses at the lower end of the recommended range for treatment of heart failure; a digitalizing dose (loading dose) may not be necessary when treating heart failure (Ross, 2001).

[2]**Do not give full total digitalizing dose (TDD) at once.** Give one-half of the total digitalizing dose (TDD) in the initial dose, then give one-quarter of the TDD in each of two subsequent doses at 6- to 8-hour intervals. Obtain ECG 6 hours after each dose to assess potential toxicity.

[3]Based on lean body weight and normal renal function for age. Decrease dose in patients with decreased renal function; digitalizing dose often not recommended in infants and children.

[4]Divided every 12 hours in infants and children <10 years of age. Given once daily to children >10 years of age and adults.

[5]I.M. not preferred due to severe injection site pain. If I.M. route is necessary, administer as deep injection followed by massage of injection site.

Adults:

Atrial fibrillation (rate control) in patients with heart failure: Loading dose: I.V.: 0.25 mg every 2 hours, up to 1.5 mg within 24 hours; for nonacute situations, may administer 0.5 mg orally once daily for 2 days followed by oral maintenance dose. Maintenance dose: I.V., Oral: 0.125-0.375 mg once daily (Fuster, 2006)

Heart failure: Daily maintenance dose (**Note:** Loading dose not recommended): Oral: 0.125-0.25 mg once daily; higher daily doses (up to 0.5 mg/day) are rarely necessary. If patient is >70 years of age, has impaired renal function, or has a low lean body mass, low doses (eg, 0.125 mg daily or every other day) should be used (Hunt, 2009).

Supraventricular tachyarrhythmias (rate control):

Initial: Total digitalizing dose:

Oral: 0.75-1.5 mg

I.V., I.M.: 0.5-1 mg (**Note:** I.M. not preferred due to severe injection site pain.)

Give 1/2 (one-half) of the total digitalizing dose (TDD) as the initial dose, then give 1/4 (one-quarter) of the TDD in each of 2 subsequent doses at 6- to 8-hour intervals. Obtain ECG 6 hours after each dose to assess potential toxicity.

Daily maintenance dose:

Oral: 0.125-0.5 mg once daily

I.V., I.M.: 0.1-0.4 mg once daily (**Note:** I.M. not preferred due to severe injection site pain.)

Elderly: Dose is based on lean body weight and normal renal function for age. Decrease dose in patients with decreased renal function (see dosing adjustment in renal impairment).

Heart failure: If patient is >70 years, low doses (eg, 0.125 mg daily or every other day) should be used (Hunt, 2009).

Dosing adjustment/interval in renal impairment:

Loading dose:

ESRD: If loading dose necessary, reduce dose by 50%

Acute renal failure: Based on expert opinion, if patient in acute renal failure requires ventricular rate control (eg, in atrial fibrillation), consider alternative therapy. If loading digoxin becomes necessary, patient volume of distribution may be increased and reduction in loading dose may not be necessary; however, maintenance dosing will require adjustment as long as renal failure persists.

Maintenance dose:

Cl_{cr} 10-50 mL/minute: Administer 25% to 75% of dose or every 36 hours

Cl_{cr} <10 mL/minute: Administer 10% to 25% of dose or every 48 hours

Hemodialysis: Not dialyzable

Dietary Considerations Maintain adequate amounts of potassium in diet to decrease risk of hypokalemia (hypokalemia may increase risk of digoxin toxicity).

Administration

I.M.: I.V. route preferred. If I.M. injection necessary, administer by deep injection followed by massage at the injection site. Inject no more than 2 mL per injection site. May cause intense pain.

I.V.: May be administered undiluted or diluted fourfold in D_5W, NS, or SWFI for direct injection. Less than fourfold dilution may lead to drug precipitation. Inject slowly over ≥5 minutes.

Monitoring Parameters

Heart rate and rhythm should be monitored along with periodic ECGs to assess desired effects and signs of toxicity; baseline and periodic serum creatinine. Periodically monitor serum potassium, magnesium, and calcium especially if on medications where these electrolyte disturbances can occur (eg, diuretics), or if patient has a history of hypokalemia or hypomagnesemia. Observe patients for noncardiac signs of toxicity, confusion, and depression.

When to draw serum digoxin concentrations: Digoxin serum concentrations are monitored because digoxin possesses a narrow therapeutic serum range; the therapeutic endpoint is difficult to quantify and digoxin toxicity may be life-threatening. Digoxin serum concentrations should be drawn **at least 6-8 hours after last dose, regardless of route of administration (optimally 12-24 hours after a dose). Note:** Serum digoxin concentrations may decrease in response to exercise due to increased skeletal muscle uptake; a period of rest (eg, ~2 hours) after exercise may be necessary prior to drawing serum digoxin concentrations.

Initiation of therapy:

If a loading dose is given: Digoxin serum concentration may be drawn within 12-24 hours after the initial loading dose administration. Concentrations drawn this early may confirm the relationship of digoxin plasma concentrations and response but are of little value in determining maintenance doses.

If a loading dose is not given: Digoxin serum concentration should be obtained after 3-5 days of therapy.

Maintenance therapy:

Trough concentrations should be followed just prior to the next dose or at a minimum of 6-8 hours after last dose.

Digoxin serum concentrations should be obtained within 5-7 days (approximate time to steady-state) after any dosage changes. Continue to obtain digoxin serum concentrations 7-14 days after any change in maintenance dose. **Note:** In patients with end-stage renal disease, it may take 15-20 days to reach steady-state.

Patients who are receiving electrolyte-depleting medications such as diuretics, serum potassium, magnesium, and calcium should be monitored closely.

Digoxin serum concentrations should be obtained whenever any of the following conditions occur:

Questionable patient compliance or to evaluate clinical deterioration following an initial good response

Changing renal function

Suspected digoxin toxicity

Initiation or discontinuation of therapy with drugs (eg, amiodarone, quinidine, verapamil) which potentially interact with digoxin.

Any disease changes (eg, thyroid disease)

Reference Range

Digoxin therapeutic serum concentrations:

Heart failure: 0.5-0.8 ng/mL

Adults: <0.5 ng/mL; probably indicates underdigitalization unless there are special circumstances

Toxic: >2 ng/mL

Digoxin-like immunoreactive substance (DLIS) may cross-react with digoxin immunoassay. DLIS has been found in patients with renal and liver disease, heart failure, neonates, and pregnant women (3rd trimester).

Test Interactions Spironolactone may interfere with digoxin radioimmunoassay.

Dosage Forms Excipient information presented when available (limited, particularly for generics); consult specific product labeling. [DSC] = Discontinued product

Injection, solution: 250 mcg/mL (2 mL)

Lanoxin®: 250 mcg/mL (2 mL) [contains ethanol 10%, propylene glycol 40%]

Injection, solution [pediatric]:

Lanoxin®: 100 mcg/mL (1 mL) [contains ethanol 10%, propylene glycol 40%]

Solution, oral: 50 mcg/mL (2.5 mL [DSC], 60 mL)

Tablet, oral: 125 mcg, 250 mcg

Lanoxin®: 125 mcg, 250 mcg [scored]

Dosage Forms: Canada Excipient information presented when available (limited, particularly for generics); consult specific product labeling.

Tablet, oral:

Apo-Digoxin®: 62.5 mcg, 125 mcg, 250 mcg

♦ **Digoxin CSD (Can)** *see* Digoxin *on page* 503

Digoxin Immune Fab (di JOKS in i MYUN fab)

Brand Names: U.S. Digibind® [DSC]; DigiFab®

Brand Names: Canada Digibind®

Index Terms Antidigoxin Fab Fragments, Ovine

Pharmacologic Category Antidote

Use Treatment of life-threatening or potentially life-threatening digoxin intoxication, including:

- acute digoxin ingestion (ie, >10 mg in adults or >4 mg in children)
- chronic ingestions leading to steady-state digoxin concentrations >6 ng/mL in adults or >4 ng/mL in children
- manifestations of digoxin toxicity due to overdose (life-threatening ventricular arrhythmias, progressive bradycardia, second- or third-degree heart block not responsive to atropine, serum potassium >5 mEq/L in adults or >6 mEq in children)

Pregnancy Risk Factor C

Pregnancy Considerations Animal reproduction studies have not been conducted. Safety and efficacy in pregnant women have not been established. Use during pregnancy only if clearly needed.

Lactation Excretion in breast milk unknown/use caution

Contraindications Hypersensitivity to digoxin immune Fab, sheep products, or any component of the formulation

Warnings/Precautions Suicidal attempts often involve multiple drugs; consider other drug toxicities as well. Hypersensitivity reactions can occur. Epinephrine should be immediately available. Serum potassium levels should be monitored, especially during the first few hours after administration. Total serum digoxin concentrations will rise precipitously following administration of this drug (has no clinical meaning; avoid monitoring serum concentrations). If digoxin was being used to treat heart failure, may see exacerbation of symptoms as digoxin level is reduced. Use with caution in renal failure (experience limited); the complex will be removed from the body more slowly. Monitor for reoccurrence of digoxin toxicity. Failure of response to adequate treatment may call diagnosis of digitalis toxicity into question. Digoxin immune Fab is processed with papain and may cause hypersensitivity reactions in patients allergic to papaya, other papaya extracts, papain, chymopapain, or the pineapple enzyme bromelain. There may also be cross allergy with dust mite and latex allergens.

Adverse Reactions Frequency not defined.

Cardiovascular: Effects (due to withdrawal of digitalis) include exacerbation of heart failure, rapid ventricular response in patients with atrial fibrillation; postural hypotension

Endocrine & metabolic: Hypokalemia

Local: Phlebitis

Miscellaneous: Allergic reactions, serum sickness

Drug Interactions

Metabolism/Transport Effects None known.

Avoid Concomitant Use There are no known interactions where it is recommended to avoid concomitant use.

Increased Effect/Toxicity There are no known significant interactions involving an increase in effect.

Decreased Effect There are no known significant interactions involving a decrease in effect.

Stability Should be refrigerated (2°C to 8°C). The following stability information has also been reported: May be stored at room temperature for up to 30 days (Cohen, 2007).

Digibind®: Reconstitute by adding 4 mL sterile water, resulting in 9.5 mg/mL for I.V. infusion. Reconstituted solutions should be used within 4 hours if refrigerated. For very small doses, reconstituted vial can be further diluted by adding an additional 34 mL of sterile isotonic saline to achieve a final concentration of 1 mg/mL.

DigiFab™: Reconstitute by adding 4 mL sterile water, resulting in 10 mg/mL for I.V. infusion. Reconstituted solutions should be used within 4 hours if refrigerated. For very small doses, reconstituted vial can be further diluted by adding an additional 36 mL of sterile isotonic saline to achieve a final concentration of 1 mg/mL.

Mechanism of Action Digoxin immune antigen-binding fragments (Fab) are specific antibodies for the treatment of digitalis intoxication in carefully selected patients; binds with molecules of digoxin or digitoxin and then is excreted by the kidneys and removed from the body

Pharmacodynamics/Kinetics

Onset of action: I.V.: Improvement in 2-30 minutes for toxicity

Half-life elimination: 15-20 hours; prolonged with renal impairment

Excretion: Urine; undetectable amounts within 5-7 days

Dosage Each vial of Digibind® 38 mg or DigiFab™ 40 mg will bind ~0.5 mg of digoxin or digitoxin.

Note: Estimation of the dose is based on the body burden of digitalis. This may be calculated if the amount ingested is known or the postdistribution serum drug level is known (round dose to the nearest whole vial). If the amount of ingestion is unknown, general dosing guidelines should be used.

Acute ingestion of *unknown* amount: I.V.: Children and Adults: 20 vials is adequate to treat most life-threatening ingestions. May give as a single dose or give 10 vials, observe response, and give a second 10-vial dose if indicated.

Acute ingestion of *known* amount: I.V.:

Based on number of tablets/capsules ingested: Children and Adults:

Step 1:

Total body load (mg) = Amount (mg) digoxin capsules/ digitoxin ingested

Step 2:

Dose (vials) = Total body load (mg) / (0.5 mg digitalis bound/vial)

Alternatively, the following table gives an estimation of the number of vials needed based on the number of digoxin tablets or capsules ingested.

Number of Digoxin Tablets or Capsules Ingested[1]	Dose of Digoxin Immune Fab (# of Vials)
25	10
50	20
75	30
100	40
150	60
200	80

[1]250 mcg tablets with 80% bioavailability or 200 mcg Lanoxicaps® capsules with 100% bioavailability.

Based on steady-state serum digoxin concentration:

Infants and Children ≤20 kg: May require smaller doses; calculate dose in milligrams, reconstitute with NS, and administer dose via tuberculin syringe

Step 1:

Dose (mg) = [(serum digoxin concentration [ng/mL] x weight [kg]) / 100] x (mg/vial)

Note: Digibind® 38 mg/vial or DigiFab™ 40 mg/vial

Alternatively, the following table gives an estimation of the amount of **Digibind®** needed based on the steady-state serum digoxin concentration.

Infants and Small Children Dose Estimates of Digibind® (in mg) From Steady-State Serum Digoxin Concentration

Patient Weight (kg)	Serum Digoxin Concentration (ng/mL)						
	1	2	4	8	12	16	20
1	0.4 mg[1]	1 mg[1]	1.5 mg[1]	3 mg[1]	5 mg	6 mg	8 mg
3	1 mg[1]	2 mg[1]	5 mg	9 mg	14 mg	18 mg	23 mg
5	2 mg[1]	4 mg	8 mg	15 mg	23 mg	30 mg	38 mg
10	4 mg	8 mg	15 mg	30 mg	46 mg	61 mg	76 mg
20	8 mg	15 mg	30 mg	61 mg	91 mg	122 mg	152 mg

[1]Dilution of reconstituted vial to 1 mg/mL may be desirable.

Alternatively, the following table gives an estimation of the amount of **DigiFab™** needed based on the steady-state serum digoxin concentration.

Infants and Small Children Dose Estimates of DigiFab™ (in mg) From Steady-State Serum Digoxin Concentration

Patient Weight (kg)	Serum Digoxin Concentration (ng/mL)						
	1	2	4	8	12	16	20
1	0.4 mg[1]	1 mg[1]	1.5 mg[1]	3 mg[1]	5 mg	6.5 mg	8 mg
3	1 mg[1]	2.5 mg[1]	5 mg	10 mg	14 mg	19 mg	24 mg
5	2 mg[1]	4 mg	8 mg	16 mg	24 mg	32 mg	40 mg
10	4 mg	8 mg	16 mg	32 mg	48 mg	64 mg	80 mg
20	8 mg	16 mg	32 mg	64 mg	96 mg	128 mg	160 mg

[1]Dilution of reconstituted vial to 1 mg/mL may be desirable.

Adults:

Step 1:

Dose (vials) = [(serum digoxin concentration [ng/mL] x weight [kg]) / 100]

Alternatively, the following table gives an estimation of the number of vials needed based on the steady-state serum digoxin concentration.

Adult Dose Estimates of Digibind® (in # of Vials) From Steady-State Serum Digoxin Concentration

Patient Weight (kg)	Serum Digoxin Concentration (ng/mL)						
	1	2	4	8	12	16	20
40	0.5 vial	1 vial	2 vials	3 vials	5 vials	7 vials	8 vials
60	0.5 vial	1 vial	3 vials	5 vials	7 vials	10 vials	12 vials
70	1 vial	2 vials	3 vials	6 vials	9 vials	11 vials	14 vials
80	1 vial	2 vials	3 vials	7 vials	10 vials	13 vials	16 vials
100	1 vial	2 vials	4 vials	8 vials	12 vials	16 vials	20 vials

Based on steady-state digitoxin concentration: Children and Adults: If the calculated dose based on the **digitoxin** concentration is different than that for the digoxin concentration, use the higher dose.

Step 1:

Dose (vials) = [serum **digitoxin** concentration (ng/mL) x weight (kg)] / 1000

Chronic toxicity (serum digoxin concentration unavailable): I.V.:

Infants and Children ≤20 kg: 1 vial is adequate to reverse most cases of toxicity

Adults: 6 vials is adequate to reverse most cases of toxicity

Administration Continuous I.V. infusion over ≥30 minutes is preferred. May give by bolus injection if cardiac arrest is imminent. Small doses (infants/small children) may be administered using tuberculin syringe. Stopping the infusion and restarting at a slower rate may help if infusion-related reactions occur.

Monitoring Parameters Serum potassium, serum digoxin concentration prior to first dose of digoxin immune Fab; **digoxin levels will greatly increase with digoxin immune Fab use and are not an accurate determination of body stores** (has no clinical meaning; avoid monitoring serum concentrations); standard digoxin concentration measurements may be misleading until Fab fragments are eliminated from the body.

Patients with renal failure should be monitored for a prolonged period for reintoxication with digoxin following the rerelease of bound digoxin into the blood.

Test Interactions Digibind® will interfere with digitalis immunoassay measurements - this will result in clinically misleading serum digoxin concentrations fragment is eliminated from the body (several days to >1 week after Digibind® administration).

Dosage Forms Excipient information presented when available (limited, particularly for generics); consult specific product labeling. [DSC] = Discontinued product

Injection, powder for reconstitution [ovine derived]:

Digibind®: 38 mg [DSC] [derived from or manufactured using papain]

DigiFab®: 40 mg [derived from or manufactured using papain]

◆ **Dihematoporphyrin Ether** *see* Porfimer *on page 1376*

◆ **Dihydroartemisinin Hemisuccinate Sodium** *see* Artesunate *on page 148*

Dihydrocodeine, Aspirin, and Caffeine

(dye hye droe KOE deen, AS pir in, & KAF een)

Brand Names: U.S. Synalgos®-DC

Index Terms Dihydrocodeine Compound

Pharmacologic Category Analgesic, Opioid

Use Management of mild-to-moderate pain that requires relaxation

Pregnancy Risk Factor B/D (prolonged use or high doses at term)

Dosage

Adults: Oral: 1-2 capsules every 4-6 hours as needed for pain

Elderly: Initial dosing should be cautious (low end of adult dosing range)

Additional Information Complete prescribing information for this medication should be consulted for additional detail.

Dosage Forms Excipient information presented when available (limited, particularly for generics); consult specific product labeling.

Capsule, oral:

Synalgos®-DC: Dihydrocodeine bitartrate 16 mg, aspirin 356.4 mg, and caffeine 30 mg

Controlled Substance C-III

Dihydrocodeine, Chlorpheniramine, and Phenylephrine

(dye hye droe KOE deen, klor fen IR a meen, & fen il EF rin)

Brand Names: U.S. Coldcough PD; DiHydro-PE [OTC]; Novahistine DH; Tusscough DHC™

Index Terms Chlorpheniramine Maleate, Dihydrocodeine Bitartrate, and Phenylephrine Hydrochloride; Phenylephrine, Chlorpheniramine, and Dihydrocodeine

Pharmacologic Category Alkylamine Derivative; Alpha-Adrenergic Agonist; Analgesic, Opioid; Antitussive; Decongestant; Histamine H_1 Antagonist; Histamine H_1 Antagonist, First Generation

Use Symptomatic relief of cough and congestion associated with the upper respiratory tract

Pregnancy Risk Factor C

Dosage Cough and congestion: Oral:

Children 2-6 years (Novahistine DH): 1.25-2.5 mL every 4-6 hours as needed (maximum: 10 mL/24 hours)

Children 6-12 years (Novahistine DH): 2.5-5 mL every 4-6 hours as needed (maximum: 20 mL/24 hours)

Children ≥12 years and Adults (Novahistine DH): 5-10 mL every 4-6 hours as needed (maximum: 40 mL/24 hours)

Additional Information Complete prescribing information for this medication should be consulted for additional detail.

Dosage Forms Excipient information presented when available (limited, particularly for generics); consult specific product labeling. [DSC] = Discontinued product

Liquid, oral:

Novahistine DH: Dihydrocodeine bitartrate 7.5 mg, chlorpheniramine maleate 2 mg and phenylephrine hydrochloride 5 mg per 5 mL (480 mL) [ethanol free, sugar free; contains propylene glycol; strawberry flavor; C-III]

Syrup, oral:

Coldcough PD: Dihydrocodeine bitartrate 3 mg, chlorpheniramine maleate 2 mg, and phenylephrine hydrochloride 7.5 mg per 5 mL (120 mL) [ethanol free, sugar free; grape flavor; C-V]

DiHydro-PE: Dihydrocodeine bitartrate 3 mg, chlorpheniramine maleate 2 mg, and phenylephrine hydrochloride 7.5 mg per 5 mL (118 mL) [grape flavor; C-V]

Tusscough DHC™: Dihydrocodeine bitartrate 3 mg, chlorpheniramine maleate 5 mg, and phenylephrine hydrochloride 20 mg per 5 mL (473 mL) [ethanol free, sugar free, dye free; contains benzoic acid, propylene glycol; grape flavor; C-III]

Controlled Substance C-III; C-V

◆ **Dihydrocodeine Compound** *see* Dihydrocodeine, Aspirin, and Caffeine *on page 508*

Dihydroergotamine (dye hye droe er GOT a meen)

Brand Names: U.S. D.H.E. 45®; Migranal®

Brand Names: Canada Migranal®

Index Terms DHE; Dihydroergotamine Mesylate

Pharmacologic Category Antimigraine Agent; Ergot Derivative

Use Treatment of migraine headache with or without aura; injection also indicated for treatment of cluster headaches

Unlabeled Use Adjunct for DVT prophylaxis for hip surgery, for orthostatic hypotension, xerostomia secondary to antidepressant use, and pelvic congestion with pain

Pregnancy Risk Factor X

Pregnancy Considerations Dihydroergotamine is oxytocic and should not be used during pregnancy.

Lactation Enters breast milk/contraindicated

Contraindications Hypersensitivity to dihydroergotamine or any component of the formulation; uncontrolled hypertension, ischemic heart disease, angina pectoris, history of MI, silent ischemia, or coronary artery vasospasm including Prinzmetal's angina; hemiplegic or basilar migraine; peripheral vascular disease; sepsis; severe hepatic or renal dysfunction; following vascular surgery; avoid use within 24 hours of sumatriptan, zolmitriptan, other serotonin agonists, or ergot-like agents; avoid during or within 2 weeks of discontinuing MAO inhibitors; concurrent use of peripheral and central vasoconstrictors; ergot alkaloids are contraindicated with potent inhibitors of CYP3A4 (includes protease inhibitors, azole antifungals, and some macrolide antibiotics); pregnancy, breast-feeding

Warnings/Precautions **[U.S. Boxed Warning]: Ergot alkaloids are contraindicated with potent inhibitors of CYP3A4 (includes protease inhibitors, azole antifungals, and some macrolide antibiotics); concomitant use associated with an increased risk of vasospasm leading to cerebral ischemia and/or ischemia of the extremities.** Do not give to patients with risk factors for CAD until a cardiovascular evaluation has been performed; if evaluation is satisfactory, the healthcare provider should administer the first dose and cardiovascular status should be periodically evaluated. May cause vasospastic reactions; persistent vasospasm may lead to gangrene or death in patients with compromised circulation. Discontinue if signs of vasoconstriction develop. Rare reports of increased blood pressure in patients without history of hypertension. Rare reports of adverse cardiac events (acute MI, life-threatening arrhythmias, death) have been reported following use of the injection. Cerebral hemorrhage, subarachnoid hemorrhage, and stroke have also occurred following use of the injection. Not for prolonged use. Pleural and peritoneal fibrosis have been reported with prolonged daily use. Cardiac valvular fibrosis has also been associated with ergot alkaloids. Use with caution in the elderly.

Migranal® Nasal Spray: Local irritation to nose and throat (usually transient and mild-moderate in severity) can occur; long-term consequences on nasal or respiratory mucosa have not been extensively evaluated.

Adverse Reactions

>10%: Nasal spray: Respiratory: Rhinitis (26%)

1% to 10%: Nasal spray:

Central nervous system: Dizziness (4%), somnolence (3%)

Endocrine & metabolic: Hot flashes (1%)

Gastrointestinal: Nausea (10%), taste disturbance (8%), vomiting (4%), diarrhea (2%)

Local: Application site reaction (6%)

Neuromuscular & skeletal: Weakness (1%), stiffness (1%)

Respiratory: Pharyngitis (3%)

<1% (Limited to important or life-threatening): Injection and nasal spray: Cerebral hemorrhage, coronary artery vasospasm, dyspnea, hypertension, MI, paresthesia, peripheral cyanosis, peripheral ischemia, stroke, subarachnoid hemorrhage, ventricular fibrillation, ventricular tachycardia. Pleural and retroperitoneal fibrosis have been reported following prolonged use of the injection; cardiac valvular fibrosis has been associated with ergot alkaloids.

Drug Interactions

Metabolism/Transport Effects Substrate of CYP3A4 (major); **Note:** Assignment of Major/Minor substrate status based on clinically relevant drug interaction potential; **Inhibits** CYP3A4 (weak)

Avoid Concomitant Use

Avoid concomitant use of Dihydroergotamine with any of the following: Alpha-/Beta-Agonists; Alpha1-Agonists; Boceprevir; Clarithromycin; Conivaptan; Crizotinib; Efavirenz; Itraconazole; Nitroglycerin; Posaconazole; Protease Inhibitors; Serotonin 5-HT1D Receptor Agonists; Telaprevir; Voriconazole

Increased Effect/Toxicity

Dihydroergotamine may increase the levels/effects of: Alpha-/Beta-Agonists; Alpha1-Agonists; Metoclopramide; Serotonin 5-HT1D Receptor Agonists; Serotonin Modulators

The levels/effects of Dihydroergotamine may be increased by: Antipsychotics; Boceprevir; Clarithromycin; Conivaptan; Crizotinib; CYP3A4 Inhibitors (Moderate); CYP3A4 Inhibitors (Strong); Dasatinib; Efavirenz; Itraconazole; Macrolide Antibiotics; Nitroglycerin; Posaconazole; Protease Inhibitors; Serotonin 5-HT1D Receptor Agonists; Telaprevir; Voriconazole

Decreased Effect

Dihydroergotamine may decrease the levels/effects of: Nitroglycerin

The levels/effects of Dihydroergotamine may be decreased by: Tocilizumab

Stability

Injection: Store below 25°C (77°F); do not refrigerate or freeze; protect from heat. Protect from light.

Nasal spray: Prior to use, store below 25°C (77°F); do not refrigerate or freeze. Once spray applicator has been prepared, use within 8 hours; discard any unused solution.

Mechanism of Action Ergot alkaloid alpha-adrenergic blocker directly stimulates vascular smooth muscle to vasoconstrict peripheral and cerebral vessels; also has effects on serotonin receptors

Pharmacodynamics/Kinetics

Onset of action: I.M.: 15-30 minutes

Duration: I.M.: 3-4 hours

Distribution: V_d: ~800 L

Protein binding: 93%

Metabolism: Extensively hepatic

Half-life elimination: ~9-10 hours

Time to peak, serum: I.M.: 24 minutes; I.V.: 1-2 minutes; Intranasal: 30-60 minutes; SubQ 15-45 minutes

Excretion: Primarily feces; urine (6% to 7% as unchanged drug)

Dosage Adults:

I.M., SubQ: 1 mg at first sign of headache; repeat hourly to a maximum dose of 3 mg/day; maximum dose: 6 mg/week

I.V.: 1 mg at first sign of headache; repeat hourly up to a maximum dose of 2 mg/day; maximum dose: 6 mg/week

Raskin protocol (unlabeled dosing): Initial test dose: 0.5 mg (following premedication with metoclopramide); subsequent dosing is titrated (range: 0.2-1 mg) every 8 hours for 2-3 days and administered with or without metoclopramide based on response and tolerance (Raskin, 1986; Raskin, 1990). **Note:** Some clinicians use modified versions of this protocol, with additional adjunctive medications and/or alternate antiemetic agents.

Intranasal: 1 spray (0.5 mg) of nasal spray should be administered into each nostril; if needed, repeat after 15 minutes, up to a total of 4 sprays (2 mg). **Note:** Do not exceed 6 sprays (3 mg) in a 24-hour period and no more than 8 sprays (4 mg) in a week.

Elderly: Patients >65 years of age were not included in controlled clinical studies

Dosing adjustment in renal impairment: Contraindicated in severe renal impairment

Dosing adjustment in hepatic impairment: Dosage reductions are probably necessary but specific guidelines are not available; contraindicated in severe hepatic dysfunction

Administration

Intranasal: Prior to administration of nasal spray, the nasal spray applicator must be primed (pumped 4 times); in order to let the drug be absorbed through the skin in the nose, patients should not inhale deeply through the nose while spraying or immediately after spraying; for best results, treatment should be initiated at the first symptom or sign of an attack; however, nasal spray can be used at any stage of a migraine attack.

I.M., SubQ: May administer by intramuscular or subcutaneous injection.

I.V.: Administer slowly over 2-3 minutes (Raskin protocol)

Reference Range Minimum concentration for vasoconstriction is reportedly 0.06 ng/mL

Dosage Forms Excipient information presented when available (limited, particularly for generics); consult specific product labeling.

Injection, solution, as mesylate: 1 mg/mL (1 mL)

D.H.E. 45®: 1 mg/mL (1 mL) [contains ethanol 6.2%]

Solution, intranasal, as mesylate [spray]:

Migranal®: 4 mg/mL (1 mL) [contains caffeine 10 mg/mL; 0.5 mg/spray]

◆ **Dihydroergotamine Mesylate** *see* Dihydroergotamine *on page 508*

◆ **Dihydrohydroxycodeinone** *see* OxyCODONE *on page 1266*

◆ **Dihydromorphinone** *see* HYDROmorphone *on page 843*

- **DiHydro-PE [OTC]** *see* Dihydrocodeine, Chlorpheniramine, and Phenylephrine *on page 508*
- **Dihydroqinghaosu Hemisuccinate Sodium** *see* Artesunate *on page 148*
- **Dihydroxyanthracenedione** *see* MitoXANtrone *on page 1145*
- **Dihydroxyanthracenedione Dihydrochloride** *see* MitoXANtrone *on page 1145*
- **1,25 Dihydroxycholecalciferol** *see* Calcitriol *on page 263*
- **Dihydroxydeoxynorvinkaleukoblastine** *see* Vinorelbine *on page 1793*
- **Diiodohydroxyquin** *see* Iodoquinol *on page 921*
- **Dilacor XR®** *see* Diltiazem *on page 510*
- **Dilantin®** *see* Phenytoin *on page 1346*
- **Dilantin-125®** *see* Phenytoin *on page 1346*
- **Dilatrate®-SR** *see* Isosorbide Dinitrate *on page 936*
- **Dilaudid®** *see* HYDROmorphone *on page 843*
- **Dilaudid-HP®** *see* HYDROmorphone *on page 843*
- **Dilaudid-HP-Plus® (Can)** *see* HYDROmorphone *on page 843*
- **Dilaudid® Sterile Powder (Can)** *see* HYDROmorphone *on page 843*
- **Dilaudid-XP® (Can)** *see* HYDROmorphone *on page 843*
- **Dilt-CD** *see* Diltiazem *on page 510*
- **Diltia XT®** *see* Diltiazem *on page 510*

Diltiazem (dil TYE a zem)

Brand Names: U.S. Cardizem®; Cardizem® CD; Cardizem® LA; Cartia XT®; Dilacor XR®; Dilt-CD; Dilt-XR; Diltia XT®; Diltzac; Matzim™ LA; Taztia XT®; Tiazac®

Brand Names: Canada Apo-Diltiaz CD®; Apo-Diltiaz SR®; Apo-Diltiaz TZ®; Apo-Diltiaz®; Apo-Diltiaz® Injectable; Ava-Diltiazem; Cardizem® CD; CO Diltiazem CD; CO Diltiazem T; Diltiazem HCl ER®; Diltiazem Hydrochloride Injection; Diltiazem TZ; Diltiazem-CD; Nu-Diltiaz; Nu-Diltiaz-CD; PMS-Diltiazem CD; ratio-Diltiazem CD; Sandoz-Diltiazem CD; Sandoz-Diltiazem T; Teva-Diltiazem; Teva-Diltiazem CD; Teva-Diltiazem HCL ER Capsules; Tiazac®; Tiazac® XC

Index Terms Diltiazem Hydrochloride

Pharmacologic Category Antianginal Agent; Antiarrhythmic Agent, Class IV; Calcium Channel Blocker; Calcium Channel Blocker, Nondihydropyridine

Additional Appendix Information

Calcium Channel Blockers *on page 1887*

Use

Oral: Essential hypertension; chronic stable angina or angina from coronary artery spasm

Injection: Control of rapid ventricular rate in patients with atrial fibrillation or atrial flutter; conversion of paroxysmal supraventricular tachycardia (PSVT)

Unlabeled Use

ACLS guidelines: Injection: Stable narrow-complex tachycardia uncontrolled or unconverted by adenosine or vagal maneuvers or if SVT is recurrent

Pediatric hypertension

Pregnancy Risk Factor C

Pregnancy Considerations Teratogenic and embryotoxic effects have been demonstrated in animal reproduction studies.

Lactation Enters breast milk/not recommended (AAP considers "compatible"; AAP 2001 update pending)

Contraindications

Oral: Hypersensitivity to diltiazem or any component of the formulation; sick sinus syndrome (except in patients with a functioning artificial pacemaker); second- or third-degree AV block (except in patients with a functioning artificial pacemaker); severe hypotension (systolic <90 mm Hg); acute MI and pulmonary congestion

Intravenous (I.V.): Hypersensitivity to diltiazem or any component of the formulation; sick sinus syndrome (except in patients with a functioning artificial pacemaker); second- or third-degree AV block (except in patients with a functioning artificial pacemaker); severe hypotension (systolic <90 mm Hg); cardiogenic shock; administration concomitantly or within a few hours of the administration of I.V. beta-blockers; atrial fibrillation or flutter associated with accessory bypass tract (eg, Wolff-Parkinson-White syndrome); ventricular tachycardia (with wide-complex tachycardia, must determine whether origin is supraventricular or ventricular)

Canadian labeling: Additional contraindications (not in U.S. labeling): I.V. and Oral: Pregnancy; use in women of child-bearing potential

Warnings/Precautions Can cause first-, second-, and third-degree AV block or sinus bradycardia and risk increases with agents known to slow cardiac conduction. The most common side effect is peripheral edema; occurs within 2-3 weeks of starting therapy. Symptomatic hypotension with or without syncope can rarely occur; blood pressure must be lowered at a rate appropriate for the patient's clinical condition. Use caution when using diltiazem together with a beta-blocker; may result in conduction disturbances, hypotension, and worsened LV function. Simultaneous administration of I.V. diltiazem and an I.V. beta-blocker or administration within a few hours of each other may result in asystole and is contraindicated. Use with other agents known to either reduce SA node function and/or AV nodal conduction (eg, digoxin) or reduce sympathetic outflow (eg, clonidine) may increase the risk of serious bradycardia. Use caution in left ventricular dysfunction (may exacerbate condition). Avoid use of diltiazem in patients with heart failure and reduced ejection fraction (Hunt, 2009). Use with caution with hypertrophic obstructive cardiomyopathy; routine use is currently not recommended due to insufficient evidence (Maron, 2003). Use with caution in hepatic or renal dysfunction. Transient dermatologic reactions have been observed with use; if reaction persists, discontinue. May (rarely) progress to erythema multiforme or exfoliative dermatitis.

Adverse Reactions Note: Frequencies represent ranges for various dosage forms. Patients with impaired ventricular function and/or conduction abnormalities may have higher incidence of adverse reactions.

>10%:

Cardiovascular: Edema (2% to 15%)

Central nervous system: Headache (5% to 12%)

2% to 10%:

Cardiovascular: AV block (first degree 2% to 8%), edema (lower limb, 2% to 8%), pain (6%), bradycardia (2% to 6%), hypotension (<2% to 4%), vasodilation (2% to 3%), extrasystoles (2%), flushing (1% to 2%), palpitation (1% to 2%)

Central nervous system: Dizziness (3% to 10%), nervousness (2%)

Dermatologic: Rash (1% to 4%)

Endocrine & metabolic: Gout (1% to 2%)

Gastrointestinal: Dyspepsia (1% to 6%), constipation (<2% to 4%), vomiting (2%), diarrhea (1% to 2%)

Local: Injection site reactions: Burning, itching (4%)

Neuromuscular & skeletal: Weakness (1% to 4%), myalgia (2%)

Respiratory: Rhinitis (<2% to 10%), pharyngitis (2% to 6%), dyspnea (1% to 6%), bronchitis (1% to 4%), cough (≤3), sinus congestion (1% to 2%)

<2% (Limited to important or life-threatening): Alkaline phosphatase increased, allergic reaction, ALT increased, AST increased, amblyopia, amnesia, arrhythmia, AV block (second or third degree), bundle branch block, CHF, depression, dysgeusia, extrapyramidal symptoms, gingival hyperplasia, hemolytic anemia, petechiae, photosensitivity, Stevens-Johnson syndrome, syncope, tachycardia, thrombocytopenia, tremor, toxic epidermal necrolysis

Drug Interactions

Metabolism/Transport Effects Substrate of CYP2C9 (minor), CYP2D6 (minor), CYP3A4 (major), P-glycoprotein; **Note:** Assignment of Major/Minor substrate status based on clinically relevant drug interaction potential; **Inhibits** CYP2C9 (weak), CYP2D6 (weak), CYP3A4 (moderate)

Avoid Concomitant Use

Avoid concomitant use of Diltiazem with any of the following: Conivaptan; Pimozide; Tolvaptan

Increased Effect/Toxicity

Diltiazem may increase the levels/effects of: Alfentanil; Amifostine; Amiodarone; Antihypertensives; Aprepitant; ARIPiprazole; Atorvastatin; Benzodiazepines (metabolized by oxidation); Beta-Blockers; Budesonide (Systemic, Oral Inhalation); BusPIRone; Calcium Channel Blockers (Dihydropyridine); CarBAMazepine; Cardiac Glycosides; Colchicine; Corticosteroids (Systemic); CycloSPORINE; CycloSPORINE (Systemic); CYP3A4 Substrates; Dronedarone; Eletriptan; Eplerenone; Everolimus; Fingolimod; Fosaprepitant; Fosphenytoin; Halofantrine; Hypotensive Agents; Lithium; Lovastatin; Lurasidone; Magnesium Salts; Midodrine; Neuromuscular-Blocking Agents (Nondepolarizing); Nitroprusside; Phenytoin; Pimecrolimus; Pimozide; Propafenone; QuiNIDine; Ranolazine; Red Yeast Rice; RiTUXimab; Rivaroxaban; Salicylates; Salmeterol; Saxagliptin; Simvastatin; Tacrolimus; Tacrolimus (Systemic); Tacrolimus (Topical); Tolvaptan; Vilazodone; Zuclopenthixol

The levels/effects of Diltiazem may be increased by: Alpha1-Blockers; Anilidopiperidine Opioids; Antifungal Agents (Azole Derivatives, Systemic); Aprepitant; Atorvastatin; Calcium Channel Blockers (Dihydropyridine); Cimetidine; Conivaptan; CycloSPORINE; CycloSPORINE (Systemic); CYP3A4 Inhibitors (Moderate); CYP3A4 Inhibitors (Strong); Dasatinib; Diazoxide; Dronedarone; Fluconazole; Fosaprepitant; Grapefruit Juice; Herbs (Hypotensive Properties); Lovastatin; Macrolide Antibiotics; Magnesium Salts; MAO Inhibitors; Pentoxifylline; P-glycoprotein/ABCB1 Inhibitors; Phosphodiesterase 5 Inhibitors; Prostacyclin Analogues; Protease Inhibitors; Simvastatin

Decreased Effect

Diltiazem may decrease the levels/effects of: Clopidogrel

The levels/effects of Diltiazem may be decreased by: Barbiturates; Calcium Salts; CarBAMazepine; Colestipol; CYP3A4 Inducers (Strong); Deferasirox; Herbs (Hypertensive Properties); Methylphenidate; Nafcillin; Peginterferon Alfa-2b; P-glycoprotein/ABCB1 Inducers; Rifamycin Derivatives; Tocilizumab; Yohimbine

Ethanol/Nutrition/Herb Interactions

Ethanol: Avoid ethanol (may increase risk of hypotension or vasodilation).

Food: Diltiazem serum levels may be elevated if taken with food. Serum concentrations were not altered by grapefruit juice in small clinical trials.

Herb/Nutraceutical: St John's wort may decrease diltiazem levels. Avoid bayberry, blue cohosh, cayenne, ephedra, ginger, ginseng (American), kola, licorice, yohimbe (may worsen hypertension). Avoid black cohosh, California poppy, coleus, garlic, golden seal, hawthorn, mistletoe, periwinkle, quinine, shepherd's purse (may have increased antihypertensive effect).

Stability

Capsule, tablet: Store at room temperature. Protect from light.

Solution for injection: Store in refrigerator at 2°C to 8°C (36°F to 46°F); do not freeze. May be stored at room temperature for up to 1 month. Following dilution to ≤1 mg/mL with $D_5{}^1/_2NS$, D_5W, or NS, solution is stable for 24 hours at room temperature or under refrigeration.

Mechanism of Action Nondihydropyridine calcium channel blocker which inhibits calcium ion from entering the "slow channels" or select voltage-sensitive areas of vascular smooth muscle and myocardium during depolarization, producing a relaxation of coronary vascular smooth muscle and coronary vasodilation; increases myocardial oxygen delivery in patients with vasospastic angina

Pharmacodynamics/Kinetics

Onset of action: Oral: Immediate release tablet: 30-60 minutes; I.V.: 3 minutes

Duration: I.V.: Bolus: 1-3 hours; Continuous infusion (after discontinuation): 0.5-10 hours

Absorption: Immediate release tablet: >90%; Extended release capsule: ~93%

Distribution: V_d: 3-13 L/kg

Protein binding: 70% to 80%

Metabolism: Hepatic (extensive first-pass effect); following single I.V. injection, plasma concentrations of N-monodesmethyldiltiazem and desacetyldiltiazem are typically undetectable; however, these metabolites accumulate to detectable concentrations following 24-hour constant rate infusion. N-monodesmethyldiltiazem appears to have 20% of the potency of diltiazem; desacetyldiltiazem is about 25% to 50% as potent as the parent compound.

Bioavailability: Oral: ~40% (undergoes extensive first-pass metabolism)

Half-life elimination: Immediate release tablet: 3-4.5 hours, may be prolonged with renal impairment; Extended release tablet: 6-9 hours; Extended release capsules: 5-10 hours; I.V.: single dose: ~3.4 hours; continuous infusion: 4-5 hours

Time to peak, serum: Immediate release tablet: 2-4 hours; Extended release tablet: 11-18 hours; Extended release capsule: 10-14 hours

Excretion: Urine (2% to 4% as unchanged drug; 6% to 7% as metabolites); feces

Dosage

Children (unlabeled use): Minimal information available; some centers use the following: Oral: Hypertension: Immediate release tablets: Initial: 1.5-2 mg/kg/day divided in 3 doses/day (maximum dose 6 mg/kg/day up to 360 mg/day) (Flynn, 2000)

Adults:

Oral:

Angina:

Capsule, extended release:

Dilacor XR®, Dilt-XR, Diltia XT®: Initial: 120 mg once daily; titrate over 7-14 days; usual dose range: 120-320 mg/day: maximum: 480 mg/day

Cardizem® CD, Cartia XT®, Dilt-CD: Initial: 120-180 mg once daily; titrate over 7-14 days; usual dose range: 120-320 mg/day; maximum: 480 mg/day

Tiazac®, Taztia XT®: Initial: 120-180 mg once daily; titrate over 7-14 days; usual dose range: 120-320 mg/day; maximum: 540 mg/day

Tablet, extended release (Cardizem® LA, Matzim™ LA, Tiazac® XC [CAN; not available in U.S.]): 180 mg once daily; may increase at 7- to 14-day intervals; usual dose range: 120-320 mg/day; maximum: 360 mg/day

Tablet, immediate release (Cardizem®): Usual starting dose: 30 mg 4 times/day; titrate dose gradually at 1- to 2-day intervals; usual dose range: 120-320 mg/day

Hypertension:

Capsule, extended release (once-daily dosing):

Cardizem® CD, Cartia XT®, Dilt-CD: Initial: 180-240 mg once daily; dose adjustment may be made after 14 days; usual dose range (JNC 7): 180-420 mg/day; maximum: 480 mg/day

Dilacor® XR, Diltia XT®, Dilt-XR: Initial: 180-240 mg once daily; dose adjustment may be made after 14 days; usual dose range (JNC 7): 180-420 mg/day; maximum: 540 mg/day

Tiazac®, Taztia XT®: Initial: 120-240 mg once daily; dose adjustment may be made after 14 days; usual dose range (JNC 7): 180-420 mg/day; maximum: 540 mg/day

Capsule, extended release (twice-daily dosing): Initial: 60-120 mg twice daily; dose adjustment may be made after 14 days; usual range: 240-360 mg/day

Note: Diltiazem is available as a generic intended for either once- or twice-daily dosing, depending on the formulation; verify appropriate extended release capsule formulation is administered.

Tablet, extended release (Cardizem® LA, Matzim™ LA, Tiazac® XC [CAN; not available in U.S.]): Initial: 180-240 mg once daily; dose adjustment may be made after 14 days; usual dose range (JNC 7): 120-540 mg/day

Note: Elderly: Consider lower initial doses (eg, 120 mg once daily using extended release capsule) and titrate to response (Aronow, 2011)

I.V.: *Atrial fibrillation, atrial flutter, PSVT:*

Initial bolus dose: 0.25 mg/kg actual body weight over 2 minutes (average adult dose: 20 mg); ACLS guideline recommends 15-20 mg

Repeat bolus dose (may be administered after 15 minutes if the response is inadequate): 0.35 mg/kg actual body weight over 2 minutes (average adult dose: 25 mg); ACLS guideline recommends 20-25 mg

Continuous infusion (infusions >24 hours or infusion rates >15 mg/hour are not recommended): Initial infusion rate of 10 mg/hour; rate may be increased in 5 mg/hour increments up to 15 mg/hour as needed; some patients may respond to an initial rate of 5 mg/hour.

If diltiazem injection is administered by continuous infusion for >24 hours, the possibility of decreased diltiazem clearance, prolonged elimination half-life, and increased diltiazem and/or diltiazem metabolite plasma concentrations should be considered.

Conversion from I.V. diltiazem to oral diltiazem:

Oral dose (mg/day) is approximately equal to [rate (mg/hour) x 3 + 3] x 10.

3 mg/hour = 120 mg/day
5 mg/hour = 180 mg/day
7 mg/hour = 240 mg/day
11 mg/hour = 360 mg/day

Dosing adjustment in renal impairment: Use with caution; no dosing adjustments recommended

Dialysis: Not removed by hemo- or peritoneal dialysis; supplemental dose is not necessary.

Dosing adjustment in hepatic impairment: Use with caution; no specific dosing recommendations available; extensively metabolized by the liver; half-life is increased in patients with cirrhosis

Administration

Oral:

Immediate release tablet (Cardizem®): Administer before meals and at bedtime.

Long acting dosage forms: Do not open, chew, or crush; swallow whole.

Cardizem® CD, Cardizem® LA, Cartia XT®, Dilt-CD, Matzim™ LA: May be administered without regards to meals.

Dilacor XR®, Dilt-XR, Diltia XT®: Administer on an empty stomach.

Taztia XT™, Tiazac®: Capsules may be opened and sprinkled on a spoonful of applesauce. Applesauce should not be hot and should be swallowed without chewing, followed by drinking a glass of water.

Tiazac® XC [CAN; not available in U.S.]: Administer at bedtime

I.V.: Bolus doses given over 2 minutes with continuous ECG and blood pressure monitoring. Continuous infusion should be via infusion pump.

Monitoring Parameters Liver function tests, blood pressure, ECG, heart rate

Dosage Forms Excipient information presented when available (limited, particularly for generics); consult specific product labeling.

Capsule, extended release, oral, as hydrochloride [once-daily dosing]: 120 mg, 180 mg, 240 mg, 300 mg, 360 mg, 420 mg

Cardizem® CD: 120 mg, 180 mg, 240 mg, 300 mg, 360 mg
Cartia XT®: 120 mg, 180 mg, 240 mg, 300 mg
Dilacor XR®: 240 mg
Dilt-CD: 120 mg, 180 mg, 240 mg, 300 mg
Dilt-XR: 120 mg, 180 mg, 240 mg
Diltia XT®: 120 mg, 180 mg, 240 mg
Diltzac: 120 mg, 180 mg, 240 mg, 300 mg, 360 mg
Taztia XT®: 120 mg, 180 mg, 240 mg, 300 mg, 360 mg
Tiazac®: 120 mg, 180 mg, 240 mg, 300 mg, 360 mg, 420 mg

Capsule, extended release, oral, as hydrochloride [twice-daily dosing]: 60 mg, 90 mg, 120 mg

Injection, powder for reconstitution, as hydrochloride: 100 mg

Injection, solution, as hydrochloride: 5 mg/mL (5 mL, 10 mL, 25 mL)

Tablet, oral, as hydrochloride: 30 mg, 60 mg, 90 mg, 120 mg

Cardizem®: 30 mg
Cardizem®: 60 mg, 90 mg, 120 mg [scored]

Tablet, extended release, oral, as hydrochloride [once-daily dosing]:

Cardizem® LA: 120 mg, 180 mg, 240 mg, 300 mg, 360 mg, 420 mg
Matzim™ LA: 180 mg, 240 mg, 300 mg, 360 mg, 420 mg

Dosage Forms: Canada Excipient information presented when available (limited, particularly for generics); consult specific product labeling.

Tablet, extended release, as hydrochloride:

Tiazac® XC: 120 mg, 180 mg, 240 mg, 300 mg, 360 mg

Extemporaneous Preparations A 12 mg/mL oral suspension may be made from tablets (regular, not extended release) and one of three different vehicles (cherry syrup, a 1:1 mixture of Ora-Sweet® and Ora-Plus®, or a 1:1 mixture of Ora-Sweet® SF and Ora-Plus®). Crush sixteen 90 mg tablets in a mortar and reduce to a fine powder. Add 10 mL of the chosen vehicle and mix to a uniform paste; mix while adding the vehicle in incremental proportions to **almost** 120 mL; transfer to a calibrated bottle, rinse mortar with vehicle, and add quantity of vehicle sufficient to make 120 mL. Label "shake well" and "protect from light". Stable for 60 days when stored in amber plastic prescription bottles in the dark at room temperature or refrigerated.

Allen LV and Erickson MA, "Stability of Baclofen, Captopril, Diltiazem Hydrochloride, Dipyridamole, and Flecainide Acetate in Extemporaneously Compounded Oral Liquids," *Am J Health Syst Pharm*, 1996, 53(18):2179-84.

◆ **Diltiazem-CD (Can)** *see* Diltiazem *on page 510*
◆ **Diltiazem HCl ER® (Can)** *see* Diltiazem *on page 510*

◆ **Diltiazem Hydrochloride** *see* Diltiazem *on page* 510
◆ **Diltiazem Hydrochloride Injection (Can)** *see* Diltiazem *on page* 510
◆ **Diltiazem TZ (Can)** *see* Diltiazem *on page* 510
◆ **Dilt-XR** *see* Diltiazem *on page* 510
◆ **Diltzac** *see* Diltiazem *on page* 510

DimenhyDRINATE (dye men HYE dri nate)

Brand Names: U.S. Dramamine® [OTC]; Driminate [OTC]; TripTone® [OTC]

Brand Names: Canada Apo-Dimenhydrinate®; Children's Motion Sickness Liquid; Dimenhydrinate Injection; Dinate®; Gravol®; Nauseatol; Novo-Dimenate; PMS-Dimenhydrinate; Sandoz-Dimenhydrinate

Pharmacologic Category Ethanolamine Derivative; Histamine H_1 Antagonist; Histamine H_1 Antagonist, First Generation

Use Treatment and prevention of nausea, vertigo, and vomiting associated with motion sickness

Pregnancy Risk Factor B

Dosage

Oral:

Children:

2-5 years: 12.5-25 mg every 6-8 hours, maximum: 75 mg/day

6-12 years: 25-50 mg every 6-8 hours, maximum: 150 mg/day

Adults: 50-100 mg every 4-6 hours, not to exceed 400 mg/day

I.M.:

Children: 1.25 mg/kg **or** 37.5 mg/m^2 4 times/day; maximum: 300 mg/day

Adults: 50 mg every 4 hours; maximum: 100 mg every 4 hours

I.V.: Adults: 50 mg every 4 hours; maximum: 100 mg every 4 hours

Additional Information Complete prescribing information for this medication should be consulted for additional detail.

Dosage Forms Excipient information presented when available (limited, particularly for generics); consult specific product labeling. [DSC] = Discontinued product

Injection, solution: 50 mg/mL (1 mL) [contains benzyl alcohol]

Tablet, oral: 50 mg [DSC]

Dramamine®: 50 mg [scored]

Driminate: 50 mg [scored]

TripTone®: 50 mg

Tablet, chewable, oral:

Dramamine®: 50 mg [scored; contains phenylalanine 0.84 mg/tablet; orange flavor]

◆ **Dimenhydrinate Injection (Can)** *see* DimenhyDRINATE *on page* 513

Dimercaprol (dye mer KAP role)

Brand Names: U.S. BAL in Oil®

Index Terms BAL; British Anti-Lewisite; Dithioglycerol

Pharmacologic Category Antidote

Use Antidote to gold, arsenic (except arsine), or acute mercury poisoning (except nonalkyl mercury); adjunct to edetate CALCIUM disodium in lead poisoning

Pregnancy Risk Factor C

Pregnancy Considerations Animal reproduction studies have not been conducted. There are no adequate and well-controlled studies in pregnant women.

Lead poisoning: Following maternal occupational exposure, lead was found to cross the placenta in amounts related to maternal plasma levels. Possible outcomes of maternal lead exposure >10 mcg/dL include spontaneous abortion, postnatal developmental delay, and reduced birth weight. Chelation therapy during pregnancy is for maternal benefit only and should be limited to the treatment of severe, symptomatic lead poisoning.

Lactation Excretion in breast milk unknown/use caution

Contraindications Hepatic insufficiency (unless due to arsenic poisoning); iron, cadmium, or selenium poisoning

Warnings/Precautions Potentially a nephrotoxic drug, use with caution in patients with oliguria; keep urine alkaline to protect kidneys (prevents dimercaprol-metal complex breakdown). Discontinue or use with extreme caution if renal insufficiency develops during treatment. Hemodialysis may be used to remove dimercaprol-metal chelate in patients with renal dysfunction. Use with caution in patients with glucose 6-phosphate dehydrogenase deficiency; may increase risk of hemolytic anemia. Administer all injections deep I.M. at different sites. Fevers may occur in ~30% of children and may persistent for the duration of therapy. Product contains peanut oil; use caution in patients with peanut allergy; medication for the treatment of hypersensitivity reactions should be available for immediate use. When used in the treatment of lead poisoning, investigate, identify, and remove sources of lead exposure prior to treatment. Primary care providers should consult experts in chemotherapy of heavy metal toxicity before using chelation drug therapy.

Adverse Reactions

Frequency not always defined.

Cardiovascular: Chest pain, hypertension (dose related), tachycardia (dose related)

Central nervous system: Anxiety, fever (children ~30%), headache, nervousness

Dermatologic: Abscess

Gastrointestinal: Abdominal pain, burning sensation (lips, mouth, throat), nausea, salivation, throat irritation/pain, vomiting

Genitourinary: Burning sensation (penis)

Hematologic: Leukopenia (polymorphonuclear)

Local: Injection site pain

Neuromuscular & skeletal: Paresthesias (hand), weakness

Ocular: Blepharospasm, conjunctivitis, lacrimation

Renal: Acute renal insufficiency

Respiratory: Rhinorrhea, throat constriction

Miscellaneous: Diaphoresis

Drug Interactions

Metabolism/Transport Effects None known.

Avoid Concomitant Use

Avoid concomitant use of Dimercaprol with any of the following: Iron Salts

Increased Effect/Toxicity

Dimercaprol may increase the levels/effects of: Iron Salts

Decreased Effect There are no known significant interactions involving a decrease in effect.

Stability Store at 20°C to 25°C (68°F to 77°F).

Mechanism of Action Sulfhydryl group combines with ions of various heavy metals to form relatively stable, nontoxic, soluble chelates which are excreted in urine

Pharmacodynamics/Kinetics

Absorption: I.M.: Rapid; Oral: Not absorbed

Distribution: To all tissues including the brain

Metabolism: Rapidly hepatic to inactive metabolites

Time to peak, serum: 0.5-1 hour

Excretion: Urine

Dosage Note: Premedication with a histamine H_1 antagonist (eg, diphenhydramine) is recommended.

Children and Adults: Deep I.M.:

Mild arsenic or gold poisoning: 2.5 mg/kg every 6 hours for 2 days, then every 12 hours for 1 day, followed by once daily for 10 days

Severe arsenic or gold poisoning: 3 mg/kg every 4 hours for 2 days, then every 6 hours for 1 day, followed every 12 hours for 10 days

Mercury poisoning: 5 mg/kg initially, followed by 2.5 mg/kg 1-2 times/day for 10 days

Lead poisoning: **Note:** For the treatment of high blood lead levels in children, the CDC recommends chelation treatment when blood lead levels are >45 mcg/dL (CDC, 2002). Combination parenteral therapy is indicated when blood lead levels are ≥70 mcg/dL or patients are symptomatic (AAP, 2005). In adults, available guidelines recommend chelation therapy with blood lead levels >50 mcg/dL and significant symptoms; chelation therapy may also be indicated with blood lead levels ≥100 mcg/dL and/or symptoms. (Kosnett, 2007).

Lead encephalopathy (in conjunction with edetate CALCIUM disodium): Dimercaprol 4 mg/kg (75 mg/m^2) loading dose, followed by dimercaprol 4 mg/kg (75 mg/m^2) every 4 hours for 2-7 days (edetate CALCIUM disodium is **not** administered with the loading dose; begin edetate CALCIUM disodium with the second dose)

Symptomatic lead poisoning or blood lead levels ≥70 mcg/dL (in conjunction with edetate CALCIUM disodium): Dimercaprol 4 mg/kg (75 mg/m^2) loading dose, followed by dimercaprol 3 mg/kg/dose (50 mg/m^2) every 4 hours for 2-7 days (edetate CALCIUM disodium is **not** administered with the loading dose; begin edetate CALCIUM disodium with the second dose)

Administration Administer all injections deep I.M. at different sites. Keep urine alkaline to protect renal function. When used in the treatment of lead poisoning, administer in a separate site from edetate CALCIUM disodium.

Monitoring Parameters Renal function, urine pH, infusion-related reactions

For lead poisoning: Blood lead levels (baseline and 7-21 days after completing chelation therapy); hemoglobin or hematocrit, iron status, free erythrocyte protoporphyrin or zinc protoporphyrin; neurodevelopmental changes

Test Interactions Iodine I^{131} thyroidal uptake values may be decreased

Dosage Forms Excipient information presented when available (limited, particularly for generics); consult specific product labeling.

Injection, oil:

BAL in Oil®: 100 mg/mL (3 mL) [contains benzyl benzoate, peanut oil]

- **Dimetapp® Children's Long Acting Cough Plus Cold [OTC]** *see* Dextromethorphan and Chlorpheniramine *on page 489*
- **Dimetapp® Children's Nighttime Cold & Congestion [OTC]** *see* Diphenhydramine and Phenylephrine *on page 518*
- **Dimethyl Triazeno Imidazole Carboxamide** *see* Dacarbazine *on page 438*
- **Dinate® (Can)** *see* DimenhyDRINATE *on page 513*

Dinoprostone (dye noe PROST one)

Brand Names: U.S. Cervidil®; Prepidil®; Prostin E2®

Brand Names: Canada Cervidil®; Prepidil®; Prostin E_2®

Index Terms PGE_2; Prostaglandin E_2

Pharmacologic Category Abortifacient; Prostaglandin

Use

Endocervical gel: Promote cervical ripening in patients at or near term in whom there is a medical or obstetrical indication for the induction of labor

Suppositories: Terminate pregnancy from 12th through 20th week of gestation; evacuate uterus in cases of missed abortion or intrauterine fetal death up to 28 weeks of gestation; manage benign hydatidiform mole (nonmetastatic gestational trophoblastic disease)

Vaginal insert: Initiation and/or continuation of cervical ripening in patients at or near term in whom there is a medical or obstetrical indication for the induction of labor

Pregnancy Risk Factor C

Pregnancy Considerations Skeletal anomalies and embryotoxicity have been observed in animal studies. Although these effects would not be expected in humans when administered after the period of organogenesis, a sustained increase in uterine tone may have increased risks of adverse events to the fetus.

Fetal distress without corresponding maternal uterine hyperstimulation was observed in 3% to 4% of infants exposed to Cervidil® *in utero*. No adverse effects on physical or psychomotor function were observed in a 3 year follow-up study of exposed infants. Abnormal fetal heart rates were observed in 17% of infants exposed to Prepidil® gel *in utero*. Deceleration, intrauterine fetal sepsis, fetal depression and fetal acidosis have also been reported with administration of the gel.

When used for termination of pregnancy, dinoprostone is not considered feticidal, but is used to terminate pregnancy due to its ability to stimulate uterine contractions; do not use if fetus has reached the stage of viability.

Lactation Excretion in breast milk unknown

Contraindications Hypersensitivity to prostaglandins or any component of the formulation

Endocervical gel *and* vaginal insert: Patients in whom oxytocic drugs are contraindicated; history of cesarean section or major uterine surgery; presence of cephalopelvic disproportion; fetal distress when delivery is not imminent; unexplained vaginal bleeding during this pregnancy. In addition:

Endocervical gel: History of difficult labor and/or traumatic delivery, ≥6 previous term pregnancies with nonvertex presentation, hyperactive or hypertonic uterine patterns, obstetric emergencies when surgical intervention would be favorable, placenta previa, when vaginal delivery is not indicated (eg, vasa previa, active herpes genitalia)

Vaginal insert: Patients already receiving I.V. oxytocic drugs, ≥6 previous term pregnancies

Suppository: Acute pelvic inflammatory disease; active cardiac, pulmonary, renal, or hepatic disease

Warnings/Precautions [U.S. Boxed Warning]: Dinoprostone should be used only by medically-trained personnel in a hospital.

Postpartum DIC has been reported following dinoprostone for labor induction. Risk may be increased in women ≥30 years of age, gestation age >40 weeks, or women with pregnancy complications. Use caution in patients with hepatic or renal impairment.

Endocervical gel: Use caution with ruptured membranes, glaucoma, or a history of asthma. Intracervical placement of gel may lead to anaphylactoid syndrome of pregnancy (rare).

Vaginal insert: Use caution with ruptured membranes; nonvertex or nonsingleton pregnancy; previous uterine hypertony; history of asthma or glaucoma. Must be removed prior to administration of oxytocin, in case of hyperstimulation or if labor begins, fetal or maternal distress, and prior to amniotomy. Intravaginal placement of insert may lead to anaphylactoid syndrome of pregnancy (rare).

Suppository: Transient pyrexia and decreased blood pressure may be observed with treatment. Use caution with history of asthma; hypotension or hypertension; cardiovascular disease; anemia; jaundice; diabetes; epilepsy;

compromised uteri; cervicitis, endocervical infections or acute vaginitis. Measures should be taken to ensure complete abortion. Commercially available suppositories should not be used for extemporaneous preparation of any other dosage form of drug. Do not use for cervical ripening or other indications in patients with term pregnancy.

Adverse Reactions

Endocervical gel:

1% to 10%:

Central nervous system: Fever (1%)

Gastrointestinal: GI upset (6%)

Genitourinary: Abnormal uterine contractions (7%), warm feeling in vagina (2%)

Neuromuscular & skeletal: Back pain (3%)

Postmarketing and/or case reports: Amnionitis, anaphylactoid syndrome of pregnancy (amniotic fluid embolism), postpartum DIC, premature rupture of membranes, uterine rupture (with intracervical administration)

Suppository:

Frequency not defined:

Cardiovascular: Arrhythmia, chest pain, chest tightness, hypotension, syncope

Central nervous system: Chills, dizziness, fever, headache, shivering, tension

Dermatologic: Rash, skin discoloration

Endocrine & metabolic: Breast tenderness, endometritis, hot flashes

Gastrointestinal: Dehydration, diarrhea, nausea, vomiting

Genitourinary: uterine rupture, urinary retention, vaginal pain, vaginismus, vaginitis, vulvitis

Neuromuscular & skeletal: Arthralgia, backache, joint inflammation/pain (new or exacerbated), leg cramps (nocturnal), muscle cramp/pain, myalgia, paresthesia, stiff neck, tremor, weakness

Ocular: Blurred vision, eye pain

Otic: Hearing impairment

Respiratory: Cough, dyspnea, laryngitis, pharyngitis, wheezing

Miscellaneous: Diaphoresis

Postmarketing and/or case reports: MI

Vaginal insert:

1% to 10%: Genitourinary: Uterine hyperstimulation *without* fetal distress (2% to 5%), uterine hyperstimulation *with* fetal distress (3%)

<1% (Limited to important or life-threatening): Anaphylactoid syndrome of pregnancy (amniotic fluid embolism), postpartum DIC, hypersensitivity reactions, hypotension, uterine rupture

Drug Interactions

Metabolism/Transport Effects None known.

Avoid Concomitant Use

Avoid concomitant use of Dinoprostone with any of the following: Carbetocin

Increased Effect/Toxicity

Dinoprostone may increase the levels/effects of: Carbetocin; Oxytocin

Decreased Effect There are no known significant interactions involving a decrease in effect.

Stability

Endocervical gel should be stored under refrigeration at 2°C to 8°C (36°F to 46°F).

Suppositories must be kept frozen; store in freezer not above -20°C (-4°F).

Vaginal insert should be stored in freezer between -20°C and -10°C (-4°F and 14°F).

Mechanism of Action A synthetic prostaglandin E_2 abortifacient that stimulates uterine contractions similar to those seen during natural labor. Prostaglandin E_2 plays a role in cervical ripening, which allows the fetus to pass through the birth canal.

Pharmacodynamics/Kinetics

Onset of action (uterine contractions): Vaginal suppository: Within 10 minutes

Duration: Vaginal insert: 0.3 mg/hour over 12 hours; Vaginal suppository: Up to 2-3 hours

Absorption: Vaginal suppository: Slow

Metabolism: Metabolized in the lungs; forms metabolites which are further metabolized in the liver and kidney

Half-life elimination: 2.5-5 minutes

Time to peak, plasma: Endocervical gel: 30-45 minutes

Excretion: Primarily urine; feces (small amounts)

Dosage Females of reproductive age:

Abortifacient: Vaginal suppository: Insert 20 mg (1 suppository) high in vagina, repeat at 3- to 5-hour intervals until abortion occurs; continued administration for longer than 2 days is not advisable

Cervical ripening:

Endocervical gel: Using catheter supplied with gel, insert 0.5 mg into the cervical canal. May repeat every 6 hours if needed. Maximum cumulative dose: 1.5 mg/24 hours

Vaginal insert: Insert 10 mg transversely into the posterior fornix of the vagina (to be removed at the onset of active labor or after 12 hours)

Administration

Endocervical gel: Bring to room temperature just prior to use. Do not force the warming process (eg, water bath, microwave). Avoid contact with skin while handling; wash hands thoroughly with soap and water after administration. For cervical ripening, patient should be supine in the dorsal position. The appropriate catheter length should be based on degree of effacement; 20 mm for no effacement; 10 mm if 50% effaced. Patient should remain supine for 15-30 minutes following administration. The manufacturer recommends waiting 6-12 hours after dinoprostone gel administration before initiating oxytocin.

Vaginal insert: One vaginal insert is placed transversely in the posterior fornix of the vagina immediately after removal from its foil package. Patients should remain in the recumbent position for 2 hours after insertion, but thereafter may be ambulatory. Do not use without retrieval system. Product does not need warmed prior to use. A water miscible lubricant may be used to facilitate insertion (avoid excessive use of lubricant). Ensure complete removal of system at completion of therapy. The manufacturer recommends waiting ≥30 minutes after removing the dinoprostone vaginal insert before initiating oxytocin.

Vaginal suppository: Insert high into vagina after removal from its foil package. Bring to room temperature just prior to use. Patient should remain supine for 10 minutes following insertion.

Monitoring Parameters

Gel, insert: Fetal heart rate, uterine activity, progression of cervical dilation and effacement

Suppository: Confirmation of fetal death

Dosage Forms Excipient information presented when available (limited, particularly for generics); consult specific product labeling.

Gel, endocervical:

Prepidil®: 0.5 mg/3 g (3 g)

Insert, vaginal:

Cervidil®: 10 mg (1s) [releases 0.3 mg/hour]

Suppository, vaginal:

Prostin E2®: 20 mg (5s)

◆ **Diocaine® (Can)** *see* Proparacaine *on page* 1421

◆ **Diocarpine (Can)** *see* Pilocarpine (Ophthalmic) *on page* 1353

◆ **Diochloram® (Can)** *see* Chloramphenicol *on page* 338

◆ **Diocto [OTC]** *see* Docusate *on page* 537

DiphenhydrAMINE (Systemic)

(dye fen HYE dra meen)

Brand Names: U.S. Aler-Cap [OTC]; Aler-Dryl [OTC]; Aler-Tab [OTC]; AllerMax® [OTC]; Altaryl [OTC]; Anti-Hist [OTC]; Banophen™ [OTC]; Benadryl® Allergy Quick Dissolve [OTC]; Benadryl® Allergy [OTC]; Benadryl® Children's Allergy FastMelt® [OTC]; Benadryl® Children's Allergy Perfect Measure™ [OTC]; Benadryl® Children's Allergy [OTC]; Benadryl® Children's Dye Free Allergy [OTC]; Benadryl® Dye-Free Allergy [OTC]; Compoz® [OTC]; Diphen [OTC]; Diphenhist® [OTC]; Geri-Dryl; Histaprin [OTC]; Nytol® Quick Caps [OTC]; Nytol® Quick Gels [OTC]; PediaCare® Children's Allergy [OTC]; PediaCare® Children's NightTime Cough [OTC]; Siladryl Allergy [OTC]; Silphen [OTC]; Simply Sleep® [OTC]; Sleep-ettes D [OTC]; Sleep-Tabs [OTC]; Sleepinal® [OTC]; Sominex® Maximum Strength [OTC]; Sominex® [OTC]; Theraflu® Thin Strips® Multi Symptom [OTC]; Triaminic Thin Strips® Children's Cough & Runny Nose [OTC]; Twilite® [OTC]; Unisom® SleepGels® Maximum Strength [OTC]; Unisom® SleepMelts™ [OTC]

Brand Names: Canada Allerdryl®; Allernix; Benadryl®; Nytol®; Nytol® Extra Strength; PMS-Diphenhydramine; Simply Sleep®; Sominex®

Index Terms Diphenhydramine Citrate; Diphenhydramine Hydrochloride; Diphenhydramine Tannate

Pharmacologic Category Ethanolamine Derivative; Histamine H_1 Antagonist; Histamine H_1 Antagonist, First Generation

Additional Appendix Information

Beers Criteria – Potentially Inappropriate Medications for Geriatrics *on page 1973*

Contrast Media Reactions, Premedication for Prophylaxis *on page 1976*

Use Symptomatic relief of allergic symptoms caused by histamine release including nasal allergies and allergic dermatosis; adjunct to epinephrine in the treatment of anaphylaxis; nighttime sleep aid; prevention or treatment of motion sickness; antitussive; management of Parkinsonian syndrome including drug-induced extrapyramidal symptoms

Pregnancy Risk Factor B

Pregnancy Considerations Teratogenic effects were not observed in animal studies. Diphenhydramine crosses the human placenta. One retrospective study showed an increased risk of cleft palate formation following maternal use of diphenhydramine during the 1st trimester of pregnancy; however, later studies have not confirmed this finding. Signs of toxicity and symptoms of withdrawal have been reported in infants following high doses or chronic maternal use close to term. Diphenhydramine has been evaluated for the treatment of hyperemesis gravidarum. It is generally not considered the antihistamine of choice for treating allergic rhinitis or nausea and vomiting during pregnancy.

Lactation Enters breast milk/contraindicated

Contraindications Hypersensitivity to diphenhydramine or any component of the formulation; acute asthma; neonates or premature infants; breast-feeding; use as a local anesthetic (injection)

Warnings/Precautions Causes sedation, caution must be used in performing tasks which require alertness (eg, operating machinery or driving). Sedative effects of CNS depressants or ethanol are potentiated. Should not be used as a hypnotic in the elderly; may cause excessive sedation and confusion; may be inappropriate in this age group when used as an antihistamine due to potent anticholinergic effects (nonanticholinergic antihistamines preferred); when used for emergency allergic reactions, use the smallest effective dose (Beers Criteria). Antihistamines may cause excitation in young children. Use with caution in patients with angle-closure glaucoma, pyloroduodenal obstruction (including stenotic peptic ulcer), urinary tract obstruction (including bladder neck obstruction and symptomatic prostatic hyperplasia), asthma, hyperthyroidism, increased intraocular pressure, and cardiovascular disease (including hypertension and tachycardia). Some preparations contain soy protein; avoid use in patients with soy protein or peanut allergies. Some products may contain phenylalanine.

Self-medication (OTC use): Do not use with other products containing diphenhydramine, even ones used on the skin. Oral products are not for OTC use in children <6 years of age.

Adverse Reactions Frequency not defined.

Cardiovascular: Chest tightness, extrasystoles, hypotension, palpitation, tachycardia

Central nervous system: Chills, confusion, convulsion, disturbed coordination, dizziness, euphoria, excitation, fatigue, headache, insomnia, irritability, nervousness, paradoxical excitement, restlessness, sedation, sleepiness, vertigo

Endocrine & metabolic: Menstrual irregularities (early menses)

Gastrointestinal: Anorexia, constipation, diarrhea, dry mucous membranes, epigastric distress, nausea, throat tightness, vomiting, xerostomia

Genitourinary: Difficult urination, urinary frequency, urinary retention
Hematologic: Agranulocytosis, hemolytic anemia, thrombocytopenia
Neuromuscular & skeletal: Neuritis, paresthesia, tremor
Ocular: Blurred vision, diplopia
Otic: Labyrinthitis (acute), tinnitus
Respiratory: Nasal stuffiness, thickening of bronchial secretions, wheezing
Miscellaneous: Anaphylactic shock, diaphoresis

Drug Interactions

Metabolism/Transport Effects Inhibits CYP2D6 (moderate)

Avoid Concomitant Use

Avoid concomitant use of DiphenhydrAMINE (Systemic) with any of the following: Thioridazine

Increased Effect/Toxicity

DiphenhydrAMINE (Systemic) may increase the levels/effects of: Alcohol (Ethyl); Anticholinergics; CNS Depressants; CYP2D6 Substrates; Fesoterodine; Methotrimeprazine; Nebivolol; Selective Serotonin Reuptake Inhibitors; Tamoxifen; Thioridazine

The levels/effects of DiphenhydrAMINE (Systemic) may be increased by: Droperidol; HydrOXYzine; Methotrimeprazine; Pramlintide; Propafenone

Decreased Effect

DiphenhydrAMINE (Systemic) may decrease the levels/effects of: Acetylcholinesterase Inhibitors (Central); Benzylpenicilloyl Polylysine; Betahistine; Codeine; TraMADol

The levels/effects of DiphenhydrAMINE (Systemic) may be decreased by: Acetylcholinesterase Inhibitors (Central); Amphetamines

Ethanol/Nutrition/Herb Interactions

Ethanol: May increase CNS depression; monitor for increased effects with coadministration. Caution patients about effects.

Herb/Nutraceutical: Avoid valerian, St John's wort, kava kava, gotu kola (may increase CNS depression).

Stability Injection: Store at room temperature of 15°C to 30°C (59°F to 86°F); protect from freezing. Protect from light.

Mechanism of Action Competes with histamine for H_1-receptor sites on effector cells in the gastrointestinal tract, blood vessels, and respiratory tract; anticholinergic and sedative effects are also seen

Pharmacodynamics/Kinetics

Onset of action: Maximum sedative effect: 1-3 hours
Duration: 4-7 hours
Distribution: V_d: 3-22 L/kg
Protein binding: 78%
Metabolism: Extensively hepatic n-demethylation via CYP2D6; minor demethylation via CYP1A2, 2C9 and 2C19; smaller degrees in pulmonary and renal systems; significant first-pass effect
Bioavailability: Oral: ~40% to 70%
Half-life elimination: 2-10 hours; Elderly: 13.5 hours
Time to peak, serum: 2-4 hours
Excretion: Urine (as unchanged drug)

Dosage Note: Dosages are expressed as the hydrochloride salt.

Children:

Allergic reactions or motion sickness: Oral, I.M., I.V.: 5 mg/kg/day or 150 mg/m²/day in divided doses every 6-8 hours, not to exceed 300 mg/day

Alternate dosing by age: Oral:

2 to <6 years: 6.25 mg every 4-6 hours; maximum: 37.5 mg/day

6 to <12 years: 12.5-25 mg every 4-6 hours; maximum: 150 mg/day

≥12 years: 25-50 mg every 4-6 hours; maximum: 300 mg/day

Night-time sleep aid: Oral: Children ≥12 years: 50 mg at bedtime

Antitussive: Oral:

2 to <6 years: 6.25 mg every 4 hours; maximum: 37.5 mg/day

6 to <12 years: 12.5 mg every 4 hours; maximum: 75 mg/day

≥12 years: 25 mg every 4 hours; maximum: 150 mg/day

Treatment of dystonic reactions: I.M., I.V.: 0.5-1 mg/kg/dose

Adults:

Allergic reactions or motion sickness: Oral: 25-50 mg every 6-8 hours

Antitussive: Oral: 25 mg every 4 hours; maximum: 150 mg/24 hours

Night-time sleep aid: Oral: 50 mg at bedtime

Allergic reactions or motion sickness: I.M., I.V.: 10-50 mg per dose; single doses up to 100 mg may be used if needed; not to exceed 400 mg/day

Dystonic reaction: I.M., I.V.: 50 mg in a single dose; may repeat in 20-30 minutes if necessary

Elderly: Initial: 25 mg 2-3 times/day increasing as needed

Dietary Considerations Some products may contain sodium and/or phenylalanine.

Administration When used to prevent motion sickness, first dose should be given 30 minutes prior to exposure. Injection solution is for I.V. or I.M. administration only; local necrosis may result with SubQ or intradermal use. For I.V. administration, inject at a rate ≤25 mg/minute.

Monitoring Parameters Relief of symptoms, mental alertness

Test Interactions May interfere with urine detection of methadone and PCP (false-positives); may cause false-positive serum TCA screen; may suppress the wheal and flare reactions to skin test antigens

Additional Information Diphenhydramine citrate 19 mg is equivalent to diphenhydramine hydrochloride 12.5 mg

Dosage Forms Excipient information presented when available (limited, particularly for generics); consult specific product labeling. [DSC] = Discontinued product

Caplet, oral, as hydrochloride:
Aler-Dryl: 50 mg
AllerMax®: 50 mg
Anti-Hist: 25 mg
Compoz®: 50 mg
Histaprin: 25 mg
Nytol® Quick Caps: 25 mg
Simply Sleep®: 25 mg [contains calcium 20 mg/caplet]
Sleep-ettes D: 50 mg
Sominex® Maximum Strength: 50 mg
Twilite®: 50 mg

Capsule, oral, as hydrochloride: 25 mg, 50 mg
Aler-Cap: 25 mg
Banophen™: 25 mg
Benadryl® Allergy: 25 mg [contains calcium 35 mg/capsule]
Diphen: 25 mg
Diphenhist®: 25 mg
Sleepinal®: 50 mg

Capsule, liquid gel, oral, as hydrochloride: 25 mg

Capsule, softgel, oral, as hydrochloride:
Benadryl® Dye-Free Allergy: 25 mg [dye free]
Compoz®: 50 mg
Nytol® Quick Gels: 50 mg
Unisom® SleepGels® Maximum Strength: 50 mg

Captab, oral, as hydrochloride:
Diphenhist®: 25 mg

Elixir, oral, as hydrochloride:
Altaryl: 12.5 mg/5 mL (120 mL [DSC], 480 mL, 3840 mL) [ethanol free; cherry flavor]
Banophen™: 12.5 mg/5 mL (120 mL)

Banophen™: 12.5 mg/5 mL (480 mL) [sugar free]
Injection, solution, as hydrochloride: 50 mg/mL (1 mL, 10 mL)
Injection, solution, as hydrochloride [preservative free]: 50 mg/mL (1 mL)
Liquid, oral, as hydrochloride:
AllerMax®: 12.5 mg/5 mL (120 mL)
Benadryl® Children's Allergy: 12.5 mg/5 mL (118 mL, 236 mL) [ethanol free; contains sodium 14 mg/5 mL, sodium benzoate; cherry flavor]
Benadryl® Children's Allergy Perfect Measure™: 12.5 mg/5 mL (5 mL) [ethanol free; contains sodium 14 mg/5 mL, sodium benzoate; cherry flavor]
Benadryl® Children's Dye Free Allergy: 12.5 mg/5 mL (118 mL) [dye free, ethanol free, sugar free; contains sodium 11 mg/5 mL, sodium benzoate; bubblegum flavor]
Siladryl Allergy: 12.5 mg/5 mL (118 mL, 237 mL, 473 mL) [ethanol free, sugar free; black-cherry flavor]
Solution, oral, as hydrochloride: 12.5 mg/5 mL (5 mL, 10 mL, 20 mL [DSC])
Diphenhist®: 12.5 mg/5 mL (120 mL, 480 mL) [ethanol free; contains sodium benzoate]
Strip, orally disintegrating, oral, as hydrochloride:
Benadryl® Allergy Quick Dissolve: 25 mg (10s) [contains sodium 4 mg/strip; vanilla-mint flavor]
Theraflu® Thin Strips® Multi Symptom: 25 mg (12s, 24s) [contains ethanol; cherry flavor]
Triaminic Thin Strips® Children's Cough & Runny Nose: 12.5 mg (14s) [contains ethanol; grape flavor]
Syrup, oral, as hydrochloride:
PediaCare® Children's Allergy: 12.5 mg/5 mL (118 mL) [contains sodium 14 mg/5 mL, sodium benzoate; cherry flavor]
PediaCare® Children's NightTime Cough: 12.5 mg/5 mL (118 mL) [ethanol free; contains sodium 15 mg/5 mL, sodium benzoate; cherry flavor]
Silphen: 12.5 mg/5 mL (118 mL, 237 mL, 473 mL) [contains ethanol 5%; strawberry flavor]
Tablet, oral, as hydrochloride: 25 mg, 50 mg
Aler-Tab: 25 mg
Banophen™: 25 mg
Benadryl® Allergy: 25 mg
Geri-Dryl: 25 mg
Sleep-Tabs: 25 mg
Sominex®: 25 mg
Tablet, orally dissolving, oral, as hydrochloride:
Benadryl® Children's Allergy FastMelt®: 12.5 mg [grape flavor]
Unisom® SleepMelts™: 25 mg [cherry flavor]
Tablet, orally dissolving, oral, as hydrochloride [strength expressed as base]:
Benadryl® Children's Allergy FastMelt®: 12.5 mg [cherry flavor]

- **Diphenhydramine and Acetaminophen** *see* Acetaminophen and Diphenhydramine *on page 31*
- **Diphenhydramine and ASA** *see* Aspirin and Diphenhydramine *on page 157*
- **Diphenhydramine and Aspirin** *see* Aspirin and Diphenhydramine *on page 157*

Diphenhydramine and Phenylephrine

(dye fen HYE dra meen & fen il EF rin)

Brand Names: U.S. Aldex® CT; Benadryl-D® Allergy & Sinus [OTC]; Benadryl-D® Children's Allergy & Sinus [OTC]; Dimetapp® Children's Nighttime Cold & Congestion [OTC]; Robitussin® Night Time Cough & Cold [OTC] [DSC]; Triaminic® Children's Night Time Cold & Cough [OTC]; Triaminic® Children's Thin Strips® Night Time Cold & Cough [OTC]

Index Terms Diphenhydramine Hydrochloride and Phenylephrine Hydrochloride; Diphenhydramine Tannate and Phenylephrine Tannate; Phenylephrine and Diphenhydramine; Phenylephrine Hydrochloride and Diphenhydramine Hydrochloride; Phenylephrine Tannate and Diphenhydramine Tannate

Pharmacologic Category Alpha-Adrenergic Agonist; Decongestant; Ethanolamine Derivative; Histamine H_1 Antagonist; Histamine H_1 Antagonist, First Generation

Use Temporary relief of symptoms of allergic rhinitis, sinusitis, and other upper respiratory conditions, including sinus/nasal congestion, sneezing, stuffy/runny nose, itchy/watery eyes, and cough

Pregnancy Risk Factor C

Dosage Oral:
Aldex® CT:
Children 6-11 years: One-half to 1 tablet every 6 hours
Children ≥12 years and Adults: 1-2 tablets every 6 hours
OTC labeling:
Children <6 years: Use not recommended
Children 6-11 years:
Benadryl-D® Children's Allergy & Sinus: 5 mL every 4 hours as needed (maximum: 6 doses/24 hours)
Dimetapp® Children's Nighttime Cold and Congestion, Triaminic® Children's Night Time Cold & Cough: 10 mL every 4 hours as needed (maximum: 6 doses/24 hours)
Triaminic® Children's Thin Strips® Night Time Cold & Cough: One strip every 4 hours as needed (maximum: 6 doses/24 hours)
Children ≥12 years and Adults: **Note:** General dosing guidelines; refer to specific product labeling:
10-20 mL every 4 hours as needed (maximum: 6 doses/24 hours) **or** 1 tablet every 4 hours as needed (maximum: 6 doses/24 hours)

Additional Information Complete prescribing information for this medication should be consulted for additional detail.

Dosage Forms Excipient information presented when available (limited, particularly for generics); consult specific product labeling. [DSC] = Discontinued product
Liquid, oral:
Benadryl-D® Children's Allergy & Sinus: Diphenhydramine hydrochloride 12.5 mg and phenylephrine hydrochloride 5 mg per 5 mL (118 mL) [ethanol free, sugar free; contains sodium 10 mg/5 mL, sodium benzoate; grape flavor]
Strip, orally disintegrating:
Triaminic® Children's Thin Strips® Night Time Cold & Cough: Diphenhydramine hydrochloride 12.5 mg and phenylephrine hydrochloride 5 mg [grape flavor]
Syrup, oral:
Dimetapp® Children's Nighttime Cold and Congestion: Diphenhydramine hydrochloride 6.25 mg and phenylephrine hydrochloride 2.5 mg per 5 mL (120 mL) [ethanol free, sugar free; contains propylene glycol, sodium 4 mg/5 mL, sodium benzoate; grape flavor]
Robitussin® Night Time Cough and Cold: Diphenhydramine hydrochloride 6.25 mg and phenylephrine hydrochloride 2.5 mg per 5 mL (120 mL) [ethanol free; contains propylene glycol, sodium 3 mg/5 mL, sodium benzoate] [DSC]
Triaminic® Children's Night Time Cold & Cough: Diphenhydramine hydrochloride 6.25 mg and phenylephrine hydrochloride 2.5 mg per 5 mL (118 mL) [contains ethanol, propylene glycol, sodium 6 mg/5 mL; grape flavor]
Tablet, oral:
Benadryl-D® Allergy & Sinus: Diphenhydramine hydrochloride 25 mg and phenylephrine hydrochloride 10 mg

Tablet, chewable, oral:

Aldex® CT: Diphenhydramine hydrochloride 12.5 mg and phenylephrine hydrochloride 5 mg [contains phenylalanine; strawberry flavor]

◆ **Diphenhydramine Citrate** *see* DiphenhydrAMINE (Systemic) *on page 516*

◆ **Diphenhydramine Citrate and Aspirin** *see* Aspirin and Diphenhydramine *on page 157*

◆ **Diphenhydramine Hydrochloride** *see* DiphenhydrAMINE (Systemic) *on page 516*

◆ **Diphenhydramine Hydrochloride and Phenylephrine Hydrochloride** *see* Diphenhydramine and Phenylephrine *on page 518*

◆ **Diphenhydramine Tannate** *see* DiphenhydrAMINE (Systemic) *on page 516*

◆ **Diphenhydramine Tannate and Phenylephrine Tannate** *see* Diphenhydramine and Phenylephrine *on page 518*

Diphenoxylate and Atropine

(dye fen OKS i late & A troe peen)

Brand Names: U.S. Lomotil®

Brand Names: Canada Lomotil®

Index Terms Atropine and Diphenoxylate

Pharmacologic Category Antidiarrheal

Use Treatment of diarrhea

Pregnancy Risk Factor C

Pregnancy Considerations Teratogenic effects were not noted in animal studies; decreased maternal weight, fertility and litter sizes were observed. There are no adequate and well-controlled studies in pregnant women.

Lactation Enters breast milk/use caution

Contraindications Hypersensitivity to diphenoxylate, atropine, or any component of the formulation; obstructive jaundice; diarrhea associated with pseudomembranous enterocolitis or enterotoxin-producing bacteria; not for use in children <2 years of age

Warnings/Precautions Use in conjunction with fluid and electrolyte therapy when appropriate. In case of severe dehydration or electrolyte imbalance, withhold diphenoxylate/atropine treatment until corrective therapy has been initiated. Inhibiting peristalsis may lead to fluid retention in the intestine aggravating dehydration and electrolyte imbalance. Reduction of intestinal motility may be deleterious in diarrhea resulting from *Shigella, Salmonella*, toxigenic strains of *E. coli*, and pseudomembranous enterocolitis associated with broad-spectrum antibiotics; use is not recommended.

Use with caution in children. Younger children may be predisposed to toxicity; signs of atropinism may occur even at recommended doses, especially in patients with Down syndrome. Overdose in children may result in severe respiratory depression, coma, and possibly permanent brain damage.

Use caution with acute ulcerative colitis, hepatic or renal dysfunction. If there is no response with 48 hours, this medication is unlikely to be effective and should be discontinued; if chronic diarrhea is not improved symptomatically within 10 days at maximum dosage, control is unlikely with further use. Physical and psychological dependence have been reported with higher than recommended dosing.

Adverse Reactions Frequency not defined.

Cardiovascular: Tachycardia

Central nervous system: Confusion, depression, dizziness, drowsiness, euphoria, flushing, headache, hyperthermia, lethargy, malaise, restlessness, sedation

Dermatologic: Angioneurotic edema, dry skin, pruritus, urticaria

Gastrointestinal: Abdominal discomfort, anorexia, gum swelling, nausea, pancreatitis, paralytic ileus, toxic megacolon, vomiting, xerostomia

Genitourinary: Urinary retention

Neuromuscular & skeletal: Numbness

Miscellaneous: Anaphylaxis

Drug Interactions

Metabolism/Transport Effects None known.

Avoid Concomitant Use There are no known interactions where it is recommended to avoid concomitant use.

Increased Effect/Toxicity

Diphenoxylate and Atropine may increase the levels/effects of: AbobotulinumtoxinA; Alcohol (Ethyl); Anticholinergics; Cannabinoids; CNS Depressants; Methotrimeprazine; OnabotulinumtoxinA; Potassium Chloride; RimabotulinumtoxinB; Selective Serotonin Reuptake Inhibitors

The levels/effects of Diphenoxylate and Atropine may be increased by: Droperidol; HydrOXYzine; Methotrimeprazine; Pramlintide

Decreased Effect

Diphenoxylate and Atropine may decrease the levels/effects of: Acetylcholinesterase Inhibitors (Central); Secretin

The levels/effects of Diphenoxylate and Atropine may be decreased by: Acetylcholinesterase Inhibitors (Central)

Ethanol/Nutrition/Herb Interactions Ethanol: May increase CNS depression; monitor for increased effects with coadministration. Caution patients about effects.

Mechanism of Action Diphenoxylate inhibits excessive GI motility and GI propulsion; commercial preparations contain a subtherapeutic amount of atropine to discourage abuse

Pharmacodynamics/Kinetics

Atropine: See Atropine monograph.

Diphenoxylate:

Onset of action: Antidiarrheal: 45-60 minutes

Duration: Antidiarrheal: 3-4 hours

Absorption: Well absorbed

Metabolism: Extensively hepatic via ester hydrolysis to diphenoxylic acid (active)

Half-life elimination: Diphenoxylate: 2.5 hours; Diphenoxylic acid: 12-14 hours

Time to peak, serum: 2 hours

Excretion: Primarily feces (49% as unchanged drug and metabolites); urine (~14%, <1% as unchanged drug)

Dosage Oral:

Children 2-12 years (use with caution in young children due to variable responses): Liquid: Diphenoxylate 0.3-0.4 mg/kg/day in 4 divided doses until control achieved (maximum: 10 mg/day), then reduce dose as needed; some patients may be controlled on doses as low as 25% of the initial daily dose

Adults: Diphenoxylate 5 mg 4 times/day until control achieved (maximum: 20 mg/day), then reduce dose as needed; some patients may be controlled on doses of 5 mg/day

Administration If there is no response within 48 hours of continuous therapy, this medication is unlikely to be effective and should be discontinued; if chronic diarrhea is not improved symptomatically within 10 days at maximum dosage, control is unlikely with further use. Use of the liquid preparation is recommended in children <13 years of age; use plastic dropper provided when measuring liquid.

Monitoring Parameters Watch for signs of atropinism (dryness of skin and mucous membranes, tachycardia, thirst, flushing); monitor number and consistency of stools; observe for signs of toxicity, fluid and electrolyte loss, hypotension, and respiratory depression

Dosage Forms Excipient information presented when available (limited, particularly for generics); consult specific product labeling. [DSC] = Discontinued product

Solution, oral: Diphenoxylate hydrochloride 2.5 mg and atropine sulfate 0.025 mg per 5 mL (5 mL, 10 mL, 60 mL)
 Lomotil®: Diphenoxylate hydrochloride 2.5 mg and atropine sulfate 0.025 mg per 5 mL (60 mL) [contains alcohol 15%; cherry flavor] [DSC]

Tablet, oral: Diphenoxylate hydrochloride 2.5 mg and atropine sulfate 0.025 mg
 Lomotil®: Diphenoxylate hydrochloride 2.5 mg and atropine sulfate 0.025 mg

Controlled Substance C-V

◆ **Diphenylhydantoin** *see* Phenytoin *on page 1346*

Diphtheria and Tetanus Toxoid

(dif THEER ee a & TET a nus TOKS oyds)

Brand Names: U.S. Decavac®

Brand Names: Canada Td Adsorbed

Index Terms DT; Td; Tetanus and Diphtheria Toxoid

Pharmacologic Category Vaccine, Inactivated (Bacterial)

Additional Appendix Information

Immunization Recommendations *on page 1922*

Use

Diphtheria and tetanus toxoids adsorbed for pediatric use (DT): Infants and children through 6 years of age: Active immunization against diphtheria and tetanus when pertussis vaccine is contraindicated

Tetanus and diphtheria toxoids adsorbed for adult use (Td) (Decavac®): Children ≥7 years of age and Adults: Active immunization against diphtheria and tetanus; tetanus prophylaxis in wound management

The Advisory Committee on Immunization Practices (ACIP) recommends routine vaccination for the following:

- Adults and children ≥7 years should receive a booster dose of Td every 10 years; may substitute a single Td booster dose with Tdap
- Children 7-10 years of age, adults, and the elderly (≥65 years) who are wounded in bombings or similar mass casualty events who have penetrating injuries or nonintact skin exposure and who cannot confirm receipt of a tetanus booster within the previous 5 years, may also receive a single dose of Td; children ≥11 years and adults may also receive Td if Tdap is unavailable

Pregnancy Risk Factor C

Pregnancy Considerations Reproduction studies have not been conducted. DT is not recommended for use in persons ≥7 years of age. Inactivated bacterial vaccines have not been shown to cause increased risks to the fetus (CDC, 60[2], 2011). The Advisory Committee on Immunization Practices (ACIP) recommends booster injections for previously vaccinated pregnant women who have not had Td vaccination within the past 10 years. Pregnant women who are not immunized or are only partially immunized should complete the primary series. Vaccination may be deferred until the postpartum period in women who are likely to have sufficient diphtheria and tetanus protection until delivery; Tdap may be substituted for Td after delivery to add extra protection against pertussis. Td should be administered during pregnancy to women who do not have sufficient tetanus immunity to protect against maternal and neonatal tetanus, and if booster protection for diphtheria is required (eg, travel to where diphtheria is endemic). Tetanus immune globulin and a tetanus toxoid containing vaccine are recommended by the ACIP as part of the standard wound management to prevent tetanus in pregnant women; the use of Td during pregnancy is recommended for wound management if ≥5 years have passed since the last Td vaccination.

Lactation Excretion in breast milk unknown/use caution

Contraindications Hypersensitivity to diphtheria, tetanus toxoid, or any component of the formulation

Warnings/Precautions Do not confuse pediatric diphtheria and tetanus (DT) with adult tetanus and diphtheria (Td). Immediate treatment for anaphylactic/anaphylactoid reaction should be available during administration. Patients with a history of severe local reaction (Arthus-type) following a previous dose should not be given further routine or emergency doses of Td more frequently than every 10 years even if using for wound management with wounds that are not clean or minor; these patients generally have high serum antitoxin levels. Continue use with caution if Guillain-Barré syndrome occurs within 6 weeks of prior tetanus toxoid. For I.M. administration; use caution with history of bleeding disorders or anticoagulant therapy. Defer administration during moderate or severe illness (with or without fever). Immune response may be decreased in immunocompromised patients; in general, household and close contacts of persons with altered immunocompetence may receive all age appropriate vaccines. Safety and efficacy of DT have not been established in children <6 weeks of age; Td should be administered to children ≥7 years of age and adults. Some products may contain natural latex/natural rubber or thimerosal. In order to maximize vaccination rates, the ACIP recommends simultaneous administration of all age-appropriate vaccines (live or inactivated) for which a person is eligible at a single clinic visit, unless contraindications exist. The use of combination vaccines is generally preferred over separate injections, taking into consideration provider assessment, patient preference, and adverse events. When using combination vaccines, the minimum age for administration is the oldest minimum age for any individual component; the minimum interval between dosing is the greatest minimum interval between any individual component.

Adverse Reactions All serious adverse reactions must be reported to the U.S. Department of Health and Human Services (DHHS) Vaccine Adverse Event Reporting System (VAERS) 1-800-822-7967 or online at https://vaers.hhs.gov/esub/index. In Canada, adverse reactions may be reported to local provincial/territorial health agencies or to the Vaccine Safety Section at Public Health Agency of Canada (1-866-844-0018).

Note: Percentages noted within 2 weeks following booster dose of Decavac® in persons ≥11 years of age:

>10%:

Central nervous system: Headache (34% to 40%), tiredness (21% to 27%), chills (7% to 13%)

Gastrointestinal: Nausea (8% to 12%), diarrhea (10% to 11%)

Local: Injection site: Pain (63% to 71%), erythema (20% to 22%), swelling (17% to 18%)

Neuromuscular & skeletal: Body ache/muscle weakness (19% to 30%), sore/swollen joints (7% to 12%)

1% to 10%:

Central nervous system: Fever (1% to 3%)

Dermatologic: Rash (2%)

Endocrine & metabolic: Lymph node swelling (4% to 5%)

Gastrointestinal: Vomiting (2% to 3%)

Postmarketing and/or case reports: Allergic reactions (angioedema, rash, urticaria), anaphylactic reactions, arthralgia, chills, dizziness, fatigue, injection site reactions (cellulitis, induration, nodules, warmth), lymphadenopathy, musculoskeletal stiffness, myalgia, pain, pain in extremities, paresthesia, peripheral edema, seizure, syncope, weakness

Drug Interactions

Metabolism/Transport Effects None known.

Avoid Concomitant Use There are no known interactions where it is recommended to avoid concomitant use.

Increased Effect/Toxicity There are no known significant interactions involving an increase in effect.

Decreased Effect

The levels/effects of Diphtheria and Tetanus Toxoids may be decreased by: Belimumab; Fingolimod; Immunosuppressants

Stability Store at 2°C to 8°C (35°F to 46°F). Do not freeze; discard if product has been frozen.

Dosage I.M.:

Children 6 weeks to <7 years (DT): Primary immunization: **Note:** For use when a pertussis-containing vaccine is contraindicated: 0.5 mL per dose, total of 5 doses administered as follows:

Three doses, usually given at 2-, 4-, and 6 months of age; may be given as early as 6 weeks of age and repeated every 4-8 weeks

Fourth dose: Given at ~15-18 months of age, but at least 6 months after third dose. The fourth dose may be given as early as 12 months of age, but at least 6 months must have elapsed between the third dose and the fourth dose.

Fifth dose: Given at 4-6 years of age, prior to starting school or kindergarten; if the fourth dose is given at ≥4 years of age, the fifth dose may be omitted

For children who start primary immunization series ≥4 months of age, refer to current ACIP "Catch-up Immunization Schedule"

Children ≥7 years and Adults (Td):

Primary immunization: Patients previously not immunized should receive 2 primary doses of 0.5 mL each, given at an interval of 4 weeks; third (reinforcing) dose of 0.5 mL 6 months later

Booster immunization: For routine booster in patients who have completed primary immunization series. The ACIP prefers Tdap for use in in some situations if no contraindications exist; refer to Diphtheria and Tetanus Toxoids, and Acellular Pertussis Vaccine monograph for additional information.

Children 11-12 years: A single dose when at least 5 years have elapsed since last dose of toxoid-containing vaccine. Subsequent routine doses are not recommended more often than every 10 years.

Adults: 0.5 mL every 10 years

Tetanus prophylaxis in wound management: Tetanus prophylaxis in patients with wounds should consider if the wound is clean or contaminated, the immunization status of the patient, proper use of tetanus toxoid and/or tetanus immune globulin (TIG), wound cleaning, and (if required) surgical debridement and the proper use of antibiotics. Patients with an uncertain or incomplete tetanus immunization status should have additional follow up to ensure a series is completed. Patients with a history of Arthus reaction following a previous dose of a tetanus toxoid-containing vaccine should not receive a tetanus toxoid-containing vaccine until >10 years after the most recent dose even if they have a wound that is neither clean nor minor. See table.

Tetanus Prophylaxis in Wound Management

History of Tetanus Immunization Doses	Clean, Minor Wounds		All Other Wounds[1]	
	Tetanus Toxoid[2]	TIG	Tetanus Toxoid[2]	TIG
Uncertain or <3 doses	Yes	No	Yes	Yes
3 or more doses	No[3]	No	No[4]	No

[1]Such as, but not limited to, wounds contaminated with dirt, feces, soil, and saliva; puncture wounds; wounds from crushing, tears, burns, and frostbite.

[2]Tetanus toxoid in this chart refers to a tetanus toxoid-containing vaccine. For children <7 years of age, DTaP (DT, if pertussis vaccine contraindicated) is preferred to tetanus toxoid alone. For children ≥7 years and adults, Td preferred to tetanus toxoid alone; Tdap may be preferred if the patient has not previously been vaccinated with Tdap.

[3]Yes, if ≥10 years since last dose.

[4]Yes, if ≥5 years since last dose.

Adapted from CDC "Yellow Book" (*Health Information for International Travel 2010*), "Routine Vaccine-Preventable Diseases, Tetanus" (available at http://www.cdc.gov/yellowbook) and *MMWR* 2006, 55 (RR-17).

Abbreviations: **DT** = Diphtheria and Tetanus Toxoids (formulation for age ≤6 years); **DTaP** = Diphtheria and Tetanus Toxoids, and Acellular Pertussis (formulation for age ≤6 years; Daptacel®, Infanrix®, Tripedia®); **Td** = Diphtheria and Tetanus Toxoids (formulation for age ≥7 years; Decavac®); **TT**= Tetanus toxoid (adsorbed [formulation for age ≥7 years]); **Tdap** = Diphtheria and Tetanus Toxoids, and Acellular Pertussis (Adacel® or Boostrix® [formulations for age ≥7 years]); **TIG** = Tetanus Immune Globulin

Administration For I.M. administration; prior to use, shake suspension well

Td: Administer in the deltoid muscle; do not inject in the gluteal area

DT: Administer in the anterolateral aspect of the thigh or the deltoid muscle; do not inject in the gluteal area

For patients at risk of hemorrhage following intramuscular injection, the ACIP recommends "it should be administered intramuscularly if, in the opinion of the physician familiar with the patients bleeding risk, the vaccine can be administered by this route with reasonable safety. If the patient receives antihemophilia or other similar therapy, intramuscular vaccination can be scheduled shortly after such therapy is administered. A fine needle (23 gauge or smaller) can be used for the vaccination and firm pressure applied to the site (without rubbing) for at least 2 minutes. The patient should be instructed concerning the risk of hematoma from the injection." Patients on anticoagulant therapy should be considered to have the same bleeding risks and treated as those with clotting factor disorders (CDC, 60[2], 2011).

Simultaneous administration of vaccines helps ensure the patients will be fully vaccinated by the appropriate age. Simultaneous administration of vaccines is defined as administering >1 vaccine on the same day at different anatomic sites. The use of licensed combination vaccines is generally preferred over separate injections of the equivalent components. Separate vaccines should not be combined in the same syringe unless indicated by product specific labeling. Separate needles and syringes should be used for each injection. The ACIP prefers each dose of a specific vaccine in a series come from the same manufacturer when possible. Adolescents and adults should be vaccinated while seated or lying down. In general, preterm infants should be vaccinated at the same chronological age as full-term infants (CDC, 60[2], 2011).

Antipyretics have not been shown to prevent febrile seizures. Antipyretics may be used to treat fever or discomfort following vaccination (CDC, 2011). One study reported that routine prophylactic administration of acetaminophen to prevent fever prior to vaccination decreased the immune response of some vaccines; the clinical significance of this reduction in immune response has not been established (Prymula, 2009).

Monitoring Parameters Monitor for syncope for ≥15 minutes following vaccination

Additional Information Pediatric dosage form should only be used in patients ≤6 years of age. Federal law requires that the name of medication, date of administration, the vaccine manufacturer, lot number of vaccine, and the administering person's name, title, and address be entered into the patient's permanent medical record.

DT contains higher proportions of diphtheria toxoid than Td.

Dosage Forms Excipient information presented when available (limited, particularly for generics); consult specific product labeling.

Injection, suspension [Td, adult; preservative free]: Diphtheria 2 Lf units and tetanus 2 Lf units per 0.5 mL (0.5 mL)

Decavac®: Diphtheria 2 Lf units and tetanus 5 Lf units per 0.5 mL (0.5 mL) [contains aluminum, may contain natural rubber/natural latex in prefilled syringe, thimerosal (may have trace amounts)]

Injection, suspension [DT, pediatric; preservative free]: Diphtheria 6.7 Lf units and tetanus 5 Lf units per 0.5 mL (0.5 mL)

Diphtheria and Tetanus Toxoids, Acellular Pertussis, and *Haemophilus influenzae* b Conjugate Vaccine

(dif THEER ee a & TET a nus TOKS oyds, ay CEL yoo lar per TUS sis & hem OF fi lus in floo EN za bee KON joo gate vak SEEN)

Brand Names: U.S. TriHIBit® [DSC]

Index Terms *Haemophilus influenzae* b Conjugate Vaccine and Diphtheria, Tetanus Toxoids, and Acellular Pertussis Vaccine; DTaP/Hib

Pharmacologic Category Vaccine, Inactivated (Bacterial)

Additional Appendix Information

Immunization Recommendations *on page 1922*

Use Active immunization of children 15-18 months of age for prevention of diphtheria, tetanus, pertussis, and invasive disease caused by *H. influenzae* type b

The Advisory Committee on Immunization Practices (ACIP) recommends the use of TriHIBit® for the fourth dose of the diphtheria, tetanus, pertussis, and *Haemophilus* vaccine series. Whenever feasible, the same manufacturer should be used to provide the pertussis component; however, vaccination should not be deferred if a specific brand is not known or is not available.

Pregnancy Risk Factor C

Dosage Children 15-18 months: I.M.: 0.5 mL: **Note:** For use as the fourth dose of the DTaP and Hib series (see individual vaccines).

Additional Information Complete prescribing information for this medication should be consulted for additional detail.

Dosage Forms Excipient information presented when available (limited, particularly for generics); consult specific product labeling.

Injection, suspension [preservative free]:

TriHIBit®: Diphtheria 6.7 Lf units, tetanus 5 Lf units, acellular pertussis antigens [inactivated pertussis toxin 23.4 mcg, filamentous hemagglutinin 23.4 mcg], and *Haemophilus* b capsular polysaccharide 10 mcg [bound to tetanus toxoid 24 mcg] per 0.5 mL (0.5 mL) [DSC] [contains aluminum, natural rubber/natural latex in packaging, polysorbate 80, sucrose, and trace amounts of thimerosal; Tripedia® vaccine used to reconstitute ActHIB® forms TriHIBit®]

Diphtheria and Tetanus Toxoids, Acellular Pertussis, and Poliovirus Vaccine

(dif THEER ee a & TET a nus TOKS oyds, ay CEL yoo lar per TUS sis & POE lee oh VYE rus vak SEEN)

Brand Names: U.S. Kinrix®

Index Terms Diphtheria and Tetanus Toxoids and Acellular Pertussis Adsorbed, and Inactivated Poliovirus Vaccine Combined; Diphtheria, Tetanus Toxoids, Acellular Pertussis (DTaP); DTaP-IPV; Poliovirus, Inactivated (IPV)

Pharmacologic Category Vaccine, Inactivated (Bacterial); Vaccine, Inactivated (Viral)

Additional Appendix Information

Immunization Recommendations *on page 1922*

Use Active immunization against diphtheria, tetanus, pertussis, and poliomyelitis, used as the 5th dose in the DTaP series and the 4th dose in the IPV series

The Advisory Committee on Immunization Practices (ACIP) recommends routine vaccination for use as the fifth dose in the DTaP series and the fourth dose in the IPV series in children who received DTaP (Infanrix®) and/or DTaP-Hepatitis B-IPV (Pediarix®) as the first 3 doses and DTaP (Infanrix®) as the fourth dose. Whenever feasible, the same manufacturer should be used to provide the pertussis component; however, vaccination should not be deferred if a specific brand is not known or is not available.

Pregnancy Risk Factor C

Dosage I.M.: Children 4-6 years: Immunization: 0.5 mL; **Note:** For use as the 5th dose in the DTaP series and the 4th dose in the IPV series

Additional Information Complete prescribing information for this medication should be consulted for additional detail.

Dosage Forms Excipient information presented when available (limited, particularly for generics); consult specific product labeling.

Injection, suspension [preservative free]:

Kinrix®: Diphtheria toxoid 25 Lf, tetanus toxoid 10 Lf, acellular pertussis antigens [inactivated pertussis toxin 25 mcg, filamentous hemagglutinin 25 mcg, pertactin 8 mcg], type 1 poliovirus 40 D-antigen units, type 2 poliovirus 8 D-antigen units, and type 3 poliovirus 32 D-antigen units per 0.5 mL (0.5 mL) [contains aluminum, neomycin sulfate, polymyxin B, polysorbate 80; may contain natural rubber/natural latex in prefilled syringe]

Diphtheria and Tetanus Toxoids, Acellular Pertussis, Poliovirus and *Haemophilus* b Conjugate Vaccine

(dif THEER ee a & TET a nus TOKS oyds ay CEL yoo lar per TUS sis POE lee oh VYE rus & hem OF fi lus bee KON joo gate vak SEEN)

Brand Names: U.S. Pentacel®

Brand Names: Canada Pediacel®; Pentacel®

Index Terms *Haemophilus* B Conjugate (Hib); *Haemophilus* B Polysaccharide; Diphtheria Toxoid; Diphtheria, Tetanus Toxoids, Acellular Pertussis (DTaP); DTaP-IPV/Hib; Pertussis, Acellular (Adsorbed); Poliovirus, Inactivated (IPV); Tetanus Toxoid

Pharmacologic Category Vaccine, Inactivated (Bacterial); Vaccine, Inactivated (Viral)

Additional Appendix Information

Immunization Recommendations *on page 1922*

Use Active immunization against diphtheria, tetanus, pertussis, poliomyelitis, and invasive disease caused by *H. influenzae* type b in children 6 weeks through 4 years of age

Advisory Committee on Immunization Practices (ACIP) recommends that Pentacel® (DTaP-IPV/Hib) may be used to provide the recommended DTaP, IPV, and Hib immunization in children <5 years of age. Whenever feasible, the same manufacturer should be used to provide the pertussis component; however, vaccination should not be deferred if a specific brand is not known or is not available. The Hib component in Pentacel® contains a tetanus toxoid conjugate. A Hib vaccine containing the PRP-OMP conjugate (PedvaxHIB®) may provide a more rapid seroconversion following the first dose and may be preferable to use in certain populations (eg, American Indian or Alaska Native children).

Pregnancy Risk Factor C

Dosage I.M.: Children:

Primary immunization: Children 6 weeks to ≤4 years: 0.5 mL per dose administered at 2, 4, 6 and 15-18 months of age (total of 4 doses). The first dose may be administered as early as 6 weeks of age. Following completion of the 4-dose series, children should receive a dose of DTaP vaccine at 4-6 years of age (Daptacel® recommended due to same pertussis antigen used in both products).

Note: Per the ACIP, polio vaccine should not be administered more frequently than 4 weeks apart. Use of the minimum age and minimum intervals during the first 6 months of life should only be done when the vaccine recipient is at risk for imminent exposure to circulating poliovirus (shorter intervals and earlier start dates may lead to lower seroconversion. Pentacel® is not indicated for the polio booster dose given at 4-6 years of age; Kinrix® or IPV should be used.

Children previously vaccinated with ≥1 dose of Daptacel® or IPV vaccines: Pentacel® may be used to complete the first 4 doses of the DTaP or IPV series in children scheduled to receive the other components in the vaccine.

Children previously vaccinated with ≥1 dose of *Haemophilus* b conjugate vaccine: Pentacel® may be used to complete the series in children scheduled to receive the other components in the vaccine; however, if different brands of *Haemophilus* b conjugate vaccine are administered to complete the series, 3 primary immunizing doses are needed, followed by a booster dose.

Note: Completion of 3 doses of Pentacel® provides primary immunization against diphtheria, tetanus, *H. influenzae* type B, and poliomyelitis. Completion of the 4-dose series with Pentacel® provides primary immunization against pertussis. It also provides a booster vaccination against diphtheria, tetanus, *H. influenzae* type B, and poliomyelitis.

Additional Information Complete prescribing information for this medication should be consulted for additional detail.

Dosage Forms Excipient information presented when available (limited, particularly for generics); consult specific product labeling.

Injection, suspension:

Pentacel®: Diphtheria toxoid 15 Lf, tetanus toxoid 5 Lf, acellular pertussis antigens [pertussis toxin detoxified 20 mcg, filamentous hemagglutinin 20 mcg, pertactin 3 mcg, fimbriae (types 2 and 3) 5 mcg], type 1poliovirus 40 D-antigen units; type 2 poliovirus 8 D-antigen units; type 3 poliovirus 32 D-antigen units, and *Haemophilus* b capsular polysaccharide 10 mcg [bound to tetanus toxoid 24 mcg] per 0.5 mL (0.5 mL) [contains albumin, aluminum, neomycin, polymyxin B sulfate, and polysorbate 80; supplied in two vials, one containing DTaP-IPV liquid and one containing Hib powder]

◆ **Diphtheria and Tetanus Toxoids and Acellular Pertussis Adsorbed, and Inactivated Poliovirus Vaccine Combined** *see* Diphtheria and Tetanus Toxoids, Acellular Pertussis, and Poliovirus Vaccine *on page 522*

◆ **Diphtheria and Tetanus Toxoids and Acellular Pertussis Adsorbed, Hepatitis B (Recombinant) and Inactivated Poliovirus Vaccine Combined** *see* Diphtheria, Tetanus Toxoids, Acellular Pertussis, Hepatitis B (Recombinant), and Poliovirus (Inactivated) Vaccine *on page 527*

Diphtheria and Tetanus Toxoids, and Acellular Pertussis Vaccine

(dif THEER ee a & TET a nus TOKS oyds & ay CEL yoo lar per TUS sis vak SEEN)

Brand Names: U.S. Adacel®; Boostrix®; Daptacel®; Infanrix®; Tripedia® [DSC]

Brand Names: Canada Adacel®; Boostrix®

Index Terms DTaP; Tdap; Tetanus Toxoid, Reduced Diphtheria Toxoid, and Acellular Pertussis, Adsorbed

Pharmacologic Category Vaccine, Inactivated (Bacterial)

Additional Appendix Information

Immunization Recommendations *on page 1922*

Use

Daptacel®, Infanrix®, Tripedia® (DTaP): Active immunization against diphtheria, tetanus, and pertussis from age 6 weeks through 6 years of age (prior to seventh birthday)

Adacel®, Boostrix® (Tdap): Active booster immunization against diphtheria, tetanus, and pertussis

The Advisory Committee on Immunization Practices (ACIP) recommends routine vaccination for the following:

Children 6 weeks to <7 years (DTaP):

- For primary immunization against diphtheria, tetanus and pertussis
- Pediatric patients who are wounded in bombings or similar mass casualty events and who have penetrating injuries or nonintact skin exposure, and have an uncertain vaccination history should receive a tetanus booster with DTaP (if no contraindications exist) (CDC, 57 [RR6], 2008)

Children 7-10 years (Tdap):

- Children not fully vaccinated against pertussis should receive a single dose of Tdap (if no contraindications exist) (CDC, 60[1], 2011)
- Children never vaccinated against diphtheria, tetanus, or pertussis, or whose vaccination status is not known should receive a series of three vaccinations containing tetanus and diphtheria toxoids and the first dose should be with Tdap (CDC, 60[1], 2011)

Adolescents 11-18 years (Tdap):

- A single dose of Tdap as a booster dose in adolescents who have completed the recommended childhood DTaP vaccination series (preferred age of administration is 11-12 years) (CDC, 60[1], 2011)

Adolescents ≥11 years and Adults (Tdap):

- Persons wounded in bombings or similar mass casualty events and who cannot confirm receipt of a tetanus booster within the previous 5 years and who have penetrating injuries or nonintact skin exposure should receive a single dose of Tdap (CDC, 57 [RR6] 2008)

Adults 19-64 years (Tdap): A single dose of Tdap should be given to replace a single dose of the 10-year Td booster in patients who have not previously received Tdap or for whom vaccine status is not known, and as soon as feasible to all:

- Postpartum women (CDC, 57[RR4], 2008; CDC, 60[4], 2011; CDC, 60[41], 2011)
- Close contacts of children <12 months of age; Tdap should ideally be administered at least 2 weeks prior to beginning close contact (CDC, 60[4], 2011; CDC, 55 [RR17], 2006; CDC, 60[41], 2011)
- Healthcare providers with direct patient contact (CDC, 60[4], 2011; CDC, 55[RR17], 2006)

Adults ≥65 years who have not previously received Tdap:
- All adults ≥65 years may receive a single dose of Tdap in place of a dose of Td (CDC, 60[1], 2011; CDC, 60 [41], 2011)
- Adults ≥65 years who anticipate close contact with children <12 months of age should receive a single dose of Tdap in place a of a dose of Td (CDC, 60[1], 2011; CDC, 60[41], 2011)

Note: Tdap is currently recommended for a single dose only (all age groups) (CDC, 60[1], 2011)

Pregnancy Risk Factor C

Pregnancy Considerations Animal reproduction studies have not been conducted. Inactivated bacterial vaccines have not been shown to cause increased risks to the fetus (CDC, 60[2], 2011). Daptacel®, Infanrix®, and Tripedia® are not recommended for use in a pregnant woman or any patient ≥7 years of age. Based on data collected from pregnancy registries, VAERS, and other small studies, the ACIP concluded that Tdap (Adacel®, Boostrix®) does not increase the risk of adverse events in pregnant women. Pregnant women not previously administered Tdap may receive a dose (preferably >20 weeks gestation) (CDC, 60[41], 2011). Alternately, administration of Tdap is to be given immediately post partum to all pregnant women who have not previously been vaccinated with Tdap in order to protect the mother and infant from pertussis (CDC, 57[RR 4], 2008; CDC, 60[41], 2011). Pregnancy registries have been established for women who may become exposed to Boostrix® (888-452-9622) or Adacel® (800-822-2463) while pregnant.

Lactation Excretion in breast milk unknown/use caution

Contraindications Hypersensitivity to diphtheria, tetanus toxoids, pertussis, or any component of the formulation; history of any of the following effects from previous administration of pertussis-containing vaccine - progressive neurologic disorder, including infantile spasms, uncontrolled epilepsy or progressive epilepsy (postpone until condition stabilized); encephalopathy occurring within 7 days of administration and not attributable to another cause

Warnings/Precautions Defer administration during moderate or severe illness (with or without fever). Carefully consider use in patients with history of any of the following effects from previous administration of any pertussis-containing vaccine: Fever ≥105°F (40.5°C) within 48 hours of unknown cause; seizures with or without fever occurring within 3 days; persistent, inconsolable crying episodes lasting ≥3 hours and occurring within 48 hours; shock or collapse within 48 hours. Carefully consider use in patients with history of Guillain-Barré syndrome occurring within 6 weeks of a vaccine containing tetanus toxoid. Td or Tdap vaccines and emergency doses of Td vaccine should not be given more frequently than every 10 years in patients who have experienced a serious Arthus-type hypersensitivity reaction following a prior use of tetanus toxoid even if using for wound management with wounds that are not clean or minor; these patients generally have high serum antitoxin levels. Apnea has been reported following I.M. vaccine administration in premature infants; consider risk versus benefit in infants born prematurely.

Use caution in patients with coagulation disorders (including thrombocytopenia) where intramuscular injections should not be used. Patients who are immunocompromised may have reduced response; may be used in patients with HIV infection. In general, household and close contacts of persons with altered immunocompetence may receive all age appropriate vaccines. Use caution in patients with history of seizure disorder, progressive neurologic disease, or conditions predisposing to seizures; ACIP and APP guidelines recommend deferring immunization until health status can be assessed and condition stabilized. Antipyretics may be considered at the time of and for 24 hours following vaccination to patients at high risk for seizures to reduce the possibility of postvaccination fever. Products may contain thimerosal or gelatin; packaging may contain natural latex rubber. Immediate treatment for anaphylactic/anaphylactoid reaction should be available during vaccine use. In order to maximize vaccination rates, the ACIP recommends simultaneous administration of all age-appropriate vaccines (live or inactivated) for which a person is eligible at a single clinic visit, unless contraindications exist. The use of combination vaccines is generally preferred over separate injections, taking into consideration provider assessment, patient preference, and adverse events. When using combination vaccines, the minimum age for administration is the oldest minimum age for any individual component; the minimum interval between dosing is the greatest minimum interval between any individual component.

Adacel® is formulated with the same antigens found in Daptacel®, but with reduced quantities of tetanus and pertussis. Safety and efficacy have not been established in children <11 years of age.

Boostrix® is formulated with the same antigens found in Infanrix®, but in reduced quantities. Safety and efficacy have not been established in patients <10 years of age. Use of Adacel® or Boostrix® in the primary immunization series or to complete the primary series has not been evaluated.

Daptacel®, Infanrix®, Tripedia®: Safety and efficacy in children <6 weeks of age or ≥7 years of age have not been established.

Adverse Reactions All serious adverse reactions must be reported to the U.S. Department of Health and Human Services (DHHS) Vaccine Adverse Event Reporting System (VAERS) 1-800-822-7967 or online at https://vaers.hhs.gov/esub/index. In Canada, adverse reactions may be reported to local provincial/territorial health agencies or to the Vaccine Safety Section at Public Health Agency of Canada (1-866-844-0018).

Daptacel®, Infanrix®, Tripedia® (incidence of erythema, swelling, and fever increases with successive doses):

Frequency not defined:

Central nervous system: Drowsiness, fever, fussiness, irritability, lethargy

Gastrointestinal: Appetite decreased, vomiting

Local: Pain, redness, swelling, tenderness

Miscellaneous: Prolonged or persistent crying, refusal to play

Postmarketing and/or case reports: Allergic reaction, anaphylactic reactions, angioedema, apnea, bronchitis, cellulitis, cough, cyanosis, diarrhea, ear pain, encephalopathy, erythema, fatigue, headache, hypersensitivity, hypotonia, hypotonic-hyporesponsive episode, idiopathic thrombocytopenic purpura, infantile spasm, injection site reaction (abscess, cellulitis, induration, mass, nodule, rash), intussusception, limb swelling, lymphadenopathy, nausea, pruritus, rash, respiratory tract infection, seizure, screaming, somnolence, sudden infant death syndrome, thrombocytopenia, urticaria

Adacel®, Boostrix®: Note: Ranges presented, actual percent varies by product and age group

>10%:

Central nervous system: Fatigue, tiredness (24% to 37%; grade 3/severe: 1% to 4%), headache (12% to 44%; grade 3/severe: 1% to 4%), chills (8% to 15%; severe: <1%)

Gastrointestinal: Gastrointestinal symptoms, includes abdominal pain, diarrhea, nausea and/or vomiting (3% to 26%; grade 3/severe: ≤3%)

Local: Injection site pain (22% to 78%; grade 3/severe: ≤5%), arm circumference increased (28%; >40 mm: 0.5%), redness (11% to 25%; ≥50 mm: 2% to 4%), swelling (8% to 21%; ≥50 mm: ≤3%)

Neuromuscular & skeletal: Body aches/muscle weakness (22% to 30%; severe: 1%), soreness/swollen joints (9% to 11%; severe: <1%)
1% to 10%:
Central nervous system: Fever ≥38°C (≥100.4°F: 1% to 5%)
Dermatologic: Rash (2% to 3%)
Miscellaneous: Lymph node swelling (7%; severe: <1%)
Postmarketing and/or case reports: Anaphylactic reaction, arthralgia, back pain, diabetes mellitus, encephalitis, exanthema, facial palsy, GBS, Henoch-Schönlein purpura, hypersensitivity reactions, hypoesthesia, injection site reaction (bruising, induration, inflammation, mass, nodule, pruritus, sterile abscess, warmth), limb swelling (extensive), lymphadenitis, lymphadenopathy, myalgia, myocarditis, myositis, nerve compression, paresthesia, pruritus, seizure, syncope, urticaria

Drug Interactions

Metabolism/Transport Effects None known.

Avoid Concomitant Use There are no known interactions where it is recommended to avoid concomitant use.

Increased Effect/Toxicity There are no known significant interactions involving an increase in effect.

Decreased Effect

The levels/effects of Diphtheria and Tetanus Toxoids, and Acellular Pertussis Vaccine may be decreased by: Belimumab; Fingolimod; Immunosuppressants

Stability Refrigerate at 2°C to 8°C (35°F to 46°F); do not freeze; discard if frozen. The following stability information has also been reported for Infanrix®: May be stored at room temperature for up to 72 hours (Cohen, 2007).

Mechanism of Action Promotes active immunity to diphtheria, tetanus, and pertussis by inducing production of specific antibodies.

Dosage Note: Tdap can be administered regardless of the interval between the last tetanus or diphtheria toxoid containing vaccine. Tdap is currently recommended for a single dose only (CDC, 60[1], 2011)

I.M.:

Children 6 weeks to <7 years: Primary immunization: **Note:** Whenever possible, the same product should be used for all doses. Interruption of recommended schedule does not require starting the series over; a delay between doses should not interfere with final immunity.

Daptacel®, Infanrix®, Tripedia®: 0.5 mL per dose, total of 5 doses administered as follows:

Three doses, usually given at 2-, 4-, and 6 months of age; may be given as early as 6 weeks of age and repeated every 4-8 weeks

Fourth dose: Given at ~15-20 months of age, but at least 6 months after third dose. The fourth dose may be given as early as 12 months of age, but at least 6 months must have elapsed between the third dose and the fourth dose.

Fifth dose: Given at 4-6 years of age, prior to starting school or kindergarten; if the fourth dose is given at ≥4 years of age, the fifth dose may be omitted

For children who start primary immunization series ≥4 months of age, refer to current ACIP "Catch-up Immunization Schedule".

Children 7-10 years: Not fully vaccinated against pertussis, or never vaccinated against diphtheria, tetanus, or pertussis, or whose vaccination status is not known: Administer a series of 3 vaccinations containing tetanus and diphtheria toxoids; the first dose should be with Tdap (CDC, 60[1], 2011).

Adolescents and Adults: Booster Immunization: ACIP recommendations:

Adolescents 11-18 years: 0.5 mL per dose. Tdap should be given as a single booster dose at age 11 or 12 years in adolescents who have completed a childhood vaccination series, followed by booster doses of Td every 10 years. Adolescents who have not received Tdap at age 11 or 12 should receive a single dose of Tdap in place of a single Td booster dose (CDC, 55[3], 2006; CDC, 60 [1], 2011).

Adults 19-64 years: 0.5 mL per dose. A single dose of Tdap should be given to replace a single dose of the 10 year Td booster in patients who have not previously received Tdap or for whom vaccine status is not known. A single dose of Tdap is recommended for health care personnel who have not previously received Tdap and who have direct patient contact (CDC, 55[17], 2006; CDC, 60[4], 2011).

Adults ≥65 years: 0.5 mL per dose. A single dose of Tdap may be given to older adults who have not previously received Tdap (CDC, 60[1], 2011)

Adolescents and Adults: Booster Immunization: Manufacturer's recommendations:

Children ≥10 years and Adults (Boostrix®): 0.5 mL as a single dose, administered 5 years after last dose of tetanus toxoid, diphtheria toxoid, and/or pertussis-containing vaccine

Children ≥11 years and Adults ≤64 years (Adacel®): 0.5 mL as a single dose, administered 5 years after last dose of tetanus toxoid, diphtheria toxoid and/or pertussis-containing vaccine

Wound management: Adacel® or Boostrix® may be used as an alternative to Td vaccine when a tetanus toxoid-containing vaccine is needed for wound management, and in whom the pertussis component is also indicated. Tetanus prophylaxis in patients with wounds should consider if the wound is clean or contaminated, the immunization status of the patient, proper use of tetanus toxoid and/or tetanus immune globulin (TIG), wound cleaning, and (if required) surgical debridement and the proper use of antibiotics. Patients with an uncertain or incomplete tetanus immunization status should have additional follow up to ensure a series is completed. Patients with a history of Arthus reaction following a previous dose of a tetanus toxoid-containing vaccine should not receive a tetanus toxoid-containing vaccine until >10 years after the most recent dose even if they have a wound that is neither clean nor minor. See table.

Tetanus Prophylaxis in Wound Management

History of Tetanus Immunization Doses	Clean, Minor Wounds		All Other Wounds[1]	
	Tetanus Toxoid[2]	TIG	Tetanus Toxoid[2]	TIG
Uncertain or <3 doses	Yes	No	Yes	Yes
3 or more doses	No[3]	No	No[4]	No

[1]Such as, but not limited to, wounds contaminated with dirt, feces, soil, and saliva; puncture wounds; wounds from crushing, tears, burns, and frostbite.

[2]Tetanus toxoid in this chart refers to a tetanus toxoid-containing vaccine. For children <7 years of age, DTaP (DT, if pertussis vaccine contraindicated) is preferred to tetanus toxoid alone. For children ≥7 years and adults, Td preferred to tetanus toxoid alone; Tdap may be preferred if the patient has not previously been vaccinated with Tdap.

[3]Yes, if ≥10 years since last dose.

[4]Yes, if ≥5 years since last dose.

Adapted from CDC "Yellow Book" (*Health Information for International Travel 2010*), "Routine Vaccine-Preventable Diseases, Tetanus" (available at http://www.cdc.gov/yellowbook) and *MMWR* 2006, 55 (RR-17).

Abbreviations: **DT** = Diphtheria and Tetanus Toxoids (formulation for age ≤6 years); **DTaP** = Diphtheria and Tetanus Toxoids, and Acellular Pertussis (formulation for age ≤6 years; Daptacel®, Infanrix®, Tripedia®); **Td** = Diphtheria and Tetanus Toxoids (formulation for age ≥7 years; Decavac®); **TT**= Tetanus toxoid (adsorbed [formulation for age ≥7 years]); **Tdap** = Diphtheria and Tetanus Toxoids, and Acellular Pertussis (Adacel® or Boostrix® [formulations for age ≥7 years]); **TIG** = Tetanus Immune Globulin

Administration Shake suspension well.

Adacel®, Boostrix®: Administer only I.M. in deltoid muscle of upper arm.

Daptacel®, Infanrix®, Tripedia®: Administer only I.M. in anterolateral aspect of thigh or deltoid muscle of upper arm.

If feasible, the same brand of DTaP should be used for all doses in the series (CDC, 60[2], 2011).

For patients at risk of hemorrhage following intramuscular injection, the ACIP recommends "it should be administered intramuscularly if, in the opinion of the physician familiar with the patients bleeding risk, the vaccine can be administered by this route with reasonable safety. If the patient receives antihemophilia or other similar therapy, intramuscular vaccination can be scheduled shortly after such therapy is administered. A fine needle (23 gauge or smaller) can be used for the vaccination and firm pressure applied to the site (without rubbing) for at least 2 minutes. The patient should be instructed concerning the risk of hematoma from the injection." Patients on anticoagulant therapy should be considered to have the same bleeding risks and treated as those with clotting factor disorders (CDC, 60[2], 2011).

Simultaneous administration of vaccines helps ensure the patients will be fully vaccinated by the appropriate age. Simultaneous administration of vaccines is defined as administering >1 vaccine on the same day at different anatomic sites. The use of licensed combination vaccines is generally preferred over separate injections of the equivalent components. Separate vaccines should not be combined in the same syringe unless indicated by product specific labeling. Separate needles and syringes should be used for each injection. The ACIP prefers each dose of a specific vaccine in a series come from the same manufacturer when possible. Adolescents and adults should be vaccinated while seated or lying down. In general, preterm infants should be vaccinated at the same chronological age as full-term infants (CDC, 60[2], 2011).

Antipyretics have not been shown to prevent febrile seizures. Antipyretics may be used to treat fever or discomfort following vaccination (CDC, 2011). One study reported that routine prophylactic administration of acetaminophen to prevent fever prior to vaccination decreased the immune response of some vaccines; the clinical significance of this reduction in immune response has not been established (Prymula, 2009).

Monitoring Parameters Monitor for syncope for ≥15 minutes following vaccination

Additional Information In patients who cannot be given pertussis vaccine, DT for pediatric use should be given to complete the series.

Adacel® is formulated with the same antigens found in Daptacel® but with reduced quantities of pertussis and tetanus. It is intended for use as a booster dose in children and adults, 11-64 years of age, and **not** for primary immunization.

Boostrix® is formulated with the same antigens found in Infanrix® but in reduced quantities. It is intended for use as a booster dose in children and adults, 10-64 years of age, and is **not** for primary immunization.

The ACIP considers Adacel® and Boostrix® to be interchangeable when administered to adolescents for childhood vaccination according to the Child and Adolescent Immunization Schedule.

The child's medical record should document that the small risk of postvaccination seizure and the benefits of the pertussis vaccination were discussed with the patient; parents or guardians should be questioned prior to administration of vaccine as to any adverse reactions from previous dose. Provide Vaccine Information Materials, as required by National Childhood Vaccine Injury Act of 1986, prior to immunization.

Federal law requires that the name of medication, date of administration, the vaccine manufacturer, lot number of vaccine, and the administering person's name, title and address be entered into the patient's permanent medical record.

Dosage Forms Excipient information presented when available (limited, particularly for generics); consult specific product labeling.

Injection, suspension [Tdap, booster formulation]:

Adacel®: Diphtheria 2 Lf units, tetanus 5 Lf units, and acellular pertussis antigens [detoxified pertussis toxin 2.5 mcg, filamentous hemagglutinin 5 mcg, pertactin 3 mcg, fimbriae (types 2 and 3) 5 mcg] per 0.5 mL (0.5 mL) [contains aluminum; may contain natural rubber/natural latex in prefilled syringe]

Boostrix®: Diphtheria 2.5 Lf units, tetanus 5 Lf units, and acellular pertussis antigens [inactivated pertussis toxin 8 mcg, filamentous hemagglutinin 8 mcg, pertactin 2.5 mcg] per 0.5 mL (0.5 mL) [contains aluminum and polysorbate 80; may contain natural rubber/natural latex in prefilled syringe]

Injection, suspension [DTaP, active immunization formulation]:

Daptacel®: Diphtheria 15 Lf units, tetanus 5 Lf units, and acellular pertussis antigens [detoxified pertussis toxin 10 mcg, filamentous hemagglutinin 5 mcg, pertactin 3 mcg, fimbriae (types 2 and 3) 5 mcg] per 0.5 mL (0.5 mL) [preservative free; contains aluminum]

Infanrix®: Diphtheria 25 Lf units, tetanus 10 Lf units, and acellular pertussis antigens [inactivated pertussis toxin 25 mcg, filamentous hemagglutinin 25 mcg, pertactin 8 mcg] per 0.5 mL (0.5 mL) [preservative free; contains aluminum and polysorbate 80]

Infanrix®: Diphtheria 25 Lf units, tetanus 10 Lf units, and acellular pertussis antigens [inactivated pertussis toxin 25 mcg, filamentous hemagglutinin 25 mcg, pertactin 8 mcg] per 0.5 mL (0.5 mL) [preservative free; contains aluminum and polysorbate 80; prefilled syringes contain natural rubber/natural latex] [DSC]

Tripedia®: Diphtheria 6.7 Lf units, tetanus 5 Lf units, and acellular pertussis antigens [inactivated pertussis toxin 23.4 mcg, filamentous hemagglutinin 23.4 mcg] per 0.5 mL (0.5 mL) [DSC] [contains aluminum, natural rubber/natural latex in packaging, polysorbate 80, and thimerosal (trace amounts)]

Note: Tripedia® vaccine is also used to reconstitute ActHIB® to prepare TriHIBit® vaccine (diphtheria, tetanus toxoids, and acellular pertussis and *Haemophilus influenzae* b conjugate vaccine combination)

◆ **Diphtheria CRM_{197} Protein** *see* Pneumococcal Conjugate Vaccine (7-Valent) *on page* 1365

◆ **Diphtheria CRM_{197} Protein** *see* Pneumococcal Conjugate Vaccine (13-Valent) *on page* 1366

◆ **Diphtheria, Tetanus Toxoids, Acellular Pertussis (DTaP)** *see* Diphtheria and Tetanus Toxoids, Acellular Pertussis, and Poliovirus Vaccine *on page* 522

◆ **Diphtheria, Tetanus Toxoids, Acellular Pertussis (DTaP)** *see* Diphtheria and Tetanus Toxoids, Acellular Pertussis, Poliovirus and *Haemophilus* b Conjugate Vaccine *on page* 522

Diphtheria, Tetanus Toxoids, Acellular Pertussis, Hepatitis B (Recombinant), and Poliovirus (Inactivated) Vaccine

(dif THEER ee a, TET a nus TOKS oyds, ay CEL yoo lar per TUS sis, hep a TYE tis bee ree KOM be nant, & POE lee oh VYE rus in ak ti VAY ted vak SEEN)

Brand Names: U.S. Pediarix®

Brand Names: Canada Pediarix®

Index Terms Diphtheria and Tetanus Toxoids and Acellular Pertussis Adsorbed, Hepatitis B (Recombinant) and Inactivated Poliovirus Vaccine Combined; Diphtheria, Tetanus Toxoids, Acellular Pertussis, Hepatitis B (Recombinant), and Poliovirus Vaccine; DTaP-HepB-IPV

Pharmacologic Category Vaccine, Inactivated (Bacterial); Vaccine, Inactivated (Viral)

Additional Appendix Information

Immunization Recommendations *on page 1922*

Use Combination vaccine for the active immunization against diphtheria, tetanus, pertussis, hepatitis B virus (all known subtypes), and poliomyelitis (caused by poliovirus types 1, 2, and 3)

The Advisory Committee on Immunization Practices (ACIP) recommends Pediarix® for the following:

- Primary vaccination for DTaP, Hep B, and IPV in children at 2, 4, and 6 months of age.
- To complete the primary vaccination series in children who have received DTaP (Infanrix®) and who are scheduled to receive the other components of the vaccine. Whenever feasible, the same manufacturer should be used to provide the pertussis component; however, vaccination should not be deferred if a specific brand is not known or is not available. HepB and IPV from different manufacturers are interchangeable.

Pregnancy Risk Factor C

Dosage I.M.: Children 6 weeks to <7 years:

Primary immunization: 0.5 mL/dose; administer as a 3-dose series at 2-, 4-, and 6 months of age in 6- to 8-week intervals (preferably 8-week intervals). Vaccination usually begins at 2 months, but may be started as early as 6 weeks of age.

Note: Pediarix® is approved for the first 3 doses of polio vaccine. Per the ACIP, polio vaccine is given at 2, 4 and 6 months of age and should not be administered more frequently than 4 weeks apart. Use of the minimum age and minimum intervals during the first 6 months of life should only be done when the vaccine recipient is at risk for imminent exposure to circulating poliovirus (shorter intervals and earlier start dates may lead to lower seroconversion).

Use in children previously vaccinated with one or more component, and who are also scheduled to receive all vaccine components:

Hepatitis B vaccine: Infants previously vaccinated with 1 or 2 doses of another hepatitis B vaccine may use Pediarix® to complete the 3-dose series. Not for use as birth dose of hepatitis B vaccine. Infants born to HB_sAg-positive women should begin dosing with DTaP-HepB-IPV by age 6-8 weeks after receiving the single antigen hepatitis B vaccine at birth.

Diphtheria and tetanus toxoids, and acellular pertussis vaccine (DTaP): Infants previously vaccinated with 1 or 2 doses of Infanrix® may use Pediarix® to complete the first 3 doses of the series; use of Pediarix® to complete DTaP vaccination started with products other than Infanrix® is not recommended.

Inactivated polio vaccine (IPV): Infants previously vaccinated with 1 or 2 doses of IPV may use Pediarix® to complete the first 3 doses of the series.

Additional Information Complete prescribing information for this medication should be consulted for additional detail.

Dosage Forms Excipient information presented when available (limited, particularly for generics); consult specific product labeling.

Injection, suspension [preservative free]:

Pediarix®: Diphtheria toxoid 25 Lf, tetanus toxoid 10 Lf, acellular pertussis antigens [inactivated pertussis toxin 25 mcg, filamentous hemagglutin 25 mcg, pertactin 8 mcg, HBsAg 10 mcg, type 1 poliovirus 40 D antigen units, type 2 poliovirus 8 D antigen units and type 3 poliovirus 32 D antigen units] per 0.5 mL (0.5 mL) [contains aluminum, neomycin sulfate (trace amounts), polymyxin B (trace amounts), polysorbate 80, and yeast protein ≤5%; may contain natural rubber/natural latex in prefilled syringe]

◆ **Diphtheria, Tetanus Toxoids, Acellular Pertussis, Hepatitis B (Recombinant), and Poliovirus Vaccine** *see* Diphtheria, Tetanus Toxoids, Acellular Pertussis, Hepatitis B (Recombinant), and Poliovirus (Inactivated) Vaccine *on page 527*

◆ **Diphtheria Toxoid** *see* Diphtheria and Tetanus Toxoids, Acellular Pertussis, Poliovirus and *Haemophilus* b Conjugate Vaccine *on page 522*

◆ **Diphtheria Toxoid Conjugate** *see* *Haemophilus* b Conjugate Vaccine *on page 815*

◆ **Dipivalyl Epinephrine** *see* Dipivefrin *on page 527*

Dipivefrin (dye PI ve frin)

Brand Names: Canada Ophtho-Dipivefrin™; PMS-Dipivefrin; Propine®

Index Terms Dipivalyl Epinephrine; Dipivefrin Hydrochloride; DPE

Pharmacologic Category Alpha/Beta Agonist; Ophthalmic Agent, Antiglaucoma; Ophthalmic Agent, Vasoconstrictor

Use Reduces elevated intraocular pressure in chronic open-angle glaucoma; also used to treat ocular hypertension, low tension, and secondary glaucomas

Pregnancy Risk Factor B

Dosage Adults: Ophthalmic: Instill 1 drop every 12 hours into the eyes

Additional Information Complete prescribing information for this medication should be consulted for additional detail.

Dosage Forms Excipient information presented when available (limited, particularly for generics); consult specific product labeling. [DSC] = Discontinued product

Solution, ophthalmic, as hydrochloride [drops]:

Propine®: 0.1% (10 mL [DSC]) [contains benzalkonium chloride]

◆ **Dipivefrin Hydrochloride** *see* Dipivefrin *on page 527*

◆ **Diprivan®** *see* Propofol *on page 1421*

◆ **Diprolene®** *see* Betamethasone *on page 208*

◆ **Diprolene® AF** *see* Betamethasone *on page 208*

◆ **Diprolene® Glycol (Can)** *see* Betamethasone *on page 208*

◆ **Dipropylacetic Acid** *see* Valproic Acid *on page 1757*

◆ **Diprosone® (Can)** *see* Betamethasone *on page 208*

Dipyridamole (dye peer ID a mole)

Brand Names: U.S. Persantine®

Brand Names: Canada Apo-Dipyridamole FC®; Dipyridamole For Injection; Persantine®

Pharmacologic Category Antiplatelet Agent; Vasodilator

Additional Appendix Information

Beers Criteria - Potentially Inappropriate Medications for Geriatrics *on page 1973*

Use

Oral: Used with warfarin to decrease thrombosis in patients after artificial heart valve replacement

I.V.: Diagnostic agent in CAD

Unlabeled Use Stroke prevention (in combination with aspirin)

Pregnancy Risk Factor B

Pregnancy Considerations Teratogenic effects were not observed in animal studies.

Lactation Enters breast milk/use caution

Contraindications Hypersensitivity to dipyridamole or any component of the formulation

Warnings/Precautions Use with caution in patients with hypotension, unstable angina, and/or recent MI. Use with caution in hepatic impairment. May be inappropriate for use in the elderly due to risk of orthostatic hypotension (Beers Criteria). Use caution in patients on other antiplatelet agents or anticoagulation. Severe adverse reactions have occurred with I.V. administration (rarely); use the I.V. form with caution in patients with bronchospastic disease or unstable angina. Aminophylline should be available in case of urgency or emergency with I.V. use.

Adverse Reactions

Oral:

>10%: Dizziness (14%)

1% to 10%:

Central nervous system: Headache (2%)

Dermatologic: Rash (2%)

Gastrointestinal: Abdominal distress (6%)

Frequency not defined: Diarrhea, vomiting, flushing, pruritus, angina pectoris, liver dysfunction

Postmarketing and/or case reports: Alopecia, arthritis, cholelithiasis, dyspepsia, fatigue, hepatitis, hypersensitivity reaction, hypotension, larynx edema, malaise, myalgia, nausea, palpitation, paresthesia, tachycardia, thrombocytopenia

I.V.:

>10%:

Cardiovascular: Exacerbation of angina pectoris (20%)

Central nervous system: Dizziness (12%), headache (12%)

1% to 10%:

Cardiovascular: Hypotension (5%), hypertension (2%), blood pressure lability (2%), ECG abnormalities (ST-T changes, extrasystoles; 5% to 8%), pain (3%), tachycardia (3%)

Central nervous system: Flushing (3%), fatigue (1%)

Gastrointestinal: Nausea (5%)

Neuromuscular & skeletal: Paresthesia (1%)

Respiratory: Dyspnea (3%)

<1% (Limited to important or life-threatening): Abdominal pain, abnormal coordination, allergic reaction (pruritus, rash, urticaria), appetite increased, arrhythmia (ventricular tachycardia, bradycardia, AV block, SVT, atrial fibrillation, asystole), arthralgia, asthenia, back pain, breast pain, bronchospasm, cardiomyopathy, cough, depersonalization, diaphoresis, dry mouth, dysgeusia, dyspepsia, dysphagia, earache, ECG abnormalities (unspecified), edema, eructation, flatulence, hypertonia, hyperventilation, injection site reaction, intermittent claudication leg cramping, malaise, MI, myalgia, orthostatic hypotension, palpitation, perineal pain, pharyngitis, pleural pain, renal pain, rhinitis, rigor, syncope, tenesmus, thirst, tinnitus, tremor, vertigo, vision abnormalities, vomiting

Drug Interactions

Metabolism/Transport Effects **Inhibits** BCRP, P-glycoprotein

Avoid Concomitant Use

Avoid concomitant use of Dipyridamole with any of the following: Silodosin; Topotecan

Increased Effect/Toxicity

Dipyridamole may increase the levels/effects of: Adenosine; Anticoagulants; Antiplatelet Agents; Beta-Blockers; Colchicine; Collagenase (Systemic); Dabigatran Etexilate; Drotrecogin Alfa (Activated); Everolimus; Hypotensive Agents; Ibritumomab; P-glycoprotein/ABCB1 Substrates; Regadenoson; Rivaroxaban; Salicylates; Silodosin; Thrombolytic Agents; Topotecan; Tositumomab and Iodine I 131 Tositumomab

The levels/effects of Dipyridamole may be increased by: Dasatinib; Glucosamine; Herbs (Anticoagulant/Antiplatelet Properties); Nonsteroidal Anti-Inflammatory Agents; Omega-3-Acid Ethyl Esters; Pentosan Polysulfate Sodium; Pentoxifylline; Prostacyclin Analogues; Vitamin E

Decreased Effect

Dipyridamole may decrease the levels/effects of: Acetylcholinesterase Inhibitors

The levels/effects of Dipyridamole may be decreased by: Nonsteroidal Anti-Inflammatory Agents

Ethanol/Nutrition/Herb Interactions Herb/Nutraceutical: Avoid cat's claw, dong quai, evening primrose, feverfew, garlic, ginger, ginkgo, red clover, horse chestnut, green tea, ginseng (all have additional antiplatelet activity).

Stability I.V.: Store between 15°C to 25°C (59°F to 77°F); do not freeze. Protect from light. Prior to administration, dilute to a ≥1:2 ratio in NS, 1/2NS, or D_5W. Total volume should be ~20-50 mL.

Mechanism of Action Inhibits the activity of adenosine deaminase and phosphodiesterase, which causes an accumulation of adenosine, adenine nucleotides, and cyclic AMP; these mediators then inhibit platelet aggregation and may cause vasodilation; may also stimulate release of prostacyclin or PGD_2; causes coronary vasodilation

Pharmacodynamics/Kinetics

Absorption: Readily, but variable

Distribution: Adults: V_d: 2-3 L/kg

Protein binding: 91% to 99%

Metabolism: Hepatic

Half-life elimination: Terminal: 10-12 hours

Time to peak, serum: 2-2.5 hours

Excretion: Feces (as glucuronide conjugates and unchanged drug)

Dosage

Oral: Children ≥12 years and Adults: Adjunctive therapy for prophylaxis of thromboembolism with cardiac valve replacement: 75-100 mg 4 times/day

I.V.: Adults: Evaluation of coronary artery disease: 0.14 mg/kg/minute for 4 minutes; maximum dose: 60 mg

Following dipyridamole infusion, inject thallium-201 within 5 minutes. **Note:** Aminophylline should be available for urgent/emergent use; dosing of 50-100 mg (range: 50-250 mg) I.V. push over 30-60 seconds.

Dietary Considerations Should be taken with water 1 hour before meals.

Administration

I.V.: Infuse diluted solution over 4 minutes.

Tablet: Administer with water 1 hour before meals.

Monitoring Parameters Blood pressure, heart rate, ECG (stress test)

Test Interactions Concurrent caffeine or theophylline use may demonstrate a false-negative result with dipyridamole-thallium myocardial imaging.

Dosage Forms Excipient information presented when available (limited, particularly for generics); consult specific product labeling. [DSC] = Discontinued product

Injection, solution: 5 mg/mL (2 mL [DSC], 10 mL)

Tablet, oral: 25 mg, 50 mg, 75 mg

Persantine®: 25 mg, 50 mg, 75 mg

Extemporaneous Preparations A 10 mg/mL oral suspension may be made with tablets and one of three different vehicles (cherry syrup, a 1:1 mixture of Ora-Sweet® and Ora-Plus®, or a 1:1 mixture of Ora-Sweet® SF and Ora-Plus®). Crush twenty-four 50 mg tablets in a mortar and reduce to a fine powder. Add 20 mL of the chosen vehicle and mix to a uniform paste; mix while adding the vehicle in incremental proportions to **almost** 120 mL; transfer to a calibrated bottle, rinse mortar with vehicle, and add quantity of vehicle sufficient to make 120 mL. Label "shake well" and "protect from light". Stable for 60 days when stored in amber plastic prescription bottles in the dark at room temperature or refrigerated.

Allen LV and Erickson III MA, "Stability of Baclofen, Captopril, Diltiazem, Hydrochloride, Dipyridamole, and Flecainide Acetate in Extemporaneously Compounded Oral Liquids," *Am J Health Syst Pharm*, 1996, 53:2179-84.

◆ **Dipyridamole and Aspirin** *see* Aspirin and Dipyridamole *on page 157*

◆ **Dipyridamole For Injection (Can)** *see* Dipyridamole *on page 527*

◆ **Disalicylic Acid** *see* Salsalate *on page 1534*

◆ **DisCoVisc®** *see* Sodium Chondroitin Sulfate and Sodium Hyaluronate *on page 1570*

◆ **Disodium Cromoglycate** *see* Cromolyn (Nasal) *on page 418*

◆ **Disodium Cromoglycate** *see* Cromolyn (Ophthalmic) *on page 418*

◆ **Disodium Thiosulfate Pentahydrate** *see* Sodium Thiosulfate *on page 1577*

◆ ***d*-Isoephedrine Hydrochloride** *see* Pseudoephedrine *on page 1430*

Disopyramide (dye soe PEER a mide)

Brand Names: U.S. Norpace®; Norpace® CR

Brand Names: Canada Norpace®; Rythmodan®; Rythmodan®-LA

Index Terms Disopyramide Phosphate

Pharmacologic Category Antiarrhythmic Agent, Class Ia

Additional Appendix Information

Beers Criteria – Potentially Inappropriate Medications for Geriatrics *on page 1973*

Use Suppression and prevention of unifocal and multifocal atrial and premature, ventricular premature complexes, coupled ventricular tachycardia; effective in the conversion of atrial fibrillation, atrial flutter, and paroxysmal atrial tachycardia to normal sinus rhythm and prevention of the recurrence of these arrhythmias after conversion by other methods

Unlabeled Use Hypertrophic obstructive cardiomyopathy (HOCM)

Pregnancy Risk Factor C

Dosage Oral:

Children:

<1 year: 10-30 mg/kg/24 hours in 4 divided doses

1-4 years: 10-20 mg/kg/24 hours in 4 divided doses

4-12 years: 10-15 mg/kg/24 hours in 4 divided doses

12-18 years: 6-15 mg/kg/24 hours in 4 divided doses

Adults:

<50 kg: 100 mg every 6 hours or 200 mg every 12 hours (controlled release)

>50 kg: 150 mg every 6 hours or 300 mg every 12 hours (controlled release); if no response, increase to 200 mg every 6 hours. Maximum dose required for patients with severe refractory ventricular tachycardia is 400 mg every 6 hours.

Hypertrophic obstructive cardiomyopathy (unlabeled use): Initial: Controlled release: 200 mg twice daily. If symptoms do not improve, increase by 100 mg/day at 2-week intervals to a maximum daily dose of 600 mg.

Elderly: Dose with caution, starting at the lower end of dosing range

Dosing adjustment in renal impairment: 100 mg (non-sustained release) given at the following intervals, based on creatinine clearance (mL/minute):

Cl_{cr} 30-40 mL/minute: Administer every 8 hours

Cl_{cr} 15-30 mL/minute: Administer every 12 hours

Cl_{cr} <15 mL/minute: Administer every 24 hours

or alter the dose as follows:

Cl_{cr} 30-<40 mL/minute: Reduce dose 50%

Cl_{cr} 15-30 mL/minute: Reduce dose 75%

Dialysis: Not dialyzable (0% to 5%) by hemo- or peritoneal methods; supplemental dose is not necessary.

Dosing interval in hepatic impairment: 100 mg every 6 hours or 200 mg every 12 hours (controlled release)

Additional Information Complete prescribing information for this medication should be consulted for additional detail.

Dosage Forms Excipient information presented when available (limited, particularly for generics); consult specific product labeling.

Capsule, oral: 100 mg, 150 mg

Norpace®: 100 mg, 150 mg

Capsule, controlled release, oral:

Norpace® CR: 100 mg, 150 mg

◆ **Disopyramide Phosphate** *see* Disopyramide *on page 529*

Disulfiram (dye SUL fi ram)

Brand Names: U.S. Antabuse®

Pharmacologic Category Aldehyde Dehydrogenase Inhibitor

Use Management of chronic alcoholism

Pregnancy Risk Factor C

Dosage Adults: Oral: Do not administer until the patient has abstained from ethanol for at least 12 hours

Initial: 500 mg/day as a single dose for 1-2 weeks; maximum daily dose is 500 mg

Average maintenance dose: 250 mg/day; range: 125-500 mg; duration of therapy is to continue until the patient is fully recovered socially and a basis for permanent self control has been established; maintenance therapy may be required for months or even years

Additional Information Complete prescribing information for this medication should be consulted for additional detail.

Dosage Forms Excipient information presented when available (limited, particularly for generics); consult specific product labeling.

Tablet, oral: 250 mg, 500 mg

Antabuse®: 250 mg, 500 mg [scored]

◆ **Dithioglycerol** *see* Dimercaprol *on page 513*

◆ **Dithranol** *see* Anthralin *on page 123*

◆ **Ditropan** *see* Oxybutynin *on page 1264*

◆ **Ditropan XL®** *see* Oxybutynin *on page 1264*

◆ **diurex® [OTC]** *see* Pamabrom *on page 1282*

◆ **diurex® Aquagels® [OTC]** *see* Pamabrom *on page 1282*

◆ **diurex® Maximum Relief [OTC]** *see* Pamabrom *on page 1282*

◆ **Diuril®** *see* Chlorothiazide *on page 344*

Divalproex (dye VAL proe ex)

Brand Names: U.S. Depakote®; Depakote® ER; Depakote® Sprinkle

Brand Names: Canada Apo-Divalproex®; Dom-Divalproex; Epival®; Mylan-Divalproex; Novo-Divalproex; Nu-Divalproex; PHL-Divalproex; PMS-Divalproex

Index Terms Divalproex Sodium; Valproate Semisodium; Valproic Acid Derivative

Pharmacologic Category Anticonvulsant, Miscellaneous; Antimanic Agent; Histone Deacetylase Inhibitor

Additional Appendix Information

Anticonvulsant Drugs of Choice *on page 1873*

Use Monotherapy and adjunctive therapy in the treatment of patients with complex partial seizures; monotherapy and adjunctive therapy of simple and complex absence seizures; adjunctive therapy in patients with multiple seizure types that include absence seizures

Depakote®, Depakote® ER: Mania associated with bipolar disorder; migraine prophylaxis

Unlabeled Use Diabetic neuropathy

Pregnancy Risk Factor D

Pregnancy Considerations [U.S. Boxed Warning]: May cause teratogenic effects such as neural tube defects (eg, spina bifida). Teratogenic effects have been reported in animals and humans. Valproic acid crosses the placenta. Neural tube, cardiac, facial (characteristic pattern of dysmorphic facial features), skeletal, multiple other defects reported. Epilepsy itself, number of medications, genetic factors, or a combination of these probably influence the teratogenicity of anticonvulsant therapy. Information from the North American Antiepileptic Drug Pregnancy Registry notes a fourfold increase in congenital malformations with exposure to valproic acid monotherapy during the 1st trimester of pregnancy when compared to monotherapy with other antiepileptic drugs (AED). The risk of neural tube defects is ~1% to 2% (general population risk estimated to be 0.14% to 0.2%). The effect of folic acid supplementation to decrease this risk is unknown, however, folic acid supplementation is recommended for all women contemplating pregnancy. An information sheet describing the teratogenic potential is available from the manufacturer.

Nonteratogenic effects have also been reported. Afibrinogenemia leading to fatal hemorrhage and hepatotoxicity have been noted in case reports of infants following *in utero* exposure to valproic acid. Developmental delay, autism and/or autism spectrum disorder have also been reported. In a prospective cohort study conducted in the U.S. and the United Kingdom, a lower Differential Ability Scale ([D.A.S.]; a battery of tests which measure cognitive development in children) score was observed in children 3 years of age with prenatal exposure to valproate compared to children with prenatal exposure to other antiepileptics (lamotrigine, carbamazepine, or phenytoin). Use in women of childbearing potential requires that benefits of use in mother be weighed against the potential risk to fetus, especially when used for conditions not associated with permanent injury or risk of death (eg, migraine).

Patients exposed to valproic acid during pregnancy are encouraged to enroll themselves into the AED Pregnancy Registry by calling 1-888-233-2334. Additional information is available at www.aedpregnancyregistry.org.

Lactation Enters breast milk/not recommended (AAP considers "compatible"; AAP 2001 update pending)

Contraindications Hypersensitivity to divalproex, derivatives, or any component of the formulation; hepatic disease or significant impairment; urea cycle disorders

Warnings/Precautions [U.S. Boxed Warning]: Hepatic failure resulting in fatalities has occurred in patients; children <2 years of age are at considerable risk. Other risk factors include organic brain disease, mental retardation with severe seizure disorders, congenital metabolic disorders, and patients on multiple anticonvulsants. Hepatotoxicity has usually been reported within 6 months of therapy initiation. Monitor patients closely for appearance of malaise, weakness, facial edema, anorexia, jaundice, and vomiting; discontinue immediately with signs/symptom of significant or suspected impairment. Liver function tests should be performed at baseline and at regular intervals after initiation of therapy, especially within the first 6 months. Hepatic dysfunction may progress despite discontinuing treatment. Should only be used as monotherapy in children <2 years of age and patients at high risk for hepatotoxicity. Contraindicated with severe impairment.

[U.S. Boxed Warning]: Cases of life-threatening pancreatitis, occurring at the start of therapy or following years of use, have been reported in adults and children. Some cases have been hemorrhagic with rapid progression of initial symptoms to death. Promptly evaluate symptoms of abdominal pain, nausea, vomiting, and/or anorexia; should generally be discontinued if pancreatitis is diagnosed.

[U.S. Boxed Warning]: May cause teratogenic effects such as neural tube defects (eg, spina bifida). Use in women of childbearing potential requires that benefits of use in mother be weighed against the potential risk to fetus, especially when used for conditions not associated with permanent injury or risk of death (eg, migraine).

May cause severe thrombocytopenia, inhibition of platelet aggregation, and bleeding. Tremors may indicate overdosage; use with caution in patients receiving other anticonvulsants. Hypersensitivity reactions affecting multiple organs have been reported in association with divalproex use; may include dermatologic and/or hematologic changes (eosinophilia, neutropenia, thrombocytopenia) or symptoms of organ dysfunction.

Hyperammonemia and/or encephalopathy, sometimes fatal, have been reported following the initiation of divalproex therapy and may be present with normal transaminase levels. Ammonia levels should be measured in patients who develop unexplained lethargy and vomiting, changes in mental status, or in patients who present with hypothermia (unintentional drop in core body temperature to <35°C/95°F). Discontinue therapy if ammonia levels are increased and evaluate for possible urea cycle disorder (UCD); contraindicated in patients with UCD. Evaluation of UCD should be considered for the following patients prior to the start of therapy: History of unexplained encephalopathy or coma; encephalopathy associated with protein load; pregnancy or postpartum encephalopathy; unexplained mental retardation; history of elevated plasma ammonia or glutamine; history of cyclical vomiting and lethargy; episodic extreme irritability, ataxia; low BUN or protein avoidance; family history of UCD or unexplained infant deaths (particularly male); or signs or symptoms of UCD (hyperammonemia, encephalopathy, respiratory alkalosis). Hypothermia has been reported with divalproex therapy; may or may not be associated with hyperammonemia; may also occur with concomitant topiramate therapy.

In vitro studies have suggested divalproex stimulates the replication of HIV and CMV viruses under experimental conditions. The clinical consequence of this is unknown, but should be considered when monitoring affected patients.

Antiepileptics are associated with an increased risk of suicidal behavior/thoughts with use (regardless of indication); patients should be monitored for signs/symptoms of depression, suicidal tendencies, and other unusual behavior changes during therapy and instructed to inform their healthcare provider immediately if symptoms occur.

Anticonvulsants should not be discontinued abruptly because of the possibility of increasing seizure frequency; divalproex should be withdrawn gradually to minimize the potential of increased seizure frequency, unless safety concerns require a more rapid withdrawal. Concomitant use with carbapenem antibiotics may reduce valproic acid levels to subtherapeutic levels; monitor levels frequently and consider alternate therapy if levels drop significantly or lack of seizure control occurs. Concomitant use with clonazepam may induce absence status. Patients treated for bipolar disorder should be monitored closely for clinical worsening or suicidality; prescriptions should be written for the smallest quantity consistent with good patient care.

CNS depression may occur with divalproex use. Patients must be cautioned about performing tasks which require mental alertness (operating machinery or driving). Effects with other sedative drugs or ethanol may be potentiated. Use with caution in the elderly.

Adverse Reactions

>10%:

Central nervous system: Headache (≤31%), somnolence (≤30%), dizziness (12% to 25%), insomnia (>1% to 15%), nervousness (>1% to 11%), pain (1% to 11%)

Dermatologic: Alopecia (>1% to 24%)

Gastrointestinal: Nausea (15% to 48%), vomiting (7% to 27%), diarrhea (7% to 23%), abdominal pain (7% to 23%), dyspepsia (7% to 23%), anorexia (>1% to 12%)

Hematologic: Thrombocytopenia (1% to 24%; dose related)

Neuromuscular & skeletal: Tremor (≤57%), weakness (6% to 27%)

Ocular: Diplopia (>1% to 16%), amblyopia/blurred vision (≤12%)

Miscellaneous: Infection (≤20%), flu-like syndrome (12%)

1% to 10%:

Cardiovascular: Peripheral edema (>1% to 8%), chest pain (>1% to <5%), edema (>1% to <5%), facial edema (>1% to <5%), hypertension (>1% to <5%), hypotension (>1% to <5%), palpitation (>1% to <5%), postural hypotension (>1% to <5%), tachycardia (>1% to <5%), vasodilation(>1% to <5%), arrhythmia

Central nervous system: Ataxia (>1% to 8%), amnesia (>1% to 7%), emotional lability (>1% to 6%), fever (>1% to 6%), abnormal thinking (≤6%), depression (>1% to 5%), abnormal dreams (>1% to <5%), agitation (>1% to <5%), anxiety (>1% to <5%), catatonia (>1% to <5%), chills (>1% to <5%), confusion (>1% to <5%), coordination abnormal (>1% to <5%), hallucination (>1% to <5%), malaise (>1% to <5%), personality disorder (>1% to <5%), speech disorder (>1% to <5%), tardive dyskinesia (>1% to <5%), vertigo (>1% to <5%), euphoria (1%), hypoesthesia (1%)

Dermatologic: Rash (>1% to 6%), bruising (>1% to 5%), discoid lupus erythematosus (>1% to <5%), dry skin (>1% to <5%), furunculosis (>1% to <5%), petechia (>1% to <5%), pruritus (>1% to <5), seborrhea (>1% to <5%)

Endocrine & metabolic: Amenorrhea (>1% to <5%), dysmenorrhea (>1% to <5%), metrorrhagia (>1% to <5%), hypoproteinemia

Gastrointestinal: Weight gain (4% to 9%), weight loss (6%), appetite increased (≤6%), constipation (>1% to 5%), xerostomia (>1% to 5%), eructation (>1% to <5%), fecal incontinence (>1% to <5%), flatulence (>1% to <5%), gastroenteritis (>1% to <5%), glossitis (>1% to <5%), hematemesis (>1% to <5%), pancreatitis (>1% to <5%), periodontal abscess (>1% to <5%), stomatitis (>1% to <5%), taste perversion (>1% to <5%), dysphagia, gum hemorrhage, mouth ulceration

Genitourinary: Cystitis (>1% to 5%), dysuria (>1% to 5%), urinary frequency (>1% to <5%), urinary incontinence (>1% to <5%), vaginal hemorrhage (>1% to 5%), vaginitis (>1% to <5%)

Hepatic: ALT increased (>1% to <5%), AST increased (>1% to <5%)

Local: Injection site pain (3%), injection site reaction (2%), injection site inflammation (1%)

Neuromuscular & skeletal: Back pain (≤8%), abnormal gait (>1% to <5%), arthralgia (>1% to <5%), arthrosis (>1% to <5%), dysarthria (>1% to <5%), hypertonia (>1% to <5%), hypokinesia (>1% to <5%), leg cramps (>1% to <5%), myalgia (>1% to <5%), myasthenia (>1% to <5%), neck pain (>1% to <5%), neck rigidity (>1% to <5%), paresthesia (>1% to <5%), reflex increased (>1% to <5%), twitching (>1% to <5%)

Ocular: Nystagmus (1% to 8%), dry eyes (>1% to 5%), eye pain (>1% to 5%), abnormal vision (>1% to <5%), conjunctivitis (>1% to <5%)

Otic: Tinnitus (1% to 7%), ear pain (>1% to 5%), deafness (>1% to <5%), otitis media (>1% to <5%)

Respiratory: Pharyngitis (2% to 8%), bronchitis (5%), rhinitis (>1% to 5%), dyspnea (1% to 5%), cough (>1% to <5%), epistaxis (>1% to <5%), pneumonia (>1% to <5%), sinusitis (>1% to <5%)

Miscellaneous: Diaphoresis (1%), hiccups

<1% (Limited to important and/or life-threatening): Aggression, agranulocytosis, allergic reaction, anaphylaxis, anemia, aplastic anemia, asterixis, behavioral deterioration, bilirubin increased, bleeding time altered, bone marrow suppression, bone pain, bradycardia, breast enlargement, cutaneous vasculitis, carnitine decreased, cerebral atrophy (reversible), coma (rare), dementia, encephalopathy (rare), enuresis, eosinophilia, erythema multiforme, Fanconi-like syndrome (rare, in children), galactorrhea, hematoma formation, hemorrhage, hepatic failure, hepatotoxicity, hostility, hyperactivity, hyperammonemia, hyperammonemic encephalopathy (in patients with UCD), hyperglycinemia, hypersensitivity reactions (severe, with multiorgan dysfunction), hypofibrinogenemia, hyponatremia, hypothermia, inappropriate ADH secretion, intermittent porphyria, LDH increased, leukopenia, lupus, lymphocytosis, macrocytosis, menstrual irregularities, pancytopenia parkinsonism, parotid gland swelling, photosensitivity, platelet aggregation inhibited, polycystic ovary disease (rare), psychosis, seeing "spots before the eyes," Stevens-Johnson syndrome, suicidal behavior/ideation, thyroid function tests abnormal, toxic epidermal necrolysis (rare), urinary tract infection

Drug Interactions

Metabolism/Transport Effects Substrate of CYP2A6 (minor), CYP2B6 (minor), CYP2C19 (minor), CYP2C9 (minor), CYP2E1 (minor); **Note:** Assignment of Major/Minor substrate status based on clinically relevant drug interaction potential; **Inhibits** CYP2C9 (weak); **Induces** CYP2A6 (weak/moderate)

Avoid Concomitant Use There are no known interactions where it is recommended to avoid concomitant use.

Increased Effect/Toxicity

Divalproex may increase the levels/effects of: Barbiturates; Ethosuximide; LamoTRIgine; LORazepam; Paliperidone; Primidone; RisperiDONE; Rufinamide; Temozolomide; Topiramate; Tricyclic Antidepressants; Vorinostat; Zidovudine

The levels/effects of Divalproex may be increased by: ChlorproMAZINE; Felbamate; GuanFACINE; Salicylates

Decreased Effect

Divalproex may decrease the levels/effects of: CarBAMazepine; Fosphenytoin; OXcarbazepine; Phenytoin

The levels/effects of Divalproex may be decreased by: Barbiturates; CarBAMazepine; Carbapenems; Cyproterone; Ethosuximide; Fosphenytoin; Methylfolate; Phenytoin; Primidone; Protease Inhibitors; Rifampin

Ethanol/Nutrition/Herb Interactions

Ethanol: Avoid ethanol (may increase CNS depression).

Food: Food may delay but does not affect the extent of absorption. Valproic acid serum concentrations may be decreased if taken with food. Milk has no effect on absorption.

Herb/Nutraceutical: Avoid evening primrose (seizure threshold decreased).

Stability

Depakote® tablet: Store below 30°C (86°F).

Depakote® Sprinkles: Store below 25°C (77°F).

Depakote® ER: Store at controlled room temperature of 25°C (77°F).

Mechanism of Action Causes increased availability of gamma-aminobutyric acid (GABA), an inhibitory neurotransmitter, to brain neurons or may enhance the action of GABA or mimic its action at postsynaptic receptor sites

Pharmacodynamics/Kinetics

Distribution: Total valproate: 11 L/1.73 m^2; Free valproate: 92 L/1.73 m^2

Protein binding (dose dependent): 80% to 90%; decreased in the elderly and with hepatic or renal dysfunction

Metabolism: Extensively hepatic via glucuronide conjugation and mitochondrial beta-oxidation. The relationship between dose and total valproate concentration is nonlinear; concentration does not increase proportionally with the dose, but increases to a lesser extent due to saturable plasma protein binding. The kinetics of unbound drug are linear.

Bioavailability: Depakote® ER: ~90% relative to I.V. dose and ~89% relative to delayed release formulation

Half-life elimination (increased in neonates and with liver disease): Children >2 months: 7-13 hours; Adults: 9-16 hours

Time to peak, serum: Depakote® tablet: ~4 hours; Depakote® ER: 4-17 hours

Excretion: Urine (30% to 50% as glucuronide conjugate, 3% as unchanged drug)

Dosage Oral: Equivalent oral dosages of divalproex and valproic acid deliver the same quantities of valproate ion.

Seizure disorders: **Note:** Administer doses >250 mg/day in divided doses.

Simple and complex absence seizures: Children and Adults: Initial: 15 mg/kg/day; increase by 5-10 mg/kg/day at weekly intervals until therapeutic levels are achieved; maximum: 60 mg/kg/day. Larger maintenance doses may be required in younger children.

Complex partial seizures: Children ≥10 years and Adults: Initial: 10-15 mg/kg/day; increase by 5-10 mg/kg/day at weekly intervals until therapeutic levels are achieved; maximum: 60 mg/kg/day. Larger maintenance doses may be required in younger children.

Note: Regular release and delayed release formulations are usually given in 2-4 divided doses/day; extended release formulation (Depakote® ER) is usually given once daily. Conversion to Depakote® ER from a stable dose of Depakote® may require an increase in the total daily dose between 8% and 20% to maintain similar serum concentrations. Depakote® ER is not recommended for use in children <10 years of age.

Mania: Adults:

Depakote® tablet: Initial: 750 mg/day in divided doses; dose should be adjusted as rapidly as possible to desired clinical effect; maximum recommended dosage: 60 mg/kg/day

Depakote® ER: Initial: 25 mg/kg/day given once daily; dose should be adjusted as rapidly as possible to desired clinical effect; maximum recommended dose: 60 mg/kg/day.

Migraine prophylaxis: Children ≥16 years and Adults:

Depakote® tablet: 250 mg twice daily; adjust dose based on patient response, up to 1000 mg/day

Depakote® ER: 500 mg once daily for 7 days, then increase to 1000 mg once daily; adjust dose based on patient response; usual dosage range: 500-1000 mg/day

Diabetic neuropathy (unlabeled use): Adults: 500-1200 mg/day (Bril, 2011)

Elderly: Elimination is decreased in the elderly. Studies of elderly patients with dementia show a high incidence of somnolence. In some patients, this was associated with weight loss. Starting doses should be lower and increases should be slow, with careful monitoring of nutritional intake and dehydration. Safety and efficacy for use in patients >65 years have not been studied for migraine prophylaxis.

Dosing adjustment in renal impairment: A 27% reduction in clearance of unbound valproate is seen in patients with Cl_{cr} <10 mL/minute. Hemodialysis reduces valproate concentrations by 20%, therefore no dose adjustment is needed in patients with renal failure. Protein binding is reduced, monitoring only total valproate concentrations may be misleading.

Dosing adjustment/comments in hepatic impairment: Reduce dose. Clearance is decreased with liver impairment. Hepatic disease is also associated with decreased albumin concentrations and 2- to 2.6-fold increase in the unbound fraction. Free concentrations of valproate may be elevated while total concentrations appear normal. Use is contraindicated in severe impairment.

Dietary Considerations Divalproex may cause GI upset; take with large amount of water or food to decrease GI upset. May need to split doses to avoid GI upset.

Depakote® Sprinkle capsule contents may be mixed with semisolid food (eg, applesauce or pudding) in patients having difficulty swallowing; particles should be swallowed and not chewed.

Administration

Depakote® ER: Swallow whole; do not crush or chew. Patients who need dose adjustments smaller than 500 mg/day for migraine prophylaxis should be changed to Depakote® delayed release tablets.

Depakote® Sprinkle capsules may be swallowed whole or open capsule and sprinkle on small amount (1 teaspoonful) of soft food and use immediately (do not store or chew).

Monitoring Parameters Liver enzymes (at baseline and during therapy), CBC with platelets (baseline and periodic intervals), PT/PTT (especially prior to surgery), serum ammonia (with symptoms of lethargy, mental status change), serum valproate levels (trough for therapeutic levels); suicidality (eg, suicidal thoughts, depression, behavioral changes)

Reference Range Note: In general, trough concentrations should be used to assess adequacy of therapy; peak concentrations may also be drawn if clinically necessary (eg, concentration-related toxicity). Within 2-4 days of initiation or dose adjustment, trough concentrations should be drawn just before the next dose (extended-release preparations) or before the morning dose (for immediate-release preparations). Patients with epilepsy should **not** delay taking their dose for >2-3 hours. Additional patient-specific factors must be taken into consideration when interpreting drug levels, including indication, age, clinical response, pregnancy status, adherence, comorbidities, adverse effects, and concomitant medications (Patsalos, 2008; Reed, 2006).

Therapeutic:

Epilepsy: 50-100 mcg/mL (SI: 350-700 micromole/L); although seizure control may improve at levels >100 mcg/mL (SI: 700 micromole/L), toxicity may occur at levels of 100-150 mcg/mL (SI: 700-1040 micromole/L)

Mania: 50-125 mcg/mL (SI: 350-875 micromole/L)

Toxic: Some laboratories may report >200 mcg/mL (SI: >1390 micromole/L) as a toxic threshold, although clinical toxicity can occur at lower concentrations. Probability of thrombocytopenia increases with total valproate levels ≥110 mcg/mL in females or ≥135 mcg/mL in males.

Epilepsy: Although seizure control may improve at levels >100 mcg/mL (SI: 700 micromole/L), toxicity may occur at levels of 100-150 mcg/mL (SI: 700-1050 micromole/L)

Mania: Clinical response seen with trough levels between 50-125 mcg/mL (SI: 350-875 micromole/L); risk of toxicity increases at levels >125 mcg/mL (SI: 875 micromole/L)

Test Interactions False-positive result for urine ketones

Additional Information Divalproex sodium is a compound of sodium valproate and valproic acid; divalproex dissociates to valproate in the GI tract.

Extended release tablets have 10% to 20% less fluctuation in serum concentration than delayed release tablets. Extended release tablets are not bioequivalent to delayed release tablets.

Dosage Forms Excipient information presented when available (limited, particularly for generics); consult specific product labeling.

Capsule, sprinkle, oral: 125 mg [strength expressed as valproic acid]

Depakote® Sprinkle: 125 mg [strength expressed as valproic acid]

Tablet, delayed release, oral: 125 mg [strength expressed as valproic acid], 250 mg [strength expressed as valproic acid], 500 mg [strength expressed as valproic acid]

Depakote®: 125 mg, 250 mg, 500 mg [strength expressed as valproic acid]

Tablet, extended release, oral: 250 mg [strength expressed as valproic acid], 500 mg [strength expressed as valproic acid]

Depakote® ER: 250 mg, 500 mg [strength expressed as valproic acid]

◆ **Divalproex Sodium** *see* Divalproex *on page* 530
◆ **Divigel®** *see* Estradiol (Systemic) *on page* 627
◆ **Dixarit® (Can)** *see* CloNIDine *on page* 392
◆ **5071-1DL(6)** *see* Megestrol *on page* 1062
◆ ***dl*-Alpha Tocopherol** *see* Vitamin E *on page* 1796
◆ **DLV** *see* Delavirdine *on page* 467
◆ ***D*-Mannitol** *see* Mannitol *on page* 1049
◆ **4-DMDR** *see* IDArubicin *on page* 865
◆ **DMSA** *see* Succimer *on page* 1595
◆ **Doan's® Extra Strength [OTC]** *see* Magnesium Salicylate *on page* 1047

DOBUTamine (doe BYOO ta meen)

Brand Names: Canada Dobutamine Injection, USP; Dobutrex®

Index Terms Dobutamine Hydrochloride

Pharmacologic Category Adrenergic Agonist Agent

Additional Appendix Information

Vasoactive Agents, Intravenous *on page* 1898

Use Short-term management of patients with cardiac decompensation

Unlabeled Use Positive inotropic agent for use in myocardial dysfunction related to sepsis; stress echocardiography

Pregnancy Risk Factor B

Pregnancy Considerations Adverse events have not been observed in animal reproduction studies.

Lactation Excretion in breast milk unknown/use caution

Contraindications Hypersensitivity to dobutamine or sulfites (some contain sodium metabisulfate), or any component of the formulation; idiopathic hypertrophic subaortic stenosis (IHSS)

Warnings/Precautions May increase heart rate. Patients with atrial fibrillation may experience an increase in ventricular response. An increase in blood pressure is more common, but occasionally a patient may become hypotensive. May exacerbate ventricular ectopy. If needed, correct hypovolemia first to optimize hemodynamics. Ineffective therapeutically in the presence of mechanical obstruction such as severe aortic stenosis. Use caution post-MI (can increase myocardial oxygen demand). Use cautiously in the elderly starting at lower end of the dosage range. Use with extreme caution in patients taking MAO inhibitors. Dobutamine in combination with stress echo may be used diagnostically. Product may contain sodium sulfite.

Adverse Reactions Incidence of adverse events is not always reported.

Cardiovascular: Increased heart rate, increased blood pressure, increased ventricular ectopic activity, hypotension, premature ventricular beats (5%, dose related), anginal pain (1% to 3%), nonspecific chest pain (1% to 3%), palpitation (1% to 3%)

Central nervous system: Fever (1% to 3%), headache (1% to 3%), paresthesia

Endocrine & metabolic: Slight decrease in serum potassium

Gastrointestinal: Nausea (1% to 3%)

Hematologic: Thrombocytopenia (isolated cases)

Local: Phlebitis, local inflammatory changes and pain from infiltration, cutaneous necrosis (isolated cases)

Neuromuscular & skeletal: Mild leg cramps

Respiratory: Dyspnea (1% to 3%)

Drug Interactions

Metabolism/Transport Effects Substrate of COMT

Avoid Concomitant Use

Avoid concomitant use of DOBUTamine with any of the following: Iobenguane I 123

Increased Effect/Toxicity

DOBUTamine may increase the levels/effects of: Sympathomimetics

The levels/effects of DOBUTamine may be increased by: Atomoxetine; Cannabinoids; COMT Inhibitors; Linezolid

Decreased Effect

DOBUTamine may decrease the levels/effects of: Iobenguane I 123

The levels/effects of DOBUTamine may be decreased by: Calcium Salts

Stability Remix solution every 24 hours. Store reconstituted solution under refrigeration for 48 hours or 6 hours at room temperature. Pink discoloration of solution indicates slight oxidation but **no** significant loss of potency.

Stability of parenteral admixture at room temperature (25°C): 48 hours; at refrigeration (4°C): 7 days.

Standard adult diluent: 250 mg/500 mL D_5W; 500 mg/500 mL D_5W.

Mechanism of Action Stimulates $beta_1$-adrenergic receptors, causing increased contractility and heart rate, with little effect on $beta_2$- or alpha-receptors

Pharmacodynamics/Kinetics

Onset of action: I.V.: 1-10 minutes

Peak effect: 10-20 minutes

Metabolism: In tissues and hepatically to inactive metabolites

Half-life elimination: 2 minutes

Excretion: Urine (as metabolites)

Dosage Administration requires the use of an infusion pump; I.V. infusion: Children and Adults: 2.5-20 mcg/kg/minute; maximum: 40 mcg/kg/minute, titrate to desired response. See table.

Infusion Rates of Various Dilutions of Dobutamine

Desired Delivery Rate (mcg/kg/min)	Infusion Rate (mL/kg/min)	
	500 mcg/mL	1000 mcg/mL
2.5	0.005	0.0025
5	0.01	0.005
7.5	0.015	0.0075
10	0.02	0.01
12.5	0.025	0.0125
15	0.03	0.015

Administration Use infusion device to control rate of flow; administer into large vein. Do not administer through same I.V. line as heparin, hydrocortisone sodium succinate, cefazolin, or penicillin.

Monitoring Parameters Blood pressure, ECG, heart rate, CVP, RAP, MAP; serum glucose, renal function; urine output; if pulmonary artery catheter is in place, monitor CI, PCWP, and SVR

Additional Information Dobutamine lowers central venous pressure and wedge pressure but has little effect on pulmonary vascular resistance.

Dobutamine therapy should be avoided in patients with stable heart failure due to an increase in mortality. In patients with intractable heart failure, dobutamine may be used as a short-term infusion to provide symptomatic benefit. It is not known whether short-term dobutamine therapy in end-stage heart failure has any outcome benefit.

Dobutamine infusion during echocardiography is used as a cardiovascular stress. Wall motion abnormalities developing with increasing doses of dobutamine may help to identify ischemic and/or hibernating myocardium.

Dosage Forms Excipient information presented when available (limited, particularly for generics); consult specific product labeling.

Infusion, premixed in D_5W, as hydrochloride: 1 mg/mL (250 mL); 2 mg/mL (250 mL); 4 mg/mL (250 mL)

Injection, solution, as hydrochloride: 12.5 mg/mL (20 mL, 40 mL)

◆ **Dobutamine Hydrochloride** *see* DOBUTamine *on page 533*

◆ **Dobutamine Injection, USP (Can)** *see* DOBUTamine *on page 533*

◆ **Dobutrex® (Can)** *see* DOBUTamine *on page 533*

◆ **Docefrez™** *see* DOCEtaxel *on page 534*

◆ **Docefrez™** *see* DOCEtaxel *on page 534*

DOCEtaxel (doe se TAKS el)

Brand Names: U.S. Docefrez™; Taxotere®

Brand Names: Canada Docetaxel for Injection; Taxotere®

Index Terms Docefrez™; RP-6976

Pharmacologic Category Antineoplastic Agent, Antimicrotubular; Antineoplastic Agent, Natural Source (Plant) Derivative; Antineoplastic Agent, Taxane Derivative

Use Treatment of breast cancer (locally advanced/metastatic or adjuvant treatment of operable node-positive); locally-advanced or metastatic nonsmall cell lung cancer (NSCLC); hormone refractory, metastatic prostate cancer; advanced gastric adenocarcinoma; locally-advanced squamous cell head and neck cancer

Unlabeled Use Treatment of bladder cancer (metastatic), ovarian cancer, cervical cancer (relapsed), esophageal cancer, small cell lung cancer (relapsed), soft tissue sarcoma, Ewing's sarcoma, osteosarcoma, and unknown-primary adenocarcinoma

Pregnancy Risk Factor D

Pregnancy Considerations Animal studies have demonstrated embryotoxicity, fetal toxicity, and maternal toxicity. There are no adequate and well-controlled studies in pregnant women; however, fetal harm may occur. Women of childbearing potential should avoid becoming pregnant. A pregnancy registry is available for all cancers diagnosed during pregnancy at Cooper Health (856-757-7876).

Lactation Excretion in breast milk unknown/not recommended

Contraindications Severe hypersensitivity to docetaxel or any component of the formulation; severe hypersensitivity to other medications containing polysorbate 80; neutrophil count <1500/mm^3

Warnings/Precautions Hazardous agent - use appropriate precautions for handling and disposal. **[U.S. Boxed Warning]: Avoid use in patients with bilirubin exceeding upper limit of normal (ULN) or AST and/or ALT >1.5 times ULN in conjunction with alkaline phosphatase >2.5 times ULN; patients with abnormal liver function are at increased risk of treatment-related adverse events,** including grade 4 neutropenia, neutropenic fever, infections, and sever thrombocytopenia, stomatitis, skin toxicity or toxic death; obtain liver function tests prior to each treatment cycle. **[U.S. Boxed Warnings]: Severe hypersensitivity reactions, characterized by generalized rash/erythema, hypotension, bronchospasms, or anaphylaxis may occur; minor reactions including flushing or localized skin reactions may also occur; do not administer to patients with a history of severe hypersensitivity to docetaxel or polysorbate 80. Severe fluid retention, characterized by pleural effusion (requiring immediate drainage, ascites, peripheral edema (poorly tolerated), dyspnea at rest, cardiac tamponade, and weight gain (2-15 kg) has been reported.** The incidence and severity of fluid retention increase sharply at cumulative doses ≥400 mg/m^2. Observe for hypersensitivity, especially with the first two infusions. Discontinue for severe reactions; do not rechallenge if severe. Patients should be premedicated with a corticosteroid (starting one day prior to administration) to prevent or reduce the severity of hypersensitivity reactions and fluid retention; severity is reduced with dexamethasone premedication starting one day prior to docetaxel administration.

[U.S. Boxed Warning]: Patients with abnormal liver function, those receiving higher doses, and patients with nonsmall cell lung cancer and a history of prior treatment with platinum derivatives who receive single-agent docetaxel at a dose of 100 mg/m^2 are at higher risk for treatment-related mortality.

Neutropenia is the dose-limiting toxicity. Patients with increased liver function tests experienced more episodes of neutropenia with a greater number of severe infections. **[U.S. Boxed Warning]: Patients with an absolute neutrophil count <1500/mm^3 should not receive docetaxel.** Platelets should recover to >100,000/mm^3 prior to treatment. When administered as sequential infusions, taxane derivatives (docetaxel, paclitaxel) should be administered before platinum derivatives (carboplatin, cisplatin) to limit myelosuppression and to enhance efficacy.

Cutaneous reactions including erythema (with edema) and desquamation have been reported; may require dose reduction. Dosage adjustment is recommended with severe neurosensory symptoms (paresthesia, dysesthesia, pain); persistent symptoms may require discontinuation; reversal of symptoms may be delayed after discontinuation. Treatment-related acute myeloid leukemia or myelodysplasia occurred in patients receiving docetaxel in combination with anthracyclines and/or cyclophosphamide. Fatigue and weakness (may be severe) have been reported; symptoms may last a few days up to several weeks; in patients with progressive disease, weakness may be associated with a decrease in performance status. Avoid concomitant use with strong CYP3A4 inhibitors; although data is limited, a 50% dose reduction is suggested if concomitant therapy with a strong CYP3A4 inhibitor is required.

Adverse Reactions Percentages reported for docetaxel monotherapy; frequency may vary depending on diagnosis, dose, liver function, prior treatment, and premedication. The incidence of adverse events was usually higher in patients with elevated liver function tests.

>10%:
- Cardiovascular: Fluid retention (13% to 60%; dose dependent)
- Central nervous system: Neurosensory events (20% to 58%; including neuropathy), fever (31% to 35%), neuromotor events (16%)
- Dermatologic: Alopecia (56% to 76%), cutaneous events (20% to 48%), nail disorder (11% to 41%)
- Gastrointestinal: Stomatitis (19% to 53%; severe 1% to 8%), diarrhea (23% to 43%; severe: 5% to 6%), nausea (34% to 42%), vomiting (22% to 23%)
- Hematologic: Neutropenia (84% to 99%; grade 4: 75% to 86%; nadir (median): 7 days, duration (severe neutropenia): 7 days; dose dependent), leukopenia (84% to 99%; grade 4: 32% to 44%), anemia (65% to 94%; dose dependent; grades 3/4: 8% to 9%), thrombocytopenia (8% to 14%; grade 4: 1%; dose dependent), febrile neutropenia (6% to 12%; dose dependent)
- Hepatic: Transaminases increased (4% to 19%)
- Neuromuscular & skeletal: Weakness (53% to 66%; severe 13% to 18%), myalgia (3% to 23%)
- Respiratory: Pulmonary events (41%)
- Miscellaneous: Infection (1% to 34%; dose dependent), hypersensitivity (1% to 21%; with premedication 15%)

1% to 10%:
- Cardiovascular: Left ventricular ejection fraction decreased (prostate cancer: 10%; metastatic breast cancer: 8%), hypotension (3%)
- Gastrointestinal: Taste perversion (6%)
- Hepatic: Bilirubin increased (9%), alkaline phosphatase increased (4% to 7%)
- Local: Infusion-site reactions (4%, including hyperpigmentation, inflammation, redness, dryness, phlebitis, extravasation, swelling of the vein)
- Neuromuscular and skeletal: Arthralgia (3% to 9%)
- Ocular: Epiphora associated with canalicular stenosis (≤77% with weekly administration; ≤1% with every 3-week administration)

<1% (Limited to important or life-threatening): Acute myeloid leukemia (AML), acute respiratory distress syndrome (ARDS), anaphylactic shock, arrhythmia, ascites, atrial fibrillation, atrial flutter, AV block, bleeding episodes, bradycardia, bronchospasm, cardiac tamponade, chest pain, chest tightness, colitis, conjunctivitis, constipation, cutaneous lupus erythematosus, deep vein thrombosis, dehydration, disseminated intravascular coagulation (DIC), drug fever, duodenal ulcer, dyspnea, dysrhythmia, ECG abnormalities, erythema multiforme, esophagitis, gastrointestinal hemorrhage, gastrointestinal obstruction, gastrointestinal perforation, hand and foot syndrome, hearing loss, heart failure, hepatitis, hypertension, ileus, interstitial pneumonia, ischemic colitis, lacrimal duct obstruction, loss of consciousness (transient), MI, multiorgan failure, myelodysplastic syndrome, myocardial ischemia, neutropenic enterocolitis, neutropenic typhlitis, ototoxicity, pericardial effusion, pleural effusion, pruritus, pulmonary edema, pulmonary embolism, pulmonary fibrosis, radiation pneumonitis, radiation recall, renal failure, renal insufficiency, scleroderma-like changes, seizure, sepsis, sinus tachycardia, Stevens-Johnson syndrome, syncope, toxic epidermal necrolysis, tachycardia, thrombophlebitis, unstable angina, visual disturbances (transient)

Drug Interactions

Metabolism/Transport Effects Substrate of CYP3A4 (major), P-glycoprotein; **Note:** Assignment of Major/Minor substrate status based on clinically relevant drug interaction potential; **Inhibits** CYP3A4 (weak)

Avoid Concomitant Use

Avoid concomitant use of DOCEtaxel with any of the following: BCG; CloZAPine; Conivaptan; Natalizumab; Pimecrolimus; Pimozide; Tacrolimus (Topical); Vaccines (Live)

Increased Effect/Toxicity

DOCEtaxel may increase the levels/effects of: Antineoplastic Agents (Anthracycline, Systemic); CloZAPine; Leflunomide; Natalizumab; Pimozide; Vaccines (Live)

The levels/effects of DOCEtaxel may be increased by: Antifungal Agents (Azole Derivatives, Systemic); Conivaptan; CYP3A4 Inhibitors (Moderate); CYP3A4 Inhibitors (Strong); Dasatinib; Denosumab; Dronedarone; P-glycoprotein/ABCB1 Inhibitors; Pimecrolimus; Platinum Derivatives; Roflumilast; SORAfenib; Tacrolimus (Topical); Trastuzumab

Decreased Effect

DOCEtaxel may decrease the levels/effects of: BCG; Coccidioidin Skin Test; Sipuleucel-T; Vaccines (Inactivated); Vaccines (Live)

The levels/effects of DOCEtaxel may be decreased by: CYP3A4 Inducers (Strong); Deferasirox; Echinacea; P-glycoprotein/ABCB1 Inducers; Tocilizumab

Ethanol/Nutrition/Herb Interactions

Ethanol: Avoid ethanol (due to GI irritation).

Herb/Nutraceutical: Avoid St John's wort (may decrease docetaxel levels).

Stability Note: Multiple concentrations: Docetaxel is available as a one-vial formulation at concentrations of 10 mg/mL (generic formulation) and 20 mg/mL (concentrate; Taxotere®), and as a lyophilized powder (Docefrez™) which is reconstituted (with provided diluent) to 20 mg/0.8 mL (20 mg vial) or 24 mg/mL (80 mg vial). Admixture errors have occurred due to the availability of various concentrations. Docetaxel was previously available as a two-vial formulation (a concentrated docetaxel vial and a diluent vial), resulting in a reconstituted concentration of 10 mg/mL; the two-vial formulation has been discontinued by the manufacturer.

Docetaxel 10 mg/mL: Store intact vials at 25°C (77°F); excursions permitted to 15°C to 30°C (59°F to 86°F). Protect from bright light. Freezing does not adversely affect the product. Multi-use vials (80 mg/8 mL and 160 mg/16 mL) are stable for up to 28 days after first entry when stored between 2°C to 8°C (36°F to 46°F) and protected from light.

Docetaxel concentrate (Taxotere®) 20 mg/mL: Store intact vials between 2°C to 25°C (36°F to 77°F). Protect from bright light. Freezing does not adversely affect the product.

Docetaxel lyophilized powder (Docefrez™): Store intact vials between 2°C to 8°C (36°F to 46°F). Protect from light. Allow vials (and provided diluent) to stand at room temperature for 5 minutes prior to reconstitution. After reconstitution, may be stored refrigerated or at room temperature for up to 8 hours.

Use appropriate precautions for handling and disposal.

One-vial formulations: Further dilute for infusion in 250-500 mL of NS or D_5W in a non-DEHP container (eg, glass, polypropylene, polyolefin) to a final concentration of 0.3-0.74 mg/mL. Gently rotate to mix thoroughly. Solutions diluted for infusion should be used within 4 hours of preparation, including infusion time.

Lyophilized powder: Dilute with the provided diluent (contains ethanol in polysorbate 80); add 1 mL to each 20 mg vial (resulting concentration is 20 mg/0.8 mL) and 4 mL to each 80 mg vial (resulting concentration is 24 mg/mL). Shake well to dissolve completely. If air bubbles are present, allow to stand for a few minutes while air bubbles dissipate. Further dilute in 250 mL of NS or D_5W in a non-DEHP container (eg, glass, polypropylene, polyolefin) to a final concentration of 0.3-0.74 mg/mL (for doses >200 mg, use a larger volume of NS or D_5W, not to exceed a final concentration of 0.74 mg/mL). Mix thoroughly by manual agitation. Solutions diluted for infusion should be used within 4 hours of preparation, including infusion time.

Two-vial formulation *(discontinued product):* Vials should be diluted with 13% (w/w) ethanol/water (provided with the drug) to a final concentration of 10 mg/mL. Do not shake. Further dilute for infusion in 250-500 mL of NS or D_5W in a non-DEHP container (eg, glass, polypropylene, polyolefin) to a final concentration of 0.3-0.74 mg/mL. Gently rotate to mix thoroughly. Reconstituted solutions of the two-vial formulation are stable in the vial for 8 hours at room temperature or under refrigeration. Solutions diluted for infusion in polyolefin containers should be used within 4 hours of preparation, including infusion time. Do not use the two-vial formulation with the one-vial formulation for the same admixture product.

Mechanism of Action Docetaxel promotes the assembly of microtubules from tubulin dimers, and inhibits the depolymerization of tubulin which stabilizes microtubules in the cell. This results in inhibition of DNA, RNA, and protein synthesis. Most activity occurs during the M phase of the cell cycle.

Pharmacodynamics/Kinetics Exhibits linear pharmacokinetics at the recommended dosage range

Distribution: Extensive extravascular distribution and/or tissue binding; V_d: 80-90 L/m^2, V_{dss}: 113 L (mean steady state)

Protein binding: ~94% to 97%, primarily to alpha$_1$-acid glycoprotein, albumin, and lipoproteins

Metabolism: Hepatic; oxidation via CYP3A4 to metabolites

Half-life elimination: Terminal: ~11 hours

Excretion: Feces (~75%, <8% as unchanged drug); urine (<5%)

Dosage Adults: I.V. infusion: **Note:** Premedicate with corticosteroids, beginning the day before docetaxel administration, (administer corticosteroids for 3 days) to reduce the severity of hypersensitivity reactions and fluid retention. Details concerning dosing in combination regimens should also be consulted.

Breast cancer:

Locally-advanced or metastatic: 60-100 mg/m^2 every 3 weeks (as a single agent)

Operable, node-positive (adjuvant treatment): 75 mg/m^2 every 3 weeks for 6 courses (in combination with doxorubicin and cyclophosphamide)

Weekly administration (unlabeled dosing): 40 mg/m^2/dose once a week (as a single agent) for 6 weeks followed by a 2-week rest, repeat until disease progression or unacceptable toxicity (Burstein, 2000) **or** 35 mg/m^2/dose once a week (in combination with trastuzumab) for 3 weeks followed by a 1-week rest; repeat until disease progression or unacceptable toxicity (Esteva, 2002)

Nonsmall cell lung cancer: 75 mg/m^2 every 3 weeks (as monotherapy or in combination with cisplatin)

Prostate cancer: 75 mg/m^2 every 3 weeks (in combination with prednisone)

Gastric adenocarcinoma: 75 mg/m^2 every 3 weeks (in combination with cisplatin and fluorouracil)

Head and neck cancer: 75 mg/m^2 every 3 weeks (in combination with cisplatin and fluorouracil) for 3 or 4 cycles, followed by radiation therapy

Bladder cancer, metastatic (unlabeled use): 100 mg/m^2 every 3 weeks (as a single agent) (McCaffrey, 1997)

Esophageal cancer (unlabeled use): 75 mg/m^2 every 3 weeks (in combination with cisplatin and fluorouracil) (Ajani, 2007; Van Cutsem, 2006)

Ovarian cancer (unlabeled use): 60 mg/m^2 every 3 weeks (in combination with carboplatin) (Markman, 2001) **or** 75 mg/m^2 every 3 weeks (in combination with carboplatin) (Vasey, 2004) **or** 35 mg/m^2 (maximum dose: 70 mg) weekly for 3 weeks followed by a 1-week rest (in combination with carboplatin) (Kushner, 2007)

Soft tissue sarcoma (unlabeled use): 100 mg/m^2 on day 8 of a 3-week treatment cycle (in combination with gemcitabine and filgrastim or pegfilgrastim) (Leu, 2004; Maki, 2007)

Unknown-primary, adenocarcinoma (unlabeled use): 65 mg/m^2 every 3 weeks (in combination with carboplatin) (Greco, 2000) **or** 75 mg/m^2 on day 8 of a 3-week treatment cycle (in combination with gemcitabine) (Pouessel, 2004)

Dosing adjustment for concomitant CYP3A4 inhibitors: Avoid the concomitant use of strong CYP3A4 inhibitors with docetaxel. If concomitant use of a strong CYP3A4 inhibitor cannot be avoided, consider reducing the docetaxel dose by 50% (based on limited pharmacokinetic data).

Dosing adjustment for toxicity:

Note: Toxicity includes febrile neutropenia, neutrophils ≤500/mm^3 for >1 week, severe or cumulative cutaneous reactions; in nonsmall cell lung cancer, this may also include platelets <25,000/mm^3 and other grade 3/4 nonhematologic toxicities.

Breast cancer (single agent): Patients dosed initially at 100 mg/m^2; reduce dose to 75 mg/m^2; **Note:** If the patient continues to experience these adverse reactions, the dosage should be reduced to 55 mg/m^2 or therapy should be discontinued; discontinue for peripheral neuropathy ≥ grade 3. Patients initiated at 60 mg/m^2 who do not develop toxicity may tolerate higher doses.

Breast cancer, adjuvant treatment (combination chemotherapy): TAC regimen should be administered when neutrophils are ≥1500/mm^3. Patients experiencing febrile neutropenia should receive G-CSF in all subsequent cycles. Patients with persistent febrile neutropenia (while on G-CSF), patients experiencing severe/cumulative cutaneous reactions, moderate neurosensory effects (signs/symptoms) or grade 3 or 4 stomatitis should receive a reduced dose (60 mg/m^2) of docetaxel. Discontinue therapy with persistent toxicities after dosage reduction.

Nonsmall cell lung cancer:

Monotherapy: Patients dosed initially at 75 mg/m^2 should have dose held until toxicity is resolved, then resume at 55 mg/m^2; discontinue for peripheral neuropathy ≥ grade 3.

Combination therapy (with cisplatin): Patients dosed initially at 75 mg/m^2 should have the docetaxel dosage reduced to 65 mg/m^2 in subsequent cycles; if further adjustment is required, dosage may be reduced to 50 mg/m^2

Prostate cancer: Reduce dose to 60 mg/m^2; discontinue therapy if toxicities persist at lower dose.

Gastric cancer, head and neck cancer: **Note:** Cisplatin may require dose reductions/therapy delays for peripheral neuropathy, ototoxicity, and/or nephrotoxicity. Patients experiencing febrile neutropenia, documented infection with neutropenia or neutropenia >7 days should receive G-CSF in all subsequent cycles. For neutropenic complications despite G-CSF use, further reduce dose to 60 mg/m^2. Neutropenic complications in subsequent cycles should be further dose reduced to 45 mg/m^2. Patients who experience grade 4 thrombocytopenia should receive a dose reduction from 75 mg/m^2 to 60 mg/m^2. Discontinue therapy for persistent toxicities.

Gastrointestinal toxicity for docetaxel in combination with cisplatin and fluorouracil for treatment of gastric cancer or head and neck cancer:

Diarrhea, grade 3:

First episode: Reduce fluorouracil dose by 20%

Second episode: Reduce docetaxel dose by 20%

Diarrhea, grade 4:

First episode: Reduce fluorouracil and docetaxel doses by 20%

Second episode: Discontinue treatment

Stomatitis, grade 3:

First episode: Reduce fluorouracil dose by 20%

Second episode: Discontinue fluorouracil for all subsequent cycles

Third episode: Reduce docetaxel dose by 20%

Stomatitis, grade 4:

First episode: Discontinue fluorouracil for all subsequent cycles

Second episode: Reduce docetaxel dose by 20%

Dosing adjustment in renal impairment: Renal excretion is minimal (<5%), therefore, the need for dosage adjustments for renal dysfunction is unlikely (Li, 2007). Not removed by hemodialysis, may be administered before or after hemodialysis (Janus, 2010).

Dosing adjustment in hepatic impairment:

The FDA-approved labeling recommends the following adjustments:

Total bilirubin greater than the ULN, or AST and/or ALT >1.5 times ULN concomitant with alkaline phosphatase >2.5 times ULN: Use is not recommended.

Hepatic impairment dosing adjustment specific for gastric adenocarcinoma:

AST/ALT >2.5 to ≤5 times ULN and alkaline phosphatase ≤2.5 times ULN: Administer 80% of dose

AST/ALT >1.5 to ≤5 times ULN and alkaline phosphatase >2.5 to ≤5 times ULN: Administer 80% of dose

AST/ALT >5 times ULN and /or alkaline phosphatase >5 times ULN: Discontinue docetaxel

The following guidelines have been used by some clinicians (Floyd, 2006):

Transaminases 1.6-6 times ULN: Administer 75% of dose

Transaminases >6 times ULN: Use clinical judgment

Administration Administer I.V. infusion over 1-hour through nonsorbing polyethylene lined (non-DEHP) tubing; in-line filter is not necessary (the use of a filter during administration is not recommended by the manufacturer). Infusion should be completed within 4 hours of final preparation. **Note:** Premedication with corticosteroids for 3 days, beginning the day before docetaxel administration, is recommended to prevent hypersensitivity reactions and fluid retention (see Additional Information).

Monitoring Parameters CBC with differential, liver function tests, bilirubin, alkaline phosphatase, renal function; monitor for hypersensitivity reactions, neurosensory symptoms, gastrointestinal toxicity (eg, diarrhea, stomatitis), cutaneous reactions, fluid retention, epiphora, and canalicular stenosis

Additional Information Premedication with oral corticosteroids is recommended to decrease the incidence and severity of fluid retention and severity of hypersensitivity reactions. The manufacturer recommends dexamethasone 16 mg/day (8 mg twice daily) orally for 3 days, starting the day before docetaxel administration; for prostate cancer, when prednisone is part of the antineoplastic regimen, dexamethasone 8 mg orally is administered at 12 hours, 3 hours, and 1 hour prior to docetaxel.

Dosage Forms Excipient information presented when available (limited, particularly for generics); consult specific product labeling. [DSC] = Discontinued product

Injection, powder for reconstitution:

Docefrez™: 20 mg, 80 mg [contains ethanol (in diluent), polysorbate 80 (in diluent); supplied with diluent]

Injection, solution: 10 mg/mL (2 mL, 8 mL, 16 mL)

Injection, solution [concentrate]:

Taxotere®: 20 mg/mL (1 mL, 4 mL) [contains dehydrated ethanol 0.395 g/mL, polysorbate 80]

Taxotere®: 20 mg/0.5 mL (0.5 mL [DSC], 2 mL [DSC]) [contains ethanol (in diluent), polysorbate 80]

◆ **Docetaxel for Injection (Can)** *see* DOCEtaxel *on page 534*

Docosanol (doe KOE san ole)

Brand Names: U.S. Abreva® [OTC]

Index Terms *n*-Docosanol; Behenyl Alcohol

Pharmacologic Category Antiviral Agent, Topical

Use Treatment of herpes simplex of the face or lips

Dosage Children ≥12 years and Adults: Topical: Apply 5 times/day to affected area of face or lips. Start at first sign of cold sore or fever blister and continue until healed.

Additional Information Complete prescribing information for this medication should be consulted for additional detail.

Dosage Forms Excipient information presented when available (limited, particularly for generics); consult specific product labeling.

Cream, topical:

Abreva®: 10% (2 g) [contains benzyl alcohol]

Docusate (DOK yoo sate)

Brand Names: U.S. Colace® [OTC]; Correctol® [OTC]; Diocto [OTC]; Docu-Soft [OTC]; DocuSoft S™ [OTC]; Dok™ [OTC]; DSS® [OTC]; Dulcolax® Stool Softener [OTC]; Dulcolax® [OTC]; Enemeez® Plus [OTC]; Enemeez® [OTC]; Fleet® Pedia-Lax™ Liquid Stool Softener [OTC]; Fleet® Sof-Lax® [OTC]; Kao-Tin [OTC]; Kaopectate® Stool Softener [OTC]; Phillips'® Liquid-Gels® [OTC]; Phillips'® Stool Softener Laxative [OTC]; Silace [OTC]

Brand Names: Canada Apo-Docusate-Sodium®; Colace®; Colax-C®; Novo-Docusate Calcium; Novo-Docusate Sodium; PMS-Docusate Calcium; PMS-Docusate Sodium; Regulex®; Selax®; Soflax™

Index Terms Dioctyl Calcium Sulfosuccinate; Dioctyl Sodium Sulfosuccinate; Docusate Calcium; Docusate Potassium; Docusate Sodium; DOSS; DSS

Pharmacologic Category Stool Softener

Additional Appendix Information

Laxatives, Classification and Properties *on page 1893*

Use Stool softener in patients who should avoid straining during defecation and constipation associated with hard, dry stools; prophylaxis for straining (Valsalva) following myocardial infarction. A safe agent to be used in elderly; some evidence that doses <200 mg are ineffective; stool softeners are unnecessary if stool is well hydrated or "mushy" and soft; shown to be ineffective used long-term.

Unlabeled Use Ceruminolytic

Pregnancy Risk Factor C

Dosage Docusate salts are interchangeable; the amount of sodium or calcium per dosage unit is clinically insignificant

Infants and Children <3 years: Oral: 10-40 mg/day in 1-4 divided doses

Children: Oral:

- 3-6 years: 20-60 mg/day in 1-4 divided doses
- 6-12 years: 40-150 mg/day in 1-4 divided doses

Adolescents and Adults: Oral: 50-500 mg/day in 1-4 divided doses

Older Children and Adults: Rectal: Add 50-100 mg of docusate liquid to enema fluid (saline or water); administer as retention or flushing enema

Ceruminolytic (unlabeled use): Intra-aural: Administer 1 mL of docusate sodium in 2 mL syringes; if no clearance in 15 minutes, irrigate with 50-100 mL normal saline (this method is 80% effective)

Additional Information Complete prescribing information for this medication should be consulted for additional detail.

Dosage Forms Excipient information presented when available (limited, particularly for generics); consult specific product labeling.

Capsule, oral, as sodium:
- Colace®: 50 mg [contains sodium 3 mg/capsule]
- Colace®: 100 mg [contains sodium 5 mg/capsule]

Capsule, liquid, oral, as sodium:
- DocuSoft S™: 100 mg [contains sodium 5 mg/capsule]

Capsule, softgel, oral, as calcium: 240 mg
- Kao-Tin: 240 mg
- Kaopectate® Stool Softener: 240 mg

Capsule, softgel, oral, as sodium: 50 mg, 100 mg, 250 mg
- Correctol®: 100 mg
- Docu-Soft: 100 mg
- Dok™: 100 mg, 250 mg
- DSS®: 100 mg, 250 mg
- Dulcolax®: 100 mg [contains sodium 5 mg/capsule]
- Dulcolax® Stool Softener: 100 mg [contains sodium 5 mg/capsule]
- Fleet® Sof-Lax®: 100 mg [contains sodium 5 mg/capsule]
- Phillips'® Liquid-Gels®: 100 mg [contains sodium 5.2 mg/capsule]
- Phillips'® Stool Softener Laxative: 100 mg [contains sodium 5.2 mg/capsule]

Liquid, oral, as sodium: 50 mg/5 mL (10 mL, 25 mL, 473 mL); 150 mg/15 mL (480 mL)
- Diocto: 50 mg/15 mL (473 mL) [contains sodium 15 mg/5 mL]
- Diocto: 150 mg/15 mL (480 mL)
- Diocto: 150 mg/15 mL (480 mL) [vanilla flavor]
- Fleet® Pedia-Lax™ Liquid Stool Softener: 50 mg/15 mL (118 mL) [contains propylene glycol, sodium 13 mg/15 mL; fruit-punch flavor]
- Silace: 150 mg/15 mL (473 mL) [lemon-vanilla flavor]

Solution, rectal, as sodium [enema]:
- Enemeez®: 283 mg/5 mL (5 mL)
- Enemeez® Plus: 283 mg/5 mL (5 mL) [contains benzocaine]

Syrup, oral, as sodium: 20 mg/5 mL (25 mL, 473 mL)
- Colace®: 60 mg/15 mL (473 mL) [ethanol free, sugar free; contains propylene glycol, sodium 34 mg/15 mL]
- Diocto: 60 mg/15 mL (480 mL) [mint flavor]
- Diocto: 60 mg/15 mL (473 mL) [contains propylene glycol, sodium 14 mg/5 mL, sodium benzoate]
- Silace: 60 mg/15 mL (480 mL) [peppermint flavor]

Tablet, oral, as sodium: 100 mg
- Dok™: 100 mg [scored]

Docusate and Senna (DOK yoo sate & SEN na)

Brand Names: U.S. Dok™ Plus [OTC]; Geri-Stool [OTC]; Peri-Colace® [OTC]; Senexon-S [OTC]; Senna Plus [OTC]; Senokot-S® [OTC]; SenoSol™-SS [OTC]

Index Terms Senna and Docusate; Senna-S

Pharmacologic Category Laxative, Stimulant; Stool Softener

Additional Appendix Information

Laxatives, Classification and Properties *on page 1893*

Use Short-term treatment of constipation

Unlabeled Use Evacuate the colon for bowel or rectal examinations; management/prevention of opiate-induced constipation

Dosage Oral: Constipation: OTC ranges:

Children:
- 2-6 years: Initial: 4.3 mg sennosides plus 25 mg docusate (1/2 tablet) once daily (maximum: 1 tablet twice daily)
- 6-12 years: Initial: 8.6 sennosides plus 50 mg docusate (1 tablet) once daily (maximum: 2 tablets twice daily)

Children ≥12 years and Adults: Initial: 2 tablets (17.2 mg sennosides plus 100 mg docusate) once daily (maximum: 4 tablets twice daily)

Elderly: Consider half the initial dose in older, debilitated patients

Additional Information Complete prescribing information for this medication should be consulted for additional detail.

Dosage Forms Excipient information presented when available (limited, particularly for generics); consult specific product labeling.

Tablet, oral: Docusate sodium 50 mg and sennosides 8.6 mg
- Dok™ Plus: Docusate sodium 50 mg and sennosides 8.6 mg
- Geri-Stool: Docusate sodium 50 mg and sennosides 8.6 mg
- Peri-Colace®: Docusate sodium 50 mg and sennosides 8.6 mg
- Senexon-S: Docusate sodium 50 mg and sennosides 8.6 mg
- Senna Plus: Docusate sodium 50 mg and sennosides 8.6 mg
- Senokot-S®: Docusate sodium 50 mg and sennosides 8.6 mg [sugar free; contains sodium 4 mg/tablet]
- SenoSol™-SS: Docusate sodium 50 mg and sennosides 8.6 mg [contains sodium 3 mg/tablet]

◆ **Docusate Calcium** *see* Docusate *on page 537*
◆ **Docusate Potassium** *see* Docusate *on page 537*
◆ **Docusate Sodium** *see* Docusate *on page 537*
◆ **Docu-Soft [OTC]** *see* Docusate *on page 537*

◆ **DocuSoft S™ [OTC]** *see* Docusate *on page 537*

Dofetilide (doe FET il ide)

Brand Names: U.S. Tikosyn®

Brand Names: Canada Tikosyn®

Pharmacologic Category Antiarrhythmic Agent, Class III

Use Maintenance of normal sinus rhythm in patients with chronic atrial fibrillation/atrial flutter of longer than 1-week duration who have been converted to normal sinus rhythm; conversion of atrial fibrillation and atrial flutter to normal sinus rhythm

Unlabeled Use Alternative antiarrhythmic for the treatment of atrial fibrillation in patients with hypertrophic cardiomyopathy (HCM)

Pregnancy Risk Factor C

Pregnancy Considerations Dofetilide has been shown to adversely affect *in utero* growth, organogenesis, and survival of rats and mice. There are no adequate and well-controlled studies in pregnant women. Dofetilide should be used with extreme caution in pregnant women and in women of childbearing age only when the benefit to the patient unequivocally justifies the potential risk to the fetus.

Lactation Excretion in breast milk unknown/not recommended

Prescribing and Access Restrictions As a requirement of the REMS program, access to this medication is restricted. Tikosyn® is only available to prescribers and hospitals that have confirmed their participation in a designated Tikosyn® Education Program. The program provides comprehensive education about the importance of in-hospital treatment initiation and individualized dosing.

T.I.P.S. is the Tikosyn® In Pharmacy System designated to allow retail pharmacies to stock and dispense Tikosyn® once they have been enrolled. A participating pharmacy must confirm receipt of the T.I.P.S. program materials and educate its pharmacy staff about the procedures required to fill an outpatient prescription for Tikosyn®. The T.I.P.S. enrollment form is available at www.tikosyn.com. Tikosyn® is only available from a special mail order pharmacy, and enrolled retail pharmacies. Pharmacists must verify that the hospital/prescriber is a confirmed participant before Tikosyn® is provided. For participant verification, the pharmacist may call 1-800-788-7353 or use the web site located at www.tikosynlist.com. Further details and directions on the program are provided at www.tikosyn.com.

Dofetilide therapy must be initiated/adjusted in a hospital setting with proper monitoring under the guidance of experienced personnel.

Medication Guide Available Yes

Contraindications Hypersensitivity to dofetilide or any component of the formulation; patients with congenital or acquired long QT syndromes, do not use if baseline QT interval or QT_c is >440 msec (500 msec in patients with ventricular conduction abnormalities); severe renal impairment (Cl_{cr} <20 mL/minute [Cockcroft-Gault method]); concurrent use with verapamil, cimetidine, hydrochlorothiazide (alone or in combinations), trimethoprim (alone or in combination with sulfamethoxazole), itraconazole (according to itraconazole prescribing information) ketoconazole, prochlorperazine, or megestrol

Warnings/Precautions [U.S. Boxed Warning]: Must be initiated (or reinitiated) in a setting with continuous monitoring and staff familiar with the recognition and treatment of life-threatening arrhythmias. Patients must be monitored with continuous ECG for a minimum of 3 days, or for a minimum of 12 hours after electrical or pharmacological cardioversion to normal sinus rhythm, whichever is greater. Patients should be readmitted for continuous monitoring if dosage is later increased. Reserve for patients who are highly symptomatic with atrial fibrillation/atrial flutter; risk of torsade de pointes (TdP) significantly increases with doses >500 mcg twice daily; hold Class I or Class III antiarrhythmics for at least three half-lives prior to starting dofetilide; use in patients previously on amiodarone therapy only if serum amiodarone level is <0.3 mg/L or if amiodarone was discontinued ≥3 months ago; correct hypokalemia or hypomagnesemia before initiating dofetilide and maintain within normal limits during treatment. The risk of TdP may be higher in certain patient subgroups (eg, patients with heart failure). Most episodes of TdP occur within the first 3 days of therapy. Risk of hypokalemia and/or hypomagnesemia may be increased by potassium-depleting diuretics, increasing the risk of TdP. Concurrent use with other drugs known to prolong QT_c interval is not recommended.

Patients with sick sinus syndrome or with second or third-degree heart block should not receive dofetilide unless a functional pacemaker is in place. Defibrillation threshold is reduced in patients with ventricular tachycardia or ventricular fibrillation undergoing implantation of a cardioverter-defibrillator device. Use with caution in renal impairment; **dose adjustment required for patients with Cl_{cr} ≤60 mL/minute.** Use with caution in patients with severe hepatic impairment; not studied.

Adverse Reactions

Supraventricular arrhythmia patients:

>10%: Central nervous system: Headache (11%)

2% to 10%:

- Central nervous system: Dizziness (8%), insomnia (4%)
- Cardiovascular: Ventricular tachycardia (2.6% to 3.7%), chest pain (10%), torsade de pointes (3.3% in HF patients and 0.9% in patients with a recent MI; up to 10.5% in patients receiving doses in excess of those recommended). Torsade de pointes occurs most frequently within the first 3 days of therapy.
- Dermatologic: Rash (3%)
- Gastrointestinal: Nausea (5%), diarrhea (3%), abdominal pain (3%)
- Neuromuscular & skeletal: Back pain (3%)
- Respiratory: Respiratory tract infection (7%), dyspnea (6%)
- Miscellaneous: Flu-like syndrome (4%)

<2%:

- Central nervous system: CVA, facial paralysis, flaccid paralysis, migraine, paralysis
- Cardiovascular: AV block (0.4% to 1.5%), bundle branch block (0.1% to 0.5%), heart block (0.1% to 0.5%), ventricular fibrillation (0% to 0.4%), bradycardia, cardiac arrest, edema, MI, sudden death, syncope
- Dermatologic: Angioedema
- Gastrointestinal: Liver damage
- Neuromuscular & skeletal: Paresthesia
- Respiratory: Cough

Drug Interactions

Metabolism/Transport Effects Substrate of CYP3A4 (minor); **Note:** Assignment of Major/Minor substrate status based on clinically relevant drug interaction potential

Avoid Concomitant Use

Avoid concomitant use of Dofetilide with any of the following: Antifungal Agents (Azole Derivatives, Systemic); Artemether; Cimetidine; Dronedarone; Lumefantrine; Megestrol; Nilotinib; Pimozide; Prochlorperazine; QUEtiapine; QuiNINE; Saquinavir; Tetrabenazine; Thiazide Diuretics; Thioridazine; Toremifene; Trimethoprim; Vandetanib; Vemurafenib; Verapamil; Ziprasidone

Increased Effect/Toxicity

Dofetilide may increase the levels/effects of: Dronedarone; Lidocaine (Topical); Pimozide; QTc-Prolonging Agents; QuiNINE; Tetrabenazine; Thioridazine; Toremifene; Vandetanib; Vemurafenib; Ziprasidone

The levels/effects of Dofetilide may be increased by: Alfuzosin; AMILoride; Antifungal Agents (Azole Derivatives, Systemic); Artemether; Chloroquine; Cimetidine; Ciprofloxacin; Ciprofloxacin (Systemic); Conivaptan; Eribulin; Fingolimod; Gadobutrol; Indacaterol; Lidocaine (Topical); Loop Diuretics; Lumefantrine; Megestrol; MetFORMIN; Nilotinib; Prochlorperazine; QUEtiapine; QuiNINE; Saquinavir; Thiazide Diuretics; Triamterene; Trimethoprim; Verapamil

Decreased Effect

The levels/effects of Dofetilide may be decreased by: Tocilizumab

Ethanol/Nutrition/Herb Interactions Herb/Nutraceutical: St John's wort may decrease dofetilide levels. Avoid ephedra (may worsen arrhythmia).

Mechanism of Action Vaughan Williams Class III antiarrhythmic activity. Blockade of the cardiac ion channel carrying the rapid component of the delayed rectifier potassium current. Dofetilide has no effect on sodium channels, adrenergic alpha-receptors, or adrenergic beta-receptors. It increases the monophasic action potential duration due to delayed repolarization. The increase in the QT interval is a function of prolongation of both effective and functional refractory periods in the His-Purkinje system and the ventricles. Changes in cardiac conduction velocity and sinus node function have not been observed in patients with or without structural heart disease. PR and QRS width remain the same in patients with pre-existing heart block and or sick sinus syndrome.

Pharmacodynamics/Kinetics

Absorption: Well absorbed

Distribution: V_d: 3 L/kg

Protein binding: 60% to 70%

Metabolism: Hepatic via CYP3A4, but low affinity for it; metabolites formed by N-dealkylation and N-oxidation

Bioavailability: >90%

Half-life elimination: ~10 hours; prolonged with renal impairment

Time to peak, serum: Fasting: 2-3 hours

Excretion: Urine (80%; 80% as unchanged drug, 20% as inactive or minimally active metabolites); renal elimination consists of glomerular filtration and active tubular secretion via cationic transport system

Dosage Adults: Oral:

Note: QT or QT_c must be determined prior to first dose. If QT_c >440 msec (>500 msec in patients with ventricular conduction abnormalities), dofetilide is contraindicated.

Initial: 500 mcg twice daily. Initial dosage must be adjusted in patients with estimated Cl_{cr} <60 mL/minute (see dosage adjustment in renal impairment). Dofetilide may be initiated at lower doses than recommended based on physician discretion.

Modification of dosage in response to **initial** dose: QT_c interval should be measured 2-3 hours after the initial dose. If the QT_c is >15% of baseline, or if the QT_c is >500 msec (550 msec in patients with ventricular conduction abnormalities), dofetilide should be reduced. If the starting dose was 500 mcg twice daily, then reduce to 250 mcg twice daily. If the starting dose was 250 mcg twice daily, then reduce to 125 mcg twice daily. If the starting dose was 125 mcg twice daily, then reduce to 125 mcg once daily. If at any time after the second dose is given the QT_c is >500 msec (550 msec in patients with ventricular conduction abnormalities), dofetilide should be discontinued.

Dosage adjustment in renal impairment: Note: Using the Modification of Diet in Renal Disease (MDRD) equation and subsequent eGFR to determine dose may lead to overestimation of creatinine clearance and overdose of medication; use only the Cockcroft-Gault equation to estimate creatinine clearance (Denetclaw, 2011). Use actual body weight when using the Cockcroft-Gault equation to calculate creatinine clearance.

Cl_{cr} >60 mL/minute: Administer 500 mcg twice daily.

Cl_{cr} 40-60 mL/minute: Administer 250 mcg twice daily.

Cl_{cr} 20-39 mL/minute: Administer 125 mcg twice daily.

Cl_{cr} <20 mL/minute: Contraindicated.

Dosage adjustment in hepatic impairment: No dosage adjustments required in Child-Pugh Class A and B. Patients with severe hepatic impairment were not studied.

Elderly: No specific dosage adjustments are recommended based on age, however, careful assessment of renal function is particularly important in this population.

Administration Swallow capsules whole, do not chew or crush; Do not use damaged or opened capsules.

Monitoring Parameters ECG monitoring with attention to QT (if heart rate <60 beats per minute) or QT_c and occurrence of ventricular arrhythmias, baseline serum creatinine and changes in serum creatinine. Upon initiation (or reinitiation) continuous ECG monitoring recommended for a minimum of 3 days, or for at least 12 hours after electrical or pharmacological conversion to normal sinus rhythm, whichever is greater. Check serum potassium and magnesium levels at baseline and throughout therapy especially if on medications where these electrolyte disturbances can occur, or if patient has a history of hypokalemia or hypomagnesemia. QT or QT_c must be monitored at baseline prior to the first dose and 2-3 hours afterwards. If at baseline, QT_c >440 msec (>500 msec in patients with ventricular conduction abnormalities), dofetilide is contraindicated. If dofetilide initiated, QT_c interval must be determined 2-3 hours after each subsequent dose of dofetilide for in-hospital doses 2-5. Thereafter, QT or QT_c and creatinine clearance should be evaluated every 3 months. If at any time during therapy after the second dose the measured QT_c is >500 msec (550 msec in patients with ventricular conduction abnormalities), dofetilide should be discontinued.

Dosage Forms Excipient information presented when available (limited, particularly for generics); consult specific product labeling.

Capsule, oral:

Tikosyn®: 125 mcg, 250 mcg, 500 mcg

◆ **Dok™ [OTC]** *see* Docusate *on page 537*

◆ **Dok™ Plus [OTC]** *see* Docusate and Senna *on page 538*

Dolasetron (dol A se tron)

Brand Names: U.S. Anzemet®

Brand Names: Canada Anzemet®

Index Terms Dolasetron Mesylate; MDL 73,147EF

Pharmacologic Category Antiemetic; Selective 5-HT_3 Receptor Antagonist

Use

U.S. labeling:

Injection: Prevention and treatment of postoperative nausea and vomiting

Oral: Prevention of nausea and vomiting associated with emetogenic cancer chemotherapy (initial and repeat courses); prevention of postoperative nausea and vomiting

Canadian labeling: Oral: Prevention of nausea and vomiting associated with emetogenic cancer chemotherapy (initial and repeat courses)

Pregnancy Risk Factor B

Pregnancy Considerations Teratogenic effects were not observed in animal studies. There are no adequate and well-controlled studies in pregnant women.

Lactation Excretion in breast milk unknown/use caution

Contraindications

U.S. labeling:

Injection: Hypersensitivity to dolasetron or any component of the formulation; use for the prevention of chemotherapy-induced nausea and vomiting

Tablet: Hypersensitivity to dolasetron or any component of the formulation

Canadian labeling: Hypersensitivity to dolasetron or any component of the formulation; use in children and adolescents <18 years of age; use for the prevention or treatment of postoperative nausea and vomiting

Warnings/Precautions Dolasetron is associated with a number of dose-dependent increases in ECG intervals (eg, PR, QRS duration, QT/QT_c, JT), usually occurring 1-2 hours after I.V. administration and usually lasting 6-8 hours; however, may last ≥24 hours and rarely lead to heart block or arrhythmia. Clinically relevant QT-interval prolongation may occur resulting in torsade de pointes, when used in conjunction with other agents that prolong the QT interval (eg, Class I and III antiarrhythmics). Avoid use in patients at greater risk for QT prolongation (eg, patients with congenital long QT syndrome, medications known to prolong QT interval, electrolyte abnormalities, and cumulative high-dose anthracycline therapy) and/or ventricular arrhythmia. Correct potassium or magnesium abnormalities prior to initiating therapy. I.V. formulations of 5-HT_3 antagonists have more association with ECG interval changes, compared to oral formulations. Reduction in heart rate may also occur with the 5-HT_3 antagonists. Use with caution in children and adolescents who have or may develop QT_c prolongation; rare cases of supraventricular and ventricular arrhythmias, cardiac arrest, and MI have been reported in this population.

Use with caution in patients allergic to other 5-HT_3 receptor antagonists; cross-reactivity has been reported with other 5-HT_3 receptor antagonists. **For chemotherapy-associated nausea and vomiting, should be used on a scheduled basis, not on an "as needed" (PRN) basis,** since data support the use of this drug only in the prevention of nausea and vomiting (due to antineoplastic therapy) and not in the rescue of nausea and vomiting. Not intended for treatment of nausea and vomiting or for chronic continuous therapy.

Adverse Reactions Adverse events may vary according to indication

>10%:

Central nervous system: Headache (7% to 24%)

Gastrointestinal: Diarrhea (2% to 12%)

1% to 10%:

Cardiovascular: Bradycardia (4% to 5%), hypertension (≤3%), tachycardia (2% to 3%)

Central nervous system: Dizziness (1% to 6%), fatigue (3% to 6%), fever (4%), pain (≤2%), chills/shivering (1% to 2%)

Gastrointestinal: Dyspepsia (≤3%), abdominal pain (≤3%)

Hepatic: Abnormal hepatic function (4%)

Renal: Oliguria (3%)

<1% (Limited to important or life-threatening): Abnormal vision, abnormal dreams, acute renal failure, alkaline phosphatase increased, ALT increased, anaphylactic reaction, anemia, anxiety, AST increased, ataxia, bronchospasm, cardiac arrest, chest pain, confusion, constipation, diaphoresis, dyspnea, dysuria, edema, epistaxis, facial edema, flushing, GGT increased, hematuria, hyperbilirubinemia, hypotension, ischemia (peripheral), local injection site reaction (pain/burning), MI, myocardial ischemia, orthostatic hypotension, palpitation, pancreatitis, paresthesia, peripheral edema, photophobia, polyuria, prothrombin time increased, PTT increased, purpura/hematoma, rash, syncope, taste alteration, thrombocytopenia, thrombophlebitis/phlebitis, tinnitus, tremor, twitching, urticaria, vertigo

Note: Cardiac conduction abnormalities (including arrhythmia [sinus, supraventricular and ventricular], atrial flutter/fibrillation, AV block, bundle branch block, extrasystoles, poor R wave progression, prolonged PR, QRS, JT, and QT_c intervals, ST, T and U wave changes, torsade de pointes, ventricular tachycardia, wide complex tachycardia and ventricular fibrillation) have also been reported.

Drug Interactions

Metabolism/Transport Effects Substrate of CYP2C9 (minor), CYP3A4 (minor); **Note:** Assignment of Major/Minor substrate status based on clinically relevant drug interaction potential; **Inhibits** CYP2D6 (weak)

Avoid Concomitant Use

Avoid concomitant use of Dolasetron with any of the following: Apomorphine; Artemether; Dronedarone; Lumefantrine; Nilotinib; Pimozide; QUEtiapine; QuiNINE; Tetrabenazine; Thioridazine; Toremifene; Vandetanib; Vemurafenib; Ziprasidone

Increased Effect/Toxicity

Dolasetron may increase the levels/effects of: Apomorphine; Dronedarone; Pimozide; QTc-Prolonging Agents; QuiNINE; Tetrabenazine; Thioridazine; Toremifene; Vandetanib; Vemurafenib; Ziprasidone

The levels/effects of Dolasetron may be increased by: Alfuzosin; Artemether; Chloroquine; Ciprofloxacin; Ciprofloxacin (Systemic); Conivaptan; Gadobutrol; Indacaterol; Lumefantrine; Nilotinib; QUEtiapine; QuiNINE

Decreased Effect

The levels/effects of Dolasetron may be decreased by: Tocilizumab

Ethanol/Nutrition/Herb Interactions Food: Food does not affect the bioavailability of oral doses.

Stability Store intact vials and tablets at room temperature of 20°C to 25°C (68°F to 77°F). Protect from light. Dilute in 50 mL of a compatible solution (ie, 0.9% NS, D_5W, $D_5 1/2$ NS, D_5LR, LR, and 10% mannitol injection). Solutions diluted for infusion are stable under normal lighting conditions at room temperature for 24 hours or under refrigeration for 48 hours.

Mechanism of Action Selective serotonin receptor (5-HT_3) antagonist, blocking serotonin both peripherally (primary site of action) and centrally at the chemoreceptor trigger zone

Pharmacodynamics/Kinetics

Absorption: Oral: Rapid and complete

Distribution: Hydrodolasetron: 5.8 L/kg

Protein binding: Hydrodolasetron: 69% to 77% (50% bound to $alpha_1$-acid glycoprotein)

Metabolism: Hepatic; rapid reduction by carbonyl reductase to hydrodolasetron (active metabolite); further metabolized by CYP2D6, CYP3A, and flavin monooxygenase

Bioavailability: Oral: ~75% (not affected by food)

Half-life elimination: Dolasetron: ≤10 minutes; hydrodolasetron: Adults: 6-8 hours; Children: 4-6 hours; Severe renal impairment: 11 hours; Severe hepatic impairment: 11 hours

Time to peak, plasma: Hydrodolasetron: I.V.: 0.6 hours; Oral: ~1 hour

Excretion: Urine ~67% (53% to 61% of the total dose as active metabolite hydrodolasetron); feces ~33%

Dosage Note: Use of dolasetron injection is contraindicated for the prevention of chemotherapy-induced nausea and vomiting. In Canada, use of dolasetron is also contraindicated in children and adolescents <18 years of age and in the prevention and treatment of postoperative nausea and vomiting in adults.

Prevention of chemotherapy-associated nausea and vomiting (including initial and repeat courses):

Children 2-16 years: Oral: 1.8 mg/kg within 1 hour before chemotherapy; maximum: 100 mg/dose

Adults: Oral: 100 mg within 1 hour before chemotherapy

Prevention of postoperative nausea and vomiting: *U.S. labeling:*

Children 2-16 years:

Oral: 1.2 mg/kg within 2 hours before surgery; maximum: 100 mg/dose

I.V.: 0.35 mg/kg ~15 minutes before cessation of anesthesia; maximum: 12.5 mg/dose

Adults:

Oral: 100 mg within 2 hours before surgery

I.V.: 12.5 mg ~15 minutes before cessation of anesthesia

Treatment of postoperative nausea and vomiting: *U.S. labeling:*

Children 2-16 years: I.V.: 0.35 mg/kg as soon as nausea or vomiting present; maximum: 12.5 mg/dose

Adults: I.V.: 12.5 mg as soon as nausea or vomiting present

Dosing adjustment in renal impairment: No dosage adjustment necessary

Dosing adjustment in hepatic impairment: No dosage adjustment necessary

Dietary Considerations May be taken without regard to meals.

Administration

I.V. injection may be given either undiluted IVP over 30 seconds or diluted in 50 mL of compatible fluid and infused over 15 minutes. Flush line before and after dolasetron administration.

Oral: When unable to administer in tablet form, dolasetron injection may be diluted in apple or apple-grape juice and taken orally; this dilution is stable for 2 hours at room temperature.

Monitoring Parameters ECG (in patients with cardiovascular disease, elderly, renally impaired, those at risk of developing hypokalemia and/or hypomagnesemia); potassium, magnesium

Additional Information Efficacy of dolasetron, for chemotherapy treatment, is enhanced with concomitant administration of dexamethasone 20 mg (increases complete response by 10% to 20%). Oral administration of the intravenous solution is equivalent to tablets.

Dosage Forms Excipient information presented when available (limited, particularly for generics); consult specific product labeling.

Injection, solution, as mesylate:

Anzemet®: 20 mg/mL (0.625 mL, 5 mL, 25 mL) [contains mannitol]

Tablet, oral, as mesylate:

Anzemet®: 50 mg, 100 mg

Extemporaneous Preparations Dolasetron injection may be diluted in apple or apple-grape juice and taken orally; this dilution is stable for 2 hours at room temperature (Anzemet® prescribing information, 2011).

A 10 mg/mL oral suspension may be prepared with tablets and either a 1:1 mixture of Ora-Plus® and Ora-Sweet® SF or a 1:1 mixture of strawberry syrup and Ora-Plus®. Crush twelve 50 mg tablets in a mortar and reduce to a fine powder. Slowly add chosen vehicle to **almost** 60 mL; transfer to a calibrated bottle, rinse mortar with vehicle, and add quantity of vehicle sufficient to make 60 mL. Label "shake well" and "refrigerate". Stable for 90 days refrigerated.

Anzemet® prescribing information, sanofi-aventis U.S. LLC, Bridgewater, NJ, 2011.

Johnson CE, Wagner DS, and Bussard WE, "Stability of Dolasetron in Two Oral Liquid Vehicles," *Am J Health Syst Pharm*, 2003, 60 (21):2242-4.

◆ **Dolasetron Mesylate** *see* Dolasetron *on page 540*

◆ **Dolgic® Plus** *see* Butalbital, Acetaminophen, and Caffeine *on page 255*

◆ **Dolobid** *see* Diflunisal *on page 502*

◆ **Dolophine®** *see* Methadone *on page 1088*

◆ **Doloral (Can)** *see* Morphine (Systemic) *on page 1153*

◆ **Dom-Alendronate (Can)** *see* Alendronate *on page 61*

◆ **Dom-Amiodarone (Can)** *see* Amiodarone *on page 90*

◆ **Dom-Amitriptyline (Can)** *see* Amitriptyline *on page 94*

◆ **Dom-Amlodipine (Can)** *see* AmLODIPine *on page 97*

◆ **Dom-Anagrelide (Can)** *see* Anagrelide *on page 119*

◆ **Dom-Atenolol (Can)** *see* Atenolol *on page 161*

◆ **Dom-Azithromycin (Can)** *see* Azithromycin (Systemic) *on page 180*

◆ **Dom-Baclofen (Can)** *see* Baclofen *on page 187*

◆ **Dom-Bicalutamide (Can)** *see* Bicalutamide *on page 217*

◆ **Dom-Bromocriptine (Can)** *see* Bromocriptine *on page 236*

◆ **Dom-Buspirone (Can)** *see* BusPIRone *on page 250*

◆ **Dom-Captopril (Can)** *see* Captopril *on page 277*

◆ **Dom-Carbamazepine (Can)** *see* CarBAMazepine *on page 280*

◆ **Dom-Carvedilol (Can)** *see* Carvedilol *on page 295*

◆ **Dom-Cephalexin (Can)** *see* Cephalexin *on page 327*

◆ **Dom-Cimetidine (Can)** *see* Cimetidine *on page 359*

◆ **Dom-Ciprofloxacin (Can)** *see* Ciprofloxacin (Systemic) *on page 362*

◆ **Dom-Citalopram (Can)** *see* Citalopram *on page 370*

◆ **Dom-Clarithromycin (Can)** *see* Clarithromycin *on page 374*

◆ **Dom-Clobazam (Can)** *see* Clobazam *on page 382*

◆ **Dom-Clonidine (Can)** *see* CloNIDine *on page 392*

◆ **Dom-Cyclobenzaprine (Can)** *see* Cyclobenzaprine *on page 419*

◆ **Dom-Diclofenac (Can)** *see* Diclofenac (Systemic) *on page 495*

◆ **Dom-Diclofenac SR (Can)** *see* Diclofenac (Systemic) *on page 495*

◆ **Dom-Divalproex (Can)** *see* Divalproex *on page 530*

◆ **Dom-Doxycycline (Can)** *see* Doxycycline *on page 557*

◆ **Domeboro® [OTC]** *see* Aluminum Sulfate and Calcium Acetate *on page 81*

◆ **Dome Paste Bandage** *see* Zinc Gelatin *on page 1817*

◆ **Dom-Fenofibrate Micro (Can)** *see* Fenofibrate *on page 693*

◆ **Dom-Fluconazole (Can)** *see* Fluconazole *on page 718*

◆ **Dom-Fluoxetine (Can)** *see* FLUoxetine *on page 731*

◆ **Dom-Furosemide (Can)** *see* Furosemide *on page 771*

◆ **Dom-Gabapentin (Can)** *see* Gabapentin *on page 773*

◆ **Dom-Glyburide (Can)** *see* GlyBURIDE *on page 799*

◆ **Dom-Hydrochlorothiazide (Can)** *see* Hydrochlorothiazide *on page 835*

◆ **Dom-Indapamide (Can)** *see* Indapamide *on page 886*

◆ **Dom-Levetiracetam (Can)** *see* LevETIRAcetam *on page 994*

◆ **Dom-Levo-Carbidopa (Can)** *see* Carbidopa and Levodopa *on page 284*

◆ **Dom-Lisinopril (Can)** *see* Lisinopril *on page 1020*

◆ **Dom-Loperamide (Can)** *see* Loperamide *on page 1026*

◆ **Dom-Lorazepam (Can)** *see* LORazepam *on page 1032*

◆ **Dom-Lovastatin (Can)** *see* Lovastatin *on page 1038*

Donepezil (doh NEP e zil)

Brand Names: U.S. Aricept®; Aricept® ODT

Brand Names: Canada Aricept®; Aricept® RDT

Index Terms E2020

Pharmacologic Category Acetylcholinesterase Inhibitor (Central)

Use Treatment of mild, moderate, or severe dementia of the Alzheimer's type

Unlabeled Use Behavioral syndromes in dementia; mild-to-moderate dementia associated with Parkinson's disease; Lewy body dementia

Pregnancy Risk Factor C

Pregnancy Considerations Teratogenic effects were not observed in animal studies. There are no adequate and well-controlled studies in pregnant women.

Lactation Excretion in breast milk unknown/not recommended

Contraindications Hypersensitivity to donepezil, piperidine derivatives, or any component of the formulation

Warnings/Precautions Cholinesterase inhibitors may have vagotonic effects which may cause bradycardia and/or heart block with or without a history of cardiac disease; syncopal episodes have been associated with donepezil. Alzheimer's treatment guidelines consider bradycardia to be a relative contraindication for use of centrally-active cholinesterase inhibitors. Use with caution with sick sinus syndrome or other supraventricular cardiac conduction abnormalities, COPD, or asthma. Use with caution in patients with a history of seizure disorder; cholinomimetics may potentially cause generalized seizures, although seizure activity may also result from Alzheimer's disease. Use with caution in patients at risk of ulcer disease (eg, previous history or NSAID use), or in patients with bladder outlet obstruction. May cause dose-related diarrhea, nausea, and/or vomiting, which usually resolves in 1-3 weeks. May cause anorexia and/or weight loss (dose-related). May exaggerate neuromuscular blockade effects of depolarizing neuromuscular-blocking agents (eg, succinylcholine).

Adverse Reactions

>10%:

Central nervous system: Insomnia (2% to 14%)

Gastrointestinal: Nausea (3% to 19%; dose related), diarrhea (5% to 15%; dose related)

Miscellaneous: Accident (7% to 13%), infection (11%)

1% to 10%:

Cardiovascular: Hypertension (3%), chest pain (2%), hemorrhage (2%), syncope (2%), hypotension, atrial fibrillation, bradycardia, ECG abnormal, edema, heart failure, hot flashes, peripheral edema, vasodilation

Central nervous system: Headache (3% to 10%), pain (3% to 9%), fatigue (1% to 8%), dizziness (2% to 8%), abnormal dreams (3%), hostility (3%), nervousness (1% to 3%), hallucinations (3%), depression (2% to 3%), confusion (2%), emotional lability (2%), personality disorder (2%), fever (2%), somnolence (2%), abnormal crying, aggression, agitation, anxiety, aphasia, delusions, irritability, restlessness, seizure, vertigo

Dermatologic: Bruising (4% to 5%), eczema (3%), pruritus, rash, skin ulcer, urticaria

Endocrine & metabolic: Dehydration (1% to 2%), hyperlipemia (2%), libido increased

Gastrointestinal: Anorexia (2% to 8%), vomiting (3% to 9%; dose related), weight loss (3% to 5%; dose related), abdominal pain, bloating, constipation, dyspepsia, epigastric pain, fecal incontinence, gastroenteritis, GI bleeding, toothache

Genitourinary: Urinary frequency (2%), urinary incontinence (1% to 3%), cystitis, hematuria, glycosuria, nocturia, UTI

Hematologic: Contusion (≤2%), anemia

Hepatic: Alkaline phosphatase increased

Neuromuscular & skeletal: Muscle cramps (3% to 8%), back pain (3%), CPK increased (3%), arthritis (1% to 2%), ataxia, bone fracture, gait abnormal, lactate dehydrogenase increased, paresthesia, tremor, weakness (1% to 2%)

Ocular: Blurred vision, cataract, eye irritation

Respiratory: Bronchitis, cough increased, dyspnea, pharyngitis, pneumonia, sore throat

Miscellaneous: Diaphoresis, fungal infection, flu symptoms, wandering

<1% (Limited to important or life-threatening): Angina, cardiomegaly, cerebrovascular accident, cholecystitis, conjunctival hemorrhage, deep vein thrombosis, diabetes

mellitus, diverticulitis, gastrointestinal ulcer, glaucoma, heart block, heart failure, hemolytic anemia, hepatitis, hyperglycemia, hypertonia, hypokalemia, hypokinesia, hyponatremia, hypoxia, intracranial hemorrhage, jaundice, LFTs increased, MI, neuroleptic malignant syndrome, pancreatitis, pleurisy, pulmonary collapse, pulmonary congestion, pyelonephritis, renal failure, retinal hemorrhage, SVT, thrombocythemia, thrombocytopenia, tongue edema, transient ischemic attack

Drug Interactions

Metabolism/Transport Effects **Substrate** of CYP2D6 (minor), CYP3A4 (minor); **Note:** Assignment of Major/Minor substrate status based on clinically relevant drug interaction potential

Avoid Concomitant Use There are no known interactions where it is recommended to avoid concomitant use.

Increased Effect/Toxicity

Donepezil may increase the levels/effects of: Antipsychotics; Beta-Blockers; Cholinergic Agonists; Succinylcholine

The levels/effects of Donepezil may be increased by: Conivaptan; Corticosteroids (Systemic)

Decreased Effect

Donepezil may decrease the levels/effects of: Anticholinergics; Neuromuscular-Blocking Agents (Nondepolarizing)

The levels/effects of Donepezil may be decreased by: Anticholinergics; Dipyridamole; Peginterferon Alfa-2b; Tocilizumab

Ethanol/Nutrition/Herb Interactions Herb/Nutraceutical: St John's wort may decrease donepezil levels. Ginkgo biloba may increase adverse effects/toxicity of acetylcholinesterase inhibitors.

Stability Store at 15°C to 30°C (59°F to 86°F).

Mechanism of Action Alzheimer's disease is characterized by cholinergic deficiency in the cortex and basal forebrain, which contributes to cognitive deficits. Donepezil reversibly and noncompetitively inhibits centrally-active acetylcholinesterase, the enzyme responsible for hydrolysis of acetylcholine. This appears to result in increased concentrations of acetylcholine available for synaptic transmission in the central nervous system.

Pharmacodynamics/Kinetics

Absorption: Well absorbed

Distribution: V_{dss}: 12-16 L/kg

Protein binding: 96%, primarily to albumin (75%) and α_1-acid glycoprotein (21%)

Metabolism: Extensively to four major metabolites (two are active) via CYP2D6 and 3A4; undergoes glucuronidation

Bioavailability: 100%

Half-life elimination: 70 hours; time to steady-state: 15 days

Time to peak, plasma: Tablet, 10 mg: 3 hours; Tablet, 23 mg: ~8 hours; **Note:** Peak plasma concentrations almost twofold higher for the 23 mg tablet compared to the 10 mg tablet

Excretion: Urine 57% (17% as unchanged drug); feces 15%

Dosage Oral:

Adults: Alzheimer's dementia:

Mild-to-moderate: Initial: 5 mg once daily; may increase to 10 mg once daily after 4-6 weeks; effective dosage range in clinical studies: 5-10 mg/day

Moderate-to-severe: Initial: 5 mg once daily; may increase to 10 mg once daily after 4-6 weeks; may increase further to 23 mg once daily after ≥3 months; effective dosage range in clinical studies: 10-23 mg/day

Elderly: Refer to adult dosing. **Note:** The Canadian labeling recommends a maximum dose of 5 mg once daily in elderly women of low body weight.

Dietary Considerations May take with or without food.

Administration Administer at bedtime without regard to food.

Aricept® 5 mg or 10 mg tablet: Swallow whole with water; do not split or crush per manufacturer's labeling. However, data available from the manufacturer showed that bioavailability was not affected by disintegration or dissolution when administered as a solution compared to a tablet during a bioequivalence study (data on file, Eisai Inc).

Aricept® 23 mg tablet: Swallow whole with water; do **NOT** crush or chew due to an increased rate of absorption. The 23 mg strength is provided in a unique film-coated formulation different from the 5 mg or 10 mg tablet strengths, which results in an altered pharmacokinetic profile.

Aricept® ODT: Allow tablet to dissolve completely on tongue and follow with water.

Monitoring Parameters Behavior, mood, bowel function, cognitive function, general function (eg, activities of daily living)

Dosage Forms Excipient information presented when available (limited, particularly for generics); consult specific product labeling.

Tablet, oral, as hydrochloride: 5 mg, 10 mg

Aricept®: 5 mg, 10 mg, 23 mg

Tablet, orally disintegrating, oral, as hydrochloride: 5 mg, 10 mg

Aricept® ODT: 5 mg, 10 mg

◆ **Donnatal®** *see* Hyoscyamine, Atropine, Scopolamine, and Phenobarbital *on page 855*

◆ **Donnatal Extentabs®** *see* Hyoscyamine, Atropine, Scopolamine, and Phenobarbital *on page 855*

DOPamine (DOE pa meen)

Index Terms Dopamine Hydrochloride; Intropin

Pharmacologic Category Adrenergic Agonist Agent

Additional Appendix Information

Vasoactive Agents, Intravenous *on page 1898*

Use Adjunct in the treatment of shock (eg, MI, open heart surgery, renal failure, cardiac decompensation) which persists after adequate fluid volume replacement

Unlabeled Use Symptomatic bradycardia or heart block unresponsive to atropine or pacing

Pregnancy Risk Factor C

Pregnancy Considerations Adverse events have been observed in some animal reproduction studies. It is not known if dopamine crosses the placenta.

Lactation Excretion in breast milk unknown/use caution

Contraindications Hypersensitivity to sulfites (commercial preparation contains sodium bisulfite); pheochromocytoma; ventricular fibrillation

Warnings/Precautions Use with caution in patients with cardiovascular disease or cardiac arrhythmias or patients with occlusive vascular disease. Correct hypovolemia and electrolytes when used in hemodynamic support. May cause increases in HR and arrhythmia. Use with caution in post-MI patients. Use with extreme caution in patients taking MAO inhibitors. Avoid extravasation; infuse into a large vein if possible. Avoid infusion into leg veins. Watch I.V. site closely. **[U.S. Boxed Warning]: If extravasation occurs, infiltrate the area with diluted phentolamine (5-10 mg in 10-15 mL of saline) with a fine hypodermic needle. Phentolamine should be administered as soon as possible after extravasation is noted.** Product may contain sodium metabisulfite.

Adverse Reactions Frequency not defined.

Most frequent:

Cardiovascular: Ectopic beats, tachycardia, anginal pain, palpitation, hypotension, vasoconstriction

Central nervous system: Headache

Gastrointestinal: Nausea and vomiting
Respiratory: Dyspnea

Infrequent:
Cardiovascular: Aberrant conduction, bradycardia, widened QRS complex, ventricular arrhythmia (high dose), gangrene (high dose), hypertension
Central nervous system: Anxiety
Endocrine & metabolic: Piloerection, serum glucose increased (usually not above normal limits)
Local: Extravasation of dopamine can cause tissue necrosis and sloughing of surrounding tissues
Ocular: Intraocular pressure increased, dilated pupils
Renal: Azotemia, polyuria

Drug Interactions

Metabolism/Transport Effects Substrate of COMT

Avoid Concomitant Use

Avoid concomitant use of DOPamine with any of the following: Inhalational Anesthetics; Iobenguane I 123; Lurasidone

Increased Effect/Toxicity

DOPamine may increase the levels/effects of: Lurasidone; Sympathomimetics

The levels/effects of DOPamine may be increased by: Atomoxetine; Cannabinoids; COMT Inhibitors; Inhalational Anesthetics; Linezolid

Decreased Effect

DOPamine may decrease the levels/effects of: Iobenguane I 123

Stability Protect from light; solutions that are darker than slightly yellow should not be used.

Mechanism of Action Stimulates both adrenergic and dopaminergic receptors, lower doses are mainly dopaminergic stimulating and produce renal and mesenteric vasodilation, higher doses also are both dopaminergic and $beta_1$-adrenergic stimulating and produce cardiac stimulation and renal vasodilation; large doses stimulate alpha-adrenergic receptors

Pharmacodynamics/Kinetics

Children: Dopamine has exhibited nonlinear kinetics in children; with medication changes, may not achieve steady-state for ~1 hour rather than 20 minutes
Onset of action: Adults: 5 minutes
Duration: Adults: <10 minutes
Metabolism: Renal, hepatic, plasma; 75% to inactive metabolites by monoamine oxidase and 25% to norepinephrine
Half-life elimination: 2 minutes
Excretion: Urine (as metabolites)
Clearance: Neonates: Varies and appears to be age related; clearance is more prolonged with combined hepatic and renal dysfunction

Dosage I.V. infusion (administration requires the use of an infusion pump):

Children: 1-20 mcg/kg/minute, maximum: 50 mcg/kg/minute continuous infusion, titrate to desired response.

Adults: 1-5 mcg/kg/minute up to 20 mcg/kg/minute, titrate to desired response (maximum: 50 mcg/kg/minute; however, doses >20 mcg/kg/minute may not have a beneficial effect on blood pressure and increase the risk of tachyarrhythmias). Infusion may be increased by 1-4 mcg/kg/minute at 10- to 30-minute intervals until optimal response is obtained.

If dosages >20-30 mcg/kg/minute are needed, a more direct-acting pressor may be more beneficial (ie, epinephrine, norepinephrine).

The hemodynamic effects of dopamine are dose dependent (however, this is relative and there is overlap of clinical effects between dosing ranges):

Low-dose: 1-3 mcg/kg/minute, increased renal blood flow and urine output
Intermediate-dose: 3-10 mcg/kg/minute, increased renal blood flow, heart rate, cardiac contractility, and cardiac output
High-dose: >10 mcg/kg/minute, alpha-adrenergic effects begin to predominate, vasoconstriction, increased blood pressure

Administration Administer into large vein to prevent the possibility of extravasation (central line administration); monitor continuously for free flow; use infusion device to control rate of flow; administration into an umbilical arterial catheter is not recommended; when discontinuing the infusion, gradually decrease the dose of dopamine (sudden discontinuation may cause hypotension).

Extravasation management: Due to short half-life, withdrawal of drug is often only necessary treatment. Use phentolamine as antidote. Mix 5 mg with 9 mL of NS; inject a small amount of this dilution into extravasated area. Blanching should reverse immediately. Monitor site. If blanching should recur, additional injections of phentolamine may be needed.

Monitoring Parameters Blood pressure, ECG, heart rate, CVP, RAP, MAP; serum glucose, renal function; urine output; if pulmonary artery catheter is in place, monitor CI, PCWP, SVR, and PVR

Additional Information Dopamine is most frequently used for treatment of hypotension because of its peripheral vasoconstrictor action. In this regard, dopamine is often used together with dobutamine and minimizes hypotension secondary to dobutamine-induced vasodilation. Thus, pressure is maintained by increased cardiac output (from dobutamine) and vasoconstriction (by dopamine). It is critical neither dopamine nor dobutamine be used in patients in the absence of correcting any hypovolemia as a cause of hypotension.

Low-dose dopamine is often used in the intensive care setting for presumed beneficial effects on renal function. However, there is no clear evidence that low-dose dopamine confers any renal or other benefit. Indeed, dopamine may act on dopamine receptors in the carotid bodies causing chemoreflex suppression. In patients with heart failure, dopamine may inhibit breathing and cause pulmonary shunting. Both these mechanisms would act to decrease minute ventilation and oxygen saturation. This could potentially be deleterious in patients with respiratory compromise and patients being weaned from ventilators.

Dosage Forms Excipient information presented when available (limited, particularly for generics); consult specific product labeling.

Infusion, premixed in D_5W, as hydrochloride: 0.8 mg/mL (250 mL, 500 mL); 1.6 mg/mL (250 mL, 500 mL); 3.2 mg/mL (250 mL)

Injection, solution, as hydrochloride: 40 mg/mL (5 mL, 10 mL); 80 mg/mL (5 mL); 160 mg/mL (5 mL)

◆ **Dopamine Hydrochloride** *see* DOPamine *on page* 544
◆ **Dopram®** *see* Doxapram *on page* 548
◆ **Doral®** *see* Quazepam *on page* 1440
◆ **Doribax®** *see* Doripenem *on page* 545

Doripenem (dore i PEN em)

Brand Names: U.S. Doribax®
Brand Names: Canada Doribax®
Index Terms S-4661
Pharmacologic Category Antibiotic, Carbapenem

Use Treatment of complicated intra-abdominal infections and complicated urinary tract infections (including pyelonephritis) due to susceptible aerobic gram-positive, aerobic gram-negative (including *Pseudomonas aeruginosa*), and anaerobic bacteria

Canadian labeling: Additional use (not in U.S. labeling): Treatment of healthcare-associated pneumonia (including ventilator-associated pneumonia)

Unlabeled Use Treatment of intravascular catheter-related bloodstream infection due to extended-spectrum β-lactamase (ESBL)-producing *Escherichia coli* and *Klebsiella* spp

Pregnancy Risk Factor B

Pregnancy Considerations Adverse events have not been observed in animal studies; therefore, the manufacturer classifies doripenem as pregnancy category B. There are no adequate and well-controlled studies completed in pregnant women.

Lactation Excretion in breast milk unknown/use caution

Contraindications Known serious hypersensitivity to doripenem or other carbapenems (eg, ertapenem, imipenem, meropenem); anaphylactic reactions to beta-lactam antibiotics

Warnings/Precautions Serious hypersensitivity reactions, including anaphylaxis, and skin reactions have been reported in patients receiving beta-lactams. Use may result in fungal or bacterial superinfection, including *C. difficile*-associated diarrhea (CDAD) and pseudomembranous colitis; CDAD has been observed >2 months postantibiotic treatment. Not indicated for the treatment of pneumonia including ventilator-associated pneumonia; decreased efficacy and increased mortality associated with use. Use with caution in patients with renal impairment; dosage adjustment required in patients with moderate-to-severe renal dysfunction. Carbapenems have been associated with CNS adverse effects, including confusional states and seizures (myoclonic); use caution with CNS disorders (eg, brain lesions and history of seizures) and adjust dose in renal impairment to avoid drug accumulation, which may increase seizure risk. May decrease divalproex sodium/valproic acid concentrations leading to breakthrough seizures; concomitant use not recommended. Administer via intravenous infusion only. Per manufacturer's labeling, investigational experience of doripenem via inhalation resulted in pneumonitis.

Adverse Reactions

>10%:

Central nervous system: Headache (4% to 16%)

Gastrointestinal: Nausea (4% to 12%), diarrhea (6% to 11%)

1% to 10%:

Dermatologic: Rash (1% to 5%; includes allergic/bullous dermatitis, erythema, macular/papular eruptions, urticaria, and erythema multiforme), pruritus (≤3%)

Gastrointestinal: Oral candidiasis (1%)

Hematologic: Anemia (2% to 10%)

Hepatic: Transaminases increased (1% to 2%)

Local: Phlebitis (4% to 8%)

Renal: Renal impairment/failure (≤1%)

Miscellaneous: Vulvomycotic infection (1% to 2%)

Postmarketing and/or case reports: Anaphylaxis, interstitial pneumonia, leukopenia, neutropenia, Stevens-Johnson syndrome, seizure, thrombocytopenia, toxic epidermal necrolysis

Drug Interactions

Metabolism/Transport Effects None known.

Avoid Concomitant Use

Avoid concomitant use of Doripenem with any of the following: BCG; Probenecid

Increased Effect/Toxicity

The levels/effects of Doripenem may be increased by: Probenecid

Decreased Effect

Doripenem may decrease the levels/effects of: BCG; Divalproex; Typhoid Vaccine; Valproic Acid

Stability Store dry powder vials at 15°C to 30°C (59°F to 86°F). Reconstitute 250 mg vial with 10 mL of SWFI or NS, and further dilute for infusion with 50 mL or 100 mL of NS or D_5W. Reconstitute 500 mg vial with 10 mL of SWFI or NS, and further dilute for infusion with 100 mL of NS or D_5W. Shake gently until clear. Reconstituted vial may be stored for up to 1 hour prior to preparation of infusion solution. Stability of solution when diluted in NS is 12 hours at room temperature or 72 hours under refrigeration; stability in D_5W is 4 hours at room temperature and 24 hours under refrigeration. To prepare a 250 mg dose using a 500 mg vial, reconstitute the 500 mg vial with 10 mL of SWFI or NS and further dilute with 100 mL of compatible solution as above, but remove and discard 55 mL from the infusion bag to leave the remaining solution containing the 250 mg dose.

Mechanism of Action Inhibits bacterial cell wall synthesis by binding to several of the penicillin-binding proteins (PBP-2, PBP-3, PBP-4), which in turn inhibits the final transpeptidation step of peptidoglycan synthesis in bacterial cell walls, thus inhibiting cell wall biosynthesis; bacteria eventually lyse due to ongoing activity of cell wall autolytic enzymes (autolysins and murein hydrolases) while cell wall assembly is arrested.

Pharmacodynamics/Kinetics **Note:** As with other time-dependent antibiotics, doripenem shows bacteriostatic effects at T> MIC <40% and bactericidal effects at T> MIC >40%. Of note, prolonged infusion time (over 4 hours) was more effective in increasing T>MIC over 40% to up to 81%. Pharmacokinetics are linear (AUC directly proportional to dose) at doses administered over 1 hour.

Distribution: Penetrates well into body fluids and tissues, including peritoneal and retroperitoneal fluids, gallbladder, bile, and urine

V_d: 16.8 L

Protein binding: 8% to 9%

Metabolism: Non-CYP-mediated metabolism via hydrolysis by dehydropeptidase-I to doripenem-M1 (inactive metabolite)

Half-life elimination: ~1 hour

Excretion: Urine (70% as unchanged drug; 15% as doripenem-M1 metabolite); feces (<1%)

Dialyzable with reduction in systemic levels by 48% to 62%.

Dosage

Note: A switch to appropriate oral antimicrobial therapy may be considered after 3 days of parenteral therapy and demonstrated clinical improvement.

Usual dosage: Adults: I.V.: 500 mg every 8 hours

Indication-specific dosing: Adults: I.V.:

Intra-abdominal infection, complicated, severe: 500 mg every 8 hours for 5-14 days. **Note:** 2010 IDSA guidelines recommend treatment duration of 4-7 days (provided source controlled). Not recommended for mild-to-moderate, community-acquired intra-abdominal infections due to risk of toxicity and the development of resistant organisms (Solomkin, 2010).

Pneumonia (healthcare-associated [HAP], including ventilator-associated [VAP]): Canadian labeling (U.S. unlabeled use [Chastre, 2008; Rea-Neto, 2008]): 500 mg every 8 hours for 7-14 days. **Note:** A VAP trial showed numerically lower cure rate (versus a comparator antibiotic) and increased mortality; doses were twofold higher than the Canadian approved dose (FDA communication, 2012).

Urinary tract infection (complicated) or pyelonephritis: 500 mg every 8 hours for 10-14 days

Intravenous catheter-related bloodstream infection (unlabeled use): 500 mg every 8 hours for 7-14 days (IDSA, 2009)

Dosing adjustment in renal impairment:

Cl_{cr} >50 mL/minute: No adjustment necessary

Cl_{cr} 30-50 mL/minute: 250 mg every 8 hours

Cl_{cr} 11-29 mL/minute: 250 mg every 12 hours

Hemodialysis: Dialyzable (~52% of dose removed during 4-hour session in ESRD patients)
Intermittent HD: 250 mg every 24 hours; if treating infections caused by ***Pseudomonas aeruginosa***, administer 500 mg every 12 hours on day 1, followed by 500 mg every 24 hours (Tanoue, 2011)
CVVHDF: 250 mg every 12 hours (Hidaka, 2010).

Administration Infuse intravenously over 1 hour. Use of 4-hour infusion has been shown to increase %T>MIC. **Note:** The Canadian labeling recommends a 4-hour infusion in late-onset ventilator-associated pneumonia (>5 days ventilation [not an approved indication in the U.S. labeling])

Monitoring Parameters Monitor for signs of anaphylaxis during first dose; periodic renal assessment; consider hematologic monitoring during prolonged therapy

Additional Information
One mechanism of resistance to doripenem is production of the Ambler's class B metallo-beta-lactamase, a potent carbapenemase produced by *Stenotrophomonas maltophilia*.

Dosage Forms Excipient information presented when available (limited, particularly for generics); consult specific product labeling.
Injection, powder for reconstitution:
Doribax®: 250 mg, 500 mg

Dornase Alfa (DOOR nase AL fa)

Brand Names: U.S. Pulmozyme®
Brand Names: Canada Pulmozyme®
Index Terms Recombinant Human Deoxyribonuclease; rhDNase
Pharmacologic Category Enzyme; Mucolytic Agent
Use Management of cystic fibrosis patients to reduce the frequency of respiratory infections that require parenteral antibiotics in patients with FVC ≥40% of predicted; in conjunction with standard therapies, to improve pulmonary function in patients with cystic fibrosis
Pregnancy Risk Factor B
Pregnancy Considerations Teratogenic effects were not observed in animal studies. There are no adequate and well-controlled studies in pregnant women.
Lactation Excretion in breast milk unknown/use caution
Contraindications Hypersensitivity to dornase alfa, Chinese hamster ovary cell products, or any component of the formulation
Warnings/Precautions Safety and efficacy have not been established for daily administration >12 months. In patients with pulmonary function <40% of normal, dornase alfa does not significantly reduce the risk of respiratory infections that require parenteral antibiotics. Safety studies included children ≥3 months, however experience is limited in children <5 years of age
Adverse Reactions Adverse events were similar in children using the PARI BABY™ nebulizer (facemask as opposed to mouthpiece) with the addition of cough (45% in children 3 months to <5 years; 30% in children 5 to ≤10 years).

>10%:
Cardiovascular: Chest pain (18% to 25%)
Central nervous system: Fever (32% in patients with FVC <40%)
Dermatologic: Rash (3% to 12%)
Respiratory: Pharyngitis (32% to 40%), rhinitis (30% in patients with FVC <40%); FVC decrease ≥10% of predicted (22% in patients with FVC <40%), dyspnea (17% in patients with FVC <40%)
Miscellaneous: Voice alteration (12% to 18%)

1% to 10%:
Gastrointestinal: Dyspepsia (≤3%)
Ocular: Conjunctivitis (1% to 5%)
Respiratory: Laryngitis (3% to 4%)
Miscellaneous: Dornase alfa serum antibodies (2% to 4%)

Postmarketing and/or case reports: Headache, urticaria

Drug Interactions
Metabolism/Transport Effects None known.
Avoid Concomitant Use There are no known interactions where it is recommended to avoid concomitant use.
Increased Effect/Toxicity There are no known significant interactions involving an increase in effect.
Decreased Effect There are no known significant interactions involving a decrease in effect.

Stability Must be stored in the refrigerator at 2°C to 8°C (36°F to 46°F) and protected from strong light.
Mechanism of Action The hallmark of cystic fibrosis lung disease is the presence of abundant, purulent airway secretions composed primarily of highly polymerized DNA. The principal source of this DNA is the nuclei of degenerating neutrophils, which is present in large concentrations in infected lung secretions. The presence of this DNA produces a viscous mucous that may contribute to the decreased mucociliary transport and persistent infections that are commonly seen in this population. Dornase alfa is a deoxyribonuclease (DNA) enzyme produced by recombinant gene technology. Dornase selectively cleaves DNA, thus reducing mucous viscosity and as a result, airflow in the lung is improved and the risk of bacterial infection may be decreased.
Pharmacodynamics/Kinetics
Onset of action: Nebulization: Enzyme levels are measured in sputum in ~15 minutes
Duration: Rapidly declines
Dosage Inhalation:
Children ≥3 months to Adults: 2.5 mg once daily through selected nebulizers; experience in children <5 years is limited
Patients unable to inhale or exhale orally throughout the entire treatment period may use Pari-Baby™ nebulizer. Some patients may benefit from twice daily administration.
Administration Nebulization: Should not be diluted or mixed with any other drugs in the nebulizer, this may inactivate the drug
Dosage Forms Excipient information presented when available (limited, particularly for generics); consult specific product labeling.
Solution, for nebulization [preservative free]:
Pulmozyme®: 2.5 mg/2.5 mL (30s) [derived from or manufactured using Chinese hamster ovary cells]

◆ **Doryx®** *see* Doxycycline *on page* 557

Dorzolamide (dor ZOLE a mide)

Brand Names: U.S. Trusopt®
Brand Names: Canada Trusopt®
Index Terms Dorzolamide Hydrochloride
Pharmacologic Category Carbonic Anhydrase Inhibitor; Ophthalmic Agent, Antiglaucoma
Use Treatment of elevated intraocular pressure in patients with ocular hypertension or open-angle glaucoma
Pregnancy Risk Factor C
Dosage Children and Adults: Reduction of intraocular pressure: Instill 1 drop in the affected eye(s) 3 times/day
Additional Information Complete prescribing information for this medication should be consulted for additional detail.
Dosage Forms Excipient information presented when available (limited, particularly for generics); consult specific product labeling.
Solution, ophthalmic [drops]: 2% (10 mL)
Trusopt®: 2% (10 mL) [contains benzalkonium chloride]

Dosage Forms: Canada Excipient information presented when available (limited, particularly for generics); consult specific product labeling.
Solution, ophthalmic [drops; preservative free]:
Trusopt®: 2% (0.2 mL)

Dorzolamide and Timolol
(dor ZOLE a mide & TYE moe lole)

Brand Names: U.S. Cosopt®
Brand Names: Canada Apo-Dorzo-Timop; Cosopt®; Sandoz-Dorzolamide/Timolol
Index Terms Timolol and Dorzolamide
Pharmacologic Category Beta-Adrenergic Blocker, Nonselective; Carbonic Anhydrase Inhibitor; Ophthalmic Agent, Antiglaucoma
Use Treatment of elevated intraocular pressure in patients with ocular hypertension or open-angle glaucoma
Pregnancy Risk Factor C
Dosage Ophthalmic: Children ≥2 years and Adults: Instill 1 drop in affected eye(s) twice daily
Additional Information Complete prescribing information for this medication should be consulted for additional detail.
Dosage Forms Excipient information presented when available (limited, particularly for generics); consult specific product labeling. [DSC] = Discontinued product; **Note:** Strength expressed as base
Solution, ophthalmic [drops]: Dorzolamide hydrochloride 2% and timolol maleate 0.5% (10 mL)
Cosopt®: Dorzolamide hydrochloride 2% and timolol maleate 0.5% (5 mL [DSC]; 10 mL) [contains benzalkonium chloride]
Dosage Forms: Canada Excipient information presented when available (limited, particularly for generics); consult specific product labeling.
Solution, ophthalmic [drops; preservative free]:
Cosopt®: Dorzolamide hydrochloride 2% and timolol maleate 0.5% (0.2 mL) (15s)

◆ **Dorzolamide Hydrochloride** *see* Dorzolamide *on page 547*
◆ **DOSS** *see* Docusate *on page 537*
◆ **Dostinex® (Can)** *see* Cabergoline *on page 259*
◆ **Double Tussin DM [OTC]** *see* Guaifenesin and Dextromethorphan *on page 810*
◆ **Dovobet® (Can)** *see* Calcipotriene and Betamethasone *on page 261*
◆ **Dovonex®** *see* Calcipotriene *on page 261*

Doxapram (DOKS a pram)

Brand Names: U.S. Dopram®
Index Terms Doxapram Hydrochloride
Pharmacologic Category Respiratory Stimulant; Stimulant
Use Respiratory and CNS stimulant for respiratory depression secondary to anesthesia, drug-induced CNS depression; acute hypercapnia secondary to COPD
Pregnancy Risk Factor B
Dosage
Respiratory depression following anesthesia:
Intermittent injection: Initial: 0.5-1 mg/kg; may repeat at 5-minute intervals (only in patients who demonstrate initial response); maximum total dose: 2 mg/kg
I.V. infusion: Initial: 5 mg/minute until adequate response or adverse effects seen; decrease to 1-3 mg/minute; maximum total dose: 4 mg/kg
Drug-induced CNS depression:
Intermittent injection: Initial: Priming dose of 1-2 mg/kg, repeat after 5 minutes; may repeat at 1-2 hour intervals (until sustained consciousness); maximum: 3 g/day. May repeat in 24 hours if necessary.
I.V. infusion: Initial: Priming dose of 1-2 mg/kg, repeat after 5 minutes. If no response, wait 1-2 hours and repeat. If some stimulation is noted, initiate infusion at 1-3 mg/minute (depending on size of patient/depth of CNS depression); suspend infusion if patient begins to awaken. Infusion should not be continued for >2 hours. May reinstitute infusion as described above, including bolus, after rest interval of 30 minutes to 2 hours; maximum: 3 g/day
Acute hypercapnia secondary to COPD: I.V. infusion: Initial: Initiate infusion at 1-2 mg/minute (depending on size of patient/depth of CNS depression); may increase to maximum rate of 3 mg/minute; infusion should not be continued for >2 hours. Monitor arterial blood gases prior to initiation of infusion and at 30-minute intervals during the infusion (to identify possible development of acidosis/CO_2 retention). Additional infusions are not recommended (per manufacturer).
Additional Information Complete prescribing information for this medication should be consulted for additional detail.
Dosage Forms Excipient information presented when available (limited, particularly for generics); consult specific product labeling.
Injection, solution, as hydrochloride: 20 mg/mL (20 mL)
Dopram®: 20 mg/mL (20 mL) [contains benzyl alcohol]

◆ **Doxapram Hydrochloride** *see* Doxapram *on page 548*

Doxazosin (doks AY zoe sin)

Brand Names: U.S. Cardura®; Cardura® XL
Brand Names: Canada Alti-Doxazosin; Apo-Doxazosin®; Cardura-1™; Cardura-2™; Cardura-4™; Gen-Doxazosin; Mylan-Doxazosin; Novo-Doxazosin
Index Terms Doxazosin Mesylate
Pharmacologic Category Alpha$_1$ Blocker
Additional Appendix Information
Beers Criteria – Potentially Inappropriate Medications for Geriatrics *on page 1973*
Use
Immediate release formulation: Treatment of hypertension as monotherapy or in conjunction with diuretics, ACE inhibitors, beta-blockers, or calcium antagonists
Immediate release and extended release formulations: Treatment of urinary outflow obstruction and/or obstructive and irritative symptoms associated with benign prostatic hyperplasia (BPH)
Unlabeled Use Pediatric hypertension
Pregnancy Risk Factor C
Pregnancy Considerations Adverse events were observed in some animal reproduction studies. Delayed postnatal development was also noted. There are no adequate and well-controlled studies in pregnant women.
Lactation Excretion in breast milk unknown/use caution
Contraindications Hypersensitivity to quinazolines (prazosin, terazosin), doxazosin, or any component of the formulation
Warnings/Precautions Can cause significant orthostatic hypotension and syncope, especially with first dose; anticipate a similar effect if therapy is interrupted for a few days, if dosage is rapidly increased, or if another antihypertensive drug (particularly vasodilators) or a PDE-5 inhibitor is introduced. Discontinue if symptoms of angina occur or worsen. Patients should be cautioned about performing hazardous tasks when starting new therapy or adjusting dosage upward. Prostate cancer should be ruled out

before starting for BPH. Use with caution in mild-to-moderate hepatic impairment; not recommended in severe dysfunction. Intraoperative floppy iris syndrome has been observed in cataract surgery patients who were on or were previously treated with alpha$_1$-blockers. Causality has not been established and there appears to be no benefit in discontinuing alpha-blocker therapy prior to surgery. May be inappropriate in the elderly due to potential for dry mouth, hypotension, and urinary problems (Beers Criteria).

The extended release formulation consists of drug within a nondeformable matrix; following drug release/absorption, the matrix/shell is expelled in the stool. The use of nondeformable products in patients with known stricture/narrowing of the GI tract has been associated with symptoms of obstruction. Use caution in patients with increased GI retention (eg, chronic constipation) as doxazosin exposure may be increased. Extended release formulation is not indicated for use in women or for the treatment of hypertension.

Adverse Reactions Note: Type and frequency of adverse reactions reflect combined data from BPH and hypertension trials and immediate release and extended release products.

>10%: Central nervous system: Dizziness (5% to 19%), headache (5% to 14%)

1% to 10%:

Cardiovascular: Orthostatic hypotension (dose related; 0.3% up to 2%), edema (3% to 4%), hypotension (1% to 2%), palpitation (1% to 2%), chest pain (1% to 2%), arrhythmia (1%), syncope (2%), flushing (1%)

Central nervous system: Fatigue (8% to 12%), somnolence (1% to 5%), nervousness (2%), pain (2%), vertigo (2% to 4%), insomnia (1%), anxiety (1%), paresthesia (1%), movement disorder (1%), ataxia (1%), hypertonia (1%), depression (1%)

Dermatologic: Rash (1%), pruritus (1%)

Endocrine & metabolic: Sexual dysfunction (2%)

Gastrointestinal: Abdominal pain (2%), diarrhea (2%), dyspepsia (1% to 2%), nausea (1% to 3%), xerostomia (1% to 2%), constipation (1%), flatulence (1%)

Genitourinary: Urinary tract infection (1%), impotence (1%), polyuria (2%), incontinence (1%)

Neuromuscular & skeletal: Back pain (2% to 3%), weakness (1% to 7%), arthritis (1%), muscle weakness (1%), myalgia (≤1%), muscle cramps (1%)

Ocular: Abnormal vision (1% to 2%), conjunctivitis (1%)

Otic: Tinnitus (1%)

Respiratory: Respiratory tract infection (5%), rhinitis (3%), dyspnea (1% to 3%), respiratory disorder (1%), epistaxis (1%)

Miscellaneous: Diaphoresis increased (1%), flu-like syndrome (1%)

<1% (Limited to important or life-threatening): Abnormal thinking, agitation, allergic reaction, amnesia, angina, anorexia, appetite increased, bradycardia, breast pain, bronchospasm, cerebrovascular accident, cholestasis, confusion, depersonalization, emotional lability, fecal incontinence, fever, gastroenteritis, gout, gynecomastia, hematuria, hepatitis, hypoesthesia, hypokalemia, infection, intraoperative floppy iris syndrome (cataract surgery), jaundice, leukopenia, liver function tests increased, lymphadenopathy, MI, micturition abnormality, migraine, neutropenia, nocturia, pallor, paranoia, paresis, paresthesia, parosmia, peripheral ischemia, priapism, purpura, renal calculus, rigors stroke, syncope, tachycardia, thrombocytopenia, urticaria, vomiting

Drug Interactions

Metabolism/Transport Effects None known.

Avoid Concomitant Use

Avoid concomitant use of Doxazosin with any of the following: Alpha1-Blockers

Increased Effect/Toxicity

Doxazosin may increase the levels/effects of: Alpha1-Blockers; Amifostine; Antihypertensives; Calcium Channel Blockers; Hypotensive Agents; RiTUXimab

The levels/effects of Doxazosin may be increased by: Beta-Blockers; Diazoxide; Herbs (Hypotensive Properties); MAO Inhibitors; Pentoxifylline; Phosphodiesterase 5 Inhibitors; Prostacyclin Analogues

Decreased Effect

The levels/effects of Doxazosin may be decreased by: Herbs (Hypertensive Properties); Methylphenidate; Yohimbine

Ethanol/Nutrition/Herb Interactions Herb/Nutraceutical: Avoid dong quai if using for hypertension (has estrogenic activity). Avoid ephedra, yohimbe, ginseng (may worsen hypertension). Avoid saw palmetto when used for BPH (due to limited experience with this combination). Avoid garlic (may have increased antihypertensive effect).

Stability Store at 25°C (77°F); excursions permitted to 15°C to 30°C (59°F to 86°F).

Mechanism of Action

Hypertension: Competitively inhibits postsynaptic alpha$_1$-adrenergic receptors which results in vasodilation of veins and arterioles and a decrease in total peripheral resistance and blood pressure; ~50% as potent on a weight by weight basis as prazosin.

BPH: Competitively inhibits postsynaptic alpha$_1$-adrenergic receptors in prostatic stromal and bladder neck tissues. This reduces the sympathetic tone-induced urethral stricture causing BPH symptoms.

Pharmacodynamics/Kinetics Not significantly affected by increased age

Duration: >24 hours

Protein binding: ~98%

Metabolism: Extensively hepatic to active metabolites; primarily via CYP3A4; secondary pathways involve CYP2D6 and 2C19

Bioavailability: Immediate release: ~65%; Extended release relative to immediate release: 54% to 59%

Half-life elimination: Immediate release: ~22 hours; Extended release: 15-19 hours

Time to peak, serum: Immediate release: 2-3 hours; Extended release: 8-9 hours

Excretion: Feces (63%, primarily as metabolites); urine (9%, primarily as metabolites)

Dosage Oral:

Children (unlabeled use): Hypertension: Immediate release: Initial: 1 mg once daily; maximum: 4 mg/day

Adults:

Immediate release: 1 mg once daily in morning or evening; may be increased to 2 mg once daily. Thereafter titrate upwards, if needed, over several weeks, balancing therapeutic benefit with doxazosin-induced postural hypotension.

BPH: Goal: 4-8 mg/day; maximum dose: 8 mg/day

Hypertension: Maximum dose: 16 mg/day

Reinitiation of therapy: If therapy is discontinued for several days, restart at 1 mg dose and titrate as before

Extended release: BPH: 4 mg once daily with breakfast; titrate based on response and tolerability every 3-4 weeks to maximum recommended dose of 8 mg/day

Reinitiation of therapy: If therapy is discontinued for several days, restart at 4 mg dose and titrate as before.

Conversion to extended release from immediate release: Omit final evening dose of immediate release prior to starting morning dosing with extended release product; initiate extended release product using 4 mg once daily

Elderly: Hypertension: Consider lower initial doses (eg, immediate release: 0.5 mg once daily) and titrate to response (Aronow, 2011)

Dosing adjustment in hepatic impairment: Use with caution in mild-to-moderate hepatic dysfunction. Do not use with severe impairment.

Dietary Considerations Cardura® XL: Take with morning meal.

Administration Cardura® XL: Tablets should be swallowed whole; do not crush, chew, or divide. Administer with morning meal.

Monitoring Parameters Blood pressure, standing and sitting/supine; syncope may occur usually within 90 minutes of the initial dose

Additional Information First-dose hypotension occurs less frequently with doxazosin as compared to prazosin; this may be due to its slower onset of action.

Dosage Forms Excipient information presented when available (limited, particularly for generics); consult specific product labeling.

Tablet, oral: 1 mg, 2 mg, 4 mg, 8 mg
Cardura®: 1 mg, 2 mg, 4 mg, 8 mg [scored]
Tablet, extended release, oral:
Cardura® XL: 4 mg, 8 mg

◆ **Doxazosin Mesylate** *see* Doxazosin *on page 548*

Doxepin (Systemic) (DOKS e pin)

Brand Names: U.S. Silenor®

Brand Names: Canada Apo-Doxepin®; Doxepine; Novo-Doxepin; Sinequan®

Index Terms Doxepin Hydrochloride

Pharmacologic Category Antidepressant, Tricyclic (Tertiary Amine)

Additional Appendix Information

Antidepressant Agents *on page 1874*
Beers Criteria – Potentially Inappropriate Medications for Geriatrics *on page 1973*

Use Depression; treatment of insomnia (with difficulty of sleep maintenance)

Unlabeled Use Analgesic for certain chronic and neuropathic pain; anxiety

Pregnancy Risk Factor C

Pregnancy Considerations Decreased fetal body weight and fetal structural abnormalities were observed in animal reproduction studies at doses greater than the maximum recommended human dose. There are no adequate and well-controlled studies in pregnant women.

Lactation Enters breast milk/use caution (AAP rates "of concern"; AAP 2001 update pending)

Medication Guide Available Yes

Contraindications Hypersensitivity to doxepin, drugs from similar chemical class, or any component of the formulation; narrow-angle glaucoma; urinary retention; use of MAO inhibitors within 14 days

Warnings/Precautions [U.S. Boxed Warning]: Antidepressants increase the risk of suicidal thinking and behavior in children, adolescents, and young adults (18-24 years of age) with major depressive disorder (MDD) and other psychiatric disorders; consider risk prior to prescribing. Short-term studies did not show an increased risk in patients >24 years of age and showed a decreased risk in patients ≥65 years. Closely monitor for clinical worsening, suicidality, or unusual changes in behavior; the patient's family or caregiver should be instructed to closely observe the patient and communicate condition with healthcare provider. A medication guide should be dispensed with each prescription. **Doxepin is approved for treatment of depression in adolescents.**

The possibility of a suicide attempt is inherent in major depression and may persist until remission occurs. Monitor for worsening of depression or suicidality, especially during initiation of therapy (generally first 1-2 months) or with dose increases or decreases. Use caution in high-risk patients. Worsening depression and severe abrupt suicidality that are not part of the presenting symptoms may require discontinuation or modification of drug therapy. The patient's family or caregiver should be alerted to monitor patients for the emergence of suicidality and associated behaviors (such as agitation, irritability, hostility, impulsivity, and hypomania) and call healthcare provider.

Risk of suicidal behavior may be increased regardless of doxepin dose; antidepressant doses of doxepin are 10- to 100-fold higher than doses for insomnia.

May worsen psychosis in some patients or precipitate a shift to mania or hypomania in patients with bipolar disorder. Patients presenting with depressive symptoms should be screened for bipolar disorder. Monotherapy in patients with bipolar disorder should be avoided. **Doxepin is not FDA approved for the treatment of bipolar depression.**

Should only be used for insomnia after evaluation of potential causes of sleep disturbance. Failure of sleep disturbance to resolve after 7-10 days may indicate psychiatric or medical illness. An increased risk for hazardous sleep-related activities has been noted; discontinue use with any sleep-related episodes. The risks of sedative and anticholinergic effects are high relative to other antidepressant agents. Doxepin frequently causes sedation, which may result in impaired performance of tasks requiring alertness (eg, operating machinery or driving). Sedative effects may be additive with other CNS depressants and/or ethanol. Also use caution in patients with benign prostatic hyperplasia, xerostomia, visual problems, constipation, or history of bowel obstruction.

May cause orthostatic hypotension or conduction disturbances (risks are moderate relative to other antidepressants). Use with caution in patients with a history of cardiovascular disease (including previous MI, stroke, tachycardia, or conduction abnormalities). Use with caution in patients with respiratory compromise or sleep apnea; use is generally not recommended with severe sleep apnea. Consider discontinuation, when possible, prior to elective surgery. Therapy should not be abruptly discontinued in patients receiving high doses for prolonged periods.

Use caution in patients with a previous seizure disorder or condition predisposing to seizures such as brain damage, alcoholism, or concurrent therapy with other drugs which lower the seizure threshold. Use with caution in hyperthyroid patients or those receiving thyroid supplementation. Use with caution in patients with hepatic or renal dysfunction. Use as an antidepressant in the elderly may be inappropriate due to potent anticholinergic and sedating effects (Beers Criteria).

Adverse Reactions Actual frequency may be dependent on diagnosis.

Cardiovascular: Flushing, hypertension (<3%), hypotension, tachycardia
Central nervous system: Ataxia, chills, confusion, disorientation, dizziness, drowsiness, fatigue, hallucinations, headache, seizure, somnolence/sedation (6% to 9%)
Dermatologic: Alopecia, photosensitivity, pruritus, rash
Endocrine & metabolic: Blood sugar increased/decreased, breast enlargement, galactorrhea, gynecomastia, libido increased/decreased, SIADH

Gastrointestinal: Anorexia, aphthous stomatitis, constipation, diarrhea, gastroenteritis (≤2%), indigestion, nausea (2%), trouble with gums, unpleasant taste, vomiting, weight gain, xerostomia; lower esophageal sphincter tone decrease may cause GE reflux
Genitourinary: Testicular edema, urinary retention
Hematologic: Agranulocytosis, eosinophilia, leukopenia, purpura, thrombocytopenia, purpura
Hepatic: Jaundice
Neuromuscular & skeletal: Extrapyramidal symptoms, numbness, paresthesia, tardive dyskinesia, tremor, weakness
Ocular: Blurred vision
Otic: Tinnitus
Respiratory: Asthma exacerbation, nasopharyngitis/upper respiratory tract infection (≤4%)
Miscellaneous: Allergic reactions, diaphoresis (excessive)
<1% (Limited to important or life-threatening): Abdominal pain, anemia, arthralgia, atrioventricular block, back pain, blepharospasm, chest pain, complex sleep-related behavior (sleep-driving, cooking or eating food, making phone calls), diplopia, dyspepsia, gingival recession, hematochezia, hyperbilirubinemia, hypermagnesemia, hypersensitivity, hypoacusis, infection, lacrimation decreased, lip blister, motion sickness, myalgia, palpitations, peripheral edema, tympanic membrane perforation, ventricular extrasystoles

Drug Interactions

Metabolism/Transport Effects **Substrate** of CYP1A2 (minor), CYP2C19 (minor), CYP2D6 (major), CYP3A4 (minor); **Note:** Assignment of Major/Minor substrate status based on clinically relevant drug interaction potential

Avoid Concomitant Use

Avoid concomitant use of Doxepin (Systemic) with any of the following: Artemether; Dronedarone; Iobenguane I 123; Lumefantrine; MAO Inhibitors; Methylene Blue; Nilotinib; Pimozide; QUEtiapine; QuiNINE; Tetrabenazine; Thioridazine; Toremifene; Vandetanib; Vemurafenib; Ziprasidone

Increased Effect/Toxicity

Doxepin (Systemic) may increase the levels/effects of: Alpha-/Beta-Agonists (Direct-Acting); Alpha1-Agonists; Amphetamines; Anticholinergics; Aspirin; Beta2-Agonists; Desmopressin; Dronedarone; Methylene Blue; Metoclopramide; NSAID (COX-2 Inhibitor); NSAID (Nonselective); Pimozide; QTc-Prolonging Agents; QuiNIDine; QuiNINE; Serotonin Modulators; Sodium Phosphates; Sulfonylureas; Tetrabenazine; Thioridazine; Toremifene; TraMADol; Vandetanib; Vemurafenib; Vitamin K Antagonists; Yohimbine; Ziprasidone

The levels/effects of Doxepin (Systemic) may be increased by: Abiraterone Acetate; Alfuzosin; Altretamine; Antipsychotics; Artemether; BuPROPion; Chloroquine; Cimetidine; Cinacalcet; Ciprofloxacin; Ciprofloxacin (Systemic); Conivaptan; CYP2D6 Inhibitors (Moderate); CYP2D6 Inhibitors (Strong); Dexmethylphenidate; Divalproex; DULoxetine; Gadobutrol; Indacaterol; Linezolid; Lithium; Lumefantrine; MAO Inhibitors; Methylphenidate; Metoclopramide; Nilotinib; Pramlintide; Protease Inhibitors; QUEtiapine; QuiNIDine; QuiNINE; Selective Serotonin Reuptake Inhibitors; Terbinafine; Terbinafine (Systemic); Valproic Acid

Decreased Effect

Doxepin (Systemic) may decrease the levels/effects of: Acetylcholinesterase Inhibitors (Central); Alpha2-Agonists; Iobenguane I 123

The levels/effects of Doxepin (Systemic) may be decreased by: Acetylcholinesterase Inhibitors (Central); Barbiturates; CarBAMazepine; Cyproterone; Peginterferon Alfa-2b; St Johns Wort; Tocilizumab

Ethanol/Nutrition/Herb Interactions
Ethanol: May increase CNS depression; monitor for increased effects with coadministration. Caution patients about effects.
Food: A high-fat meal increases the bioavailability of Silenor® and delays the peak plasma concentration by ~3 hours
Herb/Nutraceutical: Avoid valerian, St John's wort, SAMe, kava kava (may increase risk of serotonin syndrome and/or excessive sedation).

Stability Store at 20°C to 25°C (68°F to 77°F). Protect from light.

Mechanism of Action Increases the synaptic concentration of serotonin and norepinephrine in the central nervous system by inhibition of their reuptake by the presynaptic neuronal membrane; antagonizes the histamine (H_1) receptor for sleep maintenance

Pharmacodynamics/Kinetics
Onset of action: Peak effect: Antidepressant: Usually >2 weeks; Anxiolytic: may occur sooner
Protein binding: ~80%
Metabolism: Hepatic via CYP2C19 and 2D6; metabolites include N-desmethyldoxepin (active)
Half-life elimination: Adults: Doxepin: ~15 hours; N-desmethyldoxepin: 31 hours
Time to peak, serum: Hypnotic: 3.5 hours
Excretion: Urine (<3% as unchanged drug or N-desmethyldoxepin)

Dosage Oral:
Depression or anxiety (entire daily dose may be given at bedtime):
Adults: Initial: 25-150 mg/day at bedtime or in 2-3 divided doses; may gradually increase up to 300 mg/day; single dose should not exceed 150 mg; select patients may respond to 25-50 mg/day
Elderly: Initial: 10-25 mg at bedtime; increase by 10-25 mg every 3 days for inpatients and weekly for outpatients if tolerated. Rarely does the maximum dose required exceed 75 mg/day; a single bedtime dose is recommended.
Insomnia (Silenor®):
Adults: 3-6 mg once daily 30 minutes prior to bedtime; maximum dose: 6 mg/day
Elderly: 3 mg once daily; increase to 6 mg once daily if clinically needed
Dosing adjustment in hepatic impairment: Use a lower dose and adjust gradually
Silenor®: Initial: 3 mg once daily

Administration Oral: Do not mix oral concentrate with carbonated beverages (physically incompatible).
Silenor®: Administer within 30 minutes prior to bedtime; do not take within 3 hours of food

Monitoring Parameters Monitor blood pressure and pulse rate prior to and during initial therapy; monitor mental status, suicidal ideation (especially at the beginning of therapy or when doses are increased or decreased); weight; ECG in older adults

Insomnia: Re-evaluate diagnosis if insomnia does not remit within 7-10 days of treatment.

Reference Range Proposed therapeutic concentration (doxepin plus desmethyldoxepin): 110-250 ng/mL. Toxic concentration (doxepin plus desmethyldoxepin): >500 ng/mL. Utility of serum level monitoring is controversial.

Test Interactions Increased glucose

Dosage Forms Excipient information presented when available (limited, particularly for generics); consult specific product labeling.
Capsule, oral: 10 mg, 25 mg, 50 mg, 75 mg, 100 mg, 150 mg
Solution, oral [concentrate]: 10 mg/mL (118 mL, 120 mL)
Tablet, oral:
Silenor®: 3 mg, 6 mg

Doxepin (Topical) (DOKS e pin)

Brand Names: U.S. Prudoxin™; Zonalon®

Brand Names: Canada Zonalon®

Index Terms Doxepin Hydrochloride

Pharmacologic Category Topical Skin Product

Use Short-term (<8 days) management of moderate pruritus in adults with atopic dermatitis or lichen simplex chronicus

Unlabeled Use Cream: Treatment of burning mouth syndrome and neuropathic pain

Pregnancy Risk Factor B

Dosage

Oral: Topical: Burning mouth syndrome (unlabeled use): Cream: Apply 3-4 times daily

Topical: Pruritus: Adults and Elderly: Apply a thin film 4 times/day with at least 3- to 4-hour interval between applications; not recommended for use >8 days. **Note:** Low-dose (25-50 mg) oral administration has also been used to treat pruritus, but systemic effects are increased.

Additional Information Complete prescribing information for this medication should be consulted for additional detail.

Dosage Forms Excipient information presented when available (limited, particularly for generics); consult specific product labeling.

Cream, topical, as hydrochloride:

Prudoxin™: 5% (45 g) [contains benzyl alcohol]

Zonalon®: 5% (30 g, 45 g) [contains benzyl alcohol]

◆ **Doxepine (Can)** *see* Doxepin (Systemic) *on page 550*

◆ **Doxepin Hydrochloride** *see* Doxepin (Systemic) *on page 550*

◆ **Doxepin Hydrochloride** *see* Doxepin (Topical) *on page 552*

Doxercalciferol (doks er kal si fe FEER ole)

Brand Names: U.S. Hectorol®

Brand Names: Canada Hectorol®

Index Terms 1α-Hydroxyergocalciferol

Pharmacologic Category Vitamin D Analog

Use Treatment of secondary hyperparathyroidism in patients with chronic kidney disease

Pregnancy Risk Factor B

Dosage

Oral:

Dialysis patients: Dose should be titrated to lower iPTH to 150-300 pg/mL; dose is adjusted at 8-week intervals (maximum dose: 20 mcg 3 times/week)

Initial dose: iPTH >400 pg/mL: 10 mcg 3 times/week at dialysis

Dose titration:

iPTH level decreased by 50% and >300 pg/mL: Dose can be increased to 12.5 mcg 3 times/week for 8 more weeks; this titration process can continue at 8-week intervals; each increase should be by 2.5 mcg/dose

iPTH level 150-300 pg/mL: Maintain current dose

iPTH level <100 pg/mL: Suspend doxercalciferol for 1 week; resume at a reduced dose; decrease each dose (not weekly dose) by at least 2.5 mcg

Predialysis patients: Dose should be titrated to lower iPTH to 35-70 pg/mL with stage 3 disease or to 70-110 pg/mL with stage 4 disease: Dose may be adjusted at 2-week intervals (maximum dose: 3.5 mcg/day)

Initial dose: 1 mcg/day

Dose titration:

iPTH level >70 pg/mL with stage 3 disease or >110 pg/mL with stage 4 disease: Increase dose by 0.5 mcg every 2 weeks as necessary

iPTH level 35-70 pg/mL with stage 3 disease or 70-110 pg/mL with stage 4 disease: Maintain current dose

iPTH level is <35 pg/mL with stage 3 disease or <70 pg/mL with stage 4 disease: Suspend doxercalciferol for 1 week, then resume at a reduced dose (at least 0.5 mcg lower)

I.V.:

Dialysis patients: Dose should be titrated to lower iPTH to 150-300 pg/mL; dose is adjusted at 8-week intervals (maximum dose: 18 mcg/week)

Initial dose: iPTH level >400 pg/mL: 4 mcg 3 times/week after dialysis, administered as a bolus dose

Dose titration:

iPTH level decreased by <50% and >300 pg/mL: Dose can be increased by 1-2 mcg at 8-week intervals, as necessary

iPTH level decreased by >50% and >300 pg/mL: Maintain current dose

iPTH level 150-300 pg/mL: Maintain current dose

iPTH level <100 pg/mL: Suspend doxercalciferol for 1 week; resume at a reduced dose (at least 1 mcg lower)

Hypercalcemia, hyperphosphatemia, or serum calcium times phosphorus product >55 mg^2/dL^2: Decrease or suspend dose and/or adjust dose of phosphate binders; if dose is suspended, resume at a reduced dose (at least 1 mcg lower)

Dosage adjustment in hepatic impairment: Use with caution; no guidelines for dosage adjustment

Additional Information Complete prescribing information for this medication should be consulted for additional detail.

Dosage Forms Excipient information presented when available (limited, particularly for generics); consult specific product labeling.

Capsule, softgel, oral:

Hectorol®: 0.5 mcg, 1 mcg, 2.5 mcg [contains coconut oil]

Injection, solution:

Hectorol®: 2 mcg/mL (1 mL, 2 mL) [contains edetate disodium, ethanol]

◆ **Doxidan® [OTC]** *see* Bisacodyl *on page 219*

◆ **Doxil®** *see* DOXOrubicin (Liposomal) *on page 555*

DOXOrubicin (doks oh ROO bi sin)

Brand Names: U.S. Adriamycin®

Brand Names: Canada Adriamycin®; Doxorubicin Hydrochloride Injection

Index Terms ADR (error-prone abbreviation); Adria; Conventional Doxorubicin; Doxorubicin Hydrochloride; Hydroxydaunomycin Hydrochloride; Hydroxyldaunorubicin Hydrochloride

Pharmacologic Category Antineoplastic Agent, Anthracycline

Use Treatment of acute lymphocytic leukemia (ALL), acute myeloid leukemia (AML), Hodgkin's disease, malignant lymphoma, soft tissue and bone sarcomas, thyroid cancer, small cell lung cancer, breast cancer, gastric cancer, ovarian cancer, bladder cancer, neuroblastoma, and Wilms' tumor

Unlabeled Use Treatment of multiple myeloma, endometrial carcinoma, uterine sarcoma, head and neck cancer, liver cancer, kidney cancer

Pregnancy Risk Factor D

Pregnancy Considerations Teratogenicity and embryotoxicity were observed in animal studies. There are no adequate and well-controlled studies in pregnant women. Advise patients to avoid becoming pregnant (females) and to avoid causing pregnancy (males) during treatment. According to the National Comprehensive Cancer Network (NCCN) breast cancer guidelines, doxorubicin, if indicated, may be administered to pregnant women with breast cancer as part of a combination chemotherapy regimen, although chemotherapy should not be administered during the first trimester or after 35 weeks gestation.

Lactation Enters breast milk/not recommended

Contraindications Hypersensitivity to doxorubicin, any component of the formulation, or to other anthracyclines or anthracenediones; recent MI, severe myocardial insufficiency, severe arrhythmia; previous therapy with high cumulative doses of doxorubicin, daunorubicin, idarubicin, or other anthracycline and anthracenediones; baseline neutrophil count <1500/mm^3; severe hepatic impairment

Warnings/Precautions Hazardous agent - use appropriate precautions for handling and disposal. **[U.S. Boxed Warning]: May cause cumulative, dose-related, myocardial toxicity (early or delayed).** Cardiotoxicity is dose-limiting. Total cumulative dose should take into account previous or concomitant treatment with cardiotoxic agents or irradiation of chest. The incidence of irreversible myocardial toxicity increases as the total cumulative (lifetime) dosages approach 450-500 mg/m^2. Although the risk increases with cumulative dose, irreversible cardiotoxicity may occur at any dose level. Patients with pre-existing heart disease, hypertension, concurrent administration of other antineoplastic agents, prior or concurrent chest irradiation, advanced age; and infants and children are at increased risk. Alternative administration schedules (weekly or continuous infusions) have are associated with less cardiotoxicity Baseline and periodic monitoring of ECG and LVEF (with either ECHO or MUGA scan) is recommended. **[U.S. Boxed Warnings]: Reduce dose in patients with impaired hepatic function; dose-limiting severe myelosuppression (primarily leukopenia and neutropenia) may occur. Secondary acute myelogenous leukemia and myelodysplastic syndrome have been reported following treatment.** May cause tumor lysis syndrome and hyperuricemia (in patients with rapidly growing tumors).

Children are at increased risk for developing delayed cardiotoxicity; follow-up cardiac function monitoring is recommended. Doxorubicin may contribute to prepubertal growth failure in children; may also contribute to gonadal impairment (usually temporary). Radiation recall pneumonitis has been reported in children receiving concomitant dactinomycin and doxorubicin. **[U.S. Boxed Warnings]: For I.V. administration only. Potent vesicant; if extravasation occurs, severe local tissue damage leading to ulceration, necrosis, and pain may occur. Should be administered under the supervision of an experienced cancer chemotherapy physician.** Use caution when selecting product for preparation and dispensing; indications, dosages and adverse event profiles differ between conventional doxorubicin hydrochloride solution and doxorubicin liposomal. Both formulations are the same concentration. As a result, serious errors have occurred.

Adverse Reactions Frequency not defined.

Cardiovascular:

Acute cardiotoxicity: Atrioventricular block, bradycardia, bundle branch block, ECG abnormalities, extrasystoles (atrial or ventricular), sinus tachycardia, ST-T wave changes, supraventricular tachycardia, tachyarrhythmia, ventricular tachycardia

Delayed cardiotoxicity: LVEF decreased, CHF (manifestations include ascites, cardiomegaly, dyspnea, edema, gallop rhythm, hepatomegaly, oliguria, pleural effusion, pulmonary edema, tachycardia); myocarditis, pericarditis

Central nervous system: Malaise

Dermatologic: Alopecia, itching, photosensitivity, radiation recall, rash; discoloration of saliva, sweat, or tears

Endocrine & metabolic: Amenorrhea, dehydration, infertility (may be temporary), hyperuricemia

Gastrointestinal: Abdominal pain, anorexia, colon necrosis, diarrhea, GI ulceration, mucositis, nausea, vomiting

Genitourinary: Discoloration of urine

Hematologic: Leukopenia/neutropenia (75%; nadir: 10-14 days; recovery: by day 21); thrombocytopenia and anemia

Local: Skin "flare" at injection site, urticaria

Neuromuscular & skeletal: Weakness

Postmarketing and/or case reports: Anaphylaxis, azoospermia, bilirubin increased, coma (when in combination with cisplatin or vincristine), conjunctivitis, fever, gonadal impairment (children), growth failure (prepubertal), hepatitis, hyperpigmentation (nail, skin & oral mucosa), infection, keratitis, lacrimation, myelodysplastic syndrome, neutropenic fever, neutropenic typhlitis, oligospermia, peripheral neurotoxicity (with intra-arterial doxorubicin), phlebosclerosis, radiation recall pneumonitis (children), secondary acute myelogenous leukemia, seizure (when in combination with cisplatin or vincristine), sepsis, shock, Stevens-Johnson syndrome, systemic hypersensitivity (including urticaria, pruritus, angioedema, dysphagia, and dyspnea), toxic epidermal necrolysis, transaminases increased, urticaria

Drug Interactions

Metabolism/Transport Effects Substrate of CYP2D6 (major), CYP3A4 (major), P-glycoprotein; **Note:** Assignment of Major/Minor substrate status based on clinically relevant drug interaction potential; **Inhibits** CYP2B6 (moderate), CYP2D6 (weak), CYP3A4 (weak); **Induces** P-glycoprotein

Avoid Concomitant Use

Avoid concomitant use of DOXOrubicin with any of the following: BCG; CloZAPine; Conivaptan; Dabigatran Etexilate; Natalizumab; Pimecrolimus; Pimozide; Tacrolimus (Topical); Vaccines (Live)

Increased Effect/Toxicity

DOXOrubicin may increase the levels/effects of: CloZAPine; CYP2B6 Substrates; Leflunomide; Natalizumab; Pimozide; Vaccines (Live); Vitamin K Antagonists; Zidovudine

The levels/effects of DOXOrubicin may be increased by: Bevacizumab; Conivaptan; CycloSPORINE; CycloSPORINE (Systemic); CYP2D6 Inhibitors (Moderate); CYP2D6 Inhibitors (Strong); CYP3A4 Inhibitors (Moderate); CYP3A4 Inhibitors (Strong); Dasatinib; Denosumab; P-glycoprotein/ABCB1 Inhibitors; Pimecrolimus; Roflumilast; SORAfenib; Tacrolimus (Topical); Taxane Derivatives; Trastuzumab

Decreased Effect

DOXOrubicin may decrease the levels/effects of: BCG; Cardiac Glycosides; Coccidioidin Skin Test; Dabigatran Etexilate; Linagliptin; P-glycoprotein/ABCB1 Substrates; Sipuleucel-T; Stavudine; Vaccines (Inactivated); Vaccines (Live); Vitamin K Antagonists; Zidovudine

The levels/effects of DOXOrubicin may be decreased by: Cardiac Glycosides; CYP3A4 Inducers (Strong); Deferasirox; Echinacea; Peginterferon Alfa-2b; P-glycoprotein/ABCB1 Inducers; Tocilizumab

Ethanol/Nutrition/Herb Interactions Herb/Nutraceutical: Avoid St John's wort (may decrease doxorubicin levels). Avoid black cohosh, dong quai in estrogen-dependent tumors.

Stability Store intact vials of solution under refrigeration (2°C to 8°C). Protect from light. Store intact vials of lyophilized powder at room temperature (15°C to 30°C). Reconstitute lyophilized powder with NS to a final concentration of 2 mg/mL. Reconstituted vials are stable for 7 days at room temperature (25°C) and 15 days under refrigeration (5°C) when protected from light. Infusions are stable for 48 hours at room temperature (25°C) when protected from light. Solutions diluted in 50-1000 mL D_5W or NS are stable for 48 hours at room temperature (25°C) when protected from light.

Unstable in solutions with a pH <3 or >7.

Mechanism of Action Inhibition of DNA and RNA synthesis by intercalation between DNA base pairs by inhibition of topoisomerase II and by steric obstruction. Doxorubicin intercalates at points of local uncoiling of the double helix. Although the exact mechanism is unclear, it appears that direct binding to DNA (intercalation) and inhibition of DNA repair (topoisomerase II inhibition) result in blockade of DNA and RNA synthesis and fragmentation of DNA. Doxorubicin is also a powerful iron chelator; the iron-doxorubicin complex can bind DNA and cell membranes and produce free radicals that immediately cleave the DNA and cell membranes.

Pharmacodynamics/Kinetics

Absorption: Oral: Poor (<50%)

Distribution: V_d: 809-1214 L/m^2; to many body tissues, particularly liver, spleen, kidney, lung, heart; does not distribute into the CNS; crosses placenta

Protein binding, plasma: 70% to 76%

Metabolism: Primarily hepatic to doxorubicinol (active), then to inactive aglycones, conjugated sulfates, and glucuronides

Half-life elimination:

- Distribution: 5-10 minutes
- Elimination: Doxorubicin: 1-3 hours; Metabolites: 3-3.5 hours
- Terminal: 17-48 hours
- Male: 54 hours; Female: 35 hours

Excretion: Feces (~40% to 50% as unchanged drug); urine (~5% to 12% as unchanged drug and metabolites)

- Clearance: Male: 113 L/hour; Female: 44 L/hour

Dosage I.V.: Refer to individual protocols. **Note:** Lower dosage should be considered for patients with inadequate marrow reserve (due to old age, prior treatment or neoplastic marrow infiltration)

Children:

- 35-75 mg/m^2/dose every 21 days **or**
- 20-30 mg/m^2/dose once weekly **or**
- 60-90 mg/m^2/dose given as a continuous infusion over 96 hours every 3-4 weeks

Adults: Usual or typical dose: 60-75 mg/m^2/dose every 21 days **or**

- 60 mg/m^2/dose every 2 weeks (dose dense) **or**
- 40-60 mg/m^2/dose every 3-4 weeks **or**
- 20-30 mg/m^2/day for 2-3 days every 4 weeks **or**
- 20 mg/m^2/dose once weekly

Dosing adjustment in toxicity: The following delays and/or dose reductions have been used:

- Neutropenic fever/infection: Consider reducing to 75% of dose in subsequent cycles
- ANC <1000/mm^3: Delay treatment until ANC recovers to ≥1000/mm^3
- Platelets <100,000/mm^3: Delay treatment until platelets recover to ≥100,000/mm^3

Dosing adjustment in renal impairment:

Adjustments are not required.

Hemodialysis: Supplemental dose is not necessary.

Dosing adjustment in hepatic impairment:

The FDA-approved labeling recommends the following adjustments:

- Serum bilirubin 1.2-3 mg/dL: Administer 50% of dose
- Serum bilirubin 3.1-5 mg/dL: Administer 25% of dose
- Severe hepatic impairment: Use is contraindicated

The following guidelines have been used by some clinicians: Floyd, 2006:

- Transaminases 2-3 times ULN: Administer 75% of dose
- Transaminases >3 times ULN or serum bilirubin 1.2-3 mg/dL: Administer 50% of dose
- Serum bilirubin 3.1-5 mg/dL: Administer 25% of dose
- Serum bilirubin >5 mg/dL: Do not administer

Administration Vesicant. Administer I.V. push over at least 3-5 minutes or by continuous infusion (infusion via central venous line recommended). May be further diluted in either NS of D_5W for I.V. administration. Avoid extravasation associated with severe ulceration and soft tissue necrosis. Flush with 5-10 mL of I.V. solution before and after drug administration. Incompatible with heparin. Monitor for local erythematous streaking along vein and/or facial flushing (may indicate rapid infusion rate).

Monitoring Parameters CBC with differential and platelet count; liver function tests (bilirubin, ALT/AST, alkaline phosphatase); serum uric acid, calcium, potassium, phosphate and creatinine; cardiac function (baseline, periodic, and followup): ECG, left ventricular ejection fraction (echocardiography [ECHO] or multigated radionuclide angiography [MUGA])

Dosage Forms Excipient information presented when available (limited, particularly for generics); consult specific product labeling.

Injection, powder for reconstitution, as hydrochloride: 10 mg, 50 mg

- Adriamycin®: 10 mg [contains lactose 50 mg]
- Adriamycin®: 20 mg [contains lactose 100 mg]
- Adriamycin®: 50 mg [contains lactose 250 mg]

Injection, solution, as hydrochloride [preservative free]: 2 mg/mL (5 mL, 10 mL, 25 mL, 75 mL, 100 mL)

- Adriamycin®: 2 mg/mL (5 mL, 10 mL, 25 mL, 100 mL)

◆ **Doxorubicin Hydrochloride** *see* DOXOrubicin *on page 552*

◆ **Doxorubicin Hydrochloride Injection (Can)** *see* DOXOrubicin *on page 552*

◆ **DOXOrubicin Hydrochloride (Liposomal)** *see* DOXOrubicin (Liposomal) *on page* 555

◆ **DOXOrubicin Hydrochloride Liposome** *see* DOXOrubicin (Liposomal) *on page* 555

DOXOrubicin (Liposomal)

(doks oh ROO bi sin lye po SO mal)

Brand Names: U.S. Doxil®

Brand Names: Canada Caelyx®; Myocet™

Index Terms DOXOrubicin Hydrochloride (Liposomal); DOXOrubicin Hydrochloride Liposome; Liposomal DOXOrubicin; Pegylated DOXOrubicin Liposomal; Pegylated Liposomal DOXOrubicin

Pharmacologic Category Antineoplastic Agent, Anthracycline

Use Treatment of ovarian cancer (progressive or recurrent), multiple myeloma (after failure of at least 1 prior therapy), and AIDS-related Kaposi's sarcoma (after failure of or intolerance to prior systemic therapy)

Unlabeled Use Treatment of metastatic breast cancer, Hodgkin's lymphoma, cutaneous T-cell lymphomas (mycosis fungoides and Sézary syndrome), advanced soft tissue sarcomas; advanced or metastatic uterine sarcoma

Pregnancy Risk Factor D

Pregnancy Considerations May cause fetal harm if administered during pregnancy. There are no adequate and well-controlled studies in pregnant women. Women of childbearing potential should avoid becoming pregnant during treatment.

Lactation Excretion in breast milk unknown/contraindicated

Contraindications Hypersensitivity to doxorubicin liposomal, conventional doxorubicin, or any component of the formulation; breast-feeding

Warnings/Precautions Hazardous agent - use appropriate precautions for handling and disposal.

[U.S. Boxed Warning]: Doxorubicin may cause cumulative, dose-related myocardial toxicity (concurrent or delayed). Doxorubicin liposomal should be used with caution in patients with high cumulative doses of any anthracycline. Total cumulative dose should also account for previous or concomitant treatment with other cardiotoxic agents or irradiation of chest. The incidence of irreversible myocardial toxicity increases as the total cumulative (lifetime) dosages approach 450-550 mg/m^2; or 400 mg/m^2 in patients who have received prior mediastinal radiation therapy or concurrent therapy with other cardiotoxic agents (eg, cyclophosphamide). Although the risk increases with cumulative dose, irreversible cardiotoxicity may occur with anthracycline treatment at any dose level. Patients with pre-existing heart disease, hypertension, concurrent administration of other antineoplastic agents, prior or concurrent chest irradiation, and advanced age are at increased risk. Evaluate left ventricular ejection fraction (LVEF) prior to treatment and periodically during treatment. The onset of symptoms of anthracycline-induced HF and/or cardiomyopathy may be delayed.

[U.S. Boxed Warning]: Acute infusion reactions may occur, some may be serious/life-threatening, including fatal allergic/anaphylactoid-like reactions. Infusion reactions typically occur with the first infusion and may include flushing, dyspnea, facial swelling, headache, chills, back pain, hypotension, and/or tightness of chest/throat. Reactions usually resolve with termination of infusion, or in some cases, slowing the infusion rate. Medication for the treatment of reactions should be readily available in the event of severe reactions. Infuse doxorubicin liposomal at 1 mg/minute initially to minimize risk of infusion reaction.

[U.S. Boxed Warning]: Use with caution in patients with hepatic impairment; dosage reduction is recommended. Use in patients with hepatic impairment has not been adequately studied; dosing adjustment recommendations in multiple myeloma patients with hepatic impairment is not available. **[U.S. Boxed Warning]: Severe myelosuppression may occur.** Palmar-plantar erythrodysesthesia (hand-foot syndrome) has been reported in up to 51% of patients with ovarian cancer, 19% of patients with multiple myeloma, and ~3% in patients with Kaposi's sarcoma. May occur early in treatment, but is usually seen after 2-3 treatment cycles. Dosage modification may be required. In severe cases, treatment discontinuation may be required. **[U.S. Boxed Warning]: Liposomal formulations of doxorubicin should NOT be substituted for conventional doxorubicin hydrochloride on a mg-per-mg basis.**

Doxorubicin may potentiate the toxicity of cyclophosphamide (hemorrhagic cystitis) and mercaptopurine (hepatotoxicity). Radiation recall reaction has been reported with doxorubicin liposomal treatment after radiation therapy. Radiation-induced toxicity (to the myocardium, mucosa, skin, and liver) may be increased by doxorubicin.

Adverse Reactions

>10%:

Cardiovascular: Peripheral edema (≤11%)

Central nervous system: Fever (8% to 21%), headache (≤11%), pain (≤21%)

Dermatologic: Palmar-plantar erythrodysesthesia/hand-foot syndrome (≤51% in ovarian cancer [grades 3/4: 24%]; 3% in Kaposi's sarcoma), rash (≤29% in ovarian cancer, ≤5% in Kaposi's sarcoma), alopecia (9% to 19%)

Gastrointestinal: Nausea (17% to 46%), stomatitis (5% to 41%), vomiting (8% to 33%), constipation (≤30%), diarrhea (5% to 21%), anorexia (≤20%), mucositis (≤14%), dyspepsia (≤12%), intestinal obstruction (≤11%)

Hematologic: Myelosuppression (onset: 7 days; nadir: 10-14 days; recovery: 21-28 days), thrombocytopenia (13% to 65%; grades 3/4: 1%), neutropenia (12% to 62%; grade 4: 4%), leukopenia (36%), anemia (6% to 74%; grade 4: <1%)

Neuromuscular & skeletal: Weakness (7% to 40%), back pain (≤12%)

Respiratory: Pharyngitis (≤16%), dyspnea (≤15%)

Miscellaneous: Infection (≤12%)

1% to 10%:

Cardiovascular: Cardiac arrest, chest pain, deep thrombophlebitis, edema, hypotension, pallor, tachycardia, vasodilation

Central nervous system: Agitation, anxiety, chills, confusion, depression, dizziness, emotional lability, insomnia, somnolence, vertigo

Dermatologic: Acne, bruising, dry skin (6%), exfoliative dermatitis, fungal dermatitis, furunculosis, maculopapular rash, pruritus, skin discoloration, vesiculobullous rash

Endocrine & metabolic: Dehydration, hypercalcemia, hyperglycemia, hypokalemia, hyponatremia

Gastrointestinal: Abdomen enlarged, anorexia, ascites, cachexia, dyspepsia, dysphagia, esophagitis, flatulence, gingivitis, glossitis, ileus, mouth ulceration, oral moniliasis, rectal bleeding, taste perversion, weight loss, xerostomia

Genitourinary: Cystitis, dysuria, leukorrhea, pelvic pain, polyuria, urinary incontinence, urinary tract infection, urinary urgency, vaginal bleeding, vaginal moniliasis
Hematologic: Hemolysis, prothrombin time increased
Hepatic: ALT increased, alkaline phosphatase increased, hyperbilirubinemia
Local: Thrombophlebitis
Neuromuscular & skeletal: Arthralgia, hypertonia, myalgia, neuralgia, neuritis (peripheral), neuropathy, paresthesia (≤10%), pathological fracture
Ocular: Conjunctivitis, dry eyes, retinitis
Otic: Ear pain
Renal: Albuminuria, hematuria
Respiratory: Apnea, cough (≤10%), epistaxis, pleural effusion, pneumonia, rhinitis, sinusitis
Miscellaneous: Allergic reaction; infusion-related reactions (7%; includes bronchospasm, chest tightness, chills, dyspnea, facial edema, flushing, headache, herpes simplex/zoster, hypotension, pruritus); moniliasis, diaphoresis

<1% (Limited to important or life-threatening): Abscess, acute brain syndrome, abnormal vision, acute myeloid leukemia (secondary), alkaline phosphatase increased, anaphylactic or anaphylactoid reaction, asthma, balanitis, blindness, bronchitis, BUN increased, bundle branch block, cardiomegaly, cardiomyopathy, cellulitis, CHF, colitis, creatinine increased, cryptococcosis, diabetes mellitus, erythema multiforme, erythema nodosum, eosinophilia, fecal impaction, flu-like syndrome, gastritis, glucosuria, hemiplegia, hemorrhage, hepatic failure, hepatitis, hepatosplenomegaly, hyperkalemia, hypernatremia, hyperuricemia, hyperventilation, hypoglycemia, hypolipidemia, hypomagnesemia, hypophosphatemia, hypoproteinemia, hypothermia, injection site hemorrhage, injection site pain, jaundice, ketosis, lactic dehydrogenase increased, lymphadenopathy, lymphangitis, migraine, myositis, optic neuritis, oral cancers (squamous cell; long-term use), palpitation, pancreatitis, pericardial effusion, petechia, pneumothorax, pulmonary embolism, radiation injury, renal failure, sclerosing cholangitis, seizure, sepsis, skin necrosis, skin ulcer, syncope, Stevens-Johnson syndrome, tenesmus, thromboplastin decreased, thrombosis, tinnitus, toxic epidermal necrolysis, urticaria, visual field defect, ventricular arrhythmia

Drug Interactions

Metabolism/Transport Effects Substrate of CYP2D6 (major), CYP3A4 (major); **Note:** Assignment of Major/Minor substrate status based on clinically relevant drug interaction potential; **Inhibits** CYP2B6 (moderate)

Avoid Concomitant Use

Avoid concomitant use of DOXOrubicin (Liposomal) with any of the following: BCG; CloZAPine; Conivaptan; Natalizumab; Pimecrolimus; Tacrolimus (Topical); Vaccines (Live)

Increased Effect/Toxicity

DOXOrubicin (Liposomal) may increase the levels/effects of: CloZAPine; CYP2B6 Substrates; Leflunomide; Natalizumab; Vaccines (Live); Zidovudine

The levels/effects of DOXOrubicin (Liposomal) may be increased by: Abiraterone Acetate; Bevacizumab; Conivaptan; CYP2D6 Inhibitors (Moderate); CYP2D6 Inhibitors (Strong); CYP3A4 Inhibitors (Moderate); CYP3A4 Inhibitors (Strong); Darunavir; Dasatinib; Denosumab; Pimecrolimus; Roflumilast; Tacrolimus (Topical); Taxane Derivatives; Trastuzumab

Decreased Effect

DOXOrubicin (Liposomal) may decrease the levels/effects of: BCG; Cardiac Glycosides; Coccidioidin Skin Test; Sipuleucel-T; Stavudine; Vaccines (Inactivated); Vaccines (Live); Zidovudine

The levels/effects of DOXOrubicin (Liposomal) may be decreased by: Cardiac Glycosides; CYP3A4 Inducers (Strong); Deferasirox; Echinacea; Herbs (CYP3A4 Inducers); Peginterferon Alfa-2b; Tocilizumab

Ethanol/Nutrition/Herb Interactions

Ethanol: Avoid ethanol (due to GI irritation).
Herb/Nutraceutical: St John's wort may decrease doxorubicin levels.

Stability Store intact vials of solution under refrigeration at 2°C to 8°C (36°F to 46°F); avoid freezing. Prolonged freezing may adversely affect liposomal drug products, however, short-term freezing (<1 month) does not appear to have a deleterious effect.

Doses of doxorubicin liposomal ≤90 mg must be diluted in 250 mL of D_5W prior to administration. Doses >90 mg should be diluted in 500 mL D_5W. Solution is not a clear, but has a red, translucent appearance due to the liposomal dispersion. Use appropriate precautions for handling and disposal. Diluted doxorubicin hydrochloride liposome injection may be refrigerated at 2°C to 8°C (36°F to 46°F); administer within 24 hours. **Do not infuse with in-line filters.**

Mechanism of Action Doxorubicin inhibits DNA and RNA synthesis by intercalating between DNA base pairs causing steric obstruction and inhibits topoisomerase-II at the point of DNA cleavage. Doxorubicin is also a powerful iron chelator. The iron-doxorubicin complex can bind DNA and cell membranes, producing free hydroxyl (OH) radicals that cleave DNA and cell membranes. Active throughout entire cell cycle. Doxorubicin liposomal is a pegylated formulation which protects the liposomes, and thereby increases blood circulation time.

Pharmacodynamics/Kinetics

Distribution: V_{dss}: 2.7-2.8 L/m^2
Protein binding, plasma: Unknown; nonliposomal (conventional) doxorubicin: 70%
Half-life elimination: Terminal: Distribution: 4.7-5.2 hours, Elimination: 44-55 hours
Metabolism: Hepatic and in plasma to doxorubicinol and the sulfate and glucuronide conjugates of 4-demethyl,7-deoxyaglycones
Excretion: Urine (5% as doxorubicin or doxorubicinol)

Dosage Details concerning dosing in combination regimens should also be consulted. **Liposomal formulations of doxorubicin should NOT be substituted for conventional doxorubicin hydrochloride on a mg-per-mg basis.**

AIDS-related Kaposi's sarcoma: I.V.: 20 mg/m^2 every 3 weeks
Multiple myeloma: I.V.: 30 mg/m^2 on day 4 every 3 weeks (in combination with bortezomib) **or**
Unlabeled dosing: I.V.: 40 mg/m^2 every 4 weeks (in combination with vincristine and dexamethasone) (Rifkin, 2006)
Ovarian cancer: I.V.: 50 mg/m^2 every 4 weeks (minimum of 4 cycles is recommended)
Breast cancer (unlabeled use): I.V.: 50 mg/m^2 every 4 weeks (Keller, 2004)
Uterine sarcoma (unlabeled use): I.V.: 50 mg/m^2 every 4 weeks (Sutton, 2005)

Dosing adjustment in hepatic impairment: Note: Dosage adjustment information is not available in patients with multiple myeloma.
Bilirubin 1.2-3 mg/dL: Administer 50% of dose
Bilirubin >3 mg/dL: Administer 25% of dose

Dosing adjustment for toxicity:

Recommended Dose Modification Guidelines

Toxicity Grade	Dose Adjustment
HAND FOOT SYNDROME (HFS)	
1 (Mild erythema, swelling, or desquamation not interfering with daily activities)	Redose unless patient has experienced previous Grade 3 or 4 HFS toxicity. If so, delay up to 2 weeks and decrease dose by 25%; return to original dosing interval.
2 (Erythema, desquamation, or swelling interfering with, but not precluding, normal physical activities; small blisters or ulcerations <2 cm in diameter)	Delay dosing up to 2 weeks or until resolved to Grade 0-1. If after 2 weeks there is no resolution, discontinue liposomal doxorubicin. Otherwise, if no prior Grade 3-4 HFS, continue treatment at previous dose and dosage interval. If a prior Grade 3-4 HFS has occurred, continue prior dosage interval, but decrease dose by 25%.
3 (Blistering, ulceration, or swelling interfering with walking or normal daily activities; cannot wear regular clothing)	Delay dosing up to 2 weeks or until resolved to Grade 0-1. Decrease dose by 25% and return to original dosing interval; if after 2 weeks there is no resolution, discontinue liposomal doxorubicin.
4 (Diffuse or local process causing infectious complications, or a bedridden state or hospitalization)	Delay dosing up to 2 weeks or until resolved to Grade 0-1. Decrease dose by 25% and return to original dosing interval. If after 2 weeks there is no resolution, discontinue liposomal doxorubicin.
STOMATITIS	
1 (Painless ulcers, erythema, or mild soreness)	Redose unless patient has experienced previous Grade 3 or 4 toxicity. If so, delay up to 2 weeks and decrease by 25%. Return to original dosing interval.
2 (Painful erythema, edema, or ulcers, but can eat)	Delay dosing up to 2 weeks or until resolved to Grade 0-1. If after 2 weeks there is no resolution, discontinue liposomal doxorubicin. Otherwise, if not prior Grade 3-4 stomatitis, continue treatment at previous dose and dosage interval. If prior Grade 3-4 toxicity, continue treatment with previous dosage interval, but decrease dose by 25%.
3 (Painful erythema, edema, or ulcers, and cannot eat)	Delay dosing up to 2 weeks or until resolved to Grade 0-1. Decrease dose by 25% and return to original dosing interval. If after 2 weeks there is no resolution, discontinue liposomal doxorubicin.
4 (Requires parenteral or enteral support)	Delay dosing up to 2 weeks or until resolved to Grade 0-1. Decrease dose by 25% and return to original dosing interval. If after 2 weeks there is no resolution, discontinue liposomal doxorubicin.

See table: "Hematological Toxicity"

Hematological Toxicity (see below for multiple myeloma)

Grade	ANC	Platelets	Modification
1	1500-1900	75,000-150,000	Resume treatment with no dose reduction.
2	1000-<1500	50,000-<75,000	Wait until ANC ≥1500 and platelets ≥75,000; redose with no dose reduction.
3	500-999	25,000-<50,000	Wait until ANC ≥1500 and platelets ≥75,000; redose with no dose reduction.
4	<500	<25,000	Wait until ANC ≥1500 and platelets ≥75,000; redose at 25% dose reduction or continue full dose with cytokine support.

Dosing Adjustment for Toxicity in Treatment with Bortezomib (for Multiple Myeloma) (see Bortezomib monograph for bortezomib dosage reduction with toxicity guidelines):

Fever ≥38°C and ANC <1000/mm³: If prior to doxorubicin liposomal treatment (day 4), do not administer; if after doxorubicin liposomal administered, reduce dose by 25% in next cycle.

ANC <500/mm³, platelets <25,000/mm³, hemoglobin <8 g/dL: If prior to doxorubicin liposomal treatment (day 4); do not administer; if after doxorubicin liposomal administered, reduce dose by 25% in next cycle if bortezomib dose reduction occurred for hematologic toxicity.

Grade 3 or 4 nonhematologic toxicity: Delay dose until resolved to grade <2; reduce dose by 25% for all subsequent doses.

Neuropathic pain or peripheral neuropathy: No dose reductions needed for doxorubicin liposomal, refer to Bortezomib monograph for bortezomib dosing adjustment.

Administration Administer IVPB over 60 minutes; manufacturer recommends administering at initial rate of 1 mg/minute to minimize risk of infusion reactions until the absence of a reaction has been established, then increase the infusion rate for completion over 1 hour. Do **NOT** administer undiluted, as a bolus injection, or I.M. or SubQ.

Do **NOT** infuse with in-line filters. Avoid extravasation (irritant), monitor site; extravasation may occur without stinging or burning. Flush with 5-10 mL of D_5W solution before and after drug administration (do not rapidly flush through the I.V. line), incompatible with heparin flushes. Monitor for local erythematous streaking along vein and/or facial flushing (may indicate rapid infusion rate).

Monitoring Parameters CBC with differential and platelet count, liver function tests (ALT/AST, bilirubin, alkaline phosphatase); monitor for infusion reactions

Cardiac function (left ventricular ejection fraction [LVEF]), should be carefully monitored; echocardiography, or MUGA scan may be used. Endomyocardial biopsy is the most definitive test for anthracycline myocardial injury.

Dosage Forms Excipient information presented when available (limited, particularly for generics); consult specific product labeling.

Injection, solution, as hydrochloride:

Doxil®: 2 mg/mL (10 mL, 25 mL) [contains soy, sucrose]

◆ **Doxy 100™** *see* Doxycycline *on page 557*

◆ **Doxycin (Can)** *see* Doxycycline *on page 557*

Doxycycline (doks i SYE kleen)

Brand Names: U.S. Adoxa®; Adoxa® Pak™ 1/150 [DSC]; Adoxa® Pak™ 1/75 [DSC]; Alodox™; Doryx®; Doxy 100™; Monodox®; Ocudox™; Oracea®; Oraxyl™; Periostat®; Vibramycin®

Brand Names: Canada Apo-Doxy Tabs®; Apo-Doxy®; Dom-Doxycycline; Doxycin; Doxytab; Novo-Doxylin; Nu-Doxycycline; Periostat®; PHL-Doxycycline; PMS-Doxycycline; Vibra-Tabs®; Vibramycin®

Index Terms Doxycycline Calcium; Doxycycline Hyclate; Doxycycline Monohydrate

Pharmacologic Category Antibiotic, Tetracycline Derivative

Additional Appendix Information

Prevention of Wound Infection and Sepsis in Surgical Patients *on page 1954*

Use Principally in the treatment of infections caused by susceptible *Rickettsia*, *Chlamydia*, and *Mycoplasma*; alternative to mefloquine for malaria prophylaxis; treatment for syphilis, uncomplicated *Neisseria gonorrhoeae*, *Listeria*, *Actinomyces israelii*, and *Clostridium* infections in penicillin-allergic patients; used for community-acquired pneumonia and other common infections due to susceptible organisms; anthrax due to *Bacillus anthracis*, including inhalational anthrax (postexposure); treatment of infections caused by uncommon susceptible gram-negative and gram-positive organisms including *Borrelia recurrentis*, *Ureaplasma urealyticum*, *Haemophilus ducreyi*, *Yersinia pestis*, *Francisella tularensis*, *Vibrio cholerae*, *Campylobacter fetus*, *Brucella* spp, *Bartonella bacilliformis*, and *Klebsiella granulomatis*, Q fever, Lyme disease; treatment of inflammatory lesions associated with rosacea; intestinal amebiasis; severe acne

Unlabeled Use Sclerosing agent for pleural effusion injection; vancomycin-resistant enterococci (VRE); alternate treatment for MRSA infections; treatment of periodontitis (refractory); localized juvenile periodontitis (LJP)

Pregnancy Risk Factor D

Pregnancy Considerations Because use during pregnancy may cause fetal harm, doxycycline is classified as pregnancy category D. Exposure to tetracyclines during the second or third trimester may cause permanent discoloration of the teeth. Most reports do not show an increase risk for teratogenicity with the exception of a potential small increased risk for cleft palate or esophageal atresia/stenosis. When considering treatment for life-threatening infection and/or prolonged duration of therapy (such as in anthrax), the potential risk to the fetus must be balanced against the severity of the potential illness.

Lactation Enters breast milk/not recommended

Contraindications Hypersensitivity to doxycycline, tetracycline or any component of the formulation; children <8 years of age (except in treatment of anthrax exposure and tickborne rickettsial disease)

Warnings/Precautions Photosensitivity reaction may occur with this drug; avoid prolonged exposure to sunlight or tanning equipment. Antianabolic effects of tetracyclines can increase BUN (dose-related). Autoimmune syndromes have been reported. Hepatotoxicity rarely occurs; if symptomatic, conduct LFT and discontinue drug. Pseudotumor cerebri has been (rarely) reported with tetracycline use; usually resolves with discontinuation. Prolonged use may result in fungal or bacterial superinfection, including *C. difficile*-associated diarrhea (CDAD) and pseudomembranous colitis; CDAD has been observed >2 months post-antibiotic treatment. May cause tissue hyperpigmentation, enamel hypoplasia, or permanent tooth discoloration; use of tetracyclines should be avoided during tooth development (children <8 years of age) unless other drugs are not likely to be effective or are contraindicated. However, recommended in treatment of anthrax exposure and tick-borne rickettsial diseases. Do not use during pregnancy. In addition to affecting tooth development, tetracycline use has been associated with retardation of skeletal development and reduced bone growth.

Additional specific warnings: Oracea®: Should not be used for the treatment or prophylaxis of bacterial infections, since the lower dose of drug per capsule may be subefficacious and promote resistance. Syrup contains sodium metabisulfite. Effectiveness of products intended for use in periodontitis has not been established in patients with coexistent oral candidiasis; use with caution in patients with a history or predisposition to oral candidiasis.

Adverse Reactions Frequency not defined.

Cardiovascular: Intracranial hypertension, pericarditis

Dermatologic: Angioneurotic edema, erythema multiforme, exfoliative dermatitis (rare), photosensitivity, rash, skin hyperpigmentation, Stevens-Johnson syndrome, toxic epidermal necrolysis, urticaria

Endocrine & metabolic: Brown/black discoloration of thyroid gland (no dysfunction reported), hypoglycemia

Gastrointestinal: Anorexia, diarrhea, dysphagia, enterocolitis, esophagitis (rare), esophageal ulcerations (rare), glossitis, inflammatory lesions in anogenital region, nausea, oral (mucosal) pigmentation, pseudomembranous colitis, tooth discoloration (children), vomiting

Hematologic: Eosinophilia, hemolytic anemia, neutropenia, thrombocytopenia

Hepatic: Hepatotoxicity (rare)

Renal: BUN increased (dose related)

Miscellaneous: Anaphylactoid purpura, anaphylaxis, bulging fontanels (infants), serum sickness, SLE exacerbation

Note: Adverse effects in clinical trials occurring at a frequency more than 1% greater than placebo:

Periostat®: Diarrhea, dyspepsia, joint pain, menstrual cramp, nausea, dyspepsia, pain

Oracea®: Abdominal distention, abdominal pain, anxiety, AST increased, back pain, fungal infection, hyperglycemia, influenza, LDH increased, nasal congestion, nasopharyngitis, pain, sinus headache, sinusitis, xerostomia

Drug Interactions

Metabolism/Transport Effects Inhibits CYP3A4 (weak)

Avoid Concomitant Use

Avoid concomitant use of Doxycycline with any of the following: BCG; Pimozide; Retinoic Acid Derivatives

Increased Effect/Toxicity

Doxycycline may increase the levels/effects of: Neuromuscular-Blocking Agents; Pimozide; Porfimer; Retinoic Acid Derivatives; Vitamin K Antagonists

Decreased Effect

Doxycycline may decrease the levels/effects of: BCG; Penicillins; Typhoid Vaccine

The levels/effects of Doxycycline may be decreased by: Antacids; Barbiturates; Bile Acid Sequestrants; Bismuth; Bismuth Subsalicylate; Calcium Salts; CarBAMazepine; Fosphenytoin; Iron Salts; Lanthanum; Magnesium Salts; Phenytoin; Quinapril; Sucralfate

Ethanol/Nutrition/Herb Interactions

Ethanol: Chronic ethanol ingestion may reduce the serum concentration of doxycycline.

Food: Doxycycline serum levels may be slightly decreased if taken with food or milk. Administration with iron or calcium may decrease doxycycline absorption. May decrease absorption of calcium, iron, magnesium, zinc, and amino acids.

Herb/Nutraceutical: St John's wort may decrease doxycycline levels. Avoid dong quai, St John's wort (may also cause photosensitization).

Stability

Capsule, tablet: Store at controlled room temperature of 25°C (77°F); excursions permitted to 15°C to 30°C (59°F to 86°F). Protect from light.

I.V. infusion: Following reconstitution with sterile water for injection, dilute to a final concentration of 0.1-1 mg/mL using a compatible solution. Solutions for I.V. infusion may be prepared using 0.9% sodium chloride, D_5W, Ringer's injection, lactated Ringer's, D_5LR. Protect from light. Stability varies based on solution.

Mechanism of Action Inhibits protein synthesis by binding with the 30S and possibly the 50S ribosomal subunit(s) of susceptible bacteria; may also cause alterations in the cytoplasmic membrane

Periostat® capsules (proposed mechanism): Has been shown to inhibit collagenase activity *in vitro*. Also has been noted to reduce elevated collagenase activity in the gingival crevicular fluid of patients with periodontal disease. Systemic levels do not reach inhibitory concentrations against bacteria.

Pharmacodynamics/Kinetics

Absorption: Oral: Almost complete

Distribution: Widely into body tissues and fluids including synovial, pleural, prostatic, seminal fluids, and bronchial secretions; saliva, aqueous humor, and CSF penetration is poor

Protein binding: 90%

Metabolism: Not hepatic; partially inactivated in GI tract by chelate formation

Bioavailability: Reduced at high pH; may be clinically significant in patients with gastrectomy, gastric bypass surgery or who are otherwise deemed achlorhydric

Half-life elimination: 12-15 hours (usually increases to 22-24 hours with multiple doses); End-stage renal disease: 18-25 hours; Oracea®: 21 hours

Time to peak, serum: 1.5-4 hours

Excretion: Feces (30%); urine (23%)

Dosage

Usual dosage range:

Children >8 years (≤45 kg): Oral, I.V.: 2-5 mg/kg/day in 1-2 divided doses, not to exceed 200 mg/day

Children >8 years (>45 kg) and Adults: Oral, I.V.: 100-200 mg/day in 1-2 divided doses

Indication-specific dosing:

Children:

Anthrax: Doxycycline should be used in children if antibiotic susceptibility testing, exhaustion of drug supplies, or allergic reaction preclude use of penicillin or ciprofloxacin. For treatment, the consensus recommendation does not include a loading dose for doxycycline.

Inhalational (postexposure prophylaxis) (ACIP, 2010): Oral, I.V. (use oral route when possible):

≤8 years: 2.2 mg/kg every 12 hours for 60 days

>8 years and ≤45 kg: 2.2 mg/kg every 12 hours for 60 days

>8 years and >45 kg: 100 mg every 12 hours for 60 days

Cutaneous (treatment): Oral: See dosing for "Inhalational (postexposure prophylaxis)"

Note: In the presence of systemic involvement, extensive edema, and/or lesions on head/neck, doxycycline should initially be administered I.V.

Inhalational/gastrointestinal/oropharyngeal (treatment): I.V.: Refer to dosing for inhalational anthrax (postexposure prophylaxis); switch to oral therapy when clinically appropriate

Note: Initial treatment should include two or more agents predicted to be effective (CDC, 2001). Agents suggested for use in conjunction with doxycycline or ciprofloxacin include rifampin, vancomycin, imipenem, penicillin, ampicillin, chloramphenicol, clindamycin, and clarithromycin. May switch to oral antimicrobial therapy when clinically appropriate. Continue combined therapy for 60 days

Community-acquired pneumonia (CAP) (IDSA/PIDS, 2011): Oral: Children >7 years: **Note:** A beta-lactam antibiotic should be added if typical bacterial pneumonia cannot be ruled out.

Presumed atypical, mild atypical (*M. pneumoniae, C. pneumoniae, C. trachomatis*) infection or step-down therapy (alternative to azithromycin): 2-4 mg/kg/day in 2 divided doses (maximum: 200 mg/day)

Cellulitis (purulent) due to community-acquired MRSA (unlabeled use): Oral: Children >8 years and ≤45 kg: 2 mg/kg/dose every 12 hours for 5-10 days (Liu, 2011)

Localized juvenile periodontitis (LJP) (unlabeled use): Oral: 50-100 mg/day

Q fever: Oral, I.V.: 2.2 mg/kg twice/day for 15-21 days (CDC, 2009). Some clinicians may recommend trimethoprim/sulfamethoxazole for children <8 years of age (Hartzell, 2008). **Note:** Use of tetracyclines should be avoided during tooth development (children ≤8 years of age) unless other drugs are unlikely to be effective or are contraindicated.

Tickborne rickettsial disease: Oral, I.V.: Children ≤8 years: 2.2 mg/kg (maximum dose: 100 mg) every 12 hours for 5-7 days; severe or complicated disease may require longer treatment; human granulocytotropic anaplasmosis (HGA) should be treated for 10-14 days. **Note:** The American Academy of Pediatrics Committee on Infectious Diseases identifies doxycycline as the drug of choice in children of any age.

Tularemia: I.V. (may transition to oral if clinically indicated) (Dennis, 2001):

Children <45 kg: 2.2 mg/kg every 12 hours for 14-21 days

Children ≥45 kg: 100 mg every 12 hours for 14-21 days

Children ≥8 years:

Lyme disease: Oral (Halperin, 2007; Wormser, 2006):

Prevention: 4 mg/kg (maximum: 200 mg) administered as a single dose; **Note:** Initiate within 72 hours of tick removal

Treatment (early lyme disease without neurologic manifestations): 1-2 mg/kg twice daily for 10-21 days (maximum: 100 mg/dose)

Treatment (meningitis and other early neurologic manifestations): 4-8 mg/kg/day in 2 divided doses for 10-28 days (maximum: 200 mg/dose)

Malaria chemoprophylaxis: Oral: 2.2 mg/kg/day (maximum: 100 mg/day). Start 1-2 days prior to travel to endemic area; continue daily during travel and for 4 weeks after leaving endemic area (CDC, 2012)

Malaria, severe, treatment (unlabeled use): Oral, I.V.:

<45 kg: 2.2 mg/kg (maximum dose: 100 mg) every 12 hours for 7 days with quinidine gluconate. **Note:** Quinidine gluconate duration is region specific; consult CDC for current recommendations (CDC, 2011).

≥45 kg: 100 mg every 12 hours for 7 days with quinidine gluconate. **Note:** Quinidine gluconate duration is region specific; consult CDC for current recommendations (CDC, 2011).

Malaria, uncomplicated, treatment (unlabeled use): Oral: 2.2 mg/kg (maximum dose: 100 mg) every 12 hours for 7 days with quinine sulfate. **Note:** Quinine sulfate duration is region specific; consult CDC for current recommendations (CDC, 2011).

Children >8 years (and >45 kg) and Adults:

Cellulitis (purulent) due to community-acquired MRSA (unlabeled use): Oral: 100 mg twice daily for 5-10 days (Liu, 2011)

Chlamydial infections, uncomplicated: Oral: 100 mg twice daily for 7 days

Tickborne rickettsial disease: Oral, I.V.: 100 mg twice daily for 5-7 days; severe or complicated disease may require longer treatment; human granulocytotropic anaplasmosis (HGA) should be treated for 10-14 days. **Note:** The American Academy of Pediatrics Committee on Infectious Diseases identifies doxycycline as the drug of choice in children of any age.

Adults:

Anthrax:

Inhalational (postexposure prophylaxis): Oral, I.V. (use oral route when possible): 100 mg every 12 hours for 60 days (ACIP, 2010)

Cutaneous (treatment): Oral: 100 mg every 12 hours for 60 days. **Note:** In the presence of systemic involvement, extensive edema, lesions on head/neck, refer to I.V. dosing for treatment of inhalational/gastrointestinal/oropharyngeal anthrax

Inhalational/gastrointestinal/oropharyngeal (treatment): I.V.: Initial: 100 mg every 12 hours; switch to oral therapy when clinically appropriate; some recommend initial loading dose of 200 mg, followed by 100 mg every 8-12 hours (Franz, 1997). **Note:** Initial treatment should include two or more agents predicted to be effective (CDC, 2001). Agents suggested for use in conjunction with doxycycline or ciprofloxacin include rifampin, vancomycin, imipenem, penicillin, ampicillin, chloramphenicol, clindamycin, and clarithromycin. May switch to oral antimicrobial therapy when clinically appropriate. Continue combined therapy for 60 days

Brucellosis: Oral: 100 mg twice daily for 6 weeks with rifampin or streptomycin

Community-acquired pneumonia, bronchitis: Oral, I.V.: 100 mg twice daily (Ailani, 1999; Mandell, 2007)

Epididymitis: Oral: 100 mg twice daily for 10 days (in combination with ceftriaxone) (CDC, 2010)

Gonococcal infection, uncomplicated (cervix, pharynx, rectum, urethra): Oral: 100 mg twice daily for 7 days (in combination with a cephalosporin) (CDC, 2010)

Alternatively, the manufacturer recommends a single-visit dose in nonanorectal infections in men: 300 mg initially, repeat dose in 1 hour (total dose: 600 mg)

Granuloma inguinale (donovanosis): Oral: 100 mg twice daily for at least 3 weeks (and until lesions have healed) (CDC, 2010)

Lyme disease: Oral (Halperin, 2007; Wormser, 2006):

Prevention: Initiate within 72 hours of tick removal: 200 mg administered as a single dose

Treatment (early lyme disease without neurologic manifestations): 100 mg twice daily for 10-21 days

Treatment (meningitis or other early neurologic manifestations): 100-200 mg twice daily for 14 days (range: 10-28 days)

Lymphogranuloma venereum: Oral: 100 mg twice daily for 21 days (CDC, 2010)

Malaria chemoprophylaxis: Oral: 100 mg/day. Start 1-2 days prior to travel to endemic area; continue daily during travel and for 4 weeks after leaving endemic area

Malaria, severe, treatment (unlabeled use): Oral, I.V.: 100 mg every 12 hours for 7 days with quinidine gluconate. **Note:** Quinidine gluconate duration is region specific; consult CDC for current recommendations (CDC, 2011).

Malaria, uncomplicated, treatment (unlabeled use): Oral: 100 mg twice daily for 7 days with quinine sulfate. **Note:** Quinine sulfate duration is region specific; consult CDC for current recommendations (CDC, 2011).

Nongonococcal urethritis: Oral: 100 mg twice daily for 7 days (CDC, 2010)

Pelvic inflammatory disease:

Treatment, inpatient: Oral, I.V.: 100 mg twice daily (in combination with cefoxitin or cefotetan); may transition to oral doxycycline (add clindamycin or metronidazole if tubo-ovarian abscess present) to complete 14 days of treatment (CDC, 2010)

Treatment, outpatient: Oral: 100 mg twice daily for 14 days (with or without metronidazole); preceded by a single I.M. dose of cefoxitin (plus oral probenecid) or ceftriaxone (CDC, 2010)

Periodontitis: Oral (Periostat®): 20 mg twice daily as an adjunct following scaling and root planing

Periodontitis, refractory (unlabeled use): Oral: 100-200 mg daily (Jolkovsky, 2006)

Proctitis: Oral: 100 mg twice daily for 7 days (in combination with ceftriaxone) (CDC, 2010)

Q fever: Oral: 100 mg every 12 hours for 15-21days (CDC, 2009)

Rosacea (Oracea®): Oral: 40 mg once daily in the morning

Sclerosing agent for pleural effusion (unlabeled use): Intrapleural: 500 mg as a single dose in 100 mL NS (Porcel, 2006); may require a repeat dose (Kvale, 2007)

Syphilis:

Primary/secondary syphilis: Oral: 100 mg twice daily for 14 days (CDC, 2010)

Latent syphilis: Oral: 100 mg twice daily for 28 days (CDC, 2010)

Tularemia: I.V. (may transition to oral if clinically appropriate): Initial: 100 mg every 12 hours for 14-21 days (Dennis, 2001)

Vibrio cholerae: Oral: 300 mg as a single dose (WHO, 2004)

Yersinia pestis **(plague):** Oral, I.V.: 200 mg initially then 100 mg twice daily **or** 200 mg once daily for 10 days (Daya, 2005; Inglesby, 2000)

Dosing adjustment in renal impairment: No dosage adjustment necessary in renal impairment.

Poorly dialyzed; no supplemental dose or dosage adjustment necessary, including patients on intermittent hemodialysis, peritoneal dialysis, or continuous renal replacement therapy (eg, CVVHD).

Dietary Considerations

Tetracyclines (in general): Take with food if gastric irritation occurs. While administration with food may decrease GI absorption of doxycycline by up to 20%, administration on an empty stomach is not recommended due to GI intolerance. Of currently available tetracyclines, doxycycline has the least affinity for calcium.

Oracea®: Take on an empty stomach 1 hour before or 2 hours after meals.

Some products may contain sodium.

Administration Oral administration is preferable unless patient has significant nausea and vomiting; I.V. and oral routes are bioequivalent.

Oral: May give with meals to decrease GI upset. Capsule and tablet: Administer with at least 8 ounces of water and have patient sit up for at least 30 minutes after taking to reduce the risk of esophageal irritation and ulceration.

Oracea®: Take on an empty stomach 1 hour before or 2 hours after meals.

Doryx®: May be administered by carefully breaking up the tablet and sprinkling tablet contents on a spoonful of cold applesauce. The delayed release pellets must not be crushed or damaged when breaking up tablet. Should be administered immediately after preparation and without chewing.

I.V.: Infuse I.V. doxycycline over 1-4 hours; avoid extravasation

Intrapleural (unlabeled route): Add to 100 mL NS and instill into chest tube (Porcel, 2006)

Monitoring Parameters Perform culture and sensitivity testing prior to initiating therapy. CBC, renal and liver function tests periodically with prolonged therapy.

Test Interactions False-negative urine glucose using Clinistix®, Tes-Tape®; false-positive urine glucose using Clinitest®; false elevations of urinary catecholamines with fluorescence test

Additional Information Oracea® capsules are not bioequivalent to other doxycycline products.

Dosage Forms Excipient information presented when available (limited, particularly for generics); consult specific product labeling. [DSC] = Discontinued product

Capsule, oral [strength expressed as base]:

Oracea®: 40 mg [30 mg (immediate release) and 10 mg (delayed release)]

Capsule, oral, as hyclate [strength expressed as base]: 50 mg, 100 mg
  Ocudox™: 50 mg [kit includes Ocudox™ capsules (60s), Ocusoft® Lid Scrub™ Plus eyelid cleanser pads, and Tears Again® advanced spray]
  Oraxyl™: 20 mg
  Vibramycin®: 100 mg
Capsule, oral, as monohydrate [strength expressed as base]: 50 mg, 100 mg, 150 mg
  Adoxa®: 150 mg
  Monodox®: 50 mg, 75 mg, 100 mg
Injection, powder for reconstitution, as hyclate [strength expressed as base]: 100 mg
  Doxy 100™: 100 mg
Powder for suspension, oral, as monohydrate [strength expressed as base]:
  Vibramycin®: 25 mg/5 mL (60 mL) [raspberry flavor]
Syrup, oral, as calcium [strength expressed as base]:
  Vibramycin®: 50 mg/5 mL (473 mL) [contains propylene glycol, sodium metabisulfite; raspberry-apple flavor]
Tablet, oral, as hyclate [strength expressed as base]: 20 mg, 100 mg
  Alodox™: 20 mg [kit includes Alodox™ tablets (60s), Ocusoft® Lid Scrub™ pads, eyelid cleanser, and goggles]
  Periostat®: 20 mg
Tablet, oral, as monohydrate [strength expressed as base]: 50 mg, 75 mg, 100 mg, 150 mg
  Adoxa®: 50 mg [DSC], 75 mg [DSC], 100 mg [DSC]
  Adoxa® Pak™ 1/150: 150 mg [DSC] [scored]
  Adoxa® Pak™ 1/75: 75 mg [DSC]
Tablet, delayed release coated beads, oral, as hyclate [strength expressed as base]: 75 mg, 100 mg
Tablet, delayed release coated pellets, oral, as hyclate:
  Doryx®: 150 mg [scored; contains sodium 9 mg (0.392 mEq)/tablet]
Tablet, delayed release coated pellets, oral, as hyclate [strength expressed as base]:
  Doryx®: 75 mg [DSC] [scored; contains sodium 4.5 mg (0.196 mEq)/tablet]
  Doryx®: 100 mg [DSC] [scored; contains sodium 6 mg (0.261 mEq)/tablet]
  Doryx®: 150 mg [DSC] [scored; contains sodium 9 mg (0.392 mEq)/tablet]

Extemporaneous Preparations If a public health emergency is declared and liquid doxycycline is unavailable for the treatment of anthrax, emergency doses may be prepared for children or adults who cannot swallow tablets.

Add 20 mL of water to one 100 mg tablet. Allow tablet to soak in the water for 5 minutes to soften. Crush into a fine powder and stir until well mixed. Appropriate dose should be taken from this mixture. To increase palatability, mix with food or drink. If mixing with drink, add 15 mL of milk, chocolate milk, chocolate pudding, or apple juice to the appropriate dose of mixture. If using apple juice, also add 4 teaspoons of sugar. Doxycycline and water mixture may be stored at room temperature for up to 24 hours.

U.S. Food and Drug Administration, Center for Drug Evaluation and Research, "Public Health Emergency Home Preparation Instructions for Doxycycline." Available at http://www.fda.gov/Drugs/EmergencyPreparedness/BioterrorismandDrugPreparedness/ucm130996.htm

◆ **Doxycycline Calcium** *see* Doxycycline *on page 557*

◆ **Doxycycline Hyclate** *see* Doxycycline *on page 557*

◆ **Doxycycline Monohydrate** *see* Doxycycline *on page 557*

◆ **Doxytab (Can)** *see* Doxycycline *on page 557*

◆ **DPA** *see* Valproic Acid *on page 1757*

◆ **DPE** *see* Dipivefrin *on page 527*

◆ **D-Penicillamine** *see* PenicillAMINE *on page 1319*

◆ **DPH** *see* Phenytoin *on page 1346*

◆ **DPM™ [OTC]** *see* Urea *on page 1749*

◆ **Dramamine® [OTC]** *see* DimenhyDRINATE *on page 513*

◆ **Dramamine® Less Drowsy Formula [OTC]** *see* Meclizine *on page 1057*

◆ **Driminate [OTC]** *see* DimenhyDRINATE *on page 513*

◆ **Drisdol®** *see* Ergocalciferol *on page 610*

◆ **Dristan® N.D. (Can)** *see* Acetaminophen and Pseudoephedrine *on page 31*

◆ **Dristan® N.D., Extra Strength (Can)** *see* Acetaminophen and Pseudoephedrine *on page 31*

◆ **Dritho-Creme®** *see* Anthralin *on page 123*

◆ **Dritho-Scalp®** *see* Anthralin *on page 123*

◆ **Drixoral® ND (Can)** *see* Pseudoephedrine *on page 1430*

Dronabinol (droe NAB i nol)

Brand Names: Canada Marinol®

Index Terms Delta-9 THC; Delta-9-tetrahydro-cannabinol; Tetrahydrocannabinol; THC

Pharmacologic Category Antiemetic; Appetite Stimulant

Use Chemotherapy-associated nausea and vomiting refractory to other antiemetic(s); AIDS-related anorexia

Unlabeled Use Cancer-related anorexia

Pregnancy Risk Factor C

Pregnancy Considerations Adverse events have been observed in animal reproduction studies.

Lactation Enters breast milk/not recommended

Contraindications Hypersensitivity to dronabinol, cannabinoids, sesame oil, or any component of the formulation, or marijuana; should be avoided in patients with a history of schizophrenia

Warnings/Precautions Use with caution in patients with hepatic disease or seizure disorders. Reduce dosage in patients with severe hepatic impairment. May cause additive CNS effects with sedatives, hypnotics or other psychoactive agents; patients must be cautioned about performing tasks which require mental alertness (eg, operating machinery or driving).

May have potential for abuse; drug is psychoactive substance in marijuana; use caution in patients with a history of substance abuse or potential. May cause withdrawal symptoms upon abrupt discontinuation. Use with caution in patients with mania, depression, or schizophrenia; careful psychiatric monitoring is recommended. Use caution in elderly; they are more sensitive to adverse effects.

Adverse Reactions Frequency not always specified.

>1%:

Cardiovascular: Palpitations, tachycardia, vasodilation/facial flushing

Central nervous system: Euphoria (8% to 24%, dose related), abnormal thinking (3% to 10%), dizziness (3% to 10%), paranoia (3% to 10%), somnolence (3% to 10%), amnesia, anxiety, ataxia, confusion, depersonalization, hallucination

Gastrointestinal: Abdominal pain (3% to 10%), nausea (3% to 10%), vomiting (3% to 10%)

Neuromuscular & skeletal: Weakness

<1% (Limited to important or life-threatening): Conjunctivitis, depression, diarrhea, fatigue, fecal incontinence, flushing, hypotension, myalgia, nightmares, seizure, speech difficulties, tinnitus, vision difficulties

Drug Interactions

Metabolism/Transport Effects None known.

Avoid Concomitant Use There are no known interactions where it is recommended to avoid concomitant use.

Increased Effect/Toxicity

Dronabinol may increase the levels/effects of: Alcohol (Ethyl); CNS Depressants; Methotrimeprazine; Selective Serotonin Reuptake Inhibitors; Sympathomimetics

The levels/effects of Dronabinol may be increased by: Anticholinergic Agents; Cocaine; Droperidol; HydrOXYzine; MAO Inhibitors; Methotrimeprazine; Ritonavir

Decreased Effect There are no known significant interactions involving a decrease in effect.

Ethanol/Nutrition/Herb Interactions

Ethanol: May increase CNS depression; monitor for increased effects with coadministration. Caution patients about effects.

Food: Administration with high-lipid meals may increase absorption.

Herb/Nutraceutical: St John's wort may decrease dronabinol levels.

Stability Store under refrigeration (or in a cool environment) between 8°C and 15°C (46°F and 59°F); protect from freezing.

Mechanism of Action Unknown, may inhibit endorphins in the brain's emetic center, suppress prostaglandin synthesis, and/or inhibit medullary activity through an unspecified cortical action. Some pharmacologic effects appear to involve sympathimometic activity; tachyphylaxis to some effect (eg, tachycardia) may occur, but appetite-stimulating effects do not appear to wane over time. Antiemetic activity may be due to effect on cannabinoid receptors (CB1) within the central nervous system.

Pharmacodynamics/Kinetics

Onset of action: Within 1 hour

Peak effect: 2-4 hours

Duration: 24 hours (appetite stimulation)

Absorption: Oral: 90% to 95%; 10% to 20% of dose gets into systemic circulation

Distribution: V_d: 10 L/kg; dronabinol is highly lipophilic and distributes to adipose tissue

Protein binding: 97% to 99%

Metabolism: Hepatic to at least 50 metabolites, some of which are active; 11-hydroxy-delta-9-tetrahydrocannabinol (11-OH-THC) is the major metabolite; extensive first-pass effect

Half-life elimination: Dronabinol: 25-36 hours (terminal); Dronabinol metabolites: 44-59 hours

Time to peak, serum: 0.5-4 hours

Excretion: Feces (50% as unconjugated metabolites, 5% as unchanged drug); urine (10% to 15% as acid metabolites and conjugates)

Dosage Refer to individual protocols. Oral:

Antiemetic: Children and Adults: 5 mg/m^2 1-3 hours before chemotherapy, then 5 mg/m^2/dose every 2-4 hours after chemotherapy for a total of 4-6 doses/day; increase doses in increments of 2.5 mg/m^2 to a maximum of 15 mg/m^2/dose.

Appetite stimulant: Adults: Initial: 2.5 mg twice daily (before lunch and dinner); titrate up to a maximum of 20 mg/day.

Dietary Considerations Capsules contain sesame oil.

Monitoring Parameters CNS effects, heart rate, blood pressure, behavioral profile

Reference Range Antinauseant effects: 5-10 ng/mL

Test Interactions Decreased FSH, LH, growth hormone, and testosterone

Dosage Forms Excipient information presented when available (limited, particularly for generics); consult specific product labeling.

Capsule, soft gelatin, oral: 2.5 mg [contains sesame oil], 5 mg [contains sesame oil], 10 mg [contains sesame oil]

Controlled Substance C-III

Dronedarone (droe NE da rone)

Brand Names: U.S. Multaq®

Brand Names: Canada Multaq®

Index Terms Dronedarone Hydrochloride; SR33589

Pharmacologic Category Antiarrhythmic Agent, Class III

Use To reduce the risk of hospitalization for atrial fibrillation (AF) in patients in sinus rhythm with a history of paroxysmal or persistent AF

Unlabeled Use Alternative antiarrhythmic for the treatment of atrial fibrillation in patients with hypertrophic cardiomyopathy (HCM)

Pregnancy Risk Factor X

Medication Guide Available Yes

Dosage Oral: Adults: Atrial fibrillation/atrial flutter: 400 mg twice daily

Dosing adjustment in renal impairment: No dosage adjustment necessary.

Dosing adjustment in hepatic impairment:

Mild-to-moderate impairment: No dosage adjustment necessary

Severe impairment: Contraindicated

Additional Information Complete prescribing information for this medication should be consulted for additional detail.

Dosage Forms Excipient information presented when available (limited, particularly for generics); consult specific product labeling.

Tablet, oral:

Multaq®: 400 mg

◆ **Dronedarone Hydrochloride** *see* Dronedarone *on page 562*

Droperidol (droe PER i dole)

Brand Names: Canada Droperidol Injection, USP

Index Terms Dehydrobenzperidol

Pharmacologic Category Antiemetic; Antipsychotic Agent, Typical

Use Prevention and/or treatment of nausea and vomiting from surgical and diagnostic procedures

Pregnancy Risk Factor C

Pregnancy Considerations While teratogenicity has not been demonstrated in animal studies, a slight increase in fetal mortality rate has been observed in some animal studies. Droperidol crosses the placenta. Use during pregnancy only if the potential benefits outweigh potential risks to the fetus.

Lactation Excretion in breast milk unknown/use caution

Contraindications Hypersensitivity to droperidol or any component of the formulation; known or suspected QT prolongation, including congenital long QT syndrome (prolonged QT_c is defined as >440 msec in males or >450 msec in females)

Canadian labeling: Additional contraindications (not in U.S. labeling): Not for use in children ≤2 years of age

Warnings/Precautions May alter cardiac conduction. **[U.S. Boxed Warning]: Cases of QT prolongation and torsade de pointes, including some fatal cases, have been reported.** Use extreme caution in patients with bradycardia (<50 bpm), cardiac disease, concurrent MAO inhibitor therapy, Class I and Class III antiarrhythmics or other drugs known to prolong QT interval, and electrolyte disturbances (hypokalemia or hypomagnesemia), including concomitant drugs which may alter electrolytes (diuretics).

Use with caution in patients with seizures or severe liver disease. May be sedating, use with caution in disorders where CNS depression is a feature. Caution in patients with hemodynamic instability, predisposition to seizures, subcortical brain damage, pheochromocytoma or renal disease. Esophageal dysmotility and aspiration have been associated with antipsychotic use - use with caution in patients at risk of pneumonia (ie, Alzheimer's disease). Caution in breast cancer or other prolactin-dependent tumors (may elevate prolactin levels). May alter temperature regulation or mask toxicity of other drugs due to antiemetic effects. May cause orthostatic hypotension - use with caution in patients at risk of this effect or those who would tolerate transient hypotensive episodes (cerebrovascular disease, cardiovascular disease, or other medications which may predispose). Significant hypotension may occur.

May cause anticholinergic effects (confusion, agitation, constipation, xerostomia, blurred vision, urinary retention). Therefore, they should be used with caution in patients with decreased gastrointestinal motility, urinary retention, BPH, xerostomia, or visual problems. Conditions which also may be exacerbated by cholinergic blockade include narrow-angle glaucoma (screening is recommended) and worsening of myasthenia gravis. Relative to other neuroleptics, droperidol has a low potency of cholinergic blockade.

May cause extrapyramidal symptoms (EPS), including pseudoparkinsonism, acute dystonic reactions, akathisia, and tardive dyskinesia. Risk of dystonia (and possibly other EPS) may be greater with increased doses, use of conventional antipsychotics, males, and younger patients. May be associated with neuroleptic malignant syndrome (NMS). May mask toxicity of other drugs or conditions (eg, intestinal obstruction, Reye's syndrome, brain tumor) due to antiemetic effects. Use with caution in the elderly; reduce initial dose.

Adverse Reactions Frequency not defined.

Cardiovascular: Cardiac arrest, hypertension, hypotension (especially orthostatic), QT_c prolongation (dose dependent), tachycardia, torsade de pointes, ventricular tachycardia

Central nervous system: Anxiety, chills, depression (postoperative, transient), dizziness, drowsiness (postoperative) increased, dysphoria, extrapyramidal symptoms (akathisia, dystonia, oculogyric crisis), hallucinations (postoperative), hyperactivity, neuroleptic malignant syndrome (NMS) (rare), restlessness

Respiratory: Bronchospasm, laryngospasm

Miscellaneous: Anaphylaxis, shivering

Drug Interactions

Metabolism/Transport Effects None known.

Avoid Concomitant Use

Avoid concomitant use of Droperidol with any of the following: Artemether; Dronedarone; Lumefantrine; Metoclopramide; Nilotinib; Pimozide; QUEtiapine; QuiNINE; Tetrabenazine; Thioridazine; Toremifene; Vandetanib; Vemurafenib; Ziprasidone

Increased Effect/Toxicity

Droperidol may increase the levels/effects of: Alcohol (Ethyl); Anticholinergics; Anti-Parkinson's Agents (Dopamine Agonist); CNS Depressants; Dronedarone; Methylphenidate; Metoclopramide; Pimozide; QTc-Prolonging Agents; QuiNINE; Serotonin Modulators; Tetrabenazine; Thioridazine; Toremifene; Vandetanib; Vemurafenib; Ziprasidone

The levels/effects of Droperidol may be increased by: Acetylcholinesterase Inhibitors (Central); Alfuzosin; Artemether; Chloroquine; Ciprofloxacin; Ciprofloxacin (Systemic); Gadobutrol; HydrOXYzine; Indacaterol; Lithium formulations; Lumefantrine; MAO Inhibitors; Methylphenidate; Metoclopramide; Nilotinib; Pramlintide; QUEtiapine; QuiNINE; Tetrabenazine

Decreased Effect

Droperidol may decrease the levels/effects of: Amphetamines; Quinagolide

The levels/effects of Droperidol may be decreased by: Anti-Parkinson's Agents (Dopamine Agonist); Lithium formulations

Stability Store at 20°C to 25°C (68° to 77°F); excursions permitted to 15°C to 30°C (59°F to 86°F). Protect from light. Solutions diluted in NS or D_5W are stable at room temperature for up to 7 days in PVC bags or glass bottles. Solutions diluted in LR are stable at room temperature for 24 hours in PVC bags and up to 7 days in glass bottles.

Mechanism of Action Droperidol is a butyrophenone antipsychotic; antiemetic effect is a result of blockade of dopamine stimulation of the chemoreceptor trigger zone. Other effects include alpha-adrenergic blockade, peripheral vascular dilation, and reduction of the pressor effect of epinephrine resulting in hypotension and decreased peripheral vascular resistance; may also reduce pulmonary artery pressure

Pharmacodynamics/Kinetics

Onset of action: 3-10 minutes

Peak effect: ~30 minutes

Duration: 2-4 hours, may extend to 12 hours

Absorption: I.M.: Rapid

Distribution: Crosses blood-brain barrier and placenta

V_d: Children: ~0.6 L/kg; Adults: ~1.5 L/kg

Protein binding: 85% to 90%

Metabolism: Hepatic, to *p*-fluorophenylacetic acid, benzimidazolone, *p*-hydroxypiperidine

Half-life elimination: ~2.3 hours

Excretion: Urine (75%, <1% as unchanged drug); feces (22%, 11% as unchanged drug)

Dosage Note: Titrate carefully to desired effect

I.M., I.V.:

Children 2-12 years: Prevention of postoperative nausea and vomiting (PONV):

Manufacturer labeling: Maximum dose: 0.1 mg/kg; additional doses may be repeated with caution to achieve desired effect

Consensus guideline recommendations: 0.01-0.015 mg/kg (maximum: 1.25 mg) I.V. administered at the end of surgery (Gan, 2007)

Adults: Prevention of PONV:

Manufacturer labeling: Maximum initial dose: 2.5 mg; additional doses of 1.25 mg may be administered with caution to achieve desired effect

Consensus guideline recommendations: 0.625-1.25 mg I.V. administered at the end of surgery (Gan, 2007)

Canadian labeling: I.V.: Prevention and treatment of PONV:

Children >2 years and Adolescents: 0.02-0.05 mg/kg (maximum dose: 1.25 mg) 30 minutes prior to anticipated end of surgery, and then every 6 hours as needed for breakthrough PONV

Adults: 0.625-1.25 mg 30 minutes prior to anticipated end of surgery, and then every 6 hours as needed for breakthrough PONV

Elderly: PONV: 0.625 mg 30 minutes prior to anticipated end of surgery and then every 6 hours as needed for breakthrough PONV; additional dosing should be administered with caution

Dosage adjustment in renal impairment:

U.S. labeling: Specific dosing recommendations are not provided; use with caution

Canadian labeling: I.V.: 0.625 mg; additional dosing should be administered with caution

Dosage adjustment in hepatic impairment:

U.S. labeling: Specific dosing recommendations are not provided; use with caution

Canadian labeling: I.V.: 0.625 mg; additional dosing should be administered with caution

Administration Administer I.M. or I.V.; according to the manufacturer, I.V. push administration should be slow. For I.V. infusion, dilute in 50-100 mL NS or D_5W.

Monitoring Parameters To identify QT prolongation, a 12-lead ECG prior to use is recommended; continued ECG monitoring for 2-3 hours following administration is recommended. Vital signs; serum magnesium and potassium; mental status, abnormal involuntary movement scale (AIMS); observe for dystonias, extrapyramidal side effects, and temperature changes

Dosage Forms Excipient information presented when available (limited, particularly for generics); consult specific product labeling.

Injection, solution: 2.5 mg/mL (2 mL)

Injection, solution [preservative free]: 2.5 mg/mL (2 mL)

◆ **Droperidol Injection, USP (Can)** *see* Droperidol *on page 562*

◆ **Drospirenone and Ethinyl Estradiol** *see* Ethinyl Estradiol and Drospirenone *on page 654*

◆ **Drospirenone, Ethinyl Estradiol, and Levomefolate Calcium** *see* Ethinyl Estradiol, Drospirenone, and Levomefolate *on page 664*

Drotrecogin Alfa (Activated)

(dro TRE coe jin AL fa ak ti VAY ted)

Brand Names: U.S. Xigris® [DSC]

Brand Names: Canada Xigris®

Index Terms Activated Protein C, Human, Recombinant; Drotrecogin Alfa, Activated; Protein C (Activated), Human, Recombinant; rhAPC

Pharmacologic Category Protein C (Activated)

Use Reduction of mortality from severe sepsis (associated with organ dysfunction) in adults at high risk of death (eg, APACHE II score ≥25)

Note: As of October, 2011, drotrecogin alfa has been withdrawn from the market (worldwide).

Unlabeled Use Purpura fulminans

Pregnancy Risk Factor C

Pregnancy Considerations Animal reproduction studies have not been conducted. No adverse effects were seen in a limited number of case reports using drotrecogin alfa in pregnant women (Eppert, 2011; Gupta, 2011).

Lactation Excretion in breast milk unknown/not recommended

Contraindications Hypersensitivity to drotrecogin alfa or any component of the formulation; active internal bleeding; recent hemorrhagic stroke (within 3 months); severe head trauma (within 2 months); recent intracranial or intraspinal surgery (within 2 months); intracranial neoplasm or mass lesion; evidence of cerebral herniation; presence of an epidural catheter; trauma with an increased risk of life-threatening bleeding

Warnings/Precautions Increases risk of bleeding; careful evaluation of risks and benefit is required prior to initiation. Bleeding risk is increased in patients receiving concurrent therapeutic heparin, oral anticoagulants, glycoprotein IIb/IIIa antagonists, platelet aggregation inhibitors, or aspirin at a dosage of >650 mg/day (within 7 days). In addition, an increased bleeding risk is associated with prolonged INR (>3), gastrointestinal bleeding (within 6 weeks), decreased platelet count (<30,000/mm^3), thrombolytic therapy (within 3 days), recent ischemic stroke (within 3 months), intracranial AV malformation or aneurysm, known bleeding diathesis, severe hepatic disease (chronic), or other condition where bleeding is a significant hazard or difficult to manage due to its location. Discontinue if significant bleeding occurs (may consider continued use after stabilization). Treatment interruption required for invasive procedures. During treatment, aPTT cannot be used to assess coagulopathy (PT/INR not affected).

Efficacy not established in adult patients at a low risk of death. Patients with pre-existing nonsepsis-related medical conditions with a poor prognosis (anticipated survival <28 days), patients with acute pancreatitis (no established source of infection), HIV-infected patients with a CD4 count ≤50 cells/mm^3, chronic dialysis patients, pre-existing hypercoagulable conditions, and patients who had received bone marrow, liver, lung, pancreas, or small bowel transplants were excluded from the clinical trial which established benefit. In addition, patients weighing >135 kg were not evaluated. Safety and efficacy have not been established in pediatric patients.

Adverse Reactions As with all drugs which may affect hemostasis, bleeding is the major adverse effect associated with drotrecogin alfa. Hemorrhage may occur at virtually any site. Risk is dependent on multiple variables, including the dosage administered, concurrent use of multiple agents which alter hemostasis, and patient predisposition.

>10%:

Dermatologic: Bruising

Gastrointestinal: Gastrointestinal bleeding

1% to 10%: Hematologic: Bleeding (serious 2.4% during infusion vs 3.5% during 28-day study period; individual events listed as <1%)

<1% (Limited to important or life-threatening): Gastrointestinal hemorrhage, genitourinary bleeding, immune reaction (antibody production), intracranial hemorrhage (0.2%; frequencies up to 2% noted in a previous trial without placebo control), intrathoracic hemorrhage, retroperitoneal bleeding, skin/soft tissue bleeding

Drug Interactions

Metabolism/Transport Effects None known.

Avoid Concomitant Use

Avoid concomitant use of Drotrecogin Alfa (Activated) with any of the following: Rivaroxaban

Increased Effect/Toxicity

Drotrecogin Alfa (Activated) may increase the levels/effects of: Anticoagulants; Collagenase (Systemic); Deferasirox; Fondaparinux; Ibritumomab; Rivaroxaban; Tositumomab and Iodine I 131 Tositumomab

The levels/effects of Drotrecogin Alfa (Activated) may be increased by: Antiplatelet Agents; Antithrombin; Danaparoid; Dasatinib; Heparin; Heparin (Low Molecular Weight); Herbs (Anticoagulant/Antiplatelet Properties); Nonsteroidal Anti-Inflammatory Agents; Pentosan Polysulfate Sodium; Prostacyclin Analogues; Salicylates; Thrombolytic Agents; Vitamin K Antagonists

Decreased Effect There are no known significant interactions involving a decrease in effect.

Ethanol/Nutrition/Herb Interactions Herb/Nutraceutical: Recent use/intake of herbs with anticoagulant or antiplatelet activity (including cat's claw, feverfew, garlic, ginkgo, ginseng, and horse chestnut seed) may increase the risk of bleeding.

Stability Store vials under refrigeration at 2°C to 8°C (36°F to 46°F); do not freeze. Protect from light. Reconstitute 5 mg vials with 2.5 mL and 20 mg vials with 10 mL sterile water for injection (resultant solution ~2 mg/mL). Must be further diluted (within 3 hours of reconstitution) in 0.9% sodium chloride, typically to a concentration between 100 mcg/mL and 200 mcg/mL when using infusion pump and between 100 mcg/mL and 1000 mcg/mL when infused via syringe pump. Although product information states administration must be completed within 12 hours of preparation, additional studies (data on file, Lilly Research Laboratories) show that the final solution is stable for 14 hours at 15°C to 30°C (59°F to 86°F). If not used immediately, a prepared solution may be stored in the refrigerator for up to 12 hours. The total expiration time (refrigeration and administration) should be ≤24 hours from time of preparation.

Mechanism of Action Inhibits factors Va and VIIIa, limiting thrombotic effects. Additional *in vitro* data suggest inhibition of plasminogen activator inhibitor-1 (PAF-1) resulting in profibrinolytic activity, inhibition of macrophage production of tumor necrosis factor, blocking of leukocyte adhesion, and limitation of thrombin-induced inflammatory responses. Relative contribution of effects on the reduction of mortality from sepsis is not completely understood.

Pharmacodynamics/Kinetics

Duration: Plasma nondetectable within 2 hours of discontinuation

Metabolism: Inactivated by endogenous plasma protease inhibitors; mean clearance: 40 L/hour; increased with severe sepsis (~50%)

Half-life elimination: 1.6 hours

Dosage I.V.:

Children and Adults: Purpura fulminans (unlabeled use): 24 mcg/kg/**hour**

Adults: Sepsis: 24 mcg/kg/**hour** for a total of 96 hours; stop infusion **immediately** if clinically-important bleeding is identified. **Note:** Use actual body weight for dosing.

Dosage adjustment in renal impairment: No specific adjustment recommended.

Administration Infuse separately from all other medications. Only dextrose, normal saline, dextrose/saline combinations, and lactated Ringer's solution may be infused through the same line. May administer via infusion pump. Administration of prepared solution must be completed within 12 hours of preparation. Suspend administration for 2 hours prior to invasive procedures or other procedure with significant bleeding risk; may continue treatment immediately following uncomplicated, minimally-invasive procedures, but delay for 12 hours after major invasive procedures/surgery.

Monitoring Parameters Monitor for signs and symptoms of bleeding, hemoglobin/hematocrit, PT/INR, platelet count

Test Interactions May interfere with one-stage coagulation assays based on the aPTT (such as factor VIII, IX, and XI assays).

Additional Information Prepared by recombinant DNA technology in human cell line

Product Availability No longer available; withdrawn from the market (worldwide) as of October 25, 2011.

Dosage Forms Excipient information presented when available (limited, particularly for generics); consult specific product labeling. [DSC] = Discontinued product

Injection, powder for reconstitution [preservative free]:

Xigris®: 5 mg [DSC] [contains sucrose 31.8 mg]

Xigris®: 20 mg [DSC] [contains sucrose 124.9 mg]

- ◆ **Drotrecogin Alfa, Activated** *see* Drotrecogin Alfa (Activated) *on page 564*
- ◆ **Droxia®** *see* Hydroxyurea *on page 851*
- ◆ **DSCG** *see* Cromolyn (Nasal) *on page 418*
- ◆ **DSCG** *see* Cromolyn (Ophthalmic) *on page 418*
- ◆ **DSS** *see* Docusate *on page 537*
- ◆ **DSS® [OTC]** *see* Docusate *on page 537*
- ◆ **DT** *see* Diphtheria and Tetanus Toxoid *on page 520*
- ◆ **DTaP** *see* Diphtheria and Tetanus Toxoids, and Acellular Pertussis Vaccine *on page 523*
- ◆ **DTaP-HepB-IPV** *see* Diphtheria, Tetanus Toxoids, Acellular Pertussis, Hepatitis B (Recombinant), and Poliovirus (Inactivated) Vaccine *on page 527*
- ◆ **DTaP/Hib** *see* Diphtheria and Tetanus Toxoids, Acellular Pertussis, and *Haemophilus influenzae* b Conjugate Vaccine *on page 522*
- ◆ **DTaP-IPV** *see* Diphtheria and Tetanus Toxoids, Acellular Pertussis, and Poliovirus Vaccine *on page 522*
- ◆ **DTaP-IPV/Hib** *see* Diphtheria and Tetanus Toxoids, Acellular Pertussis, Poliovirus and *Haemophilus* b Conjugate Vaccine *on page 522*
- ◆ **DTC 101** *see* Cytarabine (Liposomal) *on page 432*
- ◆ **DTIC** *see* Dacarbazine *on page 438*
- ◆ **DTIC-Dome** *see* Dacarbazine *on page 438*
- ◆ **DTO (error-prone abbreviation)** *see* Opium Tincture *on page 1249*
- ◆ **D-Trp(6)-LHRH** *see* Triptorelin *on page 1742*
- ◆ **Duetact™** *see* Pioglitazone and Glimepiride *on page 1357*
- ◆ **Dulcolax® [OTC]** *see* Bisacodyl *on page 219*
- ◆ **Dulcolax® [OTC]** *see* Docusate *on page 537*
- ◆ **Dulcolax® (Can)** *see* Bisacodyl *on page 219*
- ◆ **Dulcolax Balance® [OTC]** *see* Polyethylene Glycol 3350 *on page 1372*
- ◆ **Dulcolax® Stool Softener [OTC]** *see* Docusate *on page 537*
- ◆ **Dulera®** *see* Mometasone and Formoterol *on page 1151*
- ◆ **Dull-C® [OTC]** *see* Ascorbic Acid *on page 149*

DULoxetine (doo LOX e teen)

Brand Names: U.S. Cymbalta®

Brand Names: Canada Cymbalta®

Index Terms (+)-(*S*)-*N*-Methyl-γ-(1-naphthyloxy)-2-thiophenepropylamine Hydrochloride; Duloxetine Hydrochloride; LY248686

Pharmacologic Category Antidepressant, Serotonin/Norepinephrine Reuptake Inhibitor

Additional Appendix Information

Antidepressant Agents *on page 1874*

Use Acute and maintenance treatment of major depressive disorder (MDD); treatment of generalized anxiety disorder (GAD); management of diabetic peripheral neuropathic pain (DPNP); management of fibromyalgia (FM); chronic musculoskeletal pain (eg, chronic low back pain, osteoarthritis)

Unlabeled Use Treatment of stress incontinence

Pregnancy Risk Factor C

Pregnancy Considerations Adverse events were observed in animal reproduction studies. Nonteratogenic effects in the newborn following SSRI/SNRI exposure late in the third trimester include respiratory distress, cyanosis, apnea, seizures, temperature instability, feeding difficulty, vomiting, hypoglycemia, hyper- or hypotonia, hyperreflexia, jitteriness, irritability, constant crying, and tremor. Symptoms may be due to the toxicity of the SNRIs/SSRIs or a discontinuation syndrome and may be consistent with serotonin syndrome associated with SSRI treatment. The long-term effects of *in utero* SNRI/SSRI exposure on infant development and behavior are not known.

The ACOG recommends that therapy with SSRIs or SNRIs during pregnancy be individualized; treatment of depression during pregnancy should incorporate the clinical expertise of the mental health clinician, obstetrician, primary healthcare provider, and pediatrician. According to the American Psychiatric Association (APA), the risks of medication treatment should be weighed against other treatment options and untreated depression. For women who discontinue antidepressant medications during pregnancy and who may be at high risk for postpartum depression, the medications can be restarted following delivery. Treatment algorithms have been developed by the ACOG and the APA for the management of depression in women prior to conception and during pregnancy.

Healthcare providers are encouraged to enroll women exposed to duloxetine during pregnancy in the Cymbalta® Pregnancy Registry (866-814-6975 or http://cymbalta-pregnancyregistry.com).

Lactation Enters breast milk/not recommended

Medication Guide Available Yes

Contraindications Concomitant use or within 2 weeks of MAO inhibitors; uncontrolled narrow-angle glaucoma

Note: MAO inhibitor therapy must be stopped for 14 days before duloxetine is initiated. Treatment with MAO inhibitors should not be initiated until 5 days after the discontinuation of duloxetine.

Canadian labeling: Additional contraindications (not in U.S. labeling): Hypersensitivity to duloxetine or any component of the formulation; hepatic impairment; severe renal impairment (eg, Cl_{cr} <30 mL/minute) or end-stage renal disease (ESRD); concomitant use with thioridazine or with CYP1A2 inhibitors

Warnings/Precautions [U.S. Boxed Warning]: Antidepressants increase the risk of suicidal thinking and behavior in children, adolescents, and young adults (18-24 years of age) with major depressive disorder (MDD) and other psychiatric disorders; consider risk prior to prescribing. Short-term studies did not show an increased risk in patients >24 years of age and showed a decreased risk in patients ≥65 years. Closely monitor for clinical worsening, suicidality, or unusual changes in behavior; the patient's family or caregiver should be instructed to closely observe the patient and communicate condition with healthcare provider. A medication guide concerning the use of antidepressants in children and teenagers should be dispensed with each prescription. **Duloxetine is not FDA approved for use in children.**

The possibility of a suicide attempt is inherent in major depression and may persist until remission occurs. Patients treated with antidepressants should be observed for clinical worsening and suicidality, especially during the initial (generally first 1-2 months) few months of a course of drug therapy, or at times of dose changes, either increases or decreases. Use caution in high-risk patients. Worsening depression and severe abrupt suicidality that are not part of the presenting symptoms may require discontinuation or modification of drug therapy. The patient's family or caregiver should be alerted to monitor patients for the emergence of suicidality and associated behaviors (such as agitation, irritability, hostility, impulsivity, and hypomania) and call healthcare provider.

May worsen psychosis in some patients or precipitate a shift to mania or hypomania in patients with bipolar disorder. Patients presenting with depressive symptoms should be screened for bipolar disorder. Monotherapy in patients with bipolar disorder should be avoided. **Duloxetine is not FDA approved for the treatment of bipolar depression.**

May cause orthostatic hypotension/syncope at therapeutic doses especially within the first week of therapy and after dose increases. Monitor blood pressure with initiation of therapy, dose increases (especially in patients receiving >60 mg/day), or with concomitant use of vasodilators, CYP2D6 inhibitors/substrates, or CYP1A2 inhibitors. Use caution in patients with hypertension. May increase blood pressure. Rare cases of hypertensive crisis have been reported in patients with pre-existing hypertension; evaluate blood pressure prior to initiating therapy and periodically thereafter; consider dose reduction or gradual discontinuation of therapy in individuals with sustained hypertension during therapy.

Modest increases in serum glucose and hemoglobin A_{1c} (Hb A_{1c}) levels have been observed in some diabetic patients receiving duloxetine therapy for diabetic peripheral neuropathic pain (DPNP). Duloxetine may cause increased urinary resistance; advise patient to report symptoms of urinary hesitation/difficulty. Has a low potential to impair cognitive or motor performance. Use caution with a previous seizure disorder or condition predisposing to seizures such as brain damage or alcoholism. Avoid use in patients with substantial ethanol intake, evidence of chronic liver disease, or hepatic impairment (contraindicated in Canadian labeling). Rare cases of hepatic failure (including fatalities) have been reported with use. Hepatitis with abdominal pain, hepatomegaly, elevated transaminase levels >20 times the upper limit of normal (ULN) with and without jaundice have all been observed. Discontinue therapy with the presentation of jaundice or other signs of hepatic dysfunction and do not reinitiate therapy unless another source or cause is identified. Use caution in patients with impaired gastric motility (eg, some diabetics) may affect stability of the capsule's enteric coating.

May cause hyponatremia/SIADH (elderly at increased risk); volume depletion (diuretics may increase risk). Use with caution in patients with controlled narrow angle glaucoma. May cause or exacerbate sexual dysfunction. Use caution with renal impairment (contraindicated in Canadian labeling for severe renal impairment or ESRD). Use caution with concomitant CNS depressants. May impair platelet aggregation; use caution with concomitant use of NSAIDs, ASA, or other drugs that affect coagulation; the risk of bleeding may be potentiated.

Serotonin syndrome and neuroleptic malignant syndrome (NMS)-like reactions have occurred with serotonin/norepinephrine reuptake inhibitors (SNRIs) and selective serotonin reuptake inhibitors (SSRIs) when used alone, and particularly when used in combination with serotonergic agents (eg, triptans) or antidopaminergic agents (eg, antipsychotics). Concurrent use with MAO inhibitors is contraindicated. Use caution during concurrent therapy with triptans and drugs which lower the seizure threshold; concurrent use of serotonin precursors (eg, tryptophan) is not recommended. To discontinue therapy with duloxetine, gradually taper dose. If intolerable symptoms occur following a decrease in dosage or upon discontinuation of therapy, then resuming the previous dose with a more gradual taper should be considered. May increase the risks associated with electroconvulsive therapy. Consider discontinuing, when possible, prior to elective surgery. Formulation contains sucrose; patients with fructose intolerance, glucose-galactose malabsorption, or sucrase-isomaltase deficiency should avoid use.

Adverse Reactions

>10%:

Central nervous system: Headache (13% to 14%), somnolence (10% to 12%; dose related), fatigue (10 to 11%)

Gastrointestinal: Nausea (23% to 25%), xerostomia (11% to 15%; dose related)

1% to 10%:

Cardiovascular: Palpitation (1% to 2%)

Central nervous system: Dizziness (10%), insomnia (10%; dose related), agitation (3% to 5%), anxiety (3%), dreams abnormal (1% to 2%), yawning (1% to 2%), hypoesthesia (≥1%), lethargy (≥1%), vertigo (≥1%), chills (1%), sleep disorder (1%)

Dermatologic: Hyperhydrosis (6% to 7%)

Endocrine & metabolic: Libido decreased (2% to 4%), hot flushes (1% to 3%), orgasm abnormality (1% to 3%)

Gastrointestinal: Constipation (10%; dose related), diarrhea (9% to 10%), appetite decreased (7% to 9%; dose related), abdominal pain (4% to 6%), vomiting (3% to 5%), dyspepsia (2%), weight loss (2%), flatulence (≥1%), taste abnormal (≥1%), weight gain (≥1%)

Genitourinary: Erectile dysfunction (4% to 5%), ejaculation delayed (3%; dose related), ejaculatory dysfunction (2%)
Hepatic: ALT >3x ULN (1%)
Neuromuscular & skeletal: Muscle spasms (3%), tremor (2% to 3%; dose related), musculoskeletal pain (≥1%), paresthesia (≥1%), rigors (≥1%)
Ocular: Blurred vision (1% to 3%)
Respiratory: Nasopharyngitis (5%), cough (3%)
Miscellaneous: Influenza (3%)

<1% (Limited to important or life-threatening): Alkaline phosphatase increased, anaphylactic reaction, angioneurotic edema, apathy, bruxism, contact dermatitis, dehydration, dermatitis, diastolic blood pressure increased, diplopia, disorientation, dysarthria, dyskinesia, dysuria, eructation, erythema, erythema multiforme, EPS, gastritis, gastroenteritis, glaucoma, gynecological bleeding, hallucinations, Hb A_{1c} increased, hepatic failure, hepatitis, hepatomegaly, hyperbilirubinemia, hypercholesterolemia, hyperglycemia, hyperlipidemia, hypersensitivity, hypertensive crisis, hyponatremia, hypothyroidism, jaundice, malaise, mania, MI, micturition urgency, mood swings, muscle spasm, muscle tightness, muscle twitching, night sweats, nocturia, orthostatic hypotension, peripheral coldness, photosensitivity, polyuria, rash, restless leg syndrome, seizure, serotonin syndrome, SIADH, Stevens-Johnson syndrome, stomatitis, supraventricular arrhythmia, syncope, systolic blood pressure increased, tachycardia, thirst, throat tightness, transaminases increased, trismus, urinary retention, urticaria

Drug Interactions

Metabolism/Transport Effects Substrate of CYP1A2 (major), CYP2D6 (major); **Note:** Assignment of Major/ Minor substrate status based on clinically relevant drug interaction potential; **Inhibits** CYP2D6 (moderate)

Avoid Concomitant Use

Avoid concomitant use of DULoxetine with any of the following: Iobenguane I 123; MAO Inhibitors; Methylene Blue

Increased Effect/Toxicity

DULoxetine may increase the levels/effects of: Alpha-/ Beta-Agonists; Aspirin; CYP2D6 Substrates; Fesoterodine; Methylene Blue; Metoclopramide; Nebivolol; NSAID (Nonselective); Serotonin Modulators; Tamoxifen; Tricyclic Antidepressants

The levels/effects of DULoxetine may be increased by: Abiraterone Acetate; Alcohol (Ethyl); Antipsychotics; CYP1A2 Inhibitors (Moderate); CYP1A2 Inhibitors (Strong); CYP2D6 Inhibitors (Moderate); CYP2D6 Inhibitors (Strong); Darunavir; Deferasirox; FluvoxaMINE; Linezolid; MAO Inhibitors; PARoxetine; Propafenone

Decreased Effect

DULoxetine may decrease the levels/effects of: Alpha2-Agonists; Codeine; Iobenguane I 123; Ioflupane I 123

The levels/effects of DULoxetine may be decreased by: CYP1A2 Inducers (Strong); Cyproterone; Peginterferon Alfa-2b

Ethanol/Nutrition/Herb Interactions

Ethanol: Ethanol may increase hepatotoxic potential of duloxetine. Ethanol may also increase CNS depression; monitor for increased effects with coadministration. Caution patients about effects.

Herb/Nutraceutical: Avoid valerian, St John's wort, SAMe, kava kava, and gotu kola (may increase CNS depression).

Stability Store at 25°C (77°F); excursions permitted to 15°C to 30°C (59°F to 86°F)

Mechanism of Action Duloxetine is a potent inhibitor of neuronal serotonin and norepinephrine reuptake and a weak inhibitor of dopamine reuptake. Duloxetine has no significant activity for muscarinic cholinergic, H_1-histaminergic, or alpha$_2$-adrenergic receptors. Duloxetine does not possess MAO-inhibitory activity.

Pharmacodynamics/Kinetics

Absorption: Well absorbed, 2-hour delay in absorption after ingestion; food decreases extent of absorption ~10% (no effect on C_{max})
Distribution: 1640 L (range: 701-3800 L)
Protein binding: >90%; primarily to albumin and α_1-acid glycoprotein
Metabolism: Hepatic, via CYP1A2 and CYP2D6; forms multiple metabolites (inactive)
Half-life elimination: 12 hours (range: 8-17 hours)
Time to peak: 6 hours; 10 hours when ingested with food
Excretion: Urine (~70%; <1% of total dose as unchanged drug); feces (~20%)

Dosage Oral:

Adults:

Major depressive disorder: Initial: 40-60 mg/day; dose may be divided (ie, 20 or 30 mg twice daily) or given as a single daily dose of 60 mg; maintenance: 60 mg once daily; for doses >60 mg/day, titrate dose in increments of 30 mg/day over 1 week as tolerated to a maximum dose: 120 mg/day. **Note:** Doses >60 mg/day have not been demonstrated to be more effective.

Diabetic neuropathy: 60 mg once daily; lower initial doses may be considered in patients where tolerability is a concern and/or renal impairment is present. **Note:** Doses up to 120 mg/day administered in clinical trials offered no additional benefit and were less well tolerated than dose of 60 mg/day.

Fibromyalgia: 30 mg once daily for 1 week, then increase to 60 mg once daily as tolerated. **Note:** Doses up to 120 mg/day administered in clinical trials offered no additional benefit and were less well tolerated than dose of 60 mg/day.

Generalized anxiety disorder: Initial: 30-60 mg/day as a single daily dose; patients initiated at 30 mg/day should be titrated to 60 mg/day after 1 week; maximum dose: 120 mg/day. **Note:** Doses >60 mg/day have not been demonstrated to be more effective than 60 mg/day.

Chronic musculoskeletal pain: 30 mg once daily for 1 week, then increase to 60 mg once daily as tolerated

Stress incontinence (unlabeled use): 40 mg twice daily (Dmochowski, 2003)

Note: Upon discontinuation of duloxetine therapy, gradually taper dose. If intolerable symptoms occur following a dose reduction, consider resuming the previously prescribed dose and/or decrease dose at a more gradual rate.

Elderly:

Major depressive disorder: Manufacturer does not recommend specific dosage adjustment. Conservatively, may initiate at a dose of 20 mg 1-2 times/day; increase to 40-60 mg/day as a single daily dose or in divided doses **or** initiate therapy at 30 mg/day for 1 week then increase to 60 mg/day as tolerated.

Other indications: Refer to adult dosing

Dosage adjustment in renal impairment: Not recommended for use in Cl_{cr} <30 mL/minute or ESRD (contraindicated in Canadian labeling); in mild-moderate impairment, lower initial doses may be considered with titration guided by response and tolerability

Dosage adjustment in hepatic impairment: Not recommended for use in hepatic impairment (contraindicated in Canadian labeling)

Dietary Considerations May be taken without regard to meals.

Administration Capsule should be swallowed whole; do not crush or chew. Although the manufacturer does not recommend opening the capsule to facilitate administration; the contents of capsule may be sprinkled on applesauce or in apple juice and swallowed (without chewing) immediately. Do not sprinkle contents on chocolate pudding (Wells, 2008). Administer without regard to meals.

Monitoring Parameters Blood pressure should be checked prior to initiating therapy and then regularly monitored, especially in patients with a high baseline blood pressure; mental status for depression, suicidal ideation (especially at the beginning of therapy or when doses are increased or decreased), anxiety, social functioning, mania, panic attacks; glucose levels and Hb A_{1c} levels in diabetic patients, creatinine, BUN, transaminases

For musculoskeletal pain: Pain relief

Dosage Forms Excipient information presented when available (limited, particularly for generics); consult specific product labeling.

Capsule, delayed release, enteric coated pellets, oral:

Cymbalta®: 20 mg, 30 mg, 60 mg

- **Duloxetine Hydrochloride** *see* DULoxetine *on page 565*
- **Duodopa™ (Can)** *see* Carbidopa and Levodopa *on page 284*
- **Duodote™** *see* Atropine and Pralidoxime *on page 172*
- **DuoNeb®** *see* Ipratropium and Albuterol *on page 924*
- **DuP 753** *see* Losartan *on page 1035*
- **Duraclon®** *see* CloNIDine *on page 392*
- **Duragesic®** *see* FentaNYL *on page 697*
- **Duragesic® MAT (Can)** *see* FentaNYL *on page 697*
- **Duralith® (Can)** *see* Lithium *on page 1023*
- **Duramorph** *see* Morphine (Systemic) *on page 1153*
- **Durezol®** *see* Difluprednate *on page 503*
- **Duricef** *see* Cefadroxil *on page 301*
- **Durolane® (Can)** *see* Hyaluronate and Derivatives *on page 831*

Dutasteride (doo TAS teer ide)

Brand Names: U.S. Avodart®

Brand Names: Canada Avodart®

Pharmacologic Category 5 Alpha-Reductase Inhibitor

Use Treatment of symptomatic benign prostatic hyperplasia (BPH) as monotherapy or combination therapy with tamsulosin

Unlabeled Use Treatment of male pattern baldness

Pregnancy Risk Factor X

Dosage Oral: Adults: Males: BPH: 0.5 mg once daily alone or in combination with tamsulosin

Dosage adjustment in renal impairment: No adjustment required

Dosage adjustment in hepatic impairment: Use caution; no specific adjustments recommended

Additional Information Complete prescribing information for this medication should be consulted for additional detail.

Dosage Forms Excipient information presented when available (limited, particularly for generics); consult specific product labeling.

Capsule, softgel, oral:

Avodart®: 0.5 mg

Dutasteride and Tamsulosin

(doo TAS teer ide & tam SOO loe sin)

Brand Names: U.S. Jalyn™

Index Terms Tamsulosin and Dutasteride; Tamsulosin Hydrochloride and Dutasteride

Pharmacologic Category 5 Alpha-Reductase Inhibitor; $Alpha_1$ Blocker

Use Treatment of symptomatic benign prostatic hyperplasia (BPH)

Pregnancy Risk Factor X

Dosage Oral: Adults: Males:

BPH: One capsule (0.5 mg dutasteride/0.4 mg tamsulosin) once daily ~30 minutes after the same meal each day

Dosage adjustment in renal impairment:

Cl_{cr} 10-30 mL/minute/1.73 m^2: No adjustment needed

Cl_{cr} <10 mL/minute/1.73 m^2: Not studied

Dosage adjustment in hepatic impairment: Use caution; no specific adjustments recommended

Additional Information Complete prescribing information for this medication should be consulted for additional detail.

Dosage Forms Excipient information presented when available (limited, particularly for generics); consult specific product labeling.

Capsule, oral:

Jalyn™: Dutasteride 0.5 mg and tamsulosin hydrochloride 0.4 mg

- **Duvoid® (Can)** *see* Bethanechol *on page 211*
- **DW286** *see* Gemifloxacin *on page 786*
- **DX-88** *see* Ecallantide *on page 569*
- **Dyazide®** *see* Hydrochlorothiazide and Triamterene *on page 836*
- **Dycill® (Can)** *see* Dicloxacillin *on page 499*

Dyclonine (DYE kloe neen)

Brand Names: U.S. Sucrets® Children's [OTC]; Sucrets® Maximum Strength [OTC]; Sucrets® Regular Strength [OTC]

Index Terms Dyclonine Hydrochloride

Pharmacologic Category Local Anesthetic, Oral

Use Temporary relief of pain associated with oral mucosa

Dosage Oral: Children ≥2 years and Adults: Lozenge: One lozenge every 2 hours as needed (maximum: 10 lozenges/day)

Additional Information Complete prescribing information for this medication should be consulted for additional detail.

Dosage Forms Excipient information presented when available (limited, particularly for generics); consult specific product labeling.

Lozenge, oral, as hydrochloride:

Sucrets® Children's: 1.2 mg (18s) [cherry flavor]

Sucrets® Maximum Strength: 3 mg (18s) [black-cherry flavor]

Sucrets® Maximum Strength: 3 mg (18s) [wintergreen flavor]

Sucrets® Regular Strength: 2 mg (18s)

Sucrets® Regular Strength: 2 mg (18s) [wild cherry flavor]

- **Dyclonine Hydrochloride** *see* Dyclonine *on page 568*
- **Dynacin®** *see* Minocycline *on page 1137*
- **DynaCirc CR®** *see* Isradipine *on page 941*
- **Dyna-Hex® [OTC]** *see* Chlorhexidine Gluconate *on page 341*

Dyphylline and Guaifenesin

(DYE fi lin & gwye FEN e sin)

Brand Names: U.S. COPD [DSC]; Difil-G [DSC]; Difil-G® 400; Difil®-G Forte [DSC]; Lufyllin®-GG [DSC]

Index Terms Guaifenesin and Dyphylline

Pharmacologic Category Expectorant; Theophylline Derivative

Use Treatment of bronchial asthma and reversible bronchospasm associated with chronic bronchitis and emphysema

Pregnancy Risk Factor C

Dosage Oral:

Children 6-12 years:

Elixir: Lufyllin®-GG: 15-30 mL 3 or 4 times/day

Tablet: Lufyllin®-GG: 1/2 -1 tablet 3 or 4 times/day

Children >12 years and Adults:

Elixir: Lufyllin®-GG: 30 mL 4 times/day

Liquid: Difil®-G Forte: 5-10 mL 3 or 4 times/day; may double or triple (in severe cases) according to patient response

Tablet: Difil®-G, Lufyllin®-GG: One tablet 3 or 4 times/day

Dosage adjustment in renal impairment: Dosage reduction should be considered in severe renal impairment. Half-life of dyphylline is significantly prolonged in anuria.

Additional Information Complete prescribing information for this medication should be consulted for additional detail.

Dosage Forms Excipient information presented when available (limited, particularly for generics); consult specific product labeling. [DSC] = Discontinued product

Elixir, oral: Dyphylline 100 mg and guaifenesin 100 mg per 15 mL (480 mL)

Lufyllin®-GG: Dyphylline 100 mg and guaifenesin 100 mg per 15 mL (480 mL) [contains alcohol 17%; wine-like flavor] [DSC]

Liquid, oral: Dyphylline 100 mg and guaifenesin 100 mg per 5 mL (480 mL)

Difil®-G Forte: Dyphylline 100 mg and guaifenesin 100 mg per 5 mL (240 mL) [menthol flavor] [DSC]

Tablet, oral: Dyphylline 200 mg and guaifenesin 200 mg

COPD [DSC], Lufyllin®-GG [DSC]: Dyphylline 200 mg and guaifenesin 200 mg

Difil®-G: Dyphylline 200 mg and guaifenesin 300 mg [DSC]

Difil-G® 400: Dyphylline 200 mg and guaifenesin 400 mg

◆ **Dyrenium®** *see* Triamterene *on page* 1735

◆ **Dysport™** *see* AbobotulinumtoxinA *on page* 25

◆ **7E3** *see* Abciximab *on page* 22

◆ **E2020** *see* Donepezil *on page* 543

◆ **E 2080** *see* Rufinamide *on page* 1528

◆ **E7389** *see* Eribulin *on page* 611

◆ **EACA** *see* Aminocaproic Acid *on page* 89

◆ **Ebixa® (Can)** *see* Memantine *on page* 1068

Ecallantide (e KAL lan tide)

Brand Names: U.S. Kalbitor®

Index Terms DX-88

Pharmacologic Category Kallikrein Inhibitor

Use Treatment of acute attacks of hereditary angioedema (HAE)

Pregnancy Risk Factor C

Pregnancy Considerations Adverse effects were noted in animal studies. There are no adequate and well-controlled studies in pregnant women. Use during pregnancy only if the potential benefits justify the potential risk to the fetus.

Lactation Excretion in breast milk unknown/use caution

Medication Guide Available Yes

Contraindications Hypersensitivity to ecallantide or any component of the formulation

Warnings/Precautions [U.S. Boxed Warning]: Serious hypersensitivity reactions, including anaphylaxis have been reported; administer only by healthcare provider in presence of appropriate medical support to manage anaphylaxis and hereditary angioedema. Do not administer to patients with known hypersensitivity to ecallantide. Reactions usually occur within 1 hour and may include chest discomfort, flushing, hypotension, nasal congestion, pharyngeal edema, pruritus, rash, rhinorrhea, sneezing, throat irritation, urticaria, and wheezing. Signs/symptoms of hypersensitivity reactions may be similar to those associated with hereditary angioedema attacks, therefore, consideration should be given to treatment methods; monitor patients closely.

Adverse Reactions

>10%:

Central nervous system: Headache (8% to 16%), fatigue (12%)

Gastrointestinal: Nausea (5% to 13%), diarrhea (4% to 11%)

1% to 10%:

Central nervous system: Fever (4% to 5%)

Dermatologic: Pruritus (5%), rash (3%), urticaria (2%)

Gastrointestinal: Vomiting (6%), upper abdominal pain (5%)

Local: Injection site reactions (3% to 7%; includes bruising, erythema, irritation, pain, pruritus, urticaria)

Respiratory: Upper respiratory infection (8%), nasopharyngitis (3% to 6%)

Miscellaneous: Antibody formation (5% to 7%), anaphylaxis (4%)

<1% (Limited to important or life-threatening) Hypersensitivity (chest discomfort, flushing, pharyngeal edema, rhinorrhea, sneezing, nasal congestion, wheezing, hypotension)

Drug Interactions

Metabolism/Transport Effects None known.

Avoid Concomitant Use There are no known interactions where it is recommended to avoid concomitant use.

Increased Effect/Toxicity There are no known significant interactions involving an increase in effect.

Decreased Effect There are no known significant interactions involving a decrease in effect.

Stability Store under refrigeration at 2°C to 8°C (36°F to 46°F). Protect from light. May be stored for up to 14 days at <30°C (<86°F). Do not use if solution is discolored or has particulate matter present.

Mechanism of Action Ecallantide is a recombinant protein which inhibits the conversion of high molecular weight kininogen to bradykinin by selectively and reversibly inhibiting plasma kallikrein. Unregulated bradykinin production is thought to contribute to the increased vascular permeability and angioedema observed in HAE.

Pharmacodynamics/Kinetics

Onset: 30 minutes to 4 hours

Distribution: 18.6-34.2 L

Half-life elimination: 1.5-2.5 hours

Time to peak: ~2-3 hours

Excretion: Primarily urine

Dosage SubQ: Children ≥16 years and adults: Treatment of HAE attacks: 30 mg (as three 10 mg [1 mL] injections); may repeat an additional 30 mg within 24 hours

Administration Administer as 3 (10 mg/mL each) injections subcutaneously into skin of abdomen, upper arm, or thigh (do not administer at site of attack). Recommended needle size is 27 gauge. Separate injections by 2 inches (5 cm). May inject all doses in same or different location; rotation of sites is not necessary. Monitor/observe for hypersensitivity.

Monitoring Parameters Monitor for hypersensitivity reaction

Dosage Forms Excipient information presented when available (limited, particularly for generics); consult specific product labeling.

Injection, solution [preservative free]:

Kalbitor®: 10 mg/mL (1 mL)

Echothiophate Iodide

(ek oh THYE oh fate EYE oh dide)

Brand Names: U.S. Phospholine Iodide®

Index Terms Ecostigmine Iodide

Pharmacologic Category Acetylcholinesterase Inhibitor; Ophthalmic Agent, Antiglaucoma; Ophthalmic Agent, Miotic

Use Used as miotic in treatment of chronic, open-angle glaucoma; may be useful in specific cases of angle-closure glaucoma (postiridectomy or where surgery refused/contraindicated); postcataract surgery-related glaucoma; accommodative esotropia

Pregnancy Risk Factor C

Dosage Ophthalmic:

Children: Accommodative esotropia:

Diagnosis: Instill 1 drop (0.125%) once daily into both eyes at bedtime for 2-3 weeks

Treatment: Usual dose: Instill 1 drop of 0.06% once daily or 0.125% every other day (maximum: 0.125% daily). **Note:** Use lowest concentration and frequency which gives satisfactory response; if necessary, doses >0.125% daily may be used for short periods of time.

Adults: Open-angle or secondary glaucoma:

Initial: Instill 1 drop (0.03%) twice daily into eyes with 1 dose just prior to bedtime

Maintenance: Some patients have been treated with 1 dose daily or every other day

Conversion from other ophthalmic agents: If IOP control was unsatisfactory, patients may be expected to require higher doses of echothiophate (eg, ≥0.06%); however, patients should be initially started on the 0.03% strength for a short period to better tolerance.

Additional Information Complete prescribing information for this medication should be consulted for additional detail.

Dosage Forms Excipient information presented when available (limited, particularly for generics); consult specific product labeling.

Powder for reconstitution, ophthalmic:

Phospholine Iodide®: 6.25 mg (5 mL) [0.125%]

◆ **EC-Naprosyn®** *see* Naproxen *on page* 1177

◆ ***E. coli* Asparaginase** *see* Asparaginase (*E. coli*) *on page* 151

Econazole (e KONE a zole)

Index Terms Econazole Nitrate

Pharmacologic Category Antifungal Agent, Topical

Use Topical treatment of tinea pedis (athlete's foot), tinea cruris (jock itch), tinea corporis (ringworm), tinea versicolor, and cutaneous candidiasis

Pregnancy Risk Factor C

Dosage Children and Adults: Topical:

Tinea pedis: Apply sufficient amount to cover affected areas once daily for 1 month

Tinea cruris, tinea corporis, tinea versicolor: Apply sufficient amount to cover affected areas once daily for 2 weeks

Cutaneous candidiasis: Apply sufficient quantity twice daily (morning and evening) for 2 weeks

Additional Information Complete prescribing information for this medication should be consulted for additional detail.

Dosage Forms Excipient information presented when available (limited, particularly for generics); consult specific product labeling.

Cream, topical, as nitrate: 1% (15 g, 30 g, 85 g)

◆ **Econazole Nitrate** *see* Econazole *on page* 570

◆ **Econopred** *see* PrednisoLONE (Ophthalmic) *on page* 1398

◆ **Ecostigmine Iodide** *see* Echothiophate Iodide *on page* 570

◆ **Ecotrin® [OTC]** *see* Aspirin *on page* 154

◆ **Ecotrin® Arthritis Strength [OTC]** *see* Aspirin *on page* 154

◆ **Ecotrin® Low Strength [OTC]** *see* Aspirin *on page* 154

◆ **Ectosone (Can)** *see* Betamethasone *on page* 208

Eculizumab (e kue LIZ oo mab)

Brand Names: U.S. Soliris®

Brand Names: Canada Soliris®

Index Terms h5G1.1; Monoclonal Antibody 5G1.1; Monoclonal Antibody Anti-C5

Pharmacologic Category Monoclonal Antibody; Monoclonal Antibody, Complement Inhibitor

Use Treatment of paroxysmal nocturnal hemoglobinuria (PNH) to reduce hemolysis; treatment of atypical hemolytic uremic syndrome (aHUS) to inhibit complement-mediated thrombotic microangiopathy

Note: Not indicated for the treatment of hemolytic uremic syndrome related to Shiga toxin *E. coli* (STEC-HUS)

Pregnancy Risk Factor C

Pregnancy Considerations Animal studies have demonstrated fetal abnormalities. Eculizumab is a recombinant IgG molecule with IgG2 and IgG4 sequences; human IgG is known to cross the placenta, however IgG2 may have reduced placental transfer compared to other IgG subclasses. There are no adequate and well-controlled studies in pregnant women. Pregnant women with PNH and their fetuses have high rates of morbidity and mortality during pregnancy and the postpartum period. Limited information is available related to use during pregnancy. Use during pregnancy only if clearly needed.

Lactation Excretion in breast milk unknown/use caution

Prescribing and Access Restrictions Patients and providers must enroll with Soliris® OneSource™ (1-888-765-4747) program prior to treatment initiation.

Medication Guide Available Yes

Contraindications Unresolved serious *Neisseria meningitidis* infection; patients not currently vaccinated against *Neisseria meningitidis* (unless risks of treatment delay outweigh risk of meningococcal infection)

Warnings/Precautions [U.S. Boxed Warning]: Meningococcal *(Neisseria meningitides)* infections have occurred in patients receiving eculizumab; may be fatal or life-threatening if not detected and treated promptly. Monitor for early signs of meningococcal infection; evaluate and treat promptly if suspected. Follow current meningococcal immunization recommendations for patients with complement deficiencies. Vaccinate with meningococcal vaccine at least 2 weeks prior to initiation of treatment; revaccinate according to current guidelines. Polyvalent meningococcal vaccines are recommended. If urgent treatment is necessary in an unvaccinated patient, administer meningococcal vaccine as soon as possible. Although the risk/benefits of prophylactic meningococcal antibiotic therapy have not been determined, prophylactic antibiotics were administered in clinical studies until at least 2 weeks after vaccination. Meningococcal infections developed in some patients despite vaccination. Discontinue eculizumab during the treatment of serious meningococcal infections. In addition to meningitis, the risk of other infections, especially encapsulated bacteria (eg, *Streptococcus pneumoniae, H. influenzae*) is increased with eculizumab treatment (because eculizumab blocks terminal complement activation). Children should receive vaccination for prevention of *S. pneumoniae, H. influenzae* according to current ACIP guidelines. Use caution in patients with concurrent systemic infection. Patients should be up to date with all immunizations before initiating therapy. **[U.S. Boxed Warning]: Access is restricted through a REMS program. Prescribers must be enrolled in the program; enrollment information is available at 1-888-765-4747.** Counsel patients on the risk of meningococcal infection; ensure patients are vaccinated and provide educational materials.

Infusion reactions, including anaphylaxis or hypersensitivity, may occur; interrupt infusion for severe reaction. Continue monitoring for 1 hour after completion of infusion. Patients with PNH who discontinue treatment may be at increased risk for serious hemolysis; monitor closely for at least 8 weeks after treatment discontinuation. Consider RBC transfusion, exchange transfusion, anticoagulation, corticoids or reinitiation of eculizumab for serious hemolysis after discontinuation. When used for aHUS, monitor for at least 12 weeks after treatment discontinuation for signs/symptoms of thrombotic microangiopathy (TMA) complications (angina, dyspnea, mental status changes, seizure, serum creatinine elevation, serum LDH elevation, thrombocytopenia, or thrombosis). If TMA complications occur after stopping eculizumab, consider reinitiation of treatment, plasmapheresis, plasma exchange, fresh frozen plasma infusion, and/or appropriate organ-specific measures. In clinical trials, anticoagulant therapy was continued in patients who were receiving these agents (due to history of or risk for thromboembolism) prior to initiation of eculizumab. The effect of anticoagulant therapy withdrawal is unknown; treatment with eculizumab should not alter anticoagulation management

Adverse Reactions

>10%:

Cardiovascular: Hypertension (aHUS: 35%), tachycardia (aHUS: children 21%), peripheral edema (11%)

Central nervous system: Headache (30% to 44%; serious: 2%), insomnia (14%), fatigue (11% to 12%), fever (2% to 11%; children 47%), vertigo (11%)

Gastrointestinal: Diarrhea (32%), vomiting (21% to 22%), nausea (16% to 19%), abdominal pain (11%)

Genitourinary: Urinary tract infection (16%)

Hematologic: Anemia (24%; serious: 2%), leukopenia (16%)

Neuromuscular & skeletal: Back pain (19%), limb pain (7% to 11%)

Respiratory: Respiratory tract infection (7% to 35%), cough (12% to 26%), nasopharyngitis (23%), nasal congestion (aHUS: children 21%), pharyngolaryngeal pain (14%)

1% to 10%:

Gastrointestinal: Constipation (7%)

Neuromuscular & skeletal: Myalgia (7%)

Respiratory: Sinusitis (7%)

Miscellaneous: Herpes infections (7%), flu-like syndrome (5%), viral infection (serious: 2%), meningococcal infection (≤1%)

<1% (Limited to important or life-threatening): Abdominal distention, anxiety, arthralgia, cholangitis, dizziness, endometritis, hematoma (mild), infusion reaction, pyelonephritis, renal impairment, taste alteration

Drug Interactions

Metabolism/Transport Effects None known.

Avoid Concomitant Use

Avoid concomitant use of Eculizumab with any of the following: BCG; Natalizumab; Pimecrolimus; Tacrolimus (Topical); Vaccines (Live)

Increased Effect/Toxicity

Eculizumab may increase the levels/effects of: Leflunomide; Natalizumab; Vaccines (Live)

The levels/effects of Eculizumab may be increased by: Denosumab; Pimecrolimus; Roflumilast; Tacrolimus (Topical); Trastuzumab

Decreased Effect

Eculizumab may decrease the levels/effects of: BCG; Coccidioidin Skin Test; Sipuleucel-T; Vaccines (Inactivated); Vaccines (Live)

The levels/effects of Eculizumab may be decreased by: Echinacea

Stability Prior to dilution, store vials at 2°C to 8°C (36°F to 46°F); do not freeze. Protect from light; do not shake. Add eculizumab to an infusion bag and dilute with an equal volume of D_5W, sodium chloride 0.9%, sodium chloride 0.45%, or Ringer's injection to a final concentration of 5 mg/mL (eg, 300 mg to a total volume of 60 mL, 600 mg in a total volume of 120 mL, 900 mg in a total volume of 180 mL, or 1200 mg to a total volume of 240 mL). Gently invert bag to mix thoroughly. Allow admixture to reach room temperature prior to administration (do not use a heat source or warming). Following dilution, store at room temperature or refrigerate; protect from light; use within 24 hours.

Mechanism of Action Terminal complement-mediated intravascular hemolysis is a key clinical feature of paroxysmal nocturnal hemoglobinuria (PNH); blocking the formation of membrane attack complex (MAC) results in stabilization of hemoglobin and a reduction in the need for RBC transfusions. Impairment of complement activity regulation leads to uncontrolled complement activation in atypical hemolytic uremic syndrome (aHUS). Eculizumab is a humanized monoclonal IgG antibody that binds to complement protein C5, preventing cleavage into C5a and C5b. Blocking the formation of C5b inhibits the subsequent formation of terminal complex C5b-9 or MAC.

Pharmacodynamics/Kinetics

Onset of action: PNH: Reduced hemolysis: ≤1 week

Distribution: PNH: 7.7 L; aHUS: 6.14 L

Half-life elimination: PNH: ~11 days (range: ~8-15 days); aHUS: ~12 days (during plasma exchange the half-life is reduced to 1.26 hours)

Dosage Note: Patients must receive meningococcal vaccine at least 2 weeks prior to treatment initiation; revaccinate according to current guidelines. Treatment should be administered at the recommended time interval although administration may be varied by ±2 days.

Atypical hemolytic uremic syndrome (aHUS): I.V.:

Children 5 kg to <10 kg: Induction: 300 mg weekly for 1 dose; Maintenance: 300 mg at week 2, then 300 mg every 3 weeks

Children 10 kg to <20 kg: Induction: 600 mg weekly for 1 dose; Maintenance: 300 mg at week 2, then 300 mg every 2 weeks

Children 20 kg to <30 kg: Induction: 600 mg weekly for 2 doses; Maintenance: 600 mg at week 3, then 600 mg every 2 weeks

Children 30 kg to <40 kg: Induction: 600 mg weekly for 2 doses; Maintenance: 900 mg at week 3, then 900 mg every 2 weeks

Children ≥40 kg and Adults: Induction: 900 mg weekly for 4 doses; Maintenance: 1200 mg at week 5, then 1200 mg every 2 weeks

Supplemental dosing for patients receiving plasmapheresis or plasma exchange:

If most recent dose was 300 mg, administer 300 mg within 60 minutes after each plasmapheresis or plasma exchange

If most recent dose was ≥600 mg, administer 600 mg within 60 minutes after each plasmapheresis or plasma exchange

Supplemental dosing for patients receiving fresh frozen plasma infusion: If most recent dose was ≥300 mg, administer 300 mg within 60 minutes prior to each 1 unit of fresh frozen plasma infusion

PNH: I.V.: Adults: 600 mg weekly for 4 doses, followed by 900 mg 1 week later, then 900 mg every 2 weeks

Dosage adjustment in renal impairment: No dosage adjustment is recommended in the manufacturer's labeling.

Dosage adjustment in hepatic impairment: Not studied in hepatic dysfunction

Administration I.V.: Allow to reach room temperature prior to administration. Infuse over 35 minutes. Decrease infusion rate or discontinue for infusion reactions; do not exceed a maximum 2-hour duration of infusion. Monitor for at least 1 hour following completion of infusion (for signs/symptoms of infusion reaction).

Monitoring Parameters Signs and symptoms of infusion reaction (during infusion and for 1 hour after infusion complete); CBC with differential, lactic dehydrogenase (LDH), serum creatinine, AST, urinalysis

Serum LDH levels greater than pretreatment level along with: >25% decrease in PNH clone size in ≤1 week, or hemoglobin level <5 g/dL, or a hemoglobin decrease of >4 g/dL in ≤1 week, or 50% increase in serum creatinine, or angina, mental status change, or thrombosis is indicative of serious hemolysis

After discontinuation:

aHUS: Signs/symptoms of thrombotic microangiopathy (TMA) complications (monitor for at least 12 weeks after treatment discontinuation), including angina, dyspnea, mental status changes, seizure, serum creatinine elevation, serum LDH elevation, thrombocytopenia, or thrombosis.

PNH: Signs and symptoms of intravascular hemolysis (monitor for at least 8 weeks after discontinuation), including serum LDH, hemoglobin, serum creatinine; signs of angina, mental status change, or thrombosis

Dosage Forms Excipient information presented when available (limited, particularly for generics); consult specific product labeling.

Injection, solution [preservative free]:

Soliris®: 10 mg/mL (30 mL) [contains polysorbate 80]

- **Ed A-Hist™ [DSC]** *see* Chlorpheniramine and Phenylephrine *on page 345*
- **Ed A-Hist DM [DSC]** *see* Chlorpheniramine, Phenylephrine, and Dextromethorphan *on page 346*
- **Edarbi™** *see* Azilsartan *on page 179*
- **Ed ChlorPed D** *see* Chlorpheniramine and Phenylephrine *on page 345*
- **Edecrin®** *see* Ethacrynic Acid *on page 651*

Edetate CALCIUM Disodium

(ED e tate KAL see um dye SOW dee um)

Brand Names: U.S. Calcium Disodium Versenate®

Index Terms CaEDTA; Calcium Disodium Edetate; Edetate Disodium CALCIUM; EDTA (CALCIUM Disodium) (error-prone abbreviation)

Pharmacologic Category Chelating Agent

Use Treatment of symptomatic acute and chronic lead poisoning or for symptomatic patients with high blood lead levels

Unlabeled Use Possibly useful in poisoning by zinc, manganese, and certain heavy radioisotopes

Pregnancy Risk Factor B

Pregnancy Considerations Adverse events were observed in some animal reproduction studies; there are no well controlled studies of edetate CALCIUM disodium in pregnant women. Following maternal occupational exposure, lead was found to cross the placenta in amounts related to maternal plasma levels. Possible outcomes of maternal lead exposure >10 mcg/dL includes spontaneous abortion, postnatal developmental delay, and reduced birth weight. Chelation therapy during pregnancy is for maternal benefit only and should be limited to the treatment of severe, symptomatic lead poisoning.

Lactation Excretion in breast milk unknown/use caution

Contraindications

Active renal disease or anuria; hepatitis

Warnings/Precautions [U.S. Boxed Warning]: Use with extreme caution in patients with lead encephalopathy and cerebral edema. In these patients, I.V. infusion has been associated with lethal increase in intracranial pressure; I.M. injection is preferred.

Edetate CALCIUM disodium is potentially nephrotoxic; renal tubular acidosis and fatal nephrosis may occur, especially with high doses; ECG changes may occur during therapy; do not exceed recommended daily dose. If anuria, increasing proteinuria, or hematuria occurs during therapy, discontinue edetate CALCIUM disodium. Minimize nephrotoxicity by adequate hydration, establishment of good urine output, avoidance of excessive doses, and limitation of continuous administration to ≤5 days.

Exercise caution in the ordering, dispensing, and administration of this drug. Edetate CALCIUM disodium (CaEDTA) may be confused with edetate disodium (Na_2EDTA) (not commercially available in the U.S. or Canada). The CDC and FDA recommend that edetate disodium should never be used for chelation therapy (especially in children). Death has occurred following the use of edetate disodium for chelation therapy in pediatric patients with autism. Fatal hypocalcemia may result if edetate disodium is used for the treatment of lead poisoning instead of edetate CALCIUM disodium. Investigate, identify, and remove sources of lead exposure prior to treatment. Primary care providers should consult experts in chemotherapy of lead toxicity before using chelation drug therapy.

Adverse Reactions Frequency not defined.

Cardiovascular: Arrhythmia, ECG changes, hypotension

Central nervous system: Chills, fatigue, fever, headache, malaise

Dermatologic: Cheilosis, dermatitis, rash

Endocrine & metabolic: Hypercalcemia

Gastrointestinal: Anorexia, GI upset, nausea, thirst (excessive), vomiting

Hematologic: Anemia, bone marrow suppression (transient)

Hepatic: Alkaline phosphatase decreased, liver function test increased (mild)

Local: Thrombophlebitis (I.V. infusion when concentration >5 mg/mL), pain at injection site (I.M. injection)

Neuromuscular & skeletal: Arthralgia, myalgia, numbness, tremor

Ocular: Lacrimation

Renal: Glucosuria, nephrotoxicity, renal tubular necrosis, microscopic hematuria, proteinuria, urinary frequency/urgency

Respiratory: Nasal congestion, sneezing

Miscellaneous: Iron, magnesium, and/or zinc deficiency (with chronic therapy)

Drug Interactions

Metabolism/Transport Effects None known.

Avoid Concomitant Use

Avoid concomitant use of Edetate CALCIUM Disodium with any of the following: CloZAPine

Increased Effect/Toxicity

Edetate CALCIUM Disodium may increase the levels/effects of: CloZAPine; Insulin

Decreased Effect There are no known significant interactions involving a decrease in effect.

Stability Store at controlled room temperature of 25°C (77°F); excursion permitted to 15°C to 30°C (59°F to 86°F). For I.V. infusion, dilute total daily dose into 250-500 mL of 0.9% sodium chloride or D_5W. Concentrations >0.5% (5 mg/mL) should be avoided. Procaine or lidocaine may be added to solutions given by I.M. injection.

Mechanism of Action Calcium is displaced by divalent and trivalent heavy metals, forming a nonionizing soluble complex that is excreted in urine

Pharmacodynamics/Kinetics

Onset of action: Chelation of lead: I.V.: 1 hour

Absorption: I.M., SubQ: Well absorbed; Oral: <5%

Distribution: Into extracellular fluid; minimal CSF penetration (~5%)

Metabolism: Almost none of the drug is metabolized

Half-life elimination: 20-60 minutes

Excretion: Urine (as metal chelates or unchanged drug); decreased GFR decreases elimination

Dosage

Treatment of lead poisoning: Children and Adults: **Note:** For the treatment of high blood lead levels in children, the CDC recommends chelation treatment when blood lead levels are >45 mcg/dL (CDC, 2002). In adults, available guidelines recommend chelation therapy with blood lead levels >50 mcg/dL and significant symptoms; chelation therapy may also be indicated with blood lead levels ≥100 mcg/dL and/or symptoms (Kosnett, 2007). Depending upon the blood lead level, additional courses may be necessary; at least 2-4 days, and preferably 2-4 weeks, should elapse before repeat treatment is initiated.

Asymptomatic lead poisoning with blood lead level >20 mcg/dL and <70 mcg/dL (manufacturer labeling): I.M., I.V.: 1000 mg/m^2/day (25-50 mg/kg/day) for 5 days. **Note:** The AAP recommends succimer as the drug used for initial management in asymptomatic children when blood lead levels are >45 mcg/dL and <70 mcg/dL. Edetate CALCIUM disodium can be used in children allergic to to succimer (AAP, 2005).

Symptomatic lead poisoning or blood lead levels ≥70 mcg/dL (manufacturer labeling): I.M., I.V.: 1000 mg/m^2/day (25-50 mg/kg/day) for 5 days. Edetate CALCIUM disodium should be administered 4 hours after the initial dimercaprol dose. Edetate CALCIUM disodium should be used in conjunction with dimercaprol when blood lead levels are >70 mcg/dL or when symptoms of lead poisoning are present.

Lead encephalopathy: I.M., I.V.: 1500 mg/m^2/day (50-75 mg/kg/day). Edetate CALCIUM disodium should be administered 4 hours after the initial dimercaprol dose. Edetate CALCIUM disodium should be used in conjunction with dimercaprol when blood lead levels are >70 mcg/dL or when symptoms of lead poisoning are present.

Lead nephropathy: Adults: An alternative dosing regimen reflecting the reduction in renal clearance is based upon the serum creatinine. Dose of edetate CALCIUM disodium based on serum creatinine (Morgan, 1975): **Note:** Repeat regimen monthly until lead levels are reduced to an acceptable level:

S_{cr} 2-3 mg/dL / Cl_{cr} 30-50 mL/minute: Reduce recommended dose by 50% and administer daily

S_{cr} 3-4 mg/dL / Cl_{cr} 20-30 mL/minute: Reduce recommended dose by 50% and administer every 48 hours

S_{cr} >4 mg/dL / Cl_{cr} <20 mL/minute: Reduce recommended dose by 50% and administer once weekly

Dosage adjustment in renal impairment: Dose should be reduced with pre-existing mild renal disease. Limiting daily dose to 1 g in children and 2 g in adults may decrease risk of nephrotoxicity, although larger doses may be needed in the treatment of lead encephalopathy.

Administration For I.M. or I.V. use; I.V. is generally preferred, however, I.M. route is preferred when cerebral edema is present.

I.V. infusion: Administer daily dose in diluted solution over 8-12 hours or continuously over 24 hours

For I.M. injection: Daily dose should be divided into 2-3 equal doses spaced 8-12 hours apart. Procaine hydrochloride or lidocaine may be added to edetate CALCIUM disodium to minimize pain at injection site. Administer by deep I.M. injection. When used in conjunction with dimercaprol, inject in a separate site.

Monitoring Parameters Urinary output; urinalysis; renal function, hepatic function, serum electrolytes (baseline and daily [serious] or at days 2 and 5 [less serious]); ECG changes (with I.V. therapy); blood lead levels (baseline and 7-21 days after completing chelation therapy); hemoglobin or hematocrit; iron status; free erythrocyte protoporphyrin or zinc protoporphyrin; neurodevelopmental changes

Test Interactions If edetate CALCIUM disodium is given as a continuous I.V. infusion, stop the infusion for at least 1 hour before blood is drawn for lead concentration to avoid a falsely elevated value

Dosage Forms Excipient information presented when available (limited, particularly for generics); consult specific product labeling. [DSC] = Discontinued product

Injection, solution:

Calcium Disodium Versenate®: 200 mg/mL (2.5 mL, 5 mL [DSC])

◆ **Edetate Disodium CALCIUM** *see* Edetate CALCIUM Disodium *on page* 572

◆ **Edex®** *see* Alprostadil *on page* 74

◆ **Edluar™** *see* Zolpidem *on page* 1826

Edrophonium (ed roe FOE nee um)

Brand Names: U.S. Enlon®

Brand Names: Canada Enlon®; Tensilon®

Index Terms Edrophonium Chloride

Pharmacologic Category Acetylcholinesterase Inhibitor; Antidote; Diagnostic Agent

Use Diagnosis of myasthenia gravis; differentiation of cholinergic crises from myasthenia crises; reversal of nondepolarizing neuromuscular blockers

Pregnancy Risk Factor C

Lactation Excretion in breast milk unknown

Contraindications Hypersensitivity to edrophonium, sulfites, or any component of the formulation; GI or GU obstruction

Warnings/Precautions Use with caution in patients with bronchial asthma and those receiving a cardiac glycoside; atropine sulfate should always be readily available as an antagonist. Overdosage can cause cholinergic crisis which may be fatal. I.V. atropine should be readily available for treatment of cholinergic reactions. Use with caution in patients with cardiac arrhythmias (eg, bradyarrhythmias). Avoid use in myasthenia gravis; may exacerbate muscular weakness. Products may contain sodium sulfite.

Adverse Reactions Frequency not defined.

Cardiovascular: Arrhythmias (especially bradycardia), AV block, carbon monoxide decreased, cardiac arrest, ECG changes (nonspecific), flushing, hypotension, nodal rhythm, syncope, tachycardia

Central nervous system: Convulsions, dizziness, drowsiness, dysarthria, dysphonia, headache, loss of consciousness

Dermatologic: Skin rash, thrombophlebitis (I.V.), urticaria

Gastrointestinal: Diarrhea, dysphagia, flatulence, hyperperistalsis, nausea, salivation, stomach cramps, vomiting

Genitourinary: Urinary urgency

Neuromuscular & skeletal: Arthralgias, fasciculations, muscle cramps, spasms, weakness

Ocular: Lacrimation, small pupils

Respiratory: Bronchiolar constriction, bronchospasm, dyspnea, bronchial secretions increased, laryngospasm, respiratory arrest, respiratory depression, respiratory muscle paralysis

Miscellaneous: Allergic reactions, anaphylaxis, diaphoresis increased

Drug Interactions

Metabolism/Transport Effects None known.

Avoid Concomitant Use There are no known interactions where it is recommended to avoid concomitant use.

Increased Effect/Toxicity

Edrophonium may increase the levels/effects of: Beta-Blockers; Cholinergic Agonists; Succinylcholine

The levels/effects of Edrophonium may be increased by: Corticosteroids (Systemic)

Decreased Effect

Edrophonium may decrease the levels/effects of: Neuromuscular-Blocking Agents (Nondepolarizing)

The levels/effects of Edrophonium may be decreased by: Dipyridamole

Mechanism of Action Inhibits destruction of acetylcholine by acetylcholinesterase. This facilitates transmission of impulses across myoneural junction and results in increased cholinergic responses such as miosis, increased tonus of intestinal and skeletal muscles, bronchial and ureteral constriction, bradycardia, and increased salivary and sweat gland secretions.

Pharmacodynamics/Kinetics

Onset of action: I.M.: 2-10 minutes; I.V.: 30-60 seconds

Duration: I.M.: 5-30 minutes; I.V.: 10 minutes

Distribution: V_d: Adults: 1.1 L/kg

Half-life elimination: Adults: 1.2-2.4 hours; Anephric patients: 2.4-4.4 hours

Excretion: Adults: Primarily urine (67%)

Dosage Usually administered I.V., however, if not possible, I.M. or SubQ may be used:

Infants:

I.M.: 0.5-1 mg

I.V.: Initial: 0.1 mg, followed by 0.4 mg if no response; total dose = 0.5 mg

Children:

Diagnosis: Initial: 0.04 mg/kg over 1 minute followed by 0.16 mg/kg if no response, to a maximum total dose of 5 mg for children <34 kg, or 10 mg for children >34 kg **or**

Alternative dosing (manufacturer's recommendation):

≤34 kg: 1 mg; if no response after 45 seconds, repeat dosage in 1 mg increments every 30-45 seconds, up to a total of 5 mg

>34 kg: 2 mg; if no response after 45 seconds, repeat dosage in 1 mg increments every 30-45 seconds, up to a total of 10 mg

I.M.:

<34 kg: 1 mg

>34 kg: 5 mg

Titration of oral anticholinesterase therapy: 0.04 mg/kg once given 1 hour after oral intake of the drug being used in treatment; if strength improves, an increase in neostigmine or pyridostigmine dose is indicated

Adults:

Diagnosis:

I.V.: 2 mg test dose administered over 15-30 seconds; 8 mg given 45 seconds later if no response is seen; test dose may be repeated after 30 minutes

I.M.: Initial: 10 mg; if no cholinergic reaction occurs, administer 2 mg 30 minutes later to rule out false-negative reaction

Titration of oral anticholinesterase therapy: 1-2 mg given 1 hour after oral dose of anticholinesterase; if strength improves, an increase in neostigmine or pyridostigmine dose is indicated

Reversal of nondepolarizing neuromuscular blocking agents (neostigmine with atropine usually preferred): I.V.: 10 mg over 30-45 seconds; may repeat every 5-10 minutes up to 40 mg

Termination of paroxysmal atrial tachycardia: I.V. rapid injection: 5-10 mg

Differentiation of cholinergic from myasthenic crisis: I.V.: 1 mg; may repeat after 1 minute. **Note:** Intubation and controlled ventilation may be required if patient has cholinergic crisis

Dosing adjustment in renal impairment: Dose may need to be reduced in patients with chronic renal failure

Administration Edrophonium is administered by direct I.V. injection; see Dosage

Monitoring Parameters Pre- and postinjection strength (cranial musculature is most useful); heart rate, respiratory rate, blood pressure

Test Interactions Increased aminotransferase [ALT/AST] (S), amylase (S)

Additional Information Atropine should be administered along with edrophonium when reversing the effects of nondepolarizing agents to antagonize the cholinergic effects at the muscarinic receptors, especially bradycardia. It is important to recognize the difference in dose for diagnosis of myasthenia gravis versus reversal of muscle relaxant, a much larger dose is needed for desired effect of reversal of muscle paralysis.

Dosage Forms Excipient information presented when available (limited, particularly for generics); consult specific product labeling.

Injection, solution, as chloride:

Enlon®: 10 mg/mL (15 mL) [contains natural rubber/natural latex in packaging, sodium sulfite]

Edrophonium and Atropine

(ed roe FOE nee um & A troe peen)

Brand Names: U.S. Enlon-Plus®

Index Terms Atropine Sulfate and Edrophonium Chloride; Edrophonium Chloride and Atropine Sulfate

Pharmacologic Category Acetylcholinesterase Inhibitor; Anticholinergic Agent; Antidote

Use Reversal of nondepolarizing neuromuscular blockers; adjunct treatment of respiratory depression caused by curare overdose

Pregnancy Risk Factor C

Dosage I.V.: Adults: Reversal of neuromuscular blockade: 0.05-0.1 mL/kg given over 45-60 seconds. The dose delivered is 0.5-1 mg/kg of edrophonium and 0.007-0.014 mg/kg of atropine. An edrophonium dose of 1 mg/kg should rarely be exceeded. **Note:** Monitor closely for bradyarrhythmias.

Dosage adjustment in renal impairment: Adjustment not required.

Dosage adjustment in hepatic impairment: Adjustment not required.

Additional Information Complete prescribing information for this medication should be consulted for additional detail.

Dosage Forms Excipient information presented when available (limited, particularly for generics); consult specific product labeling.

Injection, solution:

Enlon-Plus®: Edrophonium chloride 10 mg/mL and atropine sulfate 0.14 mg/mL (5 mL, 15 mL) [contains sodium sulfite; may contain natural rubber/natural latex in vial]

- ◆ **Edrophonium Chloride** *see* Edrophonium *on page 573*
- ◆ **Edrophonium Chloride and Atropine Sulfate** *see* Edrophonium and Atropine *on page 574*
- ◆ **EDTA (CALCIUM Disodium) (error-prone abbreviation)** *see* Edetate CALCIUM Disodium *on page 572*
- ◆ **Edurant™** *see* Rilpivirine *on page 1490*
- ◆ **E.E.S.®** *see* Erythromycin (Systemic) *on page 617*
- ◆ **EES® (Can)** *see* Erythromycin (Systemic) *on page 617*

Efavirenz (e FAV e renz)

Brand Names: U.S. Sustiva®

Brand Names: Canada Sustiva®

Pharmacologic Category Antiretroviral Agent, Reverse Transcriptase Inhibitor (Non-nucleoside)

Additional Appendix Information

Management of Healthcare Worker Exposures to HBV, HCV, and HIV *on page 1935*

Perinatal HIV Guidelines *on page 1946*

Use Treatment of HIV-1 infections in combination with at least two other antiretroviral agents

Pregnancy Risk Factor D

Pregnancy Considerations Teratogenic effects have been observed in primates receiving efavirenz. Efavirenz crosses the placenta. Based on data from the Antiretroviral Pregnancy Registry, an increased risk of overall birth defects has not been observed following first trimester exposure to efavirenz, however, neural tube and other CNS defects have been reported. Due to the low number of first trimester exposures and the low incidence of neural tube defects in the general population, available data are insufficient to evaluate risk. Pregnancy should be avoided and alternate therapy should be considered in women of childbearing potential. Women of childbearing potential should undergo pregnancy testing prior to initiation of efavirenz. Barrier contraception should be used in combination with other (hormonal) methods of contraception and for 12 weeks after efavirenz is discontinued. If therapy with efavirenz is administered during pregnancy, avoid use during the first trimester; use in the second and third trimesters only after considering other alternatives. For women who present in the first trimester already on an efavirenz containing regimen, change to an alternate antiretroviral medication when possible. Pharmacokinetic data from available studies do not suggest dose alterations are needed during pregnancy. Hypersensitivity reactions (including hepatic toxicity and rash) are more common in women on NNRTI therapy; it is not known if pregnancy increases this risk

Regardless of CD4 count or HIV RNA copy number, all HIV-infected pregnant women should receive a combination antepartum antiretroviral (ARV) drug regimen; this includes women who require therapy for their own health, as well as women who do not yet require therapy for their own health. ARV therapy should be started as soon as possible if required for the woman's health or immediately after the first trimester if not needed for the mother's health (although earlier initiation may be considered). Long-term follow-up is recommended for all infants exposed to ARV medications.

Healthcare providers are encouraged to enroll pregnant women exposed to antiretroviral medications in the Antiretroviral Pregnancy Registry (1-800-258-4263 or www.APRegistry.com). Healthcare providers caring for HIV-infected women and their infants may contact the National Perinatal HIV Hotline (888-448-8765) for clinical consultation (DHHS [perinatal], 2011).

Lactation Enters breast milk/contraindicated

Prescribing and Access Restrictions Efavirenz oral solution is available only through an expanded access (compassionate use) program. Enrollment information may be obtained by calling 877-372-7097.

Contraindications Hypersensitivity to efavirenz or any component of the formulation; concurrent use of bepridil, cisapride, midazolam, pimozide, triazolam, voriconazole (with standard [eg, unadjusted] voriconazole and efavirenz doses), or ergot alkaloids (includes dihydroergotamine, ergotamine, ergonovine, methylergonovine)

Warnings/Precautions Do not use as single-agent therapy; avoid pregnancy; women of childbearing potential should undergo pregnancy testing prior to initiation of therapy; use caution with other agents metabolized by cytochrome P450 isoenzyme 3A4 (see Contraindications); use caution with history of mental illness/drug abuse (predisposition to psychological reactions); may cause CNS and psychiatric symptoms, which include impaired concentration, dizziness or drowsiness (avoid potentially hazardous tasks such as driving or operating machinery if these effects are noted); CNS effects may be potentiated when used with other sedative drugs or ethanol. Serious psychiatric side effects have been associated with efavirenz, including severe depression, suicide, paranoia, and mania. May cause mild-to-moderate maculopapular rash; usually occurs within 2 weeks of starting therapy; discontinue if severe rash (involving blistering, desquamation, mucosal involvement, or fever) develops. Children are more susceptible.

Caution in patients with known or suspected hepatitis B or C infection (monitoring of liver function is recommended) or Child-Pugh class A hepatic impairment; not recommended in Child-Pugh class B or C hepatic impairment. Persistent elevations of serum transaminases >5 times the upper limit of normal should prompt evaluation - benefit of continued therapy should be weighed against possible risk of hepatotoxicity. Increases in total cholesterol and triglycerides have been reported; screening should be done prior to therapy and periodically throughout treatment. May cause redistribution of fat (eg, buffalo hump, peripheral wasting with increased abdominal girth, cushingoid appearance). Patients may develop immune reconstitution syndrome resulting in the occurrence of an inflammatory response to an indolent or residual opportunistic infection; further evaluation and treatment may be required. Use with caution in patients with a history of seizure disorder; seizures have been associated with use.

Adverse Reactions Unless otherwise noted, frequency of adverse events is as reported in adults receiving combination antiretroviral therapy.

>10%:

Central nervous system: Dizziness (2% to 28%; children 16%), fever (children 21%), depression (up to 19%; severe: 1% to 2%), insomnia (up to 16%), anxiety (2% to 13%), pain (1% to 13%; children 14%), headache (2% to 8%; children 11%)

Dermatologic: Rash (5% to 26%, grade 3/4: <1%; children up to 46%, grade 3/4: 2% to 4%)
Endocrine & metabolic: HDL increased (25% to 35%), total cholesterol increased (20% to 40%), triglycerides increased (≥751 mg/dL: 6% to 11%)
Gastrointestinal: Diarrhea (3% to 14%; children: up to 39%), nausea (2% to 12%; children 12%), vomiting (3% to 6%; children 12%)
Respiratory: Cough (children 16%)

1% to 10%:

Central nervous system: Impaired concentration (up to 8%), somnolence (up to 7%), fatigue (up to 8%), abnormal dreams (1% to 6%), nervousness (2% to 7%), hallucinations (1%)
Dermatologic: Pruritus (up to 9%)
Endocrine & metabolic: Hyperglycemia (>250 mg/dL: 2% to 5%)
Gastrointestinal: Dyspepsia (up to 4%), abdominal pain (2% to 3%), anorexia (up to 2%), amylase increased (grade 3/4: up to 6%)
Hematologic: Neutropenia (grade 3/4: 2% to 10%)
Hepatic: Transaminases increased (grade 3/4: 2% to 8%, incidence higher with hepatitis B and/or C coinfection)

<1% (Limited to important or life-threatening): Allergic reaction, aggressive reaction, agitation, arthralgia, ataxia, balance disturbances, body fat accumulation/redistribution, cerebellar coordination disturbances, constipation, coordination abnormal, delusions, dermatitis (photoallergic), dyspnea, emotional lability, erythema multiforme, flushing, gynecomastia, hepatic failure, hepatitis, hypoesthesia, immune reconstitution syndrome, malabsorption, mania, myalgia, myopathy, neuropathy, neurosis, palpitation, paranoia, paresthesia, psychosis, seizure, Stevens-Johnson syndrome, suicide attempts, suicidal ideation, tinnitus, tremor, vertigo, visual abnormality, weakness

Drug Interactions

Metabolism/Transport Effects **Substrate** of CYP2B6 (major), CYP3A4 (major); **Note:** Assignment of Major/Minor substrate status based on clinically relevant drug interaction potential; **Inhibits** CYP2C19 (moderate), CYP2C9 (moderate), CYP3A4 (moderate); **Induces** CYP2B6 (weak/moderate), CYP3A4 (strong)

Avoid Concomitant Use

Avoid concomitant use of Efavirenz with any of the following: Bepridil [Off Market]; Boceprevir; Bortezomib; Cisapride; Clopidogrel; Crizotinib; Dienogest; Dronedarone; Ergot Derivatives; Etravirine; Lapatinib; Lurasidone; Midazolam; Nevirapine; Nilotinib; Nisoldipine; Pazopanib; Pimozide; Posaconazole; Praziquantel; Ranolazine; Rilpivirine; Rivaroxaban; Roflumilast; RomiDEPsin; SORAfenib; St Johns Wort; Ticagrelor; Tolvaptan; Toremifene; Triazolam; Vandetanib

Increased Effect/Toxicity

Efavirenz may increase the levels/effects of: Alcohol (Ethyl); ARIPiprazole; Bepridil [Off Market]; Budesonide (Systemic, Oral Inhalation); Carvedilol; Cisapride; Citalopram; Clarithromycin; CNS Depressants; Colchicine; CYP2C19 Substrates; CYP2C9 Substrates; CYP3A4 Substrates; Eplerenone; Ergot Derivatives; Etravirine; FentaNYL; Fosphenytoin; Halofantrine; Lurasidone; Methotrimeprazine; Midazolam; Nevirapine; PACLitaxel; Phenytoin; Pimecrolimus; Pimozide; Propafenone; Protease Inhibitors; Ranolazine; Rilpivirine; Salmeterol; Saxagliptin; Selective Serotonin Reuptake Inhibitors; Tolvaptan; Triazolam; Vilazodone; Vitamin K Antagonists; Zuclopenthixol

The levels/effects of Efavirenz may be increased by: Boceprevir; Clarithromycin; Conivaptan; CYP2B6 Inhibitors (Moderate); CYP2B6 Inhibitors (Strong); Darunavir; Droperidol; HydrOXYzine; Methotrimeprazine; Nevirapine; Quazepam; Voriconazole

Decreased Effect

Efavirenz may decrease the levels/effects of: ARIPiprazole; Atazanavir; Atorvastatin; Boceprevir; Bortezomib; Brentuximab Vedotin; Buprenorphine; BuPROPion; Caspofungin; Clarithromycin; Clopidogrel; Crizotinib; CycloSPORINE; CycloSPORINE (Systemic); CYP3A4 Substrates; Darunavir; Dasatinib; Dienogest; Dronedarone; Etonogestrel; Etravirine; Everolimus; Exemestane; Gefitinib; GuanFACINE; Imatinib; Itraconazole; Ixabepilone; Lapatinib; Linagliptin; Lopinavir; Lovastatin; Lurasidone; Maraviroc; Methadone; NIFEdipine; Nilotinib; Nisoldipine; Norgestimate; Pazopanib; Posaconazole; Pravastatin; Praziquantel; Protease Inhibitors; Raltegravir; Ranolazine; Rifabutin; Rilpivirine; Rivaroxaban; Roflumilast; RomiDEPsin; Saxagliptin; Sertraline; Simvastatin; Sirolimus; SORAfenib; SUNItinib; Tacrolimus; Tacrolimus (Systemic); Tadalafil; Telaprevir; Ticagrelor; Tolvaptan; Toremifene; Ulipristal; Vandetanib; Vemurafenib; Vitamin K Antagonists; Voriconazole; Zuclopenthixol

The levels/effects of Efavirenz may be decreased by: CYP2B6 Inducers (Strong); CYP3A4 Inducers (Strong); Deferasirox; Fosphenytoin; Nevirapine; Phenytoin; Rifabutin; Rifampin; St Johns Wort; Telaprevir; Tocilizumab

Ethanol/Nutrition/Herb Interactions

Ethanol: Ethanol may increase hepatotoxic potential of efavirenz. Ethanol may also increase CNS depression; monitor for increased effects with coadministration. Caution patients about effects.
Food: Avoid high-fat meals (increases the absorption of efavirenz).
Herb/Nutraceutical: St John's wort may decrease efavirenz serum levels. Avoid concurrent use.

Stability Store at controlled room temperature of 25°C (77°F); excursion permitted to 15°C to 30°C (59°F to 86°F).

Mechanism of Action As a non-nucleoside reverse transcriptase inhibitor, efavirenz has activity against HIV-1 by binding to reverse transcriptase. It consequently blocks the RNA-dependent and DNA-dependent DNA polymerase activities including HIV-1 replication. It does not require intracellular phosphorylation for antiviral activity.

Pharmacodynamics/Kinetics

Absorption: Increased by fatty meals
Distribution: CSF concentrations exceed free fraction in serum
Protein binding: >99%, primarily to albumin
Metabolism: Hepatic via CYP3A4 and 2B6 to inactive hydroxylated metabolites; may induce its own metabolism
Half-life elimination: Single dose: 52-76 hours; Multiple doses: 40-55 hours
Time to peak: 3-5 hours
Excretion: Feces (16% to 61% primarily as unchanged drug); urine (14% to 34% as metabolites)

Dosage Oral: HIV infection (as part of combination therapy):

Children ≥3 years: Dosage is based on body weight:
- 10 kg to <15 kg: 200 mg once daily
- 15 kg to <20 kg: 250 mg once daily
- 20 kg to <25 kg: 300 mg once daily
- 25 kg to <32.5 kg: 350 mg once daily
- 32.5 kg to <40 kg: 400 mg once daily
- ≥40 kg: 600 mg once daily; **Note:** Dosage adjustments may be necessary if patient receives certain concomitant medications. Refer to adult dosing.

Adults: 600 mg once daily; preferred regimen for therapy-naive patients with tenofovir and emtricitabine (DHHS, 2011)

Dosage adjustment for concomitant rifampin (only if patient weighs ≥50 kg): Increase efavirenz dose to 800 mg once daily

Dosage adjustment for concomitant voriconazole: Reduce efavirenz dose to 300 mg once daily and increase voriconazole to 400 mg every 12 hours

Dosing adjustment in renal impairment: None recommended

Dosing comments in hepatic impairment:

Mild impairment (Child-Pugh class A): No dosage adjustment recommended; use with caution

Moderate-to-severe impairment (Child-Pugh class B or C): Use not recommended

Dietary Considerations Should be taken on an empty stomach.

Administration Administer on an empty stomach. Dosing at or before bedtime is recommended to limit central nervous system effects (DHHS, 2011). Tablets should not be broken. Some clinicians recommend opening capsules and adding to liquid or food for patients that cannot swallow capsules; however, no pharmacokinetic data are available and this is not recommended (DHHS [pediatric], 2010).

Monitoring Parameters Serum transaminases (discontinuation of treatment should be considered for persistent elevations greater than five times the upper limit of normal), cholesterol, triglycerides, signs and symptoms of infection

Test Interactions False-positive tests for cannabinoids have been reported when the CEDIA DAU Multilevel THC assay is used. False-positive results with other assays for cannabinoids have not been observed. False-positive tests for benzodiazepines have been reported and are likely due to the 8-hydroxy-efavirenz major metabolite.

Additional Information Early virologic failure was observed with tenofovir and didanosine delayed release capsules, plus either efavirenz or nevirapine; use caution in treatment-naive patients with high baseline viral loads.

Dosage Forms Excipient information presented when available (limited, particularly for generics); consult specific product labeling.

Capsule, oral:

Sustiva®: 50 mg, 200 mg

Tablet, oral:

Sustiva®: 600 mg

Efavirenz, Emtricitabine, and Tenofovir

(e FAV e renz, em trye SYE ta been, & te NOE fo veer)

Brand Names: U.S. Atripla®

Brand Names: Canada Atripla®

Index Terms Emtricitabine, Efavirenz, and Tenofovir; FTC, TDF, and EFV; Tenofovir Disoproxil Fumarate, Efavirenz, and Emtricitabine

Pharmacologic Category Antiretroviral Agent, Reverse Transcriptase Inhibitor (Non-nucleoside); Antiretroviral Agent, Reverse Transcriptase Inhibitor (Nucleoside); Antiretroviral Agent, Reverse Transcriptase Inhibitor (Nucleotide)

Additional Appendix Information

Management of Healthcare Worker Exposures to HBV, HCV, and HIV *on page 1935*

Use Treatment of HIV infection

Pregnancy Risk Factor D

Dosage Oral: Adults: One tablet once daily. **Note:** Recommended as an initial regimen for antiretroviral-naive patients (DHHS, 2011).

Dosage adjustment in renal impairment: Moderate-to-severe renal impairment (Cl_{cr} <50 mL/minute): Use not recommended

Dosage adjustment in hepatic impairment:

Mild hepatic impairment (Child-Pugh class A): Use with caution

Moderate or severe hepatic impairment (Child-Pugh class B, C): Not recommended

Additional Information Complete prescribing information for this medication should be consulted for additional detail.

Dosage Forms Excipient information presented when available (limited, particularly for generics); consult specific product labeling.

Tablet:

Atripla®: Efavirenz 600 mg, emtricitabine 200 mg, and tenofovir disoproxil fumarate 300 mg

- **Effer-K®** *see* Potassium Bicarbonate and Potassium Citrate *on page 1380*
- **Effexor®** *see* Venlafaxine *on page 1780*
- **Effexor XR®** *see* Venlafaxine *on page 1780*
- **Effient®** *see* Prasugrel *on page 1393*

Eflornithine (ee FLOR ni theen)

Brand Names: U.S. Vaniqa®

Brand Names: Canada Vaniqa®

Index Terms DFMO; Eflornithine Hydrochloride

Pharmacologic Category Antiprotozoal; Topical Skin Product

Use Cream: Females ≥12 years: Reduce unwanted hair from face and adjacent areas under the chin

Orphan status: Injection: Treatment of meningoencephalitic stage of *Trypanosoma brucei gambiense* infection (sleeping sickness)

Pregnancy Risk Factor C

Dosage

Children ≥12 years and Adults: Females: Topical: Apply thin layer of cream to affected areas of face and adjacent chin twice daily, at least 8 hours apart

Adults: I.V. infusion: 100 mg/kg/dose given every 6 hours (over at least 45 minutes) for 14 days

Dosing adjustment in renal impairment: Injection: Dose should be adjusted although no specific guidelines are available

Additional Information Complete prescribing information for this medication should be consulted for additional detail.

Dosage Forms Excipient information presented when available (limited, particularly for generics); consult specific product labeling.

Cream, topical, as hydrochloride:

Vaniqa®: 13.9% (30 g)

- **Eflornithine Hydrochloride** *see* Eflornithine *on page 577*
- **Eformoterol and Budesonide** *see* Budesonide and Formoterol *on page 240*
- **Efudex®** *see* Fluorouracil (Topical) *on page 731*
- **E-Gem® [OTC]** *see* Vitamin E *on page 1796*
- **E-Gem® Lip Care [OTC]** *see* Vitamin E *on page 1796*
- **E-Gems® [OTC]** *see* Vitamin E *on page 1796*
- **E-Gems® Elite [OTC]** *see* Vitamin E *on page 1796*
- **E-Gems® Plus [OTC]** *see* Vitamin E *on page 1796*
- **Egrifta™** *see* Tesamorelin *on page 1653*
- **EHDP** *see* Etidronate *on page 666*
- **EL-970** *see* Dalfampridine *on page 440*
- **Elaprase®** *see* Idursulfase *on page 867*
- **Elavil** *see* Amitriptyline *on page 94*
- **Eldepryl®** *see* Selegiline *on page 1544*
- **Eldopaque® [OTC]** *see* Hydroquinone *on page 846*
- **Eldopaque® (Can)** *see* Hydroquinone *on page 846*

- ◆ **Eldopaque Forte®** *see* Hydroquinone *on page 846*
- ◆ **Eldoquin® [OTC]** *see* Hydroquinone *on page 846*
- ◆ **Eldoquin® (Can)** *see* Hydroquinone *on page 846*
- ◆ **Eldoquin Forte®** *see* Hydroquinone *on page 846*
- ◆ **Electrolyte Lavage Solution** *see* Polyethylene Glycol-Electrolyte Solution *on page 1372*

Electrolyte Solution, Renal Replacement

(ee LEK trow lite soe LOO shun REE nil ree PLASE ment)

Brand Names: U.S. Normocarb HF® 25; Normocarb HF® 35; PrismaSol

Index Terms Continuous Renal Replacement Therapy; CRRT; Renal Replacement Solution

Pharmacologic Category Alkalinizing Agent; Electrolyte Supplement

Use Used as a replacement solution to replenish water, correct electrolytes, and adjust acid-base balance depleted by hemofiltration or hemodiafiltration (continuous renal replacement therapy [CRRT]); drug poisoning when CRRT is used to remove filterable substances

Dosage Note: If using PrismaSol™, ensure that compartment A and B are mixed.

Continuous renal replacement circuit: Children and Adults:

Pre- or post-filter: Volume of solution administered depends upon the patient's fluid balance, target fluid balance, body weight, and amount of fluid removed during hemofiltration process.

Post-filter replacement: Volume infused/hour should not be greater than 1/3 of blood flow rate (eg, blood flow rate 100 mL/minute [6000 mL/hour], post-filter replacement rate ≤2000 mL/hour)

Dosage adjustment in hepatic impairment: Ability to convert lactate to bicarbonate may be impaired; use solutions containing lactate cautiously.

Additional Information Complete prescribing information for this medication should be consulted for additional detail.

Dosage Forms Excipient information presented when available (limited, particularly for generics); consult specific product labeling.

Injection, solution [concentrate; preservative free]:

Normocarb HF® 25: Bicarbonate 25 mEq/L, chloride 116.5 mEq/L, magnesium 1.5 mEq/L, sodium 140 mEq/L (240 mL) [strength represents final solution after mixing; when diluted as directed, makes 3240 mL of infusate]

Normocarb HF® 35: Bicarbonate 35 mEq/L, chloride 106.5 mEq/L, magnesium 1.5 mEq/L, sodium 140 mEq/L (240 mL) [strength represents final solution after mixing; when diluted as directed, makes 3240 mL of infusate]

Injection, solution [preservative free]:

PrismaSol B22GK 2/0: Bicarbonate 22 mEq/L, chloride 118.5 mEq/L, dextrose 100 mg/dL, lactate 3 mEq/L, magnesium 1.5 mEq/L, potassium 2 mEq/L, sodium 140 mEq/L (5000 mL) [strength represents final solution after mixing]

PrismaSol BGK 2/0: Bicarbonate 32 mEq/L, chloride 108 mEq/L, dextrose 100 mg/dL, lactate 3 mEq/L, magnesium 1 mEq/L, potassium 2 mEq/L, sodium 140 mEq/L (5000 mL) [strength represents final solution after mixing]

PrismaSol BGK 2/3.5: Bicarbonate 32 mEq/L, calcium 3.5 mEq/L, chloride 111.5 mEq/L, dextrose 100 mg/dL, lactate 3 mEq/L, magnesium 1 mEq/L, potassium 2 mEq/L, sodium 140 mEq/L (5000 mL) [strength represents final solution after mixing]

PrismaSol BGK 4/0/1.2: Bicarbonate 32 mEq/L, chloride 110.2 mEq/L, dextrose 100 mg/dL, lactate 3 mEq/L, magnesium 1.2 mEq/L, potassium 4 mEq/L, sodium 140 mEq/L (5000 mL) [strength represents final solution after mixing]

PrismaSol BGK 4/2.5: Bicarbonate 32 mEq/L, calcium 2.5 mEq/L, chloride 113 mEq/L, dextrose 100 mg/dL, lactate 3 mEq/L, magnesium 1.5 mEq/L, potassium 4 mEq/L, sodium 140 mEq/L (5000 mL) [strength represents final solution after mixing]

PrismaSol BK 0/0/1.2: Bicarbonate 32 mEq/L, chloride 106.2 mEq/L, lactate 3 mEq/L, magnesium 1.2 mEq/L, sodium 140 mEq/L (5000 mL) [strength represents final solution after mixing]

- ◆ **Elestrin®** *see* Estradiol (Systemic) *on page 627*

Eletriptan (el e TRIP tan)

Brand Names: U.S. Relpax®

Brand Names: Canada Relpax®

Index Terms Eletriptan Hydrobromide

Pharmacologic Category Antimigraine Agent; Serotonin $5\text{-HT}_{1B,\ 1D}$ Receptor Agonist

Additional Appendix Information

Antimigraine Drugs: 5-HT_1 Receptor Agonists *on page 1878*

Use Acute treatment of migraine, with or without aura

Pregnancy Risk Factor C

Pregnancy Considerations Teratogenic effects were observed in animal studies.

Lactation Enters breast milk/use caution

Contraindications Hypersensitivity to eletriptan or any component of the formulation; ischemic heart disease (angina pectoris, history of myocardial infarction, or proven silent ischemia) or in patients with symptoms consistent with ischemic heart disease, coronary artery vasospasm, or Prinzmetal's angina; cerebrovascular syndromes (including strokes, transient ischemic attacks); peripheral vascular syndromes (including ischemic bowel disease); uncontrolled hypertension; use within 24 hours of ergotamine derivatives; use within 24 hours of another 5-HT_1 agonist; management of hemiplegic or basilar migraine; severe hepatic impairment

Warnings/Precautions Only indicated for treatment of acute migraine; not indicated for migraine prophylaxis, or for the treatment of cluster headache, hemiplegic or basilar migraine. If a patient does not respond to the first dose, the diagnosis of migraine should be reconsidered. Do not give to patients with risk factors for CAD until a cardiovascular evaluation has been performed; if evaluation is satisfactory, the healthcare provider should administer the first dose (consider ECG monitoring) and cardiovascular status should be periodically evaluated. Cardiac events (coronary artery vasospasm, transient ischemia, MI, ventricular tachycardia/fibrillation, cardiac arrest, and death), cerebral/subarachnoid hemorrhage, stroke, peripheral vascular ischemia, and colonic ischemia have been reported with 5-HT_1 agonist administration. Patients who experience sensations of chest pain/pressure/tightness or symptoms suggestive of angina following dosing should be evaluated for coronary artery disease or Prinzmetal's angina before receiving additional doses; if dosing is resumed and similar symptoms recur, monitor with ECG. Significant elevation in blood pressure, including hypertensive crisis, has also been reported on rare occasions in patients with and without a history of hypertension. Use with caution with mild-to-moderate hepatic impairment. Symptoms of agitation, confusion, hallucinations, hyper-reflexia, myoclonus, shivering, and tachycardia (serotonin syndrome) may occur with concomitant proserotonergic drugs (ie, SSRIs/SNRIs or triptans) or agents which reduce eletriptan's metabolism. Concurrent use of serotonin precursors (eg, tryptophan) is not recommended. If concomitant administration with SSRIs is warranted, monitor closely, especially at initiation and with dose increases. Use not recommended within 72 hours in patients taking strong CYP3A4 inhibitors.

Adverse Reactions

1% to 10%:

Cardiovascular: Chest pain/tightness (1% to 4%; placebo 1%), palpitation

Central nervous system: Dizziness (3% to 7%; placebo 3%), somnolence (3% to 7%; placebo 4%), headache (3% to 4%; placebo 3%), chills, pain, vertigo

Gastrointestinal: Nausea (4% to 8%; placebo 5%), xerostomia (2% to 4%, placebo 2%), dysphagia (1% to 2%), abdominal pain/discomfort (1% to 2%; placebo 1%), dyspepsia (1% to 2%; placebo 1%)

Neuromuscular & skeletal: Weakness (4% to 10%), paresthesia (3% to 4%), back pain, hypertonia, hypoesthesia

Respiratory: Pharyngitis

Miscellaneous: Diaphoresis

<1% (Limited to important or life-threatening): Agitation, allergic reaction, angina, arrhythmia, ataxia, confusion, CPK increased, depersonalization, depression, dyspnea, edema, emotional lability, esophagitis, euphoria, hyperesthesia, hyperkinesia, hypertension, impotence, incoordination, insomnia, lacrimation disorder, liver function tests abnormal, myalgia, myasthenia, peripheral vascular disorder, photophobia, polyuria, pruritus, rash, seizure, shock, speech disorder, stupor, tachycardia, thrombophlebitis, tinnitus, tongue edema, tremor, urinary frequency, vasospasm, vision abnormal

Drug Interactions

Metabolism/Transport Effects Substrate of CYP3A4 (major); **Note:** Assignment of Major/Minor substrate status based on clinically relevant drug interaction potential

Avoid Concomitant Use

Avoid concomitant use of Eletriptan with any of the following: Conivaptan; Ergot Derivatives

Increased Effect/Toxicity

Eletriptan may increase the levels/effects of: Ergot Derivatives; Metoclopramide; Serotonin Modulators

The levels/effects of Eletriptan may be increased by: Antifungal Agents (Azole Derivatives, Systemic); Antipsychotics; Calcium Channel Blockers (Nondihydropyridine); Conivaptan; CYP3A4 Inhibitors (Moderate); CYP3A4 Inhibitors (Strong); Dasatinib; Ergot Derivatives; Fluconazole; Macrolide Antibiotics

Decreased Effect

The levels/effects of Eletriptan may be decreased by: Tocilizumab

Ethanol/Nutrition/Herb Interactions Food: High-fat meal increases bioavailability.

Stability Store at 25°C (77°F); excursions permitted to 15°C to 30°C (59°F to 86°F).

Mechanism of Action Selective agonist for serotonin (5-HT_{1B} and 5-HT_{1D} receptors) in cranial arteries; causes vasoconstriction and reduces sterile inflammation associated with antidromic neuronal transmission correlating with relief of migraine

Pharmacodynamics/Kinetics

Absorption: Well absorbed

Distribution: V_d: 138 L

Protein binding: ~85%

Metabolism: Hepatic via CYP3A4; forms one metabolite (active)

Bioavailability: ~50%, increased with high-fat meal

Half-life elimination: ~4 hours (Elderly: 4.4-5.7 hours); Metabolite: ~13 hours

Time to peak, plasma: 1.5-2 hours

Dosage Oral: Adults: Acute migraine: Initial: 20-40 mg (maximum: 40 mg/dose); if the headache improves but returns, dose may be repeated after 2 hours have elapsed since first dose (maximum: 80 mg/day)

Note: If the first dose is ineffective, diagnosis needs to be re-evaluated. Safety of treating >3 headaches/month has not been established.

Dosage adjustment in renal impairment: No dosing adjustment needed; monitor for increased blood pressure

Dosage adjustment in hepatic impairment:

Mild-to-moderate impairment: No adjustment necessary

Severe impairment: Use is contraindicated

Dosage Forms Excipient information presented when available (limited, particularly for generics); consult specific product labeling.

Tablet, oral:

Relpax®: 20 mg, 40 mg

◆ **Eletriptan Hydrobromide** *see* Eletriptan *on page 578*
◆ **Elidel®** *see* Pimecrolimus *on page 1353*
◆ **Eligard®** *see* Leuprolide *on page 989*
◆ **Elimite** *see* Permethrin *on page 1336*
◆ **Eliphos™** *see* Calcium Acetate *on page 265*
◆ **Elitek®** *see* Rasburicase *on page 1467*
◆ **Elixophyllin® Elixir** *see* Theophylline *on page 1667*
◆ **ella®** *see* Ulipristal *on page 1748*
◆ **Ellence®** *see* Epirubicin *on page 597*
◆ **Elmiron®** *see* Pentosan Polysulfate Sodium *on page 1331*
◆ **Elocom® (Can)** *see* Mometasone (Topical) *on page 1151*
◆ **Elocon®** *see* Mometasone (Topical) *on page 1151*
◆ **Eloxatin®** *see* Oxaliplatin *on page 1257*
◆ **Elspar®** *see* Asparaginase (*E. coli*) *on page 151*
◆ **Eltor® (Can)** *see* Pseudoephedrine *on page 1430*

Eltrombopag (el TROM boe pag)

Brand Names: U.S. Promacta®

Brand Names: Canada Revolade™

Index Terms Eltrombopag Olamine; Revolade®; SB-497115; SB-497115-GR

Pharmacologic Category Colony Stimulating Factor; Thrombopoietic Agent

Use Treatment of thrombocytopenia in patients with chronic immune (idiopathic) thrombocytopenic purpura (ITP) at risk for bleeding who have had insufficient response to corticosteroids, immune globulin, or splenectomy

Pregnancy Risk Factor C

Pregnancy Considerations Adverse effects were observed in animal studies. There are no adequate and well-controlled studies in pregnant women. Use during pregnancy only if the potential benefit to the mother outweighs the potential risk to the fetus. A Promacta® pregnancy registry has been established to monitor outcomes of women exposed to eltrombopag during pregnancy (1-888-825-5249).

Lactation Excretion in breast milk unknown/not recommended

Medication Guide Available Yes

Contraindications There are no contraindications listed within the manufacturer's labeling.

Warnings/Precautions [U.S. Boxed Warning]: May cause hepatotoxicity; obtain ALT, AST, and bilirubin prior to treatment initiation, every 2 weeks during adjustment phase, then monthly (after stable dose established); obtain fractionation for elevated bilirubin levels. Repeat abnormal liver function tests within 3-5 days; if confirmed abnormal, monitor weekly until

resolves, stabilizes, or returns to baseline. Discontinue treatment for ALT levels ≥3 times the upper limit of normal (ULN) and which are progressive, or persistent (≥4 weeks), or accompanied by increased direct bilirubin, or accompanied by clinical signs of liver injury or evidence of hepatic decompensation. Reinitiation is not recommended; hepatotoxicity usually recurred with retreatment after therapy interruption; however, if the benefit of treatment outweighs the hepatotoxicity risk, initiate carefully, and monitor liver function tests weekly during the dose adjustment phase; permanently discontinue if hepatotoxicity recurs with rechallenge. Use with caution in patients with pre-existing hepatic impairment (clearance may be reduced); dosage reductions are recommended in patients with hepatic dysfunction; monitor closely.

May increase the risk for bone marrow reticulin formation or progression; collagen fibrosis (not associated with cytopenias) was observed in clinical trials. In an extension study, myelofibrosis (≤grade 1) was observed in a majority of bone marrow biopsies performed after 1 year of treatment. Monitor peripheral blood smear for cellular morphologic abnormalities; analyze CBC monthly; discontinue treatment with onset of new or worsening abnormalities (eg, teardrop and nucleated RBC, immature WBC) or cytopenias and consider bone marrow biopsy (with staining for fibrosis).

Thromboembolism may occur with excess increases in platelet levels. Use with caution in patients with known risk factors for thromboembolism (eg, Factor V Leiden, ATIII deficiency, antiphospholipid syndrome, chronic liver disease). Portal venous thrombosis was reported in a study of non-ITP patients with chronic liver disease (not an FDA-approved indication) receiving eltrombopag 75 mg once daily for 14 days as a preparative regimen prior to invasive procedures to reduce platelet transfusions. Stimulation of cell surface thrombopoietin (TPO) receptors may increase the risk for hematologic malignancies.

Cataract formation or worsening was observed in clinical trials. Monitor regularly for signs and symptoms of cataracts; obtain ophthalmic exam at baseline and during therapy. Use with caution in patients at risk for cataracts (eg, advanced age, long-term glucocorticoid use). Allow at least 4 hours between dosing of eltrombopag and antacids, minerals (eg, iron, calcium, aluminum, magnesium, selenium, zinc), or foods high in calcium; may reduce eltrombopag levels. Patients of East-Asian ethnicity (eg, Chinese, Japanese, Korean, Taiwanese) may have greater drug exposure (compared to non-East Asians); therapy should be initiated with lower starting doses. Use with caution in renal impairment (any degree) and monitor closely; initial dosage adjustment is not necessary.

Indicated only when the degree of thrombocytopenia and clinical conditions increase the risk for bleeding; use the lowest dose necessary to achieve and maintain platelet count ≥50,000/mm^3. Do not use to normalize platelet counts. Discontinue if platelet count does not respond to a level to avoid clinically important bleeding after 4 weeks at the maximum recommended dose.

Adverse Reactions

>10%: Hepatic: Liver function tests abnormal (11%)

1% to 10%:

- Central nervous system: Headache (10%), fatigue (4%)
- Dermatologic: Rash (3%), alopecia (2%)
- Gastrointestinal: Diarrhea (9%), nausea (4% to 9%), vomiting (6%), xerostomia (2%)
- Genitourinary: Urinary tract infection (5%)
- Hematologic: Myelofibrosis (Extension study: Grade ≤1: 93%; grade 2: 7%), rebound thrombocytopenia (8%)
- Hepatic: Hyperbilirubinemia (6%), ALT increased (5% to 6%), AST increased (4%), alkaline phosphatase increased (2%)
- Neuromuscular & skeletal: Myalgia (5%), back pain (3%), paresthesia (3%)
- Ocular: Cataract (4% to 7%)
- Respiratory: Upper respiratory infection (7%), oropharyngeal pain (4%), pharyngitis (4%)
- Miscellaneous: Influenza (3%)

<1% (Limited to important or life-threatening): Anemia, bone marrow collagen fiber deposits, bone marrow reticulin fiber deposits, hemorrhage (due to thrombocytopenia or rebound thrombocytopenia), non-Hodgkin's lymphoma, portal vein thrombosis, thrombotic/thromboembolic complications, visual acuity decreased

Drug Interactions

Metabolism/Transport Effects **Substrate** of CYP1A2 (minor), CYP2C8 (minor), UGT1A1, UGT1A3; **Note:** Assignment of Major/Minor substrate status based on clinically relevant drug interaction potential; **Inhibits** CYP2C8 (moderate), SLCO1B1, UGT1A1, UGT1A3, UGT1A4, UGT1A6, UGT1A9, UGT2B15, UGT2B7

Avoid Concomitant Use There are no known interactions where it is recommended to avoid concomitant use.

Increased Effect/Toxicity

Eltrombopag may increase the levels/effects of: CYP2C8 Substrates; Deferiprone; OATP1B1/SLCO1B1 Substrates; Rosuvastatin

Decreased Effect

The levels/effects of Eltrombopag may be decreased by: Aluminum Hydroxide; Calcium Salts; Cyproterone; Iron Salts; Magnesium Salts; Selenium; Sucralfate; Zinc Salts

Ethanol/Nutrition/Herb Interactions Food: Food, especially dairy products, may decrease the absorption of eltrombopag; allow at least 4 hours between dosing of eltrombopag and polyvalent cation intake (eg, dairy products, calcium-rich foods, multivitamins with minerals).

Stability Store at room temperature of 25°C (77°F); excursions permitted to 15°C to 30°C (59°F to 86°F).

Mechanism of Action Thrombopoietin (TPO) nonpeptide agonist which increases platelet counts by binding to and activating the human TPO receptor. Activates intracellular signal transduction pathways to increase proliferation and differentiation of marrow progenitor cells. Does not induce platelet aggregation or activation.

Pharmacodynamics/Kinetics

Onset of action: Platelet count increase: Within 1-2 weeks
Peak platelet count increase: 14-16 days

Duration: Platelets return to baseline: 1-2 weeks after last dose

Protein binding: >99%

Metabolism: Extensive hepatic metabolism; via CYP 1A2, 2C8 oxidation and UGT 1A1, 1A3 glucuronidation

Bioavailability: ~52%

Half-life elimination: ~21-32 hours in healthy individuals; ~26-35 hours in patients with ITP

Time to peak, plasma: 2-6 hours

Excretion: Feces (~59%, 20% as unchanged drug, 21% glutathione-related conjugates); urine (31%, 20% glucuronide of the phenypyrazole moiety)

Dosage Note: Use the lowest dose to achieve and maintain platelet count ≥50,000/mm^3 as needed to reduce the risk of bleeding. Adjust dose based on platelet count response; initial platelet response generally occurs within 1-2 weeks. Discontinue if platelet count does not respond to a level that avoids clinically important bleeding after 4 weeks at the maximum daily dose of 75 mg.

Oral: Adults: ITP: Initial: 50 mg once daily; adjust dose to achieve and maintain platelet count ≥50,000/mm^3 to reduce the risk of bleeding; maximum dose: 75 mg once daily

Initial dosage for patients of East-Asian ethnicity (eg, Chinese, Japanese, Korean, Taiwanese): 25 mg once daily

Dosage adjustment recommendations (based on platelet response):

Platelet count <50,000/mm^3 (after at least 2 weeks): Increase daily dose by 25 mg (if taking 12.5 mg once daily, increase dose to 25 mg once daily prior to increasing the dose amount by 25 mg/day); maximum dose: 75 mg/day

Platelet count ≥200,000/mm^3 and ≤400,000/mm^3 (at any time): Reduce daily dose by 25 mg; reassess in 2 weeks

Platelet count >400,000/mm^3: Withhold dose; assess platelet count twice weekly; when platelet count <150,000/mm^3, resume with the daily dose reduced by 25 mg (if taking 25 mg once daily, resume with 12.5 mg once daily)

Platelet count >400,000/mm^3 after 2 weeks at the lowest dose: Discontinue treatment

Dosage adjustment for toxicity:

Excessive platelet response (platelets >400,000/mm^3 after 2 weeks at the lowest dose): Discontinue treatment

New or worsening cellular abnormalities or cytopenias: Discontinue treatment

Dosage adjustment in renal impairment: No initial dosage adjustment necessary.

Dosage adjustment in hepatic impairment:

Adjustment for hepatic impairment prior to initiating treatment:

Mild, moderate, or severe impairment (Child-Pugh classes A, B, or C): Initial dose: 25 mg once daily

Patients of East-Asian ethnicity with hepatic impairment (Child-Pugh classes A, B, or C): Initial dose: 12.5 mg once daily

Adjustment for hepatic impairment during treatment:

Hepatic impairment (Child-Pugh classes A, B, or C) after treatment initiation or after dose increases: Wait 3 weeks (instead of 2 weeks) prior to increasing dose for platelet count <50,000/mm^3

ALT levels ≥3 times the upper limit of normal (ULN) **and** which are progressive, persistent (≥4 weeks), accompanied by increased direct bilirubin, or accompanied by clinical signs of liver injury or evidence of hepatic decompensation: Discontinue treatment

Dietary Considerations Take on an empty stomach (1 hour before or 2 hours after a meal). Food, especially dairy products, may decrease the absorption of eltrombopag; allow at least 4 hours between dosing of eltrombopag and polyvalent cation intake (eg, dairy products, calcium-rich foods, multivitamins with minerals).

Administration Administer on an empty stomach, 1 hour before or 2 hours after a meal. Do not administer concurrently with antacids, foods high in calcium, or minerals (eg, iron, calcium, aluminum, magnesium, selenium, zinc); separate by at least 4 hours. Do not administer more than one dose within 24 hours.

Monitoring Parameters Liver tests, including ALT, AST, and bilirubin (baseline, every 2 weeks during dosage titration, then monthly; evaluate abnormal liver function tests within 3-5 days; monitor weekly if retreating [not recommended] after therapy interruption for hepatotoxicity); bilirubin fractionation (for elevated bilirubin); CBC with differential and platelet count (weekly at initiation and during dosage titration, then monthly when stable; after cessation, monitor weekly for ≥4 weeks); peripheral blood smear (baseline and monthly when stable), bone marrow biopsy with staining for fibrosis (if peripheral blood smear reveals abnormality); ophthalmic exam (baseline and during treatment)

Reference Range Target platelet count (with treatment) of 50,000-200,000/mm^3; platelet life span: 8-11 days

Additional Information Restricted access to Promacta® was previously a REMS requirement via the Promacta® Cares™ program. Patients, prescribers, and pharmacies were required to be enrolled in this program. However, the FDA eliminated this REMS requirement in December 2011. There is currently no restricted access to obtaining Promacta®.

Product Availability

Promacta® 12.5 mg tablets (new strength): FDA approved December 2011; expected availability currently unknown.

Product labeling for Promacta® has also been updated to include dosage adjustment recommendations utilizing the new 12.5 mg strength.

Dosage Forms Excipient information presented when available (limited, particularly for generics); consult specific product labeling.

Tablet, oral:

Promacta®: 25 mg, 50 mg, 75 mg

- **Eltrombopag Olamine** *see* Eltrombopag *on page 579*
- **Eltroxin® (Can)** *see* Levothyroxine *on page 1004*
- **Embeda™** *see* Morphine and Naltrexone *on page 1158*
- **Emcyt®** *see* Estramustine *on page 636*
- **EMD 68843** *see* Vilazodone *on page 1787*
- **Emend®** *see* Aprepitant *on page 137*
- **Emend® IV (Can)** *see* Fosaprepitant *on page 759*
- **Emend® for Injection** *see* Fosaprepitant *on page 759*
- **EMLA®** *see* Lidocaine and Prilocaine *on page 1010*
- **Emo-Cort® (Can)** *see* Hydrocortisone (Topical) *on page 841*
- **Emoquette™** *see* Ethinyl Estradiol and Desogestrel *on page 653*
- **Emsam®** *see* Selegiline *on page 1544*

Emtricitabine (em trye SYE ta been)

Brand Names: U.S. Emtriva®

Brand Names: Canada Emtriva®

Index Terms BW524W91; Coviracil; FTC

Pharmacologic Category Antiretroviral Agent, Reverse Transcriptase Inhibitor (Nucleoside)

Additional Appendix Information

Management of Healthcare Worker Exposures to HBV, HCV, and HIV *on page 1935*

Perinatal HIV Guidelines *on page 1946*

Use Treatment of HIV infection in combination with at least two other antiretroviral agents

Pregnancy Risk Factor B

Pregnancy Considerations Adverse events were not observed in animal studies. Emtricitabine crosses the placenta; no increased risk of overall birth defects has been observed according to data collected by the antiretroviral pregnancy registry. Cases of lactic acidosis/hepatic steatosis syndrome related to mitochondrial toxicity have been reported in pregnant women with prolonged use of nucleoside analogues. It is not known if pregnancy itself potentiates this known side effect; however, women may be at increased risk of lactic acidosis and liver damage. In addition, these adverse events are similar to other rare but life-threatening syndromes which occur during pregnancy (eg, HELLP syndrome). Hepatic enzymes and electrolytes should be monitored in women receiving nucleoside analogues and clinicians should watch for early signs of the syndrome. In addition, mitochondrial dysfunction may develop in infants following *in utero* exposure. A pharmacokinetic study shows a slight decrease in emtricitabine serum levels during the third trimester; however, there is no clear need to adjust the dose. The DHHS Perinatal HIV Guidelines consider emtricitabine to be an alternative NRTI in dual nucleoside combination regimens. The DHHS Perinatal HIV Guidelines consider emtricitabine plus tenofovir a recommended dual NRTI/NtRTI backbone for HIV/HBV coinfected pregnant women.

Regardless of CD4 count or HIV RNA copy number, all HIV-infected pregnant women should receive a combination antepartum antiretroviral (ARV) drug regimen; this includes women who require therapy for their own health, as well as women who do not yet require therapy for their own health. ARV therapy should be started as soon as possible if required for the woman's health or immediately after the first trimester if not needed for the mother's health (although earlier initiation may be considered). Long-term follow-up is recommended for all infants exposed to ARV medications.

Healthcare providers are encouraged to enroll pregnant women exposed to antiretroviral medications in the Antiretroviral Pregnancy Registry (1-800-258-4263 or www.-APRegistry.com). Healthcare providers caring for HIV-infected women and their infants may contact the National Perinatal HIV Hotline (888-448-8765) for clinical consultation (DHHS [perinatal], 2011).

Lactation Excretion in breast milk unknown/contraindicated

Contraindications Hypersensitivity to emtricitabine or any component of the formulation

Warnings/Precautions [U.S. Boxed Warning]: Lactic acidosis, severe hepatomegaly with steatosis, and hepatic failure have occurred rarely with emtricitabine (similar to other nucleoside analogues). Some cases have been fatal; stop treatment if lactic acidosis or hepatotoxicity occur. Prior liver disease, obesity, extended duration of therapy, and female gender may represent risk factors for severe hepatic reactions. Testing for hepatitis B is recommended prior to the initiation of therapy; **[U.S. Boxed Warnings]: Hepatitis B may be exacerbated following discontinuation of emtricitabine; not indicated for treatment of chronic hepatitis B; safety and efficacy in HIV/HBV coinfected patients not established.** May be associated with fat redistribution (buffalo hump, increased abdominal girth, breast engorgement, facial atrophy, and dyslipidemia). Immune reconstitution syndrome may develop resulting in the occurrence of an inflammatory response to an indolent or residual opportunistic infection; further evaluation and treatment may be required. Use caution in patients with renal impairment (dosage adjustment required).

Adverse Reactions Clinical trials were conducted in patients receiving other antiretroviral agents, and it is not possible to correlate frequency of adverse events with emtricitabine alone. The range of frequencies of adverse events is generally comparable to comparator groups, with the exception of hyperpigmentation, which occurred more frequently in patients receiving emtricitabine. Unless otherwise noted, percentages are as reported in adults.

>10%:

- Central nervous system: Dizziness (4% to 25%), headache (6% to 22%), fever (children 18%), insomnia (5% to 16%), abnormal dreams (2% to 11%)
- Dermatologic: Hyperpigmentation (children 32%; adults 2% to 4%; primarily of palms and/or soles but may include tongue, arms, lip and nails; generally mild and nonprogressive without associated local reactions such as pruritus or rash); rash (17% to 30%; includes pruritus, maculopapular rash, vesiculobullous rash, pustular rash, and allergic reaction)
- Gastrointestinal: Diarrhea (children 20%; adults 9% to 23%), vomiting (children 23%; adults 9%), nausea (13% to 18%), abdominal pain (8% to 14%), gastroenteritis (children 11%)
- Neuromuscular & skeletal: Weakness (12% to 16%), CPK increased (grades 3/4: 11% to 12%)
- Otic: Otitis media (children 23%)
- Respiratory: Cough (children 28%; adults 14%), rhinitis (children 20%; adults 12% to 18%), pneumonia (children 15%)
- Miscellaneous: Infection (children 44%)

1% to 10%:

- Central nervous system: Depression (6% to 9%), neuropathy/neuritis (4%)
- Endocrine & metabolic: Serum triglycerides increased (grades 3/4: 4% to 10%), disordered glucose homeostasis (grades 3/4: 2% to 3%), serum amylase increased (grades 3/4: children 9%; adults 2% to 5%), serum lipase increased (grades 3/4: ≤1%)
- Gastrointestinal: Dyspepsia (4% to 8%), serum amylase increased (grades 3/4: 8%)
- Genitourinary: Hematuria (grades 3/4: 3%)
- Hematologic: Anemia (children: 7%), neutropenia (grades 3/4: children 2%; adults 5%)
- Hepatic: Transaminases increased (grades 3/4: 2% to 6%), alkaline phosphatase increased (>550 units/L: 1%), bilirubin increased (grades 3/4: 1%)
- Neuromuscular & skeletal: Creatinine kinase increased (grades 3/4: 9%), myalgia (4% to 6%), paresthesia (5% to 6%), arthralgia (3% to 5%)
- Respiratory: Upper respiratory tract infection (8%), sinusitis (8%), pharyngitis (5%)

Drug Interactions

Metabolism/Transport Effects None known.

Avoid Concomitant Use

Avoid concomitant use of Emtricitabine with any of the following: LamiVUDine

Increased Effect/Toxicity

The levels/effects of Emtricitabine may be increased by: Ganciclovir-Valganciclovir; LamiVUDine; Ribavirin

Decreased Effect There are no known significant interactions involving a decrease in effect.

Ethanol/Nutrition/Herb Interactions Food: Food decreases peak plasma concentrations, but does not alter the extent of absorption or overall systemic exposure.

Stability Store capsules at 15°C to 30°C (59°F to 86°F). Solution should be stored under refrigeration at 2°C to 8°C (36°F to 46°F). Once dispensed, may be stored at 15°C to 30°C (59°F to 86°F) if used within 3 months.

Mechanism of Action Nucleoside reverse transcriptase inhibitor; emtricitabine is a cytosine analogue which is phosphorylated intracellularly to emtricitabine 5'-triphosphate which interferes with HIV viral RNA dependent DNA polymerase resulting in inhibition of viral replication.

Pharmacodynamics/Kinetics

- Absorption: Rapid, extensive
- Protein binding: <4%
- Metabolism: Limited, via oxidation and conjugation (not via CYP isoenzymes)
- Bioavailability: Capsule: 93%; solution: 75%
- Half-life elimination: Normal renal function: Adults: 10 hours; children: 5-18 hours
- Time to peak, plasma: 1-2 hours
- Excretion: Urine (86% primarily as unchanged drug, 13% as metabolites); feces (14%)

Dosage Oral:

Children:

- 0-3 months: Solution: 3 mg/kg/day
- 3 months to 17 years:
  - Capsule: Children >33 kg: 200 mg once daily
  - Solution: 6 mg/kg once daily; maximum: 240 mg/day

Note: Emtricitabine in combination with tenofovir is recommended as a component of first line regimens (with atazanavir/ritonavir, with darunavir/ritonavir, with efavirenz, or with raltegravir) in treatment-naive patients (DHHS, 2011).

Adults:

Capsule: 200 mg once daily

Solution: 240 mg once daily

Dosage adjustment in renal impairment: Adults (consider similar adjustments in children):

Cl_{cr} 30-49 mL/minute: Capsule: 200 mg every 48 hours; solution: 120 mg every 24 hours

Cl_{cr} 15-29 mL/minute: Capsule: 200 mg every 72 hours; solution: 80 mg every 24 hours

Cl_{cr} <15 mL/minute (including hemodialysis patients): Capsule: 200 mg every 96 hours; solution: 60 mg every 24 hours; administer after dialysis

Dosage adjustment in hepatic impairment: No adjustment required.

Dietary Considerations May be taken with or without food.

Administration May be administered with or without food.

Monitoring Parameters Viral load, CD4, liver function tests; hepatitis B testing is recommended prior to initiation of therapy

Additional Information Data suggest that the combination of atazanavir/didanosine and emtricitabine is associated with inferior virologic responses; use is not recommended (DHHS, 2011). If a patient is coinfected with HIV/HBV, use of a single agent active against HBV may lead to HBV resistance; always use emtricitabine with tenofovir in these patients (DHHS, 2011).

Dosage Forms Excipient information presented when available (limited, particularly for generics); consult specific product labeling.

Capsule, oral:

Emtriva®: 200 mg

Solution, oral:

Emtriva®: 10 mg/mL (170 mL) [contains propylene glycol; cotton candy flavor]

Emtricitabine and Tenofovir

(em trye SYE ta been & te NOE fo veer)

Brand Names: U.S. Truvada®

Brand Names: Canada Truvada®

Index Terms Tenofovir and Emtricitabine

Pharmacologic Category Antiretroviral Agent, Reverse Transcriptase Inhibitor (Nucleoside); Antiretroviral Agent, Reverse Transcriptase Inhibitor (Nucleotide)

Additional Appendix Information

Management of Healthcare Worker Exposures to HBV, HCV, and HIV *on page 1935*

Use Treatment of HIV infection in combination with other antiretroviral agents

Unlabeled Use Treatment of hepatitis B in patients with antiviral-resistant HBV or coinfection with HIV; pre-exposure prophylaxis (PrEP) for prevention of HIV infection in men who have sex with men who are at high risk for acquiring HIV

Pregnancy Risk Factor B

Dosage Oral: **Note:** Avoid concurrent use with adefovir or lamivudine-containing products or other emtricitabine- and/or tenofovir-containing products.

Children ≥12 (and ≥35 kg) and Adults: HIV: One tablet (emtricitabine 200 mg and tenofovir 300 mg) once daily. **Note:** Recommended as a component of preferred regimens (in combination with atazanavir/ritonavir or darunavir/ritonavir or efavirenz or raltegravir) in antiretroviral-naive patients (DHHS, 2011).

Adults:

Treatment of hepatitis B in patients with antiviral-resistant HBV or coinfection with HIV (unlabeled use): One tablet (emtricitabine 200 mg and tenofovir 300 mg) once daily (Lok, 2009)

Pre-exposure prophylaxis (PrEP) for prevention of HIV infection in high-risk men who have sex with men (unlabeled use): One tablet (emtricitabine 200 mg and tenofovir 300 mg) once daily; in Cl_{cr} <60 mL/minute, use is not recommended(CDC interim guidance, 2011)

Dosage adjustment in renal impairment: Adults:

Cl_{cr} ≥50 mL/minute: No adjustment necessary

Cl_{cr} 30-49 mL/minute: Increase interval to every 48 hours.

Cl_{cr} <30 mL/minute or hemodialysis: Not recommended.

Dosage adjustment in hepatic impairment: No dosing adjustment necessary for tenofovir in moderate-to-severe hepatic compromise; no specific data available on emtricitabine in hepatic impairment, but given limited hepatic metabolism, dose adjustments are unlikely.

Additional Information Complete prescribing information for this medication should be consulted for additional detail.

Dosage Forms Excipient information presented when available (limited, particularly for generics); consult specific product labeling.

Tablet:

Truvada®: Emtricitabine 200 mg and tenofovir disoproxil fumarate 300 mg [equivalent to 245 mg tenofovir disoproxil]

◆ **Emtricitabine, Efavirenz, and Tenofovir** *see* Efavirenz, Emtricitabine, and Tenofovir *on page 577*

Emtricitabine, Rilpivirine, and Tenofovir

(em trye SYE ta been, ril pi VIR een, & te NOE fo veer)

Brand Names: U.S. Complera™

Brand Names: Canada Complera™

Index Terms FTC/RPV/TDF; Rilpivirine, Emtricitabine, and Tenofovir; Tenofovir Disoproxil Fumarate, Rilpivirine, and Emtricitabine; Tenofovir, Emtricitabine, and Rilpivirine

Pharmacologic Category Antiretroviral Agent, Reverse Transcriptase Inhibitor (Non-nucleoside); Antiretroviral Agent, Reverse Transcriptase Inhibitor (Nucleoside); Antiretroviral Agent, Reverse Transcriptase Inhibitor (Nucleotide)

Use Treatment of human immunodeficiency virus type 1 (HIV 1) infection in antiretroviral treatment-naive adult patients

Pregnancy Risk Factor B

Dosage Oral: Adults: HIV: One tablet once daily

Dosage adjustment in renal impairment:

Cl_{cr} ≥50 mL/minute: No dosage adjustments are recommended

Cl_{cr} <50 mL/minute: Use is not recommended

ESRD requiring dialysis: Use is not recommended

Dosage adjustment in hepatic impairment:

Mild-to-moderate hepatic impairment (Child-Pugh classes A and B): No dosage adjustments are recommended

Severe hepatic impairment (Child-Pugh class C): Use has not been studied

Additional Information Complete prescribing information for this medication should be consulted for additional detail.

Dosage Forms Excipient information presented when available (limited, particularly for generics); consult specific product labeling.

Tablet, oral:

Complera™: Emtricitabine 200 mg, rilpivirine 25 mg, and tenofovir disoproxil fumarate 300 mg

◆ **Emtriva®** *see* Emtricitabine *on page 581*
◆ **ENA 713** *see* Rivastigmine *on page 1509*
◆ **Enablex®** *see* Darifenacin *on page 450*

Enalapril (e NAL a pril)

Brand Names: U.S. Vasotec®

Brand Names: Canada Apo-Enalapril®; CO Enalapril; Mylan-Enalapril; Novo-Enalapril; PMS-Enalapril; PRO-Enalapril; RAN™-Enalapril; ratio-Enalapril; Riva-Enalapril; Sandoz-Enalapril; Sig-Enalapril; Taro-Enalapril; Teva-Enalapril; Vasotec®

Index Terms Enalapril Maleate

Pharmacologic Category Angiotensin-Converting Enzyme (ACE) Inhibitor

Additional Appendix Information

Angiotensin Agents *on page 1869*
Heart Failure (Systolic) *on page 1991*

Use Treatment of hypertension; treatment of symptomatic heart failure; treatment of asymptomatic left ventricular dysfunction

Unlabeled Use To delay the progression of nephropathy and reduce risks of cardiovascular events in hypertensive patients with type 1 or 2 diabetes mellitus; hypertensive crisis, diabetic nephropathy, hypertension secondary to scleroderma renal crisis, diagnosis of aldosteronism, idiopathic edema, Bartter's syndrome, postmyocardial infarction for prevention of ventricular failure

Pregnancy Risk Factor C (1st trimester); D (2nd and 3rd trimesters)

Pregnancy Considerations Due to adverse events observed in some animal studies, enalapril is considered pregnancy category C during the first trimester. Based on human data, enalapril is considered pregnancy category D if used during the second and third trimesters (per the manufacturer; however, one study suggests that fetal injury may occur at anytime during pregnancy). Enalaprilat, the active metabolite of enalapril, crosses the placenta. First trimester exposure to ACE inhibitors may cause major congenital malformations. An increased risk of cardiovascular and/or central nervous system malformations was observed in one study; however, an increased risk of teratogenic events was not observed in other studies. Second and third trimester use of an ACE inhibitor is associated with oligohydramnios. Oligohydramnios due to decreased fetal renal function may lead to fetal limb contractures, craniofacial deformation, and hypoplastic lung development. The use of ACE inhibitors during the second and third trimesters is also associated with anuria, hypotension, renal failure (reversible or irreversible), skull hypoplasia, and death in the fetus/neonate. Chronic maternal hypertension itself is also associated with adverse events in the fetus/infant. ACE inhibitors are not recommended during pregnancy to treat maternal hypertension or heart failure. Those who are planning a pregnancy should be considered for other medication options if an ACE inhibitor is currently prescribed or the ACE inhibitor should be discontinued as soon as possible once pregnancy is detected. The exposed fetus should be monitored for fetal growth, amniotic fluid volume, and organ formation. Infants exposed to an ACE inhibitor *in utero*, especially during the second and third trimester, should be monitored for hyperkalemia, hypotension, and oliguria.

[U.S. Boxed Warning]: Based on human data, ACE inhibitors can cause injury and death to the developing fetus when used in the second and third trimesters. ACE inhibitors should be discontinued as soon as possible once pregnancy is detected.

Lactation Enters breast milk/not recommended (AAP rates "compatible"; AAP 2001 update pending)

Contraindications Hypersensitivity to enalapril or enalaprilat; angioedema related to previous treatment with an ACE inhibitor; patients with idiopathic or hereditary angioedema

Warnings/Precautions Anaphylactic reactions may occur rarely with ACE inhibitors. At any time during treatment (especially following first dose) angioedema may occur rarely with ACE inhibitors; it may involve the head and neck (potentially compromising airway) or the intestine (presenting with abdominal pain). African-Americans may be at an increased risk. Prolonged frequent monitoring may be required especially if tongue, glottis, or larynx are involved as they are associated with airway obstruction. Patients with a history of airway surgery may have a higher risk of airway obstruction. Aggressive early and appropriate management is critical. Use in patients with idiopathic or hereditary angioedema or previous angioedema associated with ACE inhibitor therapy is contraindicated. Severe anaphylactoid reactions may be seen during hemodialysis (eg, CVVHD) with high-flux dialysis membranes (eg, AN69), and rarely, during low density lipoprotein apheresis with dextran sulfate cellulose. Rare cases of anaphylactoid reactions have been reported in patients undergoing sensitization treatment with hymenoptera (bee, wasp) venom while receiving ACE inhibitors.

Symptomatic hypotension with or without syncope can occur with ACE inhibitors (usually with the first several doses); effects are most often observed in volume depleted patients; correct volume depletion prior to initiation; close monitoring of patient is required especially with initial dosing and dosing increases; blood pressure must be lowered at a rate appropriate for the patient's clinical condition. Initiation of therapy in patients with ischemic heart disease or cerebrovascular disease warrants close observation due to the potential consequences posed by falling blood pressure (eg, MI, stroke). Use with caution in hypertrophic cardiomyopathy with outflow tract obstruction, severe aortic stenosis, or before, during, or immediately after major surgery. **[U.S. Boxed Warning]: Based on human data, ACEIs can cause injury and death to the developing fetus when used in the second and third trimesters. ACEIs should be discontinued as soon as possible once pregnancy is detected.**

Hyperkalemia may occur with ACE inhibitors; risk factors include renal dysfunction, diabetes mellitus, concomitant use of potassium-sparing diuretics, potassium supplements, and/or potassium-containing salts. Use cautiously, if at all, with these agents and monitor potassium closely. Cough may occur with ACE inhibitors. Other causes of cough should be considered (eg, pulmonary congestion in patients with heart failure) and excluded prior to discontinuation.

May be associated with deterioration of renal function and/or increases in serum creatinine, particularly in patients with low renal blood flow (eg, renal artery stenosis, heart failure) whose glomerular filtration rate (GFR) is dependent on efferent arteriolar vasoconstriction by angiotensin II; deterioration may result in oliguria, acute renal failure, and progressive azotemia. Small increases in serum creatinine may occur following initiation; consider discontinuation only in patients with progressive and/or significant deterioration in renal function. Use with caution in patients with unstented unilateral/bilateral renal artery stenosis. When unstented bilateral renal artery stenosis is present, use is generally avoided due to the elevated risk of deterioration in renal function unless possible benefits outweigh risks. Concurrent use of angiotensin receptor blockers may increase the risk of clinically-significant adverse events (eg, renal dysfunction, hyperkalemia).

Rare toxicities associated with ACE inhibitors include cholestatic jaundice (which may progress to fulminant hepatic necrosis), agranulocytosis, neutropenia or leukopenia with myeloid hypoplasia. Patients with collagen vascular diseases (especially with concomitant renal impairment) or renal impairment alone may be at increased risk for hematologic toxicity; periodically monitor CBC with differential in these patients.

Adverse Reactions Note: Frequency ranges include data from hypertension and heart failure trials. Higher rates of adverse reactions have generally been noted in patients with CHF. However, the frequency of adverse effects associated with placebo is also increased in this population.

1% to 10%: Cardiovascular: Hypotension (1% to 7%), chest pain (2%), syncope (≤2%), orthostasis (2%), orthostatic hypotension (2%)

Central nervous system: Headache (2% to 5%), dizziness (4% to 8%), fatigue (2% to 3%)

Dermatologic: Rash (2%)

Gastrointestinal: Abnormal taste, abdominal pain, vomiting, nausea, diarrhea, anorexia, constipation

Neuromuscular & skeletal: Weakness

Renal: Serum creatinine increased (≤20%), worsening of renal function (in patients with bilateral renal artery stenosis or hypovolemia)

Respiratory (1% to 2%): Bronchitis, cough, dyspnea

<1% (Limited to important or life-threatening): Agranulocytosis, alopecia, anaphylactoid reaction, angina pectoris, angioedema, ataxia, atrial fibrillation, atrial tachycardia, bone marrow suppression, bradycardia, bronchospasm, cardiac arrest, cerebral vascular accident, cholestatic jaundice, depression, eosinophilic pneumonitis, erythema multiforme, exfoliative dermatitis, flushing, giant cell arteritis, gynecomastia, hallucinations, hemolysis with G6PD, Henoch-Schönlein purpura, hepatitis, ileus, impotence, jaundice, lichen-form reaction, melena, MI, neutropenia, ototoxicity, pancreatitis, paresthesia, pemphigus, pemphigus foliaceus, peripheral neuropathy, photosensitivity, psychosis, pulmonary edema, pulmonary embolism, pulmonary infiltrates, Raynaud's phenomenon, sicca syndrome, somnolence, Stevens-Johnson syndrome, systemic lupus erythematosus, thrombocytopenia, toxic epidermal necrolysis, toxic pustuloderma, vertigo.

A syndrome which may include arthralgia, elevated ESR, eosinophilia and positive ANA, fever, interstitial nephritis, myalgia, rash, and vasculitis has been reported for enalapril and other ACE inhibitors.

Drug Interactions

Metabolism/Transport Effects None known.

Avoid Concomitant Use There are no known interactions where it is recommended to avoid concomitant use.

Increased Effect/Toxicity

Enalapril may increase the levels/effects of: Allopurinol; Amifostine; Antihypertensives; AzaTHIOprine; CycloSPORINE; CycloSPORINE (Systemic); Ferric Gluconate; Gold Sodium Thiomalate; Hypotensive Agents; Iron Dextran Complex; Lithium; Nonsteroidal Anti-Inflammatory Agents; RiTUXimab; Sodium Phosphates

The levels/effects of Enalapril may be increased by: Alfuzosin; Angiotensin II Receptor Blockers; Diazoxide; DPP-IV Inhibitors; Eplerenone; Everolimus; Herbs (Hypotensive Properties); Loop Diuretics; MAO Inhibitors; Pentoxifylline; Phosphodiesterase 5 Inhibitors; Potassium Salts; Potassium-Sparing Diuretics; Prostacyclin Analogues; Sirolimus; Temsirolimus; Thiazide Diuretics; TiZANidine; Tolvaptan; Trimethoprim

Decreased Effect

The levels/effects of Enalapril may be decreased by: Antacids; Aprotinin; Herbs (Hypertensive Properties); Icatibant; Lanthanum; Methylphenidate; Nonsteroidal Anti-Inflammatory Agents; Salicylates; Yohimbine

Ethanol/Nutrition/Herb Interactions Herb/Nutraceutical: Avoid bayberry, blue cohosh, cayenne, ephedra, ginger, ginseng (American), kola, licorice (may worsen hypertension). Avoid black cohosh, California poppy, coleus, golden seal, hawthorn, mistletoe, periwinkle, quinine, shepherd's purse (may have increased antihypertensive effect).

Mechanism of Action Competitive inhibitor of angiotensin-converting enzyme (ACE); prevents conversion of angiotensin I to angiotensin II, a potent vasoconstrictor; results in lower levels of angiotensin II which causes an increase in plasma renin activity and a reduction in aldosterone secretion

Pharmacodynamics/Kinetics

Onset of action: ~1 hour

Peak effect: 4-6 hours

Duration: 12-24 hours

Absorption: 55% to 75%

Protein binding: ~50% (Davies, 1984)

Metabolism: Prodrug, undergoes hepatic biotransformation to enalaprilat

Half-life elimination:

Enalapril: Adults: Healthy: 2 hours; Congestive heart failure: 3.4-5.8 hours

Enalaprilat: Infants 6 weeks to 8 months of age: 6-10 hours (Lloyd, 1989); Adults: ~35 hours (Till, 1984; Ulm, 1982)

Time to peak, serum: Oral: Enalapril: 0.5-1.5 hours; Enalaprilat (active metabolite): 3-4.5 hours

Excretion: Urine (61%; 18% of which was enalapril, 43% was enalaprilat); feces (33%; 6% of which was enalapril, 27% was enalaprilat) (Ulm, 1982)

Dosage Use lower listed initial dose in patients with hyponatremia, hypovolemia, severe congestive heart failure, decreased renal function, or in those receiving diuretics.

Oral:

Children 1 month to 17 years: Hypertension: Initial: 0.08 mg/kg/day (up to 5 mg) in 1-2 divided doses; adjust dosage based on patient response; doses >0.58 mg/kg (40 mg) have not been evaluated in pediatric patients

Infants and Children: Heart failure (unlabeled dosing): Initial: 0.1 mg/kg/day in 1-2 divided doses; increase as required over 2 weeks to maximum of 0.5 mg/kg/day. **Note:** Mean dose required for CHF improvement in 39 children (9 days to 17 years) was 0.36 mg/kg/day; select individuals have been treated with doses up to 0.94 mg/kg/day (Leversha, 1994).

Adults:

Asymptomatic left ventricular dysfunction: 2.5 mg twice daily, titrated as tolerated to 20 mg/day

Heart failure: Initial: 2.5 mg once or twice daily (usual range: 5-40 mg/day in 2 divided doses); titrate slowly at 1- to 2-week intervals. Target dose: 10-20 mg twice daily (ACC/AHA 2009 Heart Failure Guidelines)

Hypertension: 2.5-5 mg/day then increase as required, usually at 1- to 2-week intervals; usual dose range (JNC 7): 2.5-40 mg/day in 1-2 divided doses. **Note:** Initiate with 2.5 mg if patient is taking a diuretic which cannot be discontinued. May add a diuretic if blood pressure cannot be controlled with enalapril alone.

Conversion from I.V. **enalaprilat** to oral **enalapril** therapy: If not concurrently receiving diuretics, initiate enalapril 5 mg once daily; if concurrently receiving diuretics and responding to enalaprilat 0.625 mg I.V. every 6 hours, initiate with enalapril 2.5 mg once daily; subsequent titration as needed.

Dosing adjustment in renal impairment: Note: Use in infants and children ≤16 years of age with GFR <30 mL/minute/1.73 m^2 is not recommended (no dosing data exists).

Manufacturer's recommendations:
Cl_{cr} >30 mL/minute: No dosage adjustment necessary
Cl_{cr} ≤30 mL/minute: Administer 2.5 mg day; titrated upward until blood pressure is controlled.
Heart failure patients with sodium <130 mEq/L or serum creatinine >1.6 mg/dL: Initiate dosage with 2.5 mg/day, increasing to twice daily as needed. Increase further in increments of 2.5 mg/dose at >4-day intervals to a maximum daily dose of 40 mg.
Intermittent hemodialysis (IHD): Moderately dialyzable (20% to 50%): Initial: 2.5 mg on dialysis days; adjust dose on nondialysis days depending on blood pressure response.
Conversion from I.V. **enalaprilat** to oral **enalapril** therapy:
Cl_{cr} >30 mL/minute: May initiate enalapril 5 mg once daily.
Cl_{cr} ≤30 mL/minute: May initiate enalapril 2.5 mg once daily.
Alternate recommendations (Aronoff, 2007):
Cl_{cr} >50 mL/minute: No dosage adjustment necessary
Cl_{cr} 10-50 mL/minute: Administer 75-100% of usual dose
Cl_{cr} <10 mL/minute: Administer 50% of usual dose
Peritoneal dialysis: Supplemental dose is not necessary, although some removal of drug occurs.

Dosing adjustment in hepatic impairment: Hydrolysis of enalapril to enalaprilat may be delayed and/or impaired in patients with severe hepatic impairment, but the pharmacodynamic effects of the drug do not appear to be significantly altered; no dosage adjustment.

Dietary Considerations Limit salt substitutes or potassium-rich diet.

Monitoring Parameters Blood pressure; serum creatinine and potassium; if patient has collagen vascular disease and/or renal impairment, periodically monitor CBC with differential

Test Interactions Positive Coombs' [direct]; may cause false-positive results in urine acetone determinations using sodium nitroprusside reagent

Dosage Forms Excipient information presented when available (limited, particularly for generics); consult specific product labeling.
Tablet, oral, as maleate: 2.5 mg, 5 mg, 10 mg, 20 mg
Vasotec®: 2.5 mg, 5 mg, 10 mg, 20 mg [scored]

Extemporaneous Preparations A 1 mg/mL oral suspension may be made with tablets, Bicitra® [discontinued] or equivalent, and Ora-Sweet® SF. Place ten 20 mg tablets in a 200 mL polyethylene terephthalate bottle; add 50 mL of Bicitra® [discontinued] or equivalent and shake well for at least 2 minutes. Let stand for 1 hour then shake for 1 additional minute; add 150 mL of Ora-Sweet® SF and shake well. Label "shake well" and "refrigerate". Stable for 30 days when stored in a polyethylene terephthalate bottle and refrigerated (Vasotec® prescribing information, 2001).

A 1 mg/mL oral suspension may be made with tablets and one of three different vehicles (cherry syrup, a 1:1 mixture of Ora-Sweet® and Ora-Plus®, or a 1:1 mixture of Ora-Sweet® SF and Ora-Plus®). Crush six 20 mg tablets in a mortar and reduce to a fine powder. Add 15 mL of the chosen vehicle and mix to a uniform paste; mix while adding the vehicle in incremental proportions to **almost** 120 mL; transfer to a calibrated bottle, rinse mortar with vehicle, and add quantity of vehicle sufficient to make 120 mL. Label "shake well" and "protect from light". Stable for 60 days when stored in amber plastic prescription bottles in the dark at room temperature or refrigerated (Allen, 1998).

A 1 mg/mL oral suspension may be made with tablets and one of three different vehicles (deionized water, citrate buffer solution at pH 5.0, or a 1:1 mixture of Ora-Sweet® and Ora-Plus®). Crush twenty 10 mg tablets in a mortar and reduce to a fine powder. Add small portions of the chosen vehicle and mix to a uniform paste; mix while adding vehicle in incremental proportions to **almost** 200 mL; transfer to a graduated cylinder, rinse mortar with vehicle, and add quantity of vehicle sufficient to make 200 mL. Label "shake well" and "protect from light". Preparations made in citrate buffer solution at pH 5.0 and the 1:1 mixture of Ora-Sweet® and Ora-Plus® are stable for 91 days when stored in plastic prescription bottles in the dark at room temperature or refrigerated. Preparation made in deionized water is stable for 91 days refrigerated or 56 days at room temperature when stored in plastic prescription bottles in the dark. **Note:** To prepare the isotonic citrate buffer solution (pH 5.0), see reference (Nahata, 1998).

A more dilute, 0.1 mg/mL oral suspension may be made with tablets and an isotonic buffer solution at pH 5.0. Grind one 20 mg tablet in a glass mortar and reduce to a fine powder; mix with isotonic citrate buffer (pH 5.0) and filter; add quantity of buffer solution sufficient to make 200 mL. Label "shake well", "protect from light", and "refrigerate". Stable for 90 days (Boulton, 1994).

Allen LV Jr and Erickson MA 3rd, "Stability of Alprazolam, Chloroquine Phosphate, Cisapride, Enalapril Maleate, and Hydralazine Hydrochloride in Extemporaneously Compounded Oral Liquids," *Am J Health Syst Pharm*, 1998, 55(18):1915-20.
Boulton DW, Woods DJ, Fawcett JP, et al, "The Stability of an Enalapril Maleate Oral Solution Prepared From Tablets," *Aust J Hosp Pharm*, 1994, 24(2):151-6.
Nahata MC, Morosco RS, and Hipple TF, "Stability of Enalapril Maleate in Three Extemporaneously Prepared Oral Liquids," *Am J Health Syst Pharm*, 1998, 55(11):1155-7.
Vasotec® prescribing information, Merck & Co, Inc, West Point, PA, 2001.

Enalapril and Hydrochlorothiazide

(e NAL a pril & hye droe klor oh THYE a zide)

Brand Names: U.S. Vaseretic®
Brand Names: Canada Vaseretic®
Index Terms Enalapril Maleate and Hydrochlorothiazide; Hydrochlorothiazide and Enalapril
Pharmacologic Category Angiotensin-Converting Enzyme (ACE) Inhibitor; Diuretic, Thiazide
Use Treatment of hypertension
Pregnancy Risk Factor C/D (2nd and 3rd trimesters)
Dosage Oral: Adults: Enalapril 5-10 mg and hydrochlorothiazide 12.5-25 mg once daily (maximum: 40 mg/day [enalapril]; 50 mg/day [hydrochlorothiazide])
Additional Information Complete prescribing information for this medication should be consulted for additional detail.
Dosage Forms Excipient information presented when available (limited, particularly for generics); consult specific product labeling.
Tablet:
5/12.5: Enalapril maleate 5 mg and hydrochlorothiazide 12.5 mg
10/25: Enalapril maleate 10 mg and hydrochlorothiazide 25 mg
Vaseretic®:
10/25: Enalapril maleate 10 mg and hydrochlorothiazide 25 mg

◆ **Enalapril Maleate** *see* Enalapril *on page* 584
◆ **Enalapril Maleate and Hydrochlorothiazide** *see* Enalapril and Hydrochlorothiazide *on page* 586
◆ **Enbrel®** *see* Etanercept *on page* 649
◆ **Enbrel® SureClick®** *see* Etanercept *on page* 649
◆ **Encare® [OTC]** *see* Nonoxynol 9 *on page* 1216
◆ **Endantadine® (Can)** *see* Amantadine *on page* 82

- ◆ **Endocet®** *see* Oxycodone and Acetaminophen *on page 1269*
- ◆ **EndoCof [OTC]** *see* Chlorpheniramine, Phenylephrine, and Dextromethorphan *on page 346*
- ◆ **Endodan®** *see* Oxycodone and Aspirin *on page 1269*
- ◆ **Endo®-Levodopa/Carbidopa (Can)** *see* Carbidopa and Levodopa *on page 284*
- ◆ **Endometrin®** *see* Progesterone *on page 1414*
- ◆ **Enduron** *see* Methyclothiazide *on page 1103*
- ◆ **Enemeez® [OTC]** *see* Docusate *on page 537*
- ◆ **Enemeez® Plus [OTC]** *see* Docusate *on page 537*
- ◆ **Ener-B® [OTC]** *see* Cyanocobalamin *on page 418*
- ◆ **Enerjets [OTC]** *see* Caffeine *on page 259*

Enfuvirtide (en FYOO vir tide)

Brand Names: U.S. Fuzeon®

Brand Names: Canada Fuzeon®

Index Terms T-20

Pharmacologic Category Antiretroviral Agent, Fusion Protein Inhibitor

Additional Appendix Information

Management of Healthcare Worker Exposures to HBV, HCV, and HIV *on page 1935*

Perinatal HIV Guidelines *on page 1946*

Use Treatment of HIV-1 infection in combination with other antiretroviral agents in treatment-experienced patients with evidence of HIV-1 replication despite ongoing antiretroviral therapy

Pregnancy Risk Factor B

Pregnancy Considerations Teratogenic effects were not observed in animal studies. Limited data suggest that enfuvirtide does not cross the placenta. The DHHS Perinatal HIV Guidelines note that data are insufficient to recommend use during pregnancy.

Regardless of CD4 count or HIV RNA copy number, all HIV-infected pregnant women should receive a combination antepartum antiretroviral (ARV) drug regimen; this includes women who require therapy for their own health, as well as women who do not yet require therapy for their own health. ARV therapy should be started as soon as possible if required for the woman's health or immediately after the first trimester if not needed for the mothers health (although earlier initiation may be considered). Long-term follow-up is recommended for all infants exposed to ARV medications.

Healthcare providers are encouraged to enroll pregnant women exposed to antiretroviral medications in the Antiretroviral Pregnancy Registry (1-800-258-4263 or www.-APRegistry.com). Healthcare providers caring for HIV-infected women and their infants may contact the National Perinatal HIV Hotline (888-448-8765) for clinical consultation (DHHS [perinatal], 2011).

Lactation Excretion in breast milk unknown/contraindicated

Contraindications Hypersensitivity to enfuvirtide or any component of the formulation

Warnings/Precautions Use is not recommended in antiretroviral therapy-naive patients (DHHS, 2011). Monitor closely for signs/symptoms of pneumonia; associated with an increased incidence during clinical trials, particularly in patients with a low CD4 cell count, high initial viral load, I.V. drug use, smoking, or a history of lung disease. May cause hypersensitivity reactions (symptoms may include rash, fever, nausea, vomiting, hypotension, and elevated transaminases). In addition, local injection site reactions are common. An inflammatory response to indolent or residual opportunistic infections (immune reconstitution syndrome) has occurred with antiretroviral therapy; further investigation is warranted. Administration using a needle-free device has been associated with nerve pain (including neuralgia and/or paresthesia lasting up to 6 months), bruising, and hematomas when administered at sites where large nerves are close to the skin; only administer medication in recommended sites and use caution in patients with coagulation disorders (eg, hemophilia) or receiving anticoagulants. Safety and efficacy have not been established in children <6 years of age.

Adverse Reactions

>10%:

Central nervous system: Fatigue (20%), insomnia (11%)

Gastrointestinal: Diarrhea (32%), nausea (23%)

Local: Injection site infection (children 11%), injection site reactions (98%; may include pain, erythema, induration, pruritus, ecchymosis, nodule or cyst formation)

1% to 10%:

Dermatologic: Folliculitis (2%)

Gastrointestinal: Weight loss (7%), abdominal pain (4%), appetite decreased (3%), pancreatitis (3%), anorexia (2%), xerostomia (2%)

Hematologic: Eosinophilia (2% to 9%)

Hepatic: Transaminases increased (4%, grade 4: 1%)

Local: Injection site infection (adults 2%)

Neuromuscular & skeletal: CPK increased (3% to 7%), limb pain (3%), myalgia (3%)

Ocular: Conjunctivitis (2%)

Respiratory: Sinusitis (6%), cough (4%), bacterial pneumonia (3%)

Miscellaneous: Infections (4% to 6%), herpes simplex (4%), flu-like syndrome (2%)

<1% (Limited to important or life-threatening): Abacavir hypersensitivity worsening, amylase increased, angina, anxiety, constipation, depression, GGT increased, glomerulonephritis, Guillain-Barré syndrome, hepatic steatosis, hyperglycemia; hypersensitivity reactions (symptoms may include rash, fever, nausea, vomiting, hypotension, and transaminase increases); insomnia, lipase increased, lymphadenopathy, neutropenia, peripheral neuropathy, pneumopathy, renal failure, renal insufficiency, respiratory distress, sepsis, sixth nerve palsy, suicide attempt, taste disturbances, thrombocytopenia, toxic hepatitis, triglycerides increased, tubular necrosis, weakness

Drug Interactions

Metabolism/Transport Effects None known.

Avoid Concomitant Use There are no known interactions where it is recommended to avoid concomitant use.

Increased Effect/Toxicity

Enfuvirtide may increase the levels/effects of: Protease Inhibitors

The levels/effects of Enfuvirtide may be increased by: Protease Inhibitors

Decreased Effect There are no known significant interactions involving a decrease in effect.

Stability Store powder at 15°C to 30°C (59°F to 86°F). Reconstitute with 1.1 mL SWFI. Tap vial for 10 seconds and roll gently to ensure contact with diluent. Allow to stand until solution is completed. May require up to 45 minutes to form solution (108 mg/1.2 mL). Reconstituted solutions should be refrigerated and must be used within 24 hours.

Mechanism of Action Binds to the first heptad-repeat (HR1) in the gp41 subunit of the viral envelope glycoprotein. Inhibits the fusion of HIV-1 virus with CD4 cells by blocking the conformational change in gp41 required for membrane fusion and entry into CD4 cells

Pharmacodynamics/Kinetics

Distribution: V_d: 5.5 L; CSF concentrations (2-18 hours after administration): nondetectable (<0.025 mcg/mL)

Protein binding: 92%

Metabolism: Proteolytic hydrolysis (CYP isoenzymes do not appear to contribute to metabolism)

Clearance: Adults: 24.8 mL/hour/kg

Bioavailability: 84% ± 16%

Half-life elimination: 3.8 hours

Time to peak: 4-8 hours

Dosage Note: Use is not recommended in antiretroviral therapy naïve patients (DHHS, 2011). SubQ:

Children 6-16 years: 2 mg/kg twice daily (maximum dose: 90 mg twice daily)

Adolescents ≥16 years and Adults: 90 mg twice daily

Dosage adjustment in renal impairment:

Cl_{cr} >35 mL/minute: Clearance not affected; no dosage adjustment required.

Cl_{cr} ≤35 mL/minute: Limited data showed decreased clearance; however, no dosage adjustment recommended.

End-stage renal disease (on dialysis): Limited data showed decreased clearance; however, no dosage adjustment recommended.

Dosage adjustment in hepatic impairment: No dosage adjustment required

Administration Inject subcutaneously into upper arm, abdomen, or anterior thigh. Do not inject into moles, the navel, over a blood vessel or skin abnormalities such as scar tissue, surgical scars, bruises, or tattoos. In addition, do not inject in or near sites where large nerves are close to the skin including the elbow, knee, groin, or buttocks. Rotate injection site, give injections at a site different from the preceding injection site; do not inject into any site where an injection site reaction is evident. Bioequivalence was found to be similar in a study comparing standard administration using a needle versus a needle-free device.

Additional Information If hypersensitivity reactions occur (symptoms may include rash, fever, nausea, vomiting, hypotension, and transaminase increases), enfuvirtide rechallenge is not recommended. If changing to an oral antiretroviral, raltegravir may be considered if not used previously.

Dosage Forms Excipient information presented when available (limited, particularly for generics); consult specific product labeling.

Injection, powder for reconstitution [preservative free]:
Fuzeon®: 108 mg [90 mg/mL following reconstitution]

- **Engerix-B®** *see* Hepatitis B Vaccine (Recombinant) *on page 827*
- **Engerix-B® and Havrix®** *see* Hepatitis A and Hepatitis B Recombinant Vaccine *on page 824*
- **Enhanced-Potency Inactivated Poliovirus Vaccine** *see* Poliovirus Vaccine (Inactivated) *on page 1370*
- **Enjuvia™** *see* Estrogens (Conjugated B/Synthetic) *on page 639*
- **Enlon®** *see* Edrophonium *on page 573*
- **Enlon-Plus®** *see* Edrophonium and Atropine *on page 574*

Enoxaparin (ee noks a PA rin)

Brand Names: U.S. Lovenox®

Brand Names: Canada Enoxaparin Injection; Lovenox®; Lovenox® HP

Index Terms Enoxaparin Sodium

Pharmacologic Category Low Molecular Weight Heparin

Use

Acute coronary syndromes: Unstable angina (UA), non-ST-elevation (NSTEMI), and ST-elevation myocardial infarction (STEMI)

DVT prophylaxis: Following hip or knee replacement surgery, abdominal surgery, or in medical patients with severely-restricted mobility during acute illness who are at risk for thromboembolic complications

DVT treatment (acute): Inpatient treatment (patients with and without pulmonary embolism) and outpatient treatment (patients without pulmonary embolism)

Note: High-risk patients include those with one or more of the following risk factors: >40 years of age, obesity, general anesthesia lasting >30 minutes, malignancy, history of deep vein thrombosis or pulmonary embolism

Unlabeled Use Prophylaxis and treatment of thromboembolism in children; anticoagulant bridge therapy during temporary interruption of vitamin K antagonist therapy in patients at high risk for thromboembolism; DVT prophylaxis following moderate-risk general surgery, major gynecologic surgery and following higher-risk general surgery for cancer; management of venous thromboembolism (VTE) during pregnancy; anticoagulant used during percutaneous coronary intervention (PCI)

Pregnancy Risk Factor B

Pregnancy Considerations Animal studies have not shown teratogenic or fetotoxic effects. Pregnancy itself increases the risk of thromboembolism. Pregnant women with a history of thromboembolic disease are at increased risk of maternal and fetal complications. Enoxaparin does not cross the placenta. Use may be recommended in pregnant women for the management of VTE. Monitoring antifactor Xa levels is recommended. Risk of adverse events may be increased in pregnant women with mechanical heart valves; use is controversial and has not been adequately studied. Postmarketing reports include congenital abnormalities (cause and effect not established) and also fetal death when used in pregnant women. Multiple-dose vials contain benzyl alcohol; use caution in pregnant women.

Lactation Excretion in breast milk unknown/use caution

Contraindications Hypersensitivity to enoxaparin, heparin, or any component of the formulation; thrombocytopenia associated with a positive *in vitro* test for antiplatelet antibodies in the presence of enoxaparin; hypersensitivity to pork products; active major bleeding; not for I.M. use

Warnings/Precautions **[U.S. Boxed Warning]: Spinal or epidural hematomas, including subsequent paralysis, may occur with recent or anticipated neuraxial anesthesia (epidural or spinal anesthesia) or spinal puncture in patients anticoagulated with LMWH or heparinoids.** Consider risk versus benefit prior to spinal procedures; risk is increased by the use of concomitant agents which may alter hemostasis, the use of indwelling epidural catheters for analgesia, a history of spinal deformity or spinal surgery, as well as a history of traumatic or repeated epidural or spinal punctures. Patient should be observed closely for bleeding and signs and symptoms of neurological impairment if therapy is administered during or immediately following diagnostic lumbar puncture, epidural anesthesia, or spinal anesthesia.

Do not administer intramuscularly. Not recommended for thromboprophylaxis in patients with prosthetic heart valves (especially pregnant women). Not to be used interchangeably (unit for unit) with heparin or any other low molecular weight heparins. Use caution in patients with history of heparin-induced thrombocytopenia. Monitor patient closely for signs or symptoms of bleeding. Certain patients are at increased risk of bleeding. Risk factors include bacterial endocarditis; congenital or acquired bleeding disorders;

active ulcerative or angiodysplastic GI diseases; severe uncontrolled hypertension; history of hemorrhagic stroke; use shortly after brain, spinal, or ophthalmic surgery; patients treated concomitantly with platelet inhibitors; recent GI bleeding; thrombocytopenia or platelet defects; severe liver disease; hypertensive or diabetic retinopathy; or in patients undergoing invasive procedures. Monitor platelet count closely. Rare cases of thrombocytopenia have occurred. Discontinue therapy and consider alternative treatment if platelets are <100,000/mm^3 and/or thrombosis develops. Rare cases of thrombocytopenia with thrombosis have occurred. Use caution in patients with congenital or drug-induced thrombocytopenia or platelet defects. Risk of bleeding may be increased in women <45 kg and in men <57 kg. Use caution in patients with renal failure; dosage adjustment needed if Cl_{cr} <30 mL/minute. Use with caution in the elderly (delayed elimination may occur); dosage alteration/adjustment may be required (eg, omission of I.V. bolus in acute STEMI in patients ≥75 years of age). Monitor for hyperkalemia; can cause hyperkalemia possibly by suppressing aldosterone production. Multiple-dose vials contain benzyl alcohol (use caution in pregnant women). In neonates, large amounts of benzyl alcohol (>100 mg/kg/day) have been associated with fatal toxicity (gasping syndrome).

There is no consensus for adjusting/correcting the weight-based dosage of LMWH for patients who are morbidly obese (BMI ≥40 kg/m^2). For patients undergoing inpatient bariatric surgery, the American College of Chest Physicians Practice Guidelines suggest using a higher thromboprophylaxis dose of LMWH for obese patients (Geerts, 2008).

Adverse Reactions As with all anticoagulants, bleeding is the major adverse effect of enoxaparin. Hemorrhage may occur at virtually any site. Risk is dependent on multiple variables. At the recommended doses, single injections of enoxaparin do not significantly influence platelet aggregation or affect global clotting time (ie, PT or aPTT).

1% to 10%:

Central nervous system: Fever (5% to 8%), confusion, pain

Dermatologic: Erythema, bruising

Gastrointestinal: Nausea (3%), diarrhea

Hematologic: Hemorrhage (major, <1% to 4%; includes cases of intracranial, retroperitoneal, or intraocular hemorrhage; incidence varies with indication/population), thrombocytopenia (moderate 1%; severe 0.1% - see **"Note"**), anemia (<2%)

Hepatic: ALT increased, AST increased

Local: Injection site hematoma (9%), local reactions (irritation, pain, ecchymosis, erythema)

Renal: Hematuria (<2%)

<1% (Limited to important or life-threatening): Allergic reaction, anaphylactoid reaction, cutaneous vasculitis (hypersensitive), eczematous plaques, hematoma (see note on "Spinal or epidural hematomas"), hyperkalemia, hyperlipidemia, hypertriglyceridemia, intracranial hemorrhage (up to 0.8%), erythematous pruritic patches, pruritus, purpura, retroperitoneal bleeding, skin necrosis, thrombocytopenia with thrombosis, thrombocytosis, urticaria, vesicobullous rash

Note:

Spinal or epidural hematomas: Can occur following neuraxial anesthesia or spinal puncture, resulting in paralysis. Risk is increased in patients with indwelling epidural catheters or concomitant use of other drugs affecting hemostasis. Prosthetic valve thrombosis, including fatal cases, has been reported in pregnant women receiving enoxaparin as thromboprophylaxis.

Thrombocytopenia with thrombosis: Cases of heparin-induced thrombocytopenia (some complicated by organ infarction, limb ischemia, or death) have been reported.

Drug Interactions

Metabolism/Transport Effects None known.

Avoid Concomitant Use

Avoid concomitant use of Enoxaparin with any of the following: Rivaroxaban

Increased Effect/Toxicity

Enoxaparin may increase the levels/effects of: Anticoagulants; Collagenase (Systemic); Deferasirox; Drotrecogin Alfa (Activated); Ibritumomab; Rivaroxaban; Tositumomab and Iodine I 131 Tositumomab

The levels/effects of Enoxaparin may be increased by: 5-ASA Derivatives; Antiplatelet Agents; Dasatinib; Herbs (Anticoagulant/Antiplatelet Properties); Nonsteroidal Anti-Inflammatory Agents; Pentosan Polysulfate Sodium; Pentoxifylline; Prostacyclin Analogues; Salicylates; Thrombolytic Agents

Decreased Effect There are no known significant interactions involving a decrease in effect.

Ethanol/Nutrition/Herb Interactions Herb/Nutraceutical: Avoid cat's claw, dong quai, evening primrose, feverfew, garlic, ginger, ginkgo, red clover, horse chestnut, green tea, ginseng (all have additional antiplatelet activity).

Stability Store at 25°C (77°F); excursions permitted to 15°C to 30°C (59°F to 86°F); do not freeze.

Mechanism of Action Standard heparin consists of components with molecular weights ranging from 4000-30,000 daltons with a mean of 16,000 daltons. Heparin acts as an anticoagulant by enhancing the inhibition rate of clotting proteases by antithrombin III impairing normal hemostasis and inhibition of factor Xa. Low molecular weight heparins have a small effect on the activated partial thromboplastin time and strongly inhibit factor Xa. Enoxaparin is derived from porcine heparin that undergoes benzylation followed by alkaline depolymerization. The average molecular weight of enoxaparin is 4500 daltons which is distributed as (≤20%) 2000 daltons (≥68%) 2000-8000 daltons, and (≤15%) >8000 daltons. Enoxaparin has a higher ratio of antifactor Xa to antifactor IIa activity than unfractionated heparin.

Pharmacodynamics/Kinetics

Onset of action: Peak effect: SubQ: Antifactor Xa and antithrombin (antifactor IIa): 3-5 hours

Duration: 40 mg dose: Antifactor Xa activity: ~12 hours

Distribution: 4.3 L (based on antifactor Xa activity)

Protein binding: Does not bind to heparin binding proteins

Metabolism: Hepatic, to lower molecular weight fragments (little activity)

Half-life elimination, plasma: 2-4 times longer than standard heparin, independent of dose; based on anti-Xa activity: 4.5-7 hours

Excretion: Urine (40% of dose; 10% as active fragments)

Dosage One mg of enoxaparin is equal to 100 int. units of anti-Xa activity (World Health Organization First International Low Molecular Weight Heparin Reference Standard).

Infants and Children (unlabeled use; Monagle, 2008):

SubQ:

Infants <2 months: Initial:

Prophylaxis: 0.75 mg/kg every 12 hours

Treatment: 1.5 mg/kg every 12 hours

Infants >2 months and Children ≤18 years: Initial:

Prophylaxis: 0.5 mg/kg every 12 hours

Treatment: 1 mg/kg every 12 hours

Maintenance: See **Dosage Titration** table:

Enoxaparin Pediatric Dosage Titration

Antifactor Xa	Dose Titration	Time to Repeat Antifactor Xa Level
<0.35 units/mL	Increase dose by 25%	4 h after next dose
0.35-0.49 units/mL	Increase dose by 10%	4 h after next dose
0.5-1 unit/mL	Keep same dosage	Next day, then 1 wk later, then monthly (4 h after dose)
1.1-1.5 units/mL	Decrease dose by 20%	Before next dose
1.6-2 units/mL	Hold dose for 3 h and decrease dose by 30%	Before next dose, then 4 h after next dose
>2 units/mL	Hold all doses until antifactor Xa is 0.5 units/mL, then decrease dose by 40%	Before next dose and every 12 h until antifactor Xa <0.5 units/mL

Modified from Monagle P, Michelson AD, Bovill E, et al, "Antithrombotic Therapy in Children," *Chest*, 2001, 119:344S-70S.

Adults:

SubQ:

DVT prophylaxis: **Note:** In morbidly obese patients (BMI ≥40 kg/m^2), increasing the prophylactic dose by 30% may be appropriate for some indications (Nutescu, 2009). For bariatric surgery, dose increases may be >30% based on clinical trial data. SubQ:

Hip replacement surgery:

Twice-daily dosing: 30 mg every 12 hours, with initial dose within 12-24 hours after surgery, and every 12 hours for at least 10 days or until risk of DVT has diminished or the patient is adequately anticoagulated on warfarin.

Once-daily dosing: 40 mg once daily, with initial dose within 9-15 hours before surgery, and daily for at least 10 days (or up to 35 days postoperatively) or until risk of DVT has diminished or the patient is adequately anticoagulated on warfarin.

Knee replacement surgery: 30 mg every 12 hours, with initial dose within 12-24 hours after surgery, and every 12 hours for at least 10 days or until risk of DVT has diminished or the patient is adequately anticoagulated on warfarin.

Abdominal surgery: 40 mg once daily, with initial dose given 2 hours prior to surgery; continue until risk of DVT has diminished (usually 7-10 days).

Bariatric surgery: Roux-en-Y gastric bypass: Appropriate dosing strategies have not been clearly defined (Borkgren-Okonek, 2008; Scholten, 2002):

BMI ≤50 kg/m^2: 40 mg every 12 hours

BMI >50 kg/m^2: 60 mg every 12 hours

Note: Bariatric surgery guidelines suggest initiation 30-120 minutes before surgery and postoperatively until patient is fully mobile (Mechanick, 2009). Alternatively, limiting administration to the postoperative period may reduce perioperative bleeding.

Medical patients with severely-restricted mobility during acute illness: 40 mg once daily; continue until risk of DVT has diminished (usually 6-11 days).

DVT treatment (acute): **Note:** Start warfarin on the first treatment day and continue enoxaparin until INR is between 2 and 3 (usually 5-7 days).

Inpatient treatment (with or without pulmonary embolism): 1 mg/kg/dose every 12 hours or 1.5 mg/kg once daily.

Outpatient treatment (without pulmonary embolism): 1 mg/kg/dose every 12 hours.

Obesity: Use actual body weight to calculate dose; dose capping not recommended; use of twice daily dosing preferred (Nutescu, 2009).

ST-elevation myocardial infarction (STEMI):

Patients <75 years of age: Initial: 30 mg I.V. single bolus plus 1 mg/kg (maximum 100 mg for the first 2 doses only) SubQ every 12 hours. The first SubQ dose should be administered with the I.V. bolus. Maintenance: After first 2 doses, administer 1 mg/kg SubQ every 12 hours.

Patients ≥75 years of age: Initial: SubQ: 0.75 mg/kg every 12 hours (**Note:** No I.V. bolus is administered in this population); a maximum dose of 75 mg is recommended for the first 2 doses. Maintenance: After first 2 doses, administer 0.75 mg/kg SubQ every 12 hours

Obesity: Use weight-based dosing; a maximum dose of 100 mg is recommended for the first 2 doses (Nutescu, 2009)

Additional notes on STEMI treatment: Therapy was continued for 8 days or until hospital discharge; optimal duration not defined. Unless contraindicated, all patients received aspirin (75-325 mg daily) in clinical trials. In patients with STEMI receiving thrombolytics, initiate enoxaparin dosing between 15 minutes before and 30 minutes after fibrinolytic therapy. In patients undergoing PCI, if balloon inflation occurs ≤8 hours after the last SubQ enoxaparin dose, no additional dosing is needed. If balloon inflation occurs 8-12 hours after last SubQ enoxaparin dose, a single I.V. dose of 0.3 mg/kg should be administered (Hirsh, 2008; King, 2007).

Unstable angina or non-ST-elevation myocardial infarction (NSTEMI): 1 mg/kg every 12 hours in conjunction with oral aspirin therapy (100-325 mg once daily); continue until clinical stabilization (a minimum of at least 2 days)

Obesity: Use actual body weight to calculate dose; dose capping not recommended (Nutescu, 2009)

I.V.: Percutaneous coronary intervention (PCI), adjunctive therapy (unlabeled use): In patients treated with multiple doses of enoxaparin undergoing PCI, if PCI occurs within 8 hours after the last SubQ enoxaparin dose, no additional dosing is needed. If PCI occurs 8-12 hours after the last SubQ enoxaparin dose or the patient received only 1 therapeutic SubQ dose (eg, 1 mg/kg), a single I.V. dose of 0.3 mg/kg should be administered. If PCI occurs >12 hours after the last SubQ dose, it is prudent to use an established anticoagulation regimen (eg, unfractionated heparin or bivalirudin) (Levine, 2011).

If patient has not received prior anticoagulant therapy: 0.5-0.75 mg/kg bolus dose (Levine, 2011)

Elderly: Refer to adult dosing. Increased incidence of bleeding with doses of 1.5 mg/kg/day or 1 mg/kg every 12 hours; injection-associated bleeding and serious adverse reactions are also increased in the elderly. Careful attention should be paid to elderly patients, particularly those <45 kg. **Note:** Dosage alteration/adjustment may be required.

Dosing adjustment in renal impairment: SubQ:

Cl_{cr} ≥30 mL/minute: No specific adjustment recommended (per manufacturer); monitor closely for bleeding

Cl_{cr} <30 mL/minute:

DVT prophylaxis in abdominal surgery, hip replacement, knee replacement, or in medical patients during acute illness: 30 mg once daily

DVT treatment (inpatient or outpatient treatment in conjunction with warfarin): 1 mg/kg once daily

STEMI:

<75 years: Initial: I.V.: 30 mg as a single dose with the first dose of the SubQ maintenance regimen administered at the same time as the I.V. bolus; Maintenance: SubQ: 1 mg/kg every 24 hours

≥75 years of age: Omit I.V. bolus; Maintenance: SubQ: 1 mg/kg every 24 hours

Unstable angina, NSTEMI: SubQ: 1 mg/kg once daily

Dialysis: Enoxaparin has not been FDA approved for use in dialysis patients. It's elimination is primarily via the renal route. Serious bleeding complications have been reported with use in patients who are dialysis dependent or have severe renal failure. LMWH administration at fixed doses without monitoring has greater unpredictable anticoagulant effects in patients with chronic kidney disease. If used, dosages should be reduced and anti-Xa levels frequently monitored, as accumulation may occur with repeated doses. Many clinicians would not use enoxaparin in this population especially without timely anti-Xa levels.

Hemodialysis: Supplemental dose is not necessary.

Peritoneal dialysis: Significant drug removal is unlikely based on physiochemical characteristics.

Administration Do **not** administer I.M.; should be administered by deep SubQ injection to the left or right anterolateral and left or right posterolateral abdominal wall. A single dose may be administered I.V. as part of treatment for ST-elevation myocardial infarction (STEMI) to patients <75 years of age; no I.V. bolus is given to patients ≥75 years of age. To avoid loss of drug from the 30 mg and 40 mg syringes, do not expel the air bubble from the syringe prior to injection. In order to minimize bruising, do not rub injection site. An automatic injector (Lovenox EasyInjector™) is available with the 30 mg and 40 mg syringes to aid the patient with self-injections. **Note:** Enoxaparin is available in 100 mg/mL and 150 mg/mL concentrations.

To convert from I.V. unfractionated heparin (UFH) infusion to SubQ enoxaparin (Nutescu, 2007): Calculate specific dose for enoxaparin based on indication, discontinue UFH and begin enoxaparin within 1 hour.

To convert from SubQ enoxaparin to I.V. UFH infusion (Nutescu, 2007): Discontinue enoxaparin, calculate specific dose for I.V. UFH infusion based on indication, omit heparin bolus/loading dose:

Converting from SubQ enoxaparin dosed every 12 hours: Start I.V. UFH infusion 10-11 hours after last dose of enoxaparin

Converting from SubQ enoxaparin dosed every 24 hours: Start I.V. UFH infusion 22-23 hours after last dose of enoxaparin

Monitoring Parameters Platelets, occult blood, anti-Xa levels, serum creatinine; monitoring of PT and/or aPTT is not necessary. Routine monitoring of anti-Xa levels is not required, but has been utilized in patients with obesity and/or renal insufficiency. Monitoring anti-Xa levels is recommended in pregnant women receiving therapeutic doses of enoxaparin (Hirsh, 2008). For patients >190 kg, if anti-Xa monitoring is available, adjusting dose based on anti-Xa levels is recommended; if anti-Xa monitoring is unavailable, reduce dose if bleeding occurs (Nutescu, 2009).

Reference Range The following therapeutic ranges for anti-Xa levels have been suggested, but have not been validated in a controlled trial. Anti-Xa level measured 4 hours postdose.

DVT treatment (every-12-hour dosing): 0.6-1 units/mL

DVT treatment (once-daily dosing): 1-2 units/mL

Dosage Forms Excipient information presented when available (limited, particularly for generics); consult specific product labeling.

Injection, solution, as sodium:

Lovenox®: 100 mg/mL (3 mL) [contains benzyl alcohol; vial]

Injection, solution, as sodium [preservative free]: 30 mg/0.3 mL (0.3 mL); 40 mg/0.4 mL (0.4 mL); 60 mg/0.6 mL (0.6 mL); 80 mg/0.8 mL (0.8 mL); 100 mg/mL (1 mL); 120 mg/0.8 mL (0.8 mL); 150 mg/mL (1 mL)

Lovenox®: 30 mg/0.3 mL (0.3 mL); 40 mg/0.4 mL (0.4 mL); 60 mg/0.6 mL (0.6 mL); 80 mg/0.8 mL (0.8 mL); 100 mg/mL (1 mL); 120 mg/0.8 mL (0.8 mL); 150 mg/mL (1 mL) [prefilled syringe]

◆ **Enoxaparin Injection (Can)** *see* Enoxaparin *on page 588*

◆ **Enoxaparin Sodium** *see* Enoxaparin *on page 588*

◆ **Enpresse®** *see* Ethinyl Estradiol and Levonorgestrel *on page 656*

Entacapone (en TA ka pone)

Brand Names: U.S. Comtan®

Brand Names: Canada Comtan®

Pharmacologic Category Anti-Parkinson's Agent, COMT Inhibitor

Additional Appendix Information

Antiparkinsonian Agents *on page 1879*

Use Adjunct to levodopa/carbidopa therapy in patients with idiopathic Parkinson's disease who experience "wearing-off" symptoms at the end of a dosing interval

Pregnancy Risk Factor C

Pregnancy Considerations Not recommended

Lactation Excretion in breast milk unknown/use caution

Contraindications Hypersensitivity to entacapone or any of component of the formulation

Warnings/Precautions May cause orthostatic hypotension and syncope; Parkinson's disease patients appear to have an impaired capacity to respond to a postural challenge; use with caution in patients at risk of hypotension (such as those receiving antihypertensive drugs) or where transient hypotensive episodes would be poorly tolerated (cardiovascular disease or cerebrovascular disease). Parkinson's patients being treated with dopaminergic agonists ordinarily require careful monitoring for signs and symptoms of postural hypotension, especially during dose escalation, and should be informed of this risk. May cause hallucinations, which may improve with reduction in levodopa therapy. Use with caution in patients with pre-existing dyskinesias; exacerbation of pre-existing dyskinesia and severe rhabdomyolysis has been reported. Levodopa dosage reduction may be required, particularly in patients with levodopa dosages >600 mg daily or with moderate-to-severe dyskinesia prior to initiation. Entacapone, in conjunction with other drug therapy that alters brain biogenic amine concentrations (eg, MAO inhibitors, SSRIs), has been associated with a syndrome resembling neuroleptic malignant syndrome (hyperpyrexia and confusion - some fatal) on abrupt withdrawal or dosage reduction. Concomitant use of entacapone and nonselective MAO inhibitors should be avoided. Selegiline is a selective MAO type B inhibitor (when given orally at ≤10 mg/day) and can be taken with entacapone.

Dopaminergic agents have been associated with compulsive behaviors and/or loss of impulse control, which has manifested as pathological gambling, libido increases (hypersexuality), and/or binge eating. Causality has not been established, and controversy exists as to whether this phenomenon is related to the underlying disease, prior behaviors/addictions and/or drug therapy. Dose reduction or discontinuation of therapy has been reported to reverse these behaviors in some, but not all cases. Risk for melanoma development is increased in Parkinson's disease patients; drug causation or factors contributing to risk have not been established. Patients should be monitored closely and periodic skin examinations should be performed. Dopaminergic agents from the ergot class have also been associated with fibrotic complications, such as retroperitoneal fibrosis, pulmonary infiltrates or effusion and pleural thickening. It is unknown whether non-ergot, pro-dopaminergic agents like entacapone confer this risk. Use caution in patients with hepatic impairment or severe renal impairment. Do not withdraw therapy abruptly. Discoloration of urine, saliva, or sweat to dark colors (red, brown, black) may be observed during therapy. Use with caution in patients with lower gastrointestinal disease or an increased risk of dehydration; has been associated with delayed development of diarrhea (usual onset after 4-12 weeks). Diarrhea may be a sign of drug-induced colitis. Discontinue use with prolonged diarrhea.

Adverse Reactions

>10%:

Gastrointestinal: Nausea (14%)

Neuromuscular & skeletal: Dyskinesia (25%), placebo (15%)

1% to 10%:

Cardiovascular: Orthostatic hypotension (4.3%), syncope (1.2%)

Central nervous system: Dizziness (8%), fatigue (6%), hallucinations (4%), anxiety (2%), somnolence (2%), agitation (1%)

Dermatologic: Purpura (2%)

Gastrointestinal: Diarrhea (10%), abdominal pain (8%), constipation (6%), vomiting (4%), dry mouth (3%), dyspepsia (2%), flatulence (2%), gastritis (1%), taste perversion (1%)

Genitourinary: Brown-orange urine discoloration (10%)

Neuromuscular & skeletal: Hyperkinesia (10%), hypokinesia (9%), back pain (4%), weakness (2%)

Respiratory: Dyspnea (3%)

Miscellaneous: Diaphoresis increased (2%), bacterial infection (1%)

<1% (Limited to important or life-threatening): Hyperpyrexia and confusion (resembling neuroleptic malignant syndrome), pulmonary fibrosis, retroperitoneal fibrosis, rhabdomyolysis

Drug Interactions

Metabolism/Transport Effects Inhibits COMT, CYP1A2 (weak), CYP2A6 (weak), CYP2C19 (weak), CYP2C9 (weak), CYP2D6 (weak), CYP2E1 (weak), CYP3A4 (weak)

Avoid Concomitant Use

Avoid concomitant use of Entacapone with any of the following: Pimozide

Increased Effect/Toxicity

Entacapone may increase the levels/effects of: Alcohol (Ethyl); CNS Depressants; COMT Substrates; MAO Inhibitors; Methotrimeprazine; Pimozide; Selective Serotonin Reuptake Inhibitors

The levels/effects of Entacapone may be increased by: Droperidol; HydrOXYzine; Methotrimeprazine

Decreased Effect There are no known significant interactions involving a decrease in effect.

Ethanol/Nutrition/Herb Interactions

Ethanol: May increase CNS depression; monitor for increased effects with coadministration. Caution patients about effects.

Food: Entacapone has been reported to chelate iron and decreasing serum iron levels were noted in clinical trials; however, clinically significant anemia has not been observed.

Mechanism of Action Entacapone is a reversible and selective inhibitor of catechol-O-methyltransferase (COMT). When entacapone is taken with levodopa, the pharmacokinetics are altered, resulting in more sustained levodopa serum levels compared to levodopa taken alone. The resulting levels of levodopa provide for increased concentrations available for absorption across the blood-brain barrier, thereby providing for increased CNS levels of dopamine, the active metabolite of levodopa.

Pharmacodynamics/Kinetics

Onset of action: Rapid

Peak effect: 1 hour

Absorption: Rapid

Distribution: I.V.: V_{dss}: 20 L

Protein binding: 98%, primarily to albumin

Metabolism: Isomerization to the *cis*-isomer, followed by direct glucuronidation of the parent and *cis*-isomer

Bioavailability: 35%

Half-life elimination: Β phase: 0.4-0.7 hours; Υ phase: 2.4 hours

Time to peak, serum: 1 hour

Excretion: Feces (90%); urine (10%)

Dosage Oral: Adults: 200 mg with each dose of levodopa/carbidopa, up to a maximum of 8 times/day (maximum daily dose: 1600 mg/day). To optimize therapy, the dosage of levodopa may need reduced or the dosing interval may need extended. Patients taking levodopa ≥800 mg/day or who had moderate-to-severe dyskinesias prior to therapy required an average decrease of 25% in the daily levodopa dose.

Dosage adjustment in hepatic impairment: Treat with caution and monitor carefully; AUC and C_{max} can be possibly doubled

Dietary Considerations May be taken without regard to meals.

Administration Always administer in association with levodopa/carbidopa; can be combined with both the immediate and sustained release formulations of levodopa/carbidopa. May be administered without regard to meals. Should not be abruptly withdrawn from patient's therapy due to significant worsening of symptoms.

Monitoring Parameters Signs and symptoms of Parkinson's disease; liver function tests, blood pressure, patient's mental status; serum iron (if signs of anemia)

Dosage Forms Excipient information presented when available (limited, particularly for generics); consult specific product labeling.

Tablet, oral:

Comtan®: 200 mg

◆ **Entacapone, Carbidopa, and Levodopa** *see* Levodopa, Carbidopa, and Entacapone *on page 996*

Entecavir (en TE ka veer)

Brand Names: U.S. Baraclude®

Brand Names: Canada Baraclude®

Pharmacologic Category Antiretroviral Agent, Reverse Transcriptase Inhibitor (Nucleoside)

Use Treatment of chronic hepatitis B infection, with compensated or decompensated liver disease, in adults with evidence of active viral replication and either evidence of persistent transaminase elevations or histologically-active disease

Pregnancy Risk Factor C

Pregnancy Considerations Teratogenic effects have been observed in animal studies. There are no adequate and well-controlled studies in pregnant women. Use only if benefit outweighs risk. Pregnant women taking entecavir should enroll in the pregnancy registry by calling 1-800-258-4263.

Lactation Excretion in breast milk unknown/not recommended

Contraindications There are no contraindications listed in the manufacturer's labeling.

Warnings/Precautions Hazardous agent - use appropriate precautions for handling and disposal. **[U.S. Boxed Warning]: Lactic acidosis and severe hepatomegaly with steatosis (including fatal cases) have been reported. [U.S. Boxed Warning]: Severe, acute exacerbation of hepatitis B may occur upon discontinuation of antihepatitis B therapy, including entecavir. Monitor liver function for at least several months after stopping treatment; reinitiation of antihepatitis B therapy may be required.** Use caution in patients with renal impairment or in patients receiving concomitant therapy which may reduce renal function; dose adjustment recommended for Cl_{cr} <50 mL/minute. Cross-resistance may develop in patients failing previous therapy with lamivudine.

HIV: **[U.S. Boxed Warning]: May cause the development of HIV resistance in chronic hepatitis B patients with unrecognized or untreated HIV infection.** Determine HIV status prior to initiating treatment with entecavir. **Not recommended for HIV/HBV coinfected patients unless also receiving highly active antiretroviral therapy (HAART).** The manufacturer's labeling states that entecavir does not exhibit any clinically-relevant activity against human immunodeficiency virus (HIV type 1). However, a small number of case reports have indicated declines in virus levels during entecavir therapy. HIV resistance to a common HIV drug has been reported in an HIV/HBV-infected patient receiving entecavir as monotherapy for HBV.

Dose adjustment not required in patients with hepatic impairment. Limited data supporting treatment of chronic hepatitis B in patients with decompensated liver disease; observe for increased adverse reactions, including hepatorenal dysfunction. Safety and efficacy in liver transplant patients have not been established.

Adverse Reactions

>10%:

Cardiovascular: Peripheral edema (16% with decompensated liver disease)

Central nervous system: Pyrexia (14% with decompensated liver disease)

Hepatic: Ascites (15% with decompensated liver disease), ALT increased (>5 x ULN: 11% to 12%; post-treatment flare [lamivudine refractory]: >10 x ULN and >2 x baseline: 12%)

1% to 10%:

Central nervous system: Headache (2% to 4%), fatigue (1% to 3%), dizziness

Endocrine & metabolic: Hyperglycemia (2% to 3%), blood bicarbonate decreased (2% with decompensated liver disease)

Gastrointestinal: Lipase increased (7%), amylase increased (2% to 3%), diarrhea (≤1%), dyspepsia (≤1%), nausea

Hepatic: Hepatic encephalopathy (10% with decompensated liver disease), bilirubin increased (2% to 3%), ALT increased (>10 x ULN and >2 x baseline: 2%; post-treatment flare [nucleoside-naive]: >10 x ULN and >2 x baseline: 2% to 8%)

Renal: Hematuria (9%), glycosuria (4%), creatinine increased (1% to 2%)

Respiratory: Upper respiratory tract infection (10% with decompensated liver disease)

<1% (Limited to important or life-threatening): Alopecia, anaphylactoid reaction, hepatomegaly, hypoalbuminemia, insomnia, lactic acidosis, rash, renal failure, somnolence, thrombocytopenia, vomiting

Drug Interactions

Metabolism/Transport Effects None known.

Avoid Concomitant Use There are no known interactions where it is recommended to avoid concomitant use.

Increased Effect/Toxicity

The levels/effects of Entecavir may be increased by: Ganciclovir-Valganciclovir; Ribavirin

Decreased Effect There are no known significant interactions involving a decrease in effect.

Ethanol/Nutrition/Herb Interactions

Food: Food delays absorption and reduces AUC by 18% to 20%.

Stability Store at controlled room temperature of 25°C (77°F); excursions permitted to 15°C to 30°C (59°F to 86°F). Protect oral solution from light.

Mechanism of Action Entecavir is intracellularly phosphorylated to guanosine triphosphate which competes with natural substrates to effectively inhibit hepatitis B viral polymerase; enzyme inhibition blocks reverse transcriptase activity thereby reducing viral DNA synthesis.

Pharmacodynamics/Kinetics

Absorption: Delayed with food; C_{max} decreased 44% to 46%, AUC decreased 18% to 20%

Distribution: Extensive (V_d in excess of body water)

Protein binding: ~13%

Metabolism: Minor hepatic glucuronide/sulfate conjugation

Half-life elimination: Terminal: ~5-6 days; accumulation: ~24 hours

Time to peak, plasma: 0.5-1.5 hours

Excretion: Urine (60% to 73% as unchanged drug)

Dosage Oral: Adolescents ≥16 years and Adults:

Nucleoside treatment naive: 0.5 mg once daily

Lamivudine-refractory or -resistant viremia (or known lamivudine- or telbivudine-resistance mutations): 1 mg once daily

Decompensated liver disease: 1 mg once daily

HIV/HBV coinfection (unlabeled use):

Nucleoside treatment naive: 0.5 mg once daily

Lamivudine refractory or resistant: 1 mg once daily

Note: Only recommended in patients who cannot take tenofovir; must be used in addition to a fully suppressive antiretroviral therapy regimen. (DHHS, 2011)

Treatment duration (AASLD Practice Guidelines, 2009):

Hepatitis Be antigen (HBeAg) positive chronic hepatitis: Treat ≥1 year until HBeAg seroconversion and undetectable serum HBV DNA; continue therapy for ≥6 months after HBeAg seroconversion

HBeAg negative chronic hepatitis: Treat >1 year until hepatitis B surface antigen (HBsAg) clearance

Decompensated liver disease: Lifelong treatment is recommended

Note: Patients not achieving a primary response (<2 log decrease in serum HBV DNA) after at least 6 months of therapy should either receive additional treatment or be switched to an alternative therapy.

Dosage adjustment in renal impairment: Daily-dosage regimen preferred:

Cl_{cr} 30-49 mL/minute: Administer 50% of usual dose daily or administer the normal dose every 48 hours

Cl_{cr} 10-29 mL/minute: Administer 30% of usual dose daily or administer the normal dose every 72 hours

Cl_{cr} <10 mL/minute (including hemodialysis and CAPD): Administer 10% of usual dose daily or administer the normal dose every 7 days; administer after hemodialysis

Dosage adjustment in hepatic impairment: No adjustment necessary.

Dietary Considerations Take on an empty stomach (2 hours before or after a meal).

Administration Administer on an empty stomach (2 hours before or after a meal). Do not dilute or mix oral solution with water or other beverages; use calibrated oral dosing syringe. Oral solution and tablet are bioequivalent on a mg-to-mg basis.

Monitoring Parameters HIV status (prior to initiation of therapy); liver function tests, renal function; in HBV/HIV-coinfected patients, monitor HIV viral load and CD4 count; HBeAg, HBV DNA; in patients with lamivudine-refractory or -resistant viremia (or known lamivudine- or telbivudine-resistance mutations) entecavir resistance can develop rapidly. Monitor HBV DNA every 3 months (DHHS, 2011)

Dosage Forms Excipient information presented when available (limited, particularly for generics); consult specific product labeling.

Solution, oral:
Baraclude®: 0.05 mg/mL (210 mL) [orange flavor]

Tablet, oral:
Baraclude®: 0.5 mg, 1 mg

- **Entereg®** *see* Alvimopan *on page 81*
- **Enterex® Glutapak-10® [OTC]** *see* Glutamine *on page 799*
- **Entex® LA (Can)** *see* Guaifenesin and Pseudoephedrine *on page 813*
- **Entocort® (Can)** *see* Budesonide (Systemic) *on page 237*
- **Entocort® EC** *see* Budesonide (Systemic) *on page 237*
- **Entre-S** *see* Chlorpheniramine, Pseudoephedrine, and Dextromethorphan *on page 347*
- **Entrophen® (Can)** *see* Aspirin *on page 154*
- **Entsol® [OTC]** *see* Sodium Chloride *on page 1567*
- **Enulose** *see* Lactulose *on page 964*
- **EPEG** *see* Etoposide *on page 669*

EPHEDrine (Systemic) (e FED rin)

Index Terms Ephedrine Sulfate

Pharmacologic Category Alpha/Beta Agonist

Additional Appendix Information

Contrast Media Reactions, Premedication for Prophylaxis *on page 1976*

Use Treatment of nasal congestion, anesthesia-induced hypotension

Unlabeled Use Postoperative nausea and vomiting (PONV) refractory to traditional antiemetics; idiopathic orthostatic hypotension

Pregnancy Risk Factor C

Dosage

Children: Hypotension: Slow I.V. push: 0.2-0.3 mg/kg/dose every 4-6 hours

Adults:

Hypotension induced by anesthesia: I.V.: 5-25 mg/dose slow I.V. push repeated after 5-10 minutes as needed, then every 3-4 hours (maximum: 150 mg/24 hours)

Idiopathic orthostatic hypotension (unlabeled use): Oral: 25-50 mg 3 times/day; maximum: 150 mg/day. **Note:** Not considered first-line for this indication.

PONV refractory to traditional antiemetics (unlabeled use): I.M.: 0.5 mg/kg at the end of surgery (Gan, 2007; Hagemann, 2000)

Additional Information Complete prescribing information for this medication should be consulted for additional detail.

Dosage Forms Excipient information presented when available (limited, particularly for generics); consult specific product labeling.

Capsule, oral, as sulfate: 25 mg

Injection, solution, as sulfate [preservative free]: 50 mg/mL (1 mL)

- **Ephedrine Sulfate** *see* EPHEDrine (Systemic) *on page 594*
- **Epidoxorubicin** *see* Epirubicin *on page 597*
- **Epiduo®** *see* Adapalene and Benzoyl Peroxide *on page 44*
- **Epi E-Z Pen® (Can)** *see* EPINEPHrine (Systemic, Oral Inhalation) *on page 594*
- **Epiflur™** *see* Fluoride *on page 728*
- **Epifoam®** *see* Pramoxine and Hydrocortisone *on page 1393*
- **Epiklor™** *see* Potassium Chloride *on page 1380*
- **Epiklor™/25** *see* Potassium Chloride *on page 1380*

EPINEPHrine (Systemic, Oral Inhalation)
(ep i NEF rin)

Brand Names: U.S. Adrenalin®; EpiPen 2-Pak®; EpiPen Jr 2-Pak®; EpiPen® Jr. [DSC]; EpiPen® [DSC]; Primatene® Mist [OTC] [DSC]; S2® [OTC]; Twinject®

Brand Names: Canada Adrenalin®; Epi E-Z Pen®; EpiPen®; EpiPen® Jr; Twinject®

Index Terms Adrenaline; Epinephrine Bitartrate; Epinephrine Hydrochloride; Racemic Epinephrine; Racepinephrine

Pharmacologic Category Alpha/Beta Agonist

Additional Appendix Information

Bronchodilators *on page 1886*

Vasoactive Agents, Intravenous *on page 1898*

Use Treatment of bronchospasms, bronchial asthma, viral croup, anaphylactic reactions, cardiac arrest; added to local anesthetics to decrease systemic absorption of intraspinal and local anesthetics and increase duration of action; decrease superficial hemorrhage

Unlabeled Use ACLS guidelines: Ventricular fibrillation (VF) or pulseless ventricular tachycardia (VT) unresponsive to initial defibrillatory shocks; pulseless electrical activity; asystole; hypotension/shock unresponsive to volume resuscitation; symptomatic bradycardia unresponsive to atropine or pacing; inotropic support

Pregnancy Risk Factor C

Pregnancy Considerations Teratogenic effects have been observed in animal reproduction studies. Epinephrine crosses the placenta and may cause fetal anoxia. Use during pregnancy when the potential benefit to the mother outweighs the possible risk to the fetus.

Lactation Excretion in breast milk unknown

Contraindications There are no absolute contraindications to the use of injectable epinephrine (including EpiPen®, EpiPen® Jr, and Twinject®) in a life-threatening situation.

Oral inhalation: Concurrent use or within 2 weeks of MAO inhibitors

Injectable solution: Per the manufacturer, contraindicated in narrow-angle glaucoma; shock; during general anesthesia with halogenated hydrocarbons or cyclopropane (currently not available in U.S.); individuals with organic brain damage; with local anesthesia of the digits; during labor; heart failure; coronary insufficiency

Warnings/Precautions Use with caution in elderly patients, patients with diabetes mellitus, cardiovascular diseases (eg, coronary artery disease, hypertension), thyroid disease, cerebrovascular disease, Parkinson's disease, or patients taking tricyclic antidepressants. Some products contain sulfites as preservatives; the presence of sulfites in some products (eg, EpiPen® and Twinject®) should not deter administration during a serious allergic or other emergency situation even if the patient is sulfite-sensitive. Accidental injection into digits, hands, or feet may result in local reactions, including injection site pallor, coldness and hypoesthesia or injury, resulting in bruising, bleeding, discoloration, erythema or skeletal injury; patient should seek immediate medical attention if this occurs. Rapid I.V. administration may cause death from cerebrovascular hemorrhage or cardiac arrhythmias; however, rapid I.V. administration during pulseless arrest is necessary.

Oral inhalation: Use with caution in patients with prostate enlargement or urinary retention; may cause temporary worsening of symptoms.

Self medication (OTC use): Oral inhalation: Prior to self-medication, patients should contact healthcare provider. The product should only be used in persons with a diagnosis of asthma. If symptoms are not relieved in 20 minutes or become worse do not continue to use the product - seek immediate medical assistance. The product should not be used more frequently or at higher doses than recommended unless directed by a healthcare provider. This product should not be used in patients who have required hospitalization for asthma or if a patient is taking prescription medication for asthma. Do not use if you have taken a MAO inhibitor (certain drugs used for depression, Parkinson's disease, or other conditions) within 2 weeks.

Adverse Reactions Frequency not defined.

Cardiovascular: Angina, cardiac arrhythmia, chest pain, flushing, hypertension, pallor, palpitation, sudden death, tachycardia (parenteral), vasoconstriction, ventricular ectopy

Central nervous system: Anxiety (transient), apprehensiveness, cerebral hemorrhage, dizziness, headache, insomnia, lightheadedness, nervousness, restlessness

Gastrointestinal: Dry throat, loss of appetite, nausea, vomiting, xerostomia

Genitourinary: Acute urinary retention in patients with bladder outflow obstruction

Neuromuscular & skeletal: Tremor, weakness

Ocular: Allergic lid reaction, burning, eye pain, ocular irritation, precipitation of or exacerbation of narrow-angle glaucoma, transient stinging

Respiratory: Dyspnea, pulmonary edema

Miscellaneous: Diaphoresis

Drug Interactions

Metabolism/Transport Effects Substrate of COMT

Avoid Concomitant Use

Avoid concomitant use of EPINEPHrine (Systemic, Oral Inhalation) with any of the following: Ergot Derivatives; Iobenguane I 123; Lurasidone

Increased Effect/Toxicity

EPINEPHrine (Systemic, Oral Inhalation) may increase the levels/effects of: Bromocriptine; Lurasidone; Sympathomimetics

The levels/effects of EPINEPHrine (Systemic, Oral Inhalation) may be increased by: Antacids; Atomoxetine; Beta-Blockers; Cannabinoids; Carbonic Anhydrase Inhibitors; COMT Inhibitors; Ergot Derivatives; Inhalational Anesthetics; MAO Inhibitors; Serotonin/Norepinephrine Reuptake Inhibitors; Tricyclic Antidepressants

Decreased Effect

EPINEPHrine (Systemic, Oral Inhalation) may decrease the levels/effects of: Benzylpenicilloyl Polylysine; Iobenguane I 123

The levels/effects of EPINEPHrine (Systemic, Oral Inhalation) may be decreased by: Spironolactone

Ethanol/Nutrition/Herb Interactions Herb/Nutraceutical: Avoid ephedra, yohimbe (may cause CNS stimulation).

Stability Epinephrine is sensitive to light and air; protection from light is recommended. Oxidation turns drug pink, then a brown color. **Solutions should not be used if they are discolored or contain a precipitate.**

Adrenalin®: Store between 15°C to 25°C (59°F to 77°F); do not freeze. Protect from light. The 1:1000 solution should be discarded 30 days after initial use.

EpiPen® and EpiPen® Jr: Store at 25°C (77°F); excursions permitted to 15°C to 30°C (59°F to 86°F); do not freeze or refrigerate. Protect from light by storing in carrier tube provided.

Twinject®: Store between 20°C to 25°C (68°F to 77°F); excursions permitted to 15°C to 30°C (59°F to 86°F); do not freeze or refrigerate. Protect from light.

Primatene® Mist: Store between 20°C to 25°C (68°F to 77°F).

S2®: Store between 2°C to 20°C (36°F to 68°F). Protect from light. Dilution not required when administered via hand-bulb nebulizer; dilute with NS 3-5 mL if using jet nebulizer

Stability of injection of parenteral admixture at room temperature (25°C) or refrigeration (4°C) is 24 hours.

Standard I.V. diluent: 1 mg/250 mL NS.

Preparation of adult I.V. infusion: Dilute 1 mg in 250 mL of D_5W or NS (4 mcg/mL).

Mechanism of Action Stimulates alpha-, $beta_1$-, and $beta_2$-adrenergic receptors resulting in relaxation of smooth muscle of the bronchial tree, cardiac stimulation (increasing myocardial oxygen consumption), and dilation of skeletal muscle vasculature; small doses can cause vasodilation via $beta_2$-vascular receptors; large doses may produce constriction of skeletal and vascular smooth muscle

Pharmacodynamics/Kinetics

Onset of action: Bronchodilation: SubQ: ~5-10 minutes; Inhalation: ~1 minute

Metabolism: Taken up into the adrenergic neuron and metabolized by monoamine oxidase and catechol-o-methyltransferase; circulating drug hepatically metabolized

Excretion: Urine (as inactive metabolites, metanephrine, and sulfate and hydroxy derivatives of mandelic acid, small amounts as unchanged drug)

Dosage

Infants and Children:

Asystole/pulseless arrest, pulseless VT/VF (after failed defibrillation attempts) (PALS, 2010):

I.V., I.O.: 0.01 mg/kg (0.1 mL/kg of **1:10,000** [0.1 mg/mL] solution) (maximum single dose: 1 mg) every 3-5 minutes until return of spontaneous circulation

Endotracheal: 0.1 mg/kg (0.1 mL/kg of **1:1000** [1 mg/mL] solution) (maximum single dose: 2.5 mg) every 3-5 minutes until I.V./I.O. access established or return of spontaneous circulation. Flush with 5 mL of NS immediately after administration. May cause false-negative reading with exhaled CO_2 detectors; use second method to confirm tube placement if CO_2 is not detected (Neumar, 2010).

Postresuscitation infusion to maintain cardiac output or stabilize: I.V., I.O.: 0.1-1 mcg/kg/minute; doses <0.3 mcg/kg/minute generally produce beta-adrenergic effects and higher doses (>0.3 mcg/kg/minute) generally produce alpha-adrenergic vasoconstriction; titrate dosage to desired effect

Bradycardia (symptomatic; unresponsive to atropine or pacing):

I.V., I.O.: 0.01 mg/kg (0.1 mL/kg of **1:10,000** [0.1 mg/mL] solution) (maximum single dose: 1 mg) every 3-5 minutes as needed

Endotracheal: 0.1 mg/kg or (0.1 mL/kg of **1:1000** [1 mg/mL] solution) (maximum single dose: 2.5 mg) every 3-5 minutes as needed until I.V./I.O. access established. Flush with 5 mL of NS immediately after administration. May cause false-negative reading with exhaled CO_2 detectors; use second method to confirm tube placement if CO_2 is not detected (Neumar, 2010).

Continuous infusion: I.V., I.O.: 0.1-1 mcg/kg/minute; doses <0.3 mcg/kg/minute generally produce beta-adrenergic effects and higher doses (>0.3 mcg/kg/minute) generally produce alpha-adrenergic vasoconstriction; titrate dosage to desired effect

Bronchodilator:

SubQ: 0.01 mg/kg (0.01 mL/kg of **1:1000** [1 mg/mL] solution) (maximum single dose: 0.5 mg) every 20 minutes for 3 doses

Nebulization: S2® (racepinephrine, OTC labeling):

Children <4 years: Jet nebulizer: Croup: 0.05 mL/kg (maximum dose: 0.5 mL); dilute in 3 mL of NS. Administer over ~15 minutes; do not administer more frequently than every 2 hours

Children ≥4 years: Refer to adult dosing.

Inhalation: Children ≥4 years: Primatene® Mist: Refer to adult dosing.

Hypersensitivity reaction: **Note:** SubQ administration results in slower absorption and is less reliable. I.M. administration in the anterolateral aspect of the middle third of the thigh is preferred in the setting of anaphylaxis (ACLS guidelines, 2010; Kemp, 2008).

I.M., SubQ: 0.01 mg/kg (0.01 mL/kg of **1:1000** [1 mg/mL] solution) (maximum single dose: 0.3 mg) every 5-15 minutes; larger I.M. or SubQ doses, use of I.V. route, or continuous infusion may be needed for severe anaphylactic reactions (Kemp, 2008; Lieberman, 2010). If clinician deems appropriate, the 5-minute interval between injections may be shortened to allow for more frequent administration (Lieberman, 2010).

Self-administration following severe allergic reactions (eg, insect stings, food): **Note:** World Health Organization (WHO) and Anaphylaxis Canada recommend the availability of 1 dose for every 10-20 minutes of travel time to a medical emergency facility.

EpiPen® Jr: I.M., SubQ: Children 15-29 kg: 0.15 mg; if anaphylactic symptoms persist, dose may be repeated in 5-15 minutes using an additional EpiPen® Jr

EpiPen®: I.M., SubQ: Children ≥30 kg: 0.3 mg; if anaphylactic symptoms persist, dose may be repeated in 5-15 minutes using an additional EpiPen®

Twinject®: I.M. SubQ:

Children 15-29 kg: 0.15 mg; if anaphylactic symptoms persist, dose may be repeated in 5-15 minutes using the same device after partial disassembly

Children ≥30 kg: 0.3 mg; if anaphylactic symptoms persist, dose may be repeated in 5-15 minutes using the same device after partial disassembly

Alternate auto-injector dose: I.M. (Sicherer, 2007):

Children 10-25 kg: 0.15 mg

Children >25 kg: 0.3 mg

Hypotension/shock, fluid-resistant (unlabeled use): Continuous I.V. infusion: 0.1-1 mcg/kg/minute; doses up to 5 mcg/kg/minute may rarely be necessary (Hegenbarth, 2008)

Adults:

Asystole/pulseless arrest, pulseless VT/VF (ACLS, 2010):

I.V., I.O.: 1 mg every 3-5 minutes until return of spontaneous circulation; if this approach fails, higher doses of epinephrine (up to 0.2 mg/kg) have been used for treatment of specific problems (eg, beta-blocker or calcium channel blocker overdose)

Endotracheal: 2-2.5 mg every 3-5 minutes until I.V./I.O. access established or return of spontaneous circulation; dilute in 5-10 mL NS or sterile water. **Note:** Absorption may be greater with sterile water (Naganobu, 2000). May cause false-negative reading with exhaled CO_2 detectors; use second method to confirm tube placement if CO_2 is not detected (Neumar, 2010).

Bradycardia (symptomatic; unresponsive to atropine or pacing): I.V. infusion: 2-10 mcg/minute **or** 0.1-0.5 mcg/kg/minute (7-35 mcg/minute in a 70 kg patient); titrate to desired effect (ACLS, 2010)

Bronchodilator:

SubQ: 0.3-0.5 mg (**1:1000** [1 mg/mL] solution) every 20 minutes for 3 doses

Nebulization: S2® (racepinephrine, OTC labeling):

Hand-bulb nebulizer: Add 0.5 mL (~10 drops) to nebulizer; 1-3 inhalations up to every 3 hours if needed

Jet nebulizer: Add 0.5 mL (~10 drops) to nebulizer and dilute with 3 mL of NS; administer over ~15 minutes every 3-4 hours as needed

Inhalation: Primatene® Mist (OTC labeling): One inhalation, wait at least 1 minute; if not relieved, may use once more. Do not use again for at least 3 hours.

Hypersensitivity reaction: **Note:** SubQ administration results in slower absorption and is less reliable. I.M. administration in the anterolateral aspect of the middle third of the thigh is preferred in the setting of anaphylaxis (ACLS guidelines, 2010; Kemp, 2008).

I.M., SubQ: 0.2-0.5 mg (**1:1000** [1 mg/mL] solution) every 5-15 minutes in the absence of clinical improvement (ACLS, 2010; Kemp, 2008; Lieberman, 2010). If clinician deems appropriate, the 5-minute interval between injections may be shortened to allow for more frequent administration (Lieberman, 2010).

I.V.: 0.1 mg (**1:10,000** [0.1 mg/mL] solution) over 5 minutes; may infuse at 1-4 mcg/minute to prevent the need to repeat injections frequently **or** may initiate with an infusion at 5-15 mcg/minute (with crystalloid administration) (ACLS, 2010; Brown, 2004). In general, I.V. administration should only be done in patients who are profoundly hypotensive or are in cardiopulmonary arrest refractory to volume resuscitation and several epinephrine injections (Lieberman, 2010).

Self-administration following severe allergic reactions (eg, insect stings, food): **Note:** The World Health Organization (WHO) and Anaphylaxis Canada recommend the availability of one dose for every 10-20 minutes of travel time to a medical emergency facility. More than 2 doses should only be administered under direct medical supervision.

Twinject®: I.M., SubQ: 0.3 mg; if anaphylactic symptoms persist, dose may be repeated in 5-15 minutes using the same device after partial disassembly

EpiPen®: I.M., SubQ: 0.3 mg; if anaphylactic symptoms persist, dose may be repeated in 5-15 minutes using an additional EpiPen®

Hypotension/shock, severe and fluid resistant (unlabeled use): I.V. infusion: Initial: 0.1-0.5 mcg/kg/minute (7-35 mcg/minute in a 70 kg patient); titrate to desired response (ACLS, 2010)

Administration When administering as a continuous infusion, central line administration is preferred. I.V. infusions require an infusion pump. Epinephrine solutions for injection can be administered I.M., I.O., endotracheally, I.V., or SubQ. **Note:** EpiPen® and EpiPen® Jr Auto-Injectors contain a single, fixed-dose of epinephrine. Twinject® Auto-Injectors contain two doses; the first fixed-dose is available for auto-injection; the second dose is available for manual injection following partial disassembly of device.

Subcutaneous: SubQ administration results in slower absorption and is less reliable.

I.M.: I.M. administration into the buttocks should be avoided. I.M. administration in the anterolateral aspect of the middle third of the thigh is preferred in the setting of anaphylaxis (ACLS guidelines, 2010; Kemp, 2008).

EpiPen®, EpiPen® Jr, and Twinject® Auto-Injectors should only be injected into the anterolateral aspect of the thigh, through clothing if necessary.

Endotracheal: Dilute in NS or sterile water. Absorption may be greater with sterile water (Naganobu, 2000). Stop compressions, spray drug quickly down tube. Follow immediately with several quick insufflations and continue chest compressions. May cause false-negative reading with exhaled CO_2 detectors; use second method to confirm tube placement if CO_2 is not detected (Neumar, 2010).

Oral inhalation: S2®: If using jet nebulizer: Administer over ~15 minutes; must be diluted. If using hand-held rubber bulb nebulizer, dilution is not required.

Extravasation management: Use phentolamine as antidote. Mix 5 mg phentolamine with 9 mL of NS. Inject a small amount of this dilution into extravasated area. Blanching should reverse immediately. Monitor site. If blanching should recur, additional injections of phentolamine may be needed.

Monitoring Parameters Pulmonary function, heart rate, blood pressure, site of infusion for blanching, extravasation; cardiac monitor and blood pressure monitor required during continuous infusion. If using to treat hypotension, assess intravascular volume and support as needed.

Additional Information Twinject® and EpiPen® are not interchangeable due to packaging considerations.

Dosage Forms Excipient information presented when available (limited, particularly for generics); consult specific product labeling. [DSC] = Discontinued product

Aerosol, for oral inhalation:

Primatene® Mist: 0.22 mg/inhalation (15 mL [DSC]) [contains chlorofluorocarbon, dehydrated ethanol 34%]

Injection, solution: 0.1 mg/mL (10 mL) [1:10,000 solution]; 0.15 mg/0.15 mL (1.1 mL [DSC]) [1:1000 solution; delivers 0.15 mg per injection]; 0.3 mg/0.3 mL (1.1 mL [DSC]) [1:1000 solution; delivers 0.3 mg per injection]; 1 mg/mL (1 mL) [1:1000 solution]

EpiPen 2-Pak®: 0.3 mg/0.3 mL (2 mL) [contains sodium metabisulfite; 1:1000 solution; delivers 0.3 mg per injection]

EpiPen Jr 2-Pak®: 0.15 mg/0.3 mL (2 mL) [contains sodium metabisulfite; 1:2000 solution; delivers 0.15 mg per injection]

EpiPen®: 0.3 mg/0.3 mL (2 mL [DSC]) [contains sodium metabisulfite; 1:1000 solution; delivers 0.3 mg per injection]

EpiPen® Jr.: 0.15 mg/0.3 mL (2 mL [DSC]) [contains sodium metabisulfite; 1:2000 solution; delivers 0.15 mg per injection]

Twinject®: 0.15 mg/0.15 mL (1.1 mL) [contains chlorobutanol, sodium bisulfite; 1:1000 solution; delivers 0.15 mg per injection]

Twinject®: 0.3 mg/0.3 mL (1.1 mL) [contains chlorobutanol, sodium bisulfite; 1:1000 solution; delivers 0.3 mg per injection]

Injection, solution, as hydrochloride: 1 mg/mL (30 mL) [1:1000 solution]

Adrenalin®: 1 mg/mL (30 mL) [contains chlorobutanol, sodium bisulfite; 1:1000 solution]

Adrenalin®: 1 mg/mL (1 mL) [contains sodium bisulfite; 1:1000 solution]

Injection, solution, as hydrochloride [preservative free]: 1 mg/mL (1 mL) [1:1000 solution]

Solution, for oral inhalation [racepinephrine, preservative free]:

S2®: 2.25% (0.5 mL) [as d-epinephrine 1.125% and l-epinehrine 1.125%]

◆ **Epinephrine and Lidocaine** *see* Lidocaine and Epinephrine *on page 1010*

◆ **Epinephrine Bitartrate** *see* EPINEPHrine (Systemic, Oral Inhalation) *on page 594*

◆ **Epinephrine Hydrochloride** *see* EPINEPHrine (Systemic, Oral Inhalation) *on page 594*

◆ **EpiPen® [DSC]** *see* EPINEPHrine (Systemic, Oral Inhalation) *on page 594*

◆ **EpiPen® (Can)** *see* EPINEPHrine (Systemic, Oral Inhalation) *on page 594*

◆ **EpiPen 2-Pak®** *see* EPINEPHrine (Systemic, Oral Inhalation) *on page 594*

◆ **EpiPen® Jr. [DSC]** *see* EPINEPHrine (Systemic, Oral Inhalation) *on page 594*

◆ **EpiPen® Jr (Can)** *see* EPINEPHrine (Systemic, Oral Inhalation) *on page 594*

◆ **EpiPen Jr 2-Pak®** *see* EPINEPHrine (Systemic, Oral Inhalation) *on page 594*

◆ **Epipodophyllotoxin** *see* Etoposide *on page 669*

◆ **Epipodophyllotoxin** *see* Etoposide Phosphate *on page 671*

◆ **EpiQuin® Micro** *see* Hydroquinone *on page 846*

Epirubicin (ep i ROO bi sin)

Brand Names: U.S. Ellence®

Brand Names: Canada Ellence®; Pharmorubicin®

Index Terms Epidoxorubicin; Epirubicin Hydrochloride; Pidorubicin; Pidorubicin Hydrochloride

Pharmacologic Category Antineoplastic Agent, Anthracycline

Use Adjuvant therapy component for primary breast cancer

Unlabeled Use Treatment of esophageal cancer, gastric cancer, soft tissue sarcoma, uterine sarcoma

Pregnancy Risk Factor D

Pregnancy Considerations Teratogenic effects and embryotoxicity were noted in animal studies. If a pregnant woman is treated with epirubicin, or if a woman becomes pregnant while receiving this drug, she should be informed of the potential hazard to the fetus. Limited information is available from retrospective studies of women who received epirubicin during the second or third (prior to week 35) trimester for the treatment of pregnancy-associated breast cancer; premature births and intrauterine growth retardation have been observed (Peccatori, 2009; Ring, 2005). Women of childbearing potential should be advised to avoid becoming pregnant during treatment. Men undergoing treatment should use effective contraception. Epirubicin may cause irreversible amenorrhea in premenopausal women.

Lactation Excretion in breast milk unknown/not recommended

Contraindications Hypersensitivity to epirubicin or any component of the formulation, other anthracyclines, or anthracenediones; previous anthracycline treatment up to maximum cumulative dose; severe myocardial insufficiency, severe arrhythmias; recent myocardial infarction

Warnings/Precautions Hazardous agent - use appropriate precautions for handling and disposal.

[U.S. Boxed Warning]: Myocardial toxicity, including heart failure (HF) may occur, particularly in patients who have received prior anthracyclines, prior or concomitant radiotherapy to the mediastinal/pericardial area, who have pre-existing cardiac disease (active or dormant), or with concomitant cardiotoxic medications. Cardiotoxicity may be concurrent or delayed (months to years after treatment). The risk of HF is ~0.9% at a cumulative dose of 550 mg/m², ~1.6% at a cumulative dose of 700 mg/m², and ~3.3% at a cumulative dose of 900 mg/m². Cardiotoxicity may also occur at lower cumulative doses or without risk

factors. The risk of delayed cardiotoxicity increases more steeply with cumulative doses >900 mg/m^2 and this dose should be exceeded only with extreme caution. Acute toxicity, primarily sinus tachycardia and/or ECG abnormalities, including arrhythmia, and delayed toxicity, including decreased left ventricular ejection fraction (LVEF) and HF, have been described. Delayed toxicity usually develops late in the course of therapy or within 2-3 months after completion. Toxicity may be additive with other anthracyclines or anthracenediones, and may be increased in pediatric patients. Regular monitoring of LVEF and discontinuation at the first sign of impairment is recommended especially in patients with cardiac risk factors or impaired cardiac function. Discontinue treatment with signs of decreased LVEF. The half life of other cardiotoxic agents must be considered in sequential therapy; avoid epirubicin for up to 24 weeks after completing trastuzumab treatment.

[U.S. Boxed Warning]: May cause severe myelosuppression; neutropenia is the dose-limiting toxicity; severe thrombocytopenia or anemia may occur; obtain baseline and periodic blood counts. Patients should recover from myelosuppression due to prior chemotherapy treatment before beginning treatments. Thrombophlebitis and thromboembolic phenomena (including pulmonary embolism) have occurred.

[U.S. Boxed Warning]: Reduce dosage in patients with mild-to-moderate hepatic impairment (not recommended in severe hepatic impairment; predominantly hepatically eliminated) and in patients with serum creatinine >5 mg/dL (has not been studied in patients on dialysis); monitor hepatic and renal function at baseline and during treatment. May cause tumor lysis syndrome (TLS), although generally generally does not occur in patients with breast cancer; if TLS risk is suspected, consider monitoring serum uric acid, potassium, calcium, phosphate, and serum creatinine after initial administration; hydration and allopurinol prophylaxis may minimize potential TLS complications. Radiation recall (inflammatory) has been reported; epirubicin may have radiosensitizing activity. **[U.S. Boxed Warning]: Treatment with anthracyclines (including epirubicin) may increase the risk of secondary acute myelogenous leukemia (AML). AML is more common when given in combination with other antineoplastic agents, in patients who have received multiple courses of previous chemotherapy, or with escalated cumulative anthracycline doses (>720 mg/m^2 for epirubicin). In breast cancer patients, the risk for treatment-related AML or myelodysplastic syndrome (MDS) was estimated at 0.3% at 3 years, 0.5% at 5 years, and 0.6% at 8 years after treatment.** The latency period for secondary leukemias may be short (1-3 years).

[U.S. Boxed Warning]: For I.V. administration only, severe local tissue damage and necrosis will result if extravasation occurs (vesicant); not for I.M. or SubQ use. Injection in to a small vein or repeated administration in the same vein may result in venous sclerosis. Women ≥70 years of age should be closely monitored for toxicity. **[U.S. Boxed Warning]: Should be administered under the supervision of an experienced cancer chemotherapy physician.** Epirubicin is emetogenic; consider prophylactic antiemetics prior to administration. Patients should recover from acute toxicities (stomatitis, myelosuppression, infections) prior to initiating treatment. Assess baseline labs (blood counts, bilirubin, ALT, AST, serum creatinine) and cardiac function (with LVEF). Prophylactic antibiotics should be administered with the CDF-120 regimen. Patients should not be immunized with live viral vaccines during or shortly after treatment. Inactivated vaccines may be administered (response may be diminished).

Adverse Reactions Percentages reported as part of combination chemotherapy regimens.

>10%:

- Central nervous system: Lethargy (1% to 46%)
- Dermatologic: Alopecia (70% to 96%)
- Endocrine & metabolic: Amenorrhea (69% to 72%), hot flashes (5% to 39%)
- Gastrointestinal: Nausea/vomiting (83% to 92%; grades 3/4: 22% to 25%), mucositis (9% to 59%; grades 3/4: ≤9%), diarrhea (7% to 25%)
- Hematologic: Leukopenia (50% to 80%; grades 3/4: 2% to 59%), neutropenia (54% to 80%; grades 3/4: 11% to 67%; nadir: 10-14 days; recovery: by day 21), anemia (13% to 72%; grades 3/4: ≤6%), thrombocytopenia (5% to 49%; grades 3/4: ≤5%)
- Local: Injection site reactions (3% to 20%; grades 3/4: <1%)
- Ocular: Conjunctivitis (1% to 15%)
- Miscellaneous: Infection (15% to 22%; grades 3/4: ≤2%)

1% to 10%:

- Cardiovascular: LVEF decreased (asymptomatic; delayed: 1% to 2%), HF (0.4% to 1.5%)
- Central nervous system: Fever (1% to 5%)
- Dermatologic: Rash (1% to 9%), skin changes (1% to 5%)
- Gastrointestinal: Anorexia (2% to 3%)
- Hematologic: Neutropenic fever (grades 3/4: ≤6%)

<1%, postmarketing, case reports, and/or frequency not defined: Acute lymphoid leukemia (ALL), acute myelogenous leukemia (AML), anaphylaxis, arrhythmia, ascites, atrioventricular block, bradycardia, bundle-branch block, cardiomyopathy, chills, dehydration, dyspnea, ECG abnormalities, esophagitis, hepatomegaly, hyperpigmentation (oral mucosa, nails, skin), hypersensitivity, myelodysplastic syndrome, myocarditis, neutropenic typhlitis, photosensitivity, premature menopause, premature ventricular contractions, pulmonary edema, pulmonary embolism, radiation recall, shock, sinus tachycardia, stomatitis, ST-T wave changes (nonspecific), tachyarrhythmias, thromboembolism, thrombophlebitis, toxic megacolon, transaminases increased, urine discoloration (red), urticaria, ventricular tachycardia

Drug Interactions

Metabolism/Transport Effects None known.

Avoid Concomitant Use

Avoid concomitant use of Epirubicin with any of the following: BCG; Cimetidine; CloZAPine; Natalizumab; Pimecrolimus; Tacrolimus (Topical); Vaccines (Live)

Increased Effect/Toxicity

Epirubicin may increase the levels/effects of: CloZAPine; Leflunomide; Natalizumab; Vaccines (Live)

The levels/effects of Epirubicin may be increased by: Bevacizumab; Cimetidine; Denosumab; Pimecrolimus; Roflumilast; Tacrolimus (Topical); Taxane Derivatives; Trastuzumab

Decreased Effect

Epirubicin may decrease the levels/effects of: BCG; Cardiac Glycosides; Coccidioidin Skin Test; Sipuleucel-T; Vaccines (Inactivated); Vaccines (Live)

The levels/effects of Epirubicin may be decreased by: Cardiac Glycosides; Echinacea

Ethanol/Nutrition/Herb Interactions

Ethanol: Avoid ethanol (due to GI irritation).

Herb/Nutraceutical: Avoid black cohosh, dong quai in estrogen-dependent tumors.

Stability Use appropriate precautions for handling and disposal. Protect from light.

Solution: Store intact vials refrigerated at 2°C to 8°C (36°F to 46°F); do not freeze. Product may "gel" at refrigerated temperatures; will return to slightly viscous solution after 2-4 hours at room temperature (15°C to 30°C). Discard unused solution from single dose vials within 24 hours of entry.

Lyophilized powder: Store at room temperature of 25°C (77°F); excursions permitted to 15°C to 30°C (59°F to 86°F). Reconstitute lyophilized powder with SWFI (25 mL for the 50 mg vial or 100 mL for the 200 mg vial) to a final concentration of 2 mg/mL. Reconstituted solutions are stable for 24 hours when stored at 2°C to 8°C (36°F to 46°F) or at room temperature.

Mechanism of Action Epirubicin is an anthracycline antineoplastic agent; known to inhibit DNA and RNA synthesis by steric obstruction after intercalating between DNA base pairs; active throughout entire cell cycle. Intercalation triggers DNA cleavage by topoisomerase II, resulting in cytocidal activity. Also inhibits DNA helicase, and generates cytotoxic free radicals.

Pharmacodynamics/Kinetics

Distribution: V_{ss}: 21-27 L/kg

Protein binding: ~77% to albumin

Metabolism: Extensively via hepatic and extrahepatic (including RBCs) routes

Half-life elimination: Triphasic; Mean terminal: 33 hours

Excretion: Feces (34% to 35%); urine (20% to 27%)

Dosage Adults: I.V.: **Note:** Patients receiving 120 mg/m²/cycle as part of combination therapy (CEF-120 regimen) should also receive prophylactic therapy with sulfamethoxazole/trimethoprim or a fluoroquinolone. Details concerning dosing in combination regimens should also be consulted. Lower starting doses may be necessary for heavily pretreated patients, patients with pre-existing myelosuppression, or with bone marrow involvement.

Breast cancer, adjuvant treatment: Usual dose: 100-120 mg/m² per 3- or 4-week treatment cycle as follows:

60 mg/m² on days 1 and 8 every 28 days for 6 cycles in combination with cyclophosphamide and fluorouracil (CEF-120 regimen; Levine, 2005) **or**

100 mg/m² on day 1 every 21 days for 6 cycles in combination with cyclophosphamide and fluorouracil (FEC-100 regimen; Bonneterre, 2005) **or**

Breast cancer (unlabeled regimens; as a part of combination chemotherapy):

60 mg/m² on day 1 every 21 days for 8 cycles (EC regimen; Piccart, 2001) **or**

75 mg/m² on day 1 every 21 days for 4 cycles (FEC regimen; Buzdar, 2005) **or**

75 mg/m² on day 1 every 21 days for 6 cycles (EP or EC regimen; Langley, 2005) **or**

90 mg/m² on day 1 every 21 days for 4 or 6 cycles (FEC regimen ± paclitaxel; Martin, 2008) **or**

50 mg/m² on days 1 and 8 every 21-28 days for 6-9 cycles (CEF regimen; Ackland, 2001)

Esophageal cancer (unlabeled use; as part of combination chemotherapy):

50 mg/m² on day 1 every 21 days for up to 8 cycles (ECF, ECX, EOF, and EOX regimens; Cunningham, 2008) **or**

50 mg/m² on day 1 every 21 days for 3 preoperative and 3 postoperative cycles (ECF regimen; Cunningham, 2006)

Gastric cancer (unlabeled use; as part of combination chemotherapy):

50 mg/m² on day 1 every 21 days for up to 8 cycles (ECF, ECX, EOF, and EOX regimens [Cunningham, 2008]; ECF regimen [Waters, 1999]) **or**

50 mg/m² on day 1 every 21 days for 3 preoperative and 3 postoperative cycles (ECF regimen; Cunningham, 2006)

Dosage modifications (breast cancer; labeled dosing):

Delay day 1 dose until platelets are ≥100,000/mm³, ANC ≥1500/mm³, and nonhematologic toxicities have recovered to ≤grade 1

Reduce day 1 dose in subsequent cycles to 75% of previous day 1 dose if patient experiences nadir platelet counts <50,000/mm³, ANC <250/mm³, neutropenic fever, or grade 3/4 nonhematologic toxicity during the previous cycle

For CEF-120 regimen, reduce day 8 dose to 75% of day 1 dose if platelet counts are 75,000-100,000/mm³ and ANC is 1000-1499/mm³; omit day 8 dose if platelets are <75,000/mm³, ANC <1000/mm³, or grade 3/4 nonhematologic toxicity

Elderly: Plasma clearance of epirubicin in elderly female patients was noted to be reduced by 35%. Although no initial dosage reduction is specifically recommended, particular care should be exercised in monitoring toxicity and adjusting subsequent dosage in elderly patients (particularly females >70 years of age).

Dosage adjustment in bone marrow dysfunction: Heavily-treated patients, patients with pre-existing bone marrow depression or neoplastic bone marrow infiltration: Lower starting doses (75-90 mg/m²) should be considered.

Dosage adjustment in renal impairment: The manufacturer's labeling recommends lower doses (dose not specified) in patients with severe renal impairment (serum creatinine >5 mg/dL). Other sources (Aronoff, 2007) suggest no dosage adjustment is needed for Cl_{cr} <50 mL/minute.

Dosage adjustment in hepatic impairment: The manufacturer's labeling recommends the following adjustments (based on clinical trial information):

Bilirubin 1.2-3 mg/dL or AST 2-4 times the upper limit of normal: Administer 50% of recommended starting dose

Bilirubin >3 mg/dL or AST >4 times the upper limit of normal: Administer 25% of recommended starting dose

Severe hepatic impairment: Use is not recommended (has not been studied)

Administration I.V.: Infuse over 15-20 minutes or slow I.V. push; if lower doses due to dose reduction are administered, may reduce infusion time proportionally. Do not infuse over <3 minutes. Infuse into a free-flowing I.V. solution. Avoid the use of veins over joints or in extremities with compromised venous or lymphatic drainage. Monitor infusion site; avoid extravasation.

Monitoring Parameters Monitor injection site during infusion for possible extravasation or local reactions. Baseline and repeated measurements of CBC with differential, liver function tests, serum creatinine, ECG, and LVEF. The method used for assessment of LVEF (echocardiogram or MUGA) should be consistent during routine monitoring.

Dosage Forms Excipient information presented when available (limited, particularly for generics); consult specific product labeling.

Injection, powder for reconstitution, as hydrochloride: 50 mg

Injection, solution, as hydrochloride [preservative free]: 2 mg/mL (25 mL, 100 mL)

Ellence®: 2 mg/mL (25 mL, 100 mL)

◆ **Epirubicin Hydrochloride** *see* Epirubicin *on page 597*

◆ **Epitol®** *see* CarBAMazepine *on page 280*

◆ **Epival® (Can)** *see* Divalproex *on page 530*

◆ **Epival® I.V. (Can)** *see* Valproic Acid *on page 1757*

◆ **Epivir®** *see* LamiVUDine *on page 965*

◆ **Epivir-HBV®** *see* LamiVUDine *on page 965*

Eplerenone (e PLER en one)

Brand Names: U.S. Inspra™

Pharmacologic Category Diuretic, Potassium-Sparing; Selective Aldosterone Blocker

Use Treatment of hypertension (may be used alone or in combination with other antihypertensive agents); treatment of heart failure (HF) following acute MI

Pregnancy Risk Factor B

Pregnancy Considerations No teratogenic effects were seen in animal studies, however, there are no adequate and well-controlled studies in pregnant women. Use during pregnancy only if the potential benefit to the mother outweighs the possible risk to the fetus.

Lactation Excretion in breast milk unknown/not recommended

Contraindications Serum potassium >5.5 mEq/L at initiation; Cl_{cr} ≤30 mL/minute; concomitant use of strong CYP3A4 inhibitors (see Drug Interactions for details)

The following additional contraindications apply to patients with hypertension: Type 2 diabetes mellitus (noninsulin dependent, NIDDM) with microalbuminuria; serum creatinine >2.0 mg/dL in males or >1.8 mg/dL in females; Cl_{cr} <50 mL/minute; concomitant use with potassium supplements or potassium-sparing diuretics

Warnings/Precautions Dosage adjustment needed for patients on moderate CYP3A4 inhibitors. Monitor closely for hyperkalemia; increases in serum potassium were dose related during clinical trials and rates of hyperkalemia also increased with declining renal function. Safety and efficacy have not been established in patients with severe hepatic impairment. Use with caution in HF patients post-MI with diabetes (especially if patient has proteinuria); risk of hyperkalemia is increased. Risk of hyperkalemia is increased with declining renal function. Use with caution in patients with mild renal impairment; contraindicated with moderate-severe impairment (HTN: Cl_{cr} <50 mL/minute; other indications: Cl_{cr} ≤30 mL/minute).

Adverse Reactions

>10%: Endocrine & metabolic: Hyperkalemia ([HF post-MI: K >5.5 mEq/L: 16%; K ≥6 mEq/L: 6%] [HTN: K >5.5 mEq/L at doses ≤100 mg: ≤1%; doses >100 mg: 9%]), hypertriglyceridemia (1% to 15%, dose related)

1% to 10%:

- Central nervous system: Dizziness (3%), fatigue (2%)
- Endocrine & metabolic: Hyponatremia (2%, dose related), breast pain (males <1% to 1%), gynecomastia (males <1% to 1%), hypercholesterolemia (<1% to 1%)
- Gastrointestinal: Diarrhea (2%), abdominal pain (1%)
- Genitourinary: Abnormal vaginal bleeding (<1% to 2%)
- Renal: Creatinine increased (HF post-MI: 6%), albuminuria (1%)
- Respiratory: Cough (2%)
- Miscellaneous: Flu-like syndrome (2%)

<1%, postmarketing, and/or case reports: Angioneurotic edema, BUN increased, liver function tests increased, rash, uric acid increased

Drug Interactions

Metabolism/Transport Effects Substrate of CYP3A4 (major); **Note:** Assignment of Major/Minor substrate status based on clinically relevant drug interaction potential

Avoid Concomitant Use

Avoid concomitant use of Eplerenone with any of the following: CycloSPORINE; CycloSPORINE (Systemic); CYP3A4 Inhibitors (Strong); Itraconazole; Ketoconazole; Ketoconazole (Systemic); Posaconazole; Tacrolimus; Tacrolimus (Systemic); Voriconazole

Increased Effect/Toxicity

Eplerenone may increase the levels/effects of: ACE Inhibitors; Amifostine; Angiotensin II Receptor Blockers; Antihypertensives; CycloSPORINE; CycloSPORINE (Systemic); Hypotensive Agents; Potassium Salts; Potassium-Sparing Diuretics; RiTUXimab; Tacrolimus; Tacrolimus (Systemic)

The levels/effects of Eplerenone may be increased by: Alfuzosin; Calcium Channel Blockers (Nondihydropyridine); CYP3A4 Inhibitors (Moderate); CYP3A4 Inhibitors (Strong); Dasatinib; Diazoxide; Fluconazole; Herbs (Hypotensive Properties); Itraconazole; Ketoconazole; Ketoconazole (Systemic); Macrolide Antibiotics; MAO Inhibitors; Nitrofurantoin; Nonsteroidal Anti-Inflammatory Agents; Pentoxifylline; Phosphodiesterase 5 Inhibitors; Posaconazole; Prostacyclin Analogues; Protease Inhibitors; Trimethoprim; Voriconazole

Decreased Effect

The levels/effects of Eplerenone may be decreased by: CYP3A4 Inducers (Strong); Deferasirox; Herbs (CYP3A4 Inducers); Herbs (Hypertensive Properties); Methylphenidate; Nonsteroidal Anti-Inflammatory Agents; Tocilizumab; Yohimbine

Ethanol/Nutrition/Herb Interactions

Food: Grapefruit juice increases eplerenone AUC ~25%.

Herb/Nutraceutical: St John's wort may decrease levels of eplerenone. Avoid black cohosh, California poppy, coleus, golden seal, hawthorn, mistletoe, periwinkle, quinine, shepherd's purse (may have increased antihypertensive effect). Avoid bayberry, blue cohosh, cayenne, ephedra, ginger, ginseng (American), kola, licorice (may diminish the antihypertensive effect).

Stability Store at controlled room temperature of 25°C (77°F).

Mechanism of Action Aldosterone, a mineralocorticoid, increases blood pressure primarily by inducing sodium and water retention. Overexpression of aldosterone is thought to contribute to myocardial fibrosis (especially following myocardial infarction) and vascular fibrosis. Mineralocorticoid receptors are located in the kidney, heart, blood vessels, and brain. Eplerenone selectively blocks mineralocorticoid receptors reducing blood pressure in a dose-dependent manner and appears to prevent myocardial and vascular fibrosis.

Pharmacodynamics/Kinetics

Distribution: V_d: 43-90 L

Protein binding: ~50%; primarily to alpha$_1$-acid glycoproteins

Metabolism: Primarily hepatic via CYP3A4; metabolites inactive

Bioavailability: 69%

Half-life elimination: 4-6 hours

Time to peak, plasma: ~1.5 hours; may take up to 4 weeks for full antihypertensive effect

Excretion: Urine (~67%); feces (32%); <5% as unchanged drug in urine and feces

Dosage Oral: Adults:

Hypertension: Initial: 50 mg once daily; may increase to 50 mg twice daily if response is not adequate; may take up to 4 weeks for full therapeutic response. Doses >100 mg/day are associated with increased risk of hyperkalemia and no greater therapeutic effect.

Concurrent use with moderate CYP3A4 inhibitors: Initial: 25 mg once daily

Heart failure (post-MI): Initial: 25 mg once daily; dosage goal: Titrate to 50 mg once daily within 4 weeks, as tolerated

Dosage adjustment per serum potassium concentrations for HF (post-MI):

<5.0 mEq/L:

Increase dose from 25 mg every other day to 25 mg daily **or**

Increase dose from 25 mg daily to 50 mg daily

5.0-5.4 mEq/L: No adjustment needed

5.5-5.9 mEq/L:

Decrease dose from 50 mg daily to 25 mg daily **or**

Decrease dose from 25 mg daily to 25 mg every other day **or**

Decrease dose from 25 mg every other day to withhold medication

≥6.0 mEq/L: Withhold medication until potassium <5.5 mEq/L, then restart at 25 mg every other day

Dosage adjustment in renal impairment:

Hypertension: Cl_{cr} <50 mL/minute or serum creatinine >2.0 mg/dL in males or >1.8 mg/dL in females: Use is contraindicated; risk of hyperkalemia increases with declining renal function

All other indications: Cl_{cr} ≤30 mL/minute: Use is contraindicated.

Dosage adjustment in hepatic impairment: No dosage adjustment needed for mild-to-moderate impairment; safety and efficacy not established for severe impairment

Dietary Considerations May be taken with or without food. Do not use salt substitutes containing potassium.

Administration May be administered with or without food.

Monitoring Parameters Blood pressure; serum potassium (levels monitored prior to therapy, within the first week, and at 1 month after start of treatment or dose adjustment, then periodically [monthly in clinical trials]); renal function

Dosage Forms Excipient information presented when available (limited, particularly for generics); consult specific product labeling.

Tablet, oral: 25 mg, 50 mg

Inspra™: 25 mg, 50 mg

◆ **EPO** *see* Epoetin Alfa *on page 601*

Epoetin Alfa (e POE e tin AL fa)

Brand Names: U.S. Epogen®; Procrit®

Brand Names: Canada Eprex®

Index Terms rHuEPO; rHuEPO-α; EPO; Erythropoiesis-Stimulating Agent (ESA); Erythropoietin

Pharmacologic Category Colony Stimulating Factor; Growth Factor; Recombinant Human Erythropoietin

Use Treatment of anemia due to concurrent myelosuppressive chemotherapy in patients with cancer (nonmyeloid malignancies) receiving chemotherapy (palliative intent) for a planned minimum of 2 additional months of chemotherapy; treatment of anemia due to chronic kidney disease (including patients on dialysis and not on dialysis) to decrease the need for RBC transfusion; treatment of anemia associated with HIV (zidovudine) therapy when endogenous erythropoietin levels ≤500 mUnits/mL; reduction of allogeneic RBC transfusion for elective, noncardiac, nonvascular surgery when perioperative hemoglobin is >10 to ≤13 g/dL and there is a high risk for blood loss

Note: Epoetin is **not** indicated for use under the following conditions:

- Cancer patients receiving hormonal therapy, therapeutic biologic products, or radiation therapy unless also receiving concurrent myelosuppressive chemotherapy
- Cancer patients receiving myelosuppressive chemotherapy when the expected outcome is curative
- Surgery patients who are willing to donate autologous blood
- Surgery patients undergoing cardiac or vascular surgery
- As a substitute for RBC transfusion in patients requiring immediate correction of anemia

Note: In clinical trials (and one meta-analysis), epoetin has not demonstrated improved quality of life, fatigue, or well-being.

Unlabeled Use Treatment of symptomatic anemia in myelodysplastic syndrome (MDS)

Pregnancy Risk Factor C

Pregnancy Considerations Epoetin alfa has been shown to have adverse effects (decreased weight gain, delayed development, delayed ossification) in animal studies. Polyhydramnios and intrauterine growth retardation have been reported with use in women with chronic kidney disease. Hypospadias and pectus excavatum have been reported (case report) with first trimester exposure. Amenorrheic premenopausal women should be cautioned that menstruation may resume following treatment with rHuEPO-α and contraception should be considered if pregnancy is to be avoided. Multidose formulations containing benzyl alcohol should not be used in pregnant women. Women who become pregnant during treatment with epoetin are encouraged to enroll in Amgen's Pregnancy Surveillance Program (1-800-772-6436).

Lactation Excretion in breast milk unknown/use caution

Prescribing and Access Restrictions As a requirement of the REMS program, access to this medication is restricted. Healthcare providers and hospitals must be enrolled in the ESA APPRISE (Assisting Providers and Cancer Patients with Risk Information for the Safe use of ESAs) Oncology Program (866-284-8089; http://www.esa-apprise.com) to prescribe or dispense ESAs (ie, epoetin alfa, darbepoetin alfa) to patients with cancer.

Medication Guide Available Yes

Contraindications Hypersensitivity to epoetin or any component of the formulation; uncontrolled hypertension; pure red cell aplasia (due to epoetin or other epoetin protein drugs); multidose vials contain benzyl alcohol and are contraindicated in neonates, infants, pregnant women, and nursing women

Warnings/Precautions [U.S. Boxed Warning]: Erythropoiesis-stimulating agents (ESAs) increased the risk of serious cardiovascular events, thromboembolic events, stroke, mortality, and/or tumor progression in clinical studies when administered to target hemoglobin levels >11 g/dL (and provide no additional benefit); a rapid rise in hemoglobin (>1 g/dL over 2 weeks) may also contribute to these risks. **[U.S. Boxed Warning]: A shortened overall survival and/or increased risk of tumor progression or recurrence has been reported in studies with breast, cervical, head and neck, lymphoid, and nonsmall cell lung cancer patients.** It is of note that in these studies, patients received ESAs to a target hemoglobin of ≥12 g/dL; although risk has not been excluded when dosed to achieve a target hemoglobin of <12 g/dL. **[U.S. Boxed Warnings]: To decrease these risks, and risk of cardio- and thrombovascular events, use the lowest dose needed to avoid red blood cell transfusions. Use ESAs in cancer patients only for the treatment of anemia related to concurrent myelosuppressive chemotherapy; discontinue ESA following completion of the chemotherapy course. ESAs are not indicated for patients receiving myelosuppressive therapy when the anticipated outcome is curative.** A dosage modification is appropriate if hemoglobin levels rise >1 g/dL per 2-week time period during treatment (Rizzo, 2010). Use of ESAs has been associated with an increased risk of venous thromboembolism (VTE) without a reduction in transfusions in patients with cancer (Hershman, 2009). Improved anemia symptoms, quality of life, fatigue, or well-being have not been demonstrated in controlled clinical trials. **[U.S. Boxed Warning]: Because of the risks of decreased survival and increased risk of**

tumor growth or progression, all healthcare providers and hospitals are required to enroll and comply with the ESA APPRISE (Assisting Providers and Cancer Patients with Risk Information for the Safe use of ESAs) Oncology Program prior to prescribing or dispensing ESAs to cancer patients. Prescribers and patients will have to provide written documentation of discussed risks prior to each epoetin course.

[U.S. Boxed Warning]: An increased risk of death, serious cardiovascular events, and stroke was reported in chronic kidney disease (CKD) patients administered ESAs to target hemoglobin levels ≥11 g/dL; use the lowest dose sufficient to reduce the need for RBC transfusions. An optimal target hemoglobin level, dose or dosing strategy to reduce these risks has not been identified in clinical trials. Hemoglobin rising >1 g/dL in a 2-week period may contribute to the risk (dosage reduction recommended). Chronic kidney disease patients who exhibit an inadequate hemoglobin response to ESA therapy may be at a higher risk for cardiovascular events and mortality compared to other patients. ESA therapy may reduce dialysis efficacy (due to increase in red blood cells and decrease in plasma volume); adjustments in dialysis parameters may be needed. Patients treated with epoetin may require increased heparinization during dialysis to prevent clotting of the extracorporeal circuit. **[U.S. Boxed Warning]: DVT prophylaxis is recommended in perisurgery patients due to the risk of DVT.** Increased mortality was also observed in patients undergoing coronary artery bypass surgery who received epoetin alfa; these deaths were associated with thrombotic events. Epoetin is **not** approved for reduction of red blood cell transfusion in patients undergoing cardiac or vascular surgery and is **not** indicated for surgical patients willing to donate autologous blood.

Use with caution in patients with hypertension (contraindicated in uncontrolled hypertension) or with a history of seizures; hypertensive encephalopathy and seizures have been reported. If hypertension is difficult to control, reduce or hold epoetin alfa. An excessive rate of rise of hemoglobin is associated with hypertension or exacerbation of hypertension; decrease the epoetin dose if the hemoglobin increase exceeds 1 g/dL in any 2-week period. Blood pressure should be controlled prior to start of therapy and monitored closely throughout treatment. The risk for seizures is increased with epoetin use in patients with CKD; monitor closely for neurologic symptoms during the first several months of therapy. Due to the delayed onset of erythropoiesis, epoetin alfa is **not** recommended for acute correction of severe anemia or as a substitute for emergency transfusion.

Prior to treatment, correct or exclude deficiencies of iron, vitamin B_{12}, and/or folate, as well as other factors which may impair erythropoiesis (inflammatory conditions, infections). Prior to and periodically during therapy, iron stores must be evaluated. Supplemental iron is recommended if serum ferritin <100 mcg/L or serum transferrin saturation <20%; most patients with chronic kidney disease will require iron supplementation. Poor response should prompt evaluation of these potential factors, as well as possible malignant processes and hematologic disease (thalassemia, refractory anemia, myelodysplastic disorder), occult blood loss, hemolysis, ostetis fibrosa cystic, and/or bone marrow fibrosis. Severe anemia and pure red cell aplasia (PRCA) with associated neutralizing antibodies to erythropoietin has been reported, predominantly in patients with CKD receiving SubQ epoetin (the I.V. route is preferred for hemodialysis patients). Cases have also been reported in patients with hepatitis C who were receiving ESAs, interferon, and ribavirin. Patients with a sudden loss of response to epoetin alfa (with severe anemia and a low reticulocyte count) should be evaluated for PRCA with associated neutralizing antibodies to erythropoietin; discontinue treatment (permanently) in patients with PRCA secondary to neutralizing antibodies to epoetin.

Potentially serious allergic reactions have been reported (rarely). Discontinue immediately (and permanently) in patients who experience serious allergic/anaphylactic reactions. Some products may contain albumin. Multidose vials contain benzyl alcohol; do not use in premature infants.

Adverse Reactions

>10%:

- Cardiovascular: Hypertension (3% to 28%)
- Central nervous system: Fever (10% to 42%), headache (5% to 18%)
- Dermatologic: Pruritus (12% to 21%), rash (2% to 19%)
- Gastrointestinal: Nausea (35% to 56%), vomiting (12% to 28%)
- Local: Injection site reaction (7% to 13%)
- Neuromuscular & skeletal: Arthralgia (10% to 16%)
- Respiratory: Cough (4% to 26%)

1% to 10%:

- Cardiovascular: Deep vein thrombosis, edema, thrombosis
- Central nervous system: Chills, depression, dizziness, insomnia
- Dermatologic: Urticaria
- Endocrine & metabolic: Hyperglycemia, hypokalemia
- Gastrointestinal: Dysphagia, stomatitis, weight loss
- Hematologic: Leukopenia
- Local: Clotted vascular access
- Neuromuscular & skeletal: Bone pain, muscle spasm, myalgia
- Respiratory: Pulmonary embolism, respiratory congestion, upper respiratory infection

<1% (Limited to important or life-threatening): Allergic reaction, anaphylactic reaction, angioedema, bronchospasm, erythema, hypersensitivity reactions, hypertensive encephalopathy, microvascular thrombosis, MI, neutralizing antibodies, porphyria, pure red cell aplasia (PRCA), renal vein thrombosis, retinal artery thrombosis, seizure, stroke, tachycardia, temporal vein thrombosis, thrombophlebitis, TIA, tumor progression

Drug Interactions

Metabolism/Transport Effects None known.

Avoid Concomitant Use There are no known interactions where it is recommended to avoid concomitant use.

Increased Effect/Toxicity There are no known significant interactions involving an increase in effect.

Decreased Effect There are no known significant interactions involving a decrease in effect.

Stability

Vials should be stored at 2°C to 8°C (36°F to 46°F); **do not freeze or shake**. Protect from light.

Single-dose 1 mL vial contains no preservative: Use one dose per vial. Do not re-enter vial; discard unused portions.

Single-dose vials (except 40,000 units/mL vial) are stable for 2 weeks at room temperature (Cohen, 2007). Single-dose 40,000 units/mL vial is stable for 1 week at room temperature.

Multidose 1 mL or 2 mL vial contains preservative. Store at 2°C to 8°C after initial entry and between doses. Discard 21 days after initial entry.

Multidose vials (with preservative) are stable for 1 week at room temperature (Cohen, 2007).

Prefilled syringes containing the 20,000 units/mL formulation with preservative are stable for 6 weeks refrigerated (2°C to 8°C) (Naughton, 2003).

Dilutions of 1:10 and 1:20 (1 part epoetin:19 parts sodium chloride) are stable for 18 hours at room temperature (Ohls, 1996).

Prior to SubQ administration, preservative free solutions may be mixed with bacteriostatic NS containing benzyl alcohol 0.9% in a 1:1 ratio (Corbo, 1992). Dilutions of 1:10 in $D_{10}W$ with human albumin 0.05% or 0.1% are stable for 24 hours.

Mechanism of Action Induces erythropoiesis by stimulating the division and differentiation of committed erythroid progenitor cells; induces the release of reticulocytes from the bone marrow into the bloodstream, where they mature to erythrocytes. There is a dose response relationship with this effect. This results in an increase in reticulocyte counts followed by a rise in hematocrit and hemoglobin levels.

Pharmacodynamics/Kinetics

Onset of action: Several days

Peak effect: Hemoglobin level: 2-6 weeks

Distribution: V_d: 9 L; rapid in the plasma compartment; concentrated in liver, kidneys, and bone marrow

Metabolism: Some degradation does occur

Bioavailability: SubQ: ~21% to 31%; intraperitoneal epoetin: 3% (Macdougall, 1989)

Half-life elimination: Cancer: SubQ: 16-67 hours; Chronic kidney disease: I.V.: 4-13 hours

Time to peak, serum: Chronic kidney disease: SubQ: 5-24 hours

Excretion: Feces (majority); urine (small amounts, 10% unchanged in normal volunteers)

Dosage

Anemia associated with chronic kidney disease: Individualize dosing and use the lowest dose necessary to reduce the need for RBC transfusions.

Chronic kidney disease patients ***ON dialysis*** (I.V. route is preferred for hemodialysis patients; initiate treatment when hemoglobin is <10 g/dL; reduce dose or interrupt treatment if hemoglobin approaches or exceeds 11 g/dL):

Children 1 month to 16 years: I.V., SubQ: Initial dose: 50 units/kg 3 times/week

Adults: I.V., SubQ: Initial dose: 50-100 units/kg 3 times/week

Chronic kidney disease patients ***NOT on dialysis*** (consider initiating treatment when hemoglobin is <10 g/dL; use only if rate of hemoglobin decline would likely result in RBC transfusion and desire is to reduce risk of alloimmunization or other RBC transfusion-related risks; reduce dose or interrupt treatment if hemoglobin exceeds 10 g/dL):

Adults: I.V., SubQ: Initial dose: 50-100 units/kg 3 times/week

Dosage adjustments for chronic kidney disease patients (either on dialysis or not on dialysis):

If hemoglobin does not increase by >1 g/dL after 4 weeks: Increase dose by 25%; do not increase the dose more frequently than once every 4 weeks

If hemoglobin increases >1 g/dL in any 2-week period: Reduce dose by ≥25%; dose reductions can occur more frequently than once every 4 weeks; avoid frequent dosage adjustments

Inadequate or lack of response over a 12-week escalation period: Further increases are unlikely to improve response and may increase risks; use the minimum effective dose that will maintain a Hgb level sufficient to avoid RBC transfusions and evaluate patient for other causes of anemia. Discontinue therapy if responsiveness does not improve.

Anemia due to chemotherapy in cancer patients: Initiate treatment only if hemoglobin <10 g/dL and anticipated duration of myelosuppressive chemotherapy is ≥2 months. Titrate dosage to use the minimum effective dose that will maintain a hemoglobin level sufficient to avoid red blood cell transfusions. Discontinue erythropoietin following completion of chemotherapy.

Children ≥5 years: I.V.: Initial dose: 600 units/kg once weekly until completion of chemotherapy.

Dosage adjustments:

If hemoglobin does not increase by >1 g/dL **and** remains <10 g/dL after initial 4 weeks: Increase to 900 units/kg (maximum dose: 60,000 units); discontinue after 8 weeks of treatment if RBC transfusions are still required or there is no hemoglobin response.

If hemoglobin exceeds a level needed to avoid red blood cell transfusion: Withhold dose; resume treatment with a 25% dose reduction when hemoglobin approaches a level where transfusions may be required.

If hemoglobin increases >1 g/dL in any 2-week period **or** hemoglobin reaches a level sufficient to avoid red blood cell transfusion: Reduce dose by 25%.

Adults: SubQ: Initial dose: 150 units/kg 3 times/week or 40,000 units once weekly until completion of chemotherapy

Dosage adjustments:

If hemoglobin does not increase by >1 g/dL **and** remains below 10 g/dL after initial 4 weeks: Increase to 300 units/kg 3 times/week or 60,000 units weekly; discontinue after 8 weeks of treatment if RBC transfusions are still required or there is no hemoglobin response

If hemoglobin exceeds a level needed to avoid red blood cell transfusion: Withhold dose; resume treatment with a 25% dose reduction when hemoglobin approaches a level where transfusions may be required.

If hemoglobin increases >1 g/dL in any 2-week period **or** hemoglobin reaches a level sufficient to avoid red blood cell transfusion: Reduce dose by 25%.

Anemia due to zidovudine in HIV-infected patients: Titrate dosage to use the minimum effective dose that will maintain a hemoglobin level sufficient to avoid red blood cell transfusions. Hemoglobin levels should not exceed 12 g/dL.

Children 8 months to 17 years (based on limited data): I.V., SubQ: Reported dosing range: 50-400 units/kg 2-3 times/week

Adults (with serum erythropoietin levels ≤500 mUnits/mL and zidovudine doses ≤4200 mg/week): I.V., SubQ: Initial: 100 units/kg 3 times/week; if hemoglobin does not increase after 8 weeks, increase dose by ~50-100 units/kg at 4-8 week intervals until hemoglobin reaches a level sufficient to avoid RBC transfusion; maximum dose: 300 units/kg. Withhold dose if hemoglobin exceeds 12 g/dL, may resume treatment with a 25% dose reduction once hemoglobin <11 g/dL. Discontinue if hemoglobin increase is not achieved with 300 units/kg for 8 weeks.

Surgery patients (perioperative hemoglobin should be >10 g/dL and ≤13 g/dL; DVT prophylactic anticoagulation is recommended): Adults: SubQ: Initial dose:

300 units/kg/day beginning 10 days before surgery, on the day of surgery, and for 4 days after surgery **or**

600 units/kg once weekly for 4 doses, beginning 21-, 14-, and 7 days before surgery, and on the day of surgery

Symptomatic anemia associated with MDS (unlabeled use): Adults: SubQ: 40,000-60,000 units 1-3 times/week (NCCN MDS guidelines v.2.2011)

Administration

SubQ is the preferred route of administration **except** in patients with CKD on hemodialysis; 1:1 dilution with bacteriostatic NS (containing benzyl alcohol) acts as a local anesthetic to reduce pain at the injection site

Patients with CKD on hemodialysis: I.V. route preferred; it may be administered into the venous line at the end of the dialysis procedure

Monitoring Parameters Transferrin saturation and serum ferritin (prior to and during treatment); hemoglobin (weekly after initiation and following dose adjustments until stable and sufficient to minimize need for RBC transfusion, CKD patients should be also be monitored at least monthly following hemoglobin stability); blood pressure; seizures (CKD patients following initiation for first few months, includes new-onset or change in seizure frequency or premonitory symptoms)

Cancer patients: Examinations recommended by the ASCO/ASH guidelines (Rizzo, 2010) prior to treatment include: peripheral blood smear (in some situations a bone marrow exam may be necessary), assessment for iron, folate, or vitamin B_{12} deficiency, reticulocyte count, renal function status, and occult blood loss; during ESA treatment, assess baseline and periodic iron, total iron-binding capacity, and transferrin saturation or ferritin levels.

Reference Range Zidovudine-treated HIV patients: Available evidence indicates patients with endogenous serum erythropoietin levels >500 mU/mL are unlikely to respond

Additional Information Oncology Comment: The American Society of Clinical Oncology (ASCO) and American Society of Hematology (ASH) 2010 updates to the clinical practice guidelines for the use of erythropoiesis-stimulating agents (ESAs) in patients with cancer indicate that ESAs are most appropriate when used according to the parameters identified within the Food and Drug Administration (FDA) approved labeling for epoetin and darbepoetin (Rizzo, 2010). ESAs are an option for chemotherapy associated anemia when the hemoglobin has fallen to <10 g/dL to decrease the need for RBC transfusions. ESAs should only be used in conjunction with concurrent chemotherapy. Although the FDA label now limits ESA use to the palliative setting, the ASCO/ASH guidelines suggest using clinical judgment in weighing risks versus benefits as formal outcomes studies of ESA use defined by intent of chemotherapy treatment have not been conducted.

The ASCO/ASH guidelines continue to recommend following the FDA approved dosing (and dosing adjustment) guidelines as alternate dosing and schedules have not demonstrated consistent differences in effectiveness with regard to hemoglobin response. In patients who do not have a response within 6-8 weeks (hemoglobin rise <1-2 g/dL or no reduction in transfusions) ESA therapy should be discontinued.

Prior to the initiation of ESAs, other sources of anemia (in addition to chemotherapy or underlying hematologic malignancy) should be investigated. Examinations recommended prior to treatment include peripheral blood smear (in some situations a bone marrow exam may be necessary), assessment for iron, folate, or vitamin B_{12} deficiency, reticulocyte count, renal function status, and occult blood loss. During ESA treatment, assess baseline and periodic iron, total iron-binding capacity, and transferrin saturation or ferritin levels. Iron supplementation may be necessary

The guidelines note that patients with an increased risk of thromboembolism (generally includes previous history of thrombosis, surgery, and/or prolonged periods of immobilization) and patients receiving concomitant medications that may increase thromboembolic risk, should begin ESA therapy only after careful consideration. With the exception of low-risk myelodysplasia-associated anemia (which has evidence supporting the use of ESAs without concurrent chemotherapy), the guidelines do not support the use of ESAs in the absence of concurrent chemotherapy.

Dosage Forms Excipient information presented when available (limited, particularly for generics); consult specific product labeling.

Injection, solution:

Epogen®: 10,000 units/mL (2 mL); 20,000 units/mL (1 mL) [contains albumin (human), benzyl alcohol]

Procrit®: 10,000 units/mL (2 mL); 20,000 units/mL (1 mL) [contains albumin (human), benzyl alcohol]

Injection, solution [preservative free]:

Epogen®: 2000 units/mL (1 mL); 3000 units/mL (1 mL); 4000 units/mL (1 mL); 10,000 units/mL (1 mL) [contains albumin (human)]

Procrit®: 2000 units/mL (1 mL); 3000 units/mL (1 mL); 4000 units/mL (1 mL); 10,000 units/mL (1 mL); 40,000 units/mL (1 mL) [contains albumin (human)]

Dosage Forms: Canada Excipient information presented when available (limited, particularly for generics); consult specific product labeling.

Injection, solution [preservative free]:

Eprex®: 1000 units/0.5 mL (0.5 mL), 2000 units/0.5 mL (0.5 mL), 3000 units/0.3 mL (0.3 mL), 4000 units/0.4 mL (0.4 mL), 5000 units/0.5 mL (0.5 mL), 6000 units/0.6 mL (0.6 mL), 8000 units/0.8 mL (0.8 mL), 10,000 units/mL (1 mL), 20,000 units/0.5 mL (0.5 mL), 30,000 units/0.75 mL (0.75 mL), 40,000 units/mL (1 mL) [contains polysorbate 80; prefilled syringe, free of human serum albumin]

◆ **Epogen®** *see* Epoetin Alfa *on page 601*

Epoprostenol (e poe PROST en ole)

Brand Names: U.S. Flolan®; Veletri®

Brand Names: Canada Flolan®

Index Terms Epoprostenol Sodium; PGI_2; PGX; Prostacyclin

Pharmacologic Category Prostacyclin; Prostaglandin; Vasodilator

Use Treatment of pulmonary arterial hypertension (PAH) (WHO Group I) in patients with NYHA Class III or IV symptoms to improve exercise capacity

Unlabeled Use Acute vasodilator testing in pulmonary arterial hypertension (PAH)

Inhalation: Intraoperative treatment of pulmonary hypertension in patients undergoing cardiac surgery with cardiopulmonary bypass; post-cardiothoracic surgery pulmonary hypertension, right ventricular dysfunction, or refractory hypoxemia

Pregnancy Risk Factor B

Pregnancy Considerations Teratogenic effects were not reported in animal studies. There are no adequate and well-controlled studies in pregnant women. Women with IPAH are encouraged to avoid pregnancy.

Lactation Excretion in breast milk unknown/use caution

Prescribing and Access Restrictions Orders for epoprostenol are distributed by two sources in the United States. Information on orders or reimbursement assistance may be obtained from either Accredo Health, Inc (1-800-935-6526) or TheraCom, Inc (1-877-356-5264).

Contraindications Hypersensitivity to epoprostenol or to structurally-related compounds; chronic use in patients with heart failure due to severe left ventricular systolic dysfunction; patients who develop pulmonary edema during dose initiation

Warnings/Precautions Initiation or transition to epoprostenol requires specialized cardiopulmonary monitoring in a critical care setting where clinicians are experienced in advanced management of pulmonary arterial hypertension. Abrupt interruptions or large sudden reductions in dosage may result in rebound pulmonary hypertension; some patients with PAH have developed pulmonary edema during dosing adjustment and acute vasodilator testing (not an approved use), which may be associated with concomitant heart failure (LV systolic dysfunction with significantly elevated left heart filling pressures) or pulmonary veno-occlusive disease/pulmonary capillary hemangiomatosis. During chronic use, unless contraindicated, anticoagulants should be coadministered to reduce the risk of thromboembolism. Use cautiously in patients who have conditions that increase bleeding risk (inhibits platelet aggregation). Use with caution in patients receiving anticoagulants and antiplatelet agents. Chronic continuous I.V. infusion of epoprostenol via a chronic indwelling central venous catheter (CVC) has been associated with local infections and serious blood stream infections. Clinical studies of epoprostenol in pulmonary hypertension did not include sufficient numbers of patients ≥65 years of age to substantiate its safety and efficacy in the geriatric population. As a result, in general, dose selection for an elderly patient should be cautious usually starting at the low end of the dosing range.

Adverse Reactions Note: Adverse events reported during dose initiation and escalation include flushing (58%), headache (49%), nausea/vomiting (32%), hypotension (16%), anxiety/nervousness/agitation (11%), chest pain (11%); dizziness, abdominal pain, bradycardia, musculoskeletal pain, dyspnea, back pain, diaphoresis, dyspepsia, hypoesthesia/paresthesia, and tachycardia are also reported. Although some adverse reactions may be related to the underlying disease state, abdominal pain, anxiety/nervousness/agitation, arthralgia, bleeding, bradycardia, diarrhea, diaphoresis, flu-like syndrome, flushing, headache, hypotension, jaw pain, nausea, pain, pulmonary edema, rash, tachycardia, thrombocytopenia, and vomiting are clearly contributed to epoprostenol. The following adverse events have been reported during chronic administration for idiopathic or heritable PAH:

>10%:

Cardiovascular: Tachycardia (35% to 43%), flushing (23% to 42%), hypotension (13%)

Central nervous system: Dizziness (83%), headache (46% to 83%), chills/fever/sepsis/flu-like syndrome (25%), anxiety/nervousness/tremor (21%)

Dermatologic: Skin ulcer (39%), eczema/rash/urticaria (25%)

Gastrointestinal: Nausea/vomiting (41% to 67%), anorexia (66%), diarrhea (37% to 50%)

Local: Injection site reactions: Infection (18%), pain (11%)

Neuromuscular & skeletal: Pain/neck pain/arthralgia (84%), jaw pain (54% to 75%), arthritis (52%), myalgia (44%), musculoskeletal pain (35%), hypoesthesia/hyperesthesia/paresthesia (5% to 12%)

<1%, postmarketing, and/or case reports: Anemia, fatigue, hepatic failure, hypersplenism, hyperthyroidism, pallor, pancytopenia, pulmonary embolism, splenomegaly, thrombocytopenia

Drug Interactions

Metabolism/Transport Effects None known.

Avoid Concomitant Use There are no known interactions where it is recommended to avoid concomitant use.

Increased Effect/Toxicity

Epoprostenol may increase the levels/effects of: Anticoagulants; Antihypertensives; Antiplatelet Agents

Decreased Effect There are no known significant interactions involving a decrease in effect.

Stability Injection for reconstitution:

Flolan®: Prior to use, store vials at 15°C to 25°C (59°F to 77°F); do not freeze. Protect from light. Reconstitute only with provided sterile diluent (see table). Following reconstitution, solution must be stored under refrigeration at 2°C to 8°C (36°F to 46°F) if not used immediately; do not freeze. Protect from light. Total storage and infusion time must not exceed 48 hours for reconstituted solutions. Each reservoir of solution may be refrigerated for ≤40 hours and infused at room temperature over ≤8 hours; alternatively, each reservoir may be refrigerated for ≤24 hours and infused with the use of a cold pouch over ≤24 hours (gel packs must be changed every 12 hours).

Veletri®: Prior to use, store vials at 20°C to 25°C (68°F to 77°F); do not freeze. Protect from light. Reconstitute each vial with 5 mL of sterile water for injection or NS. Following reconstitution, vials may be stored under refrigeration at 2°C to 8°C (36°F to 46°F) up to 5 days, stored at room temperature of 25°C (77°F) up to 48 hours, or immediately diluted (see table) and added to a drug delivery reservoir.

Diluted solutions which have been immediately added to a drug delivery reservoir may be administered immediately or stored at 2°C to 8°C (36°F to 46°F) for 1-7 days (dependent on concentration and time to initiation); do not freeze. Protect from light.

If administered immediately, the following maximum durations of administration at room temperature according to solution concentration are recommended:

≥3000 to <6000 ng/mL: 12 hours
≥6000 to <30,000 ng/mL: 24 hours
≥30,000 ng/mL: 72 hours

If stored at 2°C to 8°C (36°F to 46°F) for 1 day, the following maximum durations of administration at room temperature according to solution concentration are recommended:

<6000 ng/mL: Do not use
≥6000 to <12,000 ng/mL: 12 hours
≥12,000 to <30,000 ng/mL: 24 hours
≥30,000 ng/mL: 48 hours

If stored at 2°C to 8°C (36°F to 46°F) for 7 days, the following maximum durations of administration at room temperature according to solution concentration are recommended:

<9000 ng/mL: Do not use
≥9000 to <30,000 ng/mL: 12 hours
≥30,000 ng/mL: 24 hours

If using previously reconstituted and stored vials, each vial must be further diluted (see table) prior to adding to the drug delivery reservoir. Each reservoir diluted to a concentration ≥15,000 ng/mL can be administered at room temperature for up to 24 hours; if lower concentrations are used, pump reservoirs should be changed every 12 hours.

Preparation of Epoprostenol Infusion

To make solution with concentration:	Flolan® Instructions	Veletri® Instructions
	Note: Flolan® may only be prepared with sterile diluent provided.	**Note:** Veletri® may only be prepared with sterile water for injection (SWFI) or NS.
3000 ng/mL	Dissolve one 0.5 mg vial with 5 mL supplied diluent, withdraw 3 mL, and add to a sufficient volume of supplied diluent to make a total of 100 mL.	Dissolve one 1.5 mg vial with 5 mL of SWFI or NS, withdraw 1 mL, and add to a sufficient volume of the identical diluent to make a total of 100 mL.
5000 ng/mL	Dissolve one 0.5 mg vial with 5 mL supplied diluent, withdraw entire vial contents, and add to a sufficient volume of supplied diluent to make a total of 100 mL.	
6000 ng/mL		Dissolve one 1.5 mg vial with 5 mL of SWFI or NS, withdraw 2 mL, and add to a sufficient volume of the identical diluent to make a total of 100 mL.
9000 ng/mL		Dissolve one 1.5 mg vial with 5 mL of SWFI or NS, withdraw 3 mL, and add to a sufficient volume of the identical diluent to make a total of 100 mL.
10,000 ng/mL	Dissolve two 0.5 mg vials each with 5 mL supplied diluent, withdraw entire vial contents, and add to a sufficient volume of supplied diluent to make a total of 100 mL.	
12,000 ng/mL		Dissolve one 1.5 mg vial with 5 mL of SWFI or NS, withdraw 4 mL, and add to a sufficient volume of the identical diluent to make a total of 100 mL.
15,000 ng/mL	Dissolve one 1.5 mg vial with 5 mL supplied diluent, withdraw entire vial contents, and add to a sufficient volume of supplied diluent to make a total of 100 mL.	Dissolve one 1.5 mg vial with 5 mL of SWFI or NS, withdraw entire vial contents, and add to a sufficient volume of the identical diluent to make a total of 100 mL.
20,000 ng/mL	Dissolve two 0.5 mg vials each with 5 mL supplied diluent, withdraw entire vial contents, and add to a sufficient volume of supplied diluent to make a total of **50 mL** (DeWet, 2004).	
30,000 ng/mL		Dissolve two 1.5 mg vials each with 5 mL of SWFI or NS, withdraw entire vial contents, and add to a sufficient volume of the identical diluent to make a total of 100 mL.

Mechanism of Action Epoprostenol is also known as prostacyclin and PGI_2. It is a strong vasodilator of all vascular beds. In addition, it is a potent endogenous inhibitor of platelet aggregation. The reduction in platelet aggregation results from epoprostenol's activation of intracellular adenylate cyclase and the resultant increase in cyclic adenosine monophosphate concentrations within the platelets. Additionally, it is capable of decreasing thrombogenesis and platelet clumping in the lungs by inhibiting platelet aggregation.

Pharmacodynamics/Kinetics

Metabolism: Rapidly hydrolyzed; subject to some enzymatic degradation; forms two active metabolites (6-keto-prostaglandin $F_1\alpha$ and 6,15-diketo-13,14-dihydro-prostaglandin $F_1\alpha$) with minimal activity and 14 inactive metabolites

Half-life elimination: ~6 minutes

Excretion: Urine (84%); feces (4%)

Dosage

I.V.:

Pulmonary arterial hypertension (PAH): Children (unlabeled use) and Adults: Initial: 2 ng/kg/minute; a lower initial dose may be used if patient is intolerant of starting dose. Increase dose in increments of 2 ng/kg/minute at intervals of ≥15 minutes until dose-limiting side effects (eg, flushing, jaw pain, headache, hypotension, nausea) are noted or response to epoprostenol plateaus. Usual optimal dose (monotherapy): 25-40 ng/kg/minute (McLaughlin, 2009); significant patient variability in optimal dose exists. Maximum dose with chronic therapy has not been defined; however, doses as high as 195 ng/kg/minute have been described in children (Rosenzweig, 1999).

Dose adjustment during chronic phase of treatment:

If PAH symptoms persist or recur following improvement, increase dose in 1-2 ng/kg/minute increments at intervals of ≥15 minutes. May also increase dose at intervals of 24-48 hours or longer (eg, every 1-2 weeks). **Note:** The need for increased doses should be expected with chronic use; incremental increases occur more frequently during the first few months after the drug is initiated.

In case of dose-limiting pharmacologic events (eg, hypotension, severe nausea, vomiting), decrease dose in 2 ng/kg/minute decrements at intervals of ≥15 minutes. Avoid abrupt withdrawal or sudden large dose reductions. **Note:** Adverse event may resolve without dosage adjustment.

Lung transplant: In patients receiving lung transplants, epoprostenol may be tapered after sequential lung transplantation once the allografts have been reperfused. If cardiopulmonary bypass utilized, epoprostenol may be tapered after pump perfusion has been initiated.

Acute vasodilator testing in patients with PAH (unlabeled use; McLaughlin, 2009): Adults: **Note:** Acute vasodilator testing should only be done in patients who might be considered candidates for calcium channel blocker therapy.

Initial: 2 ng/kg/minute; increase dose in increments of 2 ng/kg/minute every 10-15 minutes; dosing range during testing: 2-10 ng/kg/minute

Inhalation (unlabeled route): Adults:

Intraoperative pulmonary hypertension during cardiac surgery with cardiopulmonary bypass (CPB) (unlabeled use): **Note:** Institution-specific protocols vary.

Administration after induction of anesthesia before incision: 60 mcg (4 mL of 15,000 ng/mL concentration) via jet nebulizer; effect persists for ~25 minutes (Hache, 2003)

or

Intraoperative administration: Nebulization via ventilator circuit: Using a 15,000 ng/mL concentration and an oxygen flow of 8 L/minute, begin administration via jet nebulizer 5 minutes prior to weaning from CPB; discontinue at least 60 minutes after CPB weaned (Fattouch, 2006)

Post-cardiothoracic surgery pulmonary hypertension, right ventricular dysfunction, or refractory hypoxemia (unlabeled use) (DeWet, 2004): **Note:** May need to change ventilator filter every 2 hours due to glycine buffer diluent; may cause ventilator valve malfunction. Tidal volume delivered by ventilator may require adjustment.

Nebulization via ventilator circuit: Using a 20,000 ng/mL concentration, prime nebulizer chamber with 15 mL; administer remainder at a constant rate of 8 mL/hour; delivers ~38 ng/kg/minute (based on a 70 kg patient); set oxygen flow at 2-3 L/minute; wean as tolerated. **Note:** Although not achieved with this regimen, in general, doses >50 ng/kg/minute do not provide additional benefit and may increase the risk of hypotension.

or

Nebulization via facemask with Venturi attachment: Using a 20,000 ng/mL concentration, prime nebulizer chamber with 15 mL; set oxygen flow at 2-3 L/minute; 8 mL/hour will be nebulized; wean as tolerated.

Weaning procedure: Reduce dose by 50% every 2-4 hours (ie, 20,000 ng/mL to 10,000 ng/mL to 5000 ng/mL) until a concentration of 2500 ng/mL is reached; carefully discontinue once patient remains stable on this concentration for at least 4 hours.

Administration

I.V.: The ambulatory infusion pump should be small and lightweight, be able to adjust infusion rates in 2 ng/kg/minute increments, have occlusion, end of infusion, and low battery alarms, have ± 6% accuracy of the programmed rate, and have positive continuous or pulsatile pressure with intervals ≤3 minutes between pulses. The reservoir should be made of polyvinyl chloride, polypropylene, or glass. Immediate access to back up pump, infusion sets and medication is essential to prevent treatment interruptions.

Inhalation (unlabeled route):

Intraoperative administration: Administer via jet nebulizer connected to the inspiratory limb of the ventilator near the endotracheal tube with a bypass oxygen flow of 8 L/minute to achieve administration of a high proportion of small particles (Fattouch, 2006; Hache, 2003).

Post-cardiothoracic surgery: May also be administered via jet nebulizer connected to the inspiratory limb of the ventilator near the endotracheal tube or via face mask with a Venturi attachment for aerosolization with a bypass oxygen flow of 2-3 L/minute (De Wet, 2004). **Note:** Glycine buffer diluent may cause ventilator valve malfunction; it has been recommended that filters be changed on the ventilator every 2 hours; may also use a ventilator heating coil (De Wet, 2004).

Monitoring Parameters Monitor for improvements in pulmonary function, decreased exertional dyspnea, fatigue, syncope and chest pain, pulmonary vascular resistance, pulmonary arterial pressure and quality of life. In addition, the pump device and catheters should be monitored frequently to avoid "system" related failure. Monitor arterial pressure; assess all vital functions. Hypoxia, flushing, and tachycardia may indicate overdose.

Dosage Forms Excipient information presented when available (limited, particularly for generics); consult specific product labeling.

Injection, powder for reconstitution: 0.5 mg, 1.5 mg

Flolan®: 0.5 mg, 1.5 mg

Veletri®: 1.5 mg

- **Epoprostenol Sodium** *see* Epoprostenol *on page 604*
- **Epothilone B Lactam** *see* Ixabepilone *on page 945*
- **Eprex® (Can)** *see* Epoetin Alfa *on page 601*

Eprosartan (ep roe SAR tan)

Brand Names: U.S. Teveten®

Brand Names: Canada Teveten®

Pharmacologic Category Angiotensin II Receptor Blocker

Additional Appendix Information

Angiotensin Agents *on page 1869*

Use Treatment of hypertension; may be used alone or in combination with other antihypertensives

Pregnancy Risk Factor C (1st trimester); D (2nd and 3rd trimesters)

Pregnancy Considerations Medications which act on the renin-angiotensin system are reported to have the following fetal/neonatal effects: Hypotension, neonatal skull hypoplasia, anuria, renal failure, and death; oligohydramnios is also reported. These effects are reported to occur with exposure during the second and third trimesters. There are no adequate and well-controlled studies in pregnant women. **[U.S. Boxed Warning]: Based on human data, drugs that act on the angiotensin system can cause injury and death to the developing fetus when used in the second and third trimesters. Angiotensin receptor blockers should be discontinued as soon as possible once pregnancy is detected.**

Lactation Not recommended

Contraindications Hypersensitivity to eprosartan or any component of the formulation

Warnings/Precautions [U.S. Boxed Warning]: Based on human data, drugs that act on the angiotensin system can cause injury and death to the developing fetus when used in the second and third trimesters. Angiotensin receptor blockers should be discontinued as soon as possible once pregnancy is detected. May cause hyperkalemia; avoid potassium supplementation unless specifically required by healthcare provider. Avoid use or use a smaller dose in patients who are volume depleted; correct depletion first. May be associated with deterioration of renal function and/or increases in serum creatinine, particularly in patients with low renal blood flow (eg, renal artery stenosis, heart failure) whose glomerular filtration rate (GFR) is dependent on efferent arteriolar vasoconstriction by angiotensin II. Use with caution in unstented unilateral/bilateral renal artery stenosis. When unstented bilateral renal artery stenosis is present, use is generally avoided due to the elevated risk of deterioration in renal function unless possible benefits outweigh risks. Use with caution in pre-existing renal insufficiency; significant aortic/mitral stenosis. Concurrent use of ACE inhibitors may increase the risk of clinically-significant adverse events (eg, renal dysfunction, hyperkalemia).

Adverse Reactions

1% to 10%:

Central nervous system: Fatigue (2%), depression (1%)

Endocrine & metabolic: Hypertriglyceridemia (1%)

Gastrointestinal: Abdominal pain (2%)

Genitourinary: Urinary tract infection (1%)

Respiratory: Upper respiratory tract infection (8%), rhinitis (4%), pharyngitis (4%), cough (4%)

Miscellaneous: Viral infection (2%), injury (2%)

<1% (Limited to important or life-threatening): Abnormal ECG, angina, arthritis, asthma, ataxia, bradycardia, BUN increased, creatinine increased, eczema, edema, esophagitis, ethanol intolerance, gingivitis, gout, hypotension, influenza-like symptoms, leg cramps, leukopenia, maculopapular rash, migraine, neuritis, neutropenia, orthostasis, palpitation, paresthesia, peripheral ischemia, purpura, renal calculus, somnolence, tachycardia, tendonitis, thrombocytopenia, tinnitus, tremor, urinary incontinence, vertigo; rhabdomyolysis has been reported (rarely) with angiotensin-receptor antagonists.

Drug Interactions

Metabolism/Transport Effects Inhibits CYP2C9 (weak)

Avoid Concomitant Use There are no known interactions where it is recommended to avoid concomitant use.

Increased Effect/Toxicity

Eprosartan may increase the levels/effects of: ACE Inhibitors; Amifostine; Antihypertensives; Hypotensive Agents; Lithium; Nonsteroidal Anti-Inflammatory Agents; Potassium-Sparing Diuretics; RiTUXimab; Sodium Phosphates

The levels/effects of Eprosartan may be increased by: Alfuzosin; Diazoxide; Eplerenone; Herbs (Hypotensive Properties); MAO Inhibitors; Pentoxifylline; Phosphodiesterase 5 Inhibitors; Potassium Salts; Prostacyclin Analogues; Tolvaptan; Trimethoprim

Decreased Effect

The levels/effects of Eprosartan may be decreased by: Herbs (Hypertensive Properties); Methylphenidate; Nonsteroidal Anti-Inflammatory Agents; Yohimbine

Ethanol/Nutrition/Herb Interactions Herb/Nutraceutical: Avoid dong quai if using for hypertension (has estrogenic activity). Avoid ephedra, yohimbe, ginseng (may worsen hypertension). Avoid garlic (may have increased antihypertensive effect).

Mechanism of Action Angiotensin II is formed from angiotensin I in a reaction catalyzed by angiotensin-converting enzyme (ACE, kininase II). Angiotensin II is the principal pressor agent of the renin-angiotensin system, with effects that include vasoconstriction, stimulation of synthesis and release of aldosterone, cardiac stimulation, and renal reabsorption of sodium. Eprosartan blocks the vasoconstrictor and aldosterone-secreting effects of angiotensin II by selectively blocking the binding of angiotensin II to the AT1 receptor in many tissues, such as vascular smooth muscle and the adrenal gland. Its action is therefore independent of the pathways for angiotensin II synthesis. Blockade of the renin-angiotensin system with ACE inhibitors, which inhibit the biosynthesis of angiotensin II from angiotensin I, is widely used in the treatment of hypertension. ACE inhibitors also inhibit the degradation of bradykinin, a reaction also catalyzed by ACE. Because eprosartan does not inhibit ACE (kininase II), it does not affect the response to bradykinin. Whether this difference has clinical relevance is not yet known. Eprosartan does not bind to or block other hormone receptors or ion channels known to be important in cardiovascular regulation.

Pharmacodynamics/Kinetics

Protein binding: 98%

Metabolism: Minimally hepatic

Bioavailability: 300 mg dose: 13%

Half-life elimination: Terminal: 5-9 hours

Time to peak, serum: Fasting: 1-2 hours

Excretion: Feces (90%); urine (7%, mostly as unchanged drug)

Clearance: 7.9 L/hour

Dosage Adults: Oral: Dosage must be individualized; can administer once or twice daily with total daily doses of 400-800 mg. Usual starting dose is 600 mg once daily as monotherapy in patients who are euvolemic. Limited clinical experience with doses >800 mg.

Dosage adjustment in renal impairment: Moderate-to-severe impairment: No initial starting dosage adjustment is necessary; however, carefully monitor the patient. Maximum dose: 600 mg daily.

Hemodialysis: Poorly removed (Cl_{HD} <1 L/hour)

Dosage adjustment in hepatic impairment: No starting dosage adjustment is necessary; however, carefully monitor the patient

Elderly: No starting dosage adjustment is necessary; however, carefully monitor the patient

Monitoring Parameters Electrolytes, serum creatinine, BUN, urinalysis

Dosage Forms Excipient information presented when available (limited, particularly for generics); consult specific product labeling.

Tablet, oral: 600 mg

Teveten®: 400 mg, 600 mg

Eprosartan and Hydrochlorothiazide

(ep roe SAR tan & hye droe klor oh THYE a zide)

Brand Names: U.S. Teveten® HCT

Brand Names: Canada Teveten® HCT; Teveten® Plus

Index Terms Eprosartan Mesylate and Hydrochlorothiazide; Hydrochlorothiazide and Eprosartan

Pharmacologic Category Angiotensin II Receptor Blocker; Diuretic, Thiazide

Use Treatment of hypertension (not indicated for initial treatment)

Pregnancy Risk Factor C/D (2nd and 3rd trimesters)

Dosage Oral: Adults: Dose is individualized (combination substituted for individual components)

Usual recommended dose: Eprosartan 600 mg/hydrochlorothiazide 12.5 mg once daily (maximum dose: Eprosartan 600 mg/hydrochlorothiazide 25 mg once daily)

Dosage adjustment in renal impairment: Moderate-to-severe impairment: Initial dose adjustments are not necessary per manufacturer; however carefully monitor patient. Do not exceed a maximum dose of eprosartan 600 mg daily. Hydrochlorothiazide is ineffective in patients with Cl_{cr} <30 mL/minute.

Dosage adjustment in hepatic impairment: Initial dose adjustments not recommended by manufacturer; carefully monitor patient.

Additional Information Complete prescribing information for this medication should be consulted for additional detail.

Dosage Forms Excipient information presented when available (limited, particularly for generics); consult specific product labeling.

Tablet:

600 mg/12.5 mg: Eprosartan 600 mg and hydrochlorothiazide 12.5 mg

600 mg/25 mg: Eprosartan 600 mg and hydrochlorothiazide 25 mg

- ◆ **Eprosartan Mesylate and Hydrochlorothiazide** *see* Eprosartan and Hydrochlorothiazide *on page 608*
- ◆ **Epsilon Aminocaproic Acid** *see* Aminocaproic Acid *on page 89*
- ◆ **Epsom Salts** *see* Magnesium Sulfate *on page 1047*
- ◆ **EPT** *see* Teniposide *on page 1644*
- ◆ **Eptacog Alfa (Activated)** *see* Factor VIIa (Recombinant) *on page 681*

Eptifibatide

(ep TIF i ba tide)

Brand Names: U.S. Integrilin®

Brand Names: Canada Integrilin®

Index Terms Intrifiban

Pharmacologic Category Antiplatelet Agent, Glycoprotein IIb/IIIa Inhibitor

Use Treatment of patients with acute coronary syndrome (unstable angina/non-ST-segment elevation myocardial infarction [UA/NSTEMI]), including patients who are to be managed medically and those undergoing percutaneous coronary intervention (PCI including angioplasty, intracoronary stenting)

Unlabeled Use To support PCI during ST-elevation myocardial infarction (administered at the time of primary PCI); elective PCI for stable ischemic heart disease (in combination with unfractionated heparin)

Pregnancy Risk Factor B

Pregnancy Considerations Teratogenic effects were not observed in animal studies.

Lactation Excretion in breast milk unknown/use caution

Contraindications Hypersensitivity to eptifibatide or any component of the product; active abnormal bleeding within the previous 30 days or a history of bleeding diathesis; history of stroke within 30 days or a history of hemorrhagic stroke; severe hypertension (systolic blood pressure >200 mm Hg or diastolic blood pressure >110 mm Hg) not adequately controlled on antihypertensive therapy; major surgery within the preceding 6 weeks; current or planned administration of another parenteral GP IIb/IIIa inhibitor; dependency on hemodialysis

Canadian labeling: Additional contraindications (not in U.S. labeling): PT >1.2 times control or INR ≥2.0; known history of intracranial disease (eg, neoplasm, arteriovenous malformation, aneurysm); severe renal impairment (Cl_{cr} <30 mL/minute); thrombocytopenia (<100,000 cells/mm^3); clinically significant liver disease

Warnings/Precautions Bleeding is the most common complication. Most major bleeding occurs at the arterial access site where the cardiac catheterization was done. When bleeding can not be controlled with pressure, discontinue infusion and heparin. Patients <70 kg may be at greater risk for major and minor bleeding. Discontinue ≥2-4 hours prior to coronary artery bypass graft surgery (Hillis, 2011). Use caution in patients with hemorrhagic retinopathy or with other drugs that affect hemostasis. Use with extreme caution in patients with platelet counts <100,000/mm^3 (contraindicated in the Canadian labeling). If platelet count decreases to <100,000/mm^3 during therapy, discontinue eptifibatide and heparin if administered concurrently.

Concurrent use with thrombolytics has not been established as safe and is generally not recommended (Goodman, 2008). Minimize invasive procedures, including arterial and venous punctures, I.M. injections, and nasogastric tube insertion. Prior to sheath removal, the aPTT or ACT should be checked (do not remove unless aPTT is <45 seconds or the ACT <150 seconds). Use caution in renal dysfunction (estimated Cl_{cr} <50 mL/minute, using Cockcroft-Gault equation); dosage adjustment required. Use is contraindicated in patients dependent upon hemodialysis.

Adverse Reactions Bleeding is the major drug-related adverse effect. Access site is often primary source of bleeding complications. Incidence of bleeding is also related to heparin intensity. Patients weighing <70 kg may have an increased risk of major bleeding.

>10%: Hematologic: Bleeding (major: 1% to 11%; minor: 3% to 14%; transfusion required: 2% to 13%)

1% to 10%:
- Cardiovascular: Hypotension (up to 7%)
- Hematologic: Thrombocytopenia (1% to 3%)
- Local: Injection site reaction

<1% (Limited to important or life-threatening): Acute profound thrombocytopenia (including immune-mediated thrombocytopenia), fatal bleeding events, GI hemorrhage, pulmonary hemorrhage

Drug Interactions

Metabolism/Transport Effects None known.

Avoid Concomitant Use There are no known interactions where it is recommended to avoid concomitant use.

Increased Effect/Toxicity

Eptifibatide may increase the levels/effects of: Anticoagulants; Antiplatelet Agents; Collagenase (Systemic); Drotrecogin Alfa (Activated); Ibritumomab; Rivaroxaban; Salicylates; Thrombolytic Agents; Tositumomab and Iodine I 131 Tositumomab

The levels/effects of Eptifibatide may be increased by: Dasatinib; Glucosamine; Herbs (Anticoagulant/Antiplatelet Properties); Nonsteroidal Anti-Inflammatory Agents; Omega-3-Acid Ethyl Esters; Pentosan Polysulfate Sodium; Pentoxifylline; Prostacyclin Analogues; Vitamin E

Decreased Effect

The levels/effects of Eptifibatide may be decreased by: Nonsteroidal Anti-Inflammatory Agents

Ethanol/Nutrition/Herb Interactions Herb/Nutraceutical: Avoid alfalfa, anise, bilberry, bladderwrack, bromelain, cat's claw, celery, coleus, cordyceps, dong quai, evening primrose oil, fenugreek, feverfew, garlic, ginger, ginkgo biloba, ginseng (American), ginseng (Panax), ginseng (Siberian), grapeseed, green tea, guggul, horse chestnut seed, horseradish, licorice, prickly ash, red clover, reishi, same (s-adenosylmethionine), sweet clover, turmeric, and white willow (all have additional antiplatelet activity).

Stability Vials should be stored refrigerated at 2°C to 8°C (36°F to 46°F). Vials can be kept at room temperature for 2 months, after which they must be discarded. Protect from light until administration. Do not use beyond the expiration date. Discard any unused portion left in the vial.

Mechanism of Action Eptifibatide is a cyclic heptapeptide which blocks the platelet glycoprotein IIb/IIIa receptor, the binding site for fibrinogen, von Willebrand factor, and other ligands. Inhibition of binding at this final common receptor reversibly blocks platelet aggregation and prevents thrombosis.

Pharmacodynamics/Kinetics

Onset of action: Within 1 hour

Duration: Platelet function restored ~4 hours following discontinuation

Protein binding: ~25%

Half-life elimination: 2.5 hours

Excretion: Primarily urine (as eptifibatide and metabolites); significant renal impairment may alter disposition of this compound

Clearance: Total body: 55-58 mL/kg/hour; Renal: ~50% of total in healthy subjects

Dosage I.V.: Adults:

Acute coronary syndrome: Bolus of 180 mcg/kg (maximum: 22.6 mg) over 1-2 minutes, begun as soon as possible following diagnosis, followed by a continuous infusion of 2 mcg/kg/minute (maximum: 15 mg/hour) until hospital discharge or initiation of CABG surgery (discontinue ≥2-4 hours before surgery), up to 72 hours (if PCI performed during initial 72 hours, maintain continuous infusion at the time of PCI and continue until hospital discharge or for up to 18-24 hours, whichever comes first [total infusion time ≤96 hours]). Concurrent aspirin and heparin therapy (target aPTT 50-70 seconds) are recommended. **Note:** If UA/NSTEMI, administration ≥12 hours before angiography was shown not to be superior to provisional use at the time of PCI and has a higher incidence of bleeding (Giugliano, 2009).

Percutaneous coronary intervention (PCI) with or without stenting: Bolus of 180 mcg/kg (maximum: 22.6 mg) administered immediately before the initiation of PCI, followed by a continuous infusion of 2 mcg/kg/minute (maximum: 15 mg/hour). A second 180 mcg/kg bolus (maximum: 22.6 mg) should be administered 10 minutes after the first bolus. Infusion should be continued until hospital discharge or for up to 18-24 hours, whichever comes first; shorter infusion durations (ie, <2 hours) may be considered for nonemergent uncomplicated PCI in patients adequately pretreated with clopidogrel (Fung, 2007). Preprocedural aspirin and heparin therapy (ACT 200-250 seconds during PCI) are recommended. Heparin infusion after PCI is discouraged. In patients who undergo CABG surgery, discontinue infusion ≥2-4 hours prior to surgery.

Elderly: No dosing adjustment for the elderly appears to be necessary; adjust carefully to renal function.

Dosing adjustment in renal impairment: Dialysis is a contraindication to use.

Note: The Cockcroft-Gault equation using actual body weight should be used to estimate renal function.

Acute coronary syndrome: Cl_{cr} <50 mL/minute: 180 mcg/kg bolus (maximum: 22.6 mg) and 1 mcg/kg/minute infusion (maximum: 7.5 mg/hour)

Percutaneous coronary intervention (PCI) with or without stenting: Cl_{cr} <50 mL/minute: 180 mcg/kg bolus (maximum: 22.6 mg) administered immediately before the initiation of PCI and followed by a continuous infusion of 1 mcg/kg/minute (maximum: 7.5 mg/hour). Administer a second 180 mcg/kg (maximum: 22.6 mg) bolus 10 minutes after the first bolus.

Administration Do not shake vial. Visually inspect for discoloration or particulate matter prior to administration. The bolus dose should be withdrawn from the 10 mL vial into a syringe and administered by I.V. push over 1-2 minutes. Begin continuous infusion immediately following bolus administration, administered directly from the 100 mL vial. The 100 mL vial should be spiked with a vented infusion set.

Monitoring Parameters Coagulation parameters, signs/symptoms of excessive bleeding. Laboratory tests at baseline and monitoring during therapy: hematocrit and hemoglobin, platelet count, serum creatinine, PT/aPTT (maintain aPTT between 50-70 seconds unless PCI is to be performed), and ACT with PCI (maintain ACT between 200-300 seconds during PCI).

Assess sheath insertion site and distal pulses of affected leg every 15 minutes for the first hour and then every 1 hour for the next 6 hours. Arterial access site care is important to prevent bleeding. Care should be taken when attempting vascular access that only the anterior wall of the femoral artery is punctured, avoiding a Seldinger (through and through) technique for obtaining sheath access. Femoral vein sheath placement should be avoided unless needed. While the vascular sheath is in place, patients should be maintained on complete bedrest with the head of the bed at a 30° angle and the affected limb restrained in a straight position.

Observe patient for mental status changes, hemorrhage, assess nose and mouth mucous membranes, puncture sites for oozing, ecchymosis and hematoma formation, and examine urine, stool and emesis for presence of occult or frank blood; gentle care should be provided when removing dressings.

Dosage Forms Excipient information presented when available (limited, particularly for generics); consult specific product labeling.

Injection, solution:

Integrilin®: 0.75 mg/mL (100 mL); 2 mg/mL (10 mL, 100 mL)

◆ **Epzicom®** *see* Abacavir and Lamivudine *on page 20*

◆ **Equanil** *see* Meprobamate *on page 1077*

◆ **Equetro®** *see* CarBAMazepine *on page 280*

◆ **ER-086526** *see* Eribulin *on page 611*

◆ **Eraxis™** *see* Anidulafungin *on page 122*

◆ **Erbitux®** *see* Cetuximab *on page 332*

Ergocalciferol (er goe kal SIF e role)

Brand Names: U.S. Calciferol™ [OTC]; Drisdol®; Drisdol® [OTC]

Brand Names: Canada Drisdol®; Ostoforte®

Index Terms Activated Ergosterol; D2; Viosterol; Vitamin D2

Pharmacologic Category Vitamin D Analog

Use Treatment of refractory rickets, hypophosphatemia, hypoparathyroidism; dietary supplement

Unlabeled Use Prevention and treatment of vitamin D deficiency in patients with chronic kidney disease (CKD); osteoporosis prevention

Pregnancy Risk Factor C (manufacturer); A/C (dose exceeding RDA recommendation; per expert analysis)

Dosage Oral: **Note:** 1 mcg = 40 int. units

Dietary Reference Intake for Vitamin D:

0-12 months: Adequate intake: 400 int. units/day

1-18 years: RDA: 600 int. units/day

Adults:

19-70 years: RDA: 600 int. units/day

Female: Pregnancy/Lactating: RDA: 600 int. units/day

Elderly >70 years: RDA: 800 int. units/day

Adequate intake:

Breast-fed (fully or partially) Infants: 10 mcg/day (400 int. units/day) beginning in the first few days of life; continue supplementation until infant is weaned to ≥1 L/day or 1 quart/day of vitamin D-fortified formula or whole milk (after 12 months of age)

Nonbreast-fed Infants, Older Children ingesting <1000 mL of vitamin D-fortified formula or milk: 10 mcg/day (400 int. units/day)

Children with increased risk of vitamin D deficiency (chronic fat malabsorption, maintained on chronic anti-seizure medications): Higher doses may be required; use laboratory testing (25 [OH]D, PTH, bone mineral status) to evaluate

Osteoporosis prevention (unlabeled use): Adults ≥50 years: 800-1000 int. units/day (NOF guidelines, 2010)

Vitamin D deficiency treatment (unlabeled dose): Adults: 50,000 int. units once per week for 8 weeks, followed by 50,000 int. units every 2-4 weeks thereafter for maintenance of adequate levels (Holick, 2007) **or** 50,000 int. units twice per week for 5 weeks (Stechschulte, 2009)

Vitamin D deficiency/insufficiency in patients with CKD stages 3-4 (K/DOQI guidelines): **Note:** Dose is based on 25-hydroxyvitamin D serum level (25[OH]D):

Children (treatment duration should be a total of 3 months):

Serum 25(OH)D <5 ng/mL:

8000 int. units/day for 4 weeks, then 4000 int. units/day for 2 months **or**

50,000 int. units/week for 4 weeks, then 50,000 int. units twice a month for 2 months

Serum 25(OH)D 5-15 ng/mL:

4000 int units/day **or**

50,000 int units every other week

Serum 25(OH)D 16-30 ng/mL:

2000 int. units/day **or**

50,000 int. units every 4 weeks

Adults (treatment duration should be a total of 6 months):

Serum 25(OH)D <5 ng/mL:

50,000 int. units/week for 12 weeks, then 50,000 int. units/month

Serum 25(OH)D 5-15 ng/mL:

50,000 int. units/week for 4 weeks, then 50,000 int. units/month

Serum 25(OH)D 16-30 ng/mL:

50,000 int. units/month

Hypoparathyroidism:

Children: 1.25-5 mg/day (50,000-200,000 int. units) and calcium supplements

Adults: 625 mcg to 5 mg/day (25,000-200,000 int. units) and calcium supplements

Nutritional rickets and osteomalacia:

Children and Adults (with normal absorption): 25-125 mcg/day (1000-5000 int. units)

Children with malabsorption: 250-625 mcg/day (10,000-25,000 int. units)

Adults with malabsorption: 250-7500 mcg (10,000-300,000 int. units)

Vitamin D-*dependent* rickets:

Children: 75-125 mcg/day (3000-5000 int. units); maximum: 1500 mcg/day

Adults: 250 mcg to 1.5 mg/day (10,000-60,000 int. units)

Vitamin D-*resistant* rickets: Children and Adults: 12,000-500,000 int. units/day

Familial hypophosphatemia:

Children: 40,000-80,000 int. units plus phosphate supplements; dose may be reduced once growth is complete

Adults: 10,000-60,000 int. units plus phosphate supplements

Additional Information Complete prescribing information for this medication should be consulted for additional detail.

Dosage Forms Excipient information presented when available (limited, particularly for generics); consult specific product labeling.

Capsule, oral: 50,000 int. units

Drisdol®: 50,000 int. units [contains soybean oil, tartrazine; 1.25 mg]

Capsule, softgel, oral: 50,000 int. units, 50,000 units [1.25 mg]

Solution, oral [drops]: 8000 int. units/mL (60 mL)

Calciferol™: 8000 int. units/mL (60 mL) [contains propylene glycol; 200 mcg/mL]

Drisdol®: 8000 int. units/mL (60 mL) [contains propylene glycol; 200 mcg/mL, OTC]

Tablet, oral: 400 int. units

◆ **Ergomar®** *see* Ergotamine *on page 611*

Ergotamine (er GOT a meen)

Brand Names: U.S. Ergomar®

Index Terms Ergotamine Tartrate

Pharmacologic Category Antimigraine Agent; Ergot Derivative

Use Abort or prevent vascular headaches, such as migraine, migraine variants, or so-called "histaminic cephalalgia"

Pregnancy Risk Factor X

Dosage Sublingual: One tablet under tongue at first sign, then 1 tablet every 30 minutes if needed; maximum dose: 3 tablets/24 hours, 5 tablets/week

Additional Information Complete prescribing information for this medication should be consulted for additional detail.

Dosage Forms Excipient information presented when available (limited, particularly for generics); consult specific product labeling.

Tablet, sublingual, as tartrate:

Ergomar®: 2 mg [peppermint flavor]

◆ **Ergotamine Tartrate** *see* Ergotamine *on page 611*

Eribulin (er i BUE lin)

Brand Names: U.S. Halaven™

Index Terms B1939; E7389; ER-086526; Eribulin Mesylate; Halichondrin B Analog

Pharmacologic Category Antineoplastic Agent, Antimicrotubular

Use Treatment of metastatic breast cancer in patients who have received at least 2 prior chemotherapy regimens

Pregnancy Risk Factor D

Pregnancy Considerations Teratogenicity and fetal loss were observed in animal studies. There are no adequate and well-controlled studies in pregnant women. Based on its mechanism of action, eribulin would be expected to cause fetal harm if administered during pregnancy.

Lactation Excretion in breast milk unknown/not recommended

Contraindications There are no contraindications listed within the manufacturer's labeling.

Warnings/Precautions Hazardous agent - Use appropriate precautions for handling and disposal. Hematologic toxicity, including severe neutropenia, has occurred; may require treatment delay and dosage reduction. A higher incidence of grade 4 neutropenia and neutropenic fever occurred in patients with ALT or AST >3 x ULN or bilirubin >1.5 x ULN. Monitor complete blood counts prior to each dose; more frequently if severe cytopenias develop.

Peripheral neuropathy is a common toxicity; may be prolonged (>1 year in 5% of patients); may require treatment delay. Monitor for signs of motor or sensory neuropathy. Some patients may have pre-existing neuropathy due to prior chemotherapy; monitor closely for worsening.

QT prolongation was observed on day 8 (in an uncontrolled study); monitor ECG in patients with heart failure, bradyarrhythmia, and with concomitant medication known to prolong the QT interval; correct hypokalemia and hypomagnesemia prior to treatment; monitor electrolytes periodically during treatment. Avoid use in patients with congenital long QT syndrome.

Dosage reduction required in patients with mild-to-moderate (Child-Pugh class A or B) hepatic impairment; use has not been studied in patients with severe hepatic impairment; transaminase or bilirubin elevations are associated with a higher incidence of grade 4 neutropenia and neutropenic fever. Dosage reduction required in patients with renal impairment (Cl_{cr} 30-50 mL/minute); use has not been studied in patients with Cl_{cr} <30 mL/minute.

Adverse Reactions

>10%:

Central nervous system: Fatigue (54%), fever (21%), headache (19%)

Dermatologic: Alopecia (45%)

Gastrointestinal: Nausea (35%), stomatitis (5% to 18%), constipation (25%), weight loss (21%), anorexia (20%), diarrhea (18%), vomiting (18%)

Hematologic: Neutropenia (82%; grades 3: 28%; grade 4: 29%; nadir: 13 days; recovery: 8 days), anemia (58%; grades 3/4: 2%)

Hepatic: ALT increased (18%)

Neuromuscular & skeletal: Weakness (54%), peripheral neuropathy (35%; grades 3/4: ≤8%), arthralgia/myalgia (22%), back pain (16%), bone pain (12%), limb pain (11%)

Respiratory: Dyspnea (16%), cough (14%)

1% to 10%:

Cardiovascular: Peripheral edema

Central nervous system: Depression, dizziness, insomnia

Dermatologic: Rash

Endocrine & metabolic: Hypokalemia

Gastrointestinal: Mucosal inflammation (9%), abdominal pain, dyspepsia, taste alteration, xerostomia

Genitourinary: Urinary tract infection (10%)

Hematologic: Neutropenic fever (5%), thrombocytopenia (grades 3/4: 1%)

Neuromuscular & skeletal: Muscle spasm

Ocular: Lacrimation increased

Respiratory: Upper respiratory infection

<1% (Limited to important or life-threatening): Pharyngolaryngeal pain, sepsis

Drug Interactions

Metabolism/Transport Effects Substrate of CYP3A4 (minor); **Note:** Assignment of Major/Minor substrate status based on clinically relevant drug interaction potential; **Inhibits** CYP3A4 (weak)

Avoid Concomitant Use

Avoid concomitant use of Eribulin with any of the following: CloZAPine; Pimozide

Increased Effect/Toxicity

Eribulin may increase the levels/effects of: Antiarrhythmic Agents (Class Ia); Antiarrhythmic Agents (Class III); CloZAPine; Pimozide; Vitamin K Antagonists

The levels/effects of Eribulin may be increased by: Conivaptan

Decreased Effect

Eribulin may decrease the levels/effects of: Cardiac Glycosides; Vitamin K Antagonists

The levels/effects of Eribulin may be decreased by: Tocilizumab

Stability Store intact vials at 25°C (77°F); excursions permitted between 15°C and 30°C (59°F and 86°F); do not freeze. Store in original carton. May dilute in 100 mL normal saline. Undiluted solutions in a syringe and solutions diluted in normal saline for infusion are stable for up to 4 hours at room temperature or up to 24 hours refrigerated.

Mechanism of Action Eribulin is a non-taxane microtubule inhibitor which is a halichondrin B analog. It inhibits the growth phase of the microtubule by inhibiting formation of mitotic spindles causing mitotic blockage and arresting the cell cycle at the G_2/M phase; suppresses microtubule polymerization yet does not affect depolymerization.

Pharmacodynamics/Kinetics

Distribution: V_d: 43-114 L/m^2

Protein binding: 49% to 65%

Metabolism: Negligible

Half-life, elimination: ~40 hours

Excretion: Feces (82%; predominantly as unchanged drug); urine (9%, primarily as unchanged drug)

Dosage I.V.: Adults: Breast cancer, metastatic: 1.4 mg/m^2/dose on days 1 and 8 of a 21-day treatment cycle

Dosing adjustment in toxicity:

ANC <1000/mm^3 or platelets <75,000/mm^3 or grade 3 or 4 nonhematologic toxicity on day 1 or 8: Withhold dose; may delay day 8 dose up to 1 week. If toxicity resolves to ≤grade 2 by day 15 administer a reduced dose and wait at least 2 weeks before beginning the next cycle. Omit dose if not resolved to ≤grade 2 by day 15. Do not re-escalate dose after reduction.

Permanently reduce dose from 1.4 mg/m^2 to 1.1 mg/m^2 for the following:

- ANC <500/mm^3 for >7 days
- ANC <1000/mm^3 with fever or infection
- Platelets <25,000/mm^3
- Platelets <50,000/mm^3 requiring transfusion
- Nonhematologic toxicity of grade 3 or 4
- Dose omission or delay due to toxicity on day 8 of prior cycle

Permanently reduce dose from 1.1 mg/m^2 to 0.7 mg/m^2 for occurrence of any of the above events; discontinue treatment if the above toxicities occur at the 0.7 mg/m^2 dose level.

Dosage adjustment in renal impairment:

Cl_{cr} >50 mL/minute: No adjustment required

Cl_{cr} 30-50 mL/minute: Reduce to 1.1 mg/m^2/dose

Cl_{cr} <30 mL/minute: Use has not been studied

Dosage adjustment in hepatic impairment:

Mild hepatic impairment (Child-Pugh class A): Reduce to 1.1 mg/m^2/dose

Moderate hepatic impairment (Child-Pugh class B): Reduce to 0.7 mg/m^2/dose

Severe hepatic impairment (Child-Pugh class C): Use has not been studied

Administration I.V.: Infuse over 2-5 minutes. May be administered undiluted or diluted in 100 mL normal saline.

Monitoring Parameters CBC with differential prior to each dose; renal and liver function tests; serum electrolytes, including potassium and magnesium. Assess for peripheral neuropathy prior to each dose. Monitor ECG in patients with heart failure, bradyarrhythmia, and with concomitant medication known to prolong the QT interval, and electrolyte abnormalities (eg, hypokalemia, hypomagnesemia).

Dosage Forms Excipient information presented when available (limited, particularly for generics); consult specific product labeling.

Injection, solution, as mesylate:

Halaven™: 0.5 mg/mL (2 mL)

◆ **Eribulin Mesylate** *see* Eribulin *on page* 611

Erlotinib (er LOE tye nib)

Brand Names: U.S. Tarceva®

Brand Names: Canada Tarceva®

Index Terms CP358774; Erlotinib Hydrochloride; OSI-774

Pharmacologic Category Antineoplastic Agent, Tyrosine Kinase Inhibitor; Epidermal Growth Factor Receptor (EGFR) Inhibitor

Use Treatment of locally advanced or metastatic nonsmall cell lung cancer (NSCLC) refractory to at least 1 prior chemotherapy regimen (as monotherapy); maintenance treatment of locally advanced or metastatic NCSLC which has not progressed after 4-6 cycles of first line platinum-based chemotherapy; locally advanced, unresectable or metastatic pancreatic cancer (first-line therapy in combination with gemcitabine)

Unlabeled Use First-line treatment of NSCLC with known EGFR mutation; treatment of head and neck cancer

Pregnancy Risk Factor D

Pregnancy Considerations Animal studies have demonstrated fetal harm and abortion. There are no well-controlled studies in pregnant women. Women of childbearing potential should be advised to avoid pregnancy; adequate contraception is recommended during treatment and for 2 weeks after treatment has been completed.

Lactation Excretion in breast milk unknown/not recommended

Contraindications There are no contraindications listed within the FDA-approved manufacturer's labeling.

Canadian labeling: Hypersensitivity to erlotinib or any component of the formulation

Warnings/Precautions Hazardous agent - use appropriate precautions for handling and disposal. Rare, sometimes fatal, pulmonary toxicity, including interstitial lung disease (acute respiratory distress syndrome, interstitial pneumonia, obliterative bronchiolitis, pneumonitis, pulmonary fibrosis, and pulmonary infiltrates) has occurred; symptoms may begin within 5 days to more than 9 months after treatment initiation (median: 39 days). Interrupt therapy for unexplained pulmonary symptoms (dyspnea, cough, and fever); discontinue for confirmed ILD.

Liver enzyme elevations have been reported. Hepatic failure and hepatorenal syndrome have also been reported, particularly in patients with baseline hepatic impairment. Monitor liver function; patients with any hepatic impairment (total bilirubin >ULN; Child-Pugh class A, B, or C) should be closely monitored, including those with hepatic disease due to tumor burden; use with extreme caution in patients with total bilirubin >3 times ULN. Dosage reduction, interruption or discontinuation may be recommended for changes in hepatic function. Acute renal failure and renal insufficiency (with/without hypokalemia) have been reported; use with caution in patients with or at risk for renal impairment. Monitor closely for dehydration; monitor renal function and electrolytes in patients at risk for dehydration. Gastrointestinal perforation has been reported with use; risk for perforation is increased with concurrent antiangiogenic agents, corticosteroids, NSAIDs, and/or taxane based-therapy, and patients with history of peptic ulcers or diverticular disease; permanently discontinue in patients who develop perforation.

Bullous, blistering, or exfoliating skin conditions, some suggestive of Stevens-Johnson or toxic epidermal necrolysis (TEN) have been reported with use. Generalized or severe acneiform, erythematous or maculopapular rash may occur. Skin rash may correlate with treatment response and prolonged survival (Saif, 2008); management of skin rashes that are not serious should include alcohol-free lotions, topical antibiotics, or topical corticosteroids, or if necessary, oral antibiotics and systemic corticosteroids; avoid sunlight. Reduce dose or temporarily interrupt treatment for severe skin reactions; interrupt or discontinue treatment for bullous, blistering or exfoliative skin toxicity. Corneal perforation and ulceration have been reported with use; abnormal eyelash growth, keratoconjunctivitis sicca, or keratitis have also been reported and are known risk factors for corneal ulceration/perforation. Interrupt or discontinue treatment in patients presenting with eye pain or other acute or worsening ocular symptoms.

Use caution with cardiovascular disease; MI, CVA, and microangiopathic hemolytic anemia with thrombocytopenia have been noted in patients receiving concomitant erlotinib and gemcitabine. Elevated INR and bleeding events have been reported; use caution with concomitant anticoagulant therapy. Erlotinib levels may be lower in patients who smoke; advise patients to stop smoking. Smokers treated with 300 mg/day exhibited steady-state erlotinib levels comparable to former- and never-smokers receiving 150 mg/day (Hughes, 2009). Concurrent use with CYP3A4 inhibitors and moderate or strong CYP3A4 inducers may affect erlotinib levels; consider alternative agents to CYP3A4 inducers to avoid the potential for CYP-mediated interactions; use with caution in patients taking strong CYP3A4 inhibitors. Consider erlotinib dosage modification if concurrent use with CYP3A4 inhibitors/inducers cannot be avoided. In patients with NSCLC, EGFR mutations, specifically exon 19 deletions and exon 21 mutation (L858R), are associated with better response to erlotinib (Riely, 2006); erlotinib treatment is not recommended in patients with *K-ras* mutations; they are not likely to benefit from erlotinib treatment (Eberhard, 2005; Miller, 2008). Concurrent erlotinib plus platinum-based chemotherapy is not recommended for first line treatment of locally advanced or metastatic NSCLC due to a lack of clinical benefit. Product may contain lactose; avoid use in patients with Lapp lactase deficiency, glucose-galactose malabsorption, or glucose intolerance. Safety and efficacy have not been established in children.

Adverse Reactions

Adverse reactions reported with monotherapy:

>10%:

Central nervous system: Fatigue (9% to 52%)

Dermatologic: Rash (49% to 75%; grade 3: 6% to 8%; grade 4: <1%; median onset: 8 days), pruritus (7% to 13%), dry skin (4% to 12%)

Gastrointestinal: Diarrhea (20% to 54%; grade 3: 2% to 6%; grade 4: <1%; median onset: 12 days), anorexia (9% to 52%), nausea (33%), vomiting (23%), stomatitis (17%), abdominal pain (11%)

Ocular: Conjunctivitis (12%), keratoconjunctivitis sicca (12%)

Respiratory: Dyspnea (41%), cough (33%)

Miscellaneous: Infection (24%)

1% to 10%:

Dermatologic: Acne (6%), dermatitis acneiform (5%), paronychia (4%)

Gastrointestinal: Weight loss (4%)

Hepatic: ALT increased (grade 2: 2% to 4%; grade 3: 1%), hyperbilirubinemia (grade 2: 4%; grade 3: <1%)

Respiratory: Pneumonitis/pulmonary infiltrate (3%), pulmonary fibrosis (3%)

Adverse reactions reported with combination (erlotinib plus gemcitabine) therapy:

Cardiovascular: Edema (37%), thrombotic events (grades 3/4: 11%), deep venous thrombosis (4%), cerebrovascular accident (2%; including cerebral hemorrhage), MI/myocardial ischemia (2%), arrhythmia, syncope

Central nervous system: Fatigue (79%), fever (36%), depression (19%), dizziness (15%), headache (15%), anxiety (13%)

Dermatologic: Rash (69%), alopecia (14%)

Gastrointestinal: Nausea (60%), anorexia (52%), diarrhea (48%), abdominal pain (46%), vomiting (42%), weight loss (39%), stomatitis (22%), dyspepsia (17%), flatulence (13%), ileus, pancreatitis

Hematologic: Hemolytic anemia, microangiopathic hemolytic anemia with thrombocytopenia (1%)

Hepatic: ALT increased (grade 2: 31%, grade 3: 13%, grade 4: <1%), AST increased (grade 2: 24%, grade 3: 10%, grade 4 <1%), hyperbilirubinemia (grade 2: 17%, grade 3: 10%, grade 4: <1%)

Neuromuscular & skeletal: Bone pain (25%), myalgia (21%), neuropathy (13%), rigors (12%)

Renal: Renal insufficiency

Respiratory: Dyspnea (24%), cough (16%), interstitial lung disease (ILD)-like events (3%)

Miscellaneous: Infection (39%)

Mono- or combination therapy: <1% (Limited to important or life-threatening): Acute renal failure, bronchiolitis, blistering/bullous/exfoliative skin conditions (suggesting Stevens-Johnson syndrome or TEN), corneal perforation, corneal ulcerations, episcleritis, epistaxis, eye lash disorders (ingrown lashes, excessive growth, thickening), gastritis, gastroduodenal ulcers, GI bleeding, GI hemorrhage, GI perforation, hair/nail disorders (alopecia, brittle/loose nails, hirsutism), hearing loss, hematemesis, hematochezia, hepatic failure, hepatorenal syndrome, hepatotoxicity, hyperpigmentation, hypokalemia, keratitis, melena, peptic ulcer bleeding, rash (acneiform; sparing prior radiation field), skin fissures, tympanic membrane perforation

Drug Interactions

Metabolism/Transport Effects Substrate of CYP1A2 (minor), CYP3A4 (major); **Note:** Assignment of Major/Minor substrate status based on clinically relevant drug interaction potential

Avoid Concomitant Use

Avoid concomitant use of Erlotinib with any of the following: Conivaptan; Proton Pump Inhibitors

Increased Effect/Toxicity

Erlotinib may increase the levels/effects of: Vitamin K Antagonists

The levels/effects of Erlotinib may be increased by: Antifungal Agents (Azole Derivatives, Systemic); Ciprofloxacin; Ciprofloxacin (Systemic); Conivaptan; CYP3A4 Inhibitors (Moderate); CYP3A4 Inhibitors (Strong); Dasatinib; FluvoxaMINE

Decreased Effect

Erlotinib may decrease the levels/effects of: Cardiac Glycosides; Vitamin K Antagonists

The levels/effects of Erlotinib may be decreased by: Antacids; CYP3A4 Inducers (Strong); Cyproterone; Deferasirox; H2-Antagonists; Herbs (CYP3A4 Inducers); Proton Pump Inhibitors; Rifampin; Tocilizumab

Ethanol/Nutrition/Herb Interactions

Food: Erlotinib bioavailability is increased with food. Avoid grapefruit or grapefruit juice (may decrease the metabolism and increase erlotinib plasma concentrations).

Herb/Nutraceutical: Avoid St John's wort (may increase metabolism and decrease erlotinib concentrations).

Stability Store at room temperature of 25°C (77°F); excursions permitted to 15°C and 30°C (59°F and 86°F).

Mechanism of Action The mechanism of erlotinib's antitumor action is not fully characterized. It is known to inhibit overall epidermal growth factor receptor (HER1/EGFR) - tyrosine kinase. Active competitive inhibition of adenosine triphosphate inhibits downstream signal transduction of ligand dependent HER1/EGFR activation.

Pharmacodynamics/Kinetics

Absorption: Oral: 60% on an empty stomach; almost 100% on a full stomach

Distribution: 94-232 L

Protein binding: 92% to 95% to albumin and α_1-acid glycoprotein

Metabolism: Hepatic, via CYP3A4 (major), CYP1A1 (minor), CYP1A2 (minor), and CYP1C (minor)

Bioavailability: Almost 100% when given with food; 60% without food

Half-life elimination: 24-36 hours

Time to peak, plasma: 1-7 hours

Excretion: Primarily as metabolites: Feces (83%; 1% as unchanged drug); urine (8%)

Dosage Oral: Adults: **Note:** Details concerning dosing in combination regimens should also be consulted. Continue treatment until disease progression or unacceptable toxicity. Dose adjustments are likely to be needed when erlotinib is administered concomitantly with strong CYP3A4 inducers or inhibitors, or with continued smoking.

NSCLC, refractory: 150 mg once daily

NSCLC, maintenance therapy: 150 mg once daily

Pancreatic cancer: 100 mg once daily in combination with gemcitabine

NSCLC, first-line therapy in patients with EGFR mutations (unlabeled use): 150 mg once daily (Rosell, 2009)

Dosage adjustment for concomitant CYP3A4 inhibitors/inducers:

CYP3A4 inhibitors: Consider dose reductions for severe adverse reactions when erlotinib is administered concomitantly with strong CYP3A4 inhibitors (eg, azole antifungals, clarithromycin, erythromycin, nefazodone, protease inhibitors, telithromycin). Dose reduction (if required) should be done in decrements of 50 mg.

Concomitant CYP3A4 and CYP1A2 inhibitor (eg, ciprofloxacin): Consider dose reductions if severe adverse reactions occur.

CYP3A4 inducers: Alternatives to the enzyme-inducing agent should be utilized first. Concomitant administration with CYP3A4 inducers (eg, carbamazepine, phenobarbital, phenytoin, rifamycins, and St John's wort) may require increased erlotinib doses (increase as tolerated at 2-week intervals); doses >150 mg/day should be considered with rifampin (the maximum erlotinib dose studied in combination with rifampin was 450 mg). Immediately reduce erlotinib dose to recommended starting dose when CYP3A4 inducer is discontinued.

Dosage adjustment for concomitant smoking: A dose increase to a maximum dose of 300 mg (with careful monitoring) may be required in patients who continue to smoke; immediately reduce erlotinib dose to recommended starting dose upon smoking cessation.

Dosage adjustment for toxicity: Dose reductions should be made in 50 mg decrements

Diarrhea: Manage with loperamide; in severe diarrhea (unresponsive to loperamide) or dehydration due to diarrhea, reduce dose or temporarily interrupt treatment

Pulmonary symptoms: Acute onset (or worsening) of pulmonary symptoms (eg, dyspnea, cough, fever): Interrupt treatment and evaluate for drug-induced interstitial lung disease; discontinue permanently with development of interstitial lung disease

Severe skin reaction: Reduce dose or temporarily interrupt treatment

Bullous, blistering or exfoliative skin toxicity, acute or worsening ocular toxicities, or dehydration with risk for renal failure: Interrupt or discontinue treatment

Gastrointestinal perforation, hepatic failure: Discontinue treatment

Dosage adjustment in renal impairment: Interrupt treatment for risk of renal disease due to dehydration; may resume after euvolemia re-established.

Dosage adjustment in hepatic impairment:

The manufacturer recommends the following guidelines:

Patients with normal hepatic function at baseline: Total bilirubin >3 times ULN and/or transaminases >5 times ULN: Interrupt or discontinue treatment

Patients with baseline hepatic impairment:

Total bilirubin >3 times ULN: Use extreme caution

Worsening liver function (not yet severe): Interrupt treatment and/or reduce dose

Severe changes in liver function (eg, doubling of total bilirubin and/or tripling of transaminases): Interrupt or discontinue treatment

A reduced starting dose (75 mg once daily) has been recommended in patients with hepatic dysfunction (AST ≥3 times ULN or direct bilirubin 1-7 mg/dL), with individualized dosage escalation if tolerated (Miller, 2007).

Dietary Considerations Take this medicine an empty stomach, 1 hour before or 2 hours after a meal. Avoid grapefruit juice.

Administration The manufacturer recommends administration on an empty stomach (at least 1 hour before or 2 hours after the ingestion of food).

For patients unable to swallow whole, tablets may be dissolved in 100 mL water and administered orally or via feeding tube (silicone-based); to ensure full dose is received, rinse container with 40 mL water, administer residue and repeat rinse (data on file, Genentech; Siu, 2007; Soulieres, 2004).

Monitoring Parameters Periodic liver function tests (transaminases, bilirubin, and alkaline phosphatase); monitor more frequently with worsening liver function; periodic renal function tests and serum electrolytes (in patients at risk for dehydration); hydration status

Additional Information Oncology Comment: According to the National Comprehensive Cancer Network® (NCCN) pancreatic adenocarcinoma guidelines, gemcitabine combination therapy (including gemcitabine plus erlotinib) is an option for patients with good performance status in the treatment of locally-advanced or metastatic pancreatic cancer.

The NCCN guidelines for NSCLC recommend erlotinib as single agent treatment for disease progression after failure of first- or second-line treatment in patients with a performance status of 0-2. Erlotinib is considered a first-line single-agent therapy in patients with advanced or metastatic NSCLC who have a known active EGFR mutation or gene amplification. Erlotinib may also be used as maintenance treatment of recurrent or metastatic NCSLC which has not progressed after 4-6 cycles of first-line platinum-based chemotherapy.

Factors (in patients with NSCLC) which correlate positively with response to EGFR-tyrosine kinase inhibitor (TKI) therapy include skin rash (due to EGFR-TKI therapy), patients who have never smoked, EGFR mutation, and patients of Asian origin. EGFR mutations, specifically exon 19 deletions and exon 21 mutation (L858R) correlate with response to tyrosine kinase inhibitors (NCCN NSCLC guidelines v.2.2010; Riely, 2006). *K-ras* mutations correlated with poorer outcome with EGFR-TKI therapy in patients with NSCLC. (Cooley, 2008; Jackman, 2008; Masarelli, 2007; Shepherd, 2005).

Dosage Forms Excipient information presented when available (limited, particularly for generics); consult specific product labeling.

Tablet, oral:

Tarceva®: 25 mg, 100 mg, 150 mg

Extemporaneous Preparations A suspension for oral or feeding tube (silicone-based) administration may be prepared by dissolving tablets needed for dose in 100 mL water. To ensure full dose is received, rinse container with 40 mL water, administer residue and repeat rinse. Administer immediately after preparation; stability of solution is unknown (Tarceva® data on file from Genentech).

Siu LL, Soulieres D, Chen EX, et al, "Phase I/II Trial of Erlotinib and Cisplatin in Patients With Recurrent or Metastatic Squamous Cell Carcinoma of the Head and Neck: A Princess Margaret Hospital Phase II Consortium and National Cancer Institute of Canada Clinical Trials Group Study," *J Clin Oncol*, 2007, 25(16):2178-83.

Soulieres D, Senzer NN, Vokes EE, et al, "Multicenter Phase II Study of Erlotinib, an Oral Epidermal Growth Factor Receptor Tyrosine Kinase Inhibitor, in Patients With Recurrent or Metastatic Squamous Cell Cancer of the Head and Neck," *J Clin Oncol*, 2004, 22(1):77-85.

◆ **Erlotinib Hydrochloride** *see* Erlotinib *on page 612*

◆ **E-R-O® [OTC]** *see* Carbamide Peroxide *on page 283*

◆ **Errin®** *see* Norethindrone *on page 1217*

◆ **Ertaczo®** *see* Sertaconazole *on page 1548*

Ertapenem (er ta PEN em)

Brand Names: U.S. INVanz®

Brand Names: Canada Invanz®

Index Terms Ertapenem Sodium; L-749,345; MK0826

Pharmacologic Category Antibiotic, Carbapenem

Use Treatment of the following moderate-to-severe infections: Complicated intra-abdominal infections, complicated skin and skin structure infections (including diabetic foot infections without osteomyelitis, animal and human bites), complicated UTI (including pyelonephritis), acute pelvic infections (including postpartum endomyometritis, septic abortion, postsurgical gynecologic infections), and community-acquired pneumonia. Prophylaxis of surgical site infection following elective colorectal surgery. Antibacterial coverage includes aerobic gram-positive organisms, aerobic gram-negative organisms, and anaerobic organisms.

Note: Methicillin-resistant *Staphylococcus aureus, Enterococcus* spp, penicillin-resistant strains of *Streptococcus pneumoniae, Acinetobacter,* and *Pseudomonas aeruginosa,* are **resistant** to ertapenem while most extended-spectrum β-lactamase (ESBL)-producing bacteria remain sensitive to ertapenem.

Unlabeled Use Treatment of intravenous catheter-related bloodstream infection

Pregnancy Risk Factor B

Pregnancy Considerations With the exception of slightly decreased fetal weights in mice, teratogenic effects and fetal harm have not been shown in animal studies. Adequate and well-controlled studies have not been conducted in pregnant women and it is not known whether ertapenem can cause fetal harm.

Lactation Enters breast milk/use caution

Contraindications Hypersensitivity to ertapenem, other carbapenems (eg, doripenem, imipenem, meropenem), or any component of the formulation; anaphylactic reactions to beta-lactam antibiotics. If using intramuscularly, known hypersensitivity to local anesthetics of the amide type (lidocaine is the diluent).

Warnings/Precautions Use caution with renal impairment. Dosage adjustment required in patients with moderate-to-severe renal dysfunction; elderly patients often require lower doses (based upon renal function). Use may result in fungal or bacterial superinfection, including *C. difficile*-associated diarrhea (CDAD) and pseudomembranous colitis; CDAD has been observed >2 months postantibiotic treatment. Carbapenems have been associated with CNS adverse effects, including confusional states and seizures (myoclonic); use caution with CNS disorders (eg, brain lesions and history of seizures) and adjust dose in renal impairment to avoid drug accumulation, which may increase seizure risk. Serious hypersensitivity reactions, including anaphylaxis, have been reported (some without a history of previous allergic reactions to beta-lactams). Doses for I.M. administration are mixed with lidocaine; consult Lidocaine (Systemic) on page 1007 information for associated Warnings/Precautions. May decrease divalproex sodium/valproic acid concentrations leading to breakthrough seizures; concomitant use not recommended. Safety and efficacy have not been established in children <3 months of age.

Adverse Reactions Note: Percentages reported in adults.

1% to 10%:

Cardiovascular: Edema (3%), chest pain (1% to 2%), hypertension (1% to 2%), hypotension (1% to 2%), tachycardia (1% to 2%)

Central nervous system: Headache (6% to 7%); altered mental status (eg, agitation, confusion, disorientation, mental acuity decreased, somnolence, stupor) (3% to 5%); fever (2% to 5%), insomnia (3%), dizziness (2%), fatigue (1%), anxiety (1%)

Dermatologic: Rash (2% to 3%), pruritus (1% to 2%), erythema (1% to 2%)

Endocrine & metabolic: Hypokalemia (2%), hyperglycemia (1% to 2%), hyperkalemia (≤1%)

Gastrointestinal: Diarrhea (9% to 10%), nausea (6% to 9%), abdominal pain (4%), vomiting (4%), constipation (3% to 4%), acid regurgitation (1% to 2%), dyspepsia (1%), oral candidiasis (≤1%)

Genitourinary: Urine WBCs increased (2% to 3%), urine RBCs increased (1% to 3%), vaginitis (1% to 3%)

Hematologic: Thrombocytosis (4% to 7%), hematocrit/hemoglobin decreased (3% to 5%), eosinophils increased (1% to 2%), leukopenia (1% to 2%), neutrophils decreased (1% to 2%), thrombocytopenia (1%), prothrombin time increased (≤1%)

Hepatic: Hepatic enzyme increased (7% to 9%), alkaline phosphatase increase (4% to 7%), albumin decreased (1% to 2%), bilirubin (total) increased (1% to 2%)

Local: Infused vein complications (5% to 7%), phlebitis/thrombophlebitis (2%), extravasation (1% to 2%)

Neuromuscular & skeletal: Weakness (1%), leg pain (≤1%)

Renal: Serum creatinine increased (1%)

Respiratory: Dyspnea (1% to 3%), cough (1% to 2%), pharyngitis (1%), rales/rhonchi (1%), respiratory distress (≤1%)

<1% (Limited to important or life-threatening): Anaphylactoid reactions, anaphylaxis, arrhythmia, asthma, asystole, atrial fibrillation, bradycardia, bronchoconstriction, *C. difficile*-associated diarrhea, cardiac arrest, cholelithiasis, delirium, DRESS syndrome, dyskinesia, dysphagia, facial edema, gastritis, gastrointestinal hemorrhage, gout,

heart failure, heart murmur, hemoptysis, hypoxemia, ileus, jaundice, myoclonus, oliguria/anuria, pancreatitis, pleural effusion, renal insufficiency, seizure, septicemia, septic shock, subdural hemorrhage, syncope, ventricular tachycardia

Drug Interactions

Metabolism/Transport Effects None known.

Avoid Concomitant Use

Avoid concomitant use of Ertapenem with any of the following: BCG

Increased Effect/Toxicity

The levels/effects of Ertapenem may be increased by: Probenecid

Decreased Effect

Ertapenem may decrease the levels/effects of: BCG; Divalproex; Typhoid Vaccine; Valproic Acid

Stability Before reconstitution store at ≤25°C (77°F).

I.M.: Reconstitute 1 g vial with 3.2 mL of 1% lidocaine HCl injection (without epinephrine). Shake well. Use within 1 hour after preparation.

I.V.: Reconstitute 1 g vial with 10 mL of sterile water for injection, 0.9% sodium chloride injection, or bacteriostatic water for injection. Shake well. For adults, transfer dose to 50 mL of 0.9% sodium chloride injection; for children, dilute dose with NS to a final concentration ≤20 mg/mL. Reconstituted I.V. solution may be stored at room temperature and must be used within 6 hours **or** refrigerated, stored for up to 24 hours and used within 4 hours after removal from refrigerator. Do not freeze.

Mechanism of Action Inhibits bacterial cell wall synthesis by binding to one or more of the penicillin-binding proteins; which in turn inhibits the final transpeptidation step of peptidoglycan synthesis in bacterial cell walls, thus inhibiting cell wall biosynthesis. Bacteria eventually lyse due to ongoing activity of cell wall autolytic enzymes (autolysins and murein hydrolases) while cell wall assembly is arrested.

Pharmacodynamics/Kinetics

Absorption: I.M.: Almost complete

Distribution: V_{dss}:

Children 3 months to 12 years: ~0.2 L/kg

Children 13-17 years: ~0.16 L/kg

Adults: ~0.12 L/kg

Protein binding (concentration dependent, primarily to albumin): 85% at 300 mcg/mL, 95% at <100 mcg/mL

Metabolism: Non-CYP-mediated hydrolysis to inactive metabolite

Bioavailability: I.M.: ~90%

Half-life elimination:

Children 3 months to 12 years: ~2.5 hours

Children ≥13 years and Adults: ~4 hours

Time to peak: I.M.: ~2.3 hours

Excretion: Urine (~80% as unchanged drug and metabolite); feces (~10%)

Dosage Note: I.V. therapy may be administered for up to 14 days; I.M. therapy for up to 7 days

Usual dosage ranges:

Children 3 months to 12 years: I.M., I.V.: 15 mg/kg twice daily (maximum: 1 g/day)

Children ≥13 years and Adults: I.M., I.V.: 1 g/day

Indication-specific dosing:

Children 3 months to 12 years: I.M., I.V.:

Community-acquired pneumonia, complicated urinary tract infections (including pyelonephritis): 15 mg/kg twice daily (maximum: 1 g/day); duration of total antibiotic treatment: 10-14 days (**Note:** Duration includes possible switch to appropriate oral therapy after at least 3 days of parenteral treatment, once clinical improvement demonstrated.)

Intra-abdominal infection: 15 mg/kg twice daily (maximum: 1 g/day) for 5-14 days

Pelvic infections (acute): 15 mg/kg twice daily (maximum: 1 g/day) for 3-10 days

Skin and skin structure infections: 15 mg/kg twice daily (maximum: 1 g/day) for 7-14 days

Children ≥13 years and Adults: I.M., I.V.:

Community-acquired pneumonia, complicated urinary tract infections (including pyelonephritis): 1 g/day; duration of total antibiotic treatment: 10-14 days; duration includes possible switch to appropriate oral therapy after at least 3 days of parenteral treatment, once clinical improvement demonstrated. **Note:** The carbapenems, including ertapenem, are preferred agents for *Enterobacteriaceae, Burkholderia pseudomallei, Acinetobacter* pneumonia and considered alternative agents for anaerobes in aspiration pneumonia (IDSA, 2007).

Intra-abdominal infection: 1 g/day for 5-14 days; **Note:** 2010 IDSA guidelines recommend a treatment duration of 4-7 days (provided source controlled) for community-acquired, mild-to-moderate IAI

Pelvic infections (acute): 1 g/day for 3-10 days

Skin and skin structure infections (including moderate diabetic foot infections and animal or human bites): 1 g/day for 7-14 days (**Note:** IDSA guidelines recommend ertapenem as the preferred agent for animal bites. [IDSA, 2005].)

Adults: I.V.:

Prophylaxis of surgical site following colorectal surgery: 1 g given 1 hour preoperatively

Intravenous catheter-related bloodstream infection (unlabeled use): 1 g/day (**Note:** Carbapenems, including ertapenem, are preferred agents for extended-spectrum β-lactamase (ESBL)-positive *Escherichia coli* and *Klebsiella, Enterobacter,* and *Serratia* [IDSA, 2009].)

Dosage adjustment in renal impairment:

Children: No data available for pediatric patients with renal insufficiency.

Adults:

Cl_{cr} >30 mL/minute/1.73 m^2: No adjustment required

Cl_{cr} ≤30 mL/minute/1.73 m^2 and ESRD: 500 mg/day

Hemodialysis: Adults: When the daily dose is given within 6 hours prior to hemodialysis, a supplementary dose of 150 mg is required following hemodialysis.

CAPD: I.V.: 500 mg/day (Cardone, 2011)

Dosage adjustment in hepatic impairment: Adjustments cannot be recommended (lack of experience and research in this patient population).

Dietary Considerations Some products may contain sodium.

Administration

I.M.: Avoid injection into a blood vessel. Make sure patient does not have an allergy to lidocaine or another anesthetic of the amide type. Administer by deep I.M. injection into a large muscle mass (eg, gluteal muscle or lateral part of the thigh). Do not administer I.M. preparation or drug reconstituted for I.M. administration intravenously.

I.V.: Infuse over 30 minutes

Monitoring Parameters Periodic renal, hepatic, and hematopoietic assessment during prolonged therapy; neurological assessment

Dosage Forms Excipient information presented when available (limited, particularly for generics); consult specific product labeling.

Injection, powder for reconstitution:

INVanz®: 1 g [contains sodium ~137 mg (~6 mEq)/g]

◆ **Ertapenem Sodium** *see* Ertapenem *on page 615*

◆ **Erwinase® (Can)** *see* Asparaginase (*Erwinia*) *on page 153*

◆ **Erwinaze™** *see* Asparaginase (*Erwinia*) *on page 153*

◆ ***Erwinia chrysanthemi*** *see* Asparaginase (*Erwinia*) *on page 153*

◆ **Ery** *see* Erythromycin (Topical) *on page 619*

- ◆ **Erybid™ (Can)** *see* Erythromycin (Systemic) *on page 617*
- ◆ **Eryc® (Can)** *see* Erythromycin (Systemic) *on page 617*
- ◆ **EryPed®** *see* Erythromycin (Systemic) *on page 617*
- ◆ **Ery-Tab®** *see* Erythromycin (Systemic) *on page 617*
- ◆ **Erythrocin®** *see* Erythromycin (Systemic) *on page 617*
- ◆ **Erythrocin® Lactobionate-I.V.** *see* Erythromycin (Systemic) *on page 617*

Erythromycin (Systemic) (er ith roe MYE sin)

Brand Names: U.S. E.E.S.®; Ery-Tab®; EryPed®; Erythro-RX; Erythrocin®; Erythrocin® Lactobionate-I.V.; PCE®

Brand Names: Canada Apo-Erythro Base®; Apo-Erythro E-C®; Apo-Erythro-ES®; Apo-Erythro-S®; EES®; Erybid™; Eryc®; Novo-Rythro Estolate; Novo-Rythro Ethylsuccinate; Nu-Erythromycin-S; PCE®

Index Terms Erythromycin Base; Erythromycin Ethylsuccinate; Erythromycin Lactobionate; Erythromycin Stearate

Pharmacologic Category Antibiotic, Macrolide

Additional Appendix Information

Prevention of Wound Infection and Sepsis in Surgical Patients *on page 1954*

Use Treatment of susceptible bacterial infections including *S. pyogenes*, some *S. pneumoniae*, some *S. aureus*, *M. pneumoniae*, *Legionella pneumophila*, diphtheria, pertussis, *Chlamydia*, erythrasma, *N. gonorrhoeae*, *E. histolytica*, syphilis and nongonococcal urethritis, and *Campylobacter* gastroenteritis; used in conjunction with neomycin for decontaminating the bowel

Unlabeled Use Treatment of gastroparesis, chancroid; preoperative gut sterilization

Pregnancy Risk Factor B

Pregnancy Considerations Adverse events were not observed in animal studies; therefore, erythromycin is classified as pregnancy category B. Erythromycin crosses the placenta and low concentrations are found in the fetal serum. No increased risk for congenital abnormalities has been documented, with the exception of a possible slight increase in risk for cardiovascular anomalies. Most studies do not support a link between prenatal exposure to erythromycin and pyloric stenosis in the neonate. In general, serum concentrations of erythromycin are lower in pregnant women. Erythromycin therapy in patients with preterm, premature rupture of membranes is associated with a range of health benefits to the neonate and long-term adverse events to the child have not been observed. However, maternal use of erythromycin in women with preterm labor, intact membranes, and no documented infection does not improve neonatal health and may have adverse effects in childhood (use is not recommended). Erythromycin is the antibiotic of choice for preterm premature rupture of membranes (with membrane rupture prior to 34 weeks gestation), the treatment of granuloma inguinale and lymphogranuloma venereum in pregnancy, and the treatment of or long-term suppression of *Bartonella* infection in HIV-infected pregnant patients. Erythromycin may be appropriate as an alternative agent for the prevention of group B streptococcal disease or the treatment of chlamydial infections in pregnant women (consult current guidelines).

Lactation Enters breast milk/use caution (AAP considers "compatible"; AAP 2001 update pending)

Contraindications Hypersensitivity to erythromycin, any macrolide antibiotics, or any component of the formulation

Concomitant use with pimozide, cisapride, ergotamine or dihydroergotamine, terfenadine, astemizole

Warnings/Precautions Use caution with hepatic impairment with or without jaundice has occurred, it may be accompanied by malaise, nausea, vomiting, abdominal colic, and fever; discontinue use if these occur. Use caution with other medication relying on CYP3A4 metabolism; high potential for drug interactions exists. Prolonged use may result in fungal or bacterial superinfection, including *C. difficile*-associated diarrhea (CDAD) and pseudomembranous colitis; CDAD has been observed >2 months postantibiotic treatment. Use in infants has been associated with infantile hypertrophic pyloric stenosis (IHPS). Macrolides have been associated with rare QT_c prolongation and ventricular arrhythmias, including torsade de pointes. Use caution in elderly patients, as risk of adverse events may be increased. Use caution in myasthenia gravis patients; erythromycin may aggravate muscular weakness.

Adverse Reactions Frequency not defined. Incidence may vary with formulation.

Cardiovascular: QT_c prolongation, torsade de pointes, ventricular arrhythmia, ventricular tachycardia

Central nervous system: Seizure

Dermatologic: Erythema multiforme, pruritus, rash, Stevens-Johnson syndrome, toxic epidermal necrolysis

Gastrointestinal: Abdominal pain, anorexia, diarrhea, infantile hypertrophic pyloric stenosis, nausea, oral candidiasis, pancreatitis, pseudomembranous colitis, vomiting

Hepatic: Cholestatic jaundice (most common with estolate), hepatitis, liver function tests abnormal

Local: Phlebitis at the injection site, thrombophlebitis

Neuromuscular & skeletal: Weakness

Otic: Hearing loss

Miscellaneous: Allergic reactions, anaphylaxis, hypersensitivity reactions, interstitial nephritis, urticaria

Drug Interactions

Metabolism/Transport Effects Substrate of CYP2B6 (minor), CYP3A4 (major), P-glycoprotein; **Note:** Assignment of Major/Minor substrate status based on clinically relevant drug interaction potential; **Inhibits** CYP3A4 (moderate), P-glycoprotein

Avoid Concomitant Use

Avoid concomitant use of Erythromycin (Systemic) with any of the following: Artemether; BCG; Cisapride; Conivaptan; Disopyramide; Dronedarone; Lincosamide Antibiotics; Lumefantrine; Nilotinib; Pimozide; QUEtiapine; QuiNINE; Silodosin; Terfenadine; Tetrabenazine; Thioridazine; Topotecan; Toremifene; Vandetanib; Vemurafenib; Ziprasidone

Increased Effect/Toxicity

Erythromycin (Systemic) may increase the levels/effects of: Alfentanil; Antifungal Agents (Azole Derivatives, Systemic); Antineoplastic Agents (Vinca Alkaloids); ARIPiprazole; Benzodiazepines (metabolized by oxidation); Budesonide (Systemic, Oral Inhalation); BusPIRone; Calcium Channel Blockers; CarBAMazepine; Cardiac Glycosides; Cilostazol; Cisapride; CloZAPine; Colchicine; Corticosteroids (Systemic); CycloSPORINE; CycloSPORINE (Systemic); CYP3A4 Substrates; Dabigatran Etexilate; Disopyramide; Dronedarone; Eletriptan; Eplerenone; Ergot Derivatives; Everolimus; FentaNYL; Fexofenadine; HMG-CoA Reductase Inhibitors; Lurasidone; P-glycoprotein/ABCB1 Substrates; Pimecrolimus; Pimozide; QTc-Prolonging Agents; QuiNIDine; QuiNINE; Repaglinide; Rifamycin Derivatives; Rivaroxaban; Salmeterol; Selective Serotonin Reuptake Inhibitors; Silodosin; Sirolimus; Tacrolimus; Tacrolimus (Systemic); Tacrolimus (Topical); Temsirolimus; Terfenadine; Tetrabenazine; Theophylline Derivatives; Thioridazine; Topotecan; Toremifene; Vandetanib; Vemurafenib; Vitamin K Antagonists; Ziprasidone; Zopiclone

The levels/effects of Erythromycin (Systemic) may be increased by: Alfuzosin; Antifungal Agents (Azole Derivatives, Systemic); Artemether; Chloroquine; Ciprofloxacin; Ciprofloxacin (Systemic); Conivaptan; CYP3A4 ▶

Inhibitors (Moderate); CYP3A4 Inhibitors (Strong); Gadobutrol; Indacaterol; Lumefantrine; Nilotinib; P-glycoprotein/ABCB1 Inhibitors; QUEtiapine; QuiNINE

Decreased Effect

Erythromycin (Systemic) may decrease the levels/effects of: BCG; Clopidogrel; Typhoid Vaccine; Zafirlukast

The levels/effects of Erythromycin (Systemic) may be decreased by: CYP3A4 Inducers (Strong); Deferasirox; Etravirine; Lincosamide Antibiotics; P-glycoprotein/ABCB1 Inducers; Tocilizumab

Ethanol/Nutrition/Herb Interactions

Ethanol: Avoid ethanol (may decrease absorption of erythromycin or enhance ethanol effects).

Food: Erythromycin serum levels may be altered if taken with food (formulation-dependent).

Herb/Nutraceutical: St John's wort may decrease erythromycin levels.

Stability

Injection:

Store unreconstituted vials at 15°C to 30°C (59°F to 86°F). Erythromycin lactobionate should be reconstituted with sterile water for injection without preservatives to avoid gel formation. The reconstituted solution is stable for 2 weeks when refrigerated or for 8 hours at room temperature.

Erythromycin I.V. infusion solution is stable at pH 6-8. Stability of lactobionate is pH dependent. I.V. form has the longest stability in 0.9% sodium chloride (NS) and should be prepared in this base solution whenever possible. Do not use D_5W as a diluent unless sodium bicarbonate is added to solution. If I.V. must be prepared in D_5W, 0.5 mL of the 8.4% sodium bicarbonate solution should be added per each 100 mL of D_5W.

Stability of parenteral admixture at room temperature (25°C) and at refrigeration temperature (4°C) is 24 hours.

Standard diluent: 500 mg/250 mL D_5W/NS; 750 mg/250 mL D_5W/NS; 1 g/250 mL D_5W/NS.

Oral suspension:

Granules: Prior to mixing, store at <30°C (<86°F). After mixing, store under refrigeration and use within 10 days.

Powder: Erythromycin ethylsuccinate may be stored at room temperature if used within 14 days. Refrigerate to preserve taste.

Tablet and capsule formulations: Store at <30°C (<86°F).

Mechanism of Action Inhibits RNA-dependent protein synthesis at the chain elongation step; binds to the 50S ribosomal subunit resulting in blockage of transpeptidation

Pharmacodynamics/Kinetics

Absorption: Oral: Variable but better with salt forms than with base form; 18% to 45%; ethylsuccinate may be better absorbed with food

Distribution:

Relative diffusion from blood into CSF: Minimal even with inflammation

CSF:blood level ratio: Normal meninges: 2% to 13%; Inflamed meninges: 7% to 25%

Protein binding: Base: 73% to 81%

Metabolism: Demethylation primarily via hepatic CYP3A4

Half-life elimination: Peak: 1.5-2 hours; End-stage renal disease: 5-6 hours

Time to peak, serum: Base: 4 hours; Ethylsuccinate: 0.5-2.5 hours; delayed with food due to differences in absorption

Excretion: Primarily feces; urine (2% to 15% as unchanged drug)

Dosage Note: Due to differences in absorption, 400 mg erythromycin ethylsuccinate produces the same serum levels as 250 mg erythromycin base or stearate.

Usual dosage range:

Infants and Children:

Oral:

Base: 30-50 mg/kg/day in 2-4 divided doses; maximum: 2 g/day

Ethylsuccinate: 30-50 mg/kg/day in 2-4 divided doses; maximum: 3.2 g/day

Stearate: 30-50 mg/kg/day in 2-4 divided doses; maximum: 2 g/day

I.V.: Lactobionate: 15-50 mg/kg/day divided every 6 hours, not to exceed 4 g/day

Adults:

Oral:

Base: 250-500 mg every 6-12 hours; maximum 4 g/day

Ethylsuccinate: 400-800 mg every 6-12 hours; maximum: 4 g/day

I.V.: Lactobionate: 15-20 mg/kg/day divided every 6 hours or 500 mg to 1 g every 6 hours, or given as a continuous infusion over 24 hours; maximum: 4 g/24 hours

Indication-specific dosing:

Infants and Children:

***Bartonella sp* infections (bacillary angiomatosis [BA], peliosis hepatis [PH]) (unlabeled use):** Oral: 40 mg/kg/day (ethylsuccinate) in 4 divided doses (maximum: 2 g/day) for 3 months (BA) or 4 months (PH)

Chlamydial infection *(C. trachomatis):* Children <45 kg: Oral: 50 mg/kg/day (base or ethylsuccinate) in 4 divided doses for 14 days (CDC, 2010)

Community-acquired pneumonia (CAP) (IDSA/PIDS, 2011): Infants >3 months and Children: **Note:** A beta-lactam antibiotic should be added if typical bacterial pneumonia cannot be ruled out.

Presumed atypical *(M. pneumoniae, C. pneumoniae, C. trachomatis)* infection, mild atypical infection or step-down therapy (alternative to azithromycin): Oral: 10 mg/kg/dose every 6 hours

Moderate-to-severe atypical infection (alternative to azithromycin): I.V.: 5 mg/kg/dose every 6 hours

Mild/moderate infection: Oral: 30-50 mg/kg/day in divided doses every 6-12 hours

Pertussis: Oral: 40-50 mg/kg/day in 4 divided doses for 14 days; maximum 2 g/day (not preferred agent for infants <1 month due to IHPS)

Pharyngitis, tonsillitis (streptococcal): Oral: 20 mg (base)/kg/day or 40 mg (ethylsuccinate)/kg/day in 2 divided doses for 10 days. **Note:** No longer preferred therapy due to increased organism resistance.

Preop bowel preparation: Oral: 20 mg (base)/kg at 1, 2, and 11 PM on the day before surgery combined with mechanical cleansing of the large intestine and oral neomycin

Severe infection: I.V.: 15-50 mg/kg/day; maximum: 4 g/day

Adults:

***Bartonella sp* infections (bacillary angiomatosis [BA], peliosis hepatis [PH]) (unlabeled use):** Oral: 500 mg (base) 4 times/day for 3 months (BA) or 4 months (PH)

Chancroid (unlabeled use): Oral: 500 mg (base) 3 times/day for 7 days; **Note:** Not a preferred agent; isolates with intermediate resistance have been documented (CDC, 2010)

Gastrointestinal prokinetic (unlabeled use): I.V.: 200 mg initially followed by 250 mg (base) orally 3 times/day 30 minutes before meals. Lower dosages have been used in some trials.

Granuloma inguinale (donovanosis) (unlabeled use): Oral: 500 mg (base) 4 times/day for 21 days (CDC, 2010)

Legionnaires' disease: Oral: 1.6-4 g (ethylsuccinate)/day or 1-4 g (base)/day in divided doses for 21 days. **Note:** No longer preferred therapy and only used in nonhospitalized patients.

Lymphogranuloma venereum: Oral: 500 mg (base) 4 times/day for 21 days; **Note:** Preferred therapy for pregnant or lactating women (CDC, 2010)

Nongonococcal urethritis (including coinfection with *C. trachomatis*): Oral: 500 mg (base) 4 times/day for 7 days or 800 mg (ethylsuccinate) 4 times/day for 7 days. **Note:** May use 250 mg (base) or 400 mg (ethylsuccinate) 4 times/day for 14 days if gastrointestinal intolerance.

Pertussis: Oral: 500 mg (base) every 6 hours for 14 days

Preop bowel preparation: Oral: 1 g erythromycin base at 1, 2, and 11 PM on the day before surgery combined with mechanical cleansing of the large intestine and oral neomycin

Dosage adjustment in renal impairment: Dialysis: Slightly dialyzable (5% to 20%); no supplemental dosage necessary in hemo- or peritoneal dialysis or in continuous arteriovenous or venovenous hemofiltration

Dietary Considerations Drug may cause GI upset; may take with food. Some products may contain sodium.

Administration

Oral: Do not crush enteric coated drug product. GI upset, including diarrhea, is common. May be administered with food to decrease GI upset. Do not give with milk or acidic beverages.

I.V.: Infuse 1 g over 20-60 minutes. I.V. infusion may be very irritating to the vein. If phlebitis/pain occurs with used dilution, consider diluting further (eg, 1:5) if fluid status of the patient will tolerate, or consider administering in larger available vein. The addition of lidocaine or bicarbonate does not decrease the irritation of erythromycin infusions.

Test Interactions False-positive urinary catecholamines, 17-hydroxycorticosteroids and 17-ketosteroids

Dosage Forms Excipient information presented when available (limited, particularly for generics); consult specific product labeling.

Capsule, delayed release, enteric coated pellets, oral, as base: 250 mg

Granules for suspension, oral, as ethylsuccinate [strength expressed as base]:
- E.E.S.®: 200 mg/5 mL (200 mL) [contains sodium 25.9 mg (1.1 mEq)/5 mL; cherry flavor]
- E.E.S.®: 200 mg/5 mL (100 mL) [contains sodium 25.9 mg (1.1 mEq)/5 mL; cherry flavor]

Injection, powder for reconstitution, as lactobionate [strength expressed as base]:
- Erythrocin® Lactobionate-I.V.: 500 mg

Powder, for prescription compounding:
- Erythro-RX: USP: 100% (50 g)

Powder for suspension, oral, as ethylsuccinate [strength expressed as base]:
- EryPed®: 200 mg/5 mL (100 mL) [contains sodium 117.5 mg (5.1 mEq)/5 mL; fruit flavor]
- EryPed®: 400 mg/5 mL (100 mL) [contains sodium 117.5 mg (5.1 mEq)/5 mL; banana flavor]

Tablet, oral, as base: 250 mg, 500 mg

Tablet, oral, as ethylsuccinate [strength expressed as base]: 400 mg
- E.E.S.®: 400 mg [contains potassium 10 mg (0.3 mEq)/tablet, sodium 47 mg (2 mEq)/tablet]

Tablet, oral, as stearate [strength expressed as base]:
- Erythrocin®: 250 mg [contains potassium 5 mg (0.1 mEq)/tablet, sodium 56.7 mg (2.5 mEq)/tablet]
- Erythrocin®: 500 mg [sodium free; contains potassium 7 mg (0.2 mEq)/tablet]

Tablet, delayed release, enteric coated, oral, as base:
- Ery-Tab®: 250 mg [contains sodium 8.3 mg (0.4 mEq)/tablet]
- Ery-Tab®: 333 mg [contains sodium 11.2 mg (0.5 mEq)/tablet]
- Ery-Tab®: 500 mg [contains sodium 16.7 mg (0.7 mEq)/tablet]

Tablet, polymer coated particles, oral, as base:
- PCE®: 333 mg [contains sodium 0.5 mg (0.02mEq)/tablet]
- PCE®: 500 mg [dye free, sodium free]

Erythromycin (Ophthalmic) (er ith roe MYE sin)

Brand Names: U.S. Ilotycin™

Brand Names: Canada Diomycin®; PMS-Erythromycin

Index Terms Erythromycin Base

Pharmacologic Category Antibiotic, Macrolide; Antibiotic, Ophthalmic

Use Treatment of superficial eye infections involving the conjunctiva or cornea

Pregnancy Risk Factor B

Dosage Ophthalmic: Children and Adults: Usual dosage range: Instill 1/2" (1.25 cm) 2-6 times/day depending on the severity of the infection

Additional Information Complete prescribing information for this medication should be consulted for additional detail.

Dosage Forms Excipient information presented when available (limited, particularly for generics); consult specific product labeling.

Ointment, ophthalmic: 0.5% (1 g, 3.5 g)
- Ilotycin™: 0.5% (1 g)

Ointment, ophthalmic [preservative free]: 0.5% (1 g, 3.5 g)

Dosage Forms: Canada Excipient information presented when available (limited, particularly for generics); consult specific product labeling.

Ointment, ophthalmic: 0.5% (1 g, 3.5 g)

Erythromycin (Topical) (er ith roe MYE sin)

Brand Names: U.S. Akne-mycin®; Ery

Brand Names: Canada Sans Acne®

Pharmacologic Category Acne Products; Antibiotic, Macrolide; Antibiotic, Topical; Topical Skin Product; Topical Skin Product, Acne

Use Treatment of acne vulgaris

Pregnancy Risk Factor B

Dosage Topical: Children and Adults: Acne: Usual dosage range: Apply over the affected area twice daily after the skin has been thoroughly washed and patted dry

Additional Information Complete prescribing information for this medication should be consulted for additional detail.

Dosage Forms Excipient information presented when available (limited, particularly for generics); consult specific product labeling.

Gel, topical: 2% (30 g, 60 g)

Ointment, topical:
- Akne-mycin®: 2% (25 g)

Pledget, topical: 2% (60s)
- Ery: 2% (60s) [contains ethanol]

Solution, topical: 2% (60 mL)

Dosage Forms: Canada Excipient information presented when available (limited, particularly for generics); consult specific product labeling.

Solution, topical:
- Sans Acne®: 2% (60 mL)

Erythromycin and Benzoyl Peroxide

(er ith roe MYE sin & BEN zoe il per OKS ide)

Brand Names: U.S. Benzamycin®; Benzamycin® Pak

Index Terms Benzoyl Peroxide and Erythromycin

Pharmacologic Category Acne Products; Topical Skin Product, Acne

Use Topical control of acne vulgaris

Pregnancy Risk Factor C

Dosage Adolescents ≥12 years and Adults: Apply twice daily, morning and evening

Additional Information Complete prescribing information for this medication should be consulted for additional detail.

Dosage Forms Excipient information presented when available (limited, particularly for generics); consult specific product labeling.

Gel, topical: Erythromycin 30 mg and benzoyl peroxide 50 mg per g (23 g, 47 g)

Benzamycin®: Erythromycin 30 mg and benzoyl peroxide 50 mg per g (47 g) [contains alcohol 20%]

Benzamycin® Pak: Erythromycin 30 mg and benzoyl peroxide 50 mg per 0.8 g packet (60s) [supplied with diluent containing alcohol]

Erythromycin and Sulfisoxazole

(er ith roe MYE sin & sul fi SOKS a zole)

Brand Names: U.S. E.S.P.®

Brand Names: Canada Pediazole®

Index Terms Sulfisoxazole and Erythromycin

Pharmacologic Category Antibiotic, Macrolide; Antibiotic, Macrolide Combination; Antibiotic, Sulfonamide Derivative

Use Treatment of susceptible bacterial infections of the upper and lower respiratory tract, otitis media in children caused by susceptible strains of *Haemophilus influenzae*, and many other infections in patients allergic to penicillin

Pregnancy Risk Factor C

Dosage Oral (dosage recommendation is based on the product's erythromycin content):

Children ≥2 months: 50 mg/kg/day erythromycin and 150 mg/kg/day sulfisoxazole in divided doses every 6 hours; not to exceed 2 g erythromycin/day or 6 g sulfisoxazole/day for 10 days

Adults >45 kg: 400 mg erythromycin and 1200 mg sulfisoxazole every 6 hours

Dosing adjustment in renal impairment (sulfisoxazole must be adjusted in renal impairment):

Cl_{cr} 10-50 mL/minute: Administer every 8-12 hours

Cl_{cr} <10 mL/minute: Administer every 12-24 hours

Additional Information Complete prescribing information for this medication should be consulted for additional detail.

Dosage Forms Excipient information presented when available (limited, particularly for generics); consult specific product labeling.

Powder for oral suspension: Erythromycin ethylsuccinate 200 mg and sulfisoxazole acetyl 600 mg per 5 mL (100 mL, 150 mL, 200 mL)

E.S.P.®: Erythromycin ethylsuccinate 200 mg and sulfisoxazole acetyl 600 mg per 5 mL (100 mL, 150 mL, 200 mL) [cheri beri flavor]

◆ **Erythromycin Base** *see* Erythromycin (Ophthalmic) *on page 619*

◆ **Erythromycin Base** *see* Erythromycin (Systemic) *on page 617*

◆ **Erythromycin Ethylsuccinate** *see* Erythromycin (Systemic) *on page 617*

◆ **Erythromycin Lactobionate** *see* Erythromycin (Systemic) *on page 617*

◆ **Erythromycin Stearate** *see* Erythromycin (Systemic) *on page 617*

◆ **Erythropoiesis-Stimulating Agent (ESA)** *see* Darbepoetin Alfa *on page 447*

◆ **Erythropoiesis-Stimulating Agent (ESA)** *see* Epoetin Alfa *on page 601*

◆ **Erythropoiesis-Stimulating Protein** *see* Darbepoetin Alfa *on page 447*

◆ **Erythropoietin** *see* Epoetin Alfa *on page 601*

◆ **Erythro-RX** *see* Erythromycin (Systemic) *on page 617*

Escitalopram (es sye TAL oh pram)

Brand Names: U.S. Lexapro®

Brand Names: Canada Cipralex®

Index Terms Escitalopram Oxalate; Lu-26-054; S-Citalopram

Pharmacologic Category Antidepressant, Selective Serotonin Reuptake Inhibitor

Additional Appendix Information

Antidepressant Agents *on page 1874*

Selective Serotonin Reuptake Inhibitors (SSRIs) Pharmacokinetics *on page 1897*

Use Treatment of major depressive disorder; generalized anxiety disorders (GAD)

Unlabeled Use Treatment of mild dementia-associated agitation in nonpsychotic patients

Pregnancy Risk Factor C

Pregnancy Considerations Due to adverse effects observed in animal studies, escitalopram is classified as pregnancy category C. Escitalopram is distributed into the amniotic fluid. Limited data is available concerning the use of escitalopram during pregnancy. Nonteratogenic effects in the newborn following SSRI exposure late in the third trimester include respiratory distress, cyanosis, apnea, seizures, temperature instability, feeding difficulty, vomiting, hypoglycemia, hypo- or hypertonia, hyper-reflexia, jitteriness, irritability, constant crying, and tremor. An increased risk of low birth weight and lower Apgar scores have also been reported. Exposure to SSRIs after the twentieth week of gestation has been associated with persistent pulmonary hypertension of the newborn (PPHN). Adverse effects may be due to toxic effects of the SSRI or drug withdrawal without a taper. The long-term effects of *in utero* SSRI exposure on infant development and behavior are not known. Escitalopram is the S-enantiomer of the racemic derivative citalopram; also refer to the Citalopram monograph.

Women treated for major depression and who are euthymic prior to pregnancy are more likely to experience a relapse when medication is discontinued as compared to pregnant women who continue taking antidepressant medications. The ACOG recommends that therapy with SSRIs or SNRIs during pregnancy be individualized; treatment of depression during pregnancy should incorporate the clinical expertise of the mental health clinician, obstetrician, primary healthcare provider, and pediatrician. If treatment during pregnancy is required, consider tapering therapy during the third trimester in order to prevent withdrawal symptoms in the infant. If this is done and the woman is considered to be at risk of relapse from her major depressive disorder, the medication can be restarted following delivery, although the dose should be readjusted to that required before pregnancy. Treatment algorithms have been developed by the ACOG and the APA for the management of depression in women prior to conception and during pregnancy (Yonkers, 2009).

Lactation Enters breast milk/consider risk:benefit

Medication Guide Available Yes

Contraindications Hypersensitivity to escitalopram, citalopram, or any component of the formulation; concomitant use with pimozide; concomitant use or within 2 weeks of MAO inhibitors

Warnings/Precautions [U.S. Boxed Warning]: Antidepressants increase the risk of suicidal thinking and behavior in children, adolescents, and young adults (18-24 years of age) with major depressive disorder (MDD) and other psychiatric disorders; consider risk prior to prescribing. Short-term studies did not show an increased risk in patients >24 years of age and showed a decreased risk in patients ≥65 years. Closely monitor patients for clinical worsening, suicidality, or unusual changes in behavior, particularly during the initial 1-2 months of therapy or during periods of dosage adjustments (increases or decreases); the patient's family or caregiver should be instructed to closely observe the patient and communicate condition with healthcare provider. A medication guide concerning the use of antidepressants should be dispensed with each prescription. **Escitalopram is not FDA approved for use in children <12 years of age.**

The possibility of a suicide attempt is inherent in major depression and may persist until remission occurs. Use caution in high-risk patients. Worsening depression and severe abrupt suicidality that are not part of the presenting symptoms may require discontinuation or modification of drug therapy. The patient's family or caregiver should be alerted to monitor patients for the emergence of suicidality and associated behaviors (such as agitation, irritability, hostility, impulsivity, and hypomania) and call healthcare provider.

May worsen psychosis in some patients or precipitate a shift to mania or hypomania in patients with bipolar disorder. Patients presenting with depressive symptoms should be screened for bipolar disorder. Monotherapy in patients with bipolar disorder should be avoided. Escitalopram is not FDA approved for the treatment of bipolar depression. Escitalopram is not FDA approved for the treatment of bipolar depression.

Serotonin syndrome and neuroleptic malignant syndrome (NMS)-like reactions have occurred with serotonin/norepinephrine reuptake inhibitors (SNRIs) and selective serotonin reuptake inhibitors (SSRIs) when used alone, and particularly when used in combination with serotonergic agents (eg, triptans) or antidopaminergic agents (eg, antipsychotics). Concurrent use or within 2 weeks of an MAO inhibitor is contraindicated. May increase the risks associated with electroconvulsive therapy. Has a low potential to impair cognitive or motor performance; caution operating hazardous machinery or driving.

Use caution with a previous seizure disorder or condition predisposing to seizures such as brain damage, alcoholism, or concurrent therapy with other drugs which lower the seizure threshold. May cause hyponatremia/SIADH (elderly at increased risk); volume depletion (diuretics may increase risk) may occur. May cause or exacerbate sexual dysfunction. Use caution with severe renal impairment or liver impairment; concomitant CNS depressants; pregnancy (high doses of citalopram have been associated with teratogenicity in animals). Use caution with concomitant use of aspirin, NSAIDs, warfarin, or other drugs that affect coagulation; the risk of bleeding may be potentiated.

Upon discontinuation of escitalopram therapy, gradually taper dose. If intolerable symptoms occur following a decrease in dosage or upon discontinuation of therapy, then resuming the previous dose with a more gradual taper should be considered.

Safety and efficacy have not been established in children <12 years of age with major depressive disorder or in children <18 years with generalized anxiety disorder.

Adverse Reactions

>10%:

Central nervous system: Headache (24%), somnolence (6% to 13%), insomnia (9% to 12%)

Gastrointestinal: Nausea (15% to 18%)

Genitourinary: Ejaculation disorder (9% to 14%)

1% to 10%:

Central nervous system: Fatigue (5% to 8%), dizziness (5%), abnormal dreaming (3%), lethargy (3%), yawning (2%)

Endocrine & metabolic: Libido decreased (3% to 7%), anorgasmia (2% to 6%), menstrual disorder (2%)

Gastrointestinal: Xerostomia (6% to 9%), diarrhea (8%), constipation (3% to 5%), appetite decreased (3%), indigestion (3%), vomiting (3%), abdominal pain (2%), flatulence (2%), toothache (2%)

Genitourinary: Impotence (2% to 3%)

Neuromuscular & skeletal: Neck/shoulder pain (3%), paresthesia (2%)

Respiratory: Rhinitis (5%), sinusitis (3%)

Miscellaneous: Diaphoresis (4% to 5%), flu-like syndrome (5%)

<1% (Limited to important or life-threatening): Abdominal cramps, acute renal failure, aggression, agitation, agranulocytosis, akathisia, allergic reaction, allergy, alopecia, amnesia, anaphylaxis, anemia, anger, angioedema, anxiety, apathy, aplastic anemia, appetite increased, arthralgia, ataxia, atrial fibrillation, bilirubin increased, blurred vision, bradycardia, bronchitis, cardiac failure, cerebrovascular accident, chest pain, choreoathetosis, concentration impaired, confusion, cough, delirium, delusion, depersonalization, depression aggravated, dermatitis, diabetes mellitus, diplopia, disorientation, DVT, dysarthria, dyskinesia, dysphagia, dyspnea, dystonia, dysuria, ecchymosis, edema, epistaxis, erythema multiforme, extrapyramidal symptoms, fever, flushing, gait abnormal, gastroenhteritis, GERD, GI hemorrhage, glaucoma, hallucination, heartburn, hemolytic anemia, hepatic necrosis, hepatitis, hot flashes, hypercholesterolemia, hyper-/hypoglycemia, hypertensive crisis, hypertension, hypoesthesia, hypokalemia, hyponatremia, hypotension, INR increased, irritability, jaw stiffness, leukopenia, lightheadedness, limb pain, liver enzymes increased, liver failure, malaise, menorrhagia, menstrual cramps, migraine, mood swings, muscle cramp, muscle stiffness, muscle weakness, myalgia, mydriasis, myocardial infarction, myoclonus, nasal congestion, nervousness, neuroleptic malignant syndrome, nightmares, nystagmus, orthostasis, palpitation, pancreatitis, panic reaction, paranoia, Parkinsonism, phlebitis, photosensitivity, priapism, prolactinemia, prothrombin decreased, psychosis, pulmonary embolism, QT prolonged, rash, rectal hemorrhage, restless legs, restlessness, rhabdomyolysis, seizures, serotonin syndrome, SIADH, sinus congestion, sinus headache, spontaneous abortion, Stevens-Johnson syndrome, suicidal tendency, suicide attempt, syncope, tachycardia, tardive dyskinesia, thrombocytopenia, thrombocytopenic purpura (idiopathic), thrombosis, tinnitus, torsade de pointes, toxic epidermal necrolysis, tremor, urinary frequency, urinary retention, urinary tract infection, urticaria, ventricular arrhythmia, ventricular tachycardia, vertigo, visual disturbance, weakness, weight gain/loss, withdrawal syndrome

Drug Interactions

Metabolism/Transport Effects Substrate of CYP2C19 (major), CYP3A4 (major); **Note:** Assignment of Major/Minor substrate status based on clinically relevant drug interaction potential; **Inhibits** CYP2D6 (weak)

Avoid Concomitant Use

Avoid concomitant use of Escitalopram with any of the following: Conivaptan; Iobenguane I 123; MAO Inhibitors; Methylene Blue; Pimozide; Tryptophan

Increased Effect/Toxicity

Escitalopram may increase the levels/effects of: Alpha-/Beta-Blockers; Anticoagulants; Antidepressants (Serotonin Reuptake Inhibitor/Antagonist); Antiplatelet Agents; Aspirin; BusPIRone; CarBAMazepine; CloZAPine; Collagenase (Systemic); Desmopressin; Dextromethorphan; Drotrecogin Alfa (Activated); Ibritumomab; Lithium; Methadone; Methylene Blue; Metoclopramide; Mexiletine; NSAID (COX-2 Inhibitor); NSAID (Nonselective); Pimozide; RisperiDONE; Rivaroxaban; Salicylates; Serotonin Modulators; Thrombolytic Agents; Tositumomab and Iodine I 131 Tositumomab; TraMADol; Tricyclic Antidepressants; Vitamin K Antagonists

The levels/effects of Escitalopram may be increased by: Alcohol (Ethyl); Analgesics (Opioid); Antipsychotics; BusPIRone; Cimetidine; CNS Depressants; Conivaptan; CYP2C19 Inhibitors (Moderate); CYP2C19 Inhibitors (Strong); CYP3A4 Inhibitors (Moderate); CYP3A4 Inhibitors (Strong); Dasatinib; Glucosamine; Herbs (Anticoagulant/Antiplatelet Properties); Linezolid; Macrolide Antibiotics; MAO Inhibitors; Metoclopramide; Omega-3-Acid Ethyl Esters; Pentosan Polysulfate Sodium; Pentoxifylline; Prostacyclin Analogues; TraMADol; Tryptophan; Vitamin E

Decreased Effect

Escitalopram may decrease the levels/effects of: Iobenguane I 123; Ioflupane I 123

The levels/effects of Escitalopram may be decreased by: CarBAMazepine; CYP2C19 Inducers (Strong); CYP3A4 Inducers (Strong); Cyproheptadine; Deferasirox; NSAID (Nonselective); Telaprevir; Tocilizumab

Ethanol/Nutrition/Herb Interactions

Ethanol: May increase CNS depression; monitor for increased effects with coadministration. Caution patients about effects.

Herb/Nutraceutical: Avoid valerian, St John's wort, SAMe, kava kava, and gotu kola (may increase CNS depression).

Stability Store at 25°C (77°F); excursions permitted to 15°C to 30°C (59°F to 86°F).

Mechanism of Action Escitalopram is the S-enantiomer of the racemic derivative citalopram, which selectively inhibits the reuptake of serotonin with little to no effect on norepinephrine or dopamine reuptake. It has no or very low affinity for 5-HT_{1-7}, alpha- and beta-adrenergic, D_{1-5}, H_{1-3}, M_{1-5}, and benzodiazepine receptors. Escitalopram does not bind to or has low affinity for Na^+, K^+, Cl^-, and Ca^{++} ion channels.

Pharmacodynamics/Kinetics

Onset of action: Depression: The onset of action is within a week; however, individual response varies greatly and full response may not be seen until 8-12 weeks after initiation of treatment.

Protein binding: ~56% to plasma proteins

Metabolism: Hepatic via CYP2C19 and 3A4 to an active metabolite, S-desmethylcitalopram (S-DCT; 1/7 the activity of escitalopram); S-DCT is metabolized to S-didesmethylcitalopram (S-DDCT; active; 1/27 the activity of escitalopram) via CYP2D6

Half-life elimination: Escitalopram: 27-32 hours; S-DCT: 59 hours

Time to peak: Escitalopram: ~5 hours; S-DCT: 14 hours

Excretion: Urine (Escitalopram: 8%; S-DCT: 10%)

Dosage Oral:

Children ≥12 years: Major depressive disorder: Initial: 10 mg once daily; dose may be increased to 20 mg once daily after at least 3 weeks

Adults: Major depressive disorder, generalized anxiety disorder: Initial: 10 mg once daily; dose may be increased to 20 mg once daily after at least 1 week

Elderly: 10 mg once daily

Dosage adjustment in renal impairment:

Mild-to-moderate impairment: No dosage adjustment needed

Severe impairment: Cl_{cr} <20 mL/minute: Use with caution

Dosage adjustment in hepatic impairment: 10 mg once daily

Dietary Considerations May be taken with or without food.

Administration Administer once daily (morning or evening), with or without food.

Monitoring Parameters Mental status for depression, suicidal ideation (especially at the beginning of therapy or when doses are increased or decreased), anxiety, social functioning, mania, panic attacks; akathisia

Additional Information The tablet and oral solution dosage forms are bioequivalent. Clinically, escitalopram 20 mg is equipotent to citalopram 40 mg. Do not coadminister with citalopram.

Dosage Forms Excipient information presented when available (limited, particularly for generics); consult specific product labeling.

Solution, oral:

Lexapro®: 1 mg/mL (240 mL) [contains propylene glycol; peppermint flavor]

Tablet, oral:

Lexapro®: 5 mg

Lexapro®: 10 mg, 20 mg [scored]

Dosage Forms: Canada Excipient information presented when available (limited, particularly for generics); consult specific product labeling.

Tablet:

Cipralex®: 10 mg, 20 mg

◆ **Escitalopram Oxalate** *see* Escitalopram *on page 620*

◆ **Eserine Salicylate** *see* Physostigmine *on page 1350*

◆ **Esgic®** *see* Butalbital, Acetaminophen, and Caffeine *on page 255*

◆ **Esgic-Plus™** *see* Butalbital, Acetaminophen, and Caffeine *on page 255*

◆ **Eskalith** *see* Lithium *on page 1023*

Esmolol (ES moe lol)

Brand Names: U.S. Brevibloc

Brand Names: Canada Brevibloc®

Index Terms Esmolol Hydrochloride

Pharmacologic Category Antiarrhythmic Agent, Class II; Beta Blocker, Beta-1 Selective

Additional Appendix Information

Beta-Blockers *on page 1884*

Hypertension *on page 2001*

Use Treatment of supraventricular tachycardia (SVT) and atrial fibrillation/flutter (control ventricular rate); treatment of intraoperative and postoperative tachycardia and/or hypertension; treatment of noncompensatory sinus tachycardia

Unlabeled Use

Children: SVT and postoperative hypertension

Adults: Arrhythmia/rate control during acute coronary syndrome (eg, acute myocardial infarction, unstable angina), aortic dissection, intubation, thyroid storm, pheochromocytoma, electroconvulsive therapy

Pregnancy Risk Factor C

Pregnancy Considerations Adverse events were not observed in animal reproduction studies; therefore, esmolol is classified as pregnancy category C. In a cohort study, an increased risk of cardiovascular defects was observed following maternal use of beta-blockers during pregnancy. Intrauterine growth restriction (IUGR), small placentas, as well as fetal/neonatal bradycardia, hypoglycemia, and/or respiratory depression have been observed following *in utero* exposure to beta-blockers as a class. Adequate facilities for monitoring infants at birth should be available. Untreated chronic maternal hypertension and pre-eclampsia are also associated with adverse events in the fetus, infant, and mother. Esmolol is a short-acting beta-blocker and not intended for the chronic treatment of hypertension in pregnancy. Esmolol has been evaluated for use during intubation as an agent to offset the exaggerated pressor response observed in pregnant women with hypertension undergoing surgery.

Lactation Excretion in breast milk unknown/use with caution

Contraindications Sinus bradycardia; heart block greater than first degree (except in patients with a functioning artificial pacemaker); cardiogenic shock; uncompensated cardiac failure

Warnings/Precautions Consider pre-existing conditions such as sick sinus syndrome before initiating. Hypotension is common; patients need close blood pressure monitoring. Administer cautiously in compensated heart failure and monitor for a worsening of the condition. Can precipitate or aggravate symptoms of arterial insufficiency in patients with PVD and Raynaud's disease. Use with caution and monitor for progression of arterial obstruction. Use caution with concurrent use of digoxin, verapamil or diltiazem; bradycardia or heart block can occur. Use with caution in patients receiving inhaled anesthetic agents known to depress myocardial contractility. Use beta-blockers cautiously in patients with bronchospastic disease; monitor pulmonary status closely. Use cautiously in patients with diabetes because it can mask prominent hypoglycemic symptoms. Bradycardia may be observed more frequently in elderly patients (>65 years of age); dosage reductions may be necessary. May mask signs of hyperthyroidism (eg, tachycardia); if hyperthyroidism is suspected, carefully manage and monitor; abrupt withdrawal may exacerbate symptoms of hyperthyroidism or precipitate thyroid storm. Use with caution in patients with myasthenia gravis. Use caution in patients with renal dysfunction (active metabolite retained). Adequate alpha-blockade is required prior to use of any beta-blocker for patients with untreated pheochromocytoma. Use caution with history of severe anaphylaxis to allergens; patients taking beta-blockers may become more sensitive to repeated challenges. Treatment of anaphylaxis (eg, epinephrine) in patients taking beta-blockers may be ineffective or promote undesirable effects. Beta-blocker therapy should not be withdrawn abruptly (particularly in patients with CAD), but gradually tapered to avoid acute tachycardia, hypertension, and/or ischemia. Do not use in the treatment of hypertension associated with vasoconstriction related to hypothermia. Extravasation can lead to skin necrosis and sloughing.

Adverse Reactions

>10%:

Cardiovascular: Asymptomatic hypotension (dose related: 25% to 38%), symptomatic hypotension (dose related: 12%)

Miscellaneous: Diaphoresis (10%)

1% to 10%:

Cardiovascular: Peripheral ischemia (1%)

Central nervous system: Dizziness (3%), somnolence (3%), confusion (2%), headache (2%), agitation (2%), fatigue (1%)

Gastrointestinal: Nausea (7%), vomiting (1%)

Local: Pain on injection (8%), infusion site reaction

<1% (Limited to important or life-threatening): Abdominal discomfort, abnormal thinking, acne, alopecia, anorexia, anxiety, bradycardia, bronchospasm, chest pain, CHF, constipation, depression, dyspepsia, dyspnea, edema, erythema, exfoliative dermatitis, fever, flushing, heart block, lightheadedness, midscapular pain, nasal congestion, pallor, paresthesia, pruritus, pulmonary edema, rigors, seizure, severe bradycardia/asystole (rare), skin discoloration, skin irritation, skin necrosis (from extravasation), syncope, taste perversion, thrombophlebitis, urinary retention, vision change, weakness, wheezing, xerostomia

Drug Interactions

Metabolism/Transport Effects None known.

Avoid Concomitant Use

Avoid concomitant use of Esmolol with any of the following: Floctafenine; Methacholine

Increased Effect/Toxicity

Esmolol may increase the levels/effects of: Alpha-/Beta-Agonists (Direct-Acting); Alpha1-Blockers; Alpha2-Agonists; Amifostine; Antihypertensives; Antipsychotic Agents (Phenothiazines); Bupivacaine; Cardiac Glycosides; Cholinergic Agonists; Fingolimod; Hypotensive Agents; Insulin; Lidocaine; Lidocaine (Systemic); Lidocaine (Topical); Mepivacaine; Methacholine; Midodrine; RiTUXimab; Sulfonylureas

The levels/effects of Esmolol may be increased by: Acetylcholinesterase Inhibitors; Aminoquinolines (Antimalarial); Amiodarone; Anilidopiperidine Opioids; Antipsychotic Agents (Phenothiazines); Calcium Channel Blockers (Dihydropyridine); Calcium Channel Blockers (Nondihydropyridine); Diazoxide; Dipyridamole; Disopyramide; Dronedarone; Floctafenine; Herbs (Hypotensive Properties); MAO Inhibitors; Pentoxifylline; Phosphodiesterase 5 Inhibitors; Propafenone; Prostacyclin Analogues; QuiNIDine; Reserpine

Decreased Effect

Esmolol may decrease the levels/effects of: Beta2-Agonists; Theophylline Derivatives

The levels/effects of Esmolol may be decreased by: Barbiturates; Herbs (Hypertensive Properties); Methylphenidate; Nonsteroidal Anti-Inflammatory Agents; Rifamycin Derivatives; Yohimbine

Stability Clear, colorless to light yellow solution which should be stored at 25°C (77°F); excursions permitted to 15°C to 30°C (59°F to 86°F); do not freeze. Protect from excessive heat.

Stability of parenteral admixture at room temperature (25°C) is 24 hours.

Mechanism of Action Class II antiarrhythmic: Competitively blocks response to $beta_1$-adrenergic stimulation with little or no effect of $beta_2$-receptors except at high doses, no intrinsic sympathomimetic activity, no membrane stabilizing activity

Pharmacodynamics/Kinetics

Onset of action: Beta-blockade: I.V.: 2-10 minutes (quickest when loading doses are administered)

Duration of hemodynamic effects: 10-30 minutes; prolonged following higher cumulative doses, extended duration of use

Distribution: V_d: Esmolol: ~3.4 L/kg; Acid metabolite: ~0.4 L/kg

Protein binding: Esmolol: 55%; Acid metabolite: 10%

Metabolism: In blood by red blood cell esterases; forms acid metabolite (negligible activity; produces no clinically important effects) and methanol (does not achieve concentrations associated with methanol toxicity)

Half-life elimination: Adults: Esmolol: 9 minutes; Acid metabolite: 3.7 hours; elimination of metabolite decreases with end-stage renal disease

Excretion: Urine (~73% to 88% as acid metabolite, <2% unchanged drug)

Dosage I.V.:
Children:
SVT (unlabeled use): A limited amount of information regarding esmolol use in pediatric patients is currently available. Some centers have utilized doses of 100-500 mcg/kg given over 1 minute for control of supraventricular tachycardias.
Postoperative hypertension (unlabeled use): Loading doses of 500 mcg/kg/minute over 1 minute with maximal doses of 50-250 mcg/kg/minute (mean: 173 mcg/kg/minute) have been used in addition to nitroprusside to treat postoperative hypertension after coarctation of aorta repair.
Adults:
Intraoperative tachycardia and/or hypertension (immediate control): Initial bolus: 80 mg (~1 mg/kg) over 30 seconds, followed by a 150 mcg/kg/minute infusion, if necessary. Adjust infusion rate as needed to maintain desired heart rate and/or blood pressure, up to 300 mcg/kg/minute.
For control of postoperative hypertension, as many as one-third of patients may require higher doses (250-300 mcg/kg/minute) to control blood pressure; the safety of doses >300 mcg/kg/minute has not been studied.
Supraventricular tachycardia (SVT), gradual control of postoperative tachycardia/hypertension: Loading dose: 500 mcg/kg over 1 minute; follow with a 50 mcg/kg/minute infusion for 4 minutes; response to this initial infusion rate may be a rough indication of the responsiveness of the ventricular rate.
Infusion may be continued at 50 mcg/kg/minute or, if the response is inadequate, titrated upward in 50 mcg/kg/minute increments (increased no more frequently than every 4 minutes) to a maximum of 200 mcg/kg/minute.
To achieve more rapid response, following the initial loading dose and 50 mcg/kg/minute infusion, rebolus with a second 500 mcg/kg loading dose over 1 minute, and increase the maintenance infusion to 100 mcg/kg/minute for 4 minutes. If necessary, a third (and final) 500 mcg/kg loading dose may be administered, prior to increasing to an infusion rate of 150 mcg/kg/minute. After 4 minutes of the 150 mcg/kg/minute infusion, the infusion rate may be increased to a maximum rate of 200 mcg/kg/minute (without a bolus dose).
Acute coronary syndromes (when relative contraindications to beta-blockade exist; unlabeled use): 500 mcg/kg over 1 minute; follow with a 50 mcg/kg/minute infusion; if tolerated and response inadequate, may titrate upward in 50 mcg/kg/minute increments every 5-15 minutes to a maximum of 300 mcg/kg/minute (Mitchell, 2002); an additional bolus (500 mcg/kg over 1 minute) may be administered prior to each increase in infusion rate (Mooss, 1994)
Electroconvulsive therapy (unlabeled use): 1 mg/kg administered 1 minute prior to induction of anesthesia (Weinger, 1991)
Intubation (unlabeled use): 1-2 mg/kg I.V. given 1.5-3 minutes prior to intubation (Kindler, 1996)
Thyrotoxicosis or thyroid storm (unlabeled use): 50-100 mcg/kg/minute (Bahn, 2011)

Guidelines for transfer to oral therapy (beta-blocker, calcium channel blocker):
Infusion should be reduced by 50% 30 minutes following the first dose of the alternative agent
Manufacturer suggests following the second dose of the alternative drug, patient's response should be monitored and if control is adequate for the first hour, esmolol may be discontinued.

Dosage adjustment in renal impairment: Dialysis: Not removed by hemo- or peritoneal dialysis; supplemental dose is not necessary.

Administration Infusions must be administered with an infusion pump. Infusion into small veins or through a butterfly catheter should be avoided (can cause thrombophlebitis). Decrease or discontinue infusion if hypotension or congestive heart failure occur. Medication port of premixed bags should be used to withdraw only the initial bolus, if necessary (not to be used for withdrawal of additional bolus doses).

Monitoring Parameters Blood pressure, MAP, heart rate, continuous ECG, respiratory rate, I.V. site

Dosage Forms Excipient information presented when available (limited, particularly for generics); consult specific product labeling. [DSC] = Discontinued product
Infusion, premixed in NS, as hydrochloride [preservative free]:
Brevibloc: 2000 mg (100 mL) [20 mg/mL; double strength]
Brevibloc: 2500 mg (250 mL) [10 mg/mL]
Injection, solution, as hydrochloride [preservative free]: 10 mg/mL (10 mL)
Brevibloc: 10 mg/mL (10 mL)
Brevibloc: 20 mg/mL (5 mL [DSC]) [double strength]

◆ **Esmolol Hydrochloride** *see* Esmolol *on page 622*

Esomeprazole (es oh ME pray zol)

Brand Names: U.S. NexIUM®; NexIUM® I.V.
Brand Names: Canada Apo-Esomeprazole®; Nexium®
Index Terms Esomeprazole Magnesium; Esomeprazole Sodium
Pharmacologic Category Proton Pump Inhibitor; Substituted Benzimidazole
Use
Oral: Short-term (4-8 weeks) treatment of erosive esophagitis; maintaining symptom resolution and healing of erosive esophagitis; treatment of symptomatic gastroesophageal reflux disease (GERD); as part of a multidrug regimen for *Helicobacter pylori* eradication in patients with duodenal ulcer disease (active or history of within the past 5 years); prevention of gastric ulcers in patients at risk (age ≥60 years and/or history of gastric ulcer) associated with continuous NSAID therapy; long-term treatment of pathological hypersecretory conditions including Zollinger-Ellison syndrome
Canadian labeling: Additional use (not in U.S. labeling): Oral: Treatment of nonerosive reflux disease (NERD)
I.V.: Short-term (≤10 days) treatment of gastroesophageal reflux disease (GERD) when oral therapy is not possible or appropriate

Unlabeled Use I.V.: Prevention of recurrent peptic ulcer bleeding postendoscopy

Pregnancy Risk Factor B

Pregnancy Considerations Teratogenic effects were not observed in animal studies. However, there are no adequate and well-controlled studies in pregnant women. Congenital abnormalities have been reported sporadically following omeprazole use during pregnancy.

Lactation Excretion in breast milk unknown/not recommended

Contraindications Hypersensitivity to esomeprazole, substituted benzimidazoles (eg, omeprazole, lansoprazole), or any component of the formulation

Warnings/Precautions Use of proton pump inhibitors (PPIs) may increase the risk of gastrointestinal infections (eg, *Salmonella, Campylobacter*). Relief of symptoms does not preclude the presence of a gastric malignancy. Atrophic gastritis (by biopsy) has been noted with long-term omeprazole therapy; this may also occur with esomeprazole. No reports of enterochromaffin-like (ECL) cell carcinoids, dysplasia, or neoplasia have occurred. Severe liver dysfunction may require dosage reductions. Safety and efficacy of I.V. therapy >10 days have not been established; transition from I.V. to oral therapy as soon possible. Bioavailability may be increased in Asian populations, the elderly, and patients with hepatic dysfunction. Decreased *H. pylori* eradication rates have been observed with short-term (≤7 days) combination therapy. The American College of Gastroenterology recommends 10-14 days of therapy (triple or quadruple) for eradication of *H. pylori* (Chey, 2007).

PPIs may diminish the therapeutic effect of clopidogrel, thought to be due to reduced formation of the active metabolite of clopidogrel. The manufacturer of clopidogrel recommends either avoidance of omeprazole or use of a PPI with less potent CYP2C19 inhibition (eg, pantoprazole); avoidance of esomeprazole would appear prudent. Others have recommended the continued use of PPIs, regardless of the degree of inhibition, in patients with a history of GI bleeding or multiple risk factors for GI bleeding who are also receiving clopidogrel since no evidence has established clinically meaningful differences in outcome; however, a clinically-significant interaction cannot be excluded in those who are poor metabolizers of clopidogrel (Abraham, 2010; Levine, 2011). Avoid concurrent use of CYP3A4 and 2C19 inducers (eg, St John's wort, rifampin) as esomeprazole's efficacy may be reduced.

Increased incidence of osteoporosis-related bone fractures of the hip, spine, or wrist may occur with PPI therapy. Patients on high-dose or long-term therapy should be monitored. Use the lowest effective dose for the shortest duration of time, use vitamin D and calcium supplementation, and follow appropriate guidelines to reduce risk of fractures in patients at risk.

Hypomagnesemia, reported rarely, usually with prolonged PPI use of >3 months (most cases >1 year of therapy); may be symptomatic or asymptomatic; severe cases may cause tetany, seizures, and cardiac arrhythmias. Consider obtaining serum magnesium concentrations prior to beginning long-term therapy, especially if taking concomitant digoxin, diuretics, or other drugs known to cause hypomagnesemia; and periodically thereafter. Hypomagnesemia may be corrected by magnesium supplementation, although discontinuation of esomeprazole may be necessary; magnesium levels typically return to normal within 1 week of stopping. Serum chromogranin A levels may be increased if assessed while patient on esomeprazole; may lead to diagnostic errors related to neuroendocrine tumors.

Adverse Reactions Unless otherwise specified, percentages represent adverse reactions identified in clinical trials evaluating the oral formulation.

>10%: Central nervous system: Headache (I.V. 11%; oral ≤8%)

1% to 10%:

- Cardiovascular: Hypertension (≤3%), chest pain (>1%)
- Central nervous system: Pain (4%), dizziness (oral >1%; I.V. 3%), anxiety (2%), insomnia (2%), pyrexia (2%), fatigue (>1%)
- Dermatologic: Rash (>1%), pruritus (I.V. ≤1%)
- Endocrine & metabolic: Hypercholesterolemia (2%)
- Gastrointestinal: Flatulence (oral ≤5%; I.V. 10%), diarrhea (oral ≤7%; I.V. 4%), abdominal pain (oral ≤6%; I.V. 6%), nausea (oral 5%; I.V. 6%), dyspepsia (oral >1%; I.V. 6%), gastritis (≤6%), constipation (oral 2%; I.V. 3%), vomiting (≤3%), benign GI neoplasm (>1%), dyspepsia (>1%), duodenitis (>1%), epigastric pain (>1%), esophageal disorder (>1%), gastroenteritis (>1%), GI mucosal discoloration (>1%), serum gastrin increased (>1%), xerostomia (1%)
- Genitourinary: Urinary tract infection (4%)
- Hematologic: Anemia (>1%)
- Hepatic: Transaminases increased (>1%)
- Local: Injection site reaction (I.V. 2%)
- Neuromuscular & skeletal: Arthralgia (3%), back pain (>1%), fracture (>1%), arthropathy (1%), myalgia (1%)
- Respiratory: Respiratory infection (oral ≤9%; I.V. 1%), bronchitis (4%), sinusitis (oral ≤4%; I.V. 2%), coughing (>1%), rhinitis (>1%), dyspnea (1%)
- Miscellaneous: Accident/injury (≤8%), viral infection (4%), allergy (2%), ear infection (2%), hernia (>1%), flu-like syndrome (1%)

<1% (Limited to important or life-threatening): Abdominal rigidity, aggression, agitation, agranulocytosis, albuminuria, alkaline phosphatase increased, alopecia, anaphylactic reaction/shock, angioedema, anorexia, arthritis exacerbation, asthma exacerbation, benign polyps/nodules, bilirubinemia, blurred vision, bronchospasm, candidiasis (GI and genital), carcinoid tumor of stomach, cervical lymphadenopathy, conjunctivitis, cramps, creatinine increased, cystitis, dehydration, depression, dermatitis, dysmenorrhea, dysphagia, dysuria, edema (including facial, peripheral, and tongue), epigastric pain, epistaxis, erythema multiforme, esophageal varices, fibromyalgia syndrome, flushing, fungal infection, gastric retention, GI dysplasia, glycosuria, goiter, gynecomastia, hallucinations, hematuria, hepatic encephalopathy, hepatic failure, hepatitis, hyperhidrosis, hyperparathyroidism, hypertonia, hyperuricemia, hypoesthesia, hypokalemia, hypomagnesemia, hyponatremia, impotence, infusion site reaction (eg, erythema, edema), interstitial nephritis, jaundice, larynx edema, leukocytosis, leukopenia, malaise, microscopic colitis, micturition increased, migraine, muscular weakness, nervousness, osteoporosis, otitis media, pancreatitis, pancytopenia, paresthesia, pharyngolaryngeal pain, pharyngitis, phlebitis, photosensitivity, polymyalgia rheumatica, polyuria, proteinuria, pruritus ani, rhinorrhea, rigors, sleep disorder, somnolence, Stevens-Johnson syndrome, stomatitis, tachycardia, taste disturbances, thrombocytopenia, thrombophlebitis, thyroid-stimulating hormone increased, tinnitus, total bilirubin increased, toxic epidermal necrolysis, tremor, urticaria, vaginitis, vertigo, vitamin B_{12} deficiency, weight changes

Drug Interactions

Metabolism/Transport Effects Substrate of CYP2C19 (major), CYP3A4 (minor); **Note:** Assignment of Major/Minor substrate status based on clinically relevant drug interaction potential; **Inhibits** CYP2C19 (moderate)

Avoid Concomitant Use

Avoid concomitant use of Esomeprazole with any of the following: Delavirdine; Erlotinib; Nelfinavir; Posaconazole; Rifampin; Rilpivirine; St Johns Wort

Increased Effect/Toxicity

Esomeprazole may increase the levels/effects of: Amphetamines; Benzodiazepines (metabolized by oxidation); Cilostazol; Citalopram; CYP2C19 Substrates; Dexmethylphenidate; Methotrexate; Methylphenidate; Raltegravir; Saquinavir; Tacrolimus; Tacrolimus (Systemic); Vitamin K Antagonists; Voriconazole

The levels/effects of Esomeprazole may be increased by: Conivaptan; Fluconazole; Ketoconazole; Ketoconazole (Systemic)

Decreased Effect

Esomeprazole may decrease the levels/effects of: Atazanavir; Bisphosphonate Derivatives; Cefditoren; Clopidogrel; Dabigatran Etexilate; Dasatinib; Delavirdine; Erlotinib; Gefitinib; Indinavir; Iron Salts; Itraconazole; Ketoconazole; Ketoconazole (Systemic); Mesalamine; Mycophenolate; Nelfinavir; Posaconazole; Rilpivirine

The levels/effects of Esomeprazole may be decreased by: CYP2C19 Inducers (Strong); Rifampin; St Johns Wort; Tipranavir; Tocilizumab

Ethanol/Nutrition/Herb Interactions

Food: Absorption is decreased by 43% to 53% when taken with food.

Herb/Nutraceutical: Avoid use of St John's wort (may decrease efficacy of esomeprazole).

Stability

Capsule, granules: Store at 15°C to 30°C (59°F to 86°F). Keep container tightly closed.

Powder for injection: Store at 25°C (77°F); excursions permitted to 15°C to 30°C (59°F to 86°F). Protect from light.

For I.V. injection: Adults: Reconstitute powder with 5 mL NS.

For I.V. infusion:

Children: Initially reconstitute powder (20 mg or 40 mg) with 5 mL of NS, then further dilute to a final volume of 50 mL; withdraw the appropriate amount of the final solution to administer the intended dose.

Adults: Initially reconstitute powder with 5 mL of NS, LR, or D_5W, then further dilute to a final volume of 50 mL.

Per the manufacturer, following reconstitution, solution for injection prepared in NS, and solution for infusion prepared in NS or LR should be used within 12 hours. Following reconstitution, solution for infusion prepared in D_5W should be used within 6 hours. Refrigeration is not required following reconstitution.

Additional stability data: Following reconstitution, solutions for infusion prepared in D_5W, NS, or LR in PVC bags are chemically and physically stable for 48 hours at room temperature (25°C) and for at least 120 hours under refrigeration (4°C) (Kupiec, 2008).

Mechanism of Action Proton pump inhibitor suppresses gastric acid secretion by inhibition of the H^+/K^+-ATPase in the gastric parietal cell. Esomeprazole is the S-isomer of omeprazole.

Pharmacodynamics/Kinetics

Distribution: V_{dss}: 16 L

Protein binding: 97%

Metabolism: Hepatic via CYP2C19 primarily and (to a lesser extent) via 3A4 to hydroxy, desmethyl, and sulfone metabolites (all inactive)

Bioavailability: Oral: 90% with repeat dosing

Half-life elimination: ~1-1.5 hours

Time to peak: Oral: 1.5-2 hours

Excretion: Urine (80%, primarily as inactive metabolites; <1% as active drug); feces (20%)

Dosage

Oral:

Children 1-11 years: **Note:** Safety and efficacy of doses >1 mg/kg/day and/or therapy beyond 8 weeks have not been established.

Symptomatic GERD: 10 mg once daily for up to 8 weeks

Erosive esophagitis (healing):

<20 kg: 10 mg once daily for 8 weeks

≥20 kg: 10-20 mg once daily for 8 weeks

Nonerosive reflux disease (NERD) (Canadian labeling): 10 mg once daily for up to 8 weeks

Adolescents 12-17 years:

GERD: 20-40 mg once daily for up to 8 weeks

NERD (Canadian labeling): 20 mg once daily for 2-4 weeks; lack of symptom control after 4 weeks warrants further evaluation

Adults:

Erosive esophagitis (healing): Initial: 20-40 mg once daily for 4-8 weeks; if incomplete healing, may continue for an additional 4-8 weeks; maintenance: 20 mg once daily (controlled studies did not extend beyond 6 months)

NERD (Canadian labeling): Initial: 20 mg once daily for 2-4 weeks; lack of symptom control after 4 weeks warrants further evaluation; maintenance (in patients with successful initial therapy): 20 mg once daily as needed

Symptomatic GERD: 20 mg once daily for 4 weeks; may continue an additional 4 weeks if symptoms persist

Helicobacter pylori eradication:

Manufacturer labeling: 40 mg once daily administered with amoxicillin 1000 mg *and* clarithromycin 500 mg twice daily for 10 days

American College of Gastroenterology guidelines (Chey, 2007):

Nonpenicillin allergy: 40 mg once daily administered with amoxicillin 1000 mg *and* clarithromycin 500 mg twice daily for 10-14 days

Penicillin allergy: 40 mg once daily administered with clarithromycin 500 mg *and* metronidazole 500 mg twice daily for 10-14 days **or** 40 mg once daily administered with bismuth subsalicylate 525 mg *and* metronidazole 250 mg *plus* tetracycline 500 mg 4 times/day for 10-14 days

Canadian labeling: 20 mg twice daily for 7 days; requires combination therapy

Prevention of NSAID-induced gastric ulcers: 20-40 mg once daily for up to 6 months

Treatment of NSAID-induced gastric ulcers (Canadian labeling): 20 mg once daily for 4-8 weeks.

Pathological hypersecretory conditions (Zollinger-Ellison syndrome): 40 mg twice daily; adjust regimen to individual patient needs; doses up to 240 mg/day have been administered

I.V.:

Treatment of GERD (short-term): **Note:** Indicated only in cases where oral therapy is inappropriate or not possible; safety/efficacy ≥10 days has not been established.

Children 1-11 months: 0.5 mg/kg once daily

Children 1-17 years: <55 kg: 10 mg once daily; ≥55 kg: 20 mg once daily

Adults: 20 mg or 40 mg once daily

Prevention of recurrent peptic ulcer bleeding postendoscopy (unlabeled use; Sung, 2009): Adults: 80 mg over 30 minutes, followed by 8 mg/hour infusion for 72 hours, then 40 mg *orally* once daily for 27 additional days

Elderly: No dosage adjustment needed.

Dosage adjustment in renal impairment: No dosage adjustment needed

Dosage adjustment in hepatic impairment:

Safety and efficacy not established in children with hepatic impairment.

Mild-to-moderate hepatic impairment (Child-Pugh class A or B): No dosage adjustment needed

Severe hepatic impairment (Child-Pugh class C): Dose should not exceed 20 mg/day

Dietary Considerations Take at least 1 hour before meals; best if taken before breakfast. The contents of the capsule may be mixed in applesauce or water; pellets also remain intact when exposed to orange juice, apple juice, and yogurt.

Administration

Oral:

Capsule: Should be swallowed whole and taken at least 1 hour before eating (best if taken before breakfast). Capsule can be opened and contents mixed with 1 tablespoon of applesauce. Swallow immediately; mixture should not be chewed or warmed. For patients with difficulty swallowing, use of granules may be more appropriate.

Granules: Empty into container with 15 mL of water and stir; leave 2-3 minutes to thicken. Stir and drink within 30 minutes. If any medicine remains after drinking, add more water, stir and drink immediately.

Tablet (Canadian formulation, not available in U.S.): Swallow whole or may be dispersed in a half a glass of noncarbonated water. Stir until tablets disintegrate, leaving a liquid containing pellets. Drink contents within 30 minutes. Do not chew or crush pellets. After drinking, rinse glass with water and drink.

I.V.: Flush line prior to and after administration with NS, LR, or D_5W.

Children: Administer by intermittent infusion (10-30 minutes); the manufacturer recommends that children receive intravenous esomeprazole by intermittent infusion only.

Adults: May be administered by injection (≥3 minutes), intermittent infusion (10-30 minutes), or continuous infusion for up to 72 hours (Sung, 2009).

Nasogastric tube:

Capsule: Open capsule and place intact granules into a 60 mL catheter-tip syringe; mix with 50 mL of water. Replace plunger and shake vigorously for 15 seconds. Ensure that no granules remain in syringe tip. Do not administer if pellets dissolve or disintegrate. Use immediately after preparation. After administration, flush nasogastric tube with additional water.

Granules: Delayed release oral suspension granules can also be given by nasogastric or gastric tube. Add 15 mL of water to a catheter-tip syringe, add granules from packet. Shake the syringe, leave 2-3 minutes to thicken. Shake the syringe and administer through nasogastric or gastric tube (size 6 French or greater) within 30 minutes. Refill the syringe with 15 mL of water, shake and flush nasogastric/gastric tube.

Tablet (Canadian formulation, not available in U.S.): Disperse tablets in 50 mL of noncarbonated water. Stir until tablets disintegrate leaving a liquid containing pellets. After administration, flush with additional 25-50 mL of water to clear the syringe and tube.

Monitoring Parameters Susceptibility testing recommended in patients who fail *H. pylori* eradication regimen. Monitor for rebleeding in patients with peptic ulcer bleed.

Test Interactions Esomeprazole may falsely elevate serum chromogranin A (CgA) levels. The increased CgA level may cause false-positive results in the diagnosis of a neuroendocrine tumor. Temporarily stop esomeprazole if assessing CgA level; repeat level if initially elevated; use the same laboratory for all testing of CgA levels.

Dosage Forms Excipient information presented when available (limited, particularly for generics); consult specific product labeling.

Capsule, delayed release, oral, as magnesium [strength expressed as base]:

NexIUM®: 20 mg, 40 mg

Granules for suspension, delayed release, oral, as magnesium [strength expressed as base]:

NexIUM®: 10 mg/packet (30s); 20 mg/packet (30s); 40 mg/packet (30s)

Injection, powder for reconstitution, as sodium [strength expressed as base]:

NexIUM® I.V.: 20 mg, 40 mg [contains edetate disodium]

Dosage Forms: Canada Excipient information presented when available (limited, particularly for generics); consult specific product labeling.

Note: Strength expressed as base

Granules, for oral suspension, delayed release, as magnesium:

Nexium®: 10 mg/packet (28s)

Tablet, extended release, as magnesium:

Nexium®: 20 mg, 40 mg

◆ **Esomeprazole Magnesium** *see* Esomeprazole *on page 624*

◆ **Esomeprazole Sodium** *see* Esomeprazole *on page 624*

◆ **Esoterica® Daytime [OTC]** *see* Hydroquinone *on page 846*

◆ **Esoterica® Nighttime [OTC]** *see* Hydroquinone *on page 846*

◆ **E.S.P.®** *see* Erythromycin and Sulfisoxazole *on page 620*

◆ **Estalis® (Can)** *see* Estradiol and Norethindrone *on page 635*

◆ **Estalis-Sequi® (Can)** *see* Estradiol and Norethindrone *on page 635*

Estazolam (es TA zoe lam)

Index Terms ProSom

Pharmacologic Category Benzodiazepine

Additional Appendix Information

Benzodiazepines *on page 1882*

Use Short-term management of insomnia

Pregnancy Risk Factor X

Dosage Adults: Oral: 1 mg at bedtime, some patients may require 2 mg; start at doses of 0.5 mg in debilitated or small elderly patients

Dosing adjustment in hepatic impairment: May be necessary

Additional Information Complete prescribing information for this medication should be consulted for additional detail.

Dosage Forms Excipient information presented when available (limited, particularly for generics); consult specific product labeling.

Tablet, oral: 1 mg, 2 mg

Controlled Substance C-IV

◆ **Ester-E™ [OTC]** *see* Vitamin E *on page 1796*

◆ **Esterified Estrogens** *see* Estrogens (Esterified) *on page 645*

◆ **Estrace®** *see* Estradiol (Systemic) *on page 627*

◆ **Estrace®** *see* Estradiol (Topical) *on page 632*

◆ **Estraderm®** *see* Estradiol (Systemic) *on page 627*

◆ **Estradiol** *see* Estradiol (Systemic) *on page 627*

◆ **17β-estradiol** *see* Estradiol (Topical) *on page 632*

Estradiol (Systemic) (es tra DYE ole)

Brand Names: U.S. Alora®; Climara®; Delestrogen®; Depo®-Estradiol; Divigel®; Elestrin®; Estrace®; Estraderm®; Estrasorb®; EstroGel®; Evamist™; Femring®; Femtrace®; Menostar®; Vivelle-Dot®

Brand Names: Canada Climara®; Depo®-Estradiol; Estraderm®; Estradot®; EstroGel®; Menostar®; Oesclim®; Sandoz-Estradiol Derm 100; Sandoz-Estradiol Derm 50; Sandoz-Estradiol Derm 75

Index Terms Estradiol; Estradiol Acetate; Estradiol Transdermal; Estradiol Valerate

Pharmacologic Category Estrogen Derivative

Use Treatment of moderate-to-severe vasomotor symptoms associated with menopause; treatment of moderate-to-severe vulvar and vaginal atrophy associated with menopause; hypoestrogenism (due to hypogonadism, castration, or primary ovarian failure); advanced prostatic cancer (palliation); metastatic breast cancer (palliation) in men and postmenopausal women; postmenopausal osteoporosis (prophylaxis)

Pregnancy Risk Factor X

Pregnancy Considerations In general, the use of estrogen and progestin as in combination hormonal contraceptives has not been associated with teratogenic effects when inadvertently taken early in pregnancy. These products are contraindicated for use during pregnancy.

Lactation Enters breast milk/use caution

Contraindications Hypersensitivity to estradiol or any component of the formulation; undiagnosed abnormal vaginal bleeding; DVT or PE (current or history of); active or recent (within 1 year) arterial thromboembolic disease (eg, stroke, MI); carcinoma of the breast (known, suspected or history of), except in appropriately selected patients being treated for metastatic disease; estrogen-dependent tumor; hepatic dysfunction or disease; pregnancy

Warnings/Precautions [U.S. Boxed Warning]: Unopposed estrogens may increase the risk of endometrial carcinoma in postmenopausal women with an intact uterus. Adequate diagnostic measures, including endometrial sampling, if indicated, should be performed to rule out malignancy in all cases of undiagnosed abnormal vaginal bleeding. The use of a progestin should be considered when administering estrogens to postmenopausal women with an intact uterus. When indicated, oral progestins should be used. The use of a progestin is not generally required when low doses of estrogen are used locally for vaginal atrophy or when ultralow doses are used transdermally to prevent osteoporosis (NAMS, 2010). Estrogens may exacerbate endometriosis. Malignant transformation of residual endometrial implants has been reported posthysterectomy with estrogen only therapy. Consider adding a progestin in women with residual endometriosis posthysterectomy. Postmenopausal estrogen therapy and combined estrogen/progesterone therapy may increase the risk of ovarian cancer; however, the absolute risk to an individual woman is small. Although results from various studies are not consistent, risk does not appear to be significantly associated with the duration, route, or dose of therapy. In one study, the risk decreased after 2 years following discontinuation of therapy (Mørch, 2009). Although the risk of ovarian cancer is rare, women who are at an increased risk (eg, family history) should be counseled about the association (NAMS, 2010). **[U.S. Boxed Warning]: Estrogens may increase the risk of breast cancer. An increased risk of invasive breast cancer was observed in postmenopausal women using conjugated estrogens (CE) in combination with medroxyprogesterone acetate (MPA); a smaller increase in risk was seen with estrogen therapy alone in observational studies.** An increase in abnormal mammograms has also been reported with estrogen and progestin therapy. Estrogen use may lead to severe hypercalcemia in patients with breast cancer and bone metastases; discontinue estrogen if hypercalcemia occurs.

[U.S. Boxed Warning]: Estrogens with or without progestin should not be used to prevent coronary heart disease. Use caution with cardiovascular disease or dysfunction. May increase the risks of myocardial infarction (MI), stroke, pulmonary emboli (PE), and deep vein thrombosis (DVT); incidence of these effects was shown to be significantly increased in postmenopausal women using CE with or without MPA. Nonfatal MI, PE, and thrombophlebitis have also been reported in males taking high doses of CE (eg, for prostate cancer). Risk factors include diabetes mellitus, hypercholesterolemia, hypertension, SLE, obesity, and/or venous thromboembolism (VTE). Use caution in patients with known inherited thrombophilias (eg, protein C or S deficiency); may have increased risk of VTE (DeSancho, 2010). Use is contraindicated in patients with DVT or PE (current or history of).

[U.S. Boxed Warning]: The risk of dementia may be increased in postmenopausal women; increased incidence was observed in women ≥65 years of age taking CE alone or in combination with MPA.

[U.S. Boxed Warning]: Estrogens with or without progestin should be used for shortest duration possible at the lowest effective dose consistent with treatment goals. Before prescribing estrogen therapy to postmenopausal women, the risks and benefits must be weighed for each patient. Women should be informed of these risks and benefits, as well as possible effects of progestin when added to estrogen therapy. Conduct periodic risk:benefit assessments. **Outcomes reported from clinical trials using CE should be assumed to be similar for estradiol until comparable data becomes available. In addition, risks associated with oral CE should be assumed to be similar for other dosage forms (eg, vaginal, transdermal) until additional information is available.**

Estrogen compounds are generally associated with lipid effects such as increased HDL-cholesterol and decreased LDL-cholesterol. Triglycerides may also be increased; use with caution in patients with familial defects of lipoprotein metabolism. Estrogens may increase thyroid-binding globulin (TBG) levels leading to increased circulating total thyroid hormone levels. Women on thyroid replacement therapy may require higher doses of thyroid hormone while receiving estrogens.

Estrogens may cause retinal vascular thrombosis; discontinue if migraine, loss of vision, proptosis, diplopia, or other visual disturbances occur; discontinue permanently if papilledema or retinal vascular lesions are observed on examination. Estrogens are poorly metabolized in patients with hepatic dysfunction. Use caution with a history of cholestatic jaundice associated with prior estrogen use or pregnancy. Discontinue if jaundice develops or if acute or chronic hepatic disturbances occur. Use is contraindicated with hepatic disease. Use caution in patients with asthma, epilepsy, hepatic hemangiomas, migraine, porphyria, or SLE; may exacerbate disease. May have adverse effects on glucose tolerance; use caution in women with diabetes. Use with caution in patients with diseases which may be exacerbated by fluid retention, including cardiac or renal dysfunction. Use of postmenopausal estrogen may be associated with an increased risk of gallbladder disease requiring surgery. Use with caution in patients with severe hypocalcemia. May be inappropriate in for use in the elderly due to potential of increased risk of breast and endometrial cancers and lack of proven cardioprotection (Beers Criteria). Prior to puberty, estrogens may cause premature closure of the epiphyses, premature breast development in girls or gynecomastia in boys. Vaginal bleeding and vaginal cornification may also be induced in girls. Whenever possible, estrogens should be discontinued at least 4-6 weeks prior to elective surgery associated with an increased risk of thromboembolism or during periods of prolonged immobilization.

Estradiol may be transferred to another person following skin-to-skin contact with the application site. **[U.S. Boxed Warning]: Breast budding and breast masses in prepubertal females and gynecomastia and breast masses in prepubertal males have been reported following unintentional contact with application sites of women using topical estradiol (Evamist™). Patients should strictly adhere to instructions for use in order to prevent secondary exposure. In most cases, conditions resolved with removal of estradiol exposure.** If unexpected changes in sexual development occur in prepubertal children, the possibility of unintentional estradiol exposure should be evaluated by a healthcare provider. Discontinue if conditions for the safe use of the topical spray cannot be met.

Some products may contain chlorobutanol (a chloral derivative) as a preservative, which may be habit forming; some products may contain tartrazine.

Topical emulsion, gel, spray: Absorption of the topical emulsion (Estrasorb®) and topical gel (Elestrin®) is increased by application of sunscreen; do not apply sunscreen within close proximity of estradiol. When sunscreen is applied ~1 hour prior to the topical spray (Evamist™), no change in absorption was observed (estradiol absorption was decreased when sunscreen is applied 1 hour after Evamist™). Application of Divigel® or Estro-Gel® with sunscreen has not been evaluated.

Transdermal patch: May contain conducting metal (eg, aluminum); remove patch prior to MRI.

Vaginal ring: Use may not be appropriate in women with narrow vagina, vaginal stenosis, vaginal infections, cervical prolapse, rectoceles, cystoceles, or other conditions which may increase the risk of vaginal irritation, ulceration, or increase the risk of expulsion. Ring should be removed in case of ulceration, erosion, or adherence to vaginal wall; do not reinsert until healing is complete. Ensure proper vaginal placement of the ring to avoid inadvertent urinary bladder insertion.

Osteoporosis: For use only in women at significant risk of osteoporosis and for who other nonestrogen medications are not considered appropriate.

Vulvar and vaginal atrophy: When used solely for the treatment of vulvar and vaginal atrophy, topical vaginal products should be considered. Use caution applying topical products to severely atrophic vaginal mucosa. Use of a progestin is normally not required when low-dose estrogen is applied locally and only for this purpose (NAMS, 2007).

Adverse Reactions Frequency not defined. Some adverse reactions observed with estrogen and/or progestin combination therapy.

Cardiovascular: Chest pain, DVT, edema, hypertension, MI, stroke, syncope, TIA, vasodilation, venous thromboembolism

Central nervous system: Anxiety, dementia, dizziness, epilepsy exacerbation, headache, insomnia, irritability, mental depression, migraine, mood disturbances, nervousness

Dermatologic: Angioedema, chloasma, dermatitis, erythema multiforme, erythema nodosum, hemorrhagic eruption, hirsutism, loss of scalp hair, melasma, rash, pruritus, urticaria

Endocrine & metabolic: Breast cancer, breast enlargement, breast pain, breast tenderness, carbohydrate intolerance, fibrocystic breast changes, fluid retention, galactorrhea, hot flashes, hypocalcemia, libido changes, nipple discharge, nipple pain

Gastrointestinal: Abdominal cramps, abdominal pain, bloating, cholecystitis, cholelithiasis, constipation, diarrhea, dyspepsia, flatulence, gallbladder disease, gastritis, nausea, pancreatitis, vomiting, weight gain/loss

Genitourinary: Alterations in frequency and flow of bleeding patterns, breakthrough bleeding, cervical ectropion changes, cervical secretion changes, cystitis, dysmenorrhea, endometrial cancer, endometrial hyperplasia, genital eruption, menorrhagia, metrorrhagia, ovarian cancer, ovarian cyst, Pap smear suspicious, spotting, uterine leiomyomata size increased, leukorrhea, uterine cancer, uterine enlargement, uterine pain, urinary incontinence, urogenital pruritus, vaginal candidiasis, vaginal discharge, vaginal moniliasis, vaginitis

Hematologic: Aggravation of porphyria

Hepatic: Cholestatic jaundice, hepatic hemangioma enlargement

Local: Thrombophlebitis

Gel, spray: Application site reaction

Transdermal patches: Erythema, irritation

Neuromuscular & skeletal: Arthralgia, back pain, chorea, leg cramps, myalgia, muscle cramps, skeletal pain, weakness

Ocular: Blindness, contact lens intolerance, corneal curvature steepening, retinal vascular thrombosis

Respiratory: Asthma exacerbation, pulmonary thromboembolism

Miscellaneous: Anaphylactoid/anaphylactic reactions, hypersensitivity reactions

Postmarketing and/or case reports: Vaginal ring: Bowel obstruction, ring adherence to vaginal wall, toxic shock syndrome

Drug Interactions

Metabolism/Transport Effects Substrate of CYP1A2 (major), CYP2A6 (minor), CYP2B6 (minor), CYP2C19 (minor), CYP2C9 (minor), CYP2D6 (minor), CYP2E1 (minor), CYP3A4 (major), P-glycoprotein; **Note:** Assignment of Major/Minor substrate status based on clinically relevant drug interaction potential; **Inhibits** CYP1A2 (weak), CYP2C8 (weak); **Induces** CYP3A4 (weak/moderate)

Avoid Concomitant Use

Avoid concomitant use of Estradiol (Systemic) with any of the following: Anastrozole

Increased Effect/Toxicity

Estradiol (Systemic) may increase the levels/effects of: Corticosteroids (Systemic); ROPINIRole; Tipranavir

The levels/effects of Estradiol (Systemic) may be increased by: Ascorbic Acid; Conivaptan; Herbs (Estrogenic Properties); P-glycoprotein/ABCB1 Inhibitors

Decreased Effect

Estradiol (Systemic) may decrease the levels/effects of: Anastrozole; ARIPiprazole; Chenodiol; Saxagliptin; Somatropin; Thyroid Products; Ursodiol

The levels/effects of Estradiol (Systemic) may be decreased by: CYP1A2 Inducers (Strong); CYP3A4 Inducers (Strong); Cyproterone; Deferasirox; Peginterferon Alfa-2b; P-glycoprotein/ABCB1 Inducers; Tipranavir; Tocilizumab

Ethanol/Nutrition/Herb Interactions

Ethanol: Avoid ethanol (routine use increases estrogen level and risk of breast cancer). Ethanol may also increase the risk of osteoporosis.

Food: Folic acid absorption may be decreased

Herb/Nutraceutical: St John's wort may decrease levels. Herbs with estrogenic properties may enhance the adverse/toxic effect of estrogen derivatives; examples include alfalfa, black cohosh, bloodroot, hops, kudzu, licorice, red clover, saw palmetto, soybean, thyme, wild yam, yucca.

Stability Store all products at controlled room temperature. In addition:

Climara®, Estraderm®, Menostar®: Do not store >30°C (>86°F); store in protective pouch.

Mechanism of Action Estrogens are responsible for the development and maintenance of the female reproductive system and secondary sexual characteristics. Estradiol is the principle intracellular human estrogen and is more potent than estrone and estriol at the receptor level; it is the primary estrogen secreted prior to menopause. Following menopause, estrone and estrone sulfate are more highly produced. Estrogens modulate the pituitary secretion of gonadotropins, luteinizing hormone, and follicle-stimulating hormone through a negative feedback system; estrogen replacement reduces elevated levels of these hormones in postmenopausal women.

Pharmacodynamics/Kinetics

Absorption: Well absorbed from the gastrointestinal tract, mucous membranes, and the skin. Average serum estradiol concentrations (C_{avg}) vary by product

Oral: Femtrace®: C_{avg}: 23.5-92.1 pg/mL

Injection: Estradiol valerate and estradiol cypionate are absorbed over several weeks following I.M. injection
Topical:
Alora®: C_{avg}: 41-98 pg/mL
Climara®: C_{avg}: 22-106 pg/mL
Divigel®: C_{avg}: 9.8-30.5 pg/mL
Elestrin®: C_{avg}: 15.4-39.2 pg/mL; Exposure increased by 55% with application of sunscreen 10 minutes prior to dose
Estraderm® 0.1 mg/day: C_{avg}: 73 pg/mL
Estrasorb®: Mean serum concentration on day 22 of therapy: ~35-65 pg/mL; Exposure increased by 35% with application of sunscreen 10 minutes prior to dose
Estrogel®: C_{avg} on day 14 of therapy: 28.3 pg/mL
Evamist®: C_{avg}: 19.6-30.9 pg/mL
Menostar®: C_{avg}: 13.7 pg/mL
Vivelle-Dot®: C_{avg}: 34-104 pg/mL
Vaginal: Femring®: Rapid during the first hour following application, then declines to a steady rate over 3 months; C_{avg}: 40.6-76 pg/mL
Distribution: Widely distributed; high concentrations in the sex hormone target organs
Protein binding: Bound to sex hormone-binding globulin and albumin
Metabolism: Hepatic; partial metabolism via CYP3A4 enzymes; estradiol is reversibly converted to estrone and estriol; oral estradiol also undergoes enterohepatic recirculation by conjugation in the liver, followed by excretion of sulfate and glucuronide conjugates into the bile, then hydrolysis in the intestine and estrogen reabsorption. Sulfate conjugates are the primary form found in postmenopausal women. With transdermal application, less estradiol is metabolized leading to higher circulating concentrations of estradiol and lower concentrations of estrone and conjugates.
Half-life elimination: Femtrace®: 21-26 hours
Time to peak, plasma: Oral: Femtrace®: 0.4-0.75 hours
Excretion: Primarily urine (as estradiol, estrone, estriol and their glucuronide and sulfate conjugates)

Dosage All dosage needs to be adjusted based upon the patient's response
Oral:
Prostate cancer, advanced (androgen-dependent) (Estrace®): 1-2 mg 3 times/day
Breast cancer, metastatic (appropriately selected patients): Males and postmenopausal females (Estrace®): 10 mg 3 times/day **or** (unlabeled dosing) postmenopausal women: 2 mg 3 times/day (Ellis, 2009)
Osteoporosis prophylaxis in postmenopausal females (Estrace®): Lowest effective dose has not been determined; doses of 0.5 mg/day in a cyclic regimen for 23 days of a 28-week cycle were used in clinical studies
Female hypoestrogenism (due to hypogonadism, castration, or primary ovarian failure) (Estrace®): 1-2 mg/day; titrate as necessary to control symptoms using minimal effective dose for maintenance therapy
Vasomotor symptoms associated with menopause:
Estrace®: 1-2 mg/day, adjusted as necessary to limit symptoms; administration should be cyclic (3 weeks on, 1 week off)
Femtrace®: Initial dose: 0.45 mg/day; dosage range: 0.45-1.8 mg/day
Vulvar and vaginal atrophy associated with menopause (Estrace®): 1-2 mg/day, adjusted as necessary to limit symptoms; administration should be cyclic (3 weeks on, 1 week off)
I.M.:
Prostate cancer, advanced (androgen-dependent): Valerate (Delestrogen®): 30 mg or more every 1-2 weeks
Vasomotor symptoms associated with menopause:
Cypionate (Depo®-Estradiol): 1-5 mg every 3-4 weeks
Valerate (Delestrogen®): 10-20 mg every 4 weeks
Female hypoestrogenism (due to hypogonadism): Cypionate (Depo®-Estradiol): 1.5-2 mg monthly
Female hypoestrogenism (due to hypogonadism, castration, or primary ovarian failure): Valerate (Delestrogen®): 10-20 mg every 4 weeks
Vulvar and vaginal atrophy associated with menopause: Valerate (Delestrogen®): 10-20 mg every 4 weeks
Topical:
Emulsion: Vasomotor symptoms associated with menopause (Estrasorb®): 3.48 g applied once daily in the morning
Gel:
Vasomotor symptoms associated with menopause:
Divigel®: 0.25 g/day; adjust dose based on patient response. Dosing range: 0.25-1 g/day
Elestrin®: 0.87 g/day applied at the same time each day; adjust dose based on patient response. Dosing range: 0.87-1.7 g/day.
EstroGel®: 1.25 g/day applied at the same time each day
Vulvar and vaginal atrophy associated with menopause (EstroGel®): 1.25 g/day applied at the same time each day
Spray: Vasomotor symptoms associated with menopause (Evamist™): Initial: One spray (1.53 mg) per day. Adjust dose based on patient response. Dosing range: 1-3 sprays per day.
Transdermal patch: **Note:** Indicated dose may be used continuously in patients without an intact uterus. May be given continuously or cyclically (3 weeks on, 1 week off) in patients with an intact uterus (**exception - Menostar®, see specific dosing instructions**). When changing patients from oral to transdermal therapy, start transdermal patch 1 week after discontinuing oral hormone (may begin sooner if symptoms reappear within 1 week):
Once-weekly patch:
Vasomotor symptoms associated with menopause, vulvar and vaginal atrophy associated with menopause, female hypoestrogenism (due to hypogonadism, castration, or primary ovarian failure) (Climara®): Apply 0.025 mg/day patch once weekly. Adjust dose as necessary to control symptoms.
Osteoporosis prophylaxis in postmenopausal women:
Climara®: Apply patch once weekly; minimum effective dose 0.025 mg/day; adjust dosage based on response to therapy as indicated by biochemical markers and bone mineral density
Menostar®: Apply patch once weekly (0.014 mg/day). In women with a uterus, also administer a progestin for 14 days every 6-12 months
Twice-weekly patch:
Vasomotor symptoms associated with menopause, vulvar/vaginal atrophy associated with menopause, female hypoestrogenism (due to hypogonadism, castration, or primary ovarian failure): Titrate to lowest dose possible to control symptoms, adjusting initial dose after the first month of therapy:
Alora®, Estraderm®: Apply 0.05 mg patch twice weekly
Vivelle-Dot®: Apply 0.0375 mg patch twice weekly
Prevention of osteoporosis in postmenopausal women:
Alora®, Vivelle-Dot®: Apply 0.025 mg patch twice weekly, increase dose as necessary
Estraderm®: Apply 0.05 mg patch twice weekly
Vaginal ring: Vasomotor symptoms associated with menopause; vulvar and vaginal atrophy associated with menopause (Femring®): Initial: 0.05 mg intravaginally; following insertion, ring should remain in place for 3 months; dose may be increased to 0.1 mg if needed

Dietary Considerations Ensure adequate calcium and vitamin D intake when used for the prevention of osteoporosis.

Administration The use of a progestin should be considered when administering estrogens to postmenopausal women with an intact uterus.

Injection formulation: Intramuscular use only. Estradiol valerate should be injected into the upper outer quadrant of the gluteal muscle; administer with a dry needle (solution may become cloudy with wet needle).

Emulsion (Estrasorb®): Apply to clean, dry skin while in a sitting position. Contents of two pouches (total 3.48 g) are to be applied individually, once daily in the morning. Apply contents of first pouch to left thigh; massage into skin of left thigh and calf until thoroughly absorbed (~3 minutes). Apply excess from both hands to the buttocks. Apply contents of second pouch to the right thigh; massage into skin of right thigh and calf until thoroughly absorbed (~3 minutes). Apply excess from both hands to buttocks. Wash hands with soap and water. Allow skin to dry before covering legs with clothing. Do not apply to other areas of body. Do not apply to red or irritated skin.

Gel: Apply to clean, dry, unbroken skin at the same time each day. Allow to dry for 5 minutes prior to dressing. Gel is flammable; avoid fire or flame until dry. After application, wash hands with soap and water. Prior to the first use, pump must be primed. Do not apply gel to breast.

Divigel®: Apply entire contents of packet to right or left upper thigh each day (alternate sites). Do not apply to face, breasts, vaginal area or irritated skin. Apply over an area ~5x7 inches. Do not wash application site for 1 hour. Allow gel to dry before dressing

Elestrin®: Apply to upper arm and shoulder area using two fingers to spread gel. Apply after bath or shower; allow at least 2 hours between applying gel and going swimming. Wait at least 25 minutes before applying sunscreen to application area. Do not apply sunscreen to application area for ≥7 days (may increase absorption of gel).

EstroGel®: Apply gel to the arm, from the wrist to the shoulder. Spread gel as thinly as possible over one arm.

Spray: Evamist™: Prior to first use, prime pump by spraying 3 sprays with the cover on. To administer dose, hold container upright and vertical and rest the plastic cone flat against the skin while spraying. Spray to the inner surface of the forearm, starting near the elbow. If more than one spray is needed, apply to adjacent but not overlapping areas. Apply at the same time each day. Allow spray to dry for ~2 minutes; do not rub into skin; do not cover with clothing until dry. Do not wash application site for at least 60 minutes. Apply to clean, dry, unbroken skin. Do not apply to skin other than that of the forearm. Make sure that children do not come in contact with any skin area where the drug was applied. If contact with children is unavoidable, wear a garment with long sleeves that covers the site of application. If direct exposure should occur, wash the child in the area of exposure with soap and water as soon as possible. Solution contained in the spray is flammable; avoid fire, flame, or smoking until spray has dried. If needed, sunscreen should be applied ~1 hour prior to application of Evamist™.

Transdermal patch: Do not apply transdermal system to breasts, but place on trunk of body (preferably abdomen). Rotate application sites allowing a 1-week interval between applications at a particular site. Do not apply to oily, damaged or irritated skin; avoid waistline or other areas where tight clothing may rub the patch off. Apply patch immediately after removing from protective pouch. In general, if patch falls off, the same patch may be reapplied or a new system may be used for the remainder of the dosing interval (not recommended with all products). When replacing patch, reapply to a new site. Swimming, bathing or showering are not expected to affect use of the patch. Note the following exceptions:

Estraderm®: Do not apply to an area exposed to direct sunlight.

Climara®, Menostar®: Swimming, bathing, or wearing patch while in a sauna have not been studied; adhesion of patch may be decreased or delivery of estradiol may be affected. Remove patch slowly after use to avoid skin irritation. If any adhesive remains on the skin after removal, first allow skin to dry for 15 minutes, then gently rub area with an oil-based cream or lotion. If patch falls off, a new patch should be applied for the remainder of the dosing interval.

Vaginal ring: Exact positioning is not critical for efficacy; however, patient should not feel anything once inserted. In case of discomfort, ring should be pushed further into vagina. If ring is expelled prior to 90 days, it may be rinsed off and reinserted. Ensure proper vaginal placement of the ring to avoid inadvertent urinary bladder insertion. If vaginal infection develops, Femring® may remain in place during local treatment of a vaginal infection.

Monitoring Parameters Routine physical examination that includes blood pressure and Papanicolaou smear, breast exam, mammogram. Monitor for signs of endometrial cancer in female patients with uterus. Adequate diagnostic measures, including endometrial sampling, if indicated, should be performed to rule out malignancy in all cases of undiagnosed abnormal vaginal bleeding. Monitor for loss of vision, sudden onset of proptosis, diplopia, migraine; signs and symptoms of thromboembolic disorders; glycemic control in patients with diabetes; lipid profiles in patients being treated for hyperlipidemias; thyroid function in patients on thyroid hormone replacement therapy.

Menostar®: When used in a woman with a uterus, endometrial sampling is recommended at yearly intervals or when clinically indicated.

Menopausal symptoms, vulvar and vaginal atrophy: Assess need for therapy at 3- to 6-month intervals

Prevention of osteoporosis: Bone density measurement

Reference Range

Children 6 months to 10 years: <15 pg/mL (SI: <55 pmol/L)

Males: 10-50 pg/mL (SI: 37-184 pmol/L)

Females:

Premenopausal: 30-400 pg/mL (SI: 110-1468 pmol/L) (depending on phase of menstrual cycle)

Postmenopausal: 0-30 pg/mL (SI: 0-110 pmol/L)

Test Interactions Thyroid function tests: Estrogens may increase thyroid binding globulin and circulating total thyroid hormone (when measured by T_4 RIA, T_4 by column, or by PBI); decreases free T_3 resin uptake; concentration of free T_4 is not altered; metyrapone test: Response may be reduced

Dosage Forms Excipient information presented when available (limited, particularly for generics); consult specific product labeling.

Emulsion, topical, as hemihydrate:

Estrasorb®: 2.5 mg/g (56s) [each pouch contains estradiol hemihydrate 4.35 mg; contents of two pouches delivers estradiol 0.05 mg/day]

Gel, topical:
- Divigel®: 0.1% (30s) [delivers estradiol 0.25 mg/0.25 g packet]
- Divigel®: 0.1% (30s) [delivers estradiol 0.5 mg/0.5 g packet]
- Divigel®: 0.1% (30s) [delivers estradiol 1 mg/1 g packet]
- Elestrin®: 0.06% (35 g) [delivers estradiol 0.52 mg/0.87 g; 30 actuations]
- Elestrin®: 0.06% (70 g) [delivers estradiol 0.52 mg/0.87 g; 60 actuations; packaged as 2x35 g]
- EstroGel®: 0.06% (50 g) [contains ethanol; delivers estradiol 0.75 mg/1.25 g; 32 actuations]

Injection, oil, as cypionate:
- Depo®-Estradiol: 5 mg/mL (5 mL) [contains chlorobutanol, cottonseed oil]

Injection, oil, as valerate: 20 mg/mL (5 mL); 40 mg/mL (5 mL)
- Delestrogen®: 10 mg/mL (5 mL) [contains chlorobutanol, sesame oil]
- Delestrogen®: 20 mg/mL (5 mL); 40 mg/mL (5 mL) [contains benzyl alcohol, benzyl benzoate, castor oil]

Patch, transdermal [once-weekly patch]: 0.025 mg/24 hours (4s); 0.0375 mg/24 hours (4s); 0.05 mg/24 hours (4s); 0.06 mg/24 hours (4s); 0.075 mg/24 hours (4s); 0.1 mg/24 hours (4s)
- Climara®: 0.025 mg/24 hours (4s) [6.5 cm^2, total estradiol 2.04 mg]
- Climara®: 0.0375 mg/24 hours (4s) [9.375 cm^2, total estradiol 2.85 mg]
- Climara®: 0.05 mg/24 hours (4s) [12.5 cm^2, total estradiol 3.8 mg]
- Climara®: 0.06 mg/24 hours (4s) [15 cm^2, total estradiol 4.55 mg]
- Climara®: 0.075 mg/24 hours (4s) [18.75 cm^2, total estradiol 5.7 mg]
- Climara®: 0.1 mg/24 hours (4s) [25 cm^2, total estradiol 7.6 mg]
- Menostar®: 0.014 mg/24 hours (4s) [3.25 cm^2, total estradiol 1 mg]

Patch, transdermal [twice-weekly patch]:
- Alora®: 0.025 mg/24 hours (8s) [9 cm^2, total estradiol 0.77 mg]
- Alora®: 0.05 mg/24 hours (8s) [18 cm^2, total estradiol 1.5 mg]
- Alora®: 0.075 mg/24 hours (8s) [27 cm^2, total estradiol 2.3 mg]
- Alora®: 0.1 mg/24 hours (8s) [36 cm^2, total estradiol 3.1 mg]
- Estraderm®: 0.05 mg/24 hours (8s) [10 cm^2, total estradiol 4 mg]
- Estraderm®: 0.1 mg/24 hours (8s) [20 cm^2, total estradiol 8 mg]
- Vivelle-Dot®: 0.025 mg/24 hours (24s) [2.5 cm^2, total estradiol 0.39 mg]
- Vivelle-Dot®: 0.0375 mg/24 hours (24s) [3.75 cm^2, total estradiol 0.585 mg]
- Vivelle-Dot®: 0.05 mg/24 hours (24s) [5 cm^2, total estradiol 0.78 mg]
- Vivelle-Dot®: 0.075 mg/24 hours (24s) [7.5 cm^2, total estradiol 1.17 mg]
- Vivelle-Dot®: 0.1 mg/24 hours (24s) [10 cm^2, total estradiol 1.56 mg]

Ring, vaginal, as acetate:
- Femring®: 0.05 mg/24 hours (1s) [total estradiol 12.4 mg; releases 0.05 mg/24 hours over 3 months]
- Femring®: 0.1 mg/24 hours (1s) [total estradiol 24.8 mg; releases 0.1 mg/24 hours over 3 months]

Solution, topical [spray]:
- Evamist™: 1.53 mg/spray (8.1 mL) [contains ethanol; contains 56 sprays after priming]

Tablet, oral [micronized]: 0.5 mg, 1 mg, 2 mg
- Estrace®: 0.5 mg, 1 mg [scored]
- Estrace®: 2 mg [scored; contains tartrazine]

Tablet, oral, as acetate:
- Femtrace®: 0.45 mg, 0.9 mg, 1.8 mg

Estradiol (Topical) (es tra DYE ole)

Brand Names: U.S. Estrace®; Estring®; Vagifem®

Brand Names: Canada Estrace®; Estring®; Vagifem®; Vagifem® 10

Index Terms 17β-estradiol

Pharmacologic Category Estrogen Derivative

Use Treatment of moderate-to-severe vulvar and vaginal atrophy associated with menopause

Pregnancy Considerations In general, the use of estrogen and progestin as in combination hormonal contraceptives has not been associated with teratogenic effects when inadvertently taken early in pregnancy. These products are contraindicated for use during pregnancy.

Lactation Enters breast milk/use caution

Contraindications Hypersensitivity to estradiol or any component of the formulation; undiagnosed abnormal vaginal bleeding; DVT or PE (current or history of); active or recent (within 1 year) arterial thromboembolic disease (eg, stroke, MI); carcinoma of the breast (known, suspected or history of), except in appropriately selected patients being treated for metastatic disease; estrogen-dependent tumor; hepatic dysfunction or disease; pregnancy

Warnings/Precautions [U.S. Boxed Warning]: Unopposed estrogens may increase the risk of endometrial carcinoma in postmenopausal women with an intact uterus. Adequate diagnostic measures, including endometrial sampling, if indicated, should be performed to rule out malignancy in all cases of undiagnosed abnormal vaginal bleeding. The use of a progestin should be considered when administering estrogens to postmenopausal women with an intact uterus. Estrogens may exacerbate endometriosis. Malignant transformation of residual endometrial implants has been reported posthysterectomy with estrogen only therapy. Consider adding a progestin in women with residual endometriosis posthysterectomy. Postmenopausal estrogen therapy and combined estrogen/progesterone therapy may increase the risk of ovarian cancer; however, the absolute risk to an individual woman is small. Although results from various studies are not consistent, risk does not appear to be significantly associated with the duration, route, or dose of therapy. In one study, the risk decreased after 2 years following discontinuation of therapy (Mørch, 2009). Although the risk of ovarian cancer is rare, women who are at an increased risk (eg, family history) should be counseled about the association (NAMS, 2010). Estrogens may increase the risk of breast cancer. An increased risk of invasive breast cancer was observed in postmenopausal women using conjugated estrogens (CE) in combination with medroxyprogesterone acetate (MPA); a smaller increase in risk was seen with estrogen therapy alone in observational studies. An increase in abnormal mammograms has also been reported with estrogen and progestin therapy. Estrogen use may lead to severe hypercalcemia in patients with breast cancer and bone metastases; discontinue estrogen if hypercalcemia occurs.

[U.S. Boxed Warning]: Estrogens with or without progestin should not be used to prevent coronary heart disease. Use caution with cardiovascular disease or dysfunction. May increase the risks of myocardial infarction (MI), stroke, pulmonary emboli (PE), and deep vein thrombosis (DVT); incidence of these effects was shown to be significantly increased in postmenopausal women using CE with or without MPA. Nonfatal MI, PE, and thrombophlebitis have also been reported in males taking high doses of CE (eg, for prostate cancer). Risk factors include diabetes mellitus, hypercholesterolemia, hypertension, SLE, obesity, and/or venous thromboembolism (VTE). Use caution in patients with known inherited thrombophilias (eg, protein C or S deficiency); may have increased risk of VTE (DeSancho, 2010); use is contraindicated in patients with DVT or PE (current or history of).

[U.S. Boxed Warning]: The risk of dementia may be increased in postmenopausal women; increased incidence was observed in women ≥65 years of age taking CE alone or in combination with MPA.

[U.S. Boxed Warning]: Estrogens with or without progestin should be used for shortest duration possible at the lowest effective dose consistent with treatment goals. Before prescribing estrogen therapy to postmenopausal women, the risks and benefits must be weighed for each patient. Women should be informed of these risks and benefits, as well as possible effects of progestin when added to estrogen therapy. Conduct periodic risk:benefit assessments. Outcomes reported from clinical trials using CE should be assumed to be similar for estradiol until comparable data becomes available. In addition, risks associated with oral CE should be assumed to be similar for other dosage forms (eg, vaginal, transdermal) until additional information is available.

Estrogen compounds are generally associated with lipid effects such as increased HDL-cholesterol and decreased LDL-cholesterol. Triglycerides may also be increased; use with caution in patients with familial defects of lipoprotein metabolism. Estrogens may increase thyroid-binding globulin (TBG) levels leading to increased circulating total thyroid hormone levels. Women on thyroid replacement therapy may require higher doses of thyroid hormone while receiving estrogens.

Estrogens may cause retinal vascular thrombosis; discontinue if migraine, loss of vision, proptosis, diplopia, or other visual disturbances occur; discontinue permanently if papilledema or retinal vascular lesions are observed on examination. Estrogens are poorly metabolized in patients with hepatic dysfunction. Use caution with a history of cholestatic jaundice associated with prior estrogen use or pregnancy. Discontinue if jaundice develops or if acute or chronic hepatic disturbances occur. Use is contraindicated with hepatic disease. Use caution in patients with asthma, epilepsy, hepatic hemangiomas, migraine, porphyria, or SLE; may exacerbate disease. May have adverse effects on glucose tolerance; use caution in women with diabetes. Use with caution in patients with diseases which may be exacerbated by fluid retention, including cardiac or renal dysfunction. Use of postmenopausal estrogen may be associated with an increased risk of gallbladder disease requiring surgery. Use with caution in patients with severe hypocalcemia. Whenever possible, estrogens should be discontinued at least 4-6 weeks prior to elective surgery associated with an increased risk of thromboembolism or during periods of prolonged immobilization.

Vaginal ring: Use may not be appropriate in women with narrow vagina, vaginal stenosis, vaginal infections, cervical prolapse, rectoceles, cystoceles, or other conditions which may increase the risk of vaginal irritation, ulceration, or increase the risk of expulsion. Ring should be removed in case of ulceration, erosion, or adherence to vaginal wall; do not reinsert until healing is complete. Ensure proper vaginal placement of the ring to avoid inadvertent urinary bladder insertion.

Adverse Reactions

>10%: Central nervous system: Headache (13%)

1% to 10%:

Cardiovascular: Chest pain, edema, hypertension, leg edema, MI, stroke, syncope, venous thrombosis

Central nervous system: Insomnia (4%), anxiety, migraine

Dermatologic: Angioedema, chloasma, dermatitis, erythema multiforme, erythema nodosum, hemorrhagic eruption, hirsutism, loss of scalp hair, melasma, pruritus, rash, skin hypertrophy, urticaria

Endocrine & metabolic: Hot flashes (2%), breast pain (1%), breast cancer, breast enlargement, breast tenderness, carbohydrate tolerance decreased, endometrial carcinoma, endometrial hyperplasia, fibrocystic breast changes, galactorrhea, hypocalcemia, libido changes, nipple discharge, ovarian cancer

Gastrointestinal: Abdominal pain (4%), diarrhea (5%), nausea (3%), dyspepsia, flatulence, gastritis, hemorrhoids, toothache, weight changes

Genitourinary: Leukorrhea (7%), cervical ectropion changes, cervical secretion changes, cystitis, dysmenorrhea, dysuria, genital eruption, urinary incontinence, uterine leiomyomata change, vaginal bleeding pattern change (including abnormal flow, breakthrough bleeding, spotting)

Vaginal: Trauma from applicator insertion may occur in women with severely atrophic mucosa; burning, discomfort, hemorrhage, moniliasis, pain, pruritus, vaginitis, vulvovaginal infection

Hematologic: Porphyria aggravated

Local: Thrombophlebitis

Neuromuscular & skeletal: Back pain (6% to 7%), arthritis (4%), arthralgias (3%), skeletal pain (2%), leg cramps

Ocular: Contact lens intolerance, retinal vascular thrombosis

Otic: Otitis media

Respiratory: Respiratory tract infection: (5%), sinusitis (4%), pharyngitis (1%), asthma exacerbation, bronchitis, pulmonary embolism

Miscellaneous: Anaphylactoid/anaphylactic reactions, flu-like syndrome (3%), hypersensitivity

Postmarketing and/or case reports: Bowel obstruction (ring), ring adherence to vaginal wall (ring), toxic shock syndrome (ring)

Drug Interactions

Metabolism/Transport Effects Substrate of CYP1A2 (major), CYP2A6 (minor), CYP2B6 (minor), CYP2C19 (minor), CYP2C9 (minor), CYP2D6 (minor), CYP2E1 (minor), CYP3A4 (major), P-glycoprotein; **Note:** Assignment of Major/Minor substrate status based on clinically relevant drug interaction potential; **Inhibits** CYP1A2 (weak), CYP2C8 (weak); **Induces** CYP3A4 (weak/moderate)

Avoid Concomitant Use

Avoid concomitant use of Estradiol (Topical) with any of the following: Anastrozole

Increased Effect/Toxicity

Estradiol (Topical) may increase the levels/effects of: Corticosteroids (Systemic); ROPINIRole; Tipranavir

The levels/effects of Estradiol (Topical) may be increased by: Ascorbic Acid; Conivaptan; Herbs (Estrogenic Properties); P-glycoprotein/ABCB1 Inhibitors

Decreased Effect

Estradiol (Topical) may decrease the levels/effects of: Anastrozole; ARIPiprazole; Chenodiol; Saxagliptin; Somatropin; Thyroid Products; Ursodiol

The levels/effects of Estradiol (Topical) may be decreased by: CYP1A2 Inducers (Strong); CYP3A4 Inducers (Strong); Cyproterone; Deferasirox; Peginterferon Alfa-2b; P-glycoprotein/ABCB1 Inducers; Tipranavir; Tocilizumab

Stability

Vaginal cream (Estrace®): Store at room temperature; protect from temperatures in excess of 40°C (104°F).

Vaginal ring (Estring®): Store at 15°C to 30°C (59°F to 86°F).

Vaginal tablet (Vagifem®): Store at 25°C (77°F); do not refrigerate.

Mechanism of Action In studies for vulvar and vaginal atrophy in postmenopausal women, local estrogens have been shown to reduce vaginal pH levels and mature the vaginal and urethral mucosa after 12 weeks of therapy, thereby improving vaginal dryness and mucosal atrophy.

Pharmacodynamics/Kinetics

Absorption: Average serum estradiol concentrations (C_{avg}) vary by product

Vaginal: Vaginal absorption is typically low; any contribution to circulating estradiol concentrations via systemic absorption does not exceed normal postmenopausal ranges (Ulrich, 2010; Weisberg, 2005).

Estring®: Average steady state serum concentrations decrease from 11.2 pg/mL at 48 hours to 8 pg/mL at 12 weeks

Vagifem®: C_{avg}: 10.9 pg/mL on day 1, 5.5 pg/mL on day 83

Distribution: Widely distributed; high concentrations in the sex hormone target organs

Protein binding: Bound to sex hormone-binding globulin and albumin

Metabolism: Hepatic; partial metabolism via CYP3A4 enzymes; estradiol is reversibly converted to estrone and estriol. Sulfate conjugates are the primary form found in postmenopausal women.

Excretion: Primarily urine (as estradiol, estrone, estriol and their glucuronide and sulfate conjugates)

Dosage Adults: Topical: All dosage needs to be adjusted based upon the patient's response.

Vaginal cream: Vulvar and vaginal atrophy associated with menopause: (Estrace®): Insert 2-4 g/day intravaginally for 1-2 weeks, then gradually reduce to 1/2 the initial dose for 1-2 weeks, followed by a maintenance dose of 1 g 1-3 times/week

Vaginal ring (Estring®): Vulvar and vaginal atrophy associated with menopause: 2 mg intravaginally; following insertion, ring should remain in place for 90 days

Vaginal tablet (Vagifem®): Vulvar and vaginal atrophy associated with menopause: Initial: Insert 1 tablet (10 mcg) once daily for 2 weeks; Maintenance: Insert 1 tablet twice weekly

Administration

Vaginal ring: Exact positioning is not critical for efficacy; however, patient should not feel anything once inserted. In case of discomfort, ring should be pushed further into vagina. If ring is expelled prior to 90 days, it may be rinsed off and reinserted. Ensure proper vaginal placement of the ring to avoid inadvertent urinary bladder insertion. If vaginal infection develops, Estring® should be removed; reinsert only after infection has been appropriately treated.

Vaginal tablet: Insert tablet with supplied applicator at the same time each day. Once inserted, depress plunger until a click is heard, then remove applicator and discard. If tablet comes out of applicator prior to insertion, do not replace; use a new tablet filled applicator instead.

Monitoring Parameters Routine physical examination that includes blood pressure and Papanicolaou smear, breast exam, mammogram. Monitor for signs of endometrial cancer in female patients with uterus. Adequate diagnostic measures, including endometrial sampling, if indicated, should be performed to rule out malignancy in all cases of undiagnosed abnormal vaginal bleeding. Monitor for loss of vision, sudden onset of proptosis, diplopia, migraine; signs and symptoms of thromboembolic disorders; glycemic control in patients with diabetes; lipid profiles in patients being treated for hyperlipidemias; thyroid function in patients on thyroid hormone replacement therapy. Assess need for therapy at 3- to 6-month intervals.

Test Interactions Thyroid function tests: Estrogens may increase thyroid binding globulin and circulating total thyroid hormone (when measured by T_4 RIA, T_4 by column, or by PBI); decreases free T_3 resin uptake; concentration of free T_4 is not altered; metyrapone test: Response may be reduced.

Dosage Forms Excipient information presented when available (limited, particularly for generics); consult specific product labeling. [DSC] = Discontinued product

Cream, vaginal:

Estrace®: 0.1 mg/g (42.5 g)

Ring, vaginal, as base:

Estring®: 2 mg (1s) [total estradiol 2 mg; releases 7.5 mcg/day over 90 days]

Tablet, vaginal, as base:

Vagifem®: 10 mcg, 25 mcg [DSC]

◆ **Estradiol Acetate** *see* Estradiol (Systemic) *on page* 627

Estradiol and Dienogest

(es tra DYE ole & dye EN oh jest)

Brand Names: U.S. Natazia™

Index Terms Dienogest and Estradiol; Estradiol Valerate and Dienogest

Pharmacologic Category Contraceptive; Estrogen and Progestin Combination

Use Prevention of pregnancy

Unlabeled Use Treatment of hypermenorrhea (menorrhagia); pain associated with endometriosis; dysmenorrhea; dysfunctional uterine bleeding

Pregnancy Risk Factor X

Dosage Oral: Adults: Females: Contraception: Take 1 tablet daily in the order presented in the blister pack

Initial dosing: Start on day 1 of menstrual period (first day of bleeding). A nonhormonal contraceptive should be used for the first 9 days.

Switching from another combination oral contraceptive tablet: Take the first dark yellow tablet on the first day of withdrawal bleeding; do not continue taking tablets from previous contraceptive pack. If withdrawal bleeding does not occur, rule-out pregnancy before starting therapy. A non-hormonal contraceptive should be used for the first 9 days.

Switching from a vaginal ring or patch: Take the first dark yellow tablet on the day the ring or patch is removed. A nonhormonal contraceptive should be used for the first 9 days.

Switching from a progestin-only contraceptive: Take the first dark yellow tablet on the day the next progestin-only tablet would have been given, or the day the progestin implant or IUD is removed, or on the day the next injection would have been given. A nonhormonal contraceptive should be used for the first 9 days.

Missed doses: If ≤12 hours late, take tablet as soon as remembering and take the next tablet at the usual time. If >12 hours late, instructions vary by day of cycle and number of tablets missed:

If missed ONE dose:

Days 1-17: Take missed tablet immediately; take next tablet at usual time; use back-up (nonhormonal) contraception for the next 9 days; continue taking 1 tablet each day for the rest of the cycle

Days 18-24: Do not continue using current blister pack (throw away); take day 1 of new blister pack; use back-up (nonhormonal) contraception for the next 9 days; continue taking 1 tablet each day for the rest of the cycle

Days 25-28: Take missed tablet immediately; take next tablet at usual time; continue taking 1 tablet each day for the rest of the cycle; no backup method of contraception is needed.

If missed TWO doses in a row:

Days 1-17: Do not take missed tablets; start by taking the tablet for the day it was first noticed that the tablet was missed; use back-up (nonhormonal) contraception for the next 9 days; continue taking 1 tablet each day for the rest of the cycle. If tablets were missed on days 17 and 18, follow directions for missed tablets on days 17-25.

Days 17-25: Do not continue using current blister pack (throw away); take day 3 of new blister pack; use back-up (nonhormonal) contraception for the next 9 days; continue taking 1 tablet each day for the rest of the cycle. If tablets were missed on days 25 and 26, follow directions for missed tablets on days 25-28.

Days 25-28: Do not continue using current blister pack (throw away); start a new pack on the same day, or start a new pack the day it would normally be started; continue taking 1 tablet each day for the rest of the cycle; no backup method of contraception is needed.

Dosage adjustment in renal impairment: Safety and efficacy have not been evaluated; dose adjustment not expected to be required

Dosage adjustment in hepatic impairment: Discontinue if hepatic dysfunction occurs

Additional Information Complete prescribing information for this medication should be consulted for additional detail.

Dosage Forms Excipient information presented when available (limited, particularly for generics); consult specific product labeling.

Tablet, oral [four-phasic formulation]:

Natazia™:

Days 1-2: Estradiol valerate 3 mg [2 dark yellow tablets]

Days 3-7: Estradiol valerate 2 mg and dienogest 2 mg [5 medium red tablets]

Days 8-24: Estradiol valerate 2 mg and dienogest 3 mg [17 light yellow tablets]

Days 25-26: Estradiol valerate 1 mg [2 dark red tablets]

Days 27-28: 2 white inactive tablets (28s)

Estradiol and Levonorgestrel

(es tra DYE ole & LEE voe nor jes trel)

Brand Names: U.S. ClimaraPro®

Index Terms Levonorgestrel and Estradiol

Pharmacologic Category Estrogen and Progestin Combination

Use Women with an intact uterus: Treatment of moderate-to-severe vasomotor symptoms associated with menopause; prevention of postmenopausal osteoporosis

Dosage Topical: Adult females with an intact uterus: Treatment of moderate-to-severe vasomotor symptoms associated with menopause or prevention of postmenopausal osteoporosis:

Estradiol 0.045 mg/levonorgestrel 0.015 mg: Apply one patch weekly

Additional Information Complete prescribing information for this medication should be consulted for additional detail.

Dosage Forms Excipient information presented when available (limited, particularly for generics); consult specific product labeling.

Patch, transdermal:

ClimaraPro®: Estradiol 0.045 mg and levonorgestrel 0.015 mg per 24 hours (4s) [22 cm^2; contains estradiol 4.4 mg and levonorgestrel 1.39 mg]

Estradiol and Norethindrone

(es tra DYE ole & nor eth IN drone)

Brand Names: U.S. Activella®; CombiPatch®; Mimvey™

Brand Names: Canada Estalis-Sequi®; Estalis®

Index Terms Norethindrone and Estradiol

Pharmacologic Category Estrogen and Progestin Combination

Use Women with an intact uterus:

Tablet: Treatment of moderate-to-severe vasomotor symptoms associated with menopause; treatment of vulvar and vaginal atrophy; prophylaxis for postmenopausal osteoporosis

Transdermal patch: Treatment of moderate-to-severe vasomotor symptoms associated with menopause; treatment of vulvar and vaginal atrophy; treatment of hypoestrogenism due to hypogonadism, castration, or primary ovarian failure

Dosage Note: Patients should be treated with the lowest effective dose and for the shortest duration, consistent with treatment goals. Adults:

Oral (Activella®): One tablet daily

Transdermal patch (CombiPatch®):

Continuous combined regimen: Apply 1 patch twice weekly

Continuous sequential regimen: Apply estradiol-only patch for first 14 days of cycle, followed by one CombiPatch® applied twice weekly for the remaining 14 days of a 28-day cycle

Transdermal patch, combination pack (product-specific dosing for Canadian formulation):

Estalis®: Continuous combined regimen: Apply a new patch twice weekly during a 28-day cycle

Estalis-Sequi®: Continuous sequential regimen: Apply estradiol-only patch (Vivelle®) for first 14 days, followed by one Estalis® patch applied twice weekly during the last 14 days of a 28-day cycle

Note: In women previously receiving oral estrogens, initiate upon reappearance of menopausal symptoms following discontinuation of oral therapy.

Additional Information Complete prescribing information for this medication should be consulted for additional detail.

Dosage Forms Excipient information presented when available (limited, particularly for generics); consult specific product labeling.

Patch, transdermal:

CombiPatch®:

0.05/0.14: Estradiol 0.05 mg and norethindrone acetate 0.14 mg per day (8s) [9 sq cm]

0.05/0.25: Estradiol 0.05 mg and norethindrone acetate 0.25 mg per day (8s) [16 sq cm]

Tablet, oral: 1/0.5: Estradiol 1 mg and norethindrone acetate 0.5 mg (28s)

Activella®: 0.5/0.1: Estradiol 0.5 mg and norethindrone acetate 0.1 mg (28s)

Activella®: 1/0.5: Estradiol 1 mg and norethindrone acetate 0.5 mg (28s)

Mimvey™: 1/0.5: Estradiol 1 mg and norethindrone acetate 0.5 mg (28s)

Dosage Forms: Canada Excipient information presented when available (limited, particularly for generics); consult specific product labeling.

Combination pack:

Estalis-Sequi® 140/50:

Patch, transdermal (Vivelle®): Estradiol 50 mcg per day (4s) [14.5 sq cm; total estradiol 4.33 mg]

Patch, transdermal (Estalis®): Norethindrone acetate 140 mcg and estradiol 50 mcg per day (4s) [9 sq cm; total norethindrone acetate 2.7 mg, total estradiol 0.62 mg]

Estalis-Sequi® 250/50:
Patch, transdermal (Vivelle®): Estradiol 50 mcg per day (4s) [14.5 sq cm; total estradiol 4.33 mg]
Patch, transdermal (Estalis®): Norethindrone acetate 250 mcg and estradiol 50 mcg per day (4s) [16 sq cm; total norethindrone acetate 4.8 mg, total estradiol 0.51 mg]
Patch, transdermal:
Estalis®;
140/50: Norethindrone acetate 140 mcg and estradiol 50 mcg per day (8s) [9 sq cm; total norethindrone acetate 2.7 mg, total estradiol 0.62 mg]
250/50 Norethindrone acetate 250 mcg and estradiol 50 mcg per day (8s) [16 sq cm; total norethindrone acetate 4.8 mg, total estradiol 0.51 mg]

◆ **Estradiol Transdermal** *see* Estradiol (Systemic) *on page 627*

◆ **Estradiol Valerate** *see* Estradiol (Systemic) *on page 627*

◆ **Estradiol Valerate and Dienogest** *see* Estradiol and Dienogest *on page 634*

◆ **Estradot® (Can)** *see* Estradiol (Systemic) *on page 627*

◆ **Estragyn (Can)** *see* Estrogens (Esterified) *on page 645*

Estramustine (es tra MUS teen)

Brand Names: U.S. Emcyt®
Brand Names: Canada Emcyt®
Index Terms Estramustine Phosphate; Estramustine Phosphate Sodium; NSC-89199
Pharmacologic Category Antineoplastic Agent, Alkylating Agent; Antineoplastic Agent, Hormone; Antineoplastic Agent, Hormone (Estrogen/Nitrogen Mustard)
Use Palliative treatment of progressive or metastatic prostate cancer
Pregnancy Considerations Estramustine is not indicated for use in women. Men who were impotent on estrogen therapy have regained potency while taking estramustine; effective contraception should be used for male patients with partners of childbearing potential.
Contraindications Hypersensitivity to estramustine, estradiol, nitrogen mustard, or any component of the formulation; active thrombophlebitis or thromboembolic disorders (except where tumor mass is the cause of thromboembolic disorder and the benefit may outweigh the risk)

Canadian labeling: Additional contraindications (not in the U.S. labeling): Severe hepatic or cardiac disease

Warnings/Precautions Hazardous agent - use appropriate precautions for handling and disposal. Glucose tolerance may be decreased; use with caution in patients with diabetes. Elevated blood pressure, peripheral edema (new-onset or exacerbation), or congestive heart disease may occur; use with caution in patients where fluid accumulation may be poorly tolerated, including cardiovascular disease (HF or hypertension), migraine, seizure disorder or renal dysfunction. Estrogen treatment for prostate cancer is associated with an increased risk of thrombosis and MI; use caution with history of cardiovascular disease (eg, thrombophlebitis, thrombosis, or thromboembolic disease) and cerebrovascular or coronary artery disease. Use with caution in patients with hepatic impairment (may be metabolized poorly) or with metabolic bone diseases. Allergic reactions and angioedema, including airway involvement, have been reported with use. Patients with prostate cancer and osteoblastic metastases should have their calcium monitored regularly. Estrogen use may cause gynecomastia and/or impotence. Avoid vaccination with live vaccines during treatment (risk of infection may be increased due to immunosuppression). Although the response to vaccines may be diminished, inactivated vaccines may be administered during treatment.

Adverse Reactions
>10%:
Cardiovascular: Edema (20%)
Endocrine & metabolic: Gynecomastia (75%), breast tenderness (71%), libido decreased
Gastrointestinal: Nausea (16%), diarrhea (13%), gastrointestinal upset (12%)
Hepatic: LDH increased (2% to 33%), AST increased (2% to 33%)
Respiratory: Dyspnea (12%)
1% to 10%:
Cardiovascular: CHF (3%), MI (3%), cerebrovascular accident (2%), chest pain (1%), flushing (1%)
Central nervous system: Lethargy (4%), insomnia (3%), emotional lability (2%), anxiety (1%), headache (1%)
Dermatologic: Bruising (3%), dry skin (2%), pruritus (2%), hair thinning (1%), rash (1%), skin peeling (1%)
Gastrointestinal: Anorexia (4%), flatulence (2%), burning throat (1%), gastrointestinal bleeding (1%), thirst (1%), vomiting (1%)
Hematologic: Leukopenia (4%), thrombocytopenia (1%)
Hepatic: Bilirubin increased (1% to 2%)
Local: Thrombophlebitis (3%)
Neuromuscular & skeletal: Leg cramps (9%)
Ocular: Tearing (1%)
Respiratory: Pulmonary embolism (2%), upper respiratory discharge (1%), hoarseness (1%)
<1% (Limited to important or life-threatening): Allergic reactions, anemia, angina, angioedema, cerebrovascular ischemia, confusion, coronary ischemia, depression, glucose tolerance decreased, hyper-/hypocalcemia, hypertension, impotence, muscle weakness, venous thrombosis

Drug Interactions
Metabolism/Transport Effects None known.
Avoid Concomitant Use
Avoid concomitant use of Estramustine with any of the following: BCG; Natalizumab; Pimecrolimus; Tacrolimus (Topical); Vaccines (Live)
Increased Effect/Toxicity
Estramustine may increase the levels/effects of: Leflunomide; Natalizumab; Vaccines (Live)

The levels/effects of Estramustine may be increased by: Clodronate; Denosumab; Pimecrolimus; Roflumilast; Tacrolimus (Topical); Trastuzumab
Decreased Effect
Estramustine may decrease the levels/effects of: BCG; Coccidioidin Skin Test; Sipuleucel-T; Vaccines (Inactivated); Vaccines (Live)

The levels/effects of Estramustine may be decreased by: Calcium Salts; Echinacea

Ethanol/Nutrition/Herb Interactions Food: Estramustine serum levels may be decreased if taken with milk and other dairy products, calcium supplements, and vitamins containing calcium.
Stability Refrigerate at 2°C to 8°C (36°F to 46°F).
Mechanism of Action Combines the effects of estradiol and nitrogen mustard. It appears to bind to microtubule proteins, preventing normal tubulin function. The antitumor effect may be due solely to an estrogenic effect. Estramustine causes a marked decrease in plasma testosterone and an increase in estrogen levels.
Pharmacodynamics/Kinetics
Absorption: Oral: 75%
Metabolism:
GI tract: Initial dephosphorylation
Hepatic: Oxidation and hydrolysis; metabolites include estramustine, estrone analog, estrone, and estradiol
Half-life elimination: Terminal: 15-24 hours

Time to peak, serum: 2-3 hours
Excretion: Feces (2.9% to 4.8% as unchanged drug)

Dosage Details concerning dosing in combination regimens should also be consulted.

Oral: Adults: Males: Prostate cancer: 14 mg/kg/day (range: 10-16 mg/kg/day) in 3 or 4 divided doses

Combination therapy with docetaxel (unlabeled dose): 280 mg 3 times/day for 5 days (days 1 through 5) of a 21-day treatment cycle for up to 12 cycles (Petrylak, 2004)

Dietary Considerations Should be taken at least 1 hour before or 2 hours after eating. Milk products and calcium-rich foods or supplements may impair the oral absorption of estramustine phosphate sodium.

Administration Administer on an empty stomach, at least 1 hour before or 2 hours after eating.

Monitoring Parameters Serum calcium, liver function tests; blood pressure

Dosage Forms Excipient information presented when available (limited, particularly for generics); consult specific product labeling.

Capsule, oral, as phosphate sodium:
Emcyt®: 140 mg

◆ **Estramustine Phosphate** *see* Estramustine *on page 636*

◆ **Estramustine Phosphate Sodium** *see* Estramustine *on page 636*

◆ **Estrasorb®** *see* Estradiol (Systemic) *on page 627*

◆ **Estratab® (Can)** *see* Estrogens (Esterified) *on page 645*

◆ **Estring®** *see* Estradiol (Topical) *on page 632*

◆ **EstroGel®** *see* Estradiol (Systemic) *on page 627*

◆ **Estrogenic Substances, Conjugated** *see* Estrogens (Conjugated/Equine, Systemic) *on page 641*

◆ **Estrogenic Substances, Conjugated** *see* Estrogens (Conjugated/Equine, Topical) *on page 643*

Estrogens (Conjugated A/Synthetic)

(ES troe jenz, KON joo gate ed, aye, sin THET ik)

Brand Names: U.S. Cenestin®

Brand Names: Canada Cenestin

Pharmacologic Category Estrogen Derivative

Use Treatment of moderate-to-severe vasomotor symptoms of menopause; treatment of vulvar and vaginal atrophy

Pregnancy Considerations Use during pregnancy is contraindicated.

Lactation Enters breast milk/use caution

Contraindications Hypersensitivity to estrogens or any component of the formulation; undiagnosed abnormal vaginal bleeding; history of or current thrombophlebitis or venous thromboembolic disorders (including DVT, PE); active or recent (within 1 year) arterial thromboembolic disease (eg, stroke, MI); carcinoma of the breast; estrogen-dependent tumor; hepatic dysfunction or disease; pregnancy

Warnings/Precautions

Cardiovascular-related considerations: **[U.S. Boxed Warning]: Estrogens with or without progestin should not be used to prevent coronary heart disease.** Use caution with cardiovascular disease or dysfunction. May increase the risks of myocardial infarction (MI), stroke, pulmonary emboli (PE), and deep vein thrombosis (DVT); incidence of these effects was shown to be significantly increased in postmenopausal women using CEE in combination with MPA. Nonfatal MI, PE, and thrombophlebitis have also been reported in males taking high doses of CEE (eg, for prostate cancer). Risk factors include diabetes mellitus, hypercholesterolemia, hypertension, SLE, obesity, and/or venous thromboembolism (VTE). Estrogen compounds are generally associated with lipid effects such as increased HDL-cholesterol and decreased LDL-cholesterol. Triglycerides may also be increased; use with caution in patients with familial defects of lipoprotein metabolism. Whenever possible, estrogens should be discontinued at least 4 weeks prior to and for 2 weeks following elective surgery associated with an increased risk of thromboembolism or during periods of prolonged immobilization. Use caution in patients with known inherited thrombophilias (eg, protein C or S deficiency); may have increased risk of VTE (DeSancho, 2010); use is contraindicated in patients with DVT or PE (current or history of).

Neurological considerations: **[U.S. Boxed Warning]: The risk of dementia may be increased in postmenopausal women;** increased incidence was observed in women ≥65 years of age taking CEE alone or in combination with MPA.

Cancer-related considerations: **[U.S. Boxed Warning]: Unopposed estrogens may increase the risk of endometrial carcinoma in postmenopausal women.** Estrogens may exacerbate endometriosis. Malignant transformation of residual endometrial implants has been reported posthysterectomy with estrogen only therapy. Consider adding a progestin in women with residual endometriosis posthysterectomy. Estrogens may increase the risk of breast cancer. An increased risk of invasive breast cancer was observed in postmenopausal women using CEE in combination with MPA; a smaller increase in risk was seen with estrogen therapy alone in observational studies. An increase in abnormal mammograms has also been reported with estrogen and progestin therapy. Estrogen use may lead to severe hypercalcemia in patients with breast cancer and bone metastases; discontinue estrogen if hypercalcemia occurs. Postmenopausal estrogen therapy and combined estrogen/progesterone therapy may increase the risk of ovarian cancer; however, the absolute risk to an individual woman is small. Although results from various studies are not consistent, risk does not appear to be significantly associated with the duration, route, or dose of therapy. In one study, the risk decreased after 2 years following discontinuation of therapy.

Estrogens may cause retinal vascular thrombosis; discontinue permanently if papilledema or retinal vascular lesions are observed on examination. Use with caution in patients with diseases which may be exacerbated by fluid retention, including asthma, epilepsy, migraine, diabetes or renal dysfunction. Use with caution in patients with a history of severe hypocalcemia, SLE, hepatic hemangiomas, porphyria, endometriosis, and gallbladder disease. Use caution with history of cholestatic jaundice associated with past estrogen use or pregnancy. May be inappropriate for use in the elderly due to potential of increased risk of breast and endometrial cancers and lack of proven cardioprotection (Beers Criteria). Safety and efficacy in pediatric patients have not been established. Prior to puberty, estrogens may cause premature closure of the epiphyses, premature breast development in girls or gynecomastia in boys. Vaginal bleeding and vaginal cornification may also be induced in girls.

Before prescribing estrogen therapy to postmenopausal women, the risks and benefits must be weighed for each patient. Women should be informed of these risks and benefits, as well as possible effects of progestin when added to estrogen therapy. Estrogens with or without progestin should be used for shortest duration possible consistent with treatment goals. Conduct periodic risk: benefit assessments.

Vulvar and vaginal atrophy use: When used solely for the treatment of vulvar and vaginal atrophy, topical vaginal products should be considered.

Adverse Reactions

>10%:

Central nervous system: Headache (11% to 68%), dizziness (11%), pain (11%)
Endocrine & metabolic: Breast pain (29%), endometrial thickening (19%), metrorrhagia (14%)
Gastrointestinal: Abdominal pain (9% to 28%), nausea (9% to 18%)
Neuromuscular & skeletal: Paresthesia (8% to 33%), back pain (14%)
Respiratory: Upper respiratory tract infection (13%)
Miscellaneous: Infection (2% to 14%)

1% to 10%:

Central nervous system: Anxiety (6%), fever (1%)
Gastrointestinal: Dyspepsia (10%), vomiting (7%), constipation (6%), diarrhea (6%), weight gain (6%)
Genitourinary: Vaginitis (8%)
Neuromuscular & skeletal: Leg cramps (10%), hypertonia (6%)
Respiratory: Rhinitis (6% to 8%), cough (6%)

In addition, the following have been reported with estrogen and/or progestin therapy:

Cardiovascular: Edema, hypertension, MI, stroke, venous thromboembolism
Central nervous system: Epilepsy exacerbation, irritability, mental depression, migraine, mood disturbances, nervousness
Dermatologic: Angioedema, chloasma, erythema multiforme, erythema nodosum, hemorrhagic eruption, hirsutism, melasma, pruritus, rash, scalp hair loss, urticaria
Endocrine & metabolic: Breast cancer, breast enlargement, breast tenderness, glucose tolerance impaired, HDL-cholesterol increased, hyper-/hypocalcemia, LDL-cholesterol decreased, libido changes, serum triglycerides/phospholipids increased, thyroid-binding globulin increased, total thyroid hormone (T_4) increased
Gastrointestinal: Abdominal cramps, bloating, cholecystitis, cholelithiasis, gallbladder disease, pancreatitis, weight gain/loss
Genitourinary: Alterations in frequency and flow of menses, cervical secretion changes, endometrial cancer, endometrial hyperplasia, uterine leiomyomata size increased, vaginal candidiasis
Hematologic: Aggravation of porphyria, antithrombin III and antifactor Xa decreased, fibrinogen levels increased, platelet aggregability and platelet count increased; prothrombin and factors VII, VIII, IX, X increased
Hepatic: Cholestatic jaundice, hepatic hemangiomas enlarged
Neuromuscular & skeletal: Arthralgias, chorea, leg cramps
Local: Thrombophlebitis
Ocular: Contact lens intolerance, corneal curvature steepening, retinal vascular thrombosis
Respiratory: Asthma exacerbation, pulmonary thromboembolism
Miscellaneous: Anaphylactoid/anaphylactic reactions, carbohydrate intolerance

Drug Interactions

Metabolism/Transport Effects Substrate of CYP1A2 (major), CYP2A6 (minor), CYP2B6 (minor), CYP2C19 (minor), CYP2C9 (minor), CYP2D6 (minor), CYP2E1 (minor), CYP3A4 (major); **Note:** Assignment of Major/Minor substrate status based on clinically relevant drug interaction potential; **Inhibits** CYP1A2 (weak); **Induces** CYP3A4 (weak/moderate)

Avoid Concomitant Use

Avoid concomitant use of Estrogens (Conjugated A/Synthetic) with any of the following: Anastrozole

Increased Effect/Toxicity

Estrogens (Conjugated A/Synthetic) may increase the levels/effects of: Corticosteroids (Systemic); ROPINIRole; Tipranavir

The levels/effects of Estrogens (Conjugated A/Synthetic) may be increased by: Ascorbic Acid; Conivaptan; Herbs (Estrogenic Properties)

Decreased Effect

Estrogens (Conjugated A/Synthetic) may decrease the levels/effects of: Anastrozole; ARIPiprazole; Chenodiol; Saxagliptin; Somatropin; Thyroid Products; Ursodiol

The levels/effects of Estrogens (Conjugated A/Synthetic) may be decreased by: CYP1A2 Inducers (Strong); CYP3A4 Inducers (Strong); Cyproterone; Deferasirox; Herbs (CYP3A4 Inducers); Peginterferon Alfa-2b; Tipranavir; Tocilizumab

Ethanol/Nutrition/Herb Interactions

Ethanol: Avoid ethanol (routine use increases estrogen plasma concentrations and risk of breast cancer).
Food: Grapefruit juice may increase estrogen plasma concentrations, leading to increased adverse effects.
Herb/Nutraceutical: St John's wort may decrease levels. Herbs with estrogenic properties may enhance the adverse/toxic effect of estrogen derivatives; examples include alfalfa, black cohosh, bloodroot, hops, kudzu, licorice, red clover, saw palmetto, soybean, thyme, wild yam, yucca.

Stability Store at room temperature of 25°C (77°F).

Mechanism of Action Conjugated A/synthetic estrogens contain a mixture of 9 synthetic estrogen substances, including sodium estrone sulfate, sodium equilin sulfate, sodium 17 alpha-dihydroequilin, sodium 17 alpha-estradiol and sodium 17 beta-dihydroequilin. Estrogens are responsible for the development and maintenance of the female reproductive system and secondary sexual characteristics. Estradiol is the principle intracellular human estrogen and is more potent than estrone and estriol at the receptor level; it is the primary estrogen secreted prior to menopause. Following menopause, estrone and estrone sulfate are more highly produced. Estrogens modulate the pituitary secretion of gonadotropins, luteinizing hormone, and follicle-stimulating hormone through a negative feedback system; estrogen replacement reduces elevated levels of these hormones in postmenopausal women.

Pharmacodynamics/Kinetics

Absorption: Well absorbed over a period of several hours
Protein-binding: Sex hormone-binding globulin (SHBG) and albumin
Metabolism: Hepatic via CYP3A4; estradiol is converted to estrone and estriol; also undergoes enterohepatic recirculation; estrone sulfate is the main metabolite in postmenopausal women
Excretion: Urine (primarily estriol, also as estradiol, estrone, and conjugates)

Dosage The lowest dose that will control symptoms should be used; medication should be discontinued as soon as possible. Oral:

Adults:

Moderate-to-severe vasomotor symptoms: 0.45 mg/day; may be titrated up to 1.25 mg/day. Attempts to discontinue medication should be made at 3- to 6-month intervals.
Vulvar and vaginal atrophy: 0.3 mg/day

Elderly: Refer to adult dosing. A higher incidence of stroke and invasive breast cancer were observed in women >75 years in a WHI substudy using conjugated equine estrogen.

Monitoring Parameters Yearly physical examination that includes blood pressure and Papanicolaou smear, breast exam, mammogram. Monitor for signs of endometrial cancer in female patients with uterus. Adequate diagnostic measures, including endometrial sampling, if indicated, should be performed to rule out malignancy in all cases of undiagnosed abnormal vaginal bleeding. Monitor for loss of vision, sudden onset of proptosis, diplopia, migraine; signs and symptoms of thromboembolic disorders; glycemic control in patients with diabetes; lipid profiles in patients being treated for hyperlipidemias; thyroid function in patients on thyroid hormone replacement therapy.

Menopausal symptoms: Assess need for therapy at 3- to 6-month intervals

Test Interactions Pathologist should be advised of estrogen/progesterone therapy when specimens are submitted. Reduced response to metyrapone test observed with conjugated estrogens (equine).

Additional Information Not biologically equivalent to conjugated estrogens from equine source. Contains 9 unique estrogenic compounds (equine source contains at least 10 active estrogenic compounds).

Dosage Forms Excipient information presented when available (limited, particularly for generics); consult specific product labeling.

Tablet, oral:

Cenestin®: 0.3 mg, 0.45 mg, 0.625 mg, 0.9 mg, 1.25 mg

Estrogens (Conjugated B/Synthetic)

(ES troe jenz, KON joo gate ed, bee, sin THET ik)

Brand Names: U.S. Enjuvia™

Pharmacologic Category Estrogen Derivative

Use Treatment of moderate-to-severe vasomotor symptoms of menopause; treatment of vulvar and vaginal atrophy associated with menopause; treatment of moderate-to-severe vaginal dryness and pain with intercourse associated with menopause

Pregnancy Considerations Use during pregnancy is contraindicated.

Lactation Enters breast milk/use caution

Contraindications Hypersensitivity to estrogens or any component of the formulation; undiagnosed abnormal vaginal bleeding; history of or current thrombophlebitis or venous thromboembolic disorders (including DVT, PE); active or recent (within 1 year) arterial thromboembolic disease (eg, stroke, MI); carcinoma of the breast; estrogen-dependent tumor; hepatic dysfunction or disease; pregnancy

Warnings/Precautions

Cardiovascular-related considerations: **[U.S. Boxed Warning]: Estrogens with or without progestin should not be used to prevent coronary heart disease.** Use caution with cardiovascular disease or dysfunction. May increase the risks of myocardial infarction (MI), stroke, pulmonary emboli (PE), and deep vein thrombosis (DVT); incidence of these effects was shown to be significantly increased in postmenopausal women using CEE in combination with MPA. Nonfatal MI, PE, and thrombophlebitis have also been reported in males taking high doses of CEE (eg, for prostate cancer). Risk factors include diabetes mellitus, hypercholesterolemia, hypertension, SLE, obesity, and/or venous thromboembolism (VTE). Estrogen compounds are generally associated with lipid effects such as increased HDL-cholesterol and decreased LDL-cholesterol. Triglycerides may also be increased; use with caution in patients with familial defects of lipoprotein metabolism. Whenever possible, estrogens should be discontinued at least 4 weeks prior to and for 2 weeks following elective surgery associated with an increased risk of thromboembolism or during periods of prolonged immobilization. Use caution in patients with known inherited thrombophilias (eg, protein C or S deficiency); may have increased risk of VTE (DeSancho, 2010); use is contraindicated in patients with DVT or PE (current or history of).

Neurological considerations: **[U.S. Boxed Warning]: The risk of dementia may be increased in postmenopausal women;** increased incidence was observed in women ≥65 years of age taking CEE alone or in combination with MPA.

Cancer-related considerations: **[U.S. Boxed Warning]: Unopposed estrogens may increase the risk of endometrial carcinoma in postmenopausal women.** Estrogens may exacerbate endometriosis. Malignant transformation of residual endometrial implants has been reported posthysterectomy with estrogen only therapy. Consider adding a progestin in women with residual endometriosis posthysterectomy. Estrogens may increase the risk of breast cancer. An increased risk of invasive breast cancer was observed in postmenopausal women using CEE in combination with MPA; a smaller increase in risk was seen with estrogen therapy alone in observational studies. An increase in abnormal mammograms has also been reported with estrogen and progestin therapy. Estrogen use may lead to severe hypercalcemia in patients with breast cancer and bone metastases; discontinue estrogen if hypercalcemia occurs. Postmenopausal estrogen therapy and combined estrogen/progesterone therapy may increase the risk of ovarian cancer; however, the absolute risk to an individual woman is small. Although results from various studies are not consistent, risk does not appear to be significantly associated with the duration, route, or dose of therapy. In one study, the risk decreased after 2 years following discontinuation of therapy.

Estrogens may cause retinal vascular thrombosis; discontinue permanently if papilledema or retinal vascular lesions are observed on examination. Use with caution in patients with diseases which may be exacerbated by fluid retention, including asthma, epilepsy, migraine, diabetes or renal dysfunction. Use with caution in patients with a history of severe hypocalcemia, SLE, hepatic hemangiomas, porphyria, endometriosis, and gallbladder disease. Use caution with history of cholestatic jaundice associated with past estrogen use or pregnancy. May be inappropriate for use in the elderly due to potential of increased risk of breast and endometrial cancers and lack of proven cardioprotection (Beers Criteria). Safety and efficacy in pediatric patients have not been established. Prior to puberty, estrogens may cause premature closure of the epiphyses, premature breast development in girls or gynecomastia in boys. Vaginal bleeding and vaginal cornification may also be induced in girls.

Before prescribing estrogen therapy to postmenopausal women, the risks and benefits must be weighed for each patient. Women should be informed of these risks and benefits, as well as possible effects of progestin when added to estrogen therapy. Estrogens with or without progestin should be used for shortest duration possible consistent with treatment goals. Conduct periodic risk: benefit assessments. When used solely for the treatment of vaginal dryness and pain with intercourse, or vulvar and vaginal atrophy, topical vaginal products should be considered.

Adverse Reactions

>10%:

Central nervous system: Headache (15% to 25%), pain (10% to 19%)

Endocrine & metabolic: Breast pain (up to 14%)

Gastrointestinal: Abdominal pain (4% to 15%), nausea (7% to 12%)

1% to 10%:

Central nervous system: Dizziness (1% to 7%)

Endocrine & metabolic: Dysmenorrhea (1% to 8%)

Gastrointestinal: Flatulence (4% to 7%)

Genitourinary: Vaginitis (2% to 7%)

Neuromuscular & skeletal: Paresthesia (up to 6%)
Respiratory: Bronchitis (up to 7%), rhinitis (4% to 7%), sinusitis (3% to 7%)
Miscellaneous: Flu-like syndrome (4% to 7%)

In addition, the following have been reported with estrogen and/or progestin therapy:

Cardiovascular: Edema, hypertension, MI, stroke, venous thromboembolism

Central nervous system: Epilepsy exacerbation, irritability, mental depression, migraine, mood disturbances, nervousness

Dermatologic: Angioedema, chloasma, erythema multiforme, erythema nodosum, hemorrhagic eruption, hirsutism, loss of scalp hair, melasma, pruritus, rash, urticaria

Endocrine & metabolic: Breast cancer, breast enlargement, breast tenderness, HDL-cholesterol increased, hyper-/hypocalcemia, impaired glucose tolerance, LDL-cholesterol decreased, libido (changes in), serum triglycerides/phospholipids increased, thyroid-binding globulin increased, total thyroid hormone (T_4) increased

Gastrointestinal: Abdominal cramps, bloating, cholecystitis, cholelithiasis, gallbladder disease, pancreatitis, weight gain/loss

Genitourinary: Alterations in frequency and flow of menses, changes in cervical secretions, endometrial cancer, endometrial hyperplasia, increased size of uterine leiomyomata, vaginal candidiasis

Hematologic: Aggravation of porphyria; antithrombin III and antifactor Xa decreased; fibrinogen levels increased; platelet aggregability and platelet count increased; prothrombin and factors VII, VIII, IX, X increased

Hepatic: Cholestatic jaundice, hepatic hemangiomas enlarged

Local: Thrombophlebitis

Neuromuscular & skeletal: Arthralgias, chorea, leg cramps

Ocular: Contact lens intolerance, corneal curvature steepening, retinal vascular thrombosis

Respiratory: Asthma exacerbation, pulmonary thromboembolism

Miscellaneous: Anaphylactoid/anaphylactic reactions, carbohydrate intolerance

Drug Interactions

Metabolism/Transport Effects Substrate of CYP3A4 (major); **Note:** Assignment of Major/Minor substrate status based on clinically relevant drug interaction potential

Avoid Concomitant Use

Avoid concomitant use of Estrogens (Conjugated B/Synthetic) with any of the following: Anastrozole

Increased Effect/Toxicity

Estrogens (Conjugated B/Synthetic) may increase the levels/effects of: Corticosteroids (Systemic); ROPINIRole; Tipranavir

The levels/effects of Estrogens (Conjugated B/Synthetic) may be increased by: Ascorbic Acid; Conivaptan; Herbs (Estrogenic Properties)

Decreased Effect

Estrogens (Conjugated B/Synthetic) may decrease the levels/effects of: Anastrozole; Chenodiol; Somatropin; Thyroid Products; Ursodiol

The levels/effects of Estrogens (Conjugated B/Synthetic) may be decreased by: CYP3A4 Inducers (Strong); Deferasirox; Herbs (CYP3A4 Inducers); Tipranavir; Tocilizumab

Ethanol/Nutrition/Herb Interactions

Ethanol: Avoid ethanol (routine use increases estrogen plasma concentrations and risk of breast cancer).

Food: Grapefruit juice may increase estrogen plasma concentrations, leading to increased adverse effects.

Herb/Nutraceutical: St John's wort may decrease levels. Herbs with estrogenic properties may enhance the adverse/toxic effect of estrogen derivatives; examples include alfalfa, black cohosh, bloodroot, hops, kudzu, licorice, red clover, saw palmetto, soybean, thyme, wild yam, and yucca.

Stability Store at room temperature of 25°C (77°F).

Mechanism of Action Conjugated B/synthetic estrogens contain a mixture of 10 synthetic estrogen substances, including sodium estrone sulfate, sodium equilin sulfate, sodium 17-alpha-dihydroequilin, sodium 17-alpha-estradiol, and sodium 17-beta-dihydroequilin. Estrogens are responsible for the development and maintenance of the female reproductive system and secondary sexual characteristics. Estradiol is the principle intracellular human estrogen and is more potent than estrone and estriol at the receptor level; it is the primary estrogen secreted prior to menopause. Following menopause, estrone and estrone sulfate are more highly produced. Estrogens modulate the pituitary secretion of gonadotropins, luteinizing hormone, and follicle-stimulating hormone through a negative feedback system; estrogen replacement reduces elevated levels of these hormones in postmenopausal women.

Pharmacodynamics/Kinetics

Absorption: Well absorbed over a period of several hours

Protein-binding: Sex hormone-binding globulin (SHBG) and albumin

Metabolism: Hepatic via CYP3A4; estradiol is converted to estrone and estriol; also undergoes enterohepatic recirculation; estrone sulfate is the main metabolite in postmenopausal women

Half-life elimination: Conjugated estrone: 8-20 hours; conjugated equilin: 5-17 hours

Excretion: Urine (primarily estriol, also as estradiol, estrone, and conjugates)

Dosage The lowest dose that will control symptoms should be used; medication should be discontinued as soon as possible. Oral:

Adults:

Moderate-to-severe vasomotor symptoms associated with menopause: 0.3 mg/day; may be titrated up to 1.25 mg/day. Attempts to discontinue medication should be made at 3- to 6-month intervals.

Vaginal dryness/vulvar and vaginal atrophy associated with menopause: 0.3 mg/day. Attempts to discontinue medication should be made at 3- to 6-month intervals.

Elderly: A higher incidence of stroke and invasive breast cancer were observed in women >75 years in a WHI substudy using conjugated equine estrogen.

Monitoring Parameters Yearly physical examination that may include blood pressure and Papanicolaou smear, breast exam, mammogram. Monitor for signs of endometrial cancer in female patients with uterus. Adequate diagnostic measures, including endometrial sampling, if indicated, should be performed to rule out malignancy in all cases of undiagnosed abnormal vaginal bleeding. Monitor for loss of vision, sudden onset of proptosis, diplopia, migraine; signs and symptoms of thromboembolic disorders; glycemic control in patients with diabetes; lipid profiles in patients being treated for hyperlipidemias; thyroid function in patients on thyroid hormone replacement therapy.

Test Interactions Pathologist should be advised of estrogen/progesterone therapy when specimens are submitted. Reduced response to metyrapone test observed with conjugated estrogens (equine).

Additional Information Not biologically equivalent to conjugated estrogens from equine source. Contains 10 unique estrogenic compounds (equine source contains at least 10 active estrogenic compounds).

Dosage Forms Excipient information presented when available (limited, particularly for generics); consult specific product labeling.

Tablet, oral:

Enjuvia™: 0.3 mg, 0.45 mg, 0.625 mg, 0.9 mg, 1.25 mg

Estrogens (Conjugated/Equine, Systemic) (ES troe jenz KON joo gate ed, EE kwine)

Brand Names: U.S. Premarin®

Brand Names: Canada C.E.S.®; Congest; PMS-Conjugated Estrogens C.S.D.; Premarin®

Index Terms C.E.S.; CE; CEE; Conjugated Estrogen; Estrogenic Substances, Conjugated

Pharmacologic Category Estrogen Derivative

Use Treatment of moderate-to-severe vasomotor symptoms associated with menopause; treatment of vulvar and vaginal atrophy due to menopause; hypoestrogenism (due to hypogonadism, castration, or primary ovarian failure); prostatic cancer (palliation); breast cancer (palliation); postmenopausal osteoporosis (prophylaxis); abnormal uterine bleeding

Unlabeled Use Uremic bleeding

Pregnancy Considerations Estrogens are not indicated for use during pregnancy or immediately postpartum. In general, the use of estrogen and progestin as in combination hormonal contraceptives have not been associated with teratogenic effects when inadvertently taken early in pregnancy. These products are contraindicated for use during pregnancy.

Lactation Enters breast milk/use caution

Contraindications Angioedema or anaphylactic reaction to estrogens or any component of the formulation; undiagnosed abnormal vaginal bleeding; history of or current thrombophlebitis or venous thromboembolic disorders (including DVT, PE); active or recent (within 1 year) arterial thromboembolic disease (eg, stroke, MI); carcinoma of the breast (except in appropriately selected patients being treated for metastatic disease); known protein C, protein S, antithrombin deficiency, or other known thrombophilic disorders; pregnancy

Canadian labeling: Additional contraindications (not in U.S. labeling): Endometrial hyperplasia; partial or complete vision loss due to ophthalmic vascular disease; migraine with aura

Warnings/Precautions

Anaphylaxis requiring emergency medical management has been reported within minutes to hours of taking conjugated estrogen (CE) tablets. Angioedema involving the face, feet, hands, larynx, and tongue has also been reported. Exogenous estrogens may exacerbate symptoms in women with hereditary angioedema.

[U.S. Boxed Warning]: Estrogens may increase the risk of breast cancer. An increased risk of invasive breast cancer was observed in postmenopausal women using conjugated estrogens (CE) in combination with medroxyprogesterone acetate (MPA); a smaller increase in risk was seen with estrogen therapy alone in observational studies. An increase in abnormal mammograms has also been reported with estrogen alone or in combination with progestin therapy. Estrogen use may lead to severe hypercalcemia in patients with breast cancer and bone metastases; discontinue estrogen if hypercalcemia occurs. **[U.S. Boxed Warning]: Unopposed estrogens may increase the risk of endometrial carcinoma in postmenopausal women with an intact uterus. Adequate diagnostic measures, including endometrial sampling, if indicated, should be performed to rule out malignancy in all cases of undiagnosed abnormal vaginal bleeding. The use of a progestin should be considered when administering estrogens to postmenopausal women with an intact uterus.** When indicated, oral progestins should be used (NAMS, 2010). Estrogens may exacerbate endometriosis. Malignant transformation of residual endometrial implants has been reported posthysterectomy with estrogen only therapy. Consider adding a progestin in women with residual endometriosis posthysterectomy. Postmenopausal estrogen therapy and combined estrogen/progesterone therapy may increase the risk of ovarian cancer; however, the absolute risk to an individual woman is small. Although results from various studies are not consistent, risk does not appear to be significantly associated with the duration, route, or dose of therapy. In one study, the risk decreased after 2 years following discontinuation of therapy (Mørch, 2009). Although the risk of ovarian cancer is rare, women who are at an increased risk (eg, family history) should be counseled about the association (NAMS, 2010).

[U.S. Boxed Warning]: Estrogens with or without progestin should not be used to prevent cardiovascular disease. Use caution with cardiovascular disease or dysfunction. May increase the risks of myocardial infarction (MI), stroke, pulmonary emboli (PE), and deep vein thrombosis (DVT); incidence of these effects was shown to be significantly increased in postmenopausal women using CE with or without MPA. Nonfatal MI, PE, and thrombophlebitis have also been reported in males taking high doses of CE (eg, for prostate cancer). Risk factors include diabetes mellitus, hypercholesterolemia, hypertension, SLE, obesity, and/or venous thromboembolism (VTE). Use is contraindicated in patients with known inherited thrombophilias (eg, protein C or S deficiency); may have increased risk of VTE (DeSancho, 2010). Use is contraindicated in patients with DVT or PE (current or history of).

[U.S. Boxed Warning]: The risk of dementia may be increased in postmenopausal women; increased incidence was observed in women ≥65 years of age taking CE alone or in combination with MPA.

Estrogen compounds are generally associated with lipid effects such as increased HDL-cholesterol and decreased LDL-cholesterol. Triglycerides may also be increased; discontinue if pancreatitis occurs. Use with caution in patients with familial defects of lipoprotein metabolism. Estrogens may increase thyroid-binding globulin (TBG) levels leading to increased circulating total thyroid hormone levels. Women on thyroid replacement therapy may require higher doses of thyroid hormone while receiving estrogens. Use caution in patients with hypoparathyroidism; estrogen-induced hypocalcemia may occur. May have adverse effects on glucose tolerance; use caution in women with diabetes. Use caution in patients with asthma, epilepsy, hepatic hemangiomas, porphyria, or SLE; may exacerbate disease. Use with caution in patients with diseases which may be exacerbated by fluid retention, including cardiac or renal dysfunction. Use of postmenopausal estrogen may be associated with an increased risk of gallbladder disease requiring surgery. Use caution with migraine; may exacerbate disease. Canadian labeling contraindicates use in migraine with aura. Estrogens may cause retinal vascular thrombosis; discontinue if migraine, loss of vision, proptosis, diplopia, or other visual disturbances occur; discontinue permanently if papilledema or retinal vascular lesions are observed on examination.

Estrogens are poorly metabolized in patients with hepatic dysfunction. Use caution with a history of cholestatic jaundice associated with prior estrogen use or pregnancy. Discontinue if jaundice develops or if acute or chronic hepatic disturbances occur. Use is contraindicated with hepatic disease.

Whenever possible, estrogens should be discontinued at least 4-6 weeks prior to elective surgery associated with an increased risk of thromboembolism or during periods of prolonged immobilization. May be inappropriate for use in the elderly due to potential of increased risk of breast and endometrial cancers and lack of proven cardioprotection (Beers Criteria). Prior to puberty, estrogens may cause premature closure of the epiphyses, premature breast development in girls or gynecomastia in boys. Vaginal bleeding and vaginal cornification may also be induced in girls.

[U.S. Boxed Warning]: Estrogens with or without progestin should be used for shortest duration possible at the lowest effective dose consistent with treatment goals. Before prescribing estrogen therapy to postmenopausal women, the risks and benefits must be weighed for each patient. Women should be informed of these risks and benefits, as well as possible effects of progestin when added to estrogen therapy. Estrogens with or without progestin should be used for shortest duration possible consistent with treatment goals. Conduct periodic risk: benefit assessments.

Vulvar and vaginal atrophy use: Moderate-to-severe symptoms of vulvar and vaginal atrophy include vaginal dryness, dyspareunia, and atrophic vaginitis. When used solely for the treatment of vulvar and vaginal atrophy, topical vaginal products should be considered (NAMS, 2007).

Osteoporosis use: For use only in women at significant risk of osteoporosis and for who other nonestrogen medications are not considered appropriate.

Adverse Reactions Note: Percentages reported in postmenopausal women following oral use.

>10%:

Central nervous system: Headache (26% to 32%; placebo 28%), pain (17% to 20%; placebo 18%)
Endocrine & metabolic: Breast pain (7% to 12%; placebo 9%)
Gastrointestinal: Abdominal pain (15% to 17%), diarrhea (6% to 7%; placebo 6%)
Genitourinary: Vaginal hemorrhage (2% to 14%)
Neuromuscular & skeletal: Back pain (13% to 14%), arthralgia (7% to 14%; placebo 12%)
Respiratory: Pharyngitis (10% to 12%; placebo 11%), sinusitis: (6% to 11%; placebo 7%)

1% to 10%:

Central nervous system: Depression (5% to 8%), dizziness (4% to 6%), nervousness (2% to 5%)
Dermatologic: Pruritus (4% to 5%)
Gastrointestinal: Flatulence (6% to 7%)
Genitourinary: Vaginitis (5% to 7%), leukorrhea (4% to 7%), vaginal moniliasis (5% to 6%)
Neuromuscular & skeletal: Weakness (7% to 8%), leg cramps (3% to 7%)
Respiratory: Cough increased (4% to 7%)

Additional adverse reactions reported with injection; frequency not defined: Local: injection site: Edema, pain, phlebitis

Postmarketing and/or case reports: Alopecia, anaphylaxis, angioedema, asthma exacerbation, benign meningioma (possible growth), bloating, breast cancer, breast discharge/enlargement/tenderness, cervical secretion changes, chloasma, cholestatic jaundice, contact lens intolerance, dementia, deep vein thrombosis (DVT), dysmenorrhea, edema, endometrial cancer, endometrial hyperplasia, epilepsy exacerbation, erythema multiforme, erythema nodosum, fibrocystic breast changes, galactorrhea, gallbladder disease, glucose intolerance, gynecomastia (males), hepatic hemangiomas (enlargement), hirsutism, hypersensitivity reactions, hypertension, irritability, ischemic colitis, libido changes, melasma, MI, migraine, mood disturbances, nausea, ovarian cancer, pancreatitis, pulmonary emboli (PE), pelvic pain, porphyria exacerbation, rash, retinal vascular thrombosis, stroke, superficial venous thrombosis, thrombophlebitis, triglyceride increase, urticaria, uterine bleeding (abnormal), uterine leiomyomata (increase in size), vaginal candidiasis, vomiting, weight changes

Drug Interactions

Metabolism/Transport Effects Substrate of CYP1A2 (major), CYP2A6 (minor), CYP2B6 (minor), CYP2C19 (minor), CYP2C9 (minor), CYP2D6 (minor), CYP2E1 (minor), CYP3A4 (major); **Note:** Assignment of Major/Minor substrate status based on clinically relevant drug interaction potential; **Inhibits** CYP1A2 (weak); **Induces** CYP3A4 (weak/moderate)

Avoid Concomitant Use

Avoid concomitant use of Estrogens (Conjugated/Equine, Systemic) with any of the following: Anastrozole

Increased Effect/Toxicity

Estrogens (Conjugated/Equine, Systemic) may increase the levels/effects of: Corticosteroids (Systemic); ROPINIRole; Tipranavir

The levels/effects of Estrogens (Conjugated/Equine, Systemic) may be increased by: Ascorbic Acid; Conivaptan; Herbs (Estrogenic Properties)

Decreased Effect

Estrogens (Conjugated/Equine, Systemic) may decrease the levels/effects of: Anastrozole; ARIPiprazole; Chenodiol; Saxagliptin; Somatropin; Thyroid Products; Ursodiol

The levels/effects of Estrogens (Conjugated/Equine, Systemic) may be decreased by: CYP1A2 Inducers (Strong); CYP3A4 Inducers (Strong); Cyproterone; Deferasirox; Herbs (CYP3A4 Inducers); Peginterferon Alfa-2b; Tipranavir; Tocilizumab

Ethanol/Nutrition/Herb Interactions

Ethanol: Avoid ethanol (routine use increases estrogen plasma concentrations and risk of breast cancer). Ethanol may also increase the risk of osteoporosis.
Food: Folic acid absorption may be decreased.
Herb/Nutraceutical: St John's wort may decrease levels. Herbs with estrogenic properties may enhance the adverse/toxic effect of estrogen derivatives; examples include alfalfa, black cohosh, bloodroot, hops, kudzu, licorice, red clover, saw palmetto, soybean, thyme, wild yam, yucca.

Stability

Injection: Refrigerate at 2°C to 8°C (36°F to 46°F) prior to reconstitution. Reconstitute with sterile water for injection; slowly inject diluent against side wall of the vial. Agitate gently; do not shake violently. Use immediately following reconstitution.
Tablets: Store at room temperature 20°C to 25°C (68°F to 77°F).

Mechanism of Action Conjugated estrogens contain a mixture of estrone sulfate, equilin sulfate, 17 alpha-dihydroequilin, 17 alpha-estradiol and 17 beta-dihydroequilin. Estrogens are responsible for the development and maintenance of the female reproductive system and secondary sexual characteristics. Estradiol is the principle intracellular human estrogen and is more potent than estrone and estriol at the receptor level; it is the primary estrogen secreted prior to menopause. Following menopause, estrone and estrone sulfate are more highly produced. Estrogens modulate the pituitary secretion of gonadotropins, luteinizing hormone, and follicle-stimulating hormone through a negative feedback system; estrogen replacement reduces elevated levels of these hormones in postmenopausal women.

Pharmacodynamics/Kinetics

Absorption: Well absorbed
Protein binding: Binds to sex-hormone-binding globulin and albumin

Metabolism: Hepatic via CYP3A4; estradiol is converted to estrone and estriol; also undergoes enterohepatic recirculation (avoided with vaginal administration); estrone sulfate is the main metabolite in postmenopausal women

Half-life elimination: Total estrone: 27 hours

Time to peak, plasma: Total estrone: 7 hours

Excretion: Urine (primarily estriol, also as estradiol, estrone, and conjugates

Dosage Adults:

Males: Androgen-dependent prostate cancer palliation: Oral: 1.25-2.5 mg 3 times/day

Females:

Prevention of postmenopausal osteoporosis: Oral:

U.S. labeling: Initial: 0.3 mg/day cyclically* or daily, depending on medical assessment of patient. Dose may be adjusted based on bone mineral density and clinical response. The lowest effective dose should be used.

Canadian labeling: 0.625 mg once daily

Moderate-to-severe vasomotor symptoms associated with menopause: Oral: Initial: 0.3 mg/day, cyclically* or daily, depending on medical assessment of patient. Adjust dose based on patient's response. The lowest dose that will control symptoms should be used.

Vulvar and vaginal atrophy: Oral: Initial: 0.3 mg/day; the lowest dose that will control symptoms should be used. May be given cyclically* or daily, depending on medical assessment of patient. Adjust dose based on patient's response.

Abnormal uterine bleeding: Acute/heavy bleeding:

Oral (unlabeled route): 10-20 mg/day in 4 divided doses has been used in place of I.M./I.V. doses (ACOG, 2000)

I.M., I.V.: 25 mg, may repeat in 6-12 hours if needed (manufacturers labeling) **or** 25 mg I.V. repeated every 4 hours for 24 hours (ACOG, 2000). Patients who do not respond to 1-2 doses should be re-evaluated (ACOG, 2000).

Note: Treatment should be followed by a low-dose oral contraceptive; medroxyprogesterone acetate along with or following estrogen therapy can also be given

Female hypogonadism: Oral: 0.3-0.625 mg/day given cyclically*; dose may be titrated in 6- to 12-month intervals; progestin treatment should be added to maintain bone mineral density once skeletal maturity is achieved.

Female castration, primary ovarian failure: Oral: 1.25 mg/day given cyclically*; adjust according to severity of symptoms and patient response. For maintenance, adjust to the lowest effective dose.

***Cyclic administration:** Either 3 weeks on, 1 week off **or** 25 days on, 5 days off

Males and Females:

Breast cancer palliation, metastatic disease in selected patients: Oral: 10 mg 3 times/day for at least 3 months

Uremic bleeding (unlabeled use): I.V.: 0.6 mg/kg/day for 5 days (Livio, 1986)

Elderly: Refer to adult dosing; a higher incidence of stroke and invasive breast cancer was observed in women >75 years in a WHI substudy.

Dosage adjustment in renal impairment: No dosage adjustment provided in manufacturer's labeling (has not been studied). Use with caution; may increase risk of fluid retention.

Dosage adjustment in hepatic impairment: Use is contraindicated with hepatic dysfunction or disease.

Dietary Considerations Ensure adequate calcium and vitamin D intake when used for the prevention of osteoporosis. Powder for reconstitution for injection (25 mg) contains lactose 200 mg.

Administration

Injection: May also be administered intramuscularly; when administered I.V., drug should be administered slowly to avoid the occurrence of a flushing reaction

Oral tablet: Administer at bedtime to minimize adverse effects. May be administered without regard to meals.

Abnormal uterine bleeding: High-dose therapy (eg. 10-20 mg/day) may cause nausea; consider concomitant use of an antiemetic

Monitoring Parameters Routine physical examination that includes blood pressure and Papanicolaou smear, breast exam, mammogram. Monitor for signs of endometrial cancer in female patients with uterus. Adequate diagnostic measures, including endometrial sampling, if indicated, should be performed to rule out malignancy in all cases of undiagnosed abnormal vaginal bleeding. Monitor for loss of vision, sudden onset of proptosis, diplopia, migraine; signs and symptoms of thromboembolic disorders; glycemic control in patients with diabetes; lipid profiles in patients being treated for hyperlipidemias; thyroid function in patients on thyroid hormone replacement therapy.

Menopausal symptoms: Assess need for therapy at 3- to 6-month intervals

Prevention of osteoporosis: Bone density measurement

Uremic bleeding: Bleeding time

Reference Range

Children: <10 mcg/24 hours (SI: <35 µmol/day) (values at Mayo Medical Laboratories)

Adults:

Males: 15-40 mcg/24 hours (SI: 52-139 micromole/day)

Females:

Menstruating: 15-80 mcg/24 hours (SI: 52-277 micromole/day)

Postmenopausal: <20 mcg/24 hours (SI: <69 micromole/day)

Test Interactions Thyroid function tests: Estrogens may increase thyroid binding globulin and circulating total thyroid hormone (when measured by T_4 RIA, T_4 by column, or by PBI); decreases free T_3 resin uptake; concentration of free T_4 is not altered; metyrapone test: Response may be reduced

Dosage Forms Excipient information presented when available (limited, particularly for generics); consult specific product labeling.

Injection, powder for reconstitution:

Premarin®: 25 mg [contains benzyl alcohol (in diluent), lactose 200 mg]

Tablet, oral:

Premarin®: 0.3 mg, 0.45 mg, 0.625 mg, 0.9 mg, 1.25 mg

Estrogens (Conjugated/Equine, Topical)

(ES troe jenz KON joo gate ed, EE kwine)

Brand Names: U.S. Premarin®

Brand Names: Canada Premarin®

Index Terms C.E.S.; CE; CEE; Conjugated Estrogen; Estrogenic Substances, Conjugated

Pharmacologic Category Estrogen Derivative

Use Treatment of atrophic vaginitis and kraurosis vulvae; moderate-to-severe dyspareunia (pain during intercourse) due to vaginal/vulvar atrophy of menopause

Pregnancy Considerations Estrogens are not indicated for use during pregnancy or immediately postpartum. In general, the use of estrogen and progestin as in combination hormonal contraceptives have not been associated with teratogenic effects when inadvertently taken early in pregnancy. These products are contraindicated for use during pregnancy. Use of the vaginal cream may weaken latex found in condoms, diaphragms, or cervical caps.

Lactation Enters breast milk/use caution

Contraindications Undiagnosed abnormal vaginal bleeding; history of or current thrombophlebitis or venous thromboembolic disorders (including DVT, PE); active or recent (within 1 year) arterial thromboembolic disease (eg, stroke, MI); carcinoma of the breast; estrogen-dependent tumor; hepatic dysfunction or disease; pregnancy

Canadian labeling: Additional contraindications (not in U.S. labeling): Hypersensitivity to estrogens or any component of the formulation; endometrial hyperplasia; partial or complete vision loss due to ophthalmic vascular disease

Warnings/Precautions [U.S. Boxed Warning]: Estrogens may increase the risk of breast cancer. An increased risk of invasive breast cancer was observed in postmenopausal women using conjugated estrogens (CE) in combination with medroxyprogesterone acetate (MPA); a smaller increase in risk was seen with estrogen therapy alone in observational studies. An increase in abnormal mammograms has also been reported with estrogen alone or in combination with progestin therapy. Estrogen use may lead to severe hypercalcemia in patients with breast cancer and bone metastases; discontinue estrogen if hypercalcemia occurs. **[U.S. Boxed Warning]: Unopposed estrogens may increase the risk of endometrial carcinoma in postmenopausal women with an intact uterus. Adequate diagnostic measures, including endometrial sampling, if indicated, should be performed to rule out malignancy in all cases of undiagnosed abnormal vaginal bleeding. The use of a progestin should be considered when administering estrogens to postmenopausal women with an intact uterus.** When indicated, oral progestins should be used (NAMS, 2010). Estrogens may exacerbate endometriosis. Malignant transformation of residual endometrial implants has been reported posthysterectomy with estrogen only therapy. Consider adding a progestin in women with residual endometriosis posthysterectomy. Postmenopausal estrogen therapy and combined estrogen/progesterone therapy may increase the risk of ovarian cancer; however, the absolute risk to an individual woman is small. Although results from various studies are not consistent, risk does not appear to be significantly associated with the duration, route, or dose of therapy. In one study, the risk decreased after 2 years following discontinuation of therapy (Mørch, 2009). Although the risk of ovarian cancer is rare, women who are at an increased risk (eg, family history) should be counseled about the association (NAMS, 2010).

[U.S. Boxed Warning]: Estrogens with or without progestin should not be used to prevent cardiovascular disease. Use caution with cardiovascular disease or dysfunction. May increase the risks of myocardial infarction (MI), stroke, pulmonary emboli (PE), and deep vein thrombosis (DVT); incidence of these effects was shown to be significantly increased in postmenopausal women using CE with or without MPA. Nonfatal MI, PE, and thrombophlebitis have also been reported in males taking high doses of CE (eg, for prostate cancer). Risk factors include diabetes mellitus, hypercholesterolemia, hypertension, SLE, obesity, and/or venous thromboembolism (VTE). Use caution in patients with known inherited thrombophilias (eg, protein C or S deficiency); may have increased risk of VTE (DeSancho, 2010). Use is contraindicated in patients with DVT or PE (current or history of).

[U.S. Boxed Warning]: The risk of dementia may be increased in postmenopausal women; increased incidence was observed in women ≥65 years of age taking CE alone or in combination with MPA.

Estrogen compounds are generally associated with lipid effects such as increased HDL-cholesterol and decreased LDL-cholesterol. Triglycerides may also be increased; discontinue if pancreatitis occurs. Use with caution in patients with familial defects of lipoprotein metabolism. Estrogens may increase thyroid-binding globulin (TBG) levels leading to increased circulating total thyroid hormone levels. Women on thyroid replacement therapy may require higher doses of thyroid hormone while receiving estrogens. Use caution in patients with hypoparathyroidism; estrogen induced hypocalcemia may occur. May have adverse effects on glucose tolerance; use caution in women with diabetes. Use caution in patients with asthma, epilepsy, hepatic hemangiomas, porphyria or SLE; may exacerbate disease. Use with caution in patients with diseases which may be exacerbated by fluid retention, including cardiac or renal dysfunction. Use of postmenopausal estrogen may be associated with an increased risk of gallbladder disease requiring surgery. Estrogens may cause retinal vascular thrombosis; discontinue if migraine, loss of vision, proptosis, diplopia, or other visual disturbances occur; discontinue permanently if papilledema or retinal vascular lesions are observed on examination.

Estrogens are poorly metabolized in patients with hepatic dysfunction. Use caution with a history of cholestatic jaundice associated with prior estrogen use or pregnancy. Discontinue if jaundice develops or if acute or chronic hepatic disturbances occur. Use is contraindicated with hepatic disease.

Vulvar and vaginal atrophy use: When used solely for the treatment of vulvar and vaginal atrophy, topical vaginal products should be considered. Use caution applying topical products to severely atrophic vaginal mucosa.

Whenever possible, estrogens should be discontinued at least 4-6 weeks prior to elective surgery associated with an increased risk of thromboembolism or during periods of prolonged immobilization.

[U.S. Boxed Warning]: Estrogens with or without progestin should be used for shortest duration possible at the lowest effective dose consistent with treatment goals. Before prescribing estrogen therapy to postmenopausal women, the risks and benefits must be weighed for each patient. Women should be informed of these risks and benefits, as well as possible effects of progestin when added to estrogen therapy. Conduct periodic risk:benefit assessments.

Moderate-to-severe symptoms of vulvar and vaginal atrophy include vaginal dryness, dyspareunia, and atrophic vaginitis. When used solely for the treatment of vulvar and vaginal atrophy, topical vaginal products should be considered. Use caution applying topical products to severely atrophic vaginal mucosa. Use of a progestin is normally not required when low-dose estrogen is applied locally and only for this purpose (NAMS, 2007).

Use of the vaginal cream may weaken latex found in condoms, diaphragms or cervical caps. Systemic absorption occurs following vaginal use; warnings, precautions, and adverse events observed with oral therapy should be considered.

Adverse Reactions Due to systemic absorption, other adverse effects associated with systemic therapy may also occur. Frequency of adverse events reported with daily use:

1% to 10%:

- Central nervous system: Pain (7%)
- Endocrine & metabolic: Breast pain (6%)
- Gastrointestinal: Abdominal pain (8%)
- Genitourinary: Vaginitis (6%)
- Neuromuscular & skeletal: Back pain (5%), weakness (6%)

Postmarketing and/or case reports: Abdominal cramps, abnormal uterine bleeding/spotting, alopecia, anaphylactic reactions, application site reactions (burning, irritation, genital pruritus), arthralgia, asthma exacerbation, bloating, breast cancer; breast discharge, enlargement, tenderness; cervical secretion changes, chloasma, contact lens intolerance, cystitis-like syndrome, deep vein thrombosis (DVT), dementia, depression, dizziness, dysmenorrhea/pelvic pain, edema, endometrial cancer, endometrial hyperplasia, fibrocystic breast changes, gallbladder disease, glucose intolerance, gynecomastia (males), headache, hirsutism, hypersensitivity reactions, hypertension, irritability, leg cramps, leukorrhea, libido changes, MI, migraine, mood disturbances, nausea, nervousness, precocious puberty, pulmonary emboli (PE), rash, retinal vascular thrombosis, stroke, triglycerides increased, urticaria, uterine leiomyomata (increase in size), vomiting, weight changes

Drug Interactions

Metabolism/Transport Effects **Substrate** of CYP1A2 (major), CYP2A6 (minor), CYP2B6 (minor), CYP2C19 (minor), CYP2C9 (minor), CYP2D6 (minor), CYP2E1 (minor), CYP3A4 (major); **Note:** Assignment of Major/Minor substrate status based on clinically relevant drug interaction potential; **Inhibits** CYP1A2 (weak); **Induces** CYP3A4 (weak/moderate)

Avoid Concomitant Use

Avoid concomitant use of Estrogens (Conjugated/Equine, Topical) with any of the following: Anastrozole

Increased Effect/Toxicity

Estrogens (Conjugated/Equine, Topical) may increase the levels/effects of: Corticosteroids (Systemic); ROPINIRole; Tipranavir

The levels/effects of Estrogens (Conjugated/Equine, Topical) may be increased by: Ascorbic Acid; Conivaptan; Herbs (Estrogenic Properties)

Decreased Effect

Estrogens (Conjugated/Equine, Topical) may decrease the levels/effects of: Anastrozole; ARIPiprazole; Chenodiol; Saxagliptin; Somatropin; Thyroid Products; Ursodiol

The levels/effects of Estrogens (Conjugated/Equine, Topical) may be decreased by: CYP1A2 Inducers (Strong); CYP3A4 Inducers (Strong); Cyproterone; Deferasirox; Herbs (CYP3A4 Inducers); Peginterferon Alfa-2b; Tipranavir; Tocilizumab

Stability Vaginal cream: Store at room temperature of 20°C to 25°C (68°F to 77°F); excursions permitted to 15°C to 30°C (59°F to 86°F).

Mechanism of Action Conjugated estrogens contain a mixture of estrone sulfate, equilin sulfate, 17 alpha-dihydroequilin, 17 alpha-estradiol and 17 beta-dihydroequilin. Estrogens are responsible for the development and maintenance of the female reproductive system and secondary sexual characteristics. Estradiol is the principle intracellular human estrogen and is more potent than estrone and estriol at the receptor level; it is the primary estrogen secreted prior to menopause. Following menopause, estrone and estrone sulfate are more highly produced. Estrogens modulate the pituitary secretion of gonadotropins, luteinizing hormone, and follicle-stimulating hormone through a negative feedback system; estrogen replacement reduces elevated levels of these hormones in postmenopausal women.

Pharmacodynamics/Kinetics

Absorption: Systemic absorption occurs

Protein binding: Binds to sex-hormone-binding globulin and albumin

Metabolism: Hepatic via CYP3A4; estradiol is converted to estrone and estriol; also undergoes enterohepatic recirculation (avoided with vaginal administration); estrone sulfate is the main metabolite in postmenopausal women

Time to peak, plasma: Total estrone: 6 hours

Excretion: Urine (primarily estriol, also as estradiol, estrone, and conjugates

Dosage Adults: Females:

Atrophic vaginitis, kraurosis vulvae: Intravaginal: 0.5 g/day (range 0.5-2 g/day) administered cyclically (21 days on, 7 days off). Adjust dose based on patient response. **Note:** Canadian labeling recommends oral estrogen therapy (~1.25 mg/day for 10 days) prior to initiating topical estrogen in severe atrophic vaginitis.

Moderate-to-severe dyspareunia due to menopause: Intravaginal: 0.5 g twice weekly (eg, Monday and Thursday) **or** once daily cyclically (21 days on, 7 days off)

Dosage adjustment in renal impairment: No dosage adjustment provided in manufacturer's labeling (has not been studied). Use with caution; may increase risk of fluid retention.

Dosage adjustment in hepatic impairment: Use is contraindicated with hepatic dysfunction or disease.

Administration Administer at bedtime to minimize adverse effects. Applicator calibrated in 0.5 g increments up to 2 g. To clean applicator, remove plunger from barrel. Wash with mild soap and warm water; do not boil or use hot water.

Monitoring Parameters Routine physical examination that includes blood pressure and Papanicolaou smear, breast exam, mammogram. Monitor for signs of endometrial cancer in female patients with uterus. Adequate diagnostic measures, including endometrial sampling, if indicated, should be performed to rule out malignancy in all cases of undiagnosed abnormal vaginal bleeding. Monitor for loss of vision, sudden onset of proptosis, diplopia, migraine; signs and symptoms of thromboembolic disorders; glycemic control in patients with diabetes; lipid profiles in patients being treated for hyperlipidemias; thyroid function in patients on thyroid hormone replacement therapy.

Test Interactions Thyroid function tests: Estrogens may increase thyroid binding globulin and circulating total thyroid hormone (when measured by T_4 RIA, T_4 by column, or by PBI); decreases free T_3 resin uptake; concentration of free T_4 is not altered; metyrapone test: Response may be reduced

Dosage Forms Excipient information presented when available (limited, particularly for generics); consult specific product labeling.

Cream, vaginal:

Premarin®: 0.625 mg/g (42.5 g)

Estrogens (Esterified) (ES troe jenz, es TER i fied)

Brand Names: U.S. Menest®

Brand Names: Canada Estragyn; Estratab®; Menest®

Index Terms Esterified Estrogens

Pharmacologic Category Estrogen Derivative

Use Treatment of moderate-to-severe vasomotor symptoms associated with menopause; treatment of moderate-to-severe vulvar and vaginal atrophy associated with menopause; hypoestrogenism (due to hypogonadism, castration, or primary ovarian failure); advanced prostatic cancer (palliation), metastatic breast cancer (palliation) in men and postmenopausal women

Pregnancy Considerations In general, the use of estrogen and progestin as in combination hormonal contraceptives have not been associated with teratogenic effects when inadvertently taken early in pregnancy. This product is contraindicated for use during pregnancy.

Lactation Enters breast milk/use caution

Contraindications Hypersensitivity to estrogens or any component of the formulation; undiagnosed abnormal vaginal bleeding; DVT or PE (current or history of); active or recent (within 1 year) arterial thromboembolic disease (eg, stroke, MI); carcinoma of the breast (known, suspected or history of), except in appropriately selected patients being treated for metastatic disease; estrogen-dependent tumor; hepatic dysfunction or disease; pregnancy

Warnings/Precautions [U.S. Boxed Warning]: Unopposed estrogens may increase the risk of endometrial carcinoma in postmenopausal women with an intact uterus. Adequate diagnostic measures, including endometrial sampling, if indicated, should be performed to rule out malignancy in all cases of undiagnosed abnormal vaginal bleeding. The use of a progestin should be considered when administering estrogens to postmenopausal women with an intact uterus. When indicated, oral progestins should be used (NAMS, 2010). Estrogens may exacerbate endometriosis. Malignant transformation of residual endometrial implants has been reported posthysterectomy with estrogen only therapy. Consider adding a progestin in women with residual endometriosis posthysterectomy. Postmenopausal estrogen therapy and combined estrogen/progesterone therapy may increase the risk of ovarian cancer; however, the absolute risk to an individual woman is small. Although results from various studies are not consistent, risk does not appear to be significantly associated with the duration, route, or dose of therapy. In one study, the risk decreased after 2 years following discontinuation of therapy (Mørch, 2009). Although the risk of ovarian cancer is rare, women who are at an increased risk (eg, family history) should be counseled about the association (NAMS, 2010). Estrogens may increase the risk of breast cancer. An increased risk of invasive breast cancer was observed in postmenopausal women using conjugated equine estrogens (CEE) in combination with medroxyprogesterone acetate (MPA); a smaller increase in risk was seen with estrogen therapy alone in observational studies. An increase in abnormal mammograms has also been reported with estrogen and progestin therapy. Estrogen use may lead to severe hypercalcemia in patients with breast cancer and bone metastases; discontinue estrogen if hypercalcemia occurs.

[U.S. Boxed Warning]: Estrogens with or without progestin should not be used to prevent coronary heart disease. Use caution with cardiovascular disease or dysfunction. May increase the risks of myocardial infarction (MI), stroke, pulmonary emboli (PE), and deep vein thrombosis (DVT); incidence of these effects was shown to be significantly increased in postmenopausal women using CEE in combination with MPA. Nonfatal MI, PE, and thrombophlebitis have also been reported in males taking high doses of CEE (eg, for prostate cancer). Risk factors include diabetes mellitus, hypercholesterolemia, hypertension, SLE, obesity, and/or venous thromboembolism (VTE). Use caution in patients with known inherited thrombophilias (eg, protein C or S deficiency); may have increased risk of VTE (DeSancho, 2010); use is contraindicated in patients with DVT or PE (current or history of).

[U.S. Boxed Warning]: The risk of dementia may be increased in postmenopausal women; increased incidence was observed in women ≥65 years of age taking CEE alone or in combination with MPA.

[U.S. Boxed Warning]: Estrogens with or without progestin should be used for shortest duration possible at the lowest effective dose consistent with treatment goals. Before prescribing estrogen therapy to postmenopausal women, the risks and benefits must be weighed for each patient. Women should be informed of these risks and benefits, as well as possible effects of progestin when added to estrogen therapy. Conduct periodic risk:benefit assessments. Outcomes reported from clinical trials using CEE should be assumed to be similar for estradiol until comparable data becomes available. Moderate to severe symptoms of vulvar and vaginal atrophy include vaginal dryness, dyspareunia, and atrophic vaginitis. When used solely for the treatment of vulvar and vaginal atrophy, topical vaginal products should be considered

Estrogen compounds are generally associated with lipid effects such as increased HDL-cholesterol and decreased LDL-cholesterol. Triglycerides may also be increased; use with caution in patients with familial defects of lipoprotein metabolism. Estrogens may increase thyroid-binding globulin (TBG) levels leading to increased circulating total thyroid hormone levels. Women on thyroid replacement therapy may require higher doses of thyroid hormone while receiving estrogens.

Estrogens may cause retinal vascular thrombosis; discontinue if migraine, loss of vision, proptosis, diplopia or other visual disturbances occur; discontinue permanently if papilledema or retinal vascular lesions are observed on examination. Estrogens are poorly metabolized in patients with hepatic dysfunction. Use caution with a history of cholestatic jaundice associated with prior estrogen use or pregnancy. Discontinue if jaundice develops or if acute or chronic hepatic disturbances occur. Use is contraindicated with hepatic disease. Use caution in patients with asthma, epilepsy, hepatic hemangiomas, migraine, porphyria, or SLE; may exacerbate disease. May have adverse effects on glucose tolerance; use caution in women with diabetes. Use with caution in patients with diseases which may be exacerbated by fluid retention, including cardiac or renal dysfunction. Use of postmenopausal estrogen may be associated with an increased risk of gallbladder disease requiring surgery. Use with caution in patients with severe hypocalcemia. May be inappropriate in for use in the elderly due to potential of increased risk of breast and endometrial cancers and lack of proven cardioprotection (Beers Criteria). Prior to puberty, estrogens may cause premature closure of the epiphyses, premature breast development in girls or gynecomastia in boys. Vaginal bleeding and vaginal cornification may also be induced in girls. Whenever possible, estrogens should be discontinued at least 4-6 weeks prior to elective surgery associated with an increased risk of thromboembolism or during periods of prolonged immobilization.

Adverse Reactions Frequency not defined.

Cardiovascular: Edema, hypertension, MI, stroke, venous thromboembolism

Central nervous system: Dementia exacerbation, dizziness, epilepsy exacerbation, headache, irritability, mental depression, migraine, mood disturbances, nervousness

Dermatologic: Angioedema, chloasma, erythema multiforme, erythema nodosum, hemorrhagic eruption, hirsutism, pruritus, loss of scalp hair, melasma, rash, urticaria

Endocrine & metabolic: Breast cancer, breast enlargement, breast tenderness, carbohydrate intolerance, fibrocystic breast changes, galactorrhea, hypocalcemia, libido (changes in), nipple discharge, premenstrual like syndrome

Gastrointestinal: Abdominal cramps, bloating, gallbladder disease, nausea, pancreatitis, vomiting, weight gain/loss

Genitourinary: Alterations in frequency and flow of menstrual patterns, breakthrough bleeding, changes in cervical secretions, cervical ectropion changes, cystitis-like syndrome, dysmenorrhea, endometrial hyperplasia, endometrial cancer, increased size of uterine leiomyomata, ovarian cancer, vaginal candidiasis, vaginitis

Hematologic: Aggravation of porphyria

Hepatic: Cholestatic jaundice, hemangioma enlargement

Local: Thrombophlebitis

Neuromuscular & skeletal: Arthralgia, chorea, leg cramps

Ocular: Contact lens intolerance, corneal curvature steepening, retinal vascular thrombosis

Respiratory: Asthma exacerbation, pulmonary embolism

Miscellaneous: Anaphylactoid/anaphylactic reactions

Drug Interactions

Metabolism/Transport Effects Substrate of CYP1A2 (major), CYP2B6 (minor), CYP2C9 (minor), CYP2E1 (minor), CYP3A4 (major); **Note:** Assignment of Major/Minor substrate status based on clinically relevant drug interaction potential

Avoid Concomitant Use

Avoid concomitant use of Estrogens (Esterified) with any of the following: Anastrozole

Increased Effect/Toxicity

Estrogens (Esterified) may increase the levels/effects of: Corticosteroids (Systemic); ROPINIRole; Tipranavir

The levels/effects of Estrogens (Esterified) may be increased by: Ascorbic Acid; Conivaptan; Herbs (Estrogenic Properties)

Decreased Effect

Estrogens (Esterified) may decrease the levels/effects of: Anastrozole; Chenodiol; Somatropin; Thyroid Products; Ursodiol

The levels/effects of Estrogens (Esterified) may be decreased by: CYP1A2 Inducers (Strong); CYP3A4 Inducers (Strong); Cyproterone; Deferasirox; Herbs (CYP3A4 Inducers); Tipranavir; Tocilizumab

Ethanol/Nutrition/Herb Interactions

Ethanol: Avoid ethanol (routine use increases estrogen plasma concentrations and risk of breast cancer). Ethanol may also increase the risk of osteoporosis.

Food: Folic acid absorption may be decreased.

Herb/Nutraceutical: St John's wort may decrease levels. Herbs with estrogenic properties may enhance the adverse/toxic effect of estrogen derivatives; examples include alfalfa, black cohosh, bloodroot, hops, kudzu, licorice, red clover, saw palmetto, soybean, thyme, wild yam, yucca.

Mechanism of Action Esterified estrogens contain a mixture of estrogenic substances; the principle component is estrone. Preparations contain 75% to 85% sodium estrone sulfate and 6% to 15% sodium equilin sulfate such that the total is not <90%. Estrogens are responsible for the development and maintenance of the female reproductive system and secondary sexual characteristics. Estradiol is the principle intracellular human estrogen and is more potent than estrone and estriol at the receptor level; it is the primary estrogen secreted prior to menopause. In males and following menopause in females, estrone and estrone sulfate are more highly produced. Estrogens modulate the pituitary secretion of gonadotropins, luteinizing hormone, and follicle-stimulating hormone through a negative feedback system; estrogen replacement reduces elevated levels of these hormones.

Pharmacodynamics/Kinetics

Absorption: Readily

Distribution: Widely distributed; high concentrations in the sex hormone target organs

Protein binding: Bound to sex hormone-binding globulin and albumin

Metabolism: Hepatic; partial metabolism via CYP3A4 enzymes; estradiol is reversibly converted to estrone and estriol; oral estradiol also undergoes enterohepatic recirculation by conjugation in the liver, followed by excretion of sulfate and glucuronide conjugates into the bile, then hydrolysis in the intestine and estrogen reabsorption. Sulfate conjugates are the primary form found in postmenopausal women.

Excretion: Primarily urine (as estradiol, estrone, estriol, and their glucuronide and sulfate conjugates)

Dosage Oral: Adults:

Prostate cancer, advanced: 1.25-2.5 mg 3 times/day

Female hypoestrogenism due to hypogonadism: 2.5-7.5 mg/day in divided doses for 20 days followed by a 10-day rest period. Administer cyclically (3 weeks on and 1 week off). If bleeding does not occur by the end of the 10-day period, repeat the same dosing schedule; the number of courses is dependent upon the responsiveness of the endometrium. If bleeding occurs before the end of the 10-day period, begin an estrogen-progestin cyclic regimen of 2.5-7.5 mg/day in divided doses for 20 days; during the last 5 days of estrogen therapy, give an oral progestin. If bleeding occurs before regimen is concluded, discontinue therapy and resume on the fifth day of bleeding.

Female hypoestrogenism due to castration and primary ovarian failure: 1.25 mg/day, cyclically. Adjust dosage upward or downward, according to the severity of symptoms and patient response. For maintenance, adjust dosage to lowest level that will provide effective control.

Vasomotor symptoms associated with menopause: 1.25 mg/day administered cyclically (3 weeks on and 1 week off). If patient has not menstruated within the last 2 months or more, cyclic administration is started arbitrary. If the patient is menstruating, cyclical administration is started on day 5 of the bleeding. For short-term use only and should be discontinued as soon as possible. Re-evaluate at 3- to 6-month intervals for tapering or discontinuation of therapy.

Vulvar and vaginal atrophy associated with menopause: 0.3 to ≥1.25 mg/day, depending on the tissue response of the individual patient. Administer cyclically. For short-term use only and should be discontinued as soon as possible. Re-evaluate at 3- to 6-month intervals for tapering or discontinuation of therapy.

Breast cancer, metastatic (appropriately selected patients): Males and postmenopausal females: 10 mg 3 times/day for at least 3 months

Elderly: Refer to adult dosing.

Dietary Considerations Should be taken with food at same time each day.

Administration Administer with food at same time each day.

Monitoring Parameters Routine physical examination that includes blood pressure and Papanicolaou smear, breast exam, mammogram. Monitor for signs of endometrial cancer in female patients with uterus. Adequate diagnostic measures, including endometrial sampling, if indicated, should be performed to rule out malignancy in all cases of undiagnosed abnormal vaginal bleeding. Monitor for loss of vision, sudden onset of proptosis, diplopia, migraine; signs and symptoms of thromboembolic disorders; glycemic control in patients with diabetes; lipid profiles in patients being treated for hyperlipidemias; thyroid function in patients on thyroid hormone replacement therapy.

Menopausal symptoms; vulvar and vaginal atrophy: Assess need for therapy at 3- to 6-month intervals

Test Interactions Pathologist should be advised of estrogen/progesterone therapy when specimens are submitted. Reduced response to metyrapone test.

Prothrombin time, partial thromboplastin time, and platelet aggregation time may be accelerated; platelet count may be increased; factors II, VII antigen, VIII antigen, VII coagulant activity, IX, V, VII, VII-X complex, II-VII-X complex, and beta-thromboglobulin may be increased; anti-factor Xa and antithrombin III levels may be decreased; antithrombin III activity may be decreased; fibrinogen and fibrinogen activity may be increased; plasminogen and plasminogen activity may be increased

Thyroid-binding globulin levels may be increased; HDL and triglyceride plasma levels may be increased; LDL levels may be decreased

Dosage Forms Excipient information presented when available (limited, particularly for generics); consult specific product labeling.

Tablet, oral:

Menest®: 0.3 mg, 0.625 mg, 1.25 mg, 2.5 mg

Estropipate (ES troe pih pate)

Brand Names: Canada Ogen®

Index Terms Ortho Est; Piperazine Estrone Sulfate

Pharmacologic Category Estrogen Derivative

Use Treatment of moderate-to-severe vasomotor symptoms associated with menopause; treatment of vulvar and vaginal atrophy; hypoestrogenism (due to hypogonadism, castration, or primary ovarian failure); osteoporosis (prophylaxis, in women at significant risk only)

Pregnancy Risk Factor X

Dosage Adults:

Oral:

Moderate-to-severe vasomotor symptoms associated with menopause: Usual dosage range: 0.75-6 mg estropipate daily; use the lowest dose and regimen that will control symptoms, and discontinue as soon as possible. Attempt to discontinue or taper medication at 3- to 6-month intervals. If a patient with vasomotor symptoms has not menstruated within the last ≥2 months, start the cyclic administration arbitrarily. If the patient has menstruated, start cyclic administration on day 5 of bleeding.

Female hypogonadism: 1.5-9 mg estropipate daily for the first 3 weeks, followed by a rest period of 8-10 days; use the lowest dose and regimen that will control symptoms. Repeat if bleeding does not occur by the end of the rest period. The duration of therapy necessary to product the withdrawal bleeding will vary according to the responsiveness of the endometrium. If satisfactory withdrawal bleeding does not occur, give an oral progestin in addition to estrogen during the third week of the cycle.

Female castration or primary ovarian failure: 1.5-9 mg estropipate daily for the first 3 weeks of a theoretical cycle, followed by a rest period of 8-10 days; use the lowest dose and regimen that will control symptoms

Osteoporosis prophylaxis: 0.75 mg estropipate daily for 25 days of a 31-day cycle

Atrophic vaginitis or kraurosis vulvae: 0.75-6 mg estropipate daily; administer cyclically. Use the lowest dose and regimen that will control symptoms; discontinue as soon as possible.

Elderly: Refer to adult dosing. A higher incidence of stroke and invasive breast cancer were observed in women >75 years in a WHI substudy using conjugated equine estrogen.

Dosing adjustment in hepatic impairment:

Mild-to-moderate liver impairment: Dosage reduction of estrogens is recommended

Severe liver impairment: **Not recommended**

Additional Information Complete prescribing information for this medication should be consulted for additional detail.

Dosage Forms Excipient information presented when available (limited, particularly for generics); consult specific product labeling.

Tablet, oral: 0.625 mg [estropipate 0.75 mg], 1.25 mg [estropipate 1.5 mg], 2.5 mg [estropipate 3 mg]

◆ **Estrostep® Fe** *see* Ethinyl Estradiol and Norethindrone *on page 660*

Eszopiclone (es zoe PIK lone)

Brand Names: U.S. Lunesta®

Pharmacologic Category Hypnotic, Nonbenzodiazepine

Use Treatment of insomnia

Pregnancy Risk Factor C

Pregnancy Considerations No evidence of teratogenicity in animal models (high dose). There are no adequate or well-controlled studies in pregnant women; use only if clearly needed.

Lactation Excretion in breast milk unknown/use caution

Medication Guide Available Yes

Contraindications There are no contraindications listed within the manufacturer's labeling.

Warnings/Precautions Symptomatic treatment of insomnia should be initiated only after careful evaluation of potential causes of sleep disturbance. Tolerance did not develop over 6 months of use. Use with caution in patients with depression or a history of drug dependence. Abrupt discontinuance may lead to withdrawal symptoms. Use with caution in patients receiving other CNS depressants or psychoactive medications. Hypnotics/sedatives have been associated with abnormal thinking and behavior changes including decreased inhibition, aggression, bizarre behavior, agitation, hallucinations, and depersonalization. These changes may occur unpredictably and may indicate previously unrecognized psychiatric disorders; evaluate appropriately. Amnesia may occur. May impair physical and mental capabilities. Postmarketing studies have indicated that the use of hypnotic/sedative agents for sleep has been associated with hypersensitivity reactions including anaphylaxis as well as angioedema. An increased risk for hazardous sleep-related activities such as sleep-driving (as well as cooking and eating food and making phone calls while asleep) has also been noted. Use caution in patients with respiratory compromise, hepatic dysfunction, elderly or those taking strong CYP3A4 inhibitors. Because of the rapid onset of action, administer immediately prior to bedtime or after the patient has gone to bed and is having difficulty falling asleep.

Adverse Reactions

>10%:

Central nervous system: Headache (15% to 21%)

Gastrointestinal: Unpleasant taste (8% to 34%)

1% to 10%:

Cardiovascular: Chest pain, peripheral edema

Central nervous system: Somnolence (8% to 10%), dizziness (5% to 7%), pain (4% to 5%), nervousness (up to 5%), depression (1% to 4%), confusion (up to 3%), hallucinations (1% to 3%), anxiety (1% to 3%), abnormal dreams (1% to 3%), migraine

Dermatologic: Rash (3% to 4%), pruritus (1% to 4%)

Endocrine & metabolic: Libido decreased (up to 3%), dysmenorrhea (up to 3%), gynecomastia (males up to 3%)

Gastrointestinal: Xerostomia (3% to 7%), dyspepsia (2% to 6%), nausea (4% to 5%), diarrhea (2% to 4%), vomiting (up to 3%)

Genitourinary: Urinary tract infection (up to 3%)

Neuromuscular & skeletal: Neuralgia (up to 3%)

Miscellaneous: Infection (5% to 10%), viral infection (3%), accidental injury (up to 3%)

<1% (Limited to important or life-threatening): Abnormal gait, agitation, alopecia, allergic reaction, amenorrhea, anaphylaxis, angioedema, anorexia, asthma, ataxia, breast enlargement, breast neoplasm, bronchitis, cholelithiasis, colitis; complex sleep-related behavior (sleep-driving, cooking or eating food, making phone calls); conjunctivitis, contact dermatitis, cystitis, dehydration, diaphoresis, dry eyes, dyspnea, dysphagia, dysuria, eczema, emotional lability, epistaxis, erythema multiforme, euphoria, facial edema, fever, gout, heat stroke,

hematuria, hepatitis, hepatomegaly, herpes zoster, hostility, hypercholesterolemia, hypertension, hypokalemia, kidney calculus, kidney pain, liver damage, maculopapular rash, malaise, mastitis, melena, memory impairment, menorrhagia, myasthenia, mydriasis, myopathy, neck rigidity, neuritis, neuropathy, neurosis, nystagmus, oliguria, paresthesia, photophobia, photosensitivity, pyelonephritis, rectal hemorrhage, reflexes decreased, stomach ulcer, swelling, thrombophlebitis, tinnitus, tongue edema, tremor, twitching, ulcerative stomatitis, urinary frequency, urinary incontinence, urticaria, urethritis, vaginal hemorrhage, vaginitis, vestibular disorder, vertigo, vesiculobullous rash

Drug Interactions

Metabolism/Transport Effects **Substrate** of CYP2E1 (minor), CYP3A4 (major); **Note:** Assignment of Major/Minor substrate status based on clinically relevant drug interaction potential

Avoid Concomitant Use

Avoid concomitant use of Eszopiclone with any of the following: Conivaptan

Increased Effect/Toxicity

Eszopiclone may increase the levels/effects of: Alcohol (Ethyl); CNS Depressants; Methotrimeprazine; Selective Serotonin Reuptake Inhibitors

The levels/effects of Eszopiclone may be increased by: Antifungal Agents (Azole Derivatives, Systemic); Conivaptan; CYP3A4 Inhibitors (Moderate); CYP3A4 Inhibitors (Strong); Dasatinib; Droperidol; HydrOXYzine; Methotrimeprazine

Decreased Effect

The levels/effects of Eszopiclone may be decreased by: CYP3A4 Inducers (Strong); Cyproterone; Deferasirox; Flumazenil; Herbs (CYP3A4 Inducers); Tocilizumab

Ethanol/Nutrition/Herb Interactions

Ethanol: Ethanol: May increase CNS depression; monitor for increased effects with coadministration. Caution patients about effects.

Food: Onset of action may be reduced if taken with or immediately after a heavy meal.

Herb/Nutraceutical: Avoid valerian, St John's wort, kava kava, gotu kola (may increase CNS depression).

Stability Store at controlled room temperature of 25°C (77°F).

Mechanism of Action May interact with GABA-receptor complexes at binding domains located close to or allosterically coupled to benzodiazepine receptors.

Pharmacodynamics/Kinetics

Absorption: Rapid; high-fat/heavy meal may delay absorption

Protein binding: 52% to 59%

Metabolism: Hepatic via oxidation and demethylation (CYP2E1, 3A4); 2 primary metabolites; one with activity less than parent.

Half-life elimination: ~6 hours; Elderly (≥65 years): ~9 hours

Time to peak, plasma: ~1 hour

Excretion: Urine (up to 75%, primarily as metabolites; <10% as parent drug)

Dosage Oral:

Adults: Insomnia: Initial: 2 mg immediately before bedtime (maximum dose: 3 mg)

Concurrent use with strong CYP3A4 inhibitor: 1 mg immediately before bedtime; if needed, dose may be increased to 2 mg

Elderly:

Difficulty **falling** asleep: Initial: 1 mg immediately before bedtime; maximum dose: 2 mg

Difficulty **staying** asleep: 2 mg immediately before bedtime

Dosage adjustment in renal impairment: None required

Dosage adjustment in hepatic impairment:

Mild-to-moderate: Use with caution; dosage adjustment unnecessary

Severe: Initial dose: 1 mg; maximum dose: 2 mg

Dietary Considerations Avoid taking after a heavy meal; may delay onset.

Administration Because of the rapid onset of action, eszopiclone should be administered immediately prior to bedtime or after the patient has gone to bed and is having difficulty falling asleep. Do not take with, or immediately following, a high-fat meal; do not crush or break tablet.

Dosage Forms Excipient information presented when available (limited, particularly for generics); consult specific product labeling.

Tablet, oral:

Lunesta®: 1 mg, 2 mg, 3 mg

Controlled Substance C-IV

Etanercept (et a NER sept)

Brand Names: U.S. Enbrel®; Enbrel® SureClick®

Brand Names: Canada Enbrel®

Pharmacologic Category Antirheumatic, Disease Modifying; Tumor Necrosis Factor (TNF) Blocking Agent

Use Treatment of moderately- to severely-active rheumatoid arthritis (RA); moderately- to severely-active polyarticular juvenile idiopathic arthritis (JIA); psoriatic arthritis; active ankylosing spondylitis (AS); moderate-to-severe chronic plaque psoriasis

Pregnancy Risk Factor B

Pregnancy Considerations Developmental toxicity studies performed in animals have revealed no evidence of harm to the fetus. There are no studies in pregnant women; this drug should be used during pregnancy only if clearly needed. A pregnancy registry has been established to monitor outcomes of women exposed to etanercept during pregnancy (877-311-8972).

Lactation Excretion in breast milk unknown/not recommended

Medication Guide Available Yes

Contraindications Hypersensitivity to etanercept or any component of the formulation; patients with sepsis (mortality may be increased)

Warnings/Precautions [U.S. Boxed Warning]: Patients receiving etanercept are at increased risk for serious infections which may result in hospitalization and/or fatality; infections usually developed in patients receiving concomitant immunosuppressive agents (eg, methotrexate or corticosteroids) and may present as disseminated (rather than local) disease. Active tuberculosis (or reactivation of latent tuberculosis), invasive fungal (including aspergillosis, blastomycosis, candidiasis, coccidioidomycosis, histoplasmosis, and pneumocystosis) and bacterial, viral or other opportunistic infections (including legionellosis and listeriosis) have been reported in patients receiving TNF-blocking agents, including etanercept. Monitor closely for signs/symptoms of infection. Discontinue for serious infection or sepsis. Consider risks versus benefits prior to use in patients with a history of chronic or recurrent infection. Consider empiric antifungal therapy in patients who are at risk for invasive fungal infection and develop severe systemic illness. Caution should be exercised when considering use in the elderly or in patients with conditions that predispose them to infections (eg, diabetes) or residence/travel from areas of endemic mycoses (blastomycosis, coccidioidomycosis, histoplasmosis), or with latent or localized infections. Do not initiate etanercept therapy with clinically important active infection. Patients who develop a new infection while undergoing treatment should be monitored closely. **[U.S. Boxed Warning]: Tuberculosis (disseminated or**

extrapulmonary) has been reported in patients receiving etanercept; both reactivation of latent infection and new infections have been reported. Patients should be evaluated for tuberculosis risk factors and for latent tuberculosis infection with a tuberculin skin test prior to starting therapy. Treatment of latent tuberculosis should be initiated before etanercept therapy; consider antituberculosis treatment if adequate course of treatment cannot be confirmed in patients with a history of latent or active tuberculosis or with risk factors despite negative skin test. Some patients who tested negative prior to therapy have developed active infection; monitor for signs and symptoms of tuberculosis in all patients. Rare reactivation of hepatitis B virus (HBV) has occurred in chronic virus carriers; use with caution; evaluate prior to initiation and during treatment. Patients should be brought up to date with all immunizations before initiating therapy. Live vaccines should not be given concurrently with etanercept. Patients with a significant exposure to varicella virus should temporarily discontinue etanercept. Treatment with varicella zoster immune globulin should be considered.

[U.S. Boxed Warning]: Lymphoma and other malignancies have been reported in children and adolescent patients receiving TNF-blocking agents, including etanercept. Half of the malignancies reported in children were lymphomas (Hodgkin's and non-Hodgkin's) while other cases varied and included malignancies not typically observed in this population. The impact of etanercept on the development and course of malignancy is not fully defined. Compared to the general population, an increased risk of lymphoma has been noted in clinical trials; however, rheumatoid arthritis alone has been previously associated with an increased rate of lymphoma. Lymphomas and other malignancies were also observed (at rates higher than expected for the general population) in adult patients receiving etanercept. Etanercept is not recommended for use in patients with Wegener's granulomatosis who are receiving immunosuppressive therapy. Treatment may result in the formation of autoimmune antibodies; cases of autoimmune disease have not been described. Nonneutralizing antibodies to etanercept may also be formed. Rarely, a reversible lupus-like syndrome has occurred.

Allergic reactions may occur; if an anaphylactic reaction or other serious allergic reaction occurs, administration should be discontinued immediately and appropriate therapy initiated. Use with caution in patients with pre-existing or recent onset CNS demyelinating disorders; rare cases of new onset or exacerbation of CNS demyelinating disorders have occurred; may present with mental status changes and some may be associated with permanent disability. Optic neuritis, transverse myelitis, multiple sclerosis, and new onset or exacerbation of seizures have been reported. Use with caution in patients with heart failure or decreased left ventricular function; worsening and new-onset heart failure has been reported. Use caution in patients with a history of significant hematologic abnormalities; has been associated with pancytopenia and aplastic anemia (rare). Discontinue if significant hematologic abnormalities are confirmed. Use with caution in patients with moderate to severe alcoholic hepatitis. Compared to placebo, the mortality rate in patients treated with etanercept was similar at one month but significantly higher after 6 months

Due to a higher incidence of serious infections, concomitant use with anakinra is not recommended. Some dosage forms may contain dry natural rubber (latex). Some dosage forms may contain benzyl alcohol which has been associated with "gasping syndrome" in neonates.

Adverse Reactions Percentages reported for adults except where specified.

>10%:
- Central nervous system: Headache (17%; children 19%)
- Dermatologic: Rash (3% to 13%)
- Gastrointestinal: Abdominal pain (5%; children 19%), vomiting (3%; children 13%)
- Local: Injection site reaction (14% to 43%; bleeding, bruising, erythema, itching, pain or swelling)
- Respiratory: Respiratory tract infection (upper; 38% to 65%), rhinitis (12%)
- Miscellaneous: Infection (50% to 81%; children 62%), positive ANA (11%), positive antidouble-stranded DNA antibodies (15% by RIA, 3% by *Crithidia luciliae* assay)

≥3% to 10%:
- Central nervous system: Dizziness (7%)
- Dermatologic: Pruritus (2% to 5%)
- Gastrointestinal: Nausea (children 9%), dyspepsia (4%), diarrhea (3%)
- Neuromuscular & skeletal: Weakness (5%)
- Respiratory: Pharyngitis (7%), cough (6%), respiratory disorder (5%), sinusitis (3%)

<3%, postmarketing, and/or case reports: Abscess, adenopathy, allergic reactions, anemia, angioedema, anorexia, aplastic anemia, appendicitis, aseptic meningitis, bursitis, cerebral ischemia, chest pain, cholecystitis, coagulopathy, demyelinating CNS disorders (suggestive of multiple sclerosis, transverse myelitis, or optic neuritis), cutaneous ulcer, deep vein thrombosis, depression, dyspnea, erythema multiforme, esophagitis, fatigue, fever, flushing, flu-like syndrome, gastroenteritis, gastrointestinal hemorrhage, gastritis, heart failure, hepatitis (autoimmune), hydrocephalus (with normal pressure), hyper-/hypotension, hypersensitivity, infections (bacterial, fungal, protozoal, viral), inflammatory bowel disease, interstitial lung disease, intestinal perforation, joint pain, leukemias, leukopenia, lupus erythematous (cutaneous), lupus-like syndrome, lymphadenopathy, lymphomas, malignancies, membranous glomerulopathy, MI, mouth ulcer, multiple sclerosis, myocardial ischemia, neutropenia, ocular inflammation, optic neuritis, pancytopenia, pancreatitis, paresthesia, polymyositis, psoriasis (including new onset, palmoplantar, pustular, or exacerbation), pulmonary disease, pulmonary embolism, pyrexia, renal calculus, sarcoidosis, seizure, stroke, Stevens-Johnson syndrome, subcutaneous nodules, taste disturbances, thrombocytopenia, thrombophlebitis, toxic epidermal necrolysis, transaminases increased, tuberculosis, tuberculous arthritis, urinary tract infection, urticaria, varicella infection, vasculitis (cutaneous), weight gain, xerophthalmia, xerostomia

Drug Interactions

Metabolism/Transport Effects None known.

Avoid Concomitant Use

Avoid concomitant use of Etanercept with any of the following: Abatacept; Anakinra; BCG; Belimumab; Canakinumab; Certolizumab Pegol; Cyclophosphamide; Natalizumab; Pimecrolimus; Rilonacept; Tacrolimus (Topical); Vaccines (Live)

Increased Effect/Toxicity

Etanercept may increase the levels/effects of: Abatacept; Anakinra; Belimumab; Canakinumab; Certolizumab Pegol; Cyclophosphamide; Leflunomide; Natalizumab; Rilonacept; Vaccines (Live)

The levels/effects of Etanercept may be increased by: Denosumab; Pimecrolimus; Roflumilast; Tacrolimus (Topical); Trastuzumab

Decreased Effect

Etanercept may decrease the levels/effects of: BCG; Coccidioidin Skin Test; Sipuleucel-T; Vaccines (Inactivated); Vaccines (Live)

The levels/effects of Etanercept may be decreased by: Echinacea

Ethanol/Nutrition/Herb Interactions Herb/Nutraceutical: Echinacea may decrease the therapeutic effects of etanercept (avoid concurrent use).

Stability

Prefilled syringes, autoinjectors: Store prefilled syringes and autoinjectors at 2°C to 8°C (36°F to 46°F); do not freeze. Protect from light; do not shake. The following stability information has also been reported: May be stored at room temperature for up to 4 days (Cohen, 2007).

Powder for reconstitution: Must be refrigerated at 2°C to 8°C (36°F to 46°F); do not freeze. The following stability information has also been reported: May be stored at room temperature for up to 7 days (Cohen, 2007). Reconstitute lyophilized powder aseptically with 1 mL sterile bacteriostatic water for injection, USP (supplied); swirl gently, do not shake. Do not filter reconstituted solution during preparation or administration. Upon reconstitution of vial, administer immediately. If not administered immediately after reconstitution, vial may be stored at 2°C to 8°C (36°F to 46°F) for up to 14 days.

Mechanism of Action Etanercept is a recombinant DNA-derived protein composed of tumor necrosis factor receptor (TNFR) linked to the Fc portion of human IgG1. Etanercept binds tumor necrosis factor (TNF) and blocks its interaction with cell surface receptors. TNF plays an important role in the inflammatory processes and the resulting joint pathology of rheumatoid arthritis (RA), polyarticular-course juvenile idiopathic arthritis (JIA), ankylosing spondylitis (AS), and plaque psoriasis.

Pharmacodynamics/Kinetics

Onset of action: ~2-3 weeks; RA: 1-2 weeks

Half-life elimination: RA: SubQ: 72-132 hours

Time to peak: RA: SubQ: 35-103 hours

Dosage SubQ:

Children 2-17 years: Juvenile idiopathic arthritis:

Once-weekly dosing: 0.8 mg/kg (maximum: 50 mg/dose) once weekly

Twice-weekly dosing: 0.4 mg/kg (maximum: 25 mg/dose) twice weekly (individual doses should be separated by 72-96 hours)

Adults:

Rheumatoid arthritis, psoriatic arthritis, ankylosing spondylitis:

Once-weekly dosing: 50 mg once weekly

Twice weekly dosing: 25 mg given twice weekly (individual doses should be separated by 72-96 hours)

Plaque psoriasis:

Initial: 50 mg twice weekly, 72-96 hours apart; maintain initial dose for 3 months (starting doses of 25 or 50 mg once weekly have also been used successfully)

Maintenance dose: 50 mg once weekly

Elderly: Refer to adult dosing. Although greater sensitivity of some elderly patients cannot be ruled out, no overall differences in safety or effectiveness were observed.

Administration Administer subcutaneously. Rotate injection sites. New injections should be given at least one inch from an old site and never into areas where the skin is tender, bruised, red, or hard. **Note:** If the physician determines that it is appropriate, patients may self-inject after proper training in injection technique.

Powder for reconstitution: Follow package instructions carefully for reconstitution. The maximum amount injected at any single site should not exceed 25 mg.

Solution for injection: May be allowed to reach room temperature prior to injection.

Monitoring Parameters Monitor improvement of symptoms and physical function assessments. Latent TB screening prior to initiating and during therapy; signs/symptoms of infection (prior to, during, and following therapy); CBC with differential; signs/symptoms/worsening of heart failure; HBV screening prior to initiating (all patients), HBV carriers (during and for several months following therapy); signs and symptoms of hypersensitivity reaction; symptoms of lupus-like syndrome.

Dosage Forms Excipient information presented when available (limited, particularly for generics); consult specific product labeling.

Injection, powder for reconstitution:

Enbrel®: 25 mg [contains benzyl alcohol (in diluent), sucrose 10 mg]

Injection, solution [preservative free]:

Enbrel®: 50 mg/mL (0.51 mL, 0.98 mL) [contains natural rubber/natural latex in packaging, sucrose 1%; prefilled syringe]

Enbrel® SureClick®: 50 mg/mL (0.98 mL) [contains natural rubber/natural latex in packaging, sucrose 1%; autoinjector]

◆ **Ethacrynate Sodium** *see* Ethacrynic Acid *on page 651*

Ethacrynic Acid (eth a KRIN ik AS id)

Brand Names: U.S. Edecrin®; Sodium Edecrin®

Brand Names: Canada Edecrin®

Index Terms Ethacrynate Sodium

Pharmacologic Category Diuretic, Loop

Additional Appendix Information

Beers Criteria – Potentially Inappropriate Medications for Geriatrics *on page 1973*

Use Management of edema associated with congestive heart failure; hepatic cirrhosis or renal disease; short-term management of ascites due to malignancy, idiopathic edema, and lymphedema

Pregnancy Risk Factor B

Dosage I.V. formulation should be diluted in D_5W or NS (1 mg/mL) and infused over several minutes.

Children: Oral: 1 mg/kg/dose once daily; increase at intervals of 2-3 days as needed, to a maximum of 3 mg/kg/day.

Adults:

Oral: 50-200 mg/day in 1-2 divided doses; may increase in increments of 25-50 mg at intervals of several days; doses up to 200 mg twice daily may be required with severe, refractory edema.

I.V.: 0.5-1 mg/kg/dose (maximum: 100 mg/dose); repeat doses not routinely recommended; however, if indicated, repeat doses every 8-12 hours.

Dosing adjustment/comments in renal impairment: Cl_{cr} <10 mL/minute: Avoid use.

Dialysis: Not removed by hemo- or peritoneal dialysis; supplemental dose is not necessary.

Additional Information Complete prescribing information for this medication should be consulted for additional detail.

Dosage Forms Excipient information presented when available (limited, particularly for generics); consult specific product labeling.

Injection, powder for reconstitution, as ethacrynate sodium:

Sodium Edecrin®: 50 mg

Tablet, oral:

Edecrin®: 25 mg [scored]

Ethambutol (e THAM byoo tole)

Brand Names: U.S. Myambutol®

Brand Names: Canada Etibi®

Index Terms Ethambutol Hydrochloride

Pharmacologic Category Antitubercular Agent

Use Treatment of pulmonary tuberculosis in conjunction with other antituberculosis agents

Unlabeled Use Other mycobacterial diseases in conjunction with other antimycobacterial agents

Pregnancy Risk Factor C

Pregnancy Considerations Teratogenic effects have been seen in animals. There are no adequate and well-controlled studies in pregnant women; there have been reports of ophthalmic abnormalities in infants born to women receiving ethambutol as a component of antituberculous therapy. Use only during pregnancy if benefits outweigh risks.

Lactation Enters breast milk/use caution (AAP considers "compatible"; AAP 2001 update pending)

Contraindications Hypersensitivity to ethambutol or any component of the formulation; optic neuritis (risk vs benefit decision); use in young children, unconscious patients, or any other patient who may be unable to discern and report visual changes

Warnings/Precautions May cause optic neuritis (unilateral or bilateral), resulting in decreased visual acuity or other vision changes. Discontinue promptly in patients with changes in vision, color blindness, or visual defects (effects normally reversible, but reversal may require up to a year). Irreversible blindness has been reported. Monitor visual acuity prior to and during therapy. Evaluation of visual acuity changes may be more difficult in patients with cataracts, optic neuritis, diabetic retinopathy, and inflammatory conditions of the eye; consideration should be given to whether or not visual changes are related to disease progression or effects of therapy. Use only in children whose visual acuity can accurately be determined and monitored (not recommended for use in children <13 years of age unless the benefit outweighs the risk). Dosage modification is required in patients with renal insufficiency; monitor renal function prior to and during treatment. Hepatic toxicity has been reported, possibly due to concurrent therapy; monitor liver function prior to and during treatment.

Adverse Reactions Frequency not defined.

Cardiovascular: Myocarditis, pericarditis

Central nervous system: Confusion, disorientation, dizziness, fever, hallucinations, headache, malaise

Dermatologic: Dermatitis, erythema multiforme, exfoliative dermatitis, pruritus, rash

Endocrine & metabolic: Acute gout or hyperuricemia

Gastrointestinal: Abdominal pain, anorexia, GI upset, nausea, vomiting

Hematologic: Eosinophilia, leukopenia, lymphadenopathy, neutropenia, thrombocytopenia

Hepatic: Hepatitis, hepatotoxicity (possibly related to concurrent therapy), LFTs abnormal

Neuromuscular & skeletal: Arthralgia, peripheral neuritis

Ocular: Optic neuritis; symptoms may include decreased acuity, scotoma, color blindness, or visual defects (usually reversible with discontinuation, irreversible blindness has been described)

Renal: Nephritis

Respiratory: Infiltrates (with or without eosinophilia), pneumonitis

Miscellaneous: Anaphylaxis, anaphylactoid reaction; hypersensitivity syndrome (cutaneous reactions, eosinophilia, and organ-specific inflammation)

Drug Interactions

Metabolism/Transport Effects None known.

Avoid Concomitant Use There are no known interactions where it is recommended to avoid concomitant use.

Increased Effect/Toxicity There are no known significant interactions involving an increase in effect.

Decreased Effect

The levels/effects of Ethambutol may be decreased by: Aluminum Hydroxide

Stability Store at controlled room temperature of 20°C to 25°C (68°F to 77°F).

Mechanism of Action Inhibits arabinosyl transferase resulting in impaired mycobacterial cell wall synthesis

Pharmacodynamics/Kinetics

Absorption: ~80%

Distribution: Widely throughout body; concentrated in kidneys, lungs, saliva, and red blood cells

Relative diffusion from blood into CSF: Adequate with or without inflammation (exceeds usual MICs)

CSF:blood level ratio: Normal meninges: 0%; Inflamed meninges: 25%

Protein binding: 20% to 30%

Metabolism: Hepatic (20%) to inactive metabolite

Half-life elimination: 2.5-3.6 hours; End-stage renal disease: 7-15 hours

Time to peak, serum: 2-4 hours

Excretion: Urine (~50% as unchanged drug, 8% to 15% as metabolites); feces (~20% as unchanged drug)

Dosage

Usual dosage range: Oral:

Children: 15-20 mg/kg/day (maximum: 1 g/day) **or** 50 mg/kg/dose twice weekly (maximum: 2.5 g/dose)

Adults: 15-25 mg/kg daily (maximum dose: 1.5-2.5 g) **or** 25-30 mg/kg/dose 3 times/week (maximum: 2.4 g/dose) **or** 50 mg/kg/dose twice weekly (maximum: 4 g/dose)

Indication-specific dosing: Oral:

Infants and Children:

***Mycobacterium avium* (MAC), secondary prophylaxis or treatment: HIV-exposed/-infected:** 15-25 mg/kg/day once daily (maximum: 2.5 g/day) with clarithromycin (or azithromycin) with or without rifabutin (CDC, 2009)

Children:

Tuberculosis, active: Note: Used as part of a multidrug regimen; treatment regimens consist of an initial 2-month phase, followed by a continuation phase of 4 or 7 additional months; frequency of dosing may differ depending on phase of therapy.

HIV negative: Daily therapy: 15-20 mg/kg/day (maximum: 1 g/day); Twice weekly directly observed therapy (DOT): 50 mg/kg (maximum: 2.5 g/dose) (*MMWR*, 2003)

HIV-exposed/-infected: Daily therapy: 15-25 mg/kg/day (maximum: 2.5 g/day) (CDC, 2009)

Adolescents ≥13 years:

Tuberculosis, active: Refer to adult dosing.

Adults:

Disseminated *Mycobacterium avium* (MAC) treatment in patients with advanced HIV infection (unlabeled use; ATS/IDSA guidelines, 2007): 15 mg/kg ethambutol in combination with clarithromycin or azithromycin with/without rifabutin

Nontuberculous mycobacterium *(M. kansasii)* (unlabeled use; ATS/IDSA guidelines, 2007): 15 mg/kg/day ethambutol for duration to include 12 months of culture-negative sputum; typically used in combination with rifampin and isoniazid; **Note:** Previous recommendations stated to use 25 mg/kg/day for the initial 2 months of therapy; however, IDSA guidelines state this may be unnecessary given the success of rifampin-based regimens with ethambutol 15 mg/kg/day or omitted altogether.

Tuberculosis, active: Note: Used as part of a multidrug regimen; treatment regimens consist of an initial 2-month phase, followed by a continuation phase of 4 or 7 additional months; frequency of dosing may differ depending on phase of therapy.

FDA-approved labeling: Adolescents ≥13 years and Adults: Initial: 15 mg/kg once daily (maximum dose: 1.5 g); Retreatment (previous antituberculosis therapy): 25 mg/kg once daily (maximum dose: 2.5 g) for 60 days or until bacteriologic smears and cultures become negative, followed by 15 mg/kg daily.

Suggested doses by lean body weight (CDC, 2003):
Daily therapy: 15-25 mg/kg (maximum dose: 1.6 g)
40-55 kg: 800 mg
56-75 kg: 1200 mg
76-90 kg: 1600 mg
Twice weekly directly observed therapy (DOT): 50 mg/kg (maximum dose: 4 g)
40-55 kg: 2000 mg
56-75 kg: 2800 mg
76-90 kg: 4000 mg
Three times/week DOT: 25-30 mg/kg (maximum dose: 2.4 g)
40-55 kg: 1200 mg
56-75 kg: 2000 mg
76-90 kg: 2400 mg

Dosing interval in renal impairment:
MMWR, 2003: Cl_{cr} <30 mL/minute and hemodialysis: 15-25 mg/kg/dose 3 times weekly
Aronoff, 2007:
Cl_{cr} 10-50 mL/minute: Administer every 24-36 hours
Cl_{cr} <10 mL/minute: Administer every 48 hours
Hemodialysis: Slightly dialyzable (5% to 20%); Administer dose postdialysis
Peritoneal dialysis: Dose for Cl_{cr} <10 mL/minute: Administer every 48 hours
Continuous arteriovenous or venovenous hemofiltration: Dose for Cl_{cr} 10-50 mL/minute: Administer every 24-36 hours

Dietary Considerations May be taken with food as absorption is not affected, may cause gastric irritation.

Monitoring Parameters Baseline and periodic (monthly) visual testing (each eye individually, as well as both eyes tested together) in patients receiving >15 mg/kg/day; baseline and periodic renal, hepatic, and hematopoietic tests

Dosage Forms Excipient information presented when available (limited, particularly for generics); consult specific product labeling.
Tablet, oral, as hydrochloride: 100 mg, 400 mg
Myambutol®: 100 mg
Myambutol®: 400 mg [scored]

◆ **Ethambutol Hydrochloride** *see* Ethambutol *on page 651*

◆ **Ethamolin®** *see* Ethanolamine Oleate *on page 653*

◆ **Ethanoic Acid** *see* Acetic Acid *on page 33*

Ethanolamine Oleate (ETH a nol a meen OH lee ate)

Brand Names: U.S. Ethamolin®

Index Terms Monoethanolamine

Pharmacologic Category Sclerosing Agent

Use Orphan drug: Sclerosing agent used for bleeding esophageal varices

Pregnancy Risk Factor C

Dosage Adults: 1.5-5 mL per varix, up to 20 mL total or 0.4 mL/kg for a 50 kg patient; doses should be decreased in patients with severe hepatic dysfunction and should receive less than recommended maximum dose

Additional Information Complete prescribing information for this medication should be consulted for additional detail.

Dosage Forms Excipient information presented when available (limited, particularly for generics); consult specific product labeling.
Injection, solution:
Ethamolin®: 5% (2 mL) [contains benzyl alcohol; 50 mg/mL]

Ethinyl Estradiol and Desogestrel
(ETH in il es tra DYE ole & des oh JES trel)

Brand Names: U.S. Apri®; Azurette™; Caziant®; Cesia® [DSC]; Cyclessa®; Desogen®; Emoquette™; Kariva®; Mircette®; Ortho-Cept®; Reclipsen®; Solia® [DSC]; Velivet™

Brand Names: Canada Cyclessa®; Linessa®; Marvelon®; Ortho-Cept®

Index Terms Desogestrel and Ethinyl Estradiol; Ortho Cept

Pharmacologic Category Contraceptive; Estrogen and Progestin Combination

Use Prevention of pregnancy

Unlabeled Use Treatment of hypermenorrhea (menorrhagia); pain associated with endometriosis; dysmenorrhea; dysfunctional uterine bleeding

Pregnancy Risk Factor X

Dosage Oral: Adults: Females: Contraception:
Schedule 1 (Sunday starter): Dose begins on first Sunday after onset of menstruation; if the menstrual period starts on Sunday, take first tablet that very same day. **With a Sunday start, an additional method of contraception should be used until after the first 7 days of consecutive administration.**
For 21-tablet package: Dosage is 1 tablet daily for 21 consecutive days, followed by 7 days off of the medication; a new course begins on the 8th day after the last tablet is taken.
For 28-tablet package: Dosage is 1 tablet daily without interruption.
Schedule 2 (Day 1 starter): Dose starts on first day of menstrual cycle taking 1 tablet daily.
For 21-tablet package: Dosage is 1 tablet daily for 21 consecutive days, followed by 7 days off of the medication; a new course begins on the 8th day after the last tablet is taken.
For 28-tablet package: Dosage is 1 tablet daily without interruption.
If all doses have been taken on schedule and one menstrual period is missed, continue dosing cycle. If two consecutive menstrual periods are missed, pregnancy test is required before new dosing cycle is started.
Missed doses **monophasic formulations** (refer to package insert for complete information):
One dose missed: Take as soon as remembered or take 2 tablets next day
Two consecutive doses missed in the first 2 weeks: Take 2 tablets as soon as remembered or 2 tablets next 2 days. **An additional method of contraception should be used for 7 days after missed dose.**
Two consecutive doses missed in week 3 or three consecutive doses missed at any time:
Schedule 1 (Sunday starter): Continue to take 1 tablet daily until Sunday, then discard the rest of the pack, and a new pack is started that same day.
Schedule 2 (Day 1 starter): Current pack should be discarded, and a new pack started that same day. **An additional method of contraception should be used for 7 days after missed dose.**
Missed doses **biphasic/triphasic formulations** (refer to package insert for complete information):
One dose missed: Take as soon as remembered or take 2 tablets next day.
Two consecutive doses missed in week 1 or week 2 of the pack: Take 2 tablets as soon as remembered and 2 tablets the next day. Resume taking 1 tablet daily until the pack is empty. **An additional method of contraception should be used for 7 days after a missed dose.**

Two consecutive doses missed in week 3 of the pack; **an additional method of contraception must be used for 7 days after a missed dose**:
Schedule 1 (Sunday starter): Take 1 tablet every day until Sunday. Discard the remaining pack and start a new pack of pills on the same day.
Schedule 2 (Day 1 starter): Discard the remaining pack and start a new pack the same day.
Three or more consecutive doses missed; **an additional method of contraception must be used for 7 days after a missed dose**:
Schedule 1 (Sunday starter): Take 1 tablet every day until Sunday; on Sunday, discard the pack and start a new pack.
Schedule 2 (Day 1 starter): Discard the remaining pack and begin new pack of tablets starting on the same day.

Dosage adjustment in renal impairment: Specific guidelines not available; use with caution and monitor blood pressure closely. Consider other forms of contraception.
Dosage adjustment in hepatic impairment: Contraindicated in patients with hepatic impairment

Additional Information Complete prescribing information for this medication should be consulted for additional detail.

Dosage Forms Excipient information presented when available (limited, particularly for generics); consult specific product labeling. [DSC] = Discontinued product

Tablet, low-dose formulations:
Azurette™:
Day 1-21: Ethinyl estradiol 0.02 mg and desogestrel 0.15 mg [21 white tablets]
Day 22-23: 2 inactive green tablets
Day 24-28: Ethinyl estradiol 0.01 mg [5 blue tablets] (28s)
Kariva®:
Day 1-21: Ethinyl estradiol 0.02 mg and desogestrel 0.15 mg [21 white tablets]
Day 22-23: 2 inactive light green tablets
Day 24-28: Ethinyl estradiol 0.01 mg [5 light blue tablets] (28s)
Mircette®:
Day 1-21: Ethinyl estradiol 0.02 mg and desogestrel 0.15 mg [21 white tablets]
Day 22-23: 2 inactive green tablets
Day 24-28: Ethinyl estradiol 0.01 mg [5 yellow tablets] (28s)

Tablet, monophasic formulations:
Apri® 28: Ethinyl estradiol 0.03 mg and desogestrel 0.15 mg (28s) [21 rose tablets and 7 white inactive tablets]
Desogen®, Reclipsen®, Solia® [DSC]: Ethinyl estradiol 0.03 mg and desogestrel 0.15 mg (28s) [21 white tablets and 7 green inactive tablets]
Emoquette™: Ethinyl estradiol 0.03 mg and desogestrel 0.15 mg (28s) [21 white tablets and 7 light green inactive tablets]
Ortho-Cept® 28: Ethinyl estradiol 0.03 mg and desogestrel 0.15 mg (28s) [21 light orange tablets and 7 green inactive tablets]

Tablet, triphasic formulations:
Caziant®:
Day 1-7: Ethinyl estradiol 0.025 mg and desogestrel 0.1 mg [7 white tablets]
Day 8-14: Ethinyl estradiol 0.025 mg and desogestrel 0.125 mg [7 light blue tablets]
Day 15-21: Ethinyl estradiol 0.025 mg and desogestrel 0.15 mg [7 blue tablets]
Day 22-28: 7 green inactive tablets (28s)
Cesia® [DSC], Cyclessa®:
Day 1-7: Ethinyl estradiol 0.025 mg and desogestrel 0.1 mg [7 light yellow tablets]
Day 8-14: Ethinyl estradiol 0.025 mg and desogestrel 0.125 mg [7 orange tablets]
Day 15-21: Ethinyl estradiol 0.025 mg and desogestrel 0.15 mg [7 red tablets]
Day 22-28: 7 green inactive tablets (28s)
Velivet™:
Day 1-7: Ethinyl estradiol 0.025 mg and desogestrel 0.1 mg [7 beige tablets]
Day 8-14: Ethinyl estradiol 0.025 mg and desogestrel 0.125 mg [7 orange tablets]
Day 15-21: Ethinyl estradiol 0.025 mg and desogestrel 0.15 mg [7 pink tablets]
Day 22-28: 7 white inactive tablets (28s)

Ethinyl Estradiol and Drospirenone

(ETH in il es tra DYE ole & droh SPYE re none)

Brand Names: U.S. Gianvi™; Loryna™; Ocella™; Syeda™; Yasmin®; Yaz®; Zarah®
Brand Names: Canada Yasmin®; Yaz®
Index Terms Drospirenone and Ethinyl Estradiol
Pharmacologic Category Contraceptive; Estrogen and Progestin Combination
Use Prevention of pregnancy; treatment of premenstrual dysphoric disorder (PMDD); treatment of acne
Unlabeled Use Treatment of hypermenorrhea (menorrhagia); pain associated with endometriosis; dysmenorrhea; dysfunctional uterine bleeding
Pregnancy Risk Factor X
Dosage Oral:
Children ≥14 years and Adults: Females: Acne (Yaz®): Refer to dosing for contraception
Adults: Females: Contraception (Yasmin®, Yaz®), PMDD (Yaz®): Dosage is 1 tablet daily for 28 consecutive days. Dosing may be started on the first day of menstrual period (Day 1 starter) or on the first Sunday after the onset of the menstrual period (Sunday starter). **An additional method of contraception should be used until after the first 7 days of consecutive administration.**
Day 1 starter: Dose starts on first day of menstrual cycle taking 1 tablet daily.
Sunday starter: Dose begins on first Sunday after onset of menstruation; if the menstrual period starts on Sunday, take first tablet that very same day.
Switching from a different contraceptive:
Oral contraceptive: Start on the same day that a new pack of the previous oral contraceptive would have been taken
Transdermal patch, vaginal ring, injection: Start on the day the next dose would have been due
IUD or implant: Start on the day of removal
Use after childbirth (in women who are not breast-feeding) or after second trimester abortion: Therapy may be started ≥4 weeks postpartum. Pregnancy should be ruled out prior to treatment if menstrual periods have not restarted and an additional method of contraception (nonhormonal) should be used until after the first 7 days of consecutive administration.

Missed doses:
If all doses have been taken on schedule and one menstrual period is missed, continue dosing cycle. If two consecutive menstrual periods are missed, pregnancy test is required before new dosing cycle is started.
If doses have been missed during the first 3 weeks and the menstrual period is missed, pregnancy should be ruled out prior to continuing treatment.

Missed doses (monophasic formulations) (refer to package insert for complete information):
One dose missed: Take as soon as remembered or take 2 tablets next day
Two consecutive doses missed in the first 2 weeks: Take 2 tablets as soon as remembered or 2 tablets next 2 days. **An additional method of contraception should be used for 7 days after missed dose.**
Two consecutive doses missed in week 3 or three consecutive doses missed at any time: **An additional method of contraception must be used for 7 days after a missed dose.**
Day 1 starter: Current pack should be discarded, and a new pack should be started that same day.
Sunday starter: Continue dose of 1 tablet daily until Sunday, then discard the rest of the pack, and a new pack should be started that same day.
Any number of doses missed in week 4: Continue taking one pill each day until pack is empty; no back-up method of contraception is needed

Dosage adjustment in renal impairment: Contraindicated in patients with renal dysfunction

Dosage adjustment in hepatic impairment: Contraindicated in patients with hepatic dysfunction

Additional Information Complete prescribing information for this medication should be consulted for additional detail.

Dosage Forms Excipient information presented when available (limited, particularly for generics); consult specific product labeling.

Tablet, oral:
Gianvi™: Ethinyl estradiol 0.02 mg and drospirenone 3 mg (28s) [24 light pink active tablets and 4 white inactive tablets]
Loryna™: Ethinyl estradiol 0.02 mg and drospirenone 3 mg (28s) [24 peach active tablets and 4 white inactive tablets]
Ocella™: Ethinyl estradiol 0.03 mg and drospirenone 3 mg (28s) [21 yellow active tablets and 7 white inactive tablets]
Syeda™: Ethinyl estradiol 0.03 mg and drospirenone 3 mg (28s) [21 yellow active tablets and 7 white inactive tablets]
Yasmin®: Ethinyl estradiol 0.03 mg and drospirenone 3 mg (28s) [21 yellow active tablets and 7 white inactive tablets]
Yaz®: Ethinyl estradiol 0.02 mg and drospirenone 3 mg (28s) [24 light pink active tablets and 4 white inactive tablets]
Zarah®: Ethinyl estradiol 0.03 mg and drospirenone 3 mg (28s) [21 blue active tablets and 7 peach inactive tablets]

Ethinyl Estradiol and Ethynodiol Diacetate

(ETH in il es tra DYE ole & e thye noe DYE ole dye AS e tate)

Brand Names: U.S. Kelnor™; Zovia®

Brand Names: Canada Demulen® 30

Index Terms Ethynodiol Diacetate and Ethinyl Estradiol

Pharmacologic Category Contraceptive; Estrogen and Progestin Combination

Use Prevention of pregnancy

Unlabeled Use Treatment of hypermenorrhea (menorrhagia); pain associated with endometriosis; dysmenorrhea; dysfunctional uterine bleeding

Pregnancy Risk Factor X

Dosage Oral: Adults: Females: Contraception:
Schedule 1 (Sunday starter): Dose begins on first Sunday after onset of menstruation; if the menstrual period starts on Sunday, take first tablet that very same day. **With a Sunday start, an additional method of contraception should be used until after the first 7 days of consecutive administration.**
For 21-tablet package: 1 tablet/day for 21 consecutive days, followed by 7 days off of the medication; a new course begins on the 8th day after the last tablet is taken.
For 28-tablet package: 1 tablet/day without interruption.
Schedule 2 (Day 1 starter): Dose starts on first day of menstrual cycle taking 1 tablet daily.
For 21-tablet package: 1 tablet/day for 21 consecutive days, followed by 7 days off of the medication; a new course begins on the 8th day after the last tablet is taken.
For 28-tablet package: 1 tablet/day without interruption.
If all doses have been taken on schedule and one menstrual period is missed, continue dosing cycle. If two consecutive menstrual periods are missed, pregnancy test is required before new dosing cycle is started.
Missed doses **monophasic formulations** (refer to package insert for complete information):
One dose missed: Take as soon as remembered or take 2 tablets next day
Two consecutive doses missed in the first 2 weeks: Take 2 tablets as soon as remembered or 2 tablets next 2 days. **An additional method of contraception should be used for 7 days after missed dose.**
Two consecutive doses missed in week 3 or three consecutive doses missed at any time: **An additional method of contraception should be used for 7 days after missed dose:**
Schedule 1 (Sunday starter): Continue dose of 1 tablet daily until Sunday, then discard the rest of the pack, and a new pack should be started that same day.
Schedule 2 (Day 1 starter): Current package should be discarded, and a new pack should be started that same day.

Dosage adjustment in renal impairment: Specific guidelines not available; use with caution and monitor blood pressure closely. Consider other forms of contraception.

Dosage adjustment in hepatic impairment: Contraindicated in patients with hepatic impairment

Additional Information Complete prescribing information for this medication should be consulted for additional detail.

Dosage Forms Excipient information presented when available (limited, particularly for generics); consult specific product labeling.

Tablet, monophasic formulations:
Kelnor™ 1/35: Ethinyl estradiol 0.035 mg and ethynodiol diacetate 1 mg [21 light yellow tablets and 7 white inactive tablets] (28s)
Zovia® 1/35-28: Ethinyl estradiol 0.035 mg and ethynodiol diacetate 1 mg [21 light pink tablets and 7 white inactive tablets] (28s)
Zovia® 1/50-28: Ethinyl estradiol 0.05 mg and ethynodiol diacetate 1 mg [21 pink tablets and 7 white inactive tablets] (28s)

Ethinyl Estradiol and Etonogestrel

(ETH in il es tra DYE ole & et oh noe JES trel)

Brand Names: U.S. NuvaRing®

Brand Names: Canada NuvaRing®

Index Terms Etonogestrel and Ethinyl Estradiol

Pharmacologic Category Contraceptive; Estrogen and Progestin Combination

Use Prevention of pregnancy

Unlabeled Use Treatment of hypermenorrhea (menorrhagia); pain associated with endometriosis; dysmenorrhea; dysfunctional uterine bleeding

Pregnancy Risk Factor X

Dosage Vaginal: Adults: Females: Contraception: One ring, inserted vaginally and left in place for 3 consecutive weeks, then removed for 1 week. A new ring is inserted 7 days after the last was removed (even if bleeding is not complete) and should be inserted at approximately the same time of day the ring was removed the previous week.

Initial treatment should begin as follows (pregnancy should always be ruled out first):

No hormonal contraceptive use in the past month: Insert ring on the first day of menstrual cycle ("Day 1"). May also insert on days 2-5 even if bleeding is not complete, however, **a spermicide or barrier method of contraception should be used for the following 7 days.***

Switching from combination oral contraceptive: Ring can be inserted on any day within 7 days after the last **active** tablet in the cycle was taken and no later than the first day a new cycle of tablets would begin. Additional forms of contraception are not needed.

Switching from progestin-only contraceptive: **A spermicide or barrier method of contraception should be used for the following 7 days with any of the following.***

If previously using a progestin-only mini-pill, insert the ring on any day of the month; do not skip days between the last pill and insertion of the ring.

If previously using an implant, insert the ring on the same day of implant removal.

If previously using a progestin-containing IUD, insert the ring on day of IUD removal.

If previously using a progestin injection, insert the ring on the day the next injection would be given.

Following complete 1st trimester abortion: Insert ring within the first 5 days of abortion. If not inserted within 5 days, follow instructions for "No hormonal contraceptive use within the past month" and instruct patient to use a nonhormonal contraceptive in the interim.

Following delivery or 2nd trimester abortion: Insert ring 4 weeks postpartum (in women who are not breast-feeding) or following 2nd trimester abortion. **A spermicide or barrier method of contraception should be used for the following 7 days.***

If the ring is accidentally removed from the vagina at anytime during the 3-week period of use, it may be rinsed with cool or lukewarm water (not hot) and reinserted as soon as possible. If the ring is not reinserted within 3 hours, contraceptive effectiveness will be decreased. **A spermicide or barrier method of contraception should be used until the ring has been in place for 7 consecutive days.***

If the ring has been removed for longer than 1 week, pregnancy must be ruled out prior to restarting therapy. **A spermicide or barrier method of contraception should be used for the following 7 days.***

If the ring has been left in place for >3 weeks, a new ring should be inserted following a 1-week (ring-free) interval. Protection continues during week 4, however, if the ring is left in place >4 weeks, pregnancy must be ruled out prior to insertion and **a spermicide or barrier method of contraception should be used for the following 7 days.***

Disconnected ring: In the event the ring disconnects at the weld joint, discard and replace with a new ring.

***Note:** Diaphragms may interfere with proper ring placement, and therefore, are not recommended for use as an additional form of contraception.

Dosage adjustment in renal impairment: Specific guidelines not available; use with caution and monitor blood pressure closely. Consider other forms of contraception.

Dosage adjustment in hepatic impairment: Contraindicated in patients with hepatic impairment

Additional Information Complete prescribing information for this medication should be consulted for additional detail.

Dosage Forms Excipient information presented when available (limited, particularly for generics); consult specific product labeling.

Ring, vaginal:

NuvaRing®: Ethinyl estradiol 0.015 mg/day and etonogestrel 0.12 mg/day (1s) [3-week duration]

Ethinyl Estradiol and Levonorgestrel

(ETH in il es tra DYE ole & LEE voe nor jes trel)

Brand Names: U.S. Amethia™; Amethia™ Lo; Amethyst™; Aviane™; camrese™; Enpresse®; Introvale™; Jolessa™; Lessina®; Levora®; LoSeasonique®; Lutera®; Lybrel®; Nordette® 28; Orsythia™; Portia®; Quasense®; Seasonale®; Seasonique®; Sronyx®; Trivora®

Brand Names: Canada Alesse®; Aviane®; Min-Ovral®; Seasonale®; Triphasil®; Triquilar®

Index Terms Levonorgestrel and Ethinyl Estradiol

Pharmacologic Category Contraceptive; Estrogen and Progestin Combination

Use Prevention of pregnancy; postcoital contraception

Unlabeled Use Treatment of hypermenorrhea (menorrhagia); pain associated with endometriosis; dysmenorrhea; dysfunctional uterine bleeding

Pregnancy Risk Factor X

Pregnancy Considerations Pregnancy should be ruled out prior to treatment and discontinued if pregnancy occurs. In general, the use of combination hormonal contraceptives when inadvertently taken early in pregnancy have not been associated with teratogenic effects. Hormonal contraceptives may be less effective in obese patients. An increase in oral contraceptive failure was noted in women with a BMI >27.3 kg/m^2. Similar findings were noted in patients weighing ≥90 kg (198 lb) using the contraceptive patch.

Due to increased risk of venous thromboembolism (VTE) postpartum, combination hormonal contraceptives should not be started in any woman <21 days following delivery. Women without risk factors for VTE and who are not breast-feeding may start combination hormonal contraceptives during 21-42 days postpartum. After 42 days postpartum, restrictions for use are not related to postpartum status and should be based on other medical conditions (CDC, 2011).

Lactation Enters breast milk/not recommended

Contraindications Breast cancer or other estrogen- or progestin-dependent neoplasms (current or a history of), hepatic tumors or disease, pregnancy, undiagnosed abnormal uterine bleeding

Use is also contraindicated in women at high risk of arterial or venous thrombotic diseases including: Cerebrovascular disease, coronary artery disease, diabetes mellitus with vascular disease, DVT or PE (current or history of), hypercoagulopathies (inherited or acquired), headaches with focal neurological symptoms, hypertension (uncontrolled), migraine headaches if >35 years of age, thrombogenic valvular or rhythm diseases of the heart (eg, subacute bacterial endocarditis with valvular disease or atrial fibrillation), women >35 years of age who smoke.

Canadian-labeling: Additional contraindication: Ocular lesions due to ophthalmic vascular disease including partial or complete loss of vision or defect in visual fields; severe dyslipoproteinemia; hereditary or acquired predisposition for venous or arterial thrombosis

Warnings/Precautions Combination hormonal contraceptives do not protect against HIV infection or other sexually-transmitted diseases. **[U.S. Boxed Warning]: The risk of cardiovascular side effects is increased**

in women who smoke cigarettes; risk increases with age (especially women >35 years of age) and the number of cigarettes smoked; women who use combination hormonal contraceptives should be strongly advised not to smoke. Use is contraindicated in patients >35 years of age who smoke. Use with caution in patients with risk factors for coronary artery disease (eg, hypertension, hypercholesterolemia, morbid obesity, diabetes, or women who smoke); may lead to increased risk of myocardial infarction. May have a dose-related risk of vascular disease and hypertension; women with hypertension should be encouraged to use a nonhormonal form of contraception. May increase the risk of thromboembolism; discontinue use of combination hormonal contraceptives if an arterial or venous thrombotic event occurs. Whenever possible, combination hormonal contraceptives should be discontinued at least 4 weeks prior to and for 2 weeks following elective surgery associated with an increased risk of thromboembolism or during periods of prolonged immobilization. Combination hormonal contraceptives may have a dose-related risk of gallbladder disease and may worsen existing gallbladder disease. Women with renal disease should be encouraged to use another form of contraception. May have adverse effects on glucose tolerance; use caution in women with diabetes.

Combination hormonal contraceptives may affect serum triglyceride and lipoprotein levels. Triglycerides may also be increased; use with caution in patients with familial defects of lipoprotein metabolism. The use of combination hormonal contraceptives has been associated with a slight increase in frequency of breast cancer; however, studies are not consistent. Use is contraindicated in women with (or history of) breast cancer. Use caution with conditions that may be aggravated by fluid retention, depression, or history of migraine. Evaluate new, recurrent, severe or persistent headaches. Use with migraine headaches with or without aura if >35 years of age is contraindicated. Not for use prior to menarche. Estrogens may cause retinal vascular thrombosis; discontinue if migraine, loss of vision, proptosis, diplopia or other visual disturbances occur; discontinue permanently if papilledema or retinal vascular lesions are observed on examination. Risk of chlosasma may be increased with history of chloasma gravidarum. Women with history of chloasma should avoid exposure to sun or ultraviolet radiation during therapy. May induce or exacerbate symptoms of hereditary angioedema.

Presentation of irregular, unresolving vaginal bleeding warrants further evaluation including endometrial sampling, if indicated, to rule out malignancy; evaluate hypothalamic-pituitary-function in women with persistent (≥6 months) amenorrhea (especially associated with breast secretion) following discontinuation of therapy. Discontinue use with the onset of sudden enlargement, pain, or tenderness of fibroids (leiomyomata). Extremely rare adenomas and focal nodular hyperplasia resulting in fatal intra-abdominal hemorrhage have been reported in association with long-term oral contraceptive use. Presentation of an abdominal mass, acute abdominal pain, or intra-abdominal bleeding warrants further evaluation to rule out source. Combination hormonal contraceptives may be poorly metabolized in women with hepatic impairment. Discontinue if jaundice develops during therapy or if liver function becomes abnormal. Risk of cholestasis may be increased with previous cholestatic jaundice of pregnancy or jaundice with prior oral contraceptive use.

The minimum dosage combination of estrogen/progestin that will effectively treat the individual patient should be used. New patients should be started on products containing ≤0.035 mg of estrogen per tablet. Extended cycle regimen contraceptives provide more hormonal exposure per year than conventional monthly contraceptives.

Adverse Reactions The following reactions have been associated with oral contraceptive use:

Increased risk or evidence of association with use:

Cardiovascular: Arterial thromboembolism, cerebral hemorrhage, cerebral thrombosis, hypertension, mesenteric thrombosis, MI, venous thrombosis (with or without embolism)

Gastrointestinal: Gallbladder disease

Hepatic: Hepatic adenomas, liver tumors (benign)

Local: Thrombophlebitis

Ocular: Retinal thrombosis

Respiratory: Pulmonary embolism

Adverse reactions considered drug related:

Cardiovascular: Edema, varicose vein aggravation

Central nervous system: Depression, migraine, mood changes

Dermatologic: Chloasma, melasma, rash (allergic)

Endocrine & metabolic: Amenorrhea, breakthrough bleeding, breast changes (enlargement, pain, secretion, tenderness), carbohydrate tolerance decreased, fluid retention, infertility (temporary), lactation decreased (with use immediately postpartum), menstrual flow changes, spotting

Gastrointestinal: Abdominal bloating, abdominal cramps, abdominal pain, appetite changes, nausea, weight changes, vomiting

Genitourinary: Cervical ectropion, cervical secretion/erosion, endocervical hyperplasia, fibroid enlargement, vaginal candidiasis, vaginitis

Hematologic: Folate decreased, porphyria exacerbation

Hepatic: Cholestatic jaundice, focal nodular hyperplasia

Neuromuscular & skeletal: Chorea exacerbation

Ocular: Contact lens intolerance, corneal curvature changes (steepening)

Respiratory: Rhinitis

Miscellaneous: Anaphylactic/anaphylactoid reactions (including angioedema, circulatory collapse, respiratory collapse, urticaria), SLE exacerbation

Adverse reactions in which association is not confirmed or denied: Acne, auditory disturbances, Budd-Chiari syndrome, cataracts, cervical smear abnormal, colitis, cystitis-like syndrome, dizziness, dysmenorrhea, erythema multiforme, erythema nodosum, headache, hemolytic uremic syndrome, hemorrhagic eruption, hirsutism, libido changes, nervousness, optic neuritis (with or without partial or complete loss of vision), pancreatitis, premenstrual syndrome, renal function impaired, scalp hair loss

Drug Interactions

Metabolism/Transport Effects Refer to individual components.

Avoid Concomitant Use

Avoid concomitant use of Ethinyl Estradiol and Levonorgestrel with any of the following: Anastrozole; Griseofulvin; Pimozide

Increased Effect/Toxicity

Ethinyl Estradiol and Levonorgestrel may increase the levels/effects of: Benzodiazepines (metabolized by oxidation); Corticosteroids (Systemic); CYP1A2 Substrates; Pimozide; ROPINIRole; Selegiline; Theophylline Derivatives; Tipranavir; TiZANidine; Tranexamic Acid; Voriconazole

The levels/effects of Ethinyl Estradiol and Levonorgestrel may be increased by: Ascorbic Acid; Boceprevir; Conivaptan; Herbs (Estrogenic Properties); Herbs (Progestogenic Properties); Voriconazole

Decreased Effect

Ethinyl Estradiol and Levonorgestrel may decrease the levels/effects of: Anastrozole; Chenodiol; LamoTRIgine; Thyroid Products; Ursodiol; Vitamin K Antagonists

The levels/effects of Ethinyl Estradiol and Levonorgestrel may be decreased by: Acitretin; Aminoglutethimide; Aprepitant; Armodafinil; Artemether; Barbiturates;

Bexarotene; Bexarotene (Systemic); Bile Acid Sequestrants; Boceprevir; Bosentan; CarBAMazepine; Clobazam; Colesevelam; CYP3A4 Inducers (Strong); Deferasirox; Felbamate; Fosaprepitant; Fosphenytoin; Griseofulvin; LamoTRIgine; Modafinil; Mycophenolate; Nafcillin; Nevirapine; OXcarbazepine; Phenytoin; Protease Inhibitors; Retinoic Acid Derivatives; Rifamycin Derivatives; Rufinamide; St Johns Wort; Telaprevir; Tipranavir; Tocilizumab; Topiramate

Ethanol/Nutrition/Herb Interactions

Food: CNS effects of caffeine may be enhanced if combination hormonal contraceptives are used concurrently with caffeine. Grapefruit juice increases ethinyl estradiol plasma concentrations and would be expected to increase progesterone serum levels as well; clinical implications are unclear.

Herb/Nutraceutical: St John's wort may decrease levels. Herbs with estrogenic properties may enhance the adverse/toxic effect of estrogen derivatives; examples include alfalfa, black cohosh, bloodroot, hops, kudzu, licorice, red clover, saw palmetto, soybean, thyme, wild yam, yucca. Herbs with progestogenic properties may enhance the adverse/toxic effect of progestins; examples include bloodroot, chasteberry, damiana, oregano, yucca. Impaired folate metabolism and reduced serum levels of cyanocobalamin have been reported with oral contraceptive use; increased dietary intake or supplementation may be necessary.

Stability Store at controlled room temperature of 20°C to 25°C (68°F to 77°F).

Mechanism of Action Combination hormonal contraceptives inhibit ovulation via a negative feedback mechanism on the hypothalamus, which alters the normal pattern of gonadotropin secretion of a follicle-stimulating hormone (FSH) and luteinizing hormone by the anterior pituitary. The follicular phase FSH and midcycle surge of gonadotropins are inhibited. In addition, combination hormonal contraceptives produce alterations in the genital tract, including changes in the cervical mucus, rendering it unfavorable for sperm penetration even if ovulation occurs. Changes in the endometrium may also occur, producing an unfavorable environment for nidation. Combination hormonal contraceptive drugs may alter the tubal transport of the ova through the fallopian tubes. Progestational agents may also alter sperm fertility.

Pharmacodynamics/Kinetics

Absorption: Rapid

Distribution: Ethinyl estradiol: 4.3 L/kg; Levonorgestrel: 1.8 L/kg

Protein binding:
- Ethinyl estradiol: 95% to 97% to albumin
- Levonorgestrel: 97% to 99% primarily to sex hormone binding globulin (SHBG), lesser amounts to albumin

Metabolism:
- Ethinyl estradiol: Hepatic via CYP3A4; undergoes first-pass metabolism; forms metabolites
- Levonorgestrel: Forms conjugated in unconjugated metabolites

Bioavailability: Ethinyl estradiol: 38% to 48%; Levonorgestrel: 100%

Half-life elimination: Ethinyl estradiol: 12-23 hours; Levonorgestrel: 22-49 hours

Excretion:
- Ethinyl estradiol: Urine and feces
- Levonorgestrel: Urine (40% to 68%, parent drug and metabolites); feces (16% to 48% as metabolites)

Dosage Oral: Adults: Females:

Contraception, 28-day cycle:

Schedule 1 (Sunday starter): Dose begins on first Sunday after onset of menstruation; if the menstrual period starts on Sunday, take first tablet that very same day. With a Sunday start, an additional method of contraception should be used until after the first 7 days of consecutive administration:
- For 21-tablet package: 1 tablet/day for 21 consecutive days, followed by 7 days off of the medication; a new course begins on the 8th day after the last tablet is taken
- For 28-tablet package: 1 tablet/day without interruption

Schedule 2 (Day 1 starter): Dose starts on first day of menstrual cycle taking 1 tablet/day:
- For 21-tablet package: 1 tablet/day for 21 consecutive days, followed by 7 days off of the medication; a new course begins on the 8th day after the last tablet is taken
- For 28-tablet package: 1 tablet/day without interruption

If all doses have been taken on schedule and one menstrual period is missed, continue dosing cycle. If two consecutive menstrual periods are missed, pregnancy test is required before new dosing cycle is started.

Missed doses **monophasic formulations** (refer to package insert for complete information):
- One dose missed: Take as soon as remembered or take 2 tablets next day
- Two consecutive doses missed in the first 2 weeks: Take 2 tablets as soon as remembered or 2 tablets next 2 days. An additional method of contraception should be used for 7 days after missed dose.
- Two consecutive doses missed in week 3 or three consecutive doses missed at any time: An additional method of contraception must be used for 7 days after a missed dose:
  - Schedule 1 (Sunday starter): Continue dose of 1 tablet daily until Sunday, then discard the rest of the pack, and a new pack should be started that same day.
  - Schedule 2 (Day 1 starter): Current pack should be discarded, and a new pack should be started that same day.

Missed doses **biphasic/triphasic formulations** (refer to package insert for complete information):
- One dose missed: Take as soon as remembered or take 2 tablets next day.
- Two consecutive doses missed in week 1 or week 2 of the pack: Take 2 tablets as soon as remembered and 2 tablets the next day. Resume taking 1 tablet daily until the pack is empty. An additional method of contraception should be used for 7 days after a missed dose.
- Two consecutive doses missed in week 3 of the pack: An additional method of contraception must be used for 7 days after a missed dose.
  - Schedule 1 (Sunday starter): Take 1 tablet every day until Sunday. Discard the remaining pack and start a new pack of pills on the same day.
  - Schedule 2 (Day 1 starter): Discard the remaining pack and start a new pack the same day.
- Three or more consecutive doses missed: An additional method of contraception must be used for 7 days after a missed dose.
  - Schedule 1 (Sunday starter): Take 1 tablet every day until Sunday; on Sunday, discard the pack and start a new pack.
  - Schedule 2 (Day 1 starter): Discard the remaining pack and begin new pack of tablets starting on the same day.

Contraception, 91-day cycle (extended cycle regimen): Dose begins on first Sunday after onset of menstruation; if the menstrual period starts on Sunday, take first tablet that very same day. An additional method of contraception should be used until after the first 7 days of consecutive administration:

Seasonale®: One active tablet/day for 84 consecutive days, followed by 1 inactive tablet/day for 7 days; if all doses have been taken on schedule and one menstrual period is missed, pregnancy should be ruled out prior to continuing therapy.

Seasonique®, LoSeasonique®: One active tablet/day for 84 consecutive days, followed by 1 low dose estrogen tablet/day for 7 days; if all doses have been taken on schedule and one menstrual period is missed, pregnancy should be ruled out prior to continuing therapy.

Missed doses:

One dose missed: Take as soon as remembered or take 2 tablets the next day

Two consecutive doses missed: Take 2 tablets as soon as remembered or 2 tablets the next 2 days. An additional nonhormonal method of contraception should be used for 7 consecutive days after the missed dose.

Three or more consecutive doses missed: Do not take the missed doses; continue taking 1 tablet/day until pack is complete. Bleeding may occur during the following week. An additional nonhormonal method of contraception should be used for 7 consecutive days after the missed dose.

Any number of pills during week 13: Throw away the missed pills and keep taking scheduled pills until the pack is finished. A back-up method of contraception is not needed

Contraception, continuous use (extended cycle regimen): Lybrel®: Take one tablet daily, at the same time each day, without a tablet-free interval. Therapy should be initiated as follows:

No previous contraception: Begin on the first day of menstrual cycle. Back-up contraception is not needed.

Previously taking a 21-day or 28-day combination hormonal contraceptive: Begin on day 1 of the withdrawal bleed (at the latest, 7 days after the last active tablet). Back-up contraception is not needed.

Previously using a progestin-only pill: Begin the day after taking a progestin only pill. Back-up contraception is needed for the first 7 days of therapy.

Previously using contraceptive implant: Begin the day of implant removal. Back-up contraception is needed for the first 7 days of therapy.

Previously using contraceptive injection: Begin when the next injection is due. Back-up contraception is needed for the first 7 days of therapy.

Missed doses:

One dose missed: Take as soon as remembered then take the next tablet at the regular time (2 tablets in 1 day). An additional nonhormonal method of contraception should also be used for 7 consecutive days.

Two consecutive doses missed: If remembered the day of the second missed tablet, take 2 tablets as soon as remembered, then 1 tablet the next day. If remembered the day after the second tablet is missed, take 2 tablets the day remembered, then 2 tablets the next day. An additional nonhormonal method of contraception should also be used for 7 consecutive days.

Three or more consecutive doses missed: Take 1 tablet daily and contact healthcare provider; do not take the missed pills. An additional nonhormonal method of contraception should also be used for 7 consecutive days.

Dosage adjustment in renal impairment: Specific guidelines not available; use with caution and monitor blood pressure closely. Consider other forms of contraception.

Dosage adjustment in hepatic impairment: Contraindicated in patients with hepatic impairment

Dietary Considerations Should be taken at the same time each day.

Administration Administer at the same time each day.

Monitoring Parameters Before starting therapy, a physical exam with reference to the breasts and pelvis are recommended, including a Papanicolaou smear. Exam may be deferred if appropriate; pregnancy should be ruled out prior to use. Monitor patient closely for loss of vision, sudden onset of proptosis, diplopia, migraine; blood pressure; signs and symptoms of thromboembolic disorders; signs or symptoms of depression; glycemic control in patients with diabetes; lipid profiles in patients being treated for hyperlipidemias. Adequate diagnostic measures, including endometrial sampling, if indicated, should be performed to rule out malignancy in all cases of undiagnosed abnormal vaginal bleeding.

Test Interactions Increased prothrombin and factors VII, VIII, IX, X; increased platelet aggregability, thyroid-binding globulin, total thyroid hormone (T4), serum triglycerides/phospholipids, AST, Alkaline Phosphatase, GGT; decreased serum folate concentration; pathologist should be advised of estrogen/progesterone therapy when specimens are submitted. Oral contraceptives suppress LH and FSH levels; wait at least 2 weeks after discontinuing use of contraceptive before measuring.

Dosage Forms Excipient information presented when available (limited, particularly for generics); consult specific product labeling. [DSC] = Discontinued product

Tablet, oral [low-dose formulation]:

Aviane™: Ethinyl estradiol 0.02 mg and levonorgestrel 0.1 mg (28s) [21 orange tablets and 7 light green inactive tablets]

Lutera®, Sronyx®: Ethinyl estradiol 0.02 mg and levonorgestrel 0.1 mg (28s) [21 white tablets and 7 peach inactive tablets]

Orsythia™: Ethinyl estradiol 0.02 mg and levonorgestrel 0.1 mg (28s) [21 pink tablets and 7 light green inactive tablets]

Tablet, oral [monophasic formulation]:

Levora®: Ethinyl estradiol 0.03 mg and levonorgestrel 0.15 mg (28s) [21 white tablets and 7 peach inactive tablets]

Nordette® 28: Ethinyl estradiol 0.03 mg and levonorgestrel 0.15 mg (28s) [21 light orange tablets and 7 pink inactive tablets]

Portia® 28: Ethinyl estradiol 0.03 mg and levonorgestrel 0.15 mg (28s) [21 pink tablets and 7 white inactive tablets]

Tablet, oral [extended cycle regimen]: Ethinyl estradiol 0.02 mg and levonorgestrel 0.1 mg [84 tablets] and ethinyl estradiol 0.01 mg [7 tablets] (91s)

Amethia™: Ethinyl estradiol 0.03 mg and levonorgestrel 0.15 mg (91s) [84 white tablets] and ethinyl estradiol 0.01 mg [7 light blue tablets]

Amethia™ Lo: Ethinyl estradiol 0.02 mg and levonorgestrel 0.1 mg (91s) [84 white tablets] and ethinyl estradiol 0.01 mg [7 blue tablets]

camrese™: Ethinyl estradiol 0.03 mg and levonorgestrel 0.15 mg (91s) [84 light blue-green tablets] and ethinyl estradiol 0.01 mg [7 yellow tablets]

Introvale™: Ethinyl estradiol 0.03 mg and levonorgestrel 0.15 mg (91s) [84 peach tablets and 7 white inactive tablets]

Jolessa™, Seasonale®: Ethinyl estradiol 0.03 mg and levonorgestrel 0.15 mg (91s) [84 pink tablets and 7 white inactive tablets]

LoSeasonique®: Ethinyl estradiol 0.02 mg and levonorgestrel 0.1 mg (91s) [84 orange tablets] and ethinyl estradiol 0.01 mg [7 yellow tablets]

Quasense®: Ethinyl estradiol 0.03 mg and levonorgestrel 0.15 mg (91s) [84 white tablets and 7 peach inactive tablets]

Seasonique®: Ethinyl estradiol 0.03 mg and levonorgestrel 0.15 mg (91s) [84 light blue-green tablets] and ethinyl estradiol 0.01 mg [7 yellow tablets]

Tablet, oral [noncyclic regimen]:

Amethyst™: Ethinyl estradiol 0.02 mg and levonorgestrel 0.09 mg (28s) [28 white tablets]

Lybrel®: Ethinyl estradiol 0.02 mg and levonorgestrel 0.09 mg (28s) [28 yellow tablets]

Tablet, oral [triphasic formulation]:

Enpresse®:

Day 1-6: Ethinyl estradiol 0.03 mg and levonorgestrel 0.05 mg [6 pink tablets]

Day 7-11: Ethinyl estradiol 0.04 mg and levonorgestrel 0.075 mg [5 white tablets]

Day 12-21: Ethinyl estradiol 0.03 mg and levonorgestrel 0.125 mg [10 orange tablets]

Day 22-28: 7 light green inactive tablets (28s)

Trivora®:

Day 1-6: Ethinyl estradiol 0.03 mg and levonorgestrel 0.05 mg [6 blue tablets]

Day 7-11: Ethinyl estradiol 0.04 mg and levonorgestrel 0.075 mg [5 white tablets]

Day 12-21: Ethinyl estradiol 0.03 mg and levonorgestrel 0.125 mg [10 pink tablets]

Day 22-28: 7 peach inactive tablets (28s)

◆ **Ethinyl Estradiol and NGM** *see* Ethinyl Estradiol and Norgestimate *on page 663*

Ethinyl Estradiol and Norelgestromin

(ETH in il es tra DYE ole & nor el JES troe min)

Brand Names: U.S. Ortho Evra®

Brand Names: Canada Evra®

Index Terms Norelgestromin and Ethinyl Estradiol; Ortho-Evra

Pharmacologic Category Contraceptive; Estrogen and Progestin Combination

Use Prevention of pregnancy

Pregnancy Risk Factor X

Dosage Topical: Adults: Females:

Contraception: Apply one patch each week for 3 weeks (21 total days); followed by one week that is patch-free. Each patch should be applied on the same day each week ("patch change day") and only one patch should be worn at a time. No more than 7 days should pass during the patch-free interval.

Schedule 1 (Sunday starter): Dose begins on first Sunday after onset of menstruation; if the menstrual period starts on Sunday, apply one patch that very same day. **With a Sunday start, an additional method of contraception (nonhormonal) must be used until after the first 7 days of consecutive administration.** Each patch change will then occur on Sunday.

Schedule 2 (Day 1 starter): Dose starts on first day of menstrual cycle, applying one patch during the first 24 hours of menstrual cycle. No back-up method of contraception is needed as long as the patch is applied on the first day of cycle. Each patch change will then occur on that same day of the week.

Additional dosing considerations:

No bleeding during patch-free week/missed menstrual period: If patch has been applied as directed, continue treatment on usual "patch change day". If used correctly, no bleeding during patch-free week does not necessarily indicate pregnancy. However, if no withdrawal bleeding occurs for 2 consecutive cycles, pregnancy should be ruled out. If patch has not been applied as directed, and one menstrual period is missed, pregnancy should be ruled out prior to continuing treatment.

If a patch becomes partially or completely detached for <24 hours: Try to reapply to same place, or replace with a new patch immediately. Do not reapply if patch is no longer sticky, if it is sticking to itself or another surface, or if it has material sticking to it.

If a patch becomes partially or completely detached for >24 hours (or time period is unknown): Apply a new patch and use this day of the week as the new "patch change day" from this point on. **An additional method of contraception (nonhormonal) should be used until after the first 7 days of consecutive administration.**

Switching from oral contraceptives: Apply first patch on the first day of withdrawal bleeding. If there is no bleeding within 5 days of taking the last active tablet, pregnancy must first be ruled out. If patch is applied later than the first day of bleeding, **an additional method of contraception (nonhormonal) should be used until after the first 7 days of consecutive administration**

Use after childbirth: Therapy should not be started <4 weeks after childbirth. Pregnancy should be ruled out prior to treatment if menstrual periods have not restarted. **An additional method of contraception (nonhormonal) should be used until after the first 7 days of consecutive administration.**

Use after abortion or miscarriage: Therapy may be started immediately if abortion/miscarriage occur within the first trimester. If therapy is not started within 5 days, follow instructions for first time use. If abortion/miscarriage occur during the second trimester, therapy should not be started for at least 4 weeks. Follow directions for use after childbirth.

Dosage adjustment in renal impairment: Specific guidelines not available; use with caution and monitor blood pressure closely. Consider other forms of contraception.

Dosage adjustment in hepatic impairment: Contraindicated in patients with hepatic impairment

Additional Information Complete prescribing information for this medication should be consulted for additional detail.

Dosage Forms Excipient information presented when available (limited, particularly for generics); consult specific product labeling.

Patch, transdermal:

Ortho Evra®: Ethinyl estradiol 0.75 mg and norelgestromin 6 mg [releases ethinyl estradiol 20 mcg and norelgestromin 150 mcg per day] (1s, 3s)

Dosage Forms: Canada Excipient information presented when available (limited, particularly for generics); consult specific product labeling.

Patch, transdermal:

Evra®: Ethinyl estradiol 0.6 mg and norelgestromin 6 mg [releases ethinyl estradiol 35 mcg and norelgestromin 200 mcg per day] (1s, 3s)

Ethinyl Estradiol and Norethindrone

(ETH in il es tra DYE ole & nor eth IN drone)

Brand Names: U.S. Aranelle®; Balziva™; Brevicon®; Cyclafem™ 1/35; Cyclafem™ 7/7/7; Estrostep® Fe; Femcon® Fe; femhrt®; femhrt® Lo; Generess™ Fe; Gildess® FE 1.5/30; Gildess® FE 1/20; Jevantique™; Jinteli™; Junel® 1.5/30; Junel® 1/20; Junel® Fe 1.5/30; Junel® Fe 1/20; Leena®; Lo Loestrin™ Fe; Loestrin® 21 1.5/30; Loestrin® 21 1/20; Loestrin® 24 Fe; Loestrin® Fe 1.5/30; Loestrin® Fe 1/20; Microgestin® 1.5/30; Microgestin® 1/20; Microgestin® Fe 1.5/30; Microgestin® Fe 1/20; Modicon®; Necon® 0.5/35; Necon® 1/35; Necon® 10/11;

Necon® 7/7/7; Norinyl® 1+35; Nortrel® 0.5/35; Nortrel® 1/35; Nortrel® 7/7/7; Ortho-Novum® 1/35; Ortho-Novum® 7/7/7; Ovcon® 35; Ovcon® 50; Tilia™ Fe; Tri-Legest™ Fe; Tri-Norinyl®; Zenchent Fe™; Zenchent™; Zeosa™

Brand Names: Canada Brevicon® 0.5/35; Brevicon® 1/35; FemHRT®; Loestrin™ 1.5/30; Minestrin™ 1/20; Ortho® 0.5/35; Ortho® 1/35; Ortho® 7/7/7; Select™ 1/35; Synphasic®

Index Terms Norethindrone Acetate and Ethinyl Estradiol; Ortho Novum

Pharmacologic Category Contraceptive; Estrogen and Progestin Combination

Use Prevention of pregnancy; treatment of acne; moderate-to-severe vasomotor symptoms associated with menopause; prevention of osteoporosis (in women at significant risk only)

Unlabeled Use Treatment of hypermenorrhea (menorrhagia); pain associated with endometriosis, dysmenorrhea; dysfunctional uterine bleeding

Pregnancy Risk Factor X

Dosage Oral:

Adolescents ≥15 years and Adults: Females: Acne: Estrostep® Fe: Refer to dosing for contraception

Adults: Females:

Moderate-to-severe vasomotor symptoms associated with menopause: Initial: femhrt® 0.5/2.5: 1 tablet daily; patient should be re-evaluated at 3- to 6-month intervals to determine if treatment is still necessary; patient should be maintained at the lowest effective dose

Prevention of osteoporosis: Initial: femhrt® 0.5/2.5: 1 tablet daily; patient should be maintained on the lowest effective dose

Contraception:

Schedule 1 (Sunday starter): Dose begins on first Sunday after onset of menstruation; if the menstrual period starts on Sunday, take first tablet that very same day. This schedule is not preferred for Lo Loestrin™ Fe. With a Sunday start, an additional method of contraception should be used until after the first 7 days of consecutive administration (all products).

For 21-tablet package: Dosage is 1 tablet daily for 21 consecutive days, followed by 7 days off of the medication; a new course begins on the 8th day after the last tablet is taken.

For 28-tablet package: Dosage is 1 tablet daily without interruption.

Schedule 2 (Day 1 starter): Dose starts on first day of menstrual cycle taking 1 tablet daily.

For 21-tablet package: Dosage is 1 tablet daily for 21 consecutive days, followed by 7 days off of the medication; a new course begins on the 8th day after the last tablet is taken.

For 28-tablet package: Dosage is 1 tablet daily without interruption.

If all doses have been taken on schedule and one menstrual period is missed, continue dosing cycle. If two consecutive menstrual periods are missed, pregnancy test is required before new dosing cycle is started.

Missed doses **monophasic formulations** (refer to package insert for complete information):

One dose missed: Take as soon as remembered. Take the next tablet at your regular time. You may take 2 tablets in 1 day.

Two consecutive doses missed in the first 2 weeks: Take 2 tablets as soon as remembered and 2 tablets the next day. An additional method of contraception should be used for 7 days after missed dose.

Two consecutive doses missed in week 3 (all products) or in week 4 (Lo Loestrin™ Fe), or three consecutive doses missed at any time (all products): An additional method of contraception must be used for 7 days after a missed dose.

Schedule 1 (Sunday starter): Continue dose of 1 tablet daily until Sunday, then discard the rest of the pack, and a new pack should be started that same day.

Schedule 2 (Day 1 starter): Current pack should be discarded, and a new pack should be started that same day.

Missed doses **biphasic/triphasic formulations** (refer to package insert for complete information):

One dose missed: Take the next tablet at your regular time. You may take 2 tablets in 1 day.

Two consecutive doses missed in week 1 or week 2 of the pack: Take 2 tablets as soon as remembered and 2 tablets the next day. Resume taking 1 tablet daily until the pack is empty. An additional method of contraception should be used for 7 days after a missed dose.

Two consecutive doses missed in week 3 of the pack: An additional method of contraception must be used for 7 days after a missed dose.

Schedule 1 (Sunday Starter): Take 1 tablet every day until Sunday. Discard the remaining pack and start a new pack of pills on the same day.

Schedule 2 (Day 1 starter): Discard the remaining pack and start a new pack the same day.

Three or more consecutive doses missed: An additional method of contraception must be used for 7 days after a missed dose.

Schedule 1 (Sunday Starter): Take 1 tablet every day until Sunday; on Sunday, discard the pack and start a new pack.

Schedule 2 (Day 1 Starter): Discard the remaining pack and begin new pack of tablets starting on the same day.

Switching from a different contraceptive:

Oral contraceptive: Start on the same day that a new pack of the previous oral contraceptive would have been taken.

Transdermal patch, vaginal ring, injection: Start on the day the next dose would have been due.

IUD or implant: Start on the day of removal. A backup method of contraception may be required following IUD removal.

Use after childbirth (in women who are not breast-feeding) or after second trimester abortion: Therapy may be started ≥4 weeks postpartum. Pregnancy should be ruled out prior to treatment if menstrual periods have not restarted and an additional method of contraception (nonhormonal) should be used until after the first 7 days of consecutive administration.

Dosage adjustment in renal impairment: Specific guidelines not available; use with caution and monitor blood pressure closely. Consider other forms of contraception.

Dosage adjustment in hepatic impairment: Contraindicated in patients with hepatic impairment.

Additional Information Complete prescribing information for this medication should be consulted for additional detail.

Dosage Forms Excipient information presented when available (limited, particularly for generics); consult specific product labeling.

Tablet, oral:

femhrt® 1/5: Ethinyl estradiol 0.005 mg and norethindrone acetate 1 mg (28s, 90s) [white tablets]

femhrt® Lo 0.5/2.5: Ethinyl estradiol 0.0025 mg and norethindrone acetate 0.5 mg (28s, 90s) [white tablets]

Jevantique™ 1/5: Ethinyl estradiol 0.005 mg and norethindrone acetate 1 mg (28s, 90s) [white tablets]

Jinteli™: Ethinyl estradiol 0.005 mg and norethindrone acetate 1 mg (28s, 90s) [white tablets]

Tablet, oral, monophasic formulations:
- Balziva™: Ethinyl estradiol 0.035 mg and norethindrone 0.4 mg (28s) [21 light peach tablets and 7 white inactive tablets]
- Brevicon®: Ethinyl estradiol 0.035 mg and norethindrone 0.5 mg (28s) [21 blue tablets and 7 orange inactive tablets]
- Cyclafem™ 1/35: Ethinyl estradiol 0.035 mg and norethindrone 1 mg [21 pink tablets and 7 light green inactive tablets] (28s)
- Gildess® FE 1/20: Ethinyl estradiol 0.02 mg and norethindrone acetate 1 mg [21 white tablets] and ferrous fumarate 75 mg [7 white-speckled brown tablets] (28s)
- Gildess® FE 1.5/30: Ethinyl estradiol 0.03 mg and norethindrone acetate 1.5 mg [21 light green tablets] and ferrous fumarate 75 mg [7 white-speckled brown tablets] (28s)
- Junel® 1/20: Ethinyl estradiol 0.02 mg and norethindrone acetate 1 mg (21s) [yellow tablets]
- Junel® 1.5/30: Ethinyl estradiol 0.03 mg and norethindrone acetate 1.5 mg (21s) [pink tablets]
- Junel® Fe 1/20: Ethinyl estradiol 0.02 mg and norethindrone acetate 1 mg [21 yellow tablets] and ferrous fumarate 75 mg [7 brown tablets] (28s)
- Junel® Fe 1.5/30: Ethinyl estradiol 0.03 mg and norethindrone acetate 1.5 mg [21 pink tablets] and ferrous fumarate 75 mg [7 brown tablets] (28s)
- Loestrin® 21 1/20: Ethinyl estradiol 0.02 mg and norethindrone acetate 1 mg (21s) [light yellow tablets]
- Loestrin® 21 1.5/30: Ethinyl estradiol 0.03 mg and norethindrone acetate 1.5 mg (21s) [pink tablets]
- Lo Loestrin™ Fe: Ethinyl estradiol 0.01 mg and norethindrone acetate 1mg [24 blue tablets] and ethinyl estradiol 0.01 mg [2 white tablets] and ferrous fumarate 75 mg [2 brown tablets] (28s)
- Loestrin® 24 Fe: Ethinyl estradiol 0.02 mg and norethindrone acetate 1 mg [24 white tablets] and ferrous fumarate 75 mg [4 brown tablets] (28s)
- Loestrin® Fe 1/20: Ethinyl estradiol 0.02 mg and norethindrone acetate 1 mg [21 light yellow tablets] and ferrous fumarate 75 mg [7 brown tablets] (28s)
- Loestrin® Fe 1.5/30: Ethinyl estradiol 0.03 mg and norethindrone acetate 1.5 mg [21 pink tablets] and ferrous fumarate 75 mg [7 brown tablets] (28s)
- Microgestin® 1/20: Ethinyl estradiol 0.02 mg and norethindrone acetate 1 mg (21s) [white tablets]
- Microgestin® 1.5/30: Ethinyl estradiol 0.03 mg and norethindrone acetate 1.5 mg (21s) [green tablets]
- Microgestin® Fe 1/20: Ethinyl estradiol 0.02 mg and norethindrone acetate 1 mg [21 white tablets] and ferrous fumarate 75 mg [7 brown tablets] (28s)
- Microgestin® Fe 1.5/30: Ethinyl estradiol 0.03 mg and norethindrone acetate 1.5 mg [21 green tablets] and ferrous fumarate 75 mg [7 brown tablets] (28s)
- Modicon®: Ethinyl estradiol 0.035 mg and norethindrone 0.5 mg (28s) [21 white tablets and 7 green inactive tablets]
- Necon® 0.5/35: Ethinyl estradiol 0.035 mg and norethindrone 0.5 mg (28s) [21 light yellow tablets and 7 white inactive tablets]
- Necon® 1/35: Ethinyl estradiol 0.035 mg and norethindrone 1 mg (28s) [21 dark yellow tablets and 7 white inactive tablets]
- Norinyl® 1+35: Ethinyl estradiol 0.035 mg and norethindrone 1 mg (28s) [21 yellow-green tablets and 7 orange inactive tablets]
- Nortrel® 0.5/35: Ethinyl estradiol 0.035 mg and norethindrone 0.5 mg (28s) [21 light yellow tablets and 7 white inactive tablets]
- Nortrel® 1/35:
  - Ethinyl estradiol 0.035 mg and norethindrone 1 mg (21s) [yellow tablets]
  - Ethinyl estradiol 0.035 mg and norethindrone 1 mg (28s) [21 yellow tablets and 7 white inactive tablets]
- Ortho-Novum® 1/35: Ethinyl estradiol 0.035 mg and norethindrone 1 mg (28s) [21 peach tablets and 7 green inactive tablets]
- Ovcon® 35: Ethinyl estradiol 0.035 mg and norethindrone 0.4 mg (28s) [21 light peach tablets and 7 green inactive tablets]
- Ovcon® 50: Ethinyl estradiol 0.05 mg and norethindrone 1 mg (28s) [21 yellow tablets and 7 green inactive tablets]
- Zenchent™: Ethinyl estradiol 0.035 mg and norethindrone 0.4 mg (28s) [21 orange tablets and 7 white inactive tablets]

Tablet, chewable, oral, monophasic formulations: Ethinyl estradiol 0.035 mg and norethindrone 0.4 mg [21 tablets] and ferrous fumarate 75 mg [7 tablets] (28s)
- Femcon® Fe: Ethinyl estradiol 0.035 mg and norethindrone 0.4 mg [21 white tablets] and ferrous fumarate 75 mg [7 brown tablets] [spearmint flavor] (28s)
- Generess™ Fe: Ethinyl estradiol 0.025 mg and norethindrone 0.8 mg [24 light green tablets] and ferrous fumarate 75 mg [4 brown tablets] (28s)
- Zenchent Fe™: Ethinyl estradiol 0.035 mg and norethindrone 0.4 mg [21 light yellow tablets] and ferrous fumarate 75 mg [7 brown tablets] [spearmint flavor] (28s)
- Zeosa™: Ethinyl estradiol 0.035 mg and norethindrone 0.4 mg [21 light yellow tablets] and ferrous fumarate 75 mg [7 brown tablets] [spearmint flavor] (28s)

Tablet, oral, biphasic formulations:
- Necon® 10/11:
  - Day 1-10: Ethinyl estradiol 0.035 mg and norethindrone 0.5 mg [10 light yellow tablets]
  - Day 11-21: Ethinyl estradiol 0.035 mg and norethindrone 1 mg [11 dark yellow tablets]
  - Day 22-28: 7 white inactive tablets (28s)

Tablet, oral, triphasic formulations:
- Aranelle®:
  - Day 1-7: Ethinyl estradiol 0.035 mg and norethindrone 0.5 mg [7 light yellow tablets]
  - Day 8-16: Ethinyl estradiol 0.035 mg and norethindrone 1 mg [9 white tablets]
  - Day 17-21: Ethinyl estradiol 0.035 mg and norethindrone 0.5 mg [5 light yellow tablets]
  - Day 22-28: 7 peach inactive tablets (28s)
- Cyclafem™ 7/7/7:
  - Day 1-7: Ethinyl estradiol 0.035 mg and norethindrone 0.5 mg [7 white tablets]
  - Day 8-14: Ethinyl estradiol 0.035 mg and norethindrone 0.75 mg [7 light pink tablets]
  - Day 15-21: Ethinyl estradiol 0.035 mg and norethindrone 1 mg [7 pink tablets]
  - Day 22-28: 7 light green inactive tablets (28s)
- Estrostep® Fe:
  - Day 1-5: Ethinyl estradiol 0.02 mg and norethindrone acetate 1 mg [5 white triangular tablets]
  - Day 6-12: Ethinyl estradiol 0.03 mg and norethindrone acetate 1 mg [7 white square tablets]
  - Day 13-21: Ethinyl estradiol 0.035 mg and norethindrone acetate 1 mg [9 white round tablets]
  - Day 22-28: Ferrous fumarate 75 mg [7 brown tablets] (28s)
- Leena®:
  - Day 1-7: Ethinyl estradiol 0.035 mg and norethindrone 0.5 mg [7 light blue tablets]
  - Day 8-16: Ethinyl estradiol 0.035 mg and norethindrone 1 mg [9 light yellow-green tablets]
  - Day 17-21: Ethinyl estradiol 0.035 mg and norethindrone 0.5 mg [5 light blue tablets]
  - Day 22-28: 7 orange inactive tablets (28s)

Necon® 7/7/7, Ortho-Novum® 7/7/7:
Day 1-7: Ethinyl estradiol 0.035 mg and norethindrone 0.5 mg [7 white tablets]
Day 8-14: Ethinyl estradiol 0.035 mg and norethindrone 0.75 mg [7 light peach tablets]
Day 15-21: Ethinyl estradiol 0.035 mg and norethindrone 1 mg [7 peach tablets]
Day 22-28: 7 green inactive tablets (28s)
Nortrel® 7/7/7:
Day 1-7: Ethinyl estradiol 0.035 mg and norethindrone 0.5 mg [7 light yellow tablets]
Day 8-14: Ethinyl estradiol 0.035 mg and norethindrone 0.75 mg [7 blue tablets]
Day 15-21: Ethinyl estradiol 0.035 mg and norethindrone 1 mg [7 peach tablets]
Day 22-28: 7 white inactive tablets (28s)
Tilia™ Fe:
Day 1-5: Ethinyl estradiol 0.02 mg and norethindrone acetate 1 mg [5 white triangular tablets]
Day 6-12: Ethinyl estradiol 0.03 mg and norethindrone acetate 1 mg [7 white square tablets]
Day 13-21: Ethinyl estradiol 0.035 mg and norethindrone acetate 1 mg [9 white round tablets]
Day 22-28: Ferrous fumarate 75 mg [7 brown tablets] (28s)
Tri-Legest™ Fe:
Day 1-5: Ethinyl estradiol 0.02 mg and norethindrone acetate 1 mg [5 light pink tablets]
Day 6-12: Ethinyl estradiol 0.03 mg and norethindrone acetate 1 mg [7 light yellow tablets]
Day 13-21: Ethinyl estradiol 0.035 mg and norethindrone acetate 1 mg [9 light blue tablets]
Day 22-28: Ferrous fumarate 75 mg [7 brown tablets] (28s)
Tri-Norinyl®:
Day 1-7: Ethinyl estradiol 0.035 mg and norethindrone 0.5 mg [7 blue tablets]
Day 8-16: Ethinyl estradiol 0.035 mg and norethindrone 1 mg [9 yellow-green tablets]
Day 17-21: Ethinyl estradiol 0.035 mg and norethindrone 0.5 mg [5 blue tablets]
Day 22-28: 7 orange inactive tablets (28s)

Ethinyl Estradiol and Norgestimate

(ETH in il es tra DYE ole & nor JES ti mate)

Brand Names: U.S. MonoNessa®; Ortho Tri-Cyclen®; Ortho Tri-Cyclen® Lo; Ortho-Cyclen®; Sprintec®; Tri-Sprintec®; TriNessa®

Brand Names: Canada Cyclen®; Tri-Cyclen®; Tri-Cyclen® Lo

Index Terms Ethinyl Estradiol and NGM; Norgestimate and Ethinyl Estradiol; Ortho Cyclen; Ortho Tri Cyclen

Pharmacologic Category Contraceptive; Estrogen and Progestin Combination

Use Prevention of pregnancy; treatment of acne

Unlabeled Use Treatment of hypermenorrhea (menorrhagia); pain associated with endometriosis; dysmenorrhea; dysfunctional uterine bleeding

Pregnancy Risk Factor X

Dosage Oral:

Children ≥15 years and Adults: Females: Acne (Ortho Tri-Cyclen®): Refer to dosing for contraception

Adults: Females:
Contraception:
Schedule 1 (Sunday starter): Dose begins on first Sunday after onset of menstruation; if the menstrual period starts on Sunday, take first tablet that very same day. **With a Sunday start, an additional method of contraception should be used until after the first 7 days of consecutive administration.**
For 21-tablet package: Dosage is 1 tablet daily for 21 consecutive days, followed by 7 days off of the medication; a new course begins on the 8th day after the last tablet is taken.
For 28-tablet package: Dosage is 1 tablet daily without interruption.
Schedule 2 (Day 1 starter): Dose starts on first day of menstrual cycle taking 1 tablet daily.
For 21-tablet package: Dosage is 1 tablet daily for 21 consecutive days, followed by 7 days off of the medication; a new course begins on the 8th day after the last tablet is taken.
For 28-tablet package: Dosage is 1 tablet daily without interruption.
If all doses have been taken on schedule and one menstrual period is missed, continue dosing cycle. If two consecutive menstrual periods are missed, pregnancy test is required before new dosing cycle is started.
Missed doses **monophasic formulations** (refer to package insert for complete information):
One dose missed: Take as soon as remembered or take 2 tablets next day
Two consecutive doses missed in the first 2 weeks: Take 2 tablets as soon as remembered or 2 tablets next 2 days. **An additional method of contraception should be used for 7 days after missed dose.**
Two consecutive doses missed in week 3 or three consecutive doses missed at any time: **An additional method of contraception must be used for 7 days after a missed dose:**
Schedule 1 (Sunday starter): Continue dose of 1 tablet daily until Sunday, then discard the rest of the pack, and a new pack should be started that same day.
Schedule 2 (Day 1 starter): Current pack should be discarded, and a new pack should be started that same day.
Missed doses **biphasic/triphasic formulations** (refer to package insert for complete information):
One dose missed: Take as soon as remembered or take 2 tablets next day.
Two consecutive doses missed in week 1 or week 2 of the pack: Take 2 tablets as soon as remembered and 2 tablets the next day. Resume taking 1 tablet daily until the pack is empty. **An additional method of contraception must be used for 7 days after a missed dose.**
Two consecutive doses missed in week 3 of the pack. **An additional method of contraception must be used for 7 days after a missed dose.**
Schedule 1 (Sunday starter): Take 1 tablet every day until Sunday. Discard the remaining pack and start a new pack of pills on the same day.
Schedule 2 (Day 1 starter): Discard the remaining pack and start a new pack the same day.
Three or more consecutive doses missed. **An additional method of contraception must be used for 7 days after a missed dose.**
Schedule 1 (Sunday starter): Take 1 tablet every day until Sunday; on Sunday, discard the pack and start a new pack.
Schedule 2 (Day 1 starter): Discard the remaining pack and begin new pack of tablets starting on the same day.

Dosage adjustment in renal impairment: Specific guidelines not available; use with caution and monitor blood pressure closely. Consider other forms of contraception.

Dosage adjustment in hepatic impairment: Contraindicated in patients with hepatic impairment.

Additional Information Complete prescribing information for this medication should be consulted for additional detail.

Dosage Forms Excipient information presented when available (limited, particularly for generics); consult specific product labeling.

Tablet, monophasic formulations:

MonoNessa®, Ortho-Cyclen®: Ethinyl estradiol 0.035 mg and norgestimate 0.25 mg (28s) [21 blue tablets and 7 green inactive tablets]

Sprintec®: Ethinyl estradiol 0.035 mg and norgestimate 0.25 mg (28s) [21 blue tablets and 7 white inactive tablets]

Tablet, triphasic formulations:

Ortho Tri-Cyclen®, TriNessa®:

Day 1-7: Ethinyl estradiol 0.035 mg and norgestimate 0.18 mg [7 white tablets]

Day 8-14: Ethinyl estradiol 0.035 mg and norgestimate 0.215 mg [7 light blue tablets]

Day 15-21: Ethinyl estradiol 0.035 mg and norgestimate 0.25 mg [7 blue tablets]

Day 22-28: 7 green inactive tablets (28s)

Tri-Sprintec®:

Day 1-7: Ethinyl estradiol 0.035 mg and norgestimate 0.18 mg [7 gray tablets]

Day 8-14: Ethinyl estradiol 0.035 mg and norgestimate 0.215 mg [7 light blue tablets]

Day 15-21: Ethinyl estradiol 0.035 mg and norgestimate 0.25 mg [7 blue tablets]

Day 22-28: 7 white inactive tablets (28s)

Ortho Tri-Cyclen® Lo:

Day 1-7: Ethinyl estradiol 0.025 mg and norgestimate 0.18 mg [7 white tablets]

Day 8-14: Ethinyl estradiol 0.025 mg and norgestimate 0.215 mg [7 light blue tablets]

Day 15-21: Ethinyl estradiol 0.025 mg and norgestimate 0.25 mg [7 dark blue tablets]

Day 22-28: 7 green inactive tablets (28s)

Ethinyl Estradiol and Norgestrel

(ETH in il es tra DYE ole & nor JES trel)

Brand Names: U.S. Cryselle® 28; Lo/Ovral®-28; Low-Ogestrel®; Ogestrel®

Brand Names: Canada Lo-Femenal 21; Ovral®

Index Terms Lo Ovral; Morning After Pill; Norgestrel and Ethinyl Estradiol

Pharmacologic Category Contraceptive; Estrogen and Progestin Combination

Use Prevention of pregnancy; postcoital contraceptive or "morning after" pill

Unlabeled Use Treatment of hypermenorrhea (menorrhagia); pain associated with endometriosis; dysmenorrhea; dysfunctional uterine bleeding

Pregnancy Risk Factor X

Dosage Oral: Adults: Females:

Contraception:

Schedule 1 (Sunday starter): Dose begins on first Sunday after onset of menstruation; if the menstrual period starts on Sunday, take first tablet that very same day. **With a Sunday start, an additional method of contraception should be used until after the first 7 days of consecutive administration.**

For 21-tablet package: Dosage is 1 tablet daily for 21 consecutive days, followed by 7 days off of the medication; a new course begins on the 8th day after the last tablet is taken.

For 28-tablet package: Dosage is 1 tablet daily without interruption.

Schedule 2 (Day 1 starter): Dose starts on first day of menstrual cycle taking 1 tablet daily.

For 21-tablet package: Dosage is 1 tablet daily for 21 consecutive days, followed by 7 days off of the medication; a new course begins on the 8th day after the last tablet is taken.

For 28-tablet package: Dosage is 1 tablet daily without interruption.

If all doses have been taken on schedule and one menstrual period is missed, continue dosing cycle. If two consecutive menstrual periods are missed, pregnancy test is required before new dosing cycle is started.

Missed doses **monophasic formulations** (refer to package insert for complete information):

One dose missed: Take as soon as remembered or take 2 tablets next day

Two consecutive doses missed in the first 2 weeks: Take 2 tablets as soon as remembered or 2 tablets next 2 days. **An additional method of contraception should be used for 7 days after missed dose.**

Two consecutive doses missed in week 3 or three consecutive doses missed at any time:

Schedule 1 (Sunday starter): Continue to take 1 tablet daily until Sunday, then discard the rest of the pack, and a new pack is started that same day.

Schedule 2 (Day 1 starter): Current pack should be discarded, and a new pack started that same day. **An additional method of contraception should be used for 7 days after missed dose.**

Postcoital contraception:

Ethinyl estradiol 0.03 mg and norgestrel 0.3 mg formulation: 4 tablets within 72 hours of unprotected intercourse and 4 tablets 12 hours after first dose

Ethinyl estradiol 0.05 mg and norgestrel 0.5 mg formulation: 2 tablets within 72 hours of unprotected intercourse and 2 tablets 12 hours after first dose

Dosage adjustment in renal impairment: Specific guidelines not available; use with caution and monitor blood pressure closely. Consider other forms of contraception.

Dosage adjustment in hepatic impairment: Contraindicated in patients with hepatic impairment.

Additional Information Complete prescribing information for this medication should be consulted for additional detail.

Dosage Forms Excipient information presented when available (limited, particularly for generics); consult specific product labeling.

Tablet, monophasic formulations: Ethinyl estradiol 0.03 mg and norgestrel 0.3 mg [21 tablets and 7 inactive tablets] (28s)

Cryselle® 28: Ethinyl estradiol 0.03 mg and norgestrel 0.3 mg [21 white tablets and 7 light green inactive tablets] (28s)

Low-Ogestrel®: Ethinyl estradiol 0.03 mg and norgestrel 0.3 mg [21 white tablets and 7 peach inactive tablets] (28s)

Lo/Ovral®-28: Ethinyl estradiol 0.03 mg and norgestrel 0.3 mg [21 white tablets and 7 pink inactive tablets] (28s)

Ogestrel®: Ethinyl estradiol 0.05 mg and norgestrel 0.5 mg [21 white tablets and 7 peach inactive tablets] (28s)

Ethinyl Estradiol, Drospirenone, and Levomefolate

(ETH in il es tra DYE ole, droh SPYE re none, & lee voe me FOE late)

Brand Names: U.S. Beyaz™; Safyral™

Index Terms Drospirenone, Ethinyl Estradiol, and Levomefolate Calcium; Ethinyl Estradiol, Drospirenone, and Levomefolate Calcium; Levomefolate Calcium, Drospirenone, and Ethinyl Estradiol; Levomefolate, Drospirenone, and Ethinyl Estradiol

Pharmacologic Category Contraceptive; Estrogen and Progestin Combination

Use Prevention of pregnancy; treatment of premenstrual dysphoric disorder (PMDD); treatment of acne; folate supplementation

Unlabeled Use Treatment of hypermenorrhea (menorrhagia); pain associated with endometriosis; dysmenorrhea; dysfunctional uterine bleeding

Dosage Oral:

Children ≥14 years and Adults: Females: Acne (Beyaz™): Refer to dosing for contraception

Adults: Females: PMDD (Beyaz™): Refer to dosing for contraception

Adults: Females: Contraception (Beyaz™, Safyral™): Dosage is 1 tablet daily

Beyaz™: One pink tablet daily for 24 consecutive days, then one light orange tablet daily on days 25-28

Safyral™: One orange tablet daily for 21 consecutive days, then one light orange tablet daily on days 22-28

Dose should be taken at the same time each day, either after the evening meal or at bedtime. Dosing may be started on the first day of menstrual period (Day 1 starter) or on the first Sunday after the onset of the menstrual period (Sunday starter).

Day 1 starter: Dose starts on first day of menstrual cycle taking 1 tablet daily. If first dose is taken later than the first day of the menstrual cycle, **an additional method of contraception should be used until after the first 7 days of consecutive administration.**

Sunday starter: Dose begins on first Sunday after onset of menstruation; if the menstrual period starts on Sunday, take first tablet that very same day. **With a Sunday start, an additional method of contraception should be used until after the first 7 days of consecutive administration.**

Switching from a different contraceptive:

Oral contraceptive: Start on the same day that a new pack of the previous oral contraceptive would have been taken

Transdermal patch, vaginal ring, injection: Start on the day the next dose would have been due

IUD or implant: Start on the day of removal

Use after childbirth (in women who are not breast-feeding) or after second trimester abortion: Therapy may be started ≥4 weeks postpartum. Pregnancy should be ruled out prior to treatment if menstrual periods have not restarted and an additional method of contraception (nonhormonal) should be used until after the first 7 days of consecutive administration.

Missed doses:

If all doses have been taken on schedule and one menstrual period is missed, continue dosing cycle. If two consecutive menstrual periods are missed, rule out pregnancy and discontinue if pregnancy is confirmed.

If doses have been missed during the first 3 weeks or if active tablets (pink tablets) were started later than as directed and the menstrual period is missed, pregnancy should be ruled out prior to continuing treatment.

Missed doses (monophasic formulations) (refer to package insert for complete information):

One dose missed: Take as soon as remembered or take 2 tablets next day

Two consecutive doses missed in the first 2 weeks: Take 2 tablets as soon as remembered or 2 tablets next 2 days. **An additional method of contraception should be used for 7 days after missed dose.**

Two consecutive doses missed in week 3 or three consecutive doses missed at any time: **An additional method of contraception must be used for 7 days after a missed dose.**

Day 1 starter: Current pack should be discarded, and a new pack should be started that same day.

Sunday starter: Continue dose of 1 tablet daily until Sunday, then discard the rest of the pack, and a new pack should be started that same day.

Any number of doses missed in week 4: Throw away the pills that were missed. Continue taking one pill each day until pack is empty; no back-up method of contraception is needed

Dosage adjustment in renal impairment: Contraindicated in patients with renal dysfunction

Dosage adjustment in hepatic impairment: Contraindicated in patients with hepatic disease. Exposure to drospirenone is ~3 times higher with moderate liver impairment; information not available for severe impairment.

Additional Information Complete prescribing information for this medication should be consulted for additional detail.

Dosage Forms Excipient information presented when available (limited, particularly for generics); consult specific product labeling.

Tablet, oral:

Beyaz™: Ethinyl estradiol 0.02 mg, drospirenone 3 mg, and levomefolate calcium 0.451 mg [24 pink tablets] and levomefolate calcium 0.451 mg [4 light orange tablets] (28s)

Safyral™: Ethinyl estradiol 0.03 mg, drospirenone 3 mg, and levomefolate calcium 0.451 mg [21 orange tablets] and levomefolate calcium 0.451 mg [7 light orange tablets] (28s)

◆ **Ethinyl Estradiol, Drospirenone, and Levomefolate Calcium** *see* Ethinyl Estradiol, Drospirenone, and Levomefolate *on page 664*

◆ **Ethiofos** *see* Amifostine *on page 85*

Ethosuximide (eth oh SUKS i mide)

Brand Names: U.S. Zarontin®

Brand Names: Canada Zarontin®

Pharmacologic Category Anticonvulsant, Succinimide

Additional Appendix Information

Anticonvulsant Drugs of Choice *on page 1873*

Use Management of absence (petit mal) seizures

Medication Guide Available Yes

Dosage Oral:

Children 3-6 years: Initial: 250 mg/day; increase every 4-7 days; usual maintenance dose: 20 mg/kg/day; maximum dose: 1.5 g/day in divided doses

Children ≥6 years and Adults: Initial: 500 mg/day; increase by 250 mg as needed every 4-7 days, up to 1.5 g/day in divided doses; usual maintenance dose for most pediatric patients is 20 mg/kg/day.

Dosing comment in renal/hepatic dysfunction: Use with caution.

Additional Information Complete prescribing information for this medication should be consulted for additional detail.

Dosage Forms Excipient information presented when available (limited, particularly for generics); consult specific product labeling.

Capsule, softgel, oral: 250 mg

Zarontin®: 250 mg

Solution, oral: 250 mg/5 mL (473 mL)

Zarontin®: 250 mg/5 mL (480 mL) [contains sodium benzoate; raspberry flavor]

Syrup, oral: 250 mg/5 mL (473 mL)

◆ **Ethoxynaphthamido Penicillin Sodium** *see* Nafcillin *on page 1170*

◆ **Ethyl Aminobenzoate** *see* Benzocaine *on page 202*

◆ **Ethyl Esters of Omega-3 Fatty Acids** *see* Omega-3-Acid Ethyl Esters *on page 1241*

◆ **Ethynodiol Diacetate and Ethinyl Estradiol** *see* Ethinyl Estradiol and Ethynodiol Diacetate *on page 655*

◆ **Ethyol®** *see* Amifostine *on page 85*

◆ **Etibi® (Can)** *see* Ethambutol *on page 651*

Etidronate (e ti DROE nate)

Brand Names: U.S. Didronel®

Brand Names: Canada Co-Etidronate; Mylan-Etidronate

Index Terms EHDP; Etidronate Disodium; Sodium Etidronate

Pharmacologic Category Bisphosphonate Derivative

Use Symptomatic treatment of Paget's disease; prevention and treatment of heterotopic ossification due to spinal cord injury or after total hip replacement

Pregnancy Risk Factor C

Dosage Oral: Adults: Patients should receive supplemental calcium and vitamin D if dietary intake is inadequate.

Paget's disease:

Initial: 5-10 mg/kg/day (not to exceed 6 months) or 11-20 mg/kg/day (not to exceed 3 months). The recommended initial dose is 5 mg/kg/day (not to exceed 6 months). Higher doses should be used only when lower doses are ineffective or there is a need to suppress rapid bone turnover (ie, potential for irreversible neurologic damage) or reduce elevated cardiac output. Doses >20 mg/kg/day are **not** recommended.

Retreatment: Initiate only after etidronate-free period ≥90 days. Monitor patients every 3-6 months. Retreatment regimens are the same as for initial treatment.

Heterotopic ossification:

Caused by spinal cord injury: 20 mg/kg/day for 2 weeks, then 10 mg/kg/day for 10 weeks; total treatment period: 12 weeks

Complicating total hip replacement: 20 mg/kg/day for 1 month preoperatively then 20 mg/kg/day for 3 months postoperatively; total treatment period is 4 months

Dosing adjustment in renal impairment: Use with caution; specific guidelines are not available, however consider dose reduction.

Additional Information Complete prescribing information for this medication should be consulted for additional detail.

Dosage Forms Excipient information presented when available (limited, particularly for generics); consult specific product labeling.

Tablet, oral, as disodium: 200 mg, 400 mg

Didronel®: 400 mg [scored]

◆ **Etidronate Disodium** *see* Etidronate *on page 666*

Etodolac (ee toe DOE lak)

Brand Names: Canada Apo-Etodolac®; Utradol™

Index Terms Etodolic Acid; Lodine

Pharmacologic Category Nonsteroidal Anti-inflammatory Drug (NSAID), Oral

Use Acute and long-term use in the management of signs and symptoms of osteoarthritis; rheumatoid arthritis and juvenile idiopathic arthritis (JIA); management of acute pain

Pregnancy Risk Factor C

Pregnancy Considerations Adverse events were not observed in the initial animal reproduction studies; therefore, the manufacturer classifies etodolac as pregnancy category C. NSAID exposure during the first trimester is not strongly associated with congenital malformations; however, cardiovascular anomalies and cleft palate have been observed following NSAID exposure in some studies. The use of an NSAID close to conception may be associated with an increased risk of miscarriage. Nonteratogenic effects have been observed following NSAID administration during the third trimester including: Myocardial degenerative changes, prenatal constriction of the ductus arteriosus, fetal tricuspid regurgitation, failure of the ductus arteriosus to close postnatally; renal dysfunction or failure, oligohydramnios; gastrointestinal bleeding or perforation, increased risk of necrotizing enterocolitis; intracranial bleeding (including intraventricular hemorrhage), platelet dysfunction with resultant bleeding; pulmonary hypertension. Because they may cause premature closure of the ductus arteriosus, use of NSAIDs late in pregnancy should be avoided (use after 31 or 32 weeks gestation is not recommended by some clinicians). The chronic use of NSAIDs in women of reproductive age may be associated with infertility that is reversible upon discontinuation of the medication.

Lactation Excretion in breast milk unknown/not recommended

Medication Guide Available Yes

Contraindications Hypersensitivity to etodolac, aspirin, other NSAIDs, or any component of the formulation; perioperative pain in the setting of coronary artery bypass graft (CABG) surgery

Warnings/Precautions [U.S. Boxed Warning]: NSAIDs are associated with an increased risk of adverse cardiovascular thrombotic events, including MI and stroke. Risk may be increased with duration of use or pre-existing cardiovascular risk factors or disease. Carefully evaluate individual cardiovascular risk profiles prior to prescribing. May cause new-onset hypertension or worsening of existing hypertension. Use caution with fluid retention. Avoid use in heart failure. Concurrent administration of ibuprofen, and potentially other nonselective NSAIDs, may interfere with aspirin's cardioprotective effect. **[U.S. Boxed Warning]: Use is contraindicated for treatment of perioperative pain in the setting of coronary artery bypass graft (CABG) surgery.** Risk of MI and stroke may be increased with use following CABG surgery.

[U.S. Boxed Warning]: NSAIDs may increase risk of gastrointestinal irritation, inflammation, ulceration, bleeding, and perforation. These events may occur at any time during therapy and without warning. Use caution with a history of GI disease (bleeding or ulcers), concurrent therapy with aspirin, anticoagulants and/or corticosteroids, smoking, use of alcohol, the elderly or debilitated patients. When used concomitantly with ≤325 mg of aspirin, a substantial increase in the risk of gastrointestinal complications (eg, ulcer) occurs; concomitant gastroprotective therapy (eg, proton pump inhibitors) is recommended (Bhatt, 2008).

Platelet adhesion and aggregation may be decreased; may prolong bleeding time; patients with coagulation disorders or who are receiving anticoagulants should be monitored closely. Anemia may occur; patients on long-term NSAID therapy should be monitored for anemia. Rarely, NSAID use may cause severe blood dyscrasias (eg, agranulocytosis, aplastic anemia, thrombocytopenia).

NSAID use may compromise existing renal function; dose-dependent decreases in prostaglandin synthesis may result from NSAID use, reducing renal blood flow which may cause renal decompensation. NSAID use may increase the risk for hyperkalemia. Patients with impaired renal function, dehydration, heart failure, liver dysfunction, those taking diuretics and ACE inhibitors, and the elderly are at greater risk for renal toxicity and hyperkalemia. Rehydrate patient before starting therapy; monitor renal function closely. Not recommended for use in patients with advanced renal disease. Long-term NSAID use may result in renal papillary necrosis.

Use the lowest effective dose for the shortest duration of time, consistent with individual patient goals, to reduce risk of cardiovascular or GI adverse events. Alternate therapies should be considered for patients at high risk.

NSAIDs may cause serious skin adverse events including exfoliative dermatitis, Stevens-Johnson syndrome (SJS), and toxic epidermal necrolysis (TEN); discontinue use at first sign of skin rash or hypersensitivity. Anaphylactoid reactions may occur, even without prior exposure; patients with "aspirin triad" (bronchial asthma, aspirin intolerance, rhinitis) may be at increased risk. Do not use in patients who experience bronchospasm, asthma, rhinitis, or urticaria with NSAID or aspirin therapy. Use caution in other forms of asthma.

Use with caution in patients with decreased hepatic function. Closely monitor patients with any abnormal LFT. Severe hepatic reactions (eg, fulminant hepatitis, liver failure) have occurred with NSAID use, rarely; discontinue if signs or symptoms of liver disease develop, or if systemic manifestations occur.

NSAIDS may cause drowsiness, dizziness, blurred vision and other neurologic effects which may impair physical or mental abilities; patients must be cautioned about performing tasks which require mental alertness (eg, operating machinery or driving). Discontinue use with blurred or diminished vision and perform ophthalmologic exam. Monitor vision with long-term therapy. The elderly are at increased risk for adverse effects (especially peptic ulceration, CNS effects, renal toxicity) from NSAIDs even at low doses.

Withhold for at least 4-6 half-lives prior to surgical or dental procedures.

Use of extended release product consisting of a nondeformable matrix should be avoided in patients with stricture/narrowing of the GI tract; symptoms of obstruction have been associated with nondeformable products.

Adverse Reactions

1% to 10%:

Central nervous system: Dizziness (3% to 9%), chills/fever (1% to 3%), depression (1% to 3%), nervousness (1% to 3%)

Dermatologic: Rash (1% to 3%), pruritus (1% to 3%)

Gastrointestinal: Dyspepsia (10%), abdominal cramps (3% to 9%), diarrhea (3% to 9%), flatulence (3% to 9%), nausea (3% to 9%), vomiting (1% to 3%), constipation (1% to 3%), melena (1% to 3%), gastritis (1% to 3%)

Genitourinary: Dysuria (1% to 3%)

Neuromuscular & skeletal: Weakness (3% to 9%)

Ocular: Blurred vision (1% to 3%)

Otic: Tinnitus (1% to 3%)

Renal: Polyuria (1% to 3%)

<1% (Limited to important or life-threatening): Agranulocytosis, allergic reaction, allergic/necrotizing vasculitis, alopecia, anaphylactic/anaphylactoid reactions, anemia, angioedema, anorexia, arrhythmia, aseptic meningitis, asthma, bleeding time increased, CHF, confusion, conjunctivitis, CVA, cystitis, duodenitis, dyspnea, ecchymosis, edema, erythema multiforme, esophagitis (+/- stricture or cardiospasm), exfoliative dermatitis, GI ulceration, hallucination, headache, hearing decreased, hematemesis, hematuria, hepatic failure, hepatitis, hyperglycemia (in controlled patients with diabetes), hyperpigmentation, hypertension, infection, insomnia, interstitial nephritis, irregular uterine bleeding, jaundice, LFTs increased, leukopenia, MI, palpitation, pancreatitis, pancytopenia, paresthesia, peptic ulcer (+/- bleeding/perforation), peripheral neuropathy, photophobia, photosensitivity, pulmonary infiltration (eosinophilia), rectal bleeding, renal calculus, renal failure, renal insufficiency, shock, Stevens-Johnson syndrome, syncope, thrombocytopenia, toxic epidermal necrolysis, ulcerative stomatitis, urticaria, vesiculobullous rash, renal papillary necrosis, visual disturbances

Drug Interactions

Metabolism/Transport Effects None known.

Avoid Concomitant Use

Avoid concomitant use of Etodolac with any of the following: Floctafenine; Ketorolac; Ketorolac (Nasal); Ketorolac (Systemic)

Increased Effect/Toxicity

Etodolac may increase the levels/effects of: Aminoglycosides; Anticoagulants; Antiplatelet Agents; Bisphosphonate Derivatives; Collagenase (Systemic); CycloSPORINE; CycloSPORINE (Systemic); Deferasirox; Desmopressin; Digoxin; Drotrecogin Alfa (Activated); Eplerenone; Haloperidol; Ibritumomab; Lithium; Methotrexate; Nonsteroidal Anti-Inflammatory Agents; PEMEtrexed; Porfimer; Potassium-Sparing Diuretics; PRALAtrexate; Quinolone Antibiotics; Rivaroxaban; Salicylates; Thrombolytic Agents; Tositumomab and Iodine I 131 Tositumomab; Vancomycin; Vitamin K Antagonists

The levels/effects of Etodolac may be increased by: ACE Inhibitors; Angiotensin II Receptor Blockers; Antidepressants (Tricyclic, Tertiary Amine); Corticosteroids (Systemic); CycloSPORINE; CycloSPORINE (Systemic); Dasatinib; Floctafenine; Glucosamine; Herbs (Anticoagulant/Antiplatelet Properties); Ketorolac; Ketorolac (Nasal); Ketorolac (Systemic); Nonsteroidal Anti-Inflammatory Agents; Omega-3-Acid Ethyl Esters; Pentosan Polysulfate Sodium; Pentoxifylline; Probenecid; Prostacyclin Analogues; Selective Serotonin Reuptake Inhibitors; Serotonin/Norepinephrine Reuptake Inhibitors; Sodium Phosphates; Treprostinil; Vitamin E

Decreased Effect

Etodolac may decrease the levels/effects of: ACE Inhibitors; Angiotensin II Receptor Blockers; Antiplatelet Agents; Beta-Blockers; Eplerenone; HydrALAZINE; Loop Diuretics; Potassium-Sparing Diuretics; Salicylates; Selective Serotonin Reuptake Inhibitors; Thiazide Diuretics

The levels/effects of Etodolac may be decreased by: Bile Acid Sequestrants; Nonsteroidal Anti-Inflammatory Agents; Salicylates

Ethanol/Nutrition/Herb Interactions

Ethanol: Avoid ethanol (may enhance gastric mucosal irritation).

Food: Etodolac peak serum levels may be decreased if taken with food.

Herb/Nutraceutical: Avoid alfalfa, anise, bilberry, bladderwrack, bromelain, cat's claw, celery, chamomile, coleus, cordyceps, dong quai, evening primrose, fenugreek, feverfew, garlic, ginger, ginkgo biloba, ginseng (American, Panax, Siberian), grapeseed, green tea, guggul, horse chestnut seed, horseradish, licorice, prickly ash, red clover, reishi, SAMe (S-adenosylmethionine), sweet clover, turmeric, white willow (all have additional antiplatelet activity).

Stability Store at 20°C to 25°C (68°F to 77°F). Protect from moisture.

Mechanism of Action Reversibly inhibits cyclooxygenase-1 and 2 (COX-1 and 2) enzymes, which results in decreased formation of prostaglandin precursors; has antipyretic, analgesic, and anti-inflammatory properties

Other proposed mechanisms not fully elucidated (and possibly contributing to the anti-inflammatory effect to varying degrees), include inhibiting chemotaxis, altering lymphocyte activity, inhibiting neutrophil aggregation/activation, and decreasing proinflammatory cytokine levels.

Pharmacodynamics/Kinetics
Onset of action: Analgesic: 2-4 hours; Maximum anti-inflammatory effect: A few days
Absorption: ≥80%
Distribution: V_d:
Immediate release: Adults:0.4 L/kg
Extended release: Adults: 0.57 L/kg; Children (6-16 years): 0.08 L/kg
Protein binding: ≥99%, primarily albumin
Metabolism: Hepatic
Bioavailability: 100%
Half-life elimination: Terminal: Adults: 5-8 hours
Extended release: Children (6-16 years): 12 hours
Time to peak, serum:
Immediate release: Adults: 1-2 hours
Extended release: Extended release: 5-7 hours, increased 1.4-3.8 hours with food
Excretion: Urine 73% (1% unchanged); feces 16%

Dosage Note: For chronic conditions, response is usually observed within 2 weeks.
Children 6-16 years: Oral: Juvenile idiopathic arthritis (JIA): Extended release formulation:
20-30 kg: 400 mg once daily
31-45 kg: 600 mg once daily
46-60 kg: 800 mg once daily
>60 kg: 1000 mg once daily
Adults: Oral:
Acute pain: Immediate release formulation: 200-400 mg every 6-8 hours, as needed, not to exceed total daily doses of 1000 mg
Rheumatoid arthritis, osteoarthritis:
Immediate release formulation: 400 mg 2 times/day **or** 300 mg 2-3 times/day **or** 500 mg 2 times/day (doses >1000 mg/day have not been evaluated)
Extended release formulation: 400-1000 mg once daily
Elderly: Refer to adult dosing; in patients ≥65 years, no dosage adjustment required based on pharmacokinetics. The elderly are more sensitive to antiprostaglandin effects and may need dosage adjustments.

Dosage adjustment in renal impairment:
Mild-to-moderate: No adjustment required
Severe: Use not recommended; use with caution
Hemodialysis: Not removed
Dosage adjustment in hepatic impairment: No adjustment required.

Dietary Considerations May be taken with food to decrease GI upset.

Administration May be administered with food to decrease GI upset.

Monitoring Parameters Monitor CBC and chemistry profile, liver enzymes; in patients with an increased risk for renal failure (CHF or decreased renal function, taking ACE inhibitors or diuretics, elderly), monitor urine output and BUN/serum creatinine

Test Interactions False-positive for urinary bilirubin and ketone

Dosage Forms Excipient information presented when available (limited, particularly for generics); consult specific product labeling.
Capsule, oral: 200 mg, 300 mg
Tablet, oral: 400 mg, 500 mg
Tablet, extended release, oral: 400 mg, 500 mg, 600 mg

◆ **Etodolic Acid** *see* Etodolac *on page 666*

Etomidate (e TOM i date)

Brand Names: U.S. Amidate®
Brand Names: Canada Amidate®
Pharmacologic Category General Anesthetic
Use Induction and maintenance of general anesthesia
Unlabeled Use Sedation for diagnosis of seizure foci; procedural sedation
Pregnancy Risk Factor C
Contraindications Hypersensitivity to etomidate or any component of the formulation
Warnings/Precautions Etomidate inhibits 11-B-hydroxylase, an enzyme important in adrenal steroid production. A single induction dose blocks the normal stress-induced increase in adrenal cortisol production for 4-8 hours, up to 24 hours in elderly and debilitated patients. Continuous infusion of etomidate for sedation in the ICU may increase mortality because patients may not be able to respond to stress. No increase in mortality has been identified with a single dose for induction of anesthesia. Consider exogenous corticosteroid replacement in patients undergoing severe stress. Safety and efficacy have not been established in children <10 years of age.

Adverse Reactions
>10%:
Gastrointestinal: Nausea, vomiting on emergence from anesthesia
Local: Pain at injection site (30% to 80%)
Neuromuscular & skeletal: Myoclonus (33%), transient skeletal movements, uncontrolled eye movements
1% to 10%: Hiccups
<1% (Limited to important or life-threatening): Apnea, arrhythmia, bradycardia, decreased cortisol synthesis, hypertension, hyperventilation, hypotension, hypoventilation, laryngospasm, tachycardia

Drug Interactions
Metabolism/Transport Effects None known.
Avoid Concomitant Use There are no known interactions where it is recommended to avoid concomitant use.
Increased Effect/Toxicity There are no known significant interactions involving an increase in effect.
Decreased Effect There are no known significant interactions involving a decrease in effect.

Stability Store at room temperature.

Mechanism of Action Ultrashort-acting nonbarbiturate hypnotic (benzylimidazole) used for the induction of anesthesia; chemically, it is a carboxylated imidazole which produces a rapid induction of anesthesia with minimal cardiovascular effects; produces EEG burst suppression at high doses

Pharmacodynamics/Kinetics
Onset of action: 30-60 seconds
Peak effect: 1 minute
Duration: 3-5 minutes; terminated by redistribution
Distribution: V_d: 2-4.5 L/kg
Protein binding: 76%;
Metabolism: Hepatic and plasma esterases
Half-life elimination: Terminal: 2.6 hours

Dosage I.V.: Children >10 years and Adults:
Anesthesia: Initial: 0.2-0.6 mg/kg over 30-60 seconds for induction of anesthesia; maintenance: 5-20 mcg/kg/minute
Procedural sedation (unlabeled use): Initial: 0.1-0.2 mg/kg, followed by 0.05 mg/kg every 3-5 minutes as needed (Bahn, 2005; Miner, 2007; Vinson, 2002)

Administration Administer I.V. push over 30-60 seconds. Solution is highly irritating; avoid administration into small vessels; in some cases, preadministration of lidocaine may be considered.

Monitoring Parameters Cardiac monitoring and blood pressure required

Additional Information Etomidate decreases cerebral metabolism and cerebral blood flow while maintaining perfusion pressure. Premedication with opioids or benzodiazepines can decrease myoclonus. Etomidate can enhance somatosensory evoked potential recordings.

Dosage Forms Excipient information presented when available (limited, particularly for generics); consult specific product labeling.

Injection, solution: 2 mg/mL (10 mL, 20 mL)

Amidate®: 2 mg/mL (10 mL, 20 mL) [contains propylene glycol]

- **Etonogestrel and Ethinyl Estradiol** *see* Ethinyl Estradiol and Etonogestrel *on page 655*
- **ETOP** *see* Etoposide Phosphate *on page 671*
- **Etopophos®** *see* Etoposide Phosphate *on page 671*

Etoposide (e toe POE side)

Brand Names: U.S. Toposar®

Index Terms EPEG; Epipodophyllotoxin; VePesid; VP-16; VP-16-213

Pharmacologic Category Antineoplastic Agent, Podophyllotoxin Derivative; Antineoplastic Agent, Topoisomerase II Inhibitor

Use Treatment of refractory testicular tumors (injectable formulation); treatment of small cell lung cancer

Unlabeled Use Treatment of acute lymphocytic leukemia (ALL), refractory acute myeloid leukemia (AML), recurrent or metastatic breast cancer, central nervous system tumors, Ewing's sarcoma, gestational trophoblastic disease, Hodgkin's lymphoma, merkel cell cancer, refractory multiple myeloma, neuroblastoma, neuroendocrine tumors (adrenal gland and carcinoid tumors), non-Hodgkin's lymphomas, nonsmall-cell lung cancer (NSCLC), osteosarcoma, ovarian cancer, prostate cancer, retinoblastoma, metastatic soft tissue sarcoma, thymic malignancies, unknown-primary adenocarcinoma, Wilms' tumor; conditioning regimen for hematopoietic cell transplantation

Pregnancy Risk Factor D

Pregnancy Considerations Animal studies have demonstrated teratogenicity and fetal loss. There are no adequate and well-controlled studies in pregnant women. Women of childbearing potential should be advised to avoid pregnancy.

Lactation Excretion in breast milk unknown/not recommended

Contraindications Hypersensitivity to etoposide or any component of the formulation

Warnings/Precautions Hazardous agent - use appropriate precautions for handling and disposal. **[U.S. Boxed Warning]: Severe dose-limiting and dose-related myelosuppression with resulting infection or bleeding may occur.** Treatment should be withheld for platelets <50,000/mm^3 or absolute neutrophil count (ANC) <500/mm^3. May cause anaphylactic-like reactions manifested by chills, fever, tachycardia, bronchospasm, dyspnea, and hypotension. In addition, facial/tongue swelling, coughing, chest tightness, cyanosis, laryngospasm, diaphoresis, hypertension, and flushing have also been reported less commonly. Incidence is primarily associated with intravenous administration (up to 2%) compared to oral administration (<1%). Infusion should be interrupted and medications for the treatment of anaphylaxis should be available for immediate use. High drug concentration and rate of infusion, as well as presence of polysorbate 80 and benzyl alcohol in the etoposide intravenous formulation have been suggested as contributing factors to the development of hypersensitivity reactions. Etoposide intravenous formulations may contain polysorbate 80 and/or benzyl alcohol, while etoposide phosphate (the water soluble prodrug of etoposide) intravenous formulation does not contain either vehicle. Case reports have suggested that etoposide phosphate has been used successfully in patients with previous hypersensitivity reactions to etoposide (Collier, 2008; Siderov, 2002). The use of concentrations higher than recommended were associated with higher rates of anaphylactic-like reactions in children.

Secondary acute leukemias have been reported with etoposide, either as monotherapy or in combination with other chemotherapy agents. Must be diluted; do not give I.V. push, infuse over at least 30-60 minutes; hypotension is associated with rapid infusion. If hypotension occurs, interrupt infusion and administer I.V. hydration and supportive care; decrease infusion upon reinitiation. Dosage should be adjusted in patients with hepatic or renal impairment. Use with caution in patients with low serum albumin; may increase risk for toxicities. Use with caution in elderly patients; may be more likely to develop severe myelosuppression and/or GI effects (eg, nausea/vomiting). **[U.S. Boxed Warning]: Should be administered under the supervision of an experienced cancer chemotherapy physician.** Injectable formulation contains polysorbate 80; do not use in premature infants. May contain benzyl alcohol; do not use in newborn infants.

Adverse Reactions Note: The following may occur with higher doses used in stem cell transplantation: Alopecia, ethanol intoxication, hepatitis, hypotension (infusion-related), metabolic acidosis, mucositis, nausea and vomiting (severe), secondary malignancy, skin lesions (resembling Stevens-Johnson syndrome).

>10%:

Dermatologic: Alopecia (8% to 66%)

Gastrointestinal: Nausea/vomiting (31% to 43%), anorexia (10% to 13%), diarrhea (1% to 13%)

Hematologic: Leukopenia (60% to 91%; grade 4: 3% to 17%; nadir: 7-14 days; recovery: by day 20), thrombocytopenia (22% to 41%; grades 3/4: 1% to 20%; nadir 9-16 days; recovery: by day 20), anemia (≤33%)

1% to 10%:

Cardiovascular: Hypotension (1% to 2%; due to rapid infusion)

Gastrointestinal: Stomatitis (1% to 6%), abdominal pain (up to 2%)

Hepatic: Hepatic toxicity (up to 3%)

Neuromuscular & skeletal: Peripheral neuropathy (1% to 2%)

Miscellaneous: Anaphylactic-like reaction (I.V. infusion 1% to 2%; oral capsules <1%; including chills, fever, tachycardia, bronchospasm, dyspnea)

<1% (Limited to important or life-threatening): Amenorrhea, blindness (transient/cortical), cyanosis, extravasation (induration/necrosis), facial swelling, hypersensitivity, hypersensitivity-associated apnea, interstitial pneumonitis, laryngospasm, maculopapular rash, metabolic acidosis, MI, mucositis, myocardial ischemia, optic neuritis, perivasculitis, pruritus, pulmonary fibrosis, radiation-recall dermatitis, rash, reversible posterior leukoencephalopathy syndrome (RPLS), seizure, Stevens-Johnson syndrome, tongue swelling, toxic epidermal necrolysis, toxic megacolon, vasospasm

Drug Interactions

Metabolism/Transport Effects Substrate of CYP1A2 (minor), CYP2E1 (minor), CYP3A4 (major), P-glycoprotein; **Note:** Assignment of Major/Minor substrate status based on clinically relevant drug interaction potential; **Inhibits** CYP2C9 (weak), CYP3A4 (weak)

Avoid Concomitant Use

Avoid concomitant use of Etoposide with any of the following: BCG; CloZAPine; Conivaptan; Natalizumab; Pimecrolimus; Pimozide; Tacrolimus (Topical); Vaccines (Live)

Increased Effect/Toxicity

Etoposide may increase the levels/effects of: CloZAPine; Leflunomide; Natalizumab; Pimozide; Vaccines (Live); Vitamin K Antagonists

The levels/effects of Etoposide may be increased by: Atovaquone; Conivaptan; CycloSPORINE; CycloSPORINE (Systemic); CYP3A4 Inhibitors (Moderate); CYP3A4 Inhibitors (Strong); Dasatinib; Denosumab; P-glycoprotein/ABCB1 Inhibitors; Pimecrolimus; Roflumilast; Tacrolimus (Topical); Trastuzumab

Decreased Effect

Etoposide may decrease the levels/effects of: BCG; Coccidioidin Skin Test; Sipuleucel-T; Vaccines (Inactivated); Vaccines (Live); Vitamin K Antagonists

The levels/effects of Etoposide may be decreased by: Barbiturates; CYP3A4 Inducers (Strong); Cyproterone; Deferasirox; Echinacea; Fosphenytoin; P-glycoprotein/ABCB1 Inducers; Phenytoin; Tocilizumab

Ethanol/Nutrition/Herb Interactions

Ethanol: Avoid ethanol (may increase GI irritation).

Herb/Nutraceutical: Avoid concurrent St John's wort; may decrease etoposide levels.

Stability

Capsules: Store oral capsules under refrigeration at 2°C to 8°C (36°F to 46°F); do not freeze.

Injection: Store intact vials of injection at room temperature of 25°C (77°F); do not freeze. Protect from light. Etoposide should be diluted to a concentration of 0.2-0.4 mg/mL in D_5W or NS for administration. Diluted solutions have concentration-dependent stability; more concentrated solutions have shorter stability times. Precipitation may occur with concentrations >0.4 mg/mL. Use appropriate precautions for handling and disposal.

Solutions for infusion, at room temperature, in D_5W or NS in polyvinyl chloride, the concentration is stable as follows:

- 0.2 mg/mL: 96 hours
- 0.4 mg/mL: 24 hours

Etoposide injection contains polysorbate 80 which may cause leaching of diethylhexyl phthalate (DEHP), a plasticizer contained in polyvinyl chloride (PVC) bags and tubing. Higher concentrations and longer storage time after preparation in PVC bags may increase DEHP leaching. Preparation in glass or polyolefin containers will minimize patient exposure to DEHP. When undiluted etoposide injection is stored in acrylic or ABS (acrylonitrile, butadiene and styrene) plastic containers, may crack and leak.

Mechanism of Action Etoposide has been shown to delay transit of cells through the S phase and arrest cells in late S or early G_2 phase. The drug may inhibit mitochondrial transport at the NADH dehydrogenase level or inhibit uptake of nucleosides into HeLa cells. It is a topoisomerase II inhibitor and appears to cause DNA strand breaks. Etoposide does not inhibit microtubular assembly.

Pharmacodynamics/Kinetics

Absorption: Oral: Significant inter- and intrapatient variation

Distribution: Average V_d: 7-17 L/m^2; poor penetration across the blood-brain barrier; CSF concentrations <5% of plasma concentrations

Protein binding: 94% to 98%

Metabolism: Hepatic, via CYP3A4 and 3A5, to various metabolites; in addition, conversion of etoposide to the O-demethylated metabolites (catechol and quinine) via prostaglandin synthases or myeloperoxidase occurs, as well as glutathione and glucuronide conjugation via GSTT1/GSTP1 and UGT1A1 (Yang, 2009)

Bioavailability: Oral: ~50% (range: 25% to 75%)

Half-life elimination: Terminal: I.V.: 4-11 hours; Children: Normal renal/hepatic function: 6-8 hours

Excretion:

- Children: I.V.: Urine (~55% as unchanged drug) in 24 hours
- Adults: I.V.: Urine (56%; 45% as unchanged drug) within 120 hours; feces (44%) within 120 hours

Dosage Details concerning dosing in combination regimens should also be consulted:

Children (unlabeled uses): I.V.:

- AML induction (Woods, 1996):
  - <3 years: 3.3 mg/kg/day continuous infusion for 4 days
  - ≥3 years: 100 mg/m^2/day continuous infusion for 4 days
- Brain tumor:
  - <3 years: 6.5 mg/kg/dose days 3 and 4 of each 28-day "B" treatment cycle (Duffner, 1993)
  - ≥3 years: 100 mg/m^2/day on days 1, 2, and 3 of a 3-week treatment cycle (Taylor, 2003)
  - ≥6 years: 150 mg/m^2/day on days 3 and 4 of a 3-week treatment course (Kovnar, 1990)
- Conditioning regimen for hematopoietic stem cell transplantation: 60 mg/kg/dose over 4 hours as a single dose 3 or 4 days prior to transplantation (Horning, 1994; Snyder, 1993)
- Hodgkin's lymphoma: 200 mg/m^2/day on days 1, 2, and 3 every 3 weeks (Kelly, 2002)
- Neuroblastoma:
  - Induction: 100 mg/m^2/day on days 1-5 of each cycle (Kaneko, 2002)
  - Preconditioning regimen (prior to transplantation): 200 mg/m^2/day for 4 days beginning 8 or 9 days prior to transplantation (Kaneko, 2002)
- Sarcoma, refractory: 100 mg/m^2/day on days 1-5 of cycle; repeat cycle every 21 days (Van Winkle, 2005)

Adults:

- Small cell lung cancer (in combination with other chemotherapy agents):
  - I.V.: 35 mg/m^2/day for 4 days, up to 50 mg/m^2/day for 5 days every 3-4 weeks
  - Oral: Due to poor bioavailability, oral doses should be twice the I.V. dose (and rounded to the nearest 50 mg)
- Small cell lung cancer, limited stage (unlabeled combination chemotherapy dosing): I.V.: 120 mg/m^2/day on days 1, 2, and 3 every 3 weeks for 4 courses (Turrisi, 1999) **or** 100 mg/m^2/day on days 1, 2, and 3 for induction therapy, followed by consolidation chemotherapy (Saito, 2006) **or** 100 mg/m^2/day on days 1, 2, and 3 every 3 weeks up to a maximum of 6 cycles (Skarlos, 2001) **or** 100 mg/m^2/day I.V. on day 1, followed by 200 mg/m^2/day **orally** on days 2 through 4 every 3 weeks for a maximum of 5 courses (Sundstrom, 2002)
- Small cell lung cancer, extensive stage (unlabeled combination chemotherapy dosing): 100 mg/m^2/day I.V. on day 1, followed by 200 mg/m^2/day **orally** on days 2 through 4 every 3 weeks for a maximum of 5 courses (Sundstrom, 2002) **or** I.V.: 80 mg/m^2/day on days 1, 2, and 3 every 3 weeks up to 8 cycles (Ihede, 1994)
- Testicular cancer (in combination with other chemotherapy agents): I.V.: 50-100 mg/m^2/day for 1-5 days **or** 100 mg/m^2/day on days 1, 3, and 5 repeated every 3-4 weeks
- Testicular cancer (unlabeled combination chemotherapy dosing):
  - Nonseminoma: I.V.: 100 mg/m^2/day on days 1 through 5 every 21 days for 3-4 courses (Saxman, 1998)
  - Nonseminoma, metastatic (high-dose regimens): I.V.: 750 mg/m^2/day administered 5, 4, and 3 days before peripheral blood stem cell infusion, repeat for a second cycle after recovery of granulocyte and platelet counts (Einhorn, 2007) **or** 400 mg/m^2/day (beginning on cycle 3) on days 1, 2, and 3, with peripheral blood stem cell support, administered at 14- to 21-day intervals for 3 cycles (Kondagunta, 2007)
- Lymphoid malignancies, conditioning regimen for hematopoietic cell transplantation (unlabeled use): I.V.: 60 mg/kg over 4 hours as a single dose 3 or 4 days prior to transplantation (Horning, 1994; Snyder, 1993; Weaver, 2004)

Dosing adjustment in renal impairment:

The FDA-approved labeling recommends the following adjustments:

Cl_{cr} >50 mL/minute: No adjustment required.

Cl_{cr} 15-50 mL/minute: Administer 75% of dose

Cl_{cr} <15 mL minute: Data not available; consider further dose reductions

The following guidelines have been used by some clinicians:

Aronoff, 2007:

Cl_{cr} 10-50 mL/minute: Children and Adults: Administer 75% of dose

Cl_{cr} <10 mL minute: Children and Adults: Administer 50% of dose

Hemodialysis:

Children: Administer 50% of dose

Adults: Supplemental dose is not necessary

Peritoneal dialysis:

Children: Administer 50% of dose

Adults: Supplemental dose is not necessary

Continuous renal replacement therapy (CRRT):

Children: Administer 75% of dose and reduce for hyperbilirubinemia

Adults: Administer 75% of dose

Kintzel, 1995:

Cl_{cr} 46-60 mL/minute: Administer 85% of dose

Cl_{cr} 31-45 mL/minute: Administer 80% of dose

Cl_{cr} ≤30 mL/minute: Administer 75% of dose

Dosing adjustment in hepatic impairment: The FDA-approved labeling does not contain dosing adjustment guidelines. The following adjustments have been used by some clinicians:

Donelli, 1998: Liver dysfunction may reduce the metabolism and increase the toxicity of etoposide. Normal doses of I.V. etoposide should be given to patients with liver dysfunction (dose reductions may result in subtherapeutic concentrations); however, use caution with concomitant liver dysfunction (severe) and renal dysfunction as the decreased metabolic clearance cannot be compensated by increased renal clearance.

Floyd, 2006: Bilirubin 1.5-3 mg/dL or AST >3 times ULN: Administer 50% of dose

King, 2001; Koren, 1992: Bilirubin 1.5-3 mg/dL or AST >180 units/L: Administer 50% of dose

Administration

Oral: Doses ≤400 mg/day as a single once daily dose; doses >400 mg should be given in 2-4 divided doses. If necessary, the injection may be used for oral administration (see Extemporaneous Preparations).

I.V.: Irritant. Administer standard doses over at least 30-60 minutes to minimize the risk of hypotension. Higher (unlabeled) doses used in transplantation may be infused over longer time periods depending on the protocol. Etoposide injection contains polysorbate 80 which may cause leaching of diethylhexyl phthalate (DEHP), a plasticizer contained in polyvinyl chloride (PVC) tubing. Administration through non-PVC (low sorbing) tubing will minimize patient exposure to DEHP.

Concentrations >0.4 mg/mL are very unstable and may precipitate within a few minutes. For large doses, wher dilution to ≤0.4 mg/mL is not feasible, considerat g should be given to slow infusion of the undiluted ie/ through a running normal saline, dextrose or opo- dextrose infusion; or use of etoposide phosphate ugh a side solutions of 0.1-0.4 mg/mL may be filtered oposide 0.22 micron filter without damage to the filte n a 0.22 solutions of 0.2 mg/mL may be filtered th micron filter without significant loss of dru

Monitoring Parameters CBC with diff ial, platelet count, hemoglobin; liver function (bili , ALT, AST), albumin, renal function tests; vital sigr ood pressure)

Dosage Forms Excipient information presented when available (limited, particularly for generics); consult specific product labeling.

Capsule, softgel, oral: 50 mg

Injection, solution: 20 mg/mL (5 mL, 25 mL, 50 mL)

Toposar®: 20 mg/mL (5 mL, 25 mL, 50 mL) [contains dehydrated ethanol 33.2%, polyethylene glycol 300, polysorbate 80]

Extemporaneous Preparations Etoposide 10 mg/mL oral solution: Dilute etoposide for injection 1:1 with normal saline to a concentration of 10 mg/mL. This solution is stable in plastic oral syringes for 22 days at room temperature. Prior to oral administration, further mix with fruit juice (orange, apple, or lemon; **NOT** grapefruit juice) to a concentration of <0.4 mg/mL; once mixed with fruit juice, use within 3 hours. **Note:** Use appropriate handling precautions during preparation.

McLeod HL and Relling MV, "Stability of Etoposide Solution for Oral Use," *Am J Hosp Pharm*, 1992, 49(11):2784-5.

Etoposide Phosphate (e toe POE side FOS fate)

Brand Names: U.S. Etopophos®

Index Terms Epipodophyllotoxin; ETOP

Pharmacologic Category Antineoplastic Agent, Podophyllotoxin Derivative; Antineoplastic Agent, Topoisomerase II Inhibitor

Use Treatment of refractory testicular tumors; treatment of small cell lung cancer

Pregnancy Risk Factor D

Pregnancy Considerations Animal studies have demonstrated teratogenicity and fetal loss. There are no adequate and well-controlled studies in pregnant women. Women of childbearing potential should be advised to avoid pregnancy.

Lactation Excretion in breast milk unknown/not recommended

Contraindications Hypersensitivity to etoposide, etoposide phosphate, or any component of the formulation

Warnings/Precautions Hazardous agent - use appropriate precautions for handling and disposal. **[U.S. Boxed Warning]: Severe dose-limiting and dose-related myelosuppression with resulting infection or bleeding may occur.** Treatment should be withheld for platelets <50,000/mm³ or absolute neutrophil count (ANC) <500/mm³. May cause anaphylactic-like reactions manifested by chills, fever, tachycardia, bronchospasm, dyspnea, and hypotension. In addition, facial/tongue swelling, coughing, throat tightness, cyanosis, laryngospasm, diaphoresis, back pain, hypertension, flushing, apnea and loss of consciousness have also been reported less commonly. Anaphylactic-type reactions have occurred with the first infusion. Infusion should be interrupted and medications for the treatment of anaphylaxis should be available for immediate use. Underlying mechanisms behind the development of hypersensitivity reactions is unknown, but have been attributed to high drug concentration and rate of infusion. Another possible mechanism may be due to the differences between available etoposide intravenous formulations. Etoposide intravenous formulation contains polysorbate 80 and benzyl alcohol, while etoposide phosphate (the water soluble prodrug of etoposide) intravenous formulation does not contain either vehicle. Case reports have suggested that etoposide phosphate has been used successfully in patients with previous hypersensitivity reactions to etoposide (Collier, 2008; Siderov, 2002).

Secondary acute leukemias have been reported with etoposide, either as monotherapy or in combination with other chemotherapy agents. Dosage should be adjusted in patients with hepatic or renal impairment. Use with caution in patients with low serum albumin; may increase risk for toxicities. Doses of etoposide phosphate >175 mg/m² have not been evaluated. Use caution in elderly patients (may be more likely to develop severe myelosuppression and/or GI effects. Administer by slow I.V. infusion; hypotension has been reported with etoposide phosphate administration, generally associated with rapid I.V. infusion. Injection site reactions may occur; monitor infusion site closely. **[U.S. Boxed Warning]: Should be administered under the supervision of an experienced cancer chemotherapy physician.**

Adverse Reactions Note: Also see adverse reactions for **etoposide;** etoposide phosphate is converted to etoposide, adverse reactions experienced with etoposide would also be expected with etoposide phosphate.

>10%:
- Central nervous system: Chills/fever (24%)
- Dermatologic: Alopecia (33% to 44%)
- Gastrointestinal: Nausea/vomiting (37%), anorexia (16%), mucositis (11%)
- Hematologic: Leukopenia (91%; grade 4: 17%; nadir: day 15-22; recovery: usually by day 21), neutropenia (88%; grade 4: 37%; nadir: day 12-19; recovery: usually by day 21), anemia (72%; grades 3/4: 19%), thrombocytopenia (23%; grade 4: 9%; nadir: day 10-15; recovery: usually by day 21)
- Neuromuscular & skeletal: Weakness/malaise (39%)

1% to 10%:
- Cardiovascular: Hypotension (1% to 5%), hypertension (3%), facial flushing (2%)
- Central nervous system: Dizziness (5%)
- Dermatologic: Skin rash (3%)
- Gastrointestinal: Constipation (8%), abdominal pain (7%), diarrhea (6%), taste perversion (6%)
- Local: Extravasation/phlebitis (5%; including swelling, pain, cellulitis, necrosis, and/or skin necrosis at site of infiltration)
- Miscellaneous: Anaphylactic-type reactions (3%; including chills, diaphoresis, fever, rigor, tachycardia, bronchospasm, dyspnea, pruritus)

<1% (Limited to important or life-threatening): Acute leukemia (with/without preleukemia phase), anaphylactic-like reactions, blindness (transient, cortical), cyanosis, dysphagia, erythema, facial swelling, hepatic toxicity, hyperpigmentation, hypersensitivity-associated apnea, infection, interstitial pneumonitis, laryngospasm, maculopapular rash, neutropenic fever, optic neuritis, perivasculitis, pruritus, pulmonary fibrosis, radiation recall dermatitis, seizure, Stevens-Johnson syndrome, tongue swelling, toxic epidermal necrolysis, urticaria

Drug Interactions

Metabolism/Transport Effects Substrate of CYP1A2 (minor), CYP2E1 (minor), CYP3A4 (major), P-glycoprotein; **Note:** Assignment of Major/Minor substrate status based on clinically relevant drug interaction potential; **Inhibits** CYP2C9 (weak), CYP3A4 (weak)

Avoid Concomitant Use

Avoid concomitant use of Etoposide Phosphate with any of the following: BCG; CloZAPine; Conivaptan; Natalizumab; Pimecrolimus; Pimozide; Tacrolimus (Topical); Vaccines (Live)

Increased Effect/Toxicity

Etoposide Phosphate may increase the levels/effects of: CloZAPine; Leflunomide; Natalizumab; Pimozide; Vaccines (Live)

The levels/effects of Etoposide Phosphate may be increased by: Conivaptan; CycloSPORINE; CycloSPORINE (Systemic); CYP3A4 Inhibitors (Moderate); CYP3A4 Inhibitors (Strong); Dasatinib; Denosumab; P-glycoprotein/ABCB1 Inhibitors; Pimecrolimus; Roflumilast; Tacrolimus (Topical); Trastuzumab

Decreased Effect

Etoposide Phosphate may decrease the levels/effects of: BCG; Coccidioidin Skin Test; Sipuleucel-T; Vaccines (Inactivated); Vaccines (Live)

The levels/effects of Etoposide Phosphate may be decreased by: Barbiturates; CYP3A4 Inducers (Strong); Cyproterone; Deferasirox; Echinacea; Fosphenytoin; P-glycoprotein/ABCB1 Inducers; Phenytoin; Tocilizumab

Ethanol/Nutrition/Herb Interactions

Ethanol: Avoid ethanol (may increase GI irritation).

Herb/Nutraceutical: Avoid St John's wort (may decrease etoposide levels).

Stability Store intact vials under refrigeration at 2°C to 8°C (36°F to 46°F). Protect from light. Reconstitute vials with 5 mL or 10 mL SWFI, D_5W, NS, bacteriostatic SWFI, or bacteriostatic NS to a concentration of 20 mg/mL or 10 mg/mL etoposide equivalent. These solutions may be administered without further dilution or may be diluted in 50-500 mL of D_5W or NS to a concentration as low as 0.1 mg/mL. Use appropriate precautions for handling and disposal.

Reconstituted solution is stable refrigerated at 2°C to 8°C (36°F to 46°F) for 7 days. At room temperature of 20°C to 25°C (68°F to 77°F), reconstituted solutions are stable for 24 hours when reconstituted with SWFI, D_5W or NS, or for 48 hours when reconstituted with bacteriostatic SWFI or bacteriostatic NS. Further diluted solutions for infusion are stable at room temperature 20°C to 25°C (68°F to 77°F) or under refrigeration 2°C to 8°C (36°F to 46°F) for up to 24 hours.

Mechanism of Action Etoposide phosphate is converted *in vivo* to the active moiety, etoposide, by dephosphorylation. Etoposide inhibits mitotic activity; inhibits cells from entering prophase; inhibits DNA synthesis. Initially thought to be mitotic inhibitors similar to podophyllotoxin, but actually have no effect on microtubule assembly. However, later shown to induce DNA strand breakage and inhibition of topoisomerase II (an enzyme which breaks and repairs DNA); etoposide acts in late S or early G2 phases.

Pharmacodynamics/Kinetics

Distribution: Average V_d: 7-17 L/m^2; poor penetration across blood-brain barrier; concentrations in CSF being <10% that of plasma

Protein binding: 97%

Metabolism:
- Etoposide phosphate: Rapidly and completely converted to etoposide in plasma
- Etoposide: Hepatic, via CYP3A4 and 3A5 to various metabolites; in addition, conversion of etoposide to the O-demethylated metabolites (catechol and quinine) via prostaglandin synthases or myeloperoxidase occurs, as well as glutathione and glucuronide conjugation via GSTT1/GSTP1 and UGT1A1 (Yang, 2009)

Half-life elimination: Terminal: 4-11 hours; Children: Normal renal/hepatic function: 6-8 hours

Excretion: Urine (56%; 45% as etoposide) within 120 hours; feces (44%) within 120 hours

Children: Urine (~55% as etoposide) in 24 hours

Dosage Refer to individual protocols. Adults: **Note:** Etoposide phosphate is a prodrug of etoposide, doses should be expressed as the desired **ETOPOSIDE** dose; **not** as the etoposide phosphate dose. (eg, etoposide phosphate equivalent to ____ mg etoposide). Etoposide phosphate 1[illegible] mg is equivalent to etoposide 100 mg.

Small cell lung cancer (in combination with other approved chemotherapeutic drugs): I.V.: Etoposide 35 mg/m^2/day for 4 days up to 50 mg/m^2/day for 5 days. Courses are repeated at 3- to 4-week intervals after adequate recovery from toxicity.

Testicular cancer (in combination with other approved chemotherapeutic agents): I.V.: Etoposide 50-100 mg/m^2/day on days 1-5 to 100 mg/m^2/day on days 1, 3, and 5. Courses are repeated at 3- to 4-week intervals after adequate recovery from toxicity.

Indication-specific unlabeled dosing: Refer to Etoposide monograph.

Dosage adjustment in renal impairment:
Manufacturer recommended guidelines:
Cl_{cr} >50 mL/minute: No adjustment required
Cl_{cr} 15-50 mL/minute: Administer 75% of dose
Cl_{cr} <15 mL minute: Data are not available; consider further dose reductions
Etoposide phosphate is rapidly and completely converted to etoposide in plasma, please refer to Etoposide monograph for additional renal dosing adjustments (for etoposide).

Dosage adjustment in hepatic impairment: The FDA-approved labeling does not contain dosing adjustment guidelines. Etoposide phosphate is rapidly and completely converted to etoposide in plasma; please refer to Etoposide monograph for etoposide hepatic dosing adjustments.

Administration Infuse by slow I.V. infusion over 5-210 minutes; risk of hypotension may increase with rate of infusion. Do not administer as a bolus injection.

Monitoring Parameters CBC with differential and platelets (prior to initial treatment and each cycle), vital signs (blood pressure), bilirubin, AST/ALT, renal function

Additional Information Etoposide phosphate 113.5 mg is equivalent to etoposide 100 mg. Dosages should always be expressed, and calculated, as the desired **etoposide** dose.

Dosage Forms Excipient information presented when available (limited, particularly for generics); consult specific product labeling.
Injection, powder for reconstitution [strength expressed as base]:
Etopophos®: 100 mg

Etravirine (et ra VIR een)

Brand Names: U.S. Intelence®
Brand Names: Canada Intelence®
Index Terms TMC125
Pharmacologic Category Antiretroviral Agent, Reverse Transcriptase Inhibitor (Non-nucleoside)
Additional Appendix Information
Perinatal HIV Guidelines *on page 1946*

Use Treatment of HIV-1 infection in combination with at least two additional antiretroviral agents in treatment-experienced patients exhibiting viral replication with documented non-nucleoside reverse transcriptase inhibitor (NNRTI) resistance

Pregnancy Risk Factor B

Dosage Oral: Adults: 200 mg twice daily after meals

Dosage adjustment in renal impairment: No dosage adjustment necessary
Due to extensive protein binding, significant removal by hemodialysis or peritoneal dialysis is unlikely.

Dosage adjustment in hepatic impairment: No adjustment required for mild-to-moderate (Child-Pugh class A/B) impairment; no data in severe impairment.

Additional Information Complete prescribing information for this medication should be consulted for additional detail.

Dosage Forms Excipient information presented when available (limited, particularly for generics); consult specific product labeling.
Tablet, oral:
Intelence®: 100 mg, 200 mg

- ◆ **Euflex® (Can)** *see* Flutamide *on page 738*
- ◆ **Euflexxa®** *see* Hyaluronate and Derivatives *on page 831*
- ◆ **Euglucon® (Can)** *see* GlyBURIDE *on page 799*
- ◆ **Eulexin** *see* Flutamide *on page 738*
- ◆ **Eulexin® (Can)** *see* Flutamide *on page 738*
- ◆ **Eurax®** *see* Crotamiton *on page 418*
- ◆ **Euro-Lithium (Can)** *see* Lithium *on page 1023*
- ◆ **Euthyrox (Can)** *see* Levothyroxine *on page 1004*
- ◆ **Evamist™** *see* Estradiol (Systemic) *on page 627*

Everolimus (e ver OH li mus)

Brand Names: U.S. Afinitor®; Zortress®
Brand Names: Canada Afinitor®
Index Terms RAD001
Pharmacologic Category Antineoplastic Agent, mTOR Kinase Inhibitor; Immunosuppressant Agent; mTOR Kinase Inhibitor

Use Treatment of advanced renal cell cancer (RCC), after sunitinib or sorafenib failure (Afinitor®); treatment of subependymal giant cell astrocytoma (SEGA) associated with tuberous sclerosis, in patients who are not candidates for curative surgical resection (Afinitor®); treatment of advanced, metastatic or unresectable pancreatic neuroendocrine tumors (PNET) (Afinitor®); prophylaxis of organ rejection in patients at low-moderate immunologic risk receiving renal transplants (Zortress®)

Unlabeled Use Prophylaxis of organ rejection in heart transplant recipients; treatment of relapsed or refractory Waldenström's macroglobulinemia (WM)

Pregnancy Risk Factor D (Afinitor®) / C (Zortress®)

Pregnancy Considerations Embryotoxicity, fetotoxicity, malformations, and growth retardation were observed in animal studies with exposures lower than expected with human doses. There are no adequate and well-controlled studies in pregnant women. Based on the mechanism of action, may cause fetal harm if administered during pregnancy. Women of childbearing potential should be advised to avoid pregnancy. Women of childbearing potential should use effective birth control during treatment, and continue for 8 weeks after everolimus discontinuation.

Lactation Excretion in breast milk unknown/not recommended

Medication Guide Available Yes

Contraindications Hypersensitivity to everolimus, sirolimus, other rapamycin derivatives, or any component of the formulation.

Warnings/Precautions Hazardous agent - use appropriate precautions for handling and disposal. Noninfectious pneumonitis (sometimes fatal) has been observed with mTOR inhibitors including everolimus; symptoms include dyspnea, cough, hypoxia and/or pleural effusion; promptly evaluate worsening respiratory symptoms; may require dosage modification (pneumonitis has developed even with reduced doses) or corticosteroid therapy; severe symptoms may require discontinuation. Imaging may overestimate the incidence of clinical pneumonitis. **[U.S. Boxed Warning]: Everolimus has immunosuppressant properties which may result in infection;** the risk of developing bacterial (including mycobacterial), viral, fungal and protozoal infections and for local, opportunistic (including polyomavirus infection), systemic infections, and/or sepsis is increased. BK virus-associated nephropathy, which may result in serious cases of deteriorating renal function and renal graft loss, has been observed with use. Reactivation of hepatitis B has been observed in patients with RCC. Resolve pre-existing invasive fungal infections prior to treatment initiation. Monitor for signs and symptoms of infection during treatment. Discontinue if invasive systemic fungal infection is diagnosed (and manage with appropriate antifungal therapy).

[U.S. Boxed Warning]: Immunosuppressant use may result in the development of malignancy, including lymphoma and skin cancer. The risk is associated with treatment intensity and the duration of therapy. To minimize the risk for skin cancer, limit exposure to sunlight and ultraviolet light; wear protective clothing and use effective sunscreen.

[U.S. Boxed Warning]: Due to the increased risk for nephrotoxicity in renal transplantation, avoid standard doses of cyclosporine in combination with everolimus; reduced cyclosporine doses are recommended when everolimus is used in combination with cyclosporine. Therapeutic monitoring of cyclosporine and everolimus concentrations is recommended. Monitor for proteinuria; the risk of proteinuria is increased when everolimus is used in combination with cyclosporine, and with higher serum everolimus concentrations. Everolimus and cyclosporine combination therapy may increase the risk for thrombotic microangiopathy/thrombotic thrombocytopenic purpura/hemolytic uremic syndrome (TMA/TTP/HUS); monitor blood counts. Elevations in serum creatinine (generally mild), renal failure, and proteinuria have been also observed with everolimus use; monitor renal function (BUN, creatinine, and/or urinary protein). Avoid concomitant use with strong CYP3A4 inducers (eg, dexamethasone, phenytoin, carbamazepine, rifampin, rifabutin, rifapentine, phenobarbital) and strong CYP3A4 inhibitors (eg, ketoconazole, itraconazole, voriconazole, clarithromycin, telithromycin, atazanavir, saquinavir, ritonavir, indinavir, delavirdine, fosamprenavir, nelfinavir, nefazodone, grapefruit juice). Dosage modification may be needed if concomitant use with strong CYP3A4 inducers cannot be avoided. Use with caution with concomitant moderate CYP3A4 inhibitors and/or P-gp inhibitors; decreased everolimus doses are recommended. Use is associated with mouth ulcers, mucositis and stomatitis; avoid the use of alcohol or peroxide based mouthwashes (due to the high potential for drug interactions, avoid the use of systemic antifungals unless fungal infection has been diagnosed). In renal transplantation, avoid the use of HMG-CoA reductase inhibitors; may increase the risk for rhabdomyolysis due to the potential interaction with cyclosporine (which is given in combination with everolimus for renal transplantation). **[U.S. Boxed Warning]: An increased risk of renal arterial and venous thrombosis has been reported with use in renal transplantation, generally within the first 30 days after transplant; may result in graft loss.**

Everolimus is associated with the development of angioedema; concomitant use with other agents known to cause angioedema (eg, ACE inhibitors) may increase the risk. Everolimus use may delay wound healing and increase the occurrence of wound-related complications (eg, wound dehiscence, infection, incisional hernia, lymphocele, seroma); may require surgical intervention. Generalized edema, including peripheral edema and lymphedema, and local fluid accumulation (eg, pericardial effusion, pleural effusion, ascites) may also occur.

Everolimus exposure is increased in patients with moderate hepatic impairment; dosage reductions are recommended. Use is not recommended in patients with severe impairment (has not been studied). Use with caution in patients with hyperlipidemia; may increase serum lipids (cholesterol and triglycerides); higher serum concentrations are associated with an increased risk for hyperlipidemia; use has not been studied in patients with baseline cholesterol >350 mg/dL. Decreases in hemoglobin, neutrophils, platelets, and lymphocytes have been reported with use. Increases in serum glucose are common; may alter insulin and/or oral hypoglycemic therapy requirements in patients with diabetes; the risk for new onset diabetes is increased with everolimus use after transplantation. Patients should not be immunized with live viral vaccines during or shortly after treatment and should avoid close contact with recently vaccinated (live vaccine) individuals; consider the timing of routine immunizations prior to the start of therapy in pediatric patients treated for SEGA. Continue treatment with everolimus for renal cell cancer as long as clinical benefit is demonstrated or until occurrence of unacceptable toxicity. Safety and efficacy have not been established for the use of everolimus in the treatment of carcinoid tumors.

Azoospermia and oligospermia have been observed in males. Avoid use in patients with hereditary galactose intolerance, Lapp lactase deficiency, or glucose-galactose malabsorption; may result in diarrhea and malabsorption. The safety and efficacy of everolimus in patients with high-immunologic risk in renal transplantation or in solid organ transplant other than renal have not been established. **[U.S. Boxed Warning]: In renal transplantation, everolimus should only be used by physicians experienced in immunosuppressive therapy and management of transplant patients. Adequate laboratory and supportive medical resources must be readily available.**

Adverse Reactions

>10%:

Cardiovascular: Peripheral edema (4% to 45%), hypertension (4% to 30%)

Central nervous system: Fatigue (7% to 45%), fever (19% to 32%), headache (18% to 30%), seizure (SEGA: 29%), personality change (SEGA:18%), insomnia (9% to 17%), dizziness (7% to 14%)

Dermatologic: Rash (18% to 59%), acneiform dermatitis (SEGA: 25%; RCC: 3%), cellulitis (SEGA: 21%), nail disorders (5% to 22%), pruritus (14% to 21%), dry skin (13% to 18%), contact dermatitis (14%), excoriation (14%), acne (11%)

Endocrine & metabolic: Hypercholesterolemia (17% to 77%), hyperglycemia (12% to 75%; grades 3/4: <1% to 17%), hypertriglyceridemia (≤73%), bicarbonate decreased (≤56%), hypophosphatemia (13% to 40%), hypocalcemia (17% to 37%), hypoglycemia (≤32%), hypokalemia (12% to 23%), hyperlipidemia (renal transplant: 21%), hyperkalemia (renal transplant: 18%), dyslipidemia (renal transplant: 15%), hypomagnesemia (renal transplant: 14%), hyponatremia (≤16%), albumin decreased (≤13%)

Gastrointestinal: Stomatitis (oncology uses: 44% to 86%; grade 3: 4% to 7%; grade 4: <1%; renal transplant: 8%), diarrhea (19% to 50%; grade 3: ≤5%; grade 4: <1%), constipation (11% to 38%), abdominal pain (3% to 36%), nausea (26% to 32%: grade 3: 1% to 2%), anorexia (1% to 30%), vomiting (15% to 29%; grade 3: 1% to 2%), weight loss (9% to 28%), taste alteration (10% to 19%), gastroenteritis (1% to 18%), xerostomia (8% to 11%)

Genitourinary: Urinary tract infection (renal transplant: 16% to 22%; RCC 5%), dysuria (renal transplant: 11%)

Hematologic: Anemia (26% to 92%; grades 3/4; 13% to 15%), leukopenia (oncology uses: 26% to 54%; renal transplant 3%), lymphocytopenia (45% to 51%; grades 3/4: 16% to 18%), thrombocytopenia (21% to 45%; grade 3: 1% to 3%; renal transplant <10%), neutropenia (14% to 30%; grades 3/4: ≤4%)

Hepatic: AST increased (25% to 89%; grade 3: <4%; grade 4: <1%), alkaline phosphatase increased (PNET: 74%), ALT increased (21% to 48%; grade 3: 1%)

Neuromuscular & skeletal: Weakness (19% to 33%), arthralgia (≤15%), back pain (11% to 15%), limb pain (10% to 14%)

Otic: Otitis (SEGA: 14% to 36%)

Renal: Creatinine increased (11% to 50%), hematuria (renal transplant: 12%)

Respiratory: Upper respiratory infection (16% to 82%), sinusitis (3% to 39%), cough (7% to 30%), dyspnea (20% to 24%; grade 3: 2% to 6%; grade 4: ≤1%), epistaxis (≤22%), pneumonitis (includes alveolitis, interstitial lung disease, lung infiltrate, pulmonary alveolar hemorrhage, pulmonary toxicity; 14% to 17%; grade 3: 3% to 4%), nasal congestion (14%), rhinitis (14%), pharyngitis (4% to 11%)

Miscellaneous: Infection (RCC: All infections: 37%; grade 3: 7%; grade 4: 3%; renal transplant: 62%)

1% to 10%:

Cardiovascular: Chest pain (5%), tachycardia (3%), heart failure (1%), angina, atrial fibrillation, chest discomfort, deep vein thrombosis, edema (generalized), hypotension, palpitation, syncope

Central nervous system: Chills (4%), agitation, anxiety, depression, hallucination, hemiparesis, hypesthesia, malaise, somnolence

Dermatologic: Palmar-plantar erythrodysesthesia syndrome ([hand-foot syndrome] 5%), erythema 4%, onychoclasis (4%), pityriasis rosea (4%), skin lesions (4%), alopecia, hirsutism, incision complications, hyperhydrosis, hypertrichosis

Endocrine & metabolic: Diabetes mellitus (exacerbation: 2%; new-onset: <10%), cushingoid syndrome, dehydration, gout, hypercalcemia, hyperparathyroidism, hyperphosphatemia, hyperuricemia, iron deficiency, vitamin B_{12} deficiency

Gastrointestinal: Gastritis (7%), hemorrhoids (5%), dyspepsia (4%), dysphagia (4%), abdominal distention, epigastric discomfort, flatulence, gastroesophageal reflux, gingival hypertrophy, hematemesis, ileus, peritonitis

Genitourinary: Bladder spasm, erectile dysfunction, ovarian cysts, pollakiuria, polyuria, pyuria, scrotal edema, urinary retention, urinary urgency

Hematologic: Hemorrhage (3%), leukocytosis, lymphadenopathy, thrombocythemia

Hepatic: Bilirubin increased (3% to 10%; grades 3/4: ≤1%)

Neuromuscular & skeletal: Muscle spasm (≤10%), tremor (8%), paresthesia (5%), jaw pain (3%), joint swelling, musculoskeletal pain, myalgia, osteonecrosis, osteopenia, osteoporosis, spondylitis

Ocular: Eyelid edema (4%), ocular hyperemia (4%), conjunctivitis (2%), blurred vision, cataract

Renal: Renal failure (3%), BUN increased, hydronephrosis, interstitial nephritis, proteinuria, renal artery thrombosis, renal impairment

Respiratory: Pleural effusion (7%), nasopharyngitis (6%), pneumonia (6%), bronchitis (4%), pharyngolaryngeal pain (4%), rhinorrhea (3%), atelectasis, nasal congestion, pulmonary edema, sinus congestion, wheezing

Miscellaneous: BK virus infection, candidiasis, night sweats

<1% (Limited to important or life-threatening): Aspergillosis, azoospermia, cardiac arrest, fluid accumulation, graft thrombosis, hepatic cholestasis, hepatitis B reactivation, hypersensitivity (anaphylaxis, dyspnea, flushing, chest pain, angioedema), lymphoma, oligospermia, pancreatitis, pancytopenia, polyoma virus infection, respiratory distress, sepsis, skin cancer, synovitis (severe), testosterone levels decreased, thrombotic microangiopathy/thrombotic thrombocytopenic purpura/hemolytic uremic syndrome (TMA/TTP/HUS), wound healing complication

Drug Interactions

Metabolism/Transport Effects **Substrate** of CYP3A4 (major), P-glycoprotein; **Note:** Assignment of Major/Minor substrate status based on clinically relevant drug interaction potential

Avoid Concomitant Use

Avoid concomitant use of Everolimus with any of the following: BCG; CloZAPine; CYP3A4 Inducers (Strong); CYP3A4 Inhibitors (Strong); Grapefruit Juice; Natalizumab; Pimecrolimus; St Johns Wort; Tacrolimus (Topical); Vaccines (Live)

Increased Effect/Toxicity

Everolimus may increase the levels/effects of: ACE Inhibitors; CloZAPine; Leflunomide; Natalizumab; Vaccines (Live)

The levels/effects of Everolimus may be increased by: CycloSPORINE; CycloSPORINE (Systemic); CYP3A4 Inhibitors (Moderate); CYP3A4 Inhibitors (Strong); Dasatinib; Denosumab; Grapefruit Juice; P-glycoprotein/ABCB1 Inhibitors; Pimecrolimus; Roflumilast; Tacrolimus (Topical); Trastuzumab

Decreased Effect

Everolimus may decrease the levels/effects of: BCG; Coccidioidin Skin Test; Sipuleucel-T; Vaccines (Inactivated); Vaccines (Live)

The levels/effects of Everolimus may be decreased by: CYP3A4 Inducers (Strong); Deferasirox; Echinacea; Efavirenz; P-glycoprotein/ABCB1 Inducers; St Johns Wort; Tocilizumab

Ethanol/Nutrition/Herb Interactions

Food: Avoid grapefruit juice (may increase levels of everolimus).

Herb/Nutraceutical: Avoid St John's wort.

Stability Store at room temperature of 25°C (77°F); excursions permitted to 15°C to 30°C (59°F to 86°F). Protect from light; protect from moisture.

Mechanism of Action Everolimus is a macrolide immunosuppressant and an m-TOR inhibitor which has antiproliferative and antiangiogenic properties. Reduces protein synthesis and cell proliferation by binding to the FK binding protein-12 (FKBP-12), an intracellular protein, to form a complex that inhibits activation of mTOR (mammalian target of rapamycin) serine-threonine kinase activity. Also reduces angiogenesis by inhibiting vascular endothelial growth factor (VEGF) and hypoxia-inducible factor (HIF-1) expression.

Pharmacodynamics/Kinetics

Absorption: Rapid, but moderate

Protein binding: ~74%

Metabolism: Extensively metabolized via CYP3A4; forms 6 weak metabolites

Bioavailability: ~30%; systemic exposure reduced by 22% with a high-fat meal and by 32% with a light-fat meal

Half-life elimination: ~30 hours

Time to peak, plasma: 1-2 hours

Excretion: Feces (80%, based on solid organ transplant studies); Urine (~5%, based on solid organ transplant studies)

Dosage Oral:

Children ≥3 years of age: Subependymal giant cell astrocytoma: Refer to adult dosing

Adults:

Pancreatic neuroendocrine tumors (PNET), advanced: 10 mg once daily, continue treatment until no longer clinically benefiting or until unacceptable toxicity

Renal cell cancer (RCC), advanced: 10 mg once daily, continue treatment until no longer clinically benefiting or until unacceptable toxicity

Renal transplantation, rejection prophylaxis: Initial: 0.75 mg twice daily; adjust maintenance dose if needed at a 4- to 5-day interval (from prior dose adjustment) based on serum concentrations, tolerability, and response

Note: For use in renal transplantation, administer in combination with basiliximab induction and concurrently with cyclosporine (dose adjustment required) and corticosteroids.

Subependymal giant cell astrocytoma (SEGA): Body surface area based dosing: Initial dose (adjust maintenance dose if needed at 2-week intervals based on serum trough concentrations, tolerability, response and concomitant medications):

$0.5\ m^2$ to $1.2\ m^2$: 2.5 mg once daily
$1.3\ m^2$ to $2.1\ m^2$: 5 mg once daily
$\geq 2.2\ m^2$: 7.5 mg once daily

Note: Assess trough concentrations 2 weeks after initiation or dosage modification; target trough concentration: 5-10 ng/mL. For trough concentration between 10-15 ng/ml, may continue if tolerated; reduce dose for trough concentration >15 ng/mL. If trough <5 ng/mL, increase dose by 2.5 mg/day every 2 weeks if tolerated. Dose reductions may be made in 2.5 mg/day decrements every 2 weeks. Continue treatment until no longer clinically benefiting or until unacceptable toxicity.

Heart transplantation, rejection prophylaxis (unlabeled use): Initial: 0.75-1.5 mg twice daily in combination with cyclosporine and prednisone; adjust everolimus dose based on trough concentrations (Eisen, 2003; Vigano, 2007)

Waldenström's macroglobulinemia, relapsed or refractory (unlabeled use): 10 mg once daily (Ghobrial, 2010)

Dosage adjustment for toxicity:

PNET, RCC:

Severe/intolerable adverse reactions: Temporarily reduce dose to 5 mg once daily and/or temporarily interrupt treatment

Noninfectious pneumonitis:

Mild or asymptomatic (radiological changes suggestive of pneumonitis): Continue treatment

Moderate symptoms: Consider interrupting treatment until symptoms improve (may require corticosteroids); may reinitiate at a reduced dose of 5 mg once daily

Severe symptoms: Discontinue treatment; corticosteroids may be indicated until clinical symptoms improve; if appropriate (depending on individual circumstances) may reinitiate at a reduced dose of 5 mg once daily

SEGA:

Severe/intolerable adverse reactions: Temporarily reduce dose and/or temporarily interrupt treatment; if dose reduction is required for patients receiving 2.5 mg once daily, consider alternate day dosing.

Noninfectious pneumonitis:

Mild or asymptomatic (radiological changes suggestive of pneumonitis): Continue treatment

Moderate symptoms: Consider interrupting treatment until symptoms improve (may require corticosteroids); may reinitiate with a 50% dose reduction

Severe symptoms: Discontinue treatment and consider corticosteroids until clinical symptoms improve; if appropriate (depending on individual circumstances) may reinitiate with a 50% dose reduction

Dosage adjustment for concomitant CYP3A4 inhibitors/inducers:

PNET, RCC:

CYP3A4 inducers: Strong inducers: Avoid concomitant administration with strong CYP3A4 inducers; if concomitant use cannot be avoided, consider adjusting everolimus dose upward in 5 mg increments up to 20 mg daily, with careful monitoring. If the strong CYP3A4 enzyme inducer is discontinued, reduce the everolimus to the dose used prior to initiation of the CYP3A4 inducer.

CYP3A4 or P-gp inhibitors:

Strong inhibitors: Avoid concomitant administration with strong CYP3A4 inhibitors.

Moderate CYP3A4 and/or P-gp inhibitors: Reduce dose to 2.5 mg once daily; may consider increasing from 2.5 mg to 5 mg once daily based on patient tolerance. When the moderate inhibitor is discontinued, allow ~2-3 days to elapse prior to adjusting the everolimus upward to the dose used prior to initiation of the moderate inhibitor.

Renal transplantation: Dosage adjustments may be necessary based on everolimus serum concentrations

SEGA:

CYP3A4 inducers: Strong inducers: Avoid concomitant administration with strong CYP3A4 inducers; if concomitant use cannot be avoided, double the everolimus dose; individualize subsequent doses based on therapeutic drug monitoring. If the strong CYP3A4 enzyme inducer is discontinued, reduce the everolimus to the dose used prior to initiation of the CYP3A4 inducer; reassess trough concentration after 2 weeks.

CYP3A4 or P-gp inhibitors:

Strong inhibitors: Avoid concomitant administration with strong CYP3A4 inhibitors.

Moderate CYP3A4 and/or P-gp inhibitors: Reduce dose by 50% to maintain trough concentrations of 5-10 ng/mL (if dose reduction is required for patients receiving 2.5 mg once daily, consider alternate day dosing); assess trough concentrations after 2 weeks; individualize dosing based on therapeutic drug monitoring. When the moderate inhibitor is discontinued, adjust the everolimus upward to the dose used prior to initiation of the moderate inhibitor; reassess trough concentrations after 2 weeks.

Dosage adjustment in renal impairment: No adjustment necessary

Dosage adjustment in hepatic impairment:

Mild hepatic impairment (Child-Pugh class A): No adjustment required

Moderate hepatic impairment (Child-Pugh class B):

PNET, RCC: Reduce dose to 5 mg once daily

Renal transplantation: Reduce initial dose by 50%; monitor and adjust as appropriate

SEGA: Adjustment to initial dose may not be required; individualize subsequent dosing based on therapeutic drug monitoring

Severe hepatic impairment (Child-Pugh class C): Use is not recommended (not studied in severe hepatic impairment)

Dietary Considerations Avoid grapefruit juice. May be taken with or without food, although should be administered consistently with regard to food.

Administration May be taken with or without food; to reduce variability, take consistently with regard to food. Swallow whole with a glass of water. Do not chew or crush. If unable to swallow tablet whole, immediately prior to administration, disperse completely in 30 mL water with gentle stirring; rinse container with additional 30 mL water and swallow. Avoid contact with or exposure to crushed or broken tablets.

Pancreatic neuroendocrine tumors, renal cell cancer, subependymal giant cell astrocytoma: Administer at the same time each day.

Renal transplantation: Administer consistently ~12 hours apart; administer at the same time as cyclosporine.

Monitoring Parameters CBC with differential (baseline and periodic), liver function, serum creatinine and BUN (baseline and periodic), urinary protein, fasting serum glucose and lipid profile (baseline and periodic); monitor for signs and symptoms of infection

For renal transplantation, monitor everolimus serum concentrations, especially in patients with hepatic impairment, with concomitant CYP3A4 inhibitors and inducers, and when cyclosporine formulations or doses are changed; monitor cyclosporine concentrations; monitor for proteinuria

For SEGA, monitor everolimus trough concentrations approximately 2 weeks after treatment initiation, 2 weeks after dose modifications and after initiation or dose modification of concomitant CYP3A4 and/or P-gp inducers or inhibitors.

Reference Range Recommended range for everolimus serum concentrations:
Renal transplantation: 3-8 ng/mL
Subependymal giant cell astrocytoma: 5-10 ng/mL
Heart transplantation (unlabeled use): 3-8 ng/mL (Zuckerman, 2008)

Dosage Forms Excipient information presented when available (limited, particularly for generics); consult specific product labeling.
Tablet, oral:
Afinitor®: 2.5 mg, 5 mg, 10 mg [contains lactose]
Zortress®: 0.25 mg, 0.5 mg, 0.75 mg [contains lactose]

Extemporaneous Preparations
Hazardous agent: Use appropriate precautions for handling and disposal.

An oral liquid may be prepared using tablets. Disperse tablet in 30 mL (1 oz) of water; gently stir. Administer and rinse container with additional 30 mL (1 oz) water and administer to ensure entire dose is administered. Administer immediately after preparation.

Afinitor® prescribing information, East Hanover, NJ: Novartis Pharmaceuticals Corporation, 2011.

- ◆ **Everone® 200 (Can)** *see* Testosterone *on page 1654*
- ◆ **Evista®** *see* Raloxifene *on page 1455*
- ◆ **Evoclin®** *see* Clindamycin (Topical) *on page 381*
- ◆ **Evoxac®** *see* Cevimeline *on page 334*
- ◆ **Evra® (Can)** *see* Ethinyl Estradiol and Norelgestromin *on page 660*
- ◆ **Exactacain®** *see* Benzocaine, Butamben, and Tetracaine *on page 204*
- ◆ **Exalgo™** *see* HYDROmorphone *on page 843*
- ◆ **Excedrin® Extra Strength [OTC]** *see* Acetaminophen, Aspirin, and Caffeine *on page 32*
- ◆ **Excedrin® Migraine [OTC]** *see* Acetaminophen, Aspirin, and Caffeine *on page 32*
- ◆ **Excedrin PM® [OTC]** *see* Acetaminophen and Diphenhydramine *on page 31*
- ◆ **Excedrin® Tension Headache [OTC]** *see* Acetaminophen *on page 27*
- ◆ **ExeClear-C** *see* Guaifenesin and Codeine *on page 810*
- ◆ **ExeFen-DMX** *see* Guaifenesin, Pseudoephedrine, and Dextromethorphan *on page 814*
- ◆ **ExeFen-IR** *see* Guaifenesin and Pseudoephedrine *on page 813*
- ◆ **Exelderm®** *see* Sulconazole *on page 1599*
- ◆ **Exelon®** *see* Rivastigmine *on page 1509*

Exemestane (ex e MES tane)

Brand Names: U.S. Aromasin®
Brand Names: Canada Aromasin®
Pharmacologic Category Antineoplastic Agent, Aromatase Inactivator
Use Treatment of advanced breast cancer in postmenopausal women whose disease has progressed following tamoxifen therapy; adjuvant treatment of postmenopausal estrogen receptor-positive early breast cancer following 2-3 years of tamoxifen (for a total of 5 years of adjuvant therapy)
Unlabeled Use Risk reduction for invasive breast cancer in postmenopausal women; treatment of endometrial cancer; treatment of uterine sarcoma
Pregnancy Risk Factor X
Pregnancy Considerations According to the manufacturer, the decision to continue or discontinue breast-feeding during therapy should take into account the risk of exposure to the infant and the benefits of treatment to the mother. Not indicated for use in premenopausal women.
Lactation Excretion in breast milk unknown/not recommended
Contraindications Hypersensitivity to exemestane or any component of the formulation; use in women who are or may become pregnant; use in premenopausal women
Warnings/Precautions Hazardous agent - use appropriate precautions for handling and disposal. Due to decreased circulating estrogen levels, exemestane is associated with a reduction in bone mineral density; decreases (from baseline) in lumbar spine and femoral neck density have been observed. Grade 3 or 4 lymphopenia has been observed with exemestane use, although most patients had preexisting lower grade lymphopenia. Increases in bilirubin, alkaline phosphatase and serum creatinine have been observed. Not to be given with estrogen-containing agents. Dose adjustment recommended with concomitant CYP3A4 inducers.

Adverse Reactions
>10%:
Cardiovascular: Hypertension (5% to 15%)
Central nervous system: Fatigue (8% to 22%), insomnia (11% to 14%), pain (13%), headache (7% to 13%), depression (6% to 13%)
Dermatological: Hyperhidrosis (4% to 18%), alopecia (15%)
Endocrine & metabolic: Hot flashes (13% to 33%)
Gastrointestinal: Nausea (9% to 18%), abdominal pain (6% to 11%)
Hepatic: Alkaline phosphatase increased (14% to 15%)
Neuromuscular & skeletal: Arthralgia (15% to 29%)
1% to 10%:
Cardiovascular: Edema (6% to 7%); cardiac ischemic events (2%: MI, angina, myocardial ischemia); chest pain
Central nervous system: Dizziness (8% to 10%), anxiety (4% to 10%), fever (5%), confusion, hypoesthesia
Dermatologic: Dermatitis (8%), itching, rash
Endocrine & metabolic: Weight gain (8%)
Gastrointestinal: Diarrhea (4% to 10%), vomiting (7%), anorexia (6%), constipation (5%), appetite increased (3%), dyspepsia
Genitourinary: Urinary tract infection (2% to 5%)
Hepatic: Bilirubin increased (5% to 7%)
Neuromuscular & skeletal: Back pain (9%), limb pain (9%), myalgia (6%), osteoarthritis (6%), weakness (6%), osteoporosis (5%), pathological fracture (4%), paresthesia (3%), carpal tunnel syndrome (2%), cramps (2%)
Ocular: Visual disturbances (5%)
Renal: Creatinine increased (6%)
Respiratory: Dyspnea (10%), cough (6%), bronchitis, pharyngitis, rhinitis, sinusitis, upper respiratory infection
Miscellaneous: Flu-like syndrome (6%), lymphedema, infection

<1% (Limited to important or life-threatening): Cardiac failure, cholestatic hepatitis, endometrial hyperplasia, gastric ulcer, GGT increased, hepatitis, neuropathy, osteochondrosis, thromboembolism, transaminases increased, trigger finger, uterine polyps

A dose-dependent decrease in sex hormone-binding globulin has been observed with daily doses of ≥2.5 mg. Serum luteinizing hormone and follicle-stimulating hormone levels have increased with this medicine.

Drug Interactions

Metabolism/Transport Effects Substrate of CYP3A4 (major); **Note:** Assignment of Major/Minor substrate status based on clinically relevant drug interaction potential; **Induces** CYP3A4 (weak/moderate)

Avoid Concomitant Use There are no known interactions where it is recommended to avoid concomitant use.

Increased Effect/Toxicity

The levels/effects of Exemestane may be increased by: Conivaptan

Decreased Effect

Exemestane may decrease the levels/effects of: ARIPiprazole; Saxagliptin

The levels/effects of Exemestane may be decreased by: CYP3A4 Inducers (Strong); Deferasirox; Herbs (CYP3A4 Inducers); Rifampin; Tocilizumab

Ethanol/Nutrition/Herb Interactions

Food: Plasma levels increased by 40% when exemestane was taken with a fatty meal.

Herb/Nutraceutical: St John's wort may decrease exemestane levels. Avoid black cohosh, dong quai in estrogen-dependent tumors.

Stability Store at 25°C (77°F); excursions permitted to 15°C to 30°C (59°F to 86°F).

Mechanism of Action Exemestane is an irreversible, steroidal aromatase inactivator. It is structurally related to androstenedione, and is converted to an intermediate that irreversibly blocks the active site of the aromatase enzyme, leading to inactivation ("suicide inhibition") and thus preventing conversion of androgens to estrogens in peripheral tissues. In postmenopausal breast cancers where growth is estrogen-dependent, this medicine will lower circulating estrogens.

Pharmacodynamics/Kinetics

Absorption: Rapid and moderate (~42%) following oral administration; absorption increases ~40% following high-fat meal

Distribution: Extensive into tissues

Protein binding: 90%, primarily to albumin and α_1-acid glycoprotein

Metabolism: Extensively hepatic; oxidation (CYP3A4) of methylene group, reduction of 17-keto group with formation of many secondary metabolites; metabolites are inactive

Half-life elimination: 24 hours

Time to peak: Women with breast cancer: 1.2 hours

Excretion: Urine (<1% as unchanged drug, 39% to 45% as metabolites); feces (36% to 48%)

Dosage Oral: Adults: Females: Postmenopausal:

Breast cancer, advanced: 25 mg once daily; continue until tumor progression

Breast cancer, early (adjuvant treatment): 25 mg once daily (following 2-3 years of tamoxifen therapy) for a total duration of 5 years of endocrine therapy (in the absence of recurrence or contralateral breast cancer)

Breast cancer, risk reduction (unlabeled use): 25 mg once daily for up to 5 years (Goss, 2011)

Dosage adjustment with CYP3A4 inducers: 50 mg once daily when used with potent inducers (eg, rifampin, phenytoin)

Dosing adjustment in renal impairment: No adjustment necessary (although the safety of chronic doses in patients with moderate-to-severe renal impairment has not been studied, dosage adjustment does not appear necessary).

Dosing adjustment in hepatic impairment: No adjustment necessary (although the safety of chronic doses in patients with moderate-to-severe hepatic impairment has not been studied, dosage adjustment does not appear necessary).

Dietary Considerations Take after a meal; patients on aromatase inhibitor therapy should receive vitamin D and calcium supplements.

Administration Administer after a meal.

Additional Information Oncology Comment: The American Society of Clinical Oncology (ASCO) guidelines for adjuvant endocrine therapy in postmenopausal women with HR-positive breast cancer (Burstein, 2010) recommend considering aromatase inhibitor (AI) therapy at some point in the treatment course (primary, sequentially, or extended). Optimal duration at this time is not known; however, treatment with an AI should not exceed 5 years in primary and extended therapies, and 2-3 years if followed by tamoxifen in sequential therapy (total of 5 years). If initial therapy with AI has been discontinued before the 5 years, consideration should be taken to receive tamoxifen for a total of 5 years. The optimal time to switch to an AI is also not known, but data supports switching after 2-3 years of tamoxifen (sequential) or after 5 years of tamoxifen (extended). If patient becomes intolerant or has poor adherence, consideration should be made to switch to another AI or initiate tamoxifen.

Dosage Forms Excipient information presented when available (limited, particularly for generics); consult specific product labeling.

Tablet, oral: 25 mg

Aromasin®: 25 mg

Exenatide (ex EN a tide)

Brand Names: U.S. Byetta®

Index Terms AC 2993; AC002993; Exendin-4; LY2148568

Pharmacologic Category Antidiabetic Agent, Glucagon-Like Peptide-1 (GLP-1) Receptor Agonist

Additional Appendix Information

Diabetes Mellitus Management, Adults *on page 1983*

Use Treatment of type 2 diabetes mellitus (noninsulin dependent, NIDDM) to improve glycemic control

Pregnancy Risk Factor C

Pregnancy Considerations Due to adverse events observed in some animal studies, exenatide is classified as pregnancy category C. Based on *in vitro* data, exenatide has a low potential to cross the placenta. Maternal hyperglycemia can be associated with adverse effects in the fetus, including macrosomia, neonatal hyperglycemia, and hyperbilirubinemia; the risk of congenital malformations is increased when the Hb A_{1c} is above the normal range. Diabetes can also be associated with adverse effects in the mother. Poorly-treated diabetes may cause end-organ damage that may in turn negatively affect obstetric outcomes. Physiologic glucose levels should be maintained prior to and during pregnancy to decrease the risk of adverse events in the mother and the fetus. Until additional safety and efficacy data are obtained, the use of exenatide is generally not recommended in the routine management of diabetes mellitus during pregnancy. Insulin is the drug of choice for the control of diabetes mellitus during pregnancy. A registry has been established for women exposed to exenatide during pregnancy (1-800-633-9081).

Lactation Excretion in breast milk unknown/use caution

Medication Guide Available Yes

Contraindications Hypersensitivity to exenatide or any component of the formulation

Warnings/Precautions Mechanism requires the presence of insulin, therefore use in type 1 diabetes (insulin dependent, IDDM) or diabetic ketoacidosis is not recommended; it is not a substitute for insulin in insulin-requiring patients. Concurrent use with insulin therapy has not been evaluated. May increase the risk of hypoglycemia in patients receiving concomitant insulin secretagogues (eg, sulfonylureas, meglitinides); dosage reduction of sulfonylureas may be required. Clinicians should note that the risk of hypoglycemia is not increased when exenatide is added to metformin monotherapy.

Exenatide is frequently associated with gastrointestinal adverse effects and is not recommended for use in patients with gastroparesis or severe gastrointestinal disease. Gastrointestinal effects may be dose-related and may decrease in frequency/severity with gradual titration and continued use. Due to its effects on gastric emptying, exenatide may reduce the rate and extent of absorption of orally-administered drugs; use with caution in patients receiving medications with a narrow therapeutic window or require rapid absorption from the GI tract. Administer medications 1 hour prior to the use of exenatide when optimal drug absorption and peak levels are important to the overall therapeutic effect (eg, antibiotics, oral contraceptives). Cases of acute pancreatitis (including hemorrhagic and necrotizing with some fatalities) have been reported; monitor for unexplained severe abdominal pain and if pancreatitis suspected, discontinue use. Do not resume unless an alternative etiology of pancreatitis is confirmed. Consider alternative antidiabetic therapy in patients with a history of pancreatitis. Use may be associated with the development of anti-exenatide antibodies. Low titers are not associated with a loss of efficacy; however, high titers (observed in 6% of patients in clinical studies) may result in an attenuation of response. May be associated with weight loss (due to reduced intake) independent of the change in hemoglobin A_{1c}. Not recommended in severe renal impairment (Cl_{cr} <30 mL/minute) or end-stage renal disease (ESRD). Patients with ESRD receiving dialysis may be more susceptible to GI effects (eg, nausea, vomiting) which may result in hypovolemia and further reductions in renal function. Use with caution in patients with renal transplantation and when initiating or escalating doses in patients with moderate renal impairment (Cl_{cr} 30-50 mL/minute).

Adverse Reactions Percentages as reported for combination therapy (sulfonylurea and/or metformin; thiazolidinedione and/or metformin) unless otherwise noted:

>10%:

- Endocrine & metabolic: Hypoglycemia (monotherapy 4% to 5%; combination therapy: sulfonylurea - 14% to 36%; metformin - similar to placebo; thiazolidinedione - 11%)
- Gastrointestinal: Nausea (monotherapy 8%; combination therapy 40% to 44%; dose-dependent), vomiting (monotherapy 4%; combination therapy 13%), diarrhea (monotherapy <2%; combination therapy 6% to 13%)
- Miscellaneous: Anti-exenatide antibodies (low titers 38%, high titers 6%)

1% to 10%:

- Central nervous system: Dizziness (monotherapy <2%; combination therapy 9%), headache (9%)
- Dermatologic: Hyperhidrosis (3%)
- Endocrine & metabolic: Appetite decreased (<2%)
- Gastrointestinal: Dyspepsia (monotherapy 3%; combination therapy 6% to 7%), GERD (3%)
- Neuromuscular & skeletal: Weakness (4%)
- Miscellaneous: Feeling jittery (9%)

Postmarketing and/or case reports: Abdominal distension, abdominal pain, acute pancreatitis (including hemorrhagic and necrotizing), alopecia, anaphylactic reaction, angioedema, chest pain, chills, constipation, dehydration, dysgeusia, eructation, flatulence, hypersensitivity pneumonitis, influenza, injection site reaction, macular or papular rash, nasopharyngitis, pain (including back, extremity, and neck pain), pruritus, renal failure (exacerbation and acute; sometimes requiring hemodialysis or transplantation), renal impairment, serum creatinine increased, somnolence, upper respiratory tract infection, urticaria

Drug Interactions

Metabolism/Transport Effects None known.

Avoid Concomitant Use There are no known interactions where it is recommended to avoid concomitant use.

Increased Effect/Toxicity

Exenatide may increase the levels/effects of: Sulfonylureas; Vitamin K Antagonists

The levels/effects of Exenatide may be increased by: Pegvisomant

Decreased Effect

The levels/effects of Exenatide may be decreased by: Corticosteroids (Orally Inhaled); Corticosteroids (Systemic); Luteinizing Hormone-Releasing Hormone Analogs; Somatropin; Thiazide Diuretics

Ethanol/Nutrition/Herb Interactions Ethanol: Caution with ethanol (may cause hypoglycemia)

Stability Prior to initial use, store under refrigeration at 2°C to 8°C (36°F to 46°F); after initial use, may be stored at a temperature ≤25°C (≤77°F). Do not freeze (discard if freezing occurs). Protect from light. Pen should be discarded 30 days after initial use.

Mechanism of Action Exenatide is an analog of the hormone incretin (glucagon-like peptide 1 or GLP-1) which increases glucose-dependent insulin secretion, decreases inappropriate glucagon secretion, increases B-cell growth/replication, slows gastric emptying, and decreases food intake. Exenatide administration results in decreases in hemoglobin A_{1c} by approximately 0.5% to 1%.

Pharmacodynamics/Kinetics

Distribution: V_d: 28.3 L

Metabolism: Minimal systemic metabolism; proteolytic degradation may occur following glomerular filtration

Half-life elimination: 2.4 hours

Time to peak, plasma: SubQ: 2.1 hours

Excretion: Urine (majority of dose)

Dosage SubQ: Adults: Initial: 5 mcg twice daily within 60 minutes prior to a meal; after 1 month, may be increased to 10 mcg twice daily (based on response)

Dosage adjustment in renal impairment:

- Cl_{cr} ≥50 mL/minute: No adjustment necessary
- Cl_{cr} 30-50 mL/minute: Use caution when initiating or escalating doses.
- Cl_{cr} <30 mL/minute: Not recommended

Administration SubQ: Use only if clear, colorless, and free of particulate matter. Administer via injection in the upper arm, thigh, or abdomen. Administer within 60 minutes prior to morning and evening meal (or prior to the 2 main meals of the day, approximately ≥6 hours apart). Set up each new pen before the first use by priming it. See pen user manual for further details. Dial the dose into the dose window before each administration.

Monitoring Parameters Serum glucose, hemoglobin A_{1c}, and renal function

Reference Range Recommendations for glycemic control in adults with diabetes (ADA, 2010):

Hb A_{1c}: <7%

Preprandial capillary plasma glucose: 70-130 mg/dL

Peak postprandial capillary blood glucose: <180 mg/dL

Additional Information A dosing strategy which employs progressive dose escalation of exenatide (initiating at 0.02 mcg/kg 3 times daily and increasing in increments of 0.02 mcg/kg every 3 days) has been described, limiting the frequency and severity of gastrointestinal adverse effects. The complexity of this regimen may limit its clinical application.

In animal models, exenatide has been a useful adjunctive therapy when added to immunotherapy protocols, resulting in recovery of beta cell function and sustained remission.

Dosage Forms Excipient information presented when available (limited, particularly for generics); consult specific product labeling.

Injection, solution:

Byetta®: 250 mcg/mL (2.4 mL) [10 mcg/0.04 mL; 60 doses]

Byetta®: 250 mcg/mL (1.2 mL) [5 mcg/0.02 mL; 60 doses]

- **Exendin-4** *see* Exenatide *on page 678*
- **Exforge®** *see* Amlodipine and Valsartan *on page 100*
- **Exforge HCT®** *see* Amlodipine, Valsartan, and Hydrochlorothiazide *on page 100*
- **Exjade®** *see* Deferasirox *on page 461*
- **ex-lax® Ultra [OTC]** *see* Bisacodyl *on page 219*
- **Extavia®** *see* Interferon Beta-1b *on page 918*
- **Extended Release Epidural Morphine** *see* Morphine (Liposomal) *on page 1157*
- **Extina®** *see* Ketoconazole (Topical) *on page 953*
- **Extraneal** *see* Icodextrin *on page 865*
- **EYE001** *see* Pegaptanib *on page 1305*
- **EyeFlur** *see* Fluorescein and Benoxinate *on page 728*
- **Eyestil (Can)** *see* Hyaluronate and Derivatives *on page 831*
- **Eylea™** *see* Aflibercept *on page 48*
- **EZ-Char® [OTC]** *see* Charcoal, Activated *on page 335*

Ezetimibe (ez ET i mibe)

Brand Names: U.S. Zetia®

Brand Names: Canada Ezetrol®

Pharmacologic Category Antilipemic Agent, 2-Azetidinone

Additional Appendix Information

Hyperlipidemia Management *on page 1996*

Use Use in combination with dietary therapy for the treatment of primary hypercholesterolemia (as monotherapy or in combination with HMG-CoA reductase inhibitors); homozygous sitosterolemia; homozygous familial hypercholesterolemia (in combination with atorvastatin or simvastatin); mixed hyperlipidemia (in combination with fenofibrate)

Pregnancy Risk Factor C

Pregnancy Considerations Safety and efficacy have not been established; use during pregnancy only if the potential benefit to the mother outweighs the possible risk to the fetus.

Lactation Excretion in breast milk unknown/not recommended

Contraindications Hypersensitivity to ezetimibe or any component of the formulation; concomitant use with an HMG-CoA reductase inhibitor in patients with active hepatic disease, unexplained persistent elevations in serum transaminases; pregnancy; breast-feeding

Warnings/Precautions Secondary causes of hyperlipidemia should be ruled out prior to therapy. Use caution with severe renal (Cl_{cr} <30 mL/minute) or mild hepatic impairment (Child-Pugh class A); not recommended for use with moderate or severe hepatic impairment (Child-Pugh classes B and C). Concurrent use of ezetimibe and fibric acid derivatives may increase the risk of cholelithiasis.

Adverse Reactions

1% to 10%:

Central nervous system: Fatigue (2%)

Gastrointestinal: Diarrhea (4%)

Hepatic: Transaminases increased (with HMG-CoA reductase inhibitors) (≥3 x ULN, 1%)

Neuromuscular & skeletal: Arthralgia (3%), pain in extremity (3%)

Respiratory: Upper respiratory tract infection (4%), sinusitis (3%)

Miscellaneous: Influenza (2%)

Postmarketing and/or case reports: Abdominal pain, anaphylaxis, angioedema, autoimmune hepatitis (Stolk, 2006), cholecystitis, cholelithiasis, cholestatic hepatitis (Stolk, 2006), CPK increased, depression, dizziness, erythema multiforme, headache, hepatitis, hypersensitivity reactions, myalgia, myopathy, nausea, pancreatitis, paresthesia, rash, rhabdomyolysis, thrombocytopenia, urticaria

Drug Interactions

Metabolism/Transport Effects Substrate of SLCO1B1

Avoid Concomitant Use There are no known interactions where it is recommended to avoid concomitant use.

Increased Effect/Toxicity

Ezetimibe may increase the levels/effects of: CycloSPORINE; CycloSPORINE (Systemic)

The levels/effects of Ezetimibe may be increased by: CycloSPORINE; CycloSPORINE (Systemic); Eltrombopag; Fibric Acid Derivatives

Decreased Effect

The levels/effects of Ezetimibe may be decreased by: Bile Acid Sequestrants

Ethanol/Nutrition/Herb Interactions Food: Ezetimibe did not cause meaningful reductions in fat-soluble vitamin concentrations during a 2-week clinical trial. Effects of long-term therapy have not been evaluated.

Stability Store at controlled room temperature of 25°C (77°F). Protect from moisture.

Mechanism of Action Inhibits absorption of cholesterol at the brush border of the small intestine via the sterol transporter, Niemann-Pick C1-Like1 (NPC1L1). This leads to a decreased delivery of cholesterol to the liver, reduction of hepatic cholesterol stores and an increased clearance of cholesterol from the blood; decreases total C, LDL-cholesterol (LDL-C), ApoB, and triglycerides (TG) while increasing HDL-cholesterol (HDL-C).

Pharmacodynamics/Kinetics

Protein binding: >90% to plasma proteins

Metabolism: Undergoes glucuronide conjugation in the small intestine and liver; forms metabolite (active); may undergo enterohepatic recycling

Bioavailability: Variable

Half-life elimination: 22 hours (ezetimibe and metabolite)

Time to peak, plasma: 4-12 hours

Excretion: Feces (78%, 69% as ezetimibe); urine (11%, 9% as metabolite)

Dosage Oral:

Children ≥10 years and Adults: 10 mg/day

Elderly: Refer to adult dosing

Dosage adjustment in renal impairment: AUC increased with severe impairment (Cl_{cr} <30 mL/minute); no dosing adjustment necessary

Dosage adjustment in hepatic impairment: AUC increased with hepatic impairment

Mild impairment (Child-Pugh class A): No dosing adjustment necessary

Moderate-to-severe impairment (Child-Pugh classes B and C): Use of ezetimibe not recommended

Dietary Considerations May be taken without regard to meals. Before initiation of therapy, patients should be placed on a standard cholesterol-lowering diet for 6 weeks and the diet should be continued during drug therapy.

Administration May be administered without regard to meals. May be taken at the same time as HMG-CoA reductase inhibitors. Administer ≥2 hours before or ≥4 hours after bile acid sequestrants.

Monitoring Parameters Total cholesterol profile prior to therapy, and when clinically indicated and/or periodically thereafter. When used in combination with fenofibrate, monitor LFTs and signs and symptoms of cholelithiasis.

Additional Information When studied in combination with fenofibrate for mixed hyperlipidemia, the dose of fenofibrate was 160 mg daily.

Dosage Forms Excipient information presented when available (limited, particularly for generics); consult specific product labeling.

Tablet, oral:

Zetia®: 10 mg

Ezetimibe and Simvastatin

(ez ET i mibe & SIM va stat in)

Brand Names: U.S. Vytorin®

Index Terms Simvastatin and Ezetimibe

Pharmacologic Category Antilipemic Agent, 2-Azetidinone; Antilipemic Agent, HMG-CoA Reductase Inhibitor

Additional Appendix Information

Hyperlipidemia Management *on page 1996*

Use Used in combination with dietary modification for the treatment of primary hypercholesterolemia and homozygous familial hypercholesterolemia

Pregnancy Risk Factor X

Dosage Oral: Adults:

Note: Dosing limitation: Simvastatin 80 mg is limited to patients that have been taking this dose for >12 consecutive months without evidence of myopathy and are not currently taking or beginning to take a simvastatin dose-limiting or contraindicated interacting medication. If patient is unable to achieve low-density lipoprotein-cholesterol (LDL-C) goal using the 40 mg dose of simvastatin, increasing to 80 mg dose is not recommended. Instead, switch patient to an alternative LDL-C-lowering treatment providing greater LDL-C reduction.

Homozygous familial hypercholesterolemia: Ezetimibe 10 mg and simvastatin 40 mg once daily in the evening.

Hyperlipidemias: Initial: Ezetimibe 10 mg and simvastatin 10-20 mg once daily in the evening. Dosing range: Ezetimibe 10 mg and simvastatin 10-40 mg once daily

Patients who require less aggressive reduction in LDL-C: Initial: Ezetimibe 10 mg and simvastatin 10 mg once daily in the evening

Patients who require >55% reduction in LDL-C: Initial: Ezetimibe 10 mg and simvastatin 40 mg once daily in the evening

Dosage adjustment with concomitant medications: Note: Patients currently tolerating and requiring a dose of simvastatin 80 mg who require initiation of an interacting drug with a dose cap for simvastatin should be switched to an alternative statin with less potential for drug-drug interaction.

Amiodarone, amlodipine, or ranolazine: Simvastatin dose should **not** exceed 20 mg once daily

Diltiazem or verapamil: Simvastatin dose should **not** exceed 10 mg once daily

Dosage adjustment in Chinese patients on niacin doses ≥1 g/day: Use caution with simvastatin doses exceeding 20 mg/day; because of an increased risk of myopathy, do not administer simvastatin 80 mg

Dosage adjustment in renal impairment: Manufacturer's recommendations:

Mild-to-moderate renal impairment: No dosage adjustment necessary; neither ezetimibe or simvastatin undergo significant renal excretion

Severe renal impairment: **Note:** Degree of renal impairment (ie, creatinine clearance) not defined: Initiate therapy only if patient has already tolerated ≥5 mg daily of simvastatin; monitor closely.

Dosage adjustment in hepatic impairment: Manufacturer's recommendations:

Mild impairment: No dosage adjustment necessary.

Moderate-to-severe impairment: Use not recommended.

Additional Information Complete prescribing information for this medication should be consulted for additional detail.

Dosage Forms Excipient information presented when available (limited, particularly for generics); consult specific product labeling.

Tablet:

Vytorin® 10/10: Ezetimibe 10 mg and simvastatin 10 mg

Vytorin® 10/20: Ezetimibe 10 mg and simvastatin 20 mg

Vytorin® 10/40: Ezetimibe 10 mg and simvastatin 40 mg

Vytorin® 10/80: Ezetimibe 10 mg and simvastatin 80 mg

- **Ezetrol® (Can)** *see* Ezetimibe *on page 680*
- **F_3T** *see* Trifluridine *on page 1738*
- **FaBB** *see* Folic Acid, Cyanocobalamin, and Pyridoxine *on page 749*
- **Fabrazyme®** *see* Agalsidase Beta *on page 49*
- **Factive®** *see* Gemifloxacin *on page 786*

Factor VIIa (Recombinant)

(FAK ter SEV en aye ree KOM be nant)

Brand Names: U.S. NovoSeven® RT

Brand Names: Canada Niastase®; Niastase® RT

Index Terms Coagulation Factor VIIa; Eptacog Alfa (Activated); rFVIIa

Pharmacologic Category Antihemophilic Agent

Use Treatment of bleeding episodes and prevention of bleeding in surgical interventions in patients with either hemophilia A or B with inhibitors to factor VIII or factor IX, acquired hemophilia, or congenital factor VII deficiency

Unlabeled Use Reduction of hematoma growth in patients with acute intracerebral hemorrhage, warfarin-related intracerebral hemorrhage; treatment of refractory bleeding after cardiac surgery in nonhemophiliac patients

Pregnancy Risk Factor C

Pregnancy Considerations Animal studies have demonstrated fetal loss, but no evidence of teratogenic effects. There are no adequate and well-controlled studies in pregnant women. Use only if the potential benefit justifies the potential risk to the fetus.

Lactation Excretion in breast milk unknown/not recommended

Contraindications There are no contraindications listed within the FDA-approved labeling.

Warnings/Precautions [U.S. Boxed Warning]: Serious thrombotic events are associated with the use of factor VIIa outside labeled indications. Arterial and venous thrombotic and thromboembolic events, some fatal, following administration of factor VIIa have been reported during postmarketing surveillance. All patients receiving factor VIIa should be monitored for signs and symptoms of activation of the coagulation system or thrombosis; thrombotic events may be increased in patients with disseminated intravascular coagulation (DIC), advanced atherosclerotic disease, sepsis, crush injury, or concomitant treatment with prothrombin complex concentrates. Use with caution in patients with an increased risk of thromboembolic complications (eg, coronary heart disease, liver disease, DIC, postoperative immobilization, elderly patients, and neonates). Decreased dosage or discontinuation is warranted with confirmed intravascular coagulation or presence of clinical thrombosis. Use with caution in patients with known hypersensitivity to mouse, hamster, or bovine proteins, or factor VIIa, or any components of the product. Efficacy with prolonged infusions and data evaluating this agent's long-term adverse effects are limited.

Adverse Reactions

1% to 10%:

Cardiovascular: Hypertension (2%), bradycardia (1%), edema (1%), hypotension (1%)

Central nervous system: Fever (4%), headache (1%), pain (1%)

Dermatologic: Pruritus (1%), purpura (1%), rash (1%)

Gastrointestinal: Vomiting (1%)

Hematologic: Plasma fibrinogen decreased (2%), disseminated intravascular coagulation (1%), fibrinolysis increased (1%), prothrombin decreased (1%)

Local: Injection site reaction (1%)

Neuromuscular & skeletal: Arthrosis (1%)

Renal: Abnormal renal function (1%)

Respiratory: Pneumonia (1%)

Miscellaneous: Allergic reactions (1%)

<1% (Limited to important or life-threatening): Anaphylactic shock, angina, angioedema, antibody formation, arterial thrombosis, arterial thrombosis (limb), arthralgia, bowel infarction, cerebral artery occlusion, cerebral infarction and/or ischemia, consumptive coagulopathy, CVA, D-dimer elevation, deep vein thrombosis, fibrin degradation products increased, flushing, hepatic artery thrombosis, hypersensitivity, hypersensitivity reaction, injection site pain, intestinal infarction, I.V. site thrombosis, localized phlebitis, MI, myocardial ischemia, nausea, peripheral ischemia, portal vein thrombosis, pulmonary embolism, renal artery thrombosis, retinal artery embolism, retinal artery thrombosis, shock, thrombophlebitis, thrombosis, urticaria

Drug Interactions

Metabolism/Transport Effects None known.

Avoid Concomitant Use There are no known interactions where it is recommended to avoid concomitant use.

Increased Effect/Toxicity There are no known significant interactions involving an increase in effect.

Decreased Effect There are no known significant interactions involving a decrease in effect.

Stability NovoSeven® RT: Prior to reconstitution, store under refrigeration or between 2°C to 25°C (36°F to 77°F); do not freeze. Protect from light. Prior to reconstitution, bring vials to room temperature. Add recommended diluent along wall of vial; do not inject directly onto powder. Gently swirl until dissolved. Reconstitute each vial to a final concentration of 1 mg/mL using the provided histidine diluent as follows:

1 mg vial: 1.1 mL histidine diluent

2 mg vial: 2.1 mL histidine diluent

5 mg vial: 5.2 mL histidine diluent

Reconstituted solutions may be stored at room temperature or under refrigeration, but must be infused within 3 hours of reconstitution. Do not freeze reconstituted solutions. Do not store reconstituted solutions in syringes.

Mechanism of Action Recombinant factor VIIa, a vitamin K-dependent glycoprotein, promotes hemostasis by activating the extrinsic pathway of the coagulation cascade. It replaces deficient activated coagulation factor VII, which complexes with tissue factor and may activate coagulation factor X to Xa and factor IX to IXa. When complexed with other factors, coagulation factor Xa converts prothrombin to thrombin, a key step in the formation of a fibrin-platelet hemostatic plug.

Pharmacodynamics/Kinetics

Distribution: V_d: 103 mL/kg (range: 78-139)

Half-life elimination: 2.3 hours (range: 1.7-2.7)

Excretion: Clearance: 33 mL/kg/hour (range: 27-49)

Dosage

Children and Adults: I.V. administration only:

Hemophilia A or B with inhibitors:

Bleeding episodes: 90 mcg/kg every 2 hours until hemostasis is achieved or until the treatment is judged ineffective. Doses between 35-120 mcg/kg have been used successfully in clinical trials. The dose, interval, and duration of therapy may be adjusted based upon the severity of bleeding and the degree of hemostasis achieved. For patients experiencing severe bleeds, dosing should be continued at 3- to 6-hour intervals after hemostasis has been achieved and the duration of dosing should be minimized.

Surgical interventions: 90 mcg/kg immediately before surgery; repeat at 2-hour intervals for the duration of surgery. Continue every 2 hours for 48 hours, then every 2-6 hours until healed for minor surgery; continue every 2 hours for 5 days, then every 4 hours until healed for major surgery.

Congenital factor VII deficiency: Bleeding episodes and surgical interventions: 15-30 mcg/kg every 4-6 hours until hemostasis is achieved. Doses as low as 10 mcg/kg have been effective.

Acquired hemophilia: 70-90 mcg/kg every 2-3 hours until hemostasis is achieved

Adults: I.V.:

Intracerebral hemorrhage (warfarin-related) (unlabeled use; Freeman, 2004; Ilyas, 2008): 10-100 mcg/kg (see **"Note"**) administered concurrently with I.V. vitamin K (to correct the nonfactor VII coagulation factors).

Note: Lower doses (10-20 mcg/kg) are generally preferred given the higher risk of thromboembolic complications with higher doses; response is highly variable; monitor INR frequently after administration since rebound increases in INR occur quickly given the short half-life of rFVIIa; duration of INR correction is dose dependent.

Treatment of refractory bleeding after cardiac surgery in nonhemophiliac patients: Dosing not established; doses in the range of 35-70 mcg/kg have been recommended based on low-quality evidence (case series, observational studies) (Chapman, 2011; Ferraris, 2011; Karkouti, 2007); in patients with a left ventricular assist device, lower doses (ie, 10-20 mcg/kg) may be preferred to reduce thromboembolic events (Bruckner, 2009).

Dietary Considerations Some products may contain sodium.

Administration I.V. administration only; bolus over 2-5 minutes. Administer within 3 hours after reconstitution.

Monitoring Parameters Monitor for evidence of hemostasis; although the prothrombin time/INR, aPTT, and factor VII clotting activity have no correlation with achieving hemostasis, these parameters may be useful as adjunct tests to evaluate efficacy and guide dose or interval adjustments

Additional Information The Hemophilia and Thrombosis Research Society (HTRS) Registry surveillance program is designed to collect data on the treatment of congenital and acquired bleeding disorders. All prescribers can obtain information regarding contribution of patient data to this program by calling 1-877-362-7355 or at www.novosevensurveillance.com.

Dosage Forms Excipient information presented when available (limited, particularly for generics); consult specific product labeling.

Injection, powder for reconstitution [preservative free]:

NovoSeven® RT: 1 mg [contains polysorbate 80, sodium 0.4 mEq/mg rFVIIa, sucrose 10 mg/vial; supplied with diluent]

NovoSeven® RT: 2 mg [contains polysorbate 80, sodium 0.4 mEq/mg rFVIIa, sucrose 20 mg/vial; supplied with diluent]

NovoSeven® RT: 5 mg [contains polysorbate 80, sodium 0.4 mEq/mg rFVIIa, sucrose 50 mg/vial; supplied with diluent]
NovoSeven® RT: 8 mg [contains polysorbate 80, sodium 0.4 mEq/mg rFVIIa, sucrose 80 mg/vial; supplied with diluent]

- **Factor VIII Concentrate** *see* Antihemophilic Factor/von Willebrand Factor Complex (Human) *on page 128*
- **Factor VIII (Human)** *see* Antihemophilic Factor (Human) *on page 125*
- **Factor VIII (Human)** *see* Antihemophilic Factor/von Willebrand Factor Complex (Human) *on page 128*
- **Factor VIII (Recombinant)** *see* Antihemophilic Factor (Recombinant) *on page 127*

Factor IX (FAK ter nyne)

Brand Names: U.S. AlphaNine® SD; BeneFix®; Mononine®

Brand Names: Canada BeneFix®; Immunine® VH; Mononine®

Index Terms Factor IX Concentrate

Pharmacologic Category Antihemophilic Agent; Blood Product Derivative

Use Prevention and control of bleeding in patients with factor IX deficiency (hemophilia B or Christmas disease)

Pregnancy Risk Factor C

Pregnancy Considerations Animal reproduction studies have not been conducted. Safety and efficacy in pregnant women have not been established. Use during pregnancy only if clearly needed. Parvovirus B19 or hepatitis A, which may be present in plasma-derived products, may affect a pregnant woman more seriously than a nonpregnant woman.

Contraindications Hypersensitivity to mouse protein (Mononine®) or hamster protein (BeneFix®)

Warnings/Precautions Hypersensitivity and anaphylactic reactions have been reported with use. Delayed reactions (up to 20 days after infusion) in previously untreated patients may also occur. Due to potential for allergic reactions, the initial ~10-20 administrations should be performed under appropriate medical supervision. The development of factor IX antibodies (or inhibitors) has been reported with factor IX therapy (usually occurs within the first 10-20 exposure days); the risk of severe hypersensitivity reactions occurring may be greater in these patients. Patients experiencing allergic reactions should be evaluated for factor IX inhibitors. When clinical response is suboptimal or patient is to undergo surgical procedure, screen for inhibitors. Patients with severe gene defects (eg, gene deletion or inversion) are more likely to develop inhibitors (WFH, 2005).

Observe closely for signs or symptoms of intravascular coagulation or thrombosis; risk is generally associated with the use of factor IX complex concentrates (containing therapeutic amounts of additional factors); however, potential risk exists with use of factor IX products (containing only factor IX). Use with caution when administering to patients with liver disease, postoperatively, neonates, or patients at risk of thromboembolic phenomena, disseminated intravascular coagulation or patients with signs of fibrinolysis due to the potential risk of thromboembolic complications.

Contains either **nondetectable levels of factors II, VII, and X** (AlphaNine®, Mononine®) or **only factor IX** (BeneFIX®). Therefore, factor IX products are **NOT INDICATED** for replacement therapy of any other clotting factor besides factor IX. Factor IX is **NOT INDICATED** for the treatment or reversal of vitamin K antagonist-induced anticoagulation, hemophilia A patients with factor VIII inhibitors, or patients in a hemorrhagic state caused by reduced production of liver-dependent coagulation factors (eg, hepatitis, cirrhosis). AlphaNine® SD and Mononine® are products of human plasma and may potentially contain infectious agents which could transmit disease. Screening of donors, as well as testing and/or inactivation or removal of certain viruses, reduces the risk. Infections thought to be transmitted by this product should be reported to the manufacturer. Safety and efficacy have not been established with factor IX products in immune tolerance induction. Nephrotic syndrome has occurred following immune tolerance induction in patients with factor IX inhibitors and a history of allergic reactions to therapy.

Adverse Reactions Frequency not defined.

Cardiovascular: Cyanosis, flushing, hypotension, chest tightness, thrombosis

Central nervous system: Chills, dizziness, drowsiness, fever (including transient fever following rapid administration), headache, lethargy, lightheadedness, somnolence

Dermatologic: Angioedema, photosensitivity reaction, rash, urticaria

Gastrointestinal: Abnormal taste, diarrhea, nausea, vomiting

Hematologic: Disseminated intravascular coagulation (DIC)

Hepatic: Alkaline phosphatase increased, ALT increased, AST increased

Local: Injection site reactions: Cellulitis, discomfort, pain, phlebitis, stinging

Neuromuscular & skeletal: Neck tightness, paresthesia, rigors

Ocular: Visual disturbance

Respiratory: Allergic rhinitis, asthma, cough, dyspnea, hypoxia, laryngeal edema, lung disorder

Miscellaneous: Allergic reaction, anaphylaxis, burning sensation in jaw/skull, factor IX inhibitor development, hypersensitivity reaction

Postmarketing and/or case reports: HAV seroconversion, inadequate response/recovery, nephrotic syndrome (associated with immune tolerance induction), parvovirus B19 seroconversion, renal infarction

Drug Interactions

Metabolism/Transport Effects None known.

Avoid Concomitant Use

Avoid concomitant use of Factor IX with any of the following: Aminocaproic Acid

Increased Effect/Toxicity

The levels/effects of Factor IX may be increased by: Aminocaproic Acid

Decreased Effect There are no known significant interactions involving a decrease in effect.

Stability When stored at refrigerator temperature, 2°C to 8°C (36°F to 46°F), factor IX is stable for the period indicated by the expiration date on its label. Avoid freezing which may damage container for the diluent.

AlphaNine® SD: May also be stored at room temperature not to exceed 30°C (86°F) for up to 1 month. Reconstituted solution should be used within 3 hours of preparation.

BeneFix®: May also be stored at room temperature not to exceed 25°C (77°F) for up to 6 months. Reconstituted solution should be at room temperature and used within 3 hours of preparation.

Mononine®: May also be stored at room temperature not to exceed 25°C (77°F) for up to 1 month. Reconstituted solution should be at room temperature and used within 3 hours of preparation.

Reconstitution: Refer to instructions for individual products. Diluent and factor IX should come to room temperature before combining.

Mechanism of Action Replaces deficient clotting factor IX. Hemophilia B, or Christmas disease, is an X-linked inherited disorder of blood coagulation characterized by insufficient or abnormal synthesis of the clotting protein factor IX. Factor IX is a vitamin K-dependent coagulation factor which is synthesized in the liver. Factor IX is activated by factor XIa in the intrinsic coagulation pathway. Activated factor IX (IXa), in combination with factor VII:C activates factor X to Xa, resulting ultimately in the conversion of prothrombin to thrombin and the formation of a fibrin clot. The infusion of exogenous factor IX to replace the deficiency present in hemophilia B temporarily restores hemostasis.

Pharmacodynamics/Kinetics Half-life elimination: IX component: Adults: 21-31 hours; children: 14-28 hours

Dosage Dosage is expressed in int. units of factor IX activity; dosing must be individualized based on severity of factor IX deficiency, extent and location of bleeding, and clinical status of patient. I.V.:

Formula for int. units required to raise blood level %:

AlphaNine® SD, Mononine®: Children and Adults:

Number of factor IX int. units required = body weight (in kg) x desired factor IX level increase (as %) x 1 int. unit/kg

For example, to attain a 100% level in a 70 kg patient who has a baseline level of 20%: Number of factor IX int. units needed = 70 kg x 80% x 1 int. unit/kg = 5600 int. units

BeneFix®:

Children <15 years:

Number of factor IX int. units required = body weight (in kg) x desired factor IX level increase (as %) x 1.4 int. units/kg

Children ≥15 years and Adults:

Number of factor IX int. units required = body weight (in kg) x desired factor IX level increase (as %) x 1.3 int. units/kg

Guidelines: As a general rule, the level of factor IX required for different conditions is as follows; **Note:** The following recommendations may vary from those found within prescribing information or practitioner preference.

Primary prophylaxis: 25-40 int. units/kg twice weekly (World Federation of Hemophilia, 2005) **or** 40-100 int. units/kg 2 or 3 times weekly (National Hemophilia Foundation, MASAC recommendation, 2007); however, the optimum regimen has yet to be defined.

Minor hemorrhage (eg, bruising, cuts/scrapes, uncomplicated joint hemorrhage):

Desired levels of factor IX for hemostasis: 15% to 30%

Frequency of dosing: Every 12-24 hours if necessary

Duration of treatment: 1-2 days

Moderate hemorrhage (eg, epistaxis, oropharyngeal bleeds, dental extractions, hematuria):

Desired levels of factor IX for hemostasis: 25% to 50%

Frequency of dosing: Every 12-24 hours

Duration of treatment: 2-7 days

Major hemorrhage (eg, joint and muscle [especially large muscles] hemorrhage, intracranial or intraperitoneal hemorrhage), major trauma, or surgical prophylaxis:

Desired levels of factor IX for hemostasis: 50% to 100% (depending on the clinical situation, desired factor IX level may be reduced following active treatment period for hemorrhage or >48 hours postop)

Frequency of dosing: Every 12-24 hours or every 18-30 hours, depending on half-life and measured factor IX levels (after 3-5 days, maintain at least 20% activity)

Duration of treatment: 7-10 days, depending upon nature of insult

Administration Solution should be infused at room temperature

I.V. administration only: Should be infused **slowly**: The rate of administration should be determined by the response and comfort of the patient.

AlphaNine® SD: Administer I.V. at a rate not exceeding 10 mL/minute

BeneFix®: Administer I.V. over several minutes

Mononine®: Administer I.V. at a rate of ~2 mL/minute. Administration rates of up to 225 int. units/minute have been regularly tolerated without incident (when reconstituted as directed to ~100 int. units/mL).

Monitoring Parameters Factor IX levels, aPTT; BP, HR, signs of hypersensitivity reactions; screen for factor IX inhibitors when patient is to undergo surgery or if suboptimal response to treatment occurs

Reference Range Average normal factor IX levels are 50% to 150%; patients with severe hemophilia B will have levels <1%, often undetectable. Moderate forms of the disease have levels of 1% to 5% while some mild cases may have 5% to 49% of normal factor IX.

Dosage Forms Excipient information presented when available (limited, particularly for generics); consult specific product labeling.

Injection, powder for reconstitution [recombinant]:

BeneFix®: ~250 int. units, ~500 int. units, ~1000 int. units, ~2000 int. units [contains polysorbate 80 and sucrose 0.8%; derived from or manufactured using Chinese hamster ovary cells; exact potency labeled on each vial]

Injection, powder for reconstitution [human derived]:

AlphaNine® SD: ~500 int. units, ~1000 int. units, ~1500 int. units [contains polysorbate 80 and trace amounts of factors II, VII, and X; exact potency labeled on each vial; solvent detergent treated/virus filtered]

Mononine®: ~500 int. units, ~1000 int. units [contains polysorbate 80 and trace amounts of factors II, VII, and X; exact potency labeled on each vial; monoclonal antibody purified]

Factor IX Complex (Human)

(FAK ter nyne KOM pleks HYU man)

Brand Names: U.S. Bebulin® VH; Profilnine® SD

Index Terms PCC; Prothrombin Complex Concentrate

Pharmacologic Category Antihemophilic Agent; Blood Product Derivative; Prothrombin Complex Concentrate (PCC)

Use Prevention and control of bleeding in patients with factor IX deficiency (hemophilia B or Christmas disease)

Unlabeled Use Emergent correction of warfarin-induced coagulopathy (with clinically significant bleeding); **Note:** Products contain low or nontherapeutic levels of factor VII component; use of fresh frozen plasma (FFP) should be considered

Pregnancy Risk Factor C

Pregnancy Considerations Animal reproduction studies have not been conducted. There are no adequate and well-controlled studies in pregnant women.

Contraindications There are no contraindications listed in the manufacturer's labeling.

Warnings/Precautions Hypersensitivity and anaphylactic reactions have been reported with use. Delayed reactions (up to 20 days after infusion) in previously untreated patients may also occur. Due to potential for allergic reactions, the initial ~10-20 administrations should be performed under appropriate medical supervision. The development of factor IX antibodies (or inhibitors) has been reported with factor IX therapy (usually occurs within the first 10-20 exposure days); the risk of severe hypersensitivity reactions occurring may be greater in these patients. Patients experiencing allergic reactions should be evaluated for factor IX inhibitors. When clinical response is suboptimal or patient is to undergo surgical procedure, screen for inhibitors. Patients with severe gene defects (eg, gene deletion or inversion) are more likely to develop inhibitors (WFH, 2005).

Observe closely for signs or symptoms of intravascular coagulation or thrombosis. Use with caution when administering to patients with liver disease, postoperatively, neonates, or patients at risk of thromboembolic phenomena, disseminated intravascular coagulation or patients with signs of fibrinolysis due to the potential risk of thromboembolic complications. Use with caution in patients with liver dysfunction; may be at increased risk of developing thrombosis or DIC. Products do not contain therapeutic levels of factor VII and should not be used for the treatment of factor VII deficiency. Product of human plasma; may potentially contain infectious agents which could transmit disease. Screening of donors, as well as testing and/or inactivation or removal of certain viruses, reduces the risk. Infections thought to be transmitted by this product should be reported to the manufacturer. Some products may contain heparin. Use with caution in patients with a history of heparin-induced thrombocytopenia. Some product packaging may contain natural rubber latex.

Adverse Reactions Frequency not defined.

Cardiovascular: Flushing, thrombosis (sometimes fatal)

Central nervous system: Chills, fever, headache, lethargy, somnolence

Dermatologic: Rash, urticaria

Gastrointestinal: Nausea, vomiting

Hematologic: DIC

Neuromuscular & skeletal: Paresthesia

Respiratory: Dyspnea

Miscellaneous: Anaphylactic shock, clotting factor antibodies (development of), heparin-induced thrombocytopenia (with products containing heparin)

Drug Interactions

Metabolism/Transport Effects None known.

Avoid Concomitant Use

Avoid concomitant use of Factor IX Complex (Human) with any of the following: Aminocaproic Acid

Increased Effect/Toxicity

The levels/effects of Factor IX Complex (Human) may be increased by: Aminocaproic Acid

Decreased Effect There are no known significant interactions involving a decrease in effect.

Stability

Bebulin® VH: Prior to use, store under refrigeration at 2°C to 8°C (36°F to 46°F); avoid freezing. Bring diluent and concentrate to room temperature; gently rotate or agitate to dissolve. Following reconstitution, do not refrigerate and use within 3 hours.

Profilnine® SD: Prior to use, store under refrigeration at 2°C to 8°C (36°F to 46°F); avoid freezing; may also stored at room temperature (not to exceed 30°C) for up to 3 months. Bring diluent and concentrate to room temperature; gently rotate or agitate to dissolve. Following reconstitution, do not refrigerate and use within 3 hours.

Mechanism of Action Replaces deficient clotting factor including factor X; hemophilia B, or Christmas disease, is an X-linked recessively inherited disorder of blood coagulation characterized by insufficient or abnormal synthesis of the clotting protein factor IX. Factor IX is a vitamin K-dependent coagulation factor which is synthesized in the liver. Factor IX is activated by factor XIa in the intrinsic coagulation pathway. Activated factor IX (IXa), in combination with factor VII:C, activates factor X to Xa, resulting ultimately in the conversion of prothrombin to thrombin and the formation of a fibrin clot. The infusion of exogenous factor IX to replace the deficiency present in hemophilia B temporarily restores hemostasis.

Pharmacodynamics/Kinetics Half-life elimination: IX component: ~24 hours

Dosage Children and Adults: Dosage is expressed in international (int.) units of factor IX activity and must be individualized based on severity of factor IX deficiency, extent and location of bleeding, and clinical status of patient. When multiple doses are required, administer at 24-hour intervals unless otherwise specified. Administer I.V. only:

Formula for int. units required to raise blood level %:

Bebulin® VH: In general, factor IX 1 int. unit/kg will increase the plasma factor IX level by 0.8%

Number of Factor IX int. units required = body weight (kg) x desired factor IX increase (as %) x 1.2 int. units/kg

Profilnine® SD: In general, factor IX 1 int. unit/kg will increase the plasma factor IX level by 1%:

Number of factor IX int. units required = bodyweight (kg) x desired factor IX increase (as %) x 1 int. unit/kg

For example, to increase factor IX level to 25% of normal in a 70 kg patient: Number of factor IX int. units needed = 70 kg x 25 x 1 int. unit/kg = 1750 int. units

As a general rule, the level of factor IX required for treatment of different conditions is listed below:

Hemorrhage:

Minor bleeding (early hemarthrosis, minor epistaxis, gingival bleeding, mild hematuria):

Bebulin® VH: Raise factor IX level to 20% of normal [typical initial dose: 25-35 int. units/kg]; generally a single dose is sufficient.

Profilnine® SD: Mild-to-moderate bleeding: Raise factor IX level to 20% to 30% of normal.

Moderate bleeding (severe joint bleeding, early hematoma, major open bleeding, minor trauma, minor hemoptysis, hematemesis, melena, major hematuria):

Bebulin® VH: Raise factor IX level to 40% of normal [typical initial dose: 40-55 int. units/kg]; average duration of treatment is 2 days or until adequate wound healing.

Profilnine® SD: Mild-to-moderate bleeding: raise factor IX level to 20% to 30% of normal.

Major bleeding (severe hematoma, major trauma, severe hemoptysis, hematemesis, melena):

Bebulin® VH: Raise factor IX level to ≥60% of normal [typical initial dose: 60-70 int. units/kg]; average duration of treatment is 2-3 days or until adequate wound healing. Do not raise >60% in patients who may be predisposed to thrombosis.

Profilnine® SD: Raise factor IX level to 30% to 50% of normal.

Surgical procedures:

Dental surgery:

Bebulin® VH: Raise factor IX level to 40% to 60% of normal on day of surgery [typical dose: 50-60 int. units/kg]. One infusion, administered 1 hour prior to surgery, is generally sufficient for the extraction of one tooth; for the extraction of multiple teeth, replacement therapy may be required for up to 1 week (See dosing guidelines for *Minor surgery*).

Profilnine® SD: Raise factor IX level to 50% of normal immediately prior to procedure.

Minor surgery:

Bebulin® VH: Raise factor IX level to 40% to 60% of normal on day of surgery [typical initial dose: 50-60 int. units/kg]. Decrease factor IX level from 40% of normal to 20% of normal during initial postoperative period (1-2 weeks or until adequate wound healing) [typical dose: 55 int. units/kg decreasing to 25 int. units/kg]. The preoperative dose should be given 1 hour prior to surgery. The average dosing interval may be every 12 hours initially, then every 24 hours later in the postoperative period.

Profilnine® SD: Raise factor IX level to 30% to 50% of normal for at least 1 week following surgery.

Major surgery:

Bebulin® VH: Raise factor IX level to ≥60% of normal on day of surgery [typical initial dose: 70-95 int. units/kg]; do not raise >60% in patients who may be predisposed to thrombosis. Decrease factor IX level from 60% of normal to 20% of normal during initial postoperative period (1-2 weeks) [typical dose: 70 int. units/kg decreasing to 35 int. units/kg]; further decrease to maintain a factor IX level of 20% of normal during late postoperative period (≥3 weeks) and continuing until adequate wound healing is achieved [typical dose: 35 int. units/kg decreasing to 25 int. units/kg]. The preoperative dose should be given 1 hour prior to surgery. The average dosing interval may be every 12 hours initially, then every 24 hours later in the postoperative period.

Profilnine® SD: Raise Factor IX level to 30% to 50% of normal for at least 1 week following surgery.

Hemorrhage:

Long-term prophylactic treatment: Bebulin® VH: 20-30 int. units/kg once or twice a week may reduce frequency of spontaneous hemorrhage; dosing regimen should be individualized.

Warfarin associated hemorrhage (unlabeled use): I.V.: **Note:** Products contain low or nontherapeutic levels of factor VII component. When immediate INR reversal is required, fresh frozen plasma (FFP) should be considered to ensure acute INR reversal (Baker, 2004; Holland, 2009). Administer vitamin K (phytonadione) 10 mg by slow I.V. infusion; vitamin K may be repeated every 12 hours if INR is persistently elevated (Ansell, 2008).

Fixed-dose regimen (Yasaka, 2005; product used contained equal amounts of factors II, VII, IX, and X; also contained protein C): INR 1.5-5: 500 int. units; if INR, 10 minutes after administration, is still elevated, may repeat dose. In patients with INR >5, larger initial doses (eg, 1000-1500 int. units) may be necessary.

Adjusted-dose regimen, weight based (Makris, 2001 [recommendations based on the use of products/regimens containing adequate factor VII]):

INR 2-3.9: 25 int. units/kg

INR 4-5.9: 35 int. units/kg

INR ≥6: 50 int. units/kg

Administration I.V. administration only; should be infused **slowly**. Rate should not exceed 2 mL/minute for Bebulin® VH or 10 mL/minute for Profilnine® SD. Slowing the rate of infusion, changing the lot of medication, or administering antihistamines may relieve some adverse reactions

Monitoring Parameters Levels of factor IX; PT, PTT; INR (when used for warfarin reversal); signs and symptoms of hypersensitivity reactions, DIC, thrombosis

Reference Range Average normal factor IX levels are 50% to 150%; patients with severe hemophilia B will have factor IX levels <1%, often undetectable. Moderate forms of the disease have levels of 1% to 5% while some mild cases may have 5% to 49% of normal factor IX.

Additional Information Vaccination with hepatitis A and hepatitis B vaccines are recommended at diagnosis for patients with hemophilia.

Factor IX concentrate containing only factor IX is also available and preferable for hemophilia B (or Christmas disease). Prothrombin complex concentrates also contain factor II, factor VII, and factor X and are of intermediate purity. Heparin may be present in some products to decrease thrombotic effects.

Dosage Forms Excipient information presented when available (limited, particularly for generics); consult specific product labeling. [DSC] = Discontinued product

Injection, powder for reconstitution:

Bebulin® VH: Exact potency labeled on each vial [vapor heated; contains heparin and natural rubber/natural latex in packaging]

Profilnine® SD: ~500 int. units, ~1000 int. units, ~1500 int. units [exact potency labeled on each vial; solvent/detergent treated]

◆ **Factor IX Concentrate** *see* Factor IX *on page 683*

◆ **Factor 13** *see* Factor XIII Concentrate (Human) *on page 686*

Factor XIII Concentrate (Human)

(FAK ter THIR teen KON cen trate HYU man)

Brand Names: U.S. Corifact®

Index Terms Activated Factor XIII; Corifact®; Factor 13; FXIII

Pharmacologic Category Antihemophilic Agent; Blood Product Derivative

Use Prophylaxis against bleeding episodes in congenital factor XIII deficiency

Pregnancy Risk Factor C

Pregnancy Considerations Use in pregnant women only when benefit exceeds potential risk to the fetus. Thromboembolic events have been reported with use of factor XIII; pregnant women may be at increased risk due to hypercoagulable state.

Lactation Excretion in breast milk unknown/not recommended

Contraindications History of anaphylaxis to human blood products or hypersensitivity to any component of the formulation

Warnings/Precautions The development of factor XIII inhibitory antibodies has been reported. Factor XIII inhibitory antibodies should be measured when clinical response (breakthrough bleeding) and/or factor XIII trough levels are suboptimal. Hypersensitivity reactions have been reported with use. Thromboembolic events have been reported; pregnant women may be at increased risk. Product of human plasma; may potentially contain infectious agents which could transmit disease. Vaccination with hepatitis A and hepatitis B vaccines are recommended.

Adverse Reactions

>1%:

Central nervous system: Chills, fever, headache

Dermatologic: Bruising, erythema, pruritus, rash

Gastrointestinal: Abdominal pain, diarrhea, vomiting

Hematologic: Hematoma, thrombin-antithrombin levels increased

Hepatic: Liver function tests (increased)

Neuromuscular & skeletal: Arthralgia

Respiratory: Epistaxis, upper respiratory tract infection

Miscellaneous: Allergy, flu-like syndrome

<1% (Limited to important or life-threatening): Anaphylaxis, embolism, factor XIII inhibitory antibodies, infection, thrombosis

Drug Interactions

Metabolism/Transport Effects None known.

Avoid Concomitant Use There are no known interactions where it is recommended to avoid concomitant use.

Increased Effect/Toxicity There are no known significant interactions involving an increase in effect.

Decreased Effect There are no known significant interactions involving a decrease in effect.

Stability Store at 2°C to 8°C (36°F to 46°F); do not freeze. Protect from light. May be stored at room temperature (<25°C [<77°F]) for up to 6 months; do not return to refrigerator if stored at room temperature. Reconstitute with provided diluent (SWFI); gently swirl; do not shake. Product and diluent should be at room temperature prior to reconstitution. Reconstituted solution should be used within 4 hours; do not refrigerate or freeze.

Mechanism of Action Factor XIII (FXIII) is an endogenous plasma glycoprotein found in platelets, monocytes and macrophages that is converted to activated factor XIII (FXIIIa) in the presence of calcium ions. Once activated, FXIIIa cross-links fibrin and cross-links plasmin inhibitor to protect and strengthen the hemostatic platelet plug.

Pharmacodynamics/Kinetics

Duration of effect: Plasma levels of FXIII: ~28 days

Distribution: V_d: 51.1 mL/kg

Metabolism: Factor XIII, a proenzyme, is converted to activated factor XIII

Half-life elimination: Children (<16): 5.7 days; Adults: 7.1 days

Time to peak: 1.7 hours postinfusion

Dosage I.V.: Children and Adults:

Initial: 40 units/kg

Maintenance: Dose adjustment based on factor XIII trough levels (target level of 5% to 20% using Berichrom® activity assay) and clinical response; repeat every 4 weeks:

- One trough level of <5%: Increase dosage by 5 units/kg
- Trough level of 5% to 20%: No dosage change
- Two trough levels of >20%: Decrease dosage by 5 units/kg
- One trough level of >25%: Decrease dosage by 5 units/kg

Dosage adjustment in renal impairment: Has not been studied

Dosage adjustment in hepatic impairment: Has not been studied

Administration Administer by I.V. infusion at a rate not to exceed 4 mL/minute. Product should be brought to room temperature prior to infusing. Administer through a separate infusion line.

Monitoring Parameters Factor XIII trough levels in conjunction with clinical response to assess efficacy. Factor XIII inhibitory antibodies if inadequate clinical response and/or factor XIII trough levels are suboptimal.

Dosage Forms Excipient information presented when available (limited, particularly for generics); consult specific product labeling.

Injection, powder for reconstitution:

Corifact®: Exact potency labeled on each vial [heat treated; supplied with diluent]

Famciclovir (fam SYE kloe veer)

Brand Names: U.S. Famvir®

Brand Names: Canada Apo-Famciclovir®; Ava-Famciclovir; CO Famciclovir; Famvir®; PMS-Famciclovir; Sandoz-Famciclovir

Pharmacologic Category Antiviral Agent

Use Treatment of acute herpes zoster (shingles); treatment and suppression of recurrent episodes of genital herpes in immunocompetent patients; treatment of herpes labialis (cold sores) in immunocompetent patients; treatment of recurrent mucocutaneous/genital herpes simplex in HIV-infected patients

Pregnancy Risk Factor B

Pregnancy Considerations Teratogenic effects were not observed in animal studies. There are no adequate and well-controlled studies in pregnant women. Use only if benefit outweighs risk. A registry has been established for women exposed to famciclovir during pregnancy (888-669-6682).

Lactation Excretion in breast milk unknown/not recommended

Contraindications Hypersensitivity to famciclovir, penciclovir, or any component of the formulation

Warnings/Precautions Has not been studied in immunocompromised patients or patients with ophthalmic, disseminated zoster, or with initial episode of genital herpes. Dosage adjustment is required in patients with renal insufficiency. Tablets contain lactose; do not use with galactose intolerance, severe lactase deficiency, or glucose-galactose malabsorption syndromes.

Adverse Reactions Note: Frequencies vary with dose and duration. Single-dose treatment (herpes labialis) was associated only with headache (10%), diarrhea (2%), fatigue (1%), and dysmenorrhea (1%).

>10%:

- Central nervous system: Headache (14% to 39%)
- Gastrointestinal: Nausea (3% to 13%)

1% to 10%:

- Central nervous system: Fatigue (1% to 5%), migraine (1% to 3%)
- Dermatologic: Pruritus (≤4%), rash (≤3%)
- Endocrine & metabolic: Dysmenorrhea (≤8%)
- Gastrointestinal: Diarrhea (5% to 9%), abdominal pain (≤8%), flatulence (1% to 5%), vomiting (1% to 5%)
- Hematologic: Neutropenia (3%)
- Hepatic: Transaminases increased (2% to 3%), bilirubin increased (2%)
- Neuromuscular & skeletal: Paresthesia (≤3%)

<1% (Limited to important or life-threatening): Anemia, cholestatic jaundice, confusion, delirium, disorientation, dizziness, erythema multiforme, hallucinations, somnolence, Stevens-Johnson syndrome, thrombocytopenia, toxic epidermal necrolysis, urticaria

Drug Interactions

Metabolism/Transport Effects None known.

Avoid Concomitant Use

Avoid concomitant use of Famciclovir with any of the following: Zoster Vaccine

Increased Effect/Toxicity There are no known significant interactions involving an increase in effect.

Decreased Effect

Famciclovir may decrease the levels/effects of: Zoster Vaccine

Ethanol/Nutrition/Herb Interactions Food: Rate of absorption and/or conversion to penciclovir and peak concentration are reduced with food, but bioavailability is not affected.

Stability Store at 25°C (77°F); excursions permitted to 15°C to 30°C (59°F to 86°F).

Mechanism of Action Famciclovir undergoes rapid biotransformation to the active compound, penciclovir (prodrug), which is phosphorylated by viral thymidine kinase in HSV-1, HSV-2, and VZV-infected cells to a monophosphate form; this is then converted to penciclovir triphosphate and competes with deoxyguanosine triphosphate to inhibit HSV-2 polymerase, therefore, herpes viral DNA synthesis/replication is selectively inhibited.

Pharmacodynamics/Kinetics

Absorption: Food decreases maximum peak penciclovir concentration and delays time to penciclovir peak; AUC remains the same

Distribution: V_d: Penciclovir: 0.91-1.25 L/kg

Protein binding: Penciclovir: ≤20%

Metabolism: Famciclovir is rapidly deacetylated and oxidized to penciclovir (active prodrug); not via CYP

Bioavailability: Penciclovir: 69% to 85%

Half-life elimination: Penciclovir: 2-4 hours; Prolonged in renal impairment: Cl_{cr} 20-39 mL/minute: 5-8 hours, Cl_{cr} <20 mL/minute: 3-24 hours

Time to peak: Penciclovir: 0.9 hours; C_{max} and T_{max} are decreased and prolonged with noncompensated hepatic impairment

Excretion: Urine (73% primarily as penciclovir); feces (27%)

Dosage Adults: Oral:

Acute herpes zoster: 500 mg every 8 hours for 7 days (**Note:** Initiate therapy within 72 hours of rash onset.)

Genital herpes simplex virus (HSV) infection in immunocompetent patients:

Initial episode: 250 mg 3 times/day for 7-10 days (CDC, 2010)

Recurrence: 1000 mg twice daily for 1 day (**Note:** Initiate therapy within 6 hours of symptoms/lesions)

Alternatively, the following regimens are also recommended: 125 mg twice daily for 5 days or 500 mg as a single dose, followed by 250 mg twice daily for 2 days (CDC, 2010)

Suppressive therapy: 250 mg twice daily for up to 1 year; **Note:** Duration not established, but efficacy/safety have been demonstrated for 1 year (CDC, 2010)

Recurrent herpes labialis (cold sores): 1500 mg as a single dose; initiate therapy at first sign or symptom such as tingling, burning, or itching (initiated within 1 hour in clinical studies)

Recurrent mucocutaneous/genital HSV infection in HIV patients: 500 mg twice daily for 7 days or 5-10 days (CDC, 2010)

Prevention of HSV reactivation in HIV patients: 500 mg twice daily (CDC, 2010)

Dosing interval in renal impairment:

Herpes zoster:

Cl_{cr} 40-59 mL/minute: Administer 500 mg every 12 hours

Cl_{cr} 20-39 mL/minute: Administer 500 mg every 24 hours

Cl_{cr} <20 mL/minute: Administer 250 mg every 24 hours

Hemodialysis: Administer 250 mg after each dialysis session.

Recurrent genital herpes: Treatment (single day regimen):

Cl_{cr} 40-59 mL/minute: Administer 500 mg every 12 hours for 1 day

Cl_{cr} 20-39 mL/minute: Administer 500 mg as a single dose

Cl_{cr} <20 mL/minute: Administer 250 mg as a single dose

Hemodialysis: Administer 250 mg as a single dose after dialysis session.

Recurrent genital herpes: Suppression:

Cl_{cr} 20-39 mL/minute: Administer 125 mg every 12 hours

Cl_{cr} <20 mL/minute: Administer 125 mg every 24 hours

Hemodialysis: Administer 125 mg after each dialysis session.

Recurrent herpes labialis: Treatment (single dose regimen):

Cl_{cr} 40-59 mL/minute: Administer 750 mg as a single dose

Cl_{cr} 20-39 mL/minute: Administer 500 mg as a single dose

Cl_{cr} <20 mL/minute: Administer 250 mg as a single dose

Hemodialysis: Administer 250 mg as a single dose after dialysis session.

Recurrent orolabial or genital herpes in HIV-infected patients:

Cl_{cr} 20-39 mL/minute: Administer 500 mg every 24 hours

Cl_{cr} <20 mL/minute: Administer 250 mg every 24 hours

Hemodialysis: Administer 250 mg after each dialysis session.

Dietary Considerations May be taken without regard to meals.

Administration May be administered without regard to meals.

Monitoring Parameters Periodic CBC during long-term therapy

Additional Information Most effective for herpes zoster if therapy is initiated within 48 hours of initial lesion. Resistance may occur by alteration of thymidine kinase, resulting in loss of or reduced penciclovir phosphorylation (cross-resistance occurs between acyclovir and famciclovir). When treatment for herpes labialis is initiated within 1 hour of symptom onset, healing time is reduced by ~2 days.

Dosage Forms Excipient information presented when available (limited, particularly for generics); consult specific product labeling.

Tablet, oral: 125 mg, 250 mg, 500 mg

Famvir®: 125 mg [contains lactose 26.9 mg/tablet]

Famvir®: 250 mg [contains lactose 53.7 mg/tablet]

Famvir®: 500 mg [contains lactose 107.4 mg/tablet]

Famotidine (fa MOE ti deen)

Brand Names: U.S. Heartburn Relief Maximum Strength [OTC]; Heartburn Relief [OTC]; Pepcid®; Pepcid® AC Maximum Strength [OTC]; Pepcid® AC [OTC]

Brand Names: Canada Acid Control; Apo-Famotidine®; Apo-Famotidine® Injectable; Famotidine Omega; Mylan-Famotidine; Novo-Famotidine; Nu-Famotidine; Pepcid®; Pepcid® AC; Pepcid® I.V.; Ulcidine

Pharmacologic Category Histamine H_2 Antagonist

Use Maintenance therapy and treatment of duodenal ulcer; treatment of gastroesophageal reflux disease (GERD), active benign gastric ulcer; pathological hypersecretory conditions

OTC labeling: Relief of heartburn, acid indigestion, and sour stomach

Unlabeled Use Part of a multidrug regimen for *H. pylori* eradication to reduce the risk of duodenal ulcer recurrence; stress ulcer prophylaxis in critically-ill patients; symptomatic relief in gastritis

Pregnancy Risk Factor B

Pregnancy Considerations Adverse events have not been observed in animal reproduction studies; therefore, famotidine is classified as pregnancy category B. Famotidine crosses the placenta. An increased risk of congenital malformations or adverse events in the newborn has generally not been observed following maternal use of famotidine during pregnancy. Histamine H_2 antagonists have been evaluated for the treatment of gastroesophageal reflux disease (GERD), as well as gastric and duodenal ulcers, during pregnancy. Although if needed, famotidine is not the agent of choice. Histamine H_2 antagonists may be used for aspiration prophylaxis prior to cesarean delivery.

Lactation Enters breast milk/not recommended

Contraindications Hypersensitivity to famotidine, other H_2 antagonists, or any component of the formulation

Warnings/Precautions Modify dose in patients with moderate-to-severe renal impairment. Prolonged QT interval has been reported in patients with renal dysfunction. The FDA has received reports of torsade de pointes occurring with famotidine (Poluzzi, 2009). Relief of symptoms does not preclude the presence of a gastric malignancy. Reversible confusional states, usually clearing within 3-4 days after discontinuation, have been linked to use. Increased age (>50 years) and renal or hepatic impairment are thought to be associated. Multidose vials for injection contain benzyl alcohol.

OTC labeling: When used for self-medication, patients should be instructed not to use if they have difficulty swallowing, are vomiting blood, or have bloody or black stools. Not for use with other acid reducers.

Adverse Reactions **Note:** Agitation and vomiting have been reported in up to 14% of pediatric patients <1 year of age.

1% to 10%:

Central nervous system: Headache (5%), dizziness (1%)

Gastrointestinal: Diarrhea (2%), constipation (1%)

<1% (Limited to important or life-threatening): Abdominal discomfort, acne, agitation, agranulocytosis, allergic reaction, alopecia, anaphylaxis, angioedema, anorexia, anxiety, arrhythmia, arthralgia, AV block, bronchospasm, cholestatic jaundice, confusion, conjunctival injection, depression, dry skin, facial edema, fatigue, fever, flushing, hallucinations, hepatitis, injection site reactions, insomnia, interstitial pneumonia, leukopenia, libido decreased, liver function tests increased, muscle cramps, nausea, palpitation, pancytopenia, paresthesia, pruritus, QT-interval prolongation, rash, seizure, somnolence, Stevens-Johnson syndrome, taste disorder, tinnitus, thrombocytopenia, torsade de pointes, toxic epidermal necrolysis, urticaria, vomiting, weakness, xerostomia

Drug Interactions

Metabolism/Transport Effects None known.

Avoid Concomitant Use

Avoid concomitant use of Famotidine with any of the following: Delavirdine

Increased Effect/Toxicity

Famotidine may increase the levels/effects of: Dexmethylphenidate; Methylphenidate; Saquinavir; Varenicline

Decreased Effect

Famotidine may decrease the levels/effects of: Atazanavir; Cefditoren; Cefpodoxime; Cefuroxime; Dasatinib; Delavirdine; Erlotinib; Fosamprenavir; Gefitinib; Indinavir; Iron Salts; Itraconazole; Ketoconazole; Ketoconazole (Systemic); Mesalamine; Nelfinavir; Posaconazole; Rilpivirine

Ethanol/Nutrition/Herb Interactions

Ethanol: Avoid ethanol (may cause gastric mucosal irritation).

Food: Famotidine bioavailability may be increased if taken with food.

Stability

Oral:

Powder for oral suspension: Prior to mixing, dry powder should be stored at controlled room temperature of 25°C (77°F). Reconstituted oral suspension is stable for 30 days at room temperature; do not freeze.

Tablet: Store at controlled room temperature. Protect from moisture.

I.V.:

Solution for injection: Prior to use, store at 2°C to 8°C (36°F to 46°F). If solution freezes, allow to solubilize at controlled room temperature. May be stored at room temperature for up to 3 months (data on file [Bedford Laboratories, 2011]).

I.V. push: Dilute famotidine with NS (or another compatible solution) to a total of 5-10 mL (some centers also administer undiluted). Following preparation, solutions for I.V. push should be used immediately, or may be stored in refrigerator and used within 48 hours.

Infusion: Dilute with D_5W 100 mL or another compatible solution. Following preparation, the manufacturer states may be stored for up to 48 hours under refrigeration; however, solutions for infusion have been found to be physically and chemically stable for 7 days at room temperature.

Solution for injection, premixed bags: Store at controlled room temperature of 25°C (77°F); avoid excessive heat.

Mechanism of Action Competitive inhibition of histamine at H_2 receptors of the gastric parietal cells, which inhibits gastric acid secretion

Pharmacodynamics/Kinetics

Onset of action: Antisecretory effect: Oral: Within 1 hour; I.V.: Within 30 minutes

Peak effect: Antisecretory effect: Oral: Within 1-3 hours (dose-dependent)

Duration: Antisecretory effect: I.V., Oral: 10-12 hours

Absorption: Oral: Incompletely absorbed

Distribution: V_d:

Infants: 0-3 months: ~1.4-1.8 L/kg; >3-12 months: ~2.3 L/kg

Children: ~2 L/kg

Adults: ~1 L/kg

Protein binding: 15% to 20%

Metabolism: Minimal first-pass metabolism; forms one metabolite (S-oxide)

Bioavailability: Oral: 40% to 45%

Half-life elimination:

Infants: 0-3 months: ~8-10.5 hours; >3-12 months: ~4.5 hours

Children: 3.4 hours

Adults: 2.5-3.5 hours; prolonged with renal impairment; Oliguria: >20 hours

Time to peak, serum: Oral: ~1-3 hours

Excretion: Urine (25% to 30% [oral], 65% to 70% [I.V.] as unchanged drug)

Dosage

Children: Treatment duration and dose should be individualized

Peptic ulcer: 1-16 years:

Oral: 0.5 mg/kg/day at bedtime or divided twice daily (maximum dose: 40 mg/day); doses of up to 1 mg/kg/day have been used in clinical studies

I.V.: 0.25 mg/kg every 12 hours (maximum dose: 40 mg/day); doses of up to 0.5 mg/kg have been used in clinical studies

GERD: Oral:

<3 months: 0.5 mg/kg once daily

3-12 months: 0.5 mg/kg twice daily

1-16 years: 1 mg/kg/day divided twice daily (maximum dose: 40 mg twice daily); doses of up to 2 mg/kg/day have been used in clinical studies

Children ≥12 years and Adults: Heartburn, indigestion, sour stomach: OTC labeling: Oral: 10-20 mg every 12 hours; dose may be taken 15-60 minutes before eating foods known to cause heartburn

Adults:

Duodenal ulcer: Oral: Acute therapy: 40 mg/day at bedtime (or 20 mg twice daily) for 4-8 weeks; maintenance therapy: 20 mg/day at bedtime

Helicobacter pylori eradication (unlabeled use): Oral: 40 mg once daily; requires combination therapy with antibiotics

Gastric ulcer: Oral: Acute therapy: 40 mg/day at bedtime

Hypersecretory conditions: Oral: Initial: 20 mg every 6 hours, may increase in increments up to 160 mg every 6 hours

GERD: Oral: 20 mg twice daily for 6 weeks

Esophagitis and accompanying symptoms due to GERD: Oral: 20 mg or 40 mg twice daily for up to 12 weeks

Patients unable to take oral medication: I.V.: 20 mg every 12 hours

Dosing adjustment in renal impairment: Cl_{cr} <50 mL/minute: Manufacturer recommendation: Administer 50% of dose **or** increase the dosing interval to every 36-48 hours (to limit potential CNS adverse effects).

Dietary Considerations May be taken without regard to meals.

Administration
Oral: May administer with antacids.
Suspension: Shake vigorously before use. May be taken without regard to meals.
Tablet: May be taken without regard to meals.
I.V.:
I.V. push: Inject over at least 2 minutes.
Solution for infusion: Administer over 15-30 minutes.

Dosage Forms Excipient information presented when available (limited, particularly for generics); consult specific product labeling.
Infusion, premixed in NS [preservative free]: 20 mg (50 mL)
Injection, solution: 10 mg/mL (4 mL, 20 mL, 50 mL)
Injection, solution [preservative free]: 10 mg/mL (2 mL)
Powder for suspension, oral: 40 mg/5 mL (50 mL)
Pepcid®: 40 mg/5 mL (50 mL) [contains sodium benzoate; cherry-banana-mint flavor]
Tablet, oral: 10 mg, 20 mg, 40 mg
Heartburn Relief: 10 mg
Heartburn Relief Maximum Strength: 20 mg
Pepcid®: 20 mg, 40 mg
Pepcid® AC: 10 mg
Pepcid® AC Maximum Strength: 20 mg
Tablet, chewable, oral:
Pepcid® AC Maximum Strength: 20 mg [berries 'n' cream flavor]
Pepcid® AC Maximum Strength: 20 mg [cool mint flavor]

Extemporaneous Preparations An 8 mg/mL oral suspension may be made with tablets. Crush seventy 40 mg tablets in a mortar and reduce to a fine powder. Add small portions of sterile water and mix to a uniform paste. Mix while adding a 1:1 mixture of Ora-Plus® and Ora-Sweet® in incremental proportions to **almost** 350 mL; transfer to a calibrated bottle, rinse mortar with vehicle, and add quantity of vehicle sufficient to make 350 mL. Label "shake well". Stable for 95 days at room temperature.

Dentinger PJ, Swenson CF, and Anaizi NH, "Stability of Famotidine in an Extemporaneously Compounded Oral Liquid," *Am J Health Syst Pharm*, 2000, 57(14):1340-2.

◆ **Famotidine Omega (Can)** *see* Famotidine *on page 688*
◆ **Fampridine-SR** *see* Dalfampridine *on page 440*
◆ **Famvir®** *see* Famciclovir *on page 687*
◆ **Fanapt®** *see* Iloperidone *on page 868*
◆ **Fansidar® [DSC]** *see* Sulfadoxine and Pyrimethamine *on page 1601*
◆ **2F-ara-AMP** *see* Fludarabine *on page 721*
◆ **Fareston®** *see* Toremifene *on page 1711*
◆ **Faslodex®** *see* Fulvestrant *on page 770*
◆ **Fasturtec® (Can)** *see* Rasburicase *on page 1467*

Fat Emulsion (fat e MUL shun)

Brand Names: U.S. Intralipid®; Liposyn® III
Brand Names: Canada Intralipid®; Liposyn® II
Index Terms Intravenous Fat Emulsion
Pharmacologic Category Caloric Agent
Use Source of calories and essential fatty acids for patients requiring parenteral nutrition of extended duration; prevention and treatment of essential fatty acid deficiency (EFAD)
Unlabeled Use Local anesthetic-induced cardiac arrest unresponsive to conventional resuscitation
Pregnancy Risk Factor C
Dosage I.V.: **Note:** At the onset of therapy, the patient should be observed for any immediate allergic reactions.
Nutrition:
Premature infants: Initial dose: 0.25-0.5 g/kg/day, increase by 0.25-0.5 g/kg/day to a maximum of 3 g/kg/day depending on needs/nutritional goals; limit to 1 g/kg/day if on phototherapy; should be administered over 24 hours (A.S.P.E.N. guidelines)
Infants and Children: Initial dose: 0.5-1 g/kg/day, increase by 0.5 g/kg/day to a maximum of 3 g/kg/day depending on needs/nutritional goals; may administer over 24 hours (A.S.P.E.N. guidelines)
Note: Pediatric patients: Monitor triglycerides while receiving intralipids. If serum triglyceride levels >200 mg/dL, stop infusion and restart at 0.5-1g/kg/day. Intravenous heparin (1 unit/mL of parenteral nutrition) may enhance the clearance of lipid emulsions.
Adults: Initial dose: 1 g/kg/day, increase by 0.5-1 g/kg/day to a maximum of 2.5-3 g/kg/day
Prevention of essential fatty acid deficiency (EFAD): Adults: Administer 8% to 10% of total caloric intake as fat emulsion (may be higher in stressed patients with EFAD); may be given 2-3 times weekly to meet essential fatty acid requirements
Local anesthetic toxicity (unlabeled use): Adults: 20%: 1.5 mL/kg of lean body weight administered over 1 minute, followed immediately by an infusion of 0.25 mL/kg/minute. Continue chest compressions (lipid must circulate). Repeat bolus 1-2 times as needed for persistent asystole. Continue infusion until hemodynamic stability is restored. Increase the infusion rate to 0.5 mL/kg/minute if BP declines.

Additional Information Complete prescribing information for this medication should be consulted for additional detail.

Dosage Forms Excipient information presented when available (limited, particularly for generics); consult specific product labeling.
Injection, emulsion:
Intralipid®: 20% (100 mL, 250 mL, 500 mL, 1000 mL); 30% (500 mL) [contains aluminum, egg yolk phospholipid, soybean oil]
Liposyn® III: 10% (250 mL, 500 mL); 20% (250 mL, 500 mL); 30% (500 mL) [contains aluminum, egg yolk phospholipid, soybean oil]

◆ **Father John's® Plus [OTC]** *see* Chlorpheniramine, Phenylephrine, and Dextromethorphan *on page 346*
◆ **FazaClo®** *see* CloZAPine *on page 400*
◆ **5-FC** *see* Flucytosine *on page 720*
◆ **FC1157a** *see* Toremifene *on page 1711*
◆ **FE200486** *see* Degarelix *on page 466*

Febuxostat (feb UX oh stat)

Brand Names: U.S. Uloric®
Brand Names: Canada Uloric®
Index Terms TEI-6720; TMX-67
Pharmacologic Category Antigout Agent; Xanthine Oxidase Inhibitor
Use Chronic management of hyperuricemia in patients with gout
Pregnancy Risk Factor C
Pregnancy Considerations Animal studies have demonstrated increased neonatal mortality and reduction in weight gain, but not teratogenic effects. There are no adequate and well-controlled studies in pregnant women. Use during pregnancy only if potential benefit to the mother outweighs potential risk to the fetus.
Lactation Excretion in breast milk unknown/use caution
Contraindications Concurrent use with azathioprine or mercaptopurine

Canadian labeling: Additional contraindications (not in U.S. labeling): Hypersensitivity to febuxostat or any component of the formulation; concomitant administration with theophylline

Warnings/Precautions Administer concurrently with an NSAID or colchicine (up to 6 months) to prevent gout flare upon initiation of therapy. Do not use to treat asymptomatic or secondary hyperuricemia. Significant hepatic transaminase elevations (>3 x ULN), MI, stroke and cardiovascular deaths have been reported in controlled trials (causal relationship not established). Monitor patients for signs/symptoms of MI and stroke. Liver function tests should be monitored 2 and 4 months after initiation of therapy and then periodically. Use with caution in patients with severe hepatic impairment (Child-Pugh class C); not studied. Use with caution in patients with severe renal impairment (Cl_{cr} <30 mL/minute); insufficient data.

Adverse Reactions

1% to 10%:

Dermatologic: Rash (1% to 2%)

Hepatic: Liver function abnormalities (5% to 7%)

Neuromuscular & skeletal: Arthralgia (1%)

<1% (Limited to important or life-threatening): Aggression, agitation, alkaline phosphatase increased, alopecia, amylase increased, anaphylactic reaction, anaphylaxis, anemia, angina, angioedema, anorexia, anxiety, aPTT prolonged, atrial fibrillation/flutter, bicarbonate decreased, blurred vision, bruising, BUN increased, cardiac murmur, cerebrovascular accident, cholecystitis, cholelithiasis, constipation, CPK increased, creatinine increased, deafness, dehydration, depression, dermatitis, dermographism, diabetes mellitus, dyspepsia, dyspnea, ECG abnormal, eczema, edema, EEG abnormal, epistaxis, erectile dysfunction, flushing, gait disturbance, gastritis, gastroesophageal reflux, gingival pain, Guillain-Barré syndrome, gynecomastia, hair color change, hair growth abnormal, hematemesis, hematochezia, hematocrit decreased, hematuria, hemiparesis, hepatic steatosis, hepatitis, hepatomegaly, herpes zoster, hot flashes, hyperchlorhydria, hypercholesterolemia, hyperglycemia, hyperhidrosis, hyperkalemia, hyperlipidemia, hypernatremia, hypersensitivity, hyper/hypotension, hypertriglyceridemia, hypokalemia, idiopathic thrombocytopenic purpura, incontinence, influenza-like syndrome, joint swelling, lacunar infarction, LDH increased, lethargy, leukocytosis, leukopenia, libido decreased, lymphocytopenia, MCV increased, MI, migraine, mouth ulceration, muscle spasm/twitching, myalgia, nephrolithiasis, neutropenia, pain, palpitation, pancreatitis, pancytopenia, panic attack, paresthesia, peptic ulcer, personality change, petechiae, pharyngeal edema, photosensitivity, pollakiuria, proteinuria, PSA increased, psychotic behavior, PT prolonged, renal failure, respiratory infection, rhabdomyolysis, sinus bradycardia, skin/pigmentation discoloration, splenomegaly, Stevens-Johnson syndrome, stroke, tachycardia, taste altered, thrombocytopenia, TIA, tinnitus, tremor, TSH increased, tubulointerstitial nephritis, urinary tract infection, urine output decreased/increased, urticaria, vertigo, vomiting, weakness, weight gain/loss

Drug Interactions

Metabolism/Transport Effects None known.

Avoid Concomitant Use

Avoid concomitant use of Febuxostat with any of the following: AzaTHIOprine; Didanosine; Mercaptopurine

Increased Effect/Toxicity

Febuxostat may increase the levels/effects of: AzaTHIOprine; Didanosine; Mercaptopurine; Theophylline Derivatives

Decreased Effect There are no known significant interactions involving a decrease in effect.

Stability Store at 25°C (77°F); excursions permitted to 15°C to 30°C (59°F to 86°F). Protect from light.

Mechanism of Action Selectively inhibits xanthine oxidase, the enzyme responsible for the conversion of hypoxanthine to xanthine to uric acid thereby decreasing uric acid. At therapeutic concentration does not inhibit other enzymes involved in purine and pyrimidine synthesis.

Pharmacodynamics/Kinetics

Absorption: ≥49%

Distribution: V_{ss}: ~50 L

Protein binding: ~99%, primarily to albumin

Metabolism: Extensive conjugation via uridine diphosphate glucuronosyltransferases (UGTs) 1A1, 1A3, 1A9, and 2B7 and oxidation via cytochrome P450 (CYP) 1A2, 2C8, and 2C9 as well as non-P450 enzymes. Oxidation leads to formation of active metabolites (67M-1, 67M-2, 67M-4)

Half-life elimination: ~5-8 hours

Time to peak, plasma: 1-1.5 hours

Excretion: Urine (~49% mostly as metabolites, 3% as unchanged drug); feces (~45% mostly as metabolites, 12% as unchanged drug)

Dosage Oral: Adults: **Note:** It is recommended to take an NSAID or colchicine with initiation of therapy and may continue for up to 6 months to help prevent gout flares. If a gout flare occurs, febuxostat does not need to be discontinued.

U.S. labeling: Initial: 40 mg once daily; may increase to 80 mg once daily in patients who do not achieve a serum uric acid level <6 mg/dL after 2 weeks

Canadian labeling: 80 mg once daily

Dosing adjustment in renal impairment:

Mild-to-moderate impairment (Cl_{cr} 30-89 mL/minute): No adjustment needed

Severe impairment (Cl_{cr} <30 mL/minute): Insufficient data; use caution (use not recommended in the Canadian labeling)

Dialysis: Not studied (use not recommended in the Canadian labeling)

Dosing adjustment in hepatic impairment:

Mild-to-moderate impairment (Child-Pugh classes A and B): No adjustment needed

Severe impairment (Child-Pugh class C): Not studied; use caution (use not recommended in the Canadian labeling)

Dietary Considerations Take with or without meals or antacids.

Administration Administer with or without meals or antacids.

Monitoring Parameters Liver function tests 2 and 4 months after initiation and then periodically, serum uric acid levels (as early as 2 weeks after initiation)

Reference Range Uric acid, serum: An increase occurs during childhood

Adults:

Males: 3.4-7 mg/dL or slightly more

Females: 2.4-6 mg/dL or slightly more

Target: <6 mg/dL

Values >7 mg/dL are sometimes arbitrarily regarded as hyperuricemia, but there is no sharp line between normals on the one hand, and the serum uric acid of those with clinical gout. Normal ranges cannot be adjusted for purine ingestion, but high purine diet increases uric acid. Uric acid may be increased with body size, exercise, and stress.

Dosage Forms Excipient information presented when available (limited, particularly for generics); consult specific product labeling.

Tablet, oral:

Uloric®: 40 mg, 80 mg

◆ **Feiba NF** *see* Anti-inhibitor Coagulant Complex *on page 130*

◆ **Feiba VH [DSC]** *see* Anti-inhibitor Coagulant Complex *on page 130*

Felbamate (FEL ba mate)

Brand Names: U.S. Felbatol®

Pharmacologic Category Anticonvulsant, Miscellaneous

Additional Appendix Information

Anticonvulsant Drugs of Choice *on page 1873*

Use Not as a first-line antiepileptic treatment; only in those patients who respond inadequately to alternative treatments and whose epilepsy is so severe that a substantial risk of aplastic anemia and/or liver failure is deemed acceptable in light of the benefits conferred by its use. Patient must be fully advised of risk and provide signed written informed consent. Felbamate can be used as either monotherapy or adjunctive therapy in the treatment of partial seizures (with and without generalization) and in adults with epilepsy. Used as adjunctive therapy in the treatment of partial and generalized seizures associated with Lennox-Gastaut syndrome in children.

Pregnancy Risk Factor C

Prescribing and Access Restrictions A patient "informed consent" form should be completed and signed by the patient and physician. Copies are available from MEDA Pharmaceuticals by calling 800-526-3840.

Medication Guide Available Yes

Dosage Anticonvulsant:

Monotherapy: Children >14 years and Adults:

Initial: 1200 mg/day in divided doses 3 or 4 times/day; titrate previously untreated patients under close clinical supervision, increasing the dosage in 600 mg increments every 2 weeks to 2400 mg/day based on clinical response and thereafter to 3600 mg/day as clinically indicated

Conversion to monotherapy: Initiate at 1200 mg/day in divided doses 3 or 4 times/day, reduce the dosage of the concomitant anticonvulsant(s) by 20% to 33% at the initiation of felbamate therapy; at week 2, increase the felbamate dosage to 2400 mg/day while reducing the dosage of the other anticonvulsant(s) up to an additional 33% of their original dosage; at week 3, increase the felbamate dosage up to 3600 mg/day and continue to reduce the dosage of the other anticonvulsant(s) as clinically indicated

Adjunctive therapy: **Note:** Dose of concomitant carbamazepine, phenobarbital, phenytoin, or valproic acid should be decreased by 20% to 33% when initiating felbamate therapy. Further dosage reductions may be necessary as dose of felbamate is increased.

Children 2-14 years with Lennox-Gastaut syndrome: Initial: 15 mg/kg/day in divided doses 3 or 4 times/day; may increase once per week by 15 mg/kg/day increments up to 45 mg/kg/day in divided doses 3 or 4 times/day.

Children >14 years and Adults: Initial: 1200 mg/day in divided doses 3 or 4 times/day; may increase once per week by 1200 mg/day increments up to 3600 mg/day in divided doses 3 or 4 times/day.

Dosage adjustment in renal impairment: Use caution; reduce initial and maintenance doses by 50% (half-life prolonged by 9-15 hours)

Additional Information Complete prescribing information for this medication should be consulted for additional detail.

Dosage Forms Excipient information presented when available (limited, particularly for generics); consult specific product labeling.

Suspension, oral: 600 mg/5 mL (240 mL, 473 mL)

Felbatol®: 600 mg/5 mL (240 mL, 960 mL)

Tablet, oral: 400 mg, 600 mg

Felbatol®: 400 mg, 600 mg [scored]

◆ **Felbatol®** *see* Felbamate *on page 692*

◆ **Feldene®** *see* Piroxicam *on page 1361*

Felodipine (fe LOE di peen)

Brand Names: Canada Plendil®; Renedil®; Sandoz-Felodipine

Index Terms Plendil

Pharmacologic Category Calcium Channel Blocker; Calcium Channel Blocker, Dihydropyridine

Additional Appendix Information

Calcium Channel Blockers *on page 1887*

Use Treatment of hypertension

Unlabeled Use Pediatric hypertension

Pregnancy Risk Factor C

Pregnancy Considerations Potentially, calcium channel blockers may prolong labor. There are no adequate or well-controlled studies in pregnant women.

Lactation Excretion in breast milk unknown/not recommended

Contraindications Hypersensitivity to felodipine, any component of the formulation, or other calcium channel blocker

Warnings/Precautions Increased angina and/or MI has occurred with initiation or dosage titration of dihydropyridine calcium channel blockers, reflex tachycardia may occur resulting in angina and/or MI in patients with obstructive coronary disease especially in the absence of concurrent beta-blockade. Use with extreme caution in patients with severe aortic stenosis. Use caution in patients with heart failure and/or hypertrophic cardiomyopathy with outflow tract obstruction. Elderly patients and patients with hepatic impairment should start off with a lower dose. Peripheral edema (dose dependent) is the most common side effect (occurs within 2-3 weeks of starting therapy). Symptomatic hypotension with or without syncope can rarely occur; blood pressure must be lowered at a rate appropriate for the patient's clinical condition. Dosage titration should occur after 14 days on a given dose.

Adverse Reactions

>10%: Central nervous system: Headache (11% to 15%)

2% to 10%: Cardiovascular: Peripheral edema (2% to 17%), tachycardia (0.4% to 2.5%), flushing (4% to 7%)

<1% (Limited to important or life-threatening): Angina, angioedema, anxiety, arrhythmia, CHF, CVA, libido decreased, depression, dizziness, gingival hyperplasia, dyspnea, dysuria, gynecomastia, hypotension, impotence, insomnia, irritability, leukocytoclastic vasculitis, MI, nervousness, paresthesia, somnolence, syncope, urticaria, vomiting

Drug Interactions

Metabolism/Transport Effects Substrate of CYP3A4 (major); **Note:** Assignment of Major/Minor substrate status based on clinically relevant drug interaction potential; **Inhibits** CYP2C8 (moderate), CYP2C9 (weak), CYP2D6 (weak), CYP3A4 (weak)

Avoid Concomitant Use

Avoid concomitant use of Felodipine with any of the following: Conivaptan; Pimozide

Increased Effect/Toxicity

Felodipine may increase the levels/effects of: Amifostine; Antihypertensives; Beta-Blockers; Calcium Channel Blockers (Nondihydropyridine); CYP2C8 Substrates; Fosphenytoin; Hypotensive Agents; Magnesium Salts; Neuromuscular-Blocking Agents (Nondepolarizing); Nitroprusside; Phenytoin; Pimozide; RiTUXimab; Tacrolimus; Tacrolimus (Systemic)

The levels/effects of Felodipine may be increased by: Alpha1-Blockers; Antifungal Agents (Azole Derivatives, Systemic); Calcium Channel Blockers (Nondihydropyridine); Cimetidine; Conivaptan; CycloSPORINE;

CycloSPORINE (Systemic); CYP3A4 Inhibitors (Moderate); CYP3A4 Inhibitors (Strong); Dasatinib; Diazoxide; Fluconazole; Grapefruit Juice; Herbs (Hypotensive Properties); Macrolide Antibiotics; Magnesium Salts; MAO Inhibitors; Pentoxifylline; Phosphodiesterase 5 Inhibitors; Prostacyclin Analogues; Protease Inhibitors

Decreased Effect

Felodipine may decrease the levels/effects of: Clopidogrel

The levels/effects of Felodipine may be decreased by: Barbiturates; Calcium Salts; CarBAMazepine; CYP3A4 Inducers (Strong); Deferasirox; Herbs (CYP3A4 Inducers); Herbs (Hypertensive Properties); Methylphenidate; Nafcillin; Rifamycin Derivatives; Tocilizumab; Yohimbine

Ethanol/Nutrition/Herb Interactions

Ethanol: Increases felodipine's absorption; watch for a greater hypotensive effect.

Food: Compared to a fasted state, felodipine peak plasma concentrations are increased up to twofold when taken after a meal high in fat or carbohydrates. Grapefruit juice similarly increases felodipine C_{max} by twofold. Increased therapeutic and vasodilator side effects, including severe hypotension and myocardial ischemia, may occur. May be taken with a small meal that is low in fat and carbohydrates; avoid grapefruit juice during therapy.

Herb/Nutraceutical: St John's wort may decrease felodipine levels. Avoid dong quai if using for hypertension (has estrogenic activity). Avoid ephedra, yohimbe, ginseng (may worsen hypertension). Avoid garlic (may have increased antihypertensive effect).

Mechanism of Action Inhibits calcium ions from entering the "slow channels" or select voltage-sensitive areas of vascular smooth muscle and myocardium during depolarization, producing a relaxation of coronary vascular smooth muscle and coronary vasodilation; increases myocardial oxygen delivery in patients with vasospastic angina

Pharmacodynamics/Kinetics

Onset of action: Antihypertensive: 2-5 hours

Duration of antihypertensive effect: 24 hours

Absorption: 100%; Absolute: 20% due to first-pass effect

Protein binding: >99%

Metabolism: Hepatic; CYP3A4 substrate (major); extensive first-pass effect

Half-life elimination: Immediate release: 11-16 hours

Excretion: Urine (70% as metabolites); feces 10%

Dosage Oral: Hypertension:

Children (unlabeled use): Initial: 2.5 mg once daily; maximum: 10 mg/day

Adults: Oral: 2.5-10 mg once daily; usual initial dose: 5 mg; increase by 5 mg at 2-week intervals, as needed, to a maximum of 20 mg/day

Usual dose range (JNC 7) for hypertension: 2.5-20 mg once daily

Elderly: Consider lower initial doses (eg, 2.5 mg once daily) and titrate to response (Aronow, 2011)

Dosing adjustment/comments in hepatic impairment: Initial: 2.5 mg/day; monitor blood pressure

Dietary Considerations May be taken with a small meal that is low in fat and carbohydrates.

Administration Swallow tablet whole; tablet should not be divided, crushed, or chewed. May be administered without food or with a small meal that is low in fat and carbohydrates.

Additional Information Felodipine maintains renal and mesenteric blood flow during hemorrhagic shock in animals.

Dosage Forms Excipient information presented when available (limited, particularly for generics); consult specific product labeling.

Tablet, extended release, oral: 2.5 mg, 5 mg, 10 mg

- **Femara®** *see* Letrozole *on page 986*
- **Femcon® Fe** *see* Ethinyl Estradiol and Norethindrone *on page 660*
- **femhrt®** *see* Ethinyl Estradiol and Norethindrone *on page 660*
- **FemHRT® (Can)** *see* Ethinyl Estradiol and Norethindrone *on page 660*
- **femhrt® Lo** *see* Ethinyl Estradiol and Norethindrone *on page 660*
- **Femilax™ [OTC]** *see* Bisacodyl *on page 219*
- **Femiron® [OTC]** *see* Ferrous Fumarate *on page 706*
- **Fem-Prin® [OTC]** *see* Acetaminophen, Aspirin, and Caffeine *on page 32*
- **Femring®** *see* Estradiol (Systemic) *on page 627*
- **Femstat® One (Can)** *see* Butoconazole *on page 256*
- **Femtrace®** *see* Estradiol (Systemic) *on page 627*
- **Fenesin DM IR [OTC]** *see* Guaifenesin and Dextromethorphan *on page 810*
- **Fenesin IR [OTC]** *see* GuaiFENesin *on page 809*
- **Fenesin PE IR** *see* Guaifenesin and Phenylephrine *on page 812*

Fenofibrate (fen oh FYE brate)

Brand Names: U.S. Antara®; Fenoglide®; Lipofen®; Lofibra®; TriCor®; Triglide®

Brand Names: Canada Apo-Feno-Micro®; Apo-Feno-Super®; Apo-Fenofibrate®; Dom-Fenofibrate Micro; Feno-Micro-200; Fenofibrate Micro; Fenofibrate-S; Fenomax; Lipidil EZ®; Lipidil Micro®; Lipidil Supra®; Mylan-Fenofibrate Micro; Novo-Fenofibrate; Novo-Fenofibrate Micronized; Novo-Fenofibrate-S; Nu-Fenofibrate; PHL-Fenofibrate Micro; PHL-Fenofibrate Supra; PMS-Fenofibrate Micro; PRO-Feno-Super; ratio-Fenofibrate MC; Riva-Fenofibrate Micro; Sandoz-Fenofibrate S

Index Terms Procetofene; Proctofene

Pharmacologic Category Antilipemic Agent, Fibric Acid

Additional Appendix Information

Hyperlipidemia Management *on page 1996*

Use Adjunct to dietary therapy for the treatment of adults with elevations of serum triglyceride levels (types IV and V hyperlipidemia); adjunct to dietary therapy for the reduction of low density lipoprotein cholesterol (LDL-C), total cholesterol (total-C), triglycerides, and apolipoprotein B (apo B), and to increase high density lipoprotein cholesterol (HDL-C) in adult patients with primary hypercholesterolemia or mixed dyslipidemia (Fredrickson types IIa and IIb)

Pregnancy Risk Factor C

Pregnancy Considerations Animal studies have shown embryocidal and teratogenic effect. There are no adequate and well-controlled studies in pregnant women. Use should be avoided, if possible, in pregnant women since the neonatal glucuronide conjugation pathways are immature.

Lactation Excretion in breast milk unknown/not recommended

Contraindications Hypersensitivity to fenofibrate or any component of the formulation; hepatic dysfunction including primary biliary cirrhosis and unexplained persistent liver function abnormalities; severe renal dysfunction; pre-existing gallbladder disease; breast-feeding (only Fenoglide®)

Canadian labeling: Additional contraindications (not in U.S. labeling): Pregnancy; breast-feeding; known photoallergy or phototoxic reaction during treatment with fibrates or ketoprofen; allergy to soya lecithin or peanut or arachis oil

Warnings/Precautions Secondary causes of hyperlipidemia should be ruled out prior to therapy. Hepatic transaminases can become significantly elevated (dose-related); hepatocellular, chronic active, and cholestatic hepatitis have been reported. Regular monitoring of liver function tests is required. Increases in serum creatinine (>2 mg/dL) have been observed with use; monitor renal function in patients with renal impairment and consider monitoring patients with increased risk for developing renal impairment. May cause cholelithiasis. Use with caution in patient taking oral anticoagulants (eg, warfarin); adjustments in anticoagulation therapy may be required. Use caution with HMG-CoA reductase inhibitors (may lead to myopathy, rhabdomyolysis). In combination with HMG-CoA reductase inhibitors, fenofibrate is generally regarded as safer than gemfibrozil due to limited pharmacokinetic interaction with statins. Therapy should be withdrawn if an adequate response is not obtained after 2-3 months of therapy at the maximal daily dose. The occurrence of pancreatitis may represent a failure of efficacy in patients with severely elevated triglycerides. May cause mild-to-moderate decreases in hemoglobin, hematocrit, and WBC upon initiation of therapy which usually stabilizes with long-term therapy. Agranulocytosis and thrombocytopenia have rarely been reported. Periodic monitoring of blood counts is recommended during the first year of therapy.

Rare hypersensitivity reactions may occur. Use has been associated with pulmonary embolism (PE) and deep vein thrombosis (DVT). Use with caution in patients with risk factors for VTE. Dose adjustment is required for renal impairment and may be required for elderly patients.

Adverse Reactions

>10%: Hepatic: Liver function tests increased (dose related; 3% to 13%)

1% to 10%:

Central nervous system: Headache (3%)

Gastrointestinal: Abdominal pain (5%), constipation (2%), nausea (2%)

Neuromuscular & skeletal: Back pain (3%), CPK increased (3%)

Respiratory: Respiratory disorder (6%), rhinitis (2%)

Postmarketing and/or case reports (limited to important or life-threatening): Abnormal vision, agranulocytosis, alkaline phosphatase decreased, allergic reaction, alopecia, amblyopia, anemia, angina pectoris, anorexia, anxiety, appetite increased, arrhythmia, arthralgia, arthritis, arthrosis, asthma, atrial fibrillation, bronchitis, bruising, bursitis, cataract, cholecystitis, cholelithiasis, cholestatic hepatitis, cirrhosis, colitis, conjunctivitis, contact dermatitis, cough, creatinine increased, cyst, cystitis, deep venous thrombosis, diabetes mellitus, diarrhea, dizziness, dyspepsia, dyspnea, dysuria, edema, electrocardiogram abnormality, eosinophilia, esophagitis, extrasystoles, fatty liver deposits, fever, flatulence, gastritis, gastroenteritis, gout, gynecomastia, hepatitis, herpes simplex, herpes zoster, hyper-/hypotension, hypersensitivity reaction, hypertonia, hyperuricemia, hypoglycemia, infection, kidney function abnormality, leg cramps, leukopenia, libido decreased, lymphadenopathy, maculopapular rash, malaise, MI, migraine, myalgia, myasthenia, myopathy, myositis, neuralgia, pain, palpitation, pancreatitis, paresthesia, peptic ulcer, peripheral edema, photosensitivity reaction, pneumonia, pregnancy (unintended), prostate disorder, pruritus, pulmonary embolus, rash, rectal hemorrhage, refraction disorder, rhabdomyolysis, skin ulcer, Stevens-Johnson syndrome, tachycardia, tenosynovitis, thrombocytopenia, toxic epidermal necrolysis, urea increased, urinary frequency, urolithiasis, urticaria, vaginal moniliasis, vasodilatation, vertigo, vomiting, weakness, weight gain/loss, xerostomia

Drug Interactions

Metabolism/Transport Effects **Substrate** of CYP3A4 (minor); **Note:** Assignment of Major/Minor substrate status based on clinically relevant drug interaction potential; **Inhibits** CYP2A6 (weak), CYP2C8 (weak), CYP2C9 (weak)

Avoid Concomitant Use There are no known interactions where it is recommended to avoid concomitant use.

Increased Effect/Toxicity

Fenofibrate may increase the levels/effects of: Colchicine; Ezetimibe; HMG-CoA Reductase Inhibitors; Sulfonylureas; Vitamin K Antagonists; Warfarin

The levels/effects of Fenofibrate may be increased by: Conivaptan; CycloSPORINE; CycloSPORINE (Systemic)

Decreased Effect

Fenofibrate may decrease the levels/effects of: Chenodiol; CycloSPORINE; CycloSPORINE (Systemic); Ursodiol

The levels/effects of Fenofibrate may be decreased by: Bile Acid Sequestrants; Tocilizumab

Stability Store at 15°C to 30°C (59°F to 86°F). Protect from light and moisture. Store tablets in moisture-protective container.

Mechanism of Action Fenofibric acid, an agonist for the nuclear transcription factor peroxisome proliferator-activated receptor-alpha (PPAR-alpha), downregulates apoprotein C-III (an inhibitor of lipoprotein lipase) and upregulates the synthesis of apolipoprotein A-I, fatty acid transport protein, and lipoprotein lipase resulting in an increase in VLDL catabolism, fatty acid oxidation, and elimination of triglyceride-rich particles; as a result of a decrease in VLDL levels, total plasma triglycerides are reduced by 30% to 60%; modest increase in HDL occurs in some hypertriglyceridemic patients.

Pharmacodynamics/Kinetics

Absorption: Increased when taken with meals

Distribution: Widely to most tissues

Protein binding: >99%

Metabolism: Tissue and plasma via esterases to active form, fenofibric acid; undergoes inactivation by glucuronidation hepatically or renally

Half-life elimination: Fenofibric acid: Mean: 20 hours (range: 10-35 hours)

Time to peak: 3-8 hours

Excretion: Urine (60% as metabolites); feces (25%); hemodialysis has no effect on removal of fenofibric acid from plasma

Dosage Oral:

Adults:

Hypertriglyceridemia: Initial:

Antara® (micronized): 43-130 mg/day; maximum dose: 130 mg/day

Fenoglide®: 40-120 mg/day; maximum dose: 120 mg/day

Lipidil EZ® [CAN; not available in U.S.]: 145 mg/day; maximum dose: 145 mg/day

Lipidil Micro® [CAN; not available in U.S.]: 200 mg/day; maximum dose: 200 mg/day

Lipidil Supra® [CAN; not available in U.S.]: 160 mg/day; maximum dose: 200 mg/day

Lipofen®: 50-150 mg/day; maximum dose: 150 mg/day

Lofibra® (micronized): 67-200 mg/day with meals; maximum dose: 200 mg/day

Lofibra® (tablets): 54-160 mg/day; maximum dose: 160 mg/day

TriCor®: 48-145 mg/day; maximum dose: 145 mg/day

Triglide®: 50-160 mg/day; maximum dose: 160 mg/day

Hypercholesterolemia or mixed hyperlipidemia:
Antara® (micronized): 130 mg/day
Fenoglide®: 120 mg/day
Lipidil EZ® [CAN; not available in U.S.]: 145 mg/day; maximum dose: 145 mg/day
Lipidil Micro® [CAN; not available in U.S.]: 200 mg/day; maximum dose: 200 mg/day
Lipidil Supra® [CAN; not available in U.S.]: 160 mg/day; maximum dose: 200 mg/day
Lipofen®: 150 mg/day
Lofibra® (micronized): 200 mg/day
Lofibra® (tablets): 160 mg/day
TriCor®: 145 mg/day
Triglide®: 160 mg/day

Elderly: Initial:
Antara® (micronized): 43 mg/day
Fenoglide®: Adjust dosage based on creatinine clearance
Lipidil EZ® [CAN; not available in U.S.]: 48 mg/day
Lipidil Micro® [CAN; not available in U.S.]: Adjust dosage based on creatinine clearance
Lipidil Supra® [CAN; not available in U.S.]: Adjust dosage based on creatinine clearance
Lipofen®: 50 mg/day
Lofibra® (micronized): 67 mg/day
Lofibra® (tablets): 54 mg/day
TriCor®: Adjust dosage based on creatinine clearance
Triglide®: 50 mg/day

Dosage adjustment/interval in renal impairment: Monitor renal function and lipid panel before adjusting. Decrease dose or increase dosing interval for patients with renal failure: **Note:** Use in severe renal impairment is contraindicated (see specific product labeling):
Antara® (micronized): Initiate at 43 mg/day in patients with renal impairment
Fenoglide®:
Cl_{cr} 31-80 mL/minute: Initiate at 40 mg/day
Cl_{cr} ≤30 mL/minute: Avoid use
Lipidil EZ® [CAN; not available in U.S.]: Cl_{cr} ≥20-50 mL/minute: Initiate at 48 mg/day
Lipidil Micro® [CAN; not available in U.S.]: Cl_{cr} ≥20-100 mL/minute: Initiate at 67 mg/day; **Note:** Lipidil Micro® 67 mg capsules are discontinued in Canada. Micronized formulation at this dosage strength is available through other manufacturers in Canada.
Lipidil Supra® [CAN; not available in U.S.]: Cl_{cr} ≥20-100 mL/minute: Initiate at 100 mg/day
Lipofen®: Initiate at 50 mg/day in patients with renal impairment
Lofibra® (micronized): Initiate at 67 mg/day in patients with renal impairment
Lofibra® (tablets):
Cl_{cr} 31-80 mL/minute: Initiate at 54 mg/day
Cl_{cr} ≤30 mL/minute: Avoid use
TriCor®:
Cl_{cr} 31-80 mL/minute: Initiate at 48 mg/day
Cl_{cr} ≤30 mL/minute: Avoid use
Triglide®: Initiate at 50 mg/day in patients with renal impairment

Dietary Considerations
Fenoglide®, Lofibra® (capsules [micronized] and tablets), Lipofen®: Take with meals.
Antara®, TriCor®, Triglide®: May be taken with or without food.
Canadian products [not available in U.S.]:
Lipidil Micro®, Lipidil Supra®: Take with meals.
Lipidil EZ®: May be taken with or without food.

Administration 6-8 weeks of therapy is required to determine efficacy.
Fenoglide®, Lofibra® (capsules [micronized] and tablets), Lipofen®: Administer with meals.
Antara®, TriCor®: May be administered with or without food.
Triglide®: Do not consume chipped or broken tablets. May be administered with or without food.
Canadian products [not available in U.S.]:
Lipidil Micro®, Lipidil Supra®: Administer with meals.
Lipidil EZ®: May be administered with or without food.

Monitoring Parameters Periodic blood counts during first year of therapy. Total cholesterol, LDL-C, triglycerides, and HDL-C should be measured periodically; if only marginal changes are noted in 6-8 weeks, the drug should be discontinued. Monitor LFTs regularly and discontinue therapy if levels remain >3 times normal limits. Monitor renal function in patients with renal impairment or in those at increased risk for developing renal impairment.

Dosage Forms Excipient information presented when available (limited, particularly for generics); consult specific product labeling.
Capsule, oral:
Lipofen®: 50 mg, 150 mg
Capsule, oral [micronized]: 67 mg, 134 mg, 200 mg
Antara®: 43 mg, 130 mg
Lofibra®: 67 mg, 134 mg, 200 mg
Tablet, oral: 54 mg, 160 mg
Fenoglide®: 40 mg, 120 mg
Lofibra®: 54 mg, 160 mg
TriCor®: 48 mg, 145 mg [contains soybean lecithin]
Triglide®: 50 mg, 160 mg [contains egg lecithin]

◆ **Fenofibrate Micro (Can)** *see* Fenofibrate *on page* 693
◆ **Fenofibrate-S (Can)** *see* Fenofibrate *on page* 693

Fenofibric Acid (fen oh FYE brik AS id)

Brand Names: U.S. Fibricor®; TriLipix®
Index Terms ABT-335; Choline Fenofibrate
Pharmacologic Category Antilipemic Agent, Fibric Acid
Use Adjunct to dietary therapy for the treatment of severely elevated serum triglyceride levels; adjunct to dietary therapy for the reduction of low density lipoprotein cholesterol (LDL-C), total cholesterol (total-C), triglycerides, and apolipoprotein B (apo B) and to increase high density lipoprotein cholesterol (HDL-C) in patients with primary hypercholesterolemia or mixed dyslipidemia

TriLipix™ is also indicated as adjunct to dietary therapy concomitantly with a statin to reduce triglyceride levels and increase HDL-C levels in patients with mixed dyslipidemia and coronary heart disease (CHD) or at risk for CHD

Pregnancy Risk Factor C
Medication Guide Available Yes
Dosage Oral:
Adults:
Mixed dyslipidemia (coadministered with a statin): TriLipix™: 135 mg once daily (maximum: 135 mg/day)
Hypertriglyceridemia:
Fibricor®: Initial: 35-105 mg once daily; Maintenance: Individualize according to patient response (maximum: 105 mg/day)
TriLipix™: Initial: 45-135 mg once daily; Maintenance: Individualize according to patient response (maximum: 135 mg/day)
Primary hypercholesterolemia or mixed dyslipidemia:
Fibricor®: 105 mg once daily (maximum: 105 mg/day)
TriLipix™: 135 mg once daily (maximum: 135 mg/day)
Elderly: Dosage based on renal function

Dosage adjustment/interval in renal impairment:
Mild-to-moderate impairment (Cl_{cr} 30-80 mL/minute): Initial: Fibricor®: 35 mg once daily or TriLipix™: 45 mg once daily; only increase once effects on lipids and renal function evaluated
Severe impairment (Cl_{cr} <30 mL/minute; with or without dialysis): Contraindicated

Additional Information Complete prescribing information for this medication should be consulted for additional detail.

Dosage Forms Excipient information presented when available (limited, particularly for generics); consult specific product labeling.
Capsule, delayed release, oral:
TriLipix®: 45 mg, 135 mg
Tablet, oral: 35 mg, 105 mg
Fibricor®: 35 mg, 105 mg

◆ **Fenoglide®** *see* Fenofibrate *on page 693*

Fenoldopam (fe NOL doe pam)

Brand Names: U.S. Corlopam®
Brand Names: Canada Corlopam®
Index Terms Fenoldopam Mesylate
Pharmacologic Category Dopamine Agonist
Additional Appendix Information
Hypertension *on page 2001*

Use Treatment of severe hypertension (up to 48 hours in adults), including in patients with renal compromise; short-term (up to 4 hours) blood pressure reduction in pediatric patients

Pregnancy Risk Factor B

Pregnancy Considerations Fetal harm was not observed in animal studies; however, safety and efficacy have not been established for use during pregnancy. Use during pregnancy only if clearly needed.

Lactation Excretion in breast milk unknown/use caution

Contraindications There are no contraindications listed within the manufacturer's approved labeling.

Warnings/Precautions Use with caution in patients with open-angle glaucoma or intraocular hypertension; fenoldopam causes a dose-dependent increase in intraocular pressure. Dose-related tachycardia can occur, especially at infusion rates >0.1 mcg/kg/minute. Use with extreme caution in patients with obstructive coronary disease or ongoing angina pectoris; can increase myocardial oxygen demand due to tachycardia leading to angina pectoris. Serum potassium concentrations <3 mEq/L were observed within 6 hours of fenoldopam initiation; monitor potassium concentrations appropriately. Use with caution in patients with increased intracranial pressure; use has not been studied in this population. For continuous infusion only (no bolus doses). Contains sulfites; may cause allergic reaction in susceptible individuals.

Adverse Reactions
≥5%:
Cardiovascular: Cutaneous flushing, hypotension
Central nervous system: Headache
Gastrointestinal: Nausea
<5%:
Cardiovascular: Angina, bradycardia, chest pain, extrasystoles, heart failure, MI, palpitation, postural hypotension, ST-T abnormalities, T-wave inversion, tachycardia
Central nervous system: Anxiety, dizziness, fever, insomnia
Endocrine & metabolic: Hyperglycemia, hypokalemia, LDH increased
Gastrointestinal: Abdominal pain/fullness, constipation, diarrhea, vomiting
Genitourinary: Urinary tract infection
Hematologic: Bleeding, leukocytosis
Hepatic: Transaminases increased
Local: Injection site reactions
Neuromuscular & skeletal: Back pain, limb cramps
Ocular: Intraocular pressure increased
Renal: BUN increased, creatinine increased, oliguria
Respiratory: Dyspnea, nasal congestion
Miscellaneous: Diaphoresis

Drug Interactions
Metabolism/Transport Effects None known.
Avoid Concomitant Use There are no known interactions where it is recommended to avoid concomitant use.
Increased Effect/Toxicity There are no known significant interactions involving an increase in effect.
Decreased Effect There are no known significant interactions involving a decrease in effect.

Stability Store at 2°C to 30°C (35°F to 86°F). Must be diluted prior to infusion. Final dilution for children is 60 mcg/mL and for adults is 40 mcg/mL. Following dilution, store at room temperature and use solution within 24 hours.

Mechanism of Action A selective postsynaptic dopamine agonist (D_1-receptors) which exerts hypotensive effects by decreasing peripheral vasculature resistance with increased renal blood flow, diuresis, and natriuresis; 6 times as potent as dopamine in producing renal vasodilatation; has minimal adrenergic effects

Pharmacodynamics/Kinetics
Onset of action: I.V.: 10 minutes
Duration: I.V.: 1 hour
Distribution: V_d: 0.6 L/kg
Half-life elimination: I.V.: Children: 3-5 minutes; Adults: ~5 minutes
Metabolism: Hepatic via methylation, glucuronidation, and sulfation; the 8-sulfate metabolite may have some activity; extensive first-pass effect
Excretion: Urine (90%); feces (10%)

Dosage I.V.: Hypertension, severe:
Children: Initial: 0.2 mcg/kg/minute; may be increased to dosages of 0.3-0.5 mcg/kg/minute every 20-30 minutes (maximum dose: 0.8 mcg/kg/minute); limited to short-term (4 hours) use
Adults: Initial: 0.03-0.1 mcg/kg/minute (associated with less reflex tachycardia); may be increased in increments of 0.05-0.1 mcg/kg/minute every 15 minutes until target blood pressure is reached; the maximal infusion rate reported in clinical studies was 1.6 mcg/kg/minute
Dosing adjustment in renal impairment: No dosage adjustment required; the effects of hemodialysis on fenoldopam have not been evaluated.
Dosing adjustment in hepatic impairment: No dosage adjustment required.

Administration For continuous I.V. infusion only.

Monitoring Parameters Blood pressure, heart rate, ECG; serum potassium concentrations (eg, every 6 hours)

Dosage Forms Excipient information presented when available (limited, particularly for generics); consult specific product labeling.
Injection, solution: 10 mg/mL (1 mL, 2 mL)
Corlopam®: 10 mg/mL (1 mL, 2 mL) [contains propylene glycol, sodium metabisulfite]

◆ **Fenoldopam Mesylate** *see* Fenoldopam *on page 696*
◆ **Fenomax (Can)** *see* Fenofibrate *on page 693*
◆ **Feno-Micro-200 (Can)** *see* Fenofibrate *on page 693*

Fenoprofen (fen oh PROE fen)

Brand Names: U.S. Nalfon®
Brand Names: Canada Nalfon®
Index Terms Fenoprofen Calcium

Pharmacologic Category Nonsteroidal Anti-inflammatory Drug (NSAID), Oral

Use Symptomatic treatment of acute and chronic rheumatoid arthritis and osteoarthritis; relief of mild-to-moderate pain

Pregnancy Risk Factor C

Medication Guide Available Yes

Dosage Adults: Oral:

Rheumatoid arthritis, osteoarthritis: 300-600 mg 3-4 times/day; maximum dose: 3.2 g/day

Mild-to-moderate pain: 200 mg every 4-6 hours as needed; maximum dose: 3.2 g/day

Dosage adjustment in renal impairment: Not recommended in patients with advanced renal disease

Additional Information Complete prescribing information for this medication should be consulted for additional detail.

Dosage Forms Excipient information presented when available (limited, particularly for generics); consult specific product labeling.

Capsule, oral:

Nalfon®: 200 mg, 400 mg

Tablet, oral: 600 mg

◆ **Fenoprofen Calcium** *see* Fenoprofen *on page 696*

FentaNYL (FEN ta nil)

Brand Names: U.S. Abstral®; Actiq®; Duragesic®; Fentora®; Lazanda®; Onsolis™

Brand Names: Canada Abstral™; Actiq®; Duragesic®; Duragesic® MAT; Fentanyl Citrate Injection, USP; Novo-Fentanyl; PMS-Fentanyl MTX; RAN™-Fentanyl Matrix Patch; RAN™-Fentanyl Transdermal System; ratio-Fentanyl

Index Terms Fentanyl Citrate; Fentanyl Hydrochloride; Fentanyl Patch; OTFC (Oral Transmucosal Fentanyl Citrate); Subsys®

Pharmacologic Category Analgesic, Opioid; Anilidopiperidine Opioid; General Anesthetic

Additional Appendix Information

Opioid Analgesics *on page 1896*

Patient Information for Disposal of Unused Medications *on page 2026*

Use

Injection: Relief of pain, preoperative medication, adjunct to general or regional anesthesia

Iontophoretic transdermal system (Ionsys™): Short-term, in-hospital management of acute postoperative pain

Transdermal patch (eg, Duragesic®): Management of persistent moderate-to-severe chronic pain

Transmucosal lozenge (eg, Actiq®), buccal tablet (Fentora®), buccal film (Onsolis™), nasal spray (Lazanda®), sublingual tablet (Abstral®): Management of breakthrough cancer pain in opioid-tolerant patients

Pregnancy Risk Factor C

Pregnancy Considerations Teratogenic effects were not observed; however, embryo and fetotoxicity were noted in animal studies. Fentanyl crosses the placenta and the injectable formulation has been used safely during labor. Chronic use during pregnancy has shown detectable serum concentrations in the newborn with transient respiratory depression, behavioral changes, or seizures in the newborn infant characteristic of neonatal abstinence syndrome; transient neonatal muscular rigidity has also been observed. Transdermal patch, transmucosal lozenge, nasal spray (Lazanda®), sublingual tablet, buccal tablet (Fentora®), and buccal film (Onsolis™) are not recommended for analgesia during labor and delivery.

Lactation Enters breast milk/not recommended (AAP rates "compatible"; AAP 2001 update pending)

Prescribing and Access Restrictions As a requirement of the REMS program, access is restricted.

Abstral® (fentanyl sublingual tablet) is only available through the ABSTRAL REMS (Risk Evaluation and Mitigation Strategy) program. For outpatient use, enrollment in the ABSTRAL REMS program is required for prescribers, outpatient pharmacies, and patients. For inpatient use, enrollment in the ABSTRAL REMS program is required for inpatient pharmacies; patient and prescriber enrollment is not required for inpatient use. Distributors must also be enrolled in the program. Further information may be obtained by calling the ABSTRAL REMS program at 1-888-227-8725 or online at www.-abstralrems.com

Actiq® (fentanyl lozenge) is only available through the ACTIQ REMS program. Enrollment in the ACTIQ REMS program is required for prescribers for outpatient use, pharmacies (inpatient and outpatient), outpatients, and distributors. Further information may be obtained by calling the ACTIQ REMS program at 1-888-688-6885 or online at www.actiqandfentorarems.com.

Fentora® (fentanyl buccal tablet) is only available through the FENTORA REMS program. Enrollment in the FENTORA REMS program is required for prescribers for outpatient use, pharmacies (inpatient and outpatient), outpatients, and distributors. Further information may be obtained by calling the FENTORA REMS program at 1-888-688-6885 or online at www.actiqand-fentorarems.com.

Lazanda® (fentanyl nasal spray) is only available through the Lazanda REMS program. Enrollment in Lazanda REMS program is required for prescribers for outpatient use, pharmacies (inpatient and outpatient), outpatients, and distributors. Further information is available at 1-855-841-4234 or at www.LazandaREMS.com.

Onsolis™ (fentanyl buccal film) is only available through the restricted distribution program (FOCUS™). Enrollment in the FOCUS™ program is required for prescribers, pharmacies, and patients. Further information may be obtained from the manufacturer, Meda Pharmaceuticals, Inc (1-877-466-7654).

Medication Guide Available Yes

Contraindications Hypersensitivity to fentanyl or any component of the formulation

Transdermal system: Severe respiratory disease or depression including acute asthma (unless patient is mechanically ventilated); paralytic ileus; patients requiring short-term therapy, management of intermittent pain

Transmucosal buccal tablets (Fentora®), buccal films (Onsolis™), lozenges (eg, Actiq®), sublingual tablets (Abstral®), nasal spray (Lazanda®), and/or transdermal patches (eg, Duragesic®): Contraindicated in the management of acute or postoperative pain (including headache, migraine, dental pain, or use in emergency room), and in patients who are not opioid tolerant

Canadian labeling: Additional contraindication (not in U.S. labeling): Sublingual tablets (Abstral™): Severe respiratory depression or severe obstructive lung disease

Warnings/Precautions An opioid-containing analgesic regimen should be tailored to each patient's needs and based upon the type of pain being treated (acute versus chronic), the route of administration, degree of tolerance for opioids (naive versus chronic user), age, weight, and medical condition. The optimal analgesic dose varies widely among patients. Doses should be titrated to pain relief/prevention. May cause CNS depression, which may impair physical or mental abilities; patients must be cautioned about performing tasks which require mental alertness (eg, operating machinery or driving). When using with other CNS depressants, reduce dose of one or both agents. Fentanyl shares the toxic potentials of opiate agonists, and precautions of opiate agonist therapy should be observed; use with caution in patients with bradycardia or bradyarrhythmias; rapid I.V. infusion may result in skeletal muscle and chest wall rigidity leading to respiratory distress and/or apnea, bronchoconstriction, laryngospasm; inject slowly over 3-5 minutes. **[U.S. Boxed Warning]: Healthcare provider should be alert to problems of abuse, misuse, and diversion.** Tolerance or drug dependence may result from extended use. The elderly may be particularly susceptible to the CNS depressant and constipating effects of narcotics. Use extreme caution in patients with COPD or other chronic respiratory conditions. Use caution with head injuries, morbid obesity, renal impairment, or hepatic dysfunction. **[U.S. Boxed Warning]: Use with strong or moderate CYP3A4 inhibitors may result in increased effects and potentially fatal respiratory depression.** Use is not recommended with MAO inhibitors or within 14 days of MAO inhibitor use; severe and unpredictable adverse effects may result. Concurrent use of agonist/antagonist analgesics may precipitate withdrawal symptoms and/or reduced analgesic efficacy in patients following prolonged therapy with mu opioid agonists. Abrupt discontinuation following prolonged use may also lead to withdrawal symptoms.

[U.S. Boxed Warning]: Safety and efficacy of the transdermal patch have been limited to children ≥2 years of age who are opioid-tolerant. [U.S. Boxed Warning]: Buccal film (Onsolis™), nasal spray (Lazanda®), sublingual tablet (Abstral®): Not indicated for use in cancer patients <18 years of age. Indicated only for cancer patients who are opioid tolerant and are ≥18 years of age. [U.S. Boxed Warning]: Buccal film, buccal tablet, nasal spray, sublingual tablet, and lozenge preparations contain an amount of medication that can be fatal to children. Keep all used and unused products out of the reach of children at all times and discard products properly. Patients and caregivers should be counseled on the dangers to children including the risk of exposure to partially-consumed products.

[U.S. Boxed Warning] Abstral®, Actiq®, Duragesic®, Fentora®, Lazanda®, Onsolis™: May cause potentially life-threatening hypoventilation, respiratory depression, and/or death; Abstral®, Actiq®, Duragesic®, Fentora®, Lazanda®, or Onsolis™ should only be prescribed for opioid-tolerant patients. Risk of respiratory depression increased in elderly patients, debilitated patients, and patients with conditions associated with hypoxia or hypercapnia; usually occurs after administration of initial dose in nontolerant patients or when given with other drugs that depress respiratory function.

Nasal spray (Lazanda®): **[U.S. Boxed Warning]: Should be used only for the care of opioid-tolerant cancer patients with breakthrough pain who are already receiving opioid therapy for their underlying persistent cancer pain. Intended to be prescribed only by health care professionals who are knowledgeable in treating cancer pain. Use is contraindicated in opioid nontolerant patients or in the management of acute or postoperative pain, including headache/migraine, dental pain, or use in the ER. [U.S. Boxed Warning]: Available only through the Lazanda REMS program. Prescribers who prescribe to outpatients, pharmacies (inpatient and outpatient), outpatients, and distributors are required to enroll in the program. [U.S. Boxed Warning]: Due to differing pharmacokinetics of fentanyl in the nasal spray formulation, do not substitute Lazanda® on a mcg-per-mcg basis for any other fentanyl product. Serious adverse events, including death, may occur when used inappropriately (improper dose or patient selection). All patients must begin therapy with a 100 mcg dose and titrate, if needed. During therapy, patients must wait at least 2 hours before taking another dose of nasal spray.** Allergic rhinitis is not expected to alter fentanyl absorption following nasal administration; however, use of nasal decongestants (eg, oxymetazoline) during episodes of rhinitis may result in lower peak concentrations and delayed T_{max}, therefore, titration of the nasal spray is not recommended during use of nasal decongestants.

Transmucosal: Lozenge (eg, Actiq®), buccal tablet (Fentora®), buccal film (Onsolis™), sublingual tablet (Abstral®): **[U.S. Boxed Warning]: Should be used only for the care of opioid-tolerant cancer patients with breakthrough pain and is intended for use by specialists who are knowledgeable in treating cancer pain.** Not approved for use in management of acute or postoperative pain.

Transmucosal: Buccal film (eg, Onsolis™): **[U.S. Boxed Warning]: Available only through the FOCUS Program, a restricted distribution program with prescriber, pharmacy, and patient required enrollment. [U.S. Boxed Warning]: Onsolis™ is contraindicated in the management of acute or postoperative pain, including headache/migraine. [U.S. Boxed Warning]: Due to higher bioavailability of fentanyl in the buccal film formulation, do not substitute Onsolis™ on a mcg-per-mcg basis for any other fentanyl product. Serious adverse events, including death, may occur when used inappropriately (improper dose or patient selection). All patients must begin therapy with a 200 mcg dose and titrate, if needed. During therapy, patients must wait at least 2 hours before taking another dose.**

Transmucosal: Buccal tablet (Fentora®): **[U.S. Boxed Warning]: Available only through the FENTORA REMS program. Prescribers who prescribe to outpatients, outpatients, pharmacies, and distributors are required to enroll in the program. [U.S. Boxed Warning]: Due to the higher bioavailability of fentanyl in Fentora®, when converting patients from oral transmucosal fentanyl citrate (OTFC, Actiq®) to Fentora®, do not substitute Fentora®): on a mcg-per-mcg basis for any other fentanyl product. [U.S. Boxed Warning]: Fentora® is contraindicated in the management of acute or postoperative pain, including headache/migraine. Serious adverse events, including death, have been reported when used inappropriately (improper dose or patient selection). [U.S. Boxed Warning]: Patients using Fentora® who experience breakthrough pain may only take one additional dose using the same strength and must wait four hours before taking another dose.**

Transmucosal: Lozenge (Actiq®): **[U.S. Boxed Warning]: Available only through the ACTIQ REMS program. Prescribers who prescribe to outpatients, outpatients, pharmacies, and distributors are required to enroll in the program. [U.S. Boxed Warning]: The substitution of Actiq® for any other fentanyl product may result in a fatal overdose. Do not convert patients on a mcg-per-mcg basis to Actiq® from other fentanyl products. Do not substitute Actiq® for any other fentanyl product. [U.S. Boxed Warning]: Patients using fentanyl lozenges who experience breakthrough pain may only take 1 additional dose using the same strength and must wait 4 hours before taking another dose.**

Transmucosal: Sublingual tablet (Abstral®): **[U.S. Boxed Warning]: Available only through the ABSTRAL REMS program. Prescribers who prescribe to outpatients, outpatients, pharmacies, and distributors are required to enroll in the program. [U.S. Boxed Warning]: Abstral® is contraindicated in opioid nontolerant patients. [U.S. Boxed Warning]: Due to differing pharmacokinetics of fentanyl in the sublingual tablet formulation, do not substitute Abstral® on a mcg-per-mcg basis for any other fentanyl product. Serious adverse events, including death, may occur when used inappropriately (improper dose or patient selection). All patients must begin therapy with a 100 mcg dose. During therapy, patients must wait at least 2 hours before treating another episode of breakthrough pain.**

Transdermal patches (eg, Duragesic®): **[U.S. Boxed Warning]: Indicated for the management of persistent moderate-to-severe pain when around the clock pain control is needed for an extended time period. Should only be used in patients who are already receiving opioid therapy, are opioid tolerant, and who require a total daily dose equivalent to 25 mcg/hour transdermal patch. Contraindicated in patients who are not opioid tolerant, in the management of short-term analgesia, or in the management of postoperative pain. Should be applied only to intact skin. Use of a patch that has been cut, damaged, or altered in any way may result in overdosage.** Serum fentanyl concentrations may increase approximately one-third for patients with a body temperature of 40°C secondary to a temperature-dependent increase in fentanyl release from the patch and increased skin permeability. **[U.S. Boxed Warning]: Avoid exposure of application site and surrounding area to direct external heat sources.** Patients who experience fever or increase in core temperature should be monitored closely. Patients who experience adverse reactions should be monitored for at least 24 hours after removal of the patch. Transdermal patch may contain conducting metal (eg, aluminum); remove patch prior to MRI.

Adverse Reactions

>10%:

Cardiovascular: Bradycardia, edema

Central nervous system: CNS depression, confusion, dizziness, drowsiness, fatigue, headache, sedation

Endocrine & metabolic: Dehydration

Gastrointestinal: Constipation, nausea, vomiting, xerostomia

Local: Application-site reaction erythema

Neuromuscular & skeletal: Chest wall rigidity (high dose I.V.), muscle rigidity, weakness

Ocular: Miosis

Respiratory: Dyspnea, respiratory depression

Miscellaneous: Diaphoresis

1% to 10%:

Cardiovascular: Cardiac arrhythmia, cardiorespiratory arrest, chest pain, DVT, flushing, hyper-/hypotension, orthostatic hypotension, pallor, palpitation, peripheral edema, syncope, tachycardia, vasodilation

Central nervous system: Abnormal dreams, abnormal thinking, agitation, amnesia, anxiety, attention disturbance, depression, disorientation, dysphoria, euphoria, fever, hallucinations, hypoesthesia, insomnia, lethargy, malaise, mental status change, migraine, nervousness, paranoid reaction, somnolence, stupor, vertigo

Dermatologic: Alopecia, bruising, cellulitis, decubitus ulcer, erythema, hyperhidrosis, papules, pruritus, rash

Endocrine & metabolic: Breast pain, dehydration, hot flashes, hyper-/hypocalcemia, hyper-/hypoglycemia, hypoalbuminemia, hypokalemia, hypomagnesemia

Gastrointestinal: Abdominal pain, abnormal taste, anorexia, appetite decreased, biliary tract spasm, diarrhea, dyspepsia, dysphagia (buccal tablet/film), flatulence, gastritis, GI hemorrhage, gingival pain (buccal tablet), gingivitis (lozenge), glossitis (lozenge), ileus, intestinal obstruction (buccal film), periodontal abscess (lozenge/buccal tablet), proctalgia, stomatitis (lozenge/buccal tablet/sublingual tablet), tongue disorder (sublingual tablet), ulceration (gingival, lip, mouth; transmucosal use/nasal spray), weight loss

Genitourinary: Dysuria, erectile dysfunction, urinary incontinence, urinary retention, urinary tract infection, vaginitis, vaginal hemorrhage

Hematologic: Anemia, leukopenia, neutropenia, thrombocytopenia

Hepatic: Alkaline phosphatase increased, ascites, jaundice

Local: Application site pain, application site irritation

Neuromuscular & skeletal: Abnormal coordination, abnormal gait, arthralgia, back pain, limb pain, myalgia, neuropathy, paresthesia, rigors, tremor

Ocular: Blurred vision, diplopia, dry eye, swelling, ptosis, strabismus

Renal: Renal failure

Respiratory: Apnea, asthma, bronchitis, cough, epistaxis, hemoptysis, hypoventilation, hypoxia, nasal congestion (nasal spray), nasal discomfort (nasal spray), nasopharyngitis, pharyngolaryngeal pain, pharyngitis, pneumonia, postnasal drip (nasal spray), pulmonary embolism (nasal spray), rhinitis, rhinorrhea (nasal spray), sinusitis, upper respiratory infection, wheezing

Miscellaneous: Flu-like syndrome, hiccups, hypersensitivity, lymphadenopathy, night sweats, parosmia, speech disorder, withdrawal syndrome

<1% (Limited to important or life-threatening): Abdominal distention, amblyopia, allergic reaction, anaphylaxis, angina, anorgasmia, aphasia, bladder pain, bronchospasm, CNS excitation or delirium, cold/clammy skin, dental caries (lozenge), depersonalization, dysesthesia, emotional lability, eructation, esophageal stenosis, exfoliative dermatitis, fecal impaction, flank pain, gum line erosion (lozenge), gum hemorrhage (lozenge), hematuria, hostility, hyper-/hypotonia, laryngospasm, libido decreased, moniliasis (lozenge/buccal tablet), myasthenia, nocturia, oliguria, pancytopenia, paradoxical dizziness, physical and psychological dependence with prolonged use, pleural effusion, polyuria, pustules, speech disorder, stertorous breathing, seizure, sputum increased, tooth loss (lozenge), urinary tract spasm, urticaria, vertigo

Drug Interactions

Metabolism/Transport Effects Substrate of CYP3A4 (major); **Note:** Assignment of Major/Minor substrate status based on clinically relevant drug interaction potential; **Inhibits** CYP3A4 (weak)

Avoid Concomitant Use

Avoid concomitant use of FentaNYL with any of the following: Crizotinib; MAO Inhibitors; Pimozide

Increased Effect/Toxicity

FentaNYL may increase the levels/effects of: Alcohol (Ethyl); Alvimopan; Beta-Blockers; Calcium Channel Blockers (Nondihydropyridine); CNS Depressants; Desmopressin; MAO Inhibitors; Pimozide; Selective Serotonin Reuptake Inhibitors; Thiazide Diuretics

The levels/effects of FentaNYL may be increased by: Amphetamines; Antipsychotic Agents (Phenothiazines); Crizotinib; CYP3A4 Inhibitors (Moderate); CYP3A4 Inhibitors (Strong); Dasatinib; Droperidol; HydrOXYzine; MAO Inhibitors; Succinylcholine

Decreased Effect

FentaNYL may decrease the levels/effects of: Ioflupane I 123; Pegvisomant

The levels/effects of FentaNYL may be decreased by: Alpha-/Beta-Agonists (Indirect-Acting); Alpha1-Agonists; Ammonium Chloride; Mixed Agonist / Antagonist Opioids; Rifamycin Derivatives; Tocilizumab

Ethanol/Nutrition/Herb Interactions

Ethanol: May increase CNS depression; monitor for increased effects with coadministration. Caution patients about effects.

Food: Fentanyl concentrations may be increased by grapefruit juice; avoid concurrent intake of large quantities (>1 quart/day).

Herb/Nutraceutical: St John's wort may decrease fentanyl levels. Avoid valerian, St John's wort, kava kava, gotu kola (may increase CNS depression).

Stability

Injection formulation: Store at controlled room temperature of 20°C to 25°C (68°F to 77°F). Protect from light.

Nasal spray: Do not store above 25°C (77°F); do not freeze. Protect from light. Bottle should be stored in the provided child-resistant container when not in use and kept out of the reach of children at all times.

Transdermal patch: Do not store above 25°C (77°F). Keep out of the reach of children.

Transmucosal (buccal film, buccal tablet, lozenge, sublingual tablet): Store at controlled room temperature of 20°C to 25°C (68°F to 77°F). Protect from freezing and moisture. Keep out of the reach of children.

Mechanism of Action Binds with stereospecific receptors at many sites within the CNS, increases pain threshold, alters pain reception, inhibits ascending pain pathways

Pharmacodynamics/Kinetics

Onset of action: Analgesic: I.M.: 7-8 minutes; I.V.: Almost immediate; Transdermal (initial placement): 6 hours; Transmucosal: 5-15 minutes

Peak effect: Analgesic: Transdermal (initial placement): 12 hours; Transmucosal: 15-30 minutes

Duration: I.M.: 1-2 hours; I.V.: 0.5-1 hour; Transdermal (removal of patch/no replacement): 12 hours; Transmucosal: Related to blood level; respiratory depressant effect may last longer than analgesic effect

Absorption:

Transdermal: Initial application: Gradually absorbed for the first 12-24 hours, followed by a constant absorption for the remainder of the dosing interval. Absorption is decreased in cachectic patients (compared to normal size patients).

Transmucosal, buccal tablet and buccal film: Rapid, ~50% from the buccal mucosa; remaining 50% swallowed with saliva and slowly absorbed from GI tract.

Transmucosal, lozenge: Rapid, ~25% from the buccal mucosa; 75% swallowed with saliva and slowly absorbed from GI tract

Distribution: 4-6 L/kg; Highly lipophilic, redistributes into muscle and fat

Protein binding: 80% to 85%

Metabolism: Hepatic, primarily via CYP3A4

Bioavailability:

Buccal film: 71% (mucositis did not have a clinically significant effect on C_{max} and AUC; however, bioavailability is expected to decrease if film is inappropriately chewed and swallowed)

Buccal tablet: 65% (range: 45% to 85%)

Lozenge: 47% (range: 37% to 57%)

Sublingual tablet: 54%

Half-life elimination:

I.V.: 2-4 hours

Nasal spray: 15-25 hours

Transdermal patch: 17 hours (13-22 hours, half-life is influenced by absorption rate)

Transmucosal: Lozenge: 7 hours; Buccal film: ~14 hours; Buccal tablet: 100-200 mcg: 3-4 hours, 400-800 mcg: 11-12 hours; Sublingual tablet: 100-200 mcg: 5-7 hours; 400-800 mcg: 10-14 hours

Time to peak:

Buccal film: 0.75-4 hours (median: 1 hour)

Buccal tablet: 20-240 minutes (median: 47 minutes)

Lozenge: 20-480 minutes (median: 20-40 minutes)

Nasal spray: Median: 15-21 minutes

Sublingual tablet: 15-240 minutes (median: 30-60 minutes)

Transdermal patch: 24-72 hours, after several sequential 72-hour applications, steady state serum concentrations are reached

Excretion: Urine 75% (primarily as metabolites, <7% to 10% as unchanged drug); feces ~9%

Dosage Note: These are guidelines and do not represent the maximum doses that may be required in all patients. Doses and dosage intervals should be titrated to pain relief/prevention. Monitor vital signs routinely. Single I.M. doses have duration of 1-2 hours, single I.V. doses last 0.5-1 hour.

Minor procedures/analgesia (unlabeled use): I.V.:

Children 1-12 years: 0.5-2 mcg/kg/dose given 3 minutes prior to procedure; may repeat every 1-2 hours

Children >12 years: 0.5-2 mcg/kg/dose (maximum: 50 mcg/dose) given 3 minutes prior to procedure; may repeat in 5 minutes if necessary; if more than 2 doses are needed, repeat with a maximum of 25 mcg/dose up to 5 times

Surgery:

Children ≥2 years: Adjunct to anesthesia (induction and maintenance): Slow I.V.: 2-3 mcg/kg/dose every 1-2 hours as needed

Adults:

Premedication: I.M., slow I.V.: 50-100 mcg/dose 30-60 minutes prior to surgery

Adjunct to regional anesthesia: Slow I.V.: 25-100 mcg/dose over 1-2 minutes. **Note:** An I.V. should be in place with regional anesthesia so the I.M. route is rarely used but still maintained as an option in the package labeling.

Adjunct to general anesthesia: Slow I.V.:

Low dose: 0.5-2 mcg/kg/dose depending on the indication

Moderate dose: Initial: 2-20 mcg/kg/dose; Maintenance (bolus or infusion): 1-2 mcg/kg/**hour**. Discontinuing fentanyl infusion 30-60 minutes prior to the end of surgery will usually allow adequate ventilation upon emergence from anesthesia. For "fast-tracking" and early extubation following major surgery, total fentanyl doses are limited to 10-15 mcg/kg.

High dose: 20-50 mcg/kg/dose; **Note:** High-dose fentanyl as an adjunct to general anesthesia is rarely used, but is still described in the manufacturer's label.

Pain management:

Children (unlabeled use): I.V.: 0.5-2 mcg/kg/dose given every 1-2 hours as needed; continuous infusion: 0.5-2 mcg/kg/**hour**; titrate to desired effects

Patient-controlled analgesia (PCA) (unlabeled use; American Pain Society, 2008): Children <50 kg: **Note:** Opiate-naive: Consider lower end of dosing range:

Usual concentration: 10 mcg/mL

Demand dose: 0.5-1 mcg/kg/dose

Lockout interval: 6-8 minutes

Usual basal rate: 0-0.5 mcg/kg/**hour**

Adults:
I.V. (unlabeled use): Bolus at start of infusion: 1-2 mcg/kg **or** 25-100 mcg/dose; continuous infusion rate: 1-2 mcg/kg/**hour or** 25-200 mcg/hour
Severe pain: I.M, I.V. (unlabeled): 50-100 mcg/dose every 1-2 hours as needed; patients with prior opiate exposure may tolerate higher initial doses
Patient-controlled analgesia (PCA) (unlabeled use): I.V.:
Usual concentration: 10 mcg/mL
Demand dose: Usual: 20 mcg; range: 10-50 mcg
Lockout interval: 5-8 minutes
Usual basal rate: ≤50 mcg/hour
Critically-ill patients (unlabeled dose): Slow I.V.: 25-100 mcg (based on ~70 kg patient) **or** 0.35-1.5 mcg/kg every 30-60 minutes as needed. **Note:** More frequent dosing may be needed (eg, mechanically-ventilated patients).
Continuous infusion: 50-700 mcg/hour (based on ~70 kg patient) **or** 0.7-10 mcg/kg/**hour**
Intrathecal (I.T.) (unlabeled use; American Pain Society, 2008): **Must be preservative-free.** Doses must be adjusted for age, injection site, and patient's medical condition and degree of opioid tolerance.
Single dose: 5-25 mcg/dose; may provide adequate relief for up to 6 hours
Continuous infusion: Not recommended in acute pain management due to risk of excessive accumulation. For chronic cancer pain, infusion of very small doses may be practical (American Pain Society, 2008).
Epidural (unlabeled use; American Pain Society, 2008): **Must be preservative-free.** Doses must be adjusted for age, injection site, and patient's medical condition and degree of opioid tolerance
Single dose: 25-100 mcg/dose; may provide adequate relief for up to 8 hours
Continuous infusion: 25-100 mcg/hour

Breakthrough cancer pain: For patients who are tolerant to and currently receiving opioid therapy for persistent cancer pain; dosing should be individually titrated to provide adequate analgesia with minimal side effects. Dose titration should be done if patient requires more than 1 dose/breakthrough pain episode for several consecutive episodes. Patients experiencing >4 breakthrough pain episodes/day should have the dose of their long-term opioid re-evaluated.
Children ≥16 years and Adults: Lozenge: Initial dose: 200 mcg; the second dose may be started 15 minutes after completion of the first dose if pain unrelieved. A maximum of 1 additional dose can be given per pain episode; must wait at least 4 hours before treating another episode. Consumption should be limited to ≤4 units/day. Additional requirements suggest need for improved baseline therapy.
Adults:
Buccal film (Onsolis™): Initial dose: 200 mcg for all patients **Note:** Patients previously using another transmucosal product should be initiated at doses of 200 mcg; do **not** switch patients using any other fentanyl product on a mcg-per-mcg basis.
Dose titration: If titration required, increase dose in 200 mcg increments once per episode using multiples of the 200 mcg film; do not redose within a single episode of breakthrough pain and separate single doses by ≥2 hours. During titration, do not exceed 4 simultaneous applications of the 200 mcg films (800 mcg). If >800 mcg required, treat next episode with one 1200 mcg film (maximum dose: 1200 mcg). Once maintenance dose is determined, all other unused films should be disposed of and that strength (using a single film) should be used. During any pain episode, if adequate relief is not achieved after 30 minutes following buccal film application, a rescue medication (as determined by healthcare provider) may be used.
Maintenance: Determined dose applied as a single film once per episode and separated by ≥2 hours (dose range: 200-1200 mcg); limit to 4 applications/day. Consider increasing the around-the-clock opioid therapy in patients experiencing >4 breakthrough pain episodes/day.
Buccal tablet (Fentora®): Initial dose: 100 mcg; a second 100 mcg dose, if needed, may be started 30 minutes after the start of the first dose. **Note:** For patients previously using the transmucosal lozenge (Actiq®), the initial dose should be selected using the conversions listed below (maximum: 2 doses per breakthrough pain episode every 4 hours).
Dose titration, if required, should be done using multiples of the 100 mcg tablets. Patient can take two 100 mcg tablets (one on each side of mouth). If that dose is not successful, can use four 100 mcg tablets (two on each side of mouth). If titration requires >400 mcg/dose, then use 200 mcg tablets.
Conversion from lozenge to buccal tablet (Fentora®):
Lozenge dose 200-400 mcg, then buccal tablet 100 mcg
Lozenge dose 600-800 mcg, then buccal tablet 200 mcg
Lozenge dose 1200-1600 mcg, then buccal tablet 400 mcg
Note: Four 100 mcg buccal tablets deliver approximately 12% and 13% higher values of C_{max} and AUC, respectively, compared to one 400 mcg buccal tablet. To prevent confusion, patient should only have one strength available at a time. Using more than four buccal tablets at a time has not been studied.
Nasal spray (Lazanda®):
Initial dose: 100 mcg (one 100 mcg spray in one nostril) for all patients. **Note:** Patients previously using another fentanyl product should be initiated at a dose of 100 mcg; do not convert patients from other fentanyl products to Lazanda® on a mcg-per-mcg basis.
Dose titration: If pain is relieved within 30 minutes, that same dose should be used to treat subsequent episodes. If pain is unrelieved, may increase to a higher dose using the recommended titration steps. **Must wait at least 2 hours before treating another episode with nasal spray.** Dose titration steps: If no relief with 100 mcg dose, increase to 200 mcg dose per episode (one 100 mcg spray in each nostril); if no relief with 200 mcg dose, increase to 400 mcg per episode (one 400 mcg spray); if no relief with 400 mcg dose, increase to 800 mcg dose per episode (one 400 mcg spray in each nostril). **Note:** Single doses >800 mcg have not been evaluated. There are no data supporting the use of a combination of dose strengths.
Maintenance dose: Once maintenance dose for breakthrough pain episode has been determined, use that dose for subsequent episodes. For pain that is not relieved after 30 minutes of Lazanda® administration or if a separate breakthrough pain episode occurs within the 2 hour window before the next Lazanda® dose is permitted, a rescue medication may be used. Limit Lazanda® use to ≤4 episodes of breakthrough pain per day. If response to maintenance dose changes (increase in adverse reactions or alterations in pain relief), dose readjustment may be necessary. If patient is experiencing >4 breakthrough pain episodes/day, consider increasing the around-the-clock, long-acting opioid therapy; if long-acting opioid therapy dose is

altered, re-evaluate and retitrate Lazanda® dose as needed.

Sublingual tablet (Abstral®):

Initial dose:

U.S. labeling: 100 mcg for all patients; if pain is unrelieved, a second dose may be given 30 minutes after administration of the first dose. A maximum of 2 doses can be given per breakthrough pain episode; must wait at least 2 hours before treating another episode.

Canadian labeling: 100 mcg for all patients; if pain is unrelieved 30 minutes after administration of Abstral™, an alternative rescue medication (other than Abstral™) may be given. Administer only 1 dose of Abstral™ per breakthrough pain episode; must wait at least 2 hours before treating another episode.

Note: Patients previously using another fentanyl product should be initiated at a dose of 100 mcg; do not convert patients from other fentanyl products to Abstral® on a mcg-per-mcg basis.

Dose titration: If titration required, increase in 100 mcg increments (up to 400 mcg) over consecutive breakthrough episodes. If titration requires >400 mcg/dose, increase in increments of 200 mcg, starting with 600 mcg dose. During titration, patients may use multiples of 100 mcg and/or 200 mcg tablets for any single dose; do not exceed 4 tablets at one time; safety and efficacy of doses >800 mcg have not been evaluated.

Maintenance dose: Once maintenance dose for breakthrough pain episode has been determined, use only 1 tablet in the appropriate strength per episode; if pain is unrelieved with maintenance dose:

U.S. labeling recommendations: A second dose may be given after 30 minutes; maximum of 2 doses/episode of breakthrough pain; separate treatment of subsequent episodes by ≥2 hours; limit treatment to ≤4 breakthrough episodes/day.

Canadian labeling recommendations: Administer alternative rescue medication after 30 minutes; maximum of 1 Abstral™ dose/episode of breakthrough pain; separate treatment of subsequent episodes by ≥2 hours; limit treatment to ≤4 breakthrough episodes/day.

Consider increasing the around-the-clock long-acting opioid therapy in patients experiencing >4 breakthrough pain episodes/day; if long-acting opioid therapy dose altered, re-evaluate and retitrate Abstral® dose as needed.

Elderly >65 years: Transmucosal lozenge (eg, Actiq®): In clinical trials, patients who were >65 years of age were titrated to a mean dose that was 200 mcg less than that of younger patients.

Chronic pain management: Children ≥2 years and Adults (opioid-tolerant patients): Transdermal patch (Duragesic®):

Initial: To convert patients from oral or parenteral opioids to transdermal patch, a 24-hour analgesic requirement should be calculated (based on prior opiate use). Using the tables, the appropriate initial dose can be determined. The initial fentanyl dosage may be approximated from the 24-hour morphine dosage equivalent and titrated to minimize adverse effects and provide analgesia. With the initial application, the absorption of transdermal fentanyl requires several hours to reach plateau; therefore transdermal fentanyl is inappropriate for management of acute pain. Change patch every 72 hours.

Conversion from continuous infusion of fentanyl: In patients who have adequate pain relief with a fentanyl infusion, fentanyl may be converted to transdermal dosing at a rate equivalent to the intravenous rate. A two-step taper of the infusion to be completed over 12 hours has been recommended (Kornick, 2001) after the patch is applied. The infusion is decreased to 50% of the original rate six hours after the application of the first patch, and subsequently discontinued twelve hours after application.

Titration: Short-acting agents may be required until analgesic efficacy is established and/or as supplements for "breakthrough" pain. The amount of supplemental doses should be closely monitored. Appropriate dosage increases may be based on daily supplemental dosage using the ratio of 45 mg/24 hours of oral morphine to a 12.5 mcg/hour increase in fentanyl dosage.

Frequency of adjustment: The dosage should not be titrated more frequently than every 3 days after the initial dose or every 6 days thereafter. Patients should wear a consistent fentanyl dosage through two applications (6 days) before dosage increase based on supplemental opiate dosages can be estimated. **Note:** Upon discontinuation, ~17 hours are required for a 50% decrease in fentanyl levels.

Frequency of application: The majority of patients may be controlled on every 72-hour administration; however, a small number of patients require every 48-hour administration.

Dose conversion guidelines for transdermal fentanyl (see tables below and on next page).

Note: U.S. and Canadian dose conversion guidelines differ. Consult appropriate table.

U.S. Labeling: Dose Conversion Guidelines: Recommended Initial Duragesic® Dose Based Upon Daily Oral Morphine Dose[1,2]

Oral 24-Hour Morphine (mg/day)	Duragesic® Dose[3] (mcg/h)
60-134	25
135-224	50
225-314	75
315-404	100
405-494	125
495-584	150
585-674	175
675-764	200
765-854	225
855-944	250
945-1034	275
1035-1124	300

[1]The table should NOT be used to convert from transdermal fentanyl (Duragesic®) to other opioid analgesics. Rather, following removal of the patch, titrate the dose of the new opioid until adequate analgesia is achieved.

[2]Recommendations are based on U.S. product labeling for Duragesic®.

[3]Pediatric patients initiating therapy on a 25 mcg/hour Duragesic® system should be opioid-tolerant and receiving at least 60 mg oral morphine equivalents per day.

U.S. Labeling: Dose Conversion Guidelines[1,2]

Current Analgesic	Daily Dosage (mg/day)			
Morphine (I.M./I.V.)	10-22	23-37	38-52	53-67
Oxycodone (oral)	30-67	67.5-112	112.5-157	157.5-202
Oxycodone (I.M./I.V.)	15-33	33.1-56	56.1-78	78.1-101
Codeine (oral)	150-447	448-747	748-1047	1048-1347
Hydromorphone (oral)	8-17	17.1-28	28.1-39	39.1-51
Hydromorphone (I.V.)	1.5-3.4	3.5-5.6	5.7-7.9	8-10
Meperidine (I.M.)	75-165	166-278	279-390	391-503
Methadone (oral)	20-44	45-74	75-104	105-134
Methadone (I.M.)	10-22	23-37	38-52	53-67
Fentanyl transdermal recommended dose (mcg/h)	**25 mcg/h**	**50 mcg/h**	**75 mcg/h**	**100 mcg/h**

[1]The table should NOT be used to convert from transdermal fentanyl (Duragesic®) to other opioid analgesics. Rather, following removal of the patch, titrate the dose of the new opioid until adequate analgesia is achieved.

[2]Recommendations are based on U.S. product labeling for Duragesic®.

Transdermal patch (Duragesic® MAT [Canada; not available in U.S.]): Adults:

Canadian Labeling: Dose Conversion Guidelines (Adults): Recommended Initial Duragesic® MAT Dose Based Upon Daily Oral Morphine Dose[1,2]

Oral 24-Hour Morphine (Current Dose in mg/day)	Duragesic® MAT Dose (Initial Dose in mcg/h)
45-59	12
60-134	25
135-179	37
180-224	50
225-269	62
270-314	75
315-359	87
360-404	100
405-494	125
495-584	150
585-674	175
675-764	200
765-854	225
855-944	250
945-1034	275
1035-1124	300

[1]The table should NOT be used to convert from transdermal fentanyl (Duragesic® MAT) to other opioid analgesics. Rather, following removal of the patch, titrate the dose of the new opioid until adequate analgesia is achieved.

[2]Recommendations are based on Canadian product labeling for Duragesic® MAT.

Note: The 12 mcg/hour dose included in this table is to be used for incremental dose adjustment and is generally not recommended for initial dosing, except for patients in whom lower starting doses are deemed clinically appropriate.

Canadian Labeling: Dose Conversion Guidelines (Adults)[1,2]

Current Analgesic	Daily Dosage (mg/day)						
Morphine[3] (I.M./I.V.)	20-44	45-60	61-75	76-90	n/a[4]	n/a[4]	n/a[4]
Oxycodone (oral)	30-66	67-90	91-112	113-134	135-157	158-179	180-202
Codeine (oral)	150-447	448-597	598-747	748-897	898-1047	1048-1197	1198-1347
Hydromorphone (oral)	8-16	17-22	23-28	29-33	34-39	40-45	46-51
Hydromorphone (I.V.)	4-8.4	8.5-11.4	11.5-14.4	14.5-16.5	16.6-19.5	19.6-22.5	22.6-25.5
Fentanyl transdermal recommended dose (mcg/h)	**25 mcg/h**	**37 mcg/h**	**50 mcg/h**	**62 mcg/h**	**75 mcg/h**	**87 mcg/h**	**100 mcg/h**

[1]The table should NOT be used to convert from transdermal fentanyl (Duragesic® MAT) to other opioid analgesics. Rather, following removal of the patch, titrate the dose of the new opioid until adequate analgesia is achieved.

[2]Recommendations are based on Canadian product labeling for Duragesic® MAT.

[3]Morphine dose conversion based upon I.M to oral dose ratio of 1:3.

[4]Insufficient data available to provide specific dosing recommendations. Use caution; adjust dose conservatively.

Dosing adjustment in hepatic impairment: Actiq®: Although fentanyl kinetics may be altered in hepatic disease, Actiq® can be used successfully in the management of breakthrough cancer pain. Doses should be titrated to reach clinical effect with careful monitoring of patients with severe hepatic disease.

Dietary Considerations Transmucosal lozenge contains 2 g sugar per unit.

Administration

I.V.: Administer as slow I.V. infusion over 1-2 minutes. May also be administered as continuous infusion or PCA (unlabeled use) routes. Muscular rigidity may occur with rapid I.V. administration.

Transdermal patch (eg, Duragesic®): Apply to nonirritated and nonirradiated skin, such as chest, back, flank, or upper arm. Do not shave skin; hair at application site should be clipped. Prior to application, clean site with clear water and allow to dry completely. Do not use damaged, cut or leaking patches; patch may be less effective. Skin exposure from fentanyl gel leaking from patch may lead to serious adverse effects; thoroughly wash affected skin surfaces with water (do not use soap). Firmly press in place and hold for 30 seconds. Change patch every 72 hours. Do **not** use soap, alcohol, or other solvents to remove transdermal gel if it accidentally touches skin; use copious amounts of water. Avoid exposing application site to external heat sources (eg, heating pad, electric blanket, heat lamp, hot tub). If there is difficulty with patch adhesion, the edges of the system may be taped in place with first-aid tape. If there is continued difficulty with adhesion, an adhesive film dressing (eg, Bioclusive®, Tegaderm®) may be applied over the system.

Lozenge: Foil overwrap should be removed just prior to administration. Place the unit in mouth between the cheek and gum and allow it to dissolve. Do not chew. Lozenge may be moved from one side of the mouth to the other. The unit should be consumed over a period of 15 minutes. Handle should be removed after the lozenge is consumed; early removal should be considered if the patient has achieved an adequate response and/or shows signs of respiratory depression.

Buccal film: Foil overwrap should be removed just prior to administration. Prior to placing film, wet inside of cheek using tongue or by rinsing with water. Place film inside mouth with the pink side of the unit against the inside of the moistened cheek. With finger, press the film against cheek and hold for 5 seconds. The film should stick to the inside of cheek after 5 seconds. The film should be left in place until it dissolves (usually within 15-30 minutes after application). Liquids may be consumed after 5 minutes of application. Food can be eaten after film dissolves. If using more than 1 film simultaneously (during titration period), apply films on either side of mouth (do not apply on top of each other). Do not chew or swallow film. Do not cut or tear the film. All patients must initiate therapy using the 200 mcg film.

Buccal tablet: Patient should not open blister until ready to administer. The blister backing should be peeled back to expose the tablet; tablet should not be pushed out through the blister. Immediately use tablet once removed from blister. Place entire tablet in the buccal cavity (above a rear molar, between the upper cheek and gum). Tablet should not be broken, sucked, chewed, or swallowed. Should dissolve in about 14-25 minutes when left between the cheek and the gum. If remnants remain they may be swallowed with water.

Nasal spray: Prior to initial use, prime device by spraying 4 sprays into the provided pouch (the counting window will show a green bar when the bottle is ready for use). Insert nozzle a short distance into the nose (~1/2 inch or 1 cm) and point towards the bridge of the nose (while closing off the other nostril using 1 finger). Press on finger grips until a "click" sound is heard and the number in the counting window advances by one. The "click" sound and dose counter are the only reliable methods for ensuring a dose has been administered (spray is not always felt on the nasal mucosa). Patient should remain seated for at least 1 minute following administration. Do not blow nose for ≥30 minutes after administration. Wash hands before and after use. There are 8 full therapeutic sprays in each bottle; do not continue to use bottle after "8" sprays have been used. Dispose of bottle and contents if ≥5 days have passed since last use or if it has been ≥4 days since bottle was primed. Spray the remaining contents into the provided pouch, seal in the child-resistant container, and dispose of in the trash.

Sublingual tablet: Remove from the blister unit immediately prior to administration. Place tablet directly under the tongue on the floor of the mouth and allow to completely dissolve; do not chew, suck, or swallow. Do not eat or drink anything until tablet is completely dissolved. In patients with a dry mouth, water may be used to moisten the buccal mucosa just before administration. All patients must initiate therapy using the 100 mcg tablet.

Monitoring Parameters Respiratory and cardiovascular status, blood pressure, heart rate; signs of misuse, abuse, or addiction

Transdermal patch: Monitor for 24 hours after application of first dose

Additional Information Fentanyl is 50-100 times as potent as morphine; morphine 10 mg I.M. is equivalent to fentanyl 0.1-0.2 mg I.M.; fentanyl has less hypotensive effects than morphine due to lack of histamine release. However, fentanyl may cause rigidity with high doses. If the patient has required high-dose analgesia or has used for a prolonged period (~7 days), taper dose to prevent withdrawal; monitor for signs and symptoms of withdrawal.

Nasal spray (Lazanda®): Disposal of nasal spray: Before disposal, all unopened or partially used bottles must be completely emptied by spraying the contents into the provided pouch. After "8" therapeutic sprays has been reached on the counter, patients should continue to spray an additional four sprays into the pouch to ensure that any residual fentanyl has been expelled (an audible click will no longer be heard and the counter will not advance beyond "8"). The empty bottle and the sealed pouch must be put into the child-resistant container before placing in the trash. Wash hands with soap and water immediately after handling the pouch. If the pouch is lost, another one can be ordered by the patient or caregiver by calling 1-866-435-6775.

Transmucosal (oral lozenge, Actiq®): Disposal of lozenge units: After consumption of a complete unit, the handle may be disposed of in a trash container that is out of the reach of children. For a partially-consumed unit, or a unit that still has any drug matrix remaining on the handle, the handle should be placed under hot running tap water until the drug matrix has dissolved. Special child-resistant containers are available to temporarily store partially consumed units that cannot be disposed of immediately.

Transmucosal (buccal film, Onsolis™): Disposal of film: Remove foil overwrap from any unused, unneeded films and dispose by flushing in the toilet.

Transmucosal (sublingual tablet, Abstral®): Disposal of tablets: Remove any unused tablets from the blister cards and dispose by flushing in the toilet.

Transdermal patch (Duragesic®): Upon removal of the patch, ~17 hours are required before serum concentrations fall to 50% of their original values. Opioid withdrawal symptoms are possible. Gradual downward titration (potentially by the sequential use of lower-dose patches) is recommended. Keep transdermal patch (both used and unused) out of the reach of children. Do **not** use soap, alcohol, or other solvents to remove transdermal gel if it accidentally touches skin as they may increase transdermal absorption, use copious amounts of water. Avoid exposure of direct external heat sources (eg, heating pads, electric blankets, heat lamps, saunas, hot tubs, heated water beds) to application site.

Product Availability

Subsys® sublingual spray: FDA approved January 2012; availability is currently undetermined. Consult prescribing information for additional information.

Subsys® is a fentanyl sublingual spray formulation indicated for the management of breakthrough cancer pain in opioid-tolerant patients.

Dosage Forms Excipient information presented when available (limited, particularly for generics); consult specific product labeling.

Film, for buccal application, as citrate [strength expressed as base]:
- Onsolis™: 200 mcg (30s); 400 mcg (30s); 600 mcg (30s); 800 mcg (30s); 1200 mcg (30s)

Injection, solution, as citrate [strength expressed as base, preservative free]: 0.05 mg/mL (2 mL, 5 mL, 10 mL, 20 mL, 50 mL)

Lozenge, oral, as citrate [strength expressed as base, transmucosal]: 200 mcg (30s); 400 mcg (30s); 600 mcg (30s); 800 mcg (30s); 1200 mcg (30s); 1600 mcg (30s)
- Actiq®: 200 mcg (30s); 400 mcg (30s); 600 mcg (30s); 800 mcg (30s); 1200 mcg (30s); 1600 mcg (30s) [contains sugar 2 g/lozenge; berry flavor]

Patch, transdermal, as base: 12 [delivers 12.5 mcg/hr] (5s); 25 [delivers 25 mcg/hr] (5s); 50 [delivers 50 mcg/hr] (5s); 75 [delivers 75 mcg/hr] (5s); 100 [delivers 100 mcg/hr] (5s)
- Duragesic®: 12 [delivers 12.5 mcg/hr] (5s) [contains ethanol 0.1mL/10 cm^2; 5 cm^2]
- Duragesic®: 25 [delivers 25 mcg/hr] (5s) [contains ethanol 0.1 mL/10 cm^2; 10 cm^2]
- Duragesic®: 50 [delivers 50 mcg/hr] (5s) [contains ethanol 0.1 mL/10 cm^2; 20 cm^2]
- Duragesic®: 75 [delivers 75 mcg/hr] (5s) [contains ethanol 0.1 mL/10 cm^2; 30 cm^2]
- Duragesic®: 100 [delivers 100 mcg/hr] (5s) [contains ethanol 0.1 mL/10 cm^2; 40 cm^2]

Powder, for prescription compounding, as citrate: USP: 100% (1 g)

Solution, intranasal, as citrate [strength expressed as base, spray]:

Lazanda®: 100 mcg/spray (5 mL); 400 mcg/spray (5 mL) [delivers 8 metered sprays]

Tablet, for buccal application, as citrate [strength expressed as base]:

Fentora®: 100 mcg (28s); 200 mcg (28s); 400 mcg (28s); 600 mcg (28s); 800 mcg (28s)

Tablet, sublingual, as citrate [strength expressed as base]:

Abstral®: 100 mcg (12s, 32s); 200 mcg (12s, 32s); 300 mcg (12s, 32s); 400 mcg (12s, 32s); 600 mcg (32s); 800 mcg (32s)

Dosage Forms: Canada Excipient information presented when available (limited, particularly for generics); consult specific product labeling.

Patch, transdermal, as base: 12 mcg/hr (5s); 25 mcg/hr (5s); 50 mcg/hr (5s); 75 mcg/hr (5s); 100 mcg/hr (5s)

Duragesic® MAT: 12 mcg/hr (5s) [contains ethanol 0.1 mL/10 cm^2; 5 cm^2]

Duragesic® MAT: 25 mcg/hr (5s) [contains ethanol 0.1 mL/10 cm^2; 10 cm^2]

Duragesic® MAT: 50 mcg/hr (5s) [contains ethanol 0.1 mL/10 cm^2; 20 cm^2]

Duragesic® MAT: 75 mcg/hr (5s) [contains ethanol 0.1 mL/10 cm^2; 30 cm^2]

Duragesic® MAT: 100 mcg/hr (5s) [contains ethanol 0.1 mL/10 cm^2; 40 cm^2]

Controlled Substance C-II

- **Fentanyl Citrate** *see* FentaNYL *on page 697*
- **Fentanyl Citrate Injection, USP (Can)** *see* FentaNYL *on page 697*
- **Fentanyl Hydrochloride** *see* FentaNYL *on page 697*
- **Fentanyl Patch** *see* FentaNYL *on page 697*
- **Fentora®** *see* FentaNYL *on page 697*
- **Feosol® [OTC]** *see* Ferrous Sulfate *on page 706*
- **Feraheme®** *see* Ferumoxytol *on page 707*
- **Ferate [OTC]** *see* Ferrous Gluconate *on page 706*
- **Fergon® [OTC]** *see* Ferrous Gluconate *on page 706*
- **Fer-In-Sol® [OTC]** *see* Ferrous Sulfate *on page 706*
- **Fer-In-Sol® (Can)** *see* Ferrous Sulfate *on page 706*
- **Fer-iron [OTC]** *see* Ferrous Sulfate *on page 706*
- **Ferodan™ (Can)** *see* Ferrous Sulfate *on page 706*
- **Ferretts® [OTC]** *see* Ferrous Fumarate *on page 706*
- **Ferrex™ 150 [OTC]** *see* Polysaccharide-Iron Complex *on page 1375*
- **Ferrex™ 150 Plus [OTC]** *see* Polysaccharide-Iron Complex *on page 1375*
- **Ferric (III) Hexacyanoferrate (II)** *see* Ferric Hexacyanoferrate *on page 705*

Ferric Gluconate (FER ik GLOO koe nate)

Brand Names: U.S. Ferrlecit®; Nulecit™

Brand Names: Canada Ferrlecit®

Index Terms Sodium Ferric Gluconate

Pharmacologic Category Iron Salt

Use Repletion of total body iron content in patients with iron-deficiency anemia who are undergoing hemodialysis in conjunction with erythropoietin therapy

Unlabeled Use Cancer-/chemotherapy-associated anemia

Pregnancy Risk Factor B

Dosage

Children ≥6 years: Repletion of iron in hemodialysis patients: 1.5 mg/kg of elemental iron (maximum: 125 mg/dose) diluted in NS 25 mL, administered over 60 minutes at 8 sequential dialysis sessions

Adults:

Repletion of iron in hemodialysis patients: I.V.: 125 mg elemental iron per 10 mL (either by I.V. infusion or slow I.V. injection). Most patients will require a cumulative dose of 1 g elemental iron over approximately 8 sequential dialysis treatments to achieve a favorable response.

Note: A test dose of 2 mL diluted in NS 50 mL administered over 60 minutes was previously recommended (not in current manufacturer labeling). Doses >125 mg are associated with increased adverse events.

Cancer-/chemotherapy-associated anemia (unlabeled use): I.V. infusion: 125 mg over 1 hour; maximum: 250 mg/infusion. Repeat dose every week for 8 doses. Test doses (25 mg slow I.V. push or infusion) are recommended in patients with iron dextran hypersensitivity or those with other drug allergies (NCCN guidelines, v.2.2010)

Additional Information Complete prescribing information for this medication should be consulted for additional detail.

Dosage Forms Excipient information presented when available (limited, particularly for generics); consult specific product labeling.

Injection, solution:

Ferrlecit®: Elemental iron 12.5 mg/mL (5 mL) [contains benzyl alcohol, sucrose 20%]

Nulecit™: Elemental iron 12.5 mg/mL (5 mL) [contains benzyl alcohol, sucrose ~20%]

Ferric Hexacyanoferrate
(FER ik hex a SYE an oh fer ate)

Brand Names: U.S. Radiogardase®

Index Terms Ferric (III) Hexacyanoferrate (II); Insoluble Prussian Blue; Prussian Blue

Pharmacologic Category Antidote

Use Treatment of known or suspected internal contamination with radioactive cesium and/or radioactive or nonradioactive thallium

Pregnancy Risk Factor C

Dosage Oral: Internal contamination with radioactive cesium and/or radioactive or nonradioactive thallium:

Children 2-12 years: 1 g 3 times/day; treatment should begin as soon as possible following exposure, but is also effective if therapy is delayed

Children >12 years and Adults: 3 g 3 times/day; treatment should begin as soon as possible following exposure, but is also effective if therapy is delayed

Note: Cesium exposure: Once internal radioactivity is substantially decreased, dosage may be reduced to 1-2 g 3 times/day to improve gastrointestinal tolerance

Elderly: Refer to adult dosing

Dosage adjustment in renal impairment: Studies have not been conducted; however, ferric hexacyanoferrate is not renally eliminated.

Dosage adjustment in hepatic impairment: Studies have not been conducted; however, effectiveness may be decreased due to decreased bile excretion of cesium and thallium.

Additional Information Complete prescribing information for this medication should be consulted for additional detail.

Dosage Forms Excipient information presented when available (limited, particularly for generics); consult specific product labeling.

Capsule, oral:

Radiogardase®: 0.5 g

- **Ferriprox®** *see* Deferiprone *on page 463*
- **Ferriprox®** *see* Deferiprone *on page 463*
- **Ferrlecit®** *see* Ferric Gluconate *on page 705*
- **Ferrocite™ [OTC]** *see* Ferrous Fumarate *on page 706*
- **Ferro-Sequels® [OTC]** *see* Ferrous Fumarate *on page 706*

Ferrous Fumarate (FER us FYOO ma rate)

Brand Names: U.S. Femiron® [OTC]; Ferretts® [OTC]; Ferro-Sequels® [OTC]; Ferrocite™ [OTC]; Hemocyte® [OTC]; Ircon® [OTC]

Brand Names: Canada Palafer®

Index Terms Iron Fumarate

Pharmacologic Category Iron Salt

Use Prevention and treatment of iron-deficiency anemias

Dosage

Dietary Reference Intake: Dose is RDA presented as elemental iron unless otherwise noted:

0-6 months: 0.27 mg/day (adequate intake)

7-12 months: 11 mg/day

1-3 years: 7 mg/day

4-8 years: 10 mg/day

9-13 years: 8 mg/day

14-18 years: Males: 11 mg/day; Females: 15 mg/day; Pregnant females: 27 mg/day; Lactating females: 10 mg/day

19-50 years: Males: 8 mg/day; Females: 18 mg/day; Pregnant females: 27 mg/day; Lactating females: 9 mg/day

≥50 years: 8 mg/day

Doses expressed in terms of elemental iron; elemental iron content of ferrous fumarate is 33%. Oral:

Children:

Severe iron-deficiency anemia: 4-6 mg elemental iron/kg/day in 3 divided doses

Mild-to-moderate iron-deficiency anemia: 3 mg elemental iron/kg/day in 1-2 divided doses

Prophylaxis: 1-2 mg elemental iron/kg/day

Adults:

Iron deficiency: Usual range: 150-200 mg elemental iron/day in divided doses; 60-100 mg elemental iron twice daily, up to 60 mg elemental iron 4 times/day

Prophylaxis: 60-100 mg elemental iron/day

To avoid GI upset, start with a single daily dose and increase by 1 tablet/day each week or as tolerated until desired daily dose is achieved

Elderly: Lower doses (15-50 mg elemental iron/day) may have similar efficacy and less GI adverse events (eg, nausea,constipation) as compared to higher doses (eg, 150 mg elemental iron/day) (Rimon, 2005).

Additional Information Complete prescribing information for this medication should be consulted for additional detail.

Dosage Forms Excipient information presented when available (limited, particularly for generics); consult specific product labeling.

Tablet, oral: 324 mg [elemental iron 106 mg]

Femiron®: 63 mg [elemental iron 20 mg]

Ferretts®: 325 mg [scored; elemental iron 106 mg]

Ferrocite™: 324 mg [elemental iron 106 mg]

Hemocyte®: 324 mg [elemental iron 106 mg]

Ircon®: 200 mg [elemental iron 66 mg]

Tablet, timed release, oral:

Ferro-Sequels®: 150 mg [contains sodium benzoate; elemental iron 50 mg; with docusate sodium]

Ferrous Gluconate (FER us GLOO koe nate)

Brand Names: U.S. Ferate [OTC]; Fergon® [OTC]

Brand Names: Canada Apo-Ferrous Gluconate®; Novo-Ferrogluc

Index Terms Iron Gluconate

Pharmacologic Category Iron Salt

Use Prevention and treatment of iron-deficiency anemias

Dosage Oral:

Dietary Reference Intake: Dose is RDA presented as elemental iron unless otherwise noted:

0-6 months: 0.27 mg/day (adequate intake)

7-12 months: 11 mg/day

1-3 years: 7 mg/day

4-8 years: 10 mg/day

9-13 years: 8 mg/day

14-18 years: Males: 11 mg/day; Females: 15 mg/day; Pregnant females: 27 mg/day; Lactating females: 10 mg/day

19-50 years: Males: 8 mg/day; Females: 18 mg/day; Pregnant females: 27 mg/day; Lactating females: 9 mg/day

≥50 years: 8 mg/day

Dose expressed in terms of elemental iron:

Children:

Severe iron-deficiency anemia: 4-6 mg Fe/kg/day in 3 divided doses

Mild to moderate iron deficiency anemia: 3 mg Fe/kg/day in 1-2 divided doses

Prophylaxis: 1-2 mg Fe/kg/day

Adults:

Iron deficiency: 60 mg twice daily up to 60 mg 4 times/day

Prophylaxis: 60 mg/day

Elderly: Lower doses (15-50 mg elemental iron/day) may have similar efficacy and less GI adverse events (eg, nausea, constipation) as compared to higher doses (eg, 150 mg elemental iron/day) (Rimon, 2005).

Additional Information Complete prescribing information for this medication should be consulted for additional detail.

Dosage Forms Excipient information presented when available (limited, particularly for generics); consult specific product labeling.

Tablet, oral: 246 mg [elemental iron 28 mg], 324 mg [elemental iron 38 mg], 325 mg [elemental iron 36 mg]

Ferate: 240 mg [elemental iron 27 mg]

Fergon®: 240 mg [elemental iron 27 mg]

Ferrous Sulfate (FER us SUL fate)

Brand Names: U.S. Feosol® [OTC]; Fer-In-Sol® [OTC]; Fer-iron [OTC]; MyKidz Iron 10™ [OTC]; Slow FE® [OTC]; Slow Release [OTC]

Brand Names: Canada Apo-Ferrous Sulfate®; Fer-In-Sol®; Ferodan™

Index Terms $FeSO_4$; Iron Sulfate

Pharmacologic Category Iron Salt

Additional Appendix Information

Beers Criteria – Potentially Inappropriate Medications for Geriatrics *on page 1973*

Use Prevention and treatment of iron-deficiency anemias

Dosage Oral: **Note:** Multiple concentrations of ferrous sulfate oral liquid exist; close attention must be paid to the concentration when ordering and administering ferrous sulfate; incorrect selection or substitution of one ferrous sulfate liquid for another without proper dosage volume adjustment may result in serious over- or underdosing.

Dietary Reference Intake: Dose is RDA presented as elemental iron unless otherwise noted:
0-6 months: 0.27 mg/day (adequate intake)
7-12 months: 11 mg/day
1-3 years: 7 mg/day
4-8 years: 10 mg/day
9-13 years: 8 mg/day
14-18 years: Males: 11 mg/day; Females: 15 mg/day; Pregnant females: 27 mg/day; Lactating females: 10 mg/day
19-50 years: Males: 8 mg/day; Females: 18 mg/day; Pregnant females: 27 mg/day; Lactating females: 9 mg/day
≥50 years: 8 mg/day

Children **(dose expressed in terms of elemental iron)**:
Severe iron-deficiency anemia: 4-6 mg Fe/kg/day in 3 divided doses
Mild-to-moderate iron deficiency anemia: 3 mg Fe/kg/day in 1-2 divided doses
Prophylaxis: 1-2 mg Fe/kg/day up to a maximum of 15 mg/day

Adults **(dose expressed in terms of ferrous sulfate)**:
Iron deficiency: 300 mg twice daily up to 300 mg 4 times/day or 250 mg (extended release) 1-2 times/day
Prophylaxis: 300 mg/day

Elderly: Lower doses (15-50 mg elemental iron/day) may have similar efficacy and less GI adverse events (eg, nausea, constipation) as compared to higher doses (eg, 150 mg elemental iron/day) (Rimon, 2005).

Additional Information Complete prescribing information for this medication should be consulted for additional detail.

Dosage Forms Excipient information presented when available (limited, particularly for generics); consult specific product labeling. [DSC] = Discontinued product
Elixir, oral: 220 mg/5 mL (473 mL, 480 mL) [elemental iron 44 mg/5 mL]
Liquid, oral: 300 mg/5 mL (5 mL) [elemental iron ~60 mg/5 mL]
Liquid, oral [drops]: 75 mg/mL (50 mL) [elemental iron 15 mg/mL]; 75 mg/0.6 mL (50 mL [DSC]) [elemental iron 15 mg/0.6 mL]
Fer-In-Sol®: 75 mg/mL (50 mL) [gluten free; contains ethanol 0.2%, sodium bisulfite; elemental iron 15 mg/mL]
Fer-iron: 75 mg/mL (50 mL) [contains ethanol 0.2%, sodium bisulfite; lemon flavor; elemental iron 15 mg/mL]
Suspension, oral [drops]:
MyKidz Iron 10™: 75 mg/1.5 mL (118 mL) [dye free, ethanol free; contains propylene glycol, sodium 12 mg/1.5 mL; strawberry-banana flavor; elemental iron 15 mg/1.5 mL]
Tablet, oral: 324 mg [elemental iron 65 mg], 325 mg [elemental iron 65 mg]
Tablet, oral [exsiccated]:
Feosol®: 200 mg [elemental iron 65 mg]
Tablet, enteric coated, oral: 324 mg [elemental iron 65 mg], 325 mg [elemental iron 65 mg]
Tablet, extended release, oral: 140 mg [elemental iron 45 mg], 160 mg [DSC] [elemental iron 50 mg]
Tablet, slow release, oral: 160 mg [elemental iron 50 mg]
Slow FE®: 142 mg [elemental iron 45 mg]
Slow Release: 140 mg [elemental iron 45 mg]

◆ **Fertinorm® H.P. (Can)** *see* Urofollitropin *on page 1750*

Ferumoxytol (fer ue MOX i tol)

Brand Names: U.S. Feraheme®
Pharmacologic Category Iron Salt
Use Treatment of iron-deficiency anemia in chronic kidney disease
Pregnancy Risk Factor C
Dosage Doses expressed in mg of **elemental** iron. **Note:** Test dose: Product labeling does not indicate need for a test dose.
I.V.: Adults: Iron-deficiency anemia in chronic kidney disease: 510 mg (17 mL) as a single dose, followed by a second 510 mg dose 3-8 days after initial dose. Recommended dose may be readministered in patients with persistent or recurrent iron deficiency anemia.
Dosage adjustment in renal impairment: Hemodialysis patients should receive injection after at least 1 hour of hemodialysis has been completed and once blood pressure has stabilized.
Additional Information Complete prescribing information for this medication should be consulted for additional detail.
Dosage Forms Excipient information presented when available (limited, particularly for generics); consult specific product labeling.
Injection, solution:
Feraheme®: Elemental iron 30 mg/mL (17 mL)

◆ **FESO** *see* Fesoterodine *on page 707*
◆ **$FeSO_4$** *see* Ferrous Sulfate *on page 706*

Fesoterodine (fes oh TER oh deen)

Brand Names: U.S. Toviaz™
Index Terms FESO; Fesoterodine Fumarate
Pharmacologic Category Anticholinergic Agent
Use Treatment of patients with an overactive bladder with symptoms of urinary frequency, urgency, or urge incontinence.
Pregnancy Risk Factor C
Pregnancy Considerations Teratogenic effects were observed in some animal studies. There are no adequate and well-controlled studies in pregnant women. Use during pregnancy only if the potential benefit to the mother outweighs the possible risk to the fetus.
Lactation Excretion in breast milk unknown/not recommended
Contraindications Hypersensitivity to fesoterodine or tolterodine (both are metabolized to 5-hydroxymethyl tolterodine) or any component of the formulation; urinary retention; gastric retention; uncontrolled narrow-angle glaucoma
Warnings/Precautions Cases of angioedema involving the face, lips, tongue, and/or larynx have been reported. Immediately discontinue if tongue, hypopharynx, or larynx are involved. May cause drowsiness and/or blurred vision, which may impair physical or mental abilities; patients must be cautioned about performing tasks which require mental alertness (eg, operating machinery or driving). Patients may experience decreased sweating; caution use in hot weather or during exercise. Use is not recommended in patients with severe hepatic impairment (Child-Pugh class C). Doses >4 mg are not recommended for patients with severe renal impairment (Cl_{cr} <30 mL/minute) or patients receiving concurrent therapy with strong CYP3A4 inhibitors. Use caution in patients with bladder flow obstruction, gastrointestinal obstructive disorders, myasthenia gravis, and treated narrow-angle glaucoma. Risk of adverse effects may be increased in elderly patients.
Adverse Reactions
>10%: Gastrointestinal: Xerostomia (19% to 35%; dose related)
1% to 10%:
Central nervous system: Insomnia (1%)

Dermatological: Rash (1%)
Gastrointestinal: Constipation (4% to 6%), dyspepsia (2%), nausea (1% to 2%), abdominal pain (1%)
Genitourinary: Urinary tract infection (3% to 4%), dysuria (1% to 2%), urinary retention (1%)
Hepatic: ALT increased (1%), GGT increased (1%)
Neuromuscular & skeletal: Back pain (1% to 2%)
Ocular: Dry eyes (1% to 4%)
Respiratory: Upper respiratory tract infection (2% to 3%), cough (1% to 2%), dry throat (1% to 2%)
Miscellaneous: Peripheral edema (1%)

<1% (Limited to important or life-threatening): Angina, angioedema, diverticulitis, gastroenteritis, heat prostration, hypersensitivity reactions, irritable bowel syndrome, QT_c prolongation

Drug Interactions

Metabolism/Transport Effects Substrate of CYP2D6 (minor), CYP3A4 (major); **Note:** Assignment of Major/Minor substrate status based on clinically relevant drug interaction potential

Avoid Concomitant Use There are no known interactions where it is recommended to avoid concomitant use.

Increased Effect/Toxicity

Fesoterodine may increase the levels/effects of: AbobotulinumtoxinA; Anticholinergics; Cannabinoids; OnabotulinumtoxinA; Potassium Chloride; RimabotulinumtoxinB

The levels/effects of Fesoterodine may be increased by: CYP2D6 Inhibitors; CYP3A4 Inhibitors (Moderate); CYP3A4 Inhibitors (Strong); Dasatinib; Pramlintide

Decreased Effect

Fesoterodine may decrease the levels/effects of: Acetylcholinesterase Inhibitors (Central); Secretin

The levels/effects of Fesoterodine may be decreased by: Acetylcholinesterase Inhibitors (Central); CYP3A4 Inducers (Strong); Deferasirox; Herbs (CYP3A4 Inducers); Peginterferon Alfa-2b; Tocilizumab

Ethanol/Nutrition/Herb Interactions Ethanol: Adverse effects may be potentiated

Stability Store at 20°C to 25°C (68°F to 77°F); excursions permitted between 15°C to 30°C (59°F to 86°F). Protect from moisture.

Mechanism of Action Fesoterodine acts as a prodrug and is converted to an active metabolite, 5-hydroxymethyl tolterodine (5-HMT); 5-HMT is responsible for fesoterodine's antimuscarinic activity and acts as a competitive antagonist of muscarinic receptors.

Urinary bladder contractions are mediated by muscarinic receptors; fesoterodine inhibits the receptors in the bladder preventing symptoms of urgency and frequency.

Pharmacodynamics/Kinetics

Absorption: Well absorbed
Distribution: I.V.: 5-HMT: V_d: 169 L
Protein binding: 5-HMT: ~50% (primarily to albumin and $alpha_1$-acid glycoprotein)
Metabolism: Fesoterodine is rapidly and extensively metabolized to its active metabolite (5-hydroxymethyl tolterodine; 5-HMT) by nonspecific esterases; 5-HMT is further metabolized via CYP2D6 and CYP3A4 to inactive metabolites.
Bioavailability: 5-HMT: 52%
Half-life elimination: ~7 hours
Time to peak, plasma: 5-HMT: ~5 hours; C_{max} higher in poor CYP2D6 metabolizers
Excretion: Urine (~70%; 16% as 5-HMT, ~53% as inactive metabolites); feces (7%)

Dosage Oral: Adults: Overactive bladder: 4 mg once daily; may be increased to 8 mg once daily based on individual response and tolerability

Dosing adjustment for concomitant strong CYP3A4 inhibitors (eg, ketoconazole, itraconazole, clarithromycin): 4 mg once daily; maximum dose: 4 mg once daily

Dosing adjustment in renal impairment:
Cl_{cr} ≥30 mL/minute: No dosage adjustment necessary
Cl_{cr} <30 mL/minute: 4 mg once daily; maximum dose: 4 mg once daily

Dosing adjustment in hepatic impairment:
Mild-to-moderate impairment (Child-Pugh class A or B): No dosage adjustment necessary
Severe impairment (Child-Pugh class C): Use is not recommended; has not been studied

Dietary Considerations May be taken with or without food.

Administration May be administered with or without food. Swallow whole; do not chew, crush, or divide.

Dosage Forms Excipient information presented when available (limited, particularly for generics); consult specific product labeling.

Tablet, extended release, oral, as fumarate:
Toviaz™: 4 mg, 8 mg [contains soya lecithin]

◆ **Fesoterodine Fumarate** *see* Fesoterodine *on page 707*
◆ **Feverall® [OTC]** *see* Acetaminophen *on page 27*
◆ **Fexmid®** *see* Cyclobenzaprine *on page 419*

Fexofenadine (feks oh FEN a deen)

Brand Names: U.S. Allegra®; Allegra® Allergy 12 Hour [OTC]; Allegra® Allergy 24 Hour [OTC]; Allegra® Children's Allergy ODT [OTC]; Allegra® Children's Allergy [OTC]; Allegra® ODT [DSC]

Brand Names: Canada Allegra®

Index Terms Fexofenadine Hydrochloride

Pharmacologic Category Histamine H_1 Antagonist; Histamine H_1 Antagonist, Second Generation; Piperidine Derivative

Use Relief of symptoms associated with seasonal allergic rhinitis; treatment of chronic idiopathic urticaria

OTC labeling: Relief of symptoms associated with allergic rhinitis

Pregnancy Risk Factor C

Pregnancy Considerations Adverse events have been observed in animal reproduction studies; therefore, the manufacturer classifies fexofenadine as pregnancy category C. The use of antihistamines for the treatment of rhinitis during pregnancy is generally considered to be safe at recommended doses. Information related to the use of fexofenadine during pregnancy is limited; therefore, other agents are preferred.

Lactation Excretion in breast milk unknown/use caution (AAP rates "compatible"; AAP 2001 update pending)

Contraindications Hypersensitivity to fexofenadine or any component of the formulation

Warnings/Precautions Use with caution in patients with renal impairment; dosage adjustment recommended. Safety and efficacy in children <6 months of age have not been established; orally disintegrating tablet not recommended for use in children <6 years of age. Orally disintegrating tablet contains phenylalanine.

Adverse Reactions

>10%:
Central nervous system: Headache (5% to 11%)
Gastrointestinal: Vomiting (children 6 months to 5 years: 4% to 12%)

1% to 10%:
Central nervous system: Fatigue (1% to 3%), somnolence (1% to 3%), dizziness (2%), fever (2%), pain (2%), drowsiness (1%)
Endocrine & metabolic: Dysmenorrhea (2%)
Gastrointestinal: Diarrhea (3% to 4%), nausea (2%), dyspepsia (1% to 2%)
Neuromuscular & skeletal: Myalgia (3%), back pain (2% to 3%), pain in extremities (2%)
Otic: Otitis media (2% to 4%)

Respiratory: Upper respiratory tract infection (3% to 4%), cough (2% to 4%), rhinorrhea (1% to 2%)
Miscellaneous: Viral infection (3%)
<1% (Limited to important or life-threatening): Hypersensitivity reactions (anaphylaxis, angioedema, chest tightness, dyspnea, flushing, pruritus, rash, urticaria); insomnia, nervousness, sleep disorders, paroniria

Drug Interactions

Metabolism/Transport Effects Substrate of CYP3A4 (minor), P-glycoprotein, SLCO1B1; **Note:** Assignment of Major/Minor substrate status based on clinically relevant drug interaction potential; **Inhibits** CYP2D6 (weak)

Avoid Concomitant Use There are no known interactions where it is recommended to avoid concomitant use.

Increased Effect/Toxicity

Fexofenadine may increase the levels/effects of: Alcohol (Ethyl); Anticholinergics; CNS Depressants; Methotrimeprazine; Selective Serotonin Reuptake Inhibitors

The levels/effects of Fexofenadine may be increased by: Conivaptan; Droperidol; Eltrombopag; Erythromycin; Erythromycin (Systemic); HydrOXYzine; Itraconazole; Ketoconazole; Ketoconazole (Systemic); Methotrimeprazine; P-glycoprotein/ABCB1 Inhibitors; Pramlintide; Verapamil

Decreased Effect

Fexofenadine may decrease the levels/effects of: Acetylcholinesterase Inhibitors (Central); Benzylpenicilloyl Polylysine; Betahistine

The levels/effects of Fexofenadine may be decreased by: Acetylcholinesterase Inhibitors (Central); Amphetamines; Antacids; Grapefruit Juice; P-glycoprotein/ABCB1 Inducers; Rifampin; Tocilizumab

Ethanol/Nutrition/Herb Interactions

Ethanol: May increase CNS depression; monitor for increased effects with coadministration. Caution patients about effects.
Food: Fruit juice (apple, grapefruit, orange) may decrease bioavailability of fexofenadine by ~36%.
Herb/Nutraceutical: St John's wort may decrease fexofenadine levels.

Stability Store at controlled room temperature of 20°C to 25°C (68°F to 77°F). Protect from excessive moisture.

Mechanism of Action Fexofenadine is an active metabolite of terfenadine and like terfenadine it competes with histamine for H_1-receptor sites on effector cells in the gastrointestinal tract, blood vessels and respiratory tract; it appears that fexofenadine does not cross the blood-brain barrier to any appreciable degree, resulting in a reduced potential for sedation

Pharmacodynamics/Kinetics

Onset of action: 60 minutes
Duration: Antihistaminic effect: ≥12 hours
Absorption: Rapid
Protein binding: 60% to 70%, primarily albumin and alpha$_1$-acid glycoprotein
Metabolism: Minimal (Hepatic ~5%)
Half-life elimination: 14.4 hours (31% to 72% longer in renal impairment)
Time to peak, serum: ODT: 2 hours (4 hours with high-fat meal); Tablet: ~2.6 hours; Suspension: ~1 hour
Excretion: Feces (~80%) and urine (~11%) as unchanged drug

Dosage Oral:

Chronic idiopathic urticaria: Children 6 months to <2 years: 15 mg twice daily

Chronic idiopathic urticaria, seasonal allergic rhinitis:
- Children 2-11 years: 30 mg twice daily
- Children ≥12 years and Adults: 60 mg twice daily **or** 180 mg once daily
- Elderly: Starting dose: Use caution; adjust dose for renal impairment

Allergic rhinitis (OTC labeling):
- Children 2-11 years: 30 mg twice daily
- Children ≥12 years and Adults: 60 mg twice daily **or** 180 mg once daily

Dosing adjustment in renal impairment: Cl_{cr} <80 mL/minute:
- Children 6 months to <2 years: Initial: 15 mg once daily
- Children 2-11 years: Initial: 30 mg once daily
- Children ≥12 years and Adults: Initial: 60 mg once daily

Hemodialysis: Not effectively removed by hemodialysis

Dietary Considerations Some products may contain phenylalanine and/or sodium. Take suspension and tablets with water only; do not administer with fruit juices.

Administration

Suspension, tablet: Administer with water only; do not administer with fruit juices. Shake suspension well before use.
Orally disintegrating tablet: Take on an empty stomach. Do not remove from blister pack until administered. Using dry hands, place immediately on tongue. Tablet will dissolve within seconds, and may be swallowed with or without liquid (do not administer with fruit juices). Do not split or chew.

Monitoring Parameters Relief of symptoms

Test Interactions May suppress the wheal and flare reactions to skin test antigens

Dosage Forms Excipient information presented when available (limited, particularly for generics); consult specific product labeling. [DSC] = Discontinued product

Suspension, oral, as hydrochloride:
- Allegra®: 6 mg/mL (300 mL) [contains propylene glycol; raspberry cream flavor]
- Allegra® Children's Allergy: 6 mg/mL (120 mL) [contains propylene glycol, sodium 18 mg/5 mL; berry flavor]

Tablet, oral, as hydrochloride: 30 mg, 60 mg, 180 mg
- Allegra®: 60 mg [DSC], 180 mg [DSC]
- Allegra® Allergy 12 Hour: 60 mg
- Allegra® Allergy 24 Hour: 180 mg
- Allegra® Children's Allergy: 30 mg

Tablet, orally disintegrating, oral, as hydrochloride:
- Allegra® Children's Allergy ODT: 30 mg [contains phenylalanine 5.3 mg/tablet, sodium 5 mg/tablet; orange cream flavor]
- Allegra® ODT: 30 mg [DSC] [contains phenylalanine 5.3 mg/tablet; orange cream flavor]

Fexofenadine and Pseudoephedrine

(feks oh FEN a deen & soo doe e FED rin)

Brand Names: U.S. Allegra-D® 12 Hour; Allegra-D® 24 Hour

Brand Names: Canada Allegra-D®

Index Terms Pseudoephedrine and Fexofenadine

Pharmacologic Category Alpha/Beta Agonist; Decongestant; Histamine H_1 Antagonist; Histamine H_1 Antagonist, Second Generation; Piperidine Derivative

Use Relief of symptoms associated with seasonal allergic rhinitis in adults and children ≥12 years of age

Pregnancy Risk Factor C

Dosage Oral: Children ≥12 years and Adults:
- Allegra-D® 12 Hour: One tablet twice daily
- Allegra-D® 24 Hour: One tablet once daily

Dosage adjustment in renal impairment:
- Allegra-D® 12 Hour: Cl_{cr} <80 mL/minute (based on fexofenadine component): One tablet once daily
- Allegra-D® 24 Hour: Avoid use.

Additional Information Complete prescribing information for this medication should be consulted for additional detail.

Dosage Forms Excipient information presented when available (limited, particularly for generics); consult specific product labeling.

Tablet, extended release: Fexofenadine hydrochloride 60 mg [immediate release] and pseudoephedrine hydrochloride 120 mg [extended release]; fexofenadine hydrochloride 180 mg [immediate release] and pseudoephedrine hydrochloride 240 mg [extended release]

Allegra-D® 12 Hour: Fexofenadine hydrochloride 60 mg [immediate release] and pseudoephedrine hydrochloride 120 mg [extended release]

Allegra-D® 24 Hour: Fexofenadine hydrochloride 180 mg [immediate release] and pseudoephedrine hydrochloride 240 mg [extended release]

- **Fexofenadine Hydrochloride** *see* Fexofenadine *on page 708*
- **Fiberall® [OTC]** *see* Psyllium *on page 1432*
- **Fibricor®** *see* Fenofibric Acid *on page 695*

Fibrinogen Concentrate (Human)

(fi BRIN o gin KON suhn trate HYU man)

Brand Names: U.S. RiaSTAP®

Index Terms Coagulation Factor I

Pharmacologic Category Blood Product Derivative

Use Treatment of acute bleeding episodes in patients with congenital fibrinogen deficiency (afibrinogenemia and hypofibrinogenemia)

Pregnancy Risk Factor C

Pregnancy Considerations Animal reproduction studies have not been conducted. Increased pregnancy loss is associated with untreated congenital fibrinogen disorders.

Contraindications Severe hypersensitivity reactions to fibrinogen concentrate or any component of the formulation

Warnings/Precautions Hypersensitivity reactions (eg, urticaria, hives, wheezing, hypotension, anaphylaxis) may occur. In the event of hypersensitivity reactions, treatment should be discontinued immediately. Thrombosis may occur in patients with congenital fibrinogen deficiency with or without fibrinogen replacement therapy. Consider potential risk of thrombosis with use. Product of human plasma; may potentially contain infectious agents which could transmit disease. Screening of donors, as well as testing and/or inactivation or removal of certain viruses, reduces the risk. Infections thought to be transmitted by this product should be reported to the manufacturer. Not for the treatment of dysfibrinogenemia.

Adverse Reactions

>1%: Central nervous system: Fever, headache

Postmarketing and/or case reports: Allergic reactions, anaphylaxis, arterial thrombosis, chills, DVT, dyspnea, MI, nausea, pulmonary embolism, rash, thromboembolism, vomiting

Drug Interactions

Metabolism/Transport Effects None known.

Avoid Concomitant Use There are no known interactions where it is recommended to avoid concomitant use.

Increased Effect/Toxicity

Fibrinogen Concentrate (Human) may increase the levels/effects of: Antifibrinolytic Agents

The levels/effects of Fibrinogen Concentrate (Human) may be increased by: Antifibrinolytic Agents

Decreased Effect There are no known significant interactions involving a decrease in effect.

Stability Store at 2°C to 25°C (36°F to 77°F) in original carton; do not freeze. Protect from light. Transfer sterile water for injection 50 mL into vial. Gently swirl until dissolved; do not shake. Stable for 24 hours after reconstitution when stored at 20°C to 25°C (68°F to 77°F). Discard partially used vials.

Mechanism of Action Fibrinogen (coagulation factor I), a protein found in normal plasma, is required to clot blood. Fibrinogen concentrate made from pooled human plasma replaces this protein which is missing or reduced in patients with a congenital fibrinogen deficiency.

Pharmacodynamics/Kinetics

Distribution: V_d: 45-60 mL/kg (range 36-68 mL/kg)

Half-life elimination: 61-97 hours (range 56-117 hours); may be decreased in children <16 years of age

Dosage I.V.: Children and Adults: Congenital fibrinogen deficiency: **Note:** Adjust dose based on laboratory values and condition of patient. Maintain a target fibrinogen level of 100 mg/dL until hemostasis is achieved.

When baseline fibrinogen level is known:

Dose (mg/kg) = [Target level (mg/dL) - measured level (mg/dL)] **divided by** 1.7 (mg/dL per mg/kg body weight)

When baseline fibrinogen level is not known: 70 mg/kg

Administration For I.V. administration only; infuse at ≤5 mL/minute

Monitoring Parameters Signs and symptoms of hypersensitivity, thrombosis; fibrinogen level

Reference Range A target fibrinogen level of 100 mg/dL should be maintained until hemostasis occurs and wound healing is complete.

Normal fibrinogen levels: 200-450 mg/dL

Dosage Forms Excipient information presented when available (limited, particularly for generics); consult specific product labeling. [DSC] = Discontinued product

Injection, powder for reconstitution:

RiaSTAP®: 900-1300 mg [contains albumin (human); exact potency labeled on vial]

- **Fibro-XL [OTC]** *see* Psyllium *on page 1432*
- **Fibro-Lax [OTC]** *see* Psyllium *on page 1432*

Fidaxomicin (fye DAX oh mye sin)

Brand Names: U.S. Dificid™

Index Terms Difimicin; Lipiarrmycin; OPT-80; PAR-101; Tiacumicin B

Pharmacologic Category Antibiotic, Macrolide

Use Treatment of *Clostridium difficile*-associated diarrhea (CDAD)

Pregnancy Risk Factor B

Pregnancy Considerations Adverse events were not observed in animal reproduction studies. Due to the limited oral absorption of fidaxomicin, exposure to the fetus is expected to be low. There are no adequate and well-controlled studies in pregnant women.

Lactation Excretion in breast milk unknown/use caution

Contraindications There are no contraindications listed in the manufacturer's labeling.

Warnings/Precautions Do not use for systemic infections; fidaxomicin systemic absorption is negligible. Use only in patients with proven or strongly suspected *Clostridium difficile (C. difficile)* infections.

Adverse Reactions

>10%: Gastrointestinal: Nausea (11%)

2% to 10%:

Gastrointestinal: Gastrointestinal hemorrhage (4%), abdominal pain, vomiting

Hematologic: Anemia (2%), neutropenia (2%)

<2%: Abdominal distension, abdominal tenderness, alkaline phosphatase increased, blood bicarbonate decreased, drug eruption, dyspepsia, dysphagia, flatulence, hepatic enzymes increased, hyperglycemia, intestinal obstruction, megacolon, metabolic acidosis, platelet count decreased, pruritus, rash

Drug Interactions

Metabolism/Transport Effects None known.

Avoid Concomitant Use There are no known interactions where it is recommended to avoid concomitant use.

Increased Effect/Toxicity There are no known significant interactions involving an increase in effect.

Decreased Effect There are no known significant interactions involving a decrease in effect.

Stability Store at 20°C to 25°C (68°F to 77°F); excursions permitted to 15°C to 30°C (59°F to 86°F).

Mechanism of Action Inhibits RNA polymerase sigma subunit resulting in inhibition of protein synthesis and cell death in susceptible organisms including *C. difficile*; bactericidal

Pharmacodynamics/Kinetics

Absorption: Oral: Minimal systemic absorption

Distribution: Largely confined to the gastrointestinal tract; in single- and multiple-dose studies, fecal concentrations of fidaxomicin and its active metabolite (OP-1118) are very high while serum concentrations are minimally detectable to undetectable

Metabolism: Intestinal hydrolysis to less active metabolite (OP-1118)

Excretion: Feces (>92% as unchanged drug and metabolites); urine (<1% as metabolite)

Dosage Oral: Adults: Diarrhea due to *Clostridium difficile* (CDAD): 200 mg twice daily for 10 days

Dosing adjustment in renal impairment: Minimal systemic absorption; no dosage adjustment needed

Dosing adjustment in hepatic impairment: Not studied; minimally absorbed, so no dosage adjustment predicted

Dietary Considerations May be taken without regard to food.

Administration May be administered with or without food.

Additional Information Fidaxomicin is bactericidal against gram-positive anaerobes (including *C. difficile* NAP1/B1/027 strain) and gram-positive aerobes. Fidaxomicin spectrum does **not** include gram-negative aerobes or gram-negative anaerobes (eg, *Bacteroides spp*). At the approved dose, concentrations in feces substantially exceed the 90% MIC of *C. difficile*. Postantibiotic effects against *C. difficile* in clinical studies range from 6–10 hours. Clinical studies excluded patients with a history of >1 recurrent *C. difficile*-associated diarrhea (CDAD) episode within 3 months.

Dosage Forms Excipient information presented when available (limited, particularly for generics); consult specific product labeling.

Tablet, oral:

Dificid™: 200 mg [contains soy lecithin]

Filgrastim (fil GRA stim)

Brand Names: U.S. Neupogen®

Brand Names: Canada Neupogen®

Index Terms G-CSF; Granulocyte Colony Stimulating Factor

Pharmacologic Category Colony Stimulating Factor

Use

Cancer patients (nonmyeloid malignancies) receiving myelosuppressive chemotherapy to decrease the incidence of infection (febrile neutropenia) in regimens associated with a high incidence of neutropenia with fever

Acute myelogenous leukemia (AML) following induction or consolidation chemotherapy to shorten time to neutrophil recovery and reduce the duration of fever

Cancer patients (nonmyeloid malignancies) receiving bone marrow transplant to shorten the duration of neutropenia and neutropenia-related events (eg, neutropenic fever)

Peripheral stem cell transplantation to mobilize hematopoietic progenitor cells for leukapheresis collection

Severe chronic neutropenia (SCN; chronic administration) to reduce the incidence and duration of neutropenic complications (fever, infections, oropharyngeal ulcers) in symptomatic patients with congenital, cyclic, or idiopathic neutropenia

Unlabeled Use Treatment of anemia in myelodysplastic syndrome; mobilization of hematopoietic stem cells (HSC) for collection and subsequent autologous transplantation (in combination with plerixafor) in patients with non-Hodgkin's lymphoma (NHL) and multiple myeloma (MM); treatment of neutropenia in HIV-infected patients receiving zidovudine; hepatitis C treatment-associated neutropenia

Pregnancy Risk Factor C

Pregnancy Considerations Animal studies have demonstrated adverse effects and fetal loss. Filgrastim has been shown to cross the placenta in humans. There are no adequate and well-controlled studies in pregnant women. Use only if potential benefit to mother justifies risk to the fetus. Women who become pregnant during filgrastim treatment are encouraged to enroll in Amgen's Pregnancy Surveillance Program (1-800-772-6436).

Lactation Excretion in breast milk unknown/use caution

Contraindications Hypersensitivity to filgrastim, *E. coli*-derived proteins, or any component of the formulation

Warnings/Precautions Do not use filgrastim in the period 24 hours before to 24 hours after administration of cytotoxic chemotherapy because of the potential sensitivity of rapidly dividing myeloid cells to cytotoxic chemotherapy. May potentially act as a growth factor for any tumor type, particularly myeloid malignancies; caution should be exercised in the usage of filgrastim in any malignancy with myeloid characteristics. Increases circulating leukocytes when used in conjunction with plerixafor for stem cell mobilization; monitor WBC; use with caution in patients with neutrophil count >50,000/mm^3; tumor cells released from marrow could be collected in leukapheresis product; potential effect of tumor cell reinfusion is unknown. Reports of alveolar hemorrhage, manifested as pulmonary infiltrates and hemoptysis, have occurred in healthy donors undergoing PBPC collection (not FDA approved for use in healthy donors); hemoptysis resolved upon discontinuation. Safety and efficacy have not been established with patients receiving radiation therapy (avoid concurrent radiation therapy with filgrastim), or chemotherapy associated with delayed myelosuppression (eg, nitrosoureas, mitomycin C).

Allergic-type reactions (rash, urticaria, facial edema, wheezing, dyspnea, tachycardia, and/or hypotension) have occurred with first or subsequent doses. Reactions tended to involve ≥2 body systems and occur more frequently with intravenous administration and generally within 30 minutes of administration; may recur with rechallenge. Rare cases of acute respiratory distress syndrome (ARDS) have been reported (possibly due to influx of neutrophils to sites of lung inflammation); withhold or discontinue filgrastim if ARDS occurs; patients must be instructed to report respiratory distress; monitor for fever, infiltrates, or respiratory distress. Rare cases of splenic rupture have been reported (may be fatal); patients must be instructed to report left upper quadrant pain or shoulder tip pain. Cutaneous vasculitis has been reported, generally occurring in severe chronic neutropenia (SCN) patients on long-term therapy; symptoms generally developed with increasing absolute neutrophil count (ANC) and subsided when the ANC decreased; dose reductions may improve symptoms to allow for continued therapy. Use caution in patients with sickle cell disorders; severe sickle cell crises (sometimes resulting in fatalities) have been reported following filgrastim therapy. Filgrastim use prior to appropriate diagnosis of SCN may impair proper evaluation and treatment for neutropenia not due to SCN. Cytogenetic abnormalities, transformation to myelodysplastic syndrome (MDS) and acute myeloid leukemia (AML) have been observed in patients treated with filgrastim for congenital neutropenia; a longer duration of treatment and poorer ANC response appear to increase the risk. Carefully consider the risk of continuing filgrastim in patients who develop abnormal cytogenetics or MDS. The packaging of some forms may contain latex.

Adverse Reactions

>10%:

Central nervous system: Fever (12%)

Dermatologic: Petechiae (≤17%), rash (≤12%)

Endocrine & metabolic: LDH increased, uric acid increased

Gastrointestinal: Splenomegaly (severe chronic neutropenia: 30%; rare in other patients)

Hepatic: Alkaline phosphatase increased (21%)

Neuromuscular & skeletal: Bone/skeletal pain (22% to 33%; dose related), commonly in the lower back, posterior iliac crest, and sternum

Respiratory: Epistaxis (9% to 15%)

1% to 10%:

Cardiovascular: Hyper-/hypotension (4%), myocardial infarction/arrhythmias (3%)

Central nervous system: Headache (7%)

Gastrointestinal: Nausea (10%), vomiting (7%), peritonitis (≤2%)

Hematologic: Leukocytosis (2%)

Miscellaneous: Transfusion reaction (≤10%)

<1% (Limited to important or life-threatening): Acute respiratory distress syndrome (ARDS), allergic reactions, alopecia, alveolar hemorrhage, arthralgia, capillary leak syndrome, cerebral hemorrhage, cutaneous vasculitis, dyspnea, edema (facial), erythema nodosum, hematuria, hemoptysis, hepatomegaly, hypersensitivity reaction, injection site reaction, osteoporosis, pericarditis, proteinuria, psoriasis exacerbation, pulmonary infiltrates, renal insufficiency, sickle cell crisis, splenic rupture, Sweet's syndrome (acute febrile dermatosis), tachycardia, thrombocytopenia (in PBPC mobilization), thrombophlebitis, transient supraventricular arrhythmia, urticaria, wheezing

Drug Interactions

Metabolism/Transport Effects None known.

Avoid Concomitant Use There are no known interactions where it is recommended to avoid concomitant use.

Increased Effect/Toxicity

Filgrastim may increase the levels/effects of: Bleomycin; Topotecan

Decreased Effect There are no known significant interactions involving a decrease in effect.

Stability Intact vials and prefilled syringes should be stored under refrigeration at 2°C to 8°C (36°F to 46°F) and protected from direct sunlight. Filgrastim should be protected from freezing and temperatures >30°C to avoid aggregation. Do not shake.

Filgrastim vials and prefilled syringes are stable for 24 hours at 9°C to 30°C (47°F to 86°F).

Undiluted filgrastim is stable for 24 hours at 15°C to 30°C (59°F to 86°F) and for up to 14 days at 2°C to 8°C (36°F to 46°F) (data on file, Amgen Medical Information) in BD tuberculin syringes; however, sterility has only been assessed and maintained for up to 7 days when prepared under strict aseptic conditions (Jacobson, 1996; Singh, 1994). The manufacturer recommends using syringes within 24 hours due to the potential for bacterial contamination.

Do not dilute with saline at any time; product may precipitate. Filgrastim may be diluted with D_5W for I.V. infusion administration (5-15 mcg/mL; minimum concentration is 5 mcg/mL). This diluted solution is stable for 7 days at 2°C to 8°C (36°F to 46°F), however, should be used within 24 hours due to the possibility for bacterial contamination. Concentrations 5-15 mcg/mL require addition of albumin (final albumin concentration of 2 mg/mL) to prevent adsorption to plastics. Dilution to <5 mcg/mL is not recommended.

Mechanism of Action Stimulates the production, maturation, and activation of neutrophils; filgrastim activates neutrophils to increase both their migration and cytotoxicity.

Pharmacodynamics/Kinetics

Onset of action: ~24 hours; plateaus in 3-5 days

Duration: Neutrophil counts generally return to baseline within 4 days

Absorption: SubQ: 100%

Distribution: V_d: 150 mL/kg; no evidence of drug accumulation over a 11- to 20-day period

Metabolism: Systemically degraded

Half-life elimination: 1.8-3.5 hours

Time to peak, serum: SubQ: 2-8 hours

Dosage Details concerning dosing in combination regimens and institution protocols should also be consulted. Rounding doses to the nearest vial size may enhance patient convenience and reduce costs without compromising clinical response.

Children: Neutropenia (ANC <500/mm³) due to zidovudine treatment for HIV-infection (unlabeled use): SubQ, I.V.: 5-10 mcg/kg once daily (AIDS*info* guidelines, 2010)

Children and Adults:

Chemotherapy-induced neutropenia: SubQ, I.V.: 5 mcg/kg/day; doses may be increased by 5 mcg/kg (for each chemotherapy cycle) according to the duration and severity of the neutropenia; continue for up to 14 days or until the ANC reaches 10,000/mm³

Bone marrow transplantation (in patients with cancer; to shorten the duration of neutropenia and neutropenia-related events): SubQ, I.V.: 10 mcg/kg/day (administer ≥24 hours after chemotherapy and ≥24 hours after bone marrow infusion); adjust the dose according to the duration and severity of neutropenia; recommended steps based on neutrophil response:

When ANC >1000/mm³ for 3 consecutive days: Reduce filgrastim dose to 5 mcg/kg/day

If ANC remains >1000/mm³ for 3 more consecutive days: Discontinue filgrastim

If ANC decreases to <1000/mm³: Resume at 5 mcg/kg/day

If ANC decreases to <1000/mm³ during the 5 mcg/kg/day dose, increase filgrastim to 10 mcg/kg/day and follow the above steps

Peripheral blood progenitor cell (PBPC) collection: SubQ: 10 mcg/kg daily, usually for 6-7 days. Begin at least 4 days before the first leukapheresis and continue until the last leukapheresis; consider dose adjustment for WBC >100,000/mm³

Severe chronic neutropenia: SubQ:

Congenital: Initial: 6 mcg/kg twice daily; adjust the dose based on ANC and clinical response

Idiopathic/cyclic: Initial: 5 mcg/kg/day; adjust the dose based on ANC and clinical response

Anemia in myelodysplastic syndrome (unlabeled use; in combination with epoetin): SubQ: 30 mcg, 75 mcg, or 150 mcg once daily (Hellstrom-Lindberg, 1998) **or** 1 mcg/kg once daily (Greenberg, 2009) **or** 75 mcg, 150 mcg or 300 mcg/dose 3 times/week (Hellstrom-Lindberg, 2003) **or** 1-2 mcg/kg/dose 1-3 times/week (NCCN MDS guidelines v.2.2011)

Hematopoietic stem cell mobilization in autologous transplantation in patients with non-Hodgkin's lymphoma or multiple myeloma (in combination with plerixafor; unlabeled use): SubQ: 10 mcg/kg once daily; begin 4 days before initiation of plerixafor; continue G-CSF on each day prior to apheresis for up to 8 days (DiPersio, *JCO* 2009; DiPersio, *Blood* 2009)

Hepatitis C treatment-associated neutropenia (unlabeled use): SubQ: 150 mcg once weekly to 300 mcg 3 times/week; titrate to maintain ANC between 750-10,000/mm^3 (Younossi, 2008)

Dietary Considerations Some products may contain sodium.

Administration May be administered undiluted by SubQ injection. May also be administered by I.V. bolus, or a short infusion over 15-30 minutes in D_5W, or by continuous SubQ or I.V. infusion. Do not administer earlier than 24 hours after or in the 24 hours prior to cytotoxic chemotherapy.

Monitoring Parameters CBC with differential and platelets prior to treatment and twice weekly during filgrastim treatment for chemotherapy-induced neutropenia (3 times/week following marrow transplantation). For severe chronic neutropenia, monitor CBC with differential and platelets twice weekly during the first month of therapy and for 2 weeks following dose adjustments; once clinically stable, monthly for 1 year and quarterly thereafter; for congenital neutropenia also monitor bone marrow and karyotype prior to treatment; and monitor marrow and cytogenetics annually throughout treatment. Monitor temperature.

Reference Range No additional clinical benefit seen when filgrastim is used with ANC >10,000/mm^3

Test Interactions May interfere with bone imaging studies; increased hematopoietic activity of the bone marrow may appear as transient positive bone imaging changes

Dosage Forms Excipient information presented when available (limited, particularly for generics); consult specific product labeling.

Injection, solution [preservative free]:

Neupogen®: 300 mcg/mL (1 mL, 1.6 mL) [contains polysorbate 80, sodium 0.035 mg/mL, sorbitol; vial]

Neupogen®: 600 mcg/mL (0.5 mL, 0.8 mL) [contains natural rubber/natural latex in packaging, polysorbate 80, sodium 0.035 mg/mL, sorbitol; prefilled syringe]

◆ **Finacea®** *see* Azelaic Acid *on page 179*

◆ **Finacea® Plus™** *see* Azelaic Acid *on page 179*

Finasteride (fi NAS teer ide)

Brand Names: U.S. Propecia®; Proscar®

Brand Names: Canada CO Finasteride; JAMP-Finasteride; Mylan-Finasteride; Novo-Finasteride; PMS-Finasteride; Propecia®; Proscar®; ratio-Finasteride; Sandoz-Finasteride; Teva-Finasteride

Pharmacologic Category 5 Alpha-Reductase Inhibitor

Use

Propecia®: Treatment of male pattern hair loss in **men only**. Safety and efficacy were demonstrated in men between 18-41 years of age.

Proscar®: Treatment of symptomatic benign prostatic hyperplasia (BPH); can be used in combination with an alpha-blocker, doxazosin

Unlabeled Use Treatment of female hirsutism

Pregnancy Risk Factor X

Pregnancy Considerations Abnormalities of external male genitalia were reported in animal studies. Pregnant women are advised to avoid contact with crushed or broken tablets.

Lactation Excretion in breast milk unknown/contraindicated in women of childbearing potential

Contraindications Hypersensitivity to finasteride or any component of the formulation; pregnancy; not for use in children

Warnings/Precautions Hazardous agent - use appropriate precautions for handling and disposal. Other urological diseases (including prostate cancer) should be ruled out before initiating. For BPH, a minimum of 6 months of treatment may be necessary to determine whether an individual will respond to finasteride; for male pattern hair loss, daily use for 3 months or longer may be required before benefit is observed. Reduces prostate specific antigen (PSA) by ~50%; in patients treated for ≥6 months the PSA value should be doubled when comparing to normal ranges in untreated patients (for interpretation of serial PSAs, a new PSA baseline should be established ≥6 months after treatment initiation and PSA monitored periodically thereafter). Failure to demonstrate a meaningful PSA decrease (<50%) or a PSA increase while on this medication may be associated with an increased risk for prostate cancer (NCCN prostate cancer early detection guidelines, v.1.2011). Patients on a 5-alpha-reductase inhibitor (5-ARI) with any increase in PSA levels, even if within normal limits, should be evaluated; may indicate presence of prostate cancer. Use with caution in patients with hepatic dysfunction; finasteride is extensively metabolized in the liver. When compared to placebo, 5-ARIs have been shown to reduce the overall incidence of prostate cancer, although an increase in the incidence of high-grade prostate cancers has been observed; 5-ARIs are not FDA-approved for the prevention of prostate cancer. Carefully monitor patients with a large residual urinary volume or severely diminished urinary flow for obstructive uropathy; these patients may not be candidates for finasteride therapy. Rare reports of male breast cancer have been observed with finasteride use. Patients should promptly report any breast changes, including breast enlargement, lumps, tenderness, pain, or nipple discharge to their healthcare provider. Active ingredient can be absorbed through the skin; women should always use caution whenever handling. Pregnant women or women trying to conceive should not handle the product; finasteride may negatively impact fetal development. Not indicated for use in children.

Adverse Reactions Note: "Combination therapy" refers to finasteride and doxazosin.

>10%:

Endocrine & metabolic: Impotence (5% to 19%; combination therapy 23%), libido decreased (2% to 10%; combination therapy 12%)

Neuromuscular & skeletal: Weakness (5%; combination therapy 17%)

1% to 10%:

Cardiovascular: Postural hypotension (9%; combination therapy 18%), edema (1%; combination therapy 3%)

Central nervous system: Dizziness (7%; combination therapy 23%), somnolence (2%; combination therapy 3%)

Dermatologic: Rash (1%)

Genitourinary: Ejaculation disturbances (<1% to 7%; combination therapy 14%), decreased volume of ejaculate (2% to 4%)

Endocrine & metabolic: Gynecomastia (1% to 2%), breast tenderness (≤1%)

Respiratory: Dyspnea (1%; combination therapy 2%), rhinitis (1%; combination therapy 2%)

<1%, postmarketing and/or case reports: Breast cancer (males), depression, hypersensitivity (pruritus, rash, urticaria, swelling of face/lips), prostate cancer (high grade), testicular pain

Drug Interactions

Metabolism/Transport Effects Substrate of CYP3A4 (minor); **Note:** Assignment of Major/Minor substrate status based on clinically relevant drug interaction potential

Avoid Concomitant Use There are no known interactions where it is recommended to avoid concomitant use.

Increased Effect/Toxicity

The levels/effects of Finasteride may be increased by: Conivaptan

Decreased Effect
The levels/effects of Finasteride may be decreased by: Tocilizumab

Ethanol/Nutrition/Herb Interactions Herb/Nutraceutical: St John's wort may decrease finasteride levels. Avoid saw palmetto (concurrent use has not been adequately studied).

Stability
Propecia®: Store at 15°C to 30°C (59°F to 86°F). Protect from moisture.
Proscar®: Store below 30°C (86°F). Protect from light.

Mechanism of Action Finasteride is a competitive inhibitor of both tissue and hepatic 5-alpha reductase. This results in inhibition of the conversion of testosterone to dihydrotestosterone and markedly suppresses serum dihydrotestosterone levels

Pharmacodynamics/Kinetics
Onset of action: BPH: 6 months; Male pattern hair loss: ≥3 months of daily use
Duration:
After a single oral dose as small as 0.5 mg: 65% depression of plasma dihydrotestosterone levels persists 5-7 days
After 6 months of treatment with 5 mg/day: Circulating dihydrotestosterone levels are reduced to castrate levels without significant effects on circulating testosterone; levels return to normal within 14 days of discontinuation of treatment
Distribution: V_{dss}: 76 L
Protein binding: ~90%
Metabolism: Hepatic via CYP3A4; two active metabolites (<20% activity of finasteride)
Bioavailability: Mean: 65%
Half-life elimination, serum: 6 hours (range: 3-16 hours); Elderly: 8 hours (range: 6-15 hours)
Time to peak, serum: 1-2 hours
Excretion: Feces (57%) and urine (39%) as metabolites

Dosage Oral: Adults:
Males:
Benign prostatic hyperplasia (Proscar®): 5 mg once daily as a single dose; clinical responses occur within 12 weeks to 6 months of initiation of therapy; long-term administration is recommended for maximal response
Male pattern baldness (Propecia®): 1 mg daily
Female hirsutism (unlabeled use): 5 mg/day (Moghetti, 2000)

Dosing adjustment in renal impairment: No dosage adjustment is necessary

Dosing adjustment in hepatic impairment: Use with caution in patients with liver function abnormalities because finasteride is metabolized extensively in the liver

Dietary Considerations May be taken without regard to meals.

Administration May be administered without regard to meals. Women of childbearing age should not touch or handle broken tablets.

Monitoring Parameters Objective and subjective signs of relief of benign prostatic hyperplasia, including improvement in urinary flow, reduction in symptoms of urgency, and relief of difficulty in micturition; for interpretation of serial PSAs, establish a new PSA baseline ≥6 months after treatment initiation and monitor PSA periodically thereafter.

Test Interactions PSA levels decrease in treated patients. After 6 months of therapy, PSA levels stabilize to a new baseline that is ~50% of pretreatment values. If following serial PSAs in a patient, re-establish a new baseline after ≥6 months of use.

Dosage Forms Excipient information presented when available (limited, particularly for generics); consult specific product labeling.
Tablet, oral: 5 mg
Propecia®: 1 mg
Proscar®: 5 mg

Fingolimod (fin GOL i mod)

Brand Names: U.S. Gilenya®

Brand Names: Canada Gilenya®

Index Terms FTY720

Pharmacologic Category Sphingosine 1-Phosphate (S1P) Receptor Modulator

Use Treatment of relapsing forms of multiple sclerosis (MS) to reduce the frequency of clinical exacerbations and delay disability progression

Pregnancy Risk Factor C

Pregnancy Considerations Teratogenic and adverse effects have been observed in animal reproduction studies. Elimination of fingolimod takes approximately 2 months; to avoid potential fetal harm, women of childbearing potential should avoid pregnancy during and for 2 months after discontinuing treatment. Healthcare providers are encouraged to enroll pregnant women, or pregnant women may enroll themselves, in the Gileny™ Pregnancy Registry (1-877-598-7237).

Lactation Excretion in breast milk unknown/not recommended

Medication Guide Available Yes

Contraindications There are no contraindications listed in the manufacturers labeling.

Canadian labeling: Hypersensitivity to fingolimod or any component of the formulation; patients at increased risk for opportunistic infections (eg, immunosuppressed patients); severe active infections, active chronic bacterial, fungal or viral infections; known active malignancy (excluding basal cell carcinoma); severe hepatic impairment (Child-Pugh class C)

Warnings/Precautions Increased blood pressure may occur ~2 months after initiation of therapy; monitor blood pressure throughout treatment. Therapy may result in transient AV conduction delays; recurrence may be observed following discontinuation (>2 weeks) and subsequent resumption of therapy. Decreased heart rate may occur with initiation of therapy. Following the first dose, heart rate may decrease as soon as 1 hour postdose with the maximal decrease occurring ~6 hours postdose. Heart rate typically returns to baseline after 1 month of therapy. All patients should be monitored for 6 hours after the first dose (or in patients where therapy has been interrupted for >2 weeks) for signs and symptoms of bradycardia; in patients who develop bradycardia, initiate appropriate treatment and continue to monitor until symptoms have resolved. Due to the risk of bradycardia and AV conduction delays, ECG is recommended prior to initiation of therapy.

May increase risk of infection due to dose-dependent reduction of lymphocytes; lymphocyte counts may be decreased for up to 2 months following discontinuation of therapy. Do not initiate treatment in patients with acute or chronic infections until the infection has resolved. Use with caution in patients receiving concomitant immunosuppressant, immune modulating, or antineoplastic medications.

Use with caution and closely monitor patients with severe hepatic impairment (contraindicated in the Canadian labeling). Macular edema may occur; use with caution in patients with a history of diabetes mellitus or uveitis. Ophthalmologic exams should be performed prior to therapy and 3-4 months after treatment initiation; more frequent examination is warranted in patients with diabetes or a history of uveitis. Reductions of FEV_1 and diffusion lung capacity for carbon monoxide (DLCO) are dose-dependent and may occur within the first month of therapy. FEV_1 changes may be reversible with drug discontinuation.

Consider varicella zoster virus (VZV) vaccination prior to initiation of treatment in VZV antibody negative patients; postpone fingolimod treatment for 1 month after varicella zoster vaccination.

Adverse Reactions

>10%:
- Central nervous system: Headache (25%)
- Gastrointestinal: Diarrhea (12%)
- Hepatic: ALT increased (14%), AST increased (14%)
- Neuromuscular & skeletal: Back pain (12%)
- Miscellaneous: Flu-like syndrome (13%)

1% to 10%:
- Cardiovascular: Hypertension (6%), bradycardia (4%)
- Central nervous system: Depression (8%), dizziness (7%), migraine (5%)
- Dermatologic: Alopecia (4%), eczema (3%), pruritus (3%)
- Endocrine & metabolic: Triglycerides increased (3%)
- Gastrointestinal: Gastroenteritis (5%), weight loss (5%)
- Hematologic: Lymphopenia (4%), leukopenia (3%)
- Hepatic: GGT increased (5%)
- Neuromuscular & skeletal: Paresthesia (5%), weakness (3%)
- Ocular: Blurred vision (4%), eye pain (3%)
- Respiratory: Cough (10%), bronchitis (8%), dyspnea (8%), sinusitis (7%)
- Miscellaneous: Herpes infection (9%), tinea infection (4%)

<1% (Limited to important or life-threatening): Macular edema (incidence increased in patients with uveitis or diabetes mellitus), lymphoma

Drug Interactions

Metabolism/Transport Effects Substrate of CYP2D6 (minor), CYP2E1 (minor), CYP3A4 (minor); **Note:** Assignment of Major/Minor substrate status based on clinically relevant drug interaction potential

Avoid Concomitant Use

Avoid concomitant use of Fingolimod with any of the following: BCG; Natalizumab; Pimecrolimus; Tacrolimus (Topical); Vaccines (Live)

Increased Effect/Toxicity

Fingolimod may increase the levels/effects of: Antiarrhythmic Agents (Class Ia); Antiarrhythmic Agents (Class III); Leflunomide; Natalizumab; Vaccines (Live)

The levels/effects of Fingolimod may be increased by: Beta-Blockers; Conivaptan; Denosumab; Diltiazem; Ketoconazole; Pimecrolimus; Roflumilast; Tacrolimus (Topical); Trastuzumab; Verapamil

Decreased Effect

Fingolimod may decrease the levels/effects of: BCG; Coccidioidin Skin Test; Sipuleucel-T; Vaccines (Inactivated); Vaccines (Live)

The levels/effects of Fingolimod may be decreased by: Cyproterone; Echinacea; Peginterferon Alfa-2b; Tocilizumab

Stability Store at 25°C (77°F); excursions permitted to 15°C to 30°C (59°F to 86°F).

Mechanism of Action Fingolimod-phosphate, active metabolite of fingolimod, binds to sphingosine 1-phosphate receptors 1, 3, 4, and 5. The amount of lymphocytes available to the central nervous system are decreased which reduces central inflammation.

Pharmacodynamics/Kinetics

Distribution: V_d: 1200 ± 260 L: distributes into red blood cells (86%)

Protein binding: >99.7% (fingolimod and fingolimod-phosphate)

Metabolism: Hepatic via CYP4F2 to fingolimod-phosphate (active) and other metabolites (inactive); CYP2D6, 2E1, 3A4, and 4F12 also contribute to metabolism

Bioavailability: 93%

Half-life elimination: 6-9 days

Time to peak, plasma: 12-16 hours

Excretion: Urine (~81% as inactive metabolites); feces (fingolimod and fingolimod phosphate: <2.5% of dose)

Dosage Oral: Adults: Multiple sclerosis: 0.5 mg once daily; doses >0.5 mg/day associated with increased adverse events and no additional benefit

Dosage adjustment in hepatic impairment:

Mild-to-moderate hepatic impairment: No dosage adjustment required

Severe hepatic impairment: Use with caution and closely monitor; exposure is doubled in severe hepatic impairment. Specific dosing recommendations are not provided within the U.S. manufacturer labeling. Use is contraindicated in the Canadian labeling.

Dietary Considerations May be taken with or without food.

Administration May be administered with or without food.

Monitoring Parameters ECG (baseline); heart rate, signs and symptoms of bradycardia (for 6 hours following first dose); ophthalmologic exam at baseline and 3-4 months after initiation of treatment (continue periodic examinations for duration of therapy in patients with diabetes or history of uveitis); liver transaminase and bilirubin at least 6 months prior to treatment; respiratory function (FEV_1, DLCO); blood pressure; CBC (baseline and periodically thereafter); VZV antibodies (patients with no history of chicken pox or previous VZV vaccination)

Dosage Forms Excipient information presented when available (limited, particularly for generics); consult specific product labeling.

Capsule, oral:

Gilenya®: 0.5 mg

- ◆ **Fioricet®** *see* Butalbital, Acetaminophen, and Caffeine *on page* 255
- ◆ **Fiorinal®** *see* Butalbital, Aspirin, and Caffeine *on page* 255
- ◆ **Firazyr®** *see* Icatibant *on page* 864
- ◆ **Firmagon®** *see* Degarelix *on page* 466
- ◆ **First™-Progesterone VGS 25** *see* Progesterone *on page* 1414
- ◆ **First™-Progesterone VGS 50** *see* Progesterone *on page* 1414
- ◆ **First™-Progesterone VGS 100** *see* Progesterone *on page* 1414
- ◆ **First™-Progesterone VGS 200** *see* Progesterone *on page* 1414
- ◆ **First™-Progesterone VGS 400** *see* Progesterone *on page* 1414
- ◆ **First®-Testosterone** *see* Testosterone *on page* 1654
- ◆ **First®-Testosterone MC** *see* Testosterone *on page* 1654
- ◆ **Fisalamine** *see* Mesalamine *on page* 1081
- ◆ **Fish Oil** *see* Omega-3-Acid Ethyl Esters *on page* 1241
- ◆ **FK228** *see* RomiDEPsin *on page* 1515
- ◆ **FK506** *see* Tacrolimus (Systemic) *on page* 1615
- ◆ **Flagyl®** *see* MetroNIDAZOLE (Systemic) *on page* 1120
- ◆ **Flagyl® 375** *see* MetroNIDAZOLE (Systemic) *on page* 1120
- ◆ **Flagyl® ER** *see* MetroNIDAZOLE (Systemic) *on page* 1120
- ◆ **Flamazine® (Can)** *see* Silver Sulfadiazine *on page* 1554
- ◆ **Flarex®** *see* Fluorometholone *on page* 730

FlavoxATE (fla VOKS ate)

Brand Names: Canada Apo-Flavoxate®; Urispas®
Index Terms Flavoxate Hydrochloride; Urispas
Pharmacologic Category Antispasmodic Agent, Urinary
Use Antispasmodic to provide symptomatic relief of dysuria, nocturia, suprapubic pain, urgency, and incontinence due to detrusor instability and hyper-reflexia in elderly with cystitis, urethritis, urethrocystitis, urethrotrigonitis, and prostatitis
Pregnancy Risk Factor B
Dosage Children >12 years and Adults: Oral: 100-200 mg 3-4 times/day; reduce the dose when symptoms improve
Additional Information Complete prescribing information for this medication should be consulted for additional detail.
Dosage Forms Excipient information presented when available (limited, particularly for generics); consult specific product labeling.
Tablet, oral, as hydrochloride: 100 mg

◆ **Flavoxate Hydrochloride** *see* FlavoxATE *on page 716*
◆ **Flebogamma® DIF** *see* Immune Globulin *on page 880*

Flecainide (fle KAY nide)

Brand Names: U.S. Tambocor™
Brand Names: Canada Apo-Flecainide®; Tambocor™
Index Terms Flecainide Acetate
Pharmacologic Category Antiarrhythmic Agent, Class Ic
Use Prevention and suppression of documented life-threatening ventricular arrhythmias (eg, sustained ventricular tachycardia); controlling symptomatic, disabling supraventricular tachycardias in patients without structural heart disease in whom other agents fail
Pregnancy Risk Factor C
Pregnancy Considerations Adverse events have been observed in some animal reproduction studies.
Lactation Enters breast milk/compatible
Contraindications Hypersensitivity to flecainide or any component of the formulation; pre-existing second- or third-degree AV block or with right bundle branch block when associated with a left hemiblock (bifascicular block) (except in patients with a functioning artificial pacemaker); cardiogenic shock; coronary artery disease (based on CAST study results); concurrent use of ritonavir or amprenavir
Warnings/Precautions **[U.S. Boxed Warning]: In the Cardiac Arrhythmia Suppression Trial (CAST), recent (>6 days but <2 years ago) myocardial infarction patients with asymptomatic, non-life-threatening ventricular arrhythmias did not benefit and may have been harmed by attempts to suppress the arrhythmia with flecainide or encainide.** An increased mortality or nonfatal cardiac arrest rate (7.7%) was seen in the active treatment group compared with patients in the placebo group (3%). The applicability of the CAST results to other populations is unknown. The risks of class 1C agents and the lack of improved survival make use in patients without life-threatening arrhythmias generally unacceptable. **[U.S. Boxed Warning]: Watch for proarrhythmic effects;** monitor and adjust dose to prevent QT_c prolongation. Not recommended for patients with chronic atrial fibrillation. **[U.S. Boxed Warning]: When treating atrial flutter, 1:1 atrioventricular conduction may occur; pre-emptive negative chronotropic therapy (eg, digoxin, beta-blockers) may lower the risk.** Pre-existing hypokalemia or hyperkalemia should be corrected before initiation (can alter drug's effect). A worsening or new arrhythmia may occur (proarrhythmic effect). Use caution in heart failure (may precipitate or exacerbate HF). Dose-related increases in PR, QRS, and QT intervals occur. Use with caution in sick sinus syndrome or with permanent pacemakers or temporary pacing wires (can increase endocardial pacing thresholds). Cautious use in significant hepatic impairment.

Adverse Reactions

>10%:
- Central nervous system: Dizziness (19% to 30%)
- Ocular: Visual disturbances (16%)
- Respiratory: Dyspnea (~10%)

1% to 10%:
- Cardiovascular: Palpitation (6%), chest pain (5%), edema (3.5%), tachycardia (1% to 3%), proarrhythmic (4% to 12%), sinus node dysfunction (1.2%), syncope
- Central nervous system: Headache (4% to 10%), fatigue (8%), nervousness (5%) additional symptoms occurring at a frequency between 1% and 3%: fever, malaise, hypoesthesia, paresis, ataxia, vertigo, somnolence, tinnitus, anxiety, insomnia, depression
- Dermatologic: Rash (1% to 3%)
- Gastrointestinal: Nausea (9%), constipation (1%), abdominal pain (3%), anorexia (1% to 3%), diarrhea (0.7% to 3%)
- Neuromuscular & skeletal: Tremor (5%), weakness (5%), paresthesia (1%)
- Ocular: Diplopia (1% to 3%), blurred vision

<1% (Limited to important or life-threatening): Alopecia, alters pacing threshold, amnesia, angina, AV block, bradycardia, bronchospasm, CHF, corneal deposits, depersonalization, euphoria, exfoliative dermatitis, granulocytopenia, heart block, increased P-R, leukopenia, metallic taste, neuropathy, paradoxical increase in ventricular rate in atrial fibrillation/flutter, paresthesia, photophobia, pneumonitis, pruritus, QRS duration, swollen lips/tongue/mouth, tardive dyskinesia, thrombocytopenia, urinary retention, urticaria, ventricular arrhythmia

Drug Interactions

Metabolism/Transport Effects **Substrate** of CYP1A2 (minor), CYP2D6 (major); **Note:** Assignment of Major/Minor substrate status based on clinically relevant drug interaction potential; **Inhibits** CYP2D6 (weak)

Avoid Concomitant Use

Avoid concomitant use of Flecainide with any of the following: Artemether; Dronedarone; Lumefantrine; Nilotinib; Pimozide; QUEtiapine; QuiNINE; Ritonavir; Saquinavir; Tetrabenazine; Thioridazine; Tipranavir; Toremifene; Vandetanib; Vemurafenib; Ziprasidone

Increased Effect/Toxicity

Flecainide may increase the levels/effects of: Dronedarone; Pimozide; QTc-Prolonging Agents; QuiNINE; Tetrabenazine; Thioridazine; Toremifene; Vandetanib; Vemurafenib; Ziprasidone

The levels/effects of Flecainide may be increased by: Abiraterone Acetate; Alfuzosin; Amiodarone; Artemether; Boceprevir; Carbonic Anhydrase Inhibitors; Chloroquine; Ciprofloxacin; Ciprofloxacin (Systemic); CYP2D6 Inhibitors (Moderate); CYP2D6 Inhibitors (Strong); Darunavir; Gadobutrol; Indacaterol; Lumefantrine; Nilotinib; QUEtiapine; QuiNINE; Ritonavir; Saquinavir; Sodium Bicarbonate; Sodium Lactate; Telaprevir; Tipranavir; Tromethamine; Verapamil

Decreased Effect

The levels/effects of Flecainide may be decreased by: Cyproterone; Etravirine; Peginterferon Alfa-2b; Sodium Bicarbonate

Ethanol/Nutrition/Herb Interactions Food: Clearance may be decreased in patients following strict vegetarian diets due to urinary pH ≥8. Dairy products (milk, infant formula, yogurt) may interfere with the absorption of flecainide in infants; there is one case report of a neonate (GA 34 weeks PNA >6 days) who required extremely large doses of oral flecainide when administered every 8 hours with feedings ("milk feeds"); changing the feedings from "milk feeds" to 5% glucose feeds alone resulted in a doubling of the flecainide serum concentration and toxicity.

Mechanism of Action Class Ic antiarrhythmic; slows conduction in cardiac tissue by altering transport of ions across cell membranes; causes slight prolongation of refractory periods; decreases the rate of rise of the action potential without affecting its duration; increases electrical stimulation threshold of ventricle, His-Purkinje system; possesses local anesthetic and moderate negative inotropic effects

Pharmacodynamics/Kinetics

Absorption: Oral: Rapid

Distribution: Adults: V_d: 5-13.4 L/kg

Protein binding: Alpha$_1$ acid glycoprotein: 40% to 50%

Metabolism: Hepatic

Bioavailability: 85% to 90%

Half-life elimination: Infants: 11-12 hours; Children: 8 hours; Adults: 7-22 hours, increased with congestive heart failure or renal dysfunction; End-stage renal disease: 19-26 hours

Time to peak, serum: ~1.5-3 hours

Excretion: Urine (80% to 90%, 10% to 50% as unchanged drug and metabolites)

Dosage Oral:

Children:

Initial: 3 mg/kg/day or 50-100 mg/m^2/day in 3 divided doses

Usual: 3-6 mg/kg/day or 100-150 mg/m^2/day in 3 divided doses; up to 11 mg/kg/day or 200 mg/m^2/day for uncontrolled patients with subtherapeutic levels

Adults:

Life-threatening ventricular arrhythmias:

Initial: 100 mg every 12 hours

Increase by 50-100 mg/day (given in 2 doses/day) every 4 days; maximum: 400 mg/day.

Use of higher initial doses and more rapid dosage adjustments have resulted in an increased incidence of proarrhythmic events and congestive heart failure, particularly during the first few days. Do not use a loading dose. Use very cautiously in patients with history of congestive heart failure or myocardial infarction.

Prevention of paroxysmal supraventricular arrhythmias in patients with disabling symptoms but no structural heart disease: Initial: 50 mg every 12 hours; increase by 50 mg twice daily at 4-day intervals; maximum: 300 mg/day

Paroxysmal atrial fibrillation: Outpatient: "Pill-in-the-pocket" dose (unlabeled dose): 200 mg (weight <70 kg), 300 mg (weight ≥70 kg). May not repeat in ≤24 hours. **Note:** An initial inpatient conversion trial should have been successful before sending patient home on this approach. Patient must be taking an AV nodal-blocking agent (eg, beta-blocker, nondihydropyridine calcium channel blocker) prior to initiation of antiarrhythmic.

Dosing adjustment in severe renal impairment: GFR ≤50 mL/minute: Decrease dose by 50%; dose increases should be made cautiously at intervals >4 days and serum levels monitored frequently.

Hemodialysis: No supplemental dose recommended.

Peritoneal dialysis: No supplemental dose recommended.

Dosing adjustment/comments in hepatic impairment: Monitoring of plasma levels is recommended because of significantly increased half-life.

When transferring from another antiarrhythmic agent, allow for 2-4 half-lives of the agent to pass before initiating flecainide therapy.

Administration Administer around-the-clock to promote less variation in peak and trough serum levels

Monitoring Parameters ECG, blood pressure, pulse, periodic serum concentrations, especially in patients with renal or hepatic impairment

Reference Range Therapeutic: 0.2-1 mcg/mL; pediatric patients may respond at the lower end of the recommended therapeutic range

Dosage Forms Excipient information presented when available (limited, particularly for generics); consult specific product labeling.

Tablet, oral, as acetate: 50 mg, 100 mg, 150 mg

Tambocor™: 50 mg

Tambocor™: 100 mg, 150 mg [scored]

Extemporaneous Preparations A 20 mg/mL oral liquid suspension may be made from tablets and one of three different vehicles (cherry syrup, a 1:1 mixture of Ora-Sweet® and Ora-Plus®, or a 1:1 mixture of Ora-Sweet® SF and Ora-Plus®). Crush twenty-four 100 mg tablets in a mortar and reduce to a fine powder. Add 20 mL of the chosen vehicle and mix to a uniform paste; mix while adding the vehicle in incremental proportions to **almost** 120 mL; transfer to a calibrated bottle, rinse mortar with vehicle, and add quantity of vehicle sufficient to make 120 mL. Label "shake well" and "protect from light". Stable for 60 days when stored in amber plastic prescription bottles in the dark at room temperature or refrigerated.

Allen LV and Erickson III MA, "Stability of Baclofen, Captopril, Diltiazem, Hydrochloride, Dipyridamole, and Flecainide Acetate in Extemporaneously Compounded Oral Liquids," *Am J Health Syst Pharm*, 1996, 53:2179-84.

- **Flecainide Acetate** *see* Flecainide *on page 716*
- **Fleet® Bisacodyl [OTC]** *see* Bisacodyl *on page 219*
- **Fleet® Enema [OTC]** *see* Sodium Phosphates *on page 1573*
- **Fleet Enema® (Can)** *see* Sodium Phosphates *on page 1573*
- **Fleet® Enema Extra® [OTC]** *see* Sodium Phosphates *on page 1573*
- **Fleet® Pedia-Lax™ Chewable Tablet [OTC]** *see* Magnesium Hydroxide *on page 1045*
- **Fleet® Pedia-Lax™ Enema [OTC]** *see* Sodium Phosphates *on page 1573*
- **Fleet® Pedia-Lax™ Liquid Stool Softener [OTC]** *see* Docusate *on page 537*
- **Fleet® Sof-Lax® [OTC]** *see* Docusate *on page 537*
- **Fleet® Stimulant Laxative [OTC]** *see* Bisacodyl *on page 219*
- **Flexbumin 25%** *see* Albumin *on page 51*
- **Flexeril®** *see* Cyclobenzaprine *on page 419*
- **Flexitec (Can)** *see* Cyclobenzaprine *on page 419*
- **Flolan®** *see* Epoprostenol *on page 604*
- **Flomax®** *see* Tamsulosin *on page 1626*
- **Flomax® CR (Can)** *see* Tamsulosin *on page 1626*
- **Flonase®** *see* Fluticasone (Nasal) *on page 741*
- **Flo-Pred™** *see* PrednisoLONE (Systemic) *on page 1396*
- **Florazole® ER (Can)** *see* MetroNIDAZOLE (Systemic) *on page 1120*
- **Florical® [OTC]** *see* Calcium Carbonate *on page 266*
- **Florinef** *see* Fludrocortisone *on page 724*
- **Florinef® (Can)** *see* Fludrocortisone *on page 724*
- **Flovent** *see* Fluticasone (Systemic) *on page 738*
- **Flovent® Diskus®** *see* Fluticasone (Systemic) *on page 738*
- **Flovent® HFA** *see* Fluticasone (Systemic) *on page 738*
- **Floxin Otic Singles** *see* Ofloxacin (Otic) *on page 1233*
- **Fluad™ (Can)** *see* Influenza Virus Vaccine (Inactivated) *on page 897*

- **Fluarix®** *see* Influenza Virus Vaccine (Inactivated) *on page 897*
- **Flubenisolone** *see* Betamethasone *on page 208*
- **Flucaine** *see* Proparacaine and Fluorescein *on page 1421*

Fluconazole (floo KOE na zole)

Brand Names: U.S. Diflucan®

Brand Names: Canada Apo-Fluconazole®; CanesOral®; CO Fluconazole; Diflucan®; Dom-Fluconazole; Fluconazole Injection; Fluconazole Omega; Mylan-Fluconazole; Novo-Fluconazole; PHL-Fluconazole; PMS-Fluconazole; PRO-Fluconazole; Riva-Fluconazole; Taro-Fluconazole; ZYM-Fluconazole

Pharmacologic Category Antifungal Agent, Oral; Antifungal Agent, Parenteral

Additional Appendix Information

Antifungal Agents *on page 1876*

Use Treatment of candidiasis (vaginal, oropharyngeal, esophageal, urinary tract infections, peritonitis, pneumonia, and systemic infections); cryptococcal meningitis; antifungal prophylaxis in allogeneic bone marrow transplant recipients

Unlabeled Use Cryptococcal pneumonia; candidal intertrigo

Pregnancy Risk Factor C (single dose for vaginal candidiasis)/D (all other indications)

Pregnancy Considerations When used in high doses, fluconazole is teratogenic in animal studies. Following exposure during the first trimester, case reports have noted similar malformations in humans when used in higher doses (400 mg/day) over extended periods of time. Use of lower doses (150 mg as a single dose) does not suggest an increase risk to the fetus.

Lactation Enters breast milk/not recommended (AAP rates "compatible"; AAP 2001 update pending)

Contraindications Hypersensitivity to fluconazole or any component of the formulation (cross-reaction with other azole antifungal agents may occur, but has not been established; use caution); concomitant administration with cisapride or terfenadine

Warnings/Precautions Should be used with caution in patients with renal and hepatic dysfunction or previous hepatotoxicity from other azole derivatives. Patients who develop abnormal liver function tests during fluconazole therapy should be monitored closely and discontinued if symptoms consistent with liver disease develop. Rare exfoliative skin disorders have been observed; monitor closely if rash develops and discontinue if lesions progress. The manufacturer reports rare cases of QT_c prolongation and torsade de pointes associated with fluconazole use and advises caution in patients with concomitant medications or conditions which are arrhythmogenic. However, given the limited number of cases and the presence of multiple confounding variables, the likelihood that fluconazole causes conduction abnormalities appears remote. Oral suspension contains sucrose; avoid use in patients with fructose intolerance, glucose-galactose malabsorption, or sucrase-isomaltase insufficiency.

Adverse Reactions Frequency not always defined.

Cardiovascular: Angioedema, pallor, QT prolongation (rare, case reports), torsade de pointes(rare, case reports)

Central nervous system: Headache (2% to 13%), dizziness (1%), seizure

Dermatologic: Rash (2%), alopecia, toxic epidermal necrolysis, Stevens-Johnson syndrome

Endocrine & metabolic: Hypercholesterolemia, hypertriglyceridemia, hypokalemia

Gastrointestinal: Nausea (2% to 7%), abdominal pain (2% to 6%), vomiting (2% to 5%), diarrhea (2% to 3%), dyspepsia (1%), taste perversion (1%)

Hematologic: Agranulocytosis, leukopenia, neutropenia, thrombocytopenia

Hepatic: Alkaline phosphatase increased, ALT increased, AST increased, cholestasis, hepatic failure (rare), hepatitis, jaundice

Respiratory: Dyspnea

Miscellaneous: Anaphylactic reactions (rare)

Drug Interactions

Metabolism/Transport Effects Inhibits CYP1A2 (weak), CYP2C19 (strong), CYP2C9 (strong), CYP3A4 (moderate)

Avoid Concomitant Use

Avoid concomitant use of Fluconazole with any of the following: Artemether; Cisapride; Clopidogrel; Conivaptan; Dofetilide; Dronedarone; Lumefantrine; Nilotinib; Pimozide; QUEtiapine; QuiNIDine; QuiNINE; Ranolazine; Tetrabenazine; Thioridazine; Tolvaptan; Toremifene; Vandetanib; Vemurafenib; Voriconazole; Ziprasidone

Increased Effect/Toxicity

Fluconazole may increase the levels/effects of: Alfentanil; Aprepitant; ARIPiprazole; Benzodiazepines (metabolized by oxidation); Bosentan; Budesonide (Systemic, Oral Inhalation); BusPIRone; Busulfan; Calcium Channel Blockers; CarBAMazepine; Carvedilol; Cilostazol; Cinacalcet; Cisapride; Citalopram; Colchicine; Conivaptan; Corticosteroids (Systemic); CycloSPORINE; CycloSPORINE (Systemic); CYP2C19 Substrates; CYP2C9 Substrates; CYP3A4 Substrates; Diclofenac; DOCEtaxel; Dofetilide; Dronedarone; Eletriptan; Eplerenone; Erlotinib; Eszopiclone; Etravirine; Everolimus; FentaNYL; Fosaprepitant; Fosphenytoin; Gefitinib; HMG-CoA Reductase Inhibitors; Imatinib; Irbesartan; Irinotecan; Losartan; Lurasidone; Macrolide Antibiotics; Methadone; Phenytoin; Phosphodiesterase 5 Inhibitors; Pimecrolimus; Pimozide; Protease Inhibitors; Proton Pump Inhibitors; QTc-Prolonging Agents; QuiNIDine; QuiNINE; Ramelteon; Ranolazine; Repaglinide; Rifamycin Derivatives; Salmeterol; Saxagliptin; Sirolimus; Solifenacin; Sulfonylureas; SUNItinib; Tacrolimus; Tacrolimus (Systemic); Tacrolimus (Topical); Temsirolimus; Tetrabenazine; Thioridazine; Tolterodine; Tolvaptan; Toremifene; Vandetanib; Vemurafenib; Vilazodone; Vitamin K Antagonists; Voriconazole; Zidovudine; Ziprasidone; Zolpidem

The levels/effects of Fluconazole may be increased by: Alfuzosin; Artemether; Chloroquine; Ciprofloxacin; Ciprofloxacin (Systemic); Etravirine; Gadobutrol; Grapefruit Juice; Indacaterol; Lumefantrine; Macrolide Antibiotics; Nilotinib; Protease Inhibitors; QUEtiapine; QuiNINE

Decreased Effect

Fluconazole may decrease the levels/effects of: Amphotericin B; Clopidogrel; Saccharomyces boulardii

The levels/effects of Fluconazole may be decreased by: Didanosine; Etravirine; Fosphenytoin; Phenytoin; Rifamycin Derivatives; Sucralfate

Stability

Tablet: Store at <30°C (86°F).

Powder for oral suspension: Store dry powder at <30°C (86°F). Following reconstitution, store at 5°C to 30°C (41°F to 86°F). Discard unused portion after 2 weeks. Do not freeze.

Injection: Store injection in glass at 5°C to 30°C (41°F to 86°F). Store injection in Viaflex® at 5°C to 25°C (41°F to 77°F). Do not freeze. Do not unwrap unit until ready for use.

Mechanism of Action Interferes with fungal cytochrome P450 activity (lanosterol 14-α-demethylase), decreasing ergosterol synthesis (principal sterol in fungal cell membrane) and inhibiting cell membrane formation

Pharmacodynamics/Kinetics

Distribution: Widely throughout body with good penetration into CSF, eye, peritoneal fluid, sputum, skin, and urine

Relative diffusion blood into CSF: Adequate with or without inflammation (exceeds usual MICs)

CSF:blood level ratio: Normal meninges: 70% to 80%; Inflamed meninges: >70% to 80%

Protein binding, plasma: 11% to 12%

Bioavailability: Oral: >90%

Half-life elimination: Normal renal function: ~30 hours

Time to peak, serum: Oral: 1-2 hours

Excretion: Urine (80% as unchanged drug)

Dosage The daily dose of fluconazole is the same for oral and I.V. administration

Usual dosage ranges:

Children: Loading dose: 6-12 mg/kg; maintenance: 3-12 mg/kg/day; duration and dosage depends on severity of infection

Adults: 150 mg once **or** 200-800 mg/day; duration and dosage depends on severity of infection

Indication-specific dosing:

Children:

Candidiasis:

Oropharyngeal:

Manufacturer's recommendation: Loading dose: 6 mg/kg; maintenance: 3 mg/kg/day once daily for 2 weeks

HIV-exposed/-positive: 3-6 mg/kg/day once daily (maximum: 400 mg/day) (CDC, 2009)

Esophageal:

Manufacturer's recommendation: Loading dose: 6 mg/kg; maintenance: 3-12 mg/kg/day once daily for 21 days and at least 2 weeks following resolution of symptoms

HIV-exposed/-positive: Loading dose: 6 mg/kg once on day 1; maintenance: 3-6 mg/kg/day once daily (maximum: 400 mg/day) (CDC, 2009)

Relapse suppression (HIV-exposed/-positive): 3-6 mg/kg/day once daily (maximum: 200 mg/day) (CDC, 2009)

Invasive disease (independent of HIV status): 5-6 mg/kg every 12 hours for 28 days (maximum: 600 mg/day) (CDC, 2009)

Coccidioidomycosis (CDC, 2009):

Meningeal and disseminated disease (HIV-exposed/-positive): 5-6 mg/kg/dose every 12 hours (maximum: 800 mg/day)

Relapse suppression (HIV-exposed/-positive): 6 mg/kg/day once daily (maximum: 400 mg/day)

Histoplasmosis, relapse suppression (HIV-exposed/-positive): 3-6 mg/kg/day once daily (maximum: 200 mg/day) (CDC, 2009)

Cryptococcal disease (CDC, 2009):

Meningitis (consolidation): Loading dose: 12 mg/kg once on day 1; maintenance: 6-12 mg/kg/day once daily for a minimum of 8 weeks (maximum: 800 mg/day)

Disseminated (non-CNS) or severe pulmonary disease: Loading dose: 12 mg/kg once on day 1; maintenance: 6-12 mg/kg/day once daily (maximum: 600 mg/day)

Relapse suppression (HIV-exposed/-positive): 6 mg/kg/day once daily (maximum: 200 mg/day)

Adults:

Candidiasis (Pappas, 2009):

Candidemia (neutropenic and non-neutropenic): Loading dose: 800 mg on first day, then 400 mg/day for 14 days after first negative blood culture and resolution of signs/symptoms; **Note:** Not recommended for neutropenic patients with recent azole exposure and critical illness

Chronic, disseminated: 400 mg/day until calcification or lesion resolution

CNS candidemia: 400-800 mg/day until CSF/radiological abnormalities resolved; **Note:** Recommended as alternative therapy in patients intolerant of amphotericin B

Oropharyngeal: 100-200 mg/day for 7-14 days for uncomplicated, moderate-to-severe disease; chronic therapy of 100 mg 3 times weekly is recommended in immunocompromised patients with history of oropharyngeal candidiasis (OPC)

Osteoarticular: 400 mg/day for 6-12 months (osteomyelitis) or 6 weeks (septic arthritis)

Esophageal: 200-400 mg/day for 14-21 days

Prophylaxis:

Solid organ: 200-400 mg/day for 7-14 days

Neutropenic patients: 400 mg/day for duration of neutropenia

Urinary tract:

Fungus balls: 200-400 mg/day

Pyelonephritis: 200-400 mg/day for 2 weeks

Symptomatic cystitis: 200 mg/day for 2 weeks

Vaginal:

Uncomplicated: 150 mg as a single dose

Complicated: 150 mg every 72 hours for 3 doses

Recurrent: 150 mg daily for 10-14 days, followed by 150 mg once weekly for 6 months

Candidal intertrigo (unlabeled use; Coldiron, 1991; Nozickova, 1998; Stengel, 1994): 50 mg/day **or** 150 mg once weekly

Coccidioidomycosis (unlabeled use; Galgiani, 2005): 400-800 mg/day; doses of 800-1000 mg/day have been used for meningeal disease; usual duration of therapy ranges from 3-6 months for primary uncomplicated infections and up to 1 year for pulmonary (chronic and diffuse) infection

Endocarditis, prosthetic valve, early (unlabeled use; Pappas, 2009): 400-800 mg/day for 6 weeks after valve replacement (as step-down in stable, culture-negative patients); long-term suppression in absence of valve replacement: 400-800 mg/day

Endophthalmitis (Pappas, 2009): 400-800 mg/day for 4-6 weeks until examination indicates resolution

Meningitis, cryptococcal (Perfect, 2010):

Induction therapy: Typically consists of an amphotericin product and flucytosine for 2-6 weeks

Consolidation therapy: Fluconazole 400-800 mg/day for 8 weeks

Maintenance therapy: 200 mg/day for 6-12 months (post-transplant patients; non-HIV infected patients) **or** ≥1 year (HIV-infected patients may require lifelong therapy; CDC, 2009)

Pericarditis or myocarditis (Pappas, 2009): 400-800 mg/day

Pneumonia, cryptococcal (mild-to-moderate) (unlabeled use; Perfect, 2010): 400 mg/day for 6-12 months (HIV-infected patients may require lifelong therapy; CDC, 2009)

Dosing adjustment/interval in renal impairment:

No adjustment for vaginal candidiasis single-dose therapy

For multiple dosing, administer usual load then adjust daily doses as follows:

Cl_{cr} ≤50 mL/minute (no dialysis): Administer 50% of recommended dose or administer every 48 hours.

Intermittent hemodialysis (IHD): Dialyzable (50%): May administer 100% of daily dose (according to indication) after each dialysis session. Alternatively, doses of 200-400 mg every 48-72 hours **or** 100- 200 mg every 24 hours have been recommended (Heintz, 2009). **Note:** Dosing dependent on the assumption of 3 times/week, complete IHD sessions.

Continuous renal replacement therapy (CRRT) (Heintz, 2009; Trotman, 2005): Drug clearance is highly dependent on the method of renal replacement, filter type, and flow rate. Appropriate dosing requires close monitoring of pharmacologic response, signs of adverse reactions due to drug accumulation, as well as drug concentrations in relation to target trough (if appropriate). The following are general recommendations only (based on dialysate flow/ultrafiltration rates of 1-2 L/hour and minimal residual renal function) and should not supersede clinical judgment:

CVVH: Loading dose of 400-800 mg followed by 200-400 mg every 24 hours

CVVHD/CVVHDF: Loading dose of 400-800 mg followed by 400-800 mg every 24 hours (CVVHD or CVVHDF) **or** 800 mg every 24 hours (CVVHDF)

Note: Higher maintenance doses of 400 mg every 24 hours (CVVH), 800 mg every 24 hours (CVVHD), and 500-600 mg every 12 hours (CVVHDF) may be considered when treating resistant organisms and/or when employing combined ultrafiltration and dialysis flow rates of ≥2 L/hour for CVVHD/CVVHDF (Heintz, 2009; Trotman, 2005).

Dietary Considerations Take without regard to meals.

Administration

I.V.: Do not use if cloudy or precipitated. Infuse over approximately 1-2 hours; do not exceed 200 mg/hour.

Oral: May be administered without regard to meals.

Monitoring Parameters Periodic liver function tests (AST, ALT, alkaline phosphatase) and renal function tests, potassium

Dosage Forms Excipient information presented when available (limited, particularly for generics); consult specific product labeling. [DSC] = Discontinued product

Infusion, premixed iso-osmotic dextrose solution: 200 mg (100 mL); 400 mg (200 mL)

Diflucan®: 400 mg (200 mL [DSC])

Infusion, premixed iso-osmotic sodium chloride solution: 100 mg (50 mL); 200 mg (100 mL); 400 mg (200 mL)

Diflucan®: 200 mg (100 mL [DSC]); 400 mg (200 mL [DSC])

Infusion, premixed iso-osmotic sodium chloride solution [preservative free]: 200 mg (100 mL); 400 mg (200 mL)

Powder for suspension, oral: 10 mg/mL (35 mL); 40 mg/mL (35 mL)

Diflucan®: 10 mg/mL (35 mL); 40 mg/mL (35 mL) [contains sodium benzoate, sucrose; orange flavor]

Tablet, oral: 50 mg, 100 mg, 150 mg, 200 mg

Diflucan®: 50 mg, 100 mg, 150 mg, 200 mg

◆ **Fluconazole Injection (Can)** *see* Fluconazole *on page 718*

◆ **Fluconazole Omega (Can)** *see* Fluconazole *on page 718*

Flucytosine (floo SYE toe seen)

Brand Names: U.S. Ancobon®

Brand Names: Canada Ancobon®

Index Terms 5-FC; 5-Fluorocytosine; 5-Flurocytosine

Pharmacologic Category Antifungal Agent, Oral

Additional Appendix Information

Antifungal Agents *on page 1876*

Use Adjunctive treatment of systemic fungal infections (eg, septicemia, endocarditis, UTI, meningitis, or pulmonary) caused by susceptible strains of *Candida* or *Cryptococcus*

Pregnancy Risk Factor C

Pregnancy Considerations Teratogenic in some animal studies, however, there are no adequate and well-controlled studies in pregnant women.

Lactation Excretion in breast milk unknown/not recommended

Contraindications Hypersensitivity to flucytosine or any component of the formulation

Warnings/Precautions [U.S. Boxed Warning]: Use with extreme caution in patients with renal dysfunction; dosage adjustment required. Avoid use as monotherapy; resistance rapidly develops. Use with caution in patients with bone marrow depression; patients with hematologic disease or who have been treated with radiation or drugs that suppress the bone marrow may be at greatest risk. Bone marrow toxicity can be irreversible. **[U.S. Boxed Warning]: Closely monitor hematologic, renal, and hepatic status.** Hepatotoxicity and bone marrow toxicity appear to be dose related; monitor levels closely and adjust dose accordingly.

Adverse Reactions Frequency not defined.

Cardiovascular: Cardiac arrest, myocardial toxicity, ventricular dysfunction, chest pain

Central nervous system: Ataxia, confusion, dizziness, drowsiness, fatigue, hallucinations, headache, parkinsonism, psychosis, pyrexia, sedation, seizure, vertigo

Dermatologic: Rash, photosensitivity, pruritus, toxic epidermal necrolysis, urticaria

Endocrine & metabolic: Hypoglycemia, hypokalemia

Gastrointestinal: Abdominal pain, diarrhea, dry mouth, duodenal ulcer, hemorrhage, loss of appetite, nausea, ulcerative colitis, vomiting

Hematologic: Agranulocytosis, anemia, aplastic anemia, eosinophilia, leukopenia, pancytopenia, thrombocytopenia

Hepatic: Acute hepatic injury, bilirubin increased, hepatic dysfunction, jaundice, liver enzymes increased

Neuromuscular & skeletal: Paresthesia, peripheral neuropathy, weakness

Otic: Hearing loss

Renal: Azotemia, BUN increased, crystalluria, renal failure, serum creatinine increased

Respiratory: Dyspnea, respiratory arrest

Miscellaneous: Allergic reaction

Drug Interactions

Metabolism/Transport Effects None known.

Avoid Concomitant Use

Avoid concomitant use of Flucytosine with any of the following: CloZAPine

Increased Effect/Toxicity

Flucytosine may increase the levels/effects of: CloZAPine

The levels/effects of Flucytosine may be increased by: Amphotericin B

Decreased Effect

Flucytosine may decrease the levels/effects of: Saccharomyces boulardii

The levels/effects of Flucytosine may be decreased by: Cytarabine (Conventional)

Ethanol/Nutrition/Herb Interactions Food: Food decreases the rate, but not the extent of absorption.

Stability Store at room temperature of 15°C to 30°C (59°F to 86°F). Protect from light.

Mechanism of Action Penetrates fungal cells and is converted to fluorouracil which competes with uracil interfering with fungal RNA and protein synthesis

Pharmacodynamics/Kinetics

Absorption: 76% to 89%

Distribution: Into CSF, aqueous humor, joints, peritoneal fluid, and bronchial secretions; V_d: 0.6 L/kg

Protein binding: 3% to 4%

Metabolism: Minimally hepatic; deaminated, possibly via gut bacteria, to 5-fluorouracil

Half-life elimination:

Normal renal function: 2-5 hours

Anuria: 85 hours (range: 30-250)

End stage renal disease: 75-200 hours

Time to peak, serum: ~1-2 hours

Excretion: Urine (>90% as unchanged drug)

Dosage

Usual dosage ranges: Children (unlabeled use) and Adults: Oral: 50-150 mg/kg/day in divided doses every 6 hours

Indication-specific dosing:

Children (unlabeled use) and Adults: Oral:

Endocarditis: 25-37.5 mg/kg every 6 hours (with amphotericin B) for at least 6 weeks after valve replacement

Meningoencephalitis, cryptococcal: Induction: 25 mg/kg/dose (with amphotericin B) every 6 hours for 2 weeks; if clinical improvement, may discontinue both amphotericin and flucytosine and follow with an extended course of fluconazole (400 mg/day); alternatively, may continue flucytosine for 6-10 weeks (with amphotericin B) without conversion to fluconazole treatment

Dosing interval in renal impairment: Use lower initial dose:

Cl_{cr} 20-40 mL/minute: Administer 37.5 mg/kg every 12 hours

Cl_{cr} 10-20 mL/minute: Administer 37.5 mg/kg every 24 hours

Cl_{cr} <10 mL/minute: Administer 37.5 mg/kg every 24-48 hours, but monitor drug concentrations frequently

Hemodialysis: Dialyzable (50% to 100%); administer dose posthemodialysis

Peritoneal dialysis: Adults: Administer 0.5-1 g every 24 hours

Continuous arteriovenous or venovenous hemodiafiltration effects: Change dosing frequency to every 12-24 hours (monitor serum concentrations and adjust)

Administration Administer around-the-clock to promote less variation in peak and trough serum levels. To avoid nausea and vomiting, administer a few capsules at a time over 15 minutes until full dose is taken.

Monitoring Parameters

Pretreatment: Electrolytes (especially potassium), CBC with differential, BUN, renal function, blood culture

During treatment: CBC with differential, and LFTs (eg, alkaline phosphatase, AST/ALT) frequently, serum flucytosine concentration, renal function

Reference Range

Therapeutic: Trough: 25-50 mcg/mL; peak: 50-100 mcg/mL; peak levels should not exceed 100 mcg/mL to avoid toxic bone marrow depressive and hepatic effects

Trough: Draw just prior to dose administration

Peak: Draw 2 hours after an oral dose administration

Test Interactions Flucytosine causes markedly false elevations in serum creatinine values when the Ektachem® analyzer is used. The Jaffé reaction is recommended for determining serum creatinine.

Dosage Forms Excipient information presented when available (limited, particularly for generics); consult specific product labeling.

Capsule, oral: 250 mg, 500 mg

Ancobon®: 250 mg, 500 mg

Extemporaneous Preparations A 10 mg/mL oral suspension may be made with capsules and distilled water. Empty the contents of ten 500 mg capsules in a mortar; add small portions of distilled water and mix to a uniform paste. Mix while adding distilled water in incremental proportions to **almost** 500 mL; transfer to a 500 mL volumetric flask, rinse mortar several times with distilled water, and add sufficient quantity of distilled water to make 500 mL. Store in glass or plastic prescription bottles and label "shake well". Stable for 70 days refrigerated and 14 days at room temperature.

Wintermeyer SM and Nahata MC, "Stability of Flucytosine in an Extemporaneously Compounded Oral Liquid," *Am J Health Syst Pharm*, 1996, 53(4):407-9.

◆ **Fludara®** *see* Fludarabine *on page 721*

Fludarabine (floo DARE a been)

Brand Names: U.S. Fludara®; Oforta™ [DSC]

Brand Names: Canada Fludara®

Index Terms 2F-ara-AMP; Fludarabine Phosphate

Pharmacologic Category Antineoplastic Agent, Antimetabolite (Purine Analog)

Use Treatment of progressive or refractory B-cell chronic lymphocytic leukemia (CLL)

Canadian labeling: Second-line treatment of chronic lymphocytic leukemia (CLL); second-line treatment of low-grade, refractory non-Hodgkin's lymphoma (NHL)

Unlabeled Use Treatment of non-Hodgkin's lymphomas (NHL); acute myeloid leukemia (AML), either refractory or in poor risk patients; relapsed acute lymphocytic leukemia (ALL) or AML in pediatric patients; Waldenström's macroglobulinemia (WM); reduced-intensity conditioning regimens prior to allogeneic hematopoietic stem cell transplantation (generally administered in combination with busulfan or cyclophosphamide and antithymocyte globulin or lymphocyte immune globulin, or in combination with melphalan and alemtuzumab)

Pregnancy Risk Factor D

Pregnancy Considerations Teratogenic effects were observed in animal studies. Based on the mechanism of action, fludarabine has the potential to cause fetal harm if administered during pregnancy. There are no adequate and well-controlled studies in pregnant women. Effective contraception is recommended during and for 6 months after treatment for women and men with female partners of reproductive potential.

Lactation Excretion in breast milk unknown/not recommended

Contraindications Hypersensitivity of fludarabine or any component of the formulation

Canadian labeling: Additional contraindications (not in U.S. labeling): Severe renal impairment (Cl_{cr} <30 mL/minute); decompensated hemolytic anemia; concurrent use with pentostatin

Warnings/Precautions Hazardous agent - use appropriate precautions for handling and disposal. Use with caution in patients with renal insufficiency (clearance of the primary metabolite 2-fluoro-ara-A is reduced); dosage reductions are recommended (monitor closely for excessive toxicity); use of the I.V. formulation is not recommended if Cl_{cr} <30 mL/minute. Use with caution in patients with preexisting hematological disorders (particularly granulocytopenia) or pre-existing central nervous system disorder (epilepsy), spasticity, or peripheral neuropathy. **[U.S. Boxed Warning]: Higher than recommended doses are associated with severe neurologic toxicity (delayed blindness, coma, death); similar neurotoxicity (agitation, coma, confusion and seizure) has been reported with standard CLL doses.** Neurotoxicity symptoms due to high doses appear from 21-60 days following the last fludarabine dose, although neurotoxicity has been reported as early as 7 days and up to 225 days. Possible neurotoxic effects of chronic administration are unknown. Caution patients about performing tasks which require mental alertness (eg, operating machinery or driving). ▶

[U.S. Boxed Warning]: Life-threatening (and sometimes fatal) autoimmune effects, including hemolytic anemia, autoimmune thrombocytopenia/thrombocytopenic purpura (ITP), Evans syndrome, and acquired hemophilia have occurred; monitor closely for hemolysis; discontinue fludarabine if hemolysis occurs; the hemolytic effects usually recur with fludarabine rechallenge. **[U.S. Boxed Warning]: Severe bone marrow suppression (anemia, thrombocytopenia, and neutropenia) may occur;** may be cumulative. Severe myelosuppression (trilineage bone marrow hypoplasia/aplasia) has been reported (rare) with a duration of significant cytopenias ranging from 2 months to 1 year. First-line combination therapy is associated with prolonged cytopenias, with anemia lasting up to 7 months, neutropenia up to 9 months, and thrombocytopenia up to 10 months; increased age is predictive for prolonged cytopenias (Gill, 2010).

Use with caution in patients with documented infection, fever, immunodeficiency, or with a history of opportunistic infection; prophylactic anti-infectives should be considered for patients with an increased risk for developing opportunistic infections. Progressive multifocal leukoencephalopathy (PML) due to JC virus (usually fatal) has been reported with use; usually in patients who had received prior and/or other concurrent chemotherapy; onset ranges from a few weeks to 1 year; evaluate any neurological change promptly. Avoid vaccination with live vaccines during and after fludarabine treatment. May cause tumor lysis syndrome; risk is increased in patients with large tumor burden prior to treatment. Patients receiving blood products should only receive irradiated blood products due to the potential for transfusion related GVHD. **[U.S. Boxed Warnings]: Do not use in combination with pentostatin; may lead to severe, even fatal pulmonary toxicity. Should be administered under the supervision of an experienced cancer chemotherapy physician.**

Adverse Reactions

>10%:

- Cardiovascular: Edema (8% to 19%)
- Central nervous system: Fever (11% to 69%), fatigue (10% to 38%), pain (5% to 22%), chills (11% to 19%)
- Dermatologic: Rash (4% to 15%)
- Gastrointestinal: Nausea/vomiting (1% to 36%), anorexia (≤34%), diarrhea (5% to 15%), gastrointestinal bleeding (3% to 13%)
- Genitourinary: Urinary tract infection (2% to 15%)
- Hematologic: Myelosuppression (nadir: 10-14 days; recovery: 5-7 weeks; dose-limiting toxicity), anemia (14% to 60%), neutropenia (grade 4: 37% to 59%; nadir: ~13 days), thrombocytopenia (17% to 55%; nadir: ~16 days)
- Neuromuscular & skeletal: Weakness (9% to 65%), myalgia (4% to 16%), paresthesia (4% to 12%)
- Ocular: Visual disturbance (3% to 15%)
- Respiratory: Cough (≤44%), pneumonia (3% to 22%), dyspnea (1% to 22%), upper respiratory infection (2% to 16%), rhinitis (≤11%)
- Miscellaneous: Infection (12% to 44%), diaphoresis (≤14%)

1% to 10%:

- Cardiovascular: Peripheral edema (≤7%), angina (≤6%), chest pain (≤5%), CHF (≤3%), arrhythmia (≤3%), cerebrovascular accident (≤3%), MI (≤3%), supraventricular tachycardia (≤3%), deep vein thrombosis (1% to 3%), phlebitis (1% to 3%), aneurysm (≤1%), transient ischemic attack (≤1%)
- Central nervous system: Headache (≤9%), malaise (6% to 8%), sleep disorder (1% to 3%), cerebellar syndrome (≤1%), depression (≤1%), mentation impaired (≤1%)
- Dermatologic: Alopecia (≤3%), pruritus (1% to 3%), seborrhea (≤1%)
- Endocrine & metabolic: Hyperglycemia (1% to 6%), LDH increased (≤6%), dehydration (≤1%)
- Gastrointestinal: Abdominal pain (≤10%), stomatitis (≤9%), weight loss (≤6%), esophagitis (≤3%), constipation (1% to 3%), mucositis (≤2%), dysphagia (≤1%)
- Genitourinary: Dysuria (3% to 4%), hesitancy (≤3%)
- Hematologic: Hemorrhage (≤1%), myelodysplastic syndrome/acute myeloid leukemia (usually associated with prior or concurrent treatment with other anticancer agents)
- Hepatic: Cholelithiasis (≤3%), liver function tests abnormal (1% to 3%), liver failure (≤1%)
- Neuromuscular & skeletal: Back pain (≤9%), osteoporosis (≤2%), arthralgia (≤1%)
- Otic: Hearing loss (2% to 6%)
- Renal: Hematuria (2% to 3%), renal failure (≤1%), renal function test abnormal (≤1%), proteinuria (≤1%)
- Respiratory: Bronchitis (≤9%), pharyngitis (≤9%), allergic pneumonitis (≤6%), hemoptysis (1% to 6%), sinusitis (≤5%), epistaxis (≤1%), hypoxia (≤1%)
- Miscellaneous: Flu-like syndrome (5% to 8%), herpes simplex infection (≤8%), anaphylaxis (≤1%), tumor lysis syndrome (1%)

<1% (Limited to important or life-threatening): Acute respiratory distress syndrome, agitation, blindness, blurred vision, bone marrow fibrosis, coma, confusion, diplopia, eosinophilia, Epstein-Barr virus (EBV) associated lymphoproliferation, EBV reactivation, erythema multiforme, Evans syndrome, flank pain, hemolytic anemia (autoimmune), hemophilia (acquired), hemorrhagic cystitis, herpes zoster reactivation, hyperkalemia, hyperphosphatemia, hyperuricemia, hypocalcemia, interstitial pneumonitis, metabolic acidosis, opportunistic infection, optic neuritis, optic neuropathy, pancreatic enzymes abnormal, pancytopenia, pemphigus, pericardial effusion, peripheral neuropathy, photophobia (primarily with high doses), progressive multifocal leukoencephalopathy (PML), pulmonary fibrosis, pulmonary hemorrhage, pulmonary infiltrate, respiratory distress, respiratory failure, Richter's syndrome, seizure, skin cancer (new onset or exacerbation), Stevens-Johnson syndrome, thrombocytopenia (autoimmune), thrombocytopenic purpura (autoimmune), toxic epidermal necrolysis, trilineage bone marrow aplasia, trilineage bone marrow hypoplasia, urate crystalluria, wrist drop

Also observed: Neurologic syndrome characterized by cortical blindness, coma, and paralysis [36% at doses >96 mg/m^2 for 5-7 days; <0.2% at doses <125 mg/m^2/cycle (onset of neurologic symptoms may be delayed for 3-4 weeks)]

Drug Interactions

Metabolism/Transport Effects
None known.

Avoid Concomitant Use

Avoid concomitant use of Fludarabine with any of the following: BCG; CloZAPine; Natalizumab; Pentostatin; Pimecrolimus; Tacrolimus (Topical); Vaccines (Live)

Increased Effect/Toxicity

Fludarabine may increase the levels/effects of: CloZAPine; Leflunomide; Natalizumab; Pentostatin; Vaccines (Live)

The levels/effects of Fludarabine may be increased by: Denosumab; Pentostatin; Pimecrolimus; Roflumilast; Tacrolimus (Topical); Trastuzumab

Decreased Effect

Fludarabine may decrease the levels/effects of: BCG; Coccidioidin Skin Test; Sipuleucel-T; Vaccines (Inactivated); Vaccines (Live)

The levels/effects of Fludarabine may be decreased by: Echinacea; Imatinib

Ethanol/Nutrition/Herb Interactions Ethanol: Avoid ethanol (due to GI irritation).

Stability

I.V.: Store intact vials under refrigeration at 2°C to 8°C (36°F to 46°F). Reconstituted vials are stable for 16 days at room temperature of 15°C to 30°C (59°F to 86°F) or refrigerated, although the manufacturer recommends use within 8 hours. Solutions diluted in saline or dextrose are stable for 48 hours at room temperature or under refrigeration. Use appropriate precautions for handling and disposal. Reconstitute vials with SWI, NS, or D_5W to a concentration of 10-25 mg/mL; standard I.V. dilution: 100-125 mL D_5W or NS.

Tablet: Store at 25°C (77°F); excursions permitted to 15°C to 30°C (59°F to 86°F); should be kept within packaging until use.

Mechanism of Action Fludarabine inhibits DNA synthesis by inhibition of DNA polymerase and ribonucleotide reductase; also inhibits DNA primase and DNA ligase I

Pharmacodynamics/Kinetics

Distribution: V_d: 38-96 L/m^2; widely with extensive tissue binding

Protein binding: 2-fluoro-ara-A: ~19% to 29%

Metabolism: I.V.: Fludarabine phosphate is rapidly dephosphorylated in the plasma to 2-fluoro-ara-A (active metabolite), which subsequently enters tumor cells and is phosphorylated by deoxycytidine kinase to the active triphosphate derivative (2-fluoro-ara-ATP)

Bioavailability: Oral: 2-fluoro-ara-A: 50% to 65%

Half-life elimination: 2-fluoro-ara-A: ~20 hours

Time to peak, plasma: Oral: 1-2 hours

Excretion: Urine (60%, 23% as 2-fluoro-ara-A) within 24 hours

Dosage Details concerning dosing in combination regimens should also be consulted.

Oral: Adults: CLL: 40 mg/m^2 once daily for 5 days every 28 days

I.V.:

Children (unlabeled use):

- AML: 10.5 mg/m^2 bolus over 15 minutes followed by a continuous infusion of 30.5 mg/m^2/day for 48 hours (Lange, 2008)
- ALL or AML, relapsed: 10.5 mg/m^2 bolus over 15 minutes followed by a continuous infusion of 30.5 mg/m^2/day for 48 hours (Avramis, 1998)
- Stem cell transplant (allogeneic) conditioning regimen, reduced-intensity: 30 mg/m^2/dose for 6 doses beginning 7-10 days prior to transplant (in combination with busulfan and antithymocyte globulin) (Pulsipher, 2009)

Adults:

- CLL: 25 mg/m^2/day for 5 days every 28 days
- CLL combination regimens (unlabeled dosing):
  - CFAR: 20 mg/m^2/day for 3 days every 28 days for 6 cycles (in combination with cyclophosphamide, rituximab and alemtuzumab) (Wierda, 2008)
  - FC: 30 mg/m^2/day for 3 days every 28 days for 6 cycles (in combination with cyclophosphamide) (Eichhorst, 2006) **or** 20 mg/m^2/day for 5 days every 28 days for 6 cycles (in combination with cyclophosphamide) (Flinn, 2007)
  - FCR: 25 mg/m^2/day for 3 days every 28 days for 6 cycles (in combination with cyclophosphamide and rituximab) (Keating, 2005; Robak, 2010; Wierda, 2005)
  - FluCam: 30 mg/m^2/day for 3 days every 28 days for 4-6 cycles (in combination with alemtuzumab) (Elter, 2005)
  - FR: 25 mg/m^2/day for 5 days every 28 days for 6 cycles (in combination with rituximab) (Byrd, 2003)
  - OFAR: 30 mg/m^2/day for 2 days every 28 days for 6 cycles (in combination with oxaliplatin, cytarabine, and rituximab) (Tsimberidou, 2008)
- AML, high-risk patients (unlabeled use): 30 mg/m^2/day for 5 days induction therapy, followed by post remission therapy of 30 mg/m^2/day for 4 days every other cycle (in combination with cytarabine with or without filgrastim) (Borthakur, 2008)
- AML, refractory (unlabeled use): 30 mg/m^2/day for 5 days (in combination with cytarabine and filgrastim), may repeat once for partial remission (Montillo, 1998) **or** 30 mg/m^2/day for 5 days for 1 or 2 cycles (in combination with cytarabine, idarubicin, and filgrastim) (Virchis, 2004)
- Non-Hodgkin's lymphomas (unlabeled uses):
  - Follicular lymphoma:
    - FCR: 25 mg/m^2/day for 3 days every 21 days for 4 cycles (in combination with cyclophosphamide and rituximab) (Sacchi, 2007)
    - FCMR: 25 mg/m^2/day for 3 days every 28 days for 4 cycles (in combination with cyclophosphamide, mitoxantrone, and rituximab) (Forstpointner, 2004; Forstpointner, 2006)
    - FND: 25 mg/m^2/day for 3 days every 28 days for up to 8 cycles (in combination with mitoxantrone and dexamethasone) (McLaughlin, 1996; Tsimberidou, 2002)
    - FNDR: 25 mg/m^2/day for 3 days every 28 days for up to 8 cycles (in combination with mitoxantrone, dexamethasone, and rituximab) (McLaughlin, 2000)
    - FR: 25 mg/m^2/day for 5 days every 28 days for 6 cycles (in combination with rituximab) (Czuczman, 2005)
  - Mantle cell lymphoma:
    - FC: 20 mg/m^2/day for 4-5 days or 25 mg/m^2/day for 3-5 days (in combination with cyclophosphamide) (Cohen, 2001)
    - FCMR: 25 mg/m^2/day for 3 days every 28 days for 4 cycles (in combination with cyclophosphamide, mitoxantrone, and rituximab) (Forstpointner, 2004; Forstpointner, 2006)
- Waldenstron's macroglobulinemia (unlabeled use): 25 mg/m^2/day for 5 days every 28 days (Foran, 1999) **or** 25 mg/m^2/day for 5 days every 28 days for 6 cycles (in combination with rituximab) (Treon, 2009)
- Stem cell transplant (allogeneic) conditioning regimen, reduced-intensity, (unlabeled use): 30 mg/m^2/dose for 6 doses beginning 10 days prior to transplant **or** 30 mg/m^2/dose for 5 days beginning 6 days prior to transplant (in combination with busulfan with or without antithymocyte globulin) (Schetelig, 2003)
- Stem cell transplant (allogeneic) nonmyeloablative conditioning regimen (unlabeled use): 30 mg/m^2/dose for 3 doses beginning 5 days prior to transplant (in combination with cyclophosphamide and rituximab) (Khouri, 2008) **or** 30 mg/m^2/dose for 3 doses beginning 4 days prior to transplant (in combination with total body irradiation) (Rezvani, 2008)

Dosage adjustment for toxicity:

Hematologic or nonhematologic toxicity (other than neurotoxicity): Consider treatment delay or dosage reduction

Hemolysis: Discontinue treatment

Neurotoxicity: Consider treatment delay or discontinuation

Dosing in renal impairment:

FDA-approved labeling contains the following adjustment recommendations: Adults: CLL:

I.V.:

- Cl_{cr} 50-79 mL/minute: Decrease dose to 20 mg/m^2
- Cl_{cr} 30-49 mL/minute: Decrease dose to 15 mg/m^2
- Cl_{cr} <30 mL/minute: Avoid use

Oral:

- Cl_{cr} 30-70 mL/minute: Administer 80% of dose
- Cl_{cr} <30 mL/minute: Administer 50% of dose

Canadian labeling contains the following adjustment recommendations: CLL, NHL:
Cl_{cr} 30-70 mL/minute: Reduce dose by up to 50%
Cl_{cr} <30 mL/minute: Use is contraindicated
The following guidelines have been used by some clinicians: Aronoff, 2007: I.V.:
Children:
Cl_{cr} 30-50 mL/minute: Administer 80% of dose
Cl_{cr} <30 mL/minute: Not recommended
Hemodialysis: Administer 25% of dose
Continuous ambulatory peritoneal dialysis (CAPD): Not recommended
Continuous renal replacement therapy (CRRT): Administer 80% of dose
Adults:
Cl_{cr} 10-50 mL/minute: Administer 75% of dose
Cl_{cr} <10 mL/minute: Administer 50% of dose
Hemodialysis: Administer after dialysis
Continuous ambulatory peritoneal dialysis (CAPD): Administer 50% of dose
Continuous renal replacement therapy (CRRT): Administer 75% of dose

Dietary Considerations Tablet may be taken with or without food.

Administration
Oral: Tablet may be administered with or without food; should be swallowed whole with water; do not chew, break, or crush.
I.V.: Usually administered as a 30-minute infusion; continuous infusions (unlabeled administration rate) are occasionally used

Monitoring Parameters CBC with differential, platelet count, AST, ALT, serum creatinine, serum albumin, uric acid; monitor for signs of infection and neurotoxicity

Dosage Forms Excipient information presented when available (limited, particularly for generics); consult specific product labeling. [DSC] = Discontinued product
Injection, powder for reconstitution, as phosphate: 50 mg
Fludara®: 50 mg
Injection, solution, as phosphate [preservative free]: 25 mg/mL (2 mL)
Tablet, oral, as phosphate:
Oforta™: 10 mg [DSC]

Dosage Forms: Canada Excipient information presented when available (limited, particularly for generics); consult specific product labeling.
Tablet, as phosphate:
Fludara®: 10 mg

◆ **Fludarabine Phosphate** *see* Fludarabine *on page* 721

Fludrocortisone (floo droe KOR ti sone)

Brand Names: Canada Florinef®

Index Terms 9α-Fluorohydrocortisone Acetate; Florinef; Fludrocortisone Acetate; Fluohydrisone Acetate; Fluohydrocortisone Acetate

Pharmacologic Category Corticosteroid, Systemic

Additional Appendix Information
Corticosteroids *on page* 1888

Use Partial replacement therapy for primary and secondary adrenocortical insufficiency in Addison's disease; treatment of salt-losing adrenogenital syndrome

Pregnancy Risk Factor C

Pregnancy Considerations Animal reproduction studies have not been conducted with fludrocortisone; adverse events have been observed with corticosteroids in animal reproduction studies. Some studies have shown an association between first trimester systemic corticosteroid use and oral clefts; adverse events in the fetus/neonate have been noted in case reports following large doses of systemic corticosteroids during pregnancy.

Lactation Excretion in breast milk unknown/use caution

Contraindications Hypersensitivity to fludrocortisone or any component of the formulation; systemic fungal infections

Warnings/Precautions May cause hypercorticism or suppression of hypothalamic-pituitary-adrenal (HPA) axis, particularly in younger children or in patients receiving high doses for prolonged periods. HPA axis suppression may lead to adrenal crisis. Withdrawal and discontinuation of a corticosteroid should be done slowly and carefully. Fludrocortisone is primarily a mineralocorticoid agonist, but may also inhibit the HPA axis. May increase risk of infection and/or limit response to vaccinations; close observation is required in patients with latent tuberculosis and/or TB reactivity. Restrict use in active TB (only in conjunction with antituberculosis treatment). Use with caution in patients with sodium retention and potassium loss, hepatic impairment, myocardial infarction, osteoporosis, and/or renal impairment. Use with caution in the elderly. Withdraw therapy with gradual tapering of dose.

Adverse Reactions Frequency not defined.
Cardiovascular: CHF, edema, hypertension
Central nervous system: Dizziness, headache, seizures
Dermatologic: Acne, bruising, rash
Endocrine & metabolic: HPA suppression, hyperglycemia, hypokalemic alkalosis, suppression of growth
Gastrointestinal: Peptic ulcer
Neuromuscular & skeletal: Muscle weakness
Ocular: Cataracts
Miscellaneous: Anaphylaxis (generalized), diaphoresis

Drug Interactions

Metabolism/Transport Effects None known.

Avoid Concomitant Use
Avoid concomitant use of Fludrocortisone with any of the following: Aldesleukin; BCG; Natalizumab; Pimecrolimus; Tacrolimus (Topical)

Increased Effect/Toxicity
Fludrocortisone may increase the levels/effects of: Acetylcholinesterase Inhibitors; Amphotericin B; Deferasirox; Leflunomide; Loop Diuretics; Natalizumab; NSAID (COX-2 Inhibitor); NSAID (Nonselective); Thiazide Diuretics; Vaccines (Live); Warfarin

The levels/effects of Fludrocortisone may be increased by: Antifungal Agents (Azole Derivatives, Systemic); Aprepitant; Calcium Channel Blockers (Nondihydropyridine); Denosumab; Estrogen Derivatives; Fluconazole; Fosaprepitant; Indacaterol; Macrolide Antibiotics; Neuromuscular-Blocking Agents (Nondepolarizing); Pimecrolimus; Quinolone Antibiotics; Roflumilast; Salicylates; Tacrolimus (Topical); Telaprevir; Trastuzumab

Decreased Effect
Fludrocortisone may decrease the levels/effects of: Aldesleukin; Antidiabetic Agents; BCG; Calcitriol; Coccidioidin Skin Test; Corticorelin; Isoniazid; Salicylates; Sipuleucel-T; Telaprevir; Vaccines (Inactivated)

The levels/effects of Fludrocortisone may be decreased by: Aminoglutethimide; Antacids; Barbiturates; Bile Acid Sequestrants; Echinacea; Mitotane; Primidone; Rifamycin Derivatives

Mechanism of Action Promotes increased reabsorption of sodium and loss of potassium from renal distal tubules

Pharmacodynamics/Kinetics
Absorption: Rapid and complete
Protein binding: 42%
Metabolism: Hepatic
Half-life elimination, plasma: 30-35 minutes; Biological: 18-36 hours
Time to peak, serum: ~1.7 hours

Dosage Oral:

Infants and Children: 0.05-0.1 mg/day

Adults: 0.1-0.2 mg/day with ranges of 0.1 mg 3 times/week to 0.2 mg/day

Addison's disease: Initial: 0.1 mg/day; if transient hypertension develops, reduce the dose to 0.05 mg/day. Preferred administration with cortisone (10-37.5 mg/day) or hydrocortisone (10-30 mg/day).

Salt-losing adrenogenital syndrome: 0.1-0.2 mg/day

Dietary Considerations Systemic use of mineralocorticoids/corticosteroids may require a diet with increased potassium, vitamins A, B_6, C, D, folate, calcium, zinc, and phosphorus, and decreased sodium. With fludrocortisone, a decrease in dietary sodium is often not required as the increased retention of sodium is usually the desired therapeutic effect.

Administration Administration in conjunction with a glucocorticoid is preferable

Monitoring Parameters Monitor blood pressure and signs of edema when patient is on chronic therapy; very potent mineralocorticoid with high glucocorticoid activity; monitor serum electrolytes, serum renin activity, blood pressure, and growth in children; monitor for evidence of infection; stop treatment if a significant increase in weight or blood pressure, edema, or cardiac enlargement occurs

Additional Information In patients with salt-losing forms of congenital adrenogenital syndrome, use along with cortisone or hydrocortisone. Fludrocortisone 0.1 mg has sodium retention activity equal to DOCA® 1 mg.

Dosage Forms Excipient information presented when available (limited, particularly for generics); consult specific product labeling.

Tablet, oral, as acetate: 0.1 mg

◆ **Fludrocortisone Acetate** *see* Fludrocortisone *on page 724*

◆ **FluLaval®** *see* Influenza Virus Vaccine (Inactivated) *on page 897*

◆ **Flumadine®** *see* Rimantadine *on page 1493*

Flumazenil (FLOO may ze nil)

Brand Names: U.S. Romazicon®

Brand Names: Canada Anexate®; Flumazenil Injection; Flumazenil Injection, USP; Romazicon®

Pharmacologic Category Antidote

Use Benzodiazepine antagonist; reverses sedative effects of benzodiazepines used in conscious sedation and general anesthesia; treatment of benzodiazepine overdose

Pregnancy Risk Factor C

Pregnancy Considerations Teratogenic effects were not seen in animal studies. Embryocidal effects were seen at large doses. There are no adequate or well-controlled studies in pregnant women. Use only if clearly needed.

Lactation Excretion in breast milk unknown/use caution

Contraindications Hypersensitivity to flumazenil, benzodiazepines, or any component of the formulation; patients given benzodiazepines for control of potentially life-threatening conditions (eg, control of intracranial pressure or status epilepticus); patients who are showing signs of serious cyclic-antidepressant overdosage

Warnings/Precautions **[U.S. Boxed Warning]: Benzodiazepine reversal may result in seizures in some patients.** Patients who may develop seizures include patients on benzodiazepines for long-term sedation, tricyclic antidepressant overdose patients, concurrent major sedative-hypnotic drug withdrawal, recent therapy with repeated doses of parenteral benzodiazepines, myoclonic jerking or seizure activity prior to flumazenil administration. Flumazenil may not reliably reverse respiratory depression/hypoventilation. Flumazenil is not a substitute for evaluation of oxygenation; establishing an airway and assisting ventilation, as necessary, is always the initial step in overdose management. Resedation occurs more frequently in patients where a large single dose or cumulative dose of a benzodiazepine is administered along with a neuromuscular-blocking agent and multiple anesthetic agents. Flumazenil should be used with caution in the intensive care unit because of increased risk of unrecognized benzodiazepine dependence in such settings. Should not be used to diagnose benzodiazepine-induced sedation. Reverse neuromuscular blockade before considering use. Flumazenil does not antagonize the CNS effects of other GABA agonists (such as ethanol, barbiturates, or general anesthetics); nor does it reverse narcotics. Flumazenil does not consistently reverse amnesia; patient may not recall verbal instructions after procedure.

Use with caution in patients with a history of panic disorder; may provoke panic attacks. Use caution in drug and ethanol-dependent patients; these patients may also be dependent on benzodiazepines. Not recommended for treatment of benzodiazepine dependence. Use with caution in head injury patients. Use caution in patients with mixed drug overdoses; toxic effects of other drugs taken may emerge once benzodiazepine effects are reversed. Use caution in hepatic dysfunction and in patients relying on a benzodiazepine for seizure control. Safety and efficacy have not been established in children <1 year of age.

Adverse Reactions

>10%: Gastrointestinal: Vomiting, nausea

1% to 10%:

Cardiovascular: Vasodilation (1% to 3%), palpitation

Central nervous system: Dizziness (10%), agitation (3% to 9%), emotional lability (1% to 3%), fatigue (1% to 3%), headache (1% to 3%)

Gastrointestinal: Xerostomia

Local: Pain at injection site (3% to 9%)

Neuromuscular & skeletal: Tremor, weakness, paresthesia (1% to 3%)

Ocular: Abnormal vision, blurred vision (3% to 9%)

Respiratory: Dyspnea, hyperventilation (3% to 9%)

Miscellaneous: Diaphoresis

<1%: Abnormal hearing, altered blood pressure increased/decreased, confusion, sensation of coldness, bradycardia, chest pain, generalized seizure, hiccups, hypertension, junctional tachycardia, shivering, somnolence, tachycardia, thick tongue, ventricular tachycardia, withdrawal syndrome

Drug Interactions

Metabolism/Transport Effects None known.

Avoid Concomitant Use There are no known interactions where it is recommended to avoid concomitant use.

Increased Effect/Toxicity There are no known significant interactions involving an increase in effect.

Decreased Effect

Flumazenil may decrease the levels/effects of: Hypnotics (Nonbenzodiazepine)

Stability Store at 15°C to 30°C (59°F to 86°F). For I.V. use only. Once drawn up in the syringe or mixed with solution use within 24 hours. Discard any unused solution after 24 hours.

Mechanism of Action Competitively inhibits the activity at the benzodiazepine receptor site on the GABA/benzodiazepine receptor complex. Flumazenil does not antagonize the CNS effect of drugs affecting GABA-ergic neurons by means other than the benzodiazepine receptor (ethanol, barbiturates, general anesthetics) and does not reverse the effects of opioids

Pharmacodynamics/Kinetics

Onset of action: 1-3 minutes; 80% response within 3 minutes

Peak effect: 6-10 minutes

Duration: Resedation: ~1 hour; duration related to dose given and benzodiazepine plasma concentrations; reversal effects of flumazenil may wear off before effects of benzodiazepine
Distribution: Initial V_d: 0.5 L/kg; V_{dss}: 0.77-1.6 L/kg
Protein binding: 40% to 50%
Metabolism: Hepatic; dependent upon hepatic blood flow
Half-life elimination: Adults: Alpha: 7-15 minutes; Terminal: 41-79 minutes; Moderate hepatic dysfunction: 1.3 hours; severe hepatic impairment: 2.4 hours
Excretion: Feces; urine (0.2% as unchanged drug)

Dosage
Children and Adults: I.V.: See table.

Flumazenil

Pediatric Dosage (Children ≥1 year)	
Pediatric dosage for **reversal of conscious sedation and general anesthesia:**	
Initial dose	0.01 mg/kg over 15 seconds (maximum: 0.2 mg)
Repeat doses (maximum: 4 doses)	0.01 mg/kg (maximum: 0.2 mg) repeated at 1-minute intervals
Maximum total cumulative dose	1 mg or 0.05 mg/kg (whichever is lower)
Adult Dosage	
Adult dosage for **reversal of conscious sedation and general anesthesia:**	
Initial dose	0.2 mg over 15 seconds
Repeat doses (maximum: 4 doses)	If desired level of consciousness is not obtained, 0.2 mg may be repeated at 1-minute intervals.
Maximum total cumulative dose	1 mg (usual dose: 0.6-1 mg) **In the event of resedation:** Repeat doses may be given at 20-minute intervals with maximum of 1 mg/dose and 3 mg/hour.
Adult dosage for **suspected benzodiazepine overdose:**	
Initial dose	0.2 mg over 30 seconds; if the desired level of consciousness is not obtained, 0.3 mg can be given over 30 seconds
Repeat doses	0.5 mg over 30 seconds repeated at 1-minute intervals
Maximum total cumulative dose	3 mg (usual dose: 1-3 mg) Patients with a partial response at 3 mg may require additional titration up to a total dose of 5 mg. If a patient has not responded 5 minutes after cumulative dose of 5 mg, the major cause of sedation is not likely due to benzodiazepines.

Elderly: No differences in safety or efficacy have been reported; however, increased sensitivity may occur in some elderly patients.

Dosing in renal impairment: Not significantly affected by renal failure (Cl_{cr} <10 mL/minute) or hemodialysis beginning 1 hour after drug administration

Dosing in hepatic impairment: Initial dose is unchanged. Reduce size or frequency of repeat doses.

Administration I.V.: Administer in freely-running I.V. into large vein. Inject over 15 seconds for conscious sedation and general anesthesia and over 30 seconds for overdose.

Monitoring Parameters Monitor patients for return of sedation or respiratory depression

Dosage Forms Excipient information presented when available (limited, particularly for generics); consult specific product labeling.
Injection, solution: 0.1 mg/mL (5 mL, 10 mL)
Romazicon®: 0.1 mg/mL (5 mL, 10 mL) [contains edetate disodium]

- ◆ **Flumazenil Injection (Can)** *see* Flumazenil *on page 725*
- ◆ **Flumazenil Injection, USP (Can)** *see* Flumazenil *on page 725*
- ◆ **FluMist®** *see* Influenza Virus Vaccine (Live/Attenuated) *on page 901*

Flunisolide (Nasal) (floo NISS oh lide)

Brand Names: Canada Apo-Flunisolide®; Nasalide®; Rhinalar®

Pharmacologic Category Corticosteroid, Nasal

Use Seasonal or perennial rhinitis

Pregnancy Risk Factor C

Dosage Intranasal: Rhinitis:
Children 6-14 years: 1 spray each nostril 3 times daily **or** 2 sprays in each nostril twice daily; not to exceed 4 sprays/day in each nostril
Children ≥15 years and Adults: 2 sprays each nostril twice daily (morning and evening); may increase to 2 sprays 3 times daily; maximum dose: 8 sprays/day in each nostril

Additional Information Complete prescribing information for this medication should be consulted for additional detail.

Dosage Forms Excipient information presented when available (limited, particularly for generics); consult specific product labeling.
Solution, intranasal [spray]: 25 mcg/actuation (25 mL); 29 mcg/actuation (25 mL)

Fluocinolone (Topical) (floo oh SIN oh lone)

Brand Names: U.S. Capex®; Derma-Smoothe/FS®

Brand Names: Canada Capex®; Derma-Smoothe/FS®; Synalar®

Index Terms Fluocinolone Acetonide

Pharmacologic Category Corticosteroid, Topical

Additional Appendix Information
Corticosteroids *on page 1888*

Use Relief of susceptible inflammatory dermatosis [low, medium corticosteroid]; dermatitis or psoriasis of the scalp; atopic dermatitis in adults and children ≥3 months of age

Pregnancy Risk Factor C

Dosage Topical:
Atopic dermatitis (Derma-Smoothe/FS® body oil):
Children ≥3 months: Moisten skin; apply a thin film to affected area twice daily; do not use for longer than 4 weeks
Adults: Apply a thin film to affected area 3 times/day
Corticosteroid-responsive dermatoses: Children and Adults: Cream, ointment, solution: Apply a thin layer to affected area 2-4 times/day; may use occlusive dressings to manage psoriasis or recalcitrant conditions
Inflammatory and pruritic manifestations (dental use): Adults: Apply to oral lesion 4 times/day, after meals and at bedtime
Scalp psoriasis (Derma-Smoothe/FS® scalp oil): Adults: Massage thoroughly into wet or dampened hair/scalp; cover with shower cap. Leave on overnight (or for at least 4 hours). Remove by washing hair with shampoo and rinsing thoroughly.
Seborrheic dermatitis of the scalp (Capex®): Adults: Apply no more than 1 ounce to scalp once daily; work into lather and allow to remain on scalp for ~5 minutes. Remove from hair and scalp by rinsing thoroughly with water.

Additional Information Complete prescribing information for this medication should be consulted for additional detail.

Dosage Forms Excipient information presented when available (limited, particularly for generics); consult specific product labeling.
Cream, topical, as acetonide: 0.01% (15 g, 60 g); 0.025% (15 g, 60 g)
Oil, topical, as acetonide [body oil]: 0.01% (118 mL)
Derma-Smoothe/FS®: 0.01% (120 mL) [contains isopropyl alcohol, peanut oil]
Oil, topical, as acetonide [scalp oil]: 0.01% (118 mL)
Derma-Smoothe/FS®: 0.01% (120 mL) [contains isopropyl alcohol, peanut oil]
Ointment, topical, as acetonide: 0.025% (15 g, 60 g)
Shampoo, topical, as acetonide:
Capex®: 0.01% (120 mL)
Solution, topical, as acetonide: 0.01% (60 mL)

◆ **Fluocinolone Acetonide** *see* Fluocinolone (Topical) *on page 726*

Fluocinolone, Hydroquinone, and Tretinoin
(floo oh SIN oh lone, HYE droe kwin one, & TRET i noyn)

Brand Names: U.S. Tri-Luma®
Index Terms Hydroquinone, Fluocinolone Acetonide, and Tretinoin; Tretinoin, Fluocinolone Acetonide, and Hydroquinone
Pharmacologic Category Corticosteroid, Topical; Depigmenting Agent; Retinoic Acid Derivative
Use Short-term treatment of moderate-to-severe melasma of the face
Pregnancy Risk Factor C
Dosage Topical: Adults: Melasma: Apply a thin film once daily to affected areas; not indicated for use beyond 8 weeks
Additional Information Complete prescribing information for this medication should be consulted for additional detail.
Dosage Forms Excipient information presented when available (limited, particularly for generics); consult specific product labeling.
Cream, topical:
Tri-Luma®: Fluocinolone acetonide 0.01%, hydroquinone 4%, and tretinoin 0.05% (30 g) [contains sodium metabisulfite]

Fluocinonide (floo oh SIN oh nide)

Brand Names: U.S. Vanos®
Brand Names: Canada Lidemol®; Lidex®; Lyderm®; Tiamol®; Topactin; Topsyn®
Index Terms Lidex
Pharmacologic Category Corticosteroid, Topical
Additional Appendix Information
Corticosteroids *on page 1888*
Use Anti-inflammatory, antipruritic; treatment of plaque-type psoriasis (up to 10% of body surface area) [high-potency topical corticosteroid]
Pregnancy Risk Factor C
Dosage
Children and Adults: Pruritus and inflammation: Topical (0.05% cream): Apply thin layer to affected area 2-4 times/day depending on the severity of the condition. Therapy should be discontinued when control is achieved; if no improvement is seen, reassessment of diagnosis may be necessary.
Children ≥12 years and Adults: Plaque-type psoriasis (Vanos™): Topical (0.1% cream): Apply a thin layer once or twice daily to affected areas (limited to <10% of body surface area). **Note:** Not recommended for use >2 consecutive weeks or >60 g/week total exposure. Discontinue when control is achieved.
Additional Information Complete prescribing information for this medication should be consulted for additional detail.
Dosage Forms Excipient information presented when available (limited, particularly for generics); consult specific product labeling.
Cream, topical:
Vanos®: 0.1% (30 g, 60 g, 120 g)
Cream, anhydrous, emollient, topical: 0.05% (15 g, 30 g, 60 g, 120 g)
Cream, aqueous, emollient, topical: 0.05% (15 g, 30 g, 60 g)
Gel, topical: 0.05% (15 g, 30 g, 60 g)
Ointment, topical: 0.05% (15 g, 30 g, 60 g)
Solution, topical: 0.05% (20 mL, 60 mL)

◆ **Fluohydrisone Acetate** *see* Fludrocortisone *on page 724*
◆ **Fluohydrocortisone Acetate** *see* Fludrocortisone *on page 724*
◆ **Fluorabon™** *see* Fluoride *on page 728*
◆ **Fluor-A-Day®** *see* Fluoride *on page 728*
◆ **Fluor-A-Day (Can)** *see* Fluoride *on page 728*

Fluorescein (FLURE e seen)

Brand Names: U.S. AK-Fluor®; BioGlo™; Fluorescite®; Fluorets®; Ful-Glo®
Brand Names: Canada Fluorescite®
Index Terms Fluorescein Sodium; Sodium Fluorescein; Soluble Fluorescein
Pharmacologic Category Diagnostic Agent
Use
Injection: Diagnostic aid in ophthalmic angiography and angioscopy
Topical: To stain the anterior segment of the eye for procedures (such as fitting contact lenses), disclosing corneal injury, and in applanation tonometry
Pregnancy Risk Factor C
Dosage
Ophthalmic: Strips: Children and Adults: Moisten strip with sterile water, saline or ophthalmic fluid. Touch conjunctiva or fornix with tip of strip until adequately stained. For best results, patient should blink several times after application.
Injection:
Children: 3.5 mg/lb (7.7 mg/kg) injected rapidly into antecubital vein
Adults: 500-750 mg injected rapidly into antecubital vein
Note: Prior to use, an intradermal test dose of 0.05 mL may be used if an allergy is suspected. Evaluate 30-60 minutes following intradermal injection.
Oral: Adults: 1 g of injection solution has been administered orally in patients with inaccessible veins and when early phases of an angiogram are not needed.

Dosage adjustment in renal impairment: Injection: Dialysis patients: Decrease dose by 50%
Additional Information Complete prescribing information for this medication should be consulted for additional detail.

Dosage Forms Excipient information presented when available (limited, particularly for generics); consult specific product labeling.

Injection, solution, as sodium: 10% (5 mL); 25% (2 mL)
 AK-Fluor®: 10% (5 mL)
Injection, solution, as sodium [preservative free]:
 Fluorescite®: 10% (5 mL)
Strip, ophthalmic, as sodium:
 BioGlo™: 1 mg (100s, 300s)
 Fluorets®: 1 mg (100s)
 Ful-Glo®: 0.6 mg (300s); 1 mg (100s)

Fluorescein and Benoxinate
(FLURE e seen & ben OX i nate)

Brand Names: U.S. EyeFlur; Fluress®; Flurox™

Index Terms Benoxinate Hydrochloride and Fluorescein Sodium

Pharmacologic Category Anesthetic, Topical; Diagnostic Agent; Ophthalmic Agent

Use For use in ophthalmic procedures when a topical disclosing agent is needed along with an anesthetic

Pregnancy Risk Factor C

Dosage Ophthalmic: Adults:
 Removal of foreign bodies, sutures, or tonometry: Instill 1 or 2 drops (single instillations) into each eye before operating
 Deep ophthalmic anesthesia: Instill 2 drops into each eye every 90 seconds up to 3 doses

Additional Information Complete prescribing information for this medication should be consulted for additional detail.

Dosage Forms Excipient information presented when available (limited, particularly for generics); consult specific product labeling.

Solution, ophthalmic: Fluorescein sodium 0.25% and benoxinate hydrochloride 0.4% (5 mL)
 EyeFlur, Fluress®, Flurox™: Fluorescein sodium 0.25% and benoxinate hydrochloride 0.4% (5 mL)

◆ **Fluorescein and Proparacaine** *see* Proparacaine and Fluorescein *on page 1421*

◆ **Fluorescein Sodium** *see* Fluorescein *on page 727*

◆ **Fluorescite®** *see* Fluorescein *on page 727*

◆ **Fluorets®** *see* Fluorescein *on page 727*

Fluoride (FLOR ide)

Brand Names: U.S. Act® Kids [OTC]; Act® Restoring™ [OTC]; Act® Total Care™ [OTC]; Act® [OTC]; CaviRinse™; Clinpro™ 5000; ControlRx™; ControlRx™ Multi; Denta 5000 Plus™; DentaGel™; Epiflur™; Fluor-A-Day®; Fluorabon™; Fluorinse®; Fluoritab; Flura-Drops®; Gel-Kam® Rinse; Gel-Kam® [OTC]; Just For Kids™ [OTC]; Lozi-Flur™; NeutraCare®; NeutraGard® Advanced; Omni Gel™ [OTC]; OrthoWash™; PerioMed™; Phos-Flur®; Phos-Flur® Rinse [OTC]; PreviDent®; PreviDent® 5000 Booster; PreviDent® 5000 Dry Mouth; PreviDent® 5000 Plus®; PreviDent® 5000 Sensitive; StanGard® Perio; Stop®

Brand Names: Canada Fluor-A-Day

Index Terms Acidulated Phosphate Fluoride; Sodium Fluoride; Stannous Fluoride

Pharmacologic Category Nutritional Supplement

Use Prevention of dental caries

Pregnancy Risk Factor C

Dosage Oral:
 The recommended daily dose of oral fluoride supplement (mg), based on fluoride ion content (ppm) in drinking water (2.2 mg of sodium fluoride is equivalent to 1 mg of fluoride ion): See table.

Fluoride Ion

Fluoride Content of Drinking Water	Daily Dose, Oral (mg)
<0.3 ppm	
Birth - 6 mo	None
6 mo - 3 y	0.25
3-6 y	0.5
6-16 y	1
0.3-0.6 ppm	
Birth - 6 mo	None
6 mo - 3 y	None
3-6 y	0.25
6-16 y	0.5

Adapted from Recommended Dosage Schedule of The American Dental Association, The American Academy of Pediatric Dentistry, and The American Academy of Pediatrics.

Cream: Children ≥6 years and Adults: Brush teeth with cream once daily regardless of fluoride content of drinking water

Dental rinse or gel:
 Children 6-12 years: 5-10 mL rinse or apply to teeth and spit daily after brushing
 Adults: 10 mL rinse or apply to teeth and spit daily after brushing
 PreviDent® rinse: Children >6 years and Adults: Once weekly, rinse 10 mL vigorously around and between teeth for 1 minute, then spit; this should be done preferably at bedtime, after thoroughly brushing teeth; for maximum benefit, do not eat, drink, or rinse mouth for at least 30 minutes after treatment; do not swallow
 Fluorinse®: Children >6 years and Adults: Once weekly, vigorously swish 5-10 mL in mouth for 1 minute, then spit

Lozenge (Lozi-Flur™): Adults: One lozenge daily regardless of fluoride content of drinking water

Additional Information Complete prescribing information for this medication should be consulted for additional detail.

Dosage Forms Excipient information presented when available (limited, particularly for generics); consult specific product labeling.

Cream, oral, as sodium [toothpaste]: 1.1% (51 g) [equivalent to fluoride 2.5 mg/dose]
 Denta 5000 Plus™: 1.1% (51 g) [spearmint flavor; equivalent to fluoride 2.5 mg/dose]
 PreviDent® 5000 Plus®: 1.1% (51 g) [contains sodium benzoate; fruitastic™ flavor; equivalent to fluoride 2.5 mg/dose]
 PreviDent® 5000 Plus®: 1.1% (51 g) [contains sodium benzoate; spearmint flavor; equivalent to fluoride 2.5 mg/dose]

Gel, topical, as acidulated phosphate:
 Phos-Flur®: 1.1% (51 g) [contains propylene glycol, sodium benzoate; mint flavor; equivalent to fluoride 0.5%]

Gel, oral, as sodium [toothpaste]:
 PreviDent® 5000 Booster: 1.1% (100 mL, 106 mL) [contains sodium benzoate; fruitastic™ flavor; equivalent to fluoride 2.5 mg/dose]
 PreviDent® 5000 Booster: 1.1% (100 mL, 106 mL) [contains sodium benzoate; spearmint flavor; equivalent to fluoride 2.5 mg/dose]
 PreviDent® 5000 Dry Mouth: 1.1% (100 mL) [mint flavor; equivalent to fluoride 2.5 mg/dose]
 PreviDent® 5000 Sensitive: 1.1% (100 mL) [mild mint flavor; equivalent to fluoride 2.5 mg/dose]

Gel, topical, as sodium: 1.1% (56 g) [equivalent to fluoride 2 mg/dose]:
DentaGel™: 1.1% (56 g) [fresh mint flavor; neutral pH; equivalent to fluoride 2 mg/dose]
NeutraCare®: 1.1% (60 g) [grape flavor; neutral pH]
NeutraCare®: 1.1% (60 g) [mint flavor; neutral pH]
NeutraGard® Advanced: 1.1% (60 g) [mint flavor; neutral pH]
NeutraGard® Advanced: 1.1% (60 g) [mixed berry flavor; neutral pH]
PreviDent®: 1.1% (56 g) [mint flavor; equivalent to fluoride 2 mg/dose]
PreviDent®: 1.1% (56 g) [very berry flavor; equivalent to fluoride 2 mg/dose]
Gel, topical, as stannous flouride:
Gel-Kam®: 0.4% (129 g) [cinnamon flavor]
Gel-Kam®: 0.4% (129 g) [fruit & berry flavor]
Gel-Kam®: 0.4% (129 g) [mint flavor]
Just For Kids™: 0.4% (122 g) [bubblegum flavor]
Just For Kids™: 0.4% (122 g) [fruit-punch flavor]
Just For Kids™: 0.4% (122 g) [grapey grape flavor]
Omni Gel™: 0.4% (122 g) [cinnamon flavor]
Omni Gel™: 0.4% (122 g) [grape flavor]
Omni Gel™: 0.4% (122 g) [mint flavor]
Omni Gel™: 0.4% (122 g) [natural flavor]
Omni Gel™: 0.4% (122 g) [raspberry flavor]
Stop®: 0.4% (120 g) [bubblegum flavor]
Stop®: 0.4% (120 g) [cinnamon flavor]
Stop®: 0.4% (120 g) [grape flavor]
Stop®: 0.4% (120 g) [mint flavor]
Liquid, oral, as base:
Fluoritab: 0.125 mg/drop [dye free]
Lozenge, oral, as sodium:
Lozi-Flur™: 2.21 mg (90s) [sugar free; cherry flavor; equivalent to fluoride 1 mg]
Paste, oral, as sodium [toothpaste]:
Clinpro™ 5000: 1.1% (113 g) [vanilla-mint flavor]
ControlRx™: 1.1% (57 g) [berry flavor]
ControlRx™: 1.1% (57 g) [vanilla-mint flavor]
ControlRx™ Multi: 1.1% (57 g) [vanilla-mint flavor]
Solution, oral, as fluoride [rinse]:
Act® Total Care™: 0.02% (1000 mL) [ethanol free; contains menthol, propylene glycol, sodium benzoate, tartrazine; fresh mint flavor; equivalent to fluoride 0.009%]
Solution, oral, as sodium [drops]: 1.1 mg/mL (50 mL) [equivalent to fluoride 0.5 mg/mL]
Fluor-A-Day®: 0.278 mg/drop (30 mL) [equivalent to fluoride 0.125 mg/drop]
Fluorabon™: 0.55 mg/0.6 mL (60 mL) [dye free, sugar free; equivalent to fluoride 0.25 mg/0.6 mL]
Flura-Drops®: 0.55 mg/drop (24 mL) [dye free, sugar free; equivalent to fluoride 0.25 mg/drop]
Solution, oral, as sodium [rinse]: 0.2% (473 mL)
Act®: 0.05% (532 mL) [contains benzyl alcohol, propylene glycol, sodium benzoate, tartrazine; cinnamon flavor; equivalent to fluoride 0.02%]
Act®: 0.05% (532 mL) [contains propylene glycol, sodium benzoate, tartrazine; mint flavor; equivalent to fluoride 0.02%]
Act® Kids: 0.05% (532 mL) [ethanol free; contains benzyl alcohol, propylene glycol, sodium benzoate; bubblegum flavor; equivalent to fluoride 0.02%]
Act® Kids: 0.05% (500 mL) [ethanol free; contains benzyl alcohol, propylene glycol, sodium benzoate; ocean berry flavor; equivalent to fluoride 0.02%]
Act® Restoring™: 0.02% (1000 mL) [contains ethanol 11%, propylene glycol, sodium benzoate; Cool Splash™ mint flavor; equivalent to fluoride 0.009%]
Act® Restoring™: 0.02% (1000 mL) [contains ethanol 11%, propylene glycol, sodium benzoate; Cool Splash™ spearmint flavor; equivalent to fluoride 0.009%]
Act® Restoring™: 0.05% (532 mL) [contains ethanol 11%, propylene glycol, sodium benzoate; Cool Splash™ mint flavor; equivalent to fluoride 0.02%]
Act® Restoring™: 0.05% (532 mL) [contains ethanol 11%, propylene glycol, sodium benzoate; Cool Splash™ spearmint flavor; equivalent to fluoride 0.02%]
Act® Restoring™: 0.05% (532 mL) [contains ethanol 11%, propylene glycol, sodium benzoate; Cool Splash™ vanilla-mint flavor; equivalent to fluoride 0.02%]
Act® Total Care™: 0.02% (1000 mL) [contains ethanol 11%, propylene glycol, sodium benzoate; icy clean mint flavor; equivalent to fluoride 0.009%]
Act® Total Care™: 0.05% (88 mL, 532 mL) [contains ethanol 11%, propylene glycol, sodium benzoate; icy clean mint flavor; equivalent to fluoride 0.02%]
Act® Total Care™: 0.05% (88 mL, 532 mL) [ethanol free; contains menthol, propylene glycol, sodium benzoate, tartrazine; fresh mint flavor; equivalent to fluoride 0.02%]
CaviRinse™: 0.2% (240 mL) [mint flavor]
Fluorinse®: 0.2% (480 mL) [ethanol free; cinnamon flavor]
Fluorinse®: 0.2% (480 mL) [ethanol free; mint flavor]
OrthoWash™: 0.044% (480 mL) [contains sodium benzoate; grape flavor]
OrthoWash™: 0.044% (480 mL) [contains sodium benzoate; strawberry flavor]
Phos-Flur® Rinse: 0.044% (473 mL) [ethanol free, sugar free; bubblegum flavor]
Phos-Flur® Rinse: 0.044% (473 mL) [ethanol free, sugar free; gushing grape flavor]
Phos-Flur® Rinse: 0.044% (500 mL) [sugar free; cool mint flavor]
PreviDent®: 0.2% (473 mL) [contains benzoic acid, ethanol 6%, sodium benzoate; cool mint flavor]
Solution, oral, as stannous flouride [concentrated rinse]: 0.63% (300 mL) [equivalent to fluoride 7 mg/30 mL dose]
Gel-Kam® Rinse: 0.63% (300 mL) [mint flavor; equivalent to fluoride 7 mg/30 mL dose]
PerioMed™: 0.63% (284 mL) [ethanol free; cinnamon flavor; equivalent to fluoride 7 mg/30 mL dose]
PerioMed™: 0.63% (284 mL) [ethanol free; mint flavor; equivalent to fluoride 7 mg/30 mL dose]
PerioMed™: 0.63% (284 mL) [ethanol free; tropical fruit flavor; equivalent to fluoride 7 mg/30 mL dose]
StanGard® Perio: 0.63% (284 mL) [mint flavor]
Tablet, chewable, oral, as sodium: 0.55 mg [equivalent to fluoride 0.25 mg], 1.1 mg [equivalent to fluoride 0.5 mg], 2.2 mg [equivalent to fluoride 1 mg]
Epiflur™: 0.55 mg [sugar free; vanilla flavor; equivalent to fluoride 0.25 mg]
Epiflur™: 1.1 mg [sugar free; vanilla flavor; equivalent to fluoride 0.5 mg]
Epiflur™: 2.2 mg [sugar free; vanilla flavor; equivalent to fluoride 1 mg]
Fluor-A-Day®: 0.55 mg [raspberry flavor; equivalent to fluoride 0.25 mg]
Fluor-A-Day®: 1.1 mg [raspberry flavor; equivalent to fluoride 0.5 mg]
Fluor-A-Day®: 2.2 mg [raspberry flavor; equivalent to fluoride 1 mg]
Fluoritab: 2.2 mg [cherry flavor; equivalent to fluoride 1 mg]
Fluoritab: 1.1 mg [dye free; cherry flavor; equivalent to fluoride 0.5 mg]

◆ **Fluorinse®** *see* Fluoride *on page 728*

◆ **Fluoritab** *see* Fluoride *on page 728*

◆ **5-Fluorocytosine** *see* Flucytosine *on page 720*

◆ **9α-Fluorohydrocortisone Acetate** *see* Fludrocortisone *on page 724*

Fluorometholone (flure oh METH oh lone)

Brand Names: U.S. Flarex®; FML Forte®; FML®
Brand Names: Canada Flarex®; FML Forte®; FML®; PMS-Fluorometholone
Pharmacologic Category Corticosteroid, Ophthalmic
Use Treatment of steroid-responsive inflammatory conditions of the eye
Pregnancy Risk Factor C
Dosage Ophthalmic:

Children >2 years and Adults: Re-evaluate therapy if improvement is not seen within 2 days; use care not to discontinue prematurely; in chronic conditions, gradually decrease dosing frequency prior to discontinuing treatment

Ointment (FML®): Apply small amount (~1/2 inch ribbon) to conjunctival sac 1-3 times/day; may increase application to every 4 hours during the initial 24-48 hours

Suspension:

FML®: Instill 1 drop into conjunctival sac 2-4 times/day; may instill 1 drop every 4 hours during initial 24-48 hours

FML® Forte: Instill 1 drop into conjunctival sac 2-4 times/day

Adults: Suspension (Flarex®): Instill 1-2 drops into conjunctival sac 4 times/day; may increase application to 2 drops every 2 hours during initial 24-48 hours. Consult prescriber if no improvement after 14 days.

Additional Information Complete prescribing information for this medication should be consulted for additional detail.

Dosage Forms Excipient information presented when available (limited, particularly for generics); consult specific product labeling. [DSC] = Discontinued product

Ointment, ophthalmic, as base:

FML®: 0.1% (3.5 g)

Suspension, ophthalmic, as acetate [drops]:

Flarex®: 0.1% (5 mL) [contains benzalkonium chloride]

Suspension, ophthalmic, as base [drops]: 0.1% (5 mL, 10 mL, 15 mL)

FML Forte®: 0.25% (2 mL [DSC], 5 mL, 10 mL, 15 mL [DSC]) [contains benzalkonium chloride]

FML®: 0.1% (5 mL, 10 mL, 15 mL) [contains benzalkonium chloride]

◆ **Fluoroplex®** *see* Fluorouracil (Topical) *on page 731*
◆ **5-Fluorouracil** *see* Fluorouracil (Systemic) *on page 730*
◆ **5-Fluorouracil** *see* Fluorouracil (Topical) *on page 731*

Fluorouracil (Systemic) (flure oh YOOR a sil)

Brand Names: U.S. Adrucil®
Index Terms 5-Fluorouracil; 5-FU; FU
Pharmacologic Category Antineoplastic Agent, Antimetabolite (Pyrimidine Analog)
Use Treatment of carcinomas of the breast, colon, rectum, pancreas, or stomach
Unlabeled Use Treatment of head and neck cancer, esophageal cancer, anal cancer, cervical cancer, bladder cancer, renal cell cancer, and unknown primary cancer
Pregnancy Risk Factor D
Pregnancy Considerations Teratogenic effects have been observed with parenteral administration in animal studies; fetal defects and miscarriages have been reported following use of intravenous products in humans.
Lactation Excretion in breast milk unknown/not recommended
Contraindications Hypersensitivity to fluorouracil or any component of the formulation; poor nutritional states; depressed bone marrow function; potentially serious infections

Warnings/Precautions Hazardous agent - use appropriate precautions for handling and disposal. Use with caution in patients with impaired kidney or liver function. The drug should be discontinued if intractable vomiting or diarrhea, precipitous falls in leukocyte or platelet counts, gastrointestinal ulcer or bleeding, stomatitis, or esophagopharyngitis, hemorrhage, or myocardial ischemia occurs. Use with caution in patients who have had high-dose pelvic radiation or previous use of alkylating agents. Palmar-plantar erythrodysesthesia (hand-foot) syndrome has been associated with use.

Administration to patients with a genetic deficiency of dihydropyrimidine dehydrogenase (DPD) has been associated with prolonged clearance and increased toxicity following administration (diarrhea, neutropenia, and neurotoxicity); rechallenge has resulted in recurrent toxicity (despite dose reduction). **[U.S. Boxed Warning]: Should be administered under the supervision of an experienced cancer chemotherapy physician.**

Adverse Reactions Toxicity depends on duration of treatment

Cardiovascular: Angina, arrhythmia, heart failure, MI, myocardial ischemia, vasospasm, ventricular ectopy

Central nervous system: Acute cerebellar syndrome, confusion, disorientation, euphoria, headache, nystagmus, stroke

Dermatologic: Alopecia, dermatitis, dry skin, fissuring, palmar-plantar erythrodysesthesia syndrome, pruritic maculopapular rash, photosensitivity, Stevens-Johnson syndrome, toxic epidermal necrolysis, vein pigmentations

Gastrointestinal: Anorexia, bleeding, diarrhea, esophagopharyngitis, mesenteric ischemia (acute), nausea, sloughing, stomatitis, ulceration, vomiting

Hematologic: Myelosuppression (nadir: 9-14 days; recovery by day 30), agranulocytosis, anemia, leukopenia, pancytopenia, thrombocytopenia

Local: Thrombophlebitis

Ocular: Lacrimation, lacrimal duct stenosis, photophobia, visual changes

Respiratory: Epistaxis

Miscellaneous: Anaphylaxis, generalized allergic reactions, nail loss

Drug Interactions

Metabolism/Transport Effects Inhibits CYP2C9 (strong)

Avoid Concomitant Use

Avoid concomitant use of Fluorouracil (Systemic) with any of the following: BCG; Natalizumab; Pimecrolimus; Tacrolimus (Topical); Vaccines (Live)

Increased Effect/Toxicity

Fluorouracil (Systemic) may increase the levels/effects of: Carvedilol; CYP2C9 Substrates; Diclofenac; Fosphenytoin; Leflunomide; Natalizumab; Phenytoin; Vaccines (Live); Vitamin K Antagonists

The levels/effects of Fluorouracil (Systemic) may be increased by: Denosumab; Gemcitabine; Leucovorin Calcium-Levoleucovorin; Pimecrolimus; Roflumilast; SORAfenib; Tacrolimus (Topical); Trastuzumab

Decreased Effect

Fluorouracil (Systemic) may decrease the levels/effects of: BCG; Coccidioidin Skin Test; Sipuleucel-T; Vaccines (Inactivated); Vaccines (Live); Vitamin K Antagonists

The levels/effects of Fluorouracil (Systemic) may be decreased by: Echinacea; SORAfenib

Ethanol/Nutrition/Herb Interactions

Ethanol: Avoid ethanol (due to GI irritation).

Herb/Nutraceutical: Avoid black cohosh, dong quai in estrogen-dependent tumors.

Stability Store intact vials at room temperature. Protect from light. Slight discoloration does not usually denote decomposition. Dilute in 50-1000 mL NS, D_5W, or bacteriostatic NS for infusion. If exposed to cold, a precipitate may form; **gentle** heating to 60°C will dissolve the precipitate without impairing the potency. Solutions in 50-1000 mL NS or D_5W, or undiluted solutions in syringes are stable for 72 hours at room temperature.

Mechanism of Action A pyrimidine antimetabolite that interferes with DNA synthesis by blocking the methylation of deoxyuridylic acid; fluorouracil inhibits thymidylate synthetase (TS), or is incorporated into RNA. The reduced folate cofactor is required for tight binding to occur between the 5-FdUMP and TS.

Pharmacodynamics/Kinetics

Duration: ~3 weeks

Distribution: V_d: ~22% of total body water; penetrates extracellular fluid, CSF, and third space fluids (eg, pleural effusions and ascitic fluid)

Metabolism: Hepatic (90%); via a dehydrogenase enzyme; FU must be metabolized to be active

Half-life elimination: Biphasic: Initial: 6-20 minutes; two metabolites, FdUMP and FUTP, have prolonged half-lives depending on the type of tissue

Excretion: Lung (large amounts as CO_2); urine (5% as unchanged drug) in 6 hours

Dosage Details concerning dosing in combination regimens should be consulted: Adults:

I.V. bolus:

500 mg/m^2 once weekly **or**

500-600 mg/m^2 every 3 weeks **or**

500-600 mg/m^2/dose days 1 and 8 every 4 weeks **or**

500 mg/m^2/dose days 1 and 8 every 3 weeks **or**

500 mg/m^2/dose days 1 and 4 every 3 weeks **or**

500 mg/m^2/dose days 1, 8, 15, 22, 29, and 36 of an 8-week treatment cycle **or**

425 mg/m^2 on days 1-5 every 4 weeks

Continuous I.V. infusion:

500-750 mg/m^2/day for 5 days every 3 weeks **or**

1000 mg/m^2/day for 4-5 days every 3-4 weeks **or**

2600 mg/m^2 on day 1 every week **or**

1600 mg/m^2/day for 2 days every 2 weeks **or**

400 mg/m^2 bolus followed by 1200 mg/m^2/day for 2 days every 2 weeks **or**

200 mg/m^2/day for 21 days; can repeat 21-day cycle up to 8 cycles

Dosage adjustment for renal impairment: The FDA-approved labeling does not contain specific dosing adjustment guidelines; however, it is stated that extreme caution should be used in patients with renal impairment.

Hemodialysis: Administer dose following hemodialysis.

Aronoff, 2007: Recommends that dosage adjustment is not needed in adult patients with Cl_{cr} <50 mL/minute and patients receiving hemodialysis should be administered 50% of dose.

Dosage adjustment for hepatic impairment: The FDA-approved labeling does not contain specific dosing adjustment guidelines; however, it is stated that extreme caution should be used in patients with hepatic impairment. The following guidelines have been used by some clinicians:

Floyd, 2006: Bilirubin >5 mg/dL: Avoid use.

Koren, 1992: Hepatic impairment (degree not specified): Administer <50% of dose, then increase if toxicity does not occur.

Dietary Considerations Increase dietary intake of thiamine.

Administration I.V.: I.V. bolus as a slow push or short (5-15 minutes) bolus infusion, or as a continuous infusion. Doses >1000 mg/m^2 are usually administered as a 24-hour infusion, although some protocols may be continuous infusion with lower doses. Toxicity may be reduced by giving the drug as a constant infusion. Bolus doses may be administered by slow IVP or IVPB.

Monitoring Parameters CBC with differential and platelet count, renal function tests, liver function tests

Additional Information Oncology Comment: An investigational uridine prodrug, uridine triacetate (formerly called vistonuridine), has been studied in a limited number of cases of fluorouracil overdose. Of 17 patients receiving uridine triacetate beginning within 8-96 hours after fluorouracil overdose, all patients fully recovered (von Borstel, 2009). Updated data has described a total of 28 patients treated with uridine triacetate for fluorouracil overdose (including overdoses related to continuous infusions delivering fluorouracil at rates faster than prescribed), all of whom recovered fully (Bamat, 2010). Refer to Uridine Triacetate monograph.

Dosage Forms Excipient information presented when available (limited, particularly for generics); consult specific product labeling.

Injection, solution: 50 mg/mL (10 mL, 20 mL, 50 mL, 100 mL)

Adrucil®: 50 mg/mL (10 mL, 50 mL, 100 mL)

Fluorouracil (Topical) (flure oh YOOR a sil)

Brand Names: U.S. Carac®; Efudex®; Fluoroplex®

Brand Names: Canada Efudex®; Fluoroplex®

Index Terms 5-Fluorouracil; 5-FU; FU

Pharmacologic Category Antineoplastic Agent, Antimetabolite (Pyrimidine Analog)

Use Management of actinic or solar keratoses and superficial basal cell carcinomas

Pregnancy Risk Factor X

Dosage Topical: Refer to individual protocols: Adults:

Actinic keratoses:

Carac™: Apply thin film to lesions once daily for up to 4 weeks, as tolerated

Efudex®: Apply to lesions twice daily for 2-4 weeks; complete healing may not be evident for 1-2 months following treatment

Fluoroplex®: Apply to lesions twice daily for 2-6 weeks

Superficial basal cell carcinoma: Efudex® 5%: Apply to affected lesions twice daily for 3-6 weeks; treatment may be continued for up to 10-12 weeks

Additional Information Complete prescribing information for this medication should be consulted for additional detail.

Dosage Forms Excipient information presented when available (limited, particularly for generics); consult specific product labeling.

Cream, topical: 5% (40 g)

Carac®: 0.5% (30 g)

Efudex®: 5% (40 g)

Fluoroplex®: 1% (30 g) [contains benzyl alcohol]

Solution, topical: 2% (10 mL); 5% (10 mL)

Efudex®: 5% (10 mL)

FLUoxetine (floo OKS e teen)

Brand Names: U.S. PROzac®; PROzac® Weekly™; Sarafem®; Selfemra® [DSC]

Brand Names: Canada Apo-Fluoxetine®; CO Fluoxetine; Dom-Fluoxetine; Fluoxetine; FXT 40; Gen-Fluoxetine; Mylan-Fluoxetine; Novo-Fluoxetine; Nu-Fluoxetine; PHL-Fluoxetine; PMS-Fluoxetine; PRO-Fluoxetine; Prozac®; ratio-Fluoxetine; Riva-Fluoxetine; Sandoz-Fluoxetine; Teva-Fluoxetine; ZYM-Fluoxetine

Index Terms Fluoxetine Hydrochloride

Pharmacologic Category Antidepressant, Selective Serotonin Reuptake Inhibitor

Additional Appendix Information

Antidepressant Agents *on page 1874*

Beers Criteria – Potentially Inappropriate Medications for Geriatrics *on page 1973*

Selective Serotonin Reuptake Inhibitors (SSRIs) Pharmacokinetics *on page 1897*

Use Treatment of major depressive disorder (MDD); treatment of binge-eating and vomiting in patients with moderate-to-severe bulimia nervosa; obsessive-compulsive disorder (OCD); premenstrual dysphoric disorder (PMDD); panic disorder with or without agoraphobia; in combination with olanzapine for treatment-resistant or bipolar I depression

Unlabeled Use Selective mutism; treatment of mild dementia-associated agitation in nonpsychotic patients; post-traumatic stress disorder (PTSD); social anxiety disorder; fibromyalgia; Raynaud's phenomenon

Pregnancy Risk Factor C

Pregnancy Considerations Due to adverse effects observed in animal studies, fluoxetine is classified as pregnancy category C. Fluoxetine and its metabolite cross the human placenta. Nonteratogenic effects in the newborn following SSRIs exposure late in the third trimester include respiratory distress, cyanosis, apnea, seizures, temperature instability, feeding difficulty, vomiting, hypoglycemia, hypo- or hypertonia, hyper-reflexia, jitteriness, irritability, constant crying, and tremor. An increased risk of low birth weight, lower APGAR scores, and blunted behavioral response to pain for a prolonged period after delivery have also been reported. Exposure to SSRIs after the twentieth week of gestation has been associated with persistent pulmonary hypertension of the newborn (PPHN). Adverse effects may be due to toxic effects of the SSRI or drug withdrawal without a taper. The long term effects of *in utero* SSRI exposure on infant development and behavior are not known.

Due to pregnancy-induced physiologic changes, women who are pregnant may require increased doses of fluoxetine to achieve euthymia. Women treated for major depression and who are euthymic prior to pregnancy are more likely to experience a relapse when medication is discontinued as compared to pregnant women who continue taking antidepressant medications. The ACOG recommends that therapy with SSRIs or SNRIs during pregnancy be individualized; treatment of depression during pregnancy should incorporate the clinical expertise of the mental health clinician, obstetrician, primary healthcare provider, and pediatrician. If treatment during pregnancy is required, consider tapering therapy during the third trimester in order to prevent withdrawal symptoms in the infant. If this is done and the woman is considered to be at risk of relapse from her major depressive disorder, the medication can be restarted following delivery, although the dose should be readjusted to that required before pregnancy. Treatment algorithms have been developed by the ACOG and the APA for the management of depression in women prior to conception and during pregnancy (Yonkers, 2009).

Lactation Enters breast milk/not recommended (AAP rates "of concern"; AAP 2001 update pending)

Medication Guide Available Yes

Contraindications Hypersensitivity to fluoxetine or any component of the formulation; patients currently receiving MAO inhibitors, pimozide, or thioridazine

Note: MAO inhibitor therapy must be stopped for 14 days before fluoxetine is initiated. Treatment with MAO inhibitors or thioridazine should not be initiated until 5 weeks after the discontinuation of fluoxetine.

Warnings/Precautions [U.S. Boxed Warning]: Antidepressants increase the risk of suicidal thinking and behavior in children, adolescents, and young adults (18-24 years of age) with major depressive disorder (MDD) and other psychiatric disorders; consider risk prior to prescribing. Short-term studies did not show an increased risk in patients >24 years of age and showed a decreased risk in patients ≥65 years. Closely monitor patients for clinical worsening, suicidality, or unusual changes in behavior, particularly during the initial 1-2 months of therapy or during periods of dosage adjustments (increases or decreases); the patient's family or caregiver should be instructed to closely observe the patient and communicate condition with healthcare provider. A medication guide concerning the use of antidepressants should be dispensed with each prescription. **Fluoxetine is FDA approved for the treatment of OCD in children ≥7 years of age and MDD in children ≥8 years of age.**

The possibility of a suicide attempt is inherent in major depression and may persist until remission occurs. Use caution in high-risk patients. Worsening depression and severe abrupt suicidality that are not part of the presenting symptoms may require discontinuation or modification of drug therapy. The patient's family or caregiver should be alerted to monitor patients for the emergence of suicidality and associated behaviors (such as agitation, irritability, hostility, impulsivity, and hypomania) and call healthcare provider.

May worsen psychosis in some patients or precipitate a shift to mania or hypomania in patients with bipolar disorder. Patients presenting with depressive symptoms should be screened for bipolar disorder. Monotherapy in patients with bipolar disorder should be avoided. **Fluoxetine monotherapy is not FDA approved for the treatment of bipolar depression.** May cause insomnia, anxiety, nervousness, or anorexia. Use with caution in patients where weight loss is undesirable. May impair cognitive or motor performance; caution operating hazardous machinery or driving.

Serotonin syndrome and neuroleptic malignant syndrome (NMS)-like reactions have occurred with serotonin/norepinephrine reuptake inhibitors (SNRIs) and selective serotonin reuptake inhibitors (SSRIs) when used alone, and particularly when used in combination with serotonergic agents (eg, triptans) or antidopaminergic agents (eg, antipsychotics). Concurrent use with MAO inhibitors is contraindicated. Fluoxetine may elevate plasma levels of thioridazine or pimozide and increase the risk of QT_c interval prolongation. This may lead to serious ventricular arrhythmias, such as torsade de pointes-type arrhythmias, and sudden death. Fluoxetine use has been associated with occurrences of significant rash and allergic events, including vasculitis, lupus-like syndrome, laryngospasm, anaphylactoid reactions, and pulmonary inflammatory disease. Discontinue if underlying cause of rash cannot be identified.

Use caution in patients with a previous seizure disorder or condition predisposing to seizures such as brain damage, alcoholism, or concurrent therapy with other drugs which lower the seizure threshold. Use with caution in patients with hepatic or severe renal dysfunction and in elderly patients. Fluoxetine (daily) may be inappropriate for use in the elderly due to risk of agitation, sleep disturbances, and excessive CNS stimulation, attributed to this drug's long half-life (Beers Criteria). May cause hyponatremia/SIADH (elderly at increased risk); volume depletion (diuretics may increase risk). May increase the risks associated with electroconvulsive treatment. Use caution with concomitant use of NSAIDs, ASA, or other drugs that affect coagulation; the risk of bleeding may be potentiated. Use caution with history of MI or unstable heart disease; use in these patients is limited. May alter glycemic control in patients with diabetes. Due to the long half-life of fluoxetine and its metabolites, the effects and interactions noted may persist for prolonged periods following discontinuation. May cause or exacerbate sexual dysfunction.

May cause mydriasis; use caution in patients at risk of acute narrow-angle glaucoma or with increased intraocular pressure. Discontinuation symptoms (eg, dysphoric mood, irritability, agitation, confusion, anxiety, insomnia, hypomania) may occur upon abrupt discontinuation. Taper dose when discontinuing therapy.

Adverse Reactions Percentages listed for adverse effects as reported in placebo-controlled trials and were generally similar in adults and children; actual frequency may be dependent upon diagnosis and in some cases the range presented may be lower than or equal to placebo for a particular disorder.

>10%:

Central nervous system: Insomnia (10% to 33%), headache (21%), somnolence (5% to 17%), anxiety (6% to 15%), nervousness (8% to 14%)

Endocrine & metabolic: Libido decreased (1% to 11%)

Gastrointestinal: Nausea (12% to 29%), diarrhea (8% to 18%), anorexia (4% to 17%), xerostomia (4% to 12%)

Neuromuscular & skeletal: Weakness (7% to 21%), tremor (3% to 13%)

Respiratory: Pharyngitis (3% to 11%), yawn (≤11%)

1% to 10%:

Cardiovascular: Vasodilation (1% to 5%), chest pain, hemorrhage, hypertension, palpitation

Central nervous system: Dizziness (9%), abnormal dreams (1% to 5%), abnormal thinking (2%), agitation, amnesia, chills, confusion, emotional lability, sleep disorder

Dermatologic: Rash (2% to 6%), pruritus (4%)

Endocrine & metabolic: Ejaculation abnormal (≤7%), impotence (≤7%), menorrhagia (≥2%)

Gastrointestinal: Dyspepsia (6% to 10%), constipation (5%), flatulence (3%), vomiting (3%), thirst (≥2%), weight loss (2%), appetite increased, taste perversion, weight gain

Genitourinary: Urinary frequency

Neuromuscular & skeletal: Hyperkinesia (≥2%)

Ocular: Vision abnormal (2%)

Otic: Ear pain, tinnitus

Respiratory: Sinusitis (1% to 6%)

Miscellaneous: Flu-like syndrome (3% to 10%), diaphoresis (2% to 8%), epistaxis (≥2%)

<1% (Limited to important or life-threatening): Acne, acute abdominal syndrome, akathisia, albuminuria, allergies, alopecia, amenorrhea, anaphylactoid reactions, anemia, angina, aphthous stomatitis, aplastic anemia, arrhythmia, arthritis, asthma, ataxia, atrial fibrillation, balance disorder, bone pain, bruising, bruxism, bursitis, cardiac arrest, cataract, cerebrovascular accident, CHF, cholelithiasis, cholestatic jaundice, colitis, dehydration, delusions, depersonalization, dyskinesia, dysphagia, dysuria, ecchymosis, edema, eosinophilic pneumonia, erythema multiforme, erythema nodosum, esophagitis, euphoria, exfoliative dermatitis, extrapyramidal symptoms (rare), gastritis, gastroenteritis, GI ulcer, glossitis, gout, gynecological bleeding, gynecomastia, hallucinations, hepatic failure/necrosis, hepatitis, hiccup, hostility, hypercholesteremia, hyperprolactinemia, hypertonia, hyperventilation, hypoglycemia, hypokalemia, hyponatremia (possibly in association with SIADH), hypotension, hypothyroidism, immune-related hemolytic anemia, kidney failure, laryngospasm, laryngeal edema, leg cramps, liver function test abnormalities, lupus-like syndrome, malaise, melena, migraine, misuse/abuse, MI, mydriasis, myoclonus, neuroleptic malignant syndrome (NMS), optic neuritis, pancreatitis, pancytopenia, paranoid reaction, petechia, photosensitivity reaction, postural hypotension, priapism, pulmonary embolism, pulmonary fibrosis, pulmonary hypertension, purpuric rash, QT prolongation, serotonin syndrome, Stevens-Johnson syndrome, suicidal ideation, syncope, tachycardia, thrombocytopenia, thrombocytopenic purpura, toxic epidermal necrolysis, vasculitis, ventricular tachycardia (including torsade de pointes), violent behavior

Drug Interactions

Metabolism/Transport Effects Substrate of CYP1A2 (minor), CYP2B6 (minor), CYP2C19 (minor), CYP2C9 (major), CYP2D6 (major), CYP2E1 (minor), CYP3A4 (minor); **Note:** Assignment of Major/Minor substrate status based on clinically relevant drug interaction potential; **Inhibits** CYP1A2 (moderate), CYP2B6 (weak), CYP2C19 (moderate), CYP2C9 (weak), CYP2D6 (strong)

Avoid Concomitant Use

Avoid concomitant use of FLUoxetine with any of the following: Artemether; Clopidogrel; Dronedarone; Iobenguane I 123; Lumefantrine; MAO Inhibitors; Methylene Blue; Nilotinib; Pimozide; QUEtiapine; QuiNINE; Tamoxifen; Tetrabenazine; Thioridazine; Toremifene; Tryptophan; Vandetanib; Vemurafenib; Ziprasidone

Increased Effect/Toxicity

FLUoxetine may increase the levels/effects of: Alpha-/Beta-Blockers; Anticoagulants; Antidepressants (Serotonin Reuptake Inhibitor/Antagonist); Antiplatelet Agents; Aspirin; Atomoxetine; Benzodiazepines (metabolized by oxidation); Beta-Blockers; BusPIRone; CarBAMazepine; CloZAPine; Collagenase (Systemic); CYP1A2 Substrates; CYP2C19 Substrates; CYP2D6 Substrates; Desmopressin; Dextromethorphan; Dronedarone; Drotrecogin Alfa (Activated); Fesoterodine; Fosphenytoin; Galantamine; Haloperidol; Ibritumomab; Lithium; Methadone; Methylene Blue; Metoclopramide; Mexiletine; NIFEdipine; NiMODipine; NSAID (COX-2 Inhibitor); NSAID (Nonselective); Phenytoin; Pimozide; Propafenone; QTc-Prolonging Agents; QuiNIDine; QuiNINE; RisperiDONE; Rivaroxaban; Salicylates; Serotonin Modulators; Tamoxifen; Tetrabenazine; Thioridazine; Thrombolytic Agents; Toremifene; Tositumomab and Iodine I 131 Tositumomab; TraMADol; Tricyclic Antidepressants; Vandetanib; Vemurafenib; Vitamin K Antagonists; Ziprasidone

The levels/effects of FLUoxetine may be increased by: Abiraterone Acetate; Alcohol (Ethyl); Alfuzosin; Analgesics (Opioid); Antipsychotics; Artemether; BusPIRone; Chloroquine; Cimetidine; Ciprofloxacin; Ciprofloxacin (Systemic); CNS Depressants; Conivaptan; CYP2C9 Inhibitors (Moderate); CYP2C9 Inhibitors (Strong); CYP2D6 Inhibitors (Moderate); CYP2D6 Inhibitors (Strong); Darunavir; Gadobutrol; Glucosamine; Herbs (Anticoagulant/Antiplatelet Properties); Indacaterol; Linezolid; Lumefantrine; Macrolide Antibiotics; MAO Inhibitors; Metoclopramide; Nilotinib; Omega-3-Acid Ethyl Esters; Pentosan Polysulfate Sodium; Pentoxifylline; Prostacyclin Analogues; QUEtiapine; QuiNINE; TraMADol; Tryptophan; Vitamin E

Decreased Effect

FLUoxetine may decrease the levels/effects of: Clopidogrel; Iobenguane I 123; Ioflupane I 123

The levels/effects of FLUoxetine may be decreased by: CarBAMazepine; CYP2C9 Inducers (Strong); Cyproheptadine; Cyproterone; NSAID (Nonselective); Peginterferon Alfa-2b; Tocilizumab

Ethanol/Nutrition/Herb Interactions

Ethanol: May increase CNS depression; monitor for increased effects with coadministration. Caution patients about effects.

Herb/Nutraceutical: Avoid valerian, St John's wort, kava kava, gotu kola (may increase CNS depression).

Stability All dosage forms should be stored at controlled room temperature of 15°C to 30°C (50°F to 86°F). Oral liquid should be dispensed in a light-resistant container.

Mechanism of Action Inhibits CNS neuron serotonin reuptake; minimal or no effect on reuptake of norepinephrine or dopamine; does not significantly bind to alpha-adrenergic, histamine, or cholinergic receptors

Pharmacodynamics/Kinetics

Onset of action: Depression: The onset of action is within a week; however, individual response varies greatly and full response may not be seen until 8-12 weeks after initiation of treatment.

Absorption: Well absorbed; delayed 1-2 hours with weekly formulation

Distribution: V_d: 12-43 L/kg

Protein binding: 95% to albumin and $alpha_1$ glycoprotein

Metabolism: Hepatic, via CYP2C19 and 2D6, to norfluoxetine (activity equal to fluoxetine)

Half-life elimination: Adults:

Parent drug: 1-3 days (acute), 4-6 days (chronic), 7.6 days (cirrhosis)

Metabolite (norfluoxetine): 9.3 days (range: 4-16 days), 12 days (cirrhosis)

Time to peak, serum: 6-8 hours

Excretion: Urine (10% as norfluoxetine, 2.5% to 5% as fluoxetine)

Note: Weekly formulation results in greater fluctuations between peak and trough concentrations of fluoxetine and norfluoxetine compared to once-daily dosing (24% daily/164% weekly; 17% daily/43% weekly, respectively). Trough concentrations are 76% lower for fluoxetine and 47% lower for norfluoxetine than the concentrations maintained by 20 mg once-daily dosing. Steady-state fluoxetine concentrations are ~50% lower following the once-weekly regimen compared to 20 mg once daily. Average steady-state concentrations of once-daily dosing were highest in children ages 6 to <13 (fluoxetine 171 ng/mL; norfluoxetine 195 ng/mL), followed by adolescents ages 13 to <18 (fluoxetine 86 ng/mL; norfluoxetine 113 ng/mL); concentrations were considered to be within the ranges reported in adults (fluoxetine 91-302 ng/mL; norfluoxetine 72-258 ng/mL).

Dosage Oral: **Note:** Upon discontinuation of fluoxetine therapy, gradually taper dose. If intolerable symptoms occur following a dose reduction, consider resuming the previously prescribed dose and/or decrease dose at a more gradual rate.

Children:

Depression: 8-18 years: 10-20 mg/day; lower-weight children can be started at 10 mg/day, may increase to 20 mg/day after 1 week if needed

Obsessive-compulsive disorder: 7-17 years: Initial: 10 mg/day; may increase after 2 weeks if inadequate clinical response to 20 mg/day; further increases may be considered after several weeks to recommended range of 20-30 mg/day (lower weight children) or 20-60 mg/day (adolescents and higher weight children)

Selective mutism (unlabeled use): 5-18 years: Initial: 5-10 mg/day; titrate upwards as needed (usual maximum dose: 60 mg/day)

Adults: 20 mg/day in the morning; may increase after several weeks by 20 mg/day increments; maximum: 80 mg/day; doses >20 mg may be given once daily or divided twice daily. **Note:** Lower doses of 5-10 mg/day have been used for initial treatment.

Indication-specific dosing:

Bulimia nervosa: 60 mg/day

Depression: Initial: 20 mg/day; may increase after several weeks if inadequate response (maximum: 80 mg/day). Patients maintained on Prozac® 20 mg/day may be changed to Prozac® Weekly™ 90 mg/week, starting dose 7 days after the last 20 mg/day dose

Depression associated with bipolar disorder (in combination with olanzapine): Initial: 20 mg in the evening; adjust as tolerated to usual range of 20-50 mg/day. See **"Note"** below.

Fibromyalgia (unlabeled use): Range: 20-80 mg/day (Arnold, 2002)

Obsessive-compulsive disorder: Initial: 20 mg/day; may increase after several weeks if inadequate response; recommended range: 20-60 mg/day (maximum: 80 mg/day)

Panic disorder: Initial: 10 mg/day; after 1 week, increase to 20 mg/day; may increase after several weeks; doses >60 mg/day have not been evaluated

Post-traumatic stress disorder (PTSD) (unlabeled use): 20-40 mg/day

Premenstrual dysphoric disorder (Sarafem®): 20 mg/day continuously, **or** 20 mg/day starting 14 days prior to menstruation and through first full day of menses (repeat with each cycle)

Raynaud's phenomena (unlabeled use): 20 mg/day (Coleiro, 2001)

Social anxiety disorder (unlabeled use): Target dose: 40 mg/day; range 30-60 mg/day (Davidson, 2004)

Treatment-resistant depression (in combination with olanzapine): Initial: 20 mg in the evening; adjust as tolerated to usual range of 20-50 mg/day. See **"Note."**

Note: When using individual components of fluoxetine with olanzapine rather than fixed dose combination product (Symbyax®), approximate dosage correspondence is as follows:

Olanzapine 2.5 mg + fluoxetine 20 mg = Symbyax® 3/25

Olanzapine 5 mg + fluoxetine 20 mg = Symbyax® 6/25

Olanzapine 12.5 mg + fluoxetine 20 mg = Symbyax® 12/25

Olanzapine 5 mg + fluoxetine 50 mg = Symbyax® 6/50

Olanzapine 12.5 mg + fluoxetine 50 mg = Symbyax® 12/50

Elderly: Depression: Some patients may require an initial dose of 10 mg/day with dosage increases of 10 and 20 mg every several weeks as tolerated; should not be taken at night unless patient experiences sedation

Dosing adjustment in renal impairment:

Single dose studies: Pharmacokinetics of fluoxetine and norfluoxetine were similar among subjects with all levels of impaired renal function, including anephric patients on chronic hemodialysis

Chronic administration: Additional accumulation of fluoxetine or norfluoxetine may occur in patients with severely impaired renal function

Hemodialysis: Not removed by hemodialysis; use of lower dose or less frequent dosing is not usually necessary.

Dosing adjustment in hepatic impairment: Elimination half-life of fluoxetine is prolonged in patients with hepatic impairment; a lower or less frequent dose of fluoxetine should be used in these patients

Cirrhosis patients: Administer a lower dose or less frequent dosing interval

Compensated cirrhosis without ascites: Administer 50% of normal dose

Dietary Considerations May be taken without regard to meals.

Administration Administer without regard to meals.

Bipolar I disorder and treatment-resistant depression: Take once daily in the evening.

Major depressive disorder and obsessive compulsive disorder: Once daily doses should be taken in the morning, or twice daily (morning and noon).

Bulimia: Take once daily in the morning.

Monitoring Parameters Mental status for depression, suicidal ideation (especially at the beginning of therapy or when doses are increased or decreased), anxiety, social functioning, mania, panic attacks; akathisia, sleep status; blood glucose (for diabetic patients), baseline liver function

Reference Range Therapeutic levels have not been well established

Therapeutic: Fluoxetine: 100-800 ng/mL (SI: 289-2314 nmol/L); Norfluoxetine: 100-600 ng/mL (SI: 289-1735 nmol/L)

Toxic: Fluoxetine plus norfluoxetine: >2000 ng/mL

Additional Information ECG may reveal S-T segment depression. Not shown to be teratogenic in rodents; 15-60 mg/day, buspirone and cyproheptadine, may be useful in treatment of sexual dysfunction during treatment with a selective serotonin reuptake inhibitor.

Weekly capsules are a delayed release formulation containing enteric-coated pellets of fluoxetine hydrochloride, equivalent to 90 mg fluoxetine. Therapeutic equivalence of weekly formulation with daily formulation for delaying time to relapse has not been established.

Dosage Forms Excipient information presented when available (limited, particularly for generics); consult specific product labeling. [DSC] = Discontinued product

Capsule, oral: 10 mg, 20 mg, 40 mg
  PROzac®: 10 mg, 20 mg, 40 mg
  Selfemra®: 10 mg [DSC], 20 mg [DSC] [contains soya lecithin]

Capsule, delayed release, enteric coated pellets, oral: 90 mg
  PROzac® Weekly™: 90 mg

Solution, oral: 20 mg/5 mL (5 mL, 120 mL)

Tablet, oral: 10 mg, 20 mg
  Sarafem®: 10 mg, 15 mg, 20 mg

Extemporaneous Preparations Note: Commercial oral solution is available (4 mg/mL)

A 1 mg/mL fluoxetine oral solution may be prepared using the commercially available preparation (4 mg/mL). In separate graduated cylinders, measure 5 mL of the commercially available fluoxetine preparation and 15 mL of Simple Syrup, NF. Mix thoroughly in incremental proportions. For a 2 mg/mL solution, mix equal proportions of both the commercially available fluoxetine preparation and Simple Syrup, NF. Label "refrigerate". Both concentrations are stable for up to 56 days.

Nahata MC, Pai VB, and Hipple TF, *Pediatric Drug Formulations*, 5th ed, Cincinnati, OH: Harvey Whitney Books Co, 2004.

◆ **Fluoxetine (Can)** *see* FLUoxetine *on page 731*

◆ **Fluoxetine Hydrochloride** *see* FLUoxetine *on page 731*

Fluoxymesterone (floo oks i MES te rone)

Brand Names: U.S. Androxy™

Pharmacologic Category Androgen

Use Replacement of endogenous testicular hormone; in females, palliative treatment of breast cancer

Unlabeled Use Stimulation of erythropoiesis, angioneurotic edema

Pregnancy Risk Factor X

Dosage Adults: Oral:

Male:
  Hypogonadism: 5-20 mg/day
  Delayed puberty: 2.5-20 mg/day for 4-6 months

Female: Inoperable breast carcinoma: 10-40 mg/day in divided doses for 1-3 months

Additional Information Complete prescribing information for this medication should be consulted for additional detail.

Dosage Forms Excipient information presented when available (limited, particularly for generics); consult specific product labeling.

Tablet, oral:
  Androxy™: 10 mg [scored]

Controlled Substance C-III

FluPHENAZine (floo FEN a zeen)

Brand Names: Canada Apo-Fluphenazine Decanoate®; Apo-Fluphenazine®; Modecate®; Modecate® Concentrate; PMS-Fluphenazine Decanoate

Index Terms Fluphenazine Decanoate; Fluphenazine Hydrochloride

Pharmacologic Category Antipsychotic Agent, Typical, Phenothiazine

Additional Appendix Information

Antipsychotic Agents *on page 1880*

Use Management of manifestations of psychotic disorders and schizophrenia; depot formulation may offer improved outcome in individuals with psychosis who are nonadherent with oral antipsychotics

Unlabeled Use Psychosis/agitation related to Alzheimer's dementia

Pregnancy Considerations Jaundice or hyper-/hyporeflexia have been reported in newborn infants following maternal use of phenothiazines. Antipsychotic use during the third trimester of pregnancy has a risk for abnormal muscle movements (extrapyramidal symptoms [EPS]) and withdrawal symptoms in newborns following delivery. Symptoms in the newborn may include agitation, feeding disorder, hypertonia, hypotonia, respiratory distress, somnolence, and tremor; these effects may be self-limiting or require hospitalization.

Contraindications Hypersensitivity to fluphenazine or any component of the formulation (cross-reactivity between phenothiazines may occur); severe CNS depression; coma; subcortical brain damage; in patients receiving large doses of hypnotics; blood dyscrasias; hepatic disease

Warnings/Precautions [U.S. Boxed Warning]: Elderly patients with dementia-related psychosis treated with antipsychotics are at an increased risk of death compared to placebo. Most deaths appeared to be either cardiovascular (eg, heart failure, sudden death) or infectious (eg, pneumonia) in nature. Fluphenazine is not approved for the treatment of dementia-related psychosis. May be sedating; use with caution in disorders where CNS depression is a feature. Use with caution in Parkinson's disease. Caution in patients with hemodynamic instability; predisposition to seizures; or severe cardiac disease. Use caution in renal impairment; discontinue therapy if BUN abnormal. Use caution in hepatic impairment; use contraindicated in patients with liver damage. Esophageal dysmotility and aspiration have been associated with antipsychotic use; use with caution in patients at risk of pneumonia (ie, Alzheimer's disease). May alter temperature regulation or mask toxicity of other drugs due to antiemetic effects. May alter cardiac conduction; life-threatening arrhythmias have occurred with therapeutic doses of phenothiazines. Hypotension may occur, particularly with I.M. administration. May cause orthostatic hypotension; use with caution in patients at risk of this effect or those who would not tolerate transient hypotensive episodes (cerebrovascular disease, cardiovascular disease, or other medications which may predispose). Adverse effects of depot injections may be prolonged. Use associated with increased prolactin levels; clinical significance of hyperprolactinemia in patients with breast cancer or other prolactin-dependent tumors is unknown. May cause pigmentary retinopathy, and lenticular and corneal deposits, particularly with prolonged therapy.

Leukopenia, neutropenia, and agranulocytosis (sometimes fatal) have been reported in clinical trials and postmarketing reports with antipsychotic use; presence of risk factors (eg, pre-existing low WBC or history of drug-induced leuko-/neutropenia) should prompt periodic blood count assessment. Discontinue therapy at first signs of blood dyscrasias or if absolute neutrophil count <1000/mm^3.

Due to anticholinergic effects, use caution in patients with decreased gastrointestinal motility, urinary retention, BPH, xerostomia, visual problems, narrow-angle glaucoma, and myasthenia gravis. Relative to other antipsychotics, fluphenazine has a low potency of cholinergic blockade.

May cause extrapyramidal symptoms, including pseudoparkinsonism, acute dystonic reactions, akathisia, and tardive dyskinesia (risk of these reactions is high relative to other antipsychotics). Risk of dystonia (and possibly other EPS) may be greater with increased doses, use of conventional antipsychotics, males, and younger patients. May also be associated with neuroleptic malignant syndrome (NMS). Use caution in the elderly.

Adverse Reactions Frequency not defined.

Cardiovascular: Tachycardia, fluctuations in blood pressure, hyper-/hypotension, arrhythmia, edema

Central nervous system: Parkinsonian symptoms, akathisia, dystonias, tardive dyskinesia, dizziness, hyperreflexia, headache, cerebral edema, drowsiness, lethargy, restlessness, excitement, bizarre dreams, EEG changes, depression, seizure, NMS, altered central temperature regulation

Dermatologic: Dermatitis, eczema, erythema, itching, photosensitivity, rash, seborrhea, skin pigmentation, urticaria

Endocrine & metabolic: Menstrual cycle changes, breast pain, amenorrhea, galactorrhea, gynecomastia, libido changes, prolactin increased, SIADH

Gastrointestinal: Weight gain, appetite loss, salivation, xerostomia, constipation, paralytic ileus, laryngeal edema

Genitourinary: Ejaculatory disturbances, impotence, polyuria, bladder paralysis, enuresis

Hematologic: Agranulocytosis, leukopenia, thrombocytopenia, nonthrombocytopenic purpura, eosinophilia, pancytopenia

Hepatic: Cholestatic jaundice, hepatotoxicity

Neuromuscular & skeletal: Trembling of fingers, SLE, facial hemispasm

Ocular: Pigmentary retinopathy, cornea and lens changes, blurred vision, glaucoma

Respiratory: Nasal congestion, asthma

Drug Interactions

Metabolism/Transport Effects **Substrate** of CYP2D6 (major); **Note:** Assignment of Major/Minor substrate status based on clinically relevant drug interaction potential; **Inhibits** CYP1A2 (weak), CYP2C9 (weak), CYP2D6 (weak), CYP2E1 (weak)

Avoid Concomitant Use

Avoid concomitant use of FluPHENAZine with any of the following: Metoclopramide

Increased Effect/Toxicity

FluPHENAZine may increase the levels/effects of: Alcohol (Ethyl); Analgesics (Opioid); Anticholinergics; Antidepressants (Serotonin Reuptake Inhibitor/Antagonist); Anti-Parkinson's Agents (Dopamine Agonist); Beta-Blockers; CNS Depressants; Methotrimeprazine; Methylphenidate; Porfimer; Serotonin Modulators

The levels/effects of FluPHENAZine may be increased by: Abiraterone Acetate; Acetylcholinesterase Inhibitors (Central); Antidepressants (Serotonin Reuptake Inhibitor/Antagonist); Antimalarial Agents; Beta-Blockers; CYP2D6 Inhibitors (Moderate); CYP2D6 Inhibitors (Strong); Darunavir; Droperidol; HydrOXYzine; Lithium formulations; Methotrimeprazine; Methylphenidate; Metoclopramide; Pramlintide; Tetrabenazine

Decreased Effect

FluPHENAZine may decrease the levels/effects of: Amphetamines; Quinagolide

The levels/effects of FluPHENAZine may be decreased by: Antacids; Anti-Parkinson's Agents (Dopamine Agonist); Lithium formulations; Peginterferon Alfa-2b

Ethanol/Nutrition/Herb Interactions

Ethanol: May increase CNS depression; monitor for increased effects with coadministration. Caution patients about effects.

Herb/Nutraceutical: Avoid dong quai, St John's wort (may also cause photosensitization). Avoid kava kava, gotu kola, valerian, St John's wort (may increase CNS depression).

Stability Store at room temperature; avoid freezing and excessive heat. Protect all dosage forms from light. Clear or slightly yellow solutions may be used. Should be dispensed in amber or opaque vials/bottles. Solutions may be diluted or mixed with fruit juices or other liquids, but must be administered immediately after mixing. Do not prepare bulk dilutions or store bulk dilutions.

Mechanism of Action Fluphenazine is a piperazine phenothiazine antipsychotic which blocks postsynaptic mesolimbic dopaminergic D_1 and D_2 receptors in the brain; depresses the release of hypothalamic and hypophyseal hormones; believed to depress the reticular activating system, thus affecting basal metabolism, body temperature, wakefulness, vasomotor tone, and emesis

Pharmacodynamics/Kinetics

Onset of action: Decanoate: 24-72 hours;

Peak effect: Neuroleptic: Decanoate: 48-96 hours

Duration: Hydrochloride salt: 6-8 hours; Decanoate: ~4 weeks

Absorption: Oral: Erratic and variable

Half-life elimination (derivative dependent): Hydrochloride: ~14-16.4 hours; Decanoate: ~14 days

Time to peak, serum: Hydrochloride: Oral: 2 hours; Decanoate: 8-10 hours

Dosage

Adults: Psychoses:

Oral: Initial: 2.5-10 mg/day in divided doses at 6- to 8-hour intervals; Maintenance: 1-5 mg/day; **Note:** Some patients may require up to 40 mg/day for symptom control (long-term safety of higher doses not established)

PORT guidelines: Acute therapy: 6-20 mg/day for up to 6 weeks; Maintenance: 6-12 mg/day (Buchanan, 2009)

I.M. (hydrochloride): Initial: 1.25 mg as a single dose; depending on severity and duration, may need 2.5-10 mg/day in divided doses at 6- to 8-hour intervals (4 mg I.M. fluphenazine HCl is approximately equivalent to 10 mg oral fluphenazine HCl); use caution with doses >10 mg/day; once symptoms stabilized, transition to oral maintenance therapy

Long-acting maintenance injections (decanoate):

I.M., SubQ (decanoate): Initial: 12.5-25 mg every 2-4 weeks; response may last up to 6 weeks in some patients; titrate dose cautiously, if doses >50 mg are needed, increase in 12.5 mg increments (maximum dose: 100 mg)

Conversion from hydrochloride dosage forms to decanoate I.M.: 12.5 mg of decanoate every 2-4 weeks is approximately equivalent to 10 mg of oral hydrochloride/day; **Note:** Clinically, an every-2-week interval is frequently utilized

PORT guidelines: 6.25-25 mg every 2 weeks (Buchanan, 2009)

Elderly: Oral: Initial: 1-2.5 mg daily; titrated gradually based on patient response

Hemodialysis: Not dialyzable (0% to 5%)

Administration

I.M., SubQ: The hydrochloride or decanoate formulation may be administered intramuscularly. Watch for hypotension when administering I.M. Only the decanoate formulation may be administered subcutaneously. When administering fluphenazine decanoate, use a dry syringe and needle of ≥21 gauge to administer the fluphenazine decanoate; a wet needle/syringe may cause the solution to become cloudy.

Oral: Avoid contact of oral solution or injection with skin (contact dermatitis). Oral liquid should be diluted into at least 60 mL (2 fl oz) of the following **only**: Water, saline, homogenized milk, carbonated orange beverages, pineapple, apricot, prune, orange, tomato, and grapefruit juices. Do **not** dilute in beverages containing caffeine, tannics (eg, tea), or pectinate (eg, apple juice).

Monitoring Parameters Vital signs; lipid profile, fasting blood glucose/Hgb A_{1c}; BMI; mental status, abnormal involuntary movement scale (AIMS), extrapyramidal symptoms (EPS)

Reference Range Therapeutic: 0.3-3 ng/mL (SI: 0.6-6.0 nmol/L); correlation of serum concentrations and efficacy is controversial; most often dosed to best response

Additional Information Less sedative and hypotensive effects than chlorpromazine.

Dosage Forms Excipient information presented when available (limited, particularly for generics); consult specific product labeling.

Elixir, oral, as hydrochloride: 2.5 mg/5 mL (60 mL, 473 mL)
Injection, oil, as decanoate: 25 mg/mL (5 mL)
Injection, solution, as hydrochloride: 2.5 mg/mL (10 mL)
Solution, oral, as hydrochloride [concentrate]: 5 mg/mL (118 mL)
Tablet, oral, as hydrochloride: 1 mg, 2.5 mg, 5 mg, 10 mg

- ◆ **Fluphenazine Decanoate** *see* FluPHENAZine *on page 735*
- ◆ **Fluphenazine Hydrochloride** *see* FluPHENAZine *on page 735*
- ◆ **Flura-Drops®** *see* Fluoride *on page 728*

Flurandrenolide (flure an DREN oh lide)

Brand Names: U.S. Cordran®; Cordran® SP
Brand Names: Canada Cordran®
Index Terms Flurandrenolone
Pharmacologic Category Corticosteroid, Topical
Additional Appendix Information
Corticosteroids *on page 1888*

Use Inflammation of corticosteroid-responsive dermatoses [medium potency topical corticosteroid]

Pregnancy Risk Factor C

Dosage Topical: Therapy should be discontinued when control is achieved; if no improvement is seen, reassessment of diagnosis may be necessary.

Children:
Cream: Apply sparingly 1-2 times/day
Tape: Apply once daily
Adults: Cream, lotion: Apply sparingly 2-3 times/day

Additional Information Complete prescribing information for this medication should be consulted for additional detail.

Dosage Forms Excipient information presented when available (limited, particularly for generics); consult specific product labeling.

Cream, topical [emulsion-based]:
Cordran® SP: 0.05% (15 g, 30 g, 60 g)
Lotion, topical:
Cordran®: 0.05% (15 mL, 60 mL) [contains benzyl alcohol, menthol]
Tape, topical [roll]:
Cordran®: 4 mcg/cm^2 (24 inch, 80 inch)

- ◆ **Flurandrenolone** *see* Flurandrenolide *on page 737*

Flurazepam (flure AZ e pam)

Brand Names: Canada Apo-Flurazepam®; Dalmane®; Som Pam
Index Terms Flurazepam Hydrochloride
Pharmacologic Category Hypnotic, Benzodiazepine
Additional Appendix Information
Beers Criteria – Potentially Inappropriate Medications for Geriatrics *on page 1973*
Benzodiazepines *on page 1882*

Use Short-term treatment of insomnia

Medication Guide Available Yes

Dosage Oral: Insomnia:
Children:
<15 years: Dose not established
≥15 years: 15 mg at bedtime
Adults: 15-30 mg at bedtime
Elderly: 15 mg at bedtime; avoid use if possible

Additional Information Complete prescribing information for this medication should be consulted for additional detail.

Dosage Forms Excipient information presented when available (limited, particularly for generics); consult specific product labeling.

Capsule, oral, as hydrochloride: 15 mg, 30 mg

Controlled Substance C-IV

- ◆ **Flurazepam Hydrochloride** *see* Flurazepam *on page 737*

Flurbiprofen (Systemic) (flure BI proe fen)

Brand Names: Canada Alti-Flurbiprofen; Ansaid®; Apo-Flurbiprofen®; Froben-SR®; Froben®; Novo-Flurprofen; Nu-Flurprofen
Index Terms Flurbiprofen Sodium
Pharmacologic Category Nonsteroidal Anti-inflammatory Drug (NSAID), Oral

Use Treatment of rheumatoid arthritis and osteoarthritis

Unlabeled Use Management of postoperative pain

Pregnancy Risk Factor C

Medication Guide Available Yes

Dosage Oral:
Rheumatoid arthritis and osteoarthritis: 200-300 mg/day in 2, 3, or 4 divided doses; do not administer more than 100 mg for any single dose; maximum: 300 mg/day
Dental: Management of postoperative pain (unlabeled use): 100 mg every 12 hours
Dosage adjustment in renal impairment: Not recommended in patients with advanced renal disease.

Additional Information Complete prescribing information for this medication should be consulted for additional detail.

Dosage Forms Excipient information presented when available (limited, particularly for generics); consult specific product labeling.

Tablet, oral: 50 mg, 100 mg

Flurbiprofen (Ophthalmic) (flure BI proe fen)

Brand Names: U.S. Ocufen®
Brand Names: Canada Ocufen®
Index Terms Flurbiprofen Sodium
Pharmacologic Category Nonsteroidal Anti-inflammatory Drug (NSAID), Ophthalmic

Use Inhibition of intraoperative miosis

Pregnancy Risk Factor C

Dosage Ophthalmic: Instill 1 drop every 30 minutes, beginning 2 hours prior to surgery (total of 4 drops in each affected eye)

Additional Information Complete prescribing information for this medication should be consulted for additional detail.

Dosage Forms Excipient information presented when available (limited, particularly for generics); consult specific product labeling.

Solution, ophthalmic, as sodium [drops]: 0.03% (2.5 mL)
Ocufen®: 0.03% (2.5 mL)

◆ **Flurbiprofen Sodium** *see* Flurbiprofen (Ophthalmic) *on page 737*

◆ **Flurbiprofen Sodium** *see* Flurbiprofen (Systemic) *on page 737*

◆ **Fluress®** *see* Fluorescein and Benoxinate *on page 728*

◆ **5-Flurocytosine** *see* Flucytosine *on page 720*

◆ **Flurox™** *see* Fluorescein and Benoxinate *on page 728*

Flutamide (FLOO ta mide)

Brand Names: Canada Apo-Flutamide®; Euflex®; Eulexin®; Novo-Flutamide; PMS-Flutamide; Teva-Flutamide

Index Terms 4'-Nitro-3'-Trifluoromethylisobutyrantide; Eulexin; Niftolid; NSC-147834; SCH 13521

Pharmacologic Category Antineoplastic Agent, Antiandrogen

Use Treatment of metastatic prostatic carcinoma in combination therapy with LHRH agonist analogues

Unlabeled Use Female hirsutism

Pregnancy Risk Factor D

Dosage Oral: Adults:

Prostatic carcinoma: 250 mg 3 times/day; alternatively, once-daily doses of 0.5-1.5 g have been used (unlabeled dosing)

Female hirsutism (unlabeled use): 250 mg daily

Additional Information Complete prescribing information for this medication should be consulted for additional detail.

Dosage Forms Excipient information presented when available (limited, particularly for generics); consult specific product labeling.

Capsule, oral: 125 mg

Fluticasone (Systemic) (floo TIK a sone)

Brand Names: U.S. Flovent® Diskus®; Flovent® HFA

Brand Names: Canada Flovent® Diskus®; Flovent® HFA

Index Terms Flovent; Fluticasone Propionate

Pharmacologic Category Corticosteroid, Inhalant (Oral)

Additional Appendix Information

Asthma *on page 1967*
Corticosteroids *on page 1888*

Use Maintenance treatment of asthma as prophylactic therapy; also indicated for patients requiring oral corticosteroid therapy for asthma to assist in total discontinuation or reduction of total oral dose

Pregnancy Risk Factor C

Pregnancy Considerations Adverse events have been observed with systemic corticosteroids in animal reproduction studies. A decrease in fetal growth has not been observed with inhaled corticosteroid use during pregnancy. Inhaled corticosteroids are recommended for the treatment of asthma (most information available using budesonide) during pregnancy.

Lactation Excretion in breast milk unknown/use caution

Contraindications Hypersensitivity to fluticasone or any component of the formulation; primary treatment of status asthmaticus or acute bronchospasm

Warnings/Precautions May cause hypercorticism or suppression of hypothalamic-pituitary-adrenal (HPA) axis, particularly in younger children or in patients receiving high doses for prolonged periods. HPA axis suppression may lead to adrenal crisis. Withdrawal and discontinuation of a corticosteroid should be done slowly and carefully. Particular care is required when patients are transferred from systemic corticosteroids to inhaled products due to possible adrenal insufficiency or withdrawal from steroids, including an increase in allergic symptoms. Patients receiving ≥20 mg per day of prednisone (or equivalent) may be most susceptible. Concurrent use of ritonavir (and potentially other strong inhibitors of CYP3A4) may increase fluticasone levels and effects on HPA suppression. Fatalities have occurred due to adrenal insufficiency in asthmatic patients during and after transfer from systemic corticosteroids to aerosol steroids; aerosol steroids do **not** provide the systemic steroid needed to treat patients having trauma, surgery, or infections.

Bronchospasm may occur with wheezing after inhalation; if this occurs, stop steroid and treat with a fast-acting bronchodilator. Supplemental steroids (oral or parenteral) may be needed during stress or severe asthma attacks. Corticosteroid use may cause psychiatric disturbances, including depression, euphoria, insomnia, mood swings, and personality changes. Pre-existing psychiatric conditions may be exacerbated by corticosteroid use. Prolonged use of corticosteroids may also increase the incidence of secondary infection, mask acute infection (including fungal infections), prolong or exacerbate viral infections, or limit response to vaccines. Exposure to chickenpox should be avoided; corticosteroids should not be used to treat ocular herpes simplex. Corticosteroids should not be used for cerebral malaria. Close observation is required in patients with latent tuberculosis and/or TB reactivity; restrict use in active TB (only in conjunction with antituberculosis treatment). Rare cases of vasculitis (Churg-Strauss syndrome) or other eosinophilic conditions can occur. Prolonged treatment with corticosteroids has been associated with the development of Kaposi's sarcoma (case reports); if noted, discontinuation of therapy should be considered.

Use with caution in patients with thyroid disease, hepatic impairment, renal impairment, cardiovascular disease, diabetes, glaucoma, cataracts, myasthenia gravis, patients at risk for osteoporosis, patients at risk for seizures, or GI diseases (diverticulitis, peptic ulcer, ulcerative colitis) due to perforation risk. Use caution following acute MI (corticosteroids have been associated with myocardial rupture). Because of the risk of adverse effects, systemic corticosteroids should be used cautiously in the elderly in the smallest possible effective dose for the shortest duration.

Orally-inhaled corticosteroids may cause a reduction in growth velocity in pediatric patients (~1 centimeter per year [range: 0.3-1.8 cm per year] and related to dose and duration of exposure). To minimize the systemic effects of orally-inhaled corticosteroids, each patient should be titrated to the lowest effective dose. Growth should be routinely monitored in pediatric patients.

Not to be used in status asthmaticus or for the relief of acute bronchospasm. Flovent® Diskus® contains lactose; very rare anaphylactic reactions have been reported in patients with severe milk protein allergy. There have been reports of systemic corticosteroid withdrawal symptoms (eg, joint/muscle pain, lassitude, depression) when withdrawing oral inhalation therapy. Local yeast infections (eg, oral pharyngeal candidiasis) may occur. Lower respiratory tract infections, including pneumonia, have been reported in patients with COPD with an even higher incidence in the elderly.

Adverse Reactions

>10%:

Central nervous system: Headache (2% to 14%)

Respiratory: Upper respiratory tract infection (14% to 21%), throat irritation (3% to 22%)

3% to 10%:

Central nervous system: Fever (1% to 7%)

Gastrointestinal: Oral candidiasis (≤9%), nausea/vomiting (1% to 8%), gastrointestinal infection (including viral; 1% to 5%), gastrointestinal discomfort/pain (1% to 4%)

Neuromuscular & skeletal: Musculoskeletal pain (2% to 5%), muscle injury (1% to 5%)

Respiratory: Sinusitis/sinus infection (4% to 10%), lower respiratory tract infections/pneumonia (1% to 7%; COPD diagnosis and age >65 years increase risk), cough (1% to 6%), bronchitis (≤8%), hoarseness/dysphonia (2% to 6%), upper respiratory tract inflammation (≤5%), viral respiratory infection (1% to 5%), rhinitis (1% to 4%)

Miscellaneous: Viral infection (≤5%)

1% to 3%:

Cardiovascular: Chest symptoms, edema, palpitation

Central nervous system: Cranial nerve paralysis, dizziness, fatigue, malaise, migraine, mood disorders, pain, sleep disorder

Dermatologic: Acne, dermatitis/dermatosis, eczema, folliculitis, photodermatitis, infection (fungal, viral), pruritus, rash, urticaria

Endocrine & metabolic: Fluid disturbance, goiter, uric acid metabolism disturbance

Gastrointestinal: Abdominal discomfort/pain, appetite changes, dental caries, dental discomfort/pain, diarrhea, dyspepsia, gastroenteritis, hyposalivation, oral discomfort/pain, oral erythema/rash, oral ulcerations, oropharyngeal plaques, weight gain

Genitourinary: Reproductive organ infections (bacterial), urinary tract infection

Hematologic: Hematoma

Hepatic: Cholecystitis

Neuromuscular & skeletal: Arthralgia, articular rheumatism, muscle cramps/spasms, muscle pain, muscle stiffness/tightness/rigidity, musculoskeletal inflammation

Ocular: Blepharoconjunctivitis, conjunctivitis, keratitis

Otic: Otitis

Respiratory: Epistaxis, hoarseness/dysphonia, laryngitis, nasal sinus disorder, pharyngitis/throat infection, rhinorrhea/postnasal drip, throat constriction

Miscellaneous: Infection (bacterial, fungal); injuries (including muscle, soft tissue); polyps (ear, nose, throat); tonsillitis

Postmarketing and/or case reports: Aggression, agitation, anaphylactic reaction (rare with both products; Diskus®: some patients with severe milk allergy), angioedema, anxiety, aphonia, asthma exacerbation, behavioral changes (eg, hyperactivity and irritability in children; rare), bone mineral density decreased, bronchospasm (immediate and delayed), cataracts, chest tightness, Churg-Strauss syndrome, contusion, Cushingoid features, cutaneous hypersensitivity, depression, dyspnea, ecchymoses, eosinophilia, facial edema, growth velocity reduction in children/adolescents, HPA axis suppression, hyperglycemia, hypersensitivity reactions (immediate and delayed), oropharyngeal edema, osteoporosis, paradoxical bronchospasm, restlessness, throat soreness, tooth discoloration, vasculitis, wheeze

Drug Interactions

Metabolism/Transport Effects **Substrate** of CYP3A4 (major); **Note:** Assignment of Major/Minor substrate status based on clinically relevant drug interaction potential

Avoid Concomitant Use

Avoid concomitant use of Fluticasone (Oral Inhalation) with any of the following: Aldesleukin; BCG; CYP3A4 Inhibitors (Strong); Natalizumab; Pimecrolimus; Tacrolimus (Topical)

Increased Effect/Toxicity

Fluticasone (Oral Inhalation) may increase the levels/effects of: Amphotericin B; Deferasirox; Leflunomide; Loop Diuretics; Natalizumab; Thiazide Diuretics

The levels/effects of Fluticasone (Oral Inhalation) may be increased by: CYP3A4 Inhibitors (Moderate); CYP3A4 Inhibitors (Strong); Dasatinib; Denosumab; Pimecrolimus; Tacrolimus (Topical); Telaprevir; Trastuzumab

Decreased Effect

Fluticasone (Oral Inhalation) may decrease the levels/effects of: Aldesleukin; Antidiabetic Agents; BCG; Coccidioidin Skin Test; Corticorelin; Sipuleucel-T; Telaprevir; Vaccines (Inactivated)

The levels/effects of Fluticasone (Oral Inhalation) may be decreased by: Echinacea; Tocilizumab

Ethanol/Nutrition/Herb Interactions Herb/Nutraceutical: In theory, St John's wort may decrease serum levels of fluticasone by inducing CYP3A4 isoenzymes.

Stability

Flovent® HFA: Store at 15°C to 30°C (59°F to 86°F). Discard device when the dose counter reads "000". Store with mouthpiece down.

Flovent® Diskus®: Store at 20°C to 25°C (68°F to 77°F) in a dry place away from direct heat or sunlight. Discard after 6 weeks from removal from protective foil pouch or when the dose counter reads "0" (whichever comes first); device is not reusable.

Mechanism of Action Fluticasone belongs to a group of corticosteroids which utilizes a fluorocarbothioate ester linkage at the 17 carbon position; extremely potent vasoconstrictive and anti-inflammatory activity. The effectiveness of inhaled fluticasone is due to its direct local effect.

Pharmacodynamics/Kinetics

Onset of action: Maximal benefit may take 1-2 weeks or longer

Absorption: Absorbed systemically (Flovent® Diskus®: ~18%) primarily via lungs, minimal GI absorption (<1%) due to presystemic metabolism

Distribution: 4.2 L/kg

Protein binding: 91% to >99%

Metabolism: Hepatic via CYP3A4 to 17β-carboxylic acid (negligible activity)

Bioavailability: ~18% to 21%

Excretion: Feces (as parent drug and metabolites); urine (<5% as metabolites)

Dosage Inhalation, oral: Asthma:

Children:

Flovent® HFA:

Children 4-11 years: 88 mcg twice daily

Children ≥12 years: Refer to adult dosing.

NIH Asthma Guidelines (NIH, 2007) (administer in divided doses twice daily):

"Low" dose:

0-4 years: 176 mcg/day

5-11 years: 88-176 mcg/day

≥12 years: 88-264 mcg/day

"Medium" dose:

0-4 years: >176-352 mcg/day

5-11 years: >176-352 mcg/day

≥12 years: >264-440 mcg/day

"High" dose:

0-4 years: >352 mcg/day

5-11 years: >352 mcg/day

≥12 years: >440 mcg/day

Flovent® Diskus® *(U.S. labeling)*:

Children 4-11 years: Usual starting dose: 50 mcg twice daily; may increase to 100 mcg twice daily in patients not adequately controlled after 2 weeks of therapy. Higher starting doses may be considered in patients with poorer asthma control or those requiring high ranges of inhaled corticosteroids. Titrate to the lowest effective dose once asthma stability is achieved (maximum dose: 100 mcg twice daily)

Children >11 years: Refer to adult dosing.

Flovent® Diskus® *(Canadian labeling)*:

Children 4-16 years: Usual starting dose: 50-100 mcg twice daily; may increase to 200 mcg twice daily in patients not adequately controlled; titrate to the lowest effective dose once asthma stability is achieved

Children ≥16 years: Refer to adult dosing.

Adults: **Note:** Titrate to the lowest effective dose once asthma stability is achieved

Flovent® HFA: Manufacturers labeling: Dosing based on previous therapy

Bronchodilator alone: Recommended starting dose: 88 mcg twice daily; highest recommended dose: 440 mcg twice daily

Inhaled corticosteroids: Recommended starting dose: 88-220 mcg twice daily; highest recommended dose: 440 mcg twice daily; a higher starting dose may be considered in patients previously requiring higher doses of inhaled corticosteroids

Oral corticosteroids: Recommended starting dose: 440 mcg twice daily

Highest recommended dose: 880 mcg twice daily; starting dose is patient dependent. In patients on chronic oral corticosteroids therapy, reduce prednisone dose no faster than 2.5-5 mg/day on a weekly basis; begin taper after 1 week of fluticasone therapy.

NIH Asthma Guidelines (NIH, 2007) (administer in divided doses twice daily):

"Low" dose: 88-264 mcg/day

"Medium" dose: >264-440 mcg/day

"High" dose: >440 mcg/day

Flovent® Diskus® *(U.S. labeling)*: **Note:** May increase dose after 2 weeks of therapy in patients not adequately controlled. Higher starting doses may be considered in patients with poorer asthma control or those requiring high ranges of inhaled corticosteroids. Titrate to the lowest effective dose once asthma stability is achieved.

Bronchodilator alone: Recommended starting dose: 100 mcg twice daily; maximum recommended dose: 500 mcg twice daily

Inhaled corticosteroids: Recommended starting dose: 100-250 mcg twice daily; maximum recommended dose: 500 mcg twice daily

Oral corticosteroids: Recommended starting dose: 500-1000 mcg twice daily; maximum recommended dose: 1000 mcg twice daily. Starting dose is patient dependent. In patients on chronic oral corticosteroids therapy, reduce prednisone dose no faster than 2.5 mg/day on a weekly basis; begin taper after 1 week of fluticasone therapy.

Flovent® Diskus® *(Canadian labeling)*:

Mild asthma: 100-250 mcg twice daily

Moderate asthma: 250-500 mcg twice daily

Severe asthma: 500 mcg twice daily; may increase to 1000 mcg twice daily in very severe patients requiring high doses of corticosteroids

Elderly: No differences in safety have been observed in the elderly when compared to younger patients. Based on current data, no dosage adjustment is needed based on age.

Dosage adjustment in hepatic impairment: Fluticasone is primarily cleared in the liver. Fluticasone plasma levels may be increased in patients with hepatic impairment, use with caution; monitor.

Dietary Considerations Flovent® Diskus® contains lactose; very rare anaphylactic reactions have been reported in patients with severe milk protein allergy.

Administration

Aerosol inhalation: Flovent® HFA: Shake container thoroughly before using. Take 3-5 deep breaths. Use inhaler on inspiration. Allow 1 full minute between inhalations. Rinse mouth with water after use to reduce aftertaste and incidence of candidiasis; do not swallow. Inhaler must be primed before first use, when not used for 7 days, or if dropped. To prime the first time, release 4 sprays into air; shake well before each spray and spray away from face. If dropped or not used for 7 days, prime by releasing a single test spray. Patient should contact pharmacy for refill when the dose counter reads "020". Discard device when the dose counter reads "000". Do not use "float" test to determine contents.

Powder for oral inhalation: Flovent® Diskus®: Do not use with a spacer device. Do not exhale into Diskus®. Do not wash or take apart. Use in horizontal position. Mouth should be rinsed with water after use (do not swallow). Discard after 6 weeks once removed from protective pouch or when the dose counter reads "0", whichever comes first (device is not reusable).

Monitoring Parameters Growth (adolescents and children); signs/symptoms of HPA axis suppression/adrenal insufficiency; possible eosinophilic conditions (including Churg-Strauss syndrome); FEV_1, peak flow, and/or other pulmonary function tests; asthma symptoms

Additional Information Effects of inhaled steroids on growth have been observed in the absence of laboratory evidence of HPA axis suppression, suggesting that growth velocity is a more sensitive indicator of systemic corticosteroid exposure in pediatric patients than some commonly used tests of HPA axis function. The long-term effects of this reduction in growth velocity associated with orally-inhaled corticosteroids, including the impact on final adult height, are unknown. The potential for "catch up" growth following discontinuation of treatment with inhaled corticosteroids has not been adequately studied.

In the United States, dosage for the metered dose inhaler (Flovent® HFA) is expressed as the amount of drug which leaves the actuater and is delivered to the patient. This differs from other countries, which express the dosage as the amount of drug which leaves the valve.

Dosage Forms Excipient information presented when available (limited, particularly for generics); consult specific product labeling.

Aerosol, for oral inhalation, as propionate:

Flovent® HFA: 44 mcg/inhalation (10.6 g); 110 mcg/inhalation (12 g); 220 mcg/inhalation (12 g) [chlorofluorocarbon free; 120 metered actuations]

Powder, for oral inhalation, as propionate:

Flovent® Diskus®: 50 mcg (60s); 100 mcg (60s); 250 mcg (60s) [contains lactose]

Dosage Forms: Canada Excipient information presented when available (limited, particularly for generics); consult specific product labeling.

Powder, for oral inhalation, as propionate:

Flovent® Diskus®: 50 mcg (28s, 60s) [contains lactose; prefilled blister pack]

Flovent® Diskus®: 100 mcg (28s, 60s) [contains lactose; prefilled blister pack]

Flovent® Diskus®: 250 mcg (28s, 60s) [contains lactose; prefilled blister pack]

Flovent® Diskus®: 500 mcg (28s, 60s) [contains lactose; prefilled blister pack]

Fluticasone (Nasal) (floo TIK a sone)

Brand Names: U.S. Flonase®; Veramyst®
Brand Names: Canada Apo-Fluticasone®; Avamys®; Flonase®; ratio-Fluticasone
Index Terms Fluticasone Furoate; Fluticasone Propionate
Pharmacologic Category Corticosteroid, Nasal
Use
Flonase®: Management of seasonal and perennial allergic rhinitis and nonallergic rhinitis
Veramyst®, Avamys® [CAN]: Management of seasonal and perennial allergic rhinitis
Pregnancy Risk Factor C
Dosage
Intranasal: Rhinitis:
Children:
Flonase® (fluticasone propionate): Children ≥4 years and Adolescents: Initial: 1 spray (50 mcg/spray) per nostril once daily; patients not adequately responding or patients with more severe symptoms may use 2 sprays (100 mcg) per nostril. Depending on response, dosage may be reduced to 100 mcg daily. Total daily dosage should not exceed 2 sprays in each nostril (200 mcg)/ day. Dosing should be at regular intervals.
Veramyst® (fluticasone furoate):
Children 2-11 years: Initial: 1 spray (27.5 mcg/spray) per nostril once daily (55 mcg/day); patients not adequately responding may use 2 sprays per nostril once daily (110 mcg/day). Once symptoms are controlled, dosage may be reduced to 55 mcg once daily. Total daily dosage should not exceed 2 sprays in each nostril (110 mcg)/day.
Children ≥12 years and Adolescents: Initial: 2 sprays (27.5 mcg/spray) per nostril once daily (110 mcg/day). Once symptoms are controlled, dosage may be reduced to 1 spray per nostril once daily (55 mcg/ day). Total daily dosage should not exceed 2 sprays in each nostril (110 mcg)/day.
Avamys® [CAN] (fluticasone furoate):
Children 2-11 years: Initial: 1 spray (27.5 mcg/spray) per nostril once daily (55 mcg/day); patients not adequately responding may use 2 sprays per nostril once daily (110 mcg/day). Once symptoms are controlled, dosage may be reduced to 55 mcg once daily. Total daily dosage should not exceed 2 sprays in each nostril (110 mcg)/day.
Children ≥12 years and Adolescents: Initial: 2 sprays (27.5 mcg/spray) per nostril once daily (110 mcg/day). Total daily dosage should not exceed 2 sprays in each nostril (110 mcg)/day.
Adults:
Flonase® (fluticasone propionate): Initial: 2 sprays (50 mcg/spray) per nostril once daily; may also be divided into 100 mcg twice a day. After the first few days, dosage may be reduced to 1 spray per nostril once daily for maintenance therapy.
Veramyst® (fluticasone furoate): Initial: 2 sprays (27.5 mcg/spray) per nostril once daily (110 mcg/day). Once symptoms are controlled, may reduce dosage to 1 spray per nostril once daily (55 mcg/day) for maintenance therapy.
Avamys® [CAN] (fluticasone furoate): 2 sprays (27.5 mcg/spray) in each nostril once daily (110 mcg/day). Total daily dosage should not exceed 2 sprays in each nostril (110 mcg)/day.
Elderly: No differences in safety have been observed in the elderly when compared to younger patients. Based on current data, no dosage adjustment is needed based on age.
Additional Information Complete prescribing information for this medication should be consulted for additional detail.
Dosage Forms Excipient information presented when available (limited, particularly for generics); consult specific product labeling.
Suspension, intranasal, as furoate [spray]:
Veramyst®: 27.5 mcg/inhalation (10 g) [contains benzalkonium chloride; 120 metered actuations]
Suspension, intranasal, as propionate [spray]: 50 mcg/ inhalation (16 g)
Flonase®: 50 mcg/inhalation (16 g) [contains benzalkonium chloride; 120 metered actuations]
Dosage Forms: Canada Excipient information presented when available (limited, particularly for generics); consult specific product labeling.
Suspension, intranasal, as furoate [spray]:
Avamys®: 27.5 mcg/inhalation (4.5 g) [30 metered actuations; contains benzalkonium chloride]; (10 g) [120 metered actuations; contains benzalkonium chloride]

Fluticasone (Topical) (floo TIK a sone)

Brand Names: U.S. Cutivate®
Brand Names: Canada Cutivate™
Index Terms Fluticasone Propionate
Pharmacologic Category Corticosteroid, Topical
Additional Appendix Information
Corticosteroids *on page 1888*
Use Relief of inflammation and pruritus associated with corticosteroid-responsive dermatoses; atopic dermatitis
Pregnancy Risk Factor C
Dosage Topical:
Children:
Corticosteroid-responsive dermatoses: Children ≥3 months: Cream: Apply sparingly to affected area twice daily. If no improvement is seen within 2 weeks, reassessment of diagnosis may be necessary.
Atopic dermatitis
Children ≥3 months: Cream: Apply sparingly to affected area 1-2 times/day. If no improvement is seen within 2 weeks, reassessment of diagnosis may be necessary.
Children ≥1 year: Lotion: Apply sparingly to affected area once daily
Adults:
Corticosteroid-responsive dermatoses: Cream, lotion, ointment: Apply sparingly to affected area twice daily. If no improvement is seen within 2 weeks, reassessment of diagnosis may be necessary.
Atopic dermatitis: Cream, lotion: Apply sparingly to affected area once or twice daily. If no improvement is seen within 2 weeks, reassessment of diagnosis may be necessary.
Additional Information Complete prescribing information for this medication should be consulted for additional detail.
Dosage Forms Excipient information presented when available (limited, particularly for generics); consult specific product labeling.
Cream, topical, as propionate: 0.05% (15 g, 30 g, 60 g)
Cutivate®: 0.05% (30 g, 60 g)
Lotion, topical, as propionate:
Cutivate®: 0.05% (120 mL)
Ointment, topical, as propionate: 0.005% (15 g, 30 g, 60 g)
Cutivate®: 0.005% (30 g, 60 g)

Fluticasone and Salmeterol
(floo TIK a sone & sal ME te role)

Brand Names: U.S. Advair Diskus®; Advair® HFA
Brand Names: Canada Advair Diskus®; Advair®
Index Terms Fluticasone Propionate and Salmeterol Xinafoate; Salmeterol and Fluticasone

Pharmacologic Category Beta$_2$-Adrenergic Agonist; Beta$_2$-Adrenergic Agonist, Long-Acting; Corticosteroid, Inhalant (Oral)

Use Maintenance treatment of asthma; maintenance treatment of COPD

Pregnancy Risk Factor C

Pregnancy Considerations See individual agents.

Lactation

Fluticasone: Excretion in breast milk unknown/use caution

Salmeterol: Enters breast milk/use caution

Medication Guide Available Yes

Contraindications Hypersensitivity to fluticasone, salmeterol, or any component of the formulation; status asthmaticus; acute episodes of asthma or COPD; severe hypersensitivity to milk proteins (Advair Diskus®)

Warnings/Precautions See individual agents.

Adverse Reactions Percentages reported in patients with asthma; also see individual agents:

>10%:

Central nervous system: Headache (12% to 21%)

Respiratory: Upper respiratory tract infection (16% to 27%), pharyngitis (9% to 13%)

>3% to 10%:

Central nervous system: Dizziness (1% to 4%)

Endocrine & metabolic: Menstruation symptoms (3% to 5%)

Gastrointestinal: Nausea/vomiting (3% to 6%), diarrhea (2% to 4%), pain/discomfort (1% to 4%), oral candidiasis (1% to 4%), gastrointestinal infections (including viral, ≤4%)

Neuromuscular & skeletal: Musculoskeletal pain (2% to 7%), muscle pain (≤4%)

Respiratory: Throat irritation (7% to 9%), bronchitis (2% to 8%), upper respiratory tract inflammation (4% to 7%), lower respiratory tract infections/pneumonia (1% to 7%; COPD diagnosis and age >65 years increase risk), cough (3% to 6%), sinusitis (4% to 5%), hoarseness/dysphonia (1% to 5%), viral respiratory tract infection (3% to 5%)

1% to 3%:

Cardiovascular: Arrhythmia, chest symptoms, fluid retention, MI, palpitation, syncope, tachycardia

Central nervous system: Compressed nerve syndromes, hypnagogic effects, migraine, pain, sleep disorders, tremor

Dermatologic: Dermatitis, dermatosis, eczema, hives, skin flakiness, urticaria, viral skin infection

Endocrine & metabolic: Hypothyroidism

Gastrointestinal: Constipation, dental discomfort/pain, gastrointestinal infection, hemorrhoids, oral discomfort/pain, oral erythema/rash, oral ulcerations, unusual taste, weight gain

Genitourinary: Urinary tract infection

Hematologic: Contusions/hematomas

Hepatic: Abnormal liver function tests

Neuromuscular & skeletal: Arthralgia, articular rheumatism, bone/cartilage disorders, bone pain, cramps, fractures, muscle injuries (≤3%), muscle spasm, muscle stiffness, tightness/rigidity

Ocular: Conjunctivitis, edema, eye redness, keratitis, xerophthalmia

Respiratory: Blood in nasal mucosa, congestion, ear/nose/throat infection, epistaxis, laryngitis, lower respiratory hemorrhage, nasal irritation, rhinitis, rhinorrhea/postnasal drip, sneezing

Miscellaneous: Allergies/allergic reactions, bacterial infection, burns, candidiasis (≤3%), diaphoresis, sweat/sebum disorders, viral infection, wounds and lacerations

Postmarketing and/or case reports: Asthma exacerbation (serious and some fatal), abdominal pain, agitation, aggression, anaphylactic reaction (some in patients with severe milk allergy [Diskus®]), angioedema, aphonia, atrial fibrillation, bronchospasm, cataracts, chest congestion, chest tightness, choking, contact dermatitis, Cushing syndrome, Cushingoid features, depression, dysmenorrhea, dyspepsia, dyspnea, earache, ecchymoses, edema (facial, oropharyngeal), eosinophilic conditions, glaucoma, growth velocity reduction in children/adolescents, hyperactivity, hypercorticism, hyperglycemia, hypersensitivity reaction (immediate and delayed), hypertension, hypokalemia, hypothyroidism, influenza, intraocular pressure increased, irritability, laryngeal spasm/irritation, irregular menstruation, myositis, osteoporosis, pallor, paresthesia, paradoxical tracheitis, paranasal sinus pain, photodermatitis, PID, rash, restlessness, stridor, supraventricular tachycardia, syncope, vaginal candidiasis, vaginitis, vulvovaginitis, rare cases of vasculitis (Churg-Strauss syndrome), ventricular tachycardia, wheezing, xerostomia

Drug Interactions

Metabolism/Transport Effects Refer to individual components.

Avoid Concomitant Use

Avoid concomitant use of Fluticasone and Salmeterol with any of the following: Aldesleukin; BCG; Beta-Blockers (Nonselective); CYP3A4 Inhibitors (Strong); Iobenguane I 123; Natalizumab; Pimecrolimus; Tacrolimus (Topical); Telaprevir

Increased Effect/Toxicity

Fluticasone and Salmeterol may increase the levels/effects of: Amphotericin B; Deferasirox; Leflunomide; Loop Diuretics; Natalizumab; Sympathomimetics; Thiazide Diuretics

The levels/effects of Fluticasone and Salmeterol may be increased by: Atomoxetine; Cannabinoids; CYP3A4 Inhibitors (Moderate); CYP3A4 Inhibitors (Strong); Dasatinib; Denosumab; MAO Inhibitors; Pimecrolimus; Roflumilast; Tacrolimus (Topical); Telaprevir; Trastuzumab; Tricyclic Antidepressants

Decreased Effect

Fluticasone and Salmeterol may decrease the levels/effects of: Aldesleukin; Antidiabetic Agents; BCG; Coccidioidin Skin Test; Corticorelin; Iobenguane I 123; Sipuleucel-T; Telaprevir; Vaccines (Inactivated)

The levels/effects of Fluticasone and Salmeterol may be decreased by: Alpha-/Beta-Blockers; Beta-Blockers (Beta1 Selective); Beta-Blockers (Nonselective); Betahistine; Echinacea; Tocilizumab

Stability

Advair Diskus®: Store at controlled room temperature of 20°C to 25°C (68°F to 77°F). Store in a dry place out of direct heat or sunlight. Diskus® device should be discarded 1 month after removal from foil pouch, or when dosing indicator reads "0" (whichever comes first); device is not reusable.

Advair® HFA: Store at controlled room temperature of 25°C (77°F). Store with mouthpiece down. Discard after 120 inhalations. Discard device when the dose counter reads "000". Device is not reusable.

Mechanism of Action Combination of fluticasone (corticosteroid) and salmeterol (long-acting beta$_2$-agonist) designed to improve pulmonary function and control over what is produced by either agent when used alone. Because fluticasone and salmeterol act locally in the lung, plasma levels do not predict therapeutic effect.

Fluticasone: The mechanism of action for all topical corticosteroids is believed to be a combination of three important properties: Anti-inflammatory activity, immunosuppressive properties, and antiproliferative actions. Fluticasone has extremely potent vasoconstrictive and anti-inflammatory activity.

Salmeterol: Relaxes bronchial smooth muscle by selective action on beta$_2$-receptors with little effect on heart rate

Pharmacodynamics/Kinetics See individual agents.

Dosage Oral inhalation: **Note:** Do not use to transfer patients from systemic corticosteroid therapy.

COPD: Adults:

Advair Diskus®: Fluticasone 250 mcg/salmeterol 50 mcg twice daily, 12 hours apart. **Note:** This is the maximum dose.

Advair Diskus® [Canadian labeling; not in approved U.S. labeling]: Fluticasone 250 mcg/salmeterol 50 mcg **or** fluticasone 500 mcg/salmeterol 50 mcg twice daily, 12 hours apart.

Maximum dose: Fluticasone 500 mcg/salmeterol 50 mcg per inhalation (2 inhalations/day)

Asthma:

Children 4-11 years: Advair Diskus®: Fluticasone 100 mcg/salmeterol 50 mcg twice daily, 12 hours apart. **Note:** This is the maximum dose.

Children ≥12 years and Adults:

Advair Diskus®: One inhalation twice daily, morning and evening, 12 hours apart

Maximum dose: Fluticasone 500 mcg/salmeterol 50 mcg per inhalation (2 inhalations/day)

Advair® HFA: Two inhalations twice daily, morning and evening, 12 hours apart

Maximum dose: Fluticasone 230 mcg/salmeterol 21 mcg per inhalation (4 inhalations/day)

Advair® 125 or Advair® 250 [Canadian labeling; not in approved U.S. labeling]: Two inhalations twice daily, morning and evening, 12 hours apart

Maximum dose: Fluticasone 250 mcg/salmeterol 25 mcg per inhalation (4 inhalations/day)

Note: Initial dose prescribed should be based upon previous dose of inhaled-steroid asthma therapy. Dose should be increased after 2 weeks if adequate response is not achieved. Patients should be titrated to lowest effective dose once stable. Each suggestion below specifies the product strength to use; remember to **use 1 inhalation for Diskus® and 2 inhalations for HFA.**

Patients not currently on inhaled corticosteroids:

Advair Diskus®: Fluticasone 100 mcg/salmeterol 50 mcg **or** fluticasone 250 mcg/salmeterol 50 mcg

Advair® HFA: Fluticasone 45 mcg/salmeterol 21 mcg **or** fluticasone 115 mcg/salmeterol 21 mcg

Patients currently using inhaled beclomethasone dipropionate:

≤160 mcg/day: Fluticasone 100 mcg/salmeterol 50 mcg **or** Advair® HFA: Fluticasone 45 mcg/salmeterol 21 mcg

320 mcg/day: Fluticasone 250 mcg/salmeterol 50 mcg **or** Advair® HFA: Fluticasone 115 mcg/salmeterol 21 mcg

640 mcg/day: Fluticasone 500 mcg/salmeterol 50 mcg **or** Advair® HFA: Fluticasone 230 mcg/salmeterol 21 mcg

Patients currently using inhaled budesonide:

≤400 mcg/day: Fluticasone 100 mcg/salmeterol 50 mcg **or** Advair® HFA: Fluticasone 45 mcg/salmeterol 21 mcg

800-1200 mcg/day: Fluticasone 250 mcg/salmeterol 50 mcg **or** Advair® HFA: Fluticasone 115 mcg/salmeterol 21 mcg

1600 mcg/day: Fluticasone 500 mcg/salmeterol 50 mcg **or** Advair® HFA: Fluticasone 230 mcg/salmeterol 21 mcg

Patients currently using inhaled flunisolide CFC aerosol:

≤1000 mcg/day: Fluticasone 100 mcg/salmeterol 50 mcg **or** Advair® HFA: Fluticasone 45 mcg/salmeterol 21 mcg

1250-2000 mcg/day: Fluticasone 250 mcg/salmeterol 50 mcg **or** Advair® HFA: Fluticasone 115 mcg/salmeterol 21 mcg

Patients currently using inhaled flunisolide HFA inhalation aerosol:

≤320 mcg/day: Fluticasone 100 mcg/salmeterol 50 mcg **or** Advair® HFA: Fluticasone 45 mcg/salmeterol 21 mcg

640 mcg/day: Fluticasone 250 mcg/salmeterol 50 mcg **or** Advair® HFA: Fluticasone 115 mcg/salmeterol 21 mcg

Patients currently using inhaled fluticasone HFA aerosol:

≤176 mcg/day: Fluticasone 100 mcg/salmeterol 50 mcg **or** Advair® HFA: Fluticasone 45 mcg/salmeterol 21 mcg

440 mcg/day: Fluticasone 250 mcg/salmeterol 50 mcg **or** Advair® HFA: Fluticasone 115 mcg/salmeterol 21 mcg

660-880 mcg/day: Fluticasone 500 mcg/salmeterol 50 mcg **or** Advair® HFA: Fluticasone 230 mcg/salmeterol 21 mcg

Patients currently using inhaled fluticasone propionate powder:

≤200 mcg/day: Fluticasone 100 mcg/salmeterol 50 mcg **or** Advair® HFA: Fluticasone 45 mcg/salmeterol 21 mcg

500 mcg/day: Fluticasone 250 mcg/salmeterol 50 mcg **or** Advair® HFA: Fluticasone 115 mcg/salmeterol 21 mcg

1000 mcg/day: Fluticasone 500 mcg/salmeterol 50 mcg **or** Advair® HFA: Fluticasone 230 mcg/salmeterol 21 mcg

Patients currently using inhaled mometasone furoate powder:

220 mcg/day: Fluticasone 100 mcg/salmeterol 50 mcg **or** Advair® HFA: Fluticasone 45 mcg/salmeterol 21 mcg

440 mcg/day: Fluticasone 250 mcg/salmeterol 50 mcg **or** Advair® HFA: Fluticasone 115 mcg/salmeterol 21 mcg

880 mcg/day: Fluticasone 500 mcg/salmeterol 50 mcg **or** Advair® HFA: Fluticasone 230 mcg/salmeterol 21 mcg

Patients currently using inhaled triamcinolone acetonide:

≤1000 mcg/day: Fluticasone 100 mcg/salmeterol 50 mcg **or** Advair® HFA: Fluticasone 45 mcg/salmeterol 21 mcg

1100-1600 mcg/day: Fluticasone 250 mcg/salmeterol 50 mcg **or** Advair® HFA: Fluticasone 115 mcg/salmeterol 21 mcg

Elderly: No differences in safety or effectiveness have been seen in studies of patients ≥65 years of age. However, increased sensitivity may be seen in the elderly. Use with caution in patients with concomitant cardiovascular disease.

Dosage adjustment in renal impairment: Specific guidelines are not available

Dosage adjustment in hepatic impairment: No dosage adjustment required; manufacturer suggests close monitoring of patients with hepatic impairment.

Dietary Considerations Advair Diskus® powder for oral inhalation contains lactose; very rare anaphylactic reactions have been reported in patients with severe milk protein allergy.

Administration

Advair Diskus®: After removing from box and foil pouch, write the "Pouch opened" and "Use by" dates on the label on top of the Diskus®. The "Use by" date is 1 month from date of opening the pouch. Every time the lever is pushed back, a dose is ready to be inhaled. Do not close or tilt the Diskus® after the lever is pushed back. Do not play with the lever or move the lever more than once. The dose indicator tells you how many doses are left. When the numbers 5 to 0 appear in red, only a few doses remain. Discard device 1 month after you remove it from the foil pouch or when the dose counter reads "0" (whichever comes first). Rinse mouth with water after use and spit to reduce risk of oral candidiasis.

Advair® HFA: Shake well for 5 seconds before each spray. Prime with 4 test sprays (into air and away from face) before using for the first time. If canister is dropped or not used for >4 weeks, prime with 2 sprays. Patient should contact pharmacy for refill when the dose counter reads "020". Discard device when the dose counter reads "000". Do not spray in eyes. Rinse mouth with water after use and spit to reduce risk of oral candidiasis.

Monitoring Parameters FEV_1, peak flow, and/or other pulmonary function tests; blood pressure, heart rate; CNS stimulation. Monitor for increased use of short-acting $beta_2$-agonist inhalers; may be marker of a deteriorating asthma condition. The growth of pediatric patients receiving inhaled corticosteroids should be monitored routinely (eg, via stadiometry).

Additional Information Effects of inhaled/intranasal steroids on growth have been observed in the absence of laboratory evidence of HPA axis suppression, suggesting that growth velocity is a more sensitive indicator of systemic corticosteroid exposure in pediatric patients than some commonly used tests of HPA axis function. The long-term effects of this reduction in growth velocity associated with orally-inhaled and intranasal corticosteroids, including the impact on final adult height, are unknown. The potential for "catch up" growth following discontinuation of treatment with inhaled corticosteroids has not been adequately studied.

Advair® HFA: Salmeterol (base) 21 mcg is equivalent to 30.45 mcg of salmeterol xinafoate.

Dosage Forms Excipient information presented when available (limited, particularly for generics); consult specific product labeling. [DSC] = Discontinued product

Aerosol, for oral inhalation:

Advair® HFA:

45/21: Fluticasone propionate 45 mcg and salmeterol 21 mcg per inhalation (8 g) [chlorofluorocarbon free; 60 metered actuations]

45/21: Fluticasone propionate 45 mcg and salmeterol 21 mcg per inhalation (12 g) [chlorofluorocarbon free; 120 metered actuations]

115/21: Fluticasone propionate 115 mcg and salmeterol 21 mcg per inhalation (8 g) [chlorofluorocarbon free; 60 metered actuations]

115/21: Fluticasone propionate 115 mcg and salmeterol 21 mcg per inhalation (12 g) [chlorofluorocarbon free; 120 metered actuations]

230/21: Fluticasone propionate 230 mcg and salmeterol 21 mcg per inhalation (8 g) [chlorofluorocarbon free; 60 metered actuations]

230/21: Fluticasone propionate 230 mcg and salmeterol 21 mcg per inhalation (12 g) [chlorofluorocarbon free; 120 metered actuations]

Powder, for oral inhalation:

Advair Diskus®:

100/50: Fluticasone propionate 100 mcg and salmeterol 50 mcg (14s, 28s [DSC], 60s) [contains lactose]

250/50: Fluticasone propionate 250 mcg and salmeterol 50 mcg (14s [DSC], 60s) [contains lactose]

500/50: Fluticasone propionate 500 mcg and salmeterol 50 mcg (14s [DSC], 60s) [contains lactose]

Dosage Forms: Canada Excipient information presented when available (limited, particularly for generics); consult specific product labeling.

Aerosol, for oral inhalation:

Advair®;

125/25: Fluticasone propionate 125 mcg and salmeterol 25 mcg per inhalation (12 g) [120 metered actuations]

250/25: Fluticasone propionate 250 mcg and salmeterol 25 mcg per inhalation (12 g) [120 metered actuations]

◆ **Fluticasone Furoate** *see* Fluticasone (Nasal) *on page 741*

◆ **Fluticasone Propionate** *see* Fluticasone (Nasal) *on page 741*

◆ **Fluticasone Propionate** *see* Fluticasone (Systemic) *on page 738*

◆ **Fluticasone Propionate** *see* Fluticasone (Topical) *on page 741*

◆ **Fluticasone Propionate and Salmeterol Xinafoate** *see* Fluticasone and Salmeterol *on page 741*

Fluvastatin (FLOO va sta tin)

Brand Names: U.S. Lescol®; Lescol® XL

Brand Names: Canada Lescol®; Lescol® XL

Pharmacologic Category Antilipemic Agent, HMG-CoA Reductase Inhibitor

Additional Appendix Information

Hyperlipidemia Management *on page 1996*

Use To be used as a component of multiple risk factor intervention in patients at risk for atherosclerosis vascular disease due to hypercholesterolemia

Adjunct to dietary therapy to reduce elevated total cholesterol (total-C), LDL-C, triglyceride, and apolipoprotein B (apo-B) levels and to increase HDL-C in primary hypercholesterolemia and mixed dyslipidemia (Fredrickson types IIa and IIb); to slow the progression of coronary atherosclerosis in patients with coronary heart disease; reduce risk of coronary revascularization procedures in patients with coronary heart disease

Pregnancy Risk Factor X

Pregnancy Considerations Cholesterol biosynthesis may be important in fetal development. Contraindicated in pregnancy. Administer to women of childbearing potential only when conception is highly unlikely and patients have been informed of potential hazards.

Lactation Enters breast milk/contraindicated

Contraindications Hypersensitivity to fluvastatin or any component of the formulation; active liver disease; unexplained persistent elevations of serum transaminases; pregnancy; breast-feeding

Warnings/Precautions Secondary causes of hyperlipidemia should be ruled out prior to therapy. Liver function must be monitored by periodic laboratory assessment. Rhabdomyolysis with acute renal failure has occurred with fluvastatin and other HMG-CoA reductase inhibitors. Risk may be increased with concurrent use of other drugs which may cause rhabdomyolysis (including colchicine, gemfibrozil, fibric acid derivatives, or niacin at doses ≥1 g/day). The manufacturer recommends temporary discontinuation for elective major surgery, acute medical or surgical conditions, or in any patient experiencing an acute or serious condition predisposing to renal failure (eg, sepsis, hypotension, trauma, uncontrolled seizures). However, based upon current evidence, HMG-CoA reductase inhibitor therapy should be continued in the perioperative period unless risk outweighs cardioprotective benefit. Use with caution in patients with advanced age; these patients are predisposed to myopathy. Use caution in patients with previous liver disease or heavy ethanol use. Use caution in patients with concurrent medications or conditions which reduce steroidogenesis.

Adverse Reactions As reported with fluvastatin capsules; in general, adverse reactions reported with fluvastatin extended release tablet were similar, but the incidence was less.

1% to 10%:

Central nervous system: Headache (9%), fatigue (3%), insomnia (3%)

Gastrointestinal: Dyspepsia (8%), diarrhea (5%), abdominal pain (5%), nausea (3%)
Genitourinary: Urinary tract infection (2%)
Neuromuscular & skeletal: Myalgia (5%)
Respiratory: Sinusitis (3%), bronchitis (2%)

<1% (Limited to important or life-threatening) including additional class-related events (not necessarily reported with fluvastatin therapy): Alopecia, anaphylaxis, angioedema, arthralgia, arthritis, cataracts, cholestatic jaundice, cirrhosis, CPK increased (>10x normal), depression, dermatomyositis, dyspnea, eosinophilia, erectile dysfunction, erythema multiforme, ESR increased, facial paresis, fatty liver, fever, fulminant hepatic necrosis, gynecomastia, hemolytic anemia, hepatitis, hepatoma, hypersensitivity reaction, impotence, interstitial lung disease, leukopenia, memory loss, muscle cramps, myopathy, nodules, ophthalmoplegia, pancreatitis, paresthesia, peripheral nerve palsy, peripheral neuropathy, photosensitivity, polymyalgia rheumatica, positive ANA, pruritus, psychic disturbance, purpura, rash, renal failure (secondary to rhabdomyolysis), rhabdomyolysis, skin discoloration, Stevens-Johnson syndrome, systemic lupus erythematosus-like syndrome, taste alteration, thrombocytopenia, thyroid dysfunction, toxic epidermal necrolysis, transaminases increased, tremor, urticaria, vasculitis, vertigo

Drug Interactions

Metabolism/Transport Effects Substrate of CYP2C9 (minor), CYP2D6 (minor), CYP3A4 (minor), SLCO1B1; **Note:** Assignment of Major/Minor substrate status based on clinically relevant drug interaction potential; **Inhibits** CYP1A2 (weak), CYP2C8 (weak), CYP2C9 (moderate), CYP2D6 (weak), CYP3A4 (weak)

Avoid Concomitant Use

Avoid concomitant use of Fluvastatin with any of the following: Pimozide; Red Yeast Rice

Increased Effect/Toxicity

Fluvastatin may increase the levels/effects of: Carvedilol; CYP2C9 Substrates; DAPTOmycin; Pimozide; Trabectedin; Vitamin K Antagonists

The levels/effects of Fluvastatin may be increased by: Amiodarone; Colchicine; Conivaptan; Cyproterone; Eltrombopag; Fenofibrate; Fenofibric Acid; Fluconazole; Gemfibrozil; Niacin; Niacinamide; Red Yeast Rice

Decreased Effect

Fluvastatin may decrease the levels/effects of: Lanthanum

The levels/effects of Fluvastatin may be decreased by: Antacids; Cholestyramine Resin; Etravirine; Fosphenytoin; Peginterferon Alfa-2b; Phenytoin; Rifamycin Derivatives; Tocilizumab

Ethanol/Nutrition/Herb Interactions

Ethanol: Avoid excessive ethanol consumption (due to potential hepatic effects).

Food: Reduces rate but not the extent of absorption. Red yeast rice contains an estimated 2.4 mg lovastatin per 600 mg rice.

Stability Store at 15°C to 30°C (59°F to 86°F). Protect from light.

Mechanism of Action Acts by competitively inhibiting 3-hydroxyl-3-methylglutaryl-coenzyme A (HMG-CoA) reductase, the enzyme that catalyzes the reduction of HMG-CoA to mevalonate; this is an early rate-limiting step in cholesterol biosynthesis. HDL is increased while total, LDL, and VLDL cholesterols; apolipoprotein B; and plasma triglycerides are decreased.

Pharmacodynamics/Kinetics

Onset of action: Peak effect: Maximal LDL-C reductions achieved within 4 weeks
Distribution: V_d: 0.35 L/kg
Protein binding: >98%
Metabolism: To inactive and active metabolites (oxidative metabolism via CYP2C9 [75%], 2C8 [~5%], and 3A4 [~20%] isoenzymes); active forms do not circulate systemically; extensive (saturable) first-pass hepatic extraction
Bioavailability: Absolute: Capsule: 24%; Extended release tablet: 29%
Half-life elimination: Capsule: <3 hours; Extended release tablet: 9 hours
Time to peak: Capsule: 1 hour; Extended release tablet: 3 hours
Excretion: Feces (90%): urine (5%)

Dosage

Adolescents 10-16 years: Oral: Heterozygous familial hypercholesterolemia: Initial: 20 mg once daily; may increase every 6 weeks based on tolerability and response to a maximum recommended dose of 80 mg/day, given in 2 divided doses (immediate release capsule) or as a single daily dose (extended release tablet)

Note: Indicated only for adjunctive therapy when diet alone cannot reduce LDL-C below 190 mg/dL, or 160 mg/dL (with cardiovascular risk factors). Female patients must be 1 year postmenarche.

Adults: Oral:

Patients requiring ≥25% decrease in LDL-C: 40 mg capsule once daily in the evening, 80 mg extended release tablet once daily (anytime), or 40 mg capsule twice daily

Patients requiring <25% decrease in LDL-C: Initial: 20 mg capsule once daily in the evening; may increase based on tolerability and response to a maximum recommended dose of 80 mg/day, given in 2 divided doses (immediate release capsule) or as a single daily dose (extended release tablet)

Dosage adjustment in renal impairment: Less than 6% excreted renally; no dosage adjustment needed with mild-to-moderate renal impairment; use with caution in severe impairment

Dosage adjustment in hepatic impairment: Levels may accumulate in patients with liver disease (increased AUC and C_{max}); use caution with severe hepatic impairment or heavy ethanol ingestion; contraindicated in active liver disease or unexplained transaminase elevations; decrease dose and monitor effects carefully in patients with hepatic insufficiency

Elderly: No dosage adjustment necessary based on age

Dietary Considerations Generally, patients should be placed on a standard cholesterol-lowering diet and other lifestyle modifications for 3-6 months prior to the initiation of drug therapy. The diet should be continued during drug therapy. However, for patients with advanced risk factors (eg, known coronary heart disease), drug therapy may be initiated concurrently with diet modification. May be taken without regard to meals. Red yeast rice contains an estimated 2.4 mg lovastatin per 600 mg rice.

Administration Patient should be placed on a standard cholesterol-lowering diet before and during treatment. Fluvastatin may be taken without regard to meals. Adjust dosage as needed in response to periodic lipid determinations during the first 4 weeks after a dosage change; lipid-lowering effects are additive when fluvastatin is combined with a bile-acid binding resin or niacin, however, it must be administered at least 2 hours following these drugs. Do not break, chew, or crush extended release tablets; do not open capsules.

Monitoring Parameters Obtain baseline LFTs and total cholesterol profile; repeat tests at 12 weeks after initiation of therapy or elevation in dose, and periodically thereafter; baseline CPK (recheck CPK in any patient with symptoms suggestive of myopathy). Monitor LDL-C at intervals no less than 4 weeks.

Dosage Forms Excipient information presented when available (limited, particularly for generics); consult specific product labeling.

Capsule, oral:

Lescol®: 20 mg, 40 mg

Tablet, extended release, oral:

Lescol® XL: 80 mg

◆ **Fluviral® (Can)** *see* Influenza Virus Vaccine (Inactivated) *on page 897*

◆ **Fluvirin®** *see* Influenza Virus Vaccine (Inactivated) *on page 897*

FluvoxaMINE (floo VOKS a meen)

Brand Names: U.S. Luvox® CR

Brand Names: Canada Alti-Fluvoxamine; Apo-Fluvoxamine®; Luvox®; Novo-Fluvoxamine; Nu-Fluvoxamine; PMS-Fluvoxamine; Rhoxal-fluvoxamine; Riva-Fluvox; Sandoz-Fluvoxamine

Index Terms Luvox

Pharmacologic Category Antidepressant, Selective Serotonin Reuptake Inhibitor

Additional Appendix Information

Antidepressant Agents *on page 1874*

Selective Serotonin Reuptake Inhibitors (SSRIs) Pharmacokinetics *on page 1897*

Use Treatment of obsessive-compulsive disorder (OCD)

Unlabeled Use Treatment of major depression; panic disorder; anxiety disorders in children; treatment of mild dementia-associated agitation in nonpsychotic patients; post-traumatic stress disorder (PTSD); social anxiety disorder (SAD)

Pregnancy Risk Factor C

Pregnancy Considerations Due to adverse effects observed in animal studies, fluvoxamine is classified as pregnancy category C. Fluvoxamine crosses the human placenta. Nonteratogenic effects in the newborn following SSRI exposure late in the third trimester include respiratory distress, cyanosis, apnea, seizures, temperature instability, feeding difficulty, vomiting, hypoglycemia, hypo- or hypertonia, hyper-reflexia, jitteriness, irritability, constant crying, and tremor. An increased risk of low birth weight and low Apgar scores has also been reported. Exposure to SSRIs after the twentieth week of gestation has been associated with persistent pulmonary hypertension of the newborn (PPHN). Adverse effects may be due to toxic effects of the SSRI or drug withdrawal due to discontinuation. The long-term effects of *in utero* SSRI exposure on infant development and behavior are not known.

Women treated for major depression and who are euthymic prior to pregnancy are more likely to experience a relapse when medication is discontinued as compared to pregnant women who continue taking antidepressant medications. The ACOG recommends that therapy with SSRIs or SNRIs during pregnancy be individualized; treatment of depression during pregnancy should incorporate the clinical expertise of the mental health clinician, obstetrician, primary healthcare provider, and pediatrician. If treatment during pregnancy is required, consider tapering therapy during the third trimester in order to prevent withdrawal symptoms in the infant. If this is done and the woman is considered to be at risk of relapse from her major depressive disorder, the medication can be restarted following delivery, although the dose should be readjusted to that required before pregnancy. Treatment algorithms have been developed by the ACOG and the APA for the management of depression in women prior to conception and during pregnancy (Yonkers, 2009).

Lactation Enters breast milk/consider risk:benefit (AAP rates "of concern"; AAP 2001 update pending)

Medication Guide Available Yes

Contraindications Hypersensitivity to fluvoxamine or any component of the formulation; concurrent use with alosetron, pimozide, ramelteon, thioridazine, or tizanidine; use with or within 14 days of MAO inhibitors

Warnings/Precautions [U.S. Boxed Warning]: Antidepressants increase the risk of suicidal thinking and behavior in children, adolescents, and young adults (18-24 years of age) with major depressive disorder (MDD) and other psychiatric disorders; consider risk prior to prescribing. Short-term studies did not show an increased risk in patients >24 years of age and showed a decreased risk in patients ≥65 years. Closely monitor patients for clinical worsening, suicidality, or unusual changes in behavior, particularly during the initial 1-2 months of therapy or during periods of dosage adjustments (increases or decreases); the patient's family or caregiver should be instructed to closely observe the patient and communicate condition with healthcare provider. A medication guide concerning the use of antidepressants should be dispensed with each prescription. **Fluvoxamine is FDA approved for the treatment of OCD in children ≥8 years of age; extended release capsules are not FDA approved for use in children.**

The possibility of a suicide attempt is inherent in major depression and may persist until remission occurs. Use caution in high-risk patients. Worsening depression and severe abrupt suicidality that are not part of the presenting symptoms may require discontinuation or modification of drug therapy. The patient's family or caregiver should be alerted to monitor patients for the emergence of suicidality and associated behaviors (such as agitation, irritability, hostility, impulsivity, and hypomania) and call healthcare provider.

May worsen psychosis in some patients or precipitate a shift to mania or hypomania in patients with bipolar disorder. Patients presenting with depressive symptoms should be screened for bipolar disorder. Monotherapy in patients with bipolar disorder should be avoided. **Fluvoxamine is not FDA approved for the treatment of bipolar depression.**

Serotonin syndrome and neuroleptic malignant syndrome (NMS)-like reactions have occurred with serotonin/norepinephrine reuptake inhibitors (SNRIs) and selective serotonin reuptake inhibitors (SSRIs) when used alone, and particularly when used in combination with serotonergic agents (eg, triptans) or antidopaminergic agents (eg, antipsychotics). Concurrent use with MAO inhibitors is contraindicated. Fluvoxamine has a low potential to impair cognitive or motor performance; caution operating hazardous machinery or driving. Use caution in patients with a previous seizure disorder or condition predisposing to seizures such as brain damage, alcoholism, or concurrent therapy with other drugs which lower the seizure threshold. Fluvoxamine may significantly increase alosetron concentrations; concurrent use **contraindicated.** Potential for QT_c prolongation and arrhythmia with thioridazine and pimozide; concurrent use of fluvoxamine with either of these agents is **contraindicated.** Concomitant use with tizanidine may cause a significant decrease in blood pressure and increase in drowsiness; concurrent use is **contraindicated.** Fluvoxamine levels may be lower in patients who smoke.

May increase the risks associated with electroconvulsive therapy. Use with caution in patients with hepatic dysfunction and in elderly patients. May cause hyponatremia/SIADH (elderly at increased risk); volume depletion (diuretics may increase risk). Use with caution in patients at risk of bleeding or receiving concurrent anticoagulant therapy, although not consistently noted, fluvoxamine may cause impairment in platelet function. May cause or exacerbate sexual dysfunction.

Adverse Reactions Frequency varies by dosage form and indication. Adverse reactions reported as a composite of all indications.

>10%:

Central nervous system: Headache (22% to 35%), insomnia (21% to 35%), somnolence (22% to 27%), dizziness (11% to 15%), nervousness (10% to 12%)

Gastrointestinal: Nausea (34% to 40%), diarrhea (11% to 18%), xerostomia (10% to 14%), anorexia (6% to 14%)

Genitourinary: Ejaculation abnormal (8% to 11%)

Neuromuscular & skeletal: Weakness (14% to 26%)

1% to 10%:

Cardiovascular: Chest pain (3%), palpitation (3%), vasodilation (2% to 3%), hypertension (1% to 2%), edema (≤1%), hypotension (≤1%), syncope (≤1%), tachycardia (≤1%)

Central nervous system: Pain (10%), anxiety (5% to 8%), abnormal dreams (3%), abnormal thinking (3%), agitation (2% to 3%), apathy (≥1% to 3%), chills (2%), CNS stimulation (2%), depression (2%), neurosis (2%), amnesia, malaise, manic reaction, psychotic reaction

Dermatologic: Bruising (4%), acne (2%)

Endocrine & metabolic: Libido decreased (2% to 10%; incidence higher in males), anorgasmia (2% to 5%), sexual function abnormal (2% to 4%), menorrhagia (3%)

Gastrointestinal: Dyspepsia (8% to 10%), constipation (4% to 10%), vomiting (4% to 6%), abdominal pain (5%), flatulence (4%), taste perversion (2% to 3%), toothache and dental caries (2% to 3%), dysphagia (2%), gingivitis (2%), weight loss (≤1% to 2%), weight gain

Genitourinary: Polyuria (2% to 3%), impotence (2%), urinary tract infection (2%), urinary retention (1%)

Hepatic: Liver function tests abnormal (≥1% to 2%)

Neuromuscular & skeletal: Tremor (5% to 8%), myalgia (5%), paresthesia (3%), hypertonia (2%), twitching (2%), hyper-/hypokinesia, myoclonus

Ocular: Amblyopia (2% to 3%)

Respiratory: Upper respiratory infection (9%), pharyngitis (6%), yawn (2% to 5%), laryngitis (3%), bronchitis (2%), dyspnea (2%), epistaxis (2%), cough increased, sinusitis

Miscellaneous: Diaphoresis (6% to 7%), flu-like syndrome (3%), viral infection (2%)

<1% (Limited to important or life-threatening): Acute renal failure, agranulocytosis, akinesia, allergic reaction, anaphylactic reaction, anemia, angina, angioedema, anuria, aplastic anemia, apnea, asthma, ataxia, AV block, bradycardia, bullous eruption, cardiomyopathy, cardiorespiratory arrest, cerebrovascular accident, cholecystitis, cholelithiasis, colitis, conduction delay, coronary artery disease, diplopia, dyskinesia, dystonia, extrapyramidal syndrome, embolus, GI bleeding, goiter, hallucinations, heart failure, hematemesis, hematuria, Henoch-Schönlein purpura, hepatitis, hemoptysis, homicidal ideation, hypercholesterolemia, hyper-/hypoglycemia, hypokalemia, hyponatremia, hypothyroidism, ileus, interstitial lung disease, intestinal obstruction, jaundice, leukopenia, leukocytosis, loss of consciousness, lymphadenopathy, MI, myasthenia, myopathy, neuralgia, neuroleptic malignant syndrome, neuropathy, pancreatitis, paralysis, pericarditis, porphyria, purpura, QT prolongation, retinal detachment, rhabdomyolysis, serotonin syndrome, ST segment changes, seizure, Stevens-Johnson syndrome, suicidal tendencies, supraventricular extrasystoles, tardive dyskinesia, thrombocytopenia, toxic epidermal necrolysis, vasculitis, ventricular arrhythmia, ventricular tachycardia (including torsade de pointes), white blood cells decreased

Drug Interactions

Metabolism/Transport Effects **Substrate** of CYP1A2 (major), CYP2D6 (major); **Note:** Assignment of Major/Minor substrate status based on clinically relevant drug interaction potential; **Inhibits** CYP1A2 (strong), CYP2B6 (weak), CYP2C19 (strong), CYP2C9 (weak), CYP2D6 (weak), CYP3A4 (weak)

Avoid Concomitant Use

Avoid concomitant use of FluvoxaMINE with any of the following: Alosetron; Clopidogrel; Iobenguane I 123; MAO Inhibitors; Methylene Blue; Pimozide; Ramelteon; Thioridazine; TiZANidine; Tryptophan

Increased Effect/Toxicity

FluvoxaMINE may increase the levels/effects of: Alosetron; Anticoagulants; Antidepressants (Serotonin Reuptake Inhibitor/Antagonist); Antiplatelet Agents; Asenapine; Aspirin; Bendamustine; Benzodiazepines (metabolized by oxidation); Bromazepam; BusPIRone; CarBAMazepine; CloZAPine; Collagenase (Systemic); CYP1A2 Substrates; CYP2C19 Substrates; Desmopressin; Drotrecogin Alfa (Activated); DULoxetine; Erlotinib; Fosphenytoin; Haloperidol; Ibritumomab; Lithium; Methadone; Methylene Blue; Metoclopramide; Mexiletine; NSAID (COX-2 Inhibitor); NSAID (Nonselective); OLANZapine; Phenytoin; Pimozide; Propafenone; Propranolol; QuiNIDine; Ramelteon; Rivaroxaban; Roflumilast; Ropivacaine; Salicylates; Serotonin Modulators; Theophylline Derivatives; Thioridazine; Thrombolytic Agents; TiZANidine; Tositumomab and Iodine I 131 Tositumomab; TraMADol; Tricyclic Antidepressants; Vitamin K Antagonists

The levels/effects of FluvoxaMINE may be increased by: Abiraterone Acetate; Alcohol (Ethyl); Analgesics (Opioid); Antipsychotics; BusPIRone; Cimetidine; CNS Depressants; CYP1A2 Inhibitors (Moderate); CYP1A2 Inhibitors (Strong); CYP2D6 Inhibitors (Moderate); CYP2D6 Inhibitors (Strong); Darunavir; Dasatinib; Deferasirox; Glucosamine; Herbs (Anticoagulant/Antiplatelet Properties); Linezolid; MAO Inhibitors; Metoclopramide; Omega-3-Acid Ethyl Esters; Pentosan Polysulfate Sodium; Pentoxifylline; Prostacyclin Analogues; TraMADol; Tryptophan; Vitamin E

Decreased Effect

FluvoxaMINE may decrease the levels/effects of: Clopidogrel; Iobenguane I 123; Ioflupane I 123

The levels/effects of FluvoxaMINE may be decreased by: CarBAMazepine; CYP1A2 Inducers (Strong); Cyproheptadine; Cyproterone; NSAID (Nonselective); Peginterferon Alfa-2b

Ethanol/Nutrition/Herb Interactions

Ethanol: May increase CNS depression; monitor for increased effects with coadministration. Caution patients about effects.

Food: The bioavailability of melatonin has been reported to be increased by fluvoxamine.

Herb/Nutraceutical: Avoid valerian, St John's wort, SAMe, kava kava (may increase risk of serotonin syndrome and/or excessive sedation). Avoid alfalfa, anise, bilberry, bladderwrack, bromelain, cat's claw, celery, chamomile, coleus, cordyceps, dong quai, evening primrose, fenugreek, feverfew, garlic, ginger, ginkgo biloba, ginseng (American), ginseng (Panax), ginseng (Siberian), grape seed, green tea, guggul, horse chestnuts, horseradish, licorice, prickly ash, red clover, reishi, SAMe (S-adenosylmethionine), sweet clover, turmeric, white willow (all have additional antiplatelet activity).

Stability Protect from high humidity and store at controlled room temperature 25°C (77°F).

Mechanism of Action Inhibits CNS neuron serotonin uptake; minimal or no effect on reuptake of norepinephrine or dopamine; does not significantly bind to alpha-adrenergic, histamine or cholinergic receptors

Pharmacodynamics/Kinetics

Onset of action: Depression: The onset of action is within a week; however, individual response varies greatly and full response may not be seen until 8-12 weeks after initiation of treatment.

Absorption: Steady-state plasma concentrations have been noted to be 2-3 times higher in children than those in adolescents; female children demonstrated a significantly higher AUC than males

Distribution: V_d: ~25 L/kg

Protein binding: ~80%, primarily to albumin

Metabolism: Extensively hepatic via oxidative demethylation and deamination

Bioavailability: Immediate release: 53%; not significantly affected by food

Half-life elimination: 15-16 hours; 17-26 hours in the elderly

Time to peak, plasma: 3-8 hours

Excretion: Urine (~85% as metabolites; ~2% as unchanged drug)

Dosage Oral:

Obsessive-compulsive disorder:

Children 8-17 years: Immediate release: Initial: 25 mg once daily at bedtime; may be increased in 25 mg increments at 4- to 7-day intervals, as tolerated, to maximum therapeutic benefit; usual dose range: 50-200 mg/day. **Note:** When total daily dose exceeds 50 mg, the dose should be given in 2 divided doses with larger portion administered at bedtime.

Maximum: Children: 8-11 years: 200 mg/day, adolescents: 300 mg/day; lower doses may be effective in female versus male patients

Adults:

Immediate release: Initial: 50 mg once daily at bedtime; may be increased in 50 mg increments at 4- to 7-day intervals, as tolerated; usual dose range: 100-300 mg/day; maximum dose: 300 mg/day. **Note:** When total daily dose exceeds 100 mg, the dose should be given in 2 divided doses with larger portion administered at bedtime.

Extended release: Initial: 100 mg once daily at bedtime; may be increased in 50 mg increments at intervals of at least 1 week; usual dosage range: 100-300 mg/day; maximum dose: 300 mg/day

Social anxiety disorder (unlabeled use): Adults: Extended release: Initial: 100 mg once daily at bedtime; may be increased in 50 mg increments at intervals of at least 1 week; usual dosage range: 100-300 mg/day; maximum dose: 300 mg/day (Davidson, 2004; Stein, 2003; Westenberg, 2004)

Post-traumatic stress disorder (PTSD) (unlabeled use): Adults: Immediate release: 75 mg twice daily (Spivak, 2006)

Elderly: Reduce dose, titrate slowly

Dosage adjustment in hepatic impairment: Reduce dose, titrate slowly

Dietary Considerations May be taken with or without food.

Administration May be administered with or without food. Do not crush, open, or chew extended release capsules.

Monitoring Parameters Mental status for depression, suicide ideation (especially at the beginning of therapy or when doses are increased or decreased), anxiety, social functioning, mania, panic attacks; akathisia, weight gain or loss, nutritional intake, sleep; liver function assessment prior to beginning drug therapy

Dosage Forms Excipient information presented when available (limited, particularly for generics); consult specific product labeling.

Capsule, extended release, oral, as maleate:

Luvox® CR: 100 mg, 150 mg [gluten free]

Tablet, oral, as maleate: 25 mg, 50 mg, 100 mg

- ◆ **Fluzone®** *see* Influenza Virus Vaccine (Inactivated) *on page 897*
- ◆ **Fluzone® High-Dose** *see* Influenza Virus Vaccine (Inactivated) *on page 897*
- ◆ **Fluzone® Intradermal** *see* Influenza Virus Vaccine (Inactivated) *on page 897*
- ◆ **FML®** *see* Fluorometholone *on page 730*
- ◆ **FML Forte®** *see* Fluorometholone *on page 730*
- ◆ **Focalin®** *see* Dexmethylphenidate *on page 485*
- ◆ **Focalin XR®** *see* Dexmethylphenidate *on page 485*
- ◆ **Foille® [OTC]** *see* Benzocaine *on page 202*
- ◆ **Folacin** *see* Folic Acid *on page 748*
- ◆ **Folacin-800 [OTC]** *see* Folic Acid *on page 748*
- ◆ **Folacin, Vitamin B_{12}, and Vitamin B_6** *see* Folic Acid, Cyanocobalamin, and Pyridoxine *on page 749*
- ◆ **Folate** *see* Folic Acid *on page 748*
- ◆ **Folbee** *see* Folic Acid, Cyanocobalamin, and Pyridoxine *on page 749*
- ◆ **Folbic** *see* Folic Acid, Cyanocobalamin, and Pyridoxine *on page 749*
- ◆ **Folcaps™** *see* Folic Acid, Cyanocobalamin, and Pyridoxine *on page 749*
- ◆ **Folgard® [OTC]** *see* Folic Acid, Cyanocobalamin, and Pyridoxine *on page 749*
- ◆ **Folgard RX®** *see* Folic Acid, Cyanocobalamin, and Pyridoxine *on page 749*

Folic Acid (FOE lik AS id)

Brand Names: U.S. Folacin-800 [OTC]

Brand Names: Canada Apo-Folic®

Index Terms Folacin; Folate; Pteroylglutamic Acid

Pharmacologic Category Vitamin, Water Soluble

Use Treatment of megaloblastic and macrocytic anemias due to folate deficiency; dietary supplement to prevent neural tube defects

Unlabeled Use Adjunctive cofactor therapy in methanol toxicity (alternative to leucovorin calcium)

Pregnancy Risk Factor A

Pregnancy Considerations Folic acid requirements are increased during pregnancy; a deficiency may result in fetal harm.

Lactation Enters breast milk/compatible

Contraindications Hypersensitivity to folic acid or any component of the formulation

Warnings/Precautions Not appropriate for monotherapy with pernicious, aplastic, or normocytic anemias when anemia is present with vitamin B_{12} deficiency. Doses >0.1 mg/day may obscure pernicious anemia with continuing irreversible nerve damage progression. Resistance to treatment may occur with depressed hematopoiesis, alcoholism, and deficiencies of other vitamins. Injection contains benzyl alcohol (1.5%) as preservative (use care in administration to neonates).

Adverse Reactions Frequency not defined.

Allergic reaction, bronchospasm, erythema, flushing (slight), malaise (general), pruritus, rash

Drug Interactions

Metabolism/Transport Effects None known.

Avoid Concomitant Use

Avoid concomitant use of Folic Acid with any of the following: Raltitrexed

Increased Effect/Toxicity There are no known significant interactions involving an increase in effect.

Decreased Effect

Folic Acid may decrease the levels/effects of: Fosphenytoin; PHENobarbital; Phenytoin; Primidone; Raltitrexed

The levels/effects of Folic Acid may be decreased by: Green Tea

Stability Do not use with oxidizing and reducing agents or heavy metal ions.

Mechanism of Action Folic acid is necessary for formation of a number of coenzymes in many metabolic systems, particularly for purine and pyrimidine synthesis; required for nucleoprotein synthesis and maintenance in erythropoiesis; stimulates WBC and platelet production in folate deficiency anemia. Folic acid enhances the elimination of formic acid, the toxic metabolite of methanol (unlabeled use).

Pharmacodynamics/Kinetics

Onset of action: Peak effect: Oral: 0.5-1 hour

Absorption: Proximal part of small intestine

Metabolism: Hepatic

Excretion: Urine

Dosage

Oral, I.M., I.V., SubQ: Anemia:
- Infants: 0.1 mg/day
- Children <4 years: Up to 0.3 mg/day
- Children >4 years and Adults: 0.4 mg/day
- Pregnant and lactating women: 0.8 mg/day

Oral:
- RDA: Expressed as dietary folate equivalents:
  - Children:
    - 1-3 years: 150 mcg/day
    - 4-8 years: 200 mcg/day
    - 9-13 years: 300 mcg/day
  - Children ≥14 years and Adults: 400 mcg/day
  - Elderly: Vitamin B_{12} deficiency must be ruled out before initiating folate therapy due to frequency of combined nutritional deficiencies: RDA requirements (1999): 400 mcg/day (0.4 mg) minimum
- Prevention of neural tube defects:
  - Females of childbearing potential: 400-800 mcg/day (USPSTF)
  - Females at high risk or with family history of neural tube defects: 4 mg/day

Dietary Considerations As of January 1998, the FDA has required manufacturers of enriched flour, bread, corn meal, pasta, rice, and other grain products to add folic acid to their products. The intent is to help decrease the risk of neural tube defects by increasing folic acid intake. Other foods which contain folic acid include dark green leafy vegetables, citrus fruits and juices, and lentils.

Administration Oral preferred, but may also be administered by deep I.M., SubQ, or I.V. injection.

I.V. administration: May administer ≤5 mg dose undiluted over ≥1 minute **or** may dilute ≤5 mg in 50 mL of NS or D_5W and infuse over 30 minutes. May also be added to I.V. maintenance solutions and given as an infusion.

Reference Range Therapeutic: 0.005-0.015 mcg/mL

Test Interactions Falsely low serum concentrations may occur with the *Lactobacillus casei* assay method in patients on anti-infectives (eg, tetracycline)

Additional Information The RDA for folic acid is presented as dietary folate equivalents (DFE). DFE adjusts for the difference in bioavailability of folic acid from food as compared to dietary supplements.

Dosage Forms Excipient information presented when available (limited, particularly for generics); consult specific product labeling.

Injection, solution, as sodium folate: 5 mg/mL (10 mL)

Tablet, oral: 0.4 mg, 0.8 mg, 1 mg
- Folacin-800: 0.8 mg [scored; gluten free, sugar free]

Extemporaneous Preparations A 1 mg/mL folic acid oral solution may be made with tablets. Heat 90 mL of purified water almost to boiling. Dissolve parabens (methylparaben 200 mg and propylparaben 20 mg) in the heated water; cool to room temperature. Crush one-hundred 1 mg tablets, then dissolve folic acid in the solution. Adjust pH to 8-8.5 with sodium hydroxide 10%; add sufficient quantity of purified water to make 100 mL; mix well. Stable for 30 days at room temperature (Allen, 2007).

A 0.05 mg/mL folic acid oral solution may be prepared using the injectable formulation (5 mg/mL). Mix 1 mL of injectable folic acid with 90 mL of purified water. Adjust pH to 8-8.5 with sodium hydroxide 10%; add sufficient quantity of purified water to make 100 mL; mix well. Stable for 30 days at room temperature (Nahata, 2004).

Allen LV Jr, "Folic Acid 1-mg/mL Oral Liquid," *Int J Pharm Compound*, 2007, 11(3):244.

Nahata MC, Pai VB, and Hipple TF, *Pediatric Drug Formulations*, 5th ed, Cincinnati, OH: Harvey Whitney Books Co, 2004.

Folic Acid, Cyanocobalamin, and Pyridoxine

(FOE lik AS id, sye an oh koe BAL a min, & peer i DOKS een)

Brand Names: U.S. FaBB; Folbee; Folbic; Folcaps™; Folgard RX®; Folgard® [OTC]; Foltabs™ 800 [OTC]; Foltx®; Homocysteine Guard [OTC]; Lev-Tov [OTC]; Tri-B® [OTC]; Tricardio B; Vita-Respa®

Index Terms Cyanocobalamin, Folic Acid, and Pyridoxine; Folacin, Vitamin B_{12}, and Vitamin B_6; Pyridoxine, Folic Acid, and Cyanocobalamin

Pharmacologic Category Vitamin

Use Nutritional supplement in end-stage renal failure, dialysis, hyperhomocysteinemia, homocystinuria, malabsorption syndromes, dietary deficiencies

Dosage Oral: Adults: One tablet daily

Additional Information Complete prescribing information for this medication should be consulted for additional detail.

Dosage Forms Excipient information presented when available (limited, particularly for generics); consult specific product labeling.

Tablet, oral: Folic acid 0.8 mg, cyanocobalamin 100 mcg, and pyridoxine hydrochloride 50 mg; Folic acid 0.8 mg, cyanocobalamin 1000 mcg, and pyridoxine hydrochloride 50 mg; Folic acid 2.2 mg, cyanocobalamin 500 mcg, and pyridoxine hydrochloride 25 mg
- FaBB: Folic acid 2.2 mg, cyanocobalamin 1000 mcg, and pyridoxine hydrochloride 25 mg
- Folbee: Folic acid 2.5 mg, cyanocobalamin 1000 mcg, and pyridoxine hydrochloride 25 mg [dye free, lactose free, and sugar free]
- Folbic: Folic acid 2.5 mg, cyanocobalamin 2000 mcg, and pyridoxine hydrochloride 25 mg
- Folcaps™: Folic acid 2.2 mg, cyanocobalamin 500 mcg, and pyridoxine hydrochloride 25 mg [sugar free]
- Folgard®: Folic acid 0.8 mg, cyanocobalamin 115 mcg, and pyridoxine hydrochloride 10 mg
- Folgard RX®: Folic acid 2.2 mg, cyanocobalamin 1000 mcg, and pyridoxine hydrochloride 25 mg
- Foltabs™ 800: Folic acid 0.8 mg, cyanocobalamin 115 mcg, and pyridoxine hydrochloride 10 mg [gluten free]
- Foltx®: Folic acid 2.5 mg, cyanocobalamin 2000 mcg, and pyridoxine hydrochloride 25 mg
- Homocysteine Guard: Folic acid 0.8 mg, cyanocobalamin 400 mcg, and pyridoxine hydrochloride 25 mg
- Lev-Tov: Folic acid 0.8 mg, cyanocobalamin 250 mcg, and pyridoxine hydrochloride 25 mg
- Tri-B®: Folic acid 0.8 mg, cyanocobalamin 400 mcg, and pyridoxine hydrochloride 25 mg
- Tricardio B: Folic acid 0.4 mg, cyanocobalamin 250 mcg, and pyridoxine hydrochloride 25 mg
- Vita-Respa®: Folic acid 2.2 mg, cyanocobalamin 1300 mcg, and pyridoxine hydrochloride 25 mg [dye free and sugar free]

◆ **Folinate Calcium** *see* Leucovorin Calcium *on page* 987

- ◆ **Folinic Acid (error prone synonym)** *see* Leucovorin Calcium *on page 987*
- ◆ **Follicle-Stimulating Hormone, Human** *see* Urofollitropin *on page 1750*
- ◆ **Follicle Stimulating Hormone, Recombinant** *see* Follitropin Alfa *on page 750*
- ◆ **Follicle Stimulating Hormone, Recombinant** *see* Follitropin Beta *on page 750*
- ◆ **Follistim® AQ** *see* Follitropin Beta *on page 750*
- ◆ **Follistim® AQ Cartridge** *see* Follitropin Beta *on page 750*

Follitropin Alfa (foe li TRO pin AL fa)

Brand Names: U.S. Gonal-f®; Gonal-f® RFF; Gonal-f® RFF Pen

Brand Names: Canada Gonal-f®; Gonal-f® Pen

Index Terms Follicle Stimulating Hormone, Recombinant; FSH; rFSH-alpha; rhFSH-alpha

Pharmacologic Category Gonadotropin; Ovulation Stimulator

Use

Gonal-f®: Ovulation induction in patients in whom the cause of infertility is functional and not caused by primary ovarian failure; development of multiple follicles with Assisted Reproductive Technology (ART); spermatogenesis induction

Gonal-f® RFF: Ovulation induction in patients in whom the cause of infertility is functional and not caused by primary ovarian failure; development of multiple follicles with ART

Pregnancy Risk Factor X

Dosage Adults: **Note:** Dose should be individualized. Use the lowest dose consistent with the expectation of good results. Over the course of treatment, doses may vary depending on individual patient response.

Gonal-f®, Gonal-f® RFF: Females:

Ovulation induction: SubQ: Initial: 75 int. units/day; incremental dose adjustments of up to 37.5 int. units may be considered after 14 days; further dose increases of the same magnitude can be made, if necessary, every 7 days (maximum dose: 300 int. units/day). If response to follitropin is appropriate, hCG is given 1 day following the last dose. Withhold hCG if serum estradiol is >2000 pg/mL, if the ovaries are abnormally enlarged, or if abdominal pain occurs. In general, therapy should not exceed 35 days.

ART: SubQ: Initiate therapy with follitropin alfa in the early follicular phase (cycle day 2 or day 3) at a dose of 150 int. units/day, until sufficient follicular development is attained. In most cases, therapy should not exceed 10 days. In patients ≥35 years whose endogenous gonadotropin levels are suppressed, initiate follitropin alfa at a dose of 225 int. units/day. Continue treatment until adequate follicular development is indicated as determined by ultrasound in combination with measurement of serum estradiol levels. Consider adjustments to dose after 5 days based on the patient's response; adjust subsequent dosage every 3-5 days by ≤75-150 int. units additionally at each adjustment. Doses >450 int. units/day are not recommended. Once adequate follicular development is evident, administer hCG to induce final follicular maturation in preparation for oocyte. Withhold hCG if the ovaries are abnormally enlarged.

Gonal-f®: Males: Spermatogenesis induction: SubQ: Therapy should begin with hCG pretreatment until serum testosterone is in normal range, then 150 int. units 3 times/week with hCG 3 times/week; continue with lowest dose needed to induce spermatogenesis (maximum dose: 300 int. units 3 times/week); may be given for up to 18 months

Additional Information Complete prescribing information for this medication should be consulted for additional detail.

Dosage Forms Excipient information presented when available (limited, particularly for generics); consult specific product labeling.

Injection, powder for reconstitution [rDNA origin]:

Gonal-f®: 450 int. units, 1050 int. units [contains benzyl alcohol (in diluent), sucrose 30 mg]

Gonal-f® RFF: 75 int. units [contains sucrose 30 mg; supplied with diluent]

Injection, solution [rDNA origin]:

Gonal-f® RFF Pen: 300 int. units/0.5 mL (0.5 mL); 450 int. units/0.75 mL (0.75 mL); 900 int. units/1.5 mL (1.5 mL) [contains sucrose 60 mg/mL]

Follitropin Beta (foe li TRO pin BAY ta)

Brand Names: U.S. Follistim® AQ; Follistim® AQ Cartridge

Brand Names: Canada Puregon®

Index Terms Follicle Stimulating Hormone, Recombinant; FSH; rFSH-beta; rhFSH-beta

Pharmacologic Category Gonadotropin; Ovulation Stimulator

Use

Females: Induction of ovulation and pregnancy in anovulatory infertile patients in whom the cause of infertility is functional and not caused by primary ovarian failure; development of multiple follicles with Assisted Reproductive Technology (ART)

Males: Induction of spermatogenesis in men with primary and secondary hypogonadotropic hypogonadism in whom the cause of infertility is not due to primary testicular failure.

Pregnancy Risk Factor X

Dosage Adults: **Note:** Dose should be individualized. Use the lowest dose consistent with the expectation of good results. Over the course of treatment, doses may vary depending on individual patient response.

Females:

Ovulation induction:

Follistim® AQ: I.M., SubQ: Stepwise approach: Initiate therapy with 75 int. units/day for at least the first 7 days. Increase by 25 or 50 int. units at weekly intervals until follicular growth or serum estradiol levels indicate an adequate response. The maximum (individualized) daily dose that has been safely used for ovulation induction in patients during clinical trials is 300 int. units. If response to follitropin is appropriate, hCG is given 1 day following the last dose. Withhold hCG if the ovaries are abnormally enlarged, or if abdominal pain occurs.

Follistim® AQ Cartridge: SubQ: Stepwise approach: Initiate therapy with 50 int. units/day for at least the first 7 days. Increase by 25 or 50 int. units at weekly intervals until follicular growth or serum estradiol levels indicate an adequate response. The maximum (individualized) daily dose that has been safely used for ovulation induction in patients during clinical trials is 250 int. units. If response to follitropin is appropriate, hCG is given 1 day following the last dose. Withhold hCG if the ovaries are abnormally enlarged, or if abdominal pain occurs. See **"Note"** for dosage adjustment for this product.

ART:

Follistim® AQ: I.M., SubQ: Stepwise approach: A starting dose of 150-225 int. units is recommended for at least the first 4 days of treatment. The dose may be adjusted for the individual patient based upon their ovarian response. The maximum daily dose used in clinical studies is 600 int. units. When a sufficient number of follicles of adequate size are present, the final maturation of the follicles is induced by administering hCG. Oocyte retrieval is performed 34-36 hours later. Withhold hCG in cases where the ovaries are abnormally enlarged on the last day of follitropin beta therapy.

Follistim® AQ Cartridge: SubQ: Stepwise approach: A starting dose of 125-175 int. units is recommended for at least the first 4 days of treatment. The dose may be adjusted for the individual patient based upon their ovarian response. The maximum daily dose used in clinical studies is 500 int. units. When a sufficient number of follicles of adequate size are present, the final maturation of the follicles is induced by administering hCG. Oocyte retrieval is performed 34-36 hours later. Withhold hCG in cases where the ovaries are abnormally enlarged on the last day of follitropin beta therapy. See **"Note"** for dosage adjustment for this product.

Males: Spermatogenesis induction (Follistim® AQ, Follistim® AQ Cartridge): **Note:** Pretreatment with hCG is required prior to concomitant therapy with Follistim® AQ and hCG. Follistim® AQ therapy may be initiated after normal serum testosterone levels have been reached. SubQ: 450 int. units/week (administered as 225 int. units twice weekly or 150 int. units 3 times/weekly). A lower dose of Follistim® AQ Cartridge may be considered.

Note: Dose adjustment for Follistim® AQ Cartridge: When administered using the Follistim Pen®, the Follistim® AQ Cartridge delivers 18% more follitropin beta when compared to dissolved lyophilized follitropin beta administered by a conventional syringe. If the above starting doses were previously used when administering a recombinant lyophilized gonadotropin product via a conventional syringe, lower starting and maintenance doses should be considered when switching to Follistim® AQ Cartridge. The following dose conversion may be used:

Follistim® AQ Dosing Conversion[1]

Dose Administered Using Powder for Solution/Conventional Syringe	Follistim® AQ Dose Administered Using Follistim Pen®
75 int. units	50 int. units
150 int. units	125 int. units
225 int. units	175 int. units
300 int. units	250 int. units
375 int. units	300 int. units
450 int. units	375 int. units

[1]Values listed are rounded to the nearest 25 int. unit increment.

Additional Information Complete prescribing information for this medication should be consulted for additional detail.

Dosage Forms Excipient information presented when available (limited, particularly for generics); consult specific product labeling.

Injection, solution [rDNA origin]:

Follistim® AQ: 75 int. units/0.5 mL (0.5 mL); 150 int. units/0.5 mL (0.5 mL) [contains neomycin (may have trace amounts), streptomycin (may have trace amounts), sucrose 50 mg/mL]

Follistim® AQ Cartridge: 350 int. units/0.42 mL (0.42 mL) [contains benzyl alcohol, neomycin (may have trace amounts), streptomycin (may have trace amounts), sucrose 50 mg/mL; delivers 300 int. units]

Follistim® AQ Cartridge: 650 int. units/0.78 mL (0.78 mL) [contains benzyl alcohol, neomycin (may have trace amounts), streptomycin (may have trace amounts), sucrose 50 mg/mL; delivers 600 int. units]

Follistim® AQ Cartridge: 975 int. units/1.17 mL (1.17 mL) [contains benzyl alcohol, neomycin (may have trace amounts), streptomycin (may have trace amounts), sucrose 50 mg/mL; delivers 900 int. units]

- **Folotyn®** *see* PRALAtrexate *on page 1387*
- **Foltabs™ 800 [OTC]** *see* Folic Acid, Cyanocobalamin, and Pyridoxine *on page 749*
- **Foltx®** *see* Folic Acid, Cyanocobalamin, and Pyridoxine *on page 749*

Fomepizole (foe ME pi zole)

Brand Names: U.S. Antizol®

Index Terms 4-Methylpyrazole; 4-MP

Pharmacologic Category Antidote

Use Treatment of methanol or ethylene glycol poisoning alone or in combination with hemodialysis

Unlabeled Use Pediatric administration; treatment of propylene glycol toxicity

Pregnancy Risk Factor C

Pregnancy Considerations Reproduction studies have not been conducted; use in pregnant women only if the benefits clearly outweigh the risks.

Lactation Excretion in breast milk unknown/not recommended

Contraindications Hypersensitivity to fomepizole, other pyrazoles, or any component of the formulation

Warnings/Precautions Should not be given undiluted or by bolus injection. Fomepizole is metabolized in the liver and excreted in the urine; use caution with hepatic or renal impairment. Hemodialysis should be used in patients with renal failure, significant or worsening metabolic acidosis, or ethylene glycol/methanol levels ≥50 mg/dL. Pediatric administration is not FDA approved; however, safe and efficacious use in this patient population for ethylene glycol and methanol intoxication has been reported (Baum, 2000; Benitez, 2000; Boyer, 2001; Brown, 2001; De Brabander, 2005; Detaille, 2004; Fisher, 1998); consider consultation with a clinical toxicologist or poison control center.

Adverse Reactions

>10%:

Central nervous system: Headache (14%)

Gastrointestinal: Nausea (11%)

1% to 10% (≤3% unless otherwise noted):

Cardiovascular: Bradycardia, facial flush, hypotension, shock, tachycardia

Central nervous system: Dizziness (6%), drowsiness increased (6%), agitation, anxiety, fever, lightheadedness, seizure, vertigo

Dermatologic: Rash

Endocrine & metabolic: Liver function tests increased

Gastrointestinal: Bad/metallic taste (6%), abdominal pain, appetite decreased, diarrhea, heartburn, vomiting

Hematologic: Anemia, disseminated intravascular coagulation (DIC), eosinophilia, lymphangitis

Local: Application site reaction, injection site inflammation, pain during injection, phlebitis

Neuromuscular & skeletal: Backache

Ocular: Nystagmus, transient blurred vision, visual disturbances

Renal: Anuria

Respiratory: Abnormal smell, hiccups, pharyngitis

Miscellaneous: Multiorgan failure, speech disturbances

<1% (Limited to important or life-threatening): Mild allergic reactions (mild rash, eosinophilia)

Drug Interactions

Metabolism/Transport Effects None known.

Avoid Concomitant Use There are no known interactions where it is recommended to avoid concomitant use.

Increased Effect/Toxicity There are no known significant interactions involving an increase in effect.

Decreased Effect There are no known significant interactions involving a decrease in effect.

Ethanol/Nutrition/Herb Interactions Ethanol: Ethanol decreases the rate of fomepizole elimination by ~50%; conversely, fomepizole decreases the rate of elimination of ethanol by ~40%.

Stability Store at controlled room temperature, 20°C to 25°C (68°F to 77°F); fomepizole solidifies at temperatures <25°C (77°F). If solution becomes solid in the vial, it be should be carefully warmed by running the vial under warm water or by holding in the hand. Solidification does not affect the efficacy, safety, or stability of the drug.

Prior to administration, dilute in at least 100 mL 0.9% sodium chloride or dextrose 5% water for injection; diluted solution is stable for at least 24 hours when stored refrigerated or at room temperature. Although, it is chemically and physically stable when diluted as recommended, sterile precautions should be observed because diluents generally do not contain preservatives.

Mechanism of Action Fomepizole competitively inhibits alcohol dehydrogenase, an enzyme which catalyzes the metabolism of ethanol, ethylene glycol, and methanol to their toxic metabolites. Ethylene glycol is metabolized to glycoaldehyde, then oxidized to glycolate, glyoxylate, and oxalate. Glycolate and oxalate are responsible for metabolic acidosis and renal damage. Methanol is metabolized to formaldehyde, then oxidized to formic acid. Formic acid is responsible for metabolic acidosis and visual disturbances.

Pharmacodynamics/Kinetics

Onset of effect: Peak effect: Maximum: 1.5-2 hours

Absorption: Oral: Readily absorbed

Distribution: V_d: 0.6-1.02 L/kg; rapidly into total body water

Protein binding: Negligible

Metabolism: Hepatic to 4-carboxypyrazole (80% to 85% of dose), 4-hydroxymethylpyrazole, and their N-glucuronide conjugates; following multiple doses, induces its own metabolism via CYP oxidases after 30-40 hours

Half-life elimination: Has not been calculated; varies with dose

Excretion: Urine (1% to 3.5% as unchanged drug and metabolites)

Dosage Note: Fomepizole therapy should begin immediately upon suspicion of ethylene glycol or methanol ingestion.

Children (unlabeled use) and Adults: Ethylene glycol and methanol toxicity: I.V.: A loading dose of 15 mg/kg should be administered, followed by doses of 10 mg/kg every 12 hours for 4 doses, then 15 mg/kg every 12 hours thereafter until ethylene glycol levels have been reduced <20 mg/dL and patient is asymptomatic with normal pH

Dosage adjustment in renal impairment: I.V.: The manufacturer provides the following dosage recommendations:

Dose at the beginning of hemodialysis:

If <6 hours since last fomepizole dose: Do not administer dose

If ≥6 hours since last fomepizole dose: Administer next scheduled dose

Dosing during hemodialysis: Dose every 4 hours

Dosing at the time hemodialysis is complete, based on time between last dose and the end of hemodialysis:

<1 hour: Do not administer dose at the end of hemodialysis

1-3 hours: Administer 1/2 of next scheduled dose

>3 hours: Administer next scheduled dose

Maintenance dose when off hemodialysis: Give next scheduled dose 12 hours from last dose administered.

Alternatively, a loading dose of 10-20 mg/kg followed by 1-1.5 mg/kg/hour continuous infusion during hemodialysis has been described in case reports (Jobard, 1996).

Dosage adjustment in hepatic impairment: Fomepizole is metabolized in the liver; specific dosage adjustments have not been determined in patients with hepatic impairment

Administration The appropriate dose of fomepizole should be drawn from the vial with a syringe and injected into at least 100 mL of sterile 0.9% sodium chloride injection or dextrose 5% injection. All doses should be administered as a slow intravenous infusion (IVPB) over 30 minutes.

Monitoring Parameters Fomepizole plasma levels should be monitored; response to fomepizole; monitor plasma/urinary ethylene glycol or methanol levels, urinary oxalate (ethylene glycol), plasma/urinary osmolality, renal/hepatic function, serum electrolytes, arterial blood gases; anion and osmolar gaps, resolution of clinical signs and symptoms of ethylene glycol or methanol intoxication

Reference Range The manufacturer recommends concentrations 100-300 micromole/L (8.2-24.6 mg/L) to achieve enzyme inhibition of alcohol dehydrogenase; according to practice guidelines, serum fomepizole concentrations of ≥0.8 mg/L provide constant inhibition of alcohol dehydrogenase

Dosage Forms Excipient information presented when available (limited, particularly for generics); consult specific product labeling.

Injection, solution [preservative free]: 1 g/mL (1.5 mL)

Antizol®: 1 g/mL (1.5 mL)

Fondaparinux (fon da PARE i nuks)

Brand Names: U.S. Arixtra®

Brand Names: Canada Arixtra®

Index Terms Fondaparinux Sodium

Pharmacologic Category Factor Xa Inhibitor

Use Prophylaxis of deep vein thrombosis (DVT) in patients undergoing surgery for hip replacement, knee replacement, hip fracture (including extended prophylaxis following hip fracture surgery), or abdominal surgery (in patients at risk for thromboembolic complications); treatment of acute pulmonary embolism (PE); treatment of acute DVT without PE

Canadian labeling: Additional uses (not approved in U.S.): Unstable angina or non-ST segment elevation myocardial infarction (UA/NSTEMI) for the prevention of death and subsequent MI; ST segment elevation MI (STEMI) for the prevention of death and myocardial reinfarction

Unlabeled Use Prophylaxis of DVT in patients with a history of heparin-induced thrombocytopenia (HIT)

Pregnancy Risk Factor B

Pregnancy Considerations Reproductive animal studies have not shown fetal harm. Based on case reports, small amounts of fondaparinux have been detected in the umbilical cord following multiple doses during pregnancy. There are no adequate and well-controlled studies in pregnant women; use only if clearly needed.

Lactation Excretion in breast milk unknown/use caution

Contraindications Hypersensitivity to fondaparinux or any component of the formulation; severe renal impairment (Cl_{cr} <30 mL/minute); body weight <50 kg (prophylaxis); active major bleeding; bacterial endocarditis; thrombocytopenia associated with a positive *in vitro* test for antiplatelet antibody in the presence of fondaparinux

Warnings/Precautions **[U.S. Boxed Warning]: Spinal or epidural hematomas, including subsequent paralysis, may occur with recent or anticipated neuraxial anesthesia (epidural or spinal anesthesia) or spinal puncture in patients anticoagulated with LMWH,**

heparinoids, or fondaparinux. Consider risk versus benefit prior to spinal procedures; risk is increased by the use of concomitant agents which may alter hemostasis, the use of indwelling epidural catheters for analgesia, a history of spinal deformity or spinal surgery, as well as a history of traumatic or repeated epidural or spinal punctures. Patient should be observed closely for bleeding and signs and symptoms of neurological impairment if therapy is administered during or immediately following diagnostic lumbar puncture, epidural anesthesia, or spinal anesthesia.

Not to be used interchangeably (unit-for-unit) with heparin, low molecular weight heparins (LMWHs), or heparinoids. Use caution in patients with moderate renal dysfunction (Cl_{cr} 30-50 mL/minute); contraindicated in patients with Cl_{cr} <30 mL/minute. Discontinue if severe dysfunction or labile function develops.

Use caution in congenital or acquired bleeding disorders; bacterial endocarditis; renal impairment; hepatic impairment; active ulcerative or angiodysplastic gastrointestinal disease; hemorrhagic stroke; shortly after brain, spinal, or ophthalmologic surgery; or in patients taking platelet inhibitors. Risk of major bleeding may be increased if initial dose is administered earlier than recommended (initiation recommended at 6-8 hours following surgery). Discontinue agents that may enhance the risk of hemorrhage if possible. Although considered an insensitive measure of fondaparinux activity, there have been postmarketing reports of bleeding associated with elevated aPTT. Thrombocytopenia has occurred with administration, including reports of thrombocytopenia with thrombosis similar to heparin-induced thrombocytopenia. Monitor patients closely and discontinue therapy if platelets fall to <100,000/mm³.

For subcutaneous administration; not for I.M. administration. Do not use interchangeably (unit for unit) with low molecular weight heparins, heparin, or heparinoids. Use caution in patients <50 kg who are being treated for DVT/PE; dosage reduction recommended. Contraindicated in patients <50 kg when used for prophylactic therapy. Use with caution in the elderly. The needle guard contains natural latex rubber.

The administration of fondaparinux is **not recommended** prior to and during primary PCI in patients with STEMI, due to an increased risk for guiding-catheter thrombosis. Patients with UA/NSTEMI or STEMI undergoing any PCI should not receive fondaparinux as the sole anticoagulant. Use of an anticoagulant with antithrombin activity (eg, unfractionated heparin) is recommended as adjunctive therapy to PCI even if prior treatment with fondaparinux (must take into account whether GP IIb/IIIa antagonists have been administered) (Levine, 2011). Do not administer with other agents that increase the risk of hemorrhage unless they are essential for the management of the underlying condition (eg, warfarin for treatment of VTE).

Adverse Reactions As with all anticoagulants, bleeding is the major adverse effect. Hemorrhage may occur at any site. Risk appears increased by a number of factors including renal dysfunction, age (>75 years), and weight (<50 kg).

>10%:
- Central nervous system: Fever (4% to 14%)
- Gastrointestinal: Nausea (3% to 11%)
- Hematologic: Anemia (1% to 20%)

1% to 10%:
- Cardiovascular: Edema (9%), hypotension (4%), hypertension (2%), chest pain (1%), thrombosis PCI catheter (without heparin 1%)
- Central nervous system: Insomnia (4% to 5%), headache (2% to 5%), dizziness (4%), confusion (3%), pain (2%), anxiety (1%)
- Dermatologic: Rash (8%), purpura (4%), bullous eruption (3%), bruising (1%)
- Endocrine & metabolic: Hypokalemia (1% to 4%)
- Gastrointestinal: Constipation (5% to 9%), vomiting (1% to 6%), diarrhea (2% to 3%), dyspepsia (2%), abdominal pain (1%)
- Genitourinary: Urinary tract infection (2% to 4%), urinary retention (3%)
- Hematologic: Minor bleeding (2% to 4%), moderate thrombocytopenia (50,000-100,000/mm³: 3%), hematoma (3%), major bleeding (1% to 3%), prothrombin decreased (1%), risk of major bleeding increased as high as 5% in patients receiving initial dose <6 hours following surgery
- Hepatic: ALT increased (≤3%), AST increased (≤2%)
- Local: Injection site reaction (bleeding, rash, pruritus)
- Neuromuscular & skeletal: Back pain (1%), leg pain (1%)
- Respiratory: Cough (2%), pneumonia (2%), epistaxis (1%)
- Miscellaneous: Wound drainage increased (5%)

<1% (Limited to important or life-threatening): aPTT increased (associated with bleeding), heparin-induced thrombocytopenia (1 case report), hepatic dysfunction, severe thrombocytopenia (<50,000/mm³)

Drug Interactions

Metabolism/Transport Effects None known.

Avoid Concomitant Use

Avoid concomitant use of Fondaparinux with any of the following: Rivaroxaban

Increased Effect/Toxicity

Fondaparinux may increase the levels/effects of: Anticoagulants; Collagenase (Systemic); Deferasirox; Ibritumomab; Rivaroxaban; Tositumomab and Iodine I 131 Tositumomab

The levels/effects of Fondaparinux may be increased by: Antiplatelet Agents; Dasatinib; Drotrecogin Alfa (Activated); Herbs (Anticoagulant/Antiplatelet Properties); Nonsteroidal Anti-Inflammatory Agents; Pentosan Polysulfate Sodium; Prostacyclin Analogues; Salicylates; Thrombolytic Agents

Decreased Effect There are no known significant interactions involving a decrease in effect.

Ethanol/Nutrition/Herb Interactions Herb/Nutraceutical: Avoid alfalfa, anise, bilberry, bladderwrack, bromelain, cat's claw, celery, coleus, cordyceps, dong quai, evening primrose oil, fenugreek, feverfew, garlic, ginger, ginkgo biloba, ginseng (American/Panax/Siberian), grapeseed, green tea, guggul, horse chestnut seed, horseradish, licorice, prickly ash, red clover, reishi, sweet clover, turmeric, white willow (all possess anticoagulant or antiplatelet activity and as such, may enhance the anticoagulant effects of fondaparinux).

Stability Store at 25°C (77°F); excursions permitted to 15°C to 30°C (59°F to 86°F).

Canadian labeling: For I.V. administration: May mix with 25 mL or 50 mL NS; manufacturer recommends immediate use once diluted in NS, but is stable for up to 24 hours at 15°C to 30°C (59°F to 86°F).

Mechanism of Action Fondaparinux is a synthetic pentasaccharide that causes an antithrombin III-mediated selective inhibition of factor Xa. Neutralization of factor Xa interrupts the blood coagulation cascade and inhibits thrombin formation and thrombus development.

Pharmacodynamics/Kinetics

- Absorption: SubQ: Rapid and complete
- Distribution: V_d: 7-11 L; mainly in blood
- Protein binding: ≥94% to antithrombin III
- Bioavailability: SubQ: 100%
- Half-life elimination: 17-21 hours; prolonged with renal impairment
- Time to peak: SubQ: 2-3 hours
- Excretion: Urine (~77%, unchanged drug)

Dosage SubQ: Adults:

DVT prophylaxis: Adults ≥50 kg: 2.5 mg once daily. **Note:** Prophylactic use contraindicated in patients <50 kg. Initiate dose after hemostasis has been established, 6-8 hours postoperatively.

DVT prophylaxis with history of HIT (unlabeled use): 2.5 mg once daily

Usual duration: 5-9 days (up to 10 days following abdominal surgery or up to 11 days following hip replacement or knee replacement)

Extended prophylaxis is recommended following hip fracture surgery (has been tolerated for up to 32 days total).

Acute DVT/PE treatment: **Note:** Start warfarin on the first treatment day and continue fondaparinux until INR is between 2 and 3 (usually 5-7 days) (Hirsh, 2008):

<50 kg: 5 mg once daily

50-100 kg: 7.5 mg once daily

>100 kg: 10 mg once daily

Usual duration: 5-9 days (has been administered up to 26 days)

Canadian labeling only: Adults:

UA/NSTEMI: SubQ: 2.5 mg once daily; initiate as soon as possible after diagnosis; treat for up to 8 days or until hospital discharge.

STEMI: I.V.: 2.5 mg once; subsequent doses: SubQ: 2.5 mg once daily; treat for up to 8 days or until hospital discharge

Dosage adjustment in renal impairment:

Cl_{cr} 30-50 mL/minute: Use caution

Cl_{cr} <30 mL/minute: Contraindicated

Dosage adjustment in hepatic impairment:

Mild-to-moderate impairment: Dosage adjustment not required; monitor for signs of bleeding

Severe impairment: No data

Administration Do **not** administer I.M.; for SubQ administration only. Do not mix with other injections or infusions. Do not expel air bubble from syringe before injection. Administer according to recommended regimen; early initiation (before 6 hours after surgery) has been associated with increased bleeding.

To convert from I.V. unfractionated heparin (UFH) infusion to SubQ fondaparinux (Nutescu, 2007): Calculate specific dose for fondaparinux based on indication, discontinue UFH, and begin fondaparinux within 1 hour

To convert from SubQ fondaparinux to I.V. UFH infusion (Nutescu, 2007): Discontinue fondaparinux; calculate specific dose for I.V. UFH infusion based on indication; omit heparin bolus/loading dose

For subQ fondaparinux dosed every 24 hours: Start I.V. UFH infusion 22-23 hours after last dose of fondaparinux

Canadian labeling only: STEMI patients: I.V. push or mixed in 25-50 mL of NS and infused over 2 minutes. Flush tubing with NS after infusion to ensure complete administration of fondaparinux. Infusion bag should not be mixed with other agents.

Monitoring Parameters Periodic monitoring of CBC, serum creatinine, occult blood testing of stools recommended. Anti-Xa activity of fondaparinux can be measured by the assay if fondaparinux is used as the calibrator. PT and aPTT are insensitive measures of fondaparinux activity. If unexpected changes in coagulation parameters or major bleeding occur, discontinue fondaparinux (elevated aPTT associated with bleeding events have been reported in postmarketing data).

Test Interactions International standards of heparin or LMWH are not the appropriate calibrators for antifactor Xa activity of fondaparinux.

Dosage Forms Excipient information presented when available (limited, particularly for generics); consult specific product labeling.

Injection, solution, as sodium [preservative free]: 2.5 mg/0.5 mL (0.5 mL); 5 mg/0.4 mL (0.4 mL); 7.5 mg/0.6 mL (0.6 mL); 10 mg/0.8 mL (0.8 mL)

Arixtra®: 2.5 mg/0.5 mL (0.5 mL); 5 mg/0.4 mL (0.4 mL); 7.5 mg/0.6 mL (0.6 mL); 10 mg/0.8 mL (0.8 mL)

◆ **Fondaparinux Sodium** *see* Fondaparinux *on page 752*

◆ **Foradil® (Can)** *see* Formoterol *on page 754*

◆ **Foradil® Aerolizer®** *see* Formoterol *on page 754*

Formoterol (for MOH te rol)

Brand Names: U.S. Foradil® Aerolizer®; Perforomist®

Brand Names: Canada Foradil®; Oxeze® Turbuhaler®

Index Terms Formoterol Fumarate; Formoterol Fumarate Dihydrate

Pharmacologic Category $Beta_2$-Adrenergic Agonist; $Beta_2$-Adrenergic Agonist, Long-Acting

Additional Appendix Information

Bronchodilators *on page 1886*

Use Maintenance treatment of asthma and prevention of bronchospasm (as concomitant therapy) in patients ≥5 years of age with reversible obstructive airway disease, including patients with symptoms of nocturnal asthma; maintenance treatment of bronchoconstriction in patients with COPD; prevention of exercise-induced bronchospasm in patients ≥5 years of age (monotherapy may be indicated in patients without persistent asthma)

Canadian labeling: Oxeze®: Also approved for acute relief of symptoms ("on demand" treatment) in patients ≥6 years of age

Pregnancy Risk Factor C

Pregnancy Considerations When given orally to rats throughout organogenesis, formoterol caused delayed ossification and decreased fetal weight, but no malformations. There were no adverse events when given to pregnant rats in late pregnancy. Doses used were ≥70 times the recommended daily inhalation dose in humans. There are no adequate and well-controlled studies in pregnant women. Use only if benefit outweighs risk to the fetus. Beta-agonists interfere with uterine contractility so use during labor only if benefit outweighs risk to the fetus.

Lactation Excretion in breast milk unknown/use caution

Medication Guide Available Yes

Contraindications Hypersensitivity to formoterol or any component of the formulation (Foradil® only); monotherapy in the treatment of asthma (ie, use without a concomitant long-term asthma control medication, such as an inhaled corticosteroid)

Canadian labeling: Oxeze®: Hypersensitivity to formoterol, inhaled lactose, or any component of the formulation; presence of tachyarrhythmias

Warnings/Precautions [U.S. Boxed Warning]: Long-acting $beta_2$-agonists (LABAs) increase the risk of asthma-related deaths. Formoterol should only be used in asthma patients as adjuvant therapy in patients who are currently receiving but are not adequately controlled on a long-term asthma control medication (ie, an inhaled corticosteroid). Monotherapy with an LABA is contraindicated in the treatment of asthma. In a large, randomized, placebo-controlled U.S. clinical trial (SMART, 2006), salmeterol was associated with an increase in asthma-related deaths (when added to usual asthma therapy); risk is considered a class effect among all LABAs. Data are not available to determine if the addition of an inhaled corticosteroid lessens this increased risk of death associated with LABA use. Assess patients at regular intervals once asthma control is maintained on combination therapy to determine if step-down therapy is appropriate and the LABA can be discontinued (without loss of asthma control), and the patient can be maintained on an inhaled corticosteroid. LABAs are not appropriate in patients whose asthma is adequately controlled on low- or medium-dose inhaled corticosteroids. Do **not** use for acute bronchospasm. Short-acting beta$_2$-agonist (eg, albuterol) should be used for acute symptoms and symptoms occurring between treatments. Do **not** initiate in patients with significantly worsening or acutely deteriorating asthma; reports of severe (sometimes fatal) respiratory events have been reported when formoterol has been initiated in this situation. Corticosteroids should not be stopped or reduced when formoterol is initiated. Formoterol is not a substitute for inhaled or systemic corticosteroids and should not be used as monotherapy. During initiation, watch for signs of worsening asthma. **[U.S. Boxed Warning]: LABAs may increase the risk of asthma-related hospitalization in pediatric and adolescent patients.** In general, a combination product containing a LABA and an inhaled corticosteroid is preferred in patients <18 years of age to ensure compliance.

Because LABAs may disguise poorly controlled persistent asthma, frequent or chronic use of LABAs for exercise-induced bronchospasm is discouraged by the NIH Asthma Guidelines (NIH, 2007). The safety and efficacy of Perforomist™ in the treatment of asthma have not been established. Oxeze® is a formulation of formoterol (available outside the U.S. [eg, Canada]) approved for acute treatment of asthmatic symptoms. The labelings for U.S. approved formulations (Foradil®, Perforomist™) state that formoterol is not meant to relieve acute asthmatic symptoms.

Do **not** use for acute episodes of COPD. Do **not** initiate in patients with significantly worsening or acutely deteriorating COPD. Data are not available to determine if LABA use increases the risk of death in patients with COPD. Increased use and/or ineffectiveness of short-acting beta$_2$-agonists may indicate rapidly deteriorating disease and should prompt re-evaluation of the patient's condition.

Immediate hypersensitivity reactions (urticaria, angioedema, rash, bronchospasm) have been reported. Do not exceed recommended dose or frequency; serious adverse events (including serious asthma exacerbations and fatalities) have been associated with excessive use of inhaled sympathomimetics. Beta$_2$-agonists may increase risk of arrhythmias, decrease serum potassium, prolong QT_c interval, or increase serum glucose. These effects may be exacerbated in hypoxemia. Use caution in patients with cardiovascular disease (arrhythmia, coronary insufficiency, hypertension, or HF), seizures, diabetes, hyperthyroidism, or hypokalemia. Beta-agonists may cause elevation in blood pressure and heart rate, and result in CNS stimulation/excitation. Tolerance to the bronchodilator effect, measured by FEV_1, has been observed in studies.

Powder for oral inhalation contains lactose; very rare anaphylactic reactions have been reported in patients with severe milk protein allergy. The contents of the Foradil® capsules are for inhalation via the Aerolizer™ device. There have been reports of incorrect administration (swallowing of the capsules).

Adverse Reactions

1% to 10%:

- Cardiovascular: Chest pain (2% to 3%), palpitation
- Central nervous system: Anxiety (2%), dizziness (2%), fever (2%), insomnia (2%), dysphonia (1%), headache
- Dermatologic: Pruritus (2%), rash (1%)
- Gastrointestinal: Diarrhea (5%), nausea (5%), xerostomia (1% to 3%), vomiting (2%), abdominal pain, dyspepsia, gastroenteritis
- Neuromuscular & skeletal: Muscle cramps (2%), tremor
- Respiratory: Infection (3% to 7%), asthma exacerbation (age 5-12 years: 5% to 6%; age >12 years: <4%), bronchitis (5%), pharyngitis (3% to 4%), sinusitis (3%), dyspnea (2%), tonsillitis (1%)

<1% (Limited to important or life-threatening): Acute asthma deterioration, anaphylactic reactions (severe hypotension/angioedema), agitation, angina, arrhythmia, bronchospasm (paradoxical), fatigue, hyperglycemia, hypertension, hypokalemia, glucose intolerance, malaise, metabolic acidosis, nervousness, tachycardia

Drug Interactions

Metabolism/Transport Effects Substrate of CYP2C9 (minor); **Note:** Assignment of Major/Minor substrate status based on clinically relevant drug interaction potential

Avoid Concomitant Use

Avoid concomitant use of Formoterol with any of the following: Beta-Blockers (Nonselective); Iobenguane I 123

Increased Effect/Toxicity

Formoterol may increase the levels/effects of: Loop Diuretics; Sympathomimetics; Thiazide Diuretics

The levels/effects of Formoterol may be increased by: Atomoxetine; Caffeine; Cannabinoids; MAO Inhibitors; Theophylline Derivatives; Tricyclic Antidepressants

Decreased Effect

Formoterol may decrease the levels/effects of: Iobenguane I 123

The levels/effects of Formoterol may be decreased by: Alpha-/Beta-Blockers; Beta-Blockers (Beta1 Selective); Beta-Blockers (Nonselective); Betahistine

Stability

Foradil®: Prior to dispensing, store in refrigerator at 2°C to 8°C (36°F to 46°F). After dispensing, store at room temperature at 20°C to 25°C (68°F to 77°F). Protect from heat and moisture. Capsules should always be stored in the blister and only removed immediately before use. Always check expiration date. Use within 4 months of purchase date or product expiration date, whichever comes first.

Perforomist™: Prior to dispensing, store in refrigerator at 2°C to 8°C (36°F to 46°F). After dispensing, store at 2°C to 25°C (36°F to 77°F) for up to 3 months. Protect from heat. Unit-dose vials should always be stored in the foil pouch and only removed immediately before use.

Mechanism of Action Relaxes bronchial smooth muscle by selective action on beta$_2$ receptors with little effect on heart rate. Formoterol has a long-acting effect.

Pharmacodynamics/Kinetics

Onset of action: Powder for inhalation: Within 3 minutes

Peak effect: Powder for inhalation: 80% of peak effect within 15 minutes; Solution for nebulization: 2 hours

Duration: Improvement in FEV_1 observed for 12 hours in most patients

Absorption: Rapidly into plasma

Protein binding: 61% to 64% *in vitro* at higher concentrations than achieved with usual dosing

Metabolism: Hepatic via direct glucuronidation and O-demethylation; CYP2D6, CYP2C8/9, CYP2C19, CYP2A6 involved in O-demethylation

Half-life elimination: Powder: ~10-14 hours; Nebulized solution: ~7 hours

Time to peak: Maximum improvement in FEV_1 in 1-3 hours

Excretion:

- Children 5-12 years: Urine (7% to 9% as direct glucuronide metabolites, 6% as unchanged drug)
- Adults: Urine (15% to 18% as direct glucuronide metabolites, 2% to 10% as unchanged drug)

Dosage

Asthma maintenance treatment: Children ≥5 years and Adults: Inhalation: **Note:** For asthma control, long-acting beta$_2$-agonists (LABAs) should be used in combination with inhaled corticosteroids and **not** as monotherapy

Foradil®: 12 mcg capsule inhaled every 12 hours via Aerolizer™ device (maximum: 24 mcg/day)

Oxeze® (CAN): **Note:** Not labeled for use in the U.S.: Children ≥6 years and Adults: Inhalation: 6 mcg or 12 mcg every 12 hours (maximum dose: Children: 24 mcg/day; Adults: 48 mcg/day)

Prevention of exercise-induced bronchospasm: Children ≥5 years and Adults: Inhalation:

Foradil®:12 mcg capsule inhaled via Aerolizer™ device at least 15 minutes before exercise on an "as needed" basis; additional doses should not be used for another 12 hours. **Note:** If already using for asthma maintenance, then should not use additional doses for exercise-induced bronchospasm. Because LABAs may disguise poorly controlled persistent asthma, frequent or chronic use of LABAs for exercise-induced bronchospasm is discouraged by the NIH Asthma Guidelines (NIH, 2007).

Oxeze® (CAN): **Note:** Not labeled for use in the U.S.: Children ≥6 years and Adults: Inhalation: 6 mcg or 12 mcg at least 15 minutes before exercise.

COPD maintenance treatment: Adults: Inhalation:

Foradil®: 12 mcg capsule inhaled every 12 hours via Aerolizer™ device (maximum: 24 mcg/day)

Perforomist™: 20 mcg unit-dose vial twice daily (maximum dose: 40 mcg/day)

Additional indication for Oxeze® (approved in Canada): Acute ("on demand") relief of bronchoconstriction: Children ≥12 years and Adults: 6 mcg or 12 mcg as a single dose (maximum dose: Children: 48 mcg/24-hour period; Adults: 72 mcg/24-hour period). The prolonged use of high dosages (48 mcg/day for ≥3 consecutive days) may be a sign of suboptimal control, and should prompt the re-evaluation of therapy.

Administration

Foradil®: Remove capsule from foil blister **immediately** before use. Place capsule in the capsule-chamber in the base of the Aerolizer™ Inhaler. Must only use the Aerolizer™ Inhaler. Press both buttons **once only** and then release. Keep inhaler in a level, horizontal position. Exhale fully. Do not exhale into inhaler. Tilt head slightly back and inhale (rapidly, steadily, and deeply). Hold breath as long as possible. If any powder remains in capsule, exhale and inhale again. Repeat until capsule is empty. Throw away empty capsule; do not leave in inhaler. Do not use a spacer with the Aerolizer™ Inhaler. Always keep capsules and inhaler dry.

Perforomist™: Remove unit-dose vial from foil pouch **immediately** before use. Solution does not require dilution prior to administration; do not mix other medications with formoterol solution. Place contents of unit-dose vial into the reservoir of a standard jet nebulizer connected to an air compressor; assemble nebulizer based on the manufacturer's instructions and turn nebulizer on; breathe deeply and evenly until all of the medication has been inhaled. Discard any unused medication immediately; do not ingest contents of vial. Clean nebulizer after use.

Oxeze® Turbuhaler® [CAN; not available in U.S.]: Hold inhaler upright. Turn colored grip as far as it will go in one direction and then turn back to original position; a clicking sound should be heard which means the inhaler is ready for use. Exhale fully. Do not exhale into mouthpiece of inhaler. Place mouthpiece to lips and inhale forcefully and deeply. Do not chew or bite on mouthpiece. Clean outside of mouthpiece once weekly with a dry tissue. Avoid getting inhaler wet.

Monitoring Parameters FEV_1, peak flow, and/or other pulmonary function tests; blood pressure, heart rate; CNS stimulation; serum glucose, serum potassium

Dosage Forms Excipient information presented when available (limited, particularly for generics); consult specific product labeling.

Powder, for oral inhalation, as fumarate:

Foradil® Aerolizer®: 12 mcg/capsule (12s, 60s) [contains lactose 25 mg/capsule]

Solution, for nebulization, as fumarate dihydrate:

Perforomist®: 20 mcg/2 mL (60s)

Dosage Forms: Canada Excipient information presented when available (limited, particularly for generics); consult specific product labeling.

Powder for oral inhalation, as fumarate:

Oxeze® Turbuhaler®: 6 mcg/inhalation [delivers 60 metered doses; contains lactose 600 mcg/dose]; 12 mcg/inhalation [delivers 60 metered doses; contains lactose 600 mcg/dose]

◆ **Formoterol and Budesonide** *see* Budesonide and Formoterol *on page* 240

◆ **Formoterol and Mometasone** *see* Mometasone and Formoterol *on page* 1151

◆ **Formoterol and Mometasone Furoate** *see* Mometasone and Formoterol *on page* 1151

◆ **Formoterol Fumarate** *see* Formoterol *on page* 754

◆ **Formoterol Fumarate Dihydrate** *see* Formoterol *on page* 754

◆ **Formoterol Fumarate Dihydrate and Budesonide** *see* Budesonide and Formoterol *on page* 240

◆ **Formoterol Fumarate Dihydrate and Mometasone** *see* Mometasone and Formoterol *on page* 1151

◆ **Formulex® (Can)** *see* Dicyclomine *on page* 499

◆ **5-Formyl Tetrahydrofolate** *see* Leucovorin Calcium *on page* 987

◆ **Fortamet®** *see* MetFORMIN *on page* 1086

◆ **Fortaz®** *see* CefTAZidime *on page* 315

◆ **Forteo®** *see* Teriparatide *on page* 1651

◆ **Fortesta™** *see* Testosterone *on page* 1654

◆ **Fortical®** *see* Calcitonin *on page* 262

◆ **Fosamax®** *see* Alendronate *on page* 61

◆ **Fosamax Plus D®** *see* Alendronate and Cholecalciferol *on page* 62

Fosamprenavir (FOS am pren a veer)

Brand Names: U.S. Lexiva®

Brand Names: Canada Telzir®

Index Terms Fosamprenavir Calcium; GW433908G

Pharmacologic Category Antiretroviral Agent, Protease Inhibitor

Additional Appendix Information

Management of Healthcare Worker Exposures to HBV, HCV, and HIV *on page* 1935

Perinatal HIV Guidelines *on page* 1946

Use Treatment of HIV infections in combination with at least two other antiretroviral agents

Pregnancy Risk Factor C

Pregnancy Considerations Adverse events were observed in some animal reproduction studies. It is not known if fosamprenavir crosses the human placenta. A small increased risk of preterm birth has been associated with maternal use of protease inhibitor-based combination antiretroviral (ARV) therapy during pregnancy; however, the benefits of use generally outweigh this risk and protease inhibitors (PIs) should not be withheld if otherwise recommended. Hyperglycemia, new onset of diabetes mellitus, or diabetic ketoacidosis have been reported with PIs; it is not clear if pregnancy increases this risk. The DHHS Perinatal HIV Guidelines note there are insufficient data to recommend use during pregnancy; however, if used, they recommend that fosamprenavir be given with low-dose ritonavir boosting.

Regardless of CD4 count or HIV RNA copy number, all HIV-infected pregnant women should receive a combination antepartum ARV drug regimen; this includes women who require therapy for their own health, as well as women who do not yet require therapy for their own health. ARV therapy should be started as soon as possible if required for the woman's health or immediately after the first trimester if not needed for the mothers health (although earlier initiation may be considered). Long-term follow-up is recommended for all infants exposed to ARV medications.

Healthcare providers are encouraged to enroll pregnant women exposed to antiretroviral medications in the Antiretroviral Pregnancy Registry (1-800-258-4263 or www.-APRegistry.com). Healthcare providers caring for HIV-infected women and their infants may contact the National Perinatal HIV Hotline (888-448-8765) for clinical consultation (DHHS [perinatal], 2011).

Lactation Excretion in breast milk unknown/contraindicated

Contraindications Clinically-significant hypersensitivity (eg, Stevens-Johnson syndrome) to fosamprenavir, amprenavir, or any component of the formulation; concurrent therapy with CYP3A4 substrates with a narrow therapeutic window; concomitant use with alfuzosin, cisapride, delavirdine, ergot derivatives, lovastatin, midazolam, pimozide, rifampin, simvastatin, St John's wort, and triazolam; use of flecainide and propafenone with concomitant ritonavir therapy; sildenafil (when used for pulmonary artery hypertension [eg, Revatio®])

Warnings/Precautions Use with caution in patients taking strong CYP3A4 inhibitors, moderate or strong CYP3A4 inducers, and major CYP3A4 substrates (see Drug Interactions); consider alternative agents that avoid or lessen the potential for CYP-mediated interactions. Do not use with hormonal contraceptives. Do not coadminister colchicine in patient with renal or hepatic impairment; avoid concurrent use with salmeterol.

Use with caution in patients with diabetes mellitus or sulfonamide allergy. Use caution with hepatic impairment (dosage adjustment required) or underlying hepatitis B or C. Redistribution of fat may occur (eg, buffalo hump, peripheral wasting, cushingoid appearance). Dosage adjustment is required for combination therapies (ritonavir and/or efavirenz); in addition, the risk of hyperlipidemia may be increased during concurrent therapy. Protease inhibitors have been associated with a variety of hypersensitivity events (some severe), including rash, anaphylaxis (rare), angioedema, bronchospasm, erythema multiforme, and/or Stevens-Johnson syndrome (rare). It is generally recommended to discontinue treatment if severe rash or moderate symptoms accompanied by other systemic symptoms occur. Acute hemolytic anemia has been reported in association with amprenavir use. Cases of nephrolithiasis have been reported in postmarketing surveillance; temporary or permanent discontinuation of therapy should be considered if symptoms develop. Spontaneous bleeding has been reported in patients with hemophilia A or B following treatment with protease inhibitors; use caution. Immune reconstitution syndrome may develop resulting in the occurrence of an inflammatory response to an indolent or residual opportunistic infection; further evaluation and treatment may be necessary. Safety and efficacy have not been established in children <2 years of age.

Adverse Reactions

>10%:

Dermatologic: Rash (≤19%; onset: ~11 days; duration: ~13 days)

Endocrine & metabolic: Hypertriglyceridemia (>750 mg/dL: ≤11%)

Gastrointestinal: Diarrhea (moderate-to-severe; 5% to 13%)

1% to 10%:

Central nervous system: Headache (moderate-to-severe; 2% to 4%), fatigue (moderate-to-severe; 2% to 4%)

Dermatologic: Pruritus (7% to 8%)

Endocrine & metabolic: Hyperglycemia (>251 mg/dL: ≤2%)

Gastrointestinal: Serum lipase increased (>2 times ULN: 5% to 8%), nausea (moderate-to-severe; 3% to 7%), vomiting (moderate-to-severe; 2% to 6%), abdominal pain (moderate-to-severe; ≤2%)

Hematologic: Neutropenia (<750 cells/mm^3: 3%)

Hepatic: Transaminases increased (>5 times ULN: 4% to 8%)

<1% (Limited to important or life-threatening): Angioedema, hypercholesterolemia, myocardial infarction, nephrolithiasis, oral paresthesia, QT prolongation (with amprenavir), Stevens-Johnson syndrome, stroke

Frequency not defined: Diabetes mellitus, fat redistribution, and immune reconstitution syndrome have been associated with protease inhibitor therapy. Spontaneous bleeding has been reported in patients with hemophilia A or B following treatment with protease inhibitors. Acute hemolytic anemia has been reported in association with amprenavir use.

Drug Interactions

Metabolism/Transport Effects Substrate of CYP2C9 (minor), CYP2D6 (minor), CYP3A4 (major), P-glycoprotein; **Note:** Assignment of Major/Minor substrate status based on clinically relevant drug interaction potential; **Inhibits** CYP2C19 (weak), CYP3A4 (strong)

Avoid Concomitant Use

Avoid concomitant use of Fosamprenavir with any of the following: Alfuzosin; Amiodarone; Cisapride; Conivaptan; Crizotinib; Delavirdine; Dronedarone; Eplerenone; Ergot Derivatives; Etravirine; Everolimus; Fluticasone (Oral Inhalation); Halofantrine; Lapatinib; Lovastatin; Lurasidone; Midazolam; Nilotinib; Nisoldipine; Pimozide; QuiNIDine; Ranolazine; Rifampin; Rivaroxaban; RomiDEPsin; Salmeterol; Silodosin; Simvastatin; St Johns Wort; Tamsulosin; Telaprevir; Ticagrelor; Tolvaptan; Toremifene; Triazolam

Increased Effect/Toxicity

Fosamprenavir may increase the levels/effects of: Alfuzosin; Almotriptan; Alosetron; ALPRAZolam; Amiodarone; Antifungal Agents (Azole Derivatives, Systemic); ARIPiprazole; Bortezomib; Brentuximab Vedotin; Brinzolamide; Budesonide (Nasal); Budesonide (Systemic, Oral Inhalation); Calcium Channel Blockers (Dihydropyridine); Calcium Channel Blockers (Nondihydropyridine); CarBAMazepine; Ciclesonide; Cisapride; Clarithromycin; Clorazepate; Colchicine; Conivaptan; Corticosteroids (Orally Inhaled); Crizotinib; CycloSPORINE; CycloSPORINE (Systemic); CYP3A4 Substrates; Diazepam; Dienogest; Digoxin; Dronedarone; Dutasteride; Enfuvirtide; Eplerenone; Ergot Derivatives; Everolimus; FentaNYL; Fesoterodine; Flurazepam; Fluticasone (Nasal); Fluticasone (Oral Inhalation); Fusidic Acid; GuanFACINE; Halofantrine; HMG-CoA Reductase Inhibitors; Iloperidone; Ixabepilone; Lapatinib; Lovastatin; Lumefantrine; Lurasidone; Maraviroc; Meperidine; MethylPREDNISolone; Midazolam; Nefazodone; Nilotinib; Nisoldipine; Paricalcitol; Pazopanib; Pimecrolimus; Pimozide; Propafenone; Protease Inhibitors; QuiNIDine; Ranolazine; Rifabutin; Rivaroxaban; RomiDEPsin; Ruxolitinib; Salmeterol; Saxagliptin; Sildenafil; Silodosin;

Simvastatin; Sirolimus; SORAfenib; Tacrolimus; Tacrolimus (Systemic); Tacrolimus (Topical); Tadalafil; Tamsulosin; Temsirolimus; Tenofovir; Ticagrelor; Tolterodine; Tolvaptan; Toremifene; TraZODone; Triazolam; Tricyclic Antidepressants; Vardenafil; Vemurafenib; Vilazodone; Warfarin; Zuclopenthixol

The levels/effects of Fosamprenavir may be increased by: Antifungal Agents (Azole Derivatives, Systemic); Clarithromycin; CycloSPORINE; CycloSPORINE (Systemic); Delavirdine; Efavirenz; Enfuvirtide; Etravirine; Fosphenytoin; Fusidic Acid; P-glycoprotein/ABCB1 Inhibitors; Phenytoin; Posaconazole; Rifabutin

Decreased Effect

Fosamprenavir may decrease the levels/effects of: Abacavir; Clarithromycin; Contraceptives (Estrogens); Delavirdine; Divalproex; Fosphenytoin; Lopinavir; Meperidine; Methadone; PARoxetine; Phenytoin; Posaconazole; Prasugrel; Raltegravir; Telaprevir; Ticagrelor; Valproic Acid; Zidovudine

The levels/effects of Fosamprenavir may be decreased by: Antacids; CarBAMazepine; CYP3A4 Inducers (Strong); Deferasirox; Efavirenz; Garlic; H2-Antagonists; Nevirapine; Peginterferon Alfa-2b; P-glycoprotein/ABCB1 Inducers; Raltegravir; Rifampin; St Johns Wort; Telaprevir; Tenofovir; Tocilizumab

Ethanol/Nutrition/Herb Interactions Herb/Nutraceutical: Amprenavir serum concentration may be decreased by St John's wort; concurrent use contraindicated.

Stability

Lexiva®: Store tablets at 25°C (77°F); excursions permitted to 15°C to 30°C (59°F to 86°F). Store oral suspension at 5°C to 30°C (41°F to 86°F). Do not freeze.

Telzir®: Store tablets 2°C to 30°C; do not freeze and discard 25 days after opening.

Mechanism of Action Fosamprenavir is rapidly and almost completely converted to amprenavir by cellular phosphatases *in vivo*. Amprenavir binds to the site of HIV-1 protease activity and inhibits cleavage of viral Gag-Pol polyprotein precursors into individual functional proteins required for infectious HIV. This results in the formation of immature, noninfectious viral particles.

Pharmacodynamics/Kinetics

Absorption: 63%

Protein-binding: ~90% (to alpha$_1$-acid glycoprotein); decreased in hepatic impairment

Metabolism: Fosamprenavir is rapidly and almost completely converted to amprenavir by cellular phosphatases in gut epithelium; amprenavir is hepatically metabolized via CYP isoenzymes (primarily CYP3A4)

Bioavailability: Not established; food does not have a significant effect on absorption of tablets. Administration of oral suspension with food reduced C_{max} by 46% and AUC by 28%.

Half-life elimination: ~7.7 hours (amprenavir)

Time to peak, plasma: 1.5-4 hours (median: 2.5 hours)

Excretion: Feces (75% as metabolites, <1% as unchanged drug); urine (14% as metabolites, ~1% as unchanged drug)

Dosage Oral: HIV infection:

Children:

Antiretroviral therapy-naive patients:

Children 2-5 years of age: Fosamprenavir 30 mg/kg/dose twice daily (not to exceed adult dosage of 1400 mg twice daily without ritonavir)

Children ≥6 years of age:

Unboosted regimen: Fosamprenavir 30 mg/kg/dose twice daily (not to exceed adult dosage of 1400 mg twice daily without ritonavir)

Ritonavir-boosted regimen: Fosamprenavir 18 mg/kg/dose twice daily plus ritonavir 3 mg/kg/dose twice daily (not to exceed the adult dose of fosamprenavir 700 mg plus ritonavir 100 mg twice daily)

Protease inhibitor (PI)-experienced patients: Children ≥6 years of age: Fosamprenavir 18 mg/kg/dose plus ritonavir 3 mg/kg/dose twice daily (not to exceed the adult dose of fosamprenavir 700 mg plus ritonavir 100 mg twice daily)

Notes: The adult unboosted regimen of 1400 mg twice daily may be used for pediatric patients who weigh ≥47 kg. When combined with ritonavir, the adult regimen of fosamprenavir 700 mg plus ritonavir 100 mg twice daily can be used in children who weigh ≥39 kg while ritonavir capsules may be used for pediatric patients who weigh ≥33 kg.

Adults:

Antiretroviral therapy-naive patients:

Unboosted regimen (per manufacturer's labeling): 1400 mg twice daily (without ritonavir); **Note:** This regimen is not recommended in adults due to inferior potency compared to other protease inhibitor based regimens and the potential for cross-resistance to darunavir (DHHS, 2011).

Ritonavir-boosted regimens:

Once-daily regimen: Fosamprenavir 1400 mg plus ritonavir 100-200 mg once daily

Twice-daily regimen: Fosamprenavir 700 mg plus ritonavir 100 mg twice daily

Protease inhibitor (PI)-experienced patients: Fosamprenavir 700 mg plus ritonavir 100 mg twice daily. **Note:** Once-daily administration is not recommended in protease inhibitor-experienced patients.

Dosage adjustments for concomitant therapy: Adults:

Coadministration with bosentan:

Coadministration of bosentan in patients currently receiving fosamprenavir: For patients receiving fosamprenavir for at least 10 days, begin with bosentan 62.5 mg once daily or every other day based on tolerability

Coadministration of fosamprenavir in patients currently receiving bosentan: Discontinue bosentan 36 hours prior to the initiation of fosamprenavir. After at least 10 days of fosamprenavir, resume bosentan 62.5 mg once daily or every other day based on tolerability.

Coadministration with colchicine:

Familial Mediterranean fever (FMF):

Fosamprenavir: Maximum colchicine dose: 1.2 mg/day (0.6 mg twice daily)

Fosamprenavir with ritonavir: Maximum colchicine dose: 0.6 mg/day (0.3 mg twice daily)

Gout prophylaxis:

Fosamprenavir:

If original colchicine dose is 0.6 mg twice daily, adjust dose to 0.3 mg twice daily or 0.6 mg once daily

If original colchicine dose is 0.6 mg once daily, adjust dose to 0.3 mg once daily

Fosamprenavir with ritonavir:

If original colchicine dose is 0.6 mg twice daily, adjust dose to 0.3 mg once daily

If original colchicine dose is 0.6 mg once daily, adjust dose to 0.3 mg every other day

Gout flare treatment:

Fosamprenavir: Initial: Colchicine 1.2 mg; do not repeat for at least 3 days

Fosamprenavir with ritonavir: Initial: Colchicine 0.6 mg, followed in 1 hour by a single dose of 0.3 mg; do not repeat for at least 3 days

Combination therapy with efavirenz (ritonavir-boosted regimen):

Once-daily regimen (PI-naive patients only): Fosamprenavir 1400 mg plus ritonavir 300 mg plus efavirenz 600 mg once daily

Twice-daily regimen: Fosamprenavir 700 mg plus ritonavir 100 mg twice daily plus efavirenz 600 mg once daily

Combination therapy with maraviroc: Fosamprenavir 700 mg plus ritonavir 100 mg plus maraviroc 150 mg twice daily

Coadministration with phosphodiesterase-5 enzyme (PDE-5) inhibitor:

Pulmonary arterial hypertension: Fosamprenavir coadministered with tadalafil:

Patient receiving fosamprenavir for at least 1 week: Initiate tadalafil at 20 mg once daily; increase to 40 mg once daily based on individual tolerability

Patient receiving tadalafil when initiating fosamprenavir: Stop tadalafil at least 24 hours prior to starting fosamprenavir. After at least 1 week following the initiation of fosamprenavir, resume tadalafil at 20 mg once daily; increase to 40 mg once daily based on individual tolerability.

Erectile dysfunction:

Fosamprenavir coadministered with or without ritonavir:

Sildenafil (Viagra®): Maximum sildenafil dose: 25 mg in a 48-hour period

Tadalafil (Cialis®): Maximum tadalafil dose: 10 mg in a 72-hour period

Vardenafil:

Fosamprenavir: Maximum vardenafil dose: 2.5 mg in a 24-hour period

Fosamprenavir coadministered with ritonavir and vardenafil: Maximum vardenafil dose: 2.5 mg in a 72-hour period

Dosage adjustment in renal impairment: No dosage adjustment necessary.

Dosage adjustment in hepatic impairment:

Mild impairment (Child-Pugh score 5-6): Reduce dosage of fosamprenavir to 700 mg twice daily without concurrent ritonavir (therapy naive) **or** fosamprenavir 700 mg twice daily plus ritonavir 100 mg once daily (therapy naive or PI experienced)

Moderate impairment (Child-Pugh score 7-9): Reduce dosage of fosamprenavir to 700 mg twice daily without concurrent ritonavir (therapy naive) **or** fosamprenavir 450 mg twice daily plus ritonavir 100 mg once daily (therapy naive or PI experienced)

Severe impairment (Child-Pugh score 10-15): Reduce dosage of fosamprenavir to 350 mg twice daily without concurrent ritonavir (therapy naive) **or** fosamprenavir 300 mg twice daily plus ritonavir 100 mg once daily (therapy naive or PI experienced).

Dietary Considerations Tablets may be taken with or without food. Adults should take oral suspension **without** food; however, children should take oral suspension **with** food.

Administration

Oral suspension: Administer **without** food to adults; administer **with** food to pediatric patients. Readminister dose of suspension if emesis occurs within 30 minutes after dosing. Shake suspension vigorously prior to use.

Tablet: Administer with food if taken with ritonavir. May be administered without regard to food if not taken with ritonavir.

Monitoring Parameters Monitor viral load, CD4 count, glucose; triglycerides and cholesterol (prior to initiation and periodically during therapy)

Dosage Forms Excipient information presented when available (limited, particularly for generics); consult specific product labeling.

Suspension, oral, as calcium:

Lexiva®: 50 mg/mL (225 mL) [contains propylene glycol; grape-bubblegum-peppermint flavor; equivalent to amprenavir ~43 mg/mL]

Tablet, oral, as calcium:

Lexiva®: 700 mg [equivalent to amprenavir ~600 mg]

Dosage Forms: Canada Excipient information presented when available (limited, particularly for generics); consult specific product labeling.

Tablet, as calcium:

Telzir®: 700 mg

Suspension, oral, as calcium:

Telzir®: 50 mg/mL (225 mL)

◆ **Fosamprenavir Calcium** *see* Fosamprenavir *on page 756*

Fosaprepitant (fos a PRE pi tant)

Brand Names: U.S. Emend® for Injection

Brand Names: Canada Emend® IV

Index Terms Aprepitant Injection; Fosaprepitant Dimeglumine; L-758,298; MK 0517

Pharmacologic Category Antiemetic; Substance P/Neurokinin 1 Receptor Antagonist

Use Prevention of acute and delayed nausea and vomiting associated with moderately- and highly-emetogenic chemotherapy (in combination with other antiemetics)

Pregnancy Risk Factor B

Pregnancy Considerations Teratogenic effects were not observed in animal studies. There are no adequate and well-controlled studies in pregnant women; use only if clearly needed. Efficacy of hormonal contraceptive may be reduced; alternative or additional methods of contraception should be used both during treatment with fosaprepitant or aprepitant and for at least 1 month following the last fosaprepitant/aprepitant dose.

Lactation Excretion in breast milk unknown/not recommended

Contraindications Hypersensitivity to fosaprepitant, aprepitant, polysorbate 80, or any component of the formulation; concurrent use with pimozide or cisapride

Canadian labeling: Additional contraindications (not in U.S. labeling): Concurrent use with astemizole or terfenadine

Warnings/Precautions Fosaprepitant is rapidly converted to aprepitant, which has a high potential for drug interactions. Use caution with agents primarily metabolized via CYP3A4; aprepitant is a 3A4 inhibitor. Effect on orally administered 3A4 substrates is greater than those administered intravenously. Immediate hypersensitivity has been reported (rarely) with fosaprepitant; stop infusion with hypersensitivity symptoms (dyspnea, erythema, flushing, or anaphylaxis); do not reinitiate. Use caution with hepatic impairment; has not been studied in patients with severe hepatic impairment (Child-Pugh class C). Not studied for treatment of existing nausea and vomiting. Chronic continuous administration of fosaprepitant is not recommended.

Adverse Reactions Adverse reactions reported with aprepitant and fosaprepitant (as part of a combination chemotherapy regimen) occurring at a higher frequency than standard antiemetic therapy:

1% to 10%:

Central nervous system: Fatigue (1% to 3%), headache (2%)

Gastrointestinal: Anorexia (2%), constipation 2%), dyspepsia (2%), diarrhea (1%), eructation (1%)

Hepatic: ALT increased (1% to 3%), AST increased (1%)

Local: Injection site reactions (3%; includes erythema, induration, pain, pruritus, or thrombophlebitis)

Neuromuscular & skeletal: Weakness (3%)

Miscellaneous: Hiccups (5%)

<1% (Limited to important or life-threatening): Abdominal pain, alkaline phosphatase increased, anaphylactic reaction, anemia, angioedema, bradycardia, candidiasis, cardiovascular disorder, chest discomfort, chills, cognitive disorder, conjunctivitis, cough, disorientation, dizziness, ▶

duodenal ulcer (perforating), dyspnea, edema, erythema, flushing, gait disturbance, hematuria (microscopic), hyperglycemia, hyperhydrosis, hypersensitivity reaction, hypertension, hyponatremia, miosis, nausea, neutropenia, neutropenic colitis, neutropenic fever, palpitation, photosensitivity, pollakiuria, polyuria, pruritus, rash, sensory disturbance, somnolence, staphylococcal infection, Stevens-Johnson syndrome, stomatitis, subileus, tinnitus, urticaria, visual acuity decreased, vomiting, wheezing

Drug Interactions

Metabolism/Transport Effects **Substrate** of CYP1A2 (minor), CYP2C19 (minor), CYP3A4 (major); **Note:** Assignment of Major/Minor substrate status based on clinically relevant drug interaction potential; **Inhibits** CYP2C19 (weak), CYP2C9 (weak), CYP3A4 (moderate); **Induces** CYP2C9 (weak/moderate), CYP3A4 (weak/moderate)

Avoid Concomitant Use

Avoid concomitant use of Fosaprepitant with any of the following: Astemizole; Cisapride; Conivaptan; Pimozide; Terfenadine; Tolvaptan

Increased Effect/Toxicity

Fosaprepitant may increase the levels/effects of: ARIPiprazole; Astemizole; Benzodiazepines (metabolized by oxidation); Budesonide (Systemic, Oral Inhalation); Cisapride; Colchicine; Corticosteroids (Systemic); CYP3A4 Substrates; Diltiazem; Eplerenone; Everolimus; FentaNYL; Halofantrine; Lurasidone; Pimecrolimus; Pimozide; Propafenone; Ranolazine; Salmeterol; Saxagliptin; Terfenadine; Tolvaptan; Vilazodone; Zuclopenthixol

The levels/effects of Fosaprepitant may be increased by: Antifungal Agents (Azole Derivatives, Systemic); Conivaptan; CYP3A4 Inhibitors (Moderate); CYP3A4 Inhibitors (Strong); Dasatinib; Diltiazem

Decreased Effect

Fosaprepitant may decrease the levels/effects of: ARIPiprazole; Contraceptives (Estrogens); Contraceptives (Progestins); PARoxetine; Saxagliptin; TOLBUTamide; Warfarin

The levels/effects of Fosaprepitant may be decreased by: CYP3A4 Inducers (Strong); Cyproterone; Deferasirox; Herbs (CYP3A4 Inducers); PARoxetine; Rifampin; Tocilizumab

Ethanol/Nutrition/Herb Interactions

Food: Aprepitant serum concentration may be increased when taken with grapefruit juice; avoid concurrent use.

Herb/Nutraceutical: Avoid St John's wort (may decrease aprepitant levels).

Stability Store intact vials at 2°C to 8°C (36°F to 46°F). Reconstitute either vial size with 5 mL of sodium chloride 0.9%, directing diluent down side of vial to avoid foaming; swirl gently. Add reconstituted contents of the 150 mg vial to 145 mL sodium chloride 0.9% (add 115 mg vial to 110 mL), resulting in a final concentration of 1 mg/mL; gently invert bag to mix. Solutions diluted for infusion are stable for 24 hours at room temperature of ≤25°C (≤77°F).

Mechanism of Action Fosaprepitant is a prodrug of aprepitant, a substance P/neurokinin 1 (NK1) receptor antagonist. It is rapidly converted to aprepitant which prevents acute and delayed vomiting by inhibiting the substance P/neurokinin 1 (NK1) receptor; augments the antiemetic activity of the 5-HT_3 receptor antagonist and corticosteroid activity and inhibits chemotherapy-induced emesis.

Pharmacodynamics/Kinetics

Distribution: Fosaprepitant: ~5 L; Aprepitant: V_d: ~70 L; crosses the blood-brain barrier

Protein binding: Aprepitant: >95%

Metabolism:

Fosaprepitant: Hepatic and extrahepatic; rapidly (within 30 minutes after the end of infusion) converted to aprepitant (nearly complete conversion)

Aprepitant: Hepatic via CYP3A4 (major); CYP1A2 and CYP2C19 (minor); forms 7 weakly-active metabolites

Half-life elimination: Fosaprepitant: ~2 minutes; Aprepitant: ~9-13 hours

Time to peak, plasma: Fosaprepitant is converted to aprepitant within 30 minutes after the end of infusion

Excretion: Urine (57%); feces (45%)

Dosage I.V.: Adults: Prevention of chemotherapy-induced nausea/vomiting:

Single-dose regimen (for highly-emetogenic chemotherapy): 150 mg over 20-30 minutes ~30 minutes prior to chemotherapy on day 1 only (in combination with a 5-HT_3 antagonist on day 1 and dexamethasone on days 1 to 4)

3-day regimen (for highly-emetogenic chemotherapy): 115 mg over 15 minutes 30 minutes prior to chemotherapy on day 1, followed by aprepitant 80 mg orally on days 2 and 3 (in combination with a 5-HT_3 antagonist on day 1 and dexamethasone on days 1 to 4)

3-day regimen (for moderately-emetogenic chemotherapy): 115 mg over 15 minutes 30 minutes prior to chemotherapy on day 1, followed by aprepitant 80 mg orally on days 2 and 3 (in combination with a 5-HT_3 antagonist and dexamethasone on day 1)

Dosage adjustment in renal impairment:

Mild, moderate, or severe impairment: No adjustment required

Dialysis-dependent end-stage renal disease (ESRD): No adjustment required

Dosage adjustment in hepatic impairment:

Child-Pugh class A and B: No adjustment required

Child-Pugh class C: Has not been evaluated; use with caution

Administration

115 mg: Infuse over 15 minutes 30 minutes prior to chemotherapy

150 mg: Infuse over 20-30 minutes ~30 minutes prior to chemotherapy

Additional Information Oncology Comment: Fosaprepitant is recommended in the National Comprehensive Cancer Network® (NCCN) Clinical Practice Guidelines in Oncology for Antiemesis (version 1.2011) for use on day 1 in combination with a serotonin receptor antagonist and dexamethasone for chemotherapy with high emetic risk and for select moderately emetogenic regimens (carboplatin, cisplatin, doxorubicin, epirubicin, ifosfamide, irinotecan, or methotrexate). Either fosaprepitant 115 mg or aprepitant (125 mg orally) are administered on day 1; for day 2 and 3, patients should receive aprepitant 80 mg orally. The 1-day regimen (fosaprepitant 150 mg on day 1 only) is listed in the guidelines for highly emetogenic treatments.

Dosage Forms Excipient information presented when available (limited, particularly for generics); consult specific product labeling. [DSC] = Discontinued product

Injection, powder for reconstitution:

Emend® for Injection: 115 mg [DSC] [contains edetate disodium, lactose 287.5 mg, polysorbate 80]

Emend® for Injection: 150 mg [contains edetate disodium, lactose 375 mg, polysorbate 80]

- **Fosaprepitant Dimeglumine** *see* Fosaprepitant *on page 759*
- **Fosavance (Can)** *see* Alendronate and Cholecalciferol *on page 62*

Foscarnet (fos KAR net)

Brand Names: Canada Foscavir®

Index Terms PFA; Phosphonoformate; Phosphonoformic Acid

Pharmacologic Category Antiviral Agent

Use Treatment of acyclovir-resistant mucocutaneous herpes simplex virus (HSV) infections in immunocompromised persons (eg, with advanced AIDS); treatment of CMV retinitis in persons with HIV

Unlabeled Use Other CMV infections (eg, colitis, esophagitis, neurological disease); CMV prophylaxis for cancer patients receiving alemtuzumab therapy or allogeneic stem cell transplant

Pregnancy Risk Factor C

Pregnancy Considerations Associated with an increase in skeletal anomalies in animal studies at approximately the equivalent of 13% to 33% of the maximal daily human dose. There are no adequate and well controlled studies in pregnant women. A single case report of use during the third trimester with normal infant outcome was observed. Monitoring of amniotic fluid volumes by ultrasound is recommended weekly after 20 weeks of gestation to detect oligohydramnios.

Lactation Excretion in breast milk unknown/contraindicated

Contraindications Hypersensitivity to foscarnet or any component of the formulation

Warnings/Precautions [U.S. Boxed Warning]: Indicated only for immunocompromised patients with CMV retinitis and mucocutaneous acyclovir-resistant HSV infection. [U.S. Boxed Warning]: Renal impairment occurs to some degree in the majority of patients treated with foscarnet; renal impairment may occur at any time and is usually reversible within 1 week following dose adjustment or discontinuation of therapy, however, several patients have died with renal failure within 4 weeks of stopping foscarnet; therefore, renal function should be closely monitored. To reduce the risk of nephrotoxicity and the potential to administer a relative overdose, always calculate the creatine clearance even if serum creatinine is within the normal range. Adequate hydration may reduce the risk of nephrotoxicity; the manufacturer makes specific recommendations regarding this (see Administration).

Imbalance of serum electrolytes or minerals occurs in at least 15% of patients (hypocalcemia, low ionized calcium, hyper/hypophosphatemia, hypomagnesemia, or hypokalemia). Correct electrolytes before initiating therapy. Use caution when administering other medications that cause electrolyte imbalances. Patients who experience signs or symptoms of an electrolyte imbalance should be assessed immediately. **[U.S. Boxed Warning]: Seizures related to plasma electrolyte/mineral imbalance may occur;** incidence has been reported in up to 10% of HIV patients. Risk factors for seizures include impaired baseline renal function, low total serum calcium, and underlying CNS conditions. May cause anemia and granulocytopenia. May cause genital/vascular tissue irritation/ulceration; adequately hydrate and administer only into vein with adequate blood flow to minimize risk. Foscarnet is deposited in teeth and bone of young, growing animals; it has adversely affected tooth enamel development in rats.

Adverse Reactions

>10%:

Central nervous system: Fever (65%), headache (26%)

Endocrine & metabolic: Hypokalemia (16% to 48%), hypocalcemia (15% to 30%), hypomagnesemia (15% to 30%), hypophosphatemia (8% to 26%)

Gastrointestinal: Nausea (47%), diarrhea (30%), vomiting (26%)

Hematologic: Anemia (33%), granulocytopenia (17%)

Renal: Abnormal renal function/decreased creatinine clearance (12%; without adequate hydration 33%)

1% to 10%:

Cardiovascular: Chest pain (1% to 5%), edema (1% to 5%), facial edema (1% to 5%), flushing (1% to 5%), hyper-/hypotension (1% to 5%), palpitation (1% to 5%), ECG changes (1% to 5%)

Central nervous system: Seizure (includes grand mal; 8%), anxiety (≥5%), confusion (≥5%), depression (≥5%), dizziness (≥5%), fatigue (≥5%), hypoesthesia (≥5%), malaise (≥5%), pain (≥5%), aggressiveness (1% to 5%), agitation (1% to 5%), amnesia (1% to 5%), aphasia (1% to 5%), ataxia (1% to 5%), coordination abnormal (1% to 5%), dementia (1% to 5%), EEG abnormal (1% to 5%), hallucination (1% to 5%), insomnia (1% to 5%), meningitis (1% to 5%), nervousness (1% to 5%), somnolence (1% to 5%), stupor (1% to 5%)

Dermatologic: Rash (≥5%), erythematous rash (1% to 5%), maculopapular rash (1% to 5%), pruritus (1% to 5%), seborrhea (1% to 5%), skin discoloration (1% to 5%), skin ulceration (1% to 5%)

Endocrine & metabolic: Hyperphosphatemia (6%), acidosis (1% to 5%), hyponatremia (1% to 5%)

Gastrointestinal: Abdominal pain (≥5%), anorexia (≥5%), constipation (1% to 5%), dyspepsia (1% to 5%), dysphasia (1% to 5%), flatulence (1% to 5%), melena (1% to 5%), pancreatitis (1% to 5%), rectal hemorrhage (1% to 5%), taste perversion (1% to 5%), ulcerative stomatitis (1% to 5%), weight loss (1% to 5%), xerostomia (1% to 5%)

Genitourinary: Dysuria (1% to 5%), nocturia (1% to 5%), urinary retention (1% to 5%)

Hematologic: Leukopenia (≥5%), lymphadenopathy (1% to 5%), thrombocytopenia (1% to 5%), thrombosis (1% to 5%)

Hepatic: Alkaline phosphatase increased (1% to 5%), ALT increased (1% to 5%), AST increased (1% to 5%), hepatic function abnormal (1% to 5%), LDH increased (1% to 5%)

Local: Injection site pain/inflammation (1% to 5%)

Neuromuscular & skeletal: Paresthesia (≥5%), involuntary muscle contractions (≥5%), rigors (≥5%), neuropathy (peripheral; ≥5%), weakness (≥5%), arthralgia (1% to 5%), back pain (1% to 5%), leg cramps (1% to 5%), myalgia (1% to 5%), tremor (1% to 5%)

Ocular: Vision abnormalities (≥5%), conjunctivitis (1% to 5%), eye pain (1% to 5%)

Renal: Acute renal failure (1% to 5%), albuminuria (1% to 5%), BUN increased (1% to 5%), polyuria (1% to 5%), urinary tract infection (1% to 5%)

Respiratory: Cough (≥5%), dyspnea (≥5%), bronchospasm (1% to 5%), hemoptysis (1% to 5%), pharyngitis (1% to 5%), pneumonia (1% to 5%), pneumothorax (1% to 5%), rhinitis (1% to 5%), sinusitis (1% to 5%), stridor (1% to 5%)

Miscellaneous: Diaphoresis (≥5%), sepsis (≥5%), infection (includes bacterial and fungal; ≥5%), flu-like syndrome (1% to 5%), malignancies (lymphoma/sarcoma 1% to 5%), thirst (1% to 5%)

<1% (Limited to important or life-threatening): Amylase increased, cardiac arrest, coma, creatine phosphokinase increased, dehydration, diabetes insipidus (usually nephrogenic), erythema multiforme, GGT increased muscle weakness, hematuria, hypoproteinemia, myopathy, myositis, neutropenia, pancytopenia, QT_c prolongation, renal calculus, rhabdomyolysis, Stevens-Johnson syndrome, syndrome of inappropriate antidiuretic hormone (SIADH), toxic epidermal necrolysis, ventricular arrhythmia, vesiculobullous eruptions

Drug Interactions

Metabolism/Transport Effects None known.

Avoid Concomitant Use

Avoid concomitant use of Foscarnet with any of the following: Artemether; Dronedarone; Lumefantrine; Nilotinib; Pimozide; QUEtiapine; QuiNINE; Tetrabenazine; Thioridazine; Toremifene; Vandetanib; Vemurafenib; Ziprasidone

Increased Effect/Toxicity

Foscarnet may increase the levels/effects of: Dronedarone; Pimozide; QTc-Prolonging Agents; QuiNINE; Tetrabenazine; Thioridazine; Toremifene; Vandetanib; Vemurafenib; Ziprasidone

The levels/effects of Foscarnet may be increased by: Alfuzosin; Artemether; Chloroquine; Ciprofloxacin; Ciprofloxacin (Systemic); Gadobutrol; Indacaterol; Lumefantrine; Nilotinib; QUEtiapine; QuiNINE

Decreased Effect There are no known significant interactions involving a decrease in effect.

Stability Foscarnet injection is a clear, colorless solution. Store intact bottles at room temperature of 15°C to 30°C (59°F to 86°F) and protect from temperatures >40°C and from freezing. Diluted solution is stable for 24 hours at room temperature or under refrigeration.

Foscarnet should be diluted in D_5W or NS. For peripheral line administration, foscarnet **must** be diluted to ≤12 mg/mL with D_5W or NS. For central line administration, foscarnet may be administered undiluted.

Mechanism of Action Pyrophosphate analogue which acts as a noncompetitive inhibitor of many viral RNA and DNA polymerases as well as HIV reverse transcriptase. Similar to ganciclovir, foscarnet is a virostatic agent. Foscarnet does not require activation by thymidine kinase.

Pharmacodynamics/Kinetics

Distribution: V_d: ~0.5 L/kg; up to 28% of cumulative I.V. dose may be deposited in bone

Protein binding: 14% to 17%

Metabolism: Biotransformation does not occur

Half-life elimination: Elimination: ~3-4 hours; terminal: ~88 hours (due to bone deposition)

Excretion: Urine (≤28% as unchanged drug)

Dosage

CMV retinitis: I.V.:

Induction treatment: 60 mg/kg/dose every 8 hours **or** 90 mg/kg every 12 hours for 14-21 days

Maintenance therapy: 90-120 mg/kg/day as a single daily infusion

Herpes simplex infections (acyclovir-resistant): Induction: I.V.: 40 mg/kg/dose every 8-12 hours for 14-21 days

Therapy of CMV infection in cancer patients (unlabeled use): I.V.:

Prophylaxis: 60 mg/kg every 8-12 hours for 7 days, followed by 90-120 mg/kg daily until day 100 after HSCT

Pre-emptive treatment: 60 mg/kg every 12 hours for 14 days; if CMV still detectable, continue with 90 mg/kg daily for 5 days/week for 2 additional weeks

Treatment: 90 mg/kg every 12 hours for 2 weeks, followed by 120 mg/kg daily for ≥2 weeks

Dosage adjustment in renal impairment: Induction and maintenance dosing schedules based on creatinine clearance (mL/minute/kg): See tables.

Induction Dosing of Foscarnet in Patients With Abnormal Renal Function

Cl_{cr} (mL/min/kg)	HSV Equivalent to 40 mg/kg q12h	HSV Equivalent to 40 mg/kg q8h	CMV Equivalent to 60 mg/kg q8h	CMV Equivalent to 90 mg/kg q12h
<0.4	Not recommended	Not recommended	Not recommended	Not recommended
≥0.4-0.5	20 mg/kg every 24 hours	35 mg/kg every 24 hours	50 mg/kg every 24 hours	50 mg/kg every 24 hours
>0.5-0.6	25 mg/kg every 24 hours	40 mg/kg every 24 hours	60 mg/kg every 24 hours	60 mg/kg every 24 hours
>0.6-0.8	35 mg/kg every 24 hours	25 mg/kg every 12 hours	40 mg/kg every 12 hours	80 mg/kg every 24 hours
>0.8-1.0	20 mg/kg every 12 hours	35 mg/kg every 12 hours	50 mg/kg every 12 hours	50 mg/kg every 12 hours
>1.0-1.4	30 mg/kg every 12 hours	30 mg/kg every 8 hours	45 mg/kg every 8 hours	70 mg/kg every 12 hours
>1.4	40 mg/kg every 12 hours	40 mg/kg every 8 hours	60 mg/kg every 8 hours	90 mg/kg every 12 hours

Maintenance Dosing of Foscarnet in Patients With Abnormal Renal Function

Cl_{cr} (mL/min/kg)	CMV Equivalent to 90 mg/kg q24h	CMV Equivalent to 120 mg/kg q24h
<0.4	Not recommended	Not recommended
≥0.4-0.5	50 mg/kg every 48 hours	65 mg/kg every 48 hours
>0.5-0.6	60 mg/kg every 48 hours	80 mg/kg every 48 hours
>0.6-0.8	80 mg/kg every 48 hours	105 mg/kg every 48 hours
>0.8-1.0	50 mg/kg every 24 hours	65 mg/kg every 24 hours
>1.0-1.4	70 mg/kg every 24 hours	90 mg/kg every 24 hours
>1.4	90 mg/kg every 24 hours	120 mg/kg every 24 hours

Hemodialysis:

Foscarnet is highly removed by hemodialysis (up to ~38% in 2.5 hours HD with high-flux membrane)

Doses of 50 mg/kg/dose posthemodialysis have been found to produce similar serum concentrations as doses of 90 mg/kg twice daily in patients with normal renal function

Doses of 60-90 mg/kg/dose loading dose (posthemodialysis) followed by 45-60 mg/kg/dose posthemodialysis (3 times/week) with the monitoring of weekly plasma concentrations to maintain peak plasma concentrations in the range of 400-800 µMolar have been recommended by some clinicians

Continuous arteriovenous or venovenous hemodiafiltration effects: Dose as for Cl_{cr} 10-50 mL/minute

Administration Foscarnet is administered by intravenous infusion, using an infusion pump, at a rate not exceeding 1 mg/kg/minute. Undiluted (24 mg/mL) solution can be administered without further dilution when using a central venous catheter for infusion. For peripheral vein administration, the solution **must** be diluted to a final concentration **not to exceed** 12 mg/mL. The manufacturer recommends 750-1000 mL of NS or D_5W be administered prior to first infusion to establish diuresis. With subsequent infusions of 90-120 mg/kg, this volume would be repeated. If the dose were 40-60 mg/kg, then the volume could be reduced to 500 mL. After the first dose, the hydration fluid should be administered concurrently with foscarnet.

Monitoring Parameters 24-hour creatinine clearance at baseline and periodically thereafter. During induction therapy: Obtain complete blood counts, and electrolytes (including serum creatinine, calcium, magnesium, potassium, and phosphorus) twice weekly and then one weekly during maintenance therapy. More frequent monitoring may be required in some patients. Check hydration status before and after infusion.

Additional Information CMV retinitis maintenance treatment may be discontinued if immune reconstitution occurs as a result of ART.

Dosage Forms Excipient information presented when available (limited, particularly for generics); consult specific product labeling.

Injection, solution, as sodium [preservative free]: 24 mg/mL (250 mL, 500 mL)

◆ **Foscavir® (Can)** *see* Foscarnet *on page 760*

Fosfomycin (fos foe MYE sin)

Brand Names: U.S. Monurol®

Brand Names: Canada Monurol®

Index Terms Fosfomycin Tromethamine

Pharmacologic Category Antibiotic, Miscellaneous

Use Single oral dose in the treatment of uncomplicated urinary tract infections in women due to susceptible strains of *E. coli* and *Enterococcus faecalis*

Unlabeled Use Multiple doses have been investigated for complicated urinary tract infections in men

Pregnancy Risk Factor B

Dosage Adults: Oral:

Females: Uncomplicated UTI: Single dose of 3 g in 3-4 oz (90-120 mL) of water

Males:

Complicated UTI (unlabeled): 3 g every 2-3 days for 3 doses

Prostatitis (unlabeled): 3 g every 3 days for a total of 21 days

Dosing adjustment in hepatic impairment: No dosage decrease needed

Additional Information Complete prescribing information for this medication should be consulted for additional detail.

Dosage Forms Excipient information presented when available (limited, particularly for generics); consult specific product labeling.

Powder for solution, oral:

Monurol®: 3 g/sachet (3s) [orange flavor]

◆ **Fosfomycin Tromethamine** *see* Fosfomycin *on page 763*

Fosinopril (foe SIN oh pril)

Brand Names: Canada Apo-Fosinopril®; Jamp-Fosinopril; Monopril®; Mylan-Fosinopril; PMS-Fosinopril; RAN™-Fosinopril; Riva-Fosinopril; Teva-Fosinopril

Index Terms Fosinopril Sodium; Monopril

Pharmacologic Category Angiotensin-Converting Enzyme (ACE) Inhibitor

Additional Appendix Information

Angiotensin Agents *on page 1869*

Heart Failure (Systolic) *on page 1991*

Use Treatment of hypertension, either alone or in combination with other antihypertensive agents; treatment of heart failure (HF)

Pregnancy Risk Factor C (1st trimester); D (2nd and 3rd trimesters)

Pregnancy Considerations Due to adverse events observed in some animal studies, fosinopril is considered pregnancy category C during the first trimester. Based on human data, fosinopril is considered pregnancy category D if used during the second and third trimesters (per the manufacturer; however, one study suggests that fetal injury may occur at anytime during pregnancy). First trimester exposure to ACE inhibitors may cause major congenital malformations. An increased risk of cardiovascular and/or central nervous system malformations was observed in one study; however, an increased risk of teratogenic events was not observed in other studies. Second and third trimester use of an ACE inhibitor is associated with oligohydramnios. Oligohydramnios due to decreased fetal renal function may lead to fetal limb contractures, craniofacial deformation, and hypoplastic lung development. The use of ACE inhibitors during the second and third trimesters is also associated with anuria, hypotension, renal failure (reversible or irreversible), skull hypoplasia, and death in the fetus/neonate. Chronic maternal hypertension itself is also associated with adverse events in the fetus/infant. ACE inhibitors are not recommended during pregnancy to treat maternal hypertension or heart failure. Those who are planning a pregnancy should be considered for other medication options if an ACE inhibitor is currently prescribed or the ACE inhibitor should be discontinued as soon as possible once pregnancy is detected. The exposed fetus should be monitored for fetal growth, amniotic fluid volume, and organ formation. Infants exposed to an ACE inhibitor *in utero*, especially during the second and third trimester, should be monitored for hyperkalemia, hypotension, and oliguria.

[U.S. Boxed Warning]: Based on human data, ACE inhibitors can cause injury and death to the developing fetus when used in the second and third trimesters. ACE inhibitors should be discontinued as soon as possible once pregnancy is detected.

Lactation Enters breast milk/not recommended

Contraindications Hypersensitivity to fosinopril, any other ACE inhibitor, or any component of the formulation; angioedema related to previous treatment with an ACE inhibitor

Warnings/Precautions Anaphylactic reactions may occur rarely with ACE inhibitors. At any time during treatment (especially following first dose), angioedema may occur rarely with ACE inhibitors; it may involve the head and neck (potentially compromising airway) or the intestine (presenting with abdominal pain). African-Americans may be at an increased risk and patients with idiopathic or hereditary angioedema may be at an increased risk. Prolonged frequent monitoring may be required especially if tongue, glottis, or larynx are involved as they are associated with airway obstruction. Patients with a history of airway surgery may have a higher risk of airway obstruction. Aggressive early and appropriate management is critical. Use in patients with previous angioedema associated with ACE inhibitor therapy is contraindicated. Severe anaphylactoid reactions may be seen during hemodialysis (eg, CVVHD) with high-flux dialysis membranes (eg, AN69), and rarely, during low density lipoprotein apheresis with dextran sulfate cellulose. Rare cases of anaphylactoid reactions have been reported in patients undergoing sensitization treatment with hymenoptera (bee, wasp) venom while receiving ACE inhibitors.

Symptomatic hypotension with or without syncope can occur with ACE inhibitors (usually with the first several doses); effects are most often observed in volume-depleted patients; correct volume depletion prior to initiation; close monitoring of patient is required especially with initial dosing and dosing increases; blood pressure must be lowered at a rate appropriate for the patient's clinical condition. Initiation of therapy in patients with ischemic heart disease or cerebrovascular disease warrants close observation due to the potential consequences posed by falling blood pressure (eg, MI, stroke). Use with caution in hypertrophic cardiomyopathy with outflow tract obstruction, severe aortic stenosis, or before, during, or immediately after major surgery. **[U.S. Boxed Warning]: Based on human data, ACEIs can cause injury and death to the developing fetus when used in the second and third trimesters. ACEIs should be discontinued as soon as possible once pregnancy is detected.**

Hyperkalemia may occur with ACE inhibitors; risk factors include renal dysfunction, diabetes mellitus, concomitant use of potassium-sparing diuretics, potassium supplements, and/or potassium-containing salts. Use cautiously, if at all, with these agents and monitor potassium closely. Cough may occur with ACE inhibitors. Other causes of cough should be considered (eg, pulmonary congestion in patients with heart failure) and excluded prior to discontinuation.

May be associated with deterioration of renal function and/or increases in serum creatinine, particularly in patients with low renal blood flow (eg, renal artery stenosis, heart failure) whose glomerular filtration rate (GFR) is dependent on efferent arteriolar vasoconstriction by angiotensin II; deterioration may result in oliguria, acute renal failure, and progressive azotemia. Small increases in serum creatinine may occur following initiation; consider discontinuation only in patients with progressive and/or significant deterioration in renal function. Use with caution in patients with unstented unilateral/bilateral renal artery stenosis. When unstented bilateral renal artery stenosis is present, use is generally avoided due to the elevated risk of deterioration in renal function unless possible benefits outweigh risks. Concurrent use of angiotensin receptor blockers may increase the risk of clinically-significant adverse events (eg, renal dysfunction, hyperkalemia).

Rare toxicities associated with ACE inhibitors include cholestatic jaundice (which may progress to fulminant hepatic necrosis), agranulocytosis, neutropenia or leukopenia with myeloid hypoplasia. Patients with collagen vascular diseases (especially with concomitant renal impairment) or renal impairment alone may be at increased risk for hematologic toxicity; periodically monitor CBC with differential in these patients.

Adverse Reactions Note: Frequency ranges include data from hypertension and heart failure trials. Higher rates of adverse reactions have generally been noted in patients with CHF. However, the frequency of adverse effects associated with placebo is also increased in this population.

>10%: Central nervous system: Dizziness (1.6% to 11.9%)

1% to 10%:

- Cardiovascular: Orthostatic hypotension (1.4% to 1.9%), palpitation (1.4%)
- Central nervous system: Dizziness (1% to 2%; up to 12% in CHF patients), headache (3.2%), fatigue (1% to 2%)
- Endocrine & metabolic: Hyperkalemia (2.6%)
- Gastrointestinal: Diarrhea (2.2%), nausea/vomiting (1.2% to 2.2%)
- Hepatic: Transaminases increased
- Neuromuscular & skeletal: Musculoskeletal pain (<1% to 3.3%), noncardiac chest pain (<1% to 2.2%), weakness (1.4%)
- Renal: Serum creatinine increased, renal function worsening (in patients with bilateral renal artery stenosis or hypovolemia)
- Respiratory: Cough (2.2% to 9.7%)
- Miscellaneous: Upper respiratory infection (2.2%)

>1% but ≤ frequency in patients receiving placebo: Sexual dysfunction, fever, flu-like syndrome, dyspnea, rash, headache, insomnia

<1% (Limited to important or life-threatening): Anaphylactoid reaction, angina, angioedema, arthralgia, bronchospasm, cerebral infarction, cerebrovascular accident, gout, hepatitis, hepatomegaly, myalgia, MI, pancreatitis, paresthesia, photosensitivity, pleuritic chest pain, pruritus, rash, renal insufficiency, shock, sudden death, syncope, TIA, tinnitus, urticaria, vertigo. In a small number of patients, a symptom complex of cough, bronchospasm, and eosinophilia has been observed with fosinopril.

Other events reported with ACE inhibitors: Acute renal failure, agranulocytosis, anemia, aplastic anemia, bullous pemphigus, cardiac arrest, eosinophilic pneumonitis, exfoliative dermatitis, gynecomastia, hemolytic anemia, hepatic failure, jaundice, neutropenia, pancytopenia, Stevens-Johnson syndrome, symptomatic hyponatremia, thrombocytopenia. In addition, a syndrome which may include fever, myalgia, arthralgia, interstitial nephritis, vasculitis, rash, eosinophilia and positive ANA, and elevated ESR has been reported for other ACE inhibitors.

Drug Interactions

Metabolism/Transport Effects None known.

Avoid Concomitant Use There are no known interactions where it is recommended to avoid concomitant use.

Increased Effect/Toxicity

Fosinopril may increase the levels/effects of: Allopurinol; Amifostine; Antihypertensives; AzaTHIOprine; CycloSPORINE; CycloSPORINE (Systemic); Ferric Gluconate; Gold Sodium Thiomalate; Hypotensive Agents; Iron Dextran Complex; Lithium; Nonsteroidal Anti-Inflammatory Agents; RiTUXimab; Sodium Phosphates

The levels/effects of Fosinopril may be increased by: Alfuzosin; Angiotensin II Receptor Blockers; Diazoxide; DPP-IV Inhibitors; Eplerenone; Everolimus; Herbs (Hypotensive Properties); Loop Diuretics; MAO Inhibitors; Pentoxifylline; Phosphodiesterase 5 Inhibitors; Potassium Salts; Potassium-Sparing Diuretics; Prostacyclin Analogues; Sirolimus; Temsirolimus; Thiazide Diuretics; TiZANidine; Tolvaptan; Trimethoprim

Decreased Effect

The levels/effects of Fosinopril may be decreased by: Antacids; Aprotinin; Herbs (Hypertensive Properties); Icatibant; Lanthanum; Methylphenidate; Nonsteroidal Anti-Inflammatory Agents; Salicylates; Yohimbine

Ethanol/Nutrition/Herb Interactions Herb/Nutraceutical: Avoid bayberry, blue cohosh, cayenne, ephedra, ginger, ginseng (American), kola, licorice (may worsen hypertension). Avoid black cohosh, california poppy, coleus, golden seal, hawthorn, mistletoe, periwinkle, quinine, shepherd's purse (may have increased antihypertensive effect).

Stability Store at 25°C (77°F); excursions permitted to 15°C to 30°C (59°F to 86°F). Protect from moisture by keeping bottle tightly closed.

Mechanism of Action Competitive inhibitor of angiotensin-converting enzyme (ACE); prevents conversion of angiotensin I to angiotensin II, a potent vasoconstrictor; results in lower levels of angiotensin II which causes an increase in plasma renin activity and a reduction in aldosterone secretion; a CNS mechanism may also be involved in hypotensive effect as angiotensin II increases adrenergic outflow from CNS; vasoactive kallikreins may be decreased in conversion to active hormones by ACE inhibitors, thus reducing blood pressure

Pharmacodynamics/Kinetics

Onset of action: 1 hour

Duration: 24 hours

Absorption: 36%

Protein binding: 95%

Metabolism: Prodrug, hydrolyzed to its active metabolite fosinoprilat by intestinal wall and hepatic esterases

Bioavailability: 36%

Half-life elimination, serum (fosinoprilat): 12 hours

Time to peak, serum: ~3 hours

Excretion: Urine and feces (as fosinoprilat and other metabolites in roughly equal proportions, 45% to 50%)

Dosage Oral:

Children ≥6 years and >50 kg: Hypertension: Initial: 5-10 mg once daily (maximum: 40 mg/day)

Adults:

Heart failure: Initial: 10 mg/day (5 mg if renal dysfunction present) and increase, as needed, to a maximum of 40 mg once daily over several weeks; usual dose: 20-40 mg/day. If hypotension, orthostasis, or azotemia occur during titration, consider decreasing concomitant diuretic dose, if any.

Hypertension: Initial: 10 mg/day; most patients are maintained on 20-40 mg/day (maximum: 80 mg/day). May need to divide the dose into two if trough effect is inadequate; discontinue the diuretic, if possible 2-3 days before initiation of therapy; resume diuretic therapy carefully, if needed.

Dosing adjustment/comments in renal impairment: None needed since hepatobiliary elimination compensates adequately diminished renal elimination.

Hemodialysis: Moderately dialyzable (20% to 50%)

Dietary Considerations Should not take a potassium salt supplement without the advice of healthcare provider.

Monitoring Parameters Blood pressure; serum creatinine and potassium; if patient has collagen vascular disease and/or renal impairment, periodically monitor CBC with differential

Test Interactions Positive Coombs' (direct); may cause false-positive results in urine acetone determinations using sodium nitroprusside reagent; may cause false low serum digoxin levels with the Digi-Tab RIA kit for digoxin

Dosage Forms Excipient information presented when available (limited, particularly for generics); consult specific product labeling.

Tablet, oral, as sodium: 10 mg, 20 mg, 40 mg

◆ **Fosinopril Sodium** *see* Fosinopril *on page* 763

Fosphenytoin (FOS fen i toyn)

Brand Names: U.S. Cerebyx®

Brand Names: Canada Cerebyx®

Index Terms Fosphenytoin Sodium

Pharmacologic Category Anticonvulsant, Hydantoin

Additional Appendix Information

Status Epilepticus *on page* 2010

Use Used for the control of generalized convulsive status epilepticus and prevention and treatment of seizures occurring during neurosurgery; indicated for short-term parenteral administration when other means of phenytoin administration are unavailable, inappropriate, or deemed less advantageous (the safety and effectiveness of fosphenytoin use for more than 5 days has not been systematically evaluated)

Pregnancy Risk Factor D

Pregnancy Considerations Fosphenytoin is the prodrug of phenytoin. Refer to Phenytoin on page 1346 for additional information.

Lactation Excretion in breast milk unknown/not recommended

Contraindications Hypersensitivity to phenytoin, other hydantoins, or any component of the formulation; patients with sinus bradycardia, sinoatrial block, second- and third-degree AV block, or Adams-Stokes syndrome; occurrence of rash during treatment (should not be resumed if rash is exfoliative, purpuric, or bullous); treatment of absence seizures

Warnings/Precautions Doses of fosphenytoin are expressed as their phenytoin sodium equivalent (PE). Antiepileptic drugs should not be abruptly discontinued. Hypotension may occur, especially after I.V. administration at high doses and high rates of administration. Administration of phenytoin has been associated with atrial and ventricular conduction depression and ventricular fibrillation. Careful cardiac monitoring is needed when administering I.V. loading doses of fosphenytoin. Acute hepatotoxicity associated with a hypersensitivity syndrome characterized by fever, skin eruptions, and lymphadenopathy has been reported to occur within the first 2 months of treatment. Discontinue if skin rash or lymphadenopathy occurs. A spectrum of hematologic effects have been reported with use (eg, neutropenia, leukopenia, thrombocytopenia, pancytopenia, and anemias). Use with caution in patients with hypotension, severe myocardial insufficiency, diabetes mellitus, porphyria, hypoalbuminemia, hypothyroidism, fever, or hepatic or renal dysfunction. Effects with other sedative drugs or ethanol may be potentiated. Severe reactions, including toxic epidermal necrolysis and Stevens-Johnson syndromes, although rarely reported, have resulted in fatalities; drug should be discontinued if there are any signs of rash. Patients of Asian descent with the variant *HLA-B*1502* may be at an increased risk of developing Stevens-Johnson syndrome and/or toxic epidermal necrolysis.

Adverse Reactions The more important adverse clinical events caused by the I.V. use of fosphenytoin or phenytoin are cardiovascular collapse and/or central nervous system depression. Hypotension can occur when either drug is administered rapidly by the I.V. route. Do not exceed a rate of 150 mg phenytoin equivalent/minute when administering fosphenytoin.

The adverse clinical events most commonly observed with the use of fosphenytoin in clinical trials were nystagmus, dizziness, pruritus, paresthesia, headache, somnolence, and ataxia. Paresthesia and pruritus were seen more often following fosphenytoin (versus phenytoin) administration and occurred more often with I.V. fosphenytoin than with I.M. administration. These events were dose and rate related (doses ≥15 mg/kg at a rate of 150 mg/minute). These sensations, generally described as itching, burning, or tingling are usually not at the infusion site. The location of the discomfort varied with the groin mentioned most frequently. The paresthesia and pruritus were transient events that occurred within several minutes of the start of infusion and generally resolved within 10 minutes after completion of infusion.

Transient pruritus, tinnitus, nystagmus, somnolence, and ataxia occurred 2-3 times more often at doses ≥15 mg/kg and rates ≥150 mg/minute.

I.V. administration (maximum dose/rate):

>10%:

Central nervous system: Nystagmus, dizziness, somnolence, ataxia

Dermatologic: Pruritus

1% to 10%:

Cardiovascular: Hypotension, vasodilation, tachycardia

Central nervous system: Stupor, incoordination, paresthesia, extrapyramidal syndrome, tremor, agitation, hypoesthesia, dysarthria, vertigo, brain edema, headache

Gastrointestinal: Nausea, tongue disorder, dry mouth, vomiting

Neuromuscular & skeletal: Pelvic pain, muscle weakness, back pain

Ocular: Diplopia, amblyopia

Otic: Tinnitus, deafness

Miscellaneous: Taste perversion

I.M. administration (substitute for oral phenytoin):
1% to 10%:
Central nervous system: Nystagmus, tremor, ataxia, headache, incoordination, somnolence, dizziness, paresthesia, reflexes decreased
Dermatologic: Pruritus
Gastrointestinal: Nausea, vomiting
Hematologic/lymphatic: Ecchymosis
Neuromuscular & skeletal: Muscle weakness
<1% (Limited to important or life-threatening): Acidosis, acute hepatic failure, acute hepatotoxicity, alkalosis, anemia, atrial flutter, bundle branch block, cardiac arrest, cardiomegaly, cerebral hemorrhage, cerebral infarct, CHF, cyanosis, dehydration, hyperglycemia, hyperkalemia, hypertension, hypochromic anemia, hypokalemia, hypophosphatemia, ketosis, leukocytosis, leukopenia, lymphadenopathy, palpitation, postural hypotension, pulmonary embolus, QT interval prolongation, sinus bradycardia, syncope, Stevens-Johnson syndrome, thrombocytopenia, thrombophlebitis, toxic epidermal necrolysis, ventricular extrasystoles

Drug Interactions

Metabolism/Transport Effects Substrate of CYP2C19 (major), CYP2C9 (major), CYP3A4 (minor); **Note:** Assignment of Major/Minor substrate status based on clinically relevant drug interaction potential; **Induces** CYP2B6 (strong), CYP2C19 (strong), CYP2C8 (strong), CYP2C9 (strong), CYP3A4 (strong)

Avoid Concomitant Use

Avoid concomitant use of Fosphenytoin with any of the following: Boceprevir; Bortezomib; Crizotinib; Darunavir; Delavirdine; Dronedarone; Etravirine; Everolimus; Lapatinib; Lurasidone; Nilotinib; Pazopanib; Praziquantel; Ranolazine; Rilpivirine; Rivaroxaban; Roflumilast; RomiDEPsin; SORAfenib; Telaprevir; Ticagrelor; Tolvaptan; Toremifene; Vandetanib

Increased Effect/Toxicity

Fosphenytoin may increase the levels/effects of: Clarithromycin; CNS Depressants; Fosamprenavir; Lithium; Methotrimeprazine; Selective Serotonin Reuptake Inhibitors; Vecuronium; Vitamin K Antagonists

The levels/effects of Fosphenytoin may be increased by: Alcohol (Ethyl); Allopurinol; Amiodarone; Antifungal Agents (Azole Derivatives, Systemic); Benzodiazepines; Calcium Channel Blockers; Capecitabine; CarBAMazepine; Carbonic Anhydrase Inhibitors; CeFAZolin; Chloramphenicol; Cimetidine; Clarithromycin; Conivaptan; CYP2C19 Inhibitors (Moderate); CYP2C19 Inhibitors (Strong); CYP2C9 Inhibitors (Moderate); CYP2C9 Inhibitors (Strong); Delavirdine; Dexmethylphenidate; Disulfiram; Droperidol; Efavirenz; Ethosuximide; Felbamate; Floxuridine; Fluconazole; Fluorouracil; Fluorouracil (Systemic); Fluorouracil (Topical); FLUoxetine; FluvoxaMINE; Halothane; HydrOXYzine; Isoniazid; Methotrimeprazine; Methylphenidate; MetroNIDAZOLE; MetroNIDAZOLE (Systemic); OXcarbazepine; Proton Pump Inhibitors; Rufinamide; Sertraline; Sulfonamide Derivatives; Tacrolimus; Tacrolimus (Systemic); Telaprevir; Ticlopidine; Topiramate; TraZODone; Trimethoprim; Vitamin K Antagonists

Decreased Effect

Fosphenytoin may decrease the levels/effects of: Acetaminophen; Amiodarone; Antifungal Agents (Azole Derivatives, Systemic); ARIPiprazole; Boceprevir; Bortezomib; Brentuximab Vedotin; Busulfan; CarBAMazepine; Chloramphenicol; Clarithromycin; CloZAPine; Contraceptives (Estrogens); Contraceptives (Progestins); Crizotinib; CycloSPORINE; CycloSPORINE (Systemic); CYP2B6 Substrates; CYP2C19 Substrates; CYP2C8 Substrates; CYP2C9 Substrates; CYP3A4 Substrates; Darunavir; Dasatinib; Deferasirox; Delavirdine; Diclofenac; Disopyramide; Divalproex; Doxycycline; Dronedarone; Efavirenz; Ethosuximide; Etoposide; Etoposide Phosphate; Etravirine; Everolimus; Exemestane; Felbamate; Flunarizine; Gefitinib; GuanFACINE; HMG-CoA Reductase Inhibitors; Imatinib; Irinotecan; Ixabepilone; Lacosamide; LamoTRIgine; Lapatinib; Levodopa; Linagliptin; Loop Diuretics; Lopinavir; Lurasidone; Maraviroc; Mebendazole; Meperidine; Methadone; MetroNIDAZOLE; MetroNIDAZOLE (Systemic); Metyrapone; Mexiletine; Nelfinavir; Nilotinib; OXcarbazepine; Pazopanib; Praziquantel; Primidone; QUEtiapine; QuiNIDine; QuiNINE; Ranolazine; Rilpivirine; Ritonavir; Rivaroxaban; Roflumilast; RomiDEPsin; Rufinamide; Saxagliptin; Sertraline; Sirolimus; SORAfenib; SUNItinib; Tacrolimus; Tacrolimus (Systemic); Tadalafil; Telaprevir; Temsirolimus; Teniposide; Theophylline Derivatives; Thyroid Products; Ticagrelor; Tipranavir; Tolvaptan; Topiramate; Toremifene; TraZODone; Treprostinil; Ulipristal; Valproic Acid; Vandetanib; Vecuronium; Vemurafenib; Zonisamide; Zuclopenthixol

The levels/effects of Fosphenytoin may be decreased by: Alcohol (Ethyl); Antacids; Barbiturates; CarBAMazepine; Ciprofloxacin; Ciprofloxacin (Systemic); CISplatin; CYP2C19 Inducers (Strong); CYP2C9 Inducers (Strong); Diazoxide; Divalproex; Folic Acid; Fosamprenavir; Ketorolac; Ketorolac (Nasal); Ketorolac (Systemic); Leucovorin Calcium-Levoleucovorin; Levomefolate; Lopinavir; Mefloquine; Methylfolate; Peginterferon Alfa-2b; Pyridoxine; Rifamycin Derivatives; Ritonavir; Telaprevir; Theophylline Derivatives; Tipranavir; Tocilizumab; Valproic Acid; Vigabatrin

Ethanol/Nutrition/Herb Interactions Ethanol:
Acute use: Avoid or limit ethanol (inhibits metabolism of phenytoin). Ethanol may also increase CNS depression; monitor for increased effects with coadministration. Caution patients about effects.
Chronic use: Avoid or limit ethanol (stimulates metabolism of phenytoin).

Stability Refrigerate at 2°C to 8°C (36°F to 46°F). Do not store at room temperature for more than 48 hours. Do not use vials that develop particulate matter. Must be diluted to concentrations of 1.5-25 mg PE/mL, in normal saline or D_5W, for I.V. infusion.

Mechanism of Action Diphosphate ester salt of phenytoin which acts as a water soluble prodrug of phenytoin; after administration, plasma esterases convert fosphenytoin to phosphate, formaldehyde, and phenytoin as the active moiety; phenytoin works by stabilizing neuronal membranes and decreasing seizure activity by increasing efflux or decreasing influx of sodium ions across cell membranes in the motor cortex during generation of nerve impulses

Pharmacodynamics/Kinetics Also refer to Phenytoin monograph for additional information.
Protein binding: Fosphenytoin: 95% to 99% to albumin; can displace phenytoin and increase free fraction (up to 30% unbound) during the period required for conversion of fosphenytoin to phenytoin
Metabolism: Fosphenytoin is rapidly converted via hydrolysis to phenytoin; phenytoin is metabolized in the liver and forms metabolites
Bioavailability: I.M.: Fosphenytoin: 100%
Half-life elimination:
Fosphenytoin: 15 minutes
Phenytoin: Variable (mean: 12-29 hours); kinetics of phenytoin are saturable
Time to peak: Conversion to phenytoin: Following I.V. administration (maximum rate of administration): 15 minutes; following I.M. administration, peak phenytoin levels are reached in 3 hours
Excretion: Phenytoin: Urine (as inactive metabolites)

Dosage The dose, concentration in solutions, and infusion rates for fosphenytoin are expressed as phenytoin sodium equivalents (PE); fosphenytoin should always be prescribed and dispensed in phenytoin sodium equivalents (PE)

Infants and Children (unlabeled use): I.V.:
- Loading dose: 15-20 mg PE/kg for the treatment of generalized convulsive status epilepticus
- Maintenance dosing: Phenytoin dosing guidelines in pediatric patients are used when dosing fosphenytoin using doses in PE equal to the phenytoin doses (ie, phenytoin 1 mg = fosphenytoin 1 PE); maintenance doses may be started 8-12 hours after a loading dose

Adults:
- Status epilepticus: I.V.: Loading dose: 15-20 mg PE/kg I.V. administered at 100-150 mg PE/minute
- Nonemergent loading and maintenance dosing: I.V. or I.M.:
  - Loading dose: 10-20 mg PE/kg (I.V. rate: Infuse over 30 minutes; maximum rate: 150 mg PE/minute)
  - Initial daily maintenance dose: 4-6 mg PE/kg/day

I.M. or I.V. substitution for oral phenytoin therapy: May be substituted for oral phenytoin sodium at the same total daily dose; however, Dilantin® capsules are ~90% bioavailable by the oral route; phenytoin, supplied as fosphenytoin, is 100% bioavailable by both the I.M. and I.V. routes; for this reason, plasma phenytoin concentrations may increase when I.M. or I.V. fosphenytoin is substituted for oral phenytoin sodium therapy; in clinical trials, I.M. fosphenytoin was administered as a single daily dose utilizing either 1 or 2 injection sites; some patients may require more frequent dosing

Dosing adjustments in renal/hepatic impairment: Phenytoin clearance may be substantially reduced in cirrhosis and plasma level monitoring with dose adjustment advisable; free phenytoin levels should be monitored closely in patients with renal or hepatic disease or in those with hypoalbuminemia; furthermore, fosphenytoin clearance to phenytoin may be increased without a similar increase in phenytoin clearance in these patients leading to increased frequency and severity of adverse events

Dietary Considerations Provides phosphate 0.0037 mmol/mg PE fosphenytoin

Administration

I.M.: May be administered as a single daily dose using either 1 or 2 injection sites.

I.V.: Rates of infusion:
- Children: 1-3 mg PE/kg/minute (maximum rate: 150 mg PE/minute)
- Adults: Should not exceed 150 mg PE/minute. For nonemergent situations, may administer loading dose over 30 minutes.

Monitoring Parameters Continuous blood pressure, ECG, and respiratory function monitoring with loading dose and for 10-20 minutes following infusion; vital signs, CBC, liver function tests, plasma level monitoring (plasma levels should not be measured until conversion to phenytoin is complete, ~2 hours after an I.V. infusion or ~4 hours after an I.M. injection)

Reference Range

Therapeutic: 10-20 mcg/mL (SI: 40-79 micromole/L); toxicity is measured clinically, and some patients require levels outside the suggested therapeutic range

Toxic: 30-50 mcg/mL (SI: 120-200 micromole/L)

Lethal: >100 mcg/mL (SI: >400 micromole/L)

Manifestations of toxicity:
- Nystagmus: 20 mcg/mL (SI: 79 micromole/L)
- Ataxia: 30 mcg/mL (SI: 118.9 micromole/L)
- Decreased mental status: 40 mcg/mL (SI: 159 micromole/L)
- Coma: 50 mcg/mL (SI: 200 micromole/L)

Peak serum phenytoin level after a 375 mg I.M. fosphenytoin dose in healthy males: 5.7 mcg/mL

Peak serum fosphenytoin levels and phenytoin levels after a 1.2 g infusion (I.V.) in healthy subjects over 30 minutes were 129 mcg/mL and 17.2 mcg/mL, respectively

Test Interactions Falsely high plasma phenytoin concentrations (due to cross-reactivity with fosphenytoin) when measured by immunoanalytical techniques (eg, TD_X®, TD_XFL_X™, Emit® 2000) prior to complete conversion of fosphenytoin to phenytoin. Phenytoin may produce falsely low results for dexamethasone or metyrapone tests.

Additional Information 1.5 mg fosphenytoin is approximately equivalent to 1 mg phenytoin. Equimolar fosphenytoin dose is 375 mg (75 mg/mL solution) to phenytoin 250 mg (50 mg/mL).

Dosage Forms Excipient information presented when available (limited, particularly for generics); consult specific product labeling.

Injection, solution, as sodium: 75 mg/mL (2 mL, 10 mL) [equivalent to phenytoin sodium 50 mg/mL]
- Cerebyx®: 75 mg/mL (2 mL) [equivalent to phenytoin sodium 50 mg/mL]

Injection, solution, as sodium [preservative free]: 75 mg/mL (2 mL) [equivalent to phenytoin sodium 50 mg/mL]

◆ **Fosphenytoin Sodium** *see* Fosphenytoin *on page 765*

Fosprepofol (fos PROE po fole)

Brand Names: U.S. Lusedra™

Index Terms Aquavan; Fospropofol Disodium; GPI 15715

Pharmacologic Category Sedative

Use Monitored anesthesia care (MAC) sedation in patients undergoing diagnostic or therapeutic procedures

Pregnancy Risk Factor B

Pregnancy Considerations Adverse events were not observed in animal reproduction studies; however, fospropofol should only be used in pregnancy if clearly needed. Fospropofol is not recommended for obstetrics, including cesarean section deliveries. It is not known if fospropofol crosses the placenta. However, propofol crosses the placenta, and therefore, may be associated with neonatal CNS and respiratory depression.

Lactation Propofol (the active metabolite of fospropofol) enters breast milk/not recommended

Contraindications There are no contraindications in the manufacturer's FDA approved labeling.

Note: Applicable contraindications to propofol include: Hypersensitivity to propofol; when general anesthesia or sedation is contraindicated

Warnings/Precautions The major cardiovascular effect is hypotension; use with caution in patients who are hemodynamically unstable, hypovolemic, have abnormally low vascular tone (eg, sepsis) or compromised myocardial function (eg, heart failure). The **onset of action will be delayed** due to need for conversion to the active metabolite, propofol. If supplemental doses are administered before full effect occurs, the risk of dose-stacking may be elevated resulting in deeper sedation than intended.

Use requires careful patient monitoring; should only be administered by persons trained in the administration of general anesthesia and not involved in the conduct of the diagnostic or therapeutic procedure. Sedated patients should be continuously monitored, and facilities for maintenance of a patent airway, providing artificial ventilation, administering supplemental oxygen, and instituting cardiovascular resuscitation must be immediately available. Patients should be continuously monitored during sedation and through the recovery process for early signs of hypotension, apnea, airway obstruction, and/or oxygen desaturation. Use to induce moderate (conscious) sedation in patients warrants monitoring equivalent to that seen with general anesthesia. May cause loss of spontaneous respiration and/or hypoxemia; supplemental oxygen is recommended for all patients receiving fospropofol; monitor patient closely. The risk of these effects may be increased with the concomitant use of opioids and/or other sedatives. May cause patients to become unresponsive or minimally responsive to vigorous tactile or painful stimuli.

Use lower doses in patients ≥65 years and/or ASA-PS 3/4 patients to reduce the incidence of unwanted cardiorespiratory and neurologic depressive events. Use with caution in patients with hepatic impairment or severe renal impairment (Cl_{cr} <30 mL/minute). Use with caution in patients with respiratory disease; risk of cardiorespiratory depression may be increased. Use with caution in patients with a history of epilepsy or seizures; seizure may occur during recovery phase.

Concomitant use of opioids/sedative-hypnotics may lead to increased sedative or respiratory depressant effects of fospropofol, more pronounced decreases in systolic, diastolic, and mean arterial pressures, heart rate, and cardiac output. Fospropofol lacks analgesic properties; pain management requires specific use of analgesic agents. Fospropofol should only be used in pregnancy if clearly needed. Not recommended for use in obstetrics, including cesarean section deliveries. Safety and efficacy have not been established in patients <18 years of age.

Adverse Reactions

>10%:

Dermatologic: Pruritus (see **"Note"**; 8% to 28%)

Neuromuscular & skeletal: Paresthesia (see **"Note"**; 52% to 74%)

Respiratory: Hypoxemia (1% to 11%)

1% to 10%:

Cardiovascular: Hypotension (2% to 7%)

Central nervous system: Headache (1% to 2%)

Gastrointestinal: Nausea (≤4%), vomiting (≤3%)

Miscellaneous: Procedural pain (≤2%)

<1% (Limited to important or life-threatening): Apnea, myoclonus, systolic blood pressure increased, heart rate increased

Note: Paresthesias (including perineal discomfort or burning sensation) and pruritus (including genital, perineal, and generalized pruritus) are mostly limited to the first 5 minutes of administration and usually described as mild-moderate in intensity. No pretreatments are helpful in reducing the incidence of these adverse effects.

Drug Interactions

Metabolism/Transport Effects Substrate of CYP1A2 (minor), CYP2B6 (major), CYP2C9 (minor), CYP3A4 (minor); **Note:** Assignment of Major/Minor substrate status based on clinically relevant drug interaction potential; **Inhibits** CYP1A2 (weak), CYP2C9 (weak), CYP2E1 (weak), CYP3A4 (weak)

Avoid Concomitant Use

Avoid concomitant use of Fospropofol with any of the following: Pimozide

Increased Effect/Toxicity

Fospropofol may increase the levels/effects of: Pimozide; Ropivacaine

The levels/effects of Fospropofol may be increased by: Alfentanil; Conivaptan; CYP2B6 Inhibitors (Moderate); CYP2B6 Inhibitors (Strong); Quazepam

Decreased Effect

The levels/effects of Fospropofol may be decreased by: Cyproterone; Tocilizumab

Stability Store at controlled room temperature of 25°C (77°F); excursions permitted between 15°C and 30°C (59°F and 86°F). Single-use vials do not need to be diluted prior to administration. Draw into sterile syringes immediately after opening vials. Discard any unused portion at the end of procedure.

Mechanism of Action Fospropofol disodium is a prodrug of propofol. Propofol interacts with the $GABA_A$ receptor, which is the presumed mechanism of action whereby it produces a sedative/hypnotic effect. Propofol is an alkylphenolic compound with intravenous general anesthetic properties.

Pharmacodynamics/Kinetics

Onset of action: Bolus (dose dependent): Attainment of adequate sedation was achieved between 2-28 minutes (median: 8 minutes)

Duration of sedation: Time to fully alert: ≤1 hour (median: 5 minutes)

Distribution:

Fospropofol: V_d: 0.26-0.4 L/kg

Propofol: V_d: ~6 L/kg; decreased in the elderly

Protein binding: Fospropofol: ~98% to albumin; does not affect protein binding of propofol (also ~98% bound to albumin)

Metabolism: Fospropofol is completely metabolized by plasma alkaline phosphatases to propofol, formaldehyde (rapidly converted to formate), and phosphate. Propofol is further metabolized hepatically to water-soluble sulfate and glucuronide conjugates (~50%).

Half-life elimination:

Fospropofol: 0.8-0.96 hours

Propofol: 0.85-1.41 hours

Time to peak: Propofol (from fospropofol): Median: 12 minutes

Excretion:

Fospropofol: Urine (<0.02% unchanged)

Propofol: Urine (~88% as metabolites, 40% as glucuronide metabolite); feces (<2%)

Dosage Monitored anesthesia care (MAC) sedation: I.V.: **Note: Onset of effect is delayed as compared to propofol-emulsion due to need for conversion to active component.** If <60 kg, base dosing on 60 kg; however, lower doses may be used to achieve lower levels of sedation. If >90 kg, base dosing on 90 kg.

Healthy adults <65 years or with mild systemic disease (ASA-PS1 or -PS2): *Standard dosing regimen:* Initial: 6.5 mg/kg (maximum initial dose: 577.5 mg or 16.5 mL), followed by supplemental doses of 1.6 mg/kg (maximum supplemental dose: 140 mg or 4 mL) no more frequently than every 4 minutes as needed to achieve desired level of sedation.

Elderly patients ≥65 years or patients with severe systemic disease (ASA-PS3 or -PS4): *Modified dosing regimen:* Initial: 4.9 mg/kg (maximum initial dose: 437.5 mg or 12.5 mL), followed by supplemental doses of 1.2 mg/kg (maximum supplemental dose: 105 mg or 3 mL) no more frequently than every 4 minutes as needed to achieve desired level of sedation.

Dosage adjustment in renal impairment: No dosage adjustment recommended. Use with caution in patients with severe renal impairment (Cl_{cr} <30 mL/minute); limited safety and efficacy data available in these patients.

Dosage adjustment in hepatic impairment: No dosage adjustment recommended. Use with caution in patients with hepatic impairment; has not been adequately studied in this population.

Administration Administer as an I.V. bolus (no recommendations on rate of administration provided by manufacturer) via via a secure, freely flowing, peripheral I.V. line. Flush I.V. line with NS or other compatible fluid before and after administration. Strict aseptic technique must be maintained in handling. Discard any unused portion at the end of the procedure. Do not filter.

Monitoring Parameters ECG, blood pressure, respiration, oxygen saturation; patient responsiveness

Dosage Forms Excipient information presented when available (limited, particularly for generics); consult specific product labeling.

Injection, solution, as disodium [preservative free]:
Lusedra™: 35 mg/mL (30 mL)

Controlled Substance C-IV

- ◆ **Fospropofol Disodium** *see* Fospropofol *on page 767*
- ◆ **Fosrenol®** *see* Lanthanum *on page 975*
- ◆ **FR901228** *see* RomiDEPsin *on page 1515*
- ◆ **Fragmin®** *see* Dalteparin *on page 441*
- ◆ **Frisium® (Can)** *see* Clobazam *on page 382*
- ◆ **Froben® (Can)** *see* Flurbiprofen (Systemic) *on page 737*
- ◆ **Froben-SR® (Can)** *see* Flurbiprofen (Systemic) *on page 737*
- ◆ **Frova®** *see* Frovatriptan *on page 769*

Frovatriptan (froe va TRIP tan)

Brand Names: U.S. Frova®

Brand Names: Canada Frova®

Index Terms Frovatriptan Succinate

Pharmacologic Category Antimigraine Agent; Serotonin $5\text{-}HT_{1B,\ 1D}$ Receptor Agonist

Additional Appendix Information

Antimigraine Drugs: $5\text{-}HT_1$ Receptor Agonists *on page 1878*

Use Acute treatment of migraine with or without aura

Pregnancy Risk Factor C

Pregnancy Considerations There are no adequate and well-controlled studies using frovatriptan in pregnant women. Use only if potential benefit to the mother outweighs the potential risk to the fetus.

Lactation Excretion in breast milk unknown/use caution

Contraindications Hypersensitivity to frovatriptan or any component of the formulation; patients with ischemic heart disease or signs or symptoms of ischemic heart disease (including Prinzmetal's angina, angina pectoris, myocardial infarction, silent myocardial ischemia); cerebrovascular syndromes (including strokes, transient ischemic attacks); peripheral vascular syndromes (including ischemic bowel disease); uncontrolled hypertension; use within 24 hours of ergotamine derivatives; use within 24 hours of another $5\text{-}HT_1$ agonist; management of hemiplegic or basilar migraine

Canadian labeling: Additional contraindications (not in U.S. labeling): Cardiac arrhythmias, valvular heart disease, congenital heart disease, atherosclerotic disease; management of ophthalmoplegic migraine; severe hepatic impairment

Warnings/Precautions Not intended for migraine prophylaxis, or treatment of cluster headaches, hemiplegic or basilar migraines. Rule out underlying neurologic disease in patients with atypical headache, migraine (with no prior history of migraine) or inadequate clinical response to initial dosing. Cardiac events (coronary artery vasospasm, transient ischemia, MI, ventricular tachycardia/fibrillation, cardiac arrest, and death), cerebral/subarachnoid hemorrhage, stroke, peripheral vascular ischemia, and colonic ischemia have been reported with $5\text{-}HT_1$ agonist administration. Patients who experience sensations of chest pain/pressure/tightness or symptoms suggestive of angina following dosing should be evaluated for coronary artery disease or Prinzmetal's angina before receiving additional doses; if dosing is resumed and similar symptoms recur, monitor with ECG. May cause vasospastic reactions resulting in colonic, peripheral, or coronary ischemia. Do not give to patients with risk factors for CAD until a cardiovascular evaluation has been performed; if evaluation is satisfactory, the healthcare provider should administer the first dose (consider ECG monitoring) and cardiovascular status should be periodically evaluated. Significant elevation in blood pressure, including hypertensive crisis, has also been reported on rare occasions in patients using other $5\text{-}HT_{1D}$ agonists with and without a history of hypertension. May lower seizure threshold, use caution in epilepsy or structural brain lesions. Symptoms of agitation, confusion, hallucinations, hyper-reflexia, myoclonus, shivering, and tachycardia (serotonin syndrome) may occur with concomitant proserotonergic drugs (ie, SSRIs/SNRIs or triptans) or agents which reduce frovatriptan's metabolism. Concurrent use of serotonin precursors (eg, tryptophan) is not recommended. If concomitant administration with SSRIs is warranted, monitor closely, especially at initiation and with dose increases. Safety and efficacy in pediatric patients have not been established.

Adverse Reactions

1% to 10%:

Cardiovascular: Flushing (4%), chest pain (2%), palpitation (1%)

Central nervous system: Dizziness (8%), fatigue (5%), headache (4%), hot or cold sensation (3%), somnolence (≥2%), anxiety (1%), dysesthesia (1%), hypoesthesia (1%), insomnia (1%), pain (1%)

Gastrointestinal: Xerostomia (3%), nausea (≥2%), dyspepsia (2%), abdominal pain (1%), diarrhea (1%), vomiting (1%)

Neuromuscular & skeletal: Paresthesia (4%), skeletal pain (3%)

Ocular: Vision abnormal (1%)

Otic: Tinnitus (1%)

Respiratory: Rhinitis (1%), sinusitis (1%)

Miscellaneous: Diaphoresis (1%)

<1% (Limited to important or life-threatening): Abnormal dreaming, abnormal gait, abnormal lacrimation, abnormal reflexes, abnormal urine, agitation, amnesia, anorexia, arthralgia, arthrosis, ataxia, back pain, bowel changes, bradycardia, bullous eruption, cheilitis, concentration impaired, confusion, conjunctivitis, constipation, dehydration, depersonalization, depression, dysphagia, dyspnea, earache, ECG changes, emotional lability, epistaxis, eructation, esophagospasm, euphoria, eye pain, fever, flatulence, gastroesophageal reflux, hiccup, hot flushes, hyperacusis, hyperesthesia, hypertonia, hyperventilation, hypocalcemia, hypoglycemia, hypotonia, involuntary muscle contractions, laryngitis, leg cramps/pain, malaise, micturition, mouth edema, muscle weakness, myalgia, nervousness, nocturia, peptic ulcer, personality disorder, pharyngitis, polyuria, pruritus, purpura, renal pain, rigors, saliva increased, salivary gland pain, seizure, speech disorder, stomatitis, syncope, tachycardia, taste perversion, thirst, tongue paralysis, toothache, tremor, urinary frequency, vertigo, weakness

Drug Interactions

Metabolism/Transport Effects Substrate of CYP1A2 (minor); **Note:** Assignment of Major/Minor substrate status based on clinically relevant drug interaction potential

Avoid Concomitant Use

Avoid concomitant use of Frovatriptan with any of the following: Ergot Derivatives

Increased Effect/Toxicity

Frovatriptan may increase the levels/effects of: Ergot Derivatives; Metoclopramide; Serotonin Modulators

The levels/effects of Frovatriptan may be increased by: Antipsychotics; Ergot Derivatives

Decreased Effect

The levels/effects of Frovatriptan may be decreased by: Cyproterone

Ethanol/Nutrition/Herb Interactions Food: Food does not affect frovatriptan bioavailability.

Stability Store at controlled room temperature of 25°C (77°F); excursions permitted to 15°C to 30°C (59°F to 86°F). Protect from moisture.

Mechanism of Action Selective agonist for serotonin ($5\text{-}HT_{1B}$ and $5\text{-}HT_{1D}$ receptors) in cranial arteries; causes vasoconstriction and reduces sterile inflammation associated with antidromic neuronal transmission correlating with relief of migraine.

Pharmacodynamics/Kinetics

Distribution: Male: 4.2 L/kg; Female: 3.0 L/kg

Protein binding: ~15%

Metabolism: Primarily hepatic via CYP1A2

Bioavailability: Male: ~20%; Female: ~30%

Half-life elimination: ~26 hours

Time to peak: 2-4 hours

Excretion: Feces (62%); urine (32%; <10% as unchanged drug)

Dosage Oral: Adults: Migraine:

U.S. labeling: 2.5 mg; if headache recurs, a second dose may be given if first dose provided relief and at least 2 hours have elapsed since the first dose (maximum daily dose: 7.5 mg)

Canadian labeling: 2.5 mg; if headache recurs, a second dose may be given if first dose provided relief and at least 4 hours have elapsed since the first dose (maximum daily dose: 5 mg)

Note: The safety of treating more than 4 migraines/month has not been established.

Dosage adjustment in renal impairment: No adjustment necessary

Dosage adjustment in hepatic impairment: No adjustment necessary in mild-to-moderate hepatic impairment; use with caution in severe impairment (has not been studied in severe impairment).

Canadian labeling (not in U.S. labeling): Use is contraindicated in severe hepatic impairment.

Administration Administer with fluids.

Dosage Forms Excipient information presented when available (limited, particularly for generics); consult specific product labeling.

Tablet, oral:

Frova®: 2.5 mg

◆ **Frovatriptan Succinate** *see* Frovatriptan *on page* 769

◆ **Frusemide** *see* Furosemide *on page* 771

◆ **FSH** *see* Follitropin Alfa *on page* 750

◆ **FSH** *see* Follitropin Beta *on page* 750

◆ **FSH** *see* Urofollitropin *on page* 1750

◆ **FTC** *see* Emtricitabine *on page* 581

◆ **FTC/RPV/TDF** *see* Emtricitabine, Rilpivirine, and Tenofovir *on page* 583

◆ **FTC, TDF, and EFV** *see* Efavirenz, Emtricitabine, and Tenofovir *on page* 577

◆ **FTY720** *see* Fingolimod *on page* 714

◆ **FU** *see* Fluorouracil (Systemic) *on page* 730

◆ **FU** *see* Fluorouracil (Topical) *on page* 731

◆ **5-FU** *see* Fluorouracil (Systemic) *on page* 730

◆ **5-FU** *see* Fluorouracil (Topical) *on page* 731

◆ **Ful-Glo®** *see* Fluorescein *on page* 727

Fulvestrant (fool VES trant)

Brand Names: U.S. Faslodex®

Brand Names: Canada Faslodex®

Index Terms ICI-182,780; ZD9238

Pharmacologic Category Antineoplastic Agent, Estrogen Receptor Antagonist

Use Treatment of hormone receptor positive metastatic breast cancer in postmenopausal women with disease progression following antiestrogen therapy

Pregnancy Risk Factor D

Pregnancy Considerations Fetal loss and abnormalities were observed in animal studies. Approved for use only in postmenopausal women. If used prior to confirmed menopause, women of reproductive potential should be advised not to become pregnant.

Lactation Excretion in breast milk unknown/not recommended

Contraindications Hypersensitivity to fulvestrant or any component of the formulation

Warnings/Precautions Hazardous agent - use appropriate precautions for handling and disposal. Use caution in hepatic impairment; dosage adjustment is recommended in patients with moderate hepatic impairment. Safety and efficacy have not been established in severe hepatic impairment. Use with caution in patients with a history of bleeding disorders (including thrombocytopenia) and/or patients on anticoagulant therapy; bleeding/hematoma may occur from I.M. administration.

Adverse Reactions Adverse reactions reported with 500 mg dose.

>10%:

Endocrine & metabolic: Hot flushes (7% to 13%)

Hepatic: Alkaline phosphatase increased (>15%; grades 3/4: 1% to 2%), transaminases increased (>15%; grades 3/4: 1% to 2%)

Local: Injection site pain (12% to 14%)

Neuromuscular & skeletal: Joint disorders (14% to 19%)

1% to 10%:

Cardiovascular: Ischemic disorder (1%)

Central nervous system: Fatigue (8%), headache (8%)

Gastrointestinal: Nausea (10%), anorexia (6%), vomiting (6%), constipation (5%), weight gain (≤1%)

Genitourinary: Urinary tract infection (2% to 4%)

Neuromuscular & skeletal: Bone pain (9%), arthralgia (8%), back pain (8%), extremity pain (7%), musculoskeletal pain (6%), weakness (6%)

Respiratory: Cough (5%), dyspnea (4%)

<1% (Limited to important or life-threatening; reported with 250 mg or 500 mg dose): Angioedema, hypersensitivity reactions, leukopenia, myalgia, osteoporosis, thrombosis, urticaria, vaginal bleeding

Drug Interactions

Metabolism/Transport Effects Substrate of CYP3A4 (minor); **Note:** Assignment of Major/Minor substrate status based on clinically relevant drug interaction potential

Avoid Concomitant Use There are no known interactions where it is recommended to avoid concomitant use.

Increased Effect/Toxicity

The levels/effects of Fulvestrant may be increased by: Conivaptan

Decreased Effect

The levels/effects of Fulvestrant may be decreased by: Tocilizumab

Stability Store in original carton under refrigeration at 2°C to 8°C (36°F to 46°F). Protect from light.

Mechanism of Action Estrogen receptor antagonist; competitively binds to estrogen receptors on tumors and other tissue targets, producing a nuclear complex that causes a dose-related down-regulation of estrogen receptors and inhibits tumor growth.

Pharmacodynamics/Kinetics

Duration: I.M.: Steady state concentrations reached within first month, when administered with additional dose given 2 weeks following the initial dose; plasma levels maintained for at least 1 month

Distribution: V_d: ~3-5 L/kg

Protein binding: 99%; to plasma proteins (VLDL, LDL and HDL lipoprotein fractions)

Metabolism: Hepatic via multiple biotransformation pathways (CYP3A4 substrate involved in oxidation pathway, although relative contribution to metabolism unknown); metabolites formed are either less active or have similar activity to parent compound

Half-life elimination: 250 mg: ~40 days

Excretion: Feces (~90%); urine (<1%)

Dosage I.M.: Adults (postmenopausal women): Breast cancer, metastatic: Initial: 500 mg on days 1, 15, and 29; Maintenance: 500 mg once monthly

Dosage adjustment in hepatic impairment:

Moderate impairment (Child-Pugh class B): Decrease initial and maintenance dose to 250 mg

Severe impairment (Child-Pugh class C): Use has not been evaluated.

Administration For I.M. administration only; do not administer I.V., SubQ, or intra-arterially. Administer 500 mg dose as two 5 mL injections (one in each buttocks) slowly over 1-2 minutes per injection.

Dosage Forms Excipient information presented when available (limited, particularly for generics); consult specific product labeling.

Injection, solution:

Faslodex®: 50 mg/mL (5 mL) [contains benzyl alcohol, benzyl benzoate, castor oil, ethanol 10% w/v]

◆ **Fungizone® (Can)** *see* Amphotericin B (Conventional) *on page 109*

◆ **Fungoid® [OTC]** *see* Miconazole (Topical) *on page 1126*

◆ **Furadantin®** *see* Nitrofurantoin *on page 1210*

◆ **Furazosin** *see* Prazosin *on page 1396*

Furosemide (fyoor OH se mide)

Brand Names: U.S. Lasix®

Brand Names: Canada Apo-Furosemide®; Bio-Furosemide; Dom-Furosemide; Furosemide Injection, USP; Furosemide Special Injection; Lasix®; Lasix® Special; Novo-Semide; Nu-Furosemide; PMS-Furosemide

Index Terms Frusemide

Pharmacologic Category Diuretic, Loop

Additional Appendix Information

Heart Failure (Systolic) *on page 1991*

Use Management of edema associated with heart failure and hepatic or renal disease; acute pulmonary edema; treatment of hypertension (alone or in combination with other antihypertensives)

Canadian labeling: Additional use: Furosemide Special Injection and Lasix® Special (products not available in the U.S.): Adjunctive treatment of oliguria in patients with severe renal impairment

Pregnancy Risk Factor C

Pregnancy Considerations Animal studies have demonstrated maternal death, fetal toxicity, and fetal loss. There are no adequate and well-controlled studies in pregnant women. Crosses the placenta. Increased fetal urine production, electrolyte disturbances reported. Generally, use of diuretics during pregnancy is avoided due to risk of decreased placental perfusion. Monitor fetal growth if used during pregnancy; may increase birth weight.

Lactation Enters breast milk/use caution

Contraindications Hypersensitivity to furosemide or any component of the formulation; anuria

Canadian labeling: Additional contraindications (not in U.S. labeling): Hypersensitivity to sulfonamide-derived drugs; complete renal shutdown; hepatic coma and precoma; uncorrected states of electrolyte depletion, hypovolemia, or hypotension; jaundiced newborn infants or infants with disease(s) capable of causing hyperbilirubinemia and possibly kernicterus; breast-feeding. **Note:** Manufacturer labeling for Lasix® Special and Furosemide Special Injection also includes: GFR <5 mL/minute or GFR >20 mL/minute; hepatic cirrhosis; renal failure accompanied by hepatic coma and precoma; renal failure due to poisoning with nephrotoxic or hepatotoxic substances.

Warnings/Precautions [U.S. Boxed Warning]: If given in excessive amounts, furosemide, similar to other loop diuretics, can lead to profound diuresis, resulting in fluid and electrolyte depletion; close medical supervision and dose evaluation are required. Watch for and correct electrolyte disturbances; adjust dose to avoid dehydration. When electrolyte depletion is present, therapy should not be initiated unless serum electrolytes, especially potassium, are normalized. In cirrhosis, avoid electrolyte and acid/base imbalances that might lead to hepatic encephalopathy; correct electrolyte and acid/base imbalances prior to initiation when hepatic coma is present. Coadministration of antihypertensives may increase the risk of hypotension.

Monitor fluid status and renal function in an attempt to prevent oliguria, azotemia, and reversible increases in BUN and creatinine; close medical supervision of aggressive diuresis is required. May increase risk of contrast-induced nephropathy. Rapid I.V. administration, renal impairment, excessive doses, hypoproteinemia, and concurrent use of other ototoxins is associated with ototoxicity. Asymptomatic hyperuricemia has been reported with use; rarely, gout may precipitate. Photosensitization may occur.

Use with caution in patients with prediabetes or diabetes mellitus; may see a change in glucose control. Use with caution in patients with systemic lupus erythematosus (SLE); may cause SLE exacerbation or activation. Use with caution in patients with prostatic hyperplasia/urinary stricture; may cause urinary retention. May lead to nephrocalcinosis or nephrolithiasis in premature infants or in children <4 years of age with chronic use. May prevent closure of patent ductus arteriosus in premature infants. Chemical similarities are present among sulfonamides, sulfonylureas, carbonic anhydrase inhibitors, thiazides, and loop diuretics (except ethacrynic acid). A risk of cross-reaction exists in patients with allergy to any of these compounds; avoid use when previous reaction has been severe. Discontinue if signs of hypersensitivity are noted.

Adverse Reactions Frequency not defined.

Cardiovascular: Acute hypotension, chronic aortitis, necrotizing angiitis, orthostatic hypotension, vasculitis

Central nervous system: Dizziness, fever, headache, hepatic encephalopathy, lightheadedness, restlessness, vertigo

Dermatologic: Bullous pemphigoid, cutaneous vasculitis, erythema multiforme, exfoliative dermatitis, photosensitivity, pruritus, purpura, rash, Stevens-Johnson syndrome, toxic epidermal necrolysis, urticaria

Endocrine & metabolic: Cholesterol and triglycerides increased, glucose tolerance test altered, gout, hyperglycemia, hyperuricemia, hypocalcemia, hypochloremia, hypokalemia, hypomagnesemia, hyponatremia, metabolic alkalosis

Gastrointestinal: Anorexia, constipation, cramping, diarrhea, nausea, oral and gastric irritation, pancreatitis, vomiting

Genitourinary: Urinary bladder spasm, urinary frequency

Hematological: Agranulocytosis (rare), anemia, aplastic anemia (rare), eosinophilia, hemolytic anemia, leukopenia, thrombocytopenia

Hepatic: Intrahepatic cholestatic jaundice, ischemic hepatitis, liver enzymes increased

Local: Injection site pain (following I.M. injection), thrombophlebitis

Neuromuscular & skeletal: Muscle spasm, paresthesia, weakness
Ocular: Blurred vision, xanthopsia
Otic: Hearing impairment (reversible or permanent with rapid I.V. or I.M. administration), tinnitus
Renal: Allergic interstitial nephritis, fall in glomerular filtration rate and renal blood flow (due to overdiuresis), glycosuria, transient rise in BUN
Miscellaneous: Anaphylaxis (rare), exacerbate or activate systemic lupus erythematosus

Drug Interactions

Metabolism/Transport Effects None known.

Avoid Concomitant Use

Avoid concomitant use of Furosemide with any of the following: Chloral Hydrate; Ethacrynic Acid

Increased Effect/Toxicity

Furosemide may increase the levels/effects of: ACE Inhibitors; Allopurinol; Amifostine; Aminoglycosides; Antihypertensives; Cardiac Glycosides; Chloral Hydrate; CISplatin; Dofetilide; Ethacrynic Acid; Hypotensive Agents; Lithium; Methotrexate; Neuromuscular-Blocking Agents; RisperiDONE; RiTUXimab; Salicylates; Sodium Phosphates

The levels/effects of Furosemide may be increased by: Alfuzosin; Beta2-Agonists; Corticosteroids (Orally Inhaled); Corticosteroids (Systemic); CycloSPORINE (Systemic); Diazoxide; Herbs (Hypotensive Properties); Licorice; MAO Inhibitors; Methotrexate; Pentoxifylline; Phosphodiesterase 5 Inhibitors; Probenecid; Prostacyclin Analogues

Decreased Effect

Furosemide may decrease the levels/effects of: Lithium; Neuromuscular-Blocking Agents

The levels/effects of Furosemide may be decreased by: Aliskiren; Bile Acid Sequestrants; Fosphenytoin; Herbs (Hypertensive Properties); Methotrexate; Methylphenidate; Nonsteroidal Anti-Inflammatory Agents; Phenytoin; Probenecid; Salicylates; Sucralfate; Yohimbine

Ethanol/Nutrition/Herb Interactions

Food: Furosemide serum levels may be decreased if taken with food.
Herb/Nutraceutical: Avoid bayberry, blue cohosh, cayenne, ephedra, ginger, ginseng (American), kola, licorice (may worsen hypertension). Avoid black cohosh, California poppy, coleus, golden seal, hawthorn, mistletoe, periwinkle, quinine, shepherd's purse (may increase antihypertensive effect). Licorice may also cause or worsen hypokalemia.

Stability

Injection: Store at room temperature of 15°C to 30°C (59°F to 86°F). Protect from light. Exposure to light may cause discoloration; do not use furosemide solutions if they have a yellow color. Furosemide solutions are unstable in acidic media, but very stable in basic media. Refrigeration may result in precipitation or crystallization; however, resolubilization at room temperature or warming may be performed without affecting the drug's stability.
I.V. infusion solution mixed in NS or D_5W solution is stable for 24 hours at room temperature. May also be diluted for infusion to 1-2 mg/mL (maximum: 10 mg/mL).
Tablet: Store at 25°C (77°F); excursions permitted to 15°C to 30°C (59°F to 89°F). Protect from light.

Mechanism of Action Inhibits reabsorption of sodium and chloride in the ascending loop of Henle and distal renal tubule, interfering with the chloride-binding cotransport system, thus causing increased excretion of water, sodium, chloride, magnesium, and calcium

Pharmacodynamics/Kinetics

Onset of action: Diuresis: Oral, S.L: 30-60 minutes; I.M.: 30 minutes; I.V.: ~5 minutes
Symptomatic improvement with acute pulmonary edema: Within 15-20 minutes; occurs prior to diuretic effect
Peak effect: Oral, S.L.: 1-2 hours
Duration: Oral, S.L.: 6-8 hours; I.V.: 2 hours
Protein binding: 91% to 99%; primarily to albumin
Metabolism: Minimally hepatic
Bioavailability: Oral tablet: 47% to 64%; Oral solution: 50%; S.L. administration of oral tablet: ~60%; results of a small comparative study (n=11) showed bioavailability of S.L. administration of tablet was ~12% higher than oral administration of tablet (Haegeli, 2007)
Half-life elimination: Normal renal function: 0.5-2 hours; End-stage renal disease: 9 hours
Excretion: Urine (Oral: 50%, I.V.: 80%) within 24 hours; feces (as unchanged drug); nonrenal clearance prolonged in renal impairment

Dosage

Infants and Children: Edema, heart failure:
Oral: Initial: 2 mg/kg/dose increased in increments of 1-2 mg/kg/dose with each succeeding dose at intervals of 6-8 hours until a satisfactory response is achieved; maximum dose: 6 mg/kg/dose
I.M., I.V.: Initial: 1 mg/kg/dose; if response not adequate, may increase dose in increments of 1 mg/kg/dose and administer not sooner than 2 hours after previous dose, until a satisfactory response is achieved; may administer maintenance dose at intervals of every 6-12 hours; maximum dose: 6 mg/kg/dose
Children 1-17 years: Hypertension, resistant (unlabeled; AAP, 2004): Oral: Initial: 0.5-2 mg/kg/dose once or twice daily; maximum dose: 6 mg/kg/dose
Adults:
Edema, heart failure:
Oral: Initial: 20-80 mg/dose; if response is not adequate, may repeat the same dose or increase dose in increments of 20-40 mg/dose at intervals of 6-8 hours; may be titrated up to 600 mg/day with severe edematous states; usual maintenance dose interval is once or twice daily. **Note:** Dosing frequency may be adjusted based on patient-specific diuretic needs.
I.M., I.V.: Initial: 20-40 mg/dose; if response is not adequate, may repeat the same dose or increase dose in increments of 20 mg/dose and administer 1-2 hours after previous dose (maximum dose: 200 mg/dose). Individually determined dose should then be given once or twice daily although some patients may initially require dosing as frequent as every 6 hours. **Note:** ACC/AHA 2009 guidelines for heart failure recommend a maximum single dose of 160-200 mg.
Continuous I.V. infusion (Howard, 2001; Hunt, 2009): Initial: I.V. bolus dose 20-40 mg over 1-2 minutes, followed by continuous I.V. infusion doses of 10-40 mg/hour. If urine output is <1 mL/kg/hour, double as necessary to a maximum of 80-160 mg/hour. The risk associated with higher infusion rates (80-160 mg/hour) must be weighed against alternative strategies. **Note:** ACC/AHA 2009 guidelines for heart failure recommend 40 mg I.V. load, then 10-40 mg/hour infusion.
Acute pulmonary edema: I.V.: 40 mg over 1-2 minutes. If response not adequate within 1 hour, may increase dose to 80 mg. **Note:** ACC/AHA 2009 guidelines for heart failure recommend a maximum single dose of 160-200 mg.
Hypertension, resistant (Chobanian, 2003; JNC 7): Oral: 20-80 mg/day in 2 divided doses
Refractory heart failure: Oral, I.V.: Doses up to 8 g/day have been used.
Elderly: Oral, I.M., I.V.: Initial: 20 mg/day; increase slowly to desired response.

Dosing adjustment/comments in renal impairment: Acute renal failure: High doses (up to 1-3 g/day - oral/I.V.) have been used to initiate desired response; avoid use in oliguric states.

Dialysis: Not removed by hemo- or peritoneal dialysis; supplemental dose is not necessary.

Dosing adjustment/comments in hepatic disease: Diminished natriuretic effect with increased sensitivity to hypokalemia and volume depletion in cirrhosis; monitor effects, particularly with high doses.

Dietary Considerations May cause potassium loss; potassium supplement or dietary changes may be required.

Administration

I.V.: I.V. injections should be given slowly. In adults, undiluted direct I.V. injections may be administered at a rate of 20-40 mg per minute; maximum rate of administration for short-term intermittent infusion is 4 mg/minute; exceeding this rate increases the risk of ototoxicity. In children, a maximum rate of 0.5 mg/kg/minute has been recommended.

Oral: Administer on an empty stomach (Bard, 2004). May be administered with food or milk if GI distress occurs; however, this may reduce diuretic efficacy.

Note: When I.V. or oral administration is not possible, the sublingual route may be used. Place 1 tablet under tongue for at least 5 minutes to allow for maximal absorption. Patients should be advised not to swallow during disintegration time (Haegeli, 2007).

Monitoring Parameters Monitor weight and I & O daily; blood pressure, orthostasis; serum electrolytes, renal function; monitor hearing with high doses or rapid I.V. administration

Dosage Forms Excipient information presented when available (limited, particularly for generics); consult specific product labeling.

Injection, solution [preservative free]: 10 mg/mL (2 mL, 4 mL, 10 mL)

Solution, oral: 40 mg/5 mL (5 mL, 500 mL); 10 mg/mL (4 mL, 60 mL, 120 mL)

Tablet, oral: 20 mg, 40 mg, 80 mg

Lasix®: 20 mg

Lasix®: 40 mg, 80 mg [scored]

Dosage Forms: Canada Excipient information presented when available (limited, particularly for generics); consult specific product labeling.

Injection, solution [preservative free]:

Furosemide Special Injection: 10 mg/mL (25 mL)

Tablet, oral:

Lasix® Special: 500 mg [scored]

◆ **Furosemide Injection, USP (Can)** *see* Furosemide *on page 771*

◆ **Furosemide Special Injection (Can)** *see* Furosemide *on page 771*

◆ **Fusilev™** *see* LEVOleucovorin *on page 1000*

◆ **Fuzeon®** *see* Enfuvirtide *on page 587*

◆ **FVIII/vWF** *see* Antihemophilic Factor/von Willebrand Factor Complex (Human) *on page 128*

◆ **FXIII** *see* Factor XIII Concentrate (Human) *on page 686*

◆ **FXT 40 (Can)** *see* FLUoxetine *on page 731*

◆ **GAA** *see* Alglucosidase Alfa *on page 65*

Gabapentin (GA ba pen tin)

Brand Names: U.S. Gralise™; Neurontin®

Brand Names: Canada Apo-Gabapentin®; CO Gabapentin; Dom-Gabapentin; Mylan-Gabapentin; Neurontin®; PHL-Gabapentin; PMS-Gabapentin; PRO-Gabapentin; RAN™-Gabapentin; ratio-Gabapentin; Riva-Gabapentin; Teva-Gabapentin

Pharmacologic Category Anticonvulsant, Miscellaneous; GABA Analog

Additional Appendix Information

Anticonvulsant Drugs of Choice *on page 1873*

Use Adjunct for treatment of partial seizures with and without secondary generalized seizures in patients >12 years of age with epilepsy; adjunct for treatment of partial seizures in pediatric patients 3-12 years of age; management of postherpetic neuralgia (PHN) in adults

Unlabeled Use Neuropathic pain, diabetic peripheral neuropathy, fibromyalgia, postoperative pain, restless legs syndrome (RLS), vasomotor symptoms

Pregnancy Risk Factor C

Pregnancy Considerations Animal studies have documented teratogenic effects. There are no adequate and well-controlled studies in pregnant women. Use during pregnancy only if the potential benefit to the mother outweighs the potential risk to the fetus.

Patients exposed to gabapentin during pregnancy are encouraged to enroll in the North American Antiepileptic Drug (NAAED) Pregnancy Registry by calling 1-888-233-2334. Additional information is available at www.aedpregnancyregistry.org.

Lactation Enters breast milk/use caution

Medication Guide Available Yes

Contraindications Hypersensitivity to gabapentin or any component of the formulation

Warnings/Precautions Antiepileptics are associated with an increased risk of suicidal behavior/thoughts with use (regardless of indication); patients should be monitored for signs/symptoms of depression, suicidal tendencies, and other unusual behavior changes during therapy and instructed to inform their healthcare provider immediately if symptoms occur. Avoid abrupt withdrawal, may precipitate seizures; Gralise™ should be withdrawn over ≥1 week. Use cautiously in patients with severe renal dysfunction; male rat studies demonstrated an association with pancreatic adenocarcinoma (clinical implication unknown). May cause CNS depression, which may impair physical or mental abilities. Patients must be cautioned about performing tasks which require mental alertness (eg, operating machinery or driving). Effects with other sedative drugs or ethanol may be potentiated. Pediatric patients (3-12 years of age) have shown increased incidence of CNS-related adverse effects, including emotional lability, hostility, thought disorder, and hyperkinesia. Gabapentin immediate release and extended release (Gralise™) products are not interchangeable with each other **or** with gabapentin encarbil (Horizant™). The safety and efficacy of extended release gabapentin (Gralise™) has not been studied in patients with epilepsy. Potentially serious, sometimes fatal multiorgan hypersensitivity (also known as drug reaction with eosinophilia and systemic symptoms [DRESS]) has been reported with some antiepileptic drugs, including gabapentin; may affect lymphatic, hepatic, renal, cardiac, and/or hematologic systems; fever, rash, and eosinophilia may also be present. Discontinue immediately if suspected.

Adverse Reactions As reported for immediate release (IR) formulations in patients >12 years of age, unless otherwise noted in children (3-12 years) or with use of extended release (ER) formulation

>10%:

Central nervous system: Dizziness (IR: 17% to 28%; children 3%; ER: 11%), somnolence (IR: 19% to 21%; children 8%; ER: 5%), ataxia (3% to 13%), fatigue (11%; children 3%)

Miscellaneous: Viral infection (children 11%)

1% to 10%:

Cardiovascular: Peripheral edema (2% to 8%), vasodilatation (1%)

Central nervous system: Fever (children 10%), hostility (children 5% to 8%), emotional lability (children 4% to 6%), headache (IR: 3%; ER: 4%), abnormal thinking (2% to 3%; children 2%), amnesia (2%), depression (2%), nervousness (2%), abnormal coordination (1% to 2%), pain (ER: 1% to 2%), hyperesthesia (1%), lethargy (ER: 1%), twitching (1%), vertigo (ER: 1%)

Dermatologic: Pruritus (1%), rash (1%)

Endocrine & metabolic: Hyperglycemia (1%)

Gastrointestinal: Diarrhea (IR: 6%; ER: 3%), nausea/vomiting (3% to 4%; children 8%), abdominal pain (3%), xerostomia (2% to 5%), constipation (1% to 4%), weight gain (adults and children 2% to 3%), dyspepsia (IR: 2%; ER: 1%), flatulence (2%), dry throat (2%), dental abnormalities (2%), appetite stimulation (1%)

Genitourinary: Impotence (2%), urinary tract infection (ER: 2%)

Hematologic: Decreased WBC (1%), leukopenia (1%)

Neuromuscular & skeletal: Tremor (7%), weakness (6%), hyperkinesia (children 3% to 5%), abnormal gait (2%), back pain (2%), dysarthria (2%), myalgia (2%), fracture (1%)

Ocular: Nystagmus (8%), diplopia (1% to 6%), blurred vision (3% to 4%), conjunctivitis (1%)

Otic: Otitis media (1%)

Respiratory: Rhinitis (4%), bronchitis (children 3%), respiratory infection (children 3% to 5%), pharyngitis (1% to 3%), cough (2%)

Miscellaneous: Infection (5%)

Postmarketing and additional clinical reports (limited to important or life-threatening): Acute renal failure, anemia, angina, angioedema, aphasia, arrhythmias (various), aspiration pneumonia, blindness, bradycardia, breast enlargement, bronchospasm, cerebrovascular accident, CNS tumors, coagulation defect, colitis, Cushingoid appearance, dyspnea, encephalopathy, erythema multiforme, facial paralysis, fecal incontinence, gastroenteritis, glaucoma, glycosuria, hearing loss, heart block, heart failure, hematemesis, hematuria, hemiplegia, hemorrhage, hepatitis, hepatomegaly, hyperlipidemia, hyper-/hypotension, hyper-/hypothyroidism, hyper-/hypoventilation, hyponatremia, jaundice, leukocytosis, liver function tests increased, local myoclonus, lymphadenopathy, lymphocytosis, meningismus, MI, migraine, movement disorder, nephrosis, nerve palsy, non-Hodgkin's lymphoma, ovarian failure, palpitation, pancreatitis, paresthesia, peptic ulcer, pericardial effusion, pericardial rub, pericarditis, peripheral vascular disorder, pneumonia, psychosis, pulmonary embolus, pulmonary thrombosis, purpura, renal stone, retinopathy, skin necrosis, status epilepticus, Stevens-Johnson syndrome, subdural hematoma, suicidal behavior/ideation, syncope, tachycardia, thrombocytopenia, thrombophlebitis

Drug Interactions

Metabolism/Transport Effects None known.

Avoid Concomitant Use There are no known interactions where it is recommended to avoid concomitant use.

Increased Effect/Toxicity

Gabapentin may increase the levels/effects of: Alcohol (Ethyl); CNS Depressants; Methotrimeprazine; Selective Serotonin Reuptake Inhibitors

The levels/effects of Gabapentin may be increased by: Droperidol; HydrOXYzine; Methotrimeprazine

Decreased Effect

The levels/effects of Gabapentin may be decreased by: Antacids; Ketorolac; Ketorolac (Nasal); Ketorolac (Systemic); Mefloquine

Ethanol/Nutrition/Herb Interactions

Ethanol: May increase CNS depression; monitor for increased effects with coadministration. Caution patients about effects.

Food: Tablet, solution (immediate release): No significant effect on rate or extent of absorption; tablet (extended release): Increases rate and extent of absorption.

Herb/Nutraceutical: Avoid evening primrose (seizure threshold decreased). Avoid valerian, St John's wort, kava kava, gotu kola (may increase CNS depression).

Stability

Capsules and tablets: Store at 25°C (77°F); excursions permitted to 15°C to 30°C (59°F to 86°F).

Oral solution: Store refrigerated at 2°C to 8°C (36°F to 46°F).

Mechanism of Action Gabapentin is structurally related to GABA. However, it does not bind to $GABA_A$ or $GABA_B$ receptors, and it does not appear to influence synthesis or uptake of GABA. High affinity gabapentin binding sites have been located throughout the brain; these sites correspond to the presence of voltage-gated calcium channels specifically possessing the alpha-2-delta-1 subunit. This channel appears to be located presynaptically, and may modulate the release of excitatory neurotransmitters which participate in epileptogenesis and nociception.

Pharmacodynamics/Kinetics

Absorption: Variable, from proximal small bowel by L-amino transport system

Distribution: V_d: 58 ± 6 L

Protein binding: <3%

Bioavailability: Inversely proportional to dose due to saturable absorption:

- Immediate release:
  - 900 mg/day: 60%
  - 1200 mg/day: 47%
  - 2400 mg/day: 34%
  - 3600 mg/day: 33%
  - 4800 mg/day: 27%
- Extended release: Variable; increased with higher fat content meal

Half-life elimination: 5-7 hours; anuria 132 hours; during dialysis 3.8 hours

Time to peak: Immediate release: 2-4 hours; extended release: 8 hours

Excretion: Proportional to renal function; urine (as unchanged drug)

Dosage Oral:

Children: Immediate release: Anticonvulsant:

- 3-12 years: Initial: 10-15 mg/kg/day in 3 divided doses; titrate to effective dose over ~3 days; dosages of up to 50 mg/kg/day have been tolerated in clinical studies
  - 3-4 years: Usual dose: 40 mg/kg/day in 3 divided doses
  - ≥5-12 years: Usual dose: 25-35 mg/kg/day in 3 divided doses
- See **"Note"** in adult dosing.

Children >12 years and Adults: Immediate release: Anticonvulsant: Initial: 300 mg 3 times/day; if necessary the dose may be increased up to 1800 mg/day; Maintenance: 900-1800 mg/day administered in 3 divided doses; doses of up to 2400 mg/day have been tolerated in long-term clinical studies; up to 3600 mg/day has been tolerated in short-term studies.

Note: If gabapentin is discontinued or if another anticonvulsant is added to therapy, it should be done slowly over a minimum of 1 week

Adults:

- Immediate release:
  - Diabetic neuropathy (unlabeled use): 900-3600 mg/day (Bril, 2011)
  - Neuropathic pain (unlabeled use): 300-3600 mg/day (Attal, 2010; Dworkin, 2010)
  - Postherpetic neuralgia: Day 1: 300 mg, Day 2: 300 mg twice daily, Day 3: 300 mg 3 times/day; dose may be titrated as needed for pain relief (range: 1800-3600 mg/day in divided doses, daily doses >1800 mg do not generally show greater benefit)

Postoperative pain (unlabeled use): Usual dose: 300-1200 mg given 1-2 hours prior to surgery (Dauri, 2009)

Restless legs syndrome (RLS) (unlabeled use): Initial: 300 mg once daily 2 hours before bedtime. Doses ≥600 mg/day have been given in 2 divided doses (late afternoon and 2 hours before bedtime). Dose may be titrated every 2 weeks until symptom relief achieved (range: 300-1800 mg/day). Suggested maintenance dosing schedule: One-third of total daily dose given at 12 pm, remaining two-thirds total daily dose given at 8 pm. (Garcia-Borreguero, 2002; Happe, 2003; Saletu, 2010; Vignatelli, 2006)

Vasomotor symptoms associated with menopause (unlabeled use): Day 1: 300 mg at bedtime, Day 2: 300 mg twice daily, followed by 300 mg 3 times/day for 4 weeks and then tapered off (Butt, 2008)

Extended release (Gralise™): Postherpetic neuralgia: Day 1: 300 mg, Day 2: 600 mg, Days 3-6: 900 mg once daily, Days 7-10: 1200 mg once daily, Days 11-14: 1500 mg once daily, Days ≥15: 1800 mg once daily

Elderly: Studies in elderly patients have shown a decrease in clearance as age increases. This is most likely due to age-related decreases in renal function; dose reductions may be needed.

Dosing adjustment in renal impairment: Children ≥12 years and Adults: **Note:** Renal function may be estimated using the Cockcroft-Gault formula for dosage adjustment purposes.

Immediate release:

Cl_{cr} ≥60 mL/minute: 300-1200 mg 3 times/day

Cl_{cr} >30-59 mL/minute: 200-700 mg twice daily

Cl_{cr} >15-29 mL/minute: 200-700 mg once daily

Cl_{cr} 15 mL/minute: 100-300 mg once daily

Cl_{cr} <15 mL/minute: Reduce daily dose in proportion to creatinine clearance based on dose for creatinine clearance of 15 mL/minute (eg, reduce dose by one-half [range: 50-150 mg/day] for Cl_{cr} 7.5 mL/minute)

ESRD requiring hemodialysis: Dose for Cl_{cr} <15 mL/minute plus single supplemental dose of 125-350 mg (given after each 4 hours of hemodialysis)

Extended release: **Note:** Follow initial dose titration schedule if treatment-naive.

Cl_{cr} ≥60 mL/minute: 1800 mg once daily

Cl_{cr} >30-59 mL/minute: 600-1800 mg once daily; dependent on tolerability and clinical response

Cl_{cr} <30 mL/minute: Use is not recommended.

ESRD requiring hemodialysis: Use is not recommended.

Dosing adjustment in hepatic impairment: There are no dosage adjustments provided in the manufacturer's labeling; however, gabapentin is not hepatically metabolized.

Dietary Considerations Immediate release tablet and solution may be taken without regard to meals; extended release tablet should be taken with food.

Administration

Tablet, solution (immediate release): Administer first dose on first day at bedtime to avoid somnolence and dizziness. Dosage must be adjusted for renal function; when given 3 times daily, the maximum time between doses should not exceed 12 hours.

Tablet (extended release): Take with evening meal. Swallow whole; do not chew, crush, or split.

Monitoring Parameters Monitor serum levels of concomitant anticonvulsant therapy; suicidality (eg, suicidal thoughts, depression, behavioral changes)

Test Interactions False positives have been reported with the Ames N-Multistix SG® dipstick test for urine protein

Dosage Forms Excipient information presented when available (limited, particularly for generics); consult specific product labeling.

Capsule, oral: 100 mg, 300 mg, 400 mg

Neurontin®: 100 mg, 300 mg, 400 mg

Solution, oral: 250 mg/5 mL (470 mL)

Neurontin®: 250 mg/5 mL (470 mL) [cool strawberry-anise flavor]

Tablet, oral: 600 mg, 800 mg

Gralise™: 300 mg [contains soybean lecithin]

Gralise™: 600 mg

Neurontin®: 600 mg, 800 mg [scored]

Tablet, oral [combination package (each unit-dose starter kit contains)]:

Gralise™: 300 mg (9s) [white tablets; contains soybean lecithin] and 600 mg (69s) [beige tablets]

Extemporaneous Preparations Note: Commercial oral solution is available (50 mg/mL)

A 100 mg/mL suspension may be made with tablets (immediate release) and either a 1:1 mixture of Ora-Sweet® (100 mL) and Ora-Plus® (100 mL) or 1:1 mixture of methylcellulose 1% (100 mL) and Simple Syrup N.F. (100 mL). Crush sixty-seven 300 mg tablets in a mortar and reduce to a fine powder. Add small portions of the chosen vehicle and mix to a uniform paste; mix while adding the vehicle in incremental proportions to **almost** 200 mL; transfer to a calibrated bottle, rinse mortar with vehicle, and add sufficient quantity of vehicle to make 200 mL. Label "shake well" and "refrigerate". Stable for 91 days refrigerated (preferred) or 56 days at room temperature.

Nahata MC, Pai VB, and Hipple TF, *Pediatric Drug Formulations*, 5th ed, Cincinnati, OH: Harvey Whitney Books Co, 2004.

Gabapentin Enacarbil (gab a PEN tin en a KAR bil)

Brand Names: U.S. Horizant™

Index Terms GSK 1838262; Horizant™; Solzira; XP13512

Pharmacologic Category Anticonvulsant, Miscellaneous

Use Treatment of moderate-to-severe restless leg syndrome (RLS)

Pregnancy Risk Factor C

Pregnancy Considerations Animal studies have documented teratogenic effects. There are no adequate and well-controlled studies in pregnant women. Use during pregnancy only if the potential benefit to the mother outweighs the potential risk to the fetus.

Lactation Excretion in breast milk unknown/not recommended

Medication Guide Available Yes

Contraindications There are no contraindication listed within the manufacturer's labeling.

Warnings/Precautions Gabapentin and other antiepileptics are associated with an increased risk of suicidal behavior/thoughts with use (regardless of indication); gabapentin enacarbil is a prodrug of gabapentin and may also increase patient's risk. Patients should be monitored for signs/symptoms of depression, suicidal tendencies, and other unusual behavior changes during therapy and instructed to inform their healthcare provider immediately if symptoms occur. Doses >600 mg/day (not included in approved labeling) should be reduced to 600 mg daily for 1 week prior to stopping. Rat studies demonstrated an association with pancreatic adenocarcinoma (clinical implication unknown). May cause CNS depression, which may impair physical or mental abilities. Patients must be cautioned about performing tasks which require mental alertness (eg, operating machinery or driving). Effects with other sedative drugs or ethanol may be potentiated. Use with caution in patients with renal impairment; use not recommended in patients with severe impairment (Cl_{cr} <30 mL/minute). Gabapentin enacarbil (Horizant™) and other gabapentin products are not interchangeable due to differences in formulation, indications and pharmacokinetics.

Adverse Reactions Percentages reported are for 600 mg/day dosing.

>10%: Central nervous system: Sedation/somnolence (20%), dizziness (13%), headache (12%)

1% to 10%:

Central nervous system: Fatigue (6%), irritability (4%), balance disorder (<2%), disorientation (<2%), lethargy (<2%), drunk feeling (1%), vertigo (1%)

Gastrointestinal: Nausea (6%), flatulence (3%), xerostomia (3%), appetite increased (2%), weight gain (2%)

Ocular: Blurred vision (<2%)

<1% (Limited to important or life-threatening): Depression, feeling abnormal, libido decreased, peripheral edema

Drug Interactions

Metabolism/Transport Effects None known.

Avoid Concomitant Use There are no known interactions where it is recommended to avoid concomitant use.

Increased Effect/Toxicity

Gabapentin Enacarbil may increase the levels/effects of: Alcohol (Ethyl); CNS Depressants; Methotrimeprazine; Selective Serotonin Reuptake Inhibitors

The levels/effects of Gabapentin Enacarbil may be increased by: Droperidol; HydrOXYzine; Methotrimeprazine

Decreased Effect

The levels/effects of Gabapentin Enacarbil may be decreased by: Ketorolac; Ketorolac (Nasal); Ketorolac (Systemic); Mefloquine

Ethanol/Nutrition/Herb Interactions

Ethanol: Avoid ethanol (may increase CNS depression).

Herb/Nutraceutical: Avoid evening primrose (seizure threshold decreased). Avoid valerian, St John's wort, kava kava, gotu kola (may increase CNS depression).

Stability Store at 25°C (77°F); excursions permitted to 15°C to 30°C (59°F to 86°F). Protect from moisture. Do not remove from original container.

Mechanism of Action Gabapentin enacarbil is a prodrug of gabapentin. Gabapentin is structurally related to GABA. However, it does not bind to $GABA_A$ or $GABA_B$ receptors, and it does not appear to influence synthesis or uptake of GABA. High affinity gabapentin binding sites have been located throughout the brain; these sites correspond to the presence of voltage-gated calcium channels specifically possessing the alpha-2-delta-1 subunit. This channel appears to be located presynaptically, and may modulate the release of excitatory neurotransmitters. These effects on RLS are unknown.

Pharmacodynamics/Kinetics

Absorption: Mediated by active transport via proton-linked monocarboxylate transporter, MCT-1

Distribution: V_d: 76 L

Protein binding: <3%

Bioavailability: With food: ~75%; Fasting: 42% to 65%

Metabolism: Prodrug hydrolyzed primarily in the intestines to active metabolite

Time to peak, plasma: With food: 7.3 hours; Fasting: 5 hours

Half-life elimination: 5-6 hours

Excretion: Urine (94%); feces (5%)

Dosage Oral: Adults: Restless legs syndrome (RLS): 600 mg once daily (at ~5:00 pm); increasing to 1200 mg/day provided no additional benefit and increased side effects

Dosing adjustment in renal impairment: Note: Estimation of renal function for the purpose of drug dosing should be done using the Cockcroft-Gault formula.

Cl_{cr} >30-59 mL/minute: 600 mg/day on day 1 and day 3, then every day thereafter

Cl_{cr} <30 mL/minute: Not recommended

Dietary Considerations Take with food.

Administration Administer with food at ~5:00 pm daily; tablet should be swallowed whole; do not break, chew, cut, or crush.

Monitoring Parameters Suicidality (eg, suicidal thoughts, depression, behavioral changes)

Dosage Forms Excipient information presented when available (limited, particularly for generics); consult specific product labeling.

Tablet, extended release, oral:

Horizant™: 600 mg

◆ **Gabitril®** *see* TiaGABine *on page 1677*

◆ **Gablofen®** *see* Baclofen *on page 187*

Galantamine (ga LAN ta meen)

Brand Names: U.S. Razadyne®; Razadyne® ER

Brand Names: Canada Mylan-Galantamine ER; PAT-Galantamine ER; Reminyl®; Reminyl® ER

Index Terms Galantamine Hydrobromide

Pharmacologic Category Acetylcholinesterase Inhibitor (Central)

Use Treatment of mild-to-moderate dementia of Alzheimer's disease

Unlabeled Use Severe dementia associated with Alzheimer's disease; mild-to-moderate dementia associated with Parkinson's disease; Lewy body dementia

Pregnancy Risk Factor B

Pregnancy Considerations In animal studies, there was a slight increased in the incident of skeletal variations when given during organogenesis. Adequate, well-controlled studies in pregnant women do not exist. Should be used in pregnancy only if benefit outweighs potential risk to the fetus.

Lactation Excretion in breast milk unknown/not recommended

Contraindications Hypersensitivity to galantamine or any component of the formulation; severe liver dysfunction (Child-Pugh score 10-15); severe renal dysfunction (Cl_{cr} <9 mL/minute)

Warnings/Precautions Use caution in patients with supraventricular conduction delays (without a functional pacemaker in place); Alzheimer's treatment guidelines consider bradycardia to be a relative contraindication for use of centrally-active cholinesterase inhibitors. Use caution in patients taking medicines that slow conduction through SA or AV node. Use caution in peptic ulcer disease (or in patients at risk); seizure disorder; asthma; COPD; mild-to-moderate liver dysfunction; moderate renal dysfunction. May cause bladder outflow obstruction. May exaggerate neuromuscular blockade effects of succinylcholine and like agents. May cause nausea, vomiting, diarrhea, weight loss, and anorexia.

Adverse Reactions

>10%: Gastrointestinal: Nausea (6% to 24%), vomiting (4% to 13%), diarrhea (6% to 12%)

1% to 10%:

Cardiovascular: Bradycardia (2% to 3%), syncope (0.4% to 2.2%: dose related), chest pain (≥1%)

Central nervous system: Dizziness (9%), headache (8%), depression (7%), fatigue (5%), insomnia (5%), somnolence (4%)

Gastrointestinal: Anorexia (7% to 9%), weight loss (5% to 7%), abdominal pain (5%), dyspepsia (5%), flatulence (≥1%)

Genitourinary: Urinary tract infection (8%), hematuria (<1% to 3%), incontinence (≥1%)

Hematologic: Anemia (3%)

Neuromuscular & skeletal: Tremor (3%)

Respiratory: Rhinitis (4%)

<1% (Limited to important or life-threatening): Aggression, alkaline phosphatase increased, aphasia, apraxia, ataxia, atrial fibrillation, AV block, bundle branch block, convulsions, dehydration, delirium, diverticulitis, dysphagia, epistaxis, esophageal perforation, fever, gastrointestinal bleeding, heart failure, hyper-/hypokinesia, hypokalemia, hypotension, malaise, melena, MI, palpitation, paranoid reaction, paresthesia, paroniria, postural hypotension, purpura, QT prolongation, rectal hemorrhage, renal calculi, renal failure (due to dehydration), stroke, suicide, supraventricular tachycardia, T-wave inversion, thrombocytopenia, TIA, ventricular tachycardia, vertigo, weakness

Drug Interactions

Metabolism/Transport Effects **Substrate** of CYP2D6 (minor), CYP3A4 (minor); **Note:** Assignment of Major/Minor substrate status based on clinically relevant drug interaction potential

Avoid Concomitant Use There are no known interactions where it is recommended to avoid concomitant use.

Increased Effect/Toxicity

Galantamine may increase the levels/effects of: Antipsychotics; Beta-Blockers; Cholinergic Agonists; Succinylcholine

The levels/effects of Galantamine may be increased by: Conivaptan; Corticosteroids (Systemic); Selective Serotonin Reuptake Inhibitors

Decreased Effect

Galantamine may decrease the levels/effects of: Anticholinergics; Neuromuscular-Blocking Agents (Nondepolarizing)

The levels/effects of Galantamine may be decreased by: Anticholinergics; Dipyridamole; Peginterferon Alfa-2b; Tocilizumab

Ethanol/Nutrition/Herb Interactions

Ethanol: Avoid ethanol (may increase CNS adverse events).

Herb/Nutraceutical: St John's wort may decrease galantamine serum levels; avoid concurrent use.

Stability Store at 15°C to 30°C (59°F to 86°F). Do not freeze oral solution; protect from light.

Mechanism of Action Centrally-acting cholinesterase inhibitor (competitive and reversible). It elevates acetylcholine in cerebral cortex by slowing the degradation of acetylcholine. Modulates nicotinic acetylcholine receptor to increase acetylcholine from surviving presynaptic nerve terminals. May increase glutamate and serotonin levels.

Pharmacodynamics/Kinetics

Duration: 3 hours; maximum inhibition of erythrocyte acetylcholinesterase ~40% at 1 hour post 8 mg oral dose; levels return to baseline at 30 hours

Absorption: Rapid and complete

Distribution: 175 L; levels in the brain are 2-3 times higher than in plasma

Protein binding: 18%

Metabolism: Hepatic; linear, CYP2D6 and 3A4; metabolized to epigalanthaminone and galanthaminone both of which have acetylcholinesterase inhibitory activity 130 times less than galantamine

Bioavailability: ~90%

Half-life elimination: 7 hours

Time to peak: Immediate release: 1 hour (2.5 hours with food); extended release: 4.5-5 hours

Excretion: Urine (25%)

Dosage Oral: Adults:

Note: Oral solution and tablet should be taken with breakfast and dinner; capsule should be taken with breakfast. If therapy is interrupted for ≥3 days, restart at the lowest dose and increase to current dose.

Immediate release tablet or solution: Mild-to-moderate dementia of Alzheimer's: Initial: 4 mg twice a day for 4 weeks; if tolerated, increase to 8 mg twice daily for ≥4 weeks; if tolerated, increase to 12 mg twice daily

Range: 16-24 mg/day in 2 divided doses

Extended-release capsule: Initial: 8 mg once daily for 4 weeks; if tolerated, increase to 16 mg once daily for ≥4 weeks; if tolerated, increase to 24 mg once daily

Range: 16-24 mg once daily

Conversion to galantamine from other cholinesterase inhibitors: Patients experiencing poor tolerability with donepezil or rivastigmine should wait until side effects subside or allow a 7-day washout period prior to beginning galantamine. Patients not experiencing side effects with donepezil or rivastigmine may begin galantamine therapy the day immediately following discontinuation of previous therapy (Morris, 2001).

Elderly: No dosage adjustment needed

Dosage adjustment in renal impairment:

Moderate renal impairment: Maximum dose: 16 mg/day.

Severe renal dysfunction (Cl_{cr} <9 mL/minute): Use is not recommended

Dosage adjustment in hepatic impairment:

Moderate liver dysfunction (Child-Pugh score 7-9): Maximum dose: 16 mg/day

Severe liver dysfunction (Child-Pugh score 10-15): Use is not recommended

Dietary Considerations Administration with food is preferred, but not required; should be taken with breakfast and dinner (tablet or solution) or with breakfast (capsule).

Administration Oral: Administer solution or tablet with breakfast and dinner; administer extended release capsule with breakfast. If therapy is interrupted for ≥3 days, restart at the lowest dose and increase to current dose. If using oral solution, mix dose with 3-4 ounces of any nonalcoholic beverage; mix well and drink immediately.

Monitoring Parameters Mental status

Dosage Forms Excipient information presented when available (limited, particularly for generics); consult specific product labeling.

Capsule, extended release, oral, as hydrobromide [strength expressed as base]: 8 mg, 16 mg, 24 mg

Razadyne® ER: 8 mg, 16 mg, 24 mg [contains gelatin]

Solution, oral, as hydrobromide: 4 mg/mL (100 mL)

Razadyne®: 4 mg/mL (100 mL)

Tablet, oral, as hydrobromide [strength expressed as base]: 4 mg, 8 mg, 12 mg

Razadyne®: 4 mg, 8 mg, 12 mg

- ◆ **Galantamine Hydrobromide** *see* Galantamine *on page 776*
- ◆ **Galzin®** *see* Zinc Acetate *on page 1817*
- ◆ **GamaSTAN™ S/D** *see* Immune Globulin *on page 880*
- ◆ **Gamimune® N (Can)** *see* Immune Globulin *on page 880*
- ◆ **Gamma Benzene Hexachloride** *see* Lindane *on page 1013*
- ◆ **Gamma E-Gems® [OTC]** *see* Vitamin E *on page 1796*
- ◆ **Gamma-E PLUS [OTC]** *see* Vitamin E *on page 1796*
- ◆ **Gammagard® Liquid** *see* Immune Globulin *on page 880*
- ◆ **Gammagard Liquid (Can)** *see* Immune Globulin *on page 880*
- ◆ **Gammagard S/D®** *see* Immune Globulin *on page 880*
- ◆ **Gammagard S/D (Can)** *see* Immune Globulin *on page 880*
- ◆ **Gamma Globulin** *see* Immune Globulin *on page 880*
- ◆ **Gamma Hydroxybutyric Acid** *see* Sodium Oxybate *on page 1572*
- ◆ **Gammaked™** *see* Immune Globulin *on page 880*
- ◆ **Gammaphos** *see* Amifostine *on page 85*

◆ **Gammaplex®** *see* Immune Globulin *on page 880*
◆ **Gamunex® [DSC]** *see* Immune Globulin *on page 880*
◆ **Gamunex® (Can)** *see* Immune Globulin *on page 880*
◆ **Gamunex®-C** *see* Immune Globulin *on page 880*

Ganciclovir (Systemic) (gan SYE kloe veer)

Brand Names: U.S. Cytovene®-IV
Brand Names: Canada Cytovene®
Index Terms DHPG Sodium; GCV Sodium; Nordeoxyguanosine
Pharmacologic Category Antiviral Agent
Use Treatment of CMV retinitis in immunocompromised individuals, including patients with acquired immunodeficiency syndrome; prophylaxis of CMV infection in transplant patients
Unlabeled Use CMV retinitis: May be given in combination with foscarnet in patients who relapse after monotherapy with either drug
Pregnancy Risk Factor C
Pregnancy Considerations [U.S. Boxed Warning]: Animal studies have demonstrated carcinogenic and teratogenic effects, and inhibition of spermatogenesis. Female patients should use effective contraception during therapy; male patients should use a barrier contraceptive during and for at least 90 days after therapy.
Lactation Excretion in breast milk unknown/not recommended
Contraindications Hypersensitivity to ganciclovir, acyclovir, or any component of the formulation
Warnings/Precautions Hazardous agent - use appropriate precautions for handling and disposal. **[U.S. Boxed Warning]: Granulocytopenia (neutropenia), anemia, and thrombocytopenia may occur.** Dosage adjustment or interruption of ganciclovir therapy may be necessary in patients with neutropenia and/or thrombocytopenia and patients with impaired renal function. **[U.S. Boxed Warning]: Animal studies have demonstrated carcinogenic and teratogenic effects, and inhibition of spermatogenesis;** contraceptive precautions for female and male patients need to be followed during and for at least 90 days after therapy with the drug; take care to administer only into veins with good blood flow. **[U.S. Boxed Warning]: Indicated only for treatment of CMV retinitis in the immunocompromised patient and CMV prevention in transplant patients at risk.**
Adverse Reactions
>10%:
Central nervous system: Fever (48%)
Gastrointestinal: Diarrhea (44%), anorexia (14%), vomiting (13%)
Hematologic: Thrombocytopenia (57%), leukopenia (41%), anemia (16% to 26%), neutropenia with ANC <500/mm^3 (12% to 14%)
Ocular: Retinal detachment (11%; relationship to ganciclovir not established)
Renal: Serum creatinine increased (2% to 14%)
Miscellaneous: Sepsis (15%), diaphoresis (12%)
1% to 10%:
Central nervous system: Chills (10%), neuropathy (9%)
Dermatologic: Pruritus (5%)
<1% (Limited to important or life-threatening): Allergic reaction (including anaphylaxis), alopecia, arrhythmia, bronchospasm, cardiac arrest, cataracts, cholestasis, coma, dyspnea, edema, encephalopathy, exfoliative dermatitis, extrapyramidal symptoms, hepatitis, hepatic failure, pancreatitis, pancytopenia, pulmonary fibrosis, psychosis, rhabdomyolysis, seizure, alopecia, urticaria, eosinophilia, hemorrhage, Stevens-Johnson syndrome, torsade de pointes, renal failure, SIADH, visual loss

Drug Interactions
Metabolism/Transport Effects None known.
Avoid Concomitant Use
Avoid concomitant use of Ganciclovir (Systemic) with any of the following: Imipenem
Increased Effect/Toxicity
Ganciclovir (Systemic) may increase the levels/effects of: Imipenem; Mycophenolate; Reverse Transcriptase Inhibitors (Nucleoside); Tenofovir

The levels/effects of Ganciclovir (Systemic) may be increased by: Mycophenolate; Probenecid; Tenofovir
Decreased Effect There are no known significant interactions involving a decrease in effect.
Stability Intact vials should be stored at room temperature and protected from temperatures >40°C Reconstitute powder with unpreserved sterile water **not** bacteriostatic water because parabens may cause precipitation; dilute in 250-1000 mL D_5W or NS to a concentration ≤10 mg/mL for infusion.

Reconstituted solution is stable for 12 hours at room temperature, however, conflicting data indicates that reconstituted solution is stable for 60 days under refrigeration (4°C). Stability of parenteral admixture at room temperature (25°C) and at refrigeration temperature (4°C) is 5 days.
Mechanism of Action Ganciclovir is phosphorylated to a substrate which competitively inhibits the binding of deoxyguanosine triphosphate to DNA polymerase resulting in inhibition of viral DNA synthesis
Pharmacodynamics/Kinetics
Distribution: V_d: 15.26 L/1.73 m^2; widely to all tissues including CSF and ocular tissue
Protein binding: 1% to 2%
Half-life elimination: 1.7-5.8 hours; prolonged with renal impairment; End-stage renal disease: 5-28 hours
Excretion: Urine (80% to 99% as unchanged drug)
Dosage
CMV CNS infection in HIV-exposed/-infected patients (unlabeled use; CDC, 2009): Infants and Children: I.V.: 5 mg/kg/dose every 12 hours plus foscarnet until symptoms improve followed by chronic suppression
CMV retinitis:
I.V. (slow infusion): Children and Adults:
Induction therapy: 5 mg/kg/dose every 12 hours for 14-21 days followed by maintenance therapy
Maintenance therapy: 5 mg/kg/day as a single daily dose for 7 days/week or 6 mg/kg/day for 5 days/week
Prevention of CMV disease in HIV-exposed/-infected patients (unlabeled use; CDC, 2009): I.V.: Infants and Children: 5 mg/kg/dose daily
Prevention of CMV disease in transplant patients: I.V. (slow infusion): Children and Adults: Same initial and maintenance dose as CMV retinitis except duration of initial course is 7-14 days, duration of maintenance therapy is dependent on clinical condition and degree of immunosuppression
Varicella zoster: Progressive outer retinal necrosis in HIV-exposed/-infected patients (unlabeled use; CDC, 2009): Infants and Children: I.V.: 5 mg/kg/dose every 12 hours plus systemic foscarnet and intravitreal ganciclovir or intravitreal foscarnet

Elderly: Refer to adult dosing; in general, dose selection should be cautious, reflecting greater frequency of organ impairment

Dosing adjustment in renal impairment:
I.V. (Induction):
Cl_{cr} 50-69 mL/minute: Administer 2.5 mg/kg/dose every 12 hours
Cl_{cr} 25-49 mL/minute: Administer 2.5 mg/kg/dose every 24 hours
Cl_{cr} 10-24 mL/minute: Administer 1.25 mg/kg/dose every 24 hours
Cl_{cr} <10 mL/minute: Administer 1.25 mg/kg/dose 3 times/week following hemodialysis
I.V. (Maintenance):
Cl_{cr} 50-69 mL/minute: Administer 2.5 mg/kg/dose every 24 hours
Cl_{cr} 25-49 mL/minute: Administer 1.25 mg/kg/dose every 24 hours
Cl_{cr} 10-24 mL/minute: Administer 0.625 mg/kg/dose every 24 hours
Cl_{cr} <10 mL/minute: Administer 0.625 mg/kg/dose 3 times/week following hemodialysis

Intermittent hemodialysis (IHD) (administer after hemodialysis on dialysis days): Dialyzable (50%): CMV Infection: I.V.: Induction: 1.25 mg/kg every 48-72 hours; Maintenance: 0.625 mg/kg every 48-72 hours. **Note:** Dosing dependent on the assumption of 3 times/week, complete IHD sessions.

Peritoneal dialysis (PD): Dose as for Cl_{cr} <10 mL/minute.

Continuous renal replacement therapy (CRRT) (Heintz, 2009; Trotman, 2005): Drug clearance is highly dependent on the method of renal replacement, filter type, and flow rate. Appropriate dosing requires close monitoring of pharmacologic response, signs of adverse reactions due to drug accumulation, as well as drug concentrations in relation to target trough (if appropriate). The following are general recommendations only (based on dialysate flow/ultrafiltration rates of 1-2 L/hour and minimal residual renal function) and should not supersede clinical judgment: CMV Infection:
CVVH: I.V.: Induction: 2.5 mg/kg every 24 hours; Maintenance: 1.25 mg/kg every 24 hours
CVVHD/CVVHDF: I.V.: Induction: 2.5 mg/kg every 12 hours; Maintenance: 2.5 mg/kg every 24 hours

Dietary Considerations Some products may contain sodium.

Administration Should not be administered by I.M., SubQ, or rapid IVP; administer by slow I.V. infusion over at least 1 hour. Too rapid infusion can cause increased toxicity and excessive plasma levels.

Monitoring Parameters CBC with differential and platelet count, serum creatinine

Dosage Forms Excipient information presented when available (limited, particularly for generics); consult specific product labeling.
Injection, powder for reconstitution: 500 mg
Cytovene®-IV: 500 mg

◆ **Ganidin® NR [OTC] [DSC]** *see* GuaiFENesin *on page 809*

Ganirelix (ga ni REL ix)

Brand Names: Canada Orgalutran®

Index Terms Antagon; Ganirelix Acetate

Pharmacologic Category Gonadotropin Releasing Hormone Antagonist

Use Inhibits premature luteinizing hormone (LH) surges in women undergoing controlled ovarian hyperstimulation

Pregnancy Risk Factor X

Dosage Adult: SubQ: 250 mcg/day during the mid-to-late phase after initiating follicle-stimulating hormone on day 2 or 3 of cycle. Treatment should be continued daily until the day of chorionic gonadotropin administration.

Additional Information Complete prescribing information for this medication should be consulted for additional detail.

Dosage Forms Excipient information presented when available (limited, particularly for generics); consult specific product labeling.
Injection, solution, as acetate: 250 mcg/0.5 mL (0.5 mL) [contains natural rubber/natural latex in packaging]

◆ **Ganirelix Acetate** *see* Ganirelix *on page 779*

◆ **Gani-Tuss DM NR [DSC]** *see* Guaifenesin and Dextromethorphan *on page 810*

◆ **Gani-Tuss® NR [DSC]** *see* Guaifenesin and Codeine *on page 810*

◆ **GAR-936** *see* Tigecycline *on page 1684*

◆ **Garamycin®** *see* Gentamicin (Ophthalmic) *on page 792*

◆ **Garasone (Can)** *see* Gentamicin (Ophthalmic) *on page 792*

◆ **Gardasil®** *see* Papillomavirus (Types 6, 11, 16, 18) Vaccine (Human, Recombinant) *on page 1294*

Gatifloxacin (gat i FLOKS a sin)

Brand Names: U.S. Zymar® [DSC]; Zymaxid™

Brand Names: Canada Zymar®

Pharmacologic Category Antibiotic, Ophthalmic; Antibiotic, Quinolone

Additional Appendix Information
Prevention of Wound Infection and Sepsis in Surgical Patients *on page 1954*

Use Treatment of bacterial conjunctivitis

Pregnancy Risk Factor C

Pregnancy Considerations Gatifloxacin has been shown to be fetotoxic in animal studies. Quinolone exposure during human pregnancy has been reported with other agents (refer to Ciprofloxacin [Systemic], Ofloxacin [Systemic], and Norfloxacin monographs). Following ophthalmic administration, serum concentrations of gatifloxacin are below the limits of quantification (<5 ng/mL). Systemic absorption would be required in order for gatifloxacin to cross the placenta.

Lactation Excretion in breast milk unknown/use caution

Contraindications
Zymar®: Hypersensitivity to gatifloxacin, other quinolone antibiotics, or any component of the formulation
Zymaxid™: There are no contraindications listed in the manufacturer's labeling.

Warnings/Precautions Severe hypersensitivity reactions, including anaphylaxis, have occurred with systemic quinolone therapy. Reactions may present as typical allergic symptoms after a single dose, or may manifest as severe idiosyncratic dermatologic, vascular, pulmonary, renal, hepatic, and/or hematologic events, usually after multiple doses. Prompt discontinuation of drug should occur if skin rash or other symptoms arise. Prolonged use may result in fungal or bacterial superinfection. For topical ophthalmic use only. Do not inject ophthalmic solution subconjunctivally or introduce directly into the anterior chamber of the eye. Contact lenses should not be worn during treatment of ophthalmic infections.

Adverse Reactions 1% to 10%:
Central nervous system: Headache
Gastrointestinal: Taste disturbance
Ocular: Chemosis, conjunctival hemorrhage, conjunctival irritation, discharge, dry eye, edema, irritation, keratitis, lacrimation increased, pain, papillary conjunctivitis, visual acuity decreased

Drug Interactions
Metabolism/Transport Effects None known.
Avoid Concomitant Use There are no known interactions where it is recommended to avoid concomitant use.

Increased Effect/Toxicity There are no known significant interactions involving an increase in effect.

Decreased Effect There are no known significant interactions involving a decrease in effect.

Stability Store between 15°C to 25°C (59°F to 77°F); do not freeze.

Mechanism of Action Gatifloxacin is a DNA gyrase inhibitor, and also inhibits topoisomerase IV. DNA gyrase (topoisomerase II) is an essential bacterial enzyme that maintains the superhelical structure of DNA. DNA gyrase is required for DNA replication and transcription, DNA repair, recombination, and transposition; inhibition is bactericidal.

Pharmacodynamics/Kinetics Absorption: Ophthalmic: Not measurable (<5 ng/mL)

Dosage Ophthalmic: Children ≥1 year and Adults: Bacterial conjunctivitis:

Zymar®:

Days 1 and 2: Instill 1 drop into affected eye(s) every 2 hours while awake (maximum: 8 times/day)

Days 3-7: Instill 1 drop into affected eye(s) up to 4 times/day while awake

Zymaxid™:

Day 1: Instill 1 drop into affected eye(s) every 2 hours while awake (maximum: 8 times/day)

Days 2-7: Instill 1 drop into affected eye(s) 2-4 times/day while awake

Administration For topical ophthalmic use only; avoid touching tip of applicator to eye, fingers, or other surfaces.

Monitoring Parameters Signs of infection

Test Interactions Some quinolones may produce a false-positive urine screening result for opiates using commercially-available immunoassay kits. This has been demonstrated most consistently for levofloxacin and ofloxacin, but other quinolones have shown cross-reactivity in certain assay kits. Confirmation of positive opiate screens by more specific methods should be considered.

Dosage Forms Excipient information presented when available (limited, particularly for generics); consult specific product labeling. [DSC] = Discontinued product

Solution, ophthalmic [drops]:

Zymar®: 0.3% (5 mL [DSC]) [contains benzalkonium chloride]

Zymaxid™: 0.5% (2.5 mL) [contains benzalkonium chloride]

◆ **GaviLyte™-C** *see* Polyethylene Glycol-Electrolyte Solution *on page* 1372

◆ **GaviLyte™-G** *see* Polyethylene Glycol-Electrolyte Solution *on page* 1372

◆ **GaviLyte™-N** *see* Polyethylene Glycol-Electrolyte Solution *on page* 1372

◆ **Gaviscon® Extra Strength [OTC]** *see* Aluminum Hydroxide and Magnesium Carbonate *on page* 79

◆ **Gaviscon® Liquid [OTC]** *see* Aluminum Hydroxide and Magnesium Carbonate *on page* 79

◆ **Gaviscon® Tablet [OTC]** *see* Aluminum Hydroxide and Magnesium Trisilicate *on page* 80

◆ **G-CSF** *see* Filgrastim *on page* 711

◆ **G-CSF (PEG Conjugate)** *see* Pegfilgrastim *on page* 1307

◆ **GCV Sodium** *see* Ganciclovir (Systemic) *on page* 778

◆ **GD-Amlodipine (Can)** *see* AmLODIPine *on page* 97

◆ **GD-Atorvastatin (Can)** *see* Atorvastatin *on page* 165

◆ **GD-Azithromycin (Can)** *see* Azithromycin (Systemic) *on page* 180

◆ **GD-Latanoprost (Can)** *see* Latanoprost *on page* 978

◆ **GD-Sertraline (Can)** *see* Sertraline *on page* 1548

Gefitinib (ge FI tye nib)

Brand Names: U.S. Iressa®

Brand Names: Canada IRESSA®

Index Terms ZD1839

Pharmacologic Category Antineoplastic Agent, Tyrosine Kinase Inhibitor

Use Treatment of locally advanced or metastatic nonsmall cell lung cancer (NSCLC) after failure of platinum-based and docetaxel therapies. Treatment is limited to patients who are benefiting or have benefited from treatment with gefitinib.

Note: Due to the lack of improved survival data from clinical trials of gefitinib, and in response to positive survival data with another EGFR inhibitor, according to the U.S. labeling, physicians are advised to use treatment options other than gefitinib in patients with advanced nonsmall cell lung cancer following one or two prior chemotherapy regimens when they are refractory/intolerant to their most recent regimen.

Canada labeling: First-line treatment of locally advanced or metastatic NSCLC with activating mutations of EGFR-TK

Unlabeled Use First-line treatment of NSCLC with known EGFR mutation

Pregnancy Risk Factor D

Pregnancy Considerations Animal studies have demonstrated fetal harm; there are no well-controlled studies in pregnant women. The risk of fetal harm should be carefully weighed. Women of childbearing potential should be advised to avoid pregnancy.

Lactation Excretion in breast milk unknown/not recommended

Prescribing and Access Restrictions As of September 15, 2005, distribution of gefitinib (IRESSA®) is limited to patients enrolled in the IRESSA® Access Program. Under this program, access to gefitinib will be limited to the following groups:

Patients who are currently receiving and benefiting from gefitinib

Patients who have previously received and benefited from gefitinib

Previously-enrolled patients or new patients in non-Investigational New Drug (IND) clinical trials involving gefitinib if these protocols were approved by an IRB prior to June 17, 2005

New patients may also receive gefitinib if the manufacturer (AstraZeneca) decides to make it available under IND, and the patients meet the criteria for enrollment under the IND

Additional information on the IRESSA® Access Program, including enrollment forms, may be obtained by calling AstraZeneca at 1-800-601-8933 or via the web at www.-Iressa-access.com

Contraindications Hypersensitivity to gefitinib or any component of the formulation

Warnings/Precautions Hazardous agent - use appropriate precautions for handling and disposal. Rare, sometimes fatal, pulmonary toxicity, including interstitial lung disease (ILD) (eg, alveolitis, interstitial pneumonia, pneumonitis) has occurred. ILD has occurred in patients with prior radiation therapy, prior chemotherapy, and less commonly in treatment naïve patients. Therapy should be interrupted in patients with acute onset or worsening pulmonary symptoms (dyspnea, cough, fever); discontinue if interstitial pneumonitis is confirmed. An increase in mortality was observed in patients with concurrent idiopathic pulmonary fibrosis. Asymptomatic increases in transaminases have been reported; monitor liver function periodically and discontinue if elevations/changes are severe. Gefitinib exposure may be increased in patients with hepatic impairment. Interruption of therapy may be required in patients with poorly tolerated diarrhea or adverse skin reactions. Eye irritation should be promptly evaluated and therapy may be interrupted based on appropriate medical evaluation; may be reinitiated following resolution of symptoms or eye changes.

EGFR mutations, specifically exon 19 deletions and exon 21 mutation (L858R), are associated with better response to gefitinib in patients with NSCLC (Riely, 2006). There is a high potential for CYP3A4 mediated interactions with gefitinib. Concurrent use with CYP3A4 inducers may decrease gefitinib levels; consider increased gefitinib doses (to 500 mg) with close monitoring if concurrent use with inducers cannot be avoided. CYP3A4 inhibitors may increase gefitinib levels, use caution with concurrent administration.

Adverse Reactions

>10%:

Dermatologic: Rash (43% to 54%), acne (25% to 33%), dry skin (13% to 26%), paronychia (14%)

Gastrointestinal: Diarrhea (48% to 67%; grade 3: 1%), nausea (13% to 18%), vomiting (9% to 12%)

1% to 10%:

Cardiovascular: Peripheral edema (2%)

Dermatologic: Pruritus (8% to 9%)

Gastrointestinal: Anorexia (7% to 10%), weight loss (3% to 5%), mouth ulceration (1%)

Neuromuscular & skeletal: Weakness (4% to 6%)

Ocular: Amblyopia (2%), conjunctivitis (1%)

Respiratory: Dyspnea (2%), interstitial lung disease (1% to 2%; includes alveolitis, interstitial pneumonia, pneumonitis)

<1% (Limited to important or life-threatening): Aberrant eyelash growth, angioedema, CNS hemorrhage (pediatrics), corneal erosion/ulcer, corneal membrane sloughing, epistaxis, erythema multiforme, eye pain, fever, hematuria, hemorrhage, ocular hemorrhage, ocular ischemia, pancreatitis, toxic epidermal necrolysis, urticaria, vesiculobullous rash

Drug Interactions

Metabolism/Transport Effects Substrate of CYP2D6 (major), CYP3A4 (major); **Note:** Assignment of Major/Minor substrate status based on clinically relevant drug interaction potential; **Inhibits** BCRP, CYP2C19 (weak), CYP2D6 (weak)

Avoid Concomitant Use

Avoid concomitant use of Gefitinib with any of the following: Conivaptan

Increased Effect/Toxicity

Gefitinib may increase the levels/effects of: Topotecan; Vinorelbine; Vitamin K Antagonists

The levels/effects of Gefitinib may be increased by: Abiraterone Acetate; Antifungal Agents (Azole Derivatives, Systemic); Conivaptan; CYP2D6 Inhibitors (Moderate); CYP2D6 Inhibitors (Strong); CYP3A4 Inhibitors (Moderate); CYP3A4 Inhibitors (Strong); Darunavir; Dasatinib

Decreased Effect

Gefitinib may decrease the levels/effects of: Cardiac Glycosides; Vitamin K Antagonists

The levels/effects of Gefitinib may be decreased by: CYP3A4 Inducers (Strong); Deferasirox; H2-Antagonists; Herbs (CYP3A4 Inducers); Peginterferon Alfa-2b; Proton Pump Inhibitors; Rifamycin Derivatives; Tocilizumab

Ethanol/Nutrition/Herb Interactions

Food: Grapefruit juice may increase serum gefitinib concentrations.

Herb/Nutraceutical: St John's wort may decrease serum gefitinib concentrations.

Stability Store tablets at controlled room temperature of 20°C to 25°C (68°F to 77°F). Protect from light and moisture.

Mechanism of Action Gefitinib is a tyrosine kinase inhibitor (TKI) which inhibits numerous tyrosine kinases associated with transmembrane cell surface receptors found on both normal and cancer cells, including the tyrosine kinase associated with the epidermal growth factor receptor, EGFR. Tyrosine kinase activity appears to be vitally important to cell proliferation and survival.

Pharmacodynamics/Kinetics

Absorption: Oral: Slow

Distribution: 1400 L

Protein binding: 90%, albumin and alpha$_1$-acid glycoprotein

Metabolism: Hepatic, primarily via CYP3A4; forms metabolites

Bioavailability: 60%

Half-life elimination: Oral: 41 hours

Time to peak, plasma: Oral: 3-7 hours

Excretion: Feces (86%); urine (<4%)

Dosage Oral: Adults:

Nonsmall cell lung cancer (NSCLC): 250 mg once daily

NSCLC, first-line therapy in patients with EGFR mutations (unlabeled use): 250 mg once daily (Maemondo, 2010; Mok, 2009; Sequist, 2008)

Dosage adjustment for concomitant CYP3A4 inducers (eg, phenytoin, rifampin): Consider increasing gefitinib dose to 500 mg once daily with close monitoring

Dosage adjustment for toxicity:

Worsening pulmonary symptoms (cough dyspnea, fever): Interrupt treatment and evaluate promptly; discontinue if interstitial lung disease is confirmed

Diarrhea (poorly tolerated or associated with dehydration) or skin toxicity: Interrupt treatment for up to 14 days; may reinitiate at 250 mg once daily

Ocular symptoms (eye pain): Evaluate and interrupt treatment based on symptoms; once symptoms or eye changes have resolved, may consider reinitiating at 250 mg once daily

Dosage adjustment in renal impairment: No adjustment necessary

Dosage adjustment in hepatic impairment:

Moderate-to-severe impairment due to metastases: No adjustment necessary

Hepatotoxicity during treatment (elevations in transaminases): Discontinue if severe

Dietary Considerations Food does not affect gefitinib absorption.

Administration May administer with or without food.

For patients unable to swallow tablets or for administration via NG tube: Tablets may be dispersed in noncarbonated drinking water. Drop whole tablet (do not crush) into 1/2 glass of water; stir until tablet is dispersed (~10 minutes). Drink immediately. Rinse glass with 1/2 glass of water and drink.

Monitoring Parameters Periodic liver function tests (ALT, AST, bilirubin and alkaline phosphatase), INR or prothrombin time (with concurrently warfarin treatment), pulmonary symptoms

Additional Information Oncology Comment: Recent studies have demonstrated a subset of patients who are more likely to respond to treatment with gefitinib. This subset includes: patients of Asian origin, never-smokers, women, patients with bronchoalveolar adenocarcinoma, and patients with EGFR-mutated tumors. Deletion in exon 19 and mutation in exon 21 are the two most commonly found EGFR mutations; both mutations correlate with clinical response, resulting in increased response rates in patients with the mutation (Riely, 2006). Studies have compared gefitinib in treatment naïve patients to combination chemotherapy in the subsets of patients described above, resulting in a longer progression free survival in the gefitinib arm (Mok, 2009). Based on these data, the 2009 ASCO guidelines recommend the first-line use of gefitinib in stage IV with the known EGFR mutation (Azzoli, 2009). The NCCN guidelines recommend erlotinib as first-line therapy for EGFR mutation positive patients with stage IV NSCLC, and also states that gefitinib could be used in place of erlotinib in areas of the world where available. In patients with a kras mutation, however, EGFR-TKI therapy is not recommended.

Dosage Forms Excipient information presented when available (limited, particularly for generics); consult specific product labeling.

Tablet, oral:

Iressa®: 250 mg

Extemporaneous Preparations Hazardous agent: Use appropriate precautions for handling and disposal.

An oral suspension may be prepared by placing one tablet (whole, do not crush) in half a glass of noncarbonated drinking water. Stir until tablet is disintegrated (~10 minutes), then administer immediately. To ensure the full dose is administered, rinse with half a glass of water and administer residue.

Iressa® prescribing information, AstraZeneca Pharmaceuticals, Wilmington, DE, 2005.

◆ **Gel-Kam® [OTC]** *see* Fluoride *on page 728*

◆ **Gel-Kam® Rinse** *see* Fluoride *on page 728*

◆ **Gelnique®** *see* Oxybutynin *on page 1264*

◆ **Gelucast®** *see* Zinc Gelatin *on page 1817*

◆ **Gelusil® [OTC]** *see* Aluminum Hydroxide, Magnesium Hydroxide, and Simethicone *on page 80*

◆ **Gelusil® (Can)** *see* Aluminum Hydroxide, Magnesium Hydroxide, and Simethicone *on page 80*

◆ **Gelusil® Extra Strength (Can)** *see* Aluminum Hydroxide and Magnesium Hydroxide *on page 80*

Gemcitabine (jem SITE a been)

Brand Names: U.S. Gemzar®

Brand Names: Canada Gemcitabine For Injection, USP; Gemzar®

Index Terms dFdC; dFdCyd; Difluorodeoxycytidine Hydrochlorothiazide; Gemcitabine Hydrochloride; LY-188011

Pharmacologic Category Antineoplastic Agent, Antimetabolite (Pyrimidine Analog)

Use Treatment of metastatic breast cancer; inoperable locally-advanced or metastatic nonsmall cell lung cancer (NSCLC); locally advanced or metastatic pancreatic cancer; advanced, relapsed ovarian cancer

Unlabeled Use Treatment of biliary tract cancers (advanced), bladder cancer, cervical cancer (recurrent or persistent), Ewing's sarcoma (refractory), head and neck cancer (nasopharyngeal), Hodgkin lymphoma (relapsed), non-Hodgkin lymphomas (refractory), malignant pleural mesothelioma, osteosarcoma (refractory), renal cell cancer (metastatic), small cell lung cancer (refractory or relapsed), soft tissue sarcoma (advanced), testicular cancer (refractory germ cell tumors), thymic malignancies, uterine sarcoma, and unknown-primary adenocarcinoma

Pregnancy Risk Factor D

Pregnancy Considerations Embryotoxicity and fetal malformations (cleft palate, incomplete ossification, fused pulmonary artery, absence of gallbladder) have been reported in animal studies. There are no adequate and well-controlled studies in pregnant women. If patient becomes pregnant, she should be informed of risks. May cause fetal harm if administered during pregnancy; adverse effects in reproduction are anticipated based on the mechanism of action.

Lactation Excretion in breast milk unknown/not recommended

Contraindications Hypersensitivity to gemcitabine or any component of the formulation

Warnings/Precautions Hazardous agent - use appropriate precautions for handling and disposal. Prolongation of the infusion time >60 minutes and more frequent than weekly dosing have been shown to increase toxicity. Gemcitabine may suppress bone marrow function (leukopenia, thrombocytopenia, and anemia); myelosuppression is usually the dose-limiting toxicity; monitor blood counts; dosage adjustments are frequently required. Gemcitabine may cause fever in the absence of clinical infection. Pulmonary toxicity has occurred; discontinue if severe and institute supportive measures.

Hemolytic uremic syndrome (and/or renal failure) has been reported; monitor for evidence of microangiopathic hemolysis (elevation of bilirubin or LDH, reticulocytosis, severe thrombocytopenia, and/or renal failure); use with caution in patients with pre-existing renal impairment. Serious hepatotoxicity (including liver failure and death) has been reported (when used alone or in combination with other hepatotoxic medications). Use with caution in patients with hepatic impairment (history of cirrhosis, hepatitis, or alcoholism) or in patients with hepatic metastases; may lead to exacerbation of hepatic impairment; dose adjustments may be considered with elevated bilirubin.

Pulmonary toxicity has been observed; discontinue if severe and institute supportive measures. Use caution with concurrent radiation therapy; radiation toxicity, including tissue injury, severe mucositis, esophagitis, or pneumonitis, has been reported with concurrent and nonconcurrent administration; may have radiosensitizing activity when gemcitabine and radiation therapy are given ≤7 days apart; lower doses with concurrent radiation therapy may produce less severe toxicity; however, an optimum regimen for combination therapy has not been determined for all tumor types; radiation recall may occur when gemcitabine and radiation therapy are given >7 days apart. Prolongation of the infusion time >60 minutes and more frequent than weekly dosing have been shown to increase toxicity; has been administered at a fixed-dose rate (FDR) infusion rate of 10 mg/m^2/minute in studies (unlabeled); prolonged infusion times increase the accumulation of the active metabolite, gemcitabine triphosphate, optimizing the pharmacokinetics (Ko, 2006; Tempero, 2003); patients who receive gemcitabine FDR experience more grade 3/4 hematologic toxicity (Ko, 2006; Poplin, 2009). Use caution in the elderly; clearance is affected by age.

Adverse Reactions Frequency of adverse reactions reported for single-agent use of gemcitabine only.

>10%:

Cardiovascular: Peripheral edema (20%), edema (13%)

Central nervous system: Fever (38% to 41%), somnolence (11%)

Dermatologic: Rash (28% to 30%), alopecia (15% to 16%), pruritus (13%)

Gastrointestinal: Nausea/vomiting (69% to 71%; grade 3: 10% to 13%; grade 4: 1% to 2%), diarrhea (19% to 30%), stomatitis (10% to 11%)

Hematologic: Anemia (68% to 73%; grade 4: 1% to 2%), leukopenia (62% to 64%; grade 4: ≤1%), neutropenia (61% to 63%; grade 4: 6% to 7%), thrombocytopenia (24% to 36%; grade 4: ≤1%), hemorrhage (4% to 17%; grades 3: ≤2%; grade 4: <1%); myelosuppression is the dose-limiting toxicity

Hepatic: AST increased (67% to 78%; grade 3: 6% to 12%; grade 4: 2% to 5%), alkaline phosphatase increased (55% to 77%; grade 3: 7% to 16%; grade 4: 2% to 4%), ALT increased (68% to 72%; grade 3: 8% to 10%; grade 4: 1% to 2%), bilirubin increased (13% to 26%; grade 3: 2% to 6%; grade 4: ≤2%)

Renal: Proteinuria (32% to 45%; grades 3/4: <1%), hematuria (23% to 35%; grades 3/4: <1%), BUN increased (15% to 16%)
Respiratory: Dyspnea (10% to 23%)
Miscellaneous: Flu-like syndrome (19%), infection (10% to 16%; grade 3: 1% to 2%; grade 4: <1%)

1% to 10%:
Local: Injection site reactions (4%)
Neuromuscular & skeletal: Paresthesia (10%)
Renal: Creatinine increased (6% to 8%)
Respiratory: Bronchospasm (<2%)

<1% (Limited to important or life-threatening; reported with single-agent use or with combination therapy): Acute/adult respiratory distress syndrome, anaphylactoid reaction, arrhythmias, bullous skin eruptions, cellulitis, cerebrovascular accident, CHF, desquamation, fulminant hepatic failure, gangrene, GGT increased, hemolytic uremic syndrome (HUS), hepatic sinusoidal obstruction syndrome (SOS; veno-occlusive liver disease), hepatotoxicity (rare), hyper-/hypotension, interstitial pneumonitis, liver failure, MI, neuropathy, peripheral vasculitis, petechiae, pulmonary edema, pulmonary fibrosis, radiation recall, renal failure, respiratory failure, reversible posterior leukoencephalopathy syndrome (RPLS), sepsis, supraventricular arrhythmia, thrombotic thrombocytopenic purpura

Drug Interactions

Metabolism/Transport Effects None known.

Avoid Concomitant Use

Avoid concomitant use of Gemcitabine with any of the following: BCG; CloZAPine; Natalizumab; Pimecrolimus; Tacrolimus (Topical); Vaccines (Live)

Increased Effect/Toxicity

Gemcitabine may increase the levels/effects of: Bleomycin; CloZAPine; Fluorouracil; Fluorouracil (Systemic); Fluorouracil (Topical); Leflunomide; Natalizumab; Vaccines (Live); Vitamin K Antagonists

The levels/effects of Gemcitabine may be increased by: Denosumab; Pimecrolimus; Roflumilast; Tacrolimus (Topical); Trastuzumab

Decreased Effect

Gemcitabine may decrease the levels/effects of: BCG; Coccidioidin Skin Test; Sipuleucel-T; Vaccines (Inactivated); Vaccines (Live); Vitamin K Antagonists

The levels/effects of Gemcitabine may be decreased by: Echinacea

Ethanol/Nutrition/Herb Interactions Ethanol: Avoid ethanol (due to GI irritation).

Stability Use appropriate precautions for handling and disposal.

Lyophilized powder: Store intact vials at room temperature of 20°C to 25°C (68°F to 77°F); excursions permitted to 15°C to 30°C (59°F to 86°F). Reconstitute with preservative free NS; add 5 mL to the 200 mg vial, add 25 mL to the 1000 mg vial, or add 50 mL to the 2000 mg vial, resulting in a reconstituted concentration of 38 mg/mL (solutions must be reconstituted to ≤40 mg/mL to completely dissolve). Reconstituted vials are stable for 24 hours at room temperature. Do not refrigerate (may form crystals).

Solution for injection: Store intact vials refrigerated at 2°C to 8°C (36°F to 46°F); do not freeze.

Further dilute for infusion in NS 50-500 mL to concentrations as low as 0.1 mg/mL. Infusion solutions diluted in NS are stable for 24 hours at room temperature. Do not refrigerate.

Mechanism of Action A pyrimidine antimetabolite that inhibits DNA synthesis by inhibition of DNA polymerase and ribonucleotide reductase, cell cycle-specific for the S-phase of the cycle (also blocks cellular progression at G1/S phase). Gemcitabine is phosphorylated intracellularly by deoxycytidine kinase to gemcitabine monophosphate, which is further phosphorylated to active metabolites gemcitabine diphosphate and gemcitabine triphosphate. Gemcitabine diphosphate inhibits DNA synthesis by inhibiting ribonucleotide reductase; gemcitabine triphosphate incorporates into DNA and inhibits DNA polymerase.

Pharmacodynamics/Kinetics

Distribution: Infusions <70 minutes: 50 L/m^2; Long infusion times (70-285 minutes): 370 L/m^2

Protein binding: Negligible

Metabolism: Metabolized intracellularly by nucleoside kinases to the active diphosphate (dFdCDP) and triphosphate (dFdCTP) nucleoside metabolites

Half-life elimination:
Gemcitabine: Infusion time ≤70 minutes: 42-94 minutes; infusion time 3-4 hours: 4-10.5 hours (affected by age and gender)
Metabolite (gemcitabine triphosphate), terminal phase: 1.7-19.4 hours

Time to peak, plasma: 30 minutes after completion of infusion

Excretion: Urine (92% to 98%; primarily as inactive uracil metabolite); feces (<1%)

Dosage Details concerning dosing in combination regimens should also be consulted. **Note**: Prolongation of the infusion time >60 minutes and administration more frequently than once weekly have been shown to increase toxicity. I.V.:

Children (refer to specific references for ages of populations studied):
Germ cell tumor, refractory (unlabeled use): 1000 mg/m^2 over 30 minutes days 1, 8, and 15 every 4 weeks (in combination with paclitaxel) for up to 6 cycles (Hinton, 2002)
Hodgkin lymphoma, relapsed (unlabeled use): 1000 mg/m^2 over 100 minutes days 1 and 8; repeat cycle every 21 days (in combination with vinorelbine) (Cole; 2009) **or** 800 mg/m^2 days 1 and 4; repeat cycle every 21 days (in combination with ifosfamide, mesna, vinorelbine, and prednisolone) (Santoro, 2007)
Sarcomas (unlabeled use):
Ewing's sarcoma, refractory: 675 mg/m^2 over 90 minutes days 1 and 8; repeat cycle every 21 days (in combination with docetaxel) (Navid, 2008)
Osteosarcoma, refractory: 675 mg/m^2 over 90 minutes days 1 and 8; repeat cycle every 21 days (in combination with docetaxel) (Navid, 2008) **or** 1000 mg/m^2 weekly for 7 weeks followed by 1 week rest; then weekly for 3 weeks out of every 4 weeks (Merimsky, 2000)

Adults:
Pancreatic cancer, locally advanced or metastatic: Initial: 1000 mg/m^2 over 30 minutes once weekly for up to 7 weeks followed by 1 week rest; then once weekly for 3 weeks out of every 4 weeks
Dose escalation: Patients who complete an entire cycle of therapy may have the dose in subsequent cycles increased by 25% as long as the absolute granulocyte count (AGC) nadir is >1500/mm^3, platelet nadir is >100,000/mm^3, and nonhematologic toxicity is less than WHO Grade 1. If the increased dose is tolerated (with the same parameters) the dose in subsequent cycles may again be increased by 20%.
Pancreatic cancer, advanced (unlabeled dosing/combinations): 1000 mg/m^2 over 30 minutes weekly for up to 7 weeks followed by 1 week rest; then weekly for 3 weeks out of every 4 weeks (in combination with erlotinib) (Moore, 2007) **or** 1000 mg/m^2 over 30 minutes days 1, 8, and 15 every 4 weeks (in combination with capecitabine) (Cunningham, 2009) **or** 1000 mg/m^2 over 30 minutes days 1 and 15 every 4 weeks (in combination with cisplatin) (Heinemann, 2006) **or** 1000 mg/m^2 ▶

infused at 10 mg/m²/minute every 2 weeks (in combination with oxaliplatin) (Louvet, 2005)

Nonsmall cell lung cancer, locally advanced or metastatic (in combination with cisplatin): 1000 mg/m² over 30 minutes days 1, 8, and 15; repeat cycle every 28 days **or** 1250 mg/m² over 30 minutes days 1 and 8; repeat cycle every 21 days

Breast cancer, metastatic (AGC should be ≥1500/mm³ and platelets ≥100,000/mm³ prior to each cycle): 1250 mg/m² over 30 minutes days 1 and 8; repeat cycle every 21 days (in combination with paclitaxel) **or** (unlabeled dosing) as a single agent: 800 mg/m² over 30 minutes days 1, 8, and 15 of a 28-day treatment cycle (Carmichael, 1995)

Ovarian cancer, advanced (AGC should be ≥1500/mm³ and platelets ≥100,000/mm³ prior to each cycle): 1000 mg/m² over 30 minutes days 1 and 8; repeat cycle every 21 days (in combination with carboplatin)

Biliary tract cancer, advanced (unlabeled use): 1000 mg/m² over 30 minutes days 1 and 8; repeat cycle every 21 days (in combination with cisplatin) (Valle, 2010) **or** 1000 mg/m² over 30 minutes days 1 and 8; repeat cycle every 21 days (in combination with capecitabine) (Knox, 2005) **or** 1000 mg/m² infused at 10 mg/m²/minute every 2 weeks (in combination with oxaliplatin) (Andre, 2004)

Bladder cancer (unlabeled use):

- Advanced or metastatic: I.V.: 1000 mg/m² over 30-60 minutes days 1, 8, and 15; repeat cycle every 4 weeks (in combination with cisplatin) (von der Maase, 2000)
- Transitional cell carcinoma: Intravesicular instillation: 2000 mg (in 100 mL NS; retain for 1 hour) twice weekly for 3 weeks; repeat cycle every 4 weeks for at least 2 cycles (Dalbagni, 2006)

Cervical cancer, recurrent or persistent (unlabeled use): 1000 mg/m² days 1 and 8; repeat cycle every 21 days (in combination with cisplatin) (Monk, 2009) **or** 1250 mg/m² over 30 minutes days 1 and 8; repeat cycle every 21 days (in combination with cisplatin) (Burnett, 2000) **or** 800 mg/m² over 30 minutes days 1, 8, and 15; repeat cycle every 28 days (as a single-agent) (Schilder, 2005)

Head and neck cancer, nasopharyngeal (unlabeled use): 1000 mg/m² over 30 minutes days 1, 8, and 15 every 4 weeks (Zhang, 2008)

Hodgkin lymphoma, relapsed (unlabeled use): 1000 mg/m² (800 mg/m² for post-transplant patients) over 30 minutes days 1 and 8; repeat cycle every 21 days (in combination with vinorelbine and doxorubicin liposomal) (Bartlett, 2007) **or** 800 mg/m² days 1 and 4; repeat cycle every 21 days (in combination with ifosfamide, mesna, vinorelbine, and prednisolone) (Santoro, 2007)

Malignant pleural mesothelioma (unlabeled use; in combination with cisplatin): 1000 mg/m² over 30 minutes days 1, 8 and 15 every 4 weeks for up to 6 cycles (Nowak, 2002) **or** 1250 mg/m² over 30 minutes days 1 and 8 every 3 weeks for up to 6 cycles (van Haarst, 2002)

Non-Hodgkin lymphoma, refractory (unlabeled use): 1000 mg/m² over 30 minutes days 1 and 8; repeat cycle every 21 days (in combination with cisplatin and dexamethasone) (Crump, 2004) **or** 1000 mg/m² every 15-21days (in combination with oxaliplatin and rituximab) (Lopez, 2008)

Sarcoma (unlabeled uses):

- Ewing's sarcoma, refractory: 675 mg/m² over 90 minutes days 1 and 8; repeat cycle every 21 days (in combination with docetaxel) (Navid, 2008)
- Osteosarcoma, refractory: 675 mg/m² over 90 minutes days 1 and 8; repeat cycle every 21 days (in combination with docetaxel) (Navid, 2008) **or** 1000 mg/m² weekly for 7 weeks followed by 1 week rest; then weekly for 3 weeks out of every 4 weeks (Merimsky, 2000)
- Soft tissue sarcoma, advanced: 800 mg/m² over 90 minutes days 1 and 8; repeat cycle every 21 days (in combination with vinorelbine) (Dileo, 2007) **or** 675 mg/m² over 90 minutes days 1 and 8; repeat cycle every 21 days (in combination with docetaxel) (Leu, 2004) **or** 900 mg/m² over 90 minutes days 1 and 8; repeat cycle every 21 days (in combination with docetaxel) (Maki, 2007)

Small cell lung cancer, refractory or relapsed (unlabeled use): 1000-1250 mg/m² over 30 minutes days 1, 8, and 15 every 4 weeks (as a single agent) (Masters, 2003)

Testicular cancer, refractory germ cell (unlabeled use): 1000 mg/m² over 30 minutes days 1 and 8 every 3 weeks (in combination with oxaliplatin) (Kohllmannsberger, 2004; Pectasides, 2004) **or** 1250 mg/m² over 30 minutes days 1 and 8 every 3 weeks (in combination with oxaliplatin) (De Giorgi, 2006) **or** 1000 mg/m² over 30 minutes days 1, 8, and 15 every 4 weeks for up to 6 cycles (in combination with paclitaxel) (Hinton, 2002)

Unknown-primary, adenocarcinoma (unlabeled use): 1250 mg/m² days 1 and 8 every 3 weeks (in combination with cisplatin) (Culine, 2003) **or** 1000 mg/m² over 30 minutes days 1 and 8 every 3 weeks for up to 6 cycles (in combination with docetaxel) (Pouessel, 2004)

Uterine cancer (unlabeled use): 900 mg/m² over 90 minutes days 1 and 8 every 3 weeks (in combination with docetaxel) (Hensley, 2008) **or** 1000 mg/m² over 30 minutes days 1, 8, and 15 every 4 weeks (Look, 2004)

Dosing adjustment for toxicity:

Pancreatic cancer: Hematologic toxicity:

- AGC ≥1000/mm³ and platelet count ≥100,000/mm³: Administer 100% of full dose
- AGC 500-999/mm³ or platelet count 50,000-99,999/mm³: Administer 75% of full dose
- AGC <500/mm³ or platelet count <50,000/mm³: Hold dose

Nonsmall cell lung cancer:

- Hematologic toxicity: Refer to guidelines for pancreatic cancer. Cisplatin dosage may also need adjusted.
- Severe (grades 3 or 4) nonhematologic toxicity (except alopecia, nausea, and vomiting): Hold or decrease dose by 50%.

Breast cancer:

- Hematologic toxicity: Adjustments based on granulocyte and platelet counts on day 8:
  - AGC ≥1200/mm³ and platelet count >75,000/mm³: Administer 100% of full dose
  - AGC 1000-1199/mm³ or platelet count 50,000-75,000/mm³: Administer 75% of full dose
  - AGC 700-999/mm³ and platelet count ≥50,000/mm³: Administer 50% of full dose
  - AGC <700/mm³ or platelet count <50,000/mm³: Hold dose
- Severe (grades 3 or 4) nonhematologic toxicity (except alopecia, nausea, and vomiting): Hold or decrease dose by 50%. Paclitaxel dose may also need adjusted.

Ovarian cancer:

- Hematologic toxicity: Adjustments based on granulocyte and platelet counts on day 8:
  - AGC ≥1500/mm³ and platelet count ≥100,000/mm³: Administer 100% of full dose
  - AGC 1000-1499/mm³ and/or platelet count 75,000-99,999/mm³: Administer 50% of full dose
  - AGC <1000/mm³ and/or platelet count <75,000/mm³: Hold dose
- Severe (grades 3 or 4) nonhematologic toxicity (except nausea and vomiting): Hold or decrease dose by 50%. Carboplatin dose may also need adjusted.

Dose adjustment for subsequent cycles:

AGC <500/mm^3 for >5 days, AGC <100/mm^3 for >3 days, febrile neutropenia, platelet count <25,000/mm^3, cycle delay >1 week due to toxicity: Reduce gemcitabine to 800 mg/m^2 on days 1 and 8.

For recurrence of any of the above toxicities after initial dose reduction: Administer gemcitabine 800 mg/m^2 on day 1 only for the subsequent cycle

Dosing adjustment in renal impairment: The FDA-approved labeling does not contain dosing adjustment guidelines; use with caution in patients with pre-existing renal dysfunction. Discontinue if severe renal toxicity or hemolytic uremic syndrome (HUS) occur during gemcitabine treatment.

Mild-to-severe renal impairment: No adjustment required (Janus, 2010; Li, 2007)

ESRD (on hemodialysis): Hemodialysis should begin 6-12 hours after gemcitabine infusion (Janus 2010; Li, 2007)

Dosing adjustment in hepatic impairment: The FDA-approved labeling does not contain dosing adjustment guidelines; use with caution. Discontinue if severe hepatotoxicity occurs during treatment with gemcitabine. The following guidelines have been used by some clinicians:

Transaminases elevated (with normal bilirubin): No adjustment required (Venook, 2000)

Serum bilirubin >1.6 mg/dL: Use initial dose of 800 mg/m^2; may escalate if tolerated (Ecklund, 2005; Floyd, 2006; Venook, 2000)

Administration Infuse over 30 minutes; for unlabeled uses, infusion times may vary (refer to specific references). **Note:** Prolongation of the infusion time >60 minutes has been shown to increase toxicity. Gemcitabine has been administered at a fixed-dose rate (FDR) infusion rate of 10 mg/m^2/minute (unlabeled); prolonged infusion times increase the accumulation of the active metabolite, gemcitabine triphosphate, optimizing the pharmacokinetics (Ko, 2006; Tempero, 2003). Patients who receive gemcitabine FDR experience more grade 3/4 hematologic toxicity (Ko, 2006; Poplin, 2009).

For intravesicular (bladder) instillation, gemcitabine was diluted in 50-100 mL normal saline; patients were instructed to retain in the bladder for 1 hour (Addeo, 2010; Dalbaghi, 2006)

Monitoring Parameters CBC with differential and platelet count (prior to each dose); hepatic and renal function (prior to initiation of therapy and periodically, thereafter); monitor electrolytes, including potassium, magnesium, and calcium (when in combination therapy with cisplatin)

Dosage Forms Excipient information presented when available (limited, particularly for generics); consult specific product labeling.

Injection, powder for reconstitution: 200 mg, 1 g, 2 g

Gemzar®: 200 mg, 1 g

Injection, solution: 38 mg/mL (5.26 mL, 26.3 mL, 52.6 mL)

◆ **Gemcitabine For Injection, USP (Can)** *see* Gemcitabine *on page 782*

◆ **Gemcitabine Hydrochloride** *see* Gemcitabine *on page 782*

Gemfibrozil (jem FI broe zil)

Brand Names: U.S. Lopid®

Brand Names: Canada Apo-Gemfibrozil®; Gen-Gemfibrozil; GMD-Gemfibrozil; Lopid®; Mylan-Gemfibrozil; Novo-Gemfibrozil; Nu-Gemfibrozil; PMS-Gemfibrozil

Index Terms CI-719

Pharmacologic Category Antilipemic Agent, Fibric Acid

Use Treatment of hypertriglyceridemia in Fredrickson types IV and V hyperlipidemia for patients who are at greater risk for pancreatitis and who have not responded to dietary intervention; to reduce the risk of CHD development in Fredrickson type IIb patients without a history or symptoms of existing CHD who have not responded to dietary and other interventions (including pharmacologic treatment) and who have decreased HDL, increased LDL, and increased triglycerides

Pregnancy Risk Factor C

Pregnancy Considerations Adverse events were observed in animal reproduction studies. There are no adequate and well-controlled studies in pregnant women. Use only if benefits outweigh the risks.

Lactation Excretion in breast milk unknown/not recommended

Contraindications Hypersensitivity to gemfibrozil or any component of the formulation; hepatic or severe renal dysfunction; primary biliary cirrhosis; pre-existing gallbladder disease; concurrent use with repaglinide

Warnings/Precautions Secondary causes of hyperlipidemia should be ruled out prior to therapy. Possible increased risk of malignancy and cholelithiasis. Anemia, leukopenia, thrombocytopenia, and bone marrow hypoplasia have rarely been reported. Periodic monitoring recommended during the first year of therapy. Elevations in serum transaminases can be seen. Discontinue if lipid response not seen. Be careful in patient selection; this is not a first- or second-line choice. Other agents may be more suitable. Adjustments in warfarin therapy may be required with concurrent use. Has been associated with rare myositis or rhabdomyolysis; patients should be monitored closely. Patients should be instructed to report unexplained muscle pain, tenderness, weakness, or brown urine. Use caution when combining gemfibrozil with HMG-CoA reductase inhibitors (may lead to myopathy, rhabdomyolysis). Use with caution in patients with mild-to-moderate renal impairment; contraindicated in patients with severe impairment. Renal function deterioration has been seen when used in patients with a serum creatinine >2 mg/dL.

Adverse Reactions

>10%: Gastrointestinal: Dyspepsia (20%)

1% to 10%:

Cardiovascular: Atrial fibrillation (1%)

Central nervous system: Fatigue (4%), vertigo (2%)

Dermatologic: Eczema (2%), rash (2%)

Gastrointestinal: Abdominal pain (10%), nausea/vomiting (3%)

<1% or case reports with probable causation (limited to important or life-threatening): Alkaline phosphatase increased, anemia, angioedema, arthralgia, bilirubin increased, blurred vision, bone marrow hypoplasia, cholelithiasis, cholecystitis, cholestatic jaundice, creatine phosphokinase increased, depression, dermatitis, dermatomyositis/polymyositis, dizziness, eosinophilia, exfoliative dermatitis, headache, hypoesthesia, hypokalemia, impotence, laryngeal edema, leukopenia, libido decreased, myalgia, myasthenia, myopathy, nephrotoxicity, painful extremities, paresthesia, peripheral neuritis, pruritus, Raynaud's phenomenon, rhabdomyolysis, somnolence, synovitis, taste perversion, transaminases increased, urticaria

Reports where causal relationship has not been established: Alopecia, anaphylaxis, cataracts, colitis, confusion, decreased fertility (male), drug-induced lupus-like syndrome, extrasystoles, hepatoma, intracranial hemorrhage, pancreatitis, peripheral vascular disease, photosensitivity, positive ANA, renal dysfunction, retinal edema, seizure, syncope, thrombocytopenia, vasculitis, weight loss

Drug Interactions

Metabolism/Transport Effects Substrate of CYP3A4 (minor); **Note:** Assignment of Major/Minor substrate status based on clinically relevant drug interaction potential; **Inhibits** CYP1A2 (moderate), CYP2C19 (strong), CYP2C8 (strong), CYP2C9 (strong)

Avoid Concomitant Use

Avoid concomitant use of Gemfibrozil with any of the following: Bexarotene; Bexarotene (Systemic); Clopidogrel; Repaglinide; Simvastatin

Increased Effect/Toxicity

Gemfibrozil may increase the levels/effects of: Antidiabetic Agents (Thiazolidinedione); Atorvastatin; Bexarotene; Bexarotene (Systemic); Carvedilol; Citalopram; Colchicine; CYP1A2 Substrates; CYP2C19 Substrates; CYP2C8 Substrates; CYP2C9 Substrates; Diclofenac; Ezetimibe; Fluvastatin; Lovastatin; Pitavastatin; Pravastatin; Repaglinide; Rosuvastatin; Simvastatin; Sulfonylureas; Treprostinil; Vitamin K Antagonists

The levels/effects of Gemfibrozil may be increased by: Conivaptan; CycloSPORINE; CycloSPORINE (Systemic)

Decreased Effect

Gemfibrozil may decrease the levels/effects of: Chenodiol; Clopidogrel; CycloSPORINE; CycloSPORINE (Systemic); Ursodiol

The levels/effects of Gemfibrozil may be decreased by: Bile Acid Sequestrants; Tocilizumab

Ethanol/Nutrition/Herb Interactions

Ethanol: Avoid ethanol to decrease triglycerides.

Food: When given after meals, the AUC of gemfibrozil is decreased.

Stability Store at controlled room temperature of 20°C to 25°C (68°F to 77°F). Protect from light and moisture.

Mechanism of Action The exact mechanism of action of gemfibrozil is unknown, however, several theories exist regarding the VLDL effect; it can inhibit lipolysis and decrease subsequent hepatic fatty acid uptake as well as inhibit hepatic secretion of VLDL; together these actions decrease serum VLDL levels; increases HDL-cholesterol; the mechanism behind HDL elevation is currently unknown

Pharmacodynamics/Kinetics

Onset of action: May require several days

Absorption: Well absorbed

Protein binding: 99%

Metabolism: Hepatic via oxidation to two inactive metabolites; undergoes enterohepatic recycling

Half-life elimination: 1.5 hours

Time to peak, serum: 1-2 hours

Excretion: Urine (~70% primarily as conjugated drug); feces (6%)

Dosage Adults: Oral: 600 mg twice daily; administer 30 minutes before breakfast and dinner

Dosage adjustment in renal impairment:

Mild-to-moderate impairment: Use caution; deterioration of renal function has been reported in patients with baseline serum creatinine >2 mg/dL

Severe impairment: Use is contraindicated

Hemodialysis: Not removed by hemodialysis; supplemental dose is not necessary

Dosage adjustment in hepatic impairment: Use is contraindicated

Dietary Considerations Before initiation of therapy, patients should be placed on a standard cholesterol-lowering diet for 3-6 months and the diet should be continued during drug therapy. Should be taken 30 minutes prior to breakfast and dinner

Administration Administer 30 minutes prior to breakfast and dinner.

Monitoring Parameters Serum cholesterol, LFTs periodically, CBC periodically (first year)

Dosage Forms Excipient information presented when available (limited, particularly for generics); consult specific product labeling.

Tablet, oral: 600 mg

Lopid®: 600 mg [scored]

Gemifloxacin (je mi FLOKS a sin)

Brand Names: U.S. Factive®

Brand Names: Canada Factive®

Index Terms DW286; Gemifloxacin Mesylate; LA 20304a; SB-265805

Pharmacologic Category Antibiotic, Quinolone; Respiratory Fluoroquinolone

Use Treatment of acute exacerbation of chronic bronchitis; treatment of community-acquired pneumonia (CAP), including pneumonia caused by multidrug-resistant strains of *S. pneumoniae* (MDRSP)

Unlabeled Use Acute sinusitis

Pregnancy Risk Factor C

Pregnancy Considerations Adverse events have been observed in some animal studies; therefore, the manufacturer classifies gemifloxacin as pregnancy category C. Quinolone exposure during human pregnancy has been reported with other agents (see Ciprofloxacin [Systemic], Ofloxacin [Systemic], and Norfloxacin [Systemic] monographs). To date, no specific teratogenic effect or increased pregnancy risk has been identified; however, because of concerns of cartilage damage in immature animals exposed to quinolones and the limited gemifloxacin specific data, gemifloxacin should only be used during pregnancy if a safer option is not available.

Lactation Excretion in breast milk unknown/not recommended

Medication Guide Available Yes

Contraindications Hypersensitivity to gemifloxacin, other fluoroquinolones, or any component of the formulation

Warnings/Precautions [U.S. Boxed Warning]: There have been reports of tendon inflammation and/or rupture with quinolone antibiotics; risk may be increased with concurrent corticosteroids, organ transplant recipients, and in patients >60 years of age. Rupture of the Achilles tendon sometimes requiring surgical repair has been reported most frequently; but other tendon sites (eg, rotator cuff, biceps) have also been reported. Strenuous physical activity, rheumatoid arthritis, and renal impairment may be an independent risk factor for tendonitis. Discontinue at first sign of tendon inflammation or pain. May occur even after discontinuation of therapy. Use with caution in patients with rheumatoid arthritis; may increase risk of tendon rupture. Fluoroquinolones may prolong QT_c interval; avoid use of gemifloxacin in patients with a history of QT_c prolongation, uncorrected hypokalemia, hypomagnesemia, or concurrent administration of other medications known to prolong the QT interval (including Class Ia and Class III antiarrhythmics, cisapride, erythromycin, antipsychotics, and tricyclic antidepressants). Use with caution in patients with significant bradycardia or acute myocardial ischemia. Use with caution in individuals at risk of seizures (CNS disorders or concurrent therapy with medications which may lower seizure threshold). Potential for seizures, although very rare, may be increased with concomitant NSAID therapy. Discontinue in patients who experience significant CNS adverse effects (dizziness, hallucinations, suicidal ideation or actions). Use caution in renal dysfunction; dosage adjustment required for Cl_{cr} ≤40 mL/minute.

Fluoroquinolones have been associated with the development of serious, and sometimes fatal, hypoglycemia, most often in elderly diabetics, but also in patients without diabetes. This occurred most frequently with gatifloxacin (no longer available systemically) but may occur at a lower frequency with other quinolones.

Severe hypersensitivity reactions, including anaphylaxis, have occurred with quinolone therapy. Reactions may present as typical allergic symptoms after a single dose, or may manifest as severe idiosyncratic dermatologic, vascular, pulmonary, renal, hepatic, and/or hematologic events, usually after multiple doses. May cause maculopapular rash, usually 8-10 days after treatment initiation; risk factors may include age <40 years, female gender (including postmenopausal women on HRT), and treatment duration >7 days. Prompt discontinuation of drug should occur if skin rash or other symptoms arise. **[U.S. Boxed Warning]: Quinolones may exacerbate myasthenia gravis; avoid use (rare, potentially life-threatening weakness of respiratory muscles may occur).** Avoid excessive sunlight and take precautions to limit exposure (eg, loose fitting clothing, sunscreen); may cause moderate-to-severe phototoxicity reactions. Discontinue use if photosensitivity occurs. Prolonged use may result in fungal or bacterial superinfection, including *C. difficile*-associated diarrhea (CDAD) and pseudomembranous colitis; CDAD has been observed >2 months postantibiotic treatment. Peripheral neuropathy has been linked to the use of quinolones; these cases were rare. Hemolytic reactions may (rarely) occur with quinolone use in patients with latent or actual G6PD deficiency.

Adverse Reactions

1% to 10%:

- Central nervous system: Headache (4%), dizziness (2%)
- Dermatologic: Rash (4%)
- Gastrointestinal: Diarrhea (5%), nausea (4%), abdominal pain (2%), vomiting (2%)
- Hematologic: Neutropenia/neutrophilia (1%), platelets increased (1%), thrombocythemia (1%)
- Hepatic: Transaminases increased (1% to 4%), GGT increased (1%)
- Neuromuscular & skeletal: CPK increased (1%)

<1% (Limited to important or life-threatening): Acute renal failure, alkaline phosphatase increased, anaphylactic reaction, anemia, anorexia, arthralgia, back pain, bilirubin increased, BUN increased, constipation, cramps (leg), dermatitis, dyspepsia, dyspnea, eczema, eosinophilia, erythema multiforme, facial edema, fatigue, flatulence, flushing, fungal infection, gastritis, gastroenteritis, genital moniliasis, granulocytopenia, hematocrit decreased/increased, hemoglobin decreased/increased, hemorrhage, hot flashes, hyperglycemia, hyper-/hypocalcemia, hyper-/hypokalemia, hyper-/hyponatremia, hypoalbuminemia, INR increased, insomnia, leukopenia, moniliasis, myalgia, myasthenia gravis exacerbation, nervousness, pain, pharyngitis, photosensitivity, pneumonia, pruritus, pseudomembranous colitis, QT_c prolongation, retinal hemorrhage, serum creatinine increased, skin exfoliation, somnolence, supraventricular tachycardia, syncope, taste perversion, tendonitis, tendon rupture, thrombocytopenia, TIA, tremor, urticaria, vaginitis, vertigo, vision abnormal, weakness, xerostomia

Important adverse effects reported with other agents in this drug class include (not reported for gemifloxacin): Allergic reactions, CNS stimulation, hepatic necrosis/failure, hepatitis, hypersensitivity, jaundice, pancytopenia, peripheral neuropathy, pneumonitis (eosinophilic), seizure, sensorimotor-axonal neuropathy (paresthesia, hypoesthesias, dysesthesias, weakness), serum sickness, severe dermatologic reactions (toxic epidermal necrolysis, Stevens-Johnson syndrome), thrombotic thrombocytopenia purpura, torsade de pointes, vasculitis

Drug Interactions

Metabolism/Transport Effects None known.

Avoid Concomitant Use

Avoid concomitant use of Gemifloxacin with any of the following: BCG

Increased Effect/Toxicity

Gemifloxacin may increase the levels/effects of: Corticosteroids (Systemic); Porfimer; Sulfonylureas; Varenicline; Vitamin K Antagonists

The levels/effects of Gemifloxacin may be increased by: Insulin; Nonsteroidal Anti-Inflammatory Agents; Probenecid

Decreased Effect

Gemifloxacin may decrease the levels/effects of: BCG; Mycophenolate; Sulfonylureas; Typhoid Vaccine

The levels/effects of Gemifloxacin may be decreased by: Antacids; Calcium Salts; Didanosine; Iron Salts; Magnesium Salts; Quinapril; Sevelamer; Sucralfate; Zinc Salts

Ethanol/Nutrition/Herb Interactions Herb/Nutraceutical: Avoid dong quai, St John's wort (may also cause photosensitization).

Stability Store at 25°C (77°F). Protect from light.

Mechanism of Action Gemifloxacin is a DNA gyrase inhibitor and also inhibits topoisomerase IV. DNA gyrase (topoisomerase IV) is an essential bacterial enzyme that maintains the superhelical structure of DNA. DNA gyrase is required for DNA replication and transcription, DNA repair, recombination, and transposition; bactericidal

Pharmacodynamics/Kinetics

Absorption: Well absorbed from the GI tract

Distribution: V_{dss}: 4.2 L/kg

Protein binding: ~60% to 70%

Metabolism: Hepatic (minor); forms metabolites (CYP isoenzymes are not involved)

Bioavailability: ~71%

Half-life elimination: 7 hours (range 4-12 hours)

Time to peak, plasma: 0.5-2 hours

Excretion: Feces (61%); urine (36%)

Dosage

Usual dosage range:

Adults: Oral: 320 mg once daily

Indication-specific dosing:

Adults: Oral:

Acute exacerbations of chronic bronchitis: 320 mg once daily for 5 days

Community-acquired pneumonia (mild-to-moderate): 320 mg once daily for 5 or 7 days (decision to use 5- or 7-day regimen should be guided by initial sputum culture; 7 days are recommended for MDRSP, *Klebsiella*, or *M. catarrhalis* infection)

Sinusitis (unlabeled use): 320 mg once daily for 10 days

Elderly: Refer to adult dosing.

Dosage adjustment in renal impairment:

Cl_{cr} >40 mL/minute: No adjustment required

Cl_{cr} ≤40 mL/minute (or patients on hemodialysis/CAPD): 160 mg once daily (administer dose following hemodialysis)

Dosage adjustment in hepatic impairment: No adjustment required

Dietary Considerations May take tablets with or without food, milk, or calcium supplements. Gemifloxacin should be taken 3 hours before or 2 hours after supplements (including multivitamins) containing iron, zinc, or magnesium.

Administration May be administered with or without food, milk, or calcium supplements. Gemifloxacin should be taken 3 hours before or 2 hours after supplements (including multivitamins) containing iron, zinc, or magnesium.

Monitoring Parameters WBC, signs/symptoms of infection, renal function

Dosage Forms Excipient information presented when available (limited, particularly for generics); consult specific product labeling.

Tablet, oral:

Factive®: 320 mg [scored]

◆ **Gemifloxacin Mesylate** *see* Gemifloxacin *on page 786*

Gemtuzumab Ozogamicin

(gem TOO zoo mab oh zog a MY sin)

Index Terms CMA-676; Mylotarg

Pharmacologic Category Antineoplastic Agent, Monoclonal Antibody

Use Due to safety concerns, as well as lack of clinical benefit demonstrated in a post-approval clinical trial, gemtuzumab was withdrawn from the U.S. commercial market in 2010.

Unlabeled Use Treatment of relapsed or refractory CD33-positive acute myeloid leukemia (AML); salvage therapy for acute promyelocytic leukemia (APL)

Pregnancy Considerations Animal studies have demonstrated teratogenic effects, fetal loss, and maternal toxicity. There are no adequate and well-controlled studies in pregnant women. May cause fetal harm when administered to a pregnant woman. Women of childbearing potential should avoid becoming pregnant while receiving treatment.

Lactation Excretion in breast milk unknown/not recommended

Prescribing and Access Restrictions As of June 2010, gemtuzumab has been withdrawn from the U.S. market and is no longer commercially available to new patients; gemtuzumab is only available in the U.S. under an Investigational New Drug (IND) protocol.

In Canada, gemtuzumab is available through a special access program (access information is available from Health Canada).

Contraindications Hypersensitivity to gemtuzumab ozogamicin, calicheamicin derivatives, or any component of the formulation; patients with anti-CD33 antibody

Warnings/Precautions Hazardous agent - use appropriate precautions for handling and disposal.

Gemtuzumab has been associated with hepatotoxicity, including severe hepatic sinusoidal obstruction syndrome (SOS; formerly called veno-occlusive disease [VOD]). Symptoms of SOS include right upper quadrant pain, rapid weight gain, ascites, hepatomegaly, and bilirubin/transaminase elevations. Risk may be increased by combination chemotherapy, underlying hepatic disease, or hematopoietic stem cell transplant.

Severe hypersensitivity reactions (including anaphylaxis) and other infusion-related reactions may occur. Infusion-related events are common, generally reported to occur with the first dose after the end of the 2-hour intravenous infusion. These symptoms usually resolved after 2-4 hours with a supportive therapy of acetaminophen, diphenhydramine, and intravenous fluids. Other severe and potentially fatal infusion related pulmonary events (including dyspnea and hypoxia) have been reported infrequently. Symptomatic intrinsic lung disease or high peripheral blast counts may increase the risk of severe reactions. Fewer infusion-related events were observed after the second dose. Postinfusion reactions (may include fever, chills, hypotension, or dyspnea) may occur during the first 24 hours after administration. Consider discontinuation in patients who develop severe infusion-related reactions. In addition to infusion-related pulmonary events, gemtuzumab therapy is also associated with acute respiratory distress syndrome, pulmonary infiltrates, pleural effusion, noncardiogenic pulmonary edema, and pulmonary insufficiency.

Severe myelosuppression occurs in all patients at recommended dosages. Tumor lysis syndrome may occur as a consequence of leukemia treatment, adequate hydration and prophylactic allopurinol must be instituted prior to use. Other methods to lower WBC <30,000 cells/mm^3 may be considered (hydroxyurea or leukapheresis) to minimize the risk of tumor lysis syndrome, and/or severe infusion reactions. An increased number of deaths have been reported in patients receiving gemtuzumab in combination with chemotherapy, compared to those receiving chemotherapy alone.

Adverse Reactions Frequency not defined.

Cardiovascular: Cerebral hemorrhage, hyper-/hypotension, peripheral edema, tachycardia

Central nervous system: Anxiety, chills, depression, dizziness, fever, headache, insomnia, intracranial hemorrhage, pain

Dermatologic: Bruising, petechiae, pruritus, rash

Endocrine & metabolic: Hyperglycemia, hypocalcemia, hypokalemia, hypomagnesemia, hypophosphatemia

Gastrointestinal: Abdominal pain, anorexia, diarrhea, dyspepsia, gingival hemorrhage, melena, mucositis, nausea, stomatitis, vomiting

Genitourinary: Vaginal bleeding, vaginal hemorrhage

Hematologic: Anemia, disseminated intravascular coagulation (DIC), hemorrhage, leukopenia, lymphopenia, neutropenia (median recovery 40-51 days), neutropenic fever, thrombocytopenia (median recovery 36-51 days)

Hepatic: Alkaline phosphatase increased, ALT increased, ascites, AST increased, hyperbilirubinemia, LDH increased, prothrombin time increased, PTT increased, sinusoidal obstruction syndrome (SOS; veno-occlusive disease; higher frequency in patients with prior history of or subsequent hematopoietic stem cell transplant)

Local: Local reaction

Neuromuscular & skeletal: Arthralgia, back pain, myalgia, weakness

Renal: Creatinine increased, hematuria

Respiratory: Cough, dyspnea, epistaxis, hypoxia, pharyngitis, pneumonia, rhinitis

Miscellaneous: Cutaneous herpes simplex, infection, infusion reaction, sepsis

Infrequent and/or case reports (limited to important or life-threatening): Acute respiratory distress syndrome, anaphylaxis, bradycardia, Budd-Chiari syndrome, gastrointestinal hemorrhage, hepatic failure, hepatosplenomegaly, hypersensitivity reactions, jaundice, neutropenic sepsis, noncardiogenic pulmonary edema, portal vain thrombosis, pulmonary hemorrhage, renal impairment, renal failure (including renal failure secondary to tumor lysis syndrome)

Drug Interactions

Metabolism/Transport Effects None known.

Avoid Concomitant Use

Avoid concomitant use of Gemtuzumab Ozogamicin with any of the following: BCG; Belimumab; CloZAPine; Natalizumab; Pimecrolimus; Tacrolimus (Topical); Vaccines (Live)

Increased Effect/Toxicity

Gemtuzumab Ozogamicin may increase the levels/effects of: Belimumab; CloZAPine; Leflunomide; Natalizumab; Vaccines (Live)

The levels/effects of Gemtuzumab Ozogamicin may be increased by: Abciximab; Denosumab; Pimecrolimus; Roflumilast; Tacrolimus (Topical); Trastuzumab

Decreased Effect

Gemtuzumab Ozogamicin may decrease the levels/effects of: BCG; Coccidioidin Skin Test; Sipuleucel-T; Vaccines (Inactivated); Vaccines (Live)

The levels/effects of Gemtuzumab Ozogamicin may be decreased by: Echinacea

Stability Light sensitive; protect from light (including direct and indirect sunlight, and unshielded fluorescent light). Store intact vials under refrigeration at 2°C to 8°C (36°F to 46°F). Reconstituted solutions may be stored for up to 2 hours at room temperature or under refrigeration. Following dilution for infusion, solutions are stable for up to 16 hours at room temperature. Administration requires 2 hours; therefore, the maximum elapsed time from initial reconstitution to completion of infusion should be 20 hours.

Reconstitution: Protect from light during preparation (and administration). Prepare in biologic safety hood with shielded fluorescent light; (some institutions prepare in a darkened room with the lights in the biologic safety cabinet turned off). Allow to warm to room temperature prior to reconstitution. Reconstitute each 5 mg vial with sterile water for injection to a concentration of 1 mg/mL. Dilute in 100 mL of 0.9% sodium chloride injection. The infusion container should be placed in a UV protectant bag immediately after preparation. Hazardous agent - use appropriate precautions for handling and disposal.

Mechanism of Action Antibody to CD33 antigen, which is expressed on leukemic blasts in 80% of AML patients. Binds to the CD33 antigen, resulting in internalization of the antibody-antigen complex. Following internalization, the calicheamicin derivative is released inside the myeloid cell. The calicheamicin derivative binds to DNA resulting in double strand breaks and cell death. Pluripotent stem cells and nonhematopoietic cells are not affected.

Pharmacodynamics/Kinetics

Distribution: V_{ss}: Adults: Initial dose: 21 L; Repeat dose: 10 L

Half-life elimination: Total calicheamicin: Initial: 41-45 hours, Repeat dose: 60-64 hours; Unconjugated: 100-143 hours (no change noted in repeat dosing)

Dosage I.V.: Adults: **Note:** Patients should receive diphenhydramine 50 mg orally and acetaminophen 650-1000 mg orally 1 hour prior to administration of each dose. Acetaminophen dosage should be repeated as needed every 4 hours for 2 additional doses. Pretreatment with methylprednisolone may ameliorate infusion-related symptoms.

AML (unlabeled/investigational use):

<60 years: 9 mg/m^2 infused over 2 hours. A full treatment course is a total of 2 doses administered with 14-28 days between doses (Larson, 2005).

≥60 years: 9 mg/m^2 infused over 2 hours. A full treatment course is a total of 2 doses administered with 14-28 days between doses (Larson, 2002; Larson, 2005).

APL (unlabeled/investigational use):

Single-agent therapy: 6 mg/m^2 infused over 2 hours on days 1 and 15; for patients testing PCR negative after 2 doses, a third dose was administered (LoCoco, 2004).

Combination therapy (high-risk patients; Ravandi, 2009):

Induction: 9 mg/m^2 as a single dose on day 1 (in combination with arsenic trioxide and tretinoin)

Post remission therapy (if arsenic trioxide or tretinoin discontinued due to toxicity): 9 mg/m^2 once every 4-5 weeks until 28 weeks after complete remission

Dosage adjustment for toxicity:

Dyspnea or significant hypotension: Interrupt infusion; monitor

Anaphylaxis, pulmonary edema, acute respiratory distress syndrome: Strongly consider discontinuing treatment

Administration Do not administer as I.V. push or bolus. Administer via I.V. infusion, over at least 2 hours through a low protein-binding (0.2-1.2 micron) in-line filter. Protect from light during infusion. Premedicate with acetaminophen and diphenhydramine prior to each infusion.

Monitoring Parameters Monitor vital signs during the infusion and for 4 hours following the infusion. Monitor for signs/symptoms of postinfusion reaction. Monitor electrolytes, liver function, CBC with differential and platelets frequently. Monitor for signs and symptoms of hepatic sinusoidal obstruction syndrome (SOS; veno-occlusive disease; weight gain, right upper quadrant abdominal pain, hepatomegaly, ascites).

Product Availability No longer commercially available in the U.S. market for new patients. Available in Canada through a special access program.

◆ **Gemzar®** *see* Gemcitabine *on page 782*

◆ **Genac™ [OTC] [DSC]** *see* Triprolidine and Pseudoephedrine *on page 1741*

◆ **Gen-Acyclovir (Can)** *see* Acyclovir (Systemic) *on page 39*

◆ **Gen-Amoxicillin (Can)** *see* Amoxicillin *on page 103*

◆ **Genaphed™ [OTC] [DSC]** *see* Pseudoephedrine *on page 1430*

◆ **Genaton™ [OTC] [DSC]** *see* Aluminum Hydroxide and Magnesium Carbonate *on page 79*

◆ **Gen-Beclo (Can)** *see* Beclomethasone (Nasal) *on page 194*

◆ **Gen-Budesonide AQ (Can)** *see* Budesonide (Nasal) *on page 240*

◆ **Gen-Buspirone (Can)** *see* BusPIRone *on page 250*

◆ **Gen-Clindamycin (Can)** *see* Clindamycin (Systemic) *on page 378*

◆ **Gen-Clobetasol (Can)** *see* Clobetasol *on page 384*

◆ **Gen-Clomipramine (Can)** *see* ClomiPRAMINE *on page 388*

◆ **Gen-Clonazepam (Can)** *see* ClonazePAM *on page 390*

◆ **Gen-Clozapine (Can)** *see* CloZAPine *on page 400*

◆ **Gen-Combo Sterinebs (Can)** *see* Ipratropium and Albuterol *on page 924*

◆ **Gen-Cyclobenzaprine (Can)** *see* Cyclobenzaprine *on page 419*

◆ **Gen-Doxazosin (Can)** *see* Doxazosin *on page 548*

◆ **Gene-Activated Human Acid-Beta-Glucosidase** *see* Velaglucerase Alfa *on page 1778*

◆ **Generess™ Fe** *see* Ethinyl Estradiol and Norethindrone *on page 660*

◆ **Generlac** *see* Lactulose *on page 964*

◆ **Genfiber™ [OTC] [DSC]** *see* Psyllium *on page 1432*

◆ **Gen-Fluoxetine (Can)** *see* FLUoxetine *on page 731*

◆ **Gen-Gemfibrozil (Can)** *see* Gemfibrozil *on page 785*

◆ **Gengraf®** *see* CycloSPORINE (Systemic) *on page 422*

◆ **Gen-Hydroxychloroquine (Can)** *see* Hydroxychloroquine *on page 848*

◆ **Gen-Hydroxyurea (Can)** *see* Hydroxyurea *on page 851*

◆ **Gen-Ipratropium (Can)** *see* Ipratropium (Systemic) *on page 923*

◆ **Gen-Lovastatin (Can)** *see* Lovastatin *on page 1038*

◆ **Gen-Medroxy (Can)** *see* MedroxyPROGESTERone *on page 1058*

◆ **Gen-Nabumetone (Can)** *see* Nabumetone *on page 1167*

◆ **Gen-Nizatidine (Can)** *see* Nizatidine *on page 1215*

◆ **Gen-Nortriptyline (Can)** *see* Nortriptyline *on page 1220*

◆ **Genotropin®** *see* Somatropin *on page 1579*

◆ **Genotropin Miniquick®** *see* Somatropin *on page 1579*

◆ **Gen-Selegiline (Can)** *see* Selegiline *on page 1544*

◆ **Gentak®** *see* Gentamicin (Ophthalmic) *on page 792*

Gentamicin (Systemic) (jen ta MYE sin)

Brand Names: Canada Gentamicin Injection, USP

Index Terms Gentamicin Sulfate

Pharmacologic Category Antibiotic, Aminoglycoside

Additional Appendix Information

Antibiotic Treatment of Adults With Infective Endocarditis *on page 1956*

Prevention of Wound Infection and Sepsis in Surgical Patients *on page 1954*

Use Treatment of susceptible bacterial infections, normally gram-negative organisms, including *Pseudomonas*, *Proteus*, *Serratia*, and gram-positive *Staphylococcus*; treatment of bone infections, respiratory tract infections, skin and soft tissue infections, as well as abdominal and urinary tract infections, and septicemia; treatment of infective endocarditis

Pregnancy Risk Factor D

Pregnancy Considerations Gentamicin crosses the placenta and produces detectable serum levels in the fetus. Renal toxicity has been described in two case reports following first trimester exposure. There are several reports of total irreversible bilateral congenital deafness in children whose mothers received streptomycin during pregnancy; therefore, the manufacturer classifies gentamicin as pregnancy category D. Although ototoxicity has not been reported following maternal use of gentamicin, a potential for harm exists. **[U.S. Boxed Warning]: Aminoglycosides may cause fetal harm if administered to a pregnant woman.**

Due to pregnancy induced physiologic changes, some pharmacokinetic parameters of gentamicin may be altered. Pregnant women have an average-to-larger volume of distribution which may result in lower serum peak levels than for the same dose in nonpregnant women. Serum half-life is also shorter.

Lactation Enters breast milk/use caution (AAP rates "compatible"; AAP 2001 update pending)

Contraindications Hypersensitivity to gentamicin or other aminoglycosides

Warnings/Precautions **[U.S. Boxed Warning]: Aminoglycosides may cause neurotoxicity and/or nephrotoxicity;** usual risk factors include pre-existing renal impairment, concomitant neuro-/nephrotoxic medications, advanced age and dehydration. Ototoxicity may be directly proportional to the amount of drug given and the duration of treatment; tinnitus or vertigo are indications of vestibular injury and impending hearing loss; renal damage is usually reversible. May cause neuromuscular blockade and respiratory paralysis; especially when given soon after anesthesia or muscle relaxants.

Not intended for long-term therapy due to toxic hazards associated with extended administration; use caution in pre-existing renal insufficiency, vestibular or cochlear impairment, myasthenia gravis, hypocalcemia, conditions which depress neuromuscular transmission. Dosage modification required in patients with impaired renal function. Prolonged use may result in fungal or bacterial superinfection, including *C. difficile*-associated diarrhea (CDAD) and pseudomembranous colitis; CDAD has been observed >2 months postantibiotic treatment.

Adverse Reactions

>10%:

Central nervous system: Neurotoxicity (vertigo, ataxia)

Neuromuscular & skeletal: Gait instability

Otic: Ototoxicity (auditory), ototoxicity (vestibular)

Renal: Nephrotoxicity, decreased creatinine clearance

1% to 10%: Cardiovascular: Edema

<1% (Limited to important or life-threatening): Agranulocytosis allergic reaction, anorexia, burning, drowsiness, dyspnea, enterocolitis erythema, granulocytopenia headache, LFTs increased, muscle cramps, nausea, pseudomotor cerebri, salivation increased, thrombocytopenia, tremor, vomiting, weakness, weight loss

Drug Interactions

Metabolism/Transport Effects None known.

Avoid Concomitant Use

Avoid concomitant use of Gentamicin (Systemic) with any of the following: Agalsidase Alfa; Agalsidase Beta; BCG; Gallium Nitrate

Increased Effect/Toxicity

Gentamicin (Systemic) may increase the levels/effects of: AbobotulinumtoxinA; Bisphosphonate Derivatives; CARBOplatin; Colistimethate; CycloSPORINE; CycloSPORINE (Systemic); Gallium Nitrate; Neuromuscular-Blocking Agents; OnabotulinumtoxinA; RimabotulinumtoxinB

The levels/effects of Gentamicin (Systemic) may be increased by: Amphotericin B; Capreomycin; Cephalosporins (2nd Generation); Cephalosporins (3rd Generation); Cephalosporins (4th Generation); CISplatin; Loop Diuretics; Nonsteroidal Anti-Inflammatory Agents; Vancomycin

Decreased Effect

Gentamicin (Systemic) may decrease the levels/effects of: Agalsidase Alfa; Agalsidase Beta; BCG; Typhoid Vaccine

The levels/effects of Gentamicin (Systemic) may be decreased by: Penicillins

Stability

Gentamicin is a colorless to slightly yellow solution which should be stored between 2°C to 30°C, but refrigeration is not recommended.

I.V. infusion solutions mixed in NS or D_5W solution are stable for 24 hours at room temperature and refrigeration.

Premixed bag: Manufacturer expiration date.

Out of overwrap stability: 30 days.

Mechanism of Action Interferes with bacterial protein synthesis by binding to 30S and 50S ribosomal subunits resulting in a defective bacterial cell membrane

Pharmacodynamics/Kinetics

Absorption:

Intramuscular: Rapid and complete

Oral: None

Distribution: Primarily into extracellular fluid (highly hydrophilic); high concentration in the renal cortex; minimal penetration to ocular tissues via I.V. route

V_d: Increased by edema, ascites, fluid overload; decreased with dehydration

Neonates: 0.4-0.6 L/kg

Children: 0.3-0.35 L/kg

Adults: 0.2-0.3 L/kg

Relative diffusion from blood into CSF: Minimal even with inflammation

CSF:blood level ratio: Normal meninges: Nil; Inflamed meninges: 10% to 30%

Protein binding: <30%

Half-life elimination:

Infants: <1 week: 3-11.5 hours; 1 week to 6 months: 3-3.5 hours

Adults: 1.5-3 hours; End-stage renal disease: 36-70 hours

Time to peak, serum: I.M.: 30-90 minutes; I.V.: 30 minutes after 30-minute infusion

Excretion: Urine (as unchanged drug)

Clearance: Directly related to renal function

Dosage Note: Dosage Individualization is **critical** because of the low therapeutic index.

Use of ideal body weight (IBW) for determining the mg/kg/dose appears to be more accurate than dosing on the basis of total body weight (TBW). In morbid obesity, dosage requirement may best be estimated using a dosing weight of IBW + 0.4 (TBW - IBW).

Initial and periodic plasma drug levels (eg, peak and trough with conventional dosing) should be determined, particularly in critically-ill patients with serious infections or in disease states known to significantly alter aminoglycoside pharmacokinetics (eg, cystic fibrosis, burns, or major surgery).

Usual dosage ranges:

Infants and Children <5 years: I.M., I.V.: 2.5 mg/kg/dose every 8 hours*

Children ≥5 years: I.M., I.V.: 2-2.5 mg/kg/dose every 8 hours*

***Note:** Higher individual doses and/or more frequent intervals (eg, every 6 hours) may be required in selected clinical situations (cystic fibrosis) or serum levels document the need.

Adults:

I.M., I.V.:

Conventional: 1-2.5 mg/kg/dose every 8-12 hours; to ensure adequate peak concentrations early in therapy, higher initial dosage may be considered in selected patients when extracellular water is increased (edema, septic shock, postsurgical, or trauma)

Once daily: 4-7 mg/kg/dose once daily; some clinicians recommend this approach for all patients with normal renal function; this dose is at least as efficacious with similar, if not less, toxicity than conventional dosing

Intrathecal: 4-8 mg/day

Indication-specific dosing: Children and Adults: I.M., I.V.:

Brucellosis: 240 mg (I.M.) daily or 5 mg/kg (I.V.) daily for 7 days; either regimen recommended in combination with doxycycline

Cholangitis: 4-6 mg/kg once daily with ampicillin

Diverticulitis (complicated): 1.5-2 mg/kg every 8 hours (with ampicillin and metronidazole)

Endocarditis: Treatment: 3 mg/kg/day in 1-3 divided doses

Meningitis:

Enterococcus sp or *Pseudomonas aeruginosa*: Loading dose 2 mg/kg, then 1.7 mg/kg/dose every 8 hours (administered with another bacteriocidal drug)

Listeria: 5-7 mg/kg/day (with penicillin) for 1 week

Pelvic inflammatory disease: Loading dose: 2 mg/kg, then 1.5 mg/kg every 8 hours

Alternate therapy: 4.5 mg/kg once daily

Plague *(Yersinia pestis):* Treatment: 5 mg/kg/day, followed by postexposure prophylaxis with doxycycline

Pneumonia, hospital- or ventilator-associated: 7 mg/kg/day (with antipseudomonal beta-lactam or carbapenem)

Synergy (for gram-positive infections): 3 mg/kg/day in 1-3 divided doses (with ampicillin)

Tularemia: 5 mg/kg/day divided every 8 hours for 1-2 weeks

Urinary tract infection: 1.5 mg/kg/dose every 8 hours

Dosing interval in renal impairment:

Conventional dosing:

Cl_{cr} ≥60 mL/minute: Administer every 8 hours

Cl_{cr} 40-60 mL/minute: Administer every 12 hours

Cl_{cr} 20-40 mL/minute: Administer every 24 hours

Cl_{cr} <20 mL/minute: Loading dose, then monitor levels

High-dose therapy: Interval may be extended (eg, every 48 hours) in patients with moderate renal impairment (Cl_{cr} 30-59 mL/minute) and/or adjusted based on serum level determinations.

Intermittent hemodialysis (IHD) (administer after hemodialysis on dialysis days) (Heintz, 2009): Dialyzable (~50%; variable; dependent on filter, duration, and type of IHD): Loading dose of 2-3 mg/kg loading dose followed by:

Mild UTI or synergy: 1 mg/kg every 48-72 hours; consider redosing for pre-HD or post-HD concentrations <1 mg/L

Moderate-to-severe UTI: 1-1.5 mg/kg every 48-72 hours; consider redosing for pre-HD concentrations <1.5-2 mg/L or post-HD concentrations <1 mg/L

Systemic gram-negative rod infection: 1.5-2 mg/kg every 48-72 hours; consider redosing for pre-HD concentrations <3-5 mg/L or post-HD concentrations <2 mg/L

Note: Dosing dependent on the assumption of 3 times/week, complete IHD sessions.

Peritoneal dialysis (PD):

Administration via PD fluid:

Gram-positive infection (eg, synergy): 3-4 mg/L (3-4 mcg/mL) of PD fluid

Gram-negative infection: 4-8 mg/L (4-8 mcg/mL) of PD fluid

Administration via I.V., I.M. route during PD: Dose as for Cl_{cr} <10 mL/minute and follow levels

Continuous renal replacement therapy (CRRT) (Heintz, 2009; Trotman, 2005): Drug clearance is highly dependent on the method of renal replacement, filter type, and flow rate. Appropriate dosing requires close monitoring of pharmacologic response, signs of adverse reactions due to drug accumulation, as well as drug concentrations in relation to target trough (if appropriate). The following are general recommendations only (based on dialysate flow/ultrafiltration rates of 1-2 L/hour and minimal residual renal function) and should not supersede clinical judgment:

CVVH/CVVHD/CVVHDF: Loading dose of 2-3 mg/kg followed by:

Mild UTI or synergy: 1 mg/kg every 24-36 hours (redose when concentration <1 mg/L)

Moderate-to-severe UTI: 1-1.5 mg/kg every 24-36 hours (redose when concentration <1.5-2 mg/L)

Systemic gram-negative infection: 1.5-2.5 mg/kg every 24-48 hours (redose when concentration <3-5 mg/L)

Dosing adjustment/comments in hepatic disease: Monitor plasma concentrations

Dietary Considerations Calcium, magnesium, potassium: Renal wasting may cause hypocalcemia, hypomagnesemia, and/or hypokalemia.

Administration

I.M.: Administer by deep I.M. route if possible. Slower absorption and lower peak concentrations, probably due to poor circulation in the atrophic muscle, may occur following I.M. injection; in paralyzed patients, suggest I.V. route.

Some penicillins (eg, carbenicillin, ticarcillin, and piperacillin) have been shown to inactivate aminoglycosides *in vitro*. This has been observed to a greater extent with tobramycin and gentamicin, while amikacin has shown greater stability against inactivation. Concurrent use of these agents may pose a risk of reduced antibacterial efficacy *in vivo*, particularly in the setting of profound renal impairment. However, definitive clinical evidence is lacking. If combination penicillin/aminoglycoside therapy is desired in a patient with renal dysfunction, separation of doses (if feasible), and routine monitoring of aminoglycoside levels, CBC, and clinical response should be considered.

Monitoring Parameters Urinalysis, urine output, BUN, serum creatinine; hearing should be tested before, during, and after treatment; particularly in those at risk for ototoxicity or who will be receiving prolonged therapy (>2 weeks)

Some penicillin derivatives may accelerate the degradation of aminoglycosides *in vitro*. This may be clinically-significant for certain penicillin (ticarcillin, piperacillin, carbenicillin) and aminoglycoside (gentamicin, tobramycin) combination therapy in patients with significant renal impairment. Close monitoring of aminoglycoside levels is warranted.

Reference Range
Timing of serum samples: Draw peak 30 minutes after 30-minute infusion has been completed or 1 hour after I.M. injection; draw trough immediately before next dose
Sample size: 0.5-2 mL blood (red top tube) or 0.1-1 mL serum (separated)
Therapeutic levels:
Peak:
Serious infections: 6-8 mcg/mL (12-17 micromole/L)
Life-threatening infections: 8-10 mcg/mL (17-21 micromole/L)
Urinary tract infections: 4-6 mcg/mL
Synergy against gram-positive organisms: 3-5 mcg/mL
Trough:
Serious infections: 0.5-1 mcg/mL
Life-threatening infections: 1-2 mcg/mL
The American Thoracic Society (ATS) recommends trough levels of <1 mcg/mL for patients with hospital-acquired pneumonia.
Obtain drug levels after the third dose unless renal dysfunction/toxicity suspected

Test Interactions Some penicillin derivatives may accelerate the degradation of aminoglycosides *in vitro*, leading to a potential underestimation of aminoglycoside serum concentration.

Dosage Forms Excipient information presented when available (limited, particularly for generics); consult specific product labeling. [DSC] = Discontinued product
Infusion, premixed in NS: 60 mg (50 mL, 100 mL [DSC]); 80 mg (50 mL, 100 mL); 100 mg (50 mL, 100 mL); 120 mg (100 mL)
Injection, solution: 40 mg/mL (2 mL, 20 mL)
Injection, solution [pediatric]: 10 mg/mL (2 mL [DSC])
Injection, solution [pediatric, preservative free]: 10 mg/mL (2 mL)

Gentamicin (Ophthalmic) (jen ta MYE sin)

Brand Names: U.S. Garamycin®; Gentak®
Brand Names: Canada Diogent®; Garamycin®; Garasone; Gentak®; Gentocin; PMS-Gentamicin
Index Terms Gentamicin Sulfate
Pharmacologic Category Antibiotic, Aminoglycoside; Antibiotic, Ophthalmic
Use Treatment of ophthalmic infections caused by susceptible bacteria
Pregnancy Risk Factor C
Dosage Ophthalmic: Children and Adults:
Ointment: Instill 1/2" (1.25 cm) 2-3 times/day to every 3-4 hours
Solution: Instill 1-2 drops every 4 hours, up to 2 drops every hour for severe infections
Additional Information Complete prescribing information for this medication should be consulted for additional detail.
Dosage Forms Excipient information presented when available (limited, particularly for generics); consult specific product labeling.
Ointment, ophthalmic:
Gentak®: 0.3% (3.5 g)
Ointment, ophthalmic [preservative free]:
Garamycin®: 0.3% (3.5 g)
Solution, ophthalmic [drops]: 0.3% (5 mL, 15 mL)
Garamycin®: 0.3% (5 mL) [contains benzalkonium chloride]
Gentak®: 0.3% (5 mL) [contains benzalkonium chloride]

◆ **Gentamicin and Prednisolone** *see* Prednisolone and Gentamicin *on page 1399*
◆ **Gentamicin Injection, USP (Can)** *see* Gentamicin (Systemic) *on page 790*
◆ **Gentamicin Sulfate** *see* Gentamicin (Ophthalmic) *on page 792*
◆ **Gentamicin Sulfate** *see* Gentamicin (Systemic) *on page 790*
◆ **Gen-Temazepam (Can)** *see* Temazepam *on page 1638*

Gentian Violet (JEN shun VYE oh let)

Index Terms Crystal Violet; Methylrosaniline Chloride
Pharmacologic Category Antibiotic, Topical; Antifungal Agent, Topical
Use Treatment of cutaneous or mucocutaneous infections caused by *Candida albicans* and other superficial skin infections; external treatment of minor abrasions or cuts
Pregnancy Risk Factor C
Dosage Children and Adults: Topical: Apply to affected area once or twice daily. Solutions diluted to 0.25% to 0.5% may be less irritating. Solutions diluted to 0.01% have been recommended for use in closed cavities.
Additional Information Complete prescribing information for this medication should be consulted for additional detail.
Dosage Forms Excipient information presented when available (limited, particularly for generics); consult specific product labeling.
Solution, topical: 1% (59 mL); 2% (60 mL)

◆ **Gen-Ticlopidine (Can)** *see* Ticlopidine *on page 1682*
◆ **Gen-Tizanidine (Can)** *see* TiZANidine *on page 1695*
◆ **Gentlax® (Can)** *see* Bisacodyl *on page 219*
◆ **Gentocin (Can)** *see* Gentamicin (Ophthalmic) *on page 792*
◆ **Gen-Triazolam (Can)** *see* Triazolam *on page 1736*
◆ **Geodon®** *see* Ziprasidone *on page 1818*
◆ **Geri-Dryl** *see* DiphenhydrAMINE (Systemic) *on page 516*
◆ **Geri-Stool [OTC]** *see* Docusate and Senna *on page 538*
◆ **Geri-Tussin [OTC]** *see* GuaiFENesin *on page 809*
◆ **GF196960** *see* Tadalafil *on page 1621*
◆ **GG** *see* GuaiFENesin *on page 809*
◆ **GHB** *see* Sodium Oxybate *on page 1572*
◆ **GI87084B** *see* Remifentanil *on page 1471*
◆ **Gianvi™** *see* Ethinyl Estradiol and Drospirenone *on page 654*
◆ **Gildess® FE 1.5/30** *see* Ethinyl Estradiol and Norethindrone *on page 660*
◆ **Gildess® FE 1/20** *see* Ethinyl Estradiol and Norethindrone *on page 660*
◆ **Gilenya®** *see* Fingolimod *on page 714*
◆ **Glargine Insulin** *see* Insulin Glargine *on page 905*

Glatiramer Acetate (gla TIR a mer AS e tate)

Brand Names: U.S. Copaxone®
Brand Names: Canada Copaxone®
Index Terms Copolymer-1
Pharmacologic Category Biological, Miscellaneous

Use Management of relapsing-remitting type multiple sclerosis, including patients with a first clinical episode with MRI features consistent with multiple sclerosis

Pregnancy Risk Factor B

Pregnancy Considerations Adverse events were not observed in animal studies. There are no adequate and well-controlled studies in pregnant women. Use in pregnancy only if clearly necessary.

Lactation Excretion in breast milk unknown/use caution

Contraindications Hypersensitivity to glatiramer acetate, mannitol, or any component of the formulation

Warnings/Precautions For SubQ use only, **not for I.V. administration.** Glatiramer acetate is antigenic, and may interfere with recognition of foreign antigens affecting tumor surveillance and infection defense systems. Immediate postinjection systemic reactions occur in a substantial percentage of patients (~16% in studies); symptoms may begin within minutes of injection and are usually self-limiting. Most patients only have one reaction despite repeated administration. Chest pain (transient pain resolving in minutes) may occur as part of the postinjection systemic reaction, but can also occur alone. Lipoatrophy may occur at injection site; proper injection site rotation may prevent. Safety and efficacy has not been established in patients with renal impairment, in the elderly, or in patients <18 years of age.

Adverse Reactions

>10%:

Cardiovascular: Vasodilation (20%), chest pain (13%)

Central nervous system: Pain (20%), anxiety (13%)

Dermatologic: Rash (19%)

Gastrointestinal: Nausea (15%)

Local: Injection site reactions: Inflammation (49%), erythema (43%), pain (40%), pruritus (27%), mass (27%)

Neuromuscular & skeletal: Weakness (22%), back pain (12%)

Respiratory: Dyspnea (14%)

Miscellaneous: Infection (30%), flu-like syndrome (14%), diaphoresis (15%)

1% to 10%:

Cardiovascular: Edema (8%; includes peripheral and facial), palpitation (7%), tachycardia (5%), syncope (3%), hypertension (1%)

Central nervous system: Fever (6%), migraine (4%), chills (3%), nervousness (2%), speech disorder (2%), abnormal dreams (1%), emotional lability (1%), stupor (1%)

Dermatologic: Bruising (8%), pruritus (5%), erythema (4%), urticaria (3%), skin nodule (2%), eczema (1%), pustular rash (1%)

Endocrine & metabolic: Amenorrhea (1%), impotence (1%), menorrhagia (1%)

Gastrointestinal: Vomiting (7%), gastroenteritis (6%), weight gain (3%), dysphagia (2%), dental caries (1%)

Genitourinary: Urinary urgency (5%), vaginal moniliasis (4%)

Local: Injection site reactions: Hemorrhage (5%), hypersensitivity (4%), fibrosis (2%), lipoatrophy (2%), abscess (1%), edema (1%)

Neuromuscular & skeletal: Neck pain (8%), tremor (4%)

Ocular: Diplopia (3%), visual field defect (1%)

Respiratory: Rhinitis (7%), bronchitis (6%), cough (6%), laryngismus (5%), hyperventilation (1%)

Miscellaneous: Lymphadenopathy (7%), hypersensitivity (3%)

<1% (Limited to important or life-threatening): Allergic reaction, anaphylactoid reaction, anemia, angina, angioedema, aphasia, appetite increased, arrhythmia, arthritis, asthma, atrial fibrillation, blindness, bradycardia, carcinoma (breast, bladder, lung, ovarian), cardiomyopathy, cataract, cervical cancer, cholecystitis, cholelithiasis, cirrhosis, CNS neoplasm, colitis, corneal ulcer, Cushing's syndrome, dermatitis, dry eyes, dry skin, esophagitis, gastrointestinal carcinoma, gastrointestinal hemorrhage, gastrointestinal ulcer, glaucoma, gout, hallucination, heart failure, hepatitis, hepatomegaly, hypercholesterolemia, hypotension, injection site necrosis, leukemia, leukopenia, libido decreased, lupus erythematosus, lymphoma-like reaction, mania, meningitis, MI, mouth ulceration, neuralgia, optic neuritis, orthostatic hypotension, pancreatitis, pancytopenia, pericardial effusion, peripheral vascular disease, photophobia, pneumonia, priapism, pulmonary embolism, pyelonephritis, renal failure, seizures, sepsis, skin cancer, spasm, splenomegaly, stomatitis, stroke, thrombocytopenia, thrombophlebitis, thrombosis, urethritis

Drug Interactions

Metabolism/Transport Effects None known.

Avoid Concomitant Use

Avoid concomitant use of Glatiramer Acetate with any of the following: BCG; Natalizumab; Pimecrolimus; Tacrolimus (Topical); Vaccines (Live)

Increased Effect/Toxicity

Glatiramer Acetate may increase the levels/effects of: Leflunomide; Natalizumab; Vaccines (Live)

The levels/effects of Glatiramer Acetate may be increased by: Denosumab; Pimecrolimus; Roflumilast; Tacrolimus (Topical); Trastuzumab

Decreased Effect

Glatiramer Acetate may decrease the levels/effects of: BCG; Coccidioidin Skin Test; Sipuleucel-T; Vaccines (Inactivated); Vaccines (Live)

The levels/effects of Glatiramer Acetate may be decreased by: Echinacea

Stability Store in refrigerator at 2°C to 8°C (36°F to 46°F); excursions to room temperature for up to 1 month do not have a negative impact on potency. Avoid heat; protect from intense light.

Mechanism of Action Glatiramer is a mixture of random polymers of four amino acids; L-alanine, L-glutamic acid, L-lysine, and L-tyrosine, the resulting mixture is antigenically similar to myelin basic protein, which is an important component of the myelin sheath of nerves; glatiramer is thought to induce and activate T-lymphocyte suppressor cells specific for a myelin antigen, it is also proposed that glatiramer interferes with the antigen-presenting function of certain immune cells opposing pathogenic T-cell function

Pharmacodynamics/Kinetics

Distribution: Small amounts of intact and partial hydrolyzed drug enter lymphatic circulation

Metabolism: SubQ: Large percentage hydrolyzed locally

Dosage Adults: SubQ: 20 mg daily

Administration For SubQ administration in the arms, abdomen, hips, or thighs; rotate injection sites to prevent lipoatrophy. Bring to room temperature prior to use. Visually inspect the solution; discard if solution is cloudy or contains any particulate matter.

Dosage Forms Excipient information presented when available (limited, particularly for generics); consult specific product labeling.

Injection, solution [preservative free]:

Copaxone®: 20 mg/mL (1 mL) [contains mannitol]

◆ **GlcCerase** *see* Velaglucerase Alfa *on page* 1778

◆ **Gleevec®** *see* Imatinib *on page* 870

◆ **Gliadel®** *see* Carmustine *on page* 293

◆ **Gliadel Wafer® (Can)** *see* Carmustine *on page* 293

◆ **Glibenclamide** *see* GlyBURIDE *on page* 799

Glimepiride (GLYE me pye ride)

Brand Names: U.S. Amaryl®

Brand Names: Canada Amaryl®; Apo-Glimepiride®; CO Glimepiride; Novo-Glimepiride; PMS-Glimepiride; ratio-Glimepiride; Rhoxal-glimepiride; Sandoz-Glimepiride

Pharmacologic Category Antidiabetic Agent, Sulfonylurea

Additional Appendix Information

Diabetes Mellitus Management, Adults *on page 1983*

Use Management of type 2 diabetes mellitus (noninsulin dependent, NIDDM) as an adjunct to diet and exercise to lower blood glucose; may be used in combination with metformin or insulin in patients whose hyperglycemia cannot be controlled by diet and exercise in conjunction with a single oral hypoglycemic agent

Pregnancy Risk Factor C

Pregnancy Considerations Adverse events have been observed in animal studies; therefore, glimepiride is classified as pregnancy category C. Severe hypoglycemia lasting 4-10 days has been noted in infants born to mothers taking a sulfonylurea at the time of delivery. The manufacturer recommends that patients be switched to insulin during pregnancy. Maternal hyperglycemia can be associated with adverse effects in the fetus, including macrosomia, neonatal hyperglycemia, and hyperbilirubinemia; the risk of congenital malformations is increased when the Hb A_{1c} is above the normal range. Diabetes can also be associated with adverse effects in the mother. Poorly-treated diabetes may cause end-organ damage that may in turn negatively affect obstetric outcomes. Physiologic glucose levels should be maintained prior to and during pregnancy to decrease the risk of adverse events in the mother and the fetus. Until additional safety and efficacy data are obtained, the use of oral agents is generally not recommended as routine management of GDM or type 2 diabetes mellitus during pregnancy. Insulin is the drug of choice for the control of diabetes mellitus during pregnancy.

Lactation Excretion in breast milk unknown/not recommended

Contraindications Hypersensitivity to glimepiride, any component of the formulation, or sulfonamides; diabetic ketoacidosis (with or without coma)

Warnings/Precautions All sulfonylurea drugs are capable of producing severe hypoglycemia. Hypoglycemia is more likely to occur when caloric intake is deficient, after severe or prolonged exercise, when ethanol is ingested, or when more than one glucose-lowering drug is used. It is also more likely in elderly patients, malnourished patients and in patients with impaired renal or hepatic function; use with caution. Autonomic neuropathy, advanced age, and concomitant use of beta-blockers or other sympatholytic agents may impair the patient's ability to recognize the signs and symptoms of hypoglycemia; use with caution.

Loss of efficacy may be observed following prolonged use as a result of the progression of type 2 diabetes mellitus which results in continued beta cell destruction. In patients who were previously responding to sulfonylurea therapy, consider additional factors which may be contributing to decreased efficacy (eg, inappropriate dose, nonadherence to diet and exercise regimen). If no contributing factors can be identified, consider discontinuing use of the sulfonylurea due to secondary failure of treatment. Additional antidiabetic therapy (eg, insulin) will be required. It may be necessary to discontinue therapy and administer insulin if the patient is exposed to stress (fever, trauma, infection, surgery).

Chemical similarities are present among sulfonamides, sulfonylureas, carbonic anhydrase inhibitors, thiazides, and loop diuretics (except ethacrynic acid). Use in patients with sulfonamide allergy is not specifically contraindicated in product labeling, however, a risk of cross-reaction exists in patients with allergy to any of these compounds; avoid use when previous reaction has been severe. Patients with G6PD deficiency may be at an increased risk of sulfonylurea-induced hemolytic anemia; however, cases have also been described in patients without G6PD deficiency during postmarketing surveillance. Use with caution and consider a nonsulfonylurea alternative in patients with G6PD deficiency.

Product labeling states oral hypoglycemic drugs may be associated with an increased cardiovascular mortality as compared to treatment with diet alone or diet plus insulin. Data to support this association are limited, and several studies, including a large prospective trial (UKPDS) have not supported an association.

Adverse Reactions

1% to 10%:

- Central nervous system: Dizziness (2%), headache (2%)
- Endocrine & metabolic: Hypoglycemia (1% to 2%)
- Gastrointestinal: Nausea (1%)
- Neuromuscular & skeletal: Weakness (2%)

<1% or frequency not defined: Agranulocytosis, anorexia, aplastic anemia, cholestatic jaundice, constipation, diarrhea, disulfiram-like reaction, diuretic effect, edema, epigastric fullness, gastrointestinal pain, erythema, heartburn, hemolytic anemia, hepatitis, hypoglycemia, hyponatremia, leukopenia, liver failure, liver function tests abnormal, nausea, pancytopenia, photosensitivity, porphyria cutanea tarda, pruritus, rash (morbilliform or maculopapular), SIADH, thrombocytopenia, urticaria, vasculitis (allergic), visual accommodation changes (early treatment), vomiting

Drug Interactions

Metabolism/Transport Effects Substrate of CYP2C9 (major); **Note:** Assignment of Major/Minor substrate status based on clinically relevant drug interaction potential

Avoid Concomitant Use There are no known interactions where it is recommended to avoid concomitant use.

Increased Effect/Toxicity

Glimepiride may increase the levels/effects of: Alcohol (Ethyl); Hypoglycemic Agents; Porfimer

The levels/effects of Glimepiride may be increased by: Beta-Blockers; Chloramphenicol; Cimetidine; Cyclic Antidepressants; CYP2C9 Inhibitors (Moderate); CYP2C9 Inhibitors (Strong); Fibric Acid Derivatives; Fluconazole; GLP-1 Agonists; Herbs (Hypoglycemic Properties); Pegvisomant; Quinolone Antibiotics; Ranitidine; Salicylates; Sulfonamide Derivatives; Voriconazole

Decreased Effect

The levels/effects of Glimepiride may be decreased by: Corticosteroids (Orally Inhaled); Corticosteroids (Systemic); CYP2C9 Inducers (Strong); Luteinizing Hormone-Releasing Hormone Analogs; Peginterferon Alfa-2b; Quinolone Antibiotics; Rifampin; Somatropin; Thiazide Diuretics

Ethanol/Nutrition/Herb Interactions

Ethanol: Caution with ethanol (may cause hypoglycemia).

Herb/Nutraceutical: Caution with chromium, garlic, gymnema (may cause hypoglycemia).

Mechanism of Action Stimulates insulin release from the pancreatic beta cells; reduces glucose output from the liver; insulin sensitivity is increased at peripheral target sites

Pharmacodynamics/Kinetics

Onset of action: Peak effect: Blood glucose reductions: 2-3 hours

Duration: 24 hours

Absorption: 100%; delayed when given with food

Distribution: V_d: 8.8 L

Protein binding: >99.5%

Metabolism: Hepatic oxidation via CYP2C9 to M1 metabolite (~33% activity of parent compound); further oxidative metabolism to inactive M2 metabolite

Half-life elimination: 5-9 hours

Time to peak, plasma: 2-3 hours

Excretion: Urine (60%, 80% to 90% as M1 and M2); feces (40%, 70% as M1 and M2)

Dosage Oral:

Children 10-18 years (unlabeled use): Initial: 1 mg once daily; maintenance: 1-4 mg once daily

Adults: Initial: 1-2 mg once daily, administered with breakfast or the first main meal; usual maintenance dose: 1-4 mg once daily; after a dose of 2 mg once daily, increase in increments of 2 mg at 1- to 2-week intervals based upon the patient's blood glucose response to a maximum of 8 mg once daily. If inadequate response to maximal dose, combination therapy with metformin may be considered.

Combination with insulin therapy (fasting glucose level for instituting combination therapy is in the range of >150 mg/dL in plasma or serum depending on the patient): initial recommended dose: 8 mg once daily with the first main meal

After starting with low-dose insulin, upward adjustments of insulin can be done approximately weekly as guided by frequent measurements of fasting blood glucose. Once stable, combination-therapy patients should monitor their capillary blood glucose on an ongoing basis, preferably daily.

Conversion from therapy with long half-life agents: Observe patient carefully for 1-2 weeks when converting from a longer half-life agent (eg, chlorpropamide) to glimepiride due to overlapping hypoglycemic effects.

Dosing adjustment/comments in renal impairment: Cl_{cr} <22 mL/minute: Initial starting dose should be 1 mg and dosage increments should be based on fasting blood glucose levels

Dosing adjustment in hepatic impairment: No data available

Elderly: Initial: 1 mg/day; dose titration and maintenance dosing should be conservative to avoid hypoglycemia

Dietary Considerations Administer with breakfast or the first main meal of the day. Individualized medical nutrition therapy (MNT) based on ADA recommendations is an integral part of therapy.

Administration Administer once daily with breakfast or first main meal of the day. Patients that are NPO or require decreased caloric intake may need doses held to avoid hypoglycemia.

Monitoring Parameters Monitor for signs and symptoms of hypoglycemia (fatigue, excessive hunger, profuse sweating, numbness of extremities), fasting blood glucose, hemoglobin A_{1c}

Reference Range Recommendations for glycemic control in adults with diabetes:

Hb A_{1c}: <7%

Preprandial capillary plasma glucose: 70-130 mg/dL

Peak postprandial capillary blood glucose: <180 mg/dL

Blood pressure: <130/80 mm Hg

Dosage Forms Excipient information presented when available (limited, particularly for generics); consult specific product labeling.

Tablet, oral: 1 mg, 2 mg, 4 mg

Amaryl®: 1 mg, 2 mg, 4 mg [scored]

◆ **Glimepiride and Pioglitazone** *see* Pioglitazone and Glimepiride *on page 1357*

◆ **Glimepiride and Pioglitazone Hydrochloride** *see* Pioglitazone and Glimepiride *on page 1357*

◆ **Glimepiride and Rosiglitazone Maleate** *see* Rosiglitazone and Glimepiride *on page 1523*

GlipiZIDE (GLIP i zide)

Brand Names: U.S. Glucotrol XL®; Glucotrol®

Index Terms Glydiazinamide

Pharmacologic Category Antidiabetic Agent, Sulfonylurea

Additional Appendix Information

Diabetes Mellitus Management, Adults *on page 1983*

Use Management of type 2 diabetes mellitus (noninsulin dependent, NIDDM)

Pregnancy Risk Factor C

Pregnancy Considerations Adverse events have been observed in animal studies; therefore, glipizide is classified as pregnancy category C. Glipizide crosses the placenta. Severe hypoglycemia lasting 4-10 days has been noted in infants born to mothers taking a sulfonylurea at the time of delivery. Maternal hyperglycemia can be associated with adverse effects in the fetus, including macrosomia, neonatal hyperglycemia, and hyperbilirubinemia; the risk of congenital malformations is increased when the Hb A_{1c} is above the normal range. Diabetes can also be associated with adverse effects in the mother. Poorly-treated diabetes may cause end-organ damage that may in turn negatively affect obstetric outcomes. Physiologic glucose levels should be maintained prior to and during pregnancy to decrease the risk of adverse events in the mother and the fetus. Until additional safety and efficacy data are obtained, the use of oral agents is generally not recommended as routine management of GDM or type 2 diabetes mellitus during pregnancy. The manufacturer recommends if glipizide is used during pregnancy it should be discontinued at least 1 month before the expected delivery date. Insulin is the drug of choice for the control of diabetes mellitus during pregnancy.

Lactation Excretion in breast milk unknown/not recommended

Contraindications Hypersensitivity to glipizide or any component of the formulation, other sulfonamides; type 1 diabetes mellitus (insulin dependent, IDDM); diabetic ketoacidosis

Warnings/Precautions All sulfonylurea drugs are capable of producing severe hypoglycemia. Hypoglycemia is more likely to occur when caloric intake is deficient, after severe or prolonged exercise, when ethanol is ingested, or when more than one glucose-lowering drug is used. It is also more likely in elderly patients, malnourished patients and in patients with impaired renal or hepatic function; use with caution.

Use with caution in patients with severe hepatic disease. It may be necessary to discontinue therapy and administer insulin if the patient is exposed to stress (fever, trauma, infection, surgery). Loss of efficacy may be observed following prolonged use as a result of the progression of type 2 diabetes mellitus which results in continued beta cell destruction. In patients who were previously responding to sulfonylurea therapy, consider additional factors which may be contributing to decreased efficacy (eg, inappropriate dose, nonadherence to diet and exercise regimen). If no contributing factors can be identified, consider discontinuing use of the sulfonylurea due to secondary failure of treatment. Additional antidiabetic therapy (eg, insulin) will be required. Chemical similarities are present among sulfonamides, sulfonylureas, carbonic anhydrase inhibitors, thiazides, and loop diuretics (except ethacrynic acid). Use in patients with sulfonamide allergy is specifically contraindicated in product labeling, however, a risk of cross-reaction exists in patients with allergy to any of these compounds; avoid use when previous reaction has been severe. Patients with G6PD deficiency may be at an increased risk of sulfonylurea-induced hemolytic anemia; however, cases have also been described in patients without G6PD deficiency during postmarketing surveillance. Use with caution and consider a nonsulfonylurea alternative in patients with G6PD deficiency.

Product labeling states oral hypoglycemic drugs may be associated with an increased cardiovascular mortality as compared to treatment with diet alone or diet plus insulin. Data to support this association are limited, and several studies, including a large prospective trial (UKPDS) have not supported an association. Avoid use of extended release tablets (Glucotrol XL®) in patients with known stricture/narrowing of the GI tract.

Adverse Reactions Frequency not defined.

Cardiovascular: Edema, syncope

Central nervous system: Anxiety, depression, dizziness, drowsiness, headache, hypoesthesia, insomnia, nervousness, pain

Dermatologic: Eczema, erythema, maculopapular eruptions, morbilliform eruptions, photosensitivity, pruritus, rash, urticaria

Endocrine & metabolic: Disulfiram-like reaction, hypoglycemia, hyponatremia, SIADH (rare)

Gastrointestinal: Anorexia, constipation, diarrhea, epigastric fullness, flatulence, gastralgia, heartburn, nausea, vomiting

Hematologic: Agranulocytopenia, aplastic anemia, blood dyscrasias, hemolytic anemia, leukopenia, pancytopenia, porphyria cutanea tarda, thrombocytopenia

Hepatic: Hepatic porphyria

Neuromuscular & skeletal: Arthralgia, leg cramps, myalgia, paresthesia, tremor

Ocular: Blurred vision

Renal: Diuretic effect (minor)

Respiratory: Rhinitis

Miscellaneous: Diaphoresis

Postmarketing and/or case reports: Abdominal pain, cholestatic jaundice, liver injury

Drug Interactions

Metabolism/Transport Effects Substrate of CYP2C9 (major); **Note:** Assignment of Major/Minor substrate status based on clinically relevant drug interaction potential

Avoid Concomitant Use There are no known interactions where it is recommended to avoid concomitant use.

Increased Effect/Toxicity

GlipiZIDE may increase the levels/effects of: Alcohol (Ethyl); Hypoglycemic Agents; Porfimer

The levels/effects of GlipiZIDE may be increased by: Beta-Blockers; Chloramphenicol; Cimetidine; Clarithromycin; Cyclic Antidepressants; CYP2C9 Inhibitors (Moderate); CYP2C9 Inhibitors (Strong); Fibric Acid Derivatives; Fluconazole; GLP-1 Agonists; Herbs (Hypoglycemic Properties); Pegvisomant; Posaconazole; Quinolone Antibiotics; Ranitidine; Salicylates; Sulfonamide Derivatives; Voriconazole

Decreased Effect

The levels/effects of GlipiZIDE may be decreased by: Corticosteroids (Orally Inhaled); Corticosteroids (Systemic); CYP2C9 Inducers (Strong); Luteinizing Hormone-Releasing Hormone Analogs; Peginterferon Alfa-2b; Quinolone Antibiotics; Rifampin; Somatropin; Thiazide Diuretics

Ethanol/Nutrition/Herb Interactions

Ethanol: Caution with ethanol (may cause hypoglycemia or rare disulfiram reaction).

Food: A delayed release of insulin may occur if glipizide is taken with food. Immediate release tablets should be administered 30 minutes before meals to avoid erratic absorption.

Herb/Nutraceutical: Herbs with hypoglycemic properties may enhance the hypoglycemic effect of glipizide. This includes alfalfa, aloe, bilberry, bitter melon, burdock, celery, damiana, fenugreek, garcinia, garlic, ginger, ginseng (American), gymnema, marshmallow, stinging nettle

Mechanism of Action Stimulates insulin release from the pancreatic beta cells; reduces glucose output from the liver; insulin sensitivity is increased at peripheral target sites

Pharmacodynamics/Kinetics

Duration: 12-24 hours

Absorption: Rapid and complete; delayed with food

Distribution: 10-11 L

Protein binding: 98% to 99%; primarily to albumin

Bioavailability: 90% to 100%

Metabolism: Hepatic via CYP2C9; forms metabolites (inactive)

Half-life elimination: 2-5 hours

Time to peak: 1-3 hours; extended release tablets: 6-12 hours

Excretion: Urine (60% to 80%, 91% to 97% as metabolites); feces (11%)

Dosage

Oral: Adults:

Immediate release tablet: Initial: 5 mg once daily; titrate in 2.5-5 mg increments no more frequently than every few days based on blood glucose response; if once-daily dose is ineffective, may divide the dose; doses >15 mg/day should be administered in divided doses. Maximum recommended once-daily dose: 15 mg; maximum recommended total daily dose: 40 mg (some clinicians recommend a maximum total daily dose of 20 mg [Defronzo, 1999]).

Extended release tablet (Glucotrol XL®): Initial: 5 mg once daily; usual dose: 5-10 mg once daily; maximum recommended dose: 20 mg/day; preferred method for monitoring response to therapy and adjusting dosage is hemoglobin A_{1c} level at initiation and at ~3-month intervals; alternatively, dosage adjustments based on blood glucose monitoring should be made no more frequently than every 7 days

When transferring from immediate release to extended release glipizide: May switch the total daily dose of immediate release to the nearest equivalent daily dose of the extended release tablet and administer once daily; alternatively, may initiate extended release at 5 mg once daily and titrate accordingly.

When transferring from insulin to glipizide immediate release or extended release tablet:

Current insulin requirement ≤20 units: Discontinue insulin and initiate glipizide at usual dose

Current insulin requirement >20 units: Decrease insulin by 50% and initiate glipizide at usual dose; gradually decrease insulin dose based on patient response

Elderly:

Immediate release tablet: Initial: 2.5 mg/day; consider titrating by 2.5-5 mg/day at 1- to 2-week intervals

Extended release tablet: Initial and maintenance dosing should be on the lower end of the recommended range.

Dosing adjustment in renal impairment: The FDA-approved labeling recommends that caution should be used with initial and maintenance dosing in patients with renal impairment; however, no specific dosage adjustment guidelines are provided. The following guidelines have been used by some clinicians (Aronoff, 2007): GFR ≤50 mL/minute: Decrease dose by 50%

Dosing adjustment in hepatic impairment:

Immediate release tablet: Initial: 2.5 mg/day

Extended release tablet: There are no dosage adjustments provided in manufacturer's labeling; use of a lower initial and maintenance dose should be considered.

Dietary Considerations Take immediate release tablets 30 minutes before meals; extended release tablets should be taken with breakfast. Individualized medical nutrition therapy (MNT) based on ADA recommendations is an integral part of therapy.

Administration Administer immediate release tablets 30 minutes before a meal to achieve greatest reduction in postprandial hyperglycemia. Extended release tablets should be given with breakfast. Patients that are NPO or require decreased caloric intake may need doses held to avoid hypoglycemia.

Monitoring Parameters Signs and symptoms of hypoglycemia (fatigue, excessive hunger, profuse sweating, numbness of extremities), blood glucose, hemoglobin A_{1c}

Reference Range Recommendations for glycemic control in adults with diabetes:

Hb A_{1c}: <7%

Preprandial capillary plasma glucose: 70-130 mg/dL

Peak postprandial capillary blood glucose: <180 mg/dL

Blood pressure: <130/80 mm Hg

Dosage Forms Excipient information presented when available (limited, particularly for generics); consult specific product labeling.

Tablet, oral: 5 mg, 10 mg

Glucotrol®: 5 mg, 10 mg [scored; dye free]

Tablet, extended release, oral: 2.5 mg, 5 mg, 10 mg

Glucotrol XL®: 2.5 mg, 5 mg, 10 mg

Glipizide and Metformin

(GLIP i zide & met FOR min)

Brand Names: U.S. Metaglip™

Index Terms Glipizide and Metformin Hydrochloride; Metformin and Glipizide

Pharmacologic Category Antidiabetic Agent, Biguanide; Antidiabetic Agent, Sulfonylurea

Use Indicated as an adjunct to diet and exercise to improve glycemic control in adults with type 2 diabetes mellitus (noninsulin dependent, NIDDM)

Pregnancy Risk Factor C

Dosage Oral: Type 2 diabetes:

Adults:

Patients inadequately controlled on diet and exercise alone: Initial dose: Glipizide 2.5 mg/metformin 250 mg once daily with a meal. In patients with fasting plasma glucose (FPG) 280-320 mg/dL, initiate therapy with glipizide 2.5 mg/metformin 500 mg twice daily.

Note: Increase dose by 1 tablet/day every 2 weeks (maximum daily dose: Glipizide 10 mg/metformin 2000 mg in divided doses)

Patients inadequately controlled on a sulfonylurea and/or metformin: Initial dose: Glipizide 2.5 mg/metformin 500 mg or glipizide 5 mg/metformin 500 mg twice daily with morning and evening meals; starting dose should not exceed current daily dose of glipizide (or sulfonylurea equivalent) and/or metformin.

Note: Increase dose in increments of no more than glipizide 5 mg/metformin 500 mg (maximum daily dose: Glipizide 20 mg/metformin 2000 mg)

Elderly: Conservative doses are recommended in the elderly due to potentially decreased renal function; **do not titrate to maximum dose**; should not be used in patients ≥80 years unless renal function is verified as normal

Dosage adjustment in renal impairment: Contraindicated in the presence of renal disease or renal dysfunction (serum creatinine ≥1.5 mg/dL [males], ≥1.4 mg/dL [females], or abnormal creatinine clearance)

Dosage adjustment in hepatic impairment: Avoid use in patients with impaired liver function

Additional Information Complete prescribing information for this medication should be consulted for additional detail.

Dosage Forms Excipient information presented when available (limited, particularly for generics); consult specific product labeling. [DSC] = Discontinued product

Tablet, oral: 2.5/250: Glipizide 2.5 mg and metformin hydrochloride 250 mg; 2.5/500: Glipizide 2.5 mg and metformin hydrochloride 500 mg; 5/500: Glipizide 5 mg and metformin hydrochloride 500 mg

Metaglip™ 2.5/250: Glipizide 2.5 mg and metformin hydrochloride 250 mg [DSC]

Metaglip™ 2.5/500: Glipizide 2.5 mg and metformin hydrochloride 500 mg

Metaglip™ 5/500: Glipizide 5 mg and metformin hydrochloride 500 mg

◆ **Glipizide and Metformin Hydrochloride** *see* Glipizide and Metformin *on page 797*

◆ **Glivec** *see* Imatinib *on page 870*

◆ **Gln** *see* Glutamine *on page 799*

◆ **GlucaGen®** *see* Glucagon *on page 797*

◆ **GlucaGen® Diagnostic Kit** *see* Glucagon *on page 797*

◆ **GlucaGen® HypoKit®** *see* Glucagon *on page 797*

Glucagon (GLOO ka gon)

Brand Names: U.S. GlucaGen®; GlucaGen® Diagnostic Kit; GlucaGen® HypoKit®; Glucagon Emergency Kit

Index Terms Glucagon Hydrochloride

Pharmacologic Category Antidote; Antidote, Hypoglycemia; Diagnostic Agent

Use Management of hypoglycemia; diagnostic aid in radiologic examinations to temporarily inhibit GI tract movement

Unlabeled Use Beta-blocker- or calcium channel blocker-induced myocardial depression (with or without hypotension) unresponsive to standard measures; suspected or documented hypoglycemia secondary to insulin or sulfonylurea overdose (as adjunct to dextrose)

Pregnancy Risk Factor B

Lactation Excretion in breast milk unknown/compatible

Contraindications Hypersensitivity to glucagon or any component of the formulation; insulinoma; pheochromocytoma

Warnings/Precautions Use of glucagon is contraindicated in insulinoma; exogenous glucagon may cause an initial rise in blood glucose followed by rebound hypoglycemia. Use of glucagon is contraindicated in pheochromocytoma; exogenous glucagon may cause the release of catecholamines, resulting in an increase in blood pressure. Use caution with prolonged fasting, starvation, adrenal insufficiency or chronic hypoglycemia; levels of glucose stores in liver may be decreased. Supplemental carbohydrates should be given to patients who respond to glucagon for severe hypoglycemia to prevent secondary hypoglycemia. Monitor blood glucose levels closely.

In patients with hypoglycemia secondary to insulin or sulfonylurea overdose, dextrose should be immediately administered; if I.V. access cannot be established or if dextrose is not available, glucagon may be considered as alternative acute treatment until dextrose can be administered.

May contain lactose; avoid administration in hereditary galactose intolerance, Lapp lactase deficiency, or glucose-galactose malabsorption.

Adverse Reactions Frequency not defined.

Cardiovascular: Hypotension (up to 2 hours after GI procedures), hypertension, tachycardia

Gastrointestinal: Nausea, vomiting (high incidence with rapid administration of high doses)

Miscellaneous: Hypersensitivity reactions, anaphylaxis

Drug Interactions

Metabolism/Transport Effects None known.

Avoid Concomitant Use There are no known interactions where it is recommended to avoid concomitant use.

Increased Effect/Toxicity
Glucagon may increase the levels/effects of: Vitamin K Antagonists

Decreased Effect There are no known significant interactions involving a decrease in effect.

Ethanol/Nutrition/Herb Interactions Glucagon depletes glycogen stores.

Stability Prior to reconstitution, store at controlled room temperature of 20°C to 25°C (69°F to 77°F); do not freeze. Reconstitute powder for injection by adding 1 mL of sterile diluent to a vial containing 1 unit of the drug, to provide solutions containing 1 mg of glucagon/mL. Gently roll vial to dissolve. Use immediately after reconstitution. May be kept at 5°C for up to 48 hours if necessary. Solution for infusion may be prepared by reconstitution with and further dilution in NS or D_5W (Love, 1998).

Mechanism of Action Stimulates adenylate cyclase to produce increased cyclic AMP, which promotes hepatic glycogenolysis and gluconeogenesis, causing a raise in blood glucose levels

Pharmacodynamics/Kinetics
Onset of action: Peak effect: Blood glucose levels: Parenteral:
I.V.: 5-20 minutes
I.M.: 30 minutes
SubQ: 30-45 minutes
Duration: Glucose elevation:
SubQ: 60-90 minutes
I.V.: 30 minutes
Metabolism: Primarily hepatic; some inactivation occurring renally and in plasma
Half-life elimination, plasma: 8-18 minutes

Dosage
Hypoglycemia: I.M., I.V., SubQ:
Children <20 kg: 0.5 mg or 20-30 mcg/kg/dose; repeated in 20 minutes as needed
Children ≥20 kg and Adults: 1 mg; may repeat in 20 minutes as needed
Note: I.V. dextrose should be administered as soon as it is available; if patient fails to respond to glucagon, I.V. dextrose must be given.
Beta-blocker- or calcium channel blocker-induced myocardial depression (with or without hypotension) unresponsive to standard measures (unlabeled use): I.V.:
Children: Initial bolus of 30-150 mcg/kg followed by an infusion of 70 mcg/kg/hour (maximum: 5 mg/hour) (Hegenbarth, 2008)
Adolescents: Initial: 5-10 mg over several minutes followed by infusion of 1-5 mg/hour (Hegenbarth, 2008)
Adults: 3-10 mg (or 0.05-0.15 mg/kg) bolus followed by an infusion of 3-5 mg/hour (or 0.05-0.1 mg/kg/hour); titrate infusion rate to achieve adequate hemodynamic response (ACLS, 2010)
Diagnostic aid: Adults:
I.M.: 1-2 mg 10 minutes prior to gastrointestinal procedure
I.V.: 0.25-2 mg 10 minutes prior to gastrointestinal procedure

Dietary Considerations Administer carbohydrates to patient as soon as possible after response to treatment.

Administration I.V.: Bolus may be associated with nausea and vomiting.
Beta-blocker/calcium channel blocker toxicity: Administer bolus over 3-5 minutes; continuous infusions may be used. Ensure adequate supply available to continue therapy.

Monitoring Parameters Blood pressure, blood glucose, ECG, heart rate, mentation

Additional Information 1 unit = 1 mg

Dosage Forms Excipient information presented when available (limited, particularly for generics); consult specific product labeling.
Injection, powder for reconstitution:
Glucagon Emergency Kit: 1 mg [contains glycerin (in diluent), lactose 49 mg; equivalent to 1 unit]
Injection, powder for reconstitution, as hydrochloride:
GlucaGen®: 1 mg [contains lactose 107 mg; equivalent to 1 unit]
GlucaGen® Diagnostic Kit: 1 mg [contains lactose 107 mg; equivalent to 1 unit]
GlucaGen® HypoKit®: 1 mg [contains lactose 107 mg; equivalent to 1 unit]

◆ **Glucagon Emergency Kit** *see* Glucagon *on page* 797
◆ **Glucagon Hydrochloride** *see* Glucagon *on page* 797

Glucarpidase (gloo KAR pid ase)

Index Terms Carboxypeptidase-G2; CPDG2; CPG2; Voraxaze

Pharmacologic Category Antidote; Enzyme

Use Treatment of toxic plasma methotrexate concentrations (>1 micromole/L) in patients with delayed clearance due to renal impairment

Unlabeled Use Rescue agent to reduce methotrexate toxicity in patients with accidental intrathecal methotrexate overdose

Prescribing and Access Restrictions Glucarpidase is available for intrathecal (I.T.) use through an Emergency Use IND. Information is available from BTG International at 1-888-327-1027. For FDA Emergency Use IND information and procedures, refer to http://www.fda.gov/RegulatoryInformation/Guidances/ucm126491.htm. For further information on intrathecal use, please also refer to http://www.btgplc.com/products/voraxazeae-us-treatment-ind.

Prior to FDA approval, glucarpidase was available for I.V. use under an Open-Label Treatment protocol. Information and participation requirements are available from the Voraxaze® 24-hour access call center (Clinical Trials and Consulting Services, Inc) at 1-877-398-9829. Further information may be found at http://www.btgplc.com/products/voraxazeae-us-treatment-ind.

Warnings/Precautions Glucarpidase use for methotrexate toxicity due to delayed elimination should be accompanied with adequate hydration, urinary alkalinization, and concurrent leucovorin calcium; hemodialysis may be required. Leucovorin calcium is a substrate for glucarpidase and may compete with methotrexate for binding sites; protocols may require withholding concomitant leucovorin calcium for 2-4 hours before and 1-2 hours after glucarpidase.

Glucarpidase use for intrathecal methotrexate overdose (unlabeled use) should be used in conjunction with immediate lumbar drainage; concurrent dexamethasone (4 mg I.V. every 6 hours for 4 doses) may minimize methotrexate-induced chemical arachnoiditis; leucovorin calcium (100 mg I.V. every 6 hours for 4 doses) may prevent systemic methotrexate toxicity.

Adverse Reactions Frequency not defined.
Cardiovascular: Flushing
Central nervous system: Fever, head pressure
Dermatologic: Burning sensation (face and extremities), pruritus
Neuromuscular & skeletal: Tingling of fingers
Miscellaneous: Shaking, warmth

Stability Reconstitute immediately prior to use.
Intrathecal (unlabeled use): Reconstitute 2000 units with 12 mL preservative-free normal saline (Widemann, 2004)
I.V.: Reconstitute each 1000 units with 1 mL normal saline; prior to administration, further dilute with normal saline (Buchen, 2005)

Mechanism of Action Recombinant enzyme which rapidly hydrolyzes extracellular methotrexate into inactive metabolites, resulting in a rapid reduction of methotrexate concentrations

Pharmacodynamics/Kinetics

Distribution: V_{dss}: ~60-70 mL/kg

Half-life elimination: I.V.: Normal renal function: 9 hours; impaired renal function (Cl_{cr} <30 mL/minute): 10 hours

Dosage Children and Adults:

I.V.: Methotrexate toxicity: 50 units/kg (Buchen, 2005; Schwartz, 2007; Widemann, 1997); may require a second dose 24 hours later (Schwartz, 2007; Widemann, 1997)

Intrathecal: Intrathecal methotrexate overdose (unlabeled use): 2000 units as soon as possible after accidental overdose (Widemann, 2004)

Administration

I.V.: Infuse over 5 minutes

Intrathecal (for intrathecal methotrexate overdose; unlabeled use): Glucarpidase was administered within 3-9 hours of accidental intrathecal methotrexate overdose in conjunction with lumbar drainage or ventriculolumbar perfusion (Widemann, 2004).

Monitoring Parameters Serum methotrexate levels, CBC with differential, bilirubin, ALT, AST, serum creatinine; evaluate for signs/symptoms of methotrexate toxicity

Test Interactions Methotrexate levels: Follow specific procedures for sample handling and processing; lack of glucarpidase inactivation may allow for continued methotrexate degradation within the sample; due to potential cross reactivity between methotrexate antibodies and DAMPA (inactive methotrexate metabolite) the FPIA assay may overestimate serum methotrexate concentrations and the HPLC assay is recommended for monitoring serum methotrexate concentrations (Buchen, 2005; Widemann, 1997).

Product Availability

Voraxaze®: FDA approved January 2012; availability is currently undetermined; consult prescribing information for additional information

Prior to FDA approval, glucarpidase was available for I.V. use under an Open-Label Treatment protocol. Information and participation requirements are available from the Voraxaze® 24-hour access call center (Clinical Trials and Consulting Services, Inc) at 1-877-398-9829. Further information may be found at http://www.btgplc.com/products/voraxazeae-us-treatment-ind.

Glucarpidase is available for intrathecal (I.T.) use through an Emergency Use IND. Information is available from BTG International at 1-888-327-1027. For FDA Emergency Use IND information and procedures, refer to http://www.fda.gov/RegulatoryInformation/Guidances/ucm126491.htm. For further information on intrathecal use, please also refer to http://www.btgplc.com/products/voraxazeae-us-treatment-ind.

- **Glucobay™ (Can)** *see* Acarbose *on page* 26
- **Glucocerebrosidase** *see* Alglucerase *on page* 65
- **GlucoNorm® (Can)** *see* Repaglinide *on page* 1472
- **Glucophage®** *see* MetFORMIN *on page* 1086
- **Glucophage® XR** *see* MetFORMIN *on page* 1086
- **Glucotrol®** *see* GlipiZIDE *on page* 795
- **Glucotrol XL®** *see* GlipiZIDE *on page* 795
- **Glucovance®** *see* Glyburide and Metformin *on page* 801
- **Glulisine Insulin** *see* Insulin Glulisine *on page* 905
- **Glumetza®** *see* MetFORMIN *on page* 1086

Glutamine (GLOO ta meen)

Brand Names: U.S. Enterex® Glutapak-10® [OTC]; NutreStore™; Resource® GlutaSolve® [OTC]; Sympt-X G.I. [OTC]; Sympt-X [OTC]

Index Terms Gln; L-Glutamine

Pharmacologic Category Amino Acid; Gastrointestinal Agent, Miscellaneous

Use

NutreStore™: Treatment of short bowel syndrome (SBS) when used in combination with specialized nutritional support and growth hormone therapy

OTC products: Medical food used to promote GI tract healing and nutritional supplementation with GI disorders, HIV/AIDS, cancer, and other critical illnesses

Pregnancy Risk Factor C

Dosage Oral: Adults:

Nutritional supplement (Enterex® Glutapak-10®, Resource® GlutaSolve®, Sympt-X, Sympt-X G.I.): Average dose: 10 g 3 times/day; dosing range: 5-30 g/day

Short bowel syndrome (NutreStore™): 30 g/day administered as 5 g 6 times/day (every 2-3 hours while awake) for up to 16 weeks; to be used in combination with growth hormone and nutritional support

Additional Information Complete prescribing information for this medication should be consulted for additional detail.

Dosage Forms Excipient information presented when available (limited, particularly for generics); consult specific product labeling.

Powder for oral solution:

Enterex® Glutapak-10®: 10 g/packet (50s)

NutreStore™: 5 g/packet

Resource® GlutaSolve®: 15 g/packet (56s)

Sympt-X, Sympt-X G.I.: 10 g/packet (60s)

- **Glybenclamide** *see* GlyBURIDE *on page* 799
- **Glybenzcyclamide** *see* GlyBURIDE *on page* 799

GlyBURIDE (GLYE byoor ide)

Brand Names: U.S. DiaBeta®; Glynase® PresTab®

Brand Names: Canada Apo-Glyburide®; DiaBeta®; Dom-Glyburide; Euglucon®; Med-Glybe; Mylan-Glybe; Novo-Glyburide; Nu-Glyburide; PMS-Glyburide; PRO-Glyburide; ratio-Glyburide; Riva-Glyburide; Sandoz-Glyburide; Teva-Glyburide

Index Terms Diabeta; Glibenclamide; Glybenclamide; Glybenzcyclamide; Micronase

Pharmacologic Category Antidiabetic Agent, Sulfonylurea

Additional Appendix Information

Diabetes Mellitus Management, Adults *on page* 1983

Use Adjunct to diet and exercise for the management of type 2 diabetes mellitus (noninsulin dependent, NIDDM)

Unlabeled Use Alternative to insulin in women for the treatment of gestational diabetes mellitus (GDM) (11-33 weeks gestation)

Pregnancy Risk Factor B/C (manufacturer dependent)

Pregnancy Considerations Reproduction studies differ by manufacturer labeling. Because adverse events were not observed in animal reproduction studies, one manufacturer classifies glyburide as pregnancy category B. Because adverse events were noted in animal studies during the period of lactation, another manufacturer classifies glyburide as pregnancy category C.

Glyburide was not found to significantly cross the placenta *in vitro* and was not found in the cord serum infants of mothers taking glyburide for gestational diabetes mellitus (GDM). Nonteratogenic effects such as hypoglycemia in the neonate have been associated with maternal glyburide use. Maternal hyperglycemia can be associated with adverse effects in the fetus, including macrosomia, neonatal hyperglycemia, and hyperbilirubinemia; the risk of congenital malformations is increased when the Hb A_{1c} is above the normal range. Diabetes can also be associated with adverse effects in the mother. Poorly-treated diabetes may cause end-organ damage that may in turn negatively affect obstetric outcomes. Physiologic glucose levels should be maintained prior to and during pregnancy to decrease the risk of adverse events in the mother and the fetus. The manufacturer recommends that if glyburide is used during pregnancy, it should be discontinued at least 2 weeks before the expected delivery date. Although studies have shown positive outcomes using glyburide for the treatment of GDM, use may not be appropriate for all women. Until additional safety and efficacy data are obtained, the use of oral agents is generally not recommended as routine management of type 2 diabetes mellitus during pregnancy. Insulin is considered the drug of choice for the control of diabetes mellitus during pregnancy.

Lactation Does not enter breast milk/use caution

Contraindications Hypersensitivity to glyburide or any component of the formulation; type 1 diabetes mellitus (insulin dependent, IDDM), diabetic ketoacidosis; concomitant use with bosentan

Warnings/Precautions All sulfonylurea drugs are capable of producing severe hypoglycemia. Hypoglycemia is more likely to occur when caloric intake is deficient, after severe or prolonged exercise, when ethanol is ingested, or when more than one glucose-lowering drug is used. It is also more likely in elderly patients, malnourished patients and in patients with impaired renal or hepatic function; use with caution.

It may be necessary to discontinue therapy and administer insulin if the patient is exposed to stress (fever, trauma, infection, surgery). Loss of efficacy may be observed following prolonged use as a result of the progression of type 2 diabetes mellitus which results in continued beta cell destruction. In patients who were previously responding to sulfonylurea therapy, consider additional factors which may be contributing to decreased efficacy (eg, inappropriate dose, nonadherence to diet and exercise regimen). If no contributing factors can be identified, consider discontinuing use of the sulfonylurea due to secondary failure of treatment. Additional antidiabetic therapy (eg, insulin) will be required.

Elderly: Rapid and prolonged hypoglycemia (>12 hours) despite hypertonic glucose injections have been reported; age and hepatic and renal impairment are independent risk factors for hypoglycemia; dosage titration should be made at weekly intervals.

Chemical similarities are present among sulfonamides, sulfonylureas, carbonic anhydrase inhibitors, thiazides, and loop diuretics (except ethacrynic acid). Use in patients with sulfonamide allergy is not specifically contraindicated in product labeling, however, a risk of cross-reaction exists in patients with allergy to any of these compounds; avoid use when previous reaction has been severe.

Product labeling states oral hypoglycemic drugs may be associated with an increased cardiovascular mortality as compared to treatment with diet alone or diet plus insulin. Data to support this association are limited, and several studies, including a large prospective trial (UKPDS) have not supported an association.

Patients with G6PD deficiency may be at an increased risk of sulfonylurea-induced hemolytic anemia; however, cases have also been described in patients without G6PD deficiency during postmarketing surveillance. Use with caution and consider a nonsulfonylurea alternative in patients with G6PD deficiency.

Micronized glyburide tablets are **not** bioequivalent to *conventional* glyburide tablets; retitration should occur if patients are being transferred to a different glyburide formulation (eg, micronized-to-conventional or vice versa) or from other hypoglycemic agents.

Adverse Reactions Frequency not defined.

Cardiovascular: Vasculitis

Central nervous system: Dizziness, headache

Dermatologic: Angioedema, erythema, maculopapular eruptions, morbilliform eruptions, photosensitivity reaction, pruritus, purpura, rash, urticaria

Endocrine & metabolic: Disulfiram-like reaction, hypoglycemia, hyponatremia (SIADH reported with other sulfonylureas)

Gastrointestinal: Anorexia, constipation, diarrhea, epigastric fullness, heartburn, nausea

Genitourinary: Nocturia

Hematologic: Agranulocytosis, aplastic anemia, hemolytic anemia, leukopenia, pancytopenia, porphyria cutanea tarda, thrombocytopenia

Hepatic: Cholestatic jaundice, hepatitis, liver failure, transaminase increased

Neuromuscular & skeletal: Arthralgia, myalgia, paresthesia

Ocular: Blurred vision

Renal: Diuretic effect (minor)

Miscellaneous: Allergic reaction

Drug Interactions

Metabolism/Transport Effects Substrate of CYP2C9 (major); **Note:** Assignment of Major/Minor substrate status based on clinically relevant drug interaction potential; **Inhibits** CYP2C8 (weak), CYP3A4 (weak)

Avoid Concomitant Use

Avoid concomitant use of GlyBURIDE with any of the following: Bosentan; Pimozide

Increased Effect/Toxicity

GlyBURIDE may increase the levels/effects of: Alcohol (Ethyl); Bosentan; CycloSPORINE; CycloSPORINE (Systemic); Hypoglycemic Agents; Pimozide; Porfimer

The levels/effects of GlyBURIDE may be increased by: Beta-Blockers; Chloramphenicol; Cimetidine; Clarithromycin; Cyclic Antidepressants; CYP2C9 Inhibitors (Moderate); CYP2C9 Inhibitors (Strong); Fibric Acid Derivatives; Fluconazole; GLP-1 Agonists; Herbs (Hypoglycemic Properties); Pegvisomant; Quinolone Antibiotics; Ranitidine; Salicylates; Sulfonamide Derivatives; Voriconazole

Decreased Effect

GlyBURIDE may decrease the levels/effects of: Bosentan

The levels/effects of GlyBURIDE may be decreased by: Bosentan; Colesevelam; Corticosteroids (Orally Inhaled); Corticosteroids (Systemic); CycloSPORINE; CycloSPORINE (Systemic); CYP2C9 Inducers (Strong); Luteinizing Hormone-Releasing Hormone Analogs; Peginterferon Alfa-2b; Quinolone Antibiotics; Rifampin; Somatropin; Thiazide Diuretics

Ethanol/Nutrition/Herb Interactions

Ethanol: Caution with ethanol (may cause hypoglycemia).

Herb/Nutraceutical: Herbs with hypoglycemic properties may enhance the hypoglycemic effect of glyburide. This includes alfalfa, aloe, bilberry, bitter melon, burdock, celery, damiana, fenugreek, garcinia, garlic, ginger, ginseng (American), gymnema, marshmallow, stinging nettle

Mechanism of Action Stimulates insulin release from the pancreatic beta cells; reduces glucose output from the liver; insulin sensitivity is increased at peripheral target sites

Pharmacodynamics/Kinetics

Onset of action: Serum insulin levels begin to increase 15-60 minutes after a single dose

Duration: ≤24 hours

Absorption: Significant within 1 hour

Distribution: 9-10 L

Protein binding, plasma: >99% primarily to albumin

Metabolism: Hepatic; forms metabolites (weakly active)

Bioavailability: Variable among oral dosage forms

Half-life elimination: Diaβeta®: 10 hours; Glynase® PresTab®: ~4 hours; may be prolonged with renal or hepatic impairment

Time to peak, serum: Adults: 2-4 hours

Excretion: Feces (50%) and urine (50%) as metabolites

Dosage Oral: Micronized glyburide tablets are **not** bioequivalent to conventional glyburide tablets; retitration should occur if patients are being transferred to a different glyburide formulation (eg, micronized-to-conventional or vice versa) or from other hypoglycemic agents.

Diaβeta®: Adults:

Initial: 2.5-5 mg/day, administered with breakfast or the first main meal of the day. In patients who are more sensitive to hypoglycemic drugs, start at 1.25 mg/day.

Increase in increments of no more than 2.5 mg/day at weekly intervals based on the patient's blood glucose response

Maintenance: 1.25-20 mg/day given as single or divided doses. Some patients (especially those receiving >10 mg/day) may have a more satisfactory response with twice-daily dosing. Maximum: 20 mg/day

Elderly: Initial: 1.25-2.5 mg/day, increase by 1.25-2.5 mg/day every 1-3 weeks

Micronized tablets (Glynase® PresTab®): Adults:

Initial: 1.5-3 mg/day, administered with breakfast or the first main meal of the day in patients who are more sensitive to hypoglycemic drugs, start at 0.75 mg/day. Increase in increments of no more than 1.5 mg/day in weekly intervals based on the patient's blood glucose response.

Maintenance: 0.75-12 mg/day given as a single dose or in divided doses. Some patients (especially those receiving >6 mg/day) may have a more satisfactory response with twice-daily dosing. Maximum: 12 mg/day

Management of noninsulin-dependent diabetes mellitus in patients previously maintained on insulin: Initial dosage dependent upon previous insulin dosage, see table.

Dose Conversion: Insulin to Glyburide

Previous Daily Insulin Dosage (units/day)	Initial Glyburide Dosage *Conventional Formulation* (mg/day)	Initial Glyburide Dosage *Micronized Formulation* (mg/day)	Insulin Dosage Change (after glyburide started)
<20	2.5-5	1.5-3	Discontinue
20-40	5	3	Discontinue
>40	5 (increase in increments of 1.25-2.5 mg every 2-10 days)	3 (increase in increments of 0.75-1.5 mg every 2-10 days)	Reduce insulin dosage by 50% (gradually taper off insulin as glyburide dosage increased)

Dosing adjustment/comments in renal impairment: Cl_{cr} <50 mL/minute: **Not recommended**

Dosing adjustment in hepatic impairment: Use conservative initial and maintenance doses and avoid use in severe disease

Dietary Considerations Should be taken with meals at the same time each day (twice-daily dosing may be beneficial if conventional glyburide doses are >10 mg or micronized glyburide doses are >6 mg). Individualized medical nutrition therapy (MNT) based on ADA recommendations is an integral part of therapy.

Administration Administer with meals at the same time each day (twice-daily dosing may be beneficial if conventional glyburide doses are >10 mg or micronized glyburide doses are >6 mg). Patients that are NPO or require decreased caloric intake may need doses held to avoid hypoglycemia.

Monitoring Parameters Signs and symptoms of hypoglycemia, fasting blood glucose, hemoglobin A_{1c}

Reference Range Recommendations for glycemic control in adults with diabetes:

Hb A_{1c}: <7%

Preprandial capillary plasma glucose: 70-130 mg/dL

Peak postprandial capillary blood glucose: <180 mg/dL

Blood pressure: <130/80 mm Hg

Dosage Forms Excipient information presented when available (limited, particularly for generics); consult specific product labeling.

Tablet, oral: 1.25 mg, 2.5 mg, 5 mg

DiaBeta®: 1.25 mg, 2.5 mg, 5 mg [scored]

Tablet, oral [micronized]: 1.5 mg, 3 mg, 5 mg, 6 mg

Glynase® PresTab®: 1.5 mg, 3 mg, 6 mg [scored]

Glyburide and Metformin

(GLYE byoor ide & met FOR min)

Brand Names: U.S. Glucovance®

Index Terms Glyburide and Metformin Hydrochloride; Metformin and Glyburide

Pharmacologic Category Antidiabetic Agent, Biguanide; Antidiabetic Agent, Sulfonylurea

Use Adjunct to diet and exercise for the management of type 2 diabetes mellitus (noninsulin dependent, NIDDM)

Pregnancy Risk Factor B

Dosage Note: Dose must be individualized. Dosages expressed as glyburide/metformin components.

Adults: Oral:

Initial therapy (no prior treatment with sulfonylurea or metformin): 1.25 mg/250 mg once daily with a meal; patients with Hb A_{1c} >9% or fasting plasma glucose (FPG) >200 mg/dL may start with 1.25 mg/250 mg twice daily with meals. **Note:** Doses of 5 mg/500 mg should not be used as initial therapy, due to risk of hypoglycemia.

Dosage may be increased in increments of 1.25 mg/250 mg, at intervals of not less than 2 weeks; maximum daily dose: 10 mg/2000 mg (limited experience with higher doses)

Previously treated with a sulfonylurea or metformin alone: Initial: 2.5 mg/500 mg or 5 mg/500 mg twice daily with meals; increase in increments no greater than 5 mg/500 mg; maximum daily dose: 20 mg/2000 mg

When switching patients previously on a sulfonylurea and metformin together, do not exceed the daily dose of glyburide (or glyburide equivalent) or metformin.

Note: May combine with a thiazolidinedione in patients with an inadequate response to glyburide/metformin therapy (risk of hypoglycemia may be increased). When adding thiazolidinedione, continue glyburide and metformin at current dose and initiate thiazolidinedione at recommended starting dose.

Elderly: Oral: Conservative doses are recommended in the elderly due to potentially decreased renal function; **do not titrate to maximum dose**; should not be used in patients ≥80 years of age unless renal function is verified as normal

Dosage adjustment in renal impairment: Risk of lactic acidosis increases with degree of renal impairment; contraindicated in renal disease or renal dysfunction

Dosage adjustment in hepatic impairment: Use conservative initial and maintenance doses and avoid use in severe hepatic disease

Additional Information Complete prescribing information for this medication should be consulted for additional detail.

Dosage Forms Excipient information presented when available (limited, particularly for generics); consult specific product labeling. [DSC] = Discontinued product

Tablet: 1.25 mg/250 mg: Glyburide 1.25 mg and metformin hydrochloride 250 mg; 2.5 mg/500 mg: Glyburide 2.5 mg and metformin hydrochloride 500 mg; 5 mg/500 mg: Glyburide 5 mg and metformin hydrochloride 500 mg

Glucovance®: 1.25 mg/250 mg: Glyburide 1.25 mg and metformin hydrochloride 250 mg [DSC]

Glucovance®: 2.5 mg/500 mg: Glyburide 2.5 mg and metformin hydrochloride 500 mg

Glucovance®: 5 mg/500 mg: Glyburide 5 mg and metformin hydrochloride 500 mg

◆ **Glyburide and Metformin Hydrochloride** *see* Glyburide and Metformin *on page 801*

◆ **Glycerol Guaiacolate** *see* GuaiFENesin *on page 809*

◆ **Glyceryl Trinitrate** *see* Nitroglycerin *on page 1212*

◆ **Glycon (Can)** *see* MetFORMIN *on page 1086*

Glycopyrrolate (glye koe PYE roe late)

Brand Names: U.S. Cuvposa™; Robinul®; Robinul® Forte

Brand Names: Canada Glycopyrrolate Injection, USP

Index Terms Glycopyrronium Bromide

Pharmacologic Category Anticholinergic Agent

Use Inhibit salivation and excessive secretions of the respiratory tract preoperatively; control of upper airway secretions; intraoperatively to counteract drug-induced or vagal mediated bradyarrhythmias; adjunct in treatment of peptic ulcer (indication listed in product labeling but currently has no place in management of peptic ulcer disease)

Cuvposa™: Reduce chronic, severe drooling in those with neurologic conditions (eg, cerebral palsy) associated with drooling

Unlabeled Use Adjunct with acetylcholinesterase inhibitors (eg, neostigmine, edrophonium, pyridostigmine) to antagonize cholinergic effects

Pregnancy Risk Factor B (injection) / C (oral solution)

Pregnancy Considerations Teratogenic effects were not observed in animal studies. Small amounts of glycopyrrolate cross the human placenta.

Lactation Excretion in breast milk unknown/use caution

Contraindications Hypersensitivity to glycopyrrolate or any component of the formulation; medical conditions that preclude use of anticholinergic medication; severe ulcerative colitis, toxic megacolon complicating ulcerative colitis, paralytic ileus, obstructive disease of GI tract (eg, pyloric stenosis), intestinal atony in the elderly or debilitated patient; unstable cardiovascular status in acute hemorrhage; narrow-angle glaucoma; acute hemorrhage; tachycardia; obstructive uropathy; myasthenia gravis

Oral solution: Additional contraindication: Concomitant use of potassium chloride in a solid oral dosage form

Warnings/Precautions Diarrhea may be a sign of incomplete intestinal obstruction, treatment should be discontinued if this occurs. Use caution in elderly and in patients with autonomic neuropathy, renal disease, or ulcerative colitis; may precipitate/aggravate ileus or toxic megacolon, hyperthyroidism, CAD, CHF, arrhythmias, tachycardia, BPH, or hiatal hernia with reflux. Use of anticholinergics in gastric ulcer treatment may cause a delay in gastric emptying. Caution should be used in individuals demonstrating decreased pigmentation (skin and iris coloration, dark versus light) since there has been some evidence that these individuals have an enhanced sensitivity to the anticholinergic response. May cause drowsiness, eye sensitivity to light, or blurred vision; caution should be used when performing tasks which require mental alertness, such as driving. The risk of heat stroke with this medication may be increased during exercise or hot weather. Injection contains benzyl alcohol (associated with gasping syndrome in neonates).

Adverse Reactions

>10% (as reported with Cuvposa™):

Cardiovascular: Flushing (30%)

Central nervous system: Headache (15%)

Gastrointestinal: Vomiting (40%), xerostomia (40%), constipation (35%)

Genitourinary: Urinary retention (15%)

Respiratory: Nasal congestion (30%), sinusitis (15%), upper respiratory tract infection (15%)

<10% (frequency not always defined):

Cardiovascular: Pallor (≤2%), arrhythmias, cardiac arrest, heart block, hyper-/hypotension, malignant hyperthermia, palpitation, QT_c-interval prolongation, tachycardia

Central nervous system: Aggressiveness (≤2%), agitation (≤2%), crying (abnormal; ≤2%), irritability (≤2%), mood changes (≤2%), pain(≤2%), restlessness(≤2%), confusion, dizziness, drowsiness, excitement, insomnia, nervousness, seizure

Dermatologic: Dry skin (≤2%), pruritus (≤2%), rash (≤2%), urticaria

Endocrine & metabolic: Dehydration (≤2%), lactation suppression

Gastrointestinal: Abdominal distention (≤2%), abdominal pain (≤2%), flatulence (≤2%), retching (≤2%), bloated feeling, intestinal obstruction, loss of taste, nausea, pseudo-obstruction

Genitourinary: Urinary tract infection (≤2%), impotence, urinary hesitancy

Local: Injection site reactions (edema, erythema, pain)

Neuromuscular & skeletal: Weakness

Ocular: Nystagmus (≤2%), blurred vision, cycloplegia, mydriasis, ocular tension increased, photophobia, sensitivity to light increased

Respiratory: Bronchial secretion (thickening; ≤2%), nasal dryness (≤2%), pneumonia (≤2%), respiratory depression

Miscellaneous: Anaphylactoid reactions, diaphoresis decreased, hypersensitivity reactions

Drug Interactions

Metabolism/Transport Effects None known.

Avoid Concomitant Use

Avoid concomitant use of Glycopyrrolate with any of the following: Potassium Chloride

Increased Effect/Toxicity

Glycopyrrolate may increase the levels/effects of: AbobotulinumtoxinA; Anticholinergics; Atenolol; Cannabinoids; Digoxin; MetFORMIN; OnabotulinumtoxinA; Potassium Chloride; RimabotulinumtoxinB

The levels/effects of Glycopyrrolate may be increased by: Amantadine; MAO Inhibitors; Pramlintide

Decreased Effect

Glycopyrrolate may decrease the levels/effects of: Acetylcholinesterase Inhibitors (Central); Haloperidol; Levodopa; Secretin

The levels/effects of Glycopyrrolate may be decreased by: Acetylcholinesterase Inhibitors (Central)

Ethanol/Nutrition/Herb Interactions Food: Administration with a high-fat meal significantly reduced absorption; administer on an empty stomach.

Stability Store at 20°C to 25°C (68°F to 77°F).

Mechanism of Action Blocks the action of acetylcholine at parasympathetic sites in smooth muscle, secretory glands, and the CNS; indirectly reduces the rate of salivation by preventing the stimulation of acetylcholine receptors

Pharmacodynamics/Kinetics
Onset of action: Oral: 50 minutes; I.M.: 15-30 minutes; I.V.: ~1 minute
Peak effect: Oral: ~1 hour; I.M.: 30-45 minutes
Duration: Vagal effect: 2-3 hours; Inhibition of salivation: Up to 7 hours; Anticholinergic: Oral: 8-12 hours
Absorption: Oral tablet: Poor and erratic; Oral solution: 23% lower compared to tablet
Distribution: V_d: Children: 1.3-1.8 L/kg; Adults: 0.2-0.62 L/kg
Metabolism: Hepatic (minimal)
Bioavailability: Tablet: ~1% to 13%
Half-life elimination: Infants: 22-130 minutes; Children 19-99 minutes; Adults: ~60-75 minutes; Oral solution: Adults: 3 hours
Excretion: Urine (as unchanged drug, I.M.: 80%, I.V.: 85%); bile (as unchanged drug)

Dosage
Children:
Reduction of secretions (preanesthetic):
Oral (unlabeled): 40-100 mcg/kg/dose 3-4 times/day
I.M., I.V. (unlabeled): 4-10 mcg/kg/dose every 3-4 hours; maximum: 0.2 mg/dose or 0.8 mg/24 hours
Intraoperative: I.V.: 4 mcg/kg not to exceed 0.1 mg; repeat at 2- to 3-minute intervals as needed
Preoperative: I.M.:
<2 years: 4-9 mcg/kg 30-60 minutes before procedure
>2 years: 4 mcg/kg 30-60 minutes before procedure
Drooling, chronic: Children 3-16 years: Oral solution (Cuvposa™): Initial: 0.02 mg/kg 3 times/day; titrate in increments of 0.02 mg/kg every 5-7 days as tolerated, up to a maximum dose of 0.1 mg/kg 3 times/day, not to exceed 1.5-3 mg/dose
Children and Adults: Reverse neuromuscular blockade: I.V.: 0.2 mg for each 1 mg of neostigmine or 5 mg of pyridostigmine administered or 5-15 mcg/kg glycopyrrolate with 25-70 mcg/kg of neostigmine or 0.1-0.3 mg/kg of pyridostigmine (agents usually administered simultaneously, but glycopyrrolate may be administered first if bradycardia is present)
Adults:
Reduction of secretions:
Intraoperative: I.V.: 0.1 mg repeated as needed at 2- to 3-minute intervals
Preoperative: I.M.: 4 mcg/kg 30-60 minutes before procedure

Administration
I.V.: Administer I.V. at a rate of 0.2 mg over 1-2 minutes. May be administered I.M. or I.V. without dilution. May also be administered via the tubing of a running I.V. infusion of a compatible solution. May be administered I.V. in the same syringe with neostigmine or pyridostigmine.
Oral: Administer oral solution on an empty stomach, 1 hour before or 2 hours after meals

Monitoring Parameters Heart rate; anticholinergic effects; bowel sounds; bowel movements; effects on drooling

Dosage Forms Excipient information presented when available (limited, particularly for generics); consult specific product labeling.
Injection, solution: 0.2 mg/mL (1 mL, 2 mL, 5 mL, 20 mL)
Robinul®: 0.2 mg/mL (1 mL, 2 mL, 5 mL, 20 mL) [contains benzyl alcohol]
Solution, oral:
Cuvposa™: 1 mg/5 mL (473 mL) [contains propylene glycol; cherry flavor]
Tablet, oral: 1 mg, 2 mg
Robinul®: 1 mg [scored]
Robinul® Forte: 2 mg [scored]

Extemporaneous Preparations A 0.5 mg/mL oral suspension may be made with 1 mg tablets and a 1:1 mixture of Ora-Plus® and either Ora-Sweet® or Ora-Sweet® SF. Crush thirty 1 mg tablets in a mortar and reduce to a fine powder. Prepare diluent by mixing 30 mL of Ora-Plus® with 30 mL of either Ora-Sweet® or Ora-Sweet® SF and stir vigorously. Add 30 mL of diluent (via geometric dilution) to powder until smooth suspension is obtained. Transfer suspension to 60 mL amber bottle. Rinse contents of mortar into bottle with sufficient quantity of remaining diluent to obtain 60 mL (final volume). Label "shake well". Stable at room temperature for 90 days. Due to bitter aftertaste, chocolate syrup may be administered prior to or mixed (1:1 v/v) with suspension immediately before administration (Cober, 2011).

A 0.5 mg/mL oral solution can be made from tablets. Crush fifty 1 mg tablets in a mortar and reduce to a fine powder. Add enough distilled water to make about 90 mL, mix well. Transfer to a bottle, rinse mortar with water, and add a quantity of water sufficient to make 100 mL. Label "shake well" and "protect from light". Stable at room temperature for 25 days (Gupta, 2001).

A 0.1 mg/mL oral solution may be made using glycopyrrolate 0.2 mg/mL injection without preservatives. Withdraw 50 mL from vials with a needle and syringe, add to 50 mL of a 1:1 mixture of Ora-Sweet® and Ora-Plus® in a bottle. Label "shake well", "protect from light," and "refrigerate". Stable refrigerated for 35 days (Landry, 2005).

Cober MP, Johnson CE, Sudekum D, et al, "Stability of Extemporaneously Prepared Glycopyrrolate Oral Suspensions," *Am J Health Syst Phar*,. 2011, 68(9):843-5.
Gupta VD, "Stability of an Oral Liquid Dosage Form of Glycopyrrolate Prepared from Tablets," *IJPC* 2001, 5(6):480-1.
Landry C, "Stability and Subjective Taste Acceptability of Four Glycopyrrolate Solutions for Oral Administration," *IJPC*, 2005, 9(5):396-98.

◆ **Glycopyrrolate Injection, USP (Can)** *see* Glycopyrrolate *on page 802*
◆ **Glycopyrronium Bromide** *see* Glycopyrrolate *on page 802*
◆ **Glydiazinamide** *see* GlipiZIDE *on page 795*
◆ **Glynase® PresTab®** *see* GlyBURIDE *on page 799*
◆ **Gly-Oxide® [OTC]** *see* Carbamide Peroxide *on page 283*
◆ **Glyquin® XM (Can)** *see* Hydroquinone *on page 846*
◆ **Glyset®** *see* Miglitol *on page 1133*
◆ **GM-CSF** *see* Sargramostim *on page 1538*
◆ **GMD-Gemfibrozil (Can)** *see* Gemfibrozil *on page 785*
◆ **GnRH Agonist** *see* Histrelin *on page 830*

Golimumab (goe LIM ue mab)

Brand Names: U.S. Simponi®
Brand Names: Canada Simponi®
Index Terms CNTO-148
Pharmacologic Category Antipsoriatic Agent; Antirheumatic, Disease Modifying; Monoclonal Antibody; Tumor Necrosis Factor (TNF) Blocking Agent
Use Treatment of active rheumatoid arthritis (moderate-to-severe), active psoriatic arthritis, and active ankylosing spondylitis
Pregnancy Risk Factor B
Pregnancy Considerations In animal studies, no evidence of fetal harm has been demonstrated. There are no adequate and well-controlled studies in pregnant women. Use during pregnancy only if clearly needed.

Lactation Excretion in breast milk unknown/not recommended

Medication Guide Available Yes

Contraindications There are no contraindications listed in the FDA-approved manufacturer's labeling.

Canadian labeling: Hypersensitivity to golimumab, latex, or any other component of formulation or packaging; patients with severe infections (eg, sepsis, tuberculosis, opportunistic infections)

Warnings/Precautions [U.S. Boxed Warning]: Patients receiving golimumab are at increased risk for serious infections which may result in hospitalization and/or fatality; infections usually developed in patients receiving concomitant immunosuppressive agents (eg, methotrexate or corticosteroids) and may present as disseminated (rather than local) disease. Active tuberculosis (or reactivation of latent tuberculosis), invasive fungal (including aspergillosis, blastomycosis, candidiasis, coccidioidomycosis, histoplasmosis, and pneumocystosis) and bacterial, viral or other opportunistic infections (including legionellosis and listeriosis) have been reported in patients receiving TNF-blocking agents, including golimumab. Monitor closely for signs/symptoms of infection. Discontinue for serious infection or sepsis. Consider risks versus benefits prior to use in patients with a history of chronic or recurrent infection. Consider empiric antifungal therapy in patients who are at risk for invasive fungal infection and develop severe systemic illness. Caution should be exercised when considering use in the elderly or in patients with conditions that predispose them to infections (eg, diabetes) or residence/travel from areas of endemic mycoses (blastomycosis, coccidioidomycosis, histoplasmosis), or with latent or localized infections. Do not initiate golimumab therapy with clinically important active infection. Patients who develop a new infection while undergoing treatment should be monitored closely.

[U.S. Boxed Warning]: Tuberculosis (disseminated or extrapulmonary) has been reported in patients receiving golimumab; both reactivation of latent infection and new infections have been reported. Patients should be evaluated for tuberculosis risk factors and latent tuberculosis infection (with a tuberculin skin test) prior to therapy. Treatment of latent tuberculosis should be initiated before use. Patients with initial negative tuberculin skin tests should receive continued monitoring for tuberculosis throughout treatment; active tuberculosis has developed in this population during treatment with TNF-blocking agents. Use with caution in patients who have resided in regions where tuberculosis is endemic. Consider antituberculosis therapy if an adequate course of treatment cannot be confirmed in patients with a history of latent or active tuberculosis or for patients with risk factors despite negative skin test.

Rare reactivation of hepatitis B virus (HBV) has occurred in chronic virus carriers; use with caution; evaluate prior to initiation and during treatment. Patients should be brought up to date with all immunizations before initiating therapy. Live vaccines should not be given concurrently. In clinical trials, humoral response to pneumococcal vaccine was not suppressed in psoriatic arthritis patients.

[U.S. Boxed Warning]: Lymphoma and other malignancies have been reported in children and adolescent patients receiving TNF-blocking agents. Half of the malignancies reported in children were lymphomas (Hodgkin's and non-Hodgkin's) while other cases varied and included malignancies not typically observed in this population. The impact of golimumab on the development and course of malignancy is not fully defined. Compared to the general population, an increased risk of lymphoma has been noted in clinical trials; however, rheumatoid arthritis alone has been previously associated with an increased rate of lymphoma. Lymphomas and other malignancies were also observed (at rates higher than expected for the general population) in adult patients receiving TNF-blocking agents. Treatment may result in the formation of autoimmune antibodies; cases of autoimmune disease have not been described. Neutralizing antibodies to golimumab may also be formed. Rarely, a reversible lupus-like syndrome has occurred with use of TNF blockers.

Use with caution in patients with peripheral or central nervous system demyelinating disorders; rare cases of new onset or exacerbation of demyelinating disorders (eg, multiple sclerosis, Guillain-Barré syndrome) have occurred with use of TNF-blockers, including golimumab. Consider discontinuing use in patients who develop peripheral or central nervous system demyelinating disorders during treatment. Optic neuritis, transverse myelitis, multiple sclerosis, and new onset or exacerbation of seizures has been reported. Use with caution in patients with heart failure or decreased left ventricular function and discontinue use with new onset or worsening of symptoms. Use caution in patients with a history of significant hematologic abnormalities (cytopenias).

Avoid concomitant use with abatacept (increased incidence of serious infections) or anakinra (increased incidence of neutropenia and serious infection). Use caution when switching between biological disease-modifying antirheumatic drugs (DMARDs); overlapping of biological activity may increase the risk for infection. Use with caution in the elderly (general incidence of infection is higher). Packaging (prefilled syringe and needle cover) contains dry natural rubber (latex). Some dosage forms may contain dry natural rubber (latex) and/or polysorbate 80.

Adverse Reactions

>10%:

Respiratory: Upper respiratory tract infection (16%; includes laryngitis, nasopharyngitis, pharyngitis, and rhinitis)

Miscellaneous: Infection (28%)

1% to 10%:

Cardiovascular: Hypertension (3%)

Central nervous system: Dizziness (2%), fever (1%)

Gastrointestinal: Constipation (1%)

Hepatic: ALT increased (4%), AST increased (3%)

Local: Injection site reactions (6%)

Neuromuscular & skeletal: Paresthesia (2%)

Respiratory: Bronchitis (2%), sinusitis (2%)

Miscellaneous: Viral infection (5%; includes herpes and influenza), antibody formation (4%), fungal infection (superficial; 2%)

<1% (Limited to important or life-threatening): Anaphylaxis, aspergillosis, candidiasis, coccidioidomycosis, demyelinating disorder, HBV reactivation, histoplasmosis, hypersensitivity reactions, leukemia, leukopenia, listeriosis, lupus-like syndrome, lymphoma, malignancy (other than nonmelanoma skin cancer), pancytopenia, pneumocystosis, psoriasis (including new onset, palmoplantar, pustular, or exacerbation), pyelonephritis, sepsis, thrombocytopenia, tuberculosis (including reactivation of latent and new infection), vasculitis

Drug Interactions

Metabolism/Transport Effects None known.

Avoid Concomitant Use

Avoid concomitant use of Golimumab with any of the following: Abatacept; Anakinra; BCG; Belimumab; Canakinumab; Certolizumab Pegol; Natalizumab; Pimecrolimus; Rilonacept; Tacrolimus (Topical); Vaccines (Live)

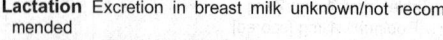

Increased Effect/Toxicity

Golimumab may increase the levels/effects of: Abatacept; Anakinra; Belimumab; Canakinumab; Certolizumab Pegol; Leflunomide; Natalizumab; Rilonacept; Vaccines (Live)

The levels/effects of Golimumab may be increased by: Abciximab; Denosumab; Pimecrolimus; Roflumilast; Tacrolimus (Topical); Trastuzumab

Decreased Effect

Golimumab may decrease the levels/effects of: BCG; Coccidioidin Skin Test; Sipuleucel-T; Vaccines (Inactivated); Vaccines (Live)

The levels/effects of Golimumab may be decreased by: Echinacea

Stability Store under refrigeration at 2°C to 8°C (36°F to 46°F); do not freeze. Do not shake. Protect from light.

Mechanism of Action Human monoclonal antibody that binds to human tumor necrosis factor alpha (TNFα), thereby interfering with endogenous TNFα activity. Biological activities of TNFα include the induction of proinflammatory cytokines (interleukin [IL]-6, IL-8, Granulocyte-colony stimulating factor, granulocyte-macrophage colony stimulating factor), expression of adhesion molecules (E-selectin, vascular cell adhesion molecule [VCAM]-1, intercellular adhesion molecule [ICAM]-1) necessary for leukocyte infiltration, activation of neutrophils and eosinophils.

Pharmacodynamics/Kinetics

Distribution: V_d: I.V.: 0.058-0.126 L/kg

Bioavailability: SubQ: ~53%

Half-life elimination: ~2 weeks

Time to peak, serum: SubQ: 2-6 days

Dosage Note: Should be administered in conjunction with methotrexate in rheumatoid arthritis; may administer with or without methotrexate or other nonbiologic disease-modifying antirheumatic drugs (DMARDs) in psoriatic arthritis or ankylosing spondylitis.

SubQ: Adults: Rheumatoid arthritis, psoriatic arthritis, ankylosing spondylitis: 50 mg once per month

Administration Subcutaneous injection: Prior to administration, allow syringe to sit at room temperature for 30 minutes. Solution should be clear to slightly opalescent and colorless to light yellow. Discard if solution is cloudy, discolored, or has foreign particles. Hold autoinjector firmly against skin and inject subcutaneously into thigh, lower abdomen (below navel), or upper arm. A loud click is heard when injection has begun. Continue to hold autoinjector against skin until second click is heard (may take 3-15 seconds). Following second click, lift autoinjector from injection site. Discard any unused portion. Rotate injection sites and avoid injecting into tender, red, hard, or bruised skin.

Monitoring Parameters Monitor improvement of symptoms and physical function assessments. Latent TB screening prior to initiating and during therapy; signs/symptoms of infection (prior to, during, and following therapy); CBC with differential; signs/symptoms/worsening of heart failure; HBV screening prior to initiating (all patients), HBV carriers (during and for several months following therapy); signs and symptoms of hypersensitivity reaction; symptoms of lupus-like syndrome.

Dosage Forms Excipient information presented when available (limited, particularly for generics); consult specific product labeling.

Injection, solution [preservative free]:

Simponi®: 50 mg/0.5 mL (0.5 mL) [contains natural rubber/natural latex in packaging, polysorbate 80; autoinjector]

Simponi®: 50 mg/0.5 mL (0.5 mL) [contains natural rubber/natural latex in packaging, polysorbate 80; prefilled syringe]

- **GoLYTELY®** *see* Polyethylene Glycol-Electrolyte Solution *on page 1372*
- **Gonal-f®** *see* Follitropin Alfa *on page 750*
- **Gonal-f® Pen (Can)** *see* Follitropin Alfa *on page 750*
- **Gonal-f® RFF** *see* Follitropin Alfa *on page 750*
- **Gonal-f® RFF Pen** *see* Follitropin Alfa *on page 750*
- **Goody's® Extra Strength Headache Powder [OTC]** *see* Acetaminophen, Aspirin, and Caffeine *on page 32*
- **Goody's® Extra Strength Pain Relief [OTC]** *see* Acetaminophen, Aspirin, and Caffeine *on page 32*
- **Goody's PM® [OTC]** *see* Acetaminophen and Diphenhydramine *on page 31*
- **Gordon Boro-Packs [OTC]** *see* Aluminum Sulfate and Calcium Acetate *on page 81*
- **Gordon's® Urea [OTC]** *see* Urea *on page 1749*
- **Gormel® [OTC]** *see* Urea *on page 1749*
- **Gormel® Ten [OTC]** *see* Urea *on page 1749*

Goserelin (GOE se rel in)

Brand Names: U.S. Zoladex®

Brand Names: Canada Zoladex®; Zoladex® LA

Index Terms Goserelin Acetate; ICI-118630; ZDX

Pharmacologic Category Antineoplastic Agent, Gonadotropin-Releasing Hormone Agonist; Gonadotropin Releasing Hormone Agonist

Use Treatment of locally confined prostate cancer; palliative treatment of advanced prostate cancer; palliative treatment of advanced breast cancer in pre- and perimenopausal women; treatment of endometriosis, including pain relief and reduction of endometriotic lesions; endometrial thinning agent as part of treatment for dysfunctional uterine bleeding

Pregnancy Risk Factor X (endometriosis, endometrial thinning); D (advanced breast cancer)

Pregnancy Considerations Goserelin has been found to be teratogenic and increases pregnancy loss in animal studies. Goserelin induces hormonal changes which increase the risk for fetal loss and use is contraindicated in pregnancy unless being used for palliative treatment of advanced breast cancer.

Breast cancer: If used for the palliative treatment of breast cancer during pregnancy, the potential for increased fetal loss should be discussed with the patient.

Endometriosis, endometrial thinning: Women of childbearing potential should not receive therapy until pregnancy has been excluded. Nonhormonal contraception is recommended for premenopausal women during therapy and for 12 weeks after therapy is discontinued. Although ovulation is usually inhibited and menstruation may stop, pregnancy prevention is not ensured during goserelin therapy. Changes in reproductive function may occur following chronic administration.

Lactation Excretion in breast milk unknown/not recommended

Contraindications Hypersensitivity to goserelin, GnRH, GnRH agonist analogues, or any component of the formulation; pregnancy (except if using for palliative treatment of advanced breast cancer)

Warnings/Precautions Hazardous agent - use appropriate precautions for handling and disposal. Allergic hypersensitivity reactions (including anaphylaxis) and antibody formation may occur; monitor. Androgen-deprivation therapy may increase the risk for cardiovascular disease (Levine, 2010). Transient increases in serum testosterone (in men with prostate cancer) and estrogen (in women with breast cancer) may result in a worsening of disease signs and symptoms (tumor flare) during the first few weeks of treatment. Urinary tract obstruction or spinal cord compression have been reported when used for prostate cancer; closely observe patients for weakness, paresthesias, and urinary tract obstruction in first few weeks of therapy. Decreased bone density has been reported in women and may be irreversible; use caution if other risk factors are present; evaluate and institute preventative treatment if necessary.

Women of childbearing potential should not receive therapy until pregnancy has been excluded. Nonhormonal contraception is recommended for premenopausal women during therapy and for 12 weeks after therapy is discontinued. Cervical resistance may be increased; use caution when dilating the cervix. The 3-month implant currently has no approved indications for use in women. Rare cases of pituitary apoplexy (frequently secondary to pituitary adenoma) have been observed with GnRH administration (onset from 1 hour to usually <2 weeks); may present as sudden headache, vomiting, visual or mental status changes, and infrequently cardiovascular collapse; immediate medical attention required. Hyperglycemia has been reported in males and may manifest as diabetes or worsening of pre-existing diabetes. Decreased AUC may be observed when using the 3-month implant in obese patients. Monitor testosterone levels if desired clinical response is not observed. Safety and efficacy have not been established in pediatric patients.

Adverse Reactions Percentages reported with the 1-month implant:

>10%:

Cardiovascular: Peripheral edema (female 21%)

Central nervous system: Headache (female 32% to 75%; male 1% to 5%), emotional lability (female 60%), depression (female 54%; male 1% to 5%), pain (female 17%; male 8%), insomnia (female 11%; male 5%)

Dermatologic: Acne (female 42%), seborrhea (female 26%)

Endocrine & metabolic: Hot flashes (female 57% to 96%; male 62%), libido decreased (female 48% to 61%), sexual dysfunction (male 21%), breast atrophy (female 33%), breast enlargement (female 18%), erections decreased (18%), libido increased (female 12%)

Gastrointestinal: Nausea (female 8% to 11%; male 5%), abdominal pain (female 7% to 11%)

Genitourinary: Vaginitis (75%), pelvic symptoms (female 9% to 18%), dyspareunia (female 14%), lower urinary symptoms (male 13%)

Neuromuscular & skeletal: Bone mineral density decreased (female 23%; ~4% decrease from baseline in 6 months; postmarketing reports in males), weakness (female 11%)

Miscellaneous: Diaphoresis (female 16% to 45%; male 6%), tumor flare (female: 23%), infection (female 13%)

1% to 10%:

Cardiovascular: Arrhythmia, chest pain, cerebrovascular accident, edema, heart failure, hypertension, MI, palpitation, peripheral vascular disorder, tachycardia

Central nervous system: Abnormal thinking, anxiety, chills, dizziness, fever, lethargy, malaise, migraine, nervousness, somnolence

Dermatologic: Alopecia, bruising, dry skin, hair disorder, hirsutism, pruritus, rash, skin discoloration

Endocrine & metabolic: Breast pain, breast swelling/tenderness, dysmenorrhea, gout, hyperglycemia

Gastrointestinal: Anorexia, appetite increased, constipation, diarrhea, dyspepsia, flatulence, ulcer, vomiting, weight gain/loss, xerostomia

Genitourinary: Urinary frequency, urinary obstruction, urinary tract infection, vaginal hemorrhage, vulvovaginitis

Hematologic: Anemia, hemorrhage

Local: Application site reaction

Neuromuscular & skeletal: Arthralgia, back pain, hypertonia, joint disorder, leg cramps, myalgia, paresthesia

Ocular: Amblyopia, dry eyes

Renal: Renal insufficiency

Respiratory: Bronchitis, COPD, cough, epistaxis, pharyngitis, rhinitis, sinusitis, upper respiratory tract infection

Miscellaneous: Allergic reaction, flu-like syndrome, voice alteration

<1% (Limited to important or life-threatening): ALT increased, anaphylaxis, AST increased, diabetes, glucose tolerance decreased, hypercalcemia, hypercholesterolemia, hyperlipidemia, hypersensitivity reactions, hypotension, ovarian cyst, pituitary apoplexy, psychotic disorders, urticaria

Drug Interactions

Metabolism/Transport Effects None known.

Avoid Concomitant Use There are no known interactions where it is recommended to avoid concomitant use.

Increased Effect/Toxicity There are no known significant interactions involving an increase in effect.

Decreased Effect

Goserelin may decrease the levels/effects of: Antidiabetic Agents

Stability Zoladex® should be stored at room temperature not to exceed 25°C or 77°F. Protect from light.

Mechanism of Action Goserelin (a gonadotropin-releasing hormone [GnRH] analog) causes an initial increase in luteinizing hormone (LH) and follicle stimulating hormone (FSH), chronic administration of goserelin results in a sustained suppression of pituitary gonadotropins. Serum testosterone falls to levels comparable to surgical castration. The exact mechanism of this effect is unknown, but may be related to changes in the control of LH or down-regulation of LH receptors.

Pharmacodynamics/Kinetics

Onset:

Females: Estradiol suppression reaches postmenopausal levels within 3 weeks and FSH and LH are suppressed to follicular phase levels within 4 weeks of initiation

Males: Testosterone suppression reaches castrate levels within 2-4 weeks after initiation

Duration:

Females: Estradiol, LH and FSH generally return to baseline levels within 12 weeks following the last monthly implant.

Males: Testosterone levels maintained at castrate levels throughout the duration of therapy.

Absorption: SubQ: Rapid and can be detected in serum in 30-60 minutes; 3.6 mg: released slowly in first 8 days, then rapid and continuous release for 28 days

Distribution: V_d: Male: 44.1 L; Female: 20.3 L

Protein binding: 27%

Time to peak, serum: SubQ: Male: 12-15 days, Female: 8-22 days

Half-life elimination: SubQ: Male: ~4 hours, Female: ~2 hours; Renal impairment: Male: 12 hours

Excretion: Urine (>90%; 20% as unchanged drug)

Dosage SubQ: Adults:

Prostate cancer, advanced:

28-day implant: 3.6 mg every 28 days

12-week implant: 10.8 mg every 12 weeks

Prostate cancer, locally confined (in combination with an antiandrogen and radiotherapy; begin 8 weeks prior to radiotherapy):

Combination 28-day/12-week implant: 3.6 mg implant, followed in 28 days by 10.8 mg implant

28-day implant (alternate dosing): 3.6 mg; repeated every 28 days for a total of 4 doses

Breast cancer, advanced: 3.6 mg every 28 days

Endometriosis: 3.6 mg every 28 days for 6 months

Endometrial thinning: 3.6 mg every 28 days for 1 or 2 doses

Dosing adjustment in renal impairment: No adjustment is necessary

Dosing adjustment in hepatic impairment: No adjustment is necessary

Administration SubQ: Administer implant by inserting needle at a 30-45 degree angle into the anterior abdominal wall below the navel line. Goserelin is an implant; therefore, do not attempt to eliminate air bubbles prior to injection (may displace implant). Do not attempt to aspirate prior to injection; if a large vessel is penetrated, blood will be visualized in the syringe chamber (if vessel is penetrated, withdraw needle and inject elsewhere with a new syringe). Do not penetrate into muscle or peritoneum. Implant may be detected by ultrasound if removal is required.

Monitoring Parameters Bone mineral density, serum calcium, cholesterol/lipids

Prostate cancer: Weakness, paresthesias, and urinary tract obstruction in first few weeks of therapy; screen for diabetes

Test Interactions Interferes with pituitary gonadotropic and gonadal function tests during and for up to 12 weeks after discontinued

Additional Information If removal is necessary, implant may be located by ultrasound.

Dosage Forms Excipient information presented when available (limited, particularly for generics); consult specific product labeling.

Implant, subcutaneous:

Zoladex®: 3.6 mg (1s) [1 month implant]

Zoladex®: 10.8 mg (1s) [3 month implant]

- **Goserelin Acetate** *see* Goserelin *on page 805*
- **GP 47680** *see* OXcarbazepine *on page 1262*
- **GPI 15715** *see* Fospropofol *on page 767*
- **GR38032R** *see* Ondansetron *on page 1246*
- **Gralise™** *see* Gabapentin *on page 773*
- **Gramicidin, Neomycin, and Polymyxin B** *see* Neomycin, Polymyxin B, and Gramicidin *on page 1189*

Granisetron (gra NI se tron)

Brand Names: U.S. Granisol™; Kytril®; Sancuso®

Brand Names: Canada Granisetron Hydrochloride Injection; Kytril®

Index Terms BRL 43694

Pharmacologic Category Antiemetic; Selective 5-HT_3 Receptor Antagonist

Use Prophylaxis of nausea and vomiting associated with emetogenic chemotherapy and radiation therapy; prophylaxis and treatment of postoperative nausea and vomiting (PONV)

Unlabeled Use Breakthrough treatment of nausea and vomiting associated with chemotherapy

Pregnancy Risk Factor B

Pregnancy Considerations There are no adequate or well-controlled studies in pregnant women. Teratogenic effects were not observed in animal studies. Injection (1 mg/mL strength) contains benzyl alcohol which may cross the placenta. Use only if benefit exceeds the risk.

Lactation Excretion in breast milk unknown/use caution

Contraindications Hypersensitivity to granisetron or any component of the formulation

Warnings/Precautions Use with caution in patients with congenital long QT syndrome or other risk factors for QT prolongation (eg, medications known to prolong QT interval, electrolyte abnormalities, and cumulative high-dose anthracycline therapy). 5-HT_3 antagonists have been associated with a number of dose-dependent increases in ECG intervals (eg, PR, QRS duration, QT/QT_c, JT), usually occurring 1-2 hours after I.V. administration. In general, these changes are not clinically relevant, however, when used in conjunction with other agents that prolong these intervals, arrhythmia may occur. When used with agents that prolong the QT interval (eg, Class I and III antiarrhythmics), clinically relevant QT interval prolongation may occur resulting in torsade de pointes. I.V. formulations of 5-HT_3 antagonists have more association with ECG interval changes, compared to oral formulations.

For chemotherapy-related emesis, **granisetron should be used on a scheduled basis, not on an "as needed" (PRN) basis**, since data support the use of this drug in the prevention of nausea and vomiting and not in the rescue of nausea and vomiting. Granisetron should be used only in the first 24-48 hours of receiving chemotherapy or radiation. Data do not support any increased efficacy of granisetron in delayed nausea and vomiting.

Use with caution in patients allergic to other 5-HT_3 receptor antagonists; cross-reactivity has been reported. Routine prophylaxis for PONV is not recommended in patients where there is little expectation of nausea and vomiting postoperatively. In patients where nausea and vomiting must be avoided postoperatively, administer to all patients even when expected incidence of nausea and vomiting is low. Use caution following abdominal surgery or in chemotherapy-induced nausea and vomiting; may mask progressive ileus or gastric distention. Application site reactions, generally mild, have occurred with transdermal patch use; if skin reaction is severe or generalized, remove patch. Cover patch application site with clothing to protect from natural or artificial sunlight exposure while patch is applied and for 10 days following removal; granisetron may potentially be affected by natural or artificial sunlight. Do not apply patch to red, irritated, or damaged skin. Injection contains benzyl alcohol (1 mg/mL) and should not be used in neonates.

Adverse Reactions

>10%:

Central nervous system: Headache (3% to 21%; transdermal patch: 1%)

Gastrointestinal: Constipation (3% to 18%)

Neuromuscular & skeletal: Weakness (5% to 18%)

1% to 10%:

Cardiovascular: QT_c prolongation (1% to 3%), hypertension (1% to 2%)

Central nervous system: Pain (10%), fever (3% to 9%), dizziness (4% to 5%), insomnia (<2% to 5%), somnolence (1% to 4%), anxiety (2%), agitation (<2%), CNS stimulation (<2%)

Dermatologic: Rash (1%)

Gastrointestinal: Diarrhea (3% to 9%), abdominal pain (4% to 6%), dyspepsia (3% to 6%), taste perversion (2%)

Hepatic: Liver enzymes increased (5% to 6%)

Renal: Oliguria (2%)

Respiratory: Cough (2%)

Miscellaneous: Infection (3%)

<1% (Limited to important or life-threatening): Agitation, allergic reactions; anaphylaxis (including hypotension, dyspnea, urticaria); angina, application site reactions (transdermal patch), arrhythmias, atrial fibrillation, extrapyramidal syndrome, hot flashes, hypotension, hypersensitivity, syncope

Drug Interactions

Metabolism/Transport Effects Substrate of CYP3A4 (minor); **Note:** Assignment of Major/Minor substrate status based on clinically relevant drug interaction potential

Avoid Concomitant Use

Avoid concomitant use of Granisetron with any of the following: Apomorphine; Artemether; Dronedarone; Lumefantrine; Nilotinib; Pimozide; QUEtiapine; QuiNINE; Tetrabenazine; Thioridazine; Toremifene; Vandetanib; Vemurafenib; Ziprasidone

Increased Effect/Toxicity

Granisetron may increase the levels/effects of: Apomorphine; Dronedarone; Pimozide; QTc-Prolonging Agents; QuiNINE; Tetrabenazine; Thioridazine; Toremifene; Vandetanib; Vemurafenib; Ziprasidone

The levels/effects of Granisetron may be increased by: Alfuzosin; Artemether; Chloroquine; Ciprofloxacin; Ciprofloxacin (Systemic); Conivaptan; Gadobutrol; Indacaterol; Lumefantrine; Nilotinib; QUEtiapine; QuiNINE

Decreased Effect

The levels/effects of Granisetron may be decreased by: Tocilizumab

Stability

I.V.: Store at 15°C to 30°C (59°F to 86°F). Stable when mixed in NS or D_5W for 7 days under refrigeration and for 3 days at room temperature. Protect from light. Do not freeze vials.

Oral: Store tablet or oral solution at 15°C to 30°C (59°F to 86°F). Protect from light.

Transdermal patch: Store at 20°C to 25°C (68°F to 77°F). Keep patch in original packaging until immediately prior to use.

Mechanism of Action Selective $5\text{-}HT_3$-receptor antagonist, blocking serotonin, both peripherally on vagal nerve terminals and centrally in the chemoreceptor trigger zone

Pharmacodynamics/Kinetics

Duration: Oral, I.V.: Generally up to 24 hours

Absorption: Oral: Tablets and oral solution are bioequivalent; Transdermal patch: ~66% over 7 days

Distribution: V_d: 2-4 L/kg; widely throughout body

Protein binding: 65%

Metabolism: Hepatic via N-demethylation, oxidation, and conjugation; some metabolites may have $5\text{-}HT_3$ antagonist activity

Half-life elimination: Oral: 6 hours; I.V.: 9 hours

Time to peak, plasma: Transdermal patch: Maximum systemic concentrations: ~48 hours after application (range: 24-168 hours)

Excretion: Urine (12% as unchanged drug, 48% to 49% as metabolites); feces (34% to 38% as metabolites)

Dosage

Oral: Adults:

Prophylaxis of chemotherapy-related emesis: 2 mg once daily up to 1 hour before chemotherapy or 1 mg twice daily; the first 1 mg dose should be given up to 1 hour before chemotherapy.

Prophylaxis of radiation therapy-associated emesis: 2 mg once daily given 1 hour before radiation therapy.

I.V.:

Children ≥2 years and Adults: Prophylaxis of chemotherapy-related emesis:

Within U.S.: 10 mcg/kg/dose (maximum: 1 mg/dose) given 30 minutes prior to chemotherapy; for some drugs (eg, carboplatin, cyclophosphamide) with a later onset of emetic action, 10 mcg/kg every 12 hours may be necessary

Outside U.S.: 40 mcg/kg/dose (or 3 mg/dose); maximum: 9 mg/24 hours

Breakthrough: Granisetron has not been shown to be effective in terminating nausea or vomiting once it occurs and should not be used for this purpose.

Adults: PONV:

Prevention: 1 mg given undiluted over 30 seconds; the manufacturer recommends administration before induction of anesthesia or immediately before reversal of anesthesia. **Note:** The Society for Ambulatory Anesthesia (SAMBA) Guidelines recommend a dosage range of 0.35-1.5 mg administered at the end of surgery (Gan, 2007). However, doses ≤1 mg are generally used since doses >1 mg are not more effective. Of note, 5 mcg/kg (~0.35 mg in a 70 kg adult) has been shown to be effective; doses >5 mcg/kg were not more effective (Mikawa, 1997).

Treatment: 1 mg given undiluted over 30 seconds

Transdermal patch: Adults: Prophylaxis of chemotherapy-related emesis: Apply 1 patch at least 24 hours prior to chemotherapy; do not apply ≥48 hours before chemotherapy. Remove patch a minimum of 24 hours after chemotherapy completion. Maximum duration: Patch may be worn up to 7 days, depending on chemotherapy regimen duration.

Dosing interval in renal impairment: No dosage adjustment required.

Dosing interval in hepatic impairment: Kinetic studies in patients with hepatic impairment showed that total clearance was approximately halved, however, standard doses were very well tolerated, and dose adjustments are not necessary.

Administration

Oral: Doses should be given up to 1 hour prior to initiation of chemotherapy/radiation

I.V.: Administer I.V. push over 30 seconds or as a 5- to 10-minute infusion

Prevention of PONV: Administer before induction of anesthesia or immediately before reversal of anesthesia.

Treatment of PONV: Administer undiluted over 30 seconds.

Transdermal (Sancuso®): Apply patch to clean, dry, intact skin on upper outer arm. Do not use on red, irritated, or damaged skin. Remove patch from pouch immediately before application. Do not cut patch.

Dosage Forms Excipient information presented when available (limited, particularly for generics); consult specific product labeling. [DSC] = Discontinued product

Injection, solution: 0.1 mg/mL (1 mL [DSC]); 1 mg/mL (1 mL, 4 mL)

Injection, solution [preservative free]: 0.1 mg/mL (1 mL); 1 mg/mL (1 mL)

Patch, transdermal:

Sancuso®: 3.1 mg/24 hours (1s) [52 cm^2, total granisetron 34.3 mg]

Solution, oral:

Granisol™: 2 mg/10 mL (30 mL) [contains sodium benzoate; orange flavor]

Tablet, oral: 1 mg

Kytril®: 1 mg

Extemporaneous Preparations Note: Commercial oral solution is available (0.2 mg/mL)

A 0.2 mg/mL oral suspension may be made with tablets. Crush twelve 1 mg tablets in a mortar and reduce to a fine powder. Add 30 mL distilled water, mix well, and transfer to a bottle. Rinse the mortar with 10 mL cherry syrup and add to bottle. Add sufficient quantity of cherry syrup to make a final volume of 60 mL. Label "shake well". Stable 14 days at room temperature or refrigerated (Quercia, 1997).

A 50 mcg/mL oral suspension may be made with tablets and one of three different vehicles (Ora-Sweet®, Ora-Plus®, or a mixture of methylcellulose 1% and Simple Syrup, N.F.). Crush one 1 mg tablet in a mortar and reduce to a fine powder. Add 20 mL of the chosen vehicle and mix to a uniform paste; transfer to a calibrated bottle. Label "shake well" and "refrigerate". Stable for 91 days refrigerated (Nahata, 1998).

Nahata MC, Morosco RS, and Hipple TF, "Stability of Granisetron Hydrochloride in Two Oral Suspensions," *Am J Health Syst Pharm*, 1998, 55(23):2511-3.

Quercia RA, Zhang J, Fan C, et al, "Stability of Granisetron Hydrochloride in an Extemporaneously Prepared Oral Liquid," *Am J Health Syst Pharm*, 1997, 54(12):1404-6.

◆ **Granisetron Hydrochloride Injection (Can)** *see* Granisetron *on page* 807

◆ **Granisol™** *see* Granisetron *on page* 807

◆ **Granulex®** *see* Trypsin, Balsam Peru, and Castor Oil *on page* 1744

◆ **Granulocyte Colony Stimulating Factor** *see* Filgrastim *on page* 711

◆ **Granulocyte Colony Stimulating Factor (PEG Conjugate)** *see* Pegfilgrastim *on page* 1307

◆ **Granulocyte-Macrophage Colony Stimulating Factor** *see* Sargramostim *on page* 1538

◆ **Gravol® (Can)** *see* DimenhyDRINATE *on page* 513

◆ **Grifulvin V®** *see* Griseofulvin *on page* 809

Griseofulvin (gri see oh FUL vin)

Brand Names: U.S. Grifulvin V®; Gris-PEG®

Index Terms Griseofulvin Microsize; Griseofulvin Ultramicrosize

Pharmacologic Category Antifungal Agent, Oral

Additional Appendix Information

Antifungal Agents *on page* 1876

Use Treatment of susceptible tinea infections of the skin, hair, and nails

Pregnancy Risk Factor C

Dosage Oral:

Children >2 years:

Microsize: 10-20 mg/kg/day in single or 2 divided doses. In the treatment of tinea capitis, higher dosages (20-25 mg/kg/day for 8-12 weeks) have been recommended by some authors (unlabeled).

Ultramicrosize: Usual: 7.3 mg/kg/day in single dose or 2 divided doses; range: 5-15 mg/kg/day in single dose or 2 divided doses (maximum: 750 mg/day)

Adults:

Microsize: 500-1000 mg/day in single or divided doses

Ultramicrosize: 375 mg/day in single or divided doses; doses up to 750 mg/day have been used for infections more difficult to eradicate such as tinea unguium and tinea pedis

Duration of therapy depends on the site of infection:

Tinea corporis: 2-4 weeks

Tinea capitis: 4-6 weeks or longer (up to 8-12 weeks)

Tinea pedis: 4-8 weeks

Tinea unguium: 3-6 months or longer

Additional Information Complete prescribing information for this medication should be consulted for additional detail.

Dosage Forms Excipient information presented when available (limited, particularly for generics); consult specific product labeling.

Suspension, oral [microsize]: 125 mg/5 mL (120 mL)

Tablet, oral [microsize]:

Grifulvin V®: 500 mg [scored]

Tablet, oral [ultramicrosize]:

Gris-PEG®: 125 mg, 250 mg [scored]

◆ **Griseofulvin Microsize** *see* Griseofulvin *on page* 809

◆ **Griseofulvin Ultramicrosize** *see* Griseofulvin *on page* 809

◆ **Gris-PEG®** *see* Griseofulvin *on page* 809

◆ **Growth Hormone, Human** *see* Somatropin *on page* 1579

◆ **GSK-580299** *see* Papillomavirus (Types 16, 18) Vaccine (Human, Recombinant) *on page* 1292

◆ **GSK 1838262** *see* Gabapentin Enacarbil *on page* 775

◆ **Guaiatussin AC** *see* Guaifenesin and Codeine *on page* 810

◆ **Guaicon DM [OTC] [DSC]** *see* Guaifenesin and Dextromethorphan *on page* 810

◆ **Guaicon DMS [OTC]** *see* Guaifenesin and Dextromethorphan *on page* 810

GuaiFENesin (gwye FEN e sin)

Brand Names: U.S. Allfen [OTC]; Bidex®-400 [OTC]; Diabetic Siltussin DAS-Na [OTC]; Diabetic Tussin® EX [OTC]; Fenesin IR [OTC]; Ganidin® NR [OTC] [DSC]; Geri-Tussin [OTC]; Humibid® Maximum Strength [OTC]; Mucinex® Kid's Mini-Melts™ [OTC]; Mucinex® Kid's [OTC]; Mucinex® Maximum Strength [OTC]; Mucinex® [OTC]; Mucus Relief [OTC]; Organidin® NR [OTC] [DSC]; Refenesen™ 400 [OTC]; Refenesen™ [OTC]; Robafen [OTC]; Scot-Tussin® Expectorant [OTC]; Siltussin SA [OTC]; Vicks® Casero™ Chest Congestion Relief [OTC]; Vicks® DayQuil® Mucus Control [OTC]; Xpect™ [OTC]

Brand Names: Canada Balminil Expectorant; Benylin® E Extra Strength; Koffex Expectorant; Robitussin®

Index Terms Cheratussin; GG; Glycerol Guaiacolate

Pharmacologic Category Expectorant

Use Help loosen phlegm and thin bronchial secretions to make coughs more productive

Pregnancy Considerations Based on the limited available data, an increased risk of adverse birth outcomes has not been observed following maternal use of guaifenesin in pregnancy. Alcohol may be present in some liquid formulations of guaifenesin. If consumed in sufficient quantities during pregnancy, fetal alcohol syndrome may result. Guaifenesin has been investigated as an agent to improve cervical mucus and improve fertility.

Lactation Excretion in breast milk unknown

Contraindications Hypersensitivity to guaifenesin or any component of the formulation

Warnings/Precautions When used for self medication (OTC) notify healthcare provider if symptoms do not improve within 7 days, or are accompanied by fever, rash, or persistent headache. Do not use for persistent or chronic cough (as with smoking, asthma, chronic bronchitis, emphysema) or if cough is accompanied by excessive phlegm unless directed to do so by healthcare provider. Not for OTC use in children <2 years of age. Some products may contain phenylalanine.

Adverse Reactions

Frequency not defined:

Central nervous system: Dizziness, drowsiness, headache

Dermatologic: Rash

Endocrine & metabolic: Uric acid levels decreased

Gastrointestinal: Nausea, stomach pain, vomiting

Postmarketing and/or case reports: Kidney stone formation (with consumption of large quantities)

Drug Interactions

Metabolism/Transport Effects None known.

Avoid Concomitant Use There are no known interactions where it is recommended to avoid concomitant use.

Increased Effect/Toxicity There are no known significant interactions involving an increase in effect.

Decreased Effect There are no known significant interactions involving a decrease in effect.

Mechanism of Action Thought to act as an expectorant by irritating the gastric mucosa and stimulating respiratory tract secretions, thereby increasing respiratory fluid volumes and decreasing mucous viscosity

Pharmacodynamics/Kinetics

Absorption: Well absorbed

Half-life elimination: ~1 hour

Excretion: Urine (as unchanged drug and metabolites)

Dosage Oral:
Children:
6 months to 2 years: 25-50 mg every 4 hours, not to exceed 300 mg/day
2-5 years: 50-100 mg every 4 hours, not to exceed 600 mg/day
6-11 years: 100-200 mg every 4 hours, not to exceed 1.2 g/day
Children >12 years and Adults: 200-400 mg every 4 hours to a maximum of 2.4 g/day
Extended release tablet: 600-1200 mg every 12 hours, not to exceed 2.4 g/day

Dietary Considerations Some products may contain phenylalanine and/or sodium.

Administration Do not crush, chew, or break extended release tablets. Administer with a full glass of water.

Test Interactions Possible color interference with determination of 5-HIAA and VMA; discontinue for 48 hours prior to test

Dosage Forms Excipient information presented when available (limited, particularly for generics); consult specific product labeling. [DSC] = Discontinued product
Caplet, oral:
Fenesin IR: 400 mg
Refenesen™ 400: 400 mg [dye free]
Granules, oral:
Mucinex® Kid's Mini-Melts™: 50 mg/packet (12s) [contains magnesium 6 mg/packet, phenylalanine 0.6 mg/packet, sodium 2 mg/packet; grape flavor]
Mucinex® Kid's Mini-Melts™: 100 mg/packet (12s) [contains magnesium 6 mg/packet, phenylalanine 1 mg/packet, sodium 3 mg/packet; bubblegum flavor]
Liquid, oral:
Diabetic Tussin® EX: 100 mg/5 mL (118 mL) [dye free, ethanol free, sugar free; contains phenylalanine 8.4 mg/5 mL]
Ganidin® NR: 100 mg/5 mL (473 mL [DSC]) [raspberry flavor]
Mucinex® Kid's: 100 mg/5 mL (118 mL) [contains propylene glycol, sodium 3 mg/5 mL; grape flavor]
Scot-Tussin® Expectorant: 100 mg/5 mL (120 mL) [dye free, ethanol free, sugar free; contains benzoic acid; grape flavor]
Vicks® Casero™ Chest Congestion Relief: 100 mg/6.25 mL (120 mL, 240 mL) [contains phenylalanine 5.5 mg/12.5 mL, sodium 32 mg/12.5 mL, sodium benzoate; honey-menthol flavor]
Vicks® DayQuil® Mucus Control: 200 mg/15 mL (295 mL) [contains propylene glycol, sodium 25 mg/15 mL, sodium benzoate; citrus blend flavor]
Syrup, oral: 100 mg/5 mL (5 mL, 10 mL, 15 mL, 118 mL, 120 mL, 240 mL, 473 mL, 480 mL)
Diabetic Siltussin DAS-Na: 100 mg/5 mL (118 mL) [ethanol free, sugar free; contains benzoic acid, phenylalanine 3 mg/5 mL, propylene glycol; strawberry flavor]
Geri-Tussin: 100 mg/5 mL (480 mL) [ethanol free, sugar free; contains sodium benzoate]
Robafen: 100 mg/5 mL (120 mL, 240 mL, 480 mL) [ethanol free; contains sodium benzoate; cherry flavor]
Siltussin SA: 100 mg/5 mL (120 mL, 240 mL, 480 mL) [ethanol free, sugar free; strawberry flavor]
Tablet, oral: 200 mg [DSC], 400 mg
Allfen: 400 mg [scored]
Bidex®-400: 400 mg
Mucus Relief: 400 mg
Organidin® NR: 200 mg [DSC] [scored]
Refenesen™: 200 mg
Xpect™: 400 mg [sugar free]
Tablet, extended release, oral:
Humibid® Maximum Strength: 1200 mg
Mucinex®: 600 mg
Mucinex® Maximum Strength: 1200 mg

Guaifenesin and Codeine

(gwye FEN e sin & KOE deen)

Brand Names: U.S. Allfen CD; Allfen CDX; Codar® GF; Dex-Tuss; ExeClear-C; Gani-Tuss® NR [DSC]; Guaiatussin AC; Iophen C-NR; Mar-Cof® CG; Robafen AC

Index Terms Codeine and Guaifenesin; Robitussin AC

Pharmacologic Category Antitussive; Cough Preparation; Expectorant

Use Temporary control of cough due to minor throat and bronchial irritation

Dosage Oral: **Note:** Also refer to specific product labeling:
Children 6-11 years:
ExeClear-C: 5 mL every 4-6 hours; maximum: 30 mL/24 hours
Dex-Tuss, Gani-Tuss® NR: 2.5 mL every 4-6 hours; maximum: 20 mL/24 hours
Children ≥12 years and Adults:
ExeClear-C: 10 mL every 4-6 hours; maximum: 60 mL/24 hours
Dex-Tuss, Gani-Tuss® NR: 5 mL every 4-6 hours; maximum 40 mL/24 hours

Additional Information Complete prescribing information for this medication should be consulted for additional detail.

Dosage Forms Excipient information presented when available (limited, particularly for generics); consult specific product labeling. [DSC] = Discontinued product
Liquid, oral:
Codar® GF: Guaifenesin 200 mg and codeine phosphate 8 mg per 5 mL (473 mL) [contains propylene glycol; cotton candy flavor]
Dex-Tuss: Guaifenesin 300 mg and codeine phosphate 10 mg per 5 mL (473 mL) [ethanol free, gluten free, sugar free; contains propylene glycol; grape flavor]
Gani-Tuss® NR: Guaifenesin 100 mg and codeine phosphate 10 mg per 5 mL (480 mL) [raspberry flavor] [DSC]
Iophen C-NR: Guaifenesin 100 mg and codeine phosphate 10 mg per 5 mL (473 mL) [contains propylene glycol, sodium benzoate; raspberry flavor]
Solution, oral: Guaifenesin 100 mg and codeine phosphate 10 mg per 5 mL (5 mL, 10 mL, 118 mL, 473 mL)
Mar-Cof® CG: Guaifenesin 225 mg and codeine phosphate 7.5 mg per 5 mL (473 ml) [ethanol free, sugar free; contains propylene glycol, sodium benzoate, sodium 6 mg/5 mL]
Syrup, oral: Guaifenesin 100 mg and codeine phosphate 10 mg per 5 mL (473 mL)
ExeClear-C: Guaifenesin 200 mg and codeine phosphate 10 mg per 5 mL (473 mL) [dye free, ethanol free, sugar free; contains propylene glycol, sodium benzoate; fruit flavor]
Guaiatussin AC: Guaifenesin 100 mg and codeine phosphate 10 mg per 5 mL (118 mL, 473 mL) [contains ethanol 3.5%, sodium 1 mg/5 mL, sodium benzoate; cherry flavor]
Robafen AC: Guaifenesin 100 mg and codeine phosphate 10 mg per 5 mL (120 mL, 480 mL) [contains ethanol 3.5%, sodium 4 mg/5 mL, sodium benzoate; cherry flavor]
Tablet, oral:
Allfen CD: Guaifenesin 400 mg and codeine phosphate 10 mg
Allfen CDX: Guaifenesin 400 mg and codeine phosphate 20 mg

Controlled Substance C-V

Guaifenesin and Dextromethorphan

(gwye FEN e sin & deks troe meth OR fan)

Brand Names: U.S. Allfen DM [OTC] [DSC]; Cheracol® D [OTC]; Cheracol® Plus [OTC]; Coricidin HBP® Chest

Congestion and Cough [OTC]; Diabetic Siltussin-DM DAS-Na Maximum Strength [OTC]; Diabetic Siltussin-DM DAS-Na [OTC]; Diabetic Tussin® DM Maximum Strength [OTC]; Diabetic Tussin® DM [OTC]; Double Tussin DM [OTC]; Fenesin DM IR [OTC]; Gani-Tuss DM NR [DSC]; Guaicon DM [OTC] [DSC]; Guaicon DMS [OTC]; Guia-D [DSC]; Guiadrine™ DX [DSC]; Kolephrin® GG/DM [OTC]; Mintab DM [DSC]; Mucinex® DM Maximum Strength [OTC]; Mucinex® DM [OTC]; Mucinex® Kid's Cough Mini-Melts™ [OTC]; Mucinex® Kid's Cough [OTC]; Refenesen™ DM [OTC]; Robafen DM Clear [OTC]; Robafen DM [OTC]; Robitussin® Cough & Chest Congestion DM Max [OTC] [DSC]; Robitussin® Cough & Chest Congestion DM [OTC] [DSC]; Robitussin® Cough & Chest Congestion Sugar-Free DM [OTC] [DSC]; Robitussin® Peak Cold Cough + Chest Congestion DM [OTC]; Robitussin® Peak Cold Maximum Strength Cough + Chest Congestion DM [OTC]; Robitussin® Peak Cold Sugar-Free Cough + Chest Congestion DM [OTC]; Safe Tussin® DM [OTC]; Scot-Tussin® Senior [OTC]; Silexin [OTC]; Siltussin DM DAS [OTC]; Siltussin DM [OTC]; Simuc-DM [DSC]; Su-Tuss DM [DSC]; Tussi-Bid® [OTC] [DSC]; Vicks® 44E [OTC]; Vicks® DayQuil® Mucus Control DM [OTC]; Vicks® Nature Fusion™ Cough & Chest Congestion [OTC]; Vicks® Pediatric Formula 44E [OTC]

Brand Names: Canada Balminil DM E; Benylin® DM-E; Koffex DM-Expectorant; Robitussin® DM

Index Terms Dextromethorphan and Guaifenesin

Pharmacologic Category Antitussive; Cough Preparation; Expectorant

Use Temporary control of cough due to minor throat and bronchial irritation

Dosage Oral:

Children 2-6 years:

General dosing guidelines: Guaifenesin 50-100 mg and dextromethorphan 2.5-5 mg every 4 hours (maximum dose: Guaifenesin 600 mg and dextromethorphan 30 mg per day)

Product-specific labeling: Vicks® Pediatric Formula 44E: 7.5 mL every 4 hours (maximum: 6 doses/24 hours)

Children: 6-12 years:

General dosing guidelines: Guaifenesin 100-200 mg and dextromethorphan 5-10 mg every 4 hours (maximum dose: Guaifenesin 1200 mg and dextromethorphan 60 mg per day)

Product-specific labeling:

Vicks® 44E: 7.5 mL every 4 hours (maximum: 6 doses/24 hours)

Vicks® Pediatric Formula 44E: 15 mL every 4 hours (maximum: 6 doses/24 hours)

Children ≥12 years and Adults:

General dosing guidelines: Guaifenesin 200-400 mg and dextromethorphan 10-20 mg every 4 hours (maximum dose: Guaifenesin 2400 mg and dextromethorphan 120 mg per day)

Product-specific labeling:

Mucinex® DM: 1-2 tablets every 12 hours (maximum: 4 tablets/24 hours)

Vicks® 44E: 15 mL every 4 hours (maximum: 6 doses/24 hours)

Vicks® Pediatric Formula 44E: 30 mL every 4 hours (maximum: 6 doses/24 hours)

Additional Information Complete prescribing information for this medication should be consulted for additional detail.

Dosage Forms Excipient information presented when available (limited, particularly for generics); consult specific product labeling. [DSC] = Discontinued product

Caplet, oral:

Fenesin DM IR: Guaifenesin 400 mg and dextromethorphan hydrobromide 15 mg

Refenesen™ DM: Guaifenesin 400 mg and dextromethorphan hydrobromide 20 mg

Capsule, softgel, oral:

Coricidin HBP® Chest Congestion and Cough: Guaifenesin 200 mg and dextromethorphan hydrobromide 10 mg

Elixir, oral:

Simuc-DM: Guaifenesin 225 mg and dextromethorphan hydrobromide 25 mg per 5 mL (480 mL) [grape flavor] [DSC]

Granules, oral:

Mucinex® Kid's Cough Mini-Melts™: Guaifenesin 100 mg and dextromethorphan hydrobromide 5 mg per packet (12s) [contains magnesium 6 mg/pack, phenylalanine 2 mg/packet, sodium 3 mg/packet; orange crème flavor]

Liquid, oral: Guaifenesin 100 mg and dextromethorphan hydrobromide 10 mg per 5 mL (480 mL)

Diabetic Tussin® DM: Guaifenesin 100 mg and dextromethorphan hydrobromide 10 mg per 5 mL (120 mL) [dye free, ethanol free, sugar free; contains phenylalanine 8.4 mg/5 mL]

Diabetic Tussin® DM Maximum Strength: Guaifenesin 200 mg and dextromethorphan hydrobromide 10 mg per 5 mL (120 mL) [dye free, ethanol free, sugar free; contains phenylalanine 8.4 mg/5 mL]

Double Tussin DM: Guaifenesin 300 mg and dextromethorphan hydrobromide 20 mg per 5 mL (120 mL, 480 mL) [dye free, ethanol free, sugar free]

Gani-Tuss DM NR: Guaifenesin 100 mg and dextromethorphan hydrobromide 10 mg per 5 mL (480 mL) [raspberry flavor] [DSC]

Guiadrine™ DX: Guaifenesin 225 mg and dextromethorphan hydrobromide 25 mg per 5 mL (473 mL) [ethanol free, sugar free; contains propylene glycol, sodium benzoate; grape flavor] [DSC]

Kolephrin® GG/DM: Guaifenesin 150 mg and dextromethorphan hydrobromide 10 mg per 5 mL (120 mL) [ethanol free; cherry flavor]

Mucinex® Kid's Cough: Guaifenesin 100 mg and dextromethorphan hydrobromide 5 mg per 5 mL (120 mL) [contains propylene glycol, sodium 3 mg/5 mL; cherry flavor]

Safe Tussin® DM: Guaifenesin 100 mg and dextromethorphan hydrobromide 15 mg per 5 mL (120 mL) [contains benzoic acid, phenylalanine 4.2 mg/5 mL, and propylene glycol; orange and mint flavors]

Scot-Tussin® Senior: Guaifenesin 200 mg and dextromethorphan hydrobromide 15 mg per 5 mL (120 mL) [ethanol free, sodium free, sugar free]

Vicks® 44E: Guaifenesin 200 mg and dextromethorphan hydrobromide 20 mg per 15 mL (120 mL, 235 mL) [contains ethanol, sodium 31 mg/15 mL, sodium benzoate]

Vicks® DayQuil® Mucus Control DM: Guaifenesin 200 mg and dextromethorphan hydrobromide 10 mg per 15 mL (295 mL) [contains propylene glycol, sodium 25 mg/15 mL, sodium benzoate; citrus blend flavor]

Vicks® Nature Fusion™ Cough & Chest Congestion: Guaifenesin 200 mg and dextromethorphan hydrobromide 20 mg per 30 mL (236 mL) [dye free, ethanol free, gluten free; contains propylene glycol, sodium 36 mg/30 mL; honey flavor]

Vicks® Pediatric Formula 44E: Guaifenesin 100 mg and dextromethorphan hydrobromide 10 mg per 15 mL (120 mL) [ethanol free; contains sodium 30 mg/15 mL, sodium benzoate; cherry flavor]

Syrup, oral: Guaifenesin 100 mg and dextromethorphan hydrobromide 10 mg per 5 mL (5 mL, 10 mL, 120 mL, 480 mL)

Cheracol® D: Guaifenesin 100 mg and dextromethorphan hydrobromide 10 mg per 5 mL (120 mL, 180 mL) [contains benzoic acid, ethanol 4.75%]

Cheracol® Plus: Guaifenesin 100 mg and dextromethorphan hydrobromide 10 mg per 5 mL (120 mL) [contains benzoic acid, ethanol 4.75%]
Diabetic Siltussin-DM DAS-Na: Guaifenesin 100 mg and dextromethorphan hydrobromide 10 mg per 5 mL (118 mL) [ethanol free, sugar free; contains benzoic acid, phenylalanine 3 mg/5 mL, propylene glycol; strawberry flavor]
Diabetic Siltussin-DM DAS-Na Maximum Strength: Guaifenesin 200 mg and dextromethorphan hydrobromide 10 mg per 5 mL (118 mL) [ethanol free, sugar free; contains benzoic acid, phenylalanine 3 mg/5 mL, propylene glycol; strawberry flavor]
Guaicon DM: Guaifenesin 100 mg and dextromethorphan hydrobromide 10 mg per 5 mL (10 mL) [ethanol free] [DSC]
Guaicon DMS: Guaifenesin 100 mg and dextromethorphan hydrobromide 10 mg per 5 mL (10 mL) [ethanol free, sugar free]
Mintab DM: Guaifenesin 200 mg and dextromethorphan hydrobromide 10 mg per 5 mL (480 mL) [dye free, ethanol free; cherry vanilla flavor] [DSC]
Robafen DM: Guaifenesin 100 mg and dextromethorphan hydrobromide 10 mg per 5 mL (120 mL, 240 mL, 480 mL) [cherry flavor]
Robafen DM Clear: Guaifenesin 100 mg and dextromethorphan hydrobromide 10 mg per 5 mL (120 mL)
Robitussin® Cough & Chest Congestion DM: Guaifenesin 100 mg and dextromethorphan hydrobromide 10 mg per 5 mL (120 mL, 240 mL, 360 mL) [ethanol free; contains propylene glycol, sodium 7 mg/5 mL, sodium benzoate] [DSC]
Robitussin® Cough & Chest Congestion DM Max: Guaifenesin 200 mg and dextromethorphan hydrobromide 10 mg per 5 mL (120 mL, 240 mL) [ethanol free; contains propylene glycol, sodium 5 mg/5 mL, sodium benzoate] [DSC]
Robitussin® Cough & Chest Congestion Sugar-Free DM: Guaifenesin 100 mg and dextromethorphan hydrobromide 10 mg per 5 mL (120 mL) [ethanol free, sugar free; contains propylene glycol, sodium 4 mg/5 mL, sodium benzoate] [DSC]
Silexin: Guaifenesin 100 mg and dextromethorphan hydrobromide 10 mg per 5 mL (45 mL) [ethanol free, sugar free)]
Siltussin DM: Guaifenesin 100 mg and dextromethorphan hydrobromide 10 mg per 5 mL (120 mL, 240 mL, 480 mL) [strawberry flavor]
Siltussin DM DAS: Guaifenesin 100 mg and dextromethorphan hydrobromide 10 mg per 5 mL (120 mL) [dye free, ethanol free, sugar free; strawberry flavor]

Tablet, oral: Guaifenesin 1000 mg and dextromethorphan hydrobromide 60 mg; guaifenesin 1200 mg and dextromethorphan hydrobromide 60 mg
Allfen DM: Guaifenesin 400 mg and dextromethorphan hydrobromide 20 mg [DSC]
Silexin: Guaifenesin 100 mg and dextromethorphan hydrobromide 10 mg

Tablet, extended release, oral:
Mucinex® DM: Guaifenesin 600 mg and dextromethorphan hydrobromide 30 mg
Mucinex® DM Maximum Strength: Guaifenesin 1200 mg and dextromethorphan hydrobromide 60 mg

Tablet, sustained release, oral
Tussi-Bid®: Guaifenesin 1200 mg and dextromethorphan hydrobromide 60 mg [DSC]

Tablet, timed release, oral [scored]: Guaifenesin 1200 mg and dextromethorphan hydrobromide 60 mg
Guia-D: Guaifenesin 1000 mg and dextromethorphan hydrobromide 60 mg [dye free] [DSC]

◆ **Guaifenesin and Dyphylline** *see* Dyphylline and Guaifenesin *on page 568*

Guaifenesin and Phenylephrine

(gwye FEN e sin & fen il EF rin)

Brand Names: U.S. Ambi 10PEH/400GFN [OTC]; Crantex® [DSC]; Donatussin Drops [DSC]; Fenesin PE IR; Guiatex PE™ [DSC]; Liquibid® D-R [OTC]; Liquibid® PD-R [OTC]; Maxiphen [OTC] [DSC]; Medent®-PEI [OTC]; Mucinex® Cold [OTC]; Mucus Relief Sinus [OTC]; Nu-COPD [OTC]; OneTab™ Congestion & Cold [OTC]; Refenesen™ PE [OTC]; Rescon GG [OTC]; Sina-12X® [DSC]; Sudafed PE® Non-Drying Sinus [OTC]; Triaminic® Children's Chest & Nasal Congestion [OTC]

Index Terms Guaifenesin and Phenylephrine Tannate; Phenylephrine Hydrochloride and Guaifenesin

Pharmacologic Category Decongestant; Expectorant

Use Temporary relief of nasal congestion, sinusitis, rhinitis, and hay fever; temporary relief of cough associated with upper respiratory tract conditions, especially when associated with dry, nonproductive cough

Dosage Oral:
Children 2-5 years (Rescon GG): 2.5 mL every 4-6 hours; maximum: 10 mL/24 hours
Children 6-11 years:
Sina-12X tablet: One-half tablet every 12 hours; maximum: 1 tablet/24 hours
Rescon GG: 5 mL every 4-6 hours; maximum: 20 mL/24 hours
Children ≥12 years (Rescon GG, Sina-12X): Refer to adult dosing
Adults:
Rescon GG: 10 mL every 4-6 hours; maximum: 40 mL/24 hours
Sina-12X tablet: 1-2 tablets every 12 hours; maximum: 4 tablets/24 hours

Additional Information Complete prescribing information for this medication should be consulted for additional detail.

Dosage Forms Excipient information presented when available (limited, particularly for generics); consult specific product labeling. [DSC] = Discontinued product

Caplet, oral:
Fenesin PE IR: Guaifenesin 400 mg and phenylephrine hydrochloride 10 mg
OneTab™ Congestion & Cold: Guaifenesin 400 mg and phenylephrine hydrochloride 10 mg
Refenesen™ PE: Guaifenesin 400 mg and phenylephrine hydrochloride 10 mg
Sudafed PE® Non-Drying Sinus: Guaifenesin 200 mg and phenylephrine hydrochloride 5 mg

Liquid, oral:
Crantex®: Guaifenesin 100 mg and phenylephrine hydrochloride 7.5 mg per 5 mL (473 mL) [dye free, ethanol free, sugar free; contains propylene glycol, sodium benzoate; orange flavor]
Mucinex® Cold: Guaifenesin 100 mg and phenylephrine hydrochloride 2.5 mg per 5 mL (480 mL) [contains propylene glycol, sodium 3 mg/5 mL; mixed berry flavor]
Nu-COPD: Guaifenesin 200 mg and phenylephrine hydrochloride 10 mg per 5 mL (480 mL)
Rescon GG: Guaifenesin 100 mg and phenylephrine hydrochloride 5 mg per 5 mL (120 mL, 480 mL) [dye free, ethanol free; contains propylene glycol; wild cherry flavor]

Liquid, oral [drops]:
Donatussin Drops: Guaifenesin 20 mg and phenylephrine hydrochloride 1.5 mg per 1 mL (30 mL) [ethanol free, sugar free; raspberry flavor] [DSC]

Syrup, oral:
Guiatex PE™: Guaifenesin 200 mg and phenylephrine hydrochloride 5 mg per 5 mL (473 mL) [ethanol free, sugar free; contains propylene glycol, sodium benzoate; strawberry flavor] [DSC]
Triaminic® Children's Chest & Nasal Congestion: Guaifenesin 50 mg and phenylephrine hydrochloride 2.5 mg per 5 mL (118 mL) [contains benzoic acid, propylene glycol, sodium 3 mg/5 mL; tropical flavor]
Tablet, oral:
Ambi 10PEH/400GFN: Guaifenesin 400 mg and phenylephrine hydrochloride 10 mg
Liquibid® D-R: Guaifenesin 400 mg and phenylephrine hydrochloride 10 mg
Liquibid® PD-R: Guaifenesin 200 mg and phenylephrine hydrochloride 5 mg
Maxiphen: Guaifenesin 400 mg and phenylephrine hydrochloride 10 mg [DSC]
Medent®-PEI: Guaifenesin 400 mg and phenylephrine hydrochloride 10 mg
Mucus Relief Sinus: Guaifenesin 400 mg and phenylephrine hydrochloride 10 mg
Nu-COPD: Guaifenesin 400 mg and phenylephrine hydrochloride 10 mg
Sina-12X®: Guaifenesin 200 mg and phenylephrine tannate 25 mg [DSC]

◆ **Guaifenesin and Phenylephrine Tannate** *see* Guaifenesin and Phenylephrine *on page* 812

Guaifenesin and Pseudoephedrine

(gwye FEN e sin & soo doe e FED rin)

Brand Names: U.S. Ambifed [OTC] [DSC]; Ambifed-G [OTC]; Congestac® [OTC]; ExeFen-IR; Maxifed [OTC]; Maxifed-G [OTC]; Mucinex® D Maximum Strength [OTC]; Mucinex® D [OTC]; Refenesen Plus [OTC]; Respaire®-30 [DSC]; SudaTex-G [OTC]; Tenar™ PSE [DSC]

Brand Names: Canada Contac® Cold-Chest Congestion, Non Drowsy, Regular Strength; Entex® LA; Novahistex® Expectorant with Decongestant

Index Terms Pseudoephedrine and Guaifenesin

Pharmacologic Category Alpha/Beta Agonist; Expectorant

Use Temporary relief of nasal congestion and to help loosen phlegm and thin bronchial secretions in the treatment of cough

Dosage Oral:
Children 2-6 years (Maxifed-G®): One-third to 1/2 tablet every 12 hours (maximum: 1 tablet/12 hours)
Children 6-12 years:
Ambifed-G, Maxifed®: One-half caplet or tablet every 12 hours (maximum: 1 tablet/24 hours)
Congestac®: One-half caplet every 4-6 hours (maximum: 2 caplets/24 hours)
Maxifed-G®: One-half to 1 tablet every 12 hours (maximum: 2 tablets/24 hours)
Children >12 years and Adults:
Ambifed-G, Mucinex® D Maximum Strength: One tablet or capsule every 12 hours (maximum: 2 tablets or capsules in 24 hours)
Congestac®: One caplet every 4-6 hours (maximum: 4 caplets in 24 hours)
Maxifed-G®, Mucinex® D: 1-2 tablets or capsules every 12 hours (maximum: 4 tablets or capsules/24 hours)
Maxifed®: One to 1 1/2 tablets every 12 hours (maximum: 3 tablets/24 hours)

Additional Information Complete prescribing information for this medication should be consulted for additional detail.

Dosage Forms Excipient information presented when available (limited, particularly for generics); consult specific product labeling. [DSC] = Discontinued product
Caplet, oral:
Congestac®, Refenesen Plus: Guaifenesin 400 mg and pseudoephedrine hydrochloride 60 mg
Capsule, oral:
Respaire®-30: Guaifenesin 150 mg and pseudoephedrine hydrochloride 30 mg [DSC]
Liquid, oral:
Tenar™ PSE: Guaifenesin 200 mg and pseudoephedrine hydrochloride 40 mg per 5 mL (473 mL) [ethanol free; contains propylene glycol, sodium benzoate; grape flavor] [DSC]
Syrup, oral: Guaifenesin 200 mg and pseudoephedrine hydrochloride 40 mg per 5 mL (480 mL) [DSC]
Tablet, oral:
Ambifed: Guaifenesin 400 mg and pseudoephedrine hydrochloride 30 mg [DSC]
Ambifed-G: Guaifenesin 400 mg and pseudoephedrine hydrochloride 20 mg
ExeFen-IR: Guaifenesin 400 mg and pseudoephedrine hydrochloride 30 mg
Maxifed: Guaifenesin 400 mg and pseudoephedrine hydrochloride 60 mg
Maxifed-G, SudaTex-G: Guaifenesin 400 mg and pseudoephedrine hydrochloride 40 mg
Tablet, extended release, oral:
Mucinex® D: Guaifenesin 600 mg and pseudoephedrine hydrochloride 60 mg
Mucinex® D Maximum Strength: Guaifenesin 1200 mg and pseudoephedrine hydrochloride 120 mg

Guaifenesin, Pseudoephedrine, and Codeine

(gwye FEN e sin, soo doe e FED rin, & KOE deen)

Brand Names: U.S. Mytussin® DAC; Tricode® GF

Brand Names: Canada Benylin® 3.3 mg-D-E; Calmylin with Codeine

Index Terms Codeine, Guaifenesin, and Pseudoephedrine; Pseudoephedrine, Guaifenesin, and Codeine

Pharmacologic Category Antitussive/Decongestant/Expectorant

Use Temporarily relieves nasal congestion and controls cough associated with upper respiratory infections and related conditions (common cold, sinusitis, bronchitis, influenza)

Pregnancy Risk Factor C

Dosage Oral: **Note:** Products listed in dosage forms may contain differing amounts of active ingredients; however, the dosing volume and frequency are the same.
Children 6-12 years: 5 mL every 4 hours (maximum: 20 mL/24 hours)
Children >12 years and Adults: 10 mL every 4 hours (maximum: 40 mL/24 hours)

Additional Information Complete prescribing information for this medication should be consulted for additional detail.

Dosage Forms Excipient information presented when available (limited, particularly for generics); consult specific product labeling.
Syrup, oral: Guaifenesin 100 mg, pseudoephedrine hydrochloride 30 mg, and codeine phosphate 10 mg per 5 mL (473 mL)
Mytussin® DAC: Guaifenesin 100 mg, pseudoephedrine hydrochloride 30 mg, and codeine phosphate 10 mg per 5 mL (118 mL, 473 mL) [sugar free; contains alcohol 1.7%; strawberry-raspberry flavor]
Tricode® GF: Guaifenesin 200 mg, pseudoephedrine hydrochloride 30 mg, and codeine phosphate 8 mg per 5 mL (473 mL) [ethanol free, dye free, gluten free, sugar free; contains propylene glycol; grape flavor]

Controlled Substance C-V

Guaifenesin, Pseudoephedrine, and Dextromethorphan

(gwye FEN e sin, soo doe e FED rin, & deks troe meth OR fan)

Brand Names: U.S. Ambifed DM; Ambifed-G DM; Donatussin DM [DSC]; ExeFen-DMX; Maxifed DM; Maxifed DMX

Brand Names: Canada Balminil DM + Decongestant + Expectorant; Benylin® DM-D-E

Index Terms Dextromethorphan, Guaifenesin, and Pseudoephedrine; Pseudoephedrine, Dextromethorphan, and Guaifenesin

Pharmacologic Category Antitussive/Decongestant/Expectorant

Use Temporarily relieves nasal congestion and controls cough due to minor throat and bronchial irritation; helps loosen phlegm and thin bronchial secretions to make coughs more productive

Dosage Note: Also refer to specific product labeling.

Syrup (Donatussin DM):

Children 6-11 years: 2.5-5 mL every 4-6 hours, not to exceed 20 mL/24 hours

Children ≥12 years and Adults: 5-10 mL every 4-6 hours, not to exceed 40 mL/24 hours

Liquid (OTC labeling; Maxifed DM):

Children 6-11 years: 2.5 mL every 4-6 hours, not to exceed 15 mL/24 hours

Children ≥12 years and Adults: 5 mL every 4-6 hours, not to exceed 30 mL/24 hours

Tablet (OTC labeling; Ambifed-G DM, Maxifed DM):

Children 6-11 years: One-half tablet every 4-6 hours, not to exceed 3 tablets/24 hours

Children ≥12 years and Adults: One tablet every 4-6 hours, not to exceed 6 tablets/24 hours

Additional Information Complete prescribing information for this medication should be consulted for additional detail.

Dosage Forms Excipient information presented when available (limited, particularly for generics); consult specific product labeling.

Liquid, oral:

Maxifed DM: Guaifenesin 200 mg, pseudoephedrine hydrochloride 20 mg, and dextromethorphan hydrobromide 10 mg per 5 mL (473 mL) [sugar free, contains ethanol 0.1%, propylene glycol; orange cream flavor]

Syrup, oral:

Donatussin DM: Guaifenesin 150 mg, pseudoephedrine hydrochloride 30 mg, and dextromethorphan hydrobromide 15 mg per 5 mL (473 mL) [ethanol free, sugar free; contains propylene glycol; cool mint flavor]

Tablet, oral:

Ambifed DM: Guaifenesin 400 mg, pseudoephedrine hydrochloride 30 mg, and dextromethorphan hydrobromide 20 mg

Ambifed-G DM: Guaifenesin 400 mg, pseudoephedrine hydrochloride 20 mg, and dextromethorphan hydrobromide 20 mg

ExeFen-DMX: Guaifenesin 400 mg, pseudoephedrine hydrochloride 60 mg, and dextromethorphan hydrobromide 20 mg

Maxifed DM: Guaifenesin 400 mg, pseudoephedrine hydrochloride 40 mg, and dextromethorphan hydrobromide 20 mg

Maxifed DMX: Guaifenesin 400 mg, pseudoephedrine hydrochloride 60 mg, and dextromethorphan hydrobromide 20 mg

Guanabenz (GWAHN a benz)

Brand Names: Canada Wytensin®

Index Terms Guanabenz Acetate

Pharmacologic Category Alpha$_2$-Adrenergic Agonist

Use Management of hypertension

Pregnancy Risk Factor C

Dosage Adults: Oral: Initial: 4 mg twice daily; increase in increments of 4-8 mg/day every 1-2 weeks to a maximum of 32 mg twice daily.

Dosing adjustment in hepatic impairment: Probably necessary

Additional Information Complete prescribing information for this medication should be consulted for additional detail.

Dosage Forms Excipient information presented when available (limited, particularly for generics); consult specific product labeling. [DSC] = Discontinued product

Tablet, oral: 4 mg, 8 mg [DSC]

◆ **Guanabenz Acetate** *see* Guanabenz *on page 814*

GuanFACINE (GWAHN fa seen)

Brand Names: U.S. Intuniv™; Tenex®

Index Terms Guanfacine Hydrochloride

Pharmacologic Category Alpha$_2$-Adrenergic Agonist

Use

Tablet, immediate release: Management of hypertension

Tablet, extended release: Treatment of attention-deficit/hyperactivity disorder (ADHD) as monotherapy or adjunctive therapy to stimulants

Unlabeled Use Tic disorder; Tourette's syndrome

Pregnancy Risk Factor B

Dosage Oral:

Children ≥6 years and Adolescents: ADHD, monotherapy or adjunct to stimulants: Extended release (Intuniv™): Initial: 1 mg once daily; may adjust by increments no larger than 1 mg/week as tolerated, based on clinical response; maximum dose: 4 mg/day. **Note:** If patient misses 2 or more consecutive doses, repeat titration of dose should be considered.

Note: Clinical response is associated with doses of 0.05-0.08 mg/kg/day. Doses up to 0.12 mg/kg/day may provide additional benefit; however, doses >4 mg/day have not been evaluated.

Children ≥12 years and Adults: Hypertension:Immediate release: 1 mg usually at bedtime, may increase if needed at 3- to 4-week intervals; usual dose range (JNC 7): 0.5-2 mg once daily

Elderly: Hypertension: Consider lower initial doses and titrate to response (Aronow, 2011)

Dosage adjustment in renal impairment: No specific dosage adjustments are recommended by the manufacturer; consider using the lower end of the dosing range in patients with renal impairment.

Hemodialysis: Dialysis clearance is ~15% of total clearance; usual doses are recommended.

Dosage adjustment in hepatic impairment: No specific dosage adjustments are recommended by the manufacturer; however, dosage adjustments may be required.

Additional Information Complete prescribing information for this medication should be consulted for additional detail.

Dosage Forms Excipient information presented when available (limited, particularly for generics); consult specific product labeling.

Tablet, oral: 1 mg, 2 mg

Tenex®: 1 mg, 2 mg

Tablet, extended release, oral:

Intuniv™: 1 mg, 2 mg, 3 mg, 4 mg

◆ **Guanfacine Hydrochloride** *see* GuanFACINE *on page 814*

◆ **Guia-D [DSC]** *see* Guaifenesin and Dextromethorphan *on page 810*

- **Guiadrine™ DX [DSC]** *see* Guaifenesin and Dextromethorphan *on page 810*
- **Guiatex PE™ [DSC]** *see* Guaifenesin and Phenylephrine *on page 812*
- **GW506U78** *see* Nelarabine *on page 1184*
- **GW433908G** *see* Fosamprenavir *on page 756*
- **GW572016** *see* Lapatinib *on page 975*
- **GW786034** *see* Pazopanib *on page 1302*
- **Gynazole-1® [DSC]** *see* Butoconazole *on page 256*
- **Gynazole-1® (Can)** *see* Butoconazole *on page 256*
- **Gyne-Lotrimin® 3 [OTC]** *see* Clotrimazole (Topical) *on page 399*
- **Gyne-Lotrimin® 7 [OTC]** *see* Clotrimazole (Topical) *on page 399*
- **Gynol II® [OTC]** *see* Nonoxynol 9 *on page 1216*
- **Gynol II® Extra Strength [OTC]** *see* Nonoxynol 9 *on page 1216*
- **H1N1 Influenza Vaccine** *see* Influenza Virus Vaccine (Inactivated) *on page 897*
- **H1N1 Influenza Vaccine** *see* Influenza Virus Vaccine (Live/Attenuated) *on page 901*
- **h5G1.1** *see* Eculizumab *on page 570*
- **H5N1 Influenza Vaccine** *see* Influenza Virus Vaccine (H5N1) *on page 896*
- **Habitrol** *see* Nicotine *on page 1200*
- **Habitrol® (Can)** *see* Nicotine *on page 1200*

Haemophilus b Conjugate and Hepatitis B Vaccine

(he MOF i lus bee KON joo gate & hep a TYE tis bee vak SEEN)

Brand Names: U.S. Comvax®

Index Terms *Haemophilus* b (meningococcal protein conjugate) Conjugate Vaccine; Hepatitis B Vaccine (Recombinant); Hib Conjugate Vaccine; Hib-HepB

Pharmacologic Category Vaccine, Inactivated (Bacterial); Vaccine, Inactivated (Viral)

Additional Appendix Information

Immunization Recommendations *on page 1922*

Use

Immunization against invasive disease caused by *H. influenzae* type b and against infection caused by all known subtypes of hepatitis B virus in infants 6 weeks to 15 months of age born of hepatitis B surface antigen (HB_sAg)-negative mothers

Infants born of HB_sAg-positive mothers or mothers of unknown HB_sAg status should receive hepatitis B vaccine (recombinant) at birth and should complete the hepatitis B vaccination series given according to a particular schedule (refer to current ACIP recommendations).

Pregnancy Risk Factor C

Dosage Infants: I.M.: 0.5 mL/dose; one dose at 2, 4, and 12-15 months of age (total of 3 doses)

If the recommended schedule cannot be followed, the interval between the first two doses should be at least 6 weeks and the interval between the second and third dose should be as close as possible to 8-11 months. Minimum age for first dose is 6 weeks.

Modified Schedule: Children who receive one dose of hepatitis B vaccine at or shortly after birth may receive Comvax® on a schedule of 2, 4, and 12-15 months of age

Additional Information Complete prescribing information for this medication should be consulted for additional detail.

Dosage Forms Excipient information presented when available (limited, particularly for generics); consult specific product labeling.

Injection, suspension [preservative free]:

Comvax®: *Haemophilus* b capsular polysaccharide 7.5 mcg (bound to *Neisseria meningitides* OMPC 125 mcg) and hepatitis B surface antigen 5 mcg per 0.5 mL (0.5 mL) [contains aluminum; contains natural rubber/natural latex in packaging]

- ***Haemophilus* B Conjugate (Hib)** *see* Diphtheria and Tetanus Toxoids, Acellular Pertussis, Poliovirus and *Haemophilus* b Conjugate Vaccine *on page 522*

Haemophilus b Conjugate Vaccine

(he MOF fi lus bee KON joo gate vak SEEN)

Brand Names: U.S. ActHIB®; Hiberix®; PedvaxHIB®

Brand Names: Canada ActHIB®; PedvaxHIB®

Index Terms *Haemophilus* b Oligosaccharide Conjugate Vaccine; *Haemophilus* b Polysaccharide Vaccine; Diphtheria Toxoid Conjugate; HbCV; Hib; Hib Conjugate Vaccine; Hib Polysaccharide Conjugate; PRP-OMP; PRP-T

Pharmacologic Category Vaccine, Inactivated (Bacterial)

Additional Appendix Information

Immunization Recommendations *on page 1922*

Use Routine immunization of children against invasive disease caused by *H. influenzae* type b

The Advisory Committee on Immunization Practices (ACIP) recommends routine vaccination of all children through age 59 months. Efficacy data are not available for use in older children and adults with chronic conditions associated with an increased risk of Hib disease. However, a single dose may also be considered for older children, adolescents, and adults who did not receive the childhood series and who have a chronic condition associated with an increased risk of Hib disease (eg, splenectomy, sickle cell disease, leukemia, HIV infection).

Pregnancy Risk Factor C

Pregnancy Considerations Reproduction studies have not been conducted.

Contraindications Hypersensitivity to *Haemophilus* b polysaccharide vaccine or any component of the formulation

Warnings/Precautions If used in persons with malignancies or those receiving immunosuppressive therapy or who are otherwise immunocompromised, the expected immune response may not be obtained; may be used in patients with HIV infection. In general, household and close contacts of persons with altered immunocompetence may receive all age appropriate vaccines. The decision to administer or delay vaccination because of current or recent febrile illness depends on the severity of symptoms and the etiology of the disease. Immunization should be delayed during the course of an acute febrile illness. Use caution in children with coagulation disorders (including thrombocytopenia) where intramuscular injections should not be used. Epinephrine 1:1000 should be readily available. Patients who develop symptoms suggestive of hypersensitivity after an injection should not receive further injections of the vaccine.

Children in whom DTP or DT vaccination is deferred: The carrier proteins used in PRP-T (ActHIB®, Hiberix®), but not PRP-OMP (PedvaxHIB®), are chemically and immunologically related to toxoids contained in DTP vaccine. Earlier or simultaneous vaccination with diphtheria or tetanus toxoids may be required to elicit an optimal anti-PRP antibody response. In contrast, the immunogenicity of

PRP-OMP is not affected by vaccination with DTP. In infants in whom DTP or DT vaccination is deferred, PRP-OMP may be advantageous for *Haemophilus influenzae* type b vaccination. Immunization with Hiberix® is not a substitute for routine tetanus immunization.

Hiberix®: Use with caution in patients with history of Guillain-Barré syndrome (GBS); carefully consider risks and benefits to vaccination in patients known to have experienced GBS within 6 weeks following previous influenza vaccination.

In order to maximize vaccination rates, the ACIP recommends simultaneous administration of all age-appropriate vaccines (live or inactivated) for which a person is eligible at a single clinic visit, unless contraindications exist. The use of combination vaccines is generally preferred over separate injections, taking into consideration provider assessment, patient preference, and adverse events. When using combination vaccines, the minimum age for administration is the oldest minimum age for any individual component; the minimum interval between dosing is the greatest minimum interval between any individual component.

Packaging may contain latex. Some products may contain lactose.

Adverse Reactions All serious adverse reactions must be reported to the U.S. Department of Health and Human Services (DHHS) Vaccine Adverse Event Reporting System (VAERS) 1-800-822-7967 or online at https://vaers.hhs.gov/esub/index. In Canada, adverse reactions may be reported to local provincial/territorial health agencies or to the Vaccine Safety Section at Public Health Agency of Canada (1-866-844-0018).

Frequency not defined:

Central nervous system: Crying (unusual, high pitched, prolonged), fever, fussiness, irritability, pain, restlessness, sleepiness

Dermatologic: Rash

Gastrointestinal: Anorexia, diarrhea, vomiting

Local: Injection site: Erythema, induration, pain, soreness, swelling

Otic: Otitis media

Respiratory: Upper respiratory tract infection

Postmarketing and/or case reports: Allergic reactions, anaphylactoid reactions, angioedema, apnea, febrile seizure, Guillain-Barré syndrome, hypersensitivity, hyporesponsive episodes, hypotonia, injection site abscess (sterile), lethargy, lymphadenopathy, malaise, mass, pneumonia, seizure, swelling (extensive) of the injected limb, syncope, urticaria, vasovagal response

Drug Interactions

Metabolism/Transport Effects None known.

Avoid Concomitant Use There are no known interactions where it is recommended to avoid concomitant use.

Increased Effect/Toxicity There are no known significant interactions involving an increase in effect.

Decreased Effect

The levels/effects of Haemophilus b Conjugate Vaccine may be decreased by: Belimumab; Fingolimod; Immunosuppressants

Stability Store under refrigeration at 2°C to 8°C (36°F to 46°F); do not freeze.

ActHIB®: Use within 24 hours following reconstitution with saline. Use within 30 minutes following reconstitution with Tripedia®.

Hiberix®: Prior to reconstitution, store powder under refrigeration at 2°C to 8°C (36°F to 46°F). Protect from light. Diluent may be stored under refrigeration or at room temperature. Do not freeze, discard diluent if frozen. Dilute with provided saline diluent only. Transfer entire contents of prefilled syringe containing diluent into the vial; with needle still inserted, shake vigorously until it becomes a clear, colorless solution. Withdraw entire contents of vial (~0.5 mL) for administration. If not used immediately after reconstitution, may store under refrigeration for up to 24 hours. Shake well prior to use. Discard any unused portion.

Mechanism of Action Stimulates production of anticapsular antibodies and provides active immunity to *Haemophilus influenzae* type b

Pharmacodynamics/Kinetics Seroconversion following one dose of Hib vaccine for children 18 months or 24 months of age or older is 75% to 90%, respectively.

Onset of action: Serum antibody response: 1-2 weeks

Duration: Immunity: 1.5 years

Dosage I.M.:

Children: 0.5 mL as a single dose should be administered to previously unvaccinated children according to one of the following "brand-specific" schedules; number of doses in series is dependent upon age at first dose. ActHIB® and PedvaxHIB® are approved for a complete vaccine series; Hiberix® is approved only as a booster (final) dose in children who have received primary immunization.

ActHIB®: *Age at first dose:*

2 months of age: Immunization consists of 3 doses (0.5 mL/dose) administered at 2-, 4-, and 6 months of age (reconstitute with provided diluent). A booster dose is given at 15-18 months of age (may reconstitute with provided diluent or Tripedia® vaccine).

7-11 months of age: Two doses (0.5 mL/dose) administered 8 weeks apart, with a booster dose at 15-18 months of age

12-14 months of age: One dose (0.5 mL) followed by a booster dose 2 months later

PedvaxHIB®: *Age at first dose:*

2-10 months of age: Two doses (0.5 mL/dose) administered 2 months apart; booster dose at 12-15 months of age

11-14 months of age: Two doses (0.5 mL/dose) administered 2 months apart

15-71 months of age: One 0.5 mL dose

Hiberix®: 15-59 months: One 0.5 mL booster dose (per manufacturer). The ACIP recommends booster dose administration at 12-15 months

Children ≥5 years of age, Adolescents, and Adults who have not received the childhood Hib series **and** are at increased risk for invasive Hib disease due to certain chronic conditions (eg, sickle cell disease, leukemia, HIV infection, or splenectomy) (ACIP recommendations): One dose (0.5 mL); may use any of the Hib conjugate vaccines

Administration For I.M. administration; do not inject I.V.

Hiberix®: Shake well prior to use. Administer into the anterolateral thigh or deltoid. If Hiberix® is inadvertently administered during the primary vaccination series, the dose can be counted as a valid PRP-T dose that does not need to be repeated if administered according to schedule. In this case, a total of 3 doses completes the primary series.

ActHIB®, PedvaxHIB®: Shake well prior to use. Administer into the anterolateral thigh or deltoid. Do not administer into buttocks due to potential risk of injury to sciatic nerve.

For patients at risk of hemorrhage following intramuscular injection, the ACIP recommends "it should be administered intramuscularly if, in the opinion of the physician familiar with the patients bleeding risk, the vaccine can be administered by this route with reasonable safety. If the patient receives antihemophilia or other similar therapy, intramuscular vaccination can be scheduled shortly after such therapy is administered. A fine needle (23 gauge or smaller) can be used for the vaccination and firm pressure applied to the site (without rubbing) for at least 2 minutes.

The patient should be instructed concerning the risk of hematoma from the injection." Patients on anticoagulant therapy should be considered to have the same bleeding risks and treated as those with clotting factor disorders (CDC, 2011).

Simultaneous administration of vaccines helps ensure the patients will be fully vaccinated by the appropriate age. Simultaneous administration of vaccines is defined as administering >1 vaccine on the same day at different anatomic sites. The use of licensed combination vaccines is generally preferred over separate injections of the equivalent components. Separate vaccines should not be combined in the same syringe unless indicated by product specific labeling. Separate needles and syringes should be used for each injection. The ACIP prefers each dose of a specific vaccine in a series come from the same manufacturer when possible. Adolescents and adults should be vaccinated while seated or lying down. In general, preterm infants should be vaccinated at the same chronological age as full-term infants (CDC, 2011).

Antipyretics have not been shown to prevent febrile seizures. Antipyretics may be used to treat fever or discomfort following vaccination (CDC, 2011). One study reported that routine prophylactic administration of acetaminophen to prevent fever prior to vaccination decreased the immune response of some vaccines; the clinical significance of this reduction in immune response has not been established (Prymula, 2009).

Test Interactions May interfere with interpretation of urine antigen detection tests; antigenuria may occur up to 2 weeks following immunization

Additional Information Federal law requires that the name of medication, date of administration, the vaccine manufacturer, lot number of vaccine, and the administering person's name, title, and address be entered into the patient's permanent medical record.

The conjugate vaccines currently available consist of *Haemophilus influenzae* type b (Hib) capsular polysaccharide (also referred to as PRP) linked to a carrier protein. PedvaxHIB® (PRP-OMP) is linked to the outer membrane protein complex from *Neisseria meningitidis*. ActHIB® and Hiberix® (PRP-T) use tetanus toxoid conjugate as the carrier protein.

Dosage Forms Excipient information presented when available (limited, particularly for generics); consult specific product labeling.

Injection, powder for reconstitution [preservative free]:

ActHIB® *Haemophilus* b capsular polysaccharide 10 mcg [bound to tetanus toxoid 24 mcg] per 0.5 mL [contains sucrose; may be reconstituted with provided diluent (forms solution; contains natural rubber/natural latex in packaging) or Tripedia® (forms suspension)]

Hiberix®: *Haemophilus* b capsular polysaccharide 10 mcg [bound to tetanus toxoid 25 mcg] per 0.5 mL (0.5 mL) [contains lactose 12.6 mg]

Injection, suspension:

PedvaxHIB®: *Haemophilus* b capsular polysaccharide 7.5 mcg [bound to *Neisseria meningitidis* OMPC 125 mcg] per 0.5 mL (0.5 mL) [contains aluminum; natural rubber/natural latex in packaging]

- ***Haemophilus* b (meningococcal protein conjugate) Conjugate Vaccine** see *Haemophilus* b Conjugate and Hepatitis B Vaccine *on page 815*
- ***Haemophilus* b Oligosaccharide Conjugate Vaccine** *see Haemophilus* b Conjugate Vaccine *on page 815*
- ***Haemophilus* B Polysaccharide** *see* Diphtheria and Tetanus Toxoids, Acellular Pertussis, Poliovirus and *Haemophilus* b Conjugate Vaccine *on page 522*
- ***Haemophilus* b Polysaccharide Vaccine** *see Haemophilus* b Conjugate Vaccine *on page 815*
- ***Haemophilus influenzae* b Conjugate Vaccine and Diphtheria, Tetanus Toxoids, and Acellular Pertussis Vaccine** *see* Diphtheria and Tetanus Toxoids, Acellular Pertussis, and *Haemophilus influenzae* b Conjugate Vaccine *on page 522*
- **Halaven™** *see* Eribulin *on page 611*

Halcinonide (hal SIN oh nide)

Brand Names: U.S. Halog®
Brand Names: Canada Halog®
Pharmacologic Category Corticosteroid, Topical
Additional Appendix Information
Corticosteroids *on page 1888*

Use Inflammation of corticosteroid-responsive dermatoses [high potency topical corticosteroid]

Pregnancy Risk Factor C

Dosage Children and Adults: Topical: Steroid-responsive dermatoses: Apply sparingly 1-3 times/day, occlusive dressing may be used for severe or resistant dermatoses; a thin film is effective; do not overuse. Therapy should be discontinued when control is achieved; if no improvement is seen, reassessment of diagnosis may be necessary.

Additional Information Complete prescribing information for this medication should be consulted for additional detail.

Dosage Forms Excipient information presented when available (limited, particularly for generics); consult specific product labeling.

Cream, topical:
Halog®: 0.1% (30 g, 60 g)
Ointment, topical:
Halog®: 0.1% (30 g, 60 g)

- **Halcion®** *see* Triazolam *on page 1736*
- **Haldol®** *see* Haloperidol *on page 818*
- **Haldol® Decanoate** *see* Haloperidol *on page 818*
- **Haley's M-O** *see* Magnesium Hydroxide and Mineral Oil *on page 1046*
- **Halfprin® [OTC]** *see* Aspirin *on page 154*
- **Halichondrin B Analog** *see* Eribulin *on page 611*

Halobetasol (hal oh BAY ta sol)

Brand Names: U.S. Ultravate®
Brand Names: Canada Ultravate®
Index Terms Halobetasol Propionate
Pharmacologic Category Corticosteroid, Topical
Additional Appendix Information
Corticosteroids *on page 1888*

Use Relief of inflammatory and pruritic manifestations of corticosteroid-response dermatoses [super high potency topical corticosteroid]

Pregnancy Risk Factor C

Dosage Children ≥12 years and Adults: Topical:

Inflammatory and pruritic manifestations (dental use):
Cream: Apply sparingly to lesion twice daily. Treatment should not exceed 2 consecutive weeks and total dosage should not exceed 50 g/week. Therapy should be discontinued when control is achieved; if no improvement is seen, reassessment of diagnosis may be necessary.

Steroid-responsive dermatoses: Apply sparingly to skin twice daily, rub in gently and completely; treatment should not exceed 2 consecutive weeks and total dosage should not exceed 50 g/week. Therapy should be discontinued when control is achieved; if no improvement is seen, reassessment of diagnosis may be necessary.

Additional Information Complete prescribing information for this medication should be consulted for additional detail.

Dosage Forms Excipient information presented when available (limited, particularly for generics); consult specific product labeling.

Cream, topical, as propionate: 0.05% (15 g, 50 g)
 Ultravate®: 0.05% (15 g, 50 g)
Ointment, topical, as propionate: 0.05% (15 g, 50 g)
 Ultravate®: 0.05% (15 g, 50 g)

◆ **Halobetasol Propionate** *see* Halobetasol *on page 817*

◆ **Halog®** *see* Halcinonide *on page 817*

Haloperidol (ha loe PER i dole)

Brand Names: U.S. Haldol®; Haldol® Decanoate

Brand Names: Canada Apo-Haloperidol LA®; Apo-Haloperidol®; Haloperidol Injection, USP; Haloperidol Long Acting; Haloperidol-LA; Haloperidol-LA Omega; Novo-Peridol; PMS-Haloperidol; PMS-Haloperidol LA

Index Terms Haloperidol Decanoate; Haloperidol Lactate

Pharmacologic Category Antipsychotic Agent, Typical

Additional Appendix Information

Antipsychotic Agents *on page 1880*

Use Management of schizophrenia; control of tics and vocal utterances of Tourette's disorder in children and adults; severe behavioral problems in children

Unlabeled Use Treatment of nonschizophrenia psychosis; may be used for the emergency sedation of severely-agitated or delirious patients; adjunctive treatment of ethanol dependence; postoperative nausea and vomiting (alternative therapy); psychosis/agitation related to Alzheimer's dementia

Pregnancy Risk Factor C

Pregnancy Considerations Adverse events were observed in animal studies. Haloperidol crosses the placenta. There are case reports of limb malformations following first trimester exposure in humans. Antipsychotic use during the third trimester of pregnancy has a risk for abnormal muscle movements (extrapyramidal symptoms [EPS]) and withdrawal symptoms in newborns following delivery. Symptoms in the newborn may include agitation, feeding disorder, hypertonia, hypotonia, respiratory distress, somnolence, and tremor; these effects may be self-limiting or require hospitalization.

Lactation Enters breast milk/not recommended (AAP rates "of concern"; AAP 2001 update pending)

Contraindications Hypersensitivity to haloperidol or any component of the formulation; Parkinson's disease; severe CNS depression; coma

Warnings/Precautions [U.S. Boxed Warning]: Elderly patients with dementia-related psychosis treated with antipsychotics are at an increased risk of death compared to placebo. Most deaths appeared to be either cardiovascular (eg, heart failure, sudden death) or infectious (eg, pneumonia) in nature. Haloperidol is not approved for the treatment of dementia-related psychosis. Hypotension may occur, particularly with parenteral administration. Although the short-acting form (lactate) is used clinically, the I.V. use of the injection is not an FDA-approved route of administration; the decanoate form should never be administered intravenously.

May alter cardiac conduction and prolong QT interval; life-threatening arrhythmias have occurred with therapeutic doses of antipsychotics but risk may be increased with doses exceeding recommendations and/or intravenous administration (unlabeled route). Use caution or avoid use in patients with electrolyte abnormalities (eg, hypokalemia, hypomagnesemia), hypothyroidism, familial long QT syndrome, concomitant medications which may augment QT prolongation, or any underlying cardiac abnormality which may also potentiate risk. Monitor ECG closely for dose-related QT effects. Adverse effects of decanoate may be prolonged. Avoid in thyrotoxicosis.

Leukopenia, neutropenia, and agranulocytosis (sometimes fatal) have been reported in clinical trials and postmarketing reports with antipsychotic use; presence of risk factors (eg, pre-existing low WBC or history of drug-induced leuko-/neutropenia) should prompt periodic blood count assessment. Discontinue therapy at first signs of blood dyscrasias or if absolute neutrophil count <1000/mm^3.

May be sedating, use with caution in disorders where CNS depression is a feature. Effects may be potentiated when used with other sedative drugs or ethanol. Caution in patients with severe cardiovascular disease, predisposition to seizures, subcortical brain damage, or renal disease. Esophageal dysmotility and aspiration have been associated with antipsychotic use - use with caution in patients at risk of pneumonia (eg, Alzheimer's disease). Use associated with increased prolactin levels; clinical significance of hyperprolactinemia in patients with breast cancer or other prolactin-dependent tumors is unknown. May alter temperature regulation or mask toxicity of other drugs due to antiemetic effects. May cause orthostatic hypotension; use with caution in patients at risk of this effect or those who would tolerate transient hypotensive episodes (cerebrovascular disease, cardiovascular disease, or other medications which may predispose). Some tablets contain tartrazine. Antipsychotics have been associated with pigmentary retinopathy.

May cause anticholinergic effects (confusion, agitation, constipation, xerostomia, blurred vision, urinary retention). Therefore, they should be used with caution in patients with decreased gastrointestinal motility, urinary retention, BPH, xerostomia, or visual problems. Conditions which also may be exacerbated by cholinergic blockade include narrow-angle glaucoma and worsening of myasthenia gravis. Relative to other neuroleptics, haloperidol has a low potency of cholinergic blockade.

May cause extrapyramidal symptoms (EPS), including pseudoparkinsonism, acute dystonic reactions, akathisia, and tardive dyskinesia. Risk of dystonia (and possibly other EPS) may be greater with increased doses, use of conventional antipsychotics, males, and younger patients. May be associated with neuroleptic malignant syndrome (NMS). Use with caution in the elderly.

Adverse Reactions Frequency not defined.

Cardiovascular: Abnormal T waves with prolonged ventricular repolarization, arrhythmia, hyper-/hypotension, QT prolongation, sudden death, tachycardia, torsade de pointes

Central nervous system: Agitation, akathisia, altered central temperature regulation, anxiety, confusion, depression, drowsiness, dystonic reactions, euphoria, extrapyramidal reactions, headache, insomnia, lethargy, neuroleptic malignant syndrome (NMS), pseudoparkinsonian signs and symptoms, restlessness, seizure, tardive dyskinesia, tardive dystonia, vertigo

Dermatologic: Alopecia, contact dermatitis, hyperpigmentation, photosensitivity (rare), pruritus, rash

Endocrine & metabolic: Amenorrhea, breast engorgement, galactorrhea, gynecomastia, hyper-/hypoglycemia, hyponatremia, lactation, mastalgia, menstrual irregularities, sexual dysfunction

Gastrointestinal: Anorexia, constipation, diarrhea, dyspepsia, hypersalivation, nausea, vomiting, xerostomia

Genitourinary: Priapism, urinary retention

Hematologic: Cholestatic jaundice, obstructive jaundice

Ocular: Blurred vision

Respiratory: Bronchospasm, laryngospasm

Miscellaneous: Diaphoresis, heat stroke

Drug Interactions

Metabolism/Transport Effects **Substrate** of CYP1A2 (minor), CYP2D6 (major), CYP3A4 (major); **Note:** Assignment of Major/Minor substrate status based on clinically relevant drug interaction potential; **Inhibits** CYP2D6 (moderate), CYP3A4 (moderate)

Avoid Concomitant Use

Avoid concomitant use of Haloperidol with any of the following: Artemether; Conivaptan; Dronedarone; Lumefantrine; Metoclopramide; Nilotinib; Pimozide; QUEtiapine; QuiNINE; Tetrabenazine; Thioridazine; Tolvaptan; Toremifene; Vandetanib; Vemurafenib; Ziprasidone

Increased Effect/Toxicity

Haloperidol may increase the levels/effects of: Alcohol (Ethyl); Anticholinergics; Anti-Parkinson's Agents (Dopamine Agonist); ARIPiprazole; Budesonide (Systemic, Oral Inhalation); ChlorproMAZINE; CNS Depressants; Colchicine; CYP2D6 Substrates; CYP3A4 Substrates; Dronedarone; Eplerenone; Everolimus; FentaNYL; Fesoterodine; Lurasidone; Methylphenidate; Nebivolol; Pimecrolimus; Pimozide; QTc-Prolonging Agents; QuiNIDine; QuiNINE; Salmeterol; Saxagliptin; Serotonin Modulators; Tamoxifen; Tetrabenazine; Thioridazine; Tolvaptan; Toremifene; Vandetanib; Vemurafenib; Ziprasidone

The levels/effects of Haloperidol may be increased by: Abiraterone Acetate; Acetylcholinesterase Inhibitors (Central); Alfuzosin; Artemether; Chloroquine; ChlorproMAZINE; Ciprofloxacin; Ciprofloxacin (Systemic); Conivaptan; CYP2D6 Inhibitors (Moderate); CYP2D6 Inhibitors (Strong); CYP3A4 Inhibitors (Moderate); CYP3A4 Inhibitors (Strong); Darunavir; FLUoxetine; FluvoxaMINE; Gadobutrol; HydrOXYzine; Indacaterol; Lithium formulations; Lumefantrine; Methylphenidate; Metoclopramide; Nilotinib; Nonsteroidal Anti-Inflammatory Agents; Pramlintide; QUEtiapine; QuiNIDine; QuiNINE; Tetrabenazine

Decreased Effect

Haloperidol may decrease the levels/effects of: Amphetamines; Codeine; Quinagolide

The levels/effects of Haloperidol may be decreased by: Anti-Parkinson's Agents (Dopamine Agonist); CarBAMazepine; CYP3A4 Inducers (Strong); Cyproterone; Deferasirox; Glycopyrrolate; Lithium formulations; Peginterferon Alfa-2b; Tocilizumab

Ethanol/Nutrition/Herb Interactions

Ethanol: May increase CNS depression; monitor for increased effects with coadministration. Caution patients about effects.

Herb/Nutraceutical: Avoid valerian, St John's wort, kava kava, gotu kola (may increase CNS depression).

Stability

Protect oral dosage forms from light.

Haloperidol lactate injection should be stored at controlled room temperature; do not freeze or expose to temperatures >40°C. Protect from light; exposure to light may cause discoloration and the development of a grayish-red precipitate over several weeks.

Haloperidol lactate may be administered IVPB or I.V. infusion in D_5W solutions. NS solutions should not be used due to reports of decreased stability and incompatibility.

Standardized dose: 0.5-100 mg/50-100 mL D_5W.

Stability of standardized solutions is 38 days at room temperature (24°C).

Mechanism of Action Haloperidol is a butyrophenone antipsychotic which blocks postsynaptic mesolimbic dopaminergic D_1 and D_2 receptors in the brain; depresses the release of hypothalamic and hypophyseal hormones; believed to depress the reticular activating system thus affecting basal metabolism, body temperature, wakefulness, vasomotor tone, and emesis

Pharmacodynamics/Kinetics

Onset of action: Sedation: I.M., I.V.: 30-60 minutes

Duration: Decanoate: 2-4 weeks

Distribution: V_d: 8-18 L/kg

Protein binding: 90%

Metabolism: Hepatic: 50% to 60% glucuronidation (inactive); 23% CYP3A4-mediated reduction to inactive metabolites (some back-oxidation to haloperidol); and 20% to 30% CYP3A4-mediated N-dealkylation, including minor oxidation pathway to toxic pyridinium derivative (Kudo, 1999)

Bioavailability: Oral: 60% to 70%

Half-life elimination: 18 hours; Decanoate: 21 days

Time to peak, serum: Oral: 2-6 hours; I.M.: 20 minutes; Decanoate: 7 days

Excretion: Urine (30%, 1% as unchanged drug); feces (15%)

Dosage

Children: 3-12 years (15-40 kg): Oral:
- Initial: 0.5 mg/day given in 2-3 divided doses; increase by 0.5 mg every 5-7 days; maximum: 0.15 mg/kg/day
- Usual maintenance:
  - Nonpsychotic disorders, Tourette's disorder: 0.05-0.075 mg/kg/day in 2-3 divided doses
  - Psychotic disorders: 0.05-0.15 mg/kg/day in 2-3 divided doses

Children 6-12 years: Sedation/psychotic disorders: I.M. (as lactate): 1-3 mg/dose every 4-8 hours to a maximum of 0.15 mg/kg/day; convert to oral therapy as soon as able

Adults:
- Psychosis:
  - Oral: 0.5-5 mg 2-3 times/day; usual maximum: 30 mg/day
  - I.M. (as lactate): 2-5 mg every 4-8 hours as needed
  - I.M. (as decanoate): Initial: 10-20 times the daily oral dose administered at 4-week intervals
  - Maintenance dose: 10-15 times initial oral dose; used to stabilize psychiatric symptoms
- Delirium in the intensive care unit (unlabeled use, unlabeled route; Jacobi, 2002): I.V.: Initial: 2-10 mg depending on degree of agitation; if inadequate response, may repeat bolus dose (with sequential doubling of initial bolus dose) every 15-30 minutes until calm achieved, then administer 25% of the last bolus dose every 6 hours; monitor ECG and QT_c interval. After the patient is controlled, haloperidol therapy should be tapered over several days. **Note:** QT_c prolongation may occur with cumulative doses ≥35 mg and torsade de pointes has been reported with single doses of ≥20 mg. The optimal dose and regimen of haloperidol for the treatment of severe agitation and/or delirium has not been established.
- Rapid tranquilization of severely-agitated patient (unlabeled use): Administer every 30-60 minutes:
  - Oral: 5-10 mg
  - I.M. (as lactate): 5 mg
  - Average total dose (oral or I.M.) for tranquilization: 10-20 mg
- Postoperative nausea and vomiting (PONV) (unlabeled use): I.M., I.V.: 0.5-2 mg (Gan, 2007)

Elderly: Nonpsychotic patient, dementia behavior (unlabeled use): Initial: Oral: 0.25-0.5 mg 1-2 times/day; increase dose at 4- to 7-day intervals by 0.25-0.5 mg/day; increase dosing intervals (twice daily, 3 times/day, etc) as necessary to control response or side effects

Hemodialysis/peritoneal dialysis: Supplemental dose is not necessary

Administration

Injection oil (decanoate): The decanoate injectable formulation should be administered I.M. only, **do not administer decanoate I.V.**

Injection solution (lactate): The lactate injectable formulation may be administered I.V. (unlabeled route) or I.M.
Oral solution (lactate): Dilute the oral concentrate with water or juice before administration. Avoid skin contact with oral solution; may cause contact dermatitis.

Monitoring Parameters Vital signs; lipid profile, fasting blood glucose/Hgb A_{1c}; BMI; mental status, abnormal involuntary movement scale (AIMS), extrapyramidal symptoms (EPS); ECG (with off-label intravenous administration)

Reference Range

Therapeutic: 5-20 ng/mL (SI: 10-40 nmol/L) (psychotic disorders - less for Tourette's and mania)
Toxic: >42 ng/mL (SI: >84 nmol/L)

Dosage Forms Excipient information presented when available (limited, particularly for generics); consult specific product labeling.

Injection, oil, as decanoate [strength expressed as base]: 50 mg/mL (1 mL, 5 mL); 100 mg/mL (1 mL, 5 mL)
Haldol® Decanoate: 50 mg/mL (1 mL); 100 mg/mL (1 mL) [contains benzyl alcohol, sesame oil]
Injection, solution, as lactate [strength expressed as base]: 5 mg/mL (1 mL, 10 mL)
Haldol®: 5 mg/mL (1 mL)
Solution, oral, as lactate [strength expressed as base, concentrate]: 2 mg/mL (5 mL, 15 mL, 120 mL)
Tablet, oral: 0.5 mg, 1 mg, 2 mg, 5 mg, 10 mg, 20 mg

- ◆ **Haloperidol Decanoate** *see* Haloperidol *on page 818*
- ◆ **Haloperidol Injection, USP (Can)** *see* Haloperidol *on page 818*
- ◆ **Haloperidol-LA (Can)** *see* Haloperidol *on page 818*
- ◆ **Haloperidol Lactate** *see* Haloperidol *on page 818*
- ◆ **Haloperidol-LA Omega (Can)** *see* Haloperidol *on page 818*
- ◆ **Haloperidol Long Acting (Can)** *see* Haloperidol *on page 818*
- ◆ **Harkoseride** *see* Lacosamide *on page 963*
- ◆ **Havrix®** *see* Hepatitis A Vaccine *on page 824*
- ◆ **HAVRIX® (Can)** *see* Hepatitis A Vaccine *on page 824*
- ◆ **Havrix® and Engerix-B®** *see* Hepatitis A and Hepatitis B Recombinant Vaccine *on page 824*
- ◆ **HbCV** *see Haemophilus* b Conjugate Vaccine *on page 815*
- ◆ **HBIG** *see* Hepatitis B Immune Globulin (Human) *on page 826*
- ◆ **hBNP** *see* Nesiritide *on page 1191*
- ◆ **hCG** *see* Chorionic Gonadotropin (Human) *on page 352*
- ◆ **HCTZ (error-prone abbreviation)** *see* Hydrochlorothiazide *on page 835*
- ◆ **HDA® Toothache [OTC]** *see* Benzocaine *on page 202*
- ◆ **HDCV** *see* Rabies Vaccine *on page 1453*
- ◆ **Head & Shoulders® Clinical Strength [OTC]** *see* Selenium Sulfide *on page 1547*
- ◆ **Healon® (Can)** *see* Hyaluronate and Derivatives *on page 831*
- ◆ **Healon GV® (Can)** *see* Hyaluronate and Derivatives *on page 831*
- ◆ **Heartburn Relief [OTC]** *see* Famotidine *on page 688*
- ◆ **Heartburn Relief Maximum Strength [OTC]** *see* Famotidine *on page 688*
- ◆ **Heather** *see* Norethindrone *on page 1217*
- ◆ **Hectorol®** *see* Doxercalciferol *on page 552*
- ◆ **Helixate® FS** *see* Antihemophilic Factor (Recombinant) *on page 127*
- ◆ **Hemabate®** *see* Carboprost Tromethamine *on page 290*
- ◆ **Hemocyte® [OTC]** *see* Ferrous Fumarate *on page 706*
- ◆ **Hemofil M** *see* Antihemophilic Factor (Human) *on page 125*
- ◆ **Hemorrhoidal HC** *see* Hydrocortisone (Topical) *on page 841*
- ◆ **Hemril® -30** *see* Hydrocortisone (Topical) *on page 841*
- ◆ **HepA** *see* Hepatitis A Vaccine *on page 824*
- ◆ **HepaGam B®** *see* Hepatitis B Immune Globulin (Human) *on page 826*
- ◆ **HepaGam B™ (Can)** *see* Hepatitis B Immune Globulin (Human) *on page 826*
- ◆ **HepA-HepB** *see* Hepatitis A and Hepatitis B Recombinant Vaccine *on page 824*
- ◆ **Hepalean® (Can)** *see* Heparin *on page 820*
- ◆ **Hepalean® Leo (Can)** *see* Heparin *on page 820*
- ◆ **Hepalean®-LOK (Can)** *see* Heparin *on page 820*

Heparin (HEP a rin)

Brand Names: U.S. Hep-Lock; Hep-Lock U/P; Hep-Flush®-10

Brand Names: Canada Hepalean®; Hepalean® Leo; Hepalean®-LOK

Index Terms Heparin Calcium; Heparin Lock Flush; Heparin Sodium

Pharmacologic Category Anticoagulant

Use Prophylaxis and treatment of thromboembolic disorders; as an anticoagulant for extracorporeal and dialysis procedures

Note: Heparin lock flush solution is intended only to maintain patency of I.V. devices and is **not** to be used for systemic anticoagulant therapy.

Unlabeled Use ST-elevation myocardial infarction (STEMI) as an adjunct to thrombolysis; unstable angina/non-STEMI (UA/NSTEMI); anticoagulant used during percutaneous coronary intervention (PCI)

Pregnancy Risk Factor C

Pregnancy Considerations Animal reproduction studies have not been conducted. Heparin does not cross the placenta. Some products contain benzyl alcohol as a preservative; their use in pregnant women is contraindicated by some manufacturers.

Lactation Does not enter breast milk

Contraindications Hypersensitivity to heparin or any component of the formulation (unless a life-threatening situation necessitates use and use of an alternative anticoagulant is not possible); severe thrombocytopenia; uncontrolled active bleeding except when due to disseminated intravascular coagulation (DIC); not for use when appropriate blood coagulation tests cannot be obtained at appropriate intervals (applies to full-dose heparin only)

Note: Some products contain benzyl alcohol as a preservative; their use in neonates, infants, or pregnant or nursing mothers is contraindicated by some manufacturers.

Warnings/Precautions Hypersensitivity reactions can occur. Only in life-threatening situations when use of an alternative anticoagulant is not possible should heparin be cautiously used in patients with a documented hypersensitivity reaction. Hemorrhage is the most common complication. Monitor for signs and symptoms of bleeding. Certain patients are at increased risk of bleeding. Risk factors for bleeding include bacterial endocarditis; congenital or acquired bleeding disorders; active ulcerative or angiodysplastic GI diseases; continuous GI tube drainage; severe uncontrolled hypertension; history of hemorrhagic stroke; or use shortly after brain, spinal, or ophthalmology surgery; patient treated concomitantly with platelet inhibitors; conditions associated with increased bleeding tendencies (hemophilia, vascular purpura); recent GI bleeding; thrombocytopenia or platelet defects; severe liver disease; hypertensive or diabetic retinopathy; renal failure; or in patients undergoing invasive procedures including spinal tap or spinal anesthesia. Many concentrations of heparin are available ranging from 1 unit/mL to 20,000 units/mL. Clinicians **must** carefully examine each prefilled syringe or vial prior to use ensuring that the correct concentration is chosen; fatal hemorrhages have occurred related to heparin overdose especially in pediatric patients. A higher incidence of bleeding has been reported in patients >60 years of age, particularly women. They are also more sensitive to the dose. Discontinue heparin if hemorrhage occurs; severe hemorrhage or overdosage may require protamine.

May cause thrombocytopenia; monitor platelet count closely. Patients who develop HIT may be at risk of developing a new thrombus (heparin-induced thrombocytopenia and thrombosis [HITT]). Discontinue therapy and consider alternatives if platelets are <100,000/mm^3 and/or thrombosis develops. HIT or HITT may be delayed and can occur up to several weeks after discontinuation of heparin. Osteoporosis may occur with prolonged use (>6 months) due to a reduction in bone mineral density. Monitor for hyperkalemia; can cause hyperkalemia by suppressing aldosterone production. Patients >60 years of age may require lower doses of heparin.

[U.S. Boxed Warning]: Some products contain benzyl alcohol as a preservative; use of these products is contraindicated in neonates. In neonates, large amounts of benzyl alcohol (>100 mg/kg/day) have been associated with fatal toxicity (gasping syndrome). Use in neonates, infants, or pregnant or nursing mothers is contraindicated by some manufacturers; the use of preservative-free heparin is, therefore, recommended in these populations. Some preparations contain sulfite which may cause allergic reactions.

Heparin resistance may occur in patients with antithrombin deficiency, increased heparin clearance, elevations in heparin-binding proteins, elevations in factor VIII and/or fibrinogen; frequently encountered in patients with fever, thrombosis, thrombophlebitis, infections with thrombosing tendencies, MI, cancer, and in postsurgical patients; measurement of anticoagulant effects using antifactor Xa levels may be of benefit.

Adverse Reactions Frequency not defined.

Cardiovascular: Allergic vasospastic reaction (possibly related to thrombosis), chest pain, hemorrhagic shock, shock, thrombosis

Central nervous system: Chills, fever, headache

Dermatologic: Alopecia (delayed, transient), bruising (unexplained), cutaneous necrosis, dysesthesia pedis, erythematous plaques (case reports), eczema, urticaria, purpura

Endocrine & metabolic: Adrenal hemorrhage, hyperkalemia (suppression of aldosterone synthesis), ovarian hemorrhage, rebound hyperlipidemia on discontinuation

Gastrointestinal: Constipation, hematemesis, nausea, tarry stools, vomiting

Genitourinary: Frequent or persistent erection

Hematologic: Bleeding from gums, epistaxis, hemorrhage, ovarian hemorrhage, retroperitoneal hemorrhage, thrombocytopenia (see **"Note"**)

Hepatic: Liver enzymes increased

Local: Irritation, erythema, pain, hematoma, and ulceration have been rarely reported with deep SubQ injections; I.M. injection (not recommended) is associated with a high incidence of these effects

Neuromuscular & skeletal: Peripheral neuropathy, osteoporosis (chronic therapy effect)

Ocular: Conjunctivitis (allergic reaction), lacrimation

Renal: Hematuria

Respiratory: Asthma, bronchospasm (case reports), hemoptysis, pulmonary hemorrhage, rhinitis

Miscellaneous: Allergic reactions, anaphylactoid reactions, heparin resistance, hypersensitivity (including chills, fever, and urticaria)

Note: Thrombocytopenia has been reported to occur at an incidence between 0% and 30%. It is often of no clinical significance. However, immunologically mediated heparin-induced thrombocytopenia (HIT) has been estimated to occur in 1% to 2% of patients, and is marked by a progressive fall in platelet counts and, in some cases, thromboembolic complications (skin necrosis, pulmonary embolism, gangrene of the extremities, stroke or MI). For recommendations regarding platelet monitoring during heparin therapy, see Monitoring Parameters.

Drug Interactions

Metabolism/Transport Effects None known.

Avoid Concomitant Use

Avoid concomitant use of Heparin with any of the following: Corticorelin; Rivaroxaban

Increased Effect/Toxicity

Heparin may increase the levels/effects of: Anticoagulants; Collagenase (Systemic); Corticorelin; Deferasirox; Drotrecogin Alfa (Activated); Ibritumomab; Rivaroxaban; Tositumomab and Iodine I 131 Tositumomab

The levels/effects of Heparin may be increased by: 5-ASA Derivatives; Antiplatelet Agents; Aspirin; Dasatinib; Herbs (Anticoagulant/Antiplatelet Properties); Nonsteroidal Anti-Inflammatory Agents; Pentosan Polysulfate Sodium; Pentoxifylline; Prostacyclin Analogues; Salicylates; Thrombolytic Agents

Decreased Effect

The levels/effects of Heparin may be decreased by: Nitroglycerin

Ethanol/Nutrition/Herb Interactions Herb/Nutraceutical: Avoid cat's claw, dong quai, evening primrose, feverfew, red clover, horse chestnut, garlic, green tea, ginseng, ginkgo (all have additional antiplatelet activity).

Stability

Heparin solutions are colorless to slightly yellow; minor color variations do not affect therapeutic efficacy.

Heparin should be stored at controlled room temperature. Protect from freezing and temperatures >40°C.

Stability at room temperature and refrigeration:

Prepared bag: 24-72 hours (specific to solution, concentration, and/or study conditions)

Premixed bag: After seal is broken, 4 days.

Out of overwrap stability: 30 days.

Standard concentration/diluent: 25,000 units/500 mL D_5W (premixed). If preparing solution, mix thoroughly prior to administration.

Minimum volume: 250 mL D_5W.

Mechanism of Action Potentiates the action of antithrombin III and thereby inactivates thrombin (as well as activated coagulation factors IX, X, XI, XII, and plasmin) and prevents the conversion of fibrinogen to fibrin; heparin also stimulates release of lipoprotein lipase (lipoprotein lipase hydrolyzes triglycerides to glycerol and free fatty acids)

Pharmacodynamics/Kinetics

Onset of action: Anticoagulation: I.V.: Immediate; SubQ: ~20-30 minutes

Absorption: Oral, rectal: Erratic at best from these routes of administration; SubQ absorption is also erratic, but considered acceptable for prophylactic use

Distribution: Does not cross placenta; does not enter breast milk

Metabolism: Hepatic; may be partially metabolized in the reticuloendothelial system

Half-life elimination:

Dose-dependent: I.V. bolus: 25 units/kg: 30 minutes; 100 units/kg: 60 minutes; 400 units/kg: 150 minutes (Hirsh, 2008)

Mean: 1.5 hours; Range: 1-2 hours; affected by obesity, renal function, malignancy, presence of pulmonary embolism, and infections

Note: At therapeutic doses, elimination occurs rapidly via nonrenal mechanisms. With very high doses, renal elimination may play more of a role; however, dosage adjustment remains unnecessary for patients with renal impairment (Hirsh, 2008).

Excretion: Urine (small amounts as unchanged drug)

Dosage Note: Many concentrations of heparin are available ranging from 1 unit/mL to 20,000 units/mL. Carefully examine each prefilled syringe or vial prior to use ensuring that the correct concentration is chosen. Heparin lock flush solution is intended only to maintain patency of I.V. devices and is not to be used for anticoagulant therapy.

Children >1 year:

Prophylaxis for cardiac catheterization (arterial approach): I.V.: Bolus: 100-150 units/kg (Monagle, 2008)

Systemic heparinization:

Intermittent I.V.: Initial: 50-100 units/kg, then 50-100 units/kg every 4 hours (**Note:** Continuous I.V. infusion is preferred)

I.V. infusion: Initial loading dose: 75 units/kg given over 10 minutes, then initial maintenance dose: 20 units/kg/hour; adjust dose to maintain aPTT of 60-85 seconds (assuming this reflects an antifactor Xa level of 0.35-0.7 units/mL); see table.

Pediatric Protocol For Systemic Heparin Adjustment

To be used after initial loading dose and maintenance I.V. infusion dose (see usual dosage listed above) to maintain aPTT of 60-85 seconds (assuming this reflects antifactor Xa level of 0.35-0.7 units/mL).

Obtain blood for aPTT 4 hours after heparin loading dose and 4 hours after every infusion rate change.

Obtain daily CBC and aPTT after aPTT is therapeutic.

aPTT (seconds)	Dosage Adjustment	Time to Repeat aPTT
<50	Give 50 units/kg bolus and increase infusion rate by 10%	4 h after rate change
50-59	Increase infusion rate by 10%	4 h after rate change
60-85	Keep rate the same	Next day
86-95	Decrease infusion rate by 10%	4 h after rate change
96-120	Hold infusion for 30 minutes and decrease infusion rate by 10%	4 h after rate change
>120	Hold infusion for 60 minutes and decrease infusion rate by 15%	4 h after rate change

Modified from Monagle P, Chalmers E, Chan A, et al, "Antithrombotic Therapy in Neonates and Children," *Chest*, 2008, 133(6 Suppl):887-968.
Note: The aPTT range of 60-85 seconds corresponds to an anti-Xa level of 0.35-0.7 units/mL.

Adults:

Thromboprophylaxis (low-dose heparin): SubQ: 5000 units every 8-12 hours

Intermittent I.V.: Initial: 10,000 units, then 50-70 units/kg (5000-10,000 units) every 4-6 hours

I.V. infusion (weight-based dosing per institutional nomogram recommended):

Acute coronary syndromes:

STEMI: Fibrinolytic therapy: *Full-dose alteplase, reteplase, or tenecteplase with dosing as follows:* Concurrent bolus of 60 units/kg (maximum: 4000 units), then 12 units/kg/hour (maximum: 1000 units/hour) as continuous infusion. Check aPTT every 4-6 hours; adjust to target of 1.5-2 times the upper limit of control (50-70 seconds in clinical trials); usual range: 10-30 units/kg/hour. Duration of heparin therapy depends on concurrent therapy and the specific patient risks for systemic or venous thromboembolism.

Percutaneous coronary intervention (Levine, 2011):

No prior anticoagulant therapy:

If no GPIIb/IIIa inhibitor use planned: Initial bolus of 70-100 units/kg (target ACT 250-300 seconds for HemoTec®, 300-350 seconds for Hemochron®)

or

If planning GPIIb/IIIa inhibitor use: Initial bolus of 50-70 units/kg (target ACT 200-250 seconds regardless of device)

Prior anticoagulant therapy:

If no GPIIb/IIIa inhibitor use planned: Additional heparin as needed (eg, 2000-5000 units) (target ACT 250-300 seconds for HemoTec®, 300-350 seconds for Hemochron®)

or

If planning GPIIb/IIIa inhibitor use: Additional heparin as needed (eg, 2000-5000 units) (target ACT 200-250 seconds regardless of device)

Treatment of unstable angina/non-ST-elevation myocardial infarction (NSTEMI): Initial bolus of 60 units/kg (maximum: 4000 units), followed by an initial infusion of 12 units/kg/hour (maximum: 1000 units/hour). The American College of Chest Physicians consensus conference has recommended dosage adjustments to correspond to a therapeutic range equivalent to heparin levels of 0.3-0.7 units/mL by antifactor Xa determinations.

Treatment of venous thromboembolism:

DVT/PE: I.V.: 80 units/kg (or alternatively 5000 units) I.V. push followed by continuous infusion of 18 units/kg/hour (or alternatively 1300 units/hour). The American College of Chest Physicians consensus conference has recommended dosage adjustments to correspond to a therapeutic range equivalent to heparin levels of 0.3-0.7 units/mL by antifactor Xa determinations.

DVT/PE: SubQ:

Monitored dosing regimen: Initial: 17,500 units or 250 units/kg then 250 units/kg every 12 hours. The American College of Chest Physicians consensus conference has recommended dosage adjustments to correspond to a therapeutic range equivalent to heparin levels of 0.3-0.7 units/mL by antifactor Xa determinations.

Unmonitored dosing regimen: Initial: 333 units/kg then 250 units/kg every 12 hours

Line flushing: When using daily flushes of heparin to maintain patency of single and double lumen central catheters, 10 units/mL is commonly used for younger infants (eg, <10 kg) while 100 units/mL is used for older infants, children, and adults. Capped PVC catheters and peripheral heparin locks require flushing more frequently (eg, every 6-8 hours). Volume of heparin flush is usually similar to volume of catheter (or slightly greater). Additional flushes should be given when stagnant blood is observed in catheter, after catheter is used for drug or blood administration, and after blood withdrawal from catheter.

Addition of heparin (0.5-3 unit/mL) to peripheral and central parenteral nutrition has not been shown to decrease catheter-related thrombosis. The final concentration of heparin used for TPN solutions may need to be decreased to 0.5 units/mL in small infants receiving larger amounts of volume in order to avoid approaching therapeutic amounts. Arterial lines are heparinized with a final concentration of 1 unit/mL.

Dosing adjustments in the elderly: Patients >60 years of age may have higher serum levels and clinical response (longer aPTTs) as compared to younger patients receiving similar dosages; lower dosages may be required

Dosage adjustment in renal impairment: No dosage adjustment required; adjust therapeutic heparin according to aPTT or anti-Xa activity.

Dosage adjustment in hepatic impairment: No dosage adjustment required; adjust therapeutic heparin according to aPTT or anti-Xa activity.

Administration SubQ: Inject in subcutaneous tissue only (not muscle tissue). Injection sites should be rotated (usually left and right portions of the abdomen, above iliac crest).

Do not administer I.M. due to pain, irritation, and hematoma formation; central venous catheters must be flushed with heparin solution when newly inserted, daily (at the time of tubing change), after blood withdrawal or transfusion, and after an intermittent infusion through an injectable cap. A volume of at least 10 mL of blood should be removed and discarded from a heparinized line before blood samples are sent for coagulation testing.

Monitoring Parameters Hemoglobin, hematocrit, signs of bleeding; fecal occult blood test; aPTT (or antifactor Xa activity levels) or ACT depending upon indication

Platelet counts should be routinely monitored when the risk of HIT is >0.1% (eg, receiving therapeutic dose heparin, postoperative antithrombotic prophylaxis), if the patient has received heparin or low molecular weight heparin (eg, enoxaparin) within the past 100 days, if pre-exposure history is uncertain, or if anaphylactoid reaction to heparin occurs. When the risk of HIT is <0.1% (eg, medical/obstetrical patients receiving heparin flushes), routine platelet count monitoring is not recommended (Hirsh, 2008).

For intermittent I.V. injections, aPTT is measured 3.5-4 hours after I.V. injection.

For SubQ injections, when used for treatment (eg, monitored dosing regimen), aPTT is measured 6 hours after injection.

Note: Continuous I.V. infusion is preferred over I.V. intermittent injections. For full-dose heparin (ie, nonlow-dose), the dose should be titrated according to aPTT results. For anticoagulation, an aPTT 1.5-2.5 times normal is usually desired. Because of variation among hospitals in the control aPTT values, nomograms should be established at each institution, designed to achieve aPTT values in the target range (eg, for a control aPTT of 30 seconds, the target range [1.5-2.5 times control] would be 45-75 seconds). Measurements should be made prior to heparin therapy, 6 hours (pediatric: 4 hours) after initiation, and 6 hours (pediatric: 4 hours) after any dosage change, and should be used to adjust the heparin infusion until the aPTT exhibits a therapeutic level. When two consecutive aPTT values are therapeutic, subsequent measurements may be made every 24 hours, and if necessary, dose adjustment carried out. In addition, a significant change in the patient's clinical condition (eg, recurrent ischemia, bleeding, hypotension) should prompt an immediate aPTT determination, followed by dose adjustment if necessary. In general, may increase or decrease infusion by 2-4 units/kg/hour dependent upon aPTT.

Heparin infusion dose adjustment: A number of dose-adjustment nomograms have been developed which target an aPTT range of 1.5-2.5 times control (Cruickshank, 1991; Flaker, 1994; Hull, 1992; Raschke, 1993). However, institution-specific and indication-specific nomograms should be consulted for dose adjustment. **Note:** aPTT values vary throughout the day with maximum values occurring during the night (Decousus, 1985).

Reference Range Venous thromboembolism: Heparin: 0.3-0.7 unit/mL anti-Xa activity (by chromogenic assay) or 0.2-0.4 unit/mL (by protamine titration); aPTT: 1.5-2.5 times control (usually reflects an aPTT of 60-85 seconds) (Hirsh, 2008; Kearon, 2008)

When used with thrombolytic therapy in patients with acute MI, a lower therapeutic range corresponding to an antiXa level of 0.2-0.5 units/mL by chromogenic assay; aPTT: 1.5-2 times control (or approximately an aPTT of 50-70 seconds) is recommended (Goodman, 2008).

Test Interactions Increased thyroxine (competitive protein binding methods); increased PT

Aprotinin significantly increases aPTT and celite Activated Clotting Time (ACT) which may not reflect the actual degree of anticoagulation by heparin. Kaolin-based ACTs are not affected by aprotinin to the same degree as celite ACTs. While institutional protocols may vary, a minimal celite ACT of 750 seconds or kaolin-ACT of 480 seconds is recommended in the presence of aprotinin. Consult the manufacturer's information on specific ACT test interpretation in the presence of aprotinin.

Dosage Forms Excipient information presented when available (limited, particularly for generics); consult specific product labeling. [DSC] = Discontinued product

Infusion, premixed in 1/2 NS, as sodium [porcine intestinal mucosa source]: 25,000 units (250 mL, 500 mL)

Infusion, premixed in D_5W, as sodium [porcine intestinal mucosa source]: 10,000 units (250 mL); 12,500 units (250 mL); 20,000 units (500 mL); 25,000 units (250 mL, 500 mL)

Infusion, premixed in D_5W, as sodium [porcine intestinal mucosa source, preservative free]: 20,000 units (500 mL [DSC]); 25,000 units (250 mL [DSC], 500 mL [DSC])

Infusion, premixed in NS, as sodium [porcine intestinal mucosa source]: 1000 units (500 mL); 2000 units (1000 mL)

Infusion, premixed in NS, as sodium [porcine intestinal mucosa source, preservative free]: 1000 units (500 mL); 2000 units (1000 mL)

Injection, solution, as sodium [lock flush preparation; porcine intestinal mucosa source]: 10 units/mL (1 mL, 2 mL, 3 mL, 5 mL, 10 mL, 30 mL [DSC]); 100 units/mL (1 mL, 2 mL, 3 mL, 5 mL, 10 mL, 30 mL)

Hep-Lock: 10 units/mL (1 mL, 2 mL, 10 mL, 30 mL); 100 units/mL (1 mL, 2 mL, 10 mL, 30 mL) [contains benzyl alcohol]

Injection, solution, as sodium [lock flush preparation; porcine intestinal mucosa source, preservative free]: 1 units/mL (2 mL, 3 mL, 5 mL); 2 units/mL (3 mL); 10 units/mL (1 mL, 2 mL, 2.5 mL, 3 mL, 5 mL, 6 mL, 10 mL); 100 units/mL (1 mL, 2 mL, 2.5 mL, 3 mL, 5 mL, 10 mL)

Hep-Lock U/P: 10 units/mL (1 mL); 100 units/mL (1 mL)

HepFlush®-10: 10 units/mL (10 mL)

Injection, solution, as sodium [porcine intestinal mucosa source]: 1000 units/mL (1 mL, 10 mL, 30 mL); 5000 units/mL (1 mL, 10 mL); 10,000 units/mL (1 mL, 4 mL, 5 mL); 20,000 units/mL (1 mL)

Injection, solution, as sodium [porcine intestinal mucosa source, preservative free]: 1000 units/mL (2 mL); 5000 units/mL (0.5 mL); 10,000 units/mL (0.5 mL)

Injection, solution, oral, as sodium [porcine intestinal mucosa source]: 10,000 units/mL (1 mL)

◆ **Heparin Calcium** *see* Heparin *on page 820*

◆ **Heparin Lock Flush** *see* Heparin *on page 820*

◆ **Heparin Sodium** *see* Heparin *on page 820*

Hepatitis A and Hepatitis B Recombinant Vaccine

(hep a TYE tis aye & hep a TYE tis bee ree KOM be nant vak SEEN)

Brand Names: U.S. Twinrix®

Brand Names: Canada Twinrix®; Twinrix® Junior

Index Terms Engerix-B® and Havrix®; Havrix® and Engerix-B®; HepA-HepB; Hepatitis B and Hepatitis A Vaccine

Pharmacologic Category Vaccine, Inactivated (Viral)

Additional Appendix Information

Immunization Recommendations *on page 1922*

Use Active immunization against disease caused by hepatitis A virus and hepatitis B virus (all known subtypes) in populations desiring protection against or at high risk of exposure to these viruses.

Populations include travelers or people living in or relocating to areas of intermediate/high endemicity for **both** HAV and HBV and are at increased risk of HBV infection due to behavioral or occupational factors; patients with chronic liver disease; laboratory workers who handle live HAV and HBV; healthcare workers, police, and other personnel who render first-aid or medical assistance; workers who come in contact with sewage; employees of day care centers and correctional facilities; patients/staff of hemodialysis units; men who have sex with men; patients frequently receiving blood products; military personnel; users of injectable illicit drugs; close household contacts of patients with hepatitis A and hepatitis B infection; residents of drug and alcohol treatment centers

Pregnancy Risk Factor C

Dosage

I.M.: Adults: Primary immunization: Three doses (1 mL each) given on a 0-, 1-, and 6-month schedule

Alternative regimen: Accelerated regimen: Four doses (1 mL each) on day 0, 7, and 21-30, followed by a booster at 12 months

Canadian labeling (not in U.S. labeling): I.M.: Children 1-18 years: Twinrix® Junior [(CAN); not available in U.S.]: Primary immunization: Three doses (0.5 mL each) given on a 0-, 1-, and 6-month schedule

Alternative regimen: Children 1-15 years: Twinrix®: One dose (1 mL) given on elected date followed by second dose (1 mL) 6-12 months later

Additional Information Complete prescribing information for this medication should be consulted for additional detail.

Dosage Forms Excipient information presented when available (limited, particularly for generics); consult specific product labeling.

Injection, suspension [preservative free]:

Twinrix®: Hepatitis A virus antigen 720 ELISA units and hepatitis B surface antigen 20 mcg per mL (1 mL) [contains aluminum, yeast protein, and trace amounts of neomycin; may contain natural rubber/natural latex in prefilled syringe]

Dosage Forms: Canada Excipient information presented when available (limited, particularly for generics); consult specific product labeling.

Injection, suspension [preservative free]:

Twinrix® Junior: Hepatitis A virus antigen 360 ELISA units and hepatitis B surface antigen 10 mcg per 0.5 mL (0.5 mL) [contains aluminum and trace amounts of neomycin]

Hepatitis A Vaccine (hep a TYE tis aye vak SEEN)

Brand Names: U.S. Havrix®; VAQTA®

Brand Names: Canada Avaxim®; Avaxim®-Pediatric; HAVRIX®; VAQTA®

Index Terms HepA

Pharmacologic Category Vaccine, Inactivated (Viral)

Additional Appendix Information

Immunization Recommendations *on page 1922*

Use

Active immunization against disease caused by hepatitis A virus (HAV)

The Advisory Committee on Immunization Practices (ACIP) recommends routine vaccination for:

- All children ≥12 months of age
- All unvaccinated adults requesting protection from HAV infection
- All unvaccinated adults at risk for HAV infection, such as:

  Behavioral risks: Men who have sex with men; injection drug users

  Occupational risks: Persons who work with HAV-infected primates or with HAV in a research laboratory setting

  Medical risks: Persons with chronic liver disease; patients who receive clotting-factor concentrates
- Other risks: International travelers to regions with high or intermediate levels of endemic HAV infection (a list of countries is available at http://wwwn.cdc.gov/travel/contentdiseases.aspx)
- Unvaccinated persons who anticipate close personal contact with international adoptee from a country of intermediate to high endemicity of HAV, during their first 60 days of arrival into the United States (eg, household contacts, babysitters)

Pregnancy Risk Factor C

Pregnancy Considerations Reproduction studies have not been conducted. The safety of vaccination during pregnancy has not been determined, however, the theoretical risk to the infant is expected to be low. Inactivated vaccines have not been shown to cause increased risks to the fetus (CDC, 2011).

Lactation Excretion in breast milk unknown/use caution

Contraindications Hypersensitivity to hepatitis A vaccine or any component of the formulation

Warnings/Precautions Use caution in patients on anticoagulants, with thrombocytopenia, or bleeding disorders (bleeding may occur following intramuscular injection). Treatment for anaphylactic reactions should be immediately available. Postpone vaccination with acute infection or febrile illness. Use with caution in severely immunocompromised patients (eg, patients receiving chemo/radiation therapy or other immunosuppressive therapy (including high dose corticosteroids)); may have a reduced response to vaccination. In general, household and close contacts of persons with altered immunocompetence may receive all age appropriate vaccines. Unrecognized hepatitis A infection may be present; immunization may not prevent infection in these patients. Patients with chronic liver disease may have decreased antibody response. Packaging may contain natural latex rubber; some products may contain neomycin. In order to maximize vaccination rates, the ACIP recommends simultaneous administration of all age-appropriate vaccines (live or inactivated) for which a person is eligible at a single clinic visit, unless contraindications exist. The use of combination vaccines is generally preferred over separate injections, taking into consideration provider assessment, patient preference, and adverse events.

Adverse Reactions All serious adverse reactions must be reported to the U.S. Department of Health and Human Services (DHHS) Vaccine Adverse Event Reporting System (VAERS) at 1-800-822-7967 or online at https://vaers.hhs.gov/esub/index.

Frequency dependent upon age, product used, and concomitant vaccine administration. In general, headache and injection site reactions were less common in younger children.

>10%:

Central nervous system: Drowsiness, fever ≥100.4°F (1-5 days post vaccination), fever >98.6°C (1-14 days post vaccination), headache, irritability

Gastrointestinal: Appetite decreased

Local: Injection site: Erythema, pain, soreness, swelling, tenderness, warmth

1% to 10%:

Central nervous system: Chills, fatigue, fever ≥102°F (1-5 days postvaccination), insomnia, malaise

Dermatologic: Rash

Endocrine & metabolic: Menstrual disorder

Gastrointestinal: Abdominal pain, anorexia, constipation, diarrhea, gastroenteritis, nausea, vomiting

Local: Injection site bruising, induration

Neuromuscular & skeletal: Arm pain, back pain, myalgia, stiffness, weakness/fatigue

Ocular: Conjunctivitis

Otic: Otitis media

Respiratory: Asthma, cough, nasopharyngitis, nasal congestion, pharyngitis, rhinorrhea, rhinitis, upper respiratory tract infection

Miscellaneous: Crying

<1% (Limited to important or life threatening): Allergic reaction, anaphylaxis, angioedema, arthralgia, bronchial constriction, bronchiolitis, cerebellar ataxia, CK increased, dehydration, dermatitis, dizziness, dyspnea, encephalitis, erythema multiforme, Guillain-Barré syndrome, hepatitis, hypoesthesia, injection site hematoma, injection site rash, jaundice, lymphadenopathy, multiple sclerosis, myelitis, neuropathy, paresthesia, photophobia, pruritus, seizure, serum sickness-like syndrome, syncope, thrombocytopenia, vasculitis, vertigo, wheezing

Drug Interactions

Metabolism/Transport Effects None known.

Avoid Concomitant Use There are no known interactions where it is recommended to avoid concomitant use.

Increased Effect/Toxicity There are no known significant interactions involving an increase in effect.

Decreased Effect

The levels/effects of Hepatitis A Vaccine may be decreased by: Belimumab; Fingolimod; Immunosuppressants

Stability Store under refrigeration at 2°C to 8°C (36°F to 46°F); do not freeze. The following stability information has also been reported for Havrix®: May be stored at room temperature for up to 72 hours (Cohen, 2007).

Mechanism of Action As an inactivated virus vaccine, hepatitis A vaccine offers active immunization against hepatitis A virus infection at an effective immune response rate in up to 99% of subjects

Pharmacodynamics/Kinetics

Onset of action (protection): 2-4 weeks after a single dose; 2 weeks after vaccine administration, 54% to 62% of patients develop neutralizing antibodies; this percentage increases to 94% to 100% at 1 month postvaccination (CDC, 2006)

Duration: Neutralizing antibodies have persisted for up to 8 years; based on kinetic models, antibodies may be present ≥14-20 years in children and ≥25 years in adults who receive the complete vaccination series (CDC, 2006; Van Damme, 2003).

Dosage I.M.: **Note:** When used for primary immunization, the vaccine should be given at least 2 weeks prior to expected HAV exposure. When used prior to an international adoption, the vaccination series should begin when adoption is being planned, but ideally ≥2 weeks prior to expected arrival of adoptee. When used for postexposure prophylaxis, the vaccine should be given as soon as possible.

HAVRIX®:

Children 12 months to 18 years: 720 ELISA units (0.5 mL) with a booster dose of 720 ELISA units to be given 6-12 months following primary immunization

Adults: 1440 ELISA units (1 mL) with a booster dose of 1440 ELISA units to be given 6-12 months following primary immunization

VAQTA®:

Children 12 months to 18 years: 25 units (0.5 mL) with a booster dose of 25 units (0.5 mL) to be given 6-18 months after primary immunization (6-12 months if initial dose was with HAVRIX®)

Adults: 50 units (1 mL) with with a booster dose of 50 units (1 mL) to be given 6-18 months after primary immunization (6-12 months if initial dose was with HAVRIX®)

Administration The deltoid muscle is the preferred site for injection for older children and adults; administer to the anterolateral aspect of the thigh in infants and young children. Do not administer to the gluteal region; may decrease efficacy. Do not administer intravenously, intradermally, or subcutaneously. Shake well prior to use; discard if the suspension is discolored or does not appear homogenous after shaking, or if there are cracks in the vial or syringe. When used for primary immunization, the vaccine should be given at least 2 weeks prior to expected HAV exposure. When used for postexposure prophylaxis, the vaccine should be given as soon as possible. For patients at risk of hemorrhage following intramuscular injection, the ACIP recommends "it should be administered intramuscularly if, in the opinion of the physician familiar with the patients bleeding risk, the vaccine can be administered by this route with reasonable safety. If the patient receives antihemophilia or other similar therapy, intramuscular vaccination can be scheduled shortly after such therapy is administered. A fine needle (23 gauge or smaller) can be used for the vaccination and firm pressure applied to the site (without rubbing) for at least 2 minutes. The patient should be instructed concerning the risk of hematoma from the injection." Patients on anticoagulant therapy should be considered to have the same bleeding risks and treated as those with clotting factor disorders (CDC, 2011).

Simultaneous administration of vaccines helps ensure the patients will be fully vaccinated by the appropriate age. Simultaneous administration of vaccines is defined as administering >1 vaccine on the same day at different anatomic sites. The use of licensed combination vaccines is generally preferred over separate injections of the equivalent components. Separate vaccines should not be combined in the same syringe unless indicated by product specific labeling. Separate needles and syringes should be used for each injection. The ACIP prefers each dose of a specific vaccine in a series come from the same manufacturer when possible. Adolescents and adults should be vaccinated while seated or lying down. In general, preterm infants should be vaccinated at the same chronological age as full-term infants (CDC, 2011).

Antipyretics have not been shown to prevent febrile seizures. Antipyretics may be used to treat fever or discomfort following vaccination (CDC, 2011). One study reported that routine prophylactic administration of acetaminophen to prevent fever prior to vaccination decreased the immune response of some vaccines; the clinical significance of this reduction in immune response has not been established (Prymula, 2009).

Monitoring Parameters Liver function tests; monitor for syncope for ≥15 minutes following vaccination

Additional Information The ACIP currently recommends that older adults, the immunocompromised, or persons with underlying medical conditions (including chronic liver disease) that are vaccinated <2 weeks from departure to an area with a high or intermediate risk of hepatitis A infection also receive immune globulin (CDC, 2007).

Federal law requires that the name of medication, date of administration, the vaccine manufacturer, lot number of vaccine, and the administering person's name, title and address be entered into the patient's permanent medical record.

Dosage Forms Excipient information presented when available (limited, particularly for generics); consult specific product labeling. [DSC] = Discontinued product

Injection, suspension [adult, preservative free]:
- Havrix®: Hepatitis A virus antigen 1440 ELISA units/mL (1 mL) [contains aluminum, neomycin (may have trace amounts); may contain natural rubber/natural latex in prefilled syringe]
- VAQTA®: Hepatitis A virus antigen 50 units/mL (1 mL) [contains aluminum, natural rubber/natural latex in packaging]

Injection, suspension [pediatric, preservative free]:
- Havrix®: Hepatitis A virus antigen 720 ELISA units/0.5 mL (0.5 mL) [contains aluminum, neomycin (may have trace amounts); may contain natural rubber/natural latex in prefilled syringe]

Injection, suspension [pediatric/adolescent, preservative free]:
- VAQTA®: Hepatitis A virus antigen 25 units/0.5 mL (0.5 mL) [contains aluminum, natural rubber/natural latex in packaging]

◆ **Hepatitis B and Hepatitis A Vaccine** *see* Hepatitis A and Hepatitis B Recombinant Vaccine *on page 824*

Hepatitis B Immune Globulin (Human)

(hep a TYE tis bee i MYUN GLOB yoo lin YU man)

Brand Names: U.S. HepaGam B®; HyperHEP B™ S/D; Nabi-HB®

Brand Names: Canada HepaGam B™; HyperHep B®

Index Terms HBIG

Pharmacologic Category Blood Product Derivative; Immune Globulin

Additional Appendix Information

Immunization Recommendations *on page 1922*

Use

Passive prophylactic immunity to hepatitis B following: Acute exposure to blood containing hepatitis B surface antigen (HBsAg); perinatal exposure of infants born to HBsAg-positive mothers; sexual exposure to HBsAg-positive persons; household exposure to persons with acute HBV infection

Prevention of hepatitis B virus recurrence after liver transplantation in HBsAg-positive transplant patients

Note: Hepatitis B immune globulin is not indicated for treatment of active hepatitis B infection and is ineffective in the treatment of chronic active hepatitis B infection.

Pregnancy Risk Factor C

Pregnancy Considerations Reproduction studies have not been conducted.

Lactation Excretion in breast milk unknown/use caution

Contraindications Hypersensitivity to hepatitis B immune globulin or any component of the formulation; severe allergy to gamma globulin or anti-immunoglobulin therapies

Warnings/Precautions Hypersensitivity and anaphylactic reactions can occur; immediate treatment (including epinephrine 1:1000) should be available. Use with caution in patients with previous systemic hypersensitivity to human immunoglobulins. Use with caution in patients with thrombocytopenia or coagulation disorders; I.M. injections may be contraindicated. Use with caution in patients with IgA deficiency. Product of human plasma; may potentially contain infectious agents which could transmit disease. Screening of donors, as well as testing and/or inactivation or removal of certain viruses, reduces the risk. Infections thought to be transmitted by this product should be reported to the manufacturer. Some products may contain maltose, which may result in falsely-elevated blood glucose readings.

Adverse Reactions Reported with postexposure prophylaxis. Adverse events reported in liver transplant patients included tremor and hypotension, were associated with a single infusion during the first week of treatment, and did not recur with additional infusions.

Central nervous system: Fainting, headache, lightheadedness, malaise
Dermatologic: Angioedema, bruising, urticaria
Gastrointestinal: Nausea, vomiting
Hematologic: WBC decreased
Hepatic: Alkaline phosphatase increased, AST increased
Local: Ache, erythema, pain, and/or tenderness at injection site
Neuromuscular & skeletal: Arthralgia, joint stiffness, myalgia
Renal: Creatinine increased
Respiratory: Cold symptoms
Miscellaneous: Anaphylaxis, flu-like syndrome

Drug Interactions

Metabolism/Transport Effects None known.

Avoid Concomitant Use There are no known interactions where it is recommended to avoid concomitant use.

Increased Effect/Toxicity There are no known significant interactions involving an increase in effect.

Decreased Effect

Hepatitis B Immune Globulin (Human) may decrease the levels/effects of: Vaccines (Live)

Stability Refrigerate at 2°C to 8°C (36°F to 46°F); do not freeze. Use within 6 hours of entering vial. Do not shake vial; avoid foaming. The following stability information has also been reported for HyperHEP B™ S/D: May be exposed to room temperature for a cumulative 7 days (Cohen, 2007).

Mechanism of Action Hepatitis B immune globulin (HBIG) is a nonpyrogenic sterile solution containing immunoglobulin G (IgG) specific to hepatitis B surface antigen (HB_sAg). HBIG differs from immune globulin in the amount of anti-HB_s. Immune globulin is prepared from plasma that is not preselected for anti-HB_s content. HBIG is prepared from plasma preselected for high titer anti-HB_s. In the U.S., HBIG has an anti-HB_s high titer >1:100,000 by IRA.

Pharmacodynamics/Kinetics

Duration: Postexposure prophylaxis: 3-6 months
Absorption: I.M.: Slow
Half-life: 17-25 days
Distribution: V_d: 7-15 L
Time to peak, serum: I.M.: 2-10 days

Dosage

I.M.:

Newborns: Perinatal exposure of infants born to HBsAg-positive mothers: 0.5 mL as soon after birth as possible (within 12 hours); active vaccination with hepatitis B vaccine may begin at the same time in a different site (if not contraindicated). If first dose of hepatitis B vaccine is delayed for as long as 3 months, dose may be repeated. If hepatitis B vaccine is refused, dose may be repeated at 3 and 6 months.

Infants <12 months: Household exposure prophylaxis: 0.5 mL (to be administered if mother or primary caregiver has acute HBV infection)

Children ≥12 months and Adults: Postexposure prophylaxis: 0.06 mL/kg as soon as possible after exposure (ie, within 24 hours of needlestick, ocular, or mucosal exposure or within 14 days of sexual exposure); usual dose: 3-5 mL; repeat at 28-30 days after exposure in nonresponders to hepatitis B vaccine or in patients who refuse vaccination

Note: HBIG may be administered at the same time (but at a different site) or up to 1 month preceding hepatitis B vaccination without impairing the active immune response

I.V.: Adults: Prevention of hepatitis B virus recurrence after liver transplantation (HepaGam B™): 20,000 int. units/dose according to the following schedule:

Anhepatic phase (Initial dose): One dose given with the liver transplant

Week 1 postop: One dose daily for 7 days (days 1-7)

Weeks 2-12 postop: One dose every 2 weeks starting day 14

Month 4 onward: One dose monthly starting on month 4

Dose adjustment: Adjust dose to reach anti-HBs levels of 500 int. units/L within the first week after transplantation. In patients with surgical bleeding, abdominal fluid drainage >500 mL or those undergoing plasmapheresis, administer 10,000 int. units/dose every 6 hours until target anti-HBs levels are reached.

Administration

I.M.: Postexposure prophylaxis: I.M. injection only in anterolateral aspect of upper thigh and deltoid muscle of upper arm; to prevent injury from injection, care should be taken when giving to patients with thrombocytopenia or bleeding disorders

I.V.:

HepaGam B™: Liver transplant: Administer at 2 mL/minute. Decrease infusion to ≤1 mL/minute for patient discomfort or infusion-related adverse events. Actual volume of infusion is dependent upon potency labeled on each individual vial.

Nabi-HB®: Although not FDA-approved for this purpose, Nabi-HB® has been administered intravenously in hepatitis B-positive liver transplant patients

Monitoring Parameters Liver transplant: Serum HBsAg; infusion-related adverse events

Test Interactions

Glucose testing: HepaGam B™ contains maltose. Falsely-elevated blood glucose levels may occur when glucose monitoring devices and test strips utilizing the glucose dehydrogenase pyrroloquinolinequinone (GDH-PQQ) based methods are used.

Serological testing: Antibodies transferred following administration of immune globulins may provide misleading positive test results (eg, Coombs' test)

Additional Information Each vial contains anti-HB_s antibody equivalent to or exceeding the potency of anti-HB_s in a U.S. reference standard hepatitis B immune globulin (FDA). The U.S. reference standard has been tested against the WHO standard hepatitis B immune globulin with listed values between 207 int. units/mL and 220 int. units/mL (included in individual product information).

Dosage Forms Excipient information presented when available (limited, particularly for generics); consult specific product labeling.

Injection, solution [preservative free]:

HepaGam B®: Anti-HBs > 312 int. units/mL (1 mL, 5 mL) [contains maltose, polysorbate 80]

HyperHEP B™ S/D: Anti-HBs ≥ 220 int. units/mL (0.5 mL, 1 mL, 5 mL)

Nabi-HB®: Anti-HBs > 312 int. units/mL (1 mL, 5 mL) [contains polysorbate 80]

◆ **Hepatitis B Inactivated Virus Vaccine (recombinant DNA)** *see* Hepatitis B Vaccine (Recombinant) *on page 827*

Hepatitis B Vaccine (Recombinant)

(hep a TYE tis bee vak SEEN ree KOM be nant)

Brand Names: U.S. Engerix-B®; Recombivax HB®

Brand Names: Canada Engerix-B®; Recombivax HB®

Index Terms Hepatitis B Inactivated Virus Vaccine (recombinant DNA); HepB

Pharmacologic Category Vaccine, Inactivated (Viral)

Additional Appendix Information

Immunization Recommendations *on page 1922*

Use Immunization against infection caused by all known subtypes of hepatitis B virus (HBV)

The Advisory Committee on Immunization Practices (ACIP) recommends routine vaccination for the following (CDC, 2005; CDC, 2006; CDC, 2011):

- All infants at birth
- All infants and children (post-birth dose; refer to recommended vaccination schedule)
- All unvaccinated adults requesting protection from HBV infection
- All unvaccinated adults at risk for HBV infection such as those with:

Behavioral risks: Sexually-active persons with >1 partner in a 6-month period; persons seeking evaluation or treatment for a sexually-transmitted disease; men who have sex with men; injection drug users

Occupational risks: Healthcare and public safety workers with reasonably anticipated risk for exposure to blood or blood contaminated body fluids

Medical risks: Persons with end-stage renal disease (including predialysis, hemodialysis, peritoneal dialysis, and home dialysis); persons with HIV infection; persons with chronic liver disease. Adults (19 through 59 years of age) with diabetes mellitus type 1 or type 2 should be vaccinated as soon as possible following diagnosis. Adults ≥60 years with diabetes mellitus may also be vaccinated at the discretion of their treating clinician.

Other risks: Household contacts and sex partners of persons with chronic HBV infection; residents and staff of facilities for developmentally disabled persons; international travelers to regions with high or intermediate levels of endemic HBV infection

In addition, the ACIP recommends vaccination for any persons who are wounded in bombings or similar mass casualty events who have penetrating injuries or nonintact skin exposure, or who have contact with mucous membranes (exception - superficial contact with intact skin), and who cannot confirm receipt of a hepatitis B vaccination (CDC, 2008).

Pregnancy Risk Factor C

Pregnancy Considerations Reproduction studies have not been conducted. The ACIP recommends HB_sAg testing for all pregnant women. Based on limited data, there is no apparent risk to the fetus when the hepatitis B vaccine is administered during pregnancy. Pregnancy itself is not a contraindication to vaccination; vaccination should be considered if otherwise indicated (CDC, 2006).

Lactation Excretion in breast milk unknown/use caution

Contraindications Hypersensitivity to yeast, hepatitis B vaccine, or any component of the formulation

Warnings/Precautions Immediate treatment for anaphylactic/anaphylactoid reaction should be available during vaccine use. Defer administration in patients with moderate or severe acute illness (with or without fever). Use caution with decreased cardiopulmonary function. Unrecognized hepatitis B infection may be present prior to vaccination; immunization may not prevent infection in these patients. Patients >65 years of age may have lower response rates. Use with caution in severely immunocompromised patients (eg, patients receiving chemo/radiation therapy or other immunosuppressive therapy [including high-dose corticosteroids]); may have a reduced response to vaccination. In general, household and close contacts of persons with altered immunocompetence may receive all age appropriate vaccines. Use caution in multiple sclerosis patients; rare exacerbations of symptoms have been observed. Apnea has been reported following I.M. vaccine administration in premature infants; consider risk versus benefit in infants born prematurely. Some dosage forms contain dry natural latex rubber. In order to maximize vaccination rates, the ACIP recommends simultaneous administration of all age-appropriate vaccines (live or inactivated) for which a person is eligible at a single clinic visit, unless contraindications exist. The use of combination vaccines is generally preferred over separate injections, taking into consideration provider assessment, patient preference, and adverse events.

Adverse Reactions All serious adverse reactions must be reported to the U.S. Department of Health and Human Services (DHHS) Vaccine Adverse Event Reporting System (VAERS) at 1-800-822-7967 or online at https://vaers.hhs.gov/esub/index.

Frequency not defined. The most common adverse effects reported with both products included injection site reactions (>10%).

Cardiovascular: Flushing, hypotension

Central nervous system: Agitation, chills, dizziness, fatigue, fever (≥37.5°C/100°F), headache, insomnia, irritability, lightheadedness, malaise, somnolence, vertigo

Dermatologic: Angioedema, petechiae, pruritus, rash, urticaria

Gastrointestinal: Abdominal pain, appetite decreased, constipation, cramps, diarrhea, dyspepsia, nausea, vomiting

Genitourinary: Dysuria

Local: Injection site reactions: Ecchymosis, erythema, induration, pain, nodule formation, soreness, swelling, tenderness, warmth

Neuromuscular & skeletal: Achiness, arthralgia, back pain, myalgia, neck pain, neck stiffness, paresthesia, shoulder pain, tingling, weakness

Otic: Earache

Respiratory: Cough, pharyngitis, rhinitis, upper respiratory tract infection

Miscellaneous: Diaphoresis, lymphadenopathy, flu-like syndrome

Postmarketing and/or case reports: Allergic reactions, alopecia, anaphylaxis, apnea, Bell's palsy, bronchospasm, encephalitis, erythema nodosum, erythema multiforme, febrile seizure, Guillain-Barré syndrome, herpes zoster, hypoesthesia, keratitis, liver enzymes increased, lupus-like syndrome, migraine, multiple sclerosis, muscle weakness, neuropathy, optic neuritis, palpitation, paralysis, paresis, polyarteritis nodosa, purpura, seizure, serum-sickness like syndrome (may be delayed days to weeks), Stevens-Johnson syndrome, SLE, syncope, tachycardia, thrombocytopenia, tinnitus, transverse myelitis, uveitis, vasculitis, visual disturbances

Drug Interactions

Metabolism/Transport Effects None known.

Avoid Concomitant Use There are no known interactions where it is recommended to avoid concomitant use.

Increased Effect/Toxicity There are no known significant interactions involving an increase in effect.

Decreased Effect

The levels/effects of Hepatitis B Vaccine (Recombinant) may be decreased by: Belimumab; Fingolimod; Immunosuppressants

Stability Refrigerate at 2°C to 8°C (36°F to 46°F); do not freeze. The following stability information has also been reported for Engerix-B®: May be stored at room temperature for up to 72 hours (Cohen, 2007).

Mechanism of Action Recombinant hepatitis B vaccine is a noninfectious subunit viral vaccine, which confers active immunity via formation of antihepatitis B antibodies. The vaccine is derived from hepatitis B surface antigen (HB_sAg) produced through recombinant DNA techniques from yeast cells. The portion of the hepatitis B gene which codes for HB_sAg is cloned into yeast which is then cultured to produce hepatitis B vaccine.

Pharmacodynamics/Kinetics Duration: Following a 3-dose series in children, up to 50% of patients will have low or undetectable anti-HB antibody 5-15 years postvaccination. However, anamnestic increases in anti-HB have been shown up to 23 years later suggesting a lifelong immune memory response.

Dosage I.M.:

Primary immunization:

Infants: 0.5 mL/dose (pediatric/adolescent formulation) for 3 total doses administered at 0, 1, and 6 months. Alternate dosing regimens are also available for children who begin vaccination ≥1 year of age.

Note: Doses are presented using the pediatric/adolescent formulations. Pediatric/adolescent formulations of hepatitis B vaccine products differ by concentration (mcg/mL). However, when dosed in terms of volume (mL), the dose of Engerix-B® and Recombivax HB® are the same (both 0.5 mL).

Note: Combination vaccines (eg, vaccines containing HepB with DTaP, HIB) should not be used for the "birth" dose but may be used to complete the course beginning after the infant is ≥6 weeks of age (CDC, 2005). Please see combination vaccine monographs for dose and schedule details.

Infants (HB_sAg-**negative** mothers):

First dose: 0.5 mL at birth or before discharge (may be delayed in certain cases)

Second dose: 0.5 mL at 1-2 months of age

Third dose: 0.5 mL at 6-18 months of age, but no sooner than 24 weeks of age

Note: Premature neonates <2 kg may have the initial dose deferred up to 30 days of chronological age or at hospital discharge (CDC, 2005).

Infants (HB_sAg-**positive** mothers):

First dose: 0.5 mL within first 12 hours of life, even if premature and regardless of birth weight (hepatitis immune globulin should also be administered at the same time at a different site)

Second dose: 0.5 mL at 1-2 months of age

Third dose: 0.5 mL at 6 months of age but no sooner than 24 weeks of age

Note: Anti-HB_s and HB_sAg levels should be checked at 9-18 months of age (ie, next well-child visit after series completion). If HB_sAg negative and anti-HB_s levels <10 mIU/mL, reimmunize with 3 doses and reassess 1-2 months after the third dose.

Note: In premature neonates <2 kg, the birth dose should not be counted as part of the 3-dose vaccine series (CDC, 2005).

Infants (mother's HB_sAg status **unknown**):

First dose: 0.5 mL within 12 hours of birth even if premature and regardless of birth weight

Second dose: 0.5 mL at 1-2 months of age

Third dose: 0.5 mL at 6 months of age but no sooner than 24 weeks of age

Note: If mother is later determined to be HB_sAg-positive, the infant should receive hepatitis immune globulin as soon as possible (no later than age 1 week).

Note: In premature neonates <2 kg, the birth dose should not be counted as part of the 3-dose vaccine series (CDC, 2005).

Children: 0.5 mL/dose (pediatric/adolescent formulation) administered at 0, 1, and 6 months (for 3 total doses).

Alternate dosing regimens are also available for children who begin vaccination ≥1 year of age.

Alternate dosing schedules (selection of schedule should optimize compliance with vaccination):

Children 1-10 years: 0.5 mL (pediatric/adolescent formulation) at the following intervals (two schedules presented):

0, 2, and 4 months (CDC, 2005)

0, 1, 2, and 12 months (Engerix-B®)

Children 5-10 years: 0.5 mL (pediatric/adolescent formulation) at 0, 12, and 24 months (Engerix-B®)

Children 11-15 years: 1 mL (adult formulation) at 0 and 4-6 months (Recombivax HB®)

Children 11-16 years: 0.5 mL (pediatric/adolescent formulation) at 0, 12, and 24 months (Engerix-B®)

Children 11-18 years: 0.5 mL (pediatric/adolescent formulation) at the following intervals (three schedules presented):

0, 1, and 4 months (CDC, 2005)

0, 2, and 4 months (CDC, 2005)

0, 12, and 24 months (CDC, 2005)

Children 11-18 years: 1 mL (adult formulation) at 0, 1, 2, and 12 months (Engerix-B®)

Adults: 1 mL/dose (adult formulation) for 3 total doses administered at 0, 1, and 6 months

Note: Adult formulations of hepatitis B vaccine products differ by concentration (mcg/mL) but when dosed in terms of volume (mL), the dose of Engerix-B® and Recombivax HB® are the same (both 1 mL).

Alternate dosing schedules (selection of schedule should optimize compliance with vaccination): All regimens use the adult formulation administered as one dose at the following intervals (three schedules presented):

0, 1, and 4 months (CDC, 2005)

0, 2, and 4 months (CDC, 2005)

0, 12, and 24 months (CDC, 2005)

Bombings or similar mass casualty events: In persons without a reliable history of vaccination against HepB and who have no known contraindications to the vaccine, vaccination should begin within 24 hours (but no later than 7 days) following the event (CDC, 2008).

Dosage adjustment for renal impairment: Adults on dialysis:

Engerix-B® 20 mcg/mL: Administer 2 mL per dose at 0, 1, 2, and 6 months

Recombivax HB® 40 mcg/mL: Administer 1 mL per dose at 0, 1, and 6 months

Note: Serologic testing is recommended 1-2 months after the final dose of the primary vaccine series and annually to determine the need for booster doses. Persons with anti-HB_s concentrations of <10 mIU/mL should be revaccinated with 3 doses of the vaccine (CDC, 2006).

Administration Pediatric/adolescent formulations of hepatitis B vaccine products differ by concentration (mcg/mL). However, when dosed in terms of volume (mL), the dose of Engerix-B® and Recombivax HB® are the same (both 0.5 mL). Adult formulations of hepatitis B vaccine products also differ by concentration (mcg/mL), but when dosed in terms of volume (mL), the dose of Engerix-B® and Recombivax HB® are the same (both 1 mL). It is possible to interchange the vaccines for completion of a series or for booster doses; the antibody produced in response to each type of vaccine is comparable, however, the quantity of the vaccine will vary.

I.M. injection only; in adults, the deltoid muscle is the preferred site; the anterolateral thigh is the recommended site in infants and young children. Not for gluteal administration. Shake well prior to withdrawal and use.

For patients at risk of hemorrhage following intramuscular injection, hepatitis B vaccine may be administered subcutaneously although lower titers and/or increased incidence of local reactions may result. The ACIP recommends "it should be administered intramuscularly if, in the opinion of the physician familiar with the patients bleeding risk, the vaccine can be administered by this route with reasonable safety. If the patient receives antihemophilia or other similar therapy, intramuscular vaccination can be scheduled shortly after such therapy is administered. A fine needle (23 gauge or smaller) can be used for the vaccination and firm pressure applied to the site (without rubbing) for at least 2 minutes. The patient should be instructed concerning the risk of hematoma from the injection." Patients on anticoagulant therapy should be considered to have the same bleeding risks and treated as those with clotting factor disorders (CDC, 2011).

Simultaneous administration of vaccines helps ensure the patients will be fully vaccinated by the appropriate age. Simultaneous administration of vaccines is defined as administering >1 vaccine on the same day at different anatomic sites. The use of licensed combination vaccines is generally preferred over separate injections of the equivalent components. Separate vaccines should not be combined in the same syringe unless indicated by product specific labeling. Separate needles and syringes should be used for each injection. The ACIP prefers each dose of a specific vaccine in a series come from the same manufacturer when possible. Adolescents and adults should be vaccinated while seated or lying down. In general, preterm infants should be vaccinated at the same chronological age as full-term infants (CDC, 2011).

Antipyretics have not been shown to prevent febrile seizures. Antipyretics may be used to treat fever or discomfort following vaccination (CDC, 2011). One study reported that routine prophylactic administration of acetaminophen to prevent fever prior to vaccination decreased the immune response of some vaccines; the clinical significance of this reduction in immune response has not been established (Prymula, 2009).

Vaccination at the time of HB_sAg testing: For persons in whom vaccination is recommended, the first dose of hepatitis B vaccine can be given after blood is drawn to test for HB_sAg.

Additional Information Federal law requires that the name of medication, date of administration, the vaccine manufacturer, lot number of vaccine, and the administering person's name, title, and address be entered into the patient's permanent medical record.

Dosage Forms Excipient information presented when available (limited, particularly for generics); consult specific product labeling. [DSC] = Discontinued product

Injection, suspension [adult, preservative free]:

Engerix-B®: Hepatitis B surface antigen 20 mcg/mL (1 mL) [contains aluminum, yeast protein, may contain natural rubber/natural latex in prefilled syringe]

Recombivax HB®: Hepatitis B surface antigen 10 mcg/mL (1 mL) [contains aluminum, natural rubber/natural latex in packaging, yeast protein]

Injection, suspension [dialysis formulation, preservative free]:

Recombivax HB®: Hepatitis B surface antigen 40 mcg/mL (1 mL) [contains aluminum, natural rubber/natural latex in packaging, yeast protein; dialysis]

Injection, suspension [pediatric/adolescent, preservative free]:

Engerix-B®: Hepatitis B surface antigen 10 mcg/0.5 mL (0.5 mL) [contains aluminum, yeast protein, may contain natural rubber/natural latex in prefilled syringe]

Recombivax HB®: Hepatitis B surface antigen 5 mcg/0.5 mL (0.5 mL) [contains aluminum, natural rubber/natural latex in packaging, yeast protein]

◆ **Hepatitis B Vaccine (Recombinant)** *see Haemophilus* b Conjugate and Hepatitis B Vaccine *on page 815*

◆ **HepB** *see* Hepatitis B Vaccine (Recombinant) *on page 827*
◆ **HepFlush®-10** *see* Heparin *on page 820*
◆ **Hep-Lock** *see* Heparin *on page 820*
◆ **Hep-Lock U/P** *see* Heparin *on page 820*
◆ **Hepsera®** *see* Adefovir *on page 44*
◆ **Hepsera™ (Can)** *see* Adefovir *on page 44*
◆ **Heptovir® (Can)** *see* LamiVUDine *on page 965*
◆ **Herceptin®** *see* Trastuzumab *on page 1722*
◆ **HES** *see* Hetastarch *on page 830*
◆ **HES** *see* Tetrastarch *on page 1663*
◆ **HES 130/0.4** *see* Tetrastarch *on page 1663*
◆ **Hespan®** *see* Hetastarch *on page 830*

Hetastarch (HET a starch)

Brand Names: U.S. Hespan®; Hextend®
Brand Names: Canada Hextend®
Index Terms HES; Hydroxyethyl Starch
Pharmacologic Category Plasma Volume Expander, Colloid
Use Blood volume expander used in treatment of hypovolemia; adjunct in leukapheresis to improve harvesting and increase the yield of granulocytes by centrifugation (Hespan®)
Unlabeled Use Priming fluid in pump oxygenators during cardiopulmonary bypass; plasma volume expansion during cardiopulmonary bypass
Pregnancy Risk Factor C
Dosage I.V. infusion: Adults:
Plasma volume expansion: 500-1000 mL (up to 1500 mL/day) or 20 mL/kg/day (up to 1500 mL/day)
Leukapheresis (Hespan®): 250-700 mL; **Note:** Citrate anticoagulant is added before use.

Dosing adjustment in renal impairment: Cl_{cr} <10 mL/minute: Initial dose is the same but subsequent doses should be reduced by 20% to 50% of normal
Additional Information Complete prescribing information for this medication should be consulted for additional detail.
Dosage Forms Excipient information presented when available (limited, particularly for generics); consult specific product labeling.
Infusion [premixed in lactated electrolyte injection]:
Hextend®: 6% (500 mL)
Infusion, premixed in NS: 6% (500 mL)
Hespan®: 6% (500 mL)

◆ **Hexachlorocyclohexane** *see* Lindane *on page 1013*
◆ **Hexamethylenetetramine** *see* Methenamine *on page 1093*
◆ **Hexit™ (Can)** *see* Lindane *on page 1013*
◆ **Hextend®** *see* Hetastarch *on page 830*
◆ **hFSH** *see* Urofollitropin *on page 1750*
◆ **hGH** *see* Somatropin *on page 1579*
◆ **Hib** *see Haemophilus* b Conjugate Vaccine *on page 815*
◆ **Hib Conjugate Vaccine** *see Haemophilus* b Conjugate and Hepatitis B Vaccine *on page 815*
◆ **Hib Conjugate Vaccine** *see Haemophilus* b Conjugate Vaccine *on page 815*
◆ **Hiberix®** *see Haemophilus* b Conjugate Vaccine *on page 815*
◆ **Hib-HepB** *see Haemophilus* b Conjugate and Hepatitis B Vaccine *on page 815*
◆ **Hibiclens® [OTC]** *see* Chlorhexidine Gluconate *on page 341*
◆ **Hibidil® 1:2000 (Can)** *see* Chlorhexidine Gluconate *on page 341*
◆ **Hibistat® [OTC]** *see* Chlorhexidine Gluconate *on page 341*
◆ **Hib Polysaccharide Conjugate** *see Haemophilus* b Conjugate Vaccine *on page 815*
◆ **High Gamma Vitamin E Complete™ [OTC]** *see* Vitamin E *on page 1796*
◆ **High-Molecular-Weight Iron Dextran (DexFerrum®)** *see* Iron Dextran Complex *on page 930*
◆ **Hiprex®** *see* Methenamine *on page 1093*
◆ **Hirulog** *see* Bivalirudin *on page 222*
◆ **Histantil (Can)** *see* Promethazine *on page 1416*
◆ **Histaprin [OTC]** *see* DiphenhydrAMINE (Systemic) *on page 516*

Histrelin (his TREL in)

Brand Names: U.S. Supprelin® LA; Vantas®
Brand Names: Canada Vantas®
Index Terms GnRH Agonist; Histrelin Acetate; LH-RH Agonist
Pharmacologic Category Gonadotropin Releasing Hormone Agonist
Use Palliative treatment of advanced prostate cancer; treatment of children with central precocious puberty (CPP)
Pregnancy Risk Factor X
Dosage SubQ:
Children ≥2 years: CPP (Supprelin® LA): 50 mg implant surgically inserted every 12 months. Discontinue at the appropriate time for the onset of puberty.
Adults: Prostate cancer, advanced (Vantas®): 50 mg implant surgically inserted every 12 months
Elderly: Refer to adult dosing
Dosage adjustment in renal impairment: Cl_{cr}: 15-60 mL/minute: Adjustment not needed
Additional Information Complete prescribing information for this medication should be consulted for additional detail.
Dosage Forms Excipient information presented when available (limited, particularly for generics); consult specific product labeling. [DSC] = Discontinued product
Implant, subcutaneous:
Supprelin® LA: 50 mg (1s) [releases ~65 mcg/day over 12 months]
Vantas®: 50 mg (1s) [Releases ~50 mcg/day over 12 months; packaged with implantation kit]
Vantas®: 50 mg (1s [DSC]) [releases 50-60 mcg/day over 12 months]

◆ **Histrelin Acetate** *see* Histrelin *on page 830*
◆ **Hizentra®** *see* Immune Globulin *on page 880*
◆ **hMG** *see* Menotropins *on page 1073*
◆ **HMR 3647** *see* Telithromycin *on page 1634*
◆ **HN_2** *see* Mechlorethamine *on page 1056*
◆ **HOE 140** *see* Icatibant *on page 864*

Homatropine (hoe MA troe peen)

Brand Names: U.S. Isopto® Homatropine
Index Terms Homatropine Hydrobromide
Pharmacologic Category Anticholinergic Agent, Ophthalmic; Ophthalmic Agent, Mydriatic
Use Producing cycloplegia and mydriasis for refraction; treatment of acute inflammatory conditions of the uveal tract; optical aid in axial lens opacities
Pregnancy Risk Factor C
Dosage Ophthalmic:

Children:

Mydriasis and cycloplegia for refraction: Instill 1 drop of 2% solution immediately before the procedure; repeat at 10-minute intervals as needed

Uveitis: Instill 1 drop of 2% solution 2-3 times/day

Adults:

Mydriasis and cycloplegia for refraction: Instill 1-2 drops of 2% solution or 1 drop of 5% solution before the procedure; repeat at 5- to 10-minute intervals as needed; maximum of 3 doses for refraction

Uveitis: Instill 1-2 drops of 2% or 5% 2-3 times/day up to every 3-4 hours as needed

Additional Information Complete prescribing information for this medication should be consulted for additional detail.

Dosage Forms Excipient information presented when available (limited, particularly for generics); consult specific product labeling.

Solution, ophthalmic, as hydrobromide [drops]:

Isopto® Homatropine: 2% (5 mL); 5% (5 mL) [contains benzalkonium chloride]

- **Homatropine and Hydrocodone** *see* Hydrocodone and Homatropine *on page 838*
- **Homatropine Hydrobromide** *see* Homatropine *on page 830*
- **Homocysteine Guard [OTC]** *see* Folic Acid, Cyanocobalamin, and Pyridoxine *on page 749*
- **Horizant™** *see* Gabapentin Enacarbil *on page 775*
- **Horizant™** *see* Gabapentin Enacarbil *on page 775*
- **Horse Antihuman Thymocyte Gamma Globulin** *see* Antithymocyte Globulin (Equine) *on page 131*
- **hpAT** *see* Antithrombin *on page 130*
- **Hp-PAC® (Can)** *see* Lansoprazole, Amoxicillin, and Clarithromycin *on page 975*
- **HPV2** *see* Papillomavirus (Types 16, 18) Vaccine (Human, Recombinant) *on page 1292*
- **HPV4** *see* Papillomavirus (Types 6, 11, 16, 18) Vaccine (Human, Recombinant) *on page 1294*
- **HPV 16/18 L1 VLP/AS04 VAC** *see* Papillomavirus (Types 16, 18) Vaccine (Human, Recombinant) *on page 1292*
- **HPV Vaccine** *see* Papillomavirus (Types 6, 11, 16, 18) Vaccine (Human, Recombinant) *on page 1294*
- **HPV Vaccine** *see* Papillomavirus (Types 16, 18) Vaccine (Human, Recombinant) *on page 1292*
- **HRIG** *see* Rabies Immune Globulin (Human) *on page 1453*
- **HumaLOG®** *see* Insulin Lispro *on page 905*
- **Humalog® (Can)** *see* Insulin Lispro *on page 905*
- **HumaLOG® KwikPen™** *see* Insulin Lispro *on page 905*
- **Humalog® Mix 25 (Can)** *see* Insulin Lispro Protamine and Insulin Lispro *on page 906*
- **HumaLOG® Mix 50/50™** *see* Insulin Lispro Protamine and Insulin Lispro *on page 906*
- **HumaLOG® Mix 50/50™ KwikPen™** *see* Insulin Lispro Protamine and Insulin Lispro *on page 906*
- **HumaLOG® Mix 75/25™** *see* Insulin Lispro Protamine and Insulin Lispro *on page 906*
- **HumaLOG® Mix 75/25™ KwikPen™** *see* Insulin Lispro Protamine and Insulin Lispro *on page 906*
- **Human Albumin Grifols® 25%** *see* Albumin *on page 51*
- **Human Antitumor Necrosis Factor Alpha** *see* Adalimumab *on page 42*
- **Human C1 Inhibitor** *see* C1 Inhibitor (Human) *on page 257*
- **Human Corticotrophin-Releasing Hormone, Analogue** *see* Corticorelin *on page 413*
- **Human Diploid Cell Cultures Rabies Vaccine** *see* Rabies Vaccine *on page 1453*
- **Human Growth Hormone** *see* Somatropin *on page 1579*
- **Humanized IgG1 Anti-CD52 Monoclonal Antibody** *see* Alemtuzumab *on page 58*
- **Human LFA-3/IgG(1) Fusion Protein** *see* Alefacept *on page 57*
- **Human Menopausal Gonadotropin** *see* Menotropins *on page 1073*
- **Human Papillomavirus Vaccine** *see* Papillomavirus (Types 6, 11, 16, 18) Vaccine (Human, Recombinant) *on page 1294*
- **Human Papillomavirus Vaccine** *see* Papillomavirus (Types 16, 18) Vaccine (Human, Recombinant) *on page 1292*
- **Human Rotavirus Vaccine, Attenuated (HRV)** *see* Rotavirus Vaccine *on page 1526*
- **Human Thyroid Stimulating Hormone** *see* Thyrotropin Alfa *on page 1677*
- **Humate-P®** *see* Antihemophilic Factor/von Willebrand Factor Complex (Human) *on page 128*
- **Humatin® (Can)** *see* Paromomycin *on page 1298*
- **Humatrope®** *see* Somatropin *on page 1579*
- **HuMax-CD20** *see* Ofatumumab *on page 1229*
- **Humibid® Maximum Strength [OTC]** *see* GuaiFENesin *on page 809*
- **Humira®** *see* Adalimumab *on page 42*
- **Humira® Pen** *see* Adalimumab *on page 42*
- **HuMist® [OTC]** *see* Sodium Chloride *on page 1567*
- **HuMist® for Kids [OTC]** *see* Sodium Chloride *on page 1567*
- **Humulin® 20/80 (Can)** *see* Insulin NPH and Insulin Regular *on page 906*
- **HumuLIN® 70/30** *see* Insulin NPH and Insulin Regular *on page 906*
- **Humulin® 70/30 (Can)** *see* Insulin NPH and Insulin Regular *on page 906*
- **HumuLIN® N** *see* Insulin NPH *on page 906*
- **Humulin® N (Can)** *see* Insulin NPH *on page 906*
- **HumuLIN® R** *see* Insulin Regular *on page 907*
- **Humulin® R (Can)** *see* Insulin Regular *on page 907*
- **HumuLIN® R U-500** *see* Insulin Regular *on page 907*
- **Hurricaine® [OTC]** *see* Benzocaine *on page 202*
- **Hyalgan®** *see* Hyaluronate and Derivatives *on page 831*
- **Hyaluronan** *see* Hyaluronate and Derivatives *on page 831*

Hyaluronate and Derivatives

(hye al yoor ON ate & dah RIV ah tives)

Brand Names: U.S. Amvisc®; Amvisc® Plus; Bionect®; Euflexxa®; Hyalgan®; Juvéderm® Ultra; Juvéderm® Ultra Plus; Juvéderm® Ultra Plus XC; Juvéderm® Ultra XC; Orthovisc®; Perlane®; Provisc®; Restylane®; Supartz®; Synvisc-One®; Synvisc®

Brand Names: Canada Cystistat®; Durolane®; Eyestil; Healon GV®; Healon®; OrthoVisc®; Suplasyn®

Index Terms Hyaluronan; Hyaluronic Acid; Hylan G-F 20; Hylan Polymers; Sodium Hyaluronate

Pharmacologic Category Antirheumatic Miscellaneous; Ophthalmic Agent, Viscoelastic; Skin and Mucous Membrane Agent, Miscellaneous

Use

Intra-articular injection: Treatment of pain in osteoarthritis in knee in patients who have failed nonpharmacologic treatment and simple analgesics

Intradermal: Correction of moderate-to-severe facial wrinkles or folds

Ophthalmic: Surgical aid in cataract extraction, intraocular implantation, corneal transplant, glaucoma filtration, and retinal attachment surgery

Topical cream, gel: Management of skin ulcers and wounds

Unlabeled Use Treatment of refractory interstitial cystitis

Pregnancy Considerations There are no adequate and well-controlled studies in pregnant women.

Lactation Excretion in breast milk unknown/not recommended

Contraindications Hypersensitivity to hyaluronate or any component of the formulation

Intradermal: Additional contraindications include history of anaphylaxis or presence of multiple severe allergies; bleeding disorders (Perlane®, Restylane®); history of hypersensitivity to gram-positive bacterial proteins or lidocaine (Juvederm® Ultra XC, Juvederm® Ultra Plus XC); implantation/injection into sites other than the anatomical spaces recommended per labeling (Perlane®, Restylane®)

Intra-articular: Additional contraindications include knee joint infections; infections or skin diseases at the site of injection; hypersensitivity to gram-positive bacterial proteins (Orthovisc®)

Intraocular: There are no contraindications in the manufacturer's labeling.

Warnings/Precautions Not for I.V. injection. Do not inject into blood vessels; may cause occlusion, infarction, embolism, or other systemic adverse events.

Intra-articular: Not for use in infected joints; do not use disinfectants containing quaternary salts for skin preparation (may cause precipitation of hyaluronate). Remove synovial fluid or effusion, if present, prior to injection. Do not inject extra-articularly or into synovium. Use with caution if venous or lymphatic stasis is present in the leg. Avoid strenuous activities for 48 hours after injection. Some products are produced from avian sources; use with caution in patients with hypersensitivity to avian proteins, feathers, or egg products.

Intradermal: Treatment may result in bruising/bleeding; use caution in patients receiving or recently exposed (≤3 weeks) to thrombolytics, anticoagulants, or platelet inhibitors. Do not inject into site of active inflammation or infection. Injection into a blood vessel may cause localized superficial necrosis or may cause occlusion and lead to embolism or infarction. Use in patients susceptible to keloid formation, hypertrophic scarring, or pigmentation disorders has not been studied; use cautiously. Use caution in patients receiving immunosuppressive treatment. Use in patients with prior herpetic eruption may result in reactivation. Delayed inflammatory papules may result from injections, necessitating evaluation and treatment as soft tissue infection. Laser treatment or chemical peeling may cause acute inflammatory reaction at the injection site if performed following intradermal treatment. Patient must avoid exposure to ultraviolet rays (sun and UV lamp) or severe cold until swelling and redness is resolved. Treatment site reactions usually improve in <1 week. Strenuous exercise and ethanol consumption should be avoided for 24 hours following use. Supplemental "touch up" treatments may be required. Use in lip augmentation has not been established.

Ophthalmic: Do not overfill the anterior chamber. Postoperative increases in intraocular pressure have occurred following use of sodium hyaluronate; monitor intraocular pressure closely.

Topical: Bionect® products (cream, gel): Do not use disinfectants containing quaternary ammonium salts for skin preparation (may cause precipitation of hyaluronate).

Adverse Reactions Frequencies and/or type of local reaction may vary by formulation and site of application/injection.

>10%:

Local: Injection site (intradermal): Erythema (75% to 93%), tenderness (61% to 92%), swelling (81% to 91%), pain (47% to 90%), firmness (86% to 89%), bruising (52% to 87%), lumps/bumps (56% to 83%), skin discoloration (33% to 78%), pruritus (25% to 36%)

Neuromuscular & skeletal: Arthralgia (intra-articular 25%)

1% to 10%:

Cardiovascular: Blood pressure increased (4%)

Central nervous system: Fatigue (1%)

Gastrointestinal: Nausea (≤2%)

Local: Injection site (intra-articular): Pain (3%)

Neuromuscular & skeletal: Back pain (intra-articular <1% to 7%), joint effusion (intra-articular 2% to 6%), tendonitis (intra-articular 2%), arthrosis (intra-articular 1%), limb pain (intra-articular 1%), parasthesia (intra-articular 1%)

Miscellaneous: Infection (intra-articular 1%)

<1% (Limited to important or life-threatening): Allergic reaction (intradermal), angioedema (intradermal), arthritis (intra-articular), dyspnea (intradermal), rash, effusion (intra-articular), facial swelling (intra-articular), gait disturbance(intra-articular), herpetic eruptions (intradermal), hives (intra-articular), infections/abscess/necrosis (injection site; intradermal), peripheral edema (intra-articular), respiratory difficulty (intra-articular), thrombocytopenia (intra-articular; rare), urticarial (intradermal), vasovagal reaction (intradermal), visual abnormalities (intradermal)

Frequency not defined: Ocular (intraocular): Postoperative inflammatory reactions (iritis, hypopyon), corneal edema, corneal decompensation, postoperative increase in IOP (transient)

Drug Interactions

Metabolism/Transport Effects None known.

Avoid Concomitant Use There are no known interactions where it is recommended to avoid concomitant use.

Increased Effect/Toxicity There are no known significant interactions involving an increase in effect.

Decreased Effect There are no known significant interactions involving a decrease in effect.

Stability

Bionect® products: Store at room temperature. Cream and gel may be stored up to 24 months.

Euflexxa™: Store refrigerated or at room temperature, 2°C to 25°C (36°F to 77°F); do not freeze. Protect from light. If refrigerated, remove from refrigeration at least 20-30 minutes before use.

Juvéderm® (all formulations), Perlane®, Restylane®: Store at up to 25°C (77°F); do not freeze. Protect from light. Do not use if gel separates or becomes cloudy.

Hyalgan®, Orthovisc®: Store below 25°C (77°F); do not freeze. Protect from light.

Provisc®: Store refrigerated at 2°C to 8°C (36°F to 46°F); do not freeze. Prior to use, allow refrigerated product to reach room temperature (~20-40 minutes). Protect from light.

Supartz®, Synvisc®, Synvisc-One®: Store at room temperature, below 30°C (86°C); do not freeze. Protect from light.

Mechanism of Action Sodium hyaluronate is a biological polysaccharide which is distributed widely in the extracellular matrix of connective tissue in man (vitreous and aqueous humor of the eye, synovial fluid, skin, and umbilical cord). Sodium hyaluronate and its derivatives form a viscoelastic solution in water (at physiological pH and ionic strength) which makes it suitable for aqueous and vitreous humor in ophthalmic surgery, and functions as a tissue and/or joint lubricant which plays an important role in modulating the interactions between adjacent tissues. Intradermal injection may decrease the depth of facial wrinkles. In the topical management of wounds and ulcers, sodium hyaluronate protects the skin against friction and abrasion.

Pharmacodynamics/Kinetics

Distribution: Intravitreous injection: Diffusion occurs slowly

Excretion: Ophthalmic: Via Canal of Schlemm

Dosage Adults:

Osteoarthritis of the knee: Intra-articular:

Euflexxa™: Inject 20 mg (2 mL) once weekly for 3 weeks (total of 3 injections)

Hyalgan®: Inject 20 mg (2 mL) once weekly for 5 weeks (total of 5 injections); some patients may benefit with a total of 3 injections

Orthovisc®: Inject 30 mg (2 mL) once weekly for 3-4 weeks (total of 3-4 injections)

Supartz®: Inject 25 mg (2.5 mL) once weekly for 5 weeks (total of 5 injections); some patients may benefit with a total of 3 injections

Synvisc®: Inject 16 mg (2 mL) once weekly for 3 weeks (total of 3 injections)

Synvisc-One®: Inject 48 mg (6 mL) once

Facial wrinkles: Intradermal:

Note: Formulations differ in terms of recommended injection depth: Juvederm® and Restylane® are intended for mid to deep intradermal injection; Perlane® is intended for injection into the deep dermis to superficial subcutis

Juvéderm® (all formulations): Inject as required for cosmetic result; typical treatment regimen requires 1.6 mL/treatment site typical volume for repeat treatment is 0.7 mL/treatment site; maximum: 20 mL/60 kg/year

Perlane®: Inject as required into deep dermis/superficial subcutis for cosmetic result; median total dose: 3 mL; maximum: 6 mL per treatment

Restylane®: Inject as required for cosmetic result; median total dose: 3 mL; maximum: 6 mL per treatment

Ophthalmic (Amvisc®, Amvisc® Plus, Provisc®): Intraocular: Depends upon procedure (slowly introduce a sufficient quantity into eye)

Topical: (Bionect® cream, gel): Apply a thin layer to clean and disinfected wound or ulcer 2-3 times/day

Interstitial cystitis, refractory (unlabeled use): Intravesical (unlabeled route): 40 mg in 50 mL saline intravesically (retain in bladder for at least 30 minutes) once weekly for 4 weeks, then monthly for up to 1 year in patients showing an initial response

Administration

Intra-articular: Inject directly into the knee joint; do not inject extra-articularly or into the synovial capsule or tissues. Do not use disinfectants containing quaternary salts for skin cleansing prior to injection. Remove synovial fluid or effusion, if present, prior to injection. If used for bilateral treatment, use a separate syringe for each knee.

Intradermal: Do not inject into a blood vessel. May apply ice pack to injection site for a short period immediately after administration if treatment area swollen.

Juvederm® and Restylane® are intended for mid to deep intradermal injection

Perlane® is intended for injection into the deep dermis to superficial subcutis

Ophthalmic: Drug may become cloudy or form a slight precipitate after administration; clinical significance unknown, but cloudy or precipitated material should be removed by irrigation or aspiration

Topical: Bionect® products: Clean and disinfect wound prior to use (do not use quaternary ammonium salts due to potential for hyaluronic acid precipitation), and debride if necessary; apply a thin layer to wound or ulcer without extensive rubbing. After application, cover the area with a sterile gauze pad and if necessary, an elastic or compressive bandage.

Monitoring Parameters Intraocular pressure (ophthalmic formulations); signs and symptoms of excess local inflammation or infection (intradermal formulations)

Additional Information Perlane® differs from Restylane® in the size of its hyaluronate particles within the gel, allowing its use in deeper injections relative to other dermal fillers.

Dosage Forms Excipient information presented when available (limited, particularly for generics); consult specific product labeling.

Cream, topical [sodium hyaluronate]:

Bionect®: 0.2% (25 g)

Gel, topical [sodium hyaluronate]:

Bionect®: 0.2% (30 g, 60 g)

Injection, gel, intradermal [hyaluronic acid]:

Juvéderm® Ultra: 24 mg/mL (0.4 mL, 0.8 mL) [derived from or manufactured from bacterial source]

Juvéderm® Ultra Plus: 24 mg/mL (0.4 mL, 0.8 mL) [derived from or manufactured from bacterial source]

Juvéderm® Ultra Plus XC: Hyaluronic acid 24 mg/mL and lidocaine 0.3% (0.4 mL, 0.8 mL) [derived from or manufactured from bacterial source]

Juvéderm® Ultra XC: Hyaluronic acid 24 mg/mL and lidocaine 0.3% (0.4 mL, 0.8 mL) [derived from or manufactured from bacterial source]

Injection, gel, intradermal [sodium hyaluronate]:

Perlane®: 20 mg/mL (1 mL) [derived from or manufactured from bacterial source]

Restylane®: 20 mg/mL (0.4 mL, 1 mL, 2 mL) [derived from or manufactured from bacterial source]

Injection, solution, intra-articular [hylan polymers A and B]:

Synvisc-One®: 8 mg/mL (6 mL) [derived from or manufactured using an avian source]

Synvisc®: 8 mg/mL (2 mL) [derived from or manufactured using an avian source]

Injection, solution, intra-articular [sodium hyaluronate]:

Euflexxa®: 10 mg/mL (2 mL)

Hyalgan®: 10 mg/mL (2 mL) [derived from or manufactured using an avian source]

Orthovisc®: 15 mg/mL (2 mL) [derived from or manufactured from bacterial source]

Supartz®: 10 mg/mL (2.5 mL) [derived from or manufactured using an avian source]

Injection, solution, intraocular [sodium hyaluronate]:

Amvisc®: 12 mg/mL (0.5 mL, 0.8 mL)

Amvisc® Plus: 16 mg/mL (0.5 mL, 0.8 mL)

Provisc®: 10 mg/mL (0.4 mL, 0.55 mL, 0.85 mL) [contains natural rubber/natural latex in packaging]

◆ **Hyaluronic Acid** *see* Hyaluronate and Derivatives *on page 831*

◆ **Hycamptamine** *see* Topotecan *on page 1709*

◆ **Hycamtin®** *see* Topotecan *on page 1709*

◆ **hycet®** *see* Hydrocodone and Acetaminophen *on page 837*

◆ **Hycodan** *see* Hydrocodone and Homatropine *on page 838*

◆ **Hycort™ (Can)** *see* Hydrocortisone (Topical) *on page 841*

◆ **Hydeltra T.B.A.® (Can)** *see* PrednisoLONE (Systemic) *on page 1396*

◆ **Hyderm (Can)** *see* Hydrocortisone (Topical) *on page 841*

HydrALAZINE (hye DRAL a zeen)

Brand Names: Canada Apo-Hydralazine®; Apresoline®; Novo-Hylazin; Nu-Hydral

Index Terms Apresoline [DSC]; Hydralazine Hydrochloride

Pharmacologic Category Vasodilator

Additional Appendix Information

Heart Failure (Systolic) *on page 1991*

Hypertension *on page 2001*

Use Management of moderate-to-severe hypertension

Unlabeled Use Heart failure; hypertension secondary to pre-eclampsia/eclampsia

Pregnancy Risk Factor C

Pregnancy Considerations Teratogenic effects were observed in animal studies at 20-30 times the maximun daily human dose. Hydralazine crosses the placenta. Hydralazine is recommended for use in the management of hypertension associated with pre-eclampsia.

Lactation Enters breast milk/use caution (AAP rates "compatible"; AAP 2001 update pending)

Contraindications Hypersensitivity to hydralazine or any component of the formulation; mitral valve rheumatic heart disease

Warnings/Precautions May cause peripheral neuritis or a drug-induced lupus-like syndrome (more likely on larger doses, longer duration). Discontinue hydralazine in patients who develop SLE-like syndrome or positive ANA. Use with caution in patients with severe renal disease or cerebral vascular accidents or with known or suspected coronary artery disease; monitor blood pressure closely with I.V. use. Slow acetylators, patients with decreased renal function, and patients receiving >200 mg/day (chronically) are at higher risk for SLE. Titrate dosage cautiously to patient's response. Hypotensive effect after I.V. administration may be delayed and unpredictable in some patients. Usually administered with diuretic and a beta-blocker to counteract side effects of sodium and water retention and reflex tachycardia.

Adjust dose in severe renal dysfunction. Use with caution in CAD (increase in tachycardia may increase myocardial oxygen demand). Use with caution in pulmonary hypertension (may cause hypotension). Patients may be poorly compliant because of frequent dosing. Hydralazine-induced fluid and sodium retention may require addition or increased dosage of a diuretic.

Adverse Reactions Frequency not defined.

Cardiovascular: Angina pectoris, flushing, orthostatic hypotension, palpitations, paradoxical hypertension, peripheral edema, tachycardia, vascular collapse

Central nervous system: Anxiety, chills, depression, disorientation, dizziness, fever, headache, increased intracranial pressure (I.V.; in patient with pre-existing increased intracranial pressure), psychotic reaction

Dermatologic: Pruritus, rash, urticaria

Gastrointestinal: Anorexia, constipation, diarrhea, nausea, paralytic ileus, vomiting

Genitourinary: Dysuria, impotence

Hematologic: Agranulocytosis, eosinophilia, erythrocyte count reduced, hemoglobin decreased, hemolytic anemia, leukopenia, thrombocytopenia (rare)

Neuromuscular & skeletal: Muscle cramps, peripheral neuritis, rheumatoid arthritis, tremor, weakness

Ocular: Conjunctivitis, lacrimation

Respiratory: Dyspnea, nasal congestion

Miscellaneous: Diaphoresis, drug-induced lupus-like syndrome (dose related; fever, arthralgia, splenomegaly, lymphadenopathy, asthenia, myalgia, malaise, pleuritic chest pain, edema, positive ANA, positive LE cells, maculopapular facial rash, positive direct Coombs' test, pericarditis, pericardial tamponade)

Drug Interactions

Metabolism/Transport Effects Inhibits CYP3A4 (weak)

Avoid Concomitant Use

Avoid concomitant use of HydrALAZINE with any of the following: Pimozide

Increased Effect/Toxicity

HydrALAZINE may increase the levels/effects of: Amifostine; Antihypertensives; Hypotensive Agents; Pimozide; RiTUXimab

The levels/effects of HydrALAZINE may be increased by: Alfuzosin; Diazoxide; Herbs (Hypotensive Properties); MAO Inhibitors; Pentoxifylline; Phosphodiesterase 5 Inhibitors; Prostacyclin Analogues

Decreased Effect

The levels/effects of HydrALAZINE may be decreased by: Herbs (Hypertensive Properties); Methylphenidate; Nonsteroidal Anti-Inflammatory Agents; Yohimbine

Ethanol/Nutrition/Herb Interactions

Ethanol: Avoid ethanol (may increase CNS depression).

Food: Food enhances bioavailability of hydralazine.

Herb/Nutraceutical: Avoid dong quai if using for hypertension (has estrogenic activity). Avoid ephedra, yohimbe, ginseng (may worsen hypertension). Avoid garlic (may have increased antihypertensive effect).

Stability Intact ampuls/vials of hydralazine should not be stored under refrigeration because of possible precipitation or crystallization. Hydralazine should be diluted in NS for IVPB administration due to decreased stability in D_5W. Stability of IVPB solution in NS is 4 days at room temperature.

Mechanism of Action Direct vasodilation of arterioles (with little effect on veins) with decreased systemic resistance

Pharmacodynamics/Kinetics

Onset of action: Oral: 20-30 minutes; I.V.: 5-20 minutes

Duration: Oral: Up to 8 hours; I.V.: 1-4 hours; **Note:** May vary depending on acetylator status of patient

Protein binding: 85% to 90%

Metabolism: Hepatically acetylated; extensive first-pass effect (oral)

Bioavailability: 30% to 50%; increased with food

Half-life elimination: Normal renal function: 2-8 hours; End-stage renal disease: 7-16 hours

Excretion: Urine (14% as unchanged drug)

Dosage

Children:

Oral: Initial: 0.75-1 mg/kg/day in 2-4 divided doses; increase over 3-4 weeks to maximum of 7.5 mg/kg/day in 2-4 divided doses; maximum daily dose: 200 mg/day

I.M., I.V.: 0.1-0.2 mg/kg/dose (not to exceed 20 mg) every 4-6 hours as needed, up to 1.7-3.5 mg/kg/day in 4-6 divided doses

Adults:

Oral:

Hypertension:

Initial dose: 10 mg 4 times/day for first 2-4 days; increase to 25 mg 4 times/day for the balance of the first week

Increase by 10-25 mg/dose gradually to 50 mg 4 times/day (maximum: 300 mg/day); usual dose range (JNC 7): 25-100 mg/day in 2 divided doses

Congestive heart failure:

Initial dose: 10-25 mg 3-4 times/day

Adjustment: Dosage must be adjusted based on individual response

Target dose: 225-300 mg/day in divided doses; use in combination with isosorbide dinitrate

I.M., I.V.:

Hypertension: Initial: 10-20 mg/dose every 4-6 hours as needed, may increase to 40 mg/dose; change to oral therapy as soon as possible.

Pre-eclampsia/eclampsia: 5 mg/dose then 5-10 mg every 20-30 minutes as needed.

Elderly: Oral: Initial: 10 mg 2-3 times/day; increase by 10-25 mg/day every 2-5 days.

Dosing interval in renal impairment:

Cl_{cr} 10-50 mL/minute: Administer every 8 hours.

Cl_{cr} <10 mL/minute: Administer every 8-16 hours in fast acetylators and every 12-24 hours in slow acetylators.

Hemodialysis: Supplemental dose is not necessary.

Peritoneal dialysis: Supplemental dose is not necessary.

Dietary Considerations Administer tablet with meals.

Administration Solution for injection: Administer as a slow I.V. push; maximum rate: 5 mg/minute

Monitoring Parameters Blood pressure (monitor closely with I.V. use), standing and sitting/supine, heart rate, ANA titer

Dosage Forms Excipient information presented when available (limited, particularly for generics); consult specific product labeling.

Injection, solution, as hydrochloride: 20 mg/mL (1 mL)

Tablet, oral, as hydrochloride: 10 mg, 25 mg, 50 mg, 100 mg

Extemporaneous Preparations A flavored suspension (1.25 mg/mL) may be made with tablets. Dissolve seventy-five 50 mg hydralazine hydrochloride tablets in 250 mL of distilled water with 2250 g of Lycasin® (75% w/w maltitol syrup vehicle). Add 3 g edetate disodium, then add 3 g sodium saccharin dissolved in 50 mL distilled water. Preserve solution with 30 mL of a solution containing methylparaben 10% (w/v) and propylparaben 2% (w/v) in propylene glycol. Flavor with 3 mL orange flavoring; add sufficient quantity of distilled water to make 3 L. Adjust to pH 3.7 with glacial acetic acid. Label "shake well" and "refrigerate". Stable for 5 days at room temperature and at least 2 weeks refrigerated (preferred).

Alexander KS, Pudipeddi M, and Parker GA, "Stability of Hydralazine Hydrochloride Syrup Compounded From Tablets," *Am J Hosp Pharm*, 1993, 50(4):683-6.

◆ **Hydralazine and Isosorbide Dinitrate** *see* Isosorbide Dinitrate and Hydralazine *on page 938*

◆ **Hydralazine Hydrochloride** *see* HydrALAZINE *on page 833*

◆ **Hydrated Chloral** *see* Chloral Hydrate *on page 336*

◆ **Hydrea®** *see* Hydroxyurea *on page 851*

◆ **Hydro 35™** *see* Urea *on page 1749*

◆ **Hydro 40™** *see* Urea *on page 1749*

Hydrochlorothiazide (hye droe klor oh THYE a zide)

Brand Names: U.S. Microzide®

Brand Names: Canada Apo-Hydro®; Bio-Hydrochlorothiazide; Dom-Hydrochlorothiazide; Novo-Hydrazide; Nu-Hydro; PMS-Hydrochlorothiazide

Index Terms HCTZ (error-prone abbreviation); Hydrodiuril

Pharmacologic Category Diuretic, Thiazide

Use Management of mild-to-moderate hypertension; treatment of edema in heart failure and nephrotic syndrome

Unlabeled Use Treatment of lithium-induced diabetes insipidus

Pregnancy Risk Factor B

Pregnancy Considerations Adverse events were not observed in animal reproduction studies. Thiazide diuretics cross the placenta and are found in cord blood. Maternal use may cause may cause fetal or neonatal jaundice, thrombocytopenia, or other adverse events observed in adults. Use of thiazide diuretics during normal pregnancies is not appropriate; use may be considered when edema is due to pathologic causes (as in the nonpregnant patient); monitor.

Lactation Enters breast milk/not recommended (AAP rates "compatible"; AAP 2001 update pending)

Contraindications Hypersensitivity to hydrochlorothiazide or any component of the formulation, thiazides, or sulfonamide-derived drugs; anuria; renal decompensation; pregnancy

Warnings/Precautions Avoid in severe renal disease (ineffective as a diuretic). Electrolyte disturbances (hypokalemia, hypochloremic alkalosis, hyponatremia) can occur. Use with caution in severe hepatic dysfunction; hepatic encephalopathy can be caused by electrolyte disturbances. Gout may be precipitated in certain patients with a history of gout, a familial predisposition to gout, or chronic renal failure. Thiazide diuretics reduce calcium excretion; pathologic changes in the parathyroid glands with hypercalcemia and hypophosphatemia have been observed with prolonged use. Use with caution in patients with prediabetes and diabetes; may alter glucose control. May cause SLE exacerbation or activation. Use with caution in patients with moderate or high cholesterol concentrations. Photosensitization may occur. Correct hypokalemia before initiating therapy. Thiazide diuretics may decrease renal calcium excretion; consider avoiding use in patients with hypercalcemia. May cause acute transient myopia and acute angle-closure glaucoma, typically occurring within hours to weeks following initiation; discontinue therapy immediately in patients with acute decreases in visual acuity or ocular pain. Risk factors may include a history of sulfonamide or penicillin allergy.

Chemical similarities are present among sulfonamides, sulfonylureas, carbonic anhydrase inhibitors, thiazides, and loop diuretics (except ethacrynic acid). Use in patients with sulfonamide allergy is specifically contraindicated in product labeling, however, a risk of cross-reaction exists in patients with allergy to any of these compounds; avoid use when previous reaction has been severe. Discontinue if signs of hypersensitivity are noted.

Adverse Reactions

Frequency not defined; adverse events reported were observed at doses ≥25 mg:

Cardiovascular: Hypotension, orthostatic hypotension

Central nervous system: Dizziness, fever, headache, vertigo

Dermatologic: Alopecia, erythema multiforme, exfoliative dermatitis, photosensitivity, purpura, rash, Stevens-Johnson syndrome, toxic epidermal necrolysis, urticaria

Endocrine & metabolic: Hyperglycemia, hypokalemia, hyperuricemia

Gastrointestinal: Anorexia, constipation, cramping, diarrhea, epigastric distress, gastric irritation, nausea, pancreatitis, sialadenitis, vomiting

Genitourinary: Glycosuria, impotence

Hematologic: Agranulocytosis, aplastic anemia, hemolytic anemia, leukopenia, thrombocytopenia

Hepatic: Jaundice

Neuromuscular & skeletal: Muscle spasm, paresthesia, restlessness, weakness

Ocular: Blurred vision (transient), xanthopsia

Renal: Interstitial nephritis, renal dysfunction, renal failure

Respiratory: Respiratory distress, pneumonitis, pulmonary edema

Miscellaneous: Anaphylactic reactions, necrotizing angiitis

<1% (Limited to important or life-threatening): Allergic myocarditis, eosinophilic pneumonitis, hepatic function impairment, hypercalcemia

Drug Interactions

Metabolism/Transport Effects None known.

Avoid Concomitant Use

Avoid concomitant use of Hydrochlorothiazide with any of the following: Dofetilide

Increased Effect/Toxicity
Hydrochlorothiazide may increase the levels/effects of: ACE Inhibitors; Allopurinol; Amifostine; Antihypertensives; Calcium Salts; CarBAMazepine; Dofetilide; Hypotensive Agents; Lithium; OXcarbazepine; Porfimer; RiTUXimab; Sodium Phosphates; Topiramate; Toremifene; Vitamin D Analogs

The levels/effects of Hydrochlorothiazide may be increased by: Alcohol (Ethyl); Alfuzosin; Analgesics (Opioid); Barbiturates; Beta2-Agonists; Corticosteroids (Orally Inhaled); Corticosteroids (Systemic); Herbs (Hypotensive Properties); Licorice; MAO Inhibitors; Pentoxifylline; Phosphodiesterase 5 Inhibitors; Prostacyclin Analogues

Decreased Effect
Hydrochlorothiazide may decrease the levels/effects of: Antidiabetic Agents

The levels/effects of Hydrochlorothiazide may be decreased by: Bile Acid Sequestrants; Herbs (Hypertensive Properties); Methylphenidate; Nonsteroidal Anti-Inflammatory Agents; Yohimbine

Ethanol/Nutrition/Herb Interactions
Food: Hydrochlorothiazide peak serum levels may be decreased if taken with food. This product may deplete potassium, sodium, and magnesium.
Herb/Nutraceutical: Avoid herbs with *hypertensive* properties (bayberry, blue cohosh, cayenne, ephedra, ginger, ginseng [American], kola, licorice); may diminish the antihypertensive effect of hydrochlorothiazide. Avoid herbs with *hypotensive* properties (black cohosh, California poppy, coleus, golden seal, hawthorn, mistletoe, periwinkle, quinine, shepherd's purse); may enhance the hypotensive effect of hydrochlorothiazide.

Mechanism of Action Inhibits sodium reabsorption in the distal tubules causing increased excretion of sodium and water as well as potassium and hydrogen ions

Pharmacodynamics/Kinetics
Onset of action: Diuresis: ~2 hours
Peak effect: 4-6 hours
Duration: 6-12 hours
Absorption: ~50% to 80%
Distribution: 3.6-7.8 L/kg
Protein binding: 68%
Metabolism: Not metabolized
Bioavailability: 50% to 80%
Half-life elimination: 5.6-14.8 hours
Time to peak: 1-2.5 hours
Excretion: Urine (as unchanged drug)

Dosage Oral (effect of drug may be decreased when used every day):
Children (in pediatric patients, chlorothiazide may be preferred over hydrochlorothiazide as there are more dosage formulations [eg, suspension] available): Edema, hypertension:
<6 months: 1-3 mg/kg/day in 2 divided doses
>6 months to 2 years: 1-3 mg/kg/day in 2 divided doses; maximum: 37.5 mg/day
>2-17 years: Initial: 1 mg/kg/day; maximum: 3 mg/kg/day (50 mg/day)
Adults:
Edema: 25-100 mg/day in 1-2 doses; maximum: 200 mg/day
Hypertension: 12.5-50 mg/day; minimal increase in response and more electrolyte disturbances are seen with doses >50 mg/day
Elderly: 12.5-25 mg once daily

Dosing adjustment/comments in renal impairment: Cl_{cr} <10 mL/minute: Avoid use. Usually ineffective with GFR <30 mL/minute. Effective at lower GFR in combination with a loop diuretic.

Note: ACC/AHA 2009 Heart Failure guidelines suggest that thiazides lose their efficacy when Cl_{cr} <40 mL/minute.

Dietary Considerations May be taken with food or milk.

Administration May be administered with food or milk. Take early in day to avoid nocturia. Take the last dose of multiple doses no later than 6 PM unless instructed otherwise.

Monitoring Parameters Assess weight, I & O reports daily to determine fluid loss; blood pressure, serum electrolytes, BUN, creatinine

Test Interactions May interfere with parathyroid function tests. Tyramine and phentolamine tests, histamine tests for pheochromocytoma.

Additional Information If given the morning of surgery, hydrochlorothiazide may render the patient volume depleted and blood pressure may be labile during general anesthesia. Effect of drug may be decreased when used every day.

Dosage Forms Excipient information presented when available (limited, particularly for generics); consult specific product labeling.
Capsule, oral: 12.5 mg
Microzide®: 12.5 mg
Tablet, oral: 12.5 mg, 25 mg, 50 mg

◆ **Hydrochlorothiazide, Aliskiren, and Amlodipine** *see* Aliskiren, Amlodipine, and Hydrochlorothiazide *on page 67*

◆ **Hydrochlorothiazide, Amlodipine, and Aliskiren** *see* Aliskiren, Amlodipine, and Hydrochlorothiazide *on page 67*

◆ **Hydrochlorothiazide, Amlodipine, and Valsartan** *see* Amlodipine, Valsartan, and Hydrochlorothiazide *on page 100*

◆ **Hydrochlorothiazide and Aliskiren** *see* Aliskiren and Hydrochlorothiazide *on page 67*

◆ **Hydrochlorothiazide and Benazepril** *see* Benazepril and Hydrochlorothiazide *on page 199*

◆ **Hydrochlorothiazide and Bisoprolol** *see* Bisoprolol and Hydrochlorothiazide *on page 221*

◆ **Hydrochlorothiazide and Candesartan** *see* Candesartan and Hydrochlorothiazide *on page 274*

◆ **Hydrochlorothiazide and Captopril** *see* Captopril and Hydrochlorothiazide *on page 280*

◆ **Hydrochlorothiazide and Enalapril** *see* Enalapril and Hydrochlorothiazide *on page 586*

◆ **Hydrochlorothiazide and Eprosartan** *see* Eprosartan and Hydrochlorothiazide *on page 608*

◆ **Hydrochlorothiazide and Irbesartan** *see* Irbesartan and Hydrochlorothiazide *on page 926*

◆ **Hydrochlorothiazide and Lisinopril** *see* Lisinopril and Hydrochlorothiazide *on page 1023*

◆ **Hydrochlorothiazide and Losartan** *see* Losartan and Hydrochlorothiazide *on page 1037*

◆ **Hydrochlorothiazide and Moexipril** *see* Moexipril and Hydrochlorothiazide *on page 1149*

◆ **Hydrochlorothiazide and Olmesartan Medoxomil** *see* Olmesartan and Hydrochlorothiazide *on page 1238*

◆ **Hydrochlorothiazide and Telmisartan** *see* Telmisartan and Hydrochlorothiazide *on page 1637*

Hydrochlorothiazide and Triamterene
(hye droe klor oh THYE a zide & trye AM ter een)

Brand Names: U.S. Dyazide®; Maxzide®; Maxzide®-25
Brand Names: Canada Apo-Triazide®; Nu-Triazide; Pro-Triazide; Riva-Zide; Teva-Triamterene HCTZ
Index Terms Triamterene and Hydrochlorothiazide

Pharmacologic Category Diuretic, Potassium-Sparing; Diuretic, Thiazide

Use Treatment of hypertension or edema (not recommended for initial treatment) when hypokalemia has developed on hydrochlorothiazide alone or when the development of hypokalemia must be avoided

Pregnancy Risk Factor C

Dosage Oral: Adults:

Hydrochlorothiazide 25 mg and triamterene 37.5 mg: 1-2 tablets/capsules once daily

Hydrochlorothiazide 50 mg and triamterene 75 mg: 1/2-1 tablet daily

Additional Information Complete prescribing information for this medication should be consulted for additional detail.

Dosage Forms Excipient information presented when available (limited, particularly for generics); consult specific product labeling.

Capsule, oral: Hydrochlorothiazide 25 mg and triamterene 37.5 mg; hydrochlorothiazide 25 mg and triamterene 50 mg

Dyazide®: Hydrochlorothiazide 25 mg and triamterene 37.5 mg

Tablet: Hydrochlorothiazide 25 mg and triamterene 37.5 mg; hydrochlorothiazide 50 mg and triamterene 75 mg

Maxzide®: Hydrochlorothiazide 50 mg and triamterene 75 mg [scored]

Maxzide®-25: Hydrochlorothiazide 25 mg and triamterene 37.5 mg [scored]

◆ **Hydrochlorothiazide and Valsartan** *see* Valsartan and Hydrochlorothiazide *on page 1763*

◆ **Hydrochlorothiazide, Olmesartan, and Amlodipine** *see* Olmesartan, Amlodipine, and Hydrochlorothiazide *on page 1238*

◆ **Hydrocil® Instant [OTC]** *see* Psyllium *on page 1432*

Hydrocodone and Acetaminophen

(hye droe KOE done & a seet a MIN oh fen)

Brand Names: U.S. hycet®; Lorcet® 10/650; Lorcet® Plus; Lortab®; Margesic® H; Maxidone®; Norco®; Stagesic™; Vicodin®; Vicodin® ES; Vicodin® HP; Xodol® 10/300; Xodol® 5/300; Xodol® 7.5/300; Zamicet™; Zolvit™; Zydone®

Index Terms Acetaminophen and Hydrocodone

Pharmacologic Category Analgesic Combination (Opioid)

Use Relief of moderate-to-severe pain

Pregnancy Risk Factor C

Dosage Oral (doses should be titrated to appropriate analgesic effect): Analgesic:

Children 2-13 years or <50 kg: Hydrocodone 0.1-0.2 mg/kg/dose every 4-6 hours; do not exceed 6 doses/day or the maximum recommended dose of acetaminophen

Children and Adults ≥50 kg: Average starting dose in opioid naive patients: Hydrocodone 5-10 mg 4 times/day; the dosage of acetaminophen should be limited to ≤4 g/day (and possibly less in patients with hepatic impairment or ethanol use).

Dosage ranges (based on specific product labeling): Hydrocodone 2.5-10 mg every 4-6 hours (maximum dose of hydrocodone may be limited by the acetaminophen content of specific product)

Elderly: Doses should be titrated to appropriate analgesic effect; 2.5-5 mg of the hydrocodone component every 4-6 hours. Do not exceed 4 g/day of acetaminophen.

Dosage adjustment in hepatic impairment: Use with caution. Limited, low-dose therapy usually well tolerated in hepatic disease/cirrhosis; however, cases of hepatotoxicity at daily acetaminophen dosages <4 g/day have been reported. Avoid chronic use in hepatic impairment.

Additional Information Complete prescribing information for this medication should be consulted for additional detail.

Dosage Forms Excipient information presented when available (limited, particularly for generics); consult specific product labeling.

Capsule, oral:

Margesic® H, Stagesic™: Hydrocodone bitartrate 5 mg and acetaminophen 500 mg

Elixir, oral:

Lortab®: Hydrocodone bitartrate 7.5 mg and acetaminophen 500 mg per 15 mL (480 mL) [contains ethanol 7%, propylene glycol; tropical fruit punch flavor]

Solution, oral: Hydrocodone bitartrate 7.5 mg and acetaminophen 325 mg per 15 mL; hydrocodone bitartrate 7.5 mg and acetaminophen 500 mg per 15 mL (5 mL, 10 mL, 15 mL, 118 mL, 473 mL); hydrocodone bitartrate 10 mg and acetaminophen 325 mg per 15 mL (7.5 mL, 15 mL)

hycet®: Hydrocodone bitartrate 7.5 mg and acetaminophen 325 mg per 15 mL (473 mL) [contains ethanol 7%, propylene glycol; fruit flavor]

Zamicet™: Hydrocodone bitartrate 10 mg and acetaminophen 325 mg per 15 mL (473 mL) [contains ethanol 6.7%, propylene glycol; fruit flavor]

Zolvit™: Hydrocodone bitartrate 10 mg and acetaminophen 300 mg per 15 mL (480 mL) [contains ethanol 7%, propylene glycol; tropical fruit-punch flavor]

Tablet, oral:

Hydrocodone bitartrate 2.5 mg and acetaminophen 500 mg

Hydrocodone bitartrate 5 mg and acetaminophen 300 mg

Hydrocodone bitartrate 5 mg and acetaminophen 325 mg

Hydrocodone bitartrate 5 mg and acetaminophen 500 mg

Hydrocodone bitartrate 7.5 mg and acetaminophen 300 mg

Hydrocodone bitartrate 7.5 mg and acetaminophen 325 mg

Hydrocodone bitartrate 7.5 mg and acetaminophen 500 mg

Hydrocodone bitartrate 7.5 mg and acetaminophen 650 mg

Hydrocodone bitartrate 7.5 mg and acetaminophen 750 mg

Hydrocodone bitartrate 10 mg and acetaminophen 300 mg

Hydrocodone bitartrate 10 mg and acetaminophen 325 mg

Hydrocodone bitartrate 10 mg and acetaminophen 500 mg

Hydrocodone bitartrate 10 mg and acetaminophen 650 mg

Hydrocodone bitartrate 10 mg and acetaminophen 660 mg

Hydrocodone bitartrate 10 mg and acetaminophen 750 mg

Lorcet® 10/650: Hydrocodone bitartrate 10 mg and acetaminophen 650 mg

Lorcet® Plus: Hydrocodone bitartrate 7.5 mg and acetaminophen 650 mg

Lortab®:
5/500: Hydrocodone bitartrate 5 mg and acetaminophen 500 mg
7.5/500: Hydrocodone bitartrate 7.5 mg and acetaminophen 500 mg
10/500: Hydrocodone bitartrate 10 mg and acetaminophen 500 mg
Maxidone®: Hydrocodone bitartrate 10 mg and acetaminophen 750 mg
Norco®:
Hydrocodone bitartrate 5 mg and acetaminophen 325 mg
Hydrocodone bitartrate 7.5 mg and acetaminophen 325 mg
Hydrocodone bitartrate 10 mg and acetaminophen 325 mg
Vicodin®: Hydrocodone bitartrate 5 mg and acetaminophen 500 mg
Vicodin® ES: Hydrocodone bitartrate 7.5 mg and acetaminophen 750 mg
Vicodin® HP: Hydrocodone bitartrate 10 mg and acetaminophen 660 mg
Xodol®:
5/300: Hydrocodone bitartrate 5 mg and acetaminophen 300 mg
7.5/300: Hydrocodone bitartrate 7.5 mg and acetaminophen 300 mg
10/300: Hydrocodone bitartrate 10 mg and acetaminophen 300 mg
Zydone®:
Hydrocodone bitartrate 5 mg and acetaminophen 400 mg
Hydrocodone bitartrate 7.5 mg and acetaminophen 400 mg
Hydrocodone bitartrate 10 mg and acetaminophen 400 mg

Controlled Substance C-III

Hydrocodone and Chlorpheniramine

(hye droe KOE done & klor fen IR a meen)

Brand Names: U.S. TussiCaps®; Tussionex®

Index Terms Chlorpheniramine Maleate and Hydrocodone Bitartrate; Hydrocodone Polistirex and Chlorpheniramine Polistirex

Pharmacologic Category Alkylamine Derivative; Alpha/Beta Agonist; Antitussive; Histamine H_1 Antagonist; Histamine H_1 Antagonist, First Generation

Use Symptomatic relief of cough and upper respiratory symptoms associated with cold and allergy

Pregnancy Risk Factor C

Dosage Oral:

Children 6-12 years
TussiCaps®: 5 mg/4 mg: One capsule every 12 hours (maximum: 2 capsules/24 hours)
Tussionex®: 2.5 mL every 12 hours; do not exceed 5 mL/24 hours
Children >12 years and Adults:
TussiCaps® 10 mg/8 mg: One capsule every 12 hours (maximum: 2 capsules/24 hours)
Tussionex®: 5 mL every 12 hours; do not exceed 10 mL/24 hours

Additional Information Complete prescribing information for this medication should be consulted for additional detail.

Dosage Forms Excipient information presented when available (limited, particularly for generics); consult specific product labeling.

Capsule, extended release, oral:
TussiCaps® 5/4: Hydrocodone polistirex [equivalent to hydrocodone bitartrate 5 mg] and chlorpheniramine polistirex [equivalent to chlorpheniramine maleate 4 mg]
TussiCaps® 10/8: Hydrocodone polistirex [equivalent to hydrocodone bitartrate 10 mg] and chlorpheniramine polistirex [equivalent to chlorpheniramine maleate 8 mg]
Suspension, extended release, oral: Hydrocodone polistirex [equivalent to hydrocodone bitartrate 10 mg] and chlorpheniramine polistirex [equivalent to chlorpheniramine maleate 8 mg] per 5 mL (480 mL)
Tussionex®: Hydrocodone polistirex [equivalent to hydrocodone bitartrate 10 mg] and chlorpheniramine polistirex [equivalent to chlorpheniramine maleate 8 mg] per 5 mL (115 mL, 480 mL [DSC]) [contains propylene glycol]

Controlled Substance C-III

Hydrocodone and Homatropine

(hye droe KOE done & hoe MA troe peen)

Brand Names: U.S. Hydromet®; Tussigon®

Index Terms Homatropine and Hydrocodone; Hycodan; Hydrocodone Bitartrate and Homatropine Methylbromide

Pharmacologic Category Antitussive

Use Symptomatic relief of cough

Pregnancy Risk Factor C

Dosage Oral:

Children 6-11 years: 1/2 tablet or 2.5 mL every 4-6 hours as needed (maximum: 3 tablets or 15 mL/24 hours)
Children ≥12 years and Adults: 1 tablet or 5 mL every 4-6 hours as needed (maximum: 6 tablets/24 hours or 30 mL/24 hours)

Additional Information Complete prescribing information for this medication should be consulted for additional detail.

Dosage Forms Excipient information presented when available (limited, particularly for generics); consult specific product labeling. [DSC] = Discontinued product

Syrup: Hydrocodone bitartrate 5 mg and homatropine methylbromide 1.5 mg per 5 mL (473 mL)
Hydromet®: Hydrocodone bitartrate 5 mg and homatropine methylbromide 1.5 mg per 5 mL (480 mL) [cherry flavor]
Tablet:
Tussigon®: Hydrocodone bitartrate 5 mg and homatropine methylbromide 1.5 mg

Controlled Substance C-III

Hydrocodone and Ibuprofen

(hye droe KOE done & eye byoo PROE fen)

Brand Names: U.S. Ibudone™; Reprexain™; Vicoprofen®

Brand Names: Canada Vicoprofen®

Index Terms Hydrocodone Bitartrate and Ibuprofen; Ibuprofen and Hydrocodone

Pharmacologic Category Analgesic, Opioid; Nonsteroidal Anti-inflammatory Drug (NSAID), Oral

Use Short-term (generally <10 days) management of moderate-to-severe acute pain; is not indicated for treatment of such conditions as osteoarthritis or rheumatoid arthritis

Pregnancy Risk Factor C/D (3rd trimester)

Medication Guide Available Yes

Dosage Oral:

Adults: 1 tablet every 4-6 hours as needed for pain; maximum: 5 tablets/day. **Note:** Short-term use is recommended (<10 days).
Elderly: Use with caution; consider reduced doses. Refer to dosing in individual monographs.

Additional Information Complete prescribing information for this medication should be consulted for additional detail.

Dosage Forms Excipient information presented when available (limited, particularly for generics); consult specific product labeling.

Tablet: Hydrocodone bitartrate 5 mg and ibuprofen 200 mg; hydrocodone bitartrate 7.5 mg and ibuprofen 200 mg

Ibudone™:

5/200: Hydrocodone bitartrate 5 mg and ibuprofen 200 mg

10/200: Hydrocodone bitartrate 10 mg and ibuprofen 200 mg

Reprexain™:

2.5/200: Hydrocodone bitartrate 2.5 mg and ibuprofen 200 mg

5/200: Hydrocodone bitartrate 5 mg and ibuprofen 200 mg

10/200: Hydrocodone bitartrate 10 mg and ibuprofen 200 mg

Vicoprofen®: 7.5/200: Hydrocodone bitartrate 7.5 mg and ibuprofen 200 mg

Controlled Substance C-III

◆ **Hydrocodone Bitartrate and Homatropine Methylbromide** *see* Hydrocodone and Homatropine *on page 838*

◆ **Hydrocodone Bitartrate and Ibuprofen** *see* Hydrocodone and Ibuprofen *on page 838*

◆ **Hydrocodone Polistirex and Chlorpheniramine Polistirex** *see* Hydrocodone and Chlorpheniramine *on page 838*

Hydrocortisone (Systemic)

(hye droe KOR ti sone)

Brand Names: U.S. A-Hydrocort®; Cortef®; Solu-CORTEF®

Brand Names: Canada Cortef®; Solu-Cortef®

Index Terms A-hydroCort; Compound F; Cortisol; Hydrocortisone Sodium Succinate

Pharmacologic Category Corticosteroid, Systemic

Additional Appendix Information

Corticosteroids *on page 1888*

Use Management of adrenocortical insufficiency; anti-inflammatory or immunosuppressive

Unlabeled Use Management of septic shock when blood pressure is poorly responsive to fluid resuscitation and vasopressor therapy; treatment of thyroid storm

Pregnancy Risk Factor C

Pregnancy Considerations Adverse events have been observed with corticosteroids in animal reproduction studies. Hydrocortisone crosses the placenta. Some studies have shown an association between first trimester systemic corticosteroid use and oral clefts; adverse events in the fetus/neonate have been noted in case reports following large doses of systemic corticosteroids during pregnancy.

Lactation Enters breast milk/use caution

Contraindications Hypersensitivity to hydrocortisone or any component of the formulation; serious infections, except septic shock or tuberculous meningitis; viral, fungal, or tubercular skin lesions; I.M. administration contraindicated in idiopathic thrombocytopenia purpura; intrathecal administration of injection

Warnings/Precautions Use with caution in patients with thyroid disease, hepatic impairment, renal impairment, heart failure, hypertension, diabetes, glaucoma, cataracts, myasthenia gravis, patients at risk for osteoporosis, patients at risk for seizures, or GI diseases (diverticulitis, peptic ulcer, ulcerative colitis) due to perforation risk. Use caution following acute MI (corticosteroids have been associated with myocardial rupture). Because of the risk of adverse effects, systemic corticosteroids should be used cautiously in the elderly in the smallest possible effective dose for the shortest duration. May affect growth velocity; growth should be routinely monitored in pediatric patients. Withdraw therapy with gradual tapering of dose.

May cause hypercorticism or suppression of hypothalamic-pituitary-adrenal (HPA) axis, particularly in younger children or in patients receiving high doses for prolonged periods. HPA axis suppression may lead to adrenal crisis. Withdrawal and discontinuation of a corticosteroid should be done slowly and carefully. Particular care is required when patients are transferred from systemic corticosteroids to inhaled products due to possible adrenal insufficiency or withdrawal from steroids, including an increase in allergic symptoms. Patients receiving >20 mg per day of prednisone (or equivalent) may be most susceptible. Fatalities have occurred due to adrenal insufficiency in asthmatic patients during and after transfer from systemic corticosteroids to aerosol steroids; aerosol steroids do not provide the systemic steroid needed to treat patients having trauma, surgery, or infections.

Acute myopathy has been reported with high dose corticosteroids, usually in patients with neuromuscular transmission disorders; may involve ocular and/or respiratory muscles; monitor creatine kinase; recovery may be delayed. Corticosteroid use may cause psychiatric disturbances, including depression, euphoria, insomnia, mood swings, and personality changes. Pre-existing psychiatric conditions may be exacerbated by corticosteroid use. Prolonged use of corticosteroids may also increase the incidence of secondary infection, mask acute infection (including fungal infections), prolong or exacerbate viral infections, or limit response to vaccines. Exposure to chickenpox should be avoided; corticosteroids should not be used to treat ocular herpes simplex. Corticosteroids should not be used for cerebral malaria or viral hepatitis. Oral steroid treatment is not recommended for the treatment of acute optic neuritis. Close observation is required in patients with latent tuberculosis and/or TB reactivity; restrict use in active TB (only in conjunction with antituberculosis treatment). Prolonged treatment with corticosteroids has been associated with the development of Kaposi's sarcoma (case reports); if noted, discontinuation of therapy should be considered. High-dose corticosteroids should not be used to manage acute head injury. Some dosage forms contain benzyl alcohol which has been associated with "gasping syndrome" in neonates.

Adverse Reactions Frequency not defined.

Cardiovascular: Arrhythmias, bradycardia, cardiac arrest, cardiomegaly, circulatory collapse, congestive heart failure, edema, fat embolism, hypertension, hypertrophic cardiomyopathy (premature infants), myocardial rupture (post MI), syncope, tachycardia, thromboembolism, vasculitis

Central nervous system: Delirium, depression, emotional instability, euphoria, hallucinations, headache, insomnia, intracranial pressure increased, malaise, mood swings, nervousness, neuritis, neuropathy, personality changes, pseudotumor cerebri, psychic disorders, psychoses, seizure, vertigo

Dermatologic: Acne, allergic dermatitis, alopecia, bruising, burning/tingling, dry scaly skin, edema, erythema, hirsutism, hyper-/hypopigmentation, impaired wound healing, petechiae, rash, skin atrophy, skin test reaction impaired, sterile abscess, striae, urticaria

Endocrine & metabolic: Adrenal suppression, alkalosis, amenorrhea, carbohydrate intolerance increased, Cushing's syndrome, diabetes mellitus, glucose intolerance, growth suppression, hyperglycemia, hyperlipidemia, hypokalemia, hypokalemic alkalosis, menstrual irregularities, negative nitrogen balance, pituitary-adrenal axis suppression, potassium loss, protein catabolism, sodium and water retention, sperm motility increased/decreased, spermatogenesis increased/decreased

Gastrointestinal: Abdominal distention, appetite increased, bowel dysfunction (intrathecal administration), indigestion, nausea, pancreatitis, peptic ulcer, gastrointestinal perforation, ulcerative esophagitis, vomiting, weight gain

Genitourinary: Bladder dysfunction (intrathecal administration)

Hematologic: Leukocytosis (transient)

Hepatic: Hepatomegaly, transaminases increased

Local: Atrophy (at injection site), postinjection flare (intra-articular use), thrombophlebitis

Neuromuscular & skeletal: Arthralgia, necrosis (femoral and humoral heads), Charcot-like arthropathy, fractures, muscle mass loss, muscle weakness, myopathy, osteoporosis, tendon rupture, vertebral compression fractures

Ocular: Cataracts, exophthalmoses, glaucoma, intraocular pressure increased

Miscellaneous: Abnormal fat deposits, anaphylaxis, avascular necrosis, diaphoresis, hiccups, hypersensitivity reactions, infection, secondary malignancy

Drug Interactions

Metabolism/Transport Effects **Substrate** of CYP3A4 (minor), P-glycoprotein; **Note:** Assignment of Major/Minor substrate status based on clinically relevant drug interaction potential; **Induces** CYP3A4 (weak/moderate)

Avoid Concomitant Use

Avoid concomitant use of Hydrocortisone (Systemic) with any of the following: Aldesleukin; BCG; Natalizumab; Pimecrolimus; Tacrolimus (Topical)

Increased Effect/Toxicity

Hydrocortisone (Systemic) may increase the levels/effects of: Acetylcholinesterase Inhibitors; Amphotericin B; Deferasirox; Leflunomide; Loop Diuretics; Natalizumab; NSAID (COX-2 Inhibitor); NSAID (Nonselective); Thiazide Diuretics; Vaccines (Live); Warfarin

The levels/effects of Hydrocortisone (Systemic) may be increased by: Antifungal Agents (Azole Derivatives, Systemic); Aprepitant; Calcium Channel Blockers (Nondihydropyridine); Conivaptan; Denosumab; Estrogen Derivatives; Fluconazole; Fosaprepitant; Indacaterol; Macrolide Antibiotics; Neuromuscular-Blocking Agents (Nondepolarizing); P-glycoprotein/ABCB1 Inhibitors; Pimecrolimus; Quinolone Antibiotics; Roflumilast; Salicylates; Tacrolimus (Topical); Telaprevir; Trastuzumab

Decreased Effect

Hydrocortisone (Systemic) may decrease the levels/effects of: Aldesleukin; Antidiabetic Agents; ARIPiprazole; BCG; Calcitriol; Coccidioidin Skin Test; Corticorelin; Isoniazid; Salicylates; Sipuleucel-T; Telaprevir; Vaccines (Inactivated)

The levels/effects of Hydrocortisone (Systemic) may be decreased by: Aminoglutethimide; Antacids; Barbiturates; Bile Acid Sequestrants; Echinacea; Mitotane; P-glycoprotein/ABCB1 Inducers; Primidone; Rifamycin Derivatives; Tocilizumab

Ethanol/Nutrition/Herb Interactions

Ethanol: Avoid ethanol (may enhance gastric mucosal irritation).

Food: Hydrocortisone interferes with calcium absorption.

Herb/Nutraceutical: St John's wort may decrease hydrocortisone levels. Avoid cat's claw, echinacea (have immunostimulant properties).

Stability Store at controlled room temperature 20°C to 25°C (68°F to 77°F). Protect from light. Hydrocortisone sodium phosphate and hydrocortisone sodium succinate are clear, light yellow solutions which are heat labile.

Sodium succinate: Reconstitute 100 mg vials with bacteriostatic water (not >2 mL). Act-O-Vial (self-contained powder for injection plus diluent) may be reconstituted by pressing the activator to force diluent into the powder compartment. Following gentle agitation, solution may be withdrawn via syringe through a needle inserted into the center of the stopper. May be administered (I.V. or I.M.) without further dilution. After initial reconstitution, hydrocortisone sodium succinate solutions are stable for 3 days at room temperature or under refrigeration when protected from light. Stability of parenteral admixture (Solu-Cortef®) at room temperature (25°C) and at refrigeration temperature (4°C) is concentration-dependent:

Stability of concentration 1 mg/mL: 24 hours.

Stability of concentration 2 mg/mL to 60 mg/mL: At least 4 hours.

Solutions for I.V. infusion: Reconstituted solutions may be added to an appropriate volume of compatible solution for infusion. Concentration should generally not exceed 1 mg/mL. However, in cases where administration of a small volume of fluid is desirable, 100-3000 mg may be added to 50 mL of D_5W or NS (stability limited to 4 hours).

Mechanism of Action Decreases inflammation by suppression of migration of polymorphonuclear leukocytes and reversal of increased capillary permeability

Pharmacodynamics/Kinetics

Onset of action: Hydrocortisone sodium succinate (water soluble): Rapid

Absorption: Rapid

Metabolism: Hepatic

Half-life elimination: Biologic: 8-12 hours

Excretion: Urine (primarily as 17-hydroxysteroids and 17-ketosteroids)

Dosage Dose should be based on severity of disease and patient response

Adrenal hyperplasia (congenital): Children: Oral: Initial: 10-20 mg/m^2/day in 3 divided doses; a variety of dosing schedules have been used. **Note:** Inconsistencies have occurred with liquid formulations; tablets may provide more reliable levels. Doses must be individualized by monitoring growth, bone age, and hormonal levels. Mineralocorticoid and sodium supplementation may be required based upon electrolyte regulation and plasma renin activity.

Adrenal insufficiency (acute): I.M., I.V.:

Infants and Young Children: 1-2 mg/kg/dose bolus, then 25-150 mg/day in divided doses every 6-8 hours

Older Children: 1-2 mg/kg bolus then 150-250 mg/day in divided doses every 6-8 hours

Adults: 100 mg I.V. bolus, then 300 mg/day in divided doses every 8 hours or as a continuous infusion for 48 hours; once patient is stable change to oral, 50 mg every 8 hours for 6 doses, then taper to 30-50 mg/day in divided doses

Adrenal insufficiency (chronic): Adults: Oral: 20-30 mg/day

Anti-inflammatory or immunosuppressive:

Infants and Children:

Oral: 2.5-10 mg/kg/day **or** 75-300 mg/m^2/day every 6-8 hours

I.M., I.V.: 1-5 mg/kg/day **or** 30-150 mg/m^2/day divided every 12-24 hours

Adolescents and Adults: Oral, I.M., I.V.: 15-240 mg every 12 hours

Physiologic replacement: Children:

Oral: 0.5-0.75 mg/kg/day **or** 20-25 mg/m^2/day divided every 8 hours

I.M.: 0.25-0.35 mg/kg/day **or** 12-15 mg/m^2/day once daily

Septic shock (unlabeled use): I.V.:
Children: Initial: 1-2 mg/kg/day (intermittent or as continuous infusion); may titrate up to 50 mg/kg/day for shock reversal (Brierley, 2009); alternative dosing suggests 50 mg/m^2/day (Dellinger, 2008). **Note:** Use recommended only in catecholamine-resistant shock and suspected or proven adrenal insufficiency.
Adults: 50 mg every 6 hours (Annane, 2002; Marik, 2008); not to exceed 300 mg/day (Dellinger, 2008). Practice guidelines also recommend alternative dosing of 100 mg bolus, followed by continuous infusion of 10 mg/hour (240 mg/day). Taper slowly (for total of 11 days) and do not stop abruptly. **Note:** Fludrocortisone is optional with use of hydrocortisone.
Status asthmaticus: Children and Adults: I.V.: 1-2 mg/kg/dose every 6 hours for 24 hours, then maintenance of 0.5-1 mg/kg every 6 hours
Stress dosing (surgery) in patients known to be adrenally-suppressed or on chronic systemic steroids: I.V.: Adults:
Minor stress (ie, inguinal herniorrhaphy): 25 mg/day for 1 day
Moderate stress (ie, joint replacement, cholecystectomy): 50-75 mg/day (25 mg every 8-12 hours) for 1-2 days
Major stress (pancreatoduodenectomy, esophagogastrectomy, cardiac surgery): 100-150 mg/day (50 mg every 8-12 hours) for 2-3 days
Thyroid storm (unlabeled use): I.V.: 300 mg loading dose, followed by 100 mg every 8 hours (Bahn, 2011)

Dietary Considerations Systemic use of corticosteroids may require a diet with increased potassium, vitamins A, B_6, C, D, folate, calcium, zinc, phosphorus, and decreased sodium. Some products may contain sodium.

Administration
Oral: Administer with food or milk to decrease GI upset
Parenteral: Hydrocortisone sodium succinate may be administered by I.M. or I.V. routes. Dermal and/or subdermal skin depression may occur at the site of injection. Avoid injection into deltoid muscle (high incidence of subcutaneous atrophy).
I.V. bolus: Dilute to 50 mg/mL and administer over 30 seconds or over 10 minutes for doses ≥500 mg
I.V. intermittent infusion: Dilute to 1 mg/mL and administer over 20-30 minutes

Monitoring Parameters Serum glucose, electrolytes; blood pressure, weight, presence of infection; monitor IOP with therapy >6 weeks; bone mineral density, growth in children

Reference Range Therapeutic: AM: 5-25 mcg/dL (SI: 138-690 nmol/L), PM: 2-9 mcg/dL (SI: 55-248 nmol/L) depending on test, assay

Test Interactions Interferes with skin tests

Dosage Forms Excipient information presented when available (limited, particularly for generics); consult specific product labeling.
Injection, powder for reconstitution, as sodium succinate [strength expressed as base]:
A-Hydrocort®: 100 mg
Solu-CORTEF®: 100 mg
Injection, powder for reconstitution, as sodium succinate [strength expressed as base, preservative free]:
Solu-CORTEF®: 100 mg, 250 mg, 500 mg, 1000 mg [supplied with diluent]
Tablet, oral, as base: 5 mg, 10 mg, 20 mg
Cortef®: 5 mg, 10 mg, 20 mg [scored]

Extemporaneous Preparations A 2.5 mg/mL oral suspension may be made with either tablets or powder and a vehicle containing sodium carboxymethylcellulose (1 g), syrup BP (10 mL), hydroxybenzoate 0.1% preservatives (0.1 g), polysorbate 80 (0.5 mL), citric acid (0.6 g), and water. To make the vehicle, dissolve the hydroxybenzoate, citric acid, and syrup BP in hot water. Cool solution and add the carboxymethylcellulose; leave overnight. Crush twelve-and-one-half 20 mg hydrocortisone tablets (or use 250 mg of powder) in a mortar and reduce to a fine powder while adding polysorbate 80. Add small portions of vehicle and mix to a uniform paste; mix while adding the vehicle in incremental proportions to **almost** 100 mL; transfer to a calibrated bottle, rinse mortar with vehicle, and add sufficient quantity of vehicle to make 100 mL. Label "shake well" and "refrigerate". Stable for 90 days.

Fawcett JP, Boulton DW, Jiang R, et al, "Stability of Hydrocortisone Oral Suspensions Prepared From Tablets and Powder," *Ann Pharmacother*, 1995, 29(10):987-90.

Hydrocortisone (Topical) (hye droe KOR ti sone)

Brand Names: U.S. Ala-Cort; Ala-Scalp; Anu-med HC; Anucort-HC™; Anusol-HC®; Aquanil HC® [OTC]; Beta-HC® [OTC]; Caldecort® [OTC]; Colocort®; Cortaid® Advanced [OTC]; Cortaid® Intensive Therapy [OTC]; Cortaid® Maximum Strength [OTC]; Cortenema®; CortiCool® [OTC]; Cortifoam®; Cortizone-10® Hydratensive Healing [OTC]; Cortizone-10® Hydratensive Soothing [OTC]; Cortizone-10® Intensive Healing Eczema [OTC]; Cortizone-10® Maximum Strength Cooling Relief [OTC]; Cortizone-10® Maximum Strength Easy Relief [OTC]; Cortizone-10® Maximum Strength Intensive Healing Formula [OTC]; Cortizone-10® Maximum Strength [OTC]; Cortizone-10® Plus Maximum Strength [OTC]; Dermarest® Eczema Medicated [OTC]; Hemril® -30; Hydrocortisone Plus [OTC]; Hydroskin® [OTC]; Locoid Lipocream®; Locoid®; Pandel®; Pediaderm™ HC; Preparation H® Hydrocortisone [OTC]; Procto-Pak™; Proctocort®; ProctoCream®-HC; Proctosol-HC®; Proctozone-HC 2.5%™; Recort [OTC]; Scalpana [OTC]; Texacort™; U-Cort®; Westcort®

Brand Names: Canada Aquacort®; Cortamed®; Cortenema®; Cortifoam™; Emo-Cort®; Hycort™; Hyderm; HydroVal®; Locoid®; Prevex® HC; Sarna® HC; Westcort®

Index Terms A-hydroCort; Compound F; Cortisol; Hemorrhoidal HC; Hydrocortisone Acetate; Hydrocortisone Butyrate; Hydrocortisone Probutate; Hydrocortisone Valerate; Nutracort

Pharmacologic Category Corticosteroid, Rectal; Corticosteroid, Topical

Additional Appendix Information
Corticosteroids *on page 1888*

Use Relief of inflammation of corticosteroid-responsive dermatoses (low and medium potency topical corticosteroid); adjunctive treatment of ulcerative colitis; mild-to-moderate atopic dermatitis; inflamed hemorrhoids, postirradiation (factitial) proctitis, and other inflammatory conditions of anorectum and pruritus ani

Pregnancy Risk Factor C

Dosage
Topical:
Children 3 months to 18 years: Atopic dermatitis: Hydrocortisone butyrate (Locoid Lipocream®): Apply thin film to affected area twice daily
Children and Adults: Dermatosis: Apply thin film to affected area 2-4 times/day. Products labeled for OTC use (self-medication) should not be used in children <2 years of age.
Children ≥12 years and Adults: External anal and genital itching: (OTC labeling): Apply to clean dry skin up to 3-4 times/day
Adults: Dermatosis:
Hydrocortisone probutate (Pandel®): Apply thin film to affected area 1-2 times/day
Hydrocortisone valerate (Westcort®): Apply thin film to affected area 2-3 times/day

Rectal: Adults:
Hemorrhoids: Suppository: One suppository (30 mg) twice daily for 2 weeks. For severe cases of proctitis, 1 suppository 3 times/day or 2 suppositories twice daily may be needed. For factitial proctitis, duration of treatment may be up to 6-8 weeks.
Ulcerative colitis:
Foam: One applicatorful (80 mg) 1-2 times/day for 2-3 weeks, and then every other day thereafter; use lowest dose to maintain clinical response; taper dose to discontinue long-term therapy
Suspension: One enema (100 mg) every night for 21 days or until remission (clinical improvement may precede improvement of mucosal integrity); 2-3 months of therapy may be required; taper dose to discontinue long-term therapy

Additional Information Complete prescribing information for this medication should be consulted for additional detail.

Dosage Forms Excipient information presented when available (limited, particularly for generics); consult specific product labeling. [DSC] = Discontinued product

Aerosol, foam, rectal, as acetate:
Cortifoam®: 10% (15 g) [90 mg/applicator]
Cream, topical, as acetate: 1% (28.4 g, 454 g); 2% (43 g)
U-Cort®: 1% (28 g) [contains sodium metabisulfite]
Cream, topical, as acetate [strength expressed as base]: 1% (30 g)
Cream, topical, as base: 0.5% (28.4 g, 30 g); 1% (1 g, 1.5 g, 15 g, 28.35 g [DSC], 28.4 g, 30 g, 114 g, 454 g); 2.5% (20 g, 28 g, 28.35 g, 30 g, 454 g)
Ala-Cort: 1% (28.4 g, 85.2 g)
Anusol-HC®: 2.5% (30 g) [contains benzyl alcohol]
Caldecort®: 1% (28.4 g) [contains aloe]
Cortaid® Advanced: 1% (42 g) [contains aloe]
Cortaid® Intensive Therapy: 1% (37 g, 56 g)
Cortaid® Maximum Strength: 1% (14 g, 28 g, 37 g, 56 g) [contains aloe]
Cortizone-10® Maximum Strength: 1% (15 g, 28 g, 56 g) [contains aloe]
Cortizone-10® Maximum Strength Intensive Healing Formula: 1% (28 g, 56 g) [contains aloe, benzyl alcohol]
Cortizone-10® Plus Maximum Strength: 1% (28 g, 56 g) [contains aloe, vitamin A, vitamin E]
Hydrocortisone Plus: 1% (28.4 g) [contains aloe, vitamin A, vitamin D, vitamin E]
Hydroskin®: 1% (28 g)
Preparation H® Hydrocortisone: 1% (26 g) [contains sodium benzoate]
Procto-Pak™: 1% (28.4 g)
Proctocort®: 1% (28.35 g)
ProctoCream®-HC: 2.5% (30 g) [contains benzyl alcohol]
Proctosol-HC®: 2.5% (28.35 g)
Proctozone-HC 2.5%™: 2.5% (30 g)
Recort: 1% (30 g)
Cream, topical, as butyrate: 0.1% (15 g, 45 g)
Locoid Lipocream®: 0.1% (15 g, 45 g, 60 g)
Locoid®: 0.1% (15 g, 45 g)
Cream, topical, as probutate:
Pandel®: 0.1% (15 g, 45 g, 80 g)
Cream, topical, as valerate: 0.2% (15 g, 45 g, 60 g)
Gel, topical, as base:
CortiCool®: 1% (0.9 g, 42.5 g) [contains ethanol 20%]
Cortizone-10® Maximum Strength Cooling Relief: 1% (28 g) [contains aloe, ethanol 15%]
Liquid, topical, as base:
Cortizone-10® Maximum Strength Easy Relief: 1% (36 mL) [contains aloe, ethanol 45%]
Scalpana: 1% (85.5 mL)
Lotion, topical, as base: 1% (114 g, 118 mL); 2.5% (59 mL, 60 mL [DSC], 118 mL)
Ala-Scalp: 2% (29.6 mL)
Aquanil HC®: 1% (120 mL) [contains benzyl alcohol]
Beta-HC®: 1% (60 mL)
Cortaid® Intensive Therapy: 1% (98 g)
Cortizone-10® Hydratensive Healing: 1% (113 g) [contains aloe]
Cortizone-10® Hydratensive Soothing: 1% (113 g) [contains aloe]
Cortizone-10® Intensive Healing Eczema: 1% (99 g) [contains aloe, vitamin A, vitamin C, vitamin E]
Dermarest® Eczema Medicated: 1% (118 mL)
Hydroskin®: 1% (118 mL)
Lotion, topical, as base [kit]:
Pediaderm™ HC: 2% (29.6 mL) [contains benzalkonium chloride, isopropyl alcohol; packaged with protective emollient]
Lotion, topical, as butyrate:
Locoid®: 0.1% (60 mL)
Ointment, topical, as acetate [strength expressed as base]: 1% (30 g)
Ointment, topical, as base: 0.5% (30 g); 1% (25 g, 30 g, 110 g, 430 g, 454 g); 2.5% (20 g, 28.35 g [DSC], 30 g, 454 g)
Cortaid® Maximum Strength: 1% (28 g, 37 g)
Cortizone-10® Maximum Strength: 1% (28 g, 56 g)
Ointment, topical, as butyrate: 0.1% (15 g, 45 g)
Locoid®: 0.1% (15 g, 45 g)
Ointment, topical, as valerate: 0.2% (15 g, 45 g, 60 g)
Westcort®: 0.2% (15 g, 45 g, 60 g)
Powder, for prescription compounding, as acetate [micronized]: USP: 100% (10 g, 25 g, 100 g)
Solution, topical, as base:
Texacort™: 2.5% (30 mL) [contains ethanol 48.8%]
Solution, topical, as base [spray]:
Cortaid® Intensive Therapy: 1% (59 mL) [contains ethanol 45%]
Solution, topical, as butyrate: 0.1% (20 mL, 60 mL)
Locoid®: 0.1% (20 mL, 60 mL) [contains isopropyl alcohol 50%]
Suppository, rectal, as acetate: 25 mg (12s); 30 mg (12s)
Anu-med HC: 25 mg (12s)
Anucort-HC™: 25 mg (12s, 24s, 100s)
Anusol-HC®: 25 mg (12s, 24s)
Hemril® -30: 30 mg (12s, 24s)
Proctocort®: 30 mg (12s, 24s)
Suspension, rectal, as base: 100 mg/60 mL (60 mL)
Colocort®: 100 mg/60 mL (60 mL)
Cortenema®: 100 mg/60 mL (60 mL)

- **Hydrocortisone Acetate** *see* Hydrocortisone (Topical) *on page 841*
- **Hydrocortisone, Acetic Acid, and Propylene Glycol Diacetate** *see* Acetic Acid, Propylene Glycol Diacetate, and Hydrocortisone *on page 33*
- **Hydrocortisone and Benzoyl Peroxide** *see* Benzoyl Peroxide and Hydrocortisone *on page 205*
- **Hydrocortisone and Ciprofloxacin** *see* Ciprofloxacin and Hydrocortisone *on page 366*
- **Hydrocortisone and Iodoquinol** *see* Iodoquinol and Hydrocortisone *on page 921*
- **Hydrocortisone and Pramoxine** *see* Pramoxine and Hydrocortisone *on page 1393*
- **Hydrocortisone and Urea** *see* Urea and Hydrocortisone *on page 1750*
- **Hydrocortisone, Bacitracin, Neomycin, and Polymyxin B** *see* Bacitracin, Neomycin, Polymyxin B, and Hydrocortisone *on page 187*
- **Hydrocortisone Butyrate** *see* Hydrocortisone (Topical) *on page 841*
- **Hydrocortisone, Neomycin, and Polymyxin B** *see* Neomycin, Polymyxin B, and Hydrocortisone *on page 1190*

HYDROmorphone (hye droe MOR fone)

Brand Names: U.S. Dilaudid-HP®; Dilaudid®; Exalgo™

Brand Names: Canada Dilaudid-HP-Plus®; Dilaudid-HP®; Dilaudid-XP®; Dilaudid®; Dilaudid® Sterile Powder; Hydromorph Contin®; Hydromorph-IR®; Hydromorphone HP; Hydromorphone HP® 10; Hydromorphone HP® 20; Hydromorphone HP® 50; Hydromorphone HP® Forte; Hydromorphone Hydrochloride Injection, USP; Jurnista™; PMS-Hydromorphone

Index Terms Dihydromorphinone; Hydromorphone Hydrochloride

Pharmacologic Category Analgesic, Opioid

Additional Appendix Information

Opioid Analgesics *on page 1896*

Patient Information for Disposal of Unused Medications *on page 2026*

Use Management of moderate-to-severe pain

Exalgo™: Management of moderate-to-severe pain in opioid-tolerant patients (requiring around-the-clock analgesia for an extended period of time)

Pregnancy Risk Factor C

Pregnancy Considerations Hydromorphone was teratogenic in some, but not all, animal studies; however, maternal toxicity was also reported. Hydromorphone crosses the placenta. Chronic opioid use during pregnancy may lead to a withdrawal syndrome in the neonate. Symptoms include irritability, hyperactivity, loss of sleep pattern, abnormal crying, tremor, vomiting, diarrhea, weight loss, or failure to gain weight.

Lactation Enters breast milk/not recommended

Prescribing and Access Restrictions Exalgo™: As a requirement of the REMS program, healthcare providers who prescribe Exalgo™ need to receive training on the proper use and potential risks of Exalgo™. For training, please refer to http://www.exalgorems.com. Prescribers will need retraining every 2 years or following any significant changes to the Exalgo™ REMS program.

Medication Guide Available Yes

Contraindications Hypersensitivity to hydromorphone, any component of the formulation; acute or severe asthma, severe respiratory depression (in absence of resuscitative equipment or ventilatory support); severe CNS depression

Additional product-specific contraindications:

Dilaudid®, Dilaudid-HP®: Obstetrical analgesia

Exalgo™: Opioid nontolerant patients, paralytic ileus, preexisting GI surgery or diseases resulting in narrowing of GI tract, loops in the GI tract or GI obstruction

Warnings/Precautions Use with caution in patients with hypersensitivity reactions to other phenanthrene derivative opioid agonists (codeine, hydrocodone, levorphanol, oxycodone, oxymorphone). Hydromorphone shares toxic potential of opiate agonists, including CNS depression and respiratory depression. Precautions associated with opiate agonist therapy should be observed. May cause CNS depression, which may impair physical or mental abilities; patients must be cautioned about performing tasks which require mental alertness (eg, operating machinery or driving). Myoclonus and seizures have been reported with high doses. Critical respiratory depression may occur, even at therapeutic dosages, particularly in elderly or debilitated patients or in patients with pre-existing respiratory compromise (hypoxia and/or hypercapnia). Use caution in COPD or other obstructive pulmonary disease. Use with caution in patients with hypersensitivity to other phenanthrene opiates, kyphoscoliosis, cardiovascular disease, morbid obesity, adrenocortical insufficiency, hypothyroidism, acute alcoholism, delirium tremens, toxic psychoses, prostatic hyperplasia and/or urinary stricture, or severe liver or renal failure. Use with caution in patients with biliary tract dysfunction. Hydromorphone may increase biliary tract pressure following spasm in sphincter of Oddi. Use caution in patients with inflammatory or obstructive bowel disorder, acute pancreatitis secondary to biliary tract disease, and patients undergoing biliary surgery. Use extreme caution in patients with head injury, intracranial lesions, or elevated intracranial pressure; exaggerated elevation of ICP may occur (in addition, hydromorphone may complicate neurologic evaluation due to pupillary dilation and CNS depressant effects). Use with caution in patients with depleted blood volume or drugs which may exaggerate hypotensive effects (including phenothiazines or general anesthetics). May obscure diagnosis or clinical course of patients with acute abdominal conditions.

[U.S. Boxed Warning]: Hydromorphone has a high potential for abuse. Those at risk for opioid abuse include patients with a history of substance abuse or mental illness. Tolerance or drug dependence may result from extended use; however, concerns for abuse should not prevent effective management of pain. In general, abrupt discontinuation of therapy in dependent patients should be avoided.

An opioid-containing analgesic regimen should be tailored to each patient's needs and based upon the type of pain being treated (acute versus chronic), the route of administration, degree of tolerance for opioids (naive versus chronic user), age, weight, and medical condition. The optimal analgesic dose varies widely among patients. Doses should be titrated to pain relief/prevention. I.M. use may result in variable absorption and a lag time to peak effect.

Dosage form specific warnings:

[U.S. Boxed Warning]: Dilaudid-HP®: Extreme caution should be taken to avoid confusing the highly-concentrated (Dilaudid-HP®) injection with the less-concentrated (Dilaudid®) injectable product. Dilaudid-HP® should only be used in patients who are opioid-tolerant.

Controlled release: Capsules should only be used when continuous analgesia is required over an extended period of time. Controlled release products are not to be used on an "as needed" (PRN) basis.

Extended release tablets (Exalgo™): **[U.S. Boxed Warning]: For use in opioid tolerant patients only; fatal respiratory depression may occur in patient who are not opioid tolerant. Indicated for the management of moderate-to-severe pain when around the clock pain control is needed for an extended time**

period. Not for use as an as-needed analgesic or for the management of acute or postoperative pain. Tablets should be swallowed whole; do not crush, break, chew, dissolve or inject; doing so may lead to rapid release and absorption of a potentially fatal dose of hydromorphone. Accidental consumption may lead to fatal overdose, especially in children. Exalgo™ tablets are nondeformable; do not administer to patients with preexisting severe gastrointestinal narrowing (eg, esophageal motility, small bowel inflammatory disease, short gut syndrome, history of peritonitis, cystic fibrosis, chronic intestinal pseudo-obstruction, Meckel's diverticulum); obstruction may occur. Exalgo™ is not recommended for use within 14 days of MAO inhibitors; severe and unpredictable potentiation by MAO inhibitors has been reported with opioid analgesics

Some dosage forms contain trace amounts of sodium metabisulfite which may cause allergic reactions in susceptible individuals.

Adverse Reactions Frequency not defined.

Cardiovascular: Bradycardia, extrasystoles, flushing of face, hyper-/hypotension, palpitation, peripheral edema, peripheral vasodilation, syncope, tachycardia

Central nervous system: Abnormal dreams, abnormal feelings, agitation, aggression, apprehension, attention disturbances, chills, coordination impaired, CNS depression, confusion, cognitive disorder, crying, dizziness, drowsiness, dysphoria, encephalopathy, euphoria, fatigue, hallucinations, headache, hyper-reflexia, hypo/hyperesthesia, hypothermia, increased intracranial pressure, insomnia, lightheadedness, listlessness, malaise, memory impairment, mental depression, mood alterations, nervousness, panic attacks, paranoia, psychomotor hyperactivity, restlessness, sedation, seizure, somnolence, suicide ideation, vertigo

Dermatologic: Hyperhidrosis, pruritus, rash, urticaria

Endocrine & metabolic: Amylase decreased, dehydration, erectile dysfunction, fluid retention, hyperuricemia, hypogonadism, hypokalemia, libido decreased, sexual dysfunction, testosterone decreased

Gastrointestinal: Abdominal distention, anal fissure, anorexia, appetite increased, bezoar (Exalgo™), biliary tract spasm, constipation, diarrhea, diverticulum, diverticulitis, duodenitis, dysgeusia, dysphagia, eructation, flatulence, gastric emptying impaired, gastrointestinal motility disorder (Exalgo™), gastroenteritis, hematochezia, ileus, intestinal obstruction (Exalgo™), large intestine perforation (Exalgo™), nausea, painful defecation, paralytic ileus, stomach cramps, taste perversion, vomiting, weight loss, xerostomia

Genitourinary: Dysuria, micturition disorder, ureteral spasm, urinary frequency, urinary hesitation, urinary retention, urinary tract spasm, urination decreased

Hepatic: LFTs increased

Local: Pain at injection site (I.M.), wheal/flare over vein (I.V.)

Neuromuscular & skeletal: Arthralgia, dysarthria, dyskinesia, muscle rigidity, muscle spasms, myalgia, myoclonus, paresthesia, trembling, tremor, uncoordinated muscle movements, weakness

Ocular: Blurred vision, diplopia, dry eyes, miosis, nystagmus

Otic: Tinnitus

Respiratory: Apnea, bronchospasm, dyspnea, hyperventilation, hypoxia, laryngospasm, oxygen saturation decreased, respiratory depression/distress, rhinorrhea

Miscellaneous: Antidiuretic effects, balance disorder, diaphoresis, difficulty walking, histamine release, physical and psychological dependence

Drug Interactions

Metabolism/Transport Effects None known.

Avoid Concomitant Use

Avoid concomitant use of HYDROmorphone with any of the following: MAO Inhibitors

Increased Effect/Toxicity

HYDROmorphone may increase the levels/effects of: Alcohol (Ethyl); Alvimopan; CNS Depressants; Desmopressin; Selective Serotonin Reuptake Inhibitors; Thiazide Diuretics

The levels/effects of HYDROmorphone may be increased by: Amphetamines; Antipsychotic Agents (Phenothiazines); Droperidol; HydrOXYzine; MAO Inhibitors; Succinylcholine

Decreased Effect

HYDROmorphone may decrease the levels/effects of: Pegvisomant

The levels/effects of HYDROmorphone may be decreased by: Ammonium Chloride; Mixed Agonist / Antagonist Opioids

Ethanol/Nutrition/Herb Interactions

Ethanol: May increase CNS depression; monitor for increased effects with coadministration. Caution patients about effects.

Herb/Nutraceutical: Avoid valerian, St John's wort, kava kava, gotu kola (may increase CNS depression).

Stability Store injection and oral dosage forms at 15°C to 30°C (59°F to 86°F). Protect tablets from light. A slightly yellowish discoloration has not been associated with a loss of potency.

Mechanism of Action Binds to opiate receptors in the CNS, causing inhibition of ascending pain pathways, altering the perception of and response to pain; causes cough supression by direct central action in the medulla; produces generalized CNS depression

Pharmacodynamics/Kinetics

Onset of action: Analgesic: Immediate release formulations:

Oral: 15-30 minutes; Peak effect: 30-60 minutes

I.V.: 5 minutes; Peak effect: 10-20 minutes

Duration: Immediate release formulations: Oral, I.V.: 4-5 hours

Absorption: I.M.: Variable and delayed

Distribution: V_d: 4 L/kg

Protein binding: ~8% to 19%

Metabolism: Hepatic via glucuronidation; to inactive metabolites

Bioavailability: 62%

Half-life elimination:

Immediate release formulations: 2-3 hours

Extended release tablets (Exalgo™): ~11 hours

Excretion: Urine (primarily as glucuronide conjugates)

Dosage

Acute pain (moderate-to-severe): Note: These are guidelines and do not represent the maximum doses that may be required in all patients. Doses should be titrated to provide adequate pain relief. When changing routes of administration, oral doses and parenteral doses are **NOT** equivalent; parenteral doses are up to 5 times more potent. Therefore, when administered parenterally, one-fifth of the oral dose will provide similar analgesia.

Children ≥6 months and <50 kg:

Oral: 0.03-0.08 mg/kg/dose every 3-4 hours as needed. **Note:** In children with severe pain, the American Pain Society recommends an initial dose of 0.06 mg/kg.

I.V.: 0.015 mg/kg/dose every 3-6 hours as needed

Patient-controlled analgesia (PCA) (American Pain Society, 2008): **Note:** Opiate-naive: Consider lower end of dosing range:
Usual concentration: 0.2 mg/mL
Demand dose: Usual: 0.003-0.004 mg/kg/dose; range: 0.003-0.005 mg/kg/dose
Lockout interval: 6-10 minutes
Usual basal rate: 0-0.004 mg/kg/hour

Children >50 kg and Adults:

Oral: Initial: Opiate-naive: 2-4 mg every 3-4 hours as needed; elderly/debilitated patients may require lower doses; patients with prior opiate exposure may require higher initial doses. **Note:** In adults with severe pain, the American Pain Society recommends an initial dose of 4-8 mg.

I.V.: Initial: Opiate-naive: 0.2-0.6 mg every 2-3 hours as needed; patients with prior opiate exposure may require higher initial doses
Mechanically ventilated/critically ill patients (unlabeled use): 0.7-4 mg (based on 70 kg patient) every 4 hours as needed. **Note:** More frequent dosing may be needed (eg, every 1-2 hours); dose should be adjusted based on patient response; elderly patients may be more sensitive (Jacobi, 2002).
Continuous infusion: Usual dosage range: 0.5-1 mg/hour (based on 70 kg patient) or 7-15 mcg/kg/**hour**

Patient-controlled analgesia (PCA): **Note:** Opiate-naive: Consider lower end of dosing range:
Usual concentration: 0.2 mg/mL
Demand dose: Usual: 0.1-0.2 mg; range: 0.05-0.4 mg
Lockout interval: 5-10 minutes

Epidural PCA (de Leon-Casasola, 1996; Liu, 2010; Smith, 2009):
Bolus dose: 0.4-1 mg
Infusion rate: 0.03-0.3 mg/**hour**
Demand dose: 0.02-0.05 mg
Lockout interval: 10-15 minutes

I.M., SubQ: **Note:** I.M. use may result in variable absorption and lag time to peak effect.
Initial: Opiate-naive: 0.8-1 mg every 4-6 hours as needed; patients with prior opiate exposure may require higher initial doses; usual dosage range: 1-2 mg every 4-6 hours as needed

Rectal: 3 mg every 6-8 hours as needed

Chronic pain: Adults: Oral: **Note:** Patients taking opioids chronically may become tolerant and require doses higher than the usual dosage range to maintain the desired effect. Tolerance can be managed by appropriate dose titration. There is no optimal or maximal dose for hydromorphone in chronic pain. The appropriate dose is one that relieves pain throughout its dosing interval without causing unmanageable side effects.

Controlled release formulation (Hydromorph Contin®, not available in U.S.): 3-30 mg every 12 hours. **Note:** A patient's hydromorphone requirement should be established using prompt release formulations; conversion to long acting products may be considered when chronic, continuous treatment is required. Higher dosages should be reserved for use only in opioid-tolerant patients.

Extended release formulation (Exalgo™): Dosing range: 8-64 mg every 24 hours. For use in opioid-tolerant patients only; discontinue all other extended release opioids when starting therapy. Suggested recommendations for converting to Exalgo™ from other analgesics are presented, but when selecting the initial dose, other characteristics (eg, patient status, degree of opioid tolerance, concurrent medications, type of pain, risk factors for addiction or diversion, etc) should also be considered.

Individualization of dose: Pain relief and adverse events should be assessed frequently. Dose increases may occur not more often than every 3-4 days; consider titrating with increases of 25% to 50% of the current daily dose. If more than 2 doses of rescue medications are needed within 24 hours for 2 consecutive days, consider increasing the dose of Exalgo™. Do not administer more frequently than every 24 hours.

Discontinuing Exalgo™: Taper by gradually decreasing the dose by 25% to 50% every 2-3 days to a dose of 8 mg every 24 hours before discontinuing therapy.

Conversion from other oral hydromorphone formulations to Exalgo™: Start with the equivalent total daily dose of hydromorphone administered once daily. May titrate every 3-4 days until adequate pain relief with tolerable side effects have been achieved.

Conversion from other opioids to Exalgo™: In general, start Exalgo™ at 50% of the calculated total daily dose every 24 hours. Titrate until adequate pain relief with tolerable side effects has been achieved. The following conversion ratios may be used to convert from **oral** opioid therapy to Exalgo™.

Conversion ratios to Exalgo™ (see table): Select the opioid, sum the total daily dose, then multiply by the conversion ratio to calculate the *approximate* oral hydromorphone equivalent; start Exalgo™ at 50% of the calculated total daily dose every 24 hours. (**Note:** The conversion ratios and approximate equivalent doses in this conversion table are only to be used for the conversion from current opioid therapy to Exalgo™).

Conversion Ratios to Exalgo™[1]

Previous Opioid	Approximate Equivalent Oral Dose	Oral Conversion Ratio[2]
Hydromorphone	12 mg	1
Codeine	200 mg	0.06
Hydrocodone	30 mg	0.4
Methadone[3]	20 mg	0.6
Morphine	60 mg	0.2
Oxycodone	30 mg	0.4
Oxymorphone	20 mg	0.6

[1] *Approximate* equivalent doses for conversion from current opioid therapy to Exalgo™.

[2]Ratio for converting oral opioid dose to approximate hydromorphone equivalent dose.

[3]Monitor closely; ratio between methadone and other opioid agonists may vary widely as a function of previous drug exposure. Methadone has a long half-life and may accumulate in the plasma.

Conversion from transdermal fentanyl to Exalgo™: Treatment with Exalgo™ can be started 18 hours after the removal of the transdermal fentanyl patch. For every fentanyl 25 mcg/hour transdermal dose, the equianalgesic dose of Exalgo™ is 12 mg every 24 hours. An appropriate starting dose is 50% of the calculated total daily dose given every 24 hours.

Dosing adjustment in renal impairment: Exalgo™:
Moderate impairment: Start with a reduced dose and monitor closely.
Severe impairment: Consider use of an alternate analgesic with better dosing flexibility.

Dosing adjustment in hepatic impairment: Dose adjustment should be considered. Exalgo™: In patients with moderate and severe hepatic impairment, start with a reduced dose and monitor closely. Consider use of an alternate analgesic with better dosing flexibility.

Administration

Parenteral: May be given SubQ or I.M.; vial stopper contains latex

I.V.: For IVP, must be given slowly over 2-3 minutes (rapid IVP has been associated with an increase in side effects, especially respiratory depression and hypotension)

Oral: Hydromorphone is available in an 8 mg immediate release tablet and an 8 mg extended release tablet. Extreme caution should be taken to avoid confusing dosage forms.

Exalgo™: Tablets should be swallowed whole; do not crush, break, chew, dissolve or inject. May be taken with or without food.

Hydromorph Contin®: Capsule should be swallowed whole; do not crush or chew; contents may be sprinkled on soft food and swallowed.

Monitoring Parameters Pain relief, respiratory and mental status, blood pressure

Test Interactions Some quinolones may produce a false-positive urine screening result for opiates using commercially-available immunoassay kits. This has been demonstrated most consistently for levofloxacin and ofloxacin, but other quinolones have shown cross-reactivity in certain assay kits. Confirmation of positive opiate screens by more specific methods should be considered.

Additional Information Equianalgesic doses: Morphine 10 mg I.M. = hydromorphone 1.5 mg I.M.

Exalgo™ is indicated for the management of moderate-to-severe pain in opioid-tolerant patients (requiring around-the-clock analgesia for an extended period of time). Patients are considered to be opioid tolerant if they have been taking oral morphine ≥60 mg/day, fentanyl transdermal ≥25 mcg/hour, oral oxycodone ≥30 mg/day, oral hydromorphone ≥8 mg/day, oral oxymorphone ≥25 mg/day, or an equianalgesic dose of another opioid for ≥1 week.

Dosage Forms Excipient information presented when available (limited, particularly for generics); consult specific product labeling.

Injection, powder for reconstitution, as hydrochloride:

Dilaudid-HP®: 250 mg [contains natural rubber/natural latex in packaging, sodium metabisulfite]

Injection, solution, as hydrochloride: 1 mg/mL (1 mL); 2 mg/mL (1 mL, 20 mL); 4 mg/mL (1 mL); 10 mg/mL (1 mL, 5 mL, 50 mL)

Dilaudid-HP®: 10 mg/mL (50 mL) [contains natural rubber/natural latex in packaging, sodium metabisulfite]

Dilaudid-HP®: 10 mg/mL (1 mL, 5 mL) [contains sodium metabisulfite]

Dilaudid®: 1 mg/mL (1 mL); 2 mg/mL (1 mL); 4 mg/mL (1 mL) [contains sodium metabisulfite]

Injection, solution, as hydrochloride [preservative free]: 10 mg/mL (1 mL, 5 mL, 50 mL)

Liquid, oral, as hydrochloride:

Dilaudid®: 1 mg/mL (473 mL) [contains sodium metabisulfite (may have trace amounts)]

Powder, for prescription compounding, as hydrochloride: USP: 100% (972 mg)

Suppository, rectal, as hydrochloride: 3 mg (6s)

Tablet, oral, as hydrochloride: 2 mg, 4 mg, 8 mg

Dilaudid®: 2 mg, 4 mg [contains sodium metabisulfite (may have trace amounts)]

Dilaudid®: 8 mg [scored; contains sodium metabisulfite (may have trace amounts)]

Tablet, extended release, oral, as hydrochloride:

Exalgo™: 8 mg, 12 mg, 16 mg [contains sodium metabisulfite]

Dosage Forms: Canada Excipient information presented when available (limited, particularly for generics); consult specific product labeling.

Capsule, controlled release:

Hydromorph Contin®: 3 mg, 6 mg, 12 mg, 18 mg, 24 mg, 30 mg

Controlled Substance C-II

- **Hydromorphone HP (Can)** *see* HYDROmorphone *on page 843*
- **Hydromorphone HP® 10 (Can)** *see* HYDROmorphone *on page 843*
- **Hydromorphone HP® 20 (Can)** *see* HYDROmorphone *on page 843*
- **Hydromorphone HP® 50 (Can)** *see* HYDROmorphone *on page 843*
- **Hydromorphone HP® Forte (Can)** *see* HYDROmorphone *on page 843*
- **Hydromorphone Hydrochloride** *see* HYDROmorphone *on page 843*
- **Hydromorphone Hydrochloride Injection, USP (Can)** *see* HYDROmorphone *on page 843*
- **Hydroquinol** *see* Hydroquinone *on page 846*

Hydroquinone (HYE droe kwin one)

Brand Names: U.S. Aclaro PD®; Aclaro®; Alphaquin HP®; Eldopaque Forte®; Eldopaque® [OTC]; Eldoquin Forte®; Eldoquin® [OTC]; EpiQuin® Micro; Esoterica® Daytime [OTC]; Esoterica® Nighttime [OTC]; Lustra-AF®; Lustra-Ultra™; Lustra®; Melanex® [DSC]; Melpaque HP®; Melquin HP®; Melquin-3®; NeoStrata® HQ Skin Lightening [OTC]; Nuquin HP®; Palmer's® Skin Success® Eventone® Fade Cream [OTC]; Palmer's® Skin Success® Eventone® Fade Milk [OTC]; Palmer's® Skin Success® Eventone® Ultra Fade Serum [OTC]

Brand Names: Canada Eldopaque®; Eldoquin®; Glyquin® XM; Lustra®; NeoStrata® HQ; Solaquin Forte®; Solaquin®; Ultraquin™

Index Terms Hydroquinol; Quinol

Pharmacologic Category Depigmenting Agent

Use Gradual bleaching of hyperpigmented skin conditions

Pregnancy Risk Factor C

Dosage Children >12 years and Adults: Topical: Apply thin layer and rub in twice daily

Additional Information Complete prescribing information for this medication should be consulted for additional detail.

Dosage Forms Excipient information presented when available (limited, particularly for generics); consult specific product labeling. [DSC] = Discontinued product

Cream, topical: 4% (28.35 g, 28.4 g, 30 g); 5% (0.25 g [DSC])

Alphaquin HP®: 4% (28.4 g, 56.7 g) [contains sodium metabisulfite, sunscreen]

Eldopaque Forte®: 4% (28.35 g) [contains sodium metabisulfite, sunscreen]

Eldopaque®: 2% (28.35 g) [contains sodium metabisulfite, sunscreen]

Eldoquin Forte®: 4% (28.4 g) [contains sodium metabisulfite]

Eldoquin®: 2% (28.35 g) [contains sodium metabisulfite]

EpiQuin® Micro: 4% (40 g) [contains benzyl alcohol, sodium metabisulfite]

Esoterica® Daytime: 2% (85 g) [contains sodium metabisulfite]

Esoterica® Daytime: 2% (70 g) [contains sodium metabisulfite, sunscreen]

Esoterica® Nighttime: 2% (85 g) [contains sodium metabisulfite]

Lustra-AF®: 4% (56.8 g) [contains benzyl alcohol, ethanol, sodium metabisulfite, sunscreen]

Lustra-Ultra™: 4% (23.4 g [DSC], 56.8 g) [contains sodium metabisulfite, sunscreen]

Lustra®: 4% (56.8 g) [contains benzyl alcohol, sodium metabisulfite]

Melpaque HP®: 4% (14.2 g, 28.4 g) [contains sodium metabisulfite, sunblock]

Melquin HP®: 4% (14.2 g, 28.4 g) [contains sodium metabisulfite]

Nuquin HP®: 4% (14.2 g, 28.4 g, 56.7 g) [contains ethanol, sodium metabisulfite, sunscreen]

Palmer's® Skin Success® Eventone® Fade Cream: 2% (75 g, 81 g [DSC], 132 g [DSC]) [contains sodium sulfite, sunscreen; dry skin formula]
Palmer's® Skin Success® Eventone® Fade Cream: 2% (75 g, 81 g [DSC], 132 g [DSC]) [contains sodium sulfite, sunscreen; oily skin formula]
Palmer's® Skin Success® Eventone® Fade Cream: 2% (75 g, 125 g) [contains sodium sulfite, sunscreen; regular skin formula]
Emulsion, topical:
Aclaro PD®: 4% (42.5 g) [contains benzyl alcohol, sunscreen]
Aclaro®: 4% (48.2 g) [contains benzyl alcohol, sodium metabisulfite, sunscreen]
Gel, topical: 4% (28.35 g)
NeoStrata® HQ Skin Lightening: 2% (30 g) [contains ethanol, sodium bisulfite, sodium sulfite]
Nuquin HP®: 4% (14.2 g, 28.4 g) [contains ethanol, sodium metabisulfite, sunscreen]
Lotion, topical:
Palmer's® Skin Success® Eventone® Fade Milk: 2% (250 mL) [contains corn oil, sodium metabisulfite, sodium sulfite, sunscreen]
Solution, topical:
Melanex®: 3% (30 mL [DSC]) [contains ethanol, sodium metabisulfite]
Melquin-3®: 3% (29.57 mL) [contains ethanol 45%, isopropyl alcohol 4%]
Palmer's® Skin Success® Eventone® Ultra Fade Serum: 2% (30 mL) [contains corn oil, shea nut derivatives, sodium metabisulfite, sodium sulfite, sunscreen]

◆ **Hydroquinone, Fluocinolone Acetonide, and Tretinoin** *see* Fluocinolone, Hydroquinone, and Tretinoin *on page 727*

◆ **Hydroskin® [OTC]** *see* Hydrocortisone (Topical) *on page 841*

◆ **HydroVal® (Can)** *see* Hydrocortisone (Topical) *on page 841*

Hydroxocobalamin (hye droks oh koe BAL a min)

Brand Names: U.S. Cyanokit®
Brand Names: Canada Cyanokit®
Index Terms Vitamin B_{12a}
Pharmacologic Category Antidote; Vitamin, Water Soluble
Use Treatment of pernicious anemia, vitamin B_{12} deficiency due to dietary deficiencies or malabsorption diseases, inadequate secretion of intrinsic factor, and inadequate utilization of B_{12} (eg, during neoplastic treatment); diagnostic agent for Schilling test

Cyanokit®: Treatment of cyanide poisoning (known or suspected)

Unlabeled Use Neuropathies
Pregnancy Risk Factor C
Pregnancy Considerations Animal studies are insufficient to determine the effect, if any, on pregnancy or fetal development. There are no adequate and well-controlled studies in pregnant women. Data on the use of hydroxocobalamin in pregnancy for the treatment of cyanide poisoning and cobalamin defects are limited.
Lactation Excretion in breast milk unknown/use caution
Contraindications Hypersensitivity to hydroxocobalamin, cyanocobalamin, cobalt, or any component of the formulation
Warnings/Precautions

Solution for I.M. injection: Treatment of severe vitamin B_{12} megaloblastic anemia may result in thrombocytosis and severe hypokalemia, sometimes fatal, due to intracellular potassium shift upon anemia resolution. Use caution in folic acid deficient megaloblastic anemia; administration of vitamin B_{12} alone is not a substitute for folic acid and might mask true diagnosis. Vitamin B_{12} deficiency masks signs of polycythemia vera; vitamin B_{12} administration may unmask this condition. Neurologic manifestations of vitamin B_{12} deficiency will not be prevented with folic acid unless vitamin B_{12} is also given; spinal cord degeneration might also occur when folic acid is used as a substitute for vitamin B_{12} in anemia prevention. Blunted therapeutic response to vitamin B_{12} may occur in certain conditions (eg, infection, uremia, concurrent iron or folic acid deficiency) or in patients on medications with bone marrow suppressant properties (eg, chloramphenicol). Approved for use as I.M. injection only.

Cyanokit®: Use caution or consider alternatives in patients with known allergic reactions, including anaphylaxis, to hydroxocobalamin or cyanocobalamin. Increased blood pressure (≥180 mm Hg systolic or ≥110 mm Hg diastolic) is associated with infusion; elevations usually noted at beginning of infusion, peak toward the end of infusion and return to baseline within 4 hours of infusion. Collection of pretreatment blood cyanide concentrations does not preclude administration and should not delay administration in the emergency management of highly suspected or confirmed cyanide toxicity. Pretreatment levels may be useful as post infusion levels may be inaccurate. Treatment of cyanide poisoning should include decontamination and supportive therapy. Use caution with concurrent use of other cyanide antidotes; safety has not been established. Photosensitivity is a potential concern; avoid direct sunlight while skin remains discolored.

Adverse Reactions

I.M. injection: Frequency not defined:
Dermatologic: Exanthema (transient), itching
Gastrointestinal: Diarrhea (mild, transient)
Local: Injection site pain
Miscellaneous: Anaphylaxis

I.V. infusion (Cyanokit®):
>10%:
Cardiovascular: Blood pressure increased (18% to 28%; systolic ≥180 mm Hg or diastolic ≥110 mm Hg)
Central nervous system: Headache (6% to 33%)
Dermatologic: Erythema (94% to 100%; may last up to 2 weeks), rash (predominantly acneiform; 20% to 44%; can appear 7-28 days after administration and usually resolves within a few weeks)
Gastrointestinal: Nausea (6% to 11%)
Genitourinary: Chromaturia (100%; may last up to 5 weeks after administration)
Hematologic: Lymphocytes decreased (8% to 17%)
Local: Infusion site reaction (6% to 39%)
Frequency not defined:
Cardiovascular: Chest discomfort, hot flashes, peripheral edema
Central nervous system: Dizziness, memory impairment, restlessness
Dermatologic: Pruritus, urticaria
Gastrointestinal: Abdominal discomfort, diarrhea, dyspepsia, dysphagia, hematochezia, vomiting
Ocular: Irritation, redness, swelling
Respiratory: Dry throat, dyspnea, throat tightness
Miscellaneous: Allergic reaction (including anaphylaxis)
Postmarketing and/or case reports: Angioneurotic edema

Drug Interactions

Metabolism/Transport Effects None known.
Avoid Concomitant Use There are no known interactions where it is recommended to avoid concomitant use.
Increased Effect/Toxicity There are no known significant interactions involving an increase in effect.
Decreased Effect There are no known significant interactions involving a decrease in effect.

Stability

Solution for I.M. injection: Store at 20°C to 25°C (68°F to 77°F). Protect from light.

I.V. infusion (Cyanokit®): Prior to reconstitution, store at 25°C (77°F): excursions permitted to 15°C to 30°C (59°F to 86°F).

Temperature variation exposure allowed for transport of lyophilized form:

Usual transport: ≤15 days at 5°C to 40°C (41°F to 104°F)

Desert transport: ≤4 days at 5°C to 60°C (41°F to 140°F)

Freezing/defrosting cycles: ≤15 days at -20°C to 40°C (-4°F to 104°F)

Reconstitute each 2.5 g vial with 100 mL of NS or 5 g vial with 200 mL of NS using provided sterile transfer spike. If NS unavailable, may use LR or D_5W. Invert or rock each 2.5 g vial for at least 30 seconds or 5 g vial for 60 seconds prior to infusion; do not shake. Discard if solution is **not** dark red. Following reconstitution, store up to 6 hours at ≤40°C (104°F); do not freeze. Discard any remaining solution after 6 hours.

Mechanism of Action Hydroxocobalamin (vitamin B_{12a}) is a precursor to cyanocobalamin (vitamin B_{12}). Cyanocobalamin acts as a coenzyme for various metabolic functions, including fat and carbohydrate metabolism and protein synthesis, used in cell replication and hematopoiesis. In the presence of cyanide, each hydroxocobalamin molecule can bind one cyanide ion by displacing it for the hydroxo ligand linked to the trivalent cobalt ion, forming cyanocobalamin.

Pharmacodynamics/Kinetics Following I.V. administration of Cyanokit®:

Protein binding: Significant; forms various cobalamin-(III) complexes

Half-life elimination: 26-31 hours

Excretion: Urine (50% to 60% within initial 72 hours)

Dosage

Vitamin B_{12} deficiency: I.M.:

Children: 100 mcg once daily for 2 or more weeks (total dose: 1-5 mg); maintenance: 30-50 mcg/month

Adults: 30 mcg/day for 5-10 days, followed by 100-200 mcg/month

Note: Larger doses may be required in critically-ill patients or if patient has neurologic disease, an infectious disease, or hyperthyroidism.

Schilling test: I.M.: Adults: 1000 mcg

Cyanide toxicity (Cyanokit®): I.V.: Adults: Initial: 5 g as single infusion; may repeat a second 5 g dose depending on severity of poisoning and clinical response. Maximum cumulative dose: 10 g. **Note:** If suspected, antidotal therapy must be given immediately.

Administration

Solution for I.M. injection: Administer 1000 mcg/mL solution I.M. only

Cyanokit®: Administer by I.V. infusion over 15 minutes; if repeat dose needed, administer second dose over 15 minutes to 2 hours

Monitoring Parameters Vitamin B_{12}, hematocrit, hemoglobin, reticulocyte count, red blood cell counts, folate and iron levels should be obtained prior to treatment and periodically during treatment.

Cyanide toxicity: Blood pressure and heart rate during and after infusion, serum lactate levels, venous-arterial PO_2 gradient. Pretreatment levels may be useful as post infusion levels may be inaccurate.

Megaloblastic anemia: In addition to normal hematological parameters, serum potassium and platelet counts should be monitored during therapy, particularly in the first 48 hours of treatment.

Test Interactions The following values may be affected, *in vitro*, following hydroxocobalamin 5 g dose. Interference following hydroxocobalamin 10 g dose can be expected to last up to an additional 24 hours. **Note:** Extent and duration of interference dependent on analyzer used and patient variability.

Falsely elevated:

Basophils, hemoglobin, MCH, and MCHC [duration: 12-16 hours]

Albumin, alkaline phosphatase, cholesterol, creatinine, glucose, total protein, and triglycerides [duration: 24 hours]

Bilirubin [duration: up to 4 days]

Urinalysis: Glucose, protein, erythrocytes, leukocytes, ketones, bilirubin, urobilinogen, nitrite [duration: 2-8 days]

Falsely decreased: ALT and amylase [duration: 24 hours]

Unpredictable:

AST, CK, CKMB, LDH, phosphate, and uric acid [duration: 24 hours]

PT (quick or INR) and aPTT [duration: 24-48 hours]

Urine pH [duration: 2-8 days]

May also interfere with colorimetric tests and cause hemodialysis machines to shut down due to false detection of a blood leak from the blood-like appearance of the solution.

Additional Information Expert advice from a regional poison control center for appropriate use may be obtained (1-800-222-1222). Cyanide is a clear colorless gas or liquid with a faint bitter almond odor. Cyanide reacts with trivalent ions in cytochrome oxidase in the mitochondria leading to histotoxic hypoxia and lactic acidosis. Signs and symptoms of cyanide toxicity include headache, altered mental status, dyspnea, mydriasis, chest tightness, nausea, vomiting, tachycardia/hypertension (initially), bradycardia/hypotension (later), seizures, cardiovascular collapse, or coma.

Dosage Forms Excipient information presented when available (limited, particularly for generics); consult specific product labeling. [DSC] = Discontinued product

Injection, powder for reconstitution:

Cyanokit®: 2.5 g [DSC], 5 g

Injection, solution: 1000 mcg/mL (30 mL)

◆ **4-Hydroxybutyrate** *see* Sodium Oxybate *on page 1572*

◆ **Hydroxycarbamide** *see* Hydroxyurea *on page 851*

Hydroxychloroquine (hye droks ee KLOR oh kwin)

Brand Names: U.S. Plaquenil®

Brand Names: Canada Apo-Hydroxyquine®; Gen-Hydroxychloroquine; Mylan-Hydroxychloroquine; Plaquenil®; PRO-Hydroxyquine

Index Terms Hydroxychloroquine Sulfate

Pharmacologic Category Aminoquinoline (Antimalarial)

Use Suppression and treatment of acute attacks of malaria; treatment of systemic lupus erythematosus (SLE) and rheumatoid arthritis

Unlabeled Use Porphyria cutanea tarda, polymorphous light eruptions

Pregnancy Considerations Malaria infection in pregnant women may be more severe than in nonpregnant women. Therefore, pregnant women and women who are likely to become pregnant are advised to avoid travel to malaria-risk areas. Hydroxychloroquine is recommended as an alternative treatment of pregnant women for uncomplicated malaria in chloroquine-sensitive regions. Women exposed to hydroxychloroquine for the treatment of rheumatoid arthritis or systemic lupus erythematosus during pregnancy may be enrolled in the Organization of Teratology Information Specialists (OTIS) Autoimmune Diseases Study pregnancy registry (877-311-8972).

Lactation Enters breast milk (AAP considers "compatible"; AAP 2001 update pending)

Contraindications Hypersensitivity to hydroxychloroquine, 4-aminoquinoline derivatives, or any component of the formulation; retinal or visual field changes attributable to 4-aminoquinolines; long-term use in children

Warnings/Precautions May cause ophthalmic adverse effects (risk factors include daily doses >6.5 mg/kg lean body weight) or neuromyopathy; perform baseline and periodic (every 3 months) ophthalmologic examinations; test periodically for muscle weakness. Rare cardiomyopathy has been associated with long-term use of hydroxychloroquine. Aminoquinolines have been associated with rare hematologic reactions, including agranulocytosis, aplastic anemia, and thrombocytopenia; monitoring (CBC) is recommended in prolonged therapy. Use with caution in patients with hepatic disease, G6PD deficiency, psoriasis, and porphyria. Use caution in children due to increased sensitivity to adverse effects (long-term use in children is contraindicated). Not effective in the treatment of malaria caused by chloroquine resistant *P. falciparum*. **[U.S. Boxed Warning]: Should be prescribed by physicians familiar with its use.**

Adverse Reactions Frequency not defined.

Cardiovascular: Cardiomyopathy (rare, relationship to hydroxychloroquine unclear)

Central nervous system: Ataxia, dizziness, emotional changes, headache, irritability, lassitude, nervousness, nightmares, psychosis, seizure, vertigo

Dermatologic: Alopecia, angioedema, bleaching of hair, pigmentation changes (skin and mucosal; black-blue color), rash (acute generalized exanthematous pustulosis, erythema annulare centrifugum, exfoliative dermatitis, lichenoid, maculopapular, morbilliform, purpuric, Stevens-Johnson syndrome, urticarial), urticaria

Gastrointestinal: Abdominal cramping, anorexia, diarrhea, nausea, vomiting, weight loss

Hematologic: Agranulocytosis, aplastic anemia, hemolysis (in patients with glucose-6-phosphate deficiency), leukopenia, thrombocytopenia

Hepatic: Abnormal liver function/hepatic failure (isolated cases)

Neuromuscular & skeletal: Myopathy, palsy, or neuromyopathy leading to progressive weakness and atrophy of proximal muscle groups (may be associated with mild sensory changes, loss of deep tendon reflexes, and abnormal nerve conduction)

Ocular: Abnormal color vision, abnormal retinal pigmentation, atrophy, attenuation of retinal arterioles, corneal changes/deposits (visual disturbances, blurred vision, photophobia [reversible on discontinuation]), decreased visual acuity, disturbance in accommodation, keratopathy, macular edema, nystagmus, optic disc pallor/atrophy, pigmentary retinopathy, retinopathy (early changes reversible [may progress despite discontinuation if advanced]), scotoma

Otic: Deafness, tinnitus

Miscellaneous: Exacerbation of porphyria and nonlight sensitive psoriasis

Respiratory: Bronchospasm, respiratory failure (myopathy-related)

Drug Interactions

Metabolism/Transport Effects None known.

Avoid Concomitant Use

Avoid concomitant use of Hydroxychloroquine with any of the following: Artemether; BCG; Lumefantrine; Mefloquine; Natalizumab; Pimecrolimus; Tacrolimus (Topical)

Increased Effect/Toxicity

Hydroxychloroquine may increase the levels/effects of: Antipsychotic Agents (Phenothiazines); Beta-Blockers; Cardiac Glycosides; Dapsone; Dapsone (Systemic); Dapsone (Topical); Leflunomide; Lumefantrine; Mefloquine; Natalizumab; Vaccines (Live)

The levels/effects of Hydroxychloroquine may be increased by: Artemether; Dapsone; Dapsone (Systemic); Denosumab; Mefloquine; Pimecrolimus; Roflumilast; Tacrolimus (Topical); Trastuzumab

Decreased Effect

Hydroxychloroquine may decrease the levels/effects of: Anthelmintics; BCG; Coccidioidin Skin Test; Sipuleucel-T; Vaccines (Inactivated)

The levels/effects of Hydroxychloroquine may be decreased by: Echinacea

Ethanol/Nutrition/Herb Interactions Ethanol: Avoid ethanol (due to GI irritation).

Mechanism of Action Interferes with digestive vacuole function within sensitive malarial parasites by increasing the pH and interfering with lysosomal degradation of hemoglobin; inhibits locomotion of neutrophils and chemotaxis of eosinophils; impairs complement-dependent antigen-antibody reactions

Pharmacodynamics/Kinetics

Onset of action: Rheumatic disease: May require 4-6 weeks to respond

Absorption: Rapid and complete

Protein binding: 55%

Metabolism: Hepatic; metabolites include desethylhydroxychloroquine and desethylchloroquine

Half-life elimination: 32-50 days

Time to peak: Rheumatic disease: Several months

Excretion: Urine (as metabolites and unchanged drug [up to 60%]); may be enhanced by urinary acidification

Dosage Note: Hydroxychloroquine sulfate 200 mg is equivalent to 155 mg hydroxychloroquine base and 250 mg chloroquine phosphate. All doses below expressed as hydroxychloroquine sulfate. Second-line alternative treatment for malaria (chloroquine is preferred).

Oral:

Children:

Malaria, chemoprophylaxis: 6.5 mg/kg once weekly (not to exceed 400 mg/dose); begin 2 weeks before exposure; continue for 4 weeks (per CDC guidelines) after leaving endemic area; if suppressive therapy is not begun prior to the exposure, double the initial dose and give in 2 doses, 6 hours apart and continue treatment for 8 weeks

Malaria, acute attack: 13 mg/kg initially (not to exceed 800 mg/dose), followed by 6.5 mg/kg (not to exceed 400 mg/dose) at 6, 24, and 48 hours

Adults:

Malaria, chemoprophylaxis: 400 mg weekly on same day each week; begin 2 weeks before exposure; continue for 4 weeks (per CDC guidelines) after leaving endemic area; if suppressive therapy is not begun prior to the exposure, double the initial dose and give in 2 doses, 6 hours apart and continue treatment for 8 weeks

Malaria, acute attack: 800 mg initially, followed by 400 mg at 6, 24, and 48 hours

Rheumatoid arthritis: Initial: 400-600 mg/day taken with food or milk; increase dose gradually until optimum response level is reached; usually after 4-12 weeks dose should be reduced by 1/2 to a maintenance dose of 200-400 mg/day

Lupus erythematosus: 400 mg every day or twice daily for several weeks-months depending on response; 200-400 mg/day for prolonged maintenance therapy

Dosage adjustment in renal impairment: Use with caution; dosage adjustment may be necessary in severe dysfunction (Bernstein, 1992); specific guidelines not available.

Dietary Considerations May be taken with food or milk.

Administration Administer with food or milk.

Monitoring Parameters Ophthalmologic exam at baseline and every 3 months during prolonged therapy (including visual acuity, slit-lamp, fundoscopic, and visual field exam); CBC at baseline and periodically; muscle strength (especially proximal, as a symptom of neuromyopathy) during long-term therapy

Dosage Forms Excipient information presented when available (limited, particularly for generics); consult specific product labeling.

Tablet, oral, as sulfate: 200 mg [equivalent to 155 mg base]

Plaquenil®: 200 mg [equivalent to 155 mg base]

Extemporaneous Preparations A 25 mg/mL hydroxychloroquine sulfate oral suspension may be made with tablets. With a towel moistened with alcohol, remove the coating from fifteen 200 mg hydroxychloroquine sulfate tablets. Crush tablets in a mortar and reduce to a fine powder. Add 15 mL of Ora-Plus® and mix to a uniform paste; add an additional 45 mL of vehicle and mix until uniform. Mix while adding sterile water for irrigation in incremental proportions to **almost** 120 mL; transfer to a calibrated bottle, rinse mortar with sterile water, and add sufficient quantity of sterile water to make 120 mL. Label "shake well". A 30-day expiration date is recommended, although stability testing has not been performed.

Pesko LJ, "Compounding: Hydroxychloroquine," *Am Druggist*, 1993, 207(4):57.

◆ **Hydroxychloroquine Sulfate** *see* Hydroxychloroquine *on page 848*

◆ **Hydroxydaunomycin Hydrochloride** *see* DOXOrubicin *on page 552*

◆ **Hydroxyethyl Starch** *see* Hetastarch *on page 830*

◆ **Hydroxyethyl Starch** *see* Tetrastarch *on page 1663*

◆ **Hydroxyldaunorubicin Hydrochloride** *see* DOXOrubicin *on page 552*

Hydroxyprogesterone Caproate

(hye droks ee proe JES te rone CAP ro ate)

Brand Names: U.S. Makena™

Index Terms 17OHPC

Pharmacologic Category Progestin

Use To reduce the risk of preterm birth in women with singleton pregnancies who have a history of spontaneous preterm birth (delivery <37 weeks gestation) with previous singleton pregnancies

Pregnancy Risk Factor B

Pregnancy Considerations Teratogenic events were not observed in animal reproduction studies; embryolethality was observed in some species. Teratogenic effects were not observed in human studies following second or third trimester exposure; first trimester data not available. *In vitro* data show hydroxyprogesterone is metabolized by the placenta and reaches the fetal circulation.

Prescribing and Access Restrictions The Makena Care Connection™ is a comprehensive program for patients and healthcare providers which provides administrative support (including insurance benefit investigation and prescription fulfillment); financial and co-pay assistance for eligible patients; and treatment support (including educational information, home health care service and scheduled treatment reminders). The Makena Care Connection™ is available by calling 1-800-847-3418, Monday-Friday, 8 AM to 9 PM EST.

Contraindications Current or history of thrombosis or thromboembolic disorders; hepatic impairment, hepatic tumors or cholestatic jaundice of pregnancy; carcinoma of the breast (known or suspected) or other hormone sensitive cancers; undiagnosed vaginal bleeding unrelated to pregnancy; uncontrolled hypertension

Warnings/Precautions Not for use in women with multiple gestations or other risk factors for preterm birth. Clinical benefits related to improved neonatal mortality or morbidity following maternal use have not been demonstrated. Not intended to stop active preterm labor. May have adverse effects on glucose tolerance; use caution in women with diabetes. Use with caution in patients with depression; discontinue if depression occurs. Use with caution in patients with diseases which may be exacerbated by fluid retention, including asthma, epilepsy, migraine, diabetes, pre-eclampsia, cardiac or renal dysfunction. Specific studies have not been conducted in patients with hepatic impairment (use is contraindicated); elimination may be decreased. Monitor women who develop hypertension during therapy; consider risk versus benefit of continuation. Use is contraindicated with uncontrolled hypertension. Monitor women who develop jaundice during therapy; consider risk versus benefit of continuation. Use is contraindicated in women with cholestatic jaundice of pregnancy. Discontinue if arterial thrombosis, DVT, or thromboembolic events occur. Use is contraindicated with current or history of thrombosis or thromboembolic disorders. Limited numbers of pregnant women between 16 and 18 years of age were included in clinical trials. Contains castor oil. Discontinue if allergic reactions (eg urticaria, pruritus, angioedema) occur.

Adverse Reactions

>10%:

Dermatologic: Urticaria (12%)

Local: Injection site: Pain (35%), swelling (17%)

1% to 10%:

Dermatologic: Pruritus (8%)

Gastrointestinal: Nausea (6%), diarrhea (2%)

Local: Injection site pruritus (6%), nodule (5%)

<1% (Limited to important or life-threatening): Injection site cellulitis, PE

Drug Interactions

Metabolism/Transport Effects Substrate of CYP3A4 (major); **Note:** Assignment of Major/Minor substrate status based on clinically relevant drug interaction potential; **Induces** CYP1A2 (weak/moderate), CYP2A6 (strong), CYP2B6 (weak/moderate)

Avoid Concomitant Use

Avoid concomitant use of Hydroxyprogesterone Caproate with any of the following: Conivaptan

Increased Effect/Toxicity

The levels/effects of Hydroxyprogesterone Caproate may be increased by: Conivaptan; CYP3A4 Inhibitors (Moderate); CYP3A4 Inhibitors (Strong); Dasatinib; Herbs (Progestogenic Properties)

Decreased Effect

Hydroxyprogesterone Caproate may decrease the levels/effects of: CYP2A6 Substrates

The levels/effects of Hydroxyprogesterone Caproate may be decreased by: Aminoglutethimide; CYP3A4 Inducers (Strong); Deferasirox; Herbs (CYP3A4 Inducers); Tocilizumab

Stability Store upright at controlled room temperature of 15°C to 30°C (59°F to 86°F); protect from light. Discard within 5 weeks of first use.

Pharmacodynamics/Kinetics

Distribution: Extensively bound to albumin and corticosteroid-binding globulins

Metabolism: Hepatic via CYP3A4 and 3A5; forms metabolites

Half-life elimination: ~8 days

Time to peak, serum: I.M.: 3-7 days

Excretion: Urine (~30%) and feces (~50%); primarily as metabolites

Dosage I.M.: Pregnant females ≥16 years: To reduce the risk of preterm birth: 250 mg once weekly (every 7 days). Treatment may begin between 16 weeks 0 days and 20 weeks 6 days of gestation. Continue weekly administration until 37 weeks gestation or until delivery, whichever comes first.

Administration For I.M. administration into the upper outer quadrant of the gluteus maximus. Withdraw dose using an 18 gauge needle; inject dose using a 21 gauge 1 1/2 inch needle. Administer by slow injection (≥1 minute). Solution is viscous and oily; do not use if solution is cloudy or contains solid particles. Apply pressure to injection site to decrease bruising and swelling.

Monitoring Parameters Signs and symptoms of thromboembolic disorders; signs or symptoms of depression; glucose in patients with diabetes; signs and symptoms of jaundice; or blood pressure

Dosage Forms Excipient information presented when available (limited, particularly for generics); consult specific product labeling.

Injection, solution:

Makena™: 250 mg/mL (5 mL) [contains benzyl alcohol, benzyl benzoate, castor oil]

◆ **9-hydroxy-risperidone** *see* Paliperidone *on page* 1277

Hydroxyurea (hye droks ee yoor EE a)

Brand Names: U.S. Droxia®; Hydrea®

Brand Names: Canada Apo-Hydroxyurea®; Gen-Hydroxyurea; Hydrea®; Mylan-Hydroxyurea

Index Terms Hydroxycarbamide; Hydurea

Pharmacologic Category Antineoplastic Agent, Antimetabolite

Use Treatment of melanoma, refractory chronic myelocytic leukemia (CML); recurrent, metastatic, or inoperable ovarian cancer; radiosensitizing agent in the treatment of squamous cell head and neck cancer (excluding lip cancer); adjunct in the management of sickle cell patients who have had at least three painful crises in the previous 12 months (to reduce frequency of these crises and the need for blood transfusions)

Unlabeled Use Treatment of essential thrombocythemia, polycythemia vera, hypereosinophilic syndrome; management of hyperleukocytosis due to acute myeloid leukemia; treatment of cervical cancer, treatment of meningiomas

Pregnancy Risk Factor D

Pregnancy Considerations Animal studies have demonstrated teratogenicity and embryotoxicity at doses lower than the usual human dose. Women of childbearing potential should be advised to avoid becoming pregnant during treatment.

Lactation Enters breast milk/not recommended

Contraindications Hypersensitivity to hydroxyurea or any component of the formulation; severe bone marrow suppression (WBC <2500/mm^3 or platelet count <100,000/mm^3) or severe anemia (in patients with sickle cell anemia; use is not recommended if neutrophils <2000/mm^3, platelets <80,000/mm^3, hemoglobin <4.5 g/dL, or reticulocytes <80,000/mm^3 when hemoglobin <9 g/dL)

Warnings/Precautions Hazardous agent - use appropriate precautions for handling and disposal; to decrease risk of exposure, wear gloves when handling and wash hands before and after contact. Leukopenia may commonly occur (thrombocytopenia and anemia are less common; reversible with treatment interruption. Use with caution in patients with a history of prior chemotherapy or radiation therapy; myelosuppression is more common. Correct severe anemia prior to initiating treatment. Patients with a history of radiation therapy are also at risk for exacerbation of post irradiation erythema. Self-limiting megaloblastic erythropoiesis may be seen early in treatment (may resemble pernicious anemia, but is unrelated to vitamin B_{12} or folic acid deficiency). Plasma iron clearance may be delayed and iron utilization rate (by erythrocytes) may be reduced. When treated concurrently with hydroxyurea and antiretroviral agents (including didanosine), HIV-infected patients are at higher risk for potentially fatal pancreatitis, hepatotoxicity, hepatic failure, and severe peripheral neuropathy. Hyperuricemia may occur with treatment; adequate hydration and initiation or dosage adjustment of uricosuric agents (eg, allopurinol) may be necessary.

In patients with sickle cell anemia, use is not recommended if neutrophils <2000/mm^3, platelets <80,000/mm^3, hemoglobin <4.5 g/dL, or reticulocytes <80,000/mm^3 when hemoglobin <9 g/dL. May cause macrocytosis, which can mask folic acid deficiency; prophylactic fold acid supplementation is recommended. **[U.S. Boxed Warning]: Hydroxyurea is mutagenic and clastogenic. Treatment of myeloproliferative disorders (eg, polycythemia vera, thrombocythemia) with long-term hydroxyurea is associated with secondary leukemia;** it is unknown if this is drug-related or disease-related. Cutaneous vasculitic toxicities (vasculitic ulceration and gangrene) have been reported with hydroxyurea treatment, most often in patients with a history of or receiving concurrent interferon therapy; discontinue hydroxyurea and consider alternate cytoreductive therapy if cutaneous vasculitic toxicity develops. Use caution with renal dysfunction; may require dose reductions. Elderly patients may be more sensitive to the effects of hydroxyurea; may require lower doses. **[U.S. Boxed Warning]: Should be administered under the supervision of a physician experienced in the treatment of sickle cell anemia** or in cancer chemotherapy.

Adverse Reactions Frequency not defined.

Cardiovascular: Edema

Central nervous system: Chills, disorientation, dizziness, drowsiness (dose-related), fever, hallucinations, headache, malaise, seizure

Dermatologic: Alopecia, cutaneous vasculitic toxicities, dermatomyositis-like skin changes, facial erythema, gangrene, hyperpigmentation, maculopapular rash, nail atrophy, nail discoloration, peripheral erythema, scaling, skin atrophy, skin cancer, skin ulcer, vasculitis ulcerations, violet papules

Endocrine & metabolic: Hyperuricemia

Gastrointestinal: Anorexia, constipation, diarrhea, gastrointestinal irritation and mucositis, (potentiated with radiation therapy), nausea, pancreatitis, stomatitis, vomiting

Genitourinary: Dysuria

Hematologic: Myelosuppression (anemia, leukopenia [common; reversal of WBC count occurs rapidly], thrombocytopenia); macrocytosis, megaloblastic erythropoiesis, secondary leukemias (long-term use)

Hepatic: Hepatic enzymes increased, hepatotoxicity

Neuromuscular & skeletal: Peripheral neuropathy, weakness

Renal: BUN increased, creatinine increased

Respiratory: Acute diffuse pulmonary infiltrates (rare), dyspnea, pulmonary fibrosis (rare)

Drug Interactions

Metabolism/Transport Effects None known.

Avoid Concomitant Use

Avoid concomitant use of Hydroxyurea with any of the following: BCG; CloZAPine; Didanosine; Natalizumab; Pimecrolimus; Stavudine; Tacrolimus (Topical); Vaccines (Live)

Increased Effect/Toxicity

Hydroxyurea may increase the levels/effects of: CloZAPine; Didanosine; Leflunomide; Natalizumab; Stavudine; Vaccines (Live)

The levels/effects of Hydroxyurea may be increased by: Denosumab; Didanosine; Pimecrolimus; Roflumilast; Stavudine; Tacrolimus (Topical); Trastuzumab

Decreased Effect

Hydroxyurea may decrease the levels/effects of: BCG; Coccidioidin Skin Test; Sipuleucel-T; Vaccines (Inactivated); Vaccines (Live)

The levels/effects of Hydroxyurea may be decreased by: Echinacea

Stability Store at room temperature of 25°C (77°F); excursions permitted between 15°C and 30°C (59°F and 86°F).

Mechanism of Action Antimetabolite which selectively inhibits ribonucleoside diphosphate reductase, preventing the conversion of ribonucleotides to deoxyribonucleotides, halting the cell cycle at the G1/S phase and therefore has radiation sensitizing activity by maintaining cells in the G_1 phase and interfering with DNA repair. In sickle cell anemia, hydroxyurea increases red blood cell (RBC) hemoglobin F levels, RBC water content, deformability of sickled cells, and alters adhesion of RBCs to endothelium.

Pharmacodynamics/Kinetics

Onset: Sickle cell anemia: Fetal hemoglobin increase: 4-12 weeks

Absorption: Readily (≥80%)

Distribution: Readily crosses blood-brain barrier; distributes into intestine, brain, lung, kidney tissues, effusions and ascites

Metabolism: 60% via hepatic and GI tract

Half-life elimination: 3-4 hours

Time to peak: 1-4 hours

Excretion: Urine (sickle cell anemia: 40% of administered dose)

Dosage Oral: Doses should be based on ideal or actual body weight, whichever is less:

Children: Sickle cell anemia (unlabeled use): 20 mg/kg once daily; increase by 5 mg/kg/day every 2-6 months to a maximum dose of 30 mg/kg/day (Ferster, 2001; Hankins, 2005; Thornburg, 2009; Wang, 2001; Zimmerman, 2004)

Adults:

Antineoplastic uses: Titrate dose to patient response; if WBC count falls to <2500/mm³, or the platelet count to <100,000/mm³, therapy should be stopped for at least 3 days and resumed when values rise toward normal

Chronic myeloid leukemia (resistant): Continuous therapy: 20-30 mg/kg once daily

Solid tumors:

Intermittent therapy: 80 mg/kg as a single dose every third day

Continuous therapy: 20-30 mg/kg once daily

Concomitant therapy with irradiation (head and neck cancer): 80 mg/kg as a single dose every third day starting at least 7 days before initiation of irradiation

Sickle cell anemia: Initial: 15 mg/kg/day; if blood counts are in an acceptable range, may increase by 5 mg/kg every 12 weeks until the maximum tolerated dose of 35 mg/kg/day is achieved or the dose that does not produce toxic effects (do not increase dose if blood counts are between acceptable and toxic ranges). Monitor for toxicity every 2 weeks; if toxicity occurs, withhold treatment until the bone marrow recovers, then restart with a dose reduction of 2.5 mg/kg/day; if no toxicity occurs over the next 12 weeks, then the subsequent dose may be increased by 2.5 mg/kg/day every 12 weeks to a maximum tolerated dose (dose which does not produce hematologic toxicity for 24 consecutive weeks). If hematologic toxicity recurs a second time at a specific dose, do not retry that dose.

Acceptable hematologic ranges: Neutrophils ≥2500/mm³; platelets ≥95,000/mm³; hemoglobin >5.3 g/dL, and reticulocytes ≥95,000/mm³ if the hemoglobin concentration is <9 g/dL

Toxic hematologic ranges: Neutrophils <2000/mm³; platelets <80,000/mm³; hemoglobin <4.5 g/dL; and reticulocytes <80,000/mm³ if the hemoglobin concentration is <9 g/dL

Cervical cancer (unlabeled use; with concurrent radiation therapy, cisplatin and fluorouracil): 2000 mg/m² (2 hours prior to radiation treatment) twice a week for 6 weeks (Rose, 2007)

Essential thrombocythemia, high-risk (unlabeled use): 500-1000 mg daily; adjust dose to maintain platelets <400,000/mm³ (Harrison, 2005)

Head and neck cancer (unlabeled dosing; with concurrent radiation therapy and fluorouracil): 1000 mg every 12 hours for 11 doses (Garden, 2004)

Hypereosinophilic syndrome (unlabeled use): 1000-3000 mg/day (Klion, 2006)

Meningioma (unlabeled use): 20 mg/kg once daily (Newton, 2000; Rosenthal, 2002)

Polycythemia vera, high-risk (unlabeled use): 15-20 mg/kg/day (Finazzi, 2007)

Dosing adjustment in renal impairment:

The FDA-approved labeling recommends the following adjustment:

Sickle cell anemia:

Cl_{cr} ≥60 mL/minute: No adjustment (of initial dose) required

Cl_{cr} <60 mL/minute: Reduce initial dose to 7.5 mg/kg/day; titrate to response/avoidance of toxicity (refer to usual dosing)

ESRD: Reduce initial dose to 7.5 mg/kg/dose (administer after dialysis on dialysis days); titrate to response/avoidance of toxicity

Other approved indications: It is recommended to reduce the initial dose; however, no specific guidelines are available.

The following guidelines have been used by some clinicians:

Aronoff, 2007: Adults:

Cl_{cr} 10-50 mL/minute: Administer 50% of dose

Cl_{cr} <10 mL/minute: Administer 20% of dose

Hemodialysis: Administer dose after dialysis on dialysis days; supplemental dose is not necessary. Hydroxyurea is a low molecular weight compound with high aqueous solubility that may be freely dialyzable, however, clinical studies confirming this hypothesis have not been performed.

Continuous renal replacement therapy (CRRT): Administer 50% of dose

Kintzel, 1995:

Cl_{cr} 46-60 mL/minute: Administer 85% of dose

Cl_{cr} 31-45 mL/minute: Administer 80% of dose

Cl_{cr} <30 mL/minute: Administer 75% of dose

Dosing adjustment in hepatic impairment: Specific guidelines are not available for dosage adjustment in hepatic impairment. The FDA-approved labeling recommends closely monitoring for bone marrow toxicity in patients with hepatic impairment.

Dietary Considerations In sickle cell patients, supplemental administration of folic acid is recommended; hydroxyurea may mask development of folic acid deficiency.

Administration The manufacturer does not recommend opening the capsules; observe proper handling procedures (eg, wear gloves)

Monitoring Parameters CBC with differential and platelets, renal function and liver function tests, serum uric acid

Sickle cell disease: Monitor for toxicity every 2 weeks. If toxicity occurs, stop treatment until the bone marrow recovers; restart at 2.5 mg/kg/day less than the dose at which toxicity occurs. If no toxicity occurs over the next 12 weeks, then the subsequent dose should be increased by 2.5 mg/kg/day. Reduced dosage of hydroxyurea alternating with erythropoietin may decrease myelotoxicity and increase levels of fetal hemoglobin in patients who have not been helped by hydroxyurea alone.

Acceptable range: Neutrophils ≥2500 cells/mm^3, platelets ≥95,000/mm^3, hemoglobin >5.3 g/dL, and reticulocytes ≥95,000/mm^3 if the hemoglobin concentration is <9 g/dL

Toxic range: Neutrophils <2000 cells/mm^3, platelets <80,000/mm^3, hemoglobin <4.5 g/dL, and reticulocytes <80,000/mm^3 if the hemoglobin concentration is <9 g/dL

Test Interactions False-negative triglyceride measurement by a glycerol oxidase method

Dosage Forms Excipient information presented when available (limited, particularly for generics); consult specific product labeling.

Capsule, oral: 500 mg

Droxia®: 200 mg, 300 mg, 400 mg

Hydrea®: 500 mg

Extemporaneous Preparations Hazardous agent: Use appropriate precautions for handling and disposal.

A 40 mg/mL oral suspension may be made with capsules and either a 1:1 mixture of Ora-Sweet® and Ora-Plus® or a 1:1 mixture of methylcellulose 1% and simple syrup NF. Empty the contents of eight 500 mg capsules into a mortar. Add small portions of chosen vehicle and mix to a uniform paste; mix while incrementally adding the vehicle to **almost** 100 mL; transfer to a calibrated bottle, rinse mortar with vehicle, and add sufficient quantity of vehicle to make 100 mL. Label "shake well" and "refrigerate". Store in plastic prescription bottles. Stable for 14 days at room temperature or refrigerated (preferred) (Nahata, 2003).

A 100 mg/mL oral solution may be made with capsules. Mix the contents of twenty 500 mg capsules with enough room temperature sterile water (~50 mL) to result in a 200 mg/mL concentration. Stir vigorously (several hours), then filter to remove insoluble contents. Add 50 mL Syrpalta® (flavored syrup, HUMCO) to filtered solution, resulting in 100 mL of a 100 mg/mL hydroxyurea solution. Stable for 1 month at room temperature or 3 months refrigerated (Heeney, 2004).

Heeney MM, Whorton MR, Howard TA, et al, "Chemical and Functional Analysis of Hydroxyurea Oral Solutions," *J Pediatr Hematol Oncol*, 2004, 26(3):179-84.

Nahata MC, Morosco RS, Boster EA, et al, "Stability of Hydroxyurea in Two Extemporaneously Prepared Oral Suspensions Stored at Two Temperatures," 2003, 38:P-161(E) [abstract from 2003 ASHP Midyear Clinical Meeting].

HydrOXYzine (hye DROKS i zeen)

Brand Names: U.S. Vistaril®

Brand Names: Canada Apo-Hydroxyzine®; Atarax®; Hydroxyzine Hydrochloride Injection, USP; Novo-Hydroxyzin; Nu-Hydroxyzine; PMS-Hydroxyzine; Riva-Hydroxyzine

Index Terms Hydroxyzine Hydrochloride; Hydroxyzine Pamoate

Pharmacologic Category Antiemetic; Histamine H_1 Antagonist; Histamine H_1 Antagonist, First Generation; Piperazine Derivative

Additional Appendix Information

Beers Criteria – Potentially Inappropriate Medications for Geriatrics *on page 1973*

Use Treatment of anxiety/agitation (including adjunctive therapy in alcoholism); adjunct to pre- and postoperative analgesia and anesthesia; antipruritic; antiemetic

Pregnancy Considerations Hydroxyzine-induced fetal abnormalities were observed at high dosages in animal studies. Neonatal withdrawal symptoms have been reported following long-term maternal use or the use of large doses near term. Use in early pregnancy is contraindicated by the manufacturer.

Lactation Excretion in breast milk unknown/not recommended

Contraindications Hypersensitivity to hydroxyzine or any component of the formulation; early pregnancy; SubQ, intra-arterial, or I.V. injection

Warnings/Precautions Causes sedation, caution must be used in performing tasks which require alertness (eg, operating machinery or driving). Sedative effects of CNS depressants or ethanol are potentiated. SubQ, I.V., and intra-arterial administration are contraindicated since tissue damage, intravascular hemolysis, thrombosis, and digital gangrene can occur. Use with caution with narrow-angle glaucoma, prostatic hyperplasia, bladder neck obstruction, asthma, or COPD. May be inappropriate for use in the elderly due to potent anticholinergic effects; nonanticholinergic antihistamines preferred for treating allergic reactions (Beers Criteria).

Adverse Reactions Frequency not defined.

Central nervous system: Dizziness, drowsiness, fatigue, hallucination, headache, nervousness, seizure

Dermatologic: Pruritus, rash, urticaria

Gastrointestinal: Xerostomia

Neuromuscular & skeletal: Involuntary movements, paresthesia, tremor

Ocular: Blurred vision

Respiratory: Respiratory depression (at higher than recommended doses)

Miscellaneous: Allergic reaction

Drug Interactions

Metabolism/Transport Effects Inhibits CYP2D6 (weak)

Avoid Concomitant Use There are no known interactions where it is recommended to avoid concomitant use.

Increased Effect/Toxicity

HydrOXYzine may increase the levels/effects of: Alcohol (Ethyl); Anticholinergics; Barbiturates; CNS Depressants; Meperidine; Methotrimeprazine; Selective Serotonin Reuptake Inhibitors

The levels/effects of HydrOXYzine may be increased by: Droperidol; Methotrimeprazine; Pramlintide

Decreased Effect

HydrOXYzine may decrease the levels/effects of: Acetylcholinesterase Inhibitors (Central); Benzylpenicilloyl Polylysine; Betahistine

The levels/effects of HydrOXYzine may be decreased by: Acetylcholinesterase Inhibitors (Central); Amphetamines

Ethanol/Nutrition/Herb Interactions

Ethanol: May increase CNS depression; monitor for increased effects with coadministration. Caution patients about effects.

Herb/Nutraceutical: Avoid valerian, St John's wort, kava kava, gotu kola (may increase CNS depression).

Stability

Injection: Store at 20°C to 25°C (68°F to 77°F); excursions permitted to 15°C to 30°C (59°F to 86°F). Protect from light.

Tablets: Store at 20°C to 25°C (68°F to 77°F).

Mechanism of Action Competes with histamine for H_1-receptor sites on effector cells in the gastrointestinal tract, blood vessels, and respiratory tract. Possesses skeletal muscle relaxing, bronchodilator, antihistamine, antiemetic, and analgesic properties.

Pharmacodynamics/Kinetics

Onset of action: Oral: 15-30 minutes; Injection: Rapid

Duration: Decreased histamine-induced wheal and flare areas: 2 to ≥36 hours; Suppression of pruritus: 1-12 hours (Simons, 1984)

Absorption: Oral: Rapid

Distribution: Adults: V_d ~16 L/kg (Simons, 1984); Elderly: ~23 L/kg (Simons K, 1989); Hepatic dysfunction: ~23 L/kg (Simons F, 1989)
Metabolism: Hepatic to multiple metabolites, including cetirizine (active) (Simons F, 1989)
Half-life elimination: Adults: ~20 hours (Simons, 1984); Elderly: ~29 hours (Simons K, 1989); Hepatic dysfunction: ~37 hours (Simons F, 1989)
Time to peak: Oral administration: Serum: ~2 hours; Peak suppression of antihistamine-induced wheal and flare: 4-12 hours (Simons, 1984)
Excretion: Urine

Dosage

Note: Adjust dose based on patient response.

Children:
- Preoperative sedation:
  - Oral: 0.6 mg/kg/dose
  - I.M.: 1.1 mg/kg/dose
- Pruritus, anxiety: Oral:
  - <6 years: 50 mg daily in divided doses
  - ≥6 years: 50-100 mg daily in divided doses
- Antiemetic: I.M.: 1.1 mg/kg/dose

Adults:
- Antiemetic: I.M.: 25-100 mg/dose
- Anxiety:
  - Oral: 50-100 mg 4 times/day
  - I.M.: Initial: 50-100 mg, then every 4-6 hours as needed
- Preoperative sedation:
  - Oral: 50-100 mg
  - I.M.: 25-100 mg
- Pruritus: Oral: 25 mg 3-4 times/day

Elderly: Initiate dosing using the lower end of the recommended dosage range due to an increased potential for anticholinergic side effects. Refer to adult dosing.

Dosing interval in hepatic impairment: Change dosing interval to every 24 hours in patients with primary biliary cirrhosis (Simons F, 1989).

Administration

Injection: For I. M. use only. Do not administer I.V., SubQ, or intra-arterially. Administer I.M. deep in large muscle. In adults, the preferred site is the upper outer quadrant of the buttock or midlateral thigh. In children, the preferred site is the midlateral thigh. The upper outer quadrant of the gluteal region should be used only when necessary to minimize potential damage to the sciatic nerve. With I.V. administration, extravasation can result in sterile abscess and marked tissue induration.

Oral: Shake suspension vigorously prior to use.

Monitoring Parameters Relief of symptoms, mental status, blood pressure

Test Interactions May cause false-positive serum TCA screen.

Dosage Forms Excipient information presented when available (limited, particularly for generics); consult specific product labeling.

Capsule, oral, as pamoate: 25 mg, 50 mg, 100 mg
Vistaril®: 25 mg, 50 mg
Injection, solution, as hydrochloride: 25 mg/mL (1 mL); 50 mg/mL (1 mL, 2 mL, 10 mL)
Solution, oral, as hydrochloride: 10 mg/5 mL (473 mL)
Syrup, oral, as hydrochloride: 10 mg/5 mL (118 mL, 473 mL)
Tablet, oral, as hydrochloride: 10 mg, 25 mg, 50 mg

◆ **Hydroxyzine Hydrochloride** *see* HydrOXYzine *on page* 853

◆ **Hydroxyzine Hydrochloride Injection, USP (Can)** *see* HydrOXYzine *on page* 853

◆ **Hydroxyzine Pamoate** *see* HydrOXYzine *on page* 853

◆ **Hydurea** *see* Hydroxyurea *on page* 851

◆ **Hygroton** *see* Chlorthalidone *on page* 350

◆ **Hylan G-F 20** *see* Hyaluronate and Derivatives *on page* 831

◆ **Hylan Polymers** *see* Hyaluronate and Derivatives *on page* 831

◆ **HyoMax™-DT** *see* Hyoscyamine *on page* 854

◆ **HyoMax™-FT** *see* Hyoscyamine *on page* 854

◆ **HyoMax®-SL** *see* Hyoscyamine *on page* 854

◆ **HyoMax® -SR** *see* Hyoscyamine *on page* 854

◆ **Hyonatol** *see* Hyoscyamine, Atropine, Scopolamine, and Phenobarbital *on page* 855

◆ **Hyophen™** *see* Methenamine, Phenyl Salicylate, Methylene Blue, Benzoic Acid, and Hyoscyamine *on page* 1094

◆ **Hyoscine Butylbromide** *see* Scopolamine (Systemic) *on page* 1542

Hyoscyamine (hye oh SYE a meen)

Brand Names: U.S. Anaspaz®; HyoMax® -SR; HyoMax®-SL; HyoMax™-DT; HyoMax™-FT; Hyosyne; Levbid®; Levsin®; Levsin®/SL; NuLev®; Oscimin; Symax® DuoTab; Symax® FasTab; Symax® SL; Symax® SR

Brand Names: Canada Levsin®

Index Terms *l*-Hyoscyamine Sulfate; Hyoscyamine Sulfate

Pharmacologic Category Anticholinergic Agent

Additional Appendix Information

Beers Criteria – Potentially Inappropriate Medications for Geriatrics *on page* 1973

Use

Oral: Adjunctive therapy for peptic ulcers, irritable bowel, neurogenic bladder/bowel; treatment of infant colic, GI tract disorders caused by spasm; to reduce rigidity, tremors, sialorrhea, and hyperhidrosis associated with parkinsonism; as a drying agent in acute rhinitis

Injection: Preoperative antimuscarinic to reduce secretions and block cardiac vagal inhibitory reflexes; to improve radiologic visibility of the kidneys; symptomatic relief of biliary and renal colic; reduce GI motility to facilitate diagnostic procedures (ie, endoscopy, hypotonic duodenography); reduce pain and hypersecretion in pancreatitis, certain cases of partial heart block associated with vagal activity; reversal of neuromuscular blockade

Pregnancy Risk Factor C

Dosage

Oral: Children: Gastrointestinal disorders: Dose as listed, based on age and weight (kg) using 0.125 mg/mL drops; repeat dose every 4 hours as needed:
- Children <2 years:
  - 3.4 kg: 4 drops; maximum: 24 drops/24 hours
  - 5 kg: 5 drops; maximum: 30 drops/24 hours
  - 7 kg: 6 drops; maximum: 36 drops/24 hours
  - 10 kg: 8 drops; maximum: 48 drops/24 hours

Oral, S.L.:
- Children 2-12 years: Gastrointestinal disorders: Dose as listed, based on age and weight (kg); repeat dose every 4 hours as needed:
  - 10 kg: 0.031-0.033 mg; maximum: 0.75 mg/24 hours
  - 20 kg: 0.0625 mg; maximum: 0.75 mg/24 hours
  - 40 kg: 0.0938 mg; maximum: 0.75 mg/24 hours
  - 50 kg: 0.125 mg; maximum: 0.75 mg/24 hours
- Children >12 years and Adults: Gastrointestinal disorders: 0.125-0.25 mg every 4 hours or as needed (before meals or food); maximum: 1.5 mg/24 hours

Oral (timed release): Children >12 years and Adults: Gastrointestinal disorders: 0.375-0.75 mg every 12 hours; maximum: 1.5 mg/24 hours

I.M., I.V., SubQ: Children >12 years and Adults: Gastrointestinal disorders: 0.25-0.5 mg; may repeat as needed up to 4 times/day, at 4-hour intervals

I.V.: Children >2 year and Adults: I.V.: Preanesthesia: 5 mcg/kg given 30-60 minutes prior to induction of anesthesia or at the time preoperative narcotics or sedatives are administered

I.V.: Adults: Diagnostic procedures: 0.25-0.5 mg given 5-10 minutes prior to procedure

To reduce drug-induced bradycardia during surgery: 0.125 mg; repeat as needed

To reverse neuromuscular blockade: 0.2 mg for every 1 mg neostigmine (or the physostigmine/pyridostigmine equivalent)

Additional Information Complete prescribing information for this medication should be consulted for additional detail.

Dosage Forms Excipient information presented when available (limited, particularly for generics); consult specific product labeling.

Elixir, oral, as sulfate: 0.125 mg/5 mL (473 mL)

Hyosyne: 0.125 mg/5 mL (473 mL) [contains ethanol 20%, sodium benzoate; orange-lemon flavor]

Injection, solution, as sulfate:

Levsin®: 0.5 mg/mL (1 mL)

Solution, oral, as sulfate [drops]: 0.125 mg/mL (15 mL)

Hyosyne: 0.125 mg/mL (15 mL) [contains ethanol 5%, sodium benzoate; orange-lemon flavor]

Tablet, oral, as sulfate: 0.125 mg

Levsin®: 0.125 mg

Tablet, sublingual, as sulfate: 0.125 mg

HyoMax®-SL: 0.125 mg [peppermint flavor]

Levsin®/SL: 0.125 mg

Oscimin: 0.125 mg [peppermint flavor]

Symax® SL: 0.125 mg

Tablet, chewable/disintegrating, oral, as sulfate:

HyoMax™-FT: 0.125 mg [mint flavor]

NuLev®: 0.125 mg [peppermint flavor]

Oscimin: 0.125 mg [peppermint flavor]

Symax® FasTab: 0.125 mg [mint flavor]

Tablet, dispersible, oral, as sulfate:

Oscimin: 0.125 mg [peppermint flavor]

Tablet, extended release, oral, as sulfate: 0.375 mg

Levbid®: 0.375 mg

Oscimin: 0.375 mg

Tablet, orally disintegrating, oral, as sulfate: 0.125 mg

Anaspaz®: 0.125 mg [scored]

Tablet, sustained release, oral, as sulfate: 0.375 mg

HyoMax® -SR: 0.375 mg [scored]

Symax® SR: 0.375 mg

Tablet, variable release, oral:

HyoMax™-DT: Hyoscyamine sulfate 0.125 mg [immediate release] and hyoscyamine sulfate 0.25 mg [sustained release]

Symax® DuoTab: Hyoscyamine sulfate 0.125 mg [immediate release] and hyoscyamine sulfate 0.25 mg [sustained release]

Hyoscyamine, Atropine, Scopolamine, and Phenobarbital

(hye oh SYE a meen, A troe peen, skoe POL a meen, & fee noe BAR bi tal)

Brand Names: U.S. Donnatal Extentabs®; Donnatal®; Hyonatol

Index Terms Atropine, Hyoscyamine, Phenobarbital, and Scopolamine; Belladonna Alkaloids With Phenobarbital; Phenobarbital, Hyoscyamine, Atropine, and Scopolamine; Scopolamine, Hyoscyamine, Atropine, and Phenobarbital

Pharmacologic Category Anticholinergic Agent; Antispasmodic Agent, Gastrointestinal

Use Adjunct in treatment of irritable bowel syndrome, acute enterocolitis, duodenal ulcer

Pregnancy Risk Factor C

Dosage Oral:

Children: Donnatal® elixir: To be given every 4-6 hours; initial dose based on weight:

4.5 kg: 0.5 mL every 4 hours **or** 0.75 mL every 6 hours

10 kg: 1 mL every 4 hours **or** 1.5 mL every 6 hours

14 kg: 1.5 mL every 4 hours **or** 2 mL every 6 hours

23 kg: 2.5 mL every 4 hours **or** 3.8 mL every 6 hours

34 kg: 3.8 mL every 4 hours **or** 5 mL every 6 hours

≥45 kg: 5 mL every 4 hours **or** 7.5 mL every 6 hours

Adults:

Donnatal®: 1-2 tablets or 5-10 mL of elixir 3-4 times/day

Donnatal Extentabs®: 1 tablet every 12 hours; may increase to 1 tablet every 8 hours if needed

Additional Information Complete prescribing information for this medication should be consulted for additional detail.

Dosage Forms Excipient information presented when available (limited, particularly for generics); consult specific product labeling. [DSC] = Discontinued product

Elixir: Hyoscyamine sulfate 0.1037 mg, atropine sulfate 0.0194 mg, scopolamine hydrobromide 0.0065 mg, and phenobarbital 16.2 mg per 5 mL (473 mL)

Donnatal®: Hyoscyamine sulfate 0.1037 mg, atropine sulfate 0.0194 mg, scopolamine hydrobromide 0.0065 mg, and phenobarbital 16.2 mg per 5 mL (120 mL, 480 mL) [contains ethanol <23.8%; citrus flavor] [DSC]

Donnatal®: Hyoscyamine sulfate 0.1037 mg, atropine sulfate 0.0194 mg, scopolamine hydrobromide 0.0065 mg, and phenobarbital 16.2 mg per 5 mL (120 mL, 480 mL) [contains ethanol <23.8%; grape flavor]

Tablet: Hyoscyamine sulfate 0.1037 mg, atropine sulfate 0.0194 mg, scopolamine hydrobromide 0.0065 mg, and phenobarbital 16.2 mg

Donnatal®: Hyoscyamine sulfate 0.1037 mg, atropine sulfate 0.0194 mg, scopolamine hydrobromide 0.0065 mg, and phenobarbital 16.2 mg

Hyonatol: Hyoscyamine sulfate 0.1037 mg, atropine sulfate 0.0194 mg, scopolamine hydrobromide 0.0065 mg, and phenobarbital 16.2 mg

Tablet, extended release:

Donnatal Extentabs®: Hyoscyamine sulfate 0.3111 mg, atropine sulfate 0.0582 mg, scopolamine hydrobromide 0.0195 mg, and phenobarbital 48.6 mg

- ◆ **Hyoscyamine, Methenamine, Benzoic Acid, Phenyl Salicylate, and Methylene Blue** *see* Methenamine, Phenyl Salicylate, Methylene Blue, Benzoic Acid, and Hyoscyamine *on page 1094*
- ◆ **Hyoscyamine, Methenamine, Methylene Blue, Phenyl Salicylate, and Sodium Biphosphate** *see* Methenamine, Sodium Biphosphate, Phenyl Salicylate, Methylene Blue, and Hyoscyamine *on page 1094*
- ◆ **Hyoscyamine, Methenamine, Sodium Biphosphate, Phenyl Salicylate, and Methylene Blue** *see* Methenamine, Sodium Biphosphate, Phenyl Salicylate, Methylene Blue, and Hyoscyamine *on page 1094*
- ◆ **Hyoscyamine Sulfate** *see* Hyoscyamine *on page 854*
- ◆ **Hyosyne** *see* Hyoscyamine *on page 854*
- ◆ **Hyperal** *see* Total Parenteral Nutrition *on page 1714*
- ◆ **Hyperalimentation** *see* Total Parenteral Nutrition *on page 1714*
- ◆ **HyperHep B® (Can)** *see* Hepatitis B Immune Globulin (Human) *on page 826*
- ◆ **HyperHEP B™ S/D** *see* Hepatitis B Immune Globulin (Human) *on page 826*
- ◆ **HyperRAB™ S/D** *see* Rabies Immune Globulin (Human) *on page 1453*
- ◆ **HyperRHO™ S/D Full Dose** *see* Rh_o(D) Immune Globulin *on page 1476*

◆ **HyperRHO™ S/D Mini-Dose** *see* Rh$_0$(D) Immune Globulin *on page 1476*

◆ **HyperSal®** *see* Sodium Chloride *on page 1567*

◆ **HyperTET™ S/D** *see* Tetanus Immune Globulin (Human) *on page 1657*

◆ **Hypertonic Saline** *see* Sodium Chloride *on page 1567*

◆ **Hytrin** *see* Terazosin *on page 1647*

◆ **Hytrin® (Can)** *see* Terazosin *on page 1647*

◆ **Hyzaar®** *see* Losartan and Hydrochlorothiazide *on page 1037*

◆ **Hyzaar® DS (Can)** *see* Losartan and Hydrochlorothiazide *on page 1037*

◆ **I^{123} Iobenguane** *see* Iobenguane I 123 *on page 920*

◆ **I-123 MIBG** *see* Iobenguane I 123 *on page 920*

Ibandronate (eye BAN droh nate)

Brand Names: U.S. Boniva®

Index Terms Ibandronate Sodium; Ibandronic Acid

Pharmacologic Category Bisphosphonate Derivative

Use Treatment and prevention of osteoporosis in postmenopausal females

Unlabeled Use Hypercalcemia of malignancy; corticosteroid-induced osteoporosis; Paget's disease; reduce bone pain and skeletal complications from metastatic bone disease

Pregnancy Risk Factor C

Pregnancy Considerations Adverse effects were demonstrated in animal studies. There are no adequate and well-controlled studies in pregnant women. Bisphosphonates are incorporated into the bone matrix and are gradually released over time. Theoretically, there may be a risk of fetal harm when pregnancy follows the completion of therapy. Based on limited case reports with pamidronate, serum calcium levels in the newborn may be altered if administered during pregnancy.

Lactation Excretion in breast milk unknown/use caution

Medication Guide Available Yes

Contraindications Hypersensitivity to ibandronate or any component of the formulation; hypocalcemia; oral tablets are also contraindicated in patients unable to stand or sit upright for at least 60 minutes and in patients with abnormalities of the esophagus which delay esophageal emptying, such as stricture or achalasia

Warnings/Precautions Hypocalcemia must be corrected before therapy initiation. Ensure adequate calcium and vitamin D intake. Osteonecrosis of the jaw (ONJ) has been reported in patients receiving bisphosphonates. Risk factors include invasive dental procedures (eg, tooth extraction, dental implants, boney surgery); a diagnosis of cancer, with concomitant chemotherapy or corticosteroids; poor oral hygiene, ill-fitting dentures; and comorbid disorders (anemia, coagulopathy, infection, pre-existing dental disease). Most reported cases occurred after I.V. bisphosphonate therapy; however, cases have been reported following oral therapy. A dental exam and preventative dentistry should be performed prior to placing patients with risk factors on chronic bisphosphonate therapy. The manufacturer's labeling states that discontinuing bisphosphonates in patients requiring invasive dental procedures may reduce the risk of ONJ. However, other experts suggest that there is no evidence that discontinuing therapy reduces the risk of developing ONJ (Assael, 2009). The benefit/risk must be assessed by the treating physician and/or dentist/surgeon prior to any invasive dental procedure. Patients developing ONJ while on bisphosphonates should receive care by an oral surgeon.

Atypical femur fractures have been reported in patients receiving bisphosphonates for treatment/prevention of osteoporosis. The fractures include subtrochanteric femur (bone just below the hip joint) and diaphyseal femur (long segment of the thigh bone). Some patients experience prodromal pain weeks or months before the fracture occurs. It is unclear if bisphosphonate therapy is the cause for these fractures, although the majority have been reported in patients taking bisphosphonates. Patients receiving long-term (>3-5 years) therapy may be at an increased risk. Discontinue bisphosphonate therapy in patients who develop a femoral shaft fracture.

Infrequently, severe (and occasionally debilitating) bone, joint, and/or muscle pain have been reported during bisphosphonate treatment. The onset of pain ranged from a single day to several months. Consider discontinuing therapy in patients who experience severe symptoms; symptoms usually resolve upon discontinuation. Some patients experienced recurrence when rechallenged with same drug or another bisphosphonate; avoid use in patients with a history of these symptoms in association with bisphosphonate therapy.

Oral bisphosphonates may cause dysphagia, esophagitis, esophageal or gastric ulcer; risk may increase in patients unable to comply with dosing instructions; discontinue use if new or worsening symptoms develop. Intravenous bisphosphonates may cause transient decreases in serum calcium and have also been associated with renal toxicity.

Use not recommended with severe renal impairment (Cl_{cr} <30 mL/minute).

Adverse Reactions Percentages vary based on frequency of administration (daily vs monthly). Unless specified, percentages are reported with oral use.

>10%:
- Gastrointestinal: Dyspepsia (6% to 12%)
- Neuromuscular & skeletal: Back pain (4% to 14%)

1% to 10%:
- Cardiovascular: Hypertension (6% to 7%)
- Central nervous system: Headache (3% to 7%), dizziness (1% to 4%), insomnia (1% to 2%)
- Dermatologic: Rash (1% to 2%)
- Endocrine & metabolic: Hypercholesterolemia (5%)
- Gastrointestinal: Abdominal pain (5% to 8%), diarrhea (4% to 7%), nausea (5%), constipation (3% to 4%), vomiting (3%)
- Genitourinary: Urinary tract infection (2% to 6%)
- Hepatic: Alkaline phosphatase decreased (frequency not defined)
- Local: Injection site reaction (<2%)
- Neuromuscular & skeletal: Pain in extremity (1% to 8%), arthralgia (4% to 6%), myalgia (1% to 6%), joint disorder (4%), osteonecrosis of the jaw (4%), weakness (4%), osteoarthritis (localized; 1% to 3%), muscle cramp (2%)
- Respiratory: Bronchitis (3% to 10%), pneumonia (6%), pharyngitis/nasopharyngitis (3% to 4%), upper respiratory infection (2%)
- Miscellaneous: Acute phase reaction (I.V. 10%; oral 3% to 9%), infection (4%), flu-like syndrome (1% to 4%), allergic reaction (3%)

Postmarketing and/or case reports: Anaphylaxis; angioedema; bronchospasm; diaphyseal femur fracture; esophageal cancer; hypocalcemia; incapacitating bone, joint, or muscle pain; iritis; ocular inflammation; scleritis; subtrochanteric femur fracture; uveitis

Drug Interactions

Metabolism/Transport Effects None known.

Avoid Concomitant Use There are no known interactions where it is recommended to avoid concomitant use.

Increased Effect/Toxicity

Ibandronate may increase the levels/effects of: Deferasirox; Phosphate Supplements

The levels/effects of Ibandronate may be increased by: Aminoglycosides; Nonsteroidal Anti-Inflammatory Agents

Decreased Effect

The levels/effects of Ibandronate may be decreased by: Antacids; Calcium Salts; Iron Salts; Magnesium Salts; Proton Pump Inhibitors

Ethanol/Nutrition/Herb Interactions

Ethanol: Avoid ethanol (may increase risk of osteoporosis).

Food: May reduce absorption; mean oral bioavailability is decreased up to 90% when given with food.

Stability Store at controlled room temperature of 25°C (77°F); excursions permitted to 15°C to 30°C (59°F to 86°F).

Mechanism of Action A bisphosphonate which inhibits bone resorption via actions on osteoclasts or on osteoclast precursors; decreases the rate of bone resorption, leading to an indirect increase in bone mineral density.

Pharmacodynamics/Kinetics

Distribution: Terminal V_d: 90 L; 40% to 50% of circulating ibandronate binds to bone

Protein binding: 85.7% to 99.5%

Metabolism: Not metabolized

Bioavailability: Oral: 2.5 mg tablet: 0.6%; Reduced by 90% following standard breakfast

Half-life elimination:

Oral: 150 mg dose: Terminal: 37-157 hours

I.V.: Terminal: ~5-25 hours

Time to peak, plasma: Oral: 0.5-2 hours

Excretion: Urine (50% to 60% of absorbed dose, excreted as unchanged drug); feces (unabsorbed drug)

Dosage

Oral:

Treatment of postmenopausal osteoporosis: 2.5 mg once daily **or** 150 mg once a month; **Note:** Patients should receive supplemental calcium and vitamin D if dietary intake is inadequate

Prevention of postmenopausal osteoporosis: 2.5 once daily **or** 150 mg once a month; **Note:** Patients should receive supplemental calcium and vitamin D if dietary intake is inadequate

Metastatic bone disease (unlabeled use): 50 mg once daily

I.V.:

Treatment of postmenopausal osteoporosis: 3 mg every 3 months; **Note:** Patients should receive supplemental calcium and vitamin D if dietary intake is inadequate

Hypercalcemia of malignancy (unlabeled use): 2-4 mg over 2 hours

Metastatic bone disease (unlabeled use): 6 mg over 1 hour every 3-4 weeks

Dosage adjustment in renal impairment:

Mild or moderate impairment: Dosing adjustment not needed

Severe impairment (Cl_{cr} <30 mL/minute): Use not recommended

Dose adjustment in renal impairment for oncologic uses (unlabeled): Severe impairment (Cl_{cr} <30 mL/minute):

Oral: 50 mg once weekly

I.V.: 2 mg over 1 hour every 3-4 weeks

Dosage adjustment in hepatic impairment: Dosing adjustment not needed

Dietary Considerations Ensure adequate calcium and vitamin D intake; women and men >50 years of age should consume 1200-1500 mg/day of elemental calcium and 800-1000 int. units/day of vitamin D. Ibandronate tablet should be taken with a full glass (6-8 oz) of plain water, at least 60 minutes prior to any food, beverages, or medications. Mineral water with a high calcium content should be avoided.

Administration

Oral: Should be administered 60 minutes before the first food or drink of the day (other than water) and prior to taking any oral medications or supplements (eg, calcium, antacids, vitamins). Ibandronate should be taken in an upright position with a full glass (6-8 oz) of plain water and the patient should avoid lying down for 60 minutes to minimize the possibility of GI side effects. Mineral water with a high calcium content should be avoided. The tablet should be swallowed whole; do not chew or suck. Do not eat or drink anything (except water) for 60 minutes following administration of ibandronate.

Once-monthly dosing: The 150 mg tablet should be taken on the same date each month. In case of a missed dose, do not take two 150 mg tablets within the same week. If the next scheduled dose is 1-7 days away, wait until the next scheduled dose to take the tablet. If the next scheduled dose is >7 days away, take the dose the morning it is remembered, and then resume taking the once-monthly dose on the originally scheduled day.

I.V.: Administer as a 15-30 second bolus. Do not mix with calcium-containing solutions or other drugs. For osteoporosis, do not administer more frequently than every 3 months. Infuse over 1 hour for metastatic bone disease and over 2 hours for hypercalcemia of malignancy.

Monitoring Parameters

Osteoporosis: Bone mineral density as measured by central dual-energy x-ray absorptiometry (DXA) of the hip or spine (prior to initiation of therapy and at least every 2 years); annual measurements of height and weight, assessment of chronic back pain; serum calcium and 25(OH)D; may consider measuring biochemical markers of bone turnover

Serum creatinine prior to each I.V. dose

Test Interactions Bisphosphonates may interfere with diagnostic imaging agents such as technetium-99m-diphosphonate in bone scans.

Dosage Forms Excipient information presented when available (limited, particularly for generics); consult specific product labeling. [DSC] = Discontinued product

Injection, solution:

Boniva®: 1 mg/mL (3 mL)

Tablet, oral:

Boniva®: 2.5 mg [DSC] [once-daily formulation]

Boniva®: 150 mg [once-monthly formulation]

◆ **Ibandronate Sodium** *see* Ibandronate *on page 856*

◆ **Ibandronic Acid** *see* Ibandronate *on page 856*

◆ **Ibidomide Hydrochloride** *see* Labetalol *on page 960*

Ibritumomab (ib ri TYOO mo mab)

Brand Names: U.S. Zevalin®

Brand Names: Canada Zevalin®

Index Terms Ibritumomab Tiuxetan; IDEC-Y2B8; In-111 Ibritumomab; In-111 Zevalin; Y-90 Ibritumomab; Y-90 Zevalin

Pharmacologic Category Antineoplastic Agent, Monoclonal Antibody; Radiopharmaceutical

Use Treatment of relapsed or refractory low-grade or follicular B-cell non-Hodgkin's lymphoma (NHL); treatment of follicular NHL in patients who achieve a response (partial or complete) to first-line chemotherapy

Pregnancy Risk Factor D

Pregnancy Considerations Animal studies have not been conducted. There are no adequate and well-controlled studies in pregnant women. Based on the radioactivity, Y-90 ibritumomab may cause fetal harm. Women of childbearing potential should avoid becoming pregnant during treatment with ibritumomab. Both males and females should use effective contraception for 12 months following treatment. The effect on future fertility is unknown.

Lactation Excretion in breast milk unknown/not recommended

Contraindications There are no contraindications listed within the manufacturer's labeling.

Warnings/Precautions Hazardous agent - use appropriate precautions for handling and disposal. **[U.S. Boxed Warning]: Severe cutaneous and mucocutaneous skin reactions have been reported (with fatalities) in post-marketing experience. Discontinue all components of the therapeutic regimen in patients experiencing severe cutaneous or mucocutaneous skin reactions,** including erythema multiforme, Stevens-Johnson syndrome, toxic epidermal necrolysis, bullous dermatitis, and exfoliative dermatitis. Onset may occur within days to 4 months following infusion.

To be used as part of the Zevalin® therapeutic regimen (in combination with rituximab). **[U.S. Boxed Warning]: Do not exceed the Y-90 ibritumomab maximum allowable dose of 32 mCi; do not administer to patients with altered biodistribution (determined by imaging with In-111 ibritumomab).** Use should be reserved to physicians and other professionals qualified and experienced in the safe handling of radiopharmaceuticals, and in monitoring and emergency treatment of infusion reactions. The contents of the kit are not radioactive until radiolabeling occurs. During and after radiolabeling, adequate shielding should be used with this product, in accordance with institutional radiation safety practices.

[U.S. Boxed Warning]: Serious fatal infusion reactions may occur with the rituximab component of the therapeutic regimen; fatalities were associated with acute respiratory distress syndrome, hypoxia, pulmonary infiltrates, cardiogenic shock, MI, or ventricular fibrillation. Immediately stop infusion and discontinue in patients who develop severe infusion reactions. Reactions typically occur with the first rituximab infusion (onset within 30-120 minutes). Reactions may also include angioedema, bronchospasm, and urticaria. Less severe reactions may be managed by slowing or interrupting infusion.

[U.S. Boxed Warning]: Delayed, prolonged, and severe cytopenias (thrombocytopenia and neutropenia) are common. Do not administer to patients with ≥25% lymphoma marrow involvement, patients with impaired bone marrow reserve (eg, prior myeloablative treatment, platelet count <100,000/mm^3, neutrophil count <1500/mm^3, hypocellular marrow), or to patients with prior stem cell collection failure. Patients with mild baseline thrombocytopenia may experience higher incidences of severe neutropenia and thrombocytopenia. Hemorrhage may occur due to thrombocytopenia; avoid concomitant use of medications interfering with coagulation or platelet function. Closely monitor patients for complications of cytopenias (eg, febrile neutropenia, hemorrhage) for up to 3 months after administration.

Secondary malignancies (acute myelogenous leukemia and/or myelodysplastic syndrome) have been reported following use; the median time to diagnosis (secondary malignancy) following ibritumomab treatment was 1.9 years (range: 0.4-6.3 years). Product contains albumin, which confers a theoretical risk of transmission of viral disease or Creutzfeldt-Jakob disease. The safety of immunization with live vaccines following ibritumomab therapy has not been studied; do not administer live viral vaccines to patients who have recently received ibritumomab treatment; the ability to generate a response to any vaccine after receiving treatment has not been studied. Safety and efficacy of repeated courses of the therapeutic regimen have not been established. Infusion site erythema and ulceration have been reported following extravasation; monitor infusion site; promptly terminate infusion with symptoms/signs of extravasation (restart in another limb). There is a case report of (delayed) erythema and ulceration, which is described as radiation necrosis following yttrium-90-ibritumomab extravasation (Williams, 2006). Delayed (up to 1 month) radiation injury has occurred in or near areas of lymphomatous involvement. Safety and efficacy have not been established in pediatric patients.

Adverse Reactions Severe, potentially life-threatening allergic reactions have occurred in association with infusions. Also refer to Rituximab monograph.

>10%:

Central nervous system: Fatigue (33%), chills (24%), fever (10% to 17%), pain (13%), headache (12%)

Gastrointestinal: Nausea (18% to 31%), abdominal pain (16% to 17%), vomiting (12%), diarrhea (9% to 11%)

Hematologic: Thrombocytopenia (62% to 95%; grades 3/4: 51% to 63%; nadir: 49-53 days), neutropenia (45% to 77%; grades 3/4: 41% to 60%; nadir: 61-62 days), anemia (22% to 61%; grades 3/4: 5% to 17%; nadir: 68-69 days), leukopenia (43%; grades 3/4: 36%), lymphopenia (26%; grades 3/4: 18%), myelosuppression (nadir: 7-9 weeks; duration: 22-35 days)

Neuromuscular & skeletal: Weakness (15% to 43%)

Respiratory: Nasopharyngitis (19%), dyspnea (14%), cough (10% to 11%)

Miscellaneous: Infection (29%; serious 1% to 5%)

1% to 10%:

Cardiovascular: Peripheral edema (8%), hypertension (7%), flushing (6%), hypotension (6%)

Central nervous system: Dizziness (7% to 10%), insomnia (5%), anxiety (4%)

Dermatologic: Pruritus (7% to 9%), rash (7% to 8%), petechiae (3% to 8%), bruising (7%), angioedema (5%; grades 3/4: <1%), urticaria (4%)

Gastrointestinal: Anorexia (8%), abdominal distension (5%), constipation (5%), dyspepsia (4%), melena (2%; life threatening in 1%), gastrointestinal hemorrhage (severe: 1%)

Genitourinary: Urinary tract infection (7%)

Hematologic: Secondary malignancies (1% to 6%; includes acute myelogenous leukemia and myelodysplastic syndrome), pancytopenia (severe: 2%)

Neuromuscular & skeletal: Myalgia (7% to 9%), back pain (8%), arthralgia (7%)

Respiratory: Throat irritation (10%), bronchitis (8%), rhinitis (6% to 8%), pharyngolaryngeal pain (7%), sinusitis (7%), bronchospasm (5%), epistaxis (3% to 5%), apnea (severe: 1%)

Miscellaneous: Flu-like syndrome (8%), night sweats (8%), diaphoresis (4%), HAMA antibody formation (4%), allergic reaction (2%), infusion reaction (severe: 1%), tumor pain (severe: 1%)

<1% (Limited to important or life-threatening: Anaphylactic reactions, arthritis, cerebral hemorrhage, cytogenetic abnormalities, encephalopathy, hematemesis, hemorrhage, hypersensitivity; infusion site erythema/ulceration (following extravasation), radiation injury/complications (delayed; in tissues in or near areas of lymphomatous involvement), meningioma (benign), pulmonary edema, pulmonary embolism, radiation necrosis (following yttrium-90-ibritumomab extravasation), stroke (hemorrhagic), subdural hematoma, tachycardia, vaginal hemorrhage

Drug Interactions

Metabolism/Transport Effects None known.

Avoid Concomitant Use

Avoid concomitant use of Ibritumomab with any of the following: BCG; CloZAPine; Natalizumab; Pimecrolimus; Tacrolimus (Topical); Vaccines (Live)

Increased Effect/Toxicity

Ibritumomab may increase the levels/effects of: CloZAPine; Leflunomide; Natalizumab; Vaccines (Live); Vitamin K Antagonists

The levels/effects of Ibritumomab may be increased by: Anticoagulants; Antiplatelet Agents; Denosumab; Pimecrolimus; Roflumilast; Tacrolimus (Topical); Trastuzumab

Decreased Effect

Ibritumomab may decrease the levels/effects of: BCG; Cardiac Glycosides; Coccidioidin Skin Test; Sipuleucel-T; Vaccines (Inactivated); Vaccines (Live); Vitamin K Antagonists

The levels/effects of Ibritumomab may be decreased by: Echinacea

Ethanol/Nutrition/Herb Interactions Herb/Nutraceutical: Avoid echinacea (may diminish therapeutic effect). Avoid cat's claw, dong quai, evening primrose, feverfew, garlic, ginger, ginkgo, red clover, horse chestnut, green tea, ginseng (all have antiplatelet activity).

Stability Store at 2°C to 8°C (36°F to 46°F); do not freeze. Administer Y-90 ibritumomab within 8 hours of radiolabeling and In-111 ibritumomab within 12 hours of radiolabeling. To prepare radiolabeled injection, follow detailed preparation guidelines provided by manufacturer (preparation procedures are different for In-111 ibritumomab and Y-90 ibritumomab).

Mechanism of Action Ibritumomab is a monoclonal antibody directed against the CD20 antigen found on B lymphocytes (normal and malignant). Ibritumomab binding induces apoptosis in B lymphocytes *in vitro*. It is combined with the chelator tiuxetan, which acts as a specific chelation site for either Indium-111 (In-111) or Yttrium-90 (Y-90). The monoclonal antibody acts as a delivery system to direct the radioactive isotope to the targeted cells, however, binding has been observed in lymphoid cells throughout the body and in lymphoid nodules in organs such as the large and small intestines. Indium-111 is a gamma-emitter used to assess biodistribution of ibritumomab, while Y-90 emits beta particles. Beta-emission induces cellular damage through the formation of free radicals (in both target cells and surrounding cells).

Pharmacodynamics/Kinetics

Duration: Beta cell recovery begins in ~12 weeks; generally in normal range within 9 months

Distribution: To lymphoid cells throughout the body and in lymphoid nodules in organs such as the large and small intestines, spleen, testes, and liver

Metabolism: Has not been characterized; the product of yttrium-90 radioactive decay is zirconium-90 (nonradioactive); Indium-111 decays to cadmium-111 (nonradioactive)

Half-life elimination: Y-90 ibritumomab: 30 hours; Indium-111 decays with a physical half-life of 67 hours; Yttrium-90 decays with a physical half-life of 64 hours

Excretion: A median of 7.2% of the radiolabeled activity was excreted in urine over 7 days

Dosage I.V.: Adults: **Note:** Premedication with oral acetaminophen 650 mg and diphenhydramine 50 mg is recommended prior to each rituximab infusion. Ibritumomab is administered **only** as part of the Zevalin® therapeutic regimen (a combined treatment regimen with rituximab). Allow at least 6 weeks, but no more than 12 weeks following first-line chemotherapy before treatment initiation; platelets should recover to ≥150,000/mm³ prior to treatment. The regimen consists of two steps:

Day 1:

Rituximab infusion: 250 mg/m² at an initial rate of 50 mg/hour. If hypersensitivity or infusion-related events do not occur, increase infusion in increments of 50 mg/hour every 30 minutes, to a maximum of 400 mg/hour. Stop rituximab and discontinue regimen for severe infusion reaction. For less severe infusion reactions, temporarily slow or interrupt; the infusion may be resumed at one-half the previous rate upon improvement of symptoms.

In-111 ibritumomab infusion: Within 4 hours of the completion of rituximab infusion, inject 5 mCi (1.6 mg total antibody dose) over 10 minutes.

Biodistribution of In-111 ibritumomab should be assessed by imaging at 48-72 hours postinjection. Optional additional imaging may be performed to resolve ambiguities. If biodistribution is not acceptable, the patient should not proceed to Step 2.

Day 7, 8, or 9:

Rituximab infusion: 250 mg/m² at an initial rate of 100 mg/hour (50 mg/hour if infusion-related events occurred with the first infusion). If hypersensitivity or infusion-related events do not occur, increase infusion in increments of 100 mg/hour every 30 minutes, to a maximum of 400 mg/hour, as tolerated (increase in 50 mg/hour increments if initial infusion rate was 50 mg/hour).

Y-90 ibritumomab infusion: Within 4 hours of the completion of rituximab infusion:

Platelet count ≥150,000 cells/mm³: Inject 0.4 mCi/kg (14.8 MBq/kg actual body weight) over 10 minutes; maximum dose: 32 mCi (1184 MBq)

Platelet count between 100,000-149,000 cells/mm³ (in relapsed or refractory patients): Inject 0.3 mCi/kg (11.1 MBq/kg actual body weight) over 10 minutes; maximum dose: 32 mCi (1184 MBq)

Platelet count <100,000 cells/mm³: Do **not** administer

Maximum dose: The prescribed, measured, and administered dose of Y-90 ibritumomab must not exceed 32 mCi (1184 MBq), regardless of the patient's body weight

Administration

Rituximab: Administer the first infusion of rituximab at an initial rate of 50 mg/hour. If hypersensitivity or infusion-related events do not occur, escalate the infusion rate in 50 mg/hour increments every 30 minutes, to a maximum of 400 mg/hour. Immediately stop infusion for severe infusion reaction (discontinue ibritumomab regimen); less severe reactions may be managed by slowing or interrupting infusion. For less severe reactions, infusion may continue at one-half the previous rate upon improvement of patient symptoms. If infusion reaction did not occur in initial rituximab infusion, subsequent rituximab infusion can be administered at an initial rate of 100 mg/hour and increased in 100 mg/hour increments at 30-minute intervals, to a maximum of 400 mg/hour as tolerated. If infusion reaction occurred with initial rituximab infusion, initiate at 50 mg/hour with increases of 50 mg/hour increments.

In-111 and Y-90 ibritumomab: Inject slowly, over 10 minutes through a 0.22 micron low protein binding in-line filter (between syringe and infusion port). After injection, flush line with at least 10 mL normal saline. Y-90 ibritumomab: Establish free-flowing I.V. line prior to administration. Avoid extravasation; if signs or symptoms of extravasation occur, stop infusion and restart in another limb.

Monitoring Parameters Patients must be monitored for infusion-related allergic reactions (typically within 30-120 minutes of administration). Monitor for extravasation during ibritumomab infusion. Obtain CBC with differential and platelet counts weekly. Platelet count must be obtained prior to Day 7, 8, or 9. Monitor for up to 3 months after use.

Biodistribution of In-111 ibritumomab should be assessed by imaging at 48-72 hours post injection. Optional additional imaging may be performed to resolve ambiguities. If biodistribution is altered, the patient should not proceed to Day 7, 8, or 9.

Additional Information Ibritumomab tiuxetan is produced in Chinese hamster ovary cell cultures. Kit is not radioactive. Radiolabeling of ibritumomab with Yttrium-90 and Indium-111 (not included in kit) must be performed by appropriate personnel in a specialized facility.

Dosage Forms Excipient information presented when available (limited, particularly for generics); consult specific product labeling.

Injection, solution [preservative free]:
Zevalin®: 1.6 mg/mL (2 mL)

◆ **Ibritumomab Tiuxetan** *see* Ibritumomab *on page 857*

◆ **Ibu®** *see* Ibuprofen *on page 860*

◆ **Ibu-200 [OTC]** *see* Ibuprofen *on page 860*

◆ **Ibudone™** *see* Hydrocodone and Ibuprofen *on page 838*

Ibuprofen (eye byoo PROE fen)

Brand Names: U.S. Addaprin [OTC]; Advil® Children's [OTC]; Advil® Infants' [OTC]; Advil® Migraine [OTC]; Advil® [OTC]; Caldolor™; I-Prin [OTC]; Ibu-200 [OTC]; Ibu®; Midol® Cramps & Body Aches [OTC]; Motrin® Children's [OTC]; Motrin® IB [OTC]; Motrin® Infants' [OTC]; Motrin® Junior [OTC]; NeoProfen®; Proprinal® [OTC]; TopCare® Junior Strength [OTC]; Ultraprin [OTC]

Brand Names: Canada Advil®; Apo-Ibuprofen®; Motrin® (Children's); Motrin® IB; Novo-Profen; Nu-Ibuprofen

Index Terms *p*-Isobutylhydratropic Acid; Ibuprofen Lysine

Pharmacologic Category Nonsteroidal Anti-inflammatory Drug (NSAID), Oral; Nonsteroidal Anti-inflammatory Drug (NSAID), Parenteral

Use

Oral: Inflammatory diseases and rheumatoid disorders including juvenile idiopathic arthritis (JIA), mild-to-moderate pain, fever, dysmenorrhea, osteoarthritis

Ibuprofen injection (Caldolor™): Management of mild-to-moderate pain; management moderate-to-severe pain when used concurrently with an opioid analgesic; reduction of fever

Ibuprofen lysine injection (NeoProfen®): To induce closure of a clinically-significant patent ductus arteriosus (PDA) in premature infants weighing between 500-1500 g and who are ≤32 weeks gestational age (GA) when usual treatments are ineffective

Unlabeled Use Cystic fibrosis, gout, ankylosing spondylitis, acute migraine headache

Pregnancy Risk Factor C/D ≥30 weeks gestation

Pregnancy Considerations Adverse events were not observed in the initial animal reproduction studies; therefore, the manufacturer classifies ibuprofen as pregnancy category C (category D: ≥30 weeks gestation). NSAID exposure during the first trimester is not strongly associated with congenital malformations; however, cardiovascular anomalies and cleft palate have been observed following NSAID exposure in some studies. The use of a NSAID close to conception may be associated with an increased risk of miscarriage. Nonteratogenic effects have been observed following NSAID administration during the third trimester including: Myocardial degenerative changes, prenatal constriction of the ductus arteriosus, fetal tricuspid regurgitation, failure of the ductus arteriosus to close postnatally; renal dysfunction or failure, oligohydramnios; gastrointestinal bleeding or perforation, increased risk of necrotizing enterocolitis; intracranial bleeding (including intraventricular hemorrhage), platelet dysfunction with resultant bleeding; pulmonary hypertension. Because they may cause premature closure of the ductus arteriosus, use of NSAIDs late in pregnancy should be avoided (use after 31 or 32 weeks gestation is not recommended by some clinicians). Product labeling for Caldolor™ specifically notes that use at ≥30 weeks gestation should be avoided and therefore classifies ibuprofen as pregnancy category D at this time. The chronic use of NSAIDs in women of reproductive age may be associated with infertility that is reversible upon discontinuation of the medication. A registry is available for pregnant women exposed to autoimmune medications including ibuprofen. For additional information contact the Organization of Teratology Information Specialists, OTIS Autoimmune Diseases Study, at 877-311-8972.

Lactation Enters breast milk/not recommended (AAP rates "compatible"; AAP 2001 update pending)

Medication Guide Available Yes

Contraindications Hypersensitivity to ibuprofen; history of asthma, urticaria, or allergic-type reaction to aspirin or other NSAIDs; aspirin triad (eg, bronchial asthma, aspirin intolerance, rhinitis); perioperative pain in the setting of coronary artery bypass graft (CABG) surgery

Ibuprofen lysine (NeoProfen®): Preterm infants with untreated proven or suspected infection; congenital heart disease where patency of the PDA is necessary for pulmonary or systemic blood flow; bleeding (especially with active intracranial hemorrhage or GI bleed); thrombocytopenia; coagulation defects; proven or suspected necrotizing enterocolitis (NEC); significant renal dysfunction

Warnings/Precautions [U.S. Boxed Warning]: NSAIDs are associated with an increased risk of adverse cardiovascular thrombotic events, including fatal MI and stroke. Risk may be increased with duration of use or pre-existing cardiovascular risk factors or disease. Carefully evaluate individual cardiovascular risk profiles prior to prescribing. May cause new-onset hypertension or worsening of existing hypertension. Response to ACE inhibitors, thiazides, or loop diuretics may be impaired with concurrent use of NSAIDs. Use caution with fluid retention. Avoid use in heart failure. Concurrent administration of ibuprofen, and potentially other nonselective NSAIDs, may interfere with aspirin's cardioprotective effect. **[U.S. Boxed Warning]: Use is contraindicated for treatment of perioperative pain in the setting of coronary artery bypass graft (CABG) surgery.** Risk of MI and stroke may be increased with use following CABG surgery.

May increase the risk of aseptic meningitis, especially in patients with systemic lupus erythematosus (SLE) and mixed connective tissue disorders. Platelet adhesion and aggregation may be decreased; may prolong bleeding time; patients with coagulation disorders or who are receiving anticoagulants should be monitored closely. Anemia may occur; patients on long-term NSAID therapy should be monitored for anemia. Rarely, NSAID use may cause severe blood dyscrasias (eg, agranulocytosis, aplastic anemia, thrombocytopenia).

NSAID use may compromise existing renal function; dose-dependent decreases in prostaglandin synthesis may result from NSAID use, reducing renal blood flow which may cause renal decompensation. NSAID use may increase the risk for hyperkalemia. Patients with impaired renal function, dehydration, heart failure, liver dysfunction, those taking diuretics, and ACE inhibitors, and the elderly are at greater risk of renal toxicity and hyperkalemia. Rehydrate patient before starting therapy; monitor renal function closely. Not recommended for use in patients with advanced renal disease. Long-term NSAID use may result in renal papillary necrosis.

NSAIDs may increase risk of gastrointestinal irritation, inflammation, ulceration, bleeding, and perforation. These events can be fatal and may occur at any time during therapy and without warning. Use caution with a history of GI disease (bleeding or ulcers), concurrent therapy with aspirin, anticoagulants and/or corticosteroids, smoking, use of ethanol, the elderly or debilitated patients. When used concomitantly with ≤325 mg of aspirin, a substantial increase in the risk of gastrointestinal complications (eg, ulcer) occurs; concomitant gastroprotective therapy (eg, proton pump inhibitors) is recommended (Bhatt, 2008).

Use the lowest effective dose for the shortest duration of time, consistent with individual patient goals, to reduce risk of cardiovascular or GI adverse events. Alternate therapies should be considered for patients at high risk.

NSAIDs may cause serious skin adverse events including exfoliative dermatitis, Stevens-Johnson Syndrome (SJS) and toxic epidermal necrolysis (TEN); discontinue use at first sign of skin rash or hypersensitivity. Anaphylactoid reactions may occur, even without prior exposure; patients with "aspirin triad" (bronchial asthma, aspirin intolerance, rhinitis) may be at increased risk. Do not use in patients who experience bronchospasm, asthma, rhinitis, or urticaria with NSAID or aspirin therapy. Use caution in other forms of asthma.

NSAIDS may cause drowsiness, dizziness, blurred vision and other neurologic effects which may impair physical or mental abilities; patients must be cautioned about performing tasks which require mental alertness (eg, operating machinery or driving). Monitor vision with long-term therapy. Blurred/diminished vision, scotomata, and changes in color vision have been reported. Discontinue use with altered vision and perform ophthalmologic exam.

Use with caution in patients with decreased hepatic function. Closely monitor patients with any abnormal LFT. Severe hepatic reactions (eg, fulminant hepatitis, liver failure) have occurred with NSAID use, rarely; discontinue if signs or symptoms of liver disease develop, or if systemic manifestations occur.

The elderly are at increased risk for adverse effects (especially serious gastrointestinal events, CNS effects, renal toxicity) from NSAIDs even at low doses.

Withhold for at least 4-6 half-lives prior to surgical or dental procedures. Some products may contain phenylalanine. Ibuprofen injection (Caldolor™) must be diluted prior to administration; hemolysis can occur if not diluted.

Ibuprofen lysine injection (NeoProfen®): Hold second or third doses if urinary output is <0.6 mL/kg/hour. May alter signs of infection. May inhibit platelet aggregation; monitor for signs of bleeding. May displace bilirubin; use caution when total bilirubin is elevated. Long-term evaluations of neurodevelopment, growth, or diseases associated with prematurity following treatment have not been conducted. A second course of treatment, alternative pharmacologic therapy or surgery may be needed if the ductus arteriosus fails to close or reopens following the initial course of therapy.

Self medication (OTC use): Prior to self-medication, patients should contact healthcare provider if they have had recurring stomach pain or upset, ulcers, bleeding problems, high blood pressure, heart or kidney disease, other serious medical problems, are currently taking a diuretic, aspirin, anticoagulant, or are ≥60 years of age. If patients are using for migraines, they should also contact healthcare provider if they have not had a migraine diagnosis by healthcare provider, a headache that is different from usual migraine, worst headache of life, fever and neck stiffness, headache from head injury or coughing, first headache at ≥50 years of age, daily headache, or migraine requiring bed rest. Recommended dosages should not be exceeded, due to an increased risk of GI bleeding. Stop use and consult a healthcare provider if symptoms get worse, newly appear, fever lasts for >3 days or pain lasts >3 days (children) and >10 days (adults). Do not give for >10 days unless instructed by healthcare provider. Consuming ≥3 alcoholic beverages/day or taking longer than recommended may increase the risk of GI bleeding.

Adverse Reactions

Oral:

1% to 10%:

Cardiovascular: Edema (1% to 3%)

Central nervous system: Dizziness (3% to 9%), headache (1% to 3%), nervousness (1% to 3%)

Dermatologic: Rash (3% to 9%), itching (1% to 3%)

Endocrine & metabolic: Fluid retention (1% to 3%)

Gastrointestinal: Epigastric pain (3% to 9%), heartburn (3% to 9%), nausea (3% to 9%), abdominal pain/cramps/distress (1% to 3%), appetite decreased (1% to 3%), constipation (1% to 3%), diarrhea (1% to 3%), dyspepsia (1% to 3%), flatulence (1% to 3%), vomiting (1% to 3%)

Otic: Tinnitus (3% to 9%)

<1% (Limited to important or life-threatening): Acute renal failure, agranulocytosis, anaphylaxis, aplastic anemia, azotemia, blurred vision, bone marrow suppression, confusion, creatinine clearance decreased, duodenal ulcer, edema, eosinophilia, epistaxis, erythema multiforme, gastric ulcer, GI bleed, GI hemorrhage, GI ulceration, hallucinations, hearing decreased, hematuria, hematocrit decreased, hemoglobin decreased, hemolytic anemia, hepatitis, hypertension, inhibition of platelet aggregation, jaundice, liver function tests abnormal, leukopenia, melena, neutropenia, pancreatitis, photosensitivity, Stevens-Johnson syndrome, thrombocytopenia, toxic amblyopia, toxic epidermal necrolysis, urticaria, vesiculobullous eruptions, vision changes

Injection: Ibuprofen (Caldolor™): Abdominal pain, anemia, BUN increased, cough, dizziness, dyspepsia, edema, flatulence, headache, hemorrhage, hypokalemia, hypernatremia, hypertension, nausea, neutropenia, pruritus, urinary retention, vomiting

Injection: Ibuprofen lysine (NeoProfen®):

>10%:

Cardiovascular: Intraventricular hemorrhage (29%; grade 3/4: 15%)

Dermatologic: Skin irritation (16%)

Endocrine & metabolic: Hypocalcemia (12%), hypoglycemia (12%)

Gastrointestinal: GI disorders, non NEC (22%)

Hematologic: Anemia (32%)

Respiratory: Apnea (28%), respiratory infection (19%)

Miscellaneous: Sepsis (43%)

1% to 10%:

Cardiovascular: Edema (4%)

Endocrine & metabolic: Adrenal insufficiency (7%), hypernatremia (7%)

Genitourinary: Urinary tract infection (9%)

Renal: Urea increased (7%), renal impairment (6%), creatinine increased (3%), urine output decreased (3%; small decrease reported on days 2-6 with compensatory increase in output on day 9), renal failure (1%)

Respiratory: Respiratory failure (10%), atelectasis (4%)

Frequency not defined: Abdominal distension, cholestasis, feeding problems, gastritis, GI reflux, heart failure, hyperglycemia, hypotension, ileus, infection, inguinal hernia, injection site reaction, jaundice, neutropenia, seizure, tachycardia, thrombocytopenia

Postmarketing and/or case reports: GI perforation, necrotizing enterocolitis

Drug Interactions

Metabolism/Transport Effects Substrate of CYP2C19 (minor), CYP2C9 (minor); **Note:** Assignment of Major/Minor substrate status based on clinically relevant drug interaction potential; **Inhibits** CYP2C9 (weak)

Avoid Concomitant Use

Avoid concomitant use of Ibuprofen with any of the following: Floctafenine; Ketorolac; Ketorolac (Nasal); Ketorolac (Systemic)

Increased Effect/Toxicity

Ibuprofen may increase the levels/effects of: Aminoglycosides; Anticoagulants; Antiplatelet Agents; Bisphosphonate Derivatives; Collagenase (Systemic); CycloSPORINE; CycloSPORINE (Systemic); Deferasirox; Desmopressin; Digoxin; Drotrecogin Alfa (Activated); Eplerenone; Haloperidol; Ibritumomab; Lithium; Methotrexate; Nonsteroidal Anti-Inflammatory Agents; PEMEtrexed; Porfimer; Potassium-Sparing Diuretics; PRALAtrexate; Quinolone Antibiotics; Rivaroxaban; Salicylates; Thrombolytic Agents; Tositumomab and Iodine I 131 Tositumomab; Vancomycin; Vitamin K Antagonists

The levels/effects of Ibuprofen may be increased by: ACE Inhibitors; Angiotensin II Receptor Blockers; Antidepressants (Tricyclic, Tertiary Amine); Corticosteroids (Systemic); CycloSPORINE; CycloSPORINE (Systemic); Dasatinib; Floctafenine; Glucosamine; Herbs (Anticoagulant/Antiplatelet Properties); Ketorolac; Ketorolac (Nasal); Ketorolac (Systemic); Nonsteroidal Anti-Inflammatory Agents; Omega-3-Acid Ethyl Esters; Pentosan Polysulfate Sodium; Pentoxifylline; Probenecid; Prostacyclin Analogues; Selective Serotonin Reuptake Inhibitors; Serotonin/Norepinephrine Reuptake Inhibitors; Sodium Phosphates; Treprostinil; Vitamin E; Voriconazole

Decreased Effect

Ibuprofen may decrease the levels/effects of: ACE Inhibitors; Angiotensin II Receptor Blockers; Antiplatelet Agents; Beta-Blockers; Eplerenone; HydrALAZINE; Loop Diuretics; Potassium-Sparing Diuretics; Salicylates; Selective Serotonin Reuptake Inhibitors; Thiazide Diuretics

The levels/effects of Ibuprofen may be decreased by: Bile Acid Sequestrants; Nonsteroidal Anti-Inflammatory Agents; Salicylates

Ethanol/Nutrition/Herb Interactions

Ethanol: Avoid ethanol (may enhance gastric mucosal irritation).

Food: Ibuprofen peak serum levels may be decreased if taken with food.

Herb/Nutraceutical: Avoid alfalfa, anise, bilberry, bladderwrack, bromelain, cat's claw, celery, chamomile, coleus, cordyceps, dong quai, evening primrose, fenugreek, feverfew, garlic, ginger, ginkgo biloba, ginseng (American, Panax, Siberian), grapeseed, green tea, guggul, horse chestnut seed, horseradish, licorice, prickly ash, red clover, reishi, SAMe (S-adenosylmethionine), sweet clover, turmeric, white willow (all have additional antiplatelet activity).

Stability

Ibuprofen injection (Caldolor™): Store intact vials at room temperature of 20°C to 25°C (68°F to 77°F). Must be diluted prior to use. Dilute with D_5W, NS or LR to a final concentration ≤4 mg/mL. Diluted solutions stable for 24 hours at room temperature.

Ibuprofen lysine injection (NeoProfen®): Store at room temperature of 20°C to 25°C (68°F to 77°F). Protect from light. Dilute with dextrose or saline to an appropriate volume. Following dilution, administer within 30 minutes of preparation.

Suspension, tablet: Store at room temperature of 20°C to 25°C (68°F to 77°F).

Mechanism of Action Reversibly inhibits cyclooxygenase-1 and 2 (COX-1 and 2) enzymes, which results in decreased formation of prostaglandin precursors; has antipyretic, analgesic, and anti-inflammatory properties

Other proposed mechanisms not fully elucidated (and possibly contributing to the anti-inflammatory effect to varying degrees), include inhibiting chemotaxis, altering lymphocyte activity, inhibiting neutrophil aggregation/activation, and decreasing proinflammatory cytokine levels.

Pharmacodynamics/Kinetics

Onset of action: Oral: Analgesic: 30-60 minutes; Anti-inflammatory: ≤7 days

Duration: Oral: 4-6 hours

Absorption: Oral: Rapid (85%)

Distribution: V_d: 6.35 L; premature infants with ductal closure (highly variable between studies):

- Day 3: 145-349 mL/kg
- Day 5: 72-222 mL/kg

Protein binding: 90% to 99%

Metabolism: Hepatic via oxidation

Half-life elimination:

- Premature infants (highly variable between studies):
  - Day 3: 35-51 hours
  - Day 5: 20-33 hours
- Children 3 months to 10 years: 1.6 ± 0.7 hours
- Adults: 2-4 hours; End-stage renal disease: Unchanged

Time to peak: Oral: ~1-2 hours

Excretion: Urine (primarily as metabolites; 1% as unchanged drug); some feces

Dosage

I.V.:

Neonates: Ibuprofen lysine (NeoProfen®): Infants between 500-1500 g and ≤32 weeks GA: Patent ductus arteriosus: Initial dose: Ibuprofen 10 mg/kg, followed by two doses of 5 mg/kg at 24 and 48 hours. Dose should be based on birth weight.

Adults (Caldolor™): **Note**: Patients should be well hydrated prior to administration

- Analgesic: 400-800 mg every 6 hours as needed (maximum: 3.2 g/day)
- Antipyretic: Initial: 400 mg, then every 4-6 hours or 100-200 mg every 4 hours as needed (maximum: 3.2 g/day)

Oral:

Children:

- Antipyretic: 6 months to 12 years: Temperature <102.5°F (39°C): 5 mg/kg/dose; temperature >102.5°F: 10 mg/kg/dose given every 6-8 hours (maximum daily dose: 40 mg/kg/day)
- Juvenile idiopathic arthritis (JIA): 30-50 mg/kg/24 hours divided every 8 hours; start at lower end of dosing range and titrate upward (maximum: 2.4 g/day)
- Analgesic: 4-10 mg/kg/dose every 6-8 hours
- Cystic fibrosis (unlabeled use): Chronic (>4 years) twice daily dosing adjusted to maintain serum concentration of 50-100 mcg/mL has been associated with slowing of disease progression in younger patients with mild lung disease

OTC labeling (analgesic, antipyretic): **Note:** Treatment for >10 days is not recommended unless directed by healthcare provider.
Children 6 months to 11 years: See table; use of weight to select dose is preferred; doses may be repeated every 6-8 hours (maximum: 4 doses/day)
Children ≥12 years: 200 mg every 4-6 hours as needed (maximum: 1200 mg/24 hours)

Ibuprofen Dosing

Weight (lb)	Age	Dosage (mg)
12-17	6-11 mo	50
18-23	12-23 mo	75
24-35	2-3 y	100
36-47	4-5 y	150
48-59	6-8 y	200
60-71	9-10 y	250
72-95	11 y	300

Adults:
Inflammatory disease: 400-800 mg/dose 3-4 times/day (maximum dose: 3.2 g/day)
Analgesia/pain/fever/dysmenorrhea: 200-400 mg/dose every 4-6 hours (maximum daily dose: 1.2 g, unless directed by physician; under physician supervision daily doses ≤2.4 g may be used)
OTC labeling (analgesic, antipyretic): 200 mg every 4-6 hours as needed (maximum: 1200 mg/24 hours); treatment for >10 days is not recommended unless directed by healthcare provider.
Migraine: 2 capsules at onset of symptoms (maximum: 400 mg/24 hours unless directed by healthcare provider)

Dosing adjustment/comments in renal impairment: If anuria or oliguria evident, hold dose until renal function returns to normal

Dosing adjustment/comments in severe hepatic impairment: Avoid use

Dietary Considerations Should be taken with food. Some products may contain phenylalanine and/or potassium.

Administration
Oral: Administer with food
I.V.:
Caldolor™: For I.V. administration only; must be diluted to a final concentration of ≤4 mg/mL prior to administration; infuse over at least 30 minutes
NeoProfen® (ibuprofen lysine): For I.V. administration only; administration via umbilical arterial line has not been evaluated. Infuse over 15 minutes through port closest to insertion site. Avoid extravasation. Do not administer simultaneously via same line with TPN. If needed, interrupt TPN for 15 minutes prior to and after ibuprofen administration, keeping line open with dextrose or saline.

Monitoring Parameters CBC, chemistry profile, occult blood loss and periodic liver function tests; monitor response (pain, range of motion, grip strength, mobility, ADL function), inflammation; observe for weight gain, edema; monitor renal function (urine output, serum BUN and creatinine); observe for bleeding, bruising; evaluate gastrointestinal effects (abdominal pain, bleeding, dyspepsia); mental confusion, disorientation; with long-term therapy, periodic ophthalmic exams; signs of infection (ibuprofen lysine)

Reference Range Plasma concentrations >200 mcg/mL may be associated with severe toxicity
PDA: Minimum effective concentration: 10-12 mg/L

Test Interactions May interfere with urine detection of PCP, cannabinoids, and barbiturates (false-positives)

Dosage Forms Excipient information presented when available (limited, particularly for generics); consult specific product labeling.
Caplet, oral: 200 mg
Advil®: 200 mg
Motrin® IB: 200 mg
Motrin® Junior: 100 mg [scored]
Capsule, liquid filled, oral: 200 mg
Advil®: 200 mg [contains potassium 20 mg/capsule; solubilized ibuprofen]
Advil® Migraine: 200 mg [contains potassium 20 mg/capsule; solubilized ibuprofen]
Capsule, softgel, oral: 200 mg
Gelcap, oral:
Advil®: 200 mg [contains coconut oil]
Injection, solution:
Caldolor™: 100 mg/mL (4 mL, 8 mL)
Injection, solution, as lysine [preservative free]:
NeoProfen®: 17.1 mg/mL (2 mL) [equivalent to ibuprofen base 10 mg/mL]
Suspension, oral: 100 mg/5 mL (5 mL, 10 mL, 120 mL, 480 mL)
Advil® Children's: 100 mg/5 mL (120 mL) [contains propylene glycol, sodium 10 mg/5 mL, sodium benzoate; blue raspberry flavor]
Advil® Children's: 100 mg/5 mL (120 mL) [contains propylene glycol, sodium 3 mg/5 mL, sodium benzoate; grape flavor]
Advil® Children's: 100 mg/5 mL (120 mL) [contains sodium 3 mg/5 mL, sodium benzoate; fruit flavor]
Motrin® Children's: 100 mg/5 mL (120 mL) [dye free, ethanol free; contains sodium 2 mg/5 mL, sodium benzoate; berry flavor]
Motrin® Children's: 100 mg/5 mL (60 mL, 120 mL) [ethanol free; contains sodium 2 mg/5 mL, sodium benzoate; berry flavor]
Motrin® Children's: 100 mg/5 mL (120 mL) [ethanol free; contains sodium 2 mg/5 mL, sodium benzoate; bubblegum flavor]
Motrin® Children's: 100 mg/5 mL (120 mL) [ethanol free; contains sodium 2 mg/5 mL, sodium benzoate; grape flavor]
Motrin® Children's: 100 mg/5 mL (120 mL) [ethanol free; contains sodium 2 mg/5 mL, sodium benzoate; tropical punch flavor]
Suspension, oral [concentrate/drops]: 40 mg/mL (15 mL)
Advil® Infants': 40 mg/mL (15 mL) [contains sodium benzoate; grape flavor]
Advil® Infants': 40 mg/mL (15 mL) [dye free; contains propylene glycol, sodium benzoate; white grape flavor]
Motrin® Infants': 40 mg/mL (15 mL) [dye free, ethanol free; contains sodium benzoate; berry flavor]
Motrin® Infants': 40 mg/mL (15 mL) [ethanol free; contains sodium benzoate; berry flavor]
Tablet, oral: 200 mg, 400 mg, 600 mg, 800 mg
Addaprin: 200 mg
Advil®: 200 mg [contains sodium benzoate]
I-Prin: 200 mg
Ibu-200: 200 mg
Ibu®: 400 mg, 600 mg, 800 mg
Midol® Cramps & Body Aches: 200 mg
Motrin® IB: 200 mg
Proprinal®: 200 mg [contains sodium benzoate]
Ultraprin: 200 mg [sugar free]
Tablet, chewable, oral:
Motrin® Junior: 100 mg [contains phenylalanine 2.8 mg/tablet; grape flavor]
Motrin® Junior: 100 mg [contains phenylalanine 2.8 mg/tablet; orange flavor]
TopCare® Junior Strength: 100 mg [scored; orange flavor]

- ◆ **Ibuprofen and Hydrocodone** *see* Hydrocodone and Ibuprofen *on page 838*
- ◆ **Ibuprofen and Oxycodone** *see* Oxycodone and Ibuprofen *on page 1269*
- ◆ **Ibuprofen and Pseudoephedrine** *see* Pseudoephedrine and Ibuprofen *on page 1432*
- ◆ **Ibuprofen Lysine** *see* Ibuprofen *on page 860*

Ibutilide (i BYOO ti lide)

Brand Names: U.S. Corvert®

Index Terms Ibutilide Fumarate

Pharmacologic Category Antiarrhythmic Agent, Class III

Use Acute termination of atrial fibrillation or flutter of recent onset; the effectiveness of ibutilide has not been determined in patients with arrhythmias >90 days in duration

Pregnancy Risk Factor C

Pregnancy Considerations Teratogenic and embryocidal in rats; avoid use in pregnancy

Lactation Enters breast milk/contraindicated

Contraindications Hypersensitivity to ibutilide or any component of the formulation; QT_c >440 msec

Warnings/Precautions [U.S. Boxed Warning]: Potentially fatal arrhythmias (eg, polymorphic ventricular tachycardia) can occur with ibutilide, usually in association with torsade de pointes (QT prolongation). Studies indicate a 1.7% incidence of arrhythmias in treated patients. The drug should be given in a setting of continuous ECG monitoring and by personnel trained in treating arrhythmias particularly polymorphic ventricular tachycardia. **[U.S. Boxed Warning]: Patients with chronic atrial fibrillation may not be the best candidates for ibutilide since they often revert after conversion and the risks of treatment may not be justified when compared to alternative management.** Dosing adjustments are not required in patients with renal or hepatic dysfunction. Safety and efficacy in children have not been established. Use caution in elderly patients. Avoid concurrent use of any drug that can prolong QT interval. Correct hyperkalemia and hypomagnesemia before using. Monitor for heart block.

Adverse Reactions

1% to 10%:

Cardiovascular: Ventricular extrasystoles (5.1%), nonsustained monomorphic ventricular tachycardia (4.9%), nonsustained polymorphic ventricular tachycardia (2.7%), tachycardia/supraventricular tachycardia (2.7%), hypotension (2%), bundle branch block (1.9%), sustained polymorphic ventricular tachycardia (eg, torsade de pointes) (1.7%, often requiring cardioversion), AV block (1.5%), bradycardia (1.2%), QT segment prolongation, hypertension (1.2%), palpitation (1%)

Central nervous system: Headache (4%)

Gastrointestinal: Nausea (>1%)

<1% (Limited to important or life-threatening): CHF, erythematous bullous lesions, idioventricular rhythm, nodal arrhythmia, renal failure, supraventricular extrasystoles, sustained monomorphic ventricular tachycardia, syncope (0.3%, not > placebo)

Drug Interactions

Metabolism/Transport Effects None known.

Avoid Concomitant Use

Avoid concomitant use of Ibutilide with any of the following: Artemether; Dronedarone; Lumefantrine; Nilotinib; Pimozide; QUEtiapine; QuiNINE; Tetrabenazine; Thioridazine; Toremifene; Vandetanib; Vemurafenib; Ziprasidone

Increased Effect/Toxicity

Ibutilide may increase the levels/effects of: Dronedarone; Lidocaine (Topical); Pimozide; QTc-Prolonging Agents; QuiNINE; Tetrabenazine; Thioridazine; Toremifene; Vandetanib; Vemurafenib; Ziprasidone

The levels/effects of Ibutilide may be increased by: Alfuzosin; Artemether; Chloroquine; Ciprofloxacin; Ciprofloxacin (Systemic); Eribulin; Fingolimod; Gadobutrol; Indacaterol; Lidocaine (Topical); Lumefantrine; Nilotinib; QUEtiapine; QuiNINE

Decreased Effect There are no known significant interactions involving a decrease in effect.

Stability Admixtures are chemically and physically stable for 24 hours at room temperature and for 48 hours at refrigerated temperatures. May be administered undiluted or diluted in 50 mL diluent (0.9% NS or D_5W).

Mechanism of Action Exact mechanism of action is unknown; prolongs the action potential in cardiac tissue

Pharmacodynamics/Kinetics

Onset of action: ~90 minutes after start of infusion (1/2 of conversions to sinus rhythm occur during infusion)

Distribution: V_d: 11 L/kg

Protein binding: 40%

Metabolism: Extensively hepatic; oxidation

Half-life elimination: 2-12 hours (average: 6 hours)

Excretion: Urine (82%; 7% as unchanged drug and metabolites); feces (19%)

Dosage I.V.: Initial:

Adults:

<60 kg: 0.01 mg/kg over 10 minutes

≥60 kg: 1 mg over 10 minutes

Note: Discontinue infusion if arrhythmia terminates, if sustained or nonsustained ventricular tachycardia occurs, or if marked prolongation of QT/QT_c occurs. If the arrhythmia does not terminate within 10 minutes after the end of the initial infusion, a second infusion of equal strength may be infused over a 10-minute period.

Elderly: Refer to adult dosing. Dose selection should be cautious, usually starting at the lower end of the dosing range.

Administration May be administered undiluted or diluted in 50 mL diluent (0.9% NS or D_5W); infuse over 10 minutes

Monitoring Parameters Electrolytes; observe patient with continuous ECG monitoring for at least 4 hours following infusion or until QT_c has returned to baseline; skilled personnel and proper equipment should be available during administration of ibutilide and subsequent monitoring of the patient

Dosage Forms Excipient information presented when available (limited, particularly for generics); consult specific product labeling.

Injection, solution, as fumarate: 0.1 mg/mL (10 mL)

Corvert®: 0.1 mg/mL (10 mL)

- ◆ **Ibutilide Fumarate** *see* Ibutilide *on page 864*
- ◆ **IC51** *see* Japanese Encephalitis Virus Vaccine (Inactivated) *on page 948*

Icatibant (eye KAT i bant)

Brand Names: U.S. Firazyr®

Index Terms HOE 140; Icatibant Acetate

Pharmacologic Category Selective Bradykinin B2 Receptor Antagonist

Use Treatment of acute attacks of hereditary angioedema (HAE)

Pregnancy Risk Factor C

Pregnancy Considerations Adverse events were observed in animal reproduction studies with doses close to or less than the recommended human dose.

Lactation Excretion unknown/use caution

Contraindications There are no contraindications listed in the manufacturer's labeling.

Warnings/Precautions Airway obstruction may occur during acute laryngeal attacks of HAE. Patients with laryngeal attacks should be instructed to seek medical attention immediately in addition to treatment with icatibant. Icatibant may potentially attenuate the antihypertensive effect of ACE inhibitors; patients taking ACE inhibitors were excluded from initial clinical trials.

Adverse Reactions

>10%: Local: Injection site reaction (97%)

1% to 10%:

Central nervous system: Pyrexia (4%), dizziness (3%)

Hepatic: Transaminase increased (4%)

<1% (Limited to important or life-threatening): Anti-icatibant antibody production (no association with efficacy observed), headache, nausea, rash

Drug Interactions

Metabolism/Transport Effects None known.

Avoid Concomitant Use There are no known interactions where it is recommended to avoid concomitant use.

Increased Effect/Toxicity There are no known significant interactions involving an increase in effect.

Decreased Effect

Icatibant may decrease the levels/effects of: ACE Inhibitors

Stability Store between 2°C to 25°C (36°F to 77°F); do not freeze. Store in original container until time of administration.

Mechanism of Action Icatibant is a selective competitive antagonist for the bradykinin B_2 receptor. Patients with HAE have an absence or dysfunction of C1-esterase-inhibitor which leads to the production of bradykinin. The presence of bradykinin may cause symptoms of localized swelling, inflammation, and pain. Icatibant inhibits bradykinin from binding at the B_2 receptor, thereby treating the symptoms associated with acute attack.

Pharmacodynamics/Kinetics

Onset: Median time to 50% decrease of symptoms: ~2 hours

Duration: Inhibits symptoms caused by bradykinin for ~6 hours

Distribution: V_{dss}: 20.3-37.7 L

Metabolism: Metabolized by proteolytic enzymes to metabolites (inactive)

Bioavailability: ~97%

Half-life elimination: 1-1.8 hours

Time to peak: 0.75 hours

Excretion: Urine (<10% unchanged)

Dosage SubQ: Adults: Hereditary angioedema (HAE): 30 mg/dose; may repeat one dose every 6 hours if response is inadequate or symptoms recur (maximum: 3 doses/24 hours)

Dosing adjustment in renal impairment: No dosage adjustments are recommended.

Dosing adjustment in hepatic impairment: No dosage adjustments are recommended.

Administration For SubQ injection only. Inject into the abdomen over ≥30 seconds, using the 25 gauge needle provided. Inject 2-4 inches below belly button and away from any scars; do not inject into an area that is bruised, swollen, or painful.

Monitoring Parameters Symptom relief; laryngeal symptoms or airway obstruction (immediate medical attention required in addition to icatibant therapy)

Dosage Forms Excipient information presented when available (limited, particularly for generics); consult specific product labeling.

Injection, solution [preservative free]:

Firazyr®: 10 mg/mL (3 mL)

◆ **Icatibant Acetate** *see* Icatibant *on page 864*

◆ **ICI-182,780** *see* Fulvestrant *on page 770*

◆ **ICI-204,219** *see* Zafirlukast *on page 1808*

◆ **ICI-46474** *see* Tamoxifen *on page 1624*

◆ **ICI-118630** *see* Goserelin *on page 805*

◆ **ICI-176334** *see* Bicalutamide *on page 217*

◆ **ICI-D1033** *see* Anastrozole *on page 121*

◆ **ICL670** *see* Deferasirox *on page 461*

Icodextrin (eye KOE dex trin)

Brand Names: U.S. Extraneal

Pharmacologic Category Adhesiolytic; Peritoneal Dialysate, Osmotic

Use

Adept®: Reduction of postsurgical adhesions in gynecologic laparoscopic procedures

Extraneal®: Daily exchange for the long dwell (8- to 16-hour) during continuous ambulatory peritoneal dialysis (CAPD) or automated peritoneal dialysis (APD) for the management of end-stage renal disease (ESRD); improvement of long-dwell ultrafiltration and clearance of creatinine and urea nitrogen (compared to 4.25% dextrose) in patients with high/average or greater transport characteristics as measured by peritoneal equilibration test (PET)

Pregnancy Risk Factor C

Medication Guide Available Yes

Dosage Intraperitoneal: Adults:

CAPD or APD (Extraneal®): Given as a single daily exchange in CAPD or APD; dwell time of 8-16 hours is suggested

Laparoscopic gynecologic surgery (Adept®): Irrigate with at least 100 mL every 30 minutes during surgery; aspirate remaining fluid after surgery is completed, then instill 1 L into the cavity

Additional Information Complete prescribing information for this medication should be consulted for additional detail.

Dosage Forms Excipient information presented when available (limited, particularly for generics); consult specific product labeling.

Solution, intraperitoneal [preservative free]:

Extraneal: 7.5% (1.5 L, 2 L, 2.5 L) [for peritoneal dialysis; contains sodium 132 mEq/L, calcium 3.5 mEq/L, magnesium 0.5 mEq/L, chloride 96 mEq/L, and lactate 40 mEq/L]

◆ **ICRF-187** *see* Dexrazoxane *on page 486*

◆ **Icy Hot® [OTC]** *see* Methyl Salicylate and Menthol *on page 1113*

◆ **Idamycin® (Can)** *see* IDArubicin *on page 865*

◆ **Idamycin PFS®** *see* IDArubicin *on page 865*

IDArubicin (eye da ROO bi sin)

Brand Names: U.S. Idamycin PFS®

Brand Names: Canada Idamycin®

Index Terms 4-Demethoxydaunorubicin; 4-DMDR; Idarubicin Hydrochloride; IDR; IMI 30; SC 33428

Pharmacologic Category Antineoplastic Agent, Anthracycline; Antineoplastic Agent, Antibiotic

Use Treatment of acute myeloid leukemia (AML)

Unlabeled Use Acute lymphocytic leukemia (ALL)

Pregnancy Risk Factor D

Lactation Excretion in breast milk unknown/not recommended

Contraindications Hypersensitivity to idarubicin, other anthracyclines, or any component of the formulation; bilirubin >5 mg/dL

Warnings/Precautions Hazardous agent - use appropriate precautions for handling and disposal. **[U.S. Boxed Warning]: May cause myocardial toxicity (HF, arrhythmias or cardiomyopathies) and is more common in patients who have previously received anthracyclines or have pre-existing cardiac disease.** The risk of myocardial toxicity is also increased in patients with concomitant or prior mediastinal/pericardial irradiation, patients with anemia, bone marrow depression, infections, leukemic pericarditis or myocarditis. Monitor cardiac function during treatment.

[U.S. Boxed Warnings]: May cause severe myelosuppression; use caution in patients with pre-existing myelosuppression from prior treatment or radiation. Use caution with renal or hepatic impairment; may required dosage reductions. For I.V. administration only; may cause severe local tissue damage and necrosis if extravasation occurs. Rapid lysis of leukemic cells may lead to hyperuricemia. Systemic infections should be managed prior to initiation of treatment. **[U.S. Boxed Warning]: Should be administered under the supervision of an experienced cancer chemotherapy physician. Safety and efficacy in children have not been established.**

Adverse Reactions

>10%:

Cardiovascular: Transient ECG abnormalities (supraventricular tachycardia, S-T wave changes, atrial or ventricular extrasystoles); generally asymptomatic and self-limiting. CHF, dose related. The relative cardiotoxicity of idarubicin compared to doxorubicin is unclear. Some investigators report no increase in cardiac toxicity at cumulative oral idarubicin doses up to 540 mg/m^2; other reports suggest a maximum cumulative intravenous dose of 150 mg/m^2.

Central nervous system: Headache

Dermatologic: Alopecia (25% to 30%), radiation recall, skin rash (11%), urticaria

Gastrointestinal: Nausea, vomiting (30% to 60%); diarrhea (9% to 22%); stomatitis (11%); GI hemorrhage (30%)

Emetic potential: Moderate (30% to 60%)

Genitourinary: Discoloration of urine (darker yellow)

Hematologic: Myelosuppression (nadir: 10-15 days; recovery: 21-28 days), primarily leukopenia; thrombocytopenia and anemia. Effects are generally less severe with oral dosing.

Hepatic: Bilirubin and transaminases increased (44%)

Local: Tissue necrosis upon extravasation, erythematous streaking

1% to 10%:

Central nervous system: Seizure

Neuromuscular & skeletal: Peripheral neuropathy

<1% (Limited to important or life-threatening): Cardiomyopathy, hyperuricemia, myocarditis, neutropenic typhlitis

Drug Interactions

Metabolism/Transport Effects Substrate of P-glycoprotein

Avoid Concomitant Use

Avoid concomitant use of IDArubicin with any of the following: BCG; CloZAPine; Natalizumab; Pimecrolimus; Tacrolimus (Topical); Vaccines (Live)

Increased Effect/Toxicity

IDArubicin may increase the levels/effects of: CloZAPine; Leflunomide; Natalizumab; Vaccines (Live)

The levels/effects of IDArubicin may be increased by: Bevacizumab; Denosumab; P-glycoprotein/ABCB1 Inhibitors; Pimecrolimus; Roflumilast; Tacrolimus (Topical); Taxane Derivatives; Trastuzumab

Decreased Effect

IDArubicin may decrease the levels/effects of: BCG; Cardiac Glycosides; Coccidioidin Skin Test; Sipuleucel-T; Vaccines (Inactivated); Vaccines (Live)

The levels/effects of IDArubicin may be decreased by: Cardiac Glycosides; Echinacea; P-glycoprotein/ABCB1 Inducers

Stability Store intact vials of solution under refrigeration at 2°C to 8°C (36°F to 46°F). Protect from light. Solutions diluted in D_5W or NS for infusion are stable for 4 weeks at room temperature, protected from light. Syringe and IVPB solutions are stable for 72 hours at room temperature and 7 days under refrigeration.

Mechanism of Action Similar to doxorubicin and daunorubicin; inhibition of DNA and RNA synthesis by intercalation between DNA base pairs

Pharmacodynamics/Kinetics

Absorption: Oral: Variable (4% to 77%; mean: ~30%)

Distribution: V_d: 64 L/kg (some reports indicate 2250 L); extensive tissue binding; CSF

Protein binding: 94% to 97%

Metabolism: Hepatic to idarubicinol (pharmacologically active)

Half-life elimination: Oral: 14-35 hours; I.V.: 12-27 hours

Time to peak, serum: 1-5 hours

Excretion:

Oral: Urine (~5% of dose; 0.5% to 0.7% as unchanged drug, 4% as idarubicinol); hepatic (8%)

I.V.: Urine (13% as idarubicinol, 3% as unchanged drug); hepatic (17%)

Dosage Refer to individual protocols. I.V.:

Children: AML (unlabeled use): 10-12 mg/m^2/day for 3 days every 3 weeks

Adults:

AML induction: 12 mg/m^2/day for 3 days

AML consolidation: 10-12 mg/m^2/day for 2 days

Dosing adjustment in renal impairment: The FDA-approved labeling does not contain specific dosing adjustment guidelines; however, it does reccomend that dosage reductions be made. Patients with S_{cr}: ≥2 mg/dL did not receive treatment in many clinical trials. The following guidelines have been used by some clinicians (Aronoff, 2007):

Children:

Cl_{cr} <50 mL/minute: Administer 75% of dose

Hemodialysis: Administer 75% of dose

Continuous ambulatory peritoneal dialysis (CAPD): Administer 75% of dose

Continuous renal replacement therapy (CRRT): Administer 75% of dose

Adults:

Cl_{cr} 10-50 mL/minute: Administer 75% of dose

Cl_{cr} <10 mL/minute: Administer 50% of dose

Hemodialysis/CAPD: Supplemental dose not needed

Dosing adjustment/comments in hepatic impairment:

Bilirubin 2.6-5 mg/dL: Administer 50% of dose

Bilirubin >5 mg/dL: Avoid use

Administration Do not administer I.M. or SubQ; administer as slow push over 3-5 minutes, preferably into the side of a freely-running saline or dextrose infusion **or** as intermittent infusion over 10-15 minutes into a free-flowing I.V. solution of NS or D_5W; also occasionally administered as a bladder lavage.

Extravasation management: Topical cooling may be achieved using ice packs or cooling pad with circulating ice water. Cooling of site for 24 hours as tolerated by the patient. Elevate and rest extremity 24-48 hours, then resume normal activity as tolerated. Application of cold inhibits vesicant's cytotoxicity. **Application of heat can be harmful and is contraindicated.** If pain, erythema, and/or swelling persist beyond 48 hours, refer patient immediately to plastic surgeon for consultation and possible debridement.

Monitoring Parameters CBC with differential, platelet count, cardiac function, serum electrolytes, creatinine, uric acid, ALT, AST, bilirubin, signs of extravasation

Dosage Forms Excipient information presented when available (limited, particularly for generics); consult specific product labeling.

Injection, solution, as hydrochloride [preservative free]:
1 mg/mL (5 mL, 10 mL, 20 mL)
Idamycin PFS®: 1 mg/mL (5 mL, 10 mL, 20 mL)

◆ **Idarubicin Hydrochloride** *see* IDArubicin *on page 865*
◆ **IDEC-C2B8** *see* RiTUXimab *on page 1503*
◆ **IDEC-Y2B8** *see* Ibritumomab *on page 857*
◆ **IDR** *see* IDArubicin *on page 865*

Idursulfase (eye dur SUL fase)

Brand Names: U.S. Elaprase®

Brand Names: Canada Elaprase®

Pharmacologic Category Enzyme

Use Replacement therapy in mucopolysaccharidosis II (MPS II, Hunter syndrome) for improvement of walking capacity

Pregnancy Risk Factor C

Dosage I.V.: MPS II:
Children ≥5 years and Adults: 0.5 mg/kg once weekly
Elderly: Studies did not include patients ≥65 years

Additional Information Complete prescribing information for this medication should be consulted for additional detail.

Dosage Forms Excipient information presented when available (limited, particularly for generics); consult specific product labeling.

Injection, solution [preservative free]:
Elaprase®: 2 mg/mL (5 mL) [extractable volume: 3 mL]

◆ **Ifex** *see* Ifosfamide *on page 867*

Ifosfamide (eye FOSS fa mide)

Brand Names: U.S. Ifex

Brand Names: Canada Ifex

Index Terms Isophosphamide; Z4942

Pharmacologic Category Antineoplastic Agent, Alkylating Agent; Antineoplastic Agent, Alkylating Agent (Nitrogen Mustard)

Use Treatment of testicular cancer

Unlabeled Use Treatment of bladder cancer, cervical cancer, ovarian cancer, nonsmall cell lung cancer, small cell lung cancer, Hodgkin's and non-Hodgkin's lymphoma; acute lymphocytic leukemia; Ewing's sarcoma, osteosarcoma, and soft tissue sarcomas

Pregnancy Risk Factor D

Pregnancy Considerations Increased resorptions and embryotoxic effects have been observed in animal studies.

Lactation Enters breast milk/not recommended

Contraindications Hypersensitivity to ifosfamide or any component of the formulation; patients with severely depressed bone marrow function

Warnings/Precautions Hazardous agent - use appropriate precautions for handling and disposal. **[U.S. Boxed Warning]: Urotoxic side effects, primarily hemorrhagic cystitis, may occur (dose-limiting toxicity).** Hydration (at least 2 L/day) and/or mesna administration will protect against hemorrhagic cystitis. **[U.S. Boxed Warning]: Severe bone marrow suppression may occur (dose-limiting toxicity);** use is contraindicated in patients with severely depressed bone marrow function. **[U.S. Boxed Warning]: May cause CNS toxicity, including confusion and coma;** usually reversible upon discontinuation of treatment. Encephalopathy, ranging from mild somnolence to hallucinations and/or coma may occur; risk factors may include hypoalbuminemia, renal dysfunction and prior history of ifosfamide-induced encephalopathy. Use with caution in patients with impaired renal function or those with compromised bone marrow reserve. May interfere with wound healing. **[U.S. Boxed Warning]: Should be administered under the supervision of an experienced cancer chemotherapy physician.** Safety and efficacy in children have not been established.

Adverse Reactions

>10%:

Central nervous system: CNS toxicity or encephalopathy (10% to 30%; includes somnolence, agitation, confusion, delirium, hallucinations, depressive psychosis, incontinence, palsy, diplopia, aphasia, or coma)
Dermatologic: Alopecia (83%)
Endocrine & metabolic: Metabolic acidosis (31%)
Gastrointestinal: Nausea/vomiting (58%), may be more common with higher doses or bolus infusion
Hematologic: Myelosuppression (onset: 7-14 days; nadir: 21-28 days; recovery: 21-28 days), leukopenia (50% to ≤100%; grade 4: ≤50%), thrombocytopenia (20%; grades 3/4: 8%)
Renal: Hematuria (6% to 92%; grade 2 [gross hematuria]: 8% to 12%)

1% to 10%:

Central nervous system: Fever
Hepatic: Bilirubin increased (3%), liver dysfunction (3%), transaminases increased (3%)
Local: Phlebitis (2%)
Renal: Renal impairment (6%)
Miscellaneous: Infection (8%)

<1% (Limited to important or life-threatening): Acidosis, acute renal failure, acute tubular necrosis, allergic reaction, anemia, arrhythmia, atrial ectopy, bradycardia, BUN increased, cardiotoxicity, CHF, chronic renal failure, coagulopathy, creatinine increased, dermatitis, diarrhea, Fanconi syndrome, hyper-/hypotension, hyperpigmentation, nonconvulsive status epilepticus, pancreatitis, polyneuropathy, proteinuria, pulmonary fibrosis, renal rickets, renal tubular acidosis, reversible posterior leukoencephalopathy syndrome (RPLS), SIADH, sterility, stomatitis

Drug Interactions

Metabolism/Transport Effects Substrate of CYP2A6 (major), CYP2B6 (minor), CYP2C19 (major), CYP2C8 (minor), CYP2C9 (minor), CYP3A4 (major); **Note:** Assignment of Major/Minor substrate status based on clinically relevant drug interaction potential; **Inhibits** CYP3A4 (weak); **Induces** CYP2C9 (weak/moderate)

Avoid Concomitant Use

Avoid concomitant use of Ifosfamide with any of the following: BCG; CloZAPine; Conivaptan; Natalizumab; Pimecrolimus; Pimozide; Tacrolimus (Topical); Vaccines (Live)

Increased Effect/Toxicity

Ifosfamide may increase the levels/effects of: CloZAPine; Leflunomide; Natalizumab; Pimozide; Vaccines (Live); Vitamin K Antagonists

The levels/effects of Ifosfamide may be increased by: Conivaptan; CYP2A6 Inhibitors (Moderate); CYP2A6 Inhibitors (Strong); CYP2C19 Inhibitors (Moderate); CYP2C19 Inhibitors (Strong); CYP3A4 Inhibitors (Moderate); CYP3A4 Inhibitors (Strong); Dasatinib; Denosumab; Pimecrolimus; Roflumilast; Tacrolimus (Topical); Trastuzumab

Decreased Effect

Ifosfamide may decrease the levels/effects of: BCG; Coccidioidin Skin Test; Sipuleucel-T; Vaccines (Inactivated); Vaccines (Live); Vitamin K Antagonists

The levels/effects of Ifosfamide may be decreased by: CYP2A6 Inducers (Strong); CYP2C19 Inducers (Strong); CYP3A4 Inducers (Strong); Deferasirox; Echinacea; Herbs (CYP3A4 Inducers); Tocilizumab

Ethanol/Nutrition/Herb Interactions Herb/Nutraceutical: St John's wort may decrease ifosfamide levels.

Stability Store intact vials of powder for injection at room temperature of 20°C to 25°C (68°F to 77°F). Store intact vials of solution under refrigeration at 2°C to 8°C (36°F to 46°F). Dilute powder with SWFI or bacteriostatic SWFI to a concentration of 50 mg/mL. Further dilution in 50-1000 mL D_5W or NS (to a final concentration of 0.6-20 mg/mL) is recommended for I.V. infusion. Reconstituted solutions may be stored under refrigeration for up to 21 days. Solutions diluted for administration are stable for 7 days at room temperature and for 6 weeks under refrigeration.

Mechanism of Action Causes cross-linking of strands of DNA by binding with nucleic acids and other intracellular structures; inhibits protein synthesis and DNA synthesis

Pharmacodynamics/Kinetics Pharmacokinetics are dose dependent

Distribution: V_d: 5.7-49 L; does penetrate CNS, but not in therapeutic levels

Protein binding: Negligible

Metabolism: Hepatic to active metabolites isofosforamide mustard, 4-hydroxy-ifosfamide, acrolein, and inactive dichloroethylated and carboxy metabolites; acrolein is the agent implicated in development of hemorrhagic cystitis

Half-life elimination:
- High dose (3800-5000 mg/m^2): ~15 hours
- Lower dose (1600-2400 mg/m^2): ~7 hours

Excretion:
- High dose (5000 mg/m^2): Urine (70% to 86%; 61% as unchanged drug)
- Lower dose (1600-2400 mg/m^2): Urine (12% to 18% as unchanged drug)

Dosage Refer to individual protocols. To prevent bladder toxicity, ifosfamide should be given with the urinary protector mesna and hydration of at least 2 L of oral or I.V. fluid per day.

Children (unlabeled use): I.V.
- 1200-1800 mg/m^2/day for 3-5 days every 21-28 days **or**
- 5 g/m^2 once every 21-28 days **or**
- 3 g/m^2/day for 2 days every 21-28 days

Adults: I.V.:
- Testicular cancer: 1200 mg/m^2/day for 5 days every 3 weeks
- Dose ranges used in other cancers (unlabeled uses):
  - 4000-5000 mg/m^2/day for 1 day every 14-28 days **or**
  - 1000-3000 mg/m^2/day for 2-5 days every 21-28 days

Dosing adjustment in renal impairment: The FDA-approved labeling does not contain dosage adjustment guidelines (has not been studied). The following guidelines have been used by some clinicians:

Aronoff, 2007:
- Cl_{cr} <10 mL/minute: Children and Adults: Administer 75% of dose
- Hemodialysis:
  - Children: 1 g/m^2 followed by hemodialysis 6-8 hours later
  - Adults: No supplemental dose needed

Kintzel, 1995:
- Cl_{cr} 46-60 mL/minute: Administer 80% of dose
- Cl_{cr} 31-45 mL/minute: Administer 75% of dose
- Cl_{cr} <30 mL/minute: Administer 70% of dose

Dosing adjustment in hepatic impairment: The FDA-approved labeling does not contain dosage adjustment guidelines (has not been studied). The following guidelines have been used by some clinicians (Floyd, 2006): Bilirubin >3 mg/dL: Administer 25% of dose

Administration Administer I.V. over 30 minutes to several hours or continuous I.V. over 5 days

Monitoring Parameters CBC with differential, hemoglobin, and platelet count, urine output, urinalysis (prior to each dose), liver function, and renal function tests

Dosage Forms Excipient information presented when available (limited, particularly for generics); consult specific product labeling.

Injection, powder for reconstitution: 1 g, 3 g
- Ifex: 1 g, 3 g

Injection, solution: 50 mg/mL (20 mL, 60 mL)

◆ **IG** *see* Immune Globulin *on page 880*

◆ **IgG4-Kappa Monoclonal Antibody** *see* Natalizumab *on page 1181*

◆ **IGIM** *see* Immune Globulin *on page 880*

◆ **IGIV** *see* Immune Globulin *on page 880*

◆ **IGIVnex® (Can)** *see* Immune Globulin *on page 880*

◆ **123I-Ioflupane** *see* Ioflupane I 123 *on page 921*

◆ **IL-1Ra** *see* Anakinra *on page 120*

◆ **IL-2** *see* Aldesleukin *on page 55*

◆ **IL-11** *see* Oprelvekin *on page 1249*

◆ **Ilaris®** *see* Canakinumab *on page 272*

Iloperidone (eye loe PER i done)

Brand Names: U.S. Fanapt®

Pharmacologic Category Antipsychotic Agent, Atypical

Additional Appendix Information

Antipsychotic Agents *on page 1880*

Use Acute treatment of schizophrenia

Pregnancy Risk Factor C

Pregnancy Considerations Animal studies have shown an increased risk of developmental toxicity and fetal mortality. Antipsychotic use during the third trimester of pregnancy has a risk for abnormal muscle movements (extrapyramidal symptoms [EPS]) and withdrawal symptoms in newborns following delivery. Symptoms in the newborn may include agitation, feeding disorder, hypertonia, hypotonia, respiratory distress, somnolence, and tremor; these effects may be self-limiting or require hospitalization.

Lactation Excretion in breast milk unknown/not recommended

Contraindications Hypersensitivity to iloperidone or any component of the formulation

Warnings/Precautions [U.S. Boxed Warning]: Elderly patients with dementia-related psychosis treated with antipsychotics are at an increased risk of death compared to placebo. Most deaths appeared to be either cardiovascular (eg, heart failure, sudden death) or infectious (eg, pneumonia) in nature. In addition, an increased incidence of cerebrovascular effects (eg, transient ischemic attack, cerebrovascular accidents) has been reported in studies of placebo-controlled trials of antipsychotics in elderly patients with dementia-related psychosis. Iloperidone is not approved for the treatment of dementia-related psychosis.

May be sedating; use with caution in disorders where CNS depression is a feature. Caution in patients with predisposition to seizures. Use is not recommended in patients with hepatic impairment. Esophageal dysmotility and aspiration have been associated with antipsychotic use; use with caution in patients at risk of aspiration pneumonia (ie, Alzheimer's disease). Use is associated with increased prolactin levels; clinical significance of hyperprolactinemia in patients with breast cancer or other prolactin-dependent tumors is unknown. May alter temperature regulation. Leukopenia, neutropenia, and agranulocytosis (sometimes fatal) have been reported in clinical trials and postmarketing reports; presence of risk factors (eg, pre-existing low

WBC or history of drug-induced leuko-/neutropenia) should prompt periodic blood count assessment and discontinuation at first signs of blood dyscrasias.

May alter cardiac conduction and prolong the QT_c interval; life-threatening arrhythmias have occurred with therapeutic doses of antipsychotics. Risks may be increased by conditions or concomitant medications which cause bradycardia, hypokalemia, and/or hypomagnesemia. Avoid use in combination with QT_c-prolonging drugs and in patients with congenital long QT syndrome, history of cardiac arrhythmia, recent MI, or uncompensated heart failure. Discontinue treatment in patients found to have persistent QT_c intervals >500 msec. Further cardiac evaluation is warranted in patients with symptoms of dizziness, palpitations, or syncope. May cause orthostatic hypotension; use with caution in patients at risk of this effect (eg, concurrent medication use which may predispose to hypotension/ bradycardia or presence of hypovolemia) or in those who would not tolerate transient hypotensive episodes. Use with caution in patients with cardiovascular diseases (eg, heart failure, history of myocardial infarction or ischemia, cerebrovascular disease, conduction abnormalities).

May cause anticholinergic effects (confusion, agitation, constipation, xerostomia, blurred vision, urinary retention); therefore, use with caution in patients with decreased gastrointestinal motility, urinary retention, BPH, xerostomia, or visual problems (including narrow-angle glaucoma). May cause extrapyramidal symptoms (EPS), including pseudoparkinsonism, acute dystonic reactions, akathisia, and tardive dyskinesia. Risk of dystonia (and probably other EPS) may be greater with increased doses, use of conventional antipsychotics, males, and younger patients. Risk of neuroleptic malignant syndrome (NMS) may be increased in patients with Parkinson's disease or Lewy body dementia. May cause hyperglycemia; in some cases may be extreme and associated with ketoacidosis, hyperosmolar coma, or death. Use with caution in patients with diabetes or other disorders of glucose regulation; monitor for worsening of glucose control. Significant weight gain has been observed with antipsychotic therapy; incidence varies with product. Monitor waist circumference and BMI. Rare cases of priapism have been reported.

Dosage adjustments are recommended for iloperidone when given concomitantly with strong CYP2D6 or CYP3A4 inhibitors or in poor metabolizers of CYP2D6. The possibility of a suicide attempt is inherent in psychotic illness; use caution in high-risk patients during initiation of therapy. Prescriptions should be written for the smallest quantity consistent with good patient care. Continued use for >6 weeks has not been evaluated.

Adverse Reactions

>10%:

Cardiovascular: Tachycardia (3% to 12%; dose related)

Central nervous system: Dizziness (10% to 20%; dose related), somnolence (9% to 15%)

1% to 10%:

Cardiovascular: Orthostatic hypotension (3% to 5%), hypotension (<1% to 3%; dose related), palpitations (≥1%)

Central nervous system: Fatigue (4% to 6%), extrapyramidal symptoms (4% to 5%), tremor (3%), lethargy (1% to 3%), akathisia (2%), aggression (≥1%), delusion (≥1%), restlessness (≥1%)

Dermatologic: Rash (2% to 3%)

Gastrointestinal: Nausea (≤10%), xerostomia (8% to 10%), weight gain (1% to 9%; dose related), diarrhea (5% to 7%), abdominal discomfort (≤3%; dose related), weight loss (≥1%)

Genitourinary: Ejaculation failure (2%), erectile dysfunction (≥1%), urinary incontinence (≥1%)

Neuromuscular & skeletal: Arthralgia (3%), stiffness (1% to 3%; dose related), dyskinesia (<2%), muscle spasm (≥1%), myalgia (≥1%)

Ocular: Blurred vision (≤3%), conjunctivitis (≥1%)

Respiratory: Nasal congestion (5% to 8%), nasopharyngitis (≤4%), upper respiratory tract infection (2% to 3%), dyspnea (2%)

<1% (Limited to important or life-threatening): Acute renal failure, amenorrhea, amnesia, anemia, anorgasmia, aphthous stomatitis, appetite increased, arrhythmia, asthma, AV block (first degree), blepharitis, bradykinesia, breast pain, bulimia nervosa, cataract, catatonia, cholelithiasis, confusion, dehydration, delirium, difficulty walking, dry eye, duodenal ulcer, dystonia, dysuria, edema, enuresis, epistaxis, esophageal reflux, eyelid edema, eye swelling, fecal incontinence, fluid retention, gastric acid secretion increased, gastritis, gynecomastia, heart failure, hematocrit/hemoglobin decreased, hiatal hernia, hostility, hyperemia, hyperthermia, hypokalemia, hypothyroidism, impulse control disorder, lenticular opacities, leukopenia, libido decreased, major depression, mania, menorrhagia, menstrual irregularities, metrorrhagia, mood swings, mouth ulceration, nasal dryness, nephrolithiasis, neutrophils increased, nystagmus, obsessive compulsive disorder, panic attack, paraesthesia, paranoia, parkinsonism, pollakiuria, polydipsia psychogenic, postmenopausal hemorrhage, prostatitis, pruritus, psychomotor hyperactivity, QT_c interval prolongation, restless leg syndrome, retrograde ejaculation, rhinorrhea, salivation, sinus congestion, sleep apnea syndrome, stomatitis, testicular pain, thirst, tinnitus, torticollis, urinary retention, urticaria, vertigo

Drug Interactions

Metabolism/Transport Effects Substrate of CYP2D6 (major), CYP3A4 (minor); **Note:** Assignment of Major/ Minor substrate status based on clinically relevant drug interaction potential

Avoid Concomitant Use

Avoid concomitant use of Iloperidone with any of the following: Artemether; Dronedarone; Lumefantrine; Metoclopramide; Nilotinib; Pimozide; QUEtiapine; QuiNINE; Tetrabenazine; Thioridazine; Toremifene; Vandetanib; Vemurafenib; Ziprasidone

Increased Effect/Toxicity

Iloperidone may increase the levels/effects of: Alcohol (Ethyl); CNS Depressants; Dronedarone; Methylphenidate; Pimozide; QTc-Prolonging Agents; QuiNINE; Serotonin Modulators; Tetrabenazine; Thioridazine; Toremifene; Vandetanib; Vemurafenib; Ziprasidone

The levels/effects of Iloperidone may be increased by: Abiraterone Acetate; Acetylcholinesterase Inhibitors (Central); Alfuzosin; Artemether; Chloroquine; Ciprofloxacin; Ciprofloxacin (Systemic); CYP2D6 Inhibitors (Moderate); CYP2D6 Inhibitors (Strong); CYP3A4 Inhibitors (Strong); Gadobutrol; HydrOXYzine; Indacaterol; Lithium formulations; Lumefantrine; MAO Inhibitors; Methylphenidate; Metoclopramide; Nilotinib; QUEtiapine; QuiNINE; Tetrabenazine

Decreased Effect

Iloperidone may decrease the levels/effects of: Amphetamines; Anti-Parkinson's Agents (Dopamine Agonist); Quinagolide

The levels/effects of Iloperidone may be decreased by: CYP2D6 Inhibitors (Strong); Lithium formulations; Peginterferon Alfa-2b; Tocilizumab

Ethanol/Nutrition/Herb Interactions

Ethanol: May increase CNS depression; monitor for increased effects with coadministration. Caution patients about effects.

Herb/Nutraceutical: Avoid St John's wort (may decrease serum levels of iloperidone). Avoid kava kava, gotu kola, valerian, St John's wort (may increase CNS depression).

Stability Store at 25°C (77°F); excursions permitted to 15°C to 30°C (59°F to 86°F). Protect from light and moisture.

Mechanism of Action Iloperidone is a piperidinyl-benzisoxazole atypical antipsychotic with mixed D_2/5-HT_2 antagonist activity. It exhibits high affinity for 5-HT_{2A}, D_2, and D_3 receptors, low to moderate affinity for D_1, D_4, H_1, 5-HT_{1A}, 5-HT_6, 5HT_7, and $NE_{\alpha1}$ receptors, and no affinity for muscarinic receptors. The addition of serotonin antagonism to dopamine antagonism (classic neuroleptic mechanism) is thought to improve negative symptoms of psychoses and reduce the incidence of extrapyramidal side effects. Iloperidone's low affinity for histamine H_1 receptors may decrease the risk for weight gain and somnolence while its affinity for $NE_{\alpha1/\alpha2C}$ may provide antidepressant and anxiolytic activity and improved cognitive function.

Pharmacodynamics/Kinetics

Absorption: Well absorbed

Distribution: V_d: 1340-2800 L

Protein binding: ~95% (iloperidone and active metabolites)

Metabolism: Hepatic via carbonyl reduction, hydroxylation (CYP2D6) and O-demethylation (CYP3A4); forms active metabolites (P88 and P95)

Bioavailability: Oral: Tablet (relative to solution): 96%

Half-life elimination:

Extensive metabolizers: Iloperidone: 18 hours; P88: 26 hours; P95: 23 hours

Poor metabolizers: Iloperidone: 33 hours; P88: 37 hours; P95: 31 hours

Time to peak, plasma: 2-4 hours

Excretion: Urine (58% extensive metabolizers, 45% poor metabolizers); feces (20% extensive metabolizers, 22% poor metabolizers)

Dosage Oral: Adults: Schizophrenia: Initial: 1 mg twice daily; recommended dosage range: 6-12 mg twice daily (maximum: 24 mg/day)

Recommended titration schedule: Increase in 2 mg increments every 24 hours on days 2-7 (eg, Day 2: 2 mg twice daily; Day 3: 4 mg twice daily; Day 4: 6 mg twice daily; Day 5: 8 mg twice daily; Day 6: 10 mg twice daily; Day 7: 12 mg twice daily)

Note: Titrate dose to effect (to avoid orthostatic hypotensive effects); treatment >6 weeks has not been evaluated; when reinitiating treatment after discontinuation (>3 days), the initial titration schedule should be followed.

Dosage adjustment in patients receiving strong CYP2D6 inhibitors (eg, paroxetine, fluoxetine, quinidine): Decrease iloperidone dose by 50%; when the CYP2D6 inhibitor is discontinued, return to previous dose.

Dosage adjustment in patients receiving strong CYP3A4 inhibitors (eg, ketoconazole, clarithromycin): Decrease iloperidone dose by 50%; when the CYP3A4 inhibitor is discontinued, return to previous dose.

Dosage adjustment in poor metabolizers of CYP2D6: Decrease iloperidone dose by 50%.

Dosing adjustment in hepatic impairment: Not recommended in patients with hepatic impairment due to lack of data

Dietary Considerations May be given with or without food.

Administration May be administered with or without food.

Monitoring Parameters Vital signs; fasting blood glucose/Hgb A_{1c} (prior to treatment and periodically during treatment); signs and symptoms of hyperglycemia; signs and symptoms of cardiac arrhythmia; CBC (frequently during first few months of therapy); serum potassium and magnesium levels (prior to treatment and periodically during treatment); orthostatic blood pressure changes; assess weight prior to and periodically during treatment

Dosage Forms Excipient information presented when available (limited, particularly for generics); consult specific product labeling.

Tablet, oral:

Fanapt®: 1 mg, 2 mg, 4 mg, 6 mg, 8 mg, 10 mg, 12 mg

Tablet, oral [combination package (each titration pack contains)]:

Fanapt®: 1 mg (2s), 2 mg (2s), 4 mg (2s), and 6 mg (2s)

Iloprost (EYE loe prost)

Brand Names: U.S. Ventavis®

Index Terms Iloprost Tromethamine; Prostacyclin PGI_2

Pharmacologic Category Prostacyclin; Prostaglandin; Vasodilator

Use Treatment of pulmonary arterial hypertension (PAH) (WHO Group I) in patients with NYHA Class III or IV symptoms to improve exercise tolerance, symptoms, and diminish clinical deterioration

Unlabeled Use WHO group III and IV pulmonary arterial hypertension (PAH)

Pregnancy Risk Factor C

Dosage Inhalation: Adults: Pulmonary arterial hypertension (PAH): Initial: 2.5 mcg/dose; if tolerated, increase to 5 mcg/dose; administer 6-9 times daily (dosing at intervals ≥2 hours while awake according to individual need and tolerability); maintenance dose: 2.5-5 mcg/dose; maximum daily dose: 45 mcg (ie, 5 mcg/dose 9 times daily)

Dosage adjustment in renal impairment: Inhaled iloprost has not been studied in renal impairment; however, according to the manufacturer, no adjustment is required in patients with renal impairment who are not on dialysis (the effect of dialysis on iloprost is unknown).

Dosage adjustment in hepatic impairment: Child-Pugh class B or C: Consider increasing dosing interval (eg, every 3-4 hours) based on response at the end of the dose interval

Additional Information Complete prescribing information for this medication should be consulted for additional detail.

Dosage Forms Excipient information presented when available (limited, particularly for generics); consult specific product labeling. [DSC] = Discontinued product

Solution, for oral inhalation [preservative free]:

Ventavis®: 10 mcg/mL (1 mL, 2 mL [DSC]); 20 mcg/mL (1 mL)

◆ **Iloprost Tromethamine** *see* Iloprost *on page 870*

◆ **Ilotycin™** *see* Erythromycin (Ophthalmic) *on page 619*

Imatinib (eye MAT eh nib)

Brand Names: U.S. Gleevec®

Brand Names: Canada Gleevec®

Index Terms CGP-57148B; Glivec; Imatinib Mesylate; STI-571

Pharmacologic Category Antineoplastic Agent, Tyrosine Kinase Inhibitor

Use Treatment of:

Gastrointestinal stromal tumors (GIST) kit-positive (CD117), including unresectable and/or metastatic malignant and adjuvant treatment following complete resection

Philadelphia chromosome-positive (Ph+) chronic myeloid leukemia (CML) in chronic phase (newly-diagnosed)

Ph+ CML in chronic phase in pediatric patients recurring following stem cell transplant or who are resistant to interferon-alpha therapy (**not** an approved use in Canada)

Ph+ CML in blast crisis, accelerated phase, or chronic phase after failure of interferon therapy

Ph+ acute lymphoblastic leukemia (ALL) (relapsed or refractory)

Aggressive systemic mastocytosis (ASM) without D816V c-Kit mutation (or c-Kit mutation status unknown)

Dermatofibrosarcoma protuberans (DFSP) (unresectable, recurrent and/or metastatic)

Hypereosinophilic syndrome (HES) and/or chronic eosinophilic leukemia (CEL)

Myelodysplastic/myeloproliferative disease (MDS/MPD) associated with platelet-derived growth factor receptor (PDGFR) gene rearrangements

Canadian labeling (not an approved indication in the U.S.): Ph+ ALL induction therapy (newly diagnosed)

Unlabeled Use Treatment of desmoid tumors (soft tissue sarcoma); post-stem cell transplant (allogeneic) follow-up treatment in CML

Pregnancy Risk Factor D

Pregnancy Considerations There are no adequate and well-controlled studies in pregnant women. Animal studies have demonstrated teratogenic effects and fetal loss. Women of childbearing potential are advised not to become pregnant (female patients and female partners of male patients). Adequate contraception is recommended. Case reports of pregnancies while on therapy (both males and females) include reports of spontaneous abortion, minor abnormalities (hypospadias, pyloric stenosis, and small intestine rotation) at or shortly after birth, and other congenital abnormalities including skeletal malformations, hypoplastic lungs, exomphalos, kidney abnormalities, hydrocephalus, cerebellar hypoplasia, and cardiac defects.

Retrospective case reports of women with CML in complete hematologic response (CHR) with cytogenic response (partial or complete) who interrupted imatinib therapy due to pregnancy, demonstrated a loss of response in some patients while off treatment. At 18 months after treatment reinitiation following delivery, CHR was again achieved in all patients and cytogenic response was achieved in some patients. Cytogenetic response rates may not be at as high as compared to patients with 18 months of uninterrupted therapy (Ault, 2006; Pye, 2008).

Lactation Enters breast milk/not recommended

Contraindications There are no contraindications listed within the FDA-approved manufacturer's labeling.

Canadian labeling: Hypersensitivity to imatinib or any component of the formulation

Warnings/Precautions Hazardous agent - use appropriate precautions for handling and disposal. Often associated with fluid retention, weight gain, and edema (probability increases with higher doses and age >65 years); occasionally leading to significant complications, including pleural effusion, pericardial effusion, pulmonary edema, and ascites. Use with caution in patients where fluid accumulation may be poorly tolerated, such as in cardiovascular disease (heart failure [HF] or hypertension) and pulmonary disease. Severe HF and left ventricular dysfunction (LVD) have been reported rarely, usually in patients with comorbidities and/or risk factors; carefully monitor patients with pre-existing cardiac disease or risk factors for HF. With initiation of imatinib treatment, cardiogenic shock and/or LVD have been reported in patients with hypereosinophilic syndrome and cardiac involvement (reversible with systemic steroids, circulatory support and temporary cessation of imatinib). Patients with high eosinophil levels and an abnormal echocardiogram or abnormal serum troponin level may benefit from prophylactic systemic steroids with the initiation of imatinib.

Severe bullous dermatologic reactions (including erythema multiforme and Stevens-Johnson syndrome) have been reported; reintroduction has been attempted following resolution. Successful resumption at a lower dose (with corticosteroids and/or antihistamine) has been described; however, some patients may experience recurrent reactions.

Hepatotoxicity may occur (may be severe); monitor; therapy interruption or dose reduction may be necessary. Transaminase and bilirubin elevations, and acute liver failure have been observed with imatinib in combination with chemotherapy. Use with caution in patients with preexisting hepatic impairment; may require dosage adjustment. Use with caution in renal impairment; may require dosage adjustment.

May cause GI irritation, severe hemorrhage (grades 3 and 4; including gastrointestinal hemorrhage and/or tumor hemorrhage; hemorrhage incidence is higher in patients with GIST), or hematologic toxicity (anemia, neutropenia, and thrombocytopenia); median duration of neutropenia is 2-3 weeks; median duration of thrombocytopenia is 3-4 weeks. Hypothyroidism has been reported in thyroidectomy patients (receiving thyroid hormone replacement therapy) during imatinib therapy; monitor. Has been associated with development of opportunistic infections. Use with caution in patients receiving concurrent therapy with drugs which alter cytochrome P450 activity or require metabolism by these isoenzymes; avoid concomitant use of strong CYP3A4 inducers. Safety and efficacy in patients <2 years of age have not been established.

Adverse Reactions Note: Adverse reactions listed as a composite of data across many trials, except where noted for a specific cancer type.

>10%:

Cardiovascular: Edema/fluid retention (33% to 86%; grades 3/4: 3% to 13%; includes aggravated edema, anasarca, ascites, pericardial effusion, peripheral edema, pleural effusion, pulmonary edema and superficial edema); facial edema (DFSP 17%), chest pain (GIST ≤7%, CML 7% to 11%)

Central nervous system: Fatigue (29% to 75%), fever (13% to 41%), headache (19% to 37%), dizziness (10% to 19%), insomnia (10% to 19%), depression (≤15%), anxiety (7% to 12%), chills (≤11%)

Dermatologic: Rash (9% to 50%; grades 3/4: 1% to 9%), pruritus (8% to 19%), alopecia (GIST 10% to 15%)

Endocrine & metabolic: Hypokalemia (6% to 13%)

Gastrointestinal: Nausea (42% to 73%), diarrhea (25% to 59%), vomiting (23% to 58%), abdominal pain (6% to 57%), anorexia (≤36%), weight gain (5% to 32%), dyspepsia (11% to 27%), constipation (9% to 16%)

Hematologic: Hemorrhage (12% to 53%; grades 3/4: 2% to 19%), neutropenia (grade 3: 7% to 27%; grade 4: 3% to 48%), thrombocytopenia (grade 3: 1% to 31%; grade 4: <1% to 33%), anemia (grade 3: 1% to 42%; grade 4: 1% to 11%), leukopenia (GIST 5% to 20%)

Hepatic: ALT increased (≤17%; grade 3: 2% to 7%; grade 4: <3%), hepatotoxicity (6% to 12%; grades 3/4: 3% to 8%)

Neuromuscular & skeletal: Muscle cramps (16% to 62%), arthralgia (≤40%), joint pain (11% to 31%), myalgia (9% to 32%), weakness (≤21%), musculoskeletal pain (children 21%; adults 12% to 49%), rigors (10% to 12%), bone pain (≤11%)

Ocular: Periorbital edema (DFSP 33%; MPD 29%; GIST ≤47%), lacrimation increased (DFSP 25%; GIST ≤10%)

Renal: Serum creatinine increased (≤12%; grade 3: ≤3%; DFSP: grade 4: 8%)

Respiratory: Nasopharyngitis (10% to 31%), cough (11% to 27%), dyspnea (≤21%), upper respiratory tract infection (3% to 21%), pharyngolaryngeal pain (7% to 18%), rhinitis (DFSP 17%), pharyngitis (CML 10% to 15%), pneumonia (CML 4% to 13%), sinusitis (4% to 11%)
Miscellaneous: Night sweats (CML 13% to 17%), infection without neutropenia (GIST ≤17%), influenza (1% to 14%), diaphoresis (GIST ≤13%)

1% to 10%:
Cardiovascular: Flushing
Central nervous system: CNS/cerebral hemorrhage (≤9%), hypoesthesia
Dermatologic: Dry skin, erythema, photosensitivity reaction
Endocrine & metabolic: Hyperglycemia (≤10%), hypocalcemia (GIST ≤6%), albumin decreased (grade 3: ≤4%)
Gastrointestinal: Flatulence (≤10%), stomatitis/mucositis (≤10%), weight loss (≤10%), gastrointestinal hemorrhage (2% to 8%), abdominal distension, gastritis, gastroesophageal reflux, mouth ulceration, taste disturbance, xerostomia
Hematologic: Lymphopenia (GIST ≤10%), neutropenic fever, pancytopenia
Hepatic: Alkaline phosphatase increased (grade 3: ≤6%; grade 4: <1%), AST increased (grade 3: 2% to 4%; grade 4: ≤3%), bilirubin increased (grade 3: 1% to 4%; grade 4: ≤3%)
Neuromuscular & skeletal: Back pain (GIST ≤7%), limb pain (GIST ≤7%), peripheral neuropathy, joint swelling, paresthesia
Ocular: Blurred vision, conjunctival hemorrhage, conjunctivitis, dry eyes, eyelid edema
Respiratory: Epistaxis

<1% (Limited to important or life-threatening): Acute febrile neutropenic dermatosis (Sweet's syndrome), amylase increased, anaphylactic shock, angina, angioedema, aplastic anemia, arrhythmia, ascites, atrial fibrillation, avascular necrosis, blepharitis, breast enlargement, bullous eruption, cardiac arrest, cardiac failure, cardiac tamponade, cardiogenic shock, cataract, cellulitis, cerebral edema, cheilitis, CHF (severe), colitis, confusion, CPK increased, dehydration, diverticulitis, dysphagia, embolism, eosinophilia, erythema multiforme, esophagitis, exanthematous pustulosis (acute generalized), exfoliative dermatitis, fungal infection, gastric ulcer, gastroenteritis, gastrointestinal obstruction, gastrointestinal perforation, glaucoma, gout, hearing loss, hematoma, hematemesis, hematuria, hemolytic anemia, hemorrhagic corpus luteum, hemorrhagic ovarian cyst, hepatic failure, hepatic necrosis, hepatitis, herpes simplex, herpes zoster, hip osteonecrosis, hypercalcemia, hyperkalemia, hyperuricemia, hyper-/hypotension, hypomagnesemia, hyponatremia, hypophosphatemia, ileus, inflammatory bowel disease, interstitial lung disease, interstitial pneumonitis, intracranial pressure increased, jaundice, LDH increased, left ventricular dysfunction, leukocytoclastic vasculitis, libido decreased, lichen planus, lichenoid keratosis, lymphadenopathy, macular edema, melena, memory impairment, menorrhagia, MI, migraine, myopathy, optic neuritis, palpitation, pancreatitis, papilledema, pericarditis, petechiae, pleural effusion, pleuritic pain, pulmonary fibrosis, pulmonary hemorrhage, pulmonary hypertension, purpura, pustular rash, Raynaud's phenomenon, renal failure, respiratory failure, respiratory tract (lower) infection, retinal hemorrhage, rhabdomyolysis, sciatica, scleral hemorrhage, seizure, sepsis, sexual dysfunction, skin pigment changes, somnolence, Stevens-Johnson syndrome, syncope, tachycardia, thrombocythemia, thrombosis, tinnitus, toxic epidermal necrolysis, tremor, tumor hemorrhage (GIST), tumor necrosis, urinary tract infection, urticaria, vertigo, vesicular rash, vitreous hemorrhage

Drug Interactions

Metabolism/Transport Effects Substrate of CYP1A2 (minor), CYP2C19 (minor), CYP2C9 (minor), CYP2D6 (minor), CYP3A4 (major), P-glycoprotein; **Note:** Assignment of Major/Minor substrate status based on clinically relevant drug interaction potential; **Inhibits** BCRP, CYP2C9 (weak), CYP2D6 (moderate), CYP3A4 (strong), P-glycoprotein

Avoid Concomitant Use

Avoid concomitant use of Imatinib with any of the following: Alfuzosin; BCG; CloZAPine; Conivaptan; Crizotinib; Dronedarone; Eplerenone; Everolimus; Fluticasone (Oral Inhalation); Halofantrine; Lapatinib; Lovastatin; Lurasidone; Natalizumab; Nilotinib; Nisoldipine; Pimecrolimus; Pimozide; Ranolazine; Rivaroxaban; RomiDEPsin; Salmeterol; Silodosin; Simvastatin; Tacrolimus (Topical); Tamsulosin; Thioridazine; Ticagrelor; Tolvaptan; Toremifene; Vaccines (Live)

Increased Effect/Toxicity

Imatinib may increase the levels/effects of: Acetaminophen; Alfuzosin; Almotriptan; Alosetron; ARIPiprazole; Bortezomib; Brentuximab Vedotin; Brinzolamide; Budesonide (Nasal); Budesonide (Systemic, Oral Inhalation); Ciclesonide; CloZAPine; Colchicine; Conivaptan; Corticosteroids (Orally Inhaled); Crizotinib; CycloSPORINE; CycloSPORINE (Systemic); CYP2D6 Substrates; CYP3A4 Substrates; Dienogest; Dronedarone; Dutasteride; Eplerenone; Everolimus; FentaNYL; Fesoterodine; Fluticasone (Nasal); Fluticasone (Oral Inhalation); GuanFACINE; Halofantrine; Iloperidone; Ixabepilone; Lapatinib; Leflunomide; Lovastatin; Lumefantrine; Lurasidone; Maraviroc; MethylPREDNISolone; Natalizumab; Nebivolol; Nilotinib; Nisoldipine; Paricalcitol; Pazopanib; Pimecrolimus; Pimozide; Propafenone; Ranolazine; Rivaroxaban; RomiDEPsin; Ruxolitinib; Salmeterol; Saxagliptin; Sildenafil; Silodosin; Simvastatin; SORAfenib; Tadalafil; Tamsulosin; Thioridazine; Ticagrelor; Tolterodine; Tolvaptan; Topotecan; Toremifene; Vaccines (Live); Vardenafil; Vemurafenib; Vilazodone; Vitamin K Antagonists; Warfarin; Zuclopenthixol

The levels/effects of Imatinib may be increased by: Acetaminophen; Antifungal Agents (Azole Derivatives, Systemic); CYP3A4 Inhibitors (Moderate); CYP3A4 Inhibitors (Strong); Dasatinib; Denosumab; Lansoprazole; P-glycoprotein/ABCB1 Inhibitors; Pimecrolimus; Roflumilast; Tacrolimus (Topical); Trastuzumab

Decreased Effect

Imatinib may decrease the levels/effects of: BCG; Cardiac Glycosides; Coccidioidin Skin Test; Codeine; Fludarabine; Prasugrel; Sipuleucel-T; Ticagrelor; TraMADol; Vaccines (Inactivated); Vaccines (Live); Vitamin K Antagonists

The levels/effects of Imatinib may be decreased by: CYP3A4 Inducers (Strong); Cyproterone; Deferasirox; Echinacea; Peginterferon Alfa-2b; P-glycoprotein/ABCB1 Inducers; Rifamycin Derivatives; St Johns Wort; Tocilizumab

Ethanol/Nutrition/Herb Interactions

Ethanol: Avoid ethanol.

Food: Food may reduce gastrointestinal irritation. Avoid grapefruit juice (may increase imatinib plasma concentration).

Herb/Nutraceutical: Avoid St John's wort (may increase metabolism and decrease imatinib plasma concentration).

Stability Store at 25°C (77°F); excursions permitted between 15°C to 30°C (59°F to 86°F). Protect from moisture.

Mechanism of Action Inhibits Bcr-Abl tyrosine kinase, the constitutive abnormal gene product of the Philadelphia chromosome in chronic myeloid leukemia (CML). Inhibition of this enzyme blocks proliferation and induces apoptosis in Bcr-Abl positive cell lines as well as in fresh leukemic cells in Philadelphia chromosome positive CML. Also inhibits tyrosine kinase for platelet-derived growth factor (PDGF), stem cell factor (SCF), c-Kit, and cellular events mediated by PDGF and SCF.

Pharmacodynamics/Kinetics

Absorption: Rapid

Protein binding: Parent drug and metabolite: ~95% to albumin and alpha$_1$-acid glycoprotein

Metabolism: Hepatic via CYP3A4 (minor metabolism via CYP1A2, CYP2D6, CYP2C9, CYP2C19); primary metabolite (active): N-demethylated piperazine derivative (CGP74588); severe hepatic impairment (bilirubin >3-10 times ULN) increases AUC by 45% to 55% for imatinib and its active metabolite, respectively

Bioavailability: 98%

Half-life elimination: Adults: Parent drug: ~18 hours; N-desmethyl metabolite: ~40 hours; Children: Parent drug: ~15 hours

Time to peak: 2-4 hours

Excretion: Feces (68% primarily as metabolites, 20% as unchanged drug); urine (13% primarily as metabolites, 5% as unchanged drug)

Dosage Oral: **Note:** For concurrent use with a strong CYP3A4 enzyme-inducing agent (eg, rifampin, phenytoin), imatinib dosage should be increased by at least 50%. The optimal duration of therapy for CML is not yet determined, discontinuing treatment is not recommended after achieving remission due to the potential for relapse (NCCN CML guidelines v.2.2010).

Children ≥2 years: **Note:** May be administered once daily or in 2 divided doses.

Ph+ CML (chronic phase, recurrent or resistant): 260 mg/m^2/day

Ph+ CML (chronic phase, newly diagnosed): 340 mg/m^2/day; maximum: 600 mg/day

Adults: **Note:** Doses ≤600 mg should be administered once daily, 800 mg doses should be administered as 400 mg twice a day.

Ph+ CML:

Chronic phase: 400 mg once daily; may be increased to 600 mg/day, if tolerated, for disease progression, lack of hematologic response after 3 months, lack of cytogenetic response after 6-12 months, or loss of previous hematologic or cytogenetic response

Canadian labeling and NCCN CML guidelines (v.2.2010): Includes range up to 800 mg/day (400 mg twice daily)

Accelerated phase or blast crisis: 600 mg once daily; may be increased to 800 mg/day (400 mg twice daily), if tolerated, for disease progression, lack of hematologic response after 3 months, lack of cytogenetic response after 6-12 months, or loss of previous hematologic or cytogenetic response

Ph+ ALL (relapsed or refractory): 600 mg once daily

GIST (adjuvant treatment following complete resection): 400 mg once daily

GIST (unresectable and/or metastatic malignant): 400 mg once daily; may be increased up to 800 mg/day (400 mg twice daily), if tolerated, for disease progression. **Note:** Significant improvement (progression-free survival, objective response rate) was demonstrated in patients with KIT exon 9 mutation with 800 mg (versus 400 mg), although overall survival (OS) was not impacted. The higher dose did not demonstrate a difference in time to progression or OS patients with Kit exon 11 mutation or wild-type status (Debiec-Rychter, 2006; Heinrich, 2009).

ASM with eosinophilia: Initiate at 100 mg once daily; titrate up to a maximum of 400 mg once daily (if tolerated) for insufficient response to lower dose

ASM without D816V c-Kit mutation or c-Kit mutation status unknown: 400 mg once daily

DFSP: 400 mg twice daily

HES/CEL: 400 mg once daily

HES/CEL with FIP1L1-PDGFRα fusion kinase: Initiate at 100 mg once daily; titrate up to a maximum of 400 mg once daily (if tolerated) if insufficient response to lower dose

MDS/MPD: 400 mg once daily

Ph+ ALL (induction, newly diagnosed): *Canadian labeling (not an approved use in the U.S.):* 600 mg once daily

Dosage adjustment with concomitant strong CYP3A4 inducers: Avoid concomitant use of strong CYP3A4 inducers (eg, dexamethasone, carbamazepine, phenobarbital, phenytoin, rifampin); if concomitant use can not be avoided, increase imatinib dose by at least 50% with careful monitoring.

Dosage adjustment for renal impairment:

Recommendation in the FDA-approved labeling:

Mild impairment (Cl_{cr} 40-59 mL/minute): Maximum recommended dose: 600 mg

Moderate impairment (Cl_{cr} 20-39 mL/minute): Decrease recommended starting dose by 50%; dose may be increased as tolerated; maximum recommended dose: 400 mg

Severe impairment (Cl_{cr} <20 mL/minute): Use caution; a dose of 100 mg/day has been tolerated in severe impairment (Gibbons, 2008)

Canadian labeling recommendation:

Mild impairment (Cl_{cr} 40-59 mL/minute): Use caution; usual minimum recommended effective dose: 400 mg once daily; titrate to efficacy and tolerability

Moderate impairment (Cl_{cr} 20-39 mL/minute): Use caution; usual minimum recommended effective dose: 400 mg once daily; titrate to efficacy and tolerability; the use of 800 mg dose is not recommended

Severe impairment (Cl_{cr} <20 mL/minute): Use is not recommended

Dosage adjustment for hepatic impairment:

Mild-to-moderate impairment: No adjustment necessary

Canadian labeling: GIST: Minimum effective dose: 400 mg once daily

Severe impairment:

Manufacturer's FDA-approved labeling: Reduce dose by 25%

Canadian labeling: GIST: 200 mg dose once daily with titration to 300 mg once daily in the absence of severe toxicity

NCCN soft tissue sarcoma guidelines (v.2.2009): GIST: Reduce dose by 25% to 50%

Dosage adjustment for hepatotoxicity (during therapy) or other nonhematologic adverse reactions: Withhold treatment until toxicity resolves; may resume if appropriate (depending on initial severity of adverse event)

NCCN soft tissue sarcoma guidelines (v.2.2009): GIST: Superficial edema: Manage with supportive care, diuretics, or dosage reduction

Hepatotoxicity (during therapy): If elevations of bilirubin >3 times upper limit of normal (ULN) or transaminases >5 times ULN occur, withhold treatment until bilirubin <1.5 times ULN and transaminases <2.5 times ULN. Resume treatment at a reduced dose as follows:

Children ≥2 years:

If current dose 260 mg/m²/day, reduce dose to 200 mg/m²/day

If current dose 340 mg/m²/day, reduce dose to 260 mg/m²/day

Adults:

If current dose 400 mg, reduce dose to 300 mg

If current dose 600 mg, reduce dose to 400 mg

If current dose 800 mg, reduce dose to 600 mg

Dosage adjustment for hematologic adverse reactions:

Chronic phase CML (initial dose 400 mg/day in adults or 260-340 mg/m²/day in children), ASM, MDS/MPD, and HES/CEL (initial dose 400 mg/day), or GIST (initial dose 400 mg): If ANC <1 x 10^9/L and/or platelets <50 x 10^9/L: Withhold until ANC ≥1.5 x 10^9/L and platelets ≥75 x 10^9/L; resume treatment at original starting dose. For recurrent neutropenia or thrombocytopenia, withhold until recovery, and reinstitute treatment at a reduced dose as follows:

Children ≥2 years:

If initial dose 260 mg/m²/day, reduce dose to 200 mg/m²/day

If initial dose 340 mg/m²/day, reduce dose to 260 mg/m²/day

Adults: If initial dose 400 mg, reduce dose to 300 mg

CML (accelerated phase or blast crisis) and PH+ ALL: Adults (initial dose 600 mg): If ANC <0.5 x 10^9/L and/or platelets <10 x 10^9/L, establish whether cytopenia is related to leukemia (bone marrow aspirate or biopsy). If unrelated to leukemia, reduce dose to 400 mg. If cytopenia persists for an additional 2 weeks, further reduce dose to 300 mg. If cytopenia persists for 4 weeks and is still unrelated to leukemia, withhold treatment until ANC ≥1 x 10^9/L and platelets ≥20 x 10^9/L, then resume treatment at 300 mg.

ASM associated with eosinophilia and HES/CEL with FIP1L1-PDGFRα fusion kinase (starting dose 100 mg/day): If ANC <1 x 10^9/L and/or platelets <50 x 10^9/L: Withhold until ANC ≥1.5 x 10^9/L and platelets ≥75 x 10^9/L; resume treatment at previous dose.

DFSP (initial dose 800 mg/day): If ANC <1 x 10^9/L and/or platelets <50 x 10^9/L, withhold until ANC ≥1.5 x 10^9/L and platelets ≥75 x 10^9/L; resume treatment at reduced dose of 600 mg/day. If depression in neutrophils or platelets recurs, withhold until recovery, and reinstitute treatment with a further dose reduction to 400 mg/day.

Dietary Considerations Should be taken with food and a large glass of water to decrease gastrointestinal irritation. Avoid grapefruit juice.

Administration Should be administered with a meal and a large glass of water. Tablets may be dispersed in water or apple juice (using ~50 mL for 100 mg tablet, ~200 mL for 400 mg tablet); stir until dissolved and use immediately. For daily dosing ≥800 mg, the 400 mg tablets should be used in order to reduce iron exposure.

Monitoring Parameters CBC (weekly for first month, biweekly for second month, then periodically thereafter), liver function tests (at baseline and monthly or as clinically indicated; more frequently [at least weekly] in patients with moderate-to-severe hepatic impairment [Ramanathan, 2008]), renal function, serum electrolytes (including calcium, phosphorus, potassium and sodium levels); thyroid function tests (in thyroidectomy patients); fatigue, weight, and edema/fluid status; consider echocardiogram and serum troponin levels in patients with HES/CEL, and in patients with MDS/MPD or ASM with high eosinophil levels; in pediatric patients, also monitor serum glucose and albumin

Monitor for signs/symptoms of CHF in patients with at risk for cardiac failure or patients with pre-existing cardiac disease. In Canada, a baseline evaluation of left ventricular ejection fraction is recommended prior to initiation of imatinib therapy in all patients with known underlying heart disease or in elderly patients.

Dosage Forms Excipient information presented when available (limited, particularly for generics); consult specific product labeling.

Tablet, oral:

Gleevec®: 100 mg, 400 mg [scored]

Extemporaneous Preparations Hazardous agent: Use appropriate precautions for handling and disposal.

An oral suspension may be prepared by placing tablets (whole, do not crush) in a glass of water or apple juice. Use ~50 mL for 100 mg tablet, or ~200 mL for 400 mg tablet. Stir until tablets are disintegrated, then administer immediately. To ensure the full dose is administered, rinse the glass and administer residue.

Gleevec® prescribing information, Novartis Pharmaceuticals Corporation, East Hanover, NJ, 2009.

◆ **Imatinib Mesylate** *see* Imatinib *on page 870*

◆ **IMC-C225** *see* Cetuximab *on page 332*

◆ **Imdur®** *see* Isosorbide Mononitrate *on page 938*

◆ **123I-Metaiodobenzylguanidine (MIBG)** *see* Iobenguane I 123 *on page 920*

◆ **Imferon** *see* Iron Dextran Complex *on page 930*

◆ **IMI 30** *see* IDArubicin *on page 865*

◆ **IMid-1** *see* Lenalidomide *on page 981*

◆ **Imidazole Carboxamide** *see* Dacarbazine *on page 438*

◆ **Imidazole Carboxamide Dimethyltriazene** *see* Dacarbazine *on page 438*

Imiglucerase (i mi GLOO ser ace)

Brand Names: U.S. Cerezyme®

Brand Names: Canada Cerezyme®

Pharmacologic Category Enzyme

Use Long-term enzyme replacement therapy for patients with Type 1 Gaucher's disease

Pregnancy Risk Factor C

Dosage I.V.: Children ≥2 years and Adults: Initial: 30-60 units/kg every 2 weeks; dosing is individualized based on disease severity. Dosing range: 2.5 units/kg 3 times/week up to as much as 60 units/kg administered as frequently as once a week or as infrequently as every 4 weeks. Average dose: 60 units/kg administered every 2 weeks

Additional Information Complete prescribing information for this medication should be consulted for additional detail.

Dosage Forms Excipient information presented when available (limited, particularly for generics); consult specific product labeling.

Injection, powder for reconstitution:

Cerezyme®: 200 units, 400 units [contains mannitol, polysorbate 80; derived from or manufactured using Chinese hamster ovary cells]

◆ **Imipemide** *see* Imipenem and Cilastatin *on page 875*

Imipenem and Cilastatin

(i mi PEN em & sye la STAT in)

Brand Names: U.S. Primaxin® I.V.

Brand Names: Canada Imipenem and Cilastatin for Injection; Primaxin® I.V. Infusion; RAN™-Imipenem-Cilastatin

Index Terms Imipemide; Primaxin® I.M. [DSC]

Pharmacologic Category Antibiotic, Carbapenem

Additional Appendix Information

Antibiotic Treatment of Adults With Infective Endocarditis *on page 1956*

Use Treatment of lower respiratory tract, urinary tract, intra-abdominal, gynecologic, bone and joint, skin and skin structure, endocarditis (caused by *Staphylococcus aureus*) and polymicrobic infections as well as bacterial septicemia. Antibacterial activity includes gram-positive bacteria (methicillin-sensitive *S. aureus* and *Streptococcus* spp), resistant gram-negative bacilli (including extended spectrum beta-lactamase-producing *Escherichia coli* and *Klebsiella* spp, *Enterobacter* spp, and *Pseudomonas aeruginosa*), and anaerobes.

Unlabeled Use Hepatic abscess; neutropenic fever; melioidosis

Pregnancy Risk Factor C

Pregnancy Considerations With the exception of slightly decreased fetal weights at the highest doses in rats and an increase in embryonic loss in cynomolgus monkeys, most animal studies have not shown an increased fetal risk or teratogenic effects. However, due to the adverse events observed in some animal studies, imipenem/cilastatin is classified as pregnancy category C. No adequate and well-controlled studies have been conducted in pregnant women and it is not known whether imipenem can cause fetal harm. Due to pregnancy induced physiologic changes, some pharmacokinetic parameters of imipenem/cilastatin may be altered. Pregnant women have a larger volume of distribution resulting in lower serum peak levels than for the same dose in nonpregnant women. Clearance is also increased.

Lactation Enters breast milk/use caution

Contraindications Hypersensitivity to imipenem/cilastatin or any component of the formulation

Warnings/Precautions Dosage adjustment required in patients with impaired renal function; elderly patients often require lower doses (adjust to renal function). Prolonged use may result in fungal or bacterial superinfection, including *C. difficile*-associated diarrhea (CDAD) and pseudomembranous colitis; CDAD has been observed >2 months postantibiotic treatment. Carbapenems have been associated with CNS adverse effects, including confusional states and seizures (myoclonic); use caution with CNS disorders (eg, brain lesions and history of seizures) and adjust dose in renal impairment to avoid drug accumulation, which may increase seizure risk. Use with caution in patients with hypersensitivity to beta-lactams (including penicillins or cephalosporins); patients with impaired renal function are at increased risk of seizures if not properly dose adjusted. May decrease divalproex sodium/valproic acid concentrations leading to breakthrough seizures; concomitant use is not recommended. Not recommended in pediatric CNS infections due to seizure risk. Serious hypersensitivity reactions, including anaphylaxis, have been reported (some without a history of previous allergic reactions to beta-lactams).

Adverse Reactions Adverse reactions reported with use for both I.V. and I.M. formulations in adults, except where noted.

1% to 10%:

Cardiovascular: Tachycardia (infants 2%; adults <1%)

Central nervous system: Seizure (infants 6%; adults <1%)

Dermatologic: Rash (≤1%, children 2%)

Gastrointestinal: Nausea (1% to 2%), diarrhea (children 3% to 4%; adults 1% to 2%), vomiting (≤2%)

Genitourinary: Oliguria/anuria (infants 2%; adults <1%)

Local: Phlebitis/thrombophlebitis (3%), pain at I.M. injection site (1.2%)

<1% (Limited to important or life-threatening): Abdominal pain, abnormal urinalysis, acute renal failure, alkaline phosphatase increased, anaphylaxis, anemia, angioneurotic edema, asthenia, bilirubin increased, bone marrow depression, BUN/creatinine increased, candidiasis, confusion, cyanosis, dizziness, drug fever, dyspnea, encephalopathy, eosinophilia, erythema multiforme, fever, flushing, gastroenteritis, glossitis, hallucinations, hearing loss, hematocrit decreased, hemoglobin decreased, hemolytic anemia, hemorrhagic colitis, hepatitis (including fulminant onset), hepatic failure, hyperchloremia, hyperhidrosis, hyperkalemia, hypersensitivity, hyperventilation, hyponatremia, hypotension, jaundice, lactate dehydrogenase increased, leukocytosis, leukopenia, myoclonus, neutropenia (including agranulocytosis), palpitation, pancytopenia, paresthesia, pharyngeal pain, polyarthralgia, polyuria, positive Coombs' test, prothrombin time increased, pruritus vulvae, pseudomembranous colitis, psychic disturbances, rash, resistant *P. aeruginosa*, somnolence, Stevens-Johnson syndrome, thoracic spine pain, thrombocythemia, thrombocytopenia, tinnitus, tongue papillar hypertrophy, toxic epidermal necrolysis, transaminases increased, tremor, urticaria, vertigo

Drug Interactions

Metabolism/Transport Effects None known.

Avoid Concomitant Use

Avoid concomitant use of Imipenem and Cilastatin with any of the following: BCG; Ganciclovir (Systemic); Ganciclovir-Valganciclovir

Increased Effect/Toxicity

Imipenem and Cilastatin may increase the levels/effects of: CycloSPORINE; CycloSPORINE (Systemic)

The levels/effects of Imipenem and Cilastatin may be increased by: CycloSPORINE; CycloSPORINE (Systemic); Ganciclovir (Systemic); Ganciclovir-Valganciclovir; Probenecid

Decreased Effect

Imipenem and Cilastatin may decrease the levels/effects of: BCG; CycloSPORINE; CycloSPORINE (Systemic); Divalproex; Typhoid Vaccine; Valproic Acid

Stability Imipenem/cilastatin powder for injection should be stored at <25°C (77°F).

I.V.: Prior to use, dilute dose into 100-250 mL of an appropriate solution. Imipenem is inactivated at acidic or alkaline pH. Final concentration should not exceed 5 mg/mL. The I.M. formulation is not buffered and cannot be used to prepare I.V. solutions. Reconstituted I.V. solutions are stable for 4 hours at room temperature and 24 hours when refrigerated. Do not freeze.

Mechanism of Action Inhibits bacterial cell wall synthesis by binding to one or more of the penicillin-binding proteins (PBPs); which in turn inhibits the final transpeptidation step of peptidoglycan synthesis in bacterial cell walls, thus inhibiting cell wall biosynthesis. Bacteria eventually lyse due to ongoing activity of cell wall autolytic enzymes (autolysins and murein hydrolases) while cell wall assembly is arrested. Cilastatin prevents renal metabolism of imipenem by competitive inhibition of dehydropeptidase along the brush border of the renal tubules.

Pharmacodynamics/Kinetics

Distribution: Rapidly and widely to most tissues and fluids including sputum, pleural fluid, peritoneal fluid, interstitial fluid, bile, aqueous humor, and bone; highest concentrations in pleural fluid, interstitial fluid, and peritoneal fluid; low concentrations in CSF

Protein binding: Imipenem: 20%; cilastatin: 40%

Metabolism: Imipenem is metabolized in the kidney by dehydropeptidase I; cilastatin prevents imipenem metabolism by this enzyme; cilastatin is partially metabolized renally

Half-life elimination: I.V.: Both drugs: 60 minutes; prolonged with renal impairment

Excretion: Both drugs: Urine (~70% as unchanged drug)

Dosage

Usual dosage ranges: Note: Dosage based on **imipenem** content:

Children >3 months: Non-CNS infections: I.V.: 15-25 mg/kg every 6 hours; maximum dosage: Susceptible infections: 2 g/day; moderately-susceptible organisms: 4 g/day

Adults: I.V.: Weight ≥70 kg: 250-1000 mg every 6-8 hours; maximum: 4 g/day. **Note:** For adults weighing <70 kg, refer to dosing adjustment in renal impairment

Indication-specific dosing: Note: Doses based on imipenem content.

Children: I.V.:

Burkholderia pseudomallei (melioidosis) (unlabeled use): I.V.: Initial: 20 mg/kg every 8 hours for at least 10 days (White, 2003) **or** 25 mg/kg (up to 1 g) every 6 hours for at least 10 days (Currie, 2003); continue parenteral therapy until clinical improvement, then switch to oral therapy if tolerated and/or appropriate

Cystic fibrosis: Children >12 years: Up to 90 mg/kg/day in divided doses has been used

Adults:

Burkholderia pseudomallei (melioidosis) (unlabeled use): Initial: 20 mg/kg every 8 hours for at least 10 days (White, 2003) **or** 25 mg/kg (up to 1 g) every 6 hours for at least 10 days (Currie, 2003); continue parenteral therapy until clinical improvement, then switch to oral therapy if tolerated and/or appropriate

Intra-abdominal infections: I.V.:

Mild infection: 250-500 mg every 6 hours

Severe infection: 500 mg every 6 hours **or** 1 g every 8 hours for 4-7 days (provided source controlled). **Note:** Not recommended for mild-to-moderate, community-acquired intra-abdominal infections due to risk of toxicity and the development of resistant organisms (Solomkin, 2010)

Liver abscess (unlabeled use): I.V.: 500 mg every 6 hours for 4-6 weeks (Ulug, 2010)

Mild infection: Note: Rarely a suitable option in mild infections; normally reserved for moderate-severe cases: I.V.:

Fully-susceptible organisms: 250 mg every 6 hours

Moderately-susceptible organisms: 500 mg every 6 hours

Moderate infection: I.V.:

Fully-susceptible organisms: 500 mg every 6-8 hours

Moderately-susceptible organisms: 500 mg every 6 hours or 1 g every 8 hours

Neutropenic fever (unlabeled use): I.V.: 500 mg every 6 hours (Paul, 2006)

***Pseudomonas* infections:** I.V.: 500 mg every 6 hours; **Note:** Higher doses may be required based on organism sensitivity.

Severe infection: I.V.:

Fully-susceptible organisms: 500 mg every 6 hours

Moderately-susceptible organisms: 1 g every 6-8 hours

Maximum daily dose should not exceed 50 mg/kg or 4 g/day, whichever is lower

Urinary tract infection: I.V.:

Uncomplicated: 250 mg every 6 hours

Complicated: 500 mg every 6 hours

Dosage adjustment in hepatic impairment: Hepatic dysfunction may further impair cilastatin clearance in patients receiving chronic renal replacement therapy; consider decreasing the dosing frequency.

Dosage adjustment in renal impairment: I.V.: **Note:**

Patients with a Cl_{cr} ≤5 mL/minute/1.73 m^2 should not receive imipenem/cilastatin unless hemodialysis is instituted within 48 hours.

Patients weighing <30 kg with impaired renal function should not receive imipenem/cilastatin.

Reduced I.V. dosage regimen based on creatinine clearance and/or body weight: See table.

Intermittent hemodialysis (IHD) (administer after hemodialysis on dialysis days): Use the dosing recommendation for patients with a Cl_{cr} 6-20 mL/minute; administer dose after dialysis session and every 12 hours thereafter **or** 250-500 mg every 12 hours (Heintz, 2009). **Note:** Dosing dependent on the assumption of 3 times/week, complete IHD sessions.

Peritoneal dialysis (unlabeled dosing): Dose as for Cl_{cr} 6-20 mL/minute (Somani, 1988)

Continuous renal replacement therapy (CRRT) (Heintz, 2009; Trotman, 2005): Drug clearance is highly dependent on the method of renal replacement, filter type, and flow rate. Appropriate dosing requires close monitoring of pharmacologic response, signs of adverse reactions due to drug accumulation, as well as drug concentrations in relation to target trough (if appropriate). The following are general recommendations only (based on dialysate flow/ultrafiltration rates of 1-2 L/hour and minimal residual renal function) and should not supersede clinical judgment:

CVVH: Loading dose of 1 g followed by either 250 mg every 6 hours **or** 500 mg every 8 hours

CVVHD: Loading dose of 1 g followed by either 250 mg every 6 hours **or** 500 mg every 6-8 hours

CVVHDF: Loading dose of 1 g followed by either 250 mg every 6 hours **or** 500 mg every 6 hours

Note: Data suggest that 500 mg every 8-12 hours may provide sufficient time above MIC to cover organisms with MIC values ≤2 mg/L; however, a higher dose of 500 mg every 6 hours is recommended for resistant organisms (particularly *Pseudomonas* spp) with MIC ≥4 mg/L or deep-seated infections (Fish, 2005).

Reduced I.V. dosage regimen based on creatinine clearance and/or body weight:

U.S. labeling: See table.

Imipenem and Cilastatin Dosage in Renal Impairment

Reduced I.V. Dosage Regimen Based on Creatinine Clearance (mL/minute/1.73 m^2) and/or Body Weight <70 kg					
	Body Weight (kg)				
	≥70	60	50	40	30
Total daily dose for normal renal function: 1 g/day					
Cl_{cr} ≥71	250 mg q6h	250 mg q8h	125 mg q6h	125 mg q6h	125 mg q8h
Cl_{cr} 41-70	250 mg q8h	125 mg q6h	125 mg q6h	125 mg q8h	125 mg q8h
Cl_{cr} 21-40	250 mg q12h	250 mg q12h	125 mg q8h	125 mg q12h	125 mg q12h
Cl_{cr} 6-20	250 mg q12h	125 mg q12h	125 mg q12h	125 mg q12h	125 mg q12h
Total daily dose for normal renal function: 1.5 g/day					
Cl_{cr} ≥71	500 mg q8h	250 mg q6h	250 mg q6h	250 mg q8h	125 mg q6h
Cl_{cr} 41-70	250 mg q6h	250 mg q8h	250 mg q8h	125 mg q6h	125 mg q8h
Cl_{cr} 21-40	250 mg q8h	250 mg q8h	250 mg q12h	125 mg q8h	125 mg q8h
Cl_{cr} 6-20	250 mg q12h	250 mg q12h	250 mg q12h	125 mg q12h	125 mg q12h
Total daily dose for normal renal function: 2 g/day					
Cl_{cr} ≥71	500 mg q6h	500 mg q8h	250 mg q6h	250 mg q6h	250 mg q8h
Cl_{cr} 41-70	500 mg q8h	250 mg q6h	250 mg q6h	250 mg q8h	125 mg q6h
Cl_{cr} 21-40	250 mg q6h	250 mg q8h	250 mg q8h	250 mg q12h	125 mg q8h
Cl_{cr} 6-20	250 mg q12h	250 mg q12h	250 mg q12h	250 mg q12h	125 mg q12h
Total daily dose for normal renal function: 3 g/day					
Cl_{cr} ≥71	1000 mg q8h	750 mg q8h	500 mg q6h	500 mg q8h	250 mg q6h
Cl_{cr} 41-70	500 mg q6h	500 mg q8h	500 mg q8h	250 mg q6h	250 mg q8h
Cl_{cr} 21-40	500 mg q8h	500 mg q8h	250 mg q6h	250 mg q8h	250 mg q8h
Cl_{cr} 6-20	500 mg q12h	500 mg q12h	250 mg q12h	250 mg q12h	250 mg q12h
Total daily dose for normal renal function: 4 g/day					
Cl_{cr} ≥71	1000 mg q6h	1000 mg q8h	750 mg q8h	500 mg q6h	500 mg q8h
Cl_{cr} 41-70	750 mg q8h	750 mg q8h	500 mg q6h	500 mg q8h	250 mg q6h
Cl_{cr} 21-40	500 mg q6h	500 mg q8h	500 mg q8h	250 mg q6h	250 mg q8h
Cl_{cr} 6-20	500 mg q12h	500 mg q12h	500 mg q12h	250 mg q12h	250 mg q12h

Canadian labeling: Reduced I.V. dosage regimen based on creatinine clearance (mL/minute/1.73 m^2) and body weight ≥70 kg (**Note:** The manufacturer labeling recommends further proportionate dose reductions for patients <70 kg, but does not provide specific dosing recommendations):

Mild renal impairment (Cl_{cr} 31-70 mL/minute/1.73 m^2):

Fully-susceptible organisms: Maximum dosage: 500 mg every 8 hours

Less susceptible organisms (primarily some *Pseudomonas* strains): Maximum dosage: 500 mg every 6 hours

Moderate renal impairment (Cl_{cr} 21-30 mL/minute/1.73 m^2):

Fully-susceptible organisms: Maximum dosage: 500 mg every 12 hours

Less susceptible organisms (primarily some *Pseudomonas* strains): Maximum dosage: 500 mg every 8 hours

Severe renal impairment (Cl_{cr} 0-20 mL/minute/1.73 m^2):

Fully-susceptible organisms: Maximum dosage: 250 mg every 12 hours

Less susceptible organisms (primarily some *Pseudomonas* strains): Maximum dosage: 500 mg every 12 hours

Note: Patients with Cl_{cr} 6-20 mL/minute/1.73 m^2 should receive 250 mg every 12 hours or 3.5 mg/kg (whichever is lower) every 12 hours for most pathogens; seizure risk may increase with higher dosing.

Dietary Considerations Some products may contain sodium.

Administration I.V.: Do not administer I.V. push. Infuse doses ≤500 mg over 20-30 minutes; infuse doses ≥750 mg over 40-60 minutes.

Monitoring Parameters Periodic renal, hepatic, and hematologic function tests; monitor for signs of anaphylaxis during first dose

Test Interactions Interferes with urinary glucose determination using Clinitest®; positive Coombs' [direct]

Dosage Forms Excipient information presented when available (limited, particularly for generics); consult specific product labeling.

Injection, powder for reconstitution: Imipenem 250 mg and cilastatin 250 mg; imipenem 500 mg and cilastatin 500 mg

Primaxin® I.V.: Imipenem 250 mg and cilastatin 250 mg [contains sodium 18.8 mg (0.8 mEq)]; imipenem 500 mg and cilastatin 500 mg [contains sodium 37.5 mg (1.6 mEq)]

◆ **Imipenem and Cilastatin for Injection (Can)** *see* Imipenem and Cilastatin *on page 875*

Imipramine (im IP ra meen)

Brand Names: U.S. Tofranil-PM®; Tofranil®

Brand Names: Canada Apo-Imipramine®; Novo-Pramine; Tofranil®

Index Terms Imipramine Hydrochloride; Imipramine Pamoate

Pharmacologic Category Antidepressant, Tricyclic (Tertiary Amine)

Additional Appendix Information

Antidepressant Agents *on page 1874*

Use Treatment of depression; treatment of nocturnal enuresis in children

Unlabeled Use Analgesic for certain chronic and neuropathic pain (including diabetic neuropathy); panic disorder; attention-deficit/hyperactivity disorder (ADHD); post-traumatic stress disorder (PTSD)

Pregnancy Considerations Animal reproduction studies are inconclusive. Congenital abnormalities have been reported in humans; however, a casual relationship has not been established. Due to pregnancy-induced physiologic changes, women who are pregnant may require dose adjustments late in pregnancy to achieve euthymia.

Lactation Enters breast milk/not recommended (AAP rates "of concern"; AAP 2001 update pending)

Medication Guide Available Yes

Contraindications Hypersensitivity to imipramine (cross-reactivity with other dibenzodiazepines may occur) or any component of the formulation; concurrent use of MAO inhibitors (within 14 days); in a patient during acute recovery phase of MI; pregnancy

Warnings/Precautions [U.S. Boxed Warning]: Antidepressants increase the risk of suicidal thinking and behavior in children, adolescents, and young adults (18-24 years of age) with major depressive disorder (MDD) and other psychiatric disorders; consider risk prior to prescribing. Short-term studies did not show an increased risk in patients >24 years of age and showed a decreased risk in patients ≥65 years. Closely monitor for clinical worsening, suicidality, or unusual changes in behavior; the patient's family or caregiver should be instructed to closely observe the patient and communicate condition with healthcare provider. A medication guide should be dispensed with each prescription. **Imipramine is FDA approved for the treatment of nocturnal enuresis in children ≥6 years of age.**

The possibility of a suicide attempt is inherent in major depression and may persist until remission occurs. Monitor for worsening of depression or suicidality, especially during initiation of therapy (generally first 1-2 months) or with dose increases or decreases. Use caution in high-risk patients. Worsening depression and severe abrupt suicidality that are not part of the presenting symptoms may require discontinuation or modification of drug therapy. The patient's family or caregiver should be alerted to monitor patients for the emergence of suicidality and associated behaviors (such as agitation, irritability, hostility, impulsivity, and hypomania) and notify healthcare provider.

May worsen psychosis in some patients or precipitate a shift to mania or hypomania in patients with bipolar disorder. Patients presenting with depressive symptoms should be screened for bipolar disorder. Monotherapy in patients with bipolar disorder should be avoided. **Imipramine is not FDA approved for the treatment of bipolar depression.**

TCAs may rarely cause bone marrow suppression; monitor for any signs of infection and obtain CBC if symptoms (eg, fever, sore throat) evident. The degree of sedation, anticholinergic effects, orthostasis, and conduction abnormalities are high relative to other antidepressants. Imipramine often causes drowsiness/sedation, resulting in impaired performance of tasks requiring alertness (eg, operating machinery or driving). Sedative effects may be additive with other CNS depressants and/or ethanol. Use with caution in patients with a history of cardiovascular disease (including previous MI, stroke, tachycardia, or conduction abnormalities). Use with caution in patients with urinary retention, benign prostatic hyperplasia, narrow-angle glaucoma, xerostomia, visual problems, constipation, or a history of bowel obstruction.

Consider discontinuing, when possible, prior to elective surgery. Therapy should not be abruptly discontinued in patients receiving high doses for prolonged periods. May lower seizure threshold - use caution in patients with a previous seizure disorder or condition predisposing to seizures such as brain damage, alcoholism, or concurrent therapy with other drugs which lower the seizure threshold. May increase the risks associated with electroconvulsive therapy. Use with caution in hyperthyroid patients or those receiving thyroid supplementation. Use with caution in patients with diabetes mellitus; may alter glucose regulation. Use with caution in patients with hepatic or renal dysfunction and in elderly patients. Has been associated with photosensitization.

Adverse Reactions Reported for tricyclic antidepressants in general. Frequency not defined.

Cardiovascular: Arrhythmia, CHF, ECG changes, heart block, hypertension, MI, orthostatic hypotension, palpitation, stroke, tachycardia

Central nervous system: Agitation, anxiety, confusion, delusions, disorientation, dizziness, drowsiness, fatigue, hallucination, headache, hypomania, insomnia, nightmares, psychosis, restlessness, seizure

Dermatologic: Alopecia, itching, petechiae, photosensitivity, purpura, rash, urticaria

Endocrine & metabolic: Breast enlargement, galactorrhea, gynecomastia, increase or decrease in blood sugar, increase or decrease in libido, SIADH

Gastrointestinal: Abdominal cramps, anorexia, black tongue, constipation, diarrhea, epigastric disorders, ileus, nausea, stomatitis, taste disturbance, vomiting, weight gain/loss, xerostomia

Genitourinary: Impotence, testicular swelling, urinary retention

Hematologic: Agranulocytosis, eosinophilia, thrombocytopenia

Hepatic: Cholestatic jaundice, transaminases increased

Neuromuscular & skeletal: Ataxia, extrapyramidal symptoms, incoordination, numbness, paresthesia, peripheral neuropathy, tingling, tremor, weakness

Ocular: Blurred vision, disturbances of accommodation, mydriasis

Otic: Tinnitus

Miscellaneous: Diaphoresis, falling, hypersensitivity (eg, drug fever, edema)

Drug Interactions

Metabolism/Transport Effects Substrate of CYP1A2 (minor), CYP2B6 (minor), CYP2C19 (major), CYP2D6 (major), CYP3A4 (minor); **Note:** Assignment of Major/Minor substrate status based on clinically relevant drug interaction potential; **Inhibits** CYP1A2 (weak), CYP2C19 (weak), CYP2D6 (moderate), CYP2E1 (weak)

Avoid Concomitant Use

Avoid concomitant use of Imipramine with any of the following: Artemether; Dronedarone; Iobenguane I 123; Lumefantrine; MAO Inhibitors; Methylene Blue; Nilotinib; Pimozide; QUEtiapine; QuiNINE; Tetrabenazine; Thioridazine; Toremifene; Vandetanib; Vemurafenib; Ziprasidone

Increased Effect/Toxicity

Imipramine may increase the levels/effects of: Alpha-/Beta-Agonists (Direct-Acting); Alpha1-Agonists; Amphetamines; Anticholinergics; Aspirin; Beta2-Agonists; CYP2D6 Substrates; Desmopressin; Dronedarone; Fesoterodine; Methylene Blue; Metoclopramide; Nebivolol; NSAID (COX-2 Inhibitor); NSAID (Nonselective); Pimozide; QTc-Prolonging Agents; QuiNIDine; QuiNINE; Serotonin Modulators; Sodium Phosphates; Sulfonylureas; Tamoxifen; Tetrabenazine; Thioridazine; Toremifene; TraMADol; Vandetanib; Vemurafenib; Vitamin K Antagonists; Yohimbine; Ziprasidone

The levels/effects of Imipramine may be increased by: Abiraterone Acetate; Alfuzosin; Altretamine; Antipsychotics; Artemether; BuPROPion; Chloroquine; Cimetidine; Cinacalcet; Ciprofloxacin; Ciprofloxacin (Systemic); Conivaptan; CYP2C19 Inhibitors (Moderate); CYP2C19 Inhibitors (Strong); CYP2D6 Inhibitors (Moderate); CYP2D6 Inhibitors (Strong); Dexmethylphenidate; Divalproex; DULoxetine; Gadobutrol; Indacaterol; Linezolid; Lithium; Lumefantrine; MAO Inhibitors; Methylphenidate; Metoclopramide; Nilotinib; Pramlintide; Protease Inhibitors; QUEtiapine; QuiNIDine; QuiNINE; Selective Serotonin Reuptake Inhibitors; Terbinafine; Terbinafine (Systemic); Valproic Acid

Decreased Effect

Imipramine may decrease the levels/effects of: Acetylcholinesterase Inhibitors (Central); Alpha2-Agonists; Codeine; Iobenguane I 123

The levels/effects of Imipramine may be decreased by: Acetylcholinesterase Inhibitors (Central); Barbiturates; CarBAMazepine; CYP2C19 Inducers (Strong); Cyproterone; Peginterferon Alfa-2b; St Johns Wort; Tocilizumab

Ethanol/Nutrition/Herb Interactions

Ethanol: May increase CNS depression; monitor for increased effects with coadministration. Caution patients about effects.

Herb/Nutraceutical: St John's wort may decrease imipramine levels. Avoid valerian, St John's wort, SAMe, kava kava (may increase risk of serotonin syndrome and/or excessive sedation).

Mechanism of Action Traditionally believed to increase the synaptic concentration of serotonin and/or norepinephrine in the central nervous system by inhibition of their reuptake by the presynaptic neuronal membrane. However, additional receptor effects have been found including desensitization of adenyl cyclase, down regulation of beta-adrenergic receptors, and down regulation of serotonin receptors.

Pharmacodynamics/Kinetics

Onset of action: Peak antidepressant effect: Usually after ≥2 weeks

Absorption: Well absorbed

Metabolism: Hepatic, primarily via CYP2D6 to desipramine (active) and other metabolites; significant first-pass effect

Half-life elimination: 6-18 hours

Excretion: Urine (as metabolites)

Dosage Oral:

Children:

Depression (unlabeled use): 1.5 mg/kg/day with dosage increments of 1 mg/kg every 3-4 days to a maximum dose of 5 mg/kg/day in 1-4 divided doses; monitor carefully especially with doses ≥3.5 mg/kg/day

Enuresis: ≥6 years: Initial: 25 mg at bedtime, if inadequate response still seen after 1 week of therapy, increase by 25 mg/day; dose should not exceed 2.5 mg/kg/day or 50 mg at bedtime if 6-12 years of age or 75 mg at bedtime if ≥12 years of age

Adjunct in the treatment of cancer pain (unlabeled use): Initial: 0.2-0.4 mg/kg at bedtime; dose may be increased by 50% every 2-3 days up to 1-3 mg/kg/dose at bedtime

Adolescents: Depression: Initial: 25-50 mg/day; increase gradually; maximum: 100 mg/day in single or divided doses

Adults:

Depression:

Outpatients: Initial: 75 mg/day; may increase gradually to 150 mg/day. May be given in divided doses or as a single bedtime dose; maximum: 200 mg/day

Inpatients: Initial: 100-150 mg/day; may increase gradually to 200 mg/day; if no response after 2 weeks, may further increase to 250-300 mg/day. May be given in divided doses or as a single bedtime dose; maximum: 300 mg/day.

Post-traumatic stress disorder (PTSD) (unlabeled use): 75-200 mg/day

Elderly: Depression: Initial: 25-50 mg at bedtime; may increase every 3 days for inpatients and weekly for outpatients if tolerated to a recommended maximum of 100 mg/day.

Monitoring Parameters Monitor blood pressure and pulse rate prior to and during initial therapy; ECG in older adults, with high doses, and/or in patients with pre-existing cardiovascular disease; evaluate mental status, suicide ideation (especially at the beginning of therapy or when doses are increased or decreased); blood levels are useful for therapeutic monitoring

Reference Range Therapeutic: Imipramine and desipramine: 150-250 ng/mL (SI: 530-890 nmol/L); desipramine: 150-300 ng/mL (SI: 560-1125 nmol/L); Toxic: >500 ng/mL (SI: 446-893 nmol/L); utility of serum level monitoring controversial

Dosage Forms Excipient information presented when available (limited, particularly for generics); consult specific product labeling.

Capsule, oral, as pamoate: 75 mg, 100 mg, 125 mg, 150 mg

Tofranil-PM®: 75 mg, 100 mg, 125 mg, 150 mg

Tablet, oral, as hydrochloride: 10 mg, 25 mg, 50 mg

Tofranil®: 10 mg, 25 mg, 50 mg

◆ **Imipramine Hydrochloride** *see* Imipramine *on page 877*

◆ **Imipramine Pamoate** *see* Imipramine *on page 877*

Imiquimod (i mi KWI mod)

Brand Names: U.S. Aldara®; Zyclara®

Brand Names: Canada Aldara®; Vyloma™; Zyclara®

Pharmacologic Category Skin and Mucous Membrane Agent; Topical Skin Product

Use Treatment of external genital and perianal warts/condyloma acuminata; nonhyperkeratotic actinic keratosis on face or scalp; superficial basal cell carcinoma (sBCC) with a maximum tumor diameter of 2 cm located on the trunk, neck, or extremities (excluding hands or feet)

Unlabeled Use Treatment of common warts

Pregnancy Risk Factor C

Dosage Topical: **Note:** A rest period of several days may be taken if required by the patient's discomfort or severity of the local skin reaction. Treatment may resume once the reaction subsides. Imiquimod treatment should not be prolonged beyond recommended period due to missed doses or rest periods.

Children ≥12 years and Adults (Aldara®): External genital and/or perianal warts/condyloma acuminata: Apply a thin layer 3 times/week prior to bedtime and leave on skin for 6-10 hours. Remove with mild soap and water. Examples of 3 times/week application schedules are: Monday, Wednesday, Friday; or Tuesday, Thursday, Saturday. Continue treatment until there is total clearance of the warts (maximum duration of therapy: 16 weeks).

Adults:

Aldara®:

Actinic keratosis: Apply twice weekly for 16 weeks to a treatment area on face or scalp (but not both concurrently); no more than 1 packet should be applied at each application and no more than 36 packets applied per 16 weeks; apply prior to bedtime and leave on skin for 8 hours. Remove with mild soap and water.

Common oral warts (dental use; unlabeled use): Apply once daily prior to bedtime

Common warts (unlabeled use): Apply once daily prior to bedtime for 5 days/week for up to 16 weeks (Hengge, 2000) or apply twice daily for up to 24 weeks (Grussendorf-Conen, 2002)

Superficial basal cell carcinoma: Apply once daily prior to bedtime, 5 days/week for 6 weeks. No more than 36 packets should be used during the 6-week treatment period. Treatment area should include a 1 cm margin of skin around the tumor. Leave on skin for 8 hours. Remove with mild soap and water.

Zyclara® 3.75%: Actinic keratosis: Treatment consists of 2 cycles (14 days each) separated by 1 rest period (14 days) with no treatment. Apply up to 2 packets once daily at bedtime to affected area on either face or balding scalp (but not both concurrently); apply no more than 2 packets at each application and no more than 56 packets per 2 cycles of treatment. Leave on skin for 8 hours. Remove with mild soap and water. **Note:** Canadian labeling recommends avoiding application to areas larger than the face or balding scalp (~200 cm^2).

Additional Information Complete prescribing information for this medication should be consulted for additional detail.

Dosage Forms Excipient information presented when available (limited, particularly for generics); consult specific product labeling.

Cream, topical: 5% (24s) [0.25 g/packet]

Aldara®: 5% (24s) [contains benzyl alcohol; 0.25 g/packet]

Zyclara®: 3.75% (28s) [contains benzyl alcohol; 0.25 g/packet]

◆ **Imitrex®** *see* SUMAtriptan *on page 1609*

◆ **Imitrex® DF (Can)** *see* SUMAtriptan *on page 1609*

◆ **Imitrex® Injection (Can)** *see* SUMAtriptan *on page 1609*

◆ **Imitrex® Nasal Spray (Can)** *see* SUMAtriptan *on page 1609*

◆ **ImmuCyst® (Can)** *see* BCG *on page 191*

Immune Globulin (i MYUN GLOB yoo lin)

Brand Names: U.S. Carimune® NF; Flebogamma® DIF; GamaSTAN™ S/D; Gammagard S/D®; Gammagard® Liquid; Gammaked™; Gammaplex®; Gamunex® [DSC]; Gamunex®-C; Hizentra®; Octagam®; Privigen®; Vivaglobin® [DSC]

Brand Names: Canada BayGam®; Gamimune® N; Gammagard Liquid; Gammagard S/D; Gamunex®; IGIVnex®; Privigen®; Vivaglobin®

Index Terms Gamma Globulin; IG; IGIM; IGIV; Immune Globulin Subcutaneous (Human); Immune Serum Globulin; ISG; IV Immune Globulin; IVIG; Panglobulin; SCIG

Pharmacologic Category Blood Product Derivative; Immune Globulin

Additional Appendix Information

Immune Globulin Products *on page 1891*

Immunization Recommendations *on page 1922*

Use

Treatment of primary humoral immunodeficiency syndromes (congenital agammaglobulinemia, severe combined immunodeficiency syndromes [SCIDS], common variable immunodeficiency, X-linked immunodeficiency, Wiskott-Aldrich syndrome) (Carimune® NF, Flebogamma® DIF, Gammagard® Liquid, Gammagard S/D®, Gammaplex®, Gamunex®, Gamunex®-C, Hizentra®, Octagam®, Privigen®, Vivaglobin®)

Treatment of acute and chronic immune (idiopathic) thrombocytopenic purpura (ITP) (Carimune® NF, Gammagard S/D®, Gamunex®, Gamunex®-C, Privigen® [chronic only])

Treatment of chronic inflammatory demyelinating polyneuropathy (CIDP) (Gamunex®, Gamunex®-C)

Prevention of coronary artery aneurysms associated with Kawasaki syndrome (in combination with aspirin) (Gammagard S/D®)

Prevention of bacterial infection in patients with hypogammaglobulinemia and/or recurrent bacterial infections with B-cell chronic lymphocytic leukemia (CLL) (Gammagard S/D®)

Prevention of serious infection in immunoglobulin deficiency (select agammaglobulinemias) (GamaSTAN™ S/D)

Provision of passive immunity in the following susceptible individuals (GamaSTAN™ S/D):

Hepatitis A: Pre-exposure prophylaxis; postexposure: within 14 days and/or prior to manifestation of disease

Measles: For use within 6 days of exposure in an unvaccinated person, who has not previously had measles

Rubella: Postexposure prophylaxis (within 72 hours) to reduce the risk of infection and fetal damage in exposed pregnant women who will not consider therapeutic abortion

Varicella: For immunosuppressed patients when varicella zoster immune globulin is not available

Unlabeled Use Acquired hypogammaglobulinemia secondary to malignancy; Guillain-Barré syndrome; hematopoietic stem cell transplantation (HSCT), to prevent bacterial infections among allogeneic recipients with severe hypogammaglobulinemia (IgG <400 mg/dL) at <100 days post transplant (CDC guidelines); HIV-associated thrombocytopenia; multiple sclerosis (relapsing, remitting when other therapies cannot be used); myasthenia gravis; refractory dermatomyositis/polymyositis

Pregnancy Risk Factor C

Pregnancy Considerations Reproduction studies have not been conducted. Immune globulins cross the placenta in increased amounts after 30 weeks gestation. Intravenous immune globulin has been recommended for use in fetal-neonatal alloimmune thrombocytopenia and pregnancy-associated ITP. May also be used in postexposure prophylaxis for rubella (within 72 hours) to reduce the risk of infection and fetal damage in exposed pregnant women who will not consider therapeutic abortion.

Lactation Excretion in breast milk unknown/use caution

Contraindications Hypersensitivity to immune globulin or any component of the formulation; selective IgA deficiency; hyperprolinemia (Hizentra®, Privigen®); severe thrombocytopenia or coagulation disorders; severe thrombocytopenia or coagulation disorders where IM injections are contraindicated

Warnings/Precautions [U.S. Boxed Warning]: I.V. formulation only: Acute renal dysfunction (increased serum creatinine, oliguria, acute renal failure, osmotic nephrosis) can rarely occur; usually within 7 days of use (more likely with products stabilized with sucrose). Use with caution in the elderly, patients with renal disease, diabetes mellitus, volume depletion, sepsis, paraproteinemia, and nephrotoxic medications due to risk of renal dysfunction. In patients at risk of renal dysfunction, the rate of infusion and concentration of solution should be minimized. Discontinue if renal function deteriorates. High-dose regimens (1 g/kg for 1-2 days) are not recommended for individuals with fluid overload or where fluid volume may be of concern. Hypersensitivity and anaphylactic reactions can occur; a severe fall in blood pressure may rarely occur with anaphylactic reaction; immediate treatment (including epinephrine 1:1000) should be available. Product of human plasma; may potentially contain infectious agents which could transmit disease. Screening of donors, as well as testing and/or inactivation or removal of certain viruses, reduces the risk. Infections thought to be transmitted by this product should be reported to the manufacturer. Aseptic meningitis may occur with high doses (≥1-2 g/kg [product-dependent]) and/or rapid infusion; syndrome usually appears within several hours to 2 days following treatment; usually resolves within several days after product is discontinued; patients with a migraine history may be at higher risk for AMS. Increased risk of hypersensitivity, especially in patients with anti-IgA antibodies. Increased risk of hematoma formation when administered subcutaneously for the treatment of ITP.

Intravenous immune globulin has been associated with antiglobulin hemolysis; monitor for signs of hemolytic anemia. Patients should be adequately hydrated prior to initiation of therapy. Hyperproteinemia, increased serum viscosity and hyponatremia may occur; distinguish hyponatremia from pseudohyponatremia to prevent volume depletion, a further increase in serum viscosity, and a higher risk of thrombotic events. Use caution in patients with a history of thrombotic events or a history of atherosclerosis or cardiovascular disease or patients with known/suspected hyperviscosity; there is clinical evidence of a possible association between thrombotic events and administration of intravenous immune globulin and subcutaneous immune globulin. Consider a baseline assessment of blood viscosity in patients at risk for hyperviscosity. Patients should be monitored for adverse events during and after the infusion. Stop administration with signs of infusion reaction (fever, chills, nausea, vomiting, and rarely shock). Risk may be increased with initial treatment, when switching brands of immune globulin, and with treatment interruptions of >8 weeks. Monitor for transfusion-related acute lung injury (TRALI); noncardiogenic pulmonary edema has been reported with intravenous immune globulin use. TRALI is characterized by severe respiratory distress, pulmonary edema, hypoxemia, and fever (in the presence of normal left ventricular function) and usually occurs within 1-6 hours after infusion. Response to live vaccinations may be impaired. Some clinicians may administer intravenous immune globulin products as a subcutaneous infusion based on patient tolerability and clinical judgment. SubQ infusion should begin 1 week after the last I.V. dose; dose should be individualized based on clinical response and serum IgG trough concentrations; consider premedicating with acetaminophen and diphenhydramine.

Some products may contain maltose, which may result in falsely-elevated blood glucose readings; maltose-containing products are contraindicated in patients with an allergy to corn. Some products may contain polysorbate 80, sodium, and/or sucrose. Some products may contain sorbitol; do not use in patients with fructose intolerance. Hizentra® and Privigen® contain the stabilizer L-proline and are contraindicated in patients with hyperprolinemia. Packaging of some products may contain natural latex/natural rubber; skin testing should not be performed with GamaSTAN™ S/D as local irritation can occur and be misinterpreted as a positive reaction.

Adverse Reactions Frequency not defined.

Cardiovascular: Angioedema, chest tightness, edema, flushing of the face, hyper-/hypotension, palpitation, tachycardia

Central nervous system: Anxiety, aseptic meningitis syndrome, chills, dizziness, drowsiness, fatigue, fever, headache, irritability, lethargy, lightheadedness, malaise, migraine, pain

Dermatologic: Bruising, contact dermatitis, eczema, erythema, hyperhidrosis, petechiae, pruritus, purpura, rash, urticaria

Gastrointestinal: Abdominal cramps, abdominal pain, diarrhea, discomfort, dyspepsia, gastroenteritis, nausea, sore throat, toothache, vomiting

Hematologic: Anemia, autoimmune hemolytic anemia, hematocrit decreased, hematoma, hemolysis (mild), hemorrhage, thrombocytopenia

Hepatic: Bilirubin increased, LDH increased, liver function test increased

Local: Muscle stiffness at I.M. site; pain, swelling, redness or irritation at the infusion site

Neuromuscular & skeletal: Arthralgia, back or hip pain, leg cramps, muscle cramps, myalgia, neck pain, rigors, weakness

Ocular: Conjunctivitis

Otic: Ear pain

Renal: Acute renal failure, acute tubular necrosis, anuria, BUN increased, creatinine increased, oliguria, proximal tubular nephropathy, osmotic nephrosis

Respiratory: Asthma aggravated, bronchitis, cough, dyspnea, epistaxis, nasal congestion, oropharyngeal pain, pharyngeal pain, pharyngitis, rhinitis, rhinorrhea, sinus headache, sinusitis, upper respiratory infection, wheezing

Miscellaneous: Anaphylaxis, diaphoresis, flu-like syndrome, hypersensitivity reactions, infusion reaction, thermal burn

Postmarketing and/or case reports: Apnea, ARDS, autoimmune pure red cell aplasia (PRCA) exacerbation, bronchopneumonia, bronchospasm, bullous dermatitis, cardiac arrest, chest pain, coma, Coombs' test positive, cyanosis, epidermolysis, erythema multiforme, hepatic dysfunction, hypoxemia, leukopenia, loss of consciousness, pancytopenia, papular rash, phlebitis, pulmonary edema, pulmonary embolism, seizures, Stevens-Johnson syndrome, thromboembolism, transfusion-related acute lung injury (TRALI), tremor, vascular collapse

Drug Interactions

Metabolism/Transport Effects None known.

Avoid Concomitant Use There are no known interactions where it is recommended to avoid concomitant use.

Increased Effect/Toxicity There are no known significant interactions involving an increase in effect.

Decreased Effect

Immune Globulin may decrease the levels/effects of: Vaccines (Live)

Stability Stability is dependent upon the manufacturer and brand. Do not freeze. Dilution is dependent upon the manufacturer and brand. Gently swirl; do not shake; avoid foaming. Do not mix products from different manufacturers together. Discard unused portion of vials.

Carimune® NF: Prior to reconstitution, store at or below 30°C (86°F). Reconstitute with NS, D_5W, or SWFI. Following reconstitution in a sterile laminar air flow environment, store under refrigeration. Begin infusion within 24 hours.

Flebogamma® DIF: Store at 2°C to 25°C (36°F to 77°F); do not freeze. Dilution is not recommended.

GamaSTAN™ S/D: Store under refrigeration at 2°C to 8°C (36°F to 46°F). The following stability information has also been reported for GamaSTAN™ S/D: May be exposed to room temperature for a cumulative 7 days (Cohen, 2007).

Gammagard® Liquid: May dilute in D_5W only. Prior to use, store at 2°C to 8°C (36°F to 46°F); do not freeze. May store at room temperature of 25°C (77°F) within the first 24 months of manufacturing. Storage time at room temperature varies with length of time previously refrigerated; refer to product labeling for details.

Gammagard S/D®: Store at ≤25°C (≤77°F). Reconstitute with SWFI; may store diluted solution under refrigeration at 2°C to 8°C (36°F to 46°F) for up to 24 hours if originally prepared in a sterile laminar air flow environment.

Gammaplex®: Store at 2°C to 25°C (36°F to 77°F); do not freeze. Protect from light.

Gamunex®, Gamunex®-C: Store at 2°C to 8°C (36°F to 46°F); may be stored at ≤25°C (≤77°F) for up to 6 months. Dilute in D_5W only.

Hizentra®: Store at ≤25°C (≤77°F); do not freeze or use product if previously frozen. Do not shake.

Octagam®: Store at 2°C to 25°C (36°F to 77°F).

Privigen®: Store at ≤25°C (≤77°F); do not freeze (do not use if previously frozen). Protect from light. If necessary to further dilute, D_5W may be used.

Vivaglobin®: Store at 2°C to 8°C (36°F to 46°F); do not freeze or use product if previously frozen. Do not shake.

Mechanism of Action Replacement therapy for primary and secondary immunodeficiencies, and IgG antibodies against bacteria, viral, parasitic and mycoplasma antigens; interference with F_c receptors on the cells of the reticuloendothelial system for autoimmune cytopenias and ITP; provides passive immunity by increasing the antibody titer and antigen-antibody reaction potential

Pharmacodynamics/Kinetics

Onset of action: I.V.: Provides immediate antibody levels

Duration: I.M., I.V.: Immune effect: 3-4 weeks (variable)

Distribution: V_d: 0.09-0.13 L/kg

Intravascular portion (primarily): Healthy subjects: 41% to 57%; Patients with congenital humoral immunodeficiencies: ~70%

Bioavailability: SubQ: Vivaglobin®: 73%

Half-life elimination: I.M.: ~23 days; I.V.: IgG (variable among patients): Healthy subjects: 14-24 days; Patients with congenital humoral immunodeficiencies: 26-40 days; hypermetabolism associated with fever and infection have coincided with a shortened half-life

Time to peak:

Plasma: SubQ: Gammagard® Liquid: 2.9 days; Hizentra®: 2.9 days; Vivaglobin®: 2.5 days

Serum: I.M.: ~48 hours

Dosage Note: Some clinicians may administer IVIG formulations FDA approved only for intravenous administration as a subcutaneous infusion based on clinical judgment and patient tolerability. Also, some clinicians dose IVIG on ideal body weight or an adjusted ideal body weight in morbidly-obese patients (Siegel, 2010).

Children and Adults:

B-cell chronic lymphocytic leukemia (CLL) (Gammagard S/D®): I.V.: 400 mg/kg every 3-4 weeks

Chronic inflammatory demyelinating polyneuropathy (CIDP) (Gamunex®, Gamunex-C®): I.V.: Loading dose: 2000 mg/kg (given in divided doses over 2-4 consecutive days); Maintenance: 1000 mg/kg every 3 weeks. Alternatively, administer 500 mg/kg/day for 2 consecutive days every 3 weeks.

Hepatitis A (GamaSTAN™ S/D): I.M.:

Pre-exposure prophylaxis upon travel into endemic areas (hepatitis A vaccine preferred):

0.02 mL/kg for anticipated risk of exposure <3 months

0.06 mL/kg for anticipated risk of exposure ≥3 months; repeat every 4-6 months.

Postexposure prophylaxis: 0.02 mL/kg given within 14 days of exposure and/or prior to manifestation of disease; not needed if at least 1 dose of hepatitis A vaccine was given at ≥1 month before exposure

Immunoglobulin deficiency (GamaSTAN™ S/D): I.M.: 0.66 mL/kg (minimum dose should be 100 mg/kg) every 3-4 weeks. Administer a double dose at onset of therapy; some patients may require more frequent injections.

Immune (idiopathic) thrombocytopenic purpura (ITP):

Carimune® NF: I.V.: Initial: 400 mg/kg/day for 2-5 days; Maintenance: 400 mg/kg as needed to maintain platelet count ≥30,000/mm^3 and/or to control significant bleeding; may increase dose if needed (range: 800-1000 mg/kg)

Gammagard S/D®: I.V.: 1000 mg/kg; up to 3 additional doses may be given based on patient response and/or platelet count. **Note:** Additional doses should be given on alternate days.

Gamunex®, Gamunex-C®: I.V.: 1000 mg/kg/day for 2 consecutive days (second dose may be withheld if adequate platelet response in 24 hours) **or** 400 mg/kg once daily for 5 consecutive days

Privigen®: I.V.: 1000 mg/kg/day for 2 consecutive days

Kawasaki syndrome: I.V.:

Gammagard S/D®: 1000 mg/kg as a single dose **or** 400 mg/kg/day for 4 consecutive days. Begin within 7 days of onset of fever.

AHA guidelines (2004): 2000 mg/kg as a single dose within 10 days of disease onset

Note: Must be used in combination with aspirin: 80-100 mg/kg/day orally, divided every 6 hours for up to 14 days (until fever resolves for at least 48 hours); then decrease dose to 3-5 mg/kg/day once daily. In patients without coronary artery abnormalities, give lower dose for 6-8 weeks. In patients with coronary artery abnormalities, low-dose aspirin should be continued indefinitely.

Measles:

GamaSTAN™ S/D: I.M.:

Immunocompetent: 0.25 mL/kg given within 6 days of exposure followed by live attenuated measles vaccine in 5-6 months when indicated (CDC, 1998)

Immunocompromised children: 0.5 mL/kg (maximum dose: 15 mL) immediately following exposure

Gamunex-C®, Octagam®: I.V.:

Prophylaxis in patients with primary humoral immunodeficiency (**ONLY** if routine dose is <400 mg/kg): ≥400 mg/kg immediately before expected exposure

Treatment in patients with primary immunodeficiency: 400 mg/kg administered as soon as possible after exposure

Hizentra®: SubQ infusion: Measles exposure in patients with primary humoral immunodeficiency: Weekly dose: ≥200 mg/kg for 2 consecutive weeks for patients at risk of measles exposure (eg, during an outbreak; travel to endemic area). In patients who have been exposed to measles, administer the minimum dose as soon as possible following exposure.

Primary humoral immunodeficiency disorders:

Carimune® NF: I.V.: 400-800 mg/kg every 3-4 weeks

Flebogamma® DIF, Gammagard® Liquid, Gammagard S/D®, Gamunex®, Gamunex-C®, Octagam®: I.V.: 300-600 mg/kg every 3-4 weeks; adjusted based on dosage and interval in conjunction with monitored serum IgG concentrations and clinical response

Gammaplex®: I.V.: 300-800 mg/kg every 3-4 weeks

Gammagard® Liquid, Gamunex-C®, Vivaglobin®: SubQ infusion: Begin 1 week after last I.V. dose. **Note:** Vivaglobin®: Patient should have received an I.V. immune globulin routinely for at least 3 months before switching to SubQ. Use the following equation to calculate initial dose:

Initial weekly dose (grams) = [1.37 x IGIV dose (grams)] divided by [I.V. dose interval (weeks)]

Note: For subsequent dose adjustments, refer to product labeling.

Hizentra®: SubQ infusion: Begin 1 week after last I.V. dose. **Note:** Patient should have received an I.V. immune globulin routinely for at least 3 months before switching to SubQ. Use the following equation to calculate initial dose:

Initial weekly dose (grams) = [1.53 x IGIV dose (grams)] divided by [I.V. dose interval (weeks)]

Note: For subsequent dose adjustments, refer to product labeling.

Privigen®: I.V.: 200-800 mg/kg every 3-4 weeks; adjusted based on dosage and interval in conjunction with monitored serum IgG concentrations and clinical response

Rubella (GamaSTAN™ S/D): I.M.: Prophylaxis during pregnancy: 0.55 mL/kg within 72 hours of exposure (CDC, 1998)

Varicella (GamaSTAN™ S/D): I.M.: Prophylaxis: 0.6-1.2 mL/kg (varicella zoster immune globulin preferred) within 72 hours of exposure

Unlabeled uses: I.V.:

Acquired hypogammaglobulinemia secondary to malignancy (unlabeled use): Adults: 400 mg/kg/dose every 3 weeks; reevaluate every 4-6 months (Anderson, 2007)

Guillain-Barré syndrome (unlabeled use): Children and Adults: Various regimens have been used, including:

400 mg/kg/day for 5 days (Hughes, 2003)

or

2000 mg/kg in divided doses administered over 2-5 days (Feasby, 2007)

Hematopoietic stem cell transplantation with hypogammaglobulinemia (CDC guidelines, 2000; unlabeled use):
Children: 400 mg/kg per month; increase dose or frequency to maintain IgG levels >400 mg/dL
Adolescents and Adults: 500 mg/kg/week
HIV-associated thrombocytopenia (unlabeled use): Adults: 1000 mg/kg/day for 2 days (Anderson, 2007)
Multiple sclerosis (relapsing-remitting, when other therapies cannot be used) (unlabeled use): Children and Adults: 1000 mg/kg per month, with or without an induction of 400 mg/kg/day for 5 days (Feasby, 2007)
Myasthenia gravis (severe exacerbation) (unlabeled use): Children and Adults: Total dose of 2000 mg/kg over 2-5 days (Feasby, 2007)
Refractory dermatomyositis/polymyositis (unlabeled uses): Children and Adults: 2000 mg/kg per treatment course administered over 2-5 days (Feasby, 2007)

Dosing adjustment/comments in renal impairment: I.V.: Cl_{cr} <10 mL/minute: Avoid use; in patients at risk of renal dysfunction, consider infusion at a rate less than maximum.

Dietary Considerations Some products may contain sodium.

Administration Note: If plasmapheresis employed for treatment of condition, administer immune globulin **after** completion of plasmapheresis session.

I.M.: Administer I.M. in the anterolateral aspects of the upper thigh or deltoid muscle of the upper arm. Avoid gluteal region due to risk of injury to sciatic nerve. Divide doses >10 mL and inject in multiple sites.
GamaSTAN™ S/D is for I.M. administration only.

I.V. infusion: Infuse over 2-24 hours; administer in separate infusion line from other medications; if using primary line, flush with saline prior to administration. Decrease dose, rate and/or concentration of infusion in patients who may be at risk of renal failure. Decreasing the rate or stopping the infusion may help relieve some adverse effects (flushing, changes in pulse rate, changes in blood pressure). Epinephrine should be available during administration. For initial treatment or in the elderly, a lower concentration and/or a slower rate of infusion should be used. Initial rate of administration and titration is specific to each IVIG product. Consult specific product prescribing information for detailed recommendations. Refrigerated product should be warmed to room temperature prior to infusion. Some products require filtration; refer to individual product labeling. Antecubital veins should be used, especially with concentrations ≥10% to prevent injection site discomfort.

SubQ infusion: Initial dose should be administered in a healthcare setting capable of providing monitoring and treatment in the event of hypersensitivity. Using aseptic technique, follow the infusion device manufacturer's instructions for filling the reservoir and preparing the pump. Remove air from administration set and needle by priming. Appropriate injection sites include the abdomen, thigh, upper arm, lower back, and/or lateral hip; dose may be infused into multiple sites (spaced ≥2 inches apart) simultaneously. After the sites are clean and dry, insert subcutaneous needle and prime administration set. Attach sterile needle to administration set, gently pull back on the syringe to assure a blood vessel has not been inadvertently accessed (do not use needle and tubing if blood present). Repeat for each injection site; deliver the dose following instructions for the infusion device. Rotate the site(s) weekly. Treatment may be transitioned to the home/home care setting in the absence of adverse reactions.

Gammagard® Liquid:
Injection sites: ≤8 simultaneous injection sites
Initial infusion rate:
<40 kg: 15 mL/hour per injection site (maximum volume: 20 mL per injection site)
≥40 kg: 20 mL/hour per injection site (maximum volume: 30 mL per injection site)
Maintenance infusion rate:
<40 kg: 15-20 mL/hour per injection site (maximum volume: 20 mL per injection site)
≥40 kg: 20-30 mL/hour per injection site (maximum volume: 30 mL per injection site)

Gamunex-C®:
Injection sites: ≤8 simultaneous injection sites
Recommended infusion rate: 20 mL/hour per injection site

Hizentra®:
Injection sites: ≤4 simultaneous injection sites
Maximum infusion rate: First infusion: 15 mL/hour per injection site; subsequent infusions: 25 mL/hour per injection site (maximum: 50 mL/hour for all simultaneous sites combined)
Maximum infusion volume: First 4 infusions: 15 mL per injection site; subsequent infusions: 20 mL per injection site (maximum: 25 mL per site as tolerated)

Vivaglobin®:
Injection sites: Children <45 kg: ≤3 simultaneous injection sites; Adults ≤65 years: ≤6 simultaneous injection sites; Adults >65 years: ≤4 simultaneous injection sites
Maximum infusion rate: 20 mL/hour per injection site (maximum: 3 mg/kg/minute [1.13 mL/kg/hour] for all simultaneous sites combined)
Maximum infusion volume: 15 mL per injection site

Monitoring Parameters Renal function, urine output, IgG concentrations, hemoglobin and hematocrit, platelets (in patients with ITP); infusion- or injection-related adverse reactions, anaphylaxis, signs and symptoms of hemolysis; blood viscosity (in patients at risk for hyperviscosity); presence of antineutrophil antibodies (if TRALI is suspected); volume status; neurologic symptoms (if AMS suspected); clinical response

SubQ infusion: Monitor IgG trough levels every 2-3 months before/after conversion from I.V.; subcutaneous infusions provide more constant IgG levels than usual I.V. immune globulin treatments.

Test Interactions Octagam® contains maltose. Falsely-elevated blood glucose levels may occur when glucose monitoring devices and test strips utilizing the glucose dehydrogenase pyrroloquinolinequinone (GDH-PQQ) based methods are used. Glucose monitoring devices and test strips which utilize the glucose-specific method are recommended. Passively-transferred antibodies may yield false-positive serologic testing results; may yield false-positive direct and indirect Coombs' test. Skin testing should not be performed with GamaSTAN™ S/D as local irritation can occur and be misinterpreted as a positive reaction.

Additional Information I.M.: When administering immune globulin for hepatitis A prophylaxis, use should be considered for the following close contacts of persons with confirmed hepatitis A: unvaccinated household and sexual contacts, persons who have shared illicit drugs, regular babysitters, staff and attendees of child care centers, food handlers within the same establishment (CDC, 2006).

All household contacts of measles patients should be evaluated to receive immune globulin unless the measles vaccine has been given on or after the first birthday, unless immunocompromised (CDC, 1998).

For travelers, immune globulin is not an alternative to careful selection of foods and water; immune globulin can interfere with the antibody response to parenterally administered live virus vaccines. Frequent travelers should be tested for hepatitis A antibody, immune hemolytic anemia, and neutropenia (with ITP, I.V. route is usually used).

IgA content:
Carimune® NF: 720 mcg/mL
Flebogamma® 5% DIF: 2.9 ± 0.1 mcg/mL
Flebogamma® 10% DIF: <100 mcg/mL
Gammagard® Liquid: 37 mcg/mL
Gammagard S/D® 5% solution: <1 mcg/mL or <2.2 mcg/mL(product dependent)
Gammaplex®: <10 mcg/mL
Gamunex-C®: 46 mcg/mL
Hizentra®: ≤50 mcg/mL
Octagam®: ≤200 mcg/mL
Privigen®: ≤25 mcg/mL
Vivaglobin®: ≤1700 mcg/mL

Dosage Forms Excipient information presented when available (limited, particularly for generics); consult specific product labeling. [DSC] = Discontinued product

Injection, powder for reconstitution [preservative free]:
Carimune® NF: 3 g, 6 g, 12 g [contains sucrose]
Gammagard S/D®: 2.5 g [contains albumin (human), glucose, glycine, natural rubber/natural latex in packaging, polyethylene glycol, polysorbate 80; IgA <2.2 mcg/mL]
Gammagard S/D®: 5 g [contains albumin (human), glucose, glycine, natural rubber/natural latex in packaging, polyethylene glycol, polysorbate 80; IgA <1 mcg/mL]
Gammagard S/D®: 5 g [contains albumin (human), glucose, glycine, natural rubber/natural latex in packaging, polyethylene glycol, polysorbate 80; IgA <2.2 mcg/mL]
Gammagard S/D®: 10 g [contains albumin (human), glucose, glycine, natural rubber/natural latex in packaging, polyethylene glycol, polysorbate 80; IgA <1 mcg/mL]
Gammagard S/D®: 10 g [contains albumin (human), glucose, glycine, natural rubber/natural latex in packaging, polyethylene glycol, polysorbate 80; IgA <2.2 mcg/mL]

Injection, solution [preservative free]:
Flebogamma® DIF: 5% [50 mg/mL] (10 mL, 50 mL, 100 mL, 200 mL, 400 mL); 10% [100 mg/mL] (100 mL, 200 mL) [contains polyethylene glycol, sorbitol]
GamaSTAN™ S/D: 15% to 18% [150 to 180 mg/mL] (2 mL, 10 mL)
Gammagard® Liquid: 10% [100 mg/mL] (10 mL, 25 mL, 50 mL, 100 mL, 200 mL) [sucrose free; contains glycine]
Gammaked™: 10% [100 mg/mL] (10 mL, 25 mL, 50 mL, 100 mL, 200 mL) [sucrose free; contains glycine]
Gammaplex®: 5% [50 mg/mL] (50 mL, 100 mL, 200 mL) [sucrose free; contains glycine, natural rubber/natural latex in packaging, polysorbate 80, sorbitol]
Gamunex®: 10% [100 mg/mL] (10 mL [DSC], 25 mL [DSC], 50 mL [DSC], 100 mL [DSC], 200 mL [DSC]) [contains glycine]
Gamunex®-C: 10% [100 mg/mL] (10 mL, 25 mL, 50 mL, 100 mL, 200 mL) [contains glycine]
Hizentra®: 200 mg/mL (5 mL, 10 mL, 20 mL) [contains L-proline, polysorbate 80]
Octagam®: 5% [50 mg/mL] (20 mL, 50 mL, 100 mL, 200 mL) [sucrose free; contains maltose, sodium 30 mmol/L]
Privigen®: 10% [100 mg/mL] (50 mL, 100 mL, 200 mL) [sucrose free; contains L-proline]
Vivaglobin®: 160 mg/mL (3 mL [DSC], 10 mL [DSC], 20 mL [DSC])

◆ **Immune Globulin Subcutaneous (Human)** *see* Immune Globulin *on page 880*

◆ **Immune Serum Globulin** *see* Immune Globulin *on page 880*

◆ **Immunine® VH (Can)** *see* Factor IX *on page 683*

◆ **Imodium® (Can)** *see* Loperamide *on page 1026*

◆ **Imodium® A-D [OTC]** *see* Loperamide *on page 1026*

◆ **Imodium® A-D for children [OTC]** *see* Loperamide *on page 1026*

◆ **Imodium® Advanced Multi-Symptom (Can)** *see* Loperamide and Simethicone *on page 1027*

◆ **Imodium® Multi-Symptom Relief [OTC]** *see* Loperamide and Simethicone *on page 1027*

◆ **Imogam® Rabies-HT** *see* Rabies Immune Globulin (Human) *on page 1453*

◆ **Imogam® Rabies Pasteurized (Can)** *see* Rabies Immune Globulin (Human) *on page 1453*

◆ **Imovax® Polio (Can)** *see* Poliovirus Vaccine (Inactivated) *on page 1370*

◆ **Imovax® Rabies** *see* Rabies Vaccine *on page 1453*

◆ **Imuran®** *see* AzaTHIOprine *on page 176*

◆ **In-111 Ibritumomab** *see* Ibritumomab *on page 857*

◆ **In-111 Zevalin** *see* Ibritumomab *on page 857*

Inamrinone (eye NAM ri none)

Index Terms Amrinone Lactate

Pharmacologic Category Phosphodiesterase Enzyme Inhibitor

Use Short-term therapy in patients with intractable heart failure

Pregnancy Risk Factor C

Dosage Dosage is based on clinical response (**Note:** Dose should not exceed 10 mg/kg/24 hours).

Infants (unlabeled population), Children (unlabeled population), and Adults: 0.75 mg/kg I.V. bolus over 2-3 minutes followed by maintenance infusion of 5-10 mcg/kg/minute; I.V. bolus may need to be repeated in 30 minutes.

Dosing adjustment in renal failure:
Infants and Children:
Cl_{cr} 30-50 mL/minute: Administer 100% of dose
Cl_{cr} 10-29 mL/minute: Administer 50% of dose
Cl_{cr} <10 mL/minute: Administer 25% of dose
Intermittent hemodialysis or peritoneal dialysis: Administer 25% of dose
Adults:
Cl_{cr} ≥10 mL/minute: Administer 100% of dose
Cl_{cr} <10 mL/minute: Administer 50% to 75% of dose

Additional Information Complete prescribing information for this medication should be consulted for additional detail.

Dosage Forms Excipient information presented when available (limited, particularly for generics); consult specific product labeling. [DSC] = Discontinued product

Injection, solution: 5 mg/mL (20 mL [DSC])

◆ **INCB 18424** *see* Ruxolitinib *on page 1530*

◆ **Incivek™** *see* Telaprevir *on page 1631*

IncobotulinumtoxinA
(in kuh BOT yoo lin num TOKS in aye)

Brand Names: U.S. Xeomin®

Brand Names: Canada Xeomin®

Index Terms Botulinum Toxin Type A

Pharmacologic Category Neuromuscular Blocker Agent, Toxin; Ophthalmic Agent, Toxin

Use Treatment of blepharospasm in patients previously treated with onabotulinumtoxinA (Botox®); treatment of cervical dystonia in botulinum toxin-naïve and previously treated patients; temporary improvement in the appearance of moderate-to-severe glabellar lines associated with corrugator and/or procerus muscle activity

Canadian labeling: Treatment of hypertonicity disorders of the seventh nerve (eg, blepharospasm, hemifacial spasm); treatment of poststroke spasticity of upper limb(s); treatment of cervical dystonia (spasmodic torticollis)

Pregnancy Risk Factor C

Medication Guide Available Yes

Dosage I.M.: Adults:

Blepharospasm:

U.S. labeling: Initial: Total dose should be the same as previously administered onabotulinumtoxinA dose. If prior onabotulinumtoxinA dose is not known: 1.25-2.5 units/injection site (maximum initial dose: 35 units/eye or 70 units/both eyes). Number and location of injection sites based on disease severity and previous dose/response to onabotulinumtoxinA (in clinical trials, a mean number of 6 injections per eye were administered). Cumulative dose should not exceed 35 units/eye or 70 units/both eyes administered no more frequently than every 3 months.

Canadian labeling: Initial: 1.25-2.5 units/injection site (maximum initial dose: 25 units/eye). Dose may be increased up to twice the previous dose if the response from the initial dose lasted ≤2 months; maximum dose per site: 5 units. Cumulative dose should not exceed 35 units/eye or 70 units/both eyes administered no more frequently than every 3 months.

Cervical dystonia:

U.S. labeling: Initial total dose: 120 units (in clinical trials, similar efficacy was noted with initial total doses of 120 and 240 units and between treatment experienced and treatment naïve patients). Dose and number of injection sites should be individualized based on prior treatment, response, duration of effect, adverse events, number/location of muscle(s) to be treated and disease severity. In clinical trials most patients received a total of 2-10 injections into treated muscles. Administer no more frequently than every 3 months

Canadian labeling: Usual total dose: 200 units (maximum: 300 units; maximum dose per injection site: 50 units); administer no more frequently than every 3 months

Reduction of glabellar lines: Inject 4 units into each of the 5 sites (2 injections in each corrugator muscle and 1 injection in the procerus muscle) for a total dose of 20 units per treatment session. Administer no more frequently than every 3 months.

Spasticity of upper limb (poststroke): Canadian labeling (not in U.S. labeling): Individualize dose based on patient size, extent, and location of muscle involvement, degree of spasticity, local muscle weakness, and response to prior treatment. In clinical trials, total doses up to 400 units were administered as separate injections typically divided among selected muscles; may repeat therapy at ≥3 months with appropriate dosage based upon the clinical condition of patient at time of retreatment.

Suggested guidelines for the treatment of stroke-related upper limb spasticity: Note: The lowest recommended starting dose should be used. Dosage and number of injection sites should be individualized. Multiple injections may minimize adverse effects. Dose listed is total dose administered to site:

Biceps: 80 units
Brachialis: 50 units
Brachioradialis: 60 units
Flexor carpi radialis: 50 units
Flexor carpi ulnaris: 40 units
Flexor digitorum profundus: 40 units
Flexor digitorum superficialis: 40 units
Adductor pollicis: 10 units
Flexor pollicis brevis: 10 units
Flexor pollicis longus: 20 units
Pronator quadratus 25 units
Pronator teres: 40 units

Elderly: Initiate therapy at lowest recommended dose and titrate upward cautiously.

Dosage adjustment in renal impairment: There are no dosage adjustments provided in manufacturer's labeling.

Dosage adjustment in hepatic impairment: There are no dosage adjustments provided in manufacturer's labeling.

Additional Information Complete prescribing information for this medication should be consulted for additional detail.

Dosage Forms Excipient information presented when available (limited, particularly for generics); consult specific product labeling.

Injection, powder for reconstitution:

Xeomin®: 50 units, 100 units [contains albumin (human), sucrose 4.7 mg]

Indacaterol (in da KA ter ol)

Index Terms Arcapta™ Neohaler™; Indacaterol Maleate; OnBrez Breezehaler; QAB149

Pharmacologic Category $Beta_2$-Adrenergic Agonist; $Beta_2$-Adrenergic Agonist, Long-Acting

Use Long-term maintenance treatment of airflow obstruction in chronic obstructive pulmonary disease (COPD) including chronic bronchitis and/or emphysema

Pregnancy Risk Factor C

Pregnancy Considerations Adverse events were not observed in animal reproduction studies. Beta agonists may interfere with uterine contractility if administered during labor.

Lactation Excretion unknown/use caution

Medication Guide Available Yes

Contraindications Monotherapy in the treatment of asthma (ie, use without a concomitant long-term asthma control medication, such as an inhaled corticosteroid). **Note:** Indacaterol is not FDA approved for treatment of asthma.

Warnings/Precautions Asthma-related deaths: **[U.S. Boxed Warning]: Long-acting $beta_2$-agonists (LABAs) increase the risk of asthma-related deaths. Indacaterol is not indicated for treatment of asthma and should not be used.** In a large, randomized, placebo-controlled U.S. clinical trial (SMART, 2006), salmeterol was associated with an increase in asthma-related deaths (when added to usual asthma therapy); risk is considered a class effect among all LABAs. It is unknown if indacaterol increases asthma-related deaths. Do not use for acutely deteriorating COPD or as rescue therapy in acute episodes. Short-acting $beta_2$-agonists (eg, albuterol) should be used for acute symptoms and symptoms occurring between treatments. If deterioration develops, prompt evaluation of the COPD regimen is warranted. Do not increase the dose or frequency of indacaterol. Data are not available to determine if LABA use increases the risk of death in patients with COPD. Do not use more than once daily or at a higher dose than indicated; do not combine use with other long-acting $beta_2$-agonists. Deaths and significant cardiovascular effects have been reported with excessive sympathomimetic use. Rarely, paradoxical bronchospasm may occur with use of inhaled bronchodilators; this should be distinguished from inadequate response.

Use caution in patients with cardiovascular disease (eg, arrhythmias, coronary insufficiency, hypertension), diabetes mellitus, hyperthyroidism, seizure disorders, or hypokalemia. Beta-agonists may cause elevation in blood pressure, heart rate, CNS stimulation/excitation, increased risk of arrhythmia, increase serum glucose, or decrease serum potassium.

Adverse Reactions

>10%: Respiratory: Cough (post inhalation 7% to 24%)

1% to 10%:

Central nervous system: Headache (5%)

Gastrointestinal: Nausea (2%)

Respiratory: Nasopharyngitis (5%), oropharyngeal pain (2%)

<1% (Limited to important or life-threatening): Dizziness, palpitation, pruritus, rash, tachycardia

Drug Interactions

Metabolism/Transport Effects Substrate of CYP2D6 (minor), CYP3A4 (minor), P-glycoprotein, UGT1A1; **Note:** Assignment of Major/Minor substrate status based on clinically relevant drug interaction potential

Avoid Concomitant Use

Avoid concomitant use of Indacaterol with any of the following: Beta-Blockers (Nonselective); Iobenguane I 123

Increased Effect/Toxicity

Indacaterol may increase the levels/effects of: Corticosteroids (Systemic); Loop Diuretics; QTc-Prolonging Agents; Sympathomimetics; Thiazide Diuretics

The levels/effects of Indacaterol may be increased by: Atomoxetine; Caffeine; Cannabinoids; Conivaptan; MAO Inhibitors; Theophylline Derivatives; Tricyclic Antidepressants

Decreased Effect

Indacaterol may decrease the levels/effects of: Iobenguane I 123

The levels/effects of Indacaterol may be decreased by: Alpha-/Beta-Blockers; Beta-Blockers (Beta1 Selective); Beta-Blockers (Nonselective); Betahistine; Peginterferon Alfa-2b; Tocilizumab

Stability Store capsules at controlled room temperature of 25°C (77°F); excursions permitted to 15°C to 30°C (59°F to 86°F). Protect from direct sunlight and moisture. Remove from blister pack immediately before use; discard capsule if not used immediately.

Mechanism of Action Relaxes bronchial smooth muscle by selective action on beta$_2$-receptors with little effect on heart rate; acts locally in the lung.

Pharmacodynamics/Kinetics

Onset of action: 5 minutes

Peak effect: 1-4 hours

Duration: 24 hours

Absorption: Systemic: Inhalation: 43% to 45% bioavailable

Protein binding: ~95%

Metabolism: Hepatic; hydroxylated via CYP3A4, CYP2D6, and CYP1A1

Half-life elimination: 40-56 hours

Time to peak, serum: ~15 minutes

Excretion: Feces (>90%; 54% as unchanged drug [after oral administration]); urine (<2% as unchanged drug)

Dosage Inhalation: Adults: COPD (maintenance): One inhalation (75 mcg/inhalation) once daily; maximum: 1 inhalation once daily. **Note:** A dose of 150-300 mcg once daily is recommended by the 2010 Updated GOLD Guidelines; the 2010 update was published prior to the FDA approval of the 75 mcg dose.

Dosage adjustment in renal impairment: No dosage adjustment is required for geriatric patients, patients with mild and moderate hepatic impairment, or renally-impaired patients.

Dosage adjustment in hepatic impairment: No data is available for subjects with severe hepatic impairment.

Administration Inhalation: **For inhalation using Neohaler™ inhaler only.** Do **not** swallow indacaterol capsules. Use the new inhaler included with each prescription. Do not remove capsules from blister until immediately before use. Use at the same time each day. Not to be used for the relief of acute attacks. Not for use with a spacer device. Do not wash mouthpiece; Neohaler™ should be kept dry. Discard any capsules that are exposed to air and not used immediately.

Monitoring Parameters FEV$_1$, FVC, and/or other pulmonary function tests; serum potassium, serum glucose; blood pressure, heart rate; CNS stimulation. Monitor for increased use of short-acting beta$_2$-agonist inhalers; may be marker of a deteriorating condition. Monitor for changes in risk factors (eg, environmental exposure, smoking status).

Additional Information In November 2009, the European Medicines Agency approved indacaterol (Onbrez® Breezhaler®) at a dose of 150-300 mcg/day. Indacaterol at this dose, along with other long acting bronchodilators, is recommended by the 2010 Updated GOLD guidelines for maintenance treatment of moderate to very severe COPD. In reviewing the available data, the FDA concluded that the benefit of higher dosing (ie, >75 mcg/day) was not justified due to lack of additional benefit seen at the end of 2 weeks and a higher incidence of adverse reactions.

Product Availability Arcapta™ Neohaler™: FDA approved July 2011; expected availability first quarter 2012; consult prescribing information for additional information

◆ **Indacaterol Maleate** *see* Indacaterol *on page* 885

Indapamide (in DAP a mide)

Brand Names: Canada Apo-Indapamide®; Dom-Indapamide; Indapamide Hemihydrate; JAMP-Indapamide; Lozide®; Mylan-Indapamide; Novo-Indapamide; Nu-Indapamide; PHL-Indapamide; PMS-Indapamide; PRO-Indapamide; Riva-Indapamide

Pharmacologic Category Diuretic, Thiazide-Related

Use Management of mild-to-moderate hypertension; treatment of edema in heart failure

Unlabeled Use Nephrotic syndrome (Tanaka, 2005)

Pregnancy Risk Factor B

Pregnancy Considerations Adverse events were not observed in animal reproduction studies. Diuretics cross the placenta and are found in cord blood. Maternal use may cause may cause fetal or neonatal jaundice, thrombocytopenia, or other adverse events observed in adults. Use of diuretics during normal pregnancies is not appropriate; use may be considered when edema is due to pathologic causes (as in the nonpregnant patient); monitor.

Lactation Excretion in breast milk unknown/not recommended

Contraindications Hypersensitivity to indapamide or any component of the formulation or sulfonamide-derived drugs; anuria

Canadian labeling: Additional contraindications (not in U.S. labeling): Severe renal failure (Cl_{cr} <30 mL/minute); hepatic encephalopathy; severe hepatic impairment; hypokalemia; concomitant use with nonantiarrhythmic agents causing torsade de pointes; breast-feeding

Warnings/Precautions Use with caution in severe renal disease; Canadian labeling contraindicates use in severe renal failure (Cl_{cr} <30 mL/minute). Electrolyte disturbances including severe hyponatremia (with hypokalemia, hypochloremic alkalosis, hypomagnesemia, or hypercalcemia) can occur; risk may be dose dependent. Correct hypokalemia before initiating therapy (Canadian labeling contraindicates use in hypokalemia). Use with caution in severe hepatic dysfunction; hepatic encephalopathy can be caused by electrolyte disturbances (Canadian labeling contraindicates use in severe hepatic impairment or hepatic encephalopathy). Gout may be precipitated in certain patients with a history of gout, a familial predisposition to gout, or chronic renal failure. Use caution in patients with prediabetes or diabetes; may alter glucose control. May cause SLE exacerbation or activation. Use with caution in patients with moderate or high cholesterol concentrations. Photosensitization may occur.

Chemical similarities are present among sulfonamides, sulfonylureas, carbonic anhydrase inhibitors, thiazides, and loop diuretics (except ethacrynic acid). Use in patients with sulfonamide allergy is specifically contraindicated in product labeling, however, a risk of cross-reaction exists in patients with allergy to any of these compounds; avoid use when previous reaction has been severe. Discontinue if signs of hypersensitivity are noted. Formulation may contain lactose; Canadian labeling recommends avoiding use in patients with hereditary conditions of galactose intolerance, glucose-galactose malabsorption, or lactase deficiency.

Adverse Reactions

≥5%:

Central nervous system: Agitation, anxiety, dizziness, fatigue, headache, irritability, lethargy, malaise, nervousness (dose dependent), pain, tension, tiredness

Endocrine & metabolic: Hypokalemia (<3.5 mEq/L: 20% to 72%, dose dependent)

Neuromuscular & skeletal: Back pain, muscle cramps/spasm, paresthesia, weakness

Respiratory: Rhinitis

Miscellaneous: Infection

≥1% to <5%:

Cardiovascular: Arrhythmia, chest pain, flushing, orthostatic hypotension, palpitation, peripheral edema, PVC, vasculitis

Central nervous system: Depression, drowsiness, insomnia, lightheadedness, vertigo

Dermatologic: Hives, pruritus, rash

Endocrine & metabolic: Hyperglycemia, hyperuricemia, hypochloremia, hyponatremia, libido decreased

Gastrointestinal: Abdominal pain, anorexia, constipation, cramping, diarrhea, dyspepsia, gastric irritation, nausea, vomiting, weight loss, xerostomia

Genitourinary: Nocturia, polyuria

Neuromuscular & skeletal: Hypertonia

Ocular: Blurred vision, conjunctivitis

Renal: BUN increased, creatinine increased, glycosuria

Respiratory: Cough, pharyngitis, rhinorrhea, sinusitis

Miscellaneous: Flu-like syndrome

<1% (Limited to important or life-threatening): Agranulocytosis, anaphylactic reaction, aplastic anemia, bullous eruptions, erythema multiforme, fever, hepatitis, hypercalcemia, jaundice (cholestatic jaundice), leukopenia, liver function test abnormality, pancreatitis, photosensitivity, pneumonitis, purpura, Stevens-Johnson syndrome, thrombocytopenia, torsade de pointes

Drug Interactions

Metabolism/Transport Effects None known.

Avoid Concomitant Use

Avoid concomitant use of Indapamide with any of the following: Artemether; Dofetilide; Dronedarone; Lumefantrine; Nilotinib; Pimozide; QUEtiapine; QuiNINE; Tetrabenazine; Thioridazine; Toremifene; Vandetanib; Vemurafenib; Ziprasidone

Increased Effect/Toxicity

Indapamide may increase the levels/effects of: ACE Inhibitors; Allopurinol; Amifostine; Antihypertensives; Calcium Salts; CarBAMazepine; Dofetilide; Dronedarone; Hypotensive Agents; Lithium; OXcarbazepine; Pimozide; Porfimer; QTc-Prolonging Agents; QuiNINE; RiTUXimab; Sodium Phosphates; Tetrabenazine; Thioridazine; Topiramate; Toremifene; Vandetanib; Vemurafenib; Vitamin D Analogs; Ziprasidone

The levels/effects of Indapamide may be increased by: Alcohol (Ethyl); Alfuzosin; Analgesics (Opioid); Artemether; Barbiturates; Beta2-Agonists; Chloroquine; Ciprofloxacin; Ciprofloxacin (Systemic); Corticosteroids (Orally Inhaled); Corticosteroids (Systemic); Gadobutrol; Herbs (Hypotensive Properties); Indacaterol; Licorice; Lumefantrine; MAO Inhibitors; Nilotinib; Pentoxifylline; Phosphodiesterase 5 Inhibitors; Prostacyclin Analogues; QUEtiapine; QuiNINE

Decreased Effect

Indapamide may decrease the levels/effects of: Antidiabetic Agents

The levels/effects of Indapamide may be decreased by: Bile Acid Sequestrants; Herbs (Hypertensive Properties); Methylphenidate; Nonsteroidal Anti-Inflammatory Agents; Yohimbine

Ethanol/Nutrition/Herb Interactions Herb/Nutraceutical: Avoid herbs with *hypertensive* properties (bayberry, blue cohosh, cayenne, ephedra, ginger, ginseng [American], kola, licorice); may diminish the antihypertensive effect of indapamide. Avoid herbs with *hypotensive* properties (black cohosh, California poppy, coleus, golden seal, hawthorn, mistletoe, periwinkle, quinine, shepherd's purse); may enhance the hypotensive effect of indapamide.

Stability Store at 20°C to 25°C (68°F to 77°F).

Mechanism of Action Diuretic effect is localized at the proximal segment of the distal tubule of the nephron; it does not appear to have significant effect on glomerular filtration rate nor renal blood flow; like other diuretics, it enhances sodium, chloride, and water excretion by interfering with the transport of sodium ions across the renal tubular epithelium

Pharmacodynamics/Kinetics

Absorption: Rapid and complete

Distribution: V_d: 25 L (Grebow, 1982)

Protein binding, plasma: 71% to 79%

Metabolism: Extensively hepatic

Bioavailability: 93% (Ernst, 2009)

Half-life elimination: Biphasic: 14 and 25 hours

Time to peak: 2 hours

Excretion: Urine (~70%; 7% as unchanged drug within 48 hours); feces (23%)

Dosage Adults: Oral:

Edema: Initial: 2.5 mg/day; if inadequate response after 1 week, may increase dose to 5 mg/day. **Note:** There is little therapeutic benefit to increasing the dose >5 mg/day; there is, however, an increased risk of electrolyte disturbances

Hypertension: Initial: 1.25 mg/day; if inadequate response, may increase dose once every 4 weeks to 2.5 mg/day and then to 5 mg/day if needed. Consider adding another antihypertensive and decreasing the dose if response is not adequate. **Note:** Canadian labeling recommends a maximum dose of 2.5 mg/day.

Dietary Considerations May be taken without regard to meals (Caruso, 1983); however, administration with food or milk may to decrease GI adverse effects.

Administration May be administered without regard to meals (Caruso, 1983); however, administration with food or milk may to decrease GI adverse effects. Administer early in day to avoid nocturia.

Monitoring Parameters Blood pressure (both standing and sitting/supine); serum electrolytes, hepatic function, renal function, uric acid; assess weight, I & O reports daily to determine fluid loss

Dosage Forms Excipient information presented when available (limited, particularly for generics); consult specific product labeling.

Tablet, oral: 1.25 mg, 2.5 mg

- ◆ **Indapamide Hemihydrate (Can)** *see* Indapamide *on page 886*
- ◆ **Inderal® (Can)** *see* Propranolol *on page 1424*
- ◆ **Inderal® LA** *see* Propranolol *on page 1424*

Indinavir (in DIN a veer)

Brand Names: U.S. Crixivan®

Brand Names: Canada Crixivan®

Index Terms Indinavir Sulfate

Pharmacologic Category Antiretroviral Agent, Protease Inhibitor

Additional Appendix Information

Management of Healthcare Worker Exposures to HBV, HCV, and HIV *on page 1935*

Perinatal HIV Guidelines *on page 1946*

Use Treatment of HIV infection; should always be used as part of a multidrug regimen (at least three antiretroviral agents)

Pregnancy Risk Factor C

Pregnancy Considerations Adverse events were observed in some animal reproduction studies. Placental passage in humans is minimal. No increased risk of overall birth defects has been observed according to data collected by the antiretroviral pregnancy registry. A small increased risk of preterm birth has been associated with maternal use of protease inhibitor-based combination antiretroviral (ARV) therapy during pregnancy; however, the benefits of use generally outweigh this risk and protease inhibitors (PIs) should not be withheld if otherwise recommended. Hyperglycemia, new onset of diabetes mellitus, or diabetic ketoacidosis have been reported with PIs; it is not clear if pregnancy increases this risk. Hyperbilirubinemia may occur in neonates following *in utero* exposure to indinavir. Plasma levels of indinavir were 74% lower at weeks 30-32 of gestation when compared to the same women at 14-28 weeks of gestation in one study. Plasma levels were not measurable in some patients 8 hours post dose. Until optimal dosing during pregnancy has been established, the manufacturer does not recommend indinavir use in pregnant patients. The DHHS Perinatal HIV Guidelines consider indinavir an alternative agent if preferred and alternative agents cannot be used; however, if needed, indinavir should be used in combination with low-dose ritonavir during pregnancy (with ritonavir boosting, 82% of pregnant women reached target trough concentrations).

Regardless of CD4 count or HIV RNA copy number, all HIV-infected pregnant women should receive a combination antepartum ARV drug regimen; this includes women who require therapy for their own health, as well as women who do not yet require therapy for their own health. ARV therapy should be started as soon as possible if required for the woman's health or immediately after the first trimester if not needed for the mothers health (although earlier initiation may be considered). Long-term follow-up is recommended for all infants exposed to ARV medications.

Healthcare providers are encouraged to enroll pregnant women exposed to antiretroviral medications in the Antiretroviral Pregnancy Registry (1-800-258-4263 or www.-APRegistry.com). Healthcare providers caring for HIV-infected women and their infants may contact the National Perinatal HIV Hotline (888-448-8765) for clinical consultation (DHHS [perinatal], 2011).

Lactation Excretion in breast milk unknown/contraindicated

Contraindications Hypersensitivity to indinavir or any component of the formulation; concurrent use of alfuzosin, alprazolam, amiodarone, cisapride, triazolam, midazolam (oral), pimozide, or ergot alkaloids; sildenafil (when used for pulmonary artery hypertension [eg, Revatio®]), simvastatin, St John's wort, or triazolam

Warnings/Precautions Because indinavir may cause nephrolithiasis/urolithiasis the drug should be discontinued if signs and symptoms occur. Adequate hydration is recommended. May cause tubulointerstitial nephritis (rare); severe asymptomatic leukocyturia may warrant evaluation. Use with caution in patients taking strong CYP3A4 inhibitors, moderate or strong CYP3A4 inducers and major CYP3A4 substrates (see Drug Interactions); consider alternative agents that avoid or lessen the potential for CYP-mediated interactions. Do not coadminister colchicine in patient with renal or hepatic impairment; avoid concurrent use with salmeterol.

Patients with hepatic insufficiency due to cirrhosis should have dose reduction. Warn patients about fat redistribution that can occur. Indinavir has been associated with hemolytic anemia (discontinue if diagnosed), hepatitis, hyperbilirubinemia, and hyperglycemia (exacerbation or new-onset diabetes). Treatment may result in immune reconstitution syndrome (acute inflammatory response to indolent or residual opportunistic infections). Use caution in patients with hemophilia; spontaneous bleeding has been reported.

Adverse Reactions

>10%:

Gastrointestinal: Abdominal pain (17%), nausea (12%)

Hepatic: Hyperbilirubinemia (14%; dose dependent)

Renal: Nephrolithiasis/urolithiasis, including flank pain with/without hematuria (29%, pediatric patients; 12% adult patients; dose dependent)

1% to 10%:

Central nervous system: Headache (5%), dizziness (3%), somnolence (2%), fever (2%), malaise (2%), fatigue (2%)

Dermatologic: Pruritus (4%), rash (1%)

Endocrine & metabolic: Hyperglycemia (1%)

Gastrointestinal: Vomiting (8%), diarrhea (3%), taste perversion (3%), acid reflux (3%), anorexia (3%), appetite increased (2%), dyspepsia (2%), serum amylase increased (2%)

Hematologic: Neutropenia (2%), anemia (1%), thrombocytopenia (1%)

Hepatic: Transaminases increased (4% to 5%), jaundice (2%)

Neuromuscular & skeletal: Back pain (8%), weakness (2%)

Renal: Dysuria (2%)

Respiratory: Cough (2%)

<1% (Limited to important or life-threatening): Abdominal distention, acute renal failure, alopecia, anaphylactoid reactions, angina, arthralgia, bleeding (spontaneous in patients with hemophilia A or B), cerebrovascular disorder, cholesterol increased, crystalluria, depression, dry skin, erythema multiforme, fat redistribution, hemolytic anemia, hepatic failure, hepatitis, hydronephrosis, hyperpigmentation, immune reconstitution syndrome, interstitial nephritis (with medullary calcification and cortical atrophy), leukocyturia (severe and asymptomatic), MI, new-onset diabetes, pancreatitis, paresthesia (oral), paronychia, pharyngitis, pyelonephritis, QT prolongation, renal insufficiency, renal failure, Stevens-Johnson syndrome, torsade de pointes, triglycerides increased, upper respiratory infection, urticaria, vasculitis

Drug Interactions

Metabolism/Transport Effects Substrate of CYP2D6 (minor), CYP3A4 (major), P-glycoprotein; **Note:** Assignment of Major/Minor substrate status based on clinically relevant drug interaction potential; **Inhibits** CYP2C19 (weak), CYP2C9 (weak), CYP2D6 (weak), CYP3A4 (strong)

Avoid Concomitant Use

Avoid concomitant use of Indinavir with any of the following: Alfuzosin; ALPRAZolam; Amiodarone; Atazanavir; Cisapride; Conivaptan; Crizotinib; Dronedarone; Eplerenone; Ergot Derivatives; Everolimus; Fluticasone (Oral Inhalation); Halofantrine; Lapatinib; Lovastatin; Lurasidone; Midazolam; Nilotinib; Nisoldipine; Pimozide; QuiNIDine; Ranolazine; Rifampin; Rivaroxaban; RomiDEPsin; Salmeterol; Silodosin; Simvastatin; St Johns Wort; Tamsulosin; Ticagrelor; Tolvaptan; Toremifene; Triazolam

Increased Effect/Toxicity

Indinavir may increase the levels/effects of: Alfuzosin; Almotriptan; Alosetron; ALPRAZolam; Amiodarone; Antifungal Agents (Azole Derivatives, Systemic); ARIPiprazole; Atazanavir; Bortezomib; Bosentan; Brentuximab Vedotin; Brinzolamide; Budesonide (Nasal); Budesonide (Systemic, Oral Inhalation); Calcium Channel Blockers (Dihydropyridine); Calcium Channel Blockers (Nondihydropyridine); CarBAMazepine; Ciclesonide; Cisapride; Clarithromycin; Colchicine; Conivaptan; Corticosteroids (Orally Inhaled); Crizotinib; CycloSPORINE; CycloSPORINE (Systemic); CYP3A4 Substrates; Dienogest; Digoxin; Dronedarone; Dutasteride; Enfuvirtide; Eplerenone; Ergot Derivatives; Everolimus; FentaNYL; Fesoterodine; Fluticasone (Nasal); Fluticasone (Oral Inhalation); Fusidic Acid; GuanFACINE; Halofantrine; HMG-CoA Reductase Inhibitors; Iloperidone; Ixabepilone; Lapatinib; Lovastatin; Lumefantrine; Lurasidone; Maraviroc; Meperidine; MethylPREDNISolone; Midazolam; Nefazodone; Nilotinib; Nisoldipine; Paricalcitol; Pazopanib; Pimecrolimus; Pimozide; Propafenone; Protease Inhibitors; QuiNIDine; Ranolazine; Rifabutin; Rivaroxaban; RomiDEPsin; Ruxolitinib; Salmeterol; Saxagliptin; Sildenafil; Silodosin; Simvastatin; Sirolimus; SORAfenib; Tacrolimus; Tacrolimus (Systemic); Tacrolimus (Topical); Tadalafil; Tamsulosin; Temsirolimus; Tenofovir; Ticagrelor; Tolterodine; Tolvaptan; Toremifene; TraZODone; Triazolam; Tricyclic Antidepressants; Vardenafil; Vemurafenib; Vilazodone; Zuclopenthixol

The levels/effects of Indinavir may be increased by: Antifungal Agents (Azole Derivatives, Systemic); Atazanavir; Clarithromycin; CycloSPORINE; CycloSPORINE (Systemic); Delavirdine; Efavirenz; Enfuvirtide; Etravirine; Fusidic Acid; P-glycoprotein/ABCB1 Inhibitors

Decreased Effect

Indinavir may decrease the levels/effects of: Abacavir; Clarithromycin; Delavirdine; Divalproex; Etravirine; Meperidine; Prasugrel; Theophylline Derivatives; Ticagrelor; Valproic Acid; Zidovudine

The levels/effects of Indinavir may be decreased by: Antacids; Atovaquone; Bosentan; CarBAMazepine; CYP3A4 Inducers (Strong); Deferasirox; Didanosine; Efavirenz; Garlic; H2-Antagonists; Nevirapine; Peginterferon Alfa-2b; P-glycoprotein/ABCB1 Inducers; Proton Pump Inhibitors; Rifabutin; Rifampin; St Johns Wort; Tenofovir; Tocilizumab; Venlafaxine

Ethanol/Nutrition/Herb Interactions

Food: Indinavir bioavailability may be decreased if taken with food. Meals high in calories, fat, and protein result in a significant decrease in drug levels. Indinavir serum concentrations may be decreased by grapefruit juice.

Herb/Nutraceutical: Garlic may decrease the levels/effects of protease inhibitors. St John's wort *(Hypericum)* appears to induce CYP3A enzymes and has lead to 57% reductions in indinavir AUCs and 81% reductions in trough serum concentrations, which may lead to treatment failures; should not be used concurrently with indinavir.

Stability Medication should be stored at 15°C to 30°C (59°F to 86°F), and used in the original container and the desiccant should remain in the bottle. Capsules are sensitive to moisture.

Mechanism of Action Binds to the site of HIV-1 protease activity and inhibits cleavage of viral Gag-Pol polyprotein precursors into individual functional proteins required for infectious HIV. This results in the formation of immature, noninfectious viral particles.

Pharmacodynamics/Kinetics

Absorption: Administration with a high fat, high calorie diet resulted in a reduction in AUC and in maximum serum concentration (77% and 84% respectively); lighter meal resulted in little or no change in these parameters.

Protein binding, plasma: 60%

Metabolism: Hepatic via CYP3A4; seven metabolites of indinavir identified

Bioavailability: Good

Half-life elimination: 1.8 ± 0.4 hour; hepatic insufficiency: 2.8 ± 0.5 hour

Time to peak: 0.8 ± 0.3 hour

Excretion: Feces (83%; 19% as unchanged drug); urine (19%; 9% as unchanged drug)

Dosage

Children 4-15 years (investigational): 500 mg/m^2 every 8 hours

Adults: Oral:

Unboosted regimen: 800 mg every 8 hours

Ritonavir-boosted regimen: Ritonavir 100-200 mg twice daily plus indinavir 800 mg twice daily

Dosage adjustments for indinavir when administered in combination therapy:

Delavirdine, itraconazole, or ketoconazole: Reduce indinavir dose to 600 mg every 8 hours

Efavirenz: Increase indinavir dose to 1000 mg every 8 hours

Lopinavir and ritonavir (Kaletra™): Indinavir 600 mg twice daily

Nelfinavir: Increase indinavir dose to 1200 mg twice daily

Nevirapine: Increase indinavir dose to 1000 mg every 8 hours

Rifabutin: Reduce rifabutin to 1/2 the standard dose plus increase indinavir to 1000 mg every 8 hours

Dosage adjustments for concomitant therapy: Adults:

Coadministration with bosentan:

Coadministration of bosentan in patients currently receiving indinavir: Begin with bosentan 62.5 mg once daily or every other day based on tolerability

Coadministration of indinavir in patients currently receiving bosentan: Adjust bosentan to 62.5 mg once daily or every other day based on tolerability

Coadministration with colchicine:

Familial Mediterranean fever (FMF): Maximum colchicine dose: 0.6 mg/day (0.3 mg twice daily)

Gout prophylaxis:

If original colchicine dose is 0.6 mg twice daily, adjust dose to 0.3 mg once daily

If original colchicine dose is 0.6 mg once daily, adjust dose to 0.3 mg every other day

Gout flare treatment: Initial: Colchicine 0.6 mg, followed in 1 hour by a single dose of 0.3 mg; do not repeat for at least 3 days

Coadministration with phosphodiesterase-5 enzyme (PDE-5) inhibitor:

Pulmonary arterial hypertension: Indinavir coadministered with tadalafil:

Patient receiving indinavir when initiating tadalafil: Initiate tadalafil at 20 mg once daily; increase to 40 mg once daily based on individual tolerability

Patient receiving tadalafil when initiating indinavir: Adjust tadalafil to 20 mg once daily; increase to 40 mg once daily based on individual tolerability.

Erectile dysfunction: Indinavir coadministered with:

Sildenafil (Viagra®): Maximum sildenafil dose: 25 mg in a 48-hour period

Tadalafil (Cialis®): Maximum tadalafil dose: 10 mg in a 72-hour period

Vardenafil: Maximum vardenafil dose: 2.5 mg in a 24-hour period

Dosage adjustment in hepatic impairment: Mild-moderate impairment due to cirrhosis: 600 mg every 8 hours

Dietary Considerations Should be taken without food but with water 1 hour before or 2 hours after a meal. Administration with lighter meals (eg, dry toast, skim milk, corn flakes) resulted in little/no change in indinavir concentration. If taking with ritonavir, may take with food. Patient should drink at least 48 oz of water daily.

Administration Drink at least 48 oz of water daily. Administer with water, 1 hour before or 2 hours after a meal. May also be administered with other liquids (eg, skim milk, juice, coffee, tea) or a light meal (eg, toast, corn flakes). Administer around-the-clock to avoid significant fluctuation in serum levels. May be taken with food when administered in combination with ritonavir.

Monitoring Parameters Monitor viral load, CD4 count, triglycerides, cholesterol, glucose, liver function tests, CBC, urinalysis (severe leukocyturia should be monitored frequently).

Dosage Forms Excipient information presented when available (limited, particularly for generics); consult specific product labeling. [DSC] = Discontinued product

Capsule, oral:

Crixivan®: 100 mg, 200 mg, 333 mg [DSC], 400 mg

Extemporaneous Preparations A 10 mg/mL oral solution may be prepared using capsules. First, prepare a 100 mg/mL indinavir concentrate by adding the contents of fifteen 400 mg capsules and 60 mL purified water to a 100 mL amber glass bottle. Place bottle in an ultrasonic bath filled with water at 37°C for 60 minutes, stirring the solution every 10 minutes. Filter solution; wash bottle and filter with 6 mL purified water; cool solution to room temperature. Add 50 mL of 100 mg/mL indinavir concentrate to 360 mL viscous sweet base, 90 mL simple syrup, 1.8 g citric acid, 45 mg azorubine, 0.1M sodium hydroxide solution to pH 3, and 12 drops of lemon oil, to make a final volume of 500 mL. Mix to a uniform solution. Label "refrigerate". Stable for 2 weeks refrigerated.

Hugen PW, Burger DM, ter Hofstede HJ, et al, "Development of an Indinavir Oral Liquid for Children," *Am J Health Syst Pharm*, 2000, 57 (14):1332-9.

◆ **Indinavir Sulfate** *see* Indinavir *on page* 888

◆ **Indocid® P.D.A. (Can)** *see* Indomethacin *on page* 890

◆ **Indocin®** *see* Indomethacin *on page* 890

◆ **Indocin® I.V.** *see* Indomethacin *on page* 890

◆ **Indometacin** *see* Indomethacin *on page* 890

Indomethacin (in doe METH a sin)

Brand Names: U.S. Indocin®; Indocin® I.V.

Brand Names: Canada Apo-Indomethacin®; Indocid® P.D.A.; Novo-Methacin; Nu-Indo; Pro-Indo; ratio-Indomethacin; Sandoz-Indomethacin

Index Terms Indometacin; Indomethacin Sodium Trihydrate

Pharmacologic Category Nonsteroidal Anti-inflammatory Drug (NSAID), Oral; Nonsteroidal Anti-inflammatory Drug (NSAID), Parenteral

Additional Appendix Information

Beers Criteria − Potentially Inappropriate Medications for Geriatrics *on page* 1973

Use Acute gouty arthritis, acute bursitis/tendonitis, moderate-to-severe osteoarthritis, rheumatoid arthritis, ankylosing spondylitis; I.V. form used as alternative to surgery for closure of patent ductus arteriosus in neonates

Unlabeled Use Management of preterm labor

Pregnancy Risk Factor C

Pregnancy Considerations Adverse events have been observed in animal reproduction studies; therefore, the manufacturer classifies indomethacin as pregnancy category C. Indomethacin crosses the placenta and can be detected in fetal plasma and amniotic fluid. Indomethacin exposure during the first trimester is not strongly associated with congenital malformations; however, cardiovascular anomalies and cleft palate have been observed following NSAID exposure in some studies. The use of an NSAID close to conception may be associated with an increased risk of miscarriage. Nonteratogenic effects have been observed following NSAID administration during the third trimester, including myocardial degenerative changes, prenatal constriction of the ductus arteriosus, failure of the ductus arteriosus to close postnatally, and fetal tricuspid regurgitation; renal dysfunction or failure, oligohydramnios; gastrointestinal bleeding or perforation, increased risk of necrotizing enterocolitis; intracranial bleeding (including intraventricular hemorrhage), platelet dysfunction with resultant bleeding; and pulmonary hypertension. The risk of fetal ductal constriction following maternal use of indomethacin is increased with gestational age and duration of therapy. Because they may cause premature closure of the ductus arteriosus, use of NSAIDs late in pregnancy should be avoided (use after 31 or 32 weeks gestation is not recommended by some clinicians). Indomethacin has been used in the management of preterm labor. Indomethacin should be used with caution in pregnant women with hypertension. The chronic use of NSAIDs in women of reproductive age may be associated with infertility that is reversible upon discontinuation of the medication.

Lactation Enters breast milk/not recommended (AAP rates "compatible"; AAP 2001 update pending)

Medication Guide Available Yes

Contraindications Hypersensitivity to indomethacin, aspirin, other NSAIDs, or any component of the formulation; perioperative pain in the setting of coronary artery bypass graft (CABG) surgery; patients with a history of proctitis or recent rectal bleeding (suppositories)

Neonates: Necrotizing enterocolitis; impaired renal function; active bleeding (including intracranial hemorrhage and gastrointestinal bleeding), thrombocytopenia, coagulation defects; untreated infection; congenital heart disease where patent ductus arteriosus is necessary

Warnings/Precautions [U.S. Boxed Warning]: NSAIDs are associated with an increased risk of adverse cardiovascular thrombotic events, including MI and stroke. Risk may be increased with duration of use or pre-existing cardiovascular risk factors or disease. May cause new-onset hypertension or worsening of existing hypertension. Use caution with fluid retention. Avoid use in heart failure. Concurrent administration of ibuprofen, and potentially other nonselective NSAIDs, may interfere with aspirin's cardioprotective effect. **[U.S. Boxed Warning]: Use is contraindicated for treatment of perioperative pain in the setting of coronary artery bypass graft**

(CABG) surgery. Risk of MI and stroke may be increased with use following CABG surgery.

Platelet adhesion and aggregation may be decreased; may prolong bleeding time; patients with coagulation disorders or who are receiving anticoagulants should be monitored closely. Anemia may occur; patients on long-term NSAID therapy should be monitored for anemia. Rarely, NSAID use may cause severe blood dyscrasias (eg, agranulocytosis, aplastic anemia, thrombocytopenia).

NSAID use may compromise existing renal function; dose-dependent decreases in prostaglandin synthesis may result from NSAID use, reducing renal blood flow which may cause renal decompensation. NSAID use may increase the risk for hyperkalemia. Patients with impaired renal function, dehydration, heart failure, liver dysfunction, those taking diuretics, and ACE inhibitors are at greater risk of renal toxicity and hyperkalemia. Rehydrate patient before starting therapy; monitor renal function closely. Not recommended for use in patients with advanced renal disease. Long-term NSAID use may result in renal papillary necrosis.

The elderly are at increased risk for adverse effects (especially peptic ulceration, CNS effects, renal toxicity) from NSAIDs even at low doses. Risk of CNS adverse events may be higher with indomethacin compared to other NSAIDs; avoid use in this age group (Beers Criteria).

[U.S. Boxed Warning]: NSAIDs may increase risk of gastrointestinal irritation, inflammation, ulceration, bleeding, and perforation. Use caution with a history of GI disease (bleeding or ulcers), concurrent therapy with aspirin, anticoagulants and/or corticosteroids, smoking, use of alcohol, the elderly or debilitated patients. When used concomitantly with ≤325 mg of aspirin, a substantial increase in the risk of gastrointestinal complications (eg, ulcer) occurs; concomitant gastroprotective therapy (eg, proton pump inhibitors) is recommended (Bhatt, 2008).

Use the lowest effective dose for the shortest duration of time, consistent with individual patient goals, to reduce risk of cardiovascular or GI adverse events. Alternate therapies should be considered for patients at high risk.

NSAIDS may cause drowsiness, dizziness, blurred vision and other neurologic effects which may impair physical or mental abilities; patients must be cautioned about performing tasks which require mental alertness (eg, operating machinery or driving). Discontinue use with blurred or diminished vision and perform ophthalmologic exam. Monitor vision with long-term therapy.

NSAIDs may cause serious skin adverse events including exfoliative dermatitis, Stevens-Johnson syndrome (SJS) and toxic epidermal necrolysis (TEN); discontinue use at first sign of skin rash or hypersensitivity. Anaphylactoid reactions may occur, even without prior exposure; patients with "aspirin triad" (bronchial asthma, aspirin intolerance, rhinitis) may be at increased risk. Do not use in patients who experience bronchospasm, asthma, rhinitis, or urticaria with NSAID or aspirin therapy. Use caution in other forms of asthma.

Use with caution in patients with decreased hepatic function. Closely monitor patients with any abnormal LFT. Severe hepatic reactions (eg, fulminant hepatitis, liver failure) have occurred with NSAID use, rarely; discontinue if signs or symptoms of liver disease develop, or if systemic manifestations occur. The elderly are at increased risk for adverse effects (especially peptic ulceration, CNS effects, renal toxicity) from NSAIDs even at low doses. Prolonged use may cause corneal deposits and retinal disturbances; discontinue if visual changes are observed. Use caution with depression, epilepsy, or Parkinson's disease.

Withhold for at least 4-6 half-lives prior to surgical or dental procedures.

Oral: Safety and efficacy have not been established in children <14 years of age. Hepatotoxicity has been reported in younger children treated for juvenile idiopathic arthritis (JIA). Closely monitor if use is needed in children ≥2 years of age.

Adverse Reactions

>10%: Central nervous system: Headache (12%)

1% to 10%:

Central nervous system: Dizziness (3% to 9%), depression (<3%), fatigue (<3%), malaise (<3%), somnolence (<3%), vertigo (<3%)

Gastrointestinal: Dyspepsia (3% to 9%), epigastric pain (3% to 9%), heartburn (3% to 9%), indigestion (3% to 9%), nausea (3% to 9%), abdominal pain/cramps/distress (<3%), constipation (<3%), diarrhea (<3%), rectal irritation (suppository), tenesmus (suppository), vomiting

Otic: Tinnitus (<3%)

<1% (Limited to important or life-threatening): Acute respiratory distress, agranulocytosis, allergic rhinitis, anaphylaxis, anemia, angiitis, angioedema, aplastic anemia, arrhythmia, aseptic meningitis, asthma, bone marrow suppression, bronchospasm, chest pain, cholestatic jaundice, coma, confusion, CHF, cystitis, depersonalization, depression, diplopia, disseminated intravascular coagulation (DIC), dysarthria, dyspnea, ecchymosis, edema, epistaxis, erythema multiforme, erythema nodosum, exfoliative dermatitis, fluid retention, flushing, hair loss, gastric perforation (rare), gastritis, GI bleeding, GI ulceration, glucosuria, gynecomastia, hearing decreased, hematuria, hemolytic anemia, hepatitis (including fatal cases), hot flashes, hyperglycemia, hyperkalemia, hypersensitivity reactions, hyper-/hypotension, interstitial nephritis, intestinal strictures, involuntary muscle movements, leukopenia, lightheadedness, necrotizing fasciitis, nephrotic syndrome, oliguria, paresthesia, parkinson's exacerbation, peptic ulcer, peripheral neuropathy, proctitis, psychosis, pulmonary edema, purpura, rectal bleeding, renal insufficiency, renal failure, retinal/macular disturbances, seizure exacerbation, shock, somnolence, Stevens-Johnson syndrome, stomatitis, syncope, thrombocytopenia, thrombocytopenic purpura, thrombophlebitis, toxic amblyopia, toxic epidermal necrolysis, ulcerative stomatitis

Drug Interactions

Metabolism/Transport Effects Substrate of CYP2C19 (minor), CYP2C9 (minor); **Note:** Assignment of Major/Minor substrate status based on clinically relevant drug interaction potential; **Inhibits** CYP2C19 (weak), CYP2C9 (weak)

Avoid Concomitant Use

Avoid concomitant use of Indomethacin with any of the following: Floctafenine; Ketorolac; Ketorolac (Nasal); Ketorolac (Systemic)

Increased Effect/Toxicity

Indomethacin may increase the levels/effects of: Aminoglycosides; Anticoagulants; Antiplatelet Agents; Bisphosphonate Derivatives; Collagenase (Systemic); CycloSPORINE; CycloSPORINE (Systemic); Deferasirox; Desmopressin; Digoxin; Drotrecogin Alfa (Activated); Eplerenone; Haloperidol; Ibritumomab; Lithium; Methotrexate; Nonsteroidal Anti-Inflammatory Agents; PEMEtrexed; Porfimer; Potassium-Sparing Diuretics; PRALAtrexate; Quinolone Antibiotics; Rivaroxaban; Salicylates; Thrombolytic Agents; Tiludronate; Tositumomab and Iodine I 131 Tositumomab; Triamterene; Vancomycin; Vitamin K Antagonists

The levels/effects of Indomethacin may be increased by: ACE Inhibitors; Angiotensin II Receptor Blockers; Antidepressants (Tricyclic, Tertiary Amine); Corticosteroids (Systemic); CycloSPORINE; CycloSPORINE (Systemic); Dasatinib; Floctafenine; Glucosamine; Herbs (Anticoagulant/Antiplatelet Properties); Ketorolac; Ketorolac (Nasal); Ketorolac (Systemic); Nonsteroidal Anti-Inflammatory Agents; Omega-3-Acid Ethyl Esters; Pentosan Polysulfate Sodium; Pentoxifylline; Probenecid; Prostacyclin Analogues; Selective Serotonin Reuptake Inhibitors; Serotonin/Norepinephrine Reuptake Inhibitors; Sodium Phosphates; Treprostinil; Vitamin E

Decreased Effect

Indomethacin may decrease the levels/effects of: ACE Inhibitors; Angiotensin II Receptor Blockers; Antiplatelet Agents; Beta-Blockers; Eplerenone; HydrALAZINE; Loop Diuretics; Potassium-Sparing Diuretics; Salicylates; Selective Serotonin Reuptake Inhibitors; Thiazide Diuretics

The levels/effects of Indomethacin may be decreased by: Bile Acid Sequestrants; Nonsteroidal Anti-Inflammatory Agents; Salicylates

Ethanol/Nutrition/Herb Interactions

Ethanol: Avoid ethanol (may enhance gastric mucosal irritation).

Food: Food may decrease the rate but not the extent of absorption. Indomethacin peak serum levels may be delayed if taken with food.

Herb/Nutraceutical: Avoid alfalfa, anise, bilberry, bladderwrack, bromelain, cat's claw, celery, chamomile, coleus, cordyceps, dong quai, evening primrose, fenugreek, feverfew, garlic, ginger, ginkgo biloba, ginseng (American, Panax, Siberian), grapeseed, green tea, guggul, horse chestnut seed, horseradish, licorice, prickly ash, red clover, reishi, SAMe (S-adenosylmethionine), sweet clover, turmeric, white willow (all have additional antiplatelet activity).

Stability I.V.: Store below 30°C (86°F). Protect from light. Not stable in alkaline solution. Reconstitute with 1-2 mL preservative free NS or SWFI just prior to administration. Discard any unused portion. Do not use preservative-containing diluents for reconstitution.

Mechanism of Action Reversibly inhibits cyclooxygenase-1 and 2 (COX-1 and 2) enzymes, which results in decreased formation of prostaglandin precursors; has antipyretic, analgesic, and anti-inflammatory properties

Other proposed mechanisms not fully elucidated (and possibly contributing to the anti-inflammatory effect to varying degrees), include inhibiting chemotaxis, altering lymphocyte activity, inhibiting neutrophil aggregation/activation, and decreasing proinflammatory cytokine levels.

Pharmacodynamics/Kinetics

Onset of action: ~30 minutes

Duration: 4-6 hours

Absorption: Oral: Immediate release: Prompt and extensive; Extended release: 90% over 12 hours

Distribution: V_d: 0.34-1.57 L/kg; crosses blood-brain barrier

Protein binding: 99%

Metabolism: Hepatic; significant enterohepatic recirculation

Bioavailability: 100%

Half-life elimination: 4.5 hours; prolonged in neonates

Time to peak: Oral: Immediate release: 2 hours

Excretion: Urine (60%, primarily as glucuronide conjugates); feces (33%, primarily as metabolites)

Dosage

Patent ductus arteriosus:

Neonates: I.V.: Initial: 0.2 mg/kg, followed by 2 doses depending on postnatal age (PNA):

PNA **at time of first dose** <48 hours: 0.1 mg/kg at 12- to 24-hour intervals

PNA **at time of first dose** 2-7 days: 0.2 mg/kg at 12- to 24-hour intervals

PNA **at time of first dose** >7 days: 0.25 mg/kg at 12- to 24-hour intervals

In general, may use 12-hour dosing interval if urine output >1 mL/kg/hour after prior dose; use 24-hour dosing interval if urine output is <1 mL/kg/hour but >0.6 mL/kg/hour; doses should be withheld if patient has oliguria (urine output <0.6 mL/kg/hour) or anuria

Inflammatory/rheumatoid disorders: Oral: Use lowest effective dose.

Children ≥2 years: 1-2 mg/kg/day in 2-4 divided doses; maximum dose: 4 mg/kg/day; not to exceed 150-200 mg/day

Adults: 25-50 mg/dose 2-3 times/day; maximum dose: 200 mg/day; extended release capsule should be given on a 1-2 times/day schedule (maximum dose for extended release: 150 mg/day). In patients with arthritis and persistent night pain and/or morning stiffness may give the larger portion (up to 100 mg) of the total daily dose at bedtime.

Bursitis/tendonitis: Oral: Adults: Initial dose: 75-150 mg/day in 3-4 divided doses **or** 1-2 divided doses for extended release; usual treatment is 7-14 days

Acute gouty arthritis: Oral: Adults: 50 mg 3 times daily until pain is tolerable then reduce dose; usual treatment <3-5 days

Elderly: Refer to adult dosing. Use lowest recommended dose and frequency in elderly to initiate therapy for indications listed in adult dosing.

Dosage adjustment in renal impairment: Not recommended in patients with advanced renal disease

Dietary Considerations May cause GI upset; take with food or milk to minimize

Administration

Oral: Administer with food, milk, or antacids to decrease GI adverse effects. Extended release capsules must be swallowed whole; do not crush.

I.V.: Administer over 20-30 minutes. Reconstitute I.V. formulation just prior to administration; discard any unused portion; avoid I.V. bolus administration or infusion via an umbilical catheter into vessels near the superior mesenteric artery as these may cause vasoconstriction and can compromise blood flow to the intestines. Do not administer intra-arterially.

Monitoring Parameters Monitor response (pain, range of motion, grip strength, mobility, ADL function), inflammation; observe for weight gain, edema; monitor renal function (serum creatinine, BUN); observe for bleeding, bruising; evaluate gastrointestinal effects (abdominal pain, bleeding, dyspepsia); mental confusion, disorientation, CBC, liver function tests (particularly with pediatric use); ophthalmologic exams with prolonged therapy

Test Interactions False-negative dexamethasone suppression test

Dosage Forms Excipient information presented when available (limited, particularly for generics); consult specific product labeling.

Capsule, oral: 25 mg, 50 mg

Capsule, extended release, oral: 75 mg

Injection, powder for reconstitution: 1 mg

Indocin® I.V.: 1 mg

Suppository, rectal: 50 mg (30s)

Suspension, oral:

Indocin®: 25 mg/5 mL (237 mL) [contains ethanol 1%; pineapple-coconut-mint flavor]

◆ **Indomethacin Sodium Trihydrate** *see* Indomethacin *on page 890*

◆ **INF-alpha 2** *see* Interferon Alfa-2b *on page 912*

- **Infanrix®** *see* Diphtheria and Tetanus Toxoids, and Acellular Pertussis Vaccine *on page 523*
- **Infantaire [OTC]** *see* Acetaminophen *on page 27*
- **Infasurf®** *see* Calfactant *on page 271*
- **INFeD®** *see* Iron Dextran Complex *on page 930*
- **Infergen®** *see* Interferon Alfacon-1 *on page 916*

InFLIXimab (in FLIKS e mab)

Brand Names: U.S. Remicade®

Brand Names: Canada Remicade®

Index Terms Avakine; Infliximab, Recombinant

Pharmacologic Category Antirheumatic, Disease Modifying; Gastrointestinal Agent, Miscellaneous; Immunosuppressant Agent; Monoclonal Antibody; Tumor Necrosis Factor (TNF) Blocking Agent

Use

Treatment of moderately- to severely-active rheumatoid arthritis (with methotrexate)

Treatment of moderately- to severely-active Crohn's disease with inadequate response to conventional therapy (to reduce signs/symptoms and induce and maintain clinical remission) or to reduce the number of draining enterocutaneous and rectovaginal fistulas and maintain fistula closure

Treatment of psoriatic arthritis (to reduce signs/symptoms of active arthritis and inhibit progression of structural damage and improve physical function)

Treatment of chronic severe plaque psoriasis

Treatment of active ankylosing spondylitis (reduce signs/symptoms)

Treatment of moderately- to severely-active ulcerative colitis with inadequate response to conventional therapy (reduce signs/symptoms and induce and maintain clinical remission, mucosal healing and eliminate corticosteroid use)

Pregnancy Risk Factor B

Pregnancy Considerations Reproduction studies have not been conducted. Use during pregnancy only if clearly needed. A Rheumatoid Arthritis and Pregnancy Registry has been established for women exposed to infliximab during pregnancy (Organization of Teratology Information Services, 877-311-8972).

Lactation Excretion in breast milk unknown/not recommended

Medication Guide Available Yes

Contraindications Hypersensitivity to infliximab, murine proteins or any component of the formulation; doses >5 mg/kg in patients with moderate or severe heart failure (NYHA Class III/IV)

Canadian labeling: Additional contraindications (not in U.S. labeling): Severe infections (eg, sepsis, abscesses, tuberculosis, and opportunistic infections)

Warnings/Precautions [U.S. Boxed Warning]: Patients receiving infliximab are at increased risk for serious infections which may result in hospitalization and/or fatality; infections usually developed in patients receiving concomitant immunosuppressive agents (eg, methotrexate or corticosteroids) and may present as disseminated (rather than local) disease. Active tuberculosis (or reactivation of latent tuberculosis), invasive fungal (including aspergillosis, blastomycosis, candidiasis, coccidioidomycosis, histoplasmosis, and pneumocystosis) and bacterial, viral or other opportunistic infections (including legionellosis and listeriosis) have been reported in patients receiving TNF-blocking agents, including infliximab. Monitor closely for signs/symptoms of infection. Discontinue for serious infection or sepsis. Consider risks versus benefits prior to use in patients with a history of chronic or recurrent infection. Consider empiric antifungal therapy in patients who are at risk for invasive fungal infection and develop severe systemic illness. Caution should be exercised when considering use the elderly or in patients with conditions that predispose them to infections (eg, diabetes) or residence/travel from areas of endemic mycoses (blastomycosis, coccidioidomycosis, histoplasmosis), or with latent or localized infections. Do not initiate infliximab therapy with clinically important active infection. Patients who develop a new infection while undergoing treatment should be monitored closely. Serious infections have been reported when anakinra or abatacept have been used concurrently with other TNF-blocking agents; concurrent use of infliximab with anakinra or abatacept is not recommended. Use caution when switching from one biologic disease-modifying antirheumatic drug (DMARD) to another; overlapping biological activities may further increase the risk of infection.

[U.S. Boxed Warning]: Infliximab treatment has been associated with active tuberculosis (may be disseminated or extrapulmonary) or reactivation of latent infections; evaluate patients for tuberculosis risk factors and latent tuberculosis infection (with a tuberculin skin test) prior to and during therapy; treatment of latent tuberculosis should be initiated before use. Patients with initial negative tuberculin skin tests should receive continued monitoring for tuberculosis throughout treatment. Most cases of reactivation have been reported within the first 3-6 months of treatment. Caution should be exercised when considering the use of infliximab in patients who have been exposed to tuberculosis.

Patients should be brought up to date with all immunizations before initiating therapy. Live vaccines should not be given concurrently; there is no data available concerning secondary transmission of live vaccines in patients receiving therapy. Rare reactivation of hepatitis B virus (HBV) has occurred in chronic virus carriers; use with caution; evaluate prior to initiation and during treatment.

[U.S. Boxed Warning]: Lymphoma and other malignancies have been reported in children and adolescent patients receiving TNF-blocking agents including infliximab. Half the cases are lymphomas (Hodgkin's and non-Hodgkin's). **[U.S. Boxed Warning]: Hepatosplenic T-cell lymphoma has been reported in patients with Crohn's disease or ulcerative colitis treated with infliximab and concurrent or prior azathioprine or mercaptopurine use, usually reported in adolescent and young adult males.** The impact of infliximab on the development and course of malignancies is not fully defined, but may be dose dependent. As compared to the general population, an increased risk of lymphoma has been noted in clinical trials; however, rheumatoid arthritis alone has been previously associated with an increased rate of lymphoma. Use caution in patients with a history of COPD, higher rates of malignancy were reported in COPD patients treated with infliximab. Psoriasis patients with a history of phototherapy had a higher incidence of nonmelanoma skin cancers.

Severe hepatic reactions (including hepatitis, jaundice, acute hepatic failure, and cholestasis) have been reported during treatment; discontinue with jaundice or marked increase in liver enzymes (≥5 times ULN). Use caution with heart failure; if a decision is made to use with heart failure, monitor closely and discontinue if exacerbated or new symptoms occur. Doses >5 mg/kg should not be administered in patients with moderate-to-severe heart failure (NYHA Class III/IV). Use caution with history of hematologic abnormalities; hematologic toxicities (eg, leukopenia, neutropenia, thrombocytopenia, pancytopenia) have been reported; discontinue if significant abnormalities occur. Autoimmune antibodies and a lupus-like syndrome have been reported. If antibodies to double-stranded DNA are confirmed in a patient with lupus-like symptoms, infliximab should be discontinued. Rare cases of optic neuritis and demyelinating disease (including multiple sclerosis, systemic vasculitis, and Guillain-Barré syndrome) have been reported; use with caution in patients with pre-existing or recent onset CNS demyelinating disorders, or seizures; discontinue if significant CNS adverse reactions develop.

Acute infusion reactions may occur. Hypersensitivity reaction may occur within 2 hours of infusion. Medication and equipment for management of hypersensitivity reaction should be available for immediate use. Interruptions and/or reinstitution at a slower rate may be required (consult protocols). Pretreatment may be considered, and may be warranted in all patients with prior infusion reactions. Serum sickness-like reactions have occurred; may be associated with a decreased response to treatment. The development of antibodies to infliximab may increase the risk of hypersensitivity and/or infusion reactions; concomitant use of immunosuppressants may lessen the development of anti-infliximab antibodies. The risk of infusion reactions may be increased with retreatment after an interruption or discontinuation of prior maintenance therapy. Retreatment in psoriasis patients should be resumed as a scheduled maintenance regimen without any induction doses; use of an induction regimen should be used cautiously for retreatment of all other patients.

Efficacy was not established in a study to evaluate infliximab use in juvenile idiopathic arthritis (JIA). Safety and efficacy for use in pediatric plaque psoriasis or pediatric ulcerative colitis have not been established. **Note:** For use in Crohn's disease: Safety and efficacy have not been established in children <6 years of age (U.S. labeling) and in children <9 years of age (Canadian labeling).

Adverse Reactions Although profile is similar, frequency of adverse effects may vary with disease state. Except where noted, percentages reported in adults with rheumatoid arthritis:

>10%:

Central nervous system: Headache (18%)
Gastrointestinal: Nausea (21%), diarrhea (12%), abdominal pain (12%, Crohn's 26%)
Hepatic: ALT increased (risk increased with concomitant methotrexate)
Respiratory: Upper respiratory tract infection (32%), sinusitis (14%), cough (12%), pharyngitis (12%)
Miscellaneous: Development of antinuclear antibodies (~50%), infection (36%), infusion reactions (20%; severe <1%), development of antibodies to double-stranded DNA (20%), development of new abscess (Crohn's patients with fistulizing disease: 15%), anti-infliximab antibodies (variable; ~10% to 15% [range: 6% to 61%]; Mayer, 2006)

5% to 10%:

Cardiovascular: Hypertension (7%)
Central nervous system: Fatigue (9%), pain (8%), fever (7%)
Dermatologic: Rash (1% to 10%), pruritus (7%)
Gastrointestinal: Dyspepsia (10%)
Genitourinary: Urinary tract infection (8%)
Neuromuscular & skeletal: Arthralgia (1% to 8%), back pain (8%)
Respiratory: Bronchitis (10%), rhinitis (8%), dyspnea (6%)
Miscellaneous: Moniliasis (5%)

<5%: Abscess, adult respiratory distress syndrome, allergic reaction, anemia, arrhythmia, basal cell carcinoma, biliary pain, bradycardia, brain infarction, breast cancer, cardiac arrest, cellulitis, cholecystitis, cholelithiasis, circulatory failure, confusion, constipation, dehydration, delayed hypersensitivity (plaque psoriasis), diaphoresis increased, dizziness, edema, gastrointestinal hemorrhage, heart failure, hemolytic anemia, hepatitis, hypersensitivity reactions, hypotension, ileus, intervertebral disk herniation, intestinal obstruction, intestinal perforation, intestinal stenosis, leukopenia, lupus-like syndrome, lymphadenopathy, lymphoma, malignancies, meningitis, menstrual irregularity, MI, myalgia, neuritis, pancreatitis, pancytopenia, peripheral neuropathy, peritonitis, pleural effusion, pleurisy, proctalgia, pulmonary edema, pulmonary embolism, renal calculus, renal failure, respiratory insufficiency, seizure, sepsis, serum sickness, suicide attempt, syncope, tachycardia, tendon disorder, thrombocytopenia, thrombophlebitis (deep), ulceration

The following adverse events were reported in children with Crohn's disease and were found more frequently in children than adults:

>10%:

Hepatic: Liver enzymes increased (18%; ≥5 times ULN: 1%)
Hematologic: Anemia (11%)
Miscellaneous: Infections (56%; more common with every 8-week versus every 12-week infusions)

1% to 10%:

Central nervous system: Flushing (9%)
Gastrointestinal: Blood in stool (10%)
Hematologic: Leukopenia (9%), neutropenia (7%)
Neuromuscular & skeletal: Bone fracture (7%)
Respiratory: Respiratory tract allergic reaction (6%)
Miscellaneous: Viral infection (8%), bacterial infection (6%), antibodies to infliximab (3%)

Postmarketing and/or case reports (adults or children): Agranulocytosis, anaphylactic reactions, anaphylactic shock, angina, angioedema, autoimmune hepatitis, bronchospasm, central demyelinating disorders (eg, multiple sclerosis, optic neuritis); cholestasis, drug-induced lupus-like syndrome, erythema multiforme, heart failure (worsening), hepatic carcinoma, hepatitis B reactivation, hepatocellular damage, hepatosplenic T-cell lymphoma (HSTCL), Hodgkin's disease, idiopathic thrombocytopenia purpura, interstitial fibrosis, interstitial pneumonitis, jaundice, laryngeal/pharyngeal edema, latent tuberculosis reactivation, leiomyosarcoma, leukemias, liver failure, liver function tests increased, melanoma, neuropathy, numbness, opportunistic infection, pericardial effusion, peripheral demyelinating disorders (eg, Guillain-Barré syndrome, chronic inflammatory demyelinating polyneuropathy, multifocal motor neuropathy); pneumonia, psoriasis (including new onset, palmoplantar, pustular, or exacerbation), renal cell carcinoma, seizure, Stevens-Johnson syndrome, thrombotic thrombocytopenia purpura, taste abnormal, tingling, toxic epidermal necrolysis, transverse myelitis, tuberculosis, urticaria, vasculitis (systemic and cutaneous)

Drug Interactions

Metabolism/Transport Effects None known.

Avoid Concomitant Use

Avoid concomitant use of InFLIXimab with any of the following: Abatacept; Anakinra; BCG; Belimumab; Canakinumab; Certolizumab Pegol; Natalizumab; Pimecrolimus; Rilonacept; Tacrolimus (Topical); Vaccines (Live)

Increased Effect/Toxicity

InFLIXimab may increase the levels/effects of: Abatacept; Anakinra; Belimumab; Canakinumab; Certolizumab Pegol; Leflunomide; Natalizumab; Rilonacept; Vaccines (Live)

The levels/effects of InFLIXimab may be increased by: Abciximab; Denosumab; Pimecrolimus; Roflumilast; Tacrolimus (Topical); Trastuzumab

Decreased Effect

InFLIXimab may decrease the levels/effects of: BCG; Coccidioidin Skin Test; Sipuleucel-T; Vaccines (Inactivated); Vaccines (Live)

The levels/effects of InFLIXimab may be decreased by: Echinacea

Ethanol/Nutrition/Herb Interactions Herb/Nutraceutical: Avoid echinacea (may diminish the therapeutic effect of infliximab).

Stability Store vials at 2°C to 8°C (36°F to 46°F). Reconstitute vials with 10 mL sterile water for injection. Swirl vial gently to dissolve powder; do not shake. Allow solution to stand for 5 minutes. Total dose of reconstituted product should be further diluted to 250 mL of 0.9% sodium chloride injection to a final concentration of 0.4-4 mg/mL. Infusion of dose should begin within 3 hours of preparation.

Mechanism of Action Infliximab is a chimeric monoclonal antibody that binds to human tumor necrosis factor alpha (TNFα), thereby interfering with endogenous TNFα activity. Elevated TNFα levels have been found in involved tissues/fluids of patients with rheumatoid arthritis, ankylosing spondylitis, psoriatic arthritis, plaque psoriasis, Crohn's disease and ulcerative colitis. Biological activities of TNFα include the induction of proinflammatory cytokines (interleukins), enhancement of leukocyte migration, activation of neutrophils and eosinophils, and the induction of acute phase reactants and tissue degrading enzymes. Animal models have shown TNFα expression causes polyarthritis, and infliximab can prevent disease as well as allow diseased joints to heal.

Pharmacodynamics/Kinetics

Onset of action: Crohn's disease: ~2 weeks

Distribution: V_d: 3-6 L

Half-life elimination: 7-12 days

Dosage I.V.: **Note:** Premedication with antihistamines (H_1-antagonist +/- H_2-antagonist), acetaminophen, and/or corticosteroids may be considered to prevent and/or manage infusion-related reactions:

Children: U.S. labeling ≥6 years, Canadian labeling ≥9 years: Crohn's disease: 5 mg/kg at 0, 2, and 6 weeks, followed by 5 mg/kg every 8 weeks thereafter; if no response by week 14, consider discontinuing therapy

Children ≥6 years: Ulcerative colitis: 5 mg/kg at 0, 2, and 6 weeks, followed by 5 mg/kg every 8 weeks thereafter

Adults:

Crohn's disease: 5 mg/kg at 0, 2, and 6 weeks, followed by 5 mg/kg every 8 weeks thereafter; dose may be increased to 10 mg/kg in patients who respond but then lose their response. If no response by week 14, consider discontinuing therapy.

Psoriatic arthritis (with or without methotrexate): 5 mg/kg at 0, 2, and 6 weeks, followed by 5 mg/kg every 8 weeks thereafter

Rheumatoid arthritis (in combination with methotrexate therapy): 3 mg/kg at 0, 2, and 6 weeks, followed by 3 mg/kg every 8 weeks thereafter; doses have ranged from 3-10 mg/kg repeated at 4- to 8-week intervals

Ankylosing spondylitis: 5 mg/kg at 0, 2, and 6 weeks, followed by 5 mg/kg every 6 weeks thereafter (Canadian labeling recommends every 6-8 weeks thereafter)

Plaque psoriasis: 5 mg/kg at 0, 2, and 6 weeks, followed by 5 mg/kg every 8 weeks thereafter

Ulcerative colitis: 5 mg/kg at 0, 2, and 6 weeks, followed by 5 mg/kg every 8 weeks thereafter

Dosage adjustment with heart failure (HF): Weigh risk versus benefits for individual patient:

Moderate-to-severe HF (NYHA Class III or IV): ≤5 mg/kg

Dosage adjustment in renal impairment: No specific adjustment is recommended

Dosage adjustment in hepatic impairment: No specific adjustment is recommended

Administration Infuse over at least 2 hours; do not infuse with other agents; use in-line low protein binding filter (≤1.2 micron). Temporarily discontinue or decrease infusion rate with infusion-related reactions. Antihistamines (H_1-antagonist +/- H_2-antagonist), acetaminophen and/or corticosteroids may be used to manage reactions. Infusion may be reinitiated at a lower rate upon resolution of mild-to-moderate symptoms.

Canadian labeling (not approved in U.S. labeling): Infusion of doses ≤6 mg/kg over not less than 1 hour may be considered in patients treated for rheumatoid arthritis who have initially tolerated 3 infusions each over 2 hours. Safety of shortened infusion has not been studied with doses >6 mg/kg.

Guidelines for the treatment and prophylaxis of infusion reactions: (Note: Limited to adult patients and dosages used in Crohn's; prospective data for other populations [pediatrics, other indications/dosing] are not available).

A protocol for the treatment of infusion reactions, as well as prophylactic therapy for repeat infusions, has been published (Mayer, 2006).

Treatment of infusion reactions: Medications for the treatment of hypersensitivity reactions should be available for immediate use. For mild reactions, the rate of infusion should be decreased to 10 mL/hour. Initiate a normal saline infusion (500-1000 mL/hour) and appropriate symptomatic treatment (eg, acetaminophen and diphenhydramine); monitor vital signs every 10 minutes until normal. After 20 minutes, the infusion may be increased at 15-minute intervals, as tolerated, to completion (initial increase to 20 mL/hour, then 40 mL/hour, then 80 mL/hour, etc [maximum of 125 mL/hour]). For moderate reactions, the infusion should be stopped or slowed. Initiate a normal saline infusion (500-1000 mL/hour) and appropriate symptomatic treatment. Monitor vital signs every 5 minutes until normal. After 20 minutes, the infusion may be reinstituted at 10 mL/hour; then increased at 15-minute intervals, as tolerated, to completion (initial increase 20 mL/hour, then 40 mL/hour, then 80 mL/hour, etc [maximum of 125 mL/hour]). For severe reactions, the infusion should be stopped with administration of appropriate symptomatic treatment (eg, hydrocortisone/methylprednisolone, diphenhydramine and epinephrine) and frequent monitoring of vitals (consult institutional policies, if available). Retreatment after a severe reaction should only be done if the benefits outweigh the risks and with appropriate prophylaxis. Delayed infusion reactions typically occur 1-7 days after an infusion. Treatment should consist of appropriate symptomatic treatment (eg. acetaminophen, antihistamine, methylprednisolone).

Prophylaxis of infusion reactions: Premedication with acetaminophen and diphenhydramine 90 minutes prior to infusion may be considered in all patients with prior infusion reactions, and in patients with severe reactions corticosteroid administration is recommended. Steroid dosing may be oral (prednisone 50 mg orally every 12 hours for 3 doses prior to infusion) or intravenous (a single dose of hydrocortisone 100 mg or methylprednisolone 20-40 mg administered 20 minutes prior to the infusion). On initiation of the infusion, begin with a test dose at 10 mL/hour for 15 minutes. Thereafter, the infusion may be increased at 15-minute intervals, as tolerated, to completion (initial increase 20 mL/hour, then 40 mL/hour, then 80 mL/hour, etc). A maximum rate of 125 mL/hour is recommended in patients who experienced prior mild-moderate reactions and 100 mL/hour is recommended in patients who experienced prior severe reactions. In patients with cutaneous flushing, aspirin may be considered (Becker, 2004). For delayed infusion reactions, premedicate with acetaminophen and diphenhydramine 90 minutes prior to infusion. On initiation of the infusion, begin with a test dose at 10 mL/hour for 15 minutes. Thereafter, the infusion may be increased to infuse over 3 hours. Postinfusion therapy with acetaminophen for 3 days and an antihistamine for 7 days is recommended.

Monitoring Parameters Monitor improvement of symptoms and physical function assessments. During infusion, if reaction is noted, monitor vital signs every 2-10 minutes, depending on reaction severity, until normal. Latent TB screening prior to initiating and during therapy; signs/symptoms of infection (prior to, during, and following therapy); CBC with differential; signs/symptoms/worsening of heart failure; HBV screening prior to initiating (all patients), HBV carriers (during and for several months following therapy); signs and symptoms of hypersensitivity reaction; symptoms of lupus-like syndrome; LFTs (discontinue if >5 times ULN); signs and symptoms of malignancy (eg, splenomegaly, hepatomegaly, abdominal pain, persistent fever, night sweats, weight loss).

Psoriasis patients with history of phototherapy should be monitored for nonmelanoma skin cancer.

Dosage Forms Excipient information presented when available (limited, particularly for generics); consult specific product labeling.

Injection, powder for reconstitution:

Remicade®: 100 mg [contains polysorbate 80, sucrose 500 mg]

◆ **Infliximab, Recombinant** *see* InFLIXimab *on page 893*

◆ **Influenza Vaccine** *see* Influenza Virus Vaccine (Inactivated) *on page 897*

◆ **Influenza Vaccine** *see* Influenza Virus Vaccine (Live/Attenuated) *on page 901*

Influenza Virus Vaccine (H5N1)

(in floo EN za VYE rus vak SEEN H5N1)

Index Terms Avian Influenza Virus Vaccine; Bird Flu Vaccine; H5N1 Influenza Vaccine; Influenza Virus Vaccine (Monovalent)

Pharmacologic Category Vaccine, Inactivated (Viral)

Additional Appendix Information

Immunization Recommendations *on page 1922*

Use Active immunization of adults at increased risk of exposure to the H5N1 viral subtype of influenza

Pregnancy Risk Factor C

Pregnancy Considerations Reproduction studies have not been conducted. Vaccine should be given only if clearly needed. Inactivated viral vaccines have not been shown to cause increased risks to the fetus (CDC, 2011).

Lactation Excretion in breast milk unknown/use caution

Prescribing and Access Restrictions Commercial distribution is not planned. The vaccine will be included as part of the U.S. Strategic National Stockpile. It will be distributed by public health officials if needed.

Contraindications Manufacturer states no contraindications

Warnings/Precautions Immediate treatment (including epinephrine 1:1000) for anaphylactoid and/or hypersensitivity reactions should be available during vaccine use. Use with caution in patients with a history of Guillain-Barré syndrome (GBS); these patients may have a greater likelihood of developing GBS. If recent occurrence of GBS (≤6 weeks), decision to administer vaccine should entail careful consideration of risk:benefit. Use with caution in severely immunocompromised patients (eg, patients receiving chemo/radiation therapy or other immunosuppressive therapy [including high-dose corticosteroids]); may have a reduced response to vaccination. Safety and efficacy in children and patients >64 years of age have not been established. In general, household and close contacts of persons with altered immunocompetence may receive all age appropriate vaccines Manufactured with chicken egg protein. Contains thimerosal; hypersensitivity reactions may occur

Adverse Reactions All serious adverse reactions must be reported to the U.S. Department of Health and Human Services (DHHS) Vaccine Adverse Event Reporting System (VAERS) 1-800-822-7967 or online at https://vaers.hhs.gov/esub/index.

>10%:

Central nervous system: Headache (3% to 36%), malaise (22%)

Local: Pain (74%), tenderness (70%), erythema/redness (20%), induration/swelling (15%)

Neuromuscular & skeletal: Myalgia (16%)

1% to 10%:

Central nervous system: Fever (up to 7%)

Gastrointestinal: Nausea (10%), diarrhea (6%)

Respiratory: Nasopharyngitis (2%), upper respiratory infection (2%), nasal congestion (1%)

Additional reactions observed with other influenza vaccine formulations: Allergic reaction, anaphylaxis, angioedema, asthma, encephalopathy, facial paralysis, hives, GBS, neuropathy, optic neuritis, vasculitis

Drug Interactions

Metabolism/Transport Effects None known.

Avoid Concomitant Use There are no known interactions where it is recommended to avoid concomitant use.

Increased Effect/Toxicity There are no known significant interactions involving an increase in effect.

Decreased Effect

The levels/effects of Influenza Virus Vaccine (H5N1) may be decreased by: Belimumab; Fingolimod; Immunosuppressants

Stability Store between 2°C to 8°C (36°F to 46°F). Potency is destroyed by freezing; do not use if product has been frozen. Protect from light.

Mechanism of Action A monovalent, split virus (inactivated) preparation of the H5N1 avian strain of influenza virus (A/Vietnam/1203/2004) which promotes active immunity to avian influenza.

Pharmacodynamics/Kinetics Onset of action: Fourfold increase in antibody titers occurred in up to 58% of patients 28 days after second dose.

Dosage I.M.: Adults 18-64 years: 1 mL, followed by second 1 mL dose given 28 days later (acceptable range: 21-35 days)

Administration For I.M. administration only. Inspect for particulate matter and discoloration prior to administration. Vaccinate in the deltoid muscle using a ≥1 inch needle length. Suspension should be shaken well prior to use. **Note:** For patients at risk of hemorrhage following intramuscular injection, the ACIP recommends "it should be administered intramuscularly if, in the opinion of the physician familiar with the patients bleeding risk, the vaccine can be administered by this route with reasonable safety. If the patient receives antihemophilia or other similar therapy, intramuscular vaccination can be scheduled shortly after such therapy is administered. A fine needle (23 gauge or smaller) can be used for the vaccination and firm pressure applied to the site (without rubbing) for at least 2 minutes. The patient should be instructed concerning the risk of hematoma from the injection." Patients on anticoagulant therapy should be considered to have the same bleeding risks and treated as those with clotting factor disorders (CDC, 2011).

Simultaneous administration of vaccines helps ensure the patients will be fully vaccinated by the appropriate age.

Simultaneous administration of vaccines is defined as administering >1 vaccine on the same day at different anatomic sites. Separate vaccines should not be combined in the same syringe unless indicated by product specific labeling. Separate needles and syringes should be used for each injection. The ACIP prefers each dose of a specific vaccine in a series come from the same manufacturer when possible. Adolescents and adults should be vaccinated while seated or lying down. In general, preterm infants should be vaccinated at the same chronological age as full-term infants (CDC, 2011).

Antipyretics have not been shown to prevent febrile seizures. Antipyretics may be used to treat fever or discomfort following vaccination (CDC, 2011). One study reported that routine prophylactic administration of acetaminophen to prevent fever prior to vaccination decreased the immune response of some vaccines; the clinical significance of this reduction in immune response has not been established (Prymula, 2009).

Monitoring Parameters Monitor for syncope for ≥15 minutes following vaccination

Additional Information Federal law requires that the name of medication, date of administration, the vaccine manufacturer, lot number of vaccine, and the administering person's name, title, and address be entered into the patient's permanent medical record.

The 2-dose regimen prompted antibody response consistent with a protective titer in up to 58% of patients (Treanor, 2006). However, there are no clinical data evaluating whether vaccination protects patients against development of infection. Therefore, protection against a pandemic avian flu strain cannot be assured. A study has shown that a third dose of the vaccine further increases the antibody response (Zangwill, 2008).

Healthcare workers involved in the care of patients with known or suspected H5N1 viral subtype influenza infection should be vaccinated with the most recent seasonal human influenza vaccine in order to reduce the risk of coinfection of human influenza A viruses.

Dosage Forms Excipient information presented when available (limited, particularly for generics); consult specific product labeling.

Injection, suspension [monovalent]: Hemagglutinin (H5N1strain) 90 mcg/mL (5 mL) [contains chicken, egg, and porcine protein, and thimerosal]

Influenza Virus Vaccine (Inactivated)

(in floo EN za VYE rus vak SEEN, in ak ti VAY ted)

Brand Names: U.S. Afluria®; Fluarix®; FluLaval®; Fluvirin®; Fluzone®; Fluzone® High-Dose; Fluzone® Intradermal

Brand Names: Canada Agriflu™; Fluad™; Fluviral®; Influvac®; Intanza®; Vaxigrip®

Index Terms H1N1 Influenza Vaccine; Influenza Vaccine; Influenza Virus Vaccine (Purified Surface Antigen); Influenza Virus Vaccine (Split-Virus); TIV; Trivalent Inactivated Influenza Vaccine

Pharmacologic Category Vaccine, Inactivated (Viral)

Additional Appendix Information

Immunization Recommendations *on page 1922*

Use Provide active immunity to influenza virus strains contained in the vaccine

The Advisory Committee on Immunization Practices (ACIP) recommends annual vaccination with the seasonal trivalent inactivated influenza vaccine (TIV) (injection) for all persons ≥6 months of age.

When vaccine supply is limited, target groups for vaccination (those at higher risk of complications from influenza infection and their close contacts) include the following:

- Persons ≥50 years of age
- Residents of nursing homes and other chronic-care facilities that house persons of any age with chronic medical conditions
- Adults and children with chronic disorders of the pulmonary or cardiovascular systems (except hypertension), including asthma
- Adults and children who have chronic metabolic diseases (including diabetes mellitus), hepatic disease, renal dysfunction, hematologic disorders, or immunosuppression (including immunosuppression caused by medications or HIV)
- Adults and children with cognitive or neurologic/neuromuscular conditions (including conditions such as spinal cord injuries or seizure disorders) which may compromise respiratory function, the handling of respiratory secretions, or that can increase the risk of aspiration
- Children and adolescents (6 months to 18 years of age) who are receiving long-term aspirin therapy, and therefore, may be at risk for developing Reye's syndrome after influenza
- Women who are or will be pregnant during the influenza season
- Children 6-59 months of age
- Healthcare personnel
- Household contacts and caregivers of children <5 years (particularly children <6 months) and adults ≥50 years
- Household contacts and caregivers of persons with medical conditions which put them at high risk of complications from influenza infection
- American Indians/Alaska Natives
- Morbidly obese (BMI ≥40)

The Advisory Committee on Immunization Practices (ACIP) states that healthy, nonpregnant persons aged 2-49 years may receive vaccination with either the seasonal live, attenuated influenza vaccine (LAIV) (nasal spray) or the seasonal trivalent inactivated influenza vaccine (TIV) (injection).

Pregnancy Risk Factor B/C (manufacturer specific)

Pregnancy Considerations Reproduction studies have not been conducted with all products. When conducted, adverse events were not observed in animal studies. Inactivated influenza vaccine has not been shown to cause fetal harm and has been shown to be safe and effective when given to pregnant women. Following maternal immunization with the influenza virus vaccine, vaccine specific antibodies are observed in the newborn.

Influenza vaccination with the trivalent inactivated vaccine (TIV) is recommended for all women who are or will become pregnant during the influenza season and who do not otherwise have contraindications to the vaccine. Pregnant women should observe the same precautions as nonpregnant women to reduce the risk of exposure to influenza and other respiratory infections. When vaccine supply is limited, focus on delivering the vaccine should be given to women who are pregnant or will be pregnant during the flu season, as well as mothers of newborns and contacts or caregivers of children <5 years of age. Most available studies show a decrease in influenza-related illnesses in children <6 months of age following maternal vaccination during pregnancy, thereby supporting current recommendations that all pregnant women should be vaccinated.

Healthcare providers are encouraged to refer women exposed to the influenza vaccine during pregnancy to the *Vaccines and Medications in Pregnancy Surveillance*

System (VAMPSS) by contacting The Organization of Teratology Information Specialists (OTIS) at (877) 311-8972. Women exposed to Flulaval® or Fluarix® during pregnancy may also contact the GlaxoSmithKline registry at 888-452-9622. Healthcare providers may enroll women exposed to Fluzone® Intradermal during pregnancy in the Sanofi Pasteur vaccination registry at 800-822-2463.

Lactation Excretion in breast milk unknown/use caution

Contraindications Prior life-threatening reaction to previous influenza vaccination; hypersensitivity to any component of the formulation

Fluviral® (not available in U.S.): Canadian labeling: Additional contraindications: Presence of acute respiratory infection, other active infections, or serious febrile illness

Warnings/Precautions Anaphylactoid/hypersensitivity reactions: Immediate treatment (including epinephrine 1:1000) for anaphylactoid and/or hypersensitivity reactions should be available during vaccine use. Influenza vaccines from previous seasons must not be used. May consider deferring administration in patients with moderate or severe acute illness (with or without fever); may administer to patients with mild acute illness (with or without fever). Use with caution in patients with a history of bleeding disorders (including thrombocytopenia) and/or patients on anticoagulant therapy; bleeding/hematoma may occur from I.M. administration. Use with caution in patients with history of Guillain-Barré syndrome (GBS); patients with history of GBS have a greater likelihood of developing GBS than those without. As a precaution, the ACIP recommends that patients with a history of GBS and who are at low risk for severe influenza complications, and patients known to have experienced GBS within 6 weeks following previous vaccination should generally not be vaccinated (consider influenza antiviral chemoprophylaxis in these patients). The benefits of vaccination may outweigh the potential risks in persons with a history of GBS who are also at high risk for complications of influenza. Some Canadian product labeling recommends delaying therapy in patients with active neurologic disorders.

Use with caution in severely immunocompromised patients (eg, patients receiving chemo/radiation therapy or other immunosuppressive therapy [including high-dose corticosteroids]); may have a reduced response to vaccination. Inactivated vaccine is preferred over live virus vaccine for household members, healthcare workers and others coming in close contact with severely-immunosuppressed persons requiring care in a protected environment. Antigenic response may not be as great as expected in HIV-infected persons with CD4 cells <100/mm^3 and viral copies of HIV type 1 >30,000/mL. In order to maximize vaccination rates, the ACIP, as well as the Canadian National Advisory Committee on Immunization (NACI), recommends simultaneous administration of all age-appropriate vaccines (live or inactivated) for which a person is eligible at a single clinic visit, unless contraindications exist. Postmarketing reports of increased incidence of fever and febrile seizures in children <5 years of age has been observed with the use of the 2010 Southern Hemisphere formulation of the Afluria® vaccine; febrile events have also been reported in children 5 to <9 years of age. Some products are manufactured with gentamicin, kanamycin, neomycin, polymyxin, and/or thimerosal. Packaging may contain natural latex rubber. All products are manufactured with chicken egg protein (expressed as ovalbumin content). The ovalbumin content may vary from season to season and lot to lot of vaccine. Allergy to eggs must be distinguished from allergy to the vaccine. Recommendations are available from the CDC and NACI regarding influenza vaccination to persons who report egg allergies; however, a prior severe allergic reaction to influenza vaccine, regardless of the component suspected, is a contraindication to vaccination (CDC, 2011). The NACI no longer considers an egg allergy as a contraindication to vaccination (NACI, 2011).

Adverse Reactions All serious adverse reactions must be reported to the U.S. Department of Health and Human Services (DHHS) Vaccine Adverse Event Reporting System (VAERS) 1-800-822-7967 or online at https://vaers.hhs.gov/esub/index. In Canada, adverse reactions may be reported to local provincial/territorial health agencies or to the Vaccine Safety Section at Public Health Agency of Canada (1-866-844-0018).

Frequency not defined. Adverse reactions in adults ≥65 years of age may be greater using the high-dose vaccine, but are typically mild and transient.

Cardiovascular: Chest tightness, facial edema

Central nervous system: Chills, drowsiness, fatigue, fever, headache, irritability, malaise, migraine, shivering

Endocrine & metabolic: Dysmenorrhea

Gastrointestinal: Appetite decreased, diarrhea, nausea, sore throat, upper abdominal pain, vomiting

Local: Injection site reactions (including bruising, erythema, induration, inflammation, pain, soreness [10% to 64%; may last up to 2 days], swelling, tenderness)

Neuromuscular & skeletal: Arthralgia, back pain, myalgia (may start within 6-12 hours and last 1-2 days; incidence equal to placebo in adults; occurs more frequently than placebo in children)

Ocular: Red eyes

Otic: Earache

Respiratory: Cough, nasal congestion, nasopharyngitis, pharyngolaryngeal pain, rhinitis, upper respiratory tract infection, wheezing

Miscellaneous: Diaphoresis

Postmarketing and/or case reports (limited to important or life-threatening): Allergic reactions, anaphylaxis, angioedema, convulsions, erythema multiforme, facial palsy (Bell's palsy), Guillain-Barré syndrome (GBS), Henoch-Schönlein purpura, hypersensitivity reaction, limb paralysis, lymphadenopathy, myelitis (including encephalomyelitis and transverse myelitis), neuralgia, oculorespiratory syndrome (ORS; acute, self-limited reaction with ocular and respiratory symptoms), optic neuritis/neuropathy, paralysis, photophobia, serum sickness, Stevens-Johnson syndrome, syncope, tachycardia, thrombocytopenia, urticaria, vasculitis, vertigo

Drug Interactions

Metabolism/Transport Effects None known.

Avoid Concomitant Use There are no known interactions where it is recommended to avoid concomitant use.

Increased Effect/Toxicity There are no known significant interactions involving an increase in effect.

Decreased Effect

Influenza Virus Vaccine (Inactivated) may decrease the levels/effects of: Pneumococcal Conjugate Vaccine (13-Valent)

The levels/effects of Influenza Virus Vaccine (Inactivated) may be decreased by: Belimumab; Fingolimod; Immunosuppressants; Pneumococcal Conjugate Vaccine (13-Valent)

Stability Store all products between 2°C to 8°C (36°F to 46°F). Potency is destroyed by freezing; do not use if product has been frozen.

Agriflu™, Fluad™, Fluarix®: Protect from light.

Afluria®, FluLaval®, Fluviral®: Discard 28 days after initial entry. Protect from light.

Fluvirin®, Fluzone®, Fluzone® High Dose: Between uses, the multiple dose vial should be stored at 2°C to 8°C (36°F to 46°F).

Vaxigrip®: Between uses, the multiple dose vial should be stored at 2°C to 8°C (36°F to 46°F). Discard 7 days after initial entry. Protect from light.

Mechanism of Action Promotes immunity to seasonal influenza virus by inducing specific antibody production.

Each year the formulation is standardized according to the U.S. Public Health Service. Preparations from previous seasons must not be used.

Pharmacodynamics/Kinetics

Onset of action: Protective antibody titers achieved ~3 weeks after vaccination

Duration: Protective antibody titers persist approximately ≥6 months. Elderly: Protective antibody titers may fall ≤4 months after vaccination.

Dosage It is important to note that influenza seasons vary in their timing and duration from year to year. In general, vaccination should begin soon after the vaccine becomes available and prior to onset of influenza activity in the community. However, vaccination should continue throughout the influenza season as long as vaccine is available.

Fluarix®: I.M.:
- Children 3-8 years: 0.5 mL/dose (1 or 2 doses per season; see **"Note"**)
- Children ≥9 years and Adults: 0.5 mL/dose (1 dose per season)

Fluzone®: I.M.:
- Children 6-35 months: 0.25 mL/dose (1 or 2 doses per season; see **"Note"**)
- Children 3-8 years: 0.5 mL/dose (1 or 2 doses per season; see **"Note"**)
- Children ≥9 years and Adults: 0.5 mL/dose (1 dose per season)

Fluzone® High-Dose: I.M.: Adults ≥65 years: 0.5 mL/dose (1 dose per season). The ACIP considers this an alternative vaccine for this age group.

Fluvirin®: I.M.:
- Children 4-8 years: 0.5 mL/dose (1 or 2 doses per season; see **"Note"**)
- Children ≥9 years and Adults: 0.5 mL/dose (1 dose per season)

Afluria®: I.M.: Although approved for use in children ≥5 years of age, the ACIP does not recommend use of Afluria® in children <8 years due to an increased incidence of fever and febrile seizures noted during the 2010-2011 influenza season. However, if other age-appropriate vaccines are not available, children 5-8 years of age who are also considered at risk for influenza complications may be given Afluria®. The benefits and risks of this vaccine should be discussed with parents or caregivers prior to administration.
- Children 5-8 years: 0.5 mL/dose (1 or 2 doses per season; see **"Note"**)
- Children ≥9 years and Adults: 0.5 mL/dose (1 dose per season)

FluLaval®: I.M.: Adults: 0.5 mL/dose (1 dose per season)

Fluzone® Intradermal: Adults 18-64 years of age: 0.1 mL/dose (1 dose per season). The ACIP considers this an alternative vaccine for this age group.

Canadian labeling (products not available in U.S.):

Agriflu™, Fluviral®, Vaxigrip®: I.M.:
- Children 6-35 months: Manufacturer labeling: 0.25 mL/dose; NACI recommendation: 0.5 mL/dose (NACI, 2011) (1 or 2 doses per season; see **"Note"**)
- Children 3-8 years: 0.5 mL/dose (1 or 2 doses per season; see **"Note"**)
- Children ≥9 years and Adults: 0.5 mL/dose (1 dose per season)

Fluad™: I.M.: Adults ≥65 years: 0.5 mL/dose (1 dose per season)

Influvac®: I.M., SubQ: Adults: 0.5 mL/dose (1 per season).

Intanza® 9 mcg/strain: Intradermal: Adults 18-59 years: 0.1 mL/dose (1 per season)

Intanza® 15 mcg/strain: Intradermal: Adults ≥60 years: 0.1 mL/dose (1 per season)

Note: Children <9 years who received no doses of flu vaccine during the 2010-2011 season, or were not previously vaccinated (ie, this is their first season of vaccination) or for whom vaccination status cannot be determined should receive 2 doses separated by ≥4 weeks, in order to achieve satisfactory antibody response. Children <9 years that received at least 1 dose of the 2010-2011 seasonal influenza vaccine require only 1 dose of the 2011-2012 seasonal influenza vaccine (CDC, 2011; NACI, 2011).

Administration

Fluzone® Intradermal, Intanza® [CAN] For intradermal administration over the deltoid muscle only. Fluzone® Intradermal should be shaken gently prior to use. Intanza® should not be shaken prior to use. Hold system using the thumb and middle finger (do not place fingers on windows). Insert needle perpendicular to the skin; inject using index finger to push on plunger. Do not aspirate.

Afluria®, Agriflu™ [CAN], Fluad™ [CAN], Fluarix®, FluLaval®, Fluviral® [CAN], Fluvirin®, Fluzone®, Fluzone® High-Dose, Vaxigrip® [CAN]: For I.M. administration only. Inspect for particulate matter and discoloration prior to administration. Adults and older children should be vaccinated in the deltoid muscle using a ≥1 inch needle length. Infants and young children <12 months of age should be vaccinated in the anterolateral aspect of the thigh using a 7/8 inch to 1 inch needle length. Young children with adequate deltoid muscle mass should be vaccinated using a 7/8 inch to 1.25 inch needle. Do not inject into the gluteal region or areas where there may be a major nerve trunk. Suspensions should be shaken well prior to use.

Influvac® [CAN]: May be administered by I.M. or deep subcutaneous injection. Shake well prior to use.

If a pediatric vaccine (0.25 mL) is inadvertently administered to an adult, an additional 0.25 mL should be administered to provide the full adult dose (0.5 mL). If the error is discovered after the patient has left, an adult dose should be given as soon as the patient can return. If an adult vaccine (0.5 mL) is inadvertently given to a child, no action needs to be taken. *Agriflu™ [CAN]:* If 0.25 mL dose is to be given, discard half the contained syringe volume prior to administration.

Note: For patients at risk of hemorrhage following intramuscular injection, the ACIP recommends "it should be administered intramuscularly if, in the opinion of the physician familiar with the patients bleeding risk, the vaccine can be administered by this route with reasonable safety. If the patient receives antihemophilia or other similar therapy, intramuscular vaccination can be scheduled shortly after such therapy is administered. A fine needle (23 gauge or smaller) can be used for the vaccination and firm pressure applied to the site (without rubbing) for at least 2 minutes. The patient should be instructed concerning the risk of hematoma from the injection." Patients on anticoagulant therapy should be considered to have the same bleeding risks and treated as those with clotting factor disorders (CDC, 2011).

Simultaneous administration of vaccines helps ensure the patients will be fully vaccinated by the appropriate age. Simultaneous administration of vaccines is defined as administering >1 vaccine on the same day at different anatomic sites. Separate vaccines should not be combined in the same syringe unless indicated by product specific labeling. Separate needles and syringes should be used for each injection. However, in general, vaccination should not be deferred if the brand name or route of the previous dose is not available or not known (CDC, 2011). Adolescents and adults should be vaccinated while seated or lying down. In general, preterm infants should be vaccinated at the same chronological age as full-term infants (CDC, 2011).

Antipyretics have not been shown to prevent febrile seizures. Antipyretics may be used to treat fever or discomfort following vaccination (CDC, 2011). One study reported that routine prophylactic administration of acetaminophen to prevent fever prior to vaccination decreased the immune response of some vaccines; the clinical significance of this reduction in immune response has not been established (Prymula, 2009).

Monitoring Parameters Monitor for ≥15 minutes following vaccination; for those individuals who report a history of egg allergy but it is determined that the inactivated vaccine can be used, observe vaccine recipient for at least 30 minutes after receipt of vaccine.

Additional Information Pharmacies will stock the formulations(s) standardized according to the USPHS requirements for the season. Influenza vaccines from previous seasons must not be used. Federal law requires that the name of medication, date of administration, the vaccine manufacturer, lot number of vaccine, and the administering person's name, title, and address, and documentation of the vaccine information statement (VIS; date on VIS and date given to patient) be entered into the patient's permanent medical record.

It is important to note that influenza seasons vary in their timing and duration from year to year. In general, vaccination should begin soon after the vaccine becomes available and prior to onset of influenza activity in the community. However, vaccination should continue throughout the influenza season as long as vaccine is available.

When vaccine supply is not limited, either TIV or LAIV can be used in healthy, nonpregnant persons aged 2-49 years of age.

When vaccine supply is limited, administration should focus on the ACIP target groups. When TIV vaccine is in short supply, administering LAIV to eligible persons is encouraged to increase available TIV to those patients in whom LAIV cannot be used. During periods of inactivated influenza vaccine (TIV) shortage, the CDC and ACIP have recommended vaccination be prioritized based on the following three tiers. The grouping is based on influenza associated mortality and hospitalization rates. Those listed in group 1 should be vaccinated first, followed by persons in group 2, and then group 3. If the vaccine supply is extremely limited, group 1 has also been subdivided in three tiers, where those in group 1A should be vaccinated first, followed by 1B, then 1C.

Priority groups for vaccination with inactivated seasonal influenza vaccine during periods of vaccine shortage:

Tier 1A:
- Persons ≥65 years with comorbid conditions
- Residents of long-term-care facilities

Tier 1B:
- Persons 2-64 years with comorbid conditions
- Persons ≥65 years without comorbid conditions
- Children 6-23 months
- Pregnant women

Tier 1C:
- Healthcare personnel
- Household contacts and out-of-home caregivers of children <6 months

Tier 2:
- Household contacts of children and adults at increased risk of influenza-associated complications
- Healthy persons 50-64 years

Tier 3:
- Persons 2-49 years without high-risk conditions

Further information available at http://www.cdc.gov/mmwr/preview/mmwrhtml/mm5430a4.htm

Dosage Forms Excipient information presented when available (limited, particularly for generics); consult specific product labeling.

Injection, suspension [purified split-virus]:
- Afluria®: Hemagglutinin 45 mcg/0.5 mL (5 mL) [contains chicken egg protein, neomycin (may have trace amounts), polymyxin B (may have trace amounts), thimerosal]
- FluLaval®: Hemagglutinin 45 mcg/0.5 mL (5 mL) [contains chicken egg protein, thimerosal]
- Fluvirin®: Hemagglutinin 45 mcg/0.5 mL (5 mL) [contains chicken egg protein, neomycin (may have trace amounts), polymyxin B (may have trace amounts), thimerosal]
- Fluzone®: Hemagglutinin 45 mcg/0.5 mL (5 mL) [contains chicken egg protein, thimerosal]

Injection, suspension [purified split-virus, preservative free]:
- Afluria®: Hemagglutinin 45 mcg/0.5 mL (0.5 mL) [contains chicken egg protein, neomycin (may have trace amounts), polymyxin B (may have trace amounts)]
- Fluarix®: Hemagglutinin 45 mcg/0.5 mL (0.5 mL) [contains chicken egg protein, gentamicin (may have trace amounts), hydrocortisone (may have trace amounts), may contain natural rubber/natural latex in prefilled syringe, polysorbate 80]
- Fluvirin®: Hemagglutinin 45 mcg/0.5 mL (0.5 mL) [contains chicken egg protein, may contain natural rubber/natural latex in prefilled syringe, neomycin (may have trace amounts), polymyxin B (may have trace amounts)]
- Fluzone®: Hemagglutinin 22.5 mcg/0.25 mL (0.25 mL) [contains chicken egg protein, may contain natural rubber/natural latex in prefilled syringe]
- Fluzone®: Hemagglutinin 45 mcg/0.5 mL (0.5 mL) [contains chicken egg protein]
- Fluzone®: Hemagglutinin 45 mcg/0.5 mL (0.5 mL) [contains chicken egg protein, may contain natural rubber/natural latex in prefilled syringe]
- Fluzone® High-Dose: Hemagglutinin 180 mcg/0.5 mL (0.5 mL) [contains chicken egg protein, may contain natural rubber/natural latex in prefilled syringe]
- Fluzone® Intradermal: Hemagglutinin 27 mcg/0.1 mL (0.1 mL) [contains chicken egg protein]

Dosage Forms: Canada Excipient information presented when available (limited, particularly for generics); consult specific product labeling.

Injection, suspension [purified split-virus]:
- Fluviral®: Hemagglutinin 45 mcg/0.5 mL (5 mL) [contains chicken egg protein, thimerosal]
- Vaxigrip®: Hemagglutinin 45 mcg/0.5 mL (5 mL) [contains chicken egg protein, neomycin (may have trace amounts), thimerosal]

Injection, suspension [purified split-virus, preservative free]:
- Agriflu™: Hemagglutinin 45 mcg/0.5 mL (0.5 mL) [contains chicken egg protein, neomycin (may have trace amounts), kanamycin (may have trace amounts), polysorbate 80]
- Fluad™: Hemagglutinin 45 mcg/0.5 mL (0.5 mL) [contains chicken egg protein, neomycin (may have trace amounts), kanamycin (may have trace amounts), polysorbate 80]
- Influvac®: Hemagglutinin 45 mcg/0.5 mL (0.5 mL) [contains chicken egg protein, gentamicin (may have trace amounts), polysorbate 80]

Intanza®: Hemagglutinin 27 mcg/0.1 mL (0.1 mL) [contains chicken egg protein, neomycin (may have trace amounts)]
Intanza®: Hemagglutinin 45 mcg/0.1 mL (0.1 mL) [contains chicken egg protein, neomycin (may have trace amounts)]
Vaxigrip®: Hemagglutinin 45 mcg/0.5 mL (0.25 mL, 0.5 mL) [contains chicken egg protein, neomycin (may have trace amounts)]

Influenza Virus Vaccine (Live/Attenuated) (in floo EN za VYE rus vak SEEN)

Brand Names: U.S. FluMist®
Brand Names: Canada FluMist®
Index Terms H1N1 Influenza Vaccine; Influenza Vaccine; Influenza Virus Vaccine (Trivalent, Live); LAIV; Live Attenuated Influenza Vaccine
Pharmacologic Category Vaccine, Live (Viral)
Additional Appendix Information
Immunization Recommendations *on page 1922*
Use Provide active immunity to influenza virus strains contained in the vaccine

The Advisory Committee on Immunization Practices (ACIP) states that healthy, nonpregnant persons aged 2-49 years may receive vaccination with either the seasonal live, attenuated influenza vaccine (LAIV) (nasal spray) or the seasonal trivalent inactivated influenza vaccine (TIV) (injection).

Pregnancy Risk Factor C
Pregnancy Considerations Animal reproduction studies have not been conducted. LAIV is not recommended for use during pregnancy. Influenza vaccination with the trivalent inactivated vaccine (TIV) is recommended for all women who are or will become pregnant during the influenza season and who do not otherwise have contraindications to the vaccine.

Healthy pregnant women do not need to avoid contact with persons vaccinated with LAIV and pregnant healthcare providers may administer the LAIV. The nasal vaccine contains the same strains of influenza A and B found in the injection. Information specific to the use of LAIV in pregnancy has not been located. Refer to the Influenza Virus Vaccine (Inactivated) monograph for additional information.

Healthcare providers are encouraged to refer women exposed to the influenza vaccine during pregnancy to the Vaccines and Medications in Pregnancy Surveillance System (VAMPSS) by contacting The Organization of Teratology Information Specialists (OTIS) at (877) 311-8972.

Lactation Excretion in breast milk unknown/use caution
Contraindications Prior life-threatening reaction to previous influenza vaccination; hypersensitivity to any component of the formulation; children 2-17 years of age receiving aspirin therapy
Warnings/Precautions Immediate treatment (including epinephrine 1:1000) for anaphylactoid and/or hypersensitivity reactions should be available during vaccine use. Influenza vaccines from previous seasons must not be used. May consider deferring administration in patients with moderate or severe acute illness (with or without fever); may administer to patients with mild acute illness (with or without fever). Defer immunization if nasal congestion is present which may impede delivery of vaccine. Use with caution in patients with history of Guillain-Barré syndrome (GBS); patients with history of GBS have a greater likelihood of developing GBS than those without. As a precaution, the ACIP recommends that patients with a history of GBS and who are at low risk for severe influenza complications, and patients known to have experienced GBS within 6 weeks following previous vaccination should generally not be vaccinated (consider influenza antiviral chemoprophylaxis in these patients). Based on limited data, the benefits of vaccinating persons with a history of GBS who are also at high risk for complications of influenza, may outweigh the risks. The nasal spray should not be used in patients with asthma or children <5 years of age with recurrent wheezing; risk of wheezing following vaccination is increased. Patients with severe asthma or active wheezing were not included in clinical trials. Children <24 months of age had increased wheezing and hospitalizations following administration in clinical trials; use of the nasal spray is not approved in this age group. Because safety and efficacy information is limited, the ACIP does not recommend the use of LAIV in patients with chronic pulmonary disorders including asthma and children 2-4 years of age who have had asthma or wheezing episodes within the past year.

Because safety and efficacy information is limited, the ACIP does not recommend the use of LAIV in patients with chronic disorders of the cardiovascular system (except isolated hypertension), diabetes, with hematologic disorders and hemoglobinopathies, hepatic disease, neurologic or neuromuscular disorders, renal disease, or pregnant women. Data on the use of the nasal spray in immunocompromised patients is limited. **Avoid contact with severely immunocompromised individuals for at least 7 days following vaccination (at least 14 days per Canadian labeling).** Because safety and efficacy information is limited, the ACIP does not recommend the use of LAIV in immunosuppressed patients including patients with HIV. In order to maximize vaccination rates, the ACIP recommends simultaneous administration of all age-appropriate vaccines (live or inactivated) for which a person is eligible at a single clinic visit, unless contraindications exist. The U.S. labeling states that safety and efficacy of the nasal spray have not been established in adults ≥50 years of age; use in adults <60 years is approved in the Canadian labeling. Manufactured using arginine, chicken egg protein, gelatin, and gentamicin. Allergy to eggs must be distinguished from allergy to the vaccine. Recommendations are available from the CDC regarding influenza vaccination to persons who report egg allergies; however, a prior severe allergic reaction to influenza vaccine, regardless of the component suspected, is a contraindication to vaccination. Use of TIV is preferred over LAIV when considering vaccination in persons reporting an egg allergy (CDC, 2011).

Adverse Reactions All serious adverse reactions must be reported to the U.S. Department of Health and Human Services (DHHS) Vaccine Adverse Event Reporting System (VAERS) 1-800-822-7967 or online at https://vaers.hhs.gov/esub/index. In Canada, adverse reactions may be reported to local provincial/territorial health agencies or to the Vaccine Safety Section at Public Health Agency of Canada (1-866-844-0018).

Frequency of events reported within 10 days.

>10%:
- Central nervous system: Headache (children 3% to 9%; adults 40%), irritability (children 12% to 21%), lethargy (children 6% to 14%)
- Gastrointestinal: Appetite decreased (children 13% to 21%), abdominal pain (children 2% to 12%)
- Neuromuscular & skeletal: Tiredness/weakness (adults 26%), muscle aches (children 2% to 6%; adults 17%)
- Respiratory: Cough (adults 14%), nasal congestion/runny nose (children 51% to 58%; adults 9% to 44%), sore throat (children 5% to 11%; adults 28%)

1% to 10%:
- Central nervous system: Chills (children 2% to 4%, adults 9%), fever (100°F to 101°F: children 6% to 9%; >101°F: children 1% to 4%)

Otic: Otitis media (children 3%)
Respiratory: Sinusitis (adults 4%), sneezing (children 2%), wheezing (children 6-23 months 6%; children 24-59 months 2%)

Postmarketing and/or case reports: Anaphylactic reactions, asthma exacerbations, Bell's palsy, encephalitis (vaccine associated), epistaxis, Guillain-Barré syndrome, hypersensitivity reaction, meningitis (including eosinophilic meningitis), mitochondrial encephalomyopathy (Leigh syndrome) exacerbation, pericarditis

Drug Interactions

Metabolism/Transport Effects None known.

Avoid Concomitant Use

Avoid concomitant use of Influenza Virus Vaccine (Live/Attenuated) with any of the following: Belimumab; Fingolimod; Immunosuppressants; Salicylates

Increased Effect/Toxicity

Influenza Virus Vaccine (Live/Attenuated) may increase the levels/effects of: Salicylates

The levels/effects of Influenza Virus Vaccine (Live/Attenuated) may be increased by: AzaTHIOprine; Belimumab; Corticosteroids (Systemic); Fingolimod; Hydroxychloroquine; Immunosuppressants; Leflunomide; Mercaptopurine; Methotrexate

Decreased Effect

Influenza Virus Vaccine (Live/Attenuated) may decrease the levels/effects of: Tuberculin Tests

The levels/effects of Influenza Virus Vaccine (Live/Attenuated) may be decreased by: Antiviral Agents (Influenza A and B); Fingolimod; Immune Globulins; Immunosuppressants

Stability Store in refrigerator at 2°C to 8°C (36°F to 46°F). **Do not freeze.**

Mechanism of Action Promotes immunity to seasonal influenza virus by inducing specific antibody production. Each year the formulation is standardized according to the U.S. Public Health Service. Preparations from previous seasons must not be used.

Pharmacodynamics/Kinetics

Onset of action: Protective antibody titers achieved ~3 weeks after vaccination

Duration: Protective antibody titers persist approximately ≥6 months. Elderly: Protective antibody titers may fall ≤4 months after vaccination.

Distribution: Following nasal administration, vaccine is distributed in the nasal cavity (~90%), stomach (~3%), brain (~2%), and lung (0.4%)

Dosage It is important to note that influenza seasons vary in their timing and duration from year to year. In general, vaccination should begin soon after the vaccine becomes available and prior to onset of influenza activity in the community. However, vaccination should continue throughout the influenza season as long as vaccine is available.

Intranasal (FluMist®):

U.S. labeling:

Children 2-8 years: 0.2 mL/dose (1 or 2 doses per season; see **"Note"**)

Children ≥9 years and Adults ≤49 years: 0.2 mL/dose (1 dose per season)

Elderly: Not indicated for use in patients ≥50 years

Canadian labeling:

Children 2-8 years: 0.2 mL/dose (1 or 2 doses per season; see **"Note"**)

Children ≥9 years and Adults ≤59 years: 0.2 mL/dose (1 dose per season)

Elderly: Not indicated for use in patients ≥60 years

Note: CDC recommendations: Children <9 years who received no doses of flu vaccine during the 2010-2011 season, or were not previously vaccinated (ie, this is their first season of vaccination) or for whom vaccination status cannot be determined should receive 2 doses separated by ≥4 weeks, in order to achieve satisfactory antibody response. Children <9 years that received at least 1 dose of the 2010-2011 seasonal influenza vaccine require only 1 dose of the 2011-2012 seasonal influenza vaccine (CDC, 2011).

Administration LAIV: Intranasal: Half the dose (0.1 mL) is administered to each nostril; patient should be in upright position. A dose divider clip is provided. Severely immunocompromised persons should not administer the live vaccine. If recipient sneezes following administration, the dose should not be repeated.

Simultaneous administration of vaccines helps ensure the patients will be fully vaccinated by the appropriate age. Simultaneous administration of vaccines is defined as administering >1 vaccine on the same day at different anatomic sites. The ACIP prefers each dose of a specific vaccine in a series come from the same manufacturer when possible. However, in general, vaccination should not be deferred if the brand name or route of the previous dose is not available or not known (CDC, 2011).

Antipyretics have not been shown to prevent febrile seizures. Antipyretics may be used to treat fever or discomfort following vaccination (CDC, 2011). One study reported that routine prophylactic administration of acetaminophen to prevent fever prior to vaccination decreased the immune response of some vaccines; the clinical significance of this reduction in immune response has not been established (Prymula, 2009).

Vaccine administration with oral influenza antiviral medications: Live influenza virus vaccine (LAIV) should not be given until 48 hours after the completion of influenza antiviral therapy (influenza A and B). Influenza antiviral therapy (influenza A and B) should not be administered for 2 weeks after receiving LAIV. If influenza antiviral therapy (influenza A and B) and LAIV are administered concomitantly, revaccination should be considered.

Test Interactions Administration of the intranasal influenza virus vaccine (live, LAIV) may cause a positive result on the rapid influenza diagnostic test for the 7 days after vaccine administration; for a person with influenza-like illness during this time, the positive test could be caused by either the live attenuated vaccine or wild-type influenza virus.

Additional Information Pharmacies will stock the formulations(s) standardized according to the USPHS requirements for the season. Influenza vaccines from previous seasons must not be used. Federal law requires that the name of medication, date of administration, the vaccine manufacturer, lot number of vaccine, and the administering person's name, title, and address, and documentation of the vaccine information statement (VIS; date on VIS and date given to patient) be entered into the patient's permanent medical record.

It is important to note that influenza seasons vary in their timing and duration from year to year. In general, vaccination should begin soon after the vaccine becomes available and prior to onset of influenza activity in the community. However, vaccination should continue throughout the influenza season as long as vaccine is available.

When vaccine supply is not limited, either TIV or LAIV can be used in healthy, nonpregnant persons aged 2-49 years of age.

When vaccine supply is limited, administration should focus on the ACIP target groups. When TIV vaccine is in short supply, administering LAIV to eligible persons is encouraged to increase available TIV to those patients in whom LAIV cannot be used. During periods of inactivated influenza vaccine (TIV) shortage, the CDC and ACIP have recommended vaccination be prioritized based on the following three tiers. The grouping is based on influenza-associated mortality and hospitalization rates. Those listed in group 1 should be vaccinated first, followed by persons in group 2, and then group 3. If the vaccine supply is extremely limited, group 1 has also been subdivided in three tiers, where those in group 1A should be vaccinated first, followed by 1B, then 1C.

Priority groups for vaccination with inactivated seasonal influenza vaccine during periods of vaccine shortage:

Tier 1A:
- Persons ≥65 years with comorbid conditions
- Residents of long-term-care facilities

Tier 1B:
- Persons 2-64 years with comorbid conditions
- Persons ≥65 years without comorbid conditions
- Children 6-23 months
- Pregnant women

Tier 1C:
- Healthcare personnel
- Household contacts and out-of-home caregivers of children <6 months

Tier 2:
- Household contacts of children and adults at increased risk of influenza-associated complications
- Healthy persons 50-64 years

Tier 3:
- Persons 2-49 years without high-risk conditions

Further information available at http://www.cdc.gov/mmwr/preview/mmwrhtml/mm5430a4.htm

Dosage Forms Excipient information presented when available (limited, particularly for generics); consult specific product labeling.

Solution, intranasal [spray, preservative free]:
FluMist®: (0.2 mL) [contains arginine, chicken egg protein, gelatin, gentamicin (may have trace amounts)]

◆ **Influenza Virus Vaccine (Monovalent)** *see* Influenza Virus Vaccine (H5N1) *on page 896*

◆ **Influenza Virus Vaccine (Purified Surface Antigen)** *see* Influenza Virus Vaccine (Inactivated) *on page 897*

◆ **Influenza Virus Vaccine (Split-Virus)** *see* Influenza Virus Vaccine (Inactivated) *on page 897*

◆ **Influenza Virus Vaccine (Trivalent, Live)** *see* Influenza Virus Vaccine (Live/Attenuated) *on page 901*

◆ **Influvac® (Can)** *see* Influenza Virus Vaccine (Inactivated) *on page 897*

◆ **Infufer® (Can)** *see* Iron Dextran Complex *on page 930*

◆ **Infumorph 200** *see* Morphine (Systemic) *on page 1153*

◆ **Infumorph 500** *see* Morphine (Systemic) *on page 1153*

◆ **INH** *see* Isoniazid *on page 933*

◆ **Innohep® [DSC]** *see* Tinzaparin *on page 1688*

◆ **Innohep® (Can)** *see* Tinzaparin *on page 1688*

◆ **InnoPran XL®** *see* Propranolol *on page 1424*

◆ **Insoluble Prussian Blue** *see* Ferric Hexacyanoferrate *on page 705*

◆ **Inspra™** *see* Eplerenone *on page 600*

Insulin Aspart (IN soo lin AS part)

Brand Names: U.S. NovoLOG®; NovoLOG® FlexPen®; NovoLOG® Penfill®

Brand Names: Canada NovoRapid®

Index Terms Aspart Insulin

Pharmacologic Category Antidiabetic Agent, Insulin

Additional Appendix Information

Diabetes Mellitus and Pregnancy *on page 1978*
Diabetes Mellitus Management, Adults *on page 1983*

Use Treatment of type 1 diabetes mellitus (insulin dependent, IDDM) and type 2 diabetes mellitus (noninsulin dependent, NIDDM) to improve glycemic control

Unlabeled Use Gestational diabetes mellitus (GDM); mild-to-moderate diabetic ketoacidosis (DKA); mild-to-moderate hyperosmolar hyperglycemic state (HHS)

Pregnancy Risk Factor B

Dosage Note: When compared to insulin regular, insulin aspart has a more rapid onset and shorter duration of activity.

SubQ:
- Diabetes mellitus:
  - Type 1:
    - Children <2 years (unlabeled use): Refer to Insulin Regular on page 907
    - Children ≥2 years and Adults: Refer to Insulin Regular on page 907
  - Type 2: Children (unlabeled use) and Adults: Refer to Insulin Regular on page 907
- Diabetic ketoacidosis (DKA), mild-to-moderate (unlabeled use): Refer to Insulin Regular on page 907
- Gestational diabetes mellitus (unlabeled use): Refer to Insulin Regular on page 907
- Hyperosmolar hyperglycemic state (HHS), mild-to-moderate (unlabeled use): Refer to Insulin Regular on page 907

I.V.: Glycemic control in selected clinical situations and under appropriate medical supervision: Adults: Refer to Insulin Regular on page 907

Dosing adjustment in renal impairment: Refer to Insulin Regular on page 907

Dosing adjustment in hepatic impairment: Refer to Insulin Regular on page 907

Additional Information Complete prescribing information for this medication should be consulted for additional detail.

Dosage Forms Excipient information presented when available (limited, particularly for generics); consult specific product labeling.

Injection, solution:
- NovoLOG®: 100 units/mL (10 mL) [vial]
- NovoLOG® FlexPen®: 100 units/mL (3 mL)
- NovoLOG® Penfill®: 100 units/mL (3 mL) [cartridge]

◆ **Insulin Aspart and Insulin Aspart Protamine** *see* Insulin Aspart Protamine and Insulin Aspart *on page 903*

Insulin Aspart Protamine and Insulin Aspart (IN soo lin AS part PROE ta meen & IN soo lin AS part)

Brand Names: U.S. NovoLOG® Mix 70/30; NovoLOG® Mix 70/30 FlexPen®

Brand Names: Canada NovoMix® 30

Index Terms Insulin Aspart and Insulin Aspart Protamine; NovoLog 70/30

Pharmacologic Category Antidiabetic Agent, Insulin

Additional Appendix Information

Diabetes Mellitus and Pregnancy *on page 1978*
Diabetes Mellitus Management, Adults *on page 1983*

Use Treatment of type 1 diabetes mellitus (insulin dependent, IDDM) and type 2 diabetes mellitus (noninsulin dependent, NIDDM) to improve glycemic control

Pregnancy Risk Factor B

Dosage Note: Insulin aspart protamine and insulin aspart combination products are approximately equipotent to insulin NPH and insulin regular combination products but with a more rapid onset and similar duration of activity. The proportion of rapid-acting to long-acting insulin is fixed in the combination products; basal versus prandial dose adjustments cannot be made.

SubQ: Diabetes mellitus: **Note:** Insulin requirements vary dramatically between patients and therapy requires dosage adjustments with careful medical supervision.

Type 1: **Note:** Multiple daily injections (MDI) guided by blood glucose monitoring. Combinations of insulin formulations are commonly used.

Initial dose: 0.5-1.0 units/kg/day in divided doses. Conservative initial doses of 0.2-0.4 units/kg/day may be recommended to avoid the potential for hypoglycemia.

Division of daily insulin requirement: Generally, 50% to 75% of the total daily dose (TDD) is given as an intermediate- (eg, the insulin aspart protamine component on the product) or long-acting form of insulin (in 1-2 daily injections). The remaining portion of the TDD is divided and administered as the rapid-acting (eg, the insulin aspart component of the product) insulin.

Adjustment of dose: Dosage must be titrated to achieve glucose control and avoid hypoglycemia. Adjust dose to maintain preprandial plasma glucose between 70-130 mg/dL for most patients. Since treatment regimens often consist of multiple formulations, dosage adjustments must address the specific phase of insulin release that is primarily contributing to the patient's impaired glycemic control. Treatment and monitoring regimens must be individualized.

Usual maintenance range: 0.5-1.2 units/kg/day in divided doses. Insulin requirements are patient-specific and may vary based on age, body weight, and/or activity factors:

Adolescents: May require as much as 1.5 units/kg/day during puberty (Silverstein, 2005)

Prepuberty: 0.7-1 unit/kg/day

Type 2: The goal of therapy is to achieve an Hb A_{1c} <7% as quickly as possible using the safe titration of medications. According to a consensus statement by the ADA and European Association for the Study of Diabetes (EASD), basal insulin therapy (eg, intermediate- or long-acting insulin) should be considered in patients with type 2 diabetes who fail to achieve glycemic goals with lifestyle interventions and metformin ± a sulfonylurea. Pioglitazone or a GLP-1 agonist may also be considered prior to initiation of basal insulin therapy. In patients who continue to fail to achieve glycemic goals despite the addition of basal insulin, intensification of insulin therapy should be considered; this generally consists of multiple daily injections with a combination of insulin formulations (Nathan, 2009).

Initial basal insulin dose: 0.2 units/kg or 10 units/day (Nathan, 2009). **Note:** Current guidelines recommend that insulin therapy begin with intermediate- or long-acting insulin given at bedtime or long-acting insulin given in the morning (Nathan, 2009).

Adjustment of basal insulin dose: Increase dose by 2 units/day every 3 days until fasting glucose levels are consistently within target range (70-130 mg/dL); may increase dose in larger increments (eg, 4 units/day) if fasting glucose levels are >180 mg/dL (Nathan, 2009).

Note: If the patient experiences hypoglycemia following adjustment, reduce dose by 4 units/day or 10% of total daily dose, whichever is greater (Nathan, 2009). Additional algorithms, such as the "1-1-100", "2-4-6-8", "3-0-3", and "3-2-1" algorithms, exist to aid in the titration of basal insulin (Davies, 2005; Gerstein, 2006; Meneghini, 2007; Riddle, 2003); therapy should be individualized and based on patient-specific details.

Intensification of therapy: Add a second injection of a short-, rapid-, or intermediate-acting insulin as needed based on blood glucose monitoring; the timing of administration and type of insulin added for intensification of therapy depends on the blood glucose level that is consistently out of the target range (eg, preprandial glucose levels before lunch or dinner, postprandial glucose levels, and/or bedtime glucose levels). Additional injections and subsequent dosage adjustments must address the specific phase of insulin release that is primarily contributing to the patient's impaired glycemic control. Intensification of therapy can usually begin with a second injection of ~4 units/day followed by adjustments of ~2 units/day every 3 days until the targeted blood glucose is within range (Nathan, 2009).

In the setting of glucose toxicity (loss of beta-cell sensitivity to glucose concentrations), insulin therapy may be used for short-term management to restore sensitivity of beta-cells; in these cases, the dose may need to be rapidly reduced/withdrawn when sensitivity is re-established.

Dosing adjustment in renal impairment: Insulin requirements are reduced due to changes in insulin clearance or metabolism. Close monitoring of blood glucose and adjustment of therapy is required in renal impairment.

Cl_{cr} 10-50 mL/minute: Administer at 75% of normal dose and monitor glucose closely

Cl_{cr} <10 mL/minute: Administer at 25% to 50% of normal dose and monitor glucose closely

Hemodialysis: Because of a large molecular weight (6000 daltons), insulin is not significantly removed by hemodialysis; supplemental dose is not necessary

Peritoneal dialysis: Because of a large molecular weight (6000 daltons), insulin is not significantly removed by peritoneal dialysis; supplemental dose is not necessary

Continuous renal replacement therapy: Administer 75% of normal dose and monitor glucose closely; supplemental dose is not necessary

Dosing adjustment in hepatic impairment: Insulin requirements may be reduced. Close monitoring of blood glucose and adjustment of therapy is required in hepatic impairment.

Additional Information Complete prescribing information for this medication should be consulted for additional detail.

Dosage Forms Excipient information presented when available (limited, particularly for generics); consult specific product labeling.

Injection, suspension:

NovoLOG® Mix 70/30: Insulin aspart protamine suspension 70% [intermediate acting] and insulin aspart solution 30% [rapid acting]: 100 units/mL (10 mL)

NovoLOG® Mix 70/30 FlexPen®: Insulin aspart protamine suspension 70% [intermediate acting] and insulin aspart solution 30% [rapid acting]: 100 units/mL (3 mL)

Insulin Detemir (IN soo lin DE te mir)

Brand Names: U.S. Levemir®; Levemir® FlexPen®

Brand Names: Canada Levemir®

Index Terms Detemir Insulin

Pharmacologic Category Antidiabetic Agent, Insulin

Additional Appendix Information

Diabetes Mellitus and Pregnancy *on page 1978*

Diabetes Mellitus Management, Adults *on page 1983*

Use Treatment of type 1 diabetes mellitus (insulin dependent, IDDM) and type 2 diabetes mellitus (noninsulin dependent, NIDDM) to improve glycemic control

Pregnancy Risk Factor C

Dosage Note: When compared to insulin NPH, insulin detemir has a slower, more prolonged absorption; duration is dose-dependent. Insulin detemir may be given once or twice daily when used as the basal insulin component of therapy. Changing the basal insulin component from another insulin to insulin detemir can be done on a unit-to-unit basis.

SubQ: Diabetes mellitus:

Type 1: Children ≥6 years and Adults: Refer to Insulin Regular on page 907

Type 2: Adults: Refer to Insulin Regular on page 907

Initial basal insulin dose: Manufacturer recommendations: 0.1-0.2 units/kg once-daily **or** 10 units once- or twice daily

Dosage adjustment in renal impairment: Refer to Insulin Regular on page 907

Dosage adjustment in hepatic impairment: Refer to Insulin Regular on page 907

Additional Information Complete prescribing information for this medication should be consulted for additional detail.

Dosage Forms Excipient information presented when available (limited, particularly for generics); consult specific product labeling.

Injection, solution:

Levemir®: 100 units/mL (10 mL)

Levemir® FlexPen®: 100 units/mL (3 mL)

Insulin Glargine (IN soo lin GLAR jeen)

Brand Names: U.S. Lantus®; Lantus® Solostar®

Brand Names: Canada Lantus®; Lantus® OptiSet®

Index Terms Glargine Insulin

Pharmacologic Category Antidiabetic Agent, Insulin

Additional Appendix Information

Diabetes Mellitus and Pregnancy *on page* 1978

Diabetes Mellitus Management, Adults *on page* 1983

Use Treatment of type 1 diabetes mellitus (insulin dependent, IDDM) and type 2 diabetes mellitus (noninsulin dependent, NIDDM) to improve glycemic control

Pregnancy Risk Factor C

Dosage Note: Insulin glargine is approximately equipotent to human insulin, but has a slower onset, no pronounced peak, and a longer duration of activity. Changing the basal insulin component from another insulin to insulin glargine can be done on a unit-to-unit basis.

SubQ: Diabetes mellitus:

Type 1:

Children <6 years (unlabeled use): Refer to Insulin Regular on page 907

Children ≥6 years and Adults: Refer to Insulin Regular on page 907

Type 2:

Children (unlabeled use): Refer to Insulin Regular on page 907

Adults: Refer to Insulin Regular on page 907

Dosage adjustment in renal impairment: Refer to Insulin Regular on page 907

Dosage adjustment in hepatic impairment: Refer to Insulin Regular on page 907

Additional Information Complete prescribing information for this medication should be consulted for additional detail.

Dosage Forms Excipient information presented when available (limited, particularly for generics); consult specific product labeling.

Injection, solution:

Lantus®: 100 units/mL (3 mL) [cartridge]

Lantus®: 100 units/mL (10 mL) [vial]

Lantus® Solostar®: 100 units/mL (3 mL) [prefilled pen]

Insulin Glulisine (IN soo lin gloo LIS een)

Brand Names: U.S. Apidra®; Apidra® SoloStar®

Brand Names: Canada Apidra®

Index Terms Glulisine Insulin

Pharmacologic Category Antidiabetic Agent, Insulin

Additional Appendix Information

Diabetes Mellitus and Pregnancy *on page* 1978

Diabetes Mellitus Management, Adults *on page* 1983

Use Treatment of type 1 diabetes mellitus (insulin dependent, IDDM) and type 2 diabetes mellitus (noninsulin dependent, NIDDM) to improve glycemic control

Pregnancy Risk Factor C

Dosage Note: Insulin glulisine is equipotent to insulin regular, but has a more rapid onset and shorter duration of activity.

SubQ:

Diabetes mellitus:

Type 1:

Children <4 years (unlabeled use): Refer to Insulin Regular on page 907

Children ≥4 years and Adults: Refer to Insulin Regular on page 907

Type 2:

Children (unlabeled use): Refer to Insulin Regular on page 907

Adults: Refer to Insulin Regular on page 907

I.V.: Glycemic control in selected clinical situations and under appropriate medical supervision: Adults: Refer to Insulin Regular on page 907

Dosage adjustment in renal impairment: Refer to Insulin Regular on page 907

Dosage adjustment in hepatic impairment: Refer to Insulin Regular on page 907

Additional Information Complete prescribing information for this medication should be consulted for additional detail.

Dosage Forms Excipient information presented when available (limited, particularly for generics); consult specific product labeling.

Injection, solution:

Apidra®: 100 units/mL (3 mL) [cartridge]

Apidra®: 100 units/mL (10 mL) [vial]

Apidra® SoloStar®: 100 units/mL (3 mL) [prefilled pen]

Insulin Lispro (IN soo lin LYE sproe)

Brand Names: U.S. HumaLOG®; HumaLOG® KwikPen™

Brand Names: Canada Humalog®

Index Terms Lispro Insulin

Pharmacologic Category Antidiabetic Agent, Insulin

Additional Appendix Information

Diabetes Mellitus and Pregnancy *on page* 1978

Diabetes Mellitus Management, Adults *on page* 1983

Use Treatment of type 1 diabetes mellitus (insulin dependent, IDDM) and type 2 diabetes mellitus (noninsulin dependent, NIDDM) to improve glycemic control

Unlabeled Use Gestational diabetes mellitus (GDM); mild-to-moderate diabetic ketoacidosis (DKA); mild-to-moderate hyperosmolar hyperglycemic state (HHS)

Pregnancy Risk Factor B

Dosage Note: Insulin lispro is equipotent to insulin regular, but has a more rapid onset and shorter duration of activity.

SubQ:

Diabetes mellitus, type 1 and type 2: Children and Adults: Refer to Insulin Regular on page 907

Diabetic ketoacidosis (DKA), mild-to-moderate (unlabeled use): Children and Adults: Refer to Insulin Regular on page 907

Gestational diabetes mellitus (unlabeled use): Adults: Refer to Insulin Regular on page 907

Hyperosmolar hyperglycemic state (HHS), mild-to-moderate (unlabeled use): Children and Adults: Refer to Insulin Regular on page 907

I.V.: Glycemic control in selected clinical situations and under appropriate medical supervision (unlabeled use): Children and Adults: Refer to Insulin Regular on page 907

Dosing adjustment in renal impairment: Refer to Insulin Regular on page 907

Dosing adjustment in hepatic impairment: Refer to Insulin Regular on page 907

Additional Information Complete prescribing information for this medication should be consulted for additional detail.

Dosage Forms Excipient information presented when available (limited, particularly for generics); consult specific product labeling.

Injection, solution:

HumaLOG®: 100 units/mL (3 mL) [cartridge]

HumaLOG®: 100 units/mL (3 mL, 10 mL) [vial]

HumaLOG® KwikPen™: 100 units/mL (3 mL)

◆ **Insulin Lispro and Insulin Lispro Protamine** *see* Insulin Lispro Protamine and Insulin Lispro *on page 906*

Insulin Lispro Protamine and Insulin Lispro

(IN soo lin LYE sproe PROE ta meen & IN soo lin LYE sproe)

Brand Names: U.S. HumaLOG® Mix 50/50™; HumaLOG® Mix 50/50™ KwikPen™; HumaLOG® Mix 75/25™; HumaLOG® Mix 75/25™ KwikPen™

Brand Names: Canada Humalog® Mix 25

Index Terms Insulin Lispro and Insulin Lispro Protamine

Pharmacologic Category Antidiabetic Agent, Insulin

Additional Appendix Information

Diabetes Mellitus and Pregnancy *on page 1978*

Diabetes Mellitus Management, Adults *on page 1983*

Use Treatment of type 1 diabetes mellitus (insulin dependent, IDDM) and type 2 diabetes mellitus (noninsulin dependent, NIDDM) to improve glycemic control

Pregnancy Risk Factor B

Dosage Note: Insulin lispro protamine and insulin lispro combination products are approximately equipotent to insulin NPH and insulin regular combination products but with a more rapid onset and similar duration of activity.

SubQ: Diabetes mellitus, type 1 and type 2: Adults: Refer to Insulin Regular on page 907

Dosage adjustment in renal impairment: Refer to Insulin Regular on page 907

Dosage adjustment in hepatic impairment: Refer to Insulin Regular on page 907

Additional Information Complete prescribing information for this medication should be consulted for additional detail.

Dosage Forms Excipient information presented when available (limited, particularly for generics); consult specific product labeling.

Injection, suspension:

HumaLOG® Mix 50/50™: Insulin lispro protamine suspension 50% [intermediate acting] and insulin lispro solution 50% [rapid acting]: 100 units/mL (10 mL)

HumaLOG® Mix 50/50™ KwikPen™: Insulin lispro protamine suspension 50% [intermediate acting] and insulin lispro solution 50% [rapid acting]: 100 units/mL (3 mL)

HumaLOG® Mix 75/25™: Insulin lispro protamine suspension 75% [intermediate acting] and insulin lispro solution 25% [rapid acting]: 100 units/mL (10 mL)

HumaLOG® Mix 75/25™ KwikPen™: Insulin lispro protamine suspension 75% [intermediate acting] and insulin lispro solution 25% [rapid acting]: 100 units/mL (3 mL)

Insulin NPH (IN soo lin N P H)

Brand Names: U.S. HumuLIN® N; NovoLIN® N

Brand Names: Canada Humulin® N; Novolin® ge NPH

Index Terms Isophane Insulin; NPH Insulin

Pharmacologic Category Antidiabetic Agent, Insulin

Additional Appendix Information

Diabetes Mellitus and Pregnancy *on page 1978*

Diabetes Mellitus Management, Adults *on page 1983*

Use Treatment of type 1 diabetes mellitus (insulin dependent, IDDM) and type 2 diabetes mellitus (noninsulin dependent, NIDDM) to improve glycemic control

Unlabeled Use Gestational diabetes mellitus (GDM)

Dosage Note: When compared to insulin regular, insulin NPH has a slower onset and longer duration of activity.

SubQ:

Diabetes mellitus, type 1 and type 2: Children and Adults: Refer to Insulin Regular on page 907

Gestational diabetes mellitus (unlabeled use): Adults: Refer to Insulin Regular on page 907

Dosing adjustment in renal impairment: Refer to Insulin Regular on page 907

Dosing adjustment in hepatic impairment: Refer to Insulin Regular on page 907

Additional Information Complete prescribing information for this medication should be consulted for additional detail.

Dosage Forms Excipient information presented when available (limited, particularly for generics); consult specific product labeling.

Injection, suspension:

HumuLIN® N: 100 units/mL (3 mL) [prefilled pen]

HumuLIN® N: 100 units/mL (3 mL, 10 mL) [vial]

NovoLIN® N: 100 units/mL (10 mL) [vial]

Dosage Forms: Canada Excipient information presented when available (limited, particularly for generics); consult specific product labeling.

Injection, suspension:

Novolin® ge NPH: 100 units/mL (3 mL) [NovolinSet® prefilled syringe or PenFill® prefilled cartridge]; 10 mL [vial]

Insulin NPH and Insulin Regular

(IN soo lin N P H & IN soo lin REG yoo ler)

Brand Names: U.S. HumuLIN® 70/30; NovoLIN® 70/30

Brand Names: Canada Humulin® 20/80; Humulin® 70/30; Novolin® ge 30/70; Novolin® ge 40/60; Novolin® ge 50/50

Index Terms Insulin Regular and Insulin NPH; Isophane Insulin and Regular Insulin; NPH Insulin and Regular Insulin

Pharmacologic Category Antidiabetic Agent, Insulin

Additional Appendix Information

Diabetes Mellitus and Pregnancy *on page 1978*

Diabetes Mellitus Management, Adults *on page 1983*

Use Treatment of type 1 diabetes mellitus (insulin dependent, IDDM) and type 2 diabetes mellitus (noninsulin dependent, NIDDM) to improve glycemic control

Unlabeled Use Gestational diabetes mellitus (GDM)

Dosage Note: When compared to insulin NPH, the combination product (insulin NPH and insulin regular) has a more rapid onset of action and a similar duration of action.

SubQ:

Diabetes mellitus, type 1 and type 2: Children and Adults: Refer to Insulin Regular on page 907

Gestational diabetes mellitus (unlabeled use): Adults: Refer to Insulin Regular on page 907

Dosing adjustment in renal impairment: Refer to Insulin Regular on page 907

Dosing adjustment in hepatic impairment: Refer to Insulin Regular on page 907

Additional Information Complete prescribing information for this medication should be consulted for additional detail.

Dosage Forms Excipient information presented when available (limited, particularly for generics); consult specific product labeling.

Injection, suspension:

HumuLIN® 70/30: Insulin NPH suspension 70% [intermediate acting] and insulin regular solution 30% [short acting]: 100 units/mL (3 mL) [prefilled pen, vial]

HumuLIN® 70/30: Insulin NPH suspension 70% [intermediate acting] and insulin regular solution 30% [short acting]: 100 units/mL (10 mL) [vial]

NovoLIN® 70/30: Insulin NPH suspension 70% [intermediate acting] and insulin regular solution 30% [short acting]: 100 units/mL (10 mL) [vial]

Dosage Forms: Canada Excipient information presented when available (limited, particularly for generics); consult specific product labeling.

Injection, suspension:

Humulin® 20/80: Insulin regular solution 20% [short acting] and insulin NPH suspension 80% [intermediate acting]: 100 units/mL (3 mL) [PenFill® prefilled cartridge]

Novolin® ge 30/70: Insulin regular solution 30% [short acting] and insulin NPH suspension 70% [intermediate acting]: 100 units/mL (3 mL) [prefilled syringe or PenFill® prefilled cartridge]; (10 mL) [vial]

Novolin® ge 40/60: Insulin regular solution 40% [short acting] and insulin NPH suspension 60% [intermediate acting]: 100 units/mL (3 mL) [PenFill® prefilled cartridge]

Novolin® ge 50/50: Insulin regular solution 50% [short acting] and insulin NPH suspension 50% [intermediate acting]: 100 units/mL (3 mL) [PenFill® prefilled cartridge]

Insulin Regular (IN soo lin REG yoo ler)

Brand Names: U.S. HumuLIN® R; HumuLIN® R U-500; NovoLIN® R

Brand Names: Canada Humulin® R; Novolin® ge Toronto

Index Terms Regular Insulin

Pharmacologic Category Antidiabetic Agent, Insulin

Additional Appendix Information

Diabetes Mellitus and Pregnancy *on page 1978*

Diabetes Mellitus Management, Adults *on page 1983*

Use Treatment of type 1 diabetes mellitus (insulin dependent, IDDM) and type 2 diabetes mellitus (noninsulin dependent, NIDDM) to improve glycemic control

Unlabeled Use Hyperkalemia; gestational diabetes mellitus (GDM), diabetic ketoacidosis (DKA); hyperosmolar hyperglycemic state (HHS); adjunct of parenteral nutrition

Pregnancy Considerations Insulin has not been found to cross the placenta, but insulin bound to anti-insulin antibodies has been detected in cord blood. Maternal hyperglycemia can be associated with adverse effects in the fetus, including macrosomia, neonatal hyperglycemia, and hyperbilirubinemia; the risk of congenital malformations is increased when the Hb A_{1c} is above the normal range. Insulin requirements tend to fall during the first trimester of pregnancy and increase in the later trimesters, peaking at 28-32 weeks of gestation. Following delivery, insulin requirements decrease rapidly. Diabetes can be associated with adverse effects in the mother. Poorly-treated diabetes may cause end-organ damage that may in turn negatively affect obstetric outcomes. Physiologic glucose levels should be maintained prior to and during pregnancy to decrease the risk of adverse events in the fetus and the mother. Insulin is the drug of choice for the control of diabetes mellitus during pregnancy.

Lactation Excretion in breast milk unknown/compatible

Contraindications Hypersensitivity to regular insulin or any component of the formulation; during episodes of hypoglycemia

Warnings/Precautions Hypoglycemia is the most common adverse effect of insulin. The timing of hypoglycemia differs among various insulin formulations. Hypoglycemia may result from increased work or exercise without eating; use of long-acting insulin preparations (eg, insulin detemir, insulin glargine) may delay recovery from hypoglycemia. Profound and prolonged episodes of hypoglycemia may result in convulsions, unconsciousness, temporary or permanent brain damage or even death. Insulin requirements may be altered during illness, emotional disturbances or other stressors. Insulin may produce hypokalemia which, if left untreated, may result in respiratory paralysis, ventricular arrhythmia and even death. Use with caution in patients at risk for hypokalemia (eg, I.V. insulin use). Use with caution in renal or hepatic impairment.

Human insulin differs from animal-source insulin. Any change of insulin should be made cautiously; changing manufacturers, type, and/or method of manufacture may result in the need for a change of dosage. U-500 regular insulin is a concentrated insulin formulation which contains 500 units of insulin per mL; for SubQ administration only using a U-100 insulin syringe or tuberculin syringe; **not for I.V. administration**. To avoid dosing errors when using a U-100 insulin syringe, the prescribed dose should be written in actual insulin units and as unit markings on the U-100 insulin syringe (eg, 50 units [10 units on a U-100 insulin syringe]). To avoid dosing errors when using a tuberculin syringe, the prescribed dose should be written in actual insulin units and as a volume (eg, 50 units [0.1 mL]). Mixing U-500 regular insulin with other insulin formulations is not recommended.

Regular insulin may be administered I.V. or I.M. in selected clinical situations; close monitoring of blood glucose and serum potassium, as well as medical supervision, is required.

The general objective of exogenous insulin therapy is to approximate the physiologic pattern of insulin secretion which is characterized by two distinct phases. Phase 1 insulin secretion suppresses hepatic glucose production and phase 2 insulin secretion occurs in response to carbohydrate ingestion; therefore, exogenous insulin therapy may consist of basal insulin (eg, intermediate- or long-acting insulin or via continuous subcutaneous insulin infusion [CSII]) and/or preprandial insulin (eg, short- or rapid-acting insulin). Patients with type 1 diabetes do not produce endogenous insulin; therefore, these patients require both basal and preprandial insulin administration. Patients with type 2 diabetes retain some beta-cell function in the early stages of their disease; however, as the disease progresses, phase 1 insulin secretion may become completely impaired and phase 2 insulin secretion becomes delayed and/or inadequate in response to meals. Therefore, patients with type 2 diabetes may be treated with oral antidiabetic agents, basal insulin, and/or preprandial insulin depending on the stage of disease and current glycemic control. Since treatment regimens often consist of multiple agents, dosage adjustments must address the specific phase of insulin release that is primarily contributing to the patient's impaired glycemic control. Diabetes self-management education (DSME) is essential to maximize the effectiveness of therapy. Treatment and monitoring regimens must be individualized.

Adverse Reactions Frequency not defined.

Cardiovascular: Palpitation, pallor, peripheral edema, tachycardia

Central nervous system: Fatigue, headache, hypothermia, loss of consciousness, mental confusion
Dermatologic: Pruritus, rash, redness, urticaria
Endocrine & metabolic: Hypoglycemia, hypokalemia
Gastrointestinal: Hunger, nausea, numbness of mouth, weight gain
Local: Injection site reaction (including edema, itching, pain or warmth, stinging), lipoatrophy, lipodystrophy
Neuromuscular & skeletal: Muscle weakness, paresthesia, tremor
Ocular: Transient presbyopia or blurred vision
Miscellaneous: Anaphylaxis, antibodies to insulin (no change in efficacy), diaphoresis, local allergy, systemic allergic symptoms

Drug Interactions

Metabolism/Transport Effects None known.

Avoid Concomitant Use There are no known interactions where it is recommended to avoid concomitant use.

Increased Effect/Toxicity

Insulin Regular may increase the levels/effects of: Antidiabetic Agents (Thiazolidinedione); Hypoglycemic Agents; Quinolone Antibiotics

The levels/effects of Insulin Regular may be increased by: Beta-Blockers; Edetate CALCIUM Disodium; Edetate Disodium; Herbs (Hypoglycemic Properties); Pegvisomant

Decreased Effect

The levels/effects of Insulin Regular may be decreased by: Corticosteroids (Orally Inhaled); Corticosteroids (Systemic); Luteinizing Hormone-Releasing Hormone Analogs; Somatropin; Thiazide Diuretics

Ethanol/Nutrition/Herb Interactions

Ethanol: Use caution with ethanol; may increase risk of hypoglycemia.
Herb/Nutraceutical: Use caution with alfalfa, aloe, bilberry, bitter melon, burdock, celery, damiana, fenugreek, garcinia, garlic, ginger, ginseng (American), gymnema, marshmallow, stinging nettle; may increase risk of hypoglycemia.

Stability

Humulin® R, Humulin® R U-500: Store unopened vials in refrigerator between 2°C and 8°C (36°F to 46°F); do not freeze; keep away from heat and sunlight. Once punctured (in use), vials may be stored for up to 31 days in the refrigerator between 2°C and 8°C (36°F to 46°F) or at room temperature of ≤30°C (≤86°F).

Novolin® R: Store unopened vials in refrigerator between 2°C and 8°C (36°F to 46°F) until product expiration date or at room temperature ≤25°C (≤77°F) for up to 42 days; do not freeze; keep away from heat and sunlight. Once punctured (in use), store vials at room temperature ≤25°C (≤77°F) for up to 42 days (this includes any days stored at room temperature prior to opening vial); refrigeration of in-use vials is not recommended.

Canadian labeling (not in U.S. labeling): All products: Unopened vials, cartridges, and pens should be stored under refrigeration between 2°C and 8°C (36°F to 46°F) until the expiration date; do not freeze; keep away from heat and sunlight. Once punctured (in use), Humulin® vials, cartridges, and pens should be stored at room temperature <25°C (<77°F) for up to 4 weeks. Once punctured (in use), Novolin® ge vials, cartridges, and pens may be stored for up to 1 month at room temperature <25°C (<77°F) for vials or <30°C (<86°F) for pens/cartridges; do not refrigerate.

For SubQ administration:

Humulin® R: May be diluted with the universal diluent, Sterile Diluent for Humalog®, Humulin® N, Humulin® R, Humulin® 70/30, and Humulin® R U-500, to a concentration of 10 units/mL (U-10) or 50 units/mL (U-50). According to the manufacturer, diluted insulin should be stored at 30°C (86°F) and used within 14 days **or** at 5°C (41°F) and used within 28 days.

Novolin® R: Insulin Diluting Medium for NovoLog® is **not** intended for use with Novolin® R or any insulin product other than insulin aspart.

For I.V. infusion:

Humulin® R: May be diluted in NS or D_5W to concentrations of 0.1-1 unit/mL. Stable for 48 hours at room temperature or for 48 hours under refrigeration followed by 48 hours at room temperature.

Novolin® R: May be diluted in NS, D_5W, or $D_{10}W$ with 40 mEq/L potassium chloride at concentrations of 0.05-1 unit/mL. Stable for 24 hours at room temperature

Mechanism of Action Insulin acts via specific membrane-bound receptors on target tissues to regulate metabolism of carbohydrate, protein, and fats. Target organs for insulin include the liver, skeletal muscle, and adipose tissue.

Within the liver, insulin stimulates hepatic glycogen synthesis. Insulin promotes hepatic synthesis of fatty acids, which are released into the circulation as lipoproteins. Skeletal muscle effects of insulin include increased protein synthesis and increased glycogen synthesis. Within adipose tissue, insulin stimulates the processing of circulating lipoproteins to provide free fatty acids, facilitating triglyceride synthesis and storage by adipocytes; also directly inhibits the hydrolysis of triglycerides. In addition, insulin stimulates the cellular uptake of amino acids and increases cellular permeability to several ions, including potassium, magnesium, and phosphate. By activating sodium-potassium ATPases, insulin promotes the intracellular movement of potassium.

Normally secreted by the pancreas, insulin products are manufactured for pharmacologic use through recombinant DNA technology using either *E. coli* or *Saccharomyces cerevisiae*. Insulins are categorized based on the onset, peak, and duration of effect (eg, rapid-, short-, intermediate-, and long-acting insulin).

Pharmacodynamics/Kinetics Note: Rate of absorption, onset, and duration of activity may be affected by site of injection, exercise, presence of lipodystrophy, local blood supply, and/or temperature.

Onset of action: SubQ: 0.5 hours
Peak effect: SubQ: 2.5-5 hours
Duration: SubQ:
U-100: 4-12 hours (may increase with dose)
U-500: Up to 24 hours
Distribution: V_d: 0.26-0.36 L/kg
Bioavailability: SubQ: 55% to 77%
Half-life elimination: I.V.: ~0.5-1 hour (dose-dependent); SubQ: 1 hour
Time to peak, plasma: SubQ: 0.8-2 hours
Excretion: Urine

Dosage

Diabetes mellitus: SubQ: **Note:** Insulin requirements vary dramatically between patients and therapy requires dosage adjustments with careful medical supervision. Specific formulations may require distinct administration procedures; please see individual agents.

Type 1: Children and Adults: **Note:** Multiple daily injections (MDI) guided by blood glucose monitoring or the use of continuous subcutaneous insulin infusions (CSII) is the standard of care for patients with type 1 diabetes. Combinations of insulin formulations are commonly used.

Initial dose: 0.5-1.0 units/kg/day in divided doses. Conservative initial doses of 0.2-0.4 units/kg/day may be recommended to avoid the potential for hypoglycemia.

Division of daily insulin requirement: Generally, 50% to 75% of the total daily dose (TDD) is given as an intermediate- or long-acting form of insulin (in 1-2 daily injections). The remaining portion of the TDD is then divided and administered before or at mealtimes (depending on the formulation) as a rapid-acting or short-acting form of insulin. Premixed combinations are available that deliver the rapid- or short-acting component at the same time as the intermediate- or long-acting component. Some patients may benefit from the use of CSII which delivers rapid-acting insulin as a continuous infusion throughout the day and as boluses at mealtimes via an external pump device.

Adjustment of dose: Dosage must be titrated to achieve glucose control and avoid hypoglycemia. Adjust dose to maintain preprandial plasma glucose between 70-130 mg/dL for most patients. Since treatment regimens often consist of multiple formulations, dosage adjustments must address the specific phase of insulin release that is primarily contributing to the patient's impaired glycemic control. Treatment and monitoring regimens must be individualized. Also see Additional Information.

Usual maintenance range: 0.5-1.2 units/kg/day in divided doses. Insulin requirements are patient-specific and may vary based on age, body weight, and/or activity factors:

Adolescents: May require as much as 1.5 units/kg/day during puberty (Silverstein, 2005)

Prepuberty: 0.7-1 unit/kg/day

Type 2: Children and Adults: The goal of therapy is to achieve an Hb A_{1c} <7% as quickly as possible using the safe titration of medications. According to a consensus statement by the ADA and European Association for the Study of Diabetes (EASD), basal insulin therapy (eg, intermediate- or long-acting insulin) should be considered in patients with type 2 diabetes who fail to achieve glycemic goals with lifestyle interventions and metformin ± a sulfonylurea. Pioglitazone or a GLP-1 agonist may also be considered prior to initiation of basal insulin therapy. In patients who continue to fail to achieve glycemic goals despite the addition of basal insulin, intensification of insulin therapy should be considered; this generally consists of multiple daily injections with a combination of insulin formulations (Nathan, 2009).

Initial basal insulin dose: 0.2 units/kg or 10 units/day (Nathan, 2009). **Note:** Current guidelines recommend that insulin therapy begin with intermediate- or long-acting insulin given at bedtime or long-acting insulin given in the morning (Nathan, 2009).

Adjustment of basal insulin dose: Increase dose by 2 units/day every 3 days until fasting glucose levels are consistently within target range (70-130 mg/dL); may increase dose in larger increments (eg, 4 units/day) if fasting glucose levels are >180 mg/dL (Nathan, 2009)

Note: If the patient experiences hypoglycemia following adjustment, reduce dose by 4 units/day or 10% of total daily dose, whichever is greater (Nathan, 2009). Additional algorithms, such as the "1-1-100", "2-4-6-8", "3-0-3", and "3-2-1" algorithms, exist to aid in the titration of basal insulin (Davies, 2005; Gerstein, 2006; Meneghini, 2007; Riddle, 2003); therapy should be individualized and based on patient-specific details.

Intensification of therapy: Add a second injection of a short-, rapid-, or intermediate-acting insulin as needed based on blood glucose monitoring; the timing of administration and type of insulin added for intensification of therapy depends on the blood glucose level that is consistently out of the target range (eg, preprandial glucose levels before lunch or dinner, postprandial glucose levels, and/or bedtime glucose levels). Additional injections and subsequent dosage adjustments must address the specific phase of insulin release that is primarily contributing to the patient's impaired glycemic control. Intensification of therapy can usually begin with a second injection of ~4 units/day followed by adjustments of ~2 units/day every 3 days until the targeted blood glucose is within range (Nathan, 2009).

In the setting of glucose toxicity (loss of beta-cell sensitivity to glucose concentrations), insulin therapy may be used for short-term management to restore sensitivity of beta-cells; in these cases, the dose may need to be rapidly reduced/withdrawn when sensitivity is re-established.

Diabetic ketoacidosis (DKA) (unlabeled use): Only I.V. regular insulin should be used for severe DKA; use of SubQ rapid-acting insulin analogs (eg, aspart, lispro) may be appropriate for mild-moderate DKA (Kitabchi, 2009). Treatment should continue until reversal of acid-base derangement/ketonemia. Serum glucose is not a direct indicator of these abnormalities, and may decrease more rapidly than correction of the metabolic abnormalities. Also, refer to institution-specific protocols where appropriate.

Children and Adults <20 years (Kitabchi, 2004):

I.V.:

Infusion: 0.1 units/kg/hour

Adjustment: If serum glucose does not fall by 50 mg/dL in the first hour, check hydration status; if acceptable, double insulin dose hourly until glucose levels fall at rate of 50-75 mg/dL per hour. Once serum glucose reaches 250 mg/dL, decrease dose to 0.05-0.1 units/kg/hour; dextrose-containing I.V. fluids should be administered to maintain serum glucose between 150-250 mg/dL until the acidosis clears. After resolution of DKA, supplement I.V. insulin with SubQ insulin as needed until the patient is able to eat and transition fully to a SubQ insulin regimen. An overlap of ~1-2 hours between discontinuation of I.V. insulin and administration of SubQ insulin is recommended to ensure adequate plasma insulin levels.

SubQ, I.M. (**Note:** Only use the SubQ and I.M route if I.V. infusion access is unavailable): 0.1-0.3 units/kg SubQ bolus, followed by 0.1 units/kg given every hour SubQ or I.M. or 0.15-0.2 units/kg every 2 hours SubQ; continue until acidosis clears, then decrease to 0.05 units/kg given every hour until SubQ replacement dosing can be initiated (Kitabchi, 2004; Wolfsdorf, 2007)

Adults ≥20 years (Kitabchi, 2009):

I.V.:

Bolus: 0.1 units/kg (optional)

Infusion: 0.1-0.14 units/kg/hour. **Note:** If no I.V. bolus was administered, patients should receive a continuous infusion of 0.14 units/kg/hour; lower doses may not achieve adequate insulin concentrations to suppress hepatic ketone body production.

Adjustment: If serum glucose does not fall by at least 10% in the first hour, give an I.V. bolus of 0.14 units/kg and continue previous regimen. In addition, if serum glucose does not fall by 50-70 mg/dL in the first hour, the insulin infusion dose should be increased hourly until a steady glucose decline is achieved Once serum glucose reaches 200 mg/dL, decrease infusion dose to 0.02-0.05 units/kg/hour or switch to SubQ rapid-acting insulin (eg, aspart, lispro) at 0.1 units/kg every 2 hours; dextrose-containing I.V. fluids should be administered to maintain serum glucose between 150-250 mg/dL until the acidosis clears. After resolution of DKA, supplement I.V. insulin with SubQ insulin as needed until the patient is able to eat and transition fully to a SubQ insulin regimen. An overlap of ~1-2 hours between discontinuation of I.V. insulin and administration of SubQ insulin is recommended to ensure adequate plasma insulin levels.

SubQ, I.M.: According to the 2009 ADA consensus statement on hyperglycemic crises, a rapid-acting insulin analog (eg, aspart, lispro) given every 1-2 hours via the SubQ route may be appropriate for mild-moderate DKA; however, specific dosing recommendations are not provided (Kitabchi, 2009). If using the I.V. route for severe DKA, consider switching to SubQ rapid-acting insulin once serum glucose reaches 200 mg/dL (Kitabchi, 2009). The following dosing regimen from the 2004 ADA position statement recommends regular insulin (Kitabchi, 2004):

Bolus: 0.4 units/kg; **Note:** Give half of the dose (0.2 units/kg) as an I.V. bolus and half of the dose (0.2 units/kg) as SubQ or I.M.

Intermittent: 0.1 units/kg given every hour SubQ or I.M.

Adjustment: If serum glucose does not fall by 50-70 mg/dL in the first hour, administer 10 units hourly by I.V. bolus until glucose levels fall at a rate of 50-70 mg/dL per hour. Once serum glucose reaches 250 mg/dL, decrease dose to 5-10 units SubQ every 2 hours; dextrose-containing I.V. fluids should be administered to maintain serum glucose between 150-250 mg/dL until the acidosis clears.

Gestational diabetes mellitus (unlabeled use): Insulin therapy should be considered when medical nutrition therapy has not achieved GDM glycemic goals (fasting plasma glucose: <95 mg/dL; 1-hour postprandial levels: <130-140 mg/dL; 2-hour postprandial levels: <120 mg/dL); dose and timing of administration should be based on frequent monitoring of plasma glucose levels (ACOG, 2001; ADA, 2004). Human insulin may be preferred (ADA, 2004); however, rapid-acting insulin analogues may also be considered (ACOG, 2001).

Hyperkalemia, moderate-to-severe (unlabeled use):

I.V.:

Children: 0.1 units/kg regular insulin with dextrose 400 mg/kg infused over 15-30 minutes; ratio of ~1 unit of insulin to every 4 g of dextrose (Hegenbarth, 2008). **Note:** Dextrose monotherapy may be sufficient to correct hyperkalemia.

Adults: 10 units regular insulin mixed with 25 g dextrose (50 mL $D_{50}W$) given over 15-30 minutes (ACLS, 2010); alternatively, 50 mL $D_{50}W$ over 5 minutes followed by 10 units regular insulin I.V. push over seconds may be administered in the setting of imminent cardiac arrest. In patients with ongoing cardiac arrest (eg, PEA with presumed hyperkalemia), administration of $D_{50}W$ over <5 minutes is routine. Effects on potassium are temporary. As appropriate, consider methods of enhancing potassium removal/excretion.

Hyperosmolar hyperglycemic state (HHS) (unlabeled use): Only regular insulin should be used. Infusion should continue until reversal of mental status changes and hyperosmolality. Serum glucose is not a direct indicator of these abnormalities, and may decrease more rapidly than correction of the metabolic abnormalities. Also, refer to institution-specific protocols where appropriate.

Children and Adults <20 years (Kitabchi, 2004):

I.V.:

Infusion: 0.1 units/kg/hour

Adjustment: If serum glucose does not fall by 50 mg/dL in the first hour, check hydration status; if acceptable, double insulin dose hourly until glucose levels fall at rate of 50-75 mg/dL per hour. Once serum glucose reaches 300 mg/dL, decrease dose to 0.05-0.1 units/kg/hour; dextrose-containing I.V. fluids should be administered to maintain serum glucose between 250-300 mg/dL until hyperosmolality clears and mental status returns to normal. After resolution of HHS, supplement I.V. insulin with SubQ insulin as needed until the patient is able to eat and transition fully to a SubQ insulin regimen. An overlap of ~1-2 hours between discontinuation of I.V. insulin and administration of SubQ insulin is recommended to ensure adequate plasma insulin levels.

SubQ, I.M. (**Note:** Only use the SubQ and I.M route if I.V. infusion access is unavailable): 0.1-0.3 units/kg SubQ bolus, followed by 0.1 units/kg given every hour SubQ or I.M. or 0.15-0.2 units/kg every 2 hours SubQ; continue until resolution of hyperosmolality, then decrease to 0.05 units/kg given every hour until SubQ replacement dosing can be initiated (Kitabchi, 2004; Wolfsdorf, 2007)

Adults ≥20 years (Kitabchi, 2009):

I.V.:

Bolus: 0.1 units/kg bolus (optional)

Infusion: 0.1-0.14 units/kg/hour. **Note:** If no I.V. bolus was administered, patients should receive a continuous infusion of 0.14 units/kg/hour.

Adjustment: If serum glucose does not fall by at least 10% in the first hour, give an I.V. bolus of 0.14 units/kg and continue previous regimen. In addition, if serum glucose does not fall by 50-70 mg/dL in the first hour, the insulin infusion dose should be increased hourly until a steady glucose decline is achieved. Once serum glucose reaches 300 mg/dL, decrease dose to 0.02-0.05 units/kg/hour; dextrose-containing I.V. fluids should be administered to maintain serum glucose between 200-300 mg/dL until the patient is mentally alert. After resolution of HHS, supplement I.V. insulin with SubQ insulin as needed until the patient is able to eat and transition fully to a SubQ insulin regimen. An overlap of ~1-2 hours between discontinuation of I.V. insulin and administration of SubQ insulin is recommended to ensure adequate plasma insulin levels.

Dosing adjustment in renal impairment: Insulin requirements are reduced due to changes in insulin clearance or metabolism. Close monitoring of blood glucose and adjustment of therapy is required in renal impairment.

Cl_{cr} 10-50 mL/minute: Administer at 75% of normal dose and monitor glucose closely

Cl_{cr} <10 mL/minute: Administer at 25% to 50% of normal dose and monitor glucose closely

Hemodialysis: Because of a large molecular weight (6000 daltons), insulin is not significantly removed by hemodialysis; supplemental dose is not necessary

Peritoneal dialysis: Because of a large molecular weight (6000 daltons), insulin is not significantly removed by peritoneal dialysis; supplemental dose is not necessary

Continuous renal replacement therapy: Administer 75% of normal dose and monitor glucose closely; supplemental dose is not necessary

Dosing adjustment in hepatic impairment: Insulin requirements may be reduced. Close monitoring of blood glucose and adjustment of therapy is required in hepatic impairment.

Dietary Considerations Individualized medical nutrition therapy (MNT) based on ADA recommendations is an integral part of therapy.

Administration

SubQ administration: Do not use if solution is viscous or cloudy; use only if clear and colorless. Regular insulin should be administered within 30-60 minutes before a meal. Cold injections should be avoided. SubQ administration is usually made into the thighs, arms, buttocks, or abdomen; rotate injection sites. When mixing regular insulin with other preparations of insulin, regular insulin should be drawn into syringe first. Regular insulin is not recommended for use in external SubQ insulin infusion pump.

I.M. administration: Do not use if solution is viscous or cloudy; use only if clear and colorless. May be administered I.M. in selected clinical situations; close monitoring of blood glucose and serum potassium as well as medical supervision is required.

I.V. administration: Do not use if solution is viscous or cloudy; use only if clear and colorless. May be administered I.V. with close monitoring of blood glucose and serum potassium; appropriate medical supervision is required. If possible, avoid I.V. bolus administration in pediatric patients with DKA; may increase risk of cerebral edema. **Do not administer mixtures of insulin formulations intravenously.** I.V. administration of U-500 regular insulin is not recommended.

I.V. infusions: To minimize adsorption to I.V. solution bag (**Note:** Refer to institution-specific protocols where appropriate):

*If new tubing is **not** needed:* Wait a minimum of 30 minutes between the preparation of the solution and the initiation of the infusion.

If new tubing is needed: After receiving the insulin drip solution, the administration set should be attached to the I.V. container and the entire line should be flushed with a priming infusion of 20-50 mL of the insulin solution (Goldberg, 2006; Hirsch, 2006). Wait 30 minutes, then flush the line again with the insulin solution prior to initiating the infusion.

If insulin is required prior to the availability of the insulin drip, regular insulin should be administered by I.V. push injection.

Because of adsorption, the actual amount of insulin being administered via I.V. infusion could be substantially less than the apparent amount. Therefore, adjustment of the I.V. infusion rate should be based on effect and not solely on the apparent insulin dose. The apparent dose may be used as a starting point for determining the subsequent SubQ dosing regimen (Moghissi, 2009); however, the transition to SubQ administration requires continuous medical supervision, frequent monitoring of blood glucose, and careful adjustment of therapy. In addition, SubQ insulin should be given 1-4 hours prior to the discontinuation of I.V. insulin to prevent hyperglycemia (Moghissi, 2009).

Monitoring Parameters

Diabetes mellitus: Plasma glucose, electrolytes, Hb A_{1c}

DKA/HHS: Serum electrolytes, glucose, BUN, creatinine, osmolality, venous pH (repeat arterial blood gases are generally unnecessary), anion gap, urine output, urinalysis, mental status

Hyperkalemia: Serum potassium and glucose must be closely monitored to avoid hypokalemia, rebound hyperkalemia, and hypoglycemia.

Reference Range

Therapeutic, serum insulin (fasting): 5-20 μIU/mL (SI: 35-145 pmol/L)

Glucose, fasting:

Newborns: 60-110 mg/dL

Adults: 60-110 mg/dL

Elderly: 100-180 mg/dL

Recommendations for glycemic control in adults with diabetes mellitus (ADA, 2010):

Hb A_{1c}: <7%

Preprandial capillary plasma glucose: 70-130 mg/dL

Peak postprandial capillary plasma glucose: <180 mg/dL

Additional Information

Split-mixed or basal-bolus regimens: Combination regimens which optimize differences in the onset and duration of different insulin products are commonly used to approximate physiologic secretion. In split-mixed regimens, an intermediate-acting insulin (eg, NPH insulin) is administered once or twice daily and supplemented by short-acting (regular) or rapid-acting (lispro, aspart, or glulisine) insulin. Blood glucose measurements are completed several times daily. Dosages are adjusted emphasizing the individual component of the regimen which most directly influences the blood sugar in question (either the intermediate-acting component or the shorter-acting component). Fixed-ratio formulations (eg, 70/30 mix) may be used as twice daily injections in this scenario; however, the ability to titrate the dosage of an individual component is limited. An example of a "split-mixed" regimen would be 21 units of NPH plus 9 units of regular insulin in the morning and an evening meal dose consisting of 14 units of NPH plus 6 units of regular insulin.

Basal-bolus regimens are designed to more closely mimic physiologic secretion. These regimens employ a long-acting insulin (eg, glargine) to simulate basal insulin secretion. The basal component is frequently administered at bedtime or in the early morning. This is supplemented by multiple daily injections of rapid-acting products (lispro, aspart, or glulisine) immediately prior to a meal, which provides insulin at the time when nutrients are absorbed. An example of a basal-bolus regimen would be 30 units of glargine at bedtime and 12 units of lispro insulin prior to each meal.

Estimation of the effect per unit: A "Rule of 1500" has been frequently used as a means to estimate the change in blood sugar relative to each unit of insulin administered. In fact, the recommended values used in these calculations may vary from 1500-2200 (a value of 1500 is generally recommended for regular insulin while 1800 is recommended for "rapid-acting insulins"). The higher values lead to more conservative estimates of the effect per unit of insulin, and therefore lead to more cautious adjustments. The effect per unit of insulin is approximated by dividing the selected numerical value (eg, 1500-2200) by the number of units/day received by the patient. This may be used as a crude approximation of the patient's insulin sensitivity as adjustments to individual components of the regimen are made. Each additional unit of insulin added to the corresponding insulin dose may be expected to lower the blood glucose by this amount.

To illustrate, in the "basal-bolus" regimen example presented above, the rule of 1800 would indicate an expected change of 27 mg/dL per unit of lispro insulin (the total daily insulin dose is 66 units; using the formula: 1800/66 = 27). A patient may be instructed to add additional insulin if the preprandial glucose is >125 mg/dL. For a prelunch glucose of 195 mg/dL, this would mean the patient would administer the scheduled 12 units of lispro along with an additional "correctional" 3 units for a total of 15 units prior to the meal. If correctional doses are required on a consistent basis, an adjustment of the patients diet and/or scheduled insulin dose may be necessary.

Dosage Forms

Excipient information presented when available (limited, particularly for generics); consult specific product labeling.

Injection, solution:

HumuLIN® R: 100 units/mL (3 mL, 10 mL)

NovoLIN® R: 100 units/mL (10 mL)

Injection, solution [concentrate]:

HumuLIN® R U-500: 500 units/mL (20 mL)

◆ **Insulin Regular and Insulin NPH** *see* Insulin NPH and Insulin Regular *on page 906*

◆ **Intanza® (Can)** *see* Influenza Virus Vaccine (Inactivated) *on page 897*

◆ **Integrilin®** *see* Eptifibatide *on page 608*

◆ **Intelence®** *see* Etravirine *on page 673*
◆ **α-2-interferon** *see* Interferon Alfa-2b *on page 912*
◆ **Interferon Alfa-2a (PEG Conjugate)** *see* Peginterferon Alfa-2a *on page 1308*
◆ **Interferon Alfa-2b and Ribavirin Combination Pack** *see* Interferon Alfa-2b and Ribavirin *on page 915*
◆ **Interferon Alfa-2b (PEG Conjugate)** *see* Peginterferon Alfa-2b *on page 1311*

Interferon Alfa-2b (in ter FEER on AL fa too bee)

Brand Names: U.S. Intron® A
Brand Names: Canada Intron® A
Index Terms INF-alpha 2; Interferon Alpha-2b; rLFN-α2; α-2-interferon
Pharmacologic Category Interferon
Use
Patients ≥1 year of age: Chronic hepatitis B
Patients ≥3 years of age: Chronic hepatitis C (in combination with ribavirin)
Patients ≥18 years of age: Condyloma acuminata, chronic hepatitis B, chronic hepatitis C, hairy cell leukemia, malignant melanoma, AIDS-related Kaposi's sarcoma, follicular non-Hodgkin's lymphoma

Unlabeled Use AIDS-related thrombocytopenia, cutaneous ulcerations of Behçet's disease, neuroendocrine tumors (including carcinoid syndrome and islet cell tumor), cutaneous T-cell lymphoma, desmoid tumor, lymphomatoid granulomatosis, hepatitis D, chronic myelogenous leukemia (CML), non-Hodgkin's lymphomas (other than follicular lymphoma, see approved use), multiple myeloma, renal cell carcinoma, West Nile virus

Pregnancy Risk Factor C / X in combination with ribavirin

Pregnancy Considerations Animal studies have demonstrated abortifacient effects. Disruption of the normal menstrual cycle was also observed in animal studies; therefore, the manufacturer recommends that reliable contraception is used in women of childbearing potential. Alfa interferon is endogenous to normal amniotic fluid. *In vitro* administration studies have reported that when administered to the mother, it does not cross the placenta. Case reports of use in pregnant women are limited. The Perinatal HIV Guidelines Working Group does not recommend that interferon-alfa be used during pregnancy. Interferon alfa-2b monotherapy should only be used in pregnancy when the potential benefit to the mother justifies the possible risk to the fetus. Combination therapy with ribavirin is contraindicated in pregnancy (refer to Ribavirin monograph); two forms of contraception should be used during combination therapy and patients should have monthly pregnancy tests. A pregnancy registry has been established for women inadvertently exposed to ribavirin while pregnant (800-593-2214).

Lactation Enters breast milk/not recommended (AAP rates "compatible"; AAP 2001 update pending)

Medication Guide Available Yes

Contraindications Hypersensitivity to interferon alfa or any component of the formulation; decompensated liver disease; autoimmune hepatitis

Combination therapy with interferon alfa-2b and ribavirin is also contraindicated in pregnancy, males with pregnant partners; hemoglobinopathies (eg, thalassemia major, sickle-cell anemia); renal dysfunction (Cl_{cr} <50 mL/minute)

Warnings/Precautions Hazardous agent - use appropriate precautions for handling and disposal.

[U.S. Boxed Warning]: May cause or aggravate fatal or life-threatening autoimmune disorders, neuropsychiatric symptoms (including depression and/or suicidal thoughts/behaviors), ischemic, and/or infectious disorders; discontinue treatment for persistent severe or worsening symptoms.

Neuropsychiatric disorders: May cause severe psychiatric adverse events (eg, depression, psychosis, mania, suicidal behavior/ideation, homicidal ideation) in patients with and without previous psychiatric symptoms, avoid use in patients with pre-existing psychiatric condition, severe psychiatric disorder or history of severe depression; careful neuropsychiatric monitoring is required during and for 6 months after therapy. Suicidal ideation or attempts may occur more frequently in pediatric patients when compared to adults. Discontinue in patients developing severe depression or psychiatric disorders. Higher doses in elderly patients, or diseases other than hairy cell leukemia, may result in increased CNS toxicity.

Hepatic disease: May cause hepatotoxicity; monitor closely if abnormal liver function tests develop. A transient increase in ALT (≥2 times baseline) may occur in patients treated with interferon alfa-2b for chronic hepatitis B. Therapy generally may continue; monitor. Worsening and potentially fatal liver disease, including jaundice, hepatic encephalopathy, and hepatic failure have been reported in patients receiving interferon alfa for chronic hepatitis B and C with decompensated liver disease, autoimmune hepatitis, history of autoimmune disease, and immunosuppressed transplant recipients; avoid use in these patients. Chronic hepatitis B or C patients with a history of autoimmune disease or who are immunosuppressed transplant recipients should not receive interferon alfa-2b. Discontinue treatment (if appropriate) in any patient developing signs or symptoms of liver failure.

Bone marrow suppression: Causes bone marrow suppression, including potentially severe cytopenias, and very rarely, aplastic anemia. Discontinue treatment for severe neutropenia (ANC <500/mm^3) or thrombocytopenia (platelets <25,000/mm^3). Hemolytic anemia (hemoglobin <10 g/dL) was observed when combined with ribavirin; anemia occurred within 1-2 weeks of initiation of therapy. Use caution in patients with pre-existing myelosuppression and in patients with concomitant medications which cause myelosuppression.

Autoimmune disorders: Avoid use in patients with history of autoimmune disorders; development of autoimmune disorders (thrombocytopenia, vasculitis, Raynaud's disease, rheumatoid arthritis, lupus erythematosus and rhabdomyolysis) has been associated with use. Monitor closely; consider discontinuing. Worsening of psoriasis and sarcoidosis (and the development of new sarcoidosis) have been reported; use caution.

Cardiovascular disease/coagulation disorders: Use caution and monitor closely in patients with cardiovascular disease (ischemic or thromboembolic), arrhythmias, hypertension, and in patients with a history of MI or prior therapy with cardiotoxic drugs. Patients with pre-existing cardiac disease and/or advanced cancer should have baseline and periodic ECGs. May cause hypotension (during administration or delayed), arrhythmia, tachycardia, cardiomyopathy (~2% in AIDS-related Kaposi's Sarcoma patients) and/or MI. Hemorrhagic cerebrovascular events have been observed with therapy. Use caution in patients with coagulation disorders.

Endocrine disorders: Thyroid disorders (possibly reversible) have been reported; use caution in patients with pre-existing thyroid disease. Discontinue use in patients who cannot maintain normal ranges with thyroid medication. Diabetes mellitus has been reported; discontinue if cannot effectively manage with medication. Use with caution in patients with a history of diabetes mellitus, particularly if prone to DKA. Hypertriglyceridemia has been reported;

discontinue if persistent and severe, and/or combined with symptoms of pancreatitis.

Pulmonary disease: Dyspnea, pulmonary infiltrates, pulmonary hypertension, interstitial pneumonitis, pneumonia, bronchiolitis obliterans, and sarcoidosis may be induced or aggravated by treatment, sometimes resulting in respiratory failure or fatality. Has been reported more in patients being treated for chronic hepatitis C, although has also occurred with use for oncology indications. Patients with fever, cough, dyspnea or other respiratory symptoms should be evaluated with a chest x-ray; monitor closely and consider discontinuing treatment with evidence of impaired pulmonary function. Use with caution in patients with a history of pulmonary disease.

Ophthalmic disorders: Decreased/loss of vision, macular edema, optic neuritis, retinal hemorrhages, cotton wool spots, papilledema, retinal detachment (serous), and retinal artery or vein thrombosis have occurred (or been aggravated) in patients receiving alpha interferons. Use caution in patients with pre-existing eye disorders; monitor closely; a complete eye exam should be done promptly in patients who develop ocular symptoms; discontinue with new or worsening ophthalmic disorders.

Commonly associated with fever and flu-like symptoms; rule out other causes/infection with persistent fever; use with caution in patients with debilitating conditions. Acute hypersensitivity reactions have been reported. Do not treat patients with visceral AIDS-related Kaposi's sarcoma associated with rapidly-progressing or life-threatening disease. Some formulations contain albumin, which may carry a remote risk of viral transmission. Due to differences in dosage, patients should not change brands of interferons without the concurrence of their healthcare provider. Combination therapy with ribavirin is associated with birth defects and/or fetal mortality and hemolytic anemia. Do not use combination therapy with ribavirin in patients with renal dysfunction (Cl_{cr} <50 mL/minute).

Adverse Reactions Note: In a majority of patients, a flu-like syndrome (fever, chills, tachycardia, malaise, myalgia, headache), occurs within 1-2 hours of administration; may last up to 24 hours and may be dose limiting.

>10%:
- Cardiovascular: Chest pain (≤28%)
- Central nervous system: Fatigue (8% to 96%), fever (34% to 94%), headache (21% to 62%), chills (≤54%), depression (3% to 40%; grades 3/4: 2%), somnolence (≤33%), dizziness (≤24%), irritability (≤22%), pain (≤18%), amnesia (≤14%), concentration impaired (≤14%), malaise (≤14%), confusion (≤12%), insomnia (≤12%)
- Dermatologic: Alopecia (≤38%), rash (≤25%), pruritus (≤11%)
- Endocrine & metabolic: Amenorrhea (≤12%)
- Gastrointestinal: Anorexia (1% to 69%), nausea, (17% to 66%), diarrhea (2% to 45%), vomiting (2% to 32%), xerostomia (≤28%), taste alteration (≤24%), abdominal pain (1% to 23%), constipation (≤14%), gingivitis (≤14%), weight loss (<1% to 13%)
- Hematologic: Neutropenia (≤92%; grade 4: 1% to 4%), leukopenia (≤68%), anemia (≤32%), thrombocytopenia (≤15%)
- Hepatic: AST increased (≤63%; grades 3/4: 14%), ALT increased (≤15%), pain (upper right quadrant: up to 15%); alkaline phosphatase increased (≤13%)
- Local: Injection site reaction (≤20%)
- Neuromuscular & skeletal: Myalgia (28% to 75%), weakness (≤63%), rigors (≤42%), paresthesia (1% to 21%), skeletal pain (≤21%), arthralgia (≤19%), back pain (≤19%)
- Renal: BUN increased (≤12%)
- Respiratory: Dyspnea (≤34%), cough (≤31%), pharyngitis (≤31%), sinusitis (≤21%)
- Miscellaneous: Flu-like syndrome (≤79%), diaphoresis (1% to 21%), moniliasis (≤17%)

5% to 10%:
- Cardiovascular: Edema (≤10%), hypertension (≤9%)
- Central nervous system: Hypoesthesia (≤10%), anxiety (≤9%), vertigo (≤8%), agitation (≤7%)
- Dermatologic: Dry skin (≤10%), dermatitis (≤8%), purpura (≤5%)
- Endocrine & metabolic: Libido decreased (≤5%)
- Gastrointestinal: Loose stools (≤10%), dyspepsia (≤8%)
- Genitourinary: Urinary tract infection (≤5%)
- Renal: Polyuria (≤10%), serum creatinine increased (≤6%)
- Respiratory: Bronchitis (≤10%), nasal congestion (≤10%), epistaxis (≤7%)
- Miscellaneous: Infection (≤7%), herpes virus infections (≤5%)

<5% (Limited to important or life-threatening): Acute hypersensitivity reaction, aggression, albuminuria, alcohol intolerance, allergic reactions, anaphylaxis, angina, angioedema, aphasia, aplastic anemia (rarely), arrhythmia, ascites, asthma, ataxia, atrial fibrillation, bell's palsy, bilirubinemia, blurred vision, bradycardia, bronchiolitis obliterans, bronchoconstriction, bronchospasm, cardiac failure, cardiomegaly, cardiomyopathy, cellulitis, colitis, coma, conjunctivitis, coronary artery disorder, cotton wool spots, cyanosis, cystitis, dehydration, diabetes mellitus, dysphasia, dysuria, eczema, ejection fraction decreased, epidermal necrolysis, erythema, erythema multiforme, erythematous rash, esophagitis, extrapyramidal disorder, extrasystoles, gastrointestinal hemorrhage, granulocytopenia, hallucination, hearing loss/impairment, heart valve disorder, hematuria, hemolytic anemia, hemoptysis, hepatic encephalopathy, hepatic failure, hepatitis, hepatotoxicity, hot flashes, homicidal ideation, hyper-/hypothyroidism, hypercalcemia, hyperglycemia, hypertriglyceridemia, hypochromic anemia, hypotension, hypothermia, hypoventilation, impotence, incontinence, injection site necrosis, jaundice, lactate dehydrogenase increased, leukorrhea, liver function test abnormal, lupus erythematosus, lymphadenitis, lymphadenopathy, lymphocytosis, lymphopenia, maculopapular rash, macular edema, menorrhagia, MI, migraine, muscle atrophy, myositis, nephrotic syndrome, nervousness, neuralgia, neuropathy, neurosis, nystagmus, optic neuritis, palpitation, pancreatitis, papilledema, paranoia, peripheral ischemia, peripheral neuropathy, photophobia, photosensitivity, pleural effusion, pneumonia, pneumonitis (interstitial), pneumothorax, proteinuria, psoriasis exacerbation, psychosis, pulmonary embolism, pulmonary fibrosis, pulmonary hypertension, pulmonary infiltrates, pure red cell aplasia, raynaud's disease, renal failure, renal insufficiency, respiratory insufficiency, retinal artery thrombosis, retinal detachment (serous), retinal vein thrombosis, rhabdomyolysis, sarcoidosis exacerbation, sebaceous cyst, seizure, sepsis, sexual dysfunction, Stevens-Johnson syndrome, stomatitis, stroke, suicidal attempt/ideation, syncope, systemic lupus erythematosus, tachycardia, tendonitis, thrombocytopenia purpura (idiopathic and thrombotic), thrombosis, toxic epidermal necrolysis, upper respiratory tract infection, urticaria, uterine bleeding, vasculitis, Vogt-Koyanagi-Harada syndrome, wheezing

Drug Interactions

Metabolism/Transport Effects Inhibits CYP1A2 (weak)

Avoid Concomitant Use

Avoid concomitant use of Interferon Alfa-2b with any of the following: CloZAPine; Telbivudine

Increased Effect/Toxicity

Interferon Alfa-2b may increase the levels/effects of: Aldesleukin; CloZAPine; Methadone; Ribavirin; Telbivudine; Theophylline Derivatives; Zidovudine

Decreased Effect There are no known significant interactions involving a decrease in effect.

Stability Store powder and solution for injection (vials and pens) under refrigeration at 2°C to 8°C (36°F to 46°F); do not freeze. The manufacturer recommends reconstituting vial with the diluent provided (SWFI). To prepare solution for infusion, further dilute appropriate dose in NS 100 mL. Final concentration should be ≥10 million units/100 mL.

Powder for injection: Following reconstitution, should be used immediately, but may be stored under refrigeration for up to 24 hours.

Prefilled pens: After first use, discard unused portion after 4 weeks.

Mechanism of Action Following activation, multiple effects can be detected including induction of gene transcription. Inhibits cellular growth, alters the state of cellular differentiation, interferes with oncogene expression, alters cell surface antigen expression, increases phagocytic activity of macrophages, and augments cytotoxicity of lymphocytes for target cells

Pharmacodynamics/Kinetics

Distribution: V_d: 31 L; but has been noted to be much greater (370-720 L) in leukemia patients receiving continuous infusion IFN; IFN does not penetrate the CSF

Metabolism: Primarily renal

Bioavailability: I.M.: 83%; SubQ: 90%

Half-life elimination: I.V.: ~2 hours; I.M., SubQ: ~2-3 hours

Time to peak, serum: I.M., SubQ: ~3-12 hours

Dosage Details concerning dosing in combination regimens should also be consulted. **Note:** Withhold treatment for ANC <500/mm^3 or platelets <25,000/mm^3. Consider premedication with acetaminophen prior to administration to reduce the incidence of some adverse reactions. Not all dosage forms and strengths are appropriate for all indications; refer to product labeling for details.

Children 1-17 years: **Note:** The following dosing may also be used in **infants** in the setting of HIV-exposure/-infection (CDC, 2009).

- Chronic hepatitis B (including HIV coinfection): SubQ: 3 million units/m^2 3 times/week for 1 week, followed by 6 million units/m^2 3 times/week (maximum: 10 million units/dose) total duration of therapy 16-24 weeks (treat for 24 weeks in HIV-exposure/-infection)
- Chronic hepatitis C with HIV coinfection: I.M., SubQ: 3-5 million units/m^2 3 times/week (maximum: 3 million units/dose) with ribavirin for 48 weeks, regardless of HCV genotype (CDC, 2009)

Adults:

- Hairy cell leukemia: I.M., SubQ: 2 million units/m^2 3 times/week for up to 6 months (may continue treatment with continued treatment response)
- Lymphoma (follicular): SubQ: 5 million units 3 times/week for up to 18 months
- Malignant melanoma: Induction: 20 million units/m^2 I.V. for 5 consecutive days per week for 4 weeks, followed by maintenance dosing of 10 million units/m^2 SubQ 3 times/week for 48 weeks
- AIDS-related Kaposi's sarcoma: I.M., SubQ: 30 million units/m^2 3 times/week
- Chronic hepatitis B: I.M., SubQ: 5 million units/day or 10 million units 3 times/week for 16 weeks
- Chronic hepatitis C: I.M., SubQ: 3 million units 3 times/week. In patients with normalization of ALT at 16 weeks, continue treatment (if tolerated) for 18-24 months; consider discontinuation if normalization does not occur at 16 weeks. **Note:** May be used in combination therapy with ribavirin in previously untreated patients or in patients who relapse following alpha interferon therapy.
- Condyloma acuminata: Intralesionally: 1 million units/lesion (maximum: 5 lesions/treatment) 3 times/week (on alternate days) for 3 weeks; may administer a second course at 12-16 weeks

Dosage adjustment in renal impairment: Combination therapy with ribavirin (hepatitis C) should not be used in patients with reduced renal function (Cl_{cr} <50 mL/minute).

Dosage adjustment for toxicity:

Neuropsychiatric disorders (during treatment):

- Clinical depression or other psychiatric problem: Monitor closely during and for 6 months after treatment
- Severe depression or other psychiatric disorder: Discontinue treatment
- Persistent or worsening psychiatric symptoms, suicidal ideation, aggression towards others: Discontinue treatment and follow with appropriate psychiatric intervention

Hypersensitivity reaction (acute, serious), ophthalmic disorders (new or worsening), thyroid abnormality development (which cannot be normalized with medication), signs or symptoms of liver failure: Discontinue treatment

Liver function abnormality, pulmonary infiltrate development, evidence of pulmonary function impairment, or autoimmune disorder development: Monitor closely and discontinue if appropriate

Manufacturer-recommended adjustments, listed according to indication:

Lymphoma (follicular):

- Neutrophils >1000/mm^3 to <1500/mm^3: Reduce dose by 50%; may re-escalate to starting dose when neutrophils return to >1500/mm^3
- Severe toxicity (neutrophils <1000/mm^3 or platelets <50,000/mm^3): Temporarily withhold
- AST >5 times ULN or serum creatinine >2 mg/dL: Permanently discontinue

Hairy cell leukemia: Severe toxicity: Reduce dose by 50% or temporarily withhold and resume with 50% dose reduction; permanently discontinue if persistent or recurrent severe toxicity is noted

Chronic hepatitis B:

- WBC <1500/mm^3, granulocytes <750/mm^3, or platelet count <50,000/mm^3, or other laboratory abnormality or severe adverse reaction: Reduce dose by 50%; may re-escalate to starting dose upon resolution of hematologic toxicity. Discontinue for persistent intolerance.
- WBC <1000/mm^3, granulocytes <500/mm^3, or platelet count <25,000/mm^3: Permanently discontinue

Chronic hepatitis C: Severe toxicity: Reduce dose by 50% or temporarily withhold until subsides; permanently discontinue for persistent toxicities after dosage reduction

AIDS-related Kaposi sarcoma: Severe toxicity: Reduce dose by 50% or temporarily withhold; may resume at reduced dose with toxicity resolution; permanently discontinue for persistent/recurrent toxicities

Malignant melanoma:

- Severe toxicity (neutrophils >250/mm^3 to <500/mm^3 or ALT/AST >5-10 times ULN): Temporarily withhold; resume with a 50% dose reduction when adverse reaction abates
- Neutrophils <250/mm^3, ALT/AST >10 times ULN, or severe/persistent adverse reactions: Permanently discontinue

Administration

I.M.: Administer in evening (if possible)

I.V.: Infuse over ~20 minutes

SubQ: Suggested for those who are at risk for bleeding or are thrombocytopenic. Rotate SubQ injection site. Administer in evening (if possible). Patient should be well hydrated. Reconstitute with recommended amount of

SWFI and agitate gently; do not shake. **Note:** Different vial strengths require different amounts of diluent. Not every dosage form is appropriate for every indication; refer to manufacturer's labeling.

Intralesional: Inject at an angle nearly parallel to the plane of the skin, directing the needle to center of the base of the wart to infiltrate the lesion core and cause a small wheal. Only infiltrate the keratinized layer; avoid administration which is too deep or shallow.

Monitoring Parameters Baseline chest x-ray, ECG; CBC with differential and platelets (baseline and routinely during treatment), liver function tests, serum creatinine, electrolytes, triglycerides, thyroid function tests (baseline and periodically during treatment); weight; ophthalmic exam (baseline and periodic, or with new ocular symptoms); patients with pre-existing cardiac abnormalities or in advanced stages of cancer should have ECGs taken before and during treatment

Dosage Forms Excipient information presented when available (limited, particularly for generics); consult specific product labeling.

Injection, powder for reconstitution [preservative free]:
- Intron® A: 10 million int. units, 18 million int. units, 50 million int. units [contains albumin (human)]

Injection, solution:
- Intron® A: 6 million int. units/mL (3 mL); 10 million int. units/mL (2.5 mL) [contains edetate disodium, polysorbate 80; vial]
- Intron® A: 3 million int. units/0.2 mL (1.2 mL) [contains edetate disodium, polysorbate 80; delivers 6 doses of 0.2 mL each; 18 million int. units total per prefilled pen]
- Intron® A: 5 million int. units/0.2 mL (1.2 mL) [contains edetate disodium, polysorbate 80; delivers 6 doses of 0.2 mL each; 30 million int.units total per prefilled pen]
- Intron® A: 10 million int. units/0.2 mL (1.2 mL) [contains edetate disodium, polysorbate 80; delivers 6 doses of 0.2 mL each; 60 million int. units total per prefilled pen]

Interferon Alfa-2b and Ribavirin

(in ter FEER on AL fa too bee & rye ba VYE rin)

Brand Names: U.S. Rebetron®

Index Terms Interferon Alfa-2b and Ribavirin Combination Pack; Ribavirin and Interferon Alfa-2b Combination Pack

Pharmacologic Category Antiviral Agent; Interferon

Use Combination therapy for the treatment of chronic hepatitis C in patients with compensated liver disease previously untreated with alpha interferon or who have relapsed after alpha interferon therapy

Pregnancy Risk Factor X

Dosage

Children ≥3 years: Chronic hepatitis C: **Note:** Treatment duration may vary. Consult current guidelines and literature. Combination therapy:
- Intron® A: SubQ:
  - 25-61 kg: 3 million int. units/m^2 3 times/week
  - >61 kg: Refer to adult dosing
- Rebetol®: Oral: **Note:** Oral solution should be used in children 3-5 years of age, children ≤25 kg, or those unable to swallow capsules.
  - Capsule/solution: 15 mg/kg/day in 2 divided doses (morning and evening)
  - Capsule dosing recommendations:
    - 26-36 kg: 400 mg/day (200 mg morning and evening)
    - 37-49 kg: 600 mg/day (200 mg in the morning and two 200 mg capsules in the evening)
    - 50-61 kg: 800 mg/day (two 200 mg capsules morning and evening)
    - >61 kg: Refer to adult dosing

Adults: Chronic hepatitis C: Recommended dosage of combination therapy:
- Intron® A: SubQ: 3 million int. units 3 times/week **and**
- Rebetol® capsule: Oral:
  - ≤75 kg (165 lb): 1000 mg/day (two 200 mg capsules in the morning and three 200 mg capsules in the evening)
  - >75 kg: 1200 mg/day (three 200 mg capsules in the morning and three 200 mg capsules in the evening)
- **Note:** Treatment duration may vary. Consult current guidelines and literature.

Dosing adjustment for toxicity: Note: Recommendations (per manufacturer labeling):

Anemia (RBC depression):
- Patient **without** cardiac history:
  - Hemoglobin <10 g/dL:
    - Children: Decrease ribavirin dose by 1/2
    - Adults: Decrease ribavirin dose to 600 mg/day
  - Hemoglobin <8.5 g/dL: Permanently discontinue treatment
- Patient **with** cardiac history:
  - Hemoglobin has ≥2 g/dL decrease during any 4-week period of treatment:
    - Children: Decrease ribavirin dose by 1/2**and** decrease interferon alfa-2b to 1.5 million int. units 3 times/week
    - Adults: Decrease dose to ribavirin to 600 mg/day **and** decrease interferon-alfa 2b dose to 1.5 million int. units 3 times/week.
  - Hemoglobin <12 g/dL after 4 weeks of reduced dose: Permanently discontinue treatment

WBC, neutrophil, or platelet depression:
- WBC <1500 cells/mm^3, neutrophils <750 cells/mm^3, or platelet count <50,000 cells/mm^3 (<80,000 cells/ mm^3 in children): Reduce interferon alfa-2b dose to 1.5 million int. units 3 times/week (50% reduction)
- WBC <1000 cells/mm^3, neutrophils <500 cells/mm^3, or platelet count <25,000 cells/mm^3 (<50,000 cells/mm^3 in children): Permanently discontinue therapy

Dosage adjustment in renal impairment: Patients with Cl_{cr} <50 mL/minutes should not receive ribavirin.

Additional Information Complete prescribing information for this medication should be consulted for additional detail.

Dosage Forms Excipient information presented when available (limited, particularly for generics); consult specific product labeling.

Combination package:

For patients ≤75 kg [contains single-dose vials]:
- Injection, solution: Interferon alfa-2b (Intron® A): 3 million int. units/0.5 mL (0.5 mL) [6 vials (3 million int. units/ vial), 6 syringes, and alcohol swabs]
- Capsule: Ribavirin (Rebetol®): 200 mg (70s)

For patients ≤75 kg [contains multidose vials]:
- Injection, solution: Interferon alfa-2b (Intron® A): 3 million int. units/0.5 mL (3.8 mL) [1 multidose vial (18 million int. units/vial), 6 syringes, and alcohol swabs]
- Capsule: Ribavirin (Rebetol®): 200 mg (70s)

For patients ≤75 kg [contains multidose pen]:
- Injection, solution: Interferon alfa-2b (Intron® A): 3 million int. units/0.2 mL (1.5 mL) [1 multidose pen (18 million int. units/pen), 6 needles, and alcohol swabs]
- Capsule: Ribavirin (Rebetol®): 200 mg (70s)

For patients >75 kg [contains single-dose vials]:
- Injection, solution: Interferon alfa-2b (Intron® A): 3 million int. units/0.5 mL (0.5 mL) [6 vials (3 million int. units/ vial), 6 syringes, and alcohol swabs]
- Capsule: Ribavirin (Rebetol®): 200 mg (84s)

For patients >75 kg [contains multidose vials]:
- Injection, solution: Interferon alfa-2b (Intron® A): 3 million int. units/0.5 mL (3.8 mL) [1 multidose vial (18 million int. units/vial), 6 syringes, and alcohol swabs]
- Capsule: Ribavirin (Rebetol®): 200 mg (84s)

For patients >75 kg [contains multidose pen]:
Injection, solution: Interferon alfa-2b (Intron® A): 3 million int. units/0.2 mL (1.5 mL) [1 multidose pen (18 million int. units/pen), 6 needles, and alcohol swabs]
Capsule: Ribavirin (Rebetol®): 200 mg (84s)

For Rebetol® dose reduction [contains single-dose vials]:
Injection, solution: Interferon alfa-2b (Intron® A): 3 million int. units/0.5 mL (0.5 mL) [6 vials (3 million int. units/vial), 6 syringes, and alcohol swabs]
Capsule: Ribavirin (Rebetol®): 200 mg (42s)

For Rebetol® dose reduction [contains multidose vials]:
Injection, solution: Interferon alfa-2b (Intron® A): 3 million int. units/0.5 mL (3.8 mL) [1 multidose vial (18 million int. units/vial), 6 syringes, and alcohol swabs]
Capsule: Ribavirin (Rebetol®): 200 mg (42s)

For Rebetol® dose reduction [contains multidose pen]:
Injection, solution: Interferon alfa-2b (Intron® A): 3 million int. units/0.2 mL (1.5 mL) [1 multidose pen (18 million int. units/pen), 6 needles, and alcohol swabs]
Capsule: Ribavirin (Rebetol®): 200 mg (42s)

Interferon Alfacon-1 (in ter FEER on AL fa con one)

Brand Names: U.S. Infergen®
Pharmacologic Category Interferon
Use Treatment of chronic hepatitis C virus (HCV) infection in patients ≥18 years of age with compensated liver disease and anti-HCV serum antibodies or HCV RNA; concurrent use with ribavirin in HCV-infected patients who have failed treatment with pegylated interferon/ribavirin (Bacon, 2009)
Pregnancy Risk Factor C
Medication Guide Available Yes
Dosage Adults ≥18 years: SubQ:
Chronic HCV infection: 9 mcg 3 times/week for 24 weeks; allow 48 hours between doses
Combination therapy with ribavirin: 15 mcg/day with ribavirin for up to 48 weeks
Patients who have previously tolerated interferon therapy but did not respond or relapsed: 15 mcg 3 times/week for up to 48 weeks
Dose reduction for toxicity: Dose should be held in patients who experience a severe adverse reaction, and treatment should be stopped or decreased if the reaction does not become tolerable.
Doses were reduced from 9 mcg to 7.5 mcg in the pivotal study.
For patients receiving 15 mcg/dose, doses were reduced in 3 mcg decrements. Efficacy is decreased with doses <7.5 mcg
Elderly: No information available.

Dosage adjustment in renal impairment: Cl_{cr} <50 mL/minute: Hepatitis C: Avoid combination therapy with ribavirin

Dosage adjustment in hepatic impairment: Use in decompensated hepatic disease (Child-Pugh class B and C) is contraindicated

Additional Information Complete prescribing information for this medication should be consulted for additional detail.
Dosage Forms Excipient information presented when available (limited, particularly for generics); consult specific product labeling.
Injection, solution [preservative free]:
Infergen®: 30 mcg/mL (0.3 mL, 0.5 mL)

Interferon Alfa-n3 (in ter FEER on AL fa en three)

Brand Names: U.S. Alferon® N
Brand Names: Canada Alferon® N
Pharmacologic Category Interferon
Use Patients ≥18 years of age: Intralesional treatment of refractory or recurring genital or venereal warts (condylomata acuminata)
Pregnancy Risk Factor C
Medication Guide Available Yes
Dosage Adults: Inject 250,000 units (0.05 mL) in each wart twice weekly for a maximum of 8 weeks; therapy should not be repeated for at least 3 months after the initial 8-week course of therapy
Additional Information Complete prescribing information for this medication should be consulted for additional detail.
Dosage Forms Excipient information presented when available (limited, particularly for generics); consult specific product labeling.
Injection, solution:
Alferon® N: 5 million int. units (1 mL) [contains albumin (human), chicken egg protein, mouse protein]

◆ **Interferon Alpha-2b** *see* Interferon Alfa-2b *on page 912*

Interferon Beta-1a (in ter FEER on BAY ta won aye)

Brand Names: U.S. Avonex®; Rebif®
Brand Names: Canada Avonex®; Rebif®
Index Terms rIFN beta-1a
Pharmacologic Category Interferon
Use Treatment of relapsing forms of multiple sclerosis (MS)
Pregnancy Risk Factor C
Pregnancy Considerations There are no adequate and well-controlled studies in pregnant women. Consideration should be given to discontinue treatment if a woman becomes pregnant, or plans to become pregnant during therapy. A dose-related abortifacient activity was reported in Rhesus monkeys.

Healthcare providers are encouraged to register pregnant women receiving Rebif® during pregnancy online at www.rebifpregnancyregistry.com or by telephone at MS LifeLines 1-877-44-REBIF. A registry has been established for women who become pregnant while receiving Avonex®. Women may be enrolled in the registry by calling 1-800-456-2255.
Lactation Excretion in breast milk unknown/not recommended
Medication Guide Available Yes
Contraindications Hypersensitivity to natural or recombinant interferons, human albumin, or any other component of the formulation
Warnings/Precautions Interferons have been associated with severe psychiatric adverse events (psychosis, mania, depression, suicidal behavior/ideation) in patients with and without previous psychiatric symptoms, avoid use in severe psychiatric disorders and use caution in patients with a history of depression; patients exhibiting depressive symptoms should be closely monitored and discontinuation of therapy should be considered.

Autoimmune disorders including idiopathic thrombocytopenia, hyper- and hypothyroidism and rarely autoimmune hepatitis have been reported. Allergic reactions, including anaphylaxis, have been reported. Caution should be used in patients with hepatic impairment or in those who abuse alcohol. Rare cases of severe hepatic injury, including hepatic failure, have been reported in patients receiving interferon beta-1a; risk may be increased by ethanol use or concurrent therapy with hepatotoxic drugs. Treatment should be suspended if jaundice or symptoms of hepatic dysfunction occur. Transaminase elevations may be asymptomatic, so monitoring is important. Dose adjustment may be necessary with hepatic impairment. Hematologic effects, including pancytopenia (rare) and thrombocytopenia, have been reported. Associated with a high incidence of flu-like adverse effects; use of analgesics and/or antipyretics on treatment days may be helpful. Use caution in patients with pre-existing cardiovascular disease, including angina, HF, and/or arrythmia. Rare cases of new-onset cardiomyopathy and/or HF have been reported. Use caution in patients with seizure disorders, or myelosuppression. Safety and efficacy in patients with chronic progressive MS or in patients <18 years of age have not been established. Albumin is a component of some formulations (contraindicated in albumin-sensitive patients); rare risk of CJD or viral transmission.

Adverse Reactions Note: Adverse reactions reported as a composite of both commercially-available products. Spectrum and incidence of reactions is generally similar between products, but consult individual product labels for specific incidence.

>10%:

Central nervous system: Headache (58% to 70%), fatigue (33% to 41%), fever (20% to 28%), pain (23%), chills (19%), depression (18% to 25%), dizziness (14%)

Gastrointestinal: Nausea (23%), abdominal pain (8% to 22%)

Genitourinary: Urinary tract infection (17%)

Hematologic: Leukopenia (28% to 36%)

Hepatic: ALT increased (20% to 27%), AST increased (10% to 17%)

Local: Injection site reaction (3% to 92%)

Neuromuscular & skeletal: Myalgia (25% to 29%), back pain (23% to 25%), weakness (24%), skeletal pain (10% to 15%), rigors (6% to 13%)

Ocular: Vision abnormal (7% to 13%)

Respiratory: Sinusitis (14%), upper respiratory tract infection (14%)

Miscellaneous: Flu-like syndrome (49% to 59%), neutralizing antibodies (significance not known; Avonex® 5%; Rebif® 24%), lymphadenopathy (11% to 12%)

1% to 10%:

Cardiovascular: Chest pain (5% to 6%), vasodilation (2%)

Central nervous system: Migraine (5%), somnolence (4% to 5%), malaise (4% to 5%), seizure (1% to 5%)

Dermatologic: Erythematous rash (5% to 7%), maculopapular rash (4% to 5%), alopecia (4%), urticaria

Endocrine & metabolic: Thyroid disorder (4% to 6%)

Gastrointestinal: Xerostomia (1% to 5%), toothache (3%)

Genitourinary: Micturition frequency (2% to 7%), urinary incontinence (2% to 4%)

Hematologic: Thrombocytopenia (2% to 8%), anemia (3% to 5%)

Hepatic: Bilirubinemia (2% to 3%)

Local: Injection site pain (8%), injection site bruising (6%), injection site necrosis (1% to 3%), injection site inflammation

Neuromuscular & skeletal: Arthralgia (9%), hypertonia (6% to 7%), coordination abnormal (4% to 5%)

Ocular: Eye disorder (4%), xerophthalmia (1% to 3%)

Respiratory: Bronchitis (8%)

Miscellaneous: Infection (7%)

<1% (Limited to important and life-threatening): Anaphylaxis, autoimmune hepatitis, cardiomyopathy, CHF, hepatic failure, hepatitis, hyper-/hypothyroidism, idiopathic thrombocytopenia, injection site abscess/cellulitis, menorrhagia, metrorrhagia, pancytopenia, psychiatric disorders (new or worsening; including suicidal ideation), vesicular rash

Drug Interactions

Metabolism/Transport Effects None known.

Avoid Concomitant Use There are no known interactions where it is recommended to avoid concomitant use.

Increased Effect/Toxicity

Interferon Beta-1a may increase the levels/effects of: Theophylline Derivatives; Zidovudine

Decreased Effect There are no known significant interactions involving a decrease in effect.

Stability

Avonex®:

Prefilled syringe: Store at 2°C to 8°C (36°F to 46°F); do not freeze. Protect from light. Allow to warm to room temperature prior to use (do not use external heat source). If refrigeration is not available, product may be stored at ≤25°C (77°F) for up to 7 days.

Vial: Store unreconstituted vial at 2°C to 8°C (36°F to 46°F). If refrigeration is not available, may be stored at 25°C (77°F) for up to 30 days; do not freeze. Protect from light. Reconstitute with 1.1 mL of diluent and swirl gently to dissolve. Do not shake. The reconstituted product contains no preservative and is for single-use only; discard unused portion. Following reconstitution, use immediately, but may be stored up to 6 hours at 2°C to 8°C (36°F to 46°F); do not freeze.

Rebif®: Store at 2°C to 8°C (36°F to 46°F); do not freeze. Protect from light. May also be stored ≤25°C (77°F) for up to 30 days if protected from heat and light.

Mechanism of Action Interferon beta differs from naturally occurring human protein by a single amino acid substitution and the lack of carbohydrate side chains; alters the expression and response to surface antigens and can enhance immune cell activities. Properties of interferon beta that modify biologic responses are mediated by cell surface receptor interactions; mechanism in the treatment of MS is unknown.

Pharmacodynamics/Kinetics

Onset of action: Avonex®: 12 hours (based on biological response markers)

Duration: Avonex®: 4 days (based on biological response markers)

Half-life elimination: Avonex®: 10 hours; Rebif®: 69 hours

Time to peak, serum: Avonex® (I.M.): 3-15 hours; Rebif® (SubQ): 16 hours

Dosage Adults: **Note:** Analgesics and/or antipyretics may help decrease flu-like symptoms on treatment days:

I.M. (Avonex®): 30 mcg once weekly

SubQ (Rebif®): Doses should be separated by at least 48 hours:

Target dose 44 mcg 3 times/week:

Initial: 8.8 mcg (20 % of final dose) 3 times/week for 2 weeks

Titration: 22 mcg (50% of final dose) 3 times/week for 2 weeks

Final dose: 44 mcg 3 times/week

Target dose 22 mcg 3 times/week:

Initial: 4.4 mcg (20 % of final dose) 3 times/week for 2 weeks

Titration: 11 mcg (50% of final dose) 3 times/week for 2 weeks

Final dose: 22 mcg 3 times/week

Dosage adjustment in hepatic impairment: Rebif®: If liver function tests increase or in case of leukopenia: Decrease dose 20% to 50% until toxicity resolves

Administration

Avonex®: Must be administered by I.M. injection

Rebif®: Administer SubQ at the same time of day on the same 3 days each week (ie, late afternoon/evening Mon, Wed, Fri); rotate injection site

Monitoring Parameters Thyroid function tests, CBC with differential, transaminase levels, symptoms of autoimmune disorders, signs/symptoms of psychiatric disorder (including depression and/or suicidal ideation), signs/symptoms of new onset/worsening cardiovascular disease

Avonex®: Frequency of monitoring for patients receiving Avonex® has not been specifically defined; in clinical trials, monitoring was at 6-month intervals.

Rebif®: CBC and liver function testing at 1-, 3-, and 6 months, then periodically thereafter. Thyroid function every 6 months (in patients with pre-existing abnormalities and/or clinical indications)

Dosage Forms Excipient information presented when available (limited, particularly for generics); consult specific product labeling.

Injection, powder for reconstitution [preservative free]:
Avonex®: 33 mcg [contains albumin (human); 6.6 million units; provides 30 mcg/mL following reconstitution; supplied with diluent]

Injection, solution:
Avonex®: 30 mcg/0.5 mL (0.5 mL) [albumin free]

Injection, solution [preservative free]:
Rebif®: 22 mcg/0.5 mL (0.5 mL), 44 mcg/0.5 mL (0.5 mL) [contains albumin (human)]

Injection, solution [preservative free, combination package]:
Rebif®: Titration Pack: 22 mcg/0.5 mL (6s) and 8.8 mcg/0.2 mL (6s) [contains albumin (human)]

Interferon Beta-1b (in ter FEER on BAY ta won bee)

Brand Names: U.S. Betaseron®; Extavia®
Brand Names: Canada Betaseron®; Extavia®
Index Terms rIFN beta-1b
Pharmacologic Category Interferon
Use Treatment of relapsing forms of multiple sclerosis (MS); treatment of first clinical episode with MRI features consistent with MS

Canadian labeling: Additional use (not in U.S. labeling): Treatment of secondary-progressive MS

Pregnancy Risk Factor C
Pregnancy Considerations A dose-related abortifacient activity was reported in Rhesus monkeys. There are no adequate and well-controlled studies in pregnant women. Treatment should be discontinued if a woman becomes pregnant, or plans to become pregnant during therapy.
Lactation Excretion in breast milk unknown/not recommended
Medication Guide Available Yes
Contraindications Hypersensitivity to *E. coli*-derived products, natural or recombinant interferon beta, albumin human or any other component of the formulation

Canadian labeling: Additional contraindication (not in U.S. labeling): Pregnancy

Warnings/Precautions Anaphylaxis has been reported rarely with use. Associated with a high incidence of flu-like adverse effects; improvement in symptoms occurs over time. Hepatotoxicity has been reported with beta interferons, including rare reports of hepatitis (autoimmune) and hepatic failure requiring transplant. Interferons have been associated with severe psychiatric adverse events (psychosis, mania, depression, suicidal behavior/ideation) in patients with and without previous psychiatric symptoms, avoid use in severe psychiatric disorders and use caution in patients with a history of depression; patients exhibiting symptoms of depression should be closely monitored and discontinuation of therapy should be considered. Use caution in patients with pre-existing cardiovascular disease, pulmonary disease, seizure disorders, renal impairment or hepatic impairment. Use caution in myelosuppression; routine monitoring for leukopenia is recommended; dose reduction may be required. Thyroid dysfunction has rarely been reported with use. Severe injection site reactions (necrosis) may occur, which may or may not heal with continued therapy; patient and/or caregiver competency in injection technique should be confirmed and periodically re-evaluated. Contains albumin, which may carry a remote risk of transmitting viral diseases.

Adverse Reactions Note: Flu-like syndrome (including at least two of the following - headache, fever, chills, malaise, diaphoresis, and myalgia) are reported in the majority of patients (60%) and decrease over time (average duration ~1 week).

>10%:
- Cardiovascular: Peripheral edema (15%), chest pain (11%)
- Central nervous system: Headache (57%), fever (36%), pain (51%), chills (25%), dizziness (24%), insomnia (24%)
- Dermatologic: Rash (24%), skin disorder (12%)
- Endocrine & metabolic: Metrorrhagia (11%)
- Gastrointestinal: Nausea (27%), diarrhea (19%), abdominal pain (19%), constipation (20%), dyspepsia (14%)
- Genitourinary: Urinary urgency (13%)
- Hematologic: Lymphopenia (88%), neutropenia (14%), leukopenia (14%)
- Local: Injection site reaction (85%), inflammation (53%), pain (18%)
- Neuromuscular & skeletal: Weakness (61%), myalgia (27%), hypertonia (50%), myasthenia (46%), arthralgia (31%), incoordination (21%)
- Miscellaneous: Flu-like syndrome (decreases over treatment course; 60%), neutralizing antibodies (≤45%; significance not known)

1% to 10%:
- Cardiovascular: Palpitation (4%), vasodilation (8%), hypertension (7%), tachycardia (4%), peripheral vascular disorder (6%)
- Central nervous system: Anxiety (10%), malaise (8%), nervousness (7%)
- Dermatologic: Alopecia (4%)
- Endocrine & metabolic: Menorrhagia (8%), dysmenorrhea (7%)
- Gastrointestinal: Weight gain (7%)
- Genitourinary: Impotence (9%), pelvic pain (6%), cystitis (8%), urinary frequency (7%), prostatic disorder (3%)
- Hematologic: Lymphadenopathy (8%)
- Hepatic: ALT increased >5x baseline (10%), AST increased >5x baseline (3%)
- Local: Injection site necrosis (4% to 5%), edema (3%), mass (2%)
- Neuromuscular & skeletal: Leg cramps (4%)
- Respiratory: Dyspnea (7%)
- Miscellaneous: Diaphoresis (8%), hypersensitivity (3%)

<1% (Limited to important or life-threatening): Anorexia, apnea, arrhythmia, ataxia, autoimmune hepatitis, bronchospasm, capillary leak syndrome (in patients with pre-existing monoclonal gammopathy), cardiac arrest, cardiomegaly, cardiomyopathy, cerebral hemorrhage, coma, confusion, delirium, depersonalization, depression, DVT, emotional lability, erythema nodosum, ethanol intolerance, exfoliative dermatitis, gamma GT increase, GI hemorrhage, hallucinations, heart failure, hematemesis, hepatic failure, hepatitis, hyperthyroidism, hyperuricemia, hypocalcemia, mania, MI, pancreatitis, paresthesia, pericardial effusion, photosensitivity, pneumonia, pruritus, psychosis, pulmonary embolism, rash, seizure, sepsis, shock, skin discoloration, suicidal ideation, syncope, SIADH, thrombocytopenia, thyroid dysfunction, triglyceride increased, urinary tract infection, urosepsis, urticaria, vasculitis, vaginal hemorrhage, vomiting, weight loss

Drug Interactions
Metabolism/Transport Effects None known.
Avoid Concomitant Use There are no known interactions where it is recommended to avoid concomitant use.

Increased Effect/Toxicity

Interferon Beta-1b may increase the levels/effects of: Theophylline Derivatives; Zidovudine

Decreased Effect There are no known significant interactions involving a decrease in effect.

Stability Store at room temperature of 25°C (77°F); excursions permitted to 15°C to 30°C (59°F to 86°F). To reconstitute solution, inject 1.2 mL of diluent (provided); gently swirl to dissolve, do not shake. Reconstituted solution provides 0.25 mg/mL (8 million units). If not used immediately following reconstitution, refrigerate solution at 2°C to 8°C (36°F to 46°F) and use within 3 hours; do not freeze or shake solution. Discard unused portion of vial.

Mechanism of Action Interferon beta-1b differs from naturally occurring human protein by a single amino acid substitution and the lack of carbohydrate side chains; mechanism in the treatment of MS is unknown; however, immunomodulatory effects attributed to interferon beta-1b include enhancement of suppressor T cell activity, reduction of proinflammatory cytokines, down-regulation of antigen presentation, and reduced trafficking of lymphocytes into the central nervous system. Improves MRI lesions, decreases relapse rate, and disease severity in patients with secondary progressive MS.

Pharmacodynamics/Kinetics Limited data due to small doses used

Half-life elimination: 8 minutes to 4.3 hours

Time to peak, serum: 1-8 hours

Dosage SubQ: **Note:** Gradual dose-titration, analgesics, and/or antipyretics may help decrease flu-like symptoms on treatment days:

Children <18 years: Not recommended

Adults:

- Multiple sclerosis (relapsing): Initial: 0.0625 mg (2 million units [0.25 mL]) every other day; gradually increase dose by 0.0625 every 2 weeks
  - Target dose: 0.25 mg (8 million units [1 mL]) every other day
- Multiple sclerosis (secondary-progressive) [Canadian labeling; not in U.S. labeling]: Initial: 0.125 mg (4 million units [0.5 mL]) every other day for 2 weeks
  - Target dose: 0.25 mg (8 million units [1 mL]) every other day

Administration Withdraw dose of reconstituted solution from the vial into a sterile syringe fitted with a 27-gauge needle and inject the solution subcutaneously; sites for self-injection include outer surface of the arms, abdomen, hips, and thighs. Rotate SubQ injection site. Patient should be well hydrated.

Monitoring Parameters Complete blood chemistries (including platelet count) and liver function tests are recommended at 1, 3, and 6 months following initiation of therapy and periodically thereafter. Thyroid function should be assessed every 6 months in patients with history of thyroid dysfunction.

Canadian labeling: Additional monitoring recommendations (not in U.S. labeling): Baseline pregnancy test, chest X-ray, and ECG

Additional Information American Academy of Neurology and MS Council guidelines suggest that, based upon published data, 6 million units of Avonex® (interferon beta-1a) (30 mcg) is equivalent to approximately 7-9 million units of Betaseron® (220-280 mcg).

Dosage Forms Excipient information presented when available (limited, particularly for generics); consult specific product labeling.

Injection, powder for reconstitution:

- Betaseron®: 0.3 mg [~9.6 million int. units] [contains albumin (human)]

Injection, powder for reconstitution [preservative free]:

- Extavia®: 0.3 mg [~9.6 million int. units] [contains albumin (human)]

Interferon Gamma-1b

(in ter FEER on GAM ah won bee)

Brand Names: U.S. Actimmune®

Brand Names: Canada Actimmune®

Pharmacologic Category Interferon

Use Reduce frequency and severity of serious infections associated with chronic granulomatous disease; delay time to disease progression in patients with severe, malignant osteopetrosis

Pregnancy Risk Factor C

Pregnancy Considerations Teratogenic effects were not observed in animal studies. A dose-related abortifacient activity was reported in Rhesus monkeys. Safety and efficacy in pregnant women has not been established.

Lactation Excretion in breast milk unknown/not recommended

Contraindications Hypersensitivity to interferon gamma, *E. coli* derived proteins, or any component of the formulation

Warnings/Precautions Hypersensitivity reactions have been reported (rarely). Transient cutaneous rashes may occur. Dose-related bone marrow toxicity has been reported; use caution in patients with myelosuppression. May cause hepatotoxicity and the incidence may be increased in children <1 year of age. Doses >10 times the weekly recommended dose (used in studies for unlabeled indications) have been associated with a different pattern/frequency of adverse effects. Flu-like symptoms which may exacerbate pre-existing cardiovascular disorders (including ischemia, HF, or arrhythmias) and the development of neurologic disorders have been noted at the higher doses. Caution should also be used in patients with seizure disorders or compromised CNS function.

Adverse Reactions Based on 50 mcg/m^2 dose administered 3 times weekly for chronic granulomatous disease

>10%:

- Central nervous system: Fever (52%), headache (33%), chills (14%), fatigue (14%)
- Dermatologic: Rash (17%)
- Gastrointestinal: Diarrhea (14%), vomiting (13%)
- Local: Injection site erythema or tenderness (14%)

1% to 10%:

- Central nervous system: Depression (3%)
- Gastrointestinal: Nausea (10%), abdominal pain (8%)
- Neuromuscular & skeletal: Myalgia (6%), arthralgia (2%), back pain (2%)

Postmarketing and/or case reports: Alkaline phosphatase elevated, atopic dermatitis, granulomatous colitis, hepatomegaly, hypersensitivity reactions, hypokalemia, neutropenia, Stevens-Johnson syndrome

Additional adverse reactions noted at doses >100 mcg/m^2 administered 3 times weekly: ALT increased, AST increased, autoantibodies increased, bronchospasm, chest discomfort, confusion, dermatomyositis exacerbation, disorientation, DVT, gait disturbance, GI bleeding, hallucinations, heart block, heart failure, hepatic insufficiency, hyperglycemia, hypertriglyceridemia, hyponatremia, hypotension, interstitial pneumonitis, lupus-like syndrome, MI, neutropenia, pancreatitis (may be fatal), Parkinsonian symptoms, PE, proteinuria, renal insufficiency (reversible), seizure, syncope, tachyarrhythmia, tachypnea, thrombocytopenia, TIA

Drug Interactions

Metabolism/Transport Effects **Inhibits** CYP1A2 (weak), CYP2E1 (weak)

Avoid Concomitant Use There are no known interactions where it is recommended to avoid concomitant use.

Increased Effect/Toxicity

Interferon Gamma-1b may increase the levels/effects of: Theophylline Derivatives; Zidovudine

Decreased Effect There are no known significant interactions involving a decrease in effect.

Stability Store in refrigerator at 2°C to 8°C (36°F to 46°F); do not freeze. Do not shake. Discard if left unrefrigerated for >12 hours.

Mechanism of Action Interferon gamma participates in immunoregulation by enhancing the oxidative metabolism of macrophages; it also enhances antibody dependent cellular cytotoxicity, activates natural killer cells and has a role in the expression of Fc receptors and histocompatibility antigens. The exact mechanism of action for the treatment of chronic granulomatous disease or osteopetrosis has not been defined.

Pharmacodynamics/Kinetics

Absorption: I.M., SubQ: >89%

Half-life elimination: I.V.: 38 minutes; I.M.: ~3 hours, SubQ: ~6 hours

Time to peak, plasma: I.M.: 4 hours (1.5 ng/mL); SubQ: 7 hours (0.6 ng/mL)

Dosage If severe reactions occur, reduce dose by 50% or therapy should be interrupted until adverse reaction abates.

Children: Severe, malignant osteopetrosis: SubQ:

BSA ≤0.5 m^2: 1.5 mcg/kg/dose 3 times/week

BSA >0.5 m^2: 50 mcg/m^2 (1 million int. units/m^2) 3 times/week

Children and Adults: Chronic granulomatous disease: SubQ:

BSA ≤0.5 m^2: 1.5 mcg/kg/dose 3 times/week

BSA >0.5 m^2: 50 mcg/m^2 (1 million int. units/m^2) 3 times/week

Note: Previously expressed as 1.5 million units/m^2; 50 mcg is equivalent to 1 million int. units/m^2.

Administration Administer by SubQ injection into the right and left deltoid or anterior thigh.

Monitoring Parameters CBC with differential, platelets, LFTs (monthly in children <1 year), electrolytes, BUN, creatinine, and urinalysis prior to therapy and at 3-month intervals

Dosage Forms Excipient information presented when available (limited, particularly for generics); consult specific product labeling.

Injection, solution [preservative free]:

Actimmune®: 100 mcg (0.5 mL) [2 million int. units]

◆ **Interleukin-1 Receptor Antagonist** *see* Anakinra *on page 120*
◆ **Interleukin 2** *see* Aldesleukin *on page 55*
◆ **Interleukin-11** *see* Oprelvekin *on page 1249*
◆ **Intermezzo®** *see* Zolpidem *on page 1826*
◆ **Intralipid®** *see* Fat Emulsion *on page 690*
◆ **Intrapleural Talc** *see* Talc (Sterile) *on page 1624*
◆ **Intravenous Fat Emulsion** *see* Fat Emulsion *on page 690*
◆ **Intrifiban** *see* Eptifibatide *on page 608*
◆ **Intron® A** *see* Interferon Alfa-2b *on page 912*
◆ **Intropin** *see* DOPamine *on page 544*
◆ **Introvale™** *see* Ethinyl Estradiol and Levonorgestrel *on page 656*
◆ **Intuniv™** *see* GuanFACINE *on page 814*
◆ **INVanz®** *see* Ertapenem *on page 615*
◆ **Invanz® (Can)** *see* Ertapenem *on page 615*
◆ **Invega®** *see* Paliperidone *on page 1277*
◆ **Invega® Sustenna®** *see* Paliperidone *on page 1277*
◆ **Invirase®** *see* Saquinavir *on page 1536*

Iobenguane I 123

(eye oh BEN gwane eye one TWEN tee three)

Brand Names: U.S. AdreView™

Index Terms 123 Meta-Iodobenzlyguanidine Sulfate; 123I-Metaiodobenzylguanidine (MIBG); I-123 MIBG; I^{123} Iobenguane; Iobenguane Sulfate I 123

Pharmacologic Category Radiopharmaceutical

Use As an adjunct to other diagnostic tests, in the detection of primary or metastatic pheochromocytoma or neuroblastoma

Pregnancy Risk Factor C

Dosage Note: Thyroid protective agents (SSKI, Lugol's solution or potassium iodide), should be given at least 1 hour prior to administration. Perform whole body planar scintigraphy imaging 18-30 hours after Iobenguane I 123 administration.

Radioimaging: I.V.:

Children 1 month to 16 years and <70 kg: Dose according to body weight; see table.

Children <16 years and ≥70 kg: 10 mCi (370 MBq)

Children ≥16 years and Adults: 10 mCi (370 MBq)

Iobenguane I 123 Pediatric Dosing by Body Weight

(Children 1 Month to 16 Years and <70 kg)

Weight (kg)	mCi Dose	MBq Dose
3	1	37
4	1.4	52
6	1.9	70
8	2.3	85.1
10	2.7	99.9
12	3.2	118.4
14	3.6	133.2
16	4	148
18	4.4	162.8
20	4.6	170.2
22	5	185
24	5.3	196.1
26	5.6	207.2
28	5.8	214.6
30	6.2	229.4
32	6.5	240.5
34	6.8	251.6
36	7.1	262.7
38	7.3	270.1
40	7.6	281.2
42	7.8	288.6
44	8	296
46	8.2	303.4
48	8.5	314.5
50	8.8	325.6
52-54	9	333
56-58	9.2	340.4
60-62	9.6	355.2
64-66	9.8	362.6
68	9.9	366.3

Additional Information Complete prescribing information for this medication should be consulted for additional detail.

Dosage Forms Excipient information presented when available (limited, particularly for generics); consult specific product labeling.

Injection, solution:

AdreView™: Iobenguane sulfate 0.08 mg and I 123 74 MBq (2 mCi) per mL (5 mL) [contains benzyl alcohol]

◆ **Iobenguane Sulfate I 123** *see* Iobenguane I 123 *on page 920*

◆ **Iodine I 131 Tositumomab and Tositumomab** *see* Tositumomab and Iodine I 131 Tositumomab *on page 1714*

◆ **Iodine and Potassium Iodide** *see* Potassium Iodide and Iodine *on page 1384*

Iodoquinol (eye oh doe KWIN ole)

Brand Names: U.S. Yodoxin®

Brand Names: Canada Diodoquin®

Index Terms Diiodohydroxyquin

Pharmacologic Category Amebicide

Use Treatment of acute and chronic intestinal amebiasis; asymptomatic cyst passers; *Blastocystis hominis* infections; ineffective for amebic hepatitis or hepatic abscess

Dosage Oral:

Children: 30-40 mg/kg/day (maximum: 650 mg/dose) in 3 divided doses for 20 days; not to exceed 1.95 g/day

Adults: 650 mg 3 times/day after meals for 20 days; not to exceed 1.95 g/day

Additional Information Complete prescribing information for this medication should be consulted for additional detail.

Dosage Forms Excipient information presented when available (limited, particularly for generics); consult specific product labeling.

Tablet, oral:

Yodoxin®: 210 mg, 650 mg

Iodoquinol and Hydrocortisone

(eye oh doe KWIN ole & hye droe KOR ti sone)

Brand Names: U.S. Alcortin® A; Dermazene®

Index Terms Hydrocortisone and Iodoquinol; Vytone

Pharmacologic Category Antifungal Agent, Topical; Corticosteroid, Topical

Use Treatment of eczema (including impetiginized, nuchal, and nummular); acne urticaria; anogenital pruritus, atopic dermatitis, chronic infectious dermatitis; chronic eczematoid otitis externa; folliculitis, intertrigo; lichen simplex chronicus; moniliasis; mycotic dermatoses; neurodermatitis (localized or systemic); pyoderma, stasis dermatitis

Pregnancy Risk Factor C

Dosage Topical: Children ≥12 years and Adults: Apply 3-4 times/day

Additional Information Complete prescribing information for this medication should be consulted for additional detail.

Dosage Forms Excipient information presented when available (limited, particularly for generics); consult specific product labeling.

Cream, topical: Iodoquinol 1% and hydrocortisone acetate 1% (30 g)

Dermazene®: Iodoquinol 1% and hydrocortisone acetate 1% (30 g)

Gel, topical:

Alcortin® A: Iodoquinol 1% and hydrocortisone 2% (2 g) [contains aloe, benzyl alcohol]

◆ **Ioflupane** *see* Ioflupane I 123 *on page 921*

◆ **Ioflupane-123 I** *see* Ioflupane I 123 *on page 921*

Ioflupane I 123

(eye oh FLOO pane eye one TWEN tee three)

Brand Names: U.S. DaTscan™

Index Terms 123I-Ioflupane; DaTSCAN; Ioflupane; Ioflupane-123 I

Pharmacologic Category Radiopharmaceutical

Use Striatal dopamine transporter (DaT) visualization using single photon emission computed tomography (SPECT) brain imaging as an adjunct to other diagnostic tests to assist in the evaluation of patients with suspected Parkinsonian syndromes (PS); specifically, to differentiate essential tremor (ET) from tremor due to PS (idiopathic Parkinson's disease, multiple system atrophy, and progressive supranuclear palsy)

Unlabeled Use DaT visualization using SPECT brain imaging as an adjunct to evaluate patients with suspected Creutzfeldt–Jakob disease

Pregnancy Risk Factor C

Dosage Note: Thyroid protective agents (potassium iodide [SSKI] or Lugol's solution) equivalent to 100 mg iodide or 400 mg potassium perchlorate, should be given at least 1 hour prior to administration. Perform SPECT imaging 3-6 hours after ioflupane I 123 administration (see manufacturer's prescribing information for additional imaging information).

Adults: Radioimaging: I.V.: 3-5 mCi (111-185 MBq)

Dosage adjustment in renal impairment: No dosage adjustment provided in manufacturer's labeling. **Note:** Ioflupane I 123 is renally excreted and patients with severe renal impairment may have increased radiation exposure and altered SPECT images.

Dosage adjustment in hepatic impairment: No dosage adjustment provided in manufacturer's labeling.

Additional Information Complete prescribing information for this medication should be consulted for additional detail.

Dosage Forms Excipient information presented when available (limited, particularly for generics); consult specific product labeling.

Injection, solution [preservative free]:

DaTscan™: Ioflupane 0.07-0.13 mcg and I 123 74 MBq (2 mCi) per 1 mL (2.5 mL) [contains ethanol 5%]

Controlled Substance C-II

◆ **Iophen C-NR** *see* Guaifenesin and Codeine *on page 810*

◆ **Iopidine®** *see* Apraclonidine *on page 137*

◆ **iOSAT™ [OTC]** *see* Potassium Iodide *on page 1383*

Ipilimumab (ip i LIM u mab)

Brand Names: U.S. Yervoy™

Index Terms MDX-010; MDX-CTLA-4; MOAB-CTLA-4

Pharmacologic Category Antineoplastic Agent, Monoclonal Antibody; Monoclonal Antibody

Use Treatment of unresectable or metastatic melanoma

Pregnancy Risk Factor C

Pregnancy Considerations Adverse fetal effects were observed in animal reproduction studies. There are no adequate and well-controlled studies in pregnant women. Ipilimumab is an IgG1 immunoglobulin and human IgG1 is known to cross the placenta, therefore ipilimumab may also cross the placenta.

Lactation Excretion in breast milk unknown/not recommended

Medication Guide Available Yes

Contraindications There are no contraindications listed within the manufacturer's labeling.

Warnings/Precautions [U.S. Boxed Warning]: Severe and fatal immune-mediated adverse effects due to T-cell activation and proliferation may occur. While any organ system may be involved, common severe effects include dermatitis (including toxic epidermal necrolysis), endocrine disorder, enterocolitis, hepatitis, and neuropathy. Reactions generally occur during treatment, although some reactions have occurred weeks to months after treatment discontinuation. Discontinue treatment (permanently) and initiate high-dose corticosteroid treatment for severe immune mediated reactions. Evaluate liver function and thyroid function tests at baseline and prior to each dose. Assess for signs and symptoms of enterocolitis, dermatitis, neuropathy, and endocrine disorder at baseline and prior to each dose. Initiate prednisone 1-2 mg/kg/day (or equivalent) for severe reactions. Uncommon immune-mediated adverse effects reported include hemolytic anemia, iritis, meningitis, nephritis, pericarditis, pneumonitis, and uveitis. Administer corticosteroid ophthalmic drops in patients who develop episcleritis, iritis, or uveitis; permanently discontinue ipilimumab if unresponsive to topical ophthalmic immunosuppressive treatments. Immune-mediated enterocolitis was reported to occur at a median onset of 6-7 weeks. Monitor for signs and symptoms of enterocolitis (abdominal pain, blood in stool, diarrhea, or mucous in stool; with or without fever) and intestinal perforation. If enterocolitis develops, infectious causes should be ruled out; consider endoscopy for persistent or severe symptoms. Withhold ipilimumab treatment and administer antidiarrheals for moderate enterocolitis (diarrhea with ≤6 stools over baseline abdominal pain, mucous or blood in stool); if persists for >1 week, initiate prednisone at 0.5 mg/kg/day (or equivalent). If severe enterocolitis (diarrhea ≥7 stools above baseline, fever, ileus, peritoneal signs) develops, permanently discontinue ipilimumab and initiate prednisone 1-2 mg/kg/day (or equivalent); when resolved to ≤grade 1, taper corticosteroids slowly over ≥1 month (rapid tapering may worsen symptoms).

Severe, life-threatening or fatal hepatotoxicity and immune-mediated hepatitis have been observed. Monitor liver function tests (LFTs) and evaluate for signs of hepatotoxicity prior to each dose; if hepatotoxicity develops, infectious or malignant causes should be ruled out and liver function should be monitored more frequently. Withhold treatment for grade 2 hepatotoxicity (ALT or AST 2.5-5 times ULN or total bilirubin 1.5-3 times ULN). If severe hepatotoxicity develops (ALT or AST >5 times ULN or total bilirubin >3 times ULN), permanently discontinue ipilimumab and initiate prednisone 1-2 mg/kg/day (or equivalent); may begin tapering corticosteroid (over 1 month) when LFTs show sustained improvement or return to baseline.

Severe, life-threatening, or fatal dermatitis has been reported. The median time to onset for dermatologic toxicity is 3 weeks (range: ≤17 weeks). Monitor for rash and pruritus; dermatitis should be considered immune-mediated unless identified otherwise. Mild-to-moderate dermatitis should be treated symptomatically; topical or systemic corticosteroids should be administered if not resolved within 1 week. Withhold treatment for moderate to severe dermatologic symptoms. Permanently discontinue and initiate prednisone 1-2 mg/kg/day (or equivalent) for Stevens-Johnson syndrome, toxic epidermal necrolysis, or rash complicated by dermal ulceration (full thickness) or necrotic, bullous, or hemorrhagic manifestations; when dermatitis is controlled, taper corticosteroid over at least 1 month.

Severe or life-threatening endocrine disorders (hypopituitarism, adrenal insufficiency, hypogonadism and hypothyroidism) have been reported; may require hospitalization. Endocrine disorders of moderate severity (including hypothyroidism, adrenal insufficiency, hypopituitarism, and less commonly hyperthyroidism and Cushing's syndrome) which have required hormone replacement therapy or medical intervention have also been reported. The median onset for moderate-to-severe endocrine disorders was 11 weeks (range: ≤19 weeks); long-term hormone replacement therapy has been required in many cases. Monitor thyroid function tests and serum chemistries prior to each dose; also monitor for signs of hypophysitis, adrenal insufficiency and thyroid disorders (eg, abdominal pain, fatigue, headache, hypotension, mental status changes, unusual bowel habits); rule out other potential causes such as brain metastases. Endocrine disorders should be considered immune-mediated unless identified otherwise. If symptomatic, withhold ipilimumab treatment and initiate prednisone 1-2 mg/kg/day (or equivalent) and appropriate hormone replacement therapy.

One case each of severe peripheral motor neuropathy and fatal Guillain-Barré syndrome have been reported. Monitor for signs of motor or sensory neuropathy (unilateral or bilateral weakness, sensory changes or paresthesia). Withhold treatment in patients with neuropathy that does not interfere with daily activities (moderate neuropathy). Permanently discontinue for severe neuropathy (interferes with daily activities, including symptoms similar to Guillain-Barré syndrome). Consider initiating prednisone 1-2 mg/kg/day (or equivalent) for severe neuropathies.

Adverse Reactions

>10%:

Central nervous system: Fatigue (41% to 42%; grades 3-5: 7%), headache (14%), fever (12%)

Dermatologic: Pruritus (24% to 31%), rash (19% to 29%; grades 3-5: 2%), dermatitis (grade 2: 12%; grades 3-5: 2% to 3% [includes Stevens-Johnson syndrome, toxic epidermal necrolysis, dermal ulceration necrotic, bullous or hemorrhagic dermatitis])

Gastrointestinal: Nausea (35%), diarrhea (32% to 33%; grades 3-5: 5%), appetite decreased (27%), vomiting (24%), constipation (21%), abdominal pain (15%)

Hematologic: Anemia (12%)

Respiratory: Cough (16%), dyspnea (15%)

1% to 10%:

Dermatologic: Urticaria (2%), vitiligo (2%)

Endocrine & metabolic: Hypopituitarism (grade 2: 2%; grades 3-5: 4%), hypothyroidism (≤2%), hypophysitis (2%), adrenal insufficiency (≤2%)

Gastrointestinal: Colitis (8%; grades 3-5: 5%), enterocolitis (grade 2: 5%; grades 3-5: 7%), intestinal perforation (1%)

Hematologic: Eosinophilia (grades 3-5: 1%)

Hepatic: Hepatotoxicity (grade 2: 3%; grades 3-5: 1% to 2%), ALT increased (2%)

Renal: Nephritis (grades 3-5: 1%)

<1% (Limited to important or life-threatening): Acute respiratory distress syndrome, angiopathy, arthritis, AST increased, bilirubin increased, blepharitis, conjunctivitis, corticotrophin decreased, Cushing's syndrome, episcleritis, erythema multiforme, esophagitis, gastrointestinal ulcer, Guillain-Barré syndrome, hemolytic anemia, hepatic failure, hepatitis (immune-mediated), hypogonadism, hyperthyroidism, infusion reaction, iritis, leukocytoclastic vasculitis, meningitis, myasthenia gravis, myelofibrosis, myocarditis, neuropathy (sensory and motor), pancreatitis, pericarditis, peritonitis, pneumonitis, polymyalgia rheumatica, psoriasis, renal failure, scleritis, sepsis, temporal arteritis, thyroiditis (autoimmune), thyrotropin increased, uveitis, vascular leak syndrome, vasculitis

Drug Interactions

Metabolism/Transport Effects None known.

Avoid Concomitant Use There are no known interactions where it is recommended to avoid concomitant use.

Increased Effect/Toxicity
Ipilimumab may increase the levels/effects of: Vitamin K Antagonists

Decreased Effect
Ipilimumab may decrease the levels/effects of: Cardiac Glycosides; Vitamin K Antagonists

Stability Store intact vials refrigerated at 2°C to 8°C (36°F to 46°C); do not freeze. Protect from light. Prior to preparation, allow vials to sit at room temperature for ~5 minutes. Withdraw appropriate ipilimumab volume and transfer to I.V. bag, dilute with NS or D_5W to a final concentration between 1-2 mg/mL. Mix by gently inverting, do not shake. Solutions diluted for infusion are stable for up to 24 hours refrigerated or at room temperature.

Mechanism of Action Ipilimumab is a recombinant human IgG1 immunoglobulin monoclonal antibody which binds to the cytotoxic T-lymphocyte associated antigen 4 (CTLA-4). CTLA-4 is a down-regulator of T-cell activation pathways. Blocking CTLA-4, allows for enhanced T-cell activation and proliferation. In melanoma, ipilimumab may indirectly mediate T-cell immune responses against tumors.

Pharmacodynamics/Kinetics
Distribution: V_{ss}: 7.21 L
Half-life elimination: Terminal: 14.7 days

Dosage I.V.: Adults: Melanoma, unresectable or metastatic: 3 mg/kg every 3 weeks for 4 doses

Dosage adjustment for toxicity:
Temporarily withhold scheduled dose for the following:
Moderate immune-mediated reactions
Symptomatic endocrine disorder
Note: If receiving less than prednisone 7.5 mg/day (or equivalent), may resume with complete or partial resolution (to ≤grade 1) of symptoms. Resume ipilimumab treatment at 3 mg/kg every 3 weeks until all 4 planned doses have been administered or until 16 weeks from initial dose, whichever occurs first.
Permanently discontinue for the following:
Failure to complete treatment course within 16 weeks of initial dose
Persistent moderate adverse reactions or unable to reduce corticosteroid dose to prednisone 7.5 mg/day (or equivalent)
Severe or life-threatening adverse reactions including:
Central nervous system or neuromuscular toxicity: Severe motor or sensory neuropathy, Guillain-Barré syndrome, or myasthenia gravis
Dermatologic toxicities: Stevens-Johnson syndrome, toxic epidermal necrolysis, or rash complicated by full thickness dermal ulceration, or necrotic, bullous, or hemorrhagic manifestations
Gastrointestinal toxicities: Colitis with abdominal pain, fever, ileus, or peritoneal symptoms, increase in stool frequency (≥7 over baseline), stool incontinence, require I.V. hydration for >24 hours, or GI hemorrhage or perforation
Hepatotoxicities: ALT or AST > 5 times ULN, or total bilirubin >3 times ULN
Ophthalmic toxicities: Immune-mediated ocular disease unresponsive to topical immunosuppressive treatment
Severe immune-mediated reactions involving any organ system (eg, myocarditis [noninfectious], nephritis, pancreatitis, pneumonitis)

Administration I.V.: Infuse over 90 minutes through a low protein-binding in-line filter. Flush with NS or D_5W at the end of infusion

Monitoring Parameters Monitor liver function and evaluate for signs of hepatotoxicity prior to each dose; if hepatotoxicity develops, liver function should be monitored more frequently. Monitor thyroid function tests and serum chemistries prior to each dose; also monitor for signs of hypophysitis, adrenal insufficiency and thyroid disorders (eg, abdominal pain, fatigue, headache, hypotension, mental status changes, unusual bowel habits). Monitor for signs and symptoms of enterocolitis (abdominal pain, blood or mucus in stool or diarrhea, and intestinal perforation. Monitor for rash and pruritus. Monitor for signs of motor or sensory neuropathy (unilateral or bilateral weakness, sensory changes or paresthesia).

Dosage Forms Excipient information presented when available (limited, particularly for generics); consult specific product labeling.
Injection, solution [preservative free]:
Yervoy™: 5 mg/mL (10 mL, 40 mL) [contains polysorbate 80; derived from or manufactured using Chinese hamster ovary cells]

◆ **IPOL®** *see* Poliovirus Vaccine (Inactivated) *on page* 1370

Ipratropium (Systemic) (i pra TROE pee um)

Brand Names: U.S. Atrovent® HFA
Brand Names: Canada Atrovent® HFA; Gen-Ipratropium; Mylan-Ipratropium Sterinebs; Novo-Ipramide; Nu-Ipratropium; PMS-Ipratropium
Index Terms Ipratropium Bromide
Pharmacologic Category Anticholinergic Agent
Use Anticholinergic bronchodilator used in bronchospasm associated with COPD, bronchitis, and emphysema
Pregnancy Risk Factor B
Pregnancy Considerations Teratogenic effects were not observed in animal studies. Inhaled ipratropium is recommended for use as additional therapy for pregnant women with severe asthma exacerbations.
Lactation Excretion in breast milk unknown/use caution
Contraindications Hypersensitivity to ipratropium, atropine (and its derivatives), or any component of the formulation
Warnings/Precautions Immediate hypersensitivity reactions (urticaria, angioedema, rash, bronchospasm) have been reported. Rarely, paradoxical bronchospasm may occur with use of inhaled bronchodilating agents; this should be distinguished from inadequate response. Not indicated for the initial treatment of acute episodes of bronchospasm where rescue therapy is required for rapid response. Should only be used in acute exacerbations of asthma in conjunction with short-acting beta-adrenergic agonists for acute episodes. Use with caution in patients with myasthenia gravis, narrow-angle glaucoma, benign prostatic hyperplasia (BPH), or bladder neck obstruction

Adverse Reactions
>10%: Respiratory: Upper respiratory tract infection (9% to 34%), bronchitis (10% to 23%), sinusitis (1% to 11%)
1% to 10%:
Cardiovascular: Chest pain (3%), palpitation
Central nervous system: Headache (6% to 7%), dizziness (2% to 3%)
Gastrointestinal: Dyspepsia (1% to 5%), nausea (4%), xerostomia (2% to 4%)
Genitourinary: Urinary tract infection (2% to 10%)
Neuromuscular & skeletal: Back pain (2% to 7%)
Respiratory: Dyspnea (7% to 10%), rhinitis (2% to 6%), cough (3% to 5%), pharyngitis (4%), bronchospasm (2%), sputum increased (1%)
Miscellaneous: Flu-like syndrome (4% to 8%)
<1% (Limited to important or life-threatening): Anaphylactic reaction, angioedema, arthritis, atrial fibrillation, bitter taste, constipation, diarrhea, eye pain (acute), glaucoma, hypersensitivity reactions, hypotension, insomnia, laryngospasm, mydriasis, nervousness, pruritus, rash, tachycardia (including supraventricular), tremor, urinary retention, urticaria

Drug Interactions
Metabolism/Transport Effects None known.

Avoid Concomitant Use There are no known interactions where it is recommended to avoid concomitant use.

Increased Effect/Toxicity

Ipratropium (Oral Inhalation) may increase the levels/effects of: AbobotulinumtoxinA; Anticholinergics; Cannabinoids; OnabotulinumtoxinA; Potassium Chloride; RimabotulinumtoxinB

The levels/effects of Ipratropium (Oral Inhalation) may be increased by: Pramlintide

Decreased Effect

Ipratropium (Oral Inhalation) may decrease the levels/effects of: Acetylcholinesterase Inhibitors (Central); Secretin

The levels/effects of Ipratropium (Oral Inhalation) may be decreased by: Acetylcholinesterase Inhibitors (Central)

Stability

Aerosol: Store at controlled room temperature of 25°C (77°F). Do not store near heat or open flame.

Solution: Store at 15°C to 30°C (59°F to 86°F). Protect from light.

Mechanism of Action Blocks the action of acetylcholine at parasympathetic sites in bronchial smooth muscle causing bronchodilation; local application to nasal mucosa inhibits serous and seromucous gland secretions.

Pharmacodynamics/Kinetics

Onset of action: Bronchodilation: Within 15 minutes

Peak effect: 1-2 hours

Duration: 2-5 hours

Absorption: Negligible

Distribution: 15% of dose reaches lower airways

Protein Binding: ≤9%

Half-life elimination: 2 hours

Excretion: Urine

Dosage

Nebulization:

Children ≤12 years: Asthma exacerbation, acute (*NIH Asthma Guidelines, 2007*): 250-500 mcg every 20 minutes for 3 doses, then as needed. **Note:** Should be given in combination with a short-acting beta-adrenergic agonist.

Children >12 years and Adults:

Bronchodilator for COPD: 500 mcg (one unit-dose vial) 3-4 times/day with doses 6-8 hours apart

Asthma exacerbation, acute (*NIH Asthma Guidelines, 2007*): 500 mcg every 20 minutes for 3 doses, then as needed. **Note:** Should be given in combination with a short-acting beta-adrenergic agonist.

Oral inhalation: MDI:

Children ≤12 years: Asthma exacerbation, acute (*NIH Asthma Guidelines, 2007*): 4-8 inhalations every 20 minutes as needed for up to 3 hours. **Note:** Should be given in combination with a short-acting beta-adrenergic agonist.

Children >12 years and Adults:

Bronchodilator for COPD: 2 inhalations 4 times/day, up to 12 inhalations/24 hours

Asthma exacerbation, acute (*NIH Asthma Guidelines, 2007*): 8 inhalations every 20 minutes as needed for up to 3 hours. **Note:** Should be given in combination with a short-acting beta-adrenergic agonist.

Administration Avoid spraying into the eyes.

Atrovent® HFA: Prior to initial use, prime inhaler by releasing 2 test sprays into the air. If the inhaler has not been used for >3 days, reprime.

Dosage Forms Excipient information presented when available (limited, particularly for generics); consult specific product labeling.

Aerosol, for oral inhalation, as bromide:

Atrovent® HFA: 17 mcg/actuation (12.9 g) [chlorofluorocarbon free; 200 metered actuations]

Solution, for nebulization, as bromide: 0.02% [500 mcg/2.5 mL] (25s, 30s, 60s)

Solution, for nebulization, as bromide [preservative free]: 0.02% [500 mcg/2.5 mL] (25s, 30s, 60s)

Ipratropium (Nasal) (i pra TROE pee um)

Brand Names: U.S. Atrovent®

Brand Names: Canada Alti-Ipratropium; Apo-Ipravent®; Atrovent®; Mylan-Ipratropium Solution

Index Terms Ipratropium Bromide

Pharmacologic Category Anticholinergic Agent

Use Symptomatic relief of rhinorrhea associated with the common cold and allergic and nonallergic rhinitis

Pregnancy Risk Factor B

Dosage Intranasal: Nasal spray:

Symptomatic relief of rhinorrhea associated with the common cold (safety and efficacy of use beyond 4 days in patients with the common cold have not been established):

Children 5-11 years: 0.06%: 2 sprays in each nostril 3 times/day

Children ≥12 years and Adults: 0.06%: 2 sprays in each nostril 3-4 times/day

Symptomatic relief of rhinorrhea associated with allergic/nonallergic rhinitis: Children ≥6 years and Adults: 0.03%: 2 sprays in each nostril 2-3 times/day

Symptomatic relief of rhinorrhea associated with seasonal allergic rhinitis (safety and efficacy of use beyond 3 weeks in patients with seasonal allergic rhinitis has not been established): Children ≥5 years and Adults: 0.06%: 2 sprays in each nostril 4 times/day

Additional Information Complete prescribing information for this medication should be consulted for additional detail.

Dosage Forms Excipient information presented when available (limited, particularly for generics); consult specific product labeling.

Solution, intranasal, as bromide [spray]: 0.03% (30 mL); 0.06% (15 mL) [delivers 42 mcg/spray; 165 sprays]; 0.06% (15 mL)

Atrovent®: 0.03% (30 mL) [contains benzalkonium chloride; delivers 21 mcg/spray; 345 sprays]

Atrovent®: 0.06% (15 mL) [contains benzalkonium chloride; delivers 42 mcg/spray; 165 sprays]

Ipratropium and Albuterol
(i pra TROE pee um & al BYOO ter ole)

Brand Names: U.S. Combivent®; DuoNeb®

Brand Names: Canada CO Ipra-Sal; Combivent UDV; Gen-Combo Sterinebs; ratio-Ipra Sal UDV

Index Terms Albuterol and Ipratropium; Salbutamol and Ipratropium

Pharmacologic Category Anticholinergic Agent; Beta$_2$-Adrenergic Agonist

Use Treatment of COPD in those patients who are currently on a regular bronchodilator who continue to have bronchospasms and require a second bronchodilator

Pregnancy Risk Factor C

Dosage Adults:

Aerosol for inhalation: 2 inhalations 4 times/day (maximum: 12 inhalations/24 hours)

Solution for nebulization: Initial: 3 mL every 6 hours (maximum: 3 mL every 4 hours)

Additional Information Complete prescribing information for this medication should be consulted for additional detail.

Product Availability

Combivent® Respimat®: FDA approved October 2011; availability expected mid-2012

Combivent® Respimat® spray is a non-CFC ipratropium and albuterol inhalation formulation approved for the treatment of COPD and will replace Combivent® inhalation aerosol, which is being phased out in accordance with the Montreal Protocol on Substances that Deplete the Ozone Layer.

Dosage Forms Excipient information presented when available (limited, particularly for generics); consult specific product labeling.

Aerosol for oral inhalation:

Combivent®: Ipratropium bromide 18 mcg and albuterol (base) 90 mcg per inhalation (14.7 g) [contains chlorofluorocarbon, soya lecithin; 200 metered actuations]

Solution for nebulization: Ipratropium bromide 0.5 mg and albuterol (base) 2.5 mg per 3 mL (30s, 60s)

DuoNeb®: Ipratropium bromide 0.5 mg and albuterol (base) 2.5 mg per 3 mL (30s, 60s)

◆ **Ipratropium Bromide** *see* Ipratropium (Nasal) *on page 924*

◆ **Ipratropium Bromide** *see* Ipratropium (Systemic) *on page 923*

◆ **I-Prin [OTC]** *see* Ibuprofen *on page 860*

◆ **Iprivask®** *see* Desirudin *on page 475*

◆ **Iproveratril Hydrochloride** *see* Verapamil *on page 1783*

◆ **IPV** *see* Poliovirus Vaccine (Inactivated) *on page 1370*

◆ **Iquix®** *see* Levofloxacin (Ophthalmic) *on page 1000*

Irbesartan (ir be SAR tan)

Brand Names: U.S. Avapro®

Brand Names: Canada Avapro®; CO Irbesartan; PMS-Irbesartan; ratio-Irbesartan; Sandoz-Irbesartan; Teva-Irbesartan

Pharmacologic Category Angiotensin II Receptor Blocker

Additional Appendix Information

Angiotensin Agents *on page 1869*

Use Treatment of hypertension alone or in combination with other antihypertensives; treatment of diabetic nephropathy in patients with type 2 diabetes mellitus (noninsulin dependent, NIDDM) and hypertension

Unlabeled Use To slow the rate of progression of aortic-root dilation in pediatric patients with Marfan's syndrome

Pregnancy Risk Factor C (1st trimester); D (2nd and 3rd trimesters)

Pregnancy Considerations Medications which act on the renin-angiotensin system are reported to have the following fetal/neonatal effects: Hypotension, neonatal skull hypoplasia, anuria, renal failure, and death; oligohydramnios is also reported. These effects are reported to occur with exposure during the second and third trimesters. There are no adequate and well-controlled studies in pregnant women. **[U.S. Boxed Warning]: Based on human data, drugs that act on the angiotensin system can cause injury and death to the developing fetus when used in the second and third trimesters. Angiotensin receptor blockers should be discontinued as soon as possible once pregnancy is detected.**

Lactation Excretion in breast milk unknown/contraindicated

Contraindications Hypersensitivity to irbesartan or any component of the formulation

Warnings/Precautions [U.S. Boxed Warning]: Based on human data, drugs that act on the angiotensin system can cause injury and death to the developing fetus when used in the second and third trimesters. Angiotensin receptor blockers should be discontinued as soon as possible once pregnancy is detected. May cause hyperkalemia; avoid potassium supplementation unless specifically required by healthcare provider. May be associated with deterioration of renal function and/or increases in serum creatinine, particularly in patients with low renal blood flow (eg, renal artery stenosis, heart failure) whose glomerular filtration rate (GFR) is dependent on efferent arteriolar vasoconstriction by angiotensin II. Avoid use or use a much smaller dose in patients who are intravascularly volume-depleted; use caution in patients with unstented unilateral or bilateral renal artery stenosis. When unstented bilateral renal artery stenosis is present, use is generally avoided due to the elevated risk of deterioration in renal function unless possible benefits outweigh risks. AUCs of irbesartan (not the active metabolite) are about 50% greater in patients with Cl_{cr} <30 mL/minute and are doubled in hemodialysis patients. Concurrent use of ACE inhibitors may increase the risk of clinically-significant adverse events (eg, renal dysfunction, hyperkalemia).

Adverse Reactions Unless otherwise indicated, percentage of incidence is reported for patients with hypertension.

>10%: Endocrine & metabolic: Hyperkalemia (19%, diabetic nephropathy; rarely seen in HTN)

1% to 10%:

Cardiovascular: Orthostatic hypotension (5%, diabetic nephropathy)

Central nervous system: Fatigue (4%), dizziness (10%, diabetic nephropathy)

Gastrointestinal: Diarrhea (3%), dyspepsia (2%)

Respiratory: Upper respiratory infection (9%), cough (2.8% versus 2.7% in placebo)

<1%, postmarketing, and/or case reports (Limited to important or life-threatening): Angina, angioedema, arrhythmia, cardiopulmonary arrest, conjunctivitis, depression, dyspnea, ecchymosis, epistaxis, gout, heart failure, hepatitis, hypotension, jaundice, libido decreased, MI, orthostatic hypotension, paresthesia, renal failure, renal function impaired, sexual dysfunction, stroke, thrombocytopenia, transaminases increased, urticaria

Drug Interactions

Metabolism/Transport Effects Substrate of CYP2C9 (minor); **Note:** Assignment of Major/Minor substrate status based on clinically relevant drug interaction potential; **Inhibits** CYP2C8 (moderate), CYP2C9 (moderate), CYP2D6 (weak), CYP3A4 (weak)

Avoid Concomitant Use

Avoid concomitant use of Irbesartan with any of the following: Pimozide

Increased Effect/Toxicity

Irbesartan may increase the levels/effects of: ACE Inhibitors; Amifostine; Antihypertensives; Carvedilol; CYP2C8 Substrates; CYP2C9 Substrates; Hypotensive Agents; Lithium; Nonsteroidal Anti-Inflammatory Agents; Pimozide; Potassium-Sparing Diuretics; RiTUXimab; Sodium Phosphates

The levels/effects of Irbesartan may be increased by: Alfuzosin; Diazoxide; Eplerenone; Fluconazole; Herbs (Hypotensive Properties); MAO Inhibitors; Pentoxifylline; Phosphodiesterase 5 Inhibitors; Potassium Salts; Prostacyclin Analogues; Tolvaptan; Trimethoprim

Decreased Effect

The levels/effects of Irbesartan may be decreased by: Herbs (Hypertensive Properties); Methylphenidate; Nonsteroidal Anti-Inflammatory Agents; Rifamycin Derivatives; Yohimbine

Ethanol/Nutrition/Herb Interactions Herb/Nutraceutical: Avoid dong quai if using for hypertension (has estrogenic activity). Avoid ephedra, yohimbe, ginseng (may worsen hypertension). Avoid garlic (may have increased antihypertensive effect).

Stability Store at room temperature of 15°C to 30°C (59°F to 86°F).

Mechanism of Action Irbesartan is an angiotensin receptor antagonist. Angiotensin II acts as a vasoconstrictor. In addition to causing direct vasoconstriction, angiotensin II also stimulates the release of aldosterone. Once aldosterone is released, sodium as well as water are reabsorbed. The end result is an elevation in blood pressure. Irbesartan binds to the AT1 angiotensin II receptor. This binding prevents angiotensin II from binding to the receptor thereby blocking the vasoconstriction and the aldosterone secreting effects of angiotensin II.

Pharmacodynamics/Kinetics

Onset of action: Peak effect: 1-2 hours

Duration: >24 hours

Distribution: V_d: 53-93 L

Protein binding, plasma: 90%

Metabolism: Hepatic, primarily CYP2C9

Bioavailability: 60% to 80%

Half-life elimination: Terminal: 11-15 hours

Time to peak, serum: 1.5-2 hours

Excretion: Feces (80%); urine (20%)

Dosage Oral:

Hypertension:

Children:

<6 years: Safety and efficacy have not been established.

≥6-12 years: Initial: 75 mg once daily; may be titrated to a maximum of 150 mg once daily

Children ≥13 years and Adults: 150 mg once daily; patients may be titrated to 300 mg once daily

Note: Starting dose in volume-depleted patients should be 75 mg

Aortic-root dilation with Marfan's syndrome (unlabeled use): Children 14 months to 16 years: Initial: 1.4 mg/kg/day; can be increased to a maximum of 2 mg/kg/day (not to exceed adult maximum of 300 mg/day)

Nephropathy in patients with type 2 diabetes and hypertension: Adults: Target dose: 300 mg once daily

Dosage adjustment in renal impairment: No dosage adjustment necessary with mild to severe impairment unless the patient is also volume depleted.

Dietary Considerations May be taken with or without food.

Monitoring Parameters Electrolytes, serum creatinine, BUN, urinalysis

Dosage Forms Excipient information presented when available (limited, particularly for generics); consult specific product labeling.

Tablet, oral:

Avapro®: 75 mg, 150 mg, 300 mg

Irbesartan and Hydrochlorothiazide

(ir be SAR tan & hye droe klor oh THYE a zide)

Brand Names: U.S. Avalide®

Brand Names: Canada Avalide®; CO Irbesartan HCT; Irbesartan-HCTZ; PMS-Irbesartan HCTZ; Ran™-Irbesartan HCTZ; ratio-Irbesartan HCTZ; Sandoz-Irbesartan HCT; Teva-Irbesartan HCTZ

Index Terms Avapro® HCT; Hydrochlorothiazide and Irbesartan

Pharmacologic Category Angiotensin II Receptor Blocker; Diuretic, Thiazide

Use Combination therapy for the management of hypertension; may be used as initial therapy in patients likely to need multiple drugs to achieve blood pressure goals

Pregnancy Risk Factor D

Dosage Oral: Adults: **Note:** Maximum antihypertensive effects are attained within 2-4 weeks after initiation or a change in dose; however, if necessary, may carefully titrate dose as soon as after 1 week of treatment.

Add-on therapy: Dose must be individualized. A patient who is not controlled with either agent alone may be switched to the combination product. The lowest dosage available is irbesartan 150 mg/hydrochlorothiazide 12.5 mg.

Initial therapy: Irbesartan 150 mg/hydrochlorothiazide 12.5 mg once daily. If initial response is inadequate, may titrate dose after 1-2 weeks, to a maximum dose of irbesartan 300 mg/hydrochlorothiazide 25 mg once daily.

Dosing adjustment in renal impairment: Not recommended in patients with Cl_{cr} ≤30 mL/minute

Dosage adjustment in hepatic impairment: Use with caution

Additional Information Complete prescribing information for this medication should be consulted for additional detail.

Dosage Forms Excipient information presented when available (limited, particularly for generics); consult specific product labeling. [DSC] = Discontinued product

Tablet:

Avalide® 150/12.5: Irbesartan 150 mg and hydrochlorothiazide 12.5 mg

Avalide® 300/12.5: Irbesartan 300 mg and hydrochlorothiazide 12.5 mg

Avalide® 300/25: Irbesartan 300 mg and hydrochlorothiazide 25 mg [DSC]

◆ **Irbesartan-HCTZ (Can)** *see* Irbesartan and Hydrochlorothiazide *on page 926*

◆ **Ircon® [OTC]** *see* Ferrous Fumarate *on page 706*

◆ **Iressa®** *see* Gefitinib *on page 780*

◆ **IRESSA® (Can)** *see* Gefitinib *on page 780*

Irinotecan (eye rye no TEE kan)

Brand Names: U.S. Camptosar®

Brand Names: Canada Camptosar®; Irinotecan Hydrochloride Trihydrate

Index Terms Camptothecin-11; CPT-11; Irinotecan HCl; Irinotecan Hydrochloride

Pharmacologic Category Antineoplastic Agent, Camptothecin; Antineoplastic Agent, Natural Source (Plant) Derivative; Antineoplastic Agent, Topoisomerase I Inhibitor

Use Treatment of metastatic carcinoma of the colon or rectum

Unlabeled Use Treatment of cervical cancer (recurrent or metastatic), central nervous system tumors (recurrent glioblastoma), esophageal cancer, Ewing's sarcoma (recurrent or progressive), gastric cancer (metastatic or locally advanced), nonsmall cell lung cancer (advanced), ovarian cancer (recurrent), pancreatic cancer (advanced), small cell lung cancer (extensive stage)

Pregnancy Risk Factor D

Pregnancy Considerations Teratogenic effects were noted in animal studies. There are no adequate and well-controlled studies in pregnant women. Women of child-bearing potential should avoid becoming pregnant while receiving treatment.

Lactation Excretion in breast milk unknown/not recommended

Contraindications Hypersensitivity to irinotecan or any component of the formulation

Warnings/Precautions Hazardous agent - use appropriate precautions for handling and disposal. Severe hypersensitivity reactions (including anaphylaxis) have occurred. For I.V. use only; monitor infusion site; may cause local tissue necrosis or thrombophlebitis if extravasation occurs.

[U.S. Boxed Warning]: Severe diarrhea may be dose-limiting and potentially fatal; early-onset and late-onset diarrhea may occur. Early diarrhea occurs during or within 24 hours of receiving irinotecan and is characterized by cholinergic symptoms (eg, increased salivation, diaphoresis, flushing, abdominal cramping, lacrimation); may be prevented or treated with atropine. Late diarrhea occurs more than 24 hours after treatment which may lead to dehydration, electrolyte imbalance, or sepsis; may be life-threatening and should be promptly treated with loperamide; dose reductions may be recommended for future doses within the current cycle. Antibiotics may be necessary if patient develops ileus, fever, or severe neutropenia. Patients with diarrhea should be carefully monitored and treated promptly; may require fluid and electrolyte therapy. Colitis, complicated by ulceration, bleeding, ileus, and infection has been reported; initiate antibiotics promptly in patients with ileus.

[U.S. Boxed Warning]: May cause severe myelosuppression. Deaths due to sepsis following severe neutropenia have been reported. Complications due to neutropenia should be promptly managed with antibiotics. Therapy should be temporarily discontinued if neutropenic fever occurs or if the absolute neutrophil count is <1000/mm^3. The dose of irinotecan should be reduced if there is a clinically significant decrease in the total WBC (<200/mm^3), neutrophil count (<1500/mm^3), hemoglobin (<8 g/dL), or platelet count (<100,000/mm^3). Routine administration of a colony-stimulating factor is generally not necessary, but may be considered for patients experiencing significant neutropenia. Fatal cases of Interstitial Pulmonary Disease (IPD)-like events have been reported with single-agent and combination therapy. Promptly evaluate changes in baseline pulmonary symptoms or any new-onset pulmonary symptoms. Discontinue therapy if IPD is diagnosed.

Patients with even modest elevations in total serum bilirubin levels (1-2 mg/dL) have a significantly greater likelihood of experiencing first-course grade 3 or 4 neutropenia than those with bilirubin levels that were <1 mg/dL. Patients with abnormal glucuronidation of bilirubin, such as those with Gilbert's syndrome, may also be at greater risk of myelosuppression when receiving therapy with irinotecan. Use caution when treating patients with known hepatic dysfunction or hyperbilirubinemia exposure to the active metabolite (SN-38) is increased; toxicities may be increased. Dosage adjustments should be considered.

Patients homozygous for the UGT1A1*28 allele are at increased risk of neutropenia; initial one-level dose reduction should be considered for both single-agent and combination regimens. Heterozygous carriers of the UGT1A1*28 allele may also be at increased risk; however, most patients have tolerated normal starting doses. Avoid vaccination with live vaccines during treatment (risk of infection may be increased due to immunosuppression). Although the response to vaccines may be diminished, inactivated vaccines may be administered during treatment.

Renal impairment and acute renal failure have been reported, possibly due to dehydration secondary to diarrhea. Use with caution in patients with renal impairment; not recommended in patients on dialysis. Patients with bowel obstruction should not be treated with irinotecan until resolution of obstruction. Use caution in patients who previously received pelvic/abdominal radiation, elderly patients with comorbid conditions, or baseline performance status of 2; close monitoring and dosage adjustments are recommended. Contains sorbitol; do not use in patients with hereditary fructose intolerance. **[U.S. Boxed Warning]: Should be administered under the supervision of an experienced cancer chemotherapy physician.** Except as part of a clinical trial, use in combination with fluorouracil and leucovorin "Mayo Clinic" regimen is not recommended. Increased toxicity has also been noted in patients with a baseline performance status of 2 in other combination regimens containing irinotecan, leucovorin, and fluorouracil. High potential for CYP-mediated drug interactions; enzyme inducers may decrease exposure to irinotecan and SN-38 (active metabolite); enzyme inhibitors may increase exposure; for use in patients with CNS tumors (unlabeled use), selection of antiseizure medications which are not enzyme inducers is preferred.

Adverse Reactions Frequency of adverse reactions reported for single-agent use of irinotecan only.

>10%:

Cardiovascular: Vasodilation (9% to 11%)

Central nervous system: Cholinergic toxicity (47% - includes rhinitis, increased salivation, miosis, lacrimation, diaphoresis, flushing and intestinal hyperperistalsis); fever (44% to 45%), pain (23% to 24%), dizziness (15% to 21%), insomnia (19%), headache (17%), chills (14%)

Dermatologic: Alopecia (46% to 72%), rash (13% to 14%)

Endocrine & metabolic: Dehydration (15%)

Gastrointestinal: Diarrhea, late (83% to 88%; grade 3/4: 14% to 31%), diarrhea, early (43% to 51%; grade 3/4: 7% to 22%), nausea (70% to 86%), abdominal pain (57% to 68%), vomiting (62% to 67%), cramps (57%), anorexia (44% to 55%), constipation (30% to 32%), mucositis (30%), weight loss (30%), flatulence (12%), stomatitis (12%)

Hematologic: Anemia (60% to 97%; grades 3/4: 5% to 7%), leukopenia (63% to 96%, grades 3/4: 14% to 28%), thrombocytopenia (96%, grades 3/4: 1% to 4%), neutropenia (30% to 96%; grades 3/4: 14% to 31%)

Hepatic: Bilirubin increased (84%), alkaline phosphatase increased (13%)

Neuromuscular & skeletal: Weakness (69% to 76%), back pain (14%)

Respiratory: Dyspnea (22%), cough (17% to 20%), rhinitis (16%)

Miscellaneous: Diaphoresis (16%), infection (14%)

1% to 10%:

Cardiovascular: Edema (10%), hypotension (6%), thromboembolic events (5%)

Central nervous system: Somnolence (9%), confusion (3%)

Gastrointestinal: Abdominal fullness (10%), dyspepsia (10%)

Hematologic: Neutropenic fever (grades 3/4: 2% to 6%), hemorrhage (grades 3/4: 1% to 5%), neutropenic infection (grades 3/4: 1% to 2%)

Hepatic: AST increased (10%), ascites and/or jaundice (grades 3/4: 9%)

Respiratory: Pneumonia (4%)

<1%, postmarketing, and/or case reports: ALT increased, amylase increased, anaphylactoid reaction, anaphylaxis, angina, arterial thrombosis, bleeding, bradycardia, cardiac arrest, cerebral infarct, cerebrovascular accident, circulatory failure, colitis, dysrhythmia, embolus, gastrointestinal bleeding, gastrointestinal obstruction, hepatomegaly, hyperglycemia, hypersensitivity, hyponatremia, ileus, interstitial lung disease, intestinal perforation, ischemic colitis, lipase increased, lymphocytopenia, megacolon, MI, myocardial ischemia, neutropenic typhlitis, pancreatitis, paresthesia, peripheral vascular disorder, pulmonary embolus; pulmonary toxicity (dyspnea, fever, reticulonodular infiltrates on chest x-ray); renal failure (acute), renal impairment, thrombocytopenia (immune mediated), thrombophlebitis, thrombosis, typhlitis, ulcerative colitis

Note: In limited pediatric experience, dehydration (often associated with severe hypokalemia and hyponatremia) was among the most significant grade 3/4 adverse events, with a frequency up to 29%. In addition, grade 3/4 infection was reported in 24%.

Drug Interactions

Metabolism/Transport Effects Substrate of CYP2B6 (major), CYP3A4 (major), P-glycoprotein, SLCO1B1, UGT1A1; **Note:** Assignment of Major/Minor substrate status based on clinically relevant drug interaction potential

Avoid Concomitant Use

Avoid concomitant use of Irinotecan with any of the following: Atazanavir; BCG; CloZAPine; Conivaptan; Natalizumab; Pimecrolimus; St Johns Wort; Tacrolimus (Topical); Vaccines (Live)

Increased Effect/Toxicity

Irinotecan may increase the levels/effects of: CloZAPine; Leflunomide; Natalizumab; Vaccines (Live)

The levels/effects of Irinotecan may be increased by: Antifungal Agents (Azole Derivatives, Systemic); Atazanavir; Bevacizumab; Conivaptan; CYP2B6 Inhibitors (Moderate); CYP2B6 Inhibitors (Strong); CYP3A4 Inhibitors (Moderate); CYP3A4 Inhibitors (Strong); Dasatinib; Denosumab; Eltrombopag; P-glycoprotein/ABCB1 Inhibitors; Pimecrolimus; Quazepam; Roflumilast; SORAfenib; Tacrolimus (Topical); Trastuzumab

Decreased Effect

Irinotecan may decrease the levels/effects of: BCG; Coccidioidin Skin Test; Sipuleucel-T; Vaccines (Inactivated); Vaccines (Live)

The levels/effects of Irinotecan may be decreased by: CarBAMazepine; CYP2B6 Inducers (Strong); CYP3A4 Inducers (Strong); Deferasirox; Echinacea; Fosphenytoin; P-glycoprotein/ABCB1 Inducers; PHENobarbital; Phenytoin; St Johns Wort; Tocilizumab

Ethanol/Nutrition/Herb Interactions Herb/Nutraceutical: Avoid St John's wort (decreases the efficacy of irinotecan).

Stability Store intact vials of injection at room temperature. Protect from light. Use appropriate precautions for handling and disposal. Doses should be diluted in 250-500 mL D_5W or NS to a final concentration of 0.12-2.8 mg/mL. Due to the relatively acidic pH, irinotecan appears to be more stable in D_5W than NS. Solutions diluted in D_5W are stable for 24 hours at room temperature or 48 hours under refrigeration at 2°C to 8°C, although the manufacturer recommends use within 6 hours at room temperature and 24 hours if refrigerated. Solutions diluted in NS may precipitate if refrigerated. Do not freeze.

Mechanism of Action Irinotecan and its active metabolite (SN-38) bind reversibly to topoisomerase I-DNA complex preventing religation of the cleaved DNA strand. This results in the accumulation of cleavable complexes and double-strand DNA breaks. As mammalian cells cannot efficiently repair these breaks, cell death consistent with S-phase cell cycle specificity occurs, leading to termination of cellular replication.

Pharmacodynamics/Kinetics

Distribution: V_d: 33-150 L/m^2

Protein binding, plasma: Predominantly albumin; Irinotecan: 30% to 68%, SN-38 (active metabolite): ~95%

Metabolism: Primarily hepatic to SN-38 (active metabolite) by carboxylesterase enzymes; SN-38 undergoes conjugation by UDP- glucuronosyl transferase 1A1 (UGT1A1) to form a glucuronide metabolite. Conversion of irinotecan to SN-38 is decreased and glucuronidation of SN-38 is increased patients who smoke cigarettes, resulting in lower levels of the metabolite and overall decreased systemic exposure. SN-38 is increased by UGT1A1*28 polymorphism (10% of North Americans are homozygous for UGT1A1*28 allele). The lactones of both irinotecan and SN-38 undergo hydrolysis to inactive hydroxy acid forms.

Half-life elimination: Irinotecan: 6-12 hours; SN-38: ~10-20 hours

Time to peak: SN-38: Following 90-minute infusion: ~1 hour

Excretion: Urine: Irinotecan (11% to 20%), metabolites (SN-38 <1%, SN-38 glucuronide, 3%)

Dosage I.V.: **Note:** A reduction in the starting dose by one dose level should be considered for prior pelvic/abdominal radiotherapy, performance status of 2, or known homozygosity for UGT1A1*28 allele. Consider premedication of atropine 0.25-1 mg I.V. or SubQ in patients with cholinergic symptoms (eg, increased salivation, diaphoresis, abdominal cramping) or diarrhea. Details concerning dosage in combination regimens should also be consulted.

Children and Adults: **Ewing's sarcoma, recurrent or progressive (unlabeled use):** 20 mg/m^2/dose days 1-5 and days 8-12 every 3 weeks (in combination with temozolomide) (Casey, 2009)

Adults:

Colorectal cancer, metastatic (single-agent therapy):

Weekly regimen: 125 mg/m^2 over 90 minutes on days 1, 8, 15, and 22 of a 6-week treatment cycle (may adjust upward to 150 mg/m^2 if tolerated)
- Adjusted dose level -1: 100 mg/m^2
- Adjusted dose level -2: 75 mg/m^2
- Further adjust to 50 mg/m^2 (in decrements of 25-50 mg/m^2) if needed

Once-every-3-week regimen: 350 mg/m^2 over 90 minutes, once every 3 weeks
- Adjusted dose level -1: 300 mg/m^2
- Adjusted dose level -2: 250 mg/m^2
- Further adjust to 200 mg/m^2 (in decrements of 25-50 mg/m^2) if needed

Colorectal cancer, metastatic (in combination with fluorouracil and leucovorin): Six-week (42-day) cycle:

Regimen 1: 125 mg/m^2 over 90 minutes on days 1, 8, 15, and 22; to be given in combination with bolus leucovorin and fluorouracil (leucovorin administered immediately following irinotecan; fluorouracil immediately following leucovorin)
- Adjusted dose level -1: 100 mg/m^2
- Adjusted dose level -2: 75 mg/m^2
- Further adjust if needed in decrements of ~20%

Regimen 2: 180 mg/m² over 90 minutes on days 1, 15, and 29; to be given in combination with infusional leucovorin and bolus/infusion fluorouracil (leucovorin administered immediately following irinotecan; fluorouracil immediately following leucovorin)

Adjusted dose level -1: 150 mg/m²

Adjusted dose level -2: 120 mg/m²

Further adjust if needed in decrements of ~20%

Colorectal cancer, metastatic (unlabeled dosing): FOLFOXIRI regimen: 165 mg/m² over 1 hour once every 2 weeks (Falcone, 2007)

Cervical cancer, recurrent or metastatic (unlabeled use): 125 mg/m² over 90 minutes once weekly for 4 consecutive weeks followed by a 2-week rest during each 6 week treatment cycle (Verschraegen, 1997)

CNS tumor, recurrent glioblastoma (unlabeled use): 125 mg/m² over 90 minutes once every 2 weeks (in combination with bevacizumab). **NOTE:** in patients taking concurrent antiepileptic enzyme-inducing medications irinotecan dose was increased to 340 mg/m² (Friedman, 2009; Vredenburgh, 2007).

Esophageal cancer, metastatic or locally advanced (unlabeled use): 65 mg/m²/dose over 90 minutes days 1, 8, 15, and 22 of a 6-week treatment cycle (in combination with cisplatin) (Ajani, 2002; Ilson, 1999) **or** 80 mg/m²/dose weekly for 6 weeks of a 7-week treatment cycle (in combination with leucovorin and fluorouracil) (Dank, 2008) **or** 250 mg/m²/dose every 3 weeks (in combination with capecitabine) (Leary, 2009; Moehler, 2010)

Gastric cancer, metastatic or locally advanced (unlabeled use): 65 mg/m²/dose over 90 minutes days 1, 8, 15, and 22 of a 6-week treatment cycle (in combination with cisplatin) (Ajani, 2002) **or** 180 mg/m²/dose over 90 minutes every 2 weeks (in combination with leucovorin and fluorouracil) (Bouche, 2004) **or** 80 mg/m²/dose weekly for 6 weeks of a 7-week treatment cycle (in combination with leucovorin and fluorouracil) (Dank, 2008) **or** 250 mg/m²/dose every 3 weeks (in combination with capecitabine) (Moehler, 2010)

Nonsmall cell lung cancer, advanced (unlabeled use): 60 mg/m² days 1, 8, and 15 every 4 weeks (in combination with cisplatin) (Ohe, 2007)

Pancreatic cancer, advanced (unlabeled use): FOLFIRINOX regimen: 180 mg/m²/dose over 90 minutes every 2 weeks (Conroy, 2005; Conroy, 2010)

Small cell lung cancer, extensive stage (unlabeled use): 60 mg/m² days 1, 8, and 15 every 4 weeks (in combination with cisplatin) (Noda, 2002) **or** 65 mg/m² days 1 and 8 every 3 weeks (in combination with cisplatin) (Hanna, 2006) **or** 175 mg/m² day 1 every 3 weeks (in combination with carboplatin) (Hermes, 2008) **or** 50 mg/m² days 1, 8 and 15 every 4 weeks (in combination with carboplatin) (Schmittel, 2006)

Elderly:

Weekly dosing schedule: No dosing adjustment is recommended

Every 3-week dosing colorectal cancer schedule: Recommended initial dose is 300 mg/m²/dose for patients ≥70 years

Dosing adjustment in renal impairment: Effects have not been evaluated; use caution, not recommended for use in patients on dialysis

Dosing adjustment in hepatic impairment:

Liver metastases with normal hepatic function: No adjustment required

Bilirubin >ULN to ≤2 mg/dL: Consider reducing initial dose by one dose level

Bilirubin >2 mg/dL: Use is not recommended

The following guidelines have been used by some clinicians: Bilirubin 1.5-3 mg/dL: Administer 75% of dose (Floyd, 2006)

Dosage adjustment for toxicities: It is recommended that new courses begin only after the granulocyte count recovers to ≥1500/mm³, the platelet counts recovers to ≥100,000/mm³, and treatment-related diarrhea has fully resolved. Depending on the patient's ability to tolerate therapy, doses should be adjusted in increments of 25-50 mg/m². Treatment should be delayed 1-2 weeks to allow for recovery from treatment-related toxicities. If the patient has not recovered after a 2-week delay, consider discontinuing irinotecan. See tables below and on next page.

Colorectal Cancer: Single-Agent Schedule: Recommended Dosage Modifications[1]

Toxicity NCI Grade[2] (Value)	During a Cycle of Therapy	At Start of Subsequent Cycles of Therapy (After Adequate Recovery), Compared to Starting Dose in Previous Cycle[1]	
	Weekly	**Weekly**	**Once Every 3 Weeks**
No toxicity	Maintain dose level	↑ 25 mg/m² up to a maximum dose of 150 mg/m²	Maintain dose level
Neutropenia			
1 (1500-1999/mm³)	Maintain dose level	Maintain dose level	Maintain dose level
2 (1000-1499/mm³)	↓ 25 mg/m²	Maintain dose level	Maintain dose level
3 (500-999/mm³)	Omit dose until resolved to ≤ grade 2, then ↓ 25 mg/m²	↓ 25 mg/m²	↓ 50 mg/m²
4 (<500/mm³)	Omit dose until resolved to ≤ grade 2, then ↓ 50 mg/m²	↓ 50 mg/m²	↓ 50 mg/m²
Neutropenic Fever (grade 4 neutropenia and ≥ grade 2 fever)	Omit dose until resolved, then ↓ 50 mg/m²	↓ 50 mg/m²	↓ 50 mg/m²
Other Hematologic Toxicities	Dose modifications for leukopenia, thrombocytopenia, and anemia during a course of therapy and at the start of subsequent courses of therapy are also based on NCI toxicity criteria and are the same as recommended for neutropenia above.		
Diarrhea			
1 (2-3 stools/day > pretreatment)	Maintain dose level	Maintain dose level	Maintain dose level
2 (4-6 stools/day > pretreatment)	↓ 25 mg/m²	Maintain dose level	Maintain dose level
3 (7-9 stools/day > pretreatment)	Omit dose until resolved to ≤ grade 2, then ↓ 25 mg/m²	↓ 25 mg/m²	↓ 50 mg/m²
4 (≥10 stools/day > pretreatment)	Omit dose until resolved to ≤ grade 2, then ↓ 50 mg/m²	↓ 50 mg/m²	↓ 50 mg/m²
Other Nonhematologic Toxicities[3]			
1	Maintain dose level	Maintain dose level	Maintain dose level
2	↓ 25 mg/m²	↓ 25 mg/m²	↓ 50 mg/m²
3	Omit dose until resolved to ≤ grade 2, then ↓ 25 mg/m²	↓ 25 mg/m²	↓ 50 mg/m²
4	Omit dose until resolved to ≤ grade 2, then ↓ 50 mg/m²	↓ 50 mg/m²	↓ 50 mg/m²

[1] All dose modifications should be based on the worst preceding toxicity.

[2] National Cancer Institute Common Toxicity Criteria (version 1.0).

[3] Excludes alopecia, anorexia, asthenia.

Colorectal Cancer: Combination Schedules: Recommended Dosage Modifications[1]

Toxicity NCI[2] Grade (Value)	During a Cycle of Therapy	At the Start of Subsequent Cycles of Therapy (After Adequate Recovery), Compared to the Starting Dose in the Previous Cycle[1]
No toxicity	Maintain dose level	Maintain dose level
Neutropenia		
1 (1500-1999/mm^3)	Maintain dose level	Maintain dose level
2 (1000-1499/mm^3)	↓ 1 dose level	Maintain dose level
3 (500-999/mm^3)	Omit dose until resolved to ≤ grade 2, then ↓ 1 dose level	↓ 1 dose level
4 (<500/mm^3)	Omit dose until resolved to ≤ grade 2, then ↓ 2 dose levels	↓ 2 dose levels
Neutropenic Fever (grade 4 neutropenia and ≥ grade 2 fever)	Omit dose until resolved, then ↓ 2 dose levels	
Other Hematologic Toxicities	Dose modifications for leukopenia or thrombocytopenia during a course of therapy and at the start of subsequent courses of therapy are also based on NCI toxicity criteria and are the same as recommended for neutropenia above.	
Diarrhea		
1 (2-3 stools/day > pretreatment)	Delay dose until resolved to baseline, then give same dose	Maintain dose level
2 (4-6 stools/day > pretreatment)	Omit dose until resolved to baseline, then ↓ 1 dose level	Maintain dose level
3 (7-9 stools/day > pretreatment)	Omit dose until resolved to baseline, then ↓ by 1 dose level	↓ 1 dose level
4 (≥10 stools/day > pretreatment)	Omit dose until resolved to baseline, then ↓ 2 dose levels	↓ 2 dose levels
Other Nonhematologic Toxicities[3]		
1	Maintain dose level	Maintain dose level
2	Omit dose until resolved to ≤ grade 1, then ↓ 1 dose level	Maintain dose level
3	Omit dose until resolved to ≤ grade 2, then ↓ 1 dose level	↓ 1 dose level
4	Omit dose until resolved to ≤ grade 2, then ↓ 2 dose levels	↓ 2 dose levels
Mucositis and/or stomatitis	Decrease only 5-FU, not irinotecan	Decrease only 5-FU, not irinotecan

[1]All dose modifications should be based on the worst preceding toxicity.

[2]National Cancer Institute Common Toxicity Criteria (version 1.0).

[3]Excludes alopecia, anorexia, asthenia.

Dietary Considerations Contains sorbitol; do not use in patients with hereditary fructose intolerance.

Administration Administer by I.V. infusion, usually over 90 minutes. Premedication with dexamethasone and a 5-HT_3 blocker is recommended 30 minutes prior to administration; prochlorperazine may be considered for subsequent use. Consider premedication of atropine 0.25-1 mg I.V. or SubQ in patients with cholinergic symptoms (eg, increased salivation, diaphoresis, abdominal cramping) or diarrhea.

The recommended regimen to manage late diarrhea is loperamide 4 mg orally at onset of late diarrhea, followed by 2 mg every 2 hours (or 4 mg every 4 hours at night) until 12 hours have passed without a bowel movement. If diarrhea recurs, then repeat administration. Loperamide should not be used for more than 48 consecutive hours.

Monitoring Parameters CBC with differential, platelet count, and hemoglobin with each dose; bilirubin, electrolytes (with severe diarrhea); bowel movements and hydration status; monitor infusion site for signs of inflammation and avoid extravasation

A test is available for genotyping of UGT1A1; however, guidelines for use are not established and not recommended in patients who have experienced toxicity as a dose reduction is already recommended (NCCN Colon Cancer Guidelines v.1.2011)

Additional Information Patients who are homozygous for the UGT1A1*28 allele are at increased risk for neutropenia; a decreased dose is recommended. Clinical research of patients who are heterozygous for UGT1A1*28 have been variable for increased neutropenic risk and such patients have tolerated normal starting doses. An FDA-approved test (Invader® Molecular Assay) is available for clinical determination of UGT phenotype.

Dosage Forms Excipient information presented when available (limited, particularly for generics); consult specific product labeling.

Injection, solution, as hydrochloride: 20 mg/mL (2 mL, 5 mL, 25 mL)

Camptosar®: 20 mg/mL (2 mL, 5 mL, 15 mL) [contains sorbitol]

◆ **Irinotecan HCl** *see* Irinotecan *on page 926*

◆ **Irinotecan Hydrochloride** *see* Irinotecan *on page 926*

◆ **Irinotecan Hydrochloride Trihydrate (Can)** *see* Irinotecan *on page 926*

◆ **Iron Dextran** *see* Iron Dextran Complex *on page 930*

Iron Dextran Complex

(EYE ern DEKS tran KOM pleks)

Brand Names: U.S. Dexferrum®; INFeD®

Brand Names: Canada Dexiron™; Infufer®

Index Terms High-Molecular-Weight Iron Dextran (DexFerrum®); Imferon; Iron Dextran; Low-Molecular-Weight Iron Dextran (INFeD®)

Pharmacologic Category Iron Salt

Use Treatment of iron deficiency in patients in whom oral administration is infeasible or ineffective

Unlabeled Use Cancer-/chemotherapy-associated anemia

Pregnancy Risk Factor C

Pregnancy Considerations Adverse events have been observed in animal reproduction studies. It is not known if iron dextran (as iron dextran) crosses the placenta. It is recommended that pregnant women meet the dietary requirements of iron with diet and/or supplements in order to prevent adverse events associated with iron deficiency anemia in pregnancy. Treatment of iron deficiency anemia in pregnant women is the same as in nonpregnant women and in most cases, oral iron preparations may be used. Except in severe cases of maternal anemia, the fetus achieves normal iron stores regardless of maternal concentrations.

Lactation Enters breast milk/use caution

Contraindications Hypersensitivity to iron dextran or any component of the formulation; any anemia not associated with iron deficiency

Warnings/Precautions [U.S. Boxed Warning]: Deaths associated with parenteral administration following anaphylactic-type reactions have been reported (use only where resuscitation equipment and personnel are available). A test dose should be administered to all patients prior to the first therapeutic dose. Fatal reactions have occurred even in patients who tolerated the test dose. Monitor patients for signs/symptoms of anaphylactic reactions during any iron dextran administration. A history of drug allergy (including multiple drug allergies) and/or the concomitant use of an ACE inhibitor may increase the risk of anaphylactic-type reactions. Adverse events (including life-threatening) associated with iron dextran usually occur with the high-molecular-weight formulation (Dexferrum®), compared to low-molecular-weight (INFeD®) (Chertow, 2006). Delayed (1-2 days) infusion reaction (including arthralgia, back pain, chills, dizziness, and fever) may occur with large doses (eg, total dose infusion) of I.V. iron dextran; usually subsides within 3-4 days. Delayed reaction may also occur (less commonly) with I.M. administration; subsiding within 3-7 days. Use with caution in patients with a history of significant allergies, asthma, serious hepatic impairment, pre-existing cardiac disease (may exacerbate cardiovascular complications), and rheumatoid arthritis (may exacerbate joint pain and swelling). Avoid use during acute kidney infection.

In patients with chronic kidney disease (CKD) requiring iron supplementation, the I.V. route is preferred for hemodialysis patients; either oral iron or I.V. iron may be used for nondialysis and peritoneal dialysis CKD patients. In patients with cancer-related anemia (either due to cancer or chemotherapy-induced) requiring iron supplementation, the I.V. route is superior to oral therapy; I.M. administration is not recommended for parenteral iron supplementation.

[U.S. Boxed Warning]: Use only in patients where the iron deficient state is not amenable to oral iron therapy. Discontinue oral iron prior to initiating parenteral iron therapy. Exogenous hemosiderosis may result from excess iron stores; patients with refractory anemias and/or hemoglobinopathies may be prone to iron overload with unwarranted iron supplementation. Anemia in the elderly is often caused by "anemia of chronic disease" or associated with inflammation rather than blood loss. Iron stores are usually normal or increased, with a serum ferritin >50 ng/mL and a decreased total iron binding capacity. I.V. administration of iron dextran is often preferred over I.M. in the elderly secondary to a decreased muscle mass and the need for daily injections. Intramuscular injections of iron-carbohydrate complexes may have a risk of delayed injection site tumor development. Iron dextran products differ in chemical characteristics. The high-molecular-weight formulation (Dexferrum®) and the low-molecular-weight formulation (INFeD®) are not clinically interchangeable. Not recommended in children <4 months of age. Intramuscular iron dextran use in neonates may be associated with an increased incidence of gram-negative sepsis.

Adverse Reactions Frequency not defined. **Note:** Adverse event risk is reported to be higher with the high-molecular-weight iron dextran formulation.

Cardiovascular: Arrhythmia, bradycardia, cardiac arrest, chest pain, chest tightness, cyanosis, flushing, hyper-/hypotension, shock, syncope, tachycardia

Central nervous system: Chills, disorientation, dizziness, fever, headache, malaise, seizure, unconsciousness, unresponsiveness

Dermatologic: Pruritus, purpura, rash, urticaria

Gastrointestinal: Abdominal pain, diarrhea, nausea, taste alteration, vomiting

Genitourinary: Discoloration of urine

Hematologic: Leukocytosis, lymphadenopathy

Local: Injection site reactions (cellulitis, inflammation, pain, phlebitis, soreness, swelling), muscle atrophy/fibrosis (with I.M. injection), skin/tissue staining (at the site of I.M. injection), sterile abscess

Neuromuscular & skeletal: Arthralgia, arthritis/arthritis exacerbation, back pain, myalgia, paresthesia, weakness

Respiratory: Bronchospasm, dyspnea, respiratory arrest, wheezing

Renal: Hematuria

Miscellaneous: Anaphylactic reactions (sudden respiratory difficulty, cardiovascular collapse), diaphoresis

Postmarketing and/or case reports: Angioedema, tumor formation (at former injection site)

Drug Interactions

Metabolism/Transport Effects None known.

Avoid Concomitant Use

Avoid concomitant use of Iron Dextran Complex with any of the following: Dimercaprol

Increased Effect/Toxicity

The levels/effects of Iron Dextran Complex may be increased by: ACE Inhibitors; Dimercaprol

Decreased Effect There are no known significant interactions involving a decrease in effect.

Stability Store at controlled room temperature. Solutions for infusion should be diluted in 250-1000 mL NS.

Mechanism of Action The released iron, from the plasma, eventually replenishes the depleted iron stores in the bone marrow where it is incorporated into hemoglobin

Pharmacodynamics/Kinetics

Onset of action: I.V.: Serum ferritin peak: 7-9 days after dose

Absorption:

I.M.: 50% to 90% is promptly absorbed, balance is slowly absorbed over month

I.V.: Uptake of iron by the reticuloendothelial system appears to be constant at about 10-20 mg/hour

Excretion: Urine and feces via reticuloendothelial system

Dosage I.M. (INFeD®; Z-track method should be used for I.M. injection), I.V. (Dexferrum®, INFeD®):

A 0.5 mL test dose (0.25 mL in infants) should be given prior to starting iron dextran therapy; total dose should be divided into a daily schedule for I.M., total dose may be given as a single continuous infusion. Individual doses of ≤2 mL may be administered daily until calculated total dose is received.

Iron-deficiency anemia:

Children 5-15 kg: Should not normally be given in the first 4 months of life:

Dose (mL) = 0.0442 (desired hemoglobin - observed hemoglobin) x W + (0.26 x W)

Desired hemoglobin: Usually 12 g/dL

W = Total body weight in kg

Children >15 kg and Adults:

Dose (mL) = 0.0442 (desired hemoglobin - observed hemoglobin) x LBW + (0.26 x LBW)

Desired hemoglobin: Usually 14.8 g/dL

LBW = Lean body weight in kg

Iron replacement therapy for blood loss: Replacement iron (mg) = blood loss (mL) x hematocrit

Maximum daily dosage: Manufacturer's labeling: **Note:** Replacement of larger estimated iron deficits may be achieved by serial administration of smaller incremental dosages. Daily dosages should be limited to:

Children:

<5 kg: 25 mg iron (0.5 mL)

5-10 kg: 50 mg iron (1 mL)

Children ≥10 kg and Adults: 100 mg iron (2 mL)

Total dose infusion (unlabeled): The entire dose (estimated iron deficit) may be diluted and administered as a one-time I.V. infusion.

Cancer-/chemotherapy-associated anemia (NCCN guidelines v.2.2010) (unlabeled use): Adults: I.V.: Test dose: 25 mg slow I.V. slow push, followed 1 hour later by 100 mg over 5 minutes; larger doses (unlabeled), up to total dose infusion (over several hours) may be administered. Low-molecular-weight iron dextran preferred.

Administration Note: Test dose: A test dose should be given on the first day of therapy; patient should be observed for 1 hour for hypersensitivity reaction, then the remaining dose (dose minus test dose) should be given. Resuscitation equipment and trained personnel should be available. An uneventful test dose does not ensure an anaphylactic-type reaction will not occur during administration of the therapeutic dose.

I.M. (INFeD®): Use Z-track technique (displacement of the skin laterally prior to injection); injection should be deep into the upper outer quadrant of buttock; alternate buttocks with subsequent injections. Administer test dose at same recommended site using the same technique.

I.V.: Test dose should be given gradually over at least 30 seconds (INFeD®) or 5 minutes (Dexferrum®). Subsequent dose(s) may be administered by I.V. bolus undiluted at a rate not to exceed 50 mg/minute or diluted in 250-1000 mL NS and infused over 1-6 hours (initial 25 mL should be given slowly and patient should be observed for allergic reactions); avoid dilutions with dextrose (increased incidence of local pain and phlebitis)

Monitoring Parameters Hemoglobin, hematocrit, reticulocyte count, serum ferritin, serum iron, TIBC; monitor for anaphylaxis/hypersensitivity reaction (during test dose and therapeutic dose)

Reference Range

Hemoglobin: Adults:

Males: 13.5-16.5 g/dL

Females: 12.0-15.0 g/dL

Serum iron: 40-160 mcg/dL

Total iron binding capacity: 230-430 mcg/dL

Transferrin: 204-360 mg/dL

Percent transferrin saturation: 20% to 50%

Test Interactions May cause falsely elevated values of serum bilirubin and falsely decreased values of serum calcium. Residual iron dextran may remain in reticuloendothelial cells; may affect accuracy of examination of bone marrow iron stores. Bone scans with 99m Tc-labeled bone seeking agents may show reduced bony uptake, marked renal activity, and excess blood pooling and soft tissue accumulation following I.V. iron dextran infusion or with high serum ferritin levels. Following I.M. iron dextran, bone scans with 99m Tc-diphosphonate may show dense activity in the buttocks.

Dosage Forms Excipient information presented when available (limited, particularly for generics); consult specific product labeling.

Injection, solution:

Dexferrum®: Elemental iron 50 mg/mL (1 mL, 2 mL) [high-molecular-weight iron dextran]

INFeD®: Elemental iron 50 mg/mL (2 mL) [low-molecular-weight iron dextran]

◆ **Iron Fumarate** *see* Ferrous Fumarate *on page 706*

◆ **Iron Gluconate** *see* Ferrous Gluconate *on page 706*

◆ **Iron-Polysaccharide Complex** *see* Polysaccharide-Iron Complex *on page 1375*

Iron Sucrose (EYE ern SOO krose)

Brand Names: U.S. Venofer®

Brand Names: Canada Venofer®

Pharmacologic Category Iron Salt

Use Treatment of iron-deficiency anemia in chronic renal failure, including nondialysis-dependent patients (with or without erythropoietin therapy) and dialysis-dependent patients receiving erythropoietin therapy

Unlabeled Use Cancer-/chemotherapy-associated anemia

Pregnancy Risk Factor B

Pregnancy Considerations Teratogenic effects were not observed in animal studies. There are no adequate and well-controlled studies in pregnant women. Based on limited data, iron sucrose may be effective for the treatment of iron-deficiency anemia in pregnancy. It is recommended that pregnant women meet the dietary requirements of iron with diet and/or supplements in order to prevent adverse events associated with iron deficiency anemia in pregnancy. Treatment of iron deficiency anemia in pregnant women is the same as in nonpregnant women and in most cases, oral iron preparations may be used. Except in severe cases of maternal anemia, the fetus achieves normal iron stores regardless of maternal concentrations.

Lactation Excretion in breast milk unknown/use caution

Contraindications Hypersensitivity to iron sucrose or any component of the formulation; evidence of iron overload; anemia not caused by iron deficiency

Warnings/Precautions Hypersensitivity reactions, including rare postmarketing anaphylactic and anaphylactoid reactions, have been reported. Hypotension has been reported frequently in hemodialysis-dependent patients. Hypotension has also been reported in peritoneal dialysis and nondialysis patients. Hypotension may be related to total dose or rate of administration (avoid rapid I.V. injection), follow recommended guidelines. Withhold iron in the presence of tissue iron overload; periodic monitoring of hemoglobin, hematocrit, serum ferritin, and transferrin saturation is recommended.

Adverse Reactions

>10%:

Cardiovascular: Hypotension (1% to 7%; 39% in hemodialysis patients; may be related to total dose or rate of administration), peripheral edema (2% to 17%)

Central nervous system: Headache (3% to 13%)

Gastrointestinal: Diarrhea (1% to 17%), nausea (1% to 15%), vomiting (3% to 12%)

Neuromuscular & skeletal: Muscle cramps (1% to 3%; 29% in hemodialysis patients)

1% to 10%:

Cardiovascular: Hypertension (6% to 8%), edema (1% to 7%), chest pain (1% to 6%), murmur (<1% to 3%), heart failure (2%), myocardial infarction (1%)

Central nervous system: Dizziness (1% to 10%), fatigue (2% to 5%), fever (1% to 3%), stroke (1%)

Dermatologic: Pruritus (1% to 7%), rash (≤1%)

Endocrine & metabolic: Gout (2% to 7%), hypoglycemia (<1% to 4%), hyperglycemia (3% to 4%), fluid overload (1% to 3%)

Gastrointestinal: Taste perversion (1% to 9%), peritoneal infection (≤8%), constipation (1% to 7%), abdominal pain (1% to 4%), positive fecal occult blood (1% to 3%)

Genitourinary: Urinary tract infection (≤1%)

Local: Injection site reaction (2% to 6%), catheter site infection (≤4%)

Neuromuscular & skeletal: Arthralgia (1% to 8%), back pain (1% to 8%), muscle pain (1% to 7%), extremity pain (3% to 6%), weakness (1% to 3%)

Ocular: Conjunctivitis (<1% to 3%)

Otic: Ear pain (1% to 7%)

Respiratory: Dyspnea (1% to 10%), pharyngitis (<1% to 7%), cough (1% to 7%), sinusitis (1% to 4%), nasopharyngitis (≤3%), upper respiratory infection (1% to 3%), nasal congestion (1%), pneumonia (1%), pulmonary edema (1%), rhinitis (≤1%)

Miscellaneous: Graft complication (1% to 10%), sepsis (2%)

<1% (Limited to important or life-threatening): Anaphylactoid reactions, anaphylactic shock, bronchospasm (with dyspnea), collapse, facial rash, hypersensitivity (including wheezing),hypoesthesia, loss of consciousness, necrotizing enterocolitis (reported in premature infants, no causal relationship established), seizure, urticaria

Drug Interactions

Metabolism/Transport Effects None known.

Avoid Concomitant Use

Avoid concomitant use of Iron Sucrose with any of the following: Dimercaprol

Increased Effect/Toxicity

The levels/effects of Iron Sucrose may be increased by: Dimercaprol

Decreased Effect There are no known significant interactions involving a decrease in effect.

Stability Store vials at controlled room temperature of 25°C (77°F); do not freeze. May be administered via the dialysis line as an undiluted solution or by diluting 100 mg (5 mL) in a maximum of 100 mL normal saline. Doses ≥200 mg should be diluted in a maximum of 250 mL normal saline. Iron sucrose is stable for 7 days at room temperature or under refrigeration when undiluted in a plastic syringe or following dilution in normal saline in a plastic syringe (2-10 mg/mL) or I.V. bag (1-2 mg/mL) (data on file [American Regent, Inc, 2010]).

Mechanism of Action Iron sucrose is dissociated by the reticuloendothelial system into iron and sucrose. The released iron increases serum iron concentrations and is incorporated into hemoglobin.

Pharmacodynamics/Kinetics

Distribution: V_{dss}: Healthy adults: 7.9 L

Metabolism: Dissociated into iron and sucrose by the reticuloendothelial system

Half-life elimination: Healthy adults: 6 hours

Excretion: Healthy adults: Urine (5%) within 24 hours

Dosage Doses expressed in mg of **elemental** iron. **Note:** Test dose: Product labeling does not indicate need for a test dose in product-naive patients.

Children ≥2 years (unlabeled use): Iron-deficiency anemia in chronic renal disease (hemodialysis-dependent patients): I.V.:

Correction: 1 mg/kg/dose per dialysis session (maximum: 100 mg)

Maintenance therapy: 0.3 mg/kg/dose per dialysis session (maximum: 100 mg). **Note:** Dosing based on limited data from a study (Leijn, 2004); study used only 14 patients (2-14 years of age) with ESRD on hemodialysis. Study initially used an iron repletion dose of 3 mg/kg/dose per dialysis session which resulted in possible iron overload (ferritin >400 mcg/L); protocol dose subsequently lowered to 1 mg/kg/dose per dialysis session which resulted in a gradual increase in ferritin levels >100 mcg/L; maintenance therapy resulted in median ferritin levels between 193-250 mcg/L.

Adults:

Iron-deficiency anemia in chronic renal disease: I.V.:

Hemodialysis-dependent patient: 100 mg over 2-5 minutes administered 1-3 times/week during dialysis; administer no more than 3 times/week to a cumulative total dose of 1000 mg (10 doses); may continue to administer at lowest dose necessary to maintain target hemoglobin, hematocrit, and iron storage parameters

Peritoneal dialysis-dependent patient: Two infusions of 300 mg each over 1.5 hours 14 days apart, followed by a single 400 mg infusion over 2.5 hours 14 days later (total cumulative dose of 1000 mg in 3 divided doses)

Nondialysis-dependent patient: 200 mg slow injection (over 2-5 minutes) on 5 different occasions within a 14-day period. Total cumulative dose: 1000 mg in 14-day period. **Note:** Dosage has also been administered as 2 infusions of 500 mg in a maximum of 250 mL normal saline infused over 3.5-4 hours on day 1 and day 14 (limited experience)

Cancer-/chemotherapy-associated anemia (unlabeled use): I.V. infusion: 200 mg over 1 hour; maximum 300-400 mg/infusion. Repeat dose every 2-3 weeks. Test doses (25 mg slow I.V. push) are recommended in patients with iron dextran hypersensitivity or those with other drug allergies (NCCN guidelines, v.2.2010)

Elderly: Insufficient data to identify differences between elderly and other adults; use caution

Administration Not for rapid I.V. injection; inject slowly over 2-5 minutes. Can be administered through dialysis line. Do not mix with other medications or parenteral nutrient solutions.

Slow I.V. injection: May administer undiluted by slow I.V. injection (100 mg over 2-5 minutes in hemodialysis-dependent patients **or** 200 mg over 2-5 minutes in non-dialysis-dependent patients)

Infusion: Dilute 100 mg in maximum of 100 mL normal saline; infuse over at least 15 minutes; 300 mg/250 mL should be infused over at least 1.5 hours; 400 mg/250 mL should be infused over at least 2.5 hours; 500 mg/250 mL should be infused over at least 3.5 hours

Monitoring Parameters Hematocrit, hemoglobin, serum ferritin, transferrin, percent transferrin saturation, TIBC; takes about 4 weeks of treatment to see increased serum iron and ferritin, and decreased TIBC. Serum iron concentrations should be drawn 48 hours after last dose.

Reference Range

Hemoglobin: Adults:

Males: 13.5-16.5 g/dL

Females: 12.0-15.0 g/dL

Serum iron: 40-160 mcg/dL

Total iron binding capacity: 230-430 mcg/dL

Transferrin: 204-360 mg/dL

Percent transferrin saturation: 20% to 50%

Test Interactions May cause falsely elevated values of serum bilirubin and falsely decreased values of serum calcium.

Dosage Forms Excipient information presented when available (limited, particularly for generics); consult specific product labeling.

Injection, solution [preservative free]:

Venofer®: Elemental iron 20 mg/mL (2.5 mL, 5 mL, 10 mL)

- **Iron Sulfate** *see* Ferrous Sulfate *on page 706*
- **ISD** *see* Isosorbide Dinitrate *on page 936*
- **ISDN** *see* Isosorbide Dinitrate *on page 936*
- **Isentress®** *see* Raltegravir *on page 1456*
- **ISG** *see* Immune Globulin *on page 880*
- **ISMN** *see* Isosorbide Mononitrate *on page 938*
- **Ismo®** *see* Isosorbide Mononitrate *on page 938*
- **Isoamyl Nitrite** *see* Amyl Nitrite *on page 119*
- **Isobamate** *see* Carisoprodol *on page 291*

Isoniazid (eye soe NYE a zid)

Brand Names: Canada Isotamine®; PMS-Isoniazid

Index Terms INH; Isonicotinic Acid Hydrazide

Pharmacologic Category Antitubercular Agent

Use Treatment of susceptible tuberculosis infections; treatment of latent tuberculosis infection (LTBI)

Pregnancy Risk Factor C

Pregnancy Considerations Isoniazid was found to be embryocidal in animal studies; teratogenic effects were not noted. Isoniazid crosses the human placenta. Due to the risk of tuberculosis to the fetus, treatment is recommended when the probability of maternal disease is moderate to high. The CDC recommends isoniazid as part of the initial treatment regimen (CDC, 2003). Pyridoxine supplementation is recommended (25 mg/day).

Lactation Enters breast milk/compatible

Contraindications Hypersensitivity to isoniazid or any component of the formulation; acute liver disease; previous history of hepatic damage during isoniazid therapy; previous severe adverse reaction (drug fever, chills, arthritis) to isoniazid

Warnings/Precautions Use with caution in patients with severe renal impairment and liver disease. **[U.S. Boxed Warning]: Severe and sometimes fatal hepatitis may occur; usually occurs within the first 3 months of treatment, although may develop even after many months of treatment.** The risk of developing hepatitis is age-related, although isoniazid-induced hepatotoxicity has been reported in children; daily ethanol consumption may also increase the risk. Patients must report any prodromal symptoms of hepatitis, such as fatigue, weakness, malaise, anorexia, nausea, abdominal pain, jaundice, or vomiting. Patients should be instructed to immediately discontinue therapy if any of these symptoms occur, even if a clinical evaluation has yet to be conducted. Treatment with isoniazid for latent tuberculosis infection should be deferred in patients with acute hepatic diseases. Periodic ophthalmic examinations are recommended even when usual symptoms do not occur. Pyridoxine (10-50 mg/day) is recommended in individuals at risk for development of peripheral neuropathies (eg, HIV infection, nutritional deficiency, diabetes, pregnancy). Children with low milk and low meat intake should receive concomitant pyridoxine therapy. Multidrug regimens should be utilized for the treatment of active tuberculosis to prevent the emergence of drug resistance.

Adverse Reactions Frequency not defined.

Cardiovascular: Hypertension, palpitation, tachycardia, vasculitis

Central nervous system: Depression, dizziness, encephalopathy, fever, lethargy, memory impairment, psychosis, seizure, slurred speech, toxic encephalopathy

Dermatologic: Flushing, rash (morbilliform, maculopapular, pruritic, or exfoliative)

Endocrine & metabolic: Gynecomastia, hyperglycemia, metabolic acidosis, pellagra, pyridoxine deficiency

Gastrointestinal: Anorexia, epigastric distress, nausea, stomach pain, vomiting

Hematologic: Agranulocytosis, anemia (sideroblastic, hemolytic, or aplastic), eosinophilia, thrombocytopenia

Hepatic: LFTs mildly increased (10% to 20%), hyperbilirubinemia, bilirubinuria, jaundice, hepatic dysfunction, hepatitis (may involve progressive liver damage; risk increases with age; 2.3% in patients >50 years)

Neuromuscular & skeletal: Arthralgia, hyper-reflexia, paresthesia, peripheral neuropathy (dose-related incidence, 10% to 20% incidence with 10 mg/kg/day), weakness

Ocular: Blurred vision, loss of vision, optic neuritis and atrophy

Miscellaneous: Lupus-like syndrome, lymphadenopathy, rheumatic syndrome

Drug Interactions

Metabolism/Transport Effects **Substrate** of CYP2E1 (major); **Note:** Assignment of Major/Minor substrate status based on clinically relevant drug interaction potential; **Inhibits** CYP1A2 (weak), CYP2A6 (moderate), CYP2C19 (strong), CYP2C9 (weak), CYP2D6 (moderate), CYP2E1 (moderate), CYP3A4 (weak); **Induces** CYP2E1 (weak/moderate)

Avoid Concomitant Use

Avoid concomitant use of Isoniazid with any of the following: Clopidogrel; Pimozide; Thioridazine

Increased Effect/Toxicity

Isoniazid may increase the levels/effects of: Acetaminophen; Benzodiazepines (metabolized by oxidation); CarBAMazepine; Chlorzoxazone; Citalopram; CycloSERINE; CYP2A6 Substrates; CYP2C19 Substrates; CYP2D6 Substrates; CYP2E1 Substrates; Fesoterodine; Fosphenytoin; Nebivolol; Phenytoin; Pimozide; Tamoxifen; Theophylline Derivatives; Thioridazine

The levels/effects of Isoniazid may be increased by: Ethionamide; Propafenone; Rifamycin Derivatives

Decreased Effect

Isoniazid may decrease the levels/effects of: Clopidogrel; Codeine; TraMADol

The levels/effects of Isoniazid may be decreased by: Antacids; Corticosteroids (Systemic); Cyproterone

Ethanol/Nutrition/Herb Interactions

Ethanol: Avoid ethanol (increases the risk of hepatitis).

Food: Isoniazid should not be taken with food; serum levels may be decreased if taken with food. Has some ability to inhibit tyramine metabolism; several case reports of mild reactions (flushing, palpitations) after ingestion of cheese (with or without wine). Reactions resembling allergic symptoms following ingestion of fish high in histamine content have been reported. Isoniazid decreases folic acid absorption. Isoniazid alters pyridoxine metabolism.

Stability

Tablet: Store at 20°C to 25°C (68°F to 77°F). Protect from light.

Oral solution: Store at 15°C to 30°C (59°F to 86°F). Protect from light.

Mechanism of Action Unknown, but may include the inhibition of mycolic acid synthesis resulting in disruption of the bacterial cell wall

Pharmacodynamics/Kinetics

Absorption: Rapid and complete; rate can be slowed with food

Distribution: All body tissues and fluids including CSF; crosses placenta; enters breast milk

Protein binding: 10% to 15%

Metabolism: Hepatic with decay rate determined genetically by acetylation phenotype

Half-life elimination: Fast acetylators: 30-100 minutes; Slow acetylators: 2-5 hours; may be prolonged with hepatic or severe renal impairment

Time to peak, serum: 1-2 hours

Excretion: Urine (75% to 95%); feces; saliva

Dosage

Usual dosage ranges: Oral, I.M.:

Infants and Children: 10-15 mg/kg/day once daily (maximum: 300 mg/day) or 20-40 mg/kg given 2-3 times per week (maximum: 900 mg/dose)

Adults: 5 mg/kg/day (usual: 300 mg/day) as a single daily dose or 15 mg/kg (maximum: 900 mg/dose) given 2-3 times per week

Indication-specific dosing: Oral, I.M.: Recommendations often change due to resistant strains and newly-developed information; consult *MMWR* for current CDC recommendations. Intramuscular injection is available for patients who are unable to either take or absorb oral therapy.

Infants and Children:

Tuberculosis, active:

Daily therapy: CDC recommendations: 10-15 mg/kg/day once daily (maximum: 300 mg/day) (*MMWR*, 2003)

Directly observed therapy (DOT): CDC recommendations: 20-30 mg/kg (maximum: 900 mg/dose) twice weekly (*MMWR*, 2003); Manufacturer's labeling: 20-40 mg/kg (maximum: 900 mg/dose) twice weekly or 3 times/week

Tuberculosis, latent infection (LTBI):

Daily therapy: CDC recommendations: 10-20 mg/kg/day once daily (maximum: 300 mg/dose) (*MMWR*, 2000); Manufacturer's labeling: 10 mg/kg/day once daily (maximum: 300 mg/dose)

Directly observed therapy (DOT): CDC recommendations: 20-40 mg/kg (maximum: 900 mg/dose) twice weekly for 9 months (*MMWR*, 2000); Manufacturer's labeling: 20-30 mg/kg twice weekly (maximum: 900 mg/dose)

Adults: **Note:** Concomitant administration of 10-50 mg/day pyridoxine is recommended in malnourished patients or those prone to neuropathy (eg, alcoholics, patients with diabetes).

Nontuberculous mycobacterium *(M. kansasii)* (unlabeled use): 5 mg/kg/day (maximum: 300 mg/day) for duration to include 12 months of culture-negative sputum; typically used in combination with ethambutol and rifampin

Tuberculosis, active:

Daily therapy: CDC recommendations: 5 mg/kg/day once daily (usual dose: 300 mg/day) (*MMWR*, 2003)

Directly observed therapy (DOT): CDC recommendations: 15 mg/kg (maximum: 900 mg/dose) twice weekly or 3 times/week; **Note:** CDC guidelines state that once-weekly therapy (15 mg/kg/dose) may be considered, but only after the first 2 months of initial therapy in HIV-negative patients, and only in combination with rifapentine (*MMWR*, 2003).

Note: Treatment may be defined by the number of doses administered (eg, "six-month" therapy involves 182 doses of INH and rifampin, and 56 doses of pyrazinamide). Six months is the shortest interval of time over which these doses may be administered, assuming no interruption of therapy.

Tuberculosis, latent infection (LTBI): CDC recommendations: 5 mg/kg (maximum: 300 mg/dose) once daily or 15 mg/kg (maximum: 900 mg/dose) twice weekly by directly observed therapy (DOT) 6-9 months in patients who do not have HIV infection (9 months is optimal, 6 months may be considered to reduce costs of therapy) and 9 months in patients who have HIV infection. Extend to 12 months of therapy if interruptions in treatment occur. (*MMWR*, 2000)

Dosing adjustment in renal impairment: No adjustment necessary

Hemodialysis: Dialyzable (50% to 100%); administer dose post dialysis

Dosing adjustment in hepatic impairment: No adjustment required, however, use with caution; may accumulate and additional liver damage may occur in patients with pre-existing liver disease. For ALT or AST >3 times the ULN: discontinue or temporarily withhold treatment. Treatment with isoniazid for latent tuberculosis infection should be deferred in patients with acute hepatic diseases.

Dietary Considerations Should be taken 1 hour before or 2 hours after meals on an empty stomach; increase dietary intake of folate, niacin, magnesium. Avoid tyramine-containing foods; some examples include aged or matured cheese, air-dried or cured meats (including sausages and salamis), fava or broad bean pods, tap/draft beers, Marmite concentrate, sauerkraut, soy sauce and other soybean condiments. Avoid histamine-containing foods.

Administration Should be administered 1 hour before or 2 hours after meals on an empty stomach.

Monitoring Parameters Baseline and periodic (more frequently in patients with higher risk for hepatitis) liver function tests (ALT and AST); sputum cultures monthly (until 2 consecutive negative cultures reported); monitoring for prodromal signs of hepatitis

LTBI therapy: American Thoracic Society/Centers for Disease Control (ATS/CDC) recommendations: Monthly clinical evaluation, including brief physical exam for adverse events. Baseline serum AST or ALT and bilirubin should be considered for patients at higher risk for adverse events (eg, history of liver disease, chronic ethanol use, HIV-infected patients, women who are pregnant or postpartum ≤3 months, older adults with concomitant medications or diseases). Routine, periodic monitoring is recommended for any patient with an abnormal baseline or at increased risk for hepatotoxicity.

Test Interactions False-positive urinary glucose with Clinitest®

Additional Information The AAP recommends that pyridoxine supplementation (1-2 mg/kg/day) should be administered to malnourished patients, children or adolescents on meat or milk-deficient diets, breast-feeding infants, and those predisposed to neuritis to prevent peripheral neuropathy; administration of isoniazid syrup has been associated with diarrhea

Dosage Forms Excipient information presented when available (limited, particularly for generics); consult specific product labeling.

Injection, solution: 100 mg/mL (10 mL)

Solution, oral: 50 mg/5 mL (473 mL)

Tablet, oral: 100 mg, 300 mg

Extemporaneous Preparations Note: Commercial oral solution is available (50 mg/mL)

A 10 mg/mL oral suspension may be made with tablets, purified water, and sorbitol. Crush ten 100 mg tablets in a mortar and reduce to a fine powder. Add 10 mL of purified water and mix to a uniform paste. Mix while adding sorbitol in incremental proportions to **almost** 100 mL; transfer to a graduated cylinder, rinse mortar with sorbitol, and add quantity of sorbitol sufficient to make 100 mL (do not use sugar-based solutions). Label "shake well" and "refrigerate". Stable for 21 days refrigerated.

Nahata MC, Pai VB, and Hipple TF, *Pediatric Drug Formulations*, 5th ed, Cincinnati, OH: Harvey Whitney Books Co, 2004.

◆ **Isonicotinic Acid Hydrazide** *see* Isoniazid *on page 933*

◆ **Isonipecaine Hydrochloride** *see* Meperidine *on page 1074*

◆ **Isophane Insulin** *see* Insulin NPH *on page 906*

◆ **Isophane Insulin and Regular Insulin** *see* Insulin NPH and Insulin Regular *on page 906*

◆ **Isophosphamide** *see* Ifosfamide *on page 867*

Isoproterenol (eye soe proe TER e nole)

Brand Names: U.S. Isuprel®

Index Terms Isoproterenol Hydrochloride

Pharmacologic Category Beta$_1$- & Beta$_2$-Adrenergic Agonist Agent

Additional Appendix Information

Bronchodilators *on page 1886*

Use Manufacturer's labeled indications (see **"Note"**): Mild or transient episodes of heart block that do not require electric shock or pacemaker therapy; serious episodes of heart block and Adams-Stokes attacks (except when caused by ventricular tachycardia or fibrillation); cardiac arrest until electric shock or pacemaker therapy is available; bronchospasm during anesthesia; adjunct to fluid and electrolyte replacement therapy and other drugs and procedures in the treatment of hypovolemic or septic shock and low cardiac output states (eg, decompensated heart failure, cardiogenic shock)

Note: The use of isoproterenol in advanced cardiac life support (ACLS) has largely been supplanted by the use of other adrenergic agents (eg, epinephrine and dopamine). The use of isoproterenol for bronchospasm during anesthesia and cardiogenic, hypovolemic, or septic shock is no longer recommended. See *Unlabeled Use* for more appropriate, yet unlabeled, uses.

Unlabeled Use Pharmacologic overdrive pacing for refractory torsade de pointes; pharmacologic provocation during tilt table testing for syncope; temporary control of bradycardia in denervated heart transplant patients unresponsive to atropine; ventricular arrhythmias due to AV nodal block; beta-blocker overdose; electrical storm associated with Brugada syndrome

Pregnancy Risk Factor C

Pregnancy Considerations Animal reproduction studies have not been conducted. Adequate studies have not been conducted in pregnant women; use during pregnancy when the potential benefit to the mother outweighs the possible risk to the fetus.

Lactation Excretion in breast milk unknown

Contraindications Angina, pre-existing ventricular arrhythmias, tachyarrhythmias; cardiac glycoside intoxication

Warnings/Precautions Use with extreme caution; not currently a treatment of choice; use with caution in elderly patients, patients with diabetes, cardiovascular disease, or hyperthyroidism; excessive or prolonged use may result in decreased effectiveness. Contains sulfites; may cause allergic reaction in susceptible individuals.

Adverse Reactions Frequency not defined.

Cardiovascular: Angina, flushing, hyper-/hypotension, pallor, palpitation, paradoxical bradycardia (with tilt table testing), premature ventricular beats, Stokes-Adams attacks, tachyarrhythmia, ventricular arrhythmia

Central nervous system: Dizziness, headache, nervousness, restlessness, Stokes-Adams seizure

Endocrine & metabolic: Hypokalemia, serum glucose increased

Gastrointestinal: Nausea, vomiting

Neuromuscular & skeletal: Tremor, weakness

Ocular: Blurred vision

Respiratory: Dyspnea, pulmonary edema

Miscellaneous: Diaphoresis

Drug Interactions

Metabolism/Transport Effects Substrate of COMT

Avoid Concomitant Use

Avoid concomitant use of Isoproterenol with any of the following: Inhalational Anesthetics

Increased Effect/Toxicity

The levels/effects of Isoproterenol may be increased by: COMT Inhibitors; Inhalational Anesthetics

Decreased Effect

Isoproterenol may decrease the levels/effects of: Theophylline Derivatives

Ethanol/Nutrition/Herb Interactions Herb/Nutraceutical: Avoid ephedra, yohimbe (may cause CNS stimulation).

Stability Store undiluted solution at 20°C to 25°C (68°F to 77°F). Solution should not be used if a color or precipitate is present. Exposure to air, light, or increased temperature may cause a pink to brownish pink color to develop. Stability of parenteral admixture at room temperature (25°C) or at refrigeration (4°C) is 24 hours.

Standard admixture concentration: 1 mg/500 mL D_5W

Maximum admixture concentration: 1 mg/100 mL D_5W

Mechanism of Action Stimulates $beta_1$- and $beta_2$-receptors resulting in relaxation of bronchial, GI, and uterine smooth muscle, increased heart rate and contractility, vasodilation of peripheral vasculature

Pharmacodynamics/Kinetics

Onset of action: I.V.: Immediate

Duration: I.V.: 10-15 minutes

Metabolism: Via conjugation in many tissues including hepatic and pulmonary

Half-life elimination: 2.5-5 minutes

Excretion: Urine (primarily as sulfate conjugates)

Dosage I.V.: **Note:** Patients may exhibit dose-dependent vasodilation due to unopposed $beta_2$-agonism elicited by isoproterenol.

Bradyarrhythmias, AV nodal block, or refractory torsade de pointes:

Children: Continuous infusion: Usual range: 0.05-2 mcg/**kg**/minute; titrate to patient response

Adults: Continuous infusion: Usual range: 2-10 mcg/minute; titrate to patient response

Brugada syndrome with electrical storm (unlabeled use):

Adults: I.V. bolus: Initial: 1-2 mcg, followed by a continuous infusion of 0.15-0.3 mcg/minute for 1 day; may repeat sequence if ventricular tachycardia/fibrillation recurs (Watanabe, 2006; Zipes, 2006).

Tilt table testing for syncope (Benditt, 1996; Brignole, 2004): Adults: Continuous infusion: Initial: 1 mcg/minute; increase as necessary based on response; maximum dose: 5 mcg/minute. **Note:** Timing of initiation and dose adjustment during test may be institution-specific.

Administration I.V. infusion administration requires the use of an infusion pump.

Monitoring Parameters ECG, heart rate, respiratory rate, arterial blood gas, arterial blood pressure, CVP; serum glucose, serum potassium, serum magnesium

Dosage Forms Excipient information presented when available (limited, particularly for generics); consult specific product labeling.

Injection, solution, as hydrochloride:

Isuprel®: 0.2 mg/mL (1 mL, 5 mL) [contains sodium metabisulfite; 1:5000]

◆ **Isoproterenol Hydrochloride** *see* Isoproterenol *on page 935*

◆ **Isoptin® SR** *see* Verapamil *on page 1783*

◆ **Isopto® Atropine** *see* Atropine *on page 170*

◆ **Isopto® Carbachol** *see* Carbachol *on page 280*

◆ **Isopto® Carpine** *see* Pilocarpine (Ophthalmic) *on page 1353*

◆ **Isopto® Homatropine** *see* Homatropine *on page 830*

◆ **Isordil® Titradose™** *see* Isosorbide Dinitrate *on page 936*

◆ **Isosorbide (Can)** *see* Isosorbide Dinitrate *on page 936*

Isosorbide Dinitrate (eye soe SOR bide dye NYE trate)

Brand Names: U.S. Dilatrate®-SR; Isordil® Titradose™

Brand Names: Canada ISDN; Isosorbide; Novo-Sorbide; PMS-Isosorbide

Index Terms ISD; ISDN

Pharmacologic Category Antianginal Agent; Vasodilator

Additional Appendix Information

Heart Failure (Systolic) *on page 1991*

Nitrates *on page 1895*

Use Prevention and treatment of angina pectoris

Note: Due to slower onset of action, not the drug of choice to abort an acute anginal episode.

Unlabeled Use Patients with heart failure (HF) who do not tolerate an ACE inhibitor or an angiotensin receptor blocker (ARB); African-American (self-identified) patients with HF remaining symptomatic despite optimal standard therapy; esophageal spastic disorders

Pregnancy Risk Factor C

Pregnancy Considerations

Increased fetal mortality has been observed in animal studies using isosorbide dinitrate at doses much higher than those used in humans. There are no adequate and well-controlled studies in pregnant women.

Lactation Excretion in breast milk unknown

Contraindications Hypersensitivity to isosorbide dinitrate or any component of the formulation; hypersensitivity to organic nitrates; concurrent use with phosphodiesterase-5 (PDE-5) inhibitors (sildenafil, tadalafil, or vardenafil)

Warnings/Precautions Severe hypotension can occur; paradoxical bradycardia and increased angina pectoris can accompany hypotension. Postural hypotension can also occur; ethanol may potentiate this effect. Use with caution in volume depletion and moderate hypotension, and use with extreme caution with inferior wall MI and suspected right ventricular infarctions. Nitrates may reduce preload, exacerbating obstruction and cause hypotension or syncope and/or worsening of heart failure (Gibbons, 2003). Avoid use in patients with hypertrophic cardiomyopathy (HCM).

Use of isosorbide dinitrate sublingual tablets to treat acute angina attacks is recommended only in patients unresponsive to sublingual nitroglycerin; however, current clinical practice guidelines do not recommend use during an acute anginal episode. Avoid use of extended release formulations in acute MI or acute HF; cannot easily reverse effects if adverse events develop. Nitrates may precipitate or aggravate increased intracranial pressure and subsequently may worsen clinical outcomes in patients with neurologic injury (eg, intracranial hemorrhage, traumatic brain injury). Appropriate dosing intervals are needed to minimize tolerance development. Tolerance can only be overcome by short periods of nitrate absence from the body. Dose escalation does not overcome this effect. When used for HF in combination with hydralazine, tolerance is less of a concern (Gogia, 1995).

Avoid concurrent use with PDE-5 inhibitors (eg, sildenafil, tadalafil, vardenafil). When nitrate administration becomes medically necessary, may administer nitrates only if 24 hours have elapsed after use of sildenafil or vardenafil (48 hours after tadalafil use) (Trujillo, 2007).

Adverse Reactions Frequency not defined.

Cardiovascular: Crescendo angina (uncommon), hypotension, postural hypotension, rebound hypertension (uncommon), syncope (uncommon)

Central nervous system: Headache (most common), lightheadedness (related to blood pressure changes)

Hematologic: Methemoglobinemia (rare, overdose)

Drug Interactions

Metabolism/Transport Effects Substrate of CYP3A4 (major); **Note:** Assignment of Major/Minor substrate status based on clinically relevant drug interaction potential

Avoid Concomitant Use

Avoid concomitant use of Isosorbide Dinitrate with any of the following: Conivaptan; Phosphodiesterase 5 Inhibitors

Increased Effect/Toxicity

Isosorbide Dinitrate may increase the levels/effects of: Hypotensive Agents; Prilocaine; Rosiglitazone

The levels/effects of Isosorbide Dinitrate may be increased by: Conivaptan; CYP3A4 Inhibitors (Moderate); CYP3A4 Inhibitors (Strong); Dasatinib; Phosphodiesterase 5 Inhibitors

Decreased Effect

The levels/effects of Isosorbide Dinitrate may be decreased by: CYP3A4 Inducers (Strong); Deferasirox; Herbs (CYP3A4 Inducers); Tocilizumab

Ethanol/Nutrition/Herb Interactions

Ethanol: Caution with ethanol (may increase risk of hypotension).

Herb/Nutraceutical: Avoid black cohosh, California poppy, coleus, golden seal, hawthorn, mistletoe, periwinkle, quinine, shepherd's purse (may cause hypotension).

Mechanism of Action Stimulation of intracellular cyclic-GMP results in vascular smooth muscle relaxation of both arterial and venous vasculature with more prominent effects on the veins. Primarily reduces cardiac oxygen demand by decreasing preload (left ventricular end-diastolic pressure); may modestly reduce afterload. Additionally, coronary artery dilation improves collateral flow to ischemic regions.

Pharmacodynamics/Kinetics

Onset of action: Sublingual tablet: ~3 minutes; Oral tablet and capsule (includes extended-release formulations): ~1 hour

Duration: Sublingual tablet: 1-2 hours; Oral tablet and capsule (includes extended-release formulations): Up to 8 hours

Distribution: V_d: 2-4 L/kg

Metabolism: Extensively hepatic to conjugated metabolites, including isosorbide 5-mononitrate (active) and 2-mononitrate (active)

Bioavailability: Sublingual tablet: 40% to 50%; Oral immediate release formulations: Highly variable (10% to 90%); increases with chronic therapy

Half-life elimination: Parent drug: ~1 hour; Metabolites (5-mononitrate: 5 hours; 2-mononitrate: 2 hours)

Excretion: Urine and feces

Dosage Note: Due to slower onset of action, not the drug of choice to abort an acute anginal episode. Tolerance to nitrate effects develops with chronic exposure: Dose escalation does not overcome this effect. Tolerance can only be overcome by short periods of nitrate absence from the body. Nitrate-free intervals of ≥14 hours (immediate release products) or >18 hours (sustained release products) may help minimize tolerance.

Adults (elderly should be given lowest recommended daily doses initially and titrate upward):

Angina:

Oral:

Immediate release: Initial: 5-20 mg 2-3 times/day; Maintenance: 10-40 mg 2-3 times/day **or** 5-80 mg 2-3 times/day (Anderson, 2007; Gibbons, 2002)

Sustained release: 40-160 mg/day has been used in clinical trials (a nitrate free interval of at least 18 hours is recommended; however, a clinically efficacious dosage interval has not been clearly established) **or** 40 mg 1-2 times/day (Anderson, 2007; Gibbons, 2002)

Sublingual:

Prophylactic use: 2.5-5 mg administered 15 minutes prior to activities which may provoke an anginal episode

Treatment of acute anginal episode (use only if patient has failed sublingual nitroglycerin): 2.5-5 mg every 5-10 minutes for maximum of 3 doses in 15-30 minutes

Heart failure (unlabeled use; Cohn, 1991; HFSA, 2010; Hunt, 2009): Oral:

Immediate release (**Note:** Use in combination with hydralazine):

Initial dose: 20 mg 3-4 times per day

Target dose: 160 mg/day in 4 divided doses

Esophageal spastic disorders (unlabeled use; Goyal, 1998): Oral (immediate release), sublingual: 10-30 mg before meals

Hemodialysis: Supplemental dose is not necessary

Peritoneal dialysis: Supplemental dose is not necessary

Administration May consider administration of first dose in physician office; observe for maximal cardiovascular dynamic effects and adverse effects (orthostatic hypotension, headache). Do not administer around the clock; allow nitrate-free interval ≥14 hours (immediate release products) and >18 hours (sustained release products). Do not crush sublingual tablets or extended release formulations.

Immediate release products: When prescribed twice daily, consider administering at 8 AM and 1 PM. For 3 times/day dosing, consider 8 AM, 1 PM, and 6 PM.

Sustained release products: Consider once daily in morning or twice-daily dosing at 8 AM and between 1-2 PM.

Monitoring Parameters Blood pressure, heart rate

Dosage Forms Excipient information presented when available (limited, particularly for generics); consult specific product labeling.

Capsule, sustained release, oral:

Dilatrate®-SR: 40 mg

Tablet, oral: 5 mg, 10 mg, 20 mg, 30 mg

Isordil® Titradose™: 5 mg, 40 mg [scored]

Tablet, sublingual: 2.5 mg, 5 mg

Tablet, extended release, oral: 40 mg

Isosorbide Dinitrate and Hydralazine

(eye soe SOR bide dye NYE trate & hye DRAL a zeen)

Brand Names: U.S. BiDil®

Index Terms Hydralazine and Isosorbide Dinitrate

Pharmacologic Category Vasodilator

Use Treatment of heart failure, adjunct to standard therapy, in self-identified African-Americans

Pregnancy Risk Factor C

Dosage Oral: Adults: Initial: 1 tablet 3 times/day; may titrate to a maximum dose of 2 tablets 3 times/day

Dosage adjustment for toxicity: If patient experiences intolerable side effects, dose may be reduced to as little as one-half tablet 3 times/day; dose should be titrated upward as soon as tolerated.

Additional Information Complete prescribing information for this medication should be consulted for additional detail.

Dosage Forms

Tablet, oral:

BiDil®: Isosorbide dinitrate 20 mg and hydralazine 37.5 mg

Isosorbide Mononitrate

(eye soe SOR bide mon oh NYE trate)

Brand Names: U.S. Imdur®; Ismo®; Monoket®

Brand Names: Canada Apo-ISMN®; Imdur®; PMS-ISMN; PRO-ISMN

Index Terms ISMN

Pharmacologic Category Antianginal Agent; Vasodilator

Additional Appendix Information

Nitrates *on page 1895*

Use Prevention of angina pectoris

Pregnancy Risk Factor B/C (manufacturer dependent)

Pregnancy Considerations Teratogenic effects were not observed in animal reproduction studies. Adverse events in the offspring were observed with use later in pregnancy at doses that were also maternally toxic.

Lactation Excretion in breast milk unknown/use caution

Contraindications Hypersensitivity to isosorbide mononitrate or any component of the formulation; hypersensitivity to organic nitrates; concurrent use with phosphodiesterase-5 (PDE-5) inhibitors (sildenafil, tadalafil, or vardenafil)

Warnings/Precautions Avoid use in hypertrophic cardiomyopathy. Use with caution in volume depletion, moderate hypotension, and extreme caution with inferior wall MI and suspected right ventricular infarctions. Nitrates may precipitate or aggravate increased intracranial pressure and subsequently may worsen clinical outcomes in patients with neurologic injury (eg, intracranial hemorrhage, traumatic brain injury). Postural hypotension, transient episodes of weakness, dizziness, or syncope may occur even with small doses; ethanol accentuates these effects; tolerance and cross-tolerance to nitrate antianginal and hemodynamic effects may occur during prolonged isosorbide mononitrate therapy; (minimized by using the smallest effective dose, by alternating coronary vasodilators or offering drug-free intervals of as little as 12 hours). Excessive doses may result in severe headache, blurred vision, or xerostomia; increased anginal symptoms may be a result of dosage increases. Avoid concurrent use with PDE-5 inhibitors (eg, sildenafil, tadalafil, vardenafil). When nitrate administration becomes medically necessary, may administer nitrates only if 24 hours have elapsed after use of sildenafil or vardenafil (48 hours after tadalafil use) (O'Connor, 2010).

Adverse Reactions

>10%: Central nervous system: Headache (13% to 35%)

1% to 10%:

Cardiovascular: Angina (≤2%), flushing (≤2%)

Central nervous system: Dizziness (≤4%), fatigue (≤4%), pain (≤4%), emotional lability (≤2%)

Dermatologic: Pruritus (≤2%), rash (≤2%)

Gastrointestinal: Nausea (≤3%), abdominal pain (≤2%), diarrhea (≤2%)

Respiratory: Upper respiratory infection (≤4%), cough increased (≤2%)

Miscellaneous: Allergic reaction (≤2%)

<1% (Limited to important or life-threatening): Apoplexy, arrhythmia, bradycardia, dyspnea, edema, hyper-/hypotension, methemoglobinemia (rare, overdose), MI, pallor, palpitation, paresthesia, postural hypotension, tachycardia

Drug Interactions

Metabolism/Transport Effects Substrate of CYP3A4 (major); **Note:** Assignment of Major/Minor substrate status based on clinically relevant drug interaction potential

Avoid Concomitant Use

Avoid concomitant use of Isosorbide Mononitrate with any of the following: Conivaptan; Phosphodiesterase 5 Inhibitors

Increased Effect/Toxicity

Isosorbide Mononitrate may increase the levels/effects of: Hypotensive Agents; Prilocaine; Rosiglitazone

The levels/effects of Isosorbide Mononitrate may be increased by: Conivaptan; CYP3A4 Inhibitors (Moderate); CYP3A4 Inhibitors (Strong); Dasatinib; Phosphodiesterase 5 Inhibitors

Decreased Effect

The levels/effects of Isosorbide Mononitrate may be decreased by: CYP3A4 Inducers (Strong); Deferasirox; Herbs (CYP3A4 Inducers); Tocilizumab

Ethanol/Nutrition/Herb Interactions Ethanol: Caution with ethanol (may increase risk of hypotension).

Stability Tablets should be stored in a tight container at room temperature of 15°C to 30°C (59°F to 86°F).

Mechanism of Action Nitroglycerin and other nitrates form free radical nitric oxide. In smooth muscle, nitric oxide activates guanylate cyclase which increases guanosine 3'5' monophosphate (cGMP) leading to dephosphorylation of myosin light chains and smooth muscle relaxation. Produces a vasodilator effect on the peripheral veins and arteries with more prominent effects on the veins. Primarily reduces cardiac oxygen demand by decreasing preload (left ventricular end-diastolic pressure); may modestly reduce afterload; dilates coronary arteries and improves collateral flow to ischemic regions.

Pharmacodynamics/Kinetics

Onset of action: 30-60 minutes

Duration: Immediate release: ≥6 hours (Thadani, 1987); Extended release: ≥12-24 hours (Anderson, 2007)

Absorption: Nearly complete and low intersubject variability in its pharmacokinetic parameters and plasma concentrations

Distribution: V_d: ~0.6 L/kg

Protein binding: <5%

Metabolism: Hepatic

Bioavailability: ~100%

Half-life elimination: Mononitrate: ~5-6 hours

Excretion: Predominantly urine (2% as unchanged drug); feces (1% of dose)

Dosage Oral:

Adults:

Regular release tablet: Initial: 5-20 mg twice daily with the 2 doses given 7 hours apart (eg, 8 AM and 3 PM) to decrease tolerance development; patients initiating therapy with 5 mg twice daily (eg, small stature) should be titrated up to 10 mg twice daily in first 2-3 days.

Extended release tablet: Initial: 30-60 mg given once daily in the morning; titrate upward as needed, giving at least 3 days between increases; maximum daily single dose: 240 mg

Elderly: Start with lowest recommended adult dose.

Dosing adjustment in renal impairment: Dose adjustment not necessary

Hemodialysis: Dose supplementation is not necessary.

Peritoneal dialysis: Dose supplementation is not necessary.

Dosing adjustment in hepatic impairment: Dose adjustment not necessary

Note: Tolerance to nitrate effects develops with chronic exposure. Dose escalation does not overcome this effect. Tolerance can only be overcome by short periods of nitrate absence from the body. Short periods of nitrate withdrawal may help minimize tolerance. Recommended twice daily dosage regimens incorporate this interval. Administer sustained release tablet once daily in the morning.

Administration Do not administer around-the-clock. Immediate release tablet should be scheduled twice daily with doses 7 hours apart (8 AM and 3 PM); extended release tablet may be administered once daily in the morning upon rising with a half-glassful of fluid and should not be chewed or crushed.

Monitoring Parameters Monitor for orthostasis, increased hypotension

Dosage Forms Excipient information presented when available (limited, particularly for generics); consult specific product labeling.

Tablet, oral: 10 mg, 20 mg

Ismo®: 20 mg [scored]

Monoket®: 10 mg, 20 mg [scored]

Tablet, extended release, oral: 30 mg, 60 mg, 120 mg

Imdur®: 30 mg, 60 mg [scored]

Imdur®: 120 mg

◆ **Isotamine® (Can)** *see* Isoniazid *on page* 933

ISOtretinoin (eye soe TRET i noyn)

Brand Names: U.S. Amnesteem®; Claravis™; Sotret®

Brand Names: Canada Accutane®; Clarus™; Isotrex®

Index Terms 13-*cis*-Retinoic Acid

Pharmacologic Category Acne Products; Retinoic Acid Derivative

Use Treatment of severe recalcitrant nodular acne unresponsive to conventional therapy

Unlabeled Use Treatment of children with metastatic neuroblastoma or leukemia that does not respond to conventional therapy

Pregnancy Risk Factor X

Pregnancy Considerations Major fetal abnormalities (both internal and external), spontaneous abortion, premature births and low IQ scores in surviving infants have been reported. **[U.S. Boxed Warning]: Because of the high likelihood of teratogenic effects, all patients (male and female), prescribers, wholesalers, and dispensing pharmacists must register and be active in the iPLEDGE™ risk management program; do not prescribe isotretinoin for women who are or who are likely to become pregnant while using the drug.** This medication is contraindicated in females of childbearing potential unless they are able to comply with the guidelines of the iPLEDGE™ pregnancy prevention program. Females of childbearing potential should not become pregnant during therapy or for 1 month following discontinuation of isotretinoin. Upon discontinuation of treatment, females of childbearing potential should have a pregnancy test after their last dose and again one month after their last dose. Two forms of contraception should be continued during this time. Any pregnancies should be reported to the iPLEDGE™ program (www.ipledgeprogram.com or 866-495-0654).

Lactation Excretion in breast milk unknown/contraindicated

Prescribing and Access Restrictions As a requirement of the REMS program, access to this medication is restricted. All patients (male and female), prescribers, wholesalers, and dispensing pharmacists must register and be active in the iPLEDGE™ risk management program, designed to eliminate fetal exposures to isotretinoin. This program covers all isotretinoin products (brand and generic). The iPLEDGE™ program requires that all patients meet qualification criteria and monthly program requirements (eg, pregnancy testing). Healthcare providers can only prescribe a maximum 30-day supply at each monthly visit and must counsel patients on the iPLEDGE™ program requirements and confirm counseling via the iPLEDGE™ automated system. Registration, activation, and additional information are provided at www.ipledgeprogram.com or by calling 866-495-0654.

Medication Guide Available Yes

Contraindications Hypersensitivity to isotretinoin or any component of the formulation; sensitivity to parabens, vitamin A, or other retinoids; pregnancy

Warnings/Precautions This medication should only be prescribed by prescribers competent in treating severe recalcitrant nodular acne and experienced with the use of systemic retinoids. **[U.S. Boxed Warning]: Because of the high likelihood of teratogenic effects, all patients (male and female), prescribers, wholesalers, and dispensing pharmacists must register and be active in the iPLEDGE™ risk management program; do not prescribe isotretinoin for women who are or who are likely to become pregnant while using the drug (see Additional Information for details).** Women of childbearing potential must be capable of complying with effective contraceptive measures. Patients must select and commit to two forms of contraception. Therapy is begun after two negative pregnancy tests; effective contraception must be used for at least 1 month before beginning therapy, during therapy, and for 1 month after discontinuation of therapy. Prescriptions should be written for no more than a 30-day supply, and pregnancy testing and counseling should be repeated monthly.

May cause depression, psychosis, aggressive or violent behavior, and changes in mood; use with extreme caution in patients with psychiatric disorders. Rarely, suicidal thoughts and actions have been reported during isotretinoin usage. All patients should be observed closely for symptoms of depression or suicidal thoughts. Discontinuation of treatment alone may not be sufficient, further evaluation may be necessary. Cases of pseudotumor cerebri (benign intracranial hypertension) have been reported, some with concomitant use of tetracycline (avoid using together). Patients with papilledema, headache, nausea, vomiting, and visual disturbances should be referred to a neurologist and treatment with isotretinoin discontinued. Hearing impairment, which can continue after therapy is discontinued, may occur. Clinical hepatitis, elevated liver enzymes, inflammatory bowel disease, skeletal hyperostosis, premature epiphyseal closure, vision impairment, corneal opacities, and decreased night vision have also been reported with the use of isotretinoin. Rare postmarketing cases of severe skin reactions (eg, Stevens-Johnson syndrome, erythema multiforme) have been reported with use.

Use with caution in patients with diabetes mellitus; impaired glucose control has been reported. Use caution in patients with hypertriglyceridemia; acute pancreatitis and fatal hemorrhagic pancreatitis (rare) have been reported. Bone mineral density may decrease; use caution in patients with a genetic predisposition to bone disorders (ie osteoporosis, osteomalacia) and with disease states or concomitant medications that can induce bone disorders.

Patients may be at risk when participating in activities with repetitive impact (such as sports). Patients should be instructed not to donate blood during therapy and for 1 month following discontinuation of therapy due to risk of donated blood being given to a pregnant female. Safety of long-term use is not established and is not recommended. Safety and efficacy have not been established in children <12 years of age.

Adverse Reactions Frequency not always defined.

Cardiovascular: Chest pain, edema, flushing, palpitation, stroke, syncope, tachycardia, vascular thrombotic disease

Central nervous system: Aggressive behavior, depression, dizziness, drowsiness, emotional instability, fatigue, headache, insomnia, lethargy, malaise, nervousness, paresthesia, pseudotumor cerebri, psychosis, seizure, stroke, suicidal ideation, suicide attempts, suicide, violent behavior

Dermatologic: Abnormal wound healing acne fulminans, alopecia, bruising, cheilitis, cutaneous allergic reactions, dry nose, dry skin, eczema, eruptive xanthomas, facial erythema, fragility of skin, hair abnormalities, hirsutism, hyperpigmentation, hypopigmentation, increased sunburn susceptibility, nail dystrophy, paronychia, peeling of palms, peeling of soles, photoallergic reactions, photosensitizing reactions, pruritus, purpura, rash

Endocrine & metabolic: Triglycerides increased (25%), abnormal menses, blood glucose increased, cholesterol increased, HDL decreased, hyperuricemia

Gastrointestinal: Bleeding and inflammation of the gums, colitis, esophagitis, esophageal ulceration, inflammatory bowel disease, nausea, nonspecific gastrointestinal symptoms, pancreatitis, weight loss, xerostomia

Genitourinary: Nonspecific urogenital findings

Hematologic: Agranulocytosis (rare), anemia, neutropenia, pyogenic granuloma, thrombocytopenia

Hepatic: Alkaline phosphatase increased, ALT increased, AST increased, GGTP increased, hepatitis, LDH increased

Neuromuscular & skeletal: Back pain (29% in pediatric patients), arthralgia, arthritis, bone abnormalities, bone mineral density decreased, calcification of tendons and ligaments, CPK increased, myalgia, premature epiphyseal closure, skeletal hyperostosis, tendonitis, weakness

Ocular: Cataracts, color vision disorder, conjunctivitis, corneal opacities, dry eyes, eyelid inflammation, keratitis, night vision decreased, optic neuritis, photophobia, visual disturbances

Otic: Hearing impairment, tinnitus

Renal: Glomerulonephritis, hematuria, proteinuria, pyuria, vasculitis

Respiratory: Bronchospasms, epistaxis, respiratory infection, voice alteration, Wegener's granulomatosis

Miscellaneous: Allergic reactions, anaphylactic reactions, disseminated herpes simplex, diaphoresis, infection, lymphadenopathy

Postmarketing and/or case reports: Erythema multiforme, Stevens-Johnson syndrome, toxic epidermal necrolysis

Drug Interactions

Metabolism/Transport Effects None known.

Avoid Concomitant Use

Avoid concomitant use of ISOtretinoin with any of the following: Tetracycline Derivatives; Vitamin A

Increased Effect/Toxicity

ISOtretinoin may increase the levels/effects of: Porfimer; Vitamin A

The levels/effects of ISOtretinoin may be increased by: Alcohol (Ethyl); Tetracycline Derivatives

Decreased Effect

ISOtretinoin may decrease the levels/effects of: Contraceptives (Estrogens); Contraceptives (Progestins)

Ethanol/Nutrition/Herb Interactions

Ethanol: Avoid or limit ethanol (may increase triglyceride levels if taken in excess).

Food: Isotretinoin bioavailability increased if taken with food or milk.

Herb/Nutraceutical: Avoid dong quai, St John's wort (may also cause photosensitization and may decrease the effectiveness of oral contraceptives). Additional vitamin A supplements may lead to vitamin A toxicity (dry skin, irritation, arthralgias, myalgias, abdominal pain, hepatic changes); avoid use.

Stability Store at room temperature of 59°F to 86°F (15°C to 30°C). Protect from light.

Mechanism of Action Reduces sebaceous gland size and reduces sebum production; regulates cell proliferation and differentiation

Pharmacodynamics/Kinetics

Distribution: Crosses placenta

Protein binding: 99% to 100%; primarily albumin

Metabolism: Hepatic via CYP2B6, 2C8, 2C9, 2D6, 3A4; forms metabolites; major metabolite: 4-oxo-isotretinoin (active)

Half-life elimination: Terminal: Parent drug: 21 hours; Metabolite: 21-24 hours

Time to peak, serum: 3-5 hours

Excretion: Urine and feces (equal amounts)

Dosage Oral:

Children: Maintenance therapy for neuroblastoma (investigational): 100-250 mg/m^2/day in 2 divided doses

Children 12-17 years and Adults: Severe recalcitrant nodular acne: 0.5-1 mg/kg/day in 2 divided doses (dosages as low as 0.05 mg/kg/day have been reported to be beneficial) for 15-20 weeks or until the total cyst count decreases by 70%, whichever is sooner. Adults with very severe disease/scarring or primarily involves the trunk may require dosage adjustment up to 2 mg/kg/day. A second course of therapy may be initiated after a period of ≥2 months off therapy.

Dosing adjustment in hepatic impairment: Dose reductions empirically are recommended in hepatitis disease

Dietary Considerations Should be taken with food. Limit intake of vitamin A; avoid use of other vitamin A products. Some formulations may contain soybean oil.

Administration Administer with food. Capsules should be swallowed whole with a full glass of water. For patients unable to swallow, the Accutane® capsule may be pierced with a large-gauge needle and the contents placed in food (cottage cheese, ice cream, pudding, or oatmeal with butter) for immediate consumption (Accutane® data on file, Roche Pharmaceuticals). Use appropriate precautions for handling teratogenic capsule contents.

Monitoring Parameters CBC with differential and platelet count, baseline sedimentation rate, glucose, CPK; signs of depression, mood alteration, psychosis, aggression, severe skin reactions

Pregnancy test (for all female patients of childbearing potential): Two negative tests prior to beginning therapy (the second performed at least 19 days after the first test and performed during the first 5 days of the menstrual period immediately preceding the start of therapy); monthly tests to rule out pregnancy prior to refilling prescription.

Lipids: Prior to treatment and at weekly or biweekly intervals until response to treatment is established. Test should not be performed <36 hours after consumption of ethanol.

Liver function tests: Prior to treatment and at weekly or biweekly intervals until response to treatment is established.

Additional Information All patients (male and female), must be registered in the iPLEDGE™ risk management program. Females of childbearing potential must receive oral and written information reviewing the hazards of therapy and the effects that isotretinoin can have on a fetus. Therapy should not begin without two negative pregnancy tests at least 19 days apart. Two forms of contraception (a primary and secondary form as described in the iPLEDGE™ program materials) must be used simultaneously beginning 1 month prior to treatment, during treatment, and for 1 month after therapy is discontinued; limitations to their use must be explained. Prescriptions should be written for no more than a 30-day supply, and pregnancy testing and counseling should be repeated monthly. During therapy, pregnancy tests must be conducted by a CLIA-certified laboratory. Prescriptions must be filled and picked up from the pharmacy within 7 days of specimen collection for pregnancy test for women of childbearing potential. Prescriptions for males and females of non-childbearing potential must be filled and picked up within 30 days of prescribing.

Any cases of accidental pregnancy should be reported to the iPLEDGE™ program or FDA MedWatch. All patients (male and female) must read and sign the informed consent material provided in the pregnancy prevention program.

Dosage Forms Excipient information presented when available (limited, particularly for generics); consult specific product labeling.

Capsule, oral:
- Claravis™: 10 mg, 20 mg, 30 mg, 40 mg [contains soybean oil]

Capsule, softgel, oral:
- Amnesteem®: 10 mg, 20 mg, 40 mg [contains soybean oil]
- Sotret®: 10 mg, 20 mg, 30 mg, 40 mg [contains parabens, soybean oil]

Extemporaneous Preparations Hazardous agent: Use appropriate precautions for handling and disposal of teratogenic capsule contents.

Alternate method of administration of isotretinoin capsules, based on unpublished data (not recommended by manufacturer): An oral suspension may be made with capsules and milk. Heat 15 mL 2% reduced-fat milk to ~37°C (~97°F). Add one entire 10 mg capsule to milk; stir until capsule shell dissolves and capsule contents disperse throughout solution (approximately 10-15 minutes). Stable for ≤4 hours at controlled room temperature or under refrigeration. Milk will probably spoil if suspension is not refrigerated; therefore, refrigeration is preferred. (Suspension may also be made with one 20 mg capsule and 30 mL milk, etc, so that the concentration is maintained).

Accutane® data on file, Hoffman-La Roche Pharmaceuticals

◆ **Isotrex® (Can)** *see* ISOtretinoin *on page 939*

Isradipine (iz RA di peen)

Brand Names: U.S. DynaCirc CR®

Pharmacologic Category Calcium Channel Blocker; Calcium Channel Blocker, Dihydropyridine

Additional Appendix Information

Calcium Channel Blockers *on page 1887*

Use Treatment of hypertension

Unlabeled Use Pediatric hypertension

Pregnancy Risk Factor C

Dosage Oral:

Children (unlabeled use): Capsule: Initial: 0.15-0.2 mg/kg/day in 2-3 divided doses; maximum 0.8 mg/kg/day, up to 20 mg/day. **Note:** Controlled release formulation is administered once daily or in 2 divided doses.

Adults:
- Capsule: 2.5 mg twice daily; antihypertensive response occurs in 2-3 hours; maximal response in 2-4 weeks; increase dose at 2- to 4-week intervals at 2.5-5 mg increments; usual dose range (JNC 7): 2.5-10 mg/day in 2 divided doses. **Note:** Most patients show no improvement with doses >10 mg/day except adverse reaction rate increases; therefore, maximal dose in older adults should be 10 mg/day.
- Controlled release tablet: 5 mg once daily; antihypertensive response occurs in 2 hours. Adjust dose in increments of 5 mg at 2-4 week intervals. Maximum dose: 20 mg/day; adverse events are increased at doses >10 mg/day.

Elderly:
- Capsule: Refer to adult dosing.
- Controlled release tablet: Initial dose: 5 mg once daily

Dosage adjustment in renal impairment: Cl_{cr} 30-80 mL/minute: Bioavailability increased by 45%. Cl_{cr} <10 mL/minute on hemodialysis: Bioavailability decreased by 20% to 50%
- Capsule: Refer to adult dosing.
- Controlled release tablet: Initial dose: 5 mg once daily

Dosage adjustment in hepatic impairment: Peak serum concentrations are increased by 32% and bioavailability is increased by 52%
- Capsule: Refer to adult dosing.
- Controlled release tablet: Initial dose: 5 mg once daily

Additional Information Complete prescribing information for this medication should be consulted for additional detail.

Dosage Forms Excipient information presented when available (limited, particularly for generics); consult specific product labeling.

Capsule, oral: 2.5 mg, 5 mg

Tablet, controlled release, oral:
- DynaCirc CR®: 5 mg, 10 mg

◆ **Istalol®** *see* Timolol (Ophthalmic) *on page 1687*
◆ **Istodax®** *see* RomiDEPsin *on page 1515*
◆ **Isuprel®** *see* Isoproterenol *on page 935*

Itraconazole (i tra KOE na zole)

Brand Names: U.S. Sporanox®

Brand Names: Canada Sporanox®

Pharmacologic Category Antifungal Agent, Oral

Additional Appendix Information

Antifungal Agents *on page 1876*

Use

Oral capsules: Treatment of susceptible fungal infections in immunocompromised and immunocompetent patients including blastomycosis and histoplasmosis; indicated for aspergillosis (in patients intolerant/refractory to amphotericin B), and onychomycosis of the toenail and fingernail (in nonimmunocompromised patients)

Oral solution: Treatment of oral and esophageal candidiasis

Pregnancy Risk Factor C

Pregnancy Considerations Should not be used to treat onychomycosis during pregnancy. Effective contraception should be used during treatment and for 2 months following treatment. Congenital abnormalities have been reported during postmarketing surveillance, but a causal relationship has not been established.

Lactation Enters breast milk/not recommended

Contraindications Hypersensitivity to itraconazole (use caution in patients with a history of hypersensitivity to other azoles), any component of the formulation; concurrent administration with cisapride, dofetilide, ergot derivatives, levomethadyl, lovastatin, midazolam (oral), nisoldipine, pimozide, quinidine, simvastatin, or triazolam; treatment of onychomycosis (or other non-life-threatening indications) in patients with evidence of ventricular dysfunction, heart failure (HF) or a history of HF; treatment of onychomycosis in patients who are pregnant or intend on becoming pregnant

Warnings/Precautions [U.S. Boxed Warning]: Negative inotropic effects have been observed following intravenous administration. Discontinue or reassess use if signs or symptoms of HF (heart failure) occur during treatment. [U.S. Boxed Warning]: Not recommended for treatment of onychomycosis in patients with ventricular dysfunction or a history of HF. HF has been reported, particularly in patients receiving a total daily oral dose of 400 mg. Use with caution in patients with risk factors for HF (COPD, renal failure, edematous disorders, ischemic or valvular disease). Discontinue if signs or symptoms of HF or neuropathy occur during treatment. **[U.S. Boxed Warning]: Serious cardiovascular adverse events including, QT prolongation, ventricular tachycardia, torsade de pointes, cardiac arrest and/or sudden death have been observed due to increased cisapride, pimozide, quinidine or levomethadyl concentrations induced by itraconazole; concurrent use contraindicated.** Additionally, the following drugs metabolized by the CYP 3A4 isoenzyme system are also contraindicated: Ergot derivatives, lovastatin, midazolam (oral), simvastatin, and triazolam.

Calcium channel blockers (CCBs) may cause additive negative inotropic effects when used concurrently with itraconazole. Itraconazole may also inhibit the metabolism of CCBs. Use caution with concurrent use of itraconazole and CCBs due to an increased risk of HF. Concurrent use of itraconazole and nisoldipine is contraindicated.

Use with caution in patients with renal impairment. Rare cases of serious hepatotoxicity (including liver failure and death) have been reported (including some cases occurring within the first week of therapy); hepatotoxicity was reported in some patients without pre-existing liver disease or risk factors. Use with caution in patients with pre-existing hepatic impairment; monitor liver function closely and dosage adjustment may be warranted. Not recommended for use in patients with active liver disease, elevated liver enzymes, or prior hepatotoxic reactions to other drugs unless the expected benefit exceeds the risk of hepatotoxicity. Transient or permanent hearing loss has been reported. Quinidine (a contraindicated drug) was used concurrently in several of these cases. Hearing loss usually resolves after discontinuation, but may persist in some patients.

Large differences in itraconazole pharmacokinetic parameters have been observed in cystic fibrosis patients receiving the solution; if a patient with cystic fibrosis does not respond to therapy, alternate therapies should be considered. Due to differences in bioavailability, oral capsules and oral solution cannot be used interchangeably. Only the oral solution has proven efficacy for oral and esophageal candidiasis. Initiation of treatment with oral solution is not recommended in patients at immediate risk for systemic candidiasis (eg, patients with severe neutropenia).

Adverse Reactions

>10%: Gastrointestinal: Nausea (11%), diarrhea (3% to 11%)

1% to 10%:

Cardiovascular: Edema (4%), hypertension (3%), chest pain (3%)

Central nervous system: Fever (3% to 7%), headache (4%), fatigue (2% to 3%), dizziness (2%), depression (2%)

Dermatologic: Rash (4% to 9%), pruritus (3%)

Endocrine & metabolic: Hypokalemia (2%)

Gastrointestinal: Vomiting (5% to 7%), abdominal pain (2% to 6%), constipation (2%)

Hepatic: LFTs abnormal (3%)

Respiratory: Rhinitis (5% to 9%), cough (4%), dyspnea (2%), pneumonia (2%), sinusitis (2%), sputum increased (2%)

Miscellaneous: Diaphoresis increased (3%)

<2% (Limited to important or life-threatening): Adrenal insufficiency, albuminuria, allergic reactions, alopecia, anaphylactoid reactions, anaphylaxis, angioedema, anorexia, arrhythmia, arthralgia, asthenia, blurred vision, diplopia, dysgeusia, dyspepsia, dysphagia, erythema multiforme, exfoliative dermatitis, flatulence, gastritis, gynecomastia, hearing loss, heart failure, hematuria, hepatic failure, hepatitis, hepatotoxicity, hepatitis, hot flashes, hypertriglyceridemia, hypoesthesia, impotence, insomnia, leukocytoclastic dermatitis, leukopenia, libido decreased, malaise, menstrual disorders, myalgia, neutropenia, pancreatitis, paresthesia, peripheral neuropathy, photosensitivity, pollakiuria, pulmonary edema, pharyngitis, rigors, serum sickness, somnolence, Stevens-Johnson syndrome, stomatitis ulcerative, thrombocytopenia, taste perversion, tinnitus, toxic epidermal necrolysis, urinary incontinence, urticaria, vasculitis

Drug Interactions

Metabolism/Transport Effects Substrate of CYP3A4 (major); **Note:** Assignment of Major/Minor substrate status based on clinically relevant drug interaction potential; **Inhibits** CYP3A4 (strong), P-glycoprotein

Avoid Concomitant Use

Avoid concomitant use of Itraconazole with any of the following: Alfuzosin; Aliskiren; Cisapride; Conivaptan; Crizotinib; Dofetilide; Dronedarone; Eplerenone; Ergot Derivatives; Everolimus; Fluticasone (Oral Inhalation); Halofantrine; Lapatinib; Lovastatin; Lurasidone; Nevirapine; Nilotinib; Nisoldipine; Pimozide; QuiNIDine; Ranolazine; Rivaroxaban; RomiDEPsin; Salmeterol; Silodosin; Simvastatin; Tamsulosin; Ticagrelor; Tolvaptan; Topotecan; Toremifene

Increased Effect/Toxicity

Itraconazole may increase the levels/effects of: Alfentanil; Alfuzosin; Aliskiren; Almotriptan; Alosetron; Aprepitant; ARIPiprazole; Benzodiazepines (metabolized by oxidation); Boceprevir; Bortezomib; Bosentan; Brentuximab Vedotin; Brinzolamide; Budesonide (Nasal); Budesonide (Systemic, Oral Inhalation); BusPIRone; Busulfan; Calcium Channel Blockers; CarBAMazepine; Cardiac Glycosides; Ciclesonide; Cilostazol; Cisapride; Colchicine; Conivaptan; Corticosteroids (Orally Inhaled); Corticosteroids (Systemic); Crizotinib; CycloSPORINE; CycloSPORINE (Systemic); CYP3A4 Substrates; Dabigatran Etexilate; Dienogest; DOCEtaxel; Dofetilide; Dronedarone; Dutasteride; Eletriptan; Eplerenone; Ergot Derivatives; Erlotinib; Eszopiclone; Etravirine; Everolimus; FentaNYL; Fesoterodine; Fexofenadine; Fluticasone (Nasal); Fluticasone (Oral Inhalation); Fosaprepitant; Fosphenytoin; Gefitinib; GuanFACINE; Halofantrine; HMG-CoA Reductase Inhibitors; Iloperidone; Imatinib; Irinotecan; Ixabepilone; Lapatinib; Losartan; Lovastatin; Lumefantrine; Lurasidone; Macrolide Antibiotics; Maraviroc; Methadone; MethylPREDNISolone; Nilotinib; Nisoldipine; Paliperidone; Paricalcitol; Pazopanib; P-glycoprotein/ABCB1 Substrates; Phenytoin; Phosphodiesterase 5 Inhibitors; Pimecrolimus; Pimozide; Propafenone; Protease Inhibitors; QuiNIDine; Ramelteon; Ranolazine; Repaglinide; Rifamycin Derivatives; Rivaroxaban; RomiDEPsin; Ruxolitinib; Salmeterol; Saxagliptin; Sildenafil; Silodosin; Simvastatin; Sirolimus; Solifenacin; SORAfenib; SUNItinib; Tacrolimus; Tacrolimus (Systemic); Tacrolimus (Topical); Tadalafil; Tamsulosin; Telaprevir; Temsirolimus; Ticagrelor; Tolterodine;

Tolvaptan; Topotecan; Toremifene; Vardenafil; Vemurafenib; Vilazodone; VinBLAStine; VinCRIStine; Vinorelbine; Vitamin K Antagonists; Ziprasidone; Zolpidem; Zuclopenthixol

The levels/effects of Itraconazole may be increased by: Boceprevir; Etravirine; Grapefruit Juice; Macrolide Antibiotics; Protease Inhibitors; Telaprevir

Decreased Effect

Itraconazole may decrease the levels/effects of: Amphotericin B; Prasugrel; Saccharomyces boulardii; Ticagrelor

The levels/effects of Itraconazole may be decreased by: Antacids; CYP3A4 Inducers (Strong); Deferasirox; Didanosine; Efavirenz; Etravirine; Fosphenytoin; H2-Antagonists; Herbs (CYP3A4 Inducers); Nevirapine; Phenytoin; Proton Pump Inhibitors; Rifamycin Derivatives; Sucralfate; Tocilizumab

Ethanol/Nutrition/Herb Interactions

Food:

Capsules: Absorption enhanced by food and possibly by gastric acidity. Cola drinks have been shown to increase the absorption of the capsules in patients with achlorhydria or those taking H_2-receptor antagonists or other gastric acid suppressors. Avoid grapefruit juice.

Solution: Food decreases the bioavailability and increases the time to peak concentration.

Herb/Nutraceutical: St John's wort may decrease itraconazole levels.

Stability

Capsule: Store at room temperature, 15°C to 25°C (59°F to 77°F). Protect from light and moisture.

Oral solution: Store at ≤25°C (77°F); do not freeze.

Mechanism of Action Interferes with cytochrome P450 activity, decreasing ergosterol synthesis (principal sterol in fungal cell membrane) and inhibiting cell membrane formation

Pharmacodynamics/Kinetics

Absorption: Requires gastric acidity; capsule better absorbed with food, solution better absorbed on empty stomach

Distribution: V_d (average): 796 ± 185 L or 10 L/kg; highly lipophilic and tissue concentrations are higher than plasma concentrations. The highest concentrations: adipose, omentum, endometrium, cervical and vaginal mucus, and skin/nails. Aqueous fluids (eg, CSF and urine) contain negligible amounts.

Protein binding, plasma: 99.8%; metabolite hydroxy-itraconazole: 99.5%

Metabolism: Extensively hepatic via CYP3A4 into >30 metabolites including hydroxy-itraconazole (major metabolite); appears to have *in vitro* antifungal activity. Main metabolic pathway is oxidation; may undergo saturation metabolism with multiple dosing.

Bioavailability: Variable, ~55% (oral solution) in 1 small study; **Note:** Oral solution has a higher degree of bioavailability (149% ± 68%) relative to oral capsules; should not be interchanged

Half-life elimination: Oral: Single dose: ~21 hours, steady state: 64 hours; Cirrhosis (single dose): 37 hours (range 20-54 hours)

Time to peak, plasma: Capsules: 3-5 hours; Oral solution: 2-3 hours

Excretion: Urine (<0.03% active drug, 40% as inactive metabolites); feces (~3% to 18%)

Dosage Oral:

Usual dosage ranges:

Children: Efficacy and safety have not been established; a small number of patients 3-16 years of age have been treated with 100 mg/day for systemic fungal infections with no serious adverse effects reported. A dose of 5 mg/kg once daily was used in a pharmacokinetic study using the oral solution in patients 6 months to 12 years; duration of study was 2 weeks.

Adults: 100-400 mg/day; doses >200 mg/day are given in 2 divided doses; length of therapy varies from 1 day to >6 months depending on the condition and mycological response

Indication-specific dosing:

Infants and Children (HIV-exposed/-positive; unlabeled use; CDC, 2009):

Candidiasis:

Oropharyngeal: Oral solution: 2.5 mg/kg/dose twice daily (maximum: 200 mg/day [400 mg/day if fluconazole-refractory]) for 7-14 days

Esophageal: Oral solution: 5 mg/kg/day once daily or divided twice daily for 4-21 days

Coccidioidomycosis:

Treatment: Oral: 5-10 mg/kg/dose twice daily for 3 days, followed by 2-5 mg/kg/dose orally twice daily (maximum: 400 mg/day)

Relapse prevention: Oral: 2-5 mg/kg/dose twice daily (maximum: 400 mg/day)

Cryptococcus: *Relapse prevention:* Oral solution: 5 mg/kg/dose once daily (maximum: 200 mg/day)

Histoplasmosis:

Treatment of mild disseminated disease: Oral solution: 2-5 mg/kg/dose 3 times daily for 3 days (9 doses), followed by twice daily for 12 months (maximum: 200 mg/dose)

Consolidation treatment for moderate-severe to severe disseminated disease, including CNS infection (following appropriate induction therapy): 2-5 mg/kg/dose 3times daily for 3 days, followed by 2-5 mg/kg/dose (maximum: 200 mg/dose) twice daily for 12 months for non-CNS-disseminated disease or for ≥12 months for CNS infection

Relapse prevention: Oral solution: 5 mg/kg/dose twice daily (maximum: 400 mg/day)

Adults:

Aspergillosis, invasive (salvage therapy): Duration of therapy should be a minimum of 6-12 weeks or throughout period of immunosuppression: Oral: 200-400 mg/day; **Note:** 2008 IDSA guidelines recommend 600 mg/day for 3 days, followed by 400 mg/day

Appropriate use: Itraconazole should **NOT** be used for voriconazole-refractory aspergillosis since the same antifungal and/or resistance mechanism(s) may be shared by both agents. Itraconazole oral solution and capsule formulations are not bioequivalent or interchangeable. Due to variable bioavailability of oral preparations, therapeutic drug monitoring advisable.

Aspergillosis, allergic (ABPA, sinusitis): 200 mg/day; may be used in conjunction with corticosteroids

Blastomycosis: 200 mg 3 times/day for 3 days, then 200 mg twice daily for 6-12 months; in moderately-severe to severe infection, therapy should be initiated with ~2 weeks of amphotericin B (Chapman, 2008)

Brain abscess: Cerebral phaeohyphomycosis (dematiaceous): 200 mg twice daily for at least 6 months with amphotericin

Candidiasis:

Oropharyngeal: Oral solution: 200 mg once daily for 1-2 weeks; in patients unresponsive or refractory to fluconazole: 100 mg twice daily (clinical response expected in 1-2 weeks)

Esophageal: Oral solution: 100-200 mg once daily for a minimum of 3 weeks; continue dosing for 2 weeks after resolution of symptoms

Coccidioidomycosis: 200 mg twice daily

Histoplasmosis: 200 mg 3 times/day for 3 days, then 200 mg twice daily (or once daily in mild-moderate disease) for 6-12 weeks in mild-moderate disease or ≥12 months in progressive disseminated or chronic cavitary pulmonary histoplasmosis; in moderately-severe to severe infection, therapy should be initiated with ~2 weeks of a lipid formation of amphotericin B (Wheat, 2007)

Long-term suppression therapy: 200 mg/day (AIDS*info* guidelines, 2008)

Meningitis:

Coccidioides: 400-800 mg/day

Coccidioides, HIV-positive (unlabeled use): 200 mg 3 times/day for 3 days, then 200 mg twice daily; maintenance: 200 mg twice daily life-long (AIDS*info* guidelines, 2008)

Appropriate use: Fluconazole is preferred for meningeal infections.

Onychomycosis: 200 mg once daily for 12 consecutive weeks; alternative "pulse-dosing" may be considering for fingernail involvement only: 200 mg twice daily for 1 week; repeat 1-week course after 3-week off-time

Penicilliosis, HIV-positive (unlabeled use): 200 mg twice daily for 8-10 weeks (in severely-ill patients, initiate therapy with 2 weeks of amphotericin B); maintenance: 200 mg/day (*AIDSinfo* guidelines, 2008)

Pneumonia:

Coccidioides: Mild-to-moderate: 200 mg twice daily

Coccidioides, HIV-positive (focal pneumonia): 200 mg 3 times/day for 3 days, then 200 mg twice daily (AIDS*info* guidelines, 2008)

Protothecal infection: 200 mg once daily for 2 months

Sporotrichosis:

Lymphocutaneous: 100-200 mg/day for 3-6 months

Osteoarticular and pulmonary: 200 mg twice daily for 1-2 years (may use amphotericin B initially for stabilization)

Dosing adjustment in renal impairment: The FDA-approved labeling states to use with caution in patients with renal impairment. The following guidelines have been used by some clinicians:

Aronoff, 2007:

Cl_{cr} >10 mL/minute: No adjustment recommended

Cl_{cr} <10 mL/minute: Administer 50% of normal dose

Poorly dialyzed; no supplemental dose or dosage adjustment necessary, including patients on intermittent hemodialysis, peritoneal dialysis, or continuous renal replacement therapy (eg, CVVHD).

Dosing adjustment in hepatic impairment: Use caution in patients with hepatic impairment

Dietary Considerations

Capsule: Take with food.

Solution: Take without food, if possible.

Administration Doses >200 mg/day are given in 2 divided doses; do not administer with antacids. Capsule and oral solution formulations are not bioequivalent and thus are not interchangeable. Capsule absorption is best if taken with food, therefore, it is best to administer itraconazole after meals; solution should be taken on an empty stomach. When treating oropharyngeal and esophageal candidiasis, solution should be swished vigorously in mouth, then swallowed.

Monitoring Parameters Liver function in patients with pre-existing hepatic dysfunction, and in all patients being treated for longer than 1 month; serum concentrations particularly for oral therapy (due to erratic bioavailability with capsule formulation); renal function

Reference Range Serum concentrations may be performed to assure therapeutic levels. Itraconazole plus the metabolite hydroxyitraconazole concentrations should be >1 mcg/mL (not to exceed 10 mcg/mL).

Timing of serum samples: Obtain level after ~2 weeks of therapy, level may be drawn anytime during the dosing interval.

Additional Information Due to potential toxicity, the manufacturer recommends confirmation of diagnosis testing of nail specimens prior to treatment of onychomycosis.

Dosage Forms Excipient information presented when available (limited, particularly for generics); consult specific product labeling.

Capsule, oral: 100 mg

Sporanox®: 100 mg

Solution, oral:

Sporanox®: 10 mg/mL (150 mL) [contains propylene glycol; cherry-caramel flavor]

Extemporaneous Preparations Note: Commercial oral solution is available (10 mg/mL)

A 20 mg/mL oral suspension may be made with capsules. Empty the contents of forty 100 mg capsules and add 15 mL of Alcohol, USP. Let stand for 5 minutes. Crush the beads in a mortar and reduce to a fine powder. Mix while adding a 1:1 mixture of Ora-Sweet® and Ora-Plus® in incremental proportions to **almost** 200 mL; transfer to a calibrated bottle, rinse mortar with vehicle, and add quantity of vehicle sufficient to make 200 mL. Label "shake well" and "refrigerate". Stable for 56 days refrigerated.

Nahata MC, Pai VB, and Hipple TF, *Pediatric Drug Formulations*, 5th ed, Cincinnati, OH: Harvey Whitney Books Co, 2004.

Ivermectin (eye ver MEK tin)

Brand Names: U.S. Stromectol®

Pharmacologic Category Anthelmintic

Use Treatment of the following infections: Strongyloidiasis of the intestinal tract due to the nematode parasite *Strongyloides stercoralis*. Onchocerciasis due to the immature form of the nematode parasite *Onchocerca volvulus*

Unlabeled Use Treatment of other parasitic infections, including *Ancylostoma braziliense, Ascaris lumbricoides, Sarcoptes scabiei, Gnathostoma spinigerum, Mansonella ozzardi, Mansonella streptocerca, Pediculus humanus capitis, Pediculus humanus corporis, Phthirus pubis, Trichuris trichiura, Wucheria bancrofti*

Pregnancy Risk Factor C

Pregnancy Considerations Teratogenic effects have been observed in animal reproduction studies; therefore, the manufacturer classifies ivermectin as pregnancy category C. Ivermectin is not recommended for use in pregnancy. Although studies during pregnancy are limited, several mass treatment programs have not identified an increased risk of adverse fetal, neonatal, or maternal outcomes following ivermectin use in the first and second trimesters.

Lactation Enters breast milk/not recommended

Contraindications Hypersensitivity to ivermectin or any component of the formulation

Warnings/Precautions Data have shown that antihelmintic drugs like ivermectin may cause cutaneous and/or systemic reactions (Mazzoti reaction) of varying severity including ophthalmological reactions in patients with onchocerciasis. These reactions are probably due to allergic and inflammatory responses to the death of microfilariae. Patients with hyper-reactive onchodermatitis may be more likely than others to experience severe adverse reactions, especially edema and aggravation of the onchodermatitis. Repeated treatment may be required in immunocompromised patients (eg, HIV); control of extraintestinal strongyloidiasis may necessitate suppressive (once monthly) therapy. Pretreatment assessment for

Loa loa infection is recommended in any patient with significant exposure to endemic areas (West and Central Africa); serious and/or fatal encephalopathy has been reported (rarely) during treatment in patients with loiasis. Ivermectin has no activity against adult *Onchocerca volvulus* parasites.

Adverse Reactions

>10%: Miscellaneous: Mazzotti-type reaction (with onchocerciasis): Pruritus (28%), fever (23%), skin involvement (23%; including edema/urticarial rash), lymph node tenderness (1% to 14%), lymph node enlargement (3% to 13%), arthralgia/synovitis (9%)

1% to 10%:

Cardiovascular: Tachycardia (4%), peripheral edema (3%), facial edema (1%), orthostatic hypotension (1%)

Central nervous system: Dizziness (3%)

Dermatologic: Pruritus (3%)

Gastrointestinal: Diarrhea (2%), nausea (2%)

Hematologic: Eosinophilia (3%), leukocytes decreased (3%), hemoglobin increased (1%)

Hepatic: ALT increased (2%), AST increased (2%)

<1% (Limited to important or life-threatening): Abdominal distention, abdominal pain, anemia, anorexia, anterior uveitis, asthma exacerbation, back pain, bilirubin increased, chest discomfort, chorioretinitis, choroiditis, coma, confusion, conjunctival hemorrhage (associated with onchocerciasis), conjunctivitis, constipation, dyspnea, encephalopathy (rare; associated with loiasis), eyelid edema, eye sensation abnormal, fatigue, fecal incontinence, headache, hepatitis, hypotension, INR increased (with concomitant warfarin), keratitis, lethargy, leukopenia, mental status changes, myalgia, neck pain, rash, red eye, seizure, somnolence, standing/walking difficulty, Stevens-Johnson syndrome, stupor, toxic epidermal necrolysis, tremor, urinary incontinence, urticaria, vertigo, vision loss (transient), vomiting, weakness

Drug Interactions

Metabolism/Transport Effects Substrate of CYP3A4 (minor), P-glycoprotein; **Note:** Assignment of Major/Minor substrate status based on clinically relevant drug interaction potential

Avoid Concomitant Use

Avoid concomitant use of Ivermectin with any of the following: BCG

Increased Effect/Toxicity

Ivermectin may increase the levels/effects of: Vitamin K Antagonists

The levels/effects of Ivermectin may be increased by: Conivaptan; P-glycoprotein/ABCB1 Inhibitors

Decreased Effect

Ivermectin may decrease the levels/effects of: BCG; Typhoid Vaccine

The levels/effects of Ivermectin may be decreased by: P-glycoprotein/ABCB1 Inducers; Tocilizumab

Ethanol/Nutrition/Herb Interactions Food: Bioavailability is increased 2.5-fold when administered following a high-fat meal.

Stability Store at <30°C (86°F).

Mechanism of Action Ivermectin is a semisynthetic anthelminthic agent; it binds selectively and with strong affinity to glutamate-gated chloride ion channels which occur in invertebrate nerve and muscle cells. This leads to increased permeability of cell membranes to chloride ions then hyperpolarization of the nerve or muscle cell, and death of the parasite.

Pharmacodynamics/Kinetics

Onset of action:

Peak effect in treatment of onchocerciasis: 3-6 months

Peak effect in treatment of strongyloides: 3 months

Absorption: Well absorbed

Distribution: V_d: 3-3.5 L/kg (healthy males); does not cross blood-brain barrier

Protein binding: ~93%

Metabolism: Hepatic via CYP3A4 (major), CYP2D6 (minor), and CYP2E1 (minor)

Bioavailability: Increased with high-fat meal

Half-life elimination: ~18 hours

Time to peak, serum: ~4 hours

Excretion: Feces; urine (<1%)

Dosage Oral: Children ≥15 kg and Adults:

Onchocerciasis: 150 mcg/kg as a single dose; retreatment may be required every 3-12 months until asymptomatic

Strongyloidiasis: Manufacturer recommendations: 200 mcg/kg as a single dose; perform follow-up stool examinations. Alternative dosing: 200 mcg/kg/day for 2 days

Ascariasis due to *Ascaris lumbricoides* (unlabeled use): 150-200 mcg/kg as a single dose

Cutaneous larva migrans (CLM) due to *Ancylostoma braziliense* (unlabeled use): 200 mcg/kg daily for 1-2 days

Filariasis due to *Mansonella ozzardi* (unlabeled use): 200 mcg/kg as a single dose

Filariasis due to *Mansonella streptocerca* (unlabeled use): 150 mcg/kg as a single dose

Filariasis due to *Wucheria bancrofti* (unlabeled use): 200 mcg/kg as a single dose given in combination with albendazole

Gnathostomiasis due to *Gnathostoma spinigerum* (unlabeled use): 200 mcg/kg/day for 2 days

Lice due to *Pediculus humanus capitis, Pediculus humanus corporis, Phthirus pubis* (unlabeled use): 200 mcg/kg/dose; generally requires more than 1 dose; number of doses and dosage intervals have not been established; 200 mcg/kg/dose for 3 doses every 7 days (Foucault, 2006) and 200 mcg/kg/dose repeated once after 10 days (Jones, 2003) have been shown to be effective; alternatively 400 mcg/kg/dose on days 1 and 8 has been utilized in *Pediculus humanus capitis* (Chosidow, 2010)

Scabies due to *Sarcoptes scabiei* (unlabeled use): 200 mcg/kg as a single dose; repeat in 2 weeks (drug of choice for immunocompromised patients with crusted scabies)

Trichuriasis due to *Trichuris trichiura* (unlabeled use): 200 mcg/kg/day for 3 days

Dietary Considerations Take on an empty stomach with water.

Administration Administer on an empty stomach with water.

Monitoring Parameters Skin and eye microfilarial counts, periodic ophthalmologic exams; follow up stool examinations

Dosage Forms Excipient information presented when available (limited, particularly for generics); consult specific product labeling.

Tablet, oral:

Stromectol®: 3 mg

◆ **IVIG** *see* Immune Globulin *on page 880*

◆ **IV Immune Globulin** *see* Immune Globulin *on page 880*

◆ **Ivy Block® [OTC]** *see* Bentoquatam *on page 201*

◆ **Ivy-Rid® [OTC]** *see* Benzocaine *on page 202*

Ixabepilone (ix ab EP i lone)

Brand Names: U.S. Ixempra®

Index Terms Azaepothilone B; BMS-247550; Epothilone B Lactam

Pharmacologic Category Antineoplastic Agent, Antimicrotubular; Antineoplastic Agent, Epothilone B Analog

Use Treatment of metastatic or locally-advanced breast cancer (refractory or resistant)

Unlabeled Use Treatment (second-line) of endometrial cancer

Pregnancy Risk Factor D

Pregnancy Considerations In animal studies, ixabepilone caused maternal toxicity and embryo/fetal toxicity at doses ~1/10 the human dose. There are no adequate and well-controlled studies in pregnant women. Women of childbearing potential should be advised to use effective contraception during treatment.

Lactation Excretion in breast milk unknown/not recommended

Contraindications History of severe hypersensitivity to polyoxyethylated castor oil or its derivatives (eg, Cremophor® EL); neutrophil count <1500/mm^3 or platelet count <100,000/mm^3; combination therapy with ixabepilone and capecitabine in patients with AST or ALT >2.5 times ULN or bilirubin >1 times ULN

Warnings/Precautions Hazardous agent - use appropriate precautions for handling and disposal. **[U.S. Boxed Warning]: Due to increased risk of toxicity and neutropenia-related mortality, combination therapy with capecitabine is contraindicated in patients with AST or ALT >2.5 times ULN or bilirubin >1 times ULN.** Use (as monotherapy) is not recommended if AST or ALT >10 times ULN or bilirubin >3 times ULN; use caution in patients with AST or ALT >5 times ULN. Toxicities and serious adverse reactions are increased (in mono- and combination therapy) with hepatic dysfunction; dosage reductions are necessary. Diluent contains Cremophor® EL, which is associated with hypersensitivity reactions; use is contraindicated in patients with a history of severe hypersensitivity to Cremophor® EL or its derivatives. Medications for the treatment of reaction should be available for immediate use; reactions may also be managed with a reduction of infusion rate. Premedicate with an H_1- and H_2-antagonist 1 hour prior to infusion; patients who experience hypersensitivity (eg, bronchospasm, dyspnea, flushing, rash) should also be premedicated with a corticosteroid for all subsequent cycles if treatment is continued.

Dose-dependent myelosuppression, particularly neutropenia, may occur with mono- or combination therapy. Neutropenic fever and infection have been reported with use. The risk for neutropenia is increased with hepatic dysfunction, especially when used in combination with capecitabine. Severe neutropenia and/or thrombocytopenia may require dosage adjustment and/or treatment delay. Peripheral (sensory and motor) neuropathy occurs commonly; may require dose reductions, treatment delays or discontinuation. Usually occurs during the first 3 cycles. Use with caution in patients with pre-existing neuropathy. Patients with diabetes may have an increased risk for severe peripheral neuropathy. Use with caution in patients with a history of cardiovascular disease; the incidence of MI, ventricular dysfunction, and supraventricular arrhythmias is higher when ixabepilone is used in combination with capecitabine (as compared to capecitabine alone). Consider discontinuing ixabepilone in patients who develop cardiac ischemia or impaired cardiac function.

Avoid concurrent use with strong CYP3A4 inhibitors (eg, itraconazole, ketoconazole, voriconazole, clarithromycin, telithromycin, nefazodone, amprenavir, atazanavir, delavirdine, indinavir, nelfinavir, ritonavir, saquinavir); dosage reductions are recommended if concurrent use cannot be avoided; allow ~1 week to elapse prior to adjusting ixabepilone dose upward after a strong CYP3A4 inhibitor is discontinued. Avoid strong CYP3A4 inducers (eg, dexamethasone, phenytoin, carbamazepine, rifampin, phenobarbital); may decrease the ixabepilone level; alternative agents should be considered; dosage increases of ixabepilone (with careful monitoring) may be recommended if concomitant administration with CYP3A4 inducers cannot be avoided. Due to the ethanol content in the diluent, may cause cognitive impairment; patients must be cautioned about performing tasks which require mental alertness (eg, operating machinery or driving). Toxicities or serious adverse events with combination therapy may be increased in the elderly.

Adverse Reactions

Percentages reported with monotherapy:

>10%:

Central nervous system: Headache (11%)

Dermatologic: Alopecia (48%)

Gastrointestinal: Nausea (42%), vomiting (29%), mucositis/stomatitis (29%), diarrhea (22%), anorexia (19%), constipation (16%), abdominal pain (13%)

Hematologic: Leukopenia (grade 3: 36%; grade 4: 13%), neutropenia (grade 3: 31%; grade 4: 23%)

Neuromuscular & skeletal: Peripheral neuropathy (63%; grades 3/4: 14%; grade 3/4 median onset: cycle 4), sensory neuropathy (62%; grades 3/4: 14%), weakness (56%), myalgia/arthralgia (49%), musculoskeletal pain (20%)

1% to 10%:

Cardiovascular: Edema (9%), chest pain (5%)

Central nervous system: Fever (8%), pain (8%), dizziness (7%), insomnia (5%)

Dermatologic: Nail disorder (9%), rash (9%), palmar-plantar erythrodysesthesia/hand-and-foot syndrome (8%), pruritus (6%), skin exfoliation (2%), hyperpigmentation (2%)

Endocrine & metabolic: Hot flush (6%), dehydration (2%)

Gastrointestinal: Gastroesophageal reflux disease (6%), taste perversion (6%), weight loss (6%)

Hematologic: Anemia (grade 3: 6%; grade 4: 2%), neutropenic fever (3%; grade 3: 3%), thrombocytopenia (grade 3: 5%; grade 4: 2%)

Neuromuscular & skeletal: Motor neuropathy (10%; grade 3: 1%)

Ocular: Lacrimation increased (4%)

Respiratory: Dyspnea (9%), upper respiratory tract infection (6%), cough (2%)

Miscellaneous: Hypersensitivity (5%; grade 3: 1%), infection (5%)

Mono- and combination therapy: <1% (Limited to important or life-threatening): Alkaline phosphatase increased, angina, atrial flutter, autonomic neuropathy, cardiomyopathy, cerebral hemorrhage, coagulopathy, colitis, dysphagia, dysphonia, embolism, enterocolitis, erythema multiforme, gastrointestinal hemorrhage, gastroparesis, GGT increased, hemorrhage, hepatic failure (acute), hypokalemia, hyponatremia, hypotension, hypovolemia, hypovolemic shock, hypoxia, ileus, interstitial pneumonia, jaundice, left ventricular dysfunction, metabolic acidosis, MI, nephrolithiasis, neutropenic infection, orthostatic hypotension, pneumonia, pneumonitis, pulmonary edema (acute), radiation recall, renal failure, respiratory failure, sepsis, septic shock, supraventricular arrhythmia, syncope, thrombosis, transaminases increased, trismus, urinary tract infection, vasculitis

Drug Interactions

Metabolism/Transport Effects Substrate of CYP3A4 (major); **Note:** Assignment of Major/Minor substrate status based on clinically relevant drug interaction potential

Avoid Concomitant Use

Avoid concomitant use of Ixabepilone with any of the following: CloZAPine; St Johns Wort

Increased Effect/Toxicity

Ixabepilone may increase the levels/effects of: CloZAPine

The levels/effects of Ixabepilone may be increased by: CYP3A4 Inhibitors (Moderate); CYP3A4 Inhibitors (Strong); Dasatinib

Decreased Effect

The levels/effects of Ixabepilone may be decreased by: CYP3A4 Inducers (Strong); Deferasirox; St Johns Wort; Tocilizumab

Ethanol/Nutrition/Herb Interactions

Food: Avoid grapefruit juice (may increase plasma concentrations of ixabepilone).

Herb/Nutraceutical: Avoid St John's wort (may decrease ixabepilone levels).

Stability Store intact vials under refrigeration at 2°C to 8°C (36°F to 46°F); protect from light. Allow to reach room temperature for ~30 minutes prior to reconstitution. Diluent vial may contain a white precipitate which should dissolve upon reaching room temperature. **Reconstitute only with the provided diluent.** Dilute the 15 mg vial with 8 mL and the 45 mg vial with 23.5 mL (using provided diluent) to a concentration of 2 mg/mL (contains overfill). Gently swirl and invert vial until dissolved completely. Prior to administration, further dilute using a non-DEHP container (eg, glass, polypropylene or polyolefin), to a final concentration of 0.2-0.6 mg/mL in ~250 mL lactated Ringer's, adjusted sodium chloride 0.9% (pH adjusted prior to ixabepilone addition with 2 mEq sodium bicarbonate per 250-500 mL sodium chloride) or PLASMA-LYTE A Injection pH 7.4®. Mix thoroughly. Use appropriate precautions for handling and disposal. Reconstituted solution (in the vial) is stable for 1 hour at room temperature; infusion solution diluted in appropriate solution for infusion is stable for 6 hours at room temperature if a pH range of 6-9 is maintained.

Mechanism of Action Epothilone B analog; binds to the beta-tubulin subunit of the microtubule, stabilizing microtubular promoting tubulin polymerization and stabilizing microtubular function, thus arresting the cell cycle (at the G2/M phase) and inducing apoptosis. Activity in taxane-resistant cells has been demonstrated.

Pharmacodynamics/Kinetics

Distribution: >1000 L

Protein binding: 67% to 77%

Metabolism: Extensively hepatic, via CYP3A4; >30 metabolites (inactive) formed

Half-life elimination: ~52 hours

Time to peak, plasma: At the end of infusion (3 hours)

Excretion: Feces (65%; 2% of the total dose as unchanged drug); urine (21%; 6% of the total dose as unchanged drug)

Dosage Details concerning dosing in combination regimens should also be consulted. **Note:** Premedicate with an H_1-antagonist (eg, oral diphenhydramine 50 mg) and H_2-antagonist (eg, oral ranitidine 150-300 mg) ~1 hour prior to infusion. Patients with a history of hypersensitivity should also be premedicated with corticosteroids (orally 1 hour before or I.V. 30 minutes before infusion). For dose calculation, body surface area (BSA) is capped at a maximum of 2.2 m^2.

I.V.: Adults:

Breast cancer (metastatic or locally advanced): 40 mg/m^2/dose over 3 hours every 3 weeks (maximum dose: 88 mg) either as monotherapy or in combination with capecitabine

Endometrial cancer (unlabeled use): 40 mg/m^2/dose over 3 hours every 3 weeks (Dizon, 2009)

Dosage adjustment with concomitant strong CYP3A4 inhibitors/inducers:

CYP3A4 inhibitors: Avoid concomitant administration with strong CYP3A4 inhibitors; if concomitant administration with a strong CYP3A4 inhibitor cannot be avoided, consider a dose reduction to 20 mg/m^2. When a strong CYP3A4 inhibitor is discontinued, allow ~1 week to elapse prior to adjusting ixabepilone dose upward to the indicated dose.

CYP3A4 inducers: Avoid concomitant administration with strong CYP3A4 inducers; if concomitant administration with a strong CYP3A4 inducer cannot be avoided and after maintenance on the strong CYP3A4 inducer is established, consider adjusting the ixabepilone dose gradually up to 60 mg/m^2 (as a 4-hour infusion), with careful monitoring. If the strong CYP3A4 enzyme inducer is discontinued, reduce ixabepilone dose to the dose used prior to initiation of the CYP3A4 inducer.

Ixabepilone dosage adjustments for toxicity for monotherapy or combination therapy:

Hematologic:

Neutrophils <500/mm^3 for ≥7 days: Reduce dose by 20%

Neutropenic fever: Reduce dose by 20%

Platelets <25,000/mm^3 (or <50,000/mm^3 with bleeding): Reduce dose by 20%

Nonhematologic:

Neuropathy:

Grade 2 (moderate) for ≥7 days: Reduce dose by 20%

Grade 3 (severe) for <7 days: Reduce dose by 20%

Grade 3 (severe or disabling) for ≥7 days: Discontinue treatment

Grade 3 toxicity (severe; other than neuropathy): Reduce dose by 20%

Grade 3 arthralgia/myalgia or fatigue (transient): Continue at current dose

Grade 3 hand-foot syndrome: Continue at current dose

Grade 4 toxicity (disabling): Discontinue treatment

Note: Adjust dosage at the start of a cycle are based on toxicities (hematologic and nonhematologic) from the previous cycle; delay new cycles until neutrophils have recovered to ≥1500/mm^3, platelets have recovered to ≥100,000/mm^3 and nonhematologic toxicities have resolved or improved to at least grade 1. If toxicities persist despite initial dose reduction, reduce dose an additional 20%.

Capecitabine dosage adjustments for toxicity in combination therapy with ixabepilone:

Hematologic:

Neutrophils <500/mm^3 for ≥7 days or neutropenic fever: Hold for concurrent diarrhea or stomatitis until neutrophils recover to >1000/mm^3, then continue at same dose

Platelets <25,000/mm^3 (or <50,000/mm^3 with bleeding): Hold for concurrent diarrhea or stomatitis until platelets recover to >50,000/mm^3, then continue at same dose

Nonhematologic: Refer to Capecitabine monograph.

Dosage adjustment in renal impairment: Pharmacokinetics (monotherapy) are not affected in patients with mild-to-moderate renal insufficiency (Cl_{cr} >30 mL/minute); monotherapy has not been studied in patients with serum creatinine >1.5 times ULN. Combination therapy with capecitabine has not been studied in patients with Cl_{cr} <50 mL/minute.

Dosage adjustment in hepatic impairment:

Ixabepilone monotherapy (initial cycle; adjust doses for subsequent cycles based on toxicity):

AST and ALT ≤2.5 times ULN and bilirubin ≤1 times ULN: No adjustment necessary

AST and ALT >2.5 to ≤10 times ULN and bilirubin >1 to ≤1.5 times ULN: Reduce dose to 32 mg/m^2

AST and ALT ≤10 times ULN and bilirubin >1.5 to ≤3 times ULN: Reduce dose to 20-30 mg/m^2 (initiate treatment at 20 mg/m^2, may escalate up to a maximum of 30 mg/m^2 in subsequent cycles if tolerated)

AST or ALT >10 times ULN or bilirubin >3 times ULN: Use is not recommended

Combination therapy of ixabepilone with capecitabine:

AST and ALT ≤2.5 times ULN and bilirubin ≤1 times ULN: No adjustment necessary

AST or ALT >2.5 times ULN or bilirubin >1 times ULN: Use is contraindicated

Dietary Considerations Avoid grapefruit juice (may increase plasma concentrations of ixabepilone).

Administration I.V.: Infuse over 3 hours. Use non-DEHP administration set (eg, polyethylene); filter with a 0.2-1.2 micron inline filter. Administration should be completed within 6 hours of preparation. If the dose is increased (above 40 mg/m^2) due to concomitant CYP3A4 inducer use, infuse over 4 hours.

Monitoring Parameters CBC with differential; hepatic function (ALT, AST, bilirubin); monitor for hypersensitivity, neuropathy

Dosage Forms Excipient information presented when available (limited, particularly for generics); consult specific product labeling.

Injection, powder for reconstitution:

Ixempra®: 15 mg, 45 mg [contains dehydrated ethanol (in diluent), polyoxyethylated castor oil (in diluent)]

- **Ixempra®** *see* Ixabepilone *on page 945*
- **Ixiaro®** *see* Japanese Encephalitis Virus Vaccine (Inactivated) *on page 948*
- **Jakafi™** *see* Ruxolitinib *on page 1530*
- **Jakafi™** *see* Ruxolitinib *on page 1530*
- **Jalyn™** *see* Dutasteride and Tamsulosin *on page 568*
- **JAMP-Amlodipine (Can)** *see* AmLODIPine *on page 97*
- **JAMP-Atenolol (Can)** *see* Atenolol *on page 161*
- **JAMP-Bicalutamide (Can)** *see* Bicalutamide *on page 217*
- **JAMP-Carvedilol (Can)** *see* Carvedilol *on page 295*
- **JAMP-Citalopram (Can)** *see* Citalopram *on page 370*
- **JAMP-Finasteride (Can)** *see* Finasteride *on page 713*
- **Jamp-Fosinopril (Can)** *see* Fosinopril *on page 763*
- **JAMP-Indapamide (Can)** *see* Indapamide *on page 886*
- **JAMP-Letrozole (Can)** *see* Letrozole *on page 986*
- **JAMP-Lisinopril (Can)** *see* Lisinopril *on page 1020*
- **JAMP-Metoprolol-L (Can)** *see* Metoprolol *on page 1117*
- **JAMP-Ondansetron (Can)** *see* Ondansetron *on page 1246*
- **JAMP-Pioglitazone (Can)** *see* Pioglitazone *on page 1355*
- **JAMP-Quetiapine (Can)** *see* QUEtiapine *on page 1440*
- **JAMP-Ramipril (Can)** *see* Ramipril *on page 1459*
- **JAMP-Risperidone (Can)** *see* RisperiDONE *on page 1496*
- **JAMP-Ropinirole (Can)** *see* ROPINIRole *on page 1517*
- **JAMP-Simvastatin (Can)** *see* Simvastatin *on page 1555*
- **JAMP-Tamsulosin (Can)** *see* Tamsulosin *on page 1626*
- **JAMP-Terbinafine (Can)** *see* Terbinafine (Systemic) *on page 1648*
- **Jantoven®** *see* Warfarin *on page 1802*
- **Janumet®** *see* Sitagliptin and Metformin *on page 1562*
- **Januvia®** *see* SitaGLIPtin *on page 1560*

Japanese Encephalitis Virus Vaccine (Inactivated)

(jap a NEESE en sef a LYE tis VYE rus vak SEEN, in ak ti VAY ted)

Brand Names: U.S. Ixiaro®

Brand Names: Canada Ixiaro®

Index Terms IC51; JE-VC (Ixiaro®)

Pharmacologic Category Vaccine, Inactivated (Viral)

Use Active immunization against Japanese encephalitis

Japanese encephalitis vaccine is not recommended for all persons traveling to or residing in Asia. The Advisory Committee on Immunization Practices (ACIP) recommends vaccination for:

- Persons spending ≥1 month in endemic areas during transmission season
- Research laboratory workers who may be exposed to the Japanese encephalitis virus

Vaccination may also be considered for the following:

- Travelers to areas with an ongoing outbreak
- Travelers spending <30 days in endemic areas during the transmission season and planning to go outside of urban areas and have an increased risk of exposure. For example, high-risk activities include extensive outdoor activity in rural areas especially at night; extensive outdoor activities such as camping, hiking, etc; staying in accommodations without air conditioning, screens or bed nets.
- Travelers to endemic areas who are unsure of specific destination, activities, or duration of travel

Pregnancy Risk Factor B

Pregnancy Considerations Adverse events were not observed in animal reproduction studies. Risks of vaccine administration should be carefully considered and in general, pregnant women should only be vaccinated if they are at high risk for exposure. Infection from Japanese encephalitis during the first or second trimesters of pregnancy may increase risk of miscarriage. Intrauterine transmission of the Japanese encephalitis virus has been reported. To report inadvertent use of Ixiaro® during pregnancy, contact Novartis Vaccines (800-244-7668).

Lactation Excretion in breast milk unknown/use caution

Contraindications

Severe allergic reaction to a previous dose of the vaccine

Canadian labeling: Additional contraindications (not in U.S. labeling): Acute severe febrile conditions

Warnings/Precautions Because of the potential for severe adverse reactions, Japanese encephalitis vaccine is not recommended for all persons traveling to or residing in Asia. Use is not recommended for short-term travelers (<30 days) who will not be outside of an urban area or when the visit is outside of a well-defined Japanese encephalitis virus transmission season. Risk of exposure to the Japanese encephalitis virus may vary from year to year for a particular area. Immediate treatment for anaphylactic/anaphylactoid reaction should be available during vaccine use.

Use of vaccine should also include other means to reduce the risk of mosquito exposure (bed nets, insect repellents, protective clothing, avoidance of travel in endemic areas, and avoidance of outdoor activity during twilight and evening periods).

May contain protamine sulfate which may cause hypersensitivity reactions in certain individuals. Immunization should be completed ≥7 days prior to potential exposure. Safety and efficacy have not been established in children <17 years of age (<18 years of age per Canadian labeling).

In general, the decision to administer or delay vaccination because of current or recent febrile illness depends on the severity of symptoms and the etiology of the disease. Immunocompromised patients may have a reduced response to vaccines; information not available specific to this vaccine. In general, household and close contacts of persons with altered immunocompetence may receive all age appropriate vaccines. In order to maximize vaccination rates, the ACIP recommends simultaneous administration of all age-appropriate vaccines (live or inactivated) for which a person is eligible at a single clinic visit, unless contraindications exist. Canadian labeling recommends avoiding I.M. administration in patients with bleeding disorders (eg, thrombocytopenia, hemophilia) and suggests that SubQ administration may be considered in these patients. Clinical efficacy data regarding this route is lacking and the U.S. labeling does not recommend SubQ administration.

Adverse Reactions **Report allergic or unusual adverse reactions to the Vaccine Adverse Event Reporting System (VAERS) 1-800-822-7967 or online at https://vaers.hhs.gov/esub/index.** In Canada, adverse reactions may be reported to local provincial/territorial health agencies or to the Vaccine Safety Section at Public Health Agency of Canada (1-866-844-0018).

Percentage of adverse reactions reported over days 0-56. In general, incidence was similar to placebo.

>10%:

Central nervous system: Headache (28%), fatigue (11%)

Local: Injection site reaction: Tenderness (36%), pain (33%)

Neuromuscular & skeletal: Myalgia (16%)

Miscellaneous: Flu-like syndrome (12%)

1% to 10%:

Central nervous system: Pyrexia (3%)

Dermatologic: Rash (1%)

Gastrointestinal: Nausea (7%), diarrhea (2%), vomiting (1%)

Local: Injection site reaction: Erythema (10%), induration (8%), edema (4%), pruritus (4%)

Neuromuscular & skeletal: Back pain (1%)

Respiratory: Nasopharyngitis (5%), pharyngolaryngeal pain (2%), upper respiratory tract infection (2%), cough (1%), rhinitis (1%)

Postmarketing and/or case reports: Encephalitis, neuritis, paresthesia

Drug Interactions

Metabolism/Transport Effects None known.

Avoid Concomitant Use There are no known interactions where it is recommended to avoid concomitant use.

Increased Effect/Toxicity There are no known significant interactions involving an increase in effect.

Decreased Effect

The levels/effects of Japanese Encephalitis Virus Vaccine (Inactivated) may be decreased by: Belimumab; Fingolimod; Immunosuppressants

Stability Store in original packaging under refrigeration at 2°C to 8°C (35°F to 46°F); do not freeze.

Dosage U.S. recommended primary immunization schedule:

Adults ≥17 years: I.M.: 0.5 mL/dose; a total of 2 doses given on days 0 and 28. Series should be completed at least 1 week prior to potential exposure.

Booster dose: Booster dose may be given prior to potential re-exposure if the primary series was completed >1 year previously.

Note: If the second dose is missed, limited data from one clinical trial demonstrate a 99% seroconversion rate when the second dose was administered 11 months after the initial dose.

Elderly: Refer to adult dosing. Elderly may be at increased risk of developing neuroinvasive disease if infected with Japanese encephalitis virus.

Administration For I.M. injection into the deltoid muscle. Do not inject I.V., SubQ, or intradermally. Shake well prior to use to form a homogeneous suspension. Do not use if discolored or if particulate matter remains. Canadian labeling recommends avoiding I.M. administration in patients with bleeding disorders (eg, thrombocytopenia, hemophilia) and suggests that SubQ administration may be considered in these patients. Clinical efficacy data regarding this route is lacking and the U.S. labeling does not recommend SubQ administration. For patients at risk of hemorrhage following intramuscular injection, the ACIP recommends "it should be administered intramuscularly if, in the opinion of the physician familiar with the patients bleeding risk, the vaccine can be administered by this route with reasonable safety. If the patient receives antihemophilia or other similar therapy, intramuscular vaccination can be scheduled shortly after such therapy is administered. A fine needle (23 gauge or smaller) can be used for the vaccination and firm pressure applied to the site (without rubbing) for at least 2 minutes. The patient should be instructed concerning the risk of hematoma from the injection." Patients on anticoagulant therapy should be considered to have the same bleeding risks and treated as those with clotting factor disorders (CDC, 2011).

Simultaneous administration of vaccines helps ensure the patients will be fully vaccinated by the appropriate age. Simultaneous administration of vaccines is defined as administering >1 vaccine on the same day at different anatomic sites. Separate vaccines should not be combined in the same syringe unless indicated by product specific labeling. Separate needles and syringes should be used for each injection. The ACIP prefers each dose of a specific vaccine in a series come from the same manufacturer when possible. Adolescents and adults should be vaccinated while seated or lying down. In general, preterm infants should be vaccinated at the same chronological age as full-term infants (CDC, 2011).

Antipyretics have not been shown to prevent febrile seizures. Antipyretics may be used to treat fever or discomfort following vaccination (CDC, 2011). One study reported that routine prophylactic administration of acetaminophen to prevent fever prior to vaccination decreased the immune response of some vaccines; the clinical significance of this reduction in immune response has not been established (Prymula, 2009).

Monitoring Parameters Observe patients for 30 minutes after vaccination for anaphylactic/hypersensitivity reactions and syncope

Additional Information Federal law requires that the name of medication, date of administration, the vaccine manufacturer, lot number of vaccine, and the administering person's name, title, and address be entered into the patient's permanent medical record.

Ixiaro® is a purified Japanese encephalitis vaccine made from the SA14-14-2 strain grown in Vero cells (JE-VC). It was developed due to neurologic side effects observed with Je-Vax®, a vaccine derived from mice-brain cells (JE-MB) that contains additives which may contribute to the adverse effects effects (Je-Vax® is no longer available in the U.S. as of May 2011). In studies comparing the two vaccines, seroconversion rates were similar following two doses of Ixiaro® as opposed to three doses of Je-Vax®. Safety profile of Ixiaro® was found to be similar to placebo.

Adults who previously received Je-Vax® vaccine and require further immunization against Japanese encephalitis should be administered a 2-dose primary series of Ixiaro® (CDC, May 2011).

Safety and immunogenicity studies related to the use of Ixiaro® in children are ongoing; at present, Ixiaro® is not FDA approved for use in children. Until additional information is available, physicians may choose to enroll children 2 months to 17 years in a clinical trial (NCT01047839; http://clinicaltrials.gov/ct2/show/nct01047839), administer the vaccine off-label (additional information available from Novartis Medical Communications at 877-683-4732 or vaccineinfo.us@novartis.com), or have the vaccine administered at an international health clinic in Asia (additional information is available at http://www.cdc.gov/ncidod/dvbid/jencephalitis/resources/UpdtJEVaccChildren_Web_Table2.pdf). In addition, children should take the same precautions to reduce the risk for Japanese encephalitis and other vector-borne infectious diseases as recommended by the CDC (CDC, May 2011).

Dosage Forms Excipient information presented when available (limited, particularly for generics); consult specific product labeling.

Injection, suspension:

Ixiaro®: Inactivated JEV proteins 6 mcg/0.5 mL (0.5 mL) [contains bovine serum, protamine sulfate, sodium metabisulfite]

◆ **Jevantique™** *see* Ethinyl Estradiol and Norethindrone *on page* 660

◆ **JE-VC (Ixiaro®)** *see* Japanese Encephalitis Virus Vaccine (Inactivated) *on page* 948

◆ **Jevtana®** *see* Cabazitaxel *on page* 257

◆ **Jinteli™** *see* Ethinyl Estradiol and Norethindrone *on page* 660

◆ **Jolessa™** *see* Ethinyl Estradiol and Levonorgestrel *on page* 656

◆ **Jolivette®** *see* Norethindrone *on page* 1217

◆ **Junel® 1.5/30** *see* Ethinyl Estradiol and Norethindrone *on page* 660

◆ **Junel® 1/20** *see* Ethinyl Estradiol and Norethindrone *on page* 660

◆ **Junel® Fe 1.5/30** *see* Ethinyl Estradiol and Norethindrone *on page* 660

◆ **Junel® Fe 1/20** *see* Ethinyl Estradiol and Norethindrone *on page* 660

◆ **Jurnista™ (Can)** *see* HYDROmorphone *on page* 843

◆ **Just For Kids™ [OTC]** *see* Fluoride *on page* 728

◆ **Juvisync™** *see* Sitagliptin and Simvastatin *on page* 1562

◆ **Juvéderm® Ultra** *see* Hyaluronate and Derivatives *on page* 831

◆ **Juvéderm® Ultra XC** *see* Hyaluronate and Derivatives *on page* 831

◆ **Juvéderm® Ultra Plus** *see* Hyaluronate and Derivatives *on page* 831

◆ **Juvéderm® Ultra Plus XC** *see* Hyaluronate and Derivatives *on page* 831

◆ **K-10® (Can)** *see* Potassium Chloride *on page* 1380

◆ **Kadian®** *see* Morphine (Systemic) *on page* 1153

◆ **Kalbitor®** *see* Ecallantide *on page* 569

◆ **Kaletra®** *see* Lopinavir and Ritonavir *on page* 1028

◆ **Kalexate** *see* Sodium Polystyrene Sulfonate *on page* 1575

Kanamycin (kan a MYE sin)

Index Terms Kanamycin Sulfate

Pharmacologic Category Antibiotic, Aminoglycoside

Use Treatment of serious infections caused by susceptible strains of *E. coli*, *Proteus* species, *Enterobacter aerogenes*, *Klebsiella pneumoniae*, *Serratia marcescens*, and *Acinetobacter* species; second-line treatment of *Mycobacterium tuberculosis*

Pregnancy Risk Factor D

Dosage Note: Dosing should be based on ideal body weight

Children: Infections: I.M., I.V.: 15 mg/kg/day in divided doses every 8-12 hours

Adults:

Infections: I.M., I.V.: 5-7.5 mg/kg/dose in divided doses every 8-12 hours (<15 mg/kg/day)

Intraperitoneal: After contamination in surgery: 500 mg

Irrigating solution: 0.25%; maximum 1.5 g/day (via all administration routes)

Aerosol: 250 mg 2-4 times/day

Dosing adjustment/interval in renal impairment:

Cl_{cr} 50-80 mL/minute: Administer 60% to 90% of dose or administer every 8-12 hours

Cl_{cr} 10-50 mL/minute: Administer 30% to 70% of dose or administer every 12 hours

Cl_{cr} <10 mL/minute: Administer 20% to 30% of dose or administer every 24-48 hours

Additional Information Complete prescribing information for this medication should be consulted for additional detail.

Dosage Forms Excipient information presented when available (limited, particularly for generics); consult specific product labeling.

Injection, solution, as sulfate: 1 g/3 mL (3 mL)

◆ **Kanamycin Sulfate** *see* Kanamycin *on page* 950

◆ **Kank-A® Soft Brush [OTC]** *see* Benzocaine *on page* 202

◆ **Kaon-CL® 10** *see* Potassium Chloride *on page* 1380

◆ **Kaopectate® [OTC]** *see* Bismuth *on page* 220

◆ **Kaopectate® Extra Strength [OTC]** *see* Bismuth *on page* 220

◆ **Kaopectate® Stool Softener [OTC]** *see* Docusate *on page* 537

◆ **Kao-Tin [OTC]** *see* Bismuth *on page* 220

◆ **Kao-Tin [OTC]** *see* Docusate *on page* 537

◆ **Kapidex** *see* Dexlansoprazole *on page* 483

◆ **Kapvay™** *see* CloNIDine *on page* 392

◆ **Kariva®** *see* Ethinyl Estradiol and Desogestrel *on page* 653

◆ **Kayexalate®** *see* Sodium Polystyrene Sulfonate *on page* 1575

◆ **KCl** *see* Potassium Chloride *on page* 1380

◆ **Kdur** *see* Potassium Chloride *on page* 1380

◆ **K-Dur® (Can)** *see* Potassium Chloride *on page* 1380

◆ **Kedbumin™** *see* Albumin *on page* 51

◆ **Keflex®** *see* Cephalexin *on page* 327

◆ **Keftab® (Can)** *see* Cephalexin *on page* 327

◆ **Kelnor™** *see* Ethinyl Estradiol and Ethynodiol Diacetate *on page* 655

◆ **Kenalog®** *see* Triamcinolone (Topical) *on page* 1735

◆ **Kenalog®-10** *see* Triamcinolone (Systemic) *on page* 1732

◆ **Kenalog®-40** *see* Triamcinolone (Systemic) *on page* 1732

◆ **Keoxifene Hydrochloride** *see* Raloxifene *on page* 1455

◆ **Kepivance®** *see* Palifermin *on page* 1276

◆ **Keppra®** *see* LevETIRAcetam *on page* 994

◆ **Keppra XR™** *see* LevETIRAcetam *on page* 994

◆ **Kerafoam®** *see* Urea *on page* 1749

◆ **Kerafoam® 42** *see* Urea *on page* 1749

◆ **Keralac™** *see* Urea *on page* 1749

◆ **Keralac™ Nailstik** *see* Urea *on page* 1749

◆ **Keratol 40™ [DSC]** *see* Urea *on page* 1749

◆ **Kerlone®** *see* Betaxolol (Systemic) *on page* 211

◆ **Kerol™** *see* Urea *on page* 1749

◆ **Kerol™ AD** *see* Urea *on page* 1749

◆ **Kerol™ Redi-Cloths** *see* Urea *on page* 1749

◆ **Kerol™ ZX** *see* Urea *on page* 1749

◆ **Kerr Insta-Char® in Aqueous Base [OTC]** *see* Charcoal, Activated *on page* 335

◆ **Kerr Insta-Char® in Sorbitol Base [OTC]** *see* Charcoal, Activated *on page* 335

◆ **Ketalar®** *see* Ketamine *on page 951*

Ketamine (KEET a meen)

Brand Names: U.S. Ketalar®

Brand Names: Canada Ketalar®; Ketamine Hydrochloride Injection, USP

Index Terms Ketamine Hydrochloride

Pharmacologic Category General Anesthetic

Use Induction and maintenance of general anesthesia

Unlabeled Use Analgesia, sedation

Pregnancy Considerations Adverse events have not been observed in animal reproduction studies. Ketamine crosses the placenta and can be detected in fetal tissue. Ketamine produces dose dependent increases in uterine contractions; effects may vary by trimester. The plasma clearance of ketamine is reduced during pregnancy. Dose related neonatal depression and decreased APGAR scores have been reported with large doses administered at delivery.

Contraindications Hypersensitivity to ketamine or any component of the formulation; conditions in which an increase in blood pressure would be hazardous

Warnings/Precautions Use with caution in patients with coronary artery disease, catecholamine depletion, hypertension, and tachycardia. Cardiac function should be continuously monitored in patients with increased blood pressure or cardiac decompensation. Postanesthetic emergence reactions which can manifest as vivid dreams, hallucinations, and/or frank delirium occur; these reactions are less common in patients <15 years of age and >65 years and when given intramuscularly. Emergence reactions, confusion, or irrational behavior may occur up to 24 hours postoperatively and may be reduced by pretreatment with a benzodiazepine and the use of ketamine at the lower end of the dosing range. Rapid I.V. administration or overdose may cause respiratory depression, apnea, and enhanced pressor response. Resuscitative equipment should be available during use. Use with caution in patients with CSF pressure elevation, the chronic alcoholic or acutely alcohol-intoxicated. May cause dependence (withdrawal symptoms on discontinuation) and tolerance with prolonged use. May cause CNS depression, which may impair physical or mental abilities; patients must be cautioned about performing tasks which require mental alertness (eg, operating machinery or driving). When used for outpatient surgery, the patient be accompanied by a responsible adult. Should be administered under the supervision of a physician experienced in administering general anesthetics.

Adverse Reactions Frequency not always defined.

Cardiovascular: Arrhythmia, bradycardia/tachycardia, hyper-/hypotension

Central nervous system: CSF pressure increased

Dermatologic: Erythema (transient), morbilliform rash (transient)

Gastrointestinal: Anorexia, nausea, salivation increased, vomiting

Local: Pain at the injection site, exanthema at the injection site

Neuromuscular & skeletal: Skeletal muscle tone enhanced (tonic-clonic movements)

Ocular: Diplopia, intraocular pressure increased, nystagmus

Respiratory: Airway obstruction, apnea, bronchial secretions increased, respiratory depression, laryngospasm

Miscellaneous: Anaphylaxis, dependence with prolonged use, emergence reactions (~12%; includes confusion, delirium, dreamlike state, excitement, hallucinations, irrational behavior, vivid imagery)

Drug Interactions

Metabolism/Transport Effects Substrate of CYP2B6 (major), CYP2C9 (major), CYP3A4 (major); **Note:** Assignment of Major/Minor substrate status based on clinically relevant drug interaction potential

Avoid Concomitant Use

Avoid concomitant use of Ketamine with any of the following: Conivaptan

Increased Effect/Toxicity

The levels/effects of Ketamine may be increased by: Conivaptan; CYP2B6 Inhibitors (Moderate); CYP2B6 Inhibitors (Strong); CYP2C9 Inhibitors (Moderate); CYP2C9 Inhibitors (Strong); CYP3A4 Inhibitors (Moderate); CYP3A4 Inhibitors (Strong); Dasatinib; Quazepam

Decreased Effect

The levels/effects of Ketamine may be decreased by: CYP2C9 Inducers (Strong); Peginterferon Alfa-2b; Tocilizumab

Stability Store at 20°C to 25°C (68°F to 77°F). Protect from light. The 50 mg/mL and 100 mg/mL vials may be further diluted in D_5W or NS to prepare a maintenance infusion with a final concentration of 1 mg/mL (or 2 mg/mL in patients with fluid restrictions). The 10 mg/mL vials are not recommended to be further diluted. Do not mix with barbiturates or diazepam (precipitation may occur).

Mechanism of Action Produces a cataleptic-like state in which the patient is dissociated from the surrounding environment by direct action on the cortex and limbic system. Ketamine is a noncompetitive NMDA receptor antagonist that blocks glutamate. Low (subanesthetic) doses produce analgesia, and modulate central sensitization, hyperalgesia and opioid tolerance. Reduces polysynaptic spinal reflexes.

Pharmacodynamics/Kinetics

Onset of action:

I.V.: Anesthetic effect: 30 seconds

I.M.: Anesthetic effect: 3-4 minutes

Duration: Anesthetic effect: I.V.: 5-10 minutes; I.M.: 12-25 minutes

Distribution: V_d: 3 L/kg

Metabolism: Hepatic via hydroxylation and N-demethylation; the metabolite norketamine is 33% as potent as parent compound; greater conversion to norketamine occurs after oral administration as compared to parenteral administration

Bioavailability: Oral: 16%; Intranasal: 50%

Half-life elimination: Alpha: 10-15 minutes; Beta: 2.5 hours

Excretion: Primarily urine

Dosage May be used in combination with anticholinergic agents to decrease hypersalivation.

Children: Note: Titrate dose for desired effect.

Sedation (unlabeled use): Oral (unlabeled route): 5-8 mg/kg for 1 dose (mixed in 0.2-0.3 mL/kg of cola or other beverage) given 30 minutes before the procedure (Sacchetti, 1994; Rosenberg, 1991)

Sedation/analgesia (unlabeled use):

I.M.: 2-5 mg/kg/dose (Green, 2011; Krause, 2000; McGlone, 2004; White, 1982)

I.V.: 0.5-1 mg/kg/dose (Sacchetti, 1994; Tobias, 1990)

Continuous I.V. infusion: 5-20 mcg/kg/minute (White, 1982; Tobias, 1990)

Children ≥16 years and Adults: Note: Titrate dose for desired effect.

Sedation/analgesia (unlabeled use):

I.M.: 2-4 mg/kg (White, 1982)

I.V.: 0.2-0.75 mg/kg (White, 1982)

Continuous I.V. infusion: 2-7 mcg/kg/minute (Hocking, 2003; Remérand, 2009; Zakine, 2008)

Induction of anesthesia (unlabeled dosing):

I.M.: 4-10 mg/kg (Green, 1990; Miller, 2010; White, 1982)

I.V.: 0.5-2 mg/kg (Miller, 2010; White, 1982)

Maintenance of anesthesia: May administer supplemental doses of one-half to the full induction dose or a continuous infusion of 0.1-0.5 mg/minute (per manufacturer). **Note:** To maintain an adequate concentration of ketamine for maintenance of anesthesia, 1-2 mg/minute has been recommended (White, 1982); doses in the range of 15-90 mcg/kg/minute (~1-6 mg/minute in a 70-kg patient) have also been suggested (Miller, 2010). Concurrent use of nitric oxide reduces ketamine requirements.

Administration

Oral: Mix the appropriate dose (using the 100 mg/mL injectable solution) in cola or other beverage; drink immediately after preparation.

Parenteral: I.V.: Administer bolus doses over 1 minute; more rapid administration may result in respiratory depression and enhanced pressor response. **Note:** The 100 mg/mL concentration should not be administered I.V. unless properly diluted with an equal volume of either SWFI, NS, or D_5W.

Monitoring Parameters Heart rate, blood pressure, respiratory rate, transcutaneous O_2 saturation, emergence reactions; cardiac function should be continuously monitored in patients with increased blood pressure or cardiac decompensation

Test Interactions May interfere with urine detection of PCP (false-positive).

Additional Information May produce emergence psychosis including auditory and visual hallucinations, restlessness, disorientation, vivid dreams, and irrational behavior in ~12% of patients; pretreatment with a benzodiazepine reduces incidence of psychosis by >50%. Spontaneous involuntary movements, nystagmus, hypertonus, and vocalizations are also common.

The analgesia outlasts the general anesthetic component. Bronchodilation is beneficial in asthmatic or COPD patients. Laryngeal reflexes may remain intact or may be obtunded. The direct myocardial depressant action of ketamine can be seen in stressed, catecholamine-deficient patients. Ketamine increases cerebral metabolism and cerebral blood flow while producing a noncompetitive block of the glutaminergic postsynaptic NMDA receptor. It lowers seizure threshold and stimulates salivary secretions (atropine/scopolamine treatment is recommended).

Dosage Forms Excipient information presented when available (limited, particularly for generics); consult specific product labeling.

Injection, solution: 10 mg/mL (20 mL); 50 mg/mL (10 mL); 100 mg/mL (5 mL, 10 mL)

Ketalar®: 10 mg/mL (20 mL); 50 mg/mL (10 mL); 100 mg/mL (5 mL)

Controlled Substance C-III

◆ **Ketamine Hydrochloride** *see* Ketamine *on page 951*

◆ **Ketamine Hydrochloride Injection, USP (Can)** *see* Ketamine *on page 951*

◆ **Ketek®** *see* Telithromycin *on page 1634*

Ketoconazole (Systemic) (kee toe KOE na zole)

Brand Names: Canada Apo-Ketoconazole®; Novo-Ketoconazole

Pharmacologic Category Antifungal Agent, Oral

Use Treatment of susceptible fungal infections, including candidiasis, oral thrush, blastomycosis, histoplasmosis, paracoccidioidomycosis, coccidioidomycosis, chromomycosis, candiduria, chronic mucocutaneous candidiasis, as well as certain recalcitrant cutaneous dermatophytoses

Unlabeled Use Treatment of prostate cancer (androgen synthesis inhibitor)

Pregnancy Risk Factor C

Pregnancy Considerations Adverse effects were noted in animal reproduction studies.

Lactation Enters breast milk/not recommended

Contraindications Hypersensitivity to ketoconazole or any component of the formulation; CNS fungal infections (due to poor CNS penetration); coadministration with ergot derivatives, cisapride, or triazolam is contraindicated due to risk of potentially fatal cardiac arrhythmias

Warnings/Precautions [U.S. Boxed Warning]: Ketoconazole has been associated with hepatotoxicity, including some fatalities; use with caution in patients with impaired hepatic function and perform periodic liver function tests. **[U.S. Boxed Warning]: Concomitant use with cisapride is contraindicated due to the occurrence of ventricular arrhythmias.** High doses of ketoconazole may depress adrenocortical function.

Adverse Reactions

1% to 10%:

Dermatologic: Pruritus (2%)

Gastrointestinal: Nausea/vomiting (3% to 10%), abdominal pain (1%)

<1% (Limited to important or life-threatening): Bulging fontanelles, chills, depression, diarrhea, dizziness, fever, gynecomastia, headache, hemolytic anemia, hepatotoxicity, impotence, leukopenia, photophobia, somnolence, thrombocytopenia

Drug Interactions

Metabolism/Transport Effects Substrate of CYP3A4 (major); **Note:** Assignment of Major/Minor substrate status based on clinically relevant drug interaction potential; **Inhibits** CYP1A2 (strong), CYP2A6 (moderate), CYP2B6 (weak), CYP2C19 (moderate), CYP2C8 (weak), CYP2C9 (strong), CYP2D6 (moderate), CYP3A4 (strong), P-glycoprotein

Avoid Concomitant Use

Avoid concomitant use of Ketoconazole (Systemic) with any of the following: Alfuzosin; Cisapride; Clopidogrel; Conivaptan; Crizotinib; Dofetilide; Dronedarone; Eplerenone; Everolimus; Fluticasone (Oral Inhalation); Halofantrine; Lapatinib; Lovastatin; Lurasidone; Nilotinib; Nisoldipine; Pimozide; QuiNIDine; Ranolazine; Rivaroxaban; RomiDEPsin; Salmeterol; Silodosin; Simvastatin; Tamsulosin; Thioridazine; Ticagrelor; Tolvaptan; Topotecan; Toremifene

Increased Effect/Toxicity

Ketoconazole (Systemic) may increase the levels/effects of: Alfentanil; Alfuzosin; Aliskiren; Almotriptan; Alosetron; Aprepitant; ARIPiprazole; Bendamustine; Benzodiazepines (metabolized by oxidation); Boceprevir; Bortezomib; Bosentan; Brentuximab Vedotin; Brinzolamide; Budesonide (Nasal); Budesonide (Systemic, Oral Inhalation); BusPIRone; Busulfan; Calcium Channel Blockers; CarBAMazepine; Ciclesonide; Cilostazol; Cinacalcet; Cisapride; Citalopram; Colchicine; Conivaptan; Corticosteroids (Orally Inhaled); Corticosteroids (Systemic); Crizotinib; CycloSPORINE; CycloSPORINE (Systemic); CYP1A2 Substrates; CYP2A6 Substrates; CYP2C19 Substrates; CYP2C9 Substrates; CYP2D6 Substrates; CYP3A4 Substrates; Dabigatran Etexilate; Diclofenac; Dienogest; DOCEtaxel; Dofetilide; Dronedarone; Dutasteride; Eletriptan; Eplerenone; Erlotinib; Eszopiclone; Etravirine; Everolimus; FentaNYL; Fesoterodine; Fexofenadine; Fluticasone (Nasal); Fluticasone (Oral Inhalation); Fosaprepitant; Fosphenytoin; Gefitinib; GuanFACINE; Halofantrine; HMG-CoA Reductase Inhibitors; Iloperidone; Imatinib; Irinotecan; Ixabepilone; Lapatinib; Losartan; Lovastatin; Lumefantrine; Lurasidone; Macrolide Antibiotics; Maraviroc; Methadone; MethylPREDNISolone; Nebivolol; Nilotinib; Nisoldipine; Paricalcitol; Pazopanib; P-glycoprotein/ABCB1 Substrates; Phenytoin; Phosphodiesterase 5 Inhibitors; Pimecrolimus; Pimozide; Praziquantel; Propafenone; Protease Inhibitors; Proton Pump Inhibitors; QuiNIDine;

Ramelteon; Ranolazine; Repaglinide; Rifamycin Derivatives; Rilpivirine; Rivaroxaban; RomiDEPsin; Ruxolitinib; Salmeterol; Saxagliptin; Sildenafil; Silodosin; Simvastatin; Sirolimus; Solifenacin; SORAfenib; SUNItinib; Tacrolimus; Tacrolimus (Systemic); Tacrolimus (Topical); Tadalafil; Tamoxifen; Tamsulosin; Telaprevir; Temsirolimus; Thioridazine; Ticagrelor; Tolterodine; Tolvaptan; Topotecan; Toremifene; Vardenafil; Vemurafenib; Vilazodone; Vitamin K Antagonists; Ziprasidone; Zolpidem; Zuclopenthixol

The levels/effects of Ketoconazole (Systemic) may be increased by: Boceprevir; Etravirine; Grapefruit Juice; Macrolide Antibiotics; Protease Inhibitors; Telaprevir

Decreased Effect

Ketoconazole (Systemic) may decrease the levels/effects of: Amphotericin B; Clopidogrel; Codeine; Prasugrel; Saccharomyces boulardii; Ticagrelor; TraMADol

The levels/effects of Ketoconazole (Systemic) may be decreased by: Antacids; CYP3A4 Inducers (Strong); Deferasirox; Didanosine; Etravirine; Fosphenytoin; H2-Antagonists; Herbs (CYP3A4 Inducers); Phenytoin; Proton Pump Inhibitors; Rifamycin Derivatives; Rilpivirine; Sucralfate; Tocilizumab

Ethanol/Nutrition/Herb Interactions

Food: Ketoconazole peak serum levels may be prolonged if taken with food.

Herb/Nutraceutical: St John's wort may decrease ketoconazole levels.

Stability Store at 15°C to 25°C (59°F to 77°F).

Mechanism of Action Alters the permeability of the cell wall by blocking fungal cytochrome P450; inhibits biosynthesis of triglycerides and phospholipids by fungi; inhibits several fungal enzymes that results in a build-up of toxic concentrations of hydrogen peroxide; also inhibits androgen synthesis

Pharmacodynamics/Kinetics

Absorption: Rapid (~75%)

Distribution: Well into inflamed joint fluid, saliva, bile, urine, sebum, cerumen, feces, tendons, skin and soft tissue, and testes; crosses blood-brain barrier poorly; only negligible amounts reach CSF

Protein binding: 93% to 96%

Metabolism: Partially hepatic via CYP3A4 to inactive compounds

Bioavailability: Decreases as gastric pH increases

Half-life elimination: Biphasic: Initial: 2 hours; Terminal: 8 hours

Time to peak, serum: 1-2 hours

Excretion: Feces (57%); urine (13%)

Dosage Oral:

Fungal infections:

Children ≥2 years: 3.3-6.6 mg/kg/day as a single dose for 1-2 weeks for candidiasis, for at least 4 weeks in recalcitrant dermatophyte infections, and for up to 6 months for other systemic mycoses

Adults: 200-400 mg/day as a single daily dose for durations as stated above

Prostate cancer (unlabeled use): Adults: 400 mg 3 times/day

Dosing adjustment in renal impairment: Hemodialysis: Not dialyzable (0% to 5%)

Dosing adjustment in hepatic impairment: Dose reductions should be considered in patients with severe liver disease

Dietary Considerations May be taken with food or milk to decrease GI adverse effects.

Administration Administer oral tablets 2 hours prior to antacids to prevent decreased absorption due to the high pH of gastric contents.

Monitoring Parameters Liver function tests

Dosage Forms Excipient information presented when available (limited, particularly for generics); consult specific product labeling.

Tablet, oral: 200 mg

Extemporaneous Preparations A 20 mg/mL oral suspension may be made with tablets and one of three different vehicles (a 1:1 mixture of Ora-Sweet® and Ora-Plus®, a 1:1 mixture of Ora-Sweet® SF and Ora-Plus®, or a 1:4 mixture of cherry syrup and Simple Syrup, NF). Crush twelve 200 mg tablets in a mortar and reduce to a fine powder. Add 20 mL of chosen vehicle and mix to a uniform paste; mix while adding the vehicle in incremental proportions to **almost** 120 mL; transfer to a calibrated bottle, rinse mortar with vehicle, and add quantity of vehicle sufficient to make 120 mL. Label "shake well" and "refrigerate". Stable for 60 days.

Nahata MC, Pai VB, and Hipple TF, *Pediatric Drug Formulations*, 5th ed, Cincinnati, OH: Harvey Whitney Books Co, 2004.

Ketoconazole (Topical) (kee toe KOE na zole)

Brand Names: U.S. Extina®; Nizoral®; Nizoral® A-D [OTC]; Xolegel®

Brand Names: Canada Ketoderm®; Xolegel®

Pharmacologic Category Antifungal Agent, Topical

Additional Appendix Information

Antifungal Agents *on page 1876*

Use

Cream: Treatment of tinea corporis, tinea cruris, tinea versicolor, cutaneous candidiasis, seborrheic dermatitis

Foam, gel: Treatment of seborrheic dermatitis

Shampoo: Treatment of dandruff, seborrheic dermatitis, tinea versicolor

Unlabeled Use Cream: Treatment of susceptible fungal infections in the oral cavity including candidiasis, oral thrush, and chronic mucocutaneous candidiasis

Pregnancy Risk Factor C

Dosage

Shampoo:

Seborrheic dermatitis (ketoconazole 1%): Children ≥12 years and Adults: Apply twice weekly for up to 8 weeks with at least 3 days between each shampoo

Tinea versicolor (ketoconazole 2%): Adults: Apply to damp skin, lather, leave on 5 minutes, and rinse (one application should be sufficient)

Topical:

Tinea infections: Adults: Cream: Rub gently into the affected area once daily. Duration of treatment: Tinea corporis, cruris: 2 weeks; tinea pedis: 6 weeks

Seborrheic dermatitis: Children ≥12 years and Adults:

Cream: Rub gently into the affected area twice daily for 4 weeks or until clinical response is noted

Foam: Apply to affected area twice daily for 4 weeks

Gel: Rub gently into the affected area once daily for 2 weeks

Susceptible fungal infections in the oral cavity (candidiasis, oral thrush, and chronic mucocutaneous candidiasis) (unlabeled use): Adults: Cream: Apply locally as directed with a thin coat to inner surface of denture and affected areas after meals

Additional Information Complete prescribing information for this medication should be consulted for additional detail.

Dosage Forms Excipient information presented when available (limited, particularly for generics); consult specific product labeling. [DSC] = Discontinued product

Aerosol, foam, topical: 2% (50 g, 100 g)

Extina®: 2% (50 g, 100 g)

Cream, topical: 2% (15 g, 30 g, 60 g)

Gel, topical:

Xolegel®: 2% (15 g [DSC], 45 g) [contains dehydrated ethanol 34%]

Shampoo, topical: 2% (120 mL)
Nizoral®: 2% (120 mL)
Nizoral® A-D: 1% (6 mL [DSC], 120 mL, 210 mL)

◆ **Ketoderm® (Can)** *see* Ketoconazole (Topical) *on page 953*

Ketoprofen (kee toe PROE fen)

Brand Names: Canada Apo-Keto SR®; Apo-Keto-E®; Apo-Keto®; Ketoprofen SR; Ketoprofen-E; Nu-Ketoprofen; Nu-Ketoprofen-E; PMS-Ketoprofen; PMS-Ketoprofen-E

Pharmacologic Category Nonsteroidal Anti-inflammatory Drug (NSAID), Oral

Use Acute and long-term treatment of rheumatoid arthritis and osteoarthritis; primary dysmenorrhea; mild-to-moderate pain

Pregnancy Risk Factor C

Pregnancy Considerations Adverse events were not observed in the initial animal reproduction studies; therefore, the manufacturer classifies ketoprofen as pregnancy category C. Ketoprofen crosses the placenta. NSAID exposure during the first trimester is not strongly associated with congenital malformations; however, cardiovascular anomalies and cleft palate have been observed following NSAID exposure in some studies. The use of an NSAID close to conception may be associated with an increased risk of miscarriage. Nonteratogenic effects have been observed following NSAID administration during the third trimester including myocardial degenerative changes, prenatal constriction of the ductus arteriosus, fetal tricuspid regurgitation, failure of the ductus arteriosus to close postnatally; renal dysfunction or failure, oligohydramnios; gastrointestinal bleeding or perforation, increased risk of necrotizing enterocolitis; intracranial bleeding (including intraventricular hemorrhage), platelet dysfunction with resultant bleeding; pulmonary hypertension. Because they may cause premature closure of the ductus arteriosus, use of NSAIDs late in pregnancy should be avoided (use after 31or 32 weeks gestation is not recommended by some clinicians). The chronic use of NSAIDs in women of reproductive age may be associated with infertility that is reversible upon discontinuation of the medication.

Lactation Enters breast milk

Medication Guide Available Yes

Contraindications Hypersensitivity to ketoprofen, aspirin, other NSAIDs, or any component of the formulation; perioperative pain in the setting of coronary artery bypass graft (CABG) surgery

Warnings/Precautions [U.S. Boxed Warning]: NSAIDs are associated with an increased risk of adverse cardiovascular thrombotic events, including MI and stroke Risk may be increased with duration of use or pre-existing cardiovascular risk factors or disease. Carefully evaluate individual cardiovascular risk profiles prior to prescribing. May cause new-onset hypertension or worsening of existing hypertension. Use caution with fluid retention. Avoid use in heart failure. Concurrent administration of ibuprofen, and potentially other nonselective NSAIDs, may interfere with aspirin's cardioprotective effect. **[U.S. Boxed Warning]: Use is contraindicated for treatment of perioperative pain in the setting of coronary artery bypass graft (CABG) surgery.** Risk of MI and stroke may be increased with use following CABG surgery.

NSAID use may compromise existing renal function; dose-dependent decreases in prostaglandin synthesis may result from NSAID use, reducing renal blood flow which may cause renal decompensation. NSAID use may increase the risk for hyperkalemia. Patients with impaired renal function, dehydration, heart failure, liver dysfunction, those taking diuretics, and ACE inhibitors, and the elderly are at greater risk of renal toxicity and hyperkalemia. Rehydrate patient before starting therapy; monitor renal function closely. Not recommended for use in patients with advanced renal disease. Long-term NSAID use may result in renal papillary necrosis.

[U.S. Boxed Warning]: NSAIDs may increase risk of gastrointestinal irritation, inflammation, ulceration, bleeding, and perforation. These events may occur at any time during therapy and without warning. Use caution with a history of GI disease (bleeding or ulcers), concurrent therapy with aspirin, anticoagulants and/or corticosteroids, smoking, use of alcohol, the elderly or debilitated patients. When used concomitantly with ≤325 mg of aspirin, a substantial increase in the risk of gastrointestinal complications (eg, ulcer) occurs; concomitant gastroprotective therapy (eg, proton pump inhibitors) is recommended (Bhatt, 2008). Platelet adhesion and aggregation may be decreased; may prolong bleeding time; patients with coagulation disorders or who are receiving anticoagulants should be monitored closely. Anemia may occur; patients on long-term NSAID therapy should be monitored for anemia. Rarely, NSAID use may cause severe blood dyscrasias (eg, agranulocytosis, aplastic anemia, thrombocytopenia).

Use the lowest effective dose for the shortest duration of time, consistent with individual patient goals, to reduce risk of cardiovascular or GI adverse events. Alternate therapies should be considered for patients at high risk.

NSAIDS may cause drowsiness, dizziness, blurred vision and other neurologic effects which may impair physical or mental abilities; patients must be cautioned about performing tasks which require mental alertness (eg, operating machinery or driving). Discontinue use with blurred or diminished vision and perform ophthalmologic exam. Monitor vision with long-term therapy.

NSAIDs may cause serious skin adverse events including exfoliative dermatitis, Stevens-Johnson syndrome (SJS), and toxic epidermal necrolysis (TEN); discontinue use at first sign of skin rash or hypersensitivity. Anaphylactoid reactions may occur, even without prior exposure; patients with "aspirin triad" (bronchial asthma, aspirin intolerance, rhinitis) may be at increased risk. Do not use in patients who experience bronchospasm, asthma, rhinitis, or urticaria with NSAID or aspirin therapy. Use caution in other forms of asthma.

Use with caution in patients with decreased hepatic function. Closely monitor patients with any abnormal LFT. Severe hepatic reactions (eg, fulminant hepatitis, liver failure) have occurred with NSAID use, rarely; discontinue if signs or symptoms of liver disease develop, or if systemic manifestations occur. The elderly are at increased risk for adverse effects (especially peptic ulceration, CNS effects, renal toxicity) from NSAIDs, even at low doses.

Withhold for at least 4-6 half-lives prior to surgical or dental procedures. Safety and efficacy have not been established in pediatric patients.

Adverse Reactions

>10%:
Gastrointestinal: Dyspepsia (11%)
Hepatic: Liver function test abnormal (≤15%)

1% to 10%:
Cardiovascular: Peripheral edema (2%)
Central nervous system: Headache (3% to 9%), depression, dizziness (>1%), dreams, insomnia, malaise, nervousness, somnolence
Dermatologic: Rash (>1%)

Gastrointestinal: Abdominal pain (3% to 9%), constipation (3% to 9%), diarrhea (3% to 9%), flatulence (3% to 9%), nausea (3% to 9%), gastrointestinal bleeding (>2%), peptic ulcer (>2%), anorexia (>1%), stomatitis (>1%), vomiting (>1%)

Genitourinary: Urinary tract irritation (>1%)

Ocular: Visual disturbances (>1%)

Otic: Tinnitus (>1%)

Renal: Renal dysfunction (3% to 9%)

<1% (Limited to important or life-threatening): Agranulocytosis, allergic reaction, allergic rhinitis, alopecia, anaphylaxis, anemia, angioedema, arrhythmia, aseptic meningitis, blurred vision, bone marrow suppression, bronchospasm, buccal necrosis, bullous rash, chills, cholestatic hepatitis, confusion, CHF, conjunctivitis, cystitis, diabetes mellitus (aggravated), drowsiness, dysphoria, dyspnea, eczema, edema, epistaxis, erythema multiforme, exfoliative dermatitis, facial edema, fecal occult blood, fluid retention, gastritis, gastrointestinal perforation, GI ulceration, gynecomastia, hallucinations, hearing decreased, hematemesis, hematuria, hemolytic anemia, hemoptysis, hepatic dysfunction, hepatitis, hot flashes, hypertension, hyponatremia, impotence, infection, interstitial nephritis, intestinal ulceration, jaundice, laryngeal edema, leukopenia, libido disturbance, melena, microvesicular steatosis, migraine, myocardial infarction, nephrotic syndrome, onycholysis, palpitation, pancreatitis, peptic ulcer, peripheral neuropathy, peripheral vascular disease, photosensitivity, polydipsia, polyuria, pruritus, purpura, purpuric rash, renal failure, renal papillary necrosis, retinal hemorrhage, septicemia, shock, Stevens-Johnson syndrome, tachycardia, thrombocytopenia, toxic amblyopia, toxic epidermal necrolysis, tubulopathy, ulcerative colitis, urticaria, vasodilation, xerostomia

Drug Interactions

Metabolism/Transport Effects **Inhibits** CYP2C9 (weak)

Avoid Concomitant Use

Avoid concomitant use of Ketoprofen with any of the following: Floctafenine; Ketorolac; Ketorolac (Nasal); Ketorolac (Systemic)

Increased Effect/Toxicity

Ketoprofen may increase the levels/effects of: Aminoglycosides; Anticoagulants; Antiplatelet Agents; Bisphosphonate Derivatives; Collagenase (Systemic); CycloSPORINE; CycloSPORINE (Systemic); Deferasirox; Desmopressin; Digoxin; Drotrecogin Alfa (Activated); Eplerenone; Haloperidol; Ibritumomab; Lithium; Methotrexate; Nonsteroidal Anti-Inflammatory Agents; PEMEtrexed; Porfimer; Potassium-Sparing Diuretics; PRALAtrexate; Quinolone Antibiotics; Rivaroxaban; Salicylates; Thrombolytic Agents; Tositumomab and Iodine I 131 Tositumomab; Vancomycin; Vitamin K Antagonists

The levels/effects of Ketoprofen may be increased by: ACE Inhibitors; Angiotensin II Receptor Blockers; Antidepressants (Tricyclic, Tertiary Amine); Corticosteroids (Systemic); CycloSPORINE; CycloSPORINE (Systemic); Dasatinib; Floctafenine; Glucosamine; Herbs (Anticoagulant/Antiplatelet Properties); Ketorolac; Ketorolac (Nasal); Ketorolac (Systemic); Nonsteroidal Anti-Inflammatory Agents; Omega-3-Acid Ethyl Esters; Pentosan Polysulfate Sodium; Pentoxifylline; Probenecid; Prostacyclin Analogues; Selective Serotonin Reuptake Inhibitors; Serotonin/Norepinephrine Reuptake Inhibitors; Sodium Phosphates; Treprostinil; Vitamin E

Decreased Effect

Ketoprofen may decrease the levels/effects of: ACE Inhibitors; Angiotensin II Receptor Blockers; Antiplatelet Agents; Beta-Blockers; Eplerenone; HydrALAZINE; Loop Diuretics; Potassium-Sparing Diuretics; Salicylates; Selective Serotonin Reuptake Inhibitors; Thiazide Diuretics

The levels/effects of Ketoprofen may be decreased by: Bile Acid Sequestrants; Nonsteroidal Anti-Inflammatory Agents; Salicylates

Ethanol/Nutrition/Herb Interactions

Ethanol: Avoid ethanol (due to GI irritation).

Food: Food slows rate of absorption resulting in delayed and reduced peak serum concentrations; total bioavailability is not affected by food.

Herb/Nutraceutical: Avoid alfalfa, anise, bilberry, bladderwrack, bromelain, cat's claw, celery, chamomile, coleus, cordyceps, dong quai, evening primrose, fenugreek, feverfew, garlic, ginger, ginkgo biloba, ginseng (American, Panax, Siberian), grapeseed, green tea, guggul, horse chestnut seed, horseradish, licorice, prickly ash, red clover, reishi, SAMe (S-adenosylmethionine), sweet clover, turmeric, and white willow (all have additional antiplatelet activity).

Stability Store at room temperature of 25°C (77°F). Protect from light; avoid excessive heat and humidity.

Mechanism of Action Reversibly inhibits cyclooxygenase-1 and 2 (COX-1 and 2) enzymes, which results in decreased formation of prostaglandin precursors; has antipyretic, analgesic, and anti-inflammatory properties

Other proposed mechanisms not fully elucidated (and possibly contributing to the anti-inflammatory effect to varying degrees), include inhibiting chemotaxis, altering lymphocyte activity, inhibiting neutrophil aggregation/activation, and decreasing proinflammatory cytokine levels.

Pharmacodynamics/Kinetics

Onset of action: Regular release: <30 minutes

Duration: Regular release: Up to 6 hours

Absorption: Almost complete

Distribution: 0.1 L/kg

Protein binding: >99%, primarily to albumin; Hepatic impairment: Unbound fraction is approximately doubled

Metabolism: Hepatic via glucuronidation; metabolite (inactive) can be converted back to parent compound; may have enterohepatic recirculation

Bioavailability: ~90%

Half-life elimination:

- Regular release: 2-4 hours; Renal impairment: Mild: 3 hours; moderate-to-severe: 5-9 hours
- Extended release: ~3-7.5 hours

Time to peak, serum:

- Regular release: 0.5-2 hours
- Extended release: 6-7 hours

Excretion: Urine (~80%, primarily as glucuronide conjugates)

Dosage Note: The extended release formulation is not recommended for the treatment of acute pain. Oral:

Adults:

- Rheumatoid arthritis, osteoarthritis (lower doses may be used in small patients or in the elderly, or debilitated):
  - Regular release: 50 mg 4 times/day **or** 75 mg 3 times/day; up to a maximum of 300 mg/day
  - Extended release: 200 mg once daily
- Dysmenorrhea, mild-to-moderate pain: Regular release: 25-50 mg every 6-8 hours up to a maximum of 300 mg/day

Elderly: Initial dose should be decreased in patients >75 years; use caution when dosage changes are made

Dosage adjustment in renal impairment: In general, NSAIDs are not recommended for use in patients with advanced renal disease, but the manufacturer of ketoprofen does provide some guidelines for adjustment in renal dysfunction:

Mild impairment: Maximum dose: 150 mg/day

Severe impairment: Cl_{cr} <25 mL/minute: Maximum dose: 100 mg/day

Dosage adjustment in hepatic impairment and serum albumin <3.5 g/dL: Maximum dose: 100 mg/day

Dietary Considerations In order to minimize gastrointestinal effects, ketoprofen can be prescribed to be taken with food or milk.

Administration May take with food to reduce GI upset. Do not crush or break extended release capsules.

Monitoring Parameters CBC, chemistry profile, occult blood loss, periodic liver function; renal function (urine output, serum BUN, creatinine)

Dosage Forms Excipient information presented when available (limited, particularly for generics); consult specific product labeling.

Capsule, oral: 50 mg, 75 mg

Capsule, extended release, oral: 200 mg

◆ **Ketoprofen-E (Can)** *see* Ketoprofen *on page 954*

◆ **Ketoprofen SR (Can)** *see* Ketoprofen *on page 954*

Ketorolac (Systemic) (KEE toe role ak)

Brand Names: Canada Apo-Ketorolac Injectable®; Apo-Ketorolac®; Ketorolac Tromethamine Injection, USP; Novo-Ketorolac; Nu-Ketorolac; Toradol®; Toradol® IM

Index Terms Ketorolac Tromethamine; Toradol

Pharmacologic Category Nonsteroidal Anti-inflammatory Drug (NSAID), Oral; Nonsteroidal Anti-inflammatory Drug (NSAID), Parenteral

Additional Appendix Information

Beers Criteria – Potentially Inappropriate Medications for Geriatrics *on page 1973*

Use Short-term (≤5 days) management of moderate-to-severe acute pain requiring analgesia at the opioid level

Pregnancy Risk Factor C

Pregnancy Considerations Adverse events were not observed in the initial animal reproduction studies; therefore, the manufacturer classifies ketorolac as pregnancy category C. Ketorolac crosses the placenta. NSAID exposure during the first trimester is not strongly associated with congenital malformations; however, cardiovascular anomalies and cleft palate have been observed following NSAID exposure in some studies. The use of an NSAID close to conception may be associated with an increased risk of miscarriage. Nonteratogenic effects have been observed following NSAID administration during the third trimester including myocardial degenerative changes, prenatal constriction of the ductus arteriosus, fetal tricuspid regurgitation, failure of the ductus arteriosus to close postnatally; renal dysfunction or failure, oligohydramnios; gastrointestinal bleeding or perforation, increased risk of necrotizing enterocolitis; intracranial bleeding (including intraventricular hemorrhage), platelet dysfunction with resultant bleeding; pulmonary hypertension. Because they may cause premature closure of the ductus arteriosus, use of NSAIDs late in pregnancy should be avoided (use after 31 or 32 weeks gestation is not recommended by some clinicians). **[U.S. Boxed Warning]: Ketorolac is contraindicated during labor and delivery (may inhibit uterine contractions and adversely affect fetal circulation).** The chronic use of NSAIDs in women of reproductive age may be associated with infertility that is reversible upon discontinuation of the medication.

Lactation Enters breast milk/contraindicated (per manufacturer's labeling)

Medication Guide Available Yes

Contraindications Hypersensitivity to ketorolac, aspirin, other NSAIDs, or any component of the formulation; active or history of peptic ulcer disease; recent or history of GI bleeding or perforation; patients with advanced renal disease or risk of renal failure (due to volume depletion); prophylaxis before major surgery; suspected or confirmed cerebrovascular bleeding; hemorrhagic diathesis, incomplete hemostasis, or high risk of bleeding; concurrent ASA or other NSAIDs; concomitant probenecid or pentoxifylline; epidural or intrathecal administration; perioperative pain in the setting of coronary artery bypass graft (CABG) surgery; labor and delivery; breast-feeding

Warnings/Precautions [U.S. Boxed Warning]: May inhibit platelet function; contraindicated in patients with cerebrovascular bleeding (suspected or confirmed), hemorrhagic diathesis, incomplete hemostasis and patients at high risk for bleeding. Effects on platelet adhesion and aggregation may prolong bleeding time. Anemia may occur; patients on long-term NSAID therapy should be monitored for anemia. Rarely, NSAID use has been associated with potentially severe blood dyscrasias (eg, agranulocytosis, thrombocytopenia, aplastic anemia).

[U.S. Boxed Warning]: NSAIDs are associated with an increased risk of adverse cardiovascular thrombotic events, including MI and stroke. Risk may be increased with duration of use or pre-existing cardiovascular risk factors or disease. Carefully evaluate individual cardiovascular risk profiles prior to prescribing. May cause new-onset hypertension or worsening of existing hypertension. Use caution with fluid retention. Avoid use in heart failure. Concurrent administration of ibuprofen, and potentially other nonselective NSAIDs, may interfere with aspirin's cardioprotective effect. **[U.S. Boxed Warning]: Use is contraindicated as prophylactic analgesic before any major surgery and is contraindicated for treatment of perioperative pain in the setting of coronary artery bypass graft (CABG) surgery.** Risk of MI and stroke may be increased with use following CABG surgery. Wound bleeding and postoperative hematomas have been associated with ketorolac use in the perioperative setting. Withhold for at least 4-6 half-lives prior to surgical or dental procedures.

[U.S. Boxed Warning]: Ketorolac is contraindicated in patients with advanced renal impairment and in patients at risk for renal failure due to volume depletion. NSAID use may compromise existing renal function; dose-dependent decreases in prostaglandin synthesis may result from NSAID use, reducing renal blood flow which may cause renal decompensation. NSAID use may increase the risk for hyperkalemia. Patients with impaired renal function, dehydration, heart failure, liver dysfunction, those taking diuretics and ACE inhibitors, and the elderly are at greater risk of renal toxicity. Use with caution in patients with impaired renal function or history of kidney disease; dosage adjustment is required in patients with moderate elevation in serum creatinine. Monitor renal function closely. Acute renal failure, interstitial nephritis, and nephrotic syndrome have been reported with ketorolac use; papillary necrosis and renal injury have been reported with the use of NSAIDs. Use of NSAIDs can compromise existing renal function. Rehydrate patient before starting therapy.

[U.S. Boxed Warning]: NSAIDs may increase risk of gastrointestinal irritation, inflammation, ulceration, bleeding, and perforation. These events may occur at any time during therapy and without warning. Use caution with a history of GI disease (bleeding, ulcers, inflammatory bowel disease), concurrent therapy with aspirin, anticoagulants and/or corticosteroids, smoking, use of alcohol, the elderly, or debilitated patients. When used concomitantly with ≤325 mg of aspirin, a substantial increase in the risk of gastrointestinal complications (eg, ulcer) occurs; concomitant gastroprotective therapy (eg, proton pump inhibitors) is recommended (Bhatt, 2008).

NSAIDs may cause serious skin adverse events including exfoliative dermatitis, Stevens-Johnson syndrome (SJS), and toxic epidermal necrolysis (TEN); discontinue use at first sign of skin rash or hypersensitivity. Hypersensitivity or anaphylactoid reactions may occur, even without prior exposure; patients with "aspirin triad" (bronchial asthma, aspirin intolerance, rhinitis) may be at increased risk. Do not use in patients who experience bronchospasm, asthma, rhinitis, or urticaria with NSAID or aspirin therapy. **[U.S. Boxed Warning]: Ketorolac injection is contraindicated in patients with prior hypersensitivity reaction to aspirin or NSAIDs.** Use caution in other forms of asthma.

Use with caution in patients with hepatic impairment or a history of liver disease. Closely monitor patients with any abnormal LFT. Rarely, severe hepatic reactions (eg, fulminant hepatitis, hepatic necrosis, liver failure) have occurred with NSAID use; discontinue if signs or symptoms of liver disease develop, or if systemic manifestations occur.

[U.S. Boxed Warning]: Dosage adjustment is required for patients ≥65 years of age. The elderly are at increased risk for adverse effects (especially peptic ulceration, CNS effects, renal toxicity) from NSAIDs, even at low doses. Avoid immediate and long-term use (Beers Criteria). **[U.S. Boxed Warning]: Dosage adjustment is required for patients weighing <50 kg (<110 pounds). [U.S. Boxed Warning]: May inhibit uterine contractions and affect fetal circulation; inhibits prostaglandin synthesis in neonates; use is contraindicated in labor and delivery and breast-feeding women.** Avoid use in late pregnancy. **[U.S. Boxed Warning]: Concurrent use of ketorolac with aspirin or other NSAIDs is contraindicated due to the increased risk of adverse reactions.**

[U.S. Boxed Warning]: Contraindicated for epidural or intrathecal administration. [U.S. Boxed Warning]: Systemic ketorolac is indicated for short term (≤5 days) use in adults for treatment of moderately severe acute pain requiring opioid-level analgesia. Low doses of narcotics may be needed for breakthrough pain. **[U.S. Boxed Warning]: Oral therapy is only indicated for use as continuation treatment, following parenteral ketorolac and is not indicated for minor or chronic painful conditions. The maximum daily oral dose is 40 mg (adults); doses above 40 mg/day do not improve efficacy but may increase the risk of serious adverse effects.** The combined therapy duration (oral and parenteral) should not exceed 5 days. Use the lowest effective dose for the shortest duration of time, consistent with individual patient goals, to reduce risk of cardiovascular or GI adverse events. Alternate therapies should be considered for patients at high risk. **[U.S. Boxed Warning]: Oral ketorolac is not indicated for use in children.**

NSAIDS may cause drowsiness, dizziness, blurred vision and other neurologic effects which may impair physical or mental abilities; patients must be cautioned about performing tasks which require mental alertness (eg, operating machinery or driving). Discontinue use with blurred or diminished vision and perform ophthalmologic exam. Monitor vision with long-term therapy.

Adverse Reactions Frequencies noted for parenteral administration:

>10%:

Central nervous system: Headache (17%)

Gastrointestinal: Gastrointestinal pain (13%), dyspepsia (12%), nausea (12%)

>1% to 10%:

Cardiovascular: Edema (4%), hypertension

Central nervous system: Dizziness (7%), drowsiness (6%)

Dermatologic: Pruritus, purpura, rash

Gastrointestinal: Diarrhea (7%), constipation, flatulence, GI bleeding, GI fullness, GI perforation, GI ulcer, heartburn, stomatitis, vomiting

Hematologic: Anemia, bleeding time increased

Hepatic: Liver enzymes increased

Local: Injection site pain (2%)

Otic: Tinnitus

Renal: Renal function abnormal

Miscellaneous: Diaphoresis

<1% (Limited to important or life-threatening): Abnormal thinking, acute pancreatitis, acute renal failure, agranulocytosis, alopecia, anaphylactoid reaction, anaphylaxis, angioedema, anxiety, aplastic anemia, arrhythmia, aseptic meningitis, asthma, azotemia, blurred vision, bradycardia, bronchospasm, bruising, chest pain, CHF, cholestatic jaundice, coma, confusion, conjunctivitis, cough, cystitis, depression, dyspnea, dysuria, eosinophilia, epistaxis, eructation, erythema multiforme, esophagitis, euphoria, excessive thirst, exfoliative dermatitis, extrapyramidal symptoms, fever, flank pain, flushing, gastritis, GI hemorrhage, glossitis, hallucinations, hearing loss, hematemesis, hematuria, hemolytic anemia, hemolytic uremic syndrome, hepatitis, hyperglycemia, hyperkalemia, hyperkinesis, hypersensitivity reactions, hyponatremia, hypotension, inability to concentrate, infection, infertility, inflammatory bowel disease exacerbation, insomnia, interstitial nephritis, jaundice, laryngeal edema, leukopenia, liver failure, Lyell's syndrome, lymphadenopathy, maculopapular rash, melena, MI, nephritis, nervousness, oliguria, pallor, palpitation, pancytopenia, paresthesia, photosensitivity, pneumonia, polyuria, proteinuria, psychosis, pulmonary edema, rectal bleeding, renal failure, respiratory depression, rhinitis, seizure, sepsis, somnolence, Stevens-Johnson syndrome, stomatitis (ulcerative), stupor, syncope, tachycardia, thrombocytopenia, tongue edema, toxic epidermal necrolysis, tremor, urinary frequency increased, urinary retention, urticaria, vasculitis, vertigo, weakness, weight gain, wound hemorrhage (postoperative), xerostomia

Drug Interactions

Metabolism/Transport Effects None known.

Avoid Concomitant Use

Avoid concomitant use of Ketorolac (Systemic) with any of the following: Aspirin; Floctafenine; Ketorolac; Ketorolac (Nasal); Nonsteroidal Anti-Inflammatory Agents; Pentoxifylline; Probenecid

Increased Effect/Toxicity

Ketorolac (Systemic) may increase the levels/effects of: Aminoglycosides; Anticoagulants; Antiplatelet Agents; Aspirin; Bisphosphonate Derivatives; Collagenase (Systemic); CycloSPORINE; CycloSPORINE (Systemic); Deferasirox; Desmopressin; Digoxin; Drotrecogin Alfa (Activated); Eplerenone; Haloperidol; Ibritumomab; Lithium; Methotrexate; Neuromuscular-Blocking Agents (Nondepolarizing); Nonsteroidal Anti-Inflammatory Agents; PEMEtrexed; Pentoxifylline; Porfimer; Potassium-Sparing Diuretics; PRALAtrexate; Quinolone Antibiotics; Rivaroxaban; Salicylates; Thrombolytic Agents; Tositumomab and Iodine I 131 Tositumomab; Vancomycin; Vitamin K Antagonists

The levels/effects of Ketorolac (Systemic) may be increased by: ACE Inhibitors; Angiotensin II Receptor Blockers; Antidepressants (Tricyclic, Tertiary Amine); Corticosteroids (Systemic); CycloSPORINE; CycloSPORINE (Systemic); Dasatinib; Floctafenine; Glucosamine; Herbs (Anticoagulant/Antiplatelet Properties); Ketorolac; Ketorolac (Nasal); Omega-3-Acid Ethyl Esters; Pentosan Polysulfate Sodium; Probenecid; Prostacyclin Analogues; Selective Serotonin Reuptake Inhibitors; Serotonin/Norepinephrine Reuptake Inhibitors; Sodium Phosphates; Treprostinil; Vitamin E

Decreased Effect

Ketorolac (Systemic) may decrease the levels/effects of: ACE Inhibitors; Angiotensin II Receptor Blockers; Anticonvulsants; Antiplatelet Agents; Beta-Blockers; Eplerenone; HydrALAZINE; Loop Diuretics; Potassium-Sparing Diuretics; Salicylates; Selective Serotonin Reuptake Inhibitors; Thiazide Diuretics

The levels/effects of Ketorolac (Systemic) may be decreased by: Bile Acid Sequestrants; Salicylates

Ethanol/Nutrition/Herb Interactions

Ethanol: Avoid ethanol (may enhance gastric mucosal irritation).

Food: Oral: High-fat meals may delay time to peak (by ~1 hour) and decrease peak concentrations.

Herb/Nutraceutical: Avoid alfalfa, anise, bilberry, bladderwrack, bromelain, cat's claw, celery, chamomile, coleus, cordyceps, dong quai, evening primrose, fenugreek, feverfew, garlic, ginger, ginkgo biloba, ginseng (American, Panax, Siberian), grapeseed, green tea, guggul, horse chestnut seed, horseradish, licorice, prickly ash, red clover, reishi, SAMe (S-adenosylmethionine), sweet clover, turmeric, and white willow (all have additional antiplatelet activity).

Stability

Injection: Store at room temperature of 15°C to 30°C (59°F to 86°F). Protect from light. Injection is clear and has a slight yellow color. Precipitation may occur at relatively low pH values.

Tablet: Store at room temperature of 15°C to 30°C (59°F to 86°F).

Mechanism of Action Reversibly inhibits cyclooxygenase-1 and 2 (COX-1 and 2) enzymes, which results in decreased formation of prostaglandin precursors; has antipyretic, analgesic, and anti-inflammatory properties

Other proposed mechanisms not fully elucidated (and possibly contributing to the anti-inflammatory effect to varying degrees), include inhibiting chemotaxis, altering lymphocyte activity, inhibiting neutrophil aggregation/activation, and decreasing proinflammatory cytokine levels.

Pharmacodynamics/Kinetics

Onset of action: Analgesic: I.M.: ~10 minutes

Peak effect: Analgesic: 2-3 hours

Duration: Analgesic: 6-8 hours

Absorption: Oral: Well absorbed (100%)

Distribution: ~13 L; poor penetration into CSF; crosses placenta

Protein binding: 99%

Metabolism: Hepatic

Half-life elimination: 2-6 hours; prolonged 30% to 50% in elderly; up to 19 hours in renal impairment

Time to peak, serum: I.M.: 30-60 minutes

Excretion: Urine (92%, ~60% as unchanged drug); feces ~6%

Dosage

Children ≥16 years and Adults (pain relief usually begins within 10 minutes with parenteral forms): **Note:** The maximum combined duration of treatment (for parenteral and oral) is 5 days; do not increase dose or frequency; supplement with low-dose opioids if needed for breakthrough pain. For patients <50 kg and/or ≥65 years, see Elderly dosing.

I.M.: 60 mg as a single dose or 30 mg every 6 hours (maximum daily dose: 120 mg)

I.V.: 30 mg as a single dose or 30 mg every 6 hours (maximum daily dose: 120 mg)

Children ≥17 years and Adults: Oral: 20 mg, followed by 10 mg every 4-6 hours; do not exceed 40 mg/day; oral dosing is intended to be a continuation of I.M. or I.V. therapy only

Note: The maximum combined duration of treatment (for parenteral and oral) is 5 days; do not increase dose or frequency; supplement with low-dose opioids if needed for breakthrough pain. Therapy should not be initiated with oral formulation. For patients <50 kg and/or ≥65 years, see Elderly dosing.

Dosage adjustments in elderly (≥65 years), renal insufficiency, or low body weight (<50 kg): Note: These groups have an increased incidence of GI bleeding, ulceration, and perforation. The maximum combined duration of treatment (for parenteral and oral) is 5 days.

I.M.: 30 mg as a single dose or 15 mg every 6 hours (maximum daily dose: 60 mg)

I.V.: 15 mg as a single dose or 15 mg every 6 hours (maximum daily dose: 60 mg)

Oral: 10 mg, followed by 10 mg every 4-6 hours; do not exceed 40 mg/day; oral dosing is intended to be a continuation of I.M. or I.V. therapy only

Dosage adjustment in renal impairment: Contraindicated in patients with advanced renal impairment. Patients with moderately-elevated serum creatinine should use half the recommended dose, not to exceed 60 mg/day I.M./I.V.

Dosage adjustment in hepatic impairment: Use with caution, may cause elevation of liver enzymes; discontinue if clinical signs and symptoms of liver disease develop

Dietary Considerations Administer tablet with food or milk to decrease gastrointestinal distress.

Administration

Oral: May take with food to reduce GI upset.

I.M.: Administer slowly and deeply into the muscle. Analgesia begins in 30 minutes and maximum effect within 2 hours.

I.V.: Administer I.V. bolus over a minimum of 15 seconds; onset within 30 minutes; peak analgesia within 2 hours.

Monitoring Parameters Monitor response (pain, range of motion, grip strength, mobility, ADL function), inflammation; observe for weight gain, edema; monitor renal function (serum creatinine, BUN, urine output); CBC and platelets, liver function tests; observe for bleeding, bruising; evaluate gastrointestinal effects (abdominal pain, bleeding, dyspepsia); mental confusion, disorientation

Reference Range Serum concentration: Therapeutic: 0.3-5 mcg/mL; Toxic: >5 mcg/mL

Additional Information First parenteral NSAID for analgesia; 30 mg provides the analgesia comparable to 12 mg of morphine or 100 mg of meperidine.

Dosage Forms Excipient information presented when available (limited, particularly for generics); consult specific product labeling.

Injection, solution, as tromethamine: 15 mg/mL (1 mL, 2 mL); 30 mg/mL (1 mL, 2 mL, 10 mL)

Tablet, oral, as tromethamine: 10 mg

Ketorolac (Nasal) (KEE toe role ak)

Brand Names: U.S. Sprix®

Index Terms Ketorolac Tromethamine

Pharmacologic Category Nonsteroidal Anti-inflammatory Drug (NSAID), Nasal

Use Short-term (≤5 days) management of moderate-to-moderately-severe acute pain requiring analgesia at the opioid level

Pregnancy Risk Factor C/D ≥30 weeks gestation

Medication Guide Available Yes

Dosage Intranasal: **Note:** The maximum combined duration of treatment (for nasal spray or other ketorolac formulations) is 5 days.

Adults<65 years and ≥50 kg: One spray (15.75 mg) in each nostril (total dose: 31.5 mg) every 6-8 hours; maximum dose: 4 doses (126 mg)/day

Dosage adjustments in adults with low body weight (<50 kg): One spray (15.75 mg) in 1 nostril (total dose: 15.75 mg) every 6-8 hours; maximum dose: 4 doses (63 mg)/day

Elderly (≥65 years): Intranasal: One spray (15.75 mg) in 1 nostril (total dose: 15.75 mg) every 6-8 hours; maximum dose: 4 doses (63 mg)/day

Dosage adjustment in renal impairment:

Renal insufficiency: Intranasal: One spray (15.75 mg) in 1 nostril (total dose: 15.75 mg) every 6-8 hours; maximum dose: 4 doses (63 mg)/day

Advanced renal impairment (or at risk for renal failure due to volume depletion): Use is contraindicated

Dosage adjustment in hepatic impairment: Use with caution with hepatic impairment or history of hepatic disease; use may cause elevation of liver enzymes; discontinue if clinical signs and symptoms of liver disease develop.

Additional Information Complete prescribing information for this medication should be consulted for additional detail.

Dosage Forms Excipient information presented when available (limited, particularly for generics); consult specific product labeling.

Solution, intranasal, as tromethamine [spray, preservative free]:

Sprix®: 15.75 mg/spray (1.7 g) [delivers 8 metered sprays]

Ketorolac (Ophthalmic) (KEE toe role ak)

Brand Names: U.S. Acular LS®; Acular®; Acuvail®

Brand Names: Canada Acular LS®; Acular®; ratio-Ketorolac

Index Terms Ketorolac Tromethamine

Pharmacologic Category Nonsteroidal Anti-inflammatory Drug (NSAID), Ophthalmic

Use Temporary relief of ocular itching due to seasonal allergic conjunctivitis; postoperative inflammation following cataract extraction; reduction of ocular pain and photophobia following incisional refractive surgery; reduction of ocular pain, burning, and stinging following corneal refractive surgery

Pregnancy Risk Factor C

Dosage Ophthalmic: Children ≥3 years and Adults:

Allergic conjunctivitis (relief of ocular itching) (Acular®): Instill 1 drop (0.25 mg) 4 times/day

Inflammation following cataract extraction (Acular®): Instill 1 drop (0.25 mg) to affected eye(s) 4 times/day beginning 24 hours after surgery; continue for 2 weeks

Pain following corneal refractive surgery (Acular LS®): Instill 1 drop 4 times/day as needed to affected eye for up to 4 days

Additional Information Complete prescribing information for this medication should be consulted for additional detail.

Dosage Forms Excipient information presented when available (limited, particularly for generics); consult specific product labeling. [DSC] = Discontinued product

Solution, ophthalmic, as tromethamine [drops]: 0.4% (5 mL); 0.5% (3 mL, 5 mL, 10 mL)

Acular LS®: 0.4% (5 mL) [contains benzalkonium chloride]

Acular®: 0.5% (5 mL, 10 mL [DSC]) [contains benzalkonium chloride]

Solution, ophthalmic, as tromethamine [drops, preservative free]:

Acuvail®: 0.45% (0.4 mL)

Ketotifen (Ophthalmic) (kee toe TYE fen)

Brand Names: U.S. Alaway™ [OTC]; Claritin™ Eye [OTC]; Zaditor® [OTC]; ZyrTEC® Itchy Eye [OTC]

Brand Names: Canada Zaditor®

Index Terms Ketotifen Fumarate

Pharmacologic Category Histamine H_1 Antagonist; Histamine H_1 Antagonist, Second Generation; Mast Cell Stabilizer; Piperidine Derivative

Use Temporary relief of eye itching due to allergic conjunctivitis

Pregnancy Risk Factor C

Dosage Ophthalmic: Allergic conjunctivitis: Children ≥3 years and Adults: Instill 1 drop into the affected eye(s) twice daily, every 8-12 hours

Additional Information Complete prescribing information for this medication should be consulted for additional detail.

Dosage Forms Excipient information presented when available (limited, particularly for generics); consult specific product labeling.

Solution, ophthalmic [drops]: 0.025% (5 mL)

Alaway™: 0.025% (10 mL) [contains benzalkonium chloride]

Claritin™ Eye: 0.025% (5 mL) [contains benzalkonium chloride]

Zaditor®: 0.025% (5 mL) [contains benzalkonium chloride]

ZyrTEC® Itchy Eye: 0.025% (5 mL) [contains benzalkonium chloride]

Dosage Forms: Canada Excipient information presented when available (limited, particularly for generics); consult specific product labeling.

Solution, ophthalmic [drops]:

Zaditor®: 0.025% (5 mL) [contains benzalkonium chloride]

Solution, ophthalmic [drops], preservative free:

Zaditor®: 0.025% (0.4 mL) (30s)

- ◆ **Kivexa™ (Can)** *see* Abacavir and Lamivudine *on page 20*
- ◆ **Klaron®** *see* Sulfacetamide (Topical) *on page 1599*
- ◆ **Klean-Prep® (Can)** *see* Polyethylene Glycol-Electrolyte Solution *on page 1372*
- ◆ **KlonoPIN®** *see* ClonazePAM *on page 390*
- ◆ **Klonopin® (Can)** *see* ClonazePAM *on page 390*
- ◆ **Klor-Con®** *see* Potassium Chloride *on page 1380*
- ◆ **Klor-Con® 8** *see* Potassium Chloride *on page 1380*
- ◆ **Klor-Con® 10** *see* Potassium Chloride *on page 1380*
- ◆ **Klor-Con®/25** *see* Potassium Chloride *on page 1380*
- ◆ **Klor-Con®/EF** *see* Potassium Bicarbonate and Potassium Citrate *on page 1380*
- ◆ **Klor-Con® M10** *see* Potassium Chloride *on page 1380*
- ◆ **Klor-Con® M15** *see* Potassium Chloride *on page 1380*
- ◆ **Klor-Con® M20** *see* Potassium Chloride *on page 1380*
- ◆ **K-Lyte/Cl** *see* Potassium Bicarbonate and Potassium Chloride *on page 1380*
- ◆ **KMD 3213** *see* Silodosin *on page 1554*
- ◆ **Koffex DM-D (Can)** *see* Pseudoephedrine and Dextromethorphan *on page 1431*
- ◆ **Koffex DM-Expectorant (Can)** *see* Guaifenesin and Dextromethorphan *on page 810*
- ◆ **Koffex Expectorant (Can)** *see* GuaiFENesin *on page 809*
- ◆ **Kogenate® FS** *see* Antihemophilic Factor (Recombinant) *on page 127*
- ◆ **Kolephrin® GG/DM [OTC]** *see* Guaifenesin and Dextromethorphan *on page 810*
- ◆ **Kombiglyze™ XR** *see* Saxagliptin and Metformin *on page 1541*
- ◆ **Konakion (Can)** *see* Phytonadione *on page 1351*
- ◆ **Konsyl® [OTC]** *see* Psyllium *on page 1432*
- ◆ **Konsyl-D™ [OTC]** *see* Psyllium *on page 1432*
- ◆ **Konsyl® Easy Mix™ [OTC]** *see* Psyllium *on page 1432*
- ◆ **Konsyl® Orange [OTC]** *see* Psyllium *on page 1432*
- ◆ **Konsyl® Original [OTC]** *see* Psyllium *on page 1432*
- ◆ **Koāte®-DVI** *see* Antihemophilic Factor (Human) *on page 125*
- ◆ **K-Phos® MF** *see* Potassium Phosphate and Sodium Phosphate *on page 1386*
- ◆ **K-Phos® Neutral** *see* Potassium Phosphate and Sodium Phosphate *on page 1386*
- ◆ **K-Phos® No. 2** *see* Potassium Phosphate and Sodium Phosphate *on page 1386*
- ◆ **K-Phos® Original** *see* Potassium Acid Phosphate *on page 1379*
- ◆ **Kristalose®** *see* Lactulose *on page 964*
- ◆ **Krystexxa™** *see* Pegloticase *on page 1315*
- ◆ **K-Tab®** *see* Potassium Chloride *on page 1380*
- ◆ **Kuvan™** *see* Sapropterin *on page 1536*
- ◆ **Kwellada-P™ (Can)** *see* Permethrin *on page 1336*
- ◆ **Kytril®** *see* Granisetron *on page 807*
- ◆ **L-749,345** *see* Ertapenem *on page 615*
- ◆ **L-758,298** *see* Fosaprepitant *on page 759*
- ◆ **L-M-X® 4 [OTC]** *see* Lidocaine (Topical) *on page 1009*
- ◆ **L-M-X® 5 [OTC]** *see* Lidocaine (Topical) *on page 1009*
- ◆ **L 754030** *see* Aprepitant *on page 137*
- ◆ **LA 20304a** *see* Gemifloxacin *on page 786*

Labetalol (la BET a lole)

Brand Names: U.S. Trandate®

Brand Names: Canada Apo-Labetalol®; Labetalol Hydrochloride Injection, USP; Normodyne®; Trandate®

Index Terms Ibidomide Hydrochloride; Labetalol Hydrochloride

Pharmacologic Category Beta Blocker With Alpha-Blocking Activity

Additional Appendix Information

Beta-Blockers *on page 1884*
Hypertension *on page 2001*

Use Treatment of mild-to-severe hypertension; I.V. for severe hypertension (eg, hypertensive emergencies)

Unlabeled Use Pediatric hypertension; management of pre-eclampsia; severe hypertension in pregnancy; hypertension during acute ischemic stroke

Pregnancy Risk Factor C

Pregnancy Considerations Because adverse events were observed in some animal reproduction studies, labetalol is classified as pregnancy category C. Labetalol crosses the placenta and can be detected in cord blood and infant serum after delivery. It has been shown to decrease maternal blood pressure without significantly effecting placental blood flow. In a cohort study, an increased risk of cardiovascular defects was observed following maternal use of beta-blockers during pregnancy. Intrauterine growth restriction (IUGR), small placentas, as well as fetal/neonatal bradycardia, hypoglycemia, and/or respiratory depression have been observed following *in utero* exposure to beta-blockers as a class. Adequate facilities for monitoring infants at birth should be available. Untreated chronic maternal hypertension and pre-eclampsia are also associated with adverse events in the fetus, infant, and mother. The pharmacokinetics of labetalol are not significantly changed during the third trimester of pregnancy. Labetalol is considered an appropriate agent for the treatment of hypertension in pregnancy; intravenous labetalol is also used for the management of pre-eclampsia.

Lactation Enters breast milk/use caution (AAP rates "compatible"; AAP 2001 update pending)

Contraindications Hypersensitivity to labetalol or any component of the formulation; severe bradycardia; heart block greater than first degree (except in patients with a functioning artificial pacemaker); cardiogenic shock; bronchial asthma; uncompensated cardiac failure; conditions associated with severe and prolonged hypotension

Warnings/Precautions Consider pre-existing conditions such as sick sinus syndrome before initiating. Symptomatic hypotension with or without syncope may occur with labetalol; close monitoring of patient is required especially with initial dosing and dosing increases; blood pressure must be lowered at a rate appropriate for the patient's clinical condition. Initiation with a low dose and gradual up-titration may help to decrease the occurrence of hypotension or syncope. Patients should be advised to avoid driving or other hazardous tasks during initiation of therapy due to the risk of syncope. Orthostatic hypotension may occur with I.V. administration; patient should remain supine during and for up to 3 hours after I.V. administration. Use with caution in impaired hepatic function; bioavailability is increased due to decreased first-pass metabolism. Severe hepatic injury including some fatalities have also been rarely reported with use: periodically monitor LFTs with prolonged use. Use with caution in patients with diabetes mellitus; may potentiate hypoglycemia and/or mask signs and symptoms. Bradycardia may be observed more frequently in elderly patients (>65 years of age); dosage reductions may be necessary. May also reduce release of insulin in response to hyperglycemia; dosage of antidiabetic agents may need to be adjusted. May mask signs of hyperthyroidism (eg, tachycardia); if hyperthyroidism is suspected, carefully manage and monitor; abrupt withdrawal may exacerbate symptoms of hyperthyroidism or precipitate thyroid storm. Elimination of labetalol is reduced in elderly patients; lower maintenance doses may be required.

Use only with extreme caution in compensated heart failure and monitor for a worsening of the condition. Beta-blocker therapy should not be withdrawn abruptly (particularly in patients with CAD), but gradually tapered to avoid acute tachycardia, hypertension, and/or ischemia. Chronic beta-blocker therapy should not be routinely withdrawn prior to major surgery. Use caution with concurrent use of digoxin, verapamil, or diltiazem; bradycardia or heart block can occur. Use with caution in patients receiving inhaled anesthetic agents known to depress myocardial contractility. Patients with bronchospastic disease should not receive beta-blockers; if used at all, should be used cautiously with close monitoring. Use with caution in patients with myasthenia gravis or psychiatric disease (may cause or exacerbate CNS depression). Can precipitate or aggravate symptoms of arterial insufficiency in patients with PVD and Raynaud's disease; use with caution and monitor for progression of arterial obstruction. If possible, obtain diagnostic tests for pheochromocytoma prior to use. May induce or exacerbate psoriasis. Labetalol has been shown to be effective in lowering blood pressure and relieving symptoms in patients with pheochromocytoma. However, some patients have experienced paradoxical hypertensive responses; use with caution in patients with pheochromocytoma. Additional alpha-blockade may be required during use of labetalol. Use caution with history of severe anaphylaxis to allergens; patients taking beta-blockers may become more sensitive to repeated challenges. Treatment of anaphylaxis (eg, epinephrine) in patients taking beta-blockers may be ineffective or promote undesirable effects.

Adverse Reactions

>10%:

- Cardiovascular: Postural hypotension (I.V. use; ≤58%)
- Central nervous system: Dizziness (1% to 20%), fatigue (1% to 11%)
- Gastrointestinal: Nausea (≤19%)

1% to 10%:

- Cardiovascular: Hypotension (1% to 5%), edema (≤2%), flushing (1%), ventricular arrhythmia (I.V. use; 1%)
- Central nervous system: Somnolence (3%), headache (2%), vertigo (1% to 2%)
- Dermatologic: Scalp tingling (≤7%), pruritus (1%), rash (1%)
- Gastrointestinal: Dyspepsia (≤4%), vomiting (≤3%), taste disturbance (1%)
- Genitourinary: Ejaculatory failure (≤5%), impotence (1% to 4%)
- Hepatic: Transaminases increased (4%)
- Neuromuscular & skeletal: Paresthesia (≤5%), weakness (1%)
- Ocular: Vision abnormal (1%)
- Renal: BUN increased (≤8%)
- Respiratory: Nasal congestion (1% to 6%), dyspnea (2%)
- Miscellaneous: Diaphoresis (≤4%)

<1% (Limited to important or life-threatening): Alopecia (reversible), anaphylactoid reaction, ANA positive, angioedema, bradycardia, bronchospasm, cholestatic jaundice, CHF, diabetes insipidus, heart block, hepatic necrosis, hepatitis, hypersensitivity, Peyronie's disease, psoriaform rash, Raynaud's syndrome, syncope, systemic lupus erythematosus, toxic myopathy, urinary retention, urticaria

Other adverse reactions noted with beta-adrenergic blocking agents include mental depression, catatonia, disorientation, short-term memory loss, emotional lability, clouded sensorium, intensification of pre-existing AV block, laryngospasm, respiratory distress, agranulocytosis, thrombocytopenic purpura, nonthrombocytopenic purpura, mesenteric artery thrombosis, and ischemic colitis.

Drug Interactions

Metabolism/Transport Effects None known.

Avoid Concomitant Use

Avoid concomitant use of Labetalol with any of the following: Beta2-Agonists; Floctafenine; Methacholine

Increased Effect/Toxicity

Labetalol may increase the levels/effects of: Alpha-/Beta-Agonists (Direct-Acting); Alpha1-Blockers; Alpha2-Agonists; Amifostine; Antihypertensives; Antipsychotic Agents (Phenothiazines); Bupivacaine; Cardiac Glycosides; Cholinergic Agonists; Fingolimod; Hypotensive Agents; Insulin; Lidocaine; Lidocaine (Systemic); Lidocaine (Topical); Mepivacaine; Methacholine; Midodrine; RiTUXimab; Sulfonylureas

The levels/effects of Labetalol may be increased by: Acetylcholinesterase Inhibitors; Aminoquinolines (Antimalarial); Amiodarone; Anilidopiperidine Opioids; Antipsychotic Agents (Phenothiazines); Calcium Channel Blockers (Dihydropyridine); Calcium Channel Blockers (Nondihydropyridine); Diazoxide; Dipyridamole; Disopyramide; Dronedarone; Floctafenine; Herbs (Hypotensive Properties); MAO Inhibitors; Pentoxifylline; Phosphodiesterase 5 Inhibitors; Propafenone; Prostacyclin Analogues; QuiNIDine; Reserpine; Selective Serotonin Reuptake Inhibitors

Decreased Effect

Labetalol may decrease the levels/effects of: Beta2-Agonists; Theophylline Derivatives

The levels/effects of Labetalol may be decreased by: Barbiturates; Herbs (Hypertensive Properties); Methylphenidate; Nonsteroidal Anti-Inflammatory Agents; Rifamycin Derivatives; Yohimbine

Ethanol/Nutrition/Herb Interactions

Food: Labetalol serum concentrations may be increased if taken with food.

Herb/Nutraceutical: Avoid dong quai if using for hypertension (has estrogenic activity). Avoid ephedra, yohimbe, ginseng (may worsen hypertension). Avoid natural licorice (causes sodium and water retention and increases potassium loss). Avoid garlic (may have increased antihypertensive effect).

Stability

Tablets: Store at room temperature (refer to manufacturer's labeling for detailed storage requirements). Protect from light and excessive moisture.

Injectable: Store at room temperature (refer to manufacturer's labeling for detailed storage requirements); do not freeze. Protect from light. The solution is clear to slightly yellow.

Parenteral admixture: Stability of parenteral admixture at room temperature (25°C) and refrigeration temperature (4°C): 3 days.

Standard concentration: 500 mg/250 mL D_5W.

Minimum volume: 250 mL D_5W.

Mechanism of Action Blocks alpha-, $beta_1$-, and $beta_2$-adrenergic receptor sites; elevated renins are reduced. The ratios of alpha- to beta-blockade differ depending on the route of administration: 1:3 (oral) and 1:7 (I.V.).

Pharmacodynamics/Kinetics

Onset of action: Oral: 20 minutes to 2 hours; I.V.: 2-5 minutes

Peak effect: Oral: 1-4 hours; I.V.: 5-15 minutes

Duration: Blood pressure response:
Oral: 8-12 hours (dose dependent)
I.V.: 2-18 hours (dose dependent; based on single and multiple sequential doses of 0.25-0.5 mg/kg with cumulative dosing up to 3.25 mg/kg)
Absorption: Complete
Distribution: V_d: Adults: 3-16 L/kg; mean: <9.4 L/kg; moderately lipid soluble, therefore, can enter CNS
Protein binding: 50%
Metabolism: Hepatic, primarily via glucuronide conjugation; extensive first-pass effect
Bioavailability: Oral: 25%; increased with liver disease, elderly, and concurrent cimetidine
Half-life elimination: Oral: 6-8 hours; I.V.: ~5.5 hours
Time to peak, plasma: Oral: 1-2 hours
Excretion: Urine (55% to 60% as glucuronide conjugates, <5% as unchanged drug)
Clearance: Possibly decreased in neonates/infants

Dosage

Children: Due to limited documentation of its use, labetalol should be initiated cautiously in pediatric patients with careful dosage adjustment and blood pressure monitoring.
Oral: Hypertension (unlabeled use): Initial: 1-3 mg/kg/day, in 2 divided doses; maximum: 10-12 mg/kg/day, up to 1200 mg/day
I.V., intermittent bolus doses of 0.3-1 mg/kg/dose have been reported.
For treatment of pediatric hypertensive emergencies, initial continuous infusions of 0.4-1 mg/kg/hour with a maximum of 3 mg/kg/hour have been used. Administration requires the use of an infusion pump.
Adults:
Hypertension: Oral: Initial: 100 mg twice daily, may increase as needed every 2-3 days by 100 mg twice daily (titration increments not to exceed 200 mg twice daily) until desired response is obtained; usual dose: 100-400 mg twice daily (JNC 7); may require up to 2.4 g/day.
Acute hypertension (hypertensive emergency/urgency):
I.V. bolus: Per the manufacturer: Initial: 20 mg I.V. push over 2 minutes; may administer 40-80 mg at 10-minute intervals, up to 300 mg total cumulative dose; as appropriate, follow with oral antihypertensive regimen
I.V. infusion (acute loading): Per the manufacturer: Initial: 2 mg/minute; titrate to response up to 300 mg total cumulative dose (eg, discontinue after 2.5 hours of 2 mg/minute); usual total dose required: 50-200 mg; as appropriate, follow with oral antihypertensive regimen
Note: Although loading infusions are well described in the product labeling, the labeling is silent in specific clinical situations, such as in the patient who has an initial response to labetalol infusions but cannot be converted to an oral route for subsequent dosing. There is limited documentation of prolonged continuous infusions (ie, >300 mg/day). In rare clinical situations, higher continuous infusion doses up to 6 mg/minute have been used in the critical care setting (eg, aortic dissection) and up to 8 mg/minute (eg, hypertension with ongoing acute ischemic stroke). At these doses, it may be best to consider an alternative agent if the labetalol infusion is not meeting the goals of therapy. At the other extreme, continuous infusions at relatively low doses (0.03-0.1 mg/minute) have been used in some settings (following loading infusion in patients who are unable to be converted to oral regimens or in some cases as a continuation of outpatient oral regimens). These prolonged infusions should not be confused with loading infusions. Because of wide variation in the use of infusions, an awareness of institutional policies and practices is extremely important. Careful clarification of orders and specific infusion rates/units is required to avoid confusion. Due to the prolonged duration of action, careful monitoring should be extended for the duration of the infusion and for several hours after the infusion. Excessive administration may result in prolonged hypotension and/or bradycardia.
Arterial hypertension in acute ischemic stroke (unlabeled use [Adams, 2007; Jauch, 2010]): I.V.:
Patient otherwise eligible for reperfusion treatment (eg, alteplase): Blood pressure (BP): Systolic >185 mm Hg or diastolic >110 mm Hg: 10-20 mg over 1-2 minutes; may repeat once. If BP does not decline and remains >185/110 mm Hg, alteplase should not be administered.
Management of BP during and after reperfusion treatment (eg, alteplase): BP: Systolic ≥180 mm Hg or diastolic ≥105 mm Hg: 10 mg over 1-2 minutes; may repeat every 10-20 minutes (maximum dose: 300 mg) **or** 10 mg followed by an infusion of 2-8 mg/minute. If hypertension is refractory, consider other I.V. antihypertensives (eg, nitroprusside)
I.V. to oral conversion: Upon discontinuation of I.V. infusion, may initiate oral dose of 200 mg followed in 6-12 hours with an additional dose of 200-400 mg. Thereafter, dose patients with 400-2400 mg/day in divided doses depending on blood pressure response.
Elderly: Refer to adult dosing.
Hypertension: Oral:
Manufacturer's recommendations: Initial: 100 mg twice daily; may titrate in increments of 100 mg twice daily; usual maintenance: 100-200 mg twice daily
ACCF/AHA Expert Consensus recommendations: Consider lower initial doses and titrating to response (Aronow, 2011)

Dosage adjustment in renal impairment: Dialysis: Not removed by hemo- or peritoneal dialysis; supplemental dose is not necessary.

Dosage adjustment in hepatic impairment: Dosage reduction may be necessary.

Administration Bolus dose may be administered I.V. push at a rate of 10 mg/minute; may follow with continuous I.V. infusion

Monitoring Parameters Blood pressure, standing and sitting/supine, pulse, cardiac monitor and blood pressure monitor required for I.V. administration

Test Interactions False-positive urine catecholamines, vanillylmandelic acid (VMA) if measured by fluorometric or photometric methods; use HPLC or specific catecholamine radioenzymatic technique; false-positive amphetamine if measured by thin-layer chromatography or radioenzymatic assay (gas chromatographic-mass spectrometer technique should be used)

Dosage Forms Excipient information presented when available (limited, particularly for generics); consult specific product labeling.
Injection, solution, as hydrochloride: 5 mg/mL (4 mL, 20 mL, 40 mL)
Trandate®: 5 mg/mL (20 mL, 40 mL) [contains edetate disodium]
Tablet, oral, as hydrochloride: 100 mg, 200 mg, 300 mg
Trandate®: 100 mg [scored]
Trandate®: 200 mg [scored; contains sodium benzoate]
Trandate®: 300 mg [scored]

Extemporaneous Preparations A 40 mg/mL labetalol hydrochloride oral suspension may be made with tablets and one of three different vehicles (cherry syrup, a 1:1 mixture of Ora-Sweet® and Ora-Plus®, or a 1:1 mixture of Ora-Sweet® SF and Ora-Plus®). Crush sixteen 300 mg tablets in a mortar and reduce to a fine powder. Add 20 mL of the chosen vehicle and mix to a uniform paste; mix while adding the vehicle in incremental proportions to **almost** 120 mL; transfer to a calibrated bottle, rinse mortar with vehicle, and add quantity of vehicle sufficient to make 120 mL. Label "shake well" and "protect from light". Stable for 60 days when stored in amber plastic prescription bottles in the dark at room temperature or refrigerated (Allen, 1996).

Extemporaneously prepared solutions of labetalol hydrochloride (approximate concentrations 7-10 mg/mL) prepared in distilled water, simple syrup, apple juice, grape juice, and orange juice were stable for 4 weeks when stored in amber glass or plastic prescription bottles at room temperature or refrigerated (Nahata, 1991).

Allen LV Jr and Erickson MA 3rd, "Stability of Labetalol Hydrochloride, Metoprolol Tartrate, Verapamil Hydrochloride, and Spironolactone with Hydrochlorothiazide in Extemporaneously Compounded Oral Liquids," *Am J Health Syst Pharm*, 1996, 53(19):2304-9.

Nahata MC, "Stability of Labetalol Hydrochloride in Distilled Water, Simple Syrup, and Three Fruit Juices," *DICP*, 1991, 25(5):465-9.

◆ **Labetalol Hydrochloride** *see* Labetalol *on page 960*

◆ **Labetalol Hydrochloride Injection, USP (Can)** *see* Labetalol *on page 960*

Lacosamide (la KOE sa mide)

Brand Names: U.S. Vimpat®

Brand Names: Canada Vimpat®

Index Terms ADD 234037; Harkoseride; LCM; SPM 927

Pharmacologic Category Anticonvulsant, Miscellaneous

Additional Appendix Information

Anticonvulsant Drugs of Choice *on page 1873*

Use Adjunctive therapy in the treatment of partial-onset seizures

Pregnancy Risk Factor C

Pregnancy Considerations Developmental toxicities were observed in animal studies. There are no adequate and well-controlled studies in pregnant women; only use during pregnancy if potential benefit justifies the potential risk to the fetus. Two registries are available for women exposed to lacosamide during pregnancy:

Antiepileptic Drug Pregnancy Registry (888-233-2334 or http://www.aedpregnancyregistry.org)

UCB AED Pregnancy Registry (888-537-7734)

Lactation Excretion in breast milk unknown/not recommended

Medication Guide Available Yes

Contraindications There are no contraindications listed in manufacturer's labeling.

Warnings/Precautions Antiepileptics are associated with an increased risk of suicidal behavior/thoughts with use (regardless of indication); patients should be monitored for signs/symptoms of depression, suicidal tendencies, and other unusual behavior changes during therapy and instructed to inform their healthcare provider immediately if symptoms occur. CNS effects may occur; patients should be cautioned about performing tasks which require alertness (eg, operating machinery or driving). Lacosamide may prolong PR interval; use caution in patients with conduction problems (eg, first/second degree atrioventricular block and sick sinus syndrome without pacemaker), myocardial ischemia, heart failure, or if concurrent use with other drugs that prolong the PR interval; ECG is recommended prior to initiating therapy and when at steady state. During investigational trials, atrial fibrillation/flutter, or syncope occurred slightly more often in patients with diabetic neuropathy and/or cardiovascular disease. Use caution with renal or hepatic impairment; dosage adjustment may be necessary. Multiorgan hypersensitivity reactions can occur (rare); monitor patient and discontinue therapy if necessary. Withdraw therapy gradually (≥1 week) to minimize the potential of increased seizure frequency. Effects with ethanol may be potentiated. Some products may contain phenylalanine.

Adverse Reactions

>10%:

Central nervous system: Dizziness (31%), headache (13%)

Gastrointestinal: Nausea (11%)

Ocular: Diplopia (11%)

1% to 10%:

Cardiovascular: Syncope (1%; dose-related: >400 mg/day)

Central nervous system: Fatigue (9%), ataxia (8%), somnolence (7%), coordination impaired (4%), vertigo (4%), depression (2%), memory impairment (2%)

Dermatologic: Pruritus (2%)

Gastrointestinal: Vomiting (9%), diarrhea (4%)

Hepatic: ALT increased (1%)

Local: Contusion (3%), skin laceration (3%), injection site pain/discomfort (2.5%), irritation (1%)

Neuromuscular & skeletal: Tremor (7%), gait instability (2%), weakness (2%)

Ocular: Blurred vision (8%), nystagmus (5%)

<1% (Limited to important or life-threatening): Anemia, atrial fibrillation/flutter, atrioventricular block, attention disturbance, bradycardia, cerebellar syndrome, cognitive dysfunction, confusion, constipation, dysarthria, dyspepsia, erythema (injection site), euphoria-like subjective responses, falling, fever, hepatitis, hypoesthesia (including oral), inebriation-like feeling, irritability, mood changes, multiorgan hypersensitivity, muscle spasm, nephritis, neutropenia, palpitation, paresthesia, rash, tinnitus, xerostomia

Drug Interactions

Metabolism/Transport Effects Substrate of CYP2C19 (minor); **Note:** Assignment of Major/Minor substrate status based on clinically relevant drug interaction potential; **Inhibits** CYP2C19 (weak)

Avoid Concomitant Use There are no known interactions where it is recommended to avoid concomitant use.

Increased Effect/Toxicity There are no known significant interactions involving an increase in effect.

Decreased Effect

The levels/effects of Lacosamide may be decreased by: CarBAMazepine; Fosphenytoin; PHENobarbital; Phenytoin

Ethanol/Nutrition/Herb Interactions Ethanol: Avoid ethanol (may increase CNS depression).

Stability

Injection: Store at 20°C to 25°C (68°F to 77°F); excursions permitted between 15°C to 30°C (59°F to 86°F). Do not freeze. Can be administered without further dilution or may be mixed with compatible diluents (NS, LR, D_5W). Reconstituted solution is stable for ≤24 hours in glass or PVC at room temperature of 15°C to 30°C (59°F to 86°F). Any unused portion should be discarded.

Oral solution, tablets: Store at 20°C to 25°C (68°F to 77°F); excursions permitted between 15°C to 30°C (59°F to 86°F). Do not freeze oral solution. Discard any unused portion of oral solution after 7 weeks.

Mechanism of Action *In vitro* studies have shown that lacosamide stabilizes hyperexcitable neuronal membranes and inhibits repetitive neuronal firing by enhancing the slow inactivation of sodium channels (with no effects on fast inactivation of sodium channels).

Pharmacodynamics/Kinetics

Absorption: Oral: Completely

Distribution: V_d: ~0.6 L/kg

Protein binding: <15%

Metabolism: Hepatic; forms metabolite, O-desmethyl-lacosamide (inactive)

Bioavailability: ~100%

Half-life elimination: ~13 hours
Time to peak, plasma: Oral: 1-4 hours postdose
Excretion: Urine (95%; 40% as unchanged drug, 30% as inactive metabolite, 20% as uncharacterized metabolite); feces (<0.5%)

Dosage Oral, I.V.: Adolescents ≥17 years and Adults:
Partial onset seizure:
Initial: 50 mg twice daily; may be increased at weekly intervals by 100 mg/day
Maintenance dose: 200-400 mg/day
Note: When switching from oral to I.V. formulations, the total daily dose and frequency should be the same; I.V. therapy should only be used temporarily.

Dosing adjustment in renal impairment: Use caution when titrating dose.
Mild-to-moderate renal impairment: No dose adjustment necessary
Severe renal impairment (Cl_{cr} ≤30 mL/minute): Maximum dose: 300 mg/day
Hemodialysis: Removed by hemodialysis; after 4-hour HD treatment, a supplemental dose of up to 50% should be considered.
Dosing adjustment in hepatic impairment: Use caution when titrating dose.
Mild-to-moderate hepatic impairment: Maximum dose: 300 mg/day
Severe hepatic impairment: Use is not recommended

Dietary Considerations Oral solution and tablets may be taken with or without food. Some products may contain phenylalanine.

Administration
Injection: Administer over 30-60 minutes. Twice daily I.V. infusions have been used for up to 5 days.
Oral solution, tablets: May be administered with or without food. Oral solution should be administered with a calibrated measuring device (not a household teaspoon or tablespoon).

Monitoring Parameters Patients with conduction problems or severe cardiac disease should have ECG tracing prior to start of therapy and when at steady-state; suicidality (eg, suicidal thoughts, depression, behavioral changes)

Dosage Forms Excipient information presented when available (limited, particularly for generics); consult specific product labeling.
Injection, solution:
Vimpat®: 10 mg/mL (20 mL)
Solution, oral:
Vimpat®: 10 mg/mL (20 mL) [contains phenylalanine 0.32 mg/20 mL, propylene glycol; strawberry flavor]
Tablet, oral:
Vimpat®: 50 mg, 100 mg, 150 mg, 200 mg

Controlled Substance C-V

◆ **LaCrosse Complete [OTC]** *see* Sodium Phosphates *on page 1573*

◆ **Lactoflavin** *see* Riboflavin *on page 1483*

Lactulose (LAK tyoo lose)

Brand Names: U.S. Constulose; Enulose; Generlac; Kristalose®

Brand Names: Canada Acilac; Apo-Lactulose®; Laxilose; PMS-Lactulose

Pharmacologic Category Ammonium Detoxicant; Laxative, Osmotic

Additional Appendix Information
Laxatives, Classification and Properties *on page 1893*

Use Prevention and treatment of portal-systemic encephalopathy (including hepatic precoma and coma); treatment of constipation

Pregnancy Risk Factor B

Lactation Excretion in breast milk unknown/use caution

Contraindications Use in patients requiring a low galactose diet

Warnings/Precautions Use with caution in patients with diabetes mellitus; solution contains galactose and lactose. Monitor periodically for electrolyte imbalance when lactulose is used >6 months or in patients predisposed to electrolyte abnormalities (eg, elderly). Hepatic disease may predispose patients to electrolyte imbalance. Infants receiving lactulose may develop hyponatremia and dehydration. Patients receiving lactulose and an oral anti-infective agent should be monitored for possible inadequate response to lactulose. During proctoscopy or colonoscopy procedures involving electrocautery, a theoretical risk of reaction between H_2 gas accumulation and electrical spark may exist; thorough bowel cleansing with a nonfermentable solution is recommended.

Adverse Reactions Frequency not defined.
Endocrine & metabolic: Dehydration, hypernatremia, hypokalemia
Gastrointestinal: Abdominal discomfort, abdominal distention, belching, cramping, diarrhea (excessive dose), flatulence, nausea, vomiting

Drug Interactions
Metabolism/Transport Effects None known.
Avoid Concomitant Use There are no known interactions where it is recommended to avoid concomitant use.
Increased Effect/Toxicity There are no known significant interactions involving an increase in effect.
Decreased Effect There are no known significant interactions involving a decrease in effect.

Stability Store at room temperature; do not freeze. Protect from light. Discard solution if cloudy or very dark. Prolonged exposure to cold temperatures will cause thickening which will return to normal upon warming to room temperature.

Mechanism of Action The bacterial degradation of lactulose resulting in an acidic pH inhibits the diffusion of NH_3 into the blood by causing the conversion of NH_3 to NH_4^+; also enhances the diffusion of NH_3 from the blood into the gut where conversion to NH_4^+ occurs; produces an osmotic effect in the colon with resultant distention promoting peristalsis; reduces blood ammonia concentration to reduce the degree of portal systemic encephalopathy

Pharmacodynamics/Kinetics
Onset:
Constipation: Up to 24-48 hours to produce a normal bowel movement
Encephalopathy: At least 24-48 hours
Absorption: Not appreciable
Metabolism: Via colonic flora to lactic acid and acetic acid; requires colonic flora for drug activation
Excretion: Primarily feces; urine (≤3%)

Dosage
Constipation: Oral:
Children (unlabeled use): 0.7-2 g/kg/day (1-3 mL/kg/day) in divided doses, maximum 40 g/day (60 mL/day) (NASPGHAN, 2006)
Adults: 10-20 g (15-30 mL) daily; may increase to 40 g (60 mL) daily if necessary
Prevention of portal systemic encephalopathy (PSE): Oral:
Infants: 1.7-6.7 g/day (2.5-10 mL/day) in divided doses; adjust dosage to produce 2-3 stools/day
Children: 26.7-60 g/day (40-90 mL/day) in divided doses; adjust dosage to produce 2-3 stools/day
Adults: 20-30 g (30-45 mL) 3-4 times/day; adjust dose every 1-2 days to produce 2-3 soft stools/day

Treatment of acute PSE: Adults:

Oral: 20-30 g (30-45 mL) every 1 hour to induce rapid laxation; reduce to 20-30 g (30-45 mL) 3-4 times/day after laxation is achieved titrate to produce 2-3 soft stools/day

Rectal administration (retention enema): 200 g (300 mL) diluted with 700 mL of water or NS via rectal balloon catheter; retain for 30-60 minutes; may repeat every 4-6 hours; transition to oral treatment prior to discontinuing rectal administration

Dietary Considerations Contraindicated in patients on galactose-restricted diet; may be mixed with fruit juice, milk, water, or citrus-flavored carbonated beverages.

Administration

Oral solution: May mix with fruit juice, water or milk.

Crystals for oral solution: Dissolve contents of packet in 120 mL water.

Rectal: Mix with water or normal saline; administer as retention enema using a rectal balloon catheter; retain for 30-60 minutes. Transition to oral lactulose when appropriate (able to take oral medication and no longer a risk for aspiration) prior to discontinuing rectal administration

Monitoring Parameters Blood pressure, standing/supine; serum electrolytes, serum ammonia; bowel movement patterns, fluid status

Dosage Forms Excipient information presented when available (limited, particularly for generics); consult specific product labeling. [DSC] = Discontinued product

Crystals for solution, oral:

Kristalose®: 10 g/packet (30s); 20 g/packet (30s)

Solution, oral: 10 g/15 mL (15 mL, 30 mL, 237 mL, 473 mL, 500 mL, 946 mL, 1892 mL)

Constulose: 10 g/15 mL (237 mL [DSC], 946 mL)

Enulose: 10 g/15 mL (473 mL)

Solution, oral/rectal: 10 g/15 mL (237 mL, 473 mL, 946 mL)

Generlac: 10 g/15 mL (473 mL, 1892 mL)

- **Ladakamycin** *see* AzaCITIDine *on page 174*
- **LAIV** *see* Influenza Virus Vaccine (Live/Attenuated) *on page 901*
- **L-AmB** *see* Amphotericin B (Liposomal) *on page 113*
- **LaMICtal®** *see* LamoTRIgine *on page 967*
- **Lamictal® (Can)** *see* LamoTRIgine *on page 967*
- **LaMICtal® ODT™** *see* LamoTRIgine *on page 967*
- **LaMICtal® XR™** *see* LamoTRIgine *on page 967*
- **LamISIL®** *see* Terbinafine (Systemic) *on page 1648*
- **Lamisil® (Can)** *see* Terbinafine (Systemic) *on page 1648*
- **Lamisil® (Can)** *see* Terbinafine (Topical) *on page 1649*
- **LamISIL AT® [OTC]** *see* Terbinafine (Topical) *on page 1649*

LamiVUDine (la MI vyoo deen)

Brand Names: U.S. Epivir-HBV®; Epivir®

Brand Names: Canada 3TC®; Heptovir®

Index Terms 3TC

Pharmacologic Category Antiretroviral Agent, Reverse Transcriptase Inhibitor (Nucleoside)

Additional Appendix Information

Management of Healthcare Worker Exposures to HBV, HCV, and HIV *on page 1935*

Perinatal HIV Guidelines *on page 1946*

Use

Epivir®: Treatment of HIV infection when antiretroviral therapy is warranted; should always be used as part of a multidrug regimen (at least three antiretroviral agents)

Epivir-HBV®: Treatment of chronic hepatitis B associated with evidence of hepatitis B viral replication and active liver inflammation. Resistance develops rapidly in hepatitis B; consider use only if other anti-HBV antiviral agents with more favorable resistance patterns cannot be used.

Unlabeled Use Postexposure prophylaxis for HIV exposure as part of a multidrug regimen

Pregnancy Risk Factor C

Pregnancy Considerations Adverse events were observed in some animal reproduction studies. Lamivudine crosses the human placenta. No increased risk of overall birth defects has been observed following first trimester exposure according to data collected by the antiretroviral pregnancy registry. The pharmacokinetics of lamivudine during pregnancy are not significantly altered and dosage adjustment is not required. Cases of lactic acidosis/hepatic steatosis syndrome related to mitochondrial toxicity have been reported in pregnant women with prolonged use of nucleoside analogues. It is not known if pregnancy itself potentiates this known side effect; however, women may be at increased risk of lactic acidosis and liver damage. In addition, these adverse events are similar to other rare but life-threatening syndromes which occur during pregnancy (eg, HELLP syndrome). Hepatic enzymes and electrolytes should be monitored in women receiving nucleoside analogues and clinicians should watch for early signs of the syndrome. In addition, mitochondrial dysfunction may develop in infants following in utero exposure The DHHS Perinatal HIV Guidelines recommend lamivudine for use during pregnancy; the combination of lamivudine with zidovudine is the recommended dual combination NRTI in pregnancy. The DHHS Perinatal HIV Guidelines consider lamivudine plus tenofovir a recommended dual NRTI/NtRTI backbone for HIV/HBV coinfected pregnant women. Use caution with hepatitis B coinfection; hepatitis B flare may occur if lamivudine is discontinued postpartum.

Regardless of CD4 count or HIV RNA copy number, all HIV-infected pregnant women should receive a combination antepartum antiretroviral (ARV) drug regimen; this includes women who require therapy for their own health, as well as women who do not yet require therapy for their own health. ARV therapy should be started as soon as possible if required for the woman's health or immediately after the first trimester if not needed for the mothers health (although earlier initiation may be considered). Long-term follow-up is recommended for all infants exposed to ARV medications.

Healthcare providers are encouraged to enroll pregnant women exposed to antiretroviral medications in the Antiretroviral Pregnancy Registry (1-800-258-4263 or www.-APRegistry.com). Healthcare providers caring for HIV-infected women and their infants may contact the National Perinatal HIV Hotline (888-448-8765) for clinical consultation (DHHS [perinatal], 2011).

Lactation Enters breast milk/contraindicated

Contraindications Hypersensitivity to lamivudine or any component of the formulation

Warnings/Precautions Use caution with renal impairment; dosage reduction recommended. Use with extreme caution in children with history of pancreatitis or risk factors for development of pancreatitis. Pancreatitis has been reported, particularly in HIV-infected children with a history of nucleoside use. Do not use as monotherapy in treatment of HIV. Lamivudine combined with emtricitabine is not recommended as a dual-NRTI combination due to similar resistance patterns and negligible additive antiviral activity; lamivudine and tenofovir combination is preferred as the NRTIs in a fully suppressive antiretroviral regimen (DHHS, 2011). Treatment of HBV in patients with unrecognized/untreated HIV may lead to rapid HIV resistance. In addition, treatment of HIV in patients with unrecognized/untreated HBV may lead to rapid HBV resistance. Use with caution in combination with interferon alfa with or without ribavirin in HIV/HBV coinfected patients; monitor closely for hepatic decompensation, anemia, or neutropenia; dose reduction or discontinuation of interferon and/or ribavirin may be required if toxicity evident. In HIV/HBV coinfection, lamivudine and tenofovir are a preferred NRTI backbone in a fully suppressive antiretroviral regimen to provide activity against both HIV and HBV (DHHS, 2011). **[U.S. Boxed Warning]: Do not use Epivir-HBV® tablets or Epivir-HBV® oral solution for the treatment of HIV.**

[U.S. Boxed Warning]: Lactic acidosis and severe hepatomegaly with steatosis have been reported, including fatal cases. Use caution in hepatic impairment. Pregnancy, obesity, and/or prolonged therapy may increase the risk of lactic acidosis and liver damage.

Immune reconstitution syndrome may develop resulting in the occurrence of an inflammatory response to an indolent or residual opportunistic infection. May be associated with fat redistribution.

[U.S. Boxed Warning]: Monitor patients closely for several months following discontinuation of therapy for chronic hepatitis B; clinical exacerbations may occur.

Not recommended as first-line therapy of chronic HBV due to high rate of resistance. Consider use only if other anti-HBV antiviral regimens with more favorable resistance patterns cannot be used. May be appropriate for short-term treatment of acute HBV (Lok, 2009). Potential compliance problems, frequency of administration, and adverse effects should be discussed with patients before initiating therapy to help prevent the emergence of resistance.

Adverse Reactions Reported for treatment of HIV or HBV in adults. Incidence data include patients on combination therapy with other antiretroviral agents.

>10%:
- Central nervous system: Headache (21% to 35%), fatigue (24% to 27%), insomnia (11%)
- Gastrointestinal: Nausea (15% to 33%), diarrhea (14% to 18%), pancreatitis (range: 0.3% to 18%; higher percentage in pediatric patients), abdominal pain (9% to 16%), vomiting (13% to 15%)
- Hematologic: Neutropenia (7% to 15%)
- Hepatic: Transaminases increased (2% to 11%)
- Neuromuscular & skeletal: Myalgia (8% to 14%), neuropathy (12%), musculoskeletal pain (12%)
- Respiratory: Nasal signs and symptoms (20%), cough (18%), sore throat (13%)
- Miscellaneous: Infections (25%; includes ear, nose, and throat)

1% to 10%:
- Central nervous system: Dizziness (10%), depression (9%), fever (7% to 10%), chills (7% to 10%)
- Dermatologic: Rash (5% to 9%)
- Gastrointestinal: Anorexia (10%), lipase increased (10%), abdominal cramps (6%), dyspepsia (5%), amylase increased (<1% to 4%), heartburn
- Hematologic: Thrombocytopenia (1% to 4%), hemoglobinemia (2% to 3%)
- Neuromuscular & skeletal: Creatine phosphokinase increased (9%), arthralgia (5% to 7%)

<1% (Limited to important or life-threatening): Alopecia, anaphylaxis, anemia, body fat redistribution, hepatitis B exacerbation, hepatomegaly, hyperbilirubinemia, hyperglycemia, immune reconstitution syndrome, lactic acidosis, lymphadenopathy, muscle weakness, paresthesia, peripheral neuropathy, pruritus, red cell aplasia, rhabdomyolysis, splenomegaly, steatosis, stomatitis, urticaria, weakness, wheezing

Drug Interactions

Metabolism/Transport Effects None known.

Avoid Concomitant Use

Avoid concomitant use of LamiVUDine with any of the following: Emtricitabine

Increased Effect/Toxicity

LamiVUDine may increase the levels/effects of: Emtricitabine

The levels/effects of LamiVUDine may be increased by: Ganciclovir-Valganciclovir; Ribavirin; Trimethoprim

Decreased Effect There are no known significant interactions involving a decrease in effect.

Ethanol/Nutrition/Herb Interactions Food: Food decreases the rate of absorption and C_{max}; however, there is no change in the systemic AUC. Therefore, may be taken with or without food.

Stability

Oral solution:
- Epivir®: Store at 25°C (77°F) tightly closed.
- Epivir-HBV®: Store at 20°C to 25°C (68°F to 77°F) tightly closed.

Tablet: Store at 25°C (77°F); excursions permitted to 15°C to 30°C (59°F to 86°F).

Mechanism of Action Lamivudine is a cytosine analog. After lamivudine is triphosphorylated, the principle mode of action is inhibition of HIV reverse transcription via viral DNA chain termination; inhibits RNA- and DNA-dependent DNA polymerase activities of reverse transcriptase. The monophosphate form of lamivudine is incorporated into the viral DNA by hepatitis B virus polymerase, resulting in DNA chain termination.

Pharmacodynamics/Kinetics

Absorption: Rapid
Distribution: V_d: 1.3 L/kg
Protein binding, plasma: <36%
Metabolism: 4.2% to trans-sulfoxide metabolite
Bioavailability: Absolute; Cp_{max} decreased with food although AUC not significantly affected
- Children: 66%
- Adults: 86% to 87%

Half-life elimination: Children: 2 hours; Adults: 5-7 hours
Time to peak, plasma: Fed: 3.2 hours; Fasted: 0.9 hours
Excretion: Primarily urine (as unchanged drug)

Dosage Oral: **Note:** Use with at least two other antiretroviral agents when treating HIV.

HIV:
- Infants 1-3 months (DHHS [pediatric], 2010): 4 mg/kg/dose twice daily
- Infants and Children 3 months to 16 years: 4 mg/kg/dose twice daily (maximum: 150 mg/dose twice daily)
- *Alternate weight-based dosing using scored 150 mg tablets (DHHS [pediatric], 2010):*
  - 14-21 kg: 75 mg/dose twice daily (150 mg/day)
  - 22-29 kg: 75 mg in the morning, 150 mg in the evening (225 mg/day)
  - ≥30 kg: 150 mg/dose twice daily (300 mg/day)
- Adults: 150 mg twice daily or 300 mg once daily
  - <50 kg (DHHS [pediatric], 2010): 4 mg/kg/dose twice daily (maximum: 150 mg/dose twice daily)

Treatment of hepatitis B (Epivir-HBV®): Note: Not a preferred agent in chronic HBV treatment due to high rates of resistance; consider alternative agents:
- Children 2-17 years: 3 mg/kg/dose once daily (maximum: 100 mg/day)
- Adults: 100 mg/day
- *Treatment duration (AASLD practice guidelines):*
  - Hepatitis Be antigen (HBeAg) positive chronic hepatitis: Treat ≥1 year until HBeAg seroconversion and undetectable serum HBV DNA; continue therapy for ≥6 months after HBeAg seroconversion
  - HBeAg negative chronic hepatitis: Treat >1 year until hepatitis B surface antigen (HBsAg) clearance

Note: Patients not achieving <2 log decrease in serum HBV DNA after at least 6 months of therapy should either receive additional treatment or be switched to an alternative therapy (Lok, 2009).

Treatment of hepatitis B/HIV coinfection (in patients with both infections requiring treatment): Note: The formulation and dosage of Epivir-HBV® are not appropriate for patients infected with both HBV and HIV. Tenofovir and lamivudine are a preferred NRTI backbone in a fully suppressive antiretroviral regimen for the treatment of HIV/HBV coinfection (DHHS, 2011).

Infants and Children: 4 mg/kg/dose (maximum: 150 mg/dose) twice daily, in combination with other antiretrovirals in a HAART regimen (CDC, 2009).

Adolescents and Adults: 150 mg/dose twice daily or 300 mg/dose once daily, in combination with other antiretrovirals in a HAART regimen (DHHS, 2011)

Postexposure prophylaxis for HIV exposure (unlabeled use [CDC, 2005]): Adolescents ≥16 years and Adults: 150 mg/dose twice daily or 300 mg/dose once daily, in combination with zidovudine, tenofovir, stavudine, or didanosine, with or without a protease inhibitor depending on risk

Dosing adjustment in renal impairment: HIV:

Patients ≤16 years: Insufficient data; however, dose reduction should be considered.

Patients >16 years:

Cl_{cr} 30-49 mL/minute: Administer 150 mg once daily

Cl_{cr} 15-29 mL/minute: Administer 150 mg first dose, then 100 mg once daily

Cl_{cr} 5-14 mL/minute: Administer 150 mg first dose, then 50 mg once daily

Cl_{cr} <5 mL/minute: Administer 50 mg first dose, then 25 mg once daily

Dosing adjustment in renal impairment: Hepatitis B:

Adults:

Cl_{cr} 30-49: Administer 100 mg first dose then 50 mg once daily

Cl_{cr} 15-29: Administer 100 mg first dose then 25 mg once daily

Cl_{cr} 5-14: Administer 35 mg first dose then 15 mg once daily

Cl_{cr} <5: Administer 35 mg first dose then 10 mg once daily

Dialysis: Negligible amounts are removed by 4-hour hemodialysis or peritoneal dialysis. Supplemental dosing not needed; however, dosing after dialysis is recommended (DHHS, 2011).

Dietary Considerations May be taken without regard to meals. Some products may contain sucrose.

Administration May be administered without regard to meals. Adjust dosage in renal failure.

Monitoring Parameters Amylase, bilirubin, liver enzymes (every 3 months during therapy), hematologic parameters, HIV viral load, and CD4 count; signs/symptoms of pancreatitis, HBV DNA (every 3-6 months during therapy), HBeAg and anti-HBe (after 1 year of therapy and every 3-6 months thereafter); signs/symptoms of HBV relapse/exacerbation (every 1-3 months for 6 months after discontinuation and every 3-6 months thereafter)

Dosage Forms Excipient information presented when available (limited, particularly for generics); consult specific product labeling. [DSC] = Discontinued product

Solution, oral:

Epivir-HBV®: 5 mg/mL [contains propylene glycol, sucrose 200 mg/mL; strawberry-banana flavor]

Epivir®: 10 mg/mL [DSC] [contains propylene glycol, sucrose 200 mg/mL; strawberry-banana flavor]

Epivir®: 10 mg/mL [ethanol free; contains propylene glycol, sucrose 200 mg/mL; strawberry-banana flavor]

Tablet, oral: 150 mg, 300 mg

Epivir-HBV®: 100 mg

Epivir®: 150 mg [scored]

Epivir®: 300 mg

◆ **Lamivudine, Abacavir, and Zidovudine** *see* Abacavir, Lamivudine, and Zidovudine *on page 20*

◆ **Lamivudine and Abacavir** *see* Abacavir and Lamivudine *on page 20*

Lamivudine and Zidovudine

(la MI vyoo deen & zye DOE vyoo deen)

Brand Names: U.S. Combivir®

Brand Names: Canada Combivir®

Index Terms AZT + 3TC (error-prone abbreviation); Zidovudine and Lamivudine

Pharmacologic Category Antiretroviral Agent, Reverse Transcriptase Inhibitor (Nucleoside)

Additional Appendix Information

Management of Healthcare Worker Exposures to HBV, HCV, and HIV *on page 1935*

Use Treatment of HIV infection when therapy is warranted based on clinical and/or immunological evidence of disease progression

Pregnancy Risk Factor C

Dosage Adolescents ≥30 kg and Adults: Oral: One tablet twice daily

Note: Because this is a fixed-dose combination product, avoid use in patients requiring dosage reduction including children <30 kg, renally-impaired patients with a creatinine clearance <50 mL/minute, hepatic impairment, or those patients experiencing dose-limiting adverse effects.

Additional Information Complete prescribing information for this medication should be consulted for additional detail.

Dosage Forms Excipient information presented when available (limited, particularly for generics); consult specific product labeling.

Tablet, oral: Lamivudine 150 mg and zidovudine 300 mg

Combivir®: Lamivudine 150 mg and zidovudine 300 mg [scored]

LamoTRIgine (la MOE tri jeen)

Brand Names: U.S. LaMICtal®; LaMICtal® ODT™; LaMICtal® XR™

Brand Names: Canada Apo-Lamotrigine®; Lamictal®; Mylan-Lamotrigine; Novo-Lamotrigine; PMS-Lamotrigine; ratio-Lamotrigine; Teva-Lamotrigine

Index Terms BW-430C; LTG

Pharmacologic Category Anticonvulsant, Miscellaneous

Additional Appendix Information

Anticonvulsant Drugs of Choice *on page 1873*

Use Adjunctive therapy in the treatment of generalized seizures of Lennox-Gastaut syndrome, primary generalized tonic-clonic seizures, and partial seizures; conversion to monotherapy in patients with partial seizures who are receiving treatment with valproic acid or a single enzyme-inducing antiepileptic drug (specifically carbamazepine, phenytoin, phenobarbital or primidone); maintenance treatment of bipolar I disorder

Pregnancy Risk Factor C

Pregnancy Considerations Lamotrigine has been found to decrease folate concentrations in animal studies. Teratogenic effects in animals were not observed. Lamotrigine crosses the human placenta and can be measured in the plasma of exposed newborns. Preliminary data from the North American Antiepileptic Drug Pregnancy Registry (NAAED) suggest an increased incidence of cleft lip and/or cleft palate following first trimester exposure. Healthcare providers may enroll patients in the Lamotrigine Pregnancy Registry by calling (800) 336-2176. Patients may enroll themselves in the NAAED registry by calling (888) 233-2334. Additional information is available at www.aedpregnancyregistry.org. Dose of lamotrigine may need adjustment during pregnancy to maintain clinical response; lamotrigine serum levels may decrease during pregnancy and return to prepartum levels following delivery. Monitor frequently during pregnancy, following delivery, and when adding or discontinuing combination hormonal contraceptives.

Lactation Enters breast milk/not recommended (AAP rates "of concern"; AAP 2001 update pending)

Medication Guide Available Yes

Contraindications Hypersensitivity to lamotrigine or any component of the formulation

Warnings/Precautions [U.S. Boxed Warning]: Severe and potentially life-threatening skin rashes requiring hospitalization have been reported; incidence of serious rash is higher in pediatric patients than adults; risk may be increased by coadministration with valproic acid, higher than recommended starting doses, and exceeding recommended dose titration. The majority of cases occur in the first 8 weeks; however, isolated cases may occur after prolonged treatment or in patients without these risk factors. Discontinue at first sign of rash and do not reinitiate therapy unless rash is clearly not drug related. Rare cases of Stevens-Johnson syndrome, toxic epidermal necrolysis, and angioedema have been reported.

Antiepileptics are associated with an increased risk of suicidal behavior/thoughts with use (regardless of indication); patients should be monitored for signs/symptoms of depression, suicidal tendencies, and other unusual behavior changes during therapy and instructed to inform their healthcare provider immediately if symptoms occur.

A spectrum of hematologic effects have been reported with use (eg, neutropenia, leukopenia, thrombocytopenia, pancytopenia, anemias, and rarely, aplastic anemia and pure red cell aplasia); patients with a previous history of adverse hematologic reaction to any drug may be at increased risk. Early detection of hematologic change is important; advise patients of early signs and symptoms including fever, sore throat, mouth ulcers, infections, easy bruising, petechial or purpuric hemorrhage. May be associated with hypersensitivity syndrome (eg, anticonvulsant hypersensitivity syndrome). Multiorgan hypersensitivity reactions (drug reaction with eosinophilia and systemic symptoms [DRESS]) have been reported. Symptoms may include fever, rash, and/or lymphadenopathy; monitor for signs and symptoms of possible disparate manifestations associated with lymphatic, hepatic, renal, and/or hematologic organ systems. Evaluate patient with fever and lymphadenopathy, even if rash is not present; discontinuation and conversion to alternate therapy may be required. Increased risk of developing aseptic meningitis has been reported; symptoms (eg, headache, nuchal rigidity, fever, nausea/vomiting, rash, photophobia) have generally occurred within 1-45 days following therapy initiation. Use caution in patients with renal or hepatic impairment. Avoid abrupt cessation, taper over at least 2 weeks if possible.

May cause CNS depression, which may impair physical or mental abilities. Patients must be cautioned about performing tasks which require mental alertness (eg, operating machinery or driving). Effects with other sedative drugs or ethanol may be potentiated. Binds to melanin and may accumulate in the eye and other melanin-rich tissues; the clinical significance of this is not known. Safety and efficacy have not been established for use as initial monotherapy, conversion to monotherapy from antiepileptic drugs (AED) other than carbamazepine, phenytoin, phenobarbital, primidone or valproic acid or conversion to monotherapy from two or more AEDs. Patients treated for bipolar disorder should be monitored closely for clinical worsening or suicidality; prescriptions should be written for the smallest quantity consistent with good patient care. Hormonal contraceptives may cause a decrease in lamotrigine levels; dose adjustment of the lamotrigine maintenance dose may be required when initiating or discontinuing estrogen-containing oral contraceptives. Valproic acid may cause an increase in lamotrigine levels requiring dose adjustment. There is a potential for medication errors with similar-sounding medications and among different lamotrigine formulations; medication errors have occurred.

Adverse Reactions Percentages reported in adults on monotherapy for epilepsy or bipolar disorder.

>10%: Gastrointestinal: Nausea (7% to 14%)

1% to 10%:

Cardiovascular: Chest pain (5%), peripheral edema (2% to 5%), edema (1% to 5%)

Central nervous system: Insomnia (5% to 10%), somnolence (9%), fatigue (8%), coordination impaired (7%), dizziness (7%), anxiety (5%), pain (5%), ataxia (2% to 5%), irritability (2% to 5%), suicidal ideation (2% to 5%), agitation (1% to 5%), amnesia (1% to 5%), depression (1% to 5%), dream abnormality (1% to 5%), emotional lability (1% to 5%), fever (1% to 5%), hypoesthesia (1% to 5%), migraine (1% to 5%), thought abnormality (1% to 5%), confusion (1%)

Dermatologic: Rash (nonserious: 7%), dermatitis (2% to 5%), dry skin (2% to 5%)

Endocrine & metabolic: Dysmenorrhea (5%), libido increased (2% to 5%)

Gastrointestinal: Vomiting (5% to 9%), dyspepsia (7%), abdominal pain (6%), xerostomia (2% to 6%), constipation (5%), weight loss (5%), anorexia (2% to 5%), peptic ulcer (2% to 5%), rectal hemorrhage (2% to 5%), flatulence (1% to 5%), weight gain (1% to 5%)

Genitourinary: Urinary frequency (1% to 5%)

Neuromuscular & skeletal: Back pain (8%), weakness (2% to 5%), arthralgia (1% to 5%), myalgia (1% to 5%), neck pain (1% to 5%), paresthesia (1%)

Ocular: Nystagmus (2% to 5%), vision abnormal (2% to 5%), amblyopia (1%)

Respiratory: Rhinitis (7%), cough (5%), pharyngitis (5%), bronchitis (2% to 5%), dyspnea (2% to 5%), epistaxis (2% to 5%), sinusitis (1% to 5%)

Miscellaneous: Infection (5%), diaphoresis (2% to 5%), reflexes increased/decreased (2% to 5%), dyspraxia (1% to 5%)

<1%: Any indication (limited to important or life-threatening): Accommodation abnormality, agranulocytosis, alcohol intolerance, allergic reaction, alopecia, anemia, angina, angioedema, aphasia, aplastic anemia, apnea, appetite increased, arthritis, aseptic meningitis, atrial fibrillation, bruising, cerebellar syndrome, cerebral sinus thrombosis, cerebrovascular accident, chills, choreoathetosis, CNS depression/stimulation, conjunctivitis, deafness, deep thrombophlebitis, delirium, delusions, dermatitis (exfoliative, fungal), disseminated intravascular coagulation, dysphagia, dysphoria, dystonia, ECG abnormality, ejaculation abnormal, eructation, erythema multiforme, esophagitis, euphoria, extrapyramidal syndrome, flushing, gastritis, gingivitis, goiter, hallucinations, hematuria, hemiplegia, hemolytic anemia, hemorrhage, hepatitis, hiccup, hirsutism, hot flashes, hyperalgesia, hyperglycemia, hypersensitivity reactions, hypertension, hyperventilation, hypokinesia, hypothyroidism, hypotonia, impotence, kidney failure (acute), leg cramps, leukopenia, liver function tests abnormal, lupus-like reaction, lymphadenopathy, maculopapular rash, menorrhagia, MI,

mouth ulceration, movement disorder, multiorgan failure, muscle spasm, myasthenia, neuralgia, neurosis, neutropenia, palpitation, pancreatitis, pancytopenia, paralysis, parkinsonian exacerbation, peripheral neuritis, photophobia, polyuria, postural hypotension, progressive immunosuppression, pruritus, pure red cell aplasia, rhabdomyolysis, salivation increased, skin discoloration, status epilepticus, Stevens-Johnson syndrome, sudden unexplained death in epilepsy (SUDEP), suicidal behavior, suicide, syncope, tachycardia, taste loss/perversion, thrombocytopenia, tic, tinnitus, tongue edema, toxic epidermal necrolysis, twitching, urinary incontinence, urticaria, vasculitis, vasodilation, withdrawal seizures

Also observed: Rash requiring hospitalization: Children <16 years 0.8% (epilepsy adjunctive therapy), 1.2% (with concurrent valproic acid use); Adults 0.3% (epilepsy adjunctive therapy), 0.13% (epilepsy monotherapy), 1% (with concurrent valproic acid use), 0.8% (bipolar disorder, monotherapy)

Drug Interactions

Metabolism/Transport Effects None known.

Avoid Concomitant Use There are no known interactions where it is recommended to avoid concomitant use.

Increased Effect/Toxicity

LamoTRIgine may increase the levels/effects of: Alcohol (Ethyl); CarBAMazepine; CNS Depressants; Desmopressin; Methotrimeprazine; OLANZapine; Selective Serotonin Reuptake Inhibitors

The levels/effects of LamoTRIgine may be increased by: Divalproex; Droperidol; HydrOXYzine; Methotrimeprazine; Valproic Acid

Decreased Effect

LamoTRIgine may decrease the levels/effects of: Contraceptives (Progestins)

The levels/effects of LamoTRIgine may be decreased by: Barbiturates; CarBAMazepine; Contraceptives (Estrogens); Fosphenytoin; Ketorolac; Ketorolac (Nasal); Ketorolac (Systemic); Mefloquine; Phenytoin; Primidone; Rifampin; Ritonavir

Ethanol/Nutrition/Herb Interactions

Ethanol: May increase CNS depression; monitor for increased effects with coadministration. Caution patients about effects.

Food: Has no effect on absorption.

Herb/Nutraceutical: Avoid evening primrose (seizure threshold decreased).

Stability Store at 25°C (77°F); excursions permitted to 15°C to 30°C (59°F to 86°F). Protect from light.

Mechanism of Action A triazine derivative which inhibits release of glutamate (an excitatory amino acid) and inhibits voltage-sensitive sodium channels, which stabilizes neuronal membranes. Lamotrigine has weak inhibitory effect on the 5-HT_3 receptor; *in vitro* inhibits dihydrofolate reductase.

Pharmacodynamics/Kinetics

Absorption: Immediate release: Rapid and complete

Distribution: V_d: 0.9-1.3 L/kg

Protein binding: ~55%

Metabolism: Hepatic and renal; metabolized primarily by glucuronic acid conjugation to inactive metabolites

Bioavailability: Immediate release: 98%; **Note:** AUCs were similar for immediate release and extended release preparations in patients receiving nonenzyme-inducing AEDs. In subjects receiving concomitant enzyme-inducing AEDs, bioavailability of extended release product was ~21% lower than immediate release product; in some of these subjects, a decrease in AUC of up to 70% was observed when switching from immediate release to extended release tablets.

Half-life elimination: Immediate release: Adults: 25-33 hours, Elderly: 25-43 hours; Extended release: Similar to immediate release

Concomitant valproic acid therapy: 48-70 hours

Concomitant phenytoin, phenobarbital, primidone, or carbamazepine therapy: 13-14 hours

Chronic renal failure: 43 hours

Hemodialysis: 13 hours during dialysis; 57 hours between dialysis (~20% of a dose is eliminated in a 4-hour dialysis session)

Hepatic impairment:

Mild: 26-66 hours

Moderate: 28-116 hours

Severe without ascites: 56-78 hours

Severe with ascites: 52-148 hours

Time to peak, plasma: Immediate release: 1-1.5 hours; Extended release: 4-11 hours (dependent on adjunct therapy)

Excretion: Urine (94%, ~90% as glucuronide conjugates and ~10% unchanged); feces (2%)

Dosage Note: Only whole tablets should be used for dosing, round calculated dose down to the nearest whole tablet. Extended release formulation not approved for children ≤12 years of age. Enzyme-inducing regimens specifically refer to those containing carbamazepine, phenytoin, phenobarbital, or primidone. Oral:

Children 2-12 years: Lennox-Gastaut (adjunctive), primary generalized tonic-clonic seizures (adjunctive), or partial seizures (adjunctive): **Note:** Children <30 kg will likely require maintenance doses to be increased as much as 50% based on clinical response regardless of regimen below:

Immediate release formulations:

Regimens **not containing** carbamazepine, phenytoin, phenobarbital, primidone, or valproic acid: Initial: Week 1 and 2: 0.3 mg/kg/day in 1-2 divided doses; Week 3 and 4: 0.6 mg/kg/day in 2 divided doses; Week 5 and beyond: Increase by 0.6 mg/kg/day every 1-2 weeks; Maintenance: 4.5-7.5 mg/kg/day (maximum: 300 mg/day) in 2 divided doses

Regimens **containing** valproic acid: Initial: Week 1 and 2: 0.15 mg/kg/day in 1-2 divided doses; Week 3 and 4: 0.3 mg/kg/day in 1-2 divided doses; Week 5 and beyond: Increase by 0.3 mg/kg/day every 1-2 weeks; Maintenance: 1-5 mg/kg/day (maximum: 200 mg/day) in 1 or 2 divided doses or 1-3 mg/kg/day (maximum: 200 mg/day) (valproic acid alone)

Regimens **containing** carbamazepine, phenytoin, phenobarbital, or primidone and without valproic acid: Initial: Week 1 and 2: 0.6 mg/kg/day in 2 divided doses; Week 3 and 4: 1.2 mg/kg/day in 2 divided doses; Week 5 and beyond: Increase by 1.2 mg/kg/day every 1-2 weeks; Maintenance: 5-15 mg/kg/day (maximum: 400 mg/day) in 2 divided doses

Children ≥13 years: Lennox-Gastaut (adjunctive), primary generalized tonic-clonic seizures (adjunctive), or partial seizures (adjunctive): Refer to adult dosing.

Children: Conversion from adjunctive therapy with a single enzyme-inducing AED regimen for partial seizures to monotherapy with lamotrigine:

Children ≥13 years: *Extended release formulation:* Refer to adult dosing.

Children ≥16 years: *Immediate release formulations:* Refer to adult dosing.

Adults:

Lennox-Gastaut (adjunctive), primary generalized tonic-clonic seizures (adjunctive) or partial seizures (adjunctive): *Immediate release formulations:*

Regimens **not containing** carbamazepine, phenytoin, phenobarbital, primidone, or valproic acid: Initial: Week 1 and 2: 25 mg once daily; Week 3 and 4: 50 mg once daily; Week 5 and beyond: Increase by 50 mg/day every 1-2 weeks; Maintenance: 225-375 mg/day in 2 divided doses

Regimens **containing** valproic acid: Initial: Week 1 and 2: 25 mg every other day; Week 3 and 4: 25 mg once daily; Week 5 and beyond: Increase by 25-50 mg/day every 1-2 weeks; Maintenance: 100-200 mg/day (valproic acid alone) or 100-400 mg/day (valproic acid and other drugs that induce glucuronidation)

Regimens **containing** carbamazepine, phenytoin, phenobarbital, or primidone and without valproic acid: Initial: Week 1 and 2: 50 mg once daily; Week 3 and 4: 100 mg/day in 2 divided doses; Week 5 and beyond: Increase by 100 mg/day every 1-2 weeks; Maintenance: 300-500 mg/day in 2 divided doses; maximum daily dose: 700 mg

Partial seizures (adjunctive) and primary generalized tonic-clonic seizures (adjunctive): *Extended release formulation:* **Note:** Dose increases after week 8 should not exceed 100 mg/day at weekly intervals:

Regimens **not containing** carbamazepine, phenytoin, phenobarbital, primidone, or valproic acid: Initial: Week 1 and 2: 25 mg once daily; Week 3 and 4: 50 mg once daily; Week 5: 100 mg once daily; Week 6: 150 mg once daily; Week 7: 200 mg once daily; Maintenance: 300-400 mg once daily

Regimens **containing** valproic acid: Initial: Week 1 and 2: 25 mg every other day; Week 3 and 4: 25 mg once daily; Week 5: 50 mg once daily; Week 6: 100 mg once daily; Week 7: 150 mg once daily; Maintenance: 200-250 mg once daily

Regimens **containing** carbamazepine, phenytoin, phenobarbital, or primidone and without valproic acid: Initial: Week 1 and 2: 50 mg once daily; Week 3 and 4: 100 mg once daily; Week 5: 200 mg once daily; Week 6: 300 mg once daily; Week 7: 400 mg once daily; Maintenance: 400-600 mg once daily

Conversion from adjunctive therapy with a single enzyme-inducing AED regimen for partial seizures to monotherapy with lamotrigine: **Note:** Goal is to achieve a lamotrigine monotherapy dose of 500 mg/day in 2 divided doses for immediate release formulations and a lamotrigine monotherapy dosage range of 250-300 mg once daily for the extended release formulation.

Conversion strategy from adjunctive therapy with valproic acid:

Immediate release formulations:

- Initiate and titrate as per escalation recommendations for adjunctive therapy to a lamotrigine dose of 200 mg/day.
- Then taper valproic acid dose in decrements of not >500 mg/day/week to a valproic acid dosage of 500 mg/day; this dosage should be maintained for 1 week. The lamotrigine dosage should then be increased to 300 mg/day while valproic acid is simultaneously decreased to 250 mg/day; this dosage should be maintained for 1 week.
- Valproic acid may then be discontinued, while the lamotrigine dose is increased by 100 mg/day at weekly intervals to achieve a lamotrigine maintenance dose of 500 mg/day in 2 divided doses.

Extended release formulation:

- Initiate and titrate as per escalation recommendations for adjunctive therapy to a lamotrigine dose of 150 mg/day.
- Then taper valproic acid dose in decrements of not >500 mg/day/week to a valproic acid dose of 500 mg/day; this dosage should be maintained for 1 week. The lamotrigine dosage should then be increased to 200 mg/day while valproic acid is simultaneously decreased to 250 mg/day; this dosage should be maintained for 1 week.
- Valproic acid may then be discontinued, while the lamotrigine dose is increased to achieve a maintenance dosage range of 250-300 mg once daily.

Conversion strategy from adjunctive therapy with carbamazepine, phenytoin, phenobarbital, or primidone: *Immediate release formulations and extended release formulation:*

- Initiate and titrate as per escalation recommendations for adjunctive therapy to a lamotrigine dose of 500 mg/day.
- Concomitant enzyme-inducing AED should then be withdrawn by 20% decrements each week over a 4-week period.
- Following withdrawal of the enzyme-inducing AED, the dosage of lamotrigine extended release may be tapered in decrements of not >100 mg/day at intervals of 1 week to achieve a maintenance dosage range of 250-300 mg once daily; no further dosage reduction is required for lamotrigine immediate release formulations.

Conversion strategy from adjunctive therapy with AED other than carbamazepine, phenytoin, phenobarbital, primidone or valproic acid:

Immediate release formulations: No specific guidelines available

Extended release formulation: Initiate and titrate as per escalation recommendations for adjunctive therapy to a lamotrigine dose of 250-300 mg/day. Concomitant AED should then be withdrawn by 20% decrements each week over a 4 week period.

Bipolar disorder: *Immediate release formulations:*

Regimens **not containing** carbamazepine, phenytoin, phenobarbital, primidone, or valproic acid: Initial: Week 1 and 2: 25 mg once daily; Week 3 and 4: 50 mg once daily; Week 5: 100 mg once daily; Week 6 and maintenance: 200 mg once daily

Regimens **containing** valproic acid: Initial: Week 1 and 2: 25 mg every other day; Week 3 and 4: 25 mg once daily; Week 5: 50 mg once daily; Week 6 and maintenance: 100 mg once daily

Regimens **containing** carbamazepine, phenytoin, phenobarbital, or primidone and without valproic acid: Initial: Week 1 and 2: 50 mg once daily; Week 3 and 4: 100 mg/day in divided doses; Week 5: 200 mg/day in divided doses; Week 6: 300 mg/day in divided doses; Maintenance: up to 400 mg/day in divided doses

Adjustment following discontinuation of psychotropic medication:

Discontinuing valproic acid with current dose of lamotrigine 100 mg/day: 150 mg/day for week 1, then increase to 200 mg/day beginning week 2

Discontinuing carbamazepine, phenytoin, phenobarbital, primidone, or rifampin with current dose of lamotrigine 400 mg/day: 400 mg/day for week 1, then decrease to 300 mg/day for week 2, then decrease to 200 mg/day beginning week 3

Conversion from immediate release to extended release (Lamictal® XR™): Initial dose of the extended release tablet should match the total daily dose of the immediate-release formulation. Adjust dose as needed within the recommended dosing guidelines.

Discontinuing therapy: Children and Adults: Decrease dose by ~50% per week, over at least 2 weeks unless safety concerns require a more rapid withdrawal. Discontinuing carbamazepine, phenytoin, phenobarbital, primidone, or rifampin should prolong the half-life of lamotrigine; discontinuing valproic acid should shorten the half-life of lamotrigine

Restarting therapy after discontinuation: If lamotrigine has been withheld for >5 half-lives, consider restarting according to initial dosing recommendations. **Note:** Concomitant medications may affect the half-life of lamotrigine; consider pharmacokinetic interactions when restarting therapy.

Dosage adjustment with estrogen-containing hormonal contraceptives: Follow initial lamotrigine dosing guidelines, maintenance dose should be adjusted as follows, based on concomitant medications:

Patients taking concomitant carbamazepine, phenytoin, phenobarbital, primidone or rifampin: No dosing adjustment required

Patients **not** taking concomitant carbamazepine, phenytoin, phenobarbital, primidone or rifampin: Lamotrigine maintenance dose may need increased by twofold over target dose. If already taking a stable dose of lamotrigine and starting contraceptive, maintenance dose may need increased by twofold. Dose increases should start when contraceptive is started and titrated to clinical response increasing no more rapidly than 50-100 mg/day every week. Gradual increases of lamotrigine plasma levels may occur during the inactive "pill-free" week and will be greater when dose increases are made the week before. If increased adverse events consistently occur during "pill-free" week, overall maintenance dose adjustments may be required. When discontinuing estrogen-containing hormonal contraceptive, dose of lamotrigine may need decreased by as much as 50%; do not decrease by more than 25% of total daily dose over a 2-week period unless clinical response or plasma levels indicate otherwise. Dose adjustments during "pill-free" week are not recommended.

Dosage adjustment in renal impairment: Decreased maintenance dosage may be effective in patients with significant renal impairment; has not been adequately studied; use with caution

Dosage adjustment in hepatic impairment:

Mild impairment: No adjustment required

Moderate-to-severe impairment without ascites: Decrease initial, escalation, and maintenance doses by ~25%; adjust according to clinical response

Moderate-to-severe impairment with ascites: Decrease initial, escalation, and maintenance doses by ~50%; adjust according to clinical response

Administration Doses should be rounded down to the nearest whole tablet.

Lamictal® chewable/dispersible tablets: May be chewed, dispersed in water or diluted fruit juice, or swallowed whole. To disperse tablets, add to a small amount of liquid (just enough to cover tablet); let sit ~1 minute until dispersed; swirl solution and consume immediately. Do not administer partial amounts of liquid. If tablets are chewed, a small amount of water or diluted fruit juice should be used to aid in swallowing.

Lamictal® ODT™: Place tablets on tongue and move around in the mouth. Tablets will dissolve rapidly and can be swallowed with or without food or water.

Lamictal® XR™: Administer without regard to meals. Swallow whole; do not chew, crush, or cut.

Monitoring Parameters Seizure, frequency and duration; serum levels of concurrent anticonvulsants, hypersensitivity reactions (especially rash); suicidality (eg, suicidal thoughts, depression, behavioral changes); signs/symptoms of aseptic meningitis

Reference Range A therapeutic serum concentration range has not been established for lamotrigine. Dosing should be based on therapeutic response. Lamotrigine plasma concentrations of 0.25-29.1 mcg/mL have been reported in the literature.

Dosage Forms Excipient information presented when available (limited, particularly for generics); consult specific product labeling.

Tablet, oral: 25 mg, 100 mg, 150 mg, 200 mg

LaMICtal®: 25 mg, 100 mg, 150 mg, 200 mg [scored]

Tablet, oral [combination package (each unit-dose starter kit contains)]:

LaMICtal®: 25 mg (84s) [white tablets] and 100 mg (14s) [peach tablets] [scored; green kit; for patients taking carbamazepine, phenytoin, phenobarbital, primidone, or rifampin and **not** taking valproic acid]

LaMICtal®: 25 mg (42s) [white tablets] and 100 mg (7s) [peach tablets] [scored; orange kit; for patients **not** taking carbamazepine, phenytoin, phenobarbital, primidone, rifampin, or valproic acid]

Tablet, oral [each unit-dose starter kit contains]:

LaMICtal®: 25 mg [scored; blue kit; for patients taking valproic acid]

Tablet, chewable/dispersible, oral: 5 mg, 25 mg

LaMICtal®: 2 mg [black currant flavor]

LaMICtal®: 5 mg [scored; black currant flavor]

LaMICtal®: 25 mg [black currant flavor]

Tablet, extended release, oral:

LaMICtal® XR™: 25 mg, 50 mg, 100 mg, 200 mg, 250 mg, 300 mg

Tablet, extended release, oral [combination package (each patient titration kit contains)]:

LaMICtal® XR™: 25 mg (21s) [yellow/white tablets] and 50 mg (7s) [green/white tablets] [blue XR kit, for patients taking valproic acid]

LaMICtal® XR™: 50 mg (14s) [green/white tablets], 100 mg (14s) [orange/white tablets], and 200 mg (7s) [blue/white tablets] [green XR kit, for patients taking carbamazepine, phenytoin, phenobarbital, primidone, and **not** taking valproic acid]

LaMICtal® XR™: 25 mg (14s) [yellow/white tablets], 50 mg (14s) [green/white tablets], and 100 mg (7s) [orange/white tablets] [orange XR kit, for patients **not** taking carbamazepine, phenytoin, phenobarbital, primidone, or valproic acid]

Tablet, orally disintegrating, oral:

LaMICtal® ODT™: 25 mg, 50 mg, 100 mg, 200 mg [cherry flavor]

Tablet, orally disintegrating, oral [combination package (each patient titration kit contains)]:

LaMICtal® ODT™: 25 mg (21s) and 50 mg (7s) [cherry flavor; blue kit, for patients taking valproic acid]

LaMICtal® ODT™: 50 mg (42s) and 100 mg (14s) [cherry flavor; green kit, for patients taking carbamazepine, phenytoin, phenobarbital, primidone, or rifampin and **not** taking valproic acid]

LaMICtal® ODT™: 25 mg (14s), 50 mg (14s), and 100 mg (7s) [cherry flavor; orange kit, for patients **not** taking carbamazepine, phenytoin, phenobarbital, primidone, rifampin, or valproic acid]

Extemporaneous Preparations A 1 mg/mL oral suspension may be made with tablets and one of two different vehicles (a 1:1 mixture of Ora-Sweet® and Ora-Plus® or a 1:1 mixture of Ora-Sweet® SF and Ora-Plus®). Crush one 100 mg tablet in a mortar and reduce to a fine powder. Add small portions of the chosen vehicle and mix to a uniform paste; mix while adding the vehicle in incremental proportions to **almost** 100 mL; transfer to a graduated cylinder, rinse mortar with vehicle, and add quantity of vehicle sufficient to make 100 mL. Label "shake well" and "protect from light". Stable for 91 days when stored in amber plastic prescription bottles in the dark at room temperature or refrigerated.

Nahata M, Morosco R, Hipple T. "Stability of Lamotrigine in Two Extemporaneously Prepared Oral Suspensions at 4 and 25 Degrees C," *Am J Health Syst Pharm*, 1999, 56(3):240-2.

◆ **Lanacane® [OTC]** *see* Benzocaine *on page* 202

◆ **Lanacane® Maximum Strength [OTC]** *see* Benzocaine *on page 202*

◆ **Lanaphilic® with Urea [OTC]** *see* Urea *on page 1749*

◆ **Lanoxin®** *see* Digoxin *on page 503*

Lanreotide (lan REE oh tide)

Brand Names: U.S. Somatuline® Depot
Brand Names: Canada Somatuline® Autogel®
Index Terms Lanreotide Acetate
Pharmacologic Category Somatostatin Analog
Use Long-term treatment of acromegaly in patients who are not candidates for or are unresponsive to surgery and/or radiotherapy

Canadian labeling: Also approved in Canada for relief of symptoms of acromegaly

Pregnancy Risk Factor C
Dosage SubQ:

U.S. labeling: Adults: Acromegaly: 90 mg once every 4 weeks for 3 months; after initial 90 days of therapy, adjust dose based on clinical response of patient, growth hormone (GH) levels, and/or insulin-like growth factor 1 (IGF-1) levels as follows:

GH ≤1 ng/mL, IGF-1 normal, symptoms stable:60 mg once every 4 weeks; once stabilized on 60 mg every 4 weeks, may consider regimen of 120 mg every 6-8 weeks (extended-interval dosing)

GH >1-2.5 ng/mL, IGF-1 normal, symptoms stable: 90 mg once every 4 weeks; once stabilized on 90 mg every 4 weeks, may consider regimen of 120 mg every 6-8 weeks (extended-interval dosing)

GH >2.5 ng/mL, IGF-1 elevated and/or uncontrolled symptoms: 120 mg once every 4 weeks

Canadian labeling: Children ≥16 years and Adults: Acromegaly: 90 mg once every 4 weeks for 3 months; after initial 90 days of therapy, adjust dose based on clinical response of patient, growth hormone (GH) levels, and/or insulin-like growth factor 1 (IGF-1) levels as follows:

GH ≤1 ng/mL, IGF-1 normal, symptoms stable: 60 mg once every 4 weeks

GH >1-2.5 ng/mL, IGF-1 normal, symptoms stable: 90 mg once every 4 weeks

GH >2.5 ng/mL, IGF-1 elevated and/or uncontrolled symptoms: 120 mg once every 4 weeks

Dosing adjustment in renal impairment:

U.S. labeling: Moderate-to-severe impairment: Recommended starting dose: 60 mg; use of an extended-interval dose of 120 mg every 6-8 weeks should be done with caution

Canadian labeling: No adjustment is necessary

Dosing adjustment in hepatic impairment:

U.S. labeling: Moderate-to-severe impairment: Recommended starting dose: 60 mg; use of an extended-interval dose of 120 mg every 6-8 weeks should be done with caution

Canadian labeling: No adjustment is necessary

Additional Information Complete prescribing information for this medication should be consulted for additional detail.

Dosage Forms Excipient information presented when available (limited, particularly for generics); consult specific product labeling.

Injection, solution:

Somatuline® Depot: 60 mg/0.4 mL (0.4 mL); 90 mg/0.4 mL (0.4 mL); 120 mg/0.5 mL (0.5 mL) [contains natural rubber/natural latex in packaging; volume is expressed as an approximate value]

Dosage Forms: Canada Excipient information presented when available (limited, particularly for generics); consult specific product labeling.

Injection, solution:

Somatuline® Autogel®: 60 mg/~0.3 mL (~0.3 mL); 90 mg/~0.4 mL (~0.4 mL); 120 mg/~0.5 mL (~0.5 mL) [packaging contains natural rubber/natural latex]

◆ **Lanreotide Acetate** *see* Lanreotide *on page 972*

Lansoprazole (lan SOE pra zole)

Brand Names: U.S. Prevacid®; Prevacid® 24 HR [OTC]; Prevacid® SoluTab™
Brand Names: Canada Apo-Lansoprazole®; Mylan-Lansoprazole; Prevacid®; Prevacid® FasTab; Teva-Lansoprazole
Pharmacologic Category Proton Pump Inhibitor; Substituted Benzimidazole
Use Short-term treatment of active duodenal ulcers; maintenance treatment of healed duodenal ulcers; as part of a multidrug regimen for *H. pylori* eradication to reduce the risk of duodenal ulcer recurrence; short-term treatment of active benign gastric ulcer; treatment of NSAID-associated gastric ulcer; to reduce the risk of NSAID-associated gastric ulcer in patients with a history of gastric ulcer who require an NSAID; short-term treatment of symptomatic GERD; short-term treatment for all grades of erosive esophagitis; to maintain healing of erosive esophagitis; long-term treatment of pathological hypersecretory conditions, including Zollinger-Ellison syndrome

OTC labeling: Relief of frequent heartburn (≥2 days/week)

Pregnancy Risk Factor B
Pregnancy Considerations Animal studies have not shown teratogenic effects to the fetus. However, there are no adequate and well-controlled studies in pregnant women; use during pregnancy only if clearly needed.
Lactation Excretion in breast milk unknown/not recommended
Contraindications Hypersensitivity to lansoprazole or any component of the formulation
Warnings/Precautions Use of proton pump inhibitors (PPIs) may increase the risk of gastrointestinal infections (eg, *Salmonella, Campylobacter*). Relief of symptoms does not preclude the presence of a gastric malignancy. Atrophic gastritis (by biopsy) has been noted with long-term omeprazole therapy; this may also occur with lansoprazole. No reports of enterochromaffin-like (ECL) cell carcinoids, dysplasia, or neoplasia have occurred. Severe liver dysfunction may require dosage reductions. Decreased *H. pylori* eradication rates have been observed with short-term (≤7 days) combination therapy. The American College of Gastroenterology recommends 10-14 days of therapy (triple or quadruple) for eradication of *H. pylori* (Chey, 2007).

PPIs may diminish the therapeutic effect of clopidogrel thought to be due to reduced formation of the active metabolite of clopidogrel. The manufacturer of clopidogrel recommends either avoidance of omeprazole or use of a PPI with less potent CYP2C19 inhibition (eg, pantoprazole). Lansoprazole exhibits the most potent CYP2C19 inhibition; given the potency of lansoprazole's CYP2C19 inhibitory activity, avoidance of lansoprazole would appear prudent. Others have recommended the continued use of PPIs, regardless of the degree of inhibition, in patients with a history of GI bleeding or multiple risk factors for GI bleeding who are also receiving clopidogrel since no evidence has established clinically meaningful differences in outcome; however, a clinically-significant interaction cannot be excluded in those who are poor metabolizers of clopidogrel (Abraham, 2010; Levine, 2011).

Increased incidence of osteoporosis-related bone fractures of the hip, spine, or wrist may occur with PPI therapy. Patients on high-dose or long-term therapy should be monitored. Use the lowest effective dose for the shortest duration of time, use vitamin D and calcium supplementation, and follow appropriate guidelines to reduce risk of fractures in patients at risk. Lansoprazole has been shown to be ineffective for the treatment of symptomatic GERD in children 1 month to <1 year.

Hypomagnesemia, reported rarely, usually with prolonged PPI use of >3 months (most cases >1 year of therapy); may be symptomatic or asymptomatic; severe cases may cause tetany, seizures, and cardiac arrhythmias. Consider obtaining serum magnesium concentrations prior to beginning long-term therapy, especially if taking concomitant digoxin, diuretics, or other drugs known to cause hypomagnesemia; and periodically thereafter. Hypomagnesemia may be corrected by magnesium supplementation, although discontinuation of lansoprazole may be necessary; magnesium levels typically return to normal within 1 week of stopping.

When used for self-medication, patients should be instructed not to use if they have difficulty swallowing, are vomiting blood, or have bloody or black stools. Prior to use, patients should contact healthcare provider if they have liver disease, heartburn for >3 months, heartburn with dizziness, lightheadedness, or sweating, MI symptoms, frequent chest pain, frequent wheezing (especially with heartburn), unexplained weight loss, nausea/vomiting, stomach pain, or are taking antifungals, atazanavir, digoxin, tacrolimus, theophylline, or warfarin. Patients should stop use and consult a healthcare provider if heartburn continues or worsens, or if they need to take for >14 days or more often than every 4 months. Patients should be informed that it may take 1-4 days for full effect to be seen; should not be used for immediate relief.

Adverse Reactions

1% to 10%:

Central nervous system: Headache (children 1-11 years 3%, 12-17 years 7%), dizziness (children 12-17 years 3%; adults <1%)

Gastrointestinal: Diarrhea (1% to 5%; 60 mg/day: 7%), abdominal pain (children 12-17 years 5%; adults 2%), constipation (children 1-11 years 5%; adults 1%), nausea (children 12-17 years 3%; adults 1%)

<1% (Limited to important or life-threatening): Abdomen enlarged, abnormal dreams, abnormal menses, abnormal stools, abnormal vision, agitation, agranulocytosis, albuminuria, allergic reaction, alkaline phosphatase increased, ALT increased, alopecia, amblyopia, amnesia, anaphylactoid reaction, anemia, angina, anorexia, anxiety, aplastic anemia, appetite increased, arrhythmia, AST increased, arthralgia, arthritis, asthma, avitaminosis, bezoar, bilirubinemia, blepharitis, blurred vision, bradycardia, breast enlargement, breast pain, breast tenderness, bronchitis, candidiasis, carcinoma, cardiospasm, cataract, cerebrovascular accident, cerebral infarction, chest pain, chills, cholelithiasis, cholesterol increased/decreased, colitis, confusion, conjunctivitis, cough increased, creatinine increased, deafness, dehydration, dementia, depersonalization, depression, diabetes mellitus, diaphoresis, diplopia, dry eyes, dry skin, dyspepsia, dysphagia, dyspnea, dysmenorrhea, dysuria, edema, electrolyte imbalance, emotional lability, enteritis, eosinophilia, epistaxis, eructation, erythema multiforme, esophageal stenosis, esophageal ulcer, esophagitis, fecal discoloration, fever, fixed eruption, flatulence, flu-like syndrome, fracture, fundic gland polyps, gastric nodules, gastrin levels increased, gastritis, gastroenteritis, gastrointestinal anomaly, gastrointestinal hemorrhage, GGTP increased/decreased, glaucoma, glucocorticoid levels increased, glossitis, glycosuria, goiter, gout, gum hemorrhage, gynecomastia, halitosis, hallucinations, hematemesis, hematuria, hemiplegia, hemolysis, hemolytic anemia, hemoptysis, hepatotoxicity, hostility aggravated, hyper-/hypoglycemia, hyperkinesia, hyperlipemia, hypertonia, hypoesthesia, hyper-/hypotension, hypomagnesemia, hypothyroidism, impotence, infection, insomnia, interstitial nephritis, kidney calculus, laryngeal neoplasia, LDH increased, leg cramps, leukopenia, leukorrhea, libido decreased/increased, liver function test abnormal, lung fibrosis, lymphadenopathy, maculopapular rash, malaise, melena, menorrhagia, migraine, moniliasis (oral), mouth ulceration, musculoskeletal pain, myalgia, myasthenia, myositis, MI, nervousness, neurosis, neutropenia, pain, palpitation, pancreatitis, pancytopenia, paresthesia, parosmia, pelvic pain, peripheral edema, pharyngitis, photophobia, platelet abnormalities, pneumonia, polyuria, pruritus, ptosis, rash, rectal hemorrhage, retinal degeneration, rhinitis, salivation increased, seizure, shock, sinusitis, skin carcinoma, sleep disorder, somnolence, speech disorder, Stevens-Johnson syndrome, stomatitis, stridor, syncope, synovitis, tachycardia, taste loss, taste perversion, tenesmus, thirst, thrombocytopenia, thrombotic thrombocytopenic purpura, tinnitus, tremor, tongue disorder, toxic epidermal necrolysis, ulcerative colitis, ulcerative stomatitis, upper respiratory inflammation, upper respiratory infection, urethral pain, urinary frequency/urgency, urination impaired, urinary retention, urinary tract infection, urticaria, vaginitis, vasodilation, vertigo, visual field defect, vomiting, weakness, WBC abnormal, weight gain/loss, xerostomia

Drug Interactions

Metabolism/Transport Effects Substrate of CYP2C19 (major), CYP2C9 (minor), CYP3A4 (major); **Note:** Assignment of Major/Minor substrate status based on clinically relevant drug interaction potential; **Inhibits** CYP2C19 (moderate), CYP2C9 (weak), CYP2D6 (weak), CYP3A4 (weak); **Induces** CYP1A2 (weak/moderate)

Avoid Concomitant Use

Avoid concomitant use of Lansoprazole with any of the following: Delavirdine; Erlotinib; Nelfinavir; Pimozide; Posaconazole; Rilpivirine

Increased Effect/Toxicity

Lansoprazole may increase the levels/effects of: Amphetamines; Citalopram; CYP2C19 Substrates; Dexmethylphenidate; Imatinib; Methotrexate; Methylphenidate; Pimozide; Raltegravir; Saquinavir; Tacrolimus; Tacrolimus (Systemic); Vitamin K Antagonists; Voriconazole

The levels/effects of Lansoprazole may be increased by: Conivaptan; Fluconazole; Ketoconazole; Ketoconazole (Systemic)

Decreased Effect

Lansoprazole may decrease the levels/effects of: Atazanavir; Bisphosphonate Derivatives; Cefditoren; Clopidogrel; Dabigatran Etexilate; Dasatinib; Delavirdine; Erlotinib; Gefitinib; Indinavir; Iron Salts; Itraconazole; Ketoconazole; Ketoconazole (Systemic); Mesalamine; Mycophenolate; Nelfinavir; Posaconazole; Rilpivirine

The levels/effects of Lansoprazole may be decreased by: CYP2C19 Inducers (Strong); CYP3A4 Inducers (Strong); Deferasirox; Herbs (CYP3A4 Inducers); Tipranavir; Tocilizumab

Ethanol/Nutrition/Herb Interactions

Ethanol: Avoid ethanol (may cause gastric mucosal irritation).

Food: Lansoprazole serum concentrations may be decreased if taken with food.

Herb/Nutraceutical: Avoid St John's wort (may decrease the levels/effect of lansoprazole).

Stability Store at 25°C (77°F); excursions permitted to 15°C to 30°C (59°F to 86°F).

Mechanism of Action Decreases acid secretion in gastric parietal cells through inhibition of (H+, K+)-ATPase enzyme system, blocking the final step in gastric acid production.

Pharmacodynamics/Kinetics

Onset of action: Gastric acid suppression: Oral: 1-3 hours

Duration: Gastric acid suppression: Oral: >1 day

Absorption: Rapid

Distribution: V_d: 14-18 L

Protein binding: 97%

Metabolism: Hepatic via CYP2C19 and 3A4, and in parietal cells to two active metabolites that are not present in systemic circulation

Bioavailability: ≥80%; decreased 50% to 70% if given 30 minutes after food

Half-life elimination: 1.5 ± 1 hours; Elderly: 2-3 hours; Hepatic impairment: 3-7 hours

Time to peak, plasma: 1.7 hours

Excretion: Feces (67%); urine (33%)

Dosage Oral:

Children 1-11 years: GERD, erosive esophagitis:

≤30 kg: 15 mg once daily for up to 12 weeks

>30 kg: 30 mg once daily for up to 12 weeks

Note: Doses were increased in some pediatric patients if still symptomatic after 2 or more weeks of treatment (maximum dose: 30 mg twice daily)

Children 12-17 years:

Nonerosive GERD: 15 mg once daily for up to 8 weeks

Erosive esophagitis: 30 mg once daily for up to 8 weeks

Adults:

Duodenal ulcer: Short-term treatment: 15 mg once daily for 4 weeks; maintenance therapy: 15 mg once daily

Gastric ulcer: Short-term treatment: 30 mg once daily for up to 8 weeks

NSAID-associated gastric ulcer (healing): 30 mg once daily for 8 weeks; controlled studies did not extend past 8 weeks of therapy

NSAID-associated gastric ulcer (to reduce risk): 15 mg once daily for up to 12 weeks; controlled studies did not extend past 12 weeks of therapy

Symptomatic GERD: Short-term treatment: 15 mg once daily for up to 8 weeks

Erosive esophagitis: Short-term treatment: 30 mg once daily for up to 8 weeks; continued treatment for an additional 8 weeks may be considered for recurrence or for patients who do not heal after the first 8 weeks of therapy; maintenance therapy: 15 mg once daily

Hypersecretory conditions: Initial: 60 mg once daily; adjust dose based upon patient response and to reduce acid secretion to <10 mEq/hour (5 mEq/hour in patients with prior gastric surgery); doses of 90 mg twice daily have been used; administer doses >120 mg/day in divided doses

Helicobacter pylori eradication:

Manufacturer labeling: 30 mg 3 times/day administered with amoxicillin 1000 mg 3 times/day for 14 days **or** 30 mg twice daily administered with amoxicillin 1000 mg *and* clarithromycin 500 mg twice daily for 10-14 days

American College of Gastroenterology guidelines (Chey, 2007):

Nonpenicillin allergy: 30 mg twice daily administered with amoxicillin 1000 mg *and* clarithromycin 500 mg twice daily for 10-14 days

Penicillin allergy: 30 mg twice daily administered with clarithromycin 500 mg *and* metronidazole 500 mg twice daily for 10-14 days **or** 30 mg once or twice daily administered with bismuth subsalicylate 525 mg *and* metronidazole 250 mg *plus* tetracycline 500 mg 4 times/day for 10-14 days

Heartburn: OTC labeling: 15 mg once daily for 14 days; may repeat 14 days of therapy every 4 months. Do not take for >14 days or more often than every 4 months, unless instructed by healthcare provider.

Dosage adjustment in renal impairment: No dosage adjustment is needed

Dosing adjustment in hepatic impairment: Severe hepatic impairment: Consider dose reduction

Dietary Considerations Should be taken before eating; best if taken before breakfast. Some products may contain phenylalanine.

Administration

Oral: Administer before food; best if taken before breakfast. The intact granules should not be chewed or crushed; however, several options are available for those patients unable to swallow capsules:

Capsules may be opened and the intact granules sprinkled on 1 tablespoon of applesauce, Ensure® pudding, cottage cheese, yogurt, or strained pears. The granules should then be swallowed immediately.

Capsules may be opened and emptied into ~60 mL orange juice, apple juice, or tomato juice; mix and swallow immediately. Rinse the glass with additional juice and swallow to assure complete delivery of the dose.

Orally-disintegrating tablets: Should not be swallowed whole, broken, cut, or chewed. Place tablet on tongue; allow to dissolve (with or without water) until particles can be swallowed. Orally-disintegrating tablets may also be administered via an oral syringe: Place the 15 mg tablet in an oral syringe and draw up ~4 mL water, or place the 30 mg tablet in an oral syringe and draw up ~10 mL water. After tablet has dispersed, administer within 15 minutes. Refill the syringe with water (2 mL for the 15 mg tablet; 5 mL for the 30 mg tablet), shake gently, then administer any remaining contents.

Nasogastric tube administration:

Capsule: Capsule can be opened, the granules mixed (not crushed) with 40 mL of apple juice and then injected through the NG tube into the stomach, then flush tube with additional apple juice. Do not mix with other liquids.

Orally-disintegrating tablet: Nasogastric tube ≥8 French: Place a 15 mg tablet in a syringe and draw up ~4 mL water, or place the 30 mg tablet in a syringe and draw up ~10 mL water. After tablet has dispersed, administer within 15 minutes. Refill the syringe with ~5 mL water, shake gently, and then flush the nasogastric tube.

Monitoring Parameters Patients with Zollinger-Ellison syndrome should be monitored for gastric acid output, which should be maintained at ≤10 mEq/hour during the last hour before the next lansoprazole dose; lab monitoring should include CBC, liver function, renal function, and serum gastrin levels

Dosage Forms Excipient information presented when available (limited, particularly for generics); consult specific product labeling.

Capsule, delayed release, oral: 15 mg, 30 mg

Prevacid®: 15 mg, 30 mg

Prevacid® 24 HR: 15 mg

Tablet, delayed release, orally disintegrating, oral: 15 mg, 30 mg

Prevacid® SoluTab™: 15 mg [contains phenylalanine 2.5 mg/tablet; strawberry flavor]

Prevacid® SoluTab™: 30 mg [contains phenylalanine 5.1 mg/tablet; strawberry flavor]

Extemporaneous Preparations A 3 mg/mL oral solution (Simplified Lansoprazole Solution) may be made with capsules and sodium bicarbonate. Empty the contents of ten lansoprazole 30 mg capsules into a beaker. Add 100 mL sodium bicarbonate 8.4% and gently stir until dissolved (about 15 minutes). Transfer solution to an amber-colored syringe or bottle. Stable for 8 hours at room temperature or for 14 days refrigerated.

DiGiancinto JL, Olsen KM, Bergman KL, et al, "Stability of Suspension Formulations of Lansoprazole and Omeprazole Stored in Amber-Colored Plastic Oral Syringes," *Ann Pharmacother*, 2000, 34 (5):600-5.

Sharma V, "Comparison of 24-hour Intragastric pH Using Four Liquid Formulations of Lansoprazole and Omeprazole," *Am J Health Syst Pharm*, 1999, 56(Suppl 4):18-21.
Sharma VK, Vasudeva R, and Howden CW, "Simplified Lansoprazole Suspension - Liquid Formulations of Lansoprazole - Effectively Suppresses Intragastric Acidity When Administered Through a Gastrostomy," *Am J Gastroenterol*, 1999, 94(7):1813-7.

Lansoprazole, Amoxicillin, and Clarithromycin
(lan SOE pra zole, a moks i SIL in, & kla RITH roe mye sin)

Brand Names: U.S. Prevpac®
Brand Names: Canada Hp-PAC®
Index Terms Amoxicillin, Clarithromycin, and Lansoprazole; Clarithromycin, Lansoprazole, and Amoxicillin; Lansoprazole, Amoxicillin, and Clarithromycin
Pharmacologic Category Antibiotic, Macrolide Combination; Antibiotic, Penicillin; Gastrointestinal Agent, Miscellaneous; Proton Pump Inhibitor; Substituted Benzimidazole
Use Eradication of *H. pylori* to reduce the risk of recurrent duodenal ulcer
Pregnancy Risk Factor C (clarithromycin)
Dosage Oral: Adults: Lansoprazole 30 mg, amoxicillin 1 g, and clarithromycin 500 mg taken together twice daily for 10 or 14 days
Dosage adjustment in renal impairment: Cl_{cr} <30 mL/minute: Use is not recommended
Additional Information Complete prescribing information for this medication should be consulted for additional detail.
Dosage Forms Excipient information presented when available (limited, particularly for generics); consult specific product labeling.
Combination package [each administration card contains]:
Prevpac®:
Capsule: Amoxicillin 500 mg (4 capsules/day)
Capsule, delayed release (Prevacid®): Lansoprazole 30 mg (2 capsules/day)
Tablet (Biaxin®): Clarithromycin 500 mg (2 tablets/day)

◆ **Lansoprazole, Amoxicillin, and Clarithromycin** *see* Lansoprazole, Amoxicillin, and Clarithromycin *on page 975*

Lanthanum (LAN tha num)

Brand Names: U.S. Fosrenol®
Brand Names: Canada Fosrenol®
Index Terms Lanthanum Carbonate
Pharmacologic Category Phosphate Binder
Use Reduction of serum phosphate in patients with stage 5 chronic kidney disease (end-stage renal disease [ESRD]; kidney failure: GFR <15 mL/minute/1.73 m^2 or dialysis)
Pregnancy Risk Factor C
Medication Guide Available Yes
Dosage Oral: Adults: Reduction of serum phosphorous: Initial: 1500 mg/day divided and taken with meals; typical increases of 750 mg/day every 2-3 weeks are suggested as needed to reduce the serum phosphate level <6 mg/dL; usual dosage range: 1500-3000 mg; doses of up to 4500 mg have been evaluated
Additional Information Complete prescribing information for this medication should be consulted for additional detail.
Dosage Forms Excipient information presented when available (limited, particularly for generics); consult specific product labeling.
Tablet, chewable, oral:
Fosrenol®: 500 mg, 750 mg, 1000 mg

◆ **Lanthanum Carbonate** *see* Lanthanum *on page 975*
◆ **Lantus®** *see* Insulin Glargine *on page 905*
◆ **Lantus® OptiSet® (Can)** *see* Insulin Glargine *on page 905*
◆ **Lantus® Solostar®** *see* Insulin Glargine *on page 905*
◆ **Lanvis® (Can)** *see* Thioguanine *on page 1670*

Lapatinib (la PA ti nib)

Brand Names: U.S. Tykerb®
Brand Names: Canada Tykerb®
Index Terms GW572016; Lapatinib Ditosylate
Pharmacologic Category Antineoplastic Agent, Tyrosine Kinase Inhibitor; Epidermal Growth Factor Receptor (EGFR) Inhibitor
Use Treatment of HER2 overexpressing advanced or metastatic breast cancer (in combination with capecitabine) in patients who have received prior therapy (with an anthracycline, a taxane, and trastuzumab) and HER2 overexpressing hormone receptor positive metastatic breast cancer in postmenopausal women (in combination with letrozole)
Unlabeled Use Treatment (in combination with trastuzumab) of HER2 overexpressing metastatic breast cancer which had progressed on prior trastuzumab containing therapy
Pregnancy Risk Factor D
Pregnancy Considerations Increased pup deaths were demonstrated in animal studies. There are no adequate and well-controlled studies in pregnant women. Lapatinib may cause fetal harm if administered during pregnancy. Women of childbearing potential should be advised to avoid pregnancy during treatment.
Lactation Excretion in breast milk unknown/not recommended
Prescribing and Access Restrictions Lapatinib is available **only** at specialty pharmacies through a restricted-access program, Tykerb® CARES. Information is available at www.tykerbcares.com or 1-866-489-5372.
Contraindications Hypersensitivity to lapatinib or any component of the formulation
Warnings/Precautions Decreases in left ventricular ejection fraction (LVEF) have been reported (usually within the first 3 months of treatment); baseline and periodic LVEF evaluations are recommended; interrupt therapy or decrease dose with decreased LVEF ≥grade 2 or LVEF < LLN. QT_c prolongation has been observed; use caution in patients with a history of QT_c prolongation or with medications known to prolong the QT interval; a baseline and periodic 12-lead ECG should be considered; correct electrolyte (potassium, calcium and magnesium) abnormalities prior to and during treatment. Use with caution in conditions which may impair left ventricular function and in patients with a history of or predisposed (prior treatment with anthracyclines, chest wall irradiation) to left ventricular dysfunction. Interstitial lung disease (ILD) and pneumonitis have been reported (with lapatinib monotherapy and with combination chemotherapy); monitor for pulmonary symptoms which may indicate ILD or pneumonitis; discontinue therapy for grade 3 (or higher) pulmonary symptoms indicative of ILD or pneumonitis (eg, dyspnea, dry cough).

[U.S. Boxed Warning]: Hepatotoxicity (ALT or AST >3 times ULN and total bilirubin >2 times ULN) has been reported with lapatinib; may be severe and/or fatal. Onset of hepatotoxicity may occur within days to several months after treatment initiation; monitor (at baseline and during treatment); discontinue with severe changes in liver function; do not retreat. Use caution in patients with hepatic dysfunction; Dose reductions should be considered in patients with severe (Child-Pugh class C) preexisting hepatic impairment. Avoid concurrent use with strong CYP3A4 inhibitors or inducers; if concomitant therapy cannot be avoided, lapatinib dosage adjustments should ▶

be considered. May cause diarrhea (may be severe); manage with antidiarrheal agents; severe diarrhea may require hydration, electrolytes, and or interruption of therapy.

Adverse Reactions Percentages reported for combination therapy.

>10%:

Central nervous system: Fatigue (10% to 20%), headache (≤14%)

Dermatologic: Palmar-plantar erythrodysesthesia (hand-and-foot syndrome) (with capecitabine: 53%; grade 3: 12%), rash (28% to 44%), dry skin (10% to 13%), alopecia (≤13%), pruritus (≤12%), nail disorder (≤11%)

Gastrointestinal: Diarrhea (64% to 65%; grade 3: 9% to 13%; grade 4: ≤1%), nausea (31% to 44%), vomiting (17% to 26%), abdominal pain (≤15%), mucosal inflammation (≤15%), stomatitis (≤14%), anorexia (≤11%), dyspepsia (≤11%)

Hematologic: Anemia (with capecitabine: 56%; grade 3: <1%), neutropenia (with capecitabine: 22%; grade 3: 3%; grade 4: <1%), thrombocytopenia (with capecitabine: 18%; grade 3: <1%)

Hepatic: AST increased (49% to 53%; grade 3: 2% to 6%; grade 4: <1%), ALT increased (37% to 46%; grade 3: 2% to 5%; grade 4<1%) total bilirubin increased (22% to 45%; grade 3: ≤4%; grade 4: <1%)

Neuromuscular & skeletal: Limb pain (≤12%), weakness (≤12%), back pain (≤11%)

Respiratory:Dyspnea (≤12%), epistaxis (≤11%)

1% to 10%:

Cardiovascular: LVEF decreased (grades 1/2: 2% to 4%; grades 3/4: <1%)

Central nervous system: Insomnia (≤10%)

<1% (Limited to important or life-threatening): Anaphylaxis, hepatotoxicity, hypersensitivity, interstitial lung disease, pneumonitis, Prinzmetal's angina, QTc prolongation

Drug Interactions

Metabolism/Transport Effects **Substrate** of CYP3A4 (major), P-glycoprotein; **Note:** Assignment of Major/Minor substrate status based on clinically relevant drug interaction potential; **Inhibits** BCRP, CYP2C8 (moderate), CYP3A4 (weak), P-glycoprotein

Avoid Concomitant Use

Avoid concomitant use of Lapatinib with any of the following: Artemether; CYP3A4 Inducers (Strong); CYP3A4 Inhibitors (Strong); Dronedarone; Grapefruit Juice; Lumefantrine; Nilotinib; Pimozide; QUEtiapine; QuiNINE; Silodosin; St Johns Wort; Tetrabenazine; Thioridazine; Topotecan; Toremifene; Vandetanib; Vemurafenib; Ziprasidone

Increased Effect/Toxicity

Lapatinib may increase the levels/effects of: Colchicine; CYP2C8 Substrates; Dabigatran Etexilate; Dronedarone; Everolimus; Pazopanib; P-glycoprotein/ABCB1 Substrates; Pimozide; QTc-Prolonging Agents; QuiNINE; Rivaroxaban; Silodosin; Tetrabenazine; Thioridazine; Topotecan; Toremifene; Vandetanib; Vemurafenib; Vitamin K Antagonists; Ziprasidone

The levels/effects of Lapatinib may be increased by: Alfuzosin; Artemether; Chloroquine; Ciprofloxacin; Ciprofloxacin (Systemic); CYP3A4 Inhibitors (Moderate); CYP3A4 Inhibitors (Strong); Gadobutrol; Grapefruit Juice; Indacaterol; Lumefantrine; Nilotinib; P-glycoprotein/ABCB1 Inhibitors; QUEtiapine; QuiNINE

Decreased Effect

Lapatinib may decrease the levels/effects of: Cardiac Glycosides; Vitamin K Antagonists

The levels/effects of Lapatinib may be decreased by: CYP3A4 Inducers (Strong); Deferasirox; P-glycoprotein/ABCB1 Inducers; St Johns Wort; Tocilizumab

Ethanol/Nutrition/Herb Interactions

Food: Systemic exposure of lapatinib is increased when administered with food (AUC three- to fourfold higher). Avoid grapefruit juice (may increase the levels/effects of lapatinib).

Herb/Nutraceutical: Avoid St John's wort (may increase metabolism and decrease lapatinib concentrations).

Stability Store at room temperature of 25°C (77°F); excursions permitted between 15°C and 30°C (59°F and 86°F).

Mechanism of Action Tyrosine kinase (dual kinase) inhibitor; inhibits EGFR (ErbB1) and HER2 (ErbB2) by reversibly binding to tyrosine kinase, blocking phosphorylation and activation of downstream second messengers (Erk1/2 and Akt), regulating cellular proliferation and survival in ErbB- and ErbB2-expressing tumors. Combination therapy with lapatinib and endocrine therapy may overcome endocrine resistance occurring in HER2+ and hormone receptor positive disease.

Pharmacodynamics/Kinetics

Absorption: Incomplete and variable

Protein binding: >99% to albumin and alpha$_1$-acid glycoprotein

Metabolism: Hepatic; extensive via CYP3A4 and 3A5, and to a lesser extent via CYP2C19 and 2C8 to oxidized metabolites

Half-life elimination: ~24 hours

Time to peak, plasma: 3-6 hours

Excretion: Feces (27% as unchanged drug; range 3% to 67%); urine (<2%)

Dosage Details concerning dosing in combination regimens should also be consulted. **Note:** Dose reductions are likely to be needed when lapatinib is administered concomitantly with a strong CYP3A4 inhibitor (an alternate medication for CYP3A4 enzyme inhibitors should be investigated first).

Oral: Adults: Breast cancer:

In combination with capecitabine: 1250 mg once daily

In combination with letrozole: 1500 mg once daily

In combination with trastuzumab (unlabeled use): 1000 mg once daily (O'Shaughnessy, 2008)

Dosage adjustment for concomitant CYP3A4 inhibitors/inducers:

CYP3A4 inhibitors: Dose reductions are likely to be needed when lapatinib is administered concomitantly with a strong CYP3A4 inhibitor (an alternate medication for CYP3A4 enzyme inhibitors should be investigated first); in the event that lapatinib must be administered concomitantly with a potent enzyme inhibitor, consider reducing lapatinib to 500 mg once daily with careful monitoring. When a strong CYP3A4 inhibitor is discontinued, allow ~1 week to elapse prior to adjusting the lapatinib dose upward.

CYP3A4 inducers: Concomitant administration with CYP3A4 inducers may require increased lapatinib doses (alternatives to the enzyme-inducing agent should be utilized first); consider titrating gradually from 1250 mg/day up to 4500 mg/day (in combination with capecitabine) **or** from 1500 mg/day up to 5500 mg/day (in combination with letrozole), with careful monitoring. (If the strong CYP3A4 enzyme inducer is discontinued, reduce the lapatinib dose to the indicated dose.)

Dosage adjustment for toxicity:

Cardiac toxicity: Discontinue treatment for decreased LVEF ≥grade 2 or LVEF < LLN; may be restarted after at least 2 weeks at 1000 mg once daily (in combination with capecitabine) **or** 1250 mg once daily (in combination with letrozole) if LVEF recovers to normal and patient is asymptomatic.

Pulmonary toxicity: Discontinue treatment with pulmonary symptoms indicative of interstitial lung disease or pneumonitis which are ≥ grade 3

Other toxicities: Withhold for any toxicity (other than cardiac) ≥grade 2 until toxicity resolves to ≤grade 1 and re-initiate at 1250 mg once daily; for persistent toxicity, reduce dosage to 1000 mg once daily (in combination with capecitabine) **or** 1250 mg once daily (in combination with letrozole)

Dosage adjustment in renal impairment: Not studied in renal dysfunction, however, due to the minimal renal elimination (<2%), dosage adjustments for renal dysfunction may not be necessary.

Dosage adjustment in hepatic impairment:

Severe preexisting hepatic impairment (Child-Pugh class C):

In combination with capecitabine: Reduce dose from 1250 mg once daily to 750 mg once daily

In combination with letrozole: Reduce dose from 1500 mg once daily to 1000 mg once daily

Severe hepatotoxicity during treatment: Discontinue treatment; do not retreat

Dietary Considerations Take on an empty stomach, 1 hour before or 1 hour after a meal. (**Note:** For combination with capecitabine treatment, capecitabine should be taken with food, or within 30 minutes after a meal.) Avoid grapefruit juice.

Administration Administer once daily, on an empty stomach, 1 hour before or 1 hour after a meal. Take at the same time each day; dividing doses is not recommended.

Monitoring Parameters LVEF (baseline and periodic), CBC with differential, liver function tests, including transaminases, bilirubin, and alkaline phosphatase (baseline and every 4-6 weeks during treatment); electrolytes including calcium, potassium, magnesium; monitor for fluid retention; ECG monitoring if at risk for QT_c prolongation; symptoms of ILD or pneumonitis

Additional Information Oncology Comment: The National Comprehensive Cancer Network (NCCN) breast cancer guidelines list lapatinib (in combination with capecitabine) as an option for the treatment of HER2-positive breast cancer in patients who are refractory to anthracycline, taxane, and trastuzumab treatment. In a randomized phase III study (Geyer, 2006) of lapatinib plus capecitabine versus capecitabine alone in HER2-positive advanced breast cancer, the addition of lapatinib was associated with a 51% reduction in the risk of disease progression in heavily pretreated patients. Lapatinib shows activity in HER2-positive metastatic breast cancer that has progressed after trastuzumab treatment. The NCCN breast cancer guidelines also list lapatinib in combination with trastuzumab in metastatic HER2+ breast cancer which has progressed on trastuzumab therapy; the combination of lapatinib and trastuzumab should not be given with concurrent chemotherapy.

Dosage Forms Excipient information presented when available (limited, particularly for generics); consult specific product labeling.

Tablet, oral:

Tykerb®: 250 mg

◆ **Lapatinib Ditosylate** *see* Lapatinib *on page 975*
◆ **Largactil® (Can)** *see* ChlorproMAZINE *on page 348*
◆ **L-Arginine** *see* Arginine *on page 142*
◆ **L-Arginine Hydrochloride** *see* Arginine *on page 142*
◆ **Lariam® (Can)** *see* Mefloquine *on page 1060*

Laronidase (lair OH ni days)

Brand Names: U.S. Aldurazyme®

Brand Names: Canada Aldurazyme®

Index Terms Recombinant α-L-Iduronidase (Glycosaminoglycan α-L-Iduronohydrolase)

Pharmacologic Category Enzyme

Use Treatment of Hurler and Hurler-Scheie forms of mucopolysaccharidosis I (MPS I); treatment of Scheie form of MPS I in patients with moderate-to-severe symptoms

Pregnancy Risk Factor B

Pregnancy Considerations Teratogenic effects were not observed in animal studies; however, there are no adequate and well-controlled studies in pregnant women. Use during pregnancy only if clearly needed. Patients are encouraged to enroll in the MPS I registry.

Lactation Excretion in breast milk unknown/use caution

Contraindications There are no contraindications listed within the manufacturer's labeling.

Warnings/Precautions [U.S. Boxed Warning]: Anaphylactic reactions have been observed during infusion, immediate treatment for hypersensitivity reactions should be available during administration. Additional monitoring may be required in patients with compromised respiratory function or acute respiratory disease; may be at increased risk for acute exacerbation of respiratory symptoms due to infusion reaction. Patients with acute illness may also be at increased risk for infusion reactions. Reactions, which may include airway obstruction, bradycardia, bronchospasm, hypotension, hypoxia, respiratory distress/failure, stridor, tachypnea, and urticaria, may be severe and tend to occur during or within 3 hours after administration. Antipyretics and or antihistamines should be administered prior to infusion to reduce the incidence/severity of headache, fever, and/or flushing. In event of reaction, decrease the rate of infusion, temporarily discontinue the infusion, and/or administer additional antipyretics/antihistamines. Risks and benefits should be carefully considered prior to readministering following a severe hypersensitivity reaction. In the case of anaphylaxis, caution should be used if epinephrine is being considered; many patients with MPS I have pre-existing heart disease.

Laronidase has not been studied in patients with mild symptoms of the Scheie form of MPS I. Not indicated for the CNS manifestations of the disorder. Studies did not include children <5 years of age. A patient registry has been established and all patients are encouraged to participate. Registry information may be obtained at www.-MPSIregistry.com or by calling 800-745-4447.

Adverse Reactions Note: Percentages reported are from a placebo-controlled study (45 patients, 22 receiving laronidase).

>10%:

Cardiovascular: Vein disorder (14%)

Dermatologic: Rash (36%)

Local: Injection site reaction (18%)

Neuromuscular & skeletal: Hyper-reflexia (14%), paresthesia (14%)

Respiratory: Upper respiratory tract infection (32%)

Miscellaneous: Antibody development to laronidase (91%); infusion reactions (32%; may be severe; includes flushing [23%], fever, and headache; frequency decreased over time during open-label extension period)

1% to 10%:

Cardiovascular: Chest pain (9%), edema (9%), facial edema (9%), hypotension (9%)

Hematologic: Thrombocytopenia (9%)

Hepatic: Bilirubinemia (9%)

Local: Abscess (9%), injection site pain (9%)

Ocular: Corneal opacity (9%)

Miscellaneous: Allergic reaction (severe/serious: 1%)

<1% (Limited to important or life-threatening): Abdominal pain, airway obstruction, anaphylaxis, angioedema, arthralgia, bronchospasm, chills, cough, diarrhea, dyspnea, hypersensitivity, hypertension, nausea, oxygen saturation decreased, pruritus, tachycardia, urticaria, vomiting

Drug Interactions

Metabolism/Transport Effects None known.

Avoid Concomitant Use There are no known interactions where it is recommended to avoid concomitant use.

Increased Effect/Toxicity There are no known significant interactions involving an increase in effect.

Decreased Effect There are no known significant interactions involving a decrease in effect.

Stability Store vials under refrigeration at 2°C to 8°C (36°F to 46°F); do not freeze. Do not shake. Allow vials to come to room temperature prior to admixture. Total volume of infusion is determined by body weight. For patients weighing ≤20 kg, dilute the required dose in 100 mL NS; for patients weighing >20 kg, dilute required dose in 250 mL NS. Determine the number of vials to dilute by calculating the required dose and rounding up to the nearest whole vial. From a PVC bag, remove and discard a volume of NS equal to the volume of the calculated dose of laronidase. Slowly withdraw from vial(s) and slowly add laronidase to the NS; avoid excessive agitation, do not use filter needle. Gently rotate infusion bag to mix (do not shake).

Following dilution, solution for infusion should be used immediately; however, if not used immediately, refrigerate. Infusion of solution should be completed within 36 hours of preparation.

Mechanism of Action Laronidase is a recombinant (replacement) form of α-L-iduronidase derived from Chinese hamster cells. α-L-iduronidase is an enzyme needed to break down endogenous glycosaminoglycans (GAGs) within lysosomes. A deficiency of α-L-iduronidase leads to an accumulation of GAGs, causing cellular, tissue, and organ dysfunction as seen in MPS I. Improved pulmonary function and walking capacity have been demonstrated with the administration of laronidase to patients with Hurler, Hurler-Scheie, or Scheie (with moderate-to-severe symptoms) forms of MPS.

Pharmacodynamics/Kinetics

Distribution: V_d: 0.24-0.6 L/kg

Half-life elimination: 1.5-3.6 hours

Excretion: Clearance: 1.7 to 2.7 mL/minute/kg; during the first 12 weeks of therapy the clearance of laronidase increases proportionally to the amount of antibodies a given patient develops against the enzyme. However, with long-term use (≥26 weeks) antibody titers have no effect on laronidase clearance.

Dosage Note: Premedicate with antipyretic and/or antihistamines 1 hour prior to start of infusion.

I.V.: Children ≥5 years and Adults: 0.58 mg/kg once weekly; dose should be rounded up to the nearest whole vial

Administration Administer using PVC container and PVC infusion set with in-line, low protein-binding 0.2 micrometer filter. Antipyretics and/or antihistamines should be administered prior to infusion. Volume and infusion rate are based on body weight. Vital signs should be monitored every 15 minutes, if stable; rate may be increased as follows:

≤20 kg: Total infusion volume: 100 mL
- 2 mL/hour for 15 minutes
- 4 mL/hour for 15 minutes
- 8 mL/hour for 15 minutes
- 16 mL/hour for 15 minutes
- 32 mL/hour for remainder of infusion

>20 kg: Total infusion volume: 250 mL
- 5 mL/hour for 15 minutes
- 10 mL/hour for 15 minutes
- 20 mL/hour for 15 minutes
- 40 mL/hour for 15 minutes
- 80 mL/hour for remainder of infusion

Note: In case of infusion-related reaction, decrease the rate of infusion, temporarily discontinue the infusion, and/or administer additional antipyretics/antihistamines.

Monitoring Parameters Vital signs; injection site reactions, infusion reactions

Dosage Forms Excipient information presented when available (limited, particularly for generics); consult specific product labeling.

Injection, solution [preservative free]:

Aldurazyme®: 2.9 mg/5 mL (5 mL) [contains polysorbate 80; derived from or manufactured using hamster protein]

- ◆ **Lasix®** *see* Furosemide *on page 771*
- ◆ **Lasix® Special (Can)** *see* Furosemide *on page 771*
- ◆ **L-asparaginase (*E. coli*)** *see* Asparaginase (*E. coli*) *on page 151*
- ◆ **L-asparaginase (*Erwinia*)** *see* Asparaginase (*Erwinia*) *on page 153*
- ◆ **L-asparaginase with Polyethylene Glycol** *see* Pegaspargase *on page 1306*
- ◆ **Lassar's Zinc Paste** *see* Zinc Oxide *on page 1817*

Latanoprost (la TA noe prost)

Brand Names: U.S. Xalatan®

Brand Names: Canada Apo-Latanoprost®; CO Latanoprost; GD-Latanoprost; Xalatan®

Pharmacologic Category Ophthalmic Agent, Antiglaucoma; Prostaglandin, Ophthalmic

Use Reduction of elevated intraocular pressure in patients with open-angle glaucoma or ocular hypertension

Pregnancy Risk Factor C

Dosage Adults: Ophthalmic: 1 drop (1.5 mcg) in the affected eye(s) once daily in the evening; do not exceed the once daily dosage because it has been shown that more frequent administration may decrease the IOP lowering effect

Note: A medication delivery device (Xal-Ease™) is available for use with Xalatan®.

Additional Information Complete prescribing information for this medication should be consulted for additional detail.

Dosage Forms Excipient information presented when available (limited, particularly for generics); consult specific product labeling.

Solution, ophthalmic [drops]: 0.005% (2.5 mL)

Xalatan®: 0.005% (2.5 mL) [contains benzalkonium chloride]

- ◆ **Latisse®** *see* Bimatoprost *on page 219*
- ◆ **Latuda®** *see* Lurasidone *on page 1041*
- ◆ **Laxilose (Can)** *see* Lactulose *on page 964*
- ◆ **Lazanda®** *see* FentaNYL *on page 697*
- ◆ ***l*-Bunolol Hydrochloride** *see* Levobunolol *on page 995*
- ◆ **LCM** *see* Lacosamide *on page 963*
- ◆ **L-Deprenyl** *see* Selegiline *on page 1544*
- ◆ **LDP-341** *see* Bortezomib *on page 228*
- ◆ **LEA29Y** *see* Belatacept *on page 194*
- ◆ **Lederle Leucovorin (Can)** *see* Leucovorin Calcium *on page 987*
- ◆ **Leena®** *see* Ethinyl Estradiol and Norethindrone *on page 660*

Leflunomide (le FLOO noh mide)

Brand Names: U.S. Arava®

Brand Names: Canada Apo-Leflunomide®; Arava®; Mylan-Leflunomide; Novo-Leflunomide; PHL-Leflunomide; PMS-Leflunomide; Sandoz-Leflunomide

Pharmacologic Category Antirheumatic, Disease Modifying

Use Treatment of active rheumatoid arthritis; indicated to reduce signs and symptoms, and to inhibit structural damage and improve physical function

Unlabeled Use Treatment of cytomegalovirus (CMV) disease in transplant recipients resistant to standard antivirals; prevention of acute and chronic rejection in recipients of solid organ transplants

Pregnancy Risk Factor X

Pregnancy Considerations Has been associated with teratogenic and embryolethal effects in animal models at low doses. Leflunomide is contraindicated in pregnant women or women of childbearing potential who are not using reliable contraception. Pregnancy must be excluded prior to initiating treatment. **[U.S. Boxed Warning]: Women of childbearing potential should not receive therapy until pregnancy has been excluded,** they have been counseled concerning fetal risk, and reliable contraceptive measures have been confirmed. Following treatment, pregnancy should be avoided until undetectable serum concentrations (<0.02 mg/L) are verified. This may be accomplished by the use of an enhanced drug elimination procedure using cholestyramine. Serum concentrations <0.02 mg/L should be verified by two separate tests performed at least 14 days apart. If serum concentrations are >0.02 mg/L, additional cholestyramine treatment should be considered. Pregnant women exposed to leflunomide should be registered with the pregnancy registry (877-311-8972). It is not known if males taking leflunomide may contribute to fetal toxicity. Males taking leflunomide who wish to father a child should consider discontinuing therapy and using the cholestyramine procedure to eliminate the medication.

Lactation Excretion in breast milk unknown/not recommended

Contraindications Hypersensitivity to leflunomide or any component of the formulation; pregnancy

Warnings/Precautions Hazardous agent - use appropriate precautions for handling and disposal. **[U.S. Boxed Warning]: Use has been associated with rare reports of hepatotoxicity, hepatic failure, and death. Treatment should not be initiated in patients with pre-existing acute or chronic liver disease or ALT >2 x ULN. Use caution in patients with concurrent exposure to potentially hepatotoxic drugs. Monitor ALT levels during therapy; discontinue if ALT >3 x ULN occurs and, if hepatotoxicity is likely leflunomide-induced, start drug elimination procedures** (eg, cholestyramine, activated charcoal).

Use has been associated (rarely) with interstitial lung disease; discontinue in patients who develop new onset or worsening of pulmonary symptoms. Drug elimination procedures should be considered (eg, cholestyramine, activated charcoal) if interstitial lung disease occurs; fatal outcomes have been reported. May increase susceptibility to infection, including opportunistic pathogens. Severe infections, sepsis, and fatalities have been reported. Not recommended in patients with severe immunodeficiency, bone marrow dysplasia, or severe, uncontrolled infections. Caution should be exercised when considering the use in patients with a history of new/recurrent infections, with conditions that predispose them to infections, or with chronic, latent, or localized infections. Patients who develop a new infection while undergoing treatment should be monitored closely; consider discontinuation of therapy and drug elimination procedures if infection is serious.

Use may affect defenses against malignancies; impact on the development and course of malignancies is not fully defined. As compared to the general population, an increased risk of lymphoma has been noted in clinical trials; however, rheumatoid arthritis has been previously associated with an increased rate of lymphoma. Use with caution in patients with a prior history of significant hematologic abnormalities; avoid use with bone marrow dysplasia. Use has been associated with rare pancytopenia, agranulocytosis, and thrombocytopenia, generally when given concurrently or recently with methotrexate or other immunosuppressive agents. Monitoring of hematologic function is required; discontinue if evidence of bone marrow suppression and begin drug elimination procedures (eg, cholestyramine or activated charcoal). Rare cases of dermatologic reactions (including Stevens-Johnson syndrome and toxic epidermal necrolysis) have been reported; discontinue if evidence of severe dermatologic reaction occurs, and begin drug elimination procedures (eg, cholestyramine or activated charcoal). Cases of peripheral neuropathy have been reported; use with caution in patients >60 years of age, receiving concomitant neurotoxic medications, or patients with diabetes; discontinue if evidence of peripheral neuropathy occurs and begin drug elimination procedures (eg, cholestyramine, activated charcoal).

Safety has not been established in patients with latent tuberculosis infection. Patients should be screened for tuberculosis and if necessary, treated prior to initiating therapy. Use with caution in patients with renal impairment. **[U.S. Boxed Warning]: Women of childbearing potential should not receive therapy until pregnancy has been excluded,** they have been counseled concerning fetal risk and reliable contraceptive measures have been confirmed. Women of childbearing potential should also undergo drug elimination procedures (eg, cholestyramine, activated charcoal) following discontinuation of therapy. Patients should be brought up to date with all immunizations before initiating therapy. Live vaccines should not be given concurrently; there is no data available concerning secondary transmission of live vaccines in patients receiving therapy. Due to variations in clearance, it may take up to 2 years to reach low levels of leflunomide metabolite serum concentrations. A drug elimination procedure using cholestyramine or activated charcoal is recommended when a more rapid elimination is needed.

Adverse Reactions

>10%:

- Gastrointestinal: Diarrhea (17%)
- Respiratory: Respiratory tract infection (4% to 15%)

1% to 10%:

- Cardiovascular: Hypertension (10%), chest pain (2%), edema (peripheral), palpitation, tachycardia, vasodilation, varicose vein, vasculitis
- Central nervous system: Headache (7%), dizziness (4%), pain (2%), anxiety, depression, fever, insomnia, malaise, migraine, sleep disorder, vertigo
- Dermatologic: Alopecia (10%), rash (10%), pruritus (4%), dry skin (2%), eczema (2%), acne, bruising, dermatitis, hair discoloration, hematoma, nail disorder, skin disorder/discoloration, skin ulcer, subcutaneous nodule
- Endocrine & metabolic: Hypokalemia (1%), diabetes mellitus, hyperglycemia, hyperlipidemia, hyperthyroidism, menstrual disorder
- Gastrointestinal: Nausea (9%), abdominal pain (5% to 6%), dyspepsia (5%), weight loss (4%), anorexia (3%), gastroenteritis (3%), mouth ulceration (3%), vomiting (3%), candidiasis (oral), colitis, constipation, esophagitis, flatulence, gastritis, gingivitis, melena, salivary gland enlarged, stomatitis, taste disturbance, xerostomia
- Genitourinary: Urinary tract infection (5%), albuminuria, cystitis, dysuria, prostate disorder, urinary frequency, vaginal candidiasis
- Hematologic: Anemia
- Hepatic: Abnormal LFTs (5%), cholelithiasis
- Local: Abscess

Neuromuscular & skeletal: Back pain (5%), joint disorder (4%), weakness (3%), tenosynovitis (3%), synovitis (2%), paresthesia (2%), arthralgia (1%), leg cramps (1%), arthrosis, bone necrosis, bone pain, bursitis, CPK increased, myalgia, neck pain, neuralgia, neuritis, pelvic pain, tendon rupture

Ocular: Blurred vision, cataract, conjunctivitis, eye disorder

Renal: Hematuria

Respiratory: Bronchitis (7%), cough (3%), pharyngitis (3%), pneumonia (2%), rhinitis (2%), sinusitis (2%), asthma, dyspnea, epistaxis

Miscellaneous: Accidental injury (5%), allergic reactions (2%), flu-like syndrome (2%), cyst, diaphoresis, hernia, herpes infection

<1% (Limited to important or life-threatening): Agranulocytosis, anaphylaxis, angioedema, cholestasis, cutaneous necrotizing vasculitis, eosinophilia, erythema multiforme, hepatotoxicity (rare, including hepatic necrosis and hepatic failure, some fatalities reported), hepatitis, interstitial lung disease, jaundice, leukopenia, neutropenia, opportunistic infection, pancreatitis, pancytopenia, peripheral neuropathy, pneumonitis (interstitial), pulmonary fibrosis, sepsis, Stevens-Johnson syndrome, thrombocytopenia, toxic epidermal necrolysis, urticaria

Drug Interactions

Metabolism/Transport Effects Inhibits CYP2C9 (moderate)

Avoid Concomitant Use

Avoid concomitant use of Leflunomide with any of the following: BCG; Natalizumab; Pimecrolimus; Tacrolimus (Topical)

Increased Effect/Toxicity

Leflunomide may increase the levels/effects of: Carvedilol; CYP2C9 Substrates; Natalizumab; TOLBUTamide; Vaccines (Live); Vitamin K Antagonists

The levels/effects of Leflunomide may be increased by: Denosumab; Immunosuppressants; Methotrexate; Pimecrolimus; Rifampin; Roflumilast; Tacrolimus (Topical); TOLBUTamide; Trastuzumab

Decreased Effect

Leflunomide may decrease the levels/effects of: BCG; Coccidioidin Skin Test; Sipuleucel-T; Vaccines (Inactivated)

The levels/effects of Leflunomide may be decreased by: Bile Acid Sequestrants; Charcoal, Activated; Echinacea

Ethanol/Nutrition/Herb Interactions

Food: No interactions with food have been noted.

Herb/Nutraceutical: Echinacea may diminish the therapeutic effect of leflunomide.

Stability Store at 25°C (77°F); excursions permitted to 15°C to 30°C (59°F to 86°F). Protect from light.

Mechanism of Action Leflunomide is an immunodulatory agent that inhibits pyrimidine synthesis, resulting in antiproliferative and anti-inflammatory effects. Leflunomide is a prodrug; the active metabolite is responsible for activity. For CMV, may interfere with virion assembly.

Pharmacodynamics/Kinetics

Distribution: V_d: M1: 0.13 L/kg

Protein binding: M1: >99% to albumin

Metabolism: Hepatic to an active metabolite M1 (also known as A77 1726 or teriflunomide), which accounts for nearly all pharmacologic activity; further metabolism to multiple inactive metabolites; undergoes enterohepatic recirculation

Bioavailability: 80% (relative to oral solution)

Half-life elimination: M1: Mean: 14-15 days; enterohepatic recycling appears to contribute to the long half-life of this agent, since activated charcoal and cholestyramine substantially reduce plasma half-life

Time to peak: M1: 6-12 hours

Excretion: Feces (48%); urine (43%)

Dosage Oral:

Adults:

Rheumatoid arthritis: Loading dose: 100 mg/day for 3 days, followed by 20 mg/day; **Note:** The loading dose may be omitted in patients at increased risk of hepatic or hematologic toxicity (eg, recent concomitant methotrexate). Dosage may be decreased to 10 mg/day in patients who have difficulty tolerating the 20 mg dose. Due to the long half-life of the active metabolite, serum concentrations may require a prolonged period to decline after dosage reduction.

CMV disease, resistant to standard antivirals (unlabeled use): Some authors recommend 100-200 mg/day for 5-7 days, followed by 40-60 mg/day (Avery, 2004; Avery, 2010). Others have utilized the standard rheumatoid arthritis dosing (John, 2004). Adjust dose based on serum concentrations of metabolite and adverse events (Avery, 2008; Avery, 2010; Williams, 2002).

Elderly: Although hepatic function may decline with age, no specific dosage adjustment is recommended. Patients should be monitored closely for adverse effects which may require dosage adjustment.

Dosing adjustment in renal impairment: No specific dosage adjustment is recommended. There is no clinical experience in the use of leflunomide in patients with renal impairment. The free fraction of M1 is doubled in dialysis patients. Patients should be monitored closely for adverse effects requiring dosage adjustment.

Dosing adjustment in hepatic impairment: Not recommended for use in patients with pre-existing liver disease or in patients with significant hepatic impairment (ALT >2 times ULN). Patients should have LFTs monitored closely. Discontinue leflunomide if ALT >3 times ULN.

Dosing adjustment in hepatic toxicity: ALT elevations >3 times ULN: Discontinue leflunomide and initiate cholestyramine to enhance elimination

Drug elimination procedure: To achieve nondetectable serum concentrations (<0.02 mg/L) of the active metabolite (M1) of leflunomide administer the following:

Cholestyramine: 8 g administered 3 times/day for 11 days. The 11 days do not need to be consecutive unless plasma concentrations need to be lowered rapidly. Verify serum concentrations by 2 separate tests ≥14 days apart. If plasma concentrations are still high, additional cholestyramine treatment may be considered. In healthy volunteers, cholestyramine 8 g administered 3 times/day for 24 hours decreased M1 concentrations by 40% in 24 hours and 49% to 65% in 48 hours.

Activated charcoal: 50 g every 6 hours for 24 hours was shown to decrease plasma concentrations of M1 by 37% in 24 hours and 48% in 48 hours.

Dietary Considerations May be taken without regard to meals.

Administration Administer without regard to meals.

Monitoring Parameters A complete blood count (WBC, platelet count, hemoglobin or hematocrit), serum phosphate, as well as serum transaminase determinations should be monitored at baseline and monthly during the initial 6 months of treatment; if stable, monitoring frequency may be decreased to every 6-8 weeks thereafter (continue monthly when used in combination with other immunosuppressive agents). ALT should be monitored at least monthly for the first 6 months of treatment, then every 6-8 weeks thereafter (discontinue if ALT >3 x ULN, treat with cholestyramine, and monitor liver function at least weekly until normal). In addition, monitor for signs/symptoms of severe infection, abnormalities in hepatic function tests, symptoms of hepatotoxicity, and blood pressure. If coadministered with methotrexate, monthly transaminases (ALT, AST) and serum albumin levels are recommended. Screen for tuberculosis and pregnancy prior to therapy.

When used for CMV disease, monitor serum trough concentrations of active metabolite (also see Reference Range).

Reference Range CMV disease:

Timing of serum samples: Initial: Obtain 24 hours after last dose of loading regimen and periodically thereafter

Therapeutic concentration: Active metabolite (A77 1726, M1, or teriflunomide): Trough: 50-80 mcg/mL (Avery, 2010) or up to 100 mcg/mL (Williams, 2002)

Dosage Forms Excipient information presented when available (limited, particularly for generics); consult specific product labeling.

Tablet, oral: 10 mg, 20 mg

Arava®: 10 mg, 20 mg

◆ **Legatrin PM® [OTC]** *see* Acetaminophen and Diphenhydramine *on page 31*

Lenalidomide (le na LID oh mide)

Brand Names: U.S. Revlimid®

Brand Names: Canada Revlimid®

Index Terms CC-5013; IMid-1

Pharmacologic Category Angiogenesis Inhibitor; Antineoplastic Agent; Immunomodulator, Systemic

Use Treatment of low- or intermediate-risk myelodysplastic syndrome (MDS) in patients with deletion 5q (del 5q) cytogenetic abnormality with transfusion-dependent anemia (with or without other cytogenetic abnormalities); treatment of multiple myeloma (in combination with dexamethasone) in patients who have received at least one prior therapy

Unlabeled Use Treatment of non-Hodgkin's lymphomas; systemic amyloidosis (light chain); lower-risk myelodysplastic syndrome (MDS) in transfusion-dependent patients without deletion 5q (del 5q); maintenance treatment for multiple myeloma (following autologous stem cell transplant)

Pregnancy Risk Factor X

Pregnancy Considerations **[U.S. Boxed Warning]: Lenalidomide is an analogue of thalidomide (a human teratogen) and could potentially cause birth defects in humans; avoid pregnancy while taking lenalidomide. Distribution is restricted; physicians, pharmacists, and patients must be registered with the RevAssist® program.** Animal studies with lenalidomide in nonhuman primates have demonstrated malformations similar to those observed with thalidomide; there are no adequate and well-controlled studies in pregnant women. Women of childbearing potential should be treated only if they are able to comply with the conditions of the RevAssist® program. Female patients must commit either to abstain continuously or two forms of effective contraception are required beginning 4 weeks prior to, during, and for 4 weeks after therapy and during therapy interruptions. Pregnancy tests (sensitivity of at least 50 mIU/mL) should be performed 10-14 days and 24 hours prior to beginning therapy; weekly for the first 4 weeks and every 4 weeks (every 2 weeks if menstrual cycle irregular) thereafter and during therapy interruptions. Lenalidomide must be immediately discontinued and the patient referred to a reproductive toxicity specialist if pregnancy occurs during treatment. Males (even those vasectomized) should use a latex condom during any sexual contact with women of childbearing age. Risk to the fetus from semen of male patients is unknown. The parent or legal guardian for patients between 12 and 18 years of age must agree to ensure compliance with the required guidelines. Any suspected fetal exposure should be reported to the FDA via the MedWatch program (1-800-FDA-1088) and to Celgene Corporation (1-888-423-5436)

Lactation Excretion in breast milk unknown/not recommended

Prescribing and Access Restrictions As a requirement of the REMS program, access to this medication is restricted. Lenalidomide is approved for marketing in the U.S. only under a Food and Drug Administration (FDA) approved, restricted distribution program called RevAssist® (www.REVLIMID.com or 1-888-423-5436). In Canada, distribution is restricted through RevAid® (www.RevAid.ca or 1-888-738-2431). Physicians, pharmacies, and patients must be registered; a maximum 28-day supply may be dispensed; a new prescription is required each time it is filled; pregnancy testing is required for females of childbearing potential.

Medication Guide Available Yes

Contraindications Hypersensitivity to lenalidomide or any component of the formulation; pregnancy or women capable of becoming pregnant

Canadian labeling: Additional contraindications (not in U.S. labeling): Platelet count <50,000/mm^3; hypersensitivity to thalidomide; breast-feeding women

Warnings/Precautions Hazardous agent - use appropriate precautions for handling and disposal. **[U.S. Boxed Warning]: Hematologic toxicity (neutropenia and thrombocytopenia) occurs in a majority of patients (grade 3/4: 80% in patients with del 5q myelodysplastic syndrome) and may require dose reductions and/or delays; the use of blood product support and/or growth factors may be needed. CBC should be monitored weekly for the first 8 weeks and at least monthly thereafter in patients being treated for del 5q myelodysplastic syndromes.** In patients being treated for multiple myeloma, monitor CBC every 2 weeks for 12 weeks and monthly thereafter. **[U.S. Boxed Warning]: Lenalidomide has been associated with a significant increase in risk for thrombosis and embolism in multiple myeloma patients treated with combination therapy. Deep vein thrombosis (DVT) and pulmonary embolism (PE) have occurred; monitor for signs and symptoms of thromboembolism (shortness of breath, chest pain, or arm or leg swelling) and seek prompt medical attention with development of these symptoms.** Use caution in renal impairment; may experience an increased rate of toxicities. The NCCN multiple myeloma guidelines (v1.2011) recommend anticoagulant prophylaxis when used in combination with dexamethasone. Anticoagulant prophylaxis should be individualized and selected based on the venous thromboembolism risk of the combination treatment regimen, using the safest and easiest to administer (Palumbo, 2008).

Angioedema, Stevens-Johnson syndrome (SJS), and toxic epidermal necrolysis (TEN) have been reported; may be fatal. Consider interrupting or discontinuing treatment with grade 2 or 3 skin rash; discontinue and do not reinitiate treatment with grade 4 rash, exfoliative or bullous rash, or for suspected SJS or TEN. Patients with a history of grade 4 rash with thalidomide should not receive lenalidomide. Discontinue treatment with angioedema. Use caution in renal impairment; may experience an increased rate of toxicities (due to reduced clearance and increased half-life); initial dosage adjustments are recommended for moderate-to-severe and dialysis-dependent renal impairment. Patients with a high tumor burden may be at risk for tumor lysis syndrome.

[U.S. Boxed Warning]: Lenalidomide is an analogue of thalidomide (a human teratogen) and could potentially cause birth defects in humans; avoid pregnancy while taking lenalidomide. Distribution is restricted; physicians, pharmacists, and patients must be registered with the RevAssist® program. Patients should be advised not to donate blood during therapy and for 4 weeks following completion of therapy. May cause dizziness or fatigue; caution patients about performing tasks which require mental alertness (eg, operating machinery or driving). Formulation contains lactose; avoid use in patients with Lapp lactase deficiency, glucose-galactose malabsorption, or glucose intolerance. Lenalidomide should only be prescribed to patients (male and female) who can understand and comply with the conditions of the RevAssist® program. If used in patients between 12-18 years of age, the parent or legal guardian must agree to ensure compliance with the RevAssist® program.

Adverse Reactions

>10%:

Cardiovascular: Peripheral edema (8% to 21%)

Central nervous system: Fatigue (31% to 38%), insomnia (10% to 32%), fever (21% to 23%), dizziness (20% to 21%), headache (20% to 21%)

Dermatologic: Pruritus (42%), rash (16% to 36%; grades 3/4: 7%), dry skin (14%)

Endocrine & metabolic: Hyperglycemia (15%), hypokalemia (11%)

Gastrointestinal: Diarrhea (29% to 49%), constipation (24% to 39%), nausea (22% to 24%), weight loss (18%), dyspepsia (14%), anorexia (10% to 14%), taste perversion (6% to 13%), abdominal pain (8% to 12%)

Genitourinary: Urinary tract infection (11%)

Hematologic: Thrombocytopenia (17% to 62%; grades 3/4: 10% to 50%; onset [MDS]: 28 days [range 8-290 days]; recovery [MDS]: 22 days [range: 5-224 days]), neutropenia (28% to 59%; grades 3/4: 21% to 53%; onset [MDS]: 42 days [range 14-411 days]; recovery [MDS]: 17 days [range: 2-170 days]), anemia (12% to 24%; grades 3/4: 6% to 8%); myelosuppression is dose-dependent and reversible with treatment interruption and/or dose reduction

Neuromuscular & skeletal: Muscle cramp (18% to 30%), weakness (15% to 23%), arthralgia (10% to 22%), back pain (15% to 21%), tremor (20%), paresthesia (12%), limb pain (11%)

Ocular: Blurred vision (15%)

Respiratory: Nasopharyngitis (23%), cough (15% to 20%), dyspnea (7% to 20%), pharyngitis (16%), epistaxis (15%), upper respiratory infection (14% to 15%), pneumonia (11% to 12%)

1% to 10%:

Cardiovascular: Edema (10%), deep vein thrombosis (≤8%; grades 3/4: ≤7%), hypertension (6%), chest pain (5%), palpitation (5%), atrial fibrillation (grades 3/4: ≤3%), syncope (grade 3: 1% to 2%)

Central nervous system: Hypoesthesia (7%), pain (7%), depression (5%)

Dermatologic: Bruising (5% to 8%), cellulitis (5%), erythema (5%)

Endocrine & metabolic: Hypothyroidism (7%), hypomagnesemia (6%), hypocalcemia (grades 3/4: 4%)

Gastrointestinal: Vomiting (10%), xerostomia (7%), loose stools (6%)

Genitourinary: Dysuria (7%)

Hematologic: Leukopenia (8%; grade 3/4: ≤5%), febrile neutropenia (5%; grades 3/4: 4%), granulocytopenia (grades 3/4: 2%), lymphopenia (grade 3: 2%), pancytopenia (grades 3/4: 2%)

Hepatic: ALT increased (8%)

Neuromuscular & skeletal: Myalgia (9%), rigors (6%), peripheral neuropathy (5%)

Respiratory: Sinusitis (8%), rhinitis (7%), bronchitis (6%), pulmonary embolism (≤3%; grades 3/4: 1% to 3%), respiratory distress (grades 3/4: 2%), hypoxia (grades 3/4: 1%), pleural effusion (grades 3/4: 1%), pneumonitis (grades 3/4: 1%), pulmonary hypertension (grades 3/4: 1%)

Miscellaneous: Night sweats (8%), diaphoresis (7%), sepsis (grades 3/4: 3%)

<1% (Limited to important or life-threatening): Acute febrile neutrophilic dermatosis, acute leukemia, acute myeloid leukemia (AML), adrenal insufficiency, angioedema, atrial flutter, azotemia, Basedow's disease, biliary obstruction, blindness, bone marrow depression, bradycardia, brain edema, cardiac failure, cardiogenic shock, cardiomyopathy, cardiopulmonary arrest, cerebrovascular accident, CHF, cholecystitis, chondrocalcinosis, chronic obstructive airway disease, circulatory collapse, coagulopathy, colonic polyp, dehydration, delirium, diabetes mellitus, diabetic ketoacidosis, diverticulitis, dysphagia, encephalitis, erythema multiforme, Fanconi syndrome, gout, hematuria, hemolysis, hemolytic anemia, hemorrhage, hepatic failure, hepatitis, herpesvirus infection, hyperbilirubinemia, hypernatremia, hypersensitivity, hypoglycemia, hypotension, infection, interstitial lung disease, intestinal perforation, intracranial hemorrhage, ischemia, ischemic colitis, leukoencephalopathy, liver failure, liver function tests abnormal, lung cancer, lung infiltration, lymphoma, MI, myopathy, neutropenic sepsis, orthostatic hypotension, pancreatitis, peripheral ischemia, pseudomembraneous colitis, pulmonary edema, refractory anemia, renal calculus, renal failure, renal mass, renal tubular necrosis, respiratory failure, septic shock, serum creatinine increased, skin desquamation, small bowel obstruction, spinal cord compression, splenic infarction, Stevens-Johnson syndrome, stomatitis, supraventricular arrhythmia, tachyarrhythmia, thrombophlebitis, toxic epidermal necrolysis, troponin I increased, urinary retention, urosepsis, urticaria, ventricular dysfunction, wheezing

Drug Interactions

Metabolism/Transport Effects None known.

Avoid Concomitant Use

Avoid concomitant use of Lenalidomide with any of the following: Abatacept; Anakinra; BCG; Canakinumab; Certolizumab Pegol; CloZAPine; Natalizumab; Pimecrolimus; Rilonacept; Tacrolimus (Topical); Vaccines (Live)

Increased Effect/Toxicity

Lenalidomide may increase the levels/effects of: Abatacept; Anakinra; Canakinumab; Certolizumab Pegol; CloZAPine; Leflunomide; Natalizumab; Rilonacept; Vaccines (Live)

The levels/effects of Lenalidomide may be increased by: Denosumab; Dexamethasone; Dexamethasone (Systemic); Pimecrolimus; Roflumilast; Tacrolimus (Topical); Trastuzumab

Decreased Effect

Lenalidomide may decrease the levels/effects of: BCG; Coccidioidin Skin Test; Sipuleucel-T; Vaccines (Inactivated); Vaccines (Live)

The levels/effects of Lenalidomide may be decreased by: Echinacea

Ethanol/Nutrition/Herb Interactions Herb/Nutraceutical: Avoid echinacea (has immunostimulant properties; consider therapy modifications).

Stability Store at 25°C (77°F); excursions permitted to 15°C and 30°C (59°F and 86°F).

Mechanism of Action Immunomodulatory, antiangiogenic, and antineoplastic characteristics via multiple mechanisms. Selectively inhibits secretion of proinflammatory cytokines (potent inhibitor of tumor necrosis factor-alpha secretion); enhances cell-mediated immunity by stimulating proliferation of anti-CD3 stimulated T cells (resulting in increased IL-2 and interferon gamma secretion); inhibits trophic signals to angiogenic factors in cells. Inhibits the growth of myeloma cells by inducing cell cycle arrest and cell death.

Pharmacodynamics/Kinetics

Absorption: Rapid

Protein binding: ~30%

Half-life elimination: ~3 hours; moderate-to-severe renal impairment: ~9 hours; hemodialysis patients: ~13.5 hours

Time, to peak, plasma: Healthy volunteers: ~0.6-1.5 hours; Myeloma patients: 0.5-4 hours

Excretion: Urine (~67% as unchanged drug)

Hemodialysis effect: ~40% of a dose is removed in a single dialysis session

Dosage Oral:

Adults:

Multiple myeloma: 25 mg once daily for 21 days of a 28-day treatment cycle (in combination with dexamethasone)

Myelodysplastic syndrome (MDS) with deletion 5q: 10 mg once daily

Diffuse large B-cell lymphoma (unlabeled use): 25 mg once daily for 21 days of a 28-day treatment cycle for up to 1 year (Wiernik, 2008)

Mantle cell lymphoma, relapsed or refractory (unlabeled use): 25 mg once daily for 21 days of a 28-day treatment cycle for up to 1 year (Habermann, 2009)

Multiple myeloma, maintenance (following autologous stem cell transplant; unlabeled use): 10-15 mg once daily until relapse (Attal, 2009; McCarthy, 2009) **or** 10 mg once daily for 21 days of a 28-day treatment cycle until relapse (Palumbo, 2010)

Myelodysplastic syndrome (MDS), lower risk, without deletion 5q (unlabeled use): 10 mg once daily (Raza, 2008)

Elderly: Refer to adult dosing; due to the potential for decreased renal function in the elderly, select dose carefully and closely monitor renal function

Dosage adjustment in renal impairment:

Recommended initial dose adjustment in the FDA-approved labeling:

MDS:

Cl_{cr} ≥60 mL/minute: No adjustment required

Cl_{cr} 30-59 mL/minute: 5 mg once daily

Cl_{cr} <30 mL/minute (nondialysis dependent): 5 mg every 48 hours

Cl_{cr} <30 mL/minute (dialysis dependent): 5 mg 3 times/week (administer following each dialysis)

Multiple myeloma:

Cl_{cr} ≥60 mL/minute: No adjustment required

Cl_{cr} 30-59 mL/minute: 10 mg once daily

Cl_{cr} <30 mL/minute (nondialysis dependent): 15 mg every 48 hours

Cl_{cr} <30 mL/minute (dialysis dependent): 5 mg once daily (administer after dialysis on dialysis days)

Recommended adjustment in Canadian labeling:

MDS:

Cl_{cr} ≥50 mL/minute: No adjustment required

Cl_{cr} 30-49 mL/minute: 5 mg once daily

Cl_{cr} <30 mL/minute (nondialysis dependent): 5 mg every 48 hours

Cl_{cr} <30 mL/minute (dialysis dependent): 5 mg 3 times/week (administer following each dialysis)

Multiple myeloma:

Cl_{cr} ≥50 mL/minute: No adjustment required

Cl_{cr} 30-49 mL/minute: 10 mg once daily; (may increase to 15 mg once daily after 2 cycles if nonresponsive but tolerating treatment; Chen, 2007)

Cl_{cr} <30 mL/minute (nondialysis dependent): 15 mg every 48 hours

Cl_{cr} <30 mL/minute (dialysis dependent): 15 mg 3 times/week (administer following each dialysis)

Dosage adjustment for NONHEMATOLOGIC toxicities:

Dermatologic toxicities:

Skin rash, grade 2 or 3: Consider interrupting or discontinuing treatment

Angioedema, grade 4 rash, exfoliative or bullous rash, or suspected Stevens-Johnson syndrome or toxic epidermal necrolysis: Discontinue treatment

Other toxicities: For additional treatment-related grade 3/4 toxicities, hold treatment and restart at next lower dose level when toxicity has resolved to ≤grade 2.

Dosage adjustment for HEMATOLOGIC toxicities:

Adjustment for thrombocytopenia in MDS:

Thrombocytopenia developing within 4 weeks of beginning treatment at 10 mg/day:

Baseline platelets ≥100,000/mm^3:

If platelets <50,000/mm^3: Hold treatment

When platelets return to ≥50,000/mm^3: Resume treatment at 5 mg/day

Baseline platelets <100,000/mm^3:

If platelets fall to 50% of baseline: Hold treatment

If baseline ≥60,000/mm^3 and platelet level returns to ≥50,000/mm^3: Resume at 5 mg/day

If baseline <60,000/mm^3 and platelet level returns to ≥30,000/mm^3: Resume at 5 mg/day

Thrombocytopenia developing after 4 weeks of beginning treatment at 10 mg/day:

Platelets <30,000/mm^3 **or** <50,000/mm^3 with platelet transfusions: Hold treatment

Platelets ≥30,000/mm^3 (without hemostatic failure): Resume at 5 mg/day

Thrombocytopenia developing with treatment at 5 mg/day:

Platelets <30,000/mm^3 **or** <50,000/mm^3 with platelet transfusions: Hold treatment

Platelets ≥30,000/mm^3 (without hemostatic failure): Resume at 5 mg every other day

Adjustment for neutropenia in MDS:

Neutropenia developing within 4 weeks of beginning treatment at 10 mg/day:

For baseline absolute neutrophil count (ANC) ≥1000/mm^3:

ANC <750/mm^3: Hold treatment

When ANC returns to ≥1000/mm^3: Resume at 5 mg/day

For baseline absolute neutrophil count (ANC) <1000/mm^3:

ANC <500/mm^3: Hold treatment

When ANC returns to ≥500/mm^3: Resume at 5 mg/day

Neutropenia developing after 4 weeks of beginning treatment at 10 mg/day:

ANC <500/mm^3 for ≥7 days or associated with fever: Hold treatment

When ≥500/mm^3: Resume at 5 mg/day

Neutropenia developing with treatment at 5 mg/day:

ANC <500/mm^3 for ≥7 days or associated with fever: Hold treatment

When ≥500/mm^3: Resume at 5 mg every other day

Adjustment for thrombocytopenia in multiple myeloma:

Platelets <30,000/mm^3: Hold treatment, check CBC weekly

When platelets ≥30,000/mm^3: Resume at 15 mg daily

Additional occurrence of platelets <30,000/mm^3: Hold treatment

When platelets ≥30,000/mm^3: Resume treatment at 5 mg below previous dose; do not dose below 5 mg daily

Adjustment for neutropenia in multiple myeloma:

ANC <1000/mm^3: Hold treatment, add G-CSF, check CBC weekly

When ≥1000/mm³ (with neutropenia as only toxicity): Resume at 25 mg/day

When ≥1000/mm³ (with additional toxicities): Resume at 15 mg/day

Additional occurrence of ANC <1000/mm³: Hold treatment

When ≥1000/mm³: Resume treatment at 5 mg below previous dose; do not dose below 5 mg daily.

Administration Administer with water. Swallow capsule whole; do not break, open, or chew.

Monitoring Parameters CBC with differential (MDS: weekly for first 8 weeks; multiple myeloma: every 2 weeks for the first 3 months), then monthly thereafter; serum creatinine, liver function tests, thyroid function tests; ECG when clinically indicated; monitor for signs and symptoms of thromboembolism or tumor lysis syndrome

Women of childbearing potential: Pregnancy test 10-14 days **and** 24 hours prior to initiating therapy, weekly during the first 4 weeks of treatment, then every 2-4 weeks through 4 weeks after therapy discontinued

Additional Information Pregnancy tests are required prior to beginning therapy, throughout treatment and during therapy interruptions for all women of childbearing age. The pregnancy test must be verified by the prescriber and the pharmacist prior to dispensing. Effective contraception with at least two reliable forms of contraception (IUD, hormonal contraception, tubal ligation or partner's vasectomy plus latex condom, diaphragm, or cervical cap) should be used for 4 weeks prior to beginning therapy, during therapy, and for 4 weeks following discontinuance of therapy. Women who have undergone a hysterectomy or have been postmenopausal for at least 24 consecutive months are the only exception. Do not prescribe, administer, or dispense to women of childbearing age or males who may have intercourse with women of childbearing age unless both female and male are capable of complying with contraceptive measures. Even males who have undergone vasectomy must acknowledge these risks in writing, and must use a latex condom during any sexual contact with women of childbearing age. Oral and written warnings concerning contraception and the hazards of thalidomide must be conveyed to females and males and they must acknowledge their understanding in writing. Parents or guardians must consent and sign acknowledgment for patients 12-18 years of age following therapy. A maximum 28-day supply should be dispensed.

Dosage Forms Excipient information presented when available (limited, particularly for generics); consult specific product labeling.

Capsule, oral:

Revlimid®: 5 mg, 10 mg, 15 mg, 25 mg

Lepirudin (leh puh ROO din)

Brand Names: U.S. Refludan®

Brand Names: Canada Refludan®

Index Terms Lepirudin (rDNA); Recombinant Hirudin

Pharmacologic Category Anticoagulant, Thrombin Inhibitor

Use Indicated for anticoagulation in patients with heparin-induced thrombocytopenia (HIT) and associated thromboembolic disease in order to prevent further thromboembolic complications

Pregnancy Risk Factor B

Pregnancy Considerations Lepirudin crosses the placenta in pregnant rats; however, it is not known if lepirudin crosses the placenta in humans.

Lactation Enters breast milk/consult prescriber

Contraindications Hypersensitivity to hirudins or any component of the formulation

Warnings/Precautions Hemorrhagic events: Intracranial bleeding following concomitant thrombolytic therapy with rt-PA or streptokinase may be life threatening. For patients with an increased risk of bleeding, a careful assessment weighing the risk of lepirudin administration versus its anticipated benefit has to be made by the treating physician. In particular, this includes the following conditions: Recent puncture of large vessels or organ biopsy; anomaly of vessels or organs; recent cerebrovascular accident, stroke, intracerebral surgery, or other neuroaxial procedures; severe uncontrolled hypertension; bacterial endocarditis; advanced renal impairment; hemorrhagic diathesis; recent major surgery; and recent major bleeding (eg, intracranial, gastrointestinal, intraocular, or pulmonary bleeding). With renal impairment, relative overdose might occur even with standard dosage regimen. The bolus dose and rate of infusion must be reduced in patients with known or suspected renal insufficiency.

Formation of antihirudin antibodies may increase the anticoagulant effect of lepirudin possibly due to delayed renal elimination of active lepirudin-antihirudin complexes. Therefore, strict monitoring of aPTT is necessary also during prolonged therapy. No evidence of neutralization of lepirudin or of allergic reactions associated with positive antibody test results was found. Allergic and hypersensitivity reactions, including anaphylaxis have been reported and may occur frequently in patients treated concomitantly with streptokinase; caution is warranted during re-exposure (anaphylaxis has been reported).

Serious liver injury (eg, liver cirrhosis) may enhance the anticoagulant effect of lepirudin due to coagulation defects secondary to reduced generation of vitamin K-dependent clotting factors.

Clinical trials have provided limited information to support any recommendations for re-exposure to lepirudin (anaphylaxis has been reported). Safety and efficacy have not been established in children.

Adverse Reactions As with all anticoagulants, bleeding is the most common adverse event associated with lepirudin. Hemorrhage may occur at virtually any site. Risk is dependent on multiple variables.

HIT patients:

>10%: Hematologic: Anemia (12%), bleeding from puncture sites (11%), hematoma (11%)

1% to 10%:

Cardiovascular: Heart failure (3%), pericardial effusion (1%), ventricular fibrillation (1%)

Central nervous system: Fever (7%)

Dermatologic: Maculopapular rash (4%), eczema (3%)

Gastrointestinal: GI bleeding/rectal bleeding (5%)

Genitourinary: Vaginal bleeding (2%)

Hepatic: Transaminases increased (6%)

Renal: Hematuria (4%)

Respiratory: Epistaxis (4%)

<1% (Limited to important or life-threatening): Allergic reactions, anaphylaxis, hemoperitoneum, hemoptysis, injection site reactions, intracranial bleeding, liver bleeding, mouth bleeding, pruritus, pulmonary bleeding, retroperitoneal bleeding, thrombocytopenia, urticaria

Non-HIT populations (including those receiving thrombolytics and/or contrast media):

1% to 10%: Respiratory: Bronchospasm/stridor/dyspnea/cough

<1% (Limited to important or life-threatening): Allergic reactions (unspecified), anaphylactoid reactions, anaphylaxis, angioedema, intracranial bleeding (0.6%), laryngeal edema, thrombocytopenia, tongue edema

Drug Interactions

Metabolism/Transport Effects None known.

Avoid Concomitant Use

Avoid concomitant use of Lepirudin with any of the following: Rivaroxaban

Increased Effect/Toxicity

Lepirudin may increase the levels/effects of: Anticoagulants; Collagenase (Systemic); Deferasirox; Ibritumomab; Rivaroxaban; Tositumomab and Iodine I 131 Tositumomab

The levels/effects of Lepirudin may be increased by: Antiplatelet Agents; Dasatinib; Herbs (Anticoagulant/Antiplatelet Properties); Nonsteroidal Anti-Inflammatory Agents; Pentosan Polysulfate Sodium; Prostacyclin Analogues; Salicylates; Thrombolytic Agents

Decreased Effect There are no known significant interactions involving a decrease in effect.

Ethanol/Nutrition/Herb Interactions Herb/Nutraceutical: Avoid cat's claw, dong quai, evening primrose, feverfew, garlic, ginger, ginkgo, red clover, horse chestnut, green tea, ginseng (all have additional antiplatelet activity)

Stability

Intact vials should be stored at 2°C to 25°C (36°F to 77°F).

Intravenous bolus: Use a solution with a concentration of 5 mg/mL.

Preparation of a lepirudin solution with a concentration of 5 mg/mL: Reconstitute one vial (50 mg) of lepirudin with 1 mL of sterile water for injection or 0.9% sodium chloride injection. The final concentration of 5 mg/mL is obtained by transferring the contents of the vial into a sterile, single-use syringe (of at least 10 mL capacity) and diluting the solution to a total volume of 10 mL using sterile water for injection, 0.9% sodium chloride, or 5% dextrose in water.

Intravenous infusion: For continuous intravenous infusion, solutions with concentrations of 0.2 or 0.4 mg/mL may be used.

Preparation of a lepirudin solution with a concentration of 0.2 mg/mL or 0.4 mg/mL: Reconstitute 2 vials (50 mg each) of lepirudin with 1 mL each using either sterile water for injection or 0.9% sodium chloride injection. The final concentration of 0.2 mg/mL or 0.4 mg/mL is obtained by transferring the contents of both vials into an infusion bag containing 500 mL or 250 mL of 0.9% sodium chloride injection or 5% dextrose injection.

Reconstituted solutions of lepirudin are stable for 24 hours at room temperature. Manufacturer recommends using reconstituted solution immediately after preparation.

Mechanism of Action Lepirudin is a highly specific direct inhibitor of thrombin; lepirudin is a recombinant hirudin derived from yeast cells

Pharmacodynamics/Kinetics

Distribution: Two-compartment model; confined to extracellular fluids

Metabolism: Via release of amino acids via catabolic hydrolysis of parent drug

Half-life elimination: Initial: ~10 minutes: Terminal: Healthy volunteers: 1.3 hours; Marked renal impairment (Cl_{cr} <15 mL/minute and on hemodialysis): ≤2 days

Excretion: Urine (~48%, 35% as unchanged drug and unchanged drug fragments of parent drug); systemic clearance is proportional to glomerular filtration rate or creatinine clearance

Dosage Note: Maximum infusion dose: Do not exceed 0.21 mg/kg/hour unless an evaluation of coagulation abnormalities limiting response has been completed. Bolus doses may increase the risk of bleeding; consider omitting or reducing dose in certain populations.

Heparin-induced thrombocytopenia: Bolus dose: 0.4 mg/kg IVP (over 15-20 seconds), followed by continuous infusion at 0.15 mg/kg/hour (maximum initial bolus dose: 44 mg; maximum initial infusion dose: 16.5 mg/hour); bolus and infusion must be reduced in renal insufficiency

or

Alternate dosing regimen (unlabeled dose; Selleng, 2007; Warkentin, 2008): Bolus dose: 0.2 mg/kg (use only if life- or limb-threatening thrombosis present) followed by continuous infusion of 0.05-0.1 mg/kg/hour. Further dosage reduction may be required in patients with renal dysfunction. This alternate dosing regimen has been recommended due to higher rates of bleeding associated with the FDA-approved dosing regimen.

Concomitant use with thrombolytic therapy: Bolus dose: 0.2 mg/kg IVP (over 15-20 seconds), followed by continuous infusion at 0.1 mg/kg/hour

Dosing adjustments during infusions: Monitor first aPTT 4 hours after the start of the infusion. Subsequent determinations of aPTT should be obtained at least once daily during treatment. More frequent monitoring is recommended in renally- or hepatically-impaired patients. Any aPTT ratio measurement out of range (1.5-2.5) should be confirmed prior to adjusting dose, unless a clinical need for immediate reaction exists. If the aPTT is below target range, increase infusion by 20%. If the aPTT is in excess of the target range, stop infusion for 2 hours and when restarted the infusion rate should be decreased by 50%. A repeat aPTT should be obtained 4 hours after any dosing change.

Use in patients scheduled for switch to oral anticoagulants: Once platelets normalize, reduce lepirudin dose gradually to reach aPTT ratio just above 1.5 before starting warfarin therapy. Monitor PT/INR closely until results stabilize in therapeutic range. When lepirudin is discontinued, there may be a small reduction in INR.

Dosing adjustment in renal impairment: All patients with a creatinine clearance of <60 mL/minute or a serum creatinine of >1.5 mg/dL require dosage reduction. An alternate dosing regimen has also been recommended for patients with serum creatinine >1 mg/dL (Warkentin, 2008). There is only limited information on the therapeutic use of lepirudin in patients with HIT and significant renal impairment; the following dosage recommendations are mainly based on single-dose studies in a small number of patients with renal impairment.

Initial: Bolus dose: 0.2 mg/kg IVP (over 15-20 seconds), followed by adjusted infusion based on renal function; refer to the following infusion rate adjustments based on creatinine clearance (mL/minute) and serum creatinine (mg/dL):

Note: Acute renal failure or hemodialysis: Infusion is to be avoided or stopped. Following the bolus dose, additional bolus doses of 0.1 mg/kg may be administered every other day only if aPTT falls below lower therapeutic limit (1.5-times patient baseline [or mean laboratory] aPTT).

Lepirudin infusion rates in patients with renal impairment: See tables.

Lepirudin Infusion Rates in Patients With Renal Impairment

Creatinine Clearance (mL/min)	Serum Creatinine (mg/dL)	Adjusted Infusion Rate	
		% of Standard Initial Infusion Rate	mg/kg/h
45-60	1.6-2.0	50%	0.075
30-44	2.1-3.0	30%	0.045
15-29	3.1-6.0	15%	0.0225
<15	>6.0	***Avoid or STOP infusion***	

Alternate Dosing Regimen for Renal Impairment (based on *Chest* 2008 guidelines[1])

Serum Creatinine (mg/dL)	Adjusted Infusion Rate	
	% of Standard Initial Infusion Rate[2]	mg/kg/h
1.0-1.6	50%	0.05
1.7-4.5	10%	0.01
>4.5-6.0	5%	0.005
>6.0	***Avoid or STOP infusion***[3]	

[1]Recommendation based on low or very low-quality evidence.

[2]Recommended standard initial infusion rate: 0.1 mg/kg/hour

[3]Recommendation based on manufacturer's labeling.

Note: The initial bolus should either be omitted, or in the case of perceived life- or limb-threatening thrombosis, be given at a reduced dose of 0.2 mg/kg.

Administration Administer **only** intravenously; administer I.V. bolus over 15-20 seconds

Monitoring Parameters Monitor aPTT levels; obtain baseline aPTT, then monitor first aPTT 4 hours after the start of the infusion and every 4 hours until steady state is reached (2 consecutive aPTTs in the same range) (Warkentin, 2008). Subsequent determinations of aPTT should be obtained at least once daily during treatment. More frequent monitoring is recommended in renally- or hepatically-impaired patients. Any aPTT ratio measurement out of range (1.5-2.5) should be confirmed prior to adjusting dose, unless a clinical need for immediate reaction exists

Reference Range aPTT 1.5 to 2.5 times the control value

Test Interactions PT/INR levels may become elevated in the absence of warfarin. If warfarin is initiated, initial PT/INR goals while on lepirudin may require modification.

Dosage Forms Excipient information presented when available (limited, particularly for generics); consult specific product labeling.

Injection, powder for reconstitution:

Refludan®: 50 mg

◆ **Lepirudin (rDNA)** *see* Lepirudin *on page 984*

◆ **Lescol®** *see* Fluvastatin *on page 744*

◆ **Lescol® XL** *see* Fluvastatin *on page 744*

◆ **Lessina®** *see* Ethinyl Estradiol and Levonorgestrel *on page 656*

◆ **Letairis®** *see* Ambrisentan *on page 84*

Letrozole (LET roe zole)

Brand Names: U.S. Femara®

Brand Names: Canada Femara®; JAMP-Letrozole; Letrozole Tablets, USP; MED-Letrozole; Myl-Letrozole; PMS-Letrozole; Sandoz-Letrozole

Index Terms CGS-20267

Pharmacologic Category Antineoplastic Agent, Aromatase Inhibitor

Use For use in postmenopausal women in the adjuvant treatment of hormone receptor positive early breast cancer, extended adjuvant treatment of early breast cancer after 5 years of tamoxifen, advanced breast cancer with disease progression following antiestrogen therapy, hormone receptor positive or hormone receptor unknown, locally-advanced, or first-line (or second-line) treatment of advanced or metastatic breast cancer

Unlabeled Use Treatment of ovarian (epithelial) cancer, endometrial cancer

Pregnancy Risk Factor X

Pregnancy Considerations Letrozole may cause fetal harm when administered to pregnant women. Animal studies have demonstrated embryotoxicity and fetotoxicity. There are no adequate and well-controlled studies in pregnant women. If used in pregnancy, or if patient becomes pregnant during treatment, the patient should be apprised of potential hazard to the fetus. Letrozole is FDA indicated for postmenopausal women only (no clinical benefit for breast cancer has been demonstrated in premenopausal women). Women who are perimenopausal or recently postmenopausal should use adequate contraception until postmenopausal status is fully established.

Lactation Excretion in breast milk unknown/not recommended

Contraindications Use in women who are or may become pregnant

Canadian labeling: Additional contraindications (not in U.S. labeling): Hypersensitivity to letrozole, other aromatase inhibitors, or any component of the formulation; use in patients <18 years of age; breast-feeding

Warnings/Precautions Hazardous agent - use appropriate precautions for handling and disposal. Use caution with hepatic impairment; dose adjustment recommended in patients with cirrhosis or severe hepatic dysfunction. May cause dizziness, fatigue, and somnolence; patients should be cautioned before performing tasks which require mental alertness (eg, operating machinery or driving). May increase total serum cholesterol; in patients treated with adjuvant therapy and cholesterol levels within normal limits, an increase of >1.5 x ULN in total cholesterol has been demonstrated in 8.2% of letrozole-treated patients (25% requiring lipid-lowering medications) vs 3.2% of tamoxifen-treated patients (16% requiring medications); monitor cholesterol panel; may require antihyperlipidemics. May cause decreases in bone mineral density (BMD); a decrease in hip BMD by 3.8% from baseline in letrozole-treated patients vs 2% in placebo at 2 years has been demonstrated; however, there was no statistical difference in changes to the lumbar spine BMD scores; monitor BMD.

Adverse Reactions

>10%:

Cardiovascular: Edema (7% to 18%)

Central nervous system: Headache (4% to 20%), dizziness (3% to 14%), fatigue (8% to 13%)

Endocrine & metabolic: Hypercholesterolemia (3% to 52%), hot flashes (6% to 50%)

Gastrointestinal: Nausea (9% to 17%), weight gain (2% to 13%), constipation (2% to 11%)

Neuromuscular & skeletal: Weakness (4% to 34%), arthralgia (8% to 25%), arthritis (7% to 25%), bone pain (5% to 22%), back pain (5% to 18%), bone mineral density decreased/osteoporosis (5% to 15%), bone fracture (10% to 14%)
Respiratory: Dyspnea (6% to 18%), cough (6% to 13%)
Miscellaneous: Diaphoresis (≤24%), night sweats (15%)

1% to 10%:
Cardiovascular: Chest pain (6% to 8%), hypertension (5% to 8%), chest wall pain (6%), peripheral edema (5%), cerebrovascular accident (2% to 3%), thromboembolic event (2% to 3%), MI (1% to 2%), angina (1%)
Central nervous system: Insomnia (6% to 7%), pain (5%), anxiety (<5%), depression (<5%), vertigo (<5%), somnolence (3%)
Dermatologic: Rash (5%), alopecia (3% to 5%), pruritus (1%)
Endocrine & metabolic: Breast pain (2% to 7%), hypercalcemia (<5%)
Gastrointestinal: Diarrhea (5% to 8%), vomiting (3% to 7%), weight loss (6% to 7%), abdominal pain (6%), anorexia (1% to 5%), dyspepsia (3%)
Genitourinary: Urinary tract infection (6%), vaginal bleeding (5%), vaginal dryness (5%), vaginal hemorrhage (5%), vaginal irritation (5%)
Neuromuscular & skeletal: Limb pain (4% to 10%), myalgia (7% to 9%)
Ocular: Cataract (2%)
Renal: Renal disorder (5%)
Respiratory: Pleural effusion (<5%)
Miscellaneous: Infection (7%), influenza (6%), viral infection (6%), secondary malignancy (2% to 4%)

<1% (Limited to important or life-threatening): Anaphylactic reaction, angioedema, arterial thrombosis, blurred vision, cardiac failure, dysesthesia, endometrial cancer, endometrial hyperplasia, endometrial proliferation, erythema multiforme, hemiparesis, hemorrhagic stroke, hepatitis, hypoesthesia, leukopenia, myocardial ischemia, palpitations, paresthesia, portal vein thrombosis, pulmonary embolism, stomatitis, tachycardia, thrombocytopenia, thrombophlebitis, thromboembolic event, thrombotic stroke, toxic epidermal necrolysis, transaminases increased, transient ischemic attack, urticaria, vaginal discharge, venous thrombosis

Drug Interactions

Metabolism/Transport Effects Substrate of CYP2A6 (minor), CYP3A4 (minor); **Note:** Assignment of Major/Minor substrate status based on clinically relevant drug interaction potential; **Inhibits** CYP2A6 (strong), CYP2C19 (weak)

Avoid Concomitant Use There are no known interactions where it is recommended to avoid concomitant use.

Increased Effect/Toxicity

Letrozole may increase the levels/effects of: CYP2A6 Substrates

The levels/effects of Letrozole may be increased by: Conivaptan

Decreased Effect

The levels/effects of Letrozole may be decreased by: Tamoxifen; Tocilizumab

Stability Store at room temperature of 25°C (77°F); excursions permitted to 15°C to 30°C (59°F to 86°F).

Mechanism of Action Nonsteroidal competitive inhibitor of the aromatase enzyme system which binds to the heme group of aromatase, a cytochrome P450 enzyme which catalyzes conversion of androgens to estrogens (specifically, androstenedione to estrone and testosterone to estradiol). This leads to inhibition of the enzyme and a significant reduction in plasma estrogen (estrone, estradiol and estrone sulfate) levels. Does not affect synthesis of adrenal or thyroid hormones, aldosterone, or androgens.

Pharmacodynamics/Kinetics
Absorption: Rapid and well absorbed; not affected by food
Distribution: V_d: ~1.9 L/kg
Protein binding, plasma: Weak
Metabolism: Hepatic via CYP3A4 and 2A6 to an inactive carbinol metabolite
Half-life elimination: Terminal: ~2 days
Time to steady state, plasma: 2-6 weeks
Excretion: Urine (90%; 6% as unchanged drug, 75% as glucuronide carbinol metabolite, 9% as unidentified metabolites)

Dosage Oral: Adults: Females: Postmenopausal:
Breast cancer, advanced (first- or second-line treatment): 2.5 mg once daily; continue until tumor progression
Breast cancer, early (adjuvant treatment): 2.5 mg once daily; optimal duration unknown, duration in clinical trial is 5 years; discontinue at relapse
Breast cancer, early (extended adjuvant treatment): 2.5 mg once daily; optimal duration unknown, duration in clinical trials is 5 years (after 5 years of tamoxifen); discontinue at relapse
Ovarian (epithelial) cancer (unlabeled use): 2.5 mg once daily; continue until disease progression (Ramirez, 2008)
Elderly: No dosage adjustments required

Dosage adjustment in renal impairment: No dosage adjustment is required in patients with renal impairment if Cl_{cr} ≥10 mL/minute

Dosage adjustment in hepatic impairment:
Mild-to-moderate impairment (Child-Pugh class A and B): No adjustment recommended
Severe impairment (Child-Pugh class C) and cirrhosis: 2.5 mg every other day

Dietary Considerations May be taken without regard to meals. Calcium and vitamin D supplementation are recommended.

Administration Administer with or without food.

Monitoring Parameters Monitor periodically during therapy: Complete blood counts, thyroid function tests; serum electrolytes, cholesterol, transaminases, and creatinine; blood pressure; bone density

Additional Information Oncology Comment: The American Society of Clinical Oncology (ASCO) guidelines for adjuvant endocrine therapy in postmenopausal women with HR-positive breast cancer (Burstein, 2010) recommend considering aromatase inhibitor (AI) therapy at some point in the treatment course (primary, sequentially, or extended). Optimal duration at this time is not known; however, treatment with an AI should not exceed 5 years in primary and extended therapies, and 2-3 years if followed by tamoxifen in sequential therapy (total of 5 years). If initial therapy with AI has been discontinued before the 5 years, consideration should be taken to receive tamoxifen for a total of 5 years. The optimal time to switch to an AI is also not known, but data supports switching after 2-3 years of tamoxifen (sequential) or after 5 years of tamoxifen (extended). If patient becomes intolerant or has poor adherence, consideration should be made to switch to another AI or initiate tamoxifen.

Dosage Forms Excipient information presented when available (limited, particularly for generics); consult specific product labeling.
Tablet, oral: 2.5 mg
Femara®: 2.5 mg

◆ **Letrozole Tablets, USP (Can)** *see* Letrozole *on page 986*

◆ **Leucovorin** *see* Leucovorin Calcium *on page 987*

Leucovorin Calcium (loo koe VOR in KAL see um)

Brand Names: Canada Lederle Leucovorin

Index Terms 5-Formyl Tetrahydrofolate; Calcium Folinate; Calcium Leucovorin; Citrovorum Factor; Folinate Calcium; Folinic Acid (error prone synonym); Leucovorin

Pharmacologic Category Antidote; Chemotherapy Modulating Agent; Rescue Agent (Chemotherapy); Vitamin, Water Soluble

Use Antidote for folic acid antagonists (methotrexate, trimethoprim, pyrimethamine) and rescue therapy following high-dose methotrexate; in combination with fluorouracil in the treatment of colon cancer; treatment of megaloblastic anemias when folate is deficient as in infancy, sprue, pregnancy, and nutritional deficiency when oral folate therapy is not possible

Unlabeled Use Adjunctive cofactor therapy in methanol toxicity; prevention of pyrimethamine hematologic toxicity in HIV-positive patients

Pregnancy Risk Factor C

Pregnancy Considerations Animal reproduction studies have not been conducted. Leucovorin is a biologically active form of folic acid. Adequate amounts of folic acid are recommended during pregnancy. Refer to Folic Acid monograph.

Lactation Excretion in breast milk unknown/use caution

Contraindications Pernicious anemia or vitamin B_{12}-deficient megaloblastic anemias

Warnings/Precautions When used for the treatment of accidental weak folic acid antagonist overdose, administer as soon as possible. When used for the treatment of a methotrexate overdose, administer as soon as possible. Do not wait for the results of a methotrexate level before initiating therapy. It is important to adjust the leucovorin dose once a methotrexate level is known. When used for methotrexate rescue therapy, methotrexate serum concentrations should be monitored to determine dose and duration of leucovorin therapy. The dose may need to be increased or administration prolonged in situations where methotrexate excretion may be delayed (eg, ascites, pleural effusion, renal insufficiency, inadequate hydration); **never administer leucovorin intrathecally.** Combination of leucovorin and sulfamethoxazole-trimethoprim for the acute treatment of PCP in patients with HIV infection has been reported to cause increased rates of treatment failure. Leucovorin may increase the toxicity of 5-fluorouracil; dose of 5-fluorouracil may need decreased.

Powder for injection: When doses >10 mg/m^2 are required, reconstitute using sterile water for injection, not a solution containing benzyl alcohol.

Injection: Due to calcium content, do not administer I.V. solutions at a rate >160 mg/minute. Not intended for intrathecal use.

Adverse Reactions Frequency not defined. Toxicities (especially gastrointestinal toxicity) of fluorouracil is higher when used in combination with leucovorin.

Dermatologic: Rash, pruritus, erythema, urticaria

Hematologic: Thrombocytosis

Respiratory: Wheezing

Miscellaneous: Allergic reactions, anaphylactoid reactions

Drug Interactions

Metabolism/Transport Effects None known.

Avoid Concomitant Use

Avoid concomitant use of Leucovorin Calcium with any of the following: Raltitrexed

Increased Effect/Toxicity

Leucovorin Calcium may increase the levels/effects of: Capecitabine; Fluorouracil; Fluorouracil (Systemic); Fluorouracil (Topical)

Decreased Effect

Leucovorin Calcium may decrease the levels/effects of: Fosphenytoin; PHENobarbital; Phenytoin; Primidone; Raltitrexed; Trimethoprim

Stability

Powder for injection: Store at room temperature of 25°C (77°F). Protect from light. Reconstitute with SWFI or BWFI; dilute in 100-1000 mL NS, D_5W for infusion. When doses >10 mg/m^2 are required, reconstitute using sterile water for injection, not a solution containing benzyl alcohol. Solutions reconstituted with bacteriostatic water for injection U.S.P., must be used within 7 days. Solutions reconstituted with SWFI must be used immediately. Parenteral admixture is stable for 24 hours stored at room temperature (25°C) and for 4 days when stored under refrigeration (4°C).

Solution for injection: Prior to dilution, store vials under refrigeration at 2°C to 8°C (36°F to 46°F). Protect from light.

Tablet: Store at room temperature of 15°C to 30°C (59°F to 86°F).

Mechanism of Action A reduced form of folic acid, leucovorin supplies the necessary cofactor blocked by methotrexate. Leucovorin actively competes with methotrexate for transport sites, displaces methotrexate from intracellular binding sites, and restores active folate stores required for DNA/RNA synthesis. Stabilizes the binding of 5-dUMP and thymidylate synthetase, enhancing the activity of fluorouracil. When administered with pyrimethamine for the treatment of opportunistic infections, leucovorin reduces the risk for hematologic toxicity.

Methanol toxicity treatment: Formic acid (methanol's toxic metabolite) is normally metabolized to carbon dioxide and water by 10-formyltetrahydrofolate dehydrogenase after being bound to tetrahydrofolate. Administering a source of tetrahydrofolate may aid the body in eliminating formic acid.

Pharmacodynamics/Kinetics

Absorption: Oral, I.M.: Well absorbed

Metabolism: Intestinal mucosa and hepatically to 5-methyltetrahydrofolate (5MTHF; active)

Bioavailability: Saturable at oral doses >25 mg; 25 mg (97%), 50 mg (75%), 100 mg (37%)

Half-life elimination: ~4-8 hours

Time to peak: Oral: ~2 hours; I.V.: Total folates: 10 minutes; 5MTHF: ~1 hour

Excretion: Urine (primarily); feces

Dosage

Treatment of weak folic acid antagonist overdosage (eg, trimethoprim, pyrimethamine): Children and Adults: Oral: 5-15 mg/day

Folate-deficient megaloblastic anemia: Children and Adults: I.M.: ≤1 mg/day

High-dose methotrexate-rescue dose: Children and Adults: Initial: Oral, I.M., I.V.: 15 mg (~10 mg/m^2); start 24 hours after beginning methotrexate infusion; continue every 6 hours for 10 doses, until methotrexate level is <0.05 micromole/L. Adjust dose as follows:

Normal methotrexate elimination: Oral, I.M., I.V.: 15 mg every 6 hours

Delayed early methotrexate elimination: I.V.: 150 mg every 3 hours until methotrexate level is <1 micromole/L, then 15 mg every 3 hours until methotrexate level is <0.05 micromole/L

Methotrexate overdose: Children and Adults: **Note:** The amount of leucovorin administered should equal the amount of methotrexate inadvertently administered.

I.V.: 1 mg per mg of methotrexate inadvertently administered; 100-1000 mg/m^2 every 3-6 hours has been used; administer until methotrexate levels decrease to goal level or longer if methotrexate levels are unavailable or if patient has renal dysfunction or third-space storage (ascites, pleural effusion)

A nomogram for leucovorin rescue in cancer patients receiving high-dose methotrexate based upon a 48-hour methotrexate level may be helpful (Widemann, 2006). Methotrexate level:
≥80 micromole/L: 1000 mg/m^2 every 6 hours
≥8 to <80 micromole/L: 100 mg/m^2 every 3 hours
≥2 to <8 micromole/L: 10 mg/m^2 every 3 hours
≥0.1 to <2 micromole/L: 10 mg/m^2 every 6 hours
Use of I.T. leucovorin is not advised (Jardine, 1996; Smith, 2008).

Cofactor therapy in methanol toxicity (unlabeled use): Children and Adults: I.V.: 1 mg/kg (maximum dose: 50 mg) over 30-60 minutes every 4-6 hours. Therapy should continue until methanol and formic acid have been completely eliminated (Barceloux, 2002)

Colorectal cancer (also refer to Combination Regimens): Adults:
I.V.: 200 mg/m^2 over at least 3 minutes (used in combination with fluorouracil 370 mg/m^2)
or
I.V.: 20 mg/m^2 (used in combination with fluorouracil 425 mg/m^2)

Pemetrexed toxicity (unlabeled dose): Adults: I.V.: 100 mg/m^2 once, followed by 50 mg/m^2 every 6 hours for 8 days (used in clinical trial for CTC grade 4 leukopenia ≥3 days; CTC grade 4 neutropenia ≥3 days; immediately for CTC grade 4 thrombocytopenia, bleeding associated with grade 3 thrombocytopenia, or grade 3 or 4 mucositis)

Prevention of pyrimethamine hematologic toxicity in HIV-positive patients (unlabeled uses; CDC, 2009):
Infants and Children >1 month of age: **Note:** Leucovorin should continue for 1 week after pyrimethamine is discontinued.
Toxoplasmosis (*Toxoplasma gondii*):
Primary prophylaxis: Oral: 5 mg once every 3 days (in combination with pyrimethamine [with either dapsone or atovaquone])
Secondary prophylaxis: Oral: 5 mg once every 3 days (in combination with pyrimethamine [with either sulfadiazine, atovaquone, or clindamycin])
Treatment (congenital): Oral or I.M.: 10 mg with every pyrimethamine dose (in combination with either sulfadiazine or clindamycin); treatment duration: 12 months
Treatment (acquired): Acute induction: Oral: 10-25 mg once daily (in combination with pyrimethamine [with either sulfadiazine, clindamycin, or atovaquone]) for ≥6 weeks
Adults: Oral:
Isosporiasis (*Isospora belli*):
Treatment: 10-25 mg once daily (in combination with pyrimethamine)
Chronic maintenance (secondary prophylaxis): 5-10 mg once daily (in combination with pyrimethamine)
Pneumocystis jirovecii pneumonia (PCP): Prophylaxis (primary and secondary): 25 mg once weekly (in combination with pyrimethamine [with dapsone]) **or** 10 mg once daily (in combination with pyrimethamine [with atovaquone])
Toxoplasmosis (*Toxoplasma gondii*):
Primary prophylaxis: 25 mg once weekly (in combination with pyrimethamine [with dapsone]) **or** 10 mg once daily (in combination with pyrimethamine [with atovaquone])
Treatment: 10-25 mg once daily (in combination with pyrimethamine [with either sulfadiazine, clindamycin, atovaquone, or azithromycin]). **Note:** May increase leucovorin to 50-100 mg/day in divided doses in cases of pyrimethamine toxicity (rash, nausea, bone marrow suppression).
Chronic maintenance (secondary prophylaxis): 10-25 mg once daily (in combination with pyrimethamine [with either sulfadiazine or clindamycin]) **or** 10 mg once daily (in combination with pyrimethamine [with atovaquone])

Dietary Considerations Solutions for injection contain calcium 0.004 mEq per leucovorin 1 mg

Administration Due to calcium content, do not administer I.V. solutions at a rate >160 mg/minute; not intended for intrathecal use.
Refer to individual protocols. Should be administered I.M., I.V. push, or I.V. infusion (15 minutes to 2 hours). Leucovorin should not be administered concurrently with methotrexate. It is commonly initiated 24 hours after the start of methotrexate. Toxicity to normal tissues may be irreversible if leucovorin is not initiated by ~40 hours after the start of methotrexate.
As a rescue after folate antagonists: Administer by I.V. bolus, I.M., or orally.
Do not administer orally in the presence of nausea or vomiting. Doses >25 mg should be administered parenterally.
In combination with fluorouracil: Fluorouracil activity, the fluorouracil is usually given after, or at the midpoint, of the leucovorin infusion. Leucovorin is usually administered by I.V. bolus injection or short (10-120 minutes) I.V. infusion. Other administration schedules have been used; refer to individual protocols.

Monitoring Parameters
High-dose methotrexate therapy: Plasma methotrexate concentration; leucovorin is continued until the plasma methotrexate level <0.05 micromole/L. With 4- to 6-hour high-dose methotrexate infusions, plasma drug values in excess of 50 and 1 micromole/L at 24 and 48 hours after starting the infusion, respectively, are often predictive of delayed methotrexate clearance.
Fluorouracil therapy: CBC with differential and platelets, liver function tests, electrolytes

Dosage Forms Excipient information presented when available (limited, particularly for generics); consult specific product labeling.
Injection, powder for reconstitution [strength expressed as base]: 50 mg, 100 mg, 200 mg, 350 mg
Injection, solution [strength expressed as base, preservative free]: 10 mg/mL (50 mL)
Tablet, oral [strength expressed as base]: 5 mg, 10 mg, 15 mg, 25 mg

Extemporaneous Preparations A 5 mg/mL oral suspension may be prepared with tablets, Cologel®, and a 2:1 mixture of simple syrup and wild cherry syrup. Crush twenty-four 25 mg tablets in a glass mortar and reduce to a fine powder; transfer powder to amber bottle. Add 30 mL Cologel® and shake mixture thoroughly. Add a quantity of syrup mixture sufficient to make 120 mL. Label "shake well" and "refrigerate". Stable for 28 days refrigerated.

Lam MS, "Extemporaneous Compounding of Oral Liquid Dosage Formulations and Alternative Drug Delivery Methods for Anticancer Drugs," *Pharmacotherapy*, 2011, 31(2):164-92.

◆ **Leukeran®** *see* Chlorambucil *on page 337*
◆ **Leukine®** *see* Sargramostim *on page 1538*

Leuprolide (loo PROE lide)

Brand Names: U.S. Eligard®; Lupron Depot-Ped®; Lupron Depot®

Brand Names: Canada Eligard®; Lupron®; Lupron® Depot®

Index Terms Abbott-43818; Leuprolide Acetate; Leuprorelin Acetate; TAP-144

Pharmacologic Category Antineoplastic Agent, Gonadotropin-Releasing Hormone Agonist; Gonadotropin Releasing Hormone Agonist

Use Palliative treatment of advanced prostate cancer; management of endometriosis; treatment of anemia caused by uterine leiomyomata (fibroids); central precocious puberty

Unlabeled Use Treatment of breast cancer; infertility

Pregnancy Risk Factor X

Pregnancy Considerations Pregnancy must be excluded prior to the start of treatment. Although leuprolide usually inhibits ovulation and stops menstruation, contraception is not ensured and a nonhormonal contraceptive should be used. Fetal abnormalities and increased fetal mortality have been noted in animal studies.

Lactation Excretion in breast milk unknown/contraindicated

Contraindications Hypersensitivity to leuprolide, GnRH, GnRH-agonist analogs, or any component of the formulation; undiagnosed abnormal vaginal bleeding; pregnancy; breast-feeding

Lupron Depot® 22.5 mg, 30 mg, and 45 mg are also not indicated for use in women

Warnings/Precautions Hazardous agent - use appropriate precautions for handling and disposal. Transient increases in testosterone serum levels (~50% above baseline) occur at the start of treatment. Androgen-deprivation therapy (ADT) may increase the risk for cardiovascular disease (Levine, 2010); sudden cardiac death and stroke have been reported in men receiving GnRH agonists; long-term ADT may prolong the QT interval; consider the benefits of ADT versus the risk for QT prolongation in patients with a history of QT_c prolongation, with medications known to prolong the QT interval, or with pre-existing cardiac disease. Tumor flare, bone pain, neuropathy, urinary tract obstruction, and spinal cord compression have been reported when used for prostate cancer; closely observe patients for weakness, paresthesias, hematuria, and urinary tract obstruction in first few weeks of therapy. Observe patients with metastatic vertebral lesions or urinary obstruction closely. Exacerbation of endometriosis or uterine leiomyomata may occur initially. Decreased bone density has been reported when used for ≥6 months; use caution in patients with additional risk factors for bone loss (eg, chronic alcohol use, corticosteroid therapy). In patients with prostate cancer, androgen deprivation therapy may increase the risk for cardiovascular disease, diabetes, insulin resistance, obesity, alterations in lipids, and fractures. Use caution in patients with a history of psychiatric illness; alteration in mood, memory impairment, and depression have been associated with use. Rare cases of pituitary apoplexy (frequently secondary to pituitary adenoma) have been observed with leuprolide administration (onset from 1 hour to usually <2 weeks); may present as sudden headache, vomiting, visual or mental status changes, and infrequently cardiovascular collapse; immediate medical attention required. Females treated for precocious puberty may experience menses or spotting during the first 2 months of treatment; notify healthcare provider if bleeding continues after the second month.

Some dosage forms may contain benzyl alcohol which has been associated with "gasping syndrome" in neonates; patients with benzyl alcohol allergy may demonstrate a hypersensitivity reaction (usually local) in the form of erythema and induration at the injection site. Vehicle used in depot injectable formulations (polylactide-co-glycolide microspheres) has rarely been associated with retinal artery occlusion in patients with abnormal arteriovenous anastomosis. Due to different release properties, combinations of dosage forms or fractions of dosage forms should not be interchanged.

Adverse Reactions

Children (percentages based on 1-month and 3-month pediatric formulations combined):

>10%: Local: Injection site pain (≤20%)

2% to 10%:

Cardiovascular: Vasodilation (2%)

Central nervous system: Emotional lability (5%), mood altered (5%), headache (3% to 5%), pain (3%)

Dermatologic: Acne (3%), rash (3% including erythema multiforme), seborrhea (3%)

Gastrointestinal: Weight gain (≤7%)

Genitourinary: Vaginal bleeding (3%), vaginal discharge (3%), vaginitis (3%)

Local: Injection site reaction (≤9%)

<2% (Limited to important or life-threatening): Allergic reaction, alopecia, appetite decreased/increased, arthralgia, asthma, body odor, bradycardia, cervix disorder, constipation, cough, crying, depression, dizziness, dysmenorrhea, dyspepsia, dysphagia, epistaxis, extremity pain, feminization, fever, flu-like syndrome, gait disturbance, gingivitis, goiter, growth retarded, gynecomastia, hirsutism, hyperhidrosis, hyperkinesias, hypertension, infection, leukoderma, musculoskeletal pain, myalgia, myopathy, nausea, nervousness, obesity, pallor, peripheral edema, personality disorder, pharyngitis, purpura, rhinitis, sexual maturity accelerated, sinusitis, skin striae, somnolence, syncope, tearfulness, urinary incontinence, vision decreased, vomiting, weakness

Adults: Note: For prostate cancer treatment, an initial rise in serum testosterone concentrations may cause "tumor flare" or worsening of symptoms, including bone pain, neuropathy, hematuria, or ureteral or bladder outlet obstruction during the first 2 weeks. Similarly, an initial increase in estradiol levels, with a temporary worsening of symptoms, may occur in women treated with leuprolide.

Delayed release formulations:

>10%:

Cardiovascular: Edema (≤14%)

Central nervous system: Headache (≤65%), pain (<2% to 33%), depression (≤31%), insomnia (≤31%), fatigue (≤17%), dizziness/vertigo (≤16%)

Dermatologic: Skin reaction (≤12%)

Endocrine & metabolic: Hot flashes (25% to 98%), testicular atrophy (≤20%), hyperlipidemia (≤12%), libido decreased (≤11%)

Gastrointestinal: Nausea/vomiting (≤25%), bowel function altered (≤14%), weight gain/loss (≤13%)

Genitourinary: Vaginitis (11% to 28%), urinary disorder (13% to 15%)

Local: Injection site burning/stinging (transient: ≤35%)

Neuromuscular & skeletal: Weakness (≤18%), joint disorder (≤12%)

Miscellaneous: Flu-like syndrome (≤12%)

1% to 10% (limited to important or life-threatening):

Cardiovascular: Angina (<5%), arrhythmia (<5%), atrial fibrillation (<5%), bradycardia (<5%), CHF (<5%), deep thrombophlebitis (<5%), hyper-/hypotension (<5%), palpitation (<5%), syncope (<5%), tachycardia (<5%)

Central nervous system: Nervousness (≤8%), anxiety (≤6%), confusion (<5%), delusions (<5%), dementia (<5%), fever (<5%), seizure (<5%)

Dermatologic: Acne (≤10%), alopecia (≤5%), bruising (≤5%), cellulitis (<5%), pruritus (≤3%), rash (≤2%), hirsutism (<2%)

Endocrine & metabolic: Dehydration (≤8%), gynecomastia (≤7%), breast tenderness/pain (≤6%), bicarbonate decreased (≥5%), hyper-/hypocholesterolemia (≥5%), hyperglycemia (≥5%), hyperphosphatemia (≥5%), hyperuricemia (≥5%), hypoalbuminemia (≥5%), hypoproteinemia (≥5%), lactation (<5%), testicular pain (≤4%), menstrual disorder (≤2%)

Gastrointestinal: Dysphagia (<5%), gastrointestinal hemorrhage (<5%), intestinal obstruction (<5%), ulcer (<5%), constipation (≤3%), gastroenteritis/colitis (≤3%), diarrhea (≤2%)

Genitourinary: Prostatic acid phosphatase increased/decreased (≥5%), urine specific gravity increased/decreased (≥5%), impotence (≤5%), balanitis (<5%), incontinence (<5%), penile/testis disorder (<5%), urinary tract infection (<5%), nocturia (≤4%), polyuria (2% to 4%), dysuria (≤2%), bladder spasm (<2%), erectile dysfunction (<2%), hematuria (<2%), urinary retention (<2%), urinary urgency (<2%)

Hematologic: Eosinophilia (≥5%), leukopenia (≥5%), platelets increased (≥5%), anemia

Hepatic: Liver function tests abnormal (≥5%), partial thromboplastin time increased (≥5%), prothrombin time increased (≥5%), hepatomegaly (<5%)

Local: Injection site pain (2% to 5%), injection site erythema (1% to 3%)

Neuromuscular & skeletal: Myalgia (≤8%), paresthesia (≤8%), neuropathy (<5%), paralysis (<5%), pathologic fracture (<5%), bone pain (<2%), arthralgia (≤1%)

Renal: BUN increased (≥5%), creatinine increased (≥5%)

Respiratory: Emphysema (<5%), epistaxis (<5%), hemoptysis (<5%), pleural effusion (<5%), pulmonary edema (<5%), dyspnea (≤2%), cough (≤1%)

Miscellaneous: Diaphoresis (≤5%), allergic reaction (<5%), infection (5%), lymphadenopathy (<5%)

Immediate release formulation:

>10%:

Cardiovascular: ECG changes/ischemia (19%), peripheral edema (12%)

Central nervous system: Pain (13%)

Endocrine & metabolic: Hot flashes (55%)

1% to 10% (limited to important or life-threatening):

Cardiovascular: Hypertension (8%), murmur (3%), thrombosis/phlebitis (2%), CHF (1%), angina, arrhythmia, MI, syncope

Central nervous system: Headache (7%), insomnia (7%), dizziness/lightheadedness (5%), anxiety, depression, fatigue, fever, nervousness

Dermatologic: Dermatitis (5%), alopecia, bruising, itching, lesions, pigmentation

Endocrine & metabolic: Gynecomastia/breast tenderness/pain (7%), testicular size decreased (7%), diabetes, hypercalcemia, hypoglycemia, libido decreased, thyroid enlarged

Gastrointestinal: Constipation (7%), anorexia (6%), nausea/vomiting (5%), diarrhea, dysphagia, gastrointestinal bleeding, peptic ulcer, rectal polyps

Genitourinary: Urinary frequency/urgency (6%), impotence (4%), urinary tract infection (3%), bladder spasm, dysuria, incontinence, testicular pain, urinary obstruction

Hematologic: Anemia (5%)

Local: Injection site reaction

Neuromuscular & skeletal: Weakness (10%), bone pain (5%), peripheral neuropathy

Ocular: Blurred vision

Renal: Hematuria (6%), BUN increased, creatinine increased

Respiratory: Dyspnea (2%), cough, pneumonia, pulmonary embolus, pulmonary fibrosis

Miscellaneous: Infection, inflammation

Children and Adults: *Any formulations:* Postmarketing and/or case reports (limited to important or life-threatening): Anaphylactic/anaphylactoid reactions, asthmatic reactions, bone density decreased; coronary artery disease, diabetes, fibromyalgia-like symptoms (arthralgia/myalgia, headaches, GI distress); hemoptysis, hepatic dysfunction, hypokalemia, hypoproteinemia, injection site induration/abscess, MI, pelvic fibrosis, penile swelling, peripheral neuropathy, photosensitivity; pituitary apoplexy (cardiovascular collapse, mental status altered, ophthalmoplegia, sudden headache, visual changes, vomiting); prostate pain, pulmonary embolism, pulmonary infiltrate, seizure, spinal fracture/paralysis, stroke, suicidal ideation/attempt (rare), tenosynovitis-like symptoms, thrombocytopenia, transient ischemia attack, uric acid increased, urticaria, WBC decreased/increased

Drug Interactions

Metabolism/Transport Effects None known.

Avoid Concomitant Use There are no known interactions where it is recommended to avoid concomitant use.

Increased Effect/Toxicity There are no known significant interactions involving an increase in effect.

Decreased Effect

Leuprolide may decrease the levels/effects of: Antidiabetic Agents

Stability

Eligard®: Store at 2°C to 8°C (36°F to 46°C). Allow to reach room temperature prior to using. Once mixed, must be administered within 30 minutes. Eligard® is packaged in two syringes; one contains the Atrigel® polymer system and the second contains leuprolide acetate powder. Follow package instructions for mixing.

Lupron Depot®, Lupron Depot-Ped®: Store at room temperature of 25°C (77°F); excursions permitted to 15°C to 30°C (59°F to 86°F). Upon reconstitution, the suspension does not contain a preservative and should be used immediately; discard if not used within 2 hours. Reconstitute only with diluent provided.

Leuprolide acetate 5 mg/mL solution: Store at 20°C to 25°C (68°F to 77°F); excursions permitted to 15°C to 30°C (59°F to 86°F). Protect from light and store vial in carton until use. Do not freeze.

Mechanism of Action Leuprolide, is an agonist of luteinizing hormone-releasing hormone (LHRH). Acting as a potent inhibitor of gonadotropin secretion; continuous administration results in suppression of ovarian and testicular steroidogenesis due to decreased levels of LH and FSH with subsequent decrease in testosterone (male) and estrogen (female) levels. In males, testosterone levels are reduced to below castrate levels. Leuprolide may also have a direct inhibitory effect on the testes, and act by a different mechanism not directly related to reduction in serum testosterone.

Pharmacodynamics/Kinetics

Onset of action: Following transient increase, testosterone suppression occurs in ~2-4 weeks of continued therapy

Distribution: Males: V_d: 27 L

Protein binding: 43% to 49%

Metabolism: Major metabolite, pentapeptide (M-1)

Bioavailability: SubQ: 94%

Excretion: Urine (<5% as parent and major metabolite)

Dosage

Children: Precocious puberty (consider discontinuing by age 11 for females and by age 12 for males):

I.M.:

Lupron Depot-Ped® (monthly):

≤25 kg: 7.5 mg every month

>25-37.5 kg: 11.25 mg every month

>37.5 kg: 15 mg every month

Titrate dose upward in increments of 3.75 mg every 4 weeks if down-regulation is not achieved.

Lupron Depot-Ped® (3 month): 11.25 mg or 30 mg every 12 weeks

SubQ (leuprolide acetate 5 mg/mL solution): Initial: 50 mcg/kg/day; titrate dose upward by 10 mcg/kg/day if down-regulation is not achieved. **Note:** Higher mg/kg doses may be required in younger children.

Adults:
Prostate cancer, advanced:
I.M.:
Lupron Depot® 7.5 mg (monthly): 7.5 mg every month **or**
Lupron Depot® 22.5 mg (3 month): 22.5 mg every 12 weeks **or**
Lupron Depot® 30 mg (4 month): 30 mg every 16 weeks **or**
Lupron Depot® 45 mg (6 month): 45 mg every 24 weeks
SubQ:
Eligard®: 7.5 mg monthly **or** 22.5 mg every 3 months **or** 30 mg every 4 months **or** 45 mg every 6 months
Leuprolide acetate 5 mg/mL solution: 1 mg/day
Endometriosis: I.M.: Initial therapy may be with leuprolide alone or in combination with norethindrone; if retreatment for an additional 6 months is necessary, concomitant norethindrone should be used. Retreatment is not recommended for longer than one additional 6-month course.
Lupron Depot®: 3.75 mg every month for up to 6 months **or**
Lupron Depot®-3 month: 11.25 mg every 3 months for up to 2 doses (6 months total duration of treatment)
Uterine leiomyomata (fibroids): I.M. (in combination with iron):
Lupron Depot®: 3.75 mg every month for up to 3 months **or**
Lupron Depot®-3 month: 11.25 mg as a single injection
Breast cancer, premenopausal ovarian ablation (unlabeled use): I.M.:
Lupron Depot®: 3.75 mg every 28 days for up to 24 months (Boccardo, 1999) **or**
Lupron Depot®-3 month: 11.25 mg every 3 months for up to 24 months (Boccardo, 1999; Schmid, 2007)

Administration
I.M.: Lupron Depot®, Lupron Depot-Ped®: Administer as a single injection. Vary injection site periodically
SubQ:
Eligard®: Vary injection site; choose site with adequate subcutaneous tissue (eg, upper or mid-abdomen, upper buttocks); avoid areas that may be compressed or rubbed (eg, belt or waistband)
Leuprolide acetate 5 mg/mL solution: Vary injection site; if an alternate syringe from the syringe provided is required, insulin syringes should be used

Monitoring Parameters Bone mineral density
Precocious puberty: GnRH testing (blood LH and FSH levels), measurement of height and bone age every 6-12 months, testosterone in males and estradiol in females (I.M. [monthly] and SubQ formulations: 1-2 months after initiation of therapy or with dosage change; I.M. [3 month] formulation: 2-3 months after initiation of therapy, month 6, and as clinically indicated thereafter); Tanner staging
Prostatic cancer: LH and FSH levels, serum testosterone (~4 weeks after initiation of therapy), PSA; weakness, paresthesias, and urinary tract obstruction in first few weeks of therapy. Screen for diabetes (blood glucose and Hb A_{1c}) and cardiovascular risk prior to initiating and periodically during treatment.

Test Interactions Interferes with pituitary gonadotropic and gonadal function tests during and up to 3 months after monthly administration of leuprolide therapy.

Additional Information
Eligard® Atrigel®: A nongelatin-based, biodegradable, polymer matrix

Oncology Comment: Guidelines from the American Society of Clinical Oncology (ASCO) for hormonal management of advanced prostate cancer which is androgen-sensitive (Loblaw, 2007) recommend either orchiectomy or luteinizing hormone-releasing hormone (LHRH) agonists as initial treatment for androgen deprivation.

Product Availability
Lupron Depot-Ped® 3-month formulation: FDA approved August 2011; availability expected August 2011
Lupron Depot-Ped® 3-month formulation will be available in two strengths, 11.25 mg and 30 mg.

Dosage Forms Excipient information presented when available (limited, particularly for generics); consult specific product labeling.
Injection, powder for reconstitution, as acetate [depot formulation, preservative free]:
Eligard®: 7.5 mg (monthly), 22.5 mg (3 month), 30 mg (4 month), 45 mg (6 month) [contains polylactide-co-glycolide; supplied with diluent]
Lupron Depot-Ped®: 7.5 mg (monthly), 11.25 mg (3 month), 11.25 mg (monthly), 15 mg (monthly), 30 mg (3 month) [contains polylactide-co-glycolide, polysorbate 80]
Lupron Depot®: 3.75 mg (monthly), 7.5 mg (monthly), 11.25 mg (3 month), 22.5 mg (3 month), 30 mg (4 month), 45 mg (6 month) [contains polylactide-co-glycolide, polysorbate 80]
Injection, solution, as acetate: 5 mg/mL (2.8 mL)

◆ **Leuprolide Acetate** *see* Leuprolide *on page 989*
◆ **Leuprorelin Acetate** *see* Leuprolide *on page 989*
◆ **Leurocristine Sulfate** *see* VinCRIStine *on page 1790*
◆ **Leustatin®** *see* Cladribine *on page 372*

Levalbuterol (leve al BYOO ter ole)

Brand Names: U.S. Xopenex HFA™; Xopenex®
Brand Names: Canada Xopenex®
Index Terms Levalbuterol Hydrochloride; Levalbuterol Tartrate; R-albuterol
Pharmacologic Category Beta$_2$-Adrenergic Agonist
Additional Appendix Information
Bronchodilators *on page 1886*
Use Treatment or prevention of bronchospasm in children and adults with reversible obstructive airway disease
Pregnancy Risk Factor C
Pregnancy Considerations Teratogenic effects were not observed in animal studies; however, racemic albuterol was teratogenic in some species. There are no adequate and well-controlled studies in pregnant women. This drug should be used during pregnancy only if benefit exceeds risk. Use caution if needed for bronchospasm during labor and delivery; has potential to interfere with uterine contractions.
Lactation Excretion in breast milk unknown/use caution
Contraindications Hypersensitivity to levalbuterol, albuterol, or any component of the formulation
Warnings/Precautions Optimize anti-inflammatory treatment before initiating maintenance treatment with levalbuterol. Do not use as a component of chronic therapy without an anti-inflammatory agent. Only the mildest form of asthma (Step 1 and/or exercise-induced) would not require concurrent use based upon asthma guidelines. Patient must be instructed to seek medical attention in cases where acute symptoms are not relieved or a previous level of response is diminished. The need to increase frequency of use may indicate deterioration of asthma, and treatment must not be delayed. A spacer device or valved holding chamber is recommended when using a metered-dose inhaler.

Use caution in patients with cardiovascular disease (arrhythmia or hypertension or HF), convulsive disorders, diabetes, glaucoma, hyperthyroidism, or hypokalemia. Beta-agonists may cause elevation in blood pressure, heart rate, and result in CNS stimulation/excitation.

Beta$_2$-agonists may increase risk of arrhythmia, increase serum glucose, or decrease serum potassium.

Immediate hypersensitivity reactions (urticaria, angioedema, rash, bronchospasm) have been reported. Do not exceed recommended dose; serious adverse events including fatalities, have been associated with excessive use of inhaled sympathomimetics. Rarely, paradoxical bronchospasm may occur with use of inhaled bronchodilating agents; this should be distinguished from inadequate response. Use with caution during labor and delivery. Safety and efficacy have not been established in patients <4 years of age.

Adverse Reactions

>10%:
- Endocrine & metabolic: Serum glucose increased, serum potassium decreased
- Neuromuscular & skeletal: Tremor (≤7%)
- Respiratory: Rhinitis (3% to 11%)
- Miscellaneous: Viral infection (7% to 12%)

>2% to 10%:
- Central nervous system: Headache (8% to 12%), nervousness (3% to 10%), dizziness (1% to 3%), anxiety (≤3%), migraine (≤3%), weakness (3%)
- Cardiovascular: Tachycardia (~3%)
- Dermatologic: Rash (≤8%)
- Gastrointestinal: Diarrhea (2% to 6%), dyspepsia (1% to 3%)
- Neuromuscular & skeletal: Leg cramps (≤3%)
- Respiratory: Asthma (9%), pharyngitis (3% to 10%), cough (1% to 4%), sinusitis (1% to 4%), nasal edema (1% to 3%)
- Miscellaneous: Flu-like syndrome (1% to 4%), accidental injury (≤3%)

<2% (Limited to important or life-threatening): Abnormal ECG, acne, anaphylaxis, angina, angioedema, arrhythmia, atrial fibrillation, chest pain, chills, constipation, conjunctivitis, cough, diaphoresis, dysmenorrhea, dyspnea, epistaxis, extrasystole, gastroenteritis, hematuria, hyper-/hypotension, hypoesthesia (hand), hypokalemia, insomnia, itching eyes, lymphadenopathy, myalgia, nausea, oropharyngeal dryness, paresthesia, supraventricular arrhythmia, syncope, vaginal moniliasis, vertigo, vomiting, wheezing, xerostomia

Note: Immediate hypersensitivity reactions have occurred (including angioedema, oropharyngeal edema, urticaria, and anaphylaxis).

Drug Interactions

Metabolism/Transport Effects None known.

Avoid Concomitant Use

Avoid concomitant use of Levalbuterol with any of the following: Beta-Blockers (Nonselective); Iobenguane I 123

Increased Effect/Toxicity

Levalbuterol may increase the levels/effects of: Loop Diuretics; Sympathomimetics; Thiazide Diuretics

The levels/effects of Levalbuterol may be increased by: Atomoxetine; Cannabinoids; MAO Inhibitors; Tricyclic Antidepressants

Decreased Effect

Levalbuterol may decrease the levels/effects of: Iobenguane I 123

The levels/effects of Levalbuterol may be decreased by: Alpha-/Beta-Blockers; Beta-Blockers (Beta1 Selective); Beta-Blockers (Nonselective); Betahistine

Stability

Aerosol: Store at room temperature of 20°C to 25°C (68°F to 77°F); protect from freezing and direct sunlight. Store with mouthpiece down. Discard after 200 actuations.

Solution for nebulization: Store in protective foil pouch at room temperature of 20°C to 25°C (68°F to 77°F). Protect from light and excessive heat. Vials should be used within 2 weeks after opening protective pouch. Use within 1 week and protect from light if removed from pouch. Vials of concentrated solution should be used immediately after removing from protective pouch. Concentrated solution should be diluted with 2.5 mL NS prior to use.

Mechanism of Action Relaxes bronchial smooth muscle by action on beta$_2$-receptors with little effect on heart rate

Pharmacodynamics/Kinetics

Onset of action (as measured by a 15% increase in FEV$_1$):
- Aerosol: 5.5-10.2 minutes
  - Peak effect: ~77 minutes
- Nebulization: 10-17 minutes
  - Peak effect: 1.5 hours

Duration (as measured by a 15% increase in FEV$_1$):
- Aerosol: 3-4 hours (up to 6 hours in some patients)
- Nebulization: 5-6 hours (up to 8 hours in some patients)

Absorption: A portion of inhaled dose is absorbed to systemic circulation

Half-life elimination: 3.3-4 hours

Time to peak, serum:
- Aerosol: Children: 0.8 hours, Adults: 0.5 hours
- Nebulization: Children: 0.3-0.6 hours, Adults: 0.2 hours

Dosage

Metered-dose inhaler (45 mcg/puff):
- Children 5-11 years:
  - Bronchospasm, quick relief: 1-2 puffs every 4-6 hours as needed
  - Exacerbation of asthma (acute, severe) *(NIH Guidelines, 2007)*: 4-8 puffs every 20 minutes for 3 doses, then every 1-4 hours as needed
- Children ≥12 years and Adults:
  - Bronchospasm, quick relief: 1-2 puffs every 4-6 hours
  - Exacerbation of asthma (acute, severe) *(NIH Guidelines, 2007)*: 4-8 puffs every 20 minutes for up to 4 hours, then every 1-4 hours as needed

Solution for nebulization:
- Children: ≤4 years:
  - Bronchospasm, quick relief *(NIH Guidelines, 2007)*: 0.31-1.25 mg every 4-6 hours as needed
  - Exacerbation of asthma (acute, severe) *(NIH Guidelines, 2007)*: 0.075 mg/kg (minimum: 1.25 mg) every 20 minutes for 3 doses, then 0.075-0.15 mg/kg (maximum: 5 mg) every 1-4 hours as needed
- Children 5-11 years:
  - Bronchospasm, quick relief: 0.31-0.63 mg every 8 hours as needed
  - Exacerbation of asthma (acute severe) *(NIH Guidelines, 2007)*: 0.075 mg/kg (minimum: 1.25 mg) every 20 minutes for 3 doses, then 0.075-0.15 mg/kg (maximum: 5 mg) every 1-4 hours as needed
- Children ≥12 years and Adults:
  - Bronchospasm, quick relief: 0.63-1.25 mg every 8 hours as needed
  - Exacerbation of asthma (acute, severe) *(NIH Guidelines, 2007)*: 1.25-2.5 mg every 20 minutes for 3 doses, then 1.25-5 mg every 1-4 hours as needed

Elderly: Only a small number of patients have been studied. Although greater sensitivity of some elderly patients cannot be ruled out, no overall differences in safety or effectiveness were observed. An initial dose of 0.63 mg should be used in all patients >65 years of age.

Administration Inhalation:

Metered-dose inhaler: Shake well before use; prime with 4 test sprays prior to first use or if inhaler has not been use of more than 3 days. Clean actuator (mouthpiece) weekly. A spacer device or valved holding chamber is recommended when using a metered-dose inhaler.

Solution for nebulization: Safety and efficacy were established when administered with the following nebulizers: PARI LC Jet™, PARI LC Plus™, as well as the following compressors: PARI Master®, Dura-Neb® 2000, and Dura-Neb® 3000. Concentrated solution should be diluted prior to use. Blow-by administration is not recommended, use a mask device if patient unable to hold mouthpiece in mouth for administration.

Monitoring Parameters Asthma symptoms; FEV_1, peak flow, and/or other pulmonary function tests; heart rate, blood pressure, CNS stimulation; arterial blood gases (if condition warrants); serum potassium, serum glucose (in selected patients)

Dosage Forms Excipient information presented when available (limited, particularly for generics); consult specific product labeling. [DSC] = Discontinued product

Aerosol, for oral inhalation, as tartrate [strength expressed as base]:

Xopenex HFA™: 45 mcg/actuation (15 g) [chlorofluorocarbon free; 200 actuations]

Solution, for nebulization, as hydrochloride [strength expressed as base, preservative free]:

Xopenex®: 0.31 mg/3 mL (24s); 0.63 mg/3 mL (24s); 1.25 mg/3 mL (24s)

Solution, for nebulization, as hydrochloride [strength expressed as base, concentrate, preservative free]: 1.25 mg/0.5 mL (30s)

Xopenex®: 1.25 mg/0.5 mL (30s [DSC])

◆ **Levalbuterol Hydrochloride** *see* Levalbuterol *on page 992*
◆ **Levalbuterol Tartrate** *see* Levalbuterol *on page 992*
◆ **Levaquin®** *see* Levofloxacin (Systemic) *on page 997*
◆ **Levarterenol Bitartrate** *see* Norepinephrine *on page 1216*
◆ **Levate® (Can)** *see* Amitriptyline *on page 94*
◆ **Levbid®** *see* Hyoscyamine *on page 854*
◆ **Levemir®** *see* Insulin Detemir *on page 904*
◆ **Levemir® FlexPen®** *see* Insulin Detemir *on page 904*

LevETIRAcetam (lee va tye RA se tam)

Brand Names: U.S. Keppra XR™; Keppra®

Brand Names: Canada Apo-Levetiracetam®; Ava-Levetiracetam; CO Levetiracetam; Dom-Levetiracetam; Keppra®; PHL-Levetiracetam; PMS-Levetiracetam; PRO-Levetiracetam

Pharmacologic Category Anticonvulsant, Miscellaneous

Additional Appendix Information

Anticonvulsant Drugs of Choice *on page 1873*

Use Adjunctive therapy in the treatment of partial onset, myoclonic, and/or primary generalized tonic-clonic seizures

Unlabeled Use Bipolar disorder

Pregnancy Risk Factor C

Pregnancy Considerations Developmental toxicities were observed in animal studies. There are no adequate and well-controlled studies in pregnant women. Two registries are available for women exposed to levetiracetam during pregnancy:

Antiepileptic Drug Pregnancy Registry (888-233-2334 or http://www.mgh.harvard.edu/aed/)

UCB AED Pregnancy Registry (888-537-7734)

Lactation Enters breast milk/not recommended

Medication Guide Available Yes

Contraindications Hypersensitivity to levetiracetam or any component of the formulation

Warnings/Precautions Antiepileptics are associated with an increased risk of suicidal behavior/thoughts with use (regardless of indication); patients should be monitored for signs/symptoms of depression, suicidal tendencies, and other unusual behavior changes during therapy and instructed to inform their healthcare provider immediately if symptoms occur.

Psychotic symptoms (psychosis, hallucinations) and behavioral symptoms (including aggression, anger, anxiety, depersonalization, depression, personality disorder) may occur; incidence may be increased in children. Dose reduction may be required. Levetiracetam should be withdrawn gradually to minimize the potential of increased seizure frequency. Use caution with renal impairment; dosage adjustment may be necessary. Weakness, dizziness, and somnolence occur mostly during the first month of therapy. Although rare, decreases in red blood cell counts, hemoglobin, hematocrit, white blood cell counts and neutrophils have been observed. Safety and efficacy in children <4 years of age (oral formulation) or <16 years (I.V. formulation and extended release tablets) have not been established.

Adverse Reactions

>10%:

Central nervous system: Behavioral symptoms (agitation, aggression, anger, anxiety, apathy, depersonalization, depression, emotional lability, hostility, hyperkinesias, irritability, nervousness, neurosis and personality disorder: adults 5% to 13%; children 5% to 38%), somnolence (8% to 23%), headache (14%), hostility (2% to 12%)

Gastrointestinal: Vomiting (15%), anorexia (3% to 13%)

Neuromuscular & skeletal: Weakness (9% to 15%)

Respiratory: Pharyngitis (6% to 14%), rhinitis (4% to 13%), cough (2% to 11%)

Miscellaneous: Accidental injury (17%), infection (2% to 13%)

1% to 10%:

Cardiovascular: Facial edema (2%)

Central nervous system: Fatigue (10%), nervousness (4% to 10%), dizziness (5% to 9%), personality disorder (8%), pain (6% to 7%), agitation (6%), irritability (6% to 7%), emotional lability (2% to 6%), mood swings (5%), depression (3% to 5%), vertigo (3% to 5%), ataxia (3%), amnesia (2%), anxiety (2%), confusion (2%)

Dermatologic: Bruising (4%), pruritus (2%), rash (2%), skin discoloration (2%)

Endocrine & metabolic: Dehydration (2%)

Gastrointestinal: Diarrhea (8%), nausea (5%), gastroenteritis (4%), constipation (3%)

Genitourinary: Urine abnormality (2%)

Hematologic: Leukocytes decreased (2% to 3%)

Neuromuscular & skeletal: Neck pain (2% to 8%), paresthesia (2%), reflexes increased (2%)

Ocular: Conjunctivitis (3%), diplopia (2%), amblyopia (2%)

Otic: Ear pain (2%)

Renal: Albuminuria (4%)

Respiratory: Influenza (5%), asthma (2%), sinusitis (2%)

Miscellaneous: Flu-like syndrome (3% to 8%), viral infection (2%)

<1% (Limited to important or life-threatening): Alopecia, anemia, catatonia, hematocrit decreased, hemoglobin decreased, hepatic failure, hepatitis, leukopenia, LFTs abnormal, neutropenia, pancreatitis, pancytopenia (with bone marrow suppression), psychotic symptoms, red blood cells decreased, suicide attempt, suicide behavior, suicide ideation, thrombocytopenia, weight loss

Drug Interactions

Metabolism/Transport Effects None known.

Avoid Concomitant Use There are no known interactions where it is recommended to avoid concomitant use.

Increased Effect/Toxicity

LevETIRAcetam may increase the levels/effects of: Alcohol (Ethyl); CNS Depressants; Methotrimeprazine; Selective Serotonin Reuptake Inhibitors

The levels/effects of LevETIRAcetam may be increased by: Droperidol; HydrOXYzine; Methotrimeprazine

Decreased Effect

The levels/effects of LevETIRAcetam may be decreased by: Ketorolac; Ketorolac (Nasal); Ketorolac (Systemic); Mefloquine

Ethanol/Nutrition/Herb Interactions

Ethanol: May increase CNS depression; monitor for increased effects with coadministration. Caution patients about effects.

Food: Food may delay, but does not affect the extent of absorption.

Stability

Oral solution, tablets: Store at 25°C (77°F); excursions permitted to 15°C to 30°C (59°F to 86°F).

Injection solution: Store at 25°C (77°F); excursions permitted to 15°C to 30°C (59°F to 86°F). Must dilute dose in 100 mL of NS, LR, or D_5W. Admixed solution is stable for 24 hours in PVC bags kept at room temperature.

Mechanism of Action The precise mechanism by which levetiracetam exerts its antiepileptic effect is unknown. However, several studies have suggested the mechanism may involve one or more of the following central pharmacologic effects: inhibition of voltage-dependent N-type calcium channels; facilitation of GABA-ergic inhibitory transmission through displacement of negative modulators; reduction of delayed rectifier potassium current; and/or binding to synaptic proteins which modulate neurotransmitter release.

Pharmacodynamics/Kinetics

Absorption: Oral: Rapid and almost complete

Distribution: V_d: Similar to total body water

Protein binding: <10%

Metabolism: Not extensive; primarily by enzymatic hydrolysis; forms metabolites (inactive)

Bioavailability: 100%

Half-life elimination: ~6-8 hours; extended release tablet: ~7 hours; half-life increased in renal dysfunction

Time to peak, plasma: Oral: Immediate release: ~1 hour; Extended release: ~4 hours

Excretion: Urine (66% as unchanged drug)

Dosage

Oral:

Children 4-15 years: Partial onset seizures: Immediate release: 10 mg/kg/dose given twice daily; may increase every 2 weeks by 10 mg/kg/dose to a maximum of 30 mg/kg/dose twice daily

Children 6-15 years: Tonic-clonic seizures: Immediate release: Initial: 10 mg/kg dose given twice daily; may increase every 2 weeks by 10 mg/kg/dose to the recommended dose of 30 mg/kg twice daily. Efficacy of doses >60 mg/kg/day has not been established.

Children ≥12 years and Adults: Myoclonic seizures: Immediate release: Initial: 500 mg twice daily; may increase every 2 weeks by 500 mg/dose to the recommended dose of 1500 mg twice daily. Efficacy of doses other than 3000 mg/day has not been established.

Children ≥16 years and Adults:

Partial onset seizure:

Immediate release: Initial: 500 mg twice daily; may increase every 2 weeks by 500 mg/dose to a maximum of 1500 mg twice daily. Doses >3000 mg/day have been used in trials; however, there is no evidence of increased benefit.

Extended release: Initial: 1000 mg once daily; may increase every 2 weeks by 1000 mg/day to a maximum of 3000 mg once daily.

Tonic-clonic seizures: Immediate release: Initial: 500 mg twice daily; may increase every 2 weeks by 500 mg/dose to the recommended dose of 1500 mg twice daily. Efficacy of doses other than 3000 mg/day has not been established.

Bipolar disorder (unlabeled use): Immediate release: Initial: 500 mg twice daily; if tolerated, increase by 500 mg twice daily; dose may be increased every 3 days until target dose of 3000 mg/day is reached; maximum: 4000 mg/day

Adults: Loading dose (unlabeled): Immediate release: Initial doses of 1500-2000 mg have been well-tolerated (Betts, 2000; Koubeissi, 2008), although the necessity of a loading dose has not been established

I.V.:

Children ≥16 years and Adults: Partial onset seizure: Initial: 500 mg twice daily; may increase every 2 weeks by 500 mg/dose to a maximum of 1500 mg twice daily. Doses >3000 mg/day have been used in trials; however, there is no evidence of increased benefit.

Note: When switching from oral to I.V. formulations, the total daily dose should be the same.

Adults: Refractory status epilepticus (unlabeled use): 1000-3000 mg administered over 15 minutes (Meierkord, 2010); 2500 mg has been safely administered over 5 minutes in one report (Uges, 2009). **Note:** Levetiracetam has not been well studied in comparison to other agents routinely used in this setting.

Dosing adjustment in renal impairment: Adults:

Immediate release and I.V. formulations:

Cl_{cr} >80 mL/minute: 500-1500 mg every 12 hours

Cl_{cr} 50-80 mL/minute: 500-1000 mg every 12 hours

Cl_{cr} 30-50 mL/minute: 250-750 mg every 12 hours

Cl_{cr} <30 mL/minute: 250-500 mg every 12 hours

End-stage renal disease patients using dialysis: 500-1000 mg every 24 hours; a supplemental dose of 250-500 mg following dialysis is recommended

Extended release tablets:

Cl_{cr} >80 mL/minute: 1000-3000 mg every 24 hours

Cl_{cr} 50-80 mL/minute: 1000-2000 mg every 24 hours

Cl_{cr} 30-50 mL/minute: 500-1500 mg every 24 hours

Cl_{cr} <30 mL/minute: 500-1000 mg every 24 hours

Dosing adjustment in hepatic impairment: No adjustment required

Dietary Considerations May be taken without regard to meals.

Administration

I.V.: Infuse over 15 minutes

Oral: May be administered without regard to meals.

Oral solution: Should be administered with a calibrated measuring device (not a household teaspoon or tablespoon)

Tablet (immediate release and extended release): Only administer as whole tablet; do not crush, break or chew.

Monitoring Parameters Suicidality (eg, suicidal thoughts, depression, behavioral changes)

Dosage Forms Excipient information presented when available (limited, particularly for generics); consult specific product labeling.

Injection, solution: 100 mg/mL (5 mL)

Keppra®: 100 mg/mL (5 mL)

Solution, oral: 100 mg/mL (5 mL, 118 mL, 472 mL, 473 mL, 480 mL, 500 mL)

Keppra®: 100 mg/mL (480 mL) [dye free; grape flavor]

Tablet, oral: 250 mg, 500 mg, 750 mg, 1000 mg

Keppra®: 250 mg, 500 mg, 750 mg [scored; gluten free]

Tablet, extended release, oral: 500 mg, 750 mg

Keppra XR™: 500 mg, 750 mg

◆ **Levitra®** *see* Vardenafil *on page* 1769

Levobunolol (lee voe BYOO noe lole)

Brand Names: U.S. Betagan®

Brand Names: Canada Apo-Levobunolol®; Betagan®; Novo-Levobunolol; Optho-Bunolol®; PMS-Levobunolol; Sandoz-Levobunolol

Index Terms *l*-Bunolol Hydrochloride; Levobunolol Hydrochloride

Pharmacologic Category Beta-Adrenergic Blocker, Nonselective; Ophthalmic Agent, Antiglaucoma

Use To lower intraocular pressure in chronic open-angle glaucoma or ocular hypertension

Pregnancy Risk Factor C

Dosage Adults: Ophthalmic: Instill 1 drop in the affected eye(s) 1-2 times/day

Additional Information Complete prescribing information for this medication should be consulted for additional detail.

Dosage Forms Excipient information presented when available (limited, particularly for generics); consult specific product labeling. [DSC] = Discontinued product

Solution, ophthalmic, as hydrochloride [drops]: 0.25% (5 mL, 10 mL); 0.5% (5 mL, 10 mL, 15 mL)
Betagan®: 0.25% (5 mL [DSC], 10 mL [DSC]); 0.5% (2 mL [DSC], 5 mL, 10 mL, 15 mL) [contains benzalkonium chloride, sodium metabisulfite]

◆ **Levobunolol Hydrochloride** *see* Levobunolol *on page 995*

◆ **Levocarb CR (Can)** *see* Carbidopa and Levodopa *on page 284*

Levocetirizine (LEE vo se TI ra zeen)

Brand Names: U.S. Xyzal®

Index Terms Levocetirizine Dihydrochloride

Pharmacologic Category Histamine H_1 Antagonist; Histamine H_1 Antagonist, Second Generation; Piperazine Derivative

Use Relief of symptoms of perennial and seasonal allergic rhinitis; treatment of skin manifestations (uncomplicated) of chronic idiopathic urticaria

Pregnancy Risk Factor B

Dosage Oral:

Perennial allergic rhinitis, chronic urticaria:
Children 6 months to 5 years: 1.25 mg once daily (in the evening); maximum: 1.25 mg
Children 6-11 years: 2.5 mg once daily (in the evening); maximum: 2.5 mg/day
Children ≥12 years and Adults: 5 mg once daily (in the evening); some patients may experience relief of symptoms with 2.5 mg once daily

Seasonal allergic rhinitis:
Children 2-5 years: 1.25 mg once daily (in the evening); maximum: 1.25 mg
Children 6-11 years: 2.5 mg once daily (in the evening); maximum: 2.5 mg/day
Children ≥12 years and Adults: 5 mg once daily (in the evening); some patients may experience relief of symptoms with 2.5 mg once daily

Elderly: Refer to adult dosing; dosing should begin at the lower end of the dosing range

Dosage adjustments in renal impairment:
Children 6 months to 11 years with renal impairment: Contraindicated
Children ≥12 and Adults:
Cl_{cr} 50-80 mL/minute: 2.5 mg once daily
Cl_{cr} 30-50 mL/minute: 2.5 mg once every other day
Cl_{cr} 10-30 mL/minute: 2.5 mg twice weekly (every 3 or 4 days)
Cl_{cr} <10 mL/minute, hemodialysis patients: Contraindicated

Dosage adjustments in hepatic impairment: No adjustment required.

Additional Information Complete prescribing information for this medication should be consulted for additional detail.

Dosage Forms Excipient information presented when available (limited, particularly for generics); consult specific product labeling.

Solution, oral, as dihydrochloride: 0.5 mg/mL (150 mL)
Xyzal®: 0.5 mg/mL (150 mL)
Tablet, oral, as dihydrochloride: 5 mg
Xyzal®: 5 mg [scored]

◆ **Levocetirizine Dihydrochloride** *see* Levocetirizine *on page 996*

◆ **Levodopa and Carbidopa** *see* Carbidopa and Levodopa *on page 284*

Levodopa, Carbidopa, and Entacapone

(lee voe DOE pa, kar bi DOE pa, & en TA ka pone)

Brand Names: U.S. Stalevo®

Brand Names: Canada Stalevo®

Index Terms Carbidopa, Entacapone, and Levodopa; Carbidopa, Levodopa, and Entacapone; Entacapone, Carbidopa, and Levodopa

Pharmacologic Category Anti-Parkinson's Agent, COMT Inhibitor; Anti-Parkinson's Agent, Decarboxylase Inhibitor; Anti-Parkinson's Agent, Dopamine Precursor

Additional Appendix Information

Antiparkinsonian Agents *on page 1879*

Use Treatment of idiopathic Parkinson's disease

Pregnancy Risk Factor C

Dosage Oral: Adults: Parkinson's disease:

Note: All strengths of Stalevo® contain a carbidopa/levodopa ratio of 1:4 plus entacapone 200 mg.

Dose should be individualized based on therapeutic response; doses may be adjusted by changing strength or adjusting interval. Fractionated doses are not recommended and only 1 tablet should be given at each dosing interval; maximum daily dose: 8 tablets of Stalevo® 50, 75, 100, 125, or 150, **or** 6 tablets of Stalevo® 200.

Patients previously treated with carbidopa/levodopa immediate release tablets (ratio of 1:4):
With current entacapone therapy: May switch directly to corresponding strength of combination tablet. No data available on transferring patients from controlled release preparations or products with a 1:10 ratio of carbidopa/levodopa.
Without entacapone therapy:
If current levodopa dose is >600 mg/day: Levodopa dose reduction may be required when adding entacapone to therapy; therefore, titrate dose using individual products first (carbidopa/levodopa immediate release with a ratio of 1:4 plus entacapone 200 mg); then transfer to combination product once stabilized.
If current levodopa dose is <600 mg without dyskinesias: May transfer to corresponding dose of combination product; monitor, dose reduction of levodopa may be required.

Patients previously treated with benserazide/levodopa immediate release tablets (Canadian labeling, not in U.S. labeling): With current entacapone therapy: Prior to switching to combination product (carbidopa/levodopa/entacapone), withhold treatment for 1 night, then initiate (carbidopa/levodopa/entacapone) therapy the following morning at a dose that provides either an equivalent amount or ~5% to 10% more levodopa.

Dosage adjustment in renal impairment: Use caution with severe renal impairment; specific dosing recommendations not available

Dosage adjustment in hepatic impairment: Use with caution; specific dosing recommendations not available

Additional Information Complete prescribing information for this medication should be consulted for additional detail.

Dosage Forms Excipient information presented when available (limited, particularly for generics); consult specific product labeling.

Tablet:

Stalevo® 50: Levodopa 50 mg, carbidopa 12.5 mg, and entacapone 200 mg

Stalevo® 75: Levodopa 75 mg, carbidopa 18.75 mg, and entacapone 200 mg

Stalevo® 100: Levodopa 100 mg, carbidopa 25 mg, and entacapone 200 mg

Stalevo® 125: Levodopa 125 mg, carbidopa 31.25 mg, and entacapone 200 mg

Stalevo® 150: Levodopa 150 mg, carbidopa 37.5 mg, and entacapone 200 mg

Stalevo® 200: Levodopa 200 mg, carbidopa 50 mg, and entacapone 200 mg

◆ **Levo-Dromoran** *see* Levorphanol *on page 1003*

Levofloxacin (Systemic) (lee voe FLOKS a sin)

Brand Names: U.S. Levaquin®

Brand Names: Canada Levaquin®; Novo-Levofloxacin; PMS-Levofloxacin

Pharmacologic Category Antibiotic, Quinolone; Respiratory Fluoroquinolone

Additional Appendix Information

Prevention of Wound Infection and Sepsis in Surgical Patients *on page 1954*

Use Treatment of community-acquired pneumonia, including multidrug resistant strains of *S. pneumoniae* (MDRSP); nosocomial pneumonia; chronic bronchitis (acute bacterial exacerbation); acute bacterial sinusitis; prostatitis, urinary tract infection (uncomplicated or complicated); acute pyelonephritis; skin or skin structure infections (uncomplicated or complicated); reduce incidence or disease progression of inhalational anthrax (postexposure)

Unlabeled Use Diverticulitis, enterocolitis (*Shigella* spp), epididymitis (nongonococcal), gonococcal infections, complicated intra-abdominal infections (in combination with metronidazole), Legionnaires' disease, peritonitis, PID

Note: As of April 2007, the CDC no longer recommends the use of fluoroquinolones for the treatment of gonococcal disease.

Pregnancy Risk Factor C

Pregnancy Considerations Adverse events have been observed in some animal studies; therefore, the manufacturer classifies levofloxacin as pregnancy category C. Levofloxacin crosses the placenta. Quinolone exposure during human pregnancy has been reported with other agents (see Ciprofloxacin [Systemic], Ofloxacin [Systemic], and Norfloxacin [Systemic] monographs). To date, no specific teratogenic effect or increased pregnancy risk has been identified; however, because of concerns of cartilage damage in immature animals exposed to quinolones and the limited levofloxacin specific data, levofloxacin should only be used during pregnancy if a safer option is not available.

Lactation Enters breast milk/not recommended

Medication Guide Available Yes

Contraindications Hypersensitivity to levofloxacin, any component of the formulation, or other quinolones

Warnings/Precautions **[U.S. Boxed Warning]: There have been reports of tendon inflammation and/or rupture with quinolone antibiotics; risk may be increased with concurrent corticosteroids, organ transplant recipients, and in patients >60 years of age.** Rupture of the Achilles tendon sometimes requiring surgical repair has been reported most frequently; but other tendon sites (eg, rotator cuff, biceps) have also been reported. Strenuous physical activity, rheumatoid arthritis, and renal impairment may be an independent risk factor for tendonitis. Discontinue at first sign of tendon inflammation or pain. May occur even after discontinuation of therapy. Use with caution in patients with rheumatoid arthritis; may increase risk of tendon rupture. Systemic use is only recommended in children <18 years of age for the prevention of inhalational anthrax (postexposure); increased incidence of musculoskeletal disorders (eg, arthralgia, tendon rupture) has been observed in children; CNS stimulation may occur (tremor, restlessness, confusion, and very rarely hallucinations or seizures). Potential for seizures, although very rare, may be increased with concomitant NSAID therapy. Use with caution in individuals at risk of seizures, with known or suspected CNS disorders or renal dysfunction. Avoid excessive sunlight and take precautions to limit exposure (eg, loose fitting clothing, sunscreen); may cause moderate-to-severe phototoxicity reactions. Discontinue use if photosensitivity occurs.

Rare cases of torsade de pointes have been reported in patients receiving levofloxacin. Use caution in patients with known prolongation of QT interval, bradycardia, hypokalemia, hypomagnesemia, or in those receiving concurrent therapy with Class Ia or Class III antiarrhythmics.

Severe hypersensitivity reactions, including anaphylaxis, have occurred with quinolone therapy. Reactions may present as typical allergic symptoms after a single dose, or may manifest as severe idiosyncratic dermatologic, vascular, pulmonary, renal, hepatic, and/or hematologic events, usually after multiple doses. Prompt discontinuation of drug should occur if skin rash or other symptoms arise. Prolonged use may result in fungal or bacterial superinfection, including *C. difficile*-associated diarrhea (CDAD) and pseudomembranous colitis; CDAD has been observed >2 months postantibiotic treatment. Peripheral neuropathies have been linked to levofloxacin use; discontinue if numbness, tingling, or weakness develops. **[U.S. Boxed Warning]: Quinolones may exacerbate myasthenia gravis; avoid use (rare, potentially life-threatening weakness of respiratory muscles may occur).** Unrelated to hypersensitivity, severe hepatotoxicity (including acute hepatitis and fatalities) has been reported. Elderly patients may be at greater risk. Discontinue therapy immediately if signs and symptoms of hepatitis occur. Hemolytic reactions may (rarely) occur with quinolone use in patients with latent or actual G6PD deficiency.

Fluoroquinolones have been associated with the development of serious, and sometimes fatal, hypoglycemia, most often in elderly diabetics, but also in patients without diabetes. This occurred most frequently with gatifloxacin (no longer available systemically) but may occur at a lower frequency with other quinolones.

Adverse Reactions

1% to 10%:

Cardiovascular: Chest pain (1%), edema (1%)

Central nervous system: Headache (6%), insomnia (4%), dizziness (3%), fatigue (1%), pain (1%)

Dermatologic: Rash (2%), pruritus (1%)

Gastrointestinal: Nausea (7%), diarrhea (5%), constipation (3%), abdominal pain (2%), dyspepsia (2%), vomiting (2%)

Genitourinary: Vaginitis (1%)

Local: Injection site reaction (1%)

Respiratory: Pharyngitis (4%), dyspnea (1%)

Miscellaneous: Moniliasis (1%)

<1% (Limited to important or life-threatening): Acute renal failure, agitation, agranulocytosis; allergic reaction (including anaphylaxis, angioedema, pneumonitis rash, pneumonitis, and serum sickness); anaphylactoid

reaction, arrhythmia (including atrial/ventricular tachycardia/fibrillation and torsade de pointes), aplastic anemia, arthralgia, ascites, bradycardia, bronchospasm, carcinoma, cardiac failure, cholecystitis, cholelithiasis, confusion, depression, EEG abnormalities, encephalopathy, eosinophilia, erythema multiforme, GI hemorrhage, granulocytopenia, hallucination, heart block, hemolytic anemia, hemoptysis, hepatic failure (some fatal), hepatitis, hyper-/hypoglycemia, hyperkalemia, hyperkinesias, hyper-/hypotension, infection, INR increased, intestinal obstruction, intracranial hypertension, involuntary muscle contractions, jaundice, leukocytosis, leukopenia, leukorrhea, lymphadenopathy, MI, migraine, multiple organ failure, myalgia, myasthenia gravis exacerbation, nephritis (interstitial), palpitation, pancreatitis, pancytopenia, paralysis, paresthesia, peripheral neuropathy, photosensitivity (<0.1%), pleural effusion, pneumonitis, postural hypotension, prothrombin time increased/decreased, pseudomembraneous colitis, psychosis, pulmonary edema, pulmonary embolism, purpura, QT_c prolongation, respiratory depression, rhabdomyolysis, seizure, skin disorder, somnolence, speech disorder, Stevens-Johnson syndrome, stupor, suicide attempt/ideation, syncope, tendonitis, tendon rupture, tongue edema, toxic epidermal necrolysis, transaminases increased, thrombocythemia, thrombocytopenia, tremor, urticaria, WBC abnormality

Drug Interactions

Metabolism/Transport Effects None known.

Avoid Concomitant Use

Avoid concomitant use of Levofloxacin (Systemic) with any of the following: Artemether; BCG; Dronedarone; Lumefantrine; Nilotinib; Pimozide; QUEtiapine; QuiNINE; Tetrabenazine; Thioridazine; Toremifene; Vandetanib; Vemurafenib; Ziprasidone

Increased Effect/Toxicity

Levofloxacin (Systemic) may increase the levels/effects of: Corticosteroids (Systemic); Dronedarone; Pimozide; Porfimer; QTc-Prolonging Agents; QuiNINE; Sulfonylureas; Tetrabenazine; Thioridazine; Toremifene; Vandetanib; Varenicline; Vemurafenib; Vitamin K Antagonists; Ziprasidone

The levels/effects of Levofloxacin (Systemic) may be increased by: Alfuzosin; Artemether; Chloroquine; Ciprofloxacin; Ciprofloxacin (Systemic); Gadobutrol; Indacaterol; Insulin; Lumefantrine; Nilotinib; Nonsteroidal Anti-Inflammatory Agents; Probenecid; QUEtiapine; QuiNINE

Decreased Effect

Levofloxacin (Systemic) may decrease the levels/effects of: BCG; Mycophenolate; Sulfonylureas; Typhoid Vaccine

The levels/effects of Levofloxacin (Systemic) may be decreased by: Antacids; Calcium Salts; Didanosine; Iron Salts; Lanthanum; Magnesium Salts; Quinapril; Sevelamer; Sucralfate; Zinc Salts

Stability

Solution for injection:

Vial: Store at room temperature. Protect from light. When diluted to 5 mg/mL in a compatible I.V. fluid, solution is stable for 72 hours when stored at room temperature; stable for 14 days when stored under refrigeration. When frozen, stable for 6 months; do not refreeze. Do not thaw in microwave or by bath immersion.

Premixed: Store at ≤25°C (77°F); do not freeze. Brief exposure to 40°C (104°F) does not affect product. Protect from light.

Tablet, oral solution: Store at 25°C (77°F); excursions permitted to 15°C to 30°C (59°F to 86°F).

Mechanism of Action As the S(-) enantiomer of the fluoroquinolone, ofloxacin, levofloxacin, inhibits DNA-gyrase in susceptible organisms thereby inhibits relaxation of supercoiled DNA and promotes breakage of DNA strands. DNA gyrase (topoisomerase II), is an essential bacterial enzyme that maintains the superhelical structure of DNA and is required for DNA replication and transcription, DNA repair, recombination, and transposition.

Pharmacodynamics/Kinetics

Absorption: Rapid and complete

Distribution: V_d: 74-112 L; CSF concentrations ~15% of serum levels; high concentrations are achieved in prostate, lung, and gynecological tissues, sinus, saliva

Protein binding: ~24% to 38%; primarily to albumin

Metabolism: Minimally hepatic

Bioavailability: ~99%

Half-life elimination: ~6-8 hours

Time to peak, serum: Oral: 1-2 hours

Excretion: Urine (~87% as unchanged drug, <5% as metabolites); feces (<4%)

Dosage Note: Sequential therapy (intravenous to oral) may be instituted based on prescriber's discretion.

Usual dosage range: Adults: Oral, I.V.: 250-500 mg every 24 hours; severe or complicated infections: 750 mg every 24 hours

Indication-specific dosing:

Infants ≥6 months and Children ≤4 years:

Community-acquired pneumonia (CAP) (IDSA/PIDS, 2011): Note: May consider addition of vancomycin or clindamycin to empiric therapy if community-acquired MRSA suspected; alternative to ceftriaxone or cefotaxime in patients not fully immunized for *H. influenzae* type b and *S. pneumoniae*, or significant local resistance to penicillin in invasive pneumococcal strains.

S. pneumoniae (MICs to penicillin ≤2.0 mcg/mL), mild infection or step-down therapy (alternative to amoxicillin): Oral: 8-10 mg/kg/dose every 12 hours (maximum: 750 mg/day)

S. pneumoniae (MICs to penicillin ≥4.0 mcg/mL):

Moderate-to-severe infection (alternative to ceftriaxone): I.V.: 8-10 mg/kg/dose every 12 hours (maximum: 750 mg/day)

Mild infection, step-down therapy (preferred): Oral: 8-10 mg/kg/dose every 12 hours (maximum: 750 mg/day)

H. influenzae, moderate-to-severe infection (alternative to ampicillin, ceftriaxone, or cefotaxime): I.V.: 8-10 mg/kg/dose every 12 hours (maximum: 750 mg/day)

Atypical pathogens, moderate-to-severe infection (alternative to azithromycin) or empiric treatment (alternative to azithromycin +/- beta-lactam; should be limited to macrolide allergic/intolerant patients): Oral, I.V.: 8-10 mg/kg/dose every 12 hours (maximum: 750 mg/day)

Children 5-16 years:

Community-acquired pneumonia (CAP) (IDSA/PIDS, 2011): Note: May consider addition of vancomycin or clindamycin to empiric therapy if community-acquired MRSA suspected; alternative to ceftriaxone or cefotaxime in patients not fully immunized for *H. influenzae* type b and *S. pneumoniae*, or significant local resistance to penicillin in invasive pneumococcal strains.

S. pneumoniae (MICs to penicillin ≤2.0 mcg/mL), mild infection or step-down therapy (alternative to amoxicillin): Oral: 8-10 mg/kg/dose once daily (maximum: 750 mg/day)

S. pneumoniae (MICs to penicillin ≥4.0 mcg/mL):

Moderate-to-severe infection (alternative to ceftriaxone): I.V.: 8-10 mg/kg/dose once daily (maximum: 750 mg/day)

Mild infection, step-down therapy (preferred): Oral: 8-10 mg/kg/dose once daily (maximum: 750 mg/day)

H. influenzae, moderate-to-severe infection (alternative to ampicillin, ceftriaxone, or cefotaxime): I.V.: 8-10 mg/kg/dose once daily (maximum: 750 mg/day)

Atypical pathogens:
Moderate-to-severe infection (alternative to azithromycin): I.V.: 8-10 mg/kg/dose once daily (maximum: 750 mg/day)
Mild infection, step-down therapy (alternative to azithromycin in adolescents with skeletal maturity): Oral: 500 mg once daily

Infants ≥6 months, Children, and Adults: Oral, I.V.:
Anthrax (inhalational, postexposure):
≤50 kg: 8 mg/kg every 12 hours for 60 days (do not exceed 250 mg/dose), beginning as soon as possible after exposure
>50 kg and Adults: 500 mg every 24 hours for 60 days, beginning as soon as possible after exposure

Adults: Oral, I.V.:
Chronic bronchitis (acute bacterial exacerbation): 500 mg every 24 hours for at least 7 days
Diverticulitis, peritonitis (unlabeled use): 750 mg every 24 hours for 7-10 days; use adjunctive metronidazole therapy
Dysenteric enterocolitis, *Shigella* spp. (unlabeled use): 500 mg every 24 hours for 3-5 days
Epididymitis, nongonococcal (unlabeled use): 500 mg once daily for 10 days
Gonococcal infection (unlabeled use):
Cervicitis, urethritis: 250 mg for one dose with azithromycin or doxycycline; **Note:** As of April 2007, the CDC no longer recommends the use of fluoroquinolones for the treatment of uncomplicated gonococcal disease.
Disseminated infection: 250 mg I.V. once daily; 24 hours after symptoms improve may change to 500 mg orally every 24 hours to complete total therapy of 7 days; **Note:** As of April 2007, the CDC no longer recommends the use of fluoroquinolones for the treatment of more serious gonococcal disease, unless no other options exist and susceptibility can be confirmed via culture.
Intra-abdominal infection, complicated, community-acquired (in combination with metronidazole) (unlabeled use): I.V.: 750 mg once daily for 4-7 days (provided source controlled). **Note:** Avoid using in settings where *E. coli* susceptibility to fluoroquinolones is <90%.
Pelvic inflammatory disease (unlabeled use): 500 mg once daily for 14 days with or without adjunctive metronidazole; **Note:** The CDC recommends use only if standard cephalosporin therapy is not feasible and community prevalence of quinolone-resistant gonococcal organisms is low. Culture sensitivity must be confirmed.
Pneumonia:
Community-acquired (CAP): 500 mg every 24 hours for 7-14 days or 750 mg every 24 hours for 5 days (efficacy of 5-day regimen for MDRSP not established)
Healthcare-associated (HAP): 750 mg every 24 hours for 7-14 days
Prostatitis (chronic bacterial): 500 mg every 24 hours for 28 days
Sinusitis (acute bacterial): 500 mg every 24 hours for 10-14 days or 750 mg every 24 hours for 5 days
Skin and skin structure infections:
Uncomplicated: 500 mg every 24 hours for 7-10 days
Complicated: 750 mg every 24 hours for 7-14 days
Traveler's diarrhea (unlabeled use): 500 mg for one dose
Urinary tract infections:
Uncomplicated: 250 mg once daily for 3 days
Complicated, including pyelonephritis: 250 mg once daily for 10 days **or** 750 mg once daily for 5 days

Dosing adjustment in renal impairment:
Normal renal function dosing of 750 mg/day:
Cl_{cr} 20-49 mL/minute: Administer 750 mg every 48 hours
Cl_{cr} 10-19 mL/minute: Administer 750 mg initial dose, followed by 500 mg every 48 hours
Hemodialysis/peritoneal dialysis (PD): Administer 750 mg initial dose, followed by 500 mg every 48 hours
Normal renal function dosing of 500 mg/day:
Cl_{cr} 20-49 mL/minute: Administer 500 mg initial dose, followed by 250 mg every 24 hours
Cl_{cr} 10-19 mL/minute: Administer 500 mg initial dose, followed by 250 mg every 48 hours
Hemodialysis (administer after hemodialysis on dialysis days)/peritoneal dialysis (PD): Administer 500 mg initial dose, followed by 250 mg every 48 hours
Normal renal function dosing of 250 mg/day:
Cl_{cr} 20-49 mL/minute: No dosage adjustment required
Cl_{cr} 10-19 mL/minute: Administer 250 mg every 48 hours (except in uncomplicated UTI, where no dosage adjustment is required)
Hemodialysis (administer after hemodialysis on dialysis days)/peritoneal dialysis (PD): No information available

Continuous renal replacement therapy (CRRT) (Heintz, 2009; Trotman, 2005): Drug clearance is highly dependent on the method of renal replacement, filter type, and flow rate. Appropriate dosing requires close monitoring of pharmacologic response, signs of adverse reactions due to drug accumulation, as well as drug concentrations in relation to target trough (if appropriate). The following are general recommendations only (based on dialysate flow/ultrafiltration rates of 1-2 L/hour and minimal residual renal function) and should not supersede clinical judgment:
CVVH: Loading dose of 500-750 mg followed by 250 mg every 24 hours
CVVHD: Loading dose of 500-750 mg followed by 250-500 mg every 24 hours
CVVHDF: Loading dose of 500-750 mg followed by 250-750 mg every 24 hours

Dietary Considerations Tablets may be taken without regard to meals. Oral solution should be administered on an empty stomach (1 hour before or 2 hours after a meal). Take 2 hours before or 2 hours after multiple vitamins, antacids, or other products containing magnesium, aluminum, iron, or zinc.

Administration
Oral: Tablets may be administered without regard to meals. Oral solution should be administered 1 hour before or 2 hours after meals. Maintain adequate hydration of patient to prevent crystalluria.
I.V.: Infuse 250-500 mg I.V. solution over 60 minutes; infuse 750 mg I.V. solution over 90 minutes. Too rapid of infusion can lead to hypotension. Avoid administration through an intravenous line with a solution containing multivalent cations (eg, magnesium, calcium). Maintain adequate hydration of patient to prevent crystalluria.

Monitoring Parameters Evaluation of organ system functions (renal, hepatic, and hematopoietic) is recommended periodically during therapy; the possibility of crystalluria should be assessed; WBC and signs of infection

Test Interactions Some quinolones may produce a false-positive urine screening result for opiates using commercially-available immunoassay kits. This has been demonstrated most consistently for levofloxacin and ofloxacin, but other quinolones have shown cross-reactivity in certain assay kits. Confirmation of positive opiate screens by more specific methods should be considered.

Dosage Forms Excipient information presented when available (limited, particularly for generics); consult specific product labeling. [DSC] = Discontinued product

Infusion, premixed in D_5W [preservative free]: 250 mg (50 mL); 500 mg (100 mL); 750 mg (150 mL)

Levaquin®: 250 mg (50 mL); 500 mg (100 mL); 750 mg (150 mL)

Injection, solution [preservative free]: 25 mg/mL (20 mL, 30 mL)

Levaquin®: 25 mg/mL (20 mL [DSC], 30 mL [DSC])

Solution, oral: 25 mg/mL (100 mL, 200 mL, 480 mL)

Levaquin®: 25 mg/mL (480 mL) [contains benzyl alcohol, propylene glycol]

Tablet, oral: 250 mg, 500 mg, 750 mg

Levaquin®: 250 mg, 500 mg, 750 mg

Extemporaneous Preparations Note: Commercial oral solution is available (25 mg/mL)

A 50 mg/mL oral suspension may be made with tablets and a 1:1 mixture of Ora-Plus® and strawberry syrup NF. Crush six 500 mg levofloxacin tablets in a mortar and reduce to a fine powder. Add small portions of the vehicle and mix to a uniform paste; mix while adding the vehicle in incremental proportions to **almost** 60 mL; transfer to a graduated cylinder, rinse mortar with vehicle, and add quantity of vehicle sufficient to make 60 mL. Label "shake well". Stable for 57 days when stored in amber plastic prescription bottles at room temperature or refrigerated.

VandenBussche HL, Johnson CE, and Fontana EM, et al, "Stability of Levofloxacin in an Extemporaneously Compounded Oral Liquid," *Am J Health Syst Pharm*, 1999, 56(22):2316-8.

Levofloxacin (Ophthalmic) (lee voe FLOKS a sin)

Brand Names: U.S. Iquix®; Quixin®

Pharmacologic Category Antibiotic, Ophthalmic; Antibiotic, Quinolone

Use Treatment of bacterial conjunctivitis caused by susceptible organisms (Quixin® 0.5% ophthalmic solution); treatment of corneal ulcer caused by susceptible organisms (Iquix® 1.5% ophthalmic solution)

Pregnancy Risk Factor C

Dosage

Ophthalmic:

Usual dosage range:

Children ≥1 year: 1-2 drops every 2-6 hours

Adults: 1-2 drops every 2-6 hours

Indication-specific dosing:

Children ≥1 year and Adults:

Conjunctivitis (0.5% ophthalmic solution):

Treatment day 1 and day 2: Instill 1-2 drops into affected eye(s) every 2 hours while awake, up to 8 times/day

Treatment day 3 through day 7: Instill 1-2 drops into affected eye(s) every 4 hours while awake, up to 4 times/day

Children ≥6 years and Adults:

Corneal ulceration (1.5% ophthalmic solution):

Treatment day 1 through day 3: Instill 1-2 drops into affected eye(s) every 30 minutes to 2 hours while awake and 4-6 hours after retiring

Treatment day 4 through completion: Instill 1-2 drops into affected eye(s) every 1-4 hours while awake

Additional Information Complete prescribing information for this medication should be consulted for additional detail.

Dosage Forms Excipient information presented when available (limited, particularly for generics); consult specific product labeling.

Solution, ophthalmic [drops]: 0.5% (5 mL)

Iquix®: 1.5% (5 mL)

Quixin®: 0.5% (5 mL) [contains benzalkonium chloride]

◆ **Levo-folinic Acid** *see* LEVOleucovorin *on page 1000*

LEVOleucovorin (lee voe loo koe VOR in)

Brand Names: U.S. Fusilev™

Index Terms 6S-leucovorin; Calcium Levoleucovorin; L-leucovorin; Levo-folinic Acid; Levo-leucovorin; Levoleucovorin Calcium Pentahydrate; S-leucovorin

Pharmacologic Category Antidote; Chemotherapy Modulating Agent; Rescue Agent (Chemotherapy)

Use Treatment of advanced, metastatic colorectal cancer (palliative) in combination with fluorouracil; rescue agent after high-dose methotrexate therapy in osteosarcoma; antidote for impaired methotrexate elimination and for inadvertent overdosage of folic acid antagonists

Pregnancy Risk Factor C

Dosage Note: Levoleucovorin, when substituted in place of leucovorin calcium (the racemic form), is dosed at **one-half** the usual dose of leucovorin calcium:

Colorectal cancer: Adults I.V.: The following regimens have been used (in combination with fluorouracil; fluorouracil doses may need to be adjusted for toxicity; no adjustment required for the levoleucovorin dose):

100 mg /m²/day over at least 3 minutes (followed by fluorouracil 370 mg/m²/day) for 5 days every 4 weeks for 2 cycles, then every 4-5 weeks depending on recovery from toxicities, **or**

10 mg /m²/day (followed by fluorouracil 425 mg/m²/day) for 5 days every 4 weeks for 2 cycles, then every 4-5 weeks depending on recovery from toxicities, **or**

Alternative dosing: Levoleucovorin, when substituted in place of leucovorin calcium within a chemotherapy regimen, is dosed at **one-half** the usual dose of leucovorin calcium (Goldberg, 1997; NCCN colon cancer guidelines v.3.2011)

High-dose methotrexate rescue: Children and Adults: I.V.: Usual dose: 7.5 mg (~5 mg/m²) every 6 hours for 10 doses, beginning 24 hours after the start of the methotrexate infusion (based on a methotrexate dose of 12 g/m² I.V. over 4 hours). Levoleucovorin (and hydration and urinary alkalinization) should be continued and/or adjusted until the methotrexate level is <0.05 micromolar (5×10^{-8} M) as follows:

Normal methotrexate elimination (serum methotrexate levels ~10 micromolar at 24 hours post administration, 1 micromolar at 48 hours and <0.2 micromolar at 72 hours post infusion): 7.5 mg I.V. every 6 hours for 10 doses

Delayed late methotrexate elimination (serum methotrexate levels >0.2 micromolar at 72 hours and >0.05 micromolar at 96 hours post methotrexate infusion): Continue 7.5 mg I.V. every 6 hours until methotrexate level is <0.05 micromolar

Delayed early methotrexate elimination and/or evidence of acute renal injury (serum methotrexate level ≥50 micromolar at 24 hours, ≥5 micromolar at 48 hours or a doubling or more of the serum creatinine level at 24 hours post methotrexate infusion): 75 mg I.V. every 3 hours until methotrexate level is <1 micromolar, followed by 7.5 mg I.V. every 3 hours until methotrexate level is <0.05 micromolar

Significant clinical toxicity in the presence of less severe abnormalities in methotrexate elimination or renal function (as described above): Extend levoleucovorin treatment for an additional 24 hours (total of 14 doses) in subsequent treatment cycles.

Delayed methotrexate elimination due to third space fluid accumulation, renal insufficiency, or inadequate hydration: May require higher levoleucovorin doses or prolonged administration.

Methotrexate overdose (inadvertent): Children and Adults: I.V.: 7.5 mg (~5 mg/m^2) every 6 hours; continue until the methotrexate level is <0.01 micromolar (10^{-8} M). Initiate treatment as soon as possible after methotrexate overdose. Increase the levoleucovorin dose to 50 mg/m^2 I.V. every 3 hours if the 24 hour serum creatinine has increased 50% over baseline, or if the 24-hour methotrexate level is >5 micromolar (5×10^{-6} M), or if the 48-hour methotrexate level is >0.9 micromolar (9×10^{-7} M); continue levoleucovorin until the methotrexate level is <0.01 micromolar (10^{-8} M). Hydration (aggressive) and urinary alkalinization (with sodium bicarbonate) should also be maintained.

Additional Information Complete prescribing information for this medication should be consulted for additional detail.

Product Availability

Fusilev™ solution for injection: FDA approved April 2011; availability expected in the third quarter of 2011

Fusilev™ solution for injection is a ready-to-use formulation and will be available in 175 mg/17.5 mL and 250 mg/25 mL presentations.

Dosage Forms Excipient information presented when available (limited, particularly for generics); consult specific product labeling.

Injection, powder for reconstitution:

Fusilev™: 50 mg

- ◆ **Levo-leucovorin** *see* LEVOleucovorin *on page 1000*
- ◆ **Levoleucovorin Calcium Pentahydrate** *see* LEVOleucovorin *on page 1000*
- ◆ **Levomefolate Calcium, Drospirenone, and Ethinyl Estradiol** *see* Ethinyl Estradiol, Drospirenone, and Levomefolate *on page 664*
- ◆ **Levomefolate, Drospirenone, and Ethinyl Estradiol** *see* Ethinyl Estradiol, Drospirenone, and Levomefolate *on page 664*

Levonorgestrel (LEE voe nor jes trel)

Brand Names: U.S. Mirena®; Next Choice™; Plan B® One Step

Brand Names: Canada Mirena®; Plan B®

Index Terms LNg 20; Plan B

Pharmacologic Category Contraceptive; Progestin

Use

Intrauterine device (IUD): Prevention of pregnancy; treatment of heavy menstrual bleeding in women who also choose to use an IUD for contraception

Oral: Emergency contraception following unprotected intercourse or possible contraceptive failure

Plan B® One-Step is approved for OTC use by women ≥17 years of age and available by prescription only for women <17 years of age. Next Choice™ (generic of the original Plan-B® 2-dose regimen) is also approved for OTC use by women ≥17 years of age and by prescription only for women <17 years of age.

Pregnancy Considerations Epidemiologic studies have not shown an increased risk of birth defects when used prior to pregnancy or inadvertently during early pregnancy, although rare reports of congenital anomalies have been reported. In doses larger than those used for oral contraception, progestins have been reported to increase the risk of masculinization of female genitalia.

Intrauterine device: Pregnancy should be ruled out prior to insertion. Women who become pregnant with an IUD in place risk septic abortion (septic shock and death may occur). Removal of the device is recommended, however, removal or manipulation of IUD may result in pregnancy loss. In addition, miscarriage, premature labor, and premature delivery may occur if pregnancy is continued with IUD in place. Following pregnancy, insertion of the device should not take place until 6 weeks postpartum or until involution of the uterus is complete. Consider waiting until 12 weeks postpartum if involution is substantially delayed. The device may be inserted immediately following a first trimester abortion. Following removal of the device, ~80% of women who wished to conceive became pregnant within 12 months.

Oral tablet: A rapid return of fertility is expected following use for emergency contraception; routine contraceptive measures should be initiated or continued following use to ensure ongoing prevention of pregnancy. Barrier contraception is recommended immediately following emergency contraception. Short-term contraception (eg, oral hormonal contraceptive pills, patches, rings) may be started with barrier contraception or after the next menstrual period. Long term contraception (eg, IUD, depot medroxyprogesterone, progestin implant) should be started after the next menstrual period.

Lactation Enters breast milk/use caution

Prescribing and Access Restrictions Plan B® One-Step will be limited to pharmacies or healthcare clinics with a valid license to distribute prescription products. Because there will be one package for both OTC and prescription use, pharmacies are required to keep the product behind the counter.

Contraindications Hypersensitivity to levonorgestrel or any component of the formulation; pregnancy

Additional product-specific contraindications:

Intrauterine device: Congenital or acquired uterine anomaly, acute pelvic inflammatory disease, history of pelvic inflammatory disease (unless there has been a subsequent intrauterine pregnancy), postpartum endometritis or infected abortion within past 3 months, known or suspected uterine or cervical neoplasia, unresolved/abnormal Pap smear, untreated acute cervicitis or vaginitis, conditions which increase susceptibility to pelvic infections, unremoved IUD, undiagnosed abnormal uterine bleeding, active hepatic disease or hepatic tumors, current or history of known or suspected carcinoma of the breast

Oral: It is not known if the same contraindications associated with long term progestin only contraceptives apply to the use of levonorgestrel and the emergency 2-dose regimen. A history of ectopic pregnancy is not a contraindication to use in emergency contraception.

Warnings/Precautions These products do not protect against HIV infection or other sexually-transmitted diseases. Menstrual bleeding patterns may be altered with use of the intrauterine device; the possibility of pregnancy should be considered if menstruation does not occur within 6 weeks of the previous menstrual period. If bleeding irregularities continue with prolonged use, appropriate diagnostic measures should be taken to rule out endometrial pathology. An increase in menstrual bleeding may indicate a partial or complete expulsion of the IUD. If expulsion occurs, device may be replaced within 7 days once pregnancy is ruled out. When using the oral tablet, spotting may occur following use; the possibility of pregnancy should be considered if menstruation is delayed for >7 days of the expected menstrual period.

Patients taking progestin-only contraceptives and presenting with lower abdominal pain should be evaluated for follicular atresia and ectopic pregnancy. Use caution in patients with previous ectopic pregnancy. Women with history of ectopic pregnancy were excluded from clinical trials; women with previous ectopic pregnancy, tubal surgery, or pelvic infection may be at increased risk ectopic pregnancy. The possibility of ectopic pregnancy should be considered in patients with abdominal pain or vaginal bleeding in women with prior amenorrhea. Patients receiving hepatic enzyme-inducing medications should be evaluated for an alternative method of contraception. May have adverse effects on glucose tolerance; use caution in women with diabetes. Safety and efficacy for use in renal impairment has not been established. Not indicated for use in postmenopausal women.

The use of combination hormonal contraceptives has been associated with a slight increase in the frequency of breast cancer, however, studies are not consistent. Data is insufficient to determine if progestin only contraceptives also increase this risk. Use of the intrauterine device is contraindicated in patients who have or who have had breast cancer. The risk of cardiovascular side effects increases in women using estrogen containing combined hormonal contraceptives and who smoke cigarettes, especially those who are >35 years of age. This risk relative to progestin-only contraceptives has not been established. Women who take contraceptives should be advised not to smoke

Additional formulation-specific warnings:

Intrauterine device: Insertion should be done by a trained healthcare provider. Increased incidence of group A streptococcal sepsis and pelvic inflammatory disease (may be asymptomatic). The highest risk of pelvic inflammatory disease is within 20 days of insertion; risk is increased with multiple sexual partners. May perforate uterus or cervix; risk of perforation is increased in lactating women. Pregnancy may result if perforation occurs; delayed detection of perforation may result in migration of IUD outside of uterine cavity. Partial penetration or embedment in the myometrium may decrease effectiveness and lead to difficult removal. Use caution in patients with coagulopathy or receiving anticoagulants. Use caution in patients with congenital heart disease or other heart conditions which may increase the risk of infective endocarditis during insertion of the device (prophylactic antibiotics may be required at time of insertion). Bradycardia or syncope may occur during insertion or removal of the intrauterine device. The device should be removed for the following reasons: Bleeding which causes anemia; if the patient or her partner become HIV positive or acquire a sexually-transmitted disease; pelvic infection, endometritis, symptomatic genital actinomycosis; intractable pelvic pain, pain during intercourse; endometrial or cervical cancer; uterine or cervical perforation; pregnancy. Embedded devices should also be removed. Use caution with or consider removal of the intrauterine device if any of the following conditions occur for the first time during therapy: Migraine, severe headache, jaundice, marked increase in blood pressure, severe arterial disease (eg, stroke, MI). Use is contraindicated in patients with vaginitis or cervicitis. Postpone insertion until after treatment for infection is complete and cause of the cervicitis is proven not to be due to gonorrhea or chlamydia. Not effective for emergency contraception.

Oral tablet: Not intended to be used for routine contraception and will not terminate an existing pregnancy. Barrier contraception is recommended immediately following emergency contraception and throughout the same menstrual cycle; efficacy of hormonal contraception may be decreased.

Adverse Reactions

Intrauterine device:

>5%:

Central nervous system: Headache/migraine (8%), depression (6%)

Dermatologic: Acne (7%)

Endocrine & metabolic: Amenorrhea (24%; 20% at 1 year), enlarged follicles (12%), menorrhagia (6%), breast pain/tenderness (5%), ovarian cysts

Gastrointestinal: Abdominal pain (12%)

Genitourinary: Uterine/vaginal bleeding alterations (52%), intermenstrual bleeding/spotting (23%), pelvic pain (13%), leukorrhea (5%)

Miscellaneous: Ectopic pregnancy (≤50%), IUD expulsion (5%)

<5% (Limited to important or life-threatening): Abdominal distension, alopecia, anemia, angioedema, back pain, cervicitis, device breakage, dysmenorrhea, dyspareunia, eczema, edema, failed insertion, hirsutism, hypertension, libido decreased, nausea, nervousness, pruritus, rash, sepsis, urticaria, vaginitis, weight gain

Oral tablets:

>10%:

Central nervous system: Fatigue (13% to 17%), headache (10% to 17%), dizziness (10% to 11%)

Endocrine & metabolic: Heavier menstrual bleeding (14% to 31%), lighter menstrual bleeding (12%), breast tenderness (8% to 11%)

Gastrointestinal: Nausea (14% to 23%), abdominal pain (13% to 18%)

1% to 10%:

Endocrine & metabolic: Menses delayed (5%)

Gastrointestinal: Vomiting (6%), diarrhea (5%)

Postmarketing and/or case reports: Dysmenorrhea, menstruation irregularities, oligomenorrhea, pelvic pain

Drug Interactions

Metabolism/Transport Effects Substrate of CYP3A4 (major); **Note:** Assignment of Major/Minor substrate status based on clinically relevant drug interaction potential

Avoid Concomitant Use

Avoid concomitant use of Levonorgestrel with any of the following: Griseofulvin

Increased Effect/Toxicity

Levonorgestrel may increase the levels/effects of: Benzodiazepines (metabolized by oxidation); Selegiline; Tranexamic Acid; Voriconazole

The levels/effects of Levonorgestrel may be increased by: Boceprevir; Conivaptan; Herbs (Progestogenic Properties); Voriconazole

Decreased Effect

Levonorgestrel may decrease the levels/effects of: Vitamin K Antagonists

The levels/effects of Levonorgestrel may be decreased by: Acitretin; Aminoglutethimide; Aprepitant; Artemether; Barbiturates; Bexarotene; Bexarotene (Systemic); Bile Acid Sequestrants; Bosentan; CarBAMazepine; Clobazam; CYP3A4 Inducers (Strong); Deferasirox; Felbamate; Fosaprepitant; Fosphenytoin; Griseofulvin; LamoTRIgine; Mycophenolate; Nevirapine; OXcarbazepine; Phenytoin; Retinoic Acid Derivatives; Rifamycin Derivatives; St Johns Wort; Telaprevir; Tocilizumab; Topiramate

Ethanol/Nutrition/Herb Interactions Herb/Nutraceutical: St John's wort (an enzyme inducer) may decrease serum levels of levonorgestrel.

Stability Store at room temperature of 20°C to 25°C (68°F to 77°F).

Mechanism of Action Pregnancy may be prevented through several mechanisms: Thickening of cervical mucus, which inhibits sperm passage through the uterus and sperm survival; inhibition of ovulation, from a negative feedback mechanism on the hypothalamus, leading to reduced secretion of follicle stimulating hormone (FSH) and luteinizing hormone (LH); and inhibition of implantation. Levonorgestrel is not effective once the implantation process has begun.

Pharmacodynamics/Kinetics

Duration: Intrauterine device: Up to 5 years

Absorption: Oral: Rapid and complete

Distribution: V_d: ~1.8 L/kg

Protein binding: Highly bound to albumin (~50%) and sex hormone-binding globulin (~47%)
Metabolism: To inactive metabolites
Half-life elimination: Oral: ~24 hours
Time to peak: Oral: ~2 hours
Excretion: Urine (45%); feces (32%)

Dosage Adults: Females:

Long-term prevention of pregnancy, treatment of heavy menstrual bleeding: Intrauterine device: To be inserted into uterine cavity; should be inserted within 7 days of onset of menstruation or immediately after 1st trimester abortion; releases 20 mcg levonorgestrel/day over 5 years. May be removed and replaced with a new unit at anytime during menstrual cycle; do not leave any one system in place for >5 years

Emergency contraception: Oral: May be used at any time during menstrual cycle:

Next Choice™: One 0.75 mg tablet as soon as possible within 72 hours of unprotected sexual intercourse; a second 0.75 mg tablet should be taken 12 hours after the first dose

Plan B® One-Step: One 1.5 mg tablet as soon as possible within 72 hours of unprotected sexual intercourse

Elderly: Not indicated for use in postmenopausal women

Dosage adjustment in renal impairment: Safety and efficacy have not been established

Dosage adjustment in hepatic impairment: Safety and efficacy have not been established; use of the intrauterine device is contraindicated with active hepatic disease or hepatic tumor.

Administration

Intrauterine device: Inserted in the uterine cavity, to a depth of 6-10 cm, with the provided insertion device; should not be forced into the uterus

Oral (Plan B® One Step): Consider repeating the dose if vomiting occurs within 2 hours. If severe vomiting occurs, may consider administering the oral tablets vaginally (ACOG, 2010).

Monitoring Parameters

IUD: Re-examine 4-12 weeks following insertion and then yearly. Threads should be visible; if length of thread has changed device may have become displaced, broken, perforated the uterus, or expelled. Transvaginal ultrasound may be used to check placement. Monitor for prolonged menstrual bleeding, amenorrhea, irregularity of menses, Pap smear, blood pressure, serum glucose in patients with diabetes, LDL levels in patients with hyperlipidemias; re-examine following first menses postinsertion of IUD. Patients presenting with lower abdominal pain should be evaluated for follicular atresia and ectopic pregnancy. Signs of infection following IUD insertion, especially in patients at increased risk (eg, patients on chronic corticosteroids, patients with type 1 diabetes mellitus).

Oral tablet: Evaluate for pregnancy, spontaneous abortion or ectopic pregnancy if menses is delayed for ≥1 week following emergency contraception, or if lower abdominal pain or persistent irregular bleeding develops.

Reference Range Intrauterine device: Plasma levels range from 150-200 pg/mL which are lower than those observed with other dosage forms of levonorgestrel

Test Interactions Decreased concentrations of sex hormone-binding globulin; decreased thyroxine concentrations (slight); increased triiodothyronine uptake

Additional Information

Intrauterine device: The cumulative 5-year pregnancy rate is ~0.7 pregnancies/100 users. Over 70% of women in the trials had previously used IUDs. The reported pregnancy rate after 12 months was ≤0.2 pregnancies/100 users. Approximately 80% of women who wish to conceive have become pregnant within 12 months of device removal. The recommended patient profile for this product: A woman who has at least one child, is in a stable and mutually-monogamous relationship, no history of pelvic inflammatory disease, and no history of ectopic pregnancy or predisposition to ectopic pregnancy. Keep a copy of the consent form and record lot number of device.

Oral tablet: Treatment for emergency contraception should begin as soon as possible; however, treatment is still moderately effective if used within 5 days and should be made available to women up to 5 days after unprotected or inadequately protected intercourse. May be used in women with contraindications to conventional oral contraceptive agents (eg, cardiovascular disease, migraines, liver disease). When used as directed for emergency contraception, the expected pregnancy rate is decreased from 8% to 1%. Approximately 87% of women have their next menstrual period at approximately the expected time. A rapid return to fertility following use is expected. When using the two-dose emergency contraceptive regimen, the second dose is equally effective if taken 12-24 hours after the first.

Dosage Forms Excipient information presented when available (limited, particularly for generics); consult specific product labeling.

Intrauterine device, intrauterine:

Mirena®: 52 mg/device [releases levonorgestrel 20 mcg/day]

Tablet, oral: 0.75 mg

Next Choice™: 0.75 mg

Plan B® One Step: 1.5 mg

◆ **Levonorgestrel and Estradiol** *see* Estradiol and Levonorgestrel *on page 635*

◆ **Levonorgestrel and Ethinyl Estradiol** *see* Ethinyl Estradiol and Levonorgestrel *on page 656*

◆ **Levophed®** *see* Norepinephrine *on page 1216*

◆ **Levora®** *see* Ethinyl Estradiol and Levonorgestrel *on page 656*

Levorphanol (lee VOR fa nole)

Index Terms Levo-Dromoran; Levorphan Tartrate; Levorphanol Tartrate

Pharmacologic Category Analgesic, Opioid

Additional Appendix Information

Opioid Analgesics *on page 1896*

Use Relief of moderate-to-severe pain; preoperative sedation/analgesia; management of chronic pain (eg, cancer) requiring opioid therapy

Pregnancy Risk Factor B/D (prolonged use or high doses at term)

Dosage Adults: **Note:** These are guidelines and do not represent the maximum doses that may be required in all patients. Doses should be titrated to pain relief/prevention.

Acute pain (moderate-to-severe): Oral: Initial: Opiate-naive: 2 mg every 6-8 hours as needed; patients with prior opiate exposure may require higher initial doses; usual dosage range: 2-4 mg every 6-8 hours as needed

Note: The American Pain Society recommends an initial dose of 4 mg for severe pain in adults (APS, 6th ed)

Chronic pain: Patients taking opioids chronically may become tolerant and require doses higher than the usual dosage range to maintain the desired effect. Tolerance can be managed by appropriate dose titration. **There is no optimal or maximal dose for levorphanol in chronic pain. The appropriate dose is one that relieves pain throughout its dosing interval without causing unmanageable side effects.**

Dosing adjustment in renal impairment: Use with caution; initial dose should be reduced in severe renal impairment

Dosing adjustment in hepatic impairment: Use with caution; initial dose should be reduced in severe hepatic impairment

Additional Information Complete prescribing information for this medication should be consulted for additional detail.

Dosage Forms Excipient information presented when available (limited, particularly for generics); consult specific product labeling.

Tablet, oral, as tartrate: 2 mg

Controlled Substance C-II

◆ **Levorphanol Tartrate** *see* Levorphanol *on page* 1003

◆ **Levorphan Tartrate** *see* Levorphanol *on page* 1003

◆ **Levothroid®** *see* Levothyroxine *on page* 1004

Levothyroxine (lee voe thye ROKS een)

Brand Names: U.S. Levothroid®; Levoxyl®; Synthroid®; Tirosint®; Unithroid®

Brand Names: Canada Eltroxin®; Euthyrox; Levothyroxine Sodium; Synthroid®

Index Terms *L*-Thyroxine Sodium; Levothyroxine Sodium; T_4

Pharmacologic Category Thyroid Product

Use Replacement or supplemental therapy in hypothyroidism; pituitary TSH suppression

Unlabeled Use Management of hemodynamically unstable potential organ donors increasing the quantity of organs available for transplantation

Pregnancy Risk Factor A

Pregnancy Considerations Adverse events have not been observed following use in pregnant women; therefore, the manufacturer classifies levothyroxine as pregnancy category A.

Endogenous thyroid hormones minimally cross the placenta. Levothyroxine has not been shown to increase the risk of teratogenic or adverse effects following maternal use during pregnancy. Maternal hypothyroidism and subclinical hypothyroidism, however, can be associated with adverse effects in the fetus, including premature birth and respiratory distress. Maternal hypothyroidism has also been associated with adverse pregnancy outcomes, including hypertension, anemia, and placental abruption. Additionally, the presence of maternal thyroid antibodies may increase the risk of premature birth and miscarriage.

Adverse effects can be decreased by maintaining maternal euthyroidism during pregnancy. Physiologic thyroid hormone concentrations should be maintained prior to and during pregnancy with levothyroxine. Levothyroxine is the drug of choice for the treatment of hypothyroidism during pregnancy. Due to alterations of endogenous thyroid hormone, the Endocrine Society recommends a levothyroxine dose increase of 30% to 50% by 4-6 weeks gestation. The levothyroxine dose is usually decreased to prepregnancy doses within 4 weeks after delivery. The Endocrine Society guidelines recommend continued monitoring of T_4 and TSH during pregnancy and for at least 6 months postpartum.

Lactation Enters breast milk/use caution

Contraindications Hypersensitivity to levothyroxine sodium or any component of the formulation; acute MI; thyrotoxicosis of any etiology; uncorrected adrenal insufficiency

Capsule: Additional contraindication: Inability to swallow capsules

Warnings/Precautions [U.S. Boxed Warning]: Thyroid supplements are ineffective and potentially toxic when used for the treatment of obesity or for weight reduction, especially in euthyroid patients. High doses may produce serious or even life-threatening toxic effects particularly when used with some anorectic drugs (eg, sympathomimetic amines). Routine use of T_4 for TSH suppression is not recommended in patients with benign thyroid nodules. In patients deemed appropriate candidates, treatment should never be fully suppressive (TSH <0.1 mIU/L). Use with caution and reduce dosage in patients with angina pectoris or other cardiovascular disease; decrease initial dose. Use cautiously in the elderly since they may be more likely to have compromised cardiovascular functions. Patients with adrenal insufficiency, myxedema, diabetes mellitus and insipidus may have symptoms exaggerated or aggravated. Chronic hypothyroidism predisposes patients to coronary artery disease. Long-term therapy can decrease bone mineral density. Levoxyl® may rapidly swell and disintegrate causing choking or gagging (should be administered with a full glass of water); use caution in patients with dysphagia or other swallowing disorders.

Adverse Reactions Frequency not defined.

Cardiovascular: Angina, arrhythmia, cardiac arrest, flushing, heart failure, hypertension, MI, palpitation, pulse increased, tachycardia

Central nervous system: Anxiety, emotional lability, fatigue, fever, headache, hyperactivity, insomnia, irritability, nervousness, pseudotumor cerebri (children), seizure (rare)

Dermatologic: Alopecia

Endocrine & metabolic: Fertility impaired, menstrual irregularities

Gastrointestinal: Abdominal cramps, appetite increased, diarrhea, vomiting, weight loss

Hepatic: Liver function tests increased

Neuromuscular & skeletal: Bone mineral density decreased, muscle weakness, tremor, slipped capital femoral epiphysis (children)

Respiratory: Dyspnea

Miscellaneous: Diaphoresis, heat intolerance, hypersensitivity (to inactive ingredients, symptoms include urticaria, pruritus, rash, flushing, angioedema, GI symptoms, fever, arthralgia, serum sickness, wheezing)

Levoxyl®: Choking, dysphagia, gagging

Drug Interactions

Metabolism/Transport Effects None known.

Avoid Concomitant Use

Avoid concomitant use of Levothyroxine with any of the following: Sodium Iodide I131

Increased Effect/Toxicity

Levothyroxine may increase the levels/effects of: Vitamin K Antagonists

Decreased Effect

Levothyroxine may decrease the levels/effects of: Sodium Iodide I131; Theophylline Derivatives

The levels/effects of Levothyroxine may be decreased by: Aluminum Hydroxide; Bile Acid Sequestrants; Calcium Polystyrene Sulfonate; Calcium Salts; CarBAMazepine; Estrogen Derivatives; Fosphenytoin; Iron Salts; Lanthanum; Orlistat; Phenytoin; Raloxifene; Rifampin; Sevelamer; Sodium Polystyrene Sulfonate; Sucralfate

Ethanol/Nutrition/Herb Interactions Food: Taking levothyroxine with enteral nutrition may cause reduced bioavailability and may lower serum thyroxine levels leading to signs or symptoms of hypothyroidism. Soybean flour (infant formula), cottonseed meal, walnuts, and dietary fiber may decrease absorption of levothyroxine from the GI tract.

Stability

Capsules, tablets: Store at room temperature; excursions permitted to 15°C to 30°C (59°F to 86°F). Protect from light and moisture.

Injection: Store at room temperature; excursions permitted to 15°C to 30°C (59°F to 86°F). Dilute vials for injection with 5 mL normal saline. Reconstituted concentrations for the 100 mcg, 200 mcg, and 500 mcg vials are 20 mcg/mL, 40 mcg/mL, and 100 mcg/mL, respectively. Shake well and use immediately after reconstitution (manufacturer recommendation); discard any unused portions.

Additional stability data:

Stability in polypropylene syringes (100 mcg/mL in NS) at 5°C ± 1°C is 7 days (Gupta, 2000).

Stability in latex-free, PVC minibags protected from light and stored at 15°C to 30°C (59°F to 86°F) was 12 hours for a 2 mcg/mL concentration or 18 hours for a 0.4 mcg/mL concentration in NS. May be exposed to light; however, stability time is significantly reduced, especially for the 2 mcg/mL concentration (Strong, 2010).

Mechanism of Action Levothyroxine (T_4) is a synthetic form of thyroxine, an endogenous hormone secreted by the thyroid gland. T_4 is converted to its active metabolite, L-triiodothyronine (T_3). Thyroid hormones (T_4 and T_3) then bind to thyroid receptor proteins in the cell nucleus and exert metabolic effects through control of DNA transcription and protein synthesis; involved in normal metabolism, growth, and development; promotes gluconeogenesis, increases utilization and mobilization of glycogen stores, and stimulates protein synthesis, increases basal metabolic rate

Pharmacodynamics/Kinetics

Onset of action: Therapeutic: Oral: 3-5 days; I.V. 6-8 hours

Peak effect: I.V.: 24 hours

Absorption: Oral: Erratic (40% to 80% [per manufacturer]); may be decreased by age and specific foods and drugs

Protein binding: >99% bound to plasma proteins including thyroxine-binding globulin, thyroxine-binding prealbumin, and albumin

Metabolism: Hepatic to triiodothyronine (T_3; active); ~80% thyroxine (T_4) deiodinated in kidney and periphery; glucuronidation/conjugation also occurs; undergoes enterohepatic recirculation

Bioavailability: Oral tablets: 64% (nonfasting state) to 79% to 81% (fasting state)

Time to peak, serum: 2-4 hours

Half-life elimination: Euthyroid: 6-7 days; Hypothyroid: 9-10 days; Hyperthyroid: 3-4 days

Excretion: Urine (major route of elimination; decreases with age); feces (~20%)

Dosage Doses should be adjusted based on clinical response and laboratory parameters.

Oral:

Infants and Children: Hypothyroidism: Daily dosage based on body weight and age as listed below:

1-3 months: 10-15 mcg/kg/day; if the infant is at risk for development of cardiac failure, use a lower starting dose of 25 mcg/day; if the initial serum T_4 is very low (<5 mcg/dL) begin treatment at a higher dosage of 50 mcg/day

3-6 months: 8-10 mcg/kg/day **or** 25-50 mcg/day

6-12 months: 6-8 mcg/kg/day **or** 50-75 mcg/day

1-5 years: 5-6 mcg/kg/day **or** 75-100 mcg/day

6-12 years: 4-5 mcg/kg/day **or** 100-125 mcg/day

>12 years: 2-3 mcg/kg/day **or** ≥150 mcg/day

Growth and puberty complete: 1.7 mcg/kg/day; refer to adult dosing.

Dosing modifications:

Hyperactivity in older children may be minimized by starting at 1/4 of the recommended dose and increasing each week by that amount until the full dose is achieved (4 weeks).

Children with severe or chronic hypothyroidism should be started at 25 mcg/day; adjust dose by 25 mcg every 2-4 weeks.

Adults (including children in whom growth and puberty are complete, healthy adults <50 years of age, and older adults who have been recently treated for hyperthyroidism or who have been hypothyroid for only a few months):

Hypothyroidism: ~1.7 mcg/kg/day; usual doses are ≤200 mcg/day (range: 100-125 mcg/day [70 kg adult]); doses ≥300 mcg/day are rare (consider poor compliance, malabsorption, and/or drug interactions). Titrate dose every 6 weeks.

Patients >50 years or patients with cardiac disease: Refer to elderly dosing.

Severe hypothyroidism: Initial: 12.5-25 mcg/day; adjust dose by 25 mcg/day every 2-4 weeks as appropriate

Myxedema: Oral agents are not recommended for myxedema: Refer to I.V. dosing.

Subclinical hypothyroidism (if treated): 1 mcg/kg/day

TSH suppression:

Well-differentiated thyroid cancer: Highly individualized; Doses >2 mcg/kg/day may be needed to suppress TSH to <0.1 mIU/L in intermediate- to high-risk tumors. Low-risk tumors may be maintained at or slightly below the lower limit of normal (0.1-0.5 mIU/L) (Cooper, 2009).

Benign nodules and nontoxic multinodular goiter: Routine use of T_4 for TSH suppression is not recommended in patients with benign thyroid nodules. In patients deemed appropriate candidates, treatment should never be fully suppressive (TSH <0.1 mIU/L) (Cooper, 2009; Gharib, 2010). Avoid use if TSH is already suppressed.

Elderly: Hypothyroidism (elderly patients may require <1 mcg/kg/day):

>50 years without cardiac disease **or** <50 years with cardiac disease: Initial: 25-50 mcg/day; adjust dose by 12.5-25 mcg increments at 6- to 8-week intervals as needed

>50 years with cardiac disease: Initial: 12.5-25 mcg/day; adjust dose by 12.5-25 mcg increments at 4- to 6-week intervals (many clinicians prefer to adjust at 6- to 8-week intervals)

Note: Patients with combined hypothyroidism and cardiac disease should be monitored carefully for changes in stability.

I.M., I.V.: Children, Adults, Elderly: Hypothyroidism: 50% of the oral dose; alternatively, some clinicians administer up to 80% of the oral dose. **Note:** Bioavailability of the oral formulation is highly variable, but absorption has been measured to be ~80%, when the oral tablet formulation was administered in the recommended fasting state (Fish, 1987; Dickerson 2010).

I.V.:

Adults: Myxedema coma or stupor: 200-500 mcg, then 100-300 mcg the next day if necessary; smaller doses should be considered in patients with cardiovascular disease

Elderly: Myxedema coma: Refer to adult dosing; lower doses may be needed

Dietary Considerations Should be taken on an empty stomach, at least 30 minutes before food.

Administration

Oral: Administer in the morning on an empty stomach, at least 30 minutes before food.

Capsule: Must be swallowed whole; do not cut, crush, or attempt to dissolve capsules in water to prepare a suspension

Tablet: May be crushed and suspended in 5-10 mL of water; suspension should be used immediately. Levoxyl® should be administered with a full glass of water to prevent gagging (due to tablet swelling).

Nasogastric tube: Bioavailability of levothyroxine is reduced if administered with enteral tube feeds. Since holding feedings for at least 1 hour before and after levothyroxine administration may not completely resolve the interaction, an increase in dose (eg, additional 25 mcg) may be necessary (Dickerson, 2010).

Parenteral: Dilute vial with 5 mL normal saline; use immediately after reconstitution; should not be admixed with other solutions

Monitoring Parameters Thyroid function test (serum thyroxine, thyrotropin concentrations), resin triiodothyronine uptake (rT_3U), free thyroxine index (FTI), T_4, TSH, heart rate, blood pressure, clinical signs of hypo- and hyperthyroidism; TSH is the most reliable guide for evaluating adequacy of thyroid replacement dosage. TSH may be elevated during the first few months of thyroid replacement despite patients being clinically euthyroid. In cases where T_4 remains low and TSH is within normal limits, an evaluation of "free" (unbound) T_4 is needed to evaluate further increase in dosage

Infants: Monitor closely for cardiac overload, arrhythmias, and aspiration from avid suckling

Infants/children: Monitor closely for under/overtreatment. Undertreatment may decrease intellectual development and linear growth, and lead to poor school performance due to impaired concentration and slowed mentation. Overtreatment may adversely affect brain maturation, accelerate bone age (leading to premature closure of the epiphyses and reduced adult height); craniosynostosis has been reported in infants. Treated children may experience a period of catch-up growth. Monitor TSH and total or free T_4 at 2 and 4 weeks after starting treatment; every 1-2 months for first year of life; every 2-3 months during years 1-3; every 3-12 months until growth completed. Perform routine clinical examinations at regular intervals (to assess mental and physical growth and development).

Adults: Monitor TSH every 6-8 weeks until normalized; 8-12 weeks after dosage changes; every 6-12 months throughout therapy

Reference Range Pediatrics: Cord T_4 and values in the first few weeks are much higher, falling over the first months and years. ≥10 years: ~5.8-11 mcg/dL (SI: 75-142 nmol/L). Borderline low: ≤4.5-5.7 mcg/dL (SI: 58-73 nmol/L); low: ≤4.4 mcg/dL (SI: 57 nmol/L); results <2.5 mcg/dL (SI: <32 nmol/L) are strong evidence for hypothyroidism.

Approximate adult normal range: 4-12 mcg/dL (SI: 51-154 nmol/L). Borderline high: 11.1-13 mcg/dL (SI: 143-167 nmol/L); high: ≥13.1 mcg/dL (SI: 169 nmol/L). Normal range is increased in women on birth control pills (5.5-12 mcg/dL); normal range in pregnancy: ~5.5-16 mcg/dL (SI: ~71-206 nmol/L). TSH: 0.4-10 (for those ≥80 years) mIU/L; T_4: 4-12 mcg/dL (SI: 51-154 nmol/L); T_3 (RIA) (total T_3): 80-230 ng/dL (SI: 1.2-3.5 nmol/L); T_4 free (free T_4): 0.7-1.8 ng/dL (SI: 9-23 pmol/L).

Test Interactions Many drugs may have effects on thyroid function tests (see Additional Information). Pregnancy, infectious hepatitis, and acute intermittent porphyria may increase TBG concentrations; nephrosis, severe hypoproteinemia, severe liver disease, and acromegaly may decrease TBG concentrations.

Additional Information Equivalent doses: The following statement on relative potency of thyroid products is included in a joint statement by American Thyroid Association (ATA), American Association of Clinical Endocrinologists (AACE) and The Endocrine Society (TES): For purposes of conversion, levothyroxine sodium (T_4) 100 mcg is usually considered equivalent to desiccated thyroid 60 mg, thyroglobulin 60 mg, or liothyronine sodium (T_3) 25 mcg. However, these are rough guidelines only and do not obviate the careful re-evaluation of a patient when switching thyroid hormone preparations, including a change from one brand of levothyroxine to another. Joint position statement is available at http://www.thyroid.org/professionals/advocacy/04_12_08_thyroxine.html.

Note: Several medications have effects on thyroid production or conversion. The impact in thyroid replacement has not been specifically evaluated, but patient response should be monitored:

Methimazole: Decreases thyroid hormone secretion, while propylthiouracil decrease thyroid hormone secretion and decreases conversion of T_4 to T_3.

Beta-adrenergic antagonists: Decrease conversion of T_4 to T_3 (dose related, propranolol ≥160 mg/day); patients may be clinically euthyroid.

Iodide, iodine-containing radiographic contrast agents may decrease thyroid hormone secretion; may also increase thyroid hormone secretion, especially in patients with Graves' disease.

Other agents reported to impact on thyroid production/conversion include aminoglutethimide, amiodarone, chloral hydrate, diazepam, ethionamide, interferon-alpha, interleukin-2, lithium, lovastatin (case report), glucocorticoids (dose-related), mercaptopurine, sulfonamides, thiazide diuretics, and tolbutamide.

In addition, a number of medications have been noted to cause transient depression in TSH secretion, which may complicate interpretation of monitoring tests for levothyroxine, including corticosteroids, octreotide, and dopamine. Metoclopramide may increase TSH secretion

Dosage Forms Excipient information presented when available (limited, particularly for generics); consult specific product labeling. [DSC] = Discontinued product

Capsule, soft gelatin, oral, as sodium:
- Tirosint®: 13 mcg, 25 mcg, 50 mcg, 75 mcg, 88 mcg, 100 mcg, 112 mcg, 125 mcg, 137 mcg, 150 mcg

Injection, powder for reconstitution, as sodium: 100 mcg, 200 mcg [DSC], 500 mcg

Tablet, oral, as sodium: 25 mcg, 50 mcg, 75 mcg, 88 mcg, 100 mcg, 112 mcg, 125 mcg, 137 mcg, 150 mcg, 175 mcg, 200 mcg, 300 mcg
- Levothroid®: 25 mcg, 75 mcg, 88 mcg, 100 mcg, 112 mcg, 125 mcg, 137 mcg, 150 mcg, 175 mcg, 200 mcg, 300 mcg [scored]
- Levothroid®: 50 mcg [scored; dye free]
- Levoxyl®: 25 mcg, 75 mcg, 88 mcg, 100 mcg, 112 mcg, 125 mcg, 137 mcg, 150 mcg, 175 mcg, 200 mcg [scored]
- Levoxyl®: 50 mcg [scored; dye free]
- Synthroid®: 25 mcg, 75 mcg, 88 mcg, 100 mcg, 112 mcg, 125 mcg, 137 mcg, 150 mcg, 175 mcg, 200 mcg, 300 mcg [scored]
- Synthroid®: 50 mcg [scored; dye free]
- Unithroid®: 25 mcg, 75 mcg, 88 mcg, 100 mcg, 112 mcg, 125 mcg, 150 mcg, 175 mcg, 200 mcg, 300 mcg [scored]
- Unithroid®: 50 mcg [scored; dye free]

Extemporaneous Preparations A 25 mcg/mL oral suspension may be made with tablets and 40 mL glycerol. Crush twenty-five 0.1 mg levothyroxine tablets in a mortar and reduce to a fine powder. Add small portions of glycerol and mix to a uniform suspension. Transfer to a calibrated 100 mL amber bottle; rinse the mortar with about 10 mL of glycerol and pour into the bottle; repeat until all 40 mL of glycerol is used. Add quantity of water sufficient to make 100 mL. Label "shake well" and "refrigerate". Stable for 8 days refrigerated.

Boulton DW, Fawcett JP, and Woods DJ, "Stability of an Extemporaneously Compounded Levothyroxine Sodium Oral Liquid," *Am J Health Syst Pharm*, 1996, 53(10):1157-61.

◆ **Levothyroxine and Liothyronine** *see* Liotrix *on page 1017*

- ◆ **Levothyroxine and Liothyronine** *see* Thyroid, Desiccated *on page 1676*
- ◆ **Levothyroxine Sodium** *see* Levothyroxine *on page 1004*
- ◆ **Levoxyl®** *see* Levothyroxine *on page 1004*
- ◆ **Levsin®** *see* Hyoscyamine *on page 854*
- ◆ **Levsin®/SL** *see* Hyoscyamine *on page 854*
- ◆ **Lev-Tov [OTC]** *see* Folic Acid, Cyanocobalamin, and Pyridoxine *on page 749*
- ◆ **Levulan® Kerastick®** *see* Aminolevulinic Acid *on page 90*
- ◆ **Lexapro®** *see* Escitalopram *on page 620*
- ◆ **Lexiva®** *see* Fosamprenavir *on page 756*
- ◆ **LFA-3/IgG(1) Fusion Protein, Human** *see* Alefacept *on page 57*
- ◆ **L-Glutamine** *see* Glutamine *on page 799*
- ◆ **LH-RH Agonist** *see* Histrelin *on page 830*
- ◆ ***l*-Hyoscyamine Sulfate** *see* Hyoscyamine *on page 854*
- ◆ **Lialda®** *see* Mesalamine *on page 1081*
- ◆ **Librax®** *see* Clidinium and Chlordiazepoxide *on page 378*
- ◆ **Librium** *see* ChlordiazePOXIDE *on page 340*
- ◆ **Licide® [OTC]** *see* Pyrethrins and Piperonyl Butoxide *on page 1435*
- ◆ **LidaMantle®** *see* Lidocaine (Topical) *on page 1009*
- ◆ **Lidemol® (Can)** *see* Fluocinonide *on page 727*
- ◆ **Lidex** *see* Fluocinonide *on page 727*
- ◆ **Lidex® (Can)** *see* Fluocinonide *on page 727*

Lidocaine (Systemic) (LYE doe kane)

Brand Names: U.S. Xylocaine®; Xylocaine® Dental; Xylocaine® MPF

Brand Names: Canada Xylocard®

Index Terms Lidocaine Hydrochloride; Lignocaine Hydrochloride

Pharmacologic Category Antiarrhythmic Agent, Class Ib; Local Anesthetic

Use Local and regional anesthesia by infiltration, nerve block, epidural, or spinal techniques; acute treatment of ventricular arrhythmias from myocardial infarction or cardiac manipulation

Unlabeled Use

ACLS guidelines: Hemodynamically stable monomorphic ventricular tachycardia (VT) (preserved ventricular function); polymorphic VT (preserved ventricular function); drug-induced monomorphic VT; when amiodarone is not available, pulseless VT or ventricular fibrillation (VF) (unresponsive to defibrillation, CPR, and vasopressor administration)

PALS guidelines: When amiodarone is not available, pulseless VT or VF (unresponsive to defibrillation, CPR, and epinephrine administration); consider in patients with cocaine overdose to prevent arrhythmias secondary to MI

I.V. infusion for chronic pain syndrome

Pregnancy Risk Factor B

Pregnancy Considerations Animal studies with lidocaine have not shown teratogenic effects. Lidocaine and the MEGX metabolite cross the placenta. Use is not contraindicated during labor and delivery. Topical lidocaine is used locally to provide analgesia prior to episiotomy and during repair of obstetric lacerations. Administration by the perineal route may result in greater absorption than administration by the epidural route. Adverse events have been reported in the infant following maternal administration, however, when used in appropriate doses, the risk to the fetus is low. Cumulative exposure from all routes of administration should be considered.

Lactation Enters breast milk/use caution (AAP rates "compatible"; AAP 2001 update pending)

Contraindications Hypersensitivity to lidocaine or any component of the formulation; hypersensitivity to another local anesthetic of the amide type; Adam-Stokes syndrome; severe degrees of SA, AV, or intraventricular heart block (except in patients with a functioning artificial pacemaker); premixed injection may contain corn-derived dextrose and its use is contraindicated in patients with allergy to corn-related products

Warnings/Precautions Use caution in patients with severe hepatic dysfunction or pseudocholinesterase deficiency; may have increased risk of lidocaine toxicity.

Intravenous: Constant ECG monitoring is necessary during I.V. administration. Use cautiously in hepatic impairment, any degree of heart block, Wolff-Parkinson-White syndrome, HF, marked hypoxia, severe respiratory depression, hypovolemia, history of malignant hyperthermia, or shock. Increased ventricular rate may be seen when administered to a patient with atrial fibrillation. Correct electrolyte disturbances, especially hypokalemia or hypomagnesemia, prior to use and throughout therapy. Correct any underlying causes of ventricular arrhythmias. Monitor closely for signs and symptoms of CNS toxicity. The elderly may be prone to increased CNS and cardiovascular side effects. Reduce dose in hepatic dysfunction and CHF.

Injectable anesthetic: Follow appropriate administration techniques so as not to administer any intravascularly. Continuous intra-articular infusion of local anesthetics after arthroscopic or other surgical procedures is **not** an approved use; chondrolysis (primarily in the shoulder joint) has occurred following infusion, with some cases requiring arthroplasty or shoulder replacement. Solutions containing antimicrobial preservatives should not be used for epidural or spinal anesthesia. Some solutions contain a bisulfite; avoid in patients who are allergic to bisulfite. Resuscitative equipment, medicine and oxygen should be available in case of emergency. Use products containing epinephrine cautiously in patients with significant vascular disease, compromised blood flow, or during or following general anesthesia (increased risk of arrhythmias). Adjust the dose for the elderly, pediatric, acutely ill, and debilitated patients.

Adverse Reactions Effects vary with route of administration. Many effects are dose related.

Frequency not defined.

Cardiovascular: Arrhythmia, bradycardia, arterial spasms, cardiovascular collapse, defibrillator threshold increased, edema, flushing, heart block, hypotension, sinus node supression, vascular insufficiency (periarticular injections)

Central nervous system: Agitation, anxiety, apprehension, coma, confusion, disorientation, dizziness, drowsiness, euphoria, hallucinations, headache, hyperesthesia, hypoesthesia, lethargy, lightheadedness, nervousness, psychosis, seizure, slurred speech, somnolence, unconsciousness

Gastrointestinal: Metallic taste, nausea, vomiting

Local: Thrombophlebitis

Neuromuscular & skeletal: Paresthesia, transient radicular pain (subarachnoid administration; up to 1.9%), tremor, twitching, weakness

Otic: Tinnitus

Respiratory: Bronchospasm, dyspnea, respiratory depression or arrest

Miscellaneous: Allergic reactions, anaphylactoid reaction, sensitivity to temperature extremes

Following spinal anesthesia: Positional headache (3%), shivering (2%) nausea, peripheral nerve symptoms, respiratory inadequacy and double vision (<1%), hypotension, cauda equina syndrome

Postmarketing and/or case reports: Asystole, disorientation, methemoglobinemia, skin reaction

Drug Interactions

Metabolism/Transport Effects Substrate of CYP1A2 (minor), CYP2A6 (minor), CYP2B6 (minor), CYP2C9 (minor), CYP2D6 (major), CYP3A4 (major), P-glycoprotein; **Note:** Assignment of Major/Minor substrate status based on clinically relevant drug interaction potential; **Inhibits** CYP1A2 (strong), CYP2D6 (moderate), CYP3A4 (moderate)

Avoid Concomitant Use

Avoid concomitant use of Lidocaine (Systemic) with any of the following: Conivaptan; Pimozide; Saquinavir; Thioridazine; Tolvaptan

Increased Effect/Toxicity

Lidocaine (Systemic) may increase the levels/effects of: ARIPiprazole; Bendamustine; Budesonide (Systemic, Oral Inhalation); Colchicine; CYP1A2 Substrates; CYP2D6 Substrates; CYP3A4 Substrates; Eplerenone; Everolimus; Fesoterodine; Halofantrine; Lurasidone; Pimecrolimus; Pimozide; Prilocaine; Propafenone; Salmeterol; Saxagliptin; Thioridazine; Tolvaptan; Vilazodone; Zuclopenthixol

The levels/effects of Lidocaine (Systemic) may be increased by: Amiodarone; Beta-Blockers; Conivaptan; CYP2D6 Inhibitors (Moderate); CYP2D6 Inhibitors (Strong); CYP3A4 Inhibitors (Moderate); CYP3A4 Inhibitors (Strong); Darunavir; Dasatinib; Disopyramide; P-glycoprotein/ABCB1 Inhibitors; Propafenone; Saquinavir; Telaprevir

Decreased Effect

The levels/effects of Lidocaine (Systemic) may be decreased by: CYP3A4 Inducers (Strong); Cyproterone; Deferasirox; Etravirine; Peginterferon Alfa-2b; P-glycoprotein/ABCB1 Inducers; Tocilizumab

Ethanol/Nutrition/Herb Interactions Herb/Nutraceutical: St John's wort may decrease lidocaine levels; avoid concurrent use.

Stability Injection: Stable at room temperature. Stability of parenteral admixture at room temperature (25°C) is the expiration date on premixed bag; out of overwrap stability is 30 days.

Standard concentration/diluent: 2 g/250 mL D_5W.

Mechanism of Action Class Ib antiarrhythmic; suppresses automaticity of conduction tissue, by increasing electrical stimulation threshold of ventricle, His-Purkinje system, and spontaneous depolarization of the ventricles during diastole by a direct action on the tissues; blocks both the initiation and conduction of nerve impulses by decreasing the neuronal membrane's permeability to sodium ions, which results in inhibition of depolarization with resultant blockade of conduction

Pharmacodynamics/Kinetics

Onset of action: Single bolus dose: 45-90 seconds

Duration: 10-20 minutes

Distribution: V_d: 1.1-2.1 L/kg; alterable by many patient factors; decreased in CHF and liver disease; crosses blood-brain barrier

Protein binding: 60% to 80% to $alpha_1$ acid glycoprotein

Metabolism: 90% hepatic; active metabolites monoethylglycinexylidide (MEGX) and glycinexylidide (GX) can accumulate and may cause CNS toxicity

Half-life elimination: Biphasic: Prolonged with congestive heart failure, liver disease, shock, severe renal disease; Initial: 7-30 minutes; Terminal: Infants, premature: 3.2 hours, Adults: 1.5-2 hours

Excretion: Urine (<10% as unchanged drug, ~90% as metabolites)

Dosage

Antiarrhythmic:

Children:

I.V., intraosseous (I.O.): **Note:** For use in VF or pulseless VT if amiodarone is not available; give after defibrillation attempts, CPR, and epinephrine:

Loading dose: 1 mg/kg (maximum: 100 mg); follow with continuous infusion; may administer second bolus of 0.5-1 mg/kg if delay between bolus and start of infusion is >15 minutes (PALS, 2000; PALS, 2010)

Continuous infusion: 20-50 mcg/kg/minute (PALS, 2010). Per the manufacturer, do not exceed 20 mcg/kg/minute in patients with shock, hepatic disease, cardiac arrest, or CHF.

Intratracheal: 2-3 mg/kg; flush with 5 mL of NS and follow with 5 assisted manual ventilations (PALS, 2010)

Adults (ACLS, 2010):

VF or pulseless VT (after defibrillation attempts, CPR, and vasopressor administration) if amiodarone is not available: I.V., intraosseous (I.O.): Initial: 1-1.5 mg/kg. If refractory VF or pulseless VT, repeat with 0.5-0.75 mg/kg bolus every 5-10 minutes (maximum cumulative dose: 3 mg/kg). Follow with continuous infusion (1-4 mg/minute) after return of perfusion. Reappearance of arrhythmia during constant infusion: 0.5 mg/kg bolus and reassessment of infusion (Zipes, 2000).

Intratracheal (loading dose only): 2-3.75 mg/kg (2-2.5 times the recommended I.V. dose); dilute in 5-10 mL NS or sterile water. **Note:** Absorption is greater with sterile water and results in less impairment of PaO_2.

Hemodynamically stable monomorphic VT: I.V.: 1-1.5 mg/kg; repeat with 0.5-0.75 mg/kg every 5-10 minutes as necessary (maximum cumulative dose: 3 mg/kg). Follow with continuous infusion of 1-4 mg/minute (or 14-57 mcg/kg/minute).

Note: Reduce maintenance infusion in patients with CHF, shock, or hepatic disease; initiate infusion at 10 mcg/kg/minute (maximum dose: 1.5 mg/minute or 20 mcg/kg/minute).

Anesthetic, local injectable: Children and Adults: Varies with procedure, degree of anesthesia needed, vascularity of tissue, duration of anesthesia required, and physical condition of patient; maximum: 4.5 mg/kg/dose not to exceed 300 mg; do not repeat within 2 hours.

Dosage adjustment in renal impairment: Not dialyzable (0% to 5%) by hemo- or peritoneal dialysis; supplemental dose is not necessary.

Dosage adjustment in hepatic impairment: Reduce maintenance infusion. Initial: 0.75 mg/minute or 10 mcg/kg/minute; maximum dose: 1.5 mg/minute or 20 mcg/kg/minute. Monitor lidocaine concentrations closely and adjust infusion rate as necessary; consider alternative therapy.

Dietary Considerations Premixed injection may contain corn-derived dextrose and its use is contraindicated in patients with allergy to corn-related products.

Administration

Local infiltration: Buffered lidocaine for injectable local anesthetic may be prepared: Add 2 mL of sodium bicarbonate 8.4% to 18 mL of lidocaine 1% (Christoph, 1988)

Intratracheal (unlabeled administration route): Dilute in NS or sterile water. Absorption is greater with sterile water and results in less impairment of PaO_2 (Hahnel, 1990). Stop compressions, spray drug quickly down tube. Flush with 5 mL of NS and follow immediately with several quick insufflations and continue chest compressions.

Continuous I.V. infusion: **Infusion rates:** 2 g/250 mL D_5W:

1 mg/minute: 7.5 mL/hour

2 mg/minute: 15 mL/hour

3 mg/minute: 22.5 mL/hour

4 mg/minute: 30 mL/hour

Intraosseous (I.O.; unlabeled administration route): Intraosseous administration is a safe and effective alternative to venous access in children with cardiac arrest; the onset for most medications is similar to that of I.V. administration (PALS, 2010). In adults, I.O. administration is a reasonable alternative when quick I.V. access is not feasible (ACLS, 2010).

Reference Range

Therapeutic: 1.5-5.0 mcg/mL (SI: 6-21 micromole/L)

Potentially toxic: >6 mcg/mL (SI: >26 micromole/L)

Toxic: >9 mcg/mL (SI: >38 micromole/L)

Dosage Forms Excipient information presented when available (limited, particularly for generics); consult specific product labeling. [DSC] = Discontinued product

Infusion, premixed in D_5W, as hydrochloride: 0.4% [4 mg/mL] (250 mL, 500 mL); 0.8% [8 mg/mL] (250 mL, 500 mL [DSC])

Injection, solution, as hydrochloride: 0.5% [5 mg/mL] (50 mL [DSC]); 1% [10 mg/mL] (2 mL, 10 mL, 20 mL, 30 mL, 50 mL); 2% [20 mg/mL] (2 mL, 5 mL, 20 mL, 50 mL)

Xylocaine®: 0.5% [5 mg/mL] (50 mL); 1% [10 mg/mL] (10 mL, 20 mL, 50 mL); 2% [20 mg/mL] (10 mL, 20 mL, 50 mL) [contains methylparaben]

Injection, solution, as hydrochloride [preservative free]: 0.5% [5 mg/mL] (50 mL); 1% [10 mg/mL] (2 mL, 5 mL, 30 mL); 1.5% [15 mg/mL] (20 mL); 2% [20 mg/mL] (2 mL, 5 mL, 10 mL); 4% [40 mg/mL] (5 mL)

Xylocaine®: 2% [20 mg/mL] (5 mL)

Xylocaine® MPF: 0.5% [5 mg/mL] (50 mL); 1% [10 mg/mL] (2 mL, 5 mL, 10 mL, 30 mL); 1.5% [15 mg/mL] (10 mL, 20 mL); 2% [20 mg/mL] (2 mL, 5 mL, 10 mL); 4% [40 mg/mL] (5 mL)

Injection, solution, as hydrochloride [for dental use]:

Xylocaine® Dental: 2% [20 mg/mL] (1.8 mL)

Injection, solution, premixed in $D_{7.5}W$, as hydrochloride [preservative free]: 5% [50 mg/mL] (2 mL)

Lidocaine (Topical) (LYE doe kane)

Brand Names: U.S. AneCream™ [OTC]; Anestafoam™ [OTC]; Band-Aid® Hurt Free™ Antiseptic Wash [OTC]; Burn Jel Plus [OTC]; Burn Jel® [OTC]; L-M-X® 4 [OTC]; L-M-X® 5 [OTC]; LidaMantle®; Lidoderm®; LTA® 360; Premjact®; Regenecare®; Regenecare® HA [OTC]; Solarcaine® cool aloe Burn Relief [OTC]; Topicaine® [OTC]; Unburn® [OTC]; Xylocaine®

Brand Names: Canada Betacaine®; Lidodan™; Lidoderm®; Maxilene®; Xylocaine®

Index Terms Lidocaine Hydrochloride; Lidocaine Patch; Lignocaine Hydrochloride; Viscous Lidocaine; Xylocaine Viscous

Pharmacologic Category Analgesic, Topical; Local Anesthetic

Use

Rectal: Temporary relief of pain and itching due to anorectal disorders

Topical: Local anesthetic for oral mucous membrane; use in laser/cosmetic surgeries; minor burns, cuts, and abrasions of the skin

Oral topical solution (viscous): Topical anesthesia of irritated oral mucous membranes and pharyngeal tissue

Patch (Lidoderm®): Relief of allodynia (painful hypersensitivity) and chronic pain in postherpetic neuralgia

Pregnancy Risk Factor B

Dosage Anesthesia, topical:

Cream:

LidaMantle®: Skin irritation: Children and Adults: Apply a thin film to affected area 2-3 times/day as needed

L-M-X® 4: Skin irritation: Children ≥2 years and Adults: Apply up to 3-4 times daily to intact skin

L-M-X® 5: Relief of anorectal pain and itching: Children ≥12 years and Adults: Apply to affected area up to 6 times/day

Gel, ointment: Adults: Apply to affected area ≤4 times/day as needed (maximum dose: 4.5 mg/kg, not to exceed 300 mg)

Topical solution: Adults: Apply 1-5 mL (40-200 mg) to affected area

Jelly:

Children: Dose varies with age and weight (maximum dose: 4.5 mg/kg)

Adults (maximum dose: 30 mL [600 mg] in any 12-hour period):

Anesthesia of male urethra: 5-30 mL (100-600 mg)

Anesthesia of female urethra: 3-5 mL (60-100 mg)

Oral topical solution (viscous):

Infants and Children <3 years: 1.25 mL applied to area with a cotton-tipped applicator no more frequently than every 3 hours (maximum: 4 doses per 12-hour period)

Children ≥3 years: Should not exceed 4.5 mg/kg/dose (or 300 mg/dose); swished in the mouth and spit out no more frequently than every 3 hours (maximum: 4 doses per 12-hour period)

Adults:

Anesthesia of the mouth: 15 mL swished in the mouth and spit out no more frequently than every 3 hours (maximum: 8 doses per 24-hour period)

Anesthesia of the pharynx: 15 mL gargled no more frequently than every 3 hours (maximum: 8 doses per 24-hour period); may be swallowed

Patch: Postherpetic neuralgia: Adults: Apply patch to most painful area. Up to 3 patches may be applied in a single application. Patch(es) may remain in place for up to 12 hours in any 24-hour period.

Additional Information Complete prescribing information for this medication should be consulted for additional detail.

Dosage Forms Excipient information presented when available (limited, particularly for generics); consult specific product labeling. [DSC] = Discontinued product

Aerosol, foam, topical:

Anestafoam™: 4% (30 g) [contains benzalkonium chloride, benzyl alcohol]

Aerosol, spray, topical:

Solarcaine® cool aloe Burn Relief: 0.5% (127 g) [contains aloe, vitamin E]

Cream, rectal:

L-M-X® 5: 5% (15 g, 30 g) [contains benzyl alcohol]

Cream, topical:

AneCream™: 4% (5 g, 15 g, 30 g) [contains benzyl alcohol, soybean lecithin]

L-M-X® 4: 4% (5 g, 15 g, 30 g) [contains benzyl alcohol]

Cream, topical, as hydrochloride: 0.5% (0.9 g)

LidaMantle®: 3% (85 g)

Gel, topical:

Topicaine®: 4% (10 g, 30 g, 113 g); 5% (10 g, 30 g, 113 g) [contains aloe, benzyl alcohol, ethanol 35%, jojoba]

Gel, topical, as hydrochloride:

Burn Jel Plus: 2.5% (118 mL) [contains vitamin E]

Burn Jel®: 2% (59 mL, 118 mL); 2% (3.5 g)

Regenecare®: 2% (14 g, 85 g) [contains aloe; contains calcium alginate]

Regenecare® HA: 2% (85 g) [contains aloe; contains hyaluronic acid]

Solarcaine® cool aloe Burn Relief: 0.5% (113 g, 226 g) [contains aloe, isopropyl alcohol, menthol, tartrazine]

Unburn®: 2.5% (59 mL) [contains vitamin E]

Jelly, topical, as hydrochloride: 2% (5 mL, 30 mL)

Xylocaine®: 2% (5 mL, 30 mL)

Jelly, topical, as hydrochloride [preservative free]: 2% (5 mL, 10 mL, 20 mL)

Lotion, topical, as hydrochloride:
LidaMantle®: 3% (177 mL)
Ointment, topical: 5% (35.4 g, 50 g)
Patch, topical:
Lidoderm®: 5% (30s)
Solution, topical [spray]:
Premjact®: 9.6% (13 mL)
Solution, topical, as hydrochloride: 4% [40 mg/mL] (50 mL)
Band-Aid® Hurt Free™ Antiseptic Wash: 2% [20 mg/mL] (177 mL) [contains aloe, benzalkonium chloride]
LTA® 360: 4% [40 mg/mL] (4 mL)
Xylocaine®: 4% (50 mL); 4% [40 mg/mL] (50 mL [DSC])
Solution, topical, as hydrochloride [preservative free]: 4% [40 mg/mL] (4 mL)
Solution, viscous, oral topical, as hydrochloride: 2% [20 mg/mL] (20 mL, 100 mL)

Lidocaine and Epinephrine

(LYE doe kane & ep i NEF rin)

Brand Names: U.S. Lignospan® Forte; Lignospan® Standard; Xylocaine® MPF With Epinephrine; Xylocaine® With Epinephrine

Brand Names: Canada Xylocaine® With Epinephrine

Index Terms Epinephrine and Lidocaine

Pharmacologic Category Local Anesthetic

Use Local infiltration anesthesia; AVS for nerve block

Pregnancy Risk Factor B

Dosage Dosage varies with the anesthetic procedure, degree of anesthesia needed, vascularity of tissue, duration of anesthesia required, and physical condition of patient.

Dental anesthesia, infiltration, or conduction block:
Children <12 years: 20-30 mg (1-1.5 mL) of lidocaine hydrochloride as a 2% solution with epinephrine 1:100,000; maximum: 4.5 mg of lidocaine hydrochloride/kg of body weight or 100-150 mg as a single dose
Children ≥12 years and Adults: Do not exceed 7 mg/kg body weight up to a maximum range of 300 mg (usual dental practice) to 500 mg (approved product labeling) of lidocaine hydrochloride and 3 mcg (0.003 mg) of epinephrine/kg of body weight or 0.2 mg epinephrine per dental appointment. The effective anesthetic dose varies with procedure, intensity of anesthesia needed, duration of anesthesia required, and physical condition of the patient. Always use the lowest effective dose along with careful aspiration.
Note: For most routine dental procedures, lidocaine hydrochloride 2% with epinephrine 1:100,000 is preferred. When a more pronounced hemostasis is required, a 1:50,000 epinephrine concentration should be used.

Additional Information Complete prescribing information for this medication should be consulted for additional detail.

Dosage Forms Excipient information presented when available (limited, particularly for generics); consult specific product labeling. [DSC] = Discontinued product

Injection, solution:
0.5% / 1:200,000: Lidocaine hydrochloride 0.5% [5 mg/mL] and epinephrine 1:200,000 (50 mL)
1% / 1:100,000: Lidocaine hydrochloride 1% [10 mg/mL] and epinephrine 1:100,000 (20 mL, 30 mL, 50 mL)
2% / 1:100,000: Lidocaine hydrochloride 2% [20 mg/mL] and epinephrine 1:100,000 (30 mL, 50 mL)
Xylocaine® with Epinephrine:
0.5% / 1:200,000: Lidocaine hydrochloride 0.5% [5 mg/mL] and epinephrine 1:200,000 (50 mL) [contains methylparaben]
1% / 1:100,000: Lidocaine hydrochloride 1% [10 mg/mL] and epinephrine 1:100,000 (10 mL, 20 mL, 50 mL) [contains methylparaben]
2% / 1:100,000: Lidocaine hydrochloride 2% [20 mg/mL] and epinephrine 1:100,000 (10 mL, 20 mL, 50 mL) [contains methylparaben]

Injection, solution [preservative free]:
1.5% / 1:200,000: Lidocaine hydrochloride 1.5% [15 mg/mL] and epinephrine 1:200,000 (5 mL, 30 mL)
2% / 1:200,000: Lidocaine hydrochloride 2% [20 mg/mL] and epinephrine 1:200,000 (20 mL)
Xylocaine®-MPF with Epinephrine:
1% / 1:200,000: Lidocaine hydrochloride 1% [10 mg/mL] and epinephrine 1:200,000 (5 mL, 10 mL, 30 mL) [contains sodium metabisulfite]
1.5% / 1:200,000: Lidocaine hydrochloride 1.5% [15 mg/mL] and epinephrine 1:200,000 (5 mL, 10 mL, 30 mL) [contains sodium metabisulfite]
2% / 1:200,000: Lidocaine hydrochloride 2% [20 mg/mL] and epinephrine 1:200,000 (5 mL, 10 mL, 20 mL) [contains sodium metabisulfite]

Injection, solution [for dental use]:
2% / 1:50,000: Lidocaine hydrochloride 2% [20 mg/mL] and epinephrine 1:50,000 (1.7 mL, 1.8 mL)
2% / 1:100,000: Lidocaine hydrochloride 2% [20 mg/mL] and epinephrine 1:100,000 (1.7 mL, 1.8 mL)
Lignospan® Forte: 2% / 1:50,000: Lidocaine hydrochloride 2% [20 mg/mL] and epinephrine 1:50,000 (1.7 mL) [contains edetate disodium, potassium metabisulfite]
Lignospan® Standard: 2% / 1:100,000: Lidocaine hydrochloride 2% [20 mg/mL] and epinephrine 1:100,000 (1.7 mL) [contains edetate disodium, potassium metabisulfite]
Xylocaine® Dental with Epinephrine:
2% / 1:50,000: Lidocaine hydrochloride 2% [20 mg/mL] and epinephrine 1:50,000 (1.7 mL; 1.8 mL [DSC]) [contains sodium metabisulfite]
2% / 1:100,000: Lidocaine hydrochloride 2% [20 mg/mL] and epinephrine 1:100,000 (1.7 mL; 1.8 mL [DSC]) [contains sodium metabisulfite]

Lidocaine and Prilocaine

(LYE doe kane & PRIL oh kane)

Brand Names: U.S. EMLA®; Oraqix®

Brand Names: Canada EMLA®

Index Terms Prilocaine and Lidocaine

Pharmacologic Category Local Anesthetic

Use

Topical anesthetic for use on normal intact skin to provide local analgesia for minor procedures such as I.V. cannulation or venipuncture; has also been used for painful procedures such as lumbar puncture and skin graft harvesting; for superficial minor surgery of genital mucous membranes and as an adjunct for local infiltration anesthesia in genital mucous membranes.

Periodontal gel: Topical anesthetic for use in periodontal pockets during scaling or root planning procedures

Pregnancy Risk Factor B

Dosage Although the incidence of systemic adverse effects is very low, caution should be exercised, particularly when applying over large areas and leaving on for >2 hours

Children (intact skin):
Cream: Should **not** be used in neonates with a gestation age <37 weeks nor in infants <12 months of age who are receiving treatment with methemoglobin-inducing agents
Dosing is based on child's age and weight:
Age 0-3 months or <5 kg: Apply a maximum of 1 g over no more than 10 cm^2 of skin; leave on for no longer than 1 hour
Age 3 months to 12 months and >5 kg: Apply no more than a maximum 2 g total over no more than 20 cm^2 of skin; leave on for no longer than 4 hours

Age 1-6 years and >10 kg: Apply no more than a maximum of 10 g total over no more than 100 cm^2 of skin; leave on for no longer than 4 hours.

Age 7-12 years and >20 kg: Apply no more than a maximum 20 g total over no more than 200 cm^2 of skin; leave on for no longer than 4 hours.

Note: If a patient >3 months of age does not meet the minimum weight requirement, the maximum total dose should be restricted to the corresponding maximum based on patient weight.

Transdermal patch: Canadian labeling (not available in U.S.): **Note:** Should not be used in neonates with a gestation age <37 weeks nor in infants <12 months of age who are receiving treatment with methemoglobin-inducing agents

Dosing is based on child's age and weight: Apply patch(es) to skin area(s) <10 cm^2:

Age 0-3 months or <5 kg: Apply 1 patch and leave on for ~1 hour (do not exceed 1-hour application time); do not apply more than 1 patch at same time; safety of repeated dosing not established

Age 3 months to 12 months and >5 kg: Apply 1-2 patches for ~1 hour (maximum application time: 4 hours); do not apply more than 2 patches at the same time

Age 1-6 years and >10 kg: Apply 1or more patches for minimum of 1 hour (maximum application time: 5 hours); maximum dose: 10 patches

Age 7-12 years and >20 kg: Apply 1 or more patches for a minimum of 1 hour (maximum application time: 5 hours); maximum dose: 20 patches

Note: If a patient >3 months of age does not meet the minimum weight requirement, the maximum total dose should be restricted to that which corresponds to the patient's weight.

Adults (intact skin): **Note:** Cream: Apply a thick layer to intact skin and cover with an occlusive dressing. Transdermal patch (CAN; not available in U.S.): Apply patch or patches to intact skin.

Minor dermal procedures (eg, I.V. cannulation or venipuncture):

Cream: Apply 2.5 g of cream (1/2 of the 5 g tube) over 20-25 cm^2 of skin surface area) for at least 1 hour

Transdermal patch: (Canadian labeling; not available in U.S.): Apply 1 or more patches to skin surface area <10 cm^2 for at least 1 hour (maximum application time: 5 hours)

Major dermal procedures (eg, more painful dermatological procedures involving a larger skin area such as split thickness skin graft harvesting): Apply 2 g of cream per 10 cm^2 of skin and allow to remain in contact with the skin for at least 2 hours.

Adult male genital skin (eg, pretreatment prior to local anesthetic infiltration): Apply a thick layer of cream (1 g/ 10 cm^2) to the skin surface for 15 minutes. Local anesthetic infiltration should be performed immediately after removal of cream.

Note: Dermal analgesia can be expected to increase for up to 3 hours under occlusive dressing and persist for 1-2 hours after removal of the cream

Adult female genital mucous membranes: Minor procedures (eg, removal of condylomata acuminata, pretreatment for local anesthetic infiltration): Apply 5-10 g (thick layer) of cream for 5-10 minutes

Periodontal gel (Oraqix®): Adults: Apply on gingival margin around selected teeth using the blunt-tipped applicator included in package. Wait 30 seconds, then fill the periodontal pockets using the blunt-tipped applicator until gel becomes visible at the gingival margin. Wait another 30 seconds before starting treatment. May reapply; maximum recommended dose: One treatment session: 5 cartridges (8.5 g)

Additional Information Complete prescribing information for this medication should be consulted for additional detail.

Dosage Forms Excipient information presented when available (limited, particularly for generics); consult specific product labeling.

Cream, topical: Lidocaine 2.5% and prilocaine 2.5% (5 g, 30 g)

EMLA®: Lidocaine 2.5% and prilocaine 2.5% (5 g, 30 g)

Gel, periodontal:

Oraqix®: Lidocaine 2.5% and prilocaine 2.5% (1.7 g)

Dosage Forms: Canada Excipient information presented when available (limited, particularly for generics); consult specific product labeling.

Patch, transdermal:

EMLA® Patch: Lidocaine 2.5% and prilocaine 2.5% per patch (2s, 20s) [active contact surface area of each 1 g patch:10 cm^2; surface area of entire patch: 40 cm^2]

Lidocaine and Tetracaine

(LYE doe kane & TET ra kane)

Brand Names: U.S. Synera™

Index Terms Tetracaine and Lidocaine

Pharmacologic Category Analgesic, Topical; Local Anesthetic

Use Topical anesthetic for use on normal intact skin for minor procedures (eg, I.V. cannulation or venipuncture) and superficial dermatologic procedures

Pregnancy Risk Factor B

Dosage Transdermal patch: Children ≥3 years and Adults:

Venipuncture or intravenous cannulation: Prior to procedure, apply to intact skin for 20-30 minutes; **Note:** Adults can use another patch at a new location to facilitate venous access after a failed attempt; remove previous patch.

Superficial dermatological procedures: Prior to procedure, apply to intact skin for 30 minutes

Dosage adjustment in hepatic impairment: Use caution in patients with severe hepatic dysfunction.

Additional Information Complete prescribing information for this medication should be consulted for additional detail.

Dosage Forms Excipient information presented when available (limited, particularly for generics); consult specific product labeling.

Patch, transdermal:

Synera™: Lidocaine 70 mg and tetracaine 70 mg (10s) [contains heating component, metal; each patch is ~50 cm^2]

◆ **Lidocaine Hydrochloride** *see* Lidocaine (Systemic) *on page 1007*

◆ **Lidocaine Hydrochloride** *see* Lidocaine (Topical) *on page 1009*

◆ **Lidocaine Patch** *see* Lidocaine (Topical) *on page 1009*

◆ **Lidodan™ (Can)** *see* Lidocaine (Topical) *on page 1009*

◆ **Lidoderm®** *see* Lidocaine (Topical) *on page 1009*

◆ **LID-Pack® (Can)** *see* Bacitracin and Polymyxin B *on page 186*

◆ **Lignocaine Hydrochloride** *see* Lidocaine (Systemic) *on page 1007*

◆ **Lignocaine Hydrochloride** *see* Lidocaine (Topical) *on page 1009*

◆ **Lignospan® Forte** *see* Lidocaine and Epinephrine *on page 1010*

◆ **Lignospan® Standard** *see* Lidocaine and Epinephrine *on page 1010*

◆ **Limbitrol** *see* Amitriptyline and Chlordiazepoxide *on page 96*

Linagliptin (lin a GLIP tin)

Brand Names: U.S. Tradjenta™

Brand Names: Canada Trajenta™

Index Terms BI-1356; Trajenta

Pharmacologic Category Antidiabetic Agent, Dipeptidyl Peptidase IV (DPP-IV) Inhibitor

Additional Appendix Information

Diabetes Mellitus Management, Adults *on page 1983*

Use Management of type 2 diabetes mellitus (noninsulin dependent, NIDDM) as an adjunct to diet and exercise as monotherapy or in combination with other antidiabetic agents

Pregnancy Risk Factor B

Pregnancy Considerations Adverse events were not observed in animal reproduction studies, except with doses that were also maternally toxic. Maternal hyperglycemia can be associated with adverse effects in the fetus, including macrosomia, neonatal hyperglycemia, and hyperbilirubinemia; the risk of congenital malformations is increased when the Hb A_{1c} is above the normal range. Diabetes can also be associated with adverse effects in the mother. Poorly-treated diabetes may cause end-organ damage that may in turn negatively affect obstetric outcomes. Physiologic glucose levels should be maintained prior to and during pregnancy to decrease the risk of adverse events in the mother and the fetus. Until additional safety and efficacy data are obtained, the use of oral agents is generally not recommended as routine management of GDM or type 2 diabetes mellitus during pregnancy. Insulin is the drug of choice for the control of diabetes mellitus during pregnancy.

Lactation Excretion in breast milk unknown/use caution

Contraindications Hypersensitivity to linagliptin or any component of the formulation

Canadian labeling: Additional contraindications: Use in type 1 diabetes mellitus or diabetic ketoacidosis

Warnings/Precautions Avoid use in type 1 diabetes mellitus (insulin dependent, IDDM) and diabetic ketoacidosis (DKA) due to lack of efficacy in these populations. Use caution if used in conjunction with insulin or insulin secretagogues; risk of hypoglycemia is increased. Monitor blood glucose closely; dosage adjustments of insulin or insulin secretagogues may be necessary. Diabetes self-management education (DSME) is essential to maximize the effectiveness of therapy.

Adverse Reactions

>10%: Endocrine & metabolic: Hypoglycemia (combined with metformin/sulfonylurea [15%], metformin [<1%], pioglitazone [<1%]; monotherapy [<1%]) (Scott, 2011)

1% to 10%:

Central nervous system: Headache (6%)

Endocrine & metabolic: Hyperuricemia (3%), lipids increased (3%), triglycerides increased (2%), weight gain (2%)

Neuromuscular & skeletal: Arthralgia (6%), back pain (6%)

Respiratory: Nasopharyngitis (6%), cough (2%)

<1% (Limited to important or life-threatening): Angioedema, hypersensitivity, pancreatitis

Drug Interactions

Metabolism/Transport Effects **Substrate** of CYP3A4 (major), P-glycoprotein; **Note:** Assignment of Major/Minor substrate status based on clinically relevant drug interaction potential

Avoid Concomitant Use There are no known interactions where it is recommended to avoid concomitant use.

Increased Effect/Toxicity

Linagliptin may increase the levels/effects of: ACE Inhibitors; Hypoglycemic Agents

The levels/effects of Linagliptin may be increased by: Conivaptan; Herbs (Hypoglycemic Properties); Pegvisomant; P-glycoprotein/ABCB1 Inhibitors; Ritonavir

Decreased Effect

The levels/effects of Linagliptin may be decreased by: Corticosteroids (Orally Inhaled); Corticosteroids (Systemic); CYP3A4 Inducers (Strong); Deferasirox; Luteinizing Hormone-Releasing Hormone Analogs; P-glycoprotein/ABCB1 Inducers; Somatropin; Thiazide Diuretics; Tocilizumab

Ethanol/Nutrition/Herb Interactions

Ethanol: Caution with ethanol (may cause hypoglycemia).

Herb/Nutraceutical: Herbs with hypoglycemic properties may enhance the hypoglycemic effect of linagliptin. This includes alfalfa, aloe, bilberry, bitter melon, burdock, celery, damiana, fenugreek, garcinia, garlic, ginger, ginseng (American), gymnema, marshmallow, stinging nettle.

Stability Store at 25°C (77°F); excursions permitted between 15°C to 30°C (59°F to 86°F).

Mechanism of Action Linagliptin inhibits dipeptidyl peptidase IV (DPP-IV) enzyme resulting in prolonged active incretin levels. Incretin hormones (eg, glucagon-like peptide-1 [GLP-1] and glucose-dependent insulinotropic polypeptide [GIP]) regulate glucose homeostasis by increasing insulin synthesis and release from pancreatic beta cells and decreasing glucagon secretion from pancreatic alpha cells. Decreased glucagon secretion results in decreased hepatic glucose production. Under normal physiologic circumstances, incretin hormones are released by the intestine throughout the day and levels are increased in response to a meal; incretin hormones are rapidly inactivated by the DPP-IV enzyme.

Pharmacodynamics/Kinetics

Absorption: Rapid

Distribution: Extensive

Protein binding: 70% to 80%; concentration dependent

Metabolism: Not extensively metabolized

Bioavailability: 30%

Half-life elimination: Effective (therapeutic): ~12 hours; Terminal (DPP-IV saturable binding): >100 hours

Time to peak: 1.5 hours

Excretion: 80% feces unchanged; 5% urine unchanged

Dosage Oral: Adults: Type 2 diabetes: 5 mg once daily

Dosage adjustment in renal impairment: No dosage adjustments are recommended. **Note:** Canadian labeling does not recommend use in severe renal impairment.

Dosage adjustment in hepatic impairment: No dosage adjustments are recommended. **Note:** Canadian labeling does not recommend use in severe hepatic impairment.

Dietary Considerations May be taken without regard to food. Individualized medical nutrition therapy (MNT) based on ADA recommendations is an integral part of therapy.

Administration May be administered with or without food.

Monitoring Parameters Hb A_{1c}, serum glucose

Reference Range Recommendations for glycemic control in adults with diabetes:

Hb A_{1c}: <7%

Preprandial capillary plasma glucose: 70-130 mg/dL

Peak postprandial capillary blood glucose: <180 mg/dL

Dosage Forms Excipient information presented when available (limited, particularly for generics); consult specific product labeling.

Tablet, oral:

Tradjenta™: 5 mg

◆ **Lin-Amox (Can)** *see* Amoxicillin *on page 103*

◆ **Lin-Buspirone (Can)** *see* BusPIRone *on page 250*

Lindane (LIN dane)

Brand Names: Canada Hexit™; PMS-Lindane

Index Terms Benzene Hexachloride; Gamma Benzene Hexachloride; Hexachlorocyclohexane

Pharmacologic Category Antiparasitic Agent, Topical; Pediculocide; Scabicidal Agent

Use Treatment of *Sarcoptes scabiei* (scabies), *Pediculus capitis* (head lice), and *Phthirus pubis* (crab lice); FDA recommends reserving lindane as a second-line agent or with inadequate response to other therapies

Pregnancy Risk Factor C

Pregnancy Considerations There are no well-controlled studies in pregnant women.

Lactation Enters breast milk/contraindicated

Medication Guide Available Yes

Contraindications Hypersensitivity to lindane or any component of the formulation; uncontrolled seizure disorders; crusted (Norwegian) scabies, acutely-inflamed skin or raw, weeping surfaces or other skin conditions which may increase systemic absorption

Warnings/Precautions Hazardous agent - use appropriate precautions for handling and disposal. **[U.S. Boxed Warning]: Not considered a drug of first choice; use only in patients who have failed first-line treatments, or in patients who cannot tolerate these agents.** Because of the potential for systemic absorption and CNS side effects, lindane should be used with caution; consider permethrin or crotamiton agent first. Oil-based hair dressing may increase toxic potential.

[U.S. Boxed Warning]: May be associated with severe neurologic toxicities (contraindicated in premature infants and uncontrolled seizure disorders). Seizures and death have been reported with use; use with caution in infants, small children, patients <50 kg, or patients with a history of seizures; use caution with conditions which may increase risk of seizures or medications which decrease seizure threshold; use caution with hepatic impairment; avoid contact with face, eyes, mucous membranes, and urethral meatus.

[U.S. Boxed Warning]: A lindane medication use guide must be given to all patients along with instructions for proper use. Patients should be informed that itching may occur following successful killing of lice and re-treatment may not be indicated. Should be used as a part of an overall lice management program.

Adverse Reactions Frequency not defined (includes postmarketing and/or case reports).

Cardiovascular: Cardiac arrhythmia

Central nervous system: Ataxia, dizziness, headache, restlessness, seizure, pain

Dermatologic: Alopecia, contact dermatitis, skin and adipose tissue may act as repositories, eczematous eruptions, pruritus, urticaria

Gastrointestinal: Nausea, vomiting

Hematologic: Aplastic anemia

Hepatic: Hepatitis

Local: Burning and stinging

Neuromuscular & skeletal: Paresthesia

Renal: Hematuria

Respiratory: Pulmonary edema

Drug Interactions

Metabolism/Transport Effects None known.

Avoid Concomitant Use There are no known interactions where it is recommended to avoid concomitant use.

Increased Effect/Toxicity There are no known significant interactions involving an increase in effect.

Decreased Effect There are no known significant interactions involving a decrease in effect.

Mechanism of Action Directly absorbed by parasites and ova through the exoskeleton; stimulates the nervous system resulting in seizures and death of parasitic arthropods

Pharmacodynamics/Kinetics

Absorption: ≤13% systemically

Distribution: Stored in body fat; accumulates in brain; skin and adipose tissue may act as repositories

Metabolism: Hepatic

Half-life elimination: Children: 17-22 hours

Time to peak, serum: Children: 6 hours

Excretion: Urine and feces

Dosage Children and Adults: Topical:

Scabies: Apply a thin layer of lotion and massage it on skin from the neck to the toes; after 8-12 hours, bathe and remove the drug

Head lice, crab lice: Apply shampoo to dry hair and massage into hair for 4 minutes; add small quantities of water to hair until lather forms, then rinse hair thoroughly and comb with a fine tooth comb to remove nits. Amount of shampoo needed is based on length and density of hair; most patients will require 30 mL (maximum: 60 mL).

Administration For topical use only; never administer orally. Caregivers should apply with gloves (avoid natural latex, may be permeable to lindane). Rinse off with warm (not hot) water.

Lotion: Apply to dry, cool skin; do not apply to face or eyes. Wait at least 1 hour after bathing or showering (wet or warm skin increases absorption). Skin should be clean and free of any other lotions, creams, or oil prior to lindane application.

Shampoo: Apply to clean, dry hair. Wait at least 1 hour after washing hair before applying lindane shampoo. Hair should be washed with a shampoo not containing a conditioner; hair and skin of head and neck should be free of any lotions, oils, or creams prior to lindane application.

Dosage Forms Excipient information presented when available (limited, particularly for generics); consult specific product labeling.

Lotion, topical: 1% (60 mL)

Shampoo, topical: 1% (60 mL)

◆ **Linessa® (Can)** *see* Ethinyl Estradiol and Desogestrel *on page 653*

Linezolid (li NE zoh lid)

Brand Names: U.S. Zyvox®

Brand Names: Canada Zyvoxam®

Pharmacologic Category Antibiotic, Oxazolidinone

Use Treatment of vancomycin-resistant *Enterococcus faecium* (VRE) infections, nosocomial pneumonia caused by *Staphylococcus aureus* (including MRSA) or *Streptococcus pneumoniae* (including multidrug-resistant strains [MDRSP]), complicated and uncomplicated skin and skin structure infections (including diabetic foot infections without concomitant osteomyelitis), and community-acquired pneumonia caused by susceptible gram-positive organisms

Pregnancy Risk Factor C

Pregnancy Considerations Because adverse effects were observed in some animal studies, linezolid is classified pregnancy category C. There are no adequate and well-controlled studies in pregnant women.

Lactation Excretion in breast milk unknown/use caution

Contraindications Hypersensitivity to linezolid or any other component of the formulation; concurrent use or within 2 weeks of MAO inhibitors; patients with uncontrolled hypertension, pheochromocytoma, thyrotoxicosis, and/or taking sympathomimetics (eg, pseudoephedrine), vasopressive agents (eg, epinephrine, norepinephrine), or dopaminergic agents (eg, dopamine, dobutamine) unless closely monitored for increased blood pressure; patients with carcinoid syndrome and/or taking SSRIs, tricyclic antidepressants, serotonin 5-$HT_{1B,1D}$ receptor agonists, meperidine, or buspirone unless closely monitored for sign/symptoms of serotonin syndrome

Warnings/Precautions Myelosuppression has been reported and may be dependent on duration of therapy (generally >2 weeks of treatment); use with caution in patients with pre-existing myelosuppression, in patients receiving other drugs which may cause bone marrow suppression, or in chronic infection (previous or concurrent antibiotic therapy). Weekly CBC monitoring is recommended. Consider discontinuation in patients developing myelosuppression (or in whom myelosuppression worsens during treatment).

Lactic acidosis has been reported with use. Linezolid exhibits mild MAO inhibitor properties and has the potential to have the same interactions as other MAO inhibitors; use with caution and monitor closely in patients with uncontrolled hypertension, pheochromocytoma, carcinoid syndrome, or untreated hyperthyroidism; use is contraindicated in the absence of close monitoring. Symptoms of agitation, confusion, hallucinations, hyper-reflexia, myoclonus, shivering, and tachycardia may occur with concomitant proserotonergic drugs (eg, SSRIs/SNRIs or triptans) or agents which reduce linezolid's metabolism; concurrent use with these medications is contraindicated unless patient is closely monitored for signs/symptoms of serotonin syndrome. Unnecessary use may lead to the development of resistance to linezolid; consider alternatives before initiating outpatient treatment.

Peripheral and optic neuropathy (with vision loss) has been reported and may occur primarily with extended courses of therapy >28 days; any symptoms of visual change or impairment warrant immediate ophthalmic evaluation and possible discontinuation of therapy. Seizures have been reported; use with caution in patients with a history of seizures. Prolonged use may result in fungal or bacterial superinfection, including *C. difficile*-associated diarrhea (CDAD) and pseudomembranous colitis; CDAD has been observed >2 months postantibiotic treatment.

Due to inconsistent concentrations in the CSF, empiric use in pediatric patients with CNS infections is not recommended by the manufacturer; however, there are multiple case reports describing successful treatment of documented VRE and *Staphylococcus aureus* CNS and shunt infections in the literature. Linezolid should not be used in the empiric treatment of catheter-related bloodstream infection (CRBSI), but may be appropriate for targeted therapy (Mermel, 2009). Oral suspension contains phenylalanine.

Adverse Reactions Percentages as reported in adults; frequency similar in pediatric patients

>10%:
- Central nervous system: Headache (<1% to 11%)
- Gastrointestinal: Diarrhea (3% to 11%)

1% to 10%:
- Central nervous system: Insomnia (3%), dizziness (≤2%), fever (2%)
- Dermatologic: Rash (2%)
- Gastrointestinal: Nausea (3% to 10%), lipase increased (3% to 4%), vomiting (1% to 4%), constipation (2%), taste alteration (1% to 2%), amylase increased (<1% to 2%), tongue discoloration (≤1%), oral moniliasis (≤1%), pancreatitis
- Genitourinary: Vaginal moniliasis (1% to 2%)
- Hematologic: Thrombocytopenia (<1% to 10%), hemoglobin decreased (1% to 7%), leukopenia (<1% to 2%), neutropenia (≤1%)
- Hepatic: ALT increased (2% to 10%), AST increased (2% to 5%), alkaline phosphatase increased (<1% to 4%), bilirubin increased (≤1%)
- Renal: BUN increased (≤2%)
- Miscellaneous: Fungal infection (≤1% to 2%), lactate dehydrogenase increased (<1% to 2%)

<1% or frequency not defined (limited to important or life-threatening): Anaphylaxis, anemia, angioedema, bullous skin disorders, creatinine increased, *C. difficile*-related complications, dyspepsia, hypertension, lactic acidosis, localized abdominal pain, optic neuropathy, pancytopenia, peripheral neuropathy, pruritus, seizures, serotonin syndrome (with concurrent use of other serotonergic agents), Stevens-Johnson syndrome, tooth discoloration, vision loss

Drug Interactions

Metabolism/Transport Effects **Inhibits** Monoamine Oxidase

Avoid Concomitant Use

Avoid concomitant use of Linezolid with any of the following: Alpha-/Beta-Agonists (Indirect-Acting); Alpha1-Agonists; Alpha2-Agonists (Ophthalmic); Amphetamines; Anilidopiperidine Opioids; Antidepressants (Serotonin Reuptake Inhibitor/Antagonist); Atomoxetine; Bezafibrate; Buprenorphine; BuPROPion; BusPIRone; CarBAMazepine; CloZAPine; Cyclobenzaprine; Dexmethylphenidate; Dextromethorphan; Diethylpropion; HYDROmorphone; MAO Inhibitors; Maprotiline; Meperidine; Methyldopa; Methylene Blue; Methylphenidate; Mirtazapine; Oxymorphone; Pizotifen; Selective Serotonin Reuptake Inhibitors; Serotonin 5-HT1D Receptor Agonists; Serotonin/Norepinephrine Reuptake Inhibitors; Tapentadol; Tetrabenazine; Tetrahydrozoline; Tetrahydrozoline (Nasal); Tricyclic Antidepressants; Tryptophan

Increased Effect/Toxicity

Linezolid may increase the levels/effects of: Alpha-/Beta-Agonists (Direct-Acting); Alpha-/Beta-Agonists (Indirect-Acting); Alpha1-Agonists; Alpha2-Agonists (Ophthalmic); Amphetamines; Antidepressants (Serotonin Reuptake Inhibitor/Antagonist); Antihypertensives; Atomoxetine; Beta2-Agonists; Bezafibrate; BuPROPion; CloZAPine; Dexmethylphenidate; Dextromethorphan; Diethylpropion; Doxapram; HYDROmorphone; Lithium; Meperidine; Methadone; Methyldopa; Methylene Blue; Methylphenidate; Metoclopramide; Mirtazapine; Nefazodone; Orthostatic Hypotension Producing Agents; Pizotifen; Reserpine; Selective Serotonin Reuptake Inhibitors; Serotonin 5-HT1D Receptor Agonists; Serotonin Modulators; Serotonin/Norepinephrine Reuptake Inhibitors; Sympathomimetics; Tetrahydrozoline; Tetrahydrozoline (Nasal); TraZODone; Tricyclic Antidepressants

The levels/effects of Linezolid may be increased by: Altretamine; Anilidopiperidine Opioids; Antipsychotics; Buprenorphine; BusPIRone; CarBAMazepine; COMT Inhibitors; Cyclobenzaprine; Levodopa; MAO Inhibitors; Maprotiline; Oxymorphone; Tapentadol; Tetrabenazine; TraMADol; Tryptophan

Decreased Effect There are no known significant interactions involving a decrease in effect.

Ethanol/Nutrition/Herb Interactions

Ethanol: Avoid ethanol (based on CNS depressant effects and potential tyramine content)

Food: Concurrent ingestion of foods rich in tyramine may cause sudden and severe high blood pressure (hypertensive crisis). Avoid tyramine-containing foods with MAOIs. Food's freshness is also an important concern; improperly stored or spoiled food can create an environment where tyramine concentrations may increase.

Herb/Nutraceutical: Avoid supplements containing caffeine, tyrosine, tryptophan or phenylalanine. Ingestion of large quantities may increase the risk of severe side effects (eg, hypertensive reactions, serotonin syndrome).

Stability

Infusion: Store at 25°C (77°F); excursions permitted to 15°C to 30°C (59°F to 86°F). Protect from light. Keep infusion bags in overwrap until ready for use. Protect infusion bags from freezing.

Oral suspension: Reconstitute with 123 mL of distilled water (in 2 portions); shake vigorously. Concentration is 100 mg/5 mL. Prior to administration mix gently by inverting bottle; do not shake. Following reconstitution, store at 25°C (77°F); excursions permitted to 15°C to 30°C (59°F to 86°F). Use reconstituted suspension within 21 days. Protect from light.

Tablet: Store at 25°C (77°F); excursions permitted to 15°C to 30°C (59°F to 86°F). Protect from light; protect from moisture.

Mechanism of Action Inhibits bacterial protein synthesis by binding to bacterial 23S ribosomal RNA of the 50S subunit. This prevents the formation of a functional 70S initiation complex that is essential for the bacterial translation process. Linezolid is bacteriostatic against enterococci and staphylococci and bactericidal against most strains of streptococci.

Pharmacodynamics/Kinetics

Absorption: Rapid and extensive

Distribution: V_{dss}: Adults: 40-50 L

Protein binding: Adults: 31%

Metabolism: Hepatic via oxidation of the morpholine ring, resulting in two inactive metabolites (aminoethoxyacetic acid, hydroxyethyl glycine); minimally metabolized, may be mediated by cytochrome P450

Bioavailability: Oral: ~100%

Half-life elimination: Children ≥1 week (full-term) to 11 years: 1.5-3 hours; Adults: 4-5 hours

Time to peak: Adults: Oral: 1-2 hours

Excretion: Urine (~30% of total dose as parent drug, ~50% of total dose as metabolites); feces (~9% of total dose as metabolites)

Nonrenal clearance: Adults: ~65%

Dosage

Usual dosage: Oral, I.V.:

Children ≤11 years: 10 mg/kg (maximum: 600 mg/dose) every 8 hours

Children ≥12 years and Adults: 600 mg every 12 hours

Indication-specific dosing:

Pneumonia:

Community-acquired pneumonia (CAP):

Manufacturer's recommendation (includes concurrent bacteremia): Oral, I.V.:

Infants (excluding preterm neonates <1 week) and Children ≤11 years: 10 mg/kg/dose every 8 hours for 10-14 days

Children ≥12 years and Adults: 600 mg every 12 hours for 10-14 days. **Note**: May consider 7-day treatment course (versus manufacturer recommended 10-14 days) in patients with healthcare-, hospital-, and ventilator-associated pneumonia who have demonstrated good clinical response (ATS/IDSA, 2005).

Alternate recommendations:

Infants >3 months and Children ≤11 years (IDSA/PIDS, 2011):

S. pneumoniae (MICs to penicillin ≤2.0 mcg/mL), mild infection or step-down therapy (alternative to amoxicillin): Oral: 10 mg/kg/dose every 8 hours

S. pneumoniae (MICs to penicillin ≥4.0 mcg/mL):

Severe infection (alternative to ceftriaxone): I.V.: 10 mg/kg/dose every 8 hours

Mild infection, step-down therapy (preferred): Oral: 10 mg/kg/dose every 8 hours

S. aureus (methicillin-resistant/clindamycin-susceptible):

Severe infection (alternative to vancomycin or clindamycin): I.V.: 10 mg/kg/dose every 8 hours

Mild infection, step-down therapy (alternative to clindamycin): Oral: 10 mg/kg/dose every 8 hours

S. aureus (methicillin- and clindamycin-resistant):

Severe infection (alternative to vancomycin): I.V.: 10 mg/kg/dose every 8 hours

Mild infection, step-down therapy (preferred): Oral: 10 mg/kg/dose every 8 hours

Children ≤11 years (Liu, 2011): Oral, I.V.: *S. aureus* (methicillin-resistant): 10 mg/kg/dose every 8 hours for 7-21 days (maximum: 600 mg/dose)

Children ≥12 years (IDSA/PIDS, 2011):

S. pneumoniae (MICs to penicillin ≤2.0 mcg/mL), mild infection or step-down therapy (alternative to amoxicillin): Oral: 10 mg/kg/dose every 12 hours

S. pneumoniae (MICs to penicillin ≥4.0 mcg/mL)

Severe infection (alternative to ceftriaxone): I.V.: 10 mg/kg/dose every 12 hours

Mild infection, step-down therapy (preferred): Oral: 10 mg/kg/dose every 12 hours

S. aureus (methicillin-resistant/clindamycin-susceptible):

Severe infection (alternative to vancomycin/clindamycin): I.V.: 10 mg/kg/dose every 12 hours

Mild infection, step-down therapy (alternative to clindamycin): Oral: 10 mg/kg/dose every 12 hours

S. aureus (methicillin- and clindamycin-resistant):

Severe infection (alternative to vancomycin): I.V.: 10 mg/kg/dose every 12 hours

Mild infection, step-down therapy (preferred): Oral: 10 mg/kg/dose every 12 hours

Children ≥12 years and Adults: (Liu, 2011): Oral, I.V.: *S. aureus* (methicillin-resistant): 600 mg every 12 hours for 7-21 days

Healthcare-associated (HA) pneumonia: Oral, I.V.:

Manufacturer's recommendation:

Infants (excluding preterm neonates <1 week) and Children ≤11 years: 10 mg/kg every 8 hours for 10-14 days

Children ≥12 years and Adults: 600 mg every 12 hours for 10-14 days.

Note: May consider 7-day treatment course (versus manufacturer recommended 10-14 days) in patients with healthcare-, hospital-, and ventilator-associated pneumonia who have demonstrated good clinical response (ATS/IDSA, 2005).

Alternate recommendations (Liu, 2011): *S. aureus* (methicillin-resistant):

Children ≤11 years: 10 mg/kg/dose every 8 hours for 7-21 days (maximum: 600 mg/dose)

Children ≥12 years and Adults: 600 mg every 12 hours for 7-21 days

Skin and skin structure infections, complicated: Oral, I.V.:

Infants (excluding preterm neonates <1 week) and Children ≤11 years: 10 mg/kg every 8 hours for 10-14 days

Children ≥12 years and Adults: 600 mg every 12 hours for 10-14 days.

Skin and skin structure infections, uncomplicated: Oral:

Infants (excluding preterm neonates <1 week) and Children <5 years: 10 mg/kg every 8 hours for 10-14 days

Children 5-11 years: 10 mg/kg every 12 hours for 10-14 days

Children ≥12-18 years: 600 mg every 12 hours for 10-14 days

Adults: 400 mg every 12 hours for 10-14 days; **Note:** 400 mg dose is recommended in the product labeling; however, 600 mg dose is commonly employed clinically; consider 5- to 10-day treatment course as opposed to the manufacturer recommended 10-14 days (Liu, 2011; Stevens, 2005)

VRE infections including concurrent bacteremia: Oral, I.V.:

Infants (excluding preterm neonates <1 week) and Children ≤11 years: 10 mg/kg every 8 hours for 14-28 days

Children ≥12 years and Adults: 600 mg every 12 hours for 14-28 days

Brain abscess, subdural empyema, spinal epidural abscess (*S. aureus* [methicillin-resistant]) (unlabeled use; Liu, 2011): Oral, I.V.:

Children ≤11 years: 10 mg/kg every 8 hours for 4-6 weeks (maximum: 600 mg/dose)

Children ≥12 years and Adults: 600 mg every 12 hours for 4-6 weeks

Meningitis (*S. aureus* [methicillin-resistant]) (unlabeled use; Liu, 2011): Oral, I.V.: Children ≥12 years and Adults: 600 mg every 12 hours for 2 weeks

Osteomyelitis (*S. aureus* [methicillin-resistant]) (unlabeled use; Liu, 2011): Oral, I.V.:

Infants (excluding preterm neonates <1 week) and Children ≤11 years: 10 mg/kg every 8 hours for a minimum of 4-6 weeks (maximum: 600 mg/dose)

Children ≥12 years and Adults: 600 mg every 12 hours for a minimum of 8 weeks (some experts combine with rifampin)

Septic arthritis (*S. aureus* [methicillin-resistant]) (unlabeled use; Liu, 2011): Oral, I.V.:

Infants (excluding preterm neonates <1 week) and Children ≤11 years: 10 mg/kg every 8 hours for 3-4 weeks (maximum: 600 mg/dose)

Children ≥12 years and Adults: 600 mg every 12 hours for 3-4 weeks

Septic thrombosis of cavernous or dural venous sinus (*S. aureus* [methicillin-resistant]) (unlabeled use; Liu, 2011): Oral, I.V.:

Children ≤11 years: 10 mg/kg every 8 hours for 4-6 weeks (maximum: 600 mg/dose)

Children ≥12 years and Adults: 600 mg every 12 hours for 4-6 weeks

Elderly: No dosage adjustment required

Dosage adjustment in renal impairment: No adjustment is recommended. The two primary metabolites may accumulate in patients with renal impairment but the clinical significance is unknown. Weigh the risk of accumulation of metabolites versus the benefit of therapy. Monitor for hematopoietic (eg, anemia, leukopenia, thrombocytopenia) and neuropathic (eg, peripheral neuropathy) adverse events when administering for extended periods.

Intermittent hemodialysis (administer after hemodialysis on dialysis days): Dialyzable (~30% removed during 3-hour dialysis session): If administration time is not immediately after dialysis session, may consider administration of a supplemental dose especially early in the treatment course to maintain levels above the MIC (Brier, 2003). Others have recommended no supplemental dose or dosage adjustment for patients on intermittent hemodialysis, peritoneal dialysis, or continuous renal replacement therapy (eg, CVVHD) (Heintz, 2009; Trotman, 2005)

Dosage adjustment in hepatic impairment:

Mild-to-moderate hepatic impairment (Child-Pugh class A or B): No dosage adjustment required

Severe hepatic impairment (Child-Pugh class C): Use has not been adequately evaluated

Dietary Considerations Take without regard to meals. Some products may contain sodium and/or phenylalanine. Avoid consuming large amounts of tyramine-containing foods/beverages. Some examples include aged or matured cheese, air-dried or cured meats (including sausages and salamis), fava or broad bean pods, tap/draft beers, Marmite concentrate, sauerkraut, soy sauce, and other soybean condiments.

Administration

I.V.: Administer intravenous infusion over 30-120 minutes. Do not mix or infuse with other medications. When the same intravenous line is used for sequential infusion of other medications, flush line with D_5W, NS, or LR before and after infusing linezolid. The yellow color of the injection may intensify over time without affecting potency.

Oral suspension: Invert gently to mix prior to administration, do not shake. Administer without regard to meals.

Monitoring Parameters Weekly CBC, particularly in patients at increased risk of bleeding, with pre-existing myelosuppression, on concomitant medications that cause bone marrow suppression, in those who require >2 weeks of therapy, or in those with chronic infection who have received previous or concomitant antibiotic therapy; visual function with extended therapy (≥3 months) or in patients with new onset visual symptoms, regardless of therapy length

Dosage Forms Excipient information presented when available (limited, particularly for generics); consult specific product labeling.

Infusion, premixed:

Zyvox®: 200 mg (100 mL); 600 mg (300 mL) [contains sodium 0.38 mg/mL]

Powder for suspension, oral:

Zyvox®: 100 mg/5 mL (150 mL) [contains phenylalanine 20 mg/5 mL, sodium 8.52 mg (0.4 mEq)/5 mL, sodium benzoate; orange flavor]

Tablet, oral:

Zyvox®: 600 mg [contains sodium 2.92 mg (0.1 mEq)/tablet]

◆ **Lioresal®** *see* Baclofen *on page 187*

◆ **Liotec (Can)** *see* Baclofen *on page 187*

Liothyronine (lye oh THYE roe neen)

Brand Names: U.S. Cytomel®; Triostat®

Brand Names: Canada Cytomel®

Index Terms Liothyronine Sodium; Sodium *L*-Triiodothyronine; T_3 Sodium (error-prone abbreviation)

Pharmacologic Category Thyroid Product

Use

Oral: Replacement or supplemental therapy in hypothyroidism; management of nontoxic goiter; a diagnostic aid

I.V.: Treatment of myxedema coma/precoma

Unlabeled Use Management of hemodynamically unstable potential organ donors increasing the quantity of organs available for transplantation

Pregnancy Risk Factor A

Dosage Doses should be adjusted based on clinical response and laboratory parameters.

Children: Congenital hypothyroidism: Oral: 5 mcg/day increase by 5 mcg every 3-4 days until the desired response is achieved. Usual maintenance dose: 20 mcg/day for infants, 50 mcg/day for children 1-3 years of age, and adult dose for children >3 years.

Adults:
Hypothyroidism: Oral: 25 mcg/day increase by increments of 12.5-25 mcg/day every 1-2 weeks to a maximum of 100 mcg/day; usual maintenance dose: 25-75 mcg/day.
Patients with cardiovascular disease: Refer to elderly dosing.
T_3 suppression test: Oral: 75-100 mcg/day for 7 days; use lowest dose for elderly
Myxedema: Oral: Initial: 5 mcg/day; increase in increments of 5-10 mcg/day every 1-2 weeks. When 25 mcg/day is reached, dosage may be increased at intervals of 5-25 mcg/day every 1-2 weeks. Usual maintenance dose: 50-100 mcg/day.
Myxedema coma: I.V.: 25-50 mcg
Patients with known or suspected cardiovascular disease: 10-20 mcg
Note: Normally, at least 4 hours should be allowed between doses to adequately assess therapeutic response and no more than 12 hours should elapse between doses to avoid fluctuations in hormone levels. Oral therapy should be resumed as soon as the clinical situation has been stabilized and the patient is able to take oral medication. If levothyroxine rather than liothyronine sodium is used in initiating oral therapy, the physician should bear in mind that there is a delay of several days in the onset of levothyroxine activity and that I.V. therapy should be discontinued gradually.
Simple (nontoxic) goiter: Oral: Initial: 5 mcg/day; increase by 5-10 mcg every 1-2 weeks; after 25 mcg/day is reached, may increase dose by 12.5-25 mcg. Usual maintenance dose: 75 mcg/day
Elderly: Oral: 5 mcg/day; increase by 5 mcg/day every 2 weeks

Additional Information Complete prescribing information for this medication should be consulted for additional detail.

Dosage Forms Excipient information presented when available (limited, particularly for generics); consult specific product labeling.
Injection, solution: 10 mcg/mL (1 mL)
Triostat®: 10 mcg/mL (1 mL) [contains ethanol 6.8%]
Tablet, oral: 5 mcg, 25 mcg, 50 mcg
Cytomel®: 5 mcg
Cytomel®: 25 mcg, 50 mcg [scored]

◆ **Liothyronine and Levothyroxine** *see* Liotrix *on page 1017*

◆ **Liothyronine Sodium** *see* Liothyronine *on page 1016*

Liotrix (LYE oh triks)

Brand Names: U.S. Thyrolar®
Brand Names: Canada Thyrolar®
Index Terms Levothyroxine and Liothyronine; Liothyronine and Levothyroxine; T_3/T_4 Liotrix
Pharmacologic Category Thyroid Product
Use
Replacement or supplemental therapy in hypothyroidism (uniform mixture of T_4:T_3 in 4:1 ratio by weight)
Thyroid-stimulating hormone (TSH) suppressant therapy used in the management of thyroid cancer (levothyroxine is generally recommended for this indication); prevention or treatment of euthyroid goiters (eg, thyroid nodules, subacute or chronic lymphocytic thyroiditis [Hashimoto's], multinodular goiters)
Diagnostic agent in suppression tests to diagnose suspected mild hyperthyroidism or to demonstrate thyroid gland autonomy
Pregnancy Risk Factor A

Dosage Oral:
Congenital hypothyroidism:
Children: **Note:** In newly diagnosed infants, begin therapy with full dose.
0-6 months: Levothyroxine 12.5-25 mcg/Liothyronine 3.1-6.25 mcg once daily
6-12 months: Levothyroxine 25-37.5 mcg/Liothyronine 6.25-9.35 mcg once daily
1-5 years: Levothyroxine 37.5-50 mcg/Liothyronine 9.35-12.5 mcg once daily
6-12 years: Levothyroxine 50-75 mcg/Liothyronine 12.5-18.75 mcg once daily
>12 years: Levothyroxine 75 mcg/Liothyronine 18.75 mcg once daily
Also see individual agents.
Hypothyroidism:
Adults: Initial: Levothyroxine 25 mcg/Liothyronine 6.25 mcg once daily; may increase by levothyroxine 12.5 mcg/Liothyronine 3.1 mcg every 2-3 weeks. A lower initial dose (levothyroxine 12.5 mcg/Liothyronine 3.1 mcg) is recommended in patients with long-standing myxedema, especially if cardiovascular impairment coexists. If angina occurs, reduce dose (usual maintenance dose: levothyroxine 50-100 mcg/Liothyronine 12.5-25 mcg)
Elderly: Initial: Levothyroxine 12.5-25 mcg/Liothyronine 3.1-6.25 mcg once daily; may increase by levothyroxine 12.5 mcg/Liothyronine 3.1 mcg every 2-3 weeks

Additional Information Complete prescribing information for this medication should be consulted for additional detail.

Dosage Forms Excipient information presented when available (limited, particularly for generics); consult specific product labeling.
Tablet, oral:
Thyrolar®: 1/4 [levothyroxine sodium 12.5 mcg and liothyronine sodium 3.1 mcg]
Thyrolar®: 1/2 [levothyroxine sodium 25 mcg and liothyronine sodium 6.25 mcg]
Thyrolar®: 1 [levothyroxine sodium 50 mcg and liothyronine sodium 12.5 mcg]
Thyrolar®: 2 [levothyroxine sodium 100 mcg and liothyronine sodium 25 mcg]
Thyrolar®: 3 [levothyroxine sodium 150 mcg and liothyronine sodium 37.5 mcg]

◆ **Lipancreatin** *see* Pancrelipase *on page 1285*
◆ **Lipase, Protease, and Amylase** *see* Pancrelipase *on page 1285*
◆ **Lipiarrmycin** *see* Fidaxomicin *on page 710*
◆ **Lipidil EZ® (Can)** *see* Fenofibrate *on page 693*
◆ **Lipidil Micro® (Can)** *see* Fenofibrate *on page 693*
◆ **Lipidil Supra® (Can)** *see* Fenofibrate *on page 693*
◆ **Lipitor®** *see* Atorvastatin *on page 165*
◆ **Lipofen®** *see* Fenofibrate *on page 693*
◆ **Liposomal Cytarabine** *see* Cytarabine (Liposomal) *on page 432*
◆ **Liposomal DAUNOrubicin** *see* DAUNOrubicin (Liposomal) *on page 458*
◆ **Liposomal DOXOrubicin** *see* DOXOrubicin (Liposomal) *on page 555*
◆ **Liposyn® II (Can)** *see* Fat Emulsion *on page 690*
◆ **Liposyn® III** *see* Fat Emulsion *on page 690*
◆ **Liqua-Cal [OTC]** *see* Calcium and Vitamin D *on page 265*
◆ **Liquibid® D-R [OTC]** *see* Guaifenesin and Phenylephrine *on page 812*
◆ **Liquibid® PD-R [OTC]** *see* Guaifenesin and Phenylephrine *on page 812*

◆ **Liquid Antidote** *see* Charcoal, Activated *on page 335*

Liraglutide (lir a GLOO tide)

Brand Names: U.S. Victoza®

Brand Names: Canada Victoza®

Index Terms NN2211

Pharmacologic Category Antidiabetic Agent, Glucagon-Like Peptide-1 (GLP-1) Receptor Agonist

Use Treatment of type 2 diabetes mellitus (noninsulin dependent, NIDDM) to improve glycemic control

Pregnancy Risk Factor C

Pregnancy Considerations Teratogenic in animal studies. There are no adequate or well-controlled studies in pregnant women; use only if potential benefit outweighs possible risk to the fetus.

Lactation Excretion in breast milk unknown/not recommended

Medication Guide Available Yes

Contraindications History of or family history of medullary thyroid carcinoma (MTC); patients with multiple endocrine neoplasia syndrome type 2 (MEN2)

Warnings/Precautions [U.S. Boxed Warning] Dose and duration dependent thyroid C-cell tumors have developed in animal studies with liraglutide therapy; relevance in humans unknown. During clinical studies a few cases of thyroid C-cell hyperplasia were reported. Due to the finding in animal studies, patients were monitored with serum calcitonin or thyroid ultrasound during clinical trials; however it us unknown if this is beneficial in decreasing the risk of thyroid tumors. Consultation with an endocrinologist is recommended in patients who develop elevated calcitonin concentrations. Patients should be counseled on the risk and symptoms of thyroid tumors. Use is contraindicated in patients with or a family history of medullary thyroid cancer and in patients with multiple endocrine neoplasia syndrome type 2 (MEN2). Cases of acute and chronic pancreatitis (including one case of fatal necrotizing pancreatitis) have been reported although conclusive evidence to liraglutide therapy has not been established; monitor for unexplained severe abdominal pain, and if pancreatitis is suspected, discontinue use. Do not resume unless an alternative etiology of pancreatitis is confirmed. Use with caution in patients with a history of pancreatitis, cholelithiasis, and/or alcohol abuse. Most common reactions are gastrointestinal related; these symptoms may be dose-related and may decrease in frequency/severity with gradual titration and continued use. Use may be associated with weight loss (likely due to reduced intake) independent of the change in hemoglobin A_{1c}. Use with caution in patients with hepatic or renal impairment; cases of acute renal failure and chronic renal failure exacerbation have been reported.

Concurrent use with insulin therapy has not been evaluated. Concomitant use of an insulin secretagogue (eg, sulfonylurea, meglitinide) may increase the risk of hypoglycemia; dosage reduction of secretagogues may be required during initiation of liraglutide. Due to its effects on gastric emptying, liraglutide may reduce the rate and extent of absorption of orally-administered drugs; use with caution in patients receiving medications with a narrow therapeutic window or require rapid absorption from the GI tract. Not recommended for first-line therapy; use as adjunct to diet and exercise. Do not use in patients with type 1 diabetes mellitus or for the treatment of diabetic ketoacidosis; not a substitute for insulin. Diabetes self-management education (DSME) is essential to maximize the effectiveness of therapy.

Adverse Reactions Percentages are as reported for monotherapy.

>10%: Gastrointestinal: Nausea (28%), diarrhea (17%), vomiting (11%)

1% to 10%:

Cardiovascular: Hypertension (3%)

Central nervous system: Headache (9%), dizziness (6%)

Gastrointestinal: Constipation (10%)

Genitourinary: Urinary tract infection (6%)

Hepatic: Hyperbilirubinemia (4%)

Local: Injection site reactions (2%; includes rash, erythema)

Neuromuscular & skeletal: Back pain (5%)

Respiratory: Upper respiratory infection (10%), sinusitis (6%), nasopharyngitis (5%)

Miscellaneous: Anti-liraglutide antibodies (low titers 9%, cross-reacting 7%), influenza (7%)

<1% (Limited to important or life-threatening): Hypoglycemia (most reports in patients receiving combination therapy), pancreatitis (including acute, chronic, and necrotizing), papillary thyroid carcinoma, thyroid C-cell hyperplasia

Drug Interactions

Metabolism/Transport Effects None known.

Avoid Concomitant Use There are no known interactions where it is recommended to avoid concomitant use.

Increased Effect/Toxicity

Liraglutide may increase the levels/effects of: Sulfonylureas

The levels/effects of Liraglutide may be increased by: Pegvisomant

Decreased Effect

The levels/effects of Liraglutide may be decreased by: Corticosteroids (Orally Inhaled); Corticosteroids (Systemic); Luteinizing Hormone-Releasing Hormone Analogs; Somatropin; Thiazide Diuretics

Ethanol/Nutrition/Herb Interactions Ethanol: Caution with ethanol (may cause hypoglycemia).

Stability Prior to initial use, store under refrigeration at 2°C to 8°C (36°F to 46°F); after initial use, may be stored in refrigerator or at room temperature of 15°C to 30°C (59°F to 86°F). Do not freeze (discard if freezing occurs). Protect from heat and light. Pen should be discarded 30 days after initial use.

Mechanism of Action Liraglutide is a long acting analog of human glucagon-like peptide-1 (GLP-1) (an incretin hormone) which increases glucose-dependent insulin secretion, decreases inappropriate glucagon secretion, increases B-cell growth/replication, slows gastric emptying, and decreases food intake. Liraglutide administration results in decreases in hemoglobin A_{1c} by approximately 1%.

Pharmacodynamics/Kinetics

Distribution: V_d: SubQ: ~13 L; I.V.: 0.07 L/kg

Protein binding: >98%

Metabolism: Endogenously metabolized by dipeptidyl peptidase IV (DPP-IV) and endogenous endopeptidases (Croom, 2009); metabolism occurs slower than that seen with native GLP-1

Bioavailability: SubQ: ~55%

Half-life, elimination: ~13 hours

Time to peak, plasma: 8-12 hours

Excretion: Urine (6%, as metabolites); feces (5%, as metabolites)

Dosage Note: Initial dose is intended to reduce GI symptoms; does not provide effective glycemic control.

SubQ: Adults: Initial: 0.6 mg once daily for 1 week; then increase to 1.2 mg once daily; may increase further to 1.8 mg once daily if optimal glycemic response not achieved with 1.2 mg/day

Dosage adjustment in renal impairment: No dosage adjustment recommended; use caution, limited experience

Dosage adjustment in hepatic impairment: No dosage adjustment recommended; use caution, limited experience

Dietary Considerations Individualized medical nutrition therapy (MNT) based on ADA recommendations is an integral part of therapy.

Administration SubQ: Use only if clear, colorless, and free of particulate matter. Administer via injection in the upper arm, thigh, or abdomen. Administer without regard to meals or time of day. Change needle with each administration. Do not share pens between patients even if needle is changed.

Monitoring Parameters Plasma glucose, Hb A_{1c}

Reference Range

Recommendations for glycemic control in adults with diabetes (ADA, 2010):

Hb A_{1c}: <7%

Preprandial capillary plasma glucose: 70-130 mg/dL

Peak postprandial capillary blood glucose: <180 mg/dL

Dosage Forms Excipient information presented when available (limited, particularly for generics); consult specific product labeling.

Injection, solution [rDNA origin]:

Victoza®: 6 mg/mL (3 mL) [contains propylene glycol 14 mg/3 mL; prefilled pen]

Lisdexamfetamine (lis dex am FET a meen)

Brand Names: U.S. Vyvanse®

Brand Names: Canada Vyvanse™

Index Terms Lisdexamfetamine Dimesylate; Lisdexamphetamine; NRP104

Pharmacologic Category Stimulant

Use Treatment of attention-deficit/hyperactivity disorder (ADHD)

Pregnancy Risk Factor C

Pregnancy Considerations Animal studies have shown that amphetamines may cause embryotoxic and teratogenic effects and that pre- or early postnatal exposure to amphetamines may lead to lasting changes in behavior, including impaired learning, memory, and motor skills, as well as changes to libido. There are no adequate and well-controlled studies in pregnant women. No reproductive studies have been performed with lisdexamfetamine. Infants born to mothers dependent on amphetamines are more likely to arrive prematurely with low birth weight and may experience withdrawal symptoms including irritation, restlessness, anxiousness, weakness, listlessness, or lethargy.

Lactation Enters breast milk/not recommended

Medication Guide Available Yes

Contraindications Known hypersensitivity or idiosyncratic reaction sympathomimetic amines; advanced arteriosclerosis, symptomatic cardiovascular disease, moderate-to-severe hypertension; hyperthyroidism; glaucoma; agitated states; history of drug abuse; concurrent use or within 2 weeks of use of MAO inhibitors

Warnings/Precautions **[U.S. Boxed Warning]: Use has been associated with serious cardiovascular events including sudden death in patients with pre-existing structural cardiac abnormalities or other serious heart problems (sudden death in children and adolescents; sudden death, stroke and MI in adults.** Use of this product should be avoided in the patients with known serious structural cardiac abnormalities, cardiomyopathy, serious heart rhythm abnormalities, coronary artery disease (adults), or other serious cardiac problems that could increase the risk of sudden death that these conditions alone carry. Patients should be carefully evaluated for these cardiac disorders prior to initiation of therapy.

Use with caution in patients with psychiatric or seizure disorders. May exacerbate symptoms of behavior and thought disorder in psychotic patients. Stimulants may unmask tics in individuals with coexisting Tourette's syndrome. **[U.S. Boxed Warning]: Potential for drug dependency exists; prolonged use may lead to drug dependency.** Use is contraindicated is patients with history of ethanol or drug abuse. Prescriptions should be written for the smallest quantity consistent with good patient care to minimize the possibility of overdose. Abrupt discontinuation following high doses or for prolonged periods may result in symptoms for withdrawal. Recommended to be used as part of a comprehensive treatment program for attention deficit disorders.

May be inappropriate for use in the elderly due to CNS stimulant adverse effects (Beers Criteria). Safety and efficacy of long-term use have not yet been established. Safety and efficacy in children <6 years of age have not been established. Appetite suppression may occur; monitor weight during therapy, particularly in children. Use of stimulants has been associated with slowing of growth rate; monitor growth rate during treatment. Treatment interruption may be necessary in patients who are not growing or gaining weight as expected.

Adverse Reactions

>10%:

Central nervous system: Headache (children 12%), insomnia (19% to 27%; 4% [initially])

Gastrointestinal: Appetite decreased (27% to 39%), xerostomia (children 5%; adults 26%), abdominal pain (children 12%)

1% to 10%:

Cardiovascular: Blood pressure increased (adults 3%), heart rate increased (adults 2%)

Central nervous system: Irritability (children 10%), anxiety (adults 6%), dizziness (children 5%), jitteriness (adults 4%), affect lability (children 3%), agitation (adults 3%), restlessness (adults 3%), fever (children 2%), somnolence (children 2%), tic (children 2%)

Dermatologic: Hyperhidrosis (adults 3%), rash (children 3%)

Gastrointestinal: Vomiting (children 9%), weight loss (children 9%), diarrhea (adults 7%), nausea (6% to 7%), anorexia (adults 5%)

Genitourinary: Erectile dysfunction (adults <2%), libido decreased (adults <2%)

Neuromuscular & skeletal: Tremor (adults 2%)

Respiratory: Dyspnea (adults 2%)

Postmarketing and/or case reports: Aggression, anaphylactic reaction, angioedema, blurred vision, depression, dermatillomania, diplopia, dyskinesia, dysphoria, eosinophilic hepatitis, euphoria, fatigue, hallucination, hypersensitivity, logorrhea, mania, mydriasis, palpitation, psychotic episodes, seizure, Stevens-Johnson syndrome, urticaria

Additional adverse reaction associated with amphetamines; frequency not defined:

Cardiovascular: Cardiomyopathy, hypertension, MI, sudden death, tachycardia

Central nervous system: Exacerbation of motor and phonic tics, overstimulation, stroke, Tourette's syndrome

Dermatologic: Toxic epidermal necrolysis

Gastrointestinal: Abnormal taste, constipation

Drug Interactions

Metabolism/Transport Effects None known.

Avoid Concomitant Use

Avoid concomitant use of Lisdexamfetamine with any of the following: Iobenguane I 123; MAO Inhibitors

Increased Effect/Toxicity

Lisdexamfetamine may increase the levels/effects of: Analgesics (Opioid); Sympathomimetics

The levels/effects of Lisdexamfetamine may be increased by: Alkalinizing Agents; Antacids; Atomoxetine; Cannabinoids; Carbonic Anhydrase Inhibitors;

MAO Inhibitors; Proton Pump Inhibitors; Tricyclic Antidepressants

Decreased Effect

Lisdexamfetamine may decrease the levels/effects of: Antihistamines; Ethosuximide; Iobenguane I 123; Ioflupane I 123; PHENobarbital; Phenytoin

The levels/effects of Lisdexamfetamine may be decreased by: Ammonium Chloride; Antipsychotics; Gastrointestinal Acidifying Agents; Lithium; Methenamine

Ethanol/Nutrition/Herb Interactions

Ethanol: Avoid ethanol (may increase CNS depression).

Food: High-fat meal prolongs T_{max} by ~1 hour.

Stability Store at controlled room temperature of 25°C (77°F) excursions permitted to 15°C to 30°C (59°F to 86°F). Protect from light.

Mechanism of Action Lisdexamfetamine dimesylate is a prodrug that is converted to the active component dextroamphetamine (a noncatecholamine, sympathomimetic amine). Amphetamines are noncatecholamine, sympathomimetic amines that cause release of catecholamines (primarily dopamine and norepinephrine) from their storage sites in the presynaptic nerve terminals. A less significant mechanism may include their ability to block the reuptake of catecholamines by competitive inhibition.

Pharmacodynamics/Kinetics

Absorption: Rapid

Distribution: Dextroamphetamine: V_d: Adults: 3.5-4.6 L/kg; distributes into CNS; mean CSF concentrations are 80% of plasma; enters breast milk

Metabolism: Non-CYP-mediated hepatic or intestinal metabolism to dextroamphetamine and l-lysine

Half-life elimination: Lisdexamfetamine: <1 hour; Dextroamphetamine: 10-13 hours

Time to peak, serum: T_{max}: Lisdexamfetamine: ~1 hour; Dextroamphetamine: ~3.5 hours

Excretion: Urine (96%, 42% as amphetamine-related compounds, 2% as lisdexamfetamine, 25% hippuric acid); feces (minimal)

Dosage Oral: Individualize dosage based on patient need and response to therapy. Administer at the lowest effective dose.

Children ≥6 years and Adults: Initial: 30 mg once daily in the morning; may increase in increments of 10 mg or 20 mg/day at weekly intervals until optimal response is obtained; maximum: 70 mg/day

Dietary Considerations May be taken without regard to meals.

Administration Administer in the morning without regard to meals; swallow capsule whole, do not chew; capsule may be opened and the contents dissolved in glass of water; consume the resulting solution immediately; do not store solution.

Monitoring Parameters Cardiac evaluation should be completed on any patient who develops chest pain, unexplained syncope, and any symptom of cardiac disease during treatment with stimulants; growth and CNS activity in all patients

When used for the treatment of ADHD, thoroughly evaluate for cardiovascular risk. Monitor heart rate, blood pressure, and consider obtaining ECG prior to initiation (Vetter, 2008).

Test Interactions Amphetamines may elevate plasma corticosteroid levels; may interfere with urinary steroid determinations.

Dosage Forms Excipient information presented when available (limited, particularly for generics); consult specific product labeling.

Capsule, oral, as dimesylate:

Vyvanse®: 20 mg, 30 mg, 40 mg, 50 mg, 60 mg, 70 mg

Controlled Substance C-II

◆ **Lisdexamfetamine Dimesylate** *see* Lisdexamfetamine *on page 1019*

◆ **Lisdexamphetamine** *see* Lisdexamfetamine *on page 1019*

Lisinopril (lyse IN oh pril)

Brand Names: U.S. Prinivil®; Zestril®

Brand Names: Canada Apo-Lisinopril®; CO Lisinopril; Dom-Lisinopril; JAMP-Lisinopril; Mint-Lisinopril; Mylan-Lisinopril; PMS-Lisinopril; Prinivil®; PRO-Lisinopril; RAN™-Lisinopril; ratio-Lisinopril; ratio-Lisinopril P; ratio-Lisinopril Z; Riva-Lisinopril; Sandoz-Lisinopril; Teva-Lisinopril (Type P); Teva-Lisinopril (Type Z); Zestril®

Pharmacologic Category Angiotensin-Converting Enzyme (ACE) Inhibitor

Additional Appendix Information

Angiotensin Agents *on page 1869*

Heart Failure (Systolic) *on page 1991*

Use Treatment of hypertension, either alone or in combination with other antihypertensive agents; adjunctive therapy in treatment of heart failure (afterload reduction); treatment of acute myocardial infarction within 24 hours in hemodynamically-stable patients to improve survival; treatment of left ventricular dysfunction after myocardial infarction

Pregnancy Risk Factor C (1st trimester); D (2nd and 3rd trimesters)

Pregnancy Considerations Due to adverse events observed in some animal studies, lisinopril is considered pregnancy category C during the first trimester. Based on human data, lisinopril is considered pregnancy category D if used during the second and third trimesters (per the manufacturer; however, one study suggests that fetal injury may occur at anytime during pregnancy). Lisinopril crosses the placenta. First trimester exposure to ACE inhibitors may cause major congenital malformations. An increased risk of cardiovascular and/or central nervous system malformations was observed in one study; however, an increased risk of teratogenic events was not observed in other studies. Second and third trimester use of an ACE inhibitor is associated with oligohydramnios. Oligohydramnios due to decreased fetal renal function may lead to fetal limb contractures, craniofacial deformation, and hypoplastic lung development. The use of ACE inhibitors during the second and third trimesters is also associated with anuria, hypotension, renal failure (reversible or irreversible), skull hypoplasia, and death in the fetus/neonate. Chronic maternal hypertension itself is also associated with adverse events in the fetus/infant. ACE inhibitors are not recommended during pregnancy to treat maternal hypertension or heart failure. Those who are planning a pregnancy should be considered for other medication options if an ACE inhibitor is currently prescribed or the ACE inhibitor should be discontinued as soon as possible once pregnancy is detected. The exposed fetus should be monitored for fetal growth, amniotic fluid volume, and organ formation. Infants exposed to an ACE inhibitor *in utero*, especially during the second and third trimester, should be monitored for hyperkalemia, hypotension, and oliguria.

[U.S. Boxed Warning]: Based on human data, ACE inhibitors can cause injury and death to the developing fetus when used in the second and third trimesters. ACE inhibitors should be discontinued as soon as possible once pregnancy is detected.

Lactation Excretion in breast milk unknown/not recommended

Contraindications Hypersensitivity to lisinopril or any component of the formulation; angioedema related to previous treatment with an ACE inhibitor; patients with idiopathic or hereditary angioedema

Warnings/Precautions Anaphylactic reactions may occur rarely with ACE inhibitors. At any time during treatment (especially following first dose), angioedema may occur rarely with ACE inhibitors; it may involve the head and neck (potentially compromising airway) or the intestine (presenting with abdominal pain). African-Americans may be at an increased risk. Prolonged frequent monitoring may be required especially if tongue, glottis, or larynx are involved as they are associated with airway obstruction. Patients with a history of airway surgery may have a higher risk of airway obstruction. Aggressive early and appropriate management is critical. Use in patients with idiopathic or hereditary angioedema or previous angioedema associated with ACE inhibitor therapy is contraindicated. Severe anaphylactoid reactions may be seen during hemodialysis (eg, CVVHD) with high-flux dialysis membranes (eg, AN69), and rarely, during low density lipoprotein apheresis with dextran sulfate cellulose. Rare cases of anaphylactoid reactions have been reported in patients undergoing sensitization treatment with hymenoptera (bee, wasp) venom while receiving ACE inhibitors.

Symptomatic hypotension with or without syncope can occur with ACE inhibitors (usually with the first several doses); effects are most often observed in volume depleted patients; correct volume depletion prior to initiation; close monitoring of patient is required especially with initial dosing and dosing increases; blood pressure must be lowered at a rate appropriate for the patient's clinical condition. Initiation of therapy in patients with ischemic heart disease or cerebrovascular disease warrants close observation due to the potential consequences posed by falling blood pressure (eg, MI, stroke). Use with caution in hypertrophic cardiomyopathy with outflow tract obstruction, severe aortic stenosis, or before, during, or immediately after major surgery. **[U.S. Boxed Warning]: Based on human data, ACEIs can cause injury and death to the developing fetus when used in the second and third trimesters. ACEIs should be discontinued as soon as possible once pregnancy is detected.**

Hyperkalemia may occur with ACE inhibitors; risk factors include renal dysfunction, diabetes mellitus, concomitant use of potassium-sparing diuretics, potassium supplements, and/or potassium-containing salts. Use cautiously, if at all, with these agents and monitor potassium closely. Cough may occur with ACE inhibitors. Other causes of cough should be considered (eg, pulmonary congestion in patients with heart failure) and excluded prior to discontinuation.

May be associated with deterioration of renal function and/or increases in serum creatinine, particularly in patients with low renal blood flow (eg, renal artery stenosis, heart failure) whose glomerular filtration rate (GFR) is dependent on efferent arteriolar vasoconstriction by angiotensin II; deterioration may result in oliguria, acute renal failure, and progressive azotemia. Small increases in serum creatinine may occur following initiation; consider discontinuation only in patients with progressive and/or significant deterioration in renal function. Use with caution in patients with unstented unilateral/bilateral renal artery stenosis. When unstented bilateral renal artery stenosis is present, use is generally avoided due to the elevated risk of deterioration in renal function unless possible benefits outweigh risks. Concurrent use of angiotensin receptor blockers may increase the risk of clinically-significant adverse events (eg, renal dysfunction, hyperkalemia).

Rare toxicities associated with ACE inhibitors include cholestatic jaundice (which may progress to fulminant hepatic necrosis), agranulocytosis, neutropenia, or leukopenia with myeloid hypoplasia. Patients with collagen vascular diseases (especially with concomitant renal impairment) or renal impairment alone may be at increased risk for hematologic toxicity; periodically monitor CBC with differential in these patients. Safety and efficacy have not been established in children <6 years of age or children with a Cl_{cr} ≤30 mL/minute.

Adverse Reactions Note: Frequency ranges include data from hypertension and heart failure trials. Higher rates of adverse reactions have generally been noted in patients with CHF. However, the frequency of adverse effects associated with placebo is also increased in this population.

1% to 10%:

- Cardiovascular: Orthostatic effects (1%), hypotension (1% to 4%)
- Central nervous system: Headache (4% to 6%), dizziness (5% to 12%), fatigue (3%)
- Dermatologic: Rash (1% to 2%)
- Endocrine & metabolic: Hyperkalemia (2% to 5%)
- Gastrointestinal: Diarrhea (3% to 4%), nausea (2%), vomiting (1%), abdominal pain (2%)
- Genitourinary: Impotence (1%)
- Hematologic: Decreased hemoglobin (small)
- Neuromuscular & skeletal: Chest pain (3%), weakness (1%)
- Renal: BUN increased (2%); deterioration in renal function (in patients with bilateral renal artery stenosis or hypovolemia); serum creatinine increased (often transient)
- Respiratory: Cough (4% to 9%), upper respiratory infection (1% to 2%)

<1% (Limited to important or life-threatening): Acute renal failure, alopecia, anaphylactoid reactions, angioedema, anuria, arrhythmia, arthralgia, arthritis, asthma, ataxia, azotemia, bilirubin increased, bone marrow suppression, bronchospasm, cardiac arrest, cutaneous pseudolymphoma, decreased libido, gout, hemolytic anemia, hepatic necrosis, hepatitis, hyponatremia, leukopenia, jaundice (cholestatic), MI, mood changes, neutropenia, olfactory disturbance, oliguria, orthostatic hypotension, pancreatitis, paresthesia, pemphigus, peripheral neuropathy, photosensitivity, pleural effusion, pulmonary embolism, pulmonary infiltrates, SIADH, Stevens-Johnson syndrome, stroke, syncope, systemic lupus erythematosus, thrombocytopenia, TIA, toxic epidermal necrolysis, transaminases increased, tremor, urticaria, vasculitis, vertigo, vision loss, volume overload, weight gain/loss, wheezing, xerostomia

Drug Interactions

Metabolism/Transport Effects None known.

Avoid Concomitant Use There are no known interactions where it is recommended to avoid concomitant use.

Increased Effect/Toxicity

Lisinopril may increase the levels/effects of: Allopurinol; Amifostine; Antihypertensives; AzaTHIOprine; CycloSPORINE; CycloSPORINE (Systemic); Ferric Gluconate; Gold Sodium Thiomalate; Hypotensive Agents; Iron Dextran Complex; Lithium; Nonsteroidal Anti-Inflammatory Agents; RiTUXimab; Sodium Phosphates

The levels/effects of Lisinopril may be increased by: Alfuzosin; Angiotensin II Receptor Blockers; Diazoxide; DPP-IV Inhibitors; Eplerenone; Everolimus; Herbs (Hypotensive Properties); Loop Diuretics; MAO Inhibitors; Pentoxifylline; Phosphodiesterase 5 Inhibitors; Potassium Salts; Potassium-Sparing Diuretics; Prostacyclin Analogues; Sirolimus; Temsirolimus; Thiazide Diuretics; TiZANidine; Tolvaptan; Trimethoprim

Decreased Effect

The levels/effects of Lisinopril may be decreased by: Antacids; Aprotinin; Herbs (Hypertensive Properties); Icatibant; Lanthanum; Methylphenidate; Nonsteroidal Anti-Inflammatory Agents; Salicylates; Yohimbine

Ethanol/Nutrition/Herb Interactions

Food: Potassium-containing salt substitutes may increase risk of hyperkalemia.

Herb/Nutraceutical: Avoid bayberry, blue cohosh, cayenne, ephedra, ginger, ginseng (American), kola, licorice (may worsen hypertension). Avoid black cohosh, California poppy, coleus, golden seal, hawthorn, mistletoe, periwinkle, quinine, shepherd's purse (may have increased antihypertensive effect).

Mechanism of Action Competitive inhibitor of angiotensin-converting enzyme (ACE); prevents conversion of angiotensin I to angiotensin II, a potent vasoconstrictor; results in lower levels of angiotensin II which causes an increase in plasma renin activity and a reduction in aldosterone secretion; a CNS mechanism may also be involved in hypotensive effect as angiotensin II increases adrenergic outflow from CNS; vasoactive kallikreins may be decreased in conversion to active hormones by ACE inhibitors, thus reducing blood pressure

Pharmacodynamics/Kinetics

Onset of action: 1 hour

Peak effect: Hypotensive: Oral: ~6 hours

Duration: 24 hours

Absorption: Well absorbed; unaffected by food

Protein binding: 25%

Metabolism: Not metabolized

Bioavailability: Decreased with NYHA Class II-IV heart failure

Half-life elimination: 11-12 hours

Time to peak: ~7 hours

Excretion: Primarily urine (as unchanged drug)

Dosage Oral:

Heart failure: Adults: Initial: 2.5-5 mg once daily; then increase by no more than 10 mg increments at intervals no less than 2 weeks to a maximum daily dose of 40 mg. Usual maintenance: 5-40 mg/day as a single dose. Target dose: 20-40 mg once daily (ACC/AHA 2009 Heart Failure Guidelines)

Note: If patient has hyponatremia (serum sodium <130 mEq/L) or renal impairment (Cl_{cr} <30 mL/minute or creatinine >3 mg/dL), then initial dose should be 2.5 mg/day

Hypertension:

Children ≥6 years: Initial: 0.07 mg/kg once daily (up to 5 mg); increase dose at 1- to 2-week intervals; doses >0.61 mg/kg or >40 mg have not been evaluated.

Adults: Usual dosage range (JNC 7): 10-40 mg/day

Not maintained on diuretic: Initial: 10 mg/day

Maintained on diuretic: Initial: 5 mg/day

Note: Antihypertensive effect may diminish toward the end of the dosing interval especially with doses of 10 mg/day. An increased dose may aid in extending the duration of antihypertensive effect. Doses up to 80 mg/day have been used, but do not appear to give greater effect.

Patients taking diuretics should have them discontinued 2-3 days prior to initiating lisinopril if possible. Restart diuretic after blood pressure is stable if needed. If diuretic cannot be discontinued prior to therapy, begin with 5 mg with close supervision until stable blood pressure. In patients with hyponatremia (<130 mEq/L), start dose at 2.5 mg/day

Elderly: Consider lower initial doses (eg, 2.5-5 mg/day) and titrate to response (Aronow, 2011)

Acute myocardial infarction (within 24 hours in hemodynamically stable patients): Adults: 5 mg immediately, then 5 mg at 24 hours, 10 mg at 48 hours, and 10 mg every day thereafter for 6 weeks. Patients should continue to receive standard treatments such as thrombolytics, aspirin, and beta-blockers.

Dosing adjustment in renal impairment:

Heart failure: Adults: Cl_{cr} <30 mL/minute or creatinine >3 mg/dL: Initial: 2.5 mg/day

Hypertension:

Adults: Initial doses should be modified and upward titration should be cautious, based on response (maximum: 40 mg/day)

Cl_{cr} >30 mL/minute: Initial: 10 mg/day

Cl_{cr} 10-30 mL/minute: Initial: 5 mg/day

Hemodialysis: Initial: 2.5 mg/day; dialyzable (50%)

Children: Use in not recommended in pediatric patients with GFR <30 mL/minute/1.73 m^2

Dietary Considerations Use potassium-containing salt substitutes cautiously in patients with diabetes, patients with renal dysfunction, or those maintained on potassium supplements or potassium-sparing diuretics.

Administration Watch for hypotensive effects within 1-3 hours of first dose or new higher dose.

Monitoring Parameters BUN, serum creatinine, renal function, WBC, and potassium; if patient has collagen vascular disease and/or renal impairment, periodically monitor CBC with differential

Test Interactions May cause false-positive results in urine acetone determinations using sodium nitroprusside reagent

Dosage Forms Excipient information presented when available (limited, particularly for generics); consult specific product labeling.

Tablet, oral: 2.5 mg, 5 mg, 10 mg, 20 mg, 30 mg, 40 mg

Prinivil®: 5 mg, 10 mg, 20 mg [scored]

Zestril®: 2.5 mg

Zestril®: 5 mg [scored]

Zestril®: 10 mg, 20 mg, 30 mg, 40 mg

Extemporaneous Preparations A 1 mg/mL lisinopril oral suspension may be made with tablets and a 1:1 mixture of Ora-Plus® and Ora-Sweet®. Crush ten 10 mg tablets in a mortar and reduce to a fine powder. Add small portions of the vehicle and mix to a uniform paste; mix while adding the vehicle in incremental proportions to **almost** 100 mL; transfer to a graduated cylinder; rinse mortar with vehicle, and add quantity of vehicle sufficient to make 100 mL. Store in amber plastic prescription bottles; label "shake well". Stable for 13 weeks at room temperature or refrigerated (Nahata, 2004).

A 1 mg/mL lisinopril oral suspension also be made with tablets, methylcellulose 1% with parabens, and simple syrup NF. Crush ten 10 mg tablets in a mortar and reduce to a fine powder. Add 7.7 mL of methylcellulose gel and mix to a uniform paste; mix while adding the simple syrup in incremental proportions to **almost** 100 mL; transfer to a graduated cylinder; rinse mortar with vehicle, and add quantity of vehicle sufficient to make 100 mL. Store in amber plastic prescription bottles; label "shake well". Stable for 13 weeks refrigerated or 8 weeks at room temperature (Nahata, 2004).

A 2 mg/mL lisinopril syrup may be made with powder (Sigma Chemical Company, St. Louis, MO) and simple syrup. Dissolve 1 g of lisinopril powder in 30 mL of distilled water. Mix while adding simple syrup in incremental proportions in a quantity sufficient to make 500 mL. Label "shake well" and "refrigerate". Stable for 30 days when stored in amber plastic prescription bottles at room temperature or refrigerated. **Note:** Although no visual evidence of microbial growth was observed, the authors recommend refrigeration to inhibit microbial growth (Webster, 1997).

Nahata MC and Morosco RS, "Stability of Lisinopril in Two Liquid Dosage Forms," *Ann Pharmacother*, 2004, 38(3):396-9.

Prinivil® prescribing information, Merck & Co, Inc, Whitehouse Station, NJ, 2008.

Thompson KC, Zhao Z, Mazakas JM, et al, "Characterization of an Extemporaneous Liquid Formulation of Lisinopril," *Am J Health Syst Pharm*, 2003, 60(1):69-74.

Webster AA, English BA, and Rose DJ, "The Stability of Lisinopril as an Extemporaneous Syrup," *Intr J Pharmaceut Compound*, 1997, 1:352-3.

Zestril® prescribing information, AstraZeneca Pharmaceuticals, Wilmington, DE, 2007.

Lisinopril and Hydrochlorothiazide

(lyse IN oh pril & hye droe klor oh THYE a zide)

Brand Names: U.S. Prinzide®; Zestoretic®

Brand Names: Canada Apo-Lisinopril®/Hctz; Mylan-Lisinopril/Hctz; Novo-Lisinopril/Hctz; Prinzide®; Sandoz-Lisinopril/Hctz; Teva-Lisinopril/Hctz (Type P); Teva-Lisinopril/Hctz (Type Z); Zestoretic®

Index Terms Hydrochlorothiazide and Lisinopril

Pharmacologic Category Angiotensin-Converting Enzyme (ACE) Inhibitor; Diuretic, Thiazide

Use Treatment of hypertension

Pregnancy Risk Factor C/D (2nd and 3rd trimesters)

Dosage Adults: Oral: Dosage is individualized; see each component for appropriate dosing suggestions; doses >80 mg/day lisinopril or >50 mg/day hydrochlorothiazide are not recommended.

Additional Information Complete prescribing information for this medication should be consulted for additional detail.

Dosage Forms Excipient information presented when available (limited, particularly for generics); consult specific product labeling.

Tablet, oral: 10/12.5: Lisinopril 10 mg and hydrochlorothiazide 12.5 mg; 20/12.5: Lisinopril 20 mg and hydrochlorothiazide 12.5 mg; 20/25: Lisinopril 20 mg and hydrochlorothiazide 25 mg

- Prinzide®:
  - 10/12.5: Lisinopril 10 mg and hydrochlorothiazide 12.5 mg
  - 20/12.5: Lisinopril 20 mg and hydrochlorothiazide 12.5 mg
- Zestoretic®:
  - 10/12.5: Lisinopril 10 mg and hydrochlorothiazide 12.5 mg
  - 20/12.5: Lisinopril 20 mg and hydrochlorothiazide 12.5 mg
  - 20/25: Lisinopril 20 mg and hydrochlorothiazide 25 mg

◆ **Lispro Insulin** *see* Insulin Lispro *on page 905*

◆ **Lithane™ (Can)** *see* Lithium *on page 1023*

Lithium (LITH ee um)

Brand Names: U.S. Lithobid®

Brand Names: Canada Apo-Lithium® Carbonate; Apo-Lithium® Carbonate SR; Carbolith™; Duralith®; Euro-Lithium; Lithane™; Lithmax; PHL-Lithium Carbonate; PMS-Lithium Carbonate; PMS-Lithium Citrate

Index Terms Eskalith; Lithium Carbonate; Lithium Citrate

Pharmacologic Category Antimanic Agent

Use Management of bipolar disorders; treatment of mania in individuals with bipolar disorder (maintenance treatment prevents or diminishes intensity of subsequent episodes)

Unlabeled Use Potential augmenting agent for antidepressants; aggression, post-traumatic stress disorder, conduct disorder in children

Pregnancy Risk Factor D

Pregnancy Considerations Cardiac malformations in the infant, including Ebstein's anomaly, are associated with use of lithium during the first trimester of pregnancy. Nontoxic effects to the newborn include shallow respiration, hypotonia, lethargy, cyanosis, diabetes insipidus, thyroid depression, and nontoxic goiter when lithium is used near term. Efforts should be made to avoid lithium use during the first trimester; if an alternative therapy is not appropriate, the lowest possible dose of lithium should be used throughout the pregnancy. Fetal echocardiography and ultrasound to screen for anomalies should be conducted between 16-20 weeks of gestation. Lithium levels should be monitored in the mother and may need to be adjusted following delivery.

Lactation Enters breast milk/contraindicated

Contraindications Hypersensitivity to lithium or any component of the formulation; avoid use in patients with severe cardiovascular or renal disease, or with severe debilitation, dehydration, or sodium depletion; pregnancy

Warnings/Precautions [U.S. Boxed Warning]: Lithium toxicity is closely related to serum levels and can occur at therapeutic doses; serum lithium determinations are required to monitor therapy. Use with caution in patients with thyroid disease, mild-moderate renal impairment, or mild-moderate cardiovascular disease. Use caution in patients receiving medications which alter sodium excretion (eg, diuretics, ACE inhibitors, NSAIDs), or in patients with significant fluid loss (protracted sweating, diarrhea, or prolonged fever); temporary reduction or cessation of therapy may be warranted. Some elderly patients may be extremely sensitive to the effects of lithium, see Dosage and Reference Range. Chronic therapy results in diminished renal concentrating ability (nephrogenic DI); this is usually reversible when lithium is discontinued. Changes in renal function should be monitored, and re-evaluation of treatment may be necessary. Use caution in patients at risk of suicide (suicidal thoughts or behavior).

Use with caution in patients receiving neuroleptic medications - a syndrome resembling NMS has been associated with concurrent therapy. Lithium may impair the patient's alertness, affecting the ability to operate machinery or driving a vehicle. Neuromuscular-blocking agents should be administered with caution; the response may be prolonged.

Higher serum concentrations may be required and tolerated during an acute manic phase; however, the tolerance decreases when symptoms subside. Normal fluid and salt intake must be maintained during therapy.

Adverse Reactions Frequency not defined.

Cardiovascular: Cardiac arrhythmia, hypotension, sinus node dysfunction, flattened or inverted T waves (reversible), edema, bradycardia, syncope

Central nervous system: Blackout spells, coma, confusion, dizziness, dystonia, fatigue, headache, lethargy, pseudotumor cerebri, psychomotor retardation, restlessness, sedation, seizure, slowed intellectual functioning, slurred speech, stupor, tics, vertigo

Dermatologic: Dry or thinning of hair, folliculitis, alopecia, exacerbation of psoriasis, rash

Endocrine & metabolic: Euthyroid goiter and/or hypothyroidism, hyperthyroidism, hyperglycemia, diabetes insipidus

Gastrointestinal: Polydipsia, anorexia, nausea, vomiting, diarrhea, xerostomia, metallic taste, weight gain, salivary gland swelling, excessive salivation

Genitourinary: Incontinence, polyuria, glycosuria, oliguria, albuminuria

Hematologic: Leukocytosis

Neuromuscular & skeletal: Tremor, muscle hyperirritability, ataxia, choreoathetoid movements, hyperactive deep tendon reflexes, myasthenia gravis (rare)

Ocular: Nystagmus, blurred vision, transient scotoma

Miscellaneous: Coldness and painful discoloration of fingers and toes

Postmarketing and/or case reports: Drug-induced Brugada syndrome

Drug Interactions

Metabolism/Transport Effects None known.

Avoid Concomitant Use There are no known interactions where it is recommended to avoid concomitant use. ▶

Increased Effect/Toxicity

Lithium may increase the levels/effects of: Antipsychotics; Metoclopramide; Neuromuscular-Blocking Agents; Serotonin Modulators; Tricyclic Antidepressants

The levels/effects of Lithium may be increased by: ACE Inhibitors; Angiotensin II Receptor Blockers; Antipsychotics; Calcium Channel Blockers (Nondihydropyridine); CarBAMazepine; Desmopressin; Fosphenytoin; Loop Diuretics; MAO Inhibitors; Methyldopa; Nonsteroidal Anti-Inflammatory Agents; Phenytoin; Potassium Iodide; Selective Serotonin Reuptake Inhibitors; Thiazide Diuretics; Topiramate

Decreased Effect

Lithium may decrease the levels/effects of: Amphetamines; Antipsychotics; Desmopressin

The levels/effects of Lithium may be decreased by: Calcitonin; Calcium Polystyrene Sulfonate; Carbonic Anhydrase Inhibitors; Loop Diuretics; Sodium Bicarbonate; Sodium Chloride; Sodium Polystyrene Sulfonate; Theophylline Derivatives

Ethanol/Nutrition/Herb Interactions Food: Limit caffeine.

Mechanism of Action Alters cation transport across cell membrane in nerve and muscle cells and influences reuptake of serotonin and/or norepinephrine; second messenger systems involving the phosphatidylinositol cycle are inhibited; postsynaptic D2 receptor supersensitivity is inhibited

Pharmacodynamics/Kinetics

Absorption: Rapid and complete

Distribution: V_d: Initial: 0.3-0.4 L/kg; V_{dss}: 0.7-1 L/kg; crosses placenta; enters breast milk at 35% to 50% the concentrations in serum; distribution is complete in 6-10 hours

CSF, liver concentrations: 1/3 to 1/2 of serum concentration

Erythrocyte concentration: ~1/2 of serum concentration

Heart, lung, kidney, muscle concentrations: Equivalent to serum concentration

Saliva concentration: 2-3 times serum concentration

Thyroid, bone, brain tissue concentrations: Increase 50% over serum concentrations

Protein binding: Not protein bound

Metabolism: Not metabolized

Bioavailability: Not affected by food; Capsule, immediate release tablet: 95% to 100%; Extended release tablet: 60% to 90%; Syrup: 100%

Half-life elimination: 18-24 hours; can increase to more than 36 hours in elderly or with renal impairment

Time to peak, serum: Immediate release: ~0.5-2 hours; extended release: 4-12 hours; syrup: 15-60 minutes

Excretion: Urine (90% to 98% as unchanged drug); sweat (4% to 5%); feces (1%)

Clearance: 80% of filtered lithium is reabsorbed in the proximal convoluted tubules; therefore, clearance approximates 20% of GFR or 20-40 mL/minute

Dosage Oral: Monitor serum concentrations and clinical response (efficacy and toxicity) to determine proper dose

Children 6-12 years:

Bipolar disorder (unlabeled use): 15-60 mg/kg/day in 3-4 divided doses; dose not to exceed usual adult dosage

Conduct disorder (unlabeled use): 15-30 mg/kg/day in 3-4 divided doses; dose not to exceed usual adult dosage

Adults: Bipolar disorder: 900-2400 mg/day in 3-4 divided doses or 900-1800 mg/day (extended release) in 2 divided doses

Elderly: Bipolar disorder: Initial dose: 300 mg once or twice daily; increase weekly in increments of 300 mg/day, monitoring levels; rarely need >900-1200 mg/day

Dosing adjustment in renal impairment:

Cl_{cr} 10-50 mL/minute: Administer 50% to 75% of normal dose

Cl_{cr} <10 mL/minute: Administer 25% to 50% of normal dose

Hemodialysis: Dialyzable (50% to 100%); 4-7 times more efficient than peritoneal dialysis

Dietary Considerations May be taken with meals to avoid GI upset; maintain adequate fluid intake.

Administration Administer with meals to decrease GI upset. Extended release tablets must be swallowed whole; do not crush or chew.

Monitoring Parameters Serum lithium every 4-5 days during initial therapy; draw lithium serum concentrations 8-12 hours postdose; renal, thyroid, and cardiovascular function; fluid status; serum electrolytes; CBC with differential, urinalysis; monitor for signs of toxicity; beta-hCG pregnancy test for all females not known to be sterile

Reference Range Levels should be obtained twice weekly until both patient's clinical status and levels are stable then levels may be obtained every 1-3 months

Timing of serum samples: Draw trough just before next dose (8-12 hours after previous dose)

Therapeutic levels:

Acute mania: 0.6-1.2 mEq/L (SI: 0.6-1.2 mmol/L)

Protection against future episodes in most patients with bipolar disorder: 0.8-1 mEq/L (SI: 0.8-1.0 mmol/L); a higher rate of relapse is described in subjects who are maintained at <0.4 mEq/L (SI: 0.4 mmol/L)

Elderly patients can usually be maintained at lower end of therapeutic range (0.6-0.8 mEq/L)

Toxic concentration: >1.5 mEq/L (SI: >2 mmol/L)

Adverse effect levels:

GI complaints/tremor: 1.5-2 mEq/L

Confusion/somnolence: 2-2.5 mEq/L

Seizures/death: >2.5 mEq/L

Dosage Forms Excipient information presented when available (limited, particularly for generics); consult specific product labeling. [DSC] = Discontinued product

Capsule, oral, as carbonate: 150 mg, 300 mg, 600 mg

Solution, oral, as citrate: 300 mg/5 mL (5 mL, 473 mL [DSC], 500 mL) [equivalent to amount of lithium in lithium carbonate]

Tablet, oral, as carbonate: 300 mg, 600 mg

Tablet, extended release, oral, as carbonate: 300 mg, 450 mg

Lithobid®: 300 mg

◆ **Lithium Carbonate** *see* Lithium *on page* 1023

◆ **Lithium Citrate** *see* Lithium *on page* 1023

◆ **Lithmax (Can)** *see* Lithium *on page* 1023

◆ **Lithobid®** *see* Lithium *on page* 1023

◆ **Little Fevers™ [OTC]** *see* Acetaminophen *on page* 27

◆ **Little Noses® Saline [OTC]** *see* Sodium Chloride *on page* 1567

◆ **Little Noses® Sterile Saline Nasal Mist [OTC]** *see* Sodium Chloride *on page* 1567

◆ **Little Noses® Stuffy Nose Kit [OTC]** *see* Sodium Chloride *on page* 1567

◆ **Little Phillips'® Milk of Magnesia [OTC]** *see* Magnesium Hydroxide *on page* 1045

◆ **Little Teethers® [OTC]** *see* Benzocaine *on page* 202

◆ **Livalo®** *see* Pitavastatin *on page* 1361

◆ **Live Attenuated Influenza Vaccine** *see* Influenza Virus Vaccine (Live/Attenuated) *on page* 901

◆ **Live Smallpox Vaccine** *see* Smallpox Vaccine *on page* 1563

◆ **L-leucovorin** *see* LEVOleucovorin *on page* 1000

◆ **LM3100** *see* Plerixafor *on page* 1361

◆ **LMD®** *see* Dextran *on page 486*
◆ **10% LMD** *see* Dextran *on page 486*
◆ **L-methylfolate, Methylcobalamin, and N-acetylcysteine** *see* Methylfolate, Methylcobalamin, and Acetylcysteine *on page 1106*
◆ **LNg 20** *see* Levonorgestrel *on page 1001*
◆ **Locoid®** *see* Hydrocortisone (Topical) *on page 841*
◆ **Locoid Lipocream®** *see* Hydrocortisone (Topical) *on page 841*
◆ **Lodine** *see* Etodolac *on page 666*
◆ **Lodosyn®** *see* Carbidopa *on page 284*

Lodoxamide (loe DOKS a mide)

Brand Names: U.S. Alomide®
Brand Names: Canada Alomide®
Index Terms Lodoxamide Tromethamine
Pharmacologic Category Mast Cell Stabilizer
Use Treatment of vernal keratoconjunctivitis, vernal conjunctivitis, and vernal keratitis
Pregnancy Risk Factor B
Dosage Ophthalmic: Children >2 years and Adults: Instill 1-2 drops in eye(s) 4 times/day for up to 3 months
Additional Information Complete prescribing information for this medication should be consulted for additional detail.
Dosage Forms Excipient information presented when available (limited, particularly for generics); consult specific product labeling.
Solution, ophthalmic [drops]:
Alomide®: 0.1% (10 mL) [contains benzalkonium chloride]

◆ **Lodoxamide Tromethamine** *see* Lodoxamide *on page 1025*
◆ **Lodrane® 24 [DSC]** *see* Brompheniramine *on page 237*
◆ **Loestrin™ 1.5/30 (Can)** *see* Ethinyl Estradiol and Norethindrone *on page 660*
◆ **Loestrin® 21 1.5/30** *see* Ethinyl Estradiol and Norethindrone *on page 660*
◆ **Loestrin® 21 1/20** *see* Ethinyl Estradiol and Norethindrone *on page 660*
◆ **Loestrin® 24 Fe** *see* Ethinyl Estradiol and Norethindrone *on page 660*
◆ **Loestrin® Fe 1.5/30** *see* Ethinyl Estradiol and Norethindrone *on page 660*
◆ **Loestrin® Fe 1/20** *see* Ethinyl Estradiol and Norethindrone *on page 660*
◆ **Lo-Femenal 21 (Can)** *see* Ethinyl Estradiol and Norgestrel *on page 664*
◆ **Lofibra®** *see* Fenofibrate *on page 693*
◆ **LoHist [OTC]** *see* Chlorpheniramine and Phenylephrine *on page 345*
◆ **LoHist-12 [DSC]** *see* Brompheniramine *on page 237*
◆ **LoHist-D** *see* Chlorpheniramine and Pseudoephedrine *on page 346*
◆ **L-OHP** *see* Oxaliplatin *on page 1257*
◆ **LoKara™** *see* Desonide *on page 479*
◆ **Lo Loestrin™ Fe** *see* Ethinyl Estradiol and Norethindrone *on page 660*
◆ **Lomine (Can)** *see* Dicyclomine *on page 499*
◆ **Lomotil®** *see* Diphenoxylate and Atropine *on page 519*

Lomustine (loe MUS teen)

Brand Names: U.S. CeeNU®
Brand Names: Canada CeeNU®
Index Terms CCNU; Lomustinum
Pharmacologic Category Antineoplastic Agent; Antineoplastic Agent, Alkylating Agent; Antineoplastic Agent, Alkylating Agent (Nitrosourea)
Use Treatment of primary and metastatic brain tumors (after surgery and/or radiation therapy); treatment of relapsed or refractory Hodgkin's disease (as part of a combination chemotherapy regimen)
Unlabeled Use Treatment of gastric cancer, metastatic melanoma
Pregnancy Risk Factor D
Pregnancy Considerations Teratogenic effects and embryotoxicity have been observed in animal studies. There are no adequate and well-controlled studies in pregnant women. May cause fetal harm when administered to a pregnant woman. Women of childbearing potential should be advised to avoid pregnancy and should be advised of the potential harm to the fetus.
Lactation Enters breast milk/not recommended
Contraindications Hypersensitivity to lomustine or any component of the formulation
Warnings/Precautions Hazardous agent - use appropriate precautions for handling and disposal. **[U.S. Boxed Warnings]: Cumulative and delayed bone marrow suppression, particularly thrombocytopenia and leukopenia, commonly occur; may lead to bleeding and overwhelming infections in an already compromised patient.** Do not administer courses more frequently than every 6 weeks due to delayed myelotoxicity. Use with caution in patients with depressed platelet, leukocyte, or erythrocyte counts. Because bone marrow toxicity is cumulative, dose adjustments should be based on nadir counts from prior dose.

May cause delayed pulmonary toxicity (infiltrates and/or fibrosis); usually related to cumulative doses >1100 mg/m^2; may be delayed (has been reported up to 17 years after childhood administration in combination with radiation therapy); patients with baseline below 70% of predicted forced vital capacity or carbon monoxide diffusing capacity are in increased risk. Long-term use may be associated with the development of secondary malignancies. Reversible hepatotoxicity (transaminase, alkaline phosphatase and bilirubin elevations) has been reported; use with caution in patients with hepatic impairment. Kidney damage has been observed and azotemia, decreased kidney size and renal failure have been reported with long-term use; use with caution in patients with renal impairment; may require dosage adjustment. **[U.S. Boxed Warning]: Should be administered under the supervision of an experienced cancer chemotherapy physician.** Lomustine should only be administered as a single dose once every 6 weeks; serious errors have occurred when lomustine was inadvertently administered daily.

Adverse Reactions
>10%:
Gastrointestinal: Nausea and vomiting, (onset: 3-6 hours after oral administration; duration: <24 hours)
Hematologic: Myelosuppression (dose-limiting, delayed, cumulative); leukopenia (65%; nadir: 5-6 weeks; recovery 6-8 weeks); thrombocytopenia (nadir: 4 weeks; recovery 5-6 weeks)
Frequency not defined: Acute leukemia, alkaline phosphatase increased, alopecia, anemia, ataxia, azotemia (progressive), bilirubin increased, blindness, bone marrow dysplasia, disorientation, dysarthria, hepatotoxicity, kidney size decreased, lethargy, optic atrophy, pulmonary fibrosis, pulmonary infiltrates, renal damage, renal failure, stomatitis, transaminases increased, visual disturbances ▶

Drug Interactions

Metabolism/Transport Effects Substrate of CYP2D6 (minor); **Note:** Assignment of Major/Minor substrate status based on clinically relevant drug interaction potential; **Inhibits** CYP2D6 (weak), CYP3A4 (weak)

Avoid Concomitant Use

Avoid concomitant use of Lomustine with any of the following: BCG; CloZAPine; Natalizumab; Pimecrolimus; Pimozide; Tacrolimus (Topical); Vaccines (Live)

Increased Effect/Toxicity

Lomustine may increase the levels/effects of: CloZAPine; Leflunomide; Natalizumab; Pimozide; Vaccines (Live)

The levels/effects of Lomustine may be increased by: Denosumab; Pimecrolimus; Roflumilast; Tacrolimus (Topical); Trastuzumab

Decreased Effect

Lomustine may decrease the levels/effects of: BCG; Coccidioidin Skin Test; Sipuleucel-T; Vaccines (Inactivated); Vaccines (Live)

The levels/effects of Lomustine may be decreased by: Echinacea; Peginterferon Alfa-2b

Ethanol/Nutrition/Herb Interactions Ethanol: Avoid ethanol (due to GI irritation).

Stability Store at room temperature of 25°C (77°F); excursions permitted to 15°C to 30°C (59°F to 86°F).

Mechanism of Action Inhibits DNA and RNA synthesis via carbamylation of DNA polymerase, alkylation of DNA, and alteration of RNA, proteins, and enzymes

Pharmacodynamics/Kinetics

Duration: Marrow recovery: ~5-8 weeks

Absorption: Complete

Distribution: Crosses blood-brain barrier to a greater degree than BCNU; CNS concentrations are ≥50% of plasma concentrations

Metabolism: Rapidly hepatic via hydroxylation producing at least two active metabolites; enterohepatically recycled

Half-life elimination: Parent drug: 16-24 hours; Active metabolite: 16-48 hours

Time to peak, serum: Active metabolite: ~3 hours

Excretion: Urine (~50%, as metabolites); feces (<5%); expired air (<10%)

Dosage Note: Repeat courses should only be administered after adequate recovery of leukocytes to >4000/mm^3 and platelets to >100,000/mm^3. Details concerning dosage in combination regimens should also be consulted. Oral: Children and Adults: Brain tumors, Hodgkin's lymphoma: 130 mg/m^2 as a single dose once every 6 weeks (dosage reductions may be recommended for combination chemotherapy regimens)

Compromised marrow function: Reduce dose to 100 mg/m^2 as a single dose once every 6 weeks

Dosing adjustment (based on nadir) for subsequent cycles:

Leukocytes >3000/mm^3, platelets >75,000/mm^3: No adjustment required

Leukocytes 2000-2999/mm^3, platelets 25,000-74,999/mm^3: Administer 70% of prior dose

Leukocytes <2000/mm^3, platelets <25,000/mm^3: Administer 50% of prior dose

Dosage adjustment in renal impairment: The FDA-approved labeling does not contain renal dosing adjustment guidelines. The following guidelines have been used by some clinicians:

Aronoff, 2007: Adults:

Cl_{cr} 10-50 mL/minute: Administer 75% of dose

Cl_{cr} <10 mL/minute: Administer 25% to 50% of dose

Hemodialysis: Supplemental dose is not necessary

Continuous ambulatory peritoneal dialysis (CAPD): Administer 25% to 50% of dose

Kintzel, 1995:

Cl_{cr} 46-60 mL/minute: Administer 75% of normal dose

Cl_{cr} 31-45 mL/minute: Administer 70% of normal dose

Cl_{cr} ≤30 mL/minute: Avoid use

Dosage adjustment in hepatic impairment: The FDA-approved labeling does not contain hepatic adjustment guidelines; lomustine is hepatically metabolized and caution should be used in patients with hepatic dysfunction.

Dietary Considerations Should be taken with fluids on an empty stomach; no food or drink for 2 hours after administration to decrease nausea.

Administration Oral: Administer with fluids on an empty stomach; no food or drink for 2 hours after administration. Administering on an empty stomach will reduce the incidence of nausea and vomiting. Standard antiemetics may be administered if needed. Varying strengths of capsules may be required to obtain necessary dose.

Do not break capsules; use appropriate precautions (eg, gloves) when handling; avoid exposure to broken capsules.

Monitoring Parameters CBC with differential and platelet count (for at least 6 weeks after dose), hepatic and renal function tests (periodic), pulmonary function tests (baseline and periodic)

Dosage Forms Excipient information presented when available (limited, particularly for generics); consult specific product labeling.

Capsule, oral:

CeeNU®: 10 mg, 40 mg, 100 mg

◆ **Lomustinum** *see* Lomustine *on page 1025*

◆ **Longastatin** *see* Octreotide *on page 1226*

◆ **Loniten® (Can)** *see* Minoxidil (Systemic) *on page 1139*

◆ **Lo Ovral** *see* Ethinyl Estradiol and Norgestrel *on page 664*

◆ **Lo/Ovral®-28** *see* Ethinyl Estradiol and Norgestrel *on page 664*

◆ **Loperacap (Can)** *see* Loperamide *on page 1026*

Loperamide (loe PER a mide)

Brand Names: U.S. Anti-Diarrheal [OTC]; Diamode [OTC]; Imodium® A-D for children [OTC]; Imodium® A-D [OTC]

Brand Names: Canada Apo-Loperamide®; Diarr-Eze; Dom-Loperamide; Imodium®; Loperacap; Novo-Loperamide; PMS-Loperamine; Rhoxal-loperamide; Rho®-Loperamine; Riva-Loperamide; Sandoz-Loperamide

Index Terms Loperamide Hydrochloride

Pharmacologic Category Antidiarrheal

Use Treatment of chronic diarrhea associated with inflammatory bowel disease; acute nonspecific diarrhea; increased volume of ileostomy discharge

OTC labeling: Control of symptoms of diarrhea, including Traveler's diarrhea

Unlabeled Use Cancer treatment-induced diarrhea (eg, irinotecan induced); chronic diarrhea caused by bowel resection

Pregnancy Risk Factor C

Pregnancy Considerations Teratogenic effects were not observed in animal studies.

Lactation Enters breast milk/not recommended.

Contraindications Hypersensitivity to loperamide or any component of the formulation; abdominal pain without diarrhea; children <2 years

Avoid use as primary therapy in acute dysentery, acute ulcerative colitis, bacterial enterocolitis, pseudomembranous colitis

Warnings/Precautions Rare cases of anaphylaxis and anaphylactic shock have been reported. Should not be used if diarrhea is accompanied by high fever or blood in stool. Use caution in young children as response may be variable because of dehydration. Concurrent fluid and electrolyte replacement is often necessary in all age groups depending upon severity of diarrhea. Should not be used when inhibition of peristalsis is undesirable or dangerous. Discontinue if constipation, abdominal pain, or ileus develop. Use caution in treatment of AIDS patients; stop therapy at the sign of abdominal distention. Cases of toxic megacolon have occurred in this population. Loperamide is a symptom-directed treatment; if an underlying diagnosis is made, other disease-specific treatment may be indicated. Use caution in patients with hepatic impairment because of reduced first-pass metabolism; monitor for signs of CNS toxicity.

OTC labeling: If diarrhea lasts longer than 2 days, patient should stop taking loperamide and consult healthcare provider.

Adverse Reactions 1% to 10%:

Central nervous system: Dizziness (1%)

Gastrointestinal: Constipation (2% to 5%), abdominal cramping (<1% to 3%), nausea (<1% to 3%)

Postmarketing and/or case reports: Abdominal distention, abdominal pain, allergic reactions, anaphylactic shock, anaphylactoid reactions, angioedema, bullous eruption (rare), drowsiness, dry mouth, dyspepsia, erythema multiforme (rare), fatigue, flatulence, paralytic ileus, megacolon, pruritus, rash, Stevens-Johnson syndrome, toxic epidermal necrolysis, toxic megacolon, urinary retention, urticaria, vomiting

Drug Interactions

Metabolism/Transport Effects **Substrate** of P-glycoprotein

Avoid Concomitant Use There are no known interactions where it is recommended to avoid concomitant use.

Increased Effect/Toxicity

The levels/effects of Loperamide may be increased by: P-glycoprotein/ABCB1 Inhibitors

Decreased Effect

The levels/effects of Loperamide may be decreased by: P-glycoprotein/ABCB1 Inducers

Stability Store at 15°C to 25°C (59°F to 77°F).

Mechanism of Action Acts directly on circular and longitudinal intestinal muscles, through the opioid receptor, to inhibit peristalsis and prolong transit time; reduces fecal volume, increases viscosity, and diminishes fluid and electrolyte loss; demonstrates antisecretory activity. Loperamide increases tone on the anal sphincter

Pharmacodynamics/Kinetics

Absorption: Poor

Distribution: Poor penetration into brain; low amounts enter breast milk

Metabolism: Hepatic via oxidative N-demethylation

Half-life elimination: 7-14 hours

Time to peak, plasma: Liquid: 2.5 hours; Capsule: 5 hours

Excretion: Urine and feces (1% as metabolites, 30% to 40% as unchanged drug)

Dosage Oral:

Children:

Acute diarrhea: Initial doses (in first 24 hours):

2-5 years (13-20 kg): 1 mg 3 times/day

6-8 years (20-30 kg): 2 mg twice daily

8-12 years (>30 kg): 2 mg 3 times/day

Maintenance: After initial dosing, 0.1 mg/kg doses after each loose stool, but not exceeding initial dosage

Traveler's diarrhea:

6-8 years: 2 mg after first loose stool, followed by 1 mg after each subsequent stool (maximum dose: 4 mg/day)

9-11 years: 2 mg after first loose stool, followed by 1 mg after each subsequent stool (maximum dose: 6 mg/day)

≥12 years: See adult dosing.

Adults:

Acute diarrhea: Initial: 4 mg, followed by 2 mg after each loose stool, up to 16 mg/day

Chronic diarrhea: Initial: Follow acute diarrhea; maintenance dose should be slowly titrated downward to minimum required to control symptoms (typically, 4-8 mg/day in divided doses)

Traveler's diarrhea: Initial: 4 mg after first loose stool, followed by 2 mg after each subsequent stool (maximum dose: 8 mg/day)

Irinotecan-induced diarrhea (unlabeled use): 4 mg after first loose or frequent bowel movement, then 2 mg every 2 hours until 12 hours have passed without a bowel movement. If diarrhea recurs, then repeat administration

Dosage adjustment in hepatic impairment: No specific guidelines available.

Dietary Considerations Some products may contain sodium.

Dosage Forms Excipient information presented when available (limited, particularly for generics); consult specific product labeling.

Caplet, oral, as hydrochloride: 2 mg

Anti-Diarrheal: 2 mg

Diamode: 2 mg

Imodium® A-D: 2 mg [scored]

Capsule, oral, as hydrochloride: 2 mg

Liquid, oral, as hydrochloride: 1 mg/5 mL (118 mL, 120 mL)

Anti-Diarrheal: 1 mg/5 mL (120 mL)

Imodium® A-D: 1 mg/5 mL (60 mL, 120 mL) [contains benzoic acid, ethanol 0.5%, sodium benzoate; cherry-mint flavor]

Imodium® A-D: 1 mg/7.5 mL (120 mL) [contains sodium 10 mg/30 mL, sodium benzoate; creamy-mint flavor]

Imodium® A-D for children: 1 mg/7.5 mL (120 mL) [contains sodium 16 mg/30 mL, sodium benzoate; creamy-mint flavor]

Solution, oral, as hydrochloride: 1 mg/5 mL (5 mL, 10 mL)

Loperamide and Simethicone

(loe PER a mide & sye METH i kone)

Brand Names: U.S. Imodium® Multi-Symptom Relief [OTC]

Brand Names: Canada Imodium® Advanced Multi-Symptom

Index Terms Simethicone and Loperamide Hydrochloride

Pharmacologic Category Antidiarrheal; Antiflatulent

Use Control of symptoms of diarrhea and gas (bloating, pressure, and cramps)

Dosage Oral: Acute diarrhea (weight-based dosing is preferred):

Children:

6-8 years (48-59 lbs): 1 caplet or tablet after first loose stool, followed by 1/2 caplet/tablet with each subsequent loose stool (maximum: 2 caplets or tablets/24 hours)

9-11 years (60-95 lbs): 1 caplet or tablet after first loose stool, followed by 1/2 caplet or tablet with each subsequent loose stool (maximum: 3 caplets or tablets/24 hours)

Children >12 years and Adults: One caplet or tablet after first loose stool, followed by 1 caplet or tablet with each subsequent loose stool (maximum: 4 caplets or tablets/24 hours)

Additional Information Complete prescribing information for this medication should be consulted for additional detail.

Dosage Forms Excipient information presented when available (limited, particularly for generics); consult specific product labeling.

Caplet:

Imodium® Multi-Symptom Relief: Loperamide hydrochloride 2 mg and simethicone 125 mg [contains calcium 65 mg/caplet, sodium 4 mg/caplet]

Tablet, chewable:

Imodium® Multi-Symptom Relief: Loperamide hydrochloride 2 mg and simethicone 125 mg [contains calcium 50 mg/tablet; mint flavor]

◆ **Loperamide Hydrochloride** *see* Loperamide *on page 1026*

◆ **Lopid®** *see* Gemfibrozil *on page 785*

Lopinavir and Ritonavir

(loe PIN a veer & rit ON uh veer)

Brand Names: U.S. Kaletra®

Brand Names: Canada Kaletra®

Index Terms Ritonavir and Lopinavir

Pharmacologic Category Antiretroviral Agent, Protease Inhibitor

Additional Appendix Information

Management of Healthcare Worker Exposures to HBV, HCV, and HIV *on page 1935*

Perinatal HIV Guidelines *on page 1946*

Use Treatment of HIV infection in combination with other antiretroviral agents

Pregnancy Risk Factor C

Pregnancy Considerations Adverse events were not seen in animal reproduction studies, except at doses which were also maternally toxic. Lopinavir/ritonavir crosses the placenta; however, based on information collected by the Antiretroviral Pregnancy Registry, an increased risk of teratogenic effects has not been observed in humans. The DHHS Perinatal HIV Guidelines consider lopinavir/ritonavir to be the preferred protease inhibitor for use in antiretroviral-naive pregnant women. Due to a decrease in bioavailability, a dose increase is suggested during the second and third trimesters of pregnancy, especially in PI-experienced women. Monitor virologic response (and lopinavir serum concentrations if available) if the standard dose is used. Once-daily dosing is not recommended during pregnancy. A small increased risk of preterm birth has been associated with maternal use of protease inhibitor-based combination antiretroviral (ARV) therapy during pregnancy; however, the benefits of use generally outweigh this risk and protease inhibitors (PIs) should not be withheld if otherwise recommended. Hyperglycemia, new onset of diabetes mellitus, or diabetic ketoacidosis have been reported with PIs; it is not clear if pregnancy increases this risk.

Regardless of CD4 count or HIV RNA copy number, all HIV-infected pregnant women should receive a combination antepartum ARV drug regimen; this includes women who require therapy for their own health, as well as women who do not yet require therapy for their own health. ARV therapy should be started as soon as possible if required for the woman's health or immediately after the first trimester if not needed for the mothers health (although earlier initiation may be considered). Long-term follow-up is recommended for all infants exposed to ARV medications.

Healthcare providers are encouraged to enroll pregnant women exposed to antiretroviral medications in the Antiretroviral Pregnancy Registry (1-800-258-4263 or www.-APRegistry.com). Healthcare providers caring for HIV-infected women and their infants may contact the National Perinatal HIV Hotline (888-448-8765) for clinical consultation (DHHS [perinatal], 2011).

Lactation Excretion in breast milk unknown/contraindicated

Medication Guide Available Yes

Contraindications Hypersensitivity (eg, Stevens-Johnson syndrome, erythema multiforme, toxic epidermal necrolysis) to lopinavir, ritonavir, or any component of the formulation; coadministration with medications highly dependent upon CYP3A4 for clearance for which increased levels are associated with serious and/or life-threatening events; coadministration with alfuzosin, cisapride, ergot alkaloids (eg, dihydroergotamine, ergonovine, ergotamine, methylergonovine), lovastatin, midazolam (oral), pimozide, rifampin, sildenafil (when used for pulmonary arterial hypertension [Revatio®]), simvastatin, St John's wort, triazolam

Once-daily dosing: Patients with ≥3 lopinavir-resistance-associated substitutions (L10F/I/R/V, K20M/N/R, L24I, L33F, M36I, I47V, G48V, I54L/T/V, V82A/C/F/S/T, and I84V); those receiving amprenavir, efavirenz, nevirapine, or nelfinavir, carbamazepine, phenobarbital, phenytoin, or in children <18 years of age

Warnings/Precautions Use with caution in patients taking strong CYP3A4 inhibitors, moderate or strong CYP3A4 inducers and major CYP3A4 substrates; contraindicated with certain CYP3A4 substrates and inducers; consider alternative agents that avoid or lessen the potential for CYP-mediated interactions. Do not coadminister colchicine in patient with renal or hepatic impairment; Avoid concurrent use with salmeterol.

Cases of pancreatitis, some fatal, have been associated with lopinavir/ritonavir; use caution in patients with a history of pancreatitis. Patients with signs or symptoms of pancreatitis should be evaluated and therapy suspended as clinically appropriate. May alter cardiac conduction and prolong the QT_c and/or PR interval; second and third degree AV block and torsade de pointes have been observed. Use with caution in patients with underlying structural heart disease, preexisting conduction system abnormalities, ischemic heart disease or cardiomyopathies. Avoid use in combination with QT_c- or PR-interval prolonging drugs or in patients with hypokalemia or congenital long QT syndrome.

Changes in glucose tolerance, hyperglycemia, exacerbation of diabetes, DKA, and new-onset diabetes mellitus have been reported in patients receiving protease inhibitors. May cause hepatitis or exacerbate pre-existing hepatic dysfunction; use with caution in patients with hepatitis B or C and in hepatic disease; patients with hepatitis or elevations in transaminases prior to the start of therapy may be at increased risk for further increases in transaminases or hepatic dysfunction (rare fatalities reported postmarketing). Large increases in total cholesterol and triglycerides have been reported; screening should be done prior to therapy and periodically throughout treatment. Increased bleeding may be seen in patients with hemophilia A or B who are taking protease inhibitors. Redistribution or accumulation of body fat has been observed in patients using antiretroviral therapy. An inflammatory response to indolent or residual opportunistic infections (referred to as immune reconstitution syndrome) has occurred with the use of combination retroviral therapy, including Kaletra®; further evaluation and treatment may be required. The oral solution is highly concentrated and contains large amounts of alcohol. Healthcare providers should pay special attention to accurate calculation, measurement, and administration of dose. Overdose in a child may lead to lethal ethanol or propylene glycol toxicity. Once-daily dosing is not recommended in patients with ≥3 lopinavir-resistance-associated substitutions; those receiving amprenavir, efavirenz, nevirapine, or nelfinavir, carbamazepine, phenobarbital, phenytoin, or in children <18 years of age. Safety, efficacy, and pharmacokinetic profiles of lopinavir and ritonavir have not been established for neonates <14 days of age. Neonates <14 days of age, particularly preterm neonates, are at risk for developing propylene glycol toxicity with use of the lopinavir/ritonavir oral solution. Oral solution contains ethanol and propylene glycol; ethanol competitively inhibits propylene glycol metabolism. Postmarketing reports in preterm neonates following use of the oral solution include cardiotoxicity (complete AV block, bradycardia, cardiomyopathy), lactic acidosis, CNS depression,respiratory complications, acute renal failure, and death. The oral solution should not be used in the immediate postnatal period, including full term neonates age <14 days or preterm neonates until 14 days after their due date, unless the infant is closely monitored and benefits clearly outweigh risk.

Adverse Reactions Data presented for short- and long-term combination antiretroviral therapy in both protease inhibitor experienced and naïve patients.

>10%:
- Dermatologic: Rash (children 12%; adults ≤5%)
- Endocrine & metabolic: Hypercholesterolemia (3% to 39%), triglycerides increased (3% to 36%)
- Gastrointestinal: Diarrhea (7% to 28%; greater with once-daily dosing), abnormal taste/taste perversion (children 22%; adults <2%), vomiting (children 21%; adults 2% to 6%), nausea (5% to 16%), abdominal pain (1% to 11%)
- Hepatic: GGT increased (10% to 29%), ALT increased (grade 3/4: 1% to 11%)

>2% to 10%:
- Cardiovascular: Vasodilation (≤3%)
- Central nervous system: Headache (2% to 6%), insomnia (≤3%)
- Endocrine & metabolic: Hyperglycemia (≤5%), hyperuricemia (≤5%), sodium decreased or increased (children 3%),
- Gastrointestinal: Amylase increased (3% to 8%), dyspepsia (≤6%), lipase increased (3% to 5%), flatulence (1% to 4%), weight loss (≤3%)
- Hematologic: Platelets decreased (grade 3/4: 4% children), neutropenia (grade 3/4: 1% to 5%)
- Hepatic: AST increased (grade 3/4: 2% to 10%), bilirubin increased (children 3%; adults 1%)
- Neuromuscular & skeletal: Weakness (≤9%)

≤2% (Limited to important or life-threatening): Abdominal distension, abnormal dreams, abnormal ejaculation, abnormal thinking, abnormal vision, acne, agitation, allergic reaction, alopecia, amnesia, anemia, anorexia, anxiety, apathy, appetite increased/decreased, arthralgia, asthma, ataxia, atrial fibrillation, atrioventricular block, AV block (second and third degree), avitaminosis, back pain, bacterial infection, benign neoplasm, body fat redistribution, bone necrosis, bradyarrhythmia, breast enlargement, bronchitis, cellulitis, cerebral infarction, chest pain, chills, cholangitis, cholecystitis, confusion, constipation, cough, creatinine clearance decreased, Cushing's syndrome, cyst, deep vein thrombosis, dehydration, depression, diabetes mellitus, dizziness, dry skin, dyskinesia, dysphagia, dyspnea, eczema, edema, emotional lability, encephalopathy, enteritis, enterocolitis, eructation, erythema multiforme, esophagitis, exfoliative dermatitis, extrapyramidal symptoms, facial edema, facial paralysis, fatigue, fatty deposits, fecal incontinence, fever, flu-like syndrome, folliculitis, furunculosis, gastritis, gastroenteritis, GERD, glucose intolerance, gynecomastia, hemorrhagic colitis, hemorrhoids, hepatic dysfunction, hepatitis, hepatomegaly, hyperacusis, hyperhidrosis, hypertension, hypertonia, hypertrophy, hypogonadism (males), hypothyroidism, immune reconstitution syndrome, impotence, inorganic phosphorus decreased, jaundice, lactic acidosis, leukopenia, libido decreased, liver tenderness, lung edema, lymphadenopathy, maculopapular rash, malaise, MI, migraine, mouth ulceration, myalgia, neoplasm, nephritis, nervousness, neuropathy, obesity, otitis media, palpitation, pancreatitis, paresthesia, periodontitis, peripheral edema, peripheral neuropathy, pharyngitis, postural hypotension, propylene glycol toxicity (preterm neonates [includes cardiomyopathy, lactic acidosis, acute renal failure, respiratory complications]), PR prolongation, pruritus, QT prolongation, rhinitis, seborrhea, seizure, sialadenitis, sinusitis, skin discoloration, skin ulcer, somnolence, splenomegaly, Stevens-Johnson syndrome, stomatitis, striae, thrombophlebitis, tinnitus, torsade de pointes, tremor, vasculitis, vertigo, viral infection, weight gain, xerostomia

Drug Interactions

Metabolism/Transport Effects Refer to individual components.

Avoid Concomitant Use

Avoid concomitant use of Lopinavir and Ritonavir with any of the following: Alfuzosin; Amiodarone; Cisapride; Conivaptan; Crizotinib; Darunavir; Disulfiram; Dronedarone; Eplerenone; Ergot Derivatives; Etravirine; Everolimus; Flecainide; Fluticasone (Nasal); Fluticasone (Oral Inhalation); Halofantrine; Lapatinib; Lovastatin; Lurasidone; Midazolam; Nilotinib; Nisoldipine; Pimozide; Propafenone; QuiNIDine; QuiNINE; Ranolazine; Rifampin; Rivaroxaban; RomiDEPsin; Salmeterol; Silodosin; Simvastatin; St Johns Wort; Tamsulosin; Telaprevir; Thioridazine; Ticagrelor; Tolvaptan; Topotecan; Toremifene; Triazolam; Voriconazole

Increased Effect/Toxicity

Lopinavir and Ritonavir may increase the levels/effects of: Alfuzosin; Almotriptan; Alosetron; ALPRAZolam; Amiodarone; Antifungal Agents (Azole Derivatives, Systemic); ARIPiprazole; Atomoxetine; Bortezomib; Bosentan; Brentuximab Vedotin; Brinzolamide; Budesonide (Nasal); Budesonide (Systemic, Oral Inhalation); Calcium Channel Blockers (Dihydropyridine); Calcium Channel Blockers (Nondihydropyridine); CarBAMazepine; Ciclesonide; Cisapride; Clarithromycin; Clorazepate; Colchicine; Conivaptan; Corticosteroids (Orally Inhaled); Crizotinib; CycloSPORINE; CycloSPORINE (Systemic); CYP2C8 Substrates; CYP2D6 Substrates; CYP3A4 Substrates; Dabigatran Etexilate; Diazepam; Dienogest; Digoxin; Dronabinol; Dronedarone; Dutasteride; Enfuvirtide; Eplerenone; Ergot Derivatives; Estazolam; Everolimus; FentaNYL; Fesoterodine; Flecainide; Flurazepam; Fluticasone (Nasal); Fluticasone (Oral Inhalation); Fusidic Acid; GuanFACINE; Halofantrine; HMG-CoA Reductase Inhibitors; Iloperidone; Ixabepilone; Lapatinib; Linagliptin; Lovastatin; Lumefantrine; Lurasidone; Maraviroc; Meperidine; MethylPREDNISolone; Midazolam; Nebivolol; Nefazodone; Nelfinavir; Nilotinib; Nisoldipine; Paricalcitol; Pazopanib; P-glycoprotein/ABCB1 Substrates; Pimecrolimus; Pimozide; PrednisoLONE; PredniSONE; Propafenone; Protease Inhibitors; QuiNIDine; QuiNINE; Ranolazine; Rifabutin; Rilpivirine; Rivaroxaban; RomiDEPsin; Ruxolitinib; Salmeterol; Saxagliptin; Sildenafil; Silodosin; Simvastatin; Sirolimus; SORAfenib; Tacrolimus; Tacrolimus (Systemic); Tacrolimus (Topical); Tadalafil; Tamsulosin; Telaprevir; Temsirolimus; Tenofovir; Tetrabenazine; Thioridazine; Ticagrelor; Tolterodine; Tolvaptan; Topotecan; Toremifene; TraZODone; Treprostinil; Triazolam; Tricyclic Antidepressants; Vardenafil; Vemurafenib; Vilazodone; VinBLAStine; VinCRIStine; Zuclopenthixol

The levels/effects of Lopinavir and Ritonavir may be increased by: Antifungal Agents (Azole Derivatives, Systemic); Clarithromycin; CycloSPORINE; CycloSPORINE (Systemic); Delavirdine; Disulfiram; Efavirenz; Enfuvirtide; Etravirine; Fusidic Acid; MetroNIDAZOLE (Topical);

P-glycoprotein/ABCB1 Inhibitors; QuiNINE; Rifabutin; Rifampin

Decreased Effect

Lopinavir and Ritonavir may decrease the levels/effects of: Abacavir; ARIPiprazole; Atovaquone; BuPROPion; Clarithromycin; Codeine; Contraceptives (Estrogens); CYP2C19 Substrates; Darunavir; Deferasirox; Delavirdine; Didanosine; Divalproex; Etravirine; Fosphenytoin; LamoTRIgine; Meperidine; Methadone; Phenytoin; Prasugrel; Telaprevir; Theophylline Derivatives; Ticagrelor; TraMADol; Valproic Acid; Voriconazole; Warfarin; Zidovudine

The levels/effects of Lopinavir and Ritonavir may be decreased by: Antacids; CarBAMazepine; CYP3A4 Inducers (Strong); Cyproterone; Efavirenz; Fosamprenavir; Fosphenytoin; Garlic; Nelfinavir; Nevirapine; Peginterferon Alfa-2b; P-glycoprotein/ABCB1 Inducers; PHENobarbital; Phenytoin; Rifampin; St Johns Wort; Tenofovir; Tocilizumab

Ethanol/Nutrition/Herb Interactions

Food: Moderate- to high-fat meals increase the C_{max} and AUC of lopinavir/ritonavir oral solution; no significant changes observed with oral tablets.

Herb/Nutraceutical: St John's wort may decrease levels of protease inhibitors and lead to possible resistance; concurrent use is contraindicated.

Stability

Oral solution: Store at 2°C to 8°C (36°F to 46°F). Avoid exposure to excessive heat. If stored at room temperature (25°C or 77°F), use within 2 months.

Tablet: Store at USP controlled room temperature of 20°C to 25°C (68°F to 77°F). Exposure to high humidity outside of the original container for >2 weeks is not recommended.

Mechanism of Action A coformulation of lopinavir and ritonavir. The lopinavir component binds to the site of HIV-1 protease activity and inhibits the cleavage of viral Gag-Pol polyprotein precursors into individual functional proteins required for infectious HIV. This results in the formation of immature, noninfectious viral particles. The ritonavir component inhibits the CYP3A metabolism of lopinavir, allowing increased plasma levels of lopinavir.

Pharmacodynamics/Kinetics

Ritonavir: See Ritonavir monograph.

Lopinavir:

Protein binding: 98% to 99%; decreased with mild-to-moderate hepatic dysfunction

Metabolism: Hepatic via CYP3A4; 13 metabolites identified

Half-life elimination: 5-6 hours

Time to peak, plasma: ~4 hours

Excretion: Feces (83%, 20% as unchanged drug); urine (10%; <3% as unchanged drug)

Dosage Oral:

Children: Dosage based on weight or body surface area (BSA), **presented based on lopinavir component** (maximum dose: Lopinavir 400 mg/ritonavir 100 mg).

14 days to 6 months: 16 mg/kg or 300 mg/m^2 twice daily; **Note:** Should not be administered to neonates age <14 days (defined as postmenstrual age of 42 weeks [first day of mother's last menstrual period to birth plus postnatal age]) and a postnatal age of at least 14 days

6 months to 18 years: **Note:** FDA-approved dose is approximately equivalent to lopinavir 230 mg/m^2 per dose.

<15 kg: 12 mg/kg twice daily

15-40 kg: 10 mg/kg twice daily

>40 kg: Lopinavir 400 mg/ritonavir 100 mg twice daily

Adults:

Twice-daily dosing:

Therapy-naive or therapy-experienced: Lopinavir 400 mg/ritonavir 100 mg twice daily. **Note:** This regimen is preferred (with zidovudine and lamivudine **or** zidovudine and emtricitabine) in pregnant therapy-naive patients (DHHS, 2011)

Therapy-naive or therapy-experienced patients receiving efavirenz, fosamprenavir, nelfinavir, nevirapine: Lopinavir 500 mg/ritonavir 125 mg tablets twice daily **or** lopinavir 533 mg/ritonavir 133 mg solution twice daily

Once-daily dosing: Therapy-naive or experienced patients with <3 lopinavir resistance-associated substitutions: Lopinavir 800 mg/ritonavir 200 mg once daily

Elderly: Initial studies did not include enough elderly patients to determine effects based on age. Use with caution due to possible decreased hepatic, renal, and cardiac function.

Dosage adjustment for combination therapy with efavirenz, fosamprenavir, nelfinavir, or nevirapine:

Twice-daily dosing:

Children 14 days to 6 months: Combination therapy with these agents is not recommended due to lack of data.

Children 6 months to 18 years: Solution or tablet (**based on mg of lopinavir component**): FDA-approved dose is approximately equivalent to lopinavir 300 mg/m^2 per dose:

<15 kg: 13 mg/kg twice daily (**Note:** Tablets are not recommended)

15-45 kg: 11 mg/kg twice daily

>45 kg: Refer to adult dosing

Children >45 kg and Adults: Therapy-naive and therapy-experienced patients:

Solution: Lopinavir 533 mg/ritonavir 133 mg (6.5 mL) twice daily

Tablet: Lopinavir 500 mg/ritonavir 125 mg twice daily

Once-daily dosing:

Children: Not recommended

Adults: Not recommended in those receiving efavirenz, fosamprenavir, nevirapine, nelfinavir, carbamazepine, phenobarbital, phenytoin.

Dosage adjustments for concomitant therapy: Adults:

Combination therapy with bosentan:

Coadministration of bosentan in patients currently receiving lopinavir/ritonavir: For patients receiving lopinavir/ritonavir for at least 10 days, begin with bosentan 62.5 mg once daily or every other day based on tolerability

Coadministration of lopinavir/ritonavir in patients currently receiving bosentan: Discontinue bosentan 36 hours prior to the initiation of lopinavir/ritonavir. After at least 10 days of lopinavir/ritonavir, resume bosentan 62.5 mg once daily or every other day based on tolerability

Combination therapy with colchicine:

Familial Mediterranean fever (FMF): Maximum colchicine dose: 0.6 mg/day (0.3 mg twice daily)

Gout prophylaxis:

If original colchicine dose is 0.6 mg twice daily, adjust dose to 0.3 mg once daily

If original colchicine dose is 0.6 mg once daily, adjust dose to 0.3 mg every other day

Gout flare treatment: Initial: Colchicine 0.6 mg, followed in 1 hour by a single dose of 0.3 mg; do not repeat for at least 3 days

Coadministration with phosphodiesterase-5 enzyme (PDE-5) inhibitor:

Pulmonary arterial hypertension: Lopinavir/ritonavir coadministered with tadalafil:

Patient receiving lopinavir/ritonavir for at least 1 week: Initiate tadalafil at 20 mg once daily; increase to 40 mg once daily based on individual tolerability

Patient receiving tadalafil when initiating lopinavir/ritonavir: Stop tadalafil at least 24 hours prior to starting lopinavir/ritonavir. After at least 1 week following the initiation of lopinavir/ritonavir, resume tadalafil at 20 mg once daily; increase to 40 mg once daily based on individual tolerability.

Erectile dysfunction: Lopinavir/ritonavir coadministered with:

Sildenafil (Viagra®): Maximum sildenafil dose: 25 mg in a 48-hour period

Tadalafil (Cialis®): Maximum tadalafil dose: 10 mg in a 72-hour period

Vardenafil: Maximum vardenafil dose: 2.5 mg in a 72-hour period

Dosage adjustment in renal impairment: Has not been studied in patients with renal impairment; however, a decrease in clearance is not expected

Hemodialysis: Do not use once-daily dosing in hemodialysis patients (DHHS, 2011)

Dosage adjustment in hepatic impairment: Use caution in hepatic impairment (metabolized primarily by the liver)

Mild-to-moderate impairment: Lopinavir AUC may be increased ~30%

Severe impairment: No data available

Dietary Considerations Solution should be taken with food. Tablet may be taken with or without food

Administration

Solution: Administer with food; if using didanosine, take didanosine 1 hour before or 2 hours after lopinavir/ritonavir. Administer using calibrated dosing syringe.

Tablet: May be taken with or without food. Swallow whole, do not break, crush, or chew. May be taken with didanosine when taken without food. Tablets are not recommended in patients <15 kg.

Monitoring Parameters Triglycerides, cholesterol, LFTs, electrolytes, basic HIV monitoring, viral load and CD4 count, glucose

Dosage Forms Excipient information presented when available (limited, particularly for generics); consult specific product labeling.

Solution, oral:

Kaletra®: Lopinavir 80 mg and ritonavir 20 mg per mL (160 mL) [contains alcohol 42.4%]

Tablet:

Kaletra®:

Lopinavir 100 mg and ritonavir 25 mg

Lopinavir 200 mg and ritonavir 50 mg

◆ **Lopressor®** *see* Metoprolol *on page 1117*

◆ **Loprox®** *see* Ciclopirox *on page 356*

◆ **Loradamed [OTC]** *see* Loratadine *on page 1031*

Loratadine (lor AT a deen)

Brand Names: U.S. Alavert® Allergy 24 Hour [OTC]; Alavert® Children's Allergy [OTC]; Claritin® 24 Hour Allergy [OTC]; Claritin® Children's Allergy [OTC]; Claritin® Liqui-Gels® 24 Hour Allergy [OTC]; Claritin® RediTabs® 24 Hour Allergy [OTC]; Loradamed [OTC]; Tavist® ND Allergy [OTC]

Brand Names: Canada Apo-Loratadine®; Claritin®; Claritin® Kids

Pharmacologic Category Histamine H_1 Antagonist; Histamine H_1 Antagonist, Second Generation; Piperidine Derivative

Use Relief of nasal and non-nasal symptoms of seasonal allergic rhinitis; treatment of chronic idiopathic urticaria

Pregnancy Considerations Maternal use of loratadine has not been associated with an increased risk of major malformations. The use of antihistamines for the treatment of rhinitis during pregnancy is generally considered to be safe at recommended doses. Although safety data is limited, loratadine may be the preferred second generation antihistamine for the treatment of rhinitis or urticaria during pregnancy.

Contraindications Hypersensitivity to loratadine or any component of the formulation

Warnings/Precautions Use with caution in patients with liver or renal impairment; dosage adjustment recommended. Some products may contain phenylalanine.

Adverse Reactions

Adults:

Central nervous system: Headache (12%), somnolence (8%), fatigue (4%)

Gastrointestinal: Xerostomia (3%)

Children:

Central nervous system: Nervousness (4% ages 6-12 years), fatigue (3% ages 6-12 years, 2% to 3% ages 2-5 years), malaise (2% ages 6-12 years)

Dermatologic: Rash (2% to 3% ages 2-5 years)

Gastrointestinal: Abdominal pain (2% ages 6-12 years), stomatitis (2% to 3% ages 2-5 years)

Neuromuscular & skeletal: Hyperkinesia (3% ages 6-12 years)

Ocular: Conjunctivitis (2% ages 6-12 years)

Respiratory: Wheezing (4% ages 6-12 years), dysphonia (2% ages 6-12 years), upper respiratory infection (2% ages 6-12 years), epistaxis (2% to 3% ages 2-5 years), pharyngitis (2% to 3% ages 2-5 years)

Miscellaneous: Flu-like syndrome (2% to 3% ages 2-5 years), viral infection (2% to 3% ages 2-5 years)

Adults and Children: <2% (Limited to important or life-threatening): Abnormal hepatic function, agitation, alopecia, altered lacrimation, altered micturition, altered salivation, altered taste, amnesia, anaphylaxis, angioneurotic edema, anorexia, arthralgia, back pain, blepharospasm, blurred vision, breast enlargement, breast pain, bronchospasm, chest pain, confusion, depression, dizziness, dysmenorrhea, dyspnea, erythema multiforme, hemoptysis, hepatic necrosis, hepatitis, hypotension, impaired concentration, impotence, insomnia, irritability, jaundice, menorrhagia, migraine, nausea, palpitation, paresthesia, paroniria, peripheral edema, photosensitivity, pruritus, purpura, rigors, seizure, supraventricular tachyarrhythmia, syncope, tachycardia, tremor, urinary discoloration, urticaria, thrombocytopenia, vaginitis, vertigo, vomiting, weight gain

Drug Interactions

Metabolism/Transport Effects Substrate of CYP2D6 (minor), CYP3A4 (minor), P-glycoprotein; **Note:** Assignment of Major/Minor substrate status based on clinically relevant drug interaction potential; **Inhibits** CYP2C19 (weak), CYP2C8 (weak), CYP2D6 (weak)

Avoid Concomitant Use There are no known interactions where it is recommended to avoid concomitant use.

Increased Effect/Toxicity

Loratadine may increase the levels/effects of: Alcohol (Ethyl); Anticholinergics; CNS Depressants; Methotrimeprazine; Selective Serotonin Reuptake Inhibitors

The levels/effects of Loratadine may be increased by: Amiodarone; Conivaptan; Droperidol; HydrOXYzine; Methotrimeprazine; P-glycoprotein/ABCB1 Inhibitors; Pramlintide

Decreased Effect

Loratadine may decrease the levels/effects of: Acetylcholinesterase Inhibitors (Central); Benzylpenicilloyl Polylysine; Betahistine

The levels/effects of Loratadine may be decreased by: Acetylcholinesterase Inhibitors (Central); Amphetamines; Peginterferon Alfa-2b; P-glycoprotein/ABCB1 Inducers; Tocilizumab

Ethanol/Nutrition/Herb Interactions
Ethanol: May increase CNS depression; monitor for increased effects with coadministration. Caution patients about effects.
Food: Increases bioavailability and delays peak.
Herb/Nutraceutical: St John's wort may decrease loratadine levels.

Stability Store at 2°C to 25°C (36°F to 77°F).
Rapidly-disintegrating tablets: Use within 6 months of opening foil pouch, and immediately after opening individual tablet blister. Store in a dry place.

Mechanism of Action Long-acting tricyclic antihistamine with selective peripheral histamine H_1-receptor antagonistic properties

Pharmacodynamics/Kinetics
Onset of action: 1-3 hours
Peak effect: 8-12 hours
Duration: >24 hours
Absorption: Rapid
Metabolism: Extensively hepatic via CYP2D6 and 3A4 to active metabolite
Half-life elimination: 12-15 hours
Excretion: Urine (40%) and feces (40%) as metabolites

Dosage Oral: Seasonal allergic rhinitis, chronic idiopathic urticaria:
Children 2-5 years: 5 mg once daily
Children ≥6 years and Adults: 10 mg once daily
Elderly: Peak plasma levels are increased; elimination half-life is slightly increased; specific dosing adjustments are not available

Dosage adjustment in renal impairment: Cl_{cr} ≤30 mL/minute:
Children 2-5 years: 5 mg every other day
Children ≥6 years and Adults: 10 mg every other day

Dosage adjustment in hepatic impairment: Elimination half-life increases with severity of disease
Children 2-5 years: 5 mg every other day
Children ≥6 years and Adults: 10 mg every other day

Dietary Considerations May be taken without regard to meals. Some products may contain phenylalanine and/or sodium.

Administration May be administered without regard to meals.

Test Interactions May suppress the wheal and flare reactions to skin test antigens

Dosage Forms Excipient information presented when available (limited, particularly for generics); consult specific product labeling.
Capsule, liquid gel, oral:
Claritin® Liqui-Gels® 24 Hour Allergy: 10 mg
Solution, oral: 5 mg/5 mL (120 mL)
Syrup, oral: 5 mg/5 mL (120 mL, 240 mL)
Claritin® Children's Allergy: 5 mg/5 mL (60 mL, 120 mL) [dye free, ethanol free; contains propylene glycol, sodium benzoate; fruit flavor]
Claritin® Children's Allergy: 5 mg/5 mL (60 mL, 120 mL) [dye free, ethanol free, sugar free; contains propylene glycol, sodium 6 mg/5 mL, sodium benzoate; grape flavor]
Tablet, oral: 10 mg
Alavert® Allergy 24 Hour: 10 mg [dye free, gluten free, sucrose free]
Claritin® 24 Hour Allergy: 10 mg
Loradamed: 10 mg
Tavist® ND Allergy: 10 mg
Tablet, chewable, oral:
Claritin® Children's Allergy: 5 mg [contains phenylalanine 1.4 mg/tablet; grape flavor]
Tablet, orally disintegrating, oral: 10 mg
Alavert® Allergy 24 Hour: 10 mg [dye free, gluten free, sucrose free; contains phenylalanine 8.4 mg/tablet; Citrus Burst™ flavor]
Alavert® Allergy 24 Hour: 10 mg [dye free, gluten free, sucrose free; contains phenylalanine 8.4 mg/tablet; mint flavor]
Alavert® Children's Allergy: 10 mg [dye free, gluten free, sucrose free; contains phenylalanine 8.4 mg/tablet; Citrus Burst™ flavor]
Alavert® Children's Allergy: 10 mg [dye free, gluten free, sucrose free; contains phenylalanine 8.4 mg/tablet; bubblegum flavor]
Claritin® RediTabs® 24 Hour Allergy: 10 mg [mint flavor]

Loratadine and Pseudoephedrine
(lor AT a deen & soo doe e FED rin)

Brand Names: U.S. Alavert™ Allergy and Sinus [OTC]; Claritin-D® 12 Hour Allergy & Congestion [OTC]; Claritin-D® 24 Hour Allergy & Congestion [OTC]

Brand Names: Canada Chlor-Tripolon ND®; Claritin® Extra; Claritin® Liberator

Index Terms Pseudoephedrine and Loratadine

Pharmacologic Category Alpha/Beta Agonist; Decongestant; Histamine H_1 Antagonist; Histamine H_1 Antagonist, Second Generation; Piperidine Derivative

Use Temporary relief of symptoms of seasonal allergic rhinitis, other upper respiratory allergies, or the common cold

Dosage Children ≥12 years and Adults: Oral:
Claritin-D® 12-Hour: 1 tablet every 12 hours
Alavert™ Allergy and Sinus, Claritin-D® 24-Hour: 1 tablet daily

Dosage adjustment in renal impairment: Cl_{cr} ≤30 mL/minute:
Claritin-D® 12-Hour: 1 tablet daily
Claritin-D® 24-Hour: 1 tablet every other day

Dosage adjustment in hepatic impairment: Should be avoided

Additional Information Complete prescribing information for this medication should be consulted for additional detail.

Dosage Forms Excipient information presented when available (limited, particularly for generics); consult specific product labeling.
Tablet, extended release: Loratadine 10 mg and pseudoephedrine sulfate 240 mg
Alavert™ Allergy and Sinus: Loratadine 5 mg and pseudoephedrine sulfate 120 mg
Claritin-D® 12 Hour Allergy & Congestion: Loratadine 5 mg and pseudoephedrine sulfate 120 mg [contains calcium 30 mg/tablet]
Claritin-D® 24 Hour Allergy & Congestion: Loratadine 10 mg and pseudoephedrine sulfate 240 mg [contains calcium 25 mg/tablet]

LORazepam (lor A ze pam)

Brand Names: U.S. Ativan®; Lorazepam Intensol™

Brand Names: Canada Apo-Lorazepam®; Ativan®; Dom-Lorazepam; Lorazepam Injection, USP; Novo-Lorazem; Nu-Loraz; PHL-Lorazepam; PMS-Lorazepam; PRO-Lorazepam

Pharmacologic Category Benzodiazepine

Additional Appendix Information

Beers Criteria – Potentially Inappropriate Medications for Geriatrics *on page 1973*

Benzodiazepines *on page 1882*

Status Epilepticus *on page 2010*

Use

Oral: Management of anxiety disorders or short-term (≤4 months) relief of the symptoms of anxiety, anxiety associated with depressive symptoms, or insomnia due to anxiety or transient stress

I.V.: Status epilepticus, amnesia, sedation

Unlabeled Use Ethanol detoxification; psychogenic catatonia; partial complex seizures; agitation (I.V.); antiemetic for chemotherapy; rapid tranquilization of the agitated patient

Pregnancy Risk Factor D

Pregnancy Considerations Teratogenic effects have been observed in some animal studies. Lorazepam and its metabolite cross the human placenta. Teratogenic effects in humans have been observed with some benzodiazepines (including lorazepam); however, additional studies are needed. The incidence of premature birth and low birth weights may be increased following maternal use of benzodiazepines; hypoglycemia and respiratory problems in the neonate may occur following exposure late in pregnancy. Neonatal withdrawal symptoms may occur within days to weeks after birth and "floppy infant syndrome" (which also includes withdrawal symptoms) have been reported with some benzodiazepines (including lorazepam). Elimination of lorazepam in the newborn infant is slow; following *in utero* exposure, term infants may excrete lorazepam for up to 8 days.

Lactation Enters breast milk/not recommended (AAP rates "of concern"; AAP 2001 update pending)

Contraindications Hypersensitivity to lorazepam or any component of the formulation (cross-sensitivity with other benzodiazepines may exist); acute narrow-angle glaucoma; sleep apnea (parenteral); intra-arterial injection of parenteral formulation; severe respiratory insufficiency (except during mechanical ventilation)

Warnings/Precautions Use with caution in elderly or debilitated patients, patients with hepatic disease (including alcoholics) or renal impairment. Due to increased sensitivity in the elderly, smaller doses of benzodiazepines may be safer and as effective; in this age group, avoid using doses >3 mg daily of lorazepam (Beers Criteria). Use with caution in patients with respiratory disease (COPD or sleep apnea) or limited pulmonary reserve, or impaired gag reflex. Initial doses in elderly or debilitated patients should be at the lower end of the dosing range. May worsen hepatic encephalopathy.

Causes CNS depression (dose-related) resulting in sedation, dizziness, confusion, or ataxia which may impair physical and mental capabilities. Patients must be cautioned about performing tasks which require mental alertness (eg, operating machinery or driving). Use with caution in patients receiving other CNS depressants or psychoactive agents. Effects with other sedative drugs or ethanol may be potentiated. Benzodiazepines have been associated with falls and traumatic injury and should be used with extreme caution in patients who are at risk of these events (especially the elderly).

Lorazepam may cause anterograde amnesia. Paradoxical reactions, including hyperactive or aggressive behavior have been reported with benzodiazepines, particularly in adolescent/pediatric or psychiatric patients. Does not have analgesic, antidepressant, or antipsychotic properties.

Use caution in patients with depression, particularly if suicidal risk may be present. Pre-existing depression may worsen or emerge during therapy. Not recommended for use in primary depressive or psychotic disorders. Use with caution in patients with a history of drug dependence, alcoholism, or significant personality disorders. Benzodiazepines have been associated with dependence and acute withdrawal symptoms on discontinuation or reduction in dose. Acute withdrawal, including seizures, may be precipitated after administration of flumazenil to patients receiving long-term benzodiazepine therapy.

As a hypnotic agent, should be used only after evaluation of potential causes of sleep disturbance. Failure of sleep disturbance to resolve after 7-10 days may indicate psychiatric or medical illness. A worsening of insomnia or the emergence of new abnormalities of thought or behavior may represent unrecognized psychiatric or medical illness and requires immediate and careful evaluation.

Parenteral formulation of lorazepam contains polyethylene glycol which has resulted in toxicity during high-dose and/or longer-term infusions. Parenteral formulation also contains propylene glycol (PG); may be associated with dose-related toxicity and can occur ≥48 hours after initiation of lorazepam. Limited data suggest increased risk of PG accumulation at doses of ≥6 mg/hour for 48 hours or more (Nelson, 2008). Consider monitoring for signs of toxicity which may include acute renal failure, lactic acidosis, and/or osmol gap. In high-risk patients requiring higher doses/extended treatment durations, use of enteral delivery of lorazepam tablets may be beneficial (Jacobi, 2002). Also contains benzyl alcohol; avoid in neonates.

Adverse Reactions

>10%:

Central nervous system: Sedation

Respiratory: Respiratory depression

1% to 10%:

Cardiovascular: Hypotension

Central nervous system: Akathisia, amnesia, ataxia, confusion, depression, disorientation, dizziness, headache

Dermatologic: Dermatitis, rash

Gastrointestinal: Changes in appetite, nausea, weight gain/loss

Neuromuscular & skeletal: Weakness

Ocular: Visual disturbances

Respiratory: Apnea, hyperventilation, nasal congestion

<1% or frequency not defined (Limited to important or life-threatening): Asthenia, blood dyscrasias, disinhibition, euphoria, fatigue, increased salivation, menstrual irregularities, physical and psychological dependence (with prolonged use), reflex slowing, polyethylene glycol or propylene glycol poisoning (prolonged I.V. infusion), suicidal ideation, seizure, vertigo

Drug Interactions

Metabolism/Transport Effects None known.

Avoid Concomitant Use

Avoid concomitant use of LORazepam with any of the following: OLANZapine

Increased Effect/Toxicity

LORazepam may increase the levels/effects of: Alcohol (Ethyl); CloZAPine; CNS Depressants; Fosphenytoin; Methotrimeprazine; Phenytoin; Selective Serotonin Reuptake Inhibitors

The levels/effects of LORazepam may be increased by: Divalproex; Droperidol; HydrOXYzine; Loxapine; Methotrimeprazine; OLANZapine; Probenecid; Valproic Acid

Decreased Effect

The levels/effects of LORazepam may be decreased by: Theophylline Derivatives; Yohimbine

Ethanol/Nutrition/Herb Interactions

Ethanol: May increase CNS depression; monitor for increased effects with coadministration. Caution patients about effects.

Herb/Nutraceutical: Avoid valerian, St John's wort, kava kava, gotu kola (may increase CNS depression).

Stability

I.V.: Intact vials should be refrigerated. Protect from light. Do not use discolored or precipitate-containing solutions. May be stored at room temperature for up to 3 months [data on file (Hospira Inc, 2010)]. Parenteral admixture is stable at room temperature (25°C) for 24 hours. Dilute I.V. dose with equal volume of compatible diluent (D_5W, NS, SWFI).

Infusion: Use 2 mg/mL injectable vial to prepare; there may be decreased stability when using 4 mg/mL vial. Dilute ≤1 mg/mL and mix in glass bottle. Precipitation may develop. Can also be administered undiluted via infusion.

Tablet: Store at room temperature.

Mechanism of Action Binds to stereospecific benzodiazepine receptors on the postsynaptic GABA neuron at several sites within the central nervous system, including the limbic system, reticular formation. Enhancement of the inhibitory effect of GABA on neuronal excitability results by increased neuronal membrane permeability to chloride ions. This shift in chloride ions results in hyperpolarization (a less excitable state) and stabilization.

Pharmacodynamics/Kinetics

Onset of action:

Hypnosis: I.M.: 20-30 minutes

Sedation: I.V.: 5-20 minutes

Anticonvulsant: I.V.: 5 minutes, oral: 30-60 minutes

Duration: 6-8 hours

Absorption: Oral, I.M.: Prompt

Distribution: V_d: Neonates: 0.76 L/kg, Adults: 1.3 L/kg

Protein binding: 85%; free fraction may be significantly higher in elderly

Metabolism: Hepatic to inactive compounds

Bioavailability: Oral: 90%

Half-life elimination: Neonates: 40.2 hours; Older children: 10.5 hours; Adults: 12.9 hours; Elderly: 15.9 hours; End-stage renal disease: 32-70 hours

Time to peak: Oral: 2 hours

Excretion: Urine; feces (minimal)

Dosage

Antiemetic (unlabeled use):

Children 2-15 years: I.V.: 0.05 mg/kg (up to 2 mg/dose) prior to chemotherapy

Adults: Oral, I.V. (**Note:** May be administered sublingually; not a labeled route): 0.5-2 mg every 4-6 hours as needed

Anxiety, sedation, and procedural amnesia (unlabeled in children except for oral use in children >12 years):

Infants and Children:

Oral, I.M.: Usual: 0.05 mg/kg/dose (range: 0.02-0.09 mg/kg) every 4-8 hours

I.V.: Usual: 0.05 mg/kg/dose (range: 0.02-0.09 mg/kg) every 4-8 hours; may use smaller doses (eg, 0.01-0.03 mg/kg) and repeat every 20 minutes, as needed to titrate to effect

Adults:

Oral: 1-10 mg/day in 2-3 divided doses; usual dose: 2-6 mg/day in divided doses or 1-2 mg 1 hour before procedure

I.M.: 0.05 mg/kg administered 2 hours before surgery (maximum: 4 mg/dose)

I.V.: 0.044 mg/kg 15-20 minutes before surgery (usual dose 2 mg; maximum: 4 mg/dose)

Elderly: Oral: Initial: 1-2 mg/day in divided doses; Beers Criteria: Avoid maintenance doses >3 mg/day

Insomnia: Adults: Oral: 2-4 mg at bedtime

Status epilepticus: I.V.:

Infants and Children (unlabeled): 0.05-0.1 mg/kg (maximum: 4 mg/dose) slow I.V. (maximum rate: 2 mg/minute); may repeat every 10-15 minutes as needed (Hegenbarth, 2008; Sabo-Graham, 1998)

Adults: 4 mg/dose slow I.V. (maximum rate: 2 mg/minute); may repeat in 10-15 minutes; usual maximum dose: 8 mg. May be given I.M, but I.V. preferred.

Rapid tranquilization of agitated patient (unlabeled use):

Adults: Oral, I.M.: 1-2 mg administered every 30-60 minutes; may be administered with an antipsychotic (eg, haloperidol) (Battaglia, 2005; De Fruyt, 2004)

Average total dose for tranquilization: 4-8 mg

Agitation in the ICU patient (unlabeled): Adults:

I.V.: 0.02-0.06 mg/kg every 2-6 hours or 0.01-0.1 mg/kg/hour (Jacobi, 2002)

Dosage adjustment for lorazepam with concomitant medications: *Probenecid or valproic acid:* Reduce lorazepam dose by 50%

Alcohol withdrawal syndrome (unlabeled use): Oral: 2 mg every 6 hours for 4 doses, then 1 mg every 6 hours for 8 additional doses (Mayo-Smith, 1997)

Alcohol withdrawal delirium (unlabeled use) (Mayo-Smith, 2004):

I.V.: 1-4 mg every 5-15 minutes until calm, then every hour as needed to maintain light somnolence

I.M.: 1-4 mg every 30-60 minutes until calm, then every hour as needed to maintain light somnolence

Dosage adjustment in renal impairment: I.V.: Risk of propylene glycol toxicity. Monitor closely if using for prolonged periods of time or at high doses.

Dosage adjustment in hepatic impairment: No dose reduction necessary.

Administration

I.M.: Should be administered deep into the muscle mass

I.V.: Do not exceed 2 mg/minute or 0.05 mg/kg over 2-5 minutes; dilute I.V. dose with equal volume of compatible diluent (D_5W, NS, SWFI). Avoid intra-arterial administration. Monitor I.V. site for extravasation.

Monitoring Parameters Respiratory and cardiovascular status, blood pressure, heart rate, symptoms of anxiety

Clinical signs of propylene glycol toxicity (for continuous high-dose and/or long duration intravenous use): Serum creatinine, BUN, serum lactate, osmol gap

Reference Range Therapeutic: 50-240 ng/mL (SI: 156-746 nmol/L)

Additional Information Oral doses >0.09 mg/kg produced increased ataxia without increased sedative benefit vs lower doses; preferred anxiolytic when I.M. route needed. Abrupt discontinuation after sustained use (generally >10 days) may cause withdrawal symptoms.

Dosage Forms Excipient information presented when available (limited, particularly for generics); consult specific product labeling. [DSC] = Discontinued product

Injection, solution: 2 mg/mL (1 mL, 10 mL); 4 mg/mL (1 mL, 10 mL)

Ativan®: 2 mg/mL (1 mL, 10 mL); 4 mg/mL (1 mL, 10 mL) [contains benzyl alcohol, polyethylene glycol 400, propylene glycol]

Injection, solution [preservative free]: 2 mg/mL (1 mL [DSC]); 4 mg/mL (1 mL [DSC])

Solution, oral [concentrate]: 2 mg/mL (30 mL)

Lorazepam Intensol™: 2 mg/mL (30 mL) [dye free, ethanol free, sugar free; contains propylene glycol]

Tablet, oral: 0.5 mg, 1 mg, 2 mg

Ativan®: 0.5 mg

Ativan®: 1 mg, 2 mg [scored]

Controlled Substance C-IV

Extemporaneous Preparations Note: Commercial oral solution is available (2 mg/mL)

Two different 1 mg/mL oral suspensions may be made from different generic lorazepam tablets (Mylan Pharmaceuticals or Watson Laboratories), sterile water, Ora-Sweet®, and Ora-Plus®.

Mylan tablets: Place one-hundred-eighty 2 mg tablets in a 12-ounce amber glass bottle; add 144 mL of sterile water to disperse the tablets; shake until slurry is formed. Add 108 mL Ora-Plus® in incremental proportions; then add a quantity of Ora-Sweet® sufficient to make 360 mL. Label "shake well" and "refrigerate". Stable for 91 days when stored in amber glass prescription bottles at room temperature or refrigerated (preferred).

Watson tablets: Place one-hundred-eighty 2 mg tablets in a 12-ounce amber glass bottle; add 48 mL sterile water to disperse the tablets; shake until slurry is formed. Add 156 mL of Ora-Plus® in incremental proportions; then add a quantity of Ora-Sweet® sufficient to make 360 mL. Label "shake well" and "refrigerate". Store in amber glass prescription bottles. Stable for 63 days at room temperature or 91 days refrigerated.

Lee ME, Lugo RA, Rusho WJ, et al, "Chemical Stability of Extemporaneously Prepared Lorazepam Suspension at Two Temperatures," *J Pediatr Pharmacol Ther*, 2004, 9(4):254-58.

◆ **Lorazepam Injection, USP (Can)** *see* LORazepam *on page 1032*
◆ **Lorazepam Intensol™** *see* LORazepam *on page 1032*
◆ **Lorcet® 10/650** *see* Hydrocodone and Acetaminophen *on page 837*
◆ **Lorcet® Plus** *see* Hydrocodone and Acetaminophen *on page 837*
◆ **Lortab®** *see* Hydrocodone and Acetaminophen *on page 837*
◆ **Loryna™** *see* Ethinyl Estradiol and Drospirenone *on page 654*
◆ **Lorzone™** *see* Chlorzoxazone *on page 351*

Losartan (loe SAR tan)

Brand Names: U.S. Cozaar®
Brand Names: Canada Cozaar®
Index Terms DuP 753; Losartan Potassium; MK594
Pharmacologic Category Angiotensin II Receptor Blocker
Additional Appendix Information
Angiotensin Agents *on page 1869*
Heart Failure (Systolic) *on page 1991*

Use Treatment of hypertension (HTN); treatment of diabetic nephropathy in patients with type 2 diabetes mellitus (noninsulin dependent, NIDDM) and a history of hypertension; stroke risk reduction in patients with HTN and left ventricular hypertrophy (LVH)

Unlabeled Use To slow the rate of progression of aortic-root dilation in pediatric patients with Marfan's syndrome

Pregnancy Risk Factor C (1st trimester); D (2nd and 3rd trimesters)

Pregnancy Considerations Medications which act on the renin-angiotensin system are reported to have the following fetal/neonatal effects: Hypotension, neonatal skull hypoplasia, anuria, renal failure, and death; oligohydramnios is also reported. These effects are reported to occur with exposure during the second and third trimesters. There are no adequate and well-controlled studies in pregnant women. **[U.S. Boxed Warning]: Based on human data, drugs that act on the angiotensin system can cause injury and death to the developing fetus when used in the second and third trimesters. Angiotensin receptor blockers should be discontinued as soon as possible once pregnancy is detected.**

Lactation Excretion in breast milk unknown/not recommended

Contraindications Hypersensitivity to losartan or any component of the formulation

Warnings/Precautions [U.S. Boxed Warning]: Based on human data, drugs that act on the angiotensin system can cause injury and death to the developing fetus when used in the second and third trimesters. Angiotensin receptor blockers should be discontinued as soon as possible once pregnancy is detected. Avoid use or use a much smaller dose in patients who are volume-depleted; correct depletion first. Use with caution in patients with significant aortic/mitral stenosis. May cause hyperkalemia; avoid potassium supplementation unless specifically required by healthcare provider. May be associated with deterioration of renal function and/or increases in serum creatinine, particularly in patients with low renal blood flow (eg, renal artery stenosis, heart failure) whose glomerular filtration rate (GFR) is dependent on efferent arteriolar vasoconstriction by angiotensin II. Use caution in patients with unstented unilateral/bilateral renal artery stenosis. When unstented bilateral renal artery stenosis is present, use is generally avoided due to the elevated risk of deterioration in renal function unless possible benefits outweigh risks. Use with caution with pre-existing renal insufficiency. AUCs of losartan (not the active metabolite) are about 50% greater in patients with Cl_{cr} <30 mL/minute and are doubled in hemodialysis patients. Concurrent use of ACE inhibitors may increase the risk of clinically-significant adverse events (eg, renal dysfunction, hyperkalemia).

At any time during treatment (especially following first dose), angioedema may occur rarely; may involve the head and neck (potentially compromising airway) or the intestine (presenting with abdominal pain). Patients with idiopathic or hereditary angioedema or previous angioedema associated with ACE-inhibitor therapy may be at an increased risk. Prolonged frequent monitoring may be required, especially if tongue, glottis, or larynx are involved, as they are associated with airway obstruction. Patients with a history of airway surgery may have a higher risk of airway obstruction. Aggressive early management is critical; intramuscular (I.M.) administration of epinephrine may be necessary.

When used to reduce the risk of stroke in patients with HTN and LVH, may not be effective in African-American population. Use caution with hepatic dysfunction, dose adjustment may be needed.

Adverse Reactions Note: The incidence of some adverse reactions varied based on the underlying disease state. Notations are made, where applicable, for data derived from trials conducted in diabetic nephropathy and hypertensive patients, respectively.

>10%:
Cardiovascular: Chest pain (12% diabetic nephropathy)
Central nervous system: Fatigue (14% diabetic nephropathy)
Endocrine: Hypoglycemia (14% diabetic nephropathy)
Gastrointestinal: Diarrhea (2% hypertension to 15% diabetic nephropathy)
Genitourinary: Urinary tract infection (13% diabetic nephropathy)
Hematologic: Anemia (14% diabetic nephropathy)
Neuromuscular & skeletal: Weakness (14% diabetic nephropathy), back pain (2% hypertension to 12% diabetic nephropathy)
Respiratory: Cough (≤3% to 11%; similar to placebo; incidence higher in patients with previous cough related to ACE inhibitor therapy)

1% to 10%:
- Cardiovascular: Hypotension (7% diabetic nephropathy), orthostatic hypotension (4% hypertension to 4% diabetic nephropathy), first-dose hypotension (dose related: <1% with 50 mg, 2% with 100 mg)
- Central nervous system: Dizziness (4%), hypoesthesia (5% diabetic nephropathy), fever (4% diabetic nephropathy), insomnia (1%)
- Dermatology: Cellulitis (7% diabetic nephropathy)
- Endocrine: Hyperkalemia (<1% hypertension to 7% diabetic nephropathy)
- Gastrointestinal: Gastritis (5% diabetic nephropathy), weight gain (4% diabetic nephropathy), dyspepsia (1% to 4%), abdominal pain (2%), nausea (2%)
- Neuromuscular & skeletal: Muscular weakness (7% diabetic nephropathy), knee pain (5% diabetic nephropathy), leg pain (1% to 5%), muscle cramps (1%), myalgia (1%)
- Respiratory: Bronchitis (10% diabetic nephropathy), upper respiratory infection (8%), nasal congestion (2%), sinusitis (1% hypertension to 6% diabetic nephropathy)
- Miscellaneous: Infection (5% diabetic nephropathy), flu-like syndrome (10% diabetic nephropathy)

<1% (Limited to important or life-threatening): Acute psychosis with paranoid delusions, ageusia, allergic reaction, alopecia, anaphylactic reactions, anemia, angina, angioedema, anorexia, anxiety, arrhythmia, arthralgia, arthritis, ataxia, AV block (second degree), bilirubin increased, blurred vision, bradycardia, bronchitis, BUN increased, confusion, conjunctivitis, constipation, CVA, depression, dermatitis, dysgeusia, dyspnea, ecchymosis, epistaxis, erythroderma, erythema, facial edema, fever, flatulence, flushing, gastritis, gout, hematocrit decreased, hemoglobin decreased, Henoch-Schönlein purpura, hepatitis, hyponatremia, hypotension, impotence, joint swelling, maculopapular rash, malaise, memory impairment, MI, migraine, muscle weakness, myositis, neoplasm, nervousness, orthostatic effects, pancreatitis, paresthesia, peripheral neuropathy, pharyngitis, photosensitivity, pruritus, rash, rhabdomyolysis, rhinitis, serum creatinine increased, sleep disorder, somnolence, syncope, tachycardia, taste perversion, thrombocytopenia, tinnitus, transaminases increased, tremor, urinary frequency, urticaria, vasculitis, ventricular arrhythmia, vertigo, visual acuity decreased, vomiting, xerostomia

Drug Interactions

Metabolism/Transport Effects Substrate of CYP2C9 (major), CYP3A4 (major); **Note:** Assignment of Major/Minor substrate status based on clinically relevant drug interaction potential; **Inhibits** CYP1A2 (weak), CYP2C19 (weak), CYP2C8 (moderate), CYP2C9 (moderate), CYP3A4 (weak)

Avoid Concomitant Use

Avoid concomitant use of Losartan with any of the following: Pimozide

Increased Effect/Toxicity

Losartan may increase the levels/effects of: ACE Inhibitors; Amifostine; Antihypertensives; Carvedilol; CYP2C8 Substrates; CYP2C9 Substrates; Hypoglycemic Agents; Hypotensive Agents; Lithium; Nonsteroidal Anti-Inflammatory Agents; Pimozide; Potassium-Sparing Diuretics; RiTUXimab; Sodium Phosphates

The levels/effects of Losartan may be increased by: Alfuzosin; Antifungal Agents (Azole Derivatives, Systemic); Conivaptan; CYP2C9 Inhibitors (Moderate); CYP2C9 Inhibitors (Strong); Diazoxide; Eplerenone; Fluconazole; Herbs (Hypoglycemic Properties); Herbs (Hypotensive Properties); MAO Inhibitors; Milk Thistle; Pentoxifylline; Phosphodiesterase 5 Inhibitors; Potassium Salts; Prostacyclin Analogues; Tolvaptan; Trimethoprim

Decreased Effect

The levels/effects of Losartan may be decreased by: CYP2C9 Inducers (Strong); CYP3A4 Inducers (Strong); Deferasirox; Herbs (CYP3A4 Inducers); Herbs (Hypertensive Properties); Methylphenidate; Nonsteroidal Anti-Inflammatory Agents; Peginterferon Alfa-2b; Rifamycin Derivatives; Tocilizumab; Yohimbine

Ethanol/Nutrition/Herb Interactions Herb/Nutraceutical: St John's wort may decrease levels of losartan. Avoid bayberry, blue cohosh, ginseng (American), kola, licorice (may worsen hypertension). Avoid black cohosh; california poppy; coleus; golden seal; hawthorn; mistletoe; periwinkle; quinine; shepherd's purse (may increase risk for hypotension). Hypoglycemic effects of losartan may be enhanced by alfalfa; aloe; bilberry; bitter melon; burdock; celery; damiana; fenugreek; garcinia; garlic; ginger; ginseng (American); gymnema; marshmallow; stinging nettle.

Stability Store at 15°C to 30°C (59°F to 86°F). Protect from light.

Mechanism of Action As a selective and competitive, nonpeptide angiotensin II receptor antagonist, losartan blocks the vasoconstrictor and aldosterone-secreting effects of angiotensin II; losartan interacts reversibly at the AT1 and AT2 receptors of many tissues and has slow dissociation kinetics; its affinity for the AT1 receptor is 1000 times greater than the AT2 receptor. Angiotensin II receptor antagonists may induce a more complete inhibition of the renin-angiotensin system than ACE inhibitors, they do not affect the response to bradykinin, and are less likely to be associated with nonrenin-angiotensin effects (eg, cough and angioedema). Losartan increases urinary flow rate and in addition to being natriuretic and kaliuretic, increases excretion of chloride, magnesium, uric acid, calcium, and phosphate.

Pharmacodynamics/Kinetics

Onset of action: 6 hours

Distribution: V_d: Losartan: 34 L; E-3174: 12 L; does not cross blood-brain barrier

Protein binding, plasma: High

Metabolism: Hepatic (14%) via CYP2C9 and 3A4 to active metabolite, E-3174 (40 times more potent than losartan); extensive first-pass effect

Bioavailability: 25% to 33%; AUC of E-3174 is four times greater than that of losartan

Half-life elimination: Losartan: 1.5-2 hours; E-3174: 6-9 hours

Time to peak, serum: Losartan: 1 hour; E-3174: 3-4 hours

Excretion: Urine (4% as unchanged drug, 6% as active metabolite)

- Clearance: Plasma: Losartan: 600 mL/minute; Active metabolite: 50 mL/minute

Dosage Oral:

Hypertension:

- Children 6-16 years:
  - *U.S. labeling:* 0.7 mg/kg once daily (maximum: 50 mg/day); doses >1.4 mg/kg (maximum: 100 mg) have not been studied
  - *Canadian labeling:*
    - ≥20 kg to <50 kg: 25 mg once daily (maximum: 50 mg once daily)
    - ≥50 kg: 50 mg once daily (maximum: 100 mg once daily)
- Adults: Usual starting dose: 50 mg once daily; can be administered once or twice daily with total daily doses ranging from 25-100 mg
  - Patients receiving diuretics or with intravascular volume depletion: Usual initial dose: 25 mg once daily

Aortic-root dilation with Marfan's syndrome (unlabeled use): Children 14 months to 16 years: Initial: 0.6 mg/kg/day; can be increased to a maximum of 1.4 mg/kg/day (not to exceed adult maximum of 100 mg/day)

Nephropathy in patients with type 2 diabetes and hypertension: Adults: Initial: 50 mg once daily; can be increased to 100 mg once daily based on blood pressure response

Stroke reduction (HTN with LVH): Adults: 50 mg once daily (maximum daily dose: 100 mg); may be used in combination with a thiazide diuretic

Dosing adjustment in renal impairment:

Children: Use is not recommended if GFR <30 mL/minute/1.73 m^2

Adults: No adjustment necessary.

Dosing adjustment in hepatic impairment:

Children 6-16 years:

U.S. labeling: No specific dosing recommendations are provided in the approved labeling, however it may be advisable to initiate therapy at a reduced dosage.

Canadian labeling: Use is not recommended.

Adults: Reduce the initial dose to 25 mg/day

Dietary Considerations May be taken without regard to meals. Some products may contain potassium.

Administration May be administered without regard to meals.

Monitoring Parameters Supine blood pressure, electrolytes, serum creatinine, BUN, urinalysis, symptomatic hypotension and tachycardia, CBC

Dosage Forms Excipient information presented when available (limited, particularly for generics); consult specific product labeling.

Tablet, oral, as potassium: 25 mg, 50 mg, 100 mg

Cozaar®: 25 mg [contains potassium 2.12 mg (0.054 mEq)]

Cozaar®: 50 mg [contains potassium 4.24 mg (0.108 mEq)]

Cozaar®: 100 mg [contains potassium 8.48 mg (0.216 mEq)]

Extemporaneous Preparations A 2.5 mg/mL losartan oral suspension may be made with tablets and a 1:1 mixture of Ora-Plus® and Ora-Sweet® SF. Combine 10 mL of purified water and ten losartan 50 mg tablets in an 8-ounce amber polyethylene terephthalate bottle. Shake well for at least 2 minutes. Allow concentrate to stand for 1 hour, then shake for 1 minute. Separately, prepare 190 mL of a 1:1 mixture of Ora-Plus® and Ora-Sweet® SF; add to tablet and water mixture in the bottle and shake for 1 minute. Label "shake well" and "refrigerate". Return promptly to refrigerator after each use. Stable for 4 weeks when stored in amber polyethylene terephthalate prescription bottles and refrigerated (Cozaar® prescribing information, 2008).

Cozaar® prescribing information, Merck & Co, Inc, Whitehouse Station, NJ, 2008.

Losartan and Hydrochlorothiazide

(loe SAR tan & hye droe klor oh THYE a zide)

Brand Names: U.S. Hyzaar®

Brand Names: Canada Hyzaar®; Hyzaar® DS

Index Terms Hydrochlorothiazide and Losartan

Pharmacologic Category Angiotensin II Receptor Blocker; Diuretic, Thiazide

Use Treatment of hypertension; stroke risk reduction in patients with HTN and left ventricular hypertrophy (LVH)

Pregnancy Risk Factor C/D (2nd and 3rd trimesters)

Dosage Oral: Adults: Dose is individualized (combination substituted for individual components); dose may be titrated after 2-4 weeks of therapy

Hypertension/stroke reduction in hypertension (with LVH): Usual recommended starting dose of losartan: 50 mg once daily when used as monotherapy in patients who are not volume depleted

Dosage adjustment in renal impairment: Cl_{cr} ≤30 mL/minute: Use of combination formulation not recommended

Dosage adjustment in hepatic impairment: Use is not recommended

Additional Information Complete prescribing information for this medication should be consulted for additional detail.

Dosage Forms Excipient information presented when available (limited, particularly for generics); consult specific product labeling.

Tablet: 50/12.5: Losartan potassium 50 mg and hydrochlorothiazide 12.5 mg; 100/12.5: Losartan potassium 100 mg and hydrochlorothiazide 12.5 mg; 100/25: Losartan potassium 100 mg and hydrochlorothiazide 25 mg

Hyzaar® 50/12.5: Losartan potassium 50 mg and hydrochlorothiazide 12.5 mg [contains potassium 4.24 mg (0.108 mEq)]

Hyzaar® 100/12.5: Losartan potassium 100 mg and hydrochlorothiazide 12.5 mg [contains potassium 8.48 mg (0.216 mEq)]

Hyzaar® 100/25: Losartan potassium 100 mg and hydrochlorothiazide 25 mg [contains potassium 8.48 mg (0.216 mEq)]

◆ **Losartan Potassium** *see* Losartan *on page* 1035

◆ **LoSeasonique®** *see* Ethinyl Estradiol and Levonorgestrel *on page* 656

◆ **Losec® (Can)** *see* Omeprazole *on page* 1241

◆ **Lotemax®** *see* Loteprednol *on page* 1037

◆ **Lotensin®** *see* Benazepril *on page* 197

◆ **Lotensin HCT®** *see* Benazepril and Hydrochlorothiazide *on page* 199

Loteprednol (loe te PRED nol)

Brand Names: U.S. Alrex®; Lotemax®

Brand Names: Canada Alrex®; Lotemax®

Index Terms Loteprednol Etabonate

Pharmacologic Category Corticosteroid, Ophthalmic

Use

Ointment, 0.5% (Lotemax®): Treatment of postoperative inflammation and pain following ocular surgery

Suspension, 0.2% (Alrex®): Temporary relief of signs and symptoms of seasonal allergic conjunctivitis

Suspension, 0.5% (Lotemax®): Inflammatory conditions (treatment of steroid-responsive inflammatory conditions of the palpebral and bulbar conjunctiva, cornea, and anterior segment of the globe such as allergic conjunctivitis, acne rosacea, superficial punctate keratitis, herpes zoster keratitis, iritis, cyclitis, selected infective conjunctivitis, when the inherent hazard of steroid use is accepted to obtain an advisable diminution in edema and inflammation) and treatment of postoperative inflammation following ocular surgery

Pregnancy Risk Factor C

Dosage Adults: Ophthalmic:

Ointment, 0.5% (Lotemax®): Apply ~1/2 inch ribbon into the conjunctival sac of the affected eye(s) 4 times/day beginning 24 hours after surgery and continuing throughout the first 2 weeks of the postoperative period

Suspension, 0.2% (Alrex®): Instill 1 drop into affected eye(s) 4 times/day

Suspension, 0.5% (Lotemax®):

Inflammatory conditions: Apply 1-2 drops into the conjunctival sac of the affected eye(s) 4 times/day. During the initial treatment within the first week, the dosing may be increased up to 1 drop every hour. Advise patients not to discontinue therapy prematurely. If signs and symptoms fail to improve after 2 days, re-evaluate the patient.

Postoperative inflammation: Apply 1-2 drops into the conjunctival sac of the operated eye(s) 4 times/day beginning 24 hours after surgery and continuing throughout the first 2 weeks of the postoperative period

Additional Information Complete prescribing information for this medication should be consulted for additional detail.

Product Availability

Lotemax® 0.5% ointment: FDA approved April 2011; expected availability undetermined

Lotemax® 0.5% ointment is a topical corticosteroid approved for the treatment of postoperative inflammation and pain following ocular surgery.

Dosage Forms Excipient information presented when available (limited, particularly for generics); consult specific product labeling.

Ointment, ophthalmic, as etabonate:

Lotemax®: 0.5% (3.5 g)

Suspension, ophthalmic, as etabonate [drops]:

Alrex®: 0.2% (5 mL, 10 mL) [contains benzalkonium chloride]

Lotemax®: 0.5% (2.5 mL, 5 mL, 10 mL, 15 mL) [contains benzalkonium chloride]

Loteprednol and Tobramycin

(loe te PRED nol & toe bra MYE sin)

Brand Names: U.S. Zylet®

Index Terms Loteprednol Etabonate and Tobramycin; Tobramycin and Loteprednol Etabonate

Pharmacologic Category Antibiotic/Corticosteroid, Ophthalmic

Use Treatment of steroid-responsive ocular inflammatory conditions where either a superficial bacterial ocular infection or the risk of a superficial bacterial ocular infection exists

Pregnancy Risk Factor C

Dosage Ophthalmic: Children and Adults: Instill 1-2 drops into the affected eye(s) every 4-6 hours; may increase frequency during the first 24-48 hours to every 1-2 hours. Interval should increase as signs and symptoms improve. Further evaluation should occur for use of greater than 20 mL.

Additional Information Complete prescribing information for this medication should be consulted for additional detail.

Dosage Forms Excipient information presented when available (limited, particularly for generics); consult specific product labeling.

Suspension, ophthalmic [drops]:

Zylet®: Loteprednol etabonate 0.5% and tobramycin 0.3% (2.5 mL, 5 mL, 10 mL) [contains benzalkonium chloride]

◆ **Loteprednol Etabonate** *see* Loteprednol *on page 1037*

◆ **Loteprednol Etabonate and Tobramycin** *see* Loteprednol and Tobramycin *on page 1038*

◆ **Lotrel®** *see* Amlodipine and Benazepril *on page 99*

◆ **Lotriderm® (Can)** *see* Betamethasone and Clotrimazole *on page 210*

◆ **Lotrimin AF® [OTC]** *see* Miconazole (Topical) *on page 1126*

◆ **Lotrimin® AF Athlete's Foot [OTC]** *see* Clotrimazole (Topical) *on page 399*

◆ **Lotrimin® AF for Her [OTC]** *see* Clotrimazole (Topical) *on page 399*

◆ **Lotrimin® AF Jock Itch [OTC]** *see* Clotrimazole (Topical) *on page 399*

◆ **Lotrimin® ultra™ [OTC]** *see* Butenafine *on page 255*

◆ **Lotrisone®** *see* Betamethasone and Clotrimazole *on page 210*

Lovastatin (LOE va sta tin)

Brand Names: U.S. Altoprev®; Mevacor®

Brand Names: Canada Apo-Lovastatin®; CO Lovastatin; Dom-Lovastatin; Gen-Lovastatin; Mevacor®; Mylan-Lovastatin; Novo-Lovastatin; Nu-Lovastatin; PHL-Lovastatin; PMS-Lovastatin; PRO-Lovastatin; RAN™-Lovastatin; ratio-Lovastatin; Riva-Lovastatin; Sandoz-Lovastatin

Index Terms Mevinolin; Monacolin K

Pharmacologic Category Antilipemic Agent, HMG-CoA Reductase Inhibitor

Additional Appendix Information

Hyperlipidemia Management *on page 1996*

Use

Adjunct to dietary therapy to decrease elevated serum total and LDL-cholesterol concentrations in primary hypercholesterolemia

Primary prevention of coronary artery disease (patients without symptomatic disease with average to moderately elevated total and LDL-cholesterol and below average HDL-cholesterol); slow progression of coronary atherosclerosis in patients with coronary heart disease

Adjunct to dietary therapy in adolescent patients (10-17 years of age, females >1 year postmenarche) with heterozygous familial hypercholesterolemia having LDL >189 mg/dL, **or** LDL >160 mg/dL with positive family history of premature cardiovascular disease (CVD), **or** LDL >160 mg/dL with the presence of at least two other CVD risk factors

Pregnancy Risk Factor X

Pregnancy Considerations Cholesterol biosynthesis may be important in fetal development. Contraindicated in pregnancy. Administer to women of childbearing potential only when conception is highly unlikely and patients have been informed of potential hazards.

Lactation Excretion in breast milk unknown/contraindicated

Contraindications Hypersensitivity to lovastatin or any component of the formulation; active liver disease; unexplained persistent elevations of serum transaminases; pregnancy; breast-feeding

Warnings/Precautions Secondary causes of hyperlipidemia should be ruled out prior to therapy. Liver function must be monitored by periodic laboratory assessment. Rhabdomyolysis with or without acute renal failure has occurred. Risk is dose-related and is increased with concurrent use of lipid-lowering agents which may cause rhabdomyolysis (gemfibrozil, fibric acid derivatives, or niacin at doses ≥1 g/day) or during concurrent use with potent CYP3A4 inhibitors. Avoid concurrent use of azole antifungals, macrolide antibiotics, and protease inhibitors. Use caution/limit dose with amiodarone, cyclosporine, danazol, gemfibrozil (or other fibrates), lipid-lowering doses of niacin, or verapamil. Monitor closely if used with other drugs associated with myopathy (eg, colchicine). Patients should be instructed to report unexplained muscle pain or weakness; lovastatin should be discontinued if myopathy is suspected/confirmed. The manufacturer recommends temporary discontinuation for elective major surgery, acute medical or surgical conditions, or in any patient experiencing an acute or serious condition predisposing to renal failure (eg, sepsis, hypotension, trauma, uncontrolled seizures). However, based upon current evidence, HMG-CoA reductase inhibitor therapy should be continued in the perioperative period unless risk outweighs cardioprotective benefit. Use with caution in patients with advanced age, these patients are predisposed to myopathy. Use with caution in patients who consume large amounts of ethanol or have a history of liver disease.

Adverse Reactions Percentages as reported with immediate release tablets; similar adverse reactions seen with extended release tablets.

>10%: Neuromuscular & skeletal: CPK increased (>2x normal) (11%)

1% to 10%:

- Central nervous system: Headache (2% to 3%), dizziness (≤1%)
- Dermatologic: Rash (≤1%)
- Gastrointestinal: Flatulence (4% to 5%), constipation (2% to 4%), abdominal pain (2% to 3%), diarrhea (2% to 3%), nausea (2% to 3%), dyspepsia (1% to 2%)
- Neuromuscular & skeletal: Myalgia (2% to 3%), weakness (1% to 2%), muscle cramps (≤1%)
- Ocular: Blurred vision (≤1%)

<1% (Limited to important or life-threatening): Acid regurgitation, alopecia, arthralgia, chest pain, dermatomyositis, eye irritation, insomnia, leg pain, paresthesia, pruritus, vomiting, xerostomia

Additional class-related events or case reports (not necessarily reported with lovastatin therapy): Alkaline phosphatase increased, alteration in taste, anaphylaxis, angioedema, anorexia, anxiety, arthritis, cataracts, chills, cholestatic jaundice, cirrhosis, depression, dryness of skin/mucous membranes, dyspnea, eosinophilia, erectile dysfunction, erythema multiforme, ESR increased, facial paresis, fatty liver, fever, flushing, fulminant hepatic necrosis, GGT increased, gynecomastia, hemolytic anemia, hepatitis, hepatoma, hyperbilirubinemia, hypersensitivity reaction, impaired extraocular muscle movement, impotence, interstitial lung disease, leukopenia, libido decreased, malaise, memory loss, myopathy, nail changes, nodules, ophthalmoplegia, pancreatitis, peripheral nerve palsy, peripheral neuropathy, photosensitivity, polymyalgia rheumatica, positive ANA, psychic disturbance, purpura, renal failure (secondary to rhabdomyolysis), rhabdomyolysis, skin discoloration, Stevens-Johnson syndrome, systemic lupus erythematosus-like syndrome, thrombocytopenia, thyroid dysfunction, toxic epidermal necrolysis, transaminases increased, tremor, urticaria, vasculitis, vertigo

Drug Interactions

Metabolism/Transport Effects Substrate of CYP3A4 (major), P-glycoprotein; **Note:** Assignment of Major/Minor substrate status based on clinically relevant drug interaction potential; **Inhibits** CYP2C9 (weak), CYP3A4 (weak)

Avoid Concomitant Use

Avoid concomitant use of Lovastatin with any of the following: Boceprevir; CYP3A4 Inhibitors (Strong); Erythromycin; Pimozide; Protease Inhibitors; Red Yeast Rice; Telaprevir

Increased Effect/Toxicity

Lovastatin may increase the levels/effects of: DAPTOmycin; Diltiazem; Pimozide; Trabectedin; Vitamin K Antagonists

The levels/effects of Lovastatin may be increased by: Amiodarone; Antifungal Agents (Azole Derivatives, Systemic); Boceprevir; Colchicine; CycloSPORINE; CycloSPORINE (Systemic); CYP3A4 Inhibitors (Moderate); CYP3A4 Inhibitors (Strong); Cyproterone; Danazol; Dasatinib; Diltiazem; Dronedarone; Erythromycin; Fenofibrate; Fenofibric Acid; Fluconazole; Gemfibrozil; Grapefruit Juice; Macrolide Antibiotics; Niacin; Niacinamide; P-glycoprotein/ABCB1 Inhibitors; Protease Inhibitors; QuiNINE; Red Yeast Rice; Sildenafil; Telaprevir; Ticagrelor; Verapamil

Decreased Effect

Lovastatin may decrease the levels/effects of: Lanthanum

The levels/effects of Lovastatin may be decreased by: Antacids; Bosentan; CYP3A4 Inducers (Strong); Deferasirox; Efavirenz; Etravirine; Fosphenytoin; P-glycoprotein/ABCB1 Inducers; Phenytoin; Rifamycin Derivatives; St Johns Wort; Tocilizumab

Ethanol/Nutrition/Herb Interactions

Ethanol: Avoid excessive ethanol consumption (due to potential hepatic effects).

Food: Food **decreases** the bioavailability of lovastatin extended release tablets and **increases** the bioavailability of lovastatin immediate release tablets. Lovastatin serum concentrations may be increased if taken with grapefruit juice; avoid concurrent intake of large quantities (>1 quart/day). Red yeast rice contains an estimated 2.4 mg lovastatin per 600 mg rice.

Herb/Nutraceutical: St John's wort may decrease lovastatin levels.

Stability

Tablet, immediate release: Store at 20°C to 25°C (68°F to 77°F). Protect from light

Tablet, extended release: Store between 20°C to 25°C (68°F to 77°F); excursions permitted between 15°C to 30°C (59°F to 86°F). Avoid excessive heat and humidity.

Mechanism of Action Lovastatin acts by competitively inhibiting 3-hydroxyl-3-methylglutaryl-coenzyme A (HMG-CoA) reductase, the enzyme that catalyzes the rate-limiting step in cholesterol biosynthesis

Pharmacodynamics/Kinetics

Onset of action: LDL-cholesterol reductions: 3 days

Absorption: 30%; increased with extended release tablets when taken in the fasting state

Protein binding: >95%

Metabolism: Hepatic; extensive first-pass effect; hydrolyzed to β-hydroxyacid (active)

Bioavailability: Increased with extended release tablets

Half-life elimination: 1.1-1.7 hours

Time to peak, serum: Immediate release: 2-4 hours; extended release: 12-14 hours

Excretion: Feces (~80% to 85%); urine (10%)

Dosage Oral:

Adolescents 10-17 years: Immediate release tablet:

- LDL reduction <20%: Initial: 10 mg/day with evening meal
- LDL reduction ≥20%: Initial: 20 mg/day with evening meal
- Usual range: 10-40 mg with evening meal, then adjust dose at 4-week intervals; maximum dose per manufacturer: 40 mg/day

Adults: Initial: 20 mg with evening meal, then adjust at 4-week intervals; maximum dose: 80 mg/day immediate release tablet **or** 60 mg/day extended release tablet

Note: Doses should be individualized according to the baseline LDL-cholesterol levels, the recommended goal of therapy, and patient response.

Dosage modification/limits based on concurrent therapy:

- Cyclosporine or danazol: Initial dose: 10 mg/day with a maximum recommended dose of 20 mg/day
- Concurrent therapy with fibrates and/or lipid-lowering doses of niacin (≥1 g/day): Maximum recommended dose: 20 mg/day. Concurrent use with fibrates should be avoided unless risk to benefit favors use.
- Concurrent therapy with amiodarone or verapamil: Maximum recommended dose: 40 mg/day of immediate release or 20 mg/day with extended release.

Dosage adjustment in renal impairment: Cl_{cr} <30 mL/minute: Use doses >20 mg/day with caution.

Dietary Considerations Before initiation of therapy, patients should be placed on a standard cholesterol-lowering diet for 6 weeks and the diet should be continued during drug therapy. Avoid intake of large quantities of grapefruit juice (≥1 quart/day); may increase toxicity. Red yeast rice contains an estimated 2.4 mg lovastatin per 600 mg rice. Immediate release tablet should be taken with the evening meal.

Administration Administer immediate release tablet with the evening meal. Administer extended release tablet at bedtime; do not crush or chew.

Monitoring Parameters Obtain baseline LFTs and total cholesterol profile. LFTs should also be assessed prior to, at 6 and 12 weeks after initiation, and periodically thereafter; baseline CPK (recheck CPK in any patient with symptoms suggestive of myopathy).

Reference Range NCEP classification of pediatric patients with familial history of hypercholesterolemia or premature CVD: Acceptable total cholesterol: <170 mg/dL, LDL: <110 mg/dL

Test Interactions Altered thyroid function tests

Dosage Forms Excipient information presented when available (limited, particularly for generics); consult specific product labeling.

Tablet, oral: 10 mg, 20 mg, 40 mg
- Mevacor®: 20 mg, 40 mg

Tablet, extended release, oral:
- Altoprev®: 20 mg, 40 mg, 60 mg

◆ **Lovastatin and Niacin** *see* Niacin and Lovastatin *on page 1197*

◆ **Lovaza®** *see* Omega-3-Acid Ethyl Esters *on page 1241*

◆ **Lovenox®** *see* Enoxaparin *on page 588*

◆ **Lovenox® HP (Can)** *see* Enoxaparin *on page 588*

◆ **Low-Molecular-Weight Iron Dextran (INFeD®)** *see* Iron Dextran Complex *on page 930*

◆ **Low-Ogestrel®** *see* Ethinyl Estradiol and Norgestrel *on page 664*

◆ **Loxapac (Can)** *see* Loxapine *on page 1040*

Loxapine (LOKS a peen)

Brand Names: U.S. Loxitane®

Brand Names: Canada Apo-Loxapine®; Dom-Loxapine; Loxapac; Nu-Loxapine; PHL-Loxapine; Xylac™

Index Terms Loxapine Succinate; Oxilapine Succinate

Pharmacologic Category Antipsychotic Agent, Typical

Additional Appendix Information

Antipsychotic Agents *on page 1880*

Use Management of psychotic disorders

Unlabeled Use Psychosis/agitation related to Alzheimer's dementia

Dosage

Oral:

Adults: Initial: 10 mg twice daily (up to 50 mg/day may be considered in severely disturbed patients), increase dose until psychotic symptoms are controlled; usual maintenance: 60-100 mg/day in divided doses 2-4 times/day; satisfactory response often observed with doses of 20-60 mg/day (maximum: 250 mg/day). Therapy should be maintained at lowest effective dose.

Elderly: Reduced dosing may be indicated due to risks of adverse events associated with high-dose therapy.

I.M. (Canadian availability; not available in the U.S.): Adults: 12.5-50 mg every 4-6 hours or longer; individualize dose early in therapy; some patients respond satisfactorily to twice-daily dosing

Dosage adjustment in renal impairment: There are no dosage adjustments provided in the manufacturer's labeling.

Dosage adjustment in hepatic impairment: There are no dosage adjustments provided in the manufacturer's labeling. Canadian labeling does not recommend use in severe hepatic disease.

Additional Information Complete prescribing information for this medication should be consulted for additional detail.

Dosage Forms Excipient information presented when available (limited, particularly for generics); consult specific product labeling.

Capsule, oral: 5 mg, 10 mg, 25 mg, 50 mg
- Loxitane®: 5 mg, 10 mg, 25 mg, 50 mg

Dosage Forms: Canada Excipient information presented when available (limited, particularly for generics); consult specific product labeling.

Injection, solution, as hydrochloride [strength expressed as base]:
- Loxapac: 50 mg/mL (1 mL) [contains polysorbate 80, propylene glycol]

Solution, oral, as hydrochloride [strength expressed as base; concentrate]:
- Xylac™: 25 mg/mL (100 mL) [contains propylene glycol]

Tablet, oral, as succinate [strength expressed as base]:
- Xylac™: 2.5 mg, 5 mg, 10 mg, 25 mg, 50 mg

◆ **Loxapine Succinate** *see* Loxapine *on page 1040*

◆ **Loxitane®** *see* Loxapine *on page 1040*

◆ **Lozide® (Can)** *see* Indapamide *on page 886*

◆ **Lozi-Flur™** *see* Fluoride *on page 728*

◆ **L-PAM** *see* Melphalan *on page 1065*

◆ **L-Phenylalanine Mustard** *see* Melphalan *on page 1065*

◆ **L-Sarcolysin** *see* Melphalan *on page 1065*

◆ **LTA® 360** *see* Lidocaine (Topical) *on page 1009*

◆ **LTG** *see* LamoTRIgine *on page 967*

◆ ***L*-Thyroxine Sodium** *see* Levothyroxine *on page 1004*

◆ **Lu-26-054** *see* Escitalopram *on page 620*

Lubiprostone (loo bi PROS tone)

Brand Names: U.S. Amitiza®

Index Terms RU 0211; SPI 0211

Pharmacologic Category Chloride Channel Activator; Gastrointestinal Agent, Miscellaneous

Additional Appendix Information

Laxatives, Classification and Properties *on page 1893*

Use Treatment of chronic idiopathic constipation; treatment of irritable bowel syndrome with constipation in adult women

Pregnancy Risk Factor C

Dosage Oral:

Chronic idiopathic constipation: Adults: 24 mcg twice daily

Irritable bowel syndrome with constipation: Females ≥18 years: 8 mcg twice daily

Dosage adjustment for toxicity for chronic idiopathic constipation: May decrease dose to 24 mcg once daily in case of severe nausea

Dosage adjustment for renal impairment: No dosage adjustment required.

Dosage adjustment for hepatic impairment:

Moderate hepatic impairment (Child-Pugh class B):

Chronic idiopathic constipation: 16 mcg twice daily; may increase to 24 mcg twice daily if tolerated and an adequate response has not been obtained with lower dosage

Irritable bowel syndrome with constipation: No dosage adjustment required

Severe hepatic impairment (Child-Pugh class C):

Chronic idiopathic constipation: 8 mcg twice daily; may increase to 16-24 mcg twice daily if tolerated and an adequate response has not been obtained with lower dosage

Irritable bowel syndrome with constipation: 8 mcg once daily; may increase to 8 mcg twice daily if tolerated and an adequate response has not been obtained at lower dosage

Additional Information Complete prescribing information for this medication should be consulted for additional detail.

Dosage Forms Excipient information presented when available (limited, particularly for generics); consult specific product labeling.

Capsule, softgel, oral:

Amitiza®: 8 mcg, 24 mcg

- ♦ **Lucentis®** *see* Ranibizumab *on page 1461*
- ♦ **Ludiomil** *see* Maprotiline *on page 1052*
- ♦ **Lufyllin®-GG [DSC]** *see* Dyphylline and Guaifenesin *on page 568*
- ♦ **Lugol's Solution** *see* Potassium Iodide and Iodine *on page 1384*
- ♦ **Lumefantrine and Artemether** *see* Artemether and Lumefantrine *on page 148*
- ♦ **Lumigan®** *see* Bimatoprost *on page 219*
- ♦ **Lumigan® RC (Can)** *see* Bimatoprost *on page 219*
- ♦ **Luminal Sodium** *see* PHENobarbital *on page 1339*
- ♦ **Lumitene™ [OTC]** *see* Beta-Carotene *on page 207*
- ♦ **Lumizyme®** *see* Alglucosidase Alfa *on page 65*
- ♦ **Lunesta®** *see* Eszopiclone *on page 648*
- ♦ **Lupron® (Can)** *see* Leuprolide *on page 989*
- ♦ **Lupron Depot®** *see* Leuprolide *on page 989*
- ♦ **Lupron® Depot® (Can)** *see* Leuprolide *on page 989*
- ♦ **Lupron Depot-Ped®** *see* Leuprolide *on page 989*

Lurasidone (loo RAS i done)

Brand Names: U.S. Latuda®

Index Terms Lurasidone Hydrochloride; SM-13496

Pharmacologic Category Antipsychotic Agent, Atypical

Use Treatment of schizophrenia

Pregnancy Risk Factor B

Pregnancy Considerations No teratogenic or adverse developmental effects were observed in animal studies. Antipsychotic use during the third trimester of pregnancy has a risk for abnormal muscle movements (extrapyramidal symptoms [EPS]) and withdrawal symptoms in newborns following delivery. Symptoms in the newborn may include agitation, feeding disorder, hypertonia, hypotonia, respiratory distress, somnolence, and tremor; these effects may be self-limiting or require hospitalization. There are no adequate and well-controlled studies in pregnant women. Use in pregnancy only when potential benefit to mother outweighs possible risk to the fetus.

Lactation Excretion in breast milk unknown/not recommended

Contraindications Hypersensitivity to lurasidone or any component of the formulation; concomitant use with potent CYP3A4 inhibitors (eg, ketoconazole) and inducers (eg, rifampin)

Warnings/Precautions [U.S. Boxed Warning]: Elderly patients with dementia-related psychosis treated with antipsychotics are at an increased risk of death compared to placebo. Most deaths appeared to be either cardiovascular (eg, heart failure, sudden death) or infectious (eg, pneumonia) in nature. Lurasidone is not approved for the treatment of dementia-related psychosis. An increased incidence of cerebrovascular effects (eg, transient ischemic attack, stroke), including fatalities, has been reported in placebo-controlled trials of antipsychotics for the unapproved use in elderly patients with dementia-related psychosis.

Leukopenia, neutropenia, and agranulocytosis (sometimes fatal) have been reported in clinical trials and postmarketing reports with antipsychotic use; presence of risk factors (eg, pre-existing low WBC or history of drug-induced leuko-/neutropenia) should prompt periodic blood count assessment. Discontinue therapy at first signs of blood dyscrasias or if absolute neutrophil count <1000/mm^3.

Low to moderately sedating, use with caution in disorders where CNS depression is a feature. Use with caution in Parkinson's disease. Caution in patients with predisposition to seizures. Use with caution in renal or hepatic dysfunction; dose reduction recommended in moderate-to-severe impairment. Esophageal dysmotility and aspiration have been associated with antipsychotic use; use with caution in patients at risk of aspiration pneumonia (ie, Alzheimer's disease). Use is associated with increased prolactin levels; clinical significance of hyperprolactinemia in patients with breast cancer or other prolactin-dependent tumors is unknown. May alter temperature regulation.

Use with caution in patients with severe cardiac disease, hemodynamic instability, prior myocardial infarction or ischemic heart disease. May cause orthostatic hypotension; use with caution in patients at risk of this effect (eg, concurrent medication use which may predispose to hypotension/bradycardia or presence of hypovolemia) or in those who would not tolerate transient hypotensive episodes. Antipsychotics may alter cardiac conduction; life-threatening arrhythmias have occurred with therapeutic doses of antipsychotics. Relative to other antipsychotics, lurasidone has minimal effects on the QT_c interval and therefore, risk for arrhythmias is low. Increases in total cholesterol and triglyceride concentrations have been observed with atypical antipsychotic use; during clinical trials of lurasidone, there were no significant changes in total cholesterol or triglycerides observed. Concurrent use with strong inhibitors/inducers of CYP3A4 is contraindicated; dosage adjustment is recommended with concurrent use of moderate CYP3A4 inhibitors (eg, diltiazem).

May cause extrapyramidal symptoms (EPS), including pseudoparkinsonism, acute dystonic reactions, akathisia, and tardive dyskinesia (potentially irreversible). Risk of tardive dyskinesia may be increased in elderly patients, particularly elderly women. Risk of dystonia (and probably other EPS) may be greater with increased doses, use of conventional antipsychotics, males, and younger patients. Use may be associated with neuroleptic malignant syndrome (NMS); monitor for mental status changes, fever, muscle rigidity and/or autonomic instability (risk may be increased in patients with Parkinson's disease or Lewy body dementia). May cause hyperglycemia; in some cases may be extreme and associated with ketoacidosis, hyperosmolar coma, or death. Use with caution in patients with diabetes or other disorders of glucose regulation; monitor for worsening of glucose control. Significant weight gain has been observed with antipsychotic therapy; incidence varies with product. Monitor waist circumference and BMI.

The possibility of a suicide attempt is inherent in psychotic illness or bipolar disorder; use caution in high-risk patients during initiation of therapy. Prescriptions should be written for the smallest quantity consistent with good patient care.

Adverse Reactions

10%:

Central nervous system: Somnolence (dose-related: 19% to 23%), akathisia (dose-related: 11% to 15%)

Endocrine & metabolic: Fasting glucose increased (10% to 14%)
Gastrointestinal: Nausea (12%)
Neuromuscular & skeletal: Extrapyramidal symptoms (24% to 26%), parkinsonism (11%)

1% to 10%:
Cardiovascular: Tachycardia
Central nervous system: Insomnia (8%), agitation (6%), anxiety (6%), dizziness (5%), dystonia (5%), fatigue (4%), restlessness (3%)
Dermatologic: Pruritus, rash
Endocrine & metabolic: Prolactin increased (≥5 x ULN: females: 8%; males: 2%)
Gastrointestinal: Dyspepsia (8%), vomiting (8%), weight gain (≥7% increase in baseline body weight: 6%), salivary hypersecretion (2%), abdominal pain, appetite decreased, diarrhea
Neuromuscular & skeletal: Back pain (4%), CPK increased
Ocular: Blurred vision
Renal: Creatinine increased (3%)

<1% (Limited to important or life-threatening): Abnormal dreams, amenorrhea, anemia, angina, angioedema, AV block, bradycardia, breast enlargement, breast pain, cerebrovascular accident, dysarthria, gastritis, dysphagia, dysmenorrhea, dysuria, erectile dysfunction, galactorrhea, hypertension, leukopenia, neuroleptic malignant syndrome, orthostatic hypotension, panic attack, renal failure, rhabdomyolysis, seizure, sleep disorder, suicidal behavior, syncope, tardive dyskinesia, vertigo

Drug Interactions

Metabolism/Transport Effects Substrate of CYP3A4 (major); **Note:** Assignment of Major/Minor substrate status based on clinically relevant drug interaction potential; **Inhibits** CYP3A4 (weak)

Avoid Concomitant Use

Avoid concomitant use of Lurasidone with any of the following: CYP3A4 Inducers (Strong); CYP3A4 Inhibitors (Strong); DOPamine; EPINEPHrine; EPINEPHrine (Systemic, Oral Inhalation); Metoclopramide; Pimozide

Increased Effect/Toxicity

Lurasidone may increase the levels/effects of: Alcohol (Ethyl); CNS Depressants; Disopyramide; Methotrimeprazine; Methylphenidate; Pimozide; Procainamide; QuiNIDine; Serotonin Modulators

The levels/effects of Lurasidone may be increased by: Acetylcholinesterase Inhibitors (Central); CYP3A4 Inhibitors (Moderate); CYP3A4 Inhibitors (Strong); Dasatinib; DOPamine; Droperidol; EPINEPHrine; EPINEPHrine (Systemic, Oral Inhalation); HydrOXYzine; Lithium formulations; MAO Inhibitors; Methotrimeprazine; Methylphenidate; Metoclopramide; Tetrabenazine

Decreased Effect

Lurasidone may decrease the levels/effects of: Amphetamines; Anti-Parkinson's Agents (Dopamine Agonist); Quinagolide

The levels/effects of Lurasidone may be decreased by: CYP3A4 Inducers (Strong); Deferasirox; Lithium formulations; Tocilizumab

Ethanol/Nutrition/Herb Interactions

Ethanol: May increase CNS depression; monitor for increased effects with coadministration. Caution patients about effects.

Food: Administration with food (≥350 calories) increased C_{max} and AUC of lurasidone ~3 times and 2 times, respectively, compared to administration under fasting conditions. Lurasidone exposure was not affected by the fat content of the meal.

Stability Store at controlled room temperature of 25°C (77°F).

Mechanism of Action Lurasidone is a benzoisothiazol-derivative atypical antipsychotic with mixed serotonin-dopamine antagonist activity. It exhibits high affinity for D_2, $5\text{-}HT_{2A}$, and $5\text{-}HT_7$ receptors; moderate affinity for $alpha_{2C}$-adrenergic receptors; and is a partial agonist for $5\text{-}HT_{1A}$ receptors. Lurasidone has no significant affinity for muscarinic M_1 and histamine H_1 receptors. The addition of serotonin antagonism to dopamine antagonism (classic neuroleptic mechanism) is thought to improve negative symptoms of psychoses and reduce the incidence of extrapyramidal side effects as compared to typical antipsychotics.

Pharmacodynamics/Kinetics

Distribution: V_d: 6173 L
Protein binding: ~99%
Metabolism: Primarily via CYP3A4; two active metabolites (ID-14283 and ID-14326) and two major nonactive metabolites (ID-20219 and ID-20220) produced
Bioavailability: 9% to 19%
Half-life elimination: 18 hours; Main active metabolite, ID-14283 (exo-hydroxy metabolite), exhibits a half-life of 7.5-10 hours
Time to peak: 1-3 hours; steady state concentrations achieved within 7 days
Excretion: Urine (~9%); feces (~80%)

Dosage Oral: Adults: Schizophrenia: Initial: 40 mg once daily; titration is not required; maximum recommended dose: 80 mg/day

Concomitant CYP3A4 inhibitors/inducers:

CYP3A4 inhibitors: If concomitant administration with a moderate CYP3A4 inhibitor (eg, diltiazem) is necessary, do not exceed 40 mg/day of lurasidone. Concomitant administration with a strong CYP3A4 inhibitor (eg, ketoconazole) is contraindicated.

CYP3A4 inducers: Concomitant administration with a strong CYP3A4 inducer (eg, rifampin) is contraindicated.

Dosing adjustment in renal impairment: Exposure is increased in renal impairment; use caution
Cl_{cr} ≥50 mL/minute: No dosage adjustment required
Cl_{cr} 10-49 mL/minute: Do not exceed 40 mg/day

Dosing adjustment in hepatic impairment: Exposure is increased in hepatic impairment; use caution
Mild hepatic impairment (Child-Pugh class A): No dosage adjustment required
Moderate-to-severe hepatic impairment (Child-Pugh class B or C): Do not exceed 40 mg/day

Dietary Considerations Should be taken with food (≥350 calories).

Administration Administer with food (≥350 calories).

Monitoring Parameters Vital signs; fasting lipid profile and fasting blood glucose/Hgb A_{1c} (baseline and periodically); CBC frequently during first few months of therapy in patients with pre-existing low WBC or a history of drug-induced leukopenia/neutropenia; BMI, personal/family history of obesity, waist circumference; blood pressure; mental status, abnormal involuntary movement scale (AIMS), extrapyramidal symptoms; orthostatic blood pressure changes for 3-5 days after starting or increasing dose. Weight should be assessed prior to treatment and regularly throughout therapy. Consider titrating to a different antipsychotic agent for a weight gain ≥5% of the initial weight.

Dosage Forms Excipient information presented when available (limited, particularly for generics); consult specific product labeling.

Tablet, oral, as hydrochloride:
Latuda®: 40 mg, 80 mg

◆ **Lurasidone Hydrochloride** *see* Lurasidone *on page 1041*

◆ **Lusedra™** *see* Fospropofol *on page 767*

- ◆ **LuSonal™ [DSC]** *see* Phenylephrine (Systemic) *on page 1344*
- ◆ **Lustra®** *see* Hydroquinone *on page 846*
- ◆ **Lustra-AF®** *see* Hydroquinone *on page 846*
- ◆ **Lustra-Ultra™** *see* Hydroquinone *on page 846*
- ◆ **Lutera®** *see* Ethinyl Estradiol and Levonorgestrel *on page 656*

Lutropin Alfa (LOO troe pin AL fa)

Brand Names: U.S. Luveris®

Index Terms r-hLH; Recombinant Human Luteinizing Hormone

Pharmacologic Category Gonadotropin; Ovulation Stimulator

Use Stimulation of follicular development in infertile hypogonadotropic hypogonadal (HH) women with profound luteinizing hormone (LH) deficiency; to be used in combination with follitropin alfa

Pregnancy Risk Factor X

Dosage SubQ: Adults: Females: Infertility: 75 int. units daily until adequate follicular development is noted; maximum duration of treatment: 14 days; to be used concomitantly with follitropin alfa

Additional Information Complete prescribing information for this medication should be consulted for additional detail.

Dosage Forms Excipient information presented when available (limited, particularly for generics); consult specific product labeling.

Injection, powder for reconstitution:

Luveris®: 75 int. units [contains sucrose 48 mg]

- ◆ **Luveris®** *see* Lutropin Alfa *on page 1043*
- ◆ **Luvox** *see* FluvoxaMINE *on page 746*
- ◆ **Luvox® (Can)** *see* FluvoxaMINE *on page 746*
- ◆ **Luvox® CR** *see* FluvoxaMINE *on page 746*
- ◆ **Luxiq®** *see* Betamethasone *on page 208*
- ◆ **LY139603** *see* Atomoxetine *on page 163*
- ◆ **LY146032** *see* DAPTOmycin *on page 446*
- ◆ **LY170053** *see* OLANZapine *on page 1233*
- ◆ **LY-188011** *see* Gemcitabine *on page 782*
- ◆ **LY231514** *see* PEMEtrexed *on page 1317*
- ◆ **LY246736** *see* Alvimopan *on page 81*
- ◆ **LY248686** *see* DULoxetine *on page 565*
- ◆ **LY303366** *see* Anidulafungin *on page 122*
- ◆ **LY570310** *see* Telaprevir *on page 1631*
- ◆ **LY-640315** *see* Prasugrel *on page 1393*
- ◆ **LY2148568** *see* Exenatide *on page 678*
- ◆ **Lybrel®** *see* Ethinyl Estradiol and Levonorgestrel *on page 656*
- ◆ **Lyderm® (Can)** *see* Fluocinonide *on page 727*
- ◆ **Lymphocyte Immune Globulin** *see* Antithymocyte Globulin (Equine) *on page 131*
- ◆ **Lymphocyte Mitogenic Factor** *see* Aldesleukin *on page 55*
- ◆ **Lyrica®** *see* Pregabalin *on page 1402*
- ◆ **Lysodren®** *see* Mitotane *on page 1144*
- ◆ **Lysteda™** *see* Tranexamic Acid *on page 1719*
- ◆ **Maalox® Advanced Maximum Strength [OTC]** *see* Aluminum Hydroxide, Magnesium Hydroxide, and Simethicone *on page 80*
- ◆ **Maalox® Advanced Regular Strength [OTC]** *see* Aluminum Hydroxide, Magnesium Hydroxide, and Simethicone *on page 80*
- ◆ **Maalox® Children's [OTC]** *see* Calcium Carbonate *on page 266*
- ◆ **Maalox® Regular Strength [OTC]** *see* Calcium Carbonate *on page 266*
- ◆ **MabCampath® (Can)** *see* Alemtuzumab *on page 58*
- ◆ **Macrobid®** *see* Nitrofurantoin *on page 1210*
- ◆ **Macrodantin®** *see* Nitrofurantoin *on page 1210*
- ◆ **Macugen®** *see* Pegaptanib *on page 1305*

Mafenide (MA fe nide)

Brand Names: U.S. Sulfamylon®

Index Terms Mafenide Acetate

Pharmacologic Category Antibiotic, Topical

Use

Cream: Adjunctive antibacterial agent in the treatment of second- and third-degree burns

Solution: Adjunctive antibacterial agent for use under moist dressings over meshed autografts on excised burn wounds

Pregnancy Risk Factor C

Dosage Children and Adults: Topical:

Cream: Apply once or twice daily with a sterile-gloved hand; apply to a thickness of approximately 1/16 inch; the burned area should be covered with cream at all times

Solution: Cover graft area with 1 layer of fine mesh gauze. Wet an 8-ply burn dressing with mafenide solution and cover graft area. Keep dressing wet using syringe or irrigation tubing every 4 hours (or as necessary), or by moistening dressing every 6-8 hours (or as necessary). Irrigation dressing should be secured with bolster dressing and wrapped as appropriate. May leave dressings in place for up to 5 days.

Dosage adjustment for acidosis: Discontinuing treatment for 24-48 hours may aid in restoring acid-base balance

Additional Information Complete prescribing information for this medication should be consulted for additional detail.

Dosage Forms Excipient information presented when available (limited, particularly for generics); consult specific product labeling.

Cream, topical:

Sulfamylon®: 85 mg/g (56.7 g, 113.4 g, 453.6 g) [contains sodium metabisulfite]

Powder for solution, topical, as acetate:

Sulfamylon®: 50 g/packet (5s)

- ◆ **Mafenide Acetate** *see* Mafenide *on page 1043*
- ◆ **Mag 64™ [OTC]** *see* Magnesium Chloride *on page 1044*
- ◆ **Mag-Al [OTC]** *see* Aluminum Hydroxide and Magnesium Hydroxide *on page 80*

Magaldrate and Simethicone
(MAG al drate & sye METH i kone)

Index Terms Riopan Plus; Simethicone and Magaldrate

Pharmacologic Category Antacid; Antiflatulent

Use Relief of hyperacidity associated with peptic ulcer, gastritis, peptic esophagitis, and hiatal hernia which are accompanied by symptoms of gas

Pregnancy Risk Factor C

Dosage Adults: Oral: 5-10 mL (540-1080 mg magaldrate) between meals and at bedtime

Additional Information Complete prescribing information for this medication should be consulted for additional detail.

Dosage Forms Excipient information presented when available (limited, particularly for generics); consult specific product labeling.

Suspension, oral: Magaldrate 540 mg and simethicone 20 mg per 5 mL (360 mL)

- **Mag-Al Ultimate [OTC]** *see* Aluminum Hydroxide and Magnesium Hydroxide *on page 80*
- **Mag Citrate** *see* Magnesium Citrate *on page 1044*
- **Mag Delay [OTC]** *see* Magnesium Chloride *on page 1044*
- **Mag®-G [OTC]** *see* Magnesium Gluconate *on page 1044*
- **Maginex™ [OTC]** *see* Magnesium L-aspartate Hydrochloride *on page 1046*
- **Maginex™ DS [OTC]** *see* Magnesium L-aspartate Hydrochloride *on page 1046*
- **Magnesia Magma** *see* Magnesium Hydroxide *on page 1045*
- **Magnesium L-lactate Dihydrate** *see* Magnesium L-lactate *on page 1046*
- **Magnesium Carbonate and Aluminum Hydroxide** *see* Aluminum Hydroxide and Magnesium Carbonate *on page 79*

Magnesium Chloride (mag NEE zhum KLOR ide)

Brand Names: U.S. Chloromag®; Mag 64™ [OTC]; Mag Delay [OTC]; Slow-Mag® [OTC]

Pharmacologic Category Electrolyte Supplement, Oral; Electrolyte Supplement, Parenteral; Magnesium Salt

Use Correction or prevention of hypomagnesemia; dietary supplement

Pregnancy Risk Factor C

Dosage Note: Serum magnesium is poor reflection of repletional status as the majority of magnesium is intracellular; serum levels may be transiently normal for a few hours after a dose is given; therefore, aim for consistently high normal serum levels in patients with normal renal function for most efficient repletion.

Dietary supplement: Adults: Oral (Mag 64™, Mag Delay®, Slow-Mag®): 2 tablets once daily

Parenteral nutrition supplementation: I.V. (elemental magnesium):

Children:
- <50 kg: 0.3-0.5 mEq/kg/day
- >50 kg: 10-30 mEq/day

Adults: 8-24 mEq/day

RDA (elemental magnesium):

Children:
- 1-3 years: 80 mg/day
- 4-8 years: 130 mg/day
- 9-13 years: 240 mg/day
- 14-18 years:
  - Females: 360 mg/day
  - Pregnant females: 400 mg/day
  - Males: 410 mg/day

Adults:
- 19-30 years:
  - Females: 310 mg/day
  - Pregnant females: 350 mg/day
  - Males: 400 mg/day
- ≥31 years:
  - Females: 320 mg/day
  - Pregnant females: 360 mg/day
  - Males: 420 mg/day

Dosage adjustment in renal impairment: Cl_{cr} <30 mL/minute: Use with caution; monitor for hypermagnesemia

Additional Information Complete prescribing information for this medication should be consulted for additional detail.

Dosage Forms Excipient information presented when available (limited, particularly for generics); consult specific product labeling.

Injection, solution, as hexahydrate: 200 mg/mL (50 mL) [equivalent to elemental magnesium 1.97 mEq/mL]

Chloromag®: 200 mg/mL (50 mL) [contains benzyl alcohol; equivalent to elemental magnesium 1.97 mEq/mL]

Tablet, delayed release, enteric coated, oral:

Mag 64™: Elemental magnesium 64 mg [sugar free; contains elemental calcium 110 mg]

Mag Delay: Elemental magnesium 64 mg [contains elemental calcium 110 mg]

Tablet, enteric coated, oral:

Slow-Mag®: Elemental magnesium 64 mg [contains elemental calcium 113 mg]

Magnesium Citrate (mag NEE zhum SIT rate)

Brand Names: U.S. Citroma® [OTC]

Brand Names: Canada Citro-Mag®

Index Terms Citrate of Magnesia; Mag Citrate

Pharmacologic Category Laxative, Saline; Magnesium Salt

Additional Appendix Information

Laxatives, Classification and Properties *on page 1893*

Use Evacuation of bowel prior to certain surgical and diagnostic procedures or overdose situations

Pregnancy Risk Factor B

Dosage Cathartic: Oral:

Children:
- <6 years: 2-4 mL/kg given once or in divided doses
- 6-12 years: 100-150 mL given once or in divided doses
- ≥12 years: 150-300 mL given once or in divided doses

Adults: 150-300 mL

Additional Information Complete prescribing information for this medication should be consulted for additional detail.

Dosage Forms Excipient information presented when available (limited, particularly for generics); consult specific product labeling.

Solution, oral: 290 mg/5 mL (296 mL)

Citroma®: 290 mg/5 mL (340 mL) [contains benzoic acid, magnesium 48 mg/5 mL, sodium 0.5 mg/5 mL; grape flavor]

Citroma®: 290 mg/5 mL (296 mL) [contains magnesium 48 mg/5 mL, potassium 13 mg/5 mL; cherry flavor]

Citroma®: 290 mg/5 mL (296 mL) [contains magnesium 48 mg/5 mL, potassium 13 mg/5 mL; lemon flavor]

Citroma®: 290 mg/5 mL (296 mL) [contains magnesium 48 mg/5 mL, sodium 7.5 mg/5 mL; grape flavor]

Citroma®: 290 mg/5 mL (296 mL) [contains magnesium 48 mg/5 mL, sodium 7.5 mg/5 mL; lemon flavor]

Tablet, oral: Elemental magnesium 100 mg

Magnesium Gluconate
(mag NEE zhum GLOO koe nate)

Brand Names: U.S. Magonate® [OTC]; Magtrate® [OTC]; Mag®-G [OTC]

Pharmacologic Category Electrolyte Supplement, Oral; Magnesium Salt

Use Dietary supplement

Dosage RDA (elemental magnesium):

Children:
- 1-3 years: 80 mg/day
- 4-8 years: 130 mg/day
- 9-13 years: 240 mg/day

14-18 years:
Females: 360 mg/day
Pregnant females: 400 mg/day
Males: 410 mg/day
Adults:
19-30 years:
Females: 310 mg/day
Pregnant females: 350 mg/day
Males: 400 mg/day
≥31 years:
Females: 320 mg/day
Pregnant females: 360 mg/day
Males: 420 mg/day

Dosing in renal impairment: Cl_{cr} <30 mL/minute: Use with caution; monitor for hypermagnesemia

Additional Information Complete prescribing information for this medication should be consulted for additional detail.

Dosage Forms Excipient information presented when available (limited, particularly for generics); consult specific product labeling.
Liquid, oral:
Magonate®: 1000 mg/5 mL (355 mL) [contains sodium benzoate; melon flavor; equivalent to elemental magnesium 54 mg /5 mL]
Tablet, oral: 500 mg [equivalent to elemental magnesium 27 mg], 550 mg [equivalent to elemental magnesium 30 mg]
Magonate®: 500 mg [scored; equivalent to elemental magnesium 27 mg]
Magtrate®: 500 mg [equivalent to elemental magnesium 27 mg]
Mag®-G: 500 mg [equivalent to elemental magnesium 27 mg]

Magnesium Hydroxide

(mag NEE zhum hye DROKS ide)

Brand Names: U.S. Fleet® Pedia-Lax™ Chewable Tablet [OTC]; Little Phillips'® Milk of Magnesia [OTC]; Milk of Magnesia [OTC]; Milk of Magnesium [OTC]; Phillips'® Milk of Magnesia [OTC]

Index Terms Magnesia Magma; Milk of Magnesia; MOM

Pharmacologic Category Antacid; Laxative; Magnesium Salt

Additional Appendix Information
Laxatives, Classification and Properties *on page 1893*

Use Short-term treatment of occasional constipation and symptoms of hyperacidity, laxative

Dosage Oral:
Laxative:
Liquid:
Children: Magnesium hydroxide 400 mg/5 mL: 1-3 mL/kg/day; adjust dose to induce daily bowel movement
OTC labeling:
<2 years: Use not recommended
2-5 years: Magnesium hydroxide 400 mg/5 mL: 5-15 mL/day once daily at bedtime or in divided doses
6-11 years:
Magnesium hydroxide 400 mg/5 mL: 15-30 mL/day once daily at bedtime or in divided doses
Magnesium hydroxide 800 mg/5 mL: 7.5-15 mL/day once daily at bedtime or in divided doses
Children ≥12 years and Adults:
Magnesium hydroxide 400 mg/5 mL: 30-60 mL/day once daily at bedtime or in divided doses
Magnesium hydroxide 800 mg/5 mL: 15-30 mL/day once daily at bedtime or in divided doses
Tablet: OTC labeling:
Children:
<3 years: Use not recommended
3-5 years: Magnesium hydroxide 311 mg/tablet: 2 tablets/day once daily at bedtime or in divided doses
6-11 years: Magnesium hydroxide 311 mg/tablet: 4 tablets/day once daily at bedtime or in divided doses
Children ≥12 years and Adults: Magnesium hydroxide 311 mg/tablet: 8 tablets/day once daily at bedtime or in divided doses
Antacid: OTC labeling:
Liquid: Children ≥12 years and Adults: Magnesium hydroxide 400 mg/5 mL: 5-15 mL as needed up to 4 times/day
Tablet:
Children <12 years: Use not recommended
Children ≥12 years and Adults: Magnesium hydroxide 311 mg/tablet: 2-4 tablets every 4 hours up to 4 times/day

Dosing in renal impairment: Patients in severe renal failure should not receive magnesium due to toxicity from accumulation. Patients with a Cl_{cr} <30 mL/minute receiving magnesium should be monitored by serum magnesium levels.

Additional Information Complete prescribing information for this medication should be consulted for additional detail.

Dosage Forms Excipient information presented when available (limited, particularly for generics); consult specific product labeling.
Suspension, oral: 400 mg/5 mL (30 mL, 473 mL)
Milk of Magnesia: 400 mg/5 mL (360 mL, 480 mL)
Milk of Magnesia: 400 mg/5 mL (360 mL, 480 mL) [mint flavor]
Milk of Magnesia: 400 mg/5 mL (480 mL) [ethanol free, sugar free]
Milk of Magnesium: 400 mg/5 mL (3.78 L, 473 mL) [contains magnesium 165 mg/5 mL]
Phillips'® Milk of Magnesia: 400 mg/5 mL (120 mL, 360 mL, 780 mL) [contains magnesium 167 mg/5 mL; fresh mint flavor]
Phillips'® Milk of Magnesia: 400 mg/5 mL (120 mL, 360 mL, 780 mL) [contains magnesium 167 mg/5 mL; original flavor]
Phillips'® Milk of Magnesia: 400 mg/5 mL (120 mL, 240 mL, 360 mL, 780 mL) [contains magnesium 167 mg/5 mL, sodium 2 mg/5 mL; cherry flavor]
Suspension, oral [concentrate]: 2400 mg/10 mL (10 mL)
Little Phillips'® Milk of Magnesia: 800 mg/5 mL (120 mL) [contains magnesium 333 mg/5 mL, propylene glycol; strawberry flavor]
Milk of Magnesia: 800 mg/5 mL (100 mL, 400 mL) [contains sodium 20 mg/10 mL, sucrose 0.8 g/10 mL; lemon flavor]
Phillips'® Milk of Magnesia: 800 mg/5 mL (240 mL) [contains magnesium 333 mg/5 mL, propylene glycol; strawberry flavor]
Tablet, chewable, oral:
Fleet® Pedia-Lax™ Chewable Tablet: 400 mg [contains magnesium 170 mg/tablet; watermelon flavor]
Phillips'® Milk of Magnesia: 311 mg [mint flavor]
Phillips'® Milk of Magnesia: 311 mg [contains magnesium 130 mg/tablet; mint flavor]

◆ **Magnesium Hydroxide, Aluminum Hydroxide, and Simethicone** *see* Aluminum Hydroxide, Magnesium Hydroxide, and Simethicone *on page 80*

◆ **Magnesium Hydroxide and Aluminum Hydroxide** *see* Aluminum Hydroxide and Magnesium Hydroxide *on page 80*

◆ **Magnesium Hydroxide and Calcium Carbonate** *see* Calcium Carbonate and Magnesium Hydroxide *on page 267*

Magnesium Hydroxide and Mineral Oil
(mag NEE zhum hye DROKS ide & MIN er al oyl)

Brand Names: U.S. Phillips'® M-O [OTC]
Index Terms Haley's M-O; MOM/Mineral Oil Emulsion
Pharmacologic Category Laxative
Use Short-term treatment of occasional constipation
Dosage Oral: Laxative: OTC labeling:
Children <6 years: Use not recommended
Children 6-11 years: 20-30 mL at bedtime
Children ≥12 years and Adults: 45-60 mL at bedtime

Dosage adjustment in renal impairment: Patients in severe renal failure should not receive magnesium due to toxicity from accumulation. Patients with a Cl_{cr} <30 mL/minute should be monitored by serum magnesium levels.
Additional Information Complete prescribing information for this medication should be consulted for additional detail.
Dosage Forms Excipient information presented when available (limited, particularly for generics); consult specific product labeling.
Suspension, oral:
Phillips'® M-O: Magnesium hydroxide 300 mg and mineral oil 1.25 mL per 5 mL (360 mL, 780 mL) [contains magnesium 125 mg and sodium 1.5 mg per 5 mL mint flavors]

Magnesium L-aspartate Hydrochloride
(mag NEE zhum el as PAR tate hye droe KLOR ide)

Brand Names: U.S. Maginex™ DS [OTC]; Maginex™ [OTC]
Index Terms MAH
Pharmacologic Category Electrolyte Supplement, Oral; Magnesium Salt
Use Dietary supplement
Dosage
RDA (elemental magnesium):
Children:
1-3 years: 80 mg/day
4-8 years: 130 mg/day
9-13 years: 240 mg/day
14-18 years:
Females: 360 mg/day
Pregnant females: 400 mg/day
Males: 410 mg/day
Adults:
19-30 years:
Females: 310 mg/day
Pregnant females: 350 mg/day
Males: 400 mg/day
≥31 years:
Females: 320 mg/day
Pregnant females: 360 mg/day
Males: 420 mg/day
Dietary supplement: Adults: Oral: Magnesium-L-aspartate 1230 mg (magnesium 122 mg) up to 3 times/day

Dosage adjustment in renal impairment: Cl_{cr} <30 mL/minute: Use with caution; monitor for hypermagnesemia
Additional Information Complete prescribing information for this medication should be consulted for additional detail.
Dosage Forms Excipient information presented when available (limited, particularly for generics); consult specific product labeling.
Granules for solution, oral [preservative free]:
Maginex™ DS: 1230 mg/packet (30s) [sugar free; lemon flavor; equivalent to elemental magnesium 122 mg]
Tablet, enteric coated, oral [preservative free]:
Maginex™: 615 mg [sugar free; equivalent to elemental magnesium 61 mg]

Magnesium L-lactate (mag NEE zhum el LAK tate)

Brand Names: U.S. Mag-Tab® SR
Index Terms Magnesium L-lactate Dihydrate
Pharmacologic Category Electrolyte Supplement; Magnesium Salt
Use Dietary supplement
Dosage
Dietary supplement: Oral: Adults: 1-2 caplets every 12 hours
RDA (elemental magnesium):
Children:
1-3 years: 80 mg/day
4-8 years: 130 mg/day
9-13 years: 240 mg/day
14-18 years:
Females: 360 mg/day
Pregnant females: 400 mg/day
Males: 410 mg/day
Adults:
19-30 years:
Females: 310 mg/day
Pregnant females: 350 mg/day
Males: 400 mg/day
≥31 years:
Females: 320 mg/day
Pregnant females: 360 mg/day
Males: 420 mg/day

Dosage adjustment in renal impairment: Cl_{cr} <30 mL/minute: Use with caution; monitor for hypermagnesemia
Additional Information Complete prescribing information for this medication should be consulted for additional detail.
Dosage Forms Excipient information presented when available (limited, particularly for generics); consult specific product labeling.
Caplet, sustained release, oral:
Mag-Tab® SR: Elemental magnesium 84 mg [scored]

Magnesium Oxide (mag NEE zhum OKS ide)

Brand Names: U.S. Mag-Ox® 400 [OTC]; MAGnesium-Oxide™ [OTC]; Phillips'® Laxative Dietary Supplement Cramp-Free [OTC]; Uro-Mag® [OTC]
Index Terms Mag Oxide
Pharmacologic Category Electrolyte Supplement, Oral; Magnesium Salt
Use Electrolyte replacement
Dosage
RDA (elemental magnesium):
Children:
1-3 years: 80 mg/day
4-8 years: 130 mg/day
9-13 years: 240 mg/day
14-18 years:
Females: 360 mg/day
Pregnant females: 400 mg/day
Males: 410 mg/day
Adults:
19-30 years:
Females: 310 mg/day
Pregnant females: 350 mg/day
Males: 400 mg/day

≥31 years:
Females: 320 mg/day
Pregnant females: 360 mg/day
Males: 420 mg/day

Dietary supplement: Adults: Oral:
Mag-Ox 400®: 2 tablets daily with food
Uro-Mag®: 4-5 capsules daily with food

Dosing in renal impairment: Cl_{cr} <30 mL/minute: Use with caution; monitor for hypermagnesemia

Additional Information Complete prescribing information for this medication should be consulted for additional detail.

Dosage Forms Excipient information presented when available (limited, particularly for generics); consult specific product labeling.
Caplet, oral: Elemental magnesium 250 mg
Phillips'® Laxative Dietary Supplement Cramp-Free: Elemental magnesium 500 mg
Capsule, oral:
Uro-Mag®: 140 mg [equivalent to elemental magnesium 84.5 mg]
Tablet, oral: 400 mg [equivalent to elemental magnesium 240 mg], Elemental magnesium 500 mg
Mag-Ox® 400: 400 mg [scored; equivalent to elemental magnesium 240 mg]
MAGnesium-Oxide™: 400 mg [equivalent to elemental magnesium 240 mg]

◆ **MAGnesium-Oxide™ [OTC]** *see* Magnesium Oxide *on page 1046*

Magnesium Salicylate (mag NEE zhum sa LIS i late)

Brand Names: U.S. Doan's® Extra Strength [OTC]; Keygesic [OTC]; Momentum® [OTC]; MST 600

Pharmacologic Category Salicylate

Use Mild-to-moderate pain, fever, various inflammatory conditions; relief of pain and inflammation of rheumatoid arthritis and osteoarthritis

Pregnancy Risk Factor C

Dosage Oral:
Children ≥12 years and Adults: Relief of mild-to-moderate pain:
Doan's® Extra Strength, Momentum®: Two caplets every 6 hours as needed (maximum: 8 caplets/24 hours)
Keygesic: One tablet every 4 hours as needed (maximum: 4 tablets/24 hours)

Additional Information Complete prescribing information for this medication should be consulted for additional detail.

Dosage Forms Excipient information presented when available (limited, particularly for generics); consult specific product labeling.
Caplet, oral, as tetrahydrate:
Doan's® Extra Strength: 580 mg [equivalent to anhydrous magnesium salicylate 467.2 mg]
Momentum®: 580 mg [equivalent to anhydrous magnesium salicylate 467 mg]
Tablet, oral [chelated]:
Keygesic: 650 mg
Tablet, oral, as tetrahydrate:
MST 600: 600 mg

Magnesium Sulfate (mag NEE zhum SUL fate)

Index Terms Epsom Salts; $MgSO_4$ (error-prone abbreviation)

Pharmacologic Category Anticonvulsant, Miscellaneous; Electrolyte Supplement, Parenteral; Magnesium Salt

Use Treatment and prevention of hypomagnesemia; prevention and treatment of seizures in severe pre-eclampsia or eclampsia, pediatric acute nephritis; torsade de pointes; treatment of cardiac arrhythmias (VT/VF) caused by hypomagnesemia; soaking aid

Unlabeled Use Asthma exacerbation (life-threatening)

Pregnancy Risk Factor A/C (manufacturer dependent)

Pregnancy Considerations Magnesium crosses the placenta; serum concentrations in the fetus correlate with those in the mother. Magnesium sulfate is used during pregnancy for the treatment of eclampsia and severe pre-eclampsia.

Lactation Enters breast milk/compatible

Contraindications Hypersensitivity to any component of the formulation; heart block; myocardial damage

Warnings/Precautions Use magnesium with caution in patients with impaired renal function (accumulation of magnesium may lead to magnesium intoxication). Use with extreme caution in patients with myasthenia gravis or other neuromuscular disease. Magnesium toxicity can lead to fatal cardiovascular arrest and/or respiratory paralysis; close monitoring of serum magnesium, respiratory rate, and presence of deep tendon reflex necessary during parenteral administration, particularly with repeated dosing. Vigilant monitoring and safe administration techniques (ISMP Medication Safety Alert, 2005) recommended to avoid potential for errors resulting in toxicity when used in obstetrics; monitor patient and fetal status, and serum magnesium concentrations closely. Solution for injection may contain aluminum; toxic concentrations may occur following prolonged administration in premature neonates or patients with renal dysfunction. Concurrent hypokalemia or hypocalcemia can accompany a magnesium deficit. Unlikely to effectively terminate irregular/polymorphic VT (with normal baseline QT interval).

Adverse Reactions Adverse effects on neuromuscular function may occur at lower concentrations in patients with neuromuscular disease (eg, myasthenia gravis).
Frequency not defined:
Cardiovascular: Flushing (I.V.; dose related), hypotension (I.V.; rate related), vasodilation (I.V.; rate related)
Gastrointestinal: Diarrhea

Drug Interactions

Metabolism/Transport Effects None known.

Avoid Concomitant Use

Avoid concomitant use of Magnesium Sulfate with any of the following: Calcium Polystyrene Sulfonate; Sodium Polystyrene Sulfonate

Increased Effect/Toxicity

Magnesium Sulfate may increase the levels/effects of: Alcohol (Ethyl); Calcium Channel Blockers; Calcium Polystyrene Sulfonate; CNS Depressants; Methotrimeprazine; Neuromuscular-Blocking Agents; Selective Serotonin Reuptake Inhibitors; Sodium Polystyrene Sulfonate

The levels/effects of Magnesium Sulfate may be increased by: Alfacalcidol; Calcitriol; Calcium Channel Blockers; Droperidol; HydrOXYzine; Methotrimeprazine

Decreased Effect

Magnesium Sulfate may decrease the levels/effects of: Bisphosphonate Derivatives; Deferiprone; Eltrombopag; Mycophenolate; Phosphate Supplements; Quinolone Antibiotics; Tetracycline Derivatives; Trientine

The levels/effects of Magnesium Sulfate may be decreased by: Ketorolac; Ketorolac (Nasal); Ketorolac (Systemic); Mefloquine; Trientine

Ethanol/Nutrition/Herb Interactions Ethanol: May increase CNS depression; monitor for increased effects with coadministration. Caution patients about effects.

Stability Prior to use, store at room temperature of 20°C to 25°C (68°F to 77°F). Refrigeration of solution may result in precipitation or crystallization.

Mechanism of Action When taken orally, magnesium promotes bowel evacuation by causing osmotic retention of fluid which distends the colon with increased peristaltic activity; parenterally, magnesium decreases acetylcholine in motor nerve terminals and acts on myocardium by slowing rate of S-A node impulse formation and prolonging conduction time. Magnesium is necessary for the movement of calcium, sodium, and potassium in and out of cells, as well as stabilizing excitable membranes.

Intravenous magnesium may improve pulmonary function in patients with asthma; causes relaxation of bronchial smooth muscle independent of serum magnesium concentration.

Pharmacodynamics/Kinetics

Onset of action: Anticonvulsant: I.M.: 1 hour; I.V.: Immediate

Duration of anticonvulsant activity: I.M.: 3-4 hours; I.V.: 30 minutes

Distribution: Bone (50% to 60%); extracellular fluid (1% to 2%)

Protein binding: 30%, to albumin

Excretion: Urine (as magnesium)

Dosage Dose represented as magnesium sulfate unless stated otherwise. **Note:** Serum magnesium is poor reflection of repletional status as the majority of magnesium is intracellular; serum concentrations may be transiently normal for a few hours after a dose is given, therefore, aim for consistently high normal serum concentrations in patients with normal renal function for most efficient repletion.

Note: 1 g of magnesium sulfate = 98.6 mg elemental magnesium = 8.12 mEq elemental magnesium

Hypomagnesemia: Note: Treatment depends on severity and clinical status:

Children: I.V., I.O.: 25-50 mg/kg/dose over 10-20 minutes (over several minutes for torsade de pointes); maximum single dose: 2000 mg (PALS, 2010)

Adults:

Mild deficiency: I.M.: 1 g every 6 hours for 4 doses, or as indicated by serum magnesium concentrations

Severe deficiency:

I.M.: Up to 250 mg/kg within a 4-hour period

I.V.: Severe, non-life-threatening: 1-2 g/hour for 3-6 hours then 0.5-1 g/hour as needed to correct deficiency

Symptomatic deficiency: I.V.: 1-2 g over 5-60 minutes; maintenance infusion may be required to correct deficiency (0.5-1 g/hour).

With polymorphic VT (including torsade de pointes): I.V. push: 1-2 g (ACLS, 2010)

With seizures: I.V.: 2 g over 10 minutes; calcium administration may also be appropriate as many patients are also hypocalcemic

Asthma (life-threatening or severe exacerbation after 1 hour of intensive conventional therapy; unlabeled use): I.V.:

Children: 25-75 mg/kg (maximum: 2 g)

Adults: 2 g

Eclampsia: Adults:

I.V.: 4-5 g infusion; followed by a 1-2 g/hour continuous infusion; or may follow with I.M. doses of 4-5 g in each buttock every 4 hours. **Note:** Initial infusion may be given over 3-4 minutes if eclampsia is severe; maximum: 40 g/24 hours

ACOG Practice Bulletin 2002: 4-6 g over 15-20 minutes followed by 2 g/hour continuous infusion

Pre-eclampsia (severe): Adults: I.V. 4-5 g infusion; followed by a 1-2 g/hour continuous infusion; or may follow with I.M. doses of 4-5 g in each buttock every 4 hours; maximum: 40 g/24 hour

Torsade de pointes or VF/pulseless VT associated with torsade de pointes (unlabeled use): Adults: I.V., I.O.: 1-2 g over 15 minutes (ACLS, 2010)

Parenteral nutrition supplementation: I.V.:

Children:

<50 kg: 0.3-0.5 mEq elemental magnesium/kg/day

>50 kg: 10-30 mEq elemental magnesium/day

Adults: 8-24 mEq elemental magnesium/day

Soaking aid: Topical: Adults: Dissolve 2 cupfuls of powder per gallon of warm water

RDA:

Children:

1-3 years: 80 mg elemental magnesium/day

4-8 years: 130 mg elemental magnesium/day

9-13 years: 240 mg elemental magnesium/day

14-18 years:

Females: 360 mg elemental magnesium/day

Pregnant females: 400 mg elemental magnesium/day

Males: 410 mg elemental magnesium/day

Adults:

19-30 years:

Females: 310 mg elemental magnesium/day

Pregnant females: 350 mg elemental magnesium/day

Males: 400 mg elemental magnesium/day

≥31 years:

Females: 320 mg elemental magnesium/day

Pregnant females: 360 mg elemental magnesium/day

Males: 420 mg elemental magnesium/day

Dosage adjustment in renal impairment: Cl_{cr} <30 mL/minute: Use with caution; monitor for hypermagnesemia; do not exceed 20 g/48 hours as per manufacturer. Close monitoring is required.

Dietary Considerations Whole grains, legumes and dark-green leafy vegetables are dietary sources of magnesium.

Administration

Injection: May be administered I.M. or I.V.

I.M.: A 25% or 50% concentration may be used for adults and dilution to a ≤20% solution is recommended for children

I.V.: Magnesium should be diluted to a ≤20% solution for I.V. infusion and may be administered I.V. push, IVPB, or continuous I.V. infusion. When giving I.V. push, must dilute first and should not be given any faster than 150 mg/minute; may administer over 1-2 minutes in patients with persistent pulseless VT or VF with known hypomagnesemia (Dager, 2006). ACLS guidelines recommend administration over 15 minutes in patients with torsade de pointes (ACLS, 2010). In patients not in cardiac arrest, hypotension and asystole may occur with rapid administration.

Maximal rate of infusion: 2 g/hour to avoid hypotension; doses of 4 g/hour have been given in emergencies (eclampsia, seizures); optimally, should add magnesium to I.V. fluids, but bolus doses are also effective

Topical: Dissolve 2 cups of powder per gallon of warm water to use as a soaking aid. To make a compress, dissolve 2 cups of powder per 2 cups of hot water and use a towel to apply as a wet dressing.

Monitoring Parameters

I.V.: Rapid administration: ECG monitoring, vital signs, deep tendon reflexes; magnesium concentrations if frequent or prolonged dosing required particularly in patients with renal dysfunction, calcium, and potassium concentrations

Obstetrics: Patient status including vital signs, oxygen saturation, deep tendon reflexes, level of consciousness, fetal heart rate, maternal uterine activity.

Reference Range Serum magnesium: 1.5-2.5 mg/dL; slightly different ranges are reported by different laboratories

Dosage Forms Excipient information presented when available (limited, particularly for generics); consult specific product labeling. [DSC] = Discontinued product

Infusion, premixed in D_5W: 10 mg/mL (100 mL) [equivalent to elemental magnesium 0.99 mg (0.08 mEq)/mL]; 20 mg/mL (500 mL [DSC]) [equivalent to elemental magnesium 1.97 mg (0.16 mEq)/mL]

Infusion, premixed in water for injection: 40 mg/mL (50 mL, 100 mL, 500 mL, 1000 mL) [equivalent to elemental magnesium 3.94 mg (0.32 mEq)/mL]; 80 mg/mL (50 mL) [equivalent to elemental magnesium 7.89 mg (0.65 mEq)/mL]

Injection, solution: 500 mg/mL (20 mL) [equivalent to elemental magnesium 49.3 mg (4.06 mEq)/mL]

Injection, solution [preservative free]: 500 mg/mL (2 mL, 10 mL, 20 mL, 50 mL) [equivalent to elemental magnesium 49.3 mg (4.06 mEq)/mL]

Powder, oral/topical: USP: 100% (227 g, 454 g, 1810 g, 2720 g)

- ◆ **Magnesium Sulfate, Potassium Sulfate, and Sodium Sulfate** *see* Sodium Sulfate, Potassium Sulfate, and Magnesium Sulfate *on page* 1576
- ◆ **Magnesium Sulfate, Sodium Sulfate, and Potassium Sulfate** *see* Sodium Sulfate, Potassium Sulfate, and Magnesium Sulfate *on page* 1576
- ◆ **Magnesium Trisilicate and Aluminum Hydroxide** *see* Aluminum Hydroxide and Magnesium Trisilicate *on page* 80
- ◆ **Magonate® [OTC]** *see* Magnesium Gluconate *on page* 1044
- ◆ **Mag-Ox® 400 [OTC]** *see* Magnesium Oxide *on page* 1046
- ◆ **Mag Oxide** *see* Magnesium Oxide *on page* 1046
- ◆ **Mag-Tab® SR** *see* Magnesium L-lactate *on page* 1046
- ◆ **Magtrate® [OTC]** *see* Magnesium Gluconate *on page* 1044
- ◆ **MAH** *see* Magnesium L-aspartate Hydrochloride *on page* 1046
- ◆ **Makena™** *see* Hydroxyprogesterone Caproate *on page* 850
- ◆ **Malarone®** *see* Atovaquone and Proguanil *on page* 168
- ◆ **Malarone® Pediatric (Can)** *see* Atovaquone and Proguanil *on page* 168

Malathion (mal a THYE on)

Brand Names: U.S. Ovide®

Pharmacologic Category Antiparasitic Agent, Topical; Pediculocide; Scabicidal Agent

Use Topical treatment of *Pediculus capitis* (head lice and their ova)

Pregnancy Risk Factor B

Dosage Topical: Children ≥6 years and Adults: Apply sufficient amount to cover and thoroughly moisten dry hair and scalp; shampoo after 8-12 hours. If required, repeat with second application in 7-9 days. Further treatment is generally not necessary.

Additional Information Complete prescribing information for this medication should be consulted for additional detail.

Dosage Forms Excipient information presented when available (limited, particularly for generics); consult specific product labeling.

Lotion, topical: 0.5% (59 mL)

Ovide®: 0.5% (59 mL) [contains isopropyl alcohol 78%]

- ◆ **Mandelamine® (Can)** *see* Methenamine *on page* 1093
- ◆ **Mandrake** *see* Podophyllum Resin *on page* 1370

Manganese (MAN ga nees)

Brand Names: U.S. Mangimin [OTC]; Mn-50™ [OTC]

Index Terms Manganese Chloride; Manganese Sulfate

Pharmacologic Category Trace Element, Parenteral

Use Trace element added to total parenteral nutrition (TPN) solution to prevent manganese deficiency; orally as a dietary supplement

Pregnancy Risk Factor C

Dosage

Oral: Adequate intake:
- 0-6 months: 0.003 mg/day
- 7-12 months: 0.6 mg/day
- 1-3 years: 1.2 mg/day
- 4-8 years: 1.5 mg/day
- 9 years to Adults, Males: 1.9-2.3 mg/day
- 9 years to Adults, Females: 1.6-1.8 mg/day
  - Pregnancy: 2 mg/day
  - Lactation: 2.6 mg/day

I.V.:

Children: 2-10 mcg/kg/day usually administered in TPN solutions

Note: Use caution in premature neonates; manganese chloride solution for injection contains aluminum

Adults: 150-800 mcg/day usually administered in TPN solutions

Dosage adjustment in renal impairment: Use caution; manganese chloride solution for injection contains aluminum

Dosage adjustment in hepatic impairment: Use caution; dose may need to be decreased or withheld

Additional Information Complete prescribing information for this medication should be consulted for additional detail.

Dosage Forms Excipient information presented when available (limited, particularly for generics); consult specific product labeling.

Capsule, oral, as chelated:

Mn-50™: Elemental manganese 16.7 mg

Injection, solution, as chloride [preservative free]: Elemental manganese 0.1 mg/mL (10 mL)

Injection, solution, as sulfate [preservative free]: Elemental manganese 0.1 mg/mL (10 mL)

Tablet, oral, as aspartate: 93 mg [elemental manganese 25 mg]

Tablet, oral, as chelated: Elemental manganese 50 mg

Mangimin: Elemental manganese 10 mg

Tablet, oral, as gluconate: Elemental manganese 5.7 mg, 600 mg [elemental manganese 50 mg]

- ◆ **Manganese Chloride** *see* Manganese *on page* 1049
- ◆ **Manganese Sulfate** *see* Manganese *on page* 1049
- ◆ **Mangimin [OTC]** *see* Manganese *on page* 1049

Mannitol (MAN i tole)

Brand Names: U.S. Aridol™; Osmitrol

Brand Names: Canada Osmitrol®

Index Terms *D*-Mannitol

Pharmacologic Category Diagnostic Agent; Diuretic, Osmotic; Genitourinary Irrigant

Use

Injection: Reduction of increased intracranial pressure associated with cerebral edema; reduction of increased intraocular pressure; promoting urinary excretion of toxic substances; genitourinary irrigant in transurethral prostatic resection or other transurethral surgical procedures

Note: Although FDA-labeled indications, the use of mannitol for the prevention of acute renal failure and/or promotion of diuresis is not routinely recommended (Kellum, 2008).

Genitourinary irrigation solution: Irrigation in transurethral prostatic resection or other transurethral surgical procedures

Powder for inhalation: Assessment of bronchial hyperresponsiveness

Unlabeled Use Improve renal transplant function

Pregnancy Risk Factor C

Pregnancy Considerations Reproduction studies have not been conducted.

Lactation Excretion in breast milk unknown/use caution

Contraindications

Injection: Hypersensitivity to mannitol or any component of the formulation; severe renal disease (anuria); severe dehydration; active intracranial bleeding except during craniotomy; progressive heart failure, pulmonary congestion, or renal dysfunction after mannitol administration; severe pulmonary edema or congestion

Genitourinary irrigation solution: Anuria

Powder for inhalation: Hypersensitivity to mannitol, gelatin, or any component of the formulation; conditions that may be compromised by induced bronchospasm or repeated spirometry (eg, aortic or cerebral aneurysm, uncontrolled hypertension, recent MI or cerebral vascular accident)

Warnings/Precautions Should not be administered until adequacy of renal function and urine flow is established; use 1-2 test doses to assess renal response. Excess amounts can lead to profound diuresis with fluid and electrolyte loss; close medical supervision and dose evaluation are required. Watch for and correct electrolyte disturbances; adjust dose to avoid dehydration. May cause renal dysfunction especially with high doses; use caution in patients taking other nephrotoxic agents, with sepsis or pre-existing renal disease. To minimize adverse renal effects, adjust to keep serum osmolality less than 320 mOsm/L. Discontinue if evidence of acute tubular necrosis.

In patients being treated for cerebral edema, mannitol may accumulate in the brain (causing rebound increases in intracranial pressure) if circulating for long periods of time as with continuous infusion; intermittent boluses preferred. Cardiovascular status should also be evaluated; do not administer electrolyte-free mannitol solutions with blood. If hypotension occurs monitor cerebral perfusion pressure to ensure adequate.

[U.S. Boxed Warning] Use may result in severe bronchospasm; use only for bronchial challenge testing. Testing should only be done by trained professionals. Not for use in patients with asthma or very low baseline pulmonary function. Medications (eg, short-acting inhaled beta-agonist) and equipment for the treatment of severe bronchospasm should be readily available. Use with caution in patients with conditions that may increase sensitivity to bronchoconstriction (eg, severe cough, ventilatory impairment, spirometry-induced bronchoconstriction, hemoptysis of unknown origin, pneumothorax, recent abdominal, thoracic, or intraocular surgery, unstable angina, active upper or lower respiratory tract infection). Patients who have ≥10% reduction in FEV_1 on administration of the 0 mg capsule, patients with a positive response to bronchial challenge testing, or patients who develop significant respiratory symptoms should receive short acting inhaled beta-agonist; monitor until full recovery to baseline. Bronchial challenge testing should not be performed in children <6 years of age as these patients are unable to provide reliable spirometric results.

Adverse Reactions

Injection: Frequency not defined:

Cardiovascular: Chest pain, CHF, circulatory overload, hyper-/hypotension, peripheral edema, tachycardia

Central nervous system: Chills, convulsions, dizziness, fever, headache

Dermatologic: Bullous eruption, urticaria

Endocrine & metabolic: Fluid and electrolyte imbalance, dehydration and hypovolemia secondary to rapid diuresis, hyperglycemia, hypernatremia, hyponatremia (dilutional), hyperosmolality-induced hyperkalemia, metabolic acidosis (dilutional), osmolar gap increased, water intoxication

Gastrointestinal: Nausea, vomiting, xerostomia

Genitourinary: Dysuria, polyuria

Local: Pain, thrombophlebitis, tissue necrosis

Ocular: Blurred vision

Renal: Acute renal failure, acute tubular necrosis (>200 g/day; serum osmolality >320 mOsm/L)

Respiratory: Pulmonary edema, rhinitis

Miscellaneous: Allergic reactions

Inhalation:

1% to 10%:

Cardiovascular: Chest discomfort (1%)

Central nervous system: Headache (adults 6%; children 3%), dizziness (1%)

Gastrointestinal: Nausea (adults 2%; children 3%), throat irritation (2%), retching (1%)

Respiratory: Cough (2%), pharyngolaryngeal pain (adults 2%; children 4%), rhinorrhea (2%), dyspnea (1%), wheezing (1%)

<1% (Limited to important or life-threatening): FEV_1 decreased, gagging

Drug Interactions

Metabolism/Transport Effects None known.

Avoid Concomitant Use There are no known interactions where it is recommended to avoid concomitant use.

Increased Effect/Toxicity

Mannitol may increase the levels/effects of: Amifostine; Antihypertensives; Hypotensive Agents; RiTUXimab; Sodium Phosphates

The levels/effects of Mannitol may be increased by: Alfuzosin; Diazoxide; Herbs (Hypotensive Properties); MAO Inhibitors; Pentoxifylline; Phosphodiesterase 5 Inhibitors; Prostacyclin Analogues

Decreased Effect

The levels/effects of Mannitol may be decreased by: Herbs (Hypertensive Properties); Methylphenidate; Yohimbine

Stability

Injection: Should be stored at room temperature of 15°C to 30°C (59°F to 86°F); do not freeze. In concentrations ≥15%, crystallization may occur at low temperatures; do not use solutions that contain crystals. Heating in a hot water bath and vigorous shaking may be utilized for resolubilization. Cool solutions to body temperature before using.

Irrigation: Store at room temperature of 25°C (77°F); excursions permitted up to 40°C. Avoid excessive heat; do not warm above 150°F (66°C). Do not freeze.

Powder for inhalation: Store at <25°C (<77°F); excursions permitted between 15°C to 30°C (59°F to 86°F). Do not freeze.

Mechanism of Action Produces an osmotic diuresis by increasing the osmotic pressure of glomerular filtrate, which inhibits tubular reabsorption of water and electrolytes and increases urinary output. Mechanism of action in reduction of intracranial pressure (ICP) is controversial. However, it is thought that mannitol reduces ICP by reducing blood viscosity which transiently increases cerebral blood flow and oxygen transport. This in turn reduces cerebral blood volume and ICP. Furthermore, mannitol reduces ICP by withdrawing water from the brain parenchyma and excretes water in the urine (Allen, 2009; Bratton, 2007; Miller, 2010).

Pharmacodynamics/Kinetics

Onset of action: Diuresis: Injection: 1-3 hours; Reduction in intracranial pressure: ~15-30 minutes

Duration: Reduction in intracranial pressure: 1.5-6 hours

Distribution: 34.3 L; remains confined to extracellular space (except in extreme concentrations); does not penetrate the blood-brain barrier (generally, penetration is low)

Metabolism: Minimally hepatic to glycogen

Bioavailability: Inhaled: 59% (relative to oral administration: 96%)

Half-life elimination: Terminal: 4.7 hours

Time to peak, plasma: Inhaled: 1.5 hours

Excretion: Urine (~55% to 87% as unchanged drug)

Dosage

Children: I.V.:

Increased intracranial pressure (unlabeled dosing): 0.25-1 g/kg/dose; repeat as needed to maintain serum osmolality <300-320 mOsm/kg (Adelson, 2003; Broderick, 2007; Hegenbarth, 2008)

Reduction of intraocular pressure: 1-2 g/kg or 30-60 g/m^2 administered over 30-60 minutes 1-1.5 hours prior to surgery

Reduction of intraocular pressure (traumatic hyphema): 1.5 g/kg administered over 45 minutes twice daily for IOP >35 mm Hg; may administer every 8 hours in patients with extremely high pressure (Crouch, 1999)

Children ≥6 years and Adults: Inhalation: Assessment of bronchial hyper-responsiveness: Administer in a stepwise fashion (measuring FEV_1 in duplicate after each administration) until the patient has a positive response or 635 mg of mannitol has been administered (whichever comes first).

Positive test: 15% reduction in FEV_1 from baseline or 10% incremental reduction in FEV_1 between consecutive doses

Negative test: Administration of full dose (635 mg) without reduction in FEV_1 sufficient to meet criteria for a positive test

Administration should be as follows:

Stepwise Administration Schedule

Dose #	Dose (mg)	Cumulative Dose (mg)	Capsules/Dose
1	0	0	1
2	5	5	1
3	10	15	1
4	20	35	1
5	40	75	1
6	80	155	2 x 40 mg caps
7	160	315	4 x 40 mg caps
8	160	475	4 x 40 mg caps
9	160	635	4 x 40 mg caps

Children ≥12 years and Adults:

I.V.:

Increased intracranial pressure, cerebral edema (unlabeled dosing): 0.25-1 g/kg/dose; may repeat every 6-8 hours as needed (Adelson, 2003; Bratton, 2007); maintain serum osmolality <300-320 mOsm/kg (Adelson, 2003; Rabinstein, 2006)

Reduction of intraocular pressure: 0.25-2 g/kg administered over 30-60 minutes 1-1.5 hours prior to surgery

Reduction of intraocular pressure (traumatic hyphema): 1.5 g/kg administered over 45 minutes twice daily for IOP >35 mm Hg; may administer every 8 hours in patients with extremely high pressure (Crouch, 1999)

Severe traumatic brain injury (unlabeled use): ~1.4 g/kg as initial management prior to neurosurgery with concurrent fluid replacement (Cruz, 2001; Cruz, 2002; Cruz, 2004)

Kidney transplant:

Donor: 12.5 g (with adequate hydration) prior to nephrectomy; may repeat (Morris, 2008)

Recipient: 50 g before kidney revascularization (Sprung, 2000; Tiggeler, 1984; van Valenberg, 1987; Weimar, 1983)

Topical: Transurethral irrigation: Use 5% urogenital solution as required for irrigation

Elderly: Refer to adult dosing. Consider initiation at lower end of dosing range.

Dosage adjustment in renal impairment: Contraindicated in severe renal impairment. Use caution in patients with underlying renal disease. May be used to reduce the incidence of acute tubular necrosis when administered prior to revascularization during kidney transplantation.

Dosage adjustment in hepatic impairment: No adjustment required.

Administration

I.V.: Vesicant; avoid extravasation. Do not administer with blood. Crenation and agglutination of red blood cells may occur if administered with whole blood. Inspect for crystals prior to administration. If crystals are present, redissolve by warming solution. Use filter-type administration set for infusion solutions containing mannitol ≥20%. For cerebral edema or elevated ICP, administer over 20-30 minutes.

Inhalation (Aridol™): Administer using supplied single patient use inhaler; do not puncture capsule more than once; do not swallow capsules. A nose clip may be used if preferred. The patient should exhale completely, followed by a controlled rapid deep inspiration from the device; hold breath for 5 seconds and exhale through the mouth. Measure FEV_1 in duplicate 60 seconds after inhalation; repeat process until positive response or full dose (635 mg) has been administered.

Irrigation: Administer using only the appropriate transurethral urologic instrumentation.

Monitoring Parameters Renal function, daily fluid I & O, serum electrolytes, serum and urine osmolality; for treatment of elevated intracranial pressure, maintain serum osmolality <300-320 mOsm/kg.

Bronchial challenge test: Standard spirometry prior to bronchial challenge test; FEV_1 in duplicate 60 seconds after administration of each step of test

Additional Information May autoclave or heat to redissolve crystals; mannitol 20% has an approximate osmolarity of 1100 mOsm/L and mannitol 25% has an approximate osmolarity of 1375 mOsm/L

Bronchial challenge testing: The dose of inhaled mannitol which causes a 15% reduction in FEV_1 is expressed as PD_{15}

Dosage Forms Excipient information presented when available (limited, particularly for generics); consult specific product labeling.

Injection, solution: 20% [200 mg/mL] (250 mL, 500 mL); 25% [250 mg/mL] (50 mL)

Osmitrol: 5% [50 mg/mL] (1000 mL); 10% [100 mg/mL] (500 mL); 15% [150 mg/mL] (500 mL); 20% [200 mg/mL] (250 mL, 500 mL)

Injection, solution [preservative free]: 25% [250 mg/mL] (50 mL)

Powder, for oral inhalation [capsule/kit]:

Aridol™: 0 mg (1s) [empty], 5 mg (1s), 10 mg (1s), 20 mg (1s), 40 mg (15s) (19s)

Solution, genitourinary irrigation: 5% [50 mg/mL] (2000 mL)

- **Mantoux** *see* Tuberculin Tests *on page 1744*
- **Mapap® [OTC]** *see* Acetaminophen *on page 27*
- **Mapap® Arthritis Pain [OTC]** *see* Acetaminophen *on page 27*
- **Mapap® Children's [OTC]** *see* Acetaminophen *on page 27*
- **Mapap® Extra Strength [OTC]** *see* Acetaminophen *on page 27*
- **Mapap® Infant's [OTC]** *see* Acetaminophen *on page 27*
- **Mapap® Junior Rapid Tabs [OTC]** *see* Acetaminophen *on page 27*
- **Mapap PM [OTC]** *see* Acetaminophen and Diphenhydramine *on page 31*
- **Mapezine® (Can)** *see* CarBAMazepine *on page 280*

Maprotiline (ma PROE ti leen)

Brand Names: Canada Novo-Maprotiline; Teva-Maprotiline

Index Terms Ludiomil; Maprotiline Hydrochloride

Pharmacologic Category Antidepressant, Tetracyclic

Additional Appendix Information

Antidepressant Agents *on page 1874*

Use Treatment of major depressive disorder (MDD) or of anxiety associated with depression

Unlabeled Use Chronic pain; panic attacks

Pregnancy Risk Factor B

Medication Guide Available Yes

Dosage Oral:

Adults:

Mild-to-moderate depression/anxiety: Initial: 75 mg/day for 2 weeks (lower doses may be considered in some patients); Maintenance: Increase by 25 mg as tolerated up to 150 mg/day; given in divided doses or in a single daily dose

Severe depression: Initial: 100-150 mg/day for 2 weeks; Maintenance: Increase by 25 mg as tolerated up to 225 mg/day; given in divided doses or in a single daily dose

Elderly: Depression/anxiety: Initial: 25 mg/day for 2 weeks; Maintenance: Increase by 25 mg as tolerated; usual dose: 50-75 mg/day, higher doses may be necessary in nonresponders

Additional Information Complete prescribing information for this medication should be consulted for additional detail.

Dosage Forms Excipient information presented when available (limited, particularly for generics); consult specific product labeling.

Tablet, oral, as hydrochloride: 25 mg, 50 mg, 75 mg

- **Maprotiline Hydrochloride** *see* Maprotiline *on page 1052*

Maraviroc (mah RAV er rock)

Brand Names: U.S. Selzentry®

Brand Names: Canada Celsentri™

Index Terms UK-427,857

Pharmacologic Category Antiretroviral Agent, CCR5 Antagonist

Additional Appendix Information

Perinatal HIV Guidelines *on page 1946*

Use Treatment of CCR5-tropic HIV-1 infection, in combination with other antiretroviral agents

Pregnancy Risk Factor B

Pregnancy Considerations Adverse fetal effects were not observed in animal reproduction studies. It is not known if maraviroc crosses the placenta. The DHHS Perinatal HIV Guidelines note there are insufficient data to recommend use in pregnancy.

Regardless of CD4 count or HIV RNA copy number, all HIV-infected pregnant women should receive a combination antepartum antiretroviral (ARV) drug regimen; this includes women who require therapy for their own health, as well as women who do not yet require therapy for their own health. ARV therapy should be started as soon as possible if required for the woman's health or immediately after the first trimester if not needed for the mothers health (although earlier initiation may be considered). Long-term follow-up is recommended for all infants exposed to ARV medications.

Healthcare providers are encouraged to enroll pregnant women exposed to antiretroviral medications in the Antiretroviral Pregnancy Registry (1-800-258-4263 or www.APRegistry.com). Healthcare providers caring for HIV-infected women and their infants may contact the National Perinatal HIV Hotline (888-448-8765) for clinical consultation (DHHS [perinatal], 2011).

Lactation Excretion in breast milk unknown/contraindicated

Medication Guide Available Yes

Contraindications Patients with severe renal impairment (Cl_{cr} <30 mL/minute) or end-stage renal disease (ESRD) who are taking potent CYP3A4 inhibitors or inducers

Canadian labeling: Additional contraindications (not in U.S. labeling): Hypersensitivity to maraviroc or any component of the formulation

Warnings/Precautions [U.S. Boxed Warning] Possible drug-induced hepatotoxicity with allergic type features has been reported; hepatotoxicity (usually after 1 month of treatment) may be preceded by allergic type reactions (eg, pruritic rash, eosinophilia, fever or increased IgE) and/or hepatic adverse events (transaminase increases or signs/symptoms of hepatitis); some cases have been life-threatening; immediately evaluate patients with signs and symptoms of allergic reaction or hepatitis. Use with caution in patients with preexisting hepatic dysfunction or coinfection with HBV or HCV, however symptoms have occurred in the absence of preexisting hepatic conditions. Monitor hepatic function at baseline and as clinically indicated during treatment. Consider discontinuation in any patient with possible hepatitis or with elevated transaminases combined with systemic allergic events. Patients may develop immune reconstitution syndrome resulting in the occurrence of an inflammatory response to an indolent or residual opportunistic infection; further evaluation and treatment may be required. Monitor closely for signs/symptoms of developing infections; use associated with a small increase of certain upper respiratory tract infections and herpes virus infections during clinical trials. Use with caution in patients with cardiovascular disease or cardiac risk factors. During trials, a small increase in cardiovascular events (myocardial ischemia and/or infarction) occurred in treated patients compared to placebo, although a contributory relationship relative to therapy is unknown. Symptomatic postural hypotension has occurred; use caution in patients at risk for postural hypotension due to concomitant medication or history of condition. Adjust dose in patients with severe renal dysfunction if postural hypotension experienced.

Use caution in patients with mild-to-moderate hepatic impairment; maraviroc concentrations are increased; no dosage adjustment recommended. Maraviroc concentrations are further increased in patients with moderate hepatic impairment receiving concomitant strong CYP3A inhibitors; monitor closely for adverse events. Renal impairment may increase maraviroc concentrations. Use with caution in patients with mild-to-moderate renal impairment. Use with caution in patients taking strong CYP3A4/P-glycoprotein inhibitors and moderate or strong CYP3A4/P-glycoprotein inducers; may require dosage adjustments; avoid concurrent use in severe renal dysfunction (Cl_{cr} <30 mL/minute). Prior to therapy, tropism testing should be performed for presence of CCR5-tropic only virus HIV-1 infection. Therapy not recommended for use in patients with CXCR4- or dual/mixed tropic HIV-1 infection; efficacy not demonstrated in this population. In studies with treatment-naive patients, virologic failure and emergent lamivudine resistance was more common in maraviroc-treated patients compared to patients receiving efavirenz.

Adverse Reactions

>10%:

Central nervous system: Fever (13%)

Dermatologic: Rash (11%)

Respiratory: Upper respiratory tract infection (23%), cough (14%)

2% to 10%:

Cardiovascular: Vascular hypertensive disorder (3%)

Central nervous system: Dizziness (9%; including postural dizziness), insomnia (8%), anxiety (4%), consciousness disturbances (4%), depression (4%), pain (4%)

Dermatologic: Folliculitis (4%), pruritus (4%), skin neoplasms (benign; 3%), erythema (2%)

Endocrine & metabolic: Lipodystrophy (3%)

Gastrointestinal: Appetite disorders (8%), constipation (6%)

Genitourinary: Urinary tract/bladder symptoms (3% to 5%), genital warts (2%)

Hematologic: Neutropenia (grades 3/4: 4%)

Hepatic: Transaminases increased (grades 3/4: 3% to 5%), bilirubin increased (grades 3/4: 6%)

Neuromuscular & skeletal: Joint disorders (7%), paresthesia (5%), peripheral neuropathy (4%), sensory abnormality (4%), muscle pain (3%)

Ocular: Conjunctivitis (2%), infection/inflammation (2%)

Otic: Otitis media (2%)

Respiratory: Bronchitis (7%), sinusitis (7%), respiratory tract/sinus disorder (3% to 6%), breathing abnormality (4%)

Miscellaneous: Herpes infection (8%), sweat gland disturbances (5%), influenza (2%)

<2% (Limited to important or life-threatening): Acute cardiac failure, anal cancer, angina, basal cell carcinoma, bile duct neoplasm, bone marrow depression, cerebrovascular accident, cholestatic jaundice, coronary artery disease, coronary artery occlusion, creatine kinase increased, endocarditis, endocrine neoplasm, esophageal carcinoma, hepatic cirrhosis, hepatic failure, hepatotoxicity, hypoplastic anemia, liver metastases, lymphoma, MI, myocardial ischemia, myositis, osteonecrosis, pneumonia, portal vein thrombosis, rhabdomyolysis, seizure, septic shock, squamous cell carcinoma, Stevens-Johnson syndrome, syncope, T-cell lymphoma, tongue neoplasm, tremor, viral meningitis

Drug Interactions

Metabolism/Transport Effects Substrate of CYP3A4 (major), P-glycoprotein; **Note:** Assignment of Major/Minor substrate status based on clinically relevant drug interaction potential

Avoid Concomitant Use

Avoid concomitant use of Maraviroc with any of the following: St Johns Wort

Increased Effect/Toxicity

The levels/effects of Maraviroc may be increased by: CYP3A4 Inhibitors (Moderate); CYP3A4 Inhibitors (Strong); Dasatinib

Decreased Effect

The levels/effects of Maraviroc may be decreased by: CYP3A4 Inducers (Strong); Deferasirox; St Johns Wort; Tocilizumab

Ethanol/Nutrition/Herb Interactions Herb/Nutraceutical: St. John's wort may decrease maraviroc concentrations leading to loss of therapeutic efficacy and potentially increased risk of resistance; concomitant use not recommended.

Stability Store at 25°C (77°F); excursions permitted to 15°C to 30°C (59°F to 86°F).

Mechanism of Action Maraviroc, a CCR5 antagonist, selectively and reversibly binds to the chemokine (C-C motif receptor 5 [CCR5]) coreceptors located on human CD4 cells. CCR5 antagonism prevents interaction between the human CCR5 coreceptor and the gp120 subunit of the viral envelope glycoprotein, thereby inhibiting gp120 conformational change required for CCR5-tropic HIV-1 fusion with the CD4 cell and subsequent cell entry.

Pharmacodynamics/Kinetics

Distribution: V_d: ~194 L

Protein binding: ~76%

Metabolism: Hepatic, via CYP3A to inactive metabolites

Bioavailability: 23% to 33%

Half-life elimination: 14-18 hours

Time to peak, plasma: 0.5-4 hours

Excretion: Urine (~20%, 8% as unchanged drug); feces (76%, 25% as unchanged drug)

Dosage Oral: Adolescents ≥16 years and Adults: 300 mg twice daily

Dosage adjustment for concomitant CYP3A4 inhibitors/inducers:

CYP3A inhibitors (with or without a CYP3A4 inducer): 150 mg twice daily; dose recommended when maraviroc administered concomitantly with strong CYP3A inhibitors including (but not limited to) protease inhibitors (excluding tipranavir/ritonavir), delavirdine, ketoconazole, itraconazole, clarithromycin, nefazodone, and telithromycin.

CYP3A inducers (without a strong CYP3A4 inhibitor): 600 mg twice daily; dose recommended when maraviroc administered concomitantly with CYP3A inducers including (but not limited to) efavirenz, etravirine, rifampin, carbamazepine, phenobarbital, and phenytoin

Dosage adjustment in renal impairment:

Cl_{cr} ≥30 mL/minute:

Cl_{cr} ≥30 mL/minute and concomitant potent CYP3A4 inhibitors (with or without a CYP3A4 inducer): 150 mg twice daily

Cl_{cr} ≥30 mL/minute and concomitant potent CYP3A4 inducer (without a CYP3A4 inhibitor): 600 mg twice daily

Cl_{cr} ≥30 mL/minute and concomitant medications (eg, tipranavir/ritonavir, nevirapine, raltegravir, all NRTIs, and enfuvirtide): 300 mg twice daily

Cl_{cr} <30 mL/minute:

Cl_{cr} <30 mL/minute or ESRD and concomitant potent CYP3A inhibitors (with or without a CYP3A4 inducer) or concomitant potent CYP3A4 inducer (without a CYP3A4 inhibitor): Not recommended

Cl_{cr} <30 mL/minute or ESRD and concomitant medications (eg, tipranavir/ritonavir, nevirapine, raltegravir, all NRTIs, and enfuvirtide): 300 mg twice daily. If postural hypotension occurs, reduce dose to 150 mg twice daily

Cl_{cr} <30 mL/minute and experiencing postural hypotension: Reduce dose to 150 mg twice daily

Hemodialysis has minimal effect on clearance

Dosage adjustment in hepatic impairment:

Mild-to-moderate impairment: Use caution; maraviroc concentrations are increased although dosage adjustment is not recommended

Moderate impairment (with concomitant strong CYP3A4 inhibitor): Use caution; monitor closely for adverse events

Severe impairment: Patient population has not been studied

Dietary Considerations May be taken without regards to meals.

Administration Administer without regards to meals.

Monitoring Parameters Viral load, CD4 count, transaminases and bilirubin (prior to initiation and periodically during treatment); signs/symptoms of infection, hepatitis and/or allergic reaction; postural hypotension; tropism testing (prior to initiation)

Additional Information Maraviroc should only be used in patients with documented CCR5-tropic only virus; if it is used in mixed tropism patients, eg, with CCR5-tropic and CXCR4-tropic, the CCR5-tropic virus will be suppressed and the CXCR4-tropic virus will continue to proliferate. If a patient is receiving a stable antiretroviral regimen and their viral loads are undetectable, no routine, validated test currently exists to evaluate viral status and potential success of maraviroc therapy (DHHS, 2011).

Dosage Forms Excipient information presented when available (limited, particularly for generics); consult specific product labeling.

Tablet, oral:

Selzentry®: 150 mg, 300 mg

◆ **Marcaine®** *see* Bupivacaine *on page 242*
◆ **Marcaine® Spinal** *see* Bupivacaine *on page 242*
◆ **Mar-Cof® CG** *see* Guaifenesin and Codeine *on page 810*
◆ **Margesic** *see* Butalbital, Acetaminophen, and Caffeine *on page 255*
◆ **Margesic® H** *see* Hydrocodone and Acetaminophen *on page 837*
◆ **Marinol® (Can)** *see* Dronabinol *on page 561*
◆ **Mark 1™** *see* Atropine and Pralidoxime *on page 172*
◆ **Marvelon® (Can)** *see* Ethinyl Estradiol and Desogestrel *on page 653*
◆ **Matulane®** *see* Procarbazine *on page 1410*
◆ **Matzim™ LA** *see* Diltiazem *on page 510*
◆ **3M™ Avagard™ [OTC]** *see* Chlorhexidine Gluconate *on page 341*
◆ **Mavik®** *see* Trandolapril *on page 1718*
◆ **Maxair® Autohaler®** *see* Pirbuterol *on page 1360*
◆ **Maxalt®** *see* Rizatriptan *on page 1510*
◆ **Maxalt™ (Can)** *see* Rizatriptan *on page 1510*
◆ **Maxalt-MLT®** *see* Rizatriptan *on page 1510*
◆ **Maxalt RPD™ (Can)** *see* Rizatriptan *on page 1510*
◆ **Maxidex®** *see* Dexamethasone (Ophthalmic) *on page 483*
◆ **Maxidone®** *see* Hydrocodone and Acetaminophen *on page 837*
◆ **Maxifed [OTC]** *see* Guaifenesin and Pseudoephedrine *on page 813*
◆ **Maxifed DM** *see* Guaifenesin, Pseudoephedrine, and Dextromethorphan *on page 814*
◆ **Maxifed DMX** *see* Guaifenesin, Pseudoephedrine, and Dextromethorphan *on page 814*
◆ **Maxifed-G [OTC]** *see* Guaifenesin and Pseudoephedrine *on page 813*
◆ **Maxilene® (Can)** *see* Lidocaine (Topical) *on page 1009*
◆ **Maxiphen [OTC] [DSC]** *see* Guaifenesin and Phenylephrine *on page 812*
◆ **Maxipime®** *see* Cefepime *on page 306*
◆ **Maxitrol®** *see* Neomycin, Polymyxin B, and Dexamethasone *on page 1189*
◆ **Maxzide®** *see* Hydrochlorothiazide and Triamterene *on page 836*
◆ **Maxzide®-25** *see* Hydrochlorothiazide and Triamterene *on page 836*
◆ **May Apple** *see* Podophyllum Resin *on page 1370*
◆ **3M™ Cavilon™ Antifungal [OTC]** *see* Miconazole (Topical) *on page 1126*
◆ **MCV** *see* Meningococcal (Groups A / C / Y and W-135) Diphtheria Conjugate Vaccine *on page 1069*
◆ **MCV4** *see* Meningococcal (Groups A / C / Y and W-135) Diphtheria Conjugate Vaccine *on page 1069*
◆ **MDL 73,147EF** *see* Dolasetron *on page 540*
◆ **MDX-010** *see* Ipilimumab *on page 921*
◆ **MDX-CTLA-4** *see* Ipilimumab *on page 921*

Measles, Mumps, and Rubella Virus Vaccine (MEE zels, mumpz & roo BEL a VYE rus vak SEEN)

Brand Names: U.S. M-M-R® II

Brand Names: Canada M-M-R® II; Priorix™

Index Terms MMR; Mumps, Measles and Rubella Vaccines; Rubella, Measles and Mumps Vaccines

Pharmacologic Category Vaccine, Live (Viral)

Additional Appendix Information

Immunization Recommendations *on page 1922*

Use Measles, mumps, and rubella prophylaxis

The Advisory Committee on Immunization Practices (ACIP) recommends routine vaccination for the following:

- All children (first dose given at 12-15 months of age)
- Adults born 1957 or later (without evidence of immunity or documentation of vaccination).
- Adults at higher risk for exposure to and transmission of measles mumps and rubella should receive special consideration for vaccination, unless an acceptable evidence of immunity exists. This includes international travelers, persons attending colleges and other post-high school education, persons working in healthcare facilities.

Pregnancy Risk Factor C

Dosage SubQ:

Infants 6-11 months: *Measles outbreak:* If there is risk of exposure to measles, single-antigen measles vaccine should be administered. If single-antigen vaccine is not readily available, MMR is an acceptable alternative. Children should be revaccinated at ≥12 months with standard 2-dose series (CDC, 1998).

Children ≥12 months: 0.5 mL

Primary immunization is recommended at 12-15 months of age and repeated at 4-6 years of age; the second dose is recommended prior to elementary school. If the second dose was not received, the schedule should be completed by the 11- to 12-year old visit. (The second dose may be administered at any time provided at least 4 weeks have elapsed since the first dose.) For older children not previously vaccinated, at least 28 days should elapse between doses (CDC, 1998).

Mumps outbreak: During a mumps outbreak, children ages 1-4 years should consider a second dose of a live mumps virus vaccine; minimum interval between doses is 28 days (CDC, 2006).

Measles outbreak: Revaccination with MMR is recommended for attendees and siblings of daycare facilities or schools if they cannot provide adequate documentation of 2 previous doses of a measles-containing vaccine after their first birthday or evidence of measles immunity (CDC, 1998).

Adults: 0.5 mL

Birth year in or after 1957 without evidence of immunity: 1 or 2 doses (0.5 mL/dose); minimum interval between doses is 28 days

Adults born in or after 1957 without documentation of live vaccine on or after first birthday, or without physician-diagnosed measles or mumps, or without laboratory evidence of immunity, should be vaccinated with at least one dose; a second dose, separated by no less than 1 month, is indicated for those previously vaccinated with one dose of measles vaccine, students entering institutions of higher learning, recently exposed in an outbreak setting, healthcare workers at time of employment, and for travelers to endemic areas (CDC, 1998).

Persons vaccinated between 1963 and 1967 with a killed measles vaccine, followed by live vaccine within 3 months, or with a vaccine of unknown type should be revaccinated with live measles virus vaccine (CDC, 1998).

Women of childbearing potential, without documentation of rubella immunity, regardless of birth year, should also receive one dose of vaccine. Do not administer rubella to women who are or who may become pregnant within 1 month of receiving vaccine; administer following completion or termination of pregnancy (CDC, 1998).

Healthcare personnel (unvaccinated) born prior to 1957 and who are without laboratory evidence of measles, mumps and/or rubella immunity or laboratory confirmation of disease: Consider 2 doses of MMR vaccine at the appropriate interval. Two doses of the MMR vaccine are needed for measles and mumps, one dose is needed for rubella (CDC, 2006).

Additional Information Complete prescribing information for this medication should be consulted for additional detail.

Dosage Forms Excipient information presented when available (limited, particularly for generics); consult specific product labeling.

Injection, powder for reconstitution [preservative free]:

M-M-R® II: Measles virus ≥1000 $TCID_{50}$, mumps virus ≥20,000 $TCID_{50}$, and rubella virus ≥1000 $TCID_{50}$ [contains albumin (human), bovine serum, chicken egg protein, gelatin, neomycin, sorbitol, and sucrose 1.9 mg/vial]

Measles, Mumps, Rubella, and Varicella Virus Vaccine

(MEE zels, mumpz, roo BEL a, & var i SEL a VYE rus vak SEEN)

Brand Names: U.S. ProQuad®

Brand Names: Canada Priorix-Tetra™

Index Terms MMR-V; MMRV; Mumps, Rubella, Varicella, and Measles Vaccine; Rubella, Varicella, Measles, and Mumps Vaccine; Varicella, Measles, Mumps, and Rubella Vaccine

Pharmacologic Category Vaccine, Live (Viral)

Use To provide simultaneous active immunization against measles, mumps, rubella, and varicella

The Advisory Committee on Immunization Practices (ACIP) recommends routine vaccination against measles, mumps, rubella, and varicella in healthy children 12 months to 12 years of age. For children receiving their first dose at 12-47 months of age, either the MMRV combination vaccine or separate MMR and varicella vaccines can be used. (The ACIP prefers administration of separate MMR and varicella vaccines as the first dose in this age group unless the parent or caregiver expresses preference for the MMRV combination.) For children receiving the first dose at ≥48 months or their second dose at any age, use of MMRV is preferred.

Canadian labeling (not in U.S. labeling): MMRV combination vaccine is approved for use in healthy children 9 months to 6 years; may consider use in healthy children ≤12 years of age based upon prior experience with the separate component (live-attenuated MMR or live-attenuated varicella [OKA-strain]) vaccines.

Pregnancy Risk Factor C

Dosage *U.S. labeling:* SubQ: Children 12 months to 12 years: One dose (0.5 mL). The first dose is usually administered at 12-15 months of age. If a second dose of measles, mumps, rubella, and varicella vaccine is needed, ProQuad® can be used with the second dose usually administered at 4-6 years of age. (The second dose may be administered before age 4 if needed, as long as ≥3 months have elapsed since the first dose.)

Administer on or after the first birthday, as soon as child becomes eligible for vaccination. It may be used whenever all components of the vaccine are needed in children within this age group. (Refer to current CDC Recommended Immunization Schedule)

ACIP recommendations: For children receiving their first dose at 12-47 months of age, either the MMRV combination vaccine or separate MMR and varicella vaccines can be used. (The ACIP prefers administration of separate MMR and varicella vaccines as the first dose in this age group unless the parent or caregiver expresses preference for the MMRV combination.) For children receiving the first dose at ≥48 months or their second dose at any age, use of MMRV is preferred. The ACIP recommends that children with a personal or family history of seizures be vaccinated with separate MMR and varicella vaccines, as opposed to the MMRV combination vaccine (CDC, 2010)

Canadian labeling: I.M., SubQ: Children 9 months to 6 years: Two doses (0.5 mL each dose) administered at least 4-6 weeks apart (minimum interval between doses: 4 weeks)

Additional Information Complete prescribing information for this medication should be consulted for additional detail.

Dosage Forms Excipient information presented when available (limited, particularly for generics); consult specific product labeling.

Injection, powder for reconstitution [preservative free]:

ProQuad®: Measles virus ≥3.00 $\log_{10}$ $TCID_{50}$, mumps virus ≥4.3 $\log_{10}$ $TCID_{50}$, rubella virus ≥3.00 $\log_{10}$ $TCID_{50}$, and varicella virus ≥3.99 $\log_{10}$ PFU [contains albumin (human), bovine serum, chicken egg protein, gelatin, neomycin, sorbitol, and sucrose (≤21 mg/vial)]

Dosage Forms: Canada Excipient information presented when available (limited, particularly for generics); consult specific product labeling.

Injection, powder for reconstitution [preservative free]:

Priorix-Tetra™ (CAN): Measles virus ≥3.00 $\log_{10}$ $CCID_{50}$, mumps virus ≥4.4 $\log_{10}$ $CCID_{50}$, rubella virus ≥3.00 $\log_{10}$ $CCID_{50}$, and varicella virus ≥3.3 $\log_{10}$ PFU [contains chicken egg protein, neomycin, sorbitol, and sucrose]

◆ **Mebaral® [DSC]** *see* Mephobarbital *on page 1076*

◆ **Mebaral® (Can)** *see* Mephobarbital *on page 1076*

Mebendazole (me BEN da zole)

Brand Names: Canada Vermox®

Index Terms Vermox

Pharmacologic Category Anthelmintic

Use Treatment of *Enterobius vermicularis* (pinworms), *Trichuris trichiura* (whipworms), *Ascaris lumbricoides* (roundworms), and *Ancylostoma duodenale* or *Necator amiericanus* (hookworms)

Unlabeled Use Treatment of *Ancylostoma caninum* (eosinophilic enterocolitis), *Capillaria philippinensis* (capillariasis), *Giardia duodenalis* (giardiasis), *Mansonella perstans* (filariasis), visceral larva migrans (toxocariasis)

Pregnancy Risk Factor C

Dosage Children ≥2 years and Adults: Oral:

Ancylostoma duodenale (hookworm), *Necator americanus* (hookworm): 100 mg twice daily for 3 days **or** (unlabeled dosing) 500 mg as a single dose

Ascaris lumbricoides (roundworm): 100 mg twice daily for 3 days **or** (unlabeled dosing) 500 mg as a single dose

Enterobius vermicularis (pinworm): 100 mg as a single dose; may repeat in 2-3 weeks; treatment should include family members in close contact with patient

Trichuris trichiura (whipworm): 100 mg twice daily for 3 days **or** (unlabeled dosing) 500 mg as a single dose

Ancylostoma caninum (unlabeled use): 100 mg twice daily for 3 days

Capillaria philippinensis (capillariasis) (unlabeled use): 200 mg twice daily for 20 days

Giardia duodenalis (giardiasis) (unlabeled use): 200 mg three times a day for 5 days (Canete, 2006; Chandy, 2009)

Mansonella perstans (filariasis) (unlabeled use): 100 mg twice daily for 30 days

Visceral larva migrans (toxocariasis) (unlabeled use): 100-200 mg twice daily for 5 days

Additional Information Complete prescribing information for this medication should be consulted for additional detail.

Dosage Forms Excipient information presented when available (limited, particularly for generics); consult specific product labeling. [DSC] = Discontinued product

Tablet, chewable, oral: 100 mg [DSC]

Mechlorethamine (me klor ETH a meen)

Brand Names: U.S. Mustargen®

Brand Names: Canada Mustargen®

Index Terms Chlorethazine; Chlorethazine Mustard; HN_2; Mechlorethamine Hydrochloride; Mustine; Nitrogen Mustard

Pharmacologic Category Antineoplastic Agent, Alkylating Agent (Nitrogen Mustard)

Use Hodgkin's disease; non-Hodgkin's lymphoma; intracavitary injection for treatment of metastatic tumors; pleural and other malignant effusions

Unlabeled Use Topical treatment of mycosis fungoides

Pregnancy Risk Factor D

Pregnancy Considerations Animal studies have demonstrated teratogenic effects. There are no adequate and well-controlled studies in pregnant women. Women of childbearing potential are advised not to become pregnant. Use only when potential benefit justifies potential risk to the fetus. **[U.S. Boxed Warning]: Avoid exposure during pregnancy.**

Lactation Excretion in breast milk unknown/not recommended

Contraindications Hypersensitivity to mechlorethamine or any component of the formulation; presence of known infection

Warnings/Precautions [U.S. Boxed Warnings]: Hazardous agent - use appropriate precautions for handling and disposal. Avoid contact with skin or eyes; avoid exposure during pregnancy. Mechlorethamine is a potent vesicant; if extravasation occurs, severe tissue damage (leading to ulceration and necrosis) and pain may occur. Sodium thiosulfate should be available for treatment of extravasation. May cause lymphopenia, granulocytopenia, thrombocytopenia and anemia. Hyperuricemia may occur, especially with lymphomas; ensure adequate hydration. **[U.S. Boxed Warning]: Should be administered under the supervision of an experienced cancer chemotherapy physician.**

Adverse Reactions

>10%:

Endocrine & metabolic: Delayed menses, oligomenorrhea, temporary or permanent amenorrhea, impaired spermatogenesis; spermatogenesis may return in patients in remission several years after the discontinuation of chemotherapy, chromosomal abnormalities

Gastrointestinal: Nausea and vomiting usually occur in nearly 100% of patients and onset is within 30 minutes to 2 hours after administration

Emetic potential: Very high (>90%)

Time course of nausea/vomiting: Onset: 1-3 hours; duration 2-8 hours

Genitourinary: Azoospermia

Hematologic: Myelosuppressive: Leukopenia and thrombocytopenia can be severe; caution should be used with patients who are receiving radiotherapy, secondary leukemia

WBC: Severe

Platelets: Severe

Onset (days): 4-7

Nadir (days): 14

Recovery (days): 21

Otic: Ototoxicity

Miscellaneous: Precipitation of herpes zoster

1% to 10%:

Central nervous system: Fever, vertigo

Dermatologic: Alopecia

Endocrine & metabolic: Hyperuricemia

Gastrointestinal: Diarrhea, anorexia, metallic taste

Local: Thrombophlebitis/extravasation: May cause local vein discomfort which may be relieved by warm soaks and pain medication. A brown discoloration of veins may occur. Mechlorethamine is a strong vesicant and can cause tissue necrosis and sloughing.

Vesicant chemotherapy

Secondary malignancies: Have been reported after several years in 1% to 6% of patients treated

Neuromuscular & skeletal: Weakness

Otic: Tinnitus

Miscellaneous: Hypersensitivity, anaphylaxis

<1% (Limited to important or life-threatening): Hemolytic anemia, hepatotoxicity, myelosuppression, peripheral neuropathy

Drug Interactions

Metabolism/Transport Effects None known.

Avoid Concomitant Use

Avoid concomitant use of Mechlorethamine with any of the following: BCG; CloZAPine; Natalizumab; Pimecrolimus; Tacrolimus (Topical); Vaccines (Live)

Increased Effect/Toxicity

Mechlorethamine may increase the levels/effects of: CloZAPine; Leflunomide; Natalizumab; Vaccines (Live)

The levels/effects of Mechlorethamine may be increased by: Denosumab; Pimecrolimus; Roflumilast; Tacrolimus (Topical); Trastuzumab

Decreased Effect

Mechlorethamine may decrease the levels/effects of: BCG; Coccidioidin Skin Test; Sipuleucel-T; Vaccines (Inactivated); Vaccines (Live)

The levels/effects of Mechlorethamine may be decreased by: Echinacea

Ethanol/Nutrition/Herb Interactions Ethanol: Avoid ethanol (due to GI irritation).

Stability Store intact vials at room temperature of 15°C to 30°C (59°F to 86°F). Protect from light. **Must be prepared immediately before use**; solution is stable for only 15-60 minutes after dilution. Use appropriate precautions for handling. Dilute powder with 10 mL SWFI or 0.9% sodium chloride to a final concentration of 1 mg/mL. May be diluted in up to 100 mL NS for intracavitary or topical administration. Extemporaneous formulations for topical use have been reported to retain biologic activity for 30 days.

Mechanism of Action Bifunctional alkylating agent that inhibits DNA and RNA synthesis via formation of carbonium ions; cross-links strands of DNA, causing miscoding, breakage, and failure of replication; produces interstrand and intrastrand cross-links in DNA resulting in miscoding, breakage, and failure of replication. Although not cell phase-specific *per se,* mechlorethamine effect is most pronounced in the S phase, and cell proliferation is arrested in the G_2 phase.

Pharmacodynamics/Kinetics

Duration: Unchanged drug is undetectable in blood within a few minutes

Absorption: Intracavitary administration: Incomplete secondary to rapid deactivation by body fluids

Metabolism: Rapid hydrolysis and demethylation, possibly in plasma

Half-life elimination: <1 minute

Excretion: Urine (50% as metabolites, <0.01% as unchanged drug)

Dosage Details concerning dosing in combination regimens should also be consulted. Dosage should be based on ideal dry weight (evaluate the presence of edema or ascites so that dosage is based on actual weight unaugmented by edema/ascites).

Children and Adults (unlabeled dosing): Lymphoma: I.V.: 6 mg/m^2 on days 1 and 8 of a 28-day cycle (MOPP regimen)

Adults:

I.V.: Lymphoma: 0.4 mg/kg as a single dose or in divided doses of 0.1 mg/kg/day (for 4 days) or 0.2 mg/kg/day (for 2 days) per treatment course; repeat treatment course after hematologic recovery

Intracavitary: 0.4 mg/kg as a single dose, although 0.2 mg/kg (10-20 mg) as a single dose has been used by the *intrapericardial* route

Topical (unlabeled use): 0.01% to 0.02% solution, lotion, or ointment

Hemodialysis: Not removed; supplemental dosing is not required.

Peritoneal dialysis: Not removed; supplemental dosing is not required.

Administration

I.V.: Administer as a slow I.V. push over a few minutes into a free-flowing I.V. solution. Must be prepared immediately prior to administration. Due to the limited stability of the drug, and the increased risk of phlebitis and venous irritation and blistering with increased contact time, infusions of the drug are not recommended.

Intracavitary: May further dilute in 50-100 mL of normal saline prior to instillation; rotate patient position every 5-10 minutes for 1 hour after instillation to obtain uniform distribution.

Mechlorethamine may cause extravasation. Use within 1 hour of preparation. Avoid extravasation since mechlorethamine is a potent vesicant.

Monitoring Parameters CBC with differential, hemoglobin, and platelet count

Dosage Forms Excipient information presented when available (limited, particularly for generics); consult specific product labeling.

Injection, powder for reconstitution, as hydrochloride:

Mustargen®: 10 mg

◆ **Mechlorethamine Hydrochloride** *see* Mechlorethamine *on page 1056*

Meclizine (MEK li zeen)

Brand Names: U.S. Antivert®; Bonine® [OTC]; Dramamine® Less Drowsy Formula [OTC]; Medi-Meclizine [OTC]; Trav-L-Tabs® [OTC]

Brand Names: Canada Bonamine™; Bonine®

Index Terms Meclizine Hydrochloride; Meclozine Hydrochloride

Pharmacologic Category Antiemetic; Histamine H_1 Antagonist; Histamine H_1 Antagonist, First Generation; Piperazine Derivative

Use Prevention and treatment of symptoms of motion sickness; management of vertigo with diseases affecting the vestibular system

Pregnancy Risk Factor B

Pregnancy Considerations No data available on crossing the placenta. Probably no effect on the fetus (insufficient data). Available evidence suggests safe use during pregnancy.

Lactation Excretion in breast milk unknown/not recommended

Contraindications Hypersensitivity to meclizine or any component of the formulation

Warnings/Precautions Use with caution in patients with asthma, angle-closure glaucoma, prostatic hyperplasia, pyloric or duodenal obstruction, or bladder neck obstruction. Elderly may be at risk for anticholinergic side effects such as glaucoma, prostatic hyperplasia, constipation, GI obstructive disease. If vertigo does not respond in 1-2 weeks, it is advised to discontinue use. May be sedating, use with caution in disorders where CNS depression is a feature; patients must be cautioned about performing tasks which require mental alertness (eg, operating machinery or driving). Effects may be potentiated when used with other sedative drugs or ethanol.

Adverse Reactions

>10%:

Central nervous system: Slight to moderate drowsiness

Respiratory: Thickening of bronchial secretions

1% to 10%:

Central nervous system: Headache, fatigue, nervousness, dizziness

Gastrointestinal: Appetite increase, weight gain, nausea, diarrhea, abdominal pain, dry mouth

Respiratory: Pharyngitis

<1% (Limited to important or life-threatening): Bronchospasm, hepatitis, hypotension, palpitation

Drug Interactions

Metabolism/Transport Effects None known.

Avoid Concomitant Use There are no known interactions where it is recommended to avoid concomitant use.

Increased Effect/Toxicity

Meclizine may increase the levels/effects of: Alcohol (Ethyl); Anticholinergics; CNS Depressants; Methotrimeprazine; Selective Serotonin Reuptake Inhibitors

The levels/effects of Meclizine may be increased by: Droperidol; HydrOXYzine; Methotrimeprazine; Pramlintide

Decreased Effect

Meclizine may decrease the levels/effects of: Acetylcholinesterase Inhibitors (Central); Benzylpenicilloyl Polylysine; Betahistine

The levels/effects of Meclizine may be decreased by: Acetylcholinesterase Inhibitors (Central); Amphetamines

Ethanol/Nutrition/Herb Interactions Ethanol: May increase CNS depression; monitor for increased effects with coadministration. Caution patients about effects.

Mechanism of Action Has central anticholinergic action by blocking chemoreceptor trigger zone; decreases excitability of the middle ear labyrinth and blocks conduction in the middle ear vestibular-cerebellar pathways

Pharmacodynamics/Kinetics
Onset of action: ~1 hour
Duration: 8-24 hours
Metabolism: Hepatic
Half-life elimination: 6 hours
Excretion: Urine (as metabolites); feces (as unchanged drug)

Dosage Children >12 years and Adults: Oral:
Motion sickness: 12.5-25 mg 1 hour before travel, repeat dose every 12-24 hours if needed; doses up to 50 mg may be needed
Vertigo: 25-100 mg/day in divided doses

Dosage Forms Excipient information presented when available (limited, particularly for generics); consult specific product labeling.
Caplet, oral, as hydrochloride: 12.5 mg
Tablet, oral, as hydrochloride: 12.5 mg, 25 mg
Antivert®: 12.5 mg, 25 mg, 50 mg
Dramamine® Less Drowsy Formula: 25 mg
Medi-Meclizine: 25 mg
Trav-L-Tabs®: 25 mg
Tablet, chewable, oral, as hydrochloride: 25 mg
Bonine®: 25 mg [scored; raspberry flavor]

◆ **Meclizine Hydrochloride** *see* Meclizine *on page* 1057
◆ **Meclozine Hydrochloride** *see* Meclizine *on page* 1057
◆ **Med-Baclofen (Can)** *see* Baclofen *on page* 187
◆ **Medent®-PEI [OTC]** *see* Guaifenesin and Phenylephrine *on page* 812
◆ **Med-Glybe (Can)** *see* GlyBURIDE *on page* 799
◆ **Medicinal Carbon** *see* Charcoal, Activated *on page* 335
◆ **Medicinal Charcoal** *see* Charcoal, Activated *on page* 335
◆ **Medicone® Hemorrhoidal [OTC]** *see* Benzocaine *on page* 202
◆ **Medi-First® Sinus Decongestant [OTC]** *see* Phenylephrine (Systemic) *on page* 1344
◆ **Medi-Meclizine [OTC]** *see* Meclizine *on page* 1057
◆ **Medi-Phenyl [OTC]** *see* Phenylephrine (Systemic) *on page* 1344
◆ **Mediproxen [OTC]** *see* Naproxen *on page* 1177
◆ **MED-Letrozole (Can)** *see* Letrozole *on page* 986
◆ **Med-Metformin (Can)** *see* MetFORMIN *on page* 1086
◆ **Medrol®** *see* MethylPREDNISolone *on page* 1110
◆ **Medrol Dose Pack** *see* MethylPREDNISolone *on page* 1110
◆ **Medrol® Dosepak™** *see* MethylPREDNISolone *on page* 1110
◆ **Medroxy (Can)** *see* MedroxyPROGESTERone *on page* 1058

MedroxyPROGESTERone
(me DROKS ee proe JES te rone)

Brand Names: U.S. Depo-Provera®; Depo-Provera® Contraceptive; depo-subQ provera 104®; Provera®

Brand Names: Canada Alti-MPA; Apo-Medroxy®; Depo-Prevera®; Depo-Provera®; Dom-Medroxyprogesterone; Gen-Medroxy; Medroxy; Medroxyprogesterone Acetate Injectable Suspension USP; Novo-Medrone; PMS-Medroxyprogesterone; Provera-Pak; Provera®; Teva-Medroxyprogesterone

Index Terms Acetoxymethylprogesterone; Medroxyprogesterone Acetate; Methylacetoxyprogesterone; MPA

Pharmacologic Category Contraceptive; Progestin

Use Secondary amenorrhea or abnormal uterine bleeding due to hormonal imbalance; reduction of endometrial hyperplasia in nonhysterectomized postmenopausal women receiving conjugated estrogens; prevention of pregnancy; management of endometriosis-associated pain; adjunctive therapy and palliative treatment of recurrent and metastatic endometrial carcinoma

Unlabeled Use Treatment of low-grade endometrial stromal sarcoma

Pregnancy Risk Factor X

Pregnancy Considerations In general, there is not an increased risk of birth defects following inadvertent use of the injectable medroxyprogesterone contraceptives early in pregnancy. There is an increased risk of minor birth defects in children whose mothers take progesterones during the first 4 months of pregnancy. Hypospadias has been reported in male babies and mild masculinization of the external genitalia has been reported in female babies exposed during the first trimester. High doses are used to impair fertility. Ectopic pregnancies have been reported with use of the MPA contraceptive injection. Median time to conception/return to ovulation following discontinuation of MPA contraceptive injection is 10 months following the last injection.

Lactation Enters breast milk

Contraindications Hypersensitivity to medroxyprogesterone or any component of the formulation; history of or current thrombophlebitis or venous thromboembolic disorders (including DVT, PE); cerebral vascular disease; severe hepatic dysfunction or disease; carcinoma of the breast or other estrogen- or progesterone-dependent neoplasia; undiagnosed vaginal bleeding; missed abortion, diagnostic test for pregnancy, pregnancy

Warnings/Precautions **[U.S. Boxed Warning]: Prolonged use of medroxyprogesterone contraceptive injection may result in a loss of bone mineral density (BMD). It is not known if use during adolescence or early adulthood will decrease peak bone mass accretion or increase the risk for osteoporotic fractures later in life. Loss is related to the duration of use, may not be completely reversible on discontinuation of the drug,** and incidence is not significantly different between the SubQ and I.M. dosage forms. The impact on peak bone mass in adolescents should be weighed against the potential for unintended pregnancies in treatment decision. Consider alternative contraceptive methods in patients at risk for osteoporosis (eg, metabolic bone disease, family history of osteoporosis, chronic use of medications associated with osteoporosis such as corticosteroids). **[U.S. Boxed Warning]: Long-term use (ie, >2 years) should be limited to situations where other birth control methods are inadequate.** Consider other methods of birth control in women with (or at risk for) osteoporosis. **[U.S. Boxed Warning]: Inform patients that injectable contraceptives do not protect against HIV infection or other sexually-transmitted diseases.** When used for contraception, the possibility of ectopic pregnancy should be considered in patients with abdominal pain. Anaphylaxis or anaphylactoid reactions have been reported with use of the injection; medication for the treatment of hypersensitivity reactions should be available for immediate use.

[U.S. Boxed Warning]: Estrogens with or without progestin should not be used to prevent coronary heart disease. Use caution with cardiovascular disease or dysfunction. MPA used in combination with estrogen may increase the risks of hypertension, myocardial infarction (MI), stroke, pulmonary emboli (PE), and deep vein thrombosis; incidence of these effects was shown to be significantly increased in postmenopausal women using conjugated equine estrogens (CEE) in combination with MPA.

[U.S. Boxed Warning]: The risk of dementia may be increased in postmenopausal women; increased incidence was observed in women ≥65 years of age taking MPA in combination with CEE. An increased risk of invasive breast cancer was observed in postmenopausal women using MPA in combination with CEE. An increase in abnormal mammograms has also been reported with estrogen and progestin therapy. Use is contraindicated in patients with known or suspected breast cancer, Whenever possible, progestins in combination with estrogens should be discontinued at least 4-6 weeks prior to surgeries associated with an increased risk of thromboembolism or during periods of prolonged immobilization. If thrombosis develops with contraceptive treatment, discontinue treatment (unless no other acceptable contraceptive alternative). Progestins used in combination with estrogen should be used for shortest duration possible consistent with treatment goals. Conduct periodic risk:benefit assessments.

Discontinue pending examination in cases of sudden partial or complete vision loss, sudden onset of proptosis, diplopia, or migraine; discontinue permanently if papilledema or retinal vascular lesions are observed on examination. Use with caution in patients with diseases that may be exacerbated by fluid retention (including asthma, epilepsy, migraine, cardiac, or renal dysfunction). Contraceptive therapy with medroxyprogesterone commonly results in an average weight gain of ~2.5 kg after 1 year and ~3.7 kg after 2 years of treatment. Use caution with history of depression.

May have adverse effects on glucose tolerance; use caution in women with diabetes. MPA is extensively metabolized in the liver. Discontinue if jaundice develops or if acute or chronic hepatic disturbances occur. Use is contraindicated with severe hepatic disease. Unscheduled bleeding/spotting may occur. Presentation of irregular, unresolving vaginal bleeding following previously regular cycles warrants further evaluation including endometrial sampling, if indicated, to rule out malignancy. Not for use prior to menarche.

Adverse Reactions Adverse effects as reported with any dosage form; percent ranges presented are noted with the MPA I.M. contraceptive injection:

>5%:
- Central nervous system: Dizziness, headache, nervousness
- Endocrine & metabolic: Libido decreased, menstrual irregularities (includes bleeding, amenorrhea, or both)
- Gastrointestinal: Abdominal pain/discomfort, weight gain (>10 lbs at 24 months: 38%)

1% to 5%:
- Cardiovascular: Edema
- Central nervous system: Depression, fatigue, insomnia
- Dermatologic: Acne, alopecia, rash
- Endocrine & metabolic: Breast pain, hot flashes
- Gastrointestinal: Bloating, nausea
- Genitourinary: Dysmenorrhea, leukorrhea, vaginitis
- Local: Injection site reaction (SubQ administration): Atrophy, induration, pain
- Neuromuscular & skeletal: Arthralgia, backache, leg cramp, weakness

<1% (Limited to important or life-threatening): Allergic reaction, anaphylaxis, anaphylactoid reactions, angioedema, asthma, blood dyscrasia, bone mineral density decreased, breast cancer, breast changes, cervical cancer, chest pain, chloasma, cholestatic jaundice, deep vein thrombosis, diaphoresis, dyspnea, facial palsy, galactorrhea, glucose tolerance decreased, hirsutism, hoarseness, injection site reactions, jaundice, lack of return to fertility, lactation decreased, melasma, nipple bleeding, optic neuritis, osteoporosis, osteoporotic fractures, paralysis, paresthesia, pulmonary embolus, rectal bleeding, retinal thrombosis, scleroderma, seizure, syncope, tachycardia, thrombophlebitis, urticaria

In addition: Depo-Provera® aqueous suspension: Residual lump, sterile abscess, or skin discoloration at the injection

Drug Interactions

Metabolism/Transport Effects Substrate of CYP3A4 (major); **Note:** Assignment of Major/Minor substrate status based on clinically relevant drug interaction potential; **Induces** CYP3A4 (weak/moderate)

Avoid Concomitant Use

Avoid concomitant use of MedroxyPROGESTERone with any of the following: Griseofulvin

Increased Effect/Toxicity

MedroxyPROGESTERone may increase the levels/effects of: Benzodiazepines (metabolized by oxidation); Selegiline; Tranexamic Acid; Voriconazole

The levels/effects of MedroxyPROGESTERone may be increased by: Boceprevir; Conivaptan; Herbs (Progestogenic Properties); Voriconazole

Decreased Effect

MedroxyPROGESTERone may decrease the levels/effects of: ARIPiprazole; Saxagliptin; Vitamin K Antagonists

The levels/effects of MedroxyPROGESTERone may be decreased by: Acitretin; Aminoglutethimide; Aprepitant; Artemether; Barbiturates; Bexarotene; Bexarotene (Systemic); Bile Acid Sequestrants; Bosentan; CarBAMazepine; Clobazam; CYP3A4 Inducers (Strong); Deferasirox; Felbamate; Fosaprepitant; Fosphenytoin; Griseofulvin; LamoTRIgine; Mycophenolate; Nevirapine; OXcarbazepine; Phenytoin; Retinoic Acid Derivatives; Rifamycin Derivatives; St Johns Wort; Telaprevir; Tocilizumab; Topiramate

Ethanol/Nutrition/Herb Interactions

Ethanol: Avoid ethanol (may increase risk of osteoporosis).

Food: Bioavailability of the oral tablet is increased when taken with food; half-life is unchanged.

Herb/Nutraceutical: St John's wort may diminish the therapeutic effect of progestin contraceptives (contraceptive failure is possible).

Stability Store at controlled room temperature.

Mechanism of Action Inhibits secretion of pituitary gonadotropins, which prevents follicular maturation and ovulation; causes endometrial thinning

Pharmacodynamics/Kinetics

Absorption: Oral: Well absorbed; I.M.: Slow

Protein binding: 86% to 90% primarily to albumin; does not bind to sex hormone-binding globulin

Metabolism: Extensively hepatic via hydroxylation and conjugation; forms metabolites

Half-life elimination: Oral: 12-17 hours; I.M. (Depo-Provera® Contraceptive): ~50 days; SubQ: ~40 days

Time to peak: Oral: 2-4 hours; I.M. (Depo-Provera® Contraceptive): ~3 weeks; SubQ: ~1 week

Excretion: Urine

Dosage

Adolescents and Adults:
- Amenorrhea: Oral: 5-10 mg/day for 5-10 days
- Abnormal uterine bleeding: Oral: 5-10 mg for 5-10 days starting on day 16 or 21 of cycle
- Contraception:
  - Depo-Provera® Contraceptive: I.M.: 150 mg every 3 months
  - depo-subQ provera 104™: SubQ: 104 mg every 3 months (every 12-14 weeks)
- Endometriosis (depo-subQ provera 104™): SubQ: 104 mg every 3 months (every 12-14 weeks)

Adults:
Endometrial carcinoma, recurrent or metastatic (adjunctive/palliative treatment) (Depo-Provera®): I.M.: 400-1000 mg/week
Accompanying cyclic estrogen therapy, postmenopausal: Oral: 5-10 mg for 12-14 consecutive days each month, starting on day 1 or day 16 of the cycle; lower doses may be used if given with estrogen continuously throughout the cycle

Dosing adjustment in hepatic impairment: Use is contraindicated with severe impairment. Discontinue with jaundice or if liver function disturbances occur. Consider lower dose or less frequent administration with mild-to-moderate impairment. Use of the contraceptive injection has not been studied in patients with hepatic impairment; consideration should be given to not readminister if jaundice develops

Dietary Considerations Ensure adequate calcium and vitamin D intake

Administration
I.M.: Depo-Provera® Contraceptive: Administer first dose during the first 5 days of menstrual period, or within the first 5 days postpartum if not breast-feeding, or at the sixth week postpartum if breast-feeding exclusively. Shake vigorously prior to administration. Administer by deep I.M. injection in the gluteal or deltoid muscle.
When switching from combined hormonal contraceptives (estrogen plus progestin), the first injection should be on the day after the last active tablet or (at the latest) the day after the final inactive tablet. When switching from other contraceptive methods, ensure continuous contraceptive coverage.
SubQ: depo-subQ provera 104™: Administer first dose during the first 5 days of menstrual period, or at the sixth week postpartum if breast-feeding. Shake vigorously prior to administration. Administer by SubQ injection in the anterior thigh or abdomen; avoid boney areas and the umbilicus. Administer over 5-7 seconds. Do not rub the injection area. When switching from combined hormonal contraceptives (estrogen plus progestin), the first injection should be within 7 days after the last active pill, or removal of patch or ring. If switching from the I.M. to SubQ formulation, the next dose should be given within the prescribed dosing period for the I.M. injection to assure continuous coverage.

Monitoring Parameters Before starting therapy, a physical exam with reference to the breasts and pelvis are recommended, including a Papanicolaou smear. Exam may be deferred if appropriate prior to administration of MPA contraceptive injection; pregnancy should be ruled out prior to use. Monitor patient closely for loss of vision; sudden onset of proptosis, diplopia, or migraine; signs and symptoms of thromboembolic disorders; signs or symptoms of depression; glucose in patients with diabetes; or blood pressure. BMD with long-term use (per manufacturer).

Adequate diagnostic measures, including endometrial sampling, if indicated, should be performed to rule out malignancy in all cases of undiagnosed abnormal vaginal bleeding.

Test Interactions
The following tests may be decreased: Steroid levels (plasma and urinary), gonadotropin levels, SHBG concentration, T_3 uptake
The following tests may be increased: Protein-bound iodine, butanol extractable protein-bound iodine, Factors II, VII, VIII, IX, X
Pathologist should be advised of estrogen/progesterone therapy when specimens are submitted.

Dosage Forms Excipient information presented when available (limited, particularly for generics); consult specific product labeling.
Injection, suspension, as acetate: 150 mg/mL (1 mL)
Depo-Provera®: 400 mg/mL (2.5 mL)
Depo-Provera® Contraceptive: 150 mg/mL (1 mL) [contains polysorbate 80]
depo-subQ provera 104®: 104 mg/0.65 mL (0.65 mL) [contains polysorbate 80]
Tablet, oral, as acetate: 2.5 mg, 5 mg, 10 mg
Provera®: 2.5 mg, 5 mg, 10 mg [scored]

- **Medroxyprogesterone Acetate** *see* MedroxyPROGESTERone *on page 1058*
- **Medroxyprogesterone Acetate Injectable Suspension USP (Can)** *see* MedroxyPROGESTERone *on page 1058*
- **Med-Salbutamol (Can)** *see* Albuterol *on page 52*
- **Med-Sotalol (Can)** *see* Sotalol *on page 1586*
- **Mefenamic-250 (Can)** *see* Mefenamic Acid *on page 1060*

Mefenamic Acid (me fe NAM ik AS id)

Brand Names: U.S. Ponstel®
Brand Names: Canada Apo-Mefenamic®; Dom-Mefenamic Acid; Mefenamic-250; Nu-Mefenamic; PMS-Mefenamic Acid; Ponstan®
Pharmacologic Category Nonsteroidal Anti-inflammatory Drug (NSAID), Oral
Use Short-term relief of mild-to-moderate pain including primary dysmenorrhea
Pregnancy Risk Factor C
Medication Guide Available Yes
Dosage Children >14 years and Adults: Oral: 500 mg to start then 250 mg every 6 hours as needed; maximum therapy: 1 week

Dosing adjustment/comments in renal impairment: Not recommended for use

Additional Information Complete prescribing information for this medication should be consulted for additional detail.
Dosage Forms Excipient information presented when available (limited, particularly for generics); consult specific product labeling.
Capsule, oral: 250 mg
Ponstel®: 250 mg

Mefloquine (ME floe kwin)

Brand Names: Canada Apo-Mefloquine®; Lariam®
Index Terms Mefloquine Hydrochloride
Pharmacologic Category Antimalarial Agent
Use Treatment of mild-to-moderate acute malarial infections (including treatment of chloroquine-resistant malaria) and prevention of malaria caused by *Plasmodium falciparum* or *P. vivax*

Note: Due to geographical resistance and cross-resistance, consult current CDC guidelines.

Unlabeled Use Treatment of uncomplicated, chloroquine-resistant *P. vivax* malaria
Pregnancy Risk Factor B
Pregnancy Considerations Mefloquine crosses the placenta and is teratogenic in animals. Malaria infection in pregnant women may be more severe than in nonpregnant women. Clinical experience with mefloquine has not shown teratogenic or embryotoxic effects in humans; use with caution during pregnancy if travel to endemic areas cannot be postponed. Nonpregnant women of childbearing potential are advised to use contraception and avoid pregnancy during malaria prophylaxis and for 3 months

thereafter. In case of an unplanned pregnancy, treatment with mefloquine is not considered a reason for pregnancy termination. CDC treatment guidelines are available for the use of mefloquine in the treatment of malaria during pregnancy (CDC, 2011).

Lactation Enters breast milk/use caution

Medication Guide Available Yes

Contraindications Hypersensitivity to mefloquine, related compounds (eg, quinine and quinidine), or any component of the formulation; prophylactic use in patients with a history of seizures or psychiatric disorder (including active or recent history of depression, generalized anxiety disorder, psychosis, or schizophrenia)

Warnings/Precautions May cause a range of psychiatric symptoms (anxiety, paranoia, depression, hallucinations and psychosis). Occasionally, symptoms have been reported to persist long after mefloquine has been discontinued. Rare cases of suicidal ideation and suicide have been reported (no causal relationship established). The appearance of psychiatric symptoms such as acute anxiety, depression, restlessness or confusion may be considered a prodrome to more serious events. Use with caution in patients with a previous history of depression; prophylactic use is contraindicated in patients with active or recent history of psychiatric disorders. Discontinue if unexplained neuropsychiatric disturbances occur. Use caution in patients with significant cardiac disease, hepatic impairment, or seizure disorder. If mefloquine is to be used for a prolonged period, periodic evaluations including liver function tests and ophthalmic examinations should be performed. (Retinal abnormalities have not been observed with mefloquine in humans; however, abnormalities have been reported with long-term administration to rats.) Hypersensitivity reactions ranging from mild skin reactions to anaphylaxis have occurred. Agranulocytosis and aplastic anemia have been reported with use.

In cases of life-threatening, serious, or overwhelming malaria infections due to *Plasmodium falciparum*, patients should be treated with intravenous antimalarial drug. Mefloquine may be given orally to complete the course. In cases of acute *Plasmodium vivax* infection treated with mefloquine, patients should subsequently be treated with an 8-aminoquinoline derivative (eg, primaquine) to avoid relapse. Dizziness, loss of balance, and other CNS disorders (eg, seizures) have been reported; due to long half-life, effects may persist after mefloquine is discontinued. Use caution in activities requiring alertness and fine motor coordination (eg, driving, piloting planes, operating machinery). Concurrent use with chloroquine and quinine derivatives may increase risk of seizures. Concurrent use with quinine derivatives may increase risk of ECG abnormalities. Concurrent use with ketoconazole is not recommended due to increased risk of QT_c prolongation; do not administer within 15 weeks of the last dose of mefloquine. Early vomiting leading to treatment failure in children has been reported in some studies; consider alternate therapy if a second dose is not tolerated.

Not recommended for the treatment of malaria acquired in Southeast Asia due to drug resistance.

Adverse Reactions

1% to 10%:

- Central nervous system: Chills, dizziness, fatigue, fever, headache
- Dermatologic: Rash
- Gastrointestinal: Vomiting (3%), abdominal pain, appetite decreased, diarrhea, nausea
- Neuromuscular & skeletal: Myalgia
- Otic: Tinnitus

<1% (Limited to important or life-threatening): Abnormal dreams, abnormal T waves, ataxia, aggressive behavior, agitation, anxiety, arrhythmia, arthralgia, AV block, cardiac arrest (with concomitant use of propranolol), chest pain, conduction abnormalities (transient), confusion, depression, diaphoresis increased, dyspepsia, dyspnea, edema, encephalopathy, erythema, erythema multiforme, exanthema, flushing, forgetfulness, hallucinations, hearing impairment, hematocrit decreased, hyper-/hypotension, insomnia, irregular pulse, leukocytosis, leukopenia, liver function tests increased, loss of balance, malaise, mood changes, muscle cramps/weakness, palpitation, panic attacks, paranoia, paresthesia, pneumonitis (allergic etiology), psychosis, QT prolongation, restlessness, somnolence, Stevens-Johnson syndrome, suicidal ideation and behavior (causal relationship not established), tachycardia, thrombocytopenia, tremor, urticaria, vertigo, visual disturbances

Drug Interactions

Metabolism/Transport Effects **Substrate** of CYP3A4 (major); **Note:** Assignment of Major/Minor substrate status based on clinically relevant drug interaction potential; **Inhibits** CYP2D6 (weak), CYP3A4 (weak), P-glycoprotein

Avoid Concomitant Use

Avoid concomitant use of Mefloquine with any of the following: Aminoquinolines (Antimalarial); Artemether; Conivaptan; Dronedarone; Halofantrine; Lumefantrine; Nilotinib; Pimozide; QUEtiapine; QuiNIDine; QuiNINE; Silodosin; Tetrabenazine; Thioridazine; Topotecan; Toremifene; Vandetanib; Vemurafenib; Ziprasidone

Increased Effect/Toxicity

Mefloquine may increase the levels/effects of: Aminoquinolines (Antimalarial); Antipsychotic Agents (Phenothiazines); Colchicine; Dabigatran Etexilate; Dapsone; Dapsone (Systemic); Dapsone (Topical); Dronedarone; Everolimus; Halofantrine; Lumefantrine; P-glycoprotein/ABCB1 Substrates; Pimozide; QTc-Prolonging Agents; QuiNINE; Rivaroxaban; Silodosin; Tetrabenazine; Thioridazine; Topotecan; Toremifene; Vandetanib; Vemurafenib; Ziprasidone

The levels/effects of Mefloquine may be increased by: Alfuzosin; Aminoquinolines (Antimalarial); Artemether; Chloroquine; Ciprofloxacin; Ciprofloxacin (Systemic); Conivaptan; CYP3A4 Inhibitors (Moderate); CYP3A4 Inhibitors (Strong); Dapsone; Dapsone (Systemic); Gadobutrol; Indacaterol; Lumefantrine; Nilotinib; QUEtiapine; QuiNIDine; QuiNINE

Decreased Effect

Mefloquine may decrease the levels/effects of: Anticonvulsants; Lumefantrine

The levels/effects of Mefloquine may be decreased by: CYP3A4 Inducers (Strong); Deferasirox; Herbs (CYP3A4 Inducers); Tocilizumab

Ethanol/Nutrition/Herb Interactions

Food: Food increases bioavailability by ~40%.

Herb/Nutraceutical: Mefloquine serum concentration may be decreased by St John's wort; avoid concurrent use.

Stability Store at controlled room temperature of 25°C (77°F); excursions permitted to 15°C to 30°C (59°F to 86°F).

Mechanism of Action Mefloquine is a quinoline-methanol compound structurally similar to quinine; mefloquine's effectiveness in the treatment and prophylaxis of malaria is due to the destruction of the asexual blood forms of the malarial pathogens that affect humans, *Plasmodium falciparum, P. vivax*

Pharmacodynamics/Kinetics

Absorption: Well absorbed

Distribution: V_d: ~20 L/kg; blood, urine, CSF, tissues

Protein binding: ~98%

Metabolism: Extensively hepatic to 2,8-bis-trifluoromethyl-4-quinoline carboxylic acid (inactive) and other metabolites

Bioavailability: Increased by food

Half-life elimination: ~3 weeks (range: 2-4 weeks)

Time to peak, plasma: ~17 hours (range: 6-24 hours)
Excretion: Primarily bile and feces; urine (9% of total dose as unchanged drug, 4% of total dose as primary metabolite)

Dosage Oral (dose expressed as mg of mefloquine hydrochloride):

Malaria:

Mild-to-moderate, treatment: **Note:** If clinical improvement is not seen within 48-72 hours, an alternative therapy should be used for retreatment.

Children ≥6 months: 20-25 mg/kg/day in 2 divided doses, taken 6-8 hours apart (maximum total dose: 1250 mg)

Adults: 1250 mg (5 tablets) as a single dose

Uncomplicated, treatment (unlabeled dose):

Children ≥6 months: 15 mg/kg, followed 6-12 hours later by 10 mg/kg/dose (maximum total dose: 1250 mg) (CDC, 2011)

Adults: 750 mg (3 tablets) as initial dose, followed 6-12 hours later by 500 mg (2 tablets) (CDC, 2011)

Uncomplicated, chloroquine-resistant *P. vivax* malaria treatment (unlabeled use):

Children ≥6 months: 15 mg/kg, followed 6-12 hours later by 10 mg/kg/dose (maximum total dose: 1250 mg) with concomitant primaquine (CDC, 2011)

Adults: 750 mg (3 tablets) as initial dose, followed 6-12 hours later by 500 mg (2 tablets) with concomitant primaquine (CDC, 2011)

Chemoprophylaxis:

Children ≥6 months: 5 mg/kg/dose once weekly (maximum dose: 250 mg) starting 1 week (CDC, 2012: ≥2 weeks) before arrival in endemic area, continuing weekly during travel and for 4 weeks after leaving endemic area. **Note:** Prophylaxis may begin 2-3 weeks prior to travel to ensure tolerance.

Manufacturer's labeling:

20-30 kg: 1/2 of 250 mg tablet (125 mg) once weekly

30-45 kg: 3/4 of 250 mg tablet (187.5 mg) once weekly

>45 kg: One tablet (250 mg) once weekly

Unlabeled dosing (CDC, 2012):

≤9 kg: 5 mg/kg/dose once weekly

10-19 kg: 1/4 of 250 mg tablet (62.5 mg) once weekly

20-30 kg: 1/2 of 250 mg tablet (125 mg) once weekly

31-45 kg: 3/4 of 250 mg tablet (187.5 mg) once weekly

≥46 kg: One tablet (250 mg) once weekly

Adults: 250 mg weekly starting 1 week (CDC, 2012: ≥2 weeks) before arrival in endemic area, continuing weekly during travel and for 4 weeks after leaving endemic area. **Note:** Prophylaxis may begin 2-3 weeks prior to travel to ensure tolerance.

Dosage adjustment in renal impairment: No dosage adjustment necessary; only a small amount of mefloquine is renally eliminated.

Dosage adjustment in hepatic impairment: No dosage adjustment provided in manufacturer's labeling; however; half-life may be prolonged and plasma levels may be higher in patients with hepatic impairment

Dietary Considerations Take with food and with at least 8 oz of water.

Administration Administer with food and with at least 8 oz of water. When used for malaria prophylaxis, dose should be taken once weekly on the same day each week. If vomiting occurs within 30 minutes after the dose, an additional full dose should be given; if it occurs within 30-60 minutes after dose, an additional half-dose should be given. Tablets may be crushed and suspended in a small amount of water, milk, or another beverage for persons unable to swallow tablets.

Monitoring Parameters When use is prolonged, periodic liver function tests and ocular examinations

Dosage Forms Excipient information presented when available (limited, particularly for generics); consult specific product labeling.

Tablet, oral, as hydrochloride: 250 mg [equivalent to mefloquine base 228 mg]

◆ **Mefloquine Hydrochloride** *see* Mefloquine *on page 1060*

◆ **Mefoxin®** *see* CefOXitin *on page 311*

◆ **Megace®** *see* Megestrol *on page 1062*

◆ **Megace® ES** *see* Megestrol *on page 1062*

◆ **Megace® OS (Can)** *see* Megestrol *on page 1062*

Megestrol (me JES trole)

Brand Names: U.S. Megace®; Megace® ES

Brand Names: Canada Apo-Megestrol®; Megace®; Megace® OS; Nu-Megestrol

Index Terms 5071-1DL(6); Megestrol Acetate; NSC-71423

Pharmacologic Category Antineoplastic Agent, Hormone; Appetite Stimulant; Progestin

Use Palliative treatment of breast and endometrial carcinoma; treatment of anorexia, cachexia, or unexplained significant weight loss in patients with AIDS

Pregnancy Risk Factor D (tablet) / X (suspension)

Pregnancy Considerations Adverse effects were demonstrated in animal studies. Use during pregnancy is contraindicated (suspension).

Lactation Enters breast milk/not recommended

Contraindications Hypersensitivity to megestrol or any component of the formulation; pregnancy (suspension)

Warnings/Precautions Hazardous agent - use appropriate precautions for handling and disposal. May suppress hypothalamic-pituitary-adrenal (HPA) axis during chronic administration; consider the possibility of adrenal suppression in any patient receiving or being withdrawn from chronic therapy when signs/symptoms suggestive of hypoadrenalism are noted (during stress or in unstressed state). Laboratory evaluation and replacement/stress doses of rapid-acting glucocorticoid should be considered. New-onset diabetes and exacerbation of pre-existing diabetes have been reported with long-term use. Use with caution in patients with a history of thromboembolic disease. Vaginal bleeding or discharge may occur in females. Megace® ES suspension is not equivalent to other formulations on a mg per mg basis; Megace® ES suspension 625 mg/5 mL is equivalent to megestrol acetate suspension 800 mg/20 mL.

Adverse Reactions

Frequency not always defined.

Cardiovascular: Hypertension (≤8%), cardiomyopathy (1% to 3%), chest pain (1% to 3%), edema (1% to 3%), palpitation (1% to 3%), peripheral edema (1% to 3%), heart failure

Central nervous system: Headache (≤10%), insomnia (≤6%), fever (1% to 6%), pain (≤6%, similar to placebo), abnormal thinking (1% to 3%), confusion (1% to 3%), depression (1% to 3%), hypoesthesia (1% to 3%), seizure (1% to 3%), mood changes, malaise, lethargy

Dermatologic: Rash (2% to 12%), alopecia (1% to 3%), pruritus (1% to 3%), vesiculobullous rash (1% to 3%)

Endocrine & metabolic: Hyperglycemia (≤6%), gynecomastia (1% to 3%), adrenal insufficiency, amenorrhea, breakthrough bleeding, cervical erosion and secretions (changes), breast tenderness increased, Cushing's syndrome, diabetes, glucose intolerance, HPA axis suppression, hot flashes, hypercalcemia, menstrual flow changes, spotting, vaginal bleeding pattern changes

Gastrointestinal: Diarrhea (6% to 15%, similar to placebo), flatulence (≤10%), vomiting (≤6%), nausea (≤5%), dyspepsia (≤4%), abdominal pain (1% to 3%), constipation (1% to 3%), salivation increased (1% to 3%), xerostomia (1% to 3%), weight gain (not attributed to edema or fluid retention)

Genitourinary: Impotence (4% to 14%), decreased libido (≤5%), urinary incontinence (1% to 3%), urinary tract infection (1% to 3%), urinary frequency (≤2%)

Hematologic: Anemia (≤5%), leukopenia (1% to 3%)

Hepatic: Hepatomegaly (1% to 3%), LDH increased (1% to 3%), cholestatic jaundice, hepatotoxicity

Neuromuscular & skeletal: Weakness (2% to 6%), neuropathy (1% to 3%), paresthesia (1% to 3%), carpal tunnel syndrome

Ocular: Amblyopia (1% to 3%)

Renal: Albuminuria (1% to 3%)

Respiratory: Dyspnea (1% to 3%), cough (1% to 3%), pharyngitis (1% to 3%), pneumonia (≤2%), hyperpnea

Miscellaneous: Diaphoresis (1% to 3%), herpes infection (1% to 3%), infection (1% to 3%), moniliasis (1% to 3%), tumor flare

Postmarketing and/or case reports: Thromboembolic phenomena (including deep vein thrombosis, pulmonary embolism, thrombophlebitis)

Drug Interactions

Metabolism/Transport Effects None known.

Avoid Concomitant Use

Avoid concomitant use of Megestrol with any of the following: Dofetilide

Increased Effect/Toxicity

Megestrol may increase the levels/effects of: Dofetilide

The levels/effects of Megestrol may be increased by: Herbs (Progestogenic Properties)

Decreased Effect

The levels/effects of Megestrol may be decreased by: Aminoglutethimide

Ethanol/Nutrition/Herb Interactions Herb/Nutraceutical: Avoid herbs with progestogenic properties (eg, bloodroot, chasteberry, damiana, oregano, and yucca); may enhance the adverse/toxic effect of megestrol.

Stability

Suspension: Store at 15°C to 25°C (59°F to 77°F); protect from heat.

Tablet: Store at 25°C (77°F); excursions permitted to 15°C to 30°C (59°F to 86°F); protect from heat (temperatures >40°C [>104°F])

Mechanism of Action A synthetic progestin with antiestrogenic properties which disrupt the estrogen receptor cycle. Megestrol interferes with the normal estrogen cycle and results in a lower LH titer. May also have a direct effect on the endometrium. Megestrol is an antineoplastic progestin thought to act through an antileutenizing effect mediated via the pituitary. May stimulate appetite by antagonizing the metabolic effects of catabolic cytokines.

Pharmacodynamics/Kinetics

Absorption: Well absorbed orally

Metabolism: Hepatic (to free steroids and glucuronide conjugates)

Half-life elimination: 13-105 hours

Time to peak, serum: 1-3 hours

Excretion: Urine (57% to 78%; 5% to 8% as metabolites); feces (8% to 30%)

Dosage Adults: Oral: **Note:** Megace® ES suspension is not equivalent to other formulations on a mg-per-mg basis:

Tablet: Females (refer to individual protocols):

Breast carcinoma: 40 mg 4 times/day

Endometrial carcinoma: 40-320 mg/day in divided doses; use for 2 months to determine efficacy; maximum doses used have been up to 800 mg/day

Suspension: Males/Females: HIV-related cachexia:

Megace®: Initial dose: 800 mg/day; daily doses of 400 and 800 mg/day were found to be clinically effective

Megace® ES: 625 mg/day

Dosing adjustment in renal impairment: No data available; however, the urinary excretion of megestrol acetate administered in doses of 4-90 mg ranged from 57% to 78% within 10 days

Administration Megestrol acetate (Megace®) oral suspension is compatible with water, orange juice, apple juice, or Sustacal H.C. for immediate consumption. Shake suspension well before use.

Monitoring Parameters Observe for signs of thromboembolic events; blood pressure, weight; serum glucose

Test Interactions Altered thyroid and liver function tests

Dosage Forms Excipient information presented when available (limited, particularly for generics); consult specific product labeling.

Suspension, oral, as acetate: 40 mg/mL (10 mL, 20 mL, 237 mL, 240 mL, 473 mL, 480 mL)

Megace®: 40 mg/mL (240 mL) [contains ethanol 0.06%, sodium benzoate; lemon-lime flavor]

Megace® ES: 125 mg/mL (150 mL) [contains ethanol 0.06%, sodium benzoate; lemon-lime flavor]

Tablet, oral, as acetate: 20 mg, 40 mg

- **Megestrol Acetate** *see* Megestrol *on page 1062*
- **Melanex® [DSC]** *see* Hydroquinone *on page 846*
- **Mellaril** *see* Thioridazine *on page 1672*

Meloxicam (mel OKS i kam)

Brand Names: U.S. Mobic®

Brand Names: Canada Apo-Meloxicam®; CO Meloxicam; Dom-Meloxicam; Mobicox®; Mobic®; Mylan-Meloxicam; Novo-Meloxicam; PHL-Meloxicam; PMS-Meloxicam; ratio-Meloxicam; Teva-Meloxicam

Pharmacologic Category Nonsteroidal Anti-inflammatory Drug (NSAID), Oral

Use Relief of signs and symptoms of osteoarthritis, rheumatoid arthritis, and juvenile idiopathic arthritis (JIA)

Pregnancy Risk Factor C /D ≥30 weeks gestation

Pregnancy Considerations Adverse events were not observed in the initial animal reproduction studies; therefore, the manufacturer classifies meloxicam as pregnancy category C (category D: ≥30 weeks gestation). Meloxicam crosses the placenta. NSAID exposure during the first trimester is not strongly associated with congenital malformations; however, cardiovascular anomalies and cleft palate have been observed following NSAID exposure in some studies. The use of an NSAID close to conception may be associated with an increased risk of miscarriage. Nonteratogenic effects have been observed following NSAID administration during the third trimester including myocardial degenerative changes, prenatal constriction of the ductus arteriosus, fetal tricuspid regurgitation, failure of the ductus arteriosus to close postnatally; renal dysfunction or failure, oligohydramnios; gastrointestinal bleeding or perforation, increased risk of necrotizing enterocolitis; intracranial bleeding (including intraventricular hemorrhage), platelet dysfunction with resultant bleeding; pulmonary hypertension. Because they may cause premature closure of the ductus arteriosus, use of NSAIDs late in pregnancy should be avoided (use after 31 or 32 weeks gestation is not recommended by some clinicians). Product labeling for Mobic® specifically notes that use at ≥30 weeks gestation should be avoided and therefore classifies meloxicam as pregnancy category D at this time. The chronic use of NSAIDs in women of reproductive age may be associated with infertility that is reversible upon discontinuation of the medication.

Lactation Excretion in breast milk unknown/not recommended

Medication Guide Available Yes

Contraindications Hypersensitivity (eg, asthma, urticaria, allergic-type reactions) to meloxicam, aspirin, other NSAIDs, or any component of the formulation; perioperative pain in the setting of coronary artery bypass graft (CABG) surgery

Warnings/Precautions [U.S. Boxed Warning]: NSAIDs are associated with an increased risk of adverse cardiovascular thrombotic events, including MI and stroke. Risk may be increased with duration of use or pre-existing cardiovascular risk factors or disease. Carefully evaluate individual cardiovascular risk profiles prior to prescribing. May cause new-onset hypertension or worsening of existing hypertension. Use caution with fluid retention. Avoid use in heart failure. Concurrent administration of ibuprofen, and potentially other nonselective NSAIDs, may interfere with aspirin's cardioprotective effect. **[U.S. Boxed Warning]: Use is contraindicated for treatment of perioperative pain in the setting of coronary artery bypass graft (CABG) surgery.** Risk of MI and stroke may be increased with use within the first 10-14 days following CABG surgery.

Platelet adhesion and aggregation may be decreased; may prolong bleeding time; patients with coagulation disorders or who are receiving anticoagulants should be monitored closely. Anemia may occur; patients on long-term NSAID therapy should be monitored for anemia. Rarely, NSAID use may cause severe blood dyscrasias (eg, agranulocytosis, aplastic anemia, thrombocytopenia).

NSAID use may compromise existing renal function; dose-dependent decreases in prostaglandin synthesis may result from NSAID use, reducing renal blood flow which may cause renal decompensation. NSAID use may increase the risk for hyperkalemia. Patients with impaired renal function, dehydration, heart failure, liver dysfunction, those taking diuretics, and ACE inhibitors, and the elderly are at greater risk of renal toxicity and hyperkalemia. Rehydrate patient before starting therapy; monitor renal function closely. Not recommended for use in patients with advanced renal disease. Long-term NSAID use may result in renal papillary necrosis.

[U.S. Boxed Warning]: NSAIDs may increase risk of gastrointestinal irritation, inflammation, ulceration, bleeding, and perforation. These events may occur at any time during therapy and without warning. Use caution with a history of GI disease (bleeding or ulcers), concurrent therapy with aspirin, anticoagulants and/or corticosteroids, smoking, use of alcohol, the elderly or debilitated patients. When used concomitantly with ≤325 mg of aspirin, a substantial increase in the risk of gastrointestinal complications (eg, ulcer) occurs; concomitant gastroprotective therapy (eg, proton pump inhibitors) is recommended (Bhatt, 2008).

Use the lowest effective dose for the shortest duration of time, consistent with individual patient goals, to reduce risk of cardiovascular or GI adverse events. Alternate therapies should be considered for patients at high risk.

NSAIDs may cause serious skin adverse events including exfoliative dermatitis, Stevens-Johnson syndrome (SJS) and toxic epidermal necrolysis (TEN); discontinue use at first sign of skin rash or hypersensitivity. Anaphylactoid reactions may occur, even without prior exposure; patients with "aspirin triad" (bronchial asthma, aspirin intolerance, rhinitis) may be at increased risk. Do not use in patients who experience bronchospasm, asthma, rhinitis, or urticaria with NSAID or aspirin therapy. Use caution in other forms of asthma.

Use with caution in patients with decreased hepatic function. Closely monitor patients with any abnormal LFT. Severe hepatic reactions (eg, fulminant hepatitis, liver failure) have occurred with NSAID use, rarely; discontinue if signs or symptoms of liver disease develop, or if systemic manifestations occur.

NSAIDS may cause drowsiness, dizziness, blurred vision and other neurologic effects which may impair physical or mental abilities; patients must be cautioned about performing tasks which require mental alertness (eg, operating machinery or driving). Discontinue use with blurred or diminished vision and perform ophthalmologic exam. Monitor vision with long-term therapy.

The elderly are at increased risk for adverse effects (especially peptic ulceration, CNS effects, renal toxicity) from NSAIDs even at low doses.

Oral suspension formulation may contain sorbitol. Concomitant use with sodium polystyrene sulfonate (Kayexalate®) may cause intestinal necrosis (including fatal cases); combined use should be avoided. Withhold for at least 4-6 half-lives prior to surgical or dental procedures.

Adverse Reactions Percentages reported in adult patients; abdominal pain, diarrhea, fever, headache, pyrexia, and vomiting were reported more commonly in pediatric patients

2% to 10%:

Cardiovascular: Edema (≤5%)

Central nervous system: Headache (2% to 8%), pain (1% to 5%), dizziness (≤4%), insomnia (≤4%)

Dermatologic: Pruritus (≤2%), rash (≤3%)

Gastrointestinal: Dyspepsia (4% to 10%), diarrhea (2% to 8%), nausea (2% to 7%), abdominal pain (2% to 5%), constipation (≤3%), flatulence (≤3%), vomiting (≤3%)

Genitourinary: Urinary tract infection (≤7%), micturition (≤2%)

Hematologic: Anemia (≤4%)

Neuromuscular & skeletal: Arthralgia (≤5%), back pain (≤3%)

Respiratory: Upper respiratory infection (≤8%), cough (≤2%), pharyngitis (≤3%)

Miscellaneous: Flu-like syndrome (2% to 6%), falls (≤3%)

<2% (Limited to important or life-threatening): Abnormal dreams, abnormal vision, agranulocytosis, albuminuria, allergic reaction, alopecia, anaphylactoid reactions, angina, angioedema, anxiety, appetite increased, arrhythmia, asthma, bilirubinemia, bronchospasm, bullous eruption, BUN increased, cardiac failure, colitis, confusion, conjunctivitis, creatinine increased, dehydration, depression, diaphoresis, duodenal perforation, duodenal ulcer, dyspnea, edema (facial), eructation, erythema multiforme, esophagitis, exfoliative dermatitis, fatigue, fever, gastric perforation, gastric ulcer, gastritis, gastroesophageal reflux, gastrointestinal hemorrhage, GGT increased, hematemesis, hematuria, hepatic failure, hepatitis, hot flushes, hyper-/hypotension, interstitial nephritis, intestinal perforation, jaundice, leukopenia, malaise, melena, MI, mood alterations, nervousness, palpitation, pancreatitis, paresthesia, photosensitivity reaction, pruritus, purpura, renal failure, seizure, shock, somnolence, Stevens-Johnson syndrome, syncope, tachycardia, taste perversion, thrombocytopenia, tinnitus, toxic epidermal necrolysis, transaminases increased, tremor, ulcerative stomatitis, urinary retention (acute), urticaria, vasculitis, vertigo, xerostomia, weight gain/loss

Drug Interactions

Metabolism/Transport Effects Substrate of CYP3A4 (minor); **Note:** Assignment of Major/Minor substrate status based on clinically relevant drug interaction potential; **Inhibits** CYP2C9 (weak)

Avoid Concomitant Use

Avoid concomitant use of Meloxicam with any of the following: Calcium Polystyrene Sulfonate; Floctafenine; Ketorolac; Ketorolac (Nasal); Ketorolac (Systemic); Sodium Polystyrene Sulfonate

Increased Effect/Toxicity

Meloxicam may increase the levels/effects of: Aminoglycosides; Anticoagulants; Antiplatelet Agents; Bisphosphonate Derivatives; Calcium Polystyrene Sulfonate; Collagenase (Systemic); CycloSPORINE; CycloSPORINE (Systemic); Deferasirox; Desmopressin; Digoxin; Drotrecogin Alfa (Activated); Eplerenone; Haloperidol; Ibritumomab; Lithium; Methotrexate; Nonsteroidal Anti-Inflammatory Agents; PEMEtrexed; Porfimer; Potassium-Sparing Diuretics; PRALAtrexate; Quinolone Antibiotics; Rivaroxaban; Salicylates; Sodium Polystyrene Sulfonate; Thrombolytic Agents; Tositumomab and Iodine I 131 Tositumomab; Vancomycin; Vitamin K Antagonists

The levels/effects of Meloxicam may be increased by: ACE Inhibitors; Angiotensin II Receptor Blockers; Antidepressants (Tricyclic, Tertiary Amine); Conivaptan; Corticosteroids (Systemic); CycloSPORINE; CycloSPORINE (Systemic); Dasatinib; Floctafenine; Glucosamine; Herbs (Anticoagulant/Antiplatelet Properties); Ketorolac; Ketorolac (Nasal); Ketorolac (Systemic); Nonsteroidal Anti-Inflammatory Agents; Omega-3-Acid Ethyl Esters; Pentosan Polysulfate Sodium; Pentoxifylline; Probenecid; Prostacyclin Analogues; Selective Serotonin Reuptake Inhibitors; Serotonin/Norepinephrine Reuptake Inhibitors; Sodium Phosphates; Treprostinil; Vitamin E; Voriconazole

Decreased Effect

Meloxicam may decrease the levels/effects of: ACE Inhibitors; Angiotensin II Receptor Blockers; Antiplatelet Agents; Beta-Blockers; Eplerenone; HydrALAZINE; Loop Diuretics; Potassium-Sparing Diuretics; Salicylates; Selective Serotonin Reuptake Inhibitors; Thiazide Diuretics

The levels/effects of Meloxicam may be decreased by: Bile Acid Sequestrants; Nonsteroidal Anti-Inflammatory Agents; Salicylates; Tocilizumab

Ethanol/Nutrition/Herb Interactions

Ethanol: Avoid ethanol (may enhance gastric mucosal irritation).

Herb/Nutraceutical: Avoid alfalfa, anise, bilberry, bladderwrack, bromelain, cat's claw, celery, chamomile, coleus, cordyceps, dong quai, evening primrose, fenugreek, feverfew, garlic, ginger, ginkgo biloba, ginseng (American, Panax, Siberian), grapeseed, green tea, guggul, horse chestnut seed, horseradish, licorice, prickly ash, red clover, reishi, SAMe (S-adenosylmethionine), sweet clover, turmeric, white willow (all have additional antiplatelet activity).

Stability Store at 25°C (77°F). Protect tablets from moisture.

Mechanism of Action Reversibly inhibits cyclooxygenase-1 and 2 (COX-1 and 2) enzymes, which results in decreased formation of prostaglandin precursors; has antipyretic, analgesic, and anti-inflammatory properties

Other proposed mechanisms not fully elucidated (and possibly contributing to the anti-inflammatory effect to varying degrees), include inhibiting chemotaxis, altering lymphocyte activity, inhibiting neutrophil aggregation/activation, and decreasing proinflammatory cytokine levels.

Pharmacodynamics/Kinetics

Distribution: 10 L

Protein binding: ~99%, primarily to albumin

Metabolism: Hepatic via CYP2C9 and CYP3A4 (minor); forms 4 metabolites (inactive)

Bioavailability: 89%

Half-life elimination: Adults: 15-20 hours

Time to peak: Initial: 4-5 hours; Secondary: 12-14 hours

Excretion: Urine and feces (as inactive metabolites)

Dosage Oral:

Children ≥2 years: Juvenile idiopathic arthritis (JIA): 0.125 mg/kg/day; maximum dose: 7.5 mg/day

Adults: Osteoarthritis, rheumatoid arthritis: Initial: 7.5 mg once daily; some patients may receive additional benefit from increasing dose to 15 mg once daily; maximum dose: 15 mg/day

Elderly: Increased concentrations may occur in elderly patients (particularly in females); however, no specific dosage adjustment is recommended

Dosage adjustment in renal impairment:

Mild-to-moderate impairment: No specific dosage recommendations

Significant impairment (Cl_{cr} ≤20 mL/minute): Patients with severe renal impairment have not been adequately studied; use not recommended.

Hemodialysis: Maximum dose: 7.5 mg/day

Dosage adjustment in hepatic impairment:

Mild (Child-Pugh class A) to moderate (Child-Pugh class B) hepatic dysfunction: No dosage adjustment is necessary

Severe hepatic impairment: Patients with severe hepatic impairment have not been adequately studied

Dietary Considerations Should be taken with food or milk to minimize gastrointestinal irritation.

Administration May be administered with or without meals; take with food or milk to minimize gastrointestinal irritation. Oral suspension: Shake gently prior to use.

Monitoring Parameters Periodic CBC, serum chemistries, liver function, renal function (serum BUN and creatinine) with long-term use; signs and symptoms of bleeding

Dosage Forms Excipient information presented when available (limited, particularly for generics); consult specific product labeling.

Suspension, oral: 7.5 mg/5 mL (100 mL)

Mobic®: 7.5 mg/5 mL (100 mL) [contains sodium benzoate; raspberry flavor]

Tablet, oral: 7.5 mg, 15 mg

Mobic®: 7.5 mg, 15 mg

◆ **Melpaque HP®** *see* Hydroquinone *on page* 846

Melphalan (MEL fa lan)

Brand Names: U.S. Alkeran®

Brand Names: Canada Alkeran®

Index Terms L-PAM; L-Phenylalanine Mustard; L-Sarcolysin; Phenylalanine Mustard

Pharmacologic Category Antineoplastic Agent, Alkylating Agent

Use Palliative treatment of multiple myeloma and nonresectable epithelial ovarian carcinoma

Unlabeled Use Treatment of Hodgkin lymphoma, light chain amyloidosis; conditioning regimen for autologous hematopoietic stem cell transplantation in adults with hematologic disorders (eg, multiple myeloma) and autologous marrow or stem cell transplantation in pediatric neuroblastoma and Ewing's sarcoma

Pregnancy Risk Factor D

Pregnancy Considerations Animal studies have demonstrated embryotoxicity and teratogenicity. Therapy may suppress ovarian function leading to amenorrhea. There are no adequate and well-controlled studies in pregnant women. May cause fetal harm if administered during pregnancy. Women of childbearing potential should be advised to avoid pregnancy while on melphalan therapy.

Lactation Excretion in breast milk unknown/not recommended

Contraindications Hypersensitivity to melphalan or any component of the formulation; patients whose disease was resistant to prior melphalan therapy

Warnings/Precautions **[U.S. Boxed Warning]: Bone marrow suppression is common; may be severe and result in infection or bleeding; has been demonstrated more with the I.V. formulation (compared to oral);** myelosuppression is dose-related. Monitor blood counts; may require treatment delay or dose modification for thrombocytopenia or neutropenia. Use with caution in patients with prior bone marrow suppression, impaired renal function (consider dose reduction), or who have received prior (or concurrent) chemotherapy or irradiation. Myelotoxicity is generally reversible, although irreversible bone marrow failure has been reported. In patients who are candidates for autologous transplantation, avoid melphalan-containing regimens prior to transplant (due to the effects on stem cell reserve). Signs of infection, such as fever and WBC rise, may not occur; lethargy and confusion may be more prominent signs of infection.

[U.S. Boxed Warning]: Hypersensitivity reactions (including anaphylaxis) have occurred in ~2% of patients receiving I.V. melphalan, usually after multiple treatment cycles. Discontinue infusion and treat symptomatically. Hypersensitivity may also occur (rarely) with oral melphalan. Do not readminister (oral or I.V.) in patients who experience hypersensitivity to melphalan.

Gastrointestinal toxicities, including nausea, vomiting, diarrhea and mucositis, are common. When administering high-dose melphalan in autologous transplantation, cryotherapy is recommended to prevent mucositis (Keefe, 2007). Abnormal liver function tests may occur; hepatitis and jaundice have also been reported; hepatic sinusoidal obstruction syndrome (SOS; formerly called veno-occlusive disease) has been reported with I.V. melphalan. Pulmonary fibrosis (some fatal) and interstitial pneumonitis have been observed with treatment. Dosage reduction is recommended with I.V. melphalan in patients with renal impairment; reduced initial doses may also be recommended with oral melphalan. Closely monitor patients with azotemia.

[U.S. Boxed Warning]: Produces chromosomal changes and is leukemogenic and potentially mutagenic; secondary malignancies (including acute myeloid leukemia, myeloproliferative disease, and carcinoma) have been reported reported (some patients were receiving combination chemotherapy or radiation therapy); the risk is increased with increased treatment duration and cumulative doses. Suppresses ovarian function and produces amenorrhea; may also cause testicular suppression.

Extravasation may cause local tissue damage; administration by slow injection into a fast running I.V. solution into an injection port or via a central line is recommended; do not administer directly into a peripheral vein. **[U.S. Boxed Warning]: Should be administered under the supervision of an experienced cancer chemotherapy physician.** Avoid vaccination with live vaccines during treatment if immunocompromised. Toxicity may be increased in elderly; start with lowest recommended adult doses.

Adverse Reactions

>10%:

Gastrointestinal: Nausea/vomiting, diarrhea, oral ulceration

Hematologic: Myelosuppression, leukopenia (nadir: 14-21 days; recovery: 28-35 days), thrombocytopenia (nadir: 14-21 days; recovery: 28-35 days), anemia

Miscellaneous: Secondary malignancy (<2% to 20%; cumulative dose and duration dependent, includes acute myeloid leukemia, myeloproliferative syndrome, carcinoma)

1% to 10%: Miscellaneous: Hypersensitivity (I.V.: 2%; includes bronchospasm, dyspnea, edema, hypotension, pruritus, rash, tachycardia, urticaria)

Infrequent, frequency undefined, postmarketing, and/or case reports: Agranulocytosis, allergic reactions, alopecia, amenorrhea, anaphylaxis (rare), bleeding (with high-dose therapy),, bone marrow failure (irreversible), BUN increased, cardiac arrest, cardiotoxicity (angina, arrhythmia, hypertension, MI; with high-dose therapy), encephalopathy, hemolytic anemia, hemorrhagic cystitis, hepatic sinusoidal obstruction syndrome (SOS; veno-occlusive disease; high-dose I.V. melphalan), hepatitis, infection, injection site reactions (ulceration, necrosis), interstitial pneumonitis, jaundice, mucositis (with high-dose therapy), ovarian suppression, paralytic ileus (with high-dose therapy), pruritus, pulmonary fibrosis, radiation myelopathy, rash (maculopapular), renal toxicity (with high-dose therapy), seizure (with high-dose therapy), sepsis, SIADH, skin hypersensitivity, sterility, stomatitis, testicular suppression, tingling sensation, transaminases increased, vasculitis, warmth sensation

Drug Interactions

Metabolism/Transport Effects None known.

Avoid Concomitant Use

Avoid concomitant use of Melphalan with any of the following: BCG; CloZAPine; Nalidixic Acid; Natalizumab; Pimecrolimus; Tacrolimus (Topical); Vaccines (Live)

Increased Effect/Toxicity

Melphalan may increase the levels/effects of: Carmustine; CloZAPine; CycloSPORINE; CycloSPORINE (Systemic); Leflunomide; Natalizumab; Vaccines (Live); Vitamin K Antagonists

The levels/effects of Melphalan may be increased by: Denosumab; Nalidixic Acid; Pimecrolimus; Roflumilast; Tacrolimus (Topical); Trastuzumab

Decreased Effect

Melphalan may decrease the levels/effects of: BCG; Cardiac Glycosides; Coccidioidin Skin Test; Sipuleucel-T; Vaccines (Inactivated); Vaccines (Live); Vitamin K Antagonists

The levels/effects of Melphalan may be decreased by: Echinacea

Ethanol/Nutrition/Herb Interactions

Ethanol: Avoid ethanol (due to GI irritation).

Food: Food interferes with oral absorption.

Stability Use appropriate precautions for handling and disposal.

Tablet: Store in refrigerator at 2°C to 8°C (36°F to 46°F). Protect from light.

Injection: Store at room temperature of 15°C to 30°C (59°F to 86°F). Protect from light. Stability is limited; must be prepared fresh. **The time between reconstitution/dilution and administration of parenteral melphalan must be kept to a minimum (manufacturer recommends <60 minutes) because reconstituted and diluted solutions are unstable.** Dissolve powder initially with 10 mL of supplied diluent to a concentration of 5 mg/mL; shake immediately and vigorously to dissolve. This solution is chemically and physically stable for ≤90 minutes when stored at room temperature, although the manufacturer recommends administration be completed within 60 minutes of reconstitution. **Immediately** dilute dose in NS to a concentration of ≤0.45 mg/mL (manufacturer recommended concentration). Do not refrigerate solution; precipitation occurs.

Mechanism of Action Alkylating agent which is a derivative of mechlorethamine that inhibits DNA and RNA synthesis via formation of carbonium ions; cross-links strands of DNA; acts on both resting and rapidly dividing tumor cells.

Pharmacodynamics/Kinetics **Note:** Pharmacokinetics listed are for FDA-approved doses.

Absorption: Oral: Variable and incomplete

Distribution: V_d: 0.5 L/kg; low penetration into CSF

Protein binding: 53% to 92%; primarily to albumin (40% to 60%), ~20% to α_1-acid glycoprotein

Metabolism: Hepatic; chemical hydrolysis to monohydroxymelphalan and dihydroxymelphalan

Bioavailability: Oral: Variable; 56% to 93%; exposure is reduced with a high-fat meal

Half-life elimination: Terminal: I.V.: 75 minutes; Oral: 1-2 hours

Time to peak, serum: Oral: ~1-2 hours

Excretion: Oral: Feces (20% to 50%); urine (~10% as unchanged drug)

Dosage Details regarding dosing in combination regimens should also be consulted.

Oral: Adults (adjust dose based on patient response and weekly blood counts):

Multiple myeloma (palliative treatment): **Note:** Response is gradual; may require repeated courses to realize benefit:

Usual dose (as described in the manufacturer's labeling):

6 mg once daily for 2-3 weeks initially, followed by up to 4 weeks rest, then a maintenance dose of 2 mg daily as hematologic recovery begins **or**

10 mg daily for 7-10 days; institute 2 mg daily maintenance dose after WBC >4000 cells/mm^3 and platelets >100,000 cells/mm^3 (~4-8 weeks); titrate maintenance dose to hematologic response **or**

0.15 mg/kg/day for 7 days, with a 2-6 week rest, followed by a maintenance dose of ≤0.05 mg/kg/day as hematologic recovery begins **or**

0.25 mg/kg/day for 4 days (or 0.2 mg/kg/day for 5 days); repeat at 4- to 6-week intervals as ANC and platelet counts return to normal

Other dosing regimens in **combination therapy** (unlabeled doses):

4 mg/m^2/day for 7 days every 4 weeks (in combination with prednisone **or** with prednisone and thalidomide) (Palumbo, 2006; Palumbo, 2008) **or**

6 mg/m^2/day for 7 days every 4 weeks (in combination with prednisone) (Palumbo, 2004) **or**

0.25 mg/kg/day for 4 days every 6 weeks (in combination with prednisone [Facon, 2006; Facon, 2007] **or** with prednisone and thalidomide [Facon, 2007]) **or**

9 mg/m^2/day for 4 days every 6 weeks (in combination with prednisone **or** with prednisone and bortezomib) (Dimopoulos, 2009; San Miguel, 2008)

Ovarian carcinoma: 0.2 mg/kg/day for 5 days, repeat every 4-5 weeks **or**

Unlabeled dosing: 7 mg/m^2/day in 2 divided doses for 5 days, repeat every 28 days (Wadler, 1996)

Amyloidosis, light chain (unlabeled use): 0.22 mg/kg/day for 4 days every 28 days (in combination with oral dexamethasone) (Palladini, 2004) **or** 10 mg/m^2/day for 4 days every month (in combination with oral dexamethasone) for 12-18 treatment cycles (Jaccard, 2007)

I.V.:

Children (unlabeled use): Conditioning regimen for autologous hematopoietic stem cell transplantation:

140 mg/m^2 2 days prior to transplantation (combined with busulfan) (Canete, 2009; Oberlin, 2006) **or**

180 mg/m^2 (with pre- and posthydration) 12-30 hours prior to transplantation (Pritchard, 2005) **or**

45 mg/m^2/day for 4 days starting 8 days prior to transplantation (combined with busulfan or etoposide and carboplatin) (Berthold, 2005)

Adults:

Multiple myeloma (palliative treatment): 16 mg/m^2 administered at 2-week intervals for 4 doses, then administer at 4-week intervals after adequate hematologic recovery.

Conditioning regimen for autologous hematopoietic stem cell transplantation (unlabeled use):

200 mg/m^2 alone 2 days prior to transplantation (Fermand, 2005; Moreau, 2002) **or**

140 mg/m^2 2 days prior to transplantation (combined with busulfan) (Fermand, 2005) **or**

140 mg/m^2 2 days prior to transplantation (combined with total body irradiation [TBI]) (Moreau, 2002) **or**

140 mg/m^2 5 days prior to transplantation (combined with TBI) (Barlogie, 2006)

Hodgkin lymphoma (unlabeled use): 30 mg/m^2 on day 6 of combination chemotherapy (mini-BEAM) regimen (Colwill, 1995; Martin, 2001)

Elderly: Refer to adult dosing; use caution and begin at the lower end of dosing range

Dosage adjustment for toxicity:

Oral:

WBC <3000/mm^3: Withhold treatment until recovery

Platelets <100,000/mm^3: Withhold treatment until recovery

I.V.: Adjust dose based on nadir blood cell counts

Dosing adjustment in renal impairment:

The FDA-approved labeling contains the following adjustment recommendations (for approved dosing levels) based on route of administration:

Oral: Moderate-to-severe renal impairment: Consider a reduced dose initially

I.V.: BUN ≥30 mg/dL: Reduce dose by up to 50%

The following guidelines have been used by some clinicians:

Aronoff, 2007 (route of administration not specified): Adults (based on a 6 mg once-daily dose):

Cl_{cr} 10-50 mL/minute: Administer 75% of dose

Cl_{cr} <10 mL/minute: Administer 50% of dose

Hemodialysis: Administer dose after hemodialysis

Continuous ambulatory peritoneal dialysis (CAPD): Administer 50% of dose

Continuous renal replacement therapy (CRRT): Administer 75% of dose

Carlson, 2005: Oral (for melphalan-prednisone combination therapy; based on a study evaluating toxicity with melphalan dosed at 0.25 mg/kg/day for 4 days/cycle):

Cl_{cr} >10 to <30 mL/minute: Administer 75% of dose

Cl_{cr} ≤10 mL/minute: Data is insufficient for a recommendation

Kintzel, 1995:

Oral: Adjust dose in the presence of hematologic toxicity

I.V.:

Cl_{cr} 46-60 mL/minute: Administer 85% of normal dose

Cl_{cr} 31-45 mL/minute: Administer 75% of normal dose

Cl_{cr} <30 mL/minute: Administer 70% of normal dose

Badros, 2001: I.V.: Autologous stem cell transplant (single-agent conditioning regimen; no busulfan or irradiation): Serum creatinine >2 mg/dL: Reduce dose from 200 mg/m^2 over 2 days (as 100 mg/m^2/day for 2 days) to 140 mg/m^2 given as a single-dose infusion

Dosing adjustment in hepatic impairment: Melphalan is hepatically metabolized; however, dosage adjustment does not appear to be necessary (King, 2001).

Dietary Considerations Should be taken on an empty stomach (1 hour prior to or 2 hours after meals).

Administration

Oral: Administer on an empty stomach (1 hour prior to or 2 hours after meals)

Parenteral: Due to limited stability, complete administration of I.V. dose should occur within 60 minutes of reconstitution

I.V.: Infuse over 15-30 minutes. Extravasation may cause local tissue damage; administration by slow injection into a fast running I.V. solution into an injection port or via a central line is recommended; do not administer by direct injection into a peripheral vein.

Monitoring Parameters CBC with differential and platelet count, serum electrolytes, serum uric acid

Test Interactions False-positive Coombs' test [direct]

Dosage Forms Excipient information presented when available (limited, particularly for generics); consult specific product labeling.

Injection, powder for reconstitution: 50 mg

Alkeran®: 50 mg [contains ethanol (in diluent), propylene glycol (in diluent)]

Tablet, oral:

Alkeran®: 2 mg

◆ **Melquin-3®** *see* Hydroquinone *on page 846*

◆ **Melquin HP®** *see* Hydroquinone *on page 846*

Memantine (me MAN teen)

Brand Names: U.S. Namenda®

Brand Names: Canada Apo-Memantine; CO Memantine; Ebixa®; PMS-Memantine; ratio-Memantine; Riva-Memantine; Sandoz-Memantine

Index Terms Memantine Hydrochloride; Namenda XR

Pharmacologic Category N-Methyl-D-Aspartate Receptor Antagonist

Use Treatment of moderate-to-severe dementia of the Alzheimer's type

Unlabeled Use Treatment of mild-to-moderate vascular dementia

Pregnancy Risk Factor B

Pregnancy Considerations Teratogenic effects were not observed in animal studies. There are no studies in pregnant women.

Lactation Excretion in breast milk unknown/use caution

Contraindications Hypersensitivity to memantine or any component of the formulation

Warnings/Precautions Use with caution in patients with cardiovascular disease; an increased incidence of cardiac failure, angina, bradycardia, and hypertension (compared with placebo) was observed in clinical trials. Use caution with seizure disorders or severe hepatic impairment. Use with caution in moderate-to-severe renal impairment; dose adjustments may be required. Worsening of corneal condition has been observed in a clinical trial; periodic ophthalmic exams during use have been recommended (Canadian labeling). Clearance is significantly reduced by alkaline urine; use caution with medications, dietary changes, or patient conditions which may alter urine pH.

Adverse Reactions

1% to 10%:

Cardiovascular: Hypertension (4%), hypotension (2%), cardiac failure, cerebrovascular accident, syncope, transient ischemic attack

Central nervous system: Dizziness (5% to 7%), confusion (6%), headache (6%), anxiety (4%), depression (3%), hallucinations (3%), pain (3%), somnolence (3%), fatigue (2%), aggressive reaction (1% to 2%), ataxia, vertigo

Dermatologic: Rash

Gastrointestinal: Constipation (3% to 5%), diarrhea (5%), weight gain (3%), vomiting (2% to 3%), abdominal pain (2%), weight loss

Genitourinary: Urinary incontinence (2%), micturition

Hematologic: Anemia

Hepatic: Alkaline phosphatase increased

Neuromuscular & skeletal: Back pain (3%), hypokinesia

Ocular: Cataract, conjunctivitis

Respiratory: Cough (4%), dyspnea (2%), pneumonia

Miscellaneous: Influenza (4%)

<1% (Limited to important or life-threatening): Agranulocytosis, allergic reaction, angina, anorexia, apathy, aphasia, apnea, arthralgia, aspiration pneumonia, atrial fibrillation, AV block, blurred vision, bradycardia, cardiac arrest, cerebral hemorrhage, cerebral infarction, cholelithiasis, colitis, conjunctival hemorrhage, corneal opacity, delirium, diabetes mellitus aggravated, diplopia, DVT, dyskinesia, dysphagia, dysuria, emotional lability, encephalopathy, extrapyramidal disorder, fever, gait disturbance, gastroenteritis, gastrointestinal hemorrhage, glaucoma, hearing decreased, hematuria, hemiplegia, hepatic failure, hepatitis, hyper/hypoglycemia, hyperlipidemia, hyponatremia, ileus, INR increased, involuntary muscle contractions, leukopenia, loss of consciousness, macula lutea degeneration, MI, myoclonus, myopia, neuralgia, neuropathy, NMS, orthostatic hypotension, pancreatitis, pancytopenia, paranoid reaction, paresthesia, parkinsonism, peripheral edema, pruritus, psychosis, pulmonary edema, pulmonary embolism, QT prolongation, renal failure, retinal detachment, retinal hemorrhage, seizure, sepsis, Stevens-Johnson syndrome, suicidal ideation, suicide attempt, supraventricular tachycardia, tardive dyskinesia, thrombocytopenia, thrombophlebitis, thrombotic thrombocytopenic purpura, tinnitus, tremor, torsade de pointes, urinary retention, urticaria

Drug Interactions

Metabolism/Transport Effects None known.

Avoid Concomitant Use There are no known interactions where it is recommended to avoid concomitant use.

Increased Effect/Toxicity

Memantine may increase the levels/effects of: Trimethoprim

The levels/effects of Memantine may be increased by: Carbonic Anhydrase Inhibitors; Sodium Bicarbonate; Trimethoprim

Decreased Effect There are no known significant interactions involving a decrease in effect.

Stability Store at 25°C (77°C); excursions permitted to 15°C to 30°C (59°F to 86°F).

Mechanism of Action Glutamate, the primary excitatory amino acid in the CNS, may contribute to the pathogenesis of Alzheimer's disease (AD) by overstimulating various glutamate receptors leading to excitotoxicity and neuronal cell death. Memantine is an uncompetitive antagonist of the N-methyl-D-aspartate (NMDA) type of glutamate receptors, located ubiquitously throughout the brain. Under normal physiologic conditions, the (unstimulated) NMDA receptor ion channel is blocked by magnesium ions, which are displaced after agonist-induced depolarization. Pathologic or excessive receptor activation, as postulated to occur during AD, prevents magnesium from reentering and blocking the channel pore resulting in a chronically open state and excessive calcium influx. Memantine binds to the intra-pore magnesium site, but with longer dwell time, and thus functions as an effective receptor blocker only under conditions of excessive stimulation; memantine does not affect normal neurotransmission.

Pharmacodynamics/Kinetics

Distribution: 9-11 L/kg

Protein binding: 45%

Metabolism: Partially hepatic, primarily independent of the CYP enzyme system; forms 3 metabolites (minimal activity)

Half-life elimination: Terminal: ~60-80 hours; severe renal impairment (Cl_{cr} 5-29 mL/minute): 117-156 hours

Time to peak, serum: Immediate release: 3-7 hours; Extended release: 9-12 hours

Excretion: Urine (74%; ~48% of the total dose as unchanged drug; undergoes active tubular secretion moderated by pH-dependent tubular reabsorption; excretion reduced by alkaline urine pH)

Dosage Oral: Adults:

Alzheimer's disease:

Immediate release: Initial: 5 mg/day; increase dose by 5 mg/day to a target dose of 20 mg/day; wait ≥1 week between dosage changes. Doses >5 mg/day should be given in 2 divided doses.

Suggested titration: 5 mg/day for ≥1 week; 5 mg twice daily for ≥1 week; 15 mg/day given in 5 mg and 10 mg separated doses for ≥1 week; then 10 mg twice daily

Extended release: Initial: 7 mg once daily, increase dose by 7 mg/day to a target maximum dose of 28 mg/day; wait ≥1 week between dosage changes

Note: When switching from the immediate release product to the extended release product, begin the extended release product the day after the last dose of the immediate release product. Patients on immediate release 10 mg twice daily should be switched to extended release 28 mg once daily.

Mild-to-moderate vascular dementia (unlabeled use): Immediate release: Initial: 5 mg/day, titrated by 5 mg/day weekly to a target dose of 10 mg twice daily (Orgogozo, 2002)

Dosage adjustment in renal impairment:

Mild impairment: No adjustment required

Moderate impairment:

U.S. labeling: No adjustment required

Canadian labeling: (Cl_{cr} 30-49 mL/minute): Initial: 5 mg once daily; after at least 1 week of therapy and if tolerated, may titrate up to 5 mg twice daily; may further titrate dosage upward in weekly increments to 20 mg/day according to suggested titration schedule

Severe impairment:

U.S. labeling: Cl_{cr} 5-29 mL/minute: Immediate release: Initial: 5 mg once daily; after at least 1 week of therapy and if tolerated, may titrate up to 5 mg twice daily; Extended release: Target dose of 14 mg/day

Note: When switching from the immediate release product to the extended release product, begin the extended release product the day after the last dose of the immediate release product. Patients on immediate release 5 mg twice daily should be switched to extended release 14 mg once daily.

Canadian labeling: Cl_{cr} 15-29 mL/minute: Initial: 5 mg once daily; after at least 1 week of therapy and if tolerated, may titrate up to 5 mg twice daily

Dosage adjustment in hepatic impairment:

Mild-to-moderate impairment: No adjustment required

Severe impairment: Use caution

U.S. labeling: No specific dosing recommendations

Canadian labeling: Avoid use

Dietary Considerations May be taken without regard to meals.

Administration Administer without regard to meals. Extended release capsules may be swallowed whole or entire contents of capsule may be sprinkled on applesauce and swallowed immediately. Do not chew, crush, or divide.

Monitoring Parameters Periodic ophthalmic exam (Canadian labeling)

Product Availability

Namenda XR™: FDA approved in June 2010; anticipated availability is currently undetermined

Namenda XR™ is an extended release capsule (once-daily administration) approved for the treatment of moderate-to-severe dementia associated with Alzheimer's disease

Dosage Forms Excipient information presented when available (limited, particularly for generics); consult specific product labeling.

Combination package, oral, as hydrochloride [titration pack contains two separate tablet formulations]:

Namenda®: Tablet: 5 mg (28s) and Tablet: 10 mg (21s)

Solution, oral, as hydrochloride:

Namenda®: 2 mg/mL (360 mL) [ethanol free, sugar free; contains propylene glycol; peppermint flavor]

Tablet, oral, as hydrochloride:

Namenda®: 5 mg, 10 mg

◆ **Memantine Hydrochloride** *see* Memantine *on page 1068*

◆ **Menactra®** *see* Meningococcal (Groups A / C / Y and W-135) Diphtheria Conjugate Vaccine *on page 1069*

◆ **MenACWY-D (Menactra®)** *see* Meningococcal (Groups A / C / Y and W-135) Diphtheria Conjugate Vaccine *on page 1069*

◆ **MenACWY-CRM (Menveo®)** *see* Meningococcal (Groups A / C / Y and W-135) Diphtheria Conjugate Vaccine *on page 1069*

◆ **Menest®** *see* Estrogens (Esterified) *on page 645*

◆ **Meningococcal Conjugate Vaccine** *see* Meningococcal (Groups A / C / Y and W-135) Diphtheria Conjugate Vaccine *on page 1069*

Meningococcal (Groups A / C / Y and W-135) Diphtheria Conjugate Vaccine

(me NIN joe kok al groops aye, see, why & dubl yoo won thur tee fyve dif THEER ee a KON joo gate vak SEEN)

Brand Names: U.S. Menactra®; Menveo®

Brand Names: Canada Menactra®; Menveo®

Index Terms MCV; MCV4; MenACWY-CRM (Menveo®); MenACWY-D (Menactra®); Meningococcal Conjugate Vaccine

Pharmacologic Category Vaccine, Inactivated (Bacterial)

Use Provide active immunization of children and adults against invasive meningococcal disease caused by *N. meningitidis* serogroups A, C, Y, and W-135.

The Advisory Committee on Immunization Practices (ACIP) recommends routine vaccination of all persons at age 11 or 12 years of age, followed by a booster at age 16 years of age (CDC, 60[3], 2011).

The ACIP also recommends vaccination for:

Children 9 through 23 months of age at increased risk for meningococcal disease (CDC 60[40], 2011). Children at increased risk include:

- Children traveling to or who reside in countries where *N. meningitidis* is hyperendemic or epidemic
- Children with persistent complement component deficiencies (eg, C5-C9, properdin, factor H, or factor D)

Persons 2 through 55 years of age at increased risk for meningococcal disease (CDC, 60[3], 2011). Meningococcal conjugate vaccine (MCV4) is preferred for persons aged 2-55 years; meningococcal polysaccharide vaccine (MPSV4) is preferred in adults ≥56 years of age (CDC, 2005). Persons at increased risk include:

- Previously unvaccinated college freshmen living in dormitories
- Microbiologists routinely exposed to isolates of *N. meningitidis*
- Military recruits
- Persons traveling to or who reside in countries where *N. meningitidis* is hyperendemic or epidemic, particularly if contact with local population will be prolonged
- Persons with persistent complement component deficiencies (eg, C5-C9, properdin, factor H, or factor D)
- Persons with anatomic or functional asplenia

Use is also recommended during meningococcal outbreaks caused by vaccine preventable serogroups (all recommended age groups) (CDC, 2005; CDC 60 [40], 2011).

Pregnancy Risk Factor B/C (manufacturer dependent)

Pregnancy Considerations Animal reproduction studies have not been conducted with Menactra® (therefore classified as pregnancy category C). An isolated teratogenic effect was observed in an animal developmental toxicity study; not necessarily vaccine related. Carcinogenic or mutagenic studies have not been performed. Patients should contact the Sanofi Pasteur Inc vaccine registry at 1-800-822-2463 if they are pregnant or become aware they were pregnant at the time of Menactra® vaccination.

Adverse events were not observed in animal reproduction studies conducted with Menveo® (therefore classified as pregnancy category B). Patients should contact the Novartis Vaccines and Diagnostics Inc. pregnancy registry at 1-877-311-8972 if they are pregnant or become aware they were pregnant at the time of Menveo® vaccination.

Limited information is available following inadvertent use of meningococcal diphtheria conjugate vaccine during pregnancy; safety and effectiveness have not been established. Inactivated bacterial vaccines have not been shown to cause increased risks to the fetus (CDC, 60 [2], 2011).

Lactation Excretion in breast milk unknown/use caution

Contraindications Hypersensitivity to other meningococcal-containing vaccines or any component of the formulation including diphtheria toxoid or CRM_{197} (a diphtheria toxin carrier protein)

Warnings/Precautions Use with caution in patients with a history of bleeding disorders (including thrombocytopenia) and/or patients on anticoagulant therapy; bleeding/hematoma may occur from I.M. administration. May consider deferring administration in patients with moderate or severe acute illness (with or without fever); may administer to patients with mild acute illness (with or without fever). Not to be used to treat meningococcal infections or to provide immunity against *N. meningitidis* serogroup B or diphtheria. Immunosuppressed patients may have a reduced response to vaccination. In general, household and close contacts of persons with altered immunocompetence may receive all age appropriate vaccines. Risk of developing Guillain-Barré syndrome (GBS) may be increased following vaccination in persons previously diagnosed with GBS. The risk of developing GBS was evaluated in a study of healthcare claims of persons 11-18 years of age (n= ~9,600,000; 15% were vaccinated with Menactra®); 72 cases of GBS were confirmed and none received the vaccine within 42 days prior to symptoms; 129 reported cases of GBS could not be confirmed or excluded. Data not currently available to assess possible risk of GBS following use of Menveo®. Immediate treatment for anaphylactic reactions should be available. In order to maximize vaccination rates, the ACIP recommends simultaneous administration of all age-appropriate vaccines (live or inactivated) for which a person is eligible at a single clinic visit, unless contraindications exist.

Adverse Reactions All serious adverse reactions must be reported to the U.S. Department of Health and Human Services (DHHS) Vaccine Adverse Event Reporting System (VAERS) 1-800-822-7967 or online at https://vaers.hhs.gov/esub/index. In Canada, adverse reactions may be reported to local provincial/territorial health agencies or to the Vaccine Safety Section at Public Health Agency of Canada (1-866-844-0018).

Actual percentages may vary by product and age group:

>10%:

Central nervous system: Crying (abnormal), drowsiness, fatigue, fever, headache, irritability, malaise, sleepiness

Gastrointestinal: Anorexia, diarrhea, nausea, vomiting

Local: Injection site: Erythema, induration, pain, redness, swelling, tenderness

Neuromuscular & skeletal: Arthralgia, myalgia

1% to 10%:

Central nervous system: Chills

Dermatologic: Rash

Gastrointestinal: Eating changes

Postmarketing and/or case reports: Acute disseminated encephalomyelitis, ALT increased, anaphylactic reactions, anaphylactoid reactions, balance disorder, bone pain, breathing difficulties, dizziness, ear pain, eyelid ptosis, facial palsy, facial paresis, Guillain-Barré syndrome, hearing impaired, hypersensitivity, hypotension, injection site reactions (cellulitis, inflammation, pruritus), oropharyngeal pain, paresthesia, pruritus, seizure, skin exfoliation, syncope, tonic convulsion, transverse myelitis, upper airway swelling, urticaria, vasovagal syncope, vertigo, vestibular disorder, wheezing

Drug Interactions

Metabolism/Transport Effects None known.

Avoid Concomitant Use There are no known interactions where it is recommended to avoid concomitant use.

Increased Effect/Toxicity There are no known significant interactions involving an increase in effect.

Decreased Effect

The levels/effects of Meningococcal (Groups A / C / Y and W-135) Diphtheria Conjugate Vaccine may be decreased by: Belimumab; Fingolimod; Immunosuppressants

Stability

Menactra®: Store between 2°C to 8°C (35°F to 46°F); do not freeze. Discard product exposed to freezing. Do not mix with other vaccines in the same syringe.

Menveo®: Prior to reconstitution, store between 2°C to 8°C (36°F to 46°F); do not freeze. Protect from light. Discard product exposed to freezing. Prior to use, remove liquid contents from vial of MenCYW-135 and inject into vial containing MenA powder. Gently invert or swirl until dissolved. The resulting solution should be clear and colorless. A small amount of liquid will remain in the vial after withdrawing the 0.5 mL dose. Use immediately after reconstitution but may be stored at ≤25°C (77°F) for up to 8 hours. Do not mix with other vaccines in the same syringe.

Mechanism of Action Induces immunity against meningococcal disease via the formation of bactericidal antibodies directed toward the polysaccharide capsular components of *Neisseria meningitidis* serogroups A, C, Y and W-135.

Dosage I.M.:

Menactra®: Children 9-23 months: 0.5 mL/dose given as a 2-dose series, 3 months apart

Menactra®, Menveo®: Children ≥2 years and Adults ≤55 years: 0.5 mL/dose given as a single dose

ACIP recommendations: Routine/primary vaccination:

Children 11-18 years of age: Routine vaccination: One dose at 11 or 12 years of age with a one-time booster dose (see "Booster dose"). Children in this age group receiving routine vaccination and who are also HIV positive should initially receive two doses, 2 months apart, and a booster dose as recommended, based on age at primary dose (see "Booster dose") (CDC, 60[3], 2011).

Children 9-23 months of age at high risk for invasive meningococcal disease (except those with functional or anatomic asplenia): Two doses, 3 months apart. A booster dose should be given as recommended if still at risk for meningococcal disease (see "Booster dose") CDC 60[40], 2011).

Children ≥2 years and Adults ≤55 years with persistent complement component deficiency, or functional or anatomic asplenia: Two doses, 2 months apart. A booster dose should be given as recommended if still at risk for meningococcal disease (see "Booster dose") (CDC, 60[3], 2011; CDC 60[40], 2011). Children at high risk for invasive meningococcal disease with functional or anatomic asplenia should receive their first dose at 2 years of age and ≥4 weeks after completion of the PCV13 vaccine series (CDC 60[40], 2011).

Children ≥2 years and Adults ≤55 years with prolonged increased risk of exposure: One dose. If still at risk for meningococcal disease, a booster dose should be given as recommended based on the age at first dose (see "Booster dose") (CDC, 60[3], 2011).

College students: Persons ≤21 years of age should have documentation of vaccination ≤5 years prior to enrollment. If the primary dose was given at <16 years of age, a booster dose should be given any time after the 16th birthday and prior to college enrollment. The minimum interval between doses is 8 weeks (CDC, 60[3], 2011).

ACIP recommendations: Booster dose:

Booster dose following routine vaccination: One booster dose should be given based on age at primary vaccination: If initial dose was at 11 or 12 years of age, a one-time booster dose should be given at age 16. If primary dose was given at age 13-15 years, a one-time booster dose should be given at 16-18 years of age. If primary dose was given ≥16 years of age, no booster dose is needed (CDC, 60[3], 2011).

Booster dose for all other indications in patients with continued risk:

If first dose received at 9-23 months of age: Repeat dose 3 years after primary vaccination, and every 5 years thereafter if the person remains at increased risk (CDC 60[40], 2011).

If first dose received at 2-6 years of age: Repeat dose 3 years after primary vaccination, and every 5 years thereafter if the person remains at increased risk (CDC, 2009; CDC, 60[3], 2011; CDC 60[40], 2011).

If first dose received at ≥7 years of age: Repeat dose 5 years after primary vaccination, and every 5 years thereafter if the person remains at increased risk (CDC, 2009; CDC, 60[3], 2011).

Administration Administer by I.M. route, preferably into the upper deltoid region. Do not administer via I.V., SubQ or I.D. route. For patients at risk of hemorrhage, the ACIP recommends "it should be administered intramuscularly if, in the opinion of a physician familiar with the patient's bleeding risk, the vaccine can be administered by this route with reasonable safety. If the patient receives antihemophilia or other similar therapy, intramuscular vaccination can be scheduled shortly after such therapy is administered. A fine needle (23 gauge or smaller) can be used for the vaccination and firm pressure applied to the site (without rubbing) for at least 2 minutes. The patient or family should be instructed concerning the risk of hematoma from the injection." Patients on anticoagulant therapy should be considered to have the same bleeding risks and treated as those with clotting factor disorders (CDC, 60[2], 2011).

For I.M. administration only. Based on limited data, inadvertent SubQ administration provides a lower serologic response, however, the response is still considered to be protective. If inadvertently administered by the SubQ route, revaccination is not necessary.

Simultaneous administration of vaccines helps ensure the patients will be fully vaccinated by the appropriate age. Simultaneous administration of vaccines is defined as administering >1 vaccine on the same day at different anatomic sites. Separate vaccines should not be combined in the same syringe unless indicated by product specific labeling. Separate needles and syringes should be used for each injection. The ACIP prefers each dose of a specific vaccine in a series come from the same manufacturer when possible. Adolescents and adults should be vaccinated while seated or lying down. In general, preterm infants should be vaccinated at the same chronological age as full-term infants (CDC, 60[2], 2011).

Antipyretics have not been shown to prevent febrile seizures. Antipyretics may be used to treat fever or discomfort following vaccination (CDC, 2011). One study reported that routine prophylactic administration of acetaminophen to prevent fever prior to vaccination decreased the immune response of some vaccines; the clinical significance of this reduction in immune response has not been established (Prymula, 2009).

Monitoring Parameters Monitor for syncope for ≥15 minutes following vaccination

Additional Information Federal law requires that the name of medication, date of administration, the vaccine manufacturer, lot number of vaccine, and the administering person's name, title and address be entered into the patient's permanent medical record.

Currently, two different meningococcal (groups A/C/Y and W-135) diphtheria conjugate vaccines are available. Menveo® uses oligosaccharides of the *N. meningitidis* serogroups linked to CRM_{197} (a nontoxic diphtheria toxin carrier protein). Menactra® uses polysaccharides from the serogroups linked to diphtheria toxoid. Both products are administered by I.M. injection and provide active immunization against invasive meningococcal disease caused by *N. meningitidis* serogroups A, C, Y, and W-135.

Dosage Forms Excipient information presented when available (limited, particularly for generics); consult specific product labeling.

Injection, solution [preservative free]:

Menactra®: 4 mcg each of polysaccharide antigen groups A, C, Y, and W-135 [bound to diphtheria toxoid 48 mcg] per 0.5 mL [MCV4 or MenACWY-D]

Menveo®: MenA oligosaccharide 10 mcg, MenC oligosaccharide 5 mcg, MenY oligosaccharide 5 mcg, and MenW-135 oligosaccharide 5 mcg [bound to CRM_{197} protein 32.7-64.1 mcg] per 0.5 mL (0.5 mL) [MenACWY-CRM; supplied in two vials, one containing MenA powder and one containing MenCYW-135 liquid]

◆ **Meningococcal Polysaccharide Vaccine** *see* Meningococcal Polysaccharide Vaccine (Groups A / C / Y and W-135) *on page 1071*

Meningococcal Polysaccharide Vaccine (Groups A / C / Y and W-135)

(me NIN joe kok al pol i SAK a ride vak SEEN groops aye, see, why & dubl yoo won thur tee fyve)

Brand Names: U.S. Menomune®-A/C/Y/W-135

Brand Names: Canada Menomune®-A/C/Y/W-135

Index Terms Meningococcal Polysaccharide Vaccine; MPSV; MPSV4

Pharmacologic Category Vaccine, Inactivated (Bacterial)

Additional Appendix Information

Immunization Recommendations *on page 1922*

Use Provide active immunity to meningococcal serogroups contained in the vaccine

The Advisory Committee on Immunization Practices (ACIP) recommends routine vaccination for persons at increased risk for meningococcal disease. Meningococcal conjugate vaccine (MCV4) is preferred for persons aged 2-55 years; meningococcal polysaccharide vaccine (MPSV4) is preferred in adults ≥56 years of age (CDC, 2005).

Persons at increased risk include:

- Previously unvaccinated college freshmen living in dormitories
- Microbiologists routinely exposed to isolates of *N. meningitidis*
- Military recruits
- Persons traveling to or who reside in countries where *N. meningitidis* is hyperendemic or epidemic, particularly if contact with local population will be prolonged
- Persons with persistent complement component deficiencies (eg, C5-C9, properidin, factor H, or factor D)
- Persons with anatomic or functional asplenia
- Persons with HIV infection

Use is also recommended during meningococcal outbreaks caused by vaccine preventable serogroups.

Pregnancy Risk Factor C

Pregnancy Considerations Animal studies have not been conducted. Inactivated bacterial vaccines have not been shown to cause increased risks to the fetus (CDC, 2011).

Lactation Excretion in breast milk unknown/use caution

Contraindications Hypersensitivity to any component of the formulation

Warnings/Precautions Immediate treatment (including epinephrine 1:1000) for anaphylactoid and/or hypersensitivity reactions should be available during vaccine use. Response may not be as great as desired in immunosuppressed patients. In general, household and close contacts of persons with altered immunocompetence may receive all age appropriate vaccines. Not to be used to treat meningococcal infections or to provide immunity against *N. meningitidis* serogroup B. May consider deferring administration in patients with moderate or severe acute illness (with or without fever); may administer to patients with mild acute illness (with or without fever). Use with caution in patients with latex sensitivity; the stopper to the vial contains dry, natural latex rubber. Some dosage forms contain thimerosal. In order to maximize vaccination rates, the ACIP recommends simultaneous administration of all age-appropriate vaccines (live or inactivated) for which a person is eligible at a single clinic visit, unless contraindications exist.

Adverse Reactions All serious adverse reactions must be reported to the U.S. Department of Health and Human Services (DHHS) Vaccine Adverse Event Reporting System (VAERS) 1-800-822-7967 or online at https://vaers.hhs.gov/esub/index. In Canada, adverse reactions may be reported to local provincial/territorial health agencies or to the Vaccine Safety Section at Public Health Agency of Canada (1-866-844-0018).

>10%:

Central nervous system: Headache (29% to 42%), fatigue (25% to 32%), malaise (17% to 22%), irritability (12%), drowsiness (11%)

Gastrointestinal: Diarrhea (10% to 14%)

Local: Injection site: Pain (26% to 48%), redness (6% to 16%), induration (4% to 11%)

Neuromuscular & skeletal: Arthralgia (5% to 16%)

1% to 10%:

Central nervous system: Chills (4% to 6%), fever (≤5%)

Dermatologic: Rash (≤3%)

Gastrointestinal: Anorexia (8% to 10%), vomiting (1% to 3%)

Local: Injection site: Swelling (3% to 8%)

Postmarketing and/or case reports: Dizziness, Guillain-Barré syndrome, hypersensitivity (angioedema, dyspnea, pruritus, rash, urticaria), myalgia, nausea, paresthesia, vasovagal syncope, weakness

Drug Interactions

Metabolism/Transport Effects None known.

Avoid Concomitant Use There are no known interactions where it is recommended to avoid concomitant use.

Increased Effect/Toxicity There are no known significant interactions involving an increase in effect.

Decreased Effect

The levels/effects of Meningococcal Polysaccharide Vaccine (Groups A / C / Y and W-135) may be decreased by: Belimumab; Fingolimod; Immunosuppressants

Stability Prior to and following reconstitution, store vaccine and diluent at 2°C to 8°C (35°F to 46°F); do not freeze. Reconstitute using provided diluent; shake well. Use single-dose vial within 30 minutes of reconstitution. Use single-dose vial immediately after reconstitution. Use multi-dose vial within 35 days of reconstitution.

Mechanism of Action Induces the formation of bactericidal antibodies to meningococcal antigens; the presence of these antibodies is strongly correlated with immunity to meningococcal disease caused by *Neisseria meningitidis* groups A, C, Y and W-135.

Pharmacodynamics/Kinetics

Onset of action: Antibody levels: 7-10 days

Duration: Antibodies against group A and C polysaccharides decline markedly (to prevaccination levels) over the first 3 years following a single dose of vaccine, especially in children <4 years of age

Dosage SubQ:

Children ≥2 years and Adults: 0.5 mL/dose

ACIP recommendations:

Children <2 years: Not usually recommended. Two doses (0.5 mL/dose), 3 months apart, may be considered in children 3-18 months to elicit short-term protection against serogroup A disease. A single dose may be considered in children 19-23 months (CDC, 2005).

Children ≥2 years and Adults ≤55 years: 0.5 mL/dose; however, use is not generally recommended; meningococcal conjugate vaccine (MCV4) is preferred (CDC, 2011); If MCV4 is unavailable, meningococcal polysaccharide vaccine (MPSV4) is an acceptable alternative (CDC, 2005). Persons at prolonged increased risk for meningococcal disease should be revaccinated with MCV4 (CDC, 2009).

Adults >55 years: 0.5 mL/dose (MPSV4 preferred in this population) (CDC, 2005)

Administration Administer by SubQ injection to the deltoid region; do not administer intradermally, I.M., or I.V.

Simultaneous administration of vaccines helps ensure the patients will be fully vaccinated by the appropriate age. Simultaneous administration of vaccines is defined as administering ≥1 vaccine on the same day at different anatomic sites. Separate vaccines should not be combined in the same syringe unless indicated by product specific labeling. Separate needles and syringes should be used for each injection. The ACIP prefers each dose of a specific vaccine in a series come from the same manufacturer when possible. Adolescents and adults should be vaccinated while seated or lying down. In general, preterm infants should be vaccinated at the same chronological age as full-term infants (CDC, 2011).

Antipyretics have not been shown to prevent febrile seizures. Antipyretics may be used to treat fever or discomfort following vaccination (CDC, 2011). One study reported that routine prophylactic administration of acetaminophen to prevent fever prior to vaccination decreased the immune response of some vaccines; the clinical significance of this reduction in immune response has not been established (Prymula, 2009).

Monitoring Parameters Monitor for syncope for ≥15 minutes following vaccination.

Additional Information Federal law requires that the name of medication, date of administration, the vaccine manufacturer, lot number of vaccine, and the administering person's name, title and address be entered into the patient's permanent medical record.

Dosage Forms Excipient information presented when available (limited, particularly for generics); consult specific product labeling.

Injection, powder for reconstitution [MPSV4]:

Menomune®-A/C/Y/W-135: 50 mcg each of polysaccharide antigen groups A, C, Y, and W-135 per 0.5 mL dose [contains lactose 2.5-5 mg/0.5 mL, natural rubber/natural latex in packaging, thimerosal in diluent for multidose vial]

◆ **Menomune®-A/C/Y/W-135** *see* Meningococcal Polysaccharide Vaccine (Groups A / C / Y and W-135) *on page 1071*

◆ **Menopur®** *see* Menotropins *on page 1073*

◆ **Menostar®** *see* Estradiol (Systemic) *on page 627*

Menotropins (men oh TROE pins)

Brand Names: U.S. Menopur®; Repronex®

Brand Names: Canada Menopur®; Repronex®

Index Terms hMG; Human Menopausal Gonadotropin

Pharmacologic Category Gonadotropin; Ovulation Stimulator

Use Female:

In conjunction with hCG to induce ovulation and pregnancy in infertile females experiencing oligoanovulation or anovulation when the cause of anovulation is functional and not caused by primary ovarian failure (Repronex®)

Stimulation of multiple follicle development in ovulatory patients as part of an assisted reproductive technology (ART) (Menopur®, Repronex®)

Unlabeled Use Male: Stimulation of spermatogenesis in primary or secondary hypogonadotropic hypogonadism

Pregnancy Risk Factor X

Pregnancy Considerations Ectopic pregnancy and congenital abnormalities have been reported. The incidence of congenital abnormality is similar during natural conception.

Lactation Excretion in breast milk unknown/use caution

Contraindications Hypersensitivity to menotropins or any component of the formulation; primary ovarian failure as indicated by a high follicle-stimulating hormone (FSH) level; uncontrolled thyroid and adrenal dysfunction; abnormal bleeding of undetermined origin; intracranial lesion (ie, pituitary tumor); ovarian cyst or enlargement not due to polycystic ovary syndrome; infertility due to any cause other than anovulation (except candidates for *in vitro* fertilization); sex hormone-dependent tumors of the reproductive tract and accessory organs; pregnancy

Warnings/Precautions These medications should only be used by physicians who are thoroughly familiar with infertility problems and their management. Advise patient of frequency and potential hazards of multiple pregnancy. May cause ovarian hyperstimulation syndrome (OHSS); if severe, treatment should be discontinued and patient should be hospitalized (may become more severe if pregnancy occurs). Monitor for ovarian enlargement; to minimize the hazard of abnormal ovarian enlargement, use the lowest possible dose. Serious pulmonary conditions (atelectasis, acute respiratory distress syndrome) and arterial thromboembolism have been reported. Safety and efficacy have not been established in renal or hepatic impairment, or in pediatric and geriatric patients. Use may lead to multiple births. Products may contain lactose.

Adverse Reactions Adverse effects may vary according to specific product, route, and/or dosage.

>10%:

- Central nervous system: Headache (up to 34%)
- Gastrointestinal: Abdominal pain (up to 18%), nausea (up to 12%)
- Genitourinary: OHSS (up to 13%, dose related)
- Local: Injection site reaction (4% to 12%)

1% to 10%:

- Cardiovascular: Flushing
- Central nervous system: Dizziness, malaise, migraine
- Endocrine & metabolic: Breast tenderness, hot flashes, menstrual irregularities
- Gastrointestinal: Abdominal cramping, abdominal fullness, constipation, diarrhea, enlarged abdomen, vomiting
- Genitourinary: Ectopic pregnancy, ovarian disease, vaginal hemorrhage
- Local: Injection site edema/pain
- Neuromuscular & skeletal: Back pain
- Respiratory: Cough increased, respiratory disorder
- Miscellaneous: Infection, flu-like syndrome

Frequency not defined:

- Cardiovascular: Stroke, tachycardia, thrombosis (venous or arterial)
- Dermatologic: Angioedema, rash, urticaria
- Genitourinary: Adnexal torsion, hemoperitoneum, ovarian enlargement
- Neuromuscular & skeletal: Limb necrosis
- Respiratory: Acute respiratory distress syndrome, atelectasis, dyspnea, embolism, laryngeal edema, pulmonary infarction, tachypnea
- Miscellaneous: Allergic reactions, anaphylaxis

Drug Interactions

Metabolism/Transport Effects None known.

Avoid Concomitant Use There are no known interactions where it is recommended to avoid concomitant use.

Increased Effect/Toxicity There are no known significant interactions involving an increase in effect.

Decreased Effect There are no known significant interactions involving a decrease in effect.

Stability Lyophilized powder may be refrigerated or stored at room temperature. Protect from light. After reconstitution inject immediately; discard any unused portion.

Mechanism of Action Actions occur as a result of both follicle stimulating hormone (FSH) effects and luteinizing hormone (LH) effects; menotropins stimulate the development and maturation of the ovarian follicle (FSH), cause ovulation (LH), and stimulate the development of the corpus luteum (LH); in males it stimulates spermatogenesis (LH)

Pharmacodynamics/Kinetics Excretion: Urine (~10% as unchanged drug)

Dosage Adults:

Repronex®: I.M., SubQ:

Induction of ovulation in patients with oligoanovulation (Females): Initial: 150 int. units daily for the first 5 days of treatment. Adjustments should not be made more frequently than once every 2 days and should not exceed 75-150 int. units per adjustment. Maximum daily dose should not exceed 450 int. units and dosing beyond 12 days is not recommended. If patient's response is appropriate, hCG 5000-10,000 units should be given one day following the last dose of Repronex®. Hold dose if serum estradiol is >2000 pg/mL, if the ovaries are abnormally enlarged, or if abdominal pain occurs; the patient should also be advised to refrain from intercourse. May repeat process if follicular development is inadequate or if pregnancy does not occur.

Assisted reproductive technologies (Females): Initial (in patients who have received GnRH agonist or antagonist pituitary suppression): 225 int. units; adjustments in dose should not be made more frequently than once every 2 days and should not exceed more than 75-150 int. units per adjustment. The maximum daily doses of Repronex® given should not exceed 450 int. units and dosing beyond 12 days is not recommended. Once adequate follicular development is evident, hCG (5000-10,000 units) should be administered to induce final follicular maturation in preparation for oocyte retrieval. Withhold treatment when ovaries are abnormally enlarged on last day of therapy (to reduce chance of developing OHSS).

Menopur®: SubQ: *Assisted reproductive technologies (ART):* Initial (in patients who have received GnRH agonist for pituitary suppression): 225 int. units; adjustments in dose should not be made more frequently than once every 2 days and should not exceed more than 150 int. units per adjustment. The maximum daily dose given should not exceed 450 int. units and dosing beyond 20 days is not recommended. Once adequate follicular development is evident, hCG should be administered to induce final follicular maturation in preparation for oocyte retrieval. Withhold treatment when ovaries are abnormally enlarged on last day of therapy (to reduce chance of developing OHSS).

Spermatogenesis (Males) (unlabeled use): I.M.: Following pretreatment with hCG: 75 int. units 3 times/week and hCG 2000 units twice weekly until sperm is detected in the ejaculate (4-6 months); may then be increased to menotropins 150 int. units 3 times/week

Administration

Menopur®: SubQ: Administer to alternating sites of the abdomen; when administration to the lower abdomen is not possible, the injection may be given into the thigh.

Repronex®:

- I.M.: Administer deep in a large muscle.
- SubQ: Administer to alternating sites of the lower abdomen.

Monitoring Parameters hCG levels, serum estradiol; vaginal ultrasound; in cases of suspected OHSS, monitor fluid intake and output, weight, hematocrit, serum and urinary electrolytes, urine specific gravity, BUN and creatinine, and abdominal girth

Dosage Forms Excipient information presented when available (limited, particularly for generics); consult specific product labeling.

Injection, powder for reconstitution:

- Menopur®: Follicle stimulating hormone activity 75 int. units and luteinizing hormone activity 75 int. units [packaged with diluent; contains lactose]
- Repronex®: Follicle stimulating hormone activity 75 int. units and luteinizing hormone activity 75 int. units [packaged with diluent; contains lactose]

◆ **Mentax®** *see* Butenafine *on page 255*

◆ **Menthol and Methyl Salicylate** *see* Methyl Salicylate and Menthol *on page 1113*

◆ **Menveo®** *see* Meningococcal (Groups A / C / Y and W-135) Diphtheria Conjugate Vaccine *on page 1069*

Meperidine (me PER i deen)

Brand Names: U.S. Demerol®

Brand Names: Canada Demerol®

Index Terms Isonipecaine Hydrochloride; Meperidine Hydrochloride; Pethidine Hydrochloride

Pharmacologic Category Analgesic, Opioid

Additional Appendix Information

Beers Criteria – Potentially Inappropriate Medications for Geriatrics *on page 1973*

Opioid Analgesics *on page 1896*

Patient Information for Disposal of Unused Medications *on page 2026*

Use Management of moderate-to-severe pain; adjunct to anesthesia and preoperative sedation

Unlabeled Use Reduce postoperative shivering; reduce rigors from amphotericin B (conventional)

Pregnancy Risk Factor C

Pregnancy Considerations Animal reproduction studies have not been conducted. Meperidine is known to cross the placenta, which may result in respiratory or CNS depression in the newborn.

Lactation Enters breast milk/not recommended (AAP rates "compatible"; AAP 2001 update pending)

Contraindications Hypersensitivity to meperidine or any component of the formulation; use with or within 14 days of MAO inhibitors

Warnings/Precautions Oral meperidine is not recommended for acute/chronic pain management. Meperidine should not be used for acute/cancer pain because of the risk of neurotoxicity. Normeperidine (an active metabolite and CNS stimulant) may accumulate and precipitate anxiety, tremors, or seizures; risk increases with CNS or renal dysfunction, prolonged use (>48 hours), and cumulative dose (>600 mg/24 hours). The Institute for Safe Medication Practice recommends avoiding the use of meperidine for pain control, especially in the elderly and renally-impaired (ISMP, 2007). In the elderly; meperidine is not an effective oral analgesic at commonly used doses; may cause confusion; other opioids are preferred in the elderly (Beers Criteria).

May cause CNS depression, which may impair physical or mental abilities; patients must be cautioned about performing tasks which require mental alertness (eg, operating machinery or driving). Effects may be potentiated when used with other sedative drugs or ethanol. Use only with extreme caution (if at all) in patients with head injury or increased intracranial pressure (ICP). Use caution with pulmonary, hepatic, or renal disorders, supraventricular tachycardias (including atrial flutter), acute abdominal conditions, hypothyroidism, myxedema, toxic psychosis, kyphoscoliosis, morbid obesity, Addison's disease, pheochromocytoma, BPH, or urethral stricture. Use with caution in patients with biliary tract dysfunction; acute pancreatitis may cause constriction of sphincter of Oddi. May cause hypotension; use with caution in patients with depleted blood volume or drugs which may exaggerate hypotensive effects (including phenothiazines or general anesthetics).

An opioid-containing analgesic regimen should be tailored to each patient's needs and based upon the type of pain being treated (acute versus chronic), the route of administration, degree of tolerance for opioids (naive versus chronic user), age, weight, and medical condition. The optimal analgesic dose varies widely among patients. Some preparations contain sulfites which may cause allergic reaction. Tolerance or drug dependence may result from extended use. Healthcare provider should be alert to problems of abuse, misuse, and diversion. Concurrent use of agonist/antagonist analgesics may precipitate withdrawal symptoms and/or reduced analgesic efficacy in patients following prolonged therapy with mu opioid agonists. Abrupt discontinuation following prolonged use may also lead to withdrawal symptoms. Avoid use in the elderly.

Adverse Reactions Frequency not defined.

Cardiovascular: Bradycardia, cardiac arrest, circulatory depression, hypotension, palpitation, shock, syncope, tachycardia

Central nervous system: Agitation, confusion, disorientation, dizziness, drowsiness, dysphoria, euphoria, fatigue, flushing, hallucinations, headache, intracranial pressure increased, lightheadedness, malaise, mental depression, nervousness, paradoxical CNS stimulation, restlessness, sedation, seizure (associated with metabolite accumulation), serotonin syndrome

Dermatologic: Pruritus, rash, urticaria

Gastrointestinal: Abdominal cramps, anorexia, biliary spasm, constipation, nausea, paralytic ileus, sphincter of Oddi spasm, vomiting, xerostomia

Genitourinary: Ureteral spasms, urinary retention

Local: Injection site reaction (including pain, wheal, and flare)

Neuromuscular & skeletal: Muscle twitching, myoclonus, tremor, weakness

Ocular: Visual disturbances

Respiratory: Dyspnea, respiratory arrest, respiratory depression

Miscellaneous: Anaphylaxis, diaphoresis, histamine release, hypersensitivity reactions, physical and psychological dependence

Drug Interactions

Metabolism/Transport Effects None known.

Avoid Concomitant Use

Avoid concomitant use of Meperidine with any of the following: MAO Inhibitors

Increased Effect/Toxicity

Meperidine may increase the levels/effects of: Alcohol (Ethyl); Alvimopan; CNS Depressants; Desmopressin; Metoclopramide; Selective Serotonin Reuptake Inhibitors; Serotonin Modulators; Thiazide Diuretics

The levels/effects of Meperidine may be increased by: Amphetamines; Antipsychotic Agents (Phenothiazines); Antipsychotics; Barbiturates; HydrOXYzine; MAO Inhibitors; Protease Inhibitors; Succinylcholine

Decreased Effect

Meperidine may decrease the levels/effects of: Pegvisomant

The levels/effects of Meperidine may be decreased by: Ammonium Chloride; Fosphenytoin; Mixed Agonist / Antagonist Opioids; Phenytoin; Protease Inhibitors

Ethanol/Nutrition/Herb Interactions

Ethanol: May increase CNS depression; monitor for increased effects with coadministration. Caution patients about effects.

Herb/Nutraceutical: Avoid valerian, St John's wort, kava kava, gotu kola (may increase CNS depression).

Stability

Injection solution: Store at 20°C to 25°C (68°F to 77°F); excursions permitted to 15°C to 30°C (59°F to 86°F).

Tablets: Store at 25°C (77°F); excursions permitted to 15°C to 30°C (59°F to 86°F).

Mechanism of Action Binds to opioid receptors in the CNS, causing inhibition of ascending pain pathways, altering the perception of and response to pain; produces generalized CNS depression

Pharmacodynamics/Kinetics

Onset of action: Analgesic: Oral, SubQ: 10-15 minutes; I.V.: ~5 minutes

Peak effect: SubQ.: ~1 hour; Oral: 2 hours

Duration: Oral, SubQ.: 2-4 hours

Absorption: I.M.: Erratic and highly variable

Protein binding: 65% to 75%

Metabolism: Hepatic; hydrolyzed to meperidinic acid (inactive) or undergoes N-demethylation to normeperidine (active; has 1/2 the analgesic effect and 2-3 times the CNS effects of meperidine)

Bioavailability: ~50% to 60%; increased with liver disease

Half-life elimination:

Parent drug: Terminal phase: Adults: 2.5-4 hours, Liver disease: 7-11 hours

Normeperidine (active metabolite): 15-30 hours; can accumulate with high doses (>600 mg/day) or with decreased renal function

Excretion: Urine (as metabolites)

Dosage Note: The American Pain Society (2008) and ISMP (2007) do not recommend meperidine's use as an analgesic. If use in acute pain (in patients without renal or CNS disease) cannot be avoided, treatment should be limited to ≤48 hours and doses should not exceed 600 mg/24 hours. Oral route is not recommended for treatment of acute or chronic pain. If I.V. route is required, consider a reduced dose. Patients with prior opioid exposure may require higher initial doses.

Children: Pain: Oral, I.M., SubQ: 1.1-1.8 mg/kg/dose every 3-4 hours as needed (maximum: 50-150 mg/dose)

Preoperatively: I.M., SubQ: 1.1-2.2 mg/kg given 30-90 minutes before the beginning of anesthesia (maximum: 50-150 mg/dose)

Adults:

Pain: Oral, I.M., SubQ: 50-150 mg every 3-4 hours as needed

Preoperatively: I.M., SubQ: 50-150 mg given 30-90 minutes before the beginning of anesthesia

Obstetrical analgesia: I.M., SubQ: 50-100 mg when pain becomes regular; may repeat at every 1-3 hours

Postoperative shivering (unlabeled use): I.V.: 25-50 mg once (Crowley, 2008; Kranke, 2002; Mercandante, 1994; Wang, 1999)

Elderly: Avoid use (American Pain Society, 2008; ISMP, 2007)

Dosing adjustment in renal impairment: Avoid use in renal impairment (American Pain Society, 2008; ISMP, 2007)

Dosing adjustment in hepatic impairment: Use with caution in severe hepatic impairment; consider a lower initial dose when initiating therapy. An increased opioid effect may be seen in patients with cirrhosis; dose reduction is more important for the oral than I.V. route.

Administration

Solution for injection: Meperidine may be administered I.M., SubQ, or I.V.; I.V. push should be administered slowly using a diluted solution, use of a 10 mg/mL concentration has been recommended.

Oral solution: Administer solution in 1/2 glass of water; undiluted solution may exert topical anesthetic effect on mucous membranes

Monitoring Parameters Pain relief, respiratory and mental status, blood pressure; observe patient for excessive sedation, CNS depression, seizures, respiratory depression

Test Interactions Increased amylase (S), increased BSP retention, increased CPK (I.M. injections)

Dosage Forms Excipient information presented when available (limited, particularly for generics); consult specific product labeling.

Injection, solution, as hydrochloride: 25 mg/mL (1 mL); 50 mg/mL (1 mL); 100 mg/mL (1 mL)

Demerol®: 25 mg/mL (1 mL); 25 mg/0.5 mL (0.5 mL); 50 mg/mL (1 mL, 1.5 mL, 2 mL, 30 mL); 75 mg/mL (1 mL); 100 mg/mL (1 mL, 20 mL)

Injection, solution, as hydrochloride [for PCA pump]: 10 mg/mL (30 mL)

Solution, oral, as hydrochloride: 50 mg/5 mL (500 mL)

Tablet, oral, as hydrochloride: 50 mg, 100 mg

Demerol®: 50 mg [scored]

Demerol®: 100 mg

Controlled Substance C-II

◆ **Meperidine Hydrochloride** *see* Meperidine *on page 1074*

Mephobarbital (me foe BAR bi tal)

Brand Names: U.S. Mebaral® [DSC]
Brand Names: Canada Mebaral®
Index Terms Methylphenobarbital
Pharmacologic Category Barbiturate
Use Sedative; treatment of grand mal and petit mal epilepsy
Pregnancy Risk Factor D
Dosage Oral:

Epilepsy: **Note:** Initiate at low dose and gradually increase over 4-5 days. Taper other antiepileptics off as dose increases. When lowering or discontinuing dose, taper over 4-5 days.

Children <5 years: 16-32 mg 3-4 times/day
Children >5 years: 32-64 mg 3-4 times/day
Adults: 400-600 mg/day

Coadministration with phenobarbital: Average dose: 200-300 mg/day mephobarbital plus 50-100 mg/day of phenobarbital (doses should be approximately half the amount of those when used alone)

Coadministration with phenytoin: Use full dose of mephobarbital and reduce phenytoin dose (average dose: phenytoin 230 mg/day plus mephobarbital 600 mg/day)

Sedation:
Children: 16-32 mg 3-4 times/day
Adults: 32-100 mg 3-4 times/day

Dosing adjustment in renal or hepatic impairment: Use with caution and reduce dosages

Additional Information Complete prescribing information for this medication should be consulted for additional detail.

Dosage Forms Excipient information presented when available (limited, particularly for generics); consult specific product labeling. [DSC] = Discontinued product

Tablet, oral:
Mebaral®: 32 mg [DSC] [scored]
Mebaral®: 50 mg [DSC], 100 mg [DSC]

Controlled Substance C-IV

◆ **Mephyton®** *see* Phytonadione *on page 1351*

Mepivacaine (me PIV a kane)

Brand Names: U.S. Carbocaine®; Polocaine®; Polocaine® Dental; Polocaine® MPF; Scandonest® 3% Plain
Brand Names: Canada Carbocaine®; Polocaine®
Index Terms Mepivacaine Hydrochloride
Pharmacologic Category Local Anesthetic
Use Local or regional analgesia; anesthesia by local infiltration, peripheral and central neural techniques (epidural and caudal); **not** for use in spinal anesthesia
Pregnancy Risk Factor C
Pregnancy Considerations Animal reproduction studies have not been conducted. Mepivacaine has been used in obstetrical analgesia.
Lactation Excretion in breast milk unknown/use caution
Contraindications Hypersensitivity to mepivacaine, other amide-type local anesthetics, or any component of the formulation

Warnings/Precautions Careful and constant monitoring of the patient's state of consciousness should be done following each local anesthetic injection; at such times, restlessness, anxiety, tinnitus, dizziness, blurred vision, tremors, depression, or drowsiness may be early warning signs of CNS toxicity; treatment is primarily symptomatic and supportive. Continuous intra-articular infusion of local anesthetics after arthroscopic or other surgical procedures is **not** an approved use; chondrolysis (primarily in the shoulder joint) has occurred following infusion, with some cases requiring arthroplasty or shoulder replacement. Use with caution in patients with cardiac disease, hepatic or renal disease, or hyperthyroidism. Local anesthetics have been associated with rare occurrences of sudden respiratory arrest; convulsions due to systemic toxicity leading to cardiac arrest have been reported presumably due to intravascular injection. A test dose is recommended prior to epidural administration and all reinforcing doses with continuous catheter technique. Do not use solutions containing preservatives for caudal or epidural block. Use caution in debilitated, elderly, or acutely-ill patients; dose reduction may be required. Resuscitative equipment, oxygen, and other resuscitative drugs should be available for immediate use.

Adverse Reactions Degree of adverse effects in the CNS and cardiovascular system is directly related to the blood levels of mepivacaine, route of administration, and physical status of the patient. The effects below are more likely to occur after systemic administration rather than infiltration.

Cardiovascular: Bradycardia, cardiac arrest, cardiac output decreased, heart block, hyper-/hypotension, myocardial depression, syncope, tachycardia, ventricular arrhythmias
Central nervous system: Anxiety, chills, convulsions, depression, dizziness, excitation, restlessness, tremors
Dermatologic: Angioneurotic edema, diaphoresis, erythema, pruritus, urticaria
Gastrointestinal: Fecal incontinence, nausea, vomiting
Genitourinary: Incontinence, urinary retention
Neuromuscular & skeletal: Chondrolysis (continuous intra-articular administration), paralysis
Ocular: Blurred vision, pupil constriction
Otic: Tinnitus
Respiratory: Apnea, hypoventilation, sneezing
Miscellaneous: Allergic reaction, anaphylactoid reaction

Drug Interactions

Metabolism/Transport Effects None known.

Avoid Concomitant Use There are no known interactions where it is recommended to avoid concomitant use.

Increased Effect/Toxicity

The levels/effects of Mepivacaine may be increased by: Beta-Blockers

Decreased Effect There are no known significant interactions involving a decrease in effect.

Stability Store at controlled room temperature of 15°C to 30°C (59°F to 86°F). Brief exposure up to 40°C (104°F) does not adversely affect the product. Solutions may be sterilized. Dental solutions should be protected from light.

Mechanism of Action Mepivacaine is an amide local anesthetic similar to lidocaine; like all local anesthetics, mepivacaine acts by preventing the generation and conduction of nerve impulses

Pharmacodynamics/Kinetics

Onset of action (route and dose dependent): Range: 3-20 minutes
Duration (route and dose dependent): 2-2.5 hours
Protein binding: ~75%
Metabolism: Primarily hepatic via N-demethylation, hydroxylation, and glucuronidation
Half-life elimination: Neonates: 8.7-9 hours; Adults: 1.9-3 hours
Excretion: Urine (95% as metabolites)

Dosage

Injectable local anesthetic: Dose varies with procedure, degree of anesthesia needed, vascularity of tissue, duration of anesthesia required, and physical condition of patient. The smallest dose and concentration required to produce the desired effect should be used.

Children: Maximum dose: 5-6 mg/kg; only concentrations <2% should be used in children <3 years or <14 kg (30 lbs)

Adults: Maximum dose: 400 mg; do not exceed 1000 mg/ 24 hours

Cervical, brachial, intercostal, pudendal nerve block: 5-40 mL of a 1% solution (maximum: 400 mg) **or** 5-20 mL of a 2% solution (maximum: 400 mg). For pudenal block, inject 1/2 the total dose each side.

Transvaginal block (paracervical plus pudenal): Up to 30 mL (both sides) of a 1% solution (maximum: 300 mg). Inject 1/2 the total dose each side.

Paracervical block: Up to 20 mL (both sides) of a 1% solution (maximum: 200 mg). Inject 1/2 the total dose to each side. This is the maximum recommended dose per 90-minute procedure; inject slowly with 5 minutes between sides.

Caudal and epidural block (preservative free solutions only): 15-30 mL of a 1% solution (maximum: 300 mg) **or** 10-25 mL of a 1.5% solution (maximum: 375 mg) **or** 10-20 mL of a 2% solution (maximum: 400 mg)

Infiltration: Up to 40 mL of a 1% solution (maximum: 400 mg)

Therapeutic block (pain management): 1-5 mL of a 1% solution (maximum: 50 mg) **or** 1-5 mL of a 2% solution (maximum: 100 mg)

Dental anesthesia: Adults:

Single site in upper or lower jaw: 54 mg (1.8 mL) as a 3% solution

Infiltration and nerve block of entire oral cavity: 270 mg (9 mL) as a 3% solution. Manufacturer's maximum recommended dose is not more than 400 mg to normal healthy adults.

Administration Before injecting, withdraw syringe plunger to ensure injection is not into vein or artery

Monitoring Parameters Vital signs, state of consciousness; signs of CNS toxicity

Dosage Forms Excipient information presented when available (limited, particularly for generics); consult specific product labeling.

Injection, solution, as hydrochloride:

Carbocaine®: 1% [10 mg/mL] (50 mL); 2% [20 mg/mL] (50 mL) [contains methylparaben]

Polocaine®: 1% [10 mg/mL] (50 mL); 2% [20 mg/mL] (50 mL) [contains methylparaben]

Polocaine® MPF: 2% [20 mg/g] (20 mL)

Injection, solution, as hydrochloride [preservative free]:

Carbocaine®: 1% [10 mg/mL] (30 mL); 1.5% [15 mg/mL] (30 mL); 2% [20 mg/mL] (20 mL)

Polocaine® MPF: 1% [10 mg/mL] (30 mL); 1.5% [15 mg/mL] (30 mL); 2% [20 mg/mL] (20 mL)

Injection, solution, as hydrochloride [for dental use]: 3% [30 mg/mL] (1.8 mL)

Carbocaine®: 3% [30 mg/mL] (1.7 mL)

Polocaine® Dental: 3% [30 mg/mL] (1.7 mL)

Scandonest® 3% Plain: 3% [30 mg/mL] (1.7 mL)

◆ **Mepivacaine Hydrochloride** *see* Mepivacaine *on page 1076*

Meprobamate (me proe BA mate)

Brand Names: Canada Novo-Mepro

Index Terms Equanil

Pharmacologic Category Antianxiety Agent, Miscellaneous

Additional Appendix Information

Beers Criteria – Potentially Inappropriate Medications for Geriatrics *on page 1973*

Use Management of anxiety disorders

Unlabeled Use Demonstrated value for muscle contraction, headache, external sphincter spasticity, muscle rigidity, opisthotonos-associated with tetanus; treatment of muscle spasm associated with acute temporomandibular joint (TMJ) pain

Dosage Oral:

Anxiety:

Children 6-12 years: 200-600 mg/day in 2-3 divided doses

Adults: 1200-1600 mg/day in 3-4 divided doses, up to 2400 mg/day

Muscle spasm (TMJ) pain (unlabeled use): Adults: 1200-1600 mg/day in 3-4 divided doses, up to 2400 mg/day

Dosing interval in renal impairment:

Cl_{cr} 10-50 mL/minute: Administer every 9-12 hours

Cl_{cr} <10 mL/minute: Administer every 12-18 hours

Hemodialysis: Moderately dialyzable (20% to 50%)

Dosing adjustment in hepatic impairment: Probably necessary in patients with liver disease

Additional Information Complete prescribing information for this medication should be consulted for additional detail.

Dosage Forms Excipient information presented when available (limited, particularly for generics); consult specific product labeling.

Tablet, oral: 200 mg, 400 mg

Controlled Substance C-IV

◆ **Mepron®** *see* Atovaquone *on page 167*

◆ **Mercaptoethane Sulfonate** *see* Mesna *on page 1083*

Mercaptopurine (mer kap toe PYOOR een)

Brand Names: U.S. Purinethol®

Brand Names: Canada Purinethol®

Index Terms 6-Mercaptopurine (error-prone abbreviation); 6-MP (error-prone abbreviation)

Pharmacologic Category Antineoplastic Agent, Antimetabolite; Antineoplastic Agent, Antimetabolite (Purine Analog); Immunosuppressant Agent

Use Maintenance treatment component of acute lymphoblastic leukemia (ALL)

Unlabeled Use Steroid-sparing agent for corticosteroid-dependent Crohn's disease (CD) and ulcerative colitis (UC); maintenance of remission in CD; fistulizing Crohn's disease; maintenance treatment in acute promyelocytic leukemia (APL); treatment component for non Hodgkin lymphoma (NHL), treatment of autoimmune hepatitis

Pregnancy Risk Factor D

Pregnancy Considerations May cause fetal harm if administered during pregnancy. Case reports of fetal loss have been noted with mercaptopurine administration during the first trimester; adverse effects have also been noted with second and third trimester use. Women of child bearing potential should avoid becoming pregnant during treatment.

Lactation Enters breast milk/not recommended

Contraindications Hypersensitivity to mercaptopurine or any component of the formulation; patients whose disease showed prior resistance to mercaptopurine

Warnings/Precautions Hazardous agent - use appropriate precautions for handling and disposal.

Hepatotoxicity has been reported, including jaundice, ascites, hepatic necrosis (may be fatal), intrahepatic cholestasis, parenchymal cell necrosis, and/or hepatic encephalopathy; may be due to direct hepatic cell damage or hypersensitivity. While hepatotoxicity or hepatic injury may occur at any dose, dosages >2.5 mg/kg/day are associated with a higher incidence. Signs of jaundice generally appear early in treatment, after ~1-2 months (range: 1 week to 8 years) and may resolve following discontinuation; recurrence with rechallenge has been noted. Monitor liver function tests (monitor more frequently if used in combination with other hepatotoxic drugs or in patients with pre-existing hepatic impairment. Consider a reduced dose in patients with hepatic impairment. Withhold treatment for clinical signs of jaundice (hepatomegaly, anorexia, tenderness), deterioration in liver function tests, toxic hepatitis, or biliary stasis until hepatotoxicity is ruled out.

Dose-related leukopenia, thrombocytopenia, and anemia are common; however, may be indicative of disease progression. Hematologic toxicity may be delayed. Bone marrow may appear hypoplastic (could also appear normal). Monitor for bleeding (due to thrombocytopenia) or infection (due to neutropenia). Patients with homozygous genetic defect of thiopurine methyltransferase (TPMT) are more sensitive to myelosuppressive effects; generally associated with rapid myelosuppression. Significant mercaptopurine dose reductions will be necessary (possibly with continued concomitant chemotherapy at normal doses). Patients who are heterozygous for TPMT defects will have intermediate activity; may have increased toxicity (primarily myelosuppression) although will generally tolerate normal mercaptopurine doses. Consider TPMT testing for severe toxicities/excessive myelosuppression. Patients on concurrent therapy with drugs which may inhibit TPMT (eg, olsalazine) or xanthine oxidase (eg, allopurinol) may be sensitive to myelosuppressive effects.

May increase the risk for secondary malignancies; hepatic T-cell lymphoma (HTCL) has been reported with mercaptopurine when used for the treatment of irritable bowel disease (an unlabeled use). Because azathioprine is metabolized to mercaptopurine, concomitant use with azathioprine may result in profound myelosuppression and should be avoided. Mercaptopurine is immunosuppressive; the risk for infection is increased; common signs of infection, such as fever and leukocytosis may not occur; lethargy and confusion may be more prominent signs of infection. Immune response to vaccines may be diminished. Consider adjusting dosage in patients with renal impairment. To avoid potentially serious dosage errors, the terms "6-mercaptopurine" or "6-MP" should be avoided; use of these terms has been associated with sixfold overdosages.

Adverse Reactions Frequency not defined.

Central nervous system: Drug fever

Dermatologic: Alopecia, hyperpigmentation, rash

Endocrine & metabolic: Hyperuricemia

Gastrointestinal: Anorexia, diarrhea, intestinal ulcers, mucositis/oral lesions (rare), nausea (minimal), pancreatitis, sprue-like symptoms, stomach pain, vomiting (minimal)

Genitourinary: Oligospermia

Hematologic: Myelosuppression (onset 7-10 days; nadir 14 days; recovery: 21 days); anemia, bleeding, granulocytopenia, leukopenia, marrow hypoplasia, thrombocytopenia

Hepatic: Hepatotoxicity, ascites, biliary stasis, hepatic damage/injury, hepatic encephalopathy, hepatic necrosis, hepatomegaly, intrahepatic cholestasis, jaundice, parenchymal cell necrosis, toxic hepatitis

Renal: Hyperuricosuria, renal toxicity

Miscellaneous: Hepatosplenic T cell lymphoma, immunosuppression, infection, secondary malignancy

Drug Interactions

Metabolism/Transport Effects None known.

Avoid Concomitant Use

Avoid concomitant use of Mercaptopurine with any of the following: AzaTHIOprine; BCG; CloZAPine; Febuxostat; Natalizumab; Pimecrolimus; Tacrolimus (Topical)

Increased Effect/Toxicity

Mercaptopurine may increase the levels/effects of: CloZAPine; Leflunomide; Natalizumab; Vaccines (Live); Vitamin K Antagonists

The levels/effects of Mercaptopurine may be increased by: 5-ASA Derivatives; Allopurinol; AzaTHIOprine; Denosumab; Febuxostat; Pimecrolimus; Roflumilast; Sulfamethoxazole; Tacrolimus (Topical); Trastuzumab; Trimethoprim

Decreased Effect

Mercaptopurine may decrease the levels/effects of: BCG; Coccidioidin Skin Test; Sipuleucel-T; Vaccines (Inactivated); Vitamin K Antagonists

The levels/effects of Mercaptopurine may be decreased by: Echinacea

Stability Store at room temperature of 15°C to 25°C (59°F to 77°F). Protect from moisture.

Mechanism of Action Purine antagonist which inhibits DNA and RNA synthesis; acts as false metabolite and is incorporated into DNA and RNA, eventually inhibiting their synthesis; specific for the S phase of the cell cycle

Pharmacodynamics/Kinetics

Absorption: Variable and incomplete (~50%)

Distribution: V_d > total body water; CNS penetration is poor

Protein binding: ~19%

Metabolism: Hepatic and in GI mucosa; hepatically via xanthine oxidase and methylation via TPMT to sulfate conjugates, 6-thiouric acid, and other inactive compounds; first-pass effect

Half-life elimination (age dependent): Children: 21 minutes; Adults: 47 minutes

Time to peak, serum: ~2 hours

Excretion: Urine (46% as mercaptopurine and metabolites)

Dosage Oral (also consult details concerning dosing in combination regimens):

Children:

ALL: Maintenance: 1.5-2.5 mg/kg/day **or**

Unlabeled ALL dosing (combination chemotherapy; refer to specific reference for combinations): Adolescents ≥15 years:

Consolidation phase: 60 mg/m²/day days 0-27 days (5-week course) (Stock, 2008) **or** 60 mg/m²/day days 0-13 and days 28-41 (9-week course) (Stock, 2008)

Early intensification (two 4-week courses): 60 mg/m²/day days 1-14 (Larson, 1995; Larson, 1998; Stock, 2008)

Interim maintenance: 60 mg/m²/day days 0-41 (8-week course) (Stock, 2008) **or** 60 mg/m²/day days 1-70 (12-week course) (Larson, 1995; Larson, 1998; Stock, 2008)

Maintenance (prolonged): 50 mg 3 times/day for 2 years (Kantarjian, 2000; Thomas, 2004) **or** 60 mg/m²/day for 2 years from diagnosis (Larson, 1995; Larson, 1998; Stock, 2008) **or** 75 mg/m²/day for 2 years (girls) or 3 years (boys) from first interim maintenance (Stock, 2008)

APL maintenance (unlabeled use): Adolescents ≥15 years: 60 mg/m²/day for 1 year (in combination with tretinoin and methotrexate) (Powell, 2010)

Autoimmune hepatitis (unlabeled use): 1.5 mg/kg/day (in combination with prednisone) (Manns, 2010)

Dosage adjustment with concurrent allopurinol: Reduce mercaptopurine dosage to 25% to 33% of the usual dose.

Dosage adjustment in TPMT-deficiency: Not always established; substantial reductions are generally required only in homozygous deficiency.

Adults:

ALL: Maintenance: 1.5-2.5 mg/kg/day **or**

Unlabeled ALL dosing (combination chemotherapy; refer to specific reference for combinations):

Early intensification (two 4 week courses): 60 mg/m²/day days 1-14 (Larson, 1995; Larson, 1998)

Interim maintenance (12-week course): 60 mg/m²/day days 1-70 (Larson, 1995; Larson, 1998)

Maintenance (prolonged): 50 mg 3 times/day for 2 years (Kantarjian, 2000; Thomas, 2004) **or** 60 mg/m^2/day for 2 years from diagnosis (Larson, 1995; Larson, 1998)

APL maintenance (unlabeled use): 60 mg/mm^2/day for 1 year (in combination with tretinoin and methotrexate) (Powell, 2010)

Crohn's disease, remission maintenance or reduction of steroid use (unlabeled use): 1-1.5 mg/kg/day (Lichtenstein, 2009)

Ulcerative colitis (unlabeled use):

Initial: 50 mg once daily; titrate dose up if clinical remission not achieved or down if leukopenia occurs (Lobel, 2004) **or**

Initial: 50 mg (25 mg if heterozygous for TPMT activity) once daily; titrate up to goal of 1.5 mg/kg (0.75 mg/kg if heterozygous for TPMT activity) if WBC >4000/mm^3 (and at least 50% of baseline) and LFTs and amylase are stable (Siegel, 2005) **or**

Maintenance: 1-1.5 mg/kg/day (Carter, 2004) **or**

Remission maintenance: 1.5 mg/kg/day (Danese, 2011)

Dosage adjustment with concurrent allopurinol: Reduce mercaptopurine dosage to 25% to 33% of the usual dose.

Dosage adjustment in TPMT-deficiency: Not always established; substantial reductions are generally required only in homozygous deficiency.

Elderly: Due to renal decline with age, initiate treatment at the low end of recommended dose range

Dosing adjustment in renal impairment: The manufacturer's labeling recommends starting with reduced doses in patients with renal impairment to avoid accumulation; however, no specific dosage adjustment is provided. The following adjustments have been used by some clinicians (Aronoff, 2007): Children:

Cl_{cr} <50 mL/minute/1.73 m^2: Administer every 48 hours

Hemodialysis: Administer every 48 hours

Continuous ambulatory peritoneal dialysis (CAPD): Administer every 48 hours

Continuous renal replacement therapy (CRRT): Administer every 48 hours

Dosing adjustment in hepatic impairment: The manufacturer's labeling recommends considering a reduced dose in patients with hepatic impairment; however, no specific dosage adjustment is provided.

Dietary Considerations Should not be administered with meals.

Administration Preferably on an empty stomach (1 hour before or 2 hours after meals)

For the treatment of ALL in children (Schmiegelow, 1997): Administration in the evening has demonstration superior outcome; administration with food did not significantly affect outcome.

Monitoring Parameters CBC with differential (weekly initially, although clinical status may require increased frequency), bone marrow exam (to evaluate marrow status), liver function tests (weekly initially, then monthly; monitor more frequently if on concomitant hepatotoxic agents), renal function, urinalysis; consider TPMT genotyping to identify TPMT defect (if severe toxicity occurs)

For use as immunomodulatory therapy in CD or UC, monitor CBC with differential weekly for 1 month, then biweekly for 1 month, followed by monitoring every 1-2 months throughout the course of therapy. LFTs should be assessed every 3 months.

Test Interactions TPMT testing: Recent transfusions may result in a misinterpretation of the actual TPMT activity. Concomitant drugs may influence TPMT activity in the blood.

Dosage Forms Excipient information presented when available (limited, particularly for generics); consult specific product labeling.

Tablet, oral: 50 mg

Purinethol®: 50 mg [scored]

Extemporaneous Preparations Hazardous agent: Use appropriate precautions for handling and disposal.

A 50 mg/mL oral suspension may be prepared in a vertical flow hood with tablets and a 1:1 mixture of methylcellulose 1% and simple syrup. Crush thirty 50 mg tablets in a mortar and reduce to a fine powder. Add small portions of the vehicle and mix to a uniform paste; mix while adding the vehicle in incremental proportions to a final volume of 30 mL; transfer to a calibrated bottle. **Note:** May use ultrasonication dispersal. Label "shake well" and "caution chemotherapy". Stable for 35 days at room temperature.

Dressman JB and Poust RI, "Stability of Allopurinol and of Five Antineoplastics in Suspension," *Am J Hosp Pharm*, 1983, 40(4):616-8.

◆ **6-Mercaptopurine (error-prone abbreviation)** *see* Mercaptopurine *on page 1077*

◆ **Mercapturic Acid** *see* Acetylcysteine *on page 34*

Meropenem (mer oh PEN em)

Brand Names: U.S. Merrem® I.V.

Brand Names: Canada Merrem®

Pharmacologic Category Antibiotic, Carbapenem

Use

Treatment of intra-abdominal infections (complicated appendicitis and peritonitis); treatment of bacterial meningitis in pediatric patients ≥3 months of age caused by *S. pneumoniae*, *H. influenzae*, and *N. meningitidis*; treatment of complicated skin and skin structure infections caused by susceptible organisms

Canadian labeling: Additional indications (not in U.S. labeling): Treatment of lower respiratory tract infections (community-acquired and nosocomial pneumonias), complicated urinary tract infections, gynecologic infections (excluding chlamydia), and septicemia; treatment of bacterial meningitis in adults caused by *S. pneumoniae*, *H. influenzae*, and *N. meningitidis* (use in adult meningitis based on pediatric data)

Unlabeled Use *Burkholderia pseudomallei* (melioidosis), febrile neutropenia, liver abscess, otitis externa

Pregnancy Risk Factor B

Pregnancy Considerations Meropenem is classified as pregnancy category B because no evidence of impaired fertility or fetal harm has been found in animals. Adequate and well-controlled studies have not been conducted in pregnant women and it is not known whether meropenem can cause fetal harm.

Lactation Excretion in breast milk unknown/use caution

Contraindications Hypersensitivity to meropenem, any component of the formulation, or other carbapenems (eg, doripenem, ertapenem, imipenem); patients who have experienced anaphylactic reactions to other beta-lactams

Warnings/Precautions Serious hypersensitivity reactions, including anaphylaxis, have been reported (some without a history of previous allergic reactions to beta-lactams). Carbapenems have been associated with CNS adverse effects, including confusional states and seizures (myoclonic); use caution with CNS disorders (eg, brain lesions and history of seizures) and adjust dose in renal impairment to avoid drug accumulation, which may increase seizure risk. Prolonged use may result in fungal or bacterial superinfection, including *C. difficile*-associated diarrhea (CDAD) and pseudomembranous colitis; CDAD has been observed >2 months postantibiotic treatment. Use with caution in patients with renal impairment; dosage adjustment required in patients with moderate-to-severe renal dysfunction. Thrombocytopenia has been reported in patients with renal dysfunction. Lower doses (based upon renal function) are often required in the elderly. May decrease divalproex sodium/valproic acid concentrations leading to breakthrough seizures; concomitant use not recommended. Alternative antimicrobial agents should be considered; if concurrent meropenem is necessary, consider additional antiseizure medication.

Adverse Reactions

1% to 10%:

Central nervous system: Headache (2% to 8%), pain (≤5%)

Dermatologic: Rash (2% to 3%, includes diaper-area moniliasis in pediatrics), pruritus (1%)

Endocrine & metabolic: Hypoglycemia

Gastrointestinal: Diarrhea (4% to 7%), nausea/vomiting (1% to 8%), constipation (1% to 7%), oral moniliasis (up to 2% in pediatric patients), glossitis (1%)

Hematologic: Anemia (≤6%)

Local: Inflammation at the injection site (2%), phlebitis/thrombophlebitis (1%), injection site reaction (1%)

Respiratory: Apnea (1%), pharyngitis, pneumonia

Miscellaneous: Sepsis (2%), shock (1%)

<1% (Limited to important or life-threatening): Abdominal enlargement, abdominal pain, agitation/delirium, agranulocytosis, alkaline phosphatase increased, ALT increased, AST increased, anemia (hypochromic), angioedema, anorexia, anxiety, aPTT decreased, asthma, back pain, bilirubin increased, bradycardia, BUN increased, cardiac arrest, chest pain, chills, cholestatic jaundice/jaundice, confusion, cough, creatinine increased, depression, diaphoresis, dizziness, dyspepsia, dyspnea, dysuria, eosinophilia, epistaxis, erythema multiforme, fever, flatulence, gastrointestinal hemorrhage, hallucinations, heart failure, hematuria, hemoglobin/hematocrit decreased, hemolytic anemia, hemoperitoneum, hepatic failure, hyper-/hypotension, hypervolemia, hypokalemia, hypoxia, ileus, injection site edema, injection site pain, insomnia, intestinal obstruction, LDH increased, leukocytosis, leukopenia, melena, MI, nervousness, neutropenia, paresthesia, pelvic pain, peripheral edema, platelets decreased/increased, pleural effusion, PT decreased, pulmonary edema, positive Coombs test, pulmonary embolism, renal failure, respiratory disorder, seizure, skin ulcer, somnolence, Stevens-Johnson syndrome, syncope, tachycardia, toxic epidermal necrolysis, urinary incontinence, urticaria, vaginal moniliasis, weakness, WBC decreased, whole body pain

Drug Interactions

Metabolism/Transport Effects None known.

Avoid Concomitant Use

Avoid concomitant use of Meropenem with any of the following: BCG; Probenecid

Increased Effect/Toxicity

The levels/effects of Meropenem may be increased by: Probenecid

Decreased Effect

Meropenem may decrease the levels/effects of: BCG; Divalproex; Typhoid Vaccine; Valproic Acid

Stability Dry powder should be stored at controlled room temperature 20°C to 25°C (68°F to 77°F). Meropenem infusion vials may be reconstituted with SWFI or a compatible diluent (eg, NS). The 500 mg vials should be reconstituted with 10 mL, and 1 g vials with 20 mL. May be further diluted with compatible solutions for infusion. Consult detailed reference/product labeling for compatibility.

Injection reconstitution: Stability in vial when constituted (up to 50 mg/mL) with:

SWFI: Stable for up to 2 hours at controlled room temperature of 15°C to 25°C (59°F to 77°F) or for up to 12 hours under refrigeration.

Sodium chloride: Stable for up to 2 hours at controlled room temperature of 15°C to 25°C (59°F to 77°F) or for up to 18 hours under refrigeration.

Dextrose 5% injection: Stable for 1 hour at controlled room temperature of 15°C to 25°C (59°F to 77°F) or for 8 hours under refrigeration.

Infusion admixture (1-20 mg/mL): Solution stability when diluted in NS is 4 hours at controlled room temperature of 15°C to 25°C (59°F to 77°F) or 24 hours under refrigeration. Stability in D_5W is 1 hour at controlled room temperature of 15°C to 25°C (59°F to 77°F) or 4 hours under refrigeration. For other diluents, see prescribing information.

Mechanism of Action Inhibits bacterial cell wall synthesis by binding to several of the penicillin-binding proteins, which in turn inhibit the final transpeptidation step of peptidoglycan synthesis in bacterial cell walls, thus inhibiting cell wall biosynthesis; bacteria eventually lyse due to ongoing activity of cell wall autolytic enzymes (autolysins and murein hydrolases) while cell wall assembly is arrested

Pharmacodynamics/Kinetics

Distribution: V_d: Adults: 15-20 L, Children: 0.3-0.4 L/kg; penetrates well into most body fluids and tissues; CSF concentrations approximate those of the plasma

Protein binding: ~2%

Metabolism: Hepatic; metabolized to open beta-lactam form (inactive)

Half-life elimination:

Normal renal function: 1-1.5 hours

Cl_{cr} 30-80 mL/minute: 1.9-3.3 hours

Cl_{cr} 2-30 mL/minute: 3.82-5.7 hours

Time to peak, tissue: 1 hour following infusion

Excretion: Urine (~70% as unchanged drug)

Dosage

Usual dosage ranges:

Children ≥3 months: I.V.: 30-120 mg/kg/day divided every 8 hours (maximum dose: 6 g/day)

Adults: I.V.: 1.5-6 g/day divided every 8 hours

Extended infusion method (unlabeled dosing): I.V.: 0.5-2 g over 3 hours every 8 hours (Crandon, 2011; Dandekar, 2003). **Note:** Dosing used at some centers and is based on pharmacokinetic/pharmacodynamic modeling and not clinical efficacy data.

Indication-specific dosing:

Children ≥3 months (<50 kg): I.V.:

Febrile neutropenia (unlabeled use): 20 mg/kg every 8 hours (maximum dose: 1 g every 8 hours)

Intra-abdominal infections (complicated): 20 mg/kg every 8 hours (maximum dose: 1 g every 8 hours)

Meningitis: 40 mg/kg every 8 hours (maximum dose: 2 g every 8 hours)

Pneumonia (community-acquired): Canadian labeling (not in U.S. labeling): 10-20 mg/kg every 8 hours (maximum dose: 1 g every 8 hours)

Skin and skin structure infections:

Complicated: U.S. labeling: 10 mg/kg every 8 hours (maximum dose: 500 mg every 8 hours)

Uncomplicated: Canadian labeling (not in U.S. labeling): 10-20 mg/kg every 8 hours (maximum dose: 1 g every 8 hours)

Urinary tract infection (complicated): Canadian labeling (not in U.S. labeling): 10 mg/kg every 8 hours (maximum dose: 500 mg every 8 hours)

Children >50 kg and Adults: I.V.:

Burkholderia pseudomallei* (melioidosis) (unlabeled use), *Pseudomonas: 1 g every 8 hours

Cholangitis, intra-abdominal infections, complicated: 1 g every 8 hours. **Note:** 2010 IDSA guidelines recommend treatment duration of 4-7 days (provided source controlled). Not recommended for mild-to-moderate, community-acquired intra-abdominal infections due to risk of toxicity and the development of resistant organisms (Solomkin, 2010).

Febrile neutropenia, otitis externa, pneumonia (unlabeled uses): 1 g every 8 hours

Liver abscess (unlabeled use): 1 g every 8 hours for 2-3 weeks, then oral therapy for duration of 4-6 weeks

Meningitis: Canadian labeling (not in U.S. labeling): 2 g every 8 hours

Mild-to-moderate infection, other severe infections (unlabeled use): 1.5-3 g/day divided every 8 hours

Pneumonia (community-acquired): Canadian labeling (not in U.S. labeling): 500 mg every 8 hours

Skin and skin structure infections:

Complicated: U.S. labeling: 500 mg every 8 hours; diabetic foot: 1 g every 8 hours

Uncomplicated: Canadian labeling (not in U.S. labeling): 500 mg every 8 hours

Urinary tract infections (complicated): Canadian labeling (not in U.S. labeling): 500 mg every 8 hours. **Note:** Up to 1 g every 8 hours may be administered (Pallett, 2010).

Adults: Canadian labeling (not in U.S. labeling): I.V.:

Gynecologic and pelvic inflammatory disease: 500 mg every 8 hours

Pneumonia (nosocomial): 1 g every 8 hours

Septicemia: 1 g every 8 hours

Dosing adjustment in renal impairment:

Children (unlabeled dosing; Aronoff, 2007):

GFR 30-50 mL/minute: Administer 20-40 mg/kg every 12 hours

GFR 10-29 mL/minute: Administer 10-20 mg/kg every 12 hours

GFR <10 mL/minute: Administer 10-20 mg/kg every 24 hours

Intermittent hemodialysis (IHD): 10-20 mg/kg every 24 hours (administer after hemodialysis on dialysis days)

Peritoneal dialysis (PD): 10-20 mg/kg every 24 hours

Continuous renal replacement therapy (CRRT): 20-40 mg/kg every 12 hours

Adults:

Cl_{cr} 26-50 mL/minute: Administer recommended dose based on indication every 12 hours

Cl_{cr} 10-25 mL/minute: Administer one-half recommended dose based on indication every 12 hours

Cl_{cr} <10 mL/minute: Administer one-half recommended dose based on indication every 24 hours

Alternative dosing recommendations: (unlabeled dosing; Aronoff, 2007):

GFR 10-50 mL/minute: Administer recommended dose (based on indication) every 12 hours

GFR <10 mL/minute: Administer recommended dose (based on indication) every 24 hours

Intermittent hemodialysis (IHD) (administer after hemodialysis on dialysis days): Meropenem and its metabolite are readily dialyzable: 500 mg every 24 hours. **Note:** Dosing dependent on the assumption of 3 times/week, complete IHD sessions.

Peritoneal dialysis (unlabeled dose): Administer recommended dose (based on indication) every 24 hours (Aronoff, 2007).

Continuous renal replacement therapy (CRRT) (Heintz, 2009; Trotman, 2005): Drug clearance is highly dependent on the method of renal replacement, filter type, and flow rate. Appropriate dosing requires close monitoring of pharmacologic response, signs of adverse reactions due to drug accumulation, as well as drug concentrations in relation to target trough (if appropriate). The following are general recommendations only (based on dialysate flow/ultrafiltration rates of 1-2 L/hour and minimal residual renal function) and should not supersede clinical judgment:

CVVH: Loading dose of 1 g followed by either 0.5 g every 8 hours **or** 1 g every 12 hours

CVVHD/CVVHDF: Loading dose of 1 g followed by either 0.5 g every 6-8 hours **or** 1 g every 8-12 hours

Note: Consider giving patients receiving CVVHDF dosages of 750 mg every 8 hours **or** 1500 mg every 12 hours (Heintz, 2009). Substantial variability exists in various published recommendations, ranging from 1-3 g/day in 2-3 divided doses. One gram every 12 hours achieves a target trough of ~4 mg/L.

Dietary Considerations Some products may contain sodium.

Administration Administer I.V. infusion over 15-30 minutes; I.V. bolus injection (5-20 mL) over 3-5 minutes

Extended infusion administration (unlabeled dosing): Administer over 3 hours (Crandon 2011; Dandekar, 2003). **Note:** Must consider meropenem's limited room temperature stability if using extended infusions

Monitoring Parameters Perform culture and sensitivity testing prior to initiating therapy. Monitor for signs of anaphylaxis during first dose. During prolonged therapy, monitor renal function, liver function, CBC.

Test Interactions Positive Coombs' [direct]

Dosage Forms Excipient information presented when available (limited, particularly for generics); consult specific product labeling.

Injection, powder for reconstitution: 500 mg, 1 g

Merrem® I.V.: 500 mg [contains sodium 45.1 mg as sodium carbonate (1.96 mEq)]

Merrem® I.V.: 1 g [contains sodium 90.2 mg as sodium carbonate (3.92 mEq)]

◆ **Merrem® (Can)** *see* Meropenem *on page* 1079

◆ **Merrem® I.V.** *see* Meropenem *on page* 1079

Mesalamine (me SAL a meen)

Brand Names: U.S. Apriso™; Asacol®; Asacol® HD; Canasa®; Lialda®; Pentasa®; Rowasa®; sfRowasa™

Brand Names: Canada 5-ASA; Asacol®; Asacol® 800; Mesasal®; Mezavant®; Novo-5 ASA; Novo-5 ASA-ECT; Pentasa®; Salofalk®; Salofalk® 5-ASA

Index Terms 5-Aminosalicylic Acid; 5-ASA; Fisalamine; Mesalazine

Pharmacologic Category 5-Aminosalicylic Acid Derivative

Use

Oral:

Asacol®, Lialda®, Pentasa®: Treatment and maintenance of remission of mildly- to moderately-active ulcerative colitis

Apriso™: Maintenance of remission of ulcerative colitis

Asacol® HD: Treatment of moderately-active ulcerative colitis

Rectal: Treatment of active mild-to-moderate distal ulcerative colitis, proctosigmoiditis, or proctitis

Pregnancy Risk Factor B/C (product specific)

Pregnancy Considerations Animal reproduction studies with mesalamine have not demonstrated teratogenicity or fertility impairment. Dibutyl phthalate (DBP) is an inactive ingredient in the enteric coating of Asacol® and Asacol® HD; adverse effects in male rats were noted at doses greater than the recommended human dose. Mesalamine is known to cross the placenta. An increased rate of congenital malformations has not been observed in human studies. Preterm birth, still birth and decreased birth weight have been observed; however, these events may also be due to maternal disease.

Lactation Enters breast milk/use caution

Contraindications Hypersensitivity to mesalamine, aminosalicylates, salicylates, or any component of the formulation

Warnings/Precautions May cause an acute intolerance syndrome (cramping, acute abdominal pain, bloody diarrhea; sometimes fever, headache, rash); discontinue if this occurs. Use caution in patients with active peptic ulcers. Patients with pyloric stenosis may have prolonged gastric retention of tablets, delaying the release of mesalamine in the colon. Pericarditis or myocarditis should be considered in patients with chest pain; use with caution in patients predisposed to these conditions. Pancreatitis should be considered in patients with new abdominal discomfort. Symptomatic worsening of colitis/IBD may occur following initiation of therapy. Oligospermia (rare, reversible) has been reported in males. Use caution in patients with sulfasalazine hypersensitivity. Use caution in patients with impaired hepatic function; hepatic failure has been reported. Renal impairment (including minimal change nephropathy and acute/chronic interstitial nephritis) and rarely failure have been reported; use caution in patients with renal impairment. Use caution with other medications converted to mesalamine. Postmarketing reports suggest an increased incidence of blood dyscrasias in patients >65 years of age. In addition, elderly may have difficulty administering and retaining rectal suppositories or may have decreased renal function; use with caution and monitor.

Apriso™ contains phenylalanine. The Asacol® HD 800 mg tablet has not been shown to be bioequivalent to 2 Asacol® 400 mg tablets. Canasa® suppositories contain saturated vegetable fatty acid esters (contraindicated in patients with allergy to these components). Rowasa® enema contains potassium metabisulfite; may cause severe hypersensitivity reactions (ie, anaphylaxis) in patients with sulfite allergies.

Adverse Reactions Adverse effects vary depending upon dosage form. Incidence usually on lower end with enema and suppository dosage forms.

>10%:

- Central nervous system: Headache (2% to 35%), pain (≤14%)
- Gastrointestinal: Abdominal pain (1% to 18%), eructation (16%), nausea (3% to 13%)
- Respiratory: Pharyngitis (11%)

1% to 10%:

- Cardiovascular: Chest pain (3%), peripheral edema (3%), vasodilation (≥2%)
- Central nervous system: Dizziness (2% to 8%), fever (1% to 6%), chills (3%), malaise (2% to 3%), fatigue (<3%), vertigo (<3%), anxiety (≥2%), migraine (≥2%), nervousness (≥2%), insomnia (2%),
- Dermatologic: Rash (1% to 6%), pruritus (1% to 3%), alopecia (<3%), acne (1% to 2%)
- Endocrine & metabolic: Triglyceride increased (<3%)
- Gastrointestinal: Diarrhea (2% to 8%), dyspepsia (1% to 6%), flatulence (1% to 6%), constipation (5%), vomiting (1% to 5%), colitis exacerbation (1% to 3%), rectal bleeding (<3%), abdominal distention (≥2%), gastroenteritis (≥2%), gastrointestinal bleeding (≥2%), stool abnormalities (≥2%), tenesmus (≥2%), rectal pain (1% to 2%), hemorrhoids (1%)
- Genitourinary: Polyuria (≥2%)
- Hematologic: Hematocrit/hemoglobin decreased (<3%)
- Hepatic: Cholestatic hepatitis (<3%), transaminases increased (<3%), ALT increased (1%)
- Local: Pain on insertion of enema tip (1%)
- Neuromuscular & skeletal: Back pain (1% to 7%), arthralgia (≤5%), hypertonia (5%), myalgia (3%), paresthesia (≥2%), weakness (≥2%), arthritis (2%), leg/joint pain (2%)
- Ocular: Vision abnormalities (≥2%), conjunctivitis (2%)
- Otic: Tinnitus (<3%), ear pain (≥2%)
- Renal: Creatinine clearance decreased (<3%), hematuria (<3%)
- Respiratory: Nasopharyngitis (1% to 4%), dyspnea (<3%), bronchitis (≥2%), sinusitis (≥2%), cough (≤2%)
- Miscellaneous: Flu-like syndrome (1% to 5%), infection (≥2%), diaphoresis (3%), intolerance syndrome (3%)

<1% (Limited to important or life-threatening): Agranulocytosis, albuminuria, alkaline phosphatase increased, anxiety, anemia, angioedema, aplastic anemia, asthma exacerbation, bilirubin increased, bloody diarrhea, BUN increased, cholestatic jaundice, cholecystitis, drug fever, dysuria, edema, eosinophilia, eosinophilic pneumonia, erythema nodosum, facial edema, fibrosing alveolitis, gastrointestinal bleeding, GGT increased, granulocytopenia, Guillain-Barré syndrome, hepatic failure, hepatic necrosis, hepatitis, hepatocellular damage, hepatotoxicity, hypersensitivity pneumonitis, hyper-/hypotension, interstitial nephritis, interstitial pneumonia, jaundice, Kawasaki-like syndrome, LDH increased, leukopenia, lupus-like syndrome, lymphadenopathy, metrorrhagia, minimal change nephrotic syndrome, myocarditis, nephropathy, nephrotoxicity, neutropenia, oligospermia, palpitation, pancreatitis, pancytopenia, paresthesia, perforated peptic ulcer, pericardial effusion, pericarditis, peripheral neuropathy, pharyngolaryngeal pain, photosensitivity, pleuritis, pneumonitis, pyoderma gangrenosum, rectal polyp, renal failure, serum creatinine increased, systemic lupus erythematosus, tachycardia, tenesmus, thrombocythemia, thrombocytopenia, transverse myelitis, T-wave abnormalities, vasodilation

Drug Interactions

Metabolism/Transport Effects None known.

Avoid Concomitant Use There are no known interactions where it is recommended to avoid concomitant use.

Increased Effect/Toxicity

Mesalamine may increase the levels/effects of: Heparin; Heparin (Low Molecular Weight); Thiopurine Analogs; Varicella Virus-Containing Vaccines

Decreased Effect

Mesalamine may decrease the levels/effects of: Cardiac Glycosides

The levels/effects of Mesalamine may be decreased by: Antacids; H2-Antagonists; Proton Pump Inhibitors

Stability

Capsule:

- Apriso™: Store at controlled room temperature of 20°C to 25°C (68°F to 77°F)
- Pentasa®: Store at controlled room temperature of 15°C to 30°C (59°F to 86°F). Protect from light.

Enema: Store at controlled room temperature. Use promptly once foil wrap is removed. Contents may darken with time (do not use if dark brown).

Suppository: Store below 25°C (below 77°F). May store under refrigeration; do not freeze. Protect from direct heat, light, and humidity.

Tablet: Store at controlled room temperature:

- Asacol®, Asacol® HD: 20°C to 25°C (68°F to 77°F)
- Lialda®: 15°C to 30°C (59°F to 86°F)
- Mezavant®: 15°C to 25°C (59°F to 77°F)

Mechanism of Action Mesalamine (5-aminosalicylic acid) is the active component of sulfasalazine; the specific mechanism of action of mesalamine is unknown; however, it is thought that it modulates local chemical mediators of the inflammatory response, especially leukotrienes, and is also postulated to be a free radical scavenger or an inhibitor of tumor necrosis factor (TNF); action appears topical rather than systemic

Pharmacodynamics/Kinetics

Absorption: Rectal: Variable and dependent upon retention time, underlying GI disease, and colonic pH; Oral: Tablet: ~20% to 28%, Capsule: ~20% to 40%

Distribution: ~18 L

Protein binding: Mesalamine (5-ASA): ~43%; N-acetyl-5-ASA: ~78%

Metabolism: Hepatic and via GI tract to N-acetyl-5-aminosalicylic acid

Half-life elimination: 5-ASA: 0.5-10 hours; N-acetyl-5-ASA: 2-15 hours

Time to peak, serum:

Capsule: Apriso™: ~4 hours; Pentasa®: 3 hours

Rectal: 4-7 hours

Tablet: Asacol®: 4-12 hours; Asacol® HD: 10-16 hours; Lialda®: 9-12 hours; Mezavant®: 8 hours

Excretion: Urine (primarily as metabolites, <8% as unchanged drug); feces (<2%)

Dosage Adults:

Oral:

Treatment of ulcerative colitis (usual course of therapy is 3-8 weeks):

Capsule (Pentasa®): 1 g 4 times/day; **Note:** Apriso™ capsules are approved for maintenance of remission only.

Tablet: Initial:

Asacol®: 800 mg 3 times/day for 6 weeks

Asacol® HD: 1.6 g 3 times/day for 6 weeks

Lialda®, Mezavant®: 2.4-4.8 g once daily for up to 8 weeks

Maintenance of remission of ulcerative colitis:

Capsule:

Apriso™: 1.5 g once daily in the morning

Pentasa®: 1 g 4 times/day

Tablet:

Asacol®): 1.6 g/day in divided doses

Lialda®: 2.4 g once daily

Note: Asacol® HD and Mezavant® tablets are approved for treatment only.

Rectal:

Active mild-to-moderate distal ulcerative colitis, proctosigmoiditis, or proctitis: Retention enema: 60 mL (4 g) at bedtime, retained overnight, approximately 8 hours

Active ulcerative proctitis: Rectal suppository (Canasa®): Insert one 1000 mg suppository in rectum daily at bedtime; retained for at least 1-3 hours to achieve maximum benefit

Note: Duration of rectal therapy is 3-6 weeks; some patients may require rectal and oral therapy concurrently.

Elderly: See adult dosing; use with caution

Dietary Considerations Some products may contain phenylalanine.

Apriso™: Take with or without food; do not administer with antacids.

Asacol® HD: Take with or without food.

Canasa® rectal suppository contains saturated vegetable fatty acid esters.

Administration Oral: Swallow capsules or tablets whole, do not break, chew, or crush.

Capsules:

Apriso™: Administer with or without food; do not administer with antacids. The capsule should be swallowed whole per the manufacturer's labeling; however, opening the capsule and placing the contents (delayed release granules) on food with a pH <6 is not expected to affect the release of mesalamine once ingested (data on file, Salix Pharmaceuticals Medical Information). There is no safety/efficacy information regarding this practice. The contents of the capsules should not be chewed or crushed.

Pentasa®: Administer with or without food. Although the manufacturer recommends swallowing the capsule whole, if a patient is unable to swallow the capsule, some clinicians support opening the capsules and placing the contents (controlled-release beads) on yogurt or peanut butter (Crohn's & Colitis Foundation of America). There are currently no published data evaluating the safety/efficacy of this practice. The contents of the capsules should not be chewed or crushed.

Tablets:

Asacol®: Do not break outer coating.

Asacol® HD: Do not break outer coating; administer with or without food.

Lialda®: Do not break outer coating; should be administered once daily with a meal

Mezavant®: Do not break outer coating; should be administered once daily with a meal

Rectal enema: Shake bottle well. Retain enemas for 8 hours or as long as practical.

Suppository: Remove foil wrapper; avoid excessive handling. Should be retained for at least 1-3 hours to achieve maximum benefit.

Monitoring Parameters Renal function (prior to and periodically during therapy); CBC (particularly in elderly patients)

Dosage Forms Excipient information presented when available (limited, particularly for generics); consult specific product labeling.

Capsule, controlled release, oral:

Pentasa®: 250 mg, 500 mg

Capsule, delayed and extended release, oral:

Apriso™: 0.375 g [contains phenylalanine 0.56 mg/capsule]

Suppository, rectal:

Canasa®: 1000 mg (30s, 42s) [contains saturated vegetable fatty esters]

Suspension, rectal: 4 g/60 mL (7s, 28s)

Rowasa®: 4 g/60 mL (7s) [contains potassium metabisulfite, sodium benzoate; packaged with wipes]

Rowasa®: 4 g/60 mL (28s) [contains potassium metabisulfite, sodium benzoate; packaged with wipes]

sfRowasa™: 4 g/60 mL (7s, 28s) [contains sodium benzoate]

Tablet, delayed release, enteric coated, oral:

Asacol®: 400 mg

Asacol® HD: 800 mg

Lialda®: 1.2 g

Dosage Forms: Canada Excipient information presented when available (limited, particularly for generics); consult specific product labeling.

Tablet, delayed and extended release:

Mezavant®: 1.2 g

◆ **Mesalazine** *see* Mesalamine *on page 1081*

◆ **Mesasal® (Can)** *see* Mesalamine *on page 1081*

◆ **M-Eslon® (Can)** *see* Morphine (Systemic) *on page 1153*

Mesna (MES na)

Brand Names: U.S. Mesnex®

Brand Names: Canada Mesna for injection; Uromitexan

Index Terms Mercaptoethane Sulfonate; Sodium 2-Mercaptoethane Sulfonate

Pharmacologic Category Antidote; Uroprotectant

Use Preventative agent to reduce the incidence of ifosfamide-induced hemorrhagic cystitis

Unlabeled Use Preventative agent to reduce the incidence of cyclophosphamide-induced hemorrhagic cystitis with high-dose cyclophosphamide

Pregnancy Risk Factor B

Pregnancy Considerations Teratogenic effects were not observed in animal studies. There are no adequate and well-controlled studies in pregnant women. Use during pregnancy only if clearly needed.

Lactation Excretion in breast milk unknown/not recommended

Contraindications Hypersensitivity to mesna or other thiol compounds, or any component of the formulation

Warnings/Precautions Examine morning urine specimen for hematuria prior to ifosfamide or cyclophosphamide treatment; if hematuria (>50 RBC/HPF) develops, reduce the ifosfamide/cyclophosphamide dose or discontinue the drug; will not prevent or alleviate other toxicities associated with ifosfamide or cyclophosphamide and will not prevent hemorrhagic cystitis in all patients. Mesna will not reduce the risk of thrombocytopenia-related hematuria. Allergic reactions have been reported; symptoms ranged from mild hypersensitivity to systemic anaphylactic reactions and may include fever, hypotension, and/or tachycardia; patients with autoimmune disorders receiving cyclophosphamide and mesna may be at increased risk. Patients should receive adequate hydration during treatment. I.V. formulation contains benzyl alcohol; do not use in neonates or infants (associated with "gasping syndrome").

Adverse Reactions

Mesna alone (frequency not defined):

Cardiovascular: Flushing

Central nervous system: Dizziness, fever, headache, hyperesthesia, somnolence

Dermatologic: Rash

Gastrointestinal: Anorexia, constipation, diarrhea, flatulence, nausea, taste alteration/bad taste (with oral administration), vomiting

Local: Injection site reactions

Neuromuscular: Arthralgia, back pain, rigors

Ocular: Conjunctivitis

Respiratory: Cough, pharyngitis, rhinitis

Miscellaneous: Flu-like syndrome

Mesna alone or in combination: Postmarketing and/or case reports: Allergic reaction, anaphylactic reaction, hypersensitivity, hyper-/hypotension, injection site erythema, injection site pain, limb pain, malaise, myalgia, platelets decreased, ST-segment increased, tachycardia, tachypnea, transaminases increased

Drug Interactions

Metabolism/Transport Effects None known.

Avoid Concomitant Use There are no known interactions where it is recommended to avoid concomitant use.

Increased Effect/Toxicity There are no known significant interactions involving an increase in effect.

Decreased Effect There are no known significant interactions involving a decrease in effect.

Stability Store intact vials and tablets at room temperature of 20°C to 25°C (68°F to 77°F). Opened multidose vials may be stored and used for up to 8 days after opening. Dilute injection in 50-1000 mL D_5W, NS, $D_5$1/4NS, $D_5$1/3NS, $D_5$1/2NS, or lactated Ringer's for infusion (the manufacturer recommends a final concentration of 20 mg/mL). Solutions diluted for infusion are stable for at least 24 hours at room temperature. Solutions in plastic syringes are stable for 9 days under refrigeration, or at room or body temperature. Solutions of mesna and ifosfamide in lactated Ringer's are stable for 7 days in a PVC ambulatory infusion pump reservoir. Solutions of mesna (0.5-3.2 mg/mL) and cyclophosphamide (1.8-10.8 mg/mL) in D_5W are stable for 48 hours refrigerated or 6 hours at room temperature (Menard, 2003). Mesna injection is stable for at least 7 days when diluted 1:2 or 1:5 with grape- and orange-flavored syrups or 11:1 to 1:100 in carbonated beverages for oral administration.

Mechanism of Action In blood, mesna is oxidized to dimesna which in turn is reduced in the kidney back to mesna, supplying a free thiol group which binds to and inactivates acrolein, the urotoxic metabolite of ifosfamide and cyclophosphamide

Pharmacodynamics/Kinetics

Distribution: No tissue penetration

Protein binding: 69% to 75%

Metabolism: Rapidly oxidized intravascularly to mesna disulfide (dimesna); dimesna is reduced in renal tubules back to mesna following glomerular filtration

Bioavailability: Oral: 45% to 79%

Half-life elimination:

I.V.: Mesna: ~22 minutes; Dimesna: ~70 minutes

I.V. followed by oral: 1-8 hours

Time to peak, plasma: 2-3 hours

Excretion: Urine (18% to 32% as mesna; 33% as dimesna)

Dosage Children and Adults: **Note:** Details concerning dosing in combination regimens should also be consulted. Mesna dosing schedule should be repeated each day ifosfamide is received. If ifosfamide dose is adjusted, the mesna dose should also be modified to maintain the mesna-to-ifosfamide ratio.

I.V.: Prevention of ifosfamide-induced hemorrhagic cystitis:

Short infusion standard-dose ifosfamide (<2.5 g/m^2/day): Mesna dose is equal to 60% of the ifosfamide dose given in 3 divided doses (0, 4, and 8 hours after the start of ifosfamide)

Continuous infusion standard-dose ifosfamide (<2.5 g/m^2/day): ASCO guidelines: Mesna dose (as an I.V. bolus) is equal to 20% of the ifosfamide dose, followed by a continuous infusion of mesna at 40% of the ifosfamide dose, continue mesna infusion for 12-24 hours after completion of ifosfamide infusion (Hensley, 2008)

High-dose ifosfamide (>2.5 g/m^2/day): ASCO guidelines: Evidence for use is inadequate; more frequent and prolonged mesna administration regimens may be required.

I.V. followed by oral (for ifosfamide doses ≤2 g/m^2/day): Mesna dose is equal to 100% of the ifosfamide dose, given as 20% of the ifosfamide dose I.V. at hour 0, followed by 40% of the ifosfamide dose given orally 2- and 6 hours after start of ifosfamide

Administration

Oral: Administer orally in tablet formulation or parenteral solution diluted in water, milk, juice, or carbonated beverages; patients who vomit within 2 hours after taking oral mesna should repeat the dose or receive I.V. mesna

I.V.: Administer by short (15-30 minutes) infusion or continuous infusion (maintain continuous infusion for 12-24 after completion of ifosfamide infusion) (Hensley, 2008)

Monitoring Parameters Urinalysis

Test Interactions False-positive urinary ketones with Chemstrip®, Multistix®, or Labstix®

Additional Information Oncology Comment: Guidelines from the American Society of Clinical Oncology (ASCO) for the use of chemotherapy and radiotherapy protectants (Hensley, 2008 [update]; Schuchter, 2002) recommend mesna to decrease the incidence of ifosfamide-induced urotoxicity associated with short infusion and continuous infusion standard-dose ifosfamide (<2.5 g/m^2/day). Although evidence is inadequate regarding mesna's uroprotective effects in high-dose ifosfamide (>2.5 g/m^2/day), the guidelines suggest more frequent and prolonged mesna administration times may be required. For prevention high-dose cyclophosphamide-induced urotoxicity (associated with stem cell transplantation), the guidelines recommend mesna in conjunction with saline diuresis (or forced saline diuresis alone).

Dosage Forms Excipient information presented when available (limited, particularly for generics); consult specific product labeling.

Injection, solution: 100 mg/mL (10 mL)

Mesnex®: 100 mg/mL (10 mL)

Tablet, oral:

Mesnex®: 400 mg [scored]

Dosage Forms: Canada Excipient information presented when available (limited, particularly for generics); consult specific product labeling.

Injection, solution:

Mesna for injection: 100 mg/mL (10 mL)

- **Mesna for injection (Can)** *see* Mesna *on page 1083*
- **Mesnex®** *see* Mesna *on page 1083*
- **Mestinon®** *see* Pyridostigmine *on page 1436*
- **Mestinon®-SR (Can)** *see* Pyridostigmine *on page 1436*
- **Mestinon® Timespan®** *see* Pyridostigmine *on page 1436*
- **Mestranol and Norethindrone** *see* Norethindrone and Mestranol *on page 1219*
- **Metadate CD®** *see* Methylphenidate *on page 1107*
- **Metadate® ER** *see* Methylphenidate *on page 1107*
- **Metadol™ (Can)** *see* Methadone *on page 1088*
- **Metadol-D™ (Can)** *see* Methadone *on page 1088*
- **Metaglip™** *see* Glipizide and Metformin *on page 797*
- **123 Meta-Iodobenzlyguanidine Sulfate** *see* Iobenguane I 123 *on page 920*
- **Metamucil® [OTC]** *see* Psyllium *on page 1432*
- **Metamucil® (Can)** *see* Psyllium *on page 1432*
- **Metamucil® Plus Calcium [OTC]** *see* Psyllium *on page 1432*
- **Metamucil® Smooth Texture [OTC]** *see* Psyllium *on page 1432*

Metaproterenol (met a proe TER e nol)

Brand Names: Canada Apo-Orciprenaline®; ratio-Orciprenaline®; Tanta-Orciprenaline®

Index Terms Alupent; Metaproterenol Sulfate; Orciprenaline Sulfate

Pharmacologic Category Beta$_2$-Adrenergic Agonist

Use Bronchodilator in reversible airway obstruction due to asthma or COPD

Pregnancy Risk Factor C

Dosage Oral:

Children:

<6 years (limited experience): 1.3-2.6 mg/kg/day divided every 6-8 hours

6-9 years (or <27 kg): 10 mg/dose 3-4 times/day

Children >9 years (or ≥27 kg) and Adults: 20 mg 3-4 times/day

Elderly: Refer to adult dosing.

Additional Information Complete prescribing information for this medication should be consulted for additional detail.

Dosage Forms Excipient information presented when available (limited, particularly for generics); consult specific product labeling.

Syrup, oral, as sulfate: 10 mg/5 mL (473 mL)

Tablet, oral, as sulfate: 10 mg, 20 mg

- **Metaproterenol Sulfate** *see* Metaproterenol *on page 1085*
- **Metastron®** *see* Strontium-89 *on page 1595*

Metaxalone (me TAKS a lone)

Brand Names: U.S. Skelaxin®

Brand Names: Canada Skelaxin®

Pharmacologic Category Skeletal Muscle Relaxant

Use Relief of discomfort associated with acute, painful musculoskeletal conditions

Pregnancy Considerations Teratogenic effects were not observed in animal studies. There are no adequate and well-controlled studies in pregnant women. Use during pregnancy (especially first trimester) only if benefits outweigh risks.

Lactation Excretion in breast milk unknown/not recommended

Contraindications Hypersensitivity to metaxalone or any component of the formulation; significantly impaired hepatic or renal function, history of drug-induced hemolytic anemias or other anemias

Warnings/Precautions May cause CNS depression. CNS depressant effects may be augmented when used in conjunction with other depressants (eg, barbiturates, ethanol), when taken with food, or in the elderly. May impair mental and/or physical ability to perform hazardous tasks such as operating machinery or driving a motor vehicle. Use with caution in patients with impaired renal or hepatic function (contraindicated if significant impairment); routine monitoring of transaminases is recommended. An increase in bioavailability and half-life have been observed in female patients. This class of medication is poorly tolerated by the elderly due to anticholinergic effects, sedation, and weakness. Efficacy is questionable at dosages tolerated by elderly patients (Beers Criteria). Safety and efficacy have not been established in children ≤12 years of age.

Adverse Reactions Frequency not defined.

Central nervous system: Dizziness, drowsiness, headache, irritability, nervousness

Dermatologic: Rash (with or without pruritus)

Gastrointestinal: Gastrointestinal upset, nausea, vomiting

Hematologic: Hemolytic anemia, leukopenia

Hepatic: Jaundice

Miscellaneous: Hypersensitivity (including rare anaphylactoid reactions)

Drug Interactions

Metabolism/Transport Effects Substrate of CYP1A2 (minor), CYP2C19 (minor), CYP2C8 (minor), CYP2C9 (minor), CYP2D6 (minor), CYP2E1 (minor), CYP3A4 (minor); **Note:** Assignment of Major/Minor substrate status based on clinically relevant drug interaction potential

Avoid Concomitant Use There are no known interactions where it is recommended to avoid concomitant use.

Increased Effect/Toxicity

Metaxalone may increase the levels/effects of: Alcohol (Ethyl); CNS Depressants; Methotrimeprazine; Selective Serotonin Reuptake Inhibitors

The levels/effects of Metaxalone may be increased by: Conivaptan; Droperidol; HydrOXYzine; Methotrimeprazine

Decreased Effect

The levels/effects of Metaxalone may be decreased by: Cyproterone; Peginterferon Alfa-2b; Tocilizumab

Ethanol/Nutrition/Herb Interactions

Ethanol: May increase CNS depression; monitor for increased effects with coadministration. Caution patients about effects.

Food: Bioavailability may be increased (may increase CNS depression).

Herb/Nutraceutical: Avoid valerian, St John's wort, kava kava, gotu kola (may increase CNS depression).

Stability Store at controlled room temperature of 15°C to 30°C (59°F to 86°F).

Mechanism of Action Precise mechanism has not been established; however, efficacy appears to result from disruption of the spasm-pain-spasm cycle, probably by a general CNS depressant effect. Does not have a direct effect on skeletal muscle.

Pharmacodynamics/Kinetics

Onset of action: ~1 hour

Duration: ~4-6 hours

Distribution: V_d: ~800 L

Metabolism: Hepatic via CYP1A2, CYP2D6, CYP2E1, CYP3A4 and to lesser extent CYP2C8, CPY2C9, and CYP2C19

Bioavailability: Not established; food may increase

Half-life elimination: 4-14 hours

Time to peak: T_{max}: ~3 hours

Excretion: Urine (as metabolites)

Dosage Oral: Children >12 years and Adults: Muscle discomfort: 800 mg 3-4 times/day

Dosage adjustment in renal impairment: Use caution in patients with mild-to-moderate renal impairment; contraindicated with significant impairment. No specific recommendation are provided in approved labeling.

Dosage adjustment in hepatic impairment: Use caution in patients with mild-to-moderate hepatic impairment; contraindicated with significant impairment. No specific recommendation are provided in approved labeling.

Dietary Considerations Administration with food may increase serum concentrations.

Administration May be administered with or without food. However, serum concentrations may be increased when administered with food; clinical significance has not been established. Patients should be monitored.

Test Interactions False-positive Benedict's test

Dosage Forms Excipient information presented when available (limited, particularly for generics); consult specific product labeling.

Tablet, oral: 800 mg

Skelaxin®: 800 mg [scored]

MetFORMIN (met FOR min)

Brand Names: U.S. Fortamet®; Glucophage®; Glucophage® XR; Glumetza®; Riomet®

Brand Names: Canada Apo-Metformin®; CO Metformin; Dom-Metformin; Glucophage®; Glumetza®; Glycon; Med-Metformin; Mylan-Metformin; Novo-Metformin; Nu-Metformin; PHL-Metformin; PMS-Metformin; PRO-Metformin; RAN™-Metformin; ratio-Metformin; Riva-Metformin; Sandoz-Metformin FC

Index Terms Metformin Hydrochloride

Pharmacologic Category Antidiabetic Agent, Biguanide

Additional Appendix Information

Diabetes Mellitus Management, Adults *on page 1983*

Use Management of type 2 diabetes mellitus (noninsulin dependent, NIDDM) when hyperglycemia cannot be managed with diet and exercise alone.

Unlabeled Use Gestational diabetes mellitus (GDM); polycystic ovary syndrome (PCOS); prevention of type 2 diabetes mellitus

Pregnancy Risk Factor B

Pregnancy Considerations Adverse events have not been observed in animal studies; therefore, metformin is classified as pregnancy category B. Metformin has been found to cross the placenta in concentrations which may be comparable to those found in the maternal plasma. Pharmacokinetic studies suggest that clearance of metformin may be increased during pregnancy and dosing may need adjusted in some women when used during the third trimester.

Fetal, neonatal, and maternal outcomes have been evaluated following maternal use of metformin for the treatment of GDM and type 2 diabetes. Available information suggests that metformin use during pregnancy may be safe as long as good glycemic control is maintained; however, many studies used metformin during the second or third trimester only. Maternal hyperglycemia can be associated with adverse effects in the fetus, including macrosomia, neonatal hyperglycemia, and hyperbilirubinemia; the risk of congenital malformations is increased when the Hb A_{1c} is above the normal range. Diabetes can also be associated with adverse effects in the mother. Poorly-treated diabetes may cause end-organ damage that may negatively affect obstetric outcomes. Physiologic glucose levels should be maintained prior to and during pregnancy to decrease the risk of adverse events in the mother and the fetus. Until additional safety and efficacy data are obtained, the use of oral agents is generally not recommended as routine management of GDM or type 2 diabetes mellitus during pregnancy. Insulin is the drug of choice for the control of diabetes mellitus during pregnancy.

Metformin has also been evaluated for the treatment of PCOS, a syndrome which may exhibit oligomenorrhea and, in some women, hyperinsulinemia. It is not recommended as first-line therapy; when used to treat infertility related to PCOS, current guidelines restrict the use of metformin to women with glucose intolerance. Because ovulation rates will likely improve in women with PCOS who are taking metformin, appropriate contraceptive measures should be discussed in women who are not attempting to conceive.

Lactation Enters breast milk/not recommended

Contraindications Hypersensitivity to metformin or any component of the formulation; renal disease or renal dysfunction (serum creatinine ≥1.5 mg/dL in males or ≥1.4 mg/dL in females) or abnormal creatinine clearance from any cause, including shock, acute myocardial infarction, or septicemia; acute or chronic metabolic acidosis with or without coma (including diabetic ketoacidosis)

Note: Temporarily discontinue in patients undergoing radiologic studies in which intravascular iodinated contrast media are utilized.

Warnings/Precautions [U.S. Boxed Warning]: Lactic acidosis is a rare, but potentially severe consequence of therapy with metformin. Lactic acidosis should be suspected in any patient with diabetes receiving metformin with evidence of acidosis but without evidence of ketoacidosis. Discontinue metformin in clinical situations predisposing to hypoxemia, including conditions such as cardiovascular collapse, respiratory failure, acute myocardial infarction, acute congestive heart failure, and septicemia. Use caution in patients with congestive heart failure requiring pharmacologic management, particularly in patients with unstable or acute CHF; risk of lactic acidosis may be increased secondary to hypoperfusion.

Metformin is substantially excreted by the kidney. The risk of accumulation and lactic acidosis increases with the degree of impairment of renal function. Patients with renal function below the limit of normal for their age should not receive metformin. In elderly patients, renal function should be monitored regularly; should not be initiated in patients ≥80 years of age unless normal renal function is confirmed. Use of concomitant medications that may affect renal function (ie, affect tubular secretion) may also affect metformin disposition. Metformin should be withheld in patients with dehydration and/or prerenal azotemia. Therapy should be suspended for any surgical procedures (resume only after normal oral intake resumed and normal renal function is verified). Therapy should be temporarily discontinued prior to or at the time of intravascular administration of iodinated contrast media (potential for acute alteration in renal function). Metformin should be withheld for 48 hours after the radiologic study and restarted only after renal function has been confirmed as normal. It may be necessary to discontinue metformin and administer insulin if the patient is exposed to stress (fever, trauma, infection, surgery).

Avoid use in patients with impaired liver function. Patient must be instructed to avoid excessive acute or chronic ethanol use; ethanol may potentiate metformin's effect on lactate metabolism. Administration of oral antidiabetic drugs has been reported to be associated with increased cardiovascular mortality; metformin does not appear to share this risk. Insoluble tablet shell of Glumetza® 1000 mg extended release tablet may remain intact and be visible in the stool. Other extended released tablets (Fortamet®, Glucophage® XR, Glumetza® 500 mg) may appear in the stool as a soft mass resembling the tablet.

Adverse Reactions

>10%:

Gastrointestinal: Diarrhea (10% to 53%), nausea/vomiting (7% to 26%), flatulence (12%)

Neuromuscular & skeletal: Weakness (9%)

1% to 10%:

Cardiovascular: Chest discomfort, flushing, palpitation

Central nervous system: Headache (6%), chills, dizziness, lightheadedness

Dermatologic: Rash

Endocrine & metabolic: Hypoglycemia

Gastrointestinal: Indigestion (7%), abdominal discomfort (6%), abdominal distention, abnormal stools, constipation, dyspepsia/ heartburn, taste disorder

Neuromuscular & skeletal: Myalgia

Respiratory: Dyspnea, upper respiratory tract infection

Miscellaneous: Decreased vitamin B_{12} levels (7%), increased diaphoresis, flu-like syndrome, nail disorder

<1% (Limited to important or life-threatening): Lactic acidosis, leukocytoclastic vasculitis, megaloblastic anemia, pneumonitis

Drug Interactions

Metabolism/Transport Effects None known.

Avoid Concomitant Use There are no known interactions where it is recommended to avoid concomitant use.

Increased Effect/Toxicity

MetFORMIN may increase the levels/effects of: Dofetilide

The levels/effects of MetFORMIN may be increased by: Cephalexin; Cimetidine; Glycopyrrolate; Iodinated Contrast Agents; Pegvisomant

Decreased Effect

MetFORMIN may decrease the levels/effects of: Trospium

The levels/effects of MetFORMIN may be decreased by: Corticosteroids (Orally Inhaled); Corticosteroids (Systemic); Luteinizing Hormone-Releasing Hormone Analogs; Somatropin; Thiazide Diuretics

Ethanol/Nutrition/Herb Interactions

Ethanol: Avoid or limit ethanol (incidence of lactic acidosis may be increased; may cause hypoglycemia).

Food: Food decreases the extent and slightly delays the absorption. May decrease absorption of vitamin B_{12} and/ or folic acid.

Herb/Nutraceutical: Caution with chromium, garlic, gymnema (may cause hypoglycemia).

Stability

Oral solution: Store at 15°C to 30°C (59°F to 86°F).

Tablets: Store at 20°C to 25°C (68°F to 77°F); excursion permitted to 15°C to 30°C (59°F to 86°F). Protect from light and moisture.

Mechanism of Action Decreases hepatic glucose production, decreasing intestinal absorption of glucose and improves insulin sensitivity (increases peripheral glucose uptake and utilization)

Pharmacodynamics/Kinetics

Onset of action: Within days; maximum effects up to 2 weeks

Distribution: V_d: 654 ± 358 L; partitions into erythrocytes

Protein binding: Negligible

Metabolism: Not metabolized by the liver

Bioavailability: Absolute: Fasting: 50% to 60%

Half-life elimination: Plasma: 4-9 hours

Time to peak, serum: Immediate release: 2-3 hours; Extended release: 7 hours (range: 4-8 hours)

Excretion: Urine (90% as unchanged drug; active secretion)

Dosage

Type 2 diabetes management: **Note:** Allow 1-2 weeks between dose titrations: Generally, clinically significant responses are not seen at doses <1500 mg daily; however, a lower recommended starting dose and gradual increased dosage is recommended to minimize gastrointestinal symptoms.

Immediate release tablet or solution: Oral:

Children 10-16 years: Initial: 500 mg twice daily; increases in daily dosage should be made in increments of 500 mg at weekly intervals, given in divided doses, up to a maximum of 2000 mg/day

Children ≥17 years and Adults: Initial: 500 mg twice daily **or** 850 mg once daily; titrate in increments of 500 mg weekly or 850 mg every other week; may also titrate from 500 mg twice a day to 850 mg twice a day after 2 weeks

Doses of up to 2000 mg/day may be given twice daily. If a dose >2000 mg/day is required, it may be better tolerated in three divided doses. Maximum recommended dose 2550 mg/day.

Extended release tablet: Oral: **Note:** If glycemic control is not achieved at maximum dose, may divide dose and administer twice daily.

Children ≥17 years and Adults:

Fortamet®: Initial: 500-1000 mg once daily; dosage may be increased by 500 mg weekly; maximum dose: 2500 mg once daily

Glucophage® XR: Initial: 500 mg once daily; dosage may be increased by 500 mg weekly; maximum dose: 2000 mg once daily

Adults: Glumetza®: Initial: 1000 mg once daily; dosage may be increased by 500 mg weekly; maximum dose: 2000 mg once daily

Elderly: The initial and maintenance dosing should be conservative, due to the potential for decreased renal function. Generally, elderly patients should not be titrated to the maximum dose of metformin. Do not use in patients ≥80 years of age unless normal renal function has been established.

Transfer from other antidiabetic agents: No transition period is generally necessary except when transferring from chlorpropamide. When transferring from chlorpropamide, care should be exercised during the first 2 weeks because of the prolonged retention of chlorpropamide in the body, leading to overlapping drug effects and possible hypoglycemia.

Concomitant metformin and oral sulfonylurea therapy: If patients have not responded to 4 weeks of the maximum dose of metformin monotherapy, consider a gradual addition of an oral sulfonylurea, even if prior primary or secondary failure to a sulfonylurea has occurred. Continue metformin at the maximum dose. If adequate response has not occurred following 3 months of metformin and sulfonylurea combination therapy, consider switching to insulin with or without metformin.

Failed sulfonylurea therapy: Patients with prior failure on glyburide may be treated by gradual addition of metformin. Initiate with glyburide 20 mg and metformin 500 mg daily. Metformin dosage may be increased by 500 mg/day at weekly intervals, up to a maximum metformin dose (dosage of glyburide maintained at 20 mg/day).

Concomitant metformin and insulin therapy: Initial: 500 mg metformin once daily, continue current insulin dose; increase by 500 mg metformin weekly until adequate glycemic control is achieved

Maximum daily dose: Immediate release and solution: 2550 mg metformin; Extended release: 2000-2500 mg (varies by product)

Decrease insulin dose 10% to 25% when FPG <120 mg/dL; monitor and make further adjustments as needed

Type 2 diabetes prevention (unlabeled use): **Immediate release tablet or solution:** Oral: Adults: Initial: 850 mg once daily; Target: 850 mg twice daily (Knowler, 2002)

Dosing adjustment/comments in renal impairment: The plasma and blood half-life of metformin is prolonged and the renal clearance is decreased in proportion to the decrease in creatinine clearance. Per the manufacturer, metformin is contraindicated in the presence of renal dysfunction defined as a serum creatinine ≥1.5 mg/dL in males, or ≥1.4 mg/dL in females and in patients with abnormal clearance. The Canadian labeling recommends that metformin be avoided in patients with Cl_{cr} <60 mL/minute.

Dosing adjustment in hepatic impairment: Avoid metformin; liver disease is a risk factor for the development of lactic acidosis during metformin therapy.

Dietary Considerations Drug may cause GI upset; take with food (to decrease GI upset). Take at the same time(s) each day. Dietary modification based on ADA recommendations is a part of therapy. Monitor for signs and symptoms of vitamin B_{12} and/or folic acid deficiency; supplementation may be required.

Administration Administer with a meal (to decrease GI upset).

Extended release: Swallow whole; do not crush, break, or chew. Administer once daily doses with the evening meal. Fortamet® should also be administered with a full glass of water.

Monitoring Parameters Urine for glucose and ketones, fasting blood glucose, and hemoglobin A_{1c}. Initial and periodic monitoring of hematologic parameters (eg, hemoglobin/hematocrit and red blood cell indices) and renal function should be performed, at least annually. Check vitamin B_{12} and folate if anemia is present.

Reference Range Recommendations for glycemic control in adults with diabetes:

Hb A_{1c}: <7%

Preprandial capillary plasma glucose: 70-130 mg/dL

Peak postprandial capillary blood glucose: <180 mg/dL

Blood pressure: <130/80 mm Hg

Dosage Forms Excipient information presented when available (limited, particularly for generics); consult specific product labeling.

Solution, oral, as hydrochloride:

Riomet®: 100 mg/mL (118 mL, 473 mL) [dye free, ethanol free, sugar free; contains saccharin; cherry flavor]

Tablet, oral, as hydrochloride: 500 mg, 850 mg, 1000 mg

Glucophage®: 500 mg, 850 mg

Glucophage®: 1000 mg [scored]

Tablet, extended release, oral, as hydrochloride: 500 mg, 750 mg

Fortamet®: 500 mg, 1000 mg

Glucophage® XR: 500 mg, 750 mg

Glumetza®: 500 mg, 1000 mg

◆ **Metformin and Glipizide** *see* Glipizide and Metformin *on page 797*

◆ **Metformin and Glyburide** *see* Glyburide and Metformin *on page 801*

◆ **Metformin and Repaglinide** *see* Repaglinide and Metformin *on page 1474*

◆ **Metformin and Rosiglitazone** *see* Rosiglitazone and Metformin *on page 1523*

◆ **Metformin and Saxagliptin** *see* Saxagliptin and Metformin *on page 1541*

◆ **Metformin and Sitagliptin** *see* Sitagliptin and Metformin *on page 1562*

◆ **Metformin Hydrochloride** *see* MetFORMIN *on page 1086*

◆ **Metformin Hydrochloride and Pioglitazone Hydrochloride** *see* Pioglitazone and Metformin *on page 1357*

◆ **Metformin Hydrochloride and Rosiglitazone Maleate** *see* Rosiglitazone and Metformin *on page 1523*

◆ **Metformin Hydrochloride and Saxagliptin** *see* Saxagliptin and Metformin *on page 1541*

Methacholine (meth a KOLE leen)

Brand Names: U.S. Provocholine®

Brand Names: Canada Methacholine Omega; Provocholine®

Index Terms Methacholine Chloride

Pharmacologic Category Diagnostic Agent

Use Diagnosis of bronchial airway hyperactivity

Pregnancy Risk Factor C

Dosage Note: For inhalation only: Children ≥5 years and Adults:

Before inhalation challenge, perform baseline pulmonary function tests; the patient must have an FEV_1 of at least 70% of the predicted value. The following is a suggested schedule for administration of methacholine challenge. Calculate cumulative units by multiplying number of breaths by concentration given. Total cumulative units is the sum of cumulative units for each concentration given. See table.

Methacholine

Vial	Serial Concentration (mg/mL)	No. of Breaths	Cumulative Units per Concentration	Total Cumulative Units
E	0.025	5	0.125	0.125
D	0.25	5	1.25	1.375
C	2.5	5	12.5	13.88
B	10	5	50	63.88
A	25	5	125	188.88

Determine FEV_1 within 5 minutes of challenge, a positive challenge is a 20% reduction in FEV_1

Additional Information Complete prescribing information for this medication should be consulted for additional detail.

Dosage Forms Excipient information presented when available (limited, particularly for generics); consult specific product labeling.

Powder for reconstitution, for oral inhalation, as chloride:

Provocholine®: 100 mg

◆ **Methacholine Chloride** *see* Methacholine *on page 1088*

◆ **Methacholine Omega (Can)** *see* Methacholine *on page 1088*

Methadone (METH a done)

Brand Names: U.S. Dolophine®; Methadone Diskets®; Methadone Intensol™; Methadose®

Brand Names: Canada Metadol-D™; Metadol™

Index Terms Methadone Hydrochloride

Pharmacologic Category Analgesic, Opioid

Additional Appendix Information

Opioid Analgesics *on page 1896*

Patient Information for Disposal of Unused Medications *on page 2026*

Use Management of moderate-to-severe pain; detoxification and maintenance treatment of opioid addiction as part of an FDA-approved program

Pregnancy Risk Factor C

Pregnancy Considerations Teratogenic effects have been observed in some, but not all, animal studies. Data collected by the Teratogen Information System are complicated by maternal use of illicit drugs, nutrition, infection, and psychosocial circumstances. However, pregnant women in methadone treatment programs are reported to have improved fetal outcomes compared to pregnant women using illicit drugs. Methadone can be detected in the amniotic fluid, cord plasma, and newborn urine. Fetal growth, birth weight, length, and/or head circumference may be decreased in infants born to narcotic-addicted mothers treated with methadone during pregnancy. Growth deficits do not appear to persist; however, decreased performance on psychometric and behavioral tests has been found to continue into childhood. Abnormal fetal nonstress tests have also been reported. Withdrawal symptoms in the neonate may be observed up to 2-4 weeks after delivery. The manufacturer states that methadone should be used during pregnancy only if clearly needed. Because methadone clearance in pregnant women is increased and half-life is decreased during the 2nd and 3rd trimesters of pregnancy, withdrawal symptoms may be observed in the mother; dosage of methadone may need increased or dosing interval decreased during pregnancy.

Lactation Enters breast milk/not recommended (AAP rates "compatible"; AAP 2001 update pending)

Prescribing and Access Restrictions When used for treatment of opioid addiction: May only be dispensed in accordance to guidelines established by the Substance Abuse and Mental Health Services Administration's (SAMHSA) Center for Substance Abuse Treatment (CSAT). Regulations regarding methadone use may vary by state and/or country. Obtain advice from appropriate regulatory agencies and/or consult with pain management/palliative care specialists.

Note: Regulatory Exceptions to the General Requirement to Provide Opioid Agonist Treatment (per manufacturer's labeling):

1. During inpatient care, when the patient was admitted for any condition other than concurrent opioid addiction, to facilitate the treatment of the primary admitting diagnosis.
2. During an emergency period of no longer than 3 days while definitive care for the addiction is being sought in an appropriately licensed facility.

Contraindications Hypersensitivity to methadone or any component of the formulation; respiratory depression (in the absence of resuscitative equipment or in an unmonitored setting); acute bronchial asthma or hypercarbia; paralytic ileus; concurrent use of selegiline

Warnings/Precautions An opioid-containing analgesic regimen should be tailored to each patient's needs and based upon the type of pain being treated (acute versus chronic), the route of administration, degree of tolerance for opioids (naive versus chronic user), age, weight, and medical condition. The optimal analgesic dose varies widely among patients. Doses should be titrated to pain relief/prevention. Patients maintained on stable doses of methadone may need higher and/or more frequent doses in case of acute pain (eg, postoperative pain, physical trauma). Methadone is ineffective for the relief of anxiety.

[U.S. Boxed Warning]: May prolong the QT_c interval and increase risk for torsade de pointes. Patients should be informed of the potential arrhythmia risk, evaluated for any history of structural heart disease, arrhythmia, syncope, and for existence of potential drug interactions including drugs that possess QT_c interval-prolonging properties, promote hypokalemia, hypomagnesemia, or hypocalcemia, or reduce elimination of methadone (eg, CYP3A4 inhibitors). Obtain baseline ECG for all patients and risk stratify according to QT_c interval (see Monitoring Parameters). Use with caution in patients at risk for QT_c prolongation, with medications known to prolong the QT_c interval, promote electrolyte depletion, or inhibit CYP3A4, or history of conduction abnormalities. QT_c interval prolongation and torsade de pointes may be associated with doses >100 mg/day, but have also been observed with lower doses. May cause severe hypotension; use caution with severe volume depletion or other conditions which may compromise maintenance of normal blood pressure. Use caution with cardiovascular disease or patients predisposed to dysrhythmias.

[U.S. Boxed Warning]: May cause respiratory depression. Use caution in patients with respiratory disease or pre-existing respiratory conditions (eg, severe obesity, asthma, COPD, sleep apnea, CNS depression). Because the respiratory effects last longer than the analgesic effects, slow titration is required. Use extreme caution during treatment initiation, dose titration and conversion from other opioid agonists. Incomplete cross tolerance may occur; patients tolerant to other mu opioid agonists may not be tolerant to methadone. Abrupt cessation may precipitate withdrawal symptoms.

May cause CNS depression, which may impair physical or mental abilities. Patients must be cautioned about performing tasks which require mental alertness (eg, operating machinery or driving). Effects with other sedative drugs or ethanol may be potentiated. Use with caution in patients with depression or suicidal tendencies, or in patients with a history of drug abuse. Tolerance or psychological and physical dependence may occur with prolonged use.

Use with caution in patients with head injury or increased intracranial pressure. May obscure diagnosis or clinical course of patients with acute abdominal conditions. Elderly may be more susceptible to adverse effects (eg, CNS, respiratory, gastrointestinal). Decrease initial dose and use caution in the elderly or debilitated; with hyper/hypothyroidism, morbid obesity, adrenal insufficiency, prostatic hyperplasia, or urethral stricture; or with severe renal or hepatic failure. Use with caution in patients with biliary tract dysfunction; acute pancreatitis may cause constriction of sphincter of Oddi. Safety and efficacy have not been established in children. **[U.S. Boxed Warning]: For oral administration only;** excipients to deter use by injection are contained in tablets.

[U.S. Boxed Warning]: When used for treatment of narcotic addiction: May only be dispensed by opioid treatment programs certified by the Substance Abuse and Mental Health Services Administration (SAMHSA) and certified by the designated state authority. Exceptions include inpatient treatment of other conditions and emergency period (not >3 days) while definitive substance abuse treatment is being sought.

Adverse Reactions Frequency not defined. During prolonged administration, adverse effects may decrease over several weeks; however, constipation and sweating may persist.

Cardiovascular: Arrhythmia, bigeminal rhythms, bradycardia, cardiac arrest, cardiomyopathy, ECG changes, edema, extrasystoles, faintness, flushing, heart failure, hypotension, palpitation,peripheral vasodilation, phlebitis, orthostatic hypotension, QT interval prolonged, shock, syncope, tachycardia, torsade de pointes, T-wave inversion, ventricular fibrillation, ventricular tachycardia,

Central nervous system: Agitation, confusion, disorientation, dizziness, drowsiness, dysphoria, euphoria, hallucination, headache, insomnia, lightheadedness, sedation, seizure

Dermatologic: Hemorrhagic urticaria, pruritus, rash, urticaria

Endocrine & metabolic: Antidiuretic effect, amenorrhea, hypokalemia, hypomagnesemia, libido decreased

Gastrointestinal: Abdominal pain, anorexia, biliary tract spasm, constipation, glossitis, nausea, stomach cramps, vomiting, weight gain, xerostomia

Genitourinary: Impotence, urinary retention or hesitancy

Hematologic: Thrombocytopenia (reversible, reported in patients with chronic hepatitis)

Neuromuscular & skeletal: Weakness

Local: I.M./SubQ injection: Erythema, pain, swelling; I.V. injection: Hemorrhagic urticaria (rare), pruritus, urticaria, rash

Ocular: Miosis, visual disturbances

Respiratory: Pulmonary edema, respiratory depression, respiratory arrest

Miscellaneous: Death, diaphoresis, physical and psychological dependence

Drug Interactions

Metabolism/Transport Effects Substrate of CYP2B6 (major), CYP2C19 (minor), CYP2C9 (minor), CYP2D6 (minor), CYP3A4 (major); **Note:** Assignment of Major/Minor substrate status based on clinically relevant drug interaction potential; **Inhibits** CYP2D6 (moderate), CYP3A4 (weak)

Avoid Concomitant Use

Avoid concomitant use of Methadone with any of the following: Artemether; Conivaptan; Dronedarone; Lumefantrine; Nilotinib; Pimozide; QUEtiapine; QuiNINE; Tetrabenazine; Thioridazine; Toremifene; Vandetanib; Vemurafenib; Ziprasidone

Increased Effect/Toxicity

Methadone may increase the levels/effects of: Alcohol (Ethyl); Alvimopan; CNS Depressants; CYP2D6 Substrates; Desmopressin; Dronedarone; Fesoterodine; Nebivolol; Pimozide; QTc-Prolonging Agents; QuiNINE; Selective Serotonin Reuptake Inhibitors; Tamoxifen; Tetrabenazine; Thiazide Diuretics; Thioridazine; Toremifene; Vandetanib; Vemurafenib; Zidovudine; Ziprasidone

The levels/effects of Methadone may be increased by: Alfuzosin; Amphetamines; Antifungal Agents (Azole Derivatives, Systemic); Antipsychotic Agents (Phenothiazines); Artemether; Boceprevir; Chloroquine; Ciprofloxacin; Ciprofloxacin (Systemic); Conivaptan; CYP2B6 Inhibitors (Moderate); CYP2B6 Inhibitors (Strong); CYP3A4 Inhibitors (Moderate); CYP3A4 Inhibitors (Strong); Gadobutrol; HydrOXYzine; Indacaterol; Interferons (Alfa); Lumefantrine; MAO Inhibitors; Nilotinib; Quazepam; QUEtiapine; QuiNINE; Selective Serotonin Reuptake Inhibitors; Succinylcholine

Decreased Effect

Methadone may decrease the levels/effects of: Codeine; Didanosine; Pegvisomant; TraMADol

The levels/effects of Methadone may be decreased by: Ammonium Chloride; Barbiturates; Boceprevir; CarBAMazepine; CYP2B6 Inducers (Strong); CYP3A4 Inducers (Strong); Deferasirox; Etravirine; Fosphenytoin; Herbs (CYP3A4 Inducers); Mixed Agonist / Antagonist Opioids; Phenytoin; Protease Inhibitors; Reverse Transcriptase Inhibitors (Non-Nucleoside); Rifamycin Derivatives; Telaprevir; Tocilizumab

Ethanol/Nutrition/Herb Interactions

Ethanol: May increase CNS depression; monitor for increased effects with coadministration. Caution patients about effects.

Herb/Nutraceutical: Avoid St John's wort (may decrease methadone levels; may increase CNS depression). Avoid valerian, kava kava, gotu kola (may increase CNS depression). Methadone is metabolized by CYP3A4 in the intestines; avoid concurrent use of grapefruit juice.

Stability

Injection: Store at controlled room temperature of 15°C to 30°C (59°F to 86°F). Protect from light.

Oral concentrate, oral solution, tablet: Store at controlled room temperature of 15°C to 30°C (59°F to 86°F).

Mechanism of Action Binds to opiate receptors in the CNS, causing inhibition of ascending pain pathways, altering the perception of and response to pain; produces generalized CNS depression

Pharmacodynamics/Kinetics

Onset of action: Oral: Analgesic: 0.5-1 hour; Parenteral: 10-20 minutes

Peak effect: Parenteral: 1-2 hours; Oral: Continuous dosing: 3-5 days

Duration of analgesia: Oral: 4-8 hours, increases to 22-48 hours with repeated doses

Distribution: V_{dss}: 1-8 L/kg

Protein binding: 85% to 90%

Metabolism: Hepatic; N-demethylation primarily via CYP3A4, CYP2B6, and CYP2C19 to inactive metabolites

Bioavailability: Oral: 36% to 100%

Half-life elimination: 8-59 hours; may be prolonged with alkaline pH, decreased during pregnancy

Time to peak, plasma: 1-7.5 hours

Excretion: Urine (<10% as unchanged drug); increased with urine pH <6

Dosage Regulations regarding methadone use may vary by state and/or country. Obtain advice from appropriate regulatory agencies and/or consult with pain management/palliative care specialists. **Note:** These are guidelines and do not represent the maximum doses that may be required. Methadone accumulates with repeated doses and dosage may need reduction after 3-5 days to prevent CNS depressant effects. Some patients may benefit from every 8-12 hour dosing interval for chronic pain management. Doses should be titrated to appropriate effects.

Children (unlabeled use):

Pain (analgesia): **Note:** Should only be initiated in patients managed by an experienced pain management specialist. Not considered first-line therapy for acute pain.

Oral: Initial: 0.1-0.2 mg/kg every 4-8 hours initially for 2-3 doses, then every 6-12 hours as needed. Dosing interval may range from 4-12 hours during initial therapy; decrease in dose or frequency may be required (~days 2-5) due to accumulation with repeated doses (maximum dose: 5-10 mg)

I.V.: 0.1 mg/kg every 4-8 hours initially for 2-3 doses, then every 6-12 hours as needed. Dosing interval may range from 4-12 hours during initial therapy; decrease in dose or frequency may be required (~days 2-5) due to accumulation with repeated doses (maximum dose: 5-8 mg)

Iatrogenic narcotic dependency: Oral: General guidelines: Initial: 0.05-0.1 mg/kg/dose every 6 hours; increase by 0.05 mg/kg/dose until withdrawal symptoms are controlled; after 24-48 hours, the dosing interval can be lengthened to every 12-24 hours; to taper dose, wean by 5% to 10% every 24-48 hours; monitor for oversedation and withdrawal symptoms; adjust to patient's response (Anand, 1994; Bowens, 2010)

Adults:

Acute pain (moderate-to-severe): Opioid-naive:

Oral: Initial: 2.5-10 mg every 8-12 hours; more frequent administration may be required during initiation to maintain adequate analgesia. Dosage interval may range from 4-12 hours, since duration of analgesia is relatively short during the first days of therapy, but increases substantially with continued administration.

I.V.: Initial: 2.5 mg every 8-12 hours; titrate slowly to effect; may also be administered by SubQ or I.M. injection

Chronic pain (CPSO, 2000; VA/DoD, 2003): Oral:

Opioid-naive:

Gradual titration (for chronic noncancer pain and situations where frequent monitoring is unnecessary): Initial: 2.5 mg every 8 hours; may increase dosing interval to every 12 hours (in about 4-5 days); may increase dose by 2.5 mg per dose every 5-7 days

Faster titration (for cancer pain and situations where frequent monitoring is possible): Initial: 2.5 mg every 6-8 hours; may increase dosing interval to every 8-12 hours (in about 4-5 days); may increase dose by 2.5 mg per dose as often as every day over about 4 days.

Opioid-tolerant: **Conversion from oral morphine to oral methadone: Note:** 1) There is not a linear relationship when converting to methadone from oral morphine. The higher the daily morphine equivalent dose the more potent methadone is, and 2) conversion to methadone is more of a process than a calculation. In general, the starting methadone dose should not exceed 30-40 mg/day, even in patients on high doses of other opioids. Patient response to methadone needs to be monitored closely throughout the process of the conversion. There are several proposed ratios for converting from oral morphine to oral methadone (Ayonrinde, 2000; Mercadente, 2001; Ripamonti, 1998). The manufacturer of Dolophine® recommends the following conversion for chronic administration:

Daily oral morphine dose <100 mg: Estimated daily oral methadone dose: 20% to 30% of total daily morphine dose

Daily oral morphine dose 100-300 mg: Estimated daily oral methadone dose: 10% to 20% of total daily morphine dose

Daily oral morphine dose 300-600 mg: Estimated daily oral methadone dose: 8% to 12% of total daily morphine dose

Daily oral morphine dose 600-1000 mg: Estimated daily oral methadone dose: 5% to 10% of total daily morphine dose.

Daily oral morphine dose >1000 mg: Estimated daily oral methadone dose: <5% of total daily morphine dose.

Note: The estimated total daily methadone dose should then be divided to reflect the intended dosing schedule (eg, divide by 3 and administer every 8 hours).

Conversion from oral methadone to parenteral methadone dose: Initial dose: Parenteral:Oral ratio: 1:2 (eg, 5 mg parenteral methadone equals 10 mg oral methadone)

Detoxification: Oral:

Initial: A single dose of 20-30 mg is generally sufficient to suppress symptoms. Should not exceed 30 mg; lower doses should be considered in patients with low tolerance at initiation (eg, absence of opioids ≥5 days); an additional 5-10 mg of methadone may be provided if withdrawal symptoms have not been suppressed or if symptoms reappear after 2-4 hours; total daily dose on the first day should not exceed 40 mg, unless the program physician documents in the patient's record that 40 mg did not control opiate abstinence symptoms.

Maintenance: Titrate to a dosage which attenuates craving, blocks euphoric effects of other opiates, and tolerance to sedative effect of methadone. Usual range: 80-120 mg/day (titration should occur cautiously)

Withdrawal: Dose reductions should be <10% of the maintenance dose, every 10-14 days

Detoxification (short-term): Oral:

Initial: Titrate to ~40 mg/day in divided doses to achieve stabilization, may continue 40 mg dose for 2-3 days

Maintenance: Titrate to a dosage which prevents/attenuates euphoric effects of self-administered opioids, reduces drug craving, and withdrawal symptoms are prevented for 24 hours.

Withdrawal: Requires individualization. Decrease daily or every other day, keeping withdrawal symptoms tolerable; hospitalized patients may tolerate a 20% reduction/day; ambulatory patients may require a slower reduction

Dosage adjustment during pregnancy: Methadone dose may need to be increased, or the dosing interval decreased; see Pregnancy Considerations - use should be reserved for cases where the benefits clearly outweigh the risks

Dosage adjustment for toxicity:

QT_c >450-499 msecs: Monitor QT_c more frequently

QT_c ≥500 msecs: Consider discontinuation or reducing methadone dose **or** eliminate factors promoting QT_c prolongation (eg, potassium-wasting drugs) **or** use alternative therapy (eg, buprenorphine)

Dosage adjustment in renal impairment: Cl_{cr} <10 mL/minute: Administer 50% to 75% of normal dose

Dosage adjustment in hepatic impairment: Avoid in severe liver disease

Administration Oral dose for detoxification and maintenance may be administered in fruit juice or water. Dispersible tablet should not be chewed or swallowed; add to liquid and allow to dissolve before administering. May rinse if residual remains.

Monitoring Parameters Obtain baseline ECG (evaluate QT_c interval), within 30 days of initiation, and then annually for all patients receiving methadone. Increase ECG monitoring if patient receiving >100 mg/day or if unexplained syncope or seizure occurs while on methadone (Krantz, 2008).

If before or at anytime during therapy:

QT_c >450-499 msecs: Discuss potential risks and benefits; monitor QT_c more frequently

QT_c ≥500 msecs: Consider discontinuation or reducing methadone dose **or** eliminate factors promoting QT_c prolongation (eg, potassium-wasting drugs) **or** use alternative therapy (eg, buprenorphine)

Pain relief, respiratory and mental status, blood pressure

Reference Range Prevention of opiate withdrawal: Therapeutic: 100-400 ng/mL (SI: 0.32-1.29 micromole/L); Toxic: >2 mcg/mL (SI: >6.46 micromole/L)

Test Interactions Some quinolones may produce a false-positive urine screening result for opiates using commercially-available immunoassay kits. This has been demonstrated most consistently for levofloxacin and ofloxacin, but other quinolones have shown cross-reactivity in certain assay kits. Confirmation of positive opiate screens by more specific methods should be considered.

Dosage Forms Excipient information presented when available (limited, particularly for generics); consult specific product labeling.

Injection, solution, as hydrochloride: 10 mg/mL (20 mL)

Solution, oral, as hydrochloride: 5 mg/5 mL (500 mL); 10 mg/5 mL (500 mL)

Solution, oral, as hydrochloride [concentrate]: 10 mg/mL (946 mL, 1000 mL, 1000s)

Methadone Intensol™: 10 mg/mL (30 mL) [dye free, sugar free; contains sodium benzoate; unflavored]

Methadose®: 10 mg/mL (1000 mL) [contains propylene glycol; cherry flavor]

Methadose®: 10 mg/mL (1000 mL) [dye free, sugar free; contains sodium benzoate; unflavored]

Tablet, oral, as hydrochloride: 5 mg, 10 mg

Dolophine®: 5 mg, 10 mg [scored]

Tablet, dispersible, oral, as hydrochloride: 40 mg

Methadone Diskets®: 40 mg [scored; orange-pineapple flavor]

Methadose®: 40 mg [scored]

Controlled Substance C-II

◆ **Methadone Diskets®** *see* Methadone *on page 1088*

◆ **Methadone Hydrochloride** *see* Methadone *on page 1088*

◆ **Methadone Intensol™** *see* Methadone *on page 1088*

◆ **Methadose®** *see* Methadone *on page 1088*

◆ **Methaminodiazepoxide Hydrochloride** *see* ChlordiazePOXIDE *on page 340*

Methamphetamine (meth am FET a meen)

Brand Names: U.S. Desoxyn®

Brand Names: Canada Desoxyn®

Index Terms Desoxyephedrine Hydrochloride; Methamphetamine Hydrochloride

Pharmacologic Category Anorexiant; Stimulant; Sympathomimetic

Use Treatment of attention-deficit/hyperactivity disorder (ADHD); exogenous obesity (short-term adjunct)

Pharmacotherapy for weight loss is recommended only for obese patients with a body mass index ≥30 kg/m^2, or ≥27 kg/m^2 in the presence of other risk factors such as hypertension, diabetes, and/or dyslipidemia or a high waist circumference; therapy should be used in conjunction with a comprehensive weight management program.

Unlabeled Use Narcolepsy

Pregnancy Risk Factor C

Pregnancy Considerations Teratogenic and embryocidal effects have been observed in animal studies. Infants may deliver prematurely and suffer withdrawal symptoms. There are no adequate and well-controlled studies in pregnant women.

Lactation Enters breast milk/contraindicated

Medication Guide Available Yes

Contraindications Hypersensitivity to methamphetamine, any component of the formulation, or idiosyncrasy to amphetamines or other sympathomimetic amines; patients with advanced arteriosclerosis, symptomatic cardiovascular disease, moderate-to-severe hypertension, hyperthyroidism, glaucoma, agitated states; patients with a history of drug abuse; use during or within 14 days following MAO inhibitor therapy; stimulant medications are contraindicated for use in children with attention-deficit/hyperactivity disorders and concomitant Tourette's syndrome or tics

Warnings/Precautions Use has been associated with serious cardiovascular events including sudden death in patients with pre-existing structural cardiac abnormalities or other serious heart problems (sudden death in children and adolescents; sudden death, stroke and MI in adults). These products should be avoided in the patients with known serious structural cardiac abnormalities, cardiomyopathy, serious heart rhythm abnormalities, or other serious cardiac problems that could increase the risk of sudden death that these conditions alone carry. Patients should be carefully evaluated for cardiac disease prior to initiation of therapy. Use with caution in patients with hypertension and other cardiovascular conditions that might be exacerbated by increases in blood pressure or heart rate. Use is contraindicated in patients with moderate-to-severe hypertension. Amphetamines may impair the ability to engage in potentially hazardous activities. Difficulty in accommodation and blurred vision has been reported with the use of stimulants.

Use with caution in patients with psychiatric disorders, diabetes, or seizure disorders,. May exacerbate symptoms of behavior and thought disorder in psychotic patients. Stimulants may unmask tics in individuals with coexisting Tourette's syndrome **[U.S. Boxed Warning]: Potential for drug dependency exists; prolonged use may lead to drug dependency.** Use is contraindicated in patients with history of ethanol or drug abuse. Prescriptions should be written for the smallest quantity consistent with good patient care to minimize possibility of overdose. **[U.S. Boxed Warning]: Use in weight reduction programs only when alternative therapy has been ineffective.** Abrupt discontinuation following high doses or for prolonged periods may result in symptoms for withdrawal. Discontinue if satisfactory weight loss has not occurred within the first 4 weeks of treatment, or if tolerance develops.

May be inappropriate for use in the elderly due to the risk for causing dependence, hypertension, angina, and myocardial infarction (Beers Criteria). Safety and efficacy have not been established in children <12 years of age for obesity. Use of stimulants has been associated with suppression of growth; monitor growth rate during treatment.

Adverse Reactions Frequency not defined.

Cardiovascular: Hypertension, palpitation, tachycardia

Central nervous system: Dizziness, dysphoria, euphoria, exacerbation of motor and phonic tics and Tourette's syndrome, headache, insomnia, overstimulation, psychosis, restlessness

Dermatologic: Rash, urticaria

Endocrine & metabolic: Change in libido

Gastrointestinal: Anorexia, constipation, diarrhea, nausea, stomach cramps, unpleasant taste, vomiting, weight loss, xerostomia

Genitourinary: Impotence

Neuromuscular & skeletal: Tremor

Miscellaneous: Suppression of growth in children, tolerance and withdrawal with prolonged use

Drug Interactions

Metabolism/Transport Effects Substrate of CYP2D6 (major); **Note:** Assignment of Major/Minor substrate status based on clinically relevant drug interaction potential

Avoid Concomitant Use

Avoid concomitant use of Methamphetamine with any of the following: Iobenguane I 123; MAO Inhibitors

Increased Effect/Toxicity

Methamphetamine may increase the levels/effects of: Analgesics (Opioid); Sympathomimetics

The levels/effects of Methamphetamine may be increased by: Abiraterone Acetate; Alkalinizing Agents; Antacids; Atomoxetine; Cannabinoids; Carbonic Anhydrase Inhibitors; CYP2D6 Inhibitors (Moderate); CYP2D6 Inhibitors (Strong); Darunavir; MAO Inhibitors; Proton Pump Inhibitors; Tricyclic Antidepressants

Decreased Effect

Methamphetamine may decrease the levels/effects of: Antihistamines; Ethosuximide; Iobenguane I 123; Ioflupane I 123; PHENobarbital; Phenytoin

The levels/effects of Methamphetamine may be decreased by: Ammonium Chloride; Antipsychotics; Gastrointestinal Acidifying Agents; Lithium; Methenamine; Peginterferon Alfa-2b

Ethanol/Nutrition/Herb Interactions

Ethanol: Avoid ethanol (may cause CNS depression).

Food: Amphetamine serum levels may be altered if taken with acidic food, juices, or vitamin C. Avoid caffeine.

Herb/Nutraceutical: Avoid ephedra (may cause hypertension or arrhythmias).

Stability Store below 30°C (86°F). Protect from light.

Mechanism of Action A sympathomimetic amine related to ephedrine and amphetamine with CNS stimulant activity; causes release of catecholamines (primarily dopamine and other catecholamines) from their storage sites in the presynaptic nerve terminals. Inhibits reuptake and metabolism of catecholamines through inhibition of monoamine transporters and oxidase.

Pharmacodynamics/Kinetics

Absorption: Rapid from GI tract

Metabolism: Hepatic; forms metabolite

Half-life elimination: 4-5 hours

Excretion: Urine primarily (dependent on urine pH)

Dosage Oral:

Children ≥6 years and Adults: ADHD: 5 mg 1-2 times/day; may increase by 5 mg increments at weekly intervals until optimum response is achieved, usually 20-25 mg/day

Children ≥12 years and Adults: Exogenous obesity: 5 mg 30 minutes before each meal; treatment duration should not exceed a few weeks

Dietary Considerations Most effective when combined with a low calorie diet and behavior modification counseling.

Monitoring Parameters Heart rate, respiratory rate, blood pressure, CNS activity, body weight (BMI); growth rate in children

When used for the treatment of ADHD, thoroughly evaluate for cardiovascular risk. Monitor heart rate, blood pressure, and consider obtaining ECG prior to initiation (Vetter, 2008).

Reference Range

Adult classification of weight by BMI (kg/m^2):

Underweight: <18.5

Normal: 18.5-24.9

Overweight: 25-29.9

Obese, class I: 30-34.9

Obese, class II: 35-39.9

Extreme obesity (class III): ≥40

Waist circumference: In adults with a BMI of 25-34.9 kg/m^2, high-risk waist circumference is defined as:

Men >102 cm (>40 in)

Women >88 cm (>35 in)

Additional Information Illicit methamphetamine may contain lead; alkalinizing urine can result in longer methamphetamine half-life and elevated blood level; ephedrine is a precursor in the illicit manufacture of methamphetamine; ephedrine is extracted by dissolving ephedrine tablets in water or alcohol (50,000 tablets can result in 1 kg of ephedrine); conversion to methamphetamine occurs at a rate of 50% to 70% of the weight of ephedrine. 3,4-methylene dioxymethamphetamine (slang: XTC, Ecstasy, Adam) affects the serotonergic, dopaminergic, and noradrenergic pathways. As such, it can cause the serotonin syndrome associated with malignant hyperthermia and rhabdomyolysis.

Dosage Forms Excipient information presented when available (limited, particularly for generics); consult specific product labeling.

Tablet, oral, as hydrochloride: 5 mg

Desoxyn®: 5 mg

Controlled Substance C-II

◆ **Methamphetamine Hydrochloride** *see* Methamphetamine *on page 1092*

Methazolamide (meth a ZOE la mide)

Brand Names: U.S. Neptazane™

Brand Names: Canada Apo-Methazolamide®

Pharmacologic Category Carbonic Anhydrase Inhibitor; Diuretic, Carbonic Anhydrase Inhibitor; Ophthalmic Agent, Antiglaucoma

Use Treatment of chronic open-angle or secondary glaucoma; short-term therapy of acute angle-closure glaucoma prior to surgery

Pregnancy Risk Factor C

Dosage Adults: Oral: 50-100 mg 2-3 times/day

Additional Information Complete prescribing information for this medication should be consulted for additional detail.

Dosage Forms Excipient information presented when available (limited, particularly for generics); consult specific product labeling.

Tablet, oral: 25 mg, 50 mg

Neptazane™: 25 mg

Neptazane™: 50 mg [scored]

Methenamine (meth EN a meen)

Brand Names: U.S. Hiprex®

Brand Names: Canada Dehydral®; Hiprex®; Mandelamine®; Urasal®

Index Terms Hexamethylenetetramine; Methenamine Hippurate; Methenamine Mandelate; Urex

Pharmacologic Category Antibiotic, Miscellaneous

Use Prophylaxis or suppression of recurrent urinary tract infections; urinary tract discomfort secondary to hypermotility

Pregnancy Risk Factor C (methenamine mandelate)

Dosage Oral:

Children:

>2-6 years: *Mandelate:* 50-75 mg/kg/day in 3-4 doses or 0.25 g/30 lb 4 times/day

6-12 years:

Hippurate: 0.5-1 g twice daily

Mandelate: 50-75 mg/kg/day in 3-4 doses or 0.5 g 4 times/day

>12 years and Adults:

Hippurate: 1 g twice daily

Mandelate: 1 g 4 times/day after meals and at bedtime

Dosing adjustment/comments in renal impairment: Cl_{cr} <50 mL/minute: Avoid use

Additional Information Complete prescribing information for this medication should be consulted for additional detail.

Dosage Forms Excipient information presented when available (limited, particularly for generics); consult specific product labeling.

Tablet, oral, as hippurate: 1 g

Hiprex®: 1 g [scored; contains tartrazine]

Tablet, oral, as mandelate: 500 mg, 1 g

Methenamine and Sodium Acid Phosphate

(meth EN a meen & SOW dee um AS id FOS fate)

Brand Names: U.S. Uroqid-Acid® No. 2

Index Terms Methenamine Mandelate and Sodium Acid Phosphate; Sodium Acid Phosphate and Methenamine

Pharmacologic Category Antibiotic, Miscellaneous

Use Prophylaxis or suppression of bacteriuria associated with recurrent urinary tract infections

Pregnancy Risk Factor C

Dosage Oral: Adults: Initial: 2 tablets 4 times daily; maintenance: 2-4 tablets daily in divided doses

Additional Information Complete prescribing information for this medication should be consulted for additional detail.

Dosage Forms Excipient information presented when available (limited, particularly for generics); consult specific product labeling.

Tablet: Methenamine mandelate 500 mg and sodium acid phosphate 500 mg [contains 83 mg sodium]

◆ **Methenamine Hippurate** *see* Methenamine *on page 1093*

◆ **Methenamine Mandelate** *see* Methenamine *on page 1093*

◆ **Methenamine Mandelate and Sodium Acid Phosphate** *see* Methenamine and Sodium Acid Phosphate *on page 1094*

Methenamine, Phenyl Salicylate, Methylene Blue, Benzoic Acid, and Hyoscyamine

(meth EN a meen, fen nil sa LIS i late, METH i leen bloo, ben ZOE ik AS id & hye oh SYE a meen)

Brand Names: U.S. Hyophen™; Prosed®/DS

Index Terms Benzoic Acid, Hyoscyamine, Methenamine, Methylene Blue, and Phenyl Salicylate; Benzoic Acid, Methenamine, Methylene Blue, Phenyl Salicylate, and Hyoscyamine; Hyoscyamine, Methenamine, Benzoic Acid, Phenyl Salicylate, and Methylene Blue; Methylene Blue, Methenamine, Benzoic Acid, Phenyl Salicylate, and Hyoscyamine; Phenyl Salicylate, Methenamine, Methylene Blue, Benzoic Acid, and Hyoscyamine

Pharmacologic Category Antibiotic, Miscellaneous

Use Urinary tract discomfort secondary to hypermotility resulting from infection or diagnostic procedures

Pregnancy Risk Factor C

Dosage Oral:

Children >6 years: Dosage must be individualized

Adults: One tablet 4 times/day

Additional Information Complete prescribing information for this medication should be consulted for additional detail.

Dosage Forms Excipient information presented when available (limited, particularly for generics); consult specific product labeling.

Tablet, oral:

Hyophen™: Methenamine 81.6 mg, phenyl salicylate 36.2 mg, methylene blue 10.8 mg, benzoic acid 9 mg, hyoscyamine sulfate 0.12 mg

Prosed®/DS: Methenamine 81.6 mg, phenyl salicylate 36.2 mg, methylene blue 10.8 mg, benzoic acid 9 mg, hyoscyamine sulfate 0.12 mg

Methenamine, Sodium Biphosphate, Phenyl Salicylate, Methylene Blue, and Hyoscyamine

(meth EN a meen, SOW dee um bye FOS fate, fen nil sa LIS i late, METH i leen bloo, & hye oh SYE a meen)

Brand Names: U.S. Phosphasal™; Urelle®; Uribel™; Uta®

Index Terms Hyoscyamine, Methenamine, Methylene Blue, Phenyl Salicylate, and Sodium Biphosphate; Hyoscyamine, Methenamine, Sodium Biphosphate, Phenyl Salicylate, and Methylene Blue; Methylene Blue, Methenamine, Sodium Biphosphate, Phenyl Salicylate, and Hyoscyamine; Phenyl Salicylate, Methenamine, Methylene Blue, Sodium Biphosphate, and Hyoscyamine; Sodium Biphosphate, Methenamine, Methylene Blue, Phenyl Salicylate, and Hyoscyamine

Pharmacologic Category Antibiotic, Miscellaneous

Use Treatment of symptoms of irritative voiding; relief of local symptoms associated with urinary tract infections; relief of urinary tract symptoms caused by diagnostic procedures

Pregnancy Risk Factor C

Lactation Enters breast milk/use caution

Contraindications Hypersensitivity to methenamine, hyoscyamine, methylene blue, or any component of the formulation

Warnings/Precautions Use caution in patients with a history of intolerance to belladonna alkaloids or salicylates. Use caution in patients with cardiovascular disease (cardiac arrhythmias, HF, coronary heart disease, mitral stenosis), gastrointestinal tract obstruction, glaucoma, myasthenia gravis, or obstructive uropathy (bladder neck obstruction or prostatic hyperplasia). Discontinue use immediately if tachycardia, dizziness, or blurred vision occur. Elderly may be more sensitive to anticholinergic effects of hyoscyamine; use caution. May cause urinary discoloration (blue). Prolonged use may result in fungal or bacterial superinfection, including *C. difficile*-associated diarrhea and pseudomembranous colitis. Safety and efficacy have not been established in children ≤6 years of age.

Adverse Reactions Frequency not defined.

Cardiovascular: Tachycardia, flushing

Central nervous system: Dizziness

Gastrointestinal: Xerostomia, nausea, vomiting

Genitourinary: Urinary retention (acute), micturition difficulty, discoloration of urine (blue)

Ocular: Blurred vision

Respiratory: Dyspnea

Drug Interactions

Metabolism/Transport Effects None known.

Avoid Concomitant Use

Avoid concomitant use of Methenamine, Sodium Biphosphate, Phenyl Salicylate, Methylene Blue, and Hyoscyamine with any of the following: BCG; BuPROPion; BusPIRone; MAO Inhibitors; Maprotiline; Mirtazapine; Nefazodone; Selective Serotonin Reuptake Inhibitors; Serotonin/Norepinephrine Reuptake Inhibitors; Sulfonamide Derivatives; TraZODone; Tricyclic Antidepressants

Increased Effect/Toxicity

Methenamine, Sodium Biphosphate, Phenyl Salicylate, Methylene Blue, and Hyoscyamine may increase the levels/effects of: AbobotulinumtoxinA; Anticholinergics; Cannabinoids; Metoclopramide; OnabotulinumtoxinA; Potassium Chloride; RimabotulinumtoxinB; Serotonin Modulators; Sulfonamide Derivatives

The levels/effects of Methenamine, Sodium Biphosphate, Phenyl Salicylate, Methylene Blue, and Hyoscyamine may be increased by: Antipsychotics; BuPROPion; BusPIRone; MAO Inhibitors; Maprotiline; Mirtazapine;

Nefazodone; Pramlintide; Selective Serotonin Reuptake Inhibitors; Serotonin/Norepinephrine Reuptake Inhibitors; TraZODone; Tricyclic Antidepressants

Decreased Effect

Methenamine, Sodium Biphosphate, Phenyl Salicylate, Methylene Blue, and Hyoscyamine may decrease the levels/effects of: Acetylcholinesterase Inhibitors (Central); Amphetamines; BCG; Secretin; Typhoid Vaccine

The levels/effects of Methenamine, Sodium Biphosphate, Phenyl Salicylate, Methylene Blue, and Hyoscyamine may be decreased by: Acetylcholinesterase Inhibitors (Central); Antacids; Carbonic Anhydrase Inhibitors

Stability Store at controlled room temperature of 15°C to 30°C (59°F to 86°F).

Dosage Oral:

Children >6 years: Dosage must be individualized

Adults: One tablet 4 times daily (followed by liberal fluid intake)

Dosage Forms Excipient information presented when available (limited, particularly for generics); consult specific product labeling.

Capsule, oral:

Uribel™: Methenamine 118 mg, sodium biphosphate 40.8 mg, phenyl salicylate 36 mg, methylene blue 10 mg, hyoscyamine sulfate 0.12 mg

Uta®: Methenamine 120 mg, sodium biphosphate 40.8 mg, phenyl salicylate 36 mg, methylene blue 10 mg, hyoscyamine sulfate 0.12 mg

Tablet, oral:

Phosphasal™: Methenamine 81.6 mg, sodium biphosphate 40.8 mg, phenyl salicylate 36.2 mg, methylene blue 10.8 mg, hyoscyamine sulfate 0.12 mg

Urelle®: Methenamine 81 mg, sodium biphosphate 40.8 mg, phenyl salicylate 32.4 mg, methylene blue 10.8 mg, hyoscyamine sulfate 0.12 mg

◆ **Methergine®** *see* Methylergonovine *on page 1105*

Methimazole (meth IM a zole)

Brand Names: U.S. Tapazole®

Brand Names: Canada Dom-Methimazole; PHL-Methimazole; Tapazole®

Index Terms Thiamazole

Pharmacologic Category Antithyroid Agent; Thioamide

Use Treatment of hyperthyroidism; improve hyperthyroidism prior to thyroidectomy or radioactive iodine therapy

Unlabeled Use Treatment of Graves' disease

Pregnancy Risk Factor D

Pregnancy Considerations Studies in pregnant women have demonstrated a risk to the fetus. Methimazole has been found to readily cross the placenta. Congenital anomalies, including esophageal atresia, choanal atresia, aplasia cutis, and iridic and retinal coloboma, have been observed in neonates born to mothers taking methimazole during pregnancy. Nonteratogenic adverse events, including fetal and neonatal hypothyroidism or hyperthyroidism have been observed following maternal methimazole use. The transfer of thyroid-stimulating immunoglobulins can stimulate the fetal thyroid *in utero* and transiently after delivery and may increase the risk of fetal or neonatal hyperthyroidism.

Pharmacokinetic studies with methimazole are not available; however, the clearance of carbimazole, a prodrug of methimazole, may be increased during pregnancy. The severity of hyperthyroidism may fluctuate throughout pregnancy and may result in decreased dose requirements or discontinuation of methimazole 2-3 weeks prior to delivery. Possible exacerbation of hyperthyroidism after delivery may require the reinitiation of antithyroid therapy.

Uncontrolled maternal hyperthyroidism may result in adverse neonatal outcomes (eg, prematurity, low birth weight, infants born small for gestational age) and adverse maternal outcomes (eg, pre-eclampsia, congestive heart failure). To prevent adverse fetal and maternal events, normal maternal thyroid function should be maintained prior to conception and throughout pregnancy. Antithyroid treatment is recommended for the control of hyperthyroidism during pregnancy. Propylthiouracil is considered first-line therapy, especially during the first trimester of pregnancy. Due to an increased risk of congenital anomalies, the use of methimazole is an option during the second and third trimesters of pregnancy.

Lactation Enters breast milk/contraindicated (per manufacturer's labeling) (AAP rates "compatible"; AAP 2001 update pending)

Contraindications Hypersensitivity to methimazole or any component of the formulation; breast-feeding (per manufacturer)

Warnings/Precautions Antithyroid agents have been associated (rarely) with significant bone marrow depression. The most severe manifestation is agranulocytosis. Aplastic anemia, thrombocytopenia, and leukopenia may also occur. Use with extreme caution in patients receiving other drugs known to cause myelosuppression (particularly agranulocytosis) and in patients >40 years of age; avoid doses ≥40 mg/day (increased myelosuppression). Monitor patients closely; discontinue if significant bone marrow suppression occurs, particularly agranulocytosis or aplastic anemia.

May cause hypoprothrombinemia and bleeding. Rare, severe hepatic reactions (hepatic necrosis, hepatitis, encephalopathy) may occur; possibly fatal. Symptoms suggestive of hepatic dysfunction should prompt evaluation. Discontinue in the presence of hepatitis (transaminase >3 times upper limit of normal). In addition, other rare hypersensitivity reactions to antithyroid agents have been reported, including the development of ANCA-positive vasculitis, drug fever, exfoliative dermatitis, glomerulonephritis, leukocytoclastic vasculitis, and a lupus-like syndrome; prompt discontinuation is warranted in patients who develop symptoms consistent with a form of autoimmunity or other hypersensitivity during therapy. Minor dermatologic reactions may not require discontinuation, depending on severity.

Adverse Reactions Frequency not defined.

Cardiovascular: ANCA-positive vasculitis, edema, leukocytoclastic vasculitis, periarteritis

Central nervous system: Drowsiness, fever, headache, neuritis, vertigo

Dermatologic: Alopecia, exfoliative dermatitis, pruritus, skin pigmentation, skin rash, urticaria

Endocrine & metabolic: Goiter, hypoglycemic coma

Gastrointestinal: Constipation, epigastric distress, loss of taste perception, nausea, salivary gland swelling, vomiting, weight gain

Hematologic: Agranulocytosis, aplastic anemia, granulocytopenia, hypoprothrombinemia, leukopenia, thrombocytopenia

Hepatic: Hepatic necrosis, hepatitis, jaundice

Neuromuscular & skeletal: Arthralgia, myalgia, paresthesia

Renal: Nephritis

Miscellaneous: Insulin autoimmune syndrome, lymphadenopathy, SLE-like syndrome

Drug Interactions

Metabolism/Transport Effects Inhibits CYP1A2 (weak), CYP2A6 (weak), CYP2B6 (weak), CYP2C19 (weak), CYP2C9 (weak), CYP2D6 (weak), CYP2E1 (weak), CYP3A4 (weak)

Avoid Concomitant Use

Avoid concomitant use of Methimazole with any of the following: CloZAPine; Pimozide; Sodium Iodide I131

Increased Effect/Toxicity
Methimazole may increase the levels/effects of: Cardiac Glycosides; CloZAPine; Pimozide; Theophylline Derivatives

Decreased Effect
Methimazole may decrease the levels/effects of: Sodium Iodide I131; Vitamin K Antagonists

Stability Store at 20°C to 25°C (68°F to 77°F); excursion permitted to 15°C to 30°C (59°F to 86°F). Protect from light.

Mechanism of Action Inhibits the synthesis of thyroid hormones by blocking the oxidation of iodine in the thyroid gland. As a result, methimazole inhibits the ability of iodine to combine with tyrosine to form thyroxine and triiodothyronine (T_3); does not inactivate circulating T_4 and T_3

Pharmacodynamics/Kinetics
Onset of action: Antithyroid: Oral: 12-18 hours
Duration: 36-72 hours
Distribution: Concentrated in thyroid gland
Protein binding, plasma: None
Metabolism: Hepatic
Bioavailability: ~93%
Half-life elimination: 4-6 hours
Time to peak, serum concentration: 1-2 hours
Excretion: Urine

Dosage Oral: Administer in equally divided doses every 8 hours
Children:
Hyperthyroidism: Initial: 0.4 mg/kg/day in 3 divided doses; maintenance: 0.2 mg/kg/day in 3 divided doses
Graves' disease (unlabeled use): 0.2-0.5 mg/kg once daily (range: 0.1-1 mg/kg/day) to restore euthyroidism, then reduce dose by 50% or more and continue for a total of 1-2 years; may then discontinue or dose reduce to assess if patient is in remission. **Note:** In severe cases, initial doses that are 50% to 100% higher may be used (Bahn, 2011).
The following dosing approach may also be used (Bahn, 2011):
Infants: 1.25 mg/day
Children 1-5 years: 2.5-5 mg/day
Children 5-10 years: 5-10 mg/day
Children 10-18 years: 10-20 mg/day
Adults:
Hyperthyroidism: Initial: 15 mg/day in 3 divided doses for mild hyperthyroidism; 30-40 mg/day in 3 divided doses for moderately-severe hyperthyroidism; 60 mg/day in 3 divided doses for severe hyperthyroidism; maintenance: 5-15 mg/day (may be given as a single daily dose in many cases)
Adjust dosage as required to achieve and maintain serum T_3, T_4, and TSH levels in the normal range. An elevated T_3 may be the sole indicator of inadequate treatment. An elevated TSH indicates excessive antithyroid treatment.
Graves' disease (unlabeled use): Initial: 10-20 mg once daily to restore euthyroidism; maintenance: 5-10 mg once daily for a total of 12-18 months, then tapered or discontinued if TSH is normal at that time (Bahn, 2011)
Iodine-induced thyrotoxicosis (unlabeled use): 20-40 mg/day given either once or twice daily (Bahn, 2011)
Thyrotoxic crisis (unlabeled use): **Note:** Recommendations vary; use in combination with other specific agents. Dosages of 20-25 mg every 6 hours have been used; once stable, dosing frequency may be reduced to once or twice daily (Nayak, 2006). The American Thyroid Association and the American Association of Clinical Endocrinologists recommend 60-80 mg/day (Bahn, 2011). Rectal administration has also been described (Nabil, 1982).
Thyrotoxicosis (type I amiodarone-induced; unlabeled use): 40 mg once daily to restore euthyroidism (generally 3-6 months). **Note:** If high doses continue to be required, dividing the dose may be more effective (Bahn, 2011).

Dosing adjustment in renal impairment: Adjustment is not necessary

Dietary Considerations Administer with meals.

Administration Administer consistently in relation to meals every day. In thyrotoxic crisis, rectal administration has been described (Nabil, 1982).

Monitoring Parameters Monitor for signs of hypothyroidism, hyperthyroidism, T_4, T_3; CBC with differential, liver function (baseline and as needed), serum thyroxine, free thyroxine index; prothrombin time

Additional Information A potency ratio of methimazole to propylthiouracil of at least 20-30:1 is recommended when changing from one drug to another (eg, 300 mg of propylthiouracil would be roughly equivalent to 10-15 mg of methimazole) (Bahn, 2011).

Dosage Forms Excipient information presented when available (limited, particularly for generics); consult specific product labeling.
Tablet, oral: 5 mg, 10 mg
Tapazole®: 5 mg, 10 mg [scored]

Extemporaneous Preparations Suppositories can be made from methimazole tablets; dissolve 1200 mg methimazole in 12 mL of water and add to 52 mL cocoa butter containing 2 drops of Span 80. Stir the resulting mixture to form a water-oil emulsion and pour into 2.6 mL suppository molds to cool.

Nabil N, Miner DJ, and Amatruda JM, "Methimazole: An Alternative Route of Administration," *J Clin Endo Metab*, 1982, 54(1):180-1.

◆ **Methitest™** *see* MethylTESTOSTERone *on page 1114*

Methocarbamol (meth oh KAR ba mole)

Brand Names: U.S. Robaxin®; Robaxin®-750
Brand Names: Canada Robaxin®
Pharmacologic Category Skeletal Muscle Relaxant
Additional Appendix Information
Beers Criteria – Potentially Inappropriate Medications for Geriatrics *on page 1973*

Use Adjunctive treatment of muscle spasm associated with acute painful musculoskeletal conditions (eg, tetanus)

Pregnancy Risk Factor C

Pregnancy Considerations Animal reproduction studies have not been conducted. The manufacturer notes that fetal and congenital abnormalities have been rarely reported following *in utero* exposure. Use during pregnancy only if clearly needed.

Lactation Excretion in breast milk unknown/use caution

Contraindications Hypersensitivity to methocarbamol or any component of the formulation; renal impairment (injection formulation)

Warnings/Precautions May cause CNS depression, which may impair physical or mental abilities; patients must be cautioned about performing tasks which require mental alertness (eg, operating machinery or driving). Effects may be potentiated when used with other sedative drugs or ethanol. Plasma protein binding and clearance are decreased and the half-life is increased in patients with hepatic impairment. This class of medication is poorly tolerated by the elderly due to anticholinergic effects, sedation, and weakness. Efficacy is questionable at dosages tolerated by elderly patients (Beers Criteria).

Injection: Contraindicated in renal impairment. Contains polyethylene glycol. Rate of injection should not exceed 3 mL/minute; solution is hypertonic; avoid extravasation. Use with caution in patients with a history of seizures. Use caution with hepatic impairment. Vial stopper contains latex. Recommended only for the treatment of tetanus in pediatric patients.

Adverse Reactions Frequency not defined.

Cardiovascular: Bradycardia, flushing, hypotension, syncope

Central nervous system: Amnesia, confusion, coordination impaired (mild), dizziness, drowsiness, fever, headache, insomnia, lightheadedness, sedation, seizures, vertigo

Dermatologic: Angioneurotic edema, pruritus, rash, urticaria

Gastrointestinal: Dyspepsia, metallic taste, nausea, vomiting

Hematologic: Leukopenia

Hepatic: Jaundice

Local: Pain at injection site, thrombophlebitis

Ocular: Blurred vision, conjunctivitis, diplopia, nystagmus

Respiratory: Nasal congestion

Miscellaneous: Hypersensitivity reactions including anaphylaxis

Drug Interactions

Metabolism/Transport Effects None known.

Avoid Concomitant Use There are no known interactions where it is recommended to avoid concomitant use.

Increased Effect/Toxicity

Methocarbamol may increase the levels/effects of: Alcohol (Ethyl); CNS Depressants; Methotrimeprazine; Selective Serotonin Reuptake Inhibitors

The levels/effects of Methocarbamol may be increased by: Droperidol; HydrOXYzine; Methotrimeprazine

Decreased Effect

Methocarbamol may decrease the levels/effects of: Pyridostigmine

Ethanol/Nutrition/Herb Interactions

Ethanol: May increase CNS depression; monitor for increased effects with coadministration. Caution patients about effects.

Herb/Nutraceutical: Avoid valerian, St John's wort, kava kava, gotu kola (may increase CNS depression).

Stability

Injection: Prior to dilution, store at controlled room temperature of 20°C to 25°C (68°F to 77°F); excursions permitted to 15°C to 30°C (59°F to 86°F).

Tablet: Store at controlled room temperature of 20°C to 25°C (68°F to 77°F).

Mechanism of Action Causes skeletal muscle relaxation by general CNS depression

Pharmacodynamics/Kinetics

Onset of action: Muscle relaxation: Oral: ~30 minutes

Protein binding: 46% to 50%

Metabolism: Hepatic via dealkylation and hydroxylation

Half-life elimination: 1-2 hours

Time to peak, serum: Oral: 1-2 hours

Excretion: Urine (primarily as metabolites)

Dosage

Tetanus: I.V.:

Children: Recommended **only** for use in tetanus: 15 mg/kg/dose or 500 mg/m^2/dose, may repeat every 6 hours if needed; maximum dose: 1.8 g/m^2/day for 3 days only

Adults: Initial dose: 1-2 g by direct I.V. injection, which may be followed by an additional 1-2 g by infusion (maximum initial dose: 3 g total); followed by 1-2 g every 6 hours until oral administration by mouth or via NG tube is possible; total oral daily doses of up to 24 g may be needed; injection should not be used for more than 3 consecutive days

Muscle spasm:

Oral: Children ≥16 years and Adults: 1.5 g 4 times/day for 2-3 days (up to 8 g/day may be given in severe conditions), then decrease to 4-4.5 g/day in 3-6 divided doses

I.M., I.V.: Adults: Initial: 1 g; may repeat every 8 hours if oral administration not possible; maximum dose: 3 g/day for no more than 3 consecutive days. If condition persists, may repeat course of therapy after a drug-free interval of 48 hours.

Dosing adjustment/comments in renal impairment: Administration of the parenteral formulation is contraindicated in patients with renal dysfunction due to the presence of polyethylene glycol.

Dosing adjustment in hepatic impairment: Specific dosing guidelines are not available.

Administration

Injection:

I.M.: A maximum of 5 mL can be administered into each gluteal region.

I.V.: Maximum rate: 3 mL/minute; may be administered undiluted or mixed with 5% dextrose or 0.9% saline (1 vial/≤250 mL diluent). Monitor closely for extravasation. Administer I.V. while in recumbent position. Maintain position for at least 10-15 minutes following infusion.

Tablet: May be crushed and mixed with food or liquid if needed.

Monitoring Parameters Monitor closely for extravasation (I.V. administration).

Test Interactions May cause color interference in certain screening tests for 5-HIAA using nitrosonaphthol reagent and in screening tests for urinary VMA using the Gitlow method.

Dosage Forms Excipient information presented when available (limited, particularly for generics); consult specific product labeling.

Injection, solution:

Robaxin®: 100 mg/mL (10 mL) [contains natural rubber/natural latex in packaging, polyethylene glycol 300]

Tablet, oral: 500 mg, 750 mg

Robaxin®: 500 mg [scored]

Robaxin®-750: 750 mg

Methohexital (meth oh HEKS i tal)

Brand Names: U.S. Brevital® Sodium

Brand Names: Canada Brevital®

Index Terms Methohexital Sodium

Pharmacologic Category Barbiturate; General Anesthetic

Use Induction of anesthesia; procedural sedation

Unlabeled Use Wada test

Pregnancy Risk Factor B

Dosage Doses must be titrated to effect.

Infants <1 month: Safety and efficacy not established.

Infants ≥1 month and Children:

Anesthesia induction:

I.M.: 6.6-10 mg/kg of a 5% solution

Rectal: Usual: 25 mg/kg of a 1% solution

I.V. (unlabeled dose): 1-2 mg/kg/dose of a 1% solution

Procedural sedation (unlabeled dose):

I.V.: Initial: 0.5 mg/kg; may repeat 0.5 mg/kg to a maximum total dose of 2 mg/kg

Rectal: 25 mg/kg of a 10% (100 mg/mL) solution given 5-15 minutes prior to procedure; maximum dose 500 mg

Adults: I.V.:

Induction: 1-1.5 mg/kg

Procedural sedation (unlabeled dose): 0.75-1 mg/kg; can redose 0.5 mg/kg every 2-5 minutes as needed (Bahn, 2005)

Wada test (unlabeled use): 3-4 mg over 3 seconds; following signs of recovery, administer a second dose of 2 mg over 2 seconds (Buchtel, 2002)

Elderly: I.V.: Refer to adult dosing. Reduce dose or administer at the low end of the dosage range.

Dosing adjustment/comments in hepatic impairment: Lower dosage and monitor closely.

Additional Information Complete prescribing information for this medication should be consulted for additional detail.

Dosage Forms Excipient information presented when available (limited, particularly for generics); consult specific product labeling.

Injection, powder for reconstitution, as sodium:

Brevital® Sodium: 500 mg, 2.5 g

Controlled Substance C-IV

◆ **Methohexital Sodium** *see* Methohexital *on page 1097*

Methotrexate (meth oh TREKS ate)

Brand Names: U.S. Rheumatrex®; Trexall™

Brand Names: Canada Apo-Methotrexate®; ratio-Methotrexate

Index Terms Amethopterin; Methotrexate Sodium; Methotrexatum; MTX (error-prone abbreviation)

Pharmacologic Category Antineoplastic Agent, Antimetabolite (Antifolate); Antirheumatic, Disease Modifying; Immunosuppressant Agent

Use

Oncology-related uses: Treatment of trophoblastic neoplasms (gestational choriocarcinoma, chorioadenoma destruens and hydatidiform mole), acute lymphocytic leukemia (ALL), meningeal leukemia, breast cancer, head and neck cancer (epidermoid), cutaneous T-Cell lymphoma (advanced mycosis fungoides), lung cancer (squamous cell and small cell), advanced non-Hodgkin's lymphomas (NHL), osteosarcoma

Nononcology uses: Treatment of psoriasis (severe, recalcitrant, disabling) and severe rheumatoid arthritis (RA), including polyarticular-course juvenile idiopathic arthritis (JIA)

Unlabeled Use Treatment and maintenance of remission in Crohn's disease; ectopic pregnancy; dermatomyositis/polymyositis; bladder cancer, central nervous system tumors (including nonleukemic meningeal cancers), acute promyelocytic leukemia (maintenance treatment), soft tissue sarcoma (desmoid tumors); acute graft-versus-host disease (GVHD) prophylaxis; medical management of abortion; systemic lupus erythematosus; Takayasu arteritis

Pregnancy Risk Factor X (psoriasis, rheumatoid arthritis)

Pregnancy Considerations **[U.S. Boxed Warning]: Methotrexate may cause fetal death and/or congenital abnormalities.** Studies in animals and pregnant women have shown evidence of fetal abnormalities; therefore, the manufacturer classifies methotrexate as pregnancy category X (for psoriasis or RA). A pattern of congenital malformations associated with maternal methotrexate use is referred to as the aminopterin/methotrexate syndrome. Features of the syndrome include CNS, skeletal, and cardiac abnormalities. Low birth weight and developmental delay have also been reported. The use of methotrexate may impair fertility and cause menstrual irregularities or oligospermia during treatment and following therapy. Methotrexate is approved for the treatment of trophoblastic neoplasms (gestational choriocarcinoma, chorioadenoma destruens, and hydatidiform mole) and has been used for the medical management of ectopic pregnancy and the medical management of abortion. **[U.S. Boxed Warning]: Use is contraindicated for the treatment of psoriasis or RA in pregnant women.** Pregnancy should be excluded prior to therapy in women of childbearing potential. Use for the treatment of neoplastic diseases only when the potential benefit to the mother outweighs the possible risk to the fetus. Pregnancy should be avoided for ≥3 months following treatment in male patients and ≥1 ovulatory cycle in female patients. A registry is available for pregnant women exposed to autoimmune medications including methotrexate. For additional information contact the Organization of Teratology Information Specialists, OTIS Autoimmune Diseases Study, at 877-311-8972.

Lactation Enters breast milk/contraindicated

Contraindications Hypersensitivity to methotrexate or any component of the formulation; breast-feeding

Additional contraindications for patients with psoriasis or rheumatoid arthritis: Pregnancy, alcoholism, alcoholic liver disease or other chronic liver disease, immunodeficiency syndrome (overt or laboratory evidence); pre-existing blood dyscrasias (eg, bone marrow hypoplasia, leukopenia, thrombocytopenia, significant anemia)

Warnings/Precautions Hazardous agent - use appropriate precautions for handling and disposal.

[U.S. Boxed Warning]: Methotrexate has been associated with acute (elevated transaminases) and potentially fatal chronic (fibrosis, cirrhosis) hepatotoxicity. Risk is related to cumulative dose and prolonged exposure. Monitor closely (with liver function tests, including serum albumin) for liver toxicities. Liver enzyme elevations may be noted, but may not be predictive of hepatic disease in long term treatment for psoriasis (but generally is predictive in rheumatoid arthritis [RA] treatment). With long-term use, liver biopsy may show histologic changes, fibrosis, or cirrhosis; periodic liver biopsy is recommended with long-term use for psoriasis patients with risk factors for hepatotoxicity and for persistent abnormal liver function tests in psoriasis patients without risk factors for hepatotoxicity and in RA patients; discontinue methotrexate with moderate-to-severe change in liver biopsy. Risk factors for hepatotoxicity include history of above moderate ethanol consumption, persistent abnormal liver chemistries, history of chronic liver disease (including hepatitis B or C), family history of inheritable liver disease, diabetes, obesity, hyperlipidemia, lack of folate supplementation during methotrexate therapy, and history of significant exposure to hepatotoxic drugs. Use caution with preexisting liver impairment; may require dosage reduction. Use caution when used with other hepatotoxic agents (azathioprine, retinoids, sulfasalazine). **[U.S. Boxed Warning]: Methotrexate elimination is reduced in patients with ascites;** may require dose reduction or discontinuation. Monitor closely for toxicity.

[U.S. Boxed Warning]: May cause renal damage leading to acute renal failure, especially with high-dose methotrexate; monitor renal function and methotrexate levels closely, maintain adequate hydration and urinary alkalinization. Use caution in osteosarcoma patients treated with high-dose methotrexate in combination with nephrotoxic chemotherapy (eg, cisplatin). **[U.S. Boxed Warning]: Methotrexate elimination is reduced in patients with renal impairment;** may require dose reduction or discontinuation; monitor closely for toxicity. **[U.S. Boxed Warning]: Tumor lysis syndrome may occur in patients with high tumor burden;** use appropriate prevention and treatment.

[U.S. Boxed Warning]: May cause potentially life-threatening pneumonitis (may occur at any time during therapy and at any dosage); monitor closely for pulmonary symptoms, particularly dry, nonproductive cough. Other potential symptoms include fever, dyspnea, hypoxemia, or pulmonary infiltrate. **[U.S. Boxed Warning]: Methotrexate elimination is reduced in patients with pleural effusions;** may require dose reduction or discontinuation. Monitor closely for toxicity.

[U.S. Boxed Warning]: Bone marrow suppression may occur, resulting in anemia, aplastic anemia, pancytopenia, leukopenia, neutropenia, and/or thrombocytopenia. Use caution in patients with pre-existing bone marrow suppression. Discontinue therapy in RA or psoriasis if a significant decrease in hematologic components is noted. **[U.S. Boxed Warning]: Use of low dose methotrexate has been associated with the development of malignant lymphomas;** may regress upon discontinuation of therapy; treat lymphoma appropriately if regression is not induced by cessation of methotrexate.

[U.S. Boxed Warning]: Diarrhea and ulcerative stomatitis may require interruption of therapy; death from hemorrhagic enteritis or intestinal perforation has been reported. Use with caution in patients with peptic ulcer disease, ulcerative colitis.

May cause neurotoxicity including seizures (usually in pediatric ALL patients), leukoencephalopathy (usually with concurrent cranial irradiation) and stroke-like encephalopathy (usually with high-dose regimens). Chemical arachnoiditis (headache, back pain, nuchal rigidity, fever), myelopathy and chronic leukoencephalopathy may result from intrathecal administration.

[U.S. Boxed Warning]: Any dose level or route of administration may cause severe and potentially fatal dermatologic reactions, including toxic epidermal necrolysis, Stevens-Johnson syndrome, exfoliative dermatitis, skin necrosis, and erythema multiforme. Radiation dermatitis and sunburn may be precipitated by methotrexate administration. Psoriatic lesions may be worsened by concomitant exposure to ultraviolet radiation.

[U.S. Boxed Warning]: Concomitant administration with NSAIDs may cause severe bone marrow suppression, aplastic anemia, and GI toxicity. Do not administer NSAIDs prior to or during high dose methotrexate therapy; may increase and prolong serum methotrexate levels. Doses used for psoriasis may still lead to unexpected toxicities; use caution when administering NSAIDs or salicylates with lower doses of methotrexate for RA. Methotrexate may increase the levels and effects of mercaptopurine; may require dosage adjustments. Vitamins containing folate may decrease response to systemic methotrexate; folate deficiency may increase methotrexate toxicity. **[U.S. Boxed Warning]: Concomitant methotrexate administration with radiotherapy may increase the risk of soft tissue necrosis and osteonecrosis.**

[U.S. Boxed Warnings]: Should be administered under the supervision of a physician experienced in the use of antimetabolite therapy; serious and fatal toxicities have occurred at all dose levels. Immune suppression may lead to potentially fatal opportunistic infections. For rheumatoid arthritis and psoriasis, immunosuppressive therapy should only be used when disease is active and less toxic, traditional therapy is ineffective. Methotrexate formulations and/or diluents containing preservatives should not be used for intrathecal or high-dose therapy. May cause fetal death or congenital abnormalities; do not use for psoriasis or RA treatment in pregnant women. May cause impairment of fertility, oligospermia, and menstrual dysfunction. Toxicity from methotrexate or any immunosuppressive is increased in the elderly. Methotrexate injection may contain benzyl alcohol and should not be used in neonates. Errors have occurred (some resulting in death) when methotrexate was administered as "daily" dose instead of an intended "weekly" dose.

When used for intrathecal administration, should not be prepared during the preparation of any other agents; after preparation, store intrathecal medications in an isolated location or container clearly marked with a label identifying as "intrathecal" use only; delivery of intrathecal medications to the patient should only be with other medications intended for administration into the central nervous system (Jacobson, 2009).

Adverse Reactions Note: Adverse reactions vary by route and dosage. Hematologic and/or gastrointestinal toxicities may be common at dosages used in chemotherapy; these reactions are much less frequent when used at typical dosages for rheumatic diseases.

>10%:

Central nervous system (with I.T. administration or very high-dose therapy):

Arachnoiditis: Acute reaction manifested as severe headache, nuchal rigidity, vomiting, and fever; may be alleviated by reducing the dose

Subacute toxicity: 10% of patients treated with 12-15 mg/m^2 of I.T. methotrexate may develop this in the second or third week of therapy; consists of motor paralysis of extremities, cranial nerve palsy, seizure, or coma. This has also been seen in pediatric cases receiving very high-dose I.V. methotrexate.

Demyelinating encephalopathy: Seen months or years after receiving methotrexate; usually in association with cranial irradiation or other systemic chemotherapy

Dermatologic: Reddening of skin

Endocrine & metabolic: Hyperuricemia, defective oogenesis or spermatogenesis

Gastrointestinal: Ulcerative stomatitis, glossitis, gingivitis, nausea, vomiting, diarrhea, anorexia, intestinal perforation, mucositis (dose dependent; appears in 3-7 days after therapy, resolving within 2 weeks)

Hematologic: Leukopenia, myelosuppression (nadir: 7-10 days), thrombocytopenia

Renal: Renal failure, azotemia, nephropathy

Respiratory: Pharyngitis

1% to 10%:

Cardiovascular: Vasculitis

Central nervous system: Dizziness, malaise, encephalopathy, seizure, fever, chills

Dermatologic: Alopecia, rash, photosensitivity, depigmentation or hyperpigmentation of skin

Endocrine & metabolic: Diabetes

Genitourinary: Cystitis

Hematologic: Hemorrhage

Hepatic: Cirrhosis and portal fibrosis have been associated with chronic methotrexate therapy; acute elevation of liver enzymes are common after high-dose methotrexate, and usually resolve within 10 days.

Neuromuscular & skeletal: Arthralgia

Ocular: Blurred vision

Renal: Renal dysfunction: Manifested by an abrupt rise in serum creatinine and BUN and a fall in urine output; more common with high-dose methotrexate, and may be due to precipitation of the drug.

Respiratory: Pneumonitis: Associated with fever, cough, and interstitial pulmonary infiltrates; treatment is to withhold methotrexate during the acute reaction; interstitial pneumonitis has been reported to occur with an incidence of 1% in patients with RA (dose 7.5-15 mg/week)

<1% (Limited to important or life-threatening): Acute neurologic syndrome (at high dosages; symptoms include confusion, hemiparesis, transient blindness, and coma); acute respiratory distress syndrome, anaphylaxis, alveolitis, arrhythmia, cognitive dysfunction (has been reported at low dosage), decreased resistance to infection, erythema multiforme, hepatic failure, leukoencephalopathy (especially following craniospinal irradiation or repeated high-dose therapy), lymphoproliferative disorders, mesenteric ischemis (acute), MI, myocardial ischemia, nasal septum perforation, osteonecrosis and soft tissue necrosis (with radiotherapy), pericarditis, plaque erosions (psoriasis), reversible posterior leukoencephalopathy

syndrome (RPLS), seizure (more frequent in pediatric patients with ALL), Stevens-Johnson syndrome, stroke, thromboembolism, toxic epidermal necrolysis

Drug Interactions

Metabolism/Transport Effects Substrate of P-glycoprotein, SLCO1B1

Avoid Concomitant Use

Avoid concomitant use of Methotrexate with any of the following: Acitretin; BCG; CloZAPine; Natalizumab; Pimecrolimus; Tacrolimus (Topical)

Increased Effect/Toxicity

Methotrexate may increase the levels/effects of: CloZAPine; CycloSPORINE; CycloSPORINE (Systemic); Leflunomide; Loop Diuretics; Natalizumab; Theophylline Derivatives; Vaccines (Live); Vitamin K Antagonists

The levels/effects of Methotrexate may be increased by: Acitretin; Ciprofloxacin; Ciprofloxacin (Systemic); CycloSPORINE; CycloSPORINE (Systemic); Denosumab; Eltrombopag; Loop Diuretics; Nonsteroidal Anti-Inflammatory Agents; Penicillins; P-glycoprotein/ABCB1 Inhibitors; Pimecrolimus; Probenecid; Proton Pump Inhibitors; Roflumilast; Salicylates; SulfaSALAzine; Sulfonamide Derivatives; Tacrolimus (Topical); Trastuzumab; Trimethoprim

Decreased Effect

Methotrexate may decrease the levels/effects of: BCG; Cardiac Glycosides; Coccidioidin Skin Test; Loop Diuretics; Sapropterin; Sipuleucel-T; Vaccines (Inactivated); Vitamin K Antagonists

The levels/effects of Methotrexate may be decreased by: Bile Acid Sequestrants; Echinacea; P-glycoprotein/ABCB1 Inducers

Ethanol/Nutrition/Herb Interactions

Ethanol: Avoid ethanol (may be associated with increased liver injury).

Food: Methotrexate peak serum levels may be decreased if taken with food. Milk-rich foods may decrease methotrexate absorption. Folate may decrease drug response.

Herb/Nutraceutical: Avoid echinacea (has immunostimulant properties).

Stability Store tablets and intact vials at room temperature (15°C to 25°C). Use appropriate precautions for handling and disposal. Protect from light. **Use preservative-free preparations for intrathecal or high-dose methotrexate administration.**

I.M., I.V., SubQ: Dilute powder with D_5W or NS to a concentration of ≤25 mg/mL (20 mg and 50 mg vials) and 50 mg/mL (1 g vial). Further dilution in D_5W or NS is stable for 24 hours at room temperature (21°C to 25°C). Reconstituted solutions with a preservative may be stored under refrigeration for up to 3 months, and up to 4 weeks at room temperature.

Intrathecal: Prepare intrathecal solutions with preservative-free NS, lactated Ringer's, or Elliot's B solution to a final volume of up to 12 mL (volume generally based on institution or practitioner preference). Intrathecal methotrexate concentrations may be institution specific or based on practitioner preference, generally ranging from a final concentration of 1 mg/mL (per prescribing information; Grossman, 1993; Lin, 2008) up to ~2-4 mg/mL (de Lemos, 2009; Glantz, 1999). For triple intrathecal therapy (methotrexate 12 mg/hydrocortisone 24 mg/cytarabine 36 mg), preparation to final volume of 12 mL is reported (Lin, 2008). Intrathecal dilutions are preservative-free and should be used as soon as possible after preparation. Intrathecal medications should **NOT** be prepared during the preparation of any other agents. After preparation, store intrathecal medications (until use) in an isolated location or container clearly marked with a label identifying as "intrathecal" use only.

Mechanism of Action Methotrexate is a folate antimetabolite that inhibits DNA synthesis. Methotrexate irreversibly binds to dihydrofolate reductase, inhibiting the formation of reduced folates, and thymidylate synthetase, resulting in inhibition of purine and thymidylic acid synthesis. Methotrexate is cell cycle specific for the S phase of the cycle.

The MOA in the treatment of rheumatoid arthritis is unknown, but may affect immune function. In psoriasis, methotrexate is thought to target rapidly proliferating epithelial cells in the skin.

In Crohn's disease, it may have immune modulator and anti-inflammatory activity.

Pharmacodynamics/Kinetics

Onset of action: Antirheumatic: 3-6 weeks; additional improvement may continue longer than 12 weeks

Absorption: Oral: Dose dependent; well absorbed at low doses (<30 mg/m^2), incomplete after higher doses; I.M. injection: Complete

Distribution: Penetrates slowly into 3rd space fluids (eg, pleural effusions, ascites), exits slowly from these compartments (slower than from plasma); sustained concentrations retained in kidney and liver

V_d: 0.18 L/kg (initial); 0.4-0.8 L/kg (steady state)

Protein binding: ~50%

Metabolism: <10%; degraded by intestinal flora to DAMPA by carboxypeptidase; hepatic aldehyde oxidase converts methotrexate to 7-OH methotrexate; polyglutamates are produced intracellularly and are just as potent as methotrexate; their production is dose- and duration-dependent and they are slowly eliminated by the cell once formed. Polyglutamated forms can be converted back to methotrexate.

Bioavailability: Dose dependent; ~60% at low doses

Half-life elimination: Low dose: 3-10 hours; High dose: 8-15 hours

Time to peak, serum: Oral: 1-2 hours; I.M.: 30-60 minutes

Excretion: Urine (44% to 100%); feces (small amounts)

Dosage Details concerning dosing in combination regimens should also be consulted.

Note: Doses between 100-500 mg/m^2 **may require** leucovorin calcium rescue. Doses >500 mg/m^2 **require** leucovorin calcium rescue: Oral, I.M., I.V.: Leucovorin calcium 10-15 mg/m^2 every 6 hours for 8 or 10 doses, starting 24 hours after the start of methotrexate infusion. Continue until the methotrexate level is ≤0.1 micromolar (10^{-7} M). Some clinicians continue leucovorin calcium until the methotrexate level is <0.05 micromolar (5 x 10^{-8} M) or 0.01 micromolar (10^{-8} M).

If the 48-hour methotrexate level is >1 micromolar (10^{-6} M) or the 72-hour methotrexate level is >0.2 micromolar (2 x 10^{-7} M): I.V., I.M, Oral: Leucovorin calcium 100 mg/m^2 every 6 hours until the methotrexate level is ≤0.1 micromolar (10^{-7} M). Some clinicians continue leucovorin calcium until the methotrexate level is <0.05 micromolar (5 x 10^{-8} M) or 0.01 micromolar (10^{-8} M).

Children:

Dermatomyositis (unlabeled use): Oral: 15-20 mg/m^2/week as a single dose once weekly **or** 0.3-1 mg/kg/dose once weekly

GVHD (acute) prophylaxis (unlabeled use): I.V.: Refer to adult dosing.

Juvenile idiopathic arthritis (JIA): Oral, I.M.: 10 mg/m^2 once weekly, then 5-15 mg/m^2/week as a single dose **or** as 3 divided doses given 12 hours apart

Antineoplastic dosage range:

Oral, I.M.: 7.5-30 mg/m^2/week **or** every 2 weeks

I.V.: 10-18,000 mg/m^2 bolus dosing **or** continuous infusion over 6-42 hours

Pediatric solid tumors (high-dose): I.V.:
<12 years: 12-25 g/m²
≥12 years: 8 g/m²
Acute lymphocytic leukemia (intermediate-dose): I.V.: Loading: 100 mg/m² bolus dose, followed by 900 mg/m²/day infusion over 23-41 hours.
Meningeal leukemia: I.T.: 6-12 mg/dose based on age.
Note: Optimal intrathecal chemotherapy dosing should be based on age rather than on body surface area (BSA); CSF volume correlates with age and not to BSA (Bleyer, 1983; Kerr, 2001):
<1 year: 6 mg/dose
1 year: 8 mg/dose
2 years: 10 mg/dose
≥3 years: 12 mg/dose

Adults:
Antineoplastic dosage range: I.V.: Range is wide from 30-40 mg/m²/week to 100-12,000 mg/m² with leucovorin calcium rescue
Breast cancer: I.V.: 30-60 mg/m² days 1 and 8 every 3-4 weeks
Head and neck cancer: Oral, I.M., I.V.: 25-50 mg/m² once weekly
Lymphoma, non-Hodgkin's: I.V.:
30 mg/m² days 3 and 10 every 3 weeks **or**
120 mg/m² day 8 and 15 every 3-4 weeks **or**
200 mg/m² day 8 and 15 every 3 weeks **or**
400 mg/m² every 4 weeks for 3 cycles **or**
1 g/m² every 3 weeks **or**
1.5 g/m² every 4 weeks
Meningeal leukemia: I.T.: Usual dose: 12 mg/dose. **Note:** Optimal intrathecal chemotherapy dosing should be based on age rather than on body surface area (BSA); CSF volume correlates with age and not to BSA (Bleyer, 1983; Kerr, 2001).
Mycosis fungoides (cutaneous T-cell lymphoma): Oral, I.M.: Initial (early stages):
5-50 mg once weekly **or**
15-37.5 mg twice weekly
Osteosarcoma: I.V.: 8-12 g/m² weekly for 2-4 weeks
Psoriasis: **Note:** Some experts recommend concomitant folic acid 1-5 mg/day (except the day of methotrexate) to reduce hematologic, gastrointestinal, and hepatic adverse events related to methotrexate.
Oral: 2.5-5 mg/dose every 12 hours for 3 doses given weekly **or**
Oral, I.M., SubQ: 10-25 mg/dose given once weekly; titrate to lowest effective dose
Note: An initial test dose of 2.5-5 mg is recommended in patients with risk factors for hematologic toxicity or renal impairment (Kalb, 2009).
Rheumatoid arthritis: **Note:** Some experts recommend concomitant folic acid at a dose of least 5 mg/week (except the day of methotrexate) to reduce hematologic, gastrointestinal, and hepatic adverse events related to methotrexate.
Oral (manufacturer labeling): 7.5 mg once weekly or 2.5 mg every 12 hours for 3 doses/week (dosage exceeding 20 mg/week may cause a higher incidence and severity of adverse events); *alternatively,* 10-15 mg once weekly, increased by 5 mg every 2-4 weeks to a maximum of 20-30 mg once weekly has been recommended by some experts (Visser, 2009)
I.M., SubQ (unlabeled route): 15 mg once weekly (dosage varies, similar to oral) (Braun, 2008)
Trophoblastic neoplasms:
Oral, I.M.: 15-30 mg/day for 5 days; repeat in 7 days for 3-5 courses
I.V.: 11 mg/m² days 1 through 5 every 3 weeks

Unlabeled uses:
Active Crohn's disease (unlabeled use): Induction of remission: I.M., SubQ: 15-25 mg once weekly; remission maintenance: 15 mg once weekly
Note: Oral dosing has been reported as effective but oral absorption is highly variable. If patient relapses after a switch to oral, may consider returning to injectable.
Bladder cancer (unlabeled use): I.V.:
30 mg/m² day 1 and 8 every 3 weeks **or**
30 mg/m² day 1, 15, and 22 every 4 weeks
Dermatomyositis/polymyositis (unlabeled uses):
Oral: Initial: 7.5-15 mg/week, often adjunctively with high-dose corticosteroid therapy; may increase in weekly 2.5 mg increments to target dose of 10-25 mg/week (**Note:** Administration of folate 5-7 mg/week has been used to reduce side effects). (Briemberg, 2003; Newman, 1995; Wiendl, 2008)
I.V., I.M.: Doses of 20-60 mg/week have been employed if failure with oral therapy (doses >50 mg/week may require leucovorin calcium rescue) (Briemberg, 2003)
Ectopic pregnancy (unlabeled use): I.M.:
Single-dose regimen: Methotrexate 50 mg/m² on day 1; Measure serum hCG levels on days 4 and 7; if needed, repeat dose on day 7 (Barnhart, 2009)
Two-dose regimen: Methotrexate 50 mg/m² on day 1; Measure serum hCG levels on day 4 and administer a second dose of methotrexate 50 mg/m²; Measure serum hCG levels on day 7 and if needed, administer a third dose of 50 mg/m² (Barnhart, 2009)
Multidose regimen: Methotrexate 1 mg/kg on day 1; leucovorin calcium 0.1 mg/kg I.M. on day 2; measure serum hCG on day 2; methotrexate 1 mg/kg on day 3; leucovorin calcium 0.1 mg/kg on day 4; measure serum hCG on day 4; continue up to a total of 4 courses based on hCG concentrations (Barnhart, 2009)
GVHD (acute) prophylaxis: I.V.: 15 mg/m²/dose on day 1 and 10 mg/m²/dose on days 3 and 6 after allogeneic transplant (in combination with cyclosporine and prednisone) (Chao, 1993; Chao, 2000; Ross, 1999) **or** 15 mg/m²/dose on day 1 and 10 mg/m²/dose on days 3, 6, and 11 after allogeneic transplant (in combination with cyclosporine) (Chao, 2000)
Nonleukemic meningeal cancer (unlabeled uses): I.T.: 10-12 mg/dose twice weekly for 4 weeks, then weekly for 4 weeks, then monthly (NCCN CNS cancer guidelines v.2.2009) **or** 12 mg/dose twice weekly for 4 weeks, then weekly for 4 doses, then monthly for 4 doses (Glantz, 1998) **or** 10 mg twice weekly for 4 weeks, then weekly for 1 month, then every 2 weeks for 2 months (Glantz, 1999)
Takayasu arteritis, refractory or relapsing disease (unlabeled use): Oral: Initial dose: 0.3 mg/kg/week (maximum: 15 mg/week), titrated by 2.5 mg increments every 1-2 weeks until reaching a maximum tolerated weekly dose of 25 mg (use in combination with a corticosteroid; Hoffman, 1994)

Elderly:
Meningeal leukemia: I.T.: Consider a dose reduction (CSF volume and turnover may decrease with age)
Rheumatoid arthritis/psoriasis: Oral: Initial: 5-7.5 mg/week, not to exceed 20 mg/week

Dosing adjustment in renal impairment: The FDA-approved labeling does not contain dosage adjustment guidelines. The following guidelines have been used by some clinicians:
Cl_{cr} 61-80 mL/minute: Administer 75% of dose
Cl_{cr} 51-60 mL/minute: Administer 70% of dose
Cl_{cr} 10-50 mL/minute: Administer 30% to 50% of dose
Cl_{cr} <10 mL/minute: Avoid use

Hemodialysis: Not dialyzable (0% to 5%); supplemental dose is not necessary
Peritoneal dialysis effects: Supplemental dose is not necessary
CAVH effects: Unknown

Aronoff, 2007:
Children:
Cl_{cr} 10-50 mL/minute: Administer 50% of dose
Cl_{cr} <10 mL/minute: Administer 30% of dose
Hemodialysis: Administer 30% of dose
Continuous ambulatory peritoneal dialysis (CAPD): Administer 30% of dose
Continuous renal replacement therapy (CRRT): Administer 50% of dose
Adults:
Cl_{cr} 10-50 mL/minute: Administer 50% of dose
Cl_{cr} <10 mL/minute: Avoid use
Hemodialysis: Administer 50% of dose
Continuous renal replacement therapy (CRRT): Administer 50% of dose

Kintzel, 1995:
Cl_{cr} 46-60 mL/minute: Administer 65% of normal dose
Cl_{cr} 31-45 mL/minute: Administer 50% of normal dose
Cl_{cr} <30 mL/minute: Avoid use

Dosage adjustment in hepatic impairment: The FDA-approved labeling does not contain dosage adjustment guidelines. The following guidelines have been used by some clinicians (Floyd, 2006):
Bilirubin 3.1-5 mg/dL **or** transaminases >3 times ULN: Administer 75% of dose
Bilirubin >5 mg/dL: Avoid use

Dietary Considerations Some products may contain sodium.

Administration Methotrexate may be administered I.M., I.V., I.T., or SubQ; I.V. administration may be as slow push, short bolus infusion, or 24- to 42-hour continuous infusion

Specific dosing schemes vary, but high dose should be followed by leucovorin calcium to prevent toxicity; refer to Leucovorin Calcium monograph on page 987

Monitoring Parameters
Laboratory tests should be performed on day 5 or day 6 of the weekly methotrexate cycle (eg, psoriasis, RA) to detect the leukopenia nadir and to avoid elevated LFTs 1-2 days after taking dose.
Patients with psoriasis:
CBC with differential and platelets (baseline, 7-14 days after initiating therapy or dosage increase, every 2-4 weeks for first few months, then every 1-3 months); BUN and serum creatinine (baseline and every 2-3 months); consider PPD for latent TB screening (baseline); LFTs (baseline, monthly for first 6 months, then every 1-2 months); chest x-ray (baseline if underlying lung disease)
Liver biopsy for patients **with** risk factors for hepatotoxicity: Baseline or after 2-6 months of therapy and with each 1-1.5 g cumulative dose interval
Liver biopsy for patients **without** risk factors for hepatotoxicity: If persistent elevations in 5 of 9 AST levels during a 12-month period, or decline of serum albumin below the normal range with normal nutritional status. Consider biopsy after cumulative dose of 3.5-4 g and after each additional 1.5 g.
Patients with RA:
CBC with differential and platelets, serum creatinine and LFTs (baseline then every 2-4 weeks for initial 3 months of therapy, then every 8-12 weeks for 3-6 months of therapy and then every 12 weeks after 6 months of therapy); chest x-ray (baseline); pulmonary function test (if methotrexate-induced lung disease suspected); hepatitis B or C testing (baseline)
Liver biopsy: Baseline (if persistent abnormal baseline LFTs, history of alcoholism, or chronic hepatitis B or C) or during treatment if persistent LFT elevations (6 of 12 tests abnormal over 1 year or 5 of 9 results when LFTs performed at 6-week intervals)
Patients with cancer: Baseline and frequently during treatment: CBC with differential and platelets, serum creatinine, LFTs; chest x-ray (baseline); methotrexate levels and urine pH (with high-dose therapy); pulmonary function test (if methotrexate-induced lung disease suspected)
Ectopic pregnancy (unlabeled use): Prior to therapy, measure serum hCG, CBC with differential, liver function tests, serum creatinine. Serum hCG concentrations should decrease between treatment days 4 and 7. If hCG decreases by >15%, additional courses are not needed however, continue to measure hCG weekly until no longer detectable. If <15% decrease is observed, repeat dose per regimen (Barnhart, 2009).

Reference Range Therapeutic levels: Variable; Toxic concentration: Variable; therapeutic range is dependent upon therapeutic approach.

High-dose regimens produce drug levels that are between 0.1-1 micromole/L 24-72 hours after drug infusion
Toxic: Low-dose therapy: >0.2 micromole/L; high-dose therapy: >1 micromole/L

Additional Information Oncology Comment: Methotrexate overexposure: The investigational rescue agent, glucarpidase, is an enzyme which rapidly hydrolyzes extracellular methotrexate into inactive metabolites, resulting in a rapid reduction of methotrexate concentrations. Glucarpidase is available for intrathecal (IT) use through an Emergency Use IND and for I.V. use under an Open-Label Treatment protocol. Refer to Glucarpidase monograph.

Dosage Forms Excipient information presented when available (limited, particularly for generics); consult specific product labeling.
Injection, powder for reconstitution: 1 g
Injection, solution: 25 mg/mL (2 mL, 10 mL)
Injection, solution [preservative free]: 25 mg/mL (2 mL, 4 mL, 8 mL, 10 mL, 40 mL)
Tablet, oral: 2.5 mg
Trexall™: 5 mg, 7.5 mg, 10 mg, 15 mg [scored]
Tablet, oral [dose-pack]:
Rheumatrex®: 2.5 mg [scored]

◆ **Methotrexate Sodium** *see* Methotrexate *on page* 1098
◆ **Methotrexatum** *see* Methotrexate *on page* 1098

Methoxsalen (Systemic) (meth OKS a len)

Brand Names: U.S. 8-MOP®; Oxsoralen-Ultra®; Uvadex®
Brand Names: Canada Oxsoralen-Ultra®; Oxsoralen® Capsule; Ultramop™
Index Terms 8-Methoxypsoralen; 8-MOP; Methoxypsoralen
Pharmacologic Category Psoralen
Use
Oral: Symptomatic control of severe, recalcitrant disabling psoriasis; repigmentation of idiopathic vitiligo; palliative treatment of skin manifestations of cutaneous T-cell lymphoma (CTCL)
Extracorporeal: Palliative treatment of skin manifestations of CTCL
Pregnancy Risk Factor C/D (Uvadex®)
Dosage Adults: **Note:** Refer to treatment protocols for UVA exposure guidelines.

Psoriasis: Oral:
Initial: 10-70 mg 1.5-2 hours (Oxsoralen-Ultra®) or 2 hours (8-MOP®) before exposure to UVA light; dose may be repeated 2-3 times per week, based on UVA exposure; doses must be given at least 48 hours apart. Dosage is based upon patient's body weight and skin type:
<30 kg: 10 mg
30-50 kg: 20 mg
51-65 kg: 30 mg
66-80 kg: 40 mg
81-90 kg: 50 mg
91-115 kg: 60 mg
>115 kg: 70 mg
Note: Dosage may be increased (one time) by 10 mg after 15th treatment if minimal or no response.
Maintenance: When 95% psoriasis clearing achieved, may begin 1 treatment every week for at least 2 treatments; followed by 1 treatment every 2 weeks for at least 2 treatments; then every 3 weeks for at least 2 treatments then as needed to maintain response while minimizing UVA exposure.
Vitiligo: Oral (8-MOP®): 20 mg 2-4 hours before exposure to UVA light; dose may be repeated based on erythema and tenderness of skin; do not give on 2 consecutive days
CTCL: Extracorporeal (Uvadex®): Dose is determined by treatment volume; amount of Uvadex® needed for each treatment may be calculated using the following equation: Treatment volume x 0.017 = mL of Uvadex® needed. Inject this amount into the photoactivation bag during the collection cycle using the UVAR® photopheresis system (consult user's guide).
Treatment schedule: Two consecutive days every 4 weeks for a minimum of 7 treatment cycles, may accelerate to 2 consecutive days every 2 weeks if skin score worsens (eg, increases from baseline) after assessment during the fourth treatment cycle. If skin score improves by 25% after 4 consecutive weeks of accelerated therapy, may resume regular treatment schedule. Maximum: 20 accelerated therapy cycles.

Additional Information Complete prescribing information for this medication should be consulted for additional detail.

Dosage Forms Excipient information presented when available (limited, particularly for generics); consult specific product labeling.
Capsule, oral:
8-MOP®: 10 mg [hard-gelatin capsule]
Oxsoralen-Ultra®: 10 mg [soft-gelatin capsule]
Solution, for extracorporeal administration:
Uvadex®: 20 mcg/mL (10 mL) [contains ethanol 0.05 mL/mL; not for injection]

Methoxsalen (Topical) (meth OKS a len)

Brand Names: U.S. Oxsoralen®
Brand Names: Canada Oxsoralen® Lotion
Index Terms Methoxypsoralen
Pharmacologic Category Psoralen
Use Repigmentation of idiopathic vitiligo
Pregnancy Risk Factor C
Dosage Topical: **Note:** Refer to treatment protocols for UVA exposure guidelines.
Children ≥12 years and Adults: Vitiligo: Lotion is applied by healthcare provider prior to UVA light exposure, usually no more than once weekly; frequency is determined by erythema response

Additional Information Complete prescribing information for this medication should be consulted for additional detail.

Dosage Forms Excipient information presented when available (limited, particularly for generics); consult specific product labeling.
Lotion, topical:
Oxsoralen®: 1% (29.57 mL) [contains ethanol 71%]

◆ **Methoxypsoralen** *see* Methoxsalen (Systemic) *on page 1102*

◆ **Methoxypsoralen** *see* Methoxsalen (Topical) *on page 1103*

◆ **8-Methoxypsoralen** *see* Methoxsalen (Systemic) *on page 1102*

◆ **Methscopolamine and Pseudoephedrine** *see* Pseudoephedrine and Methscopolamine *on page 1432*

Methsuximide (meth SUKS i mide)

Brand Names: U.S. Celontin®
Brand Names: Canada Celontin®
Pharmacologic Category Anticonvulsant, Succinimide
Use Control of absence (petit mal) seizures that are refractory to other drugs
Unlabeled Use Partial complex (psychomotor) seizures
Medication Guide Available Yes
Dosage Oral: Adults: Anticonvulsant: 300 mg/day for the first week; may increase by 300 mg/day at weekly intervals up to 1.2 g/day in 2-4 divided doses/day

Additional Information Complete prescribing information for this medication should be consulted for additional detail.

Dosage Forms Excipient information presented when available (limited, particularly for generics); consult specific product labeling.
Capsule, oral:
Celontin®: 150 mg, 300 mg

Methyclothiazide (meth i kloe THYE a zide)

Index Terms Enduron
Pharmacologic Category Diuretic, Thiazide
Use Management of hypertension; adjunctive therapy of edema
Pregnancy Risk Factor B
Dosage Adults: Oral:
Edema: 2.5-10 mg/day
Hypertension: 2.5-5 mg/day; may add another antihypertensive if 5 mg is not adequate after a trial of 8-12 weeks of therapy

Additional Information Complete prescribing information for this medication should be consulted for additional detail.

Dosage Forms Excipient information presented when available (limited, particularly for generics); consult specific product labeling.
Tablet, oral: 5 mg

◆ **Methylacetoxyprogesterone** *see* MedroxyPROGESTERone *on page 1058*

Methyl Aminolevulinate
(METH il a mee noe LEV ue lin ate)

Brand Names: U.S. Metvixia™
Brand Names: Canada Metvix®
Index Terms Methyl Aminolevulinate Hydrochloride; P-1202
Pharmacologic Category Photosensitizing Agent, Topical; Topical Skin Product
Use Treatment of thin and moderately thick, nonhyperkeratotic, nonpigmented actinic keratoses of the face and scalp; to be used in conjunction with red light illumination

Pregnancy Risk Factor C

Pregnancy Considerations Teratogenic effects have been demonstrated in animal reproduction studies using intravenous doses >900-fold higher than a human topical dose of 2 g. There are no adequate and well-controlled studies in pregnant women. Use during pregnancy only if clearly needed.

Lactation Excretion in breast milk unknown/use caution

Contraindications Hypersensitivity to methyl aminolevulinate or any component of the formulation, including peanut and almond oil (has not been tested in patients with peanut allergy); individuals with cutaneous photosensitivity; allergy to porphyrins

Warnings/Precautions Treatment site will become photosensitive following application of cream and for 48 hours after. Concomitant use of other known photosensitizing agents may increase the degree of photosensitivity reaction. For external use only. Should be applied by a qualified health professional. Has not been tested in individuals with coagulation defects (acquired or inherited).

Adverse Reactions Pain and burning begin during illumination and generally resolve completely within a few minutes or hours, but may last up to a few days. Erythema and other signs generally resolve within a few days up to 3 weeks.

>10%: Dermatologic: Skin burning/pain/discomfort (86%; severe: 20%), erythema (63%; severe 6%), scabbing/crusting/blister/erosions (29%), itching (22%), skin or eyelid edema (18%), skin exfoliation (14%)

1% to 10%:

Dermatologic: Skin warm (4%), hyperpigmentation (2%), skin hemorrhage (2%), skin tightness (2%)

Local: Application site discharge (2%)

Postmarketing and/or case reports: Contact dermatitis, eczema, keratitis (ocular), macular edema, vitreous detachment

Drug Interactions

Metabolism/Transport Effects None known.

Avoid Concomitant Use There are no known interactions where it is recommended to avoid concomitant use.

Increased Effect/Toxicity There are no known significant interactions involving an increase in effect.

Decreased Effect There are no known significant interactions involving a decrease in effect.

Stability Store at 2°C to 8°C (36°F to 46°F). Use contents within 1 week after opening; discard if unrefrigerated for >24 hours.

Mechanism of Action Methyl aminolevulinate (prodrug) is metabolically converted to photoactive porphyrins (PAPs), which accumulate in the skin lesions resulting in photosensitization. When exposed to light of appropriate wavelength and energy, the accumulated PAPs produce a photodynamic reaction, releasing oxygen singlets which result in local cytotoxicity.

Pharmacodynamics/Kinetics Peak fluorescence intensity: 3 hours after application

Dosage Topical: Adults: Apply up to 1 g to prepared actinic keratoses, occlude for 3 hours, followed by red light illumination; repeat in 1 week. **Note:** If multiple lesions being treated, 1 g should not be exceeded for all lesions combined.

Administration Prepare lesions using a small dermal curette to remove scales and crusts and roughen the surface of the lesion. Wearing nitrile gloves and using a spatula, apply a layer of methyl aminolevulinate cream about 1 mm thick topically to prepared lesion and the surrounding 5 mm of normal skin. Multiple lesions may be treated during the same treatment session; do not exceed a treatment field area of 80 x 180 mm; do not exceed a total of 1 g (half tube) of methyl aminolevulinate cream per treatment session. Occlude the site(s) with a nonabsorbent dressing for 3 hours (minimum 2.5 hours, maximum 4 hours), then remove. Remove excess cream with saline and illuminate with red light following lamp manufacturer's instructions. Following illumination of cream, the treated area should be kept covered and away from bright indoor light and sunlight from 48 hours. If, for any reason, red light illumination is not done, the cream should be removed within 4 hours (from time of initial application) and the area protected from bright indoor light or sunlight for 48 hours.

Additional Information Use in conjunction with Atkilite® CL 128 lamp.

Dosage Forms Excipient information presented when available (limited, particularly for generics); consult specific product labeling.

Cream, topical:

Metvixia™: 16.8% (2 g) [contains almond oil, peanut oil]

◆ **Methyl Aminolevulinate Hydrochloride** *see* Methyl Aminolevulinate *on page 1103*

◆ **Methylcobalamin, Acetylcysteine, and Methylfolate** *see* Methylfolate, Methylcobalamin, and Acetylcysteine *on page 1106*

Methyldopa (meth il DOE pa)

Brand Names: Canada Apo-Methyldopa®; Nu-Medopa

Index Terms Aldomet; Methyldopate Hydrochloride

Pharmacologic Category Alpha-Adrenergic Inhibitor; Alpha$_2$-Adrenergic Agonist

Additional Appendix Information

Beers Criteria – Potentially Inappropriate Medications for Geriatrics *on page 1973*

Hypertension *on page 2001*

Use Management of moderate-to-severe hypertension

Pregnancy Risk Factor B

Dosage

Children:

Oral: Initial: 10 mg/kg/day in 2-4 divided doses; increase every 2 days as needed to maximum dose of 65 mg/kg/day; do not exceed 3 g/day.

I.V.: 5-10 mg/kg/dose every 6-8 hours up to a total dose of 65 mg/kg/24 hours or 3 g/24 hours

Adults:

Oral: Initial: 250 mg 2-3 times/day; increase every 2 days as needed (maximum dose: 3 g/day): usual dose range (JNC 7): 250-1000 mg/day in 2 divided doses

I.V.: 250-500 mg every 6-8 hours; maximum dose: 1 g every 6 hours

Elderly: Initiate at the lower end of the dosage range.

Dosing interval in renal impairment:

Cl_{cr} >50 mL/minute: Administer every 8 hours.

Cl_{cr} 10-50 mL/minute: Administer every 8-12 hours.

Cl_{cr} <10 mL/minute: Administer every 12-24 hours.

Hemodialysis: Slightly dialyzable (5% to 20%)

Additional Information Complete prescribing information for this medication should be consulted for additional detail.

Dosage Forms Excipient information presented when available (limited, particularly for generics); consult specific product labeling.

Injection, solution, as hydrochloride: 50 mg/mL (5 mL)

Tablet, oral: 250 mg, 500 mg

◆ **Methyldopate Hydrochloride** *see* Methyldopa *on page 1104*

Methylene Blue (METH i leen bloo)

Index Terms Methylthionine Chloride

Pharmacologic Category Antidote

Use Antidote for cyanide poisoning and drug-induced methemoglobinemia, indicator dye

Unlabeled Use Treatment/prevention of ifosfamide-induced encephalopathy; topically, in conjunction with polychromatic light to photoinactivate viruses such as herpes simplex; alone or in combination with vitamin C for the management of chronic urolithiasis

Pregnancy Risk Factor C

Dosage

Children and Adults: Methemoglobinemia: I.V.: 1-2 mg/kg or 25-50 mg/m^2 over 5-10 minutes; may be repeated in 1 hour if necessary

Adults: Ifosfamide-induced encephalopathy (unlabeled use): **Note:** Treatment may not be necessary; encephalopathy may improve spontaneously: I.V.:

Prevention: 50 mg every 6-8 hours

Treatment: 50 mg as a single dose or every 4-8 hours until symptoms resolve

Dosage adjustment in renal impairment: No dosage adjustment recommendations available; however, caution should be used in severe renal impairment.

Additional Information Complete prescribing information for this medication should be consulted for additional detail.

Dosage Forms Excipient information presented when available (limited, particularly for generics); consult specific product labeling.

Injection, solution: 10 mg/mL (1 mL, 10 mL)

- ◆ **Methylene Blue, Methenamine, Benzoic Acid, Phenyl Salicylate, and Hyoscyamine** *see* Methenamine, Phenyl Salicylate, Methylene Blue, Benzoic Acid, and Hyoscyamine *on page 1094*
- ◆ **Methylene Blue, Methenamine, Sodium Biphosphate, Phenyl Salicylate, and Hyoscyamine** *see* Methenamine, Sodium Biphosphate, Phenyl Salicylate, Methylene Blue, and Hyoscyamine *on page 1094*
- ◆ **Methylergometrine Maleate** *see* Methylergonovine *on page 1105*

Methylergonovine (meth il er goe NOE veen)

Brand Names: U.S. Methergine®

Brand Names: Canada Methergine®

Index Terms Methylergometrine Maleate; Methylergonovine Maleate

Pharmacologic Category Ergot Derivative

Use Prevention and treatment of postpartum and postabortion hemorrhage caused by uterine atony or subinvolution

Pregnancy Risk Factor C

Pregnancy Considerations Prolonged constriction of the uterine vessels and/or increased myometrial tone may lead to reduced placental blood flow. This has contributed to fetal growth retardation in animals. Methylergonovine is intended for use after delivery of the infant.

Lactation Enters breast milk/use caution

Contraindications Hypersensitivity to methylergonovine or any component of the formulation; ergot alkaloids are contraindicated with potent inhibitors of CYP3A4 (includes protease inhibitors, azole antifungals, and some macrolide antibiotics); hypertension; toxemia; pregnancy

Warnings/Precautions Use caution in patients with sepsis, obliterative vascular disease, cardiovascular disease, hepatic or renal involvement, or second stage of labor; administer with extreme caution if using intravenously. Pleural and peritoneal fibrosis have been reported with prolonged daily use of other ergot alkaloids. Cardiac valvular fibrosis has also been associated with ergot alkaloids. Ergot alkaloid use may result in ergotism (intense vasoconstriction) resulting in peripheral vascular ischemia and possible gangrene. Concomitant use with potent inhibitors of CYP3A4 (includes protease inhibitors, azole antifungals, and some macrolide antibiotics) and ergot alkaloids has been associated with acute ergot toxicity (ergotism); concurrent use of certain ergot alkaloids (eg, ergotamine and dihydroergotamine) are not recommended by the manufacturer. Use with caution in the elderly. Safety and efficacy have not been established in children.

Adverse Reactions Frequency not defined.

Cardiovascular: Acute MI, arterial spasm, bradycardia, hyper-/hypotension, palpitation, tachycardia, temporary chest pain

Central nervous system: Dizziness, hallucinations, headache, seizure

Dermatologic: Rash

Endocrine & metabolic: Water intoxication

Gastrointestinal: Diarrhea, foul taste, nausea, vomiting

Local: Thrombophlebitis

Neuromuscular & skeletal: Leg cramps

Otic: Tinnitus

Renal: Hematuria

Respiratory: Dyspnea, nasal congestion

Miscellaneous: Anaphylaxis, diaphoresis

Drug Interactions

Metabolism/Transport Effects Substrate of CYP3A4 (major); **Note:** Assignment of Major/Minor substrate status based on clinically relevant drug interaction potential

Avoid Concomitant Use

Avoid concomitant use of Methylergonovine with any of the following: Alpha-/Beta-Agonists; Alpha1-Agonists; Boceprevir; Conivaptan; Efavirenz; Itraconazole; Nitroglycerin; Posaconazole; Protease Inhibitors; Serotonin 5-HT1D Receptor Agonists; Telaprevir; Voriconazole

Increased Effect/Toxicity

Methylergonovine may increase the levels/effects of: Alpha-/Beta-Agonists; Alpha1-Agonists; Metoclopramide; Serotonin 5-HT1D Receptor Agonists; Serotonin Modulators

The levels/effects of Methylergonovine may be increased by: Antipsychotics; Boceprevir; Conivaptan; CYP3A4 Inhibitors (Moderate); CYP3A4 Inhibitors (Strong); Dasatinib; Efavirenz; Itraconazole; Macrolide Antibiotics; Nitroglycerin; Posaconazole; Protease Inhibitors; Serotonin 5-HT1D Receptor Agonists; Telaprevir; Voriconazole

Decreased Effect

Methylergonovine may decrease the levels/effects of: Nitroglycerin

The levels/effects of Methylergonovine may be decreased by: Tocilizumab

Stability

Injection: Store under refrigeration at 2°C to 8°C (36°F to 46°F). Protect from light. The following stability information has also been reported: May be stored at room temperature for up to 14 days (Cohen, 2007).

Tablet: Store below 25°C (77°F).

Mechanism of Action Similar smooth muscle actions as seen with ergotamine; however, it affects primarily uterine smooth muscles producing sustained contractions and thereby shortens the third stage of labor and reduces blood loss.

Pharmacodynamics/Kinetics

Onset of action: Oxytocic: Oral: 5-10 minutes; I.M.: 2-5 minutes; I.V.: Immediately

Duration: Oral: ~3 hours; I.M.: ~3 hours; I.V.: 45 minutes

Absorption: Rapid

Distribution: V_d: 39-73 L

Rapid; primarily to plasma and extracellular fluid following I.V. administration; tissues

Metabolism: Hepatic

Bioavailability: Oral: 60%; I.M.: 78%

Half-life elimination: Biphasic: Initial: 1-5 minutes; Terminal: 0.5-2 hours

Time to peak, serum: Oral: 0.3-2 hours; I.M.: 0.2-0.6 hours

Excretion: Urine and feces

Dosage Adults:

Oral: 0.2 mg 3-4 times/day in the puerperium for 2-7 days

I.M., I.V.: 0.2 mg after delivery of anterior shoulder, after delivery of placenta, or during puerperium; may be repeated as required at intervals of 2-4 hours

Administration Administer over ≥60 seconds. Should not be routinely administered I.V. because of possibility of inducing sudden hypertension and cerebrovascular accident.

Dosage Forms Excipient information presented when available (limited, particularly for generics); consult specific product labeling.

Injection, solution, as maleate: 0.2 mg/mL (1 mL)

Methergine®: 0.2 mg/mL (1 mL)

Tablet, oral, as maleate:

Methergine®: 0.2 mg

◆ **Methylergonovine Maleate** *see* Methylergonovine *on page 1105*

Methylfolate, Methylcobalamin, and Acetylcysteine

(meth il FO late meth il koe BAL a min & a se teel SIS teen)

Brand Names: U.S. Cerefolin® NAC

Index Terms Acetylcysteine, Methylcobalamin, and Methylfolate; Acetylcysteine, Methylfolate, and Methylcobalamin; L-methylfolate, Methylcobalamin, and N-acetylcysteine; Methylcobalamin, Acetylcysteine, and Methylfolate

Pharmacologic Category Dietary Supplement

Use Medicinal food for use in patients with neurovascular oxidative stress and/or hyperhomocysteinemia

Dosage Oral: Children ≥12 years and Adults: One caplet daily

Additional Information Complete prescribing information for this medication should be consulted for additional detail.

Dosage Forms Excipient information presented when available (limited, particularly for generics); consult specific product labeling.

Caplet, oral:

Cerefolin® NAC: L-methylfolate 5.6 mg, methylcobalamin 2 mg, and N-acetylcysteine 600 mg [gluten free, sugar free]

◆ **Methylin®** *see* Methylphenidate *on page 1107*

◆ **Methylin® ER [DSC]** *see* Methylphenidate *on page 1107*

◆ **Methylmorphine** *see* Codeine *on page 403*

Methylnaltrexone (meth il nal TREKS one)

Brand Names: U.S. Relistor®

Brand Names: Canada Relistor®

Index Terms Methylnaltrexone Bromide; N-methylnaltrexone Bromide

Pharmacologic Category Gastrointestinal Agent, Miscellaneous; Opioid Antagonist, Peripherally-Acting

Use Treatment of opioid-induced constipation in patients with advanced illness receiving palliative care with inadequate response to conventional laxative regimens

Pregnancy Risk Factor B

Pregnancy Considerations Adverse effects were not observed in animal studies. There are no adequate and well-controlled studies in pregnant women.

Lactation Excretion in breast milk unknown/use caution

Contraindications Known or suspected mechanical bowel obstruction

Canadian labeling: Additional contraindications (not in U.S. labeling): Hypersensitivity to methylnaltrexone or any component of the formulation

Warnings/Precautions Discontinue treatment for severe or persistent diarrhea. Gastrointestinal perforation of the colon, duodenum, and stomach has been reported (rarely) in patients with advanced illnesses associated with impaired structural integrity of the GI wall (eg, cancer, Ogilvie's syndrome, peptic ulcer). Use caution in patients with known or history of GI tract lesions; discontinue therapy if persistent, severe, or worsening abdominal symptoms occur. Use with caution in patients with renal impairment; dosage adjustment recommended for severe renal impairment (Cl_{cr} <30 mL/minute). Has not been studied in patients with end-stage renal impairment requiring dialysis. Discontinue methylnaltrexone if opioids are discontinued. Use has not been studied in patients with peritoneal catheters. Use beyond 4 months has not been studied.

Adverse Reactions

>10%: Gastrointestinal: Abdominal pain (29%), flatulence (13%), nausea (12%)

1% to 10%:

Central nervous system: Dizziness (7%)

Dermatologic: Hyperhidrosis (7%)

Gastrointestinal: Diarrhea (6%)

<1% (Limited to important or life-threatening): Abdominal cramps, body temperature increased, GI perforation, muscle spasm, syncope

Drug Interactions

Metabolism/Transport Effects Substrate of CYP2D6 (minor); **Note:** Assignment of Major/Minor substrate status based on clinically relevant drug interaction potential

Avoid Concomitant Use There are no known interactions where it is recommended to avoid concomitant use.

Increased Effect/Toxicity There are no known significant interactions involving an increase in effect.

Decreased Effect

The levels/effects of Methylnaltrexone may be decreased by: Peginterferon Alfa-2b

Stability Store intact vials at room temperature of 20°C to 25°C (68°F to 77°F); excursions permitted to 15°C to 30°C (59°F to 86°F); do not freeze. Protect from light. Solution for injection is stable in a syringe for 24 hours at room temperature (protection from light during this 24 hours is not necessary).

Mechanism of Action An opioid receptor antagonist which blocks opioid binding at the mu receptor, methylnaltrexone is a quaternary derivative of naltrexone with restricted ability to cross the blood-brain barrier. It therefore functions as a peripheral acting opioid antagonist, including actions on the gastrointestinal tract to inhibit opioid-induced decreased gastrointestinal motility and delay in gastrointestinal transit time, thereby decreasing opioid-induced constipation. Does not affect opioid analgesic effects or induce opioid withdrawal symptoms.

Pharmacodynamics/Kinetics

Onset of action: Usually within 30-60 minutes (in responding patients)

Absorption: SubQ: Rapid

Distribution: V_{dss}: ~1.1 L/kg

Protein binding: 11% to 15%

Metabolism: Metabolized to methyl-6-naltrexol isomers, methylnaltrexone sulfate, and other minor metabolites

Half-life elimination: Terminal: ~8 hours

Time to peak, plasma: SubQ: 30 minutes

Excretion: Urine (~50%, primarily as unchanged drug); feces (<50%, primarily as unchanged drug)

Dosage SubQ: Adults: Opioid-induced constipation: Dosing is according to body weight: Administer 1 dose every other day as needed; maximum: 1 dose/24 hours

<38 kg: 0.15 mg/kg (round dose up to nearest 0.1 mL of volume)
38 to <62 kg: 8 mg
62-114 kg: 12 mg
>114 kg: 0.15 mg/kg (round dose up to nearest 0.1 mL of volume)

Dosage adjustment in renal impairment:
Mild-to-moderate renal impairment: No adjustment required
Severe renal impairment (Cl_{cr} <30 mL/minute): Administer 50% of normal dose
End-stage renal impairment (dialysis-dependent): Has not been studied

Dosage adjustment in hepatic impairment:
Mild-to-moderate hepatic impairment (Child-Pugh class A and B): No adjustment required
Severe hepatic impairment: Has not been studied

Administration SubQ: Administer subcutaneously into upper arm, abdomen, or thigh. Rotate injection site. Do not use tender, bruised, red, or hard areas.

Additional Information In some clinical trials, patients who received methylnaltrexone were on a palliative opioid therapy equivalent to a mean daily oral morphine dose of 172 mg, at a stable dose for ≥3 days. Constipation was defined as <3 bowel movements/week or no bowel movement for >2 days. Patients maintained their regular laxative regimen for at least 3 days prior to treatment and throughout the study.

Dosage Forms Excipient information presented when available (limited, particularly for generics); consult specific product labeling.
Injection, solution:
Relistor®: 12 mg/0.6 mL (0.6 mL) [contains edetate calcium disodium]

◆ **Methylnaltrexone Bromide** *see* Methylnaltrexone *on page 1106*

Methylphenidate (meth il FEN i date)

Brand Names: U.S. Concerta®; Daytrana®; Metadate CD®; Metadate® ER; Methylin®; Methylin® ER [DSC]; Ritalin LA®; Ritalin-SR®; Ritalin®

Brand Names: Canada Apo-Methylphenidate®; Apo-Methylphenidate® SR; Biphentin®; Concerta®; Novo-Methylphenidate ER-C; PHL-Methylphenidate; PMS-Methylphenidate; ratio-Methylphenidate; Ritalin®; Ritalin® SR; Sandoz-Methylphenidate SR

Index Terms Methylphenidate Hydrochloride

Pharmacologic Category Central Nervous System Stimulant

Additional Appendix Information
Patient Information for Disposal of Unused Medications *on page 2026*

Use Treatment of attention-deficit/hyperactivity disorder (ADHD); symptomatic management of narcolepsy

Unlabeled Use Depression (especially elderly or medically ill)

Pregnancy Risk Factor C

Pregnancy Considerations Animal studies have shown teratogenic effects to the fetus. There are no adequate and well-controlled studies in pregnant women. Do not use in women of childbearing age unless the potential benefit outweighs the possible risk.

Lactation Enters breast milk/use caution

Medication Guide Available Yes

Contraindications Hypersensitivity to methylphenidate, any component of the formulation, or idiosyncratic reactions to sympathomimetic amines; marked anxiety, tension, and agitation; glaucoma; use during or within 14 days following MAO inhibitor therapy; family history or diagnosis of Tourette's syndrome or tics

Metadate CD® and Metadate® ER: Additional contraindications: Severe hypertension, heart failure, arrhythmia, hyperthyroidism, recent MI or angina; concomitant use of halogenated anesthetics

Warnings/Precautions CNS stimulant use has been associated with serious cardiovascular events (eg, sudden death in children and adolescents; sudden death, stroke, and MI in adults) in patients with pre-existing structural cardiac abnormalities or other serious heart problems. These products should be avoided in patients with known serious structural cardiac abnormalities, cardiomyopathy, serious heart rhythm abnormalities, or other serious cardiac problems that could further increase their risk of sudden death. Patients should be carefully evaluated for cardiac disease prior to initiation of therapy. Use of stimulants can cause an increase in blood pressure (average 2-4 mm Hg) and increases in heart rate (average 3-6 bpm), although some patients may have larger than average increases. Use caution with hypertension, hyperthyroidism, or other cardiovascular conditions that might be exacerbated by increases in blood pressure or heart rate. Some products are contraindicated in patients with heart failure, arrhythmias, severe hypertension, hyperthyroidism, angina, or recent MI.

Has demonstrated value as part of a comprehensive treatment program for ADHD. Use with caution in patients with bipolar disorder (may induce mixed/manic episode). May exacerbate symptoms of behavior and thought disorder in psychotic patients; new-onset psychosis or mania may occur with stimulant use; observe for symptoms of aggression and/or hostility. Use caution with seizure disorders (may reduce seizure threshold). Use caution in patients with history of ethanol or drug abuse. May exacerbate symptoms of behavior and thought disorder in psychotic patients. **[U.S. Boxed Warning]: Potential for drug dependency exists - avoid abrupt discontinuation in patients who have received for prolonged periods.** Visual disturbances have been reported (rare). Not labeled for use in children <6 years of age. Use of stimulants has been associated with suppression of growth in children; monitor growth rate during treatment.

Concerta® should not be used in patients with esophageal motility disorders or pre-existing severe gastrointestinal narrowing (small bowel disease, short gut syndrome, history of peritonitis, cystic fibrosis, chronic intestinal pseudo-obstruction, Meckel's diverticulum). Metadate CD® and Metadate® ER contain sucrose and lactose, respectively; avoid administration in hereditary galactose intolerance, Lapp lactase deficiency, or glucose-galactose malabsorption. Concomitant use with halogenated anesthetics is contraindicated; may cause sudden elevations in blood pressure; if surgery is planned, do not administer Metadate CD® or Metadate® ER on the day of surgery. Transdermal system may cause allergic contact sensitization, characterized by intense local reactions (edema, papules) that may spread beyond the patch site; sensitization may subsequently manifest systemically with other routes of methylphenidate administration; monitor closely. Avoid exposure of application site to any direct external heat sources (eg, hair dryers, heating pads, electric blankets); may increase the rate and extent of absorption and risk of overdose. Efficacy of transdermal methylphenidate therapy for >7 weeks has not been established.

Adverse Reactions

Transdermal system: Frequency of adverse events as reported in trials of 7-week duration. Incidence of some events higher with extended use.

>10%:

Central nervous system: Headache (≤15%; long-term use in children: 28%), insomnia (6% to 13%; long-term use in children: 30%), irritability (7% to 11%)

Gastrointestinal: Appetite decreased (26%), nausea (10% to 12%)

Miscellaneous: Viral infection (long-term use in children: 28%)

1% to 10%:

Cardiovascular: Tachycardia (≤1%)

Central nervous system: Tic (7%), dizziness (adolescents 6%), emotional instability (6%)

Gastrointestinal: Vomiting (3% to 10%), weight loss (6% to 9%), abdominal pain (5% to 7%), anorexia (5%; long-term use in children: 46%)

Local: Application site reaction

Respiratory: Nasal congestion (6%) nasopharyngitis (5%)

Postmarketing and/or case reports (limited to important or life-threatening): Allergic contact dermatitis/sensitization, anaphylaxis, angioedema, hallucinations, seizures

All dosage forms: Frequency not defined:

Cardiovascular: Angina, cardiac arrhythmia, cerebral arteritis, cerebral hemorrhage, cerebral occlusion, cerebrovascular accidents, vasculitis, hyper-/hypotension, MI, murmur, palpitation, pulse increased/decreased, Raynaud's phenomenon, tachycardia

Central nervous system: Aggression, agitation, anger, anxiety, confusional state, depression, dizziness, drowsiness, fatigue, fever, headache, hypervigilance, insomnia, irritability, lethargy, mood alterations, nervousness, neuroleptic malignant syndrome (NMS) (rare), restlessness, stroke, tension, Tourette's syndrome (rare), toxic psychosis, tremor, vertigo

Dermatologic: Alopecia, erythema multiforme, exfoliative dermatitis, hyperhidrosis, rash, urticaria

Endocrine & metabolic: Dysmenorrhea, growth retardation, libido decreased

Gastrointestinal: Abdominal pain, anorexia, appetite decreased, bruxism, constipation, diarrhea, dyspepsia, nausea, vomiting, weight loss, xerostomia

Genitourinary: Erectile dysfunction

Hematologic: Anemia, leukopenia, pancytopenia, thrombocytopenic purpura, thrombocytopenia

Hepatic: Bilirubin increased, liver function tests abnormal, hepatic coma, transaminases increased

Neuromuscular & skeletal: Arthralgia, dyskinesia, muscle tightness, paresthesia

Ocular: Blurred vision, dry eyes, mydriasis, visual accommodation disturbance

Renal: Necrotizing vasculitis

Respiratory: Cough increased, dyspnea, pharyngitis, pharyngolaryngeal pain, rhinitis, sinusitis, upper respiratory tract infection

Miscellaneous: Accidental injury, hypersensitivity reactions

Postmarketing and/or case reports: Alkaline phosphatase increased, angina pectoris, bradycardia, chest pain, diplopia, disorientation, extrasystole, mydriasis; hypersensitivity reactions (eg, angioedema, anaphylactic reactions, auricular swelling, bullous conditions, exfoliative conditions, urticaria, pruritus, rash, eruptions, exanthemas); migraine, muscle twitching, hallucinations, mania, erythema, obsessive-compulsive disorder, seizure, supraventricular tachycardia, ventricular extrasystole

Drug Interactions

Metabolism/Transport Effects Inhibits CYP2D6 (weak)

Avoid Concomitant Use

Avoid concomitant use of Methylphenidate with any of the following: Inhalational Anesthetics; Iobenguane I 123; MAO Inhibitors

Increased Effect/Toxicity

Methylphenidate may increase the levels/effects of: Anti-Parkinson's Agents (Dopamine Agonist); Antipsychotics; CloNIDine; Fosphenytoin; Inhalational Anesthetics; PHENobarbital; Phenytoin; Primidone; Sympathomimetics; Tricyclic Antidepressants; Vitamin K Antagonists

The levels/effects of Methylphenidate may be increased by: Antacids; Antipsychotics; Atomoxetine; Cannabinoids; H2-Antagonists; MAO Inhibitors; Proton Pump Inhibitors

Decreased Effect

Methylphenidate may decrease the levels/effects of: Antihypertensives; Iobenguane I 123; Ioflupane I 123

Ethanol/Nutrition/Herb Interactions

Ethanol: Avoid ethanol (may cause CNS depression).

Food: Food may increase oral absorption; Concerta® formulation is not affected. Food delays early peak and high-fat meals increase C_{max} and AUC of Metadate CD® formulation.

Herb/Nutraceutical: Avoid ephedra (may cause hypertension or arrhythmias) and yohimbe (also has CNS stimulatory activity).

Stability

Capsule: *Extended release:* Store at 25°C (77°F); excursions permitted to 15°C to 30°C (59°F to 86°F). Protect from light.

Solution: Store at controlled room temperature of 20°C to 25°C (68°F to 77°F).

Tablet:

Chewable: Store at controlled room temperature of 20°C to 25°C (68°F to 77°F). Protect from light and moisture.

Extended and sustained release: Store at controlled room temperature of 20°C to 25°C (68°F to 77°F). Protect from light and moisture.

Immediate release: Store at controlled room temperature of 20°C to 25°C (68°F to 77°F). Protect from light and moisture.

Osmotic controlled release (Concerta®): Store at controlled room temperature of 25°C; excursions permitted to 15°C to 30°C (59°F to 86°F). Protect from humidity.

Transdermal system: Store at 25°C (77°F); excursions permitted to 15°C to 30°C (59°F to 86°F). Keep patches stored in protective pouch. Once tray is opened, use patches within 2 months; once an individual patch has been removed from the pouch and the protective liner removed, use immediately. Do not refrigerate or freeze.

Mechanism of Action Mild CNS stimulant; blocks the reuptake of norepinephrine and dopamine into presynaptic neurons; appears to stimulate the cerebral cortex and subcortical structures similar to amphetamines

Pharmacodynamics/Kinetics

Onset of action: Peak effect:

Immediate release tablet: Cerebral stimulation: ~2 hours

Extended release capsule (Metadate CD®, Ritalin LA®): Biphasic; initial peak similar to immediate release product, followed by second rising portion (corresponding to extended release portion)

Sustained release tablet: 4-7 hours

Osmotic release tablet (Concerta®): Initial: 1-2 hours

Transdermal: ~2 hours; may be expedited by the application of external heat

Duration: Immediate release tablet: 3-6 hours; Sustained release tablet: 8 hours; Extended release tablet: Methylin® ER, Metadate® ER: 8 hours, Concerta®: 12 hours

Absorption:

Oral: Readily absorbed

Transdermal: Absorption increased when applied to inflamed skin or exposed to heat. Absorption is continuous for 9 hours after application.

Distribution: V_d: *d*-methylphenidate: 2.65 ± 1.11 L/kg, *l*-methylphenidate: 1.80 ± 0.91 L/kg

Protein binding: 10% to 33%

Metabolism: Hepatic via carboxylesterase CES1A1 to minimally active metabolite

Half-life elimination: *d*-methylphenidate: 3-4 hours; *l*-methylphenidate: 1-3 hours

Time to peak: Concerta®: C_{max}: 6-8 hours; Daytrana™: 7.5-10.5 hours

Excretion: Urine (90% as metabolites and unchanged drug)

Dosage

ADHD:

Oral:

Immediate release products Children ≥6 years and Adults: Initial: 5 mg/dose (~0.3 mg/kg/dose) given twice daily before breakfast and lunch; increase by 5-10 mg/day (0.2 mg/kg/day) at weekly intervals; maximum dose: 60 mg/day (2 mg/kg/day). **Note:** Discontinue periodically to re-evaluate or if no improvement occurs within 1 month.

Extended release products:

Children ≥6 years and Adults:

Metadate® ER, Methylin® ER, Ritalin® SR: May be given in place of immediate release products, once the daily dose is titrated and the titrated 8-hour dosage corresponds to sustained or extended release tablet size; maximum: 60 mg/day

Metadate CD®, Ritalin LA®: Initial: 20 mg once daily; may be adjusted in 10-20 mg increments at weekly intervals; maximum: 60 mg/day

Children 6-12 years and Adolescents 13-17 years:

Concerta®:

Patients not currently taking methylphenidate: Initial dose: 18 mg once daily in the morning

Patients currently taking methylphenidate: **Note:** Initial dose: Dosing based on current regimen and clinical judgment; suggested dosing listed below:

- Patients taking methylphenidate 5 mg 2-3 times/day: 18 mg once every morning
- Patients taking methylphenidate 10 mg 2-3 times/day: 36 mg once every morning
- Patients taking methylphenidate 15 mg 2-3 times/day: 54 mg once every morning

Dose adjustment: May increase dose in increments of 18 mg; dose may be adjusted at weekly intervals. A dosage strength of 27 mg is available for situations in which a dosage between 18-36 mg is desired. Maximum dose should not exceed 54 mg/day in children 6-12 years **or** 2 mg/kg/day (up to 72 mg/day) in adolescents 13-17 years.

Adults: *Concerta®:*

Patients not currently taking methylphenidate: Initial dose: 18-36 mg once daily in the morning

Patients currently taking methylphenidate: **Note:** Initial dose: Dosing based on current regimen and clinical judgment; suggested dosing listed below:

- Patients taking methylphenidate 5 mg 2-3 times/day: 18 mg once every morning
- Patients taking methylphenidate 10 mg 2-3 times/day: 36 mg once every morning
- Patients taking methylphenidate 15 mg 2-3 times/day: 54 mg once every morning
- Patients taking methylphenidate 20 mg 2-3 times/day: 72 mg once every morning

Dose adjustment: May increase dose in increments of 18 mg; dose may be adjusted at weekly intervals. A dosage strength of 27 mg is available for situations in which a dosage between 18-36 mg is desired. Maximum dose should not exceed 72 mg/day.

Transdermal (Daytrana™): Children 6-12 years and Adolescents 13-17 years: Initial: 10 mg patch once daily; remove up to 9 hours after application. Titrate based on response and tolerability; may increase to next transdermal dose no more frequently than every week. **Note:** Application should occur 2 hours prior to desired effect. Drug absorption may continue for a period of time after patch removal. The prescribing information recommends patients converting from another formulation of methylphenidate should be initiated at 10 mg regardless of their previous dose and titrated as needed due to the differences in bioavailability of the transdermal formulation. However, some clinicians have supported higher starting patch doses for patients converting from oral methylphenidate doses of >20 mg/day; for example, the 18.75 mg patch has been investigated to have the same effect as 22.5 mg/day of the immediate release preparation, 27 mg/day of the osmotic release preparation, or 20 mg/day of the encapsulated bead preparation (Arnold, 2010).

Narcolepsy: Oral: Adults: 10 mg 2-3 times/day, up to 60 mg/day

Depression (unlabeled use): Oral: Adults: Initial: 2.5 mg every morning before 9 AM; dosage may be increased by 2.5-5 mg every 2-3 days as tolerated to a maximum of 20 mg/day; may be divided (ie, 7 AM and 12 noon), but should not be given after noon; do not use sustained release product

Dietary Considerations Should be taken 30-45 minutes before meals. Concerta® is not affected by food. Some products may contain phenylalanine.

Administration

Oral: Do not crush or allow patient to chew sustained or extended release dosage form. To effectively avoid insomnia, dosing should be completed by noon.

Concerta®: Administer dose once daily in the morning. May be taken with or without food, but must be taken with water, milk, or juice.

Metadate CD®, Ritalin LA®: Capsules may be opened and the contents sprinkled onto a small amount (equal to 1 tablespoon) of cold applesauce. Swallow applesauce without chewing. Do not crush or chew capsule contents.

Methylin® chewable tablet: Administer with at least 8 ounces of water or other fluid.

Topical: Transdermal (Daytrana™): Apply to clean, dry, non-oily, intact skin to the hip area, avoiding the waistline; do not premedicate the patch site with hydrocortisone or other solutions, creams, ointments, or emollients. Apply at the same time each day to alternating hips. Press firmly for 30 seconds to ensure proper adherence. Avoid exposure of application site to external heat source, which may increase the amount of drug absorbed. If difficulty is experienced when separating the patch from the liner or if any medication (sticky substance) remains on the liner after separation; discard that patch and apply a new patch. Do not use a patch that has been damaged or torn; do not cut patch. If patch should dislodge, may replace with new patch (to different site) but total wear time should not exceed 9 hours; do not reapply with dressings, tape, or common adhesives. Patch may be removed early if a shorter duration of effect is desired or if late day side effects occur. Wash hands with soap and water after handling. Avoid touching the sticky side of the patch. If patch removal is difficult, an oil-based product (eg, petroleum jelly, olive oil) may be applied to the patch edges to aid removal; never apply acetone-based products (eg, nail polish remover) to patch. Dispose of used patch by folding adhesive side onto itself, and discard in toilet or appropriate lidded container.

Monitoring Parameters Blood pressure, heart rate, signs and symptoms of depression, aggression, or hostility; CBC, differential and platelet counts, liver function tests; growth rate in children, signs of central nervous system stimulation

Transdermal: Signs of worsening erythema, blistering or edema which does not improve within 48 hours of patch removal, or spreads beyond patch site.

When used for the treatment of ADHD, thoroughly evaluate for cardiovascular risk. Monitor heart rate, blood pressure, and consider obtaining ECG prior to initiation (Vetter, 2008).

Test Interactions May interfere with urine detection of amphetamines/methamphetamines (false-positive).

Additional Information Treatment with methylphenidate may include "drug holidays" or periodic discontinuation in order to assess the patient's requirements and to decrease tolerance and limit suppression of linear growth and weight. Specific patients may require 3 doses/day for treatment of ADHD (ie, additional dose at 4 PM).

Concerta® is an osmotic controlled release formulation (OROS®) of methylphenidate. The tablet has an immediate-release overcoat that provides an initial dose of methylphenidate within 1 hour. The overcoat covers a trilayer core. The trilayer core is composed of two layers containing the drug and excipients, and one layer of osmotic components. As water from the gastrointestinal tract enters the core, the osmotic components expand and methylphenidate is released.

Metadate CD® capsules contain a mixture of immediate release and extended release beads, designed to release 30% of the dose immediately and 70% over an extended period.

Ritalin LA® uses a combination of immediate release and enteric coated, delayed release beads.

Dosage Forms Excipient information presented when available (limited, particularly for generics); consult specific product labeling. [DSC] = Discontinued product

Capsule, extended release, oral, as hydrochloride [bi-modal release]: 20 mg [generic for Ritalin LA®], 30 mg [generic for Ritalin LA®], 40 mg [generic for Ritalin LA®]
- Metadate CD®: 10 mg [contains sucrose; 3 mg immediate release, 7 mg extended release]
- Metadate CD®: 20 mg [contains sucrose; 6 mg immediate release, 14 mg extended release]
- Metadate CD®: 30 mg [contains sucrose; 9 mg immediate release, 21 mg extended release]
- Metadate CD®: 40 mg [contains sucrose; 12 mg immediate release, 28 mg extended release]
- Metadate CD®: 50 mg [contains sucrose; 15 mg immediate release, 35 mg extended release]
- Metadate CD®: 60 mg [contains sucrose; 18 mg immediate release, 42 mg extended release]
- Ritalin LA®: 10 mg [5 mg immediate release, 5 mg extended release]
- Ritalin LA®: 20 mg [10 mg immediate release, 10 mg extended release]
- Ritalin LA®: 30 mg [15 mg immediate release, 15 mg extended release]
- Ritalin LA®: 40 mg [20 mg immediate release, 20 mg extended release]

Patch, transdermal:
- Daytrana®: 10 mg/9 hours (30s) [12.5 cm^2, total methylphenidate 27.5 mg]
- Daytrana®: 15 mg/9 hours (30s) [18.75 cm^2, total methylphenidate 41.3 mg]
- Daytrana®: 20 mg/9 hours (30s) [25 cm^2, total methylphenidate 55 mg]
- Daytrana®: 30 mg/9 hours (30s) [37.5 cm^2, total methylphenidate 82.5 mg]

Solution, oral, as hydrochloride: 5 mg/5 mL (500 mL [DSC]); 10 mg/mL (500 mL [DSC])
- Methylin®: 5 mg/5 mL (500 mL); 10 mg/5 mL (500 mL) [grape flavor]

Tablet, oral, as hydrochloride: 5 mg, 10 mg, 20 mg
- Methylin®: 5 mg [DSC]
- Methylin®: 10 mg [DSC], 20 mg [DSC] [scored]
- Ritalin®: 5 mg
- Ritalin®: 10 mg, 20 mg [scored]

Tablet, chewable, oral, as hydrochloride:
- Methylin®: 2.5 mg [contains phenylalanine 0.42 mg/tablet; grape flavor]
- Methylin®: 5 mg [contains phenylalanine 0.84 mg/tablet; grape flavor]
- Methylin®: 10 mg [scored; contains phenylalanine 1.68 mg/tablet; grape flavor]

Tablet, extended release, oral, as hydrochloride: 10 mg, 20 mg
- Metadate® ER: 20 mg [contains lactose]
- Methylin® ER: 10 mg [DSC], 20 mg [DSC]

Tablet, extended release, oral, as hydrochloride [bi-modal release]: 18 mg, 27 mg, 36 mg, 54 mg
- Concerta®: 18 mg [4 mg immediate release, 14 mg extended release]
- Concerta®: 27 mg [6 mg immediate release, 21 mg extended release]
- Concerta®: 36 mg [8 mg immediate release, 28 mg extended release]
- Concerta®: 54 mg [12 mg immediate release, 42 mg extended release]

Tablet, sustained release, oral, as hydrochloride: 20 mg
- Ritalin-SR®: 20 mg [dye free]

Controlled Substance C-II

◆ **Methylphenidate Hydrochloride** *see* Methylphenidate *on page 1107*

◆ **Methylphenobarbital** *see* Mephobarbital *on page 1076*

◆ **Methylphenoxy-Benzene Propanamine** *see* Atomoxetine *on page 163*

◆ **Methylphenyl Isoxazolyl Penicillin** *see* Oxacillin *on page 1256*

◆ **Methylphytyl Napthoquinone** *see* Phytonadione *on page 1351*

MethylPREDNISolone (meth il pred NIS oh lone)

Brand Names: U.S. A-Methapred®; Depo-Medrol®; Medrol®; Medrol® Dosepak™; Solu-MEDROL®

Brand Names: Canada Depo-Medrol®; Medrol®; Methylprednisolone Acetate; Solu-Medrol®

Index Terms 6-α-Methylprednisolone; A-Methapred; Medrol Dose Pack; Methylprednisolone Acetate; Methylprednisolone Sodium Succinate; Solumedrol

Pharmacologic Category Corticosteroid, Systemic

Additional Appendix Information

Contrast Media Reactions, Premedication for Prophylaxis *on page 1976*

Corticosteroids *on page 1888*

Use Primarily as an anti-inflammatory or immunosuppressant agent in the treatment of a variety of diseases including those of hematologic, allergic, inflammatory, neoplastic, and autoimmune origin. Prevention and treatment of graft-versus-host disease following allogeneic bone marrow transplantation.

Unlabeled Use Acute spinal cord injury

Pregnancy Considerations Adverse events have been observed with corticosteroids in animal reproduction studies. Methylprednisolone crosses the placenta. Some studies have shown an association between first trimester systemic corticosteroid use and oral clefts; adverse events in the fetus/neonate have been noted in case reports following large doses of systemic corticosteroids during pregnancy. Pregnant women exposed to methylprednisolone for antirejection therapy following a transplant may contact the National Transplantation Pregnancy Registry (NTPR) at 215-955-4820. Women exposed to methylprednisolone during pregnancy for the treatment of an autoimmune disease may contact the OTIS Autoimmune Diseases Study at 877-311-8972.

Lactation Enters breast milk/use caution

Contraindications Hypersensitivity to methylprednisolone or any component of the formulation; systemic fungal infection (except intra-articular injection in localized joint conditions); administration of live virus vaccines. methylprednisolone formulations containing benzyl alcohol preservative are contraindicated in premature infants; I.M. administration in idiopathic thrombocytopenia purpura; intrathecal administration

Warnings/Precautions Use with caution in patients with thyroid disease, hepatic impairment, renal impairment, cardiovascular disease, diabetes, glaucoma, cataracts, myasthenia gravis, patients at risk for osteoporosis, patients at risk for seizures, or GI diseases (diverticulitis, peptic ulcer, ulcerative colitis) due to perforation risk. Not recommended for the treatment of optic neuritis; may increase frequency of new episodes. Use caution following acute MI (corticosteroids have been associated with myocardial rupture). Cardiomegaly and congestive heart failure have been reported following concurrent use of amphotericin B and hydrocortisone for the management of fungal infections.

Because of the risk of adverse effects, systemic corticosteroids should be used cautiously in the elderly in the smallest possible effective dose for the shortest duration. May affect growth velocity; growth should be routinely monitored in pediatric patients. Withdraw therapy with gradual tapering of dose.

May cause hypercorticism or suppression of hypothalamic-pituitary-adrenal (HPA) axis, particularly in younger children or in patients receiving high doses for prolonged periods. HPA axis suppression may lead to adrenal crisis. Withdrawal and discontinuation of a corticosteroid should be done slowly and carefully. Particular care is required when patients are transferred from systemic corticosteroids to inhaled products due to possible adrenal insufficiency or withdrawal from steroids, including an increase in allergic symptoms. Patients receiving >20 mg per day of prednisone (or equivalent) may be most susceptible. Fatalities have occurred due to adrenal insufficiency in asthmatic patients during and after transfer from systemic corticosteroids to aerosol steroids; aerosol steroids do not provide the systemic steroid needed to treat patients having trauma, surgery, or infections.

Acute myopathy has been reported with high dose corticosteroids, usually in patients with neuromuscular transmission disorders; may involve ocular and/or respiratory muscles; monitor creatine kinase; recovery may be delayed. Corticosteroid use may cause psychiatric disturbances, including depression, euphoria, insomnia, mood swings, and personality changes. Pre-existing psychiatric conditions may be exacerbated by corticosteroid use. Prolonged use of corticosteroids may also increase the incidence of secondary infection, cause activation of latent infections, mask acute infection (including fungal infections), prolong or exacerbate viral or parasitic infections, or limit response to vaccines. Exposure to chickenpox or measles should be avoided; corticosteroids should not be used to treat ocular herpes simplex. Corticosteroids should not be used for cerebral malaria or viral hepatitis. Close observation is required in patients with latent tuberculosis and/or TB reactivity; restrict use in active TB (only in conjunction with antituberculosis treatment). Amebiasis should be ruled out in any patient with recent travel to tropic climates or unexplained diarrhea prior to initiation of corticosteroids. Prolonged treatment with corticosteroids has been associated with the development of Kaposi's sarcoma (case reports); discontinuation may result in clinical improvement.

High-dose corticosteroids should not be used to manage acute head injury. Rare cases of anaphylactoid reactions have been observed in patients receiving corticosteroids. Avoid injection or leakage into the dermis; dermal and/or subdermal skin depression may occur at the site of injection. Avoid deltoid muscle injection; subcutaneous atrophy may occur. Some dosage forms contain benzyl alcohol which has been associated with "gasping syndrome" in neonates.

Adverse Reactions Frequency not defined.

Cardiovascular: Arrhythmias, bradycardia, cardiac arrest, cardiomegaly, circulatory collapse, congestive heart failure, edema, fat embolism, hypertension, hypertrophic cardiomyopathy in premature infants, myocardial rupture (post MI), syncope, tachycardia, thromboembolism, vasculitis

Central nervous system: Delirium, depression, emotional instability, euphoria, hallucinations, headache, intracranial pressure increased, insomnia, malaise, mood swings, nervousness, neuritis, personality changes, psychic disorders, pseudotumor cerebri (usually following discontinuation), seizure, vertigo

Dermatologic: Acne, allergic dermatitis, alopecia, dry scaly skin, ecchymoses, edema, erythema, hirsutism, hyper-/hypopigmentation, hypertrichosis, impaired wound healing, petechiae, rash, skin atrophy, sterile abscess, skin test reaction impaired, striae, urticaria

Endocrine & metabolic: Adrenal suppression, amenorrhea, carbohydrate intolerance increased, Cushing's syndrome, diabetes mellitus, fluid retention, glucose intolerance, growth suppression (children), hyperglycemia, hyperlipidemia, hypokalemia, hypokalemic alkalosis, menstrual irregularities, negative nitrogen balance, pituitary-adrenal axis suppression, protein catabolism, sodium and water retention

Gastrointestinal: Abdominal distention, appetite increased, bowel/bladder dysfunction (after intrathecal administration), gastrointestinal hemorrhage, gastrointestinal perforation, nausea, pancreatitis, peptic ulcer, perforation of the small and large intestine, ulcerative esophagitis, vomiting, weight gain

Hematologic: Leukocytosis (transient)

Hepatic: Hepatomegaly, transaminases increased

Local: Postinjection flare (intra-articular use), thrombophlebitis

Neuromuscular & skeletal: Arthralgia, arthropathy, aseptic necrosis (femoral and humoral heads), fractures, muscle mass loss, muscle weakness, myopathy (particularly in conjunction with neuromuscular disease or neuromuscular-blocking agents), neuropathy, osteoporosis, parasthesia, tendon rupture, vertebral compression fractures, weakness

Ocular: Cataracts, exophthalmoses, glaucoma, intraocular pressure increased

Renal: Glycosuria

Respiratory: Pulmonary edema

Miscellaneous: Abnormal fat disposition, anaphylactoid reaction, anaphylaxis, angioedema, avascular necrosis, diaphoresis, hiccups, hypersensitivity reactions, infections, secondary malignancy

Drug Interactions

Metabolism/Transport Effects Substrate of CYP3A4 (minor); **Note:** Assignment of Major/Minor substrate status based on clinically relevant drug interaction potential; **Inhibits** CYP2C8 (weak), CYP3A4 (weak)

Avoid Concomitant Use

Avoid concomitant use of MethylPREDNISolone with any of the following: Aldesleukin; BCG; Natalizumab; Pimecrolimus; Pimozide; Tacrolimus (Topical)

Increased Effect/Toxicity

MethylPREDNISolone may increase the levels/effects of: Acetylcholinesterase Inhibitors; Amphotericin B; CycloSPORINE; CycloSPORINE (Systemic); Deferasirox; Leflunomide; Loop Diuretics; Natalizumab; NSAID (COX-2 Inhibitor); NSAID (Nonselective); Pimozide; Thiazide Diuretics; Vaccines (Live); Warfarin

The levels/effects of MethylPREDNISolone may be increased by: Antifungal Agents (Azole Derivatives, Systemic); Aprepitant; Calcium Channel Blockers (Nondihydropyridine); CycloSPORINE; CycloSPORINE (Systemic); CYP3A4 Inhibitors (Strong); Denosumab; Estrogen Derivatives; Fluconazole; Fosaprepitant; Indacaterol; Macrolide Antibiotics; Neuromuscular-Blocking Agents (Nondepolarizing); Pimecrolimus; Quinolone Antibiotics; Roflumilast; Salicylates; Tacrolimus (Topical); Telaprevir; Trastuzumab

Decreased Effect

MethylPREDNISolone may decrease the levels/effects of: Aldesleukin; Antidiabetic Agents; BCG; Calcitriol; Coccidioidin Skin Test; Corticorelin; CycloSPORINE; CycloSPORINE (Systemic); Isoniazid; Salicylates; Sipuleucel-T; Telaprevir; Vaccines (Inactivated)

The levels/effects of MethylPREDNISolone may be decreased by: Aminoglutethimide; Antacids; Barbiturates; Bile Acid Sequestrants; Echinacea; Mitotane; Primidone; Rifamycin Derivatives; Tocilizumab

Ethanol/Nutrition/Herb Interactions

Ethanol: Avoid ethanol (may increase gastric mucosal irritation).

Food: Methylprednisolone interferes with calcium absorption. Limit caffeine.

Herb/Nutraceutical: St John's wort may decrease methylprednisolone levels. Avoid cat's claw, echinacea (have immunostimulant properties).

Stability

Intact vials of methylprednisolone sodium succinate should be stored at controlled room temperature of 20°C to 25°C (68°F to 77°F). Protect from light.

Reconstituted solutions of methylprednisolone sodium succinate should be stored at room temperature of 20°C to 25°C (68°F to 77°F), and used within 48 hours.

Stability of parenteral admixture at room temperature (25°C) and at refrigeration temperature (4°C) is 48 hours.

Standard diluent (Solu-Medrol®): 40 mg/50 mL D_5W; 125 mg/50 mL D_5W.

Minimum volume (Solu-Medrol®): 50 mL D_5W.

Mechanism of Action In a tissue-specific manner, corticosteroids regulate gene expression subsequent to binding specific intracellular receptors and translocation into the nucleus. Corticosteroids exert a wide array of physiologic effects including modulation of carbohydrate, protein, and lipid metabolism and maintenance of fluid and electrolyte homeostasis. Moreover cardiovascular, immunologic, musculoskeletal, endocrine, and neurologic physiology are influenced by corticosteroids. Decreases inflammation by suppression of migration of polymorphonuclear leukocytes and reversal of increased capillary permeability.

Pharmacodynamics/Kinetics

Onset of action: Peak effect (route dependent): Oral: 1-2 hours; I.M.: 4-8 days; Intra-articular: 1 week; methylprednisolone sodium succinate is highly soluble and has a rapid effect by I.M. and I.V. routes

Duration (route dependent): Oral: 30-36 hours; I.M.: 1-4 weeks; Intra-articular: 1-5 weeks; methylprednisolone acetate has a low solubility and has a sustained I.M. effect

Distribution: V_d: 0.7-1.5 L/kg

Half-life elimination: 3-3.5 hours; reduced in obese

Excretion: Clearance: Reduced in obese

Dosage Dosing should be based on the lesser of ideal body weight or actual body weight

Only sodium succinate may be given I.V.; methylprednisolone sodium succinate is highly soluble and has a rapid effect by I.M. and I.V. routes. Methylprednisolone acetate has a low solubility and has a sustained I.M. effect.

Children:

Acute spinal cord injury (unlabeled use): I.V. (sodium succinate): 30 mg/kg over 15 minutes, followed in 45 minutes by a continuous infusion of 5.4 mg/kg/hour for 23 hours. **Note:** Due to insufficient evidence of clinical efficacy (ie, preserving or improving spinal cord function), the routine use of methylprednisolone in the treatment of acute spinal cord injury is no longer recommended. If used in this setting, methylprednisolone should not be initiated >8 hours after the injury; not effective in penetrating trauma (eg, gunshot) (Consortium for Spinal Cord Medicine, 2008).

Anti-inflammatory or immunosuppressive: Oral, I.M., I.V. (sodium succinate): 0.5-1.7 mg/kg/day **or** 5-25 mg/m²/day in divided doses every 6-12 hours; "Pulse" therapy: 15-30 mg/kg/dose over ≥30 minutes given once daily for 3 days

Asthma exacerbations, including status asthmaticus (emergency medical care or hospital doses) (NIH Asthma Guidelines, NAEPP, 2007): Children ≤12 years: Oral, I.V.: 1-2 mg/kg/day in 2 divided doses (maximum: 60 mg/day) until peak expiratory flow is 70% of predicted or personal best

Lupus nephritis: I.V. (sodium succinate): 30 mg/kg over ≥30 minutes every other day for 6 doses

Adults: **Only sodium succinate may be given I.V.;** methylprednisolone sodium succinate is highly soluble and has a rapid effect by I.M. and I.V. routes. Methylprednisolone acetate has a low solubility and has a sustained I.M. effect.

Acute spinal cord injury (unlabeled use): I.V. (sodium succinate): 30 mg/kg over 15 minutes, followed in 45 minutes by a continuous infusion of 5.4 mg/kg/hour for 23 hours. **Note:** Due to insufficient evidence of clinical efficacy (ie, preserving or improving spinal cord function), the routine use of methylprednisolone in the treatment of acute spinal cord injury is no longer recommended. If used in this setting, methylprednisolone should not be initiated >8 hours after the injury; not effective in penetrating trauma (eg, gunshot) (Consortium for Spinal Cord Medicine, 2008).

Allergic conditions: Oral: Tapered-dosage schedule (eg, dose-pack containing 21 x 4 mg tablets):

Day 1: 24 mg on day 1 administered as 8 mg (2 tablets) before breakfast, 4 mg (1 tablet) after lunch, 4 mg (1 tablet) after supper, and 8 mg (2 tablets) at bedtime **OR** 24 mg (6 tablets) as a single dose or divided into 2 or 3 doses upon initiation (regardless of time of day)

Day 2: 20 mg on day 2 administered as 4 mg (1 tablet) before breakfast, 4 mg (1 tablet) after lunch, 4 mg (1 tablet) after supper, and 8 mg (2 tablets) at bedtime

Day 3: 16 mg on day 3 administered as 4 mg (1 tablet) before breakfast, 4 mg (1 tablet) after lunch, 4 mg (1 tablet) after supper, and 4 mg (1 tablet) at bedtime

Day 4: 12 mg on day 4 administered as 4 mg (1 tablet) before breakfast, 4 mg (1 tablet) after lunch, and 4 mg (1 tablet) at bedtime

Day 5: 8 mg on day 5 administered as 4 mg (1 tablet) before breakfast and 4 mg (1 tablet) at bedtime
Day 6: 4 mg on day 6 administered as 4 mg (1 tablet) before breakfast
Anti-inflammatory or immunosuppressive:
Oral: 2-60 mg/day in 1-4 divided doses to start, followed by gradual reduction in dosage to the lowest possible level consistent with maintaining an adequate clinical response.
I.M. (sodium succinate): 10-80 mg/day once daily
I.M. (acetate): 10-80 mg every 1-2 weeks
I.V. (sodium succinate): 10-40 mg over a period of several minutes and repeated I.V. or I.M. at intervals depending on clinical response; when high dosages are needed, give 30 mg/kg over a period ≥30 minutes and may be repeated every 4-6 hours for 48 hours.
Arthritis: Intra-articular (acetate): Administer every 1-5 weeks.
Large joints (eg, knee, ankle): 20-80 mg
Medium joints (eg, elbow, wrist): 10-40 mg
Small joints: 4-10 mg
Asthma exacerbations, including status asthmaticus (emergency medical care or hospital doses): Oral, I.V.: 40-80 mg/day in 1- 2 divided doses until peak expiratory flow is 70% of predicted or personal best (NIH Asthma Guidelines, NAEPP, 2007)
Asthma, severe persistent, long-term control: Oral: 7.5-60 mg/day (or on alternate days) (NIH Asthma Guidelines, NAEPP, 2007)
Dermatitis, acute severe: I.M. (acetate): 80-120 mg as a single dose
Dermatitis, chronic: I.M. (acetate): 40-120 mg every 5-10 days
Dermatologic conditions (eg, keloids, lichen planus): Intralesional (acetate): 20-60 mg
Dermatomyositis/polymyositis: I.V. (sodium succinate): 1 g/day for 3-5 days for severe muscle weakness, followed by conversion to oral prednisone (Drake, 1996)
Lupus nephritis: High-dose "pulse" therapy: I.V. (sodium succinate): 0.5-1 g/day for 3 days (Ponticelli, 2010)
Pneumocystis pneumonia in AIDS patients: I.V.: 30 mg twice daily for 5 days, then 30 mg once daily for 5 days, then 15 mg once daily for 11 days

Dietary Considerations Take with meals to decrease GI upset.; need diet rich in pyridoxine, vitamin C, vitamin D, folate, calcium, phosphorus, and protein.

Administration
Administer with meals to decrease GI upset.
Parenteral: Methylprednisolone sodium succinate may be administered I.M. or I.V.; I.V. administration may be IVP over one to several minutes or IVPB or continuous I.V. infusion. **Acetate salt should not be given I.V.** Avoid injection into the deltoid muscle due to a high incidence of subcutaneous atrophy. Avoid injection or leakage into the dermis; dermal and/or subdermal skin depression may occur at the site of injection.
I.V.: Succinate:
Low dose: ≤1.8 mg/kg or ≤125 mg/dose: I.V. push over 3-15 minutes
Moderate dose: ≥2 mg/kg or 250 mg/dose: I.V. over 15-30 minutes
High dose: 15 mg/kg or ≥500 mg/dose: I.V. over ≥30 minutes
Doses >15 mg/kg or ≥1 g: Administer over 1 hour
Do **not** administer high-dose I.V. push; hypotension, cardiac arrhythmia, and sudden death have been reported in patients given high-dose methylprednisolone I.V. push (>0.5 g over <10 minutes); intermittent infusion over 15-60 minutes; maximum concentration: I.V. push 125 mg/mL
I.M.: Avoid injection into the deltoid muscle due to a high incidence of subcutaneous atrophy. Avoid injection or leakage into the dermis; dermal and/or subdermal skin depression may occur at the site of injection. Do not inject into areas that have evidence of acute local infection.

Monitoring Parameters Blood pressure, blood glucose, electrolytes, growth in children

Test Interactions Interferes with skin tests

Additional Information Sodium content of 1 g sodium succinate injection: 2.01 mEq; 53 mg of sodium succinate salt is equivalent to 40 mg of methylprednisolone base
Methylprednisolone acetate: Depo-Medrol®
Methylprednisolone sodium succinate: Solu-Medrol®

Dosage Forms Excipient information presented when available (limited, particularly for generics); consult specific product labeling.
Injection, powder for reconstitution, as sodium succinate [strength expressed as base]: 40 mg, 125 mg, 500 mg, 1 g
A-Methapred®: 40 mg [contains benzyl alcohol (in diluent), lactose 25 mg/vial]
A-Methapred®: 40 mg [contains lactose 25 mg/vial]
A-Methapred®: 125 mg
A-Methapred®: 125 mg [contains benzyl alcohol (in diluent)]
Solu-MEDROL®: 500 mg, 1 g
Solu-MEDROL®: 2 g [contains benzyl alcohol (in diluent)]
Injection, powder for reconstitution, as sodium succinate [strength expressed as base, preservative free]:
Solu-MEDROL®: 40 mg [contains lactose 25 mg/vial; supplied with diluent]
Solu-MEDROL®: 125 mg, 500 mg, 1 g [supplied with diluent]
Injection, suspension, as acetate: 40 mg/mL (1 mL, 5 mL, 10 mL); 80 mg/mL (1 mL, 5 mL)
Depo-Medrol®: 20 mg/mL (5 mL); 40 mg/mL (5 mL, 10 mL); 80 mg/mL (5 mL) [contains benzyl alcohol, polysorbate 80]
Injection, suspension, as acetate [preservative free]:
Depo-Medrol®: 40 mg/mL (1 mL); 80 mg/mL (1 mL)
Tablet, oral: 4 mg, 8 mg, 16 mg, 32 mg
Medrol®: 2 mg, 4 mg, 8 mg, 16 mg, 32 mg [scored]
Tablet, oral [dose-pack]: 4 mg [21s]
Medrol® Dosepak™: 4 mg [scored; 21s]

◆ **6-α-Methylprednisolone** *see* MethylPREDNISolone *on page 1110*

◆ **Methylprednisolone Acetate** *see* MethylPREDNISolone *on page 1110*

◆ **Methylprednisolone Sodium Succinate** *see* MethylPREDNISolone *on page 1110*

◆ **4-Methylpyrazole** *see* Fomepizole *on page 751*

◆ **Methylrosaniline Chloride** *see* Gentian Violet *on page 792*

Methyl Salicylate and Menthol

(METH il sa LIS i late & MEN thol)

Brand Names: U.S. BenGay® [OTC]; Icy Hot® [OTC]; Salonpas® Arthritis Pain® [OTC]; Salonpas® Pain Relief Patch® [OTC]; Salonpas® [OTC]; Thera-Gesic® Plus [OTC]; Thera-Gesic® [OTC]

Index Terms Menthol and Methyl Salicylate

Pharmacologic Category Analgesic, Topical; Salicylate; Topical Skin Product

Use Temporary relief of minor aches and pains of muscle and joints associated with arthritis, bruises, simple backache, sprains, and strains

Dosage Topical: Pain relief:
Balm, cream, stick: Children ≥12 years and Adults: Apply to affected area; may repeat up to 3-4 times/day
Gel: Children ≥2 years and Adults: Apply to affected area; may repeat up to 3-4 times/day for up to 7 days

Patch: Adults: Apply 1 patch to affected area and leave in place for up to 8-12 hours; do not exceed 1 patch/application. If pain still present, a second patch may be applied for up to 8-12 hours (maximum: 2 patches/24 hours; 3 days of consecutive use)

Additional Information Complete prescribing information for this medication should be consulted for additional detail.

Dosage Forms Excipient information presented when available (limited, particularly for generics); consult specific product labeling.

Balm, topical:

Icy Hot® Balm: Methyl salicylate 29% and menthol 7.6% (99.2 g)

Cream, topical:

BenGay® Arthritis Formula: Methyl salicylate 30% and menthol 8% (57 g, 113 g)

BenGay® Greaseless: Methyl salicylate 15% and menthol 10% (57 g, 113 g)

Icy Hot®: Methyl salicylate 30% and menthol 10% (35.4 g, 85 g)

Thera-Gesic®: Methyl salicylate 15% and menthol 1% (85 g, 142 g)

Thera-Gesic® Plus: Methyl salicylate 15% and menthol 4% (85 g) [contains aloe]

Gel, topical:

Salonpas®: Methyl salicylate 15% and menthol 7% (40 g) [contains ethanol]

Patch, topical:

Salonpas® Arthritis Pain®: Methyl salicylate 10% and menthol 3% (5s) [contains metal]

Salonpas® Pain Relief Patch®: Methyl salicylate 10% and menthol 3% (5s) [contains metal]

Stick, topical:

Icy Hot®: Methyl salicylate 30% and menthol 10% (49 g)

MethylTESTOSTERone (meth il tes TOS te rone)

Brand Names: U.S. Android®; Methitest™; Testred®

Pharmacologic Category Androgen

Additional Appendix Information

Beers Criteria – Potentially Inappropriate Medications for Geriatrics *on page 1973*

Use

Male: Hypogonadism; delayed puberty; impotence and climacteric symptoms

Female: Palliative treatment of metastatic breast cancer

Unlabeled Use Hypogonadism (male); delayed puberty (male)

Pregnancy Risk Factor X

Dosage Oral: Adults:

Males:

Hypogonadism; delayed puberty: Individualize dose based on response and tolerability.

Androgen deficiency: 10-50 mg/day

Females: Breast cancer: 50-200 mg/day

Additional Information Complete prescribing information for this medication should be consulted for additional detail.

Dosage Forms Excipient information presented when available (limited, particularly for generics); consult specific product labeling.

Capsule, oral:

Android®: 10 mg

Testred®: 10 mg

Tablet, oral:

Methitest™: 10 mg [scored]

Controlled Substance C-III

◆ **Methylthionine Chloride** *see* Methylene Blue *on page 1104*

Metipranolol (met i PRAN oh lol)

Brand Names: U.S. OptiPranolol®

Brand Names: Canada OptiPranolol®

Index Terms Metipranolol Hydrochloride

Pharmacologic Category Beta-Adrenergic Blocker, Nonselective; Ophthalmic Agent, Antiglaucoma

Use Treatment of chronic open-angle glaucoma or ocular hypertension

Pregnancy Risk Factor C

Dosage Ophthalmic: Adults: Instill 1 drop in the affected eye(s) twice daily

Additional Information Complete prescribing information for this medication should be consulted for additional detail.

Dosage Forms Excipient information presented when available (limited, particularly for generics); consult specific product labeling.

Solution, ophthalmic [drops]: 0.3% (5 mL, 10 mL)

OptiPranolol®: 0.3% (5 mL, 10 mL) [contains benzalkonium chloride]

◆ **Metipranolol Hydrochloride** *see* Metipranolol *on page 1114*

Metoclopramide (met oh KLOE pra mide)

Brand Names: U.S. Metozolv™ ODT; Reglan®

Brand Names: Canada Apo-Metoclop®; Metoclopramide Hydrochloride Injection; Metoclopramide Omega; Nu-Metoclopramide; PMS-Metoclopramide

Pharmacologic Category Antiemetic; Gastrointestinal Agent, Prokinetic

Use

Oral: Symptomatic treatment of diabetic gastroparesis; gastroesophageal reflux

I.V., I.M.: Symptomatic treatment of diabetic gastroparesis; postpyloric placement of enteral feeding tubes; prevention and/or treatment of nausea and vomiting associated with chemotherapy, or postsurgery; to stimulate gastric emptying and intestinal transit of barium during radiological examination of the stomach/small intestine

Pregnancy Risk Factor B

Pregnancy Considerations Teratogenic effects were not observed in animal studies; however, there are no adequate and well-controlled studies in pregnant women. Crosses the placenta; available evidence suggests safe use during pregnancy.

Lactation Enters breast milk/use caution

Medication Guide Available Yes

Contraindications Hypersensitivity to metoclopramide or any component of the formulation; GI obstruction, perforation or hemorrhage; pheochromocytoma; history of seizures or concomitant use of other agents likely to increase extrapyramidal reactions

Warnings/Precautions [U.S. Boxed Warning]: May cause tardive dyskinesia, which is often irreversible; duration of treatment and total cumulative dose are associated with an increased risk. Therapy durations >12 weeks should be avoided (except in rare cases following risk:benefit assessment). Risk appears to be increased in the elderly, women, and diabetics; however, it is not possible to predict which patients will develop tardive dyskinesia. Therapy should be discontinued in any patient if signs/symptoms of tardive dyskinesia appear.

May cause extrapyramidal symptoms, generally manifested as acute dystonic reactions within the initial 24-48 hours of use. Risk of these reactions is increased at higher doses, and in pediatric patients, and adults <30 years of age. Pseudoparkinsonism (eg, bradykinesia, tremor, rigidity) may also occur (usually within first 6 months of therapy) and is generally reversible following discontinuation. Use with caution or avoid in patients with Parkinson's disease. Use caution in the elderly; may have increased risk of tardive dyskinesia, particularly older women. Neuroleptic malignant syndrome (NMS) has been reported (rarely) with metoclopramide.

May cause transient increase in serum aldosterone; use caution in patients who are at risk of fluid overload (HF, cirrhosis). Use caution in patients with hypertension or following surgical anastomosis/closure. Use caution with a history of mental illness; has been associated with depression. Abrupt discontinuation may (rarely) result in withdrawal symptoms (dizziness, headache, nervousness). Use caution and adjust dose in renal impairment. Patients with NADH-cytochrome b5 reductase deficiency are at increased risk of methemoglobinemia and/or sulfhemoglobinemia. Neonates may have an increased risk of methemoglobinemia due to decreased levels of NADH-cytochrome b5 reductase deficiency and prolonged clearance of metoclopramide.

Adverse Reactions Frequency not always defined.

Cardiovascular: AV block, bradycardia, HF, fluid retention, flushing (following high I.V. doses), hyper-/hypotension, supraventricular tachycardia

Central nervous system: Drowsiness (~10% to 70%; dose related), acute dystonic reactions (<1% to 25%; dose and age related), fatigue (2% to 10%), lassitude (~10%), restlessness (~10%), headache (4% to 5%), dizziness (1% to 4%), somnolence (2% to 3%), akathisia, confusion, depression, hallucinations (rare), insomnia, neuroleptic malignant syndrome (rare), Parkinsonian-like symptoms, suicidal ideation, seizure, tardive dyskinesia

Dermatologic: Angioneurotic edema (rare), rash, urticaria

Endocrine & metabolic: Amenorrhea, galactorrhea, gynecomastia, hyperprolactinemia, impotence

Gastrointestinal: Nausea (4% to 6%), vomiting (1% to 2%), diarrhea

Genitourinary: Incontinence, urinary frequency

Hematologic: Agranulocytosis, leukopenia, neutropenia, porphyria

Hepatic: Hepatotoxicity (rare)

Ocular: Visual disturbance

Respiratory: Bronchospasm, laryngeal edema (rare), laryngospasm (rare)

Miscellaneous: Allergic reactions, methemoglobinemia, sulfhemoglobinemia

Drug Interactions

Metabolism/Transport Effects **Substrate** of CYP1A2 (minor), CYP2D6 (minor); **Note:** Assignment of Major/Minor substrate status based on clinically relevant drug interaction potential; **Inhibits** CYP2D6 (weak)

Avoid Concomitant Use

Avoid concomitant use of Metoclopramide with any of the following: Antipsychotics; Droperidol; Promethazine; Tetrabenazine

Increased Effect/Toxicity

Metoclopramide may increase the levels/effects of: Antipsychotics; CycloSPORINE; CycloSPORINE (Systemic); Prilocaine; Promethazine; Selective Serotonin Reuptake Inhibitors; Tetrabenazine; Tricyclic Antidepressants; Venlafaxine

The levels/effects of Metoclopramide may be increased by: Droperidol; Serotonin Modulators

Decreased Effect

Metoclopramide may decrease the levels/effects of: Anti-Parkinson's Agents (Dopamine Agonist); Posaconazole; Quinagolide

The levels/effects of Metoclopramide may be decreased by: Cyproterone; Peginterferon Alfa-2b

Ethanol/Nutrition/Herb Interactions Ethanol: Avoid ethanol (may increase CNS depression).

Stability

Injection: Store intact vial at controlled room temperature. Injection is photosensitive and should be protected from light during storage. Parenteral admixtures in D_5W or NS are stable for at least 24 hours and do not require light protection if used within 24 hours.

Tablet: Store at controlled room temperature of 20°C to 25°C (68°F to 77°F).

Mechanism of Action Blocks dopamine receptors and (when given in higher doses) also blocks serotonin receptors in chemoreceptor trigger zone of the CNS; enhances the response to acetylcholine of tissue in upper GI tract causing enhanced motility and accelerated gastric emptying without stimulating gastric, biliary, or pancreatic secretions; increases lower esophageal sphincter tone

Pharmacodynamics/Kinetics

Onset of action: Oral: 30-60 minutes; I.V.: 1-3 minutes; I.M.: 10-15 minutes

Duration: Therapeutic: 1-2 hours, regardless of route

Absorption: Oral: Rapid

Distribution: V_d: ~3.5 L/kg

Protein binding: ~30%

Bioavailability: Oral: Range: 65% to 95%

Half-life elimination: Normal renal function: Children: ~4 hours; Adults: 5-6 hours (may be dose dependent)

Time to peak, serum: Oral: 1-2 hours

Excretion: Urine (~85%)

Dosage

Children:

Gastroesophageal reflux (unlabeled use): Oral: 0.1-0.2 mg/kg/dose 4 times/day

Antiemetic (chemotherapy-induced emesis) (unlabeled): I.V.: 1-2 mg/kg 30 minutes before chemotherapy and every 2-4 hours (maximum: 5 doses/day); pretreatment with diphenhydramine will decrease risk of extrapyramidal reactions to this dosage

Postpyloric feeding tube placement: I.V.:

<6 years: 0.1 mg/kg as a single dose

6-14 years: 2.5-5 mg as a single dose

>14 years: Refer to adult dosing.

Adults:

Gastroesophageal reflux: Oral: 10-15 mg/dose up to 4 times/day 30 minutes before meals or food and at bedtime; single doses of 20 mg are occasionally needed prior to provoking situations. Treatment >12 weeks is not recommended.

Diabetic gastroparesis:

Oral: 10 mg/dose up to 4 times/day 30 minutes before meals or food and at bedtime for 2-8 weeks

I.M., I.V. (for severe symptoms): 10 mg over 1-2 minutes; 10 days of I.V. therapy may be necessary before symptoms are controlled to allow transition to oral administration

Chemotherapy-induced emesis prophylaxis: I.V.: 1-2 mg/kg 30 minutes before chemotherapy and repeated every 2 hours for 2 doses, then every 3 hours for 3 doses (manufacturer labeling); pretreatment with diphenhydramine will decrease risk of extrapyramidal reactions

Alternate dosing: **Note:** Metoclopramide is considered an antiemetic with a low therapeutic index; use is generally reserved for agents with low emetogenic potential or in patients intolerant/refractory to first-line antiemetics.

Low-risk chemotherapy (unlabeled): I.V., Oral: 10-40 mg prior to dose, then every 4-6 hours as needed (NCCN Antiemesis guidelines, v.4.2009)

Breakthrough treatment (unlabeled): I.V., Oral: 10-40 mg every 4-6 hours (NCCN Antiemesis guidelines, v.4.2009)

Delayed-emesis prophylaxis (unlabeled): Oral: 20-40 mg/dose (or 0.5 mg/kg/dose) 2-4 times/day for 3-4 days (in combination with dexamethasone [ASCO guidelines, 2006])
Refractory or intolerant to antiemetics with a higher therapeutic index (unlabeled; Hesketh, 2008):
I.V.: 1-2 mg/kg/dose before chemotherapy and repeat 2 hours after chemotherapy
Oral: 0.5 mg/kg every 6 hours on days 2-4
Postoperative nausea and vomiting prophylaxis: I.M., I.V. (unlabeled route): 10-20 mg near end of surgery. **Note:** Guidelines discourage use of 10 mg metoclopramide as being ineffective (Gan, 2007); comparative study indicates higher dose (20 mg) may be efficacious (Quaynor, 2002)
Postpyloric feeding tube placement, radiological exam: I.V.: 10 mg as a single dose
Elderly: Initial: Dose at the lower end of the recommended range. Refer to adult dosing.

Dosing adjustment in renal impairment: Cl_{cr} <40 mL/minute: Administer at 50% of normal dose
Hemodialysis: Not dialyzable (0% to 5%); supplemental dose is not necessary

Administration
Injection solution: May be given I.M., direct I.V. push, short infusion (15-30 minutes), or continuous infusion; lower doses (≤10 mg) of metoclopramide can be given I.V. push undiluted over 1-2 minutes; higher doses (>10 mg) to be diluted in 50 mL of compatible solution (preferably NS) and given IVPB over at least 15 minutes; continuous SubQ infusion and rectal administration have been reported. **Note:** Rapid I.V. administration may be associated with a transient (but intense) feeling of anxiety and restlessness, followed by drowsiness.
Orally-disintegrating tablets: Administer on an empty stomach at least 30 minutes prior to food. Do not remove from packaging until time of administration. If tablet breaks or crumbles while handling, discard and remove new tablet. Using dry hands, place tablet on tongue and allow to dissolve. Swallow with saliva.

Monitoring Parameters Dystonic reactions; signs of hypoglycemia in patients using insulin and those being treated for gastroparesis; agitation, and confusion

Test Interactions Increased aminotransferase [ALT/AST] (S), increased amylase (S)

Dosage Forms Excipient information presented when available (limited, particularly for generics); consult specific product labeling.
Injection, solution [preservative free]: 5 mg/mL (2 mL)
Reglan®: 5 mg/mL (2 mL, 10 mL, 30 mL)
Solution, oral: 5 mg/5 mL (0.9 mL, 10 mL, 473 mL)
Tablet, oral: 5 mg, 10 mg
Reglan®: 5 mg
Reglan®: 10 mg [scored]
Tablet, orally disintegrating, oral:
Metozolv™ ODT: 5 mg, 10 mg [mint flavor]

◆ **Metoclopramide Hydrochloride Injection (Can)** *see* Metoclopramide *on page 1114*

◆ **Metoclopramide Omega (Can)** *see* Metoclopramide *on page 1114*

Metolazone (me TOLE a zone)

Brand Names: U.S. Zaroxolyn®
Brand Names: Canada Zaroxolyn®
Pharmacologic Category Diuretic, Thiazide-Related
Additional Appendix Information
Heart Failure (Systolic) *on page 1991*
Use Management of mild-to-moderate hypertension; treatment of edema in heart failure and nephrotic syndrome, impaired renal function

Pregnancy Risk Factor B
Pregnancy Considerations Teratogenic effects were not observed in animal studies. Metolazone crosses the placenta and appears in cord blood. Hypoglycemia, hypokalemia, hyponatremia, jaundice, and thrombocytopenia are reported as complications to the fetus or newborn following maternal use of thiazide diuretics.
Lactation Enters breast milk/not recommended
Contraindications Hypersensitivity to metolazone, any component of the formulation, other thiazides, and sulfonamide derivatives; anuria; hepatic coma; pregnancy (expert analysis)
Warnings/Precautions Electrolyte disturbances (hypokalemia, hypochloremic alkalosis, hyponatremia) can occur. Large or prolonged fluid and electrolyte losses may occur with concomitant furosemide administration. Use with caution in severe hepatic dysfunction; hepatic encephalopathy can be caused by electrolyte disturbances. Gout can be precipitate in certain patients with a history of gout, a familial predisposition to gout, or chronic renal failure. Cautious use in patients with prediabetes or diabetes; may see a change in glucose control. Can cause SLE exacerbation or activation. Use caution in severe renal impairment. Use with caution in patients with moderate or high cholesterol concentrations. Photosensitization may occur.

Chemical similarities are present among sulfonamides, sulfonylureas, carbonic anhydrase inhibitors, thiazides, and loop diuretics (except ethacrynic acid). Use in patients with thiazide or sulfonamide allergy is specifically contraindicated in product labeling, however, a risk of cross-reaction exists in patients with allergy to any of these compounds; avoid use when previous reaction has been severe. Discontinue if signs of hypersensitivity are noted.

Adverse Reactions Frequency not defined.
Cardiovascular: Chest pain/discomfort, necrotizing angiitis, orthostatic hypotension, palpitation, syncope, venous thrombosis, vertigo, volume depletion
Central nervous system: Chills, depression, dizziness, drowsiness, fatigue, headache, lightheadedness, restlessness
Dermatologic: Petechiae, photosensitivity, pruritus, purpura, rash, skin necrosis, Stevens-Johnson syndrome, toxic epidermal necrolysis, urticaria
Endocrine & metabolic: Gout attacks, hypercalcemia, hyperglycemia, hyperuricemia, hypochloremia, hypochloremic alkalosis, hypokalemia, hypomagnesemia, hyponatremia, hypophosphatemia
Gastrointestinal: Abdominal bloating, abdominal pain, anorexia, constipation, diarrhea, epigastric distress, nausea, pancreatitis, vomiting, xerostomia
Genitourinary: Impotence
Hematologic: Agranulocytosis, aplastic/hypoplastic anemia, hemoconcentration, leukopenia, thrombocytopenia
Hepatic: Cholestatic jaundice, hepatitis
Neuromuscular & skeletal: Joint pain, muscle cramps/spasm, neuropathy, paresthesia, weakness
Ocular: Blurred vision (transient)
Renal: BUN increased, glucosuria

Drug Interactions
Metabolism/Transport Effects None known.
Avoid Concomitant Use
Avoid concomitant use of Metolazone with any of the following: Dofetilide
Increased Effect/Toxicity
Metolazone may increase the levels/effects of: ACE Inhibitors; Allopurinol; Amifostine; Antihypertensives; Calcium Salts; CarBAMazepine; Dofetilide; Hypotensive Agents; Lithium; OXcarbazepine; Porfimer; RiTUXimab; Sodium Phosphates; Topiramate; Toremifene; Vitamin D Analogs

The levels/effects of Metolazone may be increased by: Alcohol (Ethyl); Alfuzosin; Analgesics (Opioid); Barbiturates; Beta2-Agonists; Corticosteroids (Orally Inhaled); Corticosteroids (Systemic); Herbs (Hypotensive Properties); Licorice; MAO Inhibitors; Pentoxifylline; Phosphodiesterase 5 Inhibitors; Prostacyclin Analogues

Decreased Effect

Metolazone may decrease the levels/effects of: Antidiabetic Agents

The levels/effects of Metolazone may be decreased by: Bile Acid Sequestrants; Herbs (Hypertensive Properties); Methylphenidate; Nonsteroidal Anti-Inflammatory Agents; Yohimbine

Ethanol/Nutrition/Herb Interactions

Ethanol: May potentiate hypotensive effect of metazolone.

Herb/Nutraceutical: Avoid herbs with *hypertensive* properties (bayberry, blue cohosh, cayenne, ephedra, ginger, ginseng [American], kola, licorice); may diminish the antihypertensive effect of metolazone. Avoid herbs with *hypotensive* properties (black cohosh, California poppy, coleus, golden seal, hawthorn, mistletoe, periwinkle, quinine, shepherd's purse); may enhance the hypotensive effect of metolazone.

Mechanism of Action Inhibits sodium reabsorption in the distal tubules causing increased excretion of sodium and water, as well as, potassium and hydrogen ions

Pharmacodynamics/Kinetics

Onset of action: Diuresis: ~60 minutes

Duration: ≥24 hours

Absorption: Incomplete

Distribution: Crosses placenta; enters breast milk

Protein binding: 95%

Half-life elimination: 20 hours

Excretion: Urine (80%); bile (10%)

Dosage Oral:

Adults:

Edema: Initial: 2.5-10 mg once daily; may increase as necessary to 20 mg once daily (ACC/AHA 2009 Heart Failure Guidelines); **Note:** Dosing frequency may be adjusted based on patient-specific diuretic needs (eg, administration every other day or weekly) (Lindenfeld, 2010).

Hypertension: 2.5-5 mg/dose every 24 hours

Elderly: Initial: 2.5 mg/day or every other day

Dosage adjustment in renal impairment: Dialysis: Not dialyzable (0% to 5%) via hemo- or peritoneal dialysis; supplemental dose is not necessary

Dietary Considerations Should be taken after breakfast; may require potassium supplementation

Administration May be taken with food or milk. Take early in day to avoid nocturia. Take the last dose of multiple doses no later than 6 PM unless instructed otherwise.

Monitoring Parameters Serum electrolytes (potassium, sodium, chloride, bicarbonate), renal function, blood pressure (standing, sitting/supine)

Additional Information Metolazone 5 mg is approximately equivalent to hydrochlorothiazide 50 mg.

Dosage Forms Excipient information presented when available (limited, particularly for generics); consult specific product labeling.

Tablet, oral: 2.5 mg, 5 mg, 10 mg

Zaroxolyn®: 2.5 mg, 5 mg

Extemporaneous Preparations A 1 mg/mL oral suspension may be made by with tablets and one of three different vehicles (cherry syrup diluted 1:4 with simple syrup; a 1:1 mixture of Ora-Sweet® and Ora-Plus®; or a 1:1 mixture of Ora-Sweet® SF and Ora-Plus®). Crush twelve 10 mg tablets in a mortar and reduce to a fine powder. Add small portions of the chosen vehicle and mix to a uniform paste; mix while adding the vehicle in incremental proportions to **almost** 120 mL; transfer to a calibrated bottle, rinse mortar with vehicle, and add quantity of vehicle sufficient to make 120 mL. Label "shake well" and "refrigerate". Stable for 60 days.

A 0.25 mg/mL oral suspension may be made with tablets and a 1:1 mixture of methylcellulose 1% and simple syrup. Crush one 2.5 mg tablet in a mortar and reduce to a fine powder. Add small portions of the vehicle and mix to a uniform paste; mix while adding the vehicle in incremental proportions to **almost** 10 mL; transfer to a calibrated bottle, rinse mortar with vehicle, and add quantity of vehicle sufficient to make 10 mL. Label "shake well" and "refrigerate". Stable for 91 days refrigerated (preferred), 28 days at room temperature in plastic, and 14 days at room temperature in glass.

Nahata, MC, Pai VB, and Hipple TF, *Pediatric Drug Formulations*, 5th ed, Cincinnati, OH: Harvey Whitney Books Co, 2004.

Metoprolol (me toe PROE lole)

Brand Names: U.S. Lopressor®; Toprol-XL®

Brand Names: Canada Apo-Metoprolol (Type L®); Apo-Metoprolol SR®; Apo-Metoprolol®; Betaloc®; Dom-Metoprolol; JAMP-Metoprolol-L; Lopressor®; Metoprolol Tartrate Injection, USP; Metoprolol-25; Metoprolol-L; Mylan-Metoprolol (Type L); Nu-Metop; PHL-Metoprolol; PMS-Metoprolol; Riva-Metoprolol; Sandoz-Metoprolol (Type L); Sandoz-Metoprolol SR; Teva-Metoprolol

Index Terms Metoprolol Succinate; Metoprolol Tartrate

Pharmacologic Category Antianginal Agent; Beta Blocker, Beta-1 Selective

Additional Appendix Information

Beta-Blockers *on page 1884*

Heart Failure (Systolic) *on page 1991*

Use Treatment of angina pectoris, hypertension, or hemodynamically-stable acute myocardial infarction

Extended release: Treatment of angina pectoris or hypertension; to reduce mortality/hospitalization in patients with heart failure (stable NYHA Class II or III) already receiving ACE inhibitors, diuretics, and/or digoxin

Unlabeled Use Treatment of ventricular arrhythmias, atrial ectopy; migraine prophylaxis, essential tremor, aggressive behavior (not recommended for dementia-associated aggression); prevention of reinfarction and sudden death after myocardial infarction; prevention and treatment of atrial fibrillation and atrial flutter; multifocal atrial tachycardia; symptomatic treatment of hypertrophic obstructive cardiomyopathy; management of thyrotoxicosis

Pregnancy Risk Factor C

Pregnancy Considerations Adverse events were observed in animal studies; therefore, the manufacturer classifies metoprolol as pregnancy category C. Metoprolol crosses the placenta and can be detected in cord blood, amniotic fluid, and the serum of newborn infants. In a cohort study, an increased risk of cardiovascular defects was observed following maternal use of beta-blockers during pregnancy. Intrauterine growth restriction (IUGR), small placentas, as well as fetal/neonatal bradycardia, hypoglycemia, and/or respiratory depression have been observed following *in utero* exposure to beta-blockers as a class. Adequate facilities for monitoring infants at birth should be available. Untreated chronic maternal hypertension and pre-eclampsia are also associated with adverse events in the fetus, infant, and mother. The clearance of metoprolol is increased and serum concentrations and AUC of metoprolol are decreased during pregnancy. Metoprolol has been evaluated for the treatment of hypertension in pregnancy, but other agents may be more appropriate for use.

Lactation Enters breast milk/use caution (AAP rates "compatible"; AAP 2001 update pending)

Contraindications

Hypersensitivity to metoprolol, any component of the formulation, or other beta-blockers

Note: Additional contraindications are formulation and/or indication specific.

Immediate release tablets/injectable formulation:

Hypertension and angina: Sinus bradycardia; second- and third-degree heart block; cardiogenic shock; overt heart failure; sick sinus syndrome (except in patients with a functioning artificial pacemaker); severe peripheral arterial disease; pheochromocytoma (without alpha blockade)

Myocardial infarction: Severe sinus bradycardia (heart rate <45 beats/minute); significant first-degree heart block (P-R interval ≥0.24 seconds); second- and third-degree heart block; systolic blood pressure <100 mm Hg; moderate-to-severe cardiac failure

Extended release tablet: Severe bradycardia, second- and third degree heart block; cardiogenic shock; decompensated heart failure; sick sinus syndrome (except in patients with a functioning artificial pacemaker)

Warnings/Precautions [U.S. Boxed Warning]: Beta-blocker therapy should not be withdrawn abruptly (particularly in patients with CAD), but gradually tapered over 1-2 weeks to avoid acute tachycardia, hypertension, and/or ischemia. Consider pre-existing conditions such as sick sinus syndrome before initiating. Metoprolol commonly produces mild first-degree heart block (P-R interval >0.2-0.24 sec). May also produce severe first- (P-R interval ≥0.26 sec), second-, or third-degree heart block. Patients with acute MI (especially right ventricular MI) have a high risk of developing heart block of varying degrees. If severe heart block occurs, metoprolol should be discontinued and measures to increase heart rate should be employed. Symptomatic hypotension may occur with use. May precipitate or aggravate symptoms of arterial insufficiency in patients with PVD and Raynaud's disease; use with caution and monitor for progression of arterial obstruction. Use caution with concurrent use of digoxin, verapamil, or diltiazem; bradycardia or heart block can occur; avoid concurrent I.V. use of both agents. Use with caution in patients receiving inhaled anesthetic agents known to depress myocardial contractility. Use with caution in patients receiving CYP2D6 inhibitors (eg, bupropion, chlorpromazine, cimetidine, diphenhydramine, hydroxychloroquine, fluoxetine, paroxetine, propafenone, propoxyphene, quinidine, ritonavir, terbinafine, thioridazine); concurrent use may increase metoprolol plasma concentrations.

In general, beta-blockers should be avoided in patients with bronchospastic disease. Metoprolol, with B_1 selectivity, should be used cautiously in bronchospastic disease with close monitoring. Use cautiously in patients with diabetes because it can mask prominent hypoglycemic symptoms. May mask signs of hyperthyroidism (eg, tachycardia); if hyperthyroidism is suspected, carefully manage and monitor; abrupt withdrawal may exacerbate symptoms of hyperthyroidism or precipitate thyroid storm. Alterations in thyroid function tests may be observed. Use caution with hepatic dysfunction. Use with caution in patients with myasthenia gravis or psychiatric disease (may cause CNS depression). Although perioperative beta-blocker therapy is recommended prior to elective surgery in selected patients, use of high-dose extended release metoprolol in patients naïve to beta-blocker therapy undergoing noncardiac surgery has been associated with bradycardia, hypotension, stroke, and death. Chronic beta-blocker therapy should not be routinely withdrawn prior to major surgery. Use of beta-blockers may unmask cardiac failure in patients without a history of dysfunction. Adequate alpha-blockade is required prior to use of any beta-blocker for patients with untreated pheochromocytoma. May induce or exacerbate psoriasis. Use caution with history of severe anaphylaxis to allergens; patients taking beta-blockers may become more sensitive to repeated allergen challenges. Treatment of anaphylaxis (eg, epinephrine) in patients taking beta-blockers may be ineffective or promote undesirable effects. Bradycardia may be observed more frequently in elderly patients (>65 years of age); dosage reductions may be necessary.

Extended release: Use with caution in patients with compensated heart failure; monitor for a worsening of heart failure.

Adverse Reactions Frequency may not be defined.

Cardiovascular: Hypotension (1% to 27%), bradycardia (2% to 16%), first-degree heart block (P-R interval ≥0.26 sec; 5%), arterial insufficiency (usually Raynaud type; 1%), chest pain (1%), CHF (1%), edema (peripheral; 1%), palpitation (1%), syncope (1%)

Central nervous system: Dizziness (2% to 10%), fatigue (1% to 10%), depression (5%), confusion, hallucinations, headache, insomnia, memory loss (short-term), nightmares, sleep disturbances, somnolence, vertigo

Dermatology: Pruritus (5%), rash (5%), photosensitivity, psoriasis exacerbated

Endocrine & metabolic: Libido decreased, Peyronie's disease (<1%), diabetes exacerbated

Gastrointestinal: Diarrhea (5%), constipation (1%), flatulence (1%), gastrointestinal pain (1%), heartburn (1%), nausea (1%), xerostomia (1%), vomiting

Hematologic: Claudication

Neuromuscular & skeletal: Musculoskeletal pain

Ocular: Blurred vision, visual disturbances

Otic: Tinnitus

Respiratory: Dyspnea (1% to 3%), bronchospasm (1%), wheezing (1%), rhinitis, shortness of breath

Miscellaneous: Cold extremities (1%)

Postmarketing and/or case reports: Agranulocytosis, alkaline phosphatase increased, alopecia (reversible), anxiety, arthralgia, arthritis, cardiogenic shock, diaphoresis increased, dry eyes, gangrene, hepatitis, HDL decreased, impotence, jaundice, lactate dehydrogenase increased, nervousness, paresthesia, retroperitoneal fibrosis, second-degree heart block, taste disturbance, third-degree heart block, thrombocytopenia, transaminases increased, triglycerides increased, urticaria, vomiting, weight gain

Other events reported with beta-blockers: Catatonia, emotional lability, fever, hypersensitivity reactions, laryngospasm, nonthrombocytopenic purpura, respiratory distress, thrombocytopenic purpura

Drug Interactions

Metabolism/Transport Effects Substrate of CYP2C19 (minor), CYP2D6 (major); **Note:** Assignment of Major/Minor substrate status based on clinically relevant drug interaction potential; **Inhibits** CYP2D6 (weak)

Avoid Concomitant Use

Avoid concomitant use of Metoprolol with any of the following: Floctafenine; Methacholine

Increased Effect/Toxicity

Metoprolol may increase the levels/effects of: Alpha-/Beta-Agonists (Direct-Acting); Alpha1-Blockers; Alpha2-Agonists; Amifostine; Antihypertensives; Antipsychotic Agents (Phenothiazines); Bupivacaine; Cardiac Glycosides; Cholinergic Agonists; Fingolimod; Hypotensive Agents; Insulin; Lidocaine; Lidocaine (Systemic); Lidocaine (Topical); Mepivacaine; Methacholine; Midodrine; RiTUXimab; Sulfonylureas

The levels/effects of Metoprolol may be increased by: Abiraterone Acetate; Acetylcholinesterase Inhibitors; Aminoquinolines (Antimalarial); Amiodarone; Anilidopiperidine Opioids; Antipsychotic Agents (Phenothiazines); Calcium Channel Blockers (Dihydropyridine); Calcium Channel Blockers (Nondihydropyridine); CYP2D6 Inhibitors (Moderate); CYP2D6 Inhibitors (Strong); Darunavir;

Diazoxide; Dipyridamole; Disopyramide; Dronedarone; Floctafenine; Herbs (Hypotensive Properties); MAO Inhibitors; Pentoxifylline; Phosphodiesterase 5 Inhibitors; Propafenone; Prostacyclin Analogues; QuiNIDine; Reserpine; Selective Serotonin Reuptake Inhibitors

Decreased Effect

Metoprolol may decrease the levels/effects of: Beta2-Agonists; Theophylline Derivatives

The levels/effects of Metoprolol may be decreased by: Barbiturates; Herbs (Hypertensive Properties); Methylphenidate; Nonsteroidal Anti-Inflammatory Agents; Peginterferon Alfa-2b; Rifamycin Derivatives; Yohimbine

Ethanol/Nutrition/Herb Interactions

Food: Food increases absorption. Metoprolol serum levels may be increased if taken with food.

Herb/Nutraceutical: Avoid bayberry, blue cohosh, cayenne, ephedra, ginger, ginseng (American), gotu kola, licorice, (may worsen hypertension). Avoid black cohosh, California poppy, coleus, golden seal, hawthorn, mistletoe, periwinkle, quinine, shepherd's purse (may have increased antihypertensive effect).

Stability

Injection: Store at 25°C (77°F); excursions permitted to 15°C to 30°C (59°F to 86°F). Protect from light.

Tablet: Store at 25°C (77°F); excursions permitted to 15°C to 30°C (59°F to 86°F). Protect from moisture.

Mechanism of Action Selective inhibitor of beta$_1$-adrenergic receptors; competitively blocks beta$_1$-receptors, with little or no effect on beta$_2$-receptors at doses <100 mg; does not exhibit any membrane stabilizing or intrinsic sympathomimetic activity

Pharmacodynamics/Kinetics

Onset of action: Peak effect: Oral: 1.5-4 hours; I.V.: 20 minutes (when infused over 10 minutes)

Duration: Oral: Immediate release: 10-20 hours, Extended release: ~24 hours; I.V.: 5-8 hours

Absorption: 95%, rapid and complete

Distribution: V_d: 5.5 L/kg

Protein binding: 12% to albumin

Metabolism: Extensively hepatic via CYP2D6; significant first-pass effect (~50%)

Bioavailability: Oral: ~50%

Half-life elimination: 3-8 hours (dependent on rate of CYP2D6 metabolism)

Excretion: Urine (<5% to 10% as unchanged drug)

Dosage

Children: Hypertension: Oral:

1-17 years: Immediate release tablet: (National High Blood Pressure Education Program Working Group on High Blood Pressure in Children and Adolescents, 2004): Initial: 1-2 mg/kg/day; maximum 6 mg/kg/day (≤200 mg/day); administer in 2 divided doses

≥6 years: Extended release tablet: Initial: 1 mg/kg once daily (maximum initial dose: 50 mg/day). Adjust dose based on patient response (maximum: 2 mg/kg/day or 200 mg/day)

Adults:

Angina: Oral:

Immediate release: Initial: 50 mg twice daily; usual dosage range: 50-200 mg twice daily; maximum: 400 mg/day; increase dose at weekly intervals to desired effect

Extended release: Initial: 100 mg/day (maximum: 400 mg/day)

Atrial fibrillation/flutter (ventricular rate control), supraventricular tachycardia (SVT) (acute treatment; unlabeled use; Antman, 2004; Fuster, 2006; Neumar, 2010): I.V.: 2.5-5 mg every 2-5 minutes (maximum total dose: 15 mg over a 10-15 minute period). **Note:** Initiate cautiously in patients with concomitant heart failure; avoid in patients with decompensated heart failure.

Maintenance: Oral (immediate release): 25-100 mg twice daily

Heart failure: Oral (extended release): Initial: 25 mg once daily (reduce to 12.5 mg once daily in NYHA class higher than class II); may double dosage every 2 weeks as tolerated (target dose: 200 mg/day)

Hypertension: Oral:

Immediate release: Initial: 50 mg twice daily; effective dosage range: 100-450 mg/day in 2-3 divided doses; increase dose at weekly intervals to desired effect; maximum: 450 mg/day; usual dosage range (JNC 7): 50-100 mg/day

Extended release: Initial: 25-100 mg once daily; increase doses at weekly (or longer) intervals to desired effect; maximum: 400 mg/day; usual dosage range (JNC 7): 50-100 mg/day

Hypertension/ventricular rate control: I.V. (in patients having nonfunctioning GI tract): Initial: 1.25-5 mg every 6-12 hours; titrate initial dose to response. Initially, low doses may be appropriate to establish response; however, although not routine, up to 15 mg administered as frequently as every 3 hours has been employed in patients with refractory tachycardia.

Myocardial infarction:

Acute: I.V.: 5 mg every 2 minutes for 3 doses in early treatment of myocardial infarction; thereafter, give 50 mg orally every 6 hours beginning 15 minutes after last I.V. dose and continue for 48 hours; then administer a maintenance dose of 100 mg twice daily. **Note:** Do not initiate this regimen in those with signs of heart failure, a low output state, increased risk of cardiogenic shock, or other contraindications (eg, second- or third-degree heart block). If initial I.V. dosing is not tolerated, may give 25-50 mg orally (depending on degree of intolerance) every 6 hours beginning 15 minutes after the last I.V. dose or as soon as clinical condition permits.

Secondary prevention (unlabeled use; Olsson, 1992): Oral: Immediate release: 25-100 mg twice daily; optimize dose based on heart rate and blood pressure; continue indefinitely.

Thyrotoxicosis (unlabeled use): Oral: Immediate release: 25-50 mg every 6 hours; may also consider administering extended release formulation (Bahn, 2011)

Elderly: Hypertension: Initiate at the lower end of the dosage range and titrate to response

Note: Switching dosage forms:

When switching from immediate release metoprolol to extended release, the same total daily dose of metoprolol should be used.

When switching between oral and intravenous dosage forms, equivalent beta-blocking effect is achieved when doses in a 2.5:1 (Oral:I.V.) ratio is used. For example, if the patient is receiving an oral dose of 25 mg twice daily (50 mg/day), this would translate to 5 mg I.V. every 6 hours; consider reducing initial I.V. dose to evaluate patient response.

Dosing adjustment in renal impairment: No adjustment required.

Dosing adjustment in hepatic impairment: Reduced dose may be necessary

Dietary Considerations Regular tablets should be taken with food. Extended release tablets may be taken without regard to meals.

Administration

Oral: Extended release tablets may be divided in half; do not crush or chew.

I.V.: I.V. dose is much smaller than oral dose. When administered acutely for cardiac treatment, monitor ECG and blood pressure; may administer by rapid infusion (I.V. push) over 1 minute. May also be administered by slow infusion (ie, 5-10 mg of metoprolol in 50 mL of fluid) over ~30-60 minutes during less urgent situations (eg, substitution for oral metoprolol).

Monitoring Parameters Acute cardiac treatment: Monitor ECG and blood pressure with I.V. administration; heart rate and blood pressure with oral administration. I.V. use in a nonemergency situation: Necessary monitoring for surgical patients who are unable to take oral beta-blockers (because of prolonged ileus) has not been defined. Some institutions require monitoring of baseline and postinfusion heart rate and blood pressure when a patient's response to beta-blockade has not been characterized (ie, the patient's initial dose or following a change in dose). Consult individual institutional policies and procedures.

Dosage Forms Excipient information presented when available (limited, particularly for generics); consult specific product labeling.

Injection, solution, as tartrate: 1 mg/mL (5 mL)
  Lopressor®: 1 mg/mL (5 mL)
Injection, solution, as tartrate [preservative free]: 1 mg/mL (5 mL)
Tablet, oral, as tartrate: 25 mg, 50 mg, 100 mg
  Lopressor®: 50 mg, 100 mg [scored]
Tablet, extended release, oral, as succinate: 25 mg [expressed as mg equivalent to tartrate], 50 mg [expressed as mg equivalent to tartrate], 100 mg [expressed as mg equivalent to tartrate], 200 mg [expressed as mg equivalent to tartrate]
  Toprol-XL®: 25 mg, 50 mg, 100 mg, 200 mg [scored; expressed as mg equivalent to tartrate]

Extemporaneous Preparations A 10 mg/mL oral suspension may be made with metoprolol tartrate tablets and one of three different vehicles (cherry syrup; a 1:1 mixture of Ora-Sweet® and Ora-Plus®; or a 1:1 mixture of Ora-Sweet® SF and Ora-Plus®). Crush twelve 100 mg tablets in a mortar and reduce to a fine powder. Add 20 mL of the chosen vehicle and mix to a uniform paste; mix while adding the vehicle in incremental proportions to **almost** 120 mL; transfer to a calibrated bottle, rinse mortar with vehicle, and add quantity of vehicle sufficient to make 120 mL. Label "shake well" and "protect from light". Stable for 60 days.

Allen LV Jr and Erickson MA 3rd, "Stability of Labetalol Hydrochloride, Metoprolol Tartrate, Verapamil Hydrochloride, and Spironolactone With Hydrochlorothiazide in Extemporaneously Compounded Oral Liquids," *Am J Health Syst Pharm*, 1996, 53(19):2304-9.

- ◆ **Metoprolol-25 (Can)** *see* Metoprolol *on page 1117*
- ◆ **Metoprolol-L (Can)** *see* Metoprolol *on page 1117*
- ◆ **Metoprolol Succinate** *see* Metoprolol *on page 1117*
- ◆ **Metoprolol Tartrate** *see* Metoprolol *on page 1117*
- ◆ **Metoprolol Tartrate Injection, USP (Can)** *see* Metoprolol *on page 1117*
- ◆ **Metozolv™ ODT** *see* Metoclopramide *on page 1114*
- ◆ **MetroCream®** *see* MetroNIDAZOLE (Topical) *on page 1122*
- ◆ **MetroGel®** *see* MetroNIDAZOLE (Topical) *on page 1122*
- ◆ **Metrogel® (Can)** *see* MetroNIDAZOLE (Topical) *on page 1122*
- ◆ **MetroGel® 1% Kit [DSC]** *see* MetroNIDAZOLE (Topical) *on page 1122*
- ◆ **MetroGel-Vaginal®** *see* MetroNIDAZOLE (Topical) *on page 1122*
- ◆ **MetroLotion®** *see* MetroNIDAZOLE (Topical) *on page 1122*

MetroNIDAZOLE (Systemic)

(met roe NYE da zole)

Brand Names: U.S. Flagyl®; Flagyl® 375; Flagyl® ER

Brand Names: Canada Apo-Metronidazole®; Flagyl®; Florazole® ER

Index Terms Metronidazole Hydrochloride

Pharmacologic Category Amebicide; Antibiotic, Miscellaneous; Antiprotozoal, Nitroimidazole

Additional Appendix Information

Prevention of Wound Infection and Sepsis in Surgical Patients *on page 1954*

Use Treatment of susceptible anaerobic bacterial and protozoal infections in the following conditions: Amebiasis, symptomatic and asymptomatic trichomoniasis; skin and skin structure infections, bone and joint infections, CNS infections, endocarditis, gynecologic infections, intra-abdominal infections (as part of combination regimen), respiratory tract infections (lower), systemic anaerobic infections; treatment of antibiotic-associated pseudomembranous colitis (AAPC); as part of a multidrug regimen for *H. pylori* eradication to reduce the risk of duodenal ulcer recurrence; surgical prophylaxis (colorectal)

Unlabeled Use Crohn's disease

Pregnancy Risk Factor B

Pregnancy Considerations Teratogenic effects have not been observed in animal reproduction studies. Metronidazole crosses the placenta and rapidly distributes into the fetal circulation. Although there have been a few reports of facial anomalies after *in utero* exposure, most studies have not found an increased risk of congenital abnormalities following maternal use of metronidazole during the first trimester of pregnancy. In studies that included women taking metronidazole during all trimesters of pregnancy, an increased risk of adverse fetal and neonatal outcomes has not been observed. Because metronidazole has been carcinogenic in some animal species, concern has been raised whether metronidazole should be used during pregnancy; however, a strong carcinogenic potential in humans has not been observed, including one study of prenatal exposure.

Metronidazole pharmacokinetics are similar between pregnant and nonpregnant patients. Bacterial vaginosis has been associated with adverse pregnancy outcomes (including preterm labor); metronidazole is recommended for the treatment of symptomatic bacterial vaginosis in pregnant patients. Vaginal trichomoniasis has been also associated with adverse pregnancy outcomes (including preterm labor). Treatment may relieve symptoms and prevent further sexual transmission; however, metronidazole has not resulted in reduced perinatal morbidity and should not be used solely to prevent preterm delivery. Some clinicians consider deferring therapy in asymptomatic women until >37 weeks gestation. Use of oral metronidazole is contraindicated during the first trimester (per the FDA approved labeling). Consult current CDC guidelines for appropriate use in pregnant women.

Lactation Enters breast milk/not recommended (AAP rates "of concern"; AAP 2001 update pending)

Contraindications Hypersensitivity to metronidazole, nitroimidazole derivatives, or any component of the formulation; pregnancy (first trimester)

Warnings/Precautions Use with caution in patients with severe liver impairment due to potential accumulation, blood dyscrasias; history of seizures, CHF or other sodium-retaining states; reduce dosage in patients with severe liver impairment, CNS disease, and consider dosage reduction in longer-term therapy with severe renal failure (Cl_{cr} <10 mL/minute); if *H. pylori* is not eradicated in patients being treated with metronidazole in a regimen, it should be assumed that metronidazole-resistance has occurred and it should not again be used; aseptic meningitis, encephalopathy, seizures, and neuropathies have been reported especially with increased doses and chronic treatment; monitor and consider discontinuation of therapy if symptoms occur. **[U.S. Boxed Warning]: Possibly**

carcinogenic based on animal data. Prolonged use may result in fungal or bacterial superinfection, including *C. difficile*-associated diarrhea (CDAD) and pseudomembranous colitis; CDAD has been observed >2 months postantibiotic treatment. The Infectious Disease Society of America (IDSA) recommends the use of oral metronidazole for initial treatment of mild-to-moderate *C. difficile* infection and the use of oral vancomycin for initial treatment of severe *C. difficile* infection with or without I.V. metronidazole depending on the presence of complications. May treat recurrent mild-to-moderate infection once with oral metronidazole; avoid use beyond first reoccurrence due to potential cumulative neurotoxicity (Cohen, 2010). Candidiasis infection (known or unknown) maybe more prominent during metronidazole treatment, antifungal treatment required. Disulfiram-like reactions to ethanol have been reported with oral metronidazole; avoid alcoholic beverages during therapy

Adverse Reactions Frequency not always defined.

- Cardiovascular: Flattening of the T-wave, flushing, syncope
- Central nervous system: Aseptic meningitis, ataxia, confusion, coordination impaired, depression, dizziness, encephalopathy, fever, headache, insomnia, irritability, seizure, vertigo
- Dermatologic: Erythematous rash, pruritus, Stevens-Johnson syndrome, toxic epidermal necrolysis, urticaria
- Endocrine & metabolic: Disulfiram-like reaction, dysmenorrhea
- Gastrointestinal: Nausea (~12%), anorexia, abdominal cramping, constipation, diarrhea, epigastric distress, furry tongue, glossitis, pancreatitis (rare), proctitis, stomatitis, unusual/metallic taste, vomiting, xerostomia
- Genitourinary: Cystitis, darkened urine (rare), dyspareunia, dysuria, incontinence, libido decreased, pelvic pressure, polyuria, vaginal dryness, vaginitis
- Hematologic: Neutropenia (reversible), thrombocytopenia (reversible, rare)
- Local: Thrombophlebitis
- Neuromuscular & skeletal: Dysarthria, peripheral neuropathy, weakness
- Ocular: Optic neuropathy
- Respiratory: Nasal congestion, pharyngitis, rhinitis, sinusitis, pharyngitis
- Miscellaneous: Flu-like syndrome, joint pains resembling serum sickness, moniliasis

Drug Interactions

Metabolism/Transport Effects **Inhibits** CYP2C9 (weak), CYP3A4 (moderate)

Avoid Concomitant Use

Avoid concomitant use of MetroNIDAZOLE (Systemic) with any of the following: BCG; Pimozide; Tolvaptan

Increased Effect/Toxicity

MetroNIDAZOLE (Systemic) may increase the levels/effects of: Alcohol (Ethyl); ARIPiprazole; Budesonide (Systemic, Oral Inhalation); Busulfan; Calcineurin Inhibitors; Colchicine; CYP3A4 Substrates; Eplerenone; Everolimus; FentaNYL; Fluorouracil; Fosphenytoin; Halofantrine; Lurasidone; Phenytoin; Pimecrolimus; Pimozide; Propafenone; Ranolazine; Salmeterol; Saxagliptin; Tipranavir; Tolvaptan; Vilazodone; Vitamin K Antagonists; Zuclopenthixol

The levels/effects of MetroNIDAZOLE (Systemic) may be increased by: Disulfiram; Mebendazole

Decreased Effect

MetroNIDAZOLE (Systemic) may decrease the levels/effects of: BCG; Mycophenolate; Typhoid Vaccine

The levels/effects of MetroNIDAZOLE (Systemic) may be decreased by: Fosphenytoin; PHENobarbital; Phenytoin

Ethanol/Nutrition/Herb Interactions

- Ethanol: The manufacturer recommends to avoid all ethanol or any ethanol-containing drugs (may cause disulfiram-like reaction characterized by flushing, headache, nausea, vomiting, sweating, or tachycardia).
- Food: Peak antibiotic serum concentration lowered and delayed, but total drug absorbed not affected.

Stability

Injection: Store at controlled room temperature of 15°C to 30°C (59°F to 86°F). Protect from light. Keep in overwrap until ready to use. Product may be refrigerated but crystals may form. Crystals redissolve on warming to room temperature. Prolonged exposure to light will cause a darkening of the product. However, short-term exposure to normal room light does not adversely affect metronidazole stability. Direct sunlight should be avoided. Stability of parenteral admixture at room temperature (25°C); Out of overwrap stability: 30 days.

Standard diluent: 500 mg/100 mL NS.

Tablets: Store at room temperature. Protect from light and moisture.

Mechanism of Action After diffusing into the organism, interacts with DNA to cause a loss of helical DNA structure and strand breakage resulting in inhibition of protein synthesis and cell death in susceptible organisms

Pharmacodynamics/Kinetics

- Absorption: Oral: Well absorbed
- Distribution: To saliva, bile, seminal fluid, bone, liver, and liver abscesses, lung and vaginal secretions; crosses blood-brain barrier
  - CSF:blood level ratio: Normal meninges: 16% to 43%; Inflamed meninges: 100%
- Protein binding: <20%
- Metabolism: Hepatic (30% to 60%)
- Half-life elimination: Neonates: 25-75 hours; Others: 6-8 hours, prolonged with hepatic impairment; End-stage renal disease: 21 hours
- Time to peak, serum: Oral: Immediate release: 1-2 hours
- Excretion: Urine (60% to 80% as unchanged drug); feces (6% to 15%)

Dosage

Infants and Children:

- Amebiasis: Oral: 35-50 mg/kg/day in divided doses every 8 hours for 10 days
- Trichomoniasis: Oral: 15-30 mg/kg/day in divided doses every 8 hours for 7 days
- Anaerobic infections:
  - Oral: 15-35 mg/kg/day in divided doses every 8 hours
  - I.V.: 30 mg/kg/day in divided doses every 6 hours
- *Clostridium difficile* (antibiotic-associated colitis): Oral: 30 mg/kg/day divided every 6 hours for 7-10 days; maximum dose: 2 g/day

Adults:

- Anaerobic infections (diverticulitis, intra-abdominal, peritonitis, cholangitis, or abscess): Oral, I.V.: 500 mg every 6-8 hours, not to exceed 4 g/day; **Note:** Initial: 1 g I.V. loading dose may be administered
- Amebiasis: Oral: 500-750 mg every 8 hours for 5-10 days
- Antibiotic-associated pseudomembranous colitis: IDSA Guidelines (Cohen, 2010):
  - Mild-to-moderate infection: Oral: 500 mg 3 times/day for 10-14 days
  - Severe complicated infection: I.V.: 500 mg 3 times/day with oral vancomycin (recommended agent) for 10-14 days
  - **Note:** Due to the emergence of a new strain of *C. difficile*, some clinicians recommend converting to oral vancomycin therapy if the patient does not show a clear clinical response after 2 days of metronidazole therapy.
- Giardiasis: 500 mg twice daily for 5-7 days

Helicobacter pylori eradication: Oral: 250-500 mg with meals and at bedtime for 14 days; requires combination therapy with at least one other antibiotic and an acid-suppressing agent (proton pump inhibitor or H_2 blocker)

Intra-abdominal infection, complicated, community-acquired, mild-to-moderate (in combination with cephalosporin or fluoroquinolone): I.V.: 500 mg every 8-12 hours **or** 1.5 g every 24 hours for for 4-7 days (provided source controlled)

Bacterial vaginosis or vaginitis due to *Gardnerella*, *Mobiluncus*: Oral: 500 mg twice daily (regular release) or 750 mg once daily (extended release tablet) for 7 days

Pelvic inflammatory disease (unlabeled use): Oral: 500 mg twice daily for 14 days (in combination with a cephalosporin and doxycycline) (CDC, 2010)

Trichomoniasis: Oral: 250 mg every 8 hours for 7 days **or** 375 mg twice daily for 7 days **or** 2 g as a single dose **or** 1 g twice daily for 2 doses (on same day)

Urethritis (unlabeled use): Oral: 2 g as a single dose with azithromycin (CDC, 2010)

Surgical prophylaxis (colorectal): I.V. 15 mg/kg 1 hour prior to surgery; followed by 7.5 mg/kg 6 and 12 hours after initial dose

Elderly: Use lower end of dosing recommendations for adults, do not administer as a single dose

Dosing adjustment in renal impairment: Cl_{cr} <10 mL/minute (not on dialysis): Recommendations vary: To reduce possible accumulation in patients receiving multiple doses, consider reduction to 50% of dose or administer normal dose every 12 hours; **Note:** Dosage reduction is unnecessary in short courses of therapy. Some references do not recommend reduction at any level of renal impairment (Lamp, 1999).

Intermittent hemodialysis (IHD) (administer after hemodialysis on dialysis days): Dialyzable (50% to 100%): 500 mg every 8-12 hours. **Note:** Dosing regimen highly dependent on clinical indication (trichomoniasis vs *C. difficile* colitis) (Heintz, 2009). **Note:** Dosing dependent on the assumption of thrice weekly, complete IHD sessions.

Peritoneal dialysis (PD): Dose as for Cl_{cr} <10 mL/minute

Continuous renal replacement therapy (CRRT) (Heintz, 2009; Trotman, 2005): Drug clearance is highly dependent on the method of renal replacement, filter type, and flow rate. Appropriate dosing requires close monitoring of pharmacologic response, signs of adverse reactions due to drug accumulation, as well as drug concentrations in relation to target trough (if appropriate). The following are general recommendations only (based on dialysate flow/ultrafiltration rates of 1-2 L/hour and minimal residual renal function) and should not supersede clinical judgment:

CVVH/CVVHD/CVVHDF: 500 mg every 6-12 hours (or per clinical indication; dosage reduction generally not necessary)

Dosing adjustment/comments in hepatic disease: Unchanged in mild liver disease; reduce dosage in severe liver disease

Dietary Considerations Take on an empty stomach. Drug may cause GI upset; if GI upset occurs, take with food. Extended release tablets should be taken on an empty stomach (1 hour before or 2 hours after meals). Some products may contain sodium. The manufacturer recommends that ethanol be avoided during treatment and for 3 days after therapy is complete.

Administration

I.V.: Infuse intravenously over 30-60 minutes. Avoid contact of drug solution with equipment containing aluminum.

Oral: May be taken with food to minimize stomach upset. Extended release tablets should be taken on an empty stomach (1 hour before or 2 hours after meals).

Test Interactions May interfere with AST, ALT, triglycerides, glucose, and LDH testing

Dosage Forms Excipient information presented when available (limited, particularly for generics); consult specific product labeling.

Capsule, oral: 375 mg
 Flagyl® 375: 375 mg
Infusion, premixed iso-osmotic sodium chloride solution: 500 mg (100 mL)
Tablet, oral: 250 mg, 500 mg
 Flagyl®: 250 mg, 500 mg
Tablet, extended release, oral:
 Flagyl® ER: 750 mg

Extemporaneous Preparations A 50 mg/mL oral suspension may be made with tablets and a 1:1 mixture of Ora-Sweet® and Ora-Plus®. Crush twenty-four 250 mg tablets in a mortar and reduce to a fine powder. Add small portions of the vehicle and mix to a uniform paste; mix while adding the vehicle in incremental portions to **almost** 120 mL; transfer to a calibrated bottle, rinse mortar with vehicle, and add quantity of vehicle sufficient to make 120 mL. Label "shake well". Stable for 60 days at room temperature or refrigerated.

Allen LV Jr and Erickson MA 3rd, "Stability of Ketoconazole, Metolazone, Metronidazole, Procainamide Hydrochloride, and Spironolactone in Extemporaneously Compounded Oral Liquids," *Am J Health Syst Pharm*, 1996, 53(17):2073-8.

MetroNIDAZOLE (Topical) (met roe NYE da zole)

Brand Names: U.S. MetroCream®; MetroGel-Vaginal®; MetroGel®; MetroGel® 1% Kit [DSC]; MetroLotion®; Noritate®; Vandazole®

Brand Names: Canada MetroCream®; Metrogel®; MetroLotion®; Nidagel™; Noritate®; Rosasol®

Index Terms Metronidazole Hydrochloride

Pharmacologic Category Antibiotic, Topical

Use

Topical: Treatment of inflammatory lesions and erythema of rosacea

Vaginal gel: Bacterial vaginosis

Pregnancy Risk Factor B

Dosage Adults:

Acne rosacea: Topical:

0.75%: Apply and rub a thin film twice daily, morning and evening, to entire affected areas after washing.

1%: Apply thin film to affected area once daily

Bacterial vaginosis or vaginitis due to *Gardnerella*, *Mobiluncus*: Vaginal: One applicatorful (~37.5 mg metronidazole) intravaginally once or twice daily for 5 days; apply once in morning and evening if using twice daily, if daily, use at bedtime

Additional Information Complete prescribing information for this medication should be consulted for additional detail.

Dosage Forms Excipient information presented when available (limited, particularly for generics); consult specific product labeling. [DSC] = Discontinued product

Cream, topical: 0.75% (45 g)
 MetroCream®: 0.75% (45 g) [contains benzyl alcohol]
 Noritate®: 1% (60 g)
Gel, topical: 0.75% (45 g)
 MetroGel®: 1% (55 g, 60 g)
 MetroGel® 1% Kit: 1% (60 g [DSC])
Gel, vaginal: 0.75% (70 g)
 MetroGel-Vaginal®: 0.75% (70 g)
 Vandazole®: 0.75% (70 g)
Lotion, topical: 0.75% (59 mL, 60 mL)
 MetroLotion®: 0.75% (59 mL) [contains benzyl alcohol]

◆ **Metronidazole Hydrochloride** *see* MetroNIDAZOLE (Systemic) *on page 1120*

◆ **Metronidazole Hydrochloride** *see* MetroNIDAZOLE (Topical) *on page 1122*

◆ **MET Tyrosine Kinase Inhibitor PF-02341066** *see* Crizotinib *on page 416*

◆ **Metvix® (Can)** *see* Methyl Aminolevulinate *on page 1103*

◆ **Metvixia™** *see* Methyl Aminolevulinate *on page 1103*

Metyrosine (me TYE roe seen)

Brand Names: U.S. Demser®

Brand Names: Canada Demser®

Index Terms AMPT; OGMT

Pharmacologic Category Tyrosine Hydroxylase Inhibitor

Use Short-term management of pheochromocytoma before surgery, long-term management when surgery is contraindicated or when chronic malignant pheochromocytoma exists

Pregnancy Risk Factor C

Dosage Children >12 years and Adults: Oral: Initial: 250 mg 4 times/day, increased by 250-500 mg/day up to 4 g/day; maintenance: 2-3 g/day in 4 divided doses; for preoperative preparation, administer optimum effective dosage for 5-7 days

Dosing adjustment in renal impairment: Adjustment should be considered

Additional Information Complete prescribing information for this medication should be consulted for additional detail.

Dosage Forms Excipient information presented when available (limited, particularly for generics); consult specific product labeling.

Capsule, oral:

Demser®: 250 mg

◆ **Mevacor®** *see* Lovastatin *on page 1038*

◆ **Mevinolin** *see* Lovastatin *on page 1038*

Mexiletine (meks IL e teen)

Brand Names: Canada Novo-Mexiletine

Pharmacologic Category Antiarrhythmic Agent, Class Ib

Use Management of serious ventricular arrhythmias; suppression of PVCs

Pregnancy Risk Factor C

Lactation Enters breast milk/not recommended

Contraindications Hypersensitivity to mexiletine or any component of the formulation; cardiogenic shock; second- or third-degree AV block (except in patients with a functioning artificial pacemaker)

Warnings/Precautions [U.S. Boxed Warning]: In the Cardiac Arrhythmia Suppression Trial (CAST), recent (>6 days but <2 years ago) myocardial infarction patients with asymptomatic, non-life-threatening ventricular arrhythmias did not benefit and may have been harmed by attempts to suppress the arrhythmia with flecainide or encainide. An increased mortality or nonfatal cardiac arrest rate (7.7%) was seen in the active treatment group compared with patients in the placebo group (3%). The applicability of the CAST results to other populations is unknown. Antiarrhythmic agents should be reserved for patients with life-threatening ventricular arrhythmias. Can be proarrhythmic. Electrolyte disturbances alter response; should be corrected before initiating therapy. Use cautiously in patients with first-degree block, pre-existing sinus node dysfunction, intraventricular conduction delays, significant hepatic dysfunction, hypotension, or severe HF. Alterations in urinary pH may change urinary excretion. Rare hepatic toxicity may occur; may cause acute hepatic injury.

Adverse Reactions

>10%:

Central nervous system: Lightheadedness (11% to 25%), dizziness (20% to 25%), nervousness (5% to 10%), incoordination (10%)

Gastrointestinal: GI distress (41%), nausea/vomiting (40%)

Neuromuscular & skeletal: Trembling, unsteady gait, tremor (13%), ataxia (10% to 20%)

1% to 10%:

Cardiovascular: Chest pain (3% to 8%), premature ventricular contractions (1% to 2%), palpitation (4% to 8%), angina (2%), proarrhythmia (10% to 15% in patients with malignant arrhythmia)

Central nervous system: Confusion, headache, insomnia (5% to 7%), depression (2%)

Dermatologic: Rash (4%)

Gastrointestinal: Constipation or diarrhea (4% to 5%), xerostomia (3%), abdominal pain (1%)

Neuromuscular & skeletal: Weakness (5%), numbness of fingers or toes (2% to 4%), paresthesia (2%), arthralgia (1%)

Ocular: Blurred vision (5% to 7%), nystagmus (6%)

Otic: Tinnitus (2% to 3%)

Respiratory: Dyspnea (3%)

<1% (Limited to important or life-threatening): Agranulocytosis, alopecia, AV block, cardiogenic shock, CHF, dysphagia, exfoliative dermatitis, hallucinations, hepatic necrosis, hepatitis, hypotension, impotence, leukopenia, myelofibrosis, pancreatitis (rare), psychosis, pulmonary fibrosis, seizure, sinus arrest, SLE syndrome, Stevens-Johnson syndrome, syncope, thrombocytopenia, torsade de pointes, upper GI bleeding, urinary retention, urticaria

Drug Interactions

Metabolism/Transport Effects Substrate of CYP1A2 (major), CYP2D6 (major); **Note:** Assignment of Major/Minor substrate status based on clinically relevant drug interaction potential; **Inhibits** CYP1A2 (strong)

Avoid Concomitant Use There are no known interactions where it is recommended to avoid concomitant use.

Increased Effect/Toxicity

Mexiletine may increase the levels/effects of: Bendamustine; CYP1A2 Substrates; Theophylline Derivatives

The levels/effects of Mexiletine may be increased by: Abiraterone Acetate; CYP1A2 Inhibitors (Moderate); CYP1A2 Inhibitors (Strong); CYP2D6 Inhibitors (Moderate); CYP2D6 Inhibitors (Strong); Darunavir; Deferasirox; Selective Serotonin Reuptake Inhibitors

Decreased Effect

The levels/effects of Mexiletine may be decreased by: CYP1A2 Inducers (Strong); Cyproterone; Etravirine; Fosphenytoin; Peginterferon Alfa-2b; Phenytoin

Ethanol/Nutrition/Herb Interactions Food: Food may decrease the rate, but not the extent of oral absorption; diets which affect urine pH can increase or decrease excretion of mexiletine. Avoid dietary changes that alter urine pH.

Mechanism of Action Class IB antiarrhythmic, structurally related to lidocaine, which inhibits inward sodium current, decreases rate of rise of phase 0, increases effective refractory period/action potential duration ratio

Pharmacodynamics/Kinetics

Absorption: Well absorbed; elderly have a slightly slower rate, but extent of absorption is the same as young adults

Distribution: V_d: 5-7 L/kg

Protein binding: 50% to 60%

Metabolism: Hepatic; low first-pass effect

Bioavailability: 80% to 95%

Half-life elimination: Adults: 10-14 hours (average: elderly: 14.4 hours, younger adults: 12 hours); prolonged with hepatic impairment or heart failure

Time to peak, serum: 2-3 hours

Excretion: Urine (10% to 15% as unchanged drug); urinary acidification increases excretion, alkalinization decreases excretion

Dosage Adults: Oral: Initial: 200 mg every 8 hours (may load with 400 mg if necessary); adjust dose every 2-3 days; usual dose: 200-300 mg every 8 hours; maximum dose: 1.2 g/day (some patients respond to every 12-hour dosing). When switching from another antiarrhythmic, initiate a 200 mg dose 6-12 hours after stopping former agents, 3-6 hours after stopping procainamide.

Dosage adjustment in hepatic impairment: Reduce dose to 25% to 30% of usual dose

Dietary Considerations Take with food.

Administration Administer around-the-clock rather than 3 times/day to promote less variation in peak and trough serum levels; administer with food

Reference Range Therapeutic range: 0.5-2 mcg/mL; potentially toxic: >2 mcg/mL

Test Interactions Abnormal liver function test, positive ANA, thrombocytopenia

Dosage Forms Excipient information presented when available (limited, particularly for generics); consult specific product labeling.

Capsule, oral, as hydrochloride: 150 mg, 200 mg, 250 mg

Extemporaneous Preparations A 10 mg/mL oral suspension may be with made with capsules and either distilled water or sorbitol USP. Empty the contents of eight 150 mg capsules in a mortar and reduce to a fine powder if necessary. Add small portions of the chosen vehicle and mix to a uniform paste; mix while adding the vehicle in incremental proportions to **almost** 120 mL; transfer to a graduated cylinder, rinse mortar with vehicle, and add quantity of vehicle sufficient to make 120 mL. Label "shake well". Sorbitol suspension is stable in plastic prescription bottles for 2 weeks at room temperature and 4 weeks refrigerated; distilled water suspension is stable in plastic prescription bottles for 7 weeks at room temperature and 13 weeks refrigerated. Extended storage under refrigeration is recommended to minimize microbial contamination.

Nahata MC, Morosco RS, and Hipple TF, "Stability of Mexiletine in Two Extemporaneous Liquid Formulations Stored Under Refrigeration and at Room Temperature," *J Am Pharm Assoc (Wash)*, 2000, 40 (2):257-9.

- **Mezavant® (Can)** *see* Mesalamine *on page 1081*
- **$MgSO_4$ (error-prone abbreviation)** *see* Magnesium Sulfate *on page 1047*
- **Miacalcin®** *see* Calcitonin *on page 262*
- **Miacalcin® NS (Can)** *see* Calcitonin *on page 262*
- **Mi-Acid [OTC]** *see* Aluminum Hydroxide, Magnesium Hydroxide, and Simethicone *on page 80*
- **Mi-Acid™ Double Strength [OTC]** *see* Calcium Carbonate and Magnesium Hydroxide *on page 267*
- **Mi-Acid Maximum Strength [OTC] [DSC]** *see* Aluminum Hydroxide, Magnesium Hydroxide, and Simethicone *on page 80*
- **Micaderm® [OTC]** *see* Miconazole (Topical) *on page 1126*

Micafungin (mi ka FUN gin)

Brand Names: U.S. Mycamine®

Brand Names: Canada Mycamine®

Index Terms Micafungin Sodium

Pharmacologic Category Antifungal Agent, Parenteral; Echinocandin

Additional Appendix Information

Antifungal Agents *on page 1876*

Use Treatment of esophageal candidiasis; *Candida* prophylaxis in patients undergoing hematopoietic stem cell transplant (HSCT); treatment of candidemia, acute disseminated candidiasis, and other *Candida* infections (peritonitis and abscesses)

Unlabeled Use Treatment of infections due to *Aspergillus* spp; prophylaxis of HIV-related esophageal candidiasis

Pregnancy Risk Factor C

Pregnancy Considerations Visceral teratogenic and abortifacient effects were noted in animal studies. There are no adequate and well-controlled studies in pregnant women. Use only if benefit outweighs risk.

Lactation Excretion in breast milk unknown/use caution

Contraindications Hypersensitivity to micafungin, other echinocandins, or any component of the formulation

Warnings/Precautions Anaphylactic reactions, including shock, have been reported. New onset or worsening hepatic failure has been reported; use caution in preexisting mild-moderate hepatic impairment; safety in severe liver failure has not been evaluated. Hemolytic anemia and hemoglobinuria have been reported. Increased BUN, serum creatinine, renal dysfunction, and/or acute renal failure has been reported; use with caution in patients with pre-existing renal impairment and monitor closely.

Adverse Reactions Percentages reflect incidence across all approved indications (prophylaxis and treatment); however, in general, a higher frequency of adverse reactions was observed in studies with HSCT patients.

>10%:

Central nervous system: Fever (7% to 20%), headache (2% to 16%)

Endocrine & metabolic: Hypokalemia (14% to 18%), hypomagnesemia (6% to 13%)

Gastrointestinal: Diarrhea (8% to 23%), nausea (7% to 22%), vomiting (7% to 22%), mucosal inflammation (14%), constipation (11%)

Hematologic: Thrombocytopenia (4% to 15%), neutropenia (14%)

Local: Phlebitis (5% to 19%)

1% to 10%:

Cardiovascular: Hypotension (6% to 10%), tachycardia (3% to 8%), hypertension (3% to 5%), peripheral edema (7%), edema (5%), bradycardia (3% to 5%), atrial fibrillation (3% to 5%)

Central nervous system: Insomnia (4% to 10%), anxiety (6%), fatigue (6%)

Dermatologic: Rash (2% to 9%), pruritus (6%)

Endocrine & metabolic: Hypocalcemia (7%), hypoglycemia (6% to 7%), hyperglycemia (6%), hypernatremia (4% to 6%), hyperkalemia (4% to 5%), fluid overload (5%)

Gastrointestinal: Abdominal pain (2% to 10%), anorexia (6%), dyspepsia (6%)

Hematologic: Anemia (3% to 10%), febrile neutropenia (6%)

Hepatic: AST increased (6%), ALT increased (5%), serum alkaline phosphatase increased (6% to 8%)

Neuromuscular & skeletal: Rigors (9%), back pain (5%)

Respiratory: Cough (8%), dyspnea (6%), epistaxis (6%)

Miscellaneous: Bacteremia (5% to 9%), sepsis (5% to 6%)

<1% (Limited to important or life-threatening) or frequency not defined: Acidosis, acute renal failure, anuria, apnea, arrhythmia, arthralgia, atrial fibrillation, BUN increased, cardiac arrest, coagulopathy, creatinine increased, cyanosis, deep vein thrombosis, delirium, disseminated intravascular coagulation (DIC), encephalopathy, erythema multiforme, facial edema, hemoglobinuria, hemolysis, hemolytic anemia, hepatic dysfunction, hepatic failure, hepatocellular damage, hepatomegaly, hiccups, hyperbilirubinemia, hyponatremia, hypoxia, infection, injection site necrosis, injection site thrombosis, intracranial hemorrhage, jaundice, MI, mucosal inflammation, oliguria, pancytopenia, pneumonia, pulmonary embolism,

renal impairment, renal tubular necrosis, seizure, shock, skin necrosis, Stevens-Johnson syndrome, thrombotic thrombocytopenia purpura, thrombophlebitis, toxic epidermal necrolysis, urticaria, vasodilatation, WBC decreased

Drug Interactions

Metabolism/Transport Effects Substrate of CYP3A4 (minor); **Note:** Assignment of Major/Minor substrate status based on clinically relevant drug interaction potential; **Inhibits** CYP3A4 (weak)

Avoid Concomitant Use

Avoid concomitant use of Micafungin with any of the following: Pimozide

Increased Effect/Toxicity

Micafungin may increase the levels/effects of: Pimozide

The levels/effects of Micafungin may be increased by: Conivaptan

Decreased Effect

Micafungin may decrease the levels/effects of: Saccharomyces boulardii

The levels/effects of Micafungin may be decreased by: Tocilizumab

Stability Store at controlled room temperature of 25°C (77°F). Reconstituted and diluted solutions are stable for 24 hours at room temperature. Protect from light. Aseptically add 5 mL of NS (preservative-free) to each 50 or 100 mg vial. Swirl to dissolve; do not shake. Further dilute 50-150 mg in 100 mL NS. Protect from light. Alternatively, D_5W may be used for reconstitution and dilution.

Mechanism of Action Concentration-dependent inhibition of 1,3-beta-D-glucan synthase resulting in reduced formation of 1,3-beta-D-glucan, an essential polysaccharide comprising 30% to 60% of *Candida* cell walls (absent in mammalian cells); decreased glucan content leads to osmotic instability and cellular lysis

Pharmacodynamics/Kinetics

Distribution: 0.28-0.5 L/kg

Protein binding: >99%; primarily to albumin

Metabolism: Hepatic; forms M-1 (catechol) and M-2 (methoxy) metabolites (activity unknown)

Half-life elimination: 11-21 hours

Excretion: Primarily feces (71%); urine (<15%)

Dosage I.V.: Adults:

Candidemia, acute disseminated candidiasis, and *Candida* peritonitis and abscesses: 100 mg daily; mean duration of therapy (from clinical trials) was 15 days (range: 10-47 days)

Esophageal candidiasis: 150 mg daily; mean duration of therapy (from clinical trials) was 15 days (range: 10-30 days)

Prophylaxis of *Candida* infection in hematopoietic stem cell transplantation: 50 mg daily

Dosing adjustment in renal impairment: No dosage adjustment required in renal impairment.

Poorly dialyzed; no supplemental dose or dosage adjustment necessary, including patients on intermittent hemodialysis, peritoneal dialysis, or continuous renal replacement therapy (eg, CVVHD).

Dosing adjustment in hepatic impairment: No dosage adjustment required for moderate hepatic impairment (Child-Pugh score 7-9). Patients with severe hepatic dysfunction have not been studied.

Administration For intravenous use only; infuse over 1 hour. Flush line with NS prior to administration.

Monitoring Parameters Liver function tests

Dosage Forms Excipient information presented when available (limited, particularly for generics); consult specific product labeling.

Injection, powder for reconstitution, as sodium:

Mycamine®: 50 mg, 100 mg [contains lactose 200 mg]

- ◆ **Micafungin Sodium** *see* Micafungin *on page 1124*
- ◆ **Micanol® (Can)** *see* Anthralin *on page 123*
- ◆ **Micardis®** *see* Telmisartan *on page 1636*
- ◆ **Micardis® HCT** *see* Telmisartan and Hydrochlorothiazide *on page 1637*
- ◆ **Micardis® Plus (Can)** *see* Telmisartan and Hydrochlorothiazide *on page 1637*
- ◆ **Micatin® [OTC]** *see* Miconazole (Topical) *on page 1126*
- ◆ **Micatin® (Can)** *see* Miconazole (Topical) *on page 1126*

Miconazole (Oral) (mi KON a zole)

Brand Names: U.S. Oravig® [DSC]

Index Terms Miconazole Nitrate

Pharmacologic Category Antifungal Agent, Oral Nonabsorbed

Use Treatment of oropharyngeal candidiasis

Pregnancy Risk Factor C

Pregnancy Considerations Embryofetotoxicity has been observed in animal reproduction studies. There are no adequate and well-controlled studies in pregnant women. Use only if benefit outweighs risk.

Lactation Excretion in breast milk unknown/use caution

Contraindications Hypersensitivity to miconazole, milk protein concentrate, or any component of the formulation

Warnings/Precautions Hypersensitivity reactions have been reported. Monitor patients who have a history of azole hypersensitivity for reactions; risk of cross-reactivity is unknown. Use with caution in patients with hepatic impairment.

Adverse Reactions

>10%: Local: Application site reaction (10% to 12%; including burning, discomfort, edema, glossodynia, pain, pruritus, toothache, ulceration)

1% to 10%:

Central nervous system: Headache (5% to 8%), fatigue (3%), pain (1%)

Dermatologic: Pruritus (2%)

Gastrointestinal: Diarrhea (6% to 9%), nausea (1% to 7%), vomiting (1% to 4%), abnormal taste (3% to 4%), oral discomfort (3%), xerostomia (3%), abdominal pain (1% to 3%), ageusia (2%), gastroenteritis (1%)

Hematologic: Anemia (3%), lymphopenia (2%), neutropenia (1%)

Hepatic: GGT increased (1%)

Respiratory: Cough (3%), upper respiratory infection (2%), pharyngeal pain (1%)

Drug Interactions

Metabolism/Transport Effects Inhibits CYP2C19 (moderate), CYP2C9 (moderate), CYP2D6 (moderate), CYP3A4 (moderate)

Avoid Concomitant Use

Avoid concomitant use of Miconazole (Oral) with any of the following: Clopidogrel; Gliclazide; Pimozide; Thioridazine; Tolvaptan

Increased Effect/Toxicity

Miconazole (Oral) may increase the levels/effects of: ARIPiprazole; Budesonide (Systemic, Oral Inhalation); Carvedilol; Citalopram; Colchicine; CYP2C19 Substrates; CYP2C9 Substrates; CYP2D6 Substrates; CYP3A4 Substrates; Eplerenone; Everolimus; FentaNYL; Fesoterodine; Gliclazide; Halofantrine; Lurasidone; Nebivolol; Pimecrolimus; Pimozide; Propafenone; Ranolazine; Salmeterol; Saxagliptin; Tamoxifen; Thioridazine; Tolvaptan; Vilazodone; Warfarin; Zuclopenthixol

The levels/effects of Miconazole (Oral) may be increased by: Propafenone

Decreased Effect

Miconazole (Oral) may decrease the levels/effects of: Clopidogrel; Codeine; TraMADol

Stability Store at 20°C to 25°C (68°F to 77°F); excursions permitted to15°C to 30°C (59°F to 86°F). Protect from moisture.

Mechanism of Action Inhibits biosynthesis of ergosterol, damaging the fungal cell wall membrane, which increases permeability causing leaking of nutrients

Pharmacodynamics/Kinetics

Duration: Buccal adhesion: 15 hours

Absorption: Minimal

Dosage Buccal tablet: Children ≥16 years and Adults: Oropharyngeal candidiasis: 50 mg (1 tablet) applied to the upper gum region once daily for 14 days

Dosage adjustment in renal impairment: No dosing adjustment is required

Dosage adjustment in hepatic impairment: Use with caution in patients with hepatic impairment

Dietary Considerations Should be taken whole; do not crush, chew, or swallow. Food and drink can be taken normally; chewing gum should be avoided.

Administration Apply in the morning after brushing teeth. With dry hands, place either side of the tablet against the upper gum above the incisor tooth; hold with slight pressure over the upper lip for 30 seconds. Placing the rounded side of the tablet against the gum may be more comfortable. Alternate sides of the mouth with each application; do not crush, chew, or swallow. Avoid chewing gum while in place.

If the tablet does not adhere to the gum or falls off within 6 hours of application, the same tablet should be repositioned immediately. If the tablet does not adhere, use a new tablet. If the tablet is swallowed within 6 hours of application, the patient should drink a glass of water and apply a new tablet (only once). If the tablet falls off or is swallowed >6 hours after application, a new tablet should not be applied until the next regularly scheduled dose.

Dosage Forms Excipient information presented when available (limited, particularly for generics); consult specific product labeling. [DSC] = Discontinued product

Tablet, for buccal application:

Oravig®: 50 mg [DSC]

Miconazole (Topical) (mi KON a zole)

Brand Names: U.S. 3M™ Cavilon™ Antifungal [OTC]; Aloe Vesta® Antifungal [OTC]; Baza® Antifungal [OTC]; Carrington® Antifungal [OTC]; Critic-Aid® Clear AF [OTC]; DermaFungal [OTC]; Dermagran® AF [OTC]; DiabetAid® Antifungal Foot Bath [OTC]; Fungoid® [OTC]; Lotrimin AF® [OTC]; Micaderm® [OTC]; Micatin® [OTC]; Micro-Guard® [OTC]; Miranel AF™ [OTC]; Mitrazol® [OTC]; Monistat® 1 Day or Night [OTC]; Monistat® 1 [OTC]; Monistat® 3 [OTC]; Monistat® 7 [OTC]; Neosporin® AF [OTC]; Podactin Cream [OTC]; Secura® Antifungal Extra Thick [OTC]; Secura® Antifungal Greaseless [OTC]; Ting® Spray Powder [OTC]; Zeasorb®-AF [OTC]

Brand Names: Canada Dermazole; Micatin®; Micozole; Monistat®; Monistat® 3

Index Terms Miconazole Nitrate

Pharmacologic Category Antifungal Agent, Topical; Antifungal Agent, Vaginal

Additional Appendix Information

Antifungal Agents *on page 1876*

Use Treatment of vulvovaginal candidiasis and a variety of skin and mucous membrane fungal infections

Pregnancy Risk Factor C

Lactation Excretion in breast milk unknown/use caution

Contraindications Hypersensitivity to miconazole or any component of the formulation

Warnings/Precautions For topical use only; avoid contact with eyes. Discontinue if sensitivity or irritation develop. Petrolatum-based vaginal products may damage rubber or latex condoms or diaphragms. Separate use by 3 days. Consult with healthcare provider prior to self-medication (OTC use) of vaginal products if experiencing vaginal itching/discomfort, lower abdominal pain, back or shoulder pain, chills, nausea, vomiting, foul-smelling discharge, if this is the first vaginal yeast infection, or if exposed to HIV. Contact healthcare provider if symptoms do not begin to improve after 3 days or last longer than 7 days. Topical products are not for self-medication (OTC use) in children <2 years of age; vaginal products are not for OTC use in children <12 years of age.

Fungoid® tincture: Patients with diabetes, circulatory problems, renal or hepatic dysfunction should contact healthcare provider prior to self-medication (OTC use).

Adverse Reactions Frequency not defined.

Topical: Allergic contact dermatitis, burning, maceration

Vaginal: Abdominal cramps, burning, irritation, itching

Drug Interactions

Metabolism/Transport Effects None known.

Avoid Concomitant Use There are no known interactions where it is recommended to avoid concomitant use.

Increased Effect/Toxicity

Miconazole (Topical) may increase the levels/effects of: Vitamin K Antagonists

Decreased Effect There are no known significant interactions involving a decrease in effect.

Ethanol/Nutrition/Herb Interactions Herb/Nutraceutical: St John's wort may decrease miconazole levels.

Mechanism of Action Inhibits biosynthesis of ergosterol, damaging the fungal cell wall membrane, which increases permeability causing leaking of nutrients

Pharmacodynamics/Kinetics

Absorption: Topical: Negligible

Excretion: Feces; urine

Dosage

Topical: Children and Adults: **Note:** Not for OTC use in children <2 years:

- Tinea corporis: Apply twice daily for 4 weeks
- Tinea pedis: Apply twice daily for 4 weeks
  - Effervescent tablet: Dissolve 1 tablet in ~1 gallon of water; soak feet for 15-30 minutes; pat dry
- Tinea cruris: Apply twice daily for 2 weeks

Vaginal: Children ≥12 years and Adults: Vulvovaginal candidiasis:

- Cream, 2%: Insert 1 applicatorful at bedtime for 7 days
- Cream, 4%: Insert 1 applicatorful at bedtime for 3 days
- Suppository, 100 mg: Insert 1 suppository at bedtime for 7 days
- Suppository, 200 mg: Insert 1 suppository at bedtime for 3 days
- Suppository, 1200 mg: Insert 1 suppository (a one-time dose); may be used at bedtime or during the day

Note: Many products are available as a combination pack, with a suppository for vaginal instillation and cream to relieve external symptoms. External cream may be used twice daily, as needed, for up to 7 days.

Dosage Forms Excipient information presented when available (limited, particularly for generics); consult specific product labeling. [DSC] = Discontinued product

Aerosol, powder, topical, as nitrate:

- Lotrimin AF®: 2% (133 g)
- Lotrimin AF®: 2% (133 g) [deodorant formulation]
- Micatin®: 2% (90 g)
- Neosporin® AF: 2% (85 g)
- Ting® Spray Powder: 2% (128 g) [contains aloe, ethanol 10% w/w]

Aerosol, spray, topical, as nitrate:

- Micatin®: 2% (90 g)
- Micatin®: 2% (105 mL) [contains benzyl alcohol]
- Neosporin® AF: 2% (105 mL)

Combination package, topical/vaginal, as nitrate: Cream, topical: 2% (9 g) and Suppository, vaginal: 200 mg (3s)
Monistat® 3: Cream, topical: 2% (9 g) and Insert, vaginal: 200 mg (3s)
Monistat® 7: Cream, topical: 2% (9 g) and Cream, vaginal: 2% (45 g), Cream, topical: 2% (9 g) and Cream, vaginal: 2% (7 x 5 g) [contains benzoic acid]
Monistat® 3: Cream, topical: 2% (9 g) and Cream, vaginal: 4% (25 g), Cream, topical: 2% (9 g) and Cream, vaginal: 4% (3 x 5 g) [contains benzoic acid; vaginal cream 200 mg/applicator]
Monistat® 7: Cream, topical: 2% (9 g) and Suppository, vaginal: 100 mg (7s) [contains benzoic acid (in cream)]
Monistat® 1: Cream, topical: 2% (9 g) and Insert, vaginal: 1200 mg (1) [contains benzoic acid (in cream), soya lecithin (in insert)]
Monistat® 1 Day or Night: Cream, topical: 2% (9 g) and Insert, vaginal: 1200 mg (1) [contains benzoic acid (in cream), mineral oil (in insert), soya lecithin (in insert)]
Cream, topical, as nitrate: 2% (15 g, 30 g, 45 g)
Baza® Antifungal: 2% (4 g, 57 g, 142 g) [zinc oxide based formula]
Carrington® Antifungal: 2% (150 g)
Micaderm®: 2% (30 g)
Micatin®: 2% (14 g) [contains benzoic acid]
Micro-Guard®: 2% (60 g [DSC])
Miranel AF™: 2% (28 g) [contains ethanol]
3M™ Cavilon™ Antifungal: 2% (56 g, 141 g) [contains castor oil]
Neosporin® AF: 2% (14 g, 15 g) [contains benzoic acid]
Podactin Cream: 2% (30 g)
Secura® Antifungal Extra Thick: 2% (97.5 g) [contains zinc oxide]
Secura® Antifungal Greaseless: 2% (60 g)
Cream, vaginal, as nitrate: 2% (45 g); 4% (25 g [DSC])
Monistat® 7: 2% (45 g) [contains benzoic acid; 100 mg/applicator]
Monistat® 3: 4% (15 g, 25 g) [contains benzoic acid; 200 mg/applicator]
Gel, topical, as nitrate:
Zeasorb®-AF: 2% (24 g [DSC])
Liquid, topical, as nitrate [spray]:
Lotrimin AF®: 2% (150 g)
Ointment, topical, as nitrate:
Aloe Vesta® Antifungal: 2% (60 g, 150 g) [contains aloe]
Critic-Aid® Clear AF: 2% (57 g, 142 g, 300s)
DermaFungal: 2% (120 g)
Dermagran® AF: 2% (120 g) [zinc oxide based formula]
Powder, topical, as nitrate:
Lotrimin AF®: 2% (90 g)
Micro-Guard®: 2% (90 g)
Mitrazol®: 2% (30 g)
Zeasorb®-AF: 2% (70 g)
Suppository, vaginal, as nitrate: 100 mg (7s); 200 mg (3s)
Tablet for solution, topical, as nitrate [effervescent]:
DiabetAid® Antifungal Foot Bath: 2% (10s)
Tincture, topical, as nitrate:
Fungoid®: 2% (7.39 mL, 30 mL) [contains isopropyl alcohol 30%]

- **Miconazole Nitrate** *see* Miconazole (Oral) *on page 1125*
- **Miconazole Nitrate** *see* Miconazole (Topical) *on page 1126*
- **Micozole (Can)** *see* Miconazole (Topical) *on page 1126*
- **MICRhoGAM® UF Plus** *see* Rh_o(D) Immune Globulin *on page 1476*
- **Microgestin® 1.5/30** *see* Ethinyl Estradiol and Norethindrone *on page 660*
- **Microgestin® 1/20** *see* Ethinyl Estradiol and Norethindrone *on page 660*
- **Microgestin® Fe 1.5/30** *see* Ethinyl Estradiol and Norethindrone *on page 660*
- **Microgestin® Fe 1/20** *see* Ethinyl Estradiol and Norethindrone *on page 660*
- **Micro-Guard® [OTC]** *see* Miconazole (Topical) *on page 1126*
- **microK®** *see* Potassium Chloride *on page 1380*
- **microK® 10** *see* Potassium Chloride *on page 1380*
- **Micro-K Extencaps® (Can)** *see* Potassium Chloride *on page 1380*
- **Micronase** *see* GlyBURIDE *on page 799*
- **Micronor® (Can)** *see* Norethindrone *on page 1217*
- **Microzide®** *see* Hydrochlorothiazide *on page 835*
- **Midamor (Can)** *see* AMILoride *on page 89*

Midazolam (MID aye zoe lam)

Brand Names: Canada Apo-Midazolam®; Midazolam Injection

Index Terms Midazolam Hydrochloride; Versed

Pharmacologic Category Benzodiazepine

Additional Appendix Information
Benzodiazepines *on page 1882*
Status Epilepticus *on page 2010*

Use Preoperative sedation; moderate sedation prior to diagnostic or radiographic procedures; ICU sedation (continuous infusion); induction and maintenance of general anesthesia

Unlabeled Use Anxiety, status epilepticus, conscious sedation (intranasal route)

Pregnancy Risk Factor D

Pregnancy Considerations Adverse events were not observed in animal teratology studies. Midazolam has been found to cross the human placenta and can be detected in the serum of the umbilical vein and artery, as well as the amniotic fluid. Teratogenic effects have been observed with some benzodiazepines; however, additional studies are needed. The incidence of premature birth and low birth weights may be increased following maternal use of benzodiazepines; hypoglycemia and respiratory problems in the neonate may occur following exposure late in pregnancy. Neonatal withdrawal symptoms may occur within days to weeks after birth and "floppy infant syndrome" (which also includes withdrawal symptoms) have been reported with some benzodiazepines.

Lactation Enters breast milk/use caution (AAP rates "of concern"; AAP 2001 update pending)

Contraindications Hypersensitivity to midazolam or any component of the formulation; intrathecal or epidural injection of parenteral forms containing preservatives (ie, benzyl alcohol); acute narrow-angle glaucoma; concurrent use of potent inhibitors of CYP3A4 (amprenavir, atazanavir, or ritonavir)

Warnings/Precautions [U.S. Boxed Warning]: May cause severe respiratory depression, respiratory arrest, or apnea. Use with extreme caution, particularly in noncritical care settings. Appropriate resuscitative equipment and qualified personnel must be available for administration and monitoring. Initial dosing must be cautiously titrated and individualized, particularly in elderly or debilitated patients, patients with hepatic impairment (including alcoholics), or in renal impairment, particularly if other CNS depressants (including opiates) are used concurrently. **[U.S. Boxed Warning]: Initial doses in elderly or debilitated patients should be conservative; as little as 1 mg, but not to exceed 2.5 mg.** Use with caution in patients with respiratory disease or impaired gag reflex. Use during upper airway procedures may increase risk of hypoventilation. Prolonged responses have been noted following extended administration by continuous infusion (possibly due to metabolite accumulation) or in the presence of drugs which inhibit midazolam metabolism.

Causes CNS depression (dose-related) resulting in sedation, dizziness, confusion, or ataxia which may impair physical and mental capabilities. Patients must be cautioned about performing tasks which require mental alertness (eg, operating machinery or driving). A minimum of 1 day should elapse after midazolam administration before attempting these tasks. Use with caution in patients receiving other CNS depressants or psychoactive agents. Effects with other sedative drugs or ethanol may be potentiated. Benzodiazepines have been associated with falls and traumatic injury and should be used with extreme caution in patients who are at risk of these events (especially the elderly).

May cause hypotension - hemodynamic events are more common in pediatric patients or patients with hemodynamic instability. Hypotension and/or respiratory depression may occur more frequently in patients who have received opioid analgesics. Use with caution in obese patients, chronic renal failure, and HF. Does not protect against increases in heart rate or blood pressure during intubation. Should not be used in shock, coma, or acute alcohol intoxication. **[U.S. Boxed Warning]: Do not administer by rapid I.V. injection in neonates; severe hypotension and seizures have been reported; risk may be increased with concomitant fentanyl use.**

Avoid intra-arterial administration or extravasation of parenteral formulation. Some parenteral dosage forms may contain benzyl alcohol which has been associated with "gasping syndrome" in neonates. Some formulations may contain cherry flavoring.

Midazolam causes anterograde amnesia. Paradoxical reactions, including hyperactive or aggressive behavior have been reported with benzodiazepines, particularly in adolescent/pediatric or psychiatric patients. Does not have analgesic, antidepressant, or antipsychotic properties.

Benzodiazepines have been associated with dependence and acute withdrawal symptoms on discontinuation or reduction in dose. Acute withdrawal, including seizures, may be precipitated after administration of flumazenil to patients receiving long-term benzodiazepine therapy.

Adverse Reactions As reported in adults unless otherwise noted:

>10%: Respiratory: Decreased tidal volume and/or respiratory rate decrease, apnea (3% children)

1% to 10%:

Cardiovascular: Hypotension (3% children)

Central nervous system: Drowsiness (1%), oversedation, headache (1%), seizure-like activity (1% children)

Gastrointestinal: Nausea (3%), vomiting (3%)

Local: Pain and local reactions at injection site (4% I.M., 5% I.V.; severity less than diazepam)

Ocular: Nystagmus (1% children)

Respiratory: Cough (1%)

Miscellaneous: Physical and psychological dependence with prolonged use, hiccups (4%, 1% children), paradoxical reaction (2% children)

<1% (Limited to important or life-threatening): Agitation, amnesia, bigeminy, bronchospasm, emergence delirium, euphoria, hallucinations, laryngospasm, rash

Drug Interactions

Metabolism/Transport Effects **Substrate** of CYP2B6 (minor), CYP3A4 (major); **Note:** Assignment of Major/Minor substrate status based on clinically relevant drug interaction potential; **Inhibits** CYP2C8 (weak), CYP2C9 (weak), CYP3A4 (weak)

Avoid Concomitant Use

Avoid concomitant use of Midazolam with any of the following: Boceprevir; Conivaptan; Efavirenz; OLANZapine; Pimozide; Protease Inhibitors; Telaprevir

Increased Effect/Toxicity

Midazolam may increase the levels/effects of: Alcohol (Ethyl); CloZAPine; CNS Depressants; Fosphenytoin; Methotrimeprazine; Phenytoin; Pimozide; Propofol; Selective Serotonin Reuptake Inhibitors

The levels/effects of Midazolam may be increased by: Antifungal Agents (Azole Derivatives, Systemic); Aprepitant; Atorvastatin; Boceprevir; Calcium Channel Blockers (Nondihydropyridine); Cimetidine; Conivaptan; Contraceptives (Estrogens); Contraceptives (Progestins); CYP3A4 Inhibitors (Moderate); CYP3A4 Inhibitors (Strong); Dasatinib; Droperidol; Efavirenz; Fluconazole; Fosaprepitant; Grapefruit Juice; HydrOXYzine; Isoniazid; Macrolide Antibiotics; Methotrimeprazine; Nefazodone; OLANZapine; Propofol; Protease Inhibitors; Proton Pump Inhibitors; Selective Serotonin Reuptake Inhibitors; Telaprevir

Decreased Effect

The levels/effects of Midazolam may be decreased by: CarBAMazepine; CYP3A4 Inducers (Strong); Deferasirox; Ginkgo Biloba; Rifamycin Derivatives; St Johns Wort; Theophylline Derivatives; Tocilizumab; Yohimbine

Ethanol/Nutrition/Herb Interactions

Ethanol: May increase CNS depression; monitor for increased effects with coadministration. Caution patients about effects.

Food: Grapefruit juice may increase serum concentrations of midazolam; avoid concurrent use with oral form.

Herb/Nutraceutical: Avoid concurrent use with St John's wort (may decrease midazolam levels, may increase CNS depression). Avoid concurrent use with valerian, kava kava, gotu kola (may increase CNS depression).

Stability The manufacturer states that midazolam, at a final concentration of 0.5 mg/mL, is stable for up to 24 hours when diluted with D_5W or NS. A final concentration of 1 mg/mL in NS has been documented to be stable for up to 10 days (McMullen, 1995). Admixtures do not require protection from light for short-term storage.

Mechanism of Action Binds to stereospecific benzodiazepine receptors on the postsynaptic GABA neuron at several sites within the central nervous system, including the limbic system, reticular formation. Enhancement of the inhibitory effect of GABA on neuronal excitability results by increased neuronal membrane permeability to chloride ions. This shift in chloride ions results in hyperpolarization (a less excitable state) and stabilization.

Pharmacodynamics/Kinetics

Onset of action: I.M.: Sedation: ~15 minutes; I.V.: 3-5 minutes; Oral: 10-20 minutes; Intranasal: Children: 4-8 minutes (Lee-Kim, 2004)

Peak effect: I.M.: 0.5-1 hour

Duration: I.M.: Up to 6 hours; Mean: 2 hours; Intranasal: Children: 18-41 minutes (Lee-Kim, 2004)

Absorption: Oral: Rapid

Distribution: V_d: 1-3.1 L/kg; increased in females, elderly, and obesity

Protein binding: ~97%

Metabolism: Extensively hepatic via CYP3A4

Bioavailability: 36% (oral, children); >90% (I.M.)

Half-life elimination: 2-6 hours; prolonged in cirrhosis, congestive heart failure, obesity, and elderly

Excretion: Urine (as glucuronide conjugated metabolites); feces (~2% to 10%)

Dosage The dose of midazolam needs to be individualized based on the patient's age, underlying diseases, and concurrent medications. Decrease dose (by ~30%) if opioids or other CNS depressants are administered concomitantly.

Children: **Note:** Children <6 years may require higher doses and closer monitoring than older children; calculate dose based on ideal body weight.

Conscious sedation for procedures or preoperative sedation:

Oral, rectal: Children: 0.5-0.75 mg/kg as a single dose preprocedure (maximum: 20 mg); administer 20-30 minutes prior to procedure. Children <6 years or less cooperative patients may require as much as 1 mg/kg as a single dose; 0.25 mg/kg may suffice for children 6-16 years of age (Bozkurt, 2007).

Intranasal (unlabeled route): Children: 0.2-0.5 mg/kg (maximum total dose: 10 mg or 5 mg per nare); may be administered 10-20 minutes prior to procedure (Bozkurt, 2007; Chiaretti, 2011). **Note:** Use 5 mg/mL injectable concentrated solution to deliver dose. Due to the low pH of the solution, burning upon administration is likely to occur.

I.M.: Children: 0.1-0.15 mg/kg 30-60 minutes before surgery or procedure; range: 0.05-0.15 mg/kg; maximum total dose: 10 mg

I.V.:

Infants <6 months: Limited information is available in nonintubated infants; dosing recommendations not clear; infants <6 months are at higher risk for airway obstruction and hypoventilation; titrate dose in small increments to desired effect

Infants 6 months to Children 5 years: Initial: 0.05-0.1 mg/kg; total dose of 0.6 mg/kg may be required; maximum total dose: 6 mg

Children 6-12 years: Initial: 0.025-0.05 mg/kg; total doses of 0.4 mg/kg may be required; maximum total dose: 10 mg

Children 12-16 years: Dose as adults; maximum total dose: 10 mg

Conscious sedation during mechanical ventilation: Children: Loading dose: 0.05-0.2 mg/kg, followed by initial continuous infusion: 0.06-0.12 mg/kg/hour (1-2 mcg/kg/minute); usual range: 0.4-6 mcg/kg/minute

Status epilepticus refractory to standard therapy (unlabeled use): **Note:** Intubation required; adjust dose based on hemodynamics, seizure activity, and EEG. Infants >2 months and Children: Loading dose: 0.15 mg/kg followed by a continuous infusion of 0.06 mg/kg/hour (1 mcg/kg/minute); titrate dose upward every 5 minutes until clinical seizure activity is controlled; mean infusion rate required in 24 children was 0.14 mg/kg/hour (2.3 mcg/kg/minute) with a range of 0.06-1.1 mg/kg/hour (1-18.3 mcg/kg/minute) (Rivera, 1993).

A more aggressive approach has been demonstrated to provide control of status epilepticus within 30 minutes of initiation: Loading dose: 0.5 mg/kg followed by 0.12 mg/kg/hour (2 mcg/kg/minute). If seizures persist or recur, administer 0.5 mg/kg bolus with an increase in the infusion rate to 0.24 mg/kg/hour (4 mcg/kg/minute); if seizures continue to persist/recur, administer 0.1 mg/kg bolus and increase infusion to 0.48 mg/kg/hour (8 mcg/kg/minute); continue to repeat this last incremental increase until seizure control or a maximum dose of 1.44 mg/kg/hour (24 mcg/kg/minute) is reached; do not allow >5 minutes to elapse between each dose increment while seizures persist (dose range within clinical trial: 0.12-1.92 mg/kg/hour or 2-32 mcg/kg/minute) (Morrison, 2006).

Adults: **Note:** Consider reducing dose by 30% to 50% in elderly or debilitated patients and those receiving opioids or other CNS depressants.

Preoperative sedation:

I.M.: 0.07-0.08 mg/kg 30-60 minutes prior to surgery/procedure; usual dose: 5 mg

I.V.: 0.02-0.04 mg/kg; repeat every 5 minutes as needed to desired effect or up to 0.1-0.2 mg/kg

Intranasal (unlabeled route): 0.1 mg/kg; administer 10-20 minutes prior to surgery/procedure (Uygur-Bayramiçli, 2002). **Note:** Use 5 mg/mL injectable solution to deliver dose. Due to the low pH of the solution, burning upon administration is likely to occur.

Conscious sedation: I.V.: Initial: 0.5-2 mg slow I.V. over at least 2 minutes; slowly titrate to effect by repeating doses every 2-3 minutes if needed; usual total dose: 2.5-5 mg

Healthy adults <60 years:

Initial: Some patients respond to doses as low as 1 mg; no more than 2.5 mg should be administered over a period of 2 minutes. Additional doses of midazolam may be administered after a 2-minute waiting period and evaluation of sedation after each dose increment. A total dose >5 mg is generally not needed.

Maintenance: 25% of dose used to reach sedative effect

Adults ≥60 years, debilitated, or chronically ill: Refer to elderly dosing.

Anesthesia: I.V.:

Induction:

Unpremedicated patients: 0.3-0.35 mg/kg (up to 0.6 mg/kg in resistant cases)

Premedicated patients: 0.15-0.35 mg/kg

Maintenance: 0.05-0.3 mg/kg as needed, or continuous infusion 0.25-1.5 mcg/kg/minute

Sedation in mechanically ventilated patients: Per the manufacturer: I.V.: Initial dose: 0.01-0.05 mg/kg (~0.5-4 mg); may repeat at 5- to 15-minute intervals until adequate sedation achieved; maintenance infusion: 0.02-0.1 mg/kg/hour. Titrate to reach desired level of sedation.

or

I.V.: Initial dose: 0.02-0.08 mg/kg (~1-5 mg in 70 kg adult); may repeat at 5- to 15-minute intervals until adequate sedation achieved; maintenance infusion: 0.04-0.2 mg/kg/hour. Titrate to reach desired level of sedation (Jacobi, 2002).

Refractory status epilepticus (unlabeled use): **Note:** Intubation required; adjust dose based on hemodynamics, seizure activity, and EEG. I.V.: 0.15-0.3 mg/kg (usual dose: 5-15 mg); may repeat every 10-15 minutes as needed **or** 0.2 mg/kg bolus followed by a continuous infusion of 0.05-0.6 mg/kg/hour (Lowenstein, 2005; Meierkord, 2010)

Elderly: I.V.: Conscious sedation: Initial: 0.5 mg slow I.V.; give no more than 1.5 mg in a 2-minute period; if additional titration is needed, give no more than 1 mg over 2 minutes, waiting another 2 or more minutes to evaluate sedative effect; a total dose of >3.5 mg is rarely necessary

Dosage adjustment in renal impairment: There are no dosage adjustments provided in manufacturer's labeling; use with caution.

Hemodialysis: Supplemental dose is not necessary.

Peritoneal dialysis: Significant drug removal is unlikely based on physiochemical characteristics.

Dosage adjustment in hepatic impairment: Severe hepatic impairment: Reduce dose by 50%.

Dietary Considerations Avoid grapefruit juice with oral syrup.

Administration

Intranasal: **Note:** Due to the low pH of the solution, burning upon administration is likely to occur. Use of an atomizer, such as the MAD 300 Mucosal Atomizer which attaches to a tuberculin syringe, can reduce irritation. If possible, based upon dose to be administered, use higher concentration injectable solution to minimize volume administered intranasal. Smaller volume will reduce irritation and swallowing of administered dose. The maximum recommended dose volume per nare is 1 mL.

Using the 5 mg/mL injectable solution, draw up desired dose with a 1-3 mL needleless syringe; may attach a nasal mucosal atomization device prior to delivering dose. Deliver half of the total dose volume (of the 5 mg/mL concentration) into the first nare using the atomizer device or by dripping slowly into nostril, then deliver the other half of the dose into the second nare.

Oral: Do not mix with any liquid (such as grapefruit juice) prior to administration

Parenteral:

I.M.: Administer deep I.M. into large muscle.

I.V.: Administer by slow I.V. injection over at least 2-5 minutes at a concentration of 1-5 mg/mL or by I.V. infusion. Continuous infusions should be administered via an infusion pump.

Monitoring Parameters Respiratory and cardiovascular status, blood pressure, blood pressure monitor required during I.V. administration

Additional Information Abrupt discontinuation after sustained use (generally >10 days) may cause withdrawal symptoms. For neonates, since both concentrations of the injection contain 1% benzyl alcohol, use the 5 mg/mL injection and dilute to 0.5 mg/mL with SWI without preservatives to decrease the amount of benzyl alcohol delivered to the neonate; with continuous infusion, midazolam may accumulate in peripheral tissues; use lowest effective infusion rate to reduce accumulation effects; midazolam is 3-4 times as potent as diazepam; paradoxical reactions associated with midazolam use in children (eg, agitation, restlessness, combativeness) have been successfully treated with flumazenil (Massanari, 1997).

Dosage Forms Excipient information presented when available (limited, particularly for generics); consult specific product labeling.

Injection, solution: 1 mg/mL (2 mL, 5 mL, 10 mL); 5 mg/mL (1 mL, 2 mL, 5 mL, 10 mL)

Injection, solution [preservative free]: 1 mg/mL (2 mL, 5 mL); 5 mg/mL (1 mL, 2 mL)

Syrup, oral: 2 mg/mL (118 mL)

Controlled Substance C-IV

- **Midazolam Hydrochloride** *see* Midazolam *on page 1127*
- **Midazolam Injection (Can)** *see* Midazolam *on page 1127*

Midodrine (MI doe dreen)

Brand Names: Canada Amatine®; Apo-Midodrine®

Index Terms Midodrine Hydrochloride; ProAmatine

Pharmacologic Category Alpha$_1$ Agonist

Use Orphan drug: Treatment of symptomatic orthostatic hypotension

Unlabeled Use Management of urinary incontinence; vasovagal syncope; prevention of dialysis-induced hypotension

Pregnancy Risk Factor C

Pregnancy Considerations Increased rate of embryo resorption and decreased fetal weight were observed in animal studies. Use during pregnancy should be avoided unless the potential benefit outweighs the risk to the fetus.

Lactation Excretion in breast milk is unknown/use caution

Contraindications Hypersensitivity to midodrine or any component of the formulation; severe organic heart disease; acute renal failure; urinary retention; pheochromocytoma; thyrotoxicosis; persistent and significant supine hypertension

Warnings/Precautions [U.S. Boxed Warning]: Indicated for patients for whom orthostatic hypotension significantly impairs their daily life despite standard clinical care. May cause hypertension. Use is not recommended with supine hypertension. May slow heart rate primarily due to vagal reflex. Use caution when administered concurrently with negative chronotropes (eg, digoxin, beta blockers). Use is not recommended with supine hypertension. Use cautiously in patients with renal impairment and initiate with a reduced dose; contraindicated in patients with acute renal failure. Caution should be exercised in patients with diabetes, visual problems (especially if receiving fludrocortisone), urinary retention (reduce initial dose), or hepatic dysfunction; monitor renal and hepatic function prior to and periodically during therapy.

Adverse Reactions

>10%:

Cardiovascular: Supine hypertension (7% to 13%)

Dermatologic: Piloerection (13%), pruritus (12%)

Genitourinary: Urinary urgency, retention, or polyuria, dysuria (up to 13%)

Neuromuscular & skeletal: Paresthesia (18%)

1% to 10%:

Central nervous system: Chills (5%), pain (5%)

Dermatologic: Rash (2%)

Gastrointestinal: Abdominal pain

<1% (Limited to important or life-threatening): Anxiety, backache, canker sore, confusion, dizziness, dry skin, erythema multiforme, facial flushing, flatulence, flushing, GI distress, headache, heartburn, hyperesthesia, insomnia, ICP increased, leg cramps, nausea, somnolence, visual field defect, weakness, xerostomia

Drug Interactions

Metabolism/Transport Effects None known.

Avoid Concomitant Use

Avoid concomitant use of Midodrine with any of the following: Ergot Derivatives; Iobenguane I 123; MAO Inhibitors

Increased Effect/Toxicity

Midodrine may increase the levels/effects of: Sympathomimetics

The levels/effects of Midodrine may be increased by: Atomoxetine; Beta-Blockers; Calcium Channel Blockers (Nondihydropyridine); Cannabinoids; Cardiac Glycosides; Ergot Derivatives; MAO Inhibitors; Tricyclic Antidepressants

Decreased Effect

Midodrine may decrease the levels/effects of: Benzylpenicilloyl Polylysine; Iobenguane I 123

Mechanism of Action Midodrine forms an active metabolite, desglymidodrine, which is an alpha$_1$-agonist. This agent increases arteriolar and venous tone resulting in a rise in standing, sitting, and supine systolic and diastolic blood pressure in patients with orthostatic hypotension.

Pharmacodynamics/Kinetics

Onset of action: ~1 hour

Duration: 2-3 hours

Absorption: Rapid

Distribution: V_d (desglymidodrine): <1.6 L/kg; poorly across membrane (eg, blood-brain barrier)

Protein binding: Minimal

Metabolism: Hepatic and many other tissues; midodrine is a prodrug which undergoes rapid deglycination to desglymidodrine (active metabolite)

Bioavailability: Desglymidodrine: 93%

Half-life elimination: Desglymidodrine: ~3-4 hours; Midodrine: 25 minutes

Time to peak, serum: Desglymidodrine: 1-2 hours; Midodrine: 30 minutes

Excretion: Urine (Midodrine: Insignificant; Desglymidodrine: 80% by active renal secretion)

Dosage Adults: Oral:

Orthostatic hypotension: 10 mg 3 times/day during daytime hours (every 3-4 hours) when patient is upright (maximum: 40 mg/day)

Prevention of hemodialysis-induced hypotension (unlabeled use): 2.5-10 mg given 15-30 minutes prior to dialysis session (Cruz, 1998; KDOQI, 2005; Prakash, 2004)

Vasovagal syncope (unlabeled use): Initial: 5 mg 3 times/day during daytime hours (every 6 hours) increased up to 15 mg/dose if necessary (Perez-Lugones, 2001; Ward, 1998)

Dosing adjustment in renal impairment: Orthostatic hypotension: 2.5 mg 3 times/day, gradually increasing as tolerated

Hemodialysis: Dialyzable; dose after hemodialysis unless used for prevention of hemodialysis-induced hypotension.

Administration Doses may be given in approximately 3- to 4-hour intervals (eg, shortly before or upon rising in the morning, at midday, in the late afternoon not later than 6 PM). Avoid dosing after the evening meal or within 4 hours of bedtime. Continue therapy only in patients who appear to attain symptomatic improvement during initial treatment. Standing systolic blood pressure may be elevated 15-30 mm Hg at 1 hour after a 10 mg dose. Some effect may persist for 2-3 hours.

Monitoring Parameters Blood pressure; renal and hepatic function

Dosage Forms Excipient information presented when available (limited, particularly for generics); consult specific product labeling.

Tablet, oral, as hydrochloride: 2.5 mg, 5 mg, 10 mg

◆ **Midodrine Hydrochloride** *see* Midodrine *on page 1130*

◆ **Midol® Cramps & Body Aches [OTC]** *see* Ibuprofen *on page 860*

◆ **Midol® Extended Relief [OTC]** *see* Naproxen *on page 1177*

◆ **Mifeprex®** *see* Mifepristone *on page 1131*

Mifepristone (mi FE pris tone)

Brand Names: U.S. Mifeprex®

Index Terms RU-38486; RU-486

Pharmacologic Category Abortifacient; Antineoplastic Agent, Hormone Antagonist; Antiprogestin

Use Medical termination of intrauterine pregnancy, through day 49 of pregnancy. Patients may need treatment with misoprostol and possibly surgery to complete therapy.

Unlabeled Use Treatment of unresectable meningioma; has been studied in the treatment of breast cancer, ovarian cancer, and adrenal cortical carcinoma

Pregnancy Risk Factor X

Pregnancy Considerations This medication is used to terminate pregnancy; there are no approved treatment indications for its use during pregnancy. Prostaglandins (including mifepristone and misoprostol) may have teratogenic effects when used during pregnancy. If treatment fails, there is a risk of fetal malformation. In sexually active women, pregnancy can occur prior to the first menstrual period following treatment. Appropriate contraception can be started as soon as termination of pregnancy is confirmed or before sexual intercourse is resumed.

Lactation Excretion in breast milk unknown/contraindicated

Prescribing and Access Restrictions As a requirement of the REMS program, a medication guide must be given to the patient prior to receiving the medication. In addition, the manufacturer recommends distributing a patient agreement form which must be signed by the patient and prescriber confirming the patient's agreement to terminate her pregnancy. A signed copy of the patient agreement should be kept in the patient's medical record.

Mifeprex® is only available direct from Danco Laboratories' distributor. To obtain the product, please refer to, http://www.earlyoptionpill.com, or call 1-877-432-7596.

Investigators wishing to obtain the agent for use in oncology patients must apply for a patient-specific IND from the FDA.

Medication Guide Available Yes

Contraindications Hypersensitivity to mifepristone, misoprostol, other prostaglandins, or any component of the formulation; chronic adrenal failure; porphyrias; hemorrhagic disorder or concurrent anticoagulant therapy; pregnancy termination >49 days; intrauterine device (IUD) in place; ectopic pregnancy or undiagnosed adnexal mass; concurrent long-term corticosteroid therapy; inadequate or lack of access to emergency medical services; inability to understand effects and/or comply with treatment

Warnings/Precautions [U.S. Boxed Warning]: Patient must be instructed of the treatment procedure and expected effects. A signed agreement form must be kept in the patient's file. Physicians may obtain patient agreement forms, physician enrollment forms, and medical consultation directly from Danco Laboratories at 1-877-432-7596. Adverse effects (including blood transfusions, hospitalization, ongoing pregnancy, and other major complications) must be reported in writing to the medication distributor. To be administered only by physicians who can date pregnancy, diagnose ectopic pregnancies, provide access to surgical abortion (if needed), and can provide access to emergency care. Medication will be distributed directly to these physicians following signed agreement with the distributor. Must be administered under supervision by the qualified physician. Pregnancy is dated from day 1 of last menstrual period (presuming a 28-day cycle, ovulation occurring midcycle). Pregnancy duration can be determined using menstrual history and clinical examination. Ultrasound should be used if an ectopic pregnancy is suspected or if duration of pregnancy is uncertain. Ultrasonography may not identify all ectopic pregnancies, and healthcare providers should be alert for signs and symptoms which may be related to undiagnosed ectopic pregnancy in any patient who receives mifepristone

[U.S. Boxed Warning]: Patients should be counseled to seek medical attention in cases of excessive bleeding. Bleeding occurs and should be expected (average 9-16 days, may be ≥30 days). In some cases, bleeding may be prolonged and heavy, potentially leading to hypovolemic shock; the manufacturer cites soaking through two thick sanitary pads per hour for two consecutive hours as an example of excessive bleeding. Bleeding may require blood transfusion (rare), curettage, saline infusions, and/or vasoconstrictors. Use caution in patients with severe anemia. Confirmation of pregnancy termination by clinical exam or ultrasound must be made 14 days following treatment. Manufacturer recommends surgical termination of pregnancy when medical termination fails or is not complete. Prescriber should determine in advance whether they will provide such care themselves or through other providers. Preventative measures to prevent rhesus immunization must be taken prior to surgical abortion. Prescriber should also give the patient clear instructions on whom to call and what to do in the event of an emergency following administration of mifepristone.

[U.S. Boxed Warning]: Bacterial infections have been reported following use of this product. In rare cases, these infections may be serious and/or fatal, with septic shock as a potential complication. A causal relationship has not been established. Sustained fever, abdominal pain, or pelvic tenderness should prompt evaluation; however, healthcare professionals are warned that atypical presentations of serious infection without these symptoms have also been noted. Patients presenting with nausea, vomiting, diarrhea, or weakness, with or without abdominal pain or fever, should be evaluated for serious bacterial infection when symptoms occur >24 hours after taking misoprostol. Treatment with antibiotics, including coverage for anaerobic bacteria (eg, *Clostridium sordellii*) should be initiated. **[U.S. Boxed Warning]: Patients undergoing treatment with mifepristone should be instructed to bring their Medication Guide with them when an obtaining treatment from an emergency room or healthcare provider that did not prescribe the medication initially in order to identify that they are undergoing a medical abortion.**

Safety and efficacy have not been established for use in women with chronic cardiovascular, hypertensive, hepatic, respiratory, or renal disease, insulin-dependent diabetes mellitus, severe anemia, or heavy smokers. Women >35 years of age and smokers (>10 cigarettes/day) were excluded from clinical trials. Safety and efficacy in pediatric patients have not been established.

Adverse Reactions Vaginal bleeding and uterine cramping are expected to occur when this medication is used to terminate a pregnancy; 90% of women using this medication for this purpose also report adverse reactions. Bleeding or spotting occurs in most women for a period of 9-16 days. Up to 8% of women will experience some degree of bleeding or spotting for 30 days or more. In some cases, bleeding may be prolonged and heavy, potentially leading to hypovolemic shock.

>10%:

- Central nervous system: Headache (2% to 31%), dizziness (1% to 12%)
- Gastrointestinal: Abdominal pain (cramping) (96%), nausea (43% to 61%), vomiting (18% to 26%), diarrhea (12% to 20%)
- Genitourinary: Uterine cramping (83%)

1% to 10%:

- Cardiovascular: Syncope (1%)
- Central nervous system: Fatigue (10%), fever (4%), insomnia (3%), anxiety (2%), fainting (2%)
- Gastrointestinal: Dyspepsia (3%)
- Genitourinary: Uterine hemorrhage (5%), vaginitis (3%), pelvic pain (2%), endometriosis/salpingitis/pelvic inflammatory disease (1%)
- Hematologic: Decreased hemoglobin >2 g/dL (6%), anemia (2%), leukorrhea (2%)
- Neuromuscular & skeletal: Back pain (9%), rigors (3%), leg pain (2%), weakness (2%)
- Respiratory: Sinusitis (2%)
- Miscellaneous: Viral infection (4%)

<1% (Limited to important or life-threatening): Adult respiratory distress syndrome (ADRS), allergic reaction including urticaria and hives, bacterial infection (including an ectopic bacteria such as *Clostridium sordellii*), Crohn's disease (exacerbation), disseminated intravascular coagulopathy (DIC), dyspnea, hematometra, hypotension, lightheadedness, loss of consciousness, MI, pancreatitis (acute), pelvic infection, postabortal infection, QT prolongation, ruptured ectopic pregnancy, sepsis, septic shock, sickle cell crisis (exacerbation), tachycardia, toxic shock syndrome

In trials for unresectable meningioma, the most common adverse effects included fatigue, hot flashes, gynecomastia or breast tenderness, hair thinning, and rash. In premenopausal women, vaginal bleeding may be seen shortly after beginning therapy and cessation of menses is common. Thyroiditis and effects related to antiglucocorticoid activity have also been noted.

Drug Interactions

Metabolism/Transport Effects **Substrate** of CYP3A4 (minor); **Note:** Assignment of Major/Minor substrate status based on clinically relevant drug interaction potential; **Inhibits** CYP2D6 (weak), CYP3A4 (weak)

Avoid Concomitant Use

Avoid concomitant use of Mifepristone with any of the following: Pimozide

Increased Effect/Toxicity

Mifepristone may increase the levels/effects of: Pimozide

The levels/effects of Mifepristone may be increased by: Conivaptan

Decreased Effect

The levels/effects of Mifepristone may be decreased by: Tocilizumab

Ethanol/Nutrition/Herb Interactions

Food: Do not take with grapefruit juice; grapefruit juice may inhibit mifepristone metabolism leading to increased levels.

Herb/Nutraceutical: Avoid St John's wort (may induce mifepristone metabolism, leading to decreased levels).

Stability Store at room temperature of 25°C (77°F).

Mechanism of Action Mifepristone, a synthetic steroid, competitively binds to the intracellular progesterone receptor, blocking the effects of progesterone. When used for the termination of pregnancy, this leads to contraction-inducing activity in the myometrium. In the absence of progesterone, mifepristone acts as a partial progesterone agonist. Mifepristone also has weak antiglucocorticoid and antiandrogenic properties; it blocks the feedback effect of cortisol on corticotropin secretion.

Pharmacodynamics/Kinetics

Absorption: Oral: rapid

Protein binding: 98% to albumin and α_1-acid glycoprotein

Metabolism: Hepatic via CYP3A4 to three metabolites (may possess some antiprogestin and antiglucocorticoid activity)

Bioavailability: Oral: 69%

Half-life elimination: Terminal: 18 hours following a slower phase where 50% eliminated between 12-72 hours

Time to peak: Oral: 90 minutes

Excretion: Feces (83%); urine (9%)

Dosage Oral:

Adults:

Termination of pregnancy: Treatment consists of three office visits by the patient; the patient must read medication guide and sign patient agreement prior to treatment:

- Day 1: 600 mg (three 200 mg tablets) taken as a single dose under physician supervision
- Day 3: Patient must return to the healthcare provider 2 days following administration of mifepristone; unless abortion has occurred (confirmed using ultrasound or clinical examination): 400 mcg (two 200 mcg tablets) of misoprostol; patient may need treatment for cramps or gastrointestinal symptoms at this time
- Day 14: Patient must return to the healthcare provider ~14 days after administration of mifepristone; confirm complete termination of pregnancy by ultrasound or clinical exam. Surgical termination is recommended to manage treatment failures.

Meningioma (unlabeled use): Refer to individual protocols. The dose used in meningioma is usually 200 mg/day, continued based on toxicity and response.

Elderly: Safety and efficacy have not been established

Dosage adjustment in renal impairment: Safety and efficacy have not been established

Dosage adjustment in hepatic impairment: Safety and efficacy have not been established; use with caution due to CYP3A4 metabolism

Monitoring Parameters Clinical exam and/or ultrasound to confirm complete termination of pregnancy; hemoglobin, hematocrit, and red blood cell count in cases of heavy bleeding. Consider CBC in any patient who reports nausea, vomiting, or diarrhea and weakness with or without abdominal pain, and without fever or other signs of infection more than 24 hours after administration of misoprostol.

Test Interactions hCG levels will not be useful to confirm pregnancy termination until at least 10 days following mifepristone treatment

Additional Information Medication will be distributed directly to qualified physicians following signed agreement with the distributor, Danco Laboratories. It will not be available through pharmacies. Major adverse reactions (hospitalization, blood transfusion, ongoing pregnancy, etc) should be reported to Danco Laboratories.

Dosage Forms Excipient information presented when available (limited, particularly for generics); consult specific product labeling.

Tablet, oral:

Mifeprex®: 200 mg

Miglitol (MIG li tol)

Brand Names: U.S. Glyset®

Pharmacologic Category Antidiabetic Agent, Alpha-Glucosidase Inhibitor

Additional Appendix Information

Diabetes Mellitus Management, Adults *on page 1983*

Use Type 2 diabetes mellitus (noninsulin-dependent, NIDDM):

Monotherapy as an adjunct to diet to improve glycemic control in patients with type 2 diabetes mellitus (noninsulin-dependent, NIDDM) whose hyperglycemia cannot be managed with diet alone

Combination therapy with a sulfonylurea when diet plus either miglitol or a sulfonylurea alone do not result in adequate glycemic control. The effect of miglitol to enhance glycemic control is additive to that of sulfonylureas when used in combination.

Pregnancy Risk Factor B

Pregnancy Considerations Adverse events have not been reported in animal reproduction studies; therefore, miglitol is classified as pregnancy category B. Information specific to the use of miglitol during pregnancy has not been located. Maternal hyperglycemia can be associated with adverse effects in the fetus, including macrosomia, neonatal hyperglycemia, and hyperbilirubinemia; the risk of congenital malformations is increased when the Hb A_{1c} is above the normal range. Diabetes can also be associated with adverse effects in the mother. Poorly-treated diabetes may cause end-organ damage that may in turn negatively affect obstetric outcomes. Physiologic glucose levels should be maintained prior to and during pregnancy to decrease the risk of adverse events in the mother and the fetus. Until additional safety and efficacy data are obtained, the use of oral agents is generally not recommended as routine management of GDM or type 2 diabetes mellitus during pregnancy. Insulin is the drug of choice for the control of diabetes mellitus during pregnancy.

Lactation Enters breast milk (small amounts)/not recommended

Contraindications Hypersensitivity to miglitol or any of component of the formulation; diabetic ketoacidosis; inflammatory bowel disease; colonic ulceration; partial intestinal obstruction or predisposition to intestinal obstruction; chronic intestinal diseases associated with marked disorders of digestion or absorption or with conditions that may deteriorate as a result of increased gas formation in the intestine

Warnings/Precautions GI symptoms are the most common reactions. The incidence of abdominal pain and diarrhea tend to diminish considerably with continued treatment. Use with caution in patients with mild-to-moderate renal impairment; not recommended in severe impairment (serum creatinine >2 mg/dL); studies have not been conducted. In combination with a sulfonylurea will cause a further lowering of blood glucose and may increase the hypoglycemic potential of the sulfonylurea. It may be necessary to discontinue miglitol and administer insulin if the patient is exposed to stress (ie, fever, trauma, infection, surgery).

Adverse Reactions

>10%: Gastrointestinal: Flatulence (42%), diarrhea (29%), abdominal pain (12%)

1% to 10%: Dermatologic: Rash (4%)

Drug Interactions

Metabolism/Transport Effects None known.

Avoid Concomitant Use There are no known interactions where it is recommended to avoid concomitant use.

Increased Effect/Toxicity

Miglitol may increase the levels/effects of: Hypoglycemic Agents

The levels/effects of Miglitol may be increased by: Herbs (Hypoglycemic Properties); Pegvisomant

Decreased Effect

The levels/effects of Miglitol may be decreased by: Corticosteroids (Orally Inhaled); Corticosteroids (Systemic); Luteinizing Hormone-Releasing Hormone Analogs; Somatropin; Thiazide Diuretics

Stability Store at 25°C (77°F); excursions permitted to 15°C to 30°C (59°F to 86°F).

Mechanism of Action In contrast to sulfonylureas, miglitol does not enhance insulin secretion; the antihyperglycemic action of miglitol results from a reversible inhibition of membrane-bound intestinal alpha-glucosidases which hydrolyze oligosaccharides and disaccharides to glucose and other monosaccharides in the brush border of the small intestine. In patients with diabetes, this enzyme inhibition results in delayed glucose absorption and lowering of postprandial hyperglycemia.

Pharmacodynamics/Kinetics

Absorption: Saturable at high doses: 25 mg dose: Completely absorbed; 100 mg dose: 50% to 70% absorbed

Distribution: V_d: 0.18 L/kg

Protein binding: <4%

Metabolism: None

Half-life elimination: ~2 hours

Time to peak: 2-3 hours

Excretion: Urine (as unchanged drug)

Dosage Adults: Oral: Initial: 25 mg 3 times/day with the first bite of food at each meal; the dose may be increased to 50 mg 3 times/day after 4-8 weeks; maximum recommended dose: 100 mg 3 times/day

Dosing adjustment in renal impairment: Miglitol is primarily excreted by the kidneys; no dosage adjustment recommended in mild-moderate impairment. Not recommended in patients with a S_{cr} >2 mg/dL; studies have not been conducted.

Dosing adjustment in hepatic impairment: No adjustment necessary

Administration Should be taken orally at the start (with the first bite) of each main meal

Monitoring Parameters Monitor therapeutic response by periodic blood glucose tests; measurement of glycosylated hemoglobin is recommended for the monitoring of long-term glycemic control

Reference Range Recommendations for glycemic control in adults with diabetes:

Hb A_{1c}: <7%

Preprandial capillary plasma glucose: 70-130 mg/dL

Peak postprandial capillary blood glucose: <180 mg/dL

Blood pressure: <130/80 mm Hg

Dosage Forms Excipient information presented when available (limited, particularly for generics); consult specific product labeling.

Tablet, oral:

Glyset®: 25 mg, 50 mg, 100 mg

Miglustat (MIG loo stat)

Brand Names: U.S. Zavesca®

Brand Names: Canada Zavesca®

Index Terms OGT-918

Pharmacologic Category Enzyme Inhibitor

Use Treatment of mild-to-moderate type 1 Gaucher disease when enzyme replacement therapy is not a therapeutic option

Canadian labeling: Additional use (not in U.S. labeling): Treatment to delay the progression of neurological manifestations in Niemann-Pick Type C disease

Pregnancy Risk Factor X

Dosage Oral:

Type 1 Gaucher disease: Adults: 100 mg 3 times/day; dose may be reduced to 100 mg 1-2 times/day in patients with adverse effects (ie, tremor, GI distress)

Niemann-Pick Type C disease (Canadian labeling; not in U.S. labeling):

Children <12 years: **Note:** Children <4 years of age were not included in clinical trials; dose based on body surface area (BSA):

BSA >1.25 m^2: Miglustat 200 mg 3 times/day

BSA >0.88-1.25 m^2: Miglustat 200 mg 2 times/day

BSA >0.73-0.88 m^2: Miglustat 100 mg 3 times/day

BSA >0.47-0.73 m^2: Miglustat 100 mg 2 times/day

BSA ≤0.47 m^2: Miglustat 100 mg once daily

Children ≥12 and Adults: 200 mg 3 times/day

Dosage adjustment in renal impairment:

Gaucher disease: Adults:

Cl_{cr} 50-70 mL/minute/1.73 m^2: 100 mg twice daily

Cl_{cr} 30-50 mL/minute/1.73 m^2: 100 mg once daily

Cl_{cr} <30 mL/minute/1.73 m^2: Not recommended

Niemann-Pick Type C disease Canadian labeling (not in U.S. labeling):

Children <12 years:

Cl_{cr} 50-70 mL/minute/1.73 m^2: Administer two-thirds of regular dose in 2 equal doses (adjusted for BSA)

Cl_{cr} 30-50 mL/minute/1.73 m^2: Administer one-third of regular dose in 2 equal doses (adjusted for BSA)

Cl_{cr} <30 mL/minute/1.73 m^2: Not recommended

Children ≥12 years and Adults:

Cl_{cr} 50-70 mL/minute/1.73 m^2: 200 mg twice daily

Cl_{cr} 30-50 mL/minute/1.73 m^2: 100 mg twice daily

Cl_{cr} <30 mL/minute/1.73 m^2: Not recommended

Additional Information Complete prescribing information for this medication should be consulted for additional detail.

Dosage Forms Excipient information presented when available (limited, particularly for generics); consult specific product labeling.

Capsule, oral:

Zavesca®: 100 mg

◆ **Migranal®** *see* Dihydroergotamine *on page 508*

◆ **Mild-C® [OTC]** *see* Ascorbic Acid *on page 149*

◆ **Milk of Magnesia** *see* Magnesium Hydroxide *on page 1045*

◆ **Milk of Magnesia [OTC]** *see* Magnesium Hydroxide *on page 1045*

◆ **Milk of Magnesium [OTC]** *see* Magnesium Hydroxide *on page 1045*

◆ **Millipred™** *see* PrednisoLONE (Systemic) *on page 1396*

◆ **Millipred™ DP** *see* PrednisoLONE (Systemic) *on page 1396*

Milnacipran (mil NAY ci pran)

Brand Names: U.S. Savella®

Pharmacologic Category Antidepressant, Serotonin/Norepinephrine Reuptake Inhibitor

Additional Appendix Information

Antidepressant Agents *on page 1874*

Use Management of fibromyalgia

Pregnancy Risk Factor C

Pregnancy Considerations Adverse events were observed in some animal reproduction studies. Nonteratogenic effects in the newborn following SSRI/SNRI exposure late in the third trimester include respiratory distress, cyanosis, apnea, seizures, temperature instability, feeding difficulty, vomiting, hypoglycemia, hyper- or hypotonia, hyper-reflexia, jitteriness, irritability, constant crying, and tremor. Symptoms may be due to the toxicity of the SNRIs/SSRIs or a discontinuation syndrome and may be consistent with serotonin syndrome associated with SSRI treatment. The long-term effects of *in utero* SNRI/SSRI exposure on infant development and behavior are not known.

Women inadvertently exposed to milnacipran during pregnancy may be enrolled in the Savella Pregnancy Registry (877-643-3010 or http://www.savellapregnancyregistry.com).

Lactation Excretion in breast milk unknown/not recommended

Medication Guide Available Yes

Contraindications Concomitant use or within 2 weeks of MAO inhibitors; uncontrolled narrow-angle glaucoma

Warnings/Precautions [U.S. Boxed Warning]: Milnacipran is a serotonin/norepinephrine reuptake inhibitor (SNRI) similar to SNRIs used to treat depression and other psychiatric disorders. **Antidepressants increase the risk of suicidal thinking and behavior in children, adolescents, and young adults (18-24 years of age) with major depressive disorder (MDD) and other psychiatric disorders**; consider risk prior to prescribing. Short-term studies did not show an increased risk in patients >24 years of age and showed a decreased risk in patients ≥65 years. Closely monitor for clinical worsening, suicidality, or unusual changes in behavior; the patient's family or caregiver should be instructed to closely observe the patient and communicate condition with healthcare provider. A medication guide should be dispensed with each prescription. **Milnacipran is not FDA approved for the treatment of major depressive disorder or for use in children.**

Suicide risks should be monitored in patients treated with SNRIs regardless of the indication. The possibility of a suicide attempt is inherent in major depression and may persist until remission occurs. Monitor for worsening of depression or suicidality, especially during initiation of therapy (generally first 1-2 months) or with dose increases or decreases. Use caution in high-risk patients. Worsening depression and severe abrupt suicidality that are not part of the presenting symptoms may require discontinuation or modification of drug therapy. The patient's family or caregiver should be alerted to monitor patients for the emergence of suicidality and associated behaviors (such as agitation, irritability, hostility, impulsivity, and hypomania) and call healthcare provider.

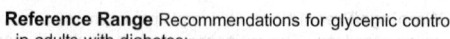

Patients with major depressive disorder were excluded from clinical trials evaluating milnacipran for fibromyalgia; however, mania has been reported in patients with mood disorders taking similar medications. May worsen psychosis in some patients or precipitate a shift to mania or hypomania in patients with bipolar disorder. Patients presenting with depressive symptoms should be screened for bipolar disorder. Monotherapy in patients with bipolar disorder should be avoided. **Milnacipran is not FDA approved for the treatment of bipolar depression.**

Serotonin syndrome and neuroleptic malignant syndrome (NMS)-like reactions have occurred with serotonin/norepinephrine reuptake inhibitors (SNRIs) and selective serotonin reuptake inhibitors (SSRIs) when used alone, and particularly when used in combination with serotonergic agents (eg, triptans) or antidopaminergic agents (eg, antipsychotics). Concurrent use with MAO inhibitors is contraindicated. May cause sustained increase in blood pressure or heart rate. Control pre-existing hypertension and cardiovascular disease prior to initiation of milnacipran. Use caution in patients with renal impairment; dose reduction required in severe renal impairment. Use caution in patients with hepatic impairment. Avoid ethanol use. May cause hyponatremia/SIADH (elderly at increased risk); volume depletion (diuretics may increase risk). Use cautiously in patients with a history of seizures. May impair platelet aggregation, resulting in bleeding. May cause increased urinary resistance. Use caution in patients with controlled narrow-angle glaucoma; use is contraindicated with uncontrolled narrow-angle glaucoma.

Abrupt discontinuation or dosage reduction after extended therapy may lead to agitation, dysphoria, anxiety, and other symptoms. When discontinuing therapy, dosage should be tapered gradually. If intolerable symptoms occur following a decrease in dosage or upon discontinuation of therapy, then resuming the previous dose with a more gradual taper should be considered.

Adverse Reactions

>10%:

Central nervous system: Headache (18%), insomnia (12%)

Endocrine & metabolic: Hot flashes (12%)

Gastrointestinal: Nausea (37%), constipation (16%)

1% to 10%:

Cardiovascular: Palpitation (7%), heart rate increased (6%), hypertension (5%), flushing (3%), blood pressure increased (3%), tachycardia (2%), peripheral edema (≥1%)

Central nervous system: Dizziness (10%), migraine (5%), chills (2%), tremor (2%), depression (≥1%), fatigue (≥1%), fever (≥1%), irritability (≥1%), somnolence (≥1%)

Dermatologic: Hyperhidrosis (9%), rash (3%)

Endocrine & metabolic: Hypercholesterolemia (≥1%)

Gastrointestinal: Vomiting (7%), xerostomia (5%), abdominal pain (3%), appetite decreased (2%), abdominal distension (≥1%), abnormal taste (≥1%), diarrhea (≥1%), dyspepsia (≥1%), flatulence (≥1%), gastroesophageal reflux disease (≥1%), weight changes (≥1%)

Genitourinary: Dysuria (≥2%), ejaculation disorder/failure (≥2%), erectile dysfunction (≥2%), libido decreased (≥2%), prostatitis (≥2%), scrotal pain (≥2%), testicular pain (≥2%), testicular swelling (≥2%), urethral pain (≥2%), urinary hesitation (≥2%), urinary retention (≥2%), urine flow decreased (≥2%), cystitis (≥1%), urinary tract infection (≥1%)

Neuromuscular & skeletal: Falling (≥1%)

Ocular: Blurred vision (2%)

Respiratory: Dyspnea (2%)

Miscellaneous: Night sweats (≥1%)

<1% (Limited to important or life-threatening): Accommodation disorder, acute renal failure, anorexia, delirium, erythema multiforme, galactorrhea, hallucination, hepatitis, hyperprolactinemia, hypertensive crisis, hyponatremia, leukopenia, loss of consciousness, neuroleptic malignant syndrome, neutropenia, parkinsonism, rhabdomyolysis, seizures, serotonin syndrome, Stevens-Johnson syndrome, supraventricular tachycardia, thrombocytopenia

Drug Interactions

Metabolism/Transport Effects None known.

Avoid Concomitant Use

Avoid concomitant use of Milnacipran with any of the following: Iobenguane I 123; MAO Inhibitors; Methylene Blue

Increased Effect/Toxicity

Milnacipran may increase the levels/effects of: Alpha-/Beta-Agonists; Aspirin; Digoxin; Methylene Blue; Metoclopramide; NSAID (Nonselective); Serotonin Modulators; Vitamin K Antagonists

The levels/effects of Milnacipran may be increased by: Alcohol (Ethyl); Antipsychotics; ClomiPRAMINE; Linezolid; MAO Inhibitors

Decreased Effect

Milnacipran may decrease the levels/effects of: Alpha2-Agonists; Iobenguane I 123; Ioflupane I 123

Ethanol/Nutrition/Herb Interactions

Ethanol: May increase CNS depression; monitor for increased effects with coadministration. Caution patients about effects.

Herb/Nutraceutical: Avoid valerian, St John's wort, SAMe, kava kava, tryptophan (may increase risk of serotonin syndrome and/or excessive sedation).

Stability Store at 25°C (77°F); excursions permitted between 15°C to 30°C (59°F to 86°F).

Mechanism of Action Potent inhibitor of norepinephrine and serotonin reuptake (3:1). Milnacipran has no significant activity for serotonergic, alpha- and beta-adrenergic, muscarinic, histaminergic, dopaminergic, opiate, benzodiazepine, and GABA receptors. It does not possess MAO-inhibitory activity.

Pharmacodynamics/Kinetics

Absorption: Well absorbed

Distribution: I.V: V_d: ~400 L

Protein binding: 13%

Metabolism: Hepatic to inactive metabolites

Bioavailability: 85% to 90%

Half-life elimination: 6-8 hours

Time to peak, plasma: Oral: 2-4 hours

Excretion: Urine (55% as unchanged drug)

Dosage Oral: Adults: 50 mg twice daily (maximum dose: 200 mg/day)

Titration schedule: 12.5 mg once on day 1, then 12.5 mg twice daily on days 2-3, 25 mg twice daily on days 4-7, then 50 mg twice daily thereafter. Dose may be increased to 100 mg twice daily, based on individual response. Doses >200 mg/day have not been studied.

Discontinuation of therapy: Gradually taper dose. If intolerable symptoms occur following a dose reduction, consider resuming the previously prescribed dose and/or decrease dose at a more gradual rate.

Dosing adjustment in renal impairment:

Mild renal impairment: No dose adjustment is recommended

Moderate renal impairment: Use with caution

Severe renal impairment (Cl_{cr} ≤29 mL/minute): Reduce maintenance dose to 25 mg twice daily; dose may be increased to 50 mg twice daily, based on individual tolerance

End-stage renal disease (ESRD): Use not recommended

Dosing adjustment in hepatic impairment:

Mild-to-moderate hepatic impairment: No dose adjustment is recommended

Severe hepatic impairment: Use with caution

Dietary Considerations May be taken with or without food; food may improve tolerability.

Administration May be administered with or without food; food may improve tolerability.

Monitoring Parameters Blood pressure and heart rate should be regularly monitored; renal function should be monitored for dosing purposes; mental status for suicidal ideation (especially at the beginning of therapy or when doses are increased or decreased); intraocular pressure should be monitored in those with baseline elevations or a history of glaucoma

Dosage Forms Excipient information presented when available (limited, particularly for generics); consult specific product labeling.

Combination package, oral [titration pack contains three separate tablet formulations]:

Savella®: Tablet: 12.5 mg (5s), Tablet: 25 mg (8s), and Tablet: 50 mg (42s)

Tablet, oral:

Savella®: 12.5 mg, 25 mg, 50 mg, 100 mg

◆ **Milophene® (Can)** *see* ClomiPHENE *on page 387*

Milrinone (MIL ri none)

Brand Names: Canada Milrinone Lactate Injection; Primacor®

Index Terms Milrinone Lactate

Pharmacologic Category Phosphodiesterase Enzyme Inhibitor

Additional Appendix Information

Vasoactive Agents, Intravenous *on page 1898*

Use Short-term I.V. therapy of acutely-decompensated heart failure

Unlabeled Use Inotropic therapy for patients unresponsive to other acute heart failure therapies (eg, dobutamine); outpatient inotropic therapy for heart transplant candidates; palliation of symptoms in end-stage heart failure patients who cannot otherwise be discharged from the hospital and are not transplant candidates

Pregnancy Risk Factor C

Pregnancy Considerations Teratogenic effects have not been observed in animal reproduction studies; however, increased resorption was reported in some studies.

Lactation Excretion in breast milk unknown/use caution

Contraindications Hypersensitivity to milrinone, inamrinone, or any component of the formulation; concurrent use of inamrinone

Warnings/Precautions Monitor closely for hypotension. Avoid in severe obstructive aortic or pulmonic valvular disease. Milrinone may aggravate outflow tract obstruction in hypertrophic subaortic stenosis. Supraventricular and ventricular arrhythmias have developed in high-risk patients. Ensure that ventricular rate controlled in atrial fibrillation/flutter prior to initiating milrinone. Not recommended for use in acute MI patients. Monitor and correct fluid and electrolyte problems. Adjust dose in renal dysfunction. Discontinue therapy if dose-related elevations in LFTs and clinical symptoms of hepatotoxicity occur.

Adverse Reactions

>10%: Cardiovascular: Ventricular arrhythmia (ectopy 9%, NSVT 3%, sustained ventricular tachycardia 1%, ventricular fibrillation <1%)

1% to 10%:

Cardiovascular: Supraventricular arrhythmia (4%), hypotension (3%), angina/chest pain (1%)

Central nervous system: Headache (3%)

<1% (Limited to important or life-threatening): Anaphylaxis, atrial fibrillation, bronchospasm, hypokalemia, injection site reaction, liver function abnormalities, MI, rash, thrombocytopenia, torsade de pointes, tremor, ventricular fibrillation

Drug Interactions

Metabolism/Transport Effects None known.

Avoid Concomitant Use There are no known interactions where it is recommended to avoid concomitant use.

Increased Effect/Toxicity There are no known significant interactions involving an increase in effect.

Decreased Effect There are no known significant interactions involving a decrease in effect.

Stability Store at 15°C to 30°C (59°F to 86°F); avoid freezing. Stable at 0.2 mg/mL in 1/2NS, NS, or D_5W for 72 hours at room temperature in normal light.

Standard dilution: For a final concentration of 0.2 mg/mL: Dilute Primacor® 1 mg/mL (20 mL) with 80 mL diluent (final volume: 100 mL). May also dilute 1 mg/mL (10 mL) with 40 mL diluent (final volume: 50 mL).

Mechanism of Action A selective phosphodiesterase inhibitor in cardiac and vascular tissue, resulting in vasodilation and inotropic effects with little chronotropic activity.

Pharmacodynamics/Kinetics

Onset of action: I.V.: 5-15 minutes

Distribution: V_{dss}: 0.32-0.45 L/kg

Protein binding, plasma: ~70%

Metabolism: Hepatic (12%)

Half-life elimination: Normal renal function: ~2.5 hours; CVVH: 20.1 hours (Taniguchi, 2000)

Excretion: Urine (85% as unchanged drug) within 24 hours; active tubular secretion is a major elimination pathway for milrinone

Dosage Adults: I.V.: Loading dose (optional; see **"Note"**): 50 mcg/kg administered over 10 minutes followed by a maintenance dose titrated according to hemodynamic and clinical response; Maintenance dose: I.V. infusion: 0.375-0.75 mcg/kg/minute; lower initial doses of 0.1 mcg/kg/minute (with final doses of 0.2-0.3 mcg/kg/minute) have also been recommended (Lindenfeld, 2010).

Note: When initiating an infusion of 0.5 mcg/kg/minute without a loading dose, significant hemodynamic changes seen at 30 minutes with similar effects on pulmonary capillary wedge pressure and cardiac index seen at 2 and 3 hours, respectively, compared to loading dose regimen (Baruch, 2011).

Dosing adjustment in renal impairment:

Manufacturer recommended adjustment:

Cl_{cr} 50 mL/minute/1.73 m²: Administer 0.43 mcg/kg/minute

Cl_{cr} 40 mL/minute/1.73 m²: Administer 0.38 mcg/kg/minute

Cl_{cr} 30 mL/minute/1.73 m²: Administer 0.33 mcg/kg/minute

Cl_{cr} 20 mL/minute/ 1.73 m^2: Administer 0.28 mcg/kg/minute
Cl_{cr} 10 mL/minute/1.73 m^2: Administer 0.23 mcg/kg/minute
Cl_{cr} 5 mL/minute/1.73 m^2: Administer 0.2 mcg/kg/minute

Alternative Dosing Adjustments in Patients with Renal Impairment[1]

		Starting dose (mcg/kg/min)		
		0.375	0.5	0.75
Cl_{cr} (mL/min)	50	0.25	0.375	0.5
	40	0.125	0.25	0.375
	30	0.0625	0.125	0.25
	20	Consider alternative therapy	0.0625	0.125
	10	Consider alternative therapy		0.0625
	5	Consider alternative therapy		

[1]Based on expert opinion.

Administration Infuse via infusion pump

Monitoring Parameters Platelet count, CBC, electrolytes (especially potassium and magnesium), liver function and renal function tests; ECG, CVP, SBP, DBP, heart rate; infusion site

If pulmonary artery catheter is in place, monitor cardiac index, stroke volume, systemic vascular resistance, pulmonary capillary wedge pressure and pulmonary vascular resistance.

Dosage Forms Excipient information presented when available (limited, particularly for generics); consult specific product labeling.

Infusion, premixed in D_5W: 200 mcg/mL (100 mL, 200 mL)
Injection, solution: 1 mg/mL (10 mL, 20 mL, 50 mL)
Injection, solution [preservative free]: 1 mg/mL (10 mL, 20 mL)

◆ **Milrinone Lactate** *see* Milrinone *on page 1136*

◆ **Milrinone Lactate Injection (Can)** *see* Milrinone *on page 1136*

◆ **Mimvey™** *see* Estradiol and Norethindrone *on page 635*

◆ **Minestrin™ 1/20 (Can)** *see* Ethinyl Estradiol and Norethindrone *on page 660*

◆ **Minipress®** *see* Prazosin *on page 1396*

◆ **Minirin® (Can)** *see* Desmopressin *on page 476*

◆ **Minitran™** *see* Nitroglycerin *on page 1212*

◆ **Minocin®** *see* Minocycline *on page 1137*

◆ **Minocin® PAC** *see* Minocycline *on page 1137*

Minocycline (mi noe SYE kleen)

Brand Names: U.S. Dynacin®; Minocin®; Minocin® PAC; Solodyn®

Brand Names: Canada Apo-Minocycline®; Arestin Microspheres; Dom-Minocycline; Minocin®; Mylan-Minocycline; Novo-Minocycline; PHL-Minocycline; PMS-Minocycline; ratio-Minocycline; Riva-Minocycline; Sandoz-Minocycline

Index Terms Minocycline Hydrochloride

Pharmacologic Category Antibiotic, Tetracycline Derivative

Use Treatment of susceptible bacterial infections of both gram-negative and gram-positive organisms; treatment of anthrax (inhalational, cutaneous, and gastrointestinal); moderate-to-severe acne; meningococcal (asymptomatic) carrier state; Rickettsial diseases (including Rocky Mountain spotted fever, Q fever); nongonococcal urethritis, gonorrhea; acute intestinal amebiasis; respiratory tract infection; skin/soft tissue infections; chlamydial infections

Extended release (Solodyn®): Only indicated for treatment of inflammatory lesions of non-nodular moderate-to-severe acne

Unlabeled Use Rheumatoid arthritis (patients with low disease activity of short duration); nocardiosis; alternative treatment for community-acquired MRSA infection

Pregnancy Risk Factor D

Pregnancy Considerations Tetracyclines, including minocycline, cross the placenta, enter fetal circulation, and may cause permanent discoloration of teeth if used during the second or third trimester. Congenital anomalies after minocycline use have been reported postmarketing. Because use during pregnancy may cause fetal harm, minocycline is classified as pregnancy category D.

Lactation Enters breast milk/not recommended

Contraindications Hypersensitivity to minocycline, other tetracyclines, or any component of the formulation; children <8 years of age

Warnings/Precautions May be associated with increases in BUN secondary to antianabolic effects; use caution in patients with renal impairment (Cl_{cr} <80 mL/minute). Hepatotoxicity has been reported; use caution in patients with hepatic insufficiency. Autoimmune syndromes (eg, lupus-like, hepatitis, and vasculitis) have been reported; discontinue if symptoms occur. CNS effects (lightheadedness, vertigo) may occur; patients must be cautioned about performing tasks which require mental alertness (eg, operating machinery or driving). Pseudotumor cerebri has been (rarely) reported with tetracycline use; usually resolves with discontinuation. May cause photosensitivity; discontinue if skin erythema occurs. Prolonged use may result in fungal or bacterial superinfection, including *C. difficile*-associated diarrhea (CDAD) and pseudomembranous colitis; CDAD has been observed >2 months postantibiotic treatment. May cause tissue hyperpigmentation, enamel hypoplasia, or permanent tooth discoloration; use of tetracyclines should be avoided during tooth development (children <8 years of age) unless other drugs are not likely to be effective or are contraindicated. Do not use during pregnancy. In addition to affecting tooth development, tetracycline use has been associated with retardation of skeletal development and reduced bone growth. Rash, along with eosinophilia, fever, and organ failure (Drug Rash with Eosinophilia and Systemic Symptoms [DRESS] syndrome) has been reported; discontinue treatment immediately if DRESS syndrome is suspected.

Adverse Reactions Frequency not defined.

Cardiovascular: Myocarditis, pericarditis, vasculitis

Central nervous system: Bulging fontanels, dizziness, fatigue, fever, headache, hypoesthesia, malaise, mood changes, paresthesia, pseudotumor cerebri, sedation, seizure, somnolence, vertigo

Dermatologic: Alopecia, angioedema, drug rash with eosinophilia and systemic symptoms (DRESS), erythema multiforme, erythema nodosum, erythematous rash, exfoliative dermatitis, hyperpigmentation of nails, maculopapular rash, photosensitivity, pigmentation of the skin and mucous membranes, pruritus, Stevens-Johnson syndrome, toxic epidermal necrolysis, urticaria

Endocrine & metabolic: Thyroid cancer, thyroid discoloration, thyroid dysfunction

Gastrointestinal: Anorexia, diarrhea, dyspepsia, dysphagia, enamel hypoplasia, enterocolitis, esophageal ulcerations, esophagitis, glossitis, inflammatory lesions (oral/anogenital), moniliasis, nausea, oral cavity discoloration, pancreatitis, pseudomembranous colitis, stomatitis, tooth discoloration, vomiting, xerostomia

Genitourinary: Balanitis, vulvovaginitis

Hematologic: Agranulocytosis, eosinophilia, hemolytic anemia, leukopenia, neutropenia, pancytopenia, thrombocytopenia
Hepatic: Autoimmune hepatitis, hepatic cholestasis, hepatic failure, hepatitis, hyperbilirubinemia, jaundice, liver enzyme increases
Local: Injection site reaction (I.V. administration)
Neuromuscular & skeletal: Arthralgia, arthritis, bone discoloration, joint stiffness, joint swelling, myalgia
Otic: Hearing loss, tinnitus
Renal: Acute renal failure, BUN increased, interstitial nephritis
Respiratory: Asthma, bronchospasm, cough, dyspnea, pneumonitis, pulmonary infiltrate (with eosinophilia)
Miscellaneous: Anaphylaxis, hypersensitivity, lupus erythematosus, lupus-like syndrome, serum sickness

Drug Interactions

Metabolism/Transport Effects None known.

Avoid Concomitant Use

Avoid concomitant use of Minocycline with any of the following: BCG; Retinoic Acid Derivatives

Increased Effect/Toxicity

Minocycline may increase the levels/effects of: Neuromuscular-Blocking Agents; Porfimer; Retinoic Acid Derivatives; Vitamin K Antagonists

Decreased Effect

Minocycline may decrease the levels/effects of: Atazanavir; BCG; Penicillins; Typhoid Vaccine

The levels/effects of Minocycline may be decreased by: Antacids; Bile Acid Sequestrants; Bismuth; Bismuth Subsalicylate; Calcium Salts; Iron Salts; Lanthanum; Magnesium Salts; Quinapril; Sucralfate; Zinc Salts

Ethanol/Nutrition/Herb Interactions

Food: Minocycline serum concentrations are not significantly altered if taken with food or dairy products.
Herb/Nutraceutical: Avoid dong quai, St John's wort (may also cause photosensitization).

Stability

Capsule (including pellet-filled), tablet: Store at 20°C to 25°C (68°F to 77°F); protect from heat. Protect from light and moisture.
Extended release tablet: Store at 15°C to 30°C (59°F to 86°F); protect from heat. Protect from light and moisture.
Injection: Store vials at 20°C to 25°C (68°F to 77°F) prior to reconstitution. Reconstitute with 5 mL of sterile water for injection, and further dilute in 500-1000 mL of NS, D_5W, D_5NS, Ringer's injection, or LR. Reconstituted solution is stable at room temperature for 24 hours. Final dilutions should be administered immediately.

Mechanism of Action Inhibits bacterial protein synthesis by binding with the 30S and possibly the 50S ribosomal subunit(s) of susceptible bacteria; cell wall synthesis is not affected

Rheumatoid arthritis: The mechanism of action of minocycline in rheumatoid arthritis is not completely understood. It is thought to have antimicrobial, anti-inflammatory, immunomodulatory, and chondroprotective effects. More specifically, it is thought to be a potent inhibitor of metalloproteinases, which are active in rheumatoid arthritis joint destruction.

Pharmacodynamics/Kinetics

Absorption: Oral: Well absorbed
Protein binding: 70% to 75%
Metabolism: Hepatic to inactive metabolites
Half-life elimination: I.V.: 15-23 hours; Oral: 16 hours (range: 11-22 hours)
Time to peak: Capsule, pellet filled: 1-4 hours; Extended release tablet: 3.5-4 hours
Excretion: Urine, feces

Dosage

Usual dosage range:

I.V.:

Children >8 years: Initial: 4 mg/kg, followed by 2 mg/kg/dose every 12 hours (maximum: 400 mg/day)
Adults: Initial: 200 mg, followed by 100 mg every 12 hours (maximum: 400 mg/day)

Oral:

Capsule or immediate release tablet:
Children >8 years: Oral: Initial: 4 mg/kg, followed by 2 mg/kg/dose every 12 hours
Adults: Oral: Initial: 200 mg, followed by 100 mg every 12 hours; more frequent dosing intervals may be used (100-200 mg initially, followed by 50 mg 4 times daily)
Extended release tablet (Solodyn®): Children ≥12 years and Adults (≥45 kg): Oral: 45-135 mg once daily (weight based)

Indication-specific dosing:

Children:

Acne *(inflammatory, non-nodular, moderate-to-severe)* (Solodyn®): Oral: Children ≥12 years:
45-54 kg: 45 mg once daily
55-77 kg: 65 mg once daily
78-102 kg: 90 mg once daily
103-125 kg: 115 mg once daily
126-136 kg: 135 mg once daily
Note: Therapy should be continued for 12 weeks. Higher doses do not confer greater efficacy and may be associated with more acute vestibular side effects. Safety of use beyond 12 weeks has not been established.

Cellulitis (purulent) infection due to community-acquired MRSA (unlabeled use): Oral: Children >8 years: Initial: 4 mg/kg (maximum: 200 mg); Maintenance: 2 mg/kg/dose (maximum: 100 mg) every 12 hours for 5-10 days (Liu, 2011)

Adults:

Acne: Oral: Capsule or immediate-release tablet: 50-100 mg twice daily
Inflammatory, non-nodular, moderate-to-severe (Solodyn®):
45-54 kg: 45 mg once daily
55-77 kg: 65 mg once daily
78-102 kg: 90 mg once daily
103-125 kg: 115 mg once daily
126-136 kg: 135 mg once daily
Note: Therapy should be continued for 12 weeks. Higher doses do not confer greater efficacy and may be associated with more acute vestibular side effects. Safety of use beyond 12 weeks has not been established.

Cellulitis (purulent) due to community-acquired MRSA (unlabeled use): Oral: Initial: 200 mg; Maintenance: 100 mg twice daily for 5-10 days (Liu, 2011)

Chlamydial or *Ureaplasma urealyticum* infection, uncomplicated: Oral, I.V.: Urethral, endocervical, or rectal: 100 mg every 12 hours for at least 7 days

Gonococcal infection, uncomplicated (males): Oral, I.V.:
Without urethritis or anorectal infection: Initial: 200 mg, followed by 100 mg every 12 hours for at least 4 days (cultures 2-3 days post-therapy)
Urethritis: 100 mg every 12 hours for 5 days

Meningococcal carrier state (manufacturer's labeling): Oral: 100 mg every 12 hours for 5 days. **Note:** CDC recommendations do not mention use of minocycline for eradicating nasopharyngeal carriage of meningococcal

***Mycobacterium marinum*:** Oral: 100 mg every 12 hours for 6-8 weeks

Nocardiosis, cutaneous (non-CNS) (unlabeled use): Oral: 100-200 mg every 12 hours

Rheumatoid arthritis (unlabeled use): Oral: 100 mg twice daily (O'Dell, 2001)

Syphilis: Oral, I.V.: Initial: 200 mg, followed by 100 mg every 12 hours for 10-15 days

Elderly: Refer to adult dosing.

Dosage adjustment in renal impairment: Use with caution; monitor BUN and creatinine clearance. Consider decreasing dose or increasing dosing interval (extended release).

Cl_{cr} <80 mL/minute: Do not exceed 200 mg/day

Dietary Considerations May be taken with or without food.

Administration

I.V.: Infuse slowly; avoid rapid administration. The manufacturer's labeling does not provide a recommended administration rate. The injectable route should be used only if the oral route is not feasible or adequate. Prolonged intravenous therapy may be associated with thrombophlebitis.

Oral: May be administered with or without food. Administer with adequate fluid to decrease the risk of esophageal irritation and ulceration. Swallow pellet-filled capsule and extended release tablet whole; do not chew, crush, or split.

Monitoring Parameters LFTs, BUN, renal function with long-term treatment; if symptomatic for autoimmune disorder, include ANA, CBC

Test Interactions May cause interference with fluorescence test for urinary catecholamines (false elevations)

Dosage Forms Excipient information presented when available (limited, particularly for generics); consult specific product labeling.

Capsule, oral: 50 mg, 75 mg, 100 mg

Capsule, pellet filled, oral:

Minocin®: 50 mg, 100 mg

Minocin® PAC: 50 mg, 100 mg

Injection, powder for reconstitution:

Minocin®: 100 mg

Tablet, oral: 50 mg, 75 mg, 100 mg

Dynacin®: 50 mg, 75 mg, 100 mg

Tablet, extended release, oral: 45 mg, 90 mg, 135 mg

Solodyn®: 45 mg, 65 mg, 90 mg, 115 mg, 135 mg

◆ **Minocycline Hydrochloride** *see* Minocycline *on page 1137*

◆ **Min-Ovral® (Can)** *see* Ethinyl Estradiol and Levonorgestrel *on page 656*

Minoxidil (Systemic) (mi NOKS i dil)

Brand Names: Canada Loniten®

Pharmacologic Category Vasodilator, Direct-Acting

Additional Appendix Information

Hypertension *on page 2001*

Use Management of severe hypertension (usually in combination with a diuretic and beta-blocker)

Pregnancy Risk Factor C

Dosage Oral:

Children <12 years: Hypertension: Initial: 0.1-0.2 mg/kg once daily; maximum: 5 mg/day; increase gradually every 3 days; usual dosage range: 0.25-1 mg/kg/day in 1-2 divided doses; maximum: 50 mg/day

Children ≥12 years and Adults: Hypertension: Initial: 5 mg once daily, increase gradually every 3 days (maximum: 100 mg/day); usual dosage range (JNC 7): 2.5-80 mg/day in 1-2 divided doses

Note: Dosage adjustment is needed when added to concomitant therapy.

Elderly: Hypertension: Initial: 2.5 mg once daily; increase gradually.

Dosing adjustment in renal impairment: Patient with renal failure and/or receiving dialysis may require dosage reduction.

Supplemental dose is not necessary after hemo- or peritoneal dialysis.

Additional Information Complete prescribing information for this medication should be consulted for additional detail.

Dosage Forms Excipient information presented when available (limited, particularly for generics); consult specific product labeling.

Tablet, oral: 2.5 mg, 10 mg

Minoxidil (Topical) (mi NOKS i dil)

Brand Names: U.S. Rogaine® Extra Strength for Men [OTC]; Rogaine® for Men [OTC]; Rogaine® for Women [OTC]

Brand Names: Canada Apo-Gain®; Rogaine®

Pharmacologic Category Topical Skin Product

Use Treatment of alopecia androgenetica in males and females

Dosage Topical: Adults: Alopecia: Apply twice daily; 4 months of therapy may be necessary for hair growth.

Additional Information Complete prescribing information for this medication should be consulted for additional detail.

Dosage Forms Excipient information presented when available (limited, particularly for generics); consult specific product labeling.

Aerosol, foam, topical:

Rogaine® for Men: 5% (60 g)

Solution, topical: 2% (60 mL); 5% (60 mL)

Rogaine® Extra Strength for Men: 5% (60 mL) [contains ethanol 30% v/v]

Rogaine® for Women: 2% (60 mL) [contains ethanol 60% v/v]

◆ **Mintab DM [DSC]** *see* Guaifenesin and Dextromethorphan *on page 810*

◆ **Mint-Amlodipine (Can)** *see* AmLODIPine *on page 97*

◆ **Mint-Atenolol (Can)** *see* Atenolol *on page 161*

◆ **Mint-Cefprozil (Can)** *see* Cefprozil *on page 314*

◆ **Mint-Ciprofloxacin (Can)** *see* Ciprofloxacin (Systemic) *on page 362*

◆ **Mint-Citalopram (Can)** *see* Citalopram *on page 370*

◆ **Mint-Lisinopril (Can)** *see* Lisinopril *on page 1020*

◆ **Mint-Ondansetron (Can)** *see* Ondansetron *on page 1246*

◆ **Mintox Plus [OTC]** *see* Aluminum Hydroxide, Magnesium Hydroxide, and Simethicone *on page 80*

◆ **Mint-Pioglitazone (Can)** *see* Pioglitazone *on page 1355*

◆ **Mint-Risperidon (Can)** *see* RisperiDONE *on page 1496*

◆ **Mint-Topiramate (Can)** *see* Topiramate *on page 1706*

◆ **Miochol®-E** *see* Acetylcholine *on page 34*

◆ **Miostat®** *see* Carbachol *on page 280*

◆ **MiraLAX® [OTC]** *see* Polyethylene Glycol 3350 *on page 1372*

◆ **Miranel AF™ [OTC]** *see* Miconazole (Topical) *on page 1126*

◆ **Mirapex®** *see* Pramipexole *on page 1389*

◆ **Mirapex® ER®** *see* Pramipexole *on page 1389*

◆ **Mircette®** *see* Ethinyl Estradiol and Desogestrel *on page 653*

◆ **Mirena®** *see* Levonorgestrel *on page 1001*

Mirtazapine (mir TAZ a peen)

Brand Names: U.S. Remeron SolTab®; Remeron®

Brand Names: Canada Apo-Mirtazapine®; CO Mirtazapine; Dom-Mirtazapine; Mylan-Mirtazapine; Novo-Mirtazapine; PHL-Mirtazapine; PMS-Mirtazapine; PRO-Mirtazapine; ratio-Mirtazapine; Remeron®; Remeron® RD; Riva-Mirtazapine; Sandoz-Mirtazapine; Sandoz-Mirtazapine FC; ZYM-Mirtazapine

Pharmacologic Category Antidepressant, Alpha-2 Antagonist

Additional Appendix Information

Antidepressant Agents *on page 1874*

Use Treatment of depression

Unlabeled Use Post-traumatic stress disorder (PTSD)

Pregnancy Risk Factor C

Pregnancy Considerations Adverse events were observed in some animal studies; therefore, the manufacturer classifies mirtazapine as pregnancy category C. A significant increase in major teratogenic effects has not been observed in humans following exposure to mirtazapine during pregnancy; however, some nonteratogenic adverse events (similar to those observed with SSRI agents) have been reported. Mirtazapine was found to cross the placenta following a maternal overdose. Pregnancy itself does not provide "protection" against depression. Women treated for major depression and who are euthymic prior to pregnancy are more likely to experience a relapse when medication is discontinued as compared to pregnant women who continue taking antidepressant medications. The ACOG recommends that therapy with antidepressants during pregnancy be individualized. According to their recommendations, treatment of depression during pregnancy should incorporate the clinical expertise of the mental health clinician, obstetrician, primary care provider, and pediatrician. If treatment during pregnancy is required, consider tapering therapy during the third trimester in order to prevent withdrawal symptoms in the infant. If this is done, and the woman is considered to be at risk of relapse from her major depressive disorder, the medication can be restarted following delivery, although the dose should be readjusted to that required before pregnancy. Treatment algorithms have been developed by the ACOG and the APA for the management of depression in women prior to conception and during pregnancy (Yonkers, 2009).

Lactation Excreted in breast milk/use caution

Medication Guide Available Yes

Contraindications Hypersensitivity to mirtazapine or any component of the formulation; use of MAO inhibitors within 14 days

Warnings/Precautions [U.S. Boxed Warning]: Antidepressants increase the risk of suicidal thinking and behavior in children, adolescents, and young adults (18-24 years of age) with major depressive disorder (MDD) and other psychiatric disorders; consider risk prior to prescribing. Short-term studies did not show an increased risk in patients >24 years of age and showed a decreased risk in patients ≥65 years. Closely monitor for clinical worsening, suicidality, or unusual changes in behavior; the patient's family or caregiver should be instructed to closely observe the patient and communicate condition with healthcare provider. A medication guide should be dispensed with each prescription. **Mirtazapine is not FDA approved for use in children.**

The possibility of a suicide attempt is inherent in major depression and may persist until remission occurs. Monitor for worsening of depression or suicidality, especially during initiation of therapy (generally first 1-2 months) or with dose increases or decreases. Use caution in high-risk patients. Worsening depression and severe abrupt suicidality that are not part of the presenting symptoms may require discontinuation or modification of drug therapy. The patient's family or caregiver should be alerted to monitor patients for the emergence of suicidality and associated behaviors (such as agitation, irritability, hostility, impulsivity, and hypomania) and call healthcare provider.

May worsen psychosis in some patients or precipitate a shift to mania or hypomania in patients with bipolar disorder. Patients presenting with depressive symptoms should be screened for bipolar disorder. Monotherapy in patients with bipolar disorder should be avoided. **Mirtazapine is not FDA approved for the treatment of bipolar depression.**

Patients should not discontinue treatment abruptly, unless significant life-threatening event, due to risk of withdrawal symptoms. A gradual reduction in the dose over several weeks is recommended.

Discontinue immediately if signs and symptoms of neutropenia/agranulocytosis occur. May cause sedation, resulting in impaired performance of tasks requiring alertness (eg, operating machinery or driving). Sedative effects may be additive with other CNS depressants and/or ethanol. The degree of sedation is moderate-high relative to other antidepressants. Conversely, may increase psychomotor restlessness within first few weeks of therapy. The risks of orthostatic hypotension or anticholinergic effects are low relative to other antidepressants. The incidence of sexual dysfunction with mirtazapine is generally lower than with SSRIs. Potential for severe reaction when used with MAO inhibitors; autonomic instability, coma, death, delirium, diaphoresis, hyperthermia, mental status changes/agitation, muscular rigidity, myoclonus, neuroleptic malignant syndrome features, and seizures may occur.

May increase appetite and stimulate weight gain. Weight gain of >7% of body weight reported in 7.5% of patients treated with mirtazapine compared to 0% for placebo; 8% of patients receiving mirtazapine discontinued treatment due to the weight gain. In an 8-week pediatric clinical trial, 49% of mirtazapine-treated patients had a weight gain of at least 7% (mean increase 4 kg) as compared to 5.7% of placebo-treated patients (mean increase 1 kg). May increase serum cholesterol and triglyceride levels.

Use caution in patients with a previous seizure disorder or condition predisposing to seizures such as brain damage, alcoholism, or concurrent therapy with other drugs which lower the seizure threshold. May cause hyponatremia.Use with caution in patients with hepatic or renal dysfunction and in elderly patients. Clinically significant transaminase elevations have been observed. SolTab® formulation contains phenylalanine.

Adverse Reactions

>10%:

Central nervous system: Somnolence (54%)
Endocrine & metabolic: Cholesterol increased
Gastrointestinal: Constipation (13%), xerostomia (25%), appetite increased (17%), weight gain (12%; weight gain of >7% reported in 8% of adults, ≤49% of pediatric patients)

1% to 10%:

Cardiovascular: Hypertension, vasodilatation, peripheral edema (2%), edema (1%)
Central nervous system: Dizziness (7%), abnormal dreams (4%), abnormal thoughts (3%), confusion (2%), malaise
Endocrine & metabolic: Triglycerides increased
Gastrointestinal: Vomiting, anorexia, abdominal pain
Genitourinary: Urinary frequency (2%)
Hepatic: SGPT increased (≥3 times ULN: 2%)
Neuromuscular & skeletal: Myalgia (2%), back pain (2%), arthralgia, tremor (2%), weakness (8%)

Respiratory: Dyspnea (1%)
Miscellaneous: Flu-like syndrome (5%), thirst (<1%)
<1% (Limited to important or life-threatening): Agranulocytosis, dehydration, liver function test increases, lymphadenopathy, neutropenia, orthostatic hypotension, seizure (1 case reported), torsade de pointes (1 case reported), weight loss

Drug Interactions

Metabolism/Transport Effects Substrate of CYP1A2 (major), CYP2C9 (minor), CYP2D6 (major), CYP3A4 (major); **Note:** Assignment of Major/Minor substrate status based on clinically relevant drug interaction potential; **Inhibits** CYP1A2 (weak), CYP3A4 (weak)

Avoid Concomitant Use

Avoid concomitant use of Mirtazapine with any of the following: Conivaptan; MAO Inhibitors; Methylene Blue

Increased Effect/Toxicity

Mirtazapine may increase the levels/effects of: Alcohol (Ethyl); CNS Depressants; Methylene Blue; Metoclopramide; Serotonin Modulators; Warfarin

The levels/effects of Mirtazapine may be increased by: Abiraterone Acetate; Antipsychotics; Conivaptan; CYP1A2 Inhibitors (Moderate); CYP1A2 Inhibitors (Strong); CYP2D6 Inhibitors (Moderate); CYP2D6 Inhibitors (Strong); CYP3A4 Inhibitors (Moderate); CYP3A4 Inhibitors (Strong); Darunavir; Dasatinib; Deferasirox; HydrOXYzine; Linezolid; MAO Inhibitors

Decreased Effect

Mirtazapine may decrease the levels/effects of: Alpha2-Agonists

The levels/effects of Mirtazapine may be decreased by: CYP1A2 Inducers (Strong); CYP3A4 Inducers (Strong); Cyproterone; Deferasirox; Peginterferon Alfa-2b; Tocilizumab

Ethanol/Nutrition/Herb Interactions

Ethanol: May increase CNS depression; monitor for increased effects with coadministration. Caution patients about effects.

Herb/Nutraceutical: Avoid St John's wort (may decrease mirtazapine levels). Avoid valerian, St John's wort, SAMe, kava kava (may increase CNS depression).

Stability Store at controlled room temperature of 25°C (77°F); excursions permitted to 15°C to 30°C (59°F to 86°F). Protect from light and moisture.

SolTab®: Protect from light and moisture. Use immediately upon opening tablet blister.

Mechanism of Action Mirtazapine is a tetracyclic antidepressant that works by its central presynaptic alpha$_2$-adrenergic antagonist effects, which results in increased release of norepinephrine and serotonin. It is also a potent antagonist of 5-HT$_2$ and 5-HT$_3$ serotonin receptors and H1 histamine receptors and a moderate peripheral alpha$_1$-adrenergic and muscarinic antagonist; it does not inhibit the reuptake of norepinephrine or serotonin.

Pharmacodynamics/Kinetics

Absorption: Rapid and complete
Distribution: 4.5 L/kg
Protein binding: 85%
Metabolism: Extensively hepatic via CYP1A2, 2C9, 2D6, 3A4 and via demethylation (forms demethylmirtazapine, an active metabolite) and hydroxylation (forms inactive metabolites)
Bioavailability: 50%
Half-life elimination: 20-40 hours; hampered with renal or hepatic impairment
Time to peak, serum: 2 hours
Excretion: Urine (75%) and feces (15%) as metabolites

Dosage Oral:

Adults:

Treatment of depression: Initial: 15 mg nightly, titrate up to 15-45 mg/day with dose increases made no more frequently than every 1-2 weeks; there is an inverse relationship between dose and sedation

Post-traumatic stress disorder (PTSD) (unlabeled use): 30-60 mg/day

Elderly: Decreased clearance seen (40% males, 10% females); no specific dosage adjustment recommended by manufacturer

Alzheimer's dementia-related depression: Initial: 7.5 mg at bedtime; may increase at 7.5-15 mg increments to 45-60 mg/day

Dosage adjustment in renal impairment:

Cl_{cr} 11-39 mL/minute: 30% decreased clearance
Cl_{cr} <10 mL/minute: 50% decreased clearance

Dosage adjustment in hepatic impairment: Clearance decreased by 30%

Dietary Considerations Some products may contain phenylalanine.

Administration SolTab®: Open blister pack and place tablet on the tongue. Do not split tablet. Tablet is formulated to dissolve on the tongue without water.

Monitoring Parameters Patients should be monitored for signs of agranulocytosis or severe neutropenia such as sore throat, stomatitis or other signs of infection or a low WBC; mental status for depression, suicide ideation (especially at the beginning of therapy or when doses are increased or decreased), anxiety, social functioning, mania, panic attacks; lipid profile

Additional Information Note: At least 14 days should elapse between discontinuation of an MAO inhibitor and initiation of therapy with mirtazapine; at least 14 days should be allowed after discontinuing mirtazapine before starting an MAO inhibitor.

Dosage Forms Excipient information presented when available (limited, particularly for generics); consult specific product labeling.

Tablet, oral: 7.5 mg, 15 mg, 30 mg, 45 mg
Remeron®: 15 mg, 30 mg [scored]
Remeron®: 45 mg

Tablet, orally disintegrating, oral: 15 mg, 30 mg, 45 mg
Remeron SolTab®: 15 mg [contains phenylalanine 2.6 mg/tablet; orange flavor]
Remeron SolTab®: 30 mg [contains phenylalanine 5.2 mg/tablet; orange flavor]
Remeron SolTab®: 45 mg [contains phenylalanine 7.8 mg/tablet; orange flavor]

Misoprostol (mye soe PROST ole)

Brand Names: U.S. Cytotec®

Brand Names: Canada Apo-Misoprostol®; Novo-Misoprostol; PMS-Misoprostol

Pharmacologic Category Prostaglandin

Use Prevention of NSAID-induced gastric ulcers; medical termination of pregnancy of ≤49 days (in conjunction with mifepristone)

Unlabeled Use Cervical ripening and labor induction (except in women with prior cesarean delivery or major uterine surgery); fat malabsorption in cystic fibrosis

Pregnancy Risk Factor X

Pregnancy Considerations Teratogenic effects were not observed in animal reproduction studies; however, congenital anomalies following first trimester exposure, fetal death, uterine perforation, and abortion have been reported after the use of misoprostol in human pregnancy. **[U.S. Boxed Warning]: Not to be used to reduce NSAID-induced ulcers in women of childbearing potential unless woman is capable of complying with**

effective contraceptive measures. Do not use in women of childbearing potential without a negative serum pregnancy test within 2 weeks prior to therapy; therapy is normally begun on the second or third day of next normal menstrual period. Use to prevent NSAID-induced ulcers is contraindicated in pregnant women. Written and verbal warnings concerning the hazards of misoprostol should be provided. During pregnancy, misoprostol may induce or augment uterine contractions; the manufacturer states that misoprostol should not be used as a cervical-ripening agent for induction of labor. However, The American College of Obstetricians and Gynecologists (ACOG) supports this off-label use in women who have not had a prior cesarean delivery or major uterine surgery. Hyperstimulation of the uterus, uterine rupture, or adverse events in the fetus or mother may occur with this use. Misoprostol is FDA approved for the medical termination of pregnancy of ≤49 days in conjunction with mifepristone.

Lactation Enters breast milk/use caution

Contraindications Hypersensitivity to prostaglandins; pregnancy (when used to reduce NSAID-induced ulcers)

Warnings/Precautions [U.S. Boxed Warning]: Due to the abortifacient property of this medication, patients must be warned not to give this drug to others. [U.S. Boxed Warning]: Not to be used to reduce NSAID-induced ulcers in pregnant women or women of childbearing potential unless woman is capable of complying with effective contraceptive measures; therapy is normally begun on the second or third day of next normal menstrual period. Uterine perforation and/or rupture have been reported in association with intravaginal use to induce labor or with combined oral/intravaginal use to induce abortion. The manufacturer states that Cytotec® should not be used as a cervical-ripening agent for induction of labor. However, The American College of Obstetricians and Gynecologists (ACOG) continues to support this off-label use. Use with caution in patients with renal impairment, cardiovascular disease and the elderly.

Adverse Reactions

>10%: Gastrointestinal: Diarrhea, abdominal pain

1% to 10%:

Central nervous system: Headache

Gastrointestinal: Constipation, dyspepsia, flatulence, nausea, vomiting

<1% (Limited to important or life-threatening): Abnormal taste, abnormal vision, alkaline phosphatase increased, alopecia, anaphylaxis, anemia, amylase increase, anxiety, appetite changes, arrhythmia, arterial thrombosis, arthralgia, back pain, breast pain, bronchitis, bronchospasm, cardiac enzymes increased, chest pain, chills, confusion, conjunctivitis, CVA, deafness, depression, dermatitis, diaphoresis, dizziness, drowsiness, dysphagia, dyspnea, dysuria, earache, edema, epistaxis, ESR increased, fatigue, fetal or infant death (when used during pregnancy), fever, GI bleeding, GI inflammation, gingivitis, glycosuria, gout; gynecological disorders (cramps, dysmenorrhea, hypermenorrhea, spotting, postmenopausal vaginal bleeding, and other menstrual disorders); hematuria, hepatobiliary function abnormal, hyper-/hypotension, impotence, loss of libido, MI, muscle cramps, myalgia, neuropathy, neurosis, nitrogen increased, pallor, phlebitis, pneumonia, polyuria, pulmonary embolism, purpura, rash, reflux, rigors, stiffness, syncope, thirst, thrombocytopenia, tinnitus, upper respiratory tract infection, urinary tract infection, uterine rupture, weakness, weight changes

Drug Interactions

Metabolism/Transport Effects None known.

Avoid Concomitant Use

Avoid concomitant use of Misoprostol with any of the following: Carbetocin

Increased Effect/Toxicity

Misoprostol may increase the levels/effects of: Carbetocin; Oxytocin

The levels/effects of Misoprostol may be increased by: Antacids

Decreased Effect There are no known significant interactions involving a decrease in effect.

Ethanol/Nutrition/Herb Interactions Food: Misoprostol peak serum concentrations may be decreased if taken with food (not clinically significant).

Stability Store at or below 25°C (77°F).

Mechanism of Action Misoprostol is a synthetic prostaglandin E_1 analog that replaces the protective prostaglandins consumed with prostaglandin-inhibiting therapies (eg, NSAIDs); has been shown to induce uterine contractions

Pharmacodynamics/Kinetics

Absorption: Rapid and extensive

Metabolism: Hepatic; rapidly de-esterified to misoprostol acid (active)

Protein binding: Misoprostol acid: <90%

Half-life elimination: Misoprostol acid: 20-40 minutes

Time to peak, serum: Misoprostol acid: Fasting: 6-22 minutes

Excretion: Urine (80%)

Dosage

Oral:

Children 8-16 years: Fat absorption in cystic fibrosis (unlabeled use): 100 mcg 4 times/day

Adults:

Prevention of NSAID-induced gastric ulcers: 200 mcg 4 times/day with food; if not tolerated, may decrease dose to 100 mcg 4 times/day with food; last dose of the day should be taken at bedtime

Medical termination of pregnancy: Refer to Mifepristone monograph.

Intravaginal: Adults: Labor induction or cervical ripening (unlabeled uses): 25 mcg (1/4 of 100 mcg tablet); may repeat at intervals no more frequent than every 3-6 hours. Do not use in patients with previous cesarean delivery or prior major uterine surgery.

Dosage adjustment in renal impairment: Half-life, maximum plasma concentration, and bioavailability may be increased; however, a correlation has not been observed with degree of dysfunction. Decrease dose if recommended dose is not tolerated. It is not known if misoprostol is removed by dialysis

Dietary Considerations Should be taken with food; incidence of diarrhea may be lessened by having patient take dose right after meals.

Administration Incidence of diarrhea may be lessened by having patient take dose right after meals and avoiding magnesium-containing antacids. When used for the prevention of NSAID-induced ulcers, therapy is usually begun on the second or third day of the next normal menstrual period in women of childbearing potential.

Monitoring Parameters Adequate diagnostic measures in all cases of undiagnosed abnormal vaginal bleeding

Dosage Forms Excipient information presented when available (limited, particularly for generics); consult specific product labeling.

Tablet, oral: 100 mcg, 200 mcg

Cytotec®: 100 mcg

Cytotec®: 200 mcg [scored]

◆ **Misoprostol and Diclofenac** *see* Diclofenac and Misoprostol *on page 498*

MitoMYcin (mye toe MYE sin)

Brand Names: Canada Mutamycin®

Index Terms Mitomycin-C; Mitomycin-X; MTC

Pharmacologic Category Antineoplastic Agent, Antibiotic

Use Treatment of adenocarcinoma of stomach or pancreas

Unlabeled Use Treatment of bladder cancer; prevention of excess scarring in glaucoma filtration procedures in patients at high risk of bleb failure

Pregnancy Risk Factor D

Pregnancy Considerations Mitomycin can cause fetal harm in humans. Animal studies show delayed fetal development, fetal external anomalies, and neonatal anomalies.

Lactation Enters breast milk/contraindicated

Contraindications Hypersensitivity to mitomycin or any component of the formulation; thrombocytopenia; coagulation disorders, increased bleeding tendency; pregnancy

Warnings/Precautions Hazardous agent - use appropriate precautions for handling and disposal. **[U.S. Boxed Warning]: May cause bone marrow suppression (thrombocytopenia and leukopenia);** monitor for infections. Use with caution in patients who have received radiation therapy or in the presence of hepatobiliary dysfunction; reduce dosage in patients who are receiving radiation therapy simultaneously. Monitor for renal toxicity; do not administer if serum creatinine is >1.7 mg/dL. **[U.S. Boxed Warning]: Hemolytic-uremic syndrome, potentially fatal, has been reported;** is correlated with total dose (single doses ≥60 mg or cumulative doses ≥50 mg/m^2) and total duration of therapy (>5-11 months). Bladder fibrosis/contraction has been reported with intravesical administration. **Mitomycin is a potent vesicant, may cause ulceration, necrosis, cellulitis, and tissue sloughing if infiltrated.** Shortness of breath and bronchospasm have been reported in patients receiving vinca alkaloids in combination with or after mitomycin; may be managed with bronchodilators, steroids and/or oxygen. Safety and efficacy in children have not been established. **[U.S. Boxed Warning]: Should be administered under the supervision of an experienced cancer chemotherapy physician.**

Adverse Reactions

>10%:

Cardiovascular: CHF (3% to 15%) (doses >30 mg/m^2)

Central nervous system: Fever (14%)

Dermatologic: Alopecia, nail banding/discoloration

Gastrointestinal: Nausea, vomiting and anorexia (14%)

Hematologic: Anemia (19% to 24%); myelosuppression, common, dose limiting, delayed

Onset: 3 weeks

Nadir: 4-6 weeks

Recovery: 6-8 weeks

1% to 10%:

Dermatologic: Rash

Gastrointestinal: Stomatitis

Neuromuscular: Paresthesia

Renal: Creatinine increase (2%)

Respiratory: Interstitial pneumonitis, infiltrates, dyspnea, cough (7%)

<1% (Limited to important or life-threatening): Extravasation reactions, hemolytic uremic syndrome, malaise, pruritus, renal failure, bladder fibrosis/contraction (intravesical administration)

Drug Interactions

Metabolism/Transport Effects Substrate of P-glycoprotein

Avoid Concomitant Use

Avoid concomitant use of MitoMYcin with any of the following: BCG; CloZAPine; Natalizumab; Pimecrolimus; Tacrolimus (Topical); Vaccines (Live)

Increased Effect/Toxicity

MitoMYcin may increase the levels/effects of: CloZAPine; Leflunomide; Natalizumab; Vaccines (Live)

The levels/effects of MitoMYcin may be increased by: Antineoplastic Agents (Vinca Alkaloids); Denosumab; P-glycoprotein/ABCB1 Inhibitors; Pimecrolimus; Roflumilast; Tacrolimus (Topical); Trastuzumab

Decreased Effect

MitoMYcin may decrease the levels/effects of: BCG; Coccidioidin Skin Test; Sipuleucel-T; Vaccines (Inactivated); Vaccines (Live)

The levels/effects of MitoMYcin may be decreased by: Echinacea; P-glycoprotein/ABCB1 Inducers

Ethanol/Nutrition/Herb Interactions Herb/Nutraceutical: Avoid black cohosh, dong quai in estrogen-dependent tumors.

Stability Store intact vials at controlled room temperature. Dilute powder with SWFI or 0.9% sodium chloride to a concentration of 0.5-1 mg/mL. Solution is stable for 7 days at room temperature and 14 days when refrigerated if protected from light. Solution of 0.5 mg/mL in a syringe is stable for 7 days at room temperature and 14 days when refrigerated and protected from light.

Further dilution to 20-40 mcg/mL:

In normal saline: Stable for 12 hours at room temperature.

In sodium lactate: Stable for 24 hours at room temperature.

Mechanism of Action Acts like an alkylating agent and produces DNA cross-linking (primarily with guanine and cytosine pairs); cell-cycle nonspecific; inhibits DNA and RNA synthesis; degrades preformed DNA, causes nuclear lysis and formation of giant cells. While not phase-specific *per se*, mitomycin has its maximum effect against cells in late G and early S phases.

Pharmacodynamics/Kinetics

Distribution: V_d: 22 L/m^2; high drug concentrations found in kidney, tongue, muscle, heart, and lung tissue; probably not distributed into the CNS

Metabolism: Hepatic

Half-life elimination: 23-78 minutes; Terminal: 50 minutes

Excretion: Urine (<10% as unchanged drug), with elevated serum concentrations

Dosage Refer to individual protocols. Children (unlabeled use) and Adults:

Single agent therapy: I.V.: 20 mg/m^2 every 6-8 weeks

Combination therapy: I.V.: 10 mg/m^2 every 6-8 weeks

Bladder carcinoma (unlabeled use): Intravesicular instillation (unapproved route): 20-40 mg instilled into the bladder and retained for 3 hours up to 3 times/week for up to 20 procedures per course

Glaucoma surgery (unlabeled use): 0.2-0.5 mg (0.2-0.5 mg/mL solution)

Dosage adjustment in renal impairment: The FDA-approved labeling states to avoid use in patients with serum creatine >1.7 mg/dL, but offers no other dosage adjustment guidelines. The following guidelines have been used by some clinicians (Aronoff, 2007): Adults:

Cl_{cr} <10 mL/minute: Administer 75% of dose

Continuous ambulatory peritoneal dialysis (CAPD): Administer 75% of dose

Dosage adjustment in hepatic impairment: Although some mitomycin may be excreted in the bile, no specific guidelines regarding dosage adjustment in hepatic impairment are available.

Administration

I.V.: Administer slow I.V. push or by slow (15-30 minute) infusion via a freely-running dextrose or saline infusion. Consider using a central venous catheter.

Intravesicular (unlabeled route): Instill into bladder for up to 3 hours (rotate patient every 15-30 minutes)

Glaucoma surgery (unlabeled route): Apply to pledget and place in contact with surgical wound for 2-5 minutes (doses and techniques may vary)

Monitoring Parameters Platelet count, CBC with differential, prothrombin time, renal and pulmonary function tests

Dosage Forms Excipient information presented when available (limited, particularly for generics); consult specific product labeling.

Injection, powder for reconstitution: 5 mg, 20 mg, 40 mg

◆ **Mitomycin-X** *see* MitoMYcin *on page 1142*

◆ **Mitomycin-C** *see* MitoMYcin *on page 1142*

Mitotane (MYE toe tane)

Brand Names: U.S. Lysodren®

Brand Names: Canada Lysodren®

Index Terms Chloditan; Chlodithane; Khloditan; Mytotan; o,p'-DDD; Ortho,para-DDD

Pharmacologic Category Antineoplastic Agent, Miscellaneous

Use Treatment of inoperable adrenocortical carcinoma

Unlabeled Use Treatment of Cushing's syndrome

Pregnancy Risk Factor C

Pregnancy Considerations Animal studies have not been conducted. There are no adequate and well-controlled studies in pregnant women. Use during pregnancy only if clearly needed.

Lactation Excretion in breast milk unknown/not recommended

Contraindications Hypersensitivity to mitotane or any component of the formulation

Warnings/Precautions Hazardous agent - use appropriate precautions for handling and disposal. Patients treated with mitotane may develop adrenal insufficiency; steroid replacement with glucocorticoid, and sometimes mineralocorticoid, is necessary. It has been recommended that steroid replacement therapy be initiated at the start of therapy, rather than waiting for evidence of adrenal insufficiency. **[U.S. Boxed Warning]: Because the primary action of mitotane is through adrenal suppression, discontinue mitotane temporarily with onset of shock or severe trauma; administer appropriate steroid coverage.** Because mitotane can increase the metabolism of exogenous steroids, higher than usual replacement steroid doses may be required. Surgically remove tumor tissues from metastatic masses prior to initiation of treatment; rapid cytotoxic effect may cause tumor hemorrhage. Observe patients for neurotoxicity with long-term (>2 years) use. Use caution with hepatic impairment; metabolism may be decreased. Other CNS adverse effects, including lethargy, sedation, and vertigo may occur; patients must be cautioned about performing tasks which require mental alertness (eg, operating machinery or driving). The manufacturer recommends initiating treatment within a hospital environment until a stabilized dose is achieved. Continue treatment as long as clinical benefit (maintenance of clinical status or metastatic lesion grown slowing) is observed. Clinical benefit is usually observed within 3 months at maximum tolerated dose, although 10% of patients may require more than 3 months for benefit. Continuous treatment at the maximum tolerated dose is generally the best approach. Some patients have been treated intermittently, restarting when severe symptoms reappear, although often response is no longer observed after 3 or 4 courses of intermittent treatment. **[U.S. Boxed Warnings]: Should be administered under the supervision of an experienced cancer chemotherapy physician.** Safety and efficacy in children have not been established.

Adverse Reactions The majority of adverse events are dose-dependent.

>10%:

Central nervous system: CNS depression (32%), lethargy/somnolence (25%), dizziness/vertigo (15%)

Dermatologic: Skin rash (15%)

Gastrointestinal: Anorexia (24%), nausea (39%), vomiting (37%), diarrhea (13%)

Neuromuscular & skeletal: Weakness (12%)

1% to 10%:

Central nervous system: Headache (5%), confusion (3%)

Neuromuscular & skeletal: Muscle tremor (3%)

<1% (Limited to important or life-threatening): Aches (generalized), adrenal insufficiency, albuminuria, anemia, ataxia, autoimmune hepatitis, bleeding time prolonged, blurred vision, cataract, diplopia, flushing, GGT increased, gynecomastia, hematuria, hemorrhagic cystitis, hormone binding globulins increased, hypercholesterolemia, hyperpyrexia, hypertension, hypertriglyceridemia, lens opacity, leukopenia, macular edema, memory decreased, mucositis, myalgia, neuropathy, orthostatic hypotension, primary hypogonadism, protein bound iodine decreased, thrombocytopenia, thyroid function tests altered, toxic retinopathy, transaminases increased

Drug Interactions

Metabolism/Transport Effects None known.

Avoid Concomitant Use There are no known interactions where it is recommended to avoid concomitant use.

Increased Effect/Toxicity

Mitotane may increase the levels/effects of: Vitamin K Antagonists

The levels/effects of Mitotane may be increased by: MAO Inhibitors

Decreased Effect

Mitotane may decrease the levels/effects of: Corticosteroids (Systemic); Vitamin K Antagonists

The levels/effects of Mitotane may be decreased by: Spironolactone

Ethanol/Nutrition/Herb Interactions Ethanol: Avoid ethanol (may increase CNS depression).

Stability Store at room temperature of 25°C (77°F); excursions permitted to 15°C to 30°C (59°F to 86°F).

Mechanism of Action Adrenolytic agent which causes adrenal cortical atrophy; affects mitochondria in adrenal cortical cells and decreases production of cortisol; also alters the peripheral metabolism of steroids

Pharmacodynamics/Kinetics

Absorption: Oral: ~5% to 40%

Distribution: Stored mainly in fat tissue but is found in all body tissues

Metabolism: Hepatic and other tissues

Half-life elimination: 18-159 days

Time to peak, serum: 3-5 hours

Excretion: Urine (~10%, as metabolites); feces (1% to 17%, as metabolites)

Dosage Oral:

Adrenocortical carcinoma:

Children (unlabeled use): 1-2 g/day in divided doses, increasing gradually to a maximum of 5-7 g/day

Adults: Start at 2-6 g/day in 3-4 divided doses, then increase incrementally to 9-10 g/day in 3-4 divided doses (maximum tolerated range: 2-16 g/day, usually 9-10 g/day; maximum dose studied: 18-19 g/day)

Cushing's syndrome (unlabeled use): Adults: Initial dose: 500 mg 3 times/day; maximum dose: 3000 mg 3 times/day (Biller, 2008)

Dosing adjustment for toxicity:

Severe side effects: Reduce dose until achieve a maximum tolerated dose

Significant neuropsychiatric adverse effects: Withhold treatment for at least 1 week and restart at a lower dose (Allolio, 2006)

Dosing adjustment in hepatic impairment: Dose may need to be decreased in patients with liver disease

Administration Oral: Administer in 3-4 divided doses/day. Do not crush tablets; wear gloves when handling; avoid exposure to crushed or broken tablets.

Monitoring Parameters Adrenal function; neurologic assessments (including behavioral) at regular intervals with chronic (>2 years) use

Dosage Forms Excipient information presented when available (limited, particularly for generics); consult specific product labeling.

Tablet, oral:

Lysodren®: 500 mg [scored]

MitoXANtrone (mye toe ZAN trone)

Brand Names: U.S. Novantrone®

Brand Names: Canada Mitoxantrone Injection®; Novantrone®

Index Terms CL-232315; DHAD; DHAQ; Dihydroxyanthracenedione; Dihydroxyanthracenedione Dihydrochloride; Mitoxantrone Dihydrochloride; Mitoxantrone HCl; Mitoxantrone Hydrochloride; Mitozantrone

Pharmacologic Category Antineoplastic Agent, Anthracenedione

Use Treatment of acute nonlymphocytic leukemias (ANLL [includes myelogenous, promyelocytic, monocytic and erythroid leukemias]); advanced hormone-refractory prostate cancer; secondary progressive or relapsing-remitting multiple sclerosis (MS)

Unlabeled Use Treatment of Hodgkin's lymphoma, non-Hodgkin's lymphomas (NHL), acute lymphocytic leukemia (ALL), myelodysplastic syndrome, breast cancer, pediatric acute myelogenous leukemia (AML), pediatric acute promyelocytic leukemia (APL); part of a conditioning regimen for autologous hematopoietic stem cell transplantation (HSCT)

Pregnancy Risk Factor D

Pregnancy Considerations Adverse effects were noted in animal studies. May cause fetal harm if administered to a pregnant woman. There are no adequate and well-controlled studies in pregnant women. Pregnancy should be avoided while on treatment. Women with multiple sclerosis and who are biologically capable of becoming pregnant should have a pregnancy test prior to each dose.

Lactation Enters breast milk/not recommended

Contraindications Hypersensitivity to mitoxantrone or any component of the formulation

Warnings/Precautions Hazardous agent - use appropriate precautions for handling and disposal.

[U.S. Boxed Warning]: Usually should not be administered if baseline neutrophil count <1500 cells/mm^3 (except for treatment of ANLL). Monitor blood counts and monitor for infection due to neutropenia. Treatment may lead to severe myelosuppression; unless the expected benefit outweighs the risk, use is generally not recommended in patients with pre-existing myelosuppression from prior chemotherapy.

[U.S. Boxed Warning]: May cause myocardial toxicity and potentially-fatal heart failure (HF); risk increases with cumulative dosing. Effects may occur during therapy or may be delayed (months or years after completion of therapy). Predisposing factors for mitoxantrone-induced cardiotoxicity include prior anthracycline or anthracenedione therapy, prior cardiovascular disease, concomitant use of cardiotoxic drugs, and mediastinal/pericardial irradiation, although may also occur in patients without risk factors. Prior to therapy initiation, evaluate all patients for cardiac-related signs/symptoms, including history, physical exam, and ECG; and evaluate baseline left ventricular ejection fraction (LVEF) with echocardiogram or multigated radionuclide angiography (MUGA) or MRI. Not recommended for use in MS patients when LVEF <50%, or baseline LVEF below the lower limit of normal (LLN). Evaluate for cardiac signs/symptoms (by history, physical exam, and ECG) and evaluate LVEF (using same method as baseline LVEF) in MS patients prior to each dose and if signs/symptoms of HF develop. Use in MS should be limited to a cumulative dose of ≤140 mg/m^2, and discontinued if LVEF falls below LLN or a significant decrease in LVEF is observed; decreases in LVEF and HF have been observed in patients with MS who have received cumulative doses <100 mg/m^2. Patients with MS should undergo annual LVEF evaluation following discontinuation of therapy to monitor for delayed cardiotoxicity.

[U.S. Boxed Warnings]: For I.V. administration only, into a free-flowing I.V.; may cause severe local tissue damage if extravasation occurs; do not administer subcutaneously, intramuscularly, or intra-arterially. Do not administer intrathecally; may cause serious and permanent neurologic damage. Extravasation resulting in burning, erythema, pain, swelling and skin discoloration (blue) has been reported; extravasation may result in tissue necrosis and require debridement for skin graft. May cause urine, saliva, tears, and sweat to turn blue-green for 24 hours postinfusion. Whites of eyes may have blue-green tinge. **[U.S. Boxed Warning]: Treatment with mitoxantrone increases the risk of developing secondary acute myelogenous leukemia (AML) in patients with cancer and in patients with MS;** acute promyelocytic leukemia (APL) has also been observed. Symptoms of acute leukemia include excessive bruising, bleeding and recurrent infections. The risk for secondary leukemia is increased in patients who are heavily pretreated, with higher doses, and with combination chemotherapy.

[U.S. Boxed Warning]: Should be administered under the supervision of a physician experienced in cancer chemotherapy agents. Dosage should be reduced in patients with impaired hepatobiliary function (clearance is reduced); not for treatment of multiple sclerosis in patients with concurrent hepatic impairment. Not for treatment of primary progressive multiple sclerosis. Rapid lysis of tumor cells may lead to hyperuricemia.

Adverse Reactions Includes events reported with any indication; incidence varies based on treatment, dose, and/or concomitant medications

>10%:

Cardiovascular: Edema (10% to 30%), arrhythmia (3% to 18%), cardiac function changes (≤18%), ECG changes (≤11%)

Central nervous system: Fever (6% to 78%), pain (8% to 41%), fatigue (≤39%), headache (6% to 13%)

Dermatologic: Alopecia (20% to 61%), nail bed changes (≤11%), petechiae/bruising (6% to 11%)

Endocrine & metabolic: Menstrual disorder (26% to 61%), amenorrhea (28% to 53%), hyperglycemia (10% to 31%)

Gastrointestinal: Nausea (26% to 76%), vomiting (6% to 72%), diarrhea (14% to 47%), mucositis (10% to 29%; onset: ≤1 week), stomatitis (8% to 29%; onset: ≤1 week), anorexia (22% to 25%), weight gain/loss (13% to 17%), constipation (10% to 16%), GI bleeding (2% to 16%), abdominal pain (9% to 15%), dyspepsia (5% to 14%)

Genitourinary: Urinary tract infection (7% to 32%), abnormal urine (5% to 11%)

Hematologic: Neutropenia (79% to 100%; onset: ≤3 weeks; grade 4: 23% to 54%), leukopenia (9% to 100%), lymphopenia (72% to 95%), anemia/hemoglobin decreased (5% to 75%) thrombocytopenia (33% to 39%; grades 3/4: 3% to 4%), neutropenic fever (≤11%)
Hepatic: Alkaline phosphatase increased (≤37%), transaminases increased (5% to 20%), GGT increased (3% to 15%)
Neuromuscular & skeletal: Weakness (≤24%)
Renal: BUN increased (≤22%), creatinine increased (≤13%), hematuria (≤11%)
Respiratory: Upper respiratory tract infection (7% to 53%), pharyngitis (≤19%), dyspnea (6% to 18%), cough (5% to 13%)
Miscellaneous: Infection (4% to 60%), sepsis (ANLL 31% to 34%), fungal infection (9% to 15%)

1% to 10%:
Cardiovascular: CHF (≤5%), ischemia (≤5%), LVEF decreased (≤5%), hypertension (≤4%)
Central nervous system: Chills (≤5%), anxiety (5%), depression (5%), seizure (2% to 4%)
Dermatologic: Cutaneous mycosis (≤10%), skin infection (≤5%)
Endocrine & metabolic: Hypocalcemia (10%), hypokalemia (7% to 10%), hyponatremia (9%), menorrhagia (7%)
Gastrointestinal: Aphthosis (≤10%)
Genitourinary: Impotence (≤7%), sterility (≤5%)
Hematologic: Granulocytopenia (6%), hemorrhage (5% to 6%), secondary acute leukemias (≤3%; includes AML, APL)
Hepatic: Jaundice (3% to 7%)
Neuromuscular & skeletal: Back pain (6% to 8%), myalgia (≤5%), arthralgia (≤5%)
Ocular: Conjunctivitis (≤5%), blurred vision (≤3%)
Renal: Renal failure (≤8%), proteinuria (≤6%)
Respiratory: Rhinitis (10%), pneumonia (≤9%), sinusitis (≤6%)
Miscellaneous: Systemic infection (≤10%), diaphoresis (≤9%)

<1% (Limited to important or life-threatening): Allergic reaction, anaphylactoid reactions, anaphylaxis, chest pain, dehydration; extravasation at injection site (may result in burning, erythema, pain, skin discoloration, swelling, or tissue necrosis); interstitial pneumonitis (with combination chemotherapy), hyperuricemia, hypotension, phlebitis at the infusion site, rash, sclera discoloration (blue), tachycardia, urine discoloration (blue-green), urticaria

Drug Interactions

Metabolism/Transport Effects **Inhibits** CYP3A4 (weak)

Avoid Concomitant Use

Avoid concomitant use of MitoXANtrone with any of the following: BCG; CloZAPine; Natalizumab; Pimecrolimus; Pimozide; Tacrolimus (Topical); Vaccines (Live)

Increased Effect/Toxicity

MitoXANtrone may increase the levels/effects of: CloZAPine; Leflunomide; Natalizumab; Pimozide; Vaccines (Live)

The levels/effects of MitoXANtrone may be increased by: Denosumab; Pimecrolimus; Roflumilast; Tacrolimus (Topical); Trastuzumab

Decreased Effect

MitoXANtrone may decrease the levels/effects of: BCG; Coccidioidin Skin Test; Sipuleucel-T; Vaccines (Inactivated); Vaccines (Live)

The levels/effects of MitoXANtrone may be decreased by: Echinacea

Ethanol/Nutrition/Herb Interactions Herb/Nutraceutical: Avoid echinacea (may diminish the immunosuppressant effect).

Stability Store intact vials at 15°C to 25°C (59°F to 77°F); do not freeze. Opened vials may be stored at room temperature for 7 days or under refrigeration for up to 14 days. Dilute in at least 50 mL of NS or D_5W. Solutions diluted for administration are stable for 7 days at room temperature or under refrigeration, although the manufacturer recommends immediate use.

Mechanism of Action Related to the anthracyclines, mitoxantrone intercalates into DNA resulting in cross-links and strand breaks; binds to nucleic acids and inhibits DNA and RNA synthesis by template disordering and steric obstruction; replication is decreased by binding to DNA topoisomerase II and seems to inhibit the incorporation of uridine into RNA and thymidine into DNA; active throughout entire cell cycle (cell-cycle nonspecific)

Pharmacodynamics/Kinetics

Absorption: Oral: Poor
Distribution: V_d: 14 L/kg; V_{dss}: >1000 L/m²; distributes extensively into tissue (pleural fluid, kidney, thyroid, liver, heart) and red blood cells
Protein binding: >95%, 76% to 78% to albumin
Metabolism: Hepatic; pathway not determined
Half-life elimination: Terminal: 23-215 hours (median: ~75 hours); may be prolonged with hepatic impairment
Excretion: Feces (25%); urine (6% to 11%; 65% as unchanged drug)

Dosage Details concerning dosing in combination regimens should also be consulted. I.V.:

Children: Acute nonlymphocytic leukemias:
AML consolidation phase (second course; unlabeled use): 10 mg/m² once daily for 5 days (Stevens, 1998)
APL consolidation phase (second course; unlabeled use): 10 mg/m² once daily for 5 days (Ortega, 2005; Sanz, 2004)

Adults:
Acute nonlymphocytic leukemias:
AML induction: 12 mg/m² once daily for 3 days (in combination with cytarabine); for incomplete response, may repeat at 12 mg/m² once daily for 2 days
AML consolidation: 12 mg/m² once daily for 2 days (in combination with cytarabine), repeat in 4 weeks
APL consolidation phase (second course; unlabeled dosing): 10 mg/m² once daily for 5 days (Sanz, 2004)
Multiple sclerosis: 12 mg/m² every 3 months (maximum lifetime cumulative dose: 140 mg/m²; discontinue use with LVEF <50% or clinically significant reduction in LVEF)
Prostate cancer (advanced, hormone-refractory): 12-14 mg/m² every 3 weeks (in combination with corticosteroids)
Hodgkin's lymphoma (unlabeled use): 10 mg/m² every 28 days as part of a combination chemotherapy regimen (Phillips, 1990)
Non-Hodgkin's lymphoma (unlabeled use; as part of combination chemotherapy regimens):
CNOP regimen: 10 mg/m² every 21 days (Bessell, 2003)
FCMR regimen: 8 mg/m² every 28 days (Forstpointner, 2004)
FMR regimen: 10 mg/m² every 21 days (Zinzani, 2004)
FND regimen: 10 mg/m² every 28 days (Tsimberidou, 2002)
MINE regimen: 8 mg/m² every 21 days (Rodriguez, 1995)
Stem cell transplantation, autologous (unlabeled use): 60 mg/m² administered 4-5 days prior to autografting (in combination with other chemotherapeutic agent[s]) (Oyan, 2006; Tarella, 2001)

Dosing adjustment for toxicity:
ANLL patients: Severe or life-threatening nonhematologic toxicity: Withhold treatment until toxicity resolves
MS patients:
Neutrophils <1500/mm^3: Use is not recommended
Signs/symptoms of HF: Evaluate for cardiac signs/symptoms and LVEF
LVEF <50% or baseline LVEF below the lower limit of normal (LLN): Use is not recommended

Dosing adjustment in renal impairment: Safety and efficacy have not been established
Hemodialysis: Supplemental dose is not necessary
Peritoneal dialysis: Supplemental dose is not necessary
Elderly: Clearance is decreased in elderly patients; use with caution

Dosing adjustment in hepatic impairment: Official dosage adjustment recommendations have not been established. Clearance is reduced in hepatic dysfunction; patients with severe hepatic dysfunction (bilirubin >3.4 mg/dL) have an AUC of 3 times greater than patients with normal hepatic function. Consider dose adjustments. **Note:** MS patients with hepatic impairment should not receive mitoxantrone.

Administration Irritant (is considered a vesicant by some institutions). For I.V. administration only; do not administer intrathecally, subcutaneously, intramuscularly or intra-arterially. Must be diluted prior to use. Avoid extravasation; may cause severe local tissue damage if extravasation occurs. Usually administered as a short I.V. infusion over 5-15 minutes; do not infuse over less then 3 minutes. High doses for bone marrow transplant (unlabeled use) are usually given as 1- to 3-hour infusions.

Monitoring Parameters CBC with differential, serum uric acid (for leukemia treatment), liver function tests; for the treatment of multiple sclerosis, obtain pregnancy test; monitor injection site for extravasation

Cardiac monitoring: Prior to initiation, evaluate all patients for cardiac-related signs/symptoms, including history, physical exam, and ECG; evaluate baseline and periodic left ventricular ejection fraction (LVEF) with echocardiogram or multigated radionuclide angiography (MUGA) or MRI. In patients with MS, evaluate for cardiac signs/symptoms (by history, physical exam, and ECG) and evaluate LVEF (using same method as baseline LVEF) prior to each dose and if signs/symptoms of HF develop. Patients with MS should undergo annual LVEF evaluation following discontinuation of therapy to monitor for delayed cardiotoxicity.

Dosage Forms Excipient information presented when available (limited, particularly for generics); consult specific product labeling.
Injection, solution [concentrate, preservative free]: 2 mg/mL (10 mL, 12.5 mL, 15 mL, 20 mL)
Novantrone®: 2 mg/mL (10 mL)

- ◆ **Mitoxantrone Dihydrochloride** *see* MitoXANtrone *on page* 1145
- ◆ **Mitoxantrone HCl** *see* MitoXANtrone *on page* 1145
- ◆ **Mitoxantrone Hydrochloride** *see* MitoXANtrone *on page* 1145
- ◆ **Mitoxantrone Injection® (Can)** *see* MitoXANtrone *on page* 1145
- ◆ **Mitozantrone** *see* MitoXANtrone *on page* 1145
- ◆ **Mitrazol® [OTC]** *see* Miconazole (Topical) *on page* 1126
- ◆ **MK-217** *see* Alendronate *on page* 61
- ◆ **MK383** *see* Tirofiban *on page* 1694
- ◆ **MK-0431** *see* SitaGLIPtin *on page* 1560
- ◆ **MK462** *see* Rizatriptan *on page* 1510
- ◆ **MK 0517** *see* Fosaprepitant *on page* 759
- ◆ **MK-0518** *see* Raltegravir *on page* 1456
- ◆ **MK594** *see* Losartan *on page* 1035
- ◆ **MK0826** *see* Ertapenem *on page* 615
- ◆ **MK 869** *see* Aprepitant *on page* 137
- ◆ **MLN341** *see* Bortezomib *on page* 228
- ◆ **MMF** *see* Mycophenolate *on page* 1162
- ◆ **MMR** *see* Measles, Mumps, and Rubella Virus Vaccine *on page* 1054
- ◆ **M-M-R® II** *see* Measles, Mumps, and Rubella Virus Vaccine *on page* 1054
- ◆ **MMR-V** *see* Measles, Mumps, Rubella, and Varicella Virus Vaccine *on page* 1055
- ◆ **MMRV** *see* Measles, Mumps, Rubella, and Varicella Virus Vaccine *on page* 1055
- ◆ **Mn-50™ [OTC]** *see* Manganese *on page* 1049
- ◆ **MOAB ABX-EGF** *see* Panitumumab *on page* 1288
- ◆ **MOAB C225** *see* Cetuximab *on page* 332
- ◆ **MoAb CD52** *see* Alemtuzumab *on page* 58
- ◆ **MOAB-CTLA-4** *see* Ipilimumab *on page* 921
- ◆ **MOAB HER2** *see* Trastuzumab *on page* 1722
- ◆ **Mobic®** *see* Meloxicam *on page* 1063
- ◆ **Mobicox® (Can)** *see* Meloxicam *on page* 1063

Modafinil (moe DAF i nil)

Brand Names: U.S. Provigil®
Brand Names: Canada Alertec®; Apo-Modafinil®
Pharmacologic Category Stimulant
Use Improve wakefulness in patients with excessive daytime sleepiness associated with narcolepsy and shift work sleep disorder (SWSD); adjunctive therapy for obstructive sleep apnea/hypopnea syndrome (OSAHS)
Unlabeled Use Attention-deficit/hyperactivity disorder (ADHD); treatment of fatigue in MS and other disorders
Pregnancy Risk Factor C
Pregnancy Considerations Embryotoxic effects have been observed in some, but not all animal studies. There are no adequate and well-controlled studies in pregnant women; use only when the potential risk of drug therapy is outweighed by the drug's benefits.

Healthcare providers are encouraged to register pregnant patients exposed to modafinil by calling 1-866-404-4106.

Efficacy of steroidal contraceptives (including depot and implantable contraceptives) may be decreased; alternate means of contraception should be considered during therapy and for 1 month after modafinil is discontinued.

Lactation Excretion in breast milk unknown/use caution
Medication Guide Available Yes
Contraindications Hypersensitivity to modafinil, armodafinil, or any component of the formulation
Warnings/Precautions For use following complete evaluation of sleepiness and in conjunction with other standard treatments (eg, CPAP). The degree of sleepiness should be reassessed frequently; some patients may not return to a normal level of wakefulness. Use is not recommended with a history of angina, cardiac ischemia, recent history of myocardial infarction, left ventricular hypertrophy, or patients with mitral valve prolapse who have developed mitral valve prolapse syndrome with previous CNS stimulant use.

Serious and life-threatening rashes (including Stevens-Johnson syndrome and toxic epidermal necrolysis) have been reported with modafinil. Most cases have occurred within the first 5 weeks of therapy; however, rare cases have occurred after long-term use. No risk factors have been identified to predict occurrence or severity. Patients should be advised to discontinue at first sign of rash. The serious nature of these dermatologic adverse effects, as well reports of psychiatric events, resulted in the FDA's Pediatric Advisory Committee unanimously recommending that a specific warning against the use of modafinil in children be added to the manufacturer's labeling. Modafinil is not FDA-approved for use in pediatrics for any indication.

In addition, rare cases of multiorgan hypersensitivity reactions in association with modafinil use, and lone cases of angioedema and anaphylactoid reactions with armodafinil, have been reported. Signs and symptoms are diverse, reflecting the involvement of specific organs. Patients typically present with fever and rash associated with organ-system dysfunction. Patients should be advised to report any signs and symptoms related to these effects; discontinuation of therapy is recommended.

Caution should be exercised when modafinil is given to patients with a history of psychosis; may impair the ability to engage in potentially hazardous activities. Stimulants may unmask tics in individuals with coexisting Tourette's syndrome. Use caution with renal or hepatic impairment (dosage adjustment in severe hepatic dysfunction is recommended).

Adverse Reactions

>10%:

Central nervous system: Headache (34%, dose related)
Gastrointestinal: Nausea (11%)

1% to 10%:

Cardiovascular: Chest pain (3%), hypertension (3%), palpitation (2%), tachycardia (2%), vasodilation (2%), edema (1%)
Central nervous system: Nervousness (7%), dizziness (5%), anxiety (5%; dose related), insomnia (5%), depression (2%), somnolence (2%), chills (1%), agitation (1%), confusion (1%), emotional lability (1%), vertigo (1%)
Dermatologic: Rash (1%; includes some severe cases requiring hospitalization)
Gastrointestinal: Diarrhea (6%), dyspepsia (5%), xerostomia (4%), anorexia (4%), constipation (2%), flatulence (1%), mouth ulceration (1%), taste perversion (1%)
Genitourinary: Abnormal urine (1%), hematuria (1%), pyuria (1%)
Hematologic: Eosinophilia (1%)
Hepatic: LFTs abnormal (2%)
Neuromuscular & skeletal: Back pain (6%), paresthesia (2%), dyskinesia (1%), hyperkinesia (1%), hypertonia (1%), neck rigidity (1%), tremor (1%)
Ocular: Amblyopia (1%), eye pain (1%), vision abnormal (1%)
Respiratory: Rhinitis (7%), pharyngitis (4%), lung disorder (2%), asthma (1%), epistaxis (1%)
Miscellaneous: Flu-like syndrome (4%), thirst (1%), diaphoresis (1%), herpes simplex infection (1%)

Postmarketing and/or case reports: Agranulocytosis, anaphylactic reaction, angioedema, DRESS syndrome, erythema multiforme, hypersensitivity syndrome (multiorgan), mania, psychosis, Stevens-Johnson syndrome, toxic epidermal necrolysis

Drug Interactions

Metabolism/Transport Effects **Substrate** of CYP3A4 (major); **Note:** Assignment of Major/Minor substrate status based on clinically relevant drug interaction potential; **Inhibits** CYP1A2 (weak), CYP2A6 (weak), CYP2C19 (strong), CYP2C9 (weak), CYP2E1 (weak), CYP3A4 (weak); **Induces** CYP1A2 (weak/moderate), CYP2B6 (weak/moderate), CYP3A4 (weak/moderate)

Avoid Concomitant Use

Avoid concomitant use of Modafinil with any of the following: Clopidogrel; Conivaptan; Iobenguane I 123; Pimozide

Increased Effect/Toxicity

Modafinil may increase the levels/effects of: Citalopram; CYP2C19 Substrates; Pimozide; Sympathomimetics

The levels/effects of Modafinil may be increased by: Atomoxetine; Cannabinoids; Conivaptan; CYP3A4 Inhibitors (Moderate); CYP3A4 Inhibitors (Strong); Dasatinib; Linezolid

Decreased Effect

Modafinil may decrease the levels/effects of: ARIPiprazole; Clopidogrel; Contraceptives (Estrogens); CycloSPORINE; CycloSPORINE (Systemic); Iobenguane I 123; Saxagliptin

The levels/effects of Modafinil may be decreased by: CYP3A4 Inducers (Strong); Deferasirox; Herbs (CYP3A4 Inducers); Tocilizumab

Ethanol/Nutrition/Herb Interactions

Ethanol: Avoid or limit ethanol.
Food: Delays absorption, but does not affect bioavailability.

Stability Store at 20°C to 25°C (68°F to 77°F).

Mechanism of Action The exact mechanism of action is unclear, it does not appear to alter the release of dopamine or norepinephrine, it may exert its stimulant effects by decreasing GABA-mediated neurotransmission, although this theory has not yet been fully evaluated; several studies also suggest that an intact central alpha-adrenergic system is required for modafinil's activity; the drug increases high-frequency alpha waves while decreasing both delta and theta wave activity, and these effects are consistent with generalized increases in mental alertness

Pharmacodynamics/Kinetics Modafinil is a racemic compound (10% *d*-isomer and 90% *l*-isomer at steady state) whose enantiomers have different pharmacokinetics

Distribution: V_d: 0.9 L/kg
Protein binding: ~60%, primarily to albumin
Metabolism: Hepatic; multiple pathways including CYP3A4
Half-life elimination: Effective half-life: 15 hours
Time to peak, serum: 2-4 hours
Excretion: Urine (as metabolites, <10% as unchanged drug)

Dosage Oral:

Adults:

ADHD (unlabeled use): 100-400 mg/day (Taylor, 2000)
Narcolepsy, obstructive sleep apnea/hypopnea syndrome (OSAHS): Initial: 200 mg as a single daily dose in the morning
Shift work sleep disorder (SWSD): Initial: 200 mg as a single dose taken ~1 hour prior to start of work shift
Note: Doses of 400 mg/day, given as a single dose, have been well tolerated, but there is no consistent evidence that this dose confers additional benefit.

Elderly: Elimination of modafinil and its metabolites may be reduced as a consequence of aging and as a result, consider initiating at lower doses in this patient population.

Dosing adjustment in renal impairment: Safety and efficacy have not been established in severe renal impairment.

Dosing adjustment in hepatic impairment: Severe hepatic impairment: Dose should be reduced to one-half of that recommended for patients with normal liver function.

Administration For the treatment of narcolepsy and obstructive sleep apnea/hypopnea syndrome (OSAHS), administer dose in the morning. For the treatment of shift work sleep disorder (SWSD), administer dose ~1 hour prior to start of work shift.

Monitoring Parameters Levels of sleepiness; blood pressure in patients with hypertension; body mass index and weight loss; development of severe skin reactions; development or exacerbation of psychiatric symptoms (eg, agitation, anxiety, depression)

When used for the treatment of ADHD, thoroughly evaluate for cardiovascular risk. Monitor heart rate, blood pressure, and consider obtaining ECG prior to initiation (Vetter, 2008).

Dosage Forms Excipient information presented when available (limited, particularly for generics); consult specific product labeling.

Tablet, oral:
- Provigil®: 100 mg
- Provigil®: 200 mg [scored]

Controlled Substance C-IV

◆ **Modecate® (Can)** *see* FluPHENAZine *on page 735*

◆ **Modecate® Concentrate (Can)** *see* FluPHENAZine *on page 735*

◆ **Modicon®** *see* Ethinyl Estradiol and Norethindrone *on page 660*

◆ **Modified Dakin's Solution** *see* Sodium Hypochlorite Solution *on page 1570*

◆ **Modified Shohl's Solution** *see* Sodium Citrate and Citric Acid *on page 1570*

Moexipril (mo EKS i pril)

Brand Names: U.S. Univasc®

Index Terms Moexipril Hydrochloride

Pharmacologic Category Angiotensin-Converting Enzyme (ACE) Inhibitor

Additional Appendix Information

Angiotensin Agents *on page 1869*

Use Treatment of hypertension, alone or in combination with thiazide diuretics

Pregnancy Risk Factor C (1st trimester); D (2nd and 3rd trimesters)

Dosage Adults: Oral: Initial: 7.5 mg once daily (in patients **not** receiving diuretics), 1 hour prior to a meal **or** 3.75 mg once daily (when combined with thiazide diuretics); maintenance dose: 7.5-30 mg/day in 1 or 2 divided doses 1 hour before meals

Dosing adjustment in renal impairment: Cl_{cr} ≤40 mL/minute: Patients may be cautiously placed on 3.75 mg once daily, then upwardly titrated to a maximum of 15 mg/day.

Additional Information Complete prescribing information for this medication should be consulted for additional detail.

Dosage Forms Excipient information presented when available (limited, particularly for generics); consult specific product labeling.

Tablet, oral, as hydrochloride: 7.5 mg, 15 mg
- Univasc®: 7.5 mg, 15 mg [scored]

Moexipril and Hydrochlorothiazide
(mo EKS i pril & hye droe klor oh THYE a zide)

Brand Names: U.S. Uniretic®

Brand Names: Canada Uniretic®

Index Terms Hydrochlorothiazide and Moexipril

Pharmacologic Category Angiotensin-Converting Enzyme (ACE) Inhibitor; Diuretic, Thiazide

Use Treatment of hypertension; not indicated for initial treatment of hypertension

Pregnancy Risk Factor C/D (2nd and 3rd trimesters)

Dosage Adults: Oral: 7.5-30 mg of moexipril, taken either in a single or divided dose 1 hour before meals; hydrochlorothiazide dose should be ≤50 mg/day

Additional Information Complete prescribing information for this medication should be consulted for additional detail.

Dosage Forms Excipient information presented when available (limited, particularly for generics); consult specific product labeling.

Tablet, oral:
- 7.5/12.5: Moexipril hydrochloride 7.5 mg and hydrochlorothiazide 12.5 mg
- 15/12.5: Moexipril hydrochloride 15 mg and hydrochlorothiazide 12.5 mg
- 15/25: Moexipril hydrochloride 15 mg and hydrochlorothiazide 25 mg

Uniretic®:
- 7.5/12.5: Moexipril hydrochloride 7.5 mg and hydrochlorothiazide 12.5 mg [scored]
- 15/12.5: Moexipril hydrochloride 15 mg and hydrochlorothiazide 12.5 mg [scored]
- 15/25: Moexipril hydrochloride 15 mg and hydrochlorothiazide 25 mg [scored]

◆ **Moexipril Hydrochloride** *see* Moexipril *on page 1149*

◆ **MOM** *see* Magnesium Hydroxide *on page 1045*

◆ **Momentum® [OTC]** *see* Magnesium Salicylate *on page 1047*

Mometasone (Oral Inhalation)
(moe MET a sone)

Brand Names: U.S. Asmanex® Twisthaler®

Index Terms Mometasone Furoate

Pharmacologic Category Corticosteroid, Inhalant (Oral)

Additional Appendix Information

Asthma *on page 1967*

Use Maintenance treatment of asthma as prophylactic therapy

Pregnancy Risk Factor C

Pregnancy Considerations Adverse events were observed in animal studies following topical and SubQ administration. Hypoadrenalism may occur in infants born to women receiving corticosteroids during pregnancy. Monitor these infants closely after birth. A decrease in fetal growth has not been observed with inhaled corticosteroid use during pregnancy. Inhaled corticosteroids are recommended for the treatment of asthma (most information available using budesonide) during pregnancy.

Lactation Excretion in breast milk unknown/use caution

Contraindications Hypersensitivity to mometasone or any component of the formulation; hypersensitivity to milk proteins; primary treatment of status asthmaticus or acute bronchospasm

Warnings/Precautions May cause hypercorticism or suppression of hypothalamic-pituitary-adrenal (HPA) axis, particularly in younger children or in patients receiving high doses for prolonged periods. HPA axis suppression may lead to adrenal crisis. Withdrawal and discontinuation of a corticosteroid should be done slowly and carefully. Particular care is required when patients are transferred from systemic corticosteroids to inhaled products due to possible adrenal insufficiency or withdrawal from steroids, including an increase in allergic symptoms. Patients receiving >20 mg per day of prednisone (or equivalent) may be most susceptible. Fatalities have occurred due to adrenal insufficiency in asthmatic patients during and after transfer from systemic corticosteroids to aerosol steroids; aerosol steroids do not provide the systemic steroid needed to treat patients having trauma, surgery, or infections. When transferring to oral inhaler, previously-suppressed allergic conditions (rhinitis, conjunctivitis, eczema) may be unmasked.

Bronchospasm may occur with wheezing after inhalation; if this occurs, stop steroid and treat with a fast-acting bronchodilator. Supplemental steroids (oral or parenteral) may be needed during stress or severe asthma attacks. Not to be used in status asthmaticus or for the relief of acute bronchospasm. Corticosteroid use may cause psychiatric disturbances, including depression, euphoria, insomnia, mood swings, and personality changes. Pre-existing psychiatric conditions may be exacerbated by corticosteroid use. Prolonged use of corticosteroids may also increase the incidence of secondary infection, mask acute infection (including fungal infections), prolong or exacerbate viral infections, or limit response to vaccines. Exposure to chickenpox should be avoided; corticosteroids should not be used to treat ocular herpes simplex. Corticosteroids should not be used for cerebral malaria or viral hepatitis. Close observation is required in patients with latent tuberculosis and/or TB reactivity; restrict use in active TB (only in conjunction with antituberculosis treatment). Prolonged treatment with corticosteroids has been associated with the development of Kaposi's sarcoma (case reports); if noted, discontinuation of therapy should be considered. Local oropharyngeal *Candida* infections have been reported; if occurs treat appropriately while continuing mometasone therapy. Patients should be instructed to rinse mouth after each use.

Reactions including, anaphylaxis, angioedema, pruritus, and rash have been reported; if these symptoms occur discontinue use. Use with caution in patients with thyroid disease, hepatic impairment, renal impairment, cardiovascular disease, diabetes, glaucoma, cataracts, myasthenia gravis, patients with or who are at risk for osteoporosis, patients at risk for seizures, or GI diseases (diverticulitis, peptic ulcer, ulcerative colitis) due to perforation risk. Use caution following acute MI (corticosteroids have been associated with myocardial rupture). Because of the risk of adverse effects, systemic corticosteroids should be used cautiously in the elderly in the smallest possible effective dose for the shortest duration.

Orally-inhaled corticosteroids may cause a reduction in growth velocity in pediatric patients (~1 centimeter per year [range: 0.3-1.8 cm per year] and related to dose and duration of exposure). To minimize the systemic effects of orally-inhaled corticosteroids, each patient should be titrated to the lowest effective dose. Growth should be routinely monitored in pediatric patients. Prior to use, the dose and duration of treatment should be based on the risk versus benefit for each individual patient. In general, use the smallest effective dose for the shortest duration of time to minimize adverse events. A gradual tapering of dose may be required prior to discontinuing therapy. There have been reports of systemic corticosteroid withdrawal symptoms (eg, joint/muscle pain, lassitude, depression) when withdrawing inhalation therapy. May contain lactose; very rare anaphylactic reactions have been reported in patients with severe milk protein allergy.

Adverse Reactions

>10%:
- Central nervous system: Headache (17% to 22%), fatigue (1% to 13%), depression (11%)
- Neuromuscular & skeletal: Musculoskeletal pain (4% to 22%), arthralgia (13%)
- Respiratory: Sinusitis (5% to 22%), rhinitis (4% to 20%), upper respiratory infection (8% to 15%), pharyngitis (8% to 13%)
- Miscellaneous: Oral candidiasis (4% to 22%)

1% to 10%:
- Central nervous system: Fever (children 7%), pain (1% to <3%)
- Dermatologic: Bruising (children 2%)
- Gastrointestinal: Abdominal pain (2% to 6%), dyspepsia (3% to 5%), nausea (1% to 3%), vomiting (1% to ≤3%), anorexia (1% to <3%), dry throat (1% to <3%), gastroenteritis (1% to <3%)
- Genitourinary: Dysmenorrhea (4% to 9%), urinary tract infection (children 2%)
- Neuromuscular & skeletal: Back pain (3% to 6%), myalgia (2% to 3%)
- Ocular: Ocular pressure increased (3%), cataracts (1%)
- Otic: Earache (1% to <3%)
- Respiratory: Sinus congestion (9%), dysphonia (1% to <3%), epistaxis (1% to <3%), nasal irritation (1% to <3%)
- Miscellaneous: Flu-like syndrome (1% to <3%), infection (1% to <3%)

Postmarketing and/or case reports: Anaphylaxis, angioedema, asthma aggravated, bronchospasm, cough, dyspnea, growth suppression, hypersensitivity, pruritus, rash, wheezing

Drug Interactions

Metabolism/Transport Effects Substrate of CYP3A4 (minor); **Note:** Assignment of Major/Minor substrate status based on clinically relevant drug interaction potential

Avoid Concomitant Use

Avoid concomitant use of Mometasone (Oral Inhalation) with any of the following: Aldesleukin

Increased Effect/Toxicity

Mometasone (Oral Inhalation) may increase the levels/effects of: Amphotericin B; Deferasirox; Loop Diuretics; Thiazide Diuretics

The levels/effects of Mometasone (Oral Inhalation) may be increased by: CYP3A4 Inhibitors (Strong); Telaprevir

Decreased Effect

Mometasone (Oral Inhalation) may decrease the levels/effects of: Aldesleukin; Antidiabetic Agents; Corticorelin; Telaprevir

The levels/effects of Mometasone (Oral Inhalation) may be decreased by: Tocilizumab

Stability Store at 25°C (77°F); excursions permitted to 15°C to 30°C (59°F to 86°F). Discard when oral dose counter reads "00" (or 45 days after opening the foil pouch).

Mechanism of Action May depress the formation, release, and activity of endogenous chemical mediators of inflammation (kinins, histamine, liposomal enzymes, prostaglandins). Leukocytes and macrophages may have to be present for the initiation of responses mediated by the above substances. Inhibits the margination and subsequent cell migration to the area of injury, and also reverses the dilatation and increased vessel permeability in the area resulting in decreased access of cells to the sites of injury.

Pharmacodynamics/Kinetics

Absorption: <1%
Protein binding: 98% to 99%
Metabolism: Hepatic via CYP3A4; forms metabolite
Half-life elimination: 5 hours
Excretion: Feces, bile, urine

Dosage Oral inhalation:

Children 4-11 years: 110 mcg once daily in the evening (maximum: 110 mcg/day)

Children ≥12 years and Adults: Previous therapy:
- Bronchodilators or inhaled corticosteroids: Initial: 1 inhalation (220 mcg) daily (maximum: 2 inhalations or 440 mcg/day); may be given in the evening or in divided doses twice daily
- Oral corticosteroids: Initial: 440 mcg twice daily (maximum: 880 mcg/day); prednisone should be reduced no faster than 2.5 mg/day on a weekly basis, beginning after at least 1 week of mometasone furoate use
- *NIH Asthma Guidelines (NIH, 2007):* Children ≥12 years and Adults:
  - "Low" dose: 220 mcg/day
  - "Medium" dose: 440 mcg/day
  - "High" dose: >440 mcg/day
- **Note:** Maximum effects may not be evident for 1-2 weeks or longer; dose should be titrated to effect, using the lowest possible dose

Dietary Considerations Asmanex® Twisthaler® contains lactose.

Administration Exhale fully prior to bringing the Twisthaler® up to the mouth. Place between lips and inhale quickly and deeply. Do not breathe out through the inhaler. Remove inhaler and hold breath for 10 seconds if possible. Rinse mouth after use.

Monitoring Parameters HPA axis suppression

Asthma: FEV_1, peak flow, and/or other pulmonary function tests

Dosage Forms Excipient information presented when available (limited, particularly for generics); consult specific product labeling.

Powder, for oral inhalation, as furoate:

Asmanex® Twisthaler®: 110 mcg (30 units) [contains lactose; delivers 100 mcg/actuation]

Asmanex® Twisthaler®: 220 mcg (14 units, 30 units, 60 units, 120 units) [contains lactose; delivers 200 mcg/actuation]

Mometasone (Nasal) (moe MET a sone)

Brand Names: U.S. Nasonex®

Brand Names: Canada Nasonex®

Index Terms Mometasone Furoate

Pharmacologic Category Corticosteroid, Nasal

Use Treatment of nasal symptoms of seasonal and perennial allergic rhinitis; prevention of nasal symptoms associated with seasonal allergic rhinitis; treatment of nasal polyps in adults

Canadian labeling: Additional use (not in U.S. labeling): Treatment of mild-to-moderate uncomplicated rhinosinusitis or as adjunctive treatment (with antimicrobials) in acute rhinosinusitis

Pregnancy Risk Factor C

Dosage Intranasal:

Allergic rhinitis (seasonal and perennial):

U.S. labeling:

Children 2-11 years: 1 spray (50 mcg) in each nostril once daily

Children ≥12 years and Adults: 2 sprays (100 mcg) in each nostril once daily; when used for the prevention of allergic rhinitis, treatment should begin 2-4 weeks prior to pollen season

Canadian labeling:

Children 3-11 years: 1 spray (50 mcg) in each nostril once daily

Children ≥12 years and Adults: Initial: 2 sprays (100 mcg) in each nostril once daily; upon symptom control, may consider dose reduction to 1 spray (50 mcg) in each nostril once daily as maintenance therapy. **Note:** If adequate symptom control is not achieved with initial dosing, may increase dose to 4 sprays (200 mcg) in each nostril once daily (total daily dose: 400 mcg). Dose reduction is recommended upon symptom control.

Nasal polyps treatment: Adults: 2 sprays (100 mcg) in each nostril twice daily; 2 sprays (100 mcg) once daily may be effective in some patients

Rhinosinusitis, adjunctive treatment (acute): Canadian labeling (not in U.S. labeling): Children ≥12 years and Adults: 2 sprays (100 mcg) in each nostril twice daily; if inadequate symptom control, may increase to 4 sprays (200 mcg) in each nostril twice daily (total daily dose: 800 mcg)

Rhinosinusitis treatment (acute, mild-to-moderate, uncomplicated): Canadian labeling (not in U.S. labeling): Children ≥12 years and Adults: 2 sprays (100 mcg) in each nostril twice daily; use beyond 15 days has not been studied.

Elderly: Refer to adult dosing.

Additional Information Complete prescribing information for this medication should be consulted for additional detail.

Dosage Forms Excipient information presented when available (limited, particularly for generics); consult specific product labeling.

Suspension, intranasal, as furoate [spray]:

Nasonex®: 50 mcg/spray (17 g) [contains benzalkonium chloride; delivers 120 sprays]

Dosage Forms: Canada Excipient information presented when available (limited, particularly for generics); consult specific product labeling.

Suspension, intranasal, as furoate [spray]:

Nasonex®: 50 mcg/spray [contains benzalkonium chloride; delivers 140 sprays]

Mometasone (Topical) (moe MET a sone)

Brand Names: U.S. Elocon®

Brand Names: Canada Elocom®; PMS-Mometasone; ratio-Mometasone; Taro-Mometasone

Index Terms Mometasone Furoate

Pharmacologic Category Corticosteroid, Topical

Additional Appendix Information

Corticosteroids *on page 1888*

Use Relief of the inflammatory and pruritic manifestations of corticosteroid-responsive dermatoses (medium potency topical corticosteroid)

Pregnancy Risk Factor C

Dosage Topical: Apply sparingly, do not use occlusive dressings. Therapy should be discontinued when control is achieved; if no improvement is seen in 2 weeks, reassessment of diagnosis may be necessary.

Cream, ointment: Children ≥2 years and Adults: Apply a thin film to affected area once daily; do not use in pediatric patients for longer than 3 weeks

Lotion: Children ≥12 years and Adults: Apply a few drops to affected area once daily

Additional Information Complete prescribing information for this medication should be consulted for additional detail.

Dosage Forms Excipient information presented when available (limited, particularly for generics); consult specific product labeling.

Cream, topical, as furoate: 0.1% (15 g, 45 g)

Elocon®: 0.1% (15 g, 45 g)

Lotion, topical, as furoate: 0.1% (30 mL, 60 mL)

Elocon®: 0.1% (30 mL, 60 mL) [contains isopropyl alcohol 40%]

Ointment, topical, as furoate: 0.1% (15 g, 45 g)

Elocon®: 0.1% (15 g, 45 g)

Mometasone and Formoterol
(moe MET a sone & for MOH te rol)

Brand Names: U.S. Dulera®

Brand Names: Canada Zenhale™

Index Terms Formoterol and Mometasone; Formoterol and Mometasone Furoate; Formoterol Fumarate Dihydrate and Mometasone

Pharmacologic Category $Beta_2$-Adrenergic Agonist; $Beta_2$-Adrenergic Agonist, Long-Acting; Corticosteroid, Inhalant (Oral)

Use Maintenance treatment of asthma where combination therapy is indicated

Pregnancy Risk Factor C

Medication Guide Available Yes

Dosage Oral inhalation: Children ≥12 years and Adults: Asthma:

Previous therapy included inhaled low-dose corticosteroids: Canadian labeling (not in U.S. labeling): Mometasone 50 mcg/formoterol 5 mcg: Two inhalations twice daily. Maximum daily dose: 4 inhalations

Previous therapy included inhaled medium-dose corticosteroids: Mometasone 100 mcg/formoterol 5 mcg: Two inhalations twice daily. Consider the higher dose combination for patients not adequately controlled on the lower combination following 1-2 weeks of therapy. Maximum daily dose: 4 inhalations

Previous therapy included inhaled high-dose corticosteroids: Mometasone 200 mcg/formoterol 5 mcg: Two inhalations twice daily. Maximum daily dose: 4 inhalations

Dosing adjustment in hepatic impairment: Mometasone systemic exposure appears to increase with increasing extent of impairment; however, there is no dosage adjustment recommended in the manufacturer labeling.

Additional Information Complete prescribing information for this medication should be consulted for additional detail.

Dosage Forms Excipient information presented when available (limited, particularly for generics); consult specific product labeling.

Aerosol, for oral inhalation:

Dulera®: Mometasone furoate 100 mcg and formoterol fumarate dihydrate 5 mcg per inhalation (13 g) [120 metered actuations]

Dulera®: Mometasone furoate 200 mcg and formoterol fumarate dihydrate 5 mcg per inhalation (13 g) [120 metered actuations]

Dosage Forms: Canada Excipient information presented when available (limited, particularly for generics); consult specific product labeling.

Aerosol, for oral inhalation:

Zenhale™: Mometasone furoate 50 mcg and formoterol fumarate dihydrate 5 mcg per inhalation [120 metered actuations]

- **Mometasone Furoate** *see* Mometasone (Nasal) *on page 1151*
- **Mometasone Furoate** *see* Mometasone (Oral Inhalation) *on page 1149*
- **Mometasone Furoate** *see* Mometasone (Topical) *on page 1151*
- **MOM/Mineral Oil Emulsion** *see* Magnesium Hydroxide and Mineral Oil *on page 1046*
- **Monacolin K** *see* Lovastatin *on page 1038*
- **Monistat® (Can)** *see* Miconazole (Topical) *on page 1126*
- **Monistat® 1 [OTC]** *see* Miconazole (Topical) *on page 1126*
- **Monistat® 1 Day or Night [OTC]** *see* Miconazole (Topical) *on page 1126*
- **Monistat® 3 [OTC]** *see* Miconazole (Topical) *on page 1126*
- **Monistat® 3 (Can)** *see* Miconazole (Topical) *on page 1126*
- **Monistat® 7 [OTC]** *see* Miconazole (Topical) *on page 1126*
- **Monoclate-P®** *see* Antihemophilic Factor (Human) *on page 125*
- **Monoclonal Antibody 5G1.1** *see* Eculizumab *on page 570*
- **Monoclonal Antibody ABX-EGF** *see* Panitumumab *on page 1288*
- **Monoclonal Antibody Anti-C5** *see* Eculizumab *on page 570*
- **Monoclonal Antibody Campath-1H** *see* Alemtuzumab *on page 58*
- **Monoclonal Antibody CD52** *see* Alemtuzumab *on page 58*
- **Monodox®** *see* Doxycycline *on page 557*
- **Monoethanolamine** *see* Ethanolamine Oleate *on page 653*
- **Monoket®** *see* Isosorbide Mononitrate *on page 938*
- **MonoNessa®** *see* Ethinyl Estradiol and Norgestimate *on page 663*
- **Mononine®** *see* Factor IX *on page 683*
- **Monopril** *see* Fosinopril *on page 763*
- **Monopril® (Can)** *see* Fosinopril *on page 763*

Montelukast (mon te LOO kast)

Brand Names: U.S. Singulair®

Brand Names: Canada PMS-Montelukast; PMS-Montelukast FC; Sandoz-Montelukast; Sandoz-Montelukast Granules; Singulair®; Teva-Montelukast

Index Terms Montelukast Sodium

Pharmacologic Category Leukotriene-Receptor Antagonist

Additional Appendix Information

Asthma *on page 1967*

Use Prophylaxis and chronic treatment of asthma; relief of symptoms of seasonal allergic rhinitis and perennial allergic rhinitis; prevention of exercise-induced bronchospasm

Unlabeled Use Acute asthma

Pregnancy Risk Factor B

Pregnancy Considerations Montelukast was not teratogenic in animal studies, however, there are no adequate and well-controlled studies in pregnant women. Based on limited data, structural defects have been reported in neonates exposed to montelukast *in utero*; however, a specific pattern and relationship to montelukast has not been established. Healthcare providers should report any prenatal exposures to the montelukast pregnancy registry at (800) 986-8999.

Lactation Excretion in breast milk unknown/use caution

Contraindications Hypersensitivity to montelukast or any component of the formulation

Warnings/Precautions Montelukast is not FDA approved for use in the reversal of bronchospasm in acute asthma attacks, including status asthmaticus; some clinicians, however, support its use as adjunctive therapy (Camargo, 2003; Cylly, 2003; Ferreira, 2001; Harmancik 2006). Appropriate rescue medication should be available. Appropriate clinical monitoring and caution are recommended when systemic corticosteroid reduction is considered in patients receiving montelukast. Patients should be instructed to notify prescriber if behavioral changes occur. Inform phenylketonuric patients that the chewable tablet contains phenylalanine.

In rare cases, patients on therapy with montelukast may present with systemic eosinophilia, sometimes presenting with clinical features of vasculitis consistent with Churg-Strauss syndrome, a condition which is often treated with systemic corticosteroid therapy. Healthcare providers should be alert to eosinophilia, vasculitic rash, worsening pulmonary symptoms, cardiac complications, and/or neuropathy presenting in their patients. A causal association between montelukast and these underlying conditions has not been established. Montelukast will not interrupt bronchoconstrictor response to aspirin or other NSAIDs; aspirin sensitive asthmatics should continue to avoid these agents. Postmarketing reports of behavior changes (agitation, aggression, depression, insomnia) have been noted in children and adults.

Adverse Reactions Note: Percentages and adverse events as reported in adults

1% to 10%:

Central nervous system: Headache (18%), dizziness (2%), fatigue (2%), fever (2%)

Dermatologic: Rash (2%)

Gastrointestinal: Dyspepsia (2%), dental pain (2%), gastroenteritis (2%)

Hepatic: AST increased (2%), ALT increased (≥1%)

Neuromuscular & skeletal: Weakness (2%)

Respiratory: Cough (≥1%), nasal congestion (2%), epistaxis (≥1%), sinusitis (≥1%), upper respiratory infection (≥1%)

Postmarketing and/or case reports: Anaphylaxis, angioedema, Churg-Strauss syndrome, depression, disorientation, eosinophilia (systemic), erythema multiforme, erythema nodosum, hallucinations, hepatic eosinophilic infiltration, hepatitis (mixed pattern, hepatocellular, and cholestatic), hypersensitivity, insomnia, pancreatitis, paresthesia, seizures, somnambulism, suicidal thinking/behavior (suicidality), suicide, thrombocytopenia, vasculitis

Drug Interactions

Metabolism/Transport Effects Substrate of CYP2C9 (major), CYP3A4 (major); **Note:** Assignment of Major/Minor substrate status based on clinically relevant drug interaction potential; **Inhibits** CYP2C8 (weak), CYP2C9 (weak)

Avoid Concomitant Use There are no known interactions where it is recommended to avoid concomitant use.

Increased Effect/Toxicity

The levels/effects of Montelukast may be increased by: Conivaptan; CYP2C9 Inhibitors (Moderate); CYP2C9 Inhibitors (Strong)

Decreased Effect

The levels/effects of Montelukast may be decreased by: CYP2C9 Inducers (Strong); CYP3A4 Inducers (Strong); Deferasirox; Herbs (CYP3A4 Inducers); Peginterferon Alfa-2b; Tocilizumab

Ethanol/Nutrition/Herb Interactions Herb/Nutraceutical: St John's wort may decrease montelukast levels.

Stability Store at room temperature of 25°C (77°F); excursions permitted to 15°C to 30°C (59°F to 86°F). Protect from moisture and light.

Granules: Store in original package; use within 15 minutes of opening packet.

Mechanism of Action Selective leukotriene receptor antagonist that inhibits the cysteinyl leukotriene receptor. Cysteinyl leukotrienes and leukotriene receptor occupation have been correlated with the pathophysiology of asthma, including airway edema, smooth muscle contraction, and altered cellular activity associated with the inflammatory process, which contribute to the signs and symptoms of asthma. Cysteinyl leukotrienes are also released from the nasal mucosa following allergen exposure leading to symptoms associated with allergic rhinitis.

Pharmacodynamics/Kinetics

Duration: >24 hours

Absorption: Rapid

Distribution: V_d: 8-11 L

Protein binding, plasma: >99%

Metabolism: Extensively hepatic via CYP3A4 and 2C9

Bioavailability: Tablet: 10 mg: Mean: 64%; 5 mg: 63% to 73%

Half-life elimination, plasma: Mean: 2.7-5.5 hours

Time to peak, serum: Tablet: 10 mg: 3-4 hours; 5 mg: 2-2.5 hours; 4 mg: 2 hours

Excretion: Feces (86%); urine (<0.2%)

Dosage Oral:

Children:

6-23 months: Perennial allergic rhinitis: 4 mg (oral granules) once daily

12-23 months: Asthma: 4 mg (oral granules) once daily, taken in the evening

2-5 years: Asthma, seasonal or perennial allergic rhinitis: 4 mg (chewable tablet or oral granules) once daily

6-14 years: Asthma, seasonal or perennial allergic rhinitis: 5 mg (chewable tablet) once daily

Children ≥15 years and Adults:

Asthma, seasonal or perennial allergic rhinitis: 10 mg once daily

Asthma, acute (unlabeled use): 10 mg as a single dose administered with first-line therapy (Camargo, 2003; Cylly, 2003)

Bronchoconstriction, exercise-induced (prevention): 10 mg at least 2 hours prior to exercise; additional doses should not be administered within 24 hours. Daily administration to prevent exercise-induced bronchoconstriction has not been evaluated.

Dosing adjustment in renal impairment: No adjustment necessary

Dosing adjustment in hepatic impairment: Mild-to-moderate: No adjustment necessary. Patients with severe hepatic disease were **not** studied.

Dietary Considerations Some products may contain phenylalanine.

Administration When treating asthma, administer dose in the evening. Patients with allergic rhinitis may individualize administration time (morning or evening). Patients with both asthma and allergic rhinitis should take their dose in the evening. Granules may be administered directly in the mouth or mixed with a spoonful of applesauce, carrots, rice, ice cream, baby formula, or breast milk; do not add to any other liquids or foods. Administer within 15 minutes of opening packet. May administer without regard to meals.

Monitoring Parameters Mood or behavior changes, including suicidal thinking/behavior

Dosage Forms Excipient information presented when available (limited, particularly for generics); consult specific product labeling.

Granules, oral:

Singulair®: 4 mg/packet (30s)

Tablet, oral:

Singulair®: 10 mg [contains lactose 89.3 mg/tablet]

Tablet, chewable, oral:

Singulair®: 4 mg [contains phenylalanine 0.67 mg/tablet; cherry flavor]

Singulair®: 5 mg [contains phenylalanine 0.84 mg/tablet; cherry flavor]

◆ **Montelukast Sodium** *see* Montelukast *on page* 1152

◆ **Monurol®** *see* Fosfomycin *on page* 763

◆ **8-MOP** *see* Methoxsalen (Systemic) *on page* 1102

◆ **8-MOP®** *see* Methoxsalen (Systemic) *on page* 1102

◆ **Morning After Pill** *see* Ethinyl Estradiol and Norgestrel *on page* 664

Morphine (Systemic) (MOR feen)

Brand Names: U.S. Astramorph®/PF; AVINza®; Duramorph; Infumorph 200; Infumorph 500; Kadian®; MS Contin®; Oramorph® SR

Brand Names: Canada Doloral; Kadian®; M-Eslon®; M.O.S.-SR®; M.O.S.-Sulfate®; M.O.S.® 10; M.O.S.® 20; M.O.S.® 30; Morphine Extra Forte Injection; Morphine Forte Injection; Morphine HP®; Morphine LP® Epidural; Morphine SR; Morphine-EPD; MS Contin SRT; MS Contin®; MS-IR®; Novo-Morphine SR; PMS-Morphine Sulfate SR; ratio-Morphine; ratio-Morphine SR; Sandoz-Morphine SR; Statex®; Teva-Morphine SR

Index Terms MS (error-prone abbreviation and should not be used); MSO_4 (error-prone abbreviation and should not be used); Roxanol

Pharmacologic Category Analgesic, Opioid

Additional Appendix Information

Opioid Analgesics *on page 1896*

Patient Information for Disposal of Unused Medications *on page 2026*

Use Relief of moderate-to-severe acute and chronic pain; relief of pain of myocardial infarction; relief of dyspnea of acute left ventricular failure and pulmonary edema; preanesthetic medication

Infumorph®: Used in continuous microinfusion devices for intrathecal or epidural administration in treatment of intractable chronic pain

Controlled, extended, or sustained release products: Only intended/indicated for use when repeated doses for an extended period of time are required. The 100 mg and 200 mg tablets or capsules of Kadian®, MS Contin®, and morphine sulfate controlled-release tablets and the 60 mg, 90 mg, and 120 mg capsules of Avinza® should only be used in opioid-tolerant patients.

Pregnancy Risk Factor C

Pregnancy Considerations Teratogenic effects were not observed in animal studies; however reduced growth and behavioral abnormalities in offspring have been observed. Morphine crosses the human placenta. The frequency of congenital malformations has not been reported to be greater than expected in children from mothers treated with morphine during pregnancy. However, following *in utero* exposure, infants may exhibit withdrawal, decreased brain volume (reversible), small size, decreased ventilatory response to CO_2, and increased risk of sudden infant death syndrome. In patients with chronic, noncancer pain, minimal (if any) opioids should be used during pregnancy. Neonates born to mothers receiving chronic opioids during pregnancy should be monitored for neonatal withdrawal syndrome.

Lactation Enters breast milk/use caution (AAP rates "compatible"; AAP 2001 update pending)

Medication Guide Available Yes

Contraindications Note: Some contraindications are product specific. For details, please see detailed product prescribing information.

Hypersensitivity to morphine sulfate or any component of the formulation; severe respiratory depression (without resuscitative equipment); acute or severe asthma; known or suspected paralytic ileus; sustained release products are not recommended with gastrointestinal obstruction or in acute/postoperative pain. Oral solutions contraindicated in patients with heart failure due to chronic lung disease, cardiac arrhythmias, head injuries, brain tumors, acute alcoholism, deliriums tremens, seizure disorders, Injectable solution contraindicated during labor when a premature birth is anticipated. Some products contraindicated in patients with head injuries or increased intracranial pressure. MS Contin® and Kadian® contraindicated in patients with hypercarbia. Some immediate release formulations (tablets and solution) contraindicated in post biliary tract surgery, suspected surgical abdomen, surgical anastomosis, MAO inhibitor use (concurrent or within 14 days), general CNS depression.

Warnings/Precautions An opioid-containing analgesic regimen should be tailored to each patient's needs and based upon the type of pain being treated (acute versus chronic), the route of administration, degree of tolerance for opioids (naive versus chronic user), age, weight, and medical condition. The optimal analgesic dose varies widely among patients. Doses should be titrated to pain relief/prevention. When used as an epidural injection, monitor for delayed sedation. **[U.S. Boxed Warning]: Healthcare provider should be alert to problems of abuse, misuse, and diversion.**

May cause respiratory depression; use with caution in patients (particularly elderly or debilitated) with impaired respiratory function, morbid obesity, adrenal insufficiency, prostatic hyperplasia, urinary stricture, renal impairment, or severe hepatic dysfunction and in patients with hypersensitivity reactions to other phenanthrene derivative opioid agonists (codeine, hydrocodone, hydromorphone, levorphanol, oxycodone, oxymorphone). Use with caution in patients with biliary tract dysfunction; acute pancreatitis may cause constriction of sphincter of Oddi. Some preparations contain sulfites which may cause allergic reactions; infants <3 months of age are more susceptible to respiratory depression, use with caution and generally in reduced doses in this age group.

May cause CNS depression, which may impair physical or mental abilities; patients must be cautioned about performing tasks which require mental alertness (eg, operating machinery or driving). Effects may be potentiated when used with other sedative drugs or ethanol. May cause hypotension in patients with acute myocardial infarction, volume depletion, or concurrent drug therapy which may exaggerate vasodilation. Use with extreme caution in patients with head injury, intracranial lesions, or elevated intracranial pressure; exaggerated elevation of ICP may occur. May cause seizures if high doses are used; use with caution in patients with seizure disorders. Tolerance or drug dependence may result from extended use. Concurrent use of agonist/antagonist analgesics may precipitate withdrawal symptoms and/or reduced analgesic efficacy in patients following prolonged therapy with mu opioid agonists. Abrupt discontinuation following prolonged use may also lead to withdrawal symptoms. Elderly may be particularly susceptible to adverse effects of narcotics. May obscure diagnosis or clinical course of patients with acute abdominal conditions.

Extended or sustained-release formulations:

[U.S. Boxed Warning]: Extended or sustained release dosage forms should not be crushed or chewed. Controlled-, extended-, or sustained-release products are not intended for "as needed (PRN)" use. **MS Contin® 100 or 200 mg tablets and Kadian® 100 mg or 200 mg capsules are for use only in opioid-tolerant patients.** Avinza®, Kadian®, MS Contin®: **[U.S. Boxed Warning]: Indicated for the management of moderate-to-severe pain when around the clock pain control is needed for an extended time period.**

[U.S. Boxed Warning]: Avinza®: Do not administer with alcoholic beverages or ethanol-containing products, which may disrupt extended-release characteristic of product.

Highly concentrated oral solutions: [U.S. Boxed Warning]: Check doses carefully when using highly concentrated oral solutions.

Injections: Note: Products are designed for administration by specific routes (I.V., intrathecal, epidural). Use caution when prescribing, dispensing, or administering to use formulations only by intended route(s).

[U.S. Boxed Warning]: Duramorph®: Due to the risk of severe and/or sustained cardiopulmonary depressant effects of Duramorph® must be administered in a fully equipped and staffed environment. Naloxone injection should be immediately available. Patient should remain in this environment for at least 24 hours following the initial dose.

[U.S. Boxed Warning]: Intrathecal dosage is usually $^{1}/_{10}$ that of epidural dosage.

Infumorph® solutions are **for use in microinfusion devices only**; not for I.V., I.M., or SubQ administration, or for single-dose administration.

When used as an epidural injection, monitor for delayed sedation.

Adverse Reactions Note: Individual patient differences are unpredictable, and percentage may differ in acute pain (surgical) treatment. Reactions may be dose, formulation, and/or route dependent.

Frequency not defined:
- Cardiovascular: Circulatory depression, flushing, shock
- Central nervous system: Dysphonia, physical and psychological dependence, sedation
- Endocrine & metabolic: Antidiuretic hormone release

>10%:
- Cardiovascular: Bradycardia, hypotension
- Central nervous system: Drowsiness (9% to 48%; tolerance usually develops to drowsiness with regular dosing for 1-2 weeks), dizziness (6% to 20%), fever (<3% to >10%), confusion, headache (following epidural or intrathecal use)
- Dermatologic: Pruritus (may be dose related)
- Gastrointestinal: Xerostomia (78%), constipation (9% to 40%; tolerance develops very slowly if at all), nausea (7% to 28%; tolerance usually develops to nausea and vomiting with chronic use), vomiting
- Genitourinary: Urinary retention (16%; may be prolonged, up to 20 hours, following epidural or intrathecal use)
- Hematologic: Anemia (following intrathecal use)
- Local: Pain at injection site
- Neuromuscular & skeletal: Weakness
- Respiratory: Oxygen saturation decreased
- Miscellaneous: Histamine release

1% to 10%:
- Cardiovascular: Atrial fibrillation (<3%), chest pain (<3%), edema, hypertension, palpitation, peripheral edema, syncope, tachycardia, vasodilation
- Central nervous system: Amnesia, agitation, anxiety, apathy, apprehension, ataxia, chills, coma, delirium, depression, dream abnormalities, euphoria, false sense of well being, hallucination, hypoesthesia, insomnia, lethargy, malaise, nervousness, restlessness, seizure, slurred speech, somnolence, vertigo
- Dermatologic: Dry skin, rash, urticaria
- Endocrine & metabolic: Gynecomastia (<3%), hypokalemia, hyponatremia, libido decreased
- Gastrointestinal: Abdominal distension, abdominal pain, anorexia, biliary colic, diarrhea, dyspepsia, dysphagia, flatulence, gastroenteritis, GERD, GI irritation, paralytic ileus, rectal disorder, taste perversion, weight loss
- Genitourinary: Bladder spasm, dysuria, ejaculation abnormal, impotence, urination decreased
- Hematologic: Leukopenia (<3%), thrombocytopenia (<3%), hematocrit decreased
- Hepatic: Liver function tests increased
- Neuromuscular & skeletal: Arthralgia, back pain, bone pain, foot drop, gait abnormalities, paresthesia, rigors, skeletal muscle rigidity, tremor
- Ocular: Amblyopia, conjunctivitis, eye pain, vision problems/disturbance
- Renal: Oliguria
- Respiratory: Asthma, atelectasis, dyspnea, hiccups, hypercapnia, hypoxia, pulmonary edema (noncardiogenic), respiratory depression, rhinitis
- Miscellaneous: Diaphoresis, flu-like syndrome, infection, thirst, voice alteration, withdrawal syndrome

<1% (Limited to important or life-threatening): Amenorrhea, anaphylaxis, apnea, biliary tract spasm, blurred vision, bronchospasm, cardiac arrest, cough reflex decreased, dehydration, diplopia, disorientation, hemorrhagic urticaria, intestinal obstruction, intracranial pressure increased, laryngospasm, menstrual irregularities, miosis, myoclonus, nystagmus, paradoxical CNS stimulation, respiratory arrest, sepsis, urinary tract spasm, thermal dysregulation, toxic psychoses

Drug Interactions

Metabolism/Transport Effects Substrate of CYP2D6 (minor); **Note:** Assignment of Major/Minor substrate status based on clinically relevant drug interaction potential

Avoid Concomitant Use There are no known interactions where it is recommended to avoid concomitant use.

Increased Effect/Toxicity

Morphine (Systemic) may increase the levels/effects of: Alcohol (Ethyl); Alvimopan; CNS Depressants; Desmopressin; Selective Serotonin Reuptake Inhibitors; Thiazide Diuretics

The levels/effects of Morphine (Systemic) may be increased by: Amphetamines; Antipsychotic Agents (Phenothiazines); Droperidol; HydrOXYzine; Succinylcholine

Decreased Effect

Morphine (Systemic) may decrease the levels/effects of: Pegvisomant

The levels/effects of Morphine (Systemic) may be decreased by: Ammonium Chloride; Mixed Agonist / Antagonist Opioids; Peginterferon Alfa-2b; Rifamycin Derivatives

Ethanol/Nutrition/Herb Interactions

Ethanol: Alcoholic beverages or ethanol-containing products may disrupt extended-release formulation resulting in rapid release of entire morphine dose. Ethanol may also increase CNS depression; monitor for increased effects with coadministration. Caution patients about effects.

Food: Administration of oral morphine solution with food may increase bioavailability (ie, a report of 34% increase in morphine AUC when morphine oral solution followed a high-fat meal). The bioavailability of Avinza®, Oramorph SR®, or Kadian® does not appear to be affected by food.

Herb/Nutraceutical: Avoid valerian, St John's wort, kava kava, gotu kola (may increase CNS depression).

Stability

Capsule, sustained release (Avinza®, Kadian®): Store at 25°C (77°F); excursions permitted to 15°C to 30°C (59°F to 86°F). Protect from light and moisture.

Injection: Store at controlled room temperature of 20°C to 25°C (68°F to 77°F); do not freeze. Protect from light. Degradation depends on pH and presence of oxygen; relatively stable in pH ≤4; darkening of solutions indicate degradation. Usual concentration for continuous I.V. infusion: 0.1-1 mg/mL in D_5W.

Oral solution: Store at controlled room temperature of 25°C (68°F to 77°F); do not freeze.

Suppositories: Store at controlled room temperature 25°C (77°F). Protect from light.

Tablet, extended release: Store at controlled room temperature of 25°C (77°F).

Tablet, immediate release: Store at controlled room temperature of 25°C (77°F). Protect from moisture.

Mechanism of Action Binds to opiate receptors in the CNS, causing inhibition of ascending pain pathways, altering the perception of and response to pain; produces generalized CNS depression

Pharmacodynamics/Kinetics

Onset of action (patient dependent; dosing must be individualized): Oral (immediate release): ~30 minutes; I.V.: 5-10 minutes

Duration (patient dependent; dosing must be individualized): Pain relief:
- Immediate release formulations: 4 hours
- Extended release capsule and tablet: 8-24 hours (formulation dependent)

Absorption: Variable

Distribution: V_d: 3-4 L/kg; binds to opioid receptors in the CNS and periphery (eg, GI tract)
Protein binding: 30% to 35%
Metabolism: Hepatic via conjugation with glucuronic acid primarily to morphine-6-glucoronide (active analgesic) morphine-3-glucuronide (inactive as analgesic); minor metabolites include morphine-3-6-diglucuronide; other minor metabolites include normorphine (active) and morphine 3-ethereal sulfate
Bioavailability: Oral: 17% to 33% (first-pass effect limits oral bioavailability; oral:parenteral effectiveness reportedly varies from 1:6 in opioid naive patients to 1:3 with chronic use)
Half-life elimination: Adults: 2-4 hours (immediate release forms)
Time to peak, plasma: Avinza®: 30 minutes (maintained for 24 hours); Kadian®: ~10 hours; Oramorph® SR: ~4 hours
Excretion: Urine (primarily as morphine-3-glucuronide, ~2% to 12% excreted unchanged); feces (~7% to 10%). It has been suggested that accumulation of morphine-6-glucuronide might cause toxicity with renal insufficiency. All of the metabolites (ie, morphine-3-glucuronide, morphine-6-glucuronide, and normorphine) have been suggested as possible causes of neurotoxicity (eg, myoclonus).

Dosage These are guidelines and do not represent the doses that may be required in all patients. Doses and dosage intervals should be titrated to pain relief/prevention.

Children >6 months and <50 kg: *Acute pain (moderate-to-severe):*
Oral (immediate release formulations): 0.15-0.3 mg/kg every 3-4 hours as needed. **Note:** The American Pain Society recommends an initial dose of 0.3 mg/kg for children with severe pain.
I.M., I.V.: 0.1-0.2 mg/kg every 3-4 hours as needed
I.V. infusion: Range: 10-60 mcg/kg/**hour**
Patient-controlled analgesia (PCA) (American Pain Society, 2008): **Note:** Opiate-naive: Consider lower end of dosing range:
Usual concentration: 1 mg/mL
Demand dose: Usual: 0.02 mg/kg/dose; range: 0.01-0.03 mg/kg/dose
Lockout interval: 6-8 minutes
Usual basal rate: 0-0.03 mg/kg/hour

Adults:
Acute pain (moderate-to-severe):
Oral (immediate release formulations): Opiate-naive: Initial: 10 mg every 4 hours as needed; patients with prior opiate exposure may require higher initial doses: usual dosage range: 10-30 mg every 4 hours as needed
I.M., SubQ: **Note:** Repeated SubQ administration causes local tissue irritation, pain, and induration.
Initial: Opiate-naive: 5-10 mg every 4 hours as needed; patients with prior opiate exposure may require higher initial doses; usual dosage range: 5-20 mg every 4 hours as needed
Rectal: 10-20 mg every 3-4 hours
I.V.: Initial: Opiate-naive: 2.5-5 mg every 3-4 hours; patients with prior opiate exposure may require higher initial doses. **Note:** Repeated doses (up to every 5 minutes if needed) in small increments (eg, 1-4 mg) may be preferred to larger and less frequent doses.
Acute myocardial infarction, analgesia (ACC/AHA 2004 guidelines): Initial management: 2-4 mg, give 2-8 mg every 5-15 minutes as needed.
Critically-ill patients (unlabeled dose): 0.7-10 mg (based on 70 kg patient) **or** 0.01-0.15 mg/kg every 1-2 hours as needed. **Note:** More frequent dosing may be needed (eg, mechanically-ventilated patients).

I.V., SubQ continuous infusion: 0.8-10 mg/hour; usual range: Up to 80 mg/hour
Continuous infusion: Usual dosage range: 5-35 mg/hour (based on 70 kg patient) **or** 0.07-0.5 mg/kg/hour
Patient-controlled analgesia (PCA): (Opiate-naive: Consider lower end of dosing range):
Usual concentration: 1 mg/mL
Demand dose: Usual: 1 mg; range: 0.5-2.5 mg
Lockout interval: 5-10 minutes
Intrathecal (I.T.): **Note: Must be preservative-free.** Administer with extreme caution and in reduced dosage to geriatric or debilitated patients. I.T. dose is usually 1/10 that of epidural dosage.
Opioid-naive: 0.2-1 mg/dose (may provide adequate relief for up to 24 hours); repeat doses are **not** recommended. **Note:** The American Pain Society recommends 0.1-0.3 mg/dose; adjust dose for age, injection site, and patient's medical condition and degree of opioid tolerance.
Continuous microinfusion (Infumorph®): Initial: 0.2-1 mg/day
Opioid-tolerant: 1-10 mg/day
Continuous microinfusion (Infumorph®): Initial: 1-10 mg/day, titrate to effect; usual maximum is ~20 mg/day
Epidural: Pain management: **Note: Must be preservative-free.** Administer with extreme caution and in reduced dosage to geriatric or debilitated patients. Vigilant monitoring is particularly important in these patients.
Single-dose (Astromorph/PF™, Duramorph®): Initial: 5 mg, if pain relief not achieved in 1 hour, careful administration of 1-2 mg at intervals sufficient to assess effectiveness may be given; maximum: 10 mg/24 hours (single doses may provide adequate relief for up to 24 hours)
Infusion: Bolus dose: 1-6 mg; infusion rate: 0.1-0.2 mg/hour; maximum dose: 10 mg/24 hours.
Note: The American Pain Society recommends 1-6 mg/dose as a single dose or an infusion of 0.1-1 mg/hour; adjust dose for age, injection site, and patient's medical condition and degree of opioid tolerance.
Continuous microinfusion (Infumorph®):
Opioid-naive: Initial: 0.2-1 mg/day
Opioid-tolerant: Initial: 1-10 mg/day, titrate to effect; usual maximum is ~20 mg/day

Chronic pain: **Note:** Patients taking opioids chronically may become tolerant and require doses higher than the usual dosage range to maintain the desired effect. Tolerance can be managed by appropriate dose titration. There is no optimal or maximal dose for morphine in chronic pain. The appropriate dose is one that relieves pain throughout its dosing interval without causing unmanageable side effects.
Oral: Controlled-, extended-, or sustained-release formulations: A patient's morphine requirement should be established using prompt-release formulations. Conversion to long-acting products may be considered when chronic, continuous treatment is required. Higher dosages should be reserved for use only in opioid-tolerant patients.
Capsules, extended release (Avinza®): Daily dose administered once daily (for best results, administer at same time each day)
Capsules, sustained release (Kadian®): Daily dose administered once daily or in 2 divided doses daily (every 12 hours)
Tablets, controlled release (MS Contin®), sustained release (Oramorph SR®), or extended release: Daily dose divided and administered every 8 or every 12 hours

Elderly or debilitated patients: Use with caution; may require dose reduction

Dosing adjustment in renal impairment:

Cl_{cr} 10-50 mL/minute: Children and Adults: Administer at 75% of normal dose

Cl_{cr} <10 mL/minute: Children and Adults: Administer at 50% of normal dose

Intermittent HD:

Children: Administer 50% of normal dose

Adults: No dosage adjustment necessary

Peritoneal dialysis: Children: Administer 50% of normal dose

CRRT: Children and Adults: Administer 75% of normal dose, titrate

Dosing adjustment/comments in hepatic disease: Unchanged in mild liver disease; substantial extrahepatic metabolism may occur; excessive sedation may occur in cirrhosis

Dietary Considerations Morphine may cause GI upset; take with food if GI upset occurs. Be consistent when taking morphine with or without meals.

Administration

Oral: Do not crush controlled release drug product, swallow whole. Kadian® and Avinza® can be opened and sprinkled on applesauce; do not crush or chew the beads. Contents of Kadian® capsules may be opened and sprinkled over 10 mL water and flushed through prewetted 16F gastrostomy tube; do not administer Kadian® through nasogastric tube.

I.V.: When giving morphine I.V. push, it is best to first dilute with sterile water or NS for a final concentration of 1-2 mg/mL and then administer slowly.

Epidural: Use preservative-free solutions for intrathecal or epidural use.

Monitoring Parameters Pain relief, respiratory and mental status, blood pressure

Astromorph/PF™, Duramorph®, Infumorph®: Patients should be observed in a fully-equipped and staffed environment for at least 24 hours following initiation, and as appropriate for the first several days after catheter implantation.

Test Interactions Some quinolones may produce a false-positive urine screening result for opiates using commercially-available immunoassay kits. This has been demonstrated most consistently for levofloxacin and ofloxacin, but other quinolones have shown cross-reactivity in certain assay kits. Confirmation of positive opiate screens by more specific methods should be considered.

Dosage Forms Excipient information presented when available (limited, particularly for generics); consult specific product labeling. [DSC] = Discontinued product

Capsule, extended release, oral, as sulfate: 10 mg, 20 mg, 30 mg, 50 mg, 60 mg, 80 mg, 100 mg, 200 mg

AVINza®: 30 mg, 45 mg, 60 mg, 75 mg, 90 mg, 120 mg

Kadian®: 10 mg, 20 mg, 30 mg, 50 mg, 60 mg, 80 mg, 100 mg, 200 mg

Injection, solution, as sulfate: 1 mg/mL (10 mL); 2 mg/mL (1 mL); 4 mg/mL (1 mL); 5 mg/mL (1 mL); 8 mg/mL (1 mL); 10 mg/mL (1 mL, 10 mL); 10 mg/0.7 mL (0.7 mL); 15 mg/mL (1 mL, 20 mL); 25 mg/mL (4 mL, 10 mL); 50 mg/mL (20 mL, 50 mL)

Injection, solution, as sulfate [preservative free]: 0.5 mg/mL (10 mL); 1 mg/mL (10 mL); 25 mg/mL (10 mL)

Injection, solution, as sulfate [epidural or intrathecal infusion via microinfusion device, preservative free]:

Infumorph 200: 10 mg/mL (20 mL)

Infumorph 500: 25 mg/mL (20 mL)

Injection, solution, as sulfate [epidural, intrathecal, or I.V. infusion, preservative free]:

Astramorph®/PF: 0.5 mg/mL (2 mL, 10 mL); 1 mg/mL (2 mL, 10 mL)

Duramorph: 0.5 mg/mL (10 mL); 1 mg/mL (10 mL)

Injection, solution, as sulfate [for PCA pump]: 1 mg/mL (30 mL)

Injection, solution, as sulfate [for PCA pump, preservative free]: 0.5 mg/mL (30 mL [DSC]); 1 mg/mL (30 mL); 5 mg/mL (30 mL)

Solution, oral, as sulfate: 10 mg/5 mL (5 mL, 100 mL, 500 mL); 20 mg/5 mL (100 mL, 500 mL)

Solution, oral, as sulfate [concentrate]: 100 mg/5 mL (15 mL, 30 mL, 120 mL, 240 mL)

Suppository, rectal, as sulfate: 5 mg (12s); 10 mg (12s); 20 mg (12s); 30 mg (12s)

Tablet, oral, as sulfate: 15 mg, 30 mg

Tablet, controlled release, oral, as sulfate:

MS Contin®: 15 mg, 30 mg, 60 mg, 100 mg, 200 mg

Tablet, extended release, oral, as sulfate: 15 mg, 30 mg, 60 mg, 100 mg, 200 mg

Tablet, sustained release, oral, as sulfate:

Oramorph® SR: 15 mg, 30 mg, 60 mg, 100 mg

Dosage Forms: Canada Excipient information presented when available (limited, particularly for generics); consult specific product labeling.

Solution, oral, as sulfate:

Doloral: 1 mg/mL (10 mL, 250 mL, 500 mL); 5 mg/mL (10 mL, 250 mL, 500 mL)

Controlled Substance C-II

Morphine (Liposomal) (MOR feen)

Brand Names: U.S. DepoDur®

Index Terms Extended Release Epidural Morphine; MS (error-prone abbreviation and should not be used); MSO_4 (error-prone abbreviation and should not be used)

Pharmacologic Category Analgesic, Opioid

Additional Appendix Information

Opioid Analgesics *on page 1896*

Use Epidural (lumbar) single-dose management of surgical pain

Pregnancy Risk Factor C

Dosage Epidural:

Adults: Surgical anesthesia: Single-dose (extended release, DepoDur®): Lumbar epidural only; not recommended in patients <18 years of age:

Cesarean section: 10 mg (after clamping umbilical cord)

Lower abdominal/pelvic surgery: 10-15 mg

Major orthopedic surgery of lower extremity: 15 mg

To minimize the pharmacokinetic interaction resulting in higher peak serum concentrations of morphine, administer the test dose of the local anesthetic at least 15 minutes prior to administration. Use of DepoDur® with epidural local anesthetics has not been studied. Other medications should not be administered into the epidural space for at least 48 hours after administration.

Note: Some patients may benefit from a 20 mg dose; however, the incidence of adverse effects may be increased.

Elderly or debilitated patients: Use with caution; may require dose reduction

Dosing adjustment in renal impairment: Dosing adjustments is not required.

Dosing adjustment/comments in hepatic disease: Dosing adjustment is not required.

Additional Information Complete prescribing information for this medication should be consulted for additional detail.

Dosage Forms Excipient information presented when available (limited, particularly for generics); consult specific product labeling.

Injection, extended release liposomal suspension, as sulfate [lumbar epidural injection, preservative free]:

DepoDur®: 10 mg/mL (1 mL, 1.5 mL)

Controlled Substance C-II

Morphine and Naltrexone

(MOR feen & nal TREKS one)

Brand Names: U.S. Embeda™

Index Terms Morphine Sulfate and Naltrexone Hydrochloride; MS (error-prone abbreviation and should not be used); MSO_4 (error-prone abbreviation and should not be used); Naltrexone and Morphine

Pharmacologic Category Analgesic, Opioid; Opioid Antagonist

Additional Appendix Information

Patient Information for Disposal of Unused Medications *on page 2026*

Use Relief of moderate-to-severe pain when continual, around-the-clock therapy is needed for an extended period of time

Pregnancy Risk Factor C

Medication Guide Available Yes

Dosage Oral: Moderate-to-severe pain: **Note:** These are guidelines and do not represent the doses that may be required in all patients. Treatment should be individualized based on patient's prior analgesic treatment experience/ tolerance and pain relief. Not intended for use as a PRN medication.

Adults: Opiate-naive: Initial: 20 mg/0.8 mg once or twice daily; 100 mg/4 mg strength for use in opioid-tolerant patients only

Titration: Do not increase dose more frequently than every other day. May supplement dose with a short-acting analgesic (<20% of total daily dose) for breakthrough pain. If once-daily dosing is inadequate may switch to twice daily dosing.

Conversion from other oral morphine products to Embeda™: Administer one-half of the patient's total daily oral morphine dose as Embeda™ every 12 hours or all of the patient's total daily oral morphine dose as Embeda™ once daily.

Conversion from other oral/parenteral opioids or parenteral morphine to Embeda™: Must first convert to oral morphine equivalent.

Conversion from parenteral to oral morphine: It may take 2-6 mg of oral morphine to provide pain relief equivalent to 1 mg of parenteral morphine. An oral dose 3 times the daily parenteral dose may be sufficient in chronic pain settings.

Conversion from other oral/parenteral opioids to oral morphine: Specific recommendations are not available; refer to published relative potency data realizing that such ratios are only approximations. It is generally safest to give half the estimated daily morphine requirement as the initial dose and manage inadequate relief with immediate release morphine.

Note: When converting from other opioid analgesics it is better to underestimate the patient's 24-hour oral requirement and provide breakthrough treatment than to overestimate and manage an adverse event.

Elderly or debilitated patients: Use with caution; may require dose reduction

Dosing adjustment in renal impairment: Use with caution in patients with severe impairment; no specific dosing recommendations are provided by the manufacturer.

Dosing adjustment/comments in hepatic disease: Use with caution in patients with severe impairment; no specific dosing recommendations are provided by the manufacturer.

Additional Information Complete prescribing information for this medication should be consulted for additional detail.

Dosage Forms Excipient information presented when available (limited, particularly for generics); consult specific product labeling.

Capsule, extended release, oral:

Embeda™ 20/0.8: Morphine sulfate 20 mg and naltrexone hydrochloride 0.8 mg

Embeda™ 30/1.2: Morphine sulfate 30 mg and naltrexone hydrochloride 1.2 mg

Embeda™ 50/2: Morphine sulfate 50 mg and naltrexone hydrochloride 2 mg

Embeda™ 60/2.4: Morphine sulfate 60 mg and naltrexone hydrochloride 2.4 mg

Embeda™ 80/3.2: Morphine sulfate 80 mg and naltrexone hydrochloride 3.2 mg

Embeda™ 100/4: Morphine sulfate 100 mg and naltrexone hydrochloride 4 mg

Controlled Substance C-II

◆ **Morphine-EPD (Can)** *see* Morphine (Systemic) *on page 1153*

◆ **Morphine Extra Forte Injection (Can)** *see* Morphine (Systemic) *on page 1153*

◆ **Morphine Forte Injection (Can)** *see* Morphine (Systemic) *on page 1153*

◆ **Morphine HP® (Can)** *see* Morphine (Systemic) *on page 1153*

◆ **Morphine LP® Epidural (Can)** *see* Morphine (Systemic) *on page 1153*

◆ **Morphine SR (Can)** *see* Morphine (Systemic) *on page 1153*

◆ **Morphine Sulfate and Naltrexone Hydrochloride** *see* Morphine and Naltrexone *on page 1158*

Morrhuate Sodium

(MOR yoo ate SOW dee um)

Pharmacologic Category Sclerosing Agent

Use Treatment of small, uncomplicated varicose veins of the lower extremities

Pregnancy Risk Factor C

Dosage I.V.: Adults:

Note: A test dose of 0.25-1 mL of a 5% injection may be given (into a varicosity) 24 hours before full-dose treatment.

Full-dose treatment: 50-250 mg, depending on the size and degree of varicosity (50-100 mg for small or medium veins, 150-250 mg for large veins); may be given as multiple injections at one time or in single doses.

Additional Information Complete prescribing information for this medication should be consulted for additional detail.

Dosage Forms Excipient information presented when available (limited, particularly for generics); consult specific product labeling.

Injection, solution: 50 mg/mL (30 mL)

◆ **M.O.S.® 10 (Can)** *see* Morphine (Systemic) *on page 1153*

◆ **M.O.S.® 20 (Can)** *see* Morphine (Systemic) *on page 1153*

◆ **M.O.S.® 30 (Can)** *see* Morphine (Systemic) *on page 1153*

◆ **M.O.S.-SR® (Can)** *see* Morphine (Systemic) *on page 1153*

◆ **M.O.S.-Sulfate® (Can)** *see* Morphine (Systemic) *on page 1153*

◆ **Motrin® Children's [OTC]** *see* Ibuprofen *on page 860*

◆ **Motrin® (Children's) (Can)** *see* Ibuprofen *on page 860*

◆ **Motrin® IB [OTC]** *see* Ibuprofen *on page 860*

◆ **Motrin® IB (Can)** *see* Ibuprofen *on page 860*

◆ **Motrin® Infants' [OTC]** *see* Ibuprofen *on page 860*

◆ **Motrin® Junior [OTC]** *see* Ibuprofen *on page 860*

◆ **MoviPrep®** *see* Polyethylene Glycol-Electrolyte Solution *on page 1372*

◆ **Moxatag™** *see* Amoxicillin *on page 103*

◆ **Moxeza™** *see* Moxifloxacin (Ophthalmic) *on page 1161*

Moxifloxacin (Systemic) (moxs i FLOKS a sin)

Brand Names: U.S. Avelox®; Avelox® ABC Pack; Avelox® I.V.

Brand Names: Canada Avelox®; Avelox® I.V.

Index Terms Moxifloxacin Hydrochloride

Pharmacologic Category Antibiotic, Quinolone; Respiratory Fluoroquinolone

Additional Appendix Information

Prevention of Wound Infection and Sepsis in Surgical Patients *on page 1954*

Use Treatment of mild-to-moderate community-acquired pneumonia, including multidrug-resistant *Streptococcus pneumoniae* (MDRSP); acute bacterial exacerbation of chronic bronchitis; acute bacterial sinusitis; complicated and uncomplicated skin and skin structure infections; complicated intra-abdominal infections

Unlabeled Use Treatment of *Legionella* pneumonia; treatment of mild-to-moderate community-acquired pneumonia (CAP), including multidrug-resistant *Streptococcus pneumoniae* (MDRSP) in adolescents with skeletal maturity

Pregnancy Risk Factor C

Pregnancy Considerations Adverse events have been observed in some animal studies; therefore, the manufacturer classifies moxifloxacin as pregnancy category C. Quinolone exposure during human pregnancy has been reported with other agents (see Ciprofloxacin [Systemic], Ofloxacin [Systemic], and Norfloxacin [Systemic] monographs). To date, no specific teratogenic effect or increased pregnancy risk has been identified; however, because of concerns of cartilage damage in immature animals exposed to quinolones and the limited moxifloxacin specific data, moxifloxacin should only be used during pregnancy if a safer option is not available.

Lactation Excretion in breast milk unknown/not recommended

Medication Guide Available Yes

Contraindications Hypersensitivity to moxifloxacin, other quinolone antibiotics, or any component of the formulation

Warnings/Precautions [U.S. Boxed Warning]: There have been reports of tendon inflammation and/or rupture with quinolone antibiotics; risk may be increased with concurrent corticosteroids, organ transplant recipients, and in patients >60 years of age. Rupture of the Achilles tendon sometimes requiring surgical repair has been reported most frequently; but other tendon sites (eg, rotator cuff, biceps) have also been reported. Strenuous physical activity, rheumatoid arthritis, and renal impairment may be an independent risk factor for tendonitis. Discontinue at first sign of tendon inflammation or pain. Tendon rupture may occur even after discontinuation of therapy. Use with caution in patients with rheumatoid arthritis or renal impairment; may increase risk of tendon rupture.

Use with caution in patients with significant bradycardia or acute myocardial ischemia. Moxifloxacin causes a concentration-dependent QT prolongation. Do not exceed recommended dose or infusion rate. Avoid use with uncorrected hypokalemia, with other drugs that prolong the QT interval or induce bradycardia, or with class Ia or III antiarrhythmic agents. Use with caution in individuals at risk of seizures (CNS disorders or concurrent therapy with medications which may lower seizure threshold). Potential for seizures, although very rare, may be increased with concomitant NSAID therapy. Discontinue in patients who experience significant CNS adverse effects (dizziness, hallucinations, suicidal ideation or actions). Use with caution in patients with mild, moderate, or severe hepatic impairment or liver cirrhosis; may increase the risk of QT prolongation. Fulminant hepatitis potentially leading to liver failure (including fatalities) has been reported with use. Use with caution in diabetes; glucose regulation may be altered.

Fluoroquinolones have been associated with the development of serious, and sometimes fatal, hypoglycemia, most often in elderly diabetics, but also in patients without diabetes. This occurred most frequently with gatifloxacin (no longer available systemically) but may occur at a lower frequency with other quinolones.

Severe hypersensitivity reactions, including anaphylaxis, have occurred with quinolone therapy. Reactions may present as typical allergic symptoms after a single dose, or may manifest as severe idiosyncratic dermatologic, vascular, pulmonary, renal, hepatic, and/or hematologic events, usually after multiple doses. Prompt discontinuation of drug should occur if skin rash or other symptoms arise. Avoid excessive sunlight and take precautions to limit exposure (eg, loose fitting clothing, sunscreen); may cause moderate-to-severe phototoxicity reactions. Discontinue use if photosensitivity occurs. Prolonged use may result in fungal or bacterial superinfection, including *C. difficile*-associated diarrhea (CDAD) and pseudomembranous colitis; CDAD has been observed >2 months post-antibiotic treatment. **[U.S. Boxed Warning]: Quinolones may exacerbate myasthenia gravis; avoid use (rare, potentially life-threatening weakness of respiratory muscles may occur).** Peripheral neuropathy may rarely occur. Hemolytic reactions may (rarely) occur with quinolone use in patients with latent or actual G6PD deficiency. Adverse effects (eg, tendon rupture, QT changes) may be increased in the elderly. Some quinolones may exacerbate myasthenia gravis, use with caution (rare, potentially life-threatening weakness of respiratory muscles may occur). Safety and efficacy of systemically administered moxifloxacin (oral, intravenous) in patients <18 years of age have not been established.

Adverse Reactions

2% to 10%:

Central nervous system: Dizziness (2%)

Endocrine & metabolic: Serum chloride increased (≥2%), serum ionized calcium increased (≥2%), serum glucose decreased (≥2%)

Gastrointestinal: Nausea (6%), diarrhea (5%), amylase decreased (≥2%)

Hematologic: Decreased serum levels of the following (≥2%): Basophils, eosinophils, hemoglobin, RBC, neutrophils; increased serum levels of the following (≥2%): MCH, neutrophils, WBC

Hepatic: Bilirubin decreased/increased (≥2%)

Renal: Serum albumin increased (≥2%)

Respiratory: PO_2 decreased (≥2%)

0.1% to <2%:

Cardiovascular: Cardiac arrhythmias, palpitation, QT_c prolongation, tachycardia, vasodilation

Central nervous system: Anxiety, headache, insomnia, malaise, nervousness, pain, somnolence, vertigo

Dermatologic: Pruritus, rash (maculopapular, purpuric, pustular), urticaria

Gastrointestinal: Abdominal pain, amylase increased, anorexia, constipation, dyspepsia, flatulence, glossitis, lactic dehydrogenase increased, stomatitis, taste perversion, vomiting, xerostomia

Genitourinary: Vaginal moniliasis, vaginitis

Hematologic: Eosinophilia, leukopenia, prothrombin time prolonged, increased INR, thrombocythemia

Hepatic: GGTP increased, liver function test abnormal

Local: Injection site reaction

Neuromuscular & skeletal: Arthralgia, myalgia, tremor, weakness

Respiratory: Pharyngitis, pneumonia, rhinitis, sinusitis
Miscellaneous: Allergic reaction, infection, diaphoresis, oral moniliasis

<0.1% (Limited to important or life-threatening): Abnormal dreams, abnormal gait, agitation, amblyopia, amnesia, anaphylactic reaction, anaphylactic shock, anemia, angioedema, aphasia, arthritis, asthma, atrial fibrillation, back pain, *C. difficile*-positive diarrhea, chest pain, cholestasis, confusion, depersonalization, depression, dysphagia, dyspnea, ECG abnormalities, emotional lability, face edema, gastritis, hallucinations, hepatic failure, hepatitis, hyperglycemia, hyperlipidemia, hyper-/hypotension, hypertonia, hyperuricemia, hypoesthesia, incoordination, INR decreased, jaundice (cholestatic), laryngeal edema, leg pain, myasthenia gravis exacerbation, nightmares, paresthesia, parosmia, pelvic pain, peripheral edema, peripheral neuropathy, photosensitivity/toxicity, prothrombin time decreased, pseudomembranous colitis, psychotic reaction, renal dysfunction, renal failure, seizure, sleep disorder, speech disorder, Stevens-Johnson syndrome, supraventricular tachycardia, syncope, taste loss, tendonitis, tendon rupture, thinking abnormal, thrombocytopenia, thromboplastin decreased, tinnitus, tongue discoloration, toxic epidermal necrolysis, ventricular tachyarrhythmias (including torsade de pointes and cardiac arrest [usually in patients with concurrent, severe proarrhythmic conditions]), vision abnormalities

Drug Interactions

Metabolism/Transport Effects None known.

Avoid Concomitant Use

Avoid concomitant use of Moxifloxacin (Systemic) with any of the following: Artemether; BCG; Dronedarone; Lumefantrine; Nilotinib; Pimozide; QUEtiapine; QuiNINE; Tetrabenazine; Thioridazine; Toremifene; Vandetanib; Vemurafenib; Ziprasidone

Increased Effect/Toxicity

Moxifloxacin (Systemic) may increase the levels/effects of: Corticosteroids (Systemic); Dronedarone; Pimozide; Porfimer; QTc-Prolonging Agents; QuiNINE; Sulfonylureas; Tetrabenazine; Thioridazine; Toremifene; Vandetanib; Varenicline; Vemurafenib; Vitamin K Antagonists; Ziprasidone

The levels/effects of Moxifloxacin (Systemic) may be increased by: Alfuzosin; Artemether; Chloroquine; Ciprofloxacin; Ciprofloxacin (Systemic); Gadobutrol; Indacaterol; Insulin; Lumefantrine; Nilotinib; Nonsteroidal Anti-Inflammatory Agents; Probenecid; QUEtiapine; QuiNINE

Decreased Effect

Moxifloxacin (Systemic) may decrease the levels/effects of: BCG; Mycophenolate; Sulfonylureas; Typhoid Vaccine

The levels/effects of Moxifloxacin (Systemic) may be decreased by: Antacids; Didanosine; Iron Salts; Lanthanum; Magnesium Salts; Quinapril; Sevelamer; Sucralfate; Zinc Salts

Ethanol/Nutrition/Herb Interactions Food: Absorption is not affected by administration with a high-fat meal or yogurt.

Stability Store at controlled room temperature of 25°C (77°F). Do not refrigerate infusion solution.

Mechanism of Action Moxifloxacin is a DNA gyrase inhibitor, and also inhibits topoisomerase IV. DNA gyrase (topoisomerase II) is an essential bacterial enzyme that maintains the superhelical structure of DNA. DNA gyrase is required for DNA replication and transcription, DNA repair, recombination, and transposition; inhibition is bactericidal.

Pharmacodynamics/Kinetics

Absorption: Well absorbed; not affected by high-fat meal or yogurt

Distribution: V_d: 1.7 to 2.7 L/kg; tissue concentrations often exceed plasma concentrations in respiratory tissues, alveolar macrophages, abdominal tissues/fluids, uterine tissue (endometrium, myometrium), and sinus tissues

Protein binding: ~30% to 50%

Metabolism: Hepatic (~52% of dose) via glucuronide (~14%) and sulfate (~38%) conjugation

Bioavailability: ~90%

Half-life elimination: Single dose: Oral: 12-16 hours; I.V.: 8-15 hours

Excretion: Urine (as unchanged drug [20%] and glucuronide conjugates); feces (as unchanged drug [25%] and sulfate conjugates)

Dosage

Adolescents (unlabeled use): **Community-acquired pneumonia (CAP) due to atypical pathogens (*M. pneumoniae, C. trachomatis, or C. pneumoniae*), mild infection or step-down therapy in adolescents with skeletal maturity, (alternative to azithromycin) (IDSA/PIDS, 2011):** Oral: 400 mg once daily

Adults: Oral, I.V.: Usual dosage range: 400 mg every 24 hours

Indication-specific dosing:

Acute bacterial sinusitis: 400 mg every 24 hours for 10 days

Chronic bronchitis, acute bacterial exacerbation: 400 mg every 24 hours for 5 days

Community-acquired pneumonia (CAP) (including MDRSP): 400 mg every 24 hours for 7-14 days

Intra-abdominal infections, complicated: 400 mg every 24 hours for 5-14 days (initiate with I.V.); **Note:** 2010 IDSA guidelines recommend a treatment duration of 4-7 days (provided source controlled) for community-acquired, mild-to-moderate IAI

Skin and skin structure infections:

Complicated: 400 mg every 24 hours for 7-21 days

Uncomplicated: 400 mg every 24 hours for 7 days

Elderly: No dosage adjustments are required based on age

Dosage adjustment in renal impairment: No dosage adjustment required in renal impairment.

Poorly dialyzed; no supplemental dose or dosage adjustment necessary, including patients on intermittent hemodialysis, peritoneal dialysis, or continuous renal replacement therapy (eg, CVVHD).

Dosage adjustment in hepatic impairment: No dosage adjustment is required in mild, moderate, or severe hepatic insufficiency (Child-Pugh class A, B, or C); however, use with caution in this patient population secondary to the risk of QT prolongation.

Dietary Considerations May be taken without regard to meals. Take 4 hours before or 8 hours after multiple vitamins, antacids, or other products containing magnesium, aluminum, iron, or zinc.

Avelox® I.V. infusion (premixed in sodium chloride 0.8%) contains sodium 34.2 mEq (~787 mg)/250 mL.

Administration Administer without regard to meals.

I.V.: Infuse over 60 minutes; do not infuse by rapid or bolus intravenous infusion

Monitoring Parameters WBC, signs of infection

Test Interactions Some quinolones may produce a false-positive urine screening result for opiates using commercially-available immunoassay kits. This has been demonstrated most consistently for levofloxacin and ofloxacin, but other quinolones have shown cross-reactivity in certain assay kits. Confirmation of positive opiate screens by more specific methods should be considered.

Dosage Forms Excipient information presented when available (limited, particularly for generics); consult specific product labeling.

Infusion, premixed in sodium chloride 0.8% [preservative free]:

Avelox® I.V.: 400 mg (250 mL) [contains sodium ~787 mg (34.2 mEq)/250 mL]

Tablet, oral:

Avelox®: 400 mg

Avelox® ABC Pack: 400 mg

Extemporaneous Preparations A 20 mg/mL oral suspension may be made using tablets. Crush three 400 mg tablets and reduce to a fine powder. Carefully sieve powder from enteric-coating remnants to improve pharmaceutical elegance. Add a small amount of a 1:1 mixture of Ora-Plus® and Ora-Sweet® or Ora-Sweet® SF and mix to a uniform paste; mix while adding the vehicle in geometric proportions to **almost** 60 mL; transfer to a calibrated bottle, rinse mortar with vehicle, and add quantity of vehicle sufficient to make 60 mL. Label "shake well". Stable 90 days at room temperature.

Hutchinson DJ, Johnson CE, and Klein KC, "Stability of Extemporaneously Prepared Moxifloxacin Oral Suspensions," *Am J Health Syst Pharm*, 2009, 66(7):665-7.

Moxifloxacin (Ophthalmic) (moxs i FLOKS a sin)

Brand Names: U.S. Moxeza™; Vigamox®

Brand Names: Canada Vigamox®

Index Terms Moxifloxacin Hydrochloride

Pharmacologic Category Antibiotic, Ophthalmic; Antibiotic, Quinolone

Use Treatment of bacterial conjunctivitis caused by susceptible organisms

Pregnancy Risk Factor C

Dosage Ophthalmic: Bacterial conjunctivitis:

Children ≥4 months and Adults (Moxeza™): Instill 1 drop into affected eye(s) 2 times/day for 7 days

Children ≥1 year and Adults (Vigamox®): Instill 1 drop into affected eye(s) 3 times/day for 7 days

Additional Information Complete prescribing information for this medication should be consulted for additional detail.

Dosage Forms Excipient information presented when available (limited, particularly for generics); consult specific product labeling.

Solution, ophthalmic [drops]:

Moxeza™: 0.5% (3 mL)

Vigamox®: 0.5% (3 mL)

Mupirocin (myoo PEER oh sin)

Brand Names: U.S. Bactroban Cream®; Bactroban Nasal®; Bactroban®; Centany®; Centany® AT

Brand Names: Canada Bactroban®

Index Terms Mupirocin Calcium; Pseudomonic Acid A

Pharmacologic Category Antibiotic, Topical

Additional Appendix Information

Prevention of Wound Infection and Sepsis in Surgical Patients *on page* 1954

Use

Intranasal: Eradication of nasal colonization with MRSA in adult patients and healthcare workers

Topical: Treatment of impetigo or secondary infected traumatic skin lesions due to *S. aureus* and *S. pyogenes*

Unlabeled Use Intranasal: Surgical prophylaxis to prevent wound infections

Pregnancy Risk Factor B

Dosage

Intranasal: Children ≥12 years and Adults: Eradication of nasal MRSA: Approximately one-half of the ointment from the single-use tube should be applied into one nostril and the other half into the other nostril twice daily for 5 days

Topical:

Children ≥2 months and Adults: Impetigo: Ointment: Apply to affected area 3 times/day; re-evaluate after 3-5 days if no clinical response

Children ≥3 months and Adults: Secondary skin infections: Cream: Apply to affected area 3 times/day for 10 days; re-evaluate after 3-5 days if no clinical response

Additional Information Complete prescribing information for this medication should be consulted for additional detail.

Dosage Forms Excipient information presented when available (limited, particularly for generics); consult specific product labeling.

Cream, topical, as calcium [strength expressed as base]:

Bactroban Cream®: 2% (15 g, 30 g) [contains benzyl alcohol]

Ointment, topical: 2% (22 g)

Bactroban®: 2% (22 g) [contains polyethylene glycol]

Centany®: 2% (30 g)

Centany® AT: 2% (1s) [kit includes Centany® ointment (30 g),12 gauze pads, and 24 cloth tape strips]

Ointment, intranasal, as calcium [strength expressed as base]:

Bactroban Nasal®: 2% (1 g)

◆ **Mupirocin Calcium** *see* Mupirocin *on page 1161*

◆ **Murine® Ear [OTC]** *see* Carbamide Peroxide *on page 283*

◆ **Murine® Ear Wax Removal Kit [OTC]** *see* Carbamide Peroxide *on page 283*

◆ **Muro 128® [OTC]** *see* Sodium Chloride *on page 1567*

◆ **Muse®** *see* Alprostadil *on page 74*

◆ **Muse® Pellet (Can)** *see* Alprostadil *on page 74*

◆ **Mustargen®** *see* Mechlorethamine *on page 1056*

◆ **Mustine** *see* Mechlorethamine *on page 1056*

◆ **Mutamycin® (Can)** *see* MitoMYcin *on page 1142*

◆ **Myambutol®** *see* Ethambutol *on page 651*

◆ **Mycamine®** *see* Micafungin *on page 1124*

◆ **Mycelex** *see* Clotrimazole (Oral) *on page 399*

◆ **Mycinettes® [OTC]** *see* Benzocaine *on page 202*

◆ **Mycobutin®** *see* Rifabutin *on page 1483*

◆ **Mycocide® NS [OTC]** *see* Tolnaftate *on page 1704*

Mycophenolate (mye koe FEN oh late)

Brand Names: U.S. CellCept®; Myfortic®

Brand Names: Canada CellCept®; Myfortic®; Novo-Mycophenolate; Sandoz-Mycophenolate

Index Terms MMF; MPA; Mycophenolate Mofetil; Mycophenolate Sodium; Mycophenolic Acid

Pharmacologic Category Immunosuppressant Agent

Use Prophylaxis of organ rejection concomitantly with cyclosporine and corticosteroids in patients receiving allogeneic renal (CellCept®, Myfortic®), cardiac (CellCept®), or hepatic (CellCept®) transplants

Unlabeled Use Treatment of rejection in liver transplant patients unable to tolerate tacrolimus or cyclosporine due to neurotoxicity; mild rejection in heart transplant patients; treatment of moderate-severe psoriasis; treatment of proliferative lupus nephritis; treatment of myasthenia gravis; prevention and treatment of graft-versus-host disease (GVHD)

Pregnancy Risk Factor D

Pregnancy Considerations **[U.S. Boxed Warning]: Mycophenolate is associated with an increased risk of congenital malformations and spontaneous abortions when used during pregnancy.** Adverse events have been reported in animal studies at doses less than the equivalent recommended human dose. Data from the National Transplantation Pregnancy Registry (NTPR) have observed an increase in structural malformations (including ear malformations) in infants born to mothers taking mycophenolate during pregnancy. Spontaneous abortions have also been noted. Females of childbearing potential should have a negative pregnancy test within 1 week prior to beginning therapy. Two reliable forms of contraception should be used beginning 4 weeks prior to, during, and for 6 weeks after therapy. The effectiveness of hormonal contraceptive agents may be affected by mycophenolate.

The National Transplantation Pregnancy Registry (NTPR, Temple University) is a registry for pregnant women taking immunosuppressants following any solid organ transplant. The NTPR encourages reporting of all immunosuppressant exposures during pregnancy in transplant recipients at 877-955-6877.

Lactation Excretion in breast milk unknown/not recommended

Medication Guide Available Yes

Contraindications Hypersensitivity to mycophenolate mofetil, mycophenolic acid, mycophenolate sodium, or any component of the formulation; intravenous formulation is contraindicated in patients who are allergic to polysorbate 80

Warnings/Precautions Hazardous agent - use appropriate precautions for handling and disposal. **[U.S. Boxed Warning]: Risk for infection and development of lymphoma and skin malignancy is increased.** Opportunistic infections, sepsis, and/or fatal infections may occur with immunosuppressive therapy. Patients should be monitored appropriately. Instruct patients to limit exposure to sunlight/UV light and give supportive treatment should these conditions occur. Pure red cell aplasia (PRCA), progressive multifocal leukoencephalopathy (PML), or BK virus-associated nephropathy (BKVAN) may occur rarely, particularly in immunosuppressed patients or those receiving immunosuppressant therapy; monitor for signs of PRCA (anemia, fatigue, lethargy, pallor, dyspnea), PML (neurologic impairment, apathy, ataxia, cognitive deficiencies, confusion, and hemiparesis), or BKVAN (deterioration of renal function, renal graft loss); may require dosage reduction or discontinuation of therapy. Neutropenia (including severe neutropenia) may occur, requiring dose reduction or interruption of treatment (risk greater from day 31-180 post-transplant). Use caution with active peptic ulcer disease; may be associated with gastric or duodenal ulcers, GI bleeding and/or perforation. Use caution in renal impairment as toxicity may be increased; may require dosage adjustment in severe impairment.

[U.S. Boxed Warning]: Mycophenolate is associated with an increased risk of congenital malformations and spontaneous abortions when used during pregnancy. Females of childbearing potential should have a negative pregnancy test within 1 week prior to beginning therapy. Two reliable forms of contraception should be used beginning 4 weeks prior to, during, and for 6 weeks after therapy. Because mycophenolate mofetil has demonstrated teratogenic effects in rats and rabbits, tablets should not be crushed, and capsules should not be opened or crushed. Avoid inhalation or direct contact with skin or mucous membranes of the powder contained in the capsules and the powder for oral suspension. Caution should be exercised in the handling and preparation of solutions of intravenous mycophenolate. Avoid skin contact with the intravenous solution and reconstituted suspension. If such contact occurs, wash thoroughly with soap and water, rinse eyes with plain water.

Theoretically, use should be avoided in patients with the rare hereditary deficiency of hypoxanthine-guanine phosphoribosyltransferase (such as Lesch-Nyhan or Kelley-Seegmiller syndrome). Intravenous solutions should be given over at least 2 hours; never administer intravenous solution by rapid or bolus injection. **[U.S. Boxed Warning]: Should be administered under the supervision of a physician experienced in immunosuppressive therapy.**

Note: CellCept® and Myfortic® dosage forms should not be used interchangeably due to differences in absorption. Some dosage forms may contain phenylalanine.

Adverse Reactions Data for incidence >20% as reported in adults following oral dosing of CellCept® alone in renal, cardiac, and hepatic allograft rejection studies. Profile in 3% to <20% range reflects use in combination with cyclosporine and corticosteroids. In general, lower doses used in renal rejection patients had less adverse effects than higher doses. Rates of adverse effects were similar for each indication, except for those unique to the specific organ involved. The type of adverse effects observed in pediatric patients was similar to those seen in adults; abdominal pain, anemia, diarrhea, fever, hypertension, infection, pharyngitis, respiratory tract infection, sepsis, and vomiting were seen in higher proportion; lymphoproliferative disorder was the only type of malignancy observed. Percentages of adverse reactions were similar in studies comparing CellCept® to Myfortic® in patients following renal transplant.

>20%:

Cardiovascular: Hypertension (28% to 78%), hypotension (33%), peripheral edema (27% to 64%), edema (27% to 28%), chest pain (26%), tachycardia (20% to 22%)

Central nervous system: Pain (31% to 76%), headache (16% to 54%), insomnia (41% to 52%), fever (21% to 52%), dizziness (29%), anxiety (28%)

Dermatologic: Rash (22%)

Endocrine & metabolic: Hyperglycemia (44% to 47%), hypercholesterolemia (41%), hypomagnesemia (39%), hypokalemia (32% to 37%), hypocalcemia (30%), hyperkalemia (22%)

Gastrointestinal: Abdominal pain (25% to 63%), nausea (20% to 55%), diarrhea (31% to 51%), constipation (19% to 41%), vomiting (33% to 34%), anorexia (25%), dyspepsia (22%)

Genitourinary: Urinary tract infection (37%)

Hematologic: Leukopenia (23% to 46%), anemia (26% to 43%; hypochromic 25%), leukocytosis (22% to 41%), thrombocytopenia (24% to 38%)

Hepatic: Liver function tests abnormal (25%), ascites (24%)

Neuromuscular & skeletal: Back pain (35% to 47%), weakness (35% to 43%), tremor (24% to 34%), paresthesia (21%)

Renal: Creatinine increased (39%), BUN increased (35%), kidney function abnormal (22% to 26%)

Respiratory: Dyspnea (31% to 37%), respiratory tract infection (22% to 37%), pleural effusion (34%), cough (31%), lung disorder (22% to 30%), sinusitis (26%)

Miscellaneous: Infection (18% to 27%), sepsis (27%), lactate dehydrogenase increased (23%), *Candida* (17% to 22%), herpes simplex (10% to 21%)

3% to <20%:

Cardiovascular: Angina, arrhythmia, arterial thrombosis, atrial fibrillation, atrial flutter, bradycardia, cardiac arrest, cardiac failure, CHF, extrasystole, facial edema, hyper-/hypovolemia, pallor, palpitation, pericardial effusion, peripheral vascular disorder, postural hypotension, supraventricular extrasystoles, supraventricular tachycardia, syncope, thrombosis, vasodilation, vasospasm, venous pressure increased, ventricular extrasystole, ventricular tachycardia

Central nervous system: Agitation, chills with fever, confusion, delirium, depression, emotional lability, hallucinations, hypoesthesia, malaise, nervousness, psychosis, seizure, somnolence, thinking abnormal, vertigo

Dermatologic: Acne, alopecia, bruising, cellulitis, fungal dermatitis, hirsutism, petechia, pruritus, skin carcinoma, skin hypertrophy, skin ulcer, vesiculobullous rash

Endocrine & metabolic: Acidosis, alkalosis, Cushing's syndrome, dehydration, diabetes mellitus, gout, hypercalcemia, hyper-hypophosphatemia, hyperlipemia, hyperuricemia, hypochloremia, hypoglycemia, hyponatremia, hypoproteinemia, hypothyroidism, parathyroid disorder

Gastrointestinal: Abdomen enlarged, dysphagia, esophagitis, flatulence, gastritis, gastroenteritis, gastrointestinal hemorrhage, gastrointestinal moniliasis, gingivitis, gum hyperplasia, ileus, melena, mouth ulceration, oral moniliasis, stomach disorder, stomach ulcer, stomatitis, xerostomia, weight gain/loss

Genitourinary: Impotence, nocturia, pelvic pain, prostatic disorder, scrotal edema, urinary frequency, urinary incontinence, urinary retention, urinary tract disorder

Hematologic: Coagulation disorder, hemorrhage, neutropenia, pancytopenia, polycythemia, prothrombin time increased, thromboplastin time increased

Hepatic: Alkaline phosphatase increased, bilirubinemia, cholangitis, cholestatic jaundice, GGT increased, hepatitis, jaundice, liver damage, transaminases increased

Local: Abscess

Neuromuscular & skeletal: Arthralgia, hypertonia, joint disorder, leg cramps, myalgia, myasthenia, neck pain, neuropathy, osteoporosis

Ocular: Amblyopia, cataract, conjunctivitis, eye hemorrhage, lacrimation disorder, vision abnormal

Otic: Deafness, ear disorder, ear pain, tinnitus

Renal: Albuminuria, creatinine increased, dysuria, hematuria, hydronephrosis, oliguria, pyelonephritis, renal failure, renal tubular necrosis

Respiratory: Apnea, asthma, atelectasis, bronchitis, epistaxis, hemoptysis, hiccup, hyperventilation, hypoxia, respiratory acidosis, pharyngitis, pneumonia, pneumothorax, pulmonary edema, pulmonary hypertension, respiratory moniliasis, rhinitis, sputum increased, voice alteration

Miscellaneous: *Candida* (mucocutaneous 16% to 18%), CMV viremia/syndrome (12% to 14%), CMV tissue invasive disease (6% to 12%), herpes zoster cutaneous disease (4% to 10%), cyst, diaphoresis, flu-like syndrome, healing abnormal, hernia, ileus infection, neoplasm, peritonitis, thirst

Postmarketing and/or case reports: Atypical mycobacterial infection, BK virus-associated nephropathy, colitis, gastrointestinal perforation, infectious endocarditis, interstitial lung disorder, intestinal villous atrophy, lymphoma, lymphoproliferative disease, malignancy, meningitis, pancreatitis, progressive multifocal leukoencephalopathy (sometimes fatal), pulmonary fibrosis (fatal), pure red cell aplasia, tuberculosis

Drug Interactions

Metabolism/Transport Effects None known.

Avoid Concomitant Use

Avoid concomitant use of Mycophenolate with any of the following: BCG; Cholestyramine Resin; Natalizumab; Pimecrolimus; Rifamycin Derivatives; Tacrolimus (Topical); Vaccines (Live)

Increased Effect/Toxicity

Mycophenolate may increase the levels/effects of: Acyclovir-Valacyclovir; Ganciclovir-Valganciclovir; Leflunomide; Natalizumab; Vaccines (Live)

The levels/effects of Mycophenolate may be increased by: Acyclovir-Valacyclovir; Belatacept; Denosumab; Ganciclovir-Valganciclovir; Pimecrolimus; Probenecid; Roflumilast; Tacrolimus (Topical); Trastuzumab

Decreased Effect

Mycophenolate may decrease the levels/effects of: BCG; Coccidioidin Skin Test; Contraceptives (Estrogens); Contraceptives (Progestins); Sipuleucel-T; Vaccines (Inactivated); Vaccines (Live)

The levels/effects of Mycophenolate may be decreased by: Antacids; Cholestyramine Resin; CycloSPORINE; CycloSPORINE (Systemic); Echinacea; Magnesium Salts; MetroNIDAZOLE; MetroNIDAZOLE (Systemic); Penicillins; Proton Pump Inhibitors; Quinolone Antibiotics; Rifamycin Derivatives; Sevelamer

Ethanol/Nutrition/Herb Interactions

Food: Decreases C_{max} of MPA by 40% following CellCept® administration and 33% following Myfortic® use; the extent of absorption is not changed

Herb/Nutraceutical: Avoid cat's claw, echinacea (have immunostimulant properties)

Stability

Capsules: Store at 25°C (77°F); excursions permitted to 15°C to 30°C (59°F to 86°F).

Tablets: Store at 25°C (77°F); excursions permitted to 15°C to 30°C (59°F to 86°F). Protect from moisture and light.

Oral suspension: Store powder for oral suspension at 25°C (77°F); excursions permitted to 15°C to 30°C (59°F to 86°F). Should be constituted prior to dispensing to the patient and **not** mixed with any other medication. Add 47 mL of water to the bottle and shake well for ~1 minute. Add another 47 mL of water to the bottle and shake well for an additional minute. Final concentration is 200 mg/mL of mycophenolate mofetil. Once reconstituted, the oral solution may be stored at room temperature or under refrigeration. Do not freeze. The mixed suspension is stable for 60 days.

I.V.: Store intact vials at 25°C (77°F); excursions permitted to 15°C to 30°C (59°F to 86°F). Reconstitute the contents of each vial with 14 mL of 5% dextrose injection; dilute the contents of a vial with 5% dextrose in water to a final concentration of 6 mg mycophenolate mofetil per mL. Begin infusion within 4 hours of reconstitution. **Note:** Vial is vacuum-sealed; if a lack of vacuum is noted during preparation, the vial should not be used. Store solutions at 25°C (77°F); excursions permitted to 15°C to 30°C (59°F to 86°F).

Mechanism of Action MPA exhibits a cytostatic effect on T and B lymphocytes. It is an inhibitor of inosine monophosphate dehydrogenase (IMPDH) which inhibits *de novo* guanosine nucleotide synthesis. T and B lymphocytes are dependent on this pathway for proliferation.

Pharmacodynamics/Kinetics

Onset of action: Peak effect: Correlation of toxicity or efficacy is still being developed, however, one study indicated that 12-hour AUCs >40 mcg/mL/hour were correlated with efficacy and decreased episodes of rejection

Absorption: AUC values for MPA are lower in the early post-transplant period versus later (>3 months) post-transplant period. The extent of absorption in pediatrics is similar to that seen in adults, although there was wide variability reported.

Oral: Myfortic®: 93%

Distribution:

CellCept®: MPA: Oral: 4 L/kg; I.V.: 3.6 L/kg

Myfortic®: MPA: Oral: 54 L (at steady state); 112 L (elimination phase)

Protein binding: MPA: >97%, MPAG 82%

Metabolism: Hepatic and via GI tract; CellCept® is completely hydrolyzed in the liver to mycophenolic acid (MPA; active metabolite); enterohepatic recirculation of MPA may occur; MPA is glucuronidated to MPAG (inactive metabolite)

Bioavailability: Oral: CellCept®: 94%; Myfortic®: 72%

Half-life elimination:

CellCept®: MPA: Oral: 18 hours; I.V.: 17 hours

Myfortic®: MPA: Oral: 8-16 hours; MPAG: 13-17 hours

Time to peak, plasma: Oral: MPA:

CellCept®: 1-1.5 hours

Myfortic®: 1.5-2.75 hours

Excretion:

CellCept®: MPA: Urine (<1%), feces (6%); MPAG: Urine (87%)

Myfortic®: MPA: Urine (3%), feces; MPAG: Urine (>60%)

Dosage

Children: Renal transplant: Oral:

CellCept® suspension: 600 mg/m^2/dose twice daily; maximum dose: 1 g twice daily

Alternatively, may use solid dosage forms according to BSA as follows:

BSA 1.25-1.5 m^2: 750 mg capsule twice daily

BSA >1.5 m^2: 1 g capsule or tablet twice daily

Myfortic®: 400 mg/m^2/dose twice daily; maximum dose: 720 mg twice daily

BSA <1.19 m^2: Use of this formulation is not recommended

BSA 1.19-1.58 m^2: 540 mg twice daily (maximum: 1080 mg/day)

BSA >1.58 m^2: 720 mg twice daily (maximum: 1440 mg/day)

Adults: **Note:** May be used I.V. for up to 14 days; transition to oral therapy as soon as tolerated.

Renal transplant:

CellCept®:

Oral: 1 g twice daily. Doses >2 g/day are not recommended.

I.V.: 1 g twice daily

Myfortic®: Oral: 720 mg twice daily (1440 mg/day)

Cardiac transplantation:

Oral (CellCept®): 1.5 g twice daily

I.V. (CellCept®): 1.5 g twice daily

Hepatic transplantation:

Oral (CellCept®): 1.5 g twice daily

I.V. (CellCept®): 1 g twice daily

Lupus nephritis (unlabeled use): Oral: 0.5-3 g/day (Contreras, 2004; Ong, 2005)

Myasthenia gravis (unlabeled use): Oral (CellCept®): 1 g twice daily (range: 1-3 g/day) (Cahoon, 2006; Ciafaloni, 2001; Merriggioli, 2003)

Psoriasis (unlabeled use): Oral: 2-3 g/day (Menter, 2009)

Elderly: Dosage is the same as younger patients, however, dosing should be cautious due to possibility of increased hepatic, renal or cardiac dysfunction; elderly patients may be at an increased risk of certain infections, gastrointestinal hemorrhage, and pulmonary edema, as compared to younger patients

Dosing adjustment for toxicity (neutropenia): Neutropenia (ANC <1.3 x 10^3/μL): Dosing should be interrupted or the dose reduced, appropriate diagnostic tests performed and patients managed appropriately

Dosing adjustment in renal impairment:

Renal transplant: GFR <25 mL/minute/1.73 m^2 in patients outside the immediate post-transplant period:

CellCept®: Doses of >1 g administered twice daily should be avoided; patients should also be carefully observed; no dose adjustments are needed in renal transplant patients experiencing delayed graft function postoperatively

Myfortic®: No dose adjustments are needed in renal transplant patients experiencing delayed graft function postoperatively; however, monitor carefully for potential concentration dependent adverse events

Cardiac or liver transplant: No data available; mycophenolate may be used in cardiac or hepatic transplant patients with severe chronic renal impairment if the potential benefit outweighs the potential risk

Hemodialysis: Not removed; supplemental dose is not necessary

Peritoneal dialysis: Supplemental dose is not necessary

Dosage adjustment in hepatic impairment: No dosage adjustment is recommended for renal patients with severe hepatic parenchymal disease; however, it is not currently known whether dosage adjustments are necessary for hepatic disease with other etiologies

Dietary Considerations Oral dosage formulations should be taken on an empty stomach to avoid variability in MPA absorption. However, in stable renal transplant patients, may be administered with food if necessary. Some products may contain phenylalanine.

Administration

Oral dosage formulations (tablet, capsule, suspension) should be administered on an empty stomach to avoid variability in MPA absorption. The oral solution may be administered via a nasogastric tube (minimum 8 French, 1.7 mm interior diameter); oral suspension should not be mixed with other medications. Delayed release tablets should not be crushed, cut, or chewed.

Intravenous solutions should be administered over at least 2 hours (either peripheral or central vein); do **not** administer intravenous solution by rapid or bolus injection.

Monitoring Parameters Complete blood count (weekly for first month, twice monthly during months 2 and 3, then monthly thereafter through the first year); renal and liver function; signs and symptoms of infection; pregnancy test (prior to initiation in females of childbearing potential)

Dosage Forms Excipient information presented when available (limited, particularly for generics); consult specific product labeling.

Capsule, oral, as mofetil: 250 mg

CellCept®: 250 mg

Injection, powder for reconstitution, as mofetil hydrochloride:

CellCept®: 500 mg [contains polysorbate 80]

Powder for suspension, oral, as mofetil:

CellCept®: 200 mg/mL (175 mL) [contains phenylalanine 0.56 mg/mL, soybean lecithin; mixed fruit flavor]

Tablet, oral, as mofetil: 500 mg

CellCept®: 500 mg [contains ethanol (may have trace amounts)]

Tablet, oral, as mycophenolic acid: 500 mg

Tablet, delayed release, oral, as mycophenolic acid:

Myfortic®: 180 mg, 360 mg [formulated as a sodium salt]

Extemporaneous Preparations Hazardous agent: Use appropriate precautions for handling and disposal.

A 50 mg/mL oral suspension may be made with mycophenolate mofetil capsules, Ora-Plus®, and cherry syrup. In a vertical flow hood, empty six 250 mg capsules into a mortar; add 7.5 mL Ora-Plus® and mix to a uniform paste. Mix while adding 15 mL of cherry syrup in incremental proportions; transfer to a calibrated bottle, rinse mortar with cherry syrup, and add sufficient quantity of cherry syrup to make 30 mL. Label "shake well". Stable for 210 days at 5°C, for 28 days at 25°C to 37°C, and for 11 days at 45°C.

Venkataramanan R, McCombs JR, Zuckerman S, et al, "Stability of Mycophenolate Mofetil as an Extemporaneous Suspension," *Ann Pharmacother*, 1998, 32(7-8):755-7.

◆ **Myl-Ranitidine (Can)** *see* Ranitidine *on page 1462*
◆ **Myobloc®** *see* RimabotulinumtoxinB *on page 1492*
◆ **Myocet™ (Can)** *see* DOXOrubicin (Liposomal) *on page 555*
◆ **Myozyme®** *see* Alglucosidase Alfa *on page 65*
◆ **Mysoline®** *see* Primidone *on page 1405*
◆ **Mytotan** *see* Mitotane *on page 1144*
◆ **Mytussin® DAC** *see* Guaifenesin, Pseudoephedrine, and Codeine *on page 813*
◆ **N-9** *see* Nonoxynol 9 *on page 1216*
◆ **NAAK** *see* Atropine and Pralidoxime *on page 172*
◆ **Nabi-HB®** *see* Hepatitis B Immune Globulin (Human) *on page 826*
◆ **nab-Paclitaxel** *see* PACLitaxel (Protein Bound) *on page 1275*

Nabumetone (na BYOO me tone)

Brand Names: Canada Apo-Nabumetone®; Gen-Nabumetone; Mylan-Nabumetone; Novo-Nabumetone; Relafen®; Rhoxal-nabumetone; Sandoz-Nabumetone

Index Terms Relafen

Pharmacologic Category Nonsteroidal Anti-inflammatory Drug (NSAID), Oral

Use Management of osteoarthritis and rheumatoid arthritis

Unlabeled Use Moderate pain

Pregnancy Risk Factor C

Pregnancy Considerations Adverse events were not observed in the initial animal reproduction studies; therefore, the manufacturer classifies nabumetone as pregnancy category C. NSAID exposure during the first trimester is not strongly associated with congenital malformations; however, cardiovascular anomalies and cleft palate have been observed following NSAID exposure in some studies. The use of an NSAID close to conception may be associated with an increased risk of miscarriage. Nonteratogenic effects have been observed following NSAID administration during the third trimester including myocardial degenerative changes, prenatal constriction of the ductus arteriosus, fetal tricuspid regurgitation, failure of the ductus arteriosus to close postnatally; renal dysfunction or failure, oligohydramnios; gastrointestinal bleeding or perforation, increased risk of necrotizing enterocolitis; intracranial bleeding (including intraventricular hemorrhage), platelet dysfunction with resultant bleeding; pulmonary hypertension. Because they may cause premature closure of the ductus arteriosus, use of NSAIDs late in pregnancy should be avoided (use after 31 or 32 weeks gestation is not recommended by some clinicians). The chronic use of NSAIDs in women of reproductive age may be associated with infertility that is reversible upon discontinuation of the medication. A registry is available for pregnant women exposed to autoimmune medications including nabumetone. For additional information contact the Organization of Teratology Information Specialists, OTIS Autoimmune Diseases Study, at 877-311-8972.

Lactation Excretion in breast milk unknown/not recommended

Medication Guide Available Yes

Contraindications Hypersensitivity to nabumetone, aspirin, other NSAIDs, or any component of the formulation; perioperative pain in the setting of coronary artery bypass graft (CABG) surgery

Warnings/Precautions **[U.S. Boxed Warning]: NSAIDs are associated with an increased risk of adverse cardiovascular thrombotic events, including MI and stroke.** Risk may be increased with duration of use or pre-existing cardiovascular risk factors or disease. Carefully evaluate individual cardiovascular risk profiles prior to prescribing. May cause new-onset hypertension or worsening of existing hypertension. Use caution with fluid retention. Avoid use in heart failure. Concurrent administration of ibuprofen, and potentially other nonselective NSAIDs, may interfere with aspirin's cardioprotective effect. **[U.S. Boxed Warning]: Use is contraindicated for treatment of perioperative pain in the setting of coronary artery bypass graft (CABG) surgery.** Risk of MI and stroke may be increased with use following CABG surgery.

Platelet adhesion and aggregation may be decreased; may prolong bleeding time; patients with coagulation disorders or who are receiving anticoagulants should be monitored closely. Anemia may occur; patients on long-term NSAID therapy should be monitored for anemia. Rarely, NSAID use may cause severe blood dyscrasias (eg, agranulocytosis, aplastic anemia, thrombocytopenia).

NSAID use may compromise existing renal function; dose-dependent decreases in prostaglandin synthesis may result from NSAID use, reducing renal blood flow which may cause renal decompensation. NSAID use may increase the risk for hyperkalemia. Patients with impaired renal function, dehydration, heart failure, liver dysfunction, those taking diuretics, and ACE inhibitors, and the elderly are at greater risk of renal toxicity and hyperkalemia. Rehydrate patient before starting therapy; monitor renal function closely. Not recommended for use in patients with advanced renal disease. Long-term NSAID use may result in renal papillary necrosis.

[U.S. Boxed Warning]: NSAIDs may increase risk of gastrointestinal irritation, inflammation, ulceration, bleeding, and perforation. These events may occur at any time during therapy and without warning. Use caution with a history of GI disease (bleeding or ulcers), concurrent therapy with aspirin, anticoagulants and/or corticosteroids, smoking, use of alcohol, the elderly or debilitated patients. When used concomitantly with ≤325 mg of aspirin, a substantial increase in the risk of gastrointestinal complications (eg, ulcer) occurs; concomitant gastroprotective therapy (eg, proton pump inhibitors) is recommended (Bhatt, 2008).

Use the lowest effective dose for the shortest duration of time, consistent with individual patient goals, to reduce risk of cardiovascular or GI adverse events. Alternate therapies should be considered for patients at high risk.

NSAIDs may cause serious skin adverse events including exfoliative dermatitis, Stevens-Johnson syndrome (SJS) and toxic epidermal necrolysis (TEN); discontinue use at first sign of skin rash or hypersensitivity. Anaphylactoid reactions may occur, even without prior exposure; patients with "aspirin triad" (bronchial asthma, aspirin intolerance, rhinitis) may be at increased risk. Do not use in patients who experience bronchospasm, asthma, rhinitis, or urticaria with NSAID or aspirin therapy. Use caution in other forms of asthma.

Use with caution in patients with decreased hepatic function. Closely monitor patients with any abnormal LFT. Severe hepatic reactions (eg, fulminant hepatitis, liver failure) have occurred with NSAID use, rarely; discontinue if signs or symptoms of liver disease develop, or if systemic manifestations occur.

NSAIDS may cause drowsiness, dizziness, blurred vision and other neurologic effects which may impair physical or mental abilities; patients must be cautioned about performing tasks which require mental alertness (eg, operating machinery or driving). Discontinue use with blurred or diminished vision and perform ophthalmologic exam. Monitor vision with long-term therapy.

The elderly are at increased risk for adverse effects (especially peptic ulceration, CNS effects, renal toxicity) from NSAIDs even at low doses.

Withhold for at least 4-6 half-lives prior to surgical or dental procedures. May cause photosensitivity reactions.

Adverse Reactions

>10%: Gastrointestinal: Diarrhea (14%), dyspepsia (13%), abdominal pain (12%)

1% to 10%:

Cardiovascular: Edema (3% to 9%)

Central nervous system: Dizziness (3% to 9%), headache (3% to 9%), fatigue (1% to 3%), insomnia (1% to 3%), nervousness (1% to 3%), somnolence (1% to 3%)

Dermatologic: Pruritus (3% to 9%), rash (3% to 9%)

Gastrointestinal: Constipation (3% to 9%), flatulence (3% to 9%), guaiac positive (3% to 9%), nausea (3% to 9%), gastritis (1% to 3%), stomatitis (1% to 3%), vomiting (1% to 3%), xerostomia (1% to 3%)

Otic: Tinnitus

Miscellaneous: Diaphoresis (1% to 3%)

<1% (Limited to important or life-threatening): Abnormal vision, acne, agitation, albuminuria, alopecia, anaphylactoid reaction, anaphylaxis, anemia, angina, angioneurotic edema, anorexia, anxiety, arrhythmia, asthma, azotemia, bilirubinemia duodenitis, bullous eruptions, CHF, chills, confusion, cough, depression, duodenal ulcer, dysphagia, dyspnea, dysuria, eosinophilic pneumonia, eructation, erythema multiforme, fever, gallstones, gastric ulcer, gastroenteritis, gingivitis, GI bleeding, glossitis, granulocytopenia, hematuria, hepatic failure, hyperglycemia, hypersensitivity pneumonitis, hypertension, hyperuricemia, hypokalemia, impotence, interstitial nephritis, interstitial pneumonitis, jaundice, leukopenia, liver function abnormalities, malaise, melena, MI, nephrotic syndrome, nightmares, palpitation, pancreatitis, paresthesia, photosensitivity, pseudoporphyria cutanea tarda, rectal bleeding, renal failure, renal stones, Stevens-Johnson syndrome, syncope, taste disorder, thrombocytopenia, thrombophlebitis, toxic epidermal necrolysis, tremor, urticaria, vasculitis, vertigo, weakness, weight gain/loss

Drug Interactions

Metabolism/Transport Effects None known.

Avoid Concomitant Use

Avoid concomitant use of Nabumetone with any of the following: Floctafenine; Ketorolac; Ketorolac (Nasal); Ketorolac (Systemic)

Increased Effect/Toxicity

Nabumetone may increase the levels/effects of: Aminoglycosides; Anticoagulants; Antiplatelet Agents; Bisphosphonate Derivatives; Collagenase (Systemic); CycloSPORINE; CycloSPORINE (Systemic); Deferasirox; Desmopressin; Digoxin; Drotrecogin Alfa (Activated); Eplerenone; Haloperidol; Ibritumomab; Lithium; Methotrexate; Nonsteroidal Anti-Inflammatory Agents; PEMEtrexed; Porfimer; Potassium-Sparing Diuretics; PRALAtrexate; Quinolone Antibiotics; Rivaroxaban; Salicylates; Thrombolytic Agents; Tositumomab and Iodine I 131 Tositumomab; Vancomycin; Vitamin K Antagonists

The levels/effects of Nabumetone may be increased by: ACE Inhibitors; Angiotensin II Receptor Blockers; Antidepressants (Tricyclic, Tertiary Amine); Corticosteroids (Systemic); CycloSPORINE; CycloSPORINE (Systemic); Dasatinib; Floctafenine; Glucosamine; Herbs (Anticoagulant/Antiplatelet Properties); Ketorolac; Ketorolac (Nasal); Ketorolac (Systemic); Nonsteroidal Anti-Inflammatory Agents; Omega-3-Acid Ethyl Esters; Pentosan Polysulfate Sodium; Pentoxifylline; Probenecid; Prostacyclin Analogues; Selective Serotonin Reuptake Inhibitors; Serotonin/Norepinephrine Reuptake Inhibitors; Sodium Phosphates; Treprostinil; Vitamin E

Decreased Effect

Nabumetone may decrease the levels/effects of: ACE Inhibitors; Angiotensin II Receptor Blockers; Antiplatelet Agents; Beta-Blockers; Eplerenone; HydrALAZINE; Loop Diuretics; Potassium-Sparing Diuretics; Salicylates; Selective Serotonin Reuptake Inhibitors; Thiazide Diuretics

The levels/effects of Nabumetone may be decreased by: Bile Acid Sequestrants; Nonsteroidal Anti-Inflammatory Agents; Salicylates

Ethanol/Nutrition/Herb Interactions

Ethanol: Avoid ethanol (may enhance gastric mucosal irritation).

Food: Nabumetone peak serum concentrations may be increased if taken with food or dairy products.

Herb/Nutraceutical: Avoid alfalfa, anise, bilberry, bladderwrack, bromelain, cat's claw, celery, chamomile, coleus, cordyceps, dong quai, evening primrose, fenugreek, feverfew, garlic, ginger, ginkgo biloba, ginseng (American, Panax, Siberian), grapeseed, green tea, guggul, horse chestnut seed, horseradish, licorice, prickly ash, red clover, reishi, SAMe (S-adenosylmethionine), sweet clover, turmeric, white willow (all have additional antiplatelet activity).

Mechanism of Action Reversibly inhibits cyclooxygenase-1 and 2 (COX-1 and 2) enzymes, which results in decreased formation of prostaglandin precursors; has antipyretic, analgesic, and anti-inflammatory properties

Other proposed mechanisms not fully elucidated (and possibly contributing to the anti-inflammatory effect to varying degrees), include inhibiting chemotaxis, altering lymphocyte activity, inhibiting neutrophil aggregation/activation, and decreasing proinflammatory cytokine levels.

Pharmacodynamics/Kinetics

Onset of action: Several days

Distribution: Diffusion occurs readily into synovial fluid

V_d: 6MNA: 29-82 L

Protein binding: 6MNA: >99%

Metabolism: Prodrug, rapidly metabolized in the liver to an active metabolite [6-methoxy-2-naphthylacetic acid (6MNA)] and inactive metabolites; extensive first-pass effect

Half-life elimination: 6MNA: ~24 hours

Time to peak, serum: 6MNA: Oral: 2.5-4 hours; Synovial fluid: 4-12 hours

Excretion: 6MNA: Urine (80%) and feces (9%)

Dosage Adults: Oral: 1000 mg/day; an additional 500-1000 mg may be needed in some patients to obtain more symptomatic relief; may be administered once or twice daily (maximum dose: 2000 mg/day)

Note: Patients <50 kg are less likely to require doses >1000 mg/day.

Dosage adjustment in renal impairment: In general, NSAIDs are not recommended for use in patients with advanced renal disease, but the manufacturer of nabumetone does provide some guidelines for adjustment in renal dysfunction:

Moderate impairment (Cl_{cr} 30-49 mL/minute): Initial dose: 750 mg/day; maximum dose: 1500 mg/day

Severe impairment (Cl_{cr} <30 mL/minute): Initial dose: 500 mg/day; maximum dose: 1000 mg/day

Monitoring Parameters Patients with renal insufficiency: Baseline renal function followed by repeat test within weeks (to determine if renal function has deteriorated)

Dosage Forms Excipient information presented when available (limited, particularly for generics); consult specific product labeling.

Tablet, oral: 500 mg, 750 mg

◆ **NAC** *see* Acetylcysteine *on page* 34

◆ ***N*-Acetyl-L-cysteine** *see* Acetylcysteine *on page* 34

- ***N* Acetylcysteine** *see* Acetylcysteine *on page* 34
- **N-Acetyl-P-Aminophenol** *see* Acetaminophen *on page* 27
- **NaCl** *see* Sodium Chloride *on page* 1567

Nadolol (NAY doe lol)

Brand Names: U.S. Corgard®

Brand Names: Canada Alti-Nadolol; Apo-Nadol®; Corgard®; Novo-Nadolol; Teva-Nadolol

Pharmacologic Category Antianginal Agent; Beta-Adrenergic Blocker, Nonselective

Additional Appendix Information
Beta-Blockers *on page* 1884

Use Treatment of hypertension and angina pectoris; prophylaxis of migraine headaches

Unlabeled Use Primary and secondary prophylaxis of variceal hemorrhage; management of thyrotoxicosis

Pregnancy Risk Factor C

Pregnancy Considerations Adverse events were observed in some animal reproduction studies; therefore, the manufacturer classifies nadolol as pregnancy category C. Nadolol crosses the placenta and is measurable in infant serum after birth. In a cohort study, an increased risk of cardiovascular defects was observed following maternal use of beta-blockers during pregnancy. Intrauterine growth restriction (IUGR), small placentas, as well as fetal/neonatal bradycardia, hypoglycemia, and/or respiratory depression have been observed following *in utero* exposure to beta-blockers as a class. Adequate facilities for monitoring infants at birth should be available. Untreated chronic maternal hypertension and pre-eclampsia are also associated with adverse events in the fetus, infant, and mother. Nadolol is indicated for the treatment of hypertension, but due to its long half-life and potential effects to the fetus, other agents may be more appropriate for use during pregnancy.

Lactation Enters breast milk/use caution consider risk: benefit (AAP rates "compatible"; AAP 2001 update pending)

Contraindications Hypersensitivity to nadolol or any component of the formulation; bronchial asthma; sinus bradycardia; sinus node dysfunction; heart block greater than first degree (except in patients with a functioning artificial pacemaker); cardiogenic shock; uncompensated cardiac failure

Warnings/Precautions Consider pre-existing conditions such as sick sinus syndrome before initiating. Administer only with extreme caution in patients with compensated heart failure, monitor for a worsening of the condition. Efficacy in heart failure has not been established for nadolol. **[U.S. Boxed Warning]: Beta-blocker therapy should not be withdrawn abruptly (particularly in patients with CAD), but gradually tapered to avoid acute tachycardia, hypertension, and/or ischemia.** Chronic beta-blocker therapy should not be routinely withdrawn prior to major surgery. Use with caution in patients on concurrent digoxin, verapamil or diltiazem; bradycardia or heart block can occur. Use with caution in patients receiving inhaled anesthetic agents known to depress myocardial contractility. In general, patients with bronchospastic disease should not receive beta-blockers. Nadolol, if used at all, should be used cautiously in bronchospastic disease with close monitoring. Use cautiously in diabetics because it can mask prominent hypoglycemic symptoms. May mask signs of hyperthyroidism (eg, tachycardia); if hyperthyroidism is suspected, carefully manage and monitor; abrupt withdrawal may exacerbate symptoms of hyperthyroidism or precipitate thyroid storm. Use cautiously in the renally impaired (dosage adjustments are required). Use with caution in patients with myasthenia gravis, peripheral vascular disease, or psychiatric disease (may cause CNS depression). Bradycardia may be observed more frequently in elderly patients (>65 years of age); dosage reductions may be necessary. Adequate alpha-blockade is required prior to use of any beta-blocker for patients with untreated pheochromocytoma. May induce or exacerbate psoriasis. Use caution with history of severe anaphylaxis to allergens; patients taking beta-blockers may become more sensitive to repeated challenges. Treatment of anaphylaxis (eg, epinephrine) in patients taking beta-blockers may be ineffective or promote undesirable effects.

Adverse Reactions
>10%:
Central nervous system: Drowsiness, insomnia
Endocrine & metabolic: Decreased sexual ability
1% to 10%:
Cardiovascular: Bradycardia, palpitation, edema, CHF, reduced peripheral circulation
Central nervous system: Mental depression
Gastrointestinal: Diarrhea or constipation, nausea, vomiting, stomach discomfort
Respiratory: Bronchospasm
Miscellaneous: Cold extremities
<1% (Limited to important or life-threatening): Arrhythmias, chest pain, confusion (especially in the elderly), depression, dyspnea, hallucinations, leukopenia, orthostatic hypotension, thrombocytopenia

Drug Interactions

Metabolism/Transport Effects Substrate of P-glycoprotein

Avoid Concomitant Use
Avoid concomitant use of Nadolol with any of the following: Beta2-Agonists; Floctafenine; Methacholine

Increased Effect/Toxicity
Nadolol may increase the levels/effects of: Alpha-/Beta-Agonists (Direct-Acting); Alpha1-Blockers; Alpha2-Agonists; Amifostine; Antihypertensives; Bupivacaine; Cardiac Glycosides; Cholinergic Agonists; Fingolimod; Hypotensive Agents; Insulin; Lidocaine; Lidocaine (Systemic); Lidocaine (Topical); Mepivacaine; Methacholine; Midodrine; RiTUXimab; Sulfonylureas

The levels/effects of Nadolol may be increased by: Acetylcholinesterase Inhibitors; Amiodarone; Anilidopiperidine Opioids; Calcium Channel Blockers (Dihydropyridine); Calcium Channel Blockers (Nondihydropyridine); Diazoxide; Dipyridamole; Disopyramide; Dronedarone; Floctafenine; Herbs (Hypotensive Properties); MAO Inhibitors; Pentoxifylline; P-glycoprotein/ABCB1 Inhibitors; Phosphodiesterase 5 Inhibitors; Prostacyclin Analogues; Reserpine

Decreased Effect
Nadolol may decrease the levels/effects of: Beta2-Agonists; Theophylline Derivatives

The levels/effects of Nadolol may be decreased by: Herbs (Hypertensive Properties); Methylphenidate; Nonsteroidal Anti-Inflammatory Agents; P-glycoprotein/ABCB1 Inducers; Yohimbine

Ethanol/Nutrition/Herb Interactions Herb/Nutraceutical: Avoid dong quai if using for hypertension (has estrogenic activity). Avoid ephedra, garlic, yohimbe, ginseng (may worsen hypertension). Avoid natural licorice (causes sodium and water retention and increases potassium loss).

Mechanism of Action Competitively blocks response to $beta_1$- and $beta_2$-adrenergic stimulation; does not exhibit any membrane stabilizing or intrinsic sympathomimetic activity. Nonselective beta-adrenergic blockers (propranolol, nadolol) reduce portal pressure by producing splanchnic vasoconstriction ($beta_2$ effect) thereby reducing portal blood flow.

Pharmacodynamics/Kinetics
Duration: 17-24 hours
Absorption: 30% to 40%

Distribution: V_d: 1.9 L/kg
Protein binding: 30%
Metabolism: Not metabolized
Half-life elimination: Adults: 10-24 hours; prolonged with renal impairment; End-stage renal disease: 45 hours
Time to peak, serum: 2-4 hours
Excretion: Urine (as unchanged drug)

Dosage Oral:
Adults:
Angina: Initial: 40 mg/day, increase dosage gradually by 40-80 mg increments at 3- to 7-day intervals until optimum clinical response is obtained with profound slowing of heart rate; doses up to 160-240 mg/day in angina
Hypertension: Initial: 40 mg/day, increase dosage gradually by 40-80 mg increments until optimum blood pressure reduction achieved. Usual dosage range (JNC 7): 40-120 mg once daily; doses up to 240-320 mg/day in hypertension may be necessary
Variceal hemorrhage prophylaxis (unlabeled use; Garcia-Tsao, 2007):
Primary prophylaxis: Initial: 40 mg once daily; adjust to maximal tolerated dose. **Note:** Risk factors for hemorrhage include Child-Pugh class B/C or variceal red wale markings on endoscopy.
Secondary prophylaxis: Initial: 40 mg once daily; adjust to maximal tolerated dose
Thyrotoxicosis (unlabeled use): 40-160 mg once daily (Bahn, 2011)
Elderly: Hypertension: Consider lower initial doses (eg, 20 mg/day) and titrate to response (Aronow, 2011)

Dosing adjustment in renal impairment:
Cl_{cr} >50 mL/minute/1.73 m^2: Administer every 24 hours
Cl_{cr} 31-50 mL/minute/1.73 m^2: Administer every 24-36 hours
Cl_{cr} 10-30 mL/minute/1.73 m^2: Administer every 24-48 hours
Cl_{cr} <10 mL/minute/1.73 m^2: Administer every 40-60 hours
Dosage adjustments for dialysis are not provided in the manufacturer's labeling; however, the following guidelines have been used by some clinicians (Aronoff, 2007):
ESRD requiring hemodialysis: Administer dose post-dialysis.
Peritoneal dialysis: Supplemental dose is not necessary.
Dosing adjustment in hepatic impairment: There are no dosage adjustments provided in the manufacturer's labeling.

Dietary Considerations May be taken without regard to meals.

Administration May be administered without regard to meals.

Dosage Forms Excipient information presented when available (limited, particularly for generics); consult specific product labeling.
Tablet, oral: 20 mg, 40 mg, 80 mg
Corgard®: 20 mg, 40 mg, 80 mg [scored]

Nafarelin (naf a REL in)

Brand Names: U.S. Synarel®
Brand Names: Canada Synarel®
Index Terms Nafarelin Acetate
Pharmacologic Category Gonadotropin Releasing Hormone Agonist
Use Treatment of endometriosis, including pain and reduction of lesions; treatment of central precocious puberty (CPP; gonadotropin-dependent precocious puberty) in children of both sexes
Pregnancy Risk Factor X

Dosage Intranasal:
Endometriosis: Adults: Females: 1 spray (200 mcg) in 1 nostril each morning and the other nostril each evening starting on days 2-4 of menstrual cycle (total: 2 sprays/day). Dose may be increased to 2 sprays (400 mcg; 1 spray in each nostril) in the morning and evening if amenorrhea is not achieved (total: 4 sprays [800 mcg]/day). Total duration of therapy should not exceed 6 months due to decreases in bone mineral density; retreatment is not recommended by the manufacturer.
Central precocious puberty: Children: Males/Females: 2 sprays (400 mcg) into each nostril in the morning and 2 sprays (400 mcg) into each nostril in the evening (total: 8 sprays [1600 mcg]/day). If inadequate suppression, may increase dose to 3 sprays (600 mcg) into alternating nostrils 3 times/day (total: 9 sprays [1800 mcg]/day).

Additional Information Complete prescribing information for this medication should be consulted for additional detail.

Dosage Forms Excipient information presented when available (limited, particularly for generics); consult specific product labeling.
Solution, intranasal [spray]:
Synarel®: 2 mg/mL (8 mL) [contains benzalkonium chloride; 200 mcg/spray; 60 metered sprays]

◆ **Nafarelin Acetate** *see* Nafarelin *on page 1170*

Nafcillin (naf SIL in)

Brand Names: Canada Nallpen®; Unipen®
Index Terms Ethoxynaphthamido Penicillin Sodium; Nafcillin Sodium; Nallpen; Sodium Nafcillin
Pharmacologic Category Antibiotic, Penicillin
Additional Appendix Information
Antibiotic Treatment of Adults With Infective Endocarditis *on page 1956*
Use Treatment of infections such as osteomyelitis, septicemia, endocarditis, and CNS infections caused by susceptible strains of staphylococci species
Pregnancy Risk Factor B
Pregnancy Considerations Adverse events have not been observed in animal studies; therefore, nafcillin is classified as pregnancy category B. There is no available data on the placental transfer of nafcillin. Human experience with the penicillins during pregnancy has not shown any positive evidence of adverse effects on the fetus.
Lactation Enters breast milk/use caution
Contraindications Hypersensitivity to nafcillin, or any component of the formulation, or penicillins; premixed injection may contain corn-derived dextrose and its use is contraindicated in patients with allergy to corn-related products
Warnings/Precautions Serious and occasionally severe or fatal hypersensitivity (anaphylactoid) reactions have been reported in patients on penicillin therapy, especially with a history of beta-lactam hypersensitivity, history of sensitivity to multiple allergens, or previous IgE-mediated reactions (eg, anaphylaxis, angioedema, urticaria). Use with caution in asthmatic patients. Extravasation of I.V. infusions should be avoided. Modification of dosage is necessary in patients with both severe renal and hepatic impairment. Elimination rate will be slow in neonates. Prolonged use may result in fungal or bacterial superinfection, including *C. difficile*-associated diarrhea (CDAD) and pseudomembranous colitis; CDAD has been observed >2 months postantibiotic treatment.
Adverse Reactions Frequency not defined.
Central nervous system: Neurotoxicity (high doses)
Gastrointestinal: Pseudomembranous colitis
Hematologic: Agranulocytosis, bone marrow depression, neutropenia

Local: Inflammation, pain, phlebitis, skin sloughing, swelling, and thrombophlebitis at the injection site; oxacillin (less likely to cause phlebitis) is often preferred in pediatric patients; tissue necrosis with sloughing (SubQ extravasation)

Renal: Interstitial nephritis (rare), renal tubular damage (rare)

Miscellaneous: Anaphylaxis, hypersensitivity reactions (immediate and delayed; general incidence of 1% to 10% for penicillins), serum sickness

Drug Interactions

Metabolism/Transport Effects **Induces** CYP3A4 (strong)

Avoid Concomitant Use

Avoid concomitant use of Nafcillin with any of the following: BCG; Bortezomib; Crizotinib; Dienogest; Dronedarone; Everolimus; Lapatinib; Lurasidone; Nilotinib; Pazopanib; Praziquantel; Ranolazine; Rivaroxaban; Roflumilast; RomiDEPsin; SORAfenib; Ticagrelor; Tolvaptan; Toremifene; Vandetanib

Increased Effect/Toxicity

Nafcillin may increase the levels/effects of: Clarithromycin; Methotrexate; Vitamin K Antagonists

The levels/effects of Nafcillin may be increased by: Clarithromycin; Probenecid

Decreased Effect

Nafcillin may decrease the levels/effects of: ARIPiprazole; BCG; Boceprevir; Bortezomib; Brentuximab Vedotin; Calcium Channel Blockers; Clarithromycin; Contraceptives (Estrogens); Crizotinib; CycloSPORINE; CycloSPORINE (Systemic); CYP3A4 Substrates; Dasatinib; Dienogest; Dronedarone; Everolimus; Exemestane; Gefitinib; GuanFACINE; Imatinib; Ixabepilone; Lapatinib; Linagliptin; Lurasidone; Maraviroc; Mycophenolate; Nilotinib; Pazopanib; Praziquantel; Ranolazine; Rivaroxaban; Roflumilast; RomiDEPsin; Saxagliptin; SORAfenib; SUNItinib; Tadalafil; Ticagrelor; Tolvaptan; Toremifene; Typhoid Vaccine; Ulipristal; Vandetanib; Vemurafenib; Vitamin K Antagonists; Zuclopenthixol

The levels/effects of Nafcillin may be decreased by: Fusidic Acid; Tetracycline Derivatives

Stability

Premixed infusions: Store in a freezer at -20°C (4°F). Thaw at room temperature or under refrigeration only. Thawed bags are stable for 21 days under refrigeration or 72 hours at room temperature. Do not refreeze.

Vials: Reconstituted parenteral solution is stable for 3 days at room temperature and 7 days when refrigerated or 12 weeks when frozen. For I.V. infusion in NS or D_5W, solution is stable for 24 hours at room temperature and 96 hours when refrigerated.

Mechanism of Action Interferes with bacterial cell wall synthesis during active multiplication, causing cell wall death and resultant bactericidal activity against susceptible bacteria

Pharmacodynamics/Kinetics

Distribution: Widely distributed; CSF penetration is poor but enhanced by meningeal inflammation

Protein binding: ~90%; primarily to albumin

Metabolism: Primarily hepatic; undergoes enterohepatic recirculation

Half-life elimination:

Neonates: <3 weeks: 2.2-5.5 hours; 4-9 weeks: 1.2-2.3 hours

Children 3 months to 14 years: 0.75-1.9 hours

Adults: Normal renal/hepatic function: 30-60 minutes

Time to peak, serum: I.M.: 30-60 minutes

Excretion: Primarily feces; urine (10% to 30% as unchanged drug)

Dosage

Usual dosage range:

Children:

I.M.: 25 mg/kg twice daily

I.V.: 50-200 mg/kg/day in divided doses every 4-6 hours (maximum: 12 g/day)

Adults:

I.M.: 500 mg every 4-6 hours

I.V.: 500-2000 mg every 4-6 hours

Indication-specific dosing:

Children:

Mild-to-moderate infections: I.M., I.V.: 50-100 mg/kg/day in divided doses every 6 hours

Severe infections: I.M., I.V.: 100-200 mg/kg/day in divided doses every 4-6 hours (maximum dose: 12 g/day)

Staphylococcal endocarditis: I.V.:

Native valve: 200 mg/kg/day in divided doses every 4-6 hours for 6 weeks

Prosthetic valve: 200 mg/kg/day in divided doses every 4-6 hours for ≥6 weeks (use with rifampin and gentamicin)

Adults: I.V.:

Endocarditis: MSSA:

Native valve: 12 g/24 hours in 4-6 divided doses for 6 weeks

Prosthetic valve: 12 g/24 hours in 6 divided doses for ≥6 weeks (use with rifampin and gentamicin)

Joint:

Bursitis, septic: 2 g every 4 hours

Prosthetic: 2 g every 4-6 hours with rifampin for 6 weeks

***Staphylococcus aureus*, methicillin-susceptible infections, including brain abscess, empyema, erysipelas, mastitis, myositis, orbital cellulitis, osteomyelitis, pneumonia, splenic abscess, toxic shock, urinary tract (perinephric abscess):** 2 g every 4 hours

Dosing adjustment in renal impairment: Not necessary unless renal impairment is in the setting of concomitant hepatic impairment

Poorly dialyzed; no supplemental dose or dosage adjustment necessary, including patients on intermittent hemodialysis, peritoneal dialysis, or continuous renal replacement therapy (eg, CVVHD).

Dosing adjustment in hepatic impairment: In patients with both hepatic and renal impairment, modification of dosage may be necessary; no data available.

Dietary Considerations Premixed injection may contain corn-derived dextrose and its use is contraindicated in patients with allergy to corn-related products. Some products may contain sodium.

Administration

I.M.: Rotate injection sites

I.V.: Vesicant. Administer around-the-clock to promote less variation in peak and trough serum levels; infuse over 30-60 minutes

Extravasation management: Use cold packs. Hyaluronidase: Add 1 mL NS to 150 unit vial to make 150 units/mL of concentration; mix 0.1 mL of above with 0.9 mL NS in 1 mL syringe to make final concentration = 15 units/mL.

Monitoring Parameters Baseline and periodic CBC with differential; periodic urinalysis, BUN, serum creatinine, AST and ALT; observe for signs and symptoms of anaphylaxis during first dose

Test Interactions Positive Coombs' test (direct), false-positive urinary and serum proteins; may inactivate aminoglycosides *in vitro*

Dosage Forms Excipient information presented when available (limited, particularly for generics); consult specific product labeling.

Infusion, premixed iso-osmotic dextrose solution: 1 g (50 mL); 2 g (100 mL)

Injection, powder for reconstitution: 1 g, 2 g, 10 g

◆ **Nafcillin Sodium** *see* Nafcillin *on page 1170*

Naftifine (NAF ti feen)

Brand Names: U.S. Naftin®

Index Terms Naftifine Hydrochloride

Pharmacologic Category Antifungal Agent, Topical

Use Topical treatment of tinea cruris (jock itch), tinea corporis (ringworm), and tinea pedis (athlete's foot)

Pregnancy Risk Factor B

Dosage Adults: Topical: Apply cream once daily and gel twice daily (morning and evening) for up to 4 weeks

Additional Information Complete prescribing information for this medication should be consulted for additional detail.

Dosage Forms Excipient information presented when available (limited, particularly for generics); consult specific product labeling.

Cream, topical, as hydrochloride:

Naftin®: 1% (30 g, 60 g, 90 g) [contains benzyl alcohol]

Gel, topical, as hydrochloride:

Naftin®: 1% (40 g, 60 g, 90 g) [contains ethanol 52%]

◆ **Naftifine Hydrochloride** *see* Naftifine *on page 1172*

◆ **Naftin®** *see* Naftifine *on page 1172*

◆ **NaHCO$_3$** *see* Sodium Bicarbonate *on page 1566*

Nalbuphine (NAL byoo feen)

Index Terms Nalbuphine Hydrochloride; Nubain

Pharmacologic Category Analgesic, Opioid; Analgesic, Opioid Partial Agonist

Additional Appendix Information

Opioid Analgesics *on page 1896*

Use Relief of moderate-to-severe pain; preoperative analgesia, postoperative and surgical anesthesia, and obstetrical analgesia during labor and delivery

Unlabeled Use Opioid-induced pruritus

Pregnancy Risk Factor C

Pregnancy Considerations Severe fetal bradycardia has been reported following use in labor/delivery. Fetal bradycardia may occur when administered earlier in pregnancy (not documented). Use only if clearly needed, with monitoring to detect and manage possible adverse fetal effects. Naloxone has been reported to reverse bradycardia. Newborn should be monitored for respiratory depression or bradycardia following nalbuphine use in labor.

Lactation Enters breast milk/use caution

Contraindications Hypersensitivity to nalbuphine or any component of the formulation

Warnings/Precautions Use caution in CNS depression. Sedation and psychomotor impairment are likely, and are additive with other CNS depressants or ethanol. May cause respiratory depression. Ambulatory patients must be cautioned about performing tasks which require mental alertness (eg, operating machinery or driving). Effects may be potentiated when used with other sedative drugs or ethanol. Use with caution in patients with recent myocardial infarction, biliary tract impairment, morbid obesity, thyroid dysfunction, head trauma, or increased intracranial pressure. Use caution in patients with prostatic hyperplasia and/or urinary stricture, adrenal insufficiency, decreased hepatic or renal function. Use with caution in patients with pre-existing respiratory compromise (hypoxia and/or hypercapnia), COPD or other obstructive pulmonary disease; critical respiratory depression may occur, even at therapeutic dosages. May cause hypotension; use with caution in patients with hypovolemia, cardiovascular disease (including acute MI), or drugs which may exaggerate hypotensive effects (including phenothiazines or general anesthetics). May obscure diagnosis or clinical course of patients with acute abdominal conditions. May result in tolerance and/or drug dependence with chronic use; use with caution in patients with a history of drug dependence. Abrupt discontinuation following prolonged use may lead to withdrawal symptoms. May precipitate withdrawal symptoms in patients following prolonged therapy with mu opioid agonists. Use with caution in pregnancy (close neonatal monitoring required when used in labor and delivery). Use with caution in the elderly and debilitated patients; may be more sensitive to adverse effects. Safety and efficacy in children have not been established.

Adverse Reactions

>10%: Central nervous system: Sedation (36%)

1% to 10%:

Central nervous system: Dizziness (5%), headache (3%)

Gastrointestinal: Nausea/vomiting (6%), xerostomia (4%)

Miscellaneous: Clamminess (9%)

<1% (Limited to important or life-threatening): Abdominal pain, agitation, allergic reaction, anaphylaxis, anaphylactoid reaction, anxiety, asthma, bitter taste, blurred vision, bradycardia, cardiac arrest, confusion, crying, delusion, depersonalization, depression, diaphoresis, dreams (abnormal), dyspepsia, dysphoria, dyspnea, euphoria, faintness, fever, floating sensation, flushing, gastrointestinal cramps, hallucinations, hostility, hypertension, hypotension, injection site reactions (pain, swelling, redness, burning); laryngeal edema, loss of consciousness, nervousness, numbness, pruritus, pulmonary edema, rash, respiratory depression, respiratory distress, restlessness, seizure, sensation of warmth/burning, somnolence, speech disorder, stridor, tachycardia, tingling, tremor, unreality, urinary urgency, urticaria

Drug Interactions

Metabolism/Transport Effects None known.

Avoid Concomitant Use There are no known interactions where it is recommended to avoid concomitant use.

Increased Effect/Toxicity

Nalbuphine may increase the levels/effects of: Alcohol (Ethyl); Alvimopan; CNS Depressants; Desmopressin; Selective Serotonin Reuptake Inhibitors; Thiazide Diuretics

The levels/effects of Nalbuphine may be increased by: Amphetamines; Antipsychotic Agents (Phenothiazines); Droperidol; HydrOXYzine; Succinylcholine

Decreased Effect

Nalbuphine may decrease the levels/effects of: Analgesics (Opioid); Pegvisomant

The levels/effects of Nalbuphine may be decreased by: Ammonium Chloride; Mixed Agonist / Antagonist Opioids

Ethanol/Nutrition/Herb Interactions

Ethanol: May increase CNS depression; monitor for increased effects with coadministration. Caution patients about effects.

Herb/Nutraceutical: Avoid valerian, St John's wort, kava kava, gotu kola (may increase CNS depression).

Stability Store at room temperature of 15°C to 30°C (59°F to 86°F). Protect from light.

Mechanism of Action Agonist of kappa opiate receptors and partial antagonist of mu opiate receptors in the CNS, causing inhibition of ascending pain pathways, altering the perception of and response to pain; produces generalized CNS depression

Pharmacodynamics/Kinetics
Onset of action: Peak effect: SubQ, I.M.: <15 minutes; I.V.: 2-3 minutes
Metabolism: Hepatic
Half-life elimination: 5 hours
Excretion: Feces; urine (~7% as metabolites)

Dosage
Children ≥1 year (unlabeled use): Pain management: I.M., I.V., SubQ: 0.1-0.2 mg/kg every 3-4 hours as needed; maximum: 20 mg/dose and/or 160 mg/day
Adults:
Pain management: I.M., I.V., SubQ: 10 mg/70 kg every 3-6 hours; maximum single dose in nonopioid-tolerant patients: 20 mg; maximum daily dose: 160 mg
Surgical anesthesia supplement: I.V.: Induction: 0.3-3 mg/kg over 10-15 minutes; maintenance doses of 0.25-0.5 mg/kg may be given as required
Opioid-induced pruritus (unlabeled use): I.V. 2.5-5 mg; may repeat dose

Dosing adjustment in renal impairment: Use with caution and reduce dose; monitor.

Dosing adjustment in hepatic impairment: Use with caution and reduce dose.

Administration Administer I.M., SubQ, or I.V.

Monitoring Parameters Relief of pain, respiratory and mental status, blood pressure

Test Interactions May interfere with certain enzymatic methods used to detect opioids, depending on sensitivity and specificity of the test (refer to test manufacturer for details)

Dosage Forms Excipient information presented when available (limited, particularly for generics); consult specific product labeling.
Injection, solution, as hydrochloride: 10 mg/mL (10 mL); 20 mg/mL (10 mL)
Injection, solution, as hydrochloride [preservative free]: 10 mg/mL (1 mL); 20 mg/mL (1 mL)

- **Nalbuphine Hydrochloride** *see* Nalbuphine *on page 1172*
- **Nalex A 12** *see* Chlorpheniramine, Pyrilamine, and Phenylephrine *on page 348*
- **Nalfon®** *see* Fenoprofen *on page 696*
- **Nallpen** *see* Nafcillin *on page 1170*
- **Nallpen® (Can)** *see* Nafcillin *on page 1170*
- ***N*-allylnoroxymorphine Hydrochloride** *see* Naloxone *on page 1173*

Naloxone (nal OKS one)

Brand Names: Canada Naloxone Hydrochloride Injection®

Index Terms *N*-allylnoroxymorphine Hydrochloride; Naloxone Hydrochloride; Narcan

Pharmacologic Category Antidote; Opioid Antagonist

Use Complete or partial reversal of opioid drug effects, including respiratory depression; management of known or suspected opioid overdose; diagnosis of suspected opioid dependence or acute opioid overdose

Unlabeled Use Opioid-induced pruritus

Pregnancy Risk Factor C

Pregnancy Considerations Consider benefit to the mother and the risk to the fetus before administering to a pregnant woman who is known or suspected to be opioid dependent. May precipitate withdrawal in both the mother and fetus.

Lactation Excretion in breast milk unknown/not recommended

Contraindications Hypersensitivity to naloxone or any component of the formulation

Warnings/Precautions Due to an association between naloxone and acute pulmonary edema, use with caution in patients with cardiovascular disease or in patients receiving medications with potential adverse cardiovascular effects (eg, hypotension, pulmonary edema, or arrhythmias). Administration of naloxone causes the release of catecholamines; may precipitate acute withdrawal or unmask pain in those who regularly take opioids. Excessive dosages should be avoided after use of opiates in surgery. Abrupt postoperative reversal may result in nausea, vomiting, sweating, tachycardia, hypertension, seizures, and other cardiovascular events (including pulmonary edema and arrhythmias). May precipitate withdrawal symptoms in patients addicted to opiates, including pain, hypertension, sweating, agitation, irritability; in neonates: shrill cry, failure to feed; carefully titrate dose to reverse hypoventilation; do not fully awaken patient or reverse analgesic effect (postoperative patient). Use caution in patients with history of seizures; avoid use in treatment of meperidine-induced seizures. Recurrence of respiratory depression is possible if the opioid involved is long-acting; observe patients until there is no reasonable risk of recurrent respiratory depression.

Adverse Reactions Adverse reactions are related to reversing dependency and precipitating withdrawal. Withdrawal symptoms are the result of sympathetic excess. Adverse events occur secondarily to reversal (withdrawal) of narcotic analgesia and sedation.
Central nervous system: Narcotic withdrawal

Drug Interactions

Metabolism/Transport Effects None known.

Avoid Concomitant Use There are no known interactions where it is recommended to avoid concomitant use.

Increased Effect/Toxicity There are no known significant interactions involving an increase in effect.

Decreased Effect There are no known significant interactions involving a decrease in effect.

Stability Store at 25°C (77°F). Protect from light. Stable in 0.9% sodium chloride and D_5W at 4 mcg/mL for 24 hours.

Mechanism of Action Pure opioid antagonist that competes and displaces narcotics at opioid receptor sites

Pharmacodynamics/Kinetics
Onset of action: Endotracheal, I.M., SubQ: 2-5 minutes; Intranasal: ~8-13 minutes (Kelley, 2005; Robertson, 2009); I.V.: ~2 minutes
Duration: ~30-120 minutes depending on route of administration; I.V. has a shorter duration of action than I.M. administration; since naloxone's action is shorter than that of most opioids, repeated doses are usually needed
Distribution: Crosses placenta
Metabolism: Primarily hepatic via glucuronidation
Half-life elimination: Neonates: 3-4 hours; Adults: 0.5-1.5 hours
Excretion: Urine (as metabolites)

Dosage Note: I.M., I.V. (preferred), intranasal (adults only), and SubQ routes may be used. Endotracheal administration is the least desirable and is supported by only anecdotal evidence (case report) (ACLS, 2010):
Infants and Children: Postoperative reversal: 0.01 mg/kg; may repeat every 2-3 minutes as needed based on response (adequate ventilation without significant pain)
Children:
Opioid overdose (with standard PALS protocols): I.V., intraosseous (I.O.), endotracheal:
Birth (including premature infants) to 5 years or ≤20 kg (unlabeled dose): 0.1 mg/kg (maximum dose: 2 mg); repeat every 2-3 minutes if needed (*Drugs for Pediatric Emergencies*, 1998; PALS, 2010)
>5 years or >20 kg: 2 mg; if no response, repeat every 2-3 minutes. If no response is observed after 10 mg total, consider other causes of respiratory depression (*Drugs for Pediatric Emergencies*, 1998; PALS, 2010).

Note: I.O. and endotracheal routes are alternative routes recommended by PALS 2010 guidelines.

Continuous infusion (unlabeled dosing): I.V.: If continuous infusion is required, calculate dosage/hour based on effective intermittent dose used and duration of adequate response seen **or** use two-thirds (2/3) of the initial effective naloxone bolus on an hourly basis; titrate dose (typically 0.04-0.16 mg/kg/hour for 2-5 days in children); one-half (1/2) of the initial bolus dose should be readministered 15 minutes after initiation of the continuous infusion to prevent a drop in naloxone levels; increase infusion rate as needed to assure adequate ventilation and prevent withdrawal symptoms.

Reversal of respiratory depression with therapeutic opioid dosing: 0.001-0.005 mg/kg; dose may be repeated as needed (PALS, 2010)

Adults:

Opioid overdose (with standard ACLS protocols):

I.V., I.M., SubQ: 2 mg; may need to repeat doses every 2-3 minutes; after reversal, may need to readminister dose(s) at a later interval (ie, 20-60 minutes) depending on type/duration of opioid. If no response is observed after 10 mg total, consider other causes of respiratory depression.

Continuous infusion (unlabeled dosing): I.V.: **Note:** For use with exposures to long-acting opioids (eg, methadone), sustained release product, and symptomatic body packers after initial naloxone response. Calculate dosage/hour based on effective intermittent dose used and duration of adequate response seen or use two-thirds (2/3) of the initial effective naloxone bolus on an hourly basis (typically 0.25-6.25 mg/hour); one-half (1/2) of the initial bolus dose should be readministered 15 minutes after initiation of the continuous infusion to prevent a drop in naloxone levels; adjust infusion rate as needed to assure adequate ventilation and prevent withdrawal symptoms (Goldfrank, 1986).

Endotracheal (unlabeled route): 0.08-5 mg (dose is 2-2.5 times I.V. dose); may repeat (ACLS, 2010)

Intranasal administration (unlabeled route): 2 mg (1 mg per nostril); may repeat in 5 minutes if respiratory depression persists. **Note:** Onset of action is slightly delayed compared to I.M. or I.V. routes (ACLS, 2010; Kelly, 2005; Robertson, 2009).

Reversal of respiratory depression with therapeutic opioid doses: I.V., I.M., SubQ.: Initial: 0.04-0.4 mg; may repeat until desired response achieved. If desired response is not observed after 0.8 mg total, consider other causes of respiratory depression.

Continuous infusion (unlabeled dosing): I.V.: **Note:** For use with exposures to long-acting opioids (eg, methadone) or sustained release products. Calculate dosage/hour based on effective intermittent dose used and duration of adequate response seen or use two-thirds (2/3) of the initial effective naloxone bolus on an hourly basis (typically 0.2-0.6 mg/hour); one-half (1/2) of the initial bolus dose should be readministered 15 minutes after initiation of the continuous infusion to prevent a drop in naloxone levels; adjust infusion rate as needed to assure adequate ventilation and prevent withdrawal symptoms (Goldfrank, 1986).

Opioid-dependent patients being treated for cancer pain (NCCN guidelines, v.2.2011): I.V.: 0.04-0.08 mg (40-80 mcg) slow I.V. push; administer every 30-60 seconds until improvement in symptoms; if no response is observed after total naloxone dose 1 mg, consider other causes of respiratory depression. **Note:** May dilute 0.4 mg/mL (1 mL) ampul into 9 mL of normal saline for a total volume of 10 mL to achieve a 0.04 mg/mL (40 mcg/mL) concentration.

Postoperative reversal: I.V.: 0.1-0.2 mg every 2-3 minutes until desired response (adequate ventilation and alertness without significant pain). **Note:** Repeat doses may be needed within 1-2 hour intervals depending on type, dose, and timing of the last dose of opioid administered.

Opioid-induced pruritus (unlabeled use): I.V. infusion: 0.25 mcg/kg/**hour**; **Note:** Monitor pain control; verify that the naloxone is not reversing analgesia (Gan, 1997)

Administration

Endotracheal (unlabeled route): There is only anecdotal support for this route of administration. May require a slightly higher dose than used in other routes. Dilute to 1-2 mL with normal saline; flush with 5 cc of saline and then administer 5 ventilations

Intranasal (unlabeled route): Administer total dose equally divided into each nostril using a mucosal atomizer device (MAD) (ACLS, 2010; Kelly, 2005; Robertson, 2009)

I.V. push: Administer over 30 seconds as undiluted preparation **or** (unlabeled) administer as diluted preparation slow I.V. push by diluting 0.4 mg (1 mL) ampul with 9 mL of normal saline for a total volume of 10 mL to achieve a concentration of 0.04 mg/mL

I.V. continuous infusion: Dilute to 4 mcg/mL in D_5W or normal saline

I.M., SubQ: May administer I.M. or SubQ if unable to obtain I.V. access

Monitoring Parameters Respiratory rate, heart rate, blood pressure, temperature, level of consciousness, ABGs or pulse oximetry

Additional Information May contain methyl and propylparabens

Dosage Forms Excipient information presented when available (limited, particularly for generics); consult specific product labeling.

Injection, solution, as hydrochloride: 0.4 mg/mL (10 mL)

Injection, solution, as hydrochloride [preservative free]: 0.4 mg/mL (1 mL); 1 mg/mL (2 mL)

◆ **Naloxone and Buprenorphine** *see* Buprenorphine and Naloxone *on page 246*

◆ **Naloxone Hydrochloride** *see* Naloxone *on page 1173*

◆ **Naloxone Hydrochloride Dihydrate and Buprenorphine Hydrochloride** *see* Buprenorphine and Naloxone *on page 246*

◆ **Naloxone Hydrochloride Injection® (Can)** *see* Naloxone *on page 1173*

Naltrexone (nal TREKS one)

Brand Names: U.S. ReVia®; Vivitrol®

Brand Names: Canada ReVia®

Index Terms Naltrexone Hydrochloride

Pharmacologic Category Antidote; Opioid Antagonist

Use Treatment of ethanol dependence; prevention of relapse in opioid dependent patients, following opioid detoxification

Pregnancy Risk Factor C

Pregnancy Considerations Evidence of early fetal loss has been observed in animal studies with oral naltrexone. Reproduction studies have not been conduced using the sustained release I.M formulation. There are no adequate and well-controlled studies of naltrexone in pregnant women.

Lactation Enters breast milk/not recommended

Medication Guide Available Yes

Contraindications Hypersensitivity to naltrexone or any component of the formulation; narcotic dependence or current use of opioid analgesics; acute opioid withdrawal; failure to pass naloxone challenge or positive urine screen for opioids; acute hepatitis; liver failure

Warnings/Precautions [U.S. Boxed Warning]: Dose-related hepatocellular injury is possible; the margin of separation between the apparent safe and hepatotoxic doses appears to be ≤ fivefold. Discontinue therapy if signs/symptoms of acute hepatitis develop. Therapy may precipitate withdrawal symptoms in patients addicted to opiates; patients should be opioid-free for a minimum of 7-10 days; use naloxone challenge test to confirm patient is opioid-free prior to therapy if there is any suspicion since urinary opioid screen may not be sufficient proof. Use of naltrexone does not eliminate or diminish withdrawal symptoms. Patients who had been treated with naltrexone may respond to lower opioid doses than previously used. This could result in potentially life-threatening opioid intoxication. Patients should be aware that they may be more sensitive to lower doses of opioids after naltrexone treatment is discontinued, after a missed dose, or near the end of the dosing interval. Warn patients that any attempt to overcome opioid blockade during naltrexone therapy, could potentially lead to fatal opioid overdose; the opioid competitive receptor blockade produced by naltrexone is potentially surmountable in the presence of large amounts of opioids. In naltrexone-treated patients requiring emergency pain management, consider alternatives to opioid therapy (eg, regional analgesia, nonopioid analgesics, general anesthesia). If opioid therapy is required for pain therapy, patients should be under the direct care of a trained anesthesia provider.

Suicidal thoughts and depression have been reported in both alcohol- and opioid-dependent patients; monitor closely. Hypersensitivity, including anaphylaxis, has been reported. Cases of eosinophilic pneumonia have been reported and should be considered in patients presenting with progressive hypoxia and dyspnea. Use with caution in patients with a history of bleeding disorders (including thrombocytopenia) and/or patients on anticoagulant therapy; bleeding/hematoma may occur from I.M. administration. Serious injection site reactions (eg, cellulitis, induration, hematoma, abscess, necrosis) have been reported with use, including severe cases requiring surgical debridement. Females appear to be at a higher risk. Patients should report any injection site pain, swelling, bruising, pruritus, or redness that does not improve (or worsens). For I.M. use only in the gluteal muscle; do **not** administer I.V., SubQ, or into fatty tissue; incorrect administration may increase the risk of injection site reactions. Use with caution in patients with hepatic or renal impairment; not studied in moderate-to-severe renal impairment or in severe hepatic impairment. Use is contraindicated in patients with acute hepatitis or hepatic failure. Vehicle used in the injectable naltrexone formulation (polylactide-co-glycolide microspheres) has rarely been associated with retinal artery occlusion in patients with abnormal arteriovenous anastomosis following injection of other drug products that also use the polylactide-co-glycolide microspheres vehicle.

Adverse Reactions Combined reporting of adverse events from oral and injectable formulations:

>10%:
- Cardiovascular: Syncope (13%)
- Central nervous system: Headache (3% to 25%), insomnia (3% to 14%), dizziness (4% to 13%), anxiety (2% to 12%), nervousness (4% to >10%)
- Gastrointestinal: Nausea (10% to 33%), vomiting (3% to 14%), appetite decreased (14%), diarrhea (13%), abdominal pain (11%), abdominal cramping
- Hepatic: ALT increased (13%)
- Local: Injection site reaction (≤69%; includes bruising, induration, nodules, pain, pruritus, swelling, tenderness)
- Neuromuscular & skeletal: Arthralgia (12%), CPK increased (11% to 39%)
- Respiratory: Pharyngitis (7% to 11%)

1% to 10%:
- Cardiovascular: Hypertension (5%)
- Central nervous system: Suicidal thoughts (≤10%), depression (8%), somnolence (2% to 4%), fatigue (4%), chills, energy increased, feeling down, irritability
- Dermatologic: Rash (6%)
- Endocrine & metabolic: Polydipsia
- Gastrointestinal: Dry mouth (5%), toothache (4%)
- Genitourinary: Delayed ejaculation, impotency
- Hepatic: AST increased (2% to 10%), GGT increased (7%)
- Neuromuscular & skeletal: Muscle cramps (8%), back pain (6%)
- Miscellaneous: Influenza (5%)

<1% (Limited to important or life-threatening): Angina, atrial fibrillation, blood pressure increased, cerebral aneurysm, chest pain, chest tightness, cholecystitis, cholelithiasis, colitis, COPD, dehydration, delirium, diaphoresis, DVT, dyspnea, ECG changes, eosinophilia (transient), eosinophilic pneumonia, GI hemorrhage, HF, hypercholesterolemia, hypersensitivity reaction (includes anaphylaxis, angioedema, and urticaria), ischemic stroke, leukocytosis, lymphadenopathy, MI, narcotic withdrawal, palpitation, pancreatitis, paralytic ileus, paranoia, PE, perirectal abscess, pneumonia, rigors, seizure, shortness of breath, suicide, tachycardia, thrombocytopenia

Drug Interactions

Metabolism/Transport Effects None known.

Avoid Concomitant Use There are no known interactions where it is recommended to avoid concomitant use.

Increased Effect/Toxicity There are no known significant interactions involving an increase in effect.

Decreased Effect There are no known significant interactions involving a decrease in effect.

Stability

Injection: Store unopened kit at 2°C to 8°C (36°F to 46°F). Kit may be kept at room temperature of ≤25°C (77°F) for ≤7 days prior to use; do not freeze.

Prior to reconstitution, allow drug vial and provided diluent to reach room temperature (~45 minutes). Using the provided 1 inch *preparation* needle, reconstitute the microsphere drug powder with 3.4 mL of the diluent and allow to dissolve by vigorously shaking the vial for ~1 minute. Mixed suspension will be milky white, free of clumps, and will move freely down the walls of the vial. Immediately after suspension, withdraw 4.2 mL of the suspension using the same preparation needle.

Prior to administration, replace the preparation needle with the appropriately size provided *administration* needle (1.5-inch Terumo® needle or 2-inch Needle-Pro® needle, depending on patient's physique). Prior to injection, remove any air bubbles and push on the plunger until 4 mL of the suspension remains in the syringe. Following reconstitution of the suspension, administer immediately.

Tablet: Store at room temperature. Protect from light.

Mechanism of Action Naltrexone (a pure opioid antagonist) is a cyclopropyl derivative of oxymorphone similar in structure to naloxone and nalorphine (a morphine derivative); it acts as a competitive antagonist at opioid receptor sites, showing the highest affinity for mu receptors.

Pharmacodynamics/Kinetics

Duration: Oral: 50 mg: 24 hours; 100 mg: 48 hours; 150 mg: 72 hours; I.M.: 4 weeks

Absorption: Oral: Almost complete

Distribution: V_d: ~1350 L; widely throughout the body but considerable interindividual variation exists

Metabolism: Extensively metabolized via noncytochrome-mediated dehydrogenase conversion to 6-beta-naltrexol (primary metabolite) and related minor metabolites; glucuronide conjugates are also formed from naltrexone and its metabolites

Oral: Extensive first-pass effect

Protein binding: 21%

Bioavailability: Oral: Variable range (5% to 40%)

Half-life elimination: Oral: 4 hours; 6-beta-naltrexol: 13 hours; I.M.: naltrexone and 6-beta-naltrexol: 5-10 days

Time to peak, serum: Oral: ~60 minutes; I.M.: Biphasic: ~2 hours (first peak), ~2-3 days (second peak)

Excretion: Primarily urine (as metabolites and small amounts of unchanged drug)

Dosage Adults: **Note:** Do not initiate therapy until patient is opioid-free for at least 7-10 days as determined by urinalysis; consider naloxone challenge test to confirm patient is opioid-free if there is any suspicion since urinary opioid screen may not be sufficient proof.

Oral: Alcohol dependence, opioid dependence: Initial: 25 mg; if no withdrawal signs occur, administer 50 mg on day 2; maintenance regimen: 50 mg/day; alternative maintenance regimens may be used and include: 50 mg on weekdays with a 100 mg dose on Saturday; 100 mg every other day; or 150 mg every 3 days (degree of blockade may be reduced with extended dosing interval regimens and doses >50 mg may increase risk of hepatocellular injury)

I.M.: Alcohol dependence, opioid dependence: 380 mg once every 4 weeks

Dosage adjustment in renal impairment: Use caution. No adjustment needed in mild impairment. Not adequately studied in moderate-to-severe renal impairment.

Dosage adjustment in hepatic impairment: Use caution. An increase in naltrexone AUC of approximately five- and 10-fold in patients with compensated or decompensated liver cirrhosis respectively, compared with normal liver function has been reported No adjustment required with mild-to-moderate hepatic impairment. Not adequately studied in severe hepatic impairment. Use is contraindicated in patients with acute hepatitis or hepatic failure.

Administration

Oral: May be administered with or without food. Administration with food or after meals may minimize adverse gastrointestinal effects. Advise patient not to self-administer opiates while receiving naltrexone therapy.

I.M.: Vivitrol®: Administer I.M. into the upper outer quadrant of the gluteal area; must inject dose using one of the provided needles for administration. Use either the 1.5-inch 20-gauge needle or the 2-inch 20-gauge needle (for patients with a larger amount of subcutaneous tissue overlying the gluteal muscle). Avoid inadvertent injection into a blood vessel; do not administer I.V., SubQ, or into fatty tissue (the risk of serious injection site reaction is increased if given incorrectly as a SubQ injection or into fatty tissue instead of the gluteal muscle). Injection should alternate between the 2 buttocks. Do not substitute any components of the dose-pack.

Monitoring Parameters For narcotic withdrawal; liver function tests; injection site reactions

Test Interactions May cause cross-reactivity with some opioid immunoassay methods.

Dosage Forms Excipient information presented when available (limited, particularly for generics); consult specific product labeling.

Injection, microspheres for suspension, extended release:

Vivitrol®: 380 mg [contains polylactide-co-glycolide; supplied with diluent]

Tablet, oral, as hydrochloride: 50 mg

ReVia®: 50 mg [scored]

◆ **Naltrexone and Morphine** *see* Morphine and Naltrexone *on page 1158*

◆ **Naltrexone Hydrochloride** *see* Naltrexone *on page 1174*

◆ **Namenda®** *see* Memantine *on page 1068*

◆ **Namenda XR** *see* Memantine *on page 1068*

◆ **Nanoparticle Albumin-Bound Paclitaxel** *see* PACLitaxel (Protein Bound) *on page 1275*

◆ **NAPA and NABZ** *see* Sodium Phenylacetate and Sodium Benzoate *on page 1572*

Naphazoline (Nasal) (naf AZ oh leen)

Brand Names: U.S. Privine® [OTC]

Index Terms Naphazoline Hydrochloride

Pharmacologic Category Alpha$_1$ Agonist

Use Temporary relief of nasal congestion associated with the common cold, upper respiratory allergies, or sinusitis

Dosage Intranasal: Children ≥12 years and Adults: 0.05% instill 1-2 drops or sprays every 6 hours if needed; therapy should not exceed 3 days

Additional Information Complete prescribing information for this medication should be consulted for additional detail.

Dosage Forms Excipient information presented when available (limited, particularly for generics); consult specific product labeling.

Solution, intranasal, as hydrochloride [drops]:

Privine®: 0.05% (25 mL) [contains benzalkonium chloride]

Solution, intranasal, as hydrochloride [spray]:

Privine®: 0.05% (20 mL) [contains benzalkonium chloride]

Naphazoline (Ophthalmic) (naf AZ oh leen)

Brand Names: U.S. AK-Con™; Clear eyes® for Dry Eyes Plus ACR Relief [OTC]; Clear eyes® for Dry Eyes plus Redness Relief [OTC]; Clear eyes® Redness Relief [OTC]; Clear eyes® Seasonal Relief [OTC]

Brand Names: Canada Naphcon Forte®; Vasocon®

Index Terms Naphazoline Hydrochloride

Pharmacologic Category Alpha$_1$ Agonist; Ophthalmic Agent, Vasoconstrictor

Use Topical ocular vasoconstrictor; relief of redness of the eye due to minor irritation

Pregnancy Risk Factor C

Dosage Ophthalmic: Adults:

0.1% solution (prescription): 1-2 drops into conjuctival sac every 3-4 hours as needed

0.012% or 0.025% solution (OTC): 1-2 drops into affected eye(s) up to 4 times/day; therapy should not exceed 3 days

Additional Information Complete prescribing information for this medication should be consulted for additional detail.

Dosage Forms Excipient information presented when available (limited, particularly for generics); consult specific product labeling.

Solution, ophthalmic, as hydrochloride [drops]:

AK-Con™: 0.1% (15 mL) [contains benzalkonium chloride]

Clear eyes® for Dry Eyes Plus ACR Relief: 0.025% (15 mL) [contains hypromellose, zinc sulfate]

Clear eyes® for Dry Eyes plus Redness Relief: 0.012% (15 mL) [contains benzalkonium chloride, glycerin, hypromellose]
Clear eyes® Redness Relief: 0.012% (6 mL, 15 mL, 30 mL) [contains benzalkonium chloride, glycerin]
Clear eyes® Seasonal Relief: 0.012% (15 mL, 30 mL) [contains benzalkonium chloride, glycerin, zinc sulfate]

Naphazoline and Pheniramine
(naf AZ oh leen & fen NIR a meen)

Brand Names: U.S. Naphcon-A® [OTC]; Opcon-A® [OTC]; Visine-A® [OTC]
Brand Names: Canada Naphcon-A®; Visine® Advanced Allergy
Index Terms Pheniramine and Naphazoline
Pharmacologic Category Alkylamine Derivative; Alpha$_1$ Agonist; Histamine H_1 Antagonist; Histamine H_1 Antagonist, First Generation; Imidazoline Derivative; Ophthalmic Agent, Vasoconstrictor
Use Treatment of ocular congestion, irritation, and itching
Pregnancy Risk Factor C
Dosage Ophthalmic: Children ≥6 years and Adults: 1-2 drops up to 4 times/day
Additional Information Complete prescribing information for this medication should be consulted for additional detail.
Dosage Forms Excipient information presented when available (limited, particularly for generics); consult specific product labeling.
Solution, ophthalmic:
Naphcon-A®: Naphazoline hydrochloride 0.025% and pheniramine maleate 0.3% (5 mL) [contains benzalkonium chloride; 2 bottles/box], (15 mL) [contains benzalkonium chloride]
Opcon-A®: Naphazoline hydrochloride 0.027% and pheniramine maleate 0.3% (15 mL) [contains benzalkonium chloride]
Visine-A®: Naphazoline hydrochloride 0.025% and pheniramine maleate 0.3% (15 mL) [contains benzalkonium chloride]

- **Naphazoline Hydrochloride** *see* Naphazoline (Nasal) *on page 1176*
- **Naphazoline Hydrochloride** *see* Naphazoline (Ophthalmic) *on page 1176*
- **Naphcon-A® [OTC]** *see* Naphazoline and Pheniramine *on page 1177*
- **Naphcon-A® (Can)** *see* Naphazoline and Pheniramine *on page 1177*
- **Naphcon Forte® (Can)** *see* Naphazoline (Ophthalmic) *on page 1176*
- **Naprelan®** *see* Naproxen *on page 1177*
- **Naprelan™ (Can)** *see* Naproxen *on page 1177*
- **Naprosyn®** *see* Naproxen *on page 1177*
- **Naprosyn® E (Can)** *see* Naproxen *on page 1177*
- **Naprosyn® SR (Can)** *see* Naproxen *on page 1177*

Naproxen (na PROKS en)

Brand Names: U.S. Aleve® [OTC]; Anaprox®; Anaprox® DS; EC-Naprosyn®; Mediproxen [OTC]; Midol® Extended Relief [OTC]; Naprelan®; Naprosyn®; Pamprin® Maximum Strength All Day Relief [OTC]
Brand Names: Canada Anaprox®; Anaprox® DS; Apo-Napro-Na DS®; Apo-Napro-Na®; Apo-Naproxen EC®; Apo-Naproxen SR®; Apo-Naproxen®; Mylan-Naproxen EC; Naprelan™; Naprosyn®; Naprosyn® E; Naprosyn® SR; Naproxen Sodium DS; Naproxen-NA; Naproxen-NA DF; PMS-Naproxen; PMS-Naproxen EC; PRO-Naproxen EC; Riva-Naproxen; Riva-Naproxen Sodium; Riva-Naproxen Sodium DS; Teva-Naproxen; Teva-Naproxen EC; Teva-Naproxen Sodium; Teva-Naproxen Sodium DS; Teva-Naproxen SR
Index Terms Naproxen Sodium
Pharmacologic Category Nonsteroidal Anti-inflammatory Drug (NSAID), Oral
Additional Appendix Information
Beers Criteria – Potentially Inappropriate Medications for Geriatrics *on page 1973*
Use Management of ankylosing spondylitis, osteoarthritis, and rheumatoid disorders (including juvenile idiopathic arthritis [JIA]); acute gout; mild-to-moderate pain; tendonitis, bursitis; dysmenorrhea; fever
Pregnancy Risk Factor C
Pregnancy Considerations Adverse events were not observed in the initial animal reproduction studies; therefore, the manufacturer classifies naproxen as pregnancy category C. Naproxen crosses the placenta and can be detected in fetal tissue and the serum of newborn infants following *in utero* exposure. NSAID exposure during the first trimester is not strongly associated with congenital malformations; however, cardiovascular anomalies and cleft palate have been observed following NSAID exposure in some studies. The use of a NSAID close to conception may be associated with an increased risk of miscarriage. Nonteratogenic effects have been observed following NSAID administration during the third trimester including: Myocardial degenerative changes, prenatal constriction of the ductus arteriosus, fetal tricuspid regurgitation, failure of the ductus arteriosus to close postnatally; renal dysfunction or failure, oligohydramnios; gastrointestinal bleeding or perforation, increased risk of necrotizing enterocolitis; intracranial bleeding (including intraventricular hemorrhage), platelet dysfunction with resultant bleeding; pulmonary hypertension. Because they may cause premature closure of the ductus arteriosus, use of NSAIDs late in pregnancy should be avoided (use after 31 or 32 weeks gestation is not recommended by some clinicians). The chronic use of NSAIDs in women of reproductive age may be associated with infertility that is reversible upon discontinuation of the medication. A registry is available for pregnant women exposed to autoimmune medications including naproxen. For additional information contact the Organization of Teratology Information Specialists, OTIS Autoimmune Diseases Study, at (877) 311-8972.
Lactation Enters breast milk/not recommended (AAP rates "compatible"; AAP 2001 update pending)
Medication Guide Available Yes
Contraindications Hypersensitivity to naproxen, aspirin, other NSAIDs, or any component of the formulation; perioperative pain in the setting of coronary artery bypass graft (CABG) surgery
Warnings/Precautions [U.S. Boxed Warning]: NSAIDs are associated with an increased risk of adverse cardiovascular thrombotic events, including MI and stroke. Risk may be increased with duration of use or pre-existing cardiovascular risk factors or disease. Carefully evaluate individual cardiovascular risk profiles prior to prescribing. May cause new-onset hypertension or worsening of existing hypertension. Use caution with fluid retention. Avoid use in heart failure. Use the lowest effective dose for the shortest duration of time, consistent with individual patient goals, to reduce risk of cardiovascular or GI adverse events. Alternate therapies should be considered for patients at high risk. Concurrent administration of ibuprofen, and potentially other nonselective NSAIDs, may interfere with aspirin's cardioprotective effect. **[U.S. Boxed Warning]: Use is contraindicated for treatment of perioperative pain in the setting of coronary artery bypass graft (CABG) surgery.** Risk of

MI and stroke may be increased with use following CABG surgery.

[U.S. Boxed Warning]: NSAIDs may increase risk of gastrointestinal irritation, inflammation, ulceration, bleeding, and perforation. These events may occur at any time during therapy and without warning. Use caution with a history of GI disease (bleeding or ulcers), concurrent therapy with aspirin, anticoagulants and/or corticosteroids, smoking, use of alcohol, the elderly or debilitated patients. When used concomitantly with ≤325 mg of aspirin, a substantial increase in the risk of gastrointestinal complications (eg, ulcer) occurs; concomitant gastroprotective therapy (eg, proton pump inhibitors) is recommended (Bhatt, 2008).

May increase the risk of aseptic meningitis, especially in patients with systemic lupus erythematosus (SLE) and mixed connective tissue disorders. Platelet adhesion and aggregation may be decreased; may prolong bleeding time; patients with coagulation disorders or who are receiving anticoagulants should be monitored closely. Anemia may occur; patients on long-term NSAID therapy should be monitored for anemia. Rarely, NSAID use may cause severe blood dyscrasias (eg, agranulocytosis, aplastic anemia, thrombocytopenia).

NSAID use may compromise existing renal function; dose-dependent decreases in prostaglandin synthesis may result from NSAID use, reducing renal blood flow which may cause renal decompensation. NSAID use may increase the risk for hyperkalemia. Patients with impaired renal function, dehydration, heart failure, liver dysfunction, those taking diuretics, and ACE inhibitors, and the elderly are at greater risk of renal toxicity and hyperkalemia. Rehydrate patient before starting therapy; monitor renal function closely. Not recommended for use in patients with advanced renal disease. Long-term NSAID use may result in renal papillary necrosis.

NSAIDs may cause serious skin adverse events including exfoliative dermatitis, Stevens-Johnson Syndrome (SJS) and toxic epidermal necrolysis (TEN); discontinue use at first sign of skin rash or hypersensitivity. Anaphylactoid reactions may occur, even without prior exposure; patients with "aspirin triad" (bronchial asthma, aspirin intolerance, rhinitis) may be at increased risk. Do not use in patients who experience bronchospasm, asthma, rhinitis, or urticaria with NSAID or aspirin therapy. Use caution in other forms of asthma.

Use with caution in patients with decreased hepatic function. Closely monitor patients with any abnormal LFT. Severe hepatic reactions (eg, fulminant hepatitis, liver failure) have occurred with NSAID use, rarely; discontinue if signs or symptoms of liver disease develop, or if systemic manifestations occur.

NSAIDS may cause drowsiness, dizziness, blurred vision and other neurologic effects which may impair physical or mental abilities; patients must be cautioned about performing tasks which require mental alertness (eg, operating machinery or driving). Discontinue use with blurred or diminished vision and perform ophthalmologic exam. Monitor vision with long-term therapy.

In the elderly, may be inappropriate for long-term use due to potential for GI bleeding, hypertension, heart failure, and renal failure (Beers Criteria).

Withhold for at least 4-6 half-lives prior to surgical or dental procedures. Safety and efficacy have not been established in children <2 years of age.

OTC labeling: Prior to self-medication, patients should contact healthcare provider if they have had recurring stomach pain or upset, ulcers, bleeding problems, asthma, high blood pressure, heart or kidney disease, other serious medical problems, are currently taking a diuretic, anticoagulant, other NSAIDs, or are ≥60 years of age. Recommended dosages and duration should not be exceeded, due to an increased risk of GI bleeding, MI, and stroke. Patients should stop use and consult a healthcare provider if symptoms get worse, newly appear, or continue; if an allergic reaction occurs; if feeling faint, vomit blood or have bloody/black stools; if having difficulty swallowing or heartburn, or if fever lasts for >3 days or pain >10 days. Consuming ≥3 alcoholic beverages/day or taking longer than recommended may increase the risk of GI bleeding. Not for self-medication (OTC use) in children <12 years of age.

Adverse Reactions

1% to 10%:

- Cardiovascular: Edema (3% to 9%), palpitations (<3%)
- Central nervous system: Dizziness (3% to 9%), drowsiness (3% to 9%), headache (3% to 9%), lightheadedness (<3%), vertigo (<3%)
- Dermatologic: Pruritus (3% to 9%), skin eruption (3% to 9%), ecchymosis (3% to 9%), purpura (<3%), rash
- Endocrine & metabolic: Fluid retention (3% to 9%)
- Gastrointestinal: Abdominal pain (3% to 9%), constipation (3% to 9%), nausea (3% to 9%), heartburn (3% to 9%), diarrhea (<3%), dyspepsia (<3%), stomatitis (<3%), flatulence, gross bleeding/perforation, indigestion, ulcers, vomiting
- Genitourinary: Abnormal renal function
- Hematologic: Hemolysis (3% to 9%), ecchymosis (3% to 9%), anemia, bleeding time increased
- Hepatic: LFTs increased
- Ocular: Visual disturbances (<3%)
- Otic: Tinnitus (3% to 9%), hearing disturbances (<3%)
- Respiratory: Dyspnea (3% to 9%)
- Miscellaneous: Diaphoresis (<3%), thirst (<3%)

<1% (Limited to important or life-threatening): Agranulocytosis, alopecia, anaphylactic/anaphylactoid reaction, angioneurotic edema, arrhythmia, aseptic meningitis, asthma, blurred vision, cognitive dysfunction, colitis, coma, confusion, CHF, conjunctivitis, cystitis, depression, dream abnormalities, dysuria, eosinophilia, eosinophilic pneumonitis, erythema multiforme, exfoliative dermatitis, glossitis, granulocytopenia, hallucinations, hematemesis, hepatitis, hyper-/hypoglycemia, hyper-/hypotension, infection, interstitial nephritis, melena, jaundice, leukopenia, liver failure, lymphadenopathy, menstrual disorders, malaise, MI, muscle weakness, myalgia, oliguria, pancreatitis, pancytopenia, paresthesia, photosensitivity, pneumonia, polyuria, proteinuria, pyrexia, rectal bleeding, renal failure, renal papillary necrosis, respiratory depression, sepsis, Stevens-Johnson syndrome, tachycardia, seizure, syncope, thrombocytopenia, toxic epidermal necrolysis ulcerative stomatitis, vasculitis

Drug Interactions

Metabolism/Transport Effects Substrate of CYP1A2 (minor), CYP2C9 (minor); **Note:** Assignment of Major/Minor substrate status based on clinically relevant drug interaction potential

Avoid Concomitant Use

Avoid concomitant use of Naproxen with any of the following: Floctafenine; Ketorolac; Ketorolac (Nasal); Ketorolac (Systemic)

Increased Effect/Toxicity

Naproxen may increase the levels/effects of: Aminoglycosides; Anticoagulants; Antiplatelet Agents; Bisphosphonate Derivatives; Collagenase (Systemic); CycloSPORINE; CycloSPORINE (Systemic); Deferasirox; Desmopressin; Digoxin; Drotrecogin Alfa (Activated); Eplerenone; Haloperidol; Ibritumomab; Lithium; Methotrexate; Nonsteroidal Anti-Inflammatory Agents; PEMEtrexed; Porfimer; Potassium-Sparing Diuretics; PRALAtrexate; Quinolone Antibiotics; Rivaroxaban;

Salicylates; Thrombolytic Agents; Tositumomab and Iodine I 131 Tositumomab; Vancomycin; Vitamin K Antagonists

The levels/effects of Naproxen may be increased by: ACE Inhibitors; Angiotensin II Receptor Blockers; Antidepressants (Tricyclic, Tertiary Amine); Corticosteroids (Systemic); CycloSPORINE; CycloSPORINE (Systemic); Dasatinib; Floctafenine; Glucosamine; Herbs (Anticoagulant/Antiplatelet Properties); Ketorolac; Ketorolac (Nasal); Ketorolac (Systemic); Nonsteroidal Anti-Inflammatory Agents; Omega-3-Acid Ethyl Esters; Pentosan Polysulfate Sodium; Pentoxifylline; Probenecid; Prostacyclin Analogues; Selective Serotonin Reuptake Inhibitors; Serotonin/Norepinephrine Reuptake Inhibitors; Sodium Phosphates; Treprostinil; Vitamin E

Decreased Effect

Naproxen may decrease the levels/effects of: ACE Inhibitors; Angiotensin II Receptor Blockers; Antiplatelet Agents; Beta-Blockers; Eplerenone; HydrALAZINE; Loop Diuretics; Potassium-Sparing Diuretics; Salicylates; Selective Serotonin Reuptake Inhibitors; Thiazide Diuretics

The levels/effects of Naproxen may be decreased by: Bile Acid Sequestrants; Cyproterone; Nonsteroidal Anti-Inflammatory Agents; Salicylates

Ethanol/Nutrition/Herb Interactions

Ethanol: Avoid ethanol (may enhance gastric mucosal irritation).

Food: Naproxen absorption rate/levels may be decreased if taken with food.

Herb/Nutraceutical: Avoid alfalfa, anise, bilberry, bladderwrack, bromelain, cat's claw, celery, chamomile, coleus, cordyceps, dong quai, evening primrose, fenugreek, feverfew, garlic, ginger, ginkgo biloba, ginseng (American, Panax, Siberian), grapeseed, green tea, guggul, horse chestnut seed, horseradish, licorice, prickly ash, red clover, reishi, SAMe (S-adenosylmethionine), sweet clover, turmeric, white willow (all have additional antiplatelet activity).

Stability Store oral suspension and tablet at 15°C to 30°C (59°F to 86°F).

Mechanism of Action Reversibly inhibits cyclooxygenase-1 and 2 (COX-1 and 2) enzymes, which results in decreased formation of prostaglandin precursors; has antipyretic, analgesic, and anti-inflammatory properties

Other proposed mechanisms not fully elucidated (and possibly contributing to the anti-inflammatory effect to varying degrees), include inhibiting chemotaxis, altering lymphocyte activity, inhibiting neutrophil aggregation/activation, and decreasing proinflammatory cytokine levels.

Pharmacodynamics/Kinetics

Onset of action: Analgesic: 1 hour; Anti-inflammatory: ~2 weeks

Peak effect: Anti-inflammatory: 2-4 weeks

Duration: Analgesic: ≤7 hours; Anti-inflammatory: ≤12 hours

Absorption: Almost 100%

Distribution: 0.16 L/kg

Protein binding: >99% to albumin; increased free fraction in elderly

Metabolism: Hepatic to metabolites

Bioavailability: 95%

Half-life elimination: Normal renal function: 12-17 hours; End-stage renal disease: No change

Time to peak, serum: 1-4 hours

Excretion: Urine (95%; primarily as metabolites); feces (≤3%)

Dosage Note: Dosage expressed as naproxen base; 200 mg naproxen base is equivalent to 220 mg naproxen sodium.

Oral:

Children >2 years: Juvenile idiopathic arthritis: 10 mg/kg/day in 2 divided doses

Adults:

Gout, acute: Initial: 750 mg, followed by 250 mg every 8 hours until attack subsides. **Note:** EC-Naprosyn® is not recommended.

Migraine, acute (unlabeled use): Initial: 500-750 mg; an additional 250-500 mg may be given if needed (maximum: 1250 mg in 24 hours). **Note:** EC-Naprosyn® is not recommended.

Pain (mild-to-moderate), dysmenorrhea, acute tendonitis, bursitis: Initial: 500 mg, then 250 mg every 6-8 hours; maximum: 1250 mg/day naproxen base

Rheumatoid arthritis, osteoarthritis, and ankylosing spondylitis: 500-1000 mg/day in 2 divided doses; may increase to 1.5 g/day of naproxen base for limited time period

OTC labeling: Pain/fever: Children ≥12 years and Adults: 200 mg naproxen base every 8-12 hours; if needed, may take 400 mg naproxen base for the initial dose; maximum: 400 mg naproxen base in any 8- to 12-hour period or 600 mg naproxen base/24 hours

Dosing adjustment in renal impairment: Cl_{cr} <30 mL/minute: Use is not recommended

Dietary Considerations Drug may cause GI upset, bleeding, ulceration, perforation; take with food or milk to minimize GI upset.

Administration Administer with food, milk, or antacids to decrease GI adverse effects

Suspension: Shake suspension well before administration.

Tablet, extended release: Swallow tablet whole; do not break, crush, or chew.

Monitoring Parameters Occult blood loss, periodic liver function test, CBC, BUN, serum creatinine; urine output

Test Interactions Naproxen may interfere with 5-HIAA urinary assays; due to an interaction with m-dinitrobenzene, naproxen should be discontinued 72 hours before adrenal function testing if the Porter-Silber test is used. May interfere with urine detection of cannabinoids and barbiturates (false-positives).

Dosage Forms Excipient information presented when available (limited, particularly for generics); consult specific product labeling.

Caplet, oral, as sodium: 220 mg [equivalent to naproxen base 200 mg]

Aleve®: 220 mg [contains sodium 20 mg; equivalent to naproxen base 200 mg]

Midol® Extended Relief: 220 mg [contains sodium 20 mg; equivalent to naproxen base 200 mg]

Pamprin® Maximum Strength All Day Relief: 220 mg [contains sodium 20 mg; equivalent to naproxen base 200 mg]

Capsule, liquid gel, oral, as sodium:

Aleve®: 220 mg [contains sodium 20 mg; equivalent to naproxen base 200 mg]

Combination package, oral, as sodium [dose-pack/each package contains]:

Naprelan®: Day 1-3: Tablet, controlled release: 825 mg [equivalent to naproxen base 750 mg] (6s) [contains sodium 75 mg] and Day 4-10: Tablet, controlled release: 550 mg [equivalent to naproxen base 500 mg] (14s) [contains sodium 50 mg]

Gelcap, oral, as sodium:

Aleve®: 220 mg [contains sodium 20 mg; equivalent to naproxen base 200 mg]

Suspension, oral: 125 mg/5 mL (500 mL)

Naprosyn®: 125 mg/5 mL (473 mL) [contains sodium 39 mg (1.5 mEq)/5 mL; orange-pineapple flavor]

Tablet, oral: 250 mg, 375 mg, 500 mg

Naprosyn®: 250 mg [scored]

Naprosyn®: 375 mg

Naprosyn®: 500 mg [scored]

Tablet, oral, as sodium: 220 mg [equivalent to naproxen base 200 mg], 220 mg, 275 mg [equivalent to naproxen base 250 mg], 550 mg [equivalent to naproxen base 500 mg]

Aleve®: 220 mg [contains sodium 20 mg; equivalent to naproxen base 200 mg]

Anaprox®: 275 mg [contains sodium 25 mg; equivalent to naproxen base 250 mg]

Anaprox® DS: 550 mg [scored; contains sodium 50 mg; equivalent to naproxen base 500 mg]

Mediproxen: 220 mg [contains sodium 20 mg; equivalent to naproxen base 200 mg]

Tablet, controlled release, oral, as sodium:

Naprelan®: 412.5 mg [contains sodium 37.5 mg; equivalent to naproxen base 375 mg]

Naprelan®: 550 mg [contains sodium 50 mg; equivalent to naproxen base 500 mg]

Naprelan®: 825 mg [contains sodium 75 mg; equivalent to naproxen base 750 mg]

Tablet, delayed release, enteric coated, oral: 375 mg, 500 mg

EC-Naprosyn®: 375 mg, 500 mg

- ◆ **Naproxen and Sumatriptan** *see* Sumatriptan and Naproxen *on page* 1612
- ◆ **Naproxen-NA (Can)** *see* Naproxen *on page* 1177
- ◆ **Naproxen-NA DF (Can)** *see* Naproxen *on page* 1177
- ◆ **Naproxen Sodium** *see* Naproxen *on page* 1177
- ◆ **Naproxen Sodium and Sumatriptan** *see* Sumatriptan and Naproxen *on page* 1612
- ◆ **Naproxen Sodium and Sumatriptan Succinate** *see* Sumatriptan and Naproxen *on page* 1612
- ◆ **Naproxen Sodium DS (Can)** *see* Naproxen *on page* 1177

Naratriptan (NAR a trip tan)

Brand Names: U.S. Amerge®

Brand Names: Canada Amerge®

Index Terms Naratriptan Hydrochloride

Pharmacologic Category Antimigraine Agent; Serotonin 5-$HT_{1B, 1D}$ Receptor Agonist

Additional Appendix Information

Antimigraine Drugs: 5-HT_1 Receptor Agonists *on page* 1878

Use Treatment of acute migraine headache with or without aura

Pregnancy Risk Factor C

Pregnancy Considerations There are no adequate and well-controlled studies using naratriptan in pregnant women. Use only if potential benefit to the mother outweighs the potential risk to the fetus. A pregnancy registry has been established to monitor outcomes of women exposed to naratriptan during pregnancy (800-336-2176). In animal studies, administration was associated with embryolethality, fetal abnormalities, and pup mortality and growth retardation. Tremors were observed in the offspring of female rats when exposed to naratriptan late in gestation.

Lactation Excretion in breast milk unknown/use caution

Contraindications Hypersensitivity to naratriptan or any component of the formulation; cerebrovascular, peripheral vascular disease (ischemic bowel disease), ischemic heart disease (angina pectoris, history of myocardial infarction, or proven silent ischemia); or in patients with symptoms consistent with ischemic heart disease, coronary artery vasospasm, or Prinzmetal's angina; uncontrolled hypertension or patients who have received within 24 hours another 5-HT agonist (sumatriptan, zolmitriptan) or ergotamine-containing product; patients with known risk factors associated with coronary artery disease; patients with severe hepatic (Child-Pugh grade C) or renal disease (Cl_{cr} <15 mL/minute); do not administer naratriptan to patients with hemiplegic or basilar migraine

Warnings/Precautions Use only if there is a clear diagnosis of migraine. Dosage reduction is required in mild-to-moderate hepatic impairment and moderate renal impairment; use is contraindicated in patients with severe hepatic or renal impairment. Do not give to patients with risk factors for CAD until a cardiovascular evaluation has been performed; if evaluation is satisfactory, the healthcare provider should administer the first dose (consider ECG monitoring) and cardiovascular status should be periodically re-evaluated. Cardiac events (coronary artery vasospasm, transient ischemia, myocardial infarction, ventricular tachycardia/fibrillation, cardiac arrest, and death), cerebral/subarachnoid hemorrhage, stroke, peripheral vascular ischemia, and colonic ischemia have been reported with 5-HT_1 agonist administration. Patients who experience sensations of chest pain/pressure/tightness or symptoms suggestive of angina following dosing should be evaluated for coronary artery disease or Prinzmetal's angina before receiving additional doses; if dosing is resumed and similar symptoms recur, monitor with ECG. Significant elevation in blood pressure, including hypertensive crisis, has also been reported on rare occasions in patients with and without a history of hypertension. Only indicated for the acute treatment of migraine; not indicated for migraine prophylaxis, or for the treatment of cluster headache, hemiplegic or basilar migraine. If a patient does not respond to the first dose, the diagnosis of migraine should be reconsidered; rule out underlying neurologic disease in patients with atypical headache and in patients with no prior history of migraine.

Symptoms of agitation, confusion, hallucinations, hyperreflexia, myoclonus, shivering, and tachycardia may occur with concomitant proserotonergic drugs (ie, SSRIs/SNRIs or triptans) or agents which reduce naratriptan's metabolism. Concurrent use of serotonin precursors (eg, tryptophan) is not recommended. If concomitant administration with SSRIs is warranted, monitor closely, especially at initiation and with dose increases.

Adverse Reactions

1% to 10%:

Central nervous system: Pain/pressure (2% to 4%), malaise/fatigue (2%), dizziness (1% to 2%), drowsiness (1% to 2%), vertigo (1%)

Gastrointestinal: Nausea (4% to 5%), hyposalivation (1%), vomiting (1%)

Neuromuscular & skeletal: Paresthesia (1% to 2%)

Ocular: Photophobia (1%)

Miscellaneous: Ear/nose/throat infection (1%), pressure/tightness/heaviness sensations (1%), warm/cold temperature sensations (1%)

<1% (Limited to important or life-threatening): Abnormal bilirubin tests, abnormal liver function tests, anaphylactoid reaction, anaphylaxis, anemia, bradycardia, cerebral infarction, colonic ischemia, coronary artery vasospasm, depression, dyspnea, ECG changes (atrial fibrillation, atrial flutter, premature ventricular contractions, PR prolongation, or QT_c prolongation), eye hemorrhage, glycosuria, hallucinations, heart murmurs, hypercholesterolemia, hyperglycemia, hyper-/hypotension, hyperlipidemia, hypothyroidism, hypersensitivity reaction, ketonuria, MI, palpitation, panic, rash, seizure, serotonin syndrome, syncope, subarachnoid hemorrhage, thrombocytopenia, TIA, transient myocardial ischemia, ventricular fibrillation, ventricular tachycardia

Drug Interactions

Metabolism/Transport Effects None known.

Avoid Concomitant Use

Avoid concomitant use of Naratriptan with any of the following: Ergot Derivatives

Increased Effect/Toxicity

Naratriptan may increase the levels/effects of: Ergot Derivatives; Metoclopramide; Serotonin Modulators

The levels/effects of Naratriptan may be increased by: Antipsychotics; Ergot Derivatives

Decreased Effect There are no known significant interactions involving a decrease in effect.

Stability Store at 20°C to 25°C (68°F to 77°F).

Mechanism of Action Selective agonist for serotonin ($5\text{-}HT_{1B}$ and $5\text{-}HT_{1D}$ receptors) in cranial arteries; causes vasoconstriction and reduces sterile inflammation associated with antidromic neuronal transmission correlating with relief of migraine

Pharmacodynamics/Kinetics

Onset of action: ~1-2 hours (Bomhof, 1999; Tfelt-Hansen, 2000)

Absorption: Well absorbed

Distribution: V_{dss}: 170 L

Protein binding, plasma: 28% to 31%

Metabolism: Hepatic via CYP

Bioavailability: ~70%

Half life, elimination: 6 hours; increased in renal impairment (moderate impairment; mean: 11 hours; range 7-20 hours); increased in hepatic impairment (moderate impairment: 8-16 hours)

Time to peak: 2-3 hours

Excretion: Urine (50% of total dose as unchanged drug; 30% of total dose as metabolites)

Dosage

Adults: Oral: 1-2.5 mg at the onset of headache; it is recommended to use the lowest possible dose to minimize adverse effects. If headache returns or does not fully resolve, the dose may be repeated after 4 hours; do not exceed 5 mg in 24 hours.

Elderly: Not recommended for use in the elderly

Dosing in renal impairment:

Mild-to-moderate renal impairment: Initial: 1 mg; do not exceed 2.5 mg in 24 hours

Severe renal impairment (Cl_{cr} <15 mL/minute): Use is contraindicated

Dosing in hepatic impairment:

Mild-to-moderate hepatic impairment (Child-Pugh grade A or B): Initial: 1 mg; do not exceed 2.5 mg in 24 hours

Severe hepatic impairment (Child-Pugh grade C): Use is contraindicated

Administration Do **not** crush or chew tablet; swallow whole with water.

Dosage Forms Excipient information presented when available (limited, particularly for generics); consult specific product labeling.

Tablet, oral: 1 mg, 2.5 mg

Amerge®: 1 mg, 2.5 mg

Extemporaneous Preparations A 0.5 mg/mL oral suspension may be made using tablets. Crush fifty 2.5 mg tablets and reduce to a fine powder. In small amounts, add 125 mL of Ora-Plus® and mix well after each addition. Transfer to a calibrated bottle, rinse mortar with vehicle, then add quantity of Ora-Sweet® or Ora-Sweet® SF sufficient to make 250 mL. Label "shake well" and "refrigerate". Stable 90 days refrigerated.

Nahata MC, Pai VB, and Hipple TF, *Pediatric Drug Formulations*, 5th ed, Cincinnati, OH: Harvey Whitney Books Co, 2004.

◆ **Naratriptan Hydrochloride** *see* Naratriptan *on page 1180*

◆ **Narcan** *see* Naloxone *on page 1173*

◆ **Nardil®** *see* Phenelzine *on page 1337*

◆ **Naropin®** *see* Ropivacaine *on page 1520*

◆ **Nasacort® AQ** *see* Triamcinolone (Nasal) *on page 1734*

◆ **NasalCrom® [OTC]** *see* Cromolyn (Nasal) *on page 418*

◆ **Nasalide® (Can)** *see* Flunisolide (Nasal) *on page 726*

◆ **Nasal Moist® Saline [OTC]** *see* Sodium Chloride *on page 1567*

◆ **Nasal Spray [OTC] [DSC]** *see* Sodium Chloride *on page 1567*

◆ **Nascobal®** *see* Cyanocobalamin *on page 418*

◆ **Nasonex®** *see* Mometasone (Nasal) *on page 1151*

◆ **Natacyn®** *see* Natamycin *on page 1182*

Natalizumab (na ta LIZ u mab)

Brand Names: U.S. Tysabri®

Brand Names: Canada Tysabri®

Index Terms AN100226; Anti-4 Alpha Integrin; IgG4-Kappa Monoclonal Antibody

Pharmacologic Category Gastrointestinal Agent, Miscellaneous; Monoclonal Antibody, Selective Adhesion-Molecule Inhibitor

Use Monotherapy for the treatment of relapsing forms of multiple sclerosis; treatment of moderately- to severely-active Crohn's disease

Canada labeling: Treatment of relapsing forms of multiple sclerosis

Pregnancy Risk Factor C

Prescribing and Access Restrictions

U.S.: Tysabri® is deemed to have an approved REMS program. As a requirement of the REMS program, access to this medication is restricted. Patients must be enrolled in the Tysabri® Outreach Unified Commitment to Health (TOUCH™) Prescribing Program (800-456-2255) to receive natalizumab (MS-TOUCH™ for multiple sclerosis or CD-TOUCH™ for Crohn's disease). Healthcare providers must also register with the program in order to prescribe, dispense or administer natalizumab. Treatment must be reauthorized every 6 months. Natalizumab is available only through infusion centers registered with the TOUCH™ program; infusion center information is available at 1-800-456-2255.

Canada: Patients receiving natalizumab therapy for multiple sclerosis are to be enrolled in the Tysabri Care Program™ (888-827-2827). This program is associated with the prescribing, administration, and monitoring of Canadian patients receiving natalizumab. Clinicians are educated on the appropriate use of natalizumab and are expected to discuss the benefits/risks of therapy. Clinicians should evaluate patients every 6 months during treatment.

Medication Guide Available Yes

Dosage I.V.: Adults:

Multiple sclerosis: 300 mg infused over 1 hour every 4 weeks

Crohn's disease: 300 mg infused over 1 hour every 4 weeks; discontinue if therapeutic benefit is not observed within initial 12 weeks of therapy

Concomitant use with corticosteroids: For patients who begin treatment while on chronic oral corticosteroids, begin tapering oral steroids when the onset of natalizumab therapeutic benefit is observed; discontinue use if patient cannot be tapered off of oral corticosteroids within 6 months of therapy initiation. If additional concomitant corticosteroids are required and exceed 3 months/year (in addition to initial corticosteroid taper), consider discontinuing therapy.

Dosage adjustment in renal impairment: Not studied

Dosage adjustment in hepatic impairment: Not studied. Discontinue use with jaundice or signs/symptoms of hepatic injury.

Additional Information Complete prescribing information for this medication should be consulted for additional detail.

Dosage Forms Excipient information presented when available (limited, particularly for generics); consult specific product labeling.

Injection, solution [preservative free]:

Tysabri®: 300 mg/15 mL (15 mL) [contains polysorbate 80]

Natamycin (na ta MYE sin)

Brand Names: U.S. Natacyn®

Brand Names: Canada Natacyn®

Index Terms Pimaricin

Pharmacologic Category Antifungal Agent, Ophthalmic

Use Treatment of blepharitis, conjunctivitis, and keratitis caused by susceptible fungi (*Aspergillus*, *Candida*, *Cephalosporium*, *Fusarium*, and *Penicillium*)

Pregnancy Risk Factor C

Dosage Adults: Ophthalmic:

Fungal keratitis: Instill 1 drop in conjunctival sac every 1-2 hours, after 3-4 days reduce to one drop 6-8 times/day; usual course of therapy is 2-3 weeks or until resolution of active fungal keratitis (may be useful to gradually reduce dosage at 4-7 day intervals to assure elimination of organism)

Fungal blepharitis or conjunctivitis: Instill 1 drop in conjunctival sac every 4-6 hours

Additional Information Complete prescribing information for this medication should be consulted for additional detail.

Dosage Forms Excipient information presented when available (limited, particularly for generics); consult specific product labeling.

Suspension, ophthalmic [drops]:

Natacyn®: 5% (15 mL) [contains benzalkonium chloride]

◆ **Natazia™** *see* Estradiol and Dienogest *on page 634*

Nateglinide (na te GLYE nide)

Brand Names: U.S. Starlix®

Brand Names: Canada Starlix®

Pharmacologic Category Antidiabetic Agent, Meglitinide Derivative

Additional Appendix Information

Diabetes Mellitus Management, Adults *on page 1983*

Use Management of type 2 diabetes mellitus (noninsulin dependent, NIDDM) as monotherapy when hyperglycemia cannot be managed by diet and exercise alone; in combination with metformin or a thiazolidinedione to lower blood glucose in patients whose hyperglycemia cannot be controlled by exercise, diet, or a single agent alone

Pregnancy Risk Factor C

Pregnancy Considerations Adverse events have been observed in animal reproduction studies; therefore, nateglinide is classified as pregnancy category C. Information describing the effects of nateglinide on pregnancy outcomes is limited. Maternal hyperglycemia can be associated with adverse effects in the fetus, including macrosomia, neonatal hyperglycemia, and hyperbilirubinemia; the risk of congenital malformations is increased when the Hb A_{1c} is above the normal range. Diabetes can also be associated with adverse effects in the mother. Poorly-treated diabetes may cause end-organ damage that may in turn negatively affect obstetric outcomes. Physiologic glucose levels should be maintained prior to and during pregnancy to decrease the risk of adverse events in the mother and the fetus. Until additional safety and efficacy data are obtained, the use of oral agents is generally not recommended as routine management of GDM or type 2 diabetes mellitus during pregnancy. Insulin is the drug of choice for the control of diabetes mellitus during pregnancy.

Lactation Excretion in breast milk unknown/not recommended

Contraindications Hypersensitivity to nateglinide or any component of the formulation; diabetic ketoacidosis, with or without coma (treat with insulin); type 1 diabetes mellitus (insulin dependent, IDDM)

Warnings/Precautions Use with caution in patients with moderate-to-severe hepatic impairment. Use caution in severe renal dysfunction, elderly, malnourished, or patients with adrenal/pituitary dysfunction; may be more susceptible to glucose-lowering effects. All oral hypoglycemic agents are capable of producing hypoglycemia. Proper patient selection, dosage, and instructions to the patients are important to avoid hypoglycemic episodes. It may be necessary to discontinue nateglinide and administer insulin if the patient is exposed to stress (ie, fever, trauma, infection, surgery). Indicated for adjunctive therapy with metformin; not to be used as a substitute for metformin monotherapy. Combination treatment with sulfonylureas is not recommended (no additional benefit). Patients not adequately controlled on oral agents which stimulate insulin release (eg, glyburide) should not be switched to nateglinide or have nateglinide added to therapy.

Adverse Reactions As reported with nateglinide monotherapy:

>10%: Respiratory: Upper respiratory infection (11%)

1% to 10%:

Central nervous system: Dizziness (4%)

Endocrine & metabolic: Hypoglycemia (2%), uric acid increased

Gastrointestinal: Diarrhea (3%), weight gain

Neuromuscular & skeletal: Back pain, (4%), arthropathy (3%)

Respiratory: Bronchitis (3%), cough (2%)

Miscellaneous: Flu-like syndrome (4%)

Postmarketing and/or case reports: Cholestatic hepatitis, hypersensitivity reactions (including pruritus, rash, urticaria), jaundice, liver enzymes increased

Drug Interactions

Metabolism/Transport Effects Substrate of CYP2C9 (major), CYP3A4 (major), SLCO1B1; **Note:** Assignment of Major/Minor substrate status based on clinically relevant drug interaction potential; **Inhibits** CYP2C9 (weak)

Avoid Concomitant Use

Avoid concomitant use of Nateglinide with any of the following: Conivaptan

Increased Effect/Toxicity

Nateglinide may increase the levels/effects of: Hypoglycemic Agents

The levels/effects of Nateglinide may be increased by: Conivaptan; CYP2C9 Inhibitors (Moderate); CYP2C9 Inhibitors (Strong); CYP3A4 Inhibitors (Moderate); CYP3A4 Inhibitors (Strong); Dasatinib; Eltrombopag; Herbs (Hypoglycemic Properties); Pegvisomant

Decreased Effect

The levels/effects of Nateglinide may be decreased by: Corticosteroids (Orally Inhaled); Corticosteroids (Systemic); CYP2C9 Inducers (Strong); CYP3A4 Inducers (Strong); Deferasirox; Herbs (CYP3A4 Inducers); Luteinizing Hormone-Releasing Hormone Analogs; Peginterferon Alfa-2b; Somatropin; Thiazide Diuretics; Tocilizumab

Ethanol/Nutrition/Herb Interactions

Ethanol: Avoid ethanol (increased risk of hypoglycemia).

Food: Rate of absorption is decreased and time to T_{max} is delayed when taken with food. Food does not affect AUC. Multiple peak plasma concentrations may be observed if fasting. Not affected by composition of meal.

Herb/Nutraceutical: Avoid alfalfa, aloe, bilberry, bitter melon, burdock, celery, damiana, fenugreek, garcinia, garlic, ginger, ginseng (American), gymnema, marshmallow, and stinging nettle (may enhance the hypoglycemic effects of antidiabetic agents). St. John's wort may decrease the levels/effect of nateglinide.

Stability Store at 25°C (77°F).

Mechanism of Action A phenylalanine derivative, nonsulfonylurea hypoglycemic agent used in the management of type 2 diabetes mellitus (noninsulin dependent, NIDDM); stimulates insulin release from the pancreatic beta cells to reduce postprandial hyperglycemia; amount of insulin release is dependent upon existing glucose levels

Pharmacodynamics/Kinetics

Onset of action: Insulin secretion: ~20 minutes

Peak effect: 1 hour

Duration: 4 hours

Absorption: Rapid

Distribution: 10 L

Protein binding: 98%, primarily to albumin

Metabolism: Hepatic via hydroxylation followed by glucuronide conjugation via CYP2C9 (70%) and CYP3A4 (30%) to metabolites

Bioavailability: 73%

Half-life elimination: 1.5 hours

Time to peak: ≤1 hour

Excretion: Urine (83%, 16% as unchanged drug); feces (10%)

Dosage

Adults: Management of type 2 diabetes mellitus: Oral: Initial and maintenance dose: 120 mg 3 times/day, 1-30 minutes before meals; may be given alone or in combination with metformin or a thiazolidinedione; patients close to Hb A_{1c} goal may be started at 60 mg 3 times/day

Elderly: No changes in safety and efficacy were seen in patients ≥65 years; however, some elderly patients may show increased sensitivity to dosing

Dosage adjustment in renal impairment: No specific dosage adjustment is recommended for patients with mild-to-severe renal disease; patients on dialysis showed reduced medication exposure and plasma protein binding. Patients with severe renal dysfunction are more susceptible to glucose-lowering effect; use with caution.

Dosage adjustment in hepatic impairment: Increased serum levels seen with mild hepatic insufficiency; no dosage adjustment is needed. Has not been studied in patients with moderate-to-severe liver disease; use with caution.

Dietary Considerations Nateglinide should be taken 1-30 minutes prior to meals. Scheduled dose should not be taken if meal is missed. Dietary modification based on ADA recommendations is a part of therapy. Decreases blood glucose concentration. Hypoglycemia may occur. Must be able to recognize symptoms of hypoglycemia (palpitations, sweaty palms, lightheadedness).

Administration Patients who are anorexic or NPO will need to have their dose held to avoid hypoglycemia.

Monitoring Parameters Glucose and Hb A_{1c} levels, weight, lipid profile

Reference Range Recommendations for glycemic control in adults with diabetes:

Hb A_{1c}: <7%

Preprandial capillary plasma glucose: 70-130 mg/dL

Peak postprandial capillary blood glucose: <180 mg/dL

Blood pressure: <130/80 mm Hg

Additional Information An increase in weight was seen in nateglinide monotherapy, which was not seen when used in combination with metformin.

Dosage Forms Excipient information presented when available (limited, particularly for generics); consult specific product labeling.

Tablet, oral: 60 mg, 120 mg

Starlix®: 60 mg, 120 mg

- ◆ **Natrecor®** *see* Nesiritide *on page 1191*
- ◆ **Natriuretic Peptide** *see* Nesiritide *on page 1191*
- ◆ **Natroba™** *see* Spinosad *on page 1590*
- ◆ **NatrOVA** *see* Spinosad *on page 1590*
- ◆ **Natulan® (Can)** *see* Procarbazine *on page 1410*
- ◆ **Natural Fiber Therapy [OTC]** *see* Psyllium *on page 1432*
- ◆ **Natural Fiber Therapy Smooth Texture [OTC]** *see* Psyllium *on page 1432*
- ◆ **Natural Lung Surfactant** *see* Beractant *on page 206*
- ◆ **Nature-Throid™** *see* Thyroid, Desiccated *on page 1676*
- ◆ **Nauseatol (Can)** *see* DimenhyDRINATE *on page 513*
- ◆ **Navane® [DSC]** *see* Thiothixene *on page 1675*
- ◆ **Navane® (Can)** *see* Thiothixene *on page 1675*
- ◆ **Navelbine®** *see* Vinorelbine *on page 1793*
- ◆ **Na-Zone® [OTC]** *see* Sodium Chloride *on page 1567*
- ◆ **N-Carbamoyl-L-Glutamic Acid** *see* Carglumic Acid *on page 291*
- ◆ **N-Carbamylglutamate** *see* Carglumic Acid *on page 291*
- ◆ ***n*-Docosanol** *see* Docosanol *on page 537*

Nebivolol (ne BIV oh lole)

Brand Names: U.S. Bystolic®

Index Terms Nebivolol Hydrochloride

Pharmacologic Category Beta Blocker, Beta-1 Selective

Additional Appendix Information

Beta-Blockers *on page 1884*

Use Treatment of hypertension, alone or in combination with other agents

Unlabeled Use Heart failure

Pregnancy Risk Factor C

Dosage Oral:

Adults:

Hypertension: Initial: 5 mg once daily; if initial response is inadequate, may be increased at 2-week intervals to a maximum dose of 40 mg once daily

Heart failure (unlabeled use): Adults ≥70 years: Initial: 1.25 mg once daily; if tolerated, may increase by 2.5 mg at 1- to 2-week intervals to a maximum dose of 10 mg once daily (Flather, 2005). **Note:** Nebivolol has not been shown to reduce morbidity or mortality in the general HF population.

Elderly: Refer to adult dosing.

Dosing adjustment in renal impairment: Severe impairment (Cl_{cr} <30 mL/minute): Initial: 2.5 mg/day; increase cautiously

Dosage adjustment in hepatic impairment: Moderate impairment (Child-Pugh class B): Initial: 2.5 mg/day; increase cautiously

Additional Information Complete prescribing information for this medication should be consulted for additional detail.

Dosage Forms Excipient information presented when available (limited, particularly for generics); consult specific product labeling.

Tablet, oral:

Bystolic®: 2.5 mg, 5 mg, 10 mg, 20 mg

- ◆ **Nebivolol Hydrochloride** *see* Nebivolol *on page 1183*
- ◆ **Nebupent®** *see* Pentamidine *on page 1327*
- ◆ **Necon® 0.5/35** *see* Ethinyl Estradiol and Norethindrone *on page 660*
- ◆ **Necon® 1/35** *see* Ethinyl Estradiol and Norethindrone *on page 660*
- ◆ **Necon® 1/50** *see* Norethindrone and Mestranol *on page 1219*

◆ **Necon® 7/7/7** *see* Ethinyl Estradiol and Norethindrone *on page 660*

◆ **Necon® 10/11** *see* Ethinyl Estradiol and Norethindrone *on page 660*

Nedocromil (ne doe KROE mil)

Brand Names: U.S. Alocril®
Brand Names: Canada Alocril®
Index Terms Nedocromil Sodium
Pharmacologic Category Mast Cell Stabilizer
Additional Appendix Information
Asthma *on page 1967*
Use Treatment of itching associated with allergic conjunctivitis
Pregnancy Risk Factor B
Dosage Ophthalmic: Children ≥3 years and Adults: 1-2 drops in each eye twice daily daily throughout the period of exposure to allergen
Additional Information Complete prescribing information for this medication should be consulted for additional detail.
Dosage Forms Excipient information presented when available (limited, particularly for generics); consult specific product labeling.
Solution, ophthalmic, as sodium [drops]:
Alocril®: 2% (5 mL) [contains benzalkonium chloride]

◆ **Nedocromil Sodium** *see* Nedocromil *on page 1184*

Nefazodone (nef AY zoe done)

Index Terms Nefazodone Hydrochloride; Serzone
Pharmacologic Category Antidepressant, Serotonin Reuptake Inhibitor/Antagonist
Additional Appendix Information
Antidepressant Agents *on page 1874*
Use Treatment of depression
Unlabeled Use Post-traumatic stress disorder (PTSD)
Pregnancy Risk Factor C
Medication Guide Available Yes
Dosage Oral:
Adults:
Depression: 200 mg/day, administered in 2 divided doses initially, with a range of 300-600 mg/day in 2 divided doses thereafter
Post-traumatic stress disorder (PTSD) (unlabeled use): Initial: 100 mg twice daily; target dose: 600 mg/day (average daily dose: 463 mg)
Elderly: Initial: 50 mg twice daily; increase dose to 100 mg twice daily in 2 weeks; usual maintenance dose: 200-400 mg/day
Additional Information Complete prescribing information for this medication should be consulted for additional detail.
Dosage Forms Excipient information presented when available (limited, particularly for generics); consult specific product labeling.
Tablet, oral, as hydrochloride: 50 mg, 100 mg, 150 mg, 200 mg, 250 mg

◆ **Nefazodone Hydrochloride** *see* Nefazodone *on page 1184*

Nelarabine (nel AY re been)

Brand Names: U.S. Arranon®
Brand Names: Canada Atriance™
Index Terms 2-Amino-6-Methoxypurine Arabinoside; 506U78; GW506U78
Pharmacologic Category Antineoplastic Agent, Antimetabolite
Use Treatment of relapsed or refractory T-cell acute lymphoblastic leukemia (ALL) and T-cell lymphoblastic lymphoma
Pregnancy Risk Factor D
Pregnancy Considerations Teratogenic effects were observed in animal studies. There are no adequate and well-controlled studies in pregnant women. May cause fetal harm if administered during pregnancy. Women of childbearing potential should be advised to use effective contraception and avoid becoming pregnant during therapy.
Lactation Excretion in breast milk unknown/not recommended
Contraindications There are no contraindications listed within the manufacturer's labeling.
Warnings/Precautions Hazardous agent - use appropriate precautions for handling and disposal. **[U.S. Boxed Warning]: Severe neurotoxicity, including severe somnolence, seizure, and peripheral neuropathy, has been reported. Observe closely for signs and symptoms of neurotoxicity; discontinue if ≥ grade 2. Adverse effects associated with demyelination or similar to Guillain-Barré syndrome (ascending peripheral neuropathies) have also been reported. Neurologic toxicities may not fully return to baseline after treatment cessation.** Neurologic toxicity is dose-limiting. Risk of neurotoxicity may increase in patients with concurrent or previous intrathecal chemotherapy or history of craniospinal irradiation. Appropriate measures must be taken to prevent hyperuricemia and tumor lysis syndrome; use extreme caution in patients with increased uric acid, gout, and history of uric acid stones; monitor, consider allopurinol and hydrate accordingly. Bone marrow suppression, including leukopenia, thrombocytopenia, anemia, neutropenia and febrile neutropenia are associated with treatment; monitor blood counts regularly. Avoid administration of live vaccines. Use caution in patients with renal impairment; ara-G clearance may be reduced with renal dysfunction. Use caution with severe hepatic impairment; risk of adverse reactions may be higher with hepatic dysfunction.
Adverse Reactions Note: Pediatric adverse reactions fell within a range similar to adults except where noted.
>10%:
Cardiovascular: Peripheral edema (15%), edema (11%)
Central nervous system: Fatigue (50%), fever (23%), somnolence (7% to 23%; grades 2-4: 1% to 6%), dizziness (21%; grade 2: 8% adults), headache (15% to 17%; grades 2-4: 4% to 8%), hypoesthesia (6% to 17%; grades 2/3: children 5%, adults 12%), pain (11%)
Dermatologic: Petechiae (12%)
Endocrine & metabolic: Hypokalemia (11%)
Gastrointestinal: Nausea (41%), diarrhea (22%), vomiting (10% to 22%), constipation (21%)
Hematologic: Anemia (95% to 99%; grade 4: 10% to 14%), neutropenia (81% to 94%; grade 4: children 62%, adults 49%), thrombocytopenia (86% to 88%; grade 4: 22% to 32%), leukopenia (38%; grade 4: 7%), febrile neutropenia (12%; grade 4: 1%)
Hepatic: Transaminases increased (12%; grade 3: 4%)
Neuromuscular & skeletal: Peripheral neuropathy (12% to 21%; grades 2/3: 11% to 14%), weakness (6% to 17%; grade 4: 1%), paresthesia (4% to 15%; grades 2/3: 3% to 4%), myalgia (13%)
Respiratory: Cough (25%), dyspnea (7% to 20%)
1% to 10%:
Cardiovascular: Hypotension (8%), sinus tachycardia (8%), chest pain (5%)

Central nervous system: Ataxia (2% to 9%; grades 2/3: children 1%, adults 8%), confusion (8%), insomnia (7%), depressed level of consciousness (6%; grades 2-4: 2%), depression (6%), seizure (grade 3: 1% adults; grade 4: 6% children), motor dysfunction (4%; grades 2/3: 2%), amnesia (3%; grade 2: 1%), balance disorder (2%; grade 2: 1%), sensory loss (1% to 2%), aphasia (grade 3: 1%), attention disturbance (1%), cerebral hemorrhage (grade 4: 1%), coma (grade 4: 1%), encephalopathy (grade 4: 1%), hemiparesis (grade 3: 1%), hydrocephalus (1%), intracranial hemorrhage (grade 4: 1%), lethargy (1%), leukoencephalopathy (grade 4: 1%), loss of consciousness (grade 3: 1%), mental impairment (1%), nerve paralysis (1%), neuropathic pain (1%), nerve palsy (1%), paralysis (1%), sciatica (1%), sensory disturbance (1%), speech disorder (1%)

Endocrine & Metabolic: Hypocalcemia (8%), dehydration (7%), hyper-/hypoglycemia (6%), hypomagnesemia (6%)

Gastrointestinal: Abdominal pain (9%), anorexia (9%), stomatitis (8%), abdominal distension (6%), taste perversion (3%)

Hepatic: Albumin decreased (10%), bilirubin increased (10%; grade 3: 7%, grade 4: 2%), AST increased (6%)

Neuromuscular & skeletal: Arthralgia (9%), back pain (8%), muscle weakness (8%), rigors (8%), limb pain (7%), abnormal gait (6%), noncardiac chest pain (5%), tremor (4% to 5%; grade 2: 2% to 3%), dysarthria (1%), hyporeflexia (1%), hypertonia (1%), incoordination (1%)

Ocular: Blurred vision (4%), nystagmus (1%)

Renal: Creatinine increased (6%)

Respiratory: Pleural effusion (10%), epistaxis (8%), pneumonia (8%), sinusitis (7%), wheezing (5%), sinus headache (1%)

Miscellaneous: Infection (5% to 9%)

<1% (Limited to important or life-threatening): Ascending peripheral neuropathy (similar to Guillain-Barré syndrome), demyelination, opportunistic infection, pneumothorax, progressive multifocal leukoencephalopathy, respiratory arrest, tumor lysis syndrome

Drug Interactions

Metabolism/Transport Effects None known.

Avoid Concomitant Use

Avoid concomitant use of Nelarabine with any of the following: BCG; CloZAPine; Natalizumab; Pentostatin; Pimecrolimus; Tacrolimus (Topical); Vaccines (Live)

Increased Effect/Toxicity

Nelarabine may increase the levels/effects of: CloZAPine; Leflunomide; Natalizumab; Vaccines (Live)

The levels/effects of Nelarabine may be increased by: Denosumab; Pimecrolimus; Roflumilast; Tacrolimus (Topical); Trastuzumab

Decreased Effect

Nelarabine may decrease the levels/effects of: BCG; Coccidioidin Skin Test; Sipuleucel-T; Vaccines (Inactivated); Vaccines (Live)

The levels/effects of Nelarabine may be decreased by: Echinacea; Pentostatin

Stability Store unopened vials at 25°C (77°F); excursions permitted to 15°C to 30°C (59°F to 86°F). Reconstitution is not required; the appropriate dose should be added to empty plastic bag or glass container. Use appropriate precautions for handling and disposal. Stable in plastic or glass containers for up to 8 hours at room temperature.

Mechanism of Action Nelarabine, a prodrug of ara-G, is demethylated by adenosine deaminase to ara-G and then converted to ara-GTP. Ara-GTP is incorporated into the DNA of the leukemic blasts, leading to inhibition of DNA synthesis and inducing apoptosis. Ara-GTP appears to accumulate at higher levels in T-cells, which correlates to clinical response.

Pharmacodynamics/Kinetics

Distribution: V_{ss}:

Nelarabine: Children: ~213 L/m^2; Adults: ~197 L/m^2

Ara-G: Children: ~33 L/m^2; Adults: ~50 L/m^2

Protein binding: Nelarabine and ara-G: <25%

Metabolism: Hepatic; demethylated by adenosine deaminase to form ara-G (active); also hydrolyzed to form methylguanine. Both ara-G and methylguanine metabolized to guanine. Guanine is deaminated into xanthine, which is further oxidized to form uric acid, which is then oxidized to form allantoin.

Half-life elimination: Children: Nelarabine: 13 minutes, Ara-G: 2 hours; Adults: Nelarabine: 18 minutes, Ara-G: 3 hours

Time to peak: Ara-G: Adults: 3-25 hours (day 1)

Excretion: Urine (nelarabine 7%, ara-G 27%) within 24 hours of infusion on day 1

Dosage I.V.: T-cell ALL, T-cell lymphoblastic lymphoma:

Children: 650 mg/m^2/dose on days 1 through 5; repeat every 21 days

Adults: 1500 mg/m^2/dose on days 1, 3, and 5; repeat every 21 days

Dosage adjustment for toxicity:

Neurologic toxicity ≥ grade 2: Discontinue treatment.

Hematologic or other (non-neurologic) toxicity: Consider treatment delay.

Dosage adjustment in renal impairment:

Cl_{cr} ≥50 mL/minute: No adjustment recommended

Cl_{cr} <50 mL/minute: Data is insufficient for a dosing recommendation; monitor closely

Dosage adjustment in hepatic impairment: Safety has not been established; closely monitor with severe impairment (bilirubin >3 times ULN)

Administration Adequate I.V. hydration recommended to prevent tumor lysis syndrome; allopurinol may be used if hyperuricemia is anticipated.

Children: Infuse over 1 hour daily for 5 consecutive days

Adults: Infuse over 2 hours on days 1, 3, and 5

Monitoring Parameters Closely monitor for neurologic toxicity (severe somnolence, seizure, peripheral neuropathy, confusion, ataxia, paresthesia, hypoesthesia, coma, or craniospinal demyelination); signs and symptoms of tumor lysis syndrome; hydration status; CBC with platelet counts, liver and kidney function

Dosage Forms Excipient information presented when available (limited, particularly for generics); consult specific product labeling.

Injection, solution:

Arranon®: 5 mg/mL (50 mL)

Dosage Forms: Canada Excipient information presented when available (limited, particularly for generics); consult specific product labeling.

Injection, solution:

Atriance™: 5 mg/mL (50 mL)

Nelfinavir (nel FIN a veer)

Brand Names: U.S. Viracept®

Brand Names: Canada Viracept®

Index Terms NFV

Pharmacologic Category Antiretroviral Agent, Protease Inhibitor

Additional Appendix Information

Management of Healthcare Worker Exposures to HBV, HCV, and HIV *on page 1935*

Perinatal HIV Guidelines *on page 1946*

Use In combination with other antiretroviral therapy in the treatment of HIV infection

Pregnancy Risk Factor B

Pregnancy Considerations Adverse events were not observed in animal reproduction studies. Nelfinavir crosses the placenta. No increased risk of overall birth defects has been observed following first trimester exposure in humans according to data collected by the antiretroviral pregnancy registry. The DHHS Perinatal HIV Guidelines recommend nelfinavir to be used only in special circumstances during pregnancy for the prophylaxis of perinatal transmission in antiretroviral-naive women when alternative agents cannot be tolerated. A dose of 1250 mg twice daily has been shown to provide adequate plasma concentrations although lower and variable levels may occur late in pregnancy. A small increased risk of preterm birth has been associated with maternal use of protease inhibitor-based combination antiretroviral (ARV) therapy during pregnancy; however, the benefits of use generally outweigh this risk and protease inhibitors (PIs) should not be withheld if otherwise recommended. Hyperglycemia, new onset of diabetes mellitus, or diabetic ketoacidosis have been reported with PIs; it is not clear if pregnancy increases this risk.

Regardless of CD4 count or HIV RNA copy number, all HIV-infected pregnant women should receive a combination antepartum ARV drug regimen; this includes women who require therapy for their own health, as well as women who do not yet require therapy for their own health. ARV therapy should be started as soon as possible if required for the woman's health or immediately after the first trimester if not needed for the mothers health (although earlier initiation may be considered). Long-term follow-up is recommended for all infants exposed to ARV medications.

Healthcare providers are encouraged to enroll pregnant women exposed to antiretroviral medications in the Antiretroviral Pregnancy Registry (1-800-258-4263 or www.-APRegistry.com). Healthcare providers caring for HIV-infected women and their infants may contact the National Perinatal HIV Hotline (888-448-8765) for clinical consultation (DHHS [perinatal], 2011).

Lactation Excretion in breast milk unknown/contraindicated

Contraindications Hypersensitivity to nelfinavir or any component of the formulation; concurrent therapy with alfuzosin, amiodarone, ergot derivatives, midazolam, pimozide, quinidine, sildenafil (when used for pulmonary artery hypertension [eg, Revatio®]), triazolam

Warnings/Precautions Use with caution in patients taking strong CYP3A4 inhibitors, moderate or strong CYP3A4 inducers and major CYP3A4 substrates and if coadministered with QT-prolonging drugs that are metabolized by CYP3A (see Drug Interactions); consider alternative agents that avoid or lessen the potential for CYP-mediated interactions. Not recommended for use with rifampin, St John's wort, lovastatin, simvastatin, phosphodiesterase-5 (PDE-5) inhibitors, or proton pump inhibitors (based on omeprazole data). Do not coadminister colchicine in patient with renal or hepatic impairment; avoid concurrent use with salmeterol.

Use caution with hepatic impairment; use not recommended with moderate-to-severe impairment. Warn patients that redistribution of body fat can occur. New-onset diabetes mellitus, exacerbation of diabetes, and hyperglycemia have been reported in HIV-infected patients receiving protease inhibitors. Use with caution in patients with hemophilia A or B; increased bleeding during protease inhibitor therapy has been reported. Immune reconstitution syndrome has been reported; may require additional evaluation and treatment. The oral powder contains phenylalanine. Safety and efficacy have not been established in children <2 years of age.

Adverse Reactions Data presented on experience in adults, unless otherwise noted.

>10%: Gastrointestinal: Diarrhea (14% to 20%; children: 39% to 47%)

2% to 10%:

Dermatologic: Rash (1% to 3%)

Gastrointestinal: Nausea (3% to 7%), flatulence (1% to 5%)

Hematologic: Lymphocytes decreased (1% to 6%), neutrophils decreased (1% to 5%)

<2% (Limited to important or life-threatening): Abdominal pain, acute iritis, alkaline phosphatase increased, allergic reaction, amylase increased, anemia, anorexia, anxiety, arthralgia, arthritis, back pain, bilirubinemia, body fat redistribution/accumulation, cramps, creatine phosphokinase increased, dehydration, depression, dermatitis, diaphoresis, dizziness, dyspepsia, dyspnea, emotional lability, epigastric pain, eye disorder, fever, folliculitis, fungal dermatitis, gastrointestinal bleeding, GGTP increased, headache, hepatitis, hyperkinesia, hyper-/hypoglycemia, hyperlipemia; hypersensitivity reaction (bronchospasm, rash, edema); hyperuricemia, immune reconstitution syndrome, insomnia, jaundice, kidney calculus, lactic dehydrogenase increased, leukopenia, lipoatrophy, lipodystrophy, liver function tests abnormal, maculopapular rash, malaise, metabolic acidosis, migraine, mouth ulceration, myalgia, myasthenia, myopathy, pain, pancreatitis, paresthesia, pharyngitis, pruritus, QT_c prolongation, rhinitis, seizure, sexual dysfunction, sinusitis, sleep disorder, somnolence, suicidal ideation, thrombocytopenia, torsade de pointes, transaminases increased, urine abnormality, urticaria, vomiting, weakness

Drug Interactions

Metabolism/Transport Effects Substrate of CYP2C19 (major), CYP2C9 (minor), CYP2D6 (minor), CYP3A4 (major), P-glycoprotein; **Note:** Assignment of Major/Minor substrate status based on clinically relevant drug interaction potential; **Inhibits** CYP1A2 (weak), CYP2B6 (weak), CYP2C19 (weak), CYP2C9 (weak), CYP2D6 (weak), CYP3A4 (strong), P-glycoprotein

Avoid Concomitant Use

Avoid concomitant use of Nelfinavir with any of the following: Alfuzosin; Amiodarone; Cisapride; Conivaptan; Crizotinib; Dronedarone; Eplerenone; Ergot Derivatives; Everolimus; Fluticasone (Oral Inhalation); Halofantrine; Lapatinib; Lovastatin; Lurasidone; Midazolam; Nilotinib; Nisoldipine; Pimozide; Proton Pump Inhibitors; QuiNIDine; Ranolazine; Rifampin; Rivaroxaban; RomiDEPsin; Salmeterol; Silodosin; Simvastatin; St Johns Wort; Tamsulosin; Ticagrelor; Tolvaptan; Topotecan; Toremifene; Triazolam

Increased Effect/Toxicity

Nelfinavir may increase the levels/effects of: Alfuzosin; Almotriptan; Alosetron; ALPRAZolam; Amiodarone; Antifungal Agents (Azole Derivatives, Systemic); ARIPiprazole; Azithromycin; Azithromycin (Systemic); Bortezomib; Bosentan; Brentuximab Vedotin; Brinzolamide; Budesonide (Nasal); Budesonide (Systemic, Oral Inhalation); Calcium Channel Blockers (Dihydropyridine); Calcium Channel Blockers (Nondihydropyridine); CarBAMazepine; Ciclesonide; Cisapride; Clarithromycin; Colchicine; Conivaptan; Corticosteroids (Orally Inhaled); Crizotinib; CycloSPORINE; CycloSPORINE (Systemic); CYP3A4 Substrates; Dabigatran Etexilate; Dienogest; Digoxin; Dronedarone; Dutasteride; Enfuvirtide; Eplerenone; Ergot Derivatives; Everolimus; FentaNYL; Fesoterodine; Fluticasone (Nasal); Fluticasone (Oral Inhalation); Fusidic Acid; GuanFACINE; Halofantrine; HMG-CoA Reductase Inhibitors; Iloperidone; Ixabepilone; Lapatinib; Lovastatin; Lumefantrine; Lurasidone; Maraviroc; Meperidine; MethylPREDNISolone; Midazolam; Nefazodone;

Nilotinib; Nisoldipine; Paricalcitol; Pazopanib; P-glycoprotein/ABCB1 Substrates; Pimecrolimus; Pimozide; Propafenone; Protease Inhibitors; QuiNIDine; Ranolazine; Rifabutin; Rivaroxaban; RomiDEPsin; Ruxolitinib; Salmeterol; Saxagliptin; Sildenafil; Silodosin; Simvastatin; Sirolimus; SORAfenib; Tacrolimus; Tacrolimus (Systemic); Tacrolimus (Topical); Tadalafil; Tamsulosin; Temsirolimus; Tenofovir; Ticagrelor; Tolterodine; Tolvaptan; Topotecan; Toremifene; TraZODone; Triazolam; Tricyclic Antidepressants; Vardenafil; Vemurafenib; Vilazodone; Warfarin; Zuclopenthixol

The levels/effects of Nelfinavir may be increased by: Antifungal Agents (Azole Derivatives, Systemic); Clarithromycin; CycloSPORINE; CycloSPORINE (Systemic); Delavirdine; Efavirenz; Enfuvirtide; Etravirine; Fusidic Acid; Lopinavir; P-glycoprotein/ABCB1 Inhibitors

Decreased Effect

Nelfinavir may decrease the levels/effects of: Abacavir; Clarithromycin; Contraceptives (Estrogens); Delavirdine; Divalproex; Etravirine; Lopinavir; Meperidine; Methadone; Phenytoin; Prasugrel; Theophylline Derivatives; Ticagrelor; Valproic Acid; Warfarin; Zidovudine

The levels/effects of Nelfinavir may be decreased by: Antacids; Bosentan; CarBAMazepine; CYP2C19 Inducers (Strong); CYP3A4 Inducers (Strong); Deferasirox; Efavirenz; Fosphenytoin; Garlic; H2-Antagonists; Nevirapine; Peginterferon Alfa-2b; P-glycoprotein/ABCB1 Inducers; Proton Pump Inhibitors; Rifabutin; Rifampin; St Johns Wort; Tenofovir; Tocilizumab

Ethanol/Nutrition/Herb Interactions

Food: Nelfinavir taken with food increases plasma concentration time curve (AUC) by two- to threefold. Do not administer with acidic food or juice (orange juice, apple juice, or applesauce) since the combination may have a bitter taste.

Herb/Nutraceutical: St John's wort may decrease the levels/effects of protease inhibitors; concurrent use should probably be avoided.

Stability Store at room temperature of 15°C to 30°C (59°F to 86°F). Oral powder (or dissolved tablets) diluted in nonacidic liquid is stable for 6 hours under refrigeration.

Mechanism of Action Binds to the site of HIV-1 protease activity and inhibits cleavage of viral Gag-Pol polyprotein precursors into individual functional proteins required for infectious HIV. This results in the formation of immature, noninfectious viral particles.

Pharmacodynamics/Kinetics

Absorption: Food increases AUC of nelfinavir by two- to fivefold

Distribution: V_d: 2-7 L/kg

Protein binding: >98%

Metabolism: Hepatic via CYP2C19 and 3A4; major metabolite has activity comparable to parent drug

Half-life elimination: 3.5-5 hours

Time to peak, serum: 2-4 hours

Excretion: Feces (98% to 99%, 78% as metabolites, 22% as unchanged drug); urine (1% to 2%)

Dosage Oral:

Children 2-13 years: 45-55 mg/kg twice daily **or** 25-35 mg/kg 3 times/day (maximum: 2500 mg/day). If tablets are unable to be taken, use oral powder in small amount of water, milk (cow's or soy), formula, or dietary supplements; do not use acidic food/juice or store for >6 hours.

Adults: 750 mg 3 times/day or 1250 mg twice daily with meals in combination with other antiretroviral therapies. **Note:** The DHHS Perinatal HIV Guidelines do not recommend the 3 times/day dosing in pregnant women (DHHS [perinatal], 2011).

Dosage adjustments for concomitant therapy: Adults:

Coadministration with bosentan:

Coadministration of bosentan in patients currently receiving nelfinavir: Begin with bosentan 62.5 mg once daily or every other day based on tolerability

Coadministration of nelfinavir in patients currently receiving bosentan: Adjust bosentan to 62.5 mg once daily or every other day based on tolerability

Coadministration with colchicine:

Familial Mediterranean fever (FMF): Maximum colchicine dose: 0.6 mg/day (0.3 mg twice daily)

Gout prophylaxis:

If original colchicine dose is 0.6 mg twice daily, adjust dose to 0.3 mg once daily

If original colchicine dose is 0.6 mg once daily, adjust dose to 0.3 mg every other day

Gout flare treatment: Initial: Colchicine 0.6 mg, followed in 1 hour by a single dose of 0.3 mg; do not repeat for at least 3 days

Coadministration with phosphodiesterase-5 enzyme (PDE-5) inhibitor:

Pulmonary arterial hypertension: Nelfinavir coadministered with tadalafil:

Patient receiving nelfinavir: Initiate tadalafil at 20 mg once daily; increase to 40 mg once daily based on individual tolerability

Patient receiving tadalafil when initiating nelfinavir: Adjust tadalafil to 20 mg once daily; increase to 40 mg once daily based on individual tolerability

Erectile dysfunction: Nelfinavir coadministered with:

Sildenafil (Viagra®): Maximum sildenafil dose: 25 mg in a 48-hour period

Tadalafil (Cialis®): Maximum tadalafil dose: 10 mg in a 72-hour period

Vardenafil: Maximum vardenafil dose: 2.5 mg in a 24-hour period

Dosing adjustment in renal impairment: No pharmacokinetic data in patients with renal impairment. However, <2% of dose excreted in urine; no dose adjustment is needed.

Dosing adjustment in hepatic impairment: No dose adjustment necessary in mild impairment (Child-Pugh class A); not recommended in patients with moderate-to-severe impairment (Child-Pugh class B or C)

Dietary Considerations Should be taken as scheduled with a meal. Some products may contain phenylalanine.

Administration

Oral powder: Administer with a meal. Mix powder in a small amount of water, milk, formula, soy milk, soy formula, pudding, ice cream, or dietary supplement. Do not reconstitute the oral powder in its original container. Be sure entire contents is consumed to receive full dose. Do not use acidic food/juice to dilute due to bitter taste. Once mixed, solution should be used immediately, but may be stored for up to 6 hours if refrigerated.

Tablets: Administer with a meal. If unable to swallow tablets, may dissolve tablets in a small amount of water; mix cloudy liquid well and consume immediately. Rinse glass with water to ensure receiving full dose. Tablets may also be crushed and mixed with pudding.

Monitoring Parameters Liver function tests, viral load, CD4 count, triglycerides, cholesterol, blood glucose, CBC with differential

Additional Information Nelfinavir (alone or in combination) is not recommended as initial therapy in the treatment of HIV infection due to inferior virologic efficacy and a high incidence of diarrhea (DHHS, 2011).

Dosage Forms Excipient information presented when available (limited, particularly for generics); consult specific product labeling. [DSC] = Discontinued product

Powder, oral:

Viracept®: 50 mg/g (144 g [DSC]) [contains phenylalanine 11.2 mg/g]

Tablet, oral:

Viracept®: 250 mg, 625 mg

- ◆ **Nembutal®** *see* PENTobarbital *on page 1329*
- ◆ **Nembutal® Sodium (Can)** *see* PENTobarbital *on page 1329*
- ◆ **Neo DM** *see* Chlorpheniramine, Phenylephrine, and Dextromethorphan *on page 346*
- ◆ **Neo-Fradin™** *see* Neomycin *on page 1188*

Neomycin (nee oh MYE sin)

Brand Names: U.S. Neo-Fradin™

Index Terms Neomycin Sulfate

Pharmacologic Category Ammonium Detoxicant; Antibiotic, Aminoglycoside; Antibiotic, Topical

Additional Appendix Information

Prevention of Wound Infection and Sepsis in Surgical Patients *on page 1954*

Use Orally to prepare GI tract for surgery; treatment of diarrhea caused by *E. coli*; adjunct in the treatment of hepatic encephalopathy

Pregnancy Risk Factor D

Pregnancy Considerations Aminoglycosides cross the placenta; however, neomycin has limited maternal absorption. Therefore the portion of an orally administered maternal dose available to cross the placenta is very low. Teratogenic effects have not been observed following maternal use of neomycin. Because of several reports of total irreversible bilateral congenital deafness in children whose mothers received another aminoglycoside (streptomycin) during pregnancy, the manufacturer classifies neomycin as pregnancy category D.

Lactation Excretion in breast milk unknown/not recommended

Contraindications Hypersensitivity to neomycin or any component of the formulation, or other aminoglycosides; intestinal obstruction, inflammatory or ulcerative gastrointestinal disease

Warnings/Precautions [U.S. Boxed Warning]: May cause neurotoxicity, nephrotoxicity, and/or neuromuscular blockade and respiratory paralysis; usual risk factors include pre-existing renal impairment, concomitant neuro-/nephrotoxic medications, advanced age and dehydration. The drug's neurotoxicity can result in respiratory paralysis from neuromuscular blockade, especially when the drug is given soon after anesthesia or muscle relaxants. Use with caution in patients with renal impairment, pre-existing hearing impairment, neuromuscular disorders; neomycin is more toxic than other aminoglycosides when given parenterally; **do not administer parenterally**; **do not use as peritoneal lavage** due to significant systemic adsorption of the drug. Prolonged use may result in fungal or bacterial superinfection, including *C. difficile*-associated diarrhea (CDAD) and pseudomembranous colitis; CDAD has been observed >2 months postantibiotic treatment.

Adverse Reactions

>10%: Gastrointestinal: Nausea, diarrhea, vomiting, irritation or soreness of the mouth or rectal area

<1% (Limited to important or life-threatening): Dyspnea, eosinophilia, nephrotoxicity, neurotoxicity, ototoxicity (auditory), ototoxicity (vestibular)

Drug Interactions

Metabolism/Transport Effects None known.

Avoid Concomitant Use

Avoid concomitant use of Neomycin with any of the following: BCG; Gallium Nitrate

Increased Effect/Toxicity

Neomycin may increase the levels/effects of: AbobotulinumtoxinA; Acarbose; Bisphosphonate Derivatives; CARBOplatin; Colistimethate; CycloSPORINE; CycloSPORINE (Systemic); Gallium Nitrate; Neuromuscular-Blocking Agents; OnabotulinumtoxinA; RimabotulinumtoxinB; Vitamin K Antagonists

The levels/effects of Neomycin may be increased by: Amphotericin B; Capreomycin; Cephalosporins (2nd Generation); Cephalosporins (3rd Generation); Cephalosporins (4th Generation); CISplatin; Loop Diuretics; Nonsteroidal Anti-Inflammatory Agents; Vancomycin

Decreased Effect

Neomycin may decrease the levels/effects of: BCG; Cardiac Glycosides; SORAfenib

The levels/effects of Neomycin may be decreased by: Penicillins

Mechanism of Action Interferes with bacterial protein synthesis by binding to 30S ribosomal subunits

Pharmacodynamics/Kinetics

Absorption: Oral, percutaneous: Poor (3%)

Distribution: 97% of an orally administered dose remains in the GI tract. Absorbed neomycin distributes to tissues and concentrates in the renal cortex. With repeated doses, accumulation also occurs in the inner ear.

V_d: 0.36 L/kg

Protein binding: 0% to 30%

Metabolism: Slightly hepatic

Half-life elimination (age and renal function dependent): 3 hours

Time to peak, serum: Oral: 1-4 hours

Excretion: Feces (97% of oral dose as unchanged drug); urine (30% to 50% of absorbed drug as unchanged drug)

Dosage

Children: Oral:

Preoperative intestinal antisepsis: 90 mg/kg/day divided every 4 hours for 2 days; or 25 mg/kg at 1 PM, 2 PM, and 11 PM on the day preceding surgery as an adjunct to mechanical cleansing of the intestine and in combination with erythromycin base

Hepatic encephalopathy: 50-100 mg/kg/day in divided doses every 6-8 hours or 2.5-7 g/m^2/day divided every 4-6 hours for 5-6 days not to exceed 12 g/day

Adults: Oral:

Preoperative intestinal antisepsis: 1 g each hour for 4 doses then 1 g every 4 hours for 5 doses; or 1 g at 1 PM, 2 PM, and 11 PM on day preceding surgery as an adjunct to mechanical cleansing of the bowel and oral erythromycin; or 6 g/day divided every 4 hours for 2-3 days

Hepatic encephalopathy: 500-2000 mg every 6-8 hours or 4-12 g/day divided every 4-6 hours for 5-6 days

Chronic hepatic insufficiency: 4 g/day for an indefinite period

Monitoring Parameters Renal function tests, audiometry in symptomatic patients

Dosage Forms Excipient information presented when available (limited, particularly for generics); consult specific product labeling.

Solution, oral, as sulfate:

Neo-Fradin™: 125 mg/5 mL (480 mL) [contains benzoic acid; cherry flavor]

Tablet, oral, as sulfate: 500 mg

Neomycin and Polymyxin B
(nee oh MYE sin & pol i MIKS in bee)

Brand Names: U.S. Neosporin® G.U. Irrigant

Brand Names: Canada Neosporin® Irrigating Solution
Index Terms Polymyxin B and Neomycin
Pharmacologic Category Antibiotic, Topical; Genitourinary Irrigant
Use Short-term as a continuous irrigant or rinse in the urinary bladder to prevent bacteriuria and gram-negative rod septicemia associated with the use of indwelling catheters
Pregnancy Risk Factor D
Dosage Children and Adults: Bladder irrigation: **Not for injection**; add 1 mL irrigant to 1 L isotonic saline solution and connect container to the inflow of lumen of 3-way catheter. Continuous irrigant or rinse in the urinary bladder for up to a maximum of 10 days with administration rate adjusted to patient's urine output; usually no more than 1 L of irrigant is used per day.
Additional Information Complete prescribing information for this medication should be consulted for additional detail.
Dosage Forms Excipient information presented when available (limited, particularly for generics); consult specific product labeling.
Solution, irrigation: Neomycin 40 mg and polymyxin B sulfate 200,000 units per 1 mL (1 mL, 20 mL)
Neosporin® G.U. Irrigant: Neomycin 40 mg and polymyxin sulfate B 200,000 units per 1 mL (1 mL, 20 mL)

◆ **Neomycin, Bacitracin, and Polymyxin B** *see* Bacitracin, Neomycin, and Polymyxin B *on page 186*
◆ **Neomycin, Bacitracin, Polymyxin B, and Hydrocortisone** *see* Bacitracin, Neomycin, Polymyxin B, and Hydrocortisone *on page 187*

Neomycin, Colistin, Hydrocortisone, and Thonzonium

(nee oh MYE sin, koe LIS tin, hye droe KOR ti sone, & thon ZOE nee um)

Brand Names: U.S. Coly-Mycin® S; Cortisporin®-TC
Index Terms Colistin, Hydrocortisone, Neomycin, and Thonzonium; Hydrocortisone, Neomycin, Colistin, and Thonzonium; Thonzonium, Neomycin, Colistin, and Hydrocortisone
Pharmacologic Category Antibiotic, Otic; Antibiotic/Corticosteroid, Otic; Corticosteroid, Otic
Use Treatment of superficial and susceptible bacterial infections of the external auditory canal; for treatment of susceptible bacterial infections of mastoidectomy and fenestration cavities
Dosage Otic:
Calibrated dropper:
Children: 4 drops in affected ear 3-4 times/day
Adults: 5 drops in affected ear 3-4 times/day
Dropper bottle:
Children: 3 drops in affected ear 3-4 times/day
Adults: 4 drops in affected ear 3-4 times/day
Note: Alternatively, a cotton wick may be inserted in the ear canal and saturated with suspension every 4 hours; wick should be replaced at least every 24 hours
Additional Information Complete prescribing information for this medication should be consulted for additional detail.
Dosage Forms Excipient information presented when available (limited, particularly for generics); consult specific product labeling.
Suspension, otic [drops]:
Coly-Mycin® S: Neomycin 0.33%, colistin 0.3%, hydrocortisone acetate 1%, and thonzonium bromide 0.05% (5 mL) [contains thimerosal]
Cortisporin®-TC: Neomycin 0.33%, colistin 0.3%, hydrocortisone acetate 1%, and thonzonium bromide 0.05% (10 mL) [contains thimerosal]

Neomycin, Polymyxin B, and Dexamethasone

(nee oh MYE sin, pol i MIKS in bee, & deks a METH a sone)

Brand Names: U.S. Maxitrol®; Poly-Dex™ [DSC]
Brand Names: Canada Dioptrol®; Maxitrol®
Index Terms Dexamethasone, Neomycin, and Polymyxin B; Polymyxin B, Neomycin, and Dexamethasone
Pharmacologic Category Antibiotic/Corticosteroid, Ophthalmic
Use Steroid-responsive inflammatory ocular conditions in which a corticosteroid is indicated and where bacterial infection or a risk of bacterial infection exists
Pregnancy Risk Factor C
Dosage Children and Adults: Ophthalmic:
Ointment: Place a small amount (~1/2") in the affected eye 3-4 times/day or apply at bedtime as an adjunct with drops
Suspension: Instill 1-2 drops into affected eye(s) every 3-4 hours; in severe disease, drops may be used hourly and tapered to discontinuation
Additional Information Complete prescribing information for this medication should be consulted for additional detail.
Dosage Forms Excipient information presented when available (limited, particularly for generics); consult specific product labeling. [DSC] = Discontinued product
Ointment, ophthalmic: Neomycin 3.5 mg, polymyxin B sulfate 10,000 units, and dexamethasone 0.1% per g (3.5 g)
Maxitrol®: Neomycin 3.5 mg, polymyxin B sulfate 10,000 units, and dexamethasone 0.1% per g (3.5 g)
Poly-Dex™: Neomycin 3.5 mg, polymyxin B sulfate 10,000 units, and dexamethasone 0.1% per g (3.5 g) [DSC]
Suspension, ophthalmic [drops]: Neomycin 3.5 mg, polymyxin B sulfate 10,000 units, and dexamethasone 0.1% per 1 mL (5 mL)
Maxitrol®: Neomycin 3.5 mg, polymyxin B sulfate 10,000 units, and dexamethasone 0.1% per 1 mL (5 mL) [contains benzalkonium chloride]
Poly-Dex™: Neomycin 3.5 mg, polymyxin B sulfate 10,000 units, and dexamethasone 0.1% per 1 mL (5 mL) [contains benzalkonium chloride] [DSC]

Neomycin, Polymyxin B, and Gramicidin

(nee oh MYE sin, pol i MIKS in bee, & gram i SYE din)

Brand Names: U.S. Neosporin® Ophthalmic Solution
Brand Names: Canada Neosporin®; Optimyxin Plus®
Index Terms Gramicidin, Neomycin, and Polymyxin B; Polymyxin B, Neomycin, and Gramicidin
Pharmacologic Category Antibiotic, Ophthalmic
Additional Appendix Information
Prevention of Wound Infection and Sepsis in Surgical Patients *on page 1954*
Use Treatment of superficial ocular infection
Pregnancy Risk Factor C
Dosage Children and Adults: Ophthalmic: Instill 1-2 drops 4-6 times/day or more frequently as required for severe infections
Additional Information Complete prescribing information for this medication should be consulted for additional detail.

Dosage Forms Excipient information presented when available (limited, particularly for generics); consult specific product labeling.

Solution, ophthalmic [drops]: Neomycin 1.75 mg, polymyxin B 10,000 units, and gramicidin 0.025 mg per 1 mL (10 mL)

Neosporin® Ophthalmic Solution: Neomycin 1.75 mg, polymyxin B 10,000 units, and gramicidin 0.025 mg per 1 mL (10 mL)

Neomycin, Polymyxin B, and Hydrocortisone

(nee oh MYE sin, pol i MIKS in bee, & hye droe KOR ti sone)

Brand Names: U.S. Cortisporin®; Cortomycin

Brand Names: Canada Cortimyxin®; Cortisporin® Otic

Index Terms Hydrocortisone, Neomycin, and Polymyxin B; Polymyxin B, Neomycin, and Hydrocortisone

Pharmacologic Category Antibiotic, Ophthalmic; Antibiotic, Otic; Antibiotic, Topical; Antibiotic/Corticosteroid, Otic; Corticosteroid, Ophthalmic; Corticosteroid, Otic; Corticosteroid, Topical

Use Steroid-responsive inflammatory condition for which a corticosteroid is indicated and where bacterial infection or a risk of bacterial infection exists

Pregnancy Risk Factor C

Dosage Note: Duration of use of ophthalmic and otic preparations should be limited to 10 days unless otherwise directed by the healthcare provider.

Ophthalmic:

Children (unlabeled use): Instill 1-2 drops 2-4 times/day, or more frequently as required for severe infections

Adults: Instill 1-2 drops 2-4 times/day, or more frequently as required for severe infections

Otic: Otic solution is used **only** for bacterial infections of external auditory canal (eg, swimmer's ear).

Children 6 months to 2 years (unlabeled use): Instill 3 drops into affected ear 3-4 times/day

Children ≥2 years: Instill 3 drops into affected ear 3-4 times/day

Adults: Instill 4 drops into affected ear 3-4 times/day; otic suspension is the preferred otic preparation

Topical:

Children (unlabeled use): Apply a thin layer 1-4 times/day. Therapy should be discontinued when control is achieved; if no improvement is seen, reassessment of diagnosis may be necessary.

Adults: Apply a thin layer 1-4 times/day. Therapy should be discontinued when control is achieved; if no improvement is seen, reassessment of diagnosis may be necessary.

Additional Information Complete prescribing information for this medication should be consulted for additional detail.

Dosage Forms Excipient information presented when available (limited, particularly for generics); consult specific product labeling.

Cream, topical

Cortisporin®: Neomycin 3.5 mg, polymyxin B 10,000 units, and hydrocortisone acetate 5 mg per g (7.5 g)

Solution, otic: Neomycin 3.5 mg, polymyxin B 10,000 units, and hydrocortisone 10 mg per 1 mL (10 mL) [contains potassium metabisulfite]

Cortisporin®: Neomycin 3.5 mg, polymyxin B 10,000 units, and hydrocortisone 10 mg per 1 mL (10 mL) [contains potassium metabisulfite]

Cortomycin: Neomycin 3.5 mg, polymyxin B 10,000 units, and hydrocortisone 10 mg per 1 mL (10 mL) [contains potassium metabisulfate]

Suspension, ophthalmic [drops]: Neomycin 3.5 mg, polymyxin B 10,000 units, and hydrocortisone 10 mg per 1 mL (7.5 mL)

Suspension, otic: Neomycin 3.5 mg, polymyxin B 10,000 units, and hydrocortisone 10 mg per 1 mL (10 mL)

Cortomycin: Neomycin 3.5 mg, polymyxin B 10,000 units, and hydrocortisone 10 mg per 1 mL (10 mL) [contains thimerosal]

- ◆ **Neomycin Sulfate** *see* Neomycin *on page* *1188*
- ◆ **Neo-Polycin™** *see* Bacitracin, Neomycin, and Polymyxin B *on page* *186*
- ◆ **Neo-Polycin™ HC** *see* Bacitracin, Neomycin, Polymyxin B, and Hydrocortisone *on page* *187*
- ◆ **NeoProfen®** *see* Ibuprofen *on page* *860*
- ◆ **Neoral®** *see* CycloSPORINE (Systemic) *on page* *422*
- ◆ **Neosar** *see* Cyclophosphamide *on page* *421*
- ◆ **Neosporin® (Can)** *see* Neomycin, Polymyxin B, and Gramicidin *on page* *1189*
- ◆ **Neosporin® AF [OTC]** *see* Miconazole (Topical) *on page* *1126*
- ◆ **Neosporin® G.U. Irrigant** *see* Neomycin and Polymyxin B *on page* *1188*
- ◆ **Neosporin® Irrigating Solution (Can)** *see* Neomycin and Polymyxin B *on page* *1188*
- ◆ **Neosporin® Neo To Go® [OTC]** *see* Bacitracin, Neomycin, and Polymyxin B *on page* *186*
- ◆ **Neosporin® Ophthalmic Solution** *see* Neomycin, Polymyxin B, and Gramicidin *on page* *1189*
- ◆ **Neosporin® Topical [OTC]** *see* Bacitracin, Neomycin, and Polymyxin B *on page* *186*

Neostigmine (nee oh STIG meen)

Brand Names: U.S. Prostigmin®

Brand Names: Canada Prostigmin®

Index Terms Neostigmine Bromide; Neostigmine Methylsulfate

Pharmacologic Category Acetylcholinesterase Inhibitor

Use Reversal of the effects of nondepolarizing neuromuscular-blocking agents; treatment of myasthenia gravis; prevention and treatment of postoperative bladder distention and urinary retention

Pregnancy Risk Factor C

Lactation Excretion in breast milk unknown/not recommended

Contraindications Hypersensitivity to neostigmine, bromides, or any component of the formulation; GI or GU obstruction

Warnings/Precautions Does **not** antagonize and may prolong the Phase I block of depolarizing muscle relaxants (eg, succinylcholine). Use with caution in patients with epilepsy, asthma, bradycardia, hyperthyroidism, cardiac arrhythmias, or peptic ulcer; not generally recommended for use in patients with vagotonia. Adequate facilities should be available for cardiopulmonary resuscitation when testing and adjusting dose for myasthenia gravis. Have atropine and epinephrine ready to treat hypersensitivity reactions. Overdosage may result in cholinergic crisis, this must be distinguished from myasthenic crisis. Anticholinesterase insensitivity can develop for brief or prolonged periods.

Adverse Reactions Frequency not defined.

Cardiovascular: Arrhythmias (especially bradycardia), AV block, cardiac arrest, flushing, hypotension, nodal rhythm, nonspecific ECG changes, syncope, tachycardia

Central nervous system: Convulsions, dizziness, drowsiness, dysarthria, dysphonia, headache, loss of consciousness

Dermatologic: Skin rash, thrombophlebitis (I.V.), urticaria

Gastrointestinal: Diarrhea, dysphagia, flatulence, hyperperistalsis, nausea, salivation, stomach cramps, vomiting
Genitourinary: Urinary urgency
Neuromuscular & skeletal: Arthralgias, fasciculations, muscle cramps, spasms, weakness
Ocular: Lacrimation, small pupils
Respiratory: Bronchiolar constriction, bronchospasm, dyspnea, increased bronchial secretions, laryngospasm, respiratory arrest, respiratory depression, respiratory muscle paralysis
Miscellaneous: Allergic reactions, anaphylaxis, diaphoresis increased

Drug Interactions

Metabolism/Transport Effects None known.

Avoid Concomitant Use There are no known interactions where it is recommended to avoid concomitant use.

Increased Effect/Toxicity

Neostigmine may increase the levels/effects of: Beta-Blockers; Cholinergic Agonists; Succinylcholine

The levels/effects of Neostigmine may be increased by: Corticosteroids (Systemic)

Decreased Effect

Neostigmine may decrease the levels/effects of: Neuromuscular-Blocking Agents (Nondepolarizing)

The levels/effects of Neostigmine may be decreased by: Dipyridamole

Mechanism of Action Inhibits destruction of acetylcholine by acetylcholinesterase which facilitates transmission of impulses across myoneural junction

Pharmacodynamics/Kinetics
Onset of action: I.M.: 20-30 minutes; I.V.: 1-20 minutes
Duration: I.M.: 2.5-4 hours; I.V.: 1-2 hours
Absorption: Oral: Poor, <2%
Metabolism: Hepatic
Half-life elimination: Normal renal function: 0.5-2.1 hours; End-stage renal disease: Prolonged
Excretion: Urine (50% as unchanged drug)

Dosage
Myasthenia gravis: Diagnosis: I.M.: **Note:** In the diagnosis of myasthenia gravis, all anticholinesterase medications should be discontinued for at least 8 hours before administering neostigmine.
Children: 0.04 mg/kg as a single dose
Adults: 0.02 mg/kg as a single dose
Myasthenia gravis: Treatment:
Children:
Oral: 2 mg/kg/day divided every 3-4 hours
I.M., I.V., SubQ: 0.01-0.04 mg/kg every 2-4 hours
Adults:
Oral: 15 mg/dose every 3-4 hours up to 375 mg/day maximum; interval between doses must be individualized to maximal response
I.M., I.V., SubQ: 0.5-2.5 mg every 1-3 hours up to 10 mg/24 hours maximum
Reversal of nondepolarizing neuromuscular blockade after surgery in conjunction with atropine (must administer atropine several minutes prior to neostigmine): I.V.:
Infants: 0.025-0.1 mg/kg/dose
Children: 0.025-0.08 mg/kg/dose
Adults: 0.5-2.5 mg; total dose not to exceed 5 mg
Bladder atony: Adults: I.M., SubQ:
Prevention: 0.25 mg every 4-6 hours for 2-3 days
Treatment: 0.5-1 mg every 3 hours for 5 doses after bladder has emptied

Dosing adjustment in renal impairment:
Cl_{cr} 10-50 mL/minute: Administer 50% of normal dose
Cl_{cr} <10 mL/minute: Administer 25% of normal dose

Administration May be administered undiluted by slow I.V. injection over several minutes.
I.M.: In the diagnosis of myasthenia gravis, all anticholinesterase medications should be discontinued for at least 8 hours before administering neostigmine.

Additional Information In the diagnosis of myasthenia gravis, all anticholinesterase medications should be discontinued for at least 8 hours before administering neostigmine.

Dosage Forms Excipient information presented when available (limited, particularly for generics); consult specific product labeling. [DSC] = Discontinued product
Injection, solution, as methylsulfate: 0.5 mg/mL (10 mL); 1 mg/mL (10 mL)
Prostigmin®: 0.5 mg/mL (1 mL [DSC], 10 mL [DSC]); 1 mg/mL (10 mL [DSC])
Tablet, oral, as bromide:
Prostigmin®: 15 mg [scored]

◆ **Neostigmine Bromide** *see* Neostigmine *on page 1190*

◆ **Neostigmine Methylsulfate** *see* Neostigmine *on page 1190*

◆ **NeoStrata® HQ (Can)** *see* Hydroquinone *on page 846*

◆ **NeoStrata® HQ Skin Lightening [OTC]** *see* Hydroquinone *on page 846*

Nepafenac (ne pa FEN ak)

Brand Names: U.S. Nevanac®

Brand Names: Canada Nevanac®

Pharmacologic Category Nonsteroidal Anti-inflammatory Drug (NSAID), Ophthalmic

Use Treatment of pain and inflammation associated with cataract surgery

Pregnancy Risk Factor C/D (3rd trimester)

Dosage Ophthalmic: Children ≥10 years and Adults: Instill 1 drop into affected eye(s) 3 times/day, beginning 1 day prior to surgery, the day of surgery, and through the first 2 weeks of the postoperative period

Additional Information Complete prescribing information for this medication should be consulted for additional detail.

Dosage Forms Excipient information presented when available (limited, particularly for generics); consult specific product labeling.
Suspension, ophthalmic [drops]:
Nevanac®: 0.1% (3 mL) [contains benzalkonium chloride]

◆ **Nephro-Calci® [OTC]** *see* Calcium Carbonate *on page 266*

◆ **Neptazane™** *see* Methazolamide *on page 1093*

◆ **Nerve Agent Antidote Kit** *see* Atropine and Pralidoxime *on page 172*

◆ **Nesacaine®** *see* Chloroprocaine *on page 342*

◆ **Nesacaine®-CE (Can)** *see* Chloroprocaine *on page 342*

◆ **Nesacaine®-MPF** *see* Chloroprocaine *on page 342*

Nesiritide (ni SIR i tide)

Brand Names: U.S. Natrecor®

Brand Names: Canada Natrecor®

Index Terms B-type Natriuretic Peptide (Human); hBNP; Natriuretic Peptide

Pharmacologic Category Natriuretic Peptide, B-Type, Human; Vasodilator

Additional Appendix Information
Vasoactive Agents, Intravenous *on page 1898*

Use Treatment of acutely decompensated heart failure (HF) with dyspnea at rest or with minimal activity

Pregnancy Risk Factor C

Pregnancy Considerations Adverse events were not observed in an animal reproduction study. Nesiritide is a recombinant B-type natriuretic peptide (rhBNP). BNP and NT-proBNP (which has been used as a marker of BNP), are endogenous peptides and NT-proBNP is measurable in the umbilical cord serum of normal pregnancies. Information related to the administration of nesiritide during pregnancy has not been located.

Lactation Excretion in breast milk unknown/use caution

Contraindications Hypersensitivity to natriuretic peptide or any component of the formulation; cardiogenic shock (when used as primary therapy); hypotension (systolic blood pressure <90 mm Hg)

Warnings/Precautions May cause hypotension; administer in clinical situations when blood pressure may be closely monitored. Use caution in patients systolic blood pressure <100 mm Hg (contraindicated if <90 mm Hg); more likely to experience hypotension. Effects may be additive with other agents capable of causing hypotension. Hypotensive effects may last for several hours.

Should not be used in patients with low cardiac filling pressures, or in patients with conditions which depend on venous return including significant valvular stenosis, restrictive or obstructive cardiomyopathy, constrictive pericarditis, and pericardial tamponade. May be associated with development of azotemia; use caution in patients with renal impairment or in patients where renal perfusion is dependent on renin-angiotensin-aldosterone system; avoid initiation at doses higher than recommended.

Monitor for allergic or anaphylactic reactions. Use caution with prolonged infusions; limited experience with infusions >48 hours.

Adverse Reactions Note: Frequencies cited below were recorded in VMAC trial at dosages similar to approved labeling. Higher frequencies have been observed in trials using higher dosages of nesiritide. The percentages marked with an asterisk (*) indicate frequency less than or equal to placebo or other standard therapy.

>10%:

- Cardiovascular: Hypotension (total: 11%; symptomatic: 4% at recommended dose, up to 17% at higher doses)
- Renal: Increased serum creatinine (28% with >0.5 mg/dL increase over baseline)

1% to 10%:

- Cardiovascular: Ventricular tachycardia (3%)*, ventricular extrasystoles (3%)*, angina (2%)*, bradycardia (1%), tachycardia, atrial fibrillation, AV node conduction abnormalities
- Central nervous system: Headache (8%)*, dizziness (3%), insomnia (2%)*, anxiety (3%), confusion, fever, paresthesia, somnolence, tremor
- Dermatologic: Pruritus, rash
- Gastrointestinal: Nausea (4%)*, abdominal pain (1%)*, vomiting (1%)*
- Hematologic: Anemia
- Local: Injection site reaction, catheter pain
- Neuromuscular & skeletal: Back pain (4%), leg cramps
- Ocular: Amblyopia
- Respiratory: Apnea, cough increased, hemoptysis
- Miscellaneous: Diaphoresis

Postmarketing and/or case reports: Hypersensitivity reactions (rare)

Drug Interactions

Metabolism/Transport Effects None known.

Avoid Concomitant Use There are no known interactions where it is recommended to avoid concomitant use.

Increased Effect/Toxicity

Nesiritide may increase the levels/effects of: Hypotensive Agents

Decreased Effect There are no known significant interactions involving a decrease in effect.

Ethanol/Nutrition/Herb Interactions Herb/Nutraceutical: Avoid bayberry, blue cohosh, cayenne, ephedra, ginger, ginseng (American), kola, and licorice (may increase blood pressure). Avoid black cohosh, California poppy, coleus, golden seal, hawthorn, mistletoe, periwinkle, quinine, and shepherd's purse (may enhance decreased blood pressure).

Stability Vials may be stored below 25°C (77°F); do not freeze. Protect from light. Following reconstitution, vials are stable at 2°C to 25°C (36°F to 77°F) for up to 24 hours. Use reconstituted solution within 24 hours.

Reconstitute 1.5 mg vial with 5 mL of diluent removed from a prefilled 250 mL plastic I.V. bag (compatible with D_5W, $D_5{}^1/_2NS$, $D_5{}^1/_4NS$, NS). Do not shake vial to dissolve (roll gently). Withdraw entire contents of vial and add to 250 mL I.V. bag. Invert several times to mix. Resultant concentration of solution is ~6 mcg/mL.

Mechanism of Action Binds to guanylate cyclase receptor on vascular smooth muscle and endothelial cells, increasing intracellular cyclic GMP, resulting in smooth muscle cell relaxation. Has been shown to produce dose-dependent reductions in pulmonary capillary wedge pressure (PCWP) and systemic arterial pressure.

Pharmacodynamics/Kinetics

Onset of action: 15 minutes (60% of 3-hour effect achieved)

Duration: >60 minutes (up to several hours) for systolic blood pressure; hemodynamic effects persist longer than serum half-life would predict

Distribution: V_{ss}: 0.19 L/kg

Metabolism: Proteolytic cleavage by vascular endopeptidases and proteolysis following binding to the membrane bound natriuretic peptide (NPR-C) and cellular internalization

Half-life elimination: Initial (distribution) 2 minutes; Terminal: 18 minutes

Time to peak: 1 hour

Excretion: Primarily eliminated by metabolism; also excreted in the urine

Dosage Adults: I.V.: Initial: 2 mcg/kg (bolus optional); followed by continuous infusion at 0.01 mcg/kg/minute. **Note:** Should not be initiated at a dosage higher than initial recommended dose. There is limited experience with increasing the dose >0.01 mcg/kg/minute; in one trial, a limited number of patients received higher doses that were increased no faster than every 3 hours by 0.005 mcg/kg/minute (preceded by a bolus of 1 mcg/kg), up to a maximum of 0.03 mcg/kg/minute. Increases beyond the initial infusion rate should be limited to selected patients and accompanied by close hemodynamic and renal function monitoring.

Patients experiencing hypotension during the infusion: Infusion dose should be reduced or discontinued. Other measures to support blood pressure should be initiated (eg, I.V. fluids, Trendelenburg position). May attempt to restart at a lower dose (reduce previous infusion dose by 30% and omit bolus).

Maximum dosing weight: According to the manufacturer, the PRECEDENT Trial capped dosing weight at 160 kg and the VMAC Trial capped dosing weight at 175 kg. There are no specific guidelines on maximum dosing weight and clinical judgment should be used.

Dosage adjustment in renal impairment: No adjustment required, but use cautiously in patients with renal impairment or those patients who rely on the renin-angiotensin-aldosterone system for renal perfusion. Monitor renal function closely.

Dosage adjustment in hepatic impairment: No dosage adjustment recommended.

Administration Do not administer through a heparin-coated catheter (concurrent administration of heparin via a separate catheter is acceptable, per manufacturer).

Prime I.V. tubing with 5 mL of infusion prior to connection with vascular access port and prior to administering bolus or starting the infusion. Withdraw bolus from the prepared infusion bag and administer over 60 seconds. Begin infusion immediately following administration of the bolus.

Monitoring Parameters Blood pressure, hemodynamic responses (PCWP, RAP, CI), BUN, creatinine; urine output

Additional Information The duration of symptomatic improvement with nesiritide following discontinuation of the infusion has been limited (generally lasting several days). Atrial natriuretic peptide, which is related to nesiritide, has been associated with increased vascular permeability. This has not been observed in clinical trials with nesiritide, but patients should be monitored for this effect.

Dosage Forms Excipient information presented when available (limited, particularly for generics); consult specific product labeling.

Injection, powder for reconstitution:

Natrecor®: 1.5 mg

- ◆ **NESP** *see* Darbepoetin Alfa *on page* 447
- ◆ **Neulasta®** *see* Pegfilgrastim *on page* 1307
- ◆ **Neumega®** *see* Oprelvekin *on page* 1249
- ◆ **Neupogen®** *see* Filgrastim *on page* 711
- ◆ **Neurontin®** *see* Gabapentin *on page* 773
- ◆ **Neut®** *see* Sodium Bicarbonate *on page* 1566
- ◆ **NeutraCare®** *see* Fluoride *on page* 728
- ◆ **NeutraGard® Advanced** *see* Fluoride *on page* 728
- ◆ **Neutrahist PDX** *see* Chlorpheniramine, Pseudoephedrine, and Dextromethorphan *on page* 347
- ◆ **Neutrahist Pediatric [OTC] [DSC]** *see* Chlorpheniramine and Pseudoephedrine *on page* 346
- ◆ **Neutra-Phos** *see* Potassium Phosphate and Sodium Phosphate *on page* 1386
- ◆ **Neutra-Phos®-K [OTC] [DSC]** *see* Potassium Phosphate *on page* 1385
- ◆ **Nevanac®** *see* Nepafenac *on page* 1191

Nevirapine (ne VYE ra peen)

Brand Names: U.S. Viramune®; Viramune® XR™

Brand Names: Canada Auro-Nevirapine; Viramune®

Index Terms NVP; Viramune® XR™

Pharmacologic Category Antiretroviral Agent, Reverse Transcriptase Inhibitor (Non-nucleoside)

Additional Appendix Information

Management of Healthcare Worker Exposures to HBV, HCV, and HIV *on page* 1935

Perinatal HIV Guidelines *on page* 1946

Use In combination therapy with other antiretroviral agents for the treatment of HIV-1

Pregnancy Risk Factor B

Pregnancy Considerations Teratogenic effects were not observed in animal reproduction studies. Nevirapine crosses the placenta. No increased risk of overall birth defects has been observed following first trimester exposure according to data collected by the antiretroviral pregnancy registry. Pharmacokinetics are not altered during pregnancy and dose adjustment is not needed. The DHHS Perinatal HIV Guidelines recommend nevirapine as the NNRTI for use during pregnancy. Nevirapine may be initiated in pregnant women with a $CD4^+$ lymphocyte count <250/mm^3 or continued in women who are virologically suppressed and tolerating therapy once pregnancy is detected (regardless of $CD4^+$ lymphocyte count); however, do not initiate therapy in pregnant women with a $CD4^+$ lymphocyte count >250/mm^3 unless the benefit of therapy clearly outweighs the risk. Monitor for liver toxicity during first 18 weeks of therapy. Hypersensitivity reactions (including hepatic toxicity and rash) are more common in women on NNRTI therapy; it is not known if pregnancy increases this risk.

Regardless of CD4 count or HIV RNA copy number, all HIV-infected pregnant women should receive a combination antepartum antiretroviral (ARV) drug regimen; this includes women who require therapy for their own health, as well as women who do not yet require therapy for their own health. ARV therapy should be started as soon as possible if required for the woman's health or immediately after the first trimester if not needed for the mother's health (although earlier initiation may be considered). Long-term follow-up is recommended for all infants exposed to ARV medications.

Healthcare providers are encouraged to enroll pregnant women exposed to antiretroviral medications in the Antiretroviral Pregnancy Registry (1-800-258-4263 or www.-APRegistry.com). Healthcare providers caring for HIV-infected women and their infants may contact the National Perinatal HIV Hotline (888-448-8765) for clinical consultation (DHHS [perinatal], 2011).

Lactation Enters breast milk/contraindicated

Medication Guide Available Yes

Contraindications Moderate-to-severe hepatic impairment (Child-Pugh class B or C); use in occupational or nonoccupational postexposure prophylaxis (PEP) regimens

Warnings/Precautions [U.S. Boxed Warning]: Severe hepatotoxic reactions may occur (fulminant and cholestatic hepatitis, hepatic necrosis) and, in some cases, have resulted in hepatic failure and death. The greatest risk of these reactions is within the initial 6 weeks of treatment. Patients with a history of chronic hepatitis (B or C) or increased baseline transaminase levels may be at increased risk of hepatotoxic reactions. Female gender and patients with increased $CD4^+$-cell counts may be at substantially greater risk of hepatic events (often associated with rash). Therapy in antiretroviral naive patients should not be started with elevated $CD4^+$-cell counts unless the benefit of therapy outweighs the risk of serious hepatotoxicity (adult/postpubertal females: $CD4^+$-cell counts >250 cells/mm^3; adult males: $CD4^+$-cell counts >400 cells/mm^3). Use with caution in patients with preexisting dysfunction; monitor closely for drug-induced hepatotoxicity; contraindicated in patients with moderate-to-severe impairment (Child-Pugh class B or C).

[U.S. Boxed Warning]: Severe life-threatening skin reactions (eg, Stevens-Johnson syndrome, toxic epidermal necrolysis, hypersensitivity reactions with rash and organ dysfunction), including fatal cases, have occurred. The greatest risk of these reactions is within the initial 6 weeks of treatment; intensive monitoring is required during the initial 18 weeks of therapy to detect potentially life-threatening dermatologic, hypersensitivity, and hepatic reactions. Risk is greatest in African-Americans, Asian, or Hispanic race/ethnicity or in females. A 14-day lead-in dosing period with immediate release formulation must be initiated to decrease the incidence of adverse effects. The lead-in dosing can be extended up to 28 days if necessary, but an alternative regimen is necessary if >28 days is required. If a severe dermatologic or hypersensitivity reaction occurs, or if signs and symptoms of hepatitis occur, nevirapine should be permanently discontinued. These events may include a severe rash, or a rash associated with fever, blisters, oral lesions, conjunctivitis, facial edema, muscle or joint aches, transaminase elevations, general malaise, hepatitis, eosinophilia, granulocytopenia, lymphadenopathy, or renal dysfunction. Coadministration of prednisone during the first 6 weeks of therapy increases incidence and severity of rash; concomitant prednisone is not recommended to prevent rash.

May cause redistribution of fat (eg, buffalo hump, peripheral wasting with increased abdominal girth, cushingoid ▶

appearance). Patients may develop immune reconstitution syndrome resulting in the occurrence of an inflammatory response to an indolent or residual opportunistic infection; further evaluation and treatment may be required. Rhabdomyolysis has been observed in conjunction with skin and/or hepatic adverse events during postmarketing surveillance. Termination of therapy is warranted with evidence of severe skin or liver toxicity.

Use with caution in patients taking strong CYP3A4 inhibitors, moderate or strong CYP3A4 inducers and major CYP3A4 substrates (see Drug Interactions); consider alternative agents that avoid or lessen the potential for CYP-mediated interactions. Concurrent use of St John's wort or efavirenz is not recommended; may decrease the therapeutic efficacy (St John's wort) or increase adverse effects (efavirenz).

Nevirapine-based initial regimens should not be used in children <3 years of age if previously exposed to nevirapine during prevention of maternal-to-child transmission of HIV due to increased risk of resistance and treatment failure. Protease inhibitor-based initial regimens preferred in this population.

Due to rapid emergence of resistance, nevirapine should not be used as monotherapy or the only agent added to a failing regimen for the treatment of HIV. Consider alteration of antiretroviral therapies if disease progression occurs while patients are receiving nevirapine. Use care when timing discontinuation of regimens containing nevirapine; levels are sustained after levels of other medications decrease, leading to nevirapine resistance. Cross-resistance may be conferred to other non-nucleoside reverse transcriptase inhibitors (DHHS, 2011).

Adverse Reactions Note: Potentially life-threatening nevirapine-associated adverse effects may present with the following symptoms: Abrupt onset of flu-like symptoms, abdominal pain, jaundice, or fever with or without rash; may progress to hepatic failure with encephalopathy. Skin rash is present in ~50% of cases.

Percentages of adverse effects vary by clinical trial and may vary by formulation; incidences reported below are based on immediate release formulation:

>10%:
- Dermatologic: Rash (grade 1/2: 13%; grade 3/4: 2%)
- Hepatic: ALT >250 units/L (5% to 14%); symptomatic hepatic events (4%, range: up to 11%)

1% to 10%:
- Central nervous system: Headache (1% to 4%), fatigue (≤5%)
- Gastrointestinal: Nausea (<1% to 9%), abdominal pain (≤2%), diarrhea (≤2%)
- Hematologic: Neutropenia (4%)
- Hepatic: AST >250 units/L (4% to 8%)

Postmarketing and/or case reports: Allergic reactions, anaphylaxis, anemia, angioedema, arthralgia, blisters, bullous eruptions, conjunctivitis, eosinophilia, facial edema, fever, fulminant and cholestatic hepatitis, granulocytopenia, hepatic failure, hepatic necrosis, hypersensitivity syndrome, jaundice, lymphadenopathy, malaise, myalgia, oral lesions, paresthesia, redistribution/accumulation of body fat, renal dysfunction, rhabdomyolysis, serum phosphorus decreased, Stevens-Johnson syndrome, somnolence, toxic epidermal necrolysis, ulcerative stomatitis, urticaria, vomiting

Drug Interactions

Metabolism/Transport Effects Substrate of CYP2B6 (minor), CYP2D6 (minor), CYP3A4 (major); **Note:** Assignment of Major/Minor substrate status based on clinically relevant drug interaction potential; **Inhibits** CYP1A2 (weak), CYP2D6 (weak), CYP3A4 (weak); **Induces** CYP2B6 (strong), CYP3A4 (strong)

Avoid Concomitant Use

Avoid concomitant use of Nevirapine with any of the following: Atazanavir; Bortezomib; Crizotinib; Dronedarone; Efavirenz; Etravirine; Everolimus; Itraconazole; Lapatinib; Lurasidone; Nilotinib; Nisoldipine; Pazopanib; Pimozide; Praziquantel; Ranolazine; Rilpivirine; Rivaroxaban; Roflumilast; RomiDEPsin; SORAfenib; St Johns Wort; Ticagrelor; Tolvaptan; Toremifene; Vandetanib

Increased Effect/Toxicity

Nevirapine may increase the levels/effects of: Clarithromycin; Efavirenz; Etravirine; PACLitaxel; Pimozide; Rifabutin; Rilpivirine

The levels/effects of Nevirapine may be increased by: Atazanavir; Clarithromycin; Conivaptan; Efavirenz; Voriconazole

Decreased Effect

Nevirapine may decrease the levels/effects of: ARIPiprazole; Atazanavir; Boceprevir; Bortezomib; Brentuximab Vedotin; Caspofungin; Clarithromycin; Contraceptives (Estrogens); Contraceptives (Progestins); Crizotinib; CYP2B6 Substrates; CYP3A4 Substrates; Dasatinib; Dronedarone; Efavirenz; Etravirine; Everolimus; Exemestane; Fosamprenavir; Gefitinib; GuanFACINE; Imatinib; Indinavir; Itraconazole; Ixabepilone; Lapatinib; Linagliptin; Lopinavir; Lurasidone; Maraviroc; Methadone; Nelfinavir; NIFEdipine; Nilotinib; Nisoldipine; Pazopanib; Praziquantel; Ranolazine; Rifabutin; Rilpivirine; Rivaroxaban; Roflumilast; RomiDEPsin; Saquinavir; Saxagliptin; SORAfenib; SUNItinib; Tadalafil; Ticagrelor; Tolvaptan; Toremifene; Ulipristal; Vandetanib; Vemurafenib; Voriconazole; Zuclopenthixol

The levels/effects of Nevirapine may be decreased by: CYP3A4 Inducers (Strong); Deferasirox; Peginterferon Alfa-2b; Rifabutin; Rifampin; St Johns Wort; Tocilizumab

Ethanol/Nutrition/Herb Interactions Herb/Nutraceutical: Nevirapine serum concentration may be decreased by St John's wort; avoid concurrent use.

Stability Store at 25°C (77°F); excursion permitted to 15°C to 30°C (59°F to 86°F).

Mechanism of Action As a non-nucleoside reverse transcriptase inhibitor, nevirapine has activity against HIV-1 by binding to reverse transcriptase. It consequently blocks the RNA-dependent and DNA-dependent DNA polymerase activities including HIV-1 replication. It does not require intracellular phosphorylation for antiviral activity.

Pharmacodynamics/Kinetics

Absorption: >90%

Distribution: Widely; V_d: 1.2 L/kg; CSF penetration approximates 40% to 50% of plasma

Protein binding, plasma: ~60%

Metabolism: Extensively hepatic via CYP3A4 and CYP2B6 (hydroxylation to inactive compounds); may undergo enterohepatic recycling

Bioavailability: 93% (immediate release tablet); ~75% (extended release tablet [relative to immediate release]); 91% (oral solution)

Half-life elimination: Decreases over 2- to 4-week time with chronic dosing due to autoinduction (ie, half-life = 45 hours initially and decreases to 25-30 hours)

Time to peak, serum: Immediate release: 4 hours; Extended release:~24 hours

Excretion: Urine (~81%, primarily as metabolites, <3% as unchanged drug); feces (~10%)

Dosage Oral:

HIV infection:

Note: If patient experiences a rash during the 14-day lead-in period, dose should not be increased until the rash has resolved. A lead-in period must always be done with immediate release formulation and regimen should not exceed 28 days; alternative treatment should be considered at that point. If a rash occurs within the first 18 weeks of therapy, immediately check serum transaminases. Discontinue if severe rash, rash with constitutional symptoms, or rash with elevated hepatic transaminases is noted. Coadministration of prednisone during the first 6 weeks of therapy increases incidence and severity of rash; concomitant prednisone is not recommended to prevent rash. Permanently discontinue if symptomatic hepatic events occur. If therapy with any formulation is interrupted for >7 days, restart with initial dose of immediate release formulation for 14 days.

Infants and Children:

Immediate release: 150 mg/m^2/dose once daily for first 14 days (maximum: 200 mg/day); increase dose to 150 mg/m^2/dose twice daily if no rash or untoward effects (maximum: 400 mg/day).

Extended release: Has not been evaluated in pediatric patients.

AIDS*info* pediatric guidelines:

Note: Children <3 years of age: Nevirapine-based initial regimens should not be used in children previously exposed to nevirapine during prevention of maternal-to-child transmission of HIV

Children <8 years: Immediate release: 200 mg/m^2/dose once daily for first 14 days (maximum dose: 200 mg); increase dose to 200 mg/m^2/dose twice daily if no rash or untoward effects (maximum: 400 mg/day)

Children ≥8 years: Immediate release: 120-150 mg/m^2/dose once daily for 14 days (maximum dose: 200 mg); increase dose to 120-150 mg/m^2/dose twice daily if no rash or untoward effects (maximum: 400 mg/day)

Adolescents and Adults: **Note:** Therapy should not be initiated in patients with elevated CD4$^+$-cell counts unless the benefit of therapy outweighs the risk of serious hepatotoxicity (adult/post-pubertal females: CD4$^+$-cell counts >250 cells/mm^3; adult males: CD4$^+$-cell counts >400 cells/mm^3)

Immediate release:

Initial: 200 mg once daily for first 14 days

Maintenance: 200 mg twice daily (in combination with additional antiretroviral agents) if there is no rash or untoward effects during initial dosing period

Adults: Extended release: Maintenance: 400 mg once daily; maintenance therapy using the extended release must follow a 14-day initial dosing period (lead-in) using the immediate release formulation unless patient is already maintained on a nevirapine immediate release regimen.

Prevention of maternal-fetal HIV transmission (DHHS [perinatal], 2011): Note: Nevirapine is used in combination with zidovudine in select situations (eg, infants born to mothers with suboptimal viral suppression at delivery, infants born to mothers with only intrapartum therapy or no therapy, or infants born to mothers with known antiretroviral drug-resistant virus).

Dosage adjustment in renal impairment:

Cl_{cr} ≥20 mL/minute: No adjustment required

Hemodialysis: Immediate release: An additional 200 mg dose is recommended following dialysis.

Dosage adjustment in hepatic impairment: Use is contraindicated with moderate-to-severe hepatic impairment (Child-Pugh Class B or C). Permanently discontinue if symptomatic hepatic events occur.

Administration Oral: May be administered with or without food; may be administered with an antacid or didanosine. Shake suspension gently prior to administration; the use of an oral dosing syringe is recommended, especially if the dose is ≤5 mL; if using a dosing cup, after administration, rinse cup with water and also administer rinse. Extended release tablets must be swallowed whole and not crushed, chewed, or divided.

Monitoring Parameters Monitor CBC and viral load. Baseline liver function tests should be obtained prior to nevirapine's initiation. DHHS adult guidelines recommend serum transaminase monitoring every 2 weeks for the first 4 weeks of therapy, monthly for the first 18 weeks, then frequently thereafter. Patients receiving maintenance immediate release nevirapine who change to the extended release formulation should adhere to their regular monitoring schedule. AIDS*info* adult guidelines recommend serum transaminase monitoring every 2 weeks for the first 4 weeks of therapy, then monthly for 3 months, followed by every 3-4 months. AIDS*info* pediatric guidelines recommend serum transaminase monitoring every 2 weeks for the first 4 weeks of therapy, followed by every 4 months. Assess/evaluate AST/ALT immediately in any patients with a rash. Permanently discontinue if patient experiences severe rash, constitutional symptoms associated with rash, rash with elevated AST/ALT, or clinical hepatitis. Mild-to-moderate rash without AST/ALT elevation may continue treatment per discretion of prescriber. If mild-to-moderate urticarial rash, do not restart if treatment is interrupted.

Additional Information Patients should never be taking more than one form (ie, immediate release or extended release) of nevirapine concomitantly. Potential compliance problems, frequency of administration, and adverse effects should be discussed with patients before initiating therapy to help prevent the emergence of resistance. Early virologic failure was observed with tenofovir and didanosine delayed release capsules, plus either efavirenz or nevirapine; use caution in treatment-naive patients with high baseline viral loads. Due to rapid emergence of resistance, nevirapine should not be used as monotherapy or as the only agent added to a failing regimen for the treatment of HIV. Use care when timing discontinuation of regimens containing nevirapine; levels of nevirapine are sustained after levels of other medications decrease, potentially leading to nevirapine resistance. Cross-resistance may be conferred to other non-nucleoside reverse transcriptase inhibitors.

Dosage Forms Excipient information presented when available (limited, particularly for generics); consult specific product labeling.

Suspension, oral:

Viramune®: 50 mg/5 mL (240 mL)

Tablet, oral:

Viramune®: 200 mg [scored]

Tablet, extended release, oral:

Viramune® XR™: 400 mg

- ◆ **New-Fill®** *see* Poly-L-Lactic Acid *on page 1374*
- ◆ **NexAVAR®** *see* SORAfenib *on page 1584*
- ◆ **Nexavar® (Can)** *see* SORAfenib *on page 1584*
- ◆ **Nexiclon™ XR** *see* CloNIDine *on page 392*
- ◆ **NexIUM®** *see* Esomeprazole *on page 624*
- ◆ **Nexium® (Can)** *see* Esomeprazole *on page 624*
- ◆ **NexIUM® I.V.** *see* Esomeprazole *on page 624*
- ◆ **Next Choice™** *see* Levonorgestrel *on page 1001*
- ◆ **Nexterone®** *see* Amiodarone *on page 90*
- ◆ **NFV** *see* Nelfinavir *on page 1185*
- ◆ **NG-Citalopram (Can)** *see* Citalopram *on page 370*

Niacin (NYE a sin)

Brand Names: U.S. Niacin-Time® [OTC]; Niacor®; Niaspan®; Slo-Niacin® [OTC]

Brand Names: Canada Niaspan®; Niaspan® FCT; Niodan

Index Terms Nicotinic Acid; Vitamin B_3

Pharmacologic Category Antilipemic Agent, Miscellaneous; Vitamin, Water Soluble

Additional Appendix Information

Hyperlipidemia Management *on page 1996*

Use Treatment of dyslipidemias (Fredrickson types IIa and IIb or primary hypercholesterolemia) as mono- or adjunctive therapy; to lower the risk of recurrent MI in patients with a history of MI and hyperlipidemia; to slow progression or promote regression of coronary artery disease; treatment of hypertriglyceridemia in patients at risk of pancreatitis

Unlabeled Use Treatment of pellagra; dietary supplement

Pregnancy Risk Factor A/C (dose exceeding RDA recommendation)

Pregnancy Considerations Animal reproduction studies have not been conducted. It is unknown whether or not niacin at lipid-lowering doses is harmful to the developing fetus. If a woman becomes pregnant while receiving niacin for primary hypercholesterolemia, niacin should be discontinued. If a woman becomes pregnant while receiving niacin for hypertriglyceridemia, the benefits and risks of continuing niacin should be assessed on an individual basis.

Lactation Enters breast milk/consider risk:benefit

Contraindications Hypersensitivity to niacin, niacinamide, or any component of the formulation; active hepatic disease or significant or unexplained persistent elevations in hepatic transaminases; active peptic ulcer; arterial hemorrhage

Warnings/Precautions Use with caution in patients with unstable angina or MI, diabetes (may interfere with glucose control), renal disease, active gallbladder disease (can exacerbate), gout, or with anticoagulants (may slightly increase prothrombin time). Use with caution in patients with a past history of hepatic impairment and/or who consume substantial amounts of ethanol; contraindicated with active liver disease or unexplained persistent transaminase elevation. Rare cases of rhabdomyolysis have occurred during concomitant use with HMG-CoA reductase inhibitors. With concurrent use or if symptoms suggestive of myopathy occur, monitor creatine phosphokinase (CPK) and potassium; use with caution in patients with renal impairment, inadequately treated hypothyroidism, patients with diabetes or the elderly; risk for myopathy and rhabdomyolysis may be increased.

Immediate and extended or sustained release products are not interchangeable. Cases of severe hepatotoxicity have occurred when immediate release (crystalline) niacin products have been substituted with sustained-release (modified release, timed-release) niacin products at equivalent doses. Patients should be initiated with low doses (eg, 500 mg at bedtime) with titration to achieve desired response. Flushing and pruritus, common adverse effects of niacin, may be attenuated with a gradual increase in dose, and/or by taking aspirin (adults: 325 mg) or an NSAID 30-60 minutes before dosing. Compliance is enhanced with twice-daily dosing (extended-release product excluded). Prior to initiation, secondary causes for hypercholesterolemia (eg, poorly controlled diabetes mellitus, hypothyroidism) should be excluded; management with diet and other nonpharmacologic measures (eg, exercise or weight reduction) should be attempted prior to initiation. Use has not been evaluated in Fredrickson type I or III dyslipidemias.

Adverse Reactions Frequency not defined.

Cardiovascular: Arrhythmias, atrial fibrillation, edema, flushing, hypotension, orthostasis, palpitation, syncope (rare), tachycardia

Central nervous system: Chills, dizziness, headache, insomnia, migraine, nervousness, pain

Dermatologic: Acanthosis nigricans, burning skin, dry skin, hyperpigmentation, maculopapular rash, pruritus, rash, skin discoloration, urticaria

Endocrine & metabolic: Glucose tolerance decreased, gout, phosphorous levels decreased, hyperuricemia

Gastrointestinal: Abdominal pain, amylase increased, diarrhea, dyspepsia, eructation, flatulence, nausea, peptic ulcers, vomiting

Hematologic: Platelet counts decreased

Hepatic: Hepatic necrosis (rare), hepatitis, jaundice, transaminases increased (dose-related), prothrombin time increased, total bilirubin increased

Neuromuscular & skeletal: CPK increased, leg cramps, myalgia, myasthenia, myopathy (with concurrent HMG-CoA reductase inhibitor), paresthesia, rhabdomyolysis (with concurrent HMG-CoA reductase inhibitor; rare), weakness

Ocular: Blurred vision, cystoid macular edema, toxic amblyopia

Respiratory: Cough, dyspnea

Miscellaneous: Diaphoresis, hypersensitivity reactions (rare; includes anaphylaxis, angioedema, laryngismus, vesiculobullous rash), LDH increased

Drug Interactions

Metabolism/Transport Effects None known.

Avoid Concomitant Use There are no known interactions where it is recommended to avoid concomitant use.

Increased Effect/Toxicity

Niacin may increase the levels/effects of: HMG-CoA Reductase Inhibitors

Decreased Effect

The levels/effects of Niacin may be decreased by: Bile Acid Sequestrants

Ethanol/Nutrition/Herb Interactions Ethanol: Avoid heavy use; avoid use around niacin dose.

Stability

Niaspan®: Store at room temperature of 20°C to 25°C (68°F to 77°F).

Niacor®: Store at controlled room temperature of 15°C to 30°C (59°F to 86°F).

Mechanism of Action Component of two coenzymes which is necessary for tissue respiration, lipid metabolism, and glycogenolysis; inhibits the synthesis of very low density lipoproteins (VLDL) and low density lipoproteins (LDL); may also increase the rate of chylomicron triglyceride removal from plasma.

Pharmacodynamics/Kinetics

Absorption: Rapid and extensive (60% to 76%)

Distribution: Mainly to hepatic, renal, and adipose tissue

Metabolism: Extensive first-pass effects; converted to nicotinamide adenine dinucleotide, nicotinuric acid, and other metabolites

Half-life elimination: 20-45 minutes

Time to peak, serum: Immediate release formulation: 30-60 minutes; extended release formulation: 4-5 hours

Excretion: Urine 60% to 88% (unchanged drug [up to 12% recovered after multiple dosing] and metabolites)

Dosage Oral: **Note:** Formulations of niacin (regular release versus extended release) are not interchangeable.

Children:

Pellagra (unlabeled use): 50-100 mg/dose 3 times/day (some experts prefer niacinamide for treatment due to more favorable side effect profile)

Adequate intake (National Academy of Sciences, 1998):

0-5 months: 2 mg/day

6-11 months: 3 mg/day

Recommended daily allowances (National Academy of Sciences, 1998):

1-3 years: 6 mg/day

4-8 years: 8 mg/day

9-13 years: 12 mg/day

14-18 years: Females: 14 mg/day; Males: 16 mg/day

≥19 years: Refer to adult dosing

Adults:
Recommended daily allowances (National Academy of Sciences, 1998):
≥19 years: Females: 14 mg/day; Males: 16 mg/day
Pregnancy (all ages): 18 mg/day
Lactation (all ages): 17 mg/day
Dietary supplement (OTC labeling): 50 mg twice daily or 100 mg once daily. **Note:** Many over-the-counter formulations exist.
Hyperlipidemia:
Regular release formulation (Niacor®): Initial: 250 mg once daily (with evening meal); increase frequency and/or dose every 4-7 days to desired response or first-level therapeutic dose (1.5-2 g/day in 2-3 divided doses); after 2 months, may increase at 2- to 4-week intervals to 3 g/day in 3 divided doses (maximum dose: 6 g/day [NCEP recommends 4.5 g/day] in 3 divided doses). Usual daily dose after titration (NCEP, 2002): 1.5-3 g/day. **Note:** Many over-the-counter formulations exist.
Sustained release (or controlled release) formulations: **Note:** Several over-the-counter formulations exist. Usual daily dose after titration (NCEP, 2002): 1-2 g/day
Extended release formulation (Niaspan®): Initial: 500 mg at bedtime for 4 weeks, then 1 g at bedtime for 4 weeks; adjust dose to response and tolerance; may increase dose every 4 weeks by 500 mg/day to a maximum of 2 g/day. Usual daily dose after titration (NCEP, 2002): 1-2 g once daily
If additional LDL-lowering is necessary with lovastatin or simvastatin: Recommended initial lovastatin or simvastatin dose: 20 mg/day (maximum lovastatin or simvastatin dose: 40 mg/day); **Note:** Lovastatin prescribing information recommends a maximum dose of 20 mg/day with concurrent use of niacin (>1 g/day).
Pellagra (unlabeled use): 50-100 mg 3-4 times/day; maximum: 500 mg/day (some experts prefer niacinamide for treatment due to more favorable side effect profile)

Dosage adjustment in renal impairment: No dosage adjustment recommended; use with caution

Dosage adjustment in hepatic impairment: Contraindicated in patients with significant or unexplained hepatic dysfunction, active liver disease or unexplained persistent transaminase elevations.

Dosage adjustment for hepatic toxicity: Transaminases rise ≥3 times ULN, either persistent or if symptoms of nausea, fever, and/or malaise occur: Discontinue therapy.

Dietary Considerations Should be taken with meal; low-fat meal if treating hyperlipidemia. Avoid hot drinks around the time of niacin dose.

Administration Administer with food.
Niaspan®: Administer at bedtime. Tablet strengths are not interchangeable. When switching from immediate release tablet, initiate Niaspan® at lower dose and titrate. If therapy is interrupted for an extended period, dose should be retitrated. Long-acting forms should not be crushed, broken, or chewed. Do not substitute long-acting forms for immediate release ones.

Monitoring Parameters Blood glucose (in diabetic patients); CPK and serum potassium (if on concurrent HMG-CoA reductase inhibitor); liver function tests pretreatment, every 6-12 weeks for first year, then periodically (approximately every 6 months), monitor liver function more frequently if history of transaminase elevation with prior use; lipid profile; platelets; PT (if on anticoagulants); uric acid (if predisposed to gout); phosphorus (if predisposed to hypophosphatemia)

Test Interactions False elevations in some fluorometric determinations of plasma or urinary catecholamines; false-positive urine glucose (Benedict's reagent)

Dosage Forms Excipient information presented when available (limited, particularly for generics); consult specific product labeling.
Caplet, timed release, oral: 500 mg
Capsule, oral: 50 mg, 250 mg
Capsule, extended release, oral: 250 mg, 500 mg
Capsule, timed release, oral: 250 mg, 400 mg, 500 mg
Tablet, oral: 50 mg, 100 mg, 250 mg, 500 mg
Niacor®: 500 mg [scored]
Tablet, controlled release, oral:
Slo-Niacin®: 250 mg, 500 mg, 750 mg [scored]
Tablet, extended release, oral:
Niaspan®: 500 mg, 750 mg, 1000 mg
Tablet, timed release, oral: 250 mg, 500 mg, 750 mg, 1000 mg
Niacin-Time®: 500 mg

Niacinamide (nye a SIN a mide)

Index Terms Nicomide-T; Nicotinamide; Nicotinic Acid Amide; Vitamin B_3

Pharmacologic Category Vitamin, Water Soluble

Use
Prophylaxis and treatment of pellagra

Pregnancy Risk Factor A/C (dose exceeding RDA recommendation)

Dosage Pellagra: Oral:
Children: 10-50 mg every 6 hours until resolution of signs and symptoms (Hegyi, 2004)
Adults: 100 mg every 6 hours for several days (or until resolution of major signs and symptoms), followed by 50 mg every 8-12 hours until skin lesions heal (Hegyi, 2004)

Additional Information Complete prescribing information for this medication should be consulted for additional detail.

Dosage Forms Excipient information presented when available (limited, particularly for generics); consult specific product labeling.
Tablet, oral: 100 mg, 250 mg, 500 mg

Niacin and Lovastatin (NYE a sin & LOE va sta tin)

Brand Names: U.S. Advicor®

Brand Names: Canada Advicor®

Index Terms Lovastatin and Niacin

Pharmacologic Category Antilipemic Agent, HMG-CoA Reductase Inhibitor; Antilipemic Agent, Miscellaneous

Additional Appendix Information
Hyperlipidemia Management *on page 1996*

Use For use when treatment with both extended-release niacin and lovastatin is appropriate in combination with a standard cholesterol-lowering diet:
Extended-release niacin: Adjunctive treatment of dyslipidemias (types IIa and IIb or primary hypercholesterolemia) to lower the risk of recurrent MI and/or slow progression of coronary artery disease, including combination therapy with other antidyslipidemic agents when additional triglyceride-lowering or HDL-increasing effects are desired; treatment of hypertriglyceridemia in patients at risk of pancreatitis
Lovastatin: Treatment of primary hypercholesterolemia (Frederickson types IIa and IIb); primary and secondary prevention of cardiovascular disease

Pregnancy Risk Factor X

Dosage Dosage forms are a fixed combination of niacin and lovastatin.

Oral: Adults: Lowest dose: Niacin 500 mg/lovastatin 20 mg; may increase by not more than 500 mg (niacin) at 4-week intervals (maximum dose: Niacin 2000 mg/ lovastatin 40 mg daily); should be taken at bedtime with a low-fat snack. **Note:** If therapy is interrupted for >7 days, reinstitution of therapy should begin with the lowest dose followed by retitration as needed.

Not for use as initial therapy of dyslipidemias. May be substituted for equivalent dose of Niaspan®, however, manufacturer does not recommend direct substitution with other niacin products.

Dosage adjustment in renal impairment:

Mild-to-moderate impairment: No dosage adjustment required

Cl_{cr} <30 mL/minute: Use doses of lovastatin >20 mg/day with caution

Dosage adjustment in hepatic impairment: Do not use in active liver disease or unexplained persistent elevations of serum transaminases.

Additional Information Complete prescribing information for this medication should be consulted for additional detail.

Dosage Forms Excipient information presented when available (limited, particularly for generics); consult specific product labeling.

Tablet, variable release (Advicor®):

500/20: Niacin 500 mg [extended release] and lovastatin 20 mg [immediate release]

750/20: Niacin 750 mg [extended release] and lovastatin 20 mg [immediate release]

1000/20: Niacin 1000 mg [extended release] and lovastatin 20 mg [immediate release]

1000/40: Niacin 1000 mg [extended release] and lovastatin 40 mg [immediate release]

◆ **Niacin-Time® [OTC]** *see* Niacin *on page 1195*

◆ **Niacor®** *see* Niacin *on page 1195*

◆ **Niaspan®** *see* Niacin *on page 1195*

◆ **Niaspan® FCT (Can)** *see* Niacin *on page 1195*

◆ **Niastase® (Can)** *see* Factor VIIa (Recombinant) *on page 681*

◆ **Niastase® RT (Can)** *see* Factor VIIa (Recombinant) *on page 681*

NiCARdipine (nye KAR de peen)

Brand Names: U.S. Cardene® I.V.; Cardene® SR

Index Terms Nicardipine Hydrochloride

Pharmacologic Category Antianginal Agent; Calcium Channel Blocker; Calcium Channel Blocker, Dihydropyridine

Additional Appendix Information

Calcium Channel Blockers *on page 1887*

Hypertension *on page 2001*

Use Chronic stable angina (immediate-release product only); management of hypertension (immediate and sustained release products); parenteral only for short-term use when oral treatment is not feasible

Unlabeled Use Congestive heart failure, control of blood pressure in acute ischemic stroke and spontaneous intracranial hemorrhage, postoperative hypertension associated with carotid endarterectomy, perioperative hypertension, prevention of migraine headaches, subarachnoid hemorrhage associated cerebral vasospasm

Pregnancy Risk Factor C

Pregnancy Considerations Adverse events were observed in some animal reproduction studies. Nicardipine has been used for the treatment of severe hypertension in pregnancy and pre-term labor. Nicardipine crosses the placenta; changes in fetal heart rate, neonatal hypotension and neonatal acidosis have been observed following maternal use (rare based on limited data). Adverse effects reported in pregnant women are generally similar to those reported in non pregnant patients; however pulmonary edema has been observed.

Lactation Enters breast milk

Contraindications Hypersensitivity to nicardipine or any component of the formulation; advanced aortic stenosis

Warnings/Precautions Symptomatic hypotension with or without syncope can rarely occur; blood pressure must be lowered at a rate appropriate for the patient's clinical condition. Close monitoring of blood pressure and heart rate is required. Reflex tachycardia may occur resulting in angina and/or MI in patients with obstructive coronary disease especially in the absence of concurrent beta blockade. The most common side effect is peripheral edema (dose-dependent); occurs within 2-3 weeks of starting therapy. Use with caution in CAD (can cause increase in angina), HF (can worsen heart failure symptoms), aortic stenosis (may reduce coronary perfusion resulting in ischemia; use is contraindicated in patients with advanced aortic stenosis), and hypertrophic cardiomyopathy with outflow tract obstruction. To minimize infusion site reactions, peripheral infusion sites (for I.V. therapy) should be changed every 12 hours; use of small peripheral veins should be avoided. Titrate I.V. dose cautiously in patients with HF, renal or hepatic dysfunction. Use the I.V. form cautiously in patients with portal hypertension (can cause increase in hepatic pressure gradient). Initiate at the low end of the dosage range in the elderly.

Adverse Reactions

1% to 10%:

Cardiovascular: Cardiovascular: Flushing (6% to 10%), peripheral edema (dose related; 6% to 8%), hypotension (I.V. 6%), increased angina (dose related; 6%), palpitation (3% to 4%), tachycardia (1% to 4%), vasodilation (1% to 5%), chest pain (I.V. 1%), ECG abnormal (I.V. 1%), extrasystoles (I.V. 1%), hemopericardium (I.V. 1%), hypertension (I.V. 1%), orthostasis (1%), supraventricular tachycardia (I.V. 1%), syncope (1%), ventricular extrasystoles (I.V. 1%), ventricular tachycardia (I.V. 1%)

Central nervous system: Headache (6% to 15%), dizziness (1% to 7%), hypoesthesia (1%), intracranial hemorrhage (1%) pain (1%), somnolence (1%)

Dermatologic: Rash (1%)

Endocrine & metabolic: Hypokalemia (I.V. 1%)

Gastrointestinal: Nausea (2% to 5%), vomiting (I.V. 5%), dyspepsia (oral 2%), abdominal pain (I.V. 1%), dry mouth (1%)

Genitourinary: Polyuria (1%)

Local: Injection site pain (I.V. 1%), injection site reaction (I.V. 1%)

Neuromuscular & skeletal: Weakness (1% to 6%), myalgia (1%), paresthesia (1%)

Renal: Hematuria (1%)

Respiratory: Dyspnea (1%)

Miscellaneous: Diaphoresis (1%)

<1% (Limited to important or life-threatening): Allergic reaction, confusion, constipation, deep vein thrombophlebitis; ECG effects (AV block, inverted T wave, ST segment depression); gingival hyperplasia, hypertonia, hypophosphatemia, insomnia, malaise, nervousness, nocturia, parotitis, thrombocytopenia, tinnitus, tremor

Drug Interactions

Metabolism/Transport Effects Substrate of CYP1A2 (minor), CYP2C9 (minor), CYP2D6 (minor), CYP2E1 (minor), CYP3A4 (major), P-glycoprotein; **Note:** Assignment of Major/Minor substrate status based on clinically relevant drug interaction potential; **Inhibits** CYP2C19 (moderate), CYP2C9 (strong), CYP2D6 (moderate), CYP3A4 (strong), P-glycoprotein

Avoid Concomitant Use

Avoid concomitant use of NiCARdipine with any of the following: Alfuzosin; Conivaptan; Crizotinib; Dronedarone; Eplerenone; Everolimus; Fluticasone (Oral Inhalation); Halofantrine; Lapatinib; Lovastatin; Lurasidone; Nilotinib; Nisoldipine; Pimozide; Ranolazine; Rivaroxaban; RomiDEPsin; Salmeterol; Silodosin; Simvastatin; Tamsulosin; Thioridazine; Ticagrelor; Tolvaptan; Topotecan; Toremifene

Increased Effect/Toxicity

NiCARdipine may increase the levels/effects of: Alfuzosin; Almotriptan; Alosetron; Amifostine; Antihypertensives; ARIPiprazole; Beta-Blockers; Bortezomib; Brentuximab Vedotin; Brinzolamide; Budesonide (Nasal); Budesonide (Systemic, Oral Inhalation); Calcium Channel Blockers (Nondihydropyridine); Ciclesonide; Citalopram; Colchicine; Conivaptan; Corticosteroids (Orally Inhaled); Crizotinib; CYP2C19 Substrates; CYP2C9 Substrates; CYP2D6 Substrates; CYP3A4 Substrates; Dabigatran Etexilate; Diclofenac; Dienogest; Dronedarone; Dutasteride; Eplerenone; Everolimus; FentaNYL; Fesoterodine; Fluticasone (Nasal); Fluticasone (Oral Inhalation); Fosphenytoin; GuanFACINE; Halofantrine; Hypotensive Agents; Iloperidone; Ixabepilone; Lapatinib; Lovastatin; Lumefantrine; Lurasidone; Magnesium Salts; Maraviroc; MethylPREDNISolone; Neuromuscular-Blocking Agents (Nondepolarizing); Nilotinib; Nisoldipine; Nitroprusside; Paricalcitol; Pazopanib; P-glycoprotein/ABCB1 Substrates; Phenytoin; Pimecrolimus; Pimozide; Propafenone; QuiNIDine; Ranolazine; RiTUXimab; Rivaroxaban; RomiDEPsin; Ruxolitinib; Salmeterol; Saxagliptin; Sildenafil; Silodosin; Simvastatin; SORAfenib; Tacrolimus; Tacrolimus (Systemic); Tadalafil; Tamsulosin; Thioridazine; Ticagrelor; Tolterodine; Tolvaptan; Topotecan; Toremifene; Vardenafil; Vemurafenib; Vilazodone; Zuclopenthixol

The levels/effects of NiCARdipine may be increased by: Alpha1-Blockers; Antifungal Agents (Azole Derivatives, Systemic); Calcium Channel Blockers (Nondihydropyridine); CycloSPORINE; CycloSPORINE (Systemic); CYP3A4 Inhibitors (Moderate); CYP3A4 Inhibitors (Strong); Dasatinib; Diazoxide; Fluconazole; Grapefruit Juice; Herbs (Hypotensive Properties); Macrolide Antibiotics; Magnesium Salts; MAO Inhibitors; Pentoxifylline; P-glycoprotein/ABCB1 Inhibitors; Prostacyclin Analogues; Protease Inhibitors; QuiNIDine

Decreased Effect

NiCARdipine may decrease the levels/effects of: Clopidogrel; Codeine; Prasugrel; QuiNIDine; Ticagrelor; TraMADol

The levels/effects of NiCARdipine may be decreased by: Barbiturates; Calcium Salts; CarBAMazepine; CYP3A4 Inducers (Strong); Cyproterone; Deferasirox; Herbs (Hypertensive Properties); Methylphenidate; Nafcillin; Peginterferon Alfa-2b; P-glycoprotein/ABCB1 Inducers; Rifamycin Derivatives; Tocilizumab; Yohimbine

Ethanol/Nutrition/Herb Interactions

Ethanol: Avoid ethanol (may increase CNS depression).

Food: Nicardipine average peak concentrations may be decreased if taken with food. Serum concentrations/toxicity of nicardipine may be increased by grapefruit juice; avoid concurrent use.

Herb/Nutraceutical: St John's wort may decrease levels. Avoid bayberry, blue cohosh, cayenne, ephedra, ginger, ginseng (American), kola, licorice (may worsen hypertension). Avoid black cohosh, California poppy, coleus, golden seal, hawthorn, mistletoe, periwinkle, quinine, shepherd's purse (may have increased antihypertensive effect).

Stability

I.V.:

Premixed bags: Store at controlled room temperature of 20°C to 25°C (68°F to 77°F). Protect from light and excessive heat. Do not freeze.

Vials: Store at controlled room temperature of 20°C to 25°C (68°F to 77°F). Protect from light. Dilute 25 mg vial with 240 mL of compatible solution to provide a 250 mL total volume solution and a final concentration of 0.1 mg/mL. Diluted solution (0.1 mg/mL) is stable at room temperature for 24 hours in glass or PVC containers. Stability has also been demonstrated at room temperature at concentrations up to 0.5 mg/mL in PVC containers for 24 hours or in glass containers for up to 7 days (Baaske, 1996).

Oral (Cardene®, Cardene SR®): Store at 15°C to 30°C (59°F to 86°F). Protect from light. Freezing does not affect stability.

Mechanism of Action Inhibits calcium ion from entering the "slow channels" or select voltage-sensitive areas of vascular smooth muscle and myocardium during depolarization, producing a relaxation of coronary vascular smooth muscle and coronary vasodilation; increases myocardial oxygen delivery in patients with vasospastic angina

Pharmacodynamics/Kinetics

Onset of action: Oral: 0.5-2 hours; I.V.: 10 minutes; Hypotension: ~20 minutes

Duration:

I.V.: ≤8 hours

Oral: Immediate release capsules: ≤8 hours; Sustained release capsules: 8-12 hours

Absorption: Oral: ~100%

Protein binding: >95%

Metabolism: Hepatic; CYP3A4 substrate (major); extensive first-pass effect (saturable)

Bioavailability: 35%

Half-life elimination: 2-4 hours

Time to peak, serum: Oral: Immediate release: 30-120 minutes; Sustained release: 60-240 minutes

Excretion: Urine (49% to 60% as metabolites); feces (43% as metabolites)

Dosage

Adults:

Oral:

Immediate release: Initial: 20 mg 3 times/day; usual: 20-40 mg 3 times/day (allow 3 days between dose increases)

Sustained release: Initial: 30 mg twice daily, titrate up to 60 mg twice daily

Note: The total daily dose of immediate-release product may not automatically be equivalent to the daily sustained-release dose; use caution in converting.

I.V.:

Acute hypertension: Initial: 5 mg/hour increased by 2.5 mg/hour every 5 minutes (for rapid titration) to every 15 minutes (for gradual titration) up to a maximum of 15 mg/hour; in rapidly titrated patients, consider reduction to 3 mg/hour after response is achieved.

Arterial hypertension in acute ischemic stroke (unlabeled use [Adams, 2007; Jauch, 2010]):

Patient otherwise eligible for reperfusion treatment (eg, alteplase): Blood pressure (BP): Systolic >185 mm Hg or diastolic >110 mm Hg: 5 mg/hour; titrate by 2.5 mg/hour at 5-15 minute intervals (maximum dose: 15 mg/hour). When goal BP obtained, reduce dose to 3 mg/hour. If BP does not decline and remains >185/110 mm Hg, alteplase should not be administered.

Management of BP during and after reperfusion treatment (eg, alteplase): BP: Systolic >230 mm Hg or diastolic >121-140 mm Hg: 5 mg/hour; titrate by 2.5 mg/hour at 5-minute intervals (maximum dose: 15 mg/hour). If hypertension is refractory, consider other I.V. antihypertensives (eg, nitroprusside).

Substitution for oral therapy (approximate equivalents):

20 mg every 8 hours oral, equivalent to 0.5 mg/hour I.V. infusion

30 mg every 8 hours oral, equivalent to 1.2 mg/hour I.V. infusion

40 mg every 8 hours oral, equivalent to 2.2 mg/hour I.V. infusion

Conversion to oral antihypertensive agent: Initiate oral antihypertensive at the same time that I.V. nicardipine is discontinued, if transitioning to oral nicardipine, start oral nicardipine 1 hour prior to I.V. discontinuation.

Elderly: Initiate at the low end of the dosage range. Specific guidelines for adjustment of nicardipine are not available, but careful monitoring is warranted and adjustment may be necessary.

Dosing adjustment in renal impairment:

Oral: Per the manufacturer: Titrate dose beginning with 20 mg 3 times/day (immediate release capsule) or 30 mg twice daily (sustained release capsule).

I.V.: Specific guidelines for adjustment of nicardipine are not available, but careful monitoring is warranted and adjustment may be necessary.

Dosing adjustment in hepatic impairment:

Oral: Per the manufacturer: Starting dose: 20 mg twice daily (immediate release) with titration. Refer to **"Note"** in adult dosing.

I.V.: Specific guidelines for adjustment of nicardipine are not available, but careful monitoring is warranted and adjustment may be necessary.

Dietary Considerations Avoid grapefruit juice.

Administration

Oral: The total daily dose of immediate-release product may not automatically be equivalent to the daily sustained-release dose; use caution in converting. Do not chew or crush the sustained release formulation, swallow whole. Do not open or cut capsules.

I.V.:

Vials must be diluted before use. Administer as a slow continuous infusion at a concentration of 0.1 mg/mL or 0.2 mg/mL. Concentrations of 0.5 mg/mL may be administered via a central line only.

Premixed bags: No further dilution needed. For single use only, discard any unused portion. Use only if solution is clear; the manufacturer recommends not to admix or run in the same line as other medications.

Monitoring Parameters Blood pressure, heart rate

Dosage Forms Excipient information presented when available (limited, particularly for generics); consult specific product labeling.

Capsule, oral, as hydrochloride: 20 mg, 30 mg

Capsule, sustained release, oral, as hydrochloride:

Cardene® SR: 30 mg, 45 mg, 60 mg

Infusion, premixed iso-osmotic dextrose solution, as hydrochloride:

Cardene® I.V.: 20 mg (200 mL); 40 mg (200 mL)

Infusion, premixed iso-osmotic sodium chloride solution, as hydrochloride:

Cardene® I.V.: 20 mg (200 mL); 40 mg (200 mL)

Injection, solution, as hydrochloride: 2.5 mg/mL (10 mL)

Cardene® I.V.: 2.5 mg/mL (10 mL)

◆ **Nicardipine Hydrochloride** *see* NiCARdipine *on page 1198*

◆ **Nicoderm® (Can)** *see* Nicotine *on page 1200*

◆ **NicoDerm® CQ® [OTC]** *see* Nicotine *on page 1200*

◆ **Nicomide-T** *see* Niacinamide *on page 1197*

◆ **Nicorelief [OTC]** *see* Nicotine *on page 1200*

◆ **Nicorette® [OTC]** *see* Nicotine *on page 1200*

◆ **Nicorette® (Can)** *see* Nicotine *on page 1200*

◆ **Nicorette® Plus (Can)** *see* Nicotine *on page 1200*

◆ **Nicotinamide** *see* Niacinamide *on page 1197*

Nicotine (nik oh TEEN)

Brand Names: U.S. Commit® [OTC]; NicoDerm® CQ® [OTC]; Nicorelief [OTC]; Nicorette® [OTC]; Nicotrol® Inhaler; Nicotrol® NS; Thrive™ [OTC]

Brand Names: Canada Habitrol®; Nicoderm®; Nicorette®; Nicorette® Plus; Nicotrol®

Index Terms Habitrol; Nicotine Patch

Pharmacologic Category Smoking Cessation Aid

Additional Appendix Information

Nicotine Products *on page 1894*

Use Treatment to aid smoking cessation for the relief of nicotine withdrawal symptoms (including nicotine craving)

Unlabeled Use Management of ulcerative colitis (transdermal)

Pregnancy Risk Factor D (nasal)

Pregnancy Considerations Nicotine is teratogenic in animal studies. Nicotine exposure via cigarette smoke may cause increased ectopic pregnancy, low birth weight, increased risk of spontaneous abortion, increased perinatal mortality; increased aortic blood flow, increased heart rate, decreased uterine blood flow, and decreased breathing have been reported in the fetus. Smoking during pregnancy is associated with sudden infant death syndrome (SIDS), an increased risk of asthma, infantile colic, and childhood obesity. Women who are pregnant should be encouraged not to smoke. The use of nicotine replacement products to aid in smoking cessation has not been adequately studied in pregnant women (amount of nicotine exposure is varied). Nonpharmacologic treatments are recommended. If the benefits of nicotine replacement therapy outweigh the unknown risks, products with intermittent dosing are suggested to be tried first. If a patch is used, it is suggested to remove it overnight while sleeping to decrease fetal exposure.

Lactation Excretion in breast milk unknown/use caution

Contraindications Hypersensitivity to nicotine or any component of the formulation; patients who are smoking during the postmyocardial infarction period; patients with life-threatening arrhythmias, or severe or worsening angina pectoris; active temporomandibular joint disease (gum); pregnancy; not for use in nonsmokers

Warnings/Precautions Hazardous agent - use appropriate precautions for handling and disposal. Use caution in patients with hyperthyroidism, pheochromocytoma, or insulin-dependent diabetes. Use with caution in oropharyngeal inflammation and in patients with history of esophagitis, peptic ulcer, coronary artery disease, recent MI, serious cardiac arrhythmias, vasospastic disease, angina, hypertension, hyperthyroidism, pheochromocytoma, diabetes, severe renal dysfunction, and hepatic dysfunction. The oral inhaler and nasal spray should be used with caution in patients with bronchospastic disease (other forms of nicotine replacement may be preferred). Use of nasal product is not recommended with chronic nasal disorders (eg, allergy, rhinitis, nasal polyps, and sinusitis). Transdermal patch may contain conducting metal (eg, aluminum); remove patch prior to MRI. Cautious use of topical nicotine in patients with certain skin diseases. Hypersensitivity to the topical products can occur. Dental problems may be worsened by chewing the gum. Urge patients to stop smoking completely when initiating therapy.

Adverse Reactions

Nasal spray/inhaler:

>10%:

Central nervous system: Headache (18% to 26%)

Gastrointestinal: Inhaler: Mouth/throat irritation (66%), dyspepsia (18%)

Respiratory: Inhaler: Cough (32%), rhinitis (23%)

1% to 10%:

Dermatologic: Acne (3%)

Endocrine & metabolic: Dysmenorrhea (3%)

Gastrointestinal: Flatulence (4%), gum problems (4%), diarrhea, hiccup, nausea, taste disturbance, tooth abrasions

Neuromuscular & skeletal: Back pain (6%), arthralgia (5%), jaw/neck pain

Respiratory: Nasal burning (nasal spray), sinusitis

Miscellaneous: Withdrawal symptoms

<1% (Limited to important or life-threatening): Allergy, amnesia, aphasia, bronchitis, bronchospasm, edema, migraine, numbness, pain, purpura, rash, sputum increased, vision abnormalities, xerostomia

Adverse events previously reported in prescription labeling for chewing gum, lozenge and/or transdermal systems. Frequency not defined; may be product or dose specific:

Central nervous system: Concentration impaired, depression, dizziness, headache, insomnia, nervousness, pain

Gastrointestinal: Aphthous stomatitis, constipation, cough, diarrhea, dyspepsia, flatulence, gingival bleeding, glossitis, hiccups, jaw pain, nausea, salivation increased, stomatitis, taste perversion, tooth abrasions, ulcerative stomatitis, xerostomia

Dermatologic: Rash

Local: Application site reaction, local edema, local erythema

Neuromuscular & skeletal: Arthralgia, myalgia, paresthesia

Respiratory: Cough, sinusitis

Miscellaneous: Allergic reaction, diaphoresis

Drug Interactions

Metabolism/Transport Effects Substrate of CYP1A2 (minor), CYP2A6 (minor), CYP2B6 (minor), CYP2C19 (minor), CYP2C9 (minor), CYP2D6 (minor), CYP2E1 (minor), CYP3A4 (minor); **Note:** Assignment of Major/Minor substrate status based on clinically relevant drug interaction potential; **Inhibits** CYP2A6 (weak), CYP2E1 (weak)

Avoid Concomitant Use There are no known interactions where it is recommended to avoid concomitant use.

Increased Effect/Toxicity

Nicotine may increase the levels/effects of: Adenosine

The levels/effects of Nicotine may be increased by: Cimetidine; Conivaptan

Decreased Effect

The levels/effects of Nicotine may be decreased by: Cyproterone; Peginterferon Alfa-2b; Tocilizumab

Ethanol/Nutrition/Herb Interactions Food: Lozenge: Acidic foods/beverages decrease absorption of nicotine.

Stability

Nicotrol®: Store inhaler cartridge at room temperature not to exceed 30°C (86°F). Protect cartridges from light.

Nicotrol® NS: Store at room temperature not to exceed 30°C (86°F).

Mechanism of Action Nicotine is one of two naturally-occurring alkaloids which exhibit their primary effects via autonomic ganglia stimulation. The other alkaloid is lobeline which has many actions similar to those of nicotine but is less potent. Nicotine is a potent ganglionic and central nervous system stimulant, the actions of which are mediated via nicotine-specific receptors. Biphasic actions are observed depending upon the dose administered. The main effect of nicotine in small doses is stimulation of all autonomic ganglia; with larger doses, initial stimulation is followed by blockade of transmission. Biphasic effects are also evident in the adrenal medulla; discharge of catecholamines occurs with small doses, whereas prevention of catecholamines release is seen with higher doses as a response to splanchnic nerve stimulation. Stimulation of the central nervous system (CNS) is characterized by tremors and respiratory excitation. However, convulsions may occur with higher doses, along with respiratory failure secondary to both central paralysis and peripheral blockade to respiratory muscles.

Pharmacodynamics/Kinetics

Onset of action: Intranasal: More closely approximate the time course of plasma nicotine levels observed after cigarette smoking than other dosage forms

Duration: Transdermal: 24 hours

Absorption: Transdermal: Slow

Metabolism: Hepatic, primarily to cotinine (1/5 as active)

Half-life elimination: 4 hours; Nasal spray: 1-2 hours

Time to peak, serum: Transdermal: 8-9 hours; Nasal spray: 10-20 minutes

Excretion: Urine

Clearance: Renal: pH dependent

Dosage

Smoking deterrent: Patients should be advised to completely stop smoking upon initiation of therapy.

Oral:

Gum: Chew 1 piece of gum when urge to smoke, up to 24 pieces/day. Patients who smoke <25 cigarettes/day should start with 2-mg strength; patients smoking ≥25 cigarettes/day should start with the 4-mg strength. Use according to the following 12-week dosing schedule:

Weeks 1-6: Chew 1 piece of gum every 1-2 hours; to increase chances of quitting, chew at least 9 pieces/day during the first 6 weeks

Weeks 7-9: Chew 1 piece of gum every 2-4 hours

Weeks 10-12: Chew 1 piece of gum every 4-8 hours

Inhaler: Usually 6 to 16 cartridges per day; best effect was achieved by frequent continuous puffing (20 minutes); recommended duration of treatment is 3 months, after which patients may be weaned from the inhaler by gradual reduction of the daily dose over 6-12 weeks

Lozenge: Patients who smoke their first cigarette within 30 minutes of waking should use the 4 mg strength; otherwise the 2 mg strength is recommended. Use according to the following 12-week dosing schedule:

Weeks 1-6: One lozenge every 1-2 hours

Weeks 7-9: One lozenge every 2-4 hours

Weeks 10-12: One lozenge every 4-8 hours

Note: Use at least 9 lozenges/day during first 6 weeks to improve chances of quitting; do not use more than one lozenge at a time (maximum: 5 lozenges every 6 hours, 20 lozenges/day)

Topical:

Transdermal patch: Apply new patch every 24 hours to nonhairy, clean, dry skin on the upper body or upper outer arm; each patch should be applied to a different site. **Note:** Adjustment may be required during initial treatment (move to higher dose if experiencing withdrawal symptoms; lower dose if side effects are experienced).

NicoDerm CQ®:

Patients smoking >10 cigarettes/day: Begin with **step 1** (21 mg/day) for 6 weeks, followed by **step 2** (14 mg/day) for 2 weeks; finish with **step 3** (7 mg/day) for 2 weeks

Patients smoking ≤10 cigarettes/day: Begin with **step 2** (14 mg/day) for 6 weeks, followed by **step 3** (7 mg/day) for 2 weeks

Note: Patients receiving >600 mg/day of cimetidine: Decrease to the next lower patch size

Note: Benefits of use of nicotine transdermal patches beyond 3 months have not been demonstrated.

Nasal: Spray: 1-2 sprays/hour; do not exceed more than 5 doses (10 sprays) per hour [maximum: 40 doses/day (80 sprays); each dose (2 sprays) contains 1 mg of nicotine]

Dietary Considerations Some products may contain phenylalanine and/or sodium.

Administration

Gum: Should be chewed slowly to avoid jaw ache and to maximize benefit. Chew slowly until it tingles, then park gum between cheek and gum until tingle is gone; repeat process until most of tingle is gone (~30 minutes).

Lozenge: Should not be chewed or swallowed; allow to dissolve slowly (~20-30 minutes)

Nasal spray: Prime pump prior to first use (pump 6-8 times until fine spray appears) or if it has not been used for 24 hours (pump 1-2 times). Blow nose prior to use. Tilt head back slightly and insert tip of bottle into nostril. Breathe through mouth and spray once in each nostril. Do not sniff, swallow, or inhale through the nose during administration. After administration, wait 2-3 minutes before blowing nose.

Oral Inhalant: Insert cartridge into inhaler and push hard until it pops into place. Replace mouthpiece and twist the top and bottom so that markings do not line up. Inhale deeply into the back of the throat or puff in short breaths. Nicotine in cartridge is used up after about 20 minutes of active puffing.

Transdermal patch: Do not cut patch; causes rapid evaporation, rendering the patch useless

Monitoring Parameters Heart rate and blood pressure periodically during therapy; discontinue therapy if signs of nicotine toxicity occur (eg, severe headache, dizziness, mental confusion, disturbed hearing and vision, abdominal pain; rapid, weak and irregular pulse; salivation, nausea, vomiting, diarrhea, cold sweat, weakness); therapy should be discontinued if rash develops; discontinuation may be considered if other adverse effects of patch occur such as myalgia, arthralgia, abnormal dreams, insomnia, nervousness, dry mouth, sweating

Additional Information A cigarette has 10-25 mg nicotine.

Dosage Forms Excipient information presented when available (limited, particularly for generics); consult specific product labeling.

Gum, chewing, oral, as polacrilex: 2 mg (20s, 40s, 50s, 100s, 110s); 4 mg (20s, 40s, 50s, 100s, 110s)

Nicorelief: 2 mg (50s, 110s)

Nicorelief: 2 mg (50s, 110s) [mint flavor]

Nicorelief: 4 mg (50s, 110s)

Nicorelief: 4 mg (50s, 110s) [mint flavor]

Nicorette®: 2 mg (40s, 100s) [fresh mint flavor]

Nicorette®: 2 mg (48s, 50s, 108s, 110s, 168s, 170s, 192s, 200s, 216s) [mint flavor]

Nicorette®: 2 mg (48s, 108s) [orange flavor]

Nicorette®: 2 mg (48s, 50s, 108s, 110s, 168s, 170s, 192s, 200s, 216s) [original flavor]

Nicorette®: 2 mg (40s, 100s) [contains calcium 94 mg/gum, sodium 11 mg/gum; fruit chill flavor]

Nicorette®: 4 mg (40s, 100s) [fresh mint flavor]

Nicorette®: 4 mg (48s, 108s, 110s, 168s, 170s, 192s, 200s, 216s) [mint flavor]

Nicorette®: 4 mg (48s, 108s, 110s) [orange flavor]

Nicorette®: 4 mg (48s, 50s, 108s, 110s, 168s, 170s, 192s, 200s, 216s) [original flavor]

Nicorette®: 4 mg (40s, 100s) [contains calcium 94 mg/gum, sodium 13 mg/gum; fruit chill flavor]

Thrive™: 2 mg (40s); 4 mg (40s) [gluten free, sucrose free; mint flavor]

Lozenge, oral, as polacrilex:

Commit®: 2 mg (48s, 72s); 4 mg (48s, 72s) [gluten free, sugar free; contains phenylalanine 3.4 mg/lozenge, sodium 18 mg/lozenge; mint flavor]

Nicorette®: 4 mg (50s) [mint flavor]

Oral inhalation system, for oral inhalation:

Nicotrol® Inhaler: 10 mg (10 mL) [contains menthol; delivering 4 mg nicotine]

Patch, transdermal: 7 mg/24 hours (7s, 14s); 14 mg/24 hours (7s, 14s); 21 mg/24 hours (7s, 14s)

NicoDerm® CQ®: 7 mg/24 hours (14s) [contains metal; step 3; clear patch]

NicoDerm® CQ®: 7 mg/24 hours (14s) [contains metal; step 3; tan patch]

NicoDerm® CQ®: 14 mg/24 hours (14s) [contains metal; step 2; clear patch]

NicoDerm® CQ®: 14 mg/24 hours (14s) [contains metal; step 2; tan patch]

NicoDerm® CQ®: 21 mg/24 hours (7s, 14s) [contains metal; step 1; clear patch]

NicoDerm® CQ®: 21 mg/24 hours (7s, 14s) [contains metal; step 1; tan patch]

Solution, intranasal [spray]:

Nicotrol® NS: 10 mg/mL (10 mL) [chlorofluorocarbon free; delivers ~0.5 mg/spray; ~200 sprays]

◆ **Nicotine Patch** *see* Nicotine *on page 1200*

◆ **Nicotinic Acid** *see* Niacin *on page 1195*

◆ **Nicotinic Acid Amide** *see* Niacinamide *on page 1197*

◆ **Nicotrol® (Can)** *see* Nicotine *on page 1200*

◆ **Nicotrol® Inhaler** *see* Nicotine *on page 1200*

◆ **Nicotrol® NS** *see* Nicotine *on page 1200*

◆ **Nidagel™ (Can)** *see* MetroNIDAZOLE (Topical) *on page 1122*

◆ **Nifediac CC®** *see* NIFEdipine *on page 1202*

◆ **Nifedical XL®** *see* NIFEdipine *on page 1202*

NIFEdipine (nye FED i peen)

Brand Names: U.S. Adalat® CC; Afeditab® CR; Nifediac CC®; Nifedical XL®; Procardia XL®; Procardia®

Brand Names: Canada Adalat® XL®; Apo-Nifed PA®; Mylan-Nifedipine Extended Release; Nu-Nifed; Nu-Nifedipine-PA; PMS-Nifedipine

Pharmacologic Category Antianginal Agent; Calcium Channel Blocker; Calcium Channel Blocker, Dihydropyridine

Additional Appendix Information

Beers Criteria – Potentially Inappropriate Medications for Geriatrics *on page 1973*

Calcium Channel Blockers *on page 1887*

Use Management of chronic stable or vasospastic angina; treatment of hypertension (sustained release products only)

Unlabeled Use Management of pulmonary hypertension, preterm labor, and Raynaud's phenomenon; prevention and treatment of high altitude pulmonary edema

Pregnancy Risk Factor C

Pregnancy Considerations Adverse events were observed in animal reproduction studies. Nifedipine crosses the placenta. Use in pregnancy only when clearly needed and when the benefits outweigh the potential hazard to the fetus. Hypotension, IUGR reported. IUGR probably related to maternal hypertension. May be used for the treatment of preterm labor.

Lactation Enters breast milk/not recommended (AAP considers "compatible"; AAP 2001 update pending)

Contraindications Hypersensitivity to nifedipine or any component of the formulation; concomitant use with strong CYP3A4 inducers (eg, rifampin); cardiogenic shock;

immediate release preparation for treatment of urgent or emergent hypertension (Chobanian, 2003); acute MI (Antman, 2004)

Warnings/Precautions Symptomatic hypotension with or without syncope can rarely occur; blood pressure must be lowered at a rate appropriate for the patient's clinical condition. **The use of immediate release nifedipine (sublingually or orally) in hypertensive emergencies and urgencies is neither safe nor effective.** Serious adverse events (eg, death, cerebrovascular ischemia, syncope, stroke, acute myocardial infarction, and fetal distress) have been reported. **Immediate release nifedipine should not be used for acute blood pressure reduction.**

Blood pressure lowering should be done at a rate appropriate for the patient's condition. Rapid drops in blood pressure can lead to arterial insufficiency. Increased angina and/or MI have occurred with initiation or dosage titration of dihydropyridine calcium channel blockers; use with caution in patients with obstructive coronary disease especially in the absence of concurrent beta-blockade. Use with caution before major surgery. Cardiopulmonary bypass, intraoperative blood loss or vasodilating anesthesia may result in severe hypotension and/or increased fluid requirements. Consider withdrawing nifedipine (>36 hours) before surgery if possible.

The most common side effect is peripheral edema; occurs within 2-3 weeks of starting therapy. Reflex tachycardia may occur with use. Use with caution in HF or severe aortic stenosis (especially with concomitant beta-adrenergic blocker), severe left ventricular dysfunction, renal impairment, hypertrophic cardiomyopathy (especially obstructive), concomitant therapy with beta-blockers or digoxin, and edema. Use caution in patients with severe hepatic impairment. Clearance of nifedipine is reduced in cirrhotic patients leading to increased systemic exposure; monitor closely for adverse effects/toxicity and consider dose adjustments. Mild and transient elevations in liver function enzymes may be apparent within 8 weeks of therapy initiation. Abrupt withdrawal may cause rebound angina in patients with CAD. Short-acting nifedipine may be inappropriate for use in the elderly due to potential to cause hypotension and constipation (Beers Criteria). Immediate release formulations should not be used to manage essential hypertension, adequate studies to evaluate outcomes have not been conducted. Avoid use of extended release tablets (Procardia XL®) in patients with known stricture/narrowing of the GI tract. Adalat® CC tablets contain lactose; do not use with galactose intolerance, Lapp lactase deficiency, or glucose-galactose malabsorption syndromes.

Use with caution in patients taking CYP3A4 inhibitors; may result in increased nifedipine concentrations; monitor for adverse effects/toxicity and consider dose adjustments. Use with strong CYP3A4 inducers (eg, rifampin, rifabutin, phenobarbital, phenytoin, carbamazepine, St John's wort) is contraindicated due to reduced bioavailability and efficacy.

Adverse Reactions

>10%:

Cardiovascular: Flushing (10% to 25%; extended release products 3% to 4%), peripheral edema (dose related 7% to 30%)

Central nervous system: Dizziness/lightheadedness/giddiness (10% to 27%), headache (10% to 23%)

Gastrointestinal: Nausea/heartburn (10% to 11%)

≥1% to 10%:

Cardiovascular: Palpitation (≤2% to 7%), transient hypotension (dose related 5%), CHF (2%)

Central nervous system: Nervousness/mood changes (≤2% to 7%), fatigue (6%), shakiness (≤2%), jitteriness (≤2%), sleep disturbances (≤2%), difficulties in balance (≤2%), fever (≤2%), chills (≤2%)

Dermatologic: Dermatitis (≤2%), pruritus (≤2%), urticaria (≤2%)

Endocrine & metabolic: Sexual difficulties (≤2%)

Gastrointestinal: Diarrhea (≤2%), constipation (≤2%), cramps (≤2%), flatulence (≤2%), gingival hyperplasia (≤10%)

Neuromuscular & skeletal: Muscle cramps/tremor (≤2% to 8%), weakness (<3%), inflammation (≤2%), joint stiffness (≤2%)

Ocular: Blurred vision (≤2%)

Respiratory: Cough/wheezing (6%), nasal congestion/sore throat (≤2% to 6%), chest congestion (≤2%), dyspnea (≤2%)

Miscellaneous: Diaphoresis (≤2%)

<1% (Limited to important or life-threatening): Agranulocytosis, allergic hepatitis, alopecia, anemia, angina, angioedema, aplastic anemia, arrhythmia, arthritis with positive ANA, bezoars (Procardia XL), cerebral ischemia, depression, dysosmia, epistaxis, EPS, erectile dysfunction, erythema multiforme, erythromelalgia, exanthematous pustulosis, exfoliative dermatitis, facial edema, gastroesophageal reflux, gastrointestinal obstruction (Procardia XL), gastrointestinal ulceration (Procardia XL), gynecomastia, hematuria, ischemia, leukopenia, memory dysfunction, migraine, myalgia, myoclonus, nocturia, paranoid syndrome, parotitis, periorbital edema, photosensitivity, polyuria, purpura, Stevens-Johnson syndrome, syncope, tachycardia, taste perversion, thrombocytopenia, tinnitus, toxic epidermal necrolysis, transient blindness, ventricular arrhythmia

Reported with use of sublingual short-acting nifedipine: Acute MI, cerebrovascular ischemia, ECG changes, fetal distress, heart block, severe hypotension, sinus arrest, stroke, syncope

Drug Interactions

Metabolism/Transport Effects Substrate of CYP2D6 (minor), CYP3A4 (major); **Note:** Assignment of Major/Minor substrate status based on clinically relevant drug interaction potential; **Inhibits** CYP1A2 (moderate), CYP2C9 (weak), CYP2D6 (weak), CYP3A4 (weak)

Avoid Concomitant Use

Avoid concomitant use of NIFEdipine with any of the following: Conivaptan; Grapefruit Juice; Pimozide

Increased Effect/Toxicity

NIFEdipine may increase the levels/effects of: Amifostine; Antihypertensives; Beta-Blockers; Calcium Channel Blockers (Nondihydropyridine); CYP1A2 Substrates; Digoxin; Fosphenytoin; Hypotensive Agents; Magnesium Salts; Neuromuscular-Blocking Agents (Nondepolarizing); Nitroprusside; Phenytoin; Pimozide; QuiNIDine; RiTUXimab; Tacrolimus; Tacrolimus (Systemic); VinCRIStine

The levels/effects of NIFEdipine may be increased by: Alcohol (Ethyl); Alpha1-Blockers; Antifungal Agents (Azole Derivatives, Systemic); Calcium Channel Blockers (Nondihydropyridine); Cimetidine; Cisapride; Conivaptan; CycloSPORINE; CycloSPORINE (Systemic); CYP3A4 Inhibitors (Moderate); CYP3A4 Inhibitors (Strong); Dasatinib; Diazoxide; Fluconazole; FLUoxetine; Grapefruit Juice; Herbs (Hypotensive Properties); Macrolide Antibiotics; Magnesium Salts; MAO Inhibitors; Pentoxifylline; Phosphodiesterase 5 Inhibitors; Prostacyclin Analogues; Protease Inhibitors; QuiNIDine

Decreased Effect

NIFEdipine may decrease the levels/effects of: Clopidogrel; QuiNIDine

The levels/effects of NIFEdipine may be decreased by: Barbiturates; Calcium Salts; CarBAMazepine; CYP3A4 Inducers (Strong); Deferasirox; Herbs (CYP3A4 Inducers); Herbs (Hypertensive Properties); Methylphenidate; Nafcillin; Peginterferon Alfa-2b; Rifamycin Derivatives; Tocilizumab; Yohimbine

Ethanol/Nutrition/Herb Interactions

Ethanol: Avoid ethanol (may increase CNS depression and may increase the effects of nifedipine). Monitor.

Food: Nifedipine serum levels may be decreased if taken with food. Food may decrease the rate but not the extent of absorption of Procardia XL®. Increased nifedipine concentrations resulting in therapeutic and vasodilator side effects, including severe hypotension and myocardial ischemia, may occur if nifedipine is taken by patients ingesting grapefruit.

Herb/Nutraceutical: St John's wort may decrease nifedipine levels (avoid use). Avoid use of bayberry, blue cohosh, cayenne, ephedra, ginger, ginseng (American), kola, licorice (may worsen hypertension). Avoid black cohosh, California poppy, coleus, golden seal, hawthorn, mistletoe, periwinkle, quinine, shepherd's purse (may have increased antihypertensive effect).

Mechanism of Action Inhibits calcium ion from entering the "slow channels" or select voltage-sensitive areas of vascular smooth muscle and myocardium during depolarization, producing a relaxation of coronary vascular smooth muscle and coronary vasodilation; increases myocardial oxygen delivery in patients with vasospastic angina; also reduces peripheral vascular resistance, producing a reduction in arterial blood pressure.

Pharmacodynamics/Kinetics

Onset of action: Immediate release: ~20 minutes

Protein binding (concentration dependent): 92% to 98%

Metabolism: Hepatic via CYP3A4 to inactive metabolites

Bioavailability: Capsule: 40% to 77%; Sustained release: 65% to 89% relative to immediate release capsules; bioavailability increased with significant hepatic disease

Half-life elimination: Adults: Healthy: 2-5 hours; Cirrhosis: 7 hours; Elderly: 7 hours (extended release tablet)

Excretion: Urine (60% to 80% as inactive metabolites); feces

Dosage Oral:

Children 1-17 years:

High altitude pulmonary edema (unlabeled use; Pollard, 2001): **Note:** Treatment with nifedipine is only necessary if response to oxygen and/or descent is unsatisfactory; extended release preparation is preferred at equivalent dose with proper frequency adjustment:

Immediate release: 0.5 mg/kg/dose (maximum: 20 mg/dose) every 8 hours

Hypertension (unlabeled use): Extended release tablet: Initial: 0.25-0.5 mg/kg/day once daily or in 2 divided doses; maximum: 3 mg/kg/day up to 120 mg/day

Adults: **Note:** Dosage adjustments should occur at 7- to 14-day intervals, to allow for adequate assessment of new dose; when switching from immediate release to sustained release formulations, use same total daily dose.

Chronic stable or vasospastic angina:

Immediate release: Initial: 10 mg 3 times/day; usual dose: 10-20 mg 3 times/day; coronary artery spasm may require up to 20-30 mg 3-4 times/day; single doses >30 mg and total daily doses >120 mg are rarely needed; maximum: 180 mg/day; **Note:** Do not use for acute anginal episodes; may precipitate myocardial infarction

Extended release: Initial: 30 or 60 mg once daily; maximum: 120-180 mg/day

Hypertension: Extended release: Initial: 30 or 60 mg once daily; maximum: 90-120 mg/day

High altitude pulmonary edema (unlabeled use; Luks, 2010):

Prevention: Extended release: 30 mg every 12 hours starting the day before ascent and may be discontinued after staying at the same elevation for 5 days or if descent initiated

Treatment: Extended release: 30 mg every 12 hours

Pulmonary hypertension (unlabeled use; Galie, 2004): Extended release: Initial: 30 mg twice daily; may increase cautiously to 120-240 mg/day

Raynaud's phenomenon (unlabeled use; Wigley, 2002): Extended release: Dosage range: 30-120 mg once daily

Elderly: Hypertension: Consider lower initial doses and titrate to response (Aronow, 2011)

Hemodialysis: Supplemental dose is not necessary

Peritoneal dialysis effects: Supplemental dose is not necessary

Dosing adjustment in hepatic impairment: Clearance of nifedipine is reduced in cirrhotic patients leading to increased systemic exposure; monitor closely for adverse effects/toxicity and consider dose adjustments.

Dietary Considerations Avoid grapefruit juice with all products.

Immediate release: Capsule is rapidly absorbed orally if it is administered without food, but may result in vasodilator side effects; if flushing is problematic, administration with low-fat meals may decrease. In general, can take with or without food.

Extended release: Adalat® CC, Afeditab® CR, Nifediac CC®: Take on an empty stomach (manufacturer recommendation). Other extended release products may not have this recommendation; consult product labeling.

Administration

Immediate release: In general, may be administered with or without food.

Extended release: Tablets should be swallowed whole; do not crush, split, or chew.

Adalat® CC, Afeditab® CR, Nifediac CC®: Administer on an empty stomach (per manufacturer). Other extended release products may not have this recommendation; consult product labeling.

Monitoring Parameters Heart rate, blood pressure, signs and symptoms of CHF, peripheral edema

Additional Information When measuring smaller doses from the liquid-filled capsules, consider the following concentrations (for Procardia®) 10 mg capsule = 10 mg/0.34 mL; 20 mg capsule = 20 mg/0.45 mL; may be used preoperative to treat hypertensive urgency.

Considerable attention has been directed to potential increases in mortality and morbidity when short-acting nifedipine is used in treating hypertension. The rapid reduction in blood pressure may precipitate adverse cardiovascular events.

Short-acting nifedipine should not be used for acute anginal episodes since this may precipitate myocardial infarction. Extended-release formulations are preferred for the management of chronic or vasospastic angina (Poole-Wilson, 2004).

Equivalency of extended release formulation (Adalat® CC): The manufacturer states that it is acceptable to interchange two 30 mg tablets with one 60 mg tablet to effectively deliver a 60 mg dose. However, it is not recommended to substitute one 90 mg tablet with three 30 mg tablets, since the resulting C_{max} is 29% higher compared to giving the single 90 mg tablet.

Dosage Forms Excipient information presented when available (limited, particularly for generics); consult specific product labeling.

Capsule, softgel, oral: 10 mg, 20 mg

Procardia®: 10 mg

Tablet, extended release, oral: 30 mg, 60 mg, 90 mg
- Adalat® CC: 30 mg, 60 mg, 90 mg
- Afeditab® CR: 30 mg, 60 mg
- Nifediac CC®: 30 mg, 60 mg
- Nifediac CC®: 90 mg [contains tartrazine]
- Nifedical XL®: 30 mg, 60 mg
- Procardia XL®: 30 mg, 60 mg, 90 mg

Extemporaneous Preparations A 4 mg/mL oral suspension may be made with liquid capsules (**Note:** Concentration inside capsule may vary depending on manufacturer. Procardia®: 10 mg capsule contains a concentration of 10 mg/0.34 mL [29.4 mg/mL]). Puncture the top of twelve 10 mg liquid capsules with one needle to create a vent. Insert a second needle attached to a syringe and extract the liquid; transfer to a calibrated bottle and add sufficient quantity of a 1:1 mixture of Ora-Sweet® and Ora-Plus® to make 30 mL. Label "shake well". Stable 90 days under refrigeration or at room temperature.

Nahata MC, Morosco RS, and Willhite EA, "Stability of Nifedipine in Two Oral Suspensions Stored at Two Temperatures," *J Am Pharm Assoc*, 2002, 42(6):865-7.

◆ **Niferex® [OTC] [DSC]** *see* Polysaccharide-Iron Complex *on page 1375*

◆ **Niftolid** *see* Flutamide *on page 738*

◆ **Nilandron®** *see* Nilutamide *on page 1205*

Nilotinib (nye LOE ti nib)

Brand Names: U.S. Tasigna®

Brand Names: Canada Tasigna®

Index Terms AMN107; Nilotinib Hydrochloride Monohydrate

Pharmacologic Category Antineoplastic Agent, Tyrosine Kinase Inhibitor

Use Treatment of newly-diagnosed Philadelphia chromosome-positive chronic myelogenous leukemia (Ph+ CML) in chronic phase; treatment of chronic and accelerated phase Ph+ CML (refractory or intolerant to prior therapy, including imatinib)

Pregnancy Risk Factor D

Medication Guide Available Yes

Dosage Oral: Adults:

Ph+ CML, newly-diagnosed (chronic phase): 300 mg twice daily

Ph+ CML, resistant or intolerant (chronic or accelerated phase): 400 mg twice daily (continue treatment until disease progression or unacceptable toxicity)

Dosage adjustment for concomitant CYP3A4 inhibitors/inducers:

CYP3A4 inhibitors: The concomitant use of a strong CYP3A4 inhibitor with nilotinib is not recommended. If a strong CYP3A4 inhibitor is required, interruption of nilotinib treatment is recommended; if therapy cannot be interrupted and concurrent use can not be avoided, consider reducing the nilotinib dose to 300 mg once daily in patients with resistant or intolerant Ph+ CML or to 200 mg once daily in newly-diagnosed Ph+ CML, with careful monitoring, especially of the QT interval. When a strong CYP3A4 inhibitor is discontinued, allow a washout period prior to adjusting nilotinib dose upward.

CYP3A4 inducers: The concomitant use of a strong CYP3A4 inducer with nilotinib is not recommended.

Dosage adjustment in renal impairment: Not studied in patients with serum creatinine >1.5 times ULN, however, nilotinib and its metabolites have minimal renal excretion; dosage adjustments for renal dysfunction may not be needed.

Dosage adjustment in hepatic impairment: Note: Dosage adjustment for impairment at treatment initiation (if possible, consider alternative therapies first); recommendations vary by indication.

Newly-diagnosed Ph+ CML: Mild-to-severe impairment (Child-Pugh class A, B, or C): Initial: 200 mg twice daily; may increase to 300 mg twice daily based on patient tolerability

Resistant or intolerant Ph+ CML:

Mild-to-moderate impairment (Child-Pugh class A or B): Initial: 300 mg twice daily; may increase to 400 mg twice daily based on patient tolerability

Severe impairment (Child-Pugh class C): Initial: 200 mg twice daily; may increase to 300 mg twice daily and then further increased to 400 mg twice daily based on patient tolerability

For hepatotoxicity during treatment:

If bilirubin >3 times ULN (≥grade 3): Withhold treatment, monitor bilirubin, resume treatment at 400 mg once daily when bilirubin returns to ≤1.5 times ULN (≤grade 1)

If ALT or AST >5 times ULN (≥grade 3): Withhold treatment, monitor transaminases, resume treatment at 400 mg once daily when ALT or AST returns to ≤2.5 times ULN (≤grade 1)

Dosage adjustment for hematologic toxicity:

ANC <1000/mm³ and/or platelets <50,000/mm³: Withhold treatment, monitor blood counts

If ANC >1000/mm³ and platelets >50,000/mm³ within 2 weeks: Resume at prior dose

If ANC <1000/mm³ and/or platelets <50,000/mm³ for >2 weeks: Reduce dose to 400 mg once daily

Dosage adjustment for nonhematologic toxicity:

Amylase or lipase >2 times ULN (≥grade 3): Withhold treatment, monitor serum amylase or lipase, resume treatment at 400 mg once daily when lipase or amylase returns to ≤1.5 times ULN (≤grade 1)

Clinically-significant moderate or severe nonhematologic toxicity: Withhold treatment, upon resolution of toxicity, resume at 400 mg once daily; may escalate back to 300 mg or 400 mg twice daily (depending on indication) if clinically appropriate.

Dosage adjustment for QT prolongation: Note: Repeat ECG ~7 days after any dosage adjustment.

QT_c >480 msec: Withhold treatment, monitor and correct potassium and magnesium levels.

If QT_cF returns to <450 msec and to within 20 msec of baseline within 2 weeks: Resume at prior dose

If QT_cF returns to 450-480 msec for >2 weeks: Reduce dose to 400 mg once daily

If QT_cF >480 msec after dosage reduction to 400 mg once daily, discontinue therapy.

Additional Information Complete prescribing information for this medication should be consulted for additional detail.

Dosage Forms Excipient information presented when available (limited, particularly for generics); consult specific product labeling.

Capsule, oral:
- Tasigna®: 150 mg, 200 mg

◆ **Nilotinib Hydrochloride Monohydrate** *see* Nilotinib *on page 1205*

Nilutamide (ni LOO ta mide)

Brand Names: U.S. Nilandron®

Brand Names: Canada Anandron®

Index Terms RU-23908

Pharmacologic Category Antiandrogen; Antineoplastic Agent, Antiandrogen

Use Treatment of metastatic prostate cancer (in combination with surgical castration)

Pregnancy Risk Factor C

Pregnancy Considerations Animal reproduction studies have not been conducted. Not indicated for use in women.

Contraindications Hypersensitivity to nilutamide or any component of the formulation; severe hepatic impairment; severe respiratory insufficiency

Warnings/Precautions Hazardous agent - use appropriate precautions for handling and disposal. **[U.S. Boxed Warning]: Interstitial pneumonitis has been reported in 2% of patients exposed to nilutamide.** Symptoms typically include exertional dyspnea, cough, chest pain and fever; interstitial changes (including pulmonary fibrosis) leading to hospitalization and fatalities have been reported (rarely). The suggestive signs of pneumonitis most often occurred within the first 3 months of treatment. X-rays showed interstitial or alveolo-interstitial changes; pulmonary function tests revealed a restrictive pattern with decreased DLco. Consider baseline pulmonary function testing. Discontinue if signs and/or symptoms of interstitial pneumonitis are noted.

Hepatitis or marked increases in liver enzymes leading to drug discontinuation occurred in 1% of nilutamide patients; rare cases of hospitalization or deaths due to severe liver injury have been reported. Discontinue treatment for jaundice or ALT >2 times the upper limit of normal (ULN).

A delay in adaptation to dark has been reported; in clinical studies, this was reported by 13% to 57% of patients; the delay ranged from seconds to a few minutes after passing from a light to a dark area (this may not abate with continued treatment although may be alleviated by wearing tinted sunglasses); caution patients who experience adaptation delay about driving at night or through tunnels. Not indicated for use in women. Patients with disease progression while receiving antiandrogen therapy may experience clinical improvement with discontinuation of the antiandrogen.

Adverse Reactions

>10%:

- Central nervous system: Insomnia (16%), headache (14%)
- Endocrine & metabolic: Hot flashes (28% to 67%)
- Gastrointestinal: Nausea (10% to 24%), constipation (7% to 20%), anorexia (11%), abdominal pain (10%)
- Genitourinary: Testicular atrophy (16%), libido decreased (11%)
- Hepatic: AST increased (8% to 13%), ALT increased (8% to 9%)
- Ocular: Impaired dark adaptation (13% to 57%)
- Respiratory: Dyspnea (6% to 11%)

1% to 10%:

- Cardiovascular: Hypertension (5% to 9%), chest pain (7%), heart failure (3%), angina (2%), edema (2%), syncope (2%)
- Central nervous system: Dizziness (7% to 10%), depression (9%), hypoesthesia (5%), malaise (2%), nervousness (2%)
- Dermatologic: Alopecia (6%), dry skin (5%), rash (5%), pruritus (2%)
- Endocrine & metabolic: Alcohol intolerance (5%), hyperglycemia (4%)
- Gastrointestinal: Vomiting (6%), diarrhea (2%), GI hemorrhage (2%), melena (2%), weight loss (2%), xerostomia (2%), dyspepsia
- Genitourinary: Nocturia (7%)
- Hematologic: Anemia (7%), haptoglobin increased (2%), leukopenia (2%)
- Hepatic: Alkaline phosphatase increased (3%)
- Neuromuscular & skeletal: Bone pain (6%), arthritis (2%), paresthesia (2%)
- Ocular: Chromatopsia (9%), impaired light adaptation (8%), abnormal vision (6% to 7%), cataract (2%), photophobia (2%)
- Renal: Hematuria (8%), BUN increased (2%), creatinine increased (2%)
- Respiratory: Pneumonia (5%), cough (2%), interstitial pneumonitis (2%), rhinitis (2%)
- Miscellaneous: Flu-like syndrome (7%), diaphoresis (6%)

<1% (Limited to important or life-threatening): Aplastic anemia, hepatitis

Drug Interactions

Metabolism/Transport Effects Substrate of CYP2C19 (major); **Note:** Assignment of Major/Minor substrate status based on clinically relevant drug interaction potential; **Inhibits** CYP2C19 (weak)

Avoid Concomitant Use There are no known interactions where it is recommended to avoid concomitant use.

Increased Effect/Toxicity

The levels/effects of Nilutamide may be increased by: CYP2C19 Inhibitors (Moderate); CYP2C19 Inhibitors (Strong)

Decreased Effect

The levels/effects of Nilutamide may be decreased by: CYP2C19 Inducers (Strong)

Ethanol/Nutrition/Herb Interactions Ethanol: Avoid ethanol (~5% of patients experience an intolerance [facial flushing, hypotension, malaise] when combined with nilutamide).

Stability Store at room temperature of 25°C (77°F); excursions permitted between 15°C to 30°C (59°F to 86°F). Protect from light.

Mechanism of Action Nonsteroidal antiandrogen which blocks testosterone effects at the androgen receptor level, preventing androgen response.

Pharmacodynamics/Kinetics

Absorption: Rapid and complete

Metabolism: Hepatic (extensive), forms active metabolites

Half-life elimination: Terminal: 38-59 hours; Metabolites: 59-126 hours

Excretion: Urine (62%; <2% as unchanged drug); feces (1% to 7%)

Dosage Oral: Adults: Prostate cancer, metastatic: 300 mg once daily (starting the same day or day after surgical castration) for 30 days, followed by 150 mg once daily

Dosage adjustment in hepatic impairment:

Prior to treatment initiation: Severe hepatic impairment: Use is contraindicated.

During treatment: ALT >2 times ULN or jaundice: Discontinue treatment.

Dietary Considerations May be taken without regard to meals.

Administration Administer without regard to meals.

Monitoring Parameters Hepatic enzymes (at baseline, regularly during the first 4 months of treatment, periodically thereafter); chest x-ray (at baseline); consider pulmonary function testing (at baseline)

Dosage Forms Excipient information presented when available (limited, particularly for generics); consult specific product labeling.

Tablet, oral:

Nilandron®: 150 mg

◆ **Nimbex®** *see* Cisatracurium *on page* 367

NiMODipine (nye MOE di peen)

Brand Names: Canada Nimotop®

Pharmacologic Category Calcium Channel Blocker; Calcium Channel Blocker, Dihydropyridine

Additional Appendix Information
Calcium Channel Blockers *on page 1887*

Use Vasospasm following subarachnoid hemorrhage from ruptured intracranial aneurysms

Unlabeled Use Prevention of migraines (inconsistent data)

Pregnancy Risk Factor C

Pregnancy Considerations Use in pregnancy only when clearly needed and when the benefits outweigh the potential hazard to the fetus. Teratogenic and embryotoxic effects have been demonstrated in small animals. No well-controlled studies have been conducted in pregnant women.

Lactation Enters breast milk/not recommended

Contraindications Hypersensitivity to nimodipine or any component of the formulation

Warnings/Precautions Increased angina and/or MI has occurred with initiation or dosage titration of calcium channel blockers. The most common side effect is peripheral edema; occurs within 2-3 weeks of starting therapy. Reflex tachycardia may occur with use. Symptomatic hypotension with or without syncope can rarely occur; blood pressure must be lowered at a rate appropriate for the patient's clinical condition. Use caution in hepatic impairment. Intestinal pseudo-obstruction and ileus have been reported during the use of nimodipine. Use caution in patients with decreased GI motility of a history of bowel obstruction. Use caution when treating patients with hypertrophic cardiomyopathy.

[U.S. Boxed Warning]: Nimodipine has inadvertently been administered I.V. when withdrawn from capsules into a syringe for subsequent nasogastric administration. Severe cardiovascular adverse events, including fatalities, have resulted; precautions (eg, adequate labeling, use of oral syringes) should be employed against such an event.

Adverse Reactions

1% to 10%:

Cardiovascular: Reductions in systemic blood pressure (1% to 8%)

Central nervous system: Headache (1% to 4%)

Dermatologic: Rash (1% to 2%)

Gastrointestinal: Diarrhea (2% to 4%), abdominal discomfort (2%)

<1% (Limited to important or life-threatening): Anemia, CHF, deep vein thrombosis, depression, disseminated intravascular coagulation, dyspnea, ECG abnormalities, GI hemorrhage, hemorrhage, hepatitis, jaundice, neurological deterioration, rebound vasospasm, thrombocytopenia, vomiting

Drug Interactions

Metabolism/Transport Effects Substrate of CYP3A4 (major); **Note:** Assignment of Major/Minor substrate status based on clinically relevant drug interaction potential

Avoid Concomitant Use

Avoid concomitant use of NiMODipine with any of the following: Conivaptan; Grapefruit Juice

Increased Effect/Toxicity

NiMODipine may increase the levels/effects of: Amifostine; Antihypertensives; Beta-Blockers; Calcium Channel Blockers (Nondihydropyridine); Fosphenytoin; Hypotensive Agents; Magnesium Salts; Neuromuscular-Blocking Agents (Nondepolarizing); Nitroprusside; Phenytoin; QuiNIDine; RiTUXimab; Tacrolimus; Tacrolimus (Systemic)

The levels/effects of NiMODipine may be increased by: Alpha1-Blockers; Antifungal Agents (Azole Derivatives, Systemic); Calcium Channel Blockers (Nondihydropyridine); Cimetidine; Conivaptan; CycloSPORINE; CycloSPORINE (Systemic); CYP3A4 Inhibitors (Moderate); CYP3A4 Inhibitors (Strong); Dasatinib; Diazoxide; Fluconazole; FLUoxetine; Grapefruit Juice; Herbs (Hypotensive Properties); Macrolide Antibiotics; Magnesium Salts; MAO Inhibitors; Pentoxifylline; Phosphodiesterase 5 Inhibitors; Prostacyclin Analogues; Protease Inhibitors; QuiNIDine

Decreased Effect

NiMODipine may decrease the levels/effects of: Clopidogrel; QuiNIDine

The levels/effects of NiMODipine may be decreased by: Barbiturates; Calcium Salts; CarBAMazepine; CYP3A4 Inducers (Strong); Deferasirox; Herbs (CYP3A4 Inducers); Herbs (Hypertensive Properties); Methylphenidate; Nafcillin; Rifamycin Derivatives; Tocilizumab; Yohimbine

Ethanol/Nutrition/Herb Interactions

Food: Nimodipine has shown a 1.5-fold increase in bioavailability when taken with grapefruit juice; avoid concurrent use.

Herb/Nutraceutical: St John's wort may decrease levels. Avoid dong quai if using for hypertension (has estrogenic activity). Avoid ephedra, yohimbe, ginseng (may worsen hypertension). Avoid garlic (may have increased antihypertensive effect).

Mechanism of Action Nimodipine shares the pharmacology of other calcium channel blockers; animal studies indicate that nimodipine has a greater effect on cerebral arterials than other arterials; this increased specificity may be due to the drug's increased lipophilicity and cerebral distribution as compared to nifedipine; inhibits calcium ion from entering the "slow channels" or select voltage sensitive areas of vascular smooth muscle and myocardium during depolarization

Pharmacodynamics/Kinetics

Protein binding: >95%

Metabolism: Extensively hepatic

Bioavailability: 13%

Half-life elimination: 1-2 hours; prolonged with renal impairment

Time to peak, serum: ~1 hour

Excretion: Urine (50%) and feces (32%) within 4 days

Dosage Note: Capsules and contents are for oral/NG tube administration **ONLY.**

Adults: Oral: 60 mg every 4 hours for 21 days, start therapy within 96 hours after subarachnoid hemorrhage.

Dialysis: Not removed by hemo- or peritoneal dialysis; supplemental dose is not necessary.

Dosing adjustment in hepatic impairment: Reduce dosage to 30 mg every 4 hours in patients with liver failure.

Administration For oral administration ONLY. Life-threatening adverse events have occurred when administered parenterally. Administer on an empty stomach.

Nasogastric (NG) tube administration: If the capsules cannot be swallowed, the liquid may be removed by making a hole in each end of the capsule with an 18-gauge needle and extracting the contents into a syringe; transfer these contents into an oral syringe (amber-colored oral syringe preferred). It is strongly recommended that preparation be done in the pharmacy. Label oral syringe with **"WARNING: For ORAL use only"** or **"Not for I.V. use."** Follow with a flush of 30 mL NS.

Dosage Forms Excipient information presented when available (limited, particularly for generics); consult specific product labeling.

Capsule, liquid filled, oral: 30 mg

Capsule, softgel, oral: 30 mg

- **Nimotop® (Can)** *see* NiMODipine *on page 1206*
- **Niodan (Can)** *see* Niacin *on page 1195*
- **Nipent®** *see* Pentostatin *on page 1331*
- **Nipride® (Can)** *see* Nitroprusside *on page 1214*

◆ **Niravam™** *see* ALPRAZolam *on page 72*

Nisoldipine (nye SOL di peen)

Brand Names: U.S. Sular®

Pharmacologic Category Calcium Channel Blocker; Calcium Channel Blocker, Dihydropyridine

Additional Appendix Information
Calcium Channel Blockers *on page 1887*

Use Management of hypertension, alone or in combination with other antihypertensive agents

Pregnancy Risk Factor C

Pregnancy Considerations Animal studies have demonstrated fetotoxic but not teratogenic effects. There are no adequate and well-controlled studies in pregnant women. Use during pregnancy only if potential benefit to the mother outweighs potential risk to the fetus.

Lactation Excretion in breast milk unknown/not recommended

Contraindications Hypersensitivity to nisoldipine, any component of the formulation, or other dihydropyridine calcium channel blockers

Warnings/Precautions With initiation or dosage titration of dihydropyridine calcium channel blockers, reflex tachycardia may occur resulting in angina and/or MI in patients with obstructive coronary disease especially in the absence of concurrent beta-blockade. Use with caution in patients with severe aortic stenosis, HF, and hypertrophic cardiomyopathy with outflow tract obstruction. Use with caution in hepatic impairment; lower starting dose required. The most common side effect is peripheral edema; occurs within 2-3 weeks of starting therapy. Symptomatic hypotension with or without syncope can rarely occur; blood pressure must be lowered at a rate appropriate for the patient's clinical condition. Some dosage forms contain tartrazine, which may cause allergic reactions in certain individuals (eg, aspirin hypersensitivity). Use with caution in patients >65 years of age; lower starting dose recommended.

Adverse Reactions

>10%:

Cardiovascular: Peripheral edema (dose related; 7% to 29%)

Central nervous system: Headache (22%)

1% to 10%:

Cardiovascular: Vasodilation (4%), palpitation (3%), angina exacerbation (2%), chest pain (2%)

Central nervous system: Dizziness (3% to 10%)

Dermatologic: Rash (2%)

Gastrointestinal: Nausea (2%)

Respiratory: Pharyngitis (5%), sinusitis (3%)

<1% (Limited to important or life-threatening): Alopecia, amblyopia, amnesia, anemia, anorexia, anxiety, appetite increased, arthralgia, arthritis, asthma, ataxia, atrial fibrillation, blepharitis, BUN increased, bruising, cellulitis, cerebral ischemia, colitis, conjunctivitis, creatinine increased, creatine kinase increased, CVA, depression, diabetes mellitus, diaphoresis, diarrhea, dreams abnormal, dyspepsia, dysphagia, dyspnea, dysuria, end inspiratory wheeze, epistaxis, exfoliative dermatitis, facial edema, fever, first-degree AV block, flu-like syndrome, gastritis, gastrointestinal hemorrhage, gingival hyperplasia, glaucoma, glossitis, gout, gynecomastia, heart failure (decompensated), hematuria, hepatomegaly, herpes simplex, herpes zoster; hypersensitivity reaction (eg, angioedema, shortness of breath, tachycardia, chest tightness, hypotension, and rash); hyper-/hypotension, hypertonia, hypoesthesia, hypokalemia, insomnia, jugular venous distention, keratoconjunctivitis, leukopenia, libido decreased, liver function tests abnormal, maculopapular rash, malaise, melena, migraine, mouth ulceration, myalgia, myasthenia, MI, myositis, nocturia, nonprotein nitrogen increased, paresthesia, petechiae, photosensitivity, pleural effusion, postural hypotension, pruritus, pustular rash, rales, retinal detachment, skin discoloration, skin ulcer, somnolence, supraventricular tachycardia, syncope, systolic ejection murmur, taste disturbance, temporary unilateral loss of vision, tenosynovitis, thyroiditis, tremor; T-wave abnormalities on ECG (flattening, inversion, nonspecific changes); urinary frequency, urticaria, vaginal hemorrhage, venous insufficiency, ventricular extrasystoles, vertigo, vitreous floater, weight gain/loss, xerostomia

Drug Interactions

Metabolism/Transport Effects Substrate of CYP3A4 (major); **Note:** Assignment of Major/Minor substrate status based on clinically relevant drug interaction potential; **Inhibits** CYP1A2 (weak), CYP3A4 (weak)

Avoid Concomitant Use

Avoid concomitant use of Nisoldipine with any of the following: CYP3A4 Inducers (Strong); CYP3A4 Inhibitors (Strong); Grapefruit Juice; Pimozide

Increased Effect/Toxicity

Nisoldipine may increase the levels/effects of: Amifostine; Antihypertensives; Beta-Blockers; Calcium Channel Blockers (Nondihydropyridine); Fosphenytoin; Hypotensive Agents; Magnesium Salts; Neuromuscular-Blocking Agents (Nondepolarizing); Nitroprusside; Phenytoin; Pimozide; RiTUXimab; Tacrolimus; Tacrolimus (Systemic)

The levels/effects of Nisoldipine may be increased by: Alpha1-Blockers; Antifungal Agents (Azole Derivatives, Systemic); Calcium Channel Blockers (Nondihydropyridine); Cimetidine; CycloSPORINE; CycloSPORINE (Systemic); CYP3A4 Inhibitors (Moderate); CYP3A4 Inhibitors (Strong); Dasatinib; Diazoxide; Fluconazole; Grapefruit Juice; Herbs (Hypotensive Properties); Macrolide Antibiotics; Magnesium Salts; MAO Inhibitors; Pentoxifylline; Phosphodiesterase 5 Inhibitors; Prostacyclin Analogues; Protease Inhibitors

Decreased Effect

Nisoldipine may decrease the levels/effects of: Clopidogrel

The levels/effects of Nisoldipine may be decreased by: Barbiturates; Calcium Salts; CarBAMazepine; CYP3A4 Inducers (Strong); Deferasirox; Herbs (CYP3A4 Inducers); Herbs (Hypertensive Properties); Methylphenidate; Nafcillin; Rifamycin Derivatives; Tocilizumab; Yohimbine

Ethanol/Nutrition/Herb Interactions

Food: Peak concentrations of nisoldipine may be significantly increased if taken with high-lipid foods; however, total exposure (AUC) may be reduced. Grapefruit juice has been shown to significantly increase the bioavailability of nisoldipine; avoid grapefruit products before and after dosing.

Herb/Nutraceutical: Avoid St John's wort (may decrease nisoldipine levels). Avoid bayberry, blue cohosh, cayenne, ephedra, ginger, ginseng (American), kola, licorice (may worsen hypertension). Avoid black cohosh, California poppy, coleus, golden seal, hawthorn, mistletoe, periwinkle, quinine, shepherd's purse (may have increased antihypertensive effect).

Stability Store at controlled room temperature of 20°C to 25°C (68°F to 77°F). Protect from light; protect from moisture.

Mechanism of Action As a dihydropyridine calcium channel blocker, structurally similar to nifedipine, nisoldipine impedes the movement of calcium ions into vascular smooth muscle and cardiac muscle. Dihydropyridines are potent vasodilators and are not as likely to suppress cardiac contractility and slow cardiac conduction as other calcium antagonists such as verapamil and diltiazem;

nisoldipine is 5-10 times as potent a vasodilator as nifedipine.

Pharmacodynamics/Kinetics

Duration: >24 hours

Absorption: Well absorbed. Peak concentrations significantly increased with high-lipid meals; however, AUC is reduced.

Protein binding: >99%

Metabolism: Extensively hepatic; 1 active metabolite (10% of activity of parent); first-pass effect

Bioavailability: ~5%

Half-life elimination: 9-18 hours

Time to peak: 4-14 hours

Excretion: Urine (60% to 80% as inactive metabolites); feces

Dosage Oral:

Sular® (Geomatrix® delivery system):

Adults: Initial: 17 mg once daily, then increase by 8.5 mg/week (or longer intervals) to attain adequate control of blood pressure

Usual dose range: 17-34 mg once daily; doses >34 mg once daily are not recommended

Elderly: Initial dose: 8.5 mg once daily, increase by 8.5 mg/week (or longer intervals) to attain adequate blood pressure control

Nisoldipine extended-release tablet (original formulation):

Adults: Oral: Initial: 20 mg once daily, then increase by 10 mg/week (or longer intervals) to attain adequate control of blood pressure

Usual dose range (JNC 7): 10-40 mg once daily; doses >60 mg once daily are not recommended

Elderly: Initial dose: 10 mg once daily, increase by 10 mg/week (or longer intervals) to attain adequate blood pressure control

Conversion from nisoldipine extended-release (original formulation) to Sular® Geomatrix® delivery system:

Nisoldipine Extended Release Dosing Equivalency

Original Extended Release Formulation	Sular® Extended Release (Geomatrix® delivery system)
10 mg	8.5 mg
20 mg	17 mg
30 mg	25.5 mg
40 mg	34 mg

Dosage adjustment in hepatic impairment:

Sular® (Geomatrix® delivery system): An initial dose exceeding 8.5 mg once daily is not recommended for patients with hepatic impairment.

Nisoldipine extended-release (original formulation): An initial dose exceeding 10 mg once daily is not recommended for patients with hepatic impairment.

Dietary Considerations Take on an empty stomach (1 hour before or 2 hours after a meal). Avoid grapefruit juice before and after dosing. Avoid grapefruit juice; avoid high-fat diet.

Administration Administer at the same time each day to ensure minimal fluctuation of serum levels. Avoid high-fat diet. Administer on an empty stomach (1 hour before or 2 hours after a meal). Swallow whole; do not crush, break, split, or chew.

Monitoring Parameters Blood pressure, heart rate

Dosage Forms Excipient information presented when available (limited, particularly for generics); consult specific product labeling.

Tablet, extended release, oral: 8.5 mg, 17 mg, 25.5 mg, 34 mg

Sular®: 8.5 mg

Sular®: 17 mg [contains tartrazine]

Sular®: 25.5 mg, 34 mg

Tablet, extended release, oral [original formula]: 20 mg, 30 mg, 40 mg

◆ **Nitalapram** *see* Citalopram *on page 370*

Nitazoxanide (nye ta ZOX a nide)

Brand Names: U.S. Alinia®

Index Terms NTZ

Pharmacologic Category Antiprotozoal

Use Treatment of diarrhea caused by *Cryptosporidium parvum* or *Giardia lamblia*

Unlabeled Use Alternative treatment for *Clostridium difficile*-associated diarrhea (CDAD)

Pregnancy Risk Factor B

Pregnancy Considerations Teratogenic effects were not observed in animal studies. There are no adequate and well-controlled studies in pregnant women.

Lactation Excretion in breast milk unknown/use caution

Contraindications Hypersensitivity to nitazoxanide or any component of the formulation

Warnings/Precautions Use caution with renal or hepatic impairment. Safety and efficacy have not been established with HIV infection, immunodeficiency, or in children <1 year of age (suspension) and <12 years of age (tablet).

Adverse Reactions Rates of adverse effects were similar to those reported with placebo.

1% to 10%:

Central nervous system: Headache (1% to 3%)

Gastrointestinal: Abdominal pain (7% to 8%), diarrhea (2% to 4%), nausea (3%), vomiting (1%)

<1% (Limited to important or life-threatening): Allergic reaction, ALT increased, anemia, anorexia, appetite increased, creatinine increased, diaphoresis, dizziness, eye discoloration (pale yellow), fever, flatulence, hypertension, infection, malaise, nausea, pruritus, rhinitis, salivary glands enlarged, tachycardia, urine discoloration

Drug Interactions

Metabolism/Transport Effects None known.

Avoid Concomitant Use There are no known interactions where it is recommended to avoid concomitant use.

Increased Effect/Toxicity There are no known significant interactions involving an increase in effect.

Decreased Effect There are no known significant interactions involving a decrease in effect.

Ethanol/Nutrition/Herb Interactions Food: Food increases AUC.

Stability

Suspension: Prior to and following reconstitution, store at room temperature of 15°C to 30°C (59°F to 86°F). For preparation at time of dispensing, add 48 mL incrementally to 60 mL bottle; shake vigorously. Resulting suspension is 20 mg/mL (100 mg per 5 mL). Following reconstitution, discard unused portion of suspension after 7 days.

Tablet: Store at room temperature.

Mechanism of Action Nitazoxanide is rapidly metabolized to the active metabolite tizoxanide *in vivo*. Activity may be due to interference with the pyruvate:ferredoxin oxidoreductase (PFOR) enzyme-dependent electron transfer reaction which is essential to anaerobic metabolism. *In vitro*, nitazoxanide and tizoxanide inhibit the growth of sporozoites and oocysts of *Cryptosporidium parvum* and trophozoites of *Giardia lamblia*.

Pharmacodynamics/Kinetics

Protein binding: Tizoxanide: >99%

Bioavailability: Relative bioavailability of suspension compared to tablet: 70%

Metabolism: Hepatic, to an active metabolite, tizoxanide. Tizoxanide undergoes conjugation to form tizoxanide glucuronide. Nitazoxanide is not detectable in the serum following oral administration.

Time to peak, plasma: Tizoxanide and tizoxanide glucuronide: 1-4 hours

Excretion: Tizoxanide: Urine, bile, and feces; Tizoxanide glucuronide: Urine and bile

Dosage Oral:

Children: Diarrhea caused by *Cryptosporidium parvum* or *Giardia lamblia*:

Children 1-3 years: 100 mg every 12 hours for 3 days; may consider increasing duration up to 14 days in HIV-exposed/-infected pediatric patients with crypotosporidiosis (CDC, 2009)

Children 4-11 years: 200 mg every 12 hours for 3 days; may consider increasing duration up to 14 days in HIV-exposed/-infected pediatric patients with crypotosporidiosis (CDC, 2009)

Children ≥12 years: Refer to adult dosing.

Adults:

Diarrhea caused by *Cryptosporidium parvum* or *Giardia lamblia*: 500 mg every 12 hours for 3 days

Clostridium difficile-associated diarrhea (unlabeled use): 500 mg every 12 hours for 10 days (Musher, 2009)

Dosage adjustment in renal/hepatic impairment: Specific recommendations are not available; use with caution

Dietary Considerations Should be taken with food.

Administration Administer with food. Shake suspension well prior to administration.

Dosage Forms Excipient information presented when available (limited, particularly for generics); consult specific product labeling.

Powder for suspension, oral:

Alinia®: 100 mg/5 mL (60 mL) [contains sodium benzoate, sucrose 1.48 g/5 mL; strawberry flavor]

Tablet, oral:

Alinia®: 500 mg [contains soy lecithin]

◆ **Nithiodote™** *see* Sodium Nitrite and Sodium Thiosulfate *on page 1570*

Nitisinone (ni TIS i known)

Brand Names: U.S. Orfadin®

Index Terms NTBC

Pharmacologic Category 4-Hydroxyphenylpyruvate Dioxygenase Inhibitor

Use Treatment of hereditary tyrosinemia type 1 (HT-1) as an adjunct to dietary restriction of tyrosine and phenylalanine

Pregnancy Risk Factor C

Prescribing and Access Restrictions Distributed by Rare Disease Therapeutics, Inc; for information regarding acquisition of product, call Accredo Health Group, Inc at 1-888-454-8860

Dosage Oral: HT-1**Note:** Must be used in conjunction with a diet restricted in tyrosine and phenylalanine.

Infants: Initial: 1 mg/kg/day in 2 divided doses

Children and Adults: Initial: 1 mg/kg/day in 2 divided doses

Dosing adjustment for inadequate response: Note: Inadequate response is defined as continued abnormal biological parameters (erythrocyte PBG-synthase activity, urine 5-ALA, and urine succinylacetone) despite treatment. If the aforementioned parameters are not available, may use urine succinylacetone, liver function tests, alpha-fetoprotein, serum tyrosine, and serum phenylalanine to evaluate response (exceptions may include during initiation of therapy and exacerbations).

Abnormal biological parameters at 1 month: Increase dose to 1.5 mg/kg/day

Abnormal biological parameters at 3 months: Further increase to maximum dose of 2 mg/kg/day

Additional Information Complete prescribing information for this medication should be consulted for additional detail.

Dosage Forms Excipient information presented when available (limited, particularly for generics); consult specific product labeling.

Capsule, oral:

Orfadin®: 2 mg, 5 mg, 10 mg

◆ **Nitoman™ (Can)** *see* Tetrabenazine *on page 1660*

◆ **4′-Nitro-3′-Trifluoromethylisobutyrantide** *see* Flutamide *on page 738*

◆ **Nitro-Bid®** *see* Nitroglycerin *on page 1212*

◆ **Nitro-Dur®** *see* Nitroglycerin *on page 1212*

Nitrofurantoin (nye troe fyoor AN toyn)

Brand Names: U.S. Furadantin®; Macrobid®; Macrodantin®

Brand Names: Canada Apo-Nitrofurantoin®; Macrobid®; Macrodantin®; Novo-Furantoin; Teva-Nitrofurantoin

Pharmacologic Category Antibiotic, Miscellaneous

Additional Appendix Information

Beers Criteria – Potentially Inappropriate Medications for Geriatrics *on page 1973*

Use Prevention and treatment of urinary tract infections caused by susceptible strains of *E. coli*, *S. aureus*, *Enterococcus*, *Klebsiella*, and *Enterobacter*

Pregnancy Risk Factor B (contraindicated at term)

Pregnancy Considerations Because adverse effects have not been observed in animals, nitrofurantoin is classified pregnancy category B. Nitrofurantoin crosses the placenta, but very little reaches the amniotic fluid. Most published experiences with nitrofurantoin use during pregnancy have failed to identify any increased obstetric or teratogenic risks. Isolated reports of a potential increased risk for cardiovascular defects and a case report of upper limb paralysis have not been replicated in other studies. Use of nitrofurantoin during pregnancy has been generally well tolerated with rare reports of maternal toxicity including severe pulmonary reactions or hematologic adverse effects. Nitrofurantoin is contraindicated in pregnant patients at term (38-42 weeks gestation), during labor and delivery, or when the onset of labor is imminent due to the possibility of hemolytic anemia in the neonate.

Lactation Enters breast milk/not recommended (infants <1 month); AAP rates "compatible" (AAP 2001 update pending)

Contraindications Hypersensitivity to nitrofurantoin or any component of the formulation; significant renal impairment (anuria, oliguria, significantly elevated serum creatinine, or Cl_{cr} <60 mL/minute); infants <1 month (due to the possibility of hemolytic anemia); pregnancy at term (38-42 weeks gestation), during labor and delivery, or when the onset of labor is imminent; use in patients with a history of cholestatic jaundice or hepatic impairment with previous nitrofurantoin therapy

Warnings/Precautions Use with caution in patients with G6PD deficiency (increased risk of hemolytic anemia). Therapeutic concentrations of nitrofurantoin are not attained in urine of patients with Cl_{cr} <60 mL/minute, therefore, use contraindicated in these patients. Use with caution if prolonged therapy is anticipated due to possible pulmonary toxicity. Acute, subacute, or chronic (usually after 6 months of therapy) pulmonary reactions (possibly fatal) have been observed in patients treated with nitrofurantoin; if these occur, discontinue therapy immediately; monitor closely for malaise, dyspnea, cough, fever, radiologic evidence of diffuse interstitial pneumonitis or fibrosis. Rare, but severe and sometimes fatal hepatic reactions (eg, cholestatic jaundice, hepatitis, hepatic necrosis) have been associated with nitrofurantoin (onset may be insidious); discontinue immediately if hepatitis occurs. Monitor liver function test periodically. Has been associated with peripheral neuropathy (rare); risk may be increased in patients with anemia, renal impairment, diabetes, vitamin B deficiency, debilitating disease, or electrolyte imbalance; use caution. Use in the elderly is not recommended due to potential for renal impairment; alternative agents preferred (Beers Criteria). Use in the elderly, particularly females receiving long-term prophylaxis for recurrent UTIs, has been associated with an increased risk of hepatic and pulmonary toxicity, and peripheral neuropathy. Avoid or use extreme caution when prescribing to elderly patients, particularly those with decreased renal function. Prolonged use may result in fungal or bacterial superinfection, including *C. difficile*-associated diarrhea (CDAD) and pseudomembranous colitis; CDAD has been observed >2 months postantibiotic treatment. Use is contraindicated in children <1 month of age (at increased risk for hemolytic anemia). Not indicated for the treatment of pyelonephritis or perinephric abscesses.

Adverse Reactions Frequency not defined.

Cardiovascular: Cyanosis, ECG changes (nonspecific ST/T wave changes, bundle branch block)

Central nervous system: Bulging fontanels (infants), chills, confusion, depression, dizziness, drowsiness, fever, headache, malaise, pseudotumor cerebri, psychotic reaction, vertigo

Dermatologic: Alopecia, angioedema, erythema multiforme, exfoliative dermatitis, pruritus, rash (eczematous, erythematous, maculopapular), Stevens-Johnson syndrome, urticaria

Endocrine & metabolic: Hyperphosphatemia

Gastrointestinal: Abdominal pain, anorexia, *C. difficile* colitis, constipation, diarrhea, dyspepsia, flatulence, nausea, pancreatitis, pseudomembranous colitis, sialadenitis, vomiting

Genitourinary: Urine discoloration (brown)

Hematologic: Agranulocytosis, aplastic anemia, eosinophilia, glucose-6-phosphate dehydrogenase deficiency anemia, granulocytopenia, hemoglobin decreased, hemolytic anemia, leukopenia, megaloblastic anemia, thrombocytopenia

Hepatic: Hepatitis, hepatic necrosis, transaminases increased, jaundice (cholestatic)

Neuromuscular & skeletal: Arthralgia, myalgia, numbness, paresthesia, peripheral neuropathy, weakness

Ocular: Amblyopia, nystagmus, optic neuritis

Respiratory: Cough, dyspnea, pneumonitis, pulmonary fibrosis (with long-term use), pulmonary infiltration

Miscellaneous: Acute pulmonary reaction (symptoms include chills, chest pain, cough, dyspnea, fever, and eosinophilia), anaphylaxis, hypersensitivity (including acute pulmonary hypersensitivity), lupus-like syndrome, superinfections (eg, *Pseudomonas* or *Candida*)

Drug Interactions

Metabolism/Transport Effects None known.

Avoid Concomitant Use

Avoid concomitant use of Nitrofurantoin with any of the following: BCG; Magnesium Trisilicate; Norfloxacin

Increased Effect/Toxicity

Nitrofurantoin may increase the levels/effects of: Eplerenone; Prilocaine; Spironolactone

The levels/effects of Nitrofurantoin may be increased by: Probenecid

Decreased Effect

Nitrofurantoin may decrease the levels/effects of: BCG; Norfloxacin; Typhoid Vaccine

The levels/effects of Nitrofurantoin may be decreased by: Magnesium Trisilicate

Ethanol/Nutrition/Herb Interactions

Ethanol: Avoid ethanol (may increase CNS depression).

Food: Nitrofurantoin serum concentrations may be increased if taken with food.

Stability Store at 20°C to 25°C (68°F to 77°F); excursions permitted to 15°C to 30°C (59°F to 86°F). Protect oral suspension from light.

Mechanism of Action Inhibits several bacterial enzyme systems including acetyl coenzyme A interfering with metabolism and possibly cell wall synthesis

Pharmacodynamics/Kinetics

Absorption: Well absorbed; macrocrystalline form absorbed more slowly due to slower dissolution (causes less GI distress)

Distribution: V_d: 0.8 L/kg

Protein binding: 60% to 90%

Metabolism: Body tissues (except plasma) metabolize 60% of drug to inactive metabolites

Bioavailability: Increased with food

Half-life elimination: 20-60 minutes; prolonged with renal impairment

Excretion:

Suspension: Urine (~40%) and feces (small amounts) as metabolites and unchanged drug

Macrocrystals: Urine (20% to 25% as unchanged drug)

Dosage Oral:

Children >1 month:

UTI treatment (Furadantin®, Macrodantin®): 5-7 mg/kg/day in divided doses every 6 hours; maximum: 400 mg/day. Administer for 7 days or at least 3 days after obtaining sterile urine

UTI prophylaxis (Furadantin®, Macrodantin®): 1-2 mg/kg/day in divided doses every 12-24 hours; maximum: 100 mg/day

Children >12 years: UTI treatment (Macrobid®): 100 mg twice daily for 7 days

Adults:

UTI treatment:

Furadantin®, Macrodantin®: 50-100 mg/dose every 6 hours; administer for 7 days or at least 3 days after obtaining sterile urine

Macrobid®: 100 mg twice daily for 7 days

UTI prophylaxis (Furadantin®, Macrodantin®): 50-100 mg/dose at bedtime

Dosing adjustment in renal impairment: Cl_{cr} <60 mL/minute: Contraindicated

Contraindicated in hemo- and peritoneal dialysis and continuous arteriovenous or venovenous hemofiltration

Dietary Considerations Take with meals to improve absorption and decrease adverse effects.

Administration Administer with meals to improve absorption and decrease adverse effects; suspension may be mixed with water, milk, fruit juice, or infant formula. Shake suspension well before use.

Monitoring Parameters Signs of pulmonary reaction; signs of numbness or tingling of the extremities; CBC, periodic liver function tests, periodic renal function tests with long-term use

Test Interactions False-positive urine glucose (Benedict's and Fehling's methods); no false positives with enzymatic tests

Dosage Forms Excipient information presented when available (limited, particularly for generics); consult specific product labeling.

Capsule, oral [macrocrystal]: 50 mg, 100 mg

Macrodantin®: 25 mg, 50 mg, 100 mg

Capsule, oral [macrocrystal/monohydrate]: 100 mg
Macrobid®: 100 mg [nitrofurantoin macrocrystal 25% and nitrofurantoin monohydrate 75%]
Suspension, oral: 25 mg/5 mL (230 mL)
Furadantin®: 25 mg/5 mL (230 mL)

◆ **Nitrogen Mustard** *see* Mechlorethamine *on page 1056*

Nitroglycerin (nye troe GLI ser in)

Brand Names: U.S. Minitran™; Nitro-Bid®; Nitro-Dur®; Nitro-Time®; Nitrolingual®; NitroMist®; Nitrostat®

Brand Names: Canada Minitran™; Mylan-Nitro Sublingual Spray; Nitro-Dur®; Nitroglycerin Injection, USP; Nitrol®; Nitrostat®; Rho®-Nitro Pump Spray; Transderm-Nitro®; Trinipatch®

Index Terms Glyceryl Trinitrate; Nitroglycerol; NTG; Rectiv™; Tridil

Pharmacologic Category Antianginal Agent; Vasodilator

Additional Appendix Information

Hypertension *on page 2001*
Nitrates *on page 1895*
Vasoactive Agents, Intravenous *on page 1898*

Use Treatment or prevention of angina pectoris

Intravenous (I.V.) administration: Treatment or prevention of angina pectoris; acute decompensated heart failure (especially when associated with acute myocardial infarction); perioperative hypertension (especially during cardiovascular surgery); induction of intraoperative hypotension

Intra-anal administration (Rectiv™ ointment): Treatment of moderate-to-severe pain associated with chronic anal fissure

Unlabeled Use Short-term management of pulmonary hypertension (I.V.); esophageal spastic disorders; uterine relaxation

Pregnancy Risk Factor C

Pregnancy Considerations Increased fetal mortality has been observed in animal studies using isosorbide mononitrate and isosorbide dinitrate at doses much higher than those used in humans. Toxic effects were not observed in animal studies following topical administration of nitroglycerin. There are no adequate and well-controlled studies in pregnant women.

Lactation Excretion in breast milk unknown/use caution

Contraindications Hypersensitivity to organic nitrates or any component of the formulation (includes adhesives for transdermal product); concurrent use with phosphodiesterase-5 (PDE-5) inhibitors (sildenafil, tadalafil, or vardenafil); increased intracranial pressure; severe anemia

Additional contraindications for I.V. product: Inadequate cerebral circulation; constrictive pericarditis; pericardial tamponade; restrictive cardiomyopathy

Note: According to the 2010 American Heart Association guidelines for the treatment of acute coronary syndromes, nitrates are considered contraindicated in the following conditions: Hypotension (SBP <90 mm Hg or ≥30 mm Hg below baseline), extreme bradycardia (<50 bpm), tachycardia in the absence of heart failure (>100 bpm), and right ventricular infarction (O'Connor, 2010).

Warnings/Precautions Severe hypotension can occur. Use with caution in volume depletion, moderate hypotension, and extreme caution with inferior wall MI and suspected right ventricular involvement. Use considered contraindicated in patients with severe hypotension (SBP <90 mm Hg or ≥30 mm Hg below baseline), extreme bradycardia (<50 bpm), and right ventricular MI (O'Connor, 2010).

Paradoxical bradycardia and increased angina pectoris can accompany hypotension. Orthostatic hypotension can also occur. Ethanol can accentuate this. Tolerance does develop to nitrates and appropriate dosing is needed to minimize this (drug-free interval). Avoid use of long-acting agents in acute MI or acute HF; cannot easily reverse effects. Nitrates may aggravate angina caused by hypertrophic cardiomyopathy. Nitroglycerin may precipitate or aggravate increased intracranial pressure and subsequently may worsen clinical outcomes in patients with neurologic injury (eg, intracranial hemorrhage, traumatic brain injury). Nitroglycerin transdermal patches may contain conducting metal (eg, aluminum); remove patch prior to MRI. Avoid concurrent use with PDE-5 inhibitors. When nitrate administration becomes medically necessary, may administer nitrates only if 24 hours have elapsed after use of sildenafil or vardenafil (48 hours after tadalafil use) (Trujillo, 2007).

Use caution when treating rectal anal fissures with nitroglycerin ointment formulation in patients with suspected or known significant cardiovascular disorders (eg, cardiomyopathies, heart failure, acute MI); intra-anal nitroglycerin administration may decrease systolic blood pressure and decrease arterial vascular resistance.

Adverse Reactions

Frequency not defined:

Cardiovascular: Flushing, hypotension, peripheral edema, postural hypotension, syncope, tachycardia
Central nervous system: Headache (common), dizziness, lightheadedness
Gastrointestinal: Nausea, vomiting, xerostomia
Neuromuscular & skeletal: Paresthesia, weakness
Respiratory: Dyspnea, pharyngitis, rhinitis
Miscellaneous: Diaphoresis

<1% (Limited to important or life-threatening): Allergic reactions, anaphylactoid reaction, application site irritation (patch), blurred vision, cardiovascular collapse, contact dermatitis (ointment, patch), crescendo angina, exfoliative dermatitis, fixed drug eruption (ointment, patch), methemoglobinemia (rare; overdose), pallor, palpitation, rash, rebound hypertension, restlessness, shock, vertigo

Drug Interactions

Metabolism/Transport Effects None known.

Avoid Concomitant Use

Avoid concomitant use of Nitroglycerin with any of the following: Ergot Derivatives; Phosphodiesterase 5 Inhibitors

Increased Effect/Toxicity

Nitroglycerin may increase the levels/effects of: Ergot Derivatives; Hypotensive Agents; Prilocaine; Rosiglitazone

The levels/effects of Nitroglycerin may be increased by: Alfuzosin; Phosphodiesterase 5 Inhibitors

Decreased Effect

Nitroglycerin may decrease the levels/effects of: Alteplase; Heparin

The levels/effects of Nitroglycerin may be decreased by: Ergot Derivatives

Ethanol/Nutrition/Herb Interactions

Ethanol: Avoid ethanol (may increase the hypotensive effects of nitroglycerin). Monitor.

Herb/Nutraceutical: Avoid bayberry, blue cohosh, cayenne, ephedra, ginger, ginseng (American), kola, licorice (may worsen hypertension). Avoid black cohosh, California poppy, coleus, golden seal, hawthorn, mistletoe, periwinkle, quinine, shepherd's purse (may cause hypotension).

Stability

I.V. solution: Doses should be made in glass bottles, EXCEL® or PAB® containers. Adsorption occurs to soft plastic (eg, PVC). Nitroglycerin diluted in D_5W or NS in glass containers is physically and chemically stable for 48 hours at room temperature and 7 days under refrigeration. In D_5W or NS in EXCEL®/PAB® containers it is physically and chemically stable for 24 hours at room temperature.

Premixed bottles are stable according to the manufacturer's expiration dating.

Standard diluent: 50 mg/250 mL D_5W; 50 mg/500 mL D_5W.

Minimum volume: 100 mg/250 mL D_5W; concentration should not exceed 400 mcg/mL.

Store sublingual tablets, topical ointment, and rectal ointment in tightly closed containers at 20°C to 25°C (68°F to 77°F); slow release capsules at 20°C to 25°C (68°F to 77°F); translingual spray and transdermal patch at 15°C to 30°C (59°F to 86°F).

Mechanism of Action Nitroglycerin forms free radical nitric oxide. In smooth muscle, nitric oxide activates guanylate cyclase which increases guanosine 3'5' monophosphate (cGMP) leading to dephosphorylation of myosin light chains and smooth muscle relaxation. Produces a vasodilator effect on the peripheral veins and arteries with more prominent effects on the veins. Primarily reduces cardiac oxygen demand by decreasing preload (left ventricular end-diastolic pressure); may modestly reduce afterload; dilates coronary arteries and improves collateral flow to ischemic regions. For use in rectal fissures, intra-anal administration results in decreased sphincter tone and intra-anal pressure.

Pharmacodynamics/Kinetics

Onset of action: Sublingual tablet: 1-3 minutes; Translingual spray: Similar to sublingual tablet; Sustained release: ~60 minutes; Topical: 15-30 minutes; Transdermal: ~30 minutes; I.V.: Immediate

Peak effect: Sublingual tablet: 5 minutes; Translingual spray: 4-10 minutes; Sustained release: 2.5-4 hours; Topical: ~60 minutes; Transdermal: 120 minutes; I.V.: Immediate

Duration: Sublingual tablet: At least 25 minutes; Translingual spray: Similar to sublingual tablet; Sustained release: 4-8 hours; Topical: 7 hours; Transdermal: 10-12 hours; I.V.: 3-5 minutes

Distribution: V_d: ~3 L/kg

Protein binding: 60%

Metabolism: Extensive first-pass effect; metabolized hepatically to glycerol di- and mononitrate metabolites via liver reductase enzyme; subsequent metabolism to glycerol and organic nitrate; nonhepatic metabolism via red blood cells and vascular walls also occurs

Half-life elimination: ~1-4 minutes

Excretion: Urine (as inactive metabolites)

Dosage Note: Hemodynamic and antianginal tolerance often develop within 24-48 hours of continuous nitrate administration. Nitrate-free interval (10-12 hours/day) is recommended to avoid tolerance development; gradually decrease dose in patients receiving NTG for prolonged period to avoid withdrawal reaction.

Adults:

Angina/coronary artery disease:

Oral: Initial: 2.5-6.5 mg 3-4 times/day; may titrate up to 26 mg 4 times/day

I.V.: 5 mcg/minute, increase by 5 mcg/minute every 3-5 minutes to 20 mcg/minute; if no response at 20 mcg/minute, may increase by 10-20 mcg/minute every 3-5 minutes (generally accepted maximum dose: 400 mcg/minute)

Sublingual: 0.3-0.6 mg every 5 minutes for maximum of 3 doses in 15 minutes; may also use prophylactically 5-10 minutes prior to activities which may provoke an attack

Topical ointment: 1/2" upon rising and 1/2" 6 hours later; if necessary, the dose may be doubled to 1" and subsequently doubled again to 2" if response is inadequate. Doses of 1/2" to 2" were used in clinical trials. Recommended maximum: 2 doses/day; include a nitrate free-interval ~10-12 hours/day.

Topical patch, transdermal: Initial: 0.2-0.4 mg/hour, titrate to 0.4-0.8 mg/hour; tolerance is minimized by using a patch-on period of 12-14 hours and patch-off period of 10-12 hours

Translingual: 1-2 sprays onto or under tongue every 3-5 minutes for maximum of 3 doses in 15 minutes, may also be used prophylactically 5-10 minutes prior to activities which may provoke an angina attack

Anal fissure, chronic (0.4% ointment): Intra-anal: 1 inch (equals 1.5 mg of nitroglycerin) every 12 hours for up to 3 weeks

Esophageal spastic disorders (unlabeled use): Sublingual: 0.3-0.6 mg (Swamy, 1977)

Uterine relaxation (unlabeled use): I.V. bolus: 100-200 mcg; may repeat dose every 2 minutes as necessary (Axemo, 1998; Chandraharan, 2005)

Elderly: In general, dose selection should be cautious, usually starting at the low end of the dosing range

Administration

I.V.: Prepare in glass bottles, EXCEL® or PAB® containers. Adsorption occurs to soft plastic (eg, PVC); use administration sets intended for nitroglycerin

Intra-anal ointment: Using a finger covering (eg, plastic wrap, surgical glove, finger cot), place finger beside 1 inch measuring guide on the box and squeeze ointment the length of the measuring line directly onto covered finger. Insert ointment into the anal canal using the covered finger up to first finger joint (do not insert further than the first finger joint) and apply ointment around the side of the anal canal. If intra-anal application is too painful, may apply the ointment to the outside of the anus. Wash hands following application.

Oral (sustained release capsule): Swallow whole. Do not chew, break, or crush. Take with a full glass of water.

Sublingual: Do not crush sublingual product (tablet). Place under tongue and allow to dissolve.

Topical ointment: Wash hands prior to and after use. Application site should be clean, dry, and hair-free. Apply to chest or back with the applicator or dose-measuring paper. Spread in a thin layer over a 2.25 x 3.5 inch area. Do not rub into skin. Tape applicator into place.

Topical patch, transdermal: Application site should be clean, dry and hair-free. Remove patch after 12-14 hours. Rotate patch sites.

Translingual spray: Do not shake container. Prior to initial use, the pump must be primed by spraying 5 times (Nitrolingual®) or 10 times (Nitromist®) into the air. Priming sprays should be directed away from patient and others. Release spray onto or under tongue. Close mouth after administration. Do not rinse the mouth for at least 5-10 minutes. The end of the pump should be covered by the fluid in the bottle. If pump is unused for 6 weeks, a single priming spray (Nitrolingual®) or 2 priming sprays (Nitromist®) should be completed.

Monitoring Parameters Blood pressure, heart rate

Test Interactions I.V. formulation: Due to propylene glycol content, triglyceride assays dependent on glycerol oxidase may be falsely elevated.

Additional Information I.V. preparations contain alcohol and/or propylene glycol; may need to use nitrate-free interval (10-12 hours/day) to avoid tolerance development. Tolerance may possibly be reversed with acetylcysteine; gradually decrease dose in patients receiving NTG for prolonged period to avoid withdrawal reaction.

Concomitant use of sildenafil (Viagra®) or other phosphodiesterase-5 enzyme inhibitors (PDE-5) may precipitate acute hypotension, myocardial infarction, or death. Nitrates used in right ventricular infarction may induce acute hypotension. Nitrate use in severe pericardial effusion may reduce cardiac filling pressure and precipitate cardiac tamponade. In the management of heart failure, the combination of isosorbide dinitrate and hydralazine confers beneficial effects on disease progression and cardiac outcomes.

Product Availability

Rectiv™: FDA approved June 2011; availability expected during the first quarter of 2012

Rectiv™ (nitroglycerin 0.4% ointment) is approved for the treatment of moderate-to-severe pain associated with chronic anal fissure.

Dosage Forms Excipient information presented when available (limited, particularly for generics); consult specific product labeling. [DSC] = Discontinued product

Aerosol, spray, translingual:
NitroMist®: 0.4 mg/spray (8.5 g) [230 metered sprays]

Capsule, extended release, oral: 2.5 mg, 6.5 mg, 9 mg
Nitro-Time®: 2.5 mg, 6.5 mg, 9 mg

Capsule, sustained release, oral: 2.5 mg [DSC], 6.5 mg [DSC], 9 mg [DSC]

Infusion, premixed in D_5W: 25 mg (250 mL) [100 mcg/mL]; 50 mg (250 mL, 500 mL) [100 mcg/mL]; 50 mg (250 mL, 500 mL) [200 mcg/mL]; 100 mg (250 mL) [400 mcg/mL]

Injection, solution: 5 mg/mL (10 mL)

Ointment, topical:
Nitro-Bid®: 2% (1 g, 30 g, 60 g) [~15 mg/inch]

Patch, transdermal: 0.1 mg/hr (30s); 0.2 mg/hr (30s); 0.4 mg/hr (30s); 0.6 mg/hr (30s)
Minitran™: 0.1 mg/hr (30s); 0.2 mg/hr (30s); 0.4 mg/hr (30s); 0.6 mg/hr (30s)
Nitro-Dur®: 0.1 mg/hr (30s); 0.2 mg/hr (30s); 0.3 mg/hr (30s); 0.4 mg/hr (30s); 0.6 mg/hr (30s); 0.8 mg/hr (30s)

Solution, translingual [spray]: 0.4 mg/spray (4.9 g, 12 g)
Nitrolingual®: 0.4 mg/spray (12 g) [contains ethanol 20%; 200 metered sprays]
Nitrolingual®: 0.4 mg/spray (4.9 g) [contains ethanol 20%; 60 metered sprays]

Tablet, sublingual:
Nitrostat®: 0.3 mg, 0.4 mg, 0.6 mg

- ◆ **Nitroglycerin Injection, USP (Can)** *see* Nitroglycerin *on page 1212*
- ◆ **Nitroglycerol** *see* Nitroglycerin *on page 1212*
- ◆ **Nitrol® (Can)** *see* Nitroglycerin *on page 1212*
- ◆ **Nitrolingual®** *see* Nitroglycerin *on page 1212*
- ◆ **NitroMist®** *see* Nitroglycerin *on page 1212*
- ◆ **Nitropress®** *see* Nitroprusside *on page 1214*

Nitroprusside (nye troe PRUS ide)

Brand Names: U.S. Nitropress®

Brand Names: Canada Nipride®

Index Terms Nitroprusside Sodium; Sodium Nitroferricyanide; Sodium Nitroprusside

Pharmacologic Category Vasodilator

Additional Appendix Information
Hypertension *on page 2001*
Vasoactive Agents, Intravenous *on page 1898*

Use Management of hypertensive crises; acute decompensated heart failure (HF); used for controlled hypotension to reduce bleeding during surgery

Pregnancy Risk Factor C

Pregnancy Considerations Animal studies have shown that nitroprusside may cross the placental barrier and result in fetal cyanide levels that are dose-related to maternal nitroprusside levels. However, information related to use in pregnancy is limited.

Lactation Excretion in breast milk unknown/not recommended

Contraindications Treatment of compensatory hypertension (aortic coarctation, arteriovenous shunting); to produce controlled hypotension during surgery in patients with known inadequate cerebral circulation or in moribund patients requiring emergency surgery; high output heart failure associated with reduced systemic vascular resistance (eg, septic shock); congenital optic atrophy or tobacco amblyopia

Warnings/Precautions [U.S. Boxed Warning] Excessive hypotension resulting in compromised perfusion of vital organs may occur; continuous blood pressure monitoring by experienced personnel is required. Except when used briefly or at low (<2 mcg/kg/minute) infusion rates, nitroprusside gives rise to large cyanide quantities. Do not use the maximum dose for more than 10 minutes; if blood pressure is not controlled by the maximum rate after 10 minutes, discontinue infusion. Monitor for cyanide toxicity via acid-base balance and venous oxygen concentration; however, clinicians should note that these indicators may not always reliably indicate cyanide toxicity. When nitroprusside is used for controlled hypotension during surgery, correct pre-existing anemia and hypovolemia prior to use when possible. Use with extreme caution in patients with elevated intracranial pressure (head trauma, cerebral hemorrhage), severe renal impairment, hepatic failure, hypothyroidism. Use the lowest end of the dosage range with renal impairment. Cyanide toxicity may occur in patients with decreased liver function. Thiocyanate toxicity occurs in patients with renal impairment or those on prolonged infusions. **[U.S. Boxed Warning]: Solution must be further diluted with 5% dextrose in water. Do not administer by direct injection.**

Adverse Reactions Frequency not defined.

Cardiovascular: Bradycardia, ECG changes, flushing, hypotension (excessive), palpitation, substernal distress, tachycardia

Central nervous system: Apprehension, dizziness, headache, intracranial pressure increased, restlessness

Dermatologic: Rash

Endocrine & metabolic: Metabolic acidosis (secondary to cyanide toxicity), hypothyroidism

Gastrointestinal: Abdominal pain, ileus, nausea, retching, vomiting

Hematologic: Methemoglobinemia, platelet aggregation decreased

Local: Injection site irritation

Neuromuscular & skeletal: Hyperreflexia (secondary to thiocyanate toxicity), muscle twitching

Ocular: Miosis (secondary to thiocyanate toxicity)

Otic: Tinnitus (secondary to thiocyanate toxicity)

Respiratory: Hyperoxemia (secondary to cyanide toxicity)

Miscellaneous: Cyanide toxicity, diaphoresis, thiocyanate toxicity

Drug Interactions

Metabolism/Transport Effects None known.

Avoid Concomitant Use There are no known interactions where it is recommended to avoid concomitant use.

Increased Effect/Toxicity

Nitroprusside may increase the levels/effects of: Amifostine; Antihypertensives; Hypotensive Agents; Prilocaine; RiTUXimab

The levels/effects of Nitroprusside may be increased by: Alfuzosin; Calcium Channel Blockers; Diazoxide; Herbs (Hypotensive Properties); MAO Inhibitors; Pentoxifylline; Phosphodiesterase 5 Inhibitors; Prostacyclin Analogues

Decreased Effect

The levels/effects of Nitroprusside may be decreased by: Herbs (Hypertensive Properties); Methylphenidate; Yohimbine

Stability Store the intact vial at 20°C to 25°C (68°F to 77°F). Protect from light.

Prior to administration, nitroprusside sodium should be further diluted by diluting 50 mg in 250-1000 mL of D_5W.

Use only clear solutions; solutions of nitroprusside exhibit a color described as brownish, brown, brownish-pink, light orange, and straw. Solutions are highly sensitive to light. Exposure to light causes decomposition, resulting in a highly colored solution of orange, dark brown or blue. **A blue color indicates almost complete decomposition.** Do not use discolored solutions (eg, blue, green, red) or solutions in which particulate matter is visible.

Prepared solutions should be wrapped with aluminum foil or other opaque material to protect from light (do as soon as possible).

Stability of parenteral admixture at room temperature (25°C) and at refrigeration temperature (4°C) is 24 hours.

Mechanism of Action Causes peripheral vasodilation by direct action on venous and arteriolar smooth muscle, thus reducing peripheral resistance; will increase cardiac output by decreasing afterload; reduces aortal and left ventricular impedance

Pharmacodynamics/Kinetics

Onset of action: Hypotensive effect: <2 minutes

Duration: Hypotensive effect: 1-10 minutes

Metabolism: Nitroprusside combines with hemoglobin to produce cyanide and cyanmethemoglobin. Cyanide detoxification occurs via rhodanase-mediated conversion of cyanide to thiocyanate; rhodanase couples cyanide molecules to sulfane sulfur groups from a sulfur donor (eg, thiosulfate, cystine, cysteine). This process has limited capacity and may become overwhelmed with large exposures once sulfur donor supplies are exhausted resulting in toxicity.

Half-life elimination: Nitroprusside, circulatory: ~2 minutes; Thiocyanate, elimination: ~3 days (may be doubled or tripled in renal failure)

Excretion: Urine (as thiocyanate)

Dosage I.V.:

Children: Acute hypertension: Initial: 0.3-0.5 mcg/kg/minute; may be titrated every few minutes to achieve desired hemodynamic effect; maximum dose: 10 mcg/kg/minute (Hegenbarth, 2008; NHBPEP, 2005). Doses ≥1.8 mcg/kg/minute are associated with increased cyanide concentration in pediatric patients (Moffett, 2008); monitor cyanide levels with prolonged use (eg, >72 hours) (NHBPEP, 2005).

Adults:

Acute hypertension: Initial: 0.25-0.3 mcg/kg/minute; may be titrated by 0.5 mcg/kg/minute every few minutes to achieve desired hemodynamic effect (JNC 7; Rhoney, 2009); usual dose: 3 mcg/kg/minute; maximum dose: 10 mcg/kg/minute. When administered in doses >3 mcg/kg/minute for prolonged periods of time (eg, 3-4 days), thiocyanate levels should be monitored daily.

Acute decompensated heart failure: Initial: 5-10 **mcg/minute**; may be titrated rapidly (eg, up to every 5 minutes) to achieve desired hemodynamic effect; usual dosage range: 5-300 **mcg/minute**. Doses >400 **mcg/minute** are not recommended due to minimal added benefit and increased risk for thiocyanate toxicity (HFSA, 2010).

Dosage adjustment in renal impairment: There are no dosage adjustments provided in manufacturer's labeling. However, use in patients with renal impairment may lead to the accumulation of thiocyanate and subsequent toxicity; limit use.

Dosage adjustment in hepatic impairment: There are no dosage adjustments provided in manufacturer's labeling; due to the risk of cyanide toxicity, use with caution.

Administration I.V. infusion only; infusion pump required. Must be diluted with D5W (preferred), LR, or NS prior to administration; not for direct injection. Due to potential for excessive hypotension, continuously monitor patient's blood pressure during therapy.

Monitoring Parameters Blood pressure, heart rate; monitor for cyanide and thiocyanate toxicity; monitor acid-base status as acidosis can be the earliest sign of cyanide toxicity; monitor thiocyanate levels if requiring prolonged infusion (>3 days) or dose >3 mcg/kg/minute or patient has renal dysfunction; monitor cyanide blood levels in patients with decreased hepatic function; cardiac monitor and blood pressure monitor required

Reference Range Serum thiocyanate levels are not helpful in detecting toxicity. A level may be confirmatory if a patient is exhibiting signs and symptoms of thiocyanate toxicity. Initial signs of toxicity (eg, tinnitus) may be observed at levels >35 mcg/mL (manufacturer suggests 60 mcg/mL), but serious toxicity typically may not occur with levels <100 mcg/mL.

Dosage Forms Excipient information presented when available (limited, particularly for generics); consult specific product labeling.

Injection, solution, as sodium:

Nitropress®: 25 mg/mL (2 mL)

- **Nitroprusside Sodium** *see* Nitroprusside *on page 1214*
- **Nitrostat®** *see* Nitroglycerin *on page 1212*
- **Nitro-Time®** *see* Nitroglycerin *on page 1212*
- **Nix® (Can)** *see* Permethrin *on page 1336*
- **Nix® Complete Lice Treatment System [OTC]** *see* Permethrin *on page 1336*
- **Nix® Creme Rinse [OTC]** *see* Permethrin *on page 1336*
- **Nix® Creme Rinse Lice Treatment [OTC]** *see* Permethrin *on page 1336*
- **Nix® Lice Control Spray [OTC]** *see* Permethrin *on page 1336*

Nizatidine (ni ZA ti deen)

Brand Names: U.S. Axid®

Brand Names: Canada Apo-Nizatidine®; Axid®; Gen-Nizatidine; Novo-Nizatidine; Nu-Nizatidine; PMS-Nizatidine

Pharmacologic Category Histamine H_2 Antagonist

Use Treatment and maintenance of duodenal ulcer; treatment of benign gastric ulcer; treatment of gastroesophageal reflux disease (GERD)

Unlabeled Use Part of a multidrug regimen for *H. pylori* eradication to reduce the risk of duodenal ulcer recurrence

Pregnancy Risk Factor B

Dosage Oral:

Children:

<12 years: GERD (unlabeled use): 10 mg/kg/day in divided doses given twice daily; may not be as effective in children <12 years

≥12 years:

GERD: Refer to adult dosing

Adults:

Duodenal ulcer:

Treatment of active ulcer: 300 mg at bedtime or 150 mg twice daily

Maintenance of healed ulcer: 150 mg/day at bedtime

Gastric ulcer: 150 mg twice daily or 300 mg at bedtime

GERD: 150 mg twice daily

Helicobacter pylori eradication (unlabeled use): 150 mg twice daily; requires combination therapy

Dosing adjustment in renal impairment:

Active treatment:

Cl_{cr} 20-50 mL/minute: 150 mg/day

Cl_{cr} <20 mL/minute: 150 mg every other day

Maintenance treatment:

Cl_{cr} 20-50 mL/minute: 150 mg every other day

Cl_{cr} <20 mL/minute: 150 mg every 3 days

Additional Information Complete prescribing information for this medication should be consulted for additional detail.

Dosage Forms Excipient information presented when available (limited, particularly for generics); consult specific product labeling.

Capsule, oral: 150 mg, 300 mg

Solution, oral: 15 mg/mL (473 mL)

Axid®: 15 mg/mL (480 mL) [bubblegum flavor]

- ◆ **Nizoral®** *see* Ketoconazole (Topical) *on page 953*
- ◆ **Nizoral® A-D [OTC]** *see* Ketoconazole (Topical) *on page 953*
- ◆ **N-Methylhydrazine** *see* Procarbazine *on page 1410*
- ◆ **N-methylnaltrexone Bromide** *see* Methylnaltrexone *on page 1106*
- ◆ **NN2211** *see* Liraglutide *on page 1018*
- ◆ **No Doz® Maximum Strength [OTC]** *see* Caffeine *on page 259*
- ◆ **NoHist [DSC]** *see* Chlorpheniramine and Phenylephrine *on page 345*
- ◆ **NoHist DM [OTC]** *see* Chlorpheniramine, Phenylephrine, and Dextromethorphan *on page 346*
- ◆ **NoHist-DMX [DSC]** *see* Chlorpheniramine, Phenylephrine, and Dextromethorphan *on page 346*
- ◆ **NoHist LQ [OTC]** *see* Chlorpheniramine and Phenylephrine *on page 345*
- ◆ **Nolvadex** *see* Tamoxifen *on page 1624*
- ◆ **Nolvadex®-D (Can)** *see* Tamoxifen *on page 1624*
- ◆ **Non-Aspirin Pain Reliever [OTC]** *see* Acetaminophen *on page 27*

Nonoxynol 9 (non OKS i nole nine)

Brand Names: U.S. Conceptrol® [OTC]; Delfen® [OTC]; Encare® [OTC]; Gynol II® Extra Strength [OTC]; Gynol II® [OTC]; Today® [OTC]; VCF® [OTC]

Index Terms N-9

Pharmacologic Category Contraceptive; Spermicide

Use Prevention of pregnancy

Dosage Adolescents and Adults: **Note:** Prior to use, refer to specific product labeling for complete instructions.

Prevention of pregnancy: Vaginal:

Conceptrol®: Insert 1 applicatorful vaginally up to 1 hour prior to intercourse

Encare®: Unwrap and insert 1 suppository vaginally at least 10 minutes prior to intercourse; effective for 1 hour

Today®: Insert 1 sponge vaginally prior to intercourse; allow to remain in place for 6 hours after intercourse before removing; effective for use up to 24 continuous hours. Do not leave in place for >30 hours.

VCF®:

Film: Insert 1 film vaginally at least 15 minutes, but no more than 3 hours, prior to intercourse. Insert new film for each act of intercourse or if more than 3 hours have elapsed.

Foam: Insert 1 applicatorful at least 15 minutes prior to intercourse; effective for up to 1 hour

Additional Information Complete prescribing information for this medication should be consulted for additional detail.

Dosage Forms Excipient information presented when available (limited, particularly for generics); consult specific product labeling.

Aerosol, foam, vaginal:

Delfen®: 12.5% (18 g) [contains benzoic acid]

VCF®: 12.5% (40 g)

Film, vaginal:

VCF®: 28% (3s, 6s, 12s)

Gel, vaginal:

Conceptrol®: 4% (2.7 g)

Encare®: 4% (2.7 g)

Gynol II®: 2% (108 g)

Gynol II® Extra Strength: 3% (81 g)

Sponge, vaginal:

Today®: 1 g (3s, 12s) [contains benzoic acid, sodium metabisulfite]

Suppository, vaginal:

Encare®: 100 mg (12s, 18s)

- ◆ **Nora-BE®** *see* Norethindrone *on page 1217*
- ◆ **Noradrenaline** *see* Norepinephrine *on page 1216*
- ◆ **Noradrenaline Acid Tartrate** *see* Norepinephrine *on page 1216*
- ◆ **Norco®** *see* Hydrocodone and Acetaminophen *on page 837*
- ◆ **Norcuron** *see* Vecuronium *on page 1777*
- ◆ **Norcuron® (Can)** *see* Vecuronium *on page 1777*
- ◆ **Nordeoxyguanosine** *see* Ganciclovir (Systemic) *on page 778*
- ◆ **Nordette® 28** *see* Ethinyl Estradiol and Levonorgestrel *on page 656*
- ◆ **Norditropin® [DSC]** *see* Somatropin *on page 1579*
- ◆ **Norditropin FlexPro®** *see* Somatropin *on page 1579*
- ◆ **Norditropin® NordiFlex®** *see* Somatropin *on page 1579*
- ◆ **Norelgestromin and Ethinyl Estradiol** *see* Ethinyl Estradiol and Norelgestromin *on page 660*

Norepinephrine (nor ep i NEF rin)

Brand Names: U.S. Levophed®

Brand Names: Canada Levophed®

Index Terms Levarterenol Bitartrate; Noradrenaline; Noradrenaline Acid Tartrate; Norepinephrine Bitartrate

Pharmacologic Category Alpha/Beta Agonist

Additional Appendix Information

Vasoactive Agents, Intravenous *on page 1898*

Use Treatment of shock which persists after adequate fluid volume replacement; severe hypotension

Pregnancy Risk Factor C

Pregnancy Considerations

Animal reproduction studies have not been conducted. Norepinephrine is an endogenous catecholamine and crosses the placenta (Minzter, 2010; Wang, 1999).

Lactation Excretion in breast milk unknown/use caution

Contraindications Hypersensitivity to norepinephrine, bisulfites (contains metabisulfite), or any component of the formulation; hypotension from hypovolemia except as an emergency measure to maintain coronary and cerebral perfusion until volume could be replaced; mesenteric or peripheral vascular thrombosis unless it is a lifesaving procedure; during anesthesia with cyclopropane (not available in U.S.) or halothane (not available in U.S.) anesthesia (risk of ventricular arrhythmias)

Warnings/Precautions Assure adequate circulatory volume to minimize need for vasoconstrictors. Avoid hypertension; monitor blood pressure closely and adjust infusion rate. Use with extreme caution in patients taking MAO-Inhibitors. Avoid extravasation; infuse into a large vein if possible. Avoid infusion into leg veins. Watch I.V. site closely. **[U.S. Boxed Warning]: If extravasation occurs, infiltrate the area with diluted phentolamine (5-10 mg in 10-15 mL of saline) with a fine hypodermic needle. Phentolamine should be administered as soon as possible after extravasation is noted.** Product may contain sodium metasulfite.

Adverse Reactions Frequency not defined.

Cardiovascular: Arrhythmias, bradycardia, peripheral (digital) ischemia

Central nervous system: Anxiety, headache (transient)

Local: Skin necrosis (with extravasation)

Respiratory: Dyspnea, respiratory difficulty

Drug Interactions

Metabolism/Transport Effects Substrate of COMT

Avoid Concomitant Use

Avoid concomitant use of Norepinephrine with any of the following: Ergot Derivatives; Inhalational Anesthetics; Iobenguane I 123

Increased Effect/Toxicity

Norepinephrine may increase the levels/effects of: Bromocriptine; Sympathomimetics

The levels/effects of Norepinephrine may be increased by: Antacids; Atomoxetine; Beta-Blockers; Cannabinoids; Carbonic Anhydrase Inhibitors; COMT Inhibitors; Ergot Derivatives; Inhalational Anesthetics; MAO Inhibitors; Serotonin/Norepinephrine Reuptake Inhibitors; Tricyclic Antidepressants

Decreased Effect

Norepinephrine may decrease the levels/effects of: Benzylpenicilloyl Polylysine; Iobenguane I 123; Ioflupane I 123

The levels/effects of Norepinephrine may be decreased by: Spironolactone

Stability Readily oxidized. Protect from light. Do not use if brown coloration. Dilute with D_5W, D_5NS, or NS; dilution in NS is not recommended by the manufacturer; however, stability in NS has been demonstrated (Tremblay, 2008). Stability of parenteral admixture at room temperature (25°C) is 24 hours.

Mechanism of Action Stimulates $beta_1$-adrenergic receptors and alpha-adrenergic receptors causing increased contractility and heart rate as well as vasoconstriction, thereby increasing systemic blood pressure and coronary blood flow; clinically, alpha effects (vasoconstriction) are greater than beta effects (inotropic and chronotropic effects)

Pharmacodynamics/Kinetics

Onset of action: I.V.: Very rapid-acting

Duration: vasopressor: 1-2 minutes

Metabolism: Via catechol-o-methyltransferase (COMT) and monoamine oxidase (MAO)

Excretion: Urine (84% to 96% as inactive metabolites)

Dosage Administration requires the use of an infusion pump.

Note: Norepinephrine dosage is stated in terms of norepinephrine base.

Continuous I.V. infusion:

Children: Initial: 0.05-0.1 mcg/kg/minute; titrate to desired effect; maximum dose: 2 mcg/kg/minute (Kleinman, 2007; AHA, 2010)

Adults: Initial: 8-12 mcg/minute; titrate to desired response. Usual maintenance range: 2-4 mcg/minute; dosage range varies greatly depending on clinical situation. If patient remains hypotensive despite large doses, evaluate for occult hypovolemia and provide fluid resuscitation as appropriate.

ACLS dosing range (weight-based dosing): Post cardiac arrest care: Initial: 0.1-0.5 mcg/**kg**/minute (7-35 mcg/minute in a 70 kg patient); titrate to desired response (AHA, 2010)

Sepsis and septic shock (weight-based dosing): Range from clinical trials: 0.01-3 mcg/**kg**/minute (0.7-210 mcg/minute in a 70 kg patient) (Hollenberg, 2004)

Administration Administer as a continuous infusion with the use of an infusion pump. Dilute prior to use. Administration via central line recommended; may cause severe ischemic necrosis if extravasated. Do not administer sodium bicarbonate (or any alkaline solution) through an I.V. line containing norepinephrine; inactivation of norepinephrine may occur.

Additional Information Norepinephrine dosage is stated in terms of norepinephrine base. Although the intravenous product vial designates the contents as norepinephrine bitartrate, the actual concentration shown is in terms of norepinephrine base 1 mg/mL.

Dosage Forms Excipient information presented when available (limited, particularly for generics); consult specific product labeling.

Injection, solution [strength expressed as base]: 1 mg/mL (4 mL)

Levophed®: 1 mg/mL (4 mL) [contains sodium metabisulfite]

◆ **Norepinephrine Bitartrate** *see* Norepinephrine *on page 1216*

Norethindrone (nor ETH in drone)

Brand Names: U.S. Aygestin®; Camila®; Errin®; Heather; Jolivette®; Nor-QD®; Nora-BE®; Ortho Micronor®

Brand Names: Canada Micronor®; Norlutate®

Index Terms Norethindrone Acetate; Norethisterone

Pharmacologic Category Contraceptive; Progestin

Use Treatment of amenorrhea; abnormal uterine bleeding; endometriosis; prevention of pregnancy

Pregnancy Risk Factor X

Pregnancy Considerations First trimester exposure may cause genital abnormalities including hypospadias in male infants and mild virilization of external female genitalia. Significant adverse events related to growth and development have not been observed (limited studies). Use is contraindicated during pregnancy. May be started immediately postpartum if not breast-feeding.

Lactation Enters breast milk/use caution

Contraindications Hypersensitivity to norethindrone or any component of the formulation; history of or current thrombophlebitis or venous thromboembolic disorders (including DVT, PE); hepatic dysfunction or tumor; known or suspected breast carcinoma; undiagnosed vaginal bleeding; pregnancy; missed abortion or as a diagnostic test for pregnancy

Warnings/Precautions Progestin only contraceptives do not protect against HIV infection or other sexually-transmitted diseases. Irregular menstrual bleeding patterns are common with progestin-only contraceptives; nonpharmacologic causes of abnormal bleeding should be ruled out. Progestin use has been associated with retinal vascular lesions; discontinue pending examination in case of sudden vision loss, complete loss of vision, sudden onset of proptosis, diplopia or migraine. May have adverse effects on glucose tolerance; use caution in women with diabetes. May have adverse effects on lipid metabolism; use caution in women with hyperlipidemias. Use with caution in patients with depression.

Use with caution in patients with diseases which may be exacerbated by fluid retention, including asthma, epilepsy, migraine, cardiac or renal dysfunction. Use caution in patients at increased risk of thromboembolism; includes elective surgery associated with an increased risk of thromboembolism or during periods of prolonged immobilization. The use of combination hormonal contraceptives has been associated with a slight increase in the frequency of breast cancer, however studies are not consistent. Data is insufficient to determine if progestin-only contraceptives also increase this risk. The risk of cardiovascular side effects increases in women using estrogen containing combined hormonal contraceptives and who smoke cigarettes, especially those who are >35 years of age. This risk relative to progestin-only contraceptives has not been established. Extremely rare hepatic adenomas and focal nodular hyperplasia resulting in fatal intra-abdominal hemorrhage have been reported in association with long-term combination oral contraceptive use. Data is insufficient to determine if progestin-only contraceptives also increase this risk. Not for use prior to menarche.

Adverse Reactions Frequency not defined.

Cardiovascular: Cerebral embolism, cerebral thrombosis, DVT, edema

Central nervous system: Depression, dizziness, headache, insomnia, migraine, mood swings

Dermatologic: Acne, chloasma, hirsutism, melasma, pruritus, rash, urticaria

Endocrine & metabolic: Amenorrhea, breakthrough bleeding, breast enlargement/tenderness, menstrual flow changes, spotting

Gastrointestinal: Nausea, weight gain/loss

Genitourinary: Cervical erosion changes, cervical secretion changes

Hepatic: Cholestatic jaundice, liver function test abnormalities

Ocular: Optic neuritis (with or without vision loss), retinal vascular thrombosis

Respiratory: Pulmonary embolism

Miscellaneous: Anaphylactic/anaphylactoid reactions

Drug Interactions

Metabolism/Transport Effects Substrate of CYP3A4 (major); **Note:** Assignment of Major/Minor substrate status based on clinically relevant drug interaction potential; **Induces** CYP2C19 (weak/moderate)

Avoid Concomitant Use

Avoid concomitant use of Norethindrone with any of the following: Griseofulvin

Increased Effect/Toxicity

Norethindrone may increase the levels/effects of: Benzodiazepines (metabolized by oxidation); Selegiline; Tranexamic Acid; Voriconazole

The levels/effects of Norethindrone may be increased by: Boceprevir; Conivaptan; Herbs (Progestogenic Properties); Voriconazole

Decreased Effect

Norethindrone may decrease the levels/effects of: Vitamin K Antagonists

The levels/effects of Norethindrone may be decreased by: Acitretin; Aminoglutethimide; Aprepitant; Artemether; Barbiturates; Bexarotene; Bexarotene (Systemic); Bile Acid Sequestrants; Bosentan; CarBAMazepine; Clobazam; Colesevelam; CYP3A4 Inducers (Strong); Darunavir; Deferasirox; Felbamate; Fosaprepitant; Fosphenytoin; Griseofulvin; LamoTRIgine; Mycophenolate; Nevirapine; OXcarbazepine; Phenytoin; Retinoic Acid Derivatives; Rifamycin Derivatives; Rufinamide; St Johns Wort; Telaprevir; Tocilizumab; Topiramate

Ethanol/Nutrition/Herb Interactions Herb/Nutraceutical: Avoid bloodroot, chasteberry, damiana, oregano, and yucca; may enhance the adverse/toxic effect of progestins. Avoid St John's wort; may diminish the therapeutic effect of progestin contraceptives; contraceptive failure is possible.

Stability Store at controlled room temperature of 25°C (77°F).

Mechanism of Action Inhibits secretion of pituitary gonadotropin (LH) which prevents follicular maturation and ovulation

Pharmacodynamics/Kinetics

Absorption: Oral: Rapidly absorbed

Distribution: V_d: 4 L/kg

Protein binding: 61% to albumin; 36% to sex hormone-binding globulin (SHBG); SHBG capacity affected by plasma ethinyl estradiol levels

Metabolism: Oral: Hepatic via reduction and conjugation; first-pass effect

Bioavailability: 64%

Half-life elimination: ~8 hours

Time to peak: 1-2 hours

Excretion: Urine (>50% as metabolites); feces (20% to 40% as metabolites)

Dosage Oral: Adolescents and Adults: Females:

Contraception: Progesterone only: Norethindrone 0.35 mg every day (no missed days)

Initial dose: Start on first day of menstrual period or the day after a miscarriage or abortion. If switching from a combined oral contraceptive, begin the day after finishing the last active combined tablet.

Missed dose: Take as soon as remembered. A back up method of contraception should be used for 48 hours if dose is taken ≥3 hours late.

Amenorrhea and abnormal uterine bleeding: Norethindrone acetate: 2.5-10 mg/day for 5-10 days during the second half of the menstrual cycle

Endometriosis: Norethindrone acetate: 5 mg/day for 14 days; increase at increments of 2.5 mg/day every 2 weeks to reach 15 mg/day; continue for 6-9 months or until breakthrough bleeding demands temporary termination

Dietary Considerations Should be taken at same time each day.

Administration Administer at the same time each day. When used for the prevention of pregnancy, a back up method of contraception should be used for 48 hours if dose is missed or taken ≥3 hours late.

Monitoring Parameters Contraception: Before starting therapy, a physical exam with reference to the breasts and pelvis are recommended, including a Papanicolaou smear. Exam may be deferred if appropriate; pregnancy should be ruled out prior to use. Monitor patient closely for loss of vision, sudden onset of proptosis, diplopia, migraine; blood pressure; signs and symptoms of thromboembolic disorders; signs or symptoms of depression; glycemic control in patients with diabetes; lipid profiles in patients being treated for hyperlipidemias. Adequate diagnostic measures, including endometrial sampling, if indicated, should be performed to rule out malignancy in all cases of undiagnosed abnormal vaginal bleeding.

Test Interactions May increase prothrombin, factors VII, VIII, IX, and X, PBI, and BEI. May decrease T_3 uptake; may decrease sex hormone-binding globulin (SHBG); may have a reduced response to metyrapone test.

Dosage Forms Excipient information presented when available (limited, particularly for generics); consult specific product labeling.

Tablet, oral: 0.35 mg

Camila®: 0.35 mg

Errin®: 0.35 mg

Heather: 0.35 mg

Jolivette®: 0.35 mg

Nor-QD®: 0.35 mg

Nora-BE®: 0.35 mg

Ortho Micronor®: 0.35 mg

Tablet, oral, as acetate: 5 mg

Aygestin®: 5 mg [scored]

◆ **Norethindrone Acetate** *see* Norethindrone *on page 1217*

◆ **Norethindrone Acetate and Ethinyl Estradiol** *see* Ethinyl Estradiol and Norethindrone *on page 660*

◆ **Norethindrone and Estradiol** *see* Estradiol and Norethindrone *on page 635*

Norethindrone and Mestranol
(nor eth IN drone & MES tra nole)

Brand Names: U.S. Necon® 1/50; Norinyl® 1+50
Brand Names: Canada Ortho-Novum® 1/50
Index Terms Mestranol and Norethindrone; Ortho Novum 1/50
Pharmacologic Category Contraceptive; Estrogen and Progestin Combination
Use Prevention of pregnancy
Unlabeled Use Treatment of hypermenorrhea (menorrhagia); pain associated with endometriosis; dysmenorrhea; dysfunctional uterine bleeding
Pregnancy Risk Factor X
Dosage Oral: Adults: Females: Contraception:

Schedule 1 (Sunday starter): Dose begins on first Sunday after onset of menstruation; if the menstrual period starts on Sunday, take first tablet that very same day. **With a Sunday start, an additional method of contraception should be used until after the first 7 days of consecutive administration.**

For 21-tablet package: Dosage is 1 tablet daily for 21 consecutive days, followed by 7 days off of the medication; a new course begins on the 8th day after the last tablet is taken.

For 28-tablet package: Dosage is 1 tablet daily without interruption.

Schedule 2 (Day 1 starter): Dose starts on first day of menstrual cycle taking 1 tablet daily.

For 21-tablet package: Dosage is 1 tablet daily for 21 consecutive days, followed by 7 days off of the medication; a new course begins on the 8th day after the last tablet is taken.

For 28-tablet package: Dosage is 1 tablet daily without interruption.

If all doses have been taken on schedule and one menstrual period is missed, continue dosing cycle. If two consecutive menstrual periods are missed, pregnancy test is required before new dosing cycle is started.

Missed doses **monophasic formulations** (refer to package insert for complete information):

One dose missed: Take as soon as remembered or take 2 tablets next day

Two consecutive doses missed in the first 2 weeks: Take 2 tablets as soon as remembered or 2 tablets next 2 days. **An additional method of contraception should be used for 7 days after missed dose.**

Two consecutive doses missed in week 3 or three consecutive doses missed at any time: **An additional method of contraception must be used for 7 days after a missed dose:**

Schedule 1 (Sunday starter): Continue dose of 1 tablet daily until Sunday, then discard the rest of the pack, and a new pack should be started that same day.

Schedule 2 (Day 1 starter): Current pack should be discarded, and a new pack should be started that same day.

Dosage adjustment in renal impairment: Specific guidelines not available; use with caution and monitor blood pressure closely. Consider other forms of contraception.

Dosage adjustment in hepatic impairment: Contraindicated in patients with hepatic impairment

Additional Information Complete prescribing information for this medication should be consulted for additional detail.

Dosage Forms Excipient information presented when available (limited, particularly for generics); consult specific product labeling.

Tablet, monophasic formulations:

Necon® 1/50: Norethindrone 1 mg and mestranol 0.05 mg [21 light blue tablets and 7 white inactive tablets] (28s)

Norinyl® 1+50: Norethindrone 1 mg and mestranol 0.05 mg [21 white tablets and 7 orange inactive tablets] (28s)

- **Norethisterone** *see* Norethindrone *on page 1217*
- **Norflex™** *see* Orphenadrine *on page 1252*

Norfloxacin (nor FLOKS a sin)

Brand Names: U.S. Noroxin®
Brand Names: Canada Apo-Norflox®; CO Norfloxacin; Norfloxacine®; Novo-Norfloxacin; PMS-Norfloxacin; Riva-Norfloxacin
Pharmacologic Category Antibiotic, Quinolone
Use Uncomplicated and complicated urinary tract infections caused by susceptible gram-negative and gram-positive bacteria; sexually-transmitted disease (eg, uncomplicated urethral and cervical gonorrhea) caused by *N. gonorrhoeae*; prostatitis due to *E. coli*

Note: As of April 2007, the CDC no longer recommends the use of fluoroquinolones for the treatment of gonococcal disease.

Pregnancy Risk Factor C
Medication Guide Available Yes
Dosage

Usual dosage range:

Adults: Oral: 400 mg every 12 hours (maximum: 800 mg/day)

Indication-specific dosing:

Adults: Oral:

Dysenteric enterocolitis *(Shigella* unlabeled use): 400 mg twice daily for 5 days

Prostatitis: 400 mg every 12 hours for 4-6 weeks

Traveler's diarrhea (unlabeled use): 400 mg twice daily for 3 days, single dose may also be effective

Uncomplicated gonorrhea: 800 mg as a single dose. **Note:** As of April 2007, the CDC no longer recommends the use of fluoroquinolones for the treatment of uncomplicated gonococcal disease.

Urinary tract infections:

Uncomplicated due to *E. coli, K. pneumoniae, P. mirabilis*: 400 mg twice daily for 3 days

Uncomplicated due to other organisms: 400 mg twice daily for 7-10 days

Complicated: 400 mg twice daily for 10-21 days

Dosing interval in renal impairment: Cl_{cr} ≤30 mL/minute/1.73 m^2: Administer 400 mg every 24 hours

Additional Information Complete prescribing information for this medication should be consulted for additional detail.

Dosage Forms Excipient information presented when available (limited, particularly for generics); consult specific product labeling.

Tablet, oral:

Noroxin®: 400 mg

- **Norfloxacine® (Can)** *see* Norfloxacin *on page 1219*
- **Norgesic** *see* Orphenadrine, Aspirin, and Caffeine *on page 1252*
- **Norgestimate and Ethinyl Estradiol** *see* Ethinyl Estradiol and Norgestimate *on page 663*
- **Norgestrel and Ethinyl Estradiol** *see* Ethinyl Estradiol and Norgestrel *on page 664*
- **Norinyl® 1+35** *see* Ethinyl Estradiol and Norethindrone *on page 660*
- **Norinyl® 1+50** *see* Norethindrone and Mestranol *on page 1219*

Nortriptyline (nor TRIP ti leen)

Brand Names: U.S. Pamelor®

Brand Names: Canada Alti-Nortriptyline; Apo-Nortriptyline®; Aventyl®; Gen-Nortriptyline; Norventyl; Novo-Nortriptyline; Nu-Nortriptyline; PMS-Nortriptyline

Index Terms Nortriptyline Hydrochloride

Pharmacologic Category Antidepressant, Tricyclic (Secondary Amine)

Additional Appendix Information

Antidepressant Agents *on page 1874*

Use Treatment of symptoms of depression

Unlabeled Use Chronic pain (including neuropathic pain), myofascial pain, burning mouth sydrome, anxiety disorders, attention-deficit/hyperactivity disorder (ADHD); enuresis; adjunctive therapy for smoking cessation

Pregnancy Considerations Animal reproduction studies are inconclusive. Nortriptyline and its metabolites cross the human placenta and can be detected in cord blood. According to the manufacturer, the decision to use nortriptyline during pregnancy or in women of childbearing potential should take into account the potential benefits and possible risks. Treatment algorithms have been developed by the ACOG and the APA for the management of depression in women prior to conception and during pregnancy.

Lactation Enters breast milk/not recommended (AAP rates "of concern"; AAP 2001 update pending)

Medication Guide Available Yes

Contraindications Hypersensitivity to nortriptyline and similar chemical class, or any component of the formulation; use of MAO inhibitors within 14 days; use in a patient during the acute recovery phase of MI

Warnings/Precautions [U.S. Boxed Warning]: Antidepressants increase the risk of suicidal thinking and behavior in children, adolescents, and young adults (18-24 years of age) with major depressive disorder (MDD) and other psychiatric disorders; consider risk prior to prescribing. Short-term studies did not show an increased risk in patients >24 years of age and showed a decreased risk in patients ≥65 years. Closely monitor for clinical worsening, suicidality, or unusual changes in behavior; the patient's family or caregiver should be instructed to closely observe the patient and communicate condition with healthcare provider. A medication guide should be dispensed with each prescription. **Nortriptyline is not FDA approved for use in children.**

The possibility of a suicide attempt is inherent in major depression and may persist until remission occurs. Monitor for worsening of depression or suicidality, especially during initiation of therapy (generally first 1-2 months) or with dose increases or decreases. Use caution in high-risk patients. Worsening depression and severe abrupt suicidality that are not part of the presenting symptoms may require discontinuation or modification of drug therapy. The patient's family or caregiver should be alerted to monitor patients for the emergence of suicidality and associated behaviors (such as agitation, irritability, hostility, impulsivity, and hypomania) and call healthcare provider.

May worsen psychosis in some patients or precipitate a shift to mania or hypomania in patients with bipolar disorder. Patients presenting with depressive symptoms should be screened for bipolar disorder. Monotherapy in patients with bipolar disorder should be avoided. **Nortriptyline is not FDA approved for the treatment of bipolar depression.**

TCAs may rarely cause bone marrow suppression; monitor for any signs of infection and obtain CBC if symptoms (eg, fever, sore throat) evident. The risk of sedation and orthostatic effects are low relative to other antidepressants. However, nortriptyline may result in impaired performance of tasks requiring alertness (eg, operating machinery or driving). Sedative effects may be additive with other CNS depressants and/or ethanol. The degree of anticholinergic blockade produced by this agent is moderate relative to other cyclic antidepressants, however, caution should still be used in patients with urinary retention, benign prostatic hyperplasia, narrow-angle glaucoma, xerostomia, visual problems, constipation, or history of bowel obstruction. May cause orthostatic hypotension (risk is low relative to other antidepressants) or conduction disturbances. Use with caution in patients with a history of cardiovascular disease (including previous MI, stroke, tachycardia, or conduction abnormalities). The risk conduction abnormalities with this agent is moderate relative to other antidepressants.

Consider discontinuing, when possible, prior to elective surgery. Therapy should not be abruptly discontinued in patients receiving high doses for prolonged periods. May alter glucose regulation - use caution in patients with diabetes. Use caution in patients with a previous seizure disorder or condition predisposing to seizures such as brain damage, alcoholism, or concurrent therapy with other drugs which lower the seizure threshold. May increase the risks associated with electroconvulsive therapy. Use with caution in hyperthyroid patients or those receiving thyroid supplementation. Use with caution in patients with hepatic or renal dysfunction and in elderly patients.

Adverse Reactions Frequency not defined.

Cardiovascular: Arrhythmia, flushing, heart block, hypertension, MI, palpitation, postural hypotension, tachycardia

Central nervous system: Agitation, anxiety, ataxia, confusion, delirium, delusions, disorientation, dizziness, drowsiness, EEG changes, exacerbation of psychosis, extrapyramidal symptoms, fatigue, hallucinations, headache, hypomania, incoordination, insomnia, nightmares, panic, restlessness, seizure

Dermatologic: Alopecia, itching, petechiae, photosensitivity, rash, urticaria

Endocrine & metabolic: Blood sugar increased/decreased, breast enlargement, galactorrhea, gynecomastia, libido increased/decreased, sexual dysfunction, SIADH

Gastrointestinal: Abdominal cramps, anorexia, black tongue, constipation, diarrhea, epigastric distress, nausea, paralytic ileus, stomatitis, taste disturbance, vomiting, weight gain/loss, xerostomia

Genitourinary: Delayed micturition, impotence, nocturia, polyuria, testicular edema, urinary retention

Hematologic: Agranulocytosis (rare), eosinophilia, purpura, thrombocytopenia

Hepatic: Cholestatic jaundice, transaminases increased

Neuromuscular & skeletal: Numbness, paresthesia, peripheral neuropathy, tingling, tremor, weakness

Ocular: Blurred vision, disturbances in accommodation, eye pain, mydriasis

Otic: Tinnitus

Miscellaneous: Allergic reactions (eg, general edema or of the face/tongue), diaphoresis (excessive), withdrawal symptoms

Drug Interactions

Metabolism/Transport Effects Substrate of CYP1A2 (minor), CYP2C19 (minor), CYP2D6 (major), CYP3A4 (minor); **Note:** Assignment of Major/Minor substrate status based on clinically relevant drug interaction potential; **Inhibits** CYP2D6 (weak), CYP2E1 (weak)

Avoid Concomitant Use

Avoid concomitant use of Nortriptyline with any of the following: Artemether; Dronedarone; Iobenguane I 123; Lumefantrine; MAO Inhibitors; Methylene Blue; Nilotinib; Pimozide; QUEtiapine; QuiNINE; Tetrabenazine; Thioridazine; Toremifene; Vandetanib; Vemurafenib; Ziprasidone

Increased Effect/Toxicity

Nortriptyline may increase the levels/effects of: Alpha-/Beta-Agonists (Direct-Acting); Alpha1-Agonists; Amphetamines; Anticholinergics; Beta2-Agonists; Desmopressin; Dronedarone; Methylene Blue; Metoclopramide; Pimozide; QTc-Prolonging Agents; QuiNIDine; QuiNINE; Serotonin Modulators; Sodium Phosphates; Sulfonylureas; Tetrabenazine; Thioridazine; Toremifene; TraMADol; Vandetanib; Vemurafenib; Vitamin K Antagonists; Yohimbine; Ziprasidone

The levels/effects of Nortriptyline may be increased by: Abiraterone Acetate; Alfuzosin; Altretamine; Antipsychotics; Artemether; BuPROPion; Chloroquine; Cimetidine; Cinacalcet; Ciprofloxacin; Ciprofloxacin (Systemic); Conivaptan; CYP2D6 Inhibitors (Moderate); CYP2D6 Inhibitors (Strong); Dexmethylphenidate; Divalproex; DULoxetine; Gadobutrol; Indacaterol; Linezolid; Lithium; Lumefantrine; MAO Inhibitors; Methylphenidate; Metoclopramide; Nilotinib; Pramlintide; Protease Inhibitors; QUEtiapine; QuiNIDine; QuiNINE; Selective Serotonin Reuptake Inhibitors; Terbinafine; Terbinafine (Systemic); Valproic Acid

Decreased Effect

Nortriptyline may decrease the levels/effects of: Acetylcholinesterase Inhibitors (Central); Alpha2-Agonists; Iobenguane I 123

The levels/effects of Nortriptyline may be decreased by: Acetylcholinesterase Inhibitors (Central); Barbiturates; CarBAMazepine; Cyproterone; Peginterferon Alfa-2b; St Johns Wort; Tocilizumab

Ethanol/Nutrition/Herb Interactions

Ethanol: May increase CNS depression; monitor for increased effects with coadministration. Caution patients about effects.

Herb/Nutraceutical: Avoid valerian, St John's wort, SAMe, kava kava (may increase risk of serotonin syndrome and/or excessive sedation).

Stability Store at 20°C to 25°C (68°F to 77°F). Protect from light.

Mechanism of Action Traditionally believed to increase the synaptic concentration of serotonin and/or norepinephrine in the central nervous system by inhibition of their reuptake by the presynaptic neuronal membrane. However, additional receptor effects have been found including desensitization of adenyl cyclase, down regulation of beta-adrenergic receptors, and down regulation of serotonin receptors.

Pharmacodynamics/Kinetics

Onset of action: Therapeutic: 1-3 weeks

Distribution: V_d: 21 L/kg

Protein binding: 93% to 95%

Metabolism: Primarily hepatic; extensive first-pass effect

Half-life elimination: 28-31 hours

Time to peak, serum: 7-8.5 hours

Excretion: Urine (as metabolites and small amounts of unchanged drug); feces (small amounts)

Dosage Oral:

Nocturnal enuresis: Children (unlabeled use): 10-20 mg/day; titrate to a maximum of 40 mg/day

Depression: Children (unlabeled use): 1-3 mg/kg/day

Depression:

Adults: 25 mg 3-4 times/day up to 150 mg/day; doses may be given once daily

Elderly: Initial: 30-50 mg/day, given as a single daily dose or in divided doses. **Note:** Nortriptyline is one of the best tolerated TCAs in the elderly)

Myofascial pain, neuralgia, burning mouth syndrome (unlabeled uses): Adults: Initial: 10-25 mg at bedtime; dosage may be increased by 25 mg/day weekly, if tolerated; usual maintenance dose: 75 mg as a single bedtime dose or 2 divided doses

Chronic urticaria, angioedema, nocturnal pruritus (unlabeled use): Adults: Oral: 75 mg/day

Smoking cessation (unlabeled use; Fiore, 2008): Adults: Initial: 25 mg/day; titrate dose to 75-100 mg/day 10-28 days prior to selected "quit" date; continue therapy for ≥12 weeks after "quit" day

Dosing adjustment in hepatic impairment: Lower doses and slower titration dependent on individualization of dosage is recommended

Monitoring Parameters Blood pressure and pulse rate (ECG, cardiac monitoring) prior to and during initial therapy in older adults; weight; blood levels are useful for therapeutic monitoring; suicide ideation (especially at the beginning of therapy or when doses are increased or decreased)

Reference Range

Plasma levels do not always correlate with clinical effectiveness

Therapeutic: 50-150 ng/mL (SI: 190-570 nmol/L)

Toxic: >500 ng/mL (SI: >1900 nmol/L)

Additional Information The maximum antidepressant effect of nortriptyline may not be seen for ≥2 weeks after initiation of therapy.

Dosage Forms Excipient information presented when available (limited, particularly for generics); consult specific product labeling. [DSC] = Discontinued product

Capsule, oral: 10 mg, 25 mg, 50 mg, 75 mg

Pamelor®: 10 mg, 25 mg

Pamelor®: 50 mg [contains sodium bisulfite (may have trace amounts)]

Pamelor®: 75 mg

Solution, oral: 10 mg/5 mL (473 mL, 480 mL)

Pamelor®: 10 mg/5 mL (480 mL [DSC]) [contains benzoic acid, ethanol 4%]

◆ **Nortriptyline Hydrochloride** *see* Nortriptyline *on page 1220*

◆ **Norvasc®** *see* AmLODIPine *on page 97*

◆ **Norventyl (Can)** *see* Nortriptyline *on page 1220*

◆ **Norvir®** *see* Ritonavir *on page 1500*

◆ **Norvir® SEC (Can)** *see* Ritonavir *on page 1500*

◆ **Novahistex® DM Decongestant (Can)** *see* Pseudoephedrine and Dextromethorphan *on page 1431*

- ◆ **Nu-Sundac (Can)** *see* Sulindac *on page 1608*
- ◆ **Nu-Temazepam (Can)** *see* Temazepam *on page 1638*
- ◆ **Nu-Terazosin (Can)** *see* Terazosin *on page 1647*
- ◆ **Nu-Terbinafine (Can)** *see* Terbinafine (Systemic) *on page 1648*
- ◆ **Nu-Tetra (Can)** *see* Tetracycline *on page 1661*
- ◆ **Nu-Ticlopidine (Can)** *see* Ticlopidine *on page 1682*
- ◆ **Nu-Timolol (Can)** *see* Timolol (Systemic) *on page 1686*
- ◆ **Nutracort** *see* Hydrocortisone (Topical) *on page 841*
- ◆ **Nutralox® [OTC]** *see* Calcium Carbonate *on page 266*
- ◆ **Nutraplus® [OTC]** *see* Urea *on page 1749*
- ◆ **Nu-Trazodone (Can)** *see* TraZODone *on page 1725*
- ◆ **Nu-Trazodone D (Can)** *see* TraZODone *on page 1725*
- ◆ **NutreStore™** *see* Glutamine *on page 799*
- ◆ **Nu-Triazide (Can)** *see* Hydrochlorothiazide and Triamterene *on page 836*
- ◆ **Nutropin®** *see* Somatropin *on page 1579*
- ◆ **Nutropin AQ®** *see* Somatropin *on page 1579*
- ◆ **Nutropin® AQ (Can)** *see* Somatropin *on page 1579*
- ◆ **Nutropin AQ® NuSpin™** *see* Somatropin *on page 1579*
- ◆ **Nutropin AQ Pen®** *see* Somatropin *on page 1579*
- ◆ **NuvaRing®** *see* Ethinyl Estradiol and Etonogestrel *on page 655*
- ◆ **Nu-Verap (Can)** *see* Verapamil *on page 1783*
- ◆ **Nu-Verap SR (Can)** *see* Verapamil *on page 1783*
- ◆ **Nuvigil®** *see* Armodafinil *on page 145*
- ◆ **NV-Clindamycin (Can)** *see* Clindamycin (Systemic) *on page 378*
- ◆ **NVP** *see* Nevirapine *on page 1193*
- ◆ **Nyaderm (Can)** *see* Nystatin (Topical) *on page 1225*
- ◆ **Nyamyc®** *see* Nystatin (Topical) *on page 1225*

Nystatin (Oral) (nye STAT in)

Brand Names: Canada PMS-Nystatin

Pharmacologic Category Antifungal Agent, Oral Nonabsorbed

Additional Appendix Information
Antifungal Agents *on page 1876*

Use Treatment of susceptible cutaneous, mucocutaneous, and oral cavity fungal infections normally caused by the *Candida* species

Pregnancy Risk Factor C

Pregnancy Considerations Animal reproduction studies have not been conducted. Adverse events in the fetus or newborn have not been reported following maternal use of vaginal nystatin during pregnancy. Absorption following oral use is poor.

Lactation Excretion in breast milk unknown/use caution

Contraindications Hypersensitivity to nystatin or any component of the formulation

Adverse Reactions
1% to 10%: Gastrointestinal: Diarrhea, nausea, stomach pain, vomiting
<1% (Limited to important or life-threatening): Hypersensitivity reactions

Drug Interactions
Metabolism/Transport Effects None known.
Avoid Concomitant Use There are no known interactions where it is recommended to avoid concomitant use.
Increased Effect/Toxicity There are no known significant interactions involving an increase in effect.
Decreased Effect
Nystatin (Oral) may decrease the levels/effects of: Saccharomyces boulardii

Stability
Tablet and suspension: Store at controlled room temperature of 15°C to 25°C (59°F to 77°F).
Powder for suspension: Store under refrigeration at 2°C to 8°C (36°F to 46°F).

Mechanism of Action Binds to sterols in fungal cell membrane, changing the cell wall permeability allowing for leakage of cellular contents

Pharmacodynamics/Kinetics
Onset of action: Symptomatic relief from candidiasis: 24-72 hours
Absorption: Poorly absorbed
Excretion: Feces (as unchanged drug)

Dosage Oral:
Oral candidiasis:
Suspension:
Premature infants: 100,000 units 4 times/day; paint suspension into recesses of the mouth
Infants: 200,000 units 4 times/day or 100,000 units to each side of mouth 4 times/day; paint suspension into recesses of the mouth
Children and Adults: 400,000-600,000 units 4 times/day; swish in the mouth and retain for as long as possible (several minutes) before swallowing
Powder for compounding: Children and Adults: 1/8 teaspoon (500,000 units) to equal approximately 1/2 cup of water; give 4 times/day
Intestinal infections: Adults: 500,000-1,000,000 units every 8 hours

Administration Suspension: Shake well before using. Should be swished about the mouth and retained in the mouth for as long as possible (several minutes) before swallowing. For neonates and infants, paint nystatin suspension into recesses of the mouth.

Dosage Forms Excipient information presented when available (limited, particularly for generics); consult specific product labeling. [DSC] = Discontinued product
Powder, for prescription compounding: 50 million units (10 g); 150 million units (30 g); 500 million units (100 g)
Suspension, oral: 100,000 units/mL (5 mL, 60 mL, 473 mL, 480 mL [DSC])
Tablet, oral: 500,000 units

Nystatin (Topical) (nye STAT in)

Brand Names: U.S. Nyamyc®; Nystop®; Pedi-Dri®; Pediaderm™ AF

Brand Names: Canada Candistatin®; Nyaderm

Pharmacologic Category Antifungal Agent, Topical; Antifungal Agent, Vaginal

Additional Appendix Information
Antifungal Agents *on page 1876*

Use Treatment of susceptible cutaneous and mucocutaneous fungal infections normally caused by the *Candida* species

Pregnancy Risk Factor A (vaginal)/C (topical)

Dosage
Mucocutaneous infections: Children and Adults: Topical: Apply 2-3 times/day to affected areas; very moist topical lesions are treated best with powder
Vaginal infections: Adults: Vaginal tablets: Insert 1 tablet/day at bedtime for 2 weeks

Additional Information Complete prescribing information for this medication should be consulted for additional detail.

Dosage Forms Excipient information presented when available (limited, particularly for generics); consult specific product labeling.
Cream, topical: 100,000 units/g (15 g, 30 g)
Cream, topical [kit]:
Pediaderm™ AF: 100,000 units/g (30 g) [packaged with protective emollient]

Ointment, topical: 100,000 units/g (15 g, 30 g)
Powder, topical: 100,000 units/g (15 g, 30 g, 60 g)
Nyamyc®: 100,000 units/g (15 g, 30 g, 60 g) [contains talc]
Nystop®: 100,000 units/g (15 g, 30 g, 60 g) [contains talc]
Pedi-Dri®: 100,000 units/g (56.7 g) [contains talc]
Tablet, vaginal: 100,000 units

Nystatin and Triamcinolone

(nye STAT in & trye am SIN oh lone)

Index Terms Triamcinolone and Nystatin

Pharmacologic Category Antifungal Agent, Topical; Corticosteroid, Topical

Use Treatment of cutaneous candidiasis

Pregnancy Risk Factor C

Dosage Children and Adults: Topical: Apply sparingly 2-4 times/day. Therapy should be discontinued when control is achieved; if no improvement is seen, reassessment of diagnosis may be necessary.

Additional Information Complete prescribing information for this medication should be consulted for additional detail.

Dosage Forms Excipient information presented when available (limited, particularly for generics); consult specific product labeling.

Cream: Nystatin 100,000 units and triamcinolone acetonide 0.1% (15 g, 30 g, 60 g)
Ointment: Nystatin 100,000 units and triamcinolone acetonide 0.1% (15 g, 30 g, 60 g)

- **Nystop®** *see* Nystatin (Topical) *on page 1225*
- **Nytol® (Can)** *see* DiphenhydrAMINE (Systemic) *on page 516*
- **Nytol® Extra Strength (Can)** *see* DiphenhydrAMINE (Systemic) *on page 516*
- **Nytol® Quick Caps [OTC]** *see* DiphenhydrAMINE (Systemic) *on page 516*
- **Nytol® Quick Gels [OTC]** *see* DiphenhydrAMINE (Systemic) *on page 516*
- **NāSal™ [OTC]** *see* Sodium Chloride *on page 1567*
- **OCBZ** *see* OXcarbazepine *on page 1262*
- **Ocean® [OTC]** *see* Sodium Chloride *on page 1567*
- **Ocean® for Kids [OTC]** *see* Sodium Chloride *on page 1567*
- **Ocella™** *see* Ethinyl Estradiol and Drospirenone *on page 654*
- **Octagam®** *see* Immune Globulin *on page 880*
- **Octostim® (Can)** *see* Desmopressin *on page 476*

Octreotide (ok TREE oh tide)

Brand Names: U.S. SandoSTATIN LAR®; SandoSTATIN®

Brand Names: Canada Octreotide Acetate Injection; Octreotide Acetate Omega; Sandostatin LAR®; Sandostatin®

Index Terms Longastatin; Octreotide Acetate

Pharmacologic Category Antidiarrheal; Antidote; Somatostatin Analog

Use Control of symptoms (diarrhea and flushing) in patients with metastatic carcinoid tumors; treatment of watery diarrhea associated with vasoactive intestinal peptide-secreting tumors (VIPomas); treatment of acromegaly

Unlabeled Use Treatment of AIDS-associated diarrhea (including *Cryptosporidiosis*), chemotherapy-induced diarrhea, graft-versus-host disease (GVHD) associated diarrhea, postgastrectomy dumping syndrome; control of bleeding of esophageal varices; second-line treatment for thymic malignancies; Cushing's syndrome (ectopic); insulinomas; small bowel fistulas; islet cell tumors; Zollinger-Ellison syndrome; congenital hyperinsulinism; hypothalamic obesity; treatment of hypoglycemia secondary to sulfonylurea poisoning; treatment of malignant bowel obstruction

Pregnancy Risk Factor B

Pregnancy Considerations Teratogenic effects were not observed in animal studies. Octreotide crosses the human placenta; data concerning use in pregnancy is limited. Women of childbearing potential should use adequate contraception during treatment with octreotide; normalization of IGF-1 and GH may restore fertility in women with acromegaly. In case reports of acromegalic women who received normal doses of octreotide during pregnancy, no congenital malformations were reported.

Lactation Excretion in breast milk unknown/use caution

Contraindications Hypersensitivity to octreotide or any component of the formulation

Warnings/Precautions May impair gallbladder function; monitor patients for cholelithiasis. The incidence of gallbladder stone or biliary sludge increases with a duration of therapy of ≥12 months. In patients with neuroendocrine tumors, the NCCN guidelines (v.1.2011) recommend considering prophylactic cholecystectomy in patients undergoing abdominal surgery if octreotide treatment is planned. Use with caution in patients with renal and/or hepatic impairment; dosage adjustment is required in patients receiving dialysis and in patients with established cirrhosis. Somatostatin analogs may affect glucose regulation. In type I diabetes, severe hypoglycemia may occur; in type II diabetes or patients without diabetes, hyperglycemia may occur. Insulin and other hypoglycemic medication requirements may change. Octreotide may worsen hypoglycemia in patients with insulinomas; use with caution. Do not use depot formulation for the treatment of sulfonylurea-induced hypoglycemia. Bradycardia, conduction abnormalities, and arrhythmia have been observed in acromegalic and carcinoid syndrome patients; use caution with CHF or concomitant medications that alter heart rate or rhythm. Cardiovascular medication requirements may change. Octreotide may enhance the adverse/toxic effects of other QT_c-prolonging agents. May alter absorption of dietary fats; monitor for pancreatitis. May reduce excessive fluid loss in patients with conditions that cause such loss; monitor for elevations in zinc levels in such patients that are maintained on total parenteral nutrition (TPN). Chronic treatment has been associated with abnormal Schillings test; monitor vitamin B_{12} levels. Suppresses secretion of TSH; monitor for hypothyroidism.

Postmarketing cases of serious and fatal events, including hypoxia and necrotizing enterocolitis, have been reported with octreotide use in children (usually with serious underlying conditions), particularly in children <2 years of age. In studies with octreotide depot, the incidence of cholelithiasis in children is higher than the reported incidences for adults and efficacy was not demonstrated. Therapy may restore fertility; females of childbearing potential should use adequate contraception. Dosage adjustment may be necessary in the elderly; significant increases in elimination half-life have been observed in older adults. Vehicle used in depot injection (polylactide-co-glycolide microspheres) has rarely been associated with retinal artery occlusion in patients with abnormal arteriovenous anastomosis.

Adverse Reactions Adverse reactions vary by route of administration and dosage form. Frequency of cardiac, endocrine, and gastrointestinal adverse reactions was generally higher in acromegalics.

>16%:

Cardiovascular: Sinus bradycardia (19% to 25%), chest pain (≤20%; non-depot formulations)

Central nervous system: Fatigue (1% to 32%), headache (6% to 30%), malaise (16% to 20%), fever (16% to 20%), dizziness (5% to 20%)

Dermatologic: Pruritus (≤18%)

Endocrine & metabolic: Hyperglycemia (2% to 27%)

Gastrointestinal: Abdominal pain (5% to 61%), loose stools (5% to 61%), nausea (5% to 61%), diarrhea (34% to 58%), flatulence (≤38%), cholelithiasis (13% to 38%; length of therapy dependent), biliary sludge (24%; length of therapy dependent), constipation (9% to 21%), vomiting (4% to 21%), biliary duct dilatation (12%)

Local: Injection site pain (2% to 50%; dose and formulation related)

Neuromuscular & skeletal: Back pain (1% to 27%), arthropathy (8% to 19%), myalgia (≤18%)

Respiratory: Upper respiratory infection (10% to 23%), dyspnea (≤20%; non-depot formulations)

Miscellaneous: Antibodies to octreotide (up to 25%; no efficacy change), flu symptoms (1% to 20%)

5% to 15%:

Cardiovascular: Hypertension (≤13%), conduction abnormalities (9% to 10%), arrhythmia (3% to 9%), palpitation, peripheral edema

Central nervous system: Pain (4% to 15%), anxiety, confusion, hypoesthesia, insomnia

Dermatologic: Rash (15%; depot formulation), alopecia (≤13%)

Endocrine & metabolic: Hypothyroidism (≤12%; non-depot formulations), goiter (≤8%; non-depot formulations)

Gastrointestinal: Anorexia, cramping, tenesmus (4% to 6%), dyspepsia (4% to 6%), steatorrhea (4% to 6%), feces discoloration (4% to 6%)

Hematologic: Anemia (≤15%; non-depot formulations: <1%)

Neuromuscular & skeletal: Arthralgia, myalgia, paresthesia, rigors, weakness

Otic: Earache

Renal: Renal calculus

Respiratory: Cough, pharyngitis, sinusitis, rhinitis

Miscellaneous: Allergy, diaphoresis

1% to 4%:

Cardiovascular: Angina, cardiac failure, edema, flushing, hematoma, phlebitis

Central nervous system: Abnormal gait, amnesia, depression, dysphonia, hallucinations, nervousness, neuralgia, somnolence, vertigo

Dermatologic: Acne, bruising, cellulitis

Endocrine & metabolic: Hypoglycemia (2% to 4%), hypokalemia, hypoproteinemia, gout, cachexia, breast pain, impotence

Gastrointestinal: Colitis, diverticulitis, dysphagia, fat malabsorption, gastritis, gastroenteritis, gingivitis, glossitis, melena, stomatitis, taste perversion, xerostomia

Genitourinary: Incontinence, pollakuria (non-depot formulations), urinary tract infection

Local: Injection site hematoma

Neuromuscular & skeletal: Hyperkinesia, hypertonia, joint pain, neuropathy, tremor

Ocular: Blurred vision, visual disturbance

Otic: Tinnitus

Renal: Albuminuria, renal abscess

Respiratory: Bronchitis, epistaxis

Miscellaneous: Bacterial infection, cold symptoms, moniliasis

<1% (Limited to important or life-threatening): Anaphylactic shock, anaphylactoid reaction, aneurysm, aphasia, appendicitis, arthritis, ascending cholangitis, ascites, atrial fibrillation, basal cell carcinoma, Bell's palsy, biliary obstruction, breast carcinoma, cardiac arrest, cerebral vascular disorder, CHF, cholecystitis, cholestatic hepatitis, CK increased, creatinine increased, deafness, diabetes insipidus, diabetes mellitus, facial edema, fatty liver, galactorrhea, gallbladder polyp, GI bleeding, GI hemorrhage, GI ulcer, glaucoma, gynecomastia, hearing loss, hematuria, hemiparesis, hemorrhoids, hepatitis, hyperesthesia, hypertensive reaction, hypoadrenalism, hypoxia (children), intestinal obstruction, intracranial hemorrhage, intraocular pressure increased, ischemia, jaundice, joint effusion, lactation, LFTs increased, libido decreased, malignant hyperpyrexia, menstrual irregularities, MI, migraine, necrotizing enterocolitis (children), nephrolithiasis, neuritis, orthostatic hypotension, pancreatitis, pancytopenia, paresis, petechiae, pituitary apoplexy, pleural effusion, pneumonia, pneumothorax, pulmonary embolism, pulmonary hypertension, pulmonary nodule, Raynaud's syndrome, rectal bleeding, renal failure, renal insufficiency, retinal vein thrombosis, scotoma, seizure, status asthmaticus, suicide attempt, syncope, tachycardia, thrombocytopenia, thrombophlebitis, thrombosis, urticaria, visual field defect, weight loss, wheal/erythema

Drug Interactions

Metabolism/Transport Effects None known.

Avoid Concomitant Use

Avoid concomitant use of Octreotide with any of the following: Artemether; Dronedarone; Lumefantrine; Nilotinib; Pimozide; QUEtiapine; QuiNINE; Tetrabenazine; Thioridazine; Toremifene; Vandetanib; Vemurafenib; Ziprasidone

Increased Effect/Toxicity

Octreotide may increase the levels/effects of: Codeine; Dronedarone; Hypoglycemic Agents; Pegvisomant; Pimozide; QTc-Prolonging Agents; QuiNINE; Tetrabenazine; Thioridazine; Toremifene; Vandetanib; Vemurafenib; Ziprasidone

The levels/effects of Octreotide may be increased by: Alfuzosin; Artemether; Chloroquine; Ciprofloxacin; Ciprofloxacin (Systemic); Gadobutrol; Herbs (Hypoglycemic Properties); Indacaterol; Lumefantrine; Nilotinib; QUEtiapine; QuiNINE

Decreased Effect

Octreotide may decrease the levels/effects of: CycloSPORINE; CycloSPORINE (Systemic)

Ethanol/Nutrition/Herb Interactions

Herb/Nutraceutical: Avoid hypoglycemic herbs, including alfalfa, aloe, bilberry, bitter melon, burdock, celery, damiana, fenugreek, garcinia, garlic, ginger, ginseng (American), gymnema, marshmallow, and stinging nettle (may enhance the hypoglycemic effect of octreotide).

Stability

Solution: Octreotide is a clear solution and should be stored at refrigerated temperatures between 2°C and 8°C (36°F and 46°F). Protect from light. May be stored at room temperature of 20°C to 30°C (68°F and 86°F) for up to 14 days when protected from light. Stable as a parenteral admixture in NS for 96 hours at room temperature (25°C) and in D_5W for 24 hours. Stable for up to 7 days in a polypropylene syringe. Discard multidose vials within 14 days after initial entry.

Suspension: Prior to dilution, store at refrigerated temperatures between 2°C and 8°C (36°F and 46°F). Protect from light. Additionally, the manufacturer reports that octreotide suspension may be stored at room temperature of 20°C to 25°C (68°F and 77°F) for up to 10 days when protected from light (data on file [Novartis, 2011]). Depot drug product kit may be at room temperature for 30-60 minutes prior to use. Use suspension immediately after preparation.

Mechanism of Action Mimics natural somatostatin by inhibiting serotonin release, and the secretion of gastrin, VIP, insulin, glucagon, secretin, motilin, and pancreatic polypeptide. Decreases growth hormone and IGF-1 in acromegaly. Octreotide provides more potent inhibition of growth hormone, glucagon, and insulin as compared to endogenous somatostatin. Also suppresses LH response to GnRH, secretion of thyroid-stimulating hormone and decreases splanchnic blood flow.

Pharmacodynamics/Kinetics

Duration: SubQ: 6-12 hours

Absorption: SubQ: Rapid and complete; I.M. (depot formulation): Released slowly (via microsphere degradation in the muscle)

Distribution: V_d: 14 L (13-30 L in acromegaly)

Protein binding: 65%, primarily to lipoprotein (41% in acromegaly)

Metabolism: Extensively hepatic

Bioavailability: SubQ: 100%; I.M: 60% to 63% of SubQ dose

Half-life elimination: 1.7-1.9 hours; Increased in elderly patients; Cirrhosis: Up to 3.7 hours; Fatty liver disease: Up to 3.4 hours; Renal impairment: Up to 3.1 hours

Time to peak, plasma: SubQ: 0.4 hours (0.7 hours acromegaly); I.M.: 1 hour

Excretion: Urine (32% as unchanged drug)

Dosage

Acromegaly: Adults:

SubQ, I.V.: Initial: 50 mcg 3 times/day; titrate to achieve growth hormone levels <5 ng/mL or IGF-I (somatomedin C) levels <1.9 units/mL in males and <2.2 units/mL in females. Usual effective dose 100-200 mcg 3 times/day; range: 300-1500 mcg/day. **Note:** Should be withdrawn yearly for a 4-week interval (8 weeks for depot injection) in patients who have received irradiation. Resume if levels increase and signs/symptoms recur.

I.M. depot injection: Patients must be stabilized on subcutaneous octreotide for at least 2 weeks before switching to the long-acting depot. Upon switch: 20 mg I.M. intragluteally every 4 weeks for 3 months, then the dose may be modified based upon response.

Dosage adjustment for acromegaly: After 3 months of depot injections, the dosage may be continued or modified as follows:

GH ≤1 ng/mL, IGF-1 normal, and symptoms controlled: Reduce octreotide depot to 10 mg I.M. every 4 weeks

GH ≤2.5 ng/mL, IGF-1 normal, and symptoms controlled: Maintain octreotide depot at 20 mg I.M. every 4 weeks

GH >2.5 ng/mL, IGF-1 elevated, and/or symptoms uncontrolled: Increase octreotide depot to 30 mg I.M. every 4 weeks

Note: Patients not adequately controlled at a dose of 30 mg may increase dose to 40 mg every 4 weeks. Dosages >40 mg are not recommended.

Carcinoid tumors: Adults:

Manufacturer labeling:

SubQ, I.V.: Initial 2 weeks: 100-600 mcg/day in 2-4 divided doses; usual range: 50-750 mcg/day (some patients may require up to 1500 mcg/day)

I.M. depot injection: Patients must be stabilized on subcutaneous octreotide for at least 2 weeks before switching to the long-acting depot. Upon switch: 20 mg I.M. intragluteally every 4 weeks for 2 months, then the dose may be modified based upon response.

NCCN guidelines (Neuroendocrine Tumor, v.1.2011):

SubQ: 150-250 mcg 3 times/day; dose and frequency may be increased if needed for symptom control

I.M. depot injection: 20-30 mg every 4 weeks; dose and frequency may be increased if needed for symptom control; SubQ octreotide may be used for breakthrough symptoms

Note: Patients should continue to receive their SubQ injections for the first 2 weeks at the same dose in order to maintain therapeutic levels (some patients may require 3-4 weeks of continued SubQ injections). Patients who experience periodic exacerbations of symptoms may require temporary SubQ injections in addition to depot injections (at their previous SubQ dosing regimen) until symptoms have resolved.

Dosage adjustment for carcinoid tumors: After 2 months of depot injections, the dosage may be continued or modified as follows:

Increase to 30 mg I.M. every 4 weeks if symptoms are inadequately controlled

Decrease to 10 mg I.M. every 4 weeks, for a trial period, if initially responsive to 20 mg dose

Dosage >30 mg is not recommended

VIPomas:

Manufacturer labeling:

SubQ, I.V.: Initial 2 weeks: 200-300 mcg/day in 2-4 divided doses; titrate dose based on response/tolerance. Range: 150-750 mcg/day (doses >450 mcg/day are rarely required)

I.M. depot injection: Patients must be stabilized on subcutaneous octreotide for at least 2 weeks before switching to the long-acting depot. Upon switch: 20 mg I.M. intragluteally every 4 weeks for 2 months, then the dose may be modified based upon response.

NCCN guidelines (Neuroendocrine Tumor, v.1.2011):

SubQ: 150-250 mcg 3 times/day; dose and frequency may be increased if needed for symptom control

I.M. depot injection: 20-30 mg every 4 weeks dose and frequency may be increased if needed for symptom control; SubQ octreotide may be used for breakthrough symptoms

Note: Patients receiving depot injection should continue to receive their SubQ injections for the first 2 weeks at the same dose in order to maintain therapeutic levels (some patients may require 3-4 weeks of continued SubQ injections). Patients who experience periodic exacerbations of symptoms may require temporary SubQ injections in addition to depot injections (at their previous SubQ dosing regimen) until symptoms have resolved.

Dosage adjustment for VIPomas: After 2 months of depot injections, the dosage may be continued or modified as follows:

Increase to 30 mg I.M. every 4 weeks if symptoms are inadequately controlled

Decrease to 10 mg I.M. every 4 weeks, for a trial period, if initially responsive to 20 mg dose

Dosage >30 mg is not recommended

Congenital hyperinsulinism (unlabeled use): Infants and Children: SubQ: Initial: 2-10 mcg/kg/day; up to 40 mcg/kg/day have been used (Stanley, 1997)

Diarrhea (unlabeled use):

Infants and Children: I.V., SubQ: Doses of 1-10 mcg/kg every 12 hours have been used in children beginning at the low end of the range and increasing by 0.3 mcg/kg/dose at 3-day intervals. Suppression of growth hormone (animal data) is of concern when used as long-term therapy.

Adults: I.V.: Initial: 50-100 mcg every 8 hours; increase by 100 mcg/dose at 48-hour intervals; maximum dose: 500 mcg every 8 hours

Diarrhea associated with chemotherapy (unlabeled use):

Low grade or uncomplicated: SubQ: 100-150 mcg every 8 hours (Benson, 2004; Kornblau, 2000)

Severe: Initial: SubQ: 100-150 mcg every 8 hours; may increase to 500-1500 mcg I.V. or SubQ every 8 hours (Kornblau, 2000)

Complicated: I.V., SubQ: Initial: 100-150 mcg 3 times/day or I.V. Infusion: 25-50 mcg/hour; may escalate to 500 mcg 3 times/day until controlled (Benson, 2004)

Diarrhea associated with GVHD (unlabeled use): I.V.: 500 mcg every 8 hours; discontinue within 24 hours of resolution; Maximum duration of therapy if diarrhea is not resolved: 7 days (Kornblau, 2000)

Esophageal varices bleeding (unlabeled use): Adults: I.V. bolus: 25-100 mcg (usual bolus dose: 50 mcg) followed by continuous I.V. infusion of 25-50 mcg/hour for 2-5 days; may repeat bolus in first hour if hemorrhage not controlled (Corley, 2001; Erstad, 2001; Garcia-Tsao, 2010)

Hypoglycemia in sulfonylurea poisoning (unlabeled use): Note: SubQ is the preferred route of administration; repeat dosing, dose escalation, or initiation of a continuous infusion may be required in patients who experience recurrent hypoglycemia. Duration of treatment may exceed 24 hours. Optimal care decisions should be made based upon patient-specific details:

Children: SubQ: 1-1.5 mcg/kg; repeat in 6-12 hours as needed based upon blood glucose concentrations (Calello, 2005; Glatstein, 2009)

Adults:

SubQ: 50-100 mcg; repeat in 6-12 hours as needed based upon blood glucose concentrations (Braatvedt, 1997; Carr, 2002; Graudins, 1997; Hung, 1997)

I.V.: Doses up to 100-125 mcg/hour have been used successfully (McLaughlin, 2000)

Islet cell tumors (unlabeled use): SubQ: 150-250 mcg 3 times/day or I.M. (depot): 20-30 mg every 4 weeks dose and frequency may be increased if needed for symptom control; SubQ octreotide may be used for breakthrough symptoms (NCCN Neuroendocrine Tumor guidelines v.1.2011)

Malignant bowel obstruction (unlabeled use):

SubQ: 100-300 mcg 2-3 times/day (Mercadante, 2007; NCCN Palliative Care guidelines v.2.2011)

Continuous SubQ/I.V. infusion: 10-40 mcg/hour (NCCN Palliative Care guidelines v.2.2011)

Elderly: Elimination half-life is increased by 46% and clearance is decreased by 26%; dose adjustment may be required. Dosing should generally begin at the lower end of dosing range.

Dosage adjustment in renal impairment:

Nondialysis-dependent renal impairment: No dosage adjustment required

Dialysis-dependent renal impairment: Depot injection: Initial dose: 10 mg I.M. every 4 weeks; titrate based upon response (clearance is reduced by ~50%)

Dosage adjustment in hepatic impairment: Patients with established cirrhosis of the liver: Depot injection: Initial dose: 10 mg I.M. every 4 weeks; titrate based upon response

Dietary Considerations Schedule injections between meals to decrease GI effects. May alter absorption of dietary fats.

Administration

Regular injection formulation (do not use if solution contains particles or is discolored): Administer SubQ or I.V.; I.V. administration may be I.V. push (undiluted over 3 minutes), intermittent I.V. infusion (over 15-30 minutes), or continuous I.V. infusion (unlabeled route).

SubQ: Use the concentration with smallest volume to deliver dose to reduce injection site pain. Rotate injection site; may bring to room temperature prior to injection.

Depot formulation: Administer I.M. intragluteal (avoid deltoid administration); alternate gluteal injection sites to avoid irritation. **Do not** administer Sandostatin LAR® intravenously or subcutaneously; must be administered immediately after mixing.

Monitoring Parameters

Acromegaly: Growth hormone, somatomedin C (IGF-1)

Carcinoid: 5-HIAA, plasma serotonin and plasma substance P

VIPomas: Vasoactive intestinal peptide

Chronic therapy: Thyroid function (baseline and periodic), vitamin B_{12} level, blood glucose, glycemic control and antidiabetic regimen (patients with diabetes mellitus), cardiac function (heart rate, ECG), zinc level (patients with excessive fluid loss maintained on TPN)

Reference Range Vasoactive intestinal peptide: <75 ng/L; levels vary considerably between laboratories

Dosage Forms Excipient information presented when available (limited, particularly for generics); consult specific product labeling.

Injection, microspheres for suspension [depot formulation]:

SandoSTATIN LAR®: 10 mg, 20 mg, 30 mg [contains polylactide-co-glycolide; supplied with diluent]

Injection, solution: 100 mcg/mL (1 mL); 200 mcg/mL (5 mL); 1000 mcg/mL (5 mL)

SandoSTATIN®: 200 mcg/mL (5 mL); 1000 mcg/mL (5 mL)

Injection, solution [preservative free]: 50 mcg/mL (1 mL); 100 mcg/mL (1 mL); 200 mcg/mL (5 mL); 500 mcg/mL (1 mL)

SandoSTATIN®: 50 mcg/mL (1 mL); 100 mcg/mL (1 mL); 500 mcg/mL (1 mL)

◆ **Octreotide Acetate** *see* Octreotide *on page 1226*

◆ **Octreotide Acetate Injection (Can)** *see* Octreotide *on page 1226*

◆ **Octreotide Acetate Omega (Can)** *see* Octreotide *on page 1226*

◆ **Ocudox™** *see* Doxycycline *on page 557*

◆ **Ocufen®** *see* Flurbiprofen (Ophthalmic) *on page 737*

◆ **Ocuflox®** *see* Ofloxacin (Ophthalmic) *on page 1232*

◆ **O-desmethylvenlafaxine** *see* Desvenlafaxine *on page 479*

◆ **ODV** *see* Desvenlafaxine *on page 479*

◆ **Oesclim® (Can)** *see* Estradiol (Systemic) *on page 627*

Ofatumumab (oh fa TOOM yoo mab)

Brand Names: U.S. Arzerra™

Index Terms HuMax-CD20

Pharmacologic Category Antineoplastic Agent, Monoclonal Antibody; Monoclonal Antibody

Use Treatment of refractory chronic lymphocytic leukemia (CLL)

Pregnancy Risk Factor C

Pregnancy Considerations Teratogenicity was not observed in animal reproduction studies, although prolonged depletion of circulating B cells was observed in animal offspring. There are no adequate and well-controlled studies in pregnant women. Use in pregnancy only if the potential benefit to the mother outweighs the potential risk to the fetus.

Lactation Excretion in breast milk unknown/use caution

Contraindications There are no contraindications listed within the manufacturer's labeling.

Warnings/Precautions May cause serious infusion reaction; reactions may include bronchospasm, dyspnea, laryngeal edema, pulmonary edema, flushing, hypertension, hypotension, syncope, cardiac ischemia/infarction, back pain, abdominal pain, fever, rash, urticaria, and/or angioedema. Premedicate prior to infusion; interrupt infusion for reaction (and institute appropriate treatment) for reaction; may require subsequent rate modification.

Severe and prolonged (≥1 week) cytopenias (neutropenia and thrombocytopenia) may occur. Monitor blood counts during treatment; more frequently if grade 3 or 4 cytopenias develop. Progressive multifocal leukoencephalopathy (PML) may occur with treatment and should be considered in any patient with new onset or worsening neurological symptoms; if PML is suspected, discontinue and evaluate promptly. Small intestine obstruction may occur with treatment; evaluate if suspected.

Reactivation of hepatitis B (including fulminant hepatitis and death) has occurred with ofatumumab; patients at high-risk for hepatitis B should be screened prior to treatment initiation. Hepatitis B carriers should be closely monitored for signs of active hepatitis B infection during and for 6-12 months after completion of treatment. Use in patients with active viral hepatitis has not been sufficiently studied; discontinue (and institute appropriate treatment) in patients who develop viral hepatitis or reactivation of viral hepatitis.

Live vaccines should not be given concurrently with ofatumumab; there is no data concerning secondary transmission; the ability to generate an immune response to any vaccine following treatment is unknown.

Adverse Reactions

>10%:

Central nervous system: Fever (20%), fatigue (15%)

Dermatologic: Rash (14%)

Gastrointestinal: Diarrhea (18%), nausea (11%)

Hematologic: Neutropenia (≥grade 3: 42%; grade 4: 18%; may be prolonged >2 weeks), anemia (16%; grades 3/4: 5%)

Respiratory: Pneumonia (23%), cough (19%), dyspnea (14%), bronchitis (11%), upper respiratory tract infection (11%)

Miscellaneous: Infection (70%; includes bacterial, fungal or viral; ≥grade 3: 29%), infusion reaction (first infusion [300 mg]: 44%; second infusion [2000 mg]: 29%)

1% to 10%:

Cardiovascular: Peripheral edema (9%), hypertension (5%), hypotension (5%), tachycardia (5%)

Central nervous system: Chills (8%), insomnia (7%), headache (6%)

Dermatologic: Urticaria (8%), hyperhidrosis (5%)

Neuromuscular & skeletal: Back pain (8%), muscle spasm (5%)

Respiratory: Nasopharyngitis (8%), sinusitis (5%)

Miscellaneous: Sepsis (8%), herpes zoster (6%)

<1% (Limited to important or life-threatening): Abdominal pain, angina, bacteremia, cytolytic hepatitis, hemolytic anemia, hypoxia, interstitial lung disease (infectious), laryngeal edema, neutropenic sepsis, peritonitis, pharyngolaryngeal pain, pruritus, rigors, septic shock, throat tightness, thrombocytopenia

Drug Interactions

Metabolism/Transport Effects None known.

Avoid Concomitant Use

Avoid concomitant use of Ofatumumab with any of the following: BCG; Belimumab; Natalizumab; Pimecrolimus; Tacrolimus (Topical); Vaccines (Live)

Increased Effect/Toxicity

Ofatumumab may increase the levels/effects of: Belimumab; Leflunomide; Natalizumab; Vaccines (Live); Vitamin K Antagonists

The levels/effects of Ofatumumab may be increased by: Abciximab; Denosumab; Pimecrolimus; Roflumilast; Tacrolimus (Topical); Trastuzumab

Decreased Effect

Ofatumumab may decrease the levels/effects of: BCG; Cardiac Glycosides; Coccidioidin Skin Test; Sipuleucel-T; Vaccines (Inactivated); Vaccines (Live); Vitamin K Antagonists

The levels/effects of Ofatumumab may be decreased by: Echinacea

Stability Store intact vials at 2°C to 8°C (36°F to 46°F); do not freeze. Protect from light. To prepare 300 mg dose, withdraw 15 mL from a 1000 mL NS bag and add contents of three ofatumumab 100 mg vials (total volume = 15 mL) to NS bag (final concentration of 0.3 mg/mL). To prepare 2000 mg dose, withdraw 100 mL from a 1000 mL NS bag and add contents of two ofatumumab 1000 mg vials (total volume = 100 mL) to NS bag (final concentration of 2 mg/mL). Gently invert to mix; do not shake. Diluted solutions for infusion must be administered within 12 hours of preparation (may store at 2°C to 8°C [36°F to 46°F] if not used immediately); discard any remaining solution 24 hours after preparation.

Mechanism of Action Ofatumumab is a monoclonal antibody which binds specifically the extracellular (large and small) loops of the CD20 molecule (which is expressed on normal B lymphocytes and in B-cell CLL) resulting in potent complement-dependent cell lysis and antibody-dependent cell-mediated toxicity in cells that overexpress CD20.

Pharmacodynamics/Kinetics

Distribution: V_{dss}: 1.7-5.1 L

Half-life elimination: Between dose 4 and dose 12: ~14 days (range: 2-62 days)

Dosage Note: Premedicate with acetaminophen, an antihistamine, and a corticosteroid 30-120 minutes prior to treatment (see Administration).

I.V.: Adults: CLL: Initial dose: 300 mg week 1, followed 1 week later by 2000 mg once weekly for 7 doses (doses 2-8), followed 4 weeks later by 2000 mg once every 4 weeks for 4 doses (doses 9-12; for a total of 12 doses)

Dosage adjustment for toxicity: Infusion reaction: Interrupt infusion for infusion reaction (any severity).

Grade 1 or 2 infusion reaction: Resume at one-half of the previous rate; may increase (see Administration) based on patient tolerance

Grade 3: Resume infusion at 12 mL/hour; may increase (see Administration) based on patient tolerance

Grade 4: Do not resume

Dosage adjustment in renal impairment: When studied in patients with creatinine clearances ranging from 33-287 mL/minute, baseline creatinine clearance did not have a clinically relevant effect.

Administration Do not administer I.V. push or as a bolus. Premedicate with acetaminophen, an antihistamine, and a corticosteroid 30-120 minutes prior to administration. Administer with an in-line filter (supplied) and polyvinyl chloride (PVC) administration sets. Do not mix with or infuse with other medications. Flush line before and after infusion with NS. Begin infusion within 12 hours of preparation. The final concentration of dose 1 is 0.3 mg/mL and final concentration of doses 2-12 is 2 mg/mL.

Premedication: Premedicate with oral acetaminophen (1000 mg), an oral or I.V. antihistamine (eg, cetirizine 10 mg orally or equivalent), and an I.V. corticosteroid. Full dose corticosteroid is recommended for doses 1, 2, and 9; in the absence of infusion reaction ≥grade 3, may gradually reduce corticosteroid dose for doses 3-8; administer full or half corticosteroid dose with doses 10-12 if ≥grade 3 did not occur with dose 9.

Doses 1 and 2: Initiate infusion at 12 mL/hour for 30 minutes, if tolerated (no infusion reaction) increase to 25 mL/hour for 30 minutes, if tolerated, increase to 50 mL/hour for 30 minutes, if tolerated, increase to 100 mL/hour for 30 minutes, if tolerated, increase to 200 mL/hour for duration of infusion.

Doses 3-12: Initiate infusion at 25 mL/hour for 30 minutes, if tolerated (no infusion reaction) increase to 50 mL/hour for 30 minutes, if tolerated, increase to 100 mL/hour for 30 minutes, if tolerated, increase to 200 mL/hour for 30 minutes, if tolerated, increase to 400 mL/hour for remainder of infusion.

Monitoring Parameters CBC with differential, hepatitis B screening (in patients at high-risk; prior to therapy initiation); signs of active hepatitis B infection (in hepatitis B carriers; during and for 6-12 months after therapy completion); signs or symptoms of infusion reaction; signs of infection

Dosage Forms Excipient information presented when available (limited, particularly for generics); consult specific product labeling.

Injection, solution [concentrate, preservative free]:
Arzerra™: 20 mg/mL (5 mL, 50 mL) [contains edetate disodium, polysorbate 80]

◆ **Ofirmev™** *see* Acetaminophen *on page 27*

Ofloxacin (Systemic) (oh FLOKS a sin)

Brand Names: Canada Apo-Oflox®; Novo-Ofloxacin

Pharmacologic Category Antibiotic, Quinolone

Additional Appendix Information

Prevention of Wound Infection and Sepsis in Surgical Patients *on page 1954*

Use Quinolone antibiotic for the treatment of acute exacerbations of chronic bronchitis, community-acquired pneumonia, skin and skin structure infections (uncomplicated), urethral and cervical gonorrhea (acute, uncomplicated), urethritis and cervicitis (nongonococcal), mixed infections of the urethra and cervix, pelvic inflammatory disease (acute), cystitis (uncomplicated), urinary tract infections (complicated), prostatitis

Note: As of April 2007, the CDC no longer recommends the use of fluoroquinolones for the treatment of gonococcal disease.

Unlabeled Use Epididymitis (nongonococcal), leprosy, Traveler's diarrhea

Pregnancy Risk Factor C

Pregnancy Considerations Adverse events have been observed in some animal studies; therefore, the manufacturer classifies ofloxacin as pregnancy category C. Ofloxacin crosses the placenta and produces measurable concentrations in the amniotic fluid. An increased risk of teratogenic effects has not been observed in animals or humans following ofloxacin use during pregnancy; however, because of concerns of cartilage damage in immature animals, ofloxacin should only be used during pregnancy if a safer option is not available. Serum concentrations of ofloxacin may be lower during pregnancy than in nonpregnant patients.

Lactation Enters breast milk/not recommended (AAP rates "compatible"; AAP 2001 update pending)

Medication Guide Available Yes

Contraindications Hypersensitivity to ofloxacin or other members of the quinolone group, such as oxolinic acid, cinoxacin, norfloxacin, and ciprofloxacin; hypersensitivity to any component of the formulation

Warnings/Precautions [U.S. Boxed Warning]: There have been reports of tendon inflammation and/or rupture with quinolone antibiotics; risk may be increased with concurrent corticosteroids, organ transplant recipients, and in patients >60 years of age. Rupture of the Achilles tendon sometimes requiring surgical repair has been reported most frequently; but other tendon sites (eg, rotator cuff, biceps) have also been reported. Strenuous physical activity, rheumatoid arthritis, and renal impairment may be an independent risk factor for tendonitis. Discontinue at first sign of tendon inflammation or pain. May occur even after discontinuation of therapy. Use with caution in patients with rheumatoid arthritis; may increase risk of tendon rupture. Use with caution in patients with epilepsy or other CNS diseases which could predispose seizures; potential for seizures, although very rare, may be increased with concomitant NSAID therapy. Tremor, restlessness, confusion, and very rarely hallucinations or seizures may occur; use with caution in patients with known or suspected CNS disorder. Discontinue in patients who experience significant CNS adverse effects (eg, dizziness, hallucinations, suicidal ideations or actions). Use with caution in patients with renal or hepatic impairment. Peripheral neuropathies have been linked to ofloxacin use; discontinue if numbness, tingling, or weakness develops.

Fluoroquinolones have been associated with the development of serious, and sometimes fatal, hypoglycemia, most often in elderly diabetics, but also in patients without diabetes. This occurred most frequently with gatifloxacin (no longer available systemically) but may occur at a lower frequency with other quinolones.

Rare cases of torsade de pointes have been reported in patients receiving ofloxacin and other quinolones. Risk may be minimized by avoiding use in patients with known prolongation of the QT interval, bradycardia, hypokalemia, hypomagnesemia, cardiomyopathy, or in those receiving concurrent therapy with Class Ia or Class III antiarrhythmics.

Severe hypersensitivity reactions, including anaphylaxis, have occurred with quinolone therapy. Reactions may present as typical allergic symptoms after a single dose, or may manifest as severe idiosyncratic dermatologic, vascular, pulmonary, renal, hepatic, and/or hematologic events, usually after multiple doses. Prompt discontinuation of drug should occur if skin rash or other symptoms arise. Prolonged use may result in fungal or bacterial superinfection, including *C. difficile*-associated diarrhea (CDAD) and pseudomembranous colitis; CDAD has been observed >2 months postantibiotic treatment. **[U.S. Boxed Warning]: Quinolones may exacerbate myasthenia gravis; avoid use (rare, potentially life-threatening weakness of respiratory muscles may occur).** Avoid excessive sunlight and take precautions to limit exposure (eg, loose fitting clothing, sunscreen); may cause moderate-to-severe phototoxicity reactions. Discontinue use if photosensitivity occurs. Since ofloxacin is ineffective in the treatment of syphilis and may mask symptoms, all patients should be tested for syphilis at the time of gonorrheal diagnosis and 3 months later. Hemolytic reactions may (rarely) occur with quinolone use in patients with latent or actual G6PD deficiency. Safety and efficacy have not been established in children.

Adverse Reactions

1% to 10%:

Cardiovascular: Chest pain (1% to 3%)

Central nervous system: Headache (1% to 9%), insomnia (3% to 7%), dizziness (1% to 5%), fatigue (1% to 3%), somnolence (1% to 3%), sleep disorders (1% to 3%), nervousness (1% to 3%), pyrexia (1% to 3%)

Dermatologic: Rash/pruritus (1% to 3%)

Gastrointestinal: Diarrhea (1% to 4%), vomiting (1% to 4%), GI distress (1% to 3%), abdominal cramps (1% to 3%), flatulence (1% to 3%), abnormal taste (1% to 3%), xerostomia (1% to 3%), appetite decreased (1% to 3%), nausea (3% to 10%), constipation (1% to 3%)

Genitourinary: Vaginitis (1% to 5%), external genital pruritus in women (1% to 3%)

Ocular: Visual disturbances (1% to 3%)

Respiratory: Pharyngitis (1% to 3%)

Miscellaneous: Trunk pain

<1%, postmarketing, and/or case reports (limited to important or life-threatening): Anaphylaxis reactions, anxiety, blurred vision, chills, cognitive change, cough, depression, dream abnormality, ecchymosis, edema, erythema nodosum, euphoria, extremity pain, hallucinations, hearing acuity decreased, hepatic dysfunction, hepatic failure (some fatal), hepatitis, hyper-/hypoglycemia, hypertension, interstitial nephritis, lightheadedness, malaise, myasthenia gravis exacerbation, palpitation, paresthesia, peripheral neuropathy, photophobia, photosensitivity, pneumonitis, psychotic reactions, rhabdomyolysis, seizure, Stevens-Johnson syndrome, syncope, tendonitis and tendon rupture, thirst, tinnitus, torsade de pointes, Tourette's syndrome, toxic epidermal necrolysis, vasculitis, vasodilation, vertigo, weakness, weight loss

Drug Interactions

Metabolism/Transport Effects **Inhibits** CYP1A2 (strong)

Avoid Concomitant Use

Avoid concomitant use of Ofloxacin (Systemic) with any of the following: BCG

Increased Effect/Toxicity

Ofloxacin (Systemic) may increase the levels/effects of: Bendamustine; Corticosteroids (Systemic); CYP1A2 Substrates; Porfimer; Sulfonylureas; Theophylline Derivatives; Varenicline; Vitamin K Antagonists

The levels/effects of Ofloxacin (Systemic) may be increased by: Insulin; Nonsteroidal Anti-Inflammatory Agents; Probenecid

Decreased Effect

Ofloxacin (Systemic) may decrease the levels/effects of: BCG; Mycophenolate; Sulfonylureas; Typhoid Vaccine

The levels/effects of Ofloxacin (Systemic) may be decreased by: Antacids; Calcium Salts; Didanosine; Iron Salts; Lanthanum; Magnesium Salts; Quinapril; Sevelamer; Sucralfate; Zinc Salts

Ethanol/Nutrition/Herb Interactions

Food: Ofloxacin average peak serum concentrations may be decreased by 20% if taken with food.

Herb/Nutraceutical: Avoid dong quai, St John's wort (may also cause photosensitization).

Stability Store at 25°C (77°F); excursions permitted to 15°C to 30°C (59°F to 86°F).

Mechanism of Action Ofloxacin is a DNA gyrase inhibitor. DNA gyrase is an essential bacterial enzyme that maintains the superhelical structure of DNA. DNA gyrase is required for DNA replication and transcription, DNA repair, recombination, and transposition; bactericidal

Pharmacodynamics/Kinetics

Absorption: Well absorbed; food causes only minor alterations

Distribution: V_d: 2.4-3.5 L/kg

Protein binding: 32%

Bioavailability: 98%

Half-life elimination: Biphasic: 4-5 hours and 20-25 hours (accounts for <5%); prolonged with renal impairment

Excretion: Primarily urine (as unchanged drug)

Dosage

Usual dosage range: Adults: Oral: 200-400 mg every 12 hours

Indication-specific dosing: Adults: Oral:

Cervicitis/urethritis:

Nongonococcal: 300 mg every 12 hours for 7 days

Gonococcal (acute, uncomplicated): 400 mg as a single dose; **Note:** As of April 2007, the CDC no longer recommends the use of fluoroquinolones for the treatment of uncomplicated gonococcal disease.

Chronic bronchitis (acute exacerbation), community-acquired pneumonia, skin and skin structure infections (uncomplicated): 400 mg every 12 hours for 10 days

Epididymitis, nongonococcal (unlabeled use): 300 mg twice daily for 10 days

Leprosy (unlabeled use): 400 mg once daily

Pelvic inflammatory disease (acute): 400 mg every 12 hours for 10-14 days with or without metronidazole; **Note:** The CDC recommends use only if standard cephalosporin therapy is not feasible and community prevalence of quinolone-resistant gonococcal organisms is low. Culture sensitivity must be confirmed.

Prostatitis:

Acute: 400 mg for 1 dose, then 300 mg twice daily for 10 days

Chronic: 200 mg every 12 hours for 6 weeks

Traveler's diarrhea (unlabeled use): 300 mg twice daily for 3 days

UTI:

Uncomplicated: 200 mg every 12 hours for 3-7 days

Complicated: 200 mg every 12 hours for 10 days

Dosing adjustment/interval in renal impairment: Adults:

Oral: After a normal initial dose, adjust as follows:

Cl_{cr} 20-50 mL/minute: Administer usual dose every 24 hours

Cl_{cr} <20 mL/minute: Administer half the usual dose every 24 hours

Continuous arteriovenous or venovenous hemodiafiltration effects: Administer 300 mg every 24 hours

Dosing adjustment in hepatic impairment: Severe impairment: Maximum dose: 400 mg/day

Administration Do not take within 2 hours of food or any antacids which contain zinc, magnesium, or aluminum.

Test Interactions Some quinolones may produce a false-positive urine screening result for opiates using commercially-available immunoassay kits. This has been demonstrated most consistently for levofloxacin and ofloxacin, but other quinolones have shown cross-reactivity in certain assay kits. Confirmation of positive opiate screens by more specific methods should be considered.

Dosage Forms Excipient information presented when available (limited, particularly for generics); consult specific product labeling.

Tablet, oral: 200 mg, 300 mg, 400 mg

Ofloxacin (Ophthalmic) (oh FLOKS a sin)

Brand Names: U.S. Ocuflox®

Brand Names: Canada Ocuflox®

Pharmacologic Category Antibiotic, Ophthalmic; Antibiotic, Quinolone

Use Treatment of superficial ocular infections involving the conjunctiva or cornea due to strains of susceptible organisms

Pregnancy Risk Factor C

Dosage

Usual dosage range: Ophthalmic:

Children >1 year: 1-2 drops every 30 minutes to 4 hours initially, decreasing to every 4-6 hours

Adults: 1-2 drops every 30 minutes to 4 hours initially, decreasing to every 4-6 hours

Indication-specific dosing: Children >1 year and Adults: Ophthalmic:

Conjunctivitis: Instill 1-2 drops in affected eye(s) every 2-4 hours for the first 2 days, then use 4 times/day for an additional 5 days

Corneal ulcer: Instill 1-2 drops every 30 minutes while awake and every 4-6 hours after retiring for the first 2 days; beginning on day 3, instill 1-2 drops every hour while awake for 4-6 additional days; thereafter, 1-2 drops 4 times/day until clinical cure.

Additional Information Complete prescribing information for this medication should be consulted for additional detail.

Dosage Forms Excipient information presented when available (limited, particularly for generics); consult specific product labeling.

Solution, ophthalmic [drops]: 0.3% (5 mL, 10 mL)

Ocuflox®: 0.3% (5 mL) [contains benzalkonium chloride]

Ofloxacin (Otic) (oh FLOKS a sin)

Index Terms Floxin Otic Singles

Pharmacologic Category Antibiotic, Quinolone

Use Otitis externa, chronic suppurative otitis media, acute otitis media

Pregnancy Risk Factor C

Dosage

Usual dosage range: Otic:

Children ≥6 months: 5 drops daily

Children >12 years: 10 drops once or twice daily

Adults: 10 drops once or twice daily

Indication-specific dosing: Otic:

Children 6 months to 13 years: **Otitis externa:** Instill 5 drops (or the contents of 1 single-dose container) into affected ear(s) once daily for 7 days

Children 1-12 years: **Acute otitis media with tympanostomy tubes:** Instill 5 drops (or the contents of 1 single-dose container) into affected ear(s) twice daily for 10 days

Children >12 years and Adults: **Otitis media, chronic suppurative with perforated tympanic membranes:** Instill 10 drops (or the contents of 2 single-dose containers) into affected ear twice daily for 14 days

Children ≥13 years and Adults: **Otitis externa:** Instill 10 drops (or the contents of 2 single-dose containers) into affected ear(s) once daily for 7 days

Additional Information Complete prescribing information for this medication should be consulted for additional detail.

Dosage Forms Excipient information presented when available (limited, particularly for generics); consult specific product labeling.

Solution, otic [drops]: 0.3% (5 mL, 10 mL)

- **Oforta™ [DSC]** *see* Fludarabine *on page 721*
- **Ogen® (Can)** *see* Estropipate *on page 648*
- **Ogestrel®** *see* Ethinyl Estradiol and Norgestrel *on page 664*
- **OGMT** *see* Metyrosine *on page 1123*
- **OGT-918** *see* Miglustat *on page 1134*
- **17OHPC** *see* Hydroxyprogesterone Caproate *on page 850*
- **9-OH-risperidone** *see* Paliperidone *on page 1277*

OLANZapine (oh LAN za peen)

Brand Names: U.S. ZyPREXA®; ZyPREXA® IntraMuscular; ZyPREXA® Relprevv™; ZyPREXA® Zydis®

Brand Names: Canada Apo-Olanzapine®; CO Olanzapine; CO Olanzapine ODT; Olanzapine ODT; PHL-Olanzapine; PHL-Olanzapine ODT; PMS-Olanzapine; PMS-Olanzapine ODT; Riva-Olanzapine; Riva-Olanzapine ODT; Sandoz-Olanzapine; Sandoz-Olanzapine ODT; Teva-Olanzapine; Teva-Olanzapine OD; Zyprexa®; Zyprexa® Intramuscular; Zyprexa® Zydis®

Index Terms LY170053; Olanzapine Pamoate; Zyprexa Zydis

Pharmacologic Category Antimanic Agent; Antipsychotic Agent, Atypical

Additional Appendix Information

Antipsychotic Agents *on page 1880*

Use

Oral: Treatment of the manifestations of schizophrenia; treatment of acute or mixed mania episodes associated with bipolar I disorder (as monotherapy or in combination with lithium or valproate); maintenance treatment of bipolar disorder; in combination with fluoxetine for treatment-resistant or bipolar I depression

I.M., extended-release (Zyprexa® Relprevv™): Treatment of schizophrenia

I.M., short-acting (Zyprexa® IntraMuscular): Treatment of acute agitation associated with schizophrenia and bipolar I mania

Unlabeled Use Treatment of psychosis/schizophrenia in children; chronic pain; prevention of chemotherapy-associated delayed nausea or vomiting; psychosis/agitation related to Alzheimer's dementia; acute treatment of delirium

Pregnancy Risk Factor C

Pregnancy Considerations No evidence of teratogenicity reported in animal studies. However, fetal toxicity and prolonged gestation have been observed. Antipsychotic use during the third trimester of pregnancy has a risk for abnormal muscle movements (extrapyramidal symptoms [EPS]) and withdrawal symptoms in newborns following delivery. Symptoms in the newborn may include agitation, feeding disorder, hypertonia, hypotonia, respiratory distress, somnolence, and tremor; these effects may be self-limiting or require hospitalization. There are no adequate and well-controlled studies in pregnant women. Healthcare providers are encouraged to enroll women 18-45 years of age exposed to olanzapine during pregnancy in the Atypical Antipsychotics Pregnancy Registry (1-866-961-2388).

Lactation Enters breast milk/not recommended

Prescribing and Access Restrictions As a requirement of the REMS program, only prescribers, healthcare facilities, and pharmacies registered with the Zyprexa® Relprevv™ Patient Care Program are able to prescribe, distribute, or dispense Zyprexa® Relprevv™ for patients who are enrolled in and meet all conditions of the program. Zyprexa® Relprevv™ must be administered at a registered healthcare facility. Prescribers will need to be recertified every 3 years. Contact the Zyprexa® Relprevv™ Patient Care Program at 1-877-772-9390.

Medication Guide Available Yes

Contraindications There are no contraindications listed in the manufacturer's labeling.

Canadian labeling: Hypersensitivity to olanzapine or any component of the formulation

Warnings/Precautions **[U.S. Boxed Warning]: Elderly patients with dementia-related psychosis treated with antipsychotics are at an increased risk of death compared to placebo.** Most deaths appeared to be either cardiovascular (eg, heart failure, sudden death) or infectious (eg, pneumonia) in nature. In addition, an increased incidence of cerebrovascular effects (eg, transient ischemic attack, stroke) has been reported in studies of placebo-controlled trials of olanzapine in elderly patients with dementia-related psychosis. Olanzapine is not approved for the treatment of dementia-related psychosis.

Moderate to highly sedating, use with caution in disorders where CNS depression is a feature; patients must be cautioned about performing tasks which require mental alertness (eg, operating machinery or driving). Use caution in patients with cardiac disease. Use with caution in Parkinson's disease, predisposition to seizures, or severe hepatic or renal disease. Life-threatening arrhythmias have occurred with therapeutic doses of some neuroleptics. May induce orthostatic hypotension; use caution with history of cardiovascular disease, hemodynamic instability, prior myocardial infarction, or ischemic heart disease. Increases in cholesterol and triglycerides have been noted. Use with caution in patients with pre-existing abnormal lipid profile. Esophageal dysmotility and aspiration have been associated with antipsychotic use; use with caution in patients at risk of aspiration pneumonia. May increase prolactin levels; clinical significance of hyperprolactinemia in patients with breast cancer or other prolactin-dependent tumors is unknown. Significant weight gain (>7% of baseline weight) may occur; monitor waist circumference and BMI. Impaired core body temperature regulation may occur; caution with strenuous exercise, heat exposure, dehydration, and concomitant medication possessing anticholinergic effects.

Leukopenia, neutropenia, and agranulocytosis (sometimes fatal) have been reported in clinical trials and postmarketing reports with antipsychotic use; presence of risk factors (eg, pre-existing low WBC or history of drug-induced leuko-/neutropenia) should prompt periodic blood count assessment. Discontinue therapy at first signs of blood dyscrasias or if absolute neutrophil count <1000/mm^3.

May cause anticholinergic effects; use with caution in patients with decreased gastrointestinal motility, urinary retention, BPH, xerostomia, or narrow-angle glaucoma. Relative to other neuroleptics, olanzapine has a moderate potency of cholinergic blockade. May cause extrapyramidal symptoms (EPS), although risk of these reactions is lower relative to other neuroleptics. Risk of dystonia (and probably other EPS) may be greater with increased doses, use of conventional antipsychotics, males, and younger patients. May be associated with neuroleptic malignant syndrome (NMS). May cause extreme and life-threatening hyperglycemia; use with caution in patients with diabetes or other disorders of glucose regulation; monitor. Olanzapine levels may be lower in patients who smoke; the manufacturer does not require dosage adjustments, although dosage adjustments may be considered. Use in adolescent patients ≥13 years of age may result in increased weight gain and sedation, as well as greater increases in LDL cholesterol, total cholesterol, triglycerides, prolactin, and liver transaminase levels when compared to adults. Adolescent patients should be maintained on the lowest dose necessary.

The possibility of a suicide attempt is inherent in psychotic illness or bipolar disorder; use caution in high-risk patients during initiation of therapy. Prescriptions should be written for the smallest quantity consistent with good patient care.

There are two Zyprexa® formulations for intramuscular injection: Zyprexa® Relprevv™ is an extended-release formulation and Zyprexa® Intramuscular is short-acting:

Extended-release I.M. injection (Zyprexa® Relprevv™): Monitor for post injection delirium/sedation syndrome; patients should be continuously watched (≥3 hours) for symptoms of olanzapine overdose. Only available through a restricted drug distribution program.

Short-acting I.M. injection (Zyprexa® IntraMuscular): Patients should remain recumbent if drowsy/dizzy until hypotension, bradycardia, and/or hypoventilation have been ruled out. Concurrent use of I.M./I.V. benzodiazepines is not recommended (fatalities have been reported, though causality not determined).

Adverse Reactions

Oral: Unless otherwise noted, adverse events are reported for placebo-controlled trials in adult patients on monotherapy:

>10%:

Central nervous system: Somnolence (dose dependent; 20% to 39%; adolescents 39% to 48%), extrapyramidal symptoms (dose dependent; ≤32%), dizziness (11% to 18%), headache (adolescents 17%), fatigue (adolescents 3% to 14%), insomnia (12%)

Endocrine & metabolic: Prolactin increased (30%; adolescents 47%)

Gastrointestinal: Weight gain (5% to 6%, has been reported as high as 40%; adolescents 29% to 31%), appetite increased (3% to 6%; adolescents 17% to 29%), xerostomia (dose dependent; 3% to 22%), constipation (9% to 11%), dyspepsia (7% to 11%)

Hepatic: ALT increased ≥3 x ULN (adolescents 12%; adults 5%)

Neuromuscular & skeletal: Weakness (dose dependent; 8% to 20%)

Miscellaneous: Accidental injury (12%)

1% to 10%:

Cardiovascular: Chest pain, hypertension, peripheral edema, postural hypotension, tachycardia

Central nervous system: Fever, personality changes, restlessness (adolescents)

Dermatologic: Bruising

Endocrine & metabolic: Breast-related events ([adolescents] discharge, enlargement, galactorrhea, gynecomastia, lactation disorder); menstrual-related events (amenorrhea, hypomenorrhea, menstruation delayed, oligomenorrhea); sexual function-related events (anorgasmia, ejaculation delayed, erectile dysfunction, changes in libido, abnormal orgasm, sexual dysfunction)

Gastrointestinal: Abdominal pain (adolescents), diarrhea (adolescents), flatulence, nausea (dose dependent), vomiting

Genitourinary: Incontinence, UTI

Hepatic: Hepatic enzymes increased

Neuromuscular & skeletal: Abnormal gait, akathisia, articulation impairment, back pain, falling, hypertonia, joint/extremity pain, muscle stiffness (adolescents), tremor (dose dependent)

Ocular: Amblyopia

Respiratory: Cough, epistaxis (adolescents), pharyngitis, respiratory tract infection (adolescents), rhinitis, sinusitis (adolescents)

<1% (Limited to important or life-threatening): Acidosis, agranulocytosis, anaphylactoid reaction, angioedema, apnea, atelectasis, atrial fibrillation, cerebrovascular accident, congestive heart failure, deafness, diabetes mellitus, diabetic ketoacidosis, diabetic coma, dystonia, encephalopathy, facial paralysis, glaucoma, heart arrest, heart failure, hemorrhage (eye, rectal, subarachnoid, vaginal), hepatitis, hypercholesterolemia, hyper-/hypoglycemia, hyper-/hypokalemia, hyperlipemia, hyper-/hyponatremia, hypertriglyceridemia, hyperuricemia, hyper-/hypoventilation, hypoproteinemia, hypoxia, jaundice, ileus, ketosis, leukocytosis (eosinophilia), leukopenia, liver damage (cholestatic or mixed), liver fatty deposit, lung edema, lymphadenopathy, myasthenia, myopathy, neuralgia, neuroleptic malignant syndrome, neutropenia, pancreatitis, paralysis, pulmonary embolus, rash, rhabdomyolysis, seizure, sudden death, suicide attempt, syncope, tardive dyskinesia, thrombocythemia, thrombocytopenia, transient ischemic attack, venous thrombotic events

Injection: Unless otherwise noted, adverse events are reported for placebo-controlled trials in adult patients on extended-release I.M. injection (Zyprexa® Relprevv™). Also refer to adverse reactions noted with oral therapy.

>10%: Central nervous system: Headache (13% to 18%), sedation (8% to 13%)

1% to 10%:

Cardiovascular: Hypertension, hypotension (short-acting), postural hypotension (short-acting), QT prolongation

Central nervous system: Abnormal dreams, abnormal thinking, auditory hallucination, dizziness, dysarthria, extrapyramidal symptoms, fatigue, fever, pain, restlessness, somnolence

Dermatologic: Acne

Gastrointestinal: Abdominal pain, appetite increased, diarrhea, flatulence, nausea, vomiting, weight gain, xerostomia

Genitourinary: Vaginal discharge

Hepatic: Liver enzymes increased

Local: Injection site pain

Neuromuscular & skeletal: Arthralgia, back pain, muscle spasms, stiffness, tremor, weakness (short-acting)

Otic: Ear pain

Respiratory: Cough, nasal congestion, nasopharyngitis, pharyngolaryngeal pain, sneezing, upper respiratory tract infection

Miscellaneous: Toothache, tooth infection, viral infection

<1% (Limited to important or life-threatening): CPK increased, post-injection delirium/sedation syndrome, syncope (short-acting)

Drug Interactions

Metabolism/Transport Effects Substrate of CYP1A2 (major), CYP2D6 (minor); **Note:** Assignment of Major/Minor substrate status based on clinically relevant drug interaction potential; **Inhibits** CYP1A2 (weak), CYP2C19 (weak), CYP2C9 (weak), CYP2D6 (weak), CYP3A4 (weak)

Avoid Concomitant Use

Avoid concomitant use of OLANZapine with any of the following: Benzodiazepines; Metoclopramide; Pimozide

Increased Effect/Toxicity

OLANZapine may increase the levels/effects of: Alcohol (Ethyl); Anticholinergics; Benzodiazepines; CNS Depressants; Methotrimeprazine; Methylphenidate; Pimozide; Serotonin Modulators

The levels/effects of OLANZapine may be increased by: Abiraterone Acetate; Acetylcholinesterase Inhibitors (Central); CYP1A2 Inhibitors (Moderate); CYP1A2 Inhibitors (Strong); Deferasirox; Droperidol; FluvoxaMINE; HydrOXYzine; LamoTRIgine; Lithium formulations; Methotrimeprazine; Methylphenidate; Metoclopramide; Pramlintide; Tetrabenazine

Decreased Effect

OLANZapine may decrease the levels/effects of: Amphetamines; Anti-Parkinson's Agents (Dopamine Agonist); Quinagolide

The levels/effects of OLANZapine may be decreased by: CYP1A2 Inducers (Strong); Cyproterone; Lithium formulations; Peginterferon Alfa-2b

Ethanol/Nutrition/Herb Interactions

Ethanol: May increase CNS depression; monitor for increased effects with coadministration. Caution patients about effects.

Herb/Nutraceutical: Avoid dong quai, St John's wort (may also cause photosensitization). Avoid kava kava, gotu kola, valerian, St John's wort (may increase CNS depression).

Stability

Injection, extended-release: Store at 20° to 25°C (68°F to 77°F); excursions permitted to 15°C to 30°C (59°F to 86°F). Dilute as directed to final concentration of 150 mg/mL. Shake vigorously to mix; will form yellow, opaque suspension. Following reconstitution, suspension may be stored at room temperature and used within 24 hours. Shake vigorously to resuspend prior to administration. Use immediately once suspension is in syringe. Suspension may be irritating to skin; wear gloves during reconstitution.

Injection, short-acting: Store at 20° to 25°C (68°F to 77°F); excursions permitted to 15°C to 30°C (59°F to 86°F); do not freeze. Protect from light. Reconstitute 10 mg vial with 2.1 mL SWFI. Resulting solution is ~5 mg/mL. Use immediately (within 1 hour) following reconstitution. Discard any unused portion.

Tablet and orally-disintegrating tablet: Store at 20° to 25°C (68°F to 77°F); excursions permitted to 15°C to 30°C (59°F to 86°F). Protect from light and moisture.

Mechanism of Action Olanzapine is a second generation thienobenzodiazepine antipsychotic which displays potent antagonism of serotonin 5-HT_{2A} and 5-HT_{2C}, dopamine D_{1-4}, histamine H_1 and alpha$_1$-adrenergic receptors. Olanzapine shows moderate antagonism of 5-HT_3 and muscarinic M_{1-5} receptors, and weak binding to GABA-A, BZD, and beta-adrenergic receptors. Although the precise mechanism of action in schizophrenia and bipolar disorder is not known, the efficacy of olanzapine is thought to be mediated through combined antagonism of dopamine and serotonin type 2 receptor sites.

Pharmacodynamics/Kinetics

Absorption:

Oral: Well absorbed; not affected by food; tablets and orally-disintegrating tablets are bioequivalent

Short-acting injection: Rapidly absorbed

Distribution: V_d: Extensive, 1000 L

Protein binding, plasma: 93% bound to albumin and alpha$_1$-glycoprotein

Metabolism: Highly metabolized via direct glucuronidation and cytochrome P450 mediated oxidation (CYP1A2, CYP2D6); 40% removed via first pass metabolism

Half-life elimination: 21-54 hours; ~1.5 times greater in elderly; Extended-release injection: ~30 days

Time to peak, plasma: Maximum plasma concentrations after I.M. administration are 5 times higher than maximum plasma concentrations produced by an oral dose.

Extended-release injection: ~7 days

Short-acting injection: 15-45 minutes

Oral: ~6 hours

Excretion: Urine (57%, 7% as unchanged drug); feces (30%)

Clearance: 40% increase in olanzapine clearance in smokers; 30% decrease in females

Dosage

Adolescents ≥13 years: Schizophrenia/bipolar disorder: Oral: Initial: 2.5-5 mg once daily; adjust by 2.5-5 mg/day to target dose of 10 mg/day; dosing range: 2.5-20 mg/day

Adults:

Agitation (acute, associated with bipolar I mania or schizophrenia): Short-acting I.M. injection: Initial dose: 10 mg (a lower dose of 5-7.5 mg may be considered when clinical factors warrant); additional doses (up to 10 mg) may be considered, however, 2-4 hours should be allowed between doses to evaluate response (maximum total daily dose: 30 mg, per manufacturer's recommendation)

Bipolar I acute mixed or manic episodes: Oral:

Monotherapy: Initial: 10-15 mg once daily; increase by 5 mg/day at intervals of not less than 24 hours. Maintenance: 5-20 mg/day; recommended maximum dose: 20 mg/day.

Combination therapy (with lithium or valproate): Initial: 10 mg once daily; dosing range: 5-20 mg/day; recommended maximum dose: 20 mg/day.

Depression:

Depression associated with bipolar disorder (in combination with fluoxetine): Oral: Initial: 5 mg in the evening; adjust as tolerated to usual range of 5-12.5 mg/day. See **"Note"**

Treatment-resistant depression (in combination with fluoxetine): Oral: Initial: 5 mg in the evening; adjust as tolerated to range of 5-20 mg/day. See **"Note"**

Note: When using individual components of fluoxetine with olanzapine rather than fixed dose combination product (Symbyax®), approximate dosage correspondence is as follows:

Olanzapine 2.5 mg + fluoxetine 20 mg = Symbyax® 3/25

Olanzapine 5 mg + fluoxetine 20 mg = Symbyax® 6/25

Olanzapine 12.5 mg + fluoxetine 20 mg = Symbyax® 12/25

Olanzapine 5 mg + fluoxetine 50 mg = Symbyax® 6/50

Olanzapine 12.5 mg + fluoxetine 50 mg = Symbyax® 12/50

Schizophrenia:

Oral: Initial: 5-10 mg once daily (increase to 10 mg once daily within 5-7 days); thereafter, adjust by 5 mg/day at 1-week intervals, up to a recommended maximum of 20 mg/day. Maintenance: 10-20 mg once daily. Doses of 30-50 mg/day have been used; however, doses >10 mg/day have not demonstrated better efficacy, and safety and efficacy of doses >20 mg/day have not been evaluated.

Extended-release I.M. injection: **Note:** Establish tolerance to oral olanzapine prior to changing to extended-release I.M. injection. Maximum dose: 300 mg/2 weeks or 405 mg/4 weeks

Patients established on oral olanzapine 10 mg/day: Initial dose: 210 mg every 2 weeks for 4 doses or 405 mg every 4 weeks for 2 doses; Maintenance dose: 150 mg every 2 weeks or 300 mg every 4 weeks

Patients established on oral olanzapine 15 mg/day: Initial dose: 300 mg every 2 weeks for 4 doses; Maintenance dose: 210 mg every 2 weeks or 405 mg every 4 weeks

Patients established on oral olanzapine 20 mg/day: Initial and maintenance dose: 300 mg every 2 weeks

Delirium (unlabeled use): Oral: 5 mg daily for up to 5 days (NICE, 2010)

Prevention of chemotherapy-associated delayed nausea or vomiting (unlabeled use; in combination with a corticosteroid and serotonin [$5HT_3$] antagonist): Oral: 10 mg once daily for 3-5 days, beginning on day 1 of chemotherapy **or** 5 mg once daily for 2 days before chemotherapy, followed by 10 mg once daily (beginning on the day of chemotherapy) for 3-8 days

Elderly:

Short-acting I.M., Oral: Consider lower starting dose of 2.5-5 mg/day for elderly or debilitated patients; may increase as clinically indicated and tolerated with close monitoring of orthostatic blood pressure

Extended release I.M.: Consider lower starting dose of 150 mg every 4 weeks for elderly or debilitated patients; increase dose with caution as clinically indicated.

Delirium (unlabeled use): Patients >60 years: 2.5 mg daily for up to 5 days (NICE, 2010)

Psychosis/agitation related to Alzheimer's dementia (unlabeled use): Oral: Initial: 2.5-5 mg/day (Sultzer, 2008)

Dosage adjustment in renal impairment: No adjustment required. Not removed by dialysis.

Dosage adjustment in hepatic impairment: Dosage adjustment may be necessary; however, there are no specific recommendations. Monitor closely.

Dietary Considerations Tablets may be taken without regard to meals. Some products may contain phenylalanine.

Administration

Short-acting I.M. injection: **For I.M. administration only**; do not administer injection intravenously or subcutaneously; inject slowly, deep into muscle. If dizziness and/or drowsiness are noted, patient should remain recumbent until examination indicates postural hypotension and/or bradycardia are not a problem.

Extended-release I.M. injection: **For I.M. gluteal injection only**; do not administer I.V. or subcutaneously. After needle insertion into muscle, aspirate to verify that no blood appears. Do not massage injection site. Use diluent, syringes, and needles provided in convenience kit; obtain a new kit if aspiration of blood occurs.

Tablet: May be administered without regard to meals.

Orally-disintegrating: Remove from foil blister by peeling back (do not push tablet through the foil); place tablet in mouth immediately upon removal; tablet dissolves rapidly in saliva and may be swallowed with or without liquid. May be administered with or without food/meals.

Monitoring Parameters Vital signs; fasting lipid profile and fasting blood glucose/Hgb A_{1c} (prior to treatment, at 3 months, then annually); periodic assessment of hepatic transaminases (in patients with hepatic disease); BMI, waist circumference; orthostatic blood pressure; mental status, abnormal involuntary movement scale (AIMS), extrapyramidal symptoms (EPS). Weight should be assessed prior to treatment, at 4 weeks, 8 weeks, 12 weeks, and then at quarterly intervals. Consider titrating to a different antipsychotic agent for a weight gain ≥5% of the initial weight.

Extended-release I.M. injection: Sedation/delirium for 3 hours after each dose

Dosage Forms Excipient information presented when available (limited, particularly for generics); consult specific product labeling.

Injection, powder for reconstitution:

ZyPREXA® IntraMuscular: 10 mg [contains lactose 50 mg]

Injection, powder for suspension, extended release:

ZyPREXA® Relprevv™: 210 mg, 300 mg, 405 mg [contains polysorbate 80 (in diluent); supplied with diluent]

Tablet, oral: 2.5 mg, 5 mg, 7.5 mg, 10 mg, 15 mg, 20 mg

ZyPREXA®: 2.5 mg, 5 mg, 7.5 mg, 10 mg, 15 mg, 20 mg

Tablet, orally disintegrating, oral: 5 mg, 10 mg, 15 mg, 20 mg

ZyPREXA® Zydis®: 5 mg [contains phenylalanine 0.34 mg/tablet]

ZyPREXA® Zydis®: 10 mg [contains phenylalanine 0.45 mg/tablet]

ZyPREXA® Zydis®: 15 mg [contains phenylalanine 0.67 mg/tablet]

ZyPREXA® Zydis®: 20 mg [contains phenylalanine 0.9 mg/tablet]

◆ **Olanzapine ODT (Can)** *see* OLANZapine *on page 1233*

◆ **Olanzapine Pamoate** *see* OLANZapine *on page 1233*

◆ **Oleovitamin A** *see* Vitamin A *on page 1795*

◆ **Oleptro™** *see* TraZODone *on page 1725*

◆ **Olestyr (Can)** *see* Cholestyramine Resin *on page 351*

Olmesartan (ole me SAR tan)

Brand Names: U.S. Benicar®

Brand Names: Canada Olmetec®

Index Terms Olmesartan Medoxomil

Pharmacologic Category Angiotensin II Receptor Blocker

Additional Appendix Information

Angiotensin Agents *on page 1869*

Use Treatment of hypertension with or without concurrent use of other antihypertensive agents

Pregnancy Risk Factor C (1st trimester); D (2nd and 3rd trimesters)

Pregnancy Considerations Medications which act on the renin-angiotensin system are reported to have the following fetal/neonatal effects: Hypotension, neonatal skull hypoplasia, anuria, renal failure, and death; oligohydramnios is also reported. These effects are reported to occur with exposure during the second and third trimesters. There are no adequate and well-controlled studies in pregnant women. **[U.S. Boxed Warning]: Based on human data, drugs that act on the angiotensin system can cause injury and death to the developing fetus when used in the second and third trimesters. Angiotensin receptor blockers should be discontinued as soon as possible once pregnancy is detected.**

Lactation Excretion in breast milk unknown/not recommended

Contraindications There are no contraindications listed in the manufacturer's labeling.

Warnings/Precautions **[U.S. Boxed Warning]: Based on human data, drugs that act on the angiotensin system can cause injury and death to the developing fetus when used in the second and third trimesters. Angiotensin receptor blockers should be discontinued as soon as possible once pregnancy is detected.** May cause hyperkalemia; avoid potassium supplementation unless specifically required by healthcare provider. Avoid use or use a smaller dose in patients who are volume depleted; correct depletion first. May be associated with deterioration of renal function and/or increases in serum creatinine, particularly in patients with low renal blood flow (eg, renal artery stenosis, heart failure) whose glomerular filtration rate (GFR) is dependent on efferent arteriolar vasoconstriction by angiotensin II. Use with caution in unstented unilateral/bilateral renal artery stenosis. When unstented bilateral renal artery stenosis is present, use is generally avoided due to the elevated risk of deterioration in renal function unless possible benefits outweigh risks. Use with caution with pre-existing renal insufficiency; significant aortic/mitral stenosis. Concurrent use of ACE inhibitors may increase the risk of clinically-significant adverse events (eg, renal dysfunction, hyperkalemia).

Adverse Reactions

1% to 10%:

- Central nervous system: Dizziness (3%), headache
- Endocrine & metabolic: Hyperglycemia, hypertriglyceridemia
- Gastrointestinal: Diarrhea
- Neuromuscular & skeletal: Back pain, CPK increased
- Renal: Hematuria
- Respiratory: Bronchitis, pharyngitis, rhinitis, sinusitis
- Miscellaneous: Flu-like syndrome

<1% (Limited to important or life-threatening): Abdominal pain, acute renal failure, alopecia, anaphylaxis, angioedema, arthralgia, arthritis, bilirubin increased, chest pain, dyspepsia, facial edema, fatigue, gastroenteritis, hypercholesterolemia, hyperkalemia, hyperlipidemia, hyperuricemia, insomnia, liver enzymes increased, myalgia, nausea, pain, peripheral edema, pruritus, rash, rhabdomyolysis, serum creatinine increased, skeletal pain, tachycardia, urinary tract infection, urticaria, vertigo, vomiting

Drug Interactions

Metabolism/Transport Effects Substrate of SLCO1B1

Avoid Concomitant Use There are no known interactions where it is recommended to avoid concomitant use.

Increased Effect/Toxicity

Olmesartan may increase the levels/effects of: ACE Inhibitors; Amifostine; Antihypertensives; Hypotensive Agents; Lithium; Nonsteroidal Anti-Inflammatory Agents; Potassium-Sparing Diuretics; RiTUXimab; Sodium Phosphates

The levels/effects of Olmesartan may be increased by: Alfuzosin; Diazoxide; Eltrombopag; Eplerenone; Herbs (Hypotensive Properties); MAO Inhibitors; Pentoxifylline; Phosphodiesterase 5 Inhibitors; Potassium Salts; Prostacyclin Analogues; Tolvaptan; Trimethoprim

Decreased Effect

The levels/effects of Olmesartan may be decreased by: Herbs (Hypertensive Properties); Methylphenidate; Nonsteroidal Anti-Inflammatory Agents; Yohimbine

Ethanol/Nutrition/Herb Interactions

Food: Does not affect olmesartan bioavailability.

Herb/Nutraceutical: Avoid bayberry, blue cohosh, cayenne, ephedra, ginger, ginseng (American), kola, licorice (may worsen hypertension). Avoid black cohosh, California poppy, coleus, golden seal, hawthorn, mistletoe, periwinkle, quinine, shepherd's purse (may have increased antihypertensive effect).

Stability Store at 20°C to 25°C (68°F to 77°F).

Mechanism of Action As a selective and competitive, nonpeptide angiotensin II receptor antagonist, olmesartan blocks the vasoconstrictor and aldosterone-secreting effects of angiotensin II; olmesartan interacts reversibly at the AT1 and AT2 receptors of many tissues and has slow dissociation kinetics; its affinity for the AT1 receptor is 12,500 times greater than the AT2 receptor. Angiotensin II receptor antagonists may induce a more complete inhibition of the renin-angiotensin system than ACE inhibitors, they do not affect the response to bradykinin, and are less likely to be associated with nonrenin-angiotensin effects (eg, cough and angioedema). Olmesartan increases urinary flow rate and, in addition to being natriuretic and kaliuretic, increases excretion of chloride, magnesium, uric acid, calcium, and phosphate.

Pharmacodynamics/Kinetics

Distribution: 17 L; does not cross the blood-brain barrier (animal studies)

Protein binding: 99%

Metabolism: Olmesartan medoxomil is hydrolyzed in the GI tract to active olmesartan. No further metabolism occurs.

Bioavailability: 26%

Half-life elimination: Terminal: 13 hours

Time to peak: 1-2 hours

Excretion: All as unchanged drug: Feces (50% to 65%); urine (35% to 50%)

Dosage Oral:

Children 6-16 years:

- 20 kg to <35 kg: Initial: 10 mg once daily; if initial response is inadequate, may be increased to 20 mg once daily after 2 weeks (maximum: 20 mg once daily)
- ≥35 kg: Initial: 20 mg once daily; if initial response is inadequate, may be increased to 40 mg once daily after 2 weeks (maximum: 40 mg once daily)

Adults: Initial: Usual starting dose is 20 mg once daily; if initial response is inadequate, may be increased to 40 mg once daily after 2 weeks. May administer with other antihypertensive agents if blood pressure inadequately controlled with olmesartan. Consider lower starting dose in patients with possible depletion of intravascular volume (eg, patients receiving diuretics).

Elderly: No initial dosage adjustment necessary per labeling; however, may consider starting at 5-10 mg/day (due to concomitant disease or age changes).

Dosage adjustment in renal impairment: No specific guidelines for dosage adjustment; patients undergoing hemodialysis have not been studied.

Dosage adjustment in hepatic impairment: No initial dosage adjustment necessary.

Dietary Considerations May be taken with or without food.

Administration May be administered with or without food.

Monitoring Parameters Blood pressure, serum potassium

Dosage Forms Excipient information presented when available (limited, particularly for generics); consult specific product labeling.

Tablet, oral, as medoxomil:

Benicar®: 5 mg, 20 mg, 40 mg

Extemporaneous Preparations A 2 mg/mL oral suspension may be made with olmesartan tablets. Combine 50 mL purified water and twenty 20 mg tablets in an 8-ounce amber bottle and allow to stand for ≥5 minutes. Shake well for ≥1 minute, then allow to stand for ≥1 minute. Repeat shaking and standing process four additional times. Add 100 mL Ora-Sweet® and 50 mL Ora-Plus® to the suspension and shake well for ≥1 minute. Label "shake well" and "refrigerate". Stable for 28 days.

Benicar® prescribing information, Daiichi Sankyo, Inc, Parsippany, NJ, 2010.

Olmesartan, Amlodipine, and Hydrochlorothiazide

(ole me SAR tan, am LOE di peen, & hye droe klor oh THYE a zide)

Brand Names: U.S. Tribenzor™

Index Terms Amlodipine Besylate, Olmesartan Medoxomil, and Hydrochlorothiazide; Amlodipine, Hydrochlorothiazide, and Olmesartan; Hydrochlorothiazide, Olmesartan, and Amlodipine; Olmesartan, Hydrochlorothiazide, and Amlodipine

Pharmacologic Category Angiotensin II Receptor Blocker; Antianginal Agent; Calcium Channel Blocker; Calcium Channel Blocker, Dihydropyridine; Diuretic, Thiazide

Use Treatment of hypertension (not for initial therapy)

Pregnancy Risk Factor C (1st trimester) / D (2nd and 3rd trimesters)

Dosage Oral: **Note:** Not for initial therapy. Dose is individualized; combination product may be substituted for individual components in patients currently maintained on all 3 agents separately or in patients not adequately controlled with any 2 of the following antihypertensive classes: Calcium channel blockers, angiotensin II receptor blockers, and diuretics.

Adults: Hypertension: Add-on/switch/replacement therapy: Amlodipine 5-10 mg, olmesartan 20-40 mg, and hydrochlorothiazide 12.5-25 mg once daily; dose may be titrated after 2 weeks of therapy. Maximum recommended daily dose: Amlodipine 10 mg/olmesartan 40 mg/hydrochlorothiazide 25 mg

Elderly: Patients ≥75 years of age should start amlodipine at 2.5 mg (combination product dosage form not available in this strength)

Dosage adjustment in renal impairment:

Cl_{cr} >30 mL/minute: No adjustment needed

Cl_{cr} ≤30 mL/minute: Use of combination not recommended; contraindicated in patients with anuria

Dosage adjustment in hepatic impairment:

Mild-to-moderate hepatic impairment: Use with caution; specific dosing recommendations are not provided in manufacturer's labeling

Severe hepatic impairment: Patients with severe hepatic impairment should start amlodipine at 2.5 mg (combination product dosage form not available)

Additional Information Complete prescribing information for this medication should be consulted for additional detail.

Dosage Forms Excipient information presented when available (limited, particularly for generics); consult specific product labeling.

Tablet, oral:

Tribenzor™:Olmesartan medoxomil 20 mg, amlodipine 5 mg, and hydrochlorothiazide 12.5 mg

Tribenzor™: Olmesartan medoxomil 40 mg, amlodipine 5 mg, and hydrochlorothiazide 12.5 mg

Tribenzor™: Olmesartan medoxomil 40 mg, amlodipine 5 mg, and hydrochlorothiazide 25 mg

Tribenzor™: Olmesartan medoxomil 40 mg, amlodipine 10 mg, and hydrochlorothiazide 12.5 mg

Tribenzor™: Olmesartan medoxomil 40 mg, amlodipine 10 mg, and hydrochlorothiazide 25 mg

◆ **Olmesartan and Amlodipine** *see* Amlodipine and Olmesartan *on page 99*

Olmesartan and Hydrochlorothiazide

(ole me SAR tan & hye droe klor oh THYE a zide)

Brand Names: U.S. Benicar HCT®

Brand Names: Canada Olmetec Plus®

Index Terms Hydrochlorothiazide and Olmesartan Medoxomil; Olmesartan Medoxomil and Hydrochlorothiazide

Pharmacologic Category Angiotensin II Receptor Blocker; Diuretic, Thiazide

Use Treatment of hypertension (not recommended for initial treatment)

Pregnancy Risk Factor C/D (2nd and 3rd trimesters)

Dosage Oral: Adults: One tablet daily; dosage must be individualized. May be titrated at 2- to 4-week intervals.

Replacement therapy: May be substituted for previously titrated dosages of the individual components.

Patients not controlled with single-agent therapy: Initiate by adding the lowest available dose of the alternative component (hydrochlorothiazide 12.5 mg or olmesartan 20 mg). Titrate to effect (maximum daily hydrochlorothiazide dose: 25 mg; maximum daily olmesartan dose: 40 mg).

Dosage adjustment in renal impairment: Not recommended in patients with Cl_{cr} <30 mL/minute

Additional Information Complete prescribing information for this medication should be consulted for additional detail.

Dosage Forms Excipient information presented when available (limited, particularly for generics); consult specific product labeling.

Tablet:

20/12.5: Olmesartan medoxomil 20 mg and hydrochlorothiazide 12.5 mg

40/12.5: Olmesartan medoxomil 40 mg and hydrochlorothiazide 12.5 mg

40/25: Olmesartan medoxomil 40 mg and hydrochlorothiazide 25 mg

◆ **Olmesartan, Hydrochlorothiazide, and Amlodipine** *see* Olmesartan, Amlodipine, and Hydrochlorothiazide *on page 1238*

◆ **Olmesartan Medoxomil** *see* Olmesartan *on page 1236*

◆ **Olmesartan Medoxomil and Hydrochlorothiazide** *see* Olmesartan and Hydrochlorothiazide *on page 1238*

◆ **Olmetec® (Can)** *see* Olmesartan *on page 1236*

◆ **Olmetec Plus® (Can)** *see* Olmesartan and Hydrochlorothiazide *on page 1238*

Olopatadine (Nasal) (oh la PAT a deen)

Brand Names: U.S. Patanase®

Index Terms Olopatadine Hydrochloride

Pharmacologic Category Histamine H_1 Antagonist; Histamine H_1 Antagonist, Second Generation; Piperidine Derivative

Use Treatment of the symptoms of seasonal allergic rhinitis

Pregnancy Risk Factor C

Dosage Intranasal: Children ≥12 years and Adults: 2 sprays into each nostril twice daily

Additional Information Complete prescribing information for this medication should be consulted for additional detail.

Dosage Forms Excipient information presented when available (limited, particularly for generics); consult specific product labeling.

Solution, intranasal [spray]:

Patanase®: 0.6% (30.5 g) [contains benzalkonium chloride; equivalent to olopatadine hydrochloride 665 mcg/100 microliters; 240 metered sprays]

Olopatadine (Ophthalmic) (oh la PAT a deen)

Brand Names: U.S. Pataday™; Patanol®

Brand Names: Canada Pataday™; Patanol®

Index Terms Olopatadine Hydrochloride

Pharmacologic Category Histamine H_1 Antagonist; Histamine H_1 Antagonist, Second Generation; Piperidine Derivative

Use Treatment of the signs and symptoms of allergic conjunctivitis

Pregnancy Risk Factor C

Pregnancy Considerations Teratogenic effects were not observed in animal studies; however, a decrease in fetal weight and a decrease in live births were observed. There are no adequate and well-controlled studies in pregnant women.

Lactation Excretion in breast milk unknown/use caution

Contraindications Hypersensitivity to olopatadine hydrochloride or any component of the formulation

Warnings/Precautions Not for use to treat contact lens-related irritation. Solution contains benzalkonium chloride; remove lens prior to administration and wait at least 10 minutes before reinserting. Do not use contact lenses if eyes are red.

Adverse Reactions

>5%:

Central nervous system: Cold syndrome (up to 10%), headache (up to 7%)

Respiratory: Pharyngitis (up to 10%)

≤5%:

Gastrointestinal: Nausea, taste perversion

Neuromuscular & skeletal: Back pain, weakness

Ocular: Blurred vision, burning, conjunctivitis, dry eyes, eye pain, eyelid edema, foreign body sensation, hyperemia, itching, keratitis, ocular pruritus, stinging

Respiratory: Cough, rhinitis, sinusitis

Miscellaneous: Flu-like syndrome, hypersensitivity, infection

Drug Interactions

Metabolism/Transport Effects None known.

Avoid Concomitant Use There are no known interactions where it is recommended to avoid concomitant use.

Increased Effect/Toxicity There are no known significant interactions involving an increase in effect.

Decreased Effect There are no known significant interactions involving a decrease in effect.

Stability Store at 2°C to 25°C (36°F to 77°F).

Mechanism of Action Selective histamine H_1-antagonist; inhibits release of histamine from mast cells. Inhibits histamine induced effects on conjunctival epithelial cells.

Pharmacodynamics/Kinetics

Absorption: Low systemic absorption

Protein binding: ~55% (primarily albumin)

Metabolism: Not extensively metabolized

Half-life elimination: ~3 hours

Excretion: Urine (60% to 70%, mostly as unchanged drug); feces (17%)

Dosage Ophthalmic: Children ≥3 years and Adults:

Patanol®: Instill 1 drop into affected eye(s) twice daily (allowing 6-8 hours between doses); results from an environmental study demonstrated that olopatadine was effective when dosed twice daily for up to 6 weeks

Pataday™: Instill 1 drop into affected eye(s) once daily

Administration For topical ophthalmic use only. After instilling drops, wait at least 10 minutes before inserting contact lenses. Do not insert contacts if eyes are red.

Dosage Forms Excipient information presented when available (limited, particularly for generics); consult specific product labeling.

Solution, ophthalmic [drops]:

Pataday™: 0.2% (2.5 mL) [contains benzalkonium chloride]

Patanol®: 0.1% (5 mL) [contains benzalkonium chloride]

◆ **Olopatadine Hydrochloride** *see* Olopatadine (Nasal) *on page 1238*

◆ **Olopatadine Hydrochloride** *see* Olopatadine (Ophthalmic) *on page 1239*

Olsalazine (ole SAL a zeen)

Brand Names: U.S. Dipentum®

Brand Names: Canada Dipentum®

Index Terms Olsalazine Sodium

Pharmacologic Category 5-Aminosalicylic Acid Derivative

Use Maintenance of remission of ulcerative colitis in patients intolerant to sulfasalazine

Pregnancy Risk Factor C

Pregnancy Considerations Animal studies have demonstrated fetal developmental toxicities. There are no well-controlled studies in pregnant women. Use during pregnancy only if clearly necessary.

Lactation Enters breast milk/not recommended

Contraindications Hypersensitivity to olsalazine, salicylates, or any component of the formulation

Warnings/Precautions Diarrhea is a common adverse effect of olsalazine. May exacerbate symptoms of colitis. Use with caution in patients with renal or hepatic impairment. Use with caution in elderly patients. Use with caution in patients with severe allergies or asthma.

Adverse Reactions

>10%: Gastrointestinal: Diarrhea (11% to 17%; dose related)

1% to 10%:

Central nervous system: Depression (2%), dizziness/vertigo (1%)

Dermatologic: Rash (2%), pruritus (1%)

Gastrointestinal: Abdominal pain/cramps (10%), nausea (5%), bloating (2%), stomatitis (1%), vomiting (1%)

Neuromuscular & skeletal: Arthralgia (4%)

Respiratory: Upper respiratory infection (2%)

<1% (Limited to important or life-threatening): Alkaline phosphatase increased, Alopecia, ALT increased, anemia, angioedema, aplastic anemia, AST increased, bilirubin increased, blood in stool, blurred vision, bronchospasm, cholestatic hepatitis, cholestatic jaundice, chest pain, chills, cirrhosis, dehydration, dry eyes, dyspnea, dysuria, eosinophilia, epigastric discomfort, erythema, erythema nodosum, fever, flare of symptoms, flatulence, GGT increased, heart block (second degree), hematuria, hemolytic anemia, hepatitis, hepatic failure, hepatic necrosis, hot flashes, hypertension, impotence, insomnia, interstitial nephritis, interstitial pneumonia,

irritability, jaundice, Kawasaki-like syndrome, LDH increased, leukopenia, lymphopenia, menorrhagia, mood swings, muscle cramps, myalgia, myocarditis, nephrotic syndrome, neutropenia, orthostatic hypotension, palpitation, pancreatitis, pancytopenia, paresthesia, pericarditis, peripheral edema, peripheral neuropathy, photosensitivity, proteinuria, rectal bleeding, rectal discomfort, reticulocytosis, rigors, tachycardia, thrombocytopenia, tinnitus, tremor, urinary frequency, watery eyes, xerostomia

Drug Interactions

Metabolism/Transport Effects None known.

Avoid Concomitant Use There are no known interactions where it is recommended to avoid concomitant use.

Increased Effect/Toxicity

Olsalazine may increase the levels/effects of: Heparin; Heparin (Low Molecular Weight); Thiopurine Analogs; Varicella Virus-Containing Vaccines

Decreased Effect

Olsalazine may decrease the levels/effects of: Cardiac Glycosides

Stability Store at 20°C to 25°C (77°F); excursions permitted to 15°C to 30°C (59°F to 86°F).

Mechanism of Action Mesalamine (5-aminosalicylic acid) is the active component of olsalazine; the specific mechanism of action of mesalamine is unknown; however, it is thought that it modulates local chemical mediators of the inflammatory response, especially leukotrienes, and is also postulated to be a free radical scavenger or an inhibitor of tumor necrosis factor (TNF); action appears topical rather than systemic.

Pharmacodynamics/Kinetics

Absorption: <3%; very little intact olsalazine is systemically absorbed

Protein binding, plasma: >99%

Metabolism: Primarily via colonic bacteria to active drug, 5-aminosalicylic acid (5-ASA)

Half-life elimination: 54 minutes

Time to peak: ~1 hour

Excretion: Primarily feces; urine (<1%)

Dosage Adults: Oral: 1 g/day in 2 divided doses

Dietary Considerations Take with food.

Administration Administer with food in evenly divided doses.

Monitoring Parameters CBC, hepatic function, renal function; stool frequency

Dosage Forms Excipient information presented when available (limited, particularly for generics); consult specific product labeling.

Capsule, oral, as sodium:

Dipentum®: 250 mg

◆ **Olsalazine Sodium** *see* Olsalazine *on page* 1239

◆ **Olux®** *see* Clobetasol *on page* 384

◆ **Olux-E™** *see* Clobetasol *on page* 384

◆ **Olux®/Olux-E™ CP [DSC]** *see* Clobetasol *on page* 384

Omalizumab (oh mah lye ZOO mab)

Brand Names: U.S. Xolair®

Brand Names: Canada Xolair®

Index Terms rhuMAb-E25

Pharmacologic Category Monoclonal Antibody, Anti-Asthmatic

Additional Appendix Information

Asthma *on page* 1967

Use Treatment of moderate-to-severe, persistent allergic asthma not adequately controlled with inhaled corticosteroids

Pregnancy Risk Factor B

Pregnancy Considerations Teratogenic effects were not observed in animal studies. There are no adequate and well-controlled studies in pregnant women. IgG molecules are known to cross the placenta; use during pregnancy only if clearly needed. A registry has been established to monitor outcomes of women exposed to omalizumab during pregnancy or within 8 weeks prior to pregnancy (866-496-5247).

Lactation Excretion in breast milk unknown/use caution

Medication Guide Available Yes

Contraindications Hypersensitivity to omalizumab or any component of the formulation; acute bronchospasm, status asthmaticus

Warnings/Precautions [U.S. Boxed Warning]: Anaphylaxis, including delayed-onset anaphylaxis, has been reported following administration; reactions usually occur within 2 hours of administration, but may occur up to 24 hours and in some cases >1 year after initiation of regular treatment. Patients should receive treatment only under direct medical supervision and be observed for a minimum of 2 hours following administration; appropriate medications for the treatment of anaphylactic reactions should be available. Hypersensitivity reactions may occur following any dose, even during chronic therapy; discontinue therapy following any severe reaction.

For use in patients with a documented reactivity to a perennial aeroallergen and with symptoms uncontrolled using inhaled corticosteroids; not used to control acute asthma symptoms. Dosing is based on pretreatment IgE serum levels and body weight. IgE levels remain elevated up to 1 year following treatment, therefore, levels taken during treatment cannot be used as a dosage guide. Corticosteroid therapy should be tapered gradually, do not discontinue abruptly. Malignant neoplasms have been reported with use in short-term studies; impact of long-term use is not known. Use caution with and monitor patients at risk for parasitic (helminth) infections (risk of infection may be increased). Safety and efficacy in children <12 years of age have not been established.

Adverse Reactions

>10%:

Central nervous system: Headache (15%)

Local: Injection site reaction (45%; placebo 43%; severe 12%). Most reactions occurred within 1 hour, lasted <8 days, and decreased in frequency with additional dosing.

Respiratory: Upper respiratory tract infection (20%), sinusitis (16%), pharyngitis (11%)

Miscellaneous: Viral infection (23%)

1% to 10%:

Central nervous system: Pain (7%), fatigue (3%), dizziness (3%)

Dermatologic: Dermatitis (2%), pruritus (2%)

Neuromuscular & skeletal: Arthralgia (8%), leg pain (4%), arm pain (2%), fracture (2%)

Otic: Earache (2%)

<1% (Limited to important or life-threatening): Alopecia; anaphylaxis (angioedema of the throat or tongue, bronchospasm, chest tightness, cough, cutaneous angioedema, dyspnea, hypotension, generalized pruritus, syncope, and urticaria); antibody formation to omalizumab, hot flushes, malignancy (0.5%; placebo 0.2%), throat edema, thrombocytopenia, tongue edema, urticaria, wheezing

Drug Interactions

Metabolism/Transport Effects None known.

Avoid Concomitant Use

Avoid concomitant use of Omalizumab with any of the following: BCG; Natalizumab; Pimecrolimus; Tacrolimus (Topical); Vaccines (Live)

Increased Effect/Toxicity

Omalizumab may increase the levels/effects of: Leflunomide; Natalizumab; Vaccines (Live)

The levels/effects of Omalizumab may be increased by: Denosumab; Pimecrolimus; Roflumilast; Tacrolimus (Topical); Trastuzumab

Decreased Effect

Omalizumab may decrease the levels/effects of: BCG; Coccidioidin Skin Test; Sipuleucel-T; Vaccines (Inactivated); Vaccines (Live)

The levels/effects of Omalizumab may be decreased by: Echinacea

Stability Prior to reconstitution, store under refrigeration at 2°C to 8°C (36°F to 46°F); product may be shipped at room temperature. Prepare using SWFI, USP only; add SWFI 1.4 mL to upright vial and swirl gently for 5-10 seconds every 5 minutes until dissolved; may take >20 minutes to dissolve completely. Resulting solution is 150 mg/1.2 mL. Do not use if powder takes >40 minutes to dissolve. Following reconstitution, protect from direct sunlight. May be stored for up to 8 hours if refrigerated or 4 hours if stored at room temperature.

Mechanism of Action Omalizumab is an IgG monoclonal antibody (recombinant DNA derived) which inhibits IgE binding to the high-affinity IgE receptor on mast cells and basophils. By decreasing bound IgE, the activation and release of mediators in the allergic response (early and late phase) is limited. Serum-free IgE levels and the number of high-affinity IgE receptors are decreased. Long-term treatment in patients with allergic asthma showed a decrease in asthma exacerbations and corticosteroid usage.

Pharmacodynamics/Kinetics

Absorption: Slow following SubQ injection

Distribution: V_d: 78 ± 32 mL/kg

Metabolism: Hepatic; IgG degradation by reticuloendothelial system and endothelial cells

Bioavailability: 62%

Half-life elimination: 26 days

Time to peak: 7-8 days

Excretion: Primarily via hepatic degradation; intact IgG may be secreted in bile

Dosage SubQ: Children ≥12 years and Adults: Asthma: Dose is based on pretreatment IgE serum levels and body weight. Dosing should not be adjusted based on IgE levels taken during treatment or <1 year following discontinuation of therapy; doses should be adjusted during treatment for significant changes in body weight.

IgE ≥30-100 int. units/mL:
- 30-90 kg: 150 mg every 4 weeks
- >90-150 kg: 300 mg every 4 weeks

IgE >100-200 int. units/mL:
- 30-90 kg: 300 mg every 4 weeks
- >90-150 kg: 225 mg every 2 weeks

IgE >200-300 int. units/mL:
- 30-60 kg: 300 mg every 4 weeks
- >60-90 kg: 225 mg every 2 weeks
- >90-150 kg: 300 mg every 2 weeks

IgE >300-400 int. units/mL:
- 30-70 kg: 225 mg every 2 weeks
- >70-90 kg: 300 mg every 2 weeks
- >90 kg: Do not administer dose

IgE >400-500 int. units/mL:
- 30-70 kg: 300 mg every 2 weeks
- >70-90 kg: 375 mg every 2 weeks
- >90 kg: Do not administer dose

IgE >500-600 int. units/mL:
- 30-60 kg: 300 mg every 2 weeks
- >60-70 kg: 375 mg every 2 weeks
- >70 kg: Do not administer dose

IgE >600-700 int. units/mL:
- 30-60 kg: 375 mg every 2 weeks
- >60 kg: Do not administer dose

Administration For SubQ injection only; doses >150 mg should divided over more than one site. Injections may take 5-10 seconds to administer. Administer only under direct medical supervision and observe patient for a minimum of 2 hours following administration of any dose given.

Monitoring Parameters Anaphylactic/hypersensitivity reactions, baseline IgE; FEV_1, peak flow, and/or other pulmonary function tests; monitor for signs of infection

Test Interactions Total IgE levels are elevated for up to 1 year following treatment. Total serum IgE may be retested after interruption of therapy for 1 year or more.

Dosage Forms Excipient information presented when available (limited, particularly for generics); consult specific product labeling.

Injection, powder for reconstitution:

Xolair®: 150 mg [contains sucrose 145.5 mg; derived from or manufactured using Chinese hamster ovary cells]

◆ **Omega 3** *see* Omega-3-Acid Ethyl Esters *on page* 1241

Omega-3-Acid Ethyl Esters

(oh MEG a three AS id ETH il ES ters)

Brand Names: U.S. Lovaza®

Index Terms Ethyl Esters of Omega-3 Fatty Acids; Fish Oil; Omega 3; P-OM3

Pharmacologic Category Antilipemic Agent, Miscellaneous

Use Lovaza®: Adjunct to diet therapy in the treatment of hypertriglyceridemia (≥500 mg/dL)

Note: A number of OTC formulations containing omega-3 fatty acids are marketed as nutritional supplements; these do not have FDA-approved indications and may not contain the same amounts of the active ingredient.

Unlabeled Use Lovaza®: Treatment of IgA nephropathy

Pregnancy Risk Factor C

Dosage Oral: Adults:

Hypertriglyceridemia: 4 g/day as a single daily dose or in 2 divided doses

Treatment of IgA nephropathy (unlabeled use): 4 g/day

Dosage adjustment in renal impairment: No dosage adjustment required.

Additional Information Complete prescribing information for this medication should be consulted for additional detail.

Dosage Forms Excipient information presented when available (limited, particularly for generics); consult specific product labeling.

Capsule, liquid gel, oral:

Lovaza®: 1 g [contains DHA ~375 mg/capsule, EPA ~465 mg/capsule, soybean oil]

Omeprazole (oh MEP ra zole)

Brand Names: U.S. PriLOSEC OTC® [OTC]; PriLOSEC®

Brand Names: Canada Apo-Omeprazole®; Losec®; Mylan-Omeprazole; PMS-Omeprazole; PMS-Omeprazole DR; ratio-Omeprazole; Sandoz-Omeprazole

Index Terms Omeprazole Magnesium

Pharmacologic Category Proton Pump Inhibitor; Substituted Benzimidazole

Use Short-term (4-8 weeks) treatment of active duodenal ulcer disease or active benign gastric ulcer; treatment of heartburn and other symptoms associated with gastroesophageal reflux disease (GERD); short-term (4-8 weeks) treatment of endoscopically-diagnosed erosive esophagitis; maintenance healing of erosive esophagitis; long-term treatment of pathological hypersecretory conditions; as part of a multidrug regimen for *H. pylori* eradication to reduce the risk of duodenal ulcer recurrence

OTC labeling: Short-term treatment of frequent, uncomplicated heartburn occurring ≥2 days/week

Unlabeled Use Healing NSAID-induced ulcers; prevention of NSAID-induced ulcer; stress-ulcer prophylaxis in the critically-ill

Pregnancy Risk Factor C

Pregnancy Considerations Adverse events were observed in some animal reproduction studies. Based on data collected by the Teratogen Information System (TERIS), it was concluded that therapeutic doses used during pregnancy would be unlikely to pose a substantial teratogenic risk (quantity/quality of data: fair). Because the possibility of harm still exists, the manufacturer recommends use during pregnancy only if the potential benefit to the mother outweighs the possible risk to the fetus.

Lactation Enters breast milk/not recommended

Contraindications Hypersensitivity to omeprazole, substituted benzimidazoles (eg, esomeprazole, lansoprazole), or any component of the formulation

Warnings/Precautions Use of proton pump inhibitors (PPIs) may increase the risk of gastrointestinal infections (eg, *Salmonella, Campylobacter*). Relief of symptoms does not preclude the presence of a gastric malignancy. Atrophic gastritis (by biopsy) has been noted with long-term omeprazole therapy. In long-term (2-year) studies in rats, omeprazole produced a dose-related increase in gastric carcinoid tumors. While available endoscopic evaluations and histologic examinations of biopsy specimens from human stomachs have not detected a risk from short-term exposure to omeprazole, further human data on the effect of sustained hypochlorhydria and hypergastrinemia are needed to rule out the possibility of an increased risk for the development of tumors in humans receiving long-term therapy.

PPIs may diminish the therapeutic effect of clopidogrel, thought to be due to reduced formation of the active metabolite of clopidogrel. The manufacturer of clopidogrel recommends either avoidance of omeprazole (even when scheduled 12 hours apart) or use of a PPI with less potent CYP2C19 inhibition (eg, pantoprazole). Others have recommended the continued use of PPIs, regardless of the degree of inhibition, in patients with a history of GI bleeding or multiple risk factors for GI bleeding who are also receiving clopidogrel since no evidence has established clinically meaningful differences in outcome; however, a clinically-significant interaction cannot be excluded in those who are poor metabolizers of clopidogrel (Abraham, 2010; Levine, 2011). Avoid concurrent use of CYP3A4 and 2C19 inducers (eg, St John's wort, rifampin) as omeprazole's efficacy may be reduced.

Increased incidence of osteoporosis-related bone fractures of the hip, spine, or wrist may occur with PPI therapy. Patients on high-dose (multiple daily doses)or long-term (≥1 year) therapy should be monitored. Use the lowest effective dose for the shortest duration of time, use vitamin D and calcium supplementation, and follow appropriate guidelines to reduce risk of fractures in patients at risk.

Hypomagnesemia, reported rarely, usually with prolonged PPI use of >3 months (most cases >1 year of therapy); may be symptomatic or asymptomatic; severe cases may cause tetany, seizures, and cardiac arrhythmias. Consider obtaining serum magnesium concentrations prior to beginning long-term therapy, especially if taking concomitant digoxin, diuretics, or other drugs known to cause hypomagnesemia; and periodically thereafter. Hypomagnesemia may be corrected by magnesium supplementation, although discontinuation of omeprazole may be necessary; magnesium levels typically return to normal within 1 week of stopping. Serum chromogranin A levels may be increased if assessed while patient on omeprazole; may lead to diagnostic errors related to neuroendocrine tumors.

Decreased *H. pylori* eradication rates have been observed with short-term (≤7 days) combination therapy. The American College of Gastroenterology recommends 10-14 days of therapy (triple or quadruple) for eradication of *H. pylori* (Chey, 2007). Bioavailability may be increased in Asian populations and patients with hepatic dysfunction; consider dosage reductions, especially for maintenance healing of erosive esophagitis. Bioavailability may be increased in the elderly. When used for self-medication (OTC), do not use for >14 days.

Adverse Reactions

1% to 10%:

Central nervous system: Headache (7%), dizziness (2%)

Dermatologic: Rash (2%)

Gastrointestinal: Abdominal pain (5%), diarrhea (4%), nausea (4%), vomiting (3%), flatulence (3%), acid regurgitation (2%), constipation (2%)

Neuromuscular & skeletal: Back pain (1%), weakness (1%)

Respiratory: Upper respiratory infection (2%), cough (1%)

≤1% (Limited to important or life-threatening; adverse event occurrence may vary based on formulation): Abdominal swelling, abnormal dreams, aggression, agitation, agranulocytosis, alkaline phosphatase increased, allergic reactions, alopecia, ALT increased, anaphylaxis, anemia, angina, angioedema, anorexia, anxiety, apathy, AST increased, atrophic gastritis, benign gastric polyps, bilirubin increased, blurred vision, bradycardia, bronchospasm, chest pain, cholestatic hepatitis, confusion, creatinine increased, depression, double vision, dry skin, epistaxis, erythema multiforme, esophageal candidiasis, fatigue, fecal discoloration, fever, fracture, gastroduodenal carcinoids, GGT increased, glycosuria, gynecomastia, hallucinations, hematuria, hemolytic anemia, hepatic encephalopathy, hepatic failure, hepatic necrosis, hepatitis, hepatocellular hepatitis, hyperhidrosis, hypersensitivity, hypertension, hypoglycemia, hypomagnesemia, hyponatremia, insomnia, interstitial nephritis, irritable colon, jaundice, joint pain, leg pain, leukocytosis, leukopenia, liver disease (hepatocellular, cholestatic, mixed), malaise, microscopic pyuria, mucosal atrophy (tongue), muscle cramps, muscle weakness, myalgia, nervousness, neutropenia, ocular irritation, optic atrophy, optic neuritis, optic neuropathy (anterior ischemic), osteoporosis-related fracture, pain, palpitation, pancreatitis, pancytopenia, paresthesia, peripheral edema, petechiae, pharyngeal pain, photosensitivity, proteinuria, pruritus, psychiatric disturbance, purpura, skin inflammation, sleep disturbance, somnolence, Stevens-Johnson syndrome, stomatitis, tachycardia, taste perversion, testicular pain, thrombocytopenia, tinnitus, toxic epidermal necrolysis, tremor, urinary frequency, urinary tract infection, urticaria, vertigo, weight gain, xerophthalmia, xerostomia

Drug Interactions

Metabolism/Transport Effects **Substrate** of CYP2A6 (minor), CYP2C19 (major), CYP2C9 (minor), CYP2D6 (minor), CYP3A4 (minor); **Note:** Assignment of Major/Minor substrate status based on clinically relevant drug interaction potential; **Inhibits** CYP1A2 (weak), CYP2C19 (moderate), CYP2C9 (moderate), CYP2D6 (weak), CYP3A4 (weak); **Induces** CYP1A2 (weak/moderate)

Avoid Concomitant Use

Avoid concomitant use of Omeprazole with any of the following: Clopidogrel; Delavirdine; Erlotinib; Nelfinavir; Pimozide; Posaconazole; Rifampin; Rilpivirine; St Johns Wort

Increased Effect/Toxicity

Omeprazole may increase the levels/effects of: Amphetamines; Benzodiazepines (metabolized by oxidation); Carvedilol; Cilostazol; Citalopram; CloZAPine; CycloSPORINE; CycloSPORINE (Systemic); CYP2C19

Substrates; CYP2C9 Substrates; Dexmethylphenidate; Fosphenytoin; Methotrexate; Methylphenidate; Phenytoin; Pimozide; Raltegravir; Saquinavir; Tacrolimus; Tacrolimus (Systemic); Vitamin K Antagonists; Voriconazole

The levels/effects of Omeprazole may be increased by: Conivaptan; Fluconazole; Ketoconazole; Ketoconazole (Systemic)

Decreased Effect

Omeprazole may decrease the levels/effects of: Atazanavir; Bisphosphonate Derivatives; Cefditoren; Clopidogrel; CloZAPine; Dabigatran Etexilate; Dasatinib; Delavirdine; Erlotinib; Gefitinib; Indinavir; Iron Salts; Itraconazole; Ketoconazole; Ketoconazole (Systemic); Mesalamine; Mycophenolate; Nelfinavir; Posaconazole; Rilpivirine

The levels/effects of Omeprazole may be decreased by: CYP2C19 Inducers (Strong); Peginterferon Alfa-2b; Rifampin; St Johns Wort; Tipranavir; Tocilizumab

Ethanol/Nutrition/Herb Interactions

Ethanol: Avoid ethanol (may cause gastric mucosal irritation).

Food: Food delays absorption.

Herb/Nutraceutical: Avoid use of St John's wort (may decrease efficacy of omeprazole).

Stability

Capsules, tablets: Store at 15°C to 30°C (59°F to 86°F). Protect from light and moisture.

Granules for oral suspension: Store at 25°C (77°F); excursions permitted to 15°C to 30°C (59°F to 86°F). For oral administration, empty the contents of the 2.5 mg packet into 5 mL of water (10 mg packet into 15 mL of water); stir. For NG administration, add 5 mL of water into a catheter-tipped syringe, and then add the contents of a 2.5 mg packet (15 mL water for the 10 mg packet); shake. **Note:** Regardless of the route of administration, the suspension should be left to thicken for 2-3 minutes prior to administration.

Mechanism of Action Proton pump inhibitor; suppresses gastric basal and stimulated acid secretion by inhibiting the parietal cell H+/K+ ATP pump

Pharmacodynamics/Kinetics

Onset of action: Antisecretory: ~1 hour

Peak effect: Within 2 hours

Duration: Up to 72 hours; 50% of maximum effect at 24 hours; after stopping treatment, secretory activity gradually returns over 3-5 days

Absorption: Rapid

Protein binding: ~95%

Metabolism: Hepatic via CYP2C19 primarily and (to a lesser extent) via 3A4 to hydroxy, desmethyl, and sulfone metabolites (all inactive); saturable first-pass effect

Bioavailability: Oral: ~30% to 40%; increased in Asian patients, elderly patients, and patients with hepatic dysfunction

Half-life elimination: 0.5-1 hour; hepatic impairment: ~3 hours

Time to peak, plasma: 0.5-3.5 hours

Excretion: Urine (~77% as metabolites, very small amount as unchanged drug); feces

Dosage Oral:

Children 1-16 years: GERD or other acid-related disorders:

- 5 kg to <10 kg: 5 mg once daily
- 10 kg to <20 kg: 10 mg once daily
- ≥20 kg: 20 mg once daily

Adults:

- Active duodenal ulcer: 20 mg once daily for 4-8 weeks
- Gastric ulcers: 40 mg once daily for 4-8 weeks
- Symptomatic GERD (without esophageal lesions): 20 mg once daily for up to 4 weeks
- Erosive esophagitis: 20 mg once daily for 4-8 weeks; maintenance of healing: 20 mg once daily for up to 12 months total therapy (including treatment period of 4-8 weeks)
- *Helicobacter pylori* eradication: Dose varies with regimen:
  - Manufacturer labeling: 40 mg once daily administered with clarithromycin 500 mg 3 times/day for 14 days **or** 20 mg twice daily administered with amoxicillin 1000 mg *and* clarithromycin 500 mg twice daily for 10 days. **Note:** Presence of ulcer at time of therapy initiation may necessitate an additional 14-18 days of omeprazole 20 mg/day (monotherapy) after completion of combination therapy.
  - American College of Gastroenterology guidelines (Chey, 2007):
    - Nonpenicillin allergy: 20 mg twice daily administered with amoxicillin 1000 mg *and* clarithromycin 500 mg twice daily for 10-14 days
    - Penicillin allergy: 20 mg twice daily administered with clarithromycin 500 mg *and* metronidazole 500 mg twice daily for 10-14 days **or** 20 mg once or twice daily administered with bismuth subsalicylate 525 mg *and* metronidazole 250 mg *plus* tetracycline 500 mg 4 times/day for 10-14 days
- Pathological hypersecretory conditions: Initial: 60 mg once daily; doses up to 120 mg 3 times/day have been administered; administer daily doses >80 mg in divided doses
- Stress-ulcer prophylaxis (ICU patients; unlabeled use): 40 mg once daily; periodically evaluate patient for continued need (Levy, 1997)
- Frequent heartburn (OTC labeling): 20 mg once daily for 14 days; treatment may be repeated after 4 months if needed

Dosage adjustment in hepatic impairment: Bioavailability is increased with chronic liver disease. Consider dosage adjustment, especially for maintenance of erosive esophagitis. Specific guidelines are not available.

Dietary Considerations Should be taken on an empty stomach; best if taken before breakfast.

Administration

Oral: Best if administered before breakfast.

Capsule: Should be swallowed whole; do not chew or crush. Delayed release capsule may be opened and contents added to 1 tablespoon of applesauce (use immediately after adding to applesauce); mixture should not be chewed or warmed.

Oral suspension: Following reconstitution, the suspension should be left to thicken for 2-3 minutes and administered within 30 minutes. If any material remains after administration, add more water, stir, and administer immediately.

Tablet: Should be swallowed whole; do not crush or chew.

Nasogastric/orogastric (NG/OG) tube administration:

Capsule: When using capsules to extemporaneously prepare a solution for NG administration, the manufacturers of Prilosec® recommend the use of an acidic juice for preparation and administration. Alternative methods have been described as follows:

NG/OG tube administration for the prevention of stress-related mucosal damage in ventilated, critically-ill patients:

Study 1 (Phillips, 1996): Pour the contents of one or two 20 mg omeprazole delayed release capsules (depending on the dose) into a syringe (after removing plunger); withdraw 10-20 mL of an 8.4% sodium bicarbonate solution into the syringe; allow 30 minutes for the enteric-coated omeprazole granules to break down. Shake the resulting milky substance prior to administration. Flush the NG tube with 5-10 mL of water and clamp for at least 1 hour.

Study 2 (Balaban, 1997): Open the omeprazole delayed release capsule (20 mg or 40 mg), then pour the intact granules into a container holding 30 mL of water. Pour one-third to one-half of the granules into a 30 mL syringe (with the plunger removed) attached to a nasogastric tube (NG). Replace the plunger with 1 cm of air between the granules and the plunger top while the plunger is depressed. Repeat this process until all the granules are flushed, then flush a final 15 mL of water through the tube.

Oral suspension: Following reconstitution in a catheter-tipped syringe, shake the suspension well and leave to thicken for 2-3 minutes. Administer within 30 minutes of reconstitution. Use an NG tube or gastric tube that is a size 6 French or larger; flush the syringe and tube with water.

Monitoring Parameters Susceptibility testing is recommended in patients who fail *H. pylori*-eradication regimen.

Test Interactions Omeprazole may falsely elevate serum chromogranin A (CgA) levels. The increased CgA level may cause false-positive results in the diagnosis of a neuroendocrine tumor. Temporarily stop omeprazole if assessing CgA level; repeat level if initially elevated; use the same laboratory for all testing of CgA levels.

Dosage Forms Excipient information presented when available (limited, particularly for generics); consult specific product labeling.

Capsule, delayed release, oral: 10 mg, 20 mg, 40 mg
PriLOSEC®: 10 mg, 20 mg, 40 mg

Granules for suspension, delayed release, oral:
PriLOSEC®: 2.5 mg/packet (30s); 10 mg/packet (30s)

Tablet, delayed release, oral: 20 mg
PriLOSEC OTC®: 20 mg

Extemporaneous Preparations A 2 mg/mL oral omeprazole solution (Simplified Omeprazole Solution) may be made with five omeprazole 20 mg delayed release capsules and 50 mL sodium bicarbonate 8.4%. Empty capsules into beaker. Add sodium bicarbonate solution. Gently stir (about 15 minutes) until a white suspension forms. Transfer to amber-colored syringe or bottle. Stable for 14 days at room temperature or for 30 days refrigerated.

DiGiacinto JL, Olsen KM, Bergman KL, et al, "Stability of Suspension Formulations of Lansoprazole and Omeprazole Stored in Amber-Colored Plastic Oral Syringes," *Ann Pharmacother*, 2000, 34 (5):600-5.

Quercia R, Fan C, Liu X, et al, "Stability of Omeprazole in an Extemporaneously Prepared Oral Liquid," *Am J Health Syst Pharm*, 1997, 54(16):1833-6.

Sharma V, "Comparison of 24-hour Intragastric pH Using Four Liquid Formulations of Lansoprazole and Omeprazole," *Am J Health Syst Pharm*, 1999, 56(23 Suppl 4):18-21.

Omeprazole and Sodium Bicarbonate

(oh MEP ra zole & SOW dee um bye KAR bun ate)

Brand Names: U.S. Zegerid OTC™ [OTC]; Zegerid®

Index Terms Sodium Bicarbonate and Omeprazole

Pharmacologic Category Proton Pump Inhibitor; Substituted Benzimidazole

Use Short-term (4-8 weeks) treatment of active duodenal ulcer or active benign gastric ulcer; treatment of heartburn and other symptoms associated with gastroesophageal reflux disease (GERD); short-term (4-8 weeks) treatment of endoscopically-diagnosed erosive esophagitis; maintenance healing of erosive esophagitis; reduction of risk of upper gastrointestinal bleeding in critically-ill patients

OTC labeling: Short-term (2 weeks) treatment of frequent (2 days/week), uncomplicated heartburn

Pregnancy Risk Factor C

Dosage Note: Both strengths of Zegerid® capsule and powder for oral suspension have identical sodium bicarbonate content, respectively. Do not substitute two 20 mg capsules/packets for one 40 mg dose.

Oral: Adults:

Active duodenal ulcer: 20 mg/day for 4-8 weeks

Gastric ulcers: 40 mg/day for 4-8 weeks

Symptomatic GERD: 20 mg/day for up to 4 weeks

Erosive esophagitis: 20 mg/day for 4-8 weeks; maintenance of healing: 20 mg/day for up to 12 months total therapy (including treatment period of 4-8 weeks)

Heartburn (OTC labeling): 20 mg once daily for 14 days. Do not take for >14 days or more often than every 4 months, unless instructed by healthcare provider.

Risk reduction of upper GI bleeding in critically-ill patients (Zegerid® powder for oral suspension):

Loading dose: Day 1: 40 mg every 6-8 hours for two doses

Maintenance dose: 40 mg/day for up to 14 days; therapy >14 days has not been evaluated

Dosage adjustment in renal impairment: No adjustment necessary

Dosage adjustment in hepatic impairment: Bioavailability is increased with chronic liver disease. Consider dosage adjustment, especially for maintenance of healing of erosive esophagitis. Specific guidelines are not available.

Additional Information Complete prescribing information for this medication should be consulted for additional detail.

Dosage Forms Excipient information presented when available (limited, particularly for generics); consult specific product labeling.

Capsule, oral: Omeprazole 20 mg [immediate release] and sodium bicarbonate 1100 mg; omeprazole 40 mg [immediate release] and sodium bicarbonate 1100 mg

Zegerid®: Omeprazole 20 mg [immediate release] and sodium bicarbonate 1100 mg [contains sodium 304 mg (13 mEq) per capsule]

Zegerid®: Omeprazole 40 mg [immediate release] and sodium bicarbonate 1100 mg [contains sodium 304 mg (13 mEq) per capsule]

Zegerid OTC™: Omeprazole 20 mg [immediate release] and sodium bicarbonate 1100 mg [contains sodium 303 mg (13 mEq) per capsule]

Powder for oral suspension:

Zegerid®: Omeprazole 20 mg and sodium bicarbonate 1680 mg per packet (30s) [contains sodium 460 mg (20 mEq) per packet]

Zegerid®: Omeprazole 40 mg and sodium bicarbonate 1680 mg per packet (30s) [contains sodium 460 mg (20 mEq) per packet]

◆ **Omeprazole Magnesium** *see* Omeprazole *on page 1241*

◆ **Omnaris™** *see* Ciclesonide (Nasal) *on page 356*

◆ **Omnicef®** *see* Cefdinir *on page 303*

◆ **Omni Gel™ [OTC]** *see* Fluoride *on page 728*

◆ **Omnipred™** *see* PrednisoLONE (Ophthalmic) *on page 1398*

◆ **Omnitrope®** *see* Somatropin *on page 1579*

OnabotulinumtoxinA

(oh nuh BOT yoo lin num TOKS in aye)

Brand Names: U.S. Botox®; Botox® Cosmetic

Brand Names: Canada Botox®; Botox® Cosmetic

Index Terms Botulinum Toxin Type A; BTX-A

Pharmacologic Category Neuromuscular Blocker Agent, Toxin; Ophthalmic Agent, Toxin

Use Treatment of strabismus and blepharospasm associated with dystonia (including benign essential blepharospasm or VII nerve disorders) in patients ≥12 years of age; treatment of cervical dystonia (spasmodic torticollis) in patients ≥16 years of age; temporary improvement in the appearance of lines/wrinkles of the face (moderate-to-severe glabellar lines associated with corrugator and/or procerus muscle activity) in adult patients ≤65 years of age; treatment of severe primary axillary hyperhidrosis in adults not adequately controlled with topical treatments; treatment of focal spasticity (specifically upper limb spasticity) in adults; prophylaxis of chronic migraine headache (≥15 days/month with ≥4 hours/day headache duration) in adults

Canadian labeling: Additional use (not in U.S. labeling): Dynamic equinus foot deformity in pediatric cerebral palsy patients; treatment of forehead, lateral canthus, and glabellar lines in adults >65 years of age

Unlabeled Use Treatment of oromandibular dystonia, spasmodic dysphonia (laryngeal dystonia) and other dystonias (ie, writer's cramp, focal task-specific dystonias); treatment of dynamic muscle contracture in pediatric cerebral palsy patients

Pregnancy Risk Factor C

Medication Guide Available Yes

Dosage Note: In adults treated for more than one indication, the maximum cumulative dose should be ≤360 units/3 months. Canadian labeling recommends a maximum cumulative dose of 6 units/kg (adults up to 360 units; children up to 200 units) over 3 months in patients receiving additional treatment for noncosmetic indications.

Blepharospasm:

Botox®: Children ≥12 years and Adults: I.M.: Initial dose: 1.25-2.5 units injected into the medial and lateral pretarsal orbicularis oculi of the upper lid and lateral pretarsal orbicularis oculi of lower lid

Dose may be increased up to twice the previous dose if the response from the initial dose lasted ≤2 months; maximum dose per site: 5 units. Tolerance may occur if treatments are given more often than every 3 months, but the effect is not usually permanent. Cumulative dose:

U.S. labeling: ≤200 units in 30-day period

Canadian labeling (not in U.S. labeling): Botox®: ≤200 units in 2-month period

Cervical dystonia:

Children ≥16 years and Adults: I.M.: For dosing guidance, the mean dose is 236 units (25th to 75th percentile range 198-300 units) divided among the affected muscles in patients previously treated with botulinum toxin (maximum: ≤50 units/site). Initial dose in previously untreated patients should be lower. Sequential dosing should be based on the patient's head and neck position, localization of pain, muscle hypertrophy, patient response, and previous adverse reactions. The total dose injected into the sternocleidomastoid muscles should be ≤100 units to decrease the occurrence of dysphagia.

Canadian labeling (not in U.S. labeling): Botox®: Children ≥16 years and Adults: I.M.: Effective range of 200-360 units has been used in clinical practice; administer no more frequently than every 2 months

Chronic migraine: Adults: I.M.: Administer 5 units/0.1 mL per site. Recommended total dose is 155 units once every 12 weeks. Each 155 unit dose should be equally divided and administered bilaterally, into 31 total sites as described below (refer to prescribing information for specific diagrams of recommended injection sites):

Corrugator: 5 units to each side (2 sites)

Procerus: 5 units (1 site only)

Frontalis: 10 units to each side (divided into 2 sites/side)

Temporalis: 20 units to each side (divided into 4 sites/side)

Occipitalis: 15 units to each side (divided into 3 sites/side)

Cervical paraspinal: 10 units to each side (divided into 2 sites/side)

Trapezius: 15 units to each side (divided into 3 sites/side)

Strabismus: Children ≥12 years and Adults: I.M.: **Note:** Several minutes prior to injection, administration of local anesthetic and ocular decongestant drops are recommended.

Initial dose:

Vertical muscles and for horizontal strabismus <20 prism diopters: 1.25-2.5 units in any one muscle

Horizontal strabismus of 20-50 prism diopters: 2.5-5 units in any one muscle

Persistent VI nerve palsy ≥1 month: 1.25-2.5 units in the medial rectus muscle

Re-examine patients 7-14 days after each injection to assess the effect of that dose. Subsequent doses for patients experiencing incomplete paralysis of the target may be increased up to twice the previous administered dose. The maximum recommended dose as a single injection for any one muscle is 25 units. Do not administer subsequent injections until the effects of the previous dose are gone.

Primary axillary hyperhidrosis: Adults ≥18 years: Intradermal: 50 units/axilla. Injection area should be defined by standard staining techniques. Injections should be evenly distributed into multiple sites (10-15), administered in 0.1-0.2 mL aliquots, ~1-2 cm apart. May repeat when clinical effect diminishes.

Spasticity (cerebral palsy related [dynamic equinus foot deformity]: Canadian labeling [not approved in U.S. labeling]): Children ≥2 years: I.M.: 4 units/kg (total dose) divided into two injections into medial and lateral heads of the gastrocnemius of affected leg; if clinically indicated, may repeat every 2 months (maximum dose: 200 units); in diplegia, the recommended dose is 6 units/kg (total dose) divided between affected limbs

Spasticity (focal): Adults ≥18 years: I.M.: Individualize dose based on patient size, extent, and location of muscle involvement, degree of spasticity, local muscle weakness, and response to prior treatment. In clinical trials, total doses up to 360 units (Botox®) were administered as separate injections typically divided among selected muscles; may repeat therapy at ≥3 months with appropriate dosage based upon the clinical condition of patient at time of retreatment.

Suggested guidelines for the treatment of upper limb spasticity. The lowest recommended starting dose should be used and ≤50 units/site should be administered. **Note:** Dose listed is total dose administered as individual or separate intramuscular injection(s):

Biceps brachii: 100-200 units (divided into 4 sites)

Flexor digitorum profundus: 30-50 units (1 site)

Flexor digitorum sublimes: 30-50 units (1 site)

Flexor carpi radialis: 12.5-50 units (1 site)

Flexor carpi ulnaris: 12.5-50 units (1 site)

Suggested guidelines for the treatment of stroke-related upper limb spasticity: Canadian labeling: **Note:** Dose listed is total dose administered as individual or separate intramuscular injection(s):

Biceps brachii: 100-200 units (up to 4 sites)

Flexor digitorum profundus: 15-50 units (1-2 sites)

Flexor digitorum sublimes: 15-50 units (1-2 sites)

Flexor carpi radialis: 15-60 units (1-2 sites)

Flexor carpi ulnaris: 10-50 units (1-2 sites)

Adductor pollicis: 20 units (1-2 sites)

Flexor pollicis longus: 20 units (1-2 sites)

Cosmetic uses:

Reduction of glabellar lines: Adults ≤65 years: I.M.: An effective dose is determined by gross observation of the patient's ability to activate the superficial muscles injected. The location, size and use of muscles may vary markedly among individuals. Inject 0.1 mL (4 units) dose into each of five sites, two in each corrugator muscle and one in the procerus muscle for a total dose 0.5 mL (20 units) administered no more frequently than every 3-4 months. **Note:** Treatment of adults >65 years is approved in the Canadian labeling.

Reduction of forehead lines (Canadian labeling; not in U.S. labeling): Adults: I.M.: Inject 2-6 units into each of four sites in the frontalis muscle every 1-2 cm along either side of forehead crease and 2-3 cm above eyebrows for total dose of 24 units.

Reduction of lateral canthus lines (Canadian labeling; not in U.S. labeling): Adults: I.M.: Inject 2-6 units into each of 1-3 injection sites, lateral to the lateral orbital rim.

Elderly: No specific adjustment recommended; initiate therapy at lowest recommended dose

Additional Information Complete prescribing information for this medication should be consulted for additional detail.

Dosage Forms Excipient information presented when available (limited, particularly for generics); consult specific product labeling. [DSC] = Discontinued product

Injection, powder for reconstitution [preservative free]:

Botox®: *Clostridium botulinum* type A neurotoxin complex 100 units, *Clostridium botulinum* type A neurotoxin complex 200 units [contains albumin (human)]

Botox® Cosmetic: *Clostridium botulinum* type A neurotoxin complex 50 units [DSC], *Clostridium botulinum* type A neurotoxin complex 100 units [contains albumin (human)]

Powder for reconstitution, for injection [preservative free]:

Botox® Cosmetic: *Clostridium botulinum* type A neurotoxin complex 50 units [contains albumin (human)]

Dosage Forms: Canada Excipient information presented when available (limited, particularly for generics); consult specific product labeling.

Injection, powder for reconstitution [preservative free]:

Botox®: Botulinum toxin A 50 units [contains albumin (human)], 100 units [contains albumin (human)], 200 units [contains albumin (human)]

Botox Cosmetic®: Botulinum toxin A 50 units [contains albumin (human)], 100 units [contains albumin (human)], 200 units [contains albumin (human)]

◆ **OnBrez Breezehaler** *see* Indacaterol *on page 885*

◆ **Oncaspar®** *see* Pegaspargase *on page 1306*

◆ **Oncotice™ (Can)** *see* BCG *on page 191*

◆ **Oncovin** *see* VinCRIStine *on page 1790*

Ondansetron (on DAN se tron)

Brand Names: U.S. Zofran®; Zofran® ODT; Zuplenz®

Brand Names: Canada Apo-Ondansetron®; CO Ondansetron; Dom-Ondansetron; JAMP-Ondansetron; Mint-Ondansetron; Mylan-Ondansetron; Ondansetron Injection; Ondansetron Injection USP; Ondansetron-Odan; Ondansetron-Omega; PHL-Ondansetron; PMS-Ondansetron; RAN™-Ondansetron; ratio-Ondansetron; Sandoz-Ondansetron; Teva-Ondansetron; Zofran®; Zofran® ODT; ZYM-Ondansetron

Index Terms GR38032R; Ondansetron Hydrochloride; Zuplenz®

Pharmacologic Category Antiemetic; Selective 5-HT_3 Receptor Antagonist

Use Prevention of nausea and vomiting associated with moderately- to highly-emetogenic cancer chemotherapy; radiotherapy; prevention of postoperative nausea and vomiting (PONV); treatment of PONV if no prophylactic dose of ondansetron received

Unlabeled Use Hyperemesis gravidarum; breakthrough treatment of nausea and vomiting associated with chemotherapy

Pregnancy Risk Factor B

Pregnancy Considerations Teratogenic effects were not observed in animal studies; however, there are no adequate and well-controlled studies in pregnant women. Use of ondansetron for the treatment of nausea and vomiting of pregnancy (NVP) has been evaluated. Additional studies are needed to determine safety to the fetus, particularly during the first trimester. Based on preliminary data, use is generally reserved for severe NVP (hyperemesis gravidarum) or when conventional treatments are not effective.

Lactation Excretion in breast milk unknown/use caution

Contraindications Hypersensitivity to ondansetron, other selective 5-HT_3 antagonists, or any component of the formulation; concomitant use of apomorphine

Warnings/Precautions Ondansetron should be used on a scheduled basis, not on an "as needed" (PRN) basis, since data support the use of this drug only in the prevention of nausea and vomiting (due to antineoplastic therapy) and not in the rescue of nausea and vomiting. Ondansetron should only be used in the first 24-48 hours of chemotherapy. Data do not support any increased efficacy of ondansetron in delayed nausea and vomiting. Does not stimulate gastric or intestinal peristalsis; may mask progressive ileus and/or gastric distension. Use with caution in patients allergic to other 5-HT_3 receptor antagonists; cross-reactivity has been reported.

Use with caution in patients with congenital long QT syndrome or other risk factors for QT prolongation (eg, medications known to prolong QT interval, electrolyte abnormalities, and cumulative high-dose anthracycline therapy). 5-HT_3 antagonists have been associated with a number of dose-dependent increases in ECG intervals (eg, PR, QRS duration, QT/QT_c, JT), usually occurring 1-2 hours after I.V. administration. In general, these changes are not clinically relevant, however, when used in conjunction with other agents that prolong these intervals, arrhythmia may occur. When used with agents that prolong the QT interval (eg, Class I and III antiarrhythmics), clinically relevant QT interval prolongation may occur resulting in torsade de pointes. I.V. formulations of 5-HT_3 antagonists have more association with ECG interval changes, compared to oral formulations. Dose recommendations provided for patients with severe hepatic impairment (Child-Pugh class C); use with caution in mild-moderate hepatic impairment; clearance is decreased and half-life increased in hepatic impairment.

Orally-disintegrating tablets contain phenylalanine.

Adverse Reactions Note: Percentages reported in adult patients.

>10%:

Central nervous system: Headache (9% to 27%), malaise/fatigue (9% to 13%)

Gastrointestinal: Constipation (6% to 11%)

1% to 10%:

Central nervous system: Drowsiness (8%), fever (2% to 8%), dizziness (4% to 7%), anxiety (6%), cold sensation (2%)

Dermatologic: Pruritus (2% to 5%), rash (1%)

Gastrointestinal: Diarrhea (2% to 7%)

Genitourinary: Gynecological disorder (7%), urinary retention (5%)

Hepatic: ALT increased (1% to 5%), AST increased (1% to 5%)

Local: Injection site reaction (4%; pain, redness, burning)

Neuromuscular & skeletal: Paresthesia (2%)

Respiratory: Hypoxia (9%)

<1% (Limited to important or life-threatening): Abnormal hepatic function, anaphylactoid reactions, anaphylaxis, angina, angioedema, arrhythmia, arthralgia, atrial fibrillation, AV block, blindness (transient/following infusion; lasting ≤48 hours), blurred vision (transient/following infusion), bradycardia, bronchospasm, cardiopulmonary arrest, chest discomfort, chills, dyspnea, dystonic reaction, ECG changes, electrocardiographic alterations (second-degree heart block and ST-segment depression), extrapyramidal symptoms, grand mal seizure, hepatic failure, hepatic necrosis, hepatitis, hypersensitivity reaction, hypokalemia, hypotension, jaundice, laryngeal edema, laryngospasm, lethargy, oculogyric crisis, palpitation, premature ventricular contractions (PVC), QT interval increased, shock, shortness of breath, stridor, supraventricular tachycardia, syncope, tachycardia, torsade de pointes, urticaria, vascular occlusive events, ventricular arrhythmia, ventricular fibrillation, ventricular tachycardia

Drug Interactions

Metabolism/Transport Effects Substrate of CYP1A2 (minor), CYP2C9 (minor), CYP2D6 (minor), CYP2E1 (minor), CYP3A4 (major), P-glycoprotein; **Note:** Assignment of Major/Minor substrate status based on clinically relevant drug interaction potential; **Inhibits** CYP1A2 (weak), CYP2C9 (weak), CYP2D6 (weak)

Avoid Concomitant Use

Avoid concomitant use of Ondansetron with any of the following: Apomorphine; Artemether; Dronedarone; Lumefantrine; Nilotinib; Pimozide; QUEtiapine; QuiNINE; Tetrabenazine; Thioridazine; Toremifene; Vandetanib; Vemurafenib; Ziprasidone

Increased Effect/Toxicity

Ondansetron may increase the levels/effects of: Apomorphine; Dronedarone; Pimozide; QTc-Prolonging Agents; QuiNINE; Tetrabenazine; Thioridazine; Toremifene; Vandetanib; Vemurafenib; Ziprasidone

The levels/effects of Ondansetron may be increased by: Alfuzosin; Artemether; Chloroquine; Ciprofloxacin; Ciprofloxacin (Systemic); Conivaptan; Gadobutrol; Indacaterol; Lumefantrine; Nilotinib; P-glycoprotein/ABCB1 Inhibitors; QUEtiapine; QuiNINE

Decreased Effect

The levels/effects of Ondansetron may be decreased by: CYP3A4 Inducers (Strong); Cyproterone; Deferasirox; Peginterferon Alfa-2b; P-glycoprotein/ABCB1 Inducers; Rifamycin Derivatives; Tocilizumab

Ethanol/Nutrition/Herb Interactions

Food: Tablet: Food slightly increases the extent of absorption.

Herb/Nutraceutical: St John's wort may decrease ondansetron levels.

Stability

Oral soluble film: Store between 20°C and 25°C (68°F and 77°F). Store pouches in cartons; keep film in individual pouch until ready to use.

Oral solution: Store between 15°C and 30°C (59°F and 86°F). Protect from light.

Premixed bag: Store between 2°C and 30°C (36°F and 86°F). Protect from light.

Tablet: Store between 2°C and 30°C (36°F and 86°F).

Vial: Store between 2°C and 30°C (36°F and 86°F). Protect from light. Prior to I.V. infusion, dilute in 50 mL D_5W or NS. Solution is stable for 48 hours at room temperature.

Mechanism of Action Selective 5-HT_3-receptor antagonist, blocking serotonin, both peripherally on vagal nerve terminals and centrally in the chemoreceptor trigger zone

Pharmacodynamics/Kinetics

Onset of action: ~30 minutes

Absorption: Oral: Well absorbed from GI tract

Distribution: V_d: Children: 1.7-3.7 L/kg; Adults: 2.2-2.5 L/kg

Protein binding, plasma: 70% to 76%

Metabolism: Extensively hepatic via hydroxylation, followed by glucuronide or sulfate conjugation; CYP1A2, CYP2D6, and CYP3A4 substrate; some demethylation occurs

Bioavailability: Oral: 56% to 71% (some first pass metabolism); Rectal: 58% to 74%

Half-life elimination: Children <15 years: 2-7 hours; Adults: 3-6 hours

Mild-to-moderate hepatic impairment (Child-Pugh classes A and B): Adults: 12 hours

Severe hepatic impairment (Child-Pugh class C): Adults: 20 hours

Time to peak: Oral: ~2 hours; Oral soluble film: ~1 hour

Excretion: Urine (44% to 60% as metabolites, ~5% as unchanged drug); feces (~25%)

Dosage

Children:

I.V.: **Note:** Premixed injection not for use in children.

Prevention of chemotherapy-induced emesis: 6 months to 18 years: 0.15 mg/kg/dose administered 30 minutes prior to chemotherapy, 4 and 8 hours after the first dose **or** 0.45 mg/kg/day as a single dose

Prevention of postoperative nausea and vomiting: 1 month to 12 years:

≤40 kg: 0.1 mg/kg as a single dose

>40 kg: 4 mg as a single dose

Oral: Prevention of moderately-emetogenic chemotherapy-induced emesis:

4-11 years: 4 mg 30 minutes before chemotherapy; repeat 4 and 8 hours after initial dose, then 4 mg every 8 hours for 1-2 days after chemotherapy completed

≥12 years: Refer to adult dosing.

Adults:

I.V.:

Prevention of chemotherapy-induced emesis:

0.15 mg/kg 3 times/day beginning 30 minutes prior to chemotherapy **or**

0.45 mg/kg once daily **or**

8-10 mg 1-2 times/day **or**

24 mg or 32 mg once daily

Treatment of hyperemesis gravidum (unlabeled use): 8 mg administered over 15 minutes every 12 hours **or** 1 mg/hour infused continuously for up to 24 hours

I.M., I.V.: Postoperative nausea and vomiting (PONV): 4 mg as a single dose approximately 30 minutes before the end of anesthesia (see **"Note"** below) or as treatment if vomiting occurs after surgery (Gan, 2007).

Note: The manufacturer recommends administration immediately before induction of anesthesia; however, this has been shown not to be as effective as administration at the end of surgery (Sun, 1997). Repeat doses given in response to inadequate control of nausea/vomiting from preoperative doses are generally ineffective.

Oral:

Chemotherapy-induced emesis prophylaxis:

Highly-emetogenic agents/single-day therapy: 24 mg given 30 minutes prior to the start of therapy

Moderately-emetogenic agents: 8 mg beginning 30 minutes before chemotherapy; repeat dose 8 hours after initial dose, then 8 mg every 12 hours for 1-2 days after chemotherapy completed

Radiation-induced nausea and vomiting prophylaxis:
Total body irradiation: 8 mg 1-2 hours before daily each fraction of radiotherapy
Single high-dose fraction radiotherapy to abdomen: 8 mg 1-2 hours before irradiation, then 8 mg every 8 hours after first dose for 1-2 days after completion of radiotherapy
Daily fractionated radiotherapy to abdomen: 8 mg 1-2 hours before irradiation, then 8 mg 8 hours after first dose for each day of radiotherapy
Postoperative nausea and vomiting: 16 mg given 1 hour prior to induction of anesthesia
Treatment of hyperemesis gravidum (unlabeled use): 8 mg every 12 hours

Elderly: No dosing adjustment required

Dosage adjustment in renal impairment: No dosing adjustment required

Dosage adjustment in hepatic impairment: Severe liver disease (Child-Pugh C): Maximum daily dose: 8 mg

Dietary Considerations Take without regard to meals. Some products may contain phenylalanine.

Administration

Oral: Oral dosage forms should be administered 30 minutes prior to chemotherapy; 1-2 hours before radiotherapy; 1 hour prior to the induction of anesthesia.

Orally-disintegrating tablets: Do not remove from blister until needed. Peel backing off the blister, do not push tablet through. Using dry hands, place tablet on tongue and allow to dissolve. Swallow with saliva.

Oral soluble film: Do not remove from pouch until immediately before use. Using dry hands, place film on top of tongue and allow to dissolve (4-20 seconds). Swallow with or without liquid. If using more than one film, each film should be allowed to dissolve completely before administering the next film.

I.M.: Should be administered undiluted.

I.V.:

IVPB: Dilute in 50 mL D_5W or NS. Infuse over 15-30 minutes; 24-hour continuous infusions have been reported, but are rarely used.

Chemotherapy-induced nausea and vomiting: Give first dose 30 minutes prior to beginning chemotherapy.

I.V. push: Prevention of postoperative nausea and vomiting: Single doses may be administered I.V. injection over 2-5 minutes as undiluted solution.

Monitoring Parameters Closely monitor patients <4 months of age

Dosage Forms Excipient information presented when available (limited, particularly for generics); consult specific product labeling. [DSC] = Discontinued product

Film, soluble, oral:
Zuplenz®: 4 mg (10s); 8 mg (10s) [peppermint flavor]

Infusion, premixed in D_5W [preservative free]: 32 mg (50 mL)
Zofran®: 32 mg (50 mL)

Infusion, premixed in NS [preservative free]: 32 mg (50 mL)

Injection, solution: 2 mg/mL (2 mL, 20 mL)
Zofran®: 2 mg/mL (20 mL)

Injection, solution [preservative free]: 2 mg/mL (2 mL)

Solution, oral: 4 mg/5 mL (5 mL, 50 mL)
Zofran®: 4 mg/5 mL (50 mL) [contains sodium benzoate; strawberry flavor]

Tablet, oral: 4 mg, 8 mg, 24 mg [DSC]
Zofran®: 4 mg, 8 mg

Tablet, orally disintegrating, oral: 4 mg, 8 mg
Zofran® ODT: 4 mg, 8 mg [contains phenylalanine <0.03 mg/tablet; strawberry flavor]

Extemporaneous Preparations Note: Commercial oral solution is available (0.8 mg/mL)

If commercial oral solution is unavailable, a 0.8 mg/mL syrup may be made with ondansetron tablets, Ora-Plus® (Paddock), and any of the the following syrups: Cherry syrup USP, Syrpalta® (HUMCO), Ora-Sweet® (Paddock), or Ora-Sweet® Sugar-Free (Paddock). Crush ten 8 mg tablets in a mortar and reduce to a fine powder (flaking of the tablet coating occurs). Add 50 mL Ora-Plus® in 5 mL increments, mixing thoroughly; mix while adding the chosen syrup in incremental proportions to **almost** 100 mL; transfer to a calibrated bottle, rinse mortar with syrup, and add sufficient quantity of syrup to make 100 mL. Label "shake well" and "refrigerate". Stable for 42 days refrigerated (Trissel, 1996).

Rectal suppositories: Calibrate a suppository mold for the base being used. Determine the displacement factor (DF) for ondansetron for the base being used (Fattibase® = 1.1; Polybase® = 0.6). Weigh the ondansetron tablet(s). Divide the tablet weight by the DF; this result is the weight of base displaced by the drug. Subtract the weight of base displaced from the calculated weight of base required for each suppository. Grind the ondansetron tablets in a mortar and reduce to a fine powder. Weigh out the appropriate weight of suppository base. Melt the base over a water bath (<55°C). Add the ondansetron powder to the suppository base and mix well. Pour the mixture into the suppository mold and cool. Stable for at least 30 days refrigerated (Tenjarla, 1998).

Tenjarla SN, Ward ES, and Fox JL, "Ondansetron Suppositories: Extemporaneous Preparation, Drug Release, Stability and Flux Through Rabbit Rectal Membrane," *Int J Pharm Compound*, 1998, 2(1):83-8.

Trissel LA, *Trissel's Stability of Compounded Formulations*, Washington, DC: American Pharmaceutical Association, 1996.

◆ **Opium and Belladonna** *see* Belladonna and Opium *on page 197*

Opium Tincture (OH pee um TING chur)

Index Terms Deodorized Tincture of Opium (error-prone synonym); DTO (error-prone abbreviation); Opium Tincture, Deodorized; Tincture of Opium

Pharmacologic Category Analgesic, Opioid; Antidiarrheal

Use Treatment of diarrhea in adults

Lactation Enters breast milk/use caution

Contraindications Hypersensitivity to opium, morphine sulfate, or any component of the formulation; diarrhea caused by poisoning prior to the toxic material being removed from the GI tract

Note: Manufacturer does not recommend use in children.

Warnings/Precautions May cause CNS depression, which may impair physical or mental abilities; patients must be cautioned about performing tasks which require mental alertness (eg, operating machinery or driving). Effects may be potentiated when used with other sedative drugs or ethanol. Opium shares the toxic potential of opiate agonists, and usual precautions of opiate agonist therapy should be observed; use with caution in patients with CNS depression or coma, morbid obesity, adrenal insufficiency, hepatic impairment, head trauma, GI hemorrhage, thyroid dysfunction, prostatic hyperplasia/urinary stricture, respiratory disease, or a history of drug abuse. Use with caution in patients with biliary tract dysfunction; acute pancreatitis may cause constriction of sphincter of Oddi. May cause hypotension; use with caution in patients with hypovolemia, cardiovascular disease (including acute MI), or with drugs which may exaggerate hypotensive effects (including phenothiazines or general anesthetics). May obscure diagnosis or clinical course of patients with acute abdominal conditions. Concurrent use of agonist/antagonist analgesics may precipitate withdrawal symptoms and/or reduced analgesic efficacy in patients following prolonged therapy with mu opioid agonists. Abrupt discontinuation following prolonged use may also lead to withdrawal symptoms. Use with caution in the elderly and debilitated patients; may be more sensitive to adverse effects. Some preparations contain sulfites which may cause allergic reactions. Infants <3 months of age are more susceptible to respiratory depression; if used, diluted doses are recommended and use with caution. Manufacturer does not recommend use in children.

Do not confuse opium tincture with paregoric; opium tincture is 25 times more potent than paregoric; opium shares the toxic potential of opiate agonists, usual precautions of opiate agonist therapy should be observed; opium may mask dehydration by producing fluid retention in the bowel; monitor patients with prolonged or severe diarrhea carefully; abrupt discontinuation after prolonged use may result in withdrawal symptoms.

Adverse Reactions Frequency not defined.

Cardiovascular: Palpitation, hypotension, bradycardia, peripheral vasodilation

Central nervous system: Drowsiness, dizziness, restlessness, headache, malaise, CNS depression, intracranial pressure increased, insomnia, mental depression

Gastrointestinal: Nausea, vomiting, constipation, anorexia, stomach cramps, biliary tract spasm

Genitourinary: Urination decreased, urinary tract spasm

Neuromuscular & skeletal: Weakness

Ocular: Miosis

Respiratory: Respiratory depression

Miscellaneous: Histamine release, physical and psychological dependence

Drug Interactions

Metabolism/Transport Effects None known.

Avoid Concomitant Use There are no known interactions where it is recommended to avoid concomitant use.

Increased Effect/Toxicity

Opium Tincture may increase the levels/effects of: Alcohol (Ethyl); Alvimopan; CNS Depressants; Desmopressin; Selective Serotonin Reuptake Inhibitors; Thiazide Diuretics

The levels/effects of Opium Tincture may be increased by: Amphetamines; Antipsychotic Agents (Phenothiazines); Droperidol; HydrOXYzine; Succinylcholine

Decreased Effect

Opium Tincture may decrease the levels/effects of: Pegvisomant

The levels/effects of Opium Tincture may be decreased by: Ammonium Chloride; Mixed Agonist / Antagonist Opioids

Ethanol/Nutrition/Herb Interactions Ethanol: May increase CNS depression; monitor for increased effects with coadministration. Caution patients about effects.

Stability Store at 68° to 77°F (20° to 25°C). Protect from light.

Mechanism of Action Contains many narcotic alkaloids including morphine; its mechanism for gastric motility inhibition is primarily due to this morphine content; it results in a decrease in digestive secretions, an increase in GI muscle tone, and therefore a reduction in GI propulsion

Pharmacodynamics/Kinetics

Duration: 4-5 hours

Absorption: Variable

Metabolism: Hepatic

Excretion: Urine

Dosage Oral: **Note:** Opium tincture 10% contains morphine 10 mg/mL. Use caution in ordering, dispensing, and/or administering. The following doses are expressed in **mg** (milligram) dosing units of morphine.

Adults: Diarrhea: Usual: 6 **mg** of undiluted opium tincture (10 mg/mL) 4 times daily

Administration May administer with food to decrease GI upset.

Monitoring Parameters Observe patient for excessive sedation, respiratory depression, implement safety measures, assist with ambulation

Test Interactions Increased aminotransferase [ALT/AST] (S)

Dosage Forms Excipient information presented when available (limited, particularly for generics); consult specific product labeling.

Tincture, oral: Anhydrous morphine 10 mg/mL (120 mL, 480 mL) [0.6 mL equivalent to morphine 6 mg; contains ethanol 19%]

Controlled Substance C-II

◆ **Opium Tincture, Deodorized** *see* Opium Tincture *on page 1249*

Oprelvekin (oh PREL ve kin)

Brand Names: U.S. Neumega®

Index Terms IL-11; Interleukin-11; Recombinant Human Interleukin-11; Recombinant Interleukin-11; rhIL-11

Pharmacologic Category Biological Response Modulator; Human Growth Factor

Use Prevention of severe thrombocytopenia; reduce the need for platelet transfusions following myelosuppressive chemotherapy for nonmyeloid malignancy

Pregnancy Risk Factor C

Pregnancy Considerations Animal studies have demonstrated adverse fetal effects. There are no adequate and well-controlled studies in pregnant women. Use during pregnancy only if the potential benefits outweigh the potential risk to the fetus.

Lactation Excretion in breast milk unknown/not recommended

Contraindications Hypersensitivity to oprelvekin or any component of the formulation

Warnings/Precautions [U.S. Boxed Warning]: Allergic or hypersensitivity reactions, including anaphylaxis have been reported. Permanently discontinue in any patient developing an allergic or hypersensitivity reaction. May occur with the first or with subsequent doses. May cause serious fluid retention (reversible) which may result in peripheral edema, capillary leak syndrome, arrhythmias, or exacerbation of pleural effusion. Use cautiously in patients with conditions where expansion of plasma volume should be avoided (eg, left ventricular dysfunction, HF, hypertension). Monitor fluid balance. Closely monitor fluid and electrolytes in patient on chronic diuretic therapy; severe hypokalemia contributing to sudden death have been reported in these patients. Reversible dilutional anemia may occur due to increased plasma volume; generally appears within 3-5 days of initiation of therapy and resolves over ~1 week following discontinuation. Atrial arrhythmias, pulmonary edema, and cardiac arrest have been reported; use in patients with a history of atrial arrhythmia only if the potential benefit exceeds possible risks. Patients experiencing arrhythmia may be at risk for stroke; use caution in patients with a history of transient ischemic attack or stroke. Ventricular arrhythmia has also been reported, occurring within 2-7 days of treatment initiation. Use caution in patients with conduction defects; history of thromboembolic problems; pre-existing pericardial effusions or ascites. May cause exacerbation of effusion; consider drainage if indicated. Use with caution in renal dysfunction; dosage adjustment required in severe renal impairment; monitor fluid balance.

Not indicated following myeloablative chemotherapy; increased toxicities were reported when used following myeloablative therapy. A higher incidence of adverse events has been reported when used following bone marrow transplantation. Begin 6-24 hours following completion of chemotherapy; use has not been adequately studied immediately before or during chemotherapy. Efficacy has not been established with chemotherapy regimens >5 days duration or with regimens associated with delayed myelosuppression (eg, nitrosoureas, mitomycin C). Safety and efficacy have not been established with chronic administration. Papilledema, more frequently associated with use in children, has occurred (usually following repeated cycles); use caution in patients with pre-existing papilledema or with tumors involving the central nervous system; may worsen pre-existing papilledema. Papilledema is dose limiting. Patients experiencing oprelvekin-related papilledema may be at risk for visual acuity changes, including blurred vision or blindness. Although used in children in clinical trials, safety and efficacy have not been established in pediatric patients. The incidence of certain adverse events may be higher in children. Use in children, especially <12 years of age, should be as part of a clinical trial.

Adverse Reactions

>10%:

Cardiovascular: Tachycardia (children 84%; adults 20%), edema (59%), cardiomegaly (children 21%), vasodilation (19%), atrial arrhythmia (12% to 15%), palpitation (14%), syncope (13%)

Central nervous system: Neutropenic fever (48%), headache (41%), dizziness (38%), fever (36%), insomnia (33%)

Dermatologic: Rash (25%)

Endocrine & metabolic: Fluid retention

Gastrointestinal: Nausea/vomiting (77%), diarrhea (43%), mucositis (43%), oral moniliasis (14%), weight gain (due to fluid retention)

Hematologic: Anemia (dilutional; onset: 3-5 days; duration: ≤1 week)

Neuromuscular & skeletal: Weakness (severe 14%), periostitis (children 11%), arthralgia

Ocular: Conjunctival injection/redness/swelling (children 57%; adults 19%), papilledema (children 16%; adults 1%)

Respiratory: Dyspnea (48%), rhinitis (42%), cough (29%), pharyngitis (25%)

1% to 10%: Respiratory: Pleural effusion (10%)

<1% (Limited to important or life-threatening): Allergic reaction, amblyopia, anaphylaxis/anaphylactoid reactions, blindness, blurred vision, capillary leak syndrome, cardiac arrest, chest pain, dehydration, dysarthria, exfoliative dermatitis, eye hemorrhage, facial edema, fibrinogen increased, fluid overload, HF, hypoalbuminemia, hypocalcemia, hypokalemia, hypotension, injection site reactions (dermatitis, pain, discoloration), loss of consciousness, mental status changes, optic neuropathy, paresthesia, pericardial effusion, peripheral edema, pneumonia, pulmonary edema, renal failure, shock, skin discoloration, stroke, urticaria, ventricular arrhythmia, visual acuity changes, visual field defect, von Willebrand factor concentration increased, wheezing

Drug Interactions

Metabolism/Transport Effects None known.

Avoid Concomitant Use There are no known interactions where it is recommended to avoid concomitant use.

Increased Effect/Toxicity There are no known significant interactions involving an increase in effect.

Decreased Effect There are no known significant interactions involving a decrease in effect.

Stability Store vials under refrigeration between 2°C to 8°C (36°F to 46°F); do not freeze. Protect from light. Reconstitute to a final concentration of 5 mg/mL with SWFI; direct diluent down side of vial, swirl gently, do not shake. Use reconstituted oprelvekin within 3 hours of reconstitution; store reconstituted solution in the vial at either 2°C to 8°C (36°F to 46°F) or room temperature of ≤25°C (77°F). Do not freeze or shake reconstituted solution.

Mechanism of Action Oprelvekin is a thrombopoietic growth factor which stimulates multiple stages of megakaryocytopoiesis and thrombopoiesis, resulting in proliferation of megakaryocyte progenitors and megakaryocyte maturation, thereby increasing platelet production.

Pharmacodynamics/Kinetics

Bioavailability: >80%

Half-life elimination: Terminal: 5-9 hours

Time to peak, serum: 1-6 hours

Excretion: Urine (primarily as metabolites)

Dosage SubQ: Administer first dose ~6-24 hours after the end of chemotherapy. Discontinue at least 48 hours before beginning the next cycle of chemotherapy.

Adults: 50 mcg/kg once daily for ~10-21 days (until postnadir platelet count ≥50,000/mm^3)

Dosage adjustment in renal impairment: Cl_{cr} <30 mL/minute: 25 mcg/kg once daily for ~10-21 days (until postnadir platelet count ≥50,000/mm^3)

Administration Subcutaneously in the abdomen, thigh, hip, or upper arm.

Monitoring Parameters Monitor electrolytes and fluid balance during therapy; obtain a CBC at regular intervals during therapy; monitor platelet counts until adequate recovery has occurred; renal function (at baseline)

Dosage Forms Excipient information presented when available (limited, particularly for generics); consult specific product labeling.

Injection, powder for reconstitution [preservative free]:

Neumega®: 5 mg [supplied with diluent]

◆ **OPT-80** *see* Fidaxomicin *on page* 710

◆ **Optase™** *see* Trypsin, Balsam Peru, and Castor Oil *on page* 1744

◆ **Optho-Bunolol® (Can)** *see* Levobunolol *on page* 995

◆ **Opticrom® (Can)** *see* Cromolyn (Ophthalmic) *on page* 418

◆ **Optimyxin® (Can)** *see* Bacitracin and Polymyxin B *on page* 186

◆ **Optimyxin Plus® (Can)** *see* Neomycin, Polymyxin B, and Gramicidin *on page* 1189

◆ **OptiPranolol®** *see* Metipranolol *on page* 1114

◆ **Optivar®** *see* Azelastine (Ophthalmic) *on page* 179

◆ **Orabase® with Benzocaine [OTC]** *see* Benzocaine *on page* 202

◆ **Oracea®** *see* Doxycycline *on page* 557

◆ **Oracit®** *see* Sodium Citrate and Citric Acid *on page* 1570

◆ **Oracort (Can)** *see* Triamcinolone (Topical) *on page* 1735

◆ **Orajel® [OTC]** *see* Benzocaine *on page* 202

◆ **Orajel® Baby Daytime and Nighttime [OTC]** *see* Benzocaine *on page* 202

◆ **Orajel® Baby Teething [OTC]** *see* Benzocaine *on page* 202

◆ **Orajel® Baby Teething Nighttime [OTC]** *see* Benzocaine *on page* 202

◆ **Orajel® Cold Sore [OTC]** *see* Benzocaine *on page* 202

◆ **Orajel® Denture Plus [OTC]** *see* Benzocaine *on page* 202

◆ **Orajel® Maximum Strength [OTC]** *see* Benzocaine *on page* 202

◆ **Orajel® Medicated Mouth Sore [OTC]** *see* Benzocaine *on page* 202

◆ **Orajel® Medicated Toothache [OTC]** *see* Benzocaine *on page* 202

◆ **Orajel® Mouth Sore [OTC]** *see* Benzocaine *on page* 202

◆ **Orajel® Multi-Action Cold Sore [OTC]** *see* Benzocaine *on page* 202

◆ **Orajel® PM Maximum Strength [OTC]** *see* Benzocaine *on page* 202

◆ **Orajel® Ultra Mouth Sore [OTC]** *see* Benzocaine *on page* 202

◆ **Oralone®** *see* Triamcinolone (Topical) *on page* 1735

◆ **Oramorph® SR** *see* Morphine (Systemic) *on page* 1153

◆ **Oranyl [OTC]** *see* Pseudoephedrine *on page* 1430

◆ **Orap®** *see* Pimozide *on page* 1354

◆ **Orapred®** *see* PrednisoLONE (Systemic) *on page* 1396

◆ **Orapred ODT®** *see* PrednisoLONE (Systemic) *on page* 1396

◆ **Oraqix®** *see* Lidocaine and Prilocaine *on page* 1010

◆ **OraVerse™** *see* Phentolamine *on page* 1343

◆ **Oravig® [DSC]** *see* Miconazole (Oral) *on page* 1125

◆ **Oraxyl™** *see* Doxycycline *on page* 557

◆ **Orazinc® 110 [OTC]** *see* Zinc Sulfate *on page* 1818

◆ **Orazinc® 220 [OTC]** *see* Zinc Sulfate *on page* 1818

◆ **Orbivan™** *see* Butalbital, Acetaminophen, and Caffeine *on page* 255

◆ **Orciprenaline Sulfate** *see* Metaproterenol *on page* 1085

◆ **Orencia®** *see* Abatacept *on page* 20

◆ **Orfadin®** *see* Nitisinone *on page* 1210

◆ **ORG 9426** *see* Rocuronium *on page* 1512

◆ **Orgalutran® (Can)** *see* Ganirelix *on page* 779

◆ **Organidin® NR [OTC] [DSC]** *see* GuaiFENesin *on page* 809

◆ **ORG NC 45** *see* Vecuronium *on page* 1777

◆ **Orinase** *see* TOLBUTamide *on page* 1702

Orlistat (OR li stat)

Brand Names: U.S. Alli® [OTC]; Xenical®

Brand Names: Canada Xenical®

Pharmacologic Category Lipase Inhibitor

Use Management of obesity, including weight loss and weight management, when used in conjunction with a reduced-calorie and low-fat diet; reduce the risk of weight regain after prior weight loss; indicated for obese patients with an initial body mass index (BMI) ≥30 kg/m^2 or ≥27 kg/m^2 in the presence of other risk factors (eg, diabetes, dyslipidemia, hypertension)

Pregnancy Risk Factor B

Pregnancy Considerations Teratogenic effects or embryotoxicity were not observed in animal studies. There are no adequate and well-controlled studies in pregnant women. Because animal reproductive studies are not always predictive of human response, orlistat is not recommended for use during pregnancy.

Lactation Excretion in breast milk unknown/not recommended

Contraindications Hypersensitivity to orlistat or any component of the formulation; chronic malabsorption syndrome or cholestasis

Warnings/Precautions Prior to use other causes for obesity (eg, hypothyroidism) should be ruled out. Cases of severe liver injury (some fatal) with hepatocellular necrosis or acute hepatic failure have been reported (rare); liver transplantation has been required in some patients. Patients should be instructed to report any symptoms of hepatic dysfunction (eg, anorexia, pruritus, jaundice, dark urine, light colored stools, right upper quadrant pain); discontinue orlistat and obtain liver function test immediately if symptoms occur. Advise patients to adhere to dietary guidelines; if taken with a diet high in fat (>30% total daily calories from fat) gastrointestinal adverse events may increase. Distribute daily fat intake over 3 main meals. If taken with any 1 meal very high in fat, the possibility of gastrointestinal effects increases. Counsel patients to take a multivitamin supplement that contains fat-soluble vitamins ≥2 hours before or after orlistat administration to ensure adequate nutrition; orlistat has been shown to reduce the absorption of some fat-soluble vitamins and beta-carotene. Increased levels of urinary oxalate following treatment may occur in some patients; use with caution in patients with a history of hyperoxaluria or calcium oxalate nephrolithiasis. The potential exists for misuse in inappropriate patient populations (eg, patients with anorexia nervosa or bulimia) similar to any weight loss agent. In general, substantial weight loss may increase the risk of cholelithiasis. Safety and efficacy with >4 years of use have not been established.

Self-medication (OTC use): Prior to use, patients should contact their healthcare provider if they have ever had kidney stones, gall bladder disease, or pancreatitis. Patients taking medications for diabetes or thyroid disease, anticoagulants, or other weight-loss products should consult their healthcare provider or pharmacist. Patients who have had an organ transplant should not use orlistat. If severe and/or continuous abdominal pain, itching, yellowing of the eyes or skin, dark urine, or loss of appetite occurs, use should be discontinued and healthcare provider consulted.

Adverse Reactions Note: The frequency of most adverse reactions (especially gastrointestinal effects) decreases over time.

>10%:

Central nervous system: Headache (≤31%)

Gastrointestinal: Oily spotting (4% to 27%), abdominal pain/discomfort (≤26%), flatus with discharge (2% to 24%), fecal urgency (3% to 22%), fatty/oily stool (6% to 20%), oily evacuation (2% to 12%), defecation increased (3% to 11%)

Neuromuscular & skeletal: Back pain (≤14%)

Respiratory: Upper respiratory infection (26% to 38%)

Miscellaneous: Influenza (≤40%)

1% to 10%:

Cardiovascular: Pedal edema (≤3%)

Central nervous system: Fatigue (3% to 7%), anxiety (3% to 5%), sleep disorder (≤4%)

Dermatologic: Dry skin (≤2%)

Endocrine & metabolic: Menstrual irregularities (≤10%)

Gastrointestinal: Nausea (4% to 8%), fecal incontinence (2% to 8%), infectious diarrhea (≤5%), rectal pain/discomfort (3% to 5%), gingival disorder (2% to 4%)

Genitourinary: Urinary tract infection (6% to 8%), vaginitis (3% to 4%)

Neuromuscular & skeletal: Myalgia (≤4%)

Otic: Otitis (3% to 4%)

Respiratory: Lower respiratory infection (≤8%)

<1% (Limited to important or life-threatening): Abdominal distension (in patients with diabetes), alkaline phosphatase increased, anaphylaxis, angioedema, bronchospasm, bullous eruption, cholelithiasis (may be caused by weight loss), coagulation parameters altered (concurrent use with warfarin), hepatic failure, hepatitis (causal relationship not established), hypersensitivity, hypoglycemia (in patients with diabetes), hypothyroidism (concurrent use with levothyroxine), kidney injury (acute), pancreatitis, pruritus, rash, transaminases increased, urinary oxalate levels increased, urticaria

Drug Interactions

Metabolism/Transport Effects None known.

Avoid Concomitant Use There are no known interactions where it is recommended to avoid concomitant use.

Increased Effect/Toxicity

Orlistat may increase the levels/effects of: Warfarin

Decreased Effect

Orlistat may decrease the levels/effects of: Amiodarone; CycloSPORINE; CycloSPORINE (Systemic); Levothyroxine; Paricalcitol; Propafenone; Vitamin D Analogs; Vitamins (Fat Soluble)

Ethanol/Nutrition/Herb Interactions Fat-soluble vitamins: Absorption of vitamins A, D, E, and K may be decreased by orlistat. A multivitamin containing the fat-soluble vitamins (A, D, E, and K) should be administered once daily at least 2 hours before or after orlistat.

Stability Store at 25°C (77°F); excursions permitted to 15°C to 30°C (59°F to 86°F).

Mechanism of Action A reversible inhibitor of gastric and pancreatic lipases, thus inhibiting absorption of dietary fats by 30% (at doses of 120 mg 3 times/day).

Pharmacodynamics/Kinetics

Onset of action: 24-48 hours

Duration: 48-72 hours

Absorption: Minimal

Metabolism: Metabolized within the gastrointestinal wall; forms inactive metabolites

Excretion: Feces (~97%, 83% as unchanged drug); urine (<2%)

Dosage Oral:

Children ≥12 years and Adults (Xenical®): 120 mg 3 times/day with each main meal containing fat (during or up to 1 hour after the meal); omit dose if meal is occasionally missed or contains no fat.

Adults (Alli™): OTC labeling: 60 mg 3 times/day with each main meal containing fat

Dietary Considerations Multivitamin supplements that contain fat-soluble vitamins should be taken once daily at least 2 hours before or after the administration of orlistat (ie, bedtime). Gastrointestinal effects of orlistat may increase if taken with any one meal very high in fat. Distribute daily intake of carbohydrates, fat (~30% of daily calories), and protein over three main meals.

Administration Administer during or up to 1 hour after each main meal containing fat.

Monitoring Parameters BMI; diet (calorie and fat intake); serum glucose in patients with diabetes; thyroid function in patient with thyroid disease; liver function tests in patients exhibiting symptoms of hepatic dysfunction; cyclosporine levels closely if taking cyclosporine

Dosage Forms Excipient information presented when available (limited, particularly for generics); consult specific product labeling.

Capsule, oral:

Alli®: 60 mg

Xenical®: 120 mg

◆ **Ornex® [OTC]** *see* Acetaminophen and Pseudoephedrine *on page 31*

◆ **Ornex® Maximum Strength [OTC]** *see* Acetaminophen and Pseudoephedrine *on page 31*

◆ **ORO-Clense (Can)** *see* Chlorhexidine Gluconate *on page 341*

◆ **Orphenace® (Can)** *see* Orphenadrine *on page 1252*

Orphenadrine (or FEN a dreen)

Brand Names: U.S. Norflex™

Brand Names: Canada Norflex™; Orphenace®; Rhoxal-orphendrine

Index Terms Orphenadrine Citrate

Pharmacologic Category Skeletal Muscle Relaxant

Additional Appendix Information

Beers Criteria – Potentially Inappropriate Medications for Geriatrics *on page 1973*

Use Treatment of muscle spasm associated with acute painful musculoskeletal conditions

Pregnancy Risk Factor C

Dosage

Adults:

Oral: 100 mg twice daily

I.M., I.V.: 60 mg every 12 hours

Elderly: Use caution; generally not recommended for use in the elderly

Additional Information Complete prescribing information for this medication should be consulted for additional detail.

Dosage Forms Excipient information presented when available (limited, particularly for generics); consult specific product labeling.

Injection, solution, as citrate: 30 mg/mL (2 mL)

Norflex™: 30 mg/mL (2 mL) [contains sodium bisulfite]

Tablet, extended release, oral, as citrate: 100 mg

Orphenadrine, Aspirin, and Caffeine

(or FEN a dreen, AS pir in, & KAF een)

Index Terms Aspirin, Caffeine, and Orphenadrine; Aspirin, Orphenadrine, and Caffeine; Caffeine, Orphenadrine, and Aspirin; Norgesic

Pharmacologic Category Skeletal Muscle Relaxant

Use Relief of discomfort associated with skeletal muscular conditions

Dosage Oral: 1-2 tablets 3-4 times/day

Additional Information Complete prescribing information for this medication should be consulted for additional detail.

Dosage Forms Excipient information presented when available (limited, particularly for generics); consult specific product labeling.

Tablet: Orphenadrine citrate 25 mg, aspirin 385 mg, and caffeine 30 mg; orphenadrine citrate 50 mg, aspirin 770 mg, and caffeine 60 mg

◆ **Orphenadrine Citrate** *see* Orphenadrine *on page 1252*

◆ **Orsythia™** *see* Ethinyl Estradiol and Levonorgestrel *on page 656*

◆ **Ortho® 0.5/35 (Can)** *see* Ethinyl Estradiol and Norethindrone *on page 660*

◆ **Ortho® 1/35 (Can)** *see* Ethinyl Estradiol and Norethindrone *on page 660*

◆ **Ortho® 7/7/7 (Can)** *see* Ethinyl Estradiol and Norethindrone *on page 660*

◆ **Ortho Cept** *see* Ethinyl Estradiol and Desogestrel *on page 653*

◆ **Ortho-Cept®** *see* Ethinyl Estradiol and Desogestrel *on page 653*

◆ **Ortho Cyclen** *see* Ethinyl Estradiol and Norgestimate *on page 663*

◆ **Ortho-Cyclen®** *see* Ethinyl Estradiol and Norgestimate *on page 663*

◆ **Ortho Est** *see* Estropipate *on page 648*

◆ **Ortho-Evra** *see* Ethinyl Estradiol and Norelgestromin *on page 660*

◆ **Ortho Evra®** *see* Ethinyl Estradiol and Norelgestromin *on page 660*

◆ **Ortho Micronor®** *see* Norethindrone *on page 1217*

◆ **Ortho Novum** *see* Ethinyl Estradiol and Norethindrone *on page 660*

◆ **Ortho-Novum® 1/35** *see* Ethinyl Estradiol and Norethindrone *on page 660*

◆ **Ortho Novum 1/50** *see* Norethindrone and Mestranol *on page 1219*

◆ **Ortho-Novum® 1/50 (Can)** *see* Norethindrone and Mestranol *on page 1219*

◆ **Ortho-Novum® 7/7/7** *see* Ethinyl Estradiol and Norethindrone *on page 660*

◆ **Ortho,para-DDD** *see* Mitotane *on page 1144*

◆ **Ortho Tri Cyclen** *see* Ethinyl Estradiol and Norgestimate *on page 663*

◆ **Ortho Tri-Cyclen®** *see* Ethinyl Estradiol and Norgestimate *on page 663*

◆ **Ortho Tri-Cyclen® Lo** *see* Ethinyl Estradiol and Norgestimate *on page 663*

◆ **Orthovisc®** *see* Hyaluronate and Derivatives *on page 831*

◆ **OrthoVisc® (Can)** *see* Hyaluronate and Derivatives *on page 831*

◆ **OrthoWash™** *see* Fluoride *on page 728*

◆ **Oscal** *see* Calcium Carbonate *on page 266*

◆ **Os-Cal® (Can)** *see* Calcium Carbonate *on page 266*

◆ **Os-Cal® 500+D [OTC]** *see* Calcium and Vitamin D *on page 265*

◆ **Oscimin** *see* Hyoscyamine *on page 854*

Oseltamivir (oh sel TAM i vir)

Brand Names: U.S. Tamiflu®

Brand Names: Canada Tamiflu®

Pharmacologic Category Antiviral Agent; Neuraminidase Inhibitor

Use Treatment of uncomplicated acute illness due to influenza (A or B) infection in children ≥1 year of age and adults who have been symptomatic for no more than 2 days; prophylaxis against influenza (A or B) infection in children ≥1 year of age and adults

The Advisory Committee on Immunization Practices (ACIP) recommends that **treatment** be considered for the following:

- Persons with severe, complicated or progressive illness
- Hospitalized persons
- Persons at higher risk for influenza complications:
  - Children <2 years of age (highest risk in children <6 months of age)
  - Adults ≥65 years of age
  - Persons with chronic disorders of the pulmonary (including asthma) or cardiovascular systems (except hypertension)
  - Persons with chronic metabolic diseases (including diabetes mellitus), hepatic disease, renal dysfunction, hematologic disorders (including sickle cell disease), or immunosuppression (including immunosuppression caused by medications or HIV)
  - Persons with neurologic/neuromuscular conditions (including conditions such as spinal cord injuries, seizure disorders, cerebral palsy, stroke, mental retardation, moderate to severe developmental delay, or muscular dystrophy) which may compromise respiratory function, the handling of respiratory secretions, or that can increase the risk of aspiration
  - Pregnant or postpartum women (≤2 weeks after delivery)
  - Persons <19 years of age on long-term aspirin therapy
  - American Indians and Alaskan Natives
  - Persons who are morbidly obese (BMI ≥40)
  - Residents of nursing homes or other chronic care facilities
- Use may also be considered for previously healthy, nonhigh-risk outpatients with confirmed or suspected influenza based on clinical judgment when treatment can be started within 48 hours of illness onset.

The ACIP recommends that **prophylaxis** be considered for the following:

- Postexposure prophylaxis may be considered for family or close contacts of suspected or confirmed cases, who are at higher risk of influenza complications, and who have not been vaccinated against the circulating strain at the time of the exposure.
- Postexposure prophylaxis may be considered for unvaccinated healthcare workers who had occupational exposure without protective equipment.
- Pre-exposure prophylaxis should only be used for persons at very high risk of influenza complications who cannot be otherwise protected at times of high risk for exposure.
- Prophylaxis should also be administered to all eligible residents of institutions that house patients at high risk when needed to control outbreaks.

The ACIP recommends that treatment and prophylaxis be given to children <1 year of age when indicated.

Pregnancy Risk Factor C

Pregnancy Considerations In animal reproduction studies, a dose-dependent increase in the rates of minor skeleton abnormalities was found in exposed offspring. The rate of each abnormality remained within the ▶

background rate of occurrence in the species studied. In an *in vitro* study, placental transfer of oseltamivir phosphate and its active metabolite oseltamivir carboxylate was found to be incomplete, resulting in minimal accumulation in the fetus. An increased risk of adverse neonatal outcomes has generally not been observed following maternal use of oseltamivir during pregnancy. Untreated influenza infection is associated with an increased risk of adverse events to the fetus and an increased risk of complications or death to the mother. Oseltamivir and zanamivir are currently recommended for the treatment or prophylaxis of influenza in pregnant women and women up to 2 weeks postpartum. Oseltamivir and zanamivir are currently recommended as an adjunct to vaccination and should not be used as a substitute for vaccination in pregnant women (consult current CDC guidelines).

Lactation Enters breast milk/not recommended

Contraindications Hypersensitivity to oseltamivir or any component of the formulation

Warnings/Precautions Oseltamivir is not a substitute for the influenza virus vaccine. It has not been shown to prevent primary or concomitant bacterial infections that may occur with influenza virus. Use caution with renal impairment; dosage adjustment is required for creatinine clearance <30 mL/minute. Safety and efficacy for use in patients with chronic cardiac and/or kidney disease, severe hepatic impairment, or for treatment or prophylaxis in immunocompromised patients have not been established. Rare but severe hypersensitivity reactions (anaphylaxis, severe dermatologic reactions) have been associated with use. Rare occurrences of neuropsychiatric events (including confusion, delirium, hallucinations, and/or self-injury) have been reported from postmarketing surveillance (primarily in pediatric patients); direct causation is difficult to establish (influenza infection may also be associated with behavioral and neurologic changes). Monitor closely for signs of any unusual behavior.

Antiviral treatment should begin within 48 hours of symptom onset. However, the CDC recommends that treatment may still be beneficial and should be started in hospitalized patients with severe, complicated or progressive illness if >48 hours. Nonhospitalized persons who are not at high risk for developing severe or complicated illness and who have a mild disease are not likely to benefit if treatment is started >48 hours after symptom onset. Nonhospitalized persons who are already beginning to recover do not need treatment.

Adverse Reactions

>10%: Gastrointestinal: Vomiting (2% to 15%)

1% to 10%:

- Gastrointestinal: Nausea (4% to 10%), abdominal pain (2% to 5%), diarrhea (1% to 3%)
- Ocular: Conjunctivitis (1%)
- Respiratory: Epistaxis (1%)

<1% (Limited to important or life-threatening): Allergy, anaphylactic/anaphylactoid reaction, angina, arrhythmia, confusion, erythema multiforme, fracture, gastrointestinal bleeding, hemorrhagic colitis, hepatitis, liver function tests abnormal, neuropsychiatric events, pseudomembranous colitis, pyrexia, seizure, Stevens-Johnson syndrome, swelling of face or tongue, toxic epidermal necrolysis

Drug Interactions

Metabolism/Transport Effects None known.

Avoid Concomitant Use There are no known interactions where it is recommended to avoid concomitant use.

Increased Effect/Toxicity

The levels/effects of Oseltamivir may be increased by: Probenecid

Decreased Effect

Oseltamivir may decrease the levels/effects of: Influenza Virus Vaccine (Live/Attenuated)

Stability

Capsules: Store at 25°C (77°F); excursions permitted to 15°C to 30°C (59°F to 86°F).

Oral suspension: Store powder for suspension at 25°C (77°F); excursions permitted to 15°C to 30°C (59°F to 86°F). Once reconstituted, store suspension under refrigeration at 2°C to 8°C (36°F to 46°F); do not freeze. Use within 10 days of preparation if stored at room temperature or within 17 days of preparation if stored under refrigeration.

New concentration (6 mg/mL): Reconstitute with 55 mL of water to a final concentration of 6 mg/mL (to make 60 mL total suspension).

Discontinued concentration (12 mg/mL): Reconstitute with 23 mL of water to a final concentration of 12 mg/mL (to make 25 mL total suspension).

Mechanism of Action Oseltamivir, a prodrug, is hydrolyzed to the active form, oseltamivir carboxylate (OC). OC inhibits influenza virus neuraminidase, an enzyme known to cleave the budding viral progeny from its cellular envelope attachment point (neuraminic acid) just prior to release.

Pharmacodynamics/Kinetics

Absorption: Well absorbed

Distribution: V_d: 23-26 L (oseltamivir carboxylate)

Protein binding, plasma: Oseltamivir carboxylate: 3%; Oseltamivir: 42%

Metabolism: Hepatic (90%) to oseltamivir carboxylate; neither the parent drug nor active metabolite has any effect on the cytochrome P450 system

Bioavailability: 75% as oseltamivir carboxylate

Half-life elimination: Oseltamivir: 1-3 hours; Oseltamivir carboxylate: 6-10 hours

Excretion: Urine (>90% as oseltamivir carboxylate); feces

Dosage Oral:

Influenza prophylaxis: Initiate prophylaxis within 48 hours of contact with an infected individual

Manufacturer's recommendation:

Children: 1-12 years:
- ≤15 kg: 30 mg once daily
- >15 kg to ≤23 kg: 45 mg once daily
- >23 kg to ≤40 kg: 60 mg once daily
- >40 kg: 75 mg once daily

Adolescents ≥13 years and Adults: 75 mg once daily

Alternate recommendations:

Children 3-11 months (unlabeled dosing; AAP, 2010): **Note:** Dosing based on age (use only if weight not available)
- 3-5 months: 20 mg once daily
- 6-11 months: 25 mg once daily

Children <12 months (unlabeled dosing, CDC 2011): **Note:** Prophylaxis is not recommended for infants <3 months of age unless clinically critical; weight-based dosing recommendations are not intended for premature neonates: 3 mg/kg/dose once daily

Children 3-23 months (unlabeled dosing, IDSA/PIDS, 2011):
- 3-8 months: 3 mg/kg/dose once daily (do not exceed maximum dose of weight-based dosing)
- 9-23 months: 3.5 mg/kg/dose once daily (do not exceed maximum dose of weight-based dosing)

Prophylaxis duration:

Individual/household exposure: 10 days

Community/institutional outbreak:

Manufacturer recommendation: May be used for up to 6 weeks

Alternate recommendations: Continue for ≥2 weeks and until ~10 days after identification of illness onset in the last patient (CDC, 2011) or until influenza activity in community subsides or immunity obtained from immunization (IDSA/PIDS, 2011). During community outbreaks, duration of protection lasts for length of dosing period; safety and efficacy have been demonstrated for use up to 6 weeks in immunocompetent patients and safety has been demonstrated for use up to 12 weeks in patients who are immunocompromised.

Influenza treatment: Initiate treatment within 48 hours of onset of symptoms; duration of treatment: 5 days unless severely ill and hospitalized. **Note:** Hospitalized patients may require longer (eg, ≥10 days) treatment courses. Some experts also recommend empirically doubling the treatment dose. Doubling the dose in adult outpatients was not associated with increased adverse events. As no double-dose studies have been published in children, use caution. Initiate as early as possible in any hospitalized patient with suspected/confirmed influenza (CDC, 2011); may be administered via naso- or orogastric tube in mechanically-ventilated patients (Taylor, 2008).

Manufacturer's recommendation: **Note:** The following dosing is also supported by some clinicians (IDSA/PIDS, 2011):
- Children: 1-12 years:
  - ≤15 kg: 30 mg twice daily
  - >15 kg to ≤23 kg: 45 mg twice daily
  - >23 kg to ≤40 kg: 60 mg twice daily
  - >40 kg: 75 mg twice daily
- Adolescents ≥13 years and Adults: 75 mg twice daily

Alternate recommendations:
- Children <12 months (unlabeled dosing, CDC 2011): **Note:** Weight-based dosing recommendations are not intended for premature neonates: 3 mg/kg/dose twice daily.
- Children <12 months (unlabeled dosing; AAP, 2010): **Note:** Dosing based on age (use only if weight not available):
  - <3 months: 12 mg twice daily
  - 3-5 months: 20 mg twice daily
  - 6-11 months: 25 mg twice daily
- Children <24 months (unlabeled dosing; IDSA/PIDS, 2011): **Note:** Do not exceed maximum dose of weight-based dosing.
  - Infants, premature: 1 mg/kg/dose twice daily
  - 0-8 months: 3 mg/kg/dose twice daily
  - 9-23 months: 3.5 mg/kg/dose twice daily

Dosage adjustment in renal impairment:

Treatment: Adults:
- U.S. labeling: Cl_{cr} 10-30 mL/minute: 75 mg once daily for 5 days
- Canadian labeling:
  - Cl_{cr} >30-60 mL/minute: 30 mg twice daily for 5 days
  - Cl_{cr} 10-30 mL/minute: 30 mg once daily for 5 days
- High-dose treatment (unlabeled [eg, severely-ill hospitalized patients with 2009 H1N1 influenza]): Currently no data are available; consider 150 mg once daily

Prophylaxis: Adults:
- U.S. labeling: Cl_{cr} 10-30 mL/minute: 75 mg every other day or 30 mg once daily
- Canadian labeling:
  - Cl_{cr} >30-60 mL/minute: 30 mg once daily for 10-14 days
  - Cl_{cr} 10-30 mL/minute: 30 mg every other day for 10-14 days

CAPD: Adults:
- Unlabeled dose: 30 mg once weekly (Robson, 2006)
- Canadian labeling (not in U.S. labeling):
  - Treatment: 30 mg prior to start of dialysis
  - Prophylaxis: 30 mg prior to start of dialysis, then 30 mg every 7 days for 10-14 days

Hemodialysis:
- Children >1 year (unlabeled dose; Schreuder, 2010):
  - ≤15 kg: 7.5 mg after each hemodialysis session
  - >15 kg to ≤23 kg: 10 mg after each hemodialysis session
  - >23 kg to ≤40 kg: 15 mg after each hemodialysis session
  - >40 kg: 30 mg after each hemodialysis session
- Adults:
  - Unlabeled dose: 30 mg after every other session (Robson, 2006)
  - Canadian labeling (not in U.S. labeling):
    - Treatment: 30 mg prior to dialysis; if symptomatic between dialysis sessions, then administer 30 mg after each dialysis session over period of 5 days
    - Prophylaxis: 30 mg prior to dialysis, then 30 mg after every other dialysis session for period of 10-14 days

Dosage adjustment in hepatic impairment:
- Mild-to-moderate impairment: No adjustment necessary
- Severe impairment: Pharmacokinetics and safety have not been evaluated

Dietary Considerations Take without regard to meals; take with food to improve tolerance.

Administration May be administered without regard to meals; take with food to improve tolerance.

Capsules may be opened and mixed with sweetened liquid (eg, chocolate syrup).

Mechanically-ventilated critically-ill patients: May administer via naso- or orogastric (NG/OG) tube. For a 150 mg dose, dissolve powder from two 75 mg capsules in 20 mL of sterile water and inject down the NG/OG tube; follow with a 10 mL sterile water flush (Taylor, 2008).

Monitoring Parameters Signs or symptoms of unusual behavior, including attempts at self-injury, confusion, and/or delirium

Critically-ill patients: Repeat rRT-PCR or viral culture may help to determine on-going viral replication

Additional Information In clinical studies of the influenza virus, 1.3% of post-treatment isolates in adults and adolescents and 8.6% of isolates in children had decreased neuraminidase susceptibility *in vitro* to oseltamivir carboxylate.

The absence of symptoms does not rule out viral influenza infection and clinical judgment should guide the decision for therapy. Treatment should not be delayed while waiting for the results of diagnostic tests. Treatment should be considered for high-risk patients with symptoms despite a negative rapid influenza test when the illness cannot be contributed to another cause. Use of oseltamivir is not a substitute for vaccination (when available); susceptibility to influenza infection returns once therapy is discontinued.

Dosage Forms Excipient information presented when available (limited, particularly for generics); consult specific product labeling. [DSC] = Discontinued product

Capsule, oral, as phosphate:
- Tamiflu®: 30 mg, 45 mg, 75 mg

Powder for suspension, oral:
- Tamiflu®: 6 mg/mL (60 mL); 12 mg/mL (25 mL [DSC]) [contains sodium benzoate; tutti frutti flavor]

Extemporaneous Preparations

If the commercially prepared oral suspension is not available, the manufacturer provides the following compounding information to prepare a **6 mg/mL** suspension in emergency situations.

1. Place the specified amount of water into a polyethyleneterephthalate (PET) or glass bottle.
2. Carefully separate the capsule body and cap and pour the contents of the required number of 75 mg capsules into the PET or glass bottle.
3. Gently swirl the suspension to ensure adequate wetting of the powder for at least 2 minutes.
4. Slowly add the specified amount of vehicle to the bottle.
5. Close the bottle using a child-resistant cap and shake well for 30 seconds to completely dissolve the active drug.
6. Label "Shake Well Before Use."

Stable for 35 days refrigerated or 5 days at room temperature. Shake gently prior to use. Do **not** dispense with dosing device provided with commercially-available product.

Preparation of Oseltamivir 6 mg/mL Suspension

Body Weight	Total Volume per Patient[1]	# of 75 mg Capsules[2]	Required Volume of Water	Required Volume of Vehicle[2,3]	Treatment Dose (wt based)[4]	Prophylactic Dose (wt based)[4]
≤15 kg	75 mL	6	5 mL	69 mL	5 mL (30 mg) twice daily for 5 days	5 mL (30 mg) once daily for 10 days
16-23 kg	100 mL	8	7 mL	91 mL	7.5 mL (45 mg) twice daily for 5 days	7.5 mL (45 mg) once daily for 10 days
24-40 kg	125 mL	10	8 mL	115 mL	10 mL (60 mg) twice daily for 5 days	10 mL (60 mg) once daily for 10 days
≥41 kg	150 mL	12	10 mL	137 mL	12.5 mL (75 mg) twice daily for 5 days	12.5 mL (75 mg) once daily for 10 days

[1]Entire course of therapy.

[2]Based on total volume per patient.

[3]Acceptable vehicles are cherry syrup, Ora-Sweet® SF, or simple syrup.

[4]Using 6 mg/mL suspension.

- ◆ **OSI-774** *see* Erlotinib *on page* 612
- ◆ **Osmitrol** *see* Mannitol *on page* 1049
- ◆ **Osmitrol® (Can)** *see* Mannitol *on page* 1049
- ◆ **OsmoPrep®** *see* Sodium Phosphates *on page* 1573
- ◆ **Osteocit® (Can)** *see* Calcium Citrate *on page* 269
- ◆ **Ostoforte® (Can)** *see* Ergocalciferol *on page* 610
- ◆ **OTFC (Oral Transmucosal Fentanyl Citrate)** *see* FentaNYL *on page* 697
- ◆ **Otix® [OTC]** *see* Carbamide Peroxide *on page* 283
- ◆ **Outgro® [OTC]** *see* Benzocaine *on page* 202
- ◆ **Ovace®** *see* Sulfacetamide (Topical) *on page* 1599
- ◆ **Ovace® Plus** *see* Sulfacetamide (Topical) *on page* 1599
- ◆ **Ovcon® 35** *see* Ethinyl Estradiol and Norethindrone *on page* 660
- ◆ **Ovcon® 50** *see* Ethinyl Estradiol and Norethindrone *on page* 660
- ◆ **Ovide®** *see* Malathion *on page* 1049
- ◆ **Ovidrel®** *see* Chorionic Gonadotropin (Recombinant) *on page* 353
- ◆ **Ovine Corticotrophin-Releasing Hormone** *see* Corticorelin *on page* 413
- ◆ **Ovral® (Can)** *see* Ethinyl Estradiol and Norgestrel *on page* 664

Oxacillin (oks a SIL in)

Index Terms Methylphenyl Isoxazolyl Penicillin; Oxacillin Sodium

Pharmacologic Category Antibiotic, Penicillin

Additional Appendix Information

Antibiotic Treatment of Adults With Infective Endocarditis *on page* 1956

Use Treatment of infections such as osteomyelitis, septicemia, endocarditis, and CNS infections caused by susceptible strains of *Staphylococcus*

Pregnancy Risk Factor B

Pregnancy Considerations Adverse events have not been observed in animal studies; therefore, oxacillin is classified as pregnancy category B. Oxacillin is distributed into the amniotic fluid and is detected in cord blood. There was not an increased risk of teratogenic effects with oxacillin observed in an epidemiologic study.

Lactation Enters breast milk/use caution

Contraindications Hypersensitivity to oxacillin or other penicillins or any component of the formulation

Warnings/Precautions Elimination rate will be slow in neonates. Modify dosage in patients with renal impairment and in the elderly. Serious and occasionally severe or fatal hypersensitivity (anaphylactoid) reactions have been reported in patients on penicillin therapy, especially with a history of beta-lactam hypersensitivity, history of sensitivity to multiple allergens, or previous IgE-mediated reactions (eg, anaphylaxis, angioedema, urticaria). Use with caution in asthmatic patients. Prolonged use may result in fungal or bacterial superinfection, including *C. difficile*-associated diarrhea (CDAD) and pseudomembranous colitis; CDAD has been observed >2 months postantibiotic treatment.

Adverse Reactions Frequency not defined.

Central nervous system: Fever

Dermatologic: Rash

Gastrointestinal: Nausea, diarrhea, vomiting

Hematologic: Eosinophilia, leukopenia, neutropenia, thrombocytopenia, agranulocytosis

Hepatic: Hepatotoxicity, AST increased

Renal: Acute interstitial nephritis, hematuria

Miscellaneous: Serum sickness-like reactions

Drug Interactions

Metabolism/Transport Effects None known.

Avoid Concomitant Use

Avoid concomitant use of Oxacillin with any of the following: BCG

Increased Effect/Toxicity

Oxacillin may increase the levels/effects of: Methotrexate; Vitamin K Antagonists

The levels/effects of Oxacillin may be increased by: Probenecid

Decreased Effect

Oxacillin may decrease the levels/effects of: BCG; Mycophenolate; Typhoid Vaccine

The levels/effects of Oxacillin may be decreased by: Fusidic Acid; Tetracycline Derivatives

Stability Reconstituted parenteral solution is stable for 3 days at room temperature and 7 days when refrigerated. For I.V. infusion in NS or D_5W, solution is stable for 24 hours at room temperature.

Mechanism of Action Inhibits bacterial cell wall synthesis by binding to one or more of the penicillin-binding proteins (PBPs); which in turn inhibits the final transpeptidation step of peptidoglycan synthesis in bacterial cell walls, thus inhibiting cell wall biosynthesis. Bacteria eventually lyse due to ongoing activity of cell wall autolytic enzymes (autolysins and murein hydrolases) while cell wall assembly is arrested.

Pharmacodynamics/Kinetics

Distribution: Into bile, synovial and pleural fluids, bronchial secretions; also distributes to peritoneal and pericardial fluids; penetrates the blood-brain barrier only when meninges are inflamed

Protein binding: ~94%

Metabolism: Hepatic to active metabolites

Half-life elimination: Children 1 week to 2 years: 0.9-1.8 hours; Adults: 23-60 minutes; prolonged in neonates and with renal impairment

Time to peak, serum: I.M.: 30-60 minutes

Excretion: Urine and feces (small amounts as unchanged drug and metabolites)

Dosage

Usual dosage range:

Infants and Children: I.M., I.V.: 100-200 mg/kg/day in divided doses every 6 hours (maximum: 12 g/day)

Adults: I.M., I.V.: 250-2000 mg every 4-6 hours

Indication-specific dosing:

Infants >3 months and Children:

Community-acquired pneumonia (CAP) (IDSA/PIDS, 2011), moderate-to-severe infection, *S. aureus* (methicillin-susceptible) (preferred): I.V.: 150-200 mg/kg/day divided every 6-8 hours

Children:

Arthritis (septic): I.V.: 37 mg/kg every 6 hours

Epiglottitis: I.V.: 150-200 mg/kg/day divided every 6 hours

Mild-to-moderate infections: I.M., I.V.: 100-150 mg/kg/day in divided doses every 6 hours (maximum: 4 g/day)

Severe infections: I.M., I.V.: 150-200 mg/kg/day in divided doses every 6 hours (maximum: 12 g/day)

Staphylococcal scalded-skin syndrome: I.V.: 150 mg/kg/day divided every 6 hours for 5-7 days

Adults:

Endocarditis: I.V.: 2 g every 4 hours with gentamicin

Mild-to-moderate infections: I.M., I.V.: 250-500 mg every 4-6 hours

Prosthetic joint infection: I.V.: 2 g every 4 hours with rifampin

Severe infections: I.M., I.V.: 1-2 g every 4-6 hours

***Staphylococcus aureus*, methicillin-susceptible infections, including brain abscess, bursitis, erysipelas, mastitis, mastoiditis, osteomyelitis, perinephric abscess, pneumonia, pyomyositis, scalded skin syndrome, toxic shock syndrome:** I.V.: 2 g every 4 hours

Dosing adjustment in renal impairment: Cl_{cr} <10 mL/minute: Clinical practice varies; some clinicians recommend adjustment to the lower range of the usual dosage as based on severity of infection.

Hemodialysis: Not dialyzable (0% to 5%)

Dietary Considerations Some products may contain sodium.

Administration Administer around-the-clock to promote less variation in peak and trough serum levels. Administer IVP over 10 minutes. Administer IVPB over 30 minutes.

Monitoring Parameters Observe for signs and symptoms of anaphylaxis during first dose; monitor periodic CBC, urinalysis, BUN, serum creatinine, AST and ALT

Test Interactions May interfere with urinary glucose tests using cupric sulfate (Benedict's solution, Clinitest®); may inactivate aminoglycosides *in vitro*; false-positive urinary and serum proteins

Dosage Forms Excipient information presented when available (limited, particularly for generics); consult specific product labeling.

Infusion, premixed iso-osmotic solution: 1 g (50 mL); 2 g (50 mL)

Injection, powder for reconstitution: 1 g, 2 g, 10 g

◆ **Oxacillin Sodium** *see* Oxacillin *on page* 1256

◆ **Oxalatoplatin** *see* Oxaliplatin *on page* 1257

◆ **Oxalatoplatinum** *see* Oxaliplatin *on page* 1257

Oxaliplatin (ox AL i pla tin)

Brand Names: U.S. Eloxatin®

Brand Names: Canada Eloxatin®

Index Terms Diaminocyclohexane Oxalatoplatinum; L-OHP; Oxalatoplatin; Oxalatoplatinum

Pharmacologic Category Antineoplastic Agent, Alkylating Agent; Antineoplastic Agent, Platinum Analog

Use Treatment of stage III colon cancer (adjuvant) and advanced colorectal cancer

Unlabeled Use Treatment of esophageal cancer, gastric cancer, hepatobiliary cancer, non-Hodgkin's lymphoma, ovarian cancer, pancreatic cancer, testicular cancer

Pregnancy Risk Factor D

Pregnancy Considerations Decreased fetal weight, decreased ossification, and increased fetal deaths were observed in animal studies at one-tenth the equivalent human dose. There are no adequate and well-controlled studies in pregnant women. Women of childbearing potential should be advised to avoid pregnancy and use effective contraception during treatment.

Canadian labeling: Use in pregnant women is contraindicated in the Canadian labeling. Males should be advised not to father children during and for up to 6 months following therapy. May cause permanent infertility in males. Prior to initiating therapy, advise males desiring to father children, to seek counseling on sperm storage.

Lactation Excretion in breast milk unknown/not recommended

Contraindications Hypersensitivity to oxaliplatin, other platinum-containing compounds, or any component of the formulation

Canadian labeling: Additional contraindications (not in U.S. labeling): Pregnancy, breast-feeding; severe renal impairment (Cl_{cr} <30 mL/minute)

Warnings/Precautions Hazardous agent - use appropriate precautions for handling and disposal. **[U.S. Boxed Warning]: Anaphylactic/anaphylactoid reactions may occur within minutes of oxaliplatin administration; symptoms may be managed with epinephrine, corticosteroids, and antihistamines.** Grade 3 or 4 hypersensitivity has been observed. Allergic reactions may occur with any cycle and may include bronchospasm (rare), erythema, hypotension (rare), pruritus, rash, and/or urticaria.

Two different types of peripheral sensory neuropathy may occur: First, an acute (within first 2 days), reversible (resolves within 14 days), with primarily peripheral symptoms that are often exacerbated by cold (may include pharyngolaryngeal dysesthesia); may recur with subsequent doses; avoid mucositis prophylaxis with ice chips during oxaliplatin infusion. Secondly, a more persistent (>14 days) presentation that often interferes with daily activities (eg, writing, buttoning, swallowing), these symptoms may improve in some patients upon discontinuing treatment.

May cause pulmonary fibrosis; withhold treatment for unexplained pulmonary symptoms (eg, crackles, dyspnea, nonproductive cough, pulmonary infiltrates) until interstitial lung disease or pulmonary fibrosis are excluded. Hepatotoxicity (including rare cases of hepatitis and hepatic failure) has been reported. Liver biopsy has revealed peliosis, nodular regenerative hyperplasia, sinusoidal alterations, perisinusoidal fibrosis, and veno-occlusive lesions; the presence of hepatic vascular disorders (including veno-occlusive disease) should be considered, especially in individuals developing portal hypertension or who present with increased liver function tests. Use caution with renal dysfunction; increased toxicity may occur. When administered as sequential infusions, taxane derivatives (docetaxel, paclitaxel) should be administered before platinum derivatives (carboplatin, cisplatin, oxaliplatin) to limit myelosuppression and enhance efficacy. Concomitant use with 5-FU may increase risk for adverse hematologic or GI effects. Elderly patients are more sensitive to some adverse events including diarrhea, dehydration, hypokalemia, leukopenia, fatigue and syncope. Safety and efficacy in children have not been established.

Adverse Reactions Percentages reported with monotherapy.

>10%:

Central nervous system: Fatigue (61%), fever (25%), pain (14%), headache (13%), insomnia (11%)

Gastrointestinal: Nausea (64%), diarrhea (46%), vomiting (37%), abdominal pain (31%), constipation (31%), anorexia (20%), stomatitis (14%)

Hematologic: Anemia (64%; grades 3/4: 1%), thrombocytopenia (30%; grades 3/4: 3%), leukopenia (13%)

Hepatic: AST increased (54%; grades 3/4: 4%), ALT increased (36%; grades 3/4: 1%), total bilirubin increased (13%; grades 3/4: 5%)

Neuromuscular & skeletal: Peripheral neuropathy (may be dose limiting; 76%; acute 65%; grades 3/4: 5%; persistent 43%; grades 3/4: 3%), back pain (11%)

Respiratory: Dyspnea (13%), cough (11%)

1% to 10%:

Cardiovascular: Edema (10%), chest pain (5%), peripheral edema (5%), flushing (3%), thromboembolism (2%)

Central nervous system: Dizziness (7%)

Dermatologic: Rash (5%), alopecia (3%), hand-foot syndrome (1%)

Endocrine & metabolic: Dehydration (5%), hypokalemia (3%)

Gastrointestinal: Dyspepsia (7%), taste perversion (5%), flatulence (3%), mucositis (2%), gastroesophageal reflux (1%), dysphagia (acute 1% to 2%)

Genitourinary: Dysuria (1%)

Hematologic: Neutropenia (7%)

Local: Injection site reaction (9%; redness/swelling/pain)

Neuromuscular & skeletal: Rigors (9%), arthralgia (7%)

Ocular: Abnormal lacrimation (1%)

Renal: Serum creatinine increased (5% to 10%)

Respiratory: URI (7%), rhinitis (6%), epistaxis (2%), pharyngitis (2%), pharyngolaryngeal dysesthesia (grades 3/4: 1% to 2%)

Miscellaneous: Allergic reactions (3%); hypersensitivity (includes urticaria, pruritus, facial flushing, shortness of breath, bronchospasm, diaphoresis, hypotension, syncope: grades 3/4: 2% to 3%); hiccup (2%)

<1% (Limited to important or life-threatening; reported with mono- and combination therapy): Acute renal failure, alkaline phosphatase increased, anaphylactic/anaphylactoid reactions, anaphylactic shock, angioedema, aphonia, ataxia, colitis, cranial nerve palsies, deep tendon reflex loss, deafness, diplopia, dysarthria, dysphonia, eosinophilic pneumonia, extravasation (including necrosis), fasciculations, gait abnormal, hematuria, hemolysis, hemolytic anemia (immuno-allergic), hemolytic uremia syndrome, hemorrhage, hepatic failure, hepatitis, hepatotoxicity, hypertension, hypomagnesemia, hypoxia, ileus, INR increased, interstitial lung diseases, interstitial nephritis (acute), intestinal obstruction, intracerebral bleeding, Lhermittes' sign, metabolic acidosis, muscle spasm, myoclonus, neutropenic fever, neutropenic sepsis, neutropenic typhlitis, nodular regenerative hyperplasia, optic neuritis, pancreatitis, peliosis, prothrombin time increased, ptosis, rectal hemorrhage, rhabdomyolysis, seizure, sepsis, thrombocytopenia (immuno-allergic), trigeminal neuralgia, tubular necrosis (acute), veno-occlusive liver disease (sinusoidal obstruction syndrome and perisinusoidal fibrosis), visual disturbance (acuity decreased, field disturbance, transient loss)

Drug Interactions

Metabolism/Transport Effects None known.

Avoid Concomitant Use

Avoid concomitant use of Oxaliplatin with any of the following: BCG; CloZAPine; Natalizumab; Pimecrolimus; Tacrolimus (Topical); Vaccines (Live)

Increased Effect/Toxicity

Oxaliplatin may increase the levels/effects of: CloZAPine; Leflunomide; Natalizumab; Taxane Derivatives; Topotecan; Vaccines (Live); Vitamin K Antagonists

The levels/effects of Oxaliplatin may be increased by: Denosumab; Pimecrolimus; Roflumilast; Tacrolimus (Topical); Trastuzumab

Decreased Effect

Oxaliplatin may decrease the levels/effects of: BCG; Cardiac Glycosides; Coccidioidin Skin Test; Sipuleucel-T; Vaccines (Inactivated); Vaccines (Live); Vitamin K Antagonists

The levels/effects of Oxaliplatin may be decreased by: Echinacea

Stability Store intact vials at room temperature of 25°C (77°F); excursions permitted to 15°C to 30°C (59°F to 86°F); do not freeze. Protect concentrated solution from light (store in original outer carton). According to the manufacturer, solutions diluted for infusion are stable up to 6 hours at room temperature of 20°C to 25°C (68°F to 77°F) or up to 24 hours under refrigeration at 2°C to 8°C (36°F to 46°F). Oxaliplatin solution diluted with D_5W to a final concentration of 0.7 mg/mL (polyolefin container) has been shown to retain >90% of it's original concentration for up to 30 days when stored at room temperature or refrigerated; artificial light did not affect the concentration (Andre, 2007). As this study did not examine sterility, refrigeration would be preferred to limit microbial growth.

Do not prepare using a chloride-containing solution such as NaCl due to rapid conversion to monochloroplatinum, dichloroplatinum, and diaquoplatinum; all highly reactive in sodium chloride (Takimoto, 2007). Use appropriate precautions for handling and disposal. Do not use needles or administration sets containing aluminum during preparation. Solutions diluted for infusion do not require protection from light.

Aqueous solution: Dilution with D_5W (250 or 500 mL) is required prior to administration.

Lyophilized powder [CAN; not available in U.S.]: Use only water for injection or D_5W to reconstitute powder. To obtain final concentration of 5 mg/mL add 10 mL of diluent to 50 mg vial or 20 mL diluent to 100 mg vial. Gently swirl vial to dissolve powder. Dilution with D_5W (250 or 500 mL) is required prior to administration. Discard unused portion of vial.

Mechanism of Action Oxaliplatin, a platinum derivative, is an alkylating agent. Following intracellular hydrolysis, the platinum compound binds to DNA forming cross-links which inhibit DNA replication and transcription, resulting in cell death. Cytotoxicity is cell-cycle nonspecific.

Pharmacodynamics/Kinetics

Distribution: V_d: 440 L

Protein binding: >90% primarily albumin and gamma globulin (irreversible binding to platinum)

Metabolism: Nonenzymatic (rapid and extensive), forms active and inactive derivatives

Half-life elimination: Terminal: 391 hours

Excretion: Urine (~54%); feces (~2%)

Dosage Details concerning dosing in combination regimens should also be consulted. Delay dosage in subsequent cycles until recovery of neutrophils ≥1.5 x 10^9/L and platelets ≥75 x 10^9/L. I.V.:

Adults:

Advanced colorectal cancer: 85 mg/m^2 every 2 weeks until disease progression or unacceptable toxicity (in combination with fluorouracil/leucovorin)

Stage III colon cancer (adjuvant): 85 mg/m^2 every 2 weeks for 12 cycles (in combination with fluorouracil/leucovorin)

Colon/colorectal cancer (unlabeled doses or combinations): 85 mg/m^2/dose on days 1, 15, and 29 of an 8-week treatment cycle in combination with fluorouracil/leucovorin (Kuebler, 2007) **or** 85 mg/m^2 every 2 weeks in combination with fluorouracil/leucovorin/irinotecan (Falcone, 2007) **or** 130 mg/m^2 every 3 weeks in combination with capecitabine (Cassidy, 2008)

Esophageal/gastric cancers (unlabeled use; as part of a combination chemotherapy regimen): 85 mg/m^2 every 2 weeks (Al-Batran, 2008) **or** 130 mg/m^2 every 3 weeks (Cunningham, 2008)

or

Gastric cancer: 100 mg/m^2 every 2 weeks (Louvet, 2002)

Hepatobiliary cancer (unlabeled use; as part of a combination chemotherapy regimen): 100 mg/m^2 every 2 weeks (Andre, 2004) **or** 130 mg/m^2 every 3 weeks (Nehls, 2008)

Non-Hodgkin's lymphoma (unlabeled use; as part of a combination chemotherapy regimen): 25 mg/m^2/day for 4 days every 4 weeks (Tsimberidou, 2008) **or** 100 mg/m^2 every 3 weeks (Lopez, 2008; Rodriguez, 2007) **or** 130 mg/m^2 every 3 weeks (Chau, 2001)

Ovarian cancer (unlabeled use): 130 mg/m^2 every 3 weeks (Dieras, 2002; Piccart, 2000)

Pancreatic cancer (unlabeled use; as part of a combination chemotherapy regimen): 85 mg/m^2 every 2 weeks (Conroy, 2005) **or** 100 mg/m^2 every 2 weeks (Louvet, 2005) **or** 110-130 mg/m^2 every 3 weeks (Xiong, 2008)

Testicular cancer (unlabeled use; in combination with gemcitabine): 130 mg/m^2 every 3 weeks (Kollmannsberger, 2004; Pectasides, 2004)

Elderly: No dosing adjustment recommended

Dosage adjustments for toxicity: Acute toxicities: Longer infusion times (up to 6 hours) may mitigate acute toxicities.

Neurosensory events:

Persistent (>7 days) grade 2 neurosensory events: Consider oxaliplatin dose reduction if symptoms do not resolve:

Adjuvant treatment of stage III colon cancer: Reduce dose to 75 mg/m^2

Advanced colorectal cancer: Reduce dose to 65 mg/m^2

Consider withholding oxaliplatin for grade 2 neuropathy lasting >7 days despite dose reduction.

Persistent grade 3 neurosensory events: Consider discontinuing oxaliplatin

Other toxicities (grade 3/4 gastrointestinal toxicity, grade 4 neutropenia, or grade 3/4 thrombocytopenia): After recovery from toxicity, oxaliplatin dose reductions are recommended:

Adjuvant treatment of stage III colon cancer: Reduce dose to 75 mg/m^2; delay next dose until neutrophils recover to ≥1500/mm^3 and platelets recover to ≥75,000/mm^3

Advanced colorectal cancer: Reduce dose to 65 mg/m^2; delay next dose until neutrophils recover to ≥1500/mm^3 and platelets recover to ≥75,000/mm^3

Dosage adjustment in renal impairment: The FDA-approved labeling does not contain renal dosing adjustment guidelines. Oxaliplatin is primarily eliminated renally; in patients with Cl_{cr} <30 mL/minute, the AUC is increased ~190%. Oxaliplatin use has been studied in 25 patients with renal dysfunction; treatment was well-tolerated in patients with mild-to-moderate impairment (Cl_{cr} 20-59 mL/minute), suggesting that dose reduction is not necessary in this patient population (Takimoto, 2003). Patients with severe renal impairment (Cl_{cr} <20 mL/minute) have not been adequately studied; consider omitting dose or changing chemotherapy regimen if Cl_{cr} <20 mL/minute.

Note: Canadian labeling: Use in patients with Cl_{cr} <30 mL/minute is contraindicated in Canadian labeling.

Dosage adjustment in hepatic impairment: Mild, moderate, or severe hepatic impairment: Dosage adjustment not necessary (Doroshow, 2003; Synold, 2007)

Administration Administer as I.V. infusion over 2-6 hours. Flush infusion line with D_5W prior to administration of any concomitant medication. Patients should receive an antiemetic premedication regimen. Avoid mucositis prophylaxis with ice chips during oxaliplatin infusion (may exacerbate acute neurological symptoms).

Monitoring Parameters CBC with differential, blood chemistries (including serum creatinine, ALT, AST, and bilirubin); INR and prothrombin time (in patients on oral anticoagulant therapy); signs of neuropathy, hypersensitivity, and/or respiratory effects

Additional Information Cold temperature may exacerbate acute neuropathy. Do not use ice for mucositis prophylaxis.

Dosage Forms Excipient information presented when available (limited, particularly for generics); consult specific product labeling. [DSC] = Discontinued product

Injection, powder for reconstitution: 50 mg, 100 mg

Injection, solution: 5 mg/mL (10 mL, 20 mL)

Injection, solution [preservative free]:

Eloxatin®: 5 mg/mL (10 mL, 20 mL, 40 mL)

Injection, solution [concentrate, preservative free]: 5 mg/mL (10 mL [DSC], 20 mL [DSC])

Dosage Forms: Canada Excipient information presented when available (limited, particularly for generics); consult specific product labeling.

Injection, powder for reconstitution:

Eloxatin®: 50 mg [contains lactose], 100 mg [contains lactose]

◆ **Oxandrin®** *see* Oxandrolone *on page 1259*

Oxandrolone (oks AN droe lone)

Brand Names: U.S. Oxandrin®

Pharmacologic Category Androgen

Use Adjunctive therapy to promote weight gain after weight loss following extensive surgery, chronic infections, or severe trauma, and in some patients who, without definite pathophysiologic reasons, fail to gain or to maintain normal weight; to offset protein catabolism with prolonged corticosteroid administration; relief of bone pain associated with osteoporosis

Pregnancy Risk Factor X

Dosage

Children: Total daily dose: ≤0.1 mg/kg **or** ≤0.045 mg/lb

Adults: 2.5-20 mg in divided doses 2-4 times/day based on individual response; a course of therapy of 2-4 weeks is usually adequate. This may be repeated intermittently as needed.

Elderly: 5 mg twice daily

Dosing adjustment in renal impairment: Caution is recommended because of the propensity of oxandrolone to cause edema and water retention

Dosing adjustment in hepatic impairment: Caution is advised but there are not specific guidelines for dosage reduction

Additional Information Complete prescribing information for this medication should be consulted for additional detail.

Dosage Forms Excipient information presented when available (limited, particularly for generics); consult specific product labeling.

Tablet, oral: 2.5 mg, 10 mg

Oxandrin®: 2.5 mg [scored]

Oxandrin®: 10 mg

Controlled Substance C-III

Oxaprozin (oks a PROE zin)

Brand Names: U.S. Daypro®

Brand Names: Canada Apo-Oxaprozin®; Daypro®

Pharmacologic Category Nonsteroidal Anti-inflammatory Drug (NSAID), Oral

Additional Appendix Information

Beers Criteria - Potentially Inappropriate Medications for Geriatrics *on page 1973*

Use Acute and long-term use in the management of signs and symptoms of osteoarthritis and rheumatoid arthritis; juvenile idiopathic arthritis (JIA)

Pregnancy Risk Factor C

Pregnancy Considerations Adverse events were not observed in the initial animal reproduction studies; therefore, the manufacturer classifies oxaprozin as pregnancy category C. NSAID exposure during the first trimester is not strongly associated with congenital malformations; however, cardiovascular anomalies and cleft palate have been observed following NSAID exposure in some studies. The use of an NSAID close to conception may be associated with an increased risk of miscarriage. Nonteratogenic effects have been observed following NSAID administration during the third trimester including myocardial degenerative changes, prenatal constriction of the ductus arteriosus, fetal tricuspid regurgitation, failure of the ductus arteriosus to close postnatally; renal dysfunction or failure, oligohydramnios; gastrointestinal bleeding or perforation, increased risk of necrotizing enterocolitis; intracranial bleeding (including intraventricular hemorrhage), platelet dysfunction with resultant bleeding; pulmonary hypertension. Because they may cause premature closure of the ductus arteriosus, use of NSAIDs late in pregnancy should be avoided (use after 31 or 32 weeks gestation is not recommended by some clinicians). The chronic use of NSAIDs in women of reproductive age may be associated with infertility that is reversible upon discontinuation of the medication. A registry is available for pregnant women exposed to autoimmune medications including oxaprozin. For additional information contact the Organization of Teratology Information Specialists, OTIS Autoimmune Diseases Study, at 877-311-8972.

Lactation Excretion in breast milk unknown/not recommended

Medication Guide Available Yes

Contraindications Hypersensitivity to oxaprozin, aspirin, other NSAIDs, or any component of the formulation; perioperative pain in the setting of coronary artery bypass graft (CABG) surgery

Warnings/Precautions [U.S. Boxed Warning]: NSAIDs are associated with an increased risk of adverse cardiovascular thrombotic events, including MI and stroke. Risk may be increased with duration of use or pre-existing cardiovascular risk factors or disease. Carefully evaluate individual cardiovascular risk profiles prior to prescribing. May cause new onset hypertension or worsening of existing hypertension. Use caution with fluid retention. Avoid use in heart failure. Concurrent administration of ibuprofen, and potentially other nonselective NSAIDs, may interfere with aspirin' s cardioprotective effect. **[U.S. Boxed Warning]: Use is contraindicated for treatment of perioperative pain in the setting of coronary artery bypass graft (CABG) surgery.** Risk of MI and stroke may be increased with use following CABG surgery.

Platelet adhesion and aggregation may be decreased; may prolong bleeding time; patients with coagulation disorders or who are receiving anticoagulants should be monitored closely. Anemia may occur; patients on long-term NSAID therapy should be monitored for anemia. Rarely, NSAID use may cause severe blood dyscrasias (eg, agranulocytosis, aplastic anemia, thrombocytopenia).

NSAID use may compromise existing renal function; dose-dependent decreases in prostaglandin synthesis may result from NSAID use, reducing renal blood flow which may cause renal decompensation. NSAID use may increase the risk for hyperkalemia. Patients with impaired renal function, dehydration, heart failure, liver dysfunction, those taking diuretics, and ACE inhibitors, and the elderly are at greater risk of renal toxicity and hyperkalemia. In the elderly, may be inappropriate for long-term use due to potential for GI bleeding, hypertension, heart failure, and renal failure (Beers Criteria). Rehydrate patient before starting therapy; monitor renal function closely. Not recommended for use in patients with advanced renal disease. Long-term NSAID use may result in renal papillary necrosis.

[U.S. Boxed Warning]: NSAIDs may increase risk of gastrointestinal irritation, inflammation, ulceration, bleeding, and perforation. These events may occur at any time during therapy and without warning. Use caution with a history of GI disease (bleeding or ulcers); concurrent therapy with aspirin, anticoagulants, and/or corticosteroids; smoking; use of alcohol; and the elderly or debilitated patients. When used concomitantly with ≤325 mg of aspirin, a substantial increase in the risk of gastrointestinal complications (eg, ulcer) occurs; concomitant gastroprotective therapy (eg, proton pump inhibitors) is recommended (Bhatt, 2008).

Use the lowest effective dose for the shortest duration of time, consistent with individual patient goals, to reduce risk of cardiovascular or GI adverse events. Alternate therapies should be considered for patients at high risk.

NSAIDs may cause serious skin adverse events including exfoliative dermatitis, Stevens-Johnson syndrome (SJS), and toxic epidermal necrolysis (TEN); discontinue use at first sign of skin rash or hypersensitivity. Anaphylactoid reactions may occur, even without prior exposure; patients with "aspirin triad" (bronchial asthma, aspirin intolerance, rhinitis) may be at increased risk. Do not use in patients who experience bronchospasm, asthma, rhinitis, or urticaria with NSAID or aspirin therapy. Use caution in other forms of asthma.

Use with caution in patients with decreased hepatic function. Closely monitor patients with any abnormal LFT. Severe hepatic reactions (eg, fulminant hepatitis, liver failure) have occurred with NSAID use, rarely; discontinue if signs or symptoms of liver disease develop, or if systemic manifestations occur.

NSAIDS may cause drowsiness, dizziness, blurred vision and other neurologic effects which may impair physical or mental abilities; patients must be cautioned about performing tasks which require mental alertness (eg, operating machinery or driving). Discontinue use with blurred or diminished vision and perform ophthalmologic exam. Monitor vision with long-term therapy.

The elderly are at increased risk for adverse effects (especially peptic ulceration, CNS effects, renal toxicity) from NSAIDs even at low doses.

Withhold for at least 4-6 half-lives prior to surgical or dental procedures. May cause mild photosensitivity reactions.

Adverse Reactions

1% to 10%:

Cardiovascular: Edema

Central nervous system: Confusion, depression, dizziness, headache, sedation, sleep disturbance, somnolence

Dermatologic: Pruritus, rash

Gastrointestinal: Abdominal distress, abdominal pain, anorexia, constipation, diarrhea, flatulence, gastrointestinal ulcer, gross bleeding with perforation, heartburn, nausea, vomiting

Hematologic: Anemia, bleeding time increased

Hepatic: Liver enzyme elevation

Otic: Tinnitus

Renal: Dysuria, renal function abnormal, urinary frequency

<1% (Limited to important or life-threatening; effects reported with oxaprozin or other NSAIDs): Acute interstitial nephritis, acute renal failure, agranulocytosis, anaphylaxis, angioedema, asthma, bruising, CHF, erythema multiforme, exfoliative dermatitis, gastritis, gastrointestinal bleeding, hearing decreased, hematemesis, hematuria, hemorrhoidal bleeding, hepatitis, hypersensitivity reaction, hypertension, jaundice, leukopenia, nephrotic syndrome, pancreatitis, peptic ulcer, photosensitivity, rectal bleeding, renal insufficiency, Stevens-Johnson syndrome, toxic epidermal necrolysis, thrombocytopenia

Drug Interactions

Metabolism/Transport Effects None known.

Avoid Concomitant Use

Avoid concomitant use of Oxaprozin with any of the following: Floctafenine; Ketorolac; Ketorolac (Nasal); Ketorolac (Systemic)

Increased Effect/Toxicity

Oxaprozin may increase the levels/effects of: Aminoglycosides; Anticoagulants; Antiplatelet Agents; Bisphosphonate Derivatives; Collagenase (Systemic); CycloSPORINE; CycloSPORINE (Systemic); Deferasirox; Desmopressin; Digoxin; Drotrecogin Alfa (Activated); Eplerenone; Haloperidol; Ibritumomab; Lithium; Methotrexate; Nonsteroidal Anti-Inflammatory Agents; PEMEtrexed; Porfimer; Potassium-Sparing Diuretics; PRALAtrexate; Quinolone Antibiotics; Rivaroxaban; Salicylates; Thrombolytic Agents; Tositumomab and Iodine I 131 Tositumomab; Vancomycin; Vitamin K Antagonists

The levels/effects of Oxaprozin may be increased by: ACE Inhibitors; Angiotensin II Receptor Blockers; Antidepressants (Tricyclic, Tertiary Amine); Corticosteroids (Systemic); CycloSPORINE; CycloSPORINE (Systemic); Dasatinib; Floctafenine; Glucosamine; Herbs (Anticoagulant/Antiplatelet Properties); Ketorolac; Ketorolac (Nasal); Ketorolac (Systemic); Nonsteroidal Anti-Inflammatory Agents; Omega-3-Acid Ethyl Esters; Pentosan Polysulfate Sodium; Pentoxifylline; Probenecid; Prostacyclin Analogues; Selective Serotonin Reuptake Inhibitors; Serotonin/Norepinephrine Reuptake Inhibitors; Sodium Phosphates; Treprostinil; Vitamin E

Decreased Effect

Oxaprozin may decrease the levels/effects of: ACE Inhibitors; Angiotensin II Receptor Blockers; Antiplatelet Agents; Beta-Blockers; Eplerenone; HydrALAZINE; Loop Diuretics; Potassium-Sparing Diuretics; Salicylates; Selective Serotonin Reuptake Inhibitors; Thiazide Diuretics

The levels/effects of Oxaprozin may be decreased by: Bile Acid Sequestrants; Nonsteroidal Anti-Inflammatory Agents; Salicylates

Ethanol/Nutrition/Herb Interactions

Ethanol: Avoid ethanol (may enhance gastric mucosal irritation).

Herb/Nutraceutical: Avoid alfalfa, anise, bilberry, bladderwrack, bromelain, cat's claw, celery, chamomile, coleus, cordyceps, dong quai, evening primrose, fenugreek, feverfew, garlic, ginger, ginkgo biloba, ginseng (American, Panax, Siberian), grapeseed, green tea, guggul, horse chestnut seed, horseradish, licorice, prickly ash, red clover, reishi, SAMe (S-adenosylmethionine), sweet clover, turmeric, white willow (all have additional antiplatelet activity).

Stability Store at 25°C (77°F). Protect from light; keep bottle tightly closed.

Mechanism of Action Reversibly inhibits cyclooxygenase-1 and 2 (COX-1 and 2) enzymes, which results in decreased formation of prostaglandin precursors; has antipyretic, analgesic, and anti-inflammatory properties.

Other proposed mechanisms not fully elucidated (and possibly contributing to the anti-inflammatory effect to varying degrees) include inhibiting chemotaxis, altering lymphocyte activity, inhibiting neutrophil aggregation/activation, and decreasing proinflammatory cytokine levels.

Pharmacodynamics/Kinetics

Absorption: Oral: 95%

Distribution: V_d: 11-17 L/70 kg

Protein binding: >99% primarily to albumin

Metabolism: Hepatic via oxidation and glucuronidation; no active metabolites

Half-life elimination: 40-50 hours

Time to peak: 2-4 hours

Excretion: Urine (5% unchanged, 65% as metabolites); feces (35% as metabolites)

Dosage Oral (individualize dosage to lowest effective dose to minimize adverse effects):

Children 6-16 years: Juvenile idiopathic arthritis (JIA):

- 22-31 kg: 600 mg once daily
- 32-54 kg: 900 mg once daily
- ≥55 kg: 1200 mg once daily

Adults:

Osteoarthritis: 600-1200 mg once daily; patients should be titrated to lowest dose possible; patients with low body weight should start with 600 mg daily

Rheumatoid arthritis: 1200 mg once daily; a one-time loading dose of up to 1800 mg/day or 26 mg/kg (whichever is lower) may be given

Maximum doses:

- Patient <50 kg: Maximum: 1200 mg/day
- Patient >50 kg with normal renal/hepatic function and low risk of peptic ulcer: Maximum: 1800 mg or 26 mg/kg (whichever is lower) in divided doses

Dosing adjustment in renal impairment: In general, NSAIDs are not recommended for use in patients with advanced renal disease but the manufacturer of oxaprozin does provide some guidelines for adjustment in renal dysfunction.

Severe renal impairment or on dialysis: 600 mg once daily; may increase cautiously to 1200 mg/day with close monitoring

Dosing adjustment in hepatic impairment: Use caution in patients with severe dysfunction

Monitoring Parameters CBC, hepatic and renal function; ocular function

Test Interactions False-positive urine immunoassay screening tests for benzodiazepines have been reported and may occur several days after discontinuing oxaprozin.

Dosage Forms Excipient information presented when available (limited, particularly for generics); consult specific product labeling.

Caplet, oral:

Daypro®: 600 mg [scored]

Tablet, oral: 600 mg

Oxazepam (oks A ze pam)

Brand Names: Canada Apo-Oxazepam®; Bio-Oxazepam; Novoxapram®; Oxpam®; Oxpram®; PMS-Oxazepam; Riva-Oxazepam

Index Terms Serax

Pharmacologic Category Benzodiazepine

Additional Appendix Information
Beers Criteria – Potentially Inappropriate Medications for Geriatrics *on page 1973*
Benzodiazepines *on page 1882*

Use Treatment of anxiety; management of ethanol withdrawal

Unlabeled Use Anticonvulsant in management of simple partial seizures; hypnotic

Dosage Oral:
Adults:
Anxiety: 10-30 mg 3-4 times/day
Ethanol withdrawal: 15-30 mg 3-4 times/day
Hypnotic: 15-30 mg
Elderly: Oral: Anxiety: 10 mg 2-3 times/day; increase gradually as needed to a total of 30-45 mg/day. Dose titration should be slow to evaluate sensitivity.
Hemodialysis: Not dialyzable (0% to 5%)

Additional Information Complete prescribing information for this medication should be consulted for additional detail.

Dosage Forms Excipient information presented when available (limited, particularly for generics); consult specific product labeling.
Capsule, oral: 10 mg, 15 mg, 30 mg

Controlled Substance C-IV

OXcarbazepine (ox car BAZ e peen)

Brand Names: U.S. Trileptal®
Brand Names: Canada Apo-Oxcarbazepine®; Trileptal®
Index Terms GP 47680; OCBZ
Pharmacologic Category Anticonvulsant, Miscellaneous
Additional Appendix Information
Anticonvulsant Drugs of Choice *on page 1873*

Use Monotherapy or adjunctive therapy in the treatment of partial seizures in adults and children ≥4 years of age with epilepsy; adjunctive therapy in the treatment of partial seizures in children ≥2 years of age with epilepsy

Unlabeled Use Bipolar disorder; treatment of neuropathic pain

Pregnancy Risk Factor C

Pregnancy Considerations Adverse events have been observed in animal reproduction studies; therefore, the manufacturer classifies oxcarbazepine as pregnancy category C. Oxcarbazepine, the active metabolite MHD and the inactive metabolite DHD, crosses the placenta and can be detected in the newborn. An increased risk in the overall rate of major congenital malformations has not been observed following maternal use of oxcarbazepine. Available studies have not been large enough to determine if there is an increased risk of specific defects. In general, the risk of teratogenic effects is higher with AED polytherapy than monotherapy. Plasma concentrations of MHD gradually decrease due to physiologic changes which occur during pregnancy; patients should be monitored during pregnancy and postpartum. Oxcarbazepine may decrease plasma concentrations of hormonal contraceptives.

Patients exposed to oxcarbazepine during pregnancy are encouraged to enroll themselves into the AED Pregnancy Registry by calling 1-888-233-2334. Additional information is available at www.aedpregnancyregistry.org.

Lactation Enters breast milk/not recommended

Medication Guide Available Yes

Contraindications Hypersensitivity to oxcarbazepine or any component of the formulation

Warnings/Precautions Antiepileptics are associated with an increased risk of suicidal behavior/thoughts with use (regardless of indication); patients should be monitored for signs/symptoms of depression, suicidal tendencies, and other unusual behavior changes during therapy and instructed to inform their healthcare provider immediately if symptoms occur.

Clinically-significant hyponatremia (serum sodium <125 mmol/L) may develop during oxcarbazepine use. Rare cases of anaphylaxis and angioedema have been reported, even after initial dosing; permanently discontinue should symptoms occur. Use caution in patients with previous hypersensitivity to carbamazepine (cross-sensitivity occurs in 25% to 30%). Potentially serious, sometimes fatal, dermatologic reactions (eg, Stevens-Johnson, toxic epidermal necrolysis) and multiorgan hypersensitivity reactions have been reported in adults and children; monitor for signs and symptoms of skin reactions and possible disparate manifestations associated with lymphatic, hepatic, renal, and/or hematologic organ systems; discontinuation and conversion to alternate therapy may be required. As with all antiepileptic drugs, oxcarbazepine should be withdrawn gradually to minimize the potential of increased seizure frequency. Use of oxcarbazepine has been associated with CNS-related adverse events, most significant of these were cognitive symptoms including psychomotor slowing, difficulty with concentration, speech or language problems, somnolence or fatigue, and coordination abnormalities, including ataxia and gait disturbances. Effects with other sedative drugs or ethanol may be potentiated. Single-dose studies show that half-life of the primary active metabolite is prolonged 3-4 fold and AUC is doubled in patients with Cl_{cr} <30 mL/minute; dose adjustment required in these patients. May reduce the efficacy of oral contraceptives (nonhormonal contraceptive measures are recommended). Agranulocytosis, leukopenia, and pancytopenia have been reported with use (rare). Discontinuation and conversion to alternate therapy may be required.

Adverse Reactions As reported in adults with doses of up to 2400 mg/day (includes patients on monotherapy, adjunctive therapy, and those not previously on AEDs); incidence in children was similar.

>10%:
Central nervous system: Dizziness (22% to 49%), somnolence (20% to 36%), headache (13% to 32%), ataxia (5% to 31%), fatigue (12% to 15%), vertigo (6% to 15%)
Gastrointestinal: Vomiting (7% to 36%), nausea (15% to 29%), abdominal pain (10% to 13%)
Neuromuscular & skeletal: Abnormal gait (5% to 17%), tremor (3% to 16%)
Ocular: Diplopia (14% to 40%), nystagmus (7% to 26%), abnormal vision (4% to 14%)

1% to 10%:
Cardiovascular: Hypotension (≤2%), leg edema (1% to 2%)
Central nervous system: Nervousness (2% to 5%), amnesia (4%), abnormal thinking (≤4%), insomnia (2% to 4%), fever (3%), speech disorder (1% to 3%), abnormal feelings (≤2%), EEG abnormalities (≤2%), agitation (1% to 2%), confusion (1% to 2%)
Dermatologic: Rash (4%), acne (1% to 2%)
Endocrine & metabolic: Hyponatremia (1% to 3%)
Gastrointestinal: Diarrhea (5% to 7%), dyspepsia (5% to 6%), constipation (2% to 6%), taste perversion (5%), xerostomia (3%), gastritis (1% to 2%), weight gain (1% to 2%)
Genitourinary: Micturition (2%)
Neuromuscular & skeletal: Weakness (3% to 6%), back pain (4%), falling down (4%), abnormal coordination (1% to 4%), dysmetria (1% to 3%), sprains/strains (≤2%), muscle weakness (1% to 2%)
Ocular: Abnormal accommodation (≤2%)
Respiratory: Upper respiratory tract infection (7%), rhinitis (2% to 5%), chest infection (4%), epistaxis (4%), sinusitis (4%)

Postmarketing and/or case reports: Aggressive reaction, alopecia, amylase increased, anaphylaxis, angioedema, anxiety, aphasia, aplastic anemia, biliary pain, bradycardia, bruising, cardiac failure, cerebral hemorrhage, chest pain, cholelithiasis, colitis, conjunctival hemorrhage, consciousness decreased, convulsions aggravated, delirium, delusion, dysphagia, dysphonia, dyspnea, dystonia, dysuria, emotional lability, enteritis, erythema multiforme, erythematosus rash, esophagitis, eye edema, extrapyramidal disorder, GGT increased, gingival bleeding, gingival hyperplasia, hematuria, hemianopia, hemiplegia, hematemesis, hypersensitivity reaction, hypertension, hypocalcemia, hypochondrium pain, hypoesthesia, hypokalemia, hysteria, laryngismus, leukopenia, leukorrhea, lipase increased, liver enzymes elevated, maculopapular rash, manic reaction, multiorgan hypersensitivity (eosinophilia, arthralgia, rash, fever, lymphadenopathy), muscle contractions (involuntary), mydriasis, neuralgia, oculogyric crisis, palpitation, pancreatitis, pancytopenia, panic disorder, paralysis, paroniria, photophobia, photosensitivity reaction, pleurisy, postural hypotension, priapism, purpura, psychosis, ptosis, renal pain, rigors, scotoma, sialoadenitis, Stevens-Johnson syndrome, stupor, suicidal behavior/ideation, syncope, systemic lupus erythematosus, tachycardia, tetany, thrombocytopenia, toxic epidermal necrolysis, ulcerative stomatitis, urinary tract pain, urticaria, vitiligo, weight loss, xerophthalmia

Drug Interactions

Metabolism/Transport Effects **Induces** CYP3A4 (strong)

Avoid Concomitant Use

Avoid concomitant use of OXcarbazepine with any of the following: Bortezomib; Crizotinib; Dronedarone; Everolimus; Lapatinib; Lurasidone; Nilotinib; Nisoldipine; Pazopanib; Praziquantel; Ranolazine; Rilpivirine; Rivaroxaban; Roflumilast; RomiDEPsin; Selegiline; SORAfenib; Ticagrelor; Tolvaptan; Toremifene; Vandetanib

Increased Effect/Toxicity

OXcarbazepine may increase the levels/effects of: Clarithromycin; Fosphenytoin; Phenytoin; Selegiline

The levels/effects of OXcarbazepine may be increased by: Clarithromycin; Thiazide Diuretics

Decreased Effect

OXcarbazepine may decrease the levels/effects of: ARIPiprazole; Boceprevir; Bortezomib; Brentuximab Vedotin; Clarithromycin; Contraceptives (Estrogens); Contraceptives (Progestins); Crizotinib; CYP3A4 Substrates; Dasatinib; Dronedarone; Everolimus; Exemestane; Gefitinib; GuanFACINE; Imatinib; Ixabepilone; Lapatinib; Linagliptin; Lurasidone; Maraviroc; NIFEdipine; Nilotinib; Nisoldipine; Pazopanib; Praziquantel; Ranolazine; Rilpivirine; Rivaroxaban; Roflumilast; RomiDEPsin; Saxagliptin; SORAfenib; SUNItinib; Tadalafil; Ticagrelor; Tolvaptan; Toremifene; Ulipristal; Vandetanib; Vemurafenib; Zuclopenthixol

The levels/effects of OXcarbazepine may be decreased by: Divalproex; Fosphenytoin; PHENobarbital; Phenytoin; Valproic Acid

Ethanol/Nutrition/Herb Interactions

Ethanol: Avoid ethanol (may increase CNS depression).

Herb/Nutraceutical: St John's wort may decrease oxcarbazepine levels. Avoid evening primrose (seizure threshold decreased). Avoid valerian, St John's wort, kava kava, gotu kola.

Stability Store tablets and suspension at 25°C (77°F). Use suspension within 7 weeks of first opening container.

Mechanism of Action Pharmacological activity results from both oxcarbazepine and its monohydroxy metabolite (MHD). Precise mechanism of anticonvulsant effect has not been defined. Oxcarbazepine and MHD block voltage-sensitive sodium channels, stabilizing hyperexcited neuronal membranes, inhibiting repetitive firing, and decreasing the propagation of synaptic impulses. These actions are believed to prevent the spread of seizures. Oxcarbazepine and MHD also increase potassium conductance and modulate the activity of high-voltage activated calcium channels.

Pharmacodynamics/Kinetics

Absorption: Complete; food has no affect on rate or extent

Distribution: MHD: V_d: 49 L

Protein binding, serum: MHD: 40%

Metabolism: Hepatic to 10-monohydroxy metabolite (MHD; active); MHD is further glucuronidated or oxidized to a 10,11-dihydroxy metabolite (DHD; inactive)

Bioavailability: Decreased in children <8 years; increased in elderly >60 years

Half-life elimination: Parent drug: 2 hours; MHD: 9 hours; renal impairment (Cl_{cr} 30 mL/minute): MHD: 19 hours

Clearance of MHD is increased in younger children (~80% in children 2-4 years of age) and approaches that of adults by ~13 years of age

Time to peak, serum (median): Tablets: 4.5 hours; oral suspension: 6 hours

Excretion: Urine (95%, <1% as unchanged oxcarbazepine, 27% as unchanged MHD, 49% as MHD glucuronides); feces (<4%)

Dosage Oral:

Children 2-3 years:

Adjunctive therapy: 8-10 mg/kg/day, not to exceed 600 mg/day, given in 2 divided daily doses. Maintenance dose should be achieved over 2 weeks, and is dependent upon patient weight.

<20 kg: Consider initiating dose at 16-20 mg/kg/day; maximum maintenance dose should be achieved over 2-4 weeks and should not exceed 60 mg/kg/day (maximum: 600 mg/day)

Children 4-16 years:

Adjunctive therapy: 8-10 mg/kg/day, not to exceed 600 mg/day, given in 2 divided daily doses. Maintenance dose should be achieved over 2 weeks, and is dependent upon patient weight, according to the following:

20-29 kg: 900 mg/day in 2 divided doses

29.1-39 kg: 1200 mg/day in 2 divided doses

>39 kg: 1800 mg/day in 2 divided doses

Children 4-16 years:

Conversion to monotherapy: Oxcarbazepine 8-10 mg/kg/day in twice daily divided doses, while simultaneously initiating the reduction of the dose of the concomitant antiepileptic drug; the concomitant drug should be withdrawn over 3-6 weeks. Oxcarbazepine dose may be increased by a maximum of 10 mg/kg/day at weekly intervals. See below for recommended total daily dose by weight.

Initiation of monotherapy: Oxcarbazepine should be initiated at 8-10 mg/kg/day in twice daily divided doses; doses may be titrated by 5 mg/kg/day every third day. See below for recommended total daily dose by weight.

Range of maintenance doses by weight during monotherapy:

20 kg: 600-900 mg/day

25-30 kg: 900-1200 mg/day

35-40 kg: 900-1500 mg/day

45 kg: 1200-1500 mg/day

50-55 kg: 1200-1800 mg/day

60-65 kg: 1200-2100 mg/day

70 kg: 1500-2100 mg/day

Adults:

Adjunctive therapy: Initial: 600 mg/day in 2 divided doses; dose may be increased by as much as 600 mg/day at weekly intervals; recommended daily dose: 1200 mg/day in 2 divided doses. Although daily doses >1200 mg/day were somewhat more efficacious, most patients were unable to tolerate 2400 mg/day (due to CNS effects).

Conversion to monotherapy: Oxcarbazepine 600 mg/day in 2 divided doses while simultaneously initiating the reduction of the dose of the concomitant antiepileptic drug. The concomitant drug should be withdrawn over 3-6 weeks, while the maximum dose of oxcarbazepine should be reached in about 2-4 weeks. Recommended daily dose: 2400 mg/day.

Initiation of monotherapy: Initial: 600 mg/day in 2 divided doses; doses may be titrated upward by 300 mg/day every third day to a final dose of 1200 mg/day given in 2 divided doses

Dosing adjustment in renal impairment: Cl_{cr} <30 mL/minute: Therapy should be initiated at one-half the usual starting dose (300 mg/day in adults) and increased slowly to achieve desired clinical response

Dosing adjustment in hepatic impairment: Adjustment not needed for mild-to-moderate impairment. No data in patients with severe impairment.

Dietary Considerations May be taken without regard to meals.

Administration All dosing should be administered twice daily.

Suspension: Prior to using for the first time, firmly insert the plastic adapter provided with the bottle. Cover adapter with child-resistant cap when not in use. Shake bottle for at least 10 seconds, remove child-resistant cap, and insert the oral dosing syringe provided to withdraw appropriate dose. Dose may be taken directly from oral syringe or may be mixed in a small glass of water immediately prior to swallowing. Rinse syringe with warm water after use and allow to dry thoroughly. Discard any unused portion after 7 weeks of first opening bottle.

Monitoring Parameters Seizure frequency, serum sodium as deemed necessary (particularly during first 3 months of therapy), symptoms of CNS depression (dizziness, headache, somnolence). Additional serum sodium monitoring recommended during maintenance treatment in patients receiving other medications known to decrease sodium levels, in patients with signs/symptoms of hyponatremia, and in patients with an increase in seizure frequency or severity. Monitor for suicidality (eg, suicidal thoughts, depression, behavioral changes). Serum levels of concomitant antiepileptic drugs during titration as necessary.

Test Interactions Thyroid function tests; may depress serum T_4 without affecting T_3 levels or TSH

Dosage Forms Excipient information presented when available (limited, particularly for generics); consult specific product labeling.

Suspension, oral: 300 mg/5 mL (250 mL)

Trileptal®: 300 mg/5 mL (250 mL) [contains ethanol, propylene glycol]

Tablet, oral: 150 mg, 300 mg, 600 mg

Trileptal®: 150 mg, 300 mg, 600 mg [scored]

- **Oxecta™** *see* OxyCODONE *on page 1266*
- **Oxeze® Turbuhaler® (Can)** *see* Formoterol *on page 754*

Oxiconazole (oks i KON a zole)

Brand Names: U.S. Oxistat®

Brand Names: Canada Oxistat®

Index Terms Oxiconazole Nitrate

Pharmacologic Category Antifungal Agent, Topical

Use Treatment of tinea pedis (athlete's foot), tinea cruris (jock itch), tinea corporis (ringworm), and tinea (pityriasis) versicolor

Pregnancy Risk Factor B

Dosage Topical: Children and Adults:

Tinea corporis/tinea cruris: Cream, lotion: Apply to affected areas 1-2 times daily for 2 weeks

Tinea pedis: Cream, lotion: Apply to affected areas 1-2 times daily for 1 month

Tinea versicolor: Cream: Apply to affected areas once daily for 2 weeks

Additional Information Complete prescribing information for this medication should be consulted for additional detail.

Dosage Forms Excipient information presented when available (limited, particularly for generics); consult specific product labeling.

Cream, topical:

Oxistat®: 1% (30 g, 60 g) [contains benzoic acid]

Lotion, topical:

Oxistat®: 1% (30 mL, 60 mL) [contains benzoic acid]

- **Oxiconazole Nitrate** *see* Oxiconazole *on page 1264*
- **Oxilapine Succinate** *see* Loxapine *on page 1040*
- **Oxistat®** *see* Oxiconazole *on page 1264*
- **Oxpam® (Can)** *see* Oxazepam *on page 1261*
- **Oxpentifylline** *see* Pentoxifylline *on page 1333*
- **Oxpram® (Can)** *see* Oxazepam *on page 1261*
- **Oxsoralen®** *see* Methoxsalen (Topical) *on page 1103*
- **Oxsoralen® Capsule (Can)** *see* Methoxsalen (Systemic) *on page 1102*
- **Oxsoralen® Lotion (Can)** *see* Methoxsalen (Topical) *on page 1103*
- **Oxsoralen-Ultra®** *see* Methoxsalen (Systemic) *on page 1102*
- **Oxybate** *see* Sodium Oxybate *on page 1572*
- **Oxybutyn (Can)** *see* Oxybutynin *on page 1264*

Oxybutynin (oks i BYOO ti nin)

Brand Names: U.S. Ditropan XL®; Gelnique®; Oxytrol®

Brand Names: Canada Apo-Oxybutynin®; Ditropan XL®; Dom-Oxybutynin; Mylan-Oxybutynin; Novo-Oxybutynin; Nu-Oxybutyn; Oxybutyn; Oxybutynine; Oxytrol®; PHL-Oxybutynin; PMS-Oxybutynin; Riva-Oxybutynin; Uromax®

Index Terms Anturol®; Ditropan; Oxybutynin Chloride

Pharmacologic Category Antispasmodic Agent, Urinary

Additional Appendix Information

Beers Criteria – Potentially Inappropriate Medications for Geriatrics *on page 1973*

Use Antispasmodic for neurogenic bladder (urgency, frequency, leakage, urge incontinence, dysuria); extended release formulation also indicated for treatment of symptoms associated with detrusor overactivity due to a neurological condition (eg, spina bifida)

Pregnancy Risk Factor B

Pregnancy Considerations Teratogenic effects were not observed in animal studies. There are no adequate and well-controlled studies in pregnant women; use during pregnancy only if clearly needed.

Lactation Excretion in breast milk unknown/use caution

Contraindications Hypersensitivity to oxybutynin or any component of the formulation; patients with or at risk for uncontrolled narrow-angle glaucoma, urinary retention, gastric retention or conditions with severely decreased GI motility

Warnings/Precautions Cases of angioedema have been reported with oral oxybutynin; some cases have occurred after a single dose. Discontinue immediately if develops. Use with caution in patients with bladder outflow obstruction, angle-closure glaucoma (treated), hyperthyroidism, reflux esophagitis (including concurrent therapy with oral bisphosphonates or drugs which may increase the risk of esophagitis), heart disease, hepatic or renal disease, prostatic hyperplasia, autonomic neuropathy, ulcerative colitis (may cause ileus and toxic megacolon), hypertension, hiatal hernia, myasthenia gravis, dementia, ulcerative colitis, or intestinal atony. May increase the risk of heat prostration. May cause anticholinergic effects (agitation, confusion, hallucinations, somnolence) which may require dose reduction or discontinuation of therapy. May cause CNS depression, which may impair physical or mental abilities; patients must be cautioned about performing tasks which require mental alertness (eg, operating machinery or driving).

This class of medication is poorly tolerated by the elderly due to anticholinergic effects, sedation, and weakness. Efficacy is questionable at dosages tolerated by elderly patients. Oxybutynin extended-release is considered an exception. (Beers Criteria).

The extended release formulation consists of drug within a nondeformable matrix; following drug release/absorption, the matrix/shell is expelled in the stool. The use of nondeformable products in patients with known stricture/narrowing of the GI tract has been associated with symptoms of obstruction. Transdermal patch may contain conducting metal (eg, aluminum); remove patch prior to MRI. When using the topical gel, cover treatment area with clothing after gel has dried to minimize transferring medication to others. Discontinue gel if skin irritation occurs. Gel contains ethanol; do not expose to open flame or smoking until gel has dried.

Adverse Reactions

Oral:

>10%:

Central nervous system: Dizziness (4% to 17%), somnolence (2% to 14%)

Gastrointestinal: Xerostomia (29% to 71%; dose related), constipation (7% to 15%), nausea (2% to 12%)

5% to 10%:

Central nervous system: Headache (6% to 10%), pain (1% to 7%), nervousness (1% to 7%), insomnia (1% to 6%)

Gastrointestinal: Diarrhea (1% to 9%), dyspepsia (5% to 7%)

Genitourinary: Urinary hesitation (9%), urinary tract infection (5% to 7%), urinary retention (6%)

Neuromuscular & skeletal: Weakness (3% to 7%)

Ocular: Blurred vision (1% to 10%), dry eyes (3% to 6%)

Respiratory: Rhinitis (2% to 6%)

1% to <5% (Limited to important or life-threatening): Abdominal pain, agitation, angioedema, aptyalism, arrhythmia, arthralgia, asthma, back pain, bronchitis, chest pain, cough, cycloplegia, cystitis, depression, dry skin, dry throat, dysgeusia, dysphagia, dysuria, edema, eructation, extremity pain, eye irritation, fatigue, flank pain, flatulence, fluid retention, flushing, fungal infection, gastrointestinal reflux disease, GI motility decreased, hallucination, hoarseness, hyperglycemia, hyper-/hypotension, impotence, keratoconjunctivitis sicca, lactation suppression, loose stools, memory impairment, mydriasis, nasal congestion, nasal dryness, nasopharyngitis, palpitation, peripheral edema, pharyngolaryngeal pain, pollakiuria, pruritus, psychotic disorder, QT_c prolongation, rash, seizure, sinus congestion, sinus headache, sinusitis, sweating decreased, tachycardia, thirst, tongue coated, upper respiratory tract infection, vomiting

Topical gel:

1% to 10%:

Central nervous system: Dizziness (2% to 3%), fatigue (2%), headache (2%)

Dermatologic: Pruritus (1%)

Gastrointestinal: Xerostomia (7% to 8%), gastroenteritis (2%), constipation (1%)

Genitourinary: Urinary tract infection (7%)

Local: Application site reaction (5%; includes anesthesia, dermatitis, erythema, irritation, pain, papules, pruritus)

Respiratory: Nasopharyngitis (3%)

Transdermal:

>10%: Local: Application site reaction (17%), pruritus (14%)

1% to 10%:

Gastrointestinal: Xerostomia (4% to 10%), diarrhea (3%), constipation (3%)

Genitourinary: Dysuria (2%)

Local: Erythema (6% to 8%), vesicles (3%), rash (3%)

Ocular: Vision changes (3%)

Postmarketing and/or case reports: Cardiac arrhythmia, cycloplegia, hallucinations, lactation suppressed, myocarditis, impotence, seizure, sweating decreased, tachycardia

Drug Interactions

Metabolism/Transport Effects Substrate of CYP3A4 (minor); **Note:** Assignment of Major/Minor substrate status based on clinically relevant drug interaction potential; **Inhibits** CYP2C8 (weak), CYP2D6 (weak), CYP3A4 (weak)

Avoid Concomitant Use

Avoid concomitant use of Oxybutynin with any of the following: Pimozide

Increased Effect/Toxicity

Oxybutynin may increase the levels/effects of: AbobotulinumtoxinA; Anticholinergics; Cannabinoids; OnabotulinumtoxinA; Pimozide; Potassium Chloride; RimabotulinumtoxinB

The levels/effects of Oxybutynin may be increased by: Conivaptan; Pramlintide

Decreased Effect

Oxybutynin may decrease the levels/effects of: Acetylcholinesterase Inhibitors (Central); Secretin

The levels/effects of Oxybutynin may be decreased by: Acetylcholinesterase Inhibitors (Central); Tocilizumab

Ethanol/Nutrition/Herb Interactions Ethanol: Use ethanol with caution (may increase CNS depression and toxicity). Watch for sedation.

Stability

Immediate release: Store at controlled room temperature of 15°C to 30°C (59°F to 86°F). Protect syrup from light.

Extended release: Store at 25°C (77°F); excursions permitted to 15°C to 30°C (59°F to 86°F). Protect from moisture and humidity.

Gel sachet, transdermal patch: Store at 25°C (77°F); excursions permitted to 15°C to 30°C (59°F to 86°F). Protect from moisture and humidity. Keel gel away from open flame. Keep patch in sealed pouch. Throw away used sachets or patches where children and pets cannot reach.

Mechanism of Action Direct antispasmodic effect on smooth muscle, also inhibits the action of acetylcholine on smooth muscle (exhibits 1/5 the anticholinergic activity of atropine, but is 4-10 times the antispasmodic activity); does not block effects at skeletal muscle or at autonomic ganglia; increases bladder capacity, decreases uninhibited contractions, and delays desire to void, therefore, decreases urgency and frequency

Pharmacodynamics/Kinetics

Onset of action: Oral: 30-60 minutes

Peak effect: 3-6 hours

Duration: 6-10 hours (up to 24 hours for extended release oral formulation)

Absorption: Oral: Rapid and well absorbed; Transdermal: High

Distribution: I.V.: V_d: 193 L

Metabolism: Hepatic via CYP3A4; Oral: High first-pass metabolism; forms active and inactive metabolites

Bioavailability: Oral: ~6%
Half-life elimination: I.V.: ~2 hours (parent drug), 7-8 hours (metabolites); Oral: ~2-3 hours
Time to peak, serum: Oral: Immediate release: ~60 minutes; Extended release: 4-6 hours; Transdermal: 24-48 hours
Excretion: Urine, as metabolites and unchanged drug (<0.1%)

Dosage
Oral:
Children:
1-5 years (unlabeled use): 0.2 mg/kg/dose 2-4 times/day
>5 years: 5 mg twice daily, up to 5 mg 3 times/day maximum
>6 years: Extended release: 5 mg once daily; adjust dose in 5 mg increments; maximum dose: 20 mg/day
Adults: 5 mg 2-3 times/day up to 5 mg 4 times/day maximum
Extended release: Initial: 5-10 mg once daily, adjust dose in 5 mg increments at weekly intervals; maximum: 30 mg daily
Elderly: Regular release: Initial dose: 2.5 mg 2-3 times/day; increase as needed to 5 mg 2-3 times/day
Topical gel: Adults: Apply contents of 1 sachet (100 mg/g) once daily
Transdermal: Adults: Apply one 3.9 mg/day patch twice weekly (every 3-4 days)

Note: Should be discontinued periodically to determine whether the patient can manage without the drug and to minimize resistance to the drug

Dietary Considerations Food causes a slight delay in the absorption of the oral solution and bioavailability is increased by ~25%. Absorption of the extended release tablet is not affected by food. May be taken without regard to meals.

Administration
Oral: Administer without regard to meals. Extended release tablets must be swallowed whole with liquid; do not crush, divide, or chew; take at approximately the same time each day.
Topical gel: For topical use only. Apply to clean, dry, intact skin on abdomen, thighs, or upper arms/shoulders. Rotate site; do not apply to same site on consecutive days. Wash hands after use. Cover treated area with clothing after gel has dried to prevent transfer of medication to others. Do not bathe, shower, or swim until 1 hour after gel applied.
Transdermal: Apply to clean, dry skin on abdomen, hip, or buttock. Select a new site for each new system (avoid reapplication to same site within 7 days).

Monitoring Parameters Incontinence episodes, postvoid residual (PVR)

Test Interactions May suppress the wheal and flare reactions to skin test antigens.

Product Availability Anturol® 3% gel: FDA approved December 2011; availability is currently undetermined. Consult prescribing information for additional information.

Dosage Forms Excipient information presented when available (limited, particularly for generics); consult specific product labeling.
Gel, topical, as chloride:
Gelnique®: 10% (1 g) [contains ethanol]
Patch, transdermal:
Oxytrol®: 3.9 mg/24 hours (8s) [39 cm^2; total oxybutynin 36 mg]
Syrup, oral, as chloride: 5 mg/5 mL (5 mL, 473 mL)
Tablet, oral, as chloride: 5 mg
Tablet, extended release, oral, as chloride: 5 mg, 10 mg, 15 mg
Ditropan XL®: 5 mg, 10 mg, 15 mg

◆ **Oxybutynin Chloride** *see* Oxybutynin *on page 1264*
◆ **Oxybutynine (Can)** *see* Oxybutynin *on page 1264*
◆ **Oxycocet® (Can)** *see* Oxycodone and Acetaminophen *on page 1269*
◆ **Oxycodan® (Can)** *see* Oxycodone and Aspirin *on page 1269*

OxyCODONE (oks i KOE done)

Brand Names: U.S. OxyCONTIN®; Roxicodone®
Brand Names: Canada Oxy.IR®; OxyContin®; Oxy-NEO™; PMS-Oxycodone; Supeudol®
Index Terms Dihydrohydroxycodeinone; Oxecta™; Oxycodone Hydrochloride
Pharmacologic Category Analgesic, Opioid
Additional Appendix Information
Opioid Analgesics *on page 1896*
Patient Information for Disposal of Unused Medications *on page 2026*

Use Management of moderate-to-severe pain, normally used in combination with nonopioid analgesics

OxyContin® is indicated for around-the-clock management of moderate-to-severe pain when an analgesic is needed for an extended period of time.

Pregnancy Risk Factor B

Pregnancy Considerations Adverse events were not observed in animal reproduction studies. Opioids cross the placenta; respiratory depression and withdrawal symptoms may occur in the neonate following use during pregnancy. Controlled release formulations should not be used immediately prior to or during labor.

Lactation Enters breast milk/not recommended

Prescribing and Access Restrictions As a requirement of the REMS program, healthcare providers who prescribe OxyContin® need to receive training on the proper use and potential risks of OxyContin®. For training, please refer to http://www.oxycontinrems.com. Prescribers will need retraining every 2 years or following any significant changes to the OxyContin® REMS program.

Medication Guide Available Yes

Contraindications Hypersensitivity to oxycodone or any component of the formulation; significant respiratory depression; hypercarbia; acute or severe bronchial asthma; paralytic ileus (known or suspected)

Warnings/Precautions May cause CNS depression, which may impair physical or mental abilities; patients must be cautioned about performing tasks which require mental alertness (eg, operating machinery or driving). Effects may be potentiated when used with other sedative drugs or ethanol. Use with caution in patients with hypersensitivity reactions to other phenanthrene derivative opioid agonists (morphine, hydrocodone, hydromorphone, levorphanol, oxymorphone), respiratory diseases including asthma, emphysema, or COPD. Use with caution in pancreatitis or biliary tract disease, acute alcoholism (including delirium tremens), morbid obesity, adrenocortical insufficiency, history of seizure disorders, CNS depression/coma, kyphoscoliosis (or other skeletal disorder which may alter respiratory function), hypothyroidism (including myxedema), prostatic hyperplasia, urethral stricture, and toxic psychosis. May obscure diagnosis or clinical course of patients with acute abdominal conditions.

Use with caution in the elderly, debilitated, and hepatic or renal function. Hemodynamic effects (hypotension, orthostasis) may be exaggerated in patients with hypovolemia, concurrent vasodilating drugs, or in patients with head injury. Respiratory depressant effects and capacity to elevate CSF pressure may be exaggerated in presence of head injury, other intracranial lesion, or pre-existing intracranial pressure.

[U.S. Boxed Warning]: Concomitant use with CYP3A4 inhibitors may result in increased effects and potentially fatal respiratory depression. Concurrent use of agonist/antagonist analgesics may precipitate withdrawal symptoms and/or reduced analgesic efficacy in patients following prolonged therapy with mu opioid agonists. Abrupt discontinuation following prolonged use may also lead to withdrawal symptoms. **[U.S. Boxed Warning]: Healthcare provider should be alert to problems of abuse, misuse, and diversion.** Tolerance or drug dependence may result from extended use. Patients should be assessed for risk of abuse or addition prior to therapy and all patients should be monitored for signs of misuse, abuse, and addiction.

Controlled-release formulations: [U.S. Boxed Warning]: OxyContin® is not intended for use as an "as needed" analgesic or for immediately-postoperative pain management (should be used postoperatively only if the patient has received it prior to surgery or if severe, persistent pain is anticipated). **[U.S. Boxed Warning]: Do NOT crush, break, or chew controlled-release tablets**; 60 mg and 80 mg strengths, a single dose >40 mg, or a total dose of >80 mg/day are for use only in opioid-tolerant patients. Tablets may be difficult to swallow and could become lodged in throat; patients with swallowing difficulties may be at increased risk. Cases of intestinal obstruction or diverticulitis exacerbation have also been reported, including cases requiring medical intervention to remove the tablet; patients with an underlying GI disease (eg, esophageal cancer, colon cancer) may be at increased risk.

Highly-concentrated oral solutions: [U.S. Boxed Warning]: Concentrated oral solutions (20 mg/mL) should only be used in opioid tolerant patients (taking ≥30 mg/day of oxycodone or equivalent for ≥1 week); orders should be clearly written to include the intended dose (in mg vs mL) and the intended product concentration to be dispensed.

Adverse Reactions Note: Percentages as reported with OxyContin®

>10%:

Central nervous system: Somnolence (23%), dizziness (13%)

Dermatologic: Pruritus (13%)

Gastrointestinal: Constipation (23%), nausea (23%), vomiting (12%)

1% to 10%:

Cardiovascular: Postural hypotension (1% to 5%)

Central nervous system: Headache (7%), abnormal dreams (1% to 5%), anxiety (1% to 5%), chills (1% to 5%), confusion (1% to 5%), dysphoria (1% to 5%), euphoria (1% to 5%), fever (1% to 5%), insomnia (1% to 5%), nervousness (1% to 5%), thought abnormalities (1% to 5%)

Dermatologic: Rash (1% to 5%)

Gastrointestinal: Xerostomia (6%), abdominal pain (1% to 5%), anorexia (1% to 5%), diarrhea (1% to 5%), dyspepsia (1% to 5%), gastritis (1% to 5%)

Neuromuscular & skeletal: Weakness (6%), twitching (1% to 5%)

Respiratory: Dyspnea (1% to 5%), hiccups (1% to 5%)

Miscellaneous: Diaphoresis (5%)

<1% (Limited to important or life-threatening): Agitation, amnesia, anaphylactoid reaction, anaphylaxis, chest pain, dehydration, depression, dysphagia, dysuria, edema, emotional lability, eructation, hallucinations, hematuria, histamine release, hyperkinesia, hypoesthesia, hyponatremia, hypotonia, ileus, intracranial pressure increased, malaise, paralytic ileus, paresthesia, seizure, SIADH, speech disorder, ST segment depression, stomatitis, stupor, syncope, tablet in stool, tremor, urinary retention, vertigo, withdrawal syndrome

Drug Interactions

Metabolism/Transport Effects Substrate of CYP2D6 (minor), CYP3A4 (major); **Note:** Assignment of Major/Minor substrate status based on clinically relevant drug interaction potential

Avoid Concomitant Use

Avoid concomitant use of OxyCODONE with any of the following: Conivaptan

Increased Effect/Toxicity

OxyCODONE may increase the levels/effects of: Alcohol (Ethyl); Alvimopan; CNS Depressants; Desmopressin; Selective Serotonin Reuptake Inhibitors; Thiazide Diuretics

The levels/effects of OxyCODONE may be increased by: Amphetamines; Antipsychotic Agents (Phenothiazines); Conivaptan; CYP3A4 Inhibitors (Moderate); CYP3A4 Inhibitors (Strong); Dasatinib; Droperidol; HydrOXYzine; Succinylcholine; Voriconazole

Decreased Effect

OxyCODONE may decrease the levels/effects of: Pegvisomant

The levels/effects of OxyCODONE may be decreased by: Ammonium Chloride; CYP3A4 Inducers (Strong); Deferasirox; Mixed Agonist / Antagonist Opioids; Rifampin; St Johns Wort; Tocilizumab

Ethanol/Nutrition/Herb Interactions

Ethanol: May increase CNS depression; monitor for increased effects with coadministration. Caution patients about effects.

Herb/Nutraceutical: Avoid valerian, St John's wort, kava kava, gotu kola (may increase CNS depression).

Stability Store at 25°C (77°F); excursions permitted between 15°C to 30°C (59°F to 86°F). Protect from light.

Mechanism of Action Binds to opiate receptors in the CNS, causing inhibition of ascending pain pathways, altering the perception of and response to pain; produces generalized CNS depression

Pharmacodynamics/Kinetics

Onset of action: Pain relief: Immediate release: 10-15 minutes

Peak effect: Immediate release: 0.5-1 hour

Duration: Immediate release: 3-6 hours; Controlled release: ≤12 hours

Distribution: V_d: 2.6 L/kg; distributed to skeletal muscle, liver, intestinal tract, lungs, spleen, and brain

Protein binding: ~45%

Metabolism: Hepatically via CYP3A4 to noroxycodone (has weak analgesic), noroxymorphone, and alpha- and beta-noroxycodol. CYP2D6 mediated metabolism produces oxymorphone (has analgesic activity; low plasma concentrations), alpha- and beta-oxymorphol.

Bioavailability: Controlled release, immediate release: 60% to 87%

Half-life elimination: Immediate release: 2-4 hours; controlled release: ~5 hours

Time to peak, plasma: Immediate release: 1.2-1.9 hours; Controlled release: 4-5 hours

Excretion: Urine (~19% as parent; >64% as metabolites)

Dosage Oral: **Note:** All doses should be titrated to appropriate effect:

Children (unlabeled use): Immediate release, initial dose: 0.1-0.2 mg/kg/dose (moderate pain) or 0.2 mg/kg/dose (severe pain) (APS 6th edition). For severe chronic pain, administer on a regularly scheduled basis, every 4-6 hours, at the lowest dose that will achieve adequate analgesia.

Adults:

Immediate release: Initial: 5-15 mg every 4-6 hours as needed; dosing range: 5-20 mg/dose (APS 6th edition). For severe chronic pain, administer on a regularly scheduled basis, every 4-6 hours, at the lowest dose that will achieve adequate analgesia.

Controlled release:

Opioid naive: 10 mg every 12 hours

Concurrent CNS depressants: Reduce usual initial oxycodone dose by 1/3 to 1/2

Conversion from transdermal fentanyl: For each 25 mcg/hour transdermal dose, substitute 10 mg controlled release oxycodone every 12 hours; should be initiated 18 hours after the removal of the transdermal fentanyl patch

Currently on opioids: Use standard conversion chart to convert daily dose to oxycodone equivalent. Divide daily dose in 2 (for twice-daily dosing, usually every 12 hours) and round down to nearest dosage form.

Dose adjustment: Doses may be adjusted by changing the total daily dose (not by changing the dosing interval). Doses may be adjusted every 1-2 days and may be increased by 25% to 50%. Dose should be gradually tapered when no longer required in order to prevent withdrawal.

Note: 60 mg and 80 mg strengths, a single dose >40 mg, or a total dose of >80 mg/day are for use only in opioid-tolerant patients.

Multiplication factors for converting the daily dose of current oral opioid to the daily dose of oral oxycodone:

Current opioid mg/day dose x factor = Oxycodone mg/day dose

Codeine mg/day oral dose **x** 0.15 = Oxycodone mg/day dose

Hydrocodone mg/day oral dose **x** 0.9 = Oxycodone mg/day dose

Hydromorphone mg/day oral dose **x** 4 = Oxycodone mg/day dose

Levorphanol mg/day oral dose **x** 7.5 = Oxycodone mg/day dose

Meperidine mg/day oral dose **x** 0.1 = Oxycodone mg/day dose

Methadone mg/day oral dose **x** 1.5 = Oxycodone mg/day dose

Morphine mg/day oral dose **x** 0.5 = Oxycodone mg/day dose

Note: Divide the oxycodone mg/day dose into the appropriate dosing interval for the specific form being used.

Dosing adjustment in hepatic impairment: Reduce dosage in patients with liver disease. Decrease the dose of controlled release tablets to 1/3 to 1/2 the usual starting dose; titrate carefully.

Dosing adjustment in renal impairment: Serum concentrations are increased ~50% in patients with Cl_{cr} <60 mL/minute; adjust dose based on clinical situation.

Dietary Considerations Instruct patient to avoid high-fat meals when taking some products (food has no effect on the reformulated OxyContin®).

Administration

Controlled release: Do not moisten, crush, break, or chew controlled release tablets. Controlled release tablets are not indicated for rectal administration; increased risk of adverse events due to better rectal absorption. Controlled release tablets should be administered one at a time and each followed with water immediately after placing in the mouth.

Immediate release (Oxecta™): Must be swallowed whole with enough water to ensure complete swallowing immediately after placing in the mouth. The tablet should not be wet prior to placing in the mouth. Do not crush, chew, or dissolve the tablets. Do not administer via feeding tubes (eg, gastric, NG) due to potential for obstruction. The formulation uses technology designed to discourage common methods of tampering to prevent misuse/abuse.

Appropriate laxatives should be administered to avoid the constipating side effects associated with use. Antiemetics may be needed for persistent nausea.

Monitoring Parameters Pain relief, respiratory and mental status, blood pressure; signs of misuse, abuse, and addiction

Reference Range Blood level of 5 mg/L associated with fatality

Test Interactions Some quinolones may produce a false-positive urine screening result for opiates using commercially-available immunoassay kits. This has been demonstrated most consistently for levofloxacin and ofloxacin, but other quinolones have shown cross-reactivity in certain assay kits. Confirmation of positive opiate screens by more specific methods should be considered.

Additional Information Oxecta™ utilizes Acura Pharmaceutical's Aversion® technology which may help discourage misuse and abuse potential. Reduced abuse potential of Oxecta™ compared to other immediate-release oxycodone tablet formulations has not been proven; the FDA is requiring Pfizer to complete a post-approval epidemiological study to determine whether the formulation actually results in a decrease of misuse/abuse. In one clinical trial in nondependent recreational opioid users, the "drug-liking" responses and safety of crushed Oxecta™ tablets were compared to crushed immediate-release oxycodone tablets following the self-administered intranasal use. A small difference in "drug-liking" scores was observed, with lower scores reported in the crushed Oxecta™ group. In regards to safety, there was an increased incidence of nasopharyngeal and facial adverse events in the Oxecta™ group. In addition, there was decreased ability in the Oxecta™ group to completely administer the two crushed Oxecta™ tablets intranasally within a set time period. However, whether these differences translate into a significant clinical difference is unknown. Of note, pharmacokinetic studies showed that Oxecta™ is bioequivalent with oxycodone immediate-release tablets with no differences in T_{max} and half-life when administered in the fasted state.

Product Availability

Oxecta™: FDA approved June 2011; availability expected late third quarter 2011 or early fourth quarter 2011.

Oxecta™ is an immediate release tablet formulation of oxycodone that uses technology designed to discourage common methods of tampering that may help decrease opioid abuse and misuse.

Dosage Forms Excipient information presented when available (limited, particularly for generics); consult specific product labeling. [DSC] = Discontinued product

Capsule, oral, as hydrochloride: 5 mg

Liquid, oral, as hydrochloride [concentrate]:

Roxicodone®: 20 mg/mL (30 mL [DSC]) [contains sodium benzoate]

Solution, oral, as hydrochloride: 5 mg/5 mL (100 mL [DSC], 500 mL [DSC])

Roxicodone®: 5 mg/5 mL (5 mL [DSC], 500 mL [DSC]) [contains ethanol]

Solution, oral, as hydrochloride [concentrate]: 20 mg/mL (30 mL)

Tablet, oral, as hydrochloride: 5 mg, 10 mg, 15 mg, 20 mg, 30 mg

Roxicodone®: 5 mg, 15 mg, 30 mg [scored]

Tablet, controlled release, oral, as hydrochloride:

OxyCONTIN®: 10 mg, 15 mg, 20 mg, 30 mg, 40 mg, 60 mg, 80 mg

Controlled Substance C-II

Oxycodone and Acetaminophen

(oks i KOE done & a seet a MIN oh fen)

Brand Names: U.S. Endocet®; Percocet®; Primlev™; Roxicet™; Roxicet™ 5/500; Tylox®

Brand Names: Canada Endocet®; Novo-Oxycodone Acet; Oxycocet®; Percocet®; Percocet®-Demi; PMS-Oxycodone-Acetaminophen

Index Terms Acetaminophen and Oxycodone

Pharmacologic Category Analgesic, Opioid

Additional Appendix Information

Patient Information for Disposal of Unused Medications *on page 2026*

Use Management of moderate-to-severe pain

Pregnancy Risk Factor C

Dosage Oral: Doses should be given every 4-6 hours as needed and titrated to appropriate analgesic effects. **Note:** Initial dose is based on the **oxycodone** content; however, the maximum daily dose is based on the **acetaminophen** content.

Children: Maximum acetaminophen dose: Children <45 kg: 90 mg/kg/day; children >45 kg: 4 g/day

Mild-to-moderate pain: Initial dose, **based on oxycodone content:** 0.05-0.1 mg/kg/dose

Severe pain: Initial dose, **based on oxycodone content:** 0.3 mg/kg/dose

Adults:

Mild-to-moderate pain: Initial dose, **based on oxycodone content:** 2.5-5 mg

Severe pain: Initial dose, **based on oxycodone content:** 10-30 mg. Do not exceed acetaminophen 4 g/day.

Elderly: Doses should be titrated to appropriate analgesic effects: Initial dose, **based on oxycodone content:** 2.5-5 mg every 6 hours. Do not exceed acetaminophen 4 g/day.

Dosage adjustment in hepatic impairment: Dose should be reduced in patients with severe liver disease.

Additional Information Complete prescribing information for this medication should be consulted for additional detail.

Dosage Forms Excipient information presented when available (limited, particularly for generics); consult specific product labeling.

Caplet:

Roxicet™ 5/500: Oxycodone hydrochloride 5 mg and acetaminophen 500 mg

Capsule: 5/500: Oxycodone hydrochloride 5 mg and acetaminophen 500 mg

Tylox®: 5/500: Oxycodone hydrochloride 5 mg and acetaminophen 500 mg [contains sodium benzoate and sodium metabisulfite]

Solution, oral:

Roxicet™: Oxycodone hydrochloride 5 mg and acetaminophen 325 mg per 5 mL (5 mL, 500 mL) [contains ethanol <0.5%; mint flavor]

Tablet: 2.5/325: Oxycodone hydrochloride 2.5 mg and acetaminophen 325 mg; 5/325: Oxycodone hydrochloride 5 mg and acetaminophen 325 mg; 7.5/325: Oxycodone hydrochloride 7.5 mg and acetaminophen 325 mg; 7.5/500: Oxycodone hydrochloride 7.5 mg and acetaminophen 500 mg; 10/325: Oxycodone hydrochloride 10 mg and acetaminophen 325 mg; 10/650: Oxycodone hydrochloride 10 mg and acetaminophen 650 mg

Endocet® 5/325 [scored]: Oxycodone hydrochloride 5 mg and acetaminophen 325 mg

Endocet® 7.5/325: Oxycodone hydrochloride 7.5 mg and acetaminophen 325 mg

Endocet® 7.5/500: Oxycodone hydrochloride 7.5 mg and acetaminophen 500 mg

Endocet® 10/325: Oxycodone hydrochloride 10 mg and acetaminophen 325 mg

Endocet® 10/650: Oxycodone hydrochloride 10 mg and acetaminophen 650 mg

Percocet® 2.5/325: Oxycodone hydrochloride 2.5 mg and acetaminophen 325 mg

Percocet® 5/325 [scored]: Oxycodone hydrochloride 5 mg and acetaminophen 325 mg

Percocet® 7.5/325: Oxycodone hydrochloride 7.5 mg and acetaminophen 325 mg

Percocet® 7.5/500: Oxycodone hydrochloride 7.5 mg and acetaminophen 500 mg

Percocet® 10/325: Oxycodone hydrochloride 10 mg and acetaminophen 325 mg

Percocet® 10/650: Oxycodone hydrochloride 10 mg and acetaminophen 650 mg

Primlev™ 5/300: Oxycodone hydrochloride 5 mg and acetaminophen 300 mg

Primlev™ 7.5/300: Oxycodone hydrochloride 7.5 mg and acetaminophen 300 mg

Primlev™ 10/300: Oxycodone hydrochloride 10 mg and acetaminophen 300 mg

Roxicet™ [scored]: Oxycodone hydrochloride 5 mg and acetaminophen 325 mg

Controlled Substance C-II

Oxycodone and Aspirin (oks i KOE done & AS pir in)

Brand Names: U.S. Endodan®; Percodan®

Brand Names: Canada Endodan®; Oxycodan®; Percodan®

Index Terms Aspirin and Oxycodone

Pharmacologic Category Analgesic, Opioid

Use Management of moderate- to moderately-severe pain

Pregnancy Risk Factor B (oxycodone); D (aspirin)

Dosage Oral:

Children (dose based on total oxycodone content): Oxycodone 0.1-0.2 mg/kg/dose (maximum oxycodone: 5 mg/dose; maximum aspirin: 4 g/day). Doses should be given every 4-6 hours as needed (American Pain Society, 2008)

Adults: One tablet every 6 hours as needed for pain; maximum aspirin dose should not exceed 4 g/day

Dosing adjustment in renal impairment: Use with caution. Avoid use of aspirin in patients with Cl_{cr} <10 mL/minute.

Dosing adjustment in hepatic impairment: Use with caution. Avoid use of aspirin-containing products in severe impairment.

Additional Information Complete prescribing information for this medication should be consulted for additional detail.

Dosage Forms Excipient information presented when available (limited, particularly for generics); consult specific product labeling.

Tablet: Oxycodone hydrochloride 4.8355 mg and aspirin 325 mg

Endodan®, Percodan®: Oxycodone hydrochloride 4.8355 mg and aspirin 325 mg

Controlled Substance C-II

Oxycodone and Ibuprofen

(oks i KOE done & eye byoo PROE fen)

Index Terms Ibuprofen and Oxycodone

Pharmacologic Category Analgesic, Opioid; Nonsteroidal Anti-inflammatory Drug (NSAID), Oral

Use Short-term (≤7 days) management of acute, moderate-to-severe pain

Pregnancy Risk Factor C/D ≥30 weeks gestation

Medication Guide Available Yes

Dosage Oral: Adults: Pain: Take 1 tablet as needed (maximum: 4 tablets/24 hours); do not take for longer than 7 days

Additional Information Complete prescribing information for this medication should be consulted for additional detail.

Dosage Forms Excipient information presented when available (limited, particularly for generics); consult specific product labeling.

Tablet: Oxycodone hydrochloride 5 mg and ibuprofen 400 mg

Controlled Substance C-II

◆ **Oxycodone Hydrochloride** *see* OxyCODONE *on page 1266*

◆ **OxyCONTIN®** *see* OxyCODONE *on page 1266*

◆ **OxyContin® (Can)** *see* OxyCODONE *on page 1266*

◆ **Oxy.IR® (Can)** *see* OxyCODONE *on page 1266*

Oxymetholone (oks i METH oh lone)

Brand Names: U.S. Anadrol®-50

Pharmacologic Category Anabolic Steroid

Use Treatment of anemias caused by deficient red cell production

Pregnancy Risk Factor X

Dosage Note: The National Kidney Foundation does not recommend the use of androgens as an adjuvant to ESA treatment in anemic patients with chronic kidney disease (KDOQI, 2006).

Oral: Children and Adults: Erythropoietic effects: 1-5 mg/kg/day once daily; usual effective dose: 1-2 mg/kg/day; give for a minimum trial of 3-6 months because response may be delayed

Dosing adjustment in hepatic impairment:

Mild-to-moderate hepatic impairment: There are no dosage adjustments provided in the manufacturer's labeling.

Severe hepatic impairment: Use is contraindicated.

Additional Information Complete prescribing information for this medication should be consulted for additional detail.

Dosage Forms Excipient information presented when available (limited, particularly for generics); consult specific product labeling.

Tablet, oral:

Anadrol®-50: 50 mg [scored]

Controlled Substance C-III

Oxymorphone (oks i MOR fone)

Brand Names: U.S. Opana®; Opana® ER

Index Terms Oxymorphone Hydrochloride

Pharmacologic Category Analgesic, Opioid

Additional Appendix Information

Opioid Analgesics *on page 1896*

Use

Parenteral: Management of moderate-to-severe acute pain; relief of anxiety in patients with dyspnea associated with pulmonary edema secondary to acute left ventricular failure

Oral, regular release: Management of moderate-to-severe acute pain

Oral, extended release: Management of moderate-to-severe pain in patients requiring around-the-clock opioid treatment for an extended period of time

Pregnancy Risk Factor C

Pregnancy Considerations Teratogenic effects were not observed in animal studies; however, decreased fetal weight, decreased litter size, increased stillbirths, and increased neonatal death were noted. Chronic opioid use during pregnancy may lead to a withdrawal syndrome in the neonate. Symptoms include irritability, hyperactivity, loss of sleep pattern, abnormal crying, tremor, vomiting, diarrhea, weight loss, or failure to gain weight.

Lactation Excretion in breast milk unknown/use caution

Medication Guide Available Yes

Contraindications Hypersensitivity to oxymorphone, other morphine analogs (phenanthrene derivatives), or any component of the formulation; paralytic ileus (known or suspected); moderate-to-severe hepatic impairment; severe respiratory depression (unless in monitored setting with resuscitative equipment); acute/severe bronchial asthma; hypercarbia

Note: Injection formulation is also contraindicated in the treatment of upper airway obstruction and pulmonary edema due to a chemical respiratory irritant.

Warnings/Precautions An opioid-containing analgesic regimen should be tailored to each patient's needs and based upon the type of pain being treated (acute versus chronic), the route of administration, degree of tolerance for opioids (naive versus chronic user), age, weight, and medical condition. The optimal analgesic dose varies widely among patients. Doses should be titrated to pain relief/prevention.

May cause CNS depression, which may impair physical or mental abilities; patients must be cautioned about performing tasks which require mental alertness (eg, operating machinery or driving). Effects may be potentiated when used with other sedative drugs or ethanol. Use not recommended within 14 days of MAO inhibitors. Use with caution in patients with hypersensitivity reactions to other phenanthrene-derivative opioid agonists (codeine, hydrocodone, hydromorphone, levorphanol, oxycodone). May cause respiratory depression. Use extreme caution in patients with COPD or other chronic respiratory conditions characterized by hypoxia, hypercapnia, or diminished respiratory reserve (myxedema, cor pulmonale, kyphoscoliosis, obstructive sleep apnea, severe obesity). Use with caution in patients (particularly elderly or debilitated) with impaired respiratory function, adrenal disease, morbid obesity, seizure disorders, toxic psychosis, thyroid dysfunction, prostatic hyperplasia, or renal impairment. Use caution in mild hepatic dysfunction; use is contraindicated in moderate-to-severe hepatic impairment. Use only with extreme caution (if at all) in patients with head injury or increased intracranial pressure (ICP); potential to elevate ICP and/or blunt papillary response may be greatly exaggerated in these patients. Use with caution in biliary tract disease or acute pancreatitis (may cause constriction of sphincter of Oddi). May obscure diagnosis or clinical course of patients with acute abdominal conditions.

Oxymorphone shares the toxic potential of opiate agonists and usual precautions of opiate agonist therapy should be observed; may cause hypotension in patients with acute myocardial infarction, volume depletion, or concurrent drug therapy which may exaggerate vasodilation. The elderly may be particularly susceptible to adverse effects of narcotics.

[U.S. Boxed Warning]: Healthcare provider should be alert to problems of abuse, misuse, and diversion. Tolerance or drug dependence may result from extended use. Use caution in patients with a history of drug dependence or abuse. Abrupt discontinuation may precipitate withdrawal syndrome.

Extended release formulation:

[U.S. Boxed Warnings]: Opana® ER is an extended release oral formulation of oxymorphone and is not suitable for use as an "as needed" analgesic. Tablets should not be broken, chewed, dissolved, or crushed;

tablets should be swallowed whole. Opana® ER is intended for use in long-term, continuous management of moderate-to-severe chronic pain. It is not indicated for use in the immediate postoperative period (12-24 hours). **[U.S. Boxed Warning]: The coingestion of ethanol or ethanol-containing medications with Opana® ER may result in accelerated release of drug from the dosage form, abruptly increasing plasma levels, which may have fatal consequences.**

Adverse Reactions Incidence usually on higher end with extended release tablet.

>10%:

Central nervous system: Somnolence (9% to 19%), dizziness (7% to 18%), fever (1% to 14%), headache (7% to 12%)

Dermatologic: Pruritus (8% to 15%)

Gastrointestinal: Nausea (19% to 33%), constipation (4% to 28%), vomiting (9% to 16%)

1% to 10%:

Cardiovascular: Hypotension (<10%), tachycardia (<10%), edema (<10%), flushing (<10%), hypertension (<10%)

Central nervous system: Anxiety (1% to <10%), sedation (1% to <10%), depression (<10%), disorientation (<10%), lethargy (<10%), nervousness (<10%), restlessness (<10%), fatigue (≤4%), insomnia (≤4%), confusion (3%)

Endocrine & metabolic: Dehydration (<10%)

Gastrointestinal: Abdominal distension (<10%), flatulence (1% to <10%), xerostomia (1% to <10%), dyspepsia (<10%), weight loss (<10%), diarrhea (≤4%), abdominal pain (≤3%), appetite decreased (≤3%)

Neuromuscular & skeletal: Weakness (<10%)

Ocular: Blurred vision (<10%)

Respiratory: Hypoxia (<10%), dyspnea (<10%)

Miscellaneous: Diaphoresis (1% to <10%)

<1% (Limited to important or life-threatening): Agitation, allergic reaction, apnea (injection), atelectasis (injection), biliary colic, bradycardia,,bronchospasm (injection), clamminess, dermatitis, diplopia (injection), dysphoria, euphoric mood, hallucination, hot flashes, hypersensitivity, ileus, injection site reaction, micturition difficulty, miosis, oliguria (injection), palpitation, physical and psychological dependence, postural hypotension, respiratory depression, syncope, uretral spasm (injection), urinary retention, urticaria

Drug Interactions

Metabolism/Transport Effects None known.

Avoid Concomitant Use

Avoid concomitant use of Oxymorphone with any of the following: MAO Inhibitors

Increased Effect/Toxicity

Oxymorphone may increase the levels/effects of: Alcohol (Ethyl); Alvimopan; CNS Depressants; Desmopressin; MAO Inhibitors; Selective Serotonin Reuptake Inhibitors; Thiazide Diuretics

The levels/effects of Oxymorphone may be increased by: Amphetamines; Antipsychotic Agents (Phenothiazines); Droperidol; HydrOXYzine; Succinylcholine

Decreased Effect

Oxymorphone may decrease the levels/effects of: Pegvisomant

The levels/effects of Oxymorphone may be decreased by: Ammonium Chloride; Mixed Agonist / Antagonist Opioids

Ethanol/Nutrition/Herb Interactions

Ethanol: Ethanol ingestion with extended-release tablets is specifically contraindicated due to possible accelerated release and potentially fatal overdose. Ethanol may also increase CNS depression; monitor for increased effects with coadministration. Caution patients about effects.

Food: When taken orally with a high-fat meal, peak concentration is 38% to 50% greater. Both immediate-release and extended-release tablets should be taken 1 hour before or 2 hours after eating.

Herb/Nutraceutical: Avoid valerian, St John's wort, kava kava, gotu kola (may increase CNS depression).

Stability Injection solution, tablet: Store at 25°C (77°F); excursions permitted to 15°C to 30°C (59°F to 86°F). Protect injection from light.

Mechanism of Action Oxymorphone hydrochloride is a potent narcotic analgesic with uses similar to those of morphine. The drug is a semisynthetic derivative of morphine (phenanthrene derivative) and is closely related to hydromorphone chemically (Dilaudid®).

Pharmacodynamics/Kinetics

Onset of action: Parenteral: 5-10 minutes

Duration: Analgesic: Parenteral: 3-6 hours

Distribution: V_d: I.V.: 1.94-4.22 L/kg

Protein binding: 10% to 12%

Metabolism: Hepatic via glucuronidation to active and inactive metabolites

Bioavailability: Oral: ~10%

Half-life elimination: Oral: Immediate release: 7-9 hours; Extended release: 9-11 hours

Excretion: Urine (<1% as unchanged drug); feces

Dosage Adults: **Note:** Dosage must be individualized.

I.M., SubQ: Initial: 1-1.5 mg; may repeat every 4-6 hours as needed

Labor analgesia: I.M.: 0.5-1 mg

I.V.: Initial: 0.5 mg

Oral:

Immediate release:

Opioid-naive: 10-20 mg every 4-6 hours as needed. Initial dosages as low as 5 mg may be considered in selected patients and/or patients with renal impairment. Dosage adjustment should be based on level of analgesia, side effects, and pain intensity. Initiation of therapy with initial dose >20 mg is **not** recommended.

Note: The American Pain Society recommends an initial dose of 5-10 mg for adult patients with severe pain.

Currently on stable dose of parenteral oxymorphone: ~10 times the daily parenteral requirement. The calculated amount should be divided and given in 4-6 equal doses.

Currently on other opioids: Use standard conversion chart to convert daily dose to oxymorphone equivalent. Generally start with 1/2 the calculated daily oxymorphone dosage and administered in divided doses every 4-6 hours.

Extended release (Opana® ER):

Opioid-naive: Initial: 5 mg every 12 hours. Supplemental doses of immediate-release oxymorphone may be used as "rescue" medication as dosage is titrated.

Note: Continued requirement for supplemental dosing may be used to titrate the dose of extended-release continuous therapy. Adjust therapy incrementally, by 5-10 mg every 12 hours at intervals of every 3-7 days. Ideally, basal dosage may be titrated to generally mild pain or no pain with the regular use of fewer than 2 supplemental doses per 24 hours.

Currently on stable dose of parenteral oxymorphone: Approximately 10 times the daily parenteral requirement. The calculated amount should be given in 2 divided doses (every 12 hours).

Currently on opioids: Use conversion chart (see **"Note"**) to convert daily dose to oxymorphone equivalent. Generally start with 1/2 the calculated daily oxymorphone dosage. Divide daily dose in 2 (for every 12-hour dosing) and round down to nearest dosage form. **Note:** Per manufacturer, the following approximate oral dosages are equivalent to oxymorphone 10 mg:

Hydrocodone 20 mg
Oxycodone 20 mg
Methadone 20 mg
Morphine 30 mg

Conversion of stable dose of immediate-release oxymorphone to extended-release oxymorphone: Administer 1/2 of the daily dose of immediate-release oxymorphone (Opana®) as the extended-release formulation (Opana® ER) every 12 hours

Elderly: Initiate dosing at the lower end of the dosage range

Dosing adjustment in renal impairment: Cl_{cr} <50 mL/minute: Reduce initial dosage of oral formulations (bioavailability increased 57% to 65%). Begin therapy at lowest dose and titrate carefully.

Dosing adjustment in hepatic impairment: Generally, contraindicated for use in patients with moderate-to-severe liver disease. Initiate with lowest possible dose and titrate slowly in mild impairment.

Dietary Considerations Immediate release and extended release tablets should be taken 1 hour before or 2 hours after eating.

Administration Administer immediate release and extended release tablets 1 hour before or 2 hours after eating. Opana® ER tablet should be swallowed; do not break, crush, or chew.

Monitoring Parameters Respiratory rate, heart rate, blood pressure, CNS activity

Test Interactions Some quinolones may produce a false-positive urine screening result for opiates using commercially-available immunoassay kits. This has been demonstrated most consistently for levofloxacin and ofloxacin, but other quinolones have shown cross-reactivity in certain assay kits. Confirmation of positive opiate screens by more specific methods should be considered. May cause elevation in amylase (due to constriction of the sphincter of Oddi).

Dosage Forms Excipient information presented when available (limited, particularly for generics); consult specific product labeling. [DSC] = Discontinued product

Injection, solution, as hydrochloride:
Opana®: 1 mg/mL (1 mL)
Tablet, oral, as hydrochloride: 5 mg, 10 mg
Opana®: 5 mg, 10 mg
Tablet, extended release, oral, as hydrochloride: 7.5 mg, 15 mg
Opana® ER: 5 mg, 7.5 mg [DSC], 10 mg, 15 mg [DSC], 20 mg, 30 mg, 40 mg

Controlled Substance C-II

◆ **Oxymorphone Hydrochloride** *see* Oxymorphone *on page 1270*

◆ **OxyNEO™ (Can)** *see* OxyCODONE *on page 1266*

Oxytocin (oks i TOE sin)

Brand Names: U.S. Pitocin®

Brand Names: Canada Oxytocin for injection

Index Terms Pit

Pharmacologic Category Oxytocic Agent

Use Induction of labor in patients with a medical indication; stimulation or reinforcement of labor; adjunctive therapy in management of abortion; to produce uterine contractions during the third stage of labor; control of postpartum bleeding

Pregnancy Risk Factor C (manufacturer specific)

Pregnancy Considerations [U.S. Boxed Warning]: To be used for medical rather than elective induction of labor. Animal reproduction studies have not been conducted. When used as indicated, teratogenic effects would not be expected. Nonteratogenic adverse reactions are reported in the neonate as well as the mother.

Lactation Excretion in breast milk unknown/use caution

Contraindications Hypersensitivity to oxytocin or any component of the formulation; significant cephalopelvic disproportion; unfavorable fetal positions; fetal distress when delivery is not imminent; hypertonic or hyperactive uterus; contraindicated vaginal delivery (invasive cervical cancer, active genital herpes, prolapse of the cord, cord presentation, total placenta previa, or vasa previa); obstetrical emergencies where surgical intervention is favored; where adequate uterine activity fails to achieve satisfactory progress

Warnings/Precautions Hazardous agent - use appropriate precautions for handling and disposal. **[U.S. Boxed Warning]: To be used for medical rather than elective induction of labor.** Medical indications for labor induction may include Rh problems, maternal diabetes, preeclampsia at or near term, when delivery is in the best interest of mother or fetus, or premature rupture of membranes when delivery is indicated. Use is generally not recommended in the following conditions: Fetal distress, hydramnios, partial placenta previa, prematurity, borderline cephalopelvic disproportion, or conditions where there is a predisposition for uterine rupture. May produce antidiuretic effect (ie, water intoxication). Severe water intoxication with convulsions, coma, and death is associated with a slow oxytocin infusion over 24 hours. High doses or hypersensitivity to oxytocin may cause uterine hypertonicity, spasm, tetanic contraction, or rupture of the uterus. Intravenous preparations should be administered by adequately trained individuals familiar with its use and able to identify complications.

Adverse Reactions Frequency not defined.

Fetus or neonate:

Cardiovascular: Arrhythmias (including premature ventricular contractions), bradycardia
Central nervous system: Brain or CNS damage (permanent), neonatal seizure
Hepatic: Neonatal jaundice
Ocular: Neonatal retinal hemorrhage
Miscellaneous: Fetal death, low Apgar score (5 minute)

Mother:

Cardiovascular: Arrhythmias (including premature ventricular contractions), hypertensive episodes
Gastrointestinal: Nausea, vomiting
Genitourinary: Pelvic hematoma, postpartum hemorrhage, uterine hypertonicity, tetanic contraction of the uterus, uterine rupture, uterine spasm
Hematologic: Afibrinogenemia (fatal)
Miscellaneous: Anaphylactic reaction, subarachnoid hemorrhage; severe water intoxication with convulsions, coma, and death is associated with a slow oxytocin infusion over 24 hours

Drug Interactions

Metabolism/Transport Effects None known.

Avoid Concomitant Use There are no known interactions where it is recommended to avoid concomitant use.

Increased Effect/Toxicity

The levels/effects of Oxytocin may be increased by: Dinoprostone; Misoprostol

Decreased Effect There are no known significant interactions involving a decrease in effect.

Stability Store at 20°C to 25°C (68°F to 77°F); excursions permitted to 15°C to 30°C (59°F to 86°F); do not freeze.

Reconstitution: I.V.:

Induction or stimulation of labor: Add oxytocin 10 units to NS or LR 1000 mL to yield a solution containing oxytocin 10 milliunits/mL. Rotate solution to mix.

Postpartum uterine bleeding: Add oxytocin 10-40 units to running I.V. infusion; maximum: 40 units/1000 mL.

Adjunctive management of abortion: Add oxytocin 10 units to 500 mL of a physiologic saline solution or D_5W.

Mechanism of Action Oxytocin stimulates uterine contraction by activating G-protein-coupled receptors that trigger increases in intracellular calcium levels in uterine myofibrils. Oxytocin also increases local prostaglandin production, further stimulating uterine contraction.

Pharmacodynamics/Kinetics

Onset of action: Uterine contractions: I.M.: 3-5 minutes; I.V.: ~1 minute

Duration: I.M.: 2-3 hour; I.V.: 1 hour

Metabolism: Rapidly hepatic and via plasma (by oxytocinase) and to a smaller degree the mammary gland

Half-life elimination: 1-6 minutes; decreased in late pregnancy and during lactation

Excretion: Urine

Dosage I.V. administration requires the use of an infusion pump. Adults:

Induction of labor: Manufacturers labeling: I.V.: 0.5-1 milliunits/minute; gradually increase dose in 30-60 minute intervals by increments of 1-2 milliunits/minute until desired contraction pattern is established; dose may be decreased after desired frequency of contractions is reached and labor has progressed to 5-6 cm dilation. Infusion rates of 6 milliunits/minute provide oxytocin levels similar to those at spontaneous labor; rates >9-10 milliunits/minute are rarely required. Higher dose regimens (example, initial dose 2-6 milliunits/minute) with larger incremental dose increases (example, 1-6 milliunits/minute) have also been proposed; decrease or discontinue dose for abnormal or excessive uterine contractions (ACOG, 2009).

Postpartum bleeding:

I.M.: Total dose of 10 units after delivery of the placenta

I.V.: 10-40 units by I.V. infusion in 1000 mL of intravenous fluid at a rate sufficient to control uterine atony

Adjunctive treatment of abortion: I.V.: 10-20 milliunits/minute; maximum total dose: 30 units/12 hours

Administration I.V.: An infusion pump is required for administration

Monitoring Parameters Fluid intake and output during administration, uterine activity, blood pressure; fetal monitoring

Dosage Forms Excipient information presented when available (limited, particularly for generics); consult specific product labeling.

Injection, solution: 10 units/mL (1 mL, 10 mL, 30 mL)

Pitocin®: 10 units/mL (1 mL, 10 mL) [contains chlorobutanol]

◆ **Oxytocin for injection (Can)** *see* Oxytocin *on page* 1272

◆ **Oxytrol®** *see* Oxybutynin *on page* 1264

◆ **Oysco D [OTC]** *see* Calcium and Vitamin D *on page* 265

◆ **Oysco 500 [OTC]** *see* Calcium Carbonate *on page* 266

◆ **Oysco 500+D [OTC]** *see* Calcium and Vitamin D *on page* 265

◆ **Oyst-Cal-D [OTC]** *see* Calcium and Vitamin D *on page* 265

◆ **Oyst-Cal-D 500 [OTC]** *see* Calcium and Vitamin D *on page* 265

◆ **Oystercal™ 500 [OTC]** *see* Calcium Carbonate *on page* 266

◆ **Ozurdex®** *see* Dexamethasone (Ophthalmic) *on page* 483

◆ **P01BE03** *see* Artesunate *on page* 148

◆ **P32** *see* Chromic Phosphate P 32 *on page* 354

◆ **P-071** *see* Cetirizine *on page* 330

◆ **P-1202** *see* Methyl Aminolevulinate *on page* 1103

◆ **Pacerone®** *see* Amiodarone *on page* 90

◆ **Pacis™ (Can)** *see* BCG *on page* 191

PACLitaxel (pac li TAKS el)

Brand Names: Canada Apo-Paclitaxel®; Paclitaxel For Injection; Taxol®

Index Terms Conventional Paclitaxel; Paclitaxel (Conventional); Taxol

Pharmacologic Category Antineoplastic Agent, Antimicrotubular; Antineoplastic Agent, Natural Source (Plant) Derivative; Antineoplastic Agent, Taxane Derivative

Use Treatment of breast, nonsmall cell lung, and ovarian cancers; treatment of AIDS-related Kaposi's sarcoma (KS)

Unlabeled Use Treatment of bladder, cervical, small cell lung, and head and neck cancers; treatment of (unknown primary) adenocarcinoma

Pregnancy Risk Factor D

Pregnancy Considerations Animal studies have demonstrated embryotoxicity, fetal toxicity, and maternal toxicity. There are no adequate and well-controlled studies in pregnant women. Women of childbearing potential should be advised to avoid becoming pregnant.

Lactation Excretion in breast milk unknown/contraindicated

Contraindications Hypersensitivity to paclitaxel, Cremophor® EL (polyoxyethylated castor oil), or any component of the formulation

Warnings/Precautions Hazardous agent - use appropriate precautions for handling and disposal. **[U.S. Boxed Warning]: Severe hypersensitivity reactions have been reported;** premedication may minimize this effect. Stop infusion and do not rechallenge for severe hypersensitivity reactions (hypotension requiring treatment, dyspnea requiring bronchodilators, angioedema, urticaria). Minor hypersensitivity reactions (flushing, skin reactions, dyspnea, hypotension, or tachycardia) do not require interruption of treatment. **[U.S. Boxed Warning]: Bone marrow suppression is the dose-limiting toxicity; do not administer if baseline absolute neutrophil count (ANC) is <1500 cells/mm^3 (<1000 cells/mm^3 for patients with AIDS-related KS);** reduce future doses by 20% for severe neutropenia (<500 cells/mm^3 for 7 days or more) and consider the use of supportive therapy, including growth factor treatment.

Use extreme caution with hepatic dysfunction (myelotoxicity may be worsened); dose reductions are recommended. Peripheral neuropathy may occur; patients with pre-existing neuropathies from chemotherapy or coexisting conditions (eg, diabetes mellitus) may be at a higher risk; reduce dose by 20% for severe neuropathy. Paclitaxel formulations contain dehydrated alcohol; may cause adverse CNS effects. Infusion-related hypotension, bradycardia, and/or hypertension may occur; frequent monitoring of vital signs is recommended, especially during the first hour of the infusion. Rare but severe conduction abnormalities have been reported; conduct cardiac monitoring during subsequent infusions for these patients. When administered as sequential infusions, taxane derivatives (docetaxel, paclitaxel) should be administered before platinum derivatives (carboplatin, cisplatin) to limit myelosuppression. Elderly patients have an increased risk of toxicity (neutropenia, neuropathy). **[U.S. Boxed Warning]: Should be administered under the supervision of an experienced cancer chemotherapy physician.** Safety and efficacy in children have not been established.

Adverse Reactions Percentages reported with single-agent therapy. **Note:** Myelosuppression is dose related, schedule related, and infusion-rate dependent (increased incidences with higher doses, more frequent doses, and longer infusion times) and, in general, rapidly reversible upon discontinuation.

>10%:

Cardiovascular: Flushing (28%), ECG abnormal (14% to 23%), edema (21%), hypotension (4% to 12%)

Dermatologic: Alopecia (87%), rash (12%)

Gastrointestinal: Nausea/vomiting (52%), diarrhea (38%), mucositis (17% to 35%; grades 3/4: up to 3%), stomatitis (15%; most common at doses >390 mg/m^2), abdominal pain (with intraperitoneal paclitaxel)

Hematologic: Neutropenia (78% to 98%; grade 4: 14% to 75%; onset 8-10 days, median nadir 11 days, recovery 15-21 days), leukopenia (90%; grade 4: 17%), anemia (47% to 90%; grades 3/4: 2% to 16%), thrombocytopenia (4% to 20%; grades 3/4: 1% to 7%), bleeding (14%)

Hepatic: Alkaline phosphatase increased (22%), AST increased (19%)

Local: Injection site reaction (erythema, tenderness, skin discoloration, swelling: 13%)

Neuromuscular & skeletal: Peripheral neuropathy (42% to 70%; grades 3/4: up to 7%), arthralgia/myalgia (60%), weakness (17%)

Renal: Creatinine increased (observed in KS patients only: 18% to 34%; severe: 5% to 7%)

Miscellaneous: Hypersensitivity reaction (31% to 45%; grades 3/4: up to 2%), infection (15% to 30%)

1% to 10%:

Cardiovascular: Bradycardia (3%), tachycardia (2%), hypertension (1%), rhythm abnormalities (1%), syncope (1%), venous thrombosis (1%)

Dermatologic: Nail changes (2%)

Hematologic: Febrile neutropenia (2%)

Hepatic: Bilirubin increased (7%)

Respiratory: Dyspnea (2%)

<1% (Limited to important or life-threatening): Anaphylaxis, arrhythmia, ataxia, atrial fibrillation, AV block, back pain, cardiac conduction abnormalities, cellulitis, CHF, chills, conjunctivitis, dehydration, enterocolitis, extravasation recall, hepatic encephalopathy, hepatic necrosis, induration, intestinal obstruction, intestinal perforation, interstitial pneumonia, ischemic colitis, lacrimation increased, maculopapular rash, malaise, MI, myocardial ischemia, necrotic changes and ulceration following extravasation, neuroencephalopathy, neutropenic enterocolitis, neutropenic typhlitis, ototoxicity (tinnitus and hearing loss), pancreatitis, paralytic ileus, phlebitis, pneumonitis, pruritus, pulmonary embolism, pulmonary fibrosis, radiation recall, radiation pneumonitis, renal insufficiency, seizure, skin exfoliation, skin fibrosis, skin necrosis, Stevens-Johnson syndrome, supraventricular tachycardia, toxic epidermal necrolysis, ventricular tachycardia (asymptomatic), visual disturbances (scintillating scotomata)

Drug Interactions

Metabolism/Transport Effects **Substrate** of CYP2C8 (major), CYP3A4 (major), P-glycoprotein; **Note:** Assignment of Major/Minor substrate status based on clinically relevant drug interaction potential; **Induces** CYP3A4 (weak/moderate)

Avoid Concomitant Use

Avoid concomitant use of PACLitaxel with any of the following: BCG; CloZAPine; Conivaptan; Natalizumab; Pimecrolimus; SORAfenib; Tacrolimus (Topical); Vaccines (Live)

Increased Effect/Toxicity

PACLitaxel may increase the levels/effects of: Antineoplastic Agents (Anthracycline, Systemic); Bexarotene; Bexarotene (Systemic); CloZAPine; DOXOrubicin; Leflunomide; Natalizumab; Trastuzumab; Vaccines (Live); Vinorelbine

The levels/effects of PACLitaxel may be increased by: Conivaptan; CYP2C8 Inhibitors (Moderate); CYP2C8 Inhibitors (Strong); CYP3A4 Inhibitors (Moderate); CYP3A4 Inhibitors (Strong); Dasatinib; Deferasirox; Denosumab; P-glycoprotein/ABCB1 Inhibitors; Pimecrolimus; Platinum Derivatives; Reverse Transcriptase Inhibitors (Non-Nucleoside); Roflumilast; SORAfenib; Tacrolimus (Topical); Trastuzumab

Decreased Effect

PACLitaxel may decrease the levels/effects of: ARIPiprazole; BCG; Coccidioidin Skin Test; Saxagliptin; Sipuleucel-T; Vaccines (Inactivated); Vaccines (Live)

The levels/effects of PACLitaxel may be decreased by: Bexarotene; Bexarotene (Systemic); CYP2C8 Inducers (Strong); CYP3A4 Inducers (Strong); Deferasirox; Echinacea; P-glycoprotein/ABCB1 Inducers; Tocilizumab; Trastuzumab

Ethanol/Nutrition/Herb Interactions Herb/Nutraceutical: Avoid black cohosh, dong quai in estrogen-dependent tumors. Avoid valerian, St John's wort (may decrease paclitaxel levels), kava kava, gotu kola (may increase CNS depression).

Stability Store intact vials at room temperature of 20°C to 25°C (68°F to 77°F) and protect from light. Dilute in 250-1000 mL D_5W, D_5LR, D_5NS, or NS to a concentration of 0.3-1.2 mg/mL. Solutions in D_5W and NS are stable for up to 3 days at room temperature (25°C). Chemotherapy dispensing devices (eg, Chemo Dispensing Pin™) should not be used to withdraw paclitaxel from the vial.

Paclitaxel should be dispensed in either glass or non-PVC containers (eg, Excel™/PAB™). Use **nonpolyvinyl** (non-PVC) tubing (eg, polyethylene) to minimize leaching. Formulated in a vehicle known as Cremophor® EL (polyoxyethylated castor oil). Cremophor® EL has been found to leach the plasticizer DEHP from polyvinyl chloride infusion bags or administration sets. Contact of the undiluted concentrate with plasticized polyvinyl chloride (PVC) equipment or devices is not recommended.

Mechanism of Action Paclitaxel promotes microtubule assembly by enhancing the action of tubulin dimers, stabilizing existing microtubules, and inhibiting their disassembly, interfering with the late G_2 mitotic phase, and inhibiting cell replication. In addition, the drug can distort mitotic spindles, resulting in the breakage of chromosomes. Paclitaxel may also suppress cell proliferation and modulate immune response.

Pharmacodynamics/Kinetics

Distribution:

V_d: Widely distributed into body fluids and tissues; affected by dose and duration of infusion

V_{dss}:

1- to 6-hour infusion: 67.1 L/m^2

24-hour infusion: 227-688 L/m^2

Protein binding: 89% to 98%

Metabolism: Hepatic via CYP2C8 and 3A4; forms metabolites (primarily 6α-hydroxypaclitaxel)

Half-life elimination:

1- to 6-hour infusion: Mean (beta): 6.4 hours

3-hour infusion: Mean (terminal): 13.1-20.2 hours

24-hour infusion: Mean (terminal): 15.7-52.7 hours

Excretion: Feces (~70%, 5% as unchanged drug); urine (14%)

Clearance: Mean: Total body: After 1- and 6-hour infusions: 5.8-16.3 L/hour/m^2; After 24-hour infusions: 14.2-17.2 L/hour/m^2

Dosage Premedication with dexamethasone (20 mg orally or I.V. at 12 and 6 hours **or** 14 and 7 hours before the dose; reduce dexamethasone dose to 10 mg orally with advanced HIV disease), diphenhydramine (50 mg I.V. 30-60 minutes prior to the dose), and cimetidine, famotidine, or ranitidine (I.V. 30-60 minutes prior to the dose) is recommended.

Adults: I.V.: Refer to individual protocols

Ovarian carcinoma: 135-175 mg/m^2 over 3 hours every 3 weeks **or**
135 mg/m^2 over 24 hours every 3 weeks **or**
50-80 mg/m^2 over 1-3 hours weekly **or**
1.4-4 mg/m^2/day continuous infusion for 14 days every 4 weeks

Metastatic breast cancer: 175-250 mg/m^2 over 3 hours every 3 weeks **or**
50-80 mg/m^2 weekly **or**
1.4-4 mg/m^2/day continuous infusion for 14 days every 4 weeks

Nonsmall cell lung carcinoma: 135 mg/m^2 over 24 hours every 3 weeks

AIDS-related Kaposi's sarcoma: 135 mg/m^2 over 3 hours every 3 weeks **or**
100 mg/m^2 over 3 hours every 2 weeks

Intraperitoneal (unlabeled route): Ovarian carcinoma: 60 mg/m^2 on day 8 of a 21-day treatment cycle for 6 cycles, in combination with I.V. paclitaxel and intraperitoneal cisplatin. **Note:** Administration of intraperitoneal paclitaxel should include the standard paclitaxel premedication regimen.

Dosage modification for toxicity (solid tumors, including ovary, breast, and lung carcinoma): Courses of paclitaxel should not be repeated until the neutrophil count is ≥1500 cells/mm^3 and the platelet count is ≥100,000 cells/mm^3; reduce dosage by 20% for patients experiencing severe peripheral neuropathy or severe neutropenia (neutrophil <500 cells/mm^3 for a week or longer)

Dosage modification for immunosuppression in advanced HIV disease: Paclitaxel should not be given to patients with HIV if the baseline or subsequent neutrophil count is <1000 cells/mm^3. Additional modifications include: Reduce dosage of dexamethasone in premedication to 10 mg orally; reduce dosage by 20% in patients experiencing severe peripheral neuropathy or severe neutropenia (neutrophil <500 cells/mm^3 for a week or longer); initiate concurrent hematopoietic growth factor (G-CSF) as clinically indicated

Dosage adjustment in renal impairment: There are no FDA-approved labeling guidelines for dosage adjustment in patients with renal impairment. Aronoff (2007) recommends no dosage adjustment necessary for adults with Cl_{cr} <50 mL/minute.

Dosage adjustment in hepatic impairment: Note: The FDA-approved labeling recommendations are based upon the patient's first course of therapy where the usual dose would be 135 mg/m^2 dose over 24 hours or the 175 mg/m^2 dose over 3 hours in patients with normal hepatic function. Dosage in subsequent courses should be based upon individual tolerance. Adjustments for other regimens are not available.

24-hour infusion:
Transaminases <2 times upper limit of normal (ULN) and bilirubin level ≤1.5 mg/dL: 135 mg/m^2
Transaminases 2-<10 times ULN and bilirubin level ≤1.5 mg/dL: 100 mg/m^2
Transaminases <10 times ULN and bilirubin level 1.6-7.5 mg/dL: 50 mg/m^2
Transaminases ≥10 times ULN **or** bilirubin level >7.5 mg/dL: Avoid use

3-hour infusion:
Transaminases <10 times ULN and bilirubin level ≤1.25 times ULN: 175 mg/m^2
Transaminases <10 times ULN and bilirubin level 1.26-2 times ULN: 135 mg/m^2
Transaminases <10 times ULN and bilirubin level 2.01-5 times ULN: 90 mg/m^2
Transaminases ≥10 times ULN **or** bilirubin level >5 times ULN: Avoid use

Administration

I.V.: Infuse over 1-96 hours. When administered as sequential infusions, taxane derivatives should be administered before platinum derivatives (cisplatin, carboplatin) to limit myelosuppression and to enhance efficacy.

Premedication with dexamethasone (20 mg orally or I.V. at 12 and 6 hours **or** 14 and 7 hours before the dose; reduce to 10 mg with advanced HIV disease), diphenhydramine (50 mg I.V. 30-60 minutes prior to the dose), and cimetidine 300 mg, famotidine 20 mg, or ranitidine 50 mg (I.V. 30-60 minutes prior to the dose) is recommended.

Administer I.V. infusion over 1-24 hours; infuse through a 0.22 micron in-line filter and nonsorbing administration set.

Intraperitoneal: 1- to 2-hour infusion

Monitoring Parameters CBC with differential and platelet count, liver and kidney function; monitor for hypersensitivity reactions, vital signs (frequently during the first hour of infusion), continuous cardiac monitoring (patients with conduction abnormalities)

Reference Range Mean maximum serum concentrations: 435-802 ng/mL following 24-hour infusions of 200-275 mg/m^2 and were approximately 10% to 30% of those following 6-hour infusions of equivalent doses

Additional Information Sensory neuropathy is almost universal at doses >250 mg/m^2; motor neuropathy is uncommon at doses <250 mg/m^2. Myopathic effects are common with doses >200 mg/m^2, generally occur within 2-3 days of treatment, and resolve over 5-6 days. Intraperitoneal administration of paclitaxel is associated with a higher incidence of chemotherapy related toxicity.

Dosage Forms Excipient information presented when available (limited, particularly for generics); consult specific product labeling.

Injection, solution: 6 mg/mL (5 mL, 16.7 mL, 25 mL, 50 mL)

- **Paclitaxel, Albumin-Bound** *see* PACLitaxel (Protein Bound) *on page* 1275
- **Paclitaxel (Conventional)** *see* PACLitaxel *on page* 1273
- **Paclitaxel For Injection (Can)** *see* PACLitaxel *on page* 1273

PACLitaxel (Protein Bound)

(pac li TAKS el PROE teen bownd)

Brand Names: U.S. Abraxane®

Brand Names: Canada Abraxane®

Index Terms ABI-007; Albumin-Bound Paclitaxel; Albumin-Stabilized Nanoparticle Paclitaxel; nab-Paclitaxel; Nanoparticle Albumin-Bound Paclitaxel; Paclitaxel, Albumin-Bound; Protein-Bound Paclitaxel

Pharmacologic Category Antineoplastic Agent, Antimicrotubular; Antineoplastic Agent, Natural Source (Plant) Derivative; Antineoplastic Agent, Taxane Derivative

Use Treatment of refractory (metastatic) or relapsed (within 6 months of adjuvant therapy) breast cancer

Unlabeled Use Treatment of advanced nonsmall cell lung cancer (NSCLC)

Pregnancy Risk Factor D

Dosage I.V.: Adults:

Breast cancer: 260 mg/m^2 every 3 weeks

Breast cancer (weekly treatment; unlabeled schedule): 100-150 mg/m^2 on days 1, 8, and 15 of a 28-day cycle (Gradishar, 2009)

NSCLC (unlabeled use): 260 mg/m^2 every 3 weeks (Green, 2006) **or** 125 mg/m^2 on days 1, 8, and 15 of a 28-day cycle (Rizvi, 2008)

Dosage adjustment for toxicity:

Severe neutropenia (<500 cells/mm^3) ≥1 week: Reduce dose to 220 mg/m^2 for subsequent courses

Recurrent severe neutropenia: Reduce dose to 180 mg/m^2

Sensory neuropathy

Grade 1 or 2: Dosage adjustment generally not required

Grade 3: Hold treatment until resolved to grade 1 or 2, then resume with reduced dose for all subsequent cycles

Severe sensory neuropathy: Reduce dose to 220 mg/m^2 for subsequent courses

Recurrent severe sensory neuropathy: Reduce dose to 180 mg/m^2

Dosage adjustment in renal impairment: Has not been studied; patients with serum creatinine >2 mg/dL were excluded from clinical trials

Dosage adjustment in hepatic impairment: Every-3-week breast cancer regimen:

Mild impairment (AST <10 times ULN and bilirubin ≤1.25 times ULN): No adjustment required

Moderate impairment (AST <10 times ULN and bilirubin 1.26-2 times ULN): Reduce dose to 200 mg/m^2

Severe impairment:

AST <10 times ULN and bilirubin 2.01-5 times ULN: Reduce dose to 130 mg/m^2; may increase up to 200 mg/m^2 in subsequent cycles (based on individual tolerance)

AST >10 times ULN or bilirubin >5 times ULN: Use is not recommended

Additional Information Complete prescribing information for this medication should be consulted for additional detail.

Dosage Forms Excipient information presented when available (limited, particularly for generics); consult specific product labeling.

Injection, powder for reconstitution:

Abraxane®: 100 mg [contains albumin (human)]

◆ **Pain Eze [OTC]** *see* Acetaminophen *on page 27*

◆ **Pain & Fever Children's [OTC]** *see* Acetaminophen *on page 27*

◆ **Pain-Off [OTC]** *see* Acetaminophen, Aspirin, and Caffeine *on page 32*

◆ **Palafer® (Can)** *see* Ferrous Fumarate *on page 706*

◆ **Palgic®** *see* Carbinoxamine *on page 287*

Palifermin (pal ee FER min)

Brand Names: U.S. Kepivance®

Brand Names: Canada Kepivance®

Index Terms AMJ 9701; rhKGF; rhu Keratinocyte Growth Factor; rHu-KGF

Pharmacologic Category Keratinocyte Growth Factor

Use Decrease the incidence and severity of severe oral mucositis associated with hematologic malignancies in patients receiving myelotoxic therapy requiring hematopoietic stem cell support

Pregnancy Risk Factor C

Pregnancy Considerations Palifermin has been shown to be embryotoxic in animal studies at doses also associated with maternal toxicity. There are no adequate and well-controlled studies in pregnant women.

Lactation Excretion in breast milk unknown/use caution

Contraindications Hypersensitivity to palifermin, *E. coli*-derived proteins, or any component of the formulation

Warnings/Precautions Hazardous agent - use appropriate precautions for handling and disposal. Edema, erythema, pruritus, rash, oral/perioral dysesthesia, taste alteration, tongue discoloration, and tongue thickening may occur; instruct patients to report mucocutaneous effects. Safety and efficacy have not been established with nonhematologic malignancies; effect on the growth of non-hematopoietic human tumors is not known. Palifermin has been shown to enhance epithelial tumor cell lines *in vitro*. Palifermin should be administered prior to and following, but not with, chemotherapy. If administered during or within 24 hours of (before or after) chemotherapy, palifermin may increase the severity and duration of mucositis due to the increased sensitivity of rapidly-dividing epithelial cells. Safety and efficacy have not been established in children.

Adverse Reactions

>10%:

Cardiovascular: Edema (28%), hypertension (7% to 14%)

Central nervous system: Fever (39%); pain (16%); dysesthesia (oral hyperesthesia, hypoesthesia, and paresthesia 12%)

Dermatologic: Rash (62%; grade 3: 3%), pruritus (35%), erythema (32%)

Gastrointestinal: Serum amylase increased (grades 3/4: 38%), mouth/tongue discoloration or thickness (17%), taste alteration (16%), serum lipase increased (grades 3/4: 11%)

Renal: Proteinuria (17%)

Respiratory: Cough (32%), rhinitis (16%)

1% to 10%:

Neuromuscular & skeletal: Arthralgia (10%)

Miscellaneous: Antibody formation (2%)

<1% (Limited to important or life-threatening): Flexural hyperpigmentation

Drug Interactions

Metabolism/Transport Effects None known.

Avoid Concomitant Use There are no known interactions where it is recommended to avoid concomitant use.

Increased Effect/Toxicity There are no known significant interactions involving an increase in effect.

Decreased Effect There are no known significant interactions involving a decrease in effect.

Stability Store intact vials under refrigeration at 2°C to 8°C (36°F to 46°F). Protect from light. To reconstitute, slowly add 1.2 mL SWFI, to a final concentration of 5 mg/mL. Swirl gently; do not shake or vigorously agitate. Do not filter during preparation or administration. Protect reconstituted solution from light. Reconstituted vials are stable for up to 72 hours refrigerated and should not be used if left at room temperature >2 hours (data on file). The product labeling, however, indicates that reconstituted vials are stable for up to 24 hours refrigerated and should not be used if left at room temperature >1 hour. Do not freeze reconstituted product.

Mechanism of Action Palifermin is a recombinant keratinocyte growth factor (KGF) produced in *E. coli*. Endogenous KGF is produced by mesenchymal cells in response to epithelial tissue injury. KGF binds to the KGF receptor resulting in proliferation, differentiation and migration of epithelial cells in multiple tissues, including (but not limited to) the tongue, buccal mucosa, esophagus, and salivary gland.

Pharmacodynamics/Kinetics

Onset of action: Epithelial cell proliferation (dose-dependent): 48 hours

Half-life elimination: 4.5 hours (range: 3.3-5.7 hours)

Dosage I.V.: Adults: 60 mcg/kg/day for 3 consecutive days before and after myelotoxic therapy; total of 6 doses

Note: Administer first 3 doses prior to myelotoxic therapy, with the 3rd dose given 24-48 hours before therapy begins. The last 3 doses should be administered after myelotoxic therapy, with the first of these doses after but on the same day as hematopoietic stem cell infusion and at least 4 days after the most recent dose of palifermin.

Dosage adjustment in renal impairment: No adjustment necessary

Administration Administer by I.V. bolus. If heparin is used to maintain the patency of the I.V. line, flush line with saline prior to and after palifermin administration. Do not administer palifermin during or within 24 hours before or after chemotherapy. Allow solution to reach room temperature prior to administration; do not use if at room temperature >1 hour. Do not filter.

Additional Information Oncology Comment: The Multinational Association of Supportive Care in Cancer and the International Society for Oral Oncology (MASCC/ISOO) guidelines for the prevention and treatment of mucositis recommend palifermin (at the FDA-approved dose) for the prevention of oral mucositis in patients with hematologic malignancies who are receiving high-dose chemotherapy and total body irradiation with autologous stem cell transplantation (Keefe, 2007).

Guidelines from the American Society of Clinical Oncology (ASCO) for the use of chemotherapy and radiotherapy protectants (Hensley, 2008) recommend the use of palifermin to decrease the incidence of severe mucositis in patients undergoing autologous stem-cell transplantation with a total body irradiation (TBI) conditioning regimen. According to the ASCO guidelines, data are insufficient to recommend palifermin when the conditioning regimen is chemotherapy only. Palifermin may be considered in patients undergoing myeloablative allogeneic stem-cell transplantation with a TBI conditioning regimen, however data are again insufficient to recommend palifermin when the conditioning regimen is chemotherapy only. Due to a lack of appropriate data, the guidelines also do not recommend palifermin use in non-stem-cell transplantation treatment regimens or for use when treating solid tumors.

Dosage Forms Excipient information presented when available (limited, particularly for generics); consult specific product labeling.

Injection, powder for reconstitution [preservative free]:

Kepivance®: 6.25 mg [contains mannitol, sucrose 25 mg]

Paliperidone (pal ee PER i done)

Brand Names: U.S. Invega®; Invega® Sustenna®

Brand Names: Canada Invega®; Invega® Sustenna®

Index Terms 9-hydroxy-risperidone; 9-OH-risperidone; Paliperidone Palmitate

Pharmacologic Category Antipsychotic Agent, Atypical

Additional Appendix Information

Antipsychotic Agents *on page 1880*

Use

Oral: Acute and maintenance treatment of schizophrenia; acute treatment of schizoaffective disorder (monotherapy or adjunctive therapy to mood stabilizers and/or antidepressants)

Injection: Acute and maintenance treatment of schizophrenia

Unlabeled Use Psychosis/agitation related to Alzheimer's dementia

Pregnancy Risk Factor C

Pregnancy Considerations Animal studies with risperidone indicate an increase in fetal mortality. Antipsychotic use during the third trimester of pregnancy has a risk for abnormal muscle movements (extrapyramidal symptoms [EPS]) and withdrawal symptoms in newborns following delivery. Symptoms in the newborn may include agitation, feeding disorder, hypertonia, hypotonia, respiratory distress, somnolence, and tremor; these effects may be self-limiting or require hospitalization. There are no adequate and well-controlled studies in pregnant women. Reversible EPS symptoms were noted in neonates following maternal use of risperidone during the last trimester. Healthcare providers are encouraged to enroll women 18-45 years of age exposed to paliperidone during pregnancy in the Atypical Antipsychotics Pregnancy Registry (1-866-961-2388).

Lactation Enters breast milk/not recommended

Contraindications Hypersensitivity to paliperidone, risperidone, or any component of the formulation

Warnings/Precautions [U.S. Boxed Warning]: Elderly patients with dementia-related psychosis treated with antipsychotics are at an increased risk of death compared to placebo. Most deaths appeared to be either cardiovascular (eg, heart failure, sudden death) or infectious (eg, pneumonia) in nature. In addition, an increased incidence of cerebrovascular adverse effects (eg, transient ischemic attack, cerebrovascular accidents) has been reported in studies of placebo-controlled trials of risperidone (paliperidone is the primary active metabolite of risperidone) in elderly patients with dementia-related psychosis. Paliperidone is not approved for the treatment of dementia-related psychosis.

Compared with risperidone, paliperidone is low to moderately sedating; use with caution in disorders where CNS depression is a feature. Use caution in patients with predisposition to seizures. Use with caution in renal dysfunction; dose reduction recommended. Esophageal dysmotility and aspiration have been associated with antipsychotic use; use with caution in patients at risk of aspiration pneumonia (eg, Alzheimer's disease).

Leukopenia, neutropenia, and agranulocytosis (sometimes fatal) have been reported in clinical trials and postmarketing reports with antipsychotic use; presence of risk factors (eg, pre-existing low WBC or history of drug-induced leuko-/neutropenia) should prompt periodic blood count assessment. Discontinue therapy at first signs of blood dyscrasias or if absolute neutrophil count <1000/mm^3.

Paliperidone is associated with increased prolactin levels; clinical significance of hyperprolactinemia in patients with breast cancer or other prolactin-dependent tumors is unknown. May alter temperature regulation. May mask toxicity of other drugs or conditions (eg intestinal obstruction, Reyes syndrome, brain tumor) due to antiemetic effects. Priapism has been reported rarely with use.

May cause orthostasis and syncope. Use with caution in patients with cardiovascular diseases (eg, heart failure, history of myocardial infarction or ischemia, cerebrovascular disease, conduction abnormalities). Use caution in patients receiving medications for hypertension (orthostatic effects may be exacerbated) or in patients with hypovolemia or dehydration. May alter cardiac conduction; life-threatening arrhythmias have occurred with therapeutic doses of neuroleptics. Avoid use in combination with QT_c-prolonging drugs. Avoid use in patients with congenital long QT syndrome and in patients with history of cardiac arrhythmia.

May cause extrapyramidal symptoms (EPS), including pseudoparkinsonism, acute dystonic reactions, akathisia, and tardive dyskinesia (risk of these reactions is low relative to other neuroleptics, and is dose dependent). Risk of dystonia (and probably other EPS) may be greater with increased doses, use of conventional antipsychotics, males, and younger patients. Risk of neuroleptic malignant syndrome (NMS) may be increased in patients with Parkinson's disease or Lewy body dementia; monitor for symptoms of confusion, obtundation, postural instability and extrapyramidal symptoms. May cause hyperglycemia; in some cases may be extreme and associated with ketoacidosis, hyperosmolar coma, or death. Use with caution in patients with diabetes (or risk factors) or other disorders of glucose regulation; monitor for worsening of glucose control. Significant weight gain has been observed with antipsychotic therapy; incidence varies with product. Monitor waist circumference and BMI. May cause lipid abnormalities (LDL and triglycerides increased; HDL decreased).

The possibility of a suicide attempt is inherent in psychotic illness or bipolar disorder; use caution in high-risk patients during initiation of therapy. Prescriptions should be written for the smallest quantity consistent with good patient care.

The tablet formulation consists of drug within a nonabsorbable shell that is expelled and may be visible in the stool. Use is not recommended in patients with pre-existing severe gastrointestinal narrowing disorders. Patients with upper GI tract alterations in transit time may have increased or decreased bioavailability of paliperidone. Do not use in patients unable to swallow the tablet whole.

Adverse Reactions Unless otherwise noted, frequency of adverse effects is reported for the oral/I.M. formulation in adults.

>10%:

Cardiovascular: Tachycardia (1% to 14%)

Central nervous system: EPS (≤26%; dose dependent), insomnia (10% to 15%), headache (6% to 15%), parkinsonism (3% to 14%; dose dependent), somnolence (adolescents 9% to 26%; adults 1% to 12%; dose dependent)

Neuromuscular & skeletal: Tremor (2% to 12%)

3% to 10%:

Cardiovascular: Orthostatic hypotension (1% to 4%; dose dependent), bundle branch block (≤3%)

Central nervous system: Agitation (4% to 10%), akathisia (adolescents 4% to 17%; adults 1% to 10%; dose dependent), anxiety (adolescents ≤9%; adults 3% to 8%), dizziness (1% to 6%), dystonia (1% to 5%; dose dependent), dysarthria (1% to 4%; dose dependent), fatigue (adolescents ≤4%), sleep disorder (≤3%), lethargy (adolescents ≤3%)

Endocrine and metabolic: Amenorrhea (adolescents ≤6%), galactorrhea (adolescents ≤4%), gynecomastia (adolescents ≤3%)

Gastrointestinal: Weight gain (1% to 9%; dose dependent), nausea (2% to 8%), dyspepsia (5% to 6%), vomiting (adolescents ≤11%; adults 2% to 5%), constipation (1% to 5%), salivation increased (adolescents ≤6%; adults ≤4%; dose dependent), appetite increased (2% to 3%), toothache (1% to 3%), abdominal pain (≤3%), diarrhea (≤3%), xerostomia (≤3%); tongue swelling (adolescents ≤3%), tongue paralysis (adolescents ≤3%)

Local: I.M. formulation: Injection site reaction (≤10%)

Neuromuscular & skeletal: Hyperkinesia (2% to 10% dose dependent), dyskinesia (1% to 9%), weakness (≤4%), myalgia (≤4% dose dependent), back pain (1% to 3%), extremity pain (≤3%)

Ocular: Blurred vision (adolescents ≤3%)

Respiratory: Nasopharyngitis (≤5%; dose dependent), upper respiratory tract infection (1% to 4%), cough (≤3%; dose dependent), rhinitis (1% to 3%; dose dependent)

≤2% (Limited to important or life-threatening): Agranulocytosis, ALT increased, amenorrhea, appetite decreased, anaphylactic reaction, angioedema, arrhythmia, arthralgia, aspiration pneumonia, AV block (first degree), blurred vision, bradycardia, breast abnormalities (includes discharge, engorgement, pain, tenderness), cerebrovascular accident, drooling, edema, erectile dysfunction, epistaxis (adolescents), fatigue, flatulence, galactorrhea, gynecomastia, hypercholesterolemia, hyperglycemia, hyper-/hypotension, hyperprolactinemia, hypertonia, intestinal obstruction, ischemia, lethargy, leukopenia, menstrual irregularities, nasal congestion, neuroleptic malignant syndrome, neutropenia, nightmares, oculogyric crisis, palpitation, peripheral edema, pharyngolaryngeal pain (dose dependent), postural dizziness, postural orthostatic tachycardia syndrome, priapism, pruritus, psychomotor hyperactivity, QT_c-interval prolongation, rash, restlessness, retrograde ejaculation, seizure, sexual dysfunction, stiffness, suicidal ideation, syncope, tardive dyskinesia, tongue swelling, transient ischemic attack, urinary incontinence, urinary retention, urinary tract infection, vertigo

Drug Interactions

Metabolism/Transport Effects **Substrate** of P-glycoprotein

Avoid Concomitant Use

Avoid concomitant use of Paliperidone with any of the following: Metoclopramide

Increased Effect/Toxicity

Paliperidone may increase the levels/effects of: Alcohol (Ethyl); CNS Depressants; Methotrimeprazine; Methylphenidate; Serotonin Modulators

The levels/effects of Paliperidone may be increased by: Acetylcholinesterase Inhibitors (Central); Divalproex; Droperidol; HydrOXYzine; Itraconazole; Lithium formulations; Methotrimeprazine; Methylphenidate; Metoclopramide; P-glycoprotein/ABCB1 Inhibitors; RisperiDONE; Tetrabenazine; Valproic Acid

Decreased Effect

Paliperidone may decrease the levels/effects of: Amphetamines; Anti-Parkinson's Agents (Dopamine Agonist); Quinagolide

The levels/effects of Paliperidone may be decreased by: CarBAMazepine; Lithium formulations; P-glycoprotein/ABCB1 Inducers

Ethanol/Nutrition/Herb Interactions

Ethanol: May increase CNS depression; monitor for increased effects with coadministration. Caution patients about effects.

Herb/Nutraceutical: Avoid kava kava, gotu kola, valerian, St John's wort (may increase CNS depression).

Stability Store at controlled room temperature of ≤25°C (77°F); excursions permitted to 15°C to 30°C (59°F to 86°F). Protect tablets from moisture.

Mechanism of Action Paliperidone is considered a benzisoxazole atypical antipsychotic as it is the primary active metabolite of risperidone. As with other atypical antipsychotics, its therapeutic efficacy is believed to result from mixed central serotonergic and dopaminergic antagonism. The addition of serotonin antagonism to dopamine antagonism (classic neuroleptic mechanism) is thought to improve negative symptoms of psychoses and reduce the incidence of extrapyramidal side effects. Similar to risperidone, paliperidone demonstrates high affinity to α_1, D_2, H_1, and 5-HT_{2C} receptors, and low affinity for muscarinic and 5-HT_{1A} receptors. In contrast to risperidone, paliperidone displays nearly 10-fold lower affinity for α_2 and 5-HT_{2A} receptors, and nearly three- to fivefold less affinity for 5-HT_{1A} and 5-HT_{1D}, respectively.

Pharmacodynamics/Kinetics

Absorption: I.M.: Slow release (begins on day 1 and continues up to 126 days)

Distribution: V_d: 391-487 L

Protein binding: 74%

Metabolism: Hepatic via CYP2D6 and 3A4 (limited role in elimination); minor metabolism (<10% each) via dealkylation, hydroxylation, dehydrogenation, and benzisoxazole scission
Bioavailability: 28%
Half-life elimination:
Oral: 23 hours; 24-51 hours with renal impairment (Cl_{cr} <80 mL/minute)
I.M. (following a single-dose administration): Range: 25-49 days
Time to peak, plasma: Oral: ~24 hours; I.M.: 13 days
Excretion: Urine (80%); feces (11%)

Dosage

U.S. labeling:

Oral:

Adolescents 12-17 years: Schizophrenia: Initial: 3 mg once daily; titration not required (no known benefit from higher doses). If exceeding 3 mg/day, increases of 3 mg/day are recommended no more frequently than every 5 days.

Adults: Schizoaffective disorder, schizophrenia: Usual: 6 mg once daily in the morning; titration not required, though some may benefit from higher or lower doses. If exceeding 6 mg/day, increases of 3 mg/day are recommended no more frequently than every 4 days in schizoaffective disorder or every 5 days in schizophrenia, up to a maximum of 12 mg/day. Some patients may require only 3 mg/day.

I.M.: Adults: Schizophrenia: **Note:** Prior to initiation of I.M therapy, tolerability should be established with oral paliperidone or oral risperidone. Previous oral antipsychotics can be discontinued at the time of initiation of I.M. therapy. **Dosing based on paliperidone palmitate.**

Initiation of therapy:

Initial: 234 mg on treatment day 1 followed by 156 mg 1 week later. The second dose may be administered 2 days before or after the weekly timepoint.

Maintenance: Following the 1-week initiation regimen, begin a maintenance dose of 117 mg every month. Some patients may benefit from higher or lower monthly maintenance doses (monthly maintenance dosage range: 39-234 mg). The monthly maintenance dose may be administered 7 days before or after the monthly timepoint.

Conversion from oral paliperidone to I.M paliperidone: Initiate I.M. therapy as described using the 1-week initiation regimen. Patients previously stabilized on oral doses can expect similar steady state exposure during maintenance treatment with I.M. therapy using the following conversion:

Oral extended release dose of 12 mg, then I.M. maintenance dose of 234 mg
Oral extended release dose of 6 mg, then I.M. maintenance dose of 117 mg
Oral extended release dose of 3 mg, then I.M. maintenance dose of 39-78 mg

Switching from other long-acting injectable antipsychotics to I.M. paliperidone: Initiate I.M. paliperidone in the place of the next scheduled injection and continue at monthly intervals. The 1-week initiation regimen is not required in these patients.

Dosage adjustments: Adjustments may be made monthly (full effect from adjustments may not be seen for several months)

Missed doses:

If <6 weeks has elapsed since the last monthly injection: Administer the missed dose as soon as possible and continue therapy at monthly intervals.

If >6 weeks and ≤6 months has elapsed since the last monthly injection: Therapy may be resumed at same dose the patient was previously stabilized on, if the maintenance dose was <234 mg. If the dose was 234 mg, then administer a 156 mg dose as soon as possible, followed by a second dose of 156 mg 1 week later, then resume monthly maintenance dosing.

If >6 months has elapsed since last monthly maintenance injection: Therapy must be reinitiated following dosing recommendations for initiation of therapy.

Canadian labeling:

Oral: Adults: Schizophrenia: Usual: 6 mg once daily in the morning; titration not required, though some may benefit from higher or lower doses. If exceeding 6 mg/day, increases of 3 mg/day are recommended no more frequently than every 5 days in schizophrenia, up to a maximum of 12 mg/day. Some patients may require only 3 mg/day.

I.M.: Adults: Schizophrenia: **Note:** Prior to initiation of I.M therapy, tolerability should be established with oral paliperidone or oral risperidone. Previous oral antipsychotics can be discontinued at the time of initiation of I.M. therapy. **Dosing based on paliperidone.**

Initiation of therapy:

Initial: 150 mg on treatment day 1 followed by 100 mg 1 week later (day 8). The second dose may be administered 2 days before or after the weekly timepoint.

Maintenance: Following the 1-week initiation regimen, begin a maintenance dose of 75 mg every month. Some patients may benefit from higher or lower monthly maintenance doses (monthly maintenance dosage range: 25-150 mg). The monthly maintenance dose may be administered 7 days before or after the monthly timepoint.

Conversion from oral paliperidone to I.M paliperidone: Initiate I.M. therapy as described using the 1-week initiation regimen. Patients previously stabilized on oral doses can expect similar steady state exposure during maintenance treatment with I.M. therapy using the following conversion:

Oral extended release dose of 12 mg, then I.M. maintenance dose of 150 mg
Oral extended release dose of 6 mg, then I.M. maintenance dose of 75 mg
Oral extended release dose of 3 mg, then I.M. maintenance dose of 25-50 mg

Switching from injectable risperidone (Risperdal® Consta®) to I.M. paliperidone:

Risperdal® Consta® dose of 25 mg every 2 weeks, then I.M. paliperidone maintenance dose of 50 mg
Risperdal® Consta® dose of 37.5 mg every 2 weeks, then I.M. paliperidone maintenance dose of 75 mg
Risperdal® Consta® dose of 50 mg every 2 weeks, then I.M. paliperidone maintenance dose of 100 mg

Switching from other long-acting injectable antipsychotics to I.M. paliperidone: Initiate I.M. paliperidone in the place of the next scheduled injection and continue at monthly intervals. The 1-week initiation regimen is not required in these patients.

Dosage adjustments: Adjustments may be made monthly (full effect from adjustments may not be seen for several months)

Missed doses:

If <6 weeks has elapsed since the last monthly injection: Administer the missed dose as soon as possible and continue therapy at monthly intervals.

If >6 weeks and ≤6 months has elapsed since the last monthly injection: Therapy may be resumed at same dose (25-100 mg) the patient was previously stabilized on and then repeated 1 week later (day 8). Resume usual monthly maintenance dosing cycle thereafter. If the dose was 150 mg, administer a 100 mg dose as soon as possible and repeat 1 week later (day 8), then resume usual monthly maintenance dosing cycle 25-150 mg.

If >6 months has elapsed since last monthly maintenance injection: Therapy must be reinitiated following dosing recommendations for initiation of therapy.

Dosage adjustment in renal impairment: Clearance is decreased in renal impairment; adjust dose according to renal function:

Oral:

Mild impairment (Cl_{cr} 50-79 mL/minute): Initial dose: 3 mg once daily; maximum dose: 6 mg once daily

Moderate-to-severe impairment (Cl_{cr} 10-49 mL/minute): Initial dose: 1.5 mg once daily; maximum dose: 3 mg once daily

Severe impairment (Cl_{cr} <10 mL/minute): Use not recommended; not studied in this population

I.M., U.S. labeling:

Mild impairment (Cl_{cr} 50-79 mL/minute): Initiation of therapy: 156 mg on treatment day 1, followed by 117 mg 1 week later, followed by a maintenance dose of 78 mg every month

Moderate-to-severe impairment (Cl_{cr} <50 mL/minute): Use not recommended

I.M., Canadian labeling:

Mild impairment (Cl_{cr} 50-79 mL/minute): Initiation of therapy: 100 mg on treatment day 1, followed by 75 mg 1 week later followed by a maintenance dose of 50 mg every month

Moderate-to-severe impairment (Cl_{cr} <50 mL/minute): Use not recommended

Dosage adjustment in hepatic impairment: Oral, I.M.: No adjustment necessary for mild-to-moderate (Child-Pugh class A and B) impairment. Not studied in severe impairment.

Dietary Considerations May be taken without regard to meals.

Administration

Oral: Administer in the morning without regard to meals. Extended release tablets should be swallowed whole with liquids; do not crush, chew, or divide.

Injection: Invega® Sustenna™ should be administered by I.M. route only as a single injection (do not divide); do not administer I.V. or subcutaneously. Avoid inadvertent injection into vasculature. Prior to injection, shake syringe for at least 10 seconds to ensure a homogenous suspension. The 2 initial injections should be administered in the deltoid muscle using a 1$^1/_2$ inch, 22-gauge needle for patients ≥90 kg, and a 1 inch, 23-gauge needle for patients <90 kg. The 2 initial deltoid intramuscular injections help attain therapeutic concentrations rapidly. Alternate deltoid injections (right and left deltoid muscle). The second dose may be administered 2 days before or after the weekly timepoint. Monthly maintenance doses can be administered in either the deltoid or gluteal muscle. Administer injections in the gluteal muscle using a 1$^1/_2$ inch, 22-gauge needle in the upper-outer quadrant of the gluteal area. Alternate gluteal injections (right and left gluteal muscle). The monthly maintenance dose may be administered 7 days before or after the monthly timepoint.

Monitoring Parameters Vital signs; fasting lipid profile and fasting blood glucose/Hgb A_{1c} (prior to treatment, at 3 months, then annually), prolactin levels, CBC frequently during first few months of therapy in patients with preexisting low WBC or a history of drug-induced leukopenia/neutropenia; BMI, personal/family history of obesity, diabetes, waist circumference; blood pressure; mental status, abnormal involuntary movement scale (AIMS), extrapyramidal symptoms; orthostatic blood pressure changes for 3-5 days after starting or increasing dose. Weight should be assessed prior to treatment, at 4 weeks, 8 weeks, 12 weeks, and then at quarterly intervals. Consider titrating to a different antipsychotic agent for a weight gain ≥5% of the initial weight.

Additional Information Invega® is an extended release tablet based on the OROS® osmotic delivery system. Water from the GI tract enters through a semipermeable membrane coating the tablet, solubilizing the drug into a gelatinous form which, through hydrophilic expansion, is then expelled through laser-drilled holes in the coating.

Dosage Forms Excipient information presented when available (limited, particularly for generics); consult specific product labeling.

Injection, suspension, extended release, as palmitate:

Invega® Sustenna®: 39 mg/0.25 mL (0.25 mL); 78 mg/0.5 mL (0.5 mL); 117 mg/0.75 mL (0.75 mL); 156 mg/mL (1 mL); 234 mg/1.5 mL (1.5 mL)

Tablet, extended release, oral:

Invega®: 1.5 mg, 3 mg, 6 mg, 9 mg [osmotic controlled release]

Dosage Forms: Canada Excipient information presented when available (limited, particularly for generics); consult specific product labeling.

Injection, suspension, extended release:

Invega® Sustenna™: 25 mg/0.25 mL (0.25 mL), 50 mg/0.5 mL (0.5 mL), 75 mg/0.75 mL (0.75 mL), 100 mg/1 mL (1 mL), 150 mg/1.5 mL (1.5 mL)

◆ **Paliperidone Palmitate** *see* Paliperidone *on page 1277*

Palivizumab (pah li VIZ u mab)

Brand Names: U.S. Synagis®

Brand Names: Canada Synagis®

Pharmacologic Category Monoclonal Antibody

Use Prevention of serious lower respiratory tract disease caused by respiratory syncytial virus (RSV) in infants and children at high risk of RSV disease

The American Academy of Pediatrics recommends RSV prophylaxis with palivizumab during RSV season for:

- Infants <3 months of age who were born between 32 and 34 6/7 weeks gestational age and have one of the following:
  - Day care attendance
  - One or more siblings <5 years of age living in the same household
- Infants <6 months of age who were born between 29 and 31 6/7 weeks gestational age
- Infants <12 months of age who were born <28 weeks gestational age
- Infants <12 months of age with congenital airway abnormality or neuromuscular disorder that decreases the ability to manage airway secretions
- Infants and children <24 months of age with chronic lung disease (CLD) necessitating medical therapy within 6 month prior to the beginning of RSV season
- Infants and children ≤24 months of age with congenital heart disease and one of the following:
  - Receiving medication to treat congestive heart failure
  - Moderate-to-severe pulmonary hypertension
  - Cyanotic heart disease

Pregnancy Risk Factor C

Pregnancy Considerations Not for adult use; reproduction studies have not been conducted

Contraindications History of severe prior reaction to palivizumab or any component of the formulation

Warnings/Precautions Very rare cases of anaphylaxis have been observed following palivizumab. Rare cases of severe acute hypersensitivity reactions have also been reported. Use with caution after mild hypersensitivity reaction; permanently discontinue for severe hypersensitivity reaction. Safety and efficacy of palivizumab have not been demonstrated in the treatment of established RSV disease. Use with caution in patients with thrombocytopenia or any coagulation disorder.

Adverse Reactions The incidence of adverse events was similar between the palivizumab and placebo groups.

>1%:

Cardiovascular: Arrhythmia, cyanosis

Central nervous system: Fever, nervousness

Dermatologic: Rash

Gastrointestinal: Diarrhea, gastroenteritis, vomiting

Hepatic: AST increased

Otic: Otitis media

Respiratory: Cough, rhinitis, upper respiratory infection, wheezing

<1% (Limited to important or life-threatening): Anaphylaxis (very rare - includes angioedema, dyspnea, hypotonia, pruritus, respiratory failure, unresponsiveness, urticaria); antibody development, hypersensitivity reactions, injection site reactions, thrombocytopenia

Drug Interactions

Metabolism/Transport Effects None known.

Avoid Concomitant Use

Avoid concomitant use of Palivizumab with any of the following: Belimumab

Increased Effect/Toxicity

Palivizumab may increase the levels/effects of: Belimumab

The levels/effects of Palivizumab may be increased by: Abciximab

Decreased Effect There are no known significant interactions involving a decrease in effect.

Stability Store in refrigerator at a temperature between 2°C to 8°C (36°F to 46°F) in original container; do not freeze. Intact vials may be exposed to room temperature for a cumulative 14 days (data on file [MedImmune, 2011]). Do not shake, vigorously agitate or dilute the solution.

Mechanism of Action Exhibits neutralizing and fusion-inhibitory activity against RSV; these activities inhibit RSV replication in laboratory and clinical studies

Pharmacodynamics/Kinetics Half-life elimination: Children <24 months: 20 days

Dosage I.M.: Infants and Children <2 years:

Prevention of RSV: 15 mg/kg of body weight, monthly throughout RSV season (first dose administered prior to commencement of RSV season)

Note: The AAP recommends a maximum of 3 doses for patients born 32-34 6/7 weeks without significant congenital heart disease or chronic lung disease; maximum of 5 doses for all others (AAP, 2009).

Cardiopulmonary bypass patients: Administer a dose as soon as possible after cardiopulmonary bypass procedure, even if <1 month from previous dose.

Administration Injection should (preferably) be in the anterolateral aspect of the thigh; gluteal muscle should not be used routinely; injection volume over 1 mL should be administered as divided doses

Monitoring Parameters Monitor for anaphylaxis or acute hypersensitivity reactions

Additional Information RSV prophylaxis should be initiated no earlier than July 1 in Southeast Florida, September 15 in North-central and Southwest Florida and November 1 in most other areas of the United States.

Dosage Forms Excipient information presented when available (limited, particularly for generics); consult specific product labeling.

Injection, solution [preservative free]:

Synagis®: 100 mg/mL (0.5 mL, 1 mL)

◆ **Palmer's® Skin Success® Eventone® Fade Cream [OTC]** *see* Hydroquinone *on page 846*

◆ **Palmer's® Skin Success® Eventone® Fade Milk [OTC]** *see* Hydroquinone *on page 846*

◆ **Palmer's® Skin Success® Eventone® Ultra Fade Serum [OTC]** *see* Hydroquinone *on page 846*

Palonosetron (pal oh NOE se tron)

Brand Names: U.S. Aloxi®

Index Terms Palonosetron Hydrochloride; RS-25259; RS-25259-197

Pharmacologic Category Antiemetic; Selective 5-HT_3 Receptor Antagonist

Use Prevention of chemotherapy-associated nausea and vomiting; indicated for prevention of acute (highly-emetogenic therapy) as well as acute and delayed (moderately-emetogenic therapy) nausea and vomiting; prevention of postoperative nausea and vomiting (PONV)

Pregnancy Risk Factor B

Pregnancy Considerations Teratogenic effects were not observed in animal studies. There are no adequate and well-controlled studies in pregnant women; use during pregnancy only if clearly needed.

Lactation Excretion in breast milk unknown/not recommended

Contraindications Hypersensitivity to palonosetron or any component of the formulation

Warnings/Precautions Hypersensitivity has been observed rarely with I.V. palonosetron. Use caution in patients allergic to other 5-HT_3 receptor antagonists; cross-reactivity is possible. Some selective 5-HT_3 receptor antagonists have been associated with dose-dependent increases in ECG intervals (eg, PR, QRS duration, QT/QT_c, JT), usually occurring 1-2 hours after I.V. administration. In general, these changes are not clinically relevant, however, when these agents are used in conjunction with other agents that prolong these intervals, arrhythmia may occur. When used with agents that prolong the QT interval (eg, Class I and III antiarrhythmics), clinically relevant QT interval prolongation could result in torsade de pointes. A number of trials have shown that 5-HT_3 antagonists produce QT interval prolongation to variable degrees. Use with caution in patients at risk of QT prolongation and/or ventricular arrhythmia. Reduction in heart rate may also occur with the 5-HT_3 antagonists. Use with caution in patients with congenital long QT syndrome or other risk factors for QT prolongation (eg, medications known to prolong QT interval, electrolyte abnormalities, and cumulative high dose anthracycline therapy).

Not intended for treatment of nausea and vomiting or for chronic continuous therapy. **For chemotherapy, should be used on a scheduled basis, not on an "as needed" (PRN) basis,** since data support the use of this drug only in the prevention of nausea and vomiting (due to antineoplastic therapy) and not in the rescue of nausea and vomiting. For PONV, may use for low expectation of PONV if it is essential to avoid nausea and vomiting in the postoperative period; use is not recommended if there is little expectation of nausea and vomiting.

Adverse Reactions Adverse events may vary according to indication.

1% to 10%:

Cardiovascular: QT prolongation (chemotherapy-associated <1%; PONV 1% to 5%), bradycardia (chemotherapy-associated 1%; PONV 4%), hypotension (≤1%), sinus bradycardia (≤1%), tachycardia (nonsustained) (≤1%)

Central nervous system: Headache (chemotherapy-associated 5% to 9%; PONV 3%), anxiety (1%), dizziness (≤1%)

Dermatologic: Pruritus (≤1%)

Endocrine & metabolic: Hyperkalemia (1%)

Gastrointestinal: Constipation (2% to 5%), diarrhea (≤1%), flatulence (≤1%)

Genitourinary: Urinary retention (≤1%)

Hepatic: ALT increased (≤1%; transient), AST increased (≤1%; transient)

Neuromuscular & skeletal: Weakness (1%)

<1% (Limited to important or life-threatening): Abdominal pain, allergic dermatitis, amblyopia, anemia, anorexia, appetite decreased, arrhythmia, arthralgia, bilirubin increased (transient), chills, dyspepsia, edema (generalized), electrolyte fluctuations, epistaxis, erythema, euphoric mood, extrasystoles, eye irritation, fatigue, fever, flu-like syndrome, glycosuria, hiccups, hot flash, hyperglycemia, hypersensitivity (rare), hypersomnia, hypertension, hypokalemia, hypoventilation, injection site reactions (burning/discomfort/induration/pain; rare), insomnia, intestinal hypomotility, laryngospasm, metabolic acidosis, motion sickness, myocardial ischemia, pain in extremities, paresthesia, platelets decreased, rash, salivation increased, seizure, sinus arrhythmia, sinus tachycardia, somnolence, supraventricular extrasystoles, tinnitus, T-wave amplitude decreased, vein discoloration, vein distention, ventricular extrasystoles, xerostomia

Drug Interactions

Metabolism/Transport Effects Substrate of CYP1A2 (minor), CYP2D6 (minor), CYP3A4 (minor); **Note:** Assignment of Major/Minor substrate status based on clinically relevant drug interaction potential

Avoid Concomitant Use

Avoid concomitant use of Palonosetron with any of the following: Apomorphine

Increased Effect/Toxicity

Palonosetron may increase the levels/effects of: Apomorphine

The levels/effects of Palonosetron may be increased by: Conivaptan

Decreased Effect

The levels/effects of Palonosetron may be decreased by: Cyproterone; Peginterferon Alfa-2b; Tocilizumab

Stability Store intact vials at room temperature of 20°C to 25°C (68°F to 77°F); excursions permitted to 15°C to 30°C (59°F to 86°F); do not freeze. Protect from light. Solutions of 5 mcg/mL and 30 mcg/mL in NS, D_5W, $D_5{}^1/_2NS$, and D_5LR injection are stable for 48 hours at room temperature and 14 days under refrigeration (Trissel, 2004).

Mechanism of Action Selective $5\text{-}HT_3$ receptor antagonist, blocking serotonin, both on vagal nerve terminals in the periphery and centrally in the chemoreceptor trigger zone

Pharmacodynamics/Kinetics

Distribution: V_d: 8.3 ± 2.5 L/kg

Protein binding: ~62%

Metabolism: ~50% metabolized via CYP enzymes (and likely other pathways) to relatively inactive metabolites (N-oxide-palonosetron and 6-S-hydroxy-palonosetron); CYP1A2, 2D6, and 3A4 contribute to its metabolism

Half-life elimination: I.V.: Terminal: ~40 hours

Excretion: Urine (80% to 93%, 40% as unchanged drug); feces (5% to 8%)

Dosage I.V.: Adults:

Chemotherapy-associated nausea and vomiting: 0.25 mg 30 minutes prior to the start of chemotherapy administration

Breakthrough: Palonosetron has not been shown to be effective in terminating nausea or vomiting once it occurs and should not be used for this purpose.

PONV: 0.075 mg immediately prior to anesthesia induction

Elderly: No dosage adjustment necessary

Dosage adjustment in renal/hepatic impairment: No dosage adjustment necessary

Administration Flush I.V. line with NS prior to and following administration.

Chemotherapy-associated nausea and vomiting: Infuse over 30 seconds, 30 minutes prior to the start of chemotherapy

PONV: Infuse over 10 seconds immediately prior to anesthesia induction

Dosage Forms Excipient information presented when available (limited, particularly for generics); consult specific product labeling.

Injection, solution:

Aloxi®: 0.05 mg/mL (1.5 mL, 5 mL) [contains edetate disodium]

◆ **Palonosetron Hydrochloride** *see* Palonosetron *on page 1281*

◆ **2-PAM** *see* Pralidoxime *on page 1388*

Pamabrom (PAM a brom)

Brand Names: U.S. Aqua-Ban® Maximum Strength [OTC]; diurex® Aquagels® [OTC]; diurex® Maximum Relief [OTC]; diurex® [OTC]

Pharmacologic Category Diuretic

Use Temporary relief of symptoms associated with premenstrual and menstrual periods (eg, bloating, water-weight gain, swelling, full feeling)

Dosage Oral: Adults: 50 mg after breakfast and then every 6 hours as needed (maximum: 200 mg/24 hours); should be taken 5-6 days prior to onset of menstrual period and continued until desired relief or end of period

Additional Information Complete prescribing information for this medication should be consulted for additional detail.

Dosage Forms Excipient information presented when available (limited, particularly for generics); consult specific product labeling.

Caplet, oral:

diurex® Maximum Relief: 50 mg

Capsule, oral:

diurex®: 50 mg

Capsule, softgel, oral:

diurex® Aquagels®: 50 mg

Tablet, oral:

Aqua-Ban® Maximum Strength: 50 mg

◆ **Pamelor®** *see* Nortriptyline *on page 1220*

Pamidronate (pa mi DROE nate)

Brand Names: U.S. Aredia®

Brand Names: Canada Aredia®; Pamidronate Disodium Omega; Pamidronate Disodium®; PMS-Pamidronate; Rhoxal-pamidronate

Index Terms Pamidronate Disodium

Pharmacologic Category Antidote; Bisphosphonate Derivative

Use Treatment of moderate or severe hypercalcemia associated with malignancy (in conjunction with adequate hydration) with or without bone metastases; treatment of osteolytic bone lesions associated with multiple myeloma or metastatic breast cancer; moderate-to-severe Paget's disease of bone

Unlabeled Use Treatment of osteogenesis imperfecta; treatment of symptomatic bone metastases of thyroid cancer; prevention of bone loss associated with androgen deprivation treatment in prostate cancer

Pregnancy Risk Factor D

Pregnancy Considerations Pamidronate has been shown to cross the placenta and cause nonteratogenic embryo/fetal effects in animals. There are no adequate and well-controlled studies in pregnant women; manufacturer states pamidronate should not be used in pregnancy. Based on limited case reports, serum calcium levels in the newborn may be altered if pamidronate is administered during pregnancy. Bisphosphonates are incorporated into the bone matrix and gradually released over time.

Theoretically, there may be a risk of fetal harm when pregnancy follows the completion of therapy. Women of childbearing potential should be advised to use effective contraception and avoid becoming pregnant during therapy.

Lactation Excretion in breast milk unknown/use caution

Contraindications Hypersensitivity to pamidronate, other bisphosphonates, or any component of the formulation

Warnings/Precautions Osteonecrosis of the jaw (ONJ) has been reported in patients receiving bisphosphonates. Risk factors include invasive dental procedures (eg, tooth extraction, dental implants, boney surgery); a diagnosis of cancer, with concomitant chemotherapy, radiotherapy, or corticosteroids; poor oral hygiene, ill-fitting dentures; and comorbid disorders (anemia, coagulopathy, infection, pre-existing dental disease). Most reported cases occurred after I.V. bisphosphonate therapy; however, cases have been reported following oral therapy. A dental exam and preventative dentistry should be performed prior to placing patients with risk factors on chronic bisphosphonate therapy. The manufacturer's labeling states that discontinuing bisphosphonates in patients requiring invasive dental procedures reduces the risk of ONJ. However, other experts suggest that there is no evidence that discontinuing therapy reduces the risk of developing ONJ (Assael, 2009). The benefit/risk must be assessed by the treating physician and/or dentist/surgeon prior to any invasive dental procedure. Patients developing ONJ while on bisphosphonates should receive care by an oral surgeon.

Infrequently, severe (and occasionally debilitating) musculoskeletal (bone, joint, and/or muscle) pain have been reported during bisphosphonate treatment. The onset of pain ranged from a single day to several months. Consider discontinuing therapy in patients who experience severe symptoms; symptoms usually resolve upon discontinuation. Some patients experienced recurrence when rechallenged with same drug or another bisphosphonate; avoid use in patients with a history of these symptoms in association with bisphosphonate therapy.

Initial or single doses have been associated with renal deterioration, progressing to renal failure and dialysis. Withhold pamidronate treatment (until renal function returns to baseline) in patients with evidence of renal deterioration. Glomerulosclerosis (focal segmental) with or without nephrotic syndrome has also been reported. Longer infusion times (>2 hours) may reduce the risk for renal toxicity, especially in patients with pre-existing renal insufficiency. Single pamidronate doses should not exceed 90 mg. Patients with serum creatinine >3 mg/dL were not studied in clinical trials; limited data are available in patients with Cl_{cr} <30 mL/minute. Evaluate serum creatinine prior to each treatment. For the treatment of bone metastases, use is not recommended in patients with severe renal impairment; for renal impairment in indications other than bone metastases, use clinical judgment to determine if benefits outweigh potential risks.

Use has been associated with asymptomatic electrolyte abnormalities (including hypophosphatemia, hypokalemia, hypomagnesemia, and hypocalcemia). Rare cases of symptomatic hypocalcemia, including tetany have been reported. Patients with a history of thyroid surgery may have relative hypoparathyroidism; predisposing them to pamidronate-related hypocalcemia. Patients with pre-existing anemia, leukopenia, or thrombocytopenia should be closely monitored during the first 2 weeks of treatment.

According to the American Society of Clinical Oncology (ASCO) guidelines for bisphosphonates in multiple myeloma, treatment with pamidronate is not recommended for asymptomatic (smoldering) or indolent myeloma or with solitary plasmacytoma (Kyle, 2007). The National Comprehensive Cancer Network® (NCCN) multiple myeloma guidelines (v.1.2011) also do not recommend pamidronate use in stage 1 or smoldering disease, unless part of a clinical trial.

Adequate hydration is required during treatment (urine output ~2 L/day); avoid overhydration, especially in patients with heart failure. Vein irritation and thrombophlebitis may occur with infusions. Women of childbearing potential should be advised to use effective contraception and avoid becoming pregnant during therapy.

Adverse Reactions Note: Actual percentages may vary by indication; treatment for multiple myeloma is associated with higher percentage.

>10%:
- Central nervous system: Fever (18% to 39%; transient), fatigue (≤37%), headache (≤26%), insomnia (≤22%)
- Endocrine & metabolic: Hypophosphatemia (≤18%), hypokalemia (4% to 18%), hypomagnesemia (4% to 12%), hypocalcemia (≤12%)
- Gastrointestinal: Nausea (≤54%), vomiting (≤36%), anorexia (≤26%), abdominal pain (≤23%), dyspepsia (≤23%)
- Genitourinary: Urinary tract infection (≤19%)
- Hematologic: Anemia (≤43%), granulocytopenia (≤20%)
- Local: Infusion site reaction (≤18%; includes induration, pain, redness and swelling)
- Neuromuscular & skeletal: Myalgia (≤26%), weakness (≤22%), arthralgia (≤14%), osteonecrosis of the jaw (cancer patients: 1% to 11%)
- Renal: Serum creatinine increased (≤19%)
- Respiratory: Dyspnea (≤30%), cough (≤26%), upper respiratory tract infection (≤24%), sinusitis (≤16%), pleural effusion (≤11%)

1% to 10%:
- Cardiovascular: Atrial fibrillation (≤6%), hypertension (≤6%), syncope (≤6%), tachycardia (≤6%), atrial flutter (≤1%), cardiac failure (≤1%), edema (≤1%)
- Central nervous system: Somnolence (≤6%), psychosis (≤4%), seizure (≤2%)
- Endocrine & metabolic: Hypothyroidism (≤6%)
- Gastrointestinal: Constipation (≤6%), gastrointestinal hemorrhage (≤6%), diarrhea (≤1%), stomatitis (≤1%)
- Hematologic: Leukopenia (≤4%), neutropenia (≤1%), thrombocytopenia (≤1%)
- Neuromuscular & skeletal: Back pain, bone pain
- Renal: Uremia (≤4%)
- Respiratory: Rales (≤6%), rhinitis (≤6%)
- Miscellaneous: Moniliasis (≤6%)

<1% (Limited to important or life-threatening): Acute renal failure, adult respiratory distress syndrome, allergic reaction, anaphylactic shock, angioedema, bronchospasm, CHF, confusion, conjunctivitis, electrolyte/mineral abnormality, episcleritis, fluid overload, flu-like syndrome, focal segmental glomerulosclerosis (including collapsing variant), hallucinations (visual), hematuria, herpes virus reactivation, hyperkalemia, hypernatremia, hypotension, injection site phlebitis/thrombophlebitis, interstitial pneumonitis, iridocyclitis, iritis, joint and/or muscle pain (sometimes severe and/or incapacitating), left ventricular failure, lymphocytopenia, malaise, nephrotic syndrome, orbital inflammation, osteonecrosis (other than jaw), paresthesia, pruritus, rash, renal deterioration, renal failure, scleritis, tetany, uveitis, xanthopsia

Drug Interactions

Metabolism/Transport Effects None known.

Avoid Concomitant Use There are no known interactions where it is recommended to avoid concomitant use.

Increased Effect/Toxicity

Pamidronate may increase the levels/effects of: Deferasirox; Phosphate Supplements

The levels/effects of Pamidronate may be increased by: Aminoglycosides; Nonsteroidal Anti-Inflammatory Agents; Thalidomide

Decreased Effect

The levels/effects of Pamidronate may be decreased by: Proton Pump Inhibitors

Stability

Powder for injection: Store below 30°C (86°F). Reconstitute by adding 10 mL of SWFI to each vial of lyophilized pamidronate disodium powder; the resulting solution will be 30 mg/10 mL or 90 mg/10 mL. The reconstituted solution is stable for 24 hours stored under refrigeration at 2°C to 8°C (36°F to 46°F).

Solution for injection: Store at 20°C to 25°C (68°F to 77°F).

Pamidronate may be further diluted in 250-1000 mL of 0.45% or 0.9% sodium chloride or 5% dextrose. (The manufacturer recommends dilution in 1000 mL for hypercalcemia of malignancy, 500 mL for Paget's disease and bone metastases of myeloma, and 250 mL for bone metastases of breast cancer.) Pamidronate solution for infusion is stable at room temperature for up to 24 hours.

Mechanism of Action A bisphosphonate which inhibits bone resorption via actions on osteoclasts and/or on osteoclast precursors. Does not appear to produce any significant effects on renal tubular calcium handling and is poorly absorbed following oral administration (high oral doses have been reported effective); therefore, I.V. therapy is preferred.

Pharmacodynamics/Kinetics

Onset of action: 24-48 hours

Peak effect: Maximum: 5-7 days

Absorption: Poor; pharmacokinetic studies lacking

Metabolism: Not metabolized

Half-life elimination: 21-35 hours

Excretion: Biphasic; urine (30% to 62% as unchanged drug; lower in patients with renal dysfunction) within 120 hours

Dosage Note: Single doses should not exceed 90 mg. I.V.:

Adults:

Hypercalcemia of malignancy:

Moderate cancer-related hypercalcemia (corrected serum calcium: 12-13.5 mg/dL): 60-90 mg, as a single dose over 2-24 hours

Severe cancer-related hypercalcemia (corrected serum calcium: >13.5 mg/dL): 90 mg, as a single dose over 2-24 hours

Retreatment in patients who show an initial complete or partial response (allow at least 7 days to elapse prior to retreatment): May retreat at the same dose if serum calcium does not return to normal or does not remain normal after initial treatment.

Multiple myeloma, osteolytic bone lesions: 90 mg over 4 hours monthly

Lytic disease: American Society of Clinical Oncology (ASCO) guidelines: 90 mg over at least 2 hours every 3-4 weeks for 2 years; discontinue after 2 years in patients with responsive and/or stable disease; resume therapy with new-onset skeletal-related events (Kyle, 2007)

Newly-diagnosed, symptomatic (unlabeled dose): 30 mg over 2.5 hours monthly for at least 3 years (Gimsing, 2010)

Breast cancer, osteolytic bone metastases: 90 mg over 2 hours every 3-4 weeks

Paget's disease (moderate-to-severe): 30 mg over 4 hours daily for 3 consecutive days (total dose = 90 mg); may retreat at initial dose if clinically indicated

Prevention of androgen deprivation-induced osteoporosis (unlabeled use): 60 mg over 2 hours every 3 months (Smith, 2001) **or** 90 mg as a single dose over 3-4 hours (Diamond, 2001)

Elderly: Begin at lower end of adult dosing range.

Dosing adjustment in renal impairment: Patients with serum creatinine >3 mg/dL were excluded from clinical trials; there are only limited pharmacokinetic data in patients with Cl_{cr} <30 mL/minute.

Manufacturer recommends the following guidelines:

Treatment of bone metastases: Use is not recommended in patients with severe renal impairment.

Renal impairment in indications other than bone metastases: Use clinical judgment to determine if benefits outweigh potential risks.

Multiple myeloma: American Society of Clinical Oncology (ASCO) guidelines (Kyle, 2007):

Severe renal impairment (serum creatinine >3 mg/dL **or** Cl_{cr} <30 mL/minute) and extensive bone disease: 90 mg over 4-6 hours. However, a reduced initial dose should be considered if renal impairment was pre-existing.

Albuminuria >500 mg/24 hours (unexplained): Withhold dose until returns to baseline, then recheck every 3-4 weeks; consider reinitiating at a dose not to exceed 90 mg every 4 weeks and with a longer infusion time of at least 4 hours

Dosing adjustment in renal toxicity: In patients with bone metastases, treatment should be withheld for deterioration in renal function (increase of serum creatinine ≥0.5 mg/dL in patients with normal baseline or ≥1.0 mg/dL in patients with abnormal baseline). Resumption of therapy may be considered when serum creatinine returns to within 10% of baseline.

Dosage adjustment in hepatic impairment: No adjustment required in patients with mild-to-moderate hepatic impairment; not studied in patients with severe hepatic impairment.

Dietary Considerations Multiple myeloma or metastatic bone lesions from solid tumors or Paget's disease: Take adequate daily calcium and vitamin D supplement (if patient is not hypercalcemic).

Administration I.V.: Infusion rate varies by indication. Longer infusion times (>2 hours) may reduce the risk for renal toxicity, especially in patients with pre-existing renal insufficiency. The manufacturer recommends infusing over 2-24 hours for hypercalcemia of malignancy; over 2 hours for osteolytic bone lesions with metastatic breast cancer; and over 4 hours for Paget's disease and for osteolytic bone lesions with multiple myeloma. The ASCO guidelines for bisphosphonate use in multiple myeloma recommend infusing pamidronate over at least 2 hours; if therapy is withheld due to renal toxicity, infuse over at least 4 hours upon reintroduction of treatment after renal recovery.

Monitoring Parameters Serum creatinine (prior to each treatment); serum electrolytes, including calcium, phosphate, magnesium, and potassium; CBC with differential; monitor for hypocalcemia for at least 2 weeks after therapy; dental exam and preventative dentistry prior to therapy for patients at risk of osteonecrosis, including all cancer patients; patients with pre-existing anemia, leukopenia, or thrombocytopenia should be closely monitored during the first 2 weeks of treatment; in addition, monitor urine albumin every 3-6 months in multiple myeloma patients

Reference Range Calcium (total): Adults: 9.0-11.0 mg/dL (SI: 2.05-2.54 mmol/L), may slightly decrease with aging; Phosphorus: 2.5-4.5 mg/dL (SI: 0.81-1.45 mmol/L)

Test Interactions Bisphosphonates may interfere with diagnostic imaging agents such as technetium-99m-diphosphonate in bone scans.

Additional Information Oncology Comment:

Metastatic breast cancer: The American Society of Clinical Oncology (ASCO) updated guidelines on the role of bone-modifying agents (BMAs) in the prevention and treatment of skeletal-related events for metastatic breast cancer patients (Van Poznak, 2011). The guidelines recommend initiating a BMA (denosumab, pamidronate, zoledronic acid) in patients with metastatic breast cancer to the bone. There is currently no literature indicating the superiority of one particular BMA. Optimal duration is not defined; however, the guidelines recommend continuing therapy until substantial decline in patient's performance status. In patients with normal Cl_{cr} (>60 mL/minute), no dosage/interval/infusion rate changes for pamidronate or zoledronic acid are necessary. For patients with Cl_{cr} <30 mL/minute, pamidronate and zoledronic acid are not recommended. While no renal dose adjustments are recommended for denosumab, close monitoring is advised for risk of hypocalcemia in patients with Cl_{cr} <30 mL/minute or on dialysis. The ASCO guidelines are in alignment with package insert guidelines for dosing, renal dose adjustments, infusion times, prevention and management of osteonecrosis of the jaw, and monitoring of laboratory parameter recommendations. BMAs are not the first-line therapy for pain. BMAs are to be used as adjunctive therapy for cancer-related bone pain associated with bone metastasis, demonstrating a modest pain control benefit. BMAs should be used in conjunction with agents such as NSAIDs, opioid and nonopioid analgesics, corticosteroids, radiation/surgery, and interventional procedures.

Multiple myeloma: The American Society of Clinical Oncology (ASCO) has also published guidelines on the use of bisphosphonates for prevention and treatment of bone disease in multiple myeloma (Kyle, 2007). Pamidronate or zoledronic acid use is recommended in multiple myeloma patients with lytic bone destruction or compression spine fracture from osteopenia. Clodronate (not available in the U.S.; available in Canada), administered orally or I.V., is an alternative treatment. The use of the bisphosphonates pamidronate and zoledronic acid may be considered in patients with pain secondary to osteolytic disease, adjunct therapy to stabilize fractures or impending fractures, and I.V. bisphosphonates for multiple myeloma patients with osteopenia but no radiographic evidence of lytic bone disease. Bisphosphonates are not recommended in patients with solitary plasmacytoma, smoldering (asymptomatic) or indolent myeloma, or monoclonal gammopathy of undetermined significance. The guidelines recommend monthly treatment for a period of 2 years. At that time, physicians need to consider discontinuing in responsive and stable patients, and reinitiate if a new-onset skeletal-related event occurs. The ASCO guidelines are in alignment with package insert guidelines for dosing, renal dose adjustments, infusion times, prevention and management of osteonecrosis of the jaw, and monitoring of laboratory parameter recommendations. The guidelines also recommend in patients with extensive bone disease with existing severe renal disease (a serum creatinine >3 mg/dL or Cl_{cr} <30 mL/minute) pamidronate at a dose of 90 mg over 4-6 hours (unless pre-existing renal disease in which a reduced initial dose should be considered). ASCO also recommends monitoring for albuminuria every 3-6 months. In patients with unexplained albuminuria >500 mg/24 hours, withhold the dose until level returns to baseline, then recheck every 3-4 weeks. Pamidronate may be reinitiated at a dose not to exceed 90 mg every 4 weeks with a longer infusion time of at least 4 hours.

Dosage Forms Excipient information presented when available (limited, particularly for generics); consult specific product labeling. [DSC] = Discontinued product

Injection, powder for reconstitution, as disodium: 30 mg, 90 mg

Aredia®: 30 mg, 90 mg [DSC]

Injection, solution, as disodium: 3 mg/mL (10 mL); 6 mg/mL (10 mL); 9 mg/mL (10 mL)

Injection, solution, as disodium [preservative free]: 3 mg/mL (10 mL); 9 mg/mL (10 mL)

◆ **Pamidronate Disodium** *see* Pamidronate *on page 1282*

◆ **Pamidronate Disodium® (Can)** *see* Pamidronate *on page 1282*

◆ **Pamidronate Disodium Omega (Can)** *see* Pamidronate *on page 1282*

◆ **p-amino-benzenesulfonamide** *see* Sulfanilamide *on page 1605*

◆ **p-Aminoclonidine** *see* Apraclonidine *on page 137*

◆ **Pamprin® Maximum Strength All Day Relief [OTC]** *see* Naproxen *on page 1177*

◆ **Pancrease® MT (Can)** *see* Pancrelipase *on page 1285*

◆ **Pancreatic Enzymes** *see* Pancrelipase *on page 1285*

◆ **Pancreaze™** *see* Pancrelipase *on page 1285*

Pancrelipase (pan kre LYE pase)

Brand Names: U.S. Creon®; Pancreaze™; Pancrelipase™; Zenpep®

Brand Names: Canada Cotazym®; Creon®; Pancrease® MT; Ultrase®; Ultrase® MT; Viokase®

Index Terms Amylase, Lipase, and Protease; Lipancreatin; Lipase, Protease, and Amylase; Pancreatic Enzymes; Protease, Lipase, and Amylase

Pharmacologic Category Enzyme

Use Treatment of exocrine pancreatic insufficiency (EPI) due to conditions such as cystic fibrosis (Creon®, Pancreaze™, Zenpep®); chronic pancreatitis (Creon®); or pancreatectomy (Creon®)

Pregnancy Risk Factor C

Pregnancy Considerations Reproduction studies have not been conducted. Nutrition should be optimized in pregnancy; in cystic fibrosis patients with malabsorption, pancreatic enzyme replacement is not considered to cause a risk to the pregnancy.

Lactation Excretion in breast milk unknown/use caution

Medication Guide Available Yes

Contraindications There are no contraindications listed in the manufacturer's labeling.

Warnings/Precautions Fibrosing colonopathy advancing to colonic strictures have been reported with doses of lipase >6000 units/kg/meal over long periods of time in children <12 years of age. Patients taking doses of lipase >6000 units/kg/meal should be examined and the dose decreased. Doses of lipase >2500 units/kg/meal (or lipase >10,000 units/kg/day) should be used with caution and only with documentation of 3-day fecal fat measures. Crushing or chewing the contents of the capsules, or mixing the contents with foods outside of product labeling, may cause early release of the enzymes, causing irritation of the oral mucosa and/or loss of enzyme activity. When mixing the contents of capsules with food, the mixture should be swallowed immediately and followed with water or juice to ensure complete ingestion. Use caution in patients with gout, hyperuricemia, or renal impairment; products contain purines which may increase uric acid concentrations. Products are derived from porcine pancreatic glands. Severe, allergic reactions (rare) have been observed; use with caution in patients hypersensitive to pork proteins. Transmission of porcine viruses is theoretically a risk; however, testing and/or inactivation or removal of certain viruses, reduces the risk. There have been no cases of transmission of an infectious illness reported. Available brand products are **not** interchangeable.

Adverse Reactions The following adverse reactions were reported in a short-term safety studies; actual frequency varies with different products; adverse events, particularly gastrointestinal events, were often greater with placebo:

10%:

Central nervous system: Headache (6% to 15%)

Gastrointestinal: Abdominal pain (4% to 18%)

1% to 10%:

Central nervous system: Dizziness (4% to 6%)

Endocrine & metabolic: Diabetes mellitus exacerbation (4%), hyperglycemia (4% to 8%), hypoglycemia (4%)

Gastrointestinal: Flatulence (4% to 9%), early satiety (6%), weight loss (3% to 6%), vomiting (6%), upper abdominal pain (≤5%), diarrhea (≤4%), feces abnormal (≤4%)

Respiratory: Cough (4% to 6%), nasopharyngitis (4%)

<1% (Limited to important or life-threatening; reported with various formulations of pancrelipase): Allergic reactions (severe), anaphylaxis, asthma, carcinoma recurrence, constipation, distal intestinal obstruction syndrome (DIOS), duodenitis, fibrosing colonopathy, gastritis, hives, hyperuricemia, muscle spasm, myalgia, nausea, neutropenia (transient), pruritus, rash, transaminases increased (asymptomatic), urticaria, vision blurred

Drug Interactions

Metabolism/Transport Effects None known.

Avoid Concomitant Use There are no known interactions where it is recommended to avoid concomitant use.

Increased Effect/Toxicity There are no known significant interactions involving an increase in effect.

Decreased Effect

Pancrelipase may decrease the levels/effects of: Iron Salts

Ethanol/Nutrition/Herb Interactions Food: Avoid placing contents of opened capsules on alkaline food; pancrelipase may impair absorption of oral iron.

Stability

Creon®: Store at room temperature of 25°C (77°F); excursions permitted between 25°C to 40°C (77°F to 104°F) for ≤30 days. Protect from moisture, and discard if moisture conditions are >70%. Keep bottle tightly closed.

Pancreaze™: Store at ≤25°C (77°F). Protect from moisture; keep bottle tightly closed.

Zenpep®: Store at room temperature 20°C to 25°C (68°F to 77°F). Protect from moisture; keep bottle tightly closed after opening.

Mechanism of Action Pancrelipase is a natural product harvested from the porcine pancreatic glands. It contains a combination of lipase, amylase, and protease. Products are formulated to dissolve in the more basic pH of the duodenum so that they may act locally to break down fats, protein, and starch.

Pharmacodynamics/Kinetics

Absorption: None; acts locally in GI tract

Excretion: Feces

Dosage Oral: **Note:** Adjust dose based on body weight, clinical symptoms, and stool fat content. Allow several days between dose adjustments. Total daily dose reflects ~3 meals/day and 2-3 snacks/day, with half the mealtime dose given with a snack. Doses of lipase >2500 units/kg/meal (or lipase >10,000 units/kg/day) should be used with caution and only with documentation of 3-day fecal fat measures. Doses of lipase >6000 units/kg/meal are associated with colonic stricture and should be decreased.

Pancreatic insufficiency:

Children:

≤1 year: Lipase 2000-4000 units per 120 mL of formula or breast milk

>1 and <4 years: Initial dose: Lipase 1000 units/kg/meal. Dosage range: Lipase 1000-2500 units/kg/meal. Maximum dose: Lipase 10,000 units/kg/day **or** lipase 4000 units/g of fat per day

≥4 years: Refer to adult dosing

Adults: Initial: Lipase 500 units/kg/meal. Dosage range: Lipase 500-2500 units/kg/meal. Maximum dose: Lipase 10,000 units/kg/day **or** lipase 4000 units/g of fat per day

Pancreatic insufficiency due to chronic pancreatitis or pancreatectomy (Creon®): Adults: Lipase 72,000 units/meal while consuming ≥100 g of fat per day; alternatively, lower initial doses of lipase 500 units/kg/meal with individualized dosage titrations have also been used

Dietary Considerations Take with meals or snacks and swallow whole with a generous amount of liquid. Vitamin supplementation should be per current guidelines for patients with cystic fibrosis.

Administration Oral: Administer with meals or snacks and swallow whole with a generous amount of liquid. Do not crush or chew; retention in the mouth before swallowing may cause mucosal irritation and stomatitis. If necessary, capsules may also be opened and contents added to a small amount of an acidic food (pH ≤4.5), such as applesauce. The food should be at room temperature and swallowed immediately after mixing. The contents of the capsule should not be crushed or chewed. Follow with water or juice to ensure complete ingestion and that no medication remains in the mouth.

When administering to infants <1 year of age, do not mix with breast milk or infant formula. Open capsule and place the contents directly into the mouth or mix with a small amount of acidic soft food (pH ≤4.5), such as applesauce or other acidic commercially prepared baby food (pears or bananas) at room temperature. Administer immediately after mixing (or within 15 minutes of mixing using Pancreaze™). Follow with infant formula or breast milk to ensure complete ingestion and that no medication remains in the mouth.

Creon®: Capsules contain enteric coated spheres which are 0.71-1.6 mm in diameter

Pancreaze™: Capsules contain enteric coated microtablets which are ~2 mm in diameter

Zenpep®: Capsules contain enteric coated beads which are 1.8-2.5 mm in diameter

Administration via gastrostomy (G) tube: An *in vitro* study demonstrated that Creon® delayed-release capsules sprinkled onto a small amount of baby food (pH<4.5; applesauce or bananas manufactured by both Gerber and Beech-Nut) stirred gently and after 15 minutes was administered through the following G-tubes without significant loss of lipase activity: Kimberly-Clark MIC Bolus® size 18 Fr, Kimberly-Clark MIC-KEY® size 16 Fr, Bard® Tri-Funnel size 18 Fr, and Bard® Button size 18 Fr (Shlieout, 2011).

Monitoring Parameters Abdominal symptoms, nutritional intake, weight, growth (in children), stool character, fecal fat

Additional Information Unapproved PEPs are no longer allowed to be distributed in the U.S. There are three PEPs with FDA approval commercially available in the U.S.: Creon®, Pancreaze™, and Zenpep®. PEPs are **not** interchangeable, and patients will require new prescriptions when changing from one product to another. However, Pancrelipase™ lipase 5000 units strength (manufactured by Eurand Pharmaceuticals and distributed by X-Gen Pharmaceuticals) is an authorized generic which may be used interchangeably with the Zenpep® lipase 5000 units product (manufactured by Eurand Pharmaceuticals).

Dosage Forms Excipient information presented when available (limited, particularly for generics); consult specific product labeling.

Capsule, delayed release, enteric coated beads [porcine derived]:

Pancrelipase™: Lipase 5000 units, protease 17,000 units, amylase 27,000 units

Zenpep®: Lipase 3000 units, protease 10,000 units, and amylase 16,000 units

Zenpep®: Lipase 5000 units, protease 17,000 units, and amylase 27,000 units

Zenpep®: Lipase 10,000 units, protease 34,000 units, and amylase 55,000 units
Zenpep®: Lipase 15,000 units, protease 51,000 units, and amylase 82,000 units
Zenpep®: Lipase 20,000 units, protease 68,000 units, and amylase 109,000 units
Zenpep®: Lipase 25,000 units, protease 85,000 units, and amylase 136,000 units

Capsule, delayed release, enteric coated microspheres [new formulation; porcine derived]:
Creon®: Lipase 3000 units, protease 9500 units, and amylase 15,000 units
Creon®: Lipase 6000 units, protease 19,000 units, and amylase 30,000 units
Creon®: Lipase 12000 units, protease 38,000 units, and amylase 60,000 units
Creon®: Lipase 24,000 units, protease 76,000 units, and amylase 120,000 units

Capsule, delayed release, enteric coated microtablets [porcine derived]:
Pancreaze™: Lipase 4200 units, protease 10,000 units, and amylase 17,500 units
Pancreaze™: Lipase 10,500 units, protease 25,000 units, and amylase 43,750 units
Pancreaze™: Lipase 16,800 units, protease 40,000 units, and amylase 70,000 units
Pancreaze™: Lipase 21,000 units, protease 37,000 units, and amylase 61,000 units

◆ **Pancrelipase™** *see* Pancrelipase *on page* 1285

Pancuronium (pan kyoo ROE nee um)

Brand Names: Canada Pancuronium Bromide®

Index Terms Pancuronium Bromide; Pavulon [DSC]

Pharmacologic Category Neuromuscular Blocker Agent, Nondepolarizing

Use Facilitation of endotracheal intubation and relaxation of skeletal muscles during surgery; facilitation of mechanical ventilation in ICU patients; does not relieve pain or produce sedation

Pregnancy Risk Factor C

Pregnancy Considerations Animal reproduction studies have not been conducted. Small amounts of pancuronium cross the placenta (Daily, 1984). May be used short-term in cesarean section; reduced doses recommended in patients also receiving magnesium sulfate due to enhanced effects.

Contraindications Hypersensitivity to pancuronium, bromide, or any component of the formulation

Warnings/Precautions Ventilation must be supported during neuromuscular blockade; use with caution in patients with renal and/or hepatic impairment (adjust dose appropriately); certain clinical conditions may result in potentiation or antagonism of neuromuscular blockade:

Potentiation: Electrolyte abnormalities, severe hyponatremia, severe hypocalcemia, severe hypokalemia, hypermagnesemia, neuromuscular diseases, acidosis, acute intermittent porphyria, renal failure, hepatic failure

Antagonism: Alkalosis, hypercalcemia, demyelinating lesions, peripheral neuropathies, diabetes mellitus

Increased sensitivity in patients with myasthenia gravis, Eaton-Lambert syndrome; resistance in burn patients (>30% of body) for period of 5-70 days postinjury; resistance in patients with muscle trauma, denervation, immobilization, infection. Cross-sensitivity with other neuromuscular-blocking agents may occur; use extreme caution in patients with previous anaphylactic reactions. Use caution in the elderly. **[U.S. Boxed Warning]: Should be administered by adequately trained individuals familiar with its use.** Some dosage forms may contain benzyl alcohol which has been associated with "gasping syndrome" in neonates.

Adverse Reactions Frequency not defined.

Cardiovascular: Elevation in pulse rate, elevated blood pressure and cardiac output, tachycardia, edema, skin flushing, circulatory collapse
Dermatologic: Rash, itching, erythema, burning sensation along the vein
Gastrointestinal: Excessive salivation
Neuromuscular & skeletal: Profound muscle weakness
Respiratory: Wheezing, bronchospasm
Miscellaneous: Hypersensitivity reaction

Postmarketing and/or case reports: Acute quadriplegic myopathy syndrome (prolonged use), anaphylactoid reactions, anaphylaxis, myositis ossificans (prolonged use)

Drug Interactions

Metabolism/Transport Effects None known.

Avoid Concomitant Use

Avoid concomitant use of Pancuronium with any of the following: QuiNINE

Increased Effect/Toxicity

Pancuronium may increase the levels/effects of: Cardiac Glycosides; Corticosteroids (Systemic); OnabotulinumtoxinA; RimabotulinumtoxinB

The levels/effects of Pancuronium may be increased by: AbobotulinumtoxinA; Aminoglycosides; Calcium Channel Blockers; Capreomycin; Colistimethate; Inhalational Anesthetics; Ketorolac; Ketorolac (Nasal); Ketorolac (Systemic); Lincosamide Antibiotics; Lithium; Loop Diuretics; Magnesium Salts; Polymyxin B; Procainamide; QuiNIDine; QuiNINE; Spironolactone; Tetracycline Derivatives; Theophylline Derivatives; Vancomycin

Decreased Effect

The levels/effects of Pancuronium may be decreased by: Acetylcholinesterase Inhibitors; Loop Diuretics; Theophylline Derivatives

Stability Refrigerate; however, stable for up to 6 months at room temperature.

Mechanism of Action Blocks neural transmission at the myoneural junction by binding with cholinergic receptor sites

Pharmacodynamics/Kinetics

Onset of effect: Peak effect: I.V.: 2-3 minutes
Duration (dose dependent): 60-100 minutes
Metabolism: Hepatic (30% to 45%); active metabolite 3-hydroxypancuronium (1/3 to 1/2 the activity of parent drug)
Half-life elimination: 110 minutes
Excretion: Urine (55% to 70% as unchanged drug)

Dosage Administer I.V.; dose to effect; doses will vary due to interpatient variability; use ideal body weight for obese patients

Surgery:

Infants >1 month, Children, and Adults: Initial: 0.06-0.1 mg/kg or 0.05 mg/kg after initial dose of succinylcholine for intubation; maintenance dose: 0.01 mg/kg administered 60-100 minutes after initial dose and then 0.01 mg/kg every 25-60 minutes

Pretreatment/priming: 10% of intubating dose given 3-5 minutes before intubating dose

ICU paralysis (eg, facilitate mechanical ventilation) in select adequately sedated patients: 0.06-0.1 mg/kg bolus followed by 1-2 mcg/kg/minute (Murray, 2002) **or** 0.1-0.2 mg/kg every 1-3 hours

Dosing adjustment in renal impairment: Elimination half-life is doubled, plasma clearance is reduced and rate of recovery is sometimes much slower

Cl_{cr} 10-50 mL/minute: Administer 50% of normal dose
Cl_{cr} <10 mL/minute: Do not use

Dosing adjustment/comments in hepatic/biliary tract disease: Elimination half-life is doubled, plasma clearance is reduced, recovery time is prolonged, volume of distribution is increased (50%) and results in a slower onset, higher total initial dosage, and prolongation of neuromuscular blockade

Administration May be administered undiluted by rapid I.V. injection

Monitoring Parameters Heart rate, blood pressure, assisted ventilation status; cardiac monitor, blood pressure monitor, and ventilator required

Additional Information Pancuronium is classified as a long-duration neuromuscular-blocking agent. Neuromuscular blockade will be prolonged in patients with decreased renal function. Pancuronium does not relieve pain or produce sedation. It may produce cumulative effect on duration of blockade. It produces tachycardia secondary to vagolytic activity and sympathetic stimulation.

Dosage Forms Excipient information presented when available (limited, particularly for generics); consult specific product labeling.

Injection, solution, as bromide: 1 mg/mL (10 mL)

◆ **Pancuronium Bromide** *see* Pancuronium *on page 1287*
◆ **Pancuronium Bromide® (Can)** *see* Pancuronium *on page 1287*
◆ **Pandel®** *see* Hydrocortisone (Topical) *on page 841*
◆ **Panglobulin** *see* Immune Globulin *on page 880*

Panitumumab (pan i TOOM yoo mab)

Brand Names: U.S. Vectibix®

Brand Names: Canada Vectibix®

Index Terms ABX-EGF; MOAB ABX-EGF; Monoclonal Antibody ABX-EGF; rHuMAb-EGFr

Pharmacologic Category Antineoplastic Agent, Monoclonal Antibody; Epidermal Growth Factor Receptor (EGFR) Inhibitor

Use Monotherapy in treatment of refractory metastatic colorectal cancer

Note: Subset analyses (retrospective) in metastatic colorectal cancer trials have not shown a benefit with EGFR inhibitor treatment in patients whose tumors have codon 12 or 13 *KRAS* mutations; use is not recommended in these patients.

Pregnancy Risk Factor C

Pregnancy Considerations Animal reproductive studies have demonstrated adverse fetal effects. Based on animal studies, panitumumab may disrupt normal menstrual cycles. There are no adequate and well-controlled studies in pregnant women. IgG is known to cross the placenta; therefore, it is possible the developing fetus may be exposed to panitumumab. Because panitumumab inhibits epidermal growth factor (EGF), a component of fetal development, adverse effects on pregnancy would be expected. Panitumumab should only be given to a pregnant woman if the potential benefit justifies the potential risk to the fetus. Women of childbearing potential should use effective contraception during and for 6 months after treatment. Women who become pregnant during panitumumab treatment are encouraged to enroll in Amgen's Pregnancy Surveillance Program (1-800-772-6436).

Lactation Excretion in breast milk unknown/not recommended

Contraindications There are no contraindications listed in manufacturer's labeling.

Warnings/Precautions [U.S. Boxed Warning]: Dermatologic toxicities have been reported in ~90% of patients (severe in 12% of patients); may include dermatitis acneiform, pruritus, erythema, rash, skin exfoliation, paronychia, dry skin and skin fissures. Severe skin toxicities may be complicated by infection, sepsis, or abscesses. The median time to development of skin (or ocular) toxicity was 2 weeks, with resolution ~7 weeks after discontinuation. Withhold treatment (and monitor) for severe or life-threatening dermatologic toxicities; may require dose reduction or permanent discontinuation. The severity of dermatologic toxicity is predictive for response; grades 2-4 skin toxicity correlates with improved progression free survival and overall survival, compared to grade 1 skin toxicity (Peeters, 2009; Van Cutsem, 2007). Patients should minimize sunlight exposure; may exacerbate skin reactions. Gastric mucosal, ocular and nail toxicities have also been reported.

[U.S. Boxed Warning]: Severe infusion reactions (anaphylactic reaction, bronchospasm, fever, chills, and hypotension) have been reported in ~1% of patients. Discontinue infusion for severe reactions; permanently discontinue in patients with persistent severe infusion reactions. Appropriate medical support for the management of infusion reactions should be readily available. Mild-to-moderate infusion reactions are managed by slowing the infusion rate.

Pulmonary fibrosis has been reported (rarely); permanently discontinue treatment if interstitial lung disease, pneumonitis or lung infiltrates develop. Use caution with lung disease; patients with underlying lung disease were excluded from clinical trials. May cause diarrhea; the incidence and severity of chemotherapy-induced diarrhea and other toxicities (rash, electrolyte abnormalities, stomatitis) is increased with combination chemotherapy; acute renal failure resulting from severe diarrhea and dehydration has also been observed in patients receiving panitumumab with combination chemotherapy. In addition to increased toxicity, studies using panitumumab in combination with chemotherapy (with or without bevacizumab) resulted in decreased progression-free survival compared to regimens without panitumumab; therefore, panitumumab is not indicated for use in combination with chemotherapy. Electrolyte depletion may occur during treatment and after treatment is discontinued; monitor for hypomagnesemia and hypocalcemia during treatment and for at least 8 weeks after completion. Patients with colorectal cancer with tumors with a codon 12 or 13 *KRAS* mutation are unlikely to benefit from EGFR inhibitor therapy and should not receive panitumumab treatment. Safety and efficacy in children have not been established.

Adverse Reactions

>10%:

Cardiovascular: Peripheral edema (12%)

Central nervous system: Fatigue (26%)

Dermatologic: Skin toxicity (90%; grades 3/4: 14% to 16%), erythema (65%; grades 3/4: 5%), acneiform rash (57%; grades 3/4: 7%), pruritus (57%; grades 3/4: 2%), exfoliation (25%; grades 3/4: 2%), paronychia (25%), rash (22%; grades 3/4: 1%), fissures (20%; grades 3/4: 1%), acne (13%; grades 3/4: 1%)

Endocrine & metabolic: Hypomagnesemia (38%; grades 3/4: 4%)

Gastrointestinal: Abdominal pain (25%), nausea (23%), diarrhea (21%; grades 3/4: 2%), constipation (21%), vomiting (19%)

Respiratory: Cough (14%)

1% to 10%:

Dermatologic: Dry skin (10%), nail disorder (other than paronychia: 9%)

Gastrointestinal: Stomatitis (7%), mucositis (6%)

Ocular: Eyelash growth (6%), conjunctivitis (4%), ocular hyperemia (3%), lacrimation increased (2%), eye/eye lid irritation (1%)

Miscellaneous: Antibody formation (≤5%), infusion reactions (3%; grades 3/4: 1%)

<1% (Limited to important or life-threatening): Abscess, allergic reaction, anaphylactoid reaction, angioedema, chills, dyspnea, fever, hypocalcemia, hypoxia, pulmonary embolism, pulmonary fibrosis, pulmonary infiltrate, sepsis, septic death

Drug Interactions

Metabolism/Transport Effects None known.

Avoid Concomitant Use There are no known interactions where it is recommended to avoid concomitant use.

Increased Effect/Toxicity There are no known significant interactions involving an increase in effect.

Decreased Effect There are no known significant interactions involving a decrease in effect.

Stability Store unopened vials under refrigeration at 2°C to 8°C (36°F to 46°F). Do not freeze; do not shake; protect from light. Dilute in 100-150 mL of normal saline to a final concentration of ≤10 mg/mL. Do not shake, invert gently to mix. Preparations in infusion containers are stable for 24 hours under refrigeration at 2°C to 8°C (36°F to 46°F) or for 6 hours at room temperature (do not freeze).

Mechanism of Action Recombinant human IgG2 monoclonal antibody which binds specifically to the epidermal growth factor receptor (EGFR, HER1, c-ErbB-1) and competitively inhibits the binding of epidermal growth factor (EGF) and other ligands. Binding to the EGFR blocks phosphorylation and activation of intracellular tyrosine kinases, resulting in inhibition of cell survival, growth, proliferation and transformation. EGFR signal transduction results in *KRAS* wild-type activation; cells with *KRAS* mutations appear to be unaffected by EGFR inhibition.

Pharmacodynamics/Kinetics Half-life elimination: ~7.5 days (range: 4-11 days)

Dosage I.V.: Adults: Metastatic colorectal cancer: 6 mg/kg every 2 weeks

Dosing adjustment for toxicity:

Infusion reactions, mild-to-moderate (grade 1 or 2): Reduce the infusion rate by 50% for the duration of infusion

Infusion reactions, severe (grade 3 or 4): Immediately and permanently discontinue treatment

Dermatologic toxicity (≥grade 3, or intolerable): Withhold treatment; if skin toxicity does not improve to ≤grade 2 within 1 month, permanently discontinue. If skin toxicity improves to ≤grade 2 within 1 month (with patient missing ≤2 doses), resume treatment at 50% of the original dose. Dose may be increased in increments of 25% of the original dose (up to 6 mg/kg) if skin toxicities do not recur. For recurrent skin toxicity, permanently discontinue.

Dosage adjustment in renal impairment: Has not been studied

Dosage adjustment in hepatic impairment: Has not been studied

Administration I.V.: Doses ≤1000 mg, infuse over 1 hour; doses >1000 mg, infuse over 90 minutes; reduce infusion rate by 50% for mild-to-moderate infusion reactions (grades 1 and 2); discontinue for severe infusion reactions (grades 3 and 4). Administer through a low protein-binding 0.2 or 0.22 micrometer in-line filter. Flush with NS before and after infusion.

Monitoring Parameters *KRAS* genotyping of tumor tissue. Monitor serum electrolytes, including magnesium and calcium (periodically during and for at least 8 weeks after therapy). Monitor vital signs and temperature before, during, and after infusion. Monitor for skin toxicity.

Additional Information Oncology Comment: The National Comprehensive Cancer Network® (NCCN) guidelines for colon cancer (v.2.2009) and the American Society of Clinical Oncology (ASCO) provisional clinical opinion (Allegra, 2009) recommend genotyping tumor tissue for *KRAS* mutation in all patients with metastatic colorectal cancer (genotyping may be done on archived specimens). Patients with known codon 12 or 13 *KRAS* gene mutations are unlikely to respond to EGFR inhibitors and should not receive panitumumab. Favorable progression-free survival and higher response rates have been demonstrated with panitumumab in patients with *KRAS* wild-type; patients with the *KRAS* mutation did not respond to panitumumab (Amado, 2008). Because EGFR testing in colorectal tumors does not correlate with response, the NCCN guidelines do not recommend routine EGFR testing in colorectal cancer. Severity of dermatologic toxicity associated with panitumumab is predictive for response; grades 2-4 skin toxicity correlates with improved progression free survival and overall survival, compared to patients with grade 1 skin toxicity (Van Cutsem, 2007). The association between dermatologic toxicity and progression free survival was not noted in patients with *KRAS* mutation (Peeters, 2009). The NCCN guidelines do not recommend the use of panitumumab after failure of cetuximab therapy.

Dosage Forms Excipient information presented when available (limited, particularly for generics); consult specific product labeling. [DSC] = Discontinued product

Injection, solution [preservative free]:

Vectibix®: 20 mg/mL (5 mL, 10 mL [DSC], 20 mL)

◆ **Panto™ I.V. (Can)** *see* Pantoprazole *on page 1289*

◆ **Pantoloc® (Can)** *see* Pantoprazole *on page 1289*

Pantoprazole (pan TOE pra zole)

Brand Names: U.S. Protonix®; Protonix® I.V.

Brand Names: Canada Apo-Pantoprazole®; Ava-Pantoprazole; CO Pantoprazole; Mylan-Pantoprazole; Pantoloc®; Pantoprazole for Injection; Panto™ I.V.; PMS-Pantoprazole; Q-Pantoprazole; RAN™-Pantoprazole; ratio-Pantoprazole; Riva-Pantoprazole; Sandoz-Pantoprazole; Tecta™; Teva-Pantoprazole

Pharmacologic Category Proton Pump Inhibitor; Substituted Benzimidazole

Use

Oral: Treatment and maintenance of healing of erosive esophagitis associated with GERD; reduction in relapse rates of daytime and nighttime heartburn symptoms in GERD; hypersecretory disorders associated with Zollinger-Ellison syndrome or other GI hypersecretory disorders

I.V.: Short-term treatment (7-10 days) of patients with gastroesophageal reflux disease (GERD) and a history of erosive esophagitis; hypersecretory disorders associated with Zollinger-Ellison syndrome or other neoplastic disorders

Unlabeled Use Peptic ulcer disease, active ulcer bleeding (parenteral formulation); adjunct treatment with antibiotics for *Helicobacter pylori* eradication; stress-ulcer prophylaxis in the critically-ill

Pregnancy Risk Factor B

Pregnancy Considerations Teratogenic effects were not observed in animal studies. There are no adequate and well-controlled studies in pregnant women. Use in pregnancy only if clearly needed.

Lactation Enters breast milk/not recommended

Contraindications Hypersensitivity to pantoprazole, substituted benzamidazoles (eg, esomeprazole, lansoprazole, omeprazole, rabeprazole), or any component of the formulation

Canadian labeling: Additional contraindication (not in U.S. labeling): Concomitant use with atazanavir

Warnings/Precautions Use of proton pump inhibitors (PPIs) may increase the risk of gastrointestinal infections (eg, *Salmonella, Campylobacter*). Relief of symptoms does not preclude the presence of a gastric malignancy. Long-term pantoprazole therapy (especially in patients who were *H. pylori* positive) has caused biopsy-proven atrophic gastritis. No reports of enterochromaffin-like

(ECL) cell carcinoids, dysplasia, or neoplasia such as those seen in rodent studies have occurred in humans. Not indicated for maintenance therapy; safety and efficacy for use beyond 16 weeks have not been established. Prolonged treatment (typically >3 years) may lead to vitamin B_{12} malabsorption and subsequent deficiency. Intravenous preparation contains edetate sodium (EDTA); use caution in patients who are at risk for zinc deficiency if other EDTA-containing solutions are coadministered. Decreased *H. pylori* eradication rates have been observed with short-term (≤7 days) combination therapy. The American College of Gastroenterology recommends 10-14 days of therapy (triple or quadruple) for eradication of *H. pylori* (Chey, 2007).

PPIs may diminish the therapeutic effect of clopidogrel, thought to be due to reduced formation of the active metabolite of clopidogrel. Of the PPIs, pantoprazole has the lowest degree of CYP2C19 inhibition. Therefore, the manufacturer of clopidogrel prefers pantoprazole if concomitant use of a PPI is necessary. Others have recommended the continued use of PPIs, regardless of the degree of inhibition, in patients with a history of GI bleeding or multiple risk factors for GI bleeding who are also receiving clopidogrel since no evidence has established clinically meaningful differences in outcome; however, a clinically-significant interaction cannot be excluded in those who are poor metabolizers of clopidogrel (Abraham, 2010; Levine, 2011).

Increased incidence of osteoporosis-related bone fractures of the hip, spine, or wrist may occur with PPI therapy. Patients on high-dose or long-term therapy should be monitored. Use the lowest effective dose for the shortest duration of time, use vitamin D and calcium supplementation, and follow appropriate guidelines to reduce risk of fractures in patients at risk.

Hypomagnesemia, reported rarely, usually with prolonged PPI use of >3 months (most cases >1 year of therapy); may be symptomatic or asymptomatic; severe cases may cause tetany, seizures, and cardiac arrhythmias. Consider obtaining serum magnesium concentrations prior to beginning long-term therapy, especially if taking concomitant digoxin, diuretics, or other drugs known to cause hypomagnesemia; and periodically thereafter. Hypomagnesemia may be corrected by magnesium supplementation, although discontinuation of pantoprazole may be necessary; magnesium levels typically return to normal within 1 week of stopping.

Adverse Reactions

1% to 10%:

- Cardiovascular: Chest pain
- Central nervous system: Headache (2% to 9%), insomnia (≤1%), anxiety, dizziness, migraine, pain
- Dermatologic: Rash (≤2%)
- Endocrine & metabolic: Hyperglycemia (≤1%), hyperlipidemia
- Gastrointestinal: Diarrhea (2% to 6%), flatulence (2% to 4%), abdominal pain (1% to 4%), nausea (≤2%), vomiting (≤2%), eructation (≤1%), constipation, dyspepsia, gastroenteritis, rectal disorder
- Genitourinary: Urinary frequency, UTI
- Hepatic: Liver function tests abnormal (≤2%)
- Local: Injection site reaction (includes thrombophlebitis and abscess)
- Neuromuscular & skeletal: Arthralgia, back pain, hypertonia, neck pain, weakness
- Respiratory: Bronchitis, cough, dyspnea, pharyngitis, rhinitis, sinusitis, upper respiratory tract infection
- Miscellaneous: Flu syndrome, infection

<1% (Limited to important or life-threatening): Abnormal dreams, acne, albuminuria, alkaline phosphatase increased, allergic reaction, alopecia, anaphylaxis, anemia, angioedema, angina pectoris, anorexia, aphthous stomatitis, appetite increased, arrhythmia, asthma exacerbation, atrial fibrillation/flutter, atrophic gastritis, balanitis, biliary pain, blurred vision, bone pain, breast pain, bursitis, cataract, CHF, chills, cholecystitis, cholelithiasis, CPK increased, colitis, confusion, contact dermatitis, creatinine increased, cystitis, deafness, decreased reflexes, dehydration, depression, diabetes mellitus, diaphoresis, diplopia, duodenitis, dysarthria, dysmenorrhea, dysphagia, dysuria, ecchymosis, ECG abnormality, eczema, eosinophilia, epididymitis, epistaxis, erythema multiforme, esophagitis, extraocular palsy, facial edema, fatigue, fever, fracture, fungal dermatitis, gastrointestinal carcinoma, gastrointestinal hemorrhage, gastrointestinal moniliasis, generalized edema, GGT increased, gingivitis, glaucoma, glossitis, glycosuria, goiter, gout, halitosis, hallucinations, heat stroke, hematemesis, hematuria, hemorrhage, hepatic failure, hepatitis, hernia, herpes simplex, herpes zoster, hiccup, hyperbilirubinemia, hyperesthesia, hyper-/hypotension, hyperkinesia, hyperuricemia, hypokinesia, hypomagnesemia, hyponatremia, impaired urination, impotence, interstitial nephritis, jaundice, kidney calculus, kidney pain, laryngitis, leg cramps, leukocytosis, leukopenia, libido decreased, lichenoid dermatitis, maculopapular rash, malaise, melena, mouth ulceration, myalgia, myocardial infarction, myocardial ischemia, neoplasm, nervousness, neuralgia, neuritis, nocturia, optic neuropathy (including anterior ischemic), otitis externa, palpitation, pancreatitis, pancytopenia, paresthesia, periodontal abscess, periodontitis, photosensitivity, pneumonia, pruritus, pyelonephritis, rectal hemorrhage, retinal vascular disorder, rhabdomyolysis, salivation increased, scrotal edema, seizure, skin ulcer, somnolence, Stevens-Johnson syndrome, stomach ulcer, stomatitis, syncope, tachycardia, taste perversion, tenosynovitis, thrombocytopenia, thrombosis, tinnitus, tongue discoloration, toxic epidermal necrolysis, tremor, urethral pain, urethritis, urticaria, vaginitis, vasodilation, vertigo, vision abnormal, weight changes, xerostomia

Drug Interactions

Metabolism/Transport Effects Substrate of CYP2C19 (major), CYP2D6 (minor), CYP3A4 (minor); **Note:** Assignment of Major/Minor substrate status based on clinically relevant drug interaction potential; **Inhibits** BCRP, CYP2C19 (moderate); **Induces** CYP1A2 (weak/moderate)

Avoid Concomitant Use

Avoid concomitant use of Pantoprazole with any of the following: Delavirdine; Erlotinib; Nelfinavir; Posaconazole; Rilpivirine

Increased Effect/Toxicity

Pantoprazole may increase the levels/effects of: Amphetamines; Citalopram; CYP2C19 Substrates; Dexmethylphenidate; Methotrexate; Methylphenidate; Raltegravir; Saquinavir; Topotecan; Voriconazole

The levels/effects of Pantoprazole may be increased by: Conivaptan; Fluconazole; Ketoconazole; Ketoconazole (Systemic)

Decreased Effect

Pantoprazole may decrease the levels/effects of: Atazanavir; Bisphosphonate Derivatives; Cefditoren; Clopidogrel; Dabigatran Etexilate; Dasatinib; Delavirdine; Erlotinib; Gefitinib; Indinavir; Iron Salts; Itraconazole; Ketoconazole; Ketoconazole (Systemic); Mesalamine; Mycophenolate; Nelfinavir; Posaconazole; Rilpivirine

The levels/effects of Pantoprazole may be decreased by: CYP2C19 Inducers (Strong); Peginterferon Alfa-2b; Tipranavir; Tocilizumab

Ethanol/Nutrition/Herb Interactions

Ethanol: Avoid ethanol (may cause gastric mucosal irritation).

Herb/Nutraceutical: Prolonged treatment (typically >3 years) may lead to vitamin B_{12} malabsorption and subsequent deficiency.

Stability

Oral: Store tablet and oral suspension at controlled room temperature of 20°C to 25°C (68°F to 77°F).

I.V.: Prior to reconstitution, store at controlled room temperature of 20°C to 25°C (68°F to 77°F). Protect from light. Reconstitute with 10 mL NS (final concentration 4 mg/mL). Reconstituted solution may be given intravenously (over 2 minutes) or may be added to 100 mL D_5W, NS, or LR (for 15-minute infusion). When reconstituted, solution is stable up to 96 hours at room temperature (Johnson, 2005). The preparation should be stored at 3°C to 5°C (37°F to 41°F) if it is stored beyond 48 hours to minimize discoloration. If further diluting in 100 mL of D_5W, LR, or NS, dilute within 6 hours of reconstitution. Diluted solution is stable at room temperature for up to 24 hours from the time of initial reconstitution; protection from light is not required.

Mechanism of Action Suppresses gastric acid secretion by inhibiting the parietal cell H^+/K^+ ATP pump

Pharmacodynamics/Kinetics

Absorption: Rapid, well absorbed

Distribution: V_d: 11-24 L

Protein binding: 98%, primarily to albumin

Metabolism: Extensively hepatic; CYP2C19 (demethylation), CYP3A4; no evidence that metabolites have pharmacologic activity

Bioavailability: 77%

Half-life elimination: 1 hour; increased to 3.5-10 hours with CYP2C19 deficiency

Time to peak: Oral: 2.5 hours

Excretion: Urine (71%); feces (18%)

Dosage

Oral:

Children ≥5 years (unlabeled use): GERD, erosive esophagitis associated with GERD: 20-40 mg once daily

Adults:

Erosive esophagitis associated with GERD:

Treatment: 40 mg once daily for up to 8 weeks; an additional 8 weeks may be used in patients who have not healed after an 8-week course

Maintenance of healing: 40 mg once daily

Note: Lower doses (20 mg once daily) have been used successfully in mild GERD treatment and maintenance of healing

Hypersecretory disorders (including Zollinger-Ellison): Initial: 40 mg twice daily; adjust dose based on patient needs; doses up to 240 mg/day have been administered

Helicobacter pylori eradication (unlabeled use): American College of Gastroenterology guidelines (Chey, 2007):

Nonpenicillin allergy: 40 mg twice daily administered with amoxicillin 1000 mg *and* clarithromycin 500 mg twice daily for 10-14 days

Penicillin allergy: 40 mg twice daily administered with clarithromycin 500 mg *and* metronidazole 500 mg twice daily for 10-14 days **or** 40 mg once or twice daily administered with bismuth subsalicylate 525 mg *and* metronidazole 250 mg *plus* tetracycline 500 mg 4 times/day for 10-14 days

I.V.:

Erosive esophagitis associated with GERD: 40 mg once daily for 7-10 days

Hypersecretory disorders: 80 mg twice daily; adjust dose based on acid output measurements; 160-240 mg/day in divided doses has been used for a limited period (up to 7 days)

Prevention of rebleeding in peptic ulcer bleed (unlabeled use): 80 mg, followed by 8 mg/hour infusion for 72 hours. **Note:** A daily infusion of 40 mg does not raise gastric pH sufficiently to enhance coagulation in active GI bleeds.

Elderly: Dosage adjustment not required

Dosage adjustment in renal impairment: Not required; pantoprazole is not removed by hemodialysis

Dosage adjustment in hepatic impairment: Not required

Dietary Considerations

Oral: May be taken with or without food; best if taken before breakfast.

I.V.: Due to EDTA in preparation, zinc supplementation may be needed in patients prone to zinc deficiency.

Administration

I.V.: Flush I.V. line before and after administration. In-line filter not required.

2-minute infusion: The volume of reconstituted solution (4 mg/mL) to be injected may be administered intravenously over at least 2 minutes.

15-minute infusion: Infuse over 15 minutes at a rate not to exceed 7 mL/minute (3 mg/minute).

Oral:

Tablet: Should be swallowed whole, do not crush or chew. Best if taken before breakfast.

Delayed-release oral suspension: Should only be administered in apple juice or applesauce and taken ~30 minutes before a meal. Do not administer with any other liquid (eg, water) or foods.

Oral administration in **applesauce**: Sprinkle intact granules on 1 tablespoon of applesauce and swallow within 10 minutes of preparation.

Oral administration in **apple juice**: Empty intact granules into 5 mL of apple juice, stir for 5 seconds, and swallow immediately after preparation. Rinse container once or twice with apple juice and swallow immediately.

Nasogastric tube administration: Separate the plunger from the barrel of a 60 mL catheter tip syringe and connect to a ≥16 French nasogastric tube. Holding the syringe attached to the tubing as high as possible, empty the contents of the packet into barrel of the syringe, add 10 mL of apple juice and gently tap/shake the barrel of the syringe to help empty the syringe. Add an additional 10 mL of apple juice and gently tap/shake the barrel to help rinse. Repeat rinse with at least 2-10 mL aliquots of apple juice. No granules should remain in the syringe.

Monitoring Parameters Hypersecretory disorders: Acid output measurements, target level <10 mEq/hour (<5 mEq/hour if prior gastric acid-reducing surgery)

Test Interactions False-positive urine screening tests for tetrahydrocannabinol (THC) have been noted in patients receiving proton pump inhibitors, including pantoprazole.

Dosage Forms Excipient information presented when available (limited, particularly for generics); consult specific product labeling.

Granules for suspension, delayed release, enteric coated, oral:

Protonix®: 40 mg/packet (30s)

Injection, powder for reconstitution:

Protonix® I.V.: 40 mg [contains edetate disodium]

Tablet, delayed release, oral: 20 mg, 40 mg

Protonix®: 20 mg, 40 mg

Dosage Forms: Canada Excipient information presented when available (limited, particularly for generics); consult specific product labeling.

Note: Strength expressed as base

Tablet, enteric coated, as magnesium:

Pantoloc®: 40 mg

Extemporaneous Preparations A 2 mg/mL pantoprazole oral suspension may be made with pantoprazole tablets, sterile water, and sodium bicarbonate powder. Remove the Protonix® imprint from twenty 40 mg tablets with a paper towel dampened with ethanol (improves the look of product). Let tablets air dry. Crush the tablets in a mortar and reduce to a fine powder. Transfer to a 600 mL beaker, and add 340 mL sterile water. Place beaker on a magnetic stirrer. Add 16.8 g of sodium bicarbonate powder and stir for about 20 minutes until the tablet remnants have disintegrated. While stirring, add another 16.8 g of sodium bicarbonate powder and stir for about 5 minutes until powder has dissolved. Add enough sterile water for irrigation to bring the final volume to 400 mL. Mix well. Transfer to amber-colored bottle. Label "shake well" and "refrigerate". Stable for 62 days refrigerated.

Dentinger PJ, Swenson CF, and Anaizi NH, "Stability of Pantoprazole in an Extemporaneously Compounded Oral Liquid," *Am J Health Syst Pharm*, 2002, 59(10):953-6.

- **Pantoprazole for Injection (Can)** *see* Pantoprazole *on page 1289*
- **Pantothenyl Alcohol** *see* Dexpanthenol *on page 486*

Papaverine (pa PAV er een)

Index Terms Papaverine Hydrochloride; Pavabid

Pharmacologic Category Vasodilator

Use Oral: Relief of peripheral and cerebral ischemia associated with arterial spasm and myocardial ischemia complicated by arrhythmias

Unlabeled Use Parenteral: Various vascular spasms associated with muscle spasms as in myocardial infarction, angina, peripheral and pulmonary embolism, peripheral vascular disease, angiospastic states, and visceral spasm (ureteral, biliary, and GI colic); testing for impotence

Pregnancy Risk Factor C

Dosage

I.M., I.V.:

Children: 6 mg/kg/day in 4 divided doses

Adults: 30-65 mg (rarely up to 120 mg); may repeat every 3 hours

Oral, sustained release: Adults: 150-300 mg every 12 hours; in difficult cases: 150 mg every 8 hours

Additional Information Complete prescribing information for this medication should be consulted for additional detail.

Dosage Forms Excipient information presented when available (limited, particularly for generics); consult specific product labeling. [DSC] = Discontinued product

Capsule, sustained release, oral, as hydrochloride: 150 mg [DSC]

Injection, solution, as hydrochloride: 30 mg/mL (2 mL, 10 mL)

- **Papaverine Hydrochloride** *see* Papaverine *on page 1292*

Papillomavirus (Types 16, 18) Vaccine (Human, Recombinant)

(pap ih LO ma VYE rus typs SIX teen AYE teen vak SEEN YU man ree KOM be nant)

Brand Names: U.S. Cervarix®

Brand Names: Canada Cervarix®

Index Terms Bivalent Human Papillomavirus Vaccine; GSK-580299; HPV 16/18 L1 VLP/AS04 VAC; HPV Vaccine; HPV2; Human Papillomavirus Vaccine; Papillomavirus Vaccine, Recombinant

Pharmacologic Category Vaccine, Inactivated (Viral)

Additional Appendix Information

Immunization Recommendations *on page 1922*

Use Females 9 through 25 years of age: Prevention of cervical cancer, cervical adenocarcinoma *in situ*, and cervical intraepithelial neoplasia caused by human papillomavirus (HPV) types 16, 18

The Advisory Committee on Immunization Practices (ACIP) recommends routine vaccination for females 11-12 years of age; catch-up vaccination is recommended for females 13-25 years of age.

Pregnancy Risk Factor B

Pregnancy Considerations Adverse events were not observed in animal reproduction studies. Vaccination with papilloma virus vaccine is not recommended in pregnant women. In clinical trials, pregnancy testing was conducted prior to each vaccine administration and vaccination was discontinued if the woman was found to be pregnant; women were also instructed to avoid pregnancy for 2 months after receiving the vaccine. Pregnancies detected within 30 days prior or 45 days after vaccination had a higher rate of spontaneous abortions. A registry has been established for women exposed to Cervarix® during pregnancy (888-452-9622).

Lactation Excretion in breast milk unknown/use caution

Contraindications Hypersensitivity to papillomavirus recombinant vaccine or any component of the formulation

Warnings/Precautions Immediate treatment (including epinephrine 1:1000) for anaphylactoid and/or hypersensitivity reactions should be available during vaccine use. Syncope may occur following vaccination and may be associated with tonic-clonic movements or other seizure-like activity; observe for 15 minutes following administration. May consider deferring administration in patients with moderate or severe acute illness (with or without fever); may administer to patients with mild acute illness (with or without fever). Use with caution in patients with a history of bleeding disorders (including thrombocytopenia) and/or patients on anticoagulant therapy; bleeding/hematoma may occur from I.M. administration. There is no evidence that individuals already exposed to or infected with HPV will be protected; those already infected with 1 or more HPV types were protected from disease in the remaining HPV types. Not for the treatment of active disease; will not protect against diseases not caused by HPV vaccine types 16 and 18. Use with caution in severely immunocompromised patients (eg, patients receiving chemo/radiation therapy or other immunosuppressive therapy [including high-dose corticosteroids]); may have a reduced response to vaccination. In general, household and close contacts of persons with altered immunocompetence may receive all age appropriate vaccines. Packaging may contain natural rubber/natural latex. Safety and efficacy have not been established in males or in females <9 years of age. Not recommended for use during pregnancy. The entire 3-dose regimen should be completed for maximum efficacy. In order to maximize vaccination rates, the ACIP recommends simultaneous administration of all age-appropriate vaccines (live or inactivated) for which a person is eligible at a single clinic visit, unless contraindications exist.

Adverse Reactions All serious adverse reactions must be reported to the U.S. Department of Health and Human Services (DHHS) Vaccine Adverse Event Reporting System (VAERS) 1-800-822-7967 or online at https://vaers.hhs.gov/esub/index. In Canada, adverse reactions may be reported to local provincial/territorial health agencies or to the Vaccine Safety Section at Public Health Agency of Canada (1-866-844-0018).

>10%:

Central nervous system: Fatigue (55%)

Local: Injection site reactions: Pain (92%), redness (48%), swelling (44%)

Neuromuscular & skeletal: Myalgia (49%), arthralgia (21%)

1% to 10%:

Dermatologic: Urticaria (7%)

Local: Injection site: Pruritus (1%)

Respiratory: Nasopharyngitis (4%), pharyngolaryngeal pain (3%), upper respiratory tract infection (2%), pharyngitis (1%)

Miscellaneous: Influenza (3%), chlamydia infection (2%), vaginal infection (1%)

<1%, postmarketing, and/or case reports: Allergic reactions, anaphylactic/anaphylactoid reactions, angioedema, erythema multiforme, lymphadenopathy, syncope (may be associated with tonic-clonic movements), vasovagal response

Drug Interactions

Metabolism/Transport Effects None known.

Avoid Concomitant Use There are no known interactions where it is recommended to avoid concomitant use.

Increased Effect/Toxicity There are no known significant interactions involving an increase in effect.

Decreased Effect

The levels/effects of Papillomavirus (Types 16, 18) Vaccine (Human, Recombinant) may be decreased by: Belimumab; Fingolimod; Immunosuppressants

Stability Store under refrigeration at 2°C to 8°C (36°F to 46°F); do not freeze; discard if frozen. May develop a fine, white deposit with a clear, colorless supernatant during storage (not a sign of deterioration).

Mechanism of Action Contains inactive human papillomavirus (HPV) proteins HPV 16 L1, and HPV 18 L1 which produce neutralizing antibodies to prevent cervical cancer, cervical adenocarcinoma, and cervical neoplasia cause by HPV.

Pharmacodynamics/Kinetics

Onset: Peak seroconversion was observed 1 month following the last dose of vaccine

Duration: Not well defined; >5 years

Dosage I.M.: Immunization: Females ≥9 years and ≤25 years: 0.5 mL followed by 0.5 mL at 1 and 6 months after initial dose

CDC recommended immunization schedule: Administer first dose to females at age 11-12 years; begin series in females aged 13-25 years if not previously vaccinated. Minimum interval between first and second doses is 4 weeks; the minimum interval between first and third doses is 24 weeks. Inadequate doses or doses received following a shorter than recommended dosing interval should be repeated. The HPV vaccine series should be completed with the same product whenever possible.

Administration Shake well prior to use. Do not use if discolored or if containing particulate matter, or if vial or syringe is cracked. Inject I.M. into the deltoid region of the upper arm. Do not administer I.V., SubQ, or intradermally.

For patients at risk of hemorrhage following intramuscular injection, the ACIP recommends "it should be administered intramuscularly if, in the opinion of the physician familiar with the patients bleeding risk, the vaccine can be administered by this route with reasonable safety. If the patient receives antihemophilia or other similar therapy, intramuscular vaccination can be scheduled shortly after such therapy is administered. A fine needle (23 gauge or smaller) can be used for the vaccination and firm pressure applied to the site (without rubbing) for at least 2 minutes. The patient should be instructed concerning the risk of hematoma from the injection." Patients on anticoagulant therapy should be considered to have the same bleeding risks and treated as those with clotting factor disorders (CDC, 2011).

Simultaneous administration of vaccines helps ensure the patients will be fully vaccinated by the appropriate age. Simultaneous administration of vaccines is defined as administering >1 vaccine on the same day at different anatomic sites. Separate vaccines should not be combined in the same syringe unless indicated by product specific labeling. Separate needles and syringes should be used for each injection. The ACIP prefers each dose of a specific vaccine in a series come from the same manufacturer when possible. Adolescents and adults should be vaccinated while seated or lying down. In general, preterm infants should be vaccinated at the same chronological age as full-term infants (CDC, 2011).

Antipyretics have not been shown to prevent febrile seizures. Antipyretics may be used to treat fever or discomfort following vaccination (CDC, 2011). One study reported that routine prophylactic administration of acetaminophen to prevent fever prior to vaccination decreased the immune response of some vaccines; the clinical significance of this reduction in immune response has not been established (Prymula, 2009).

Monitoring Parameters Gynecologic screening exam, papillomavirus test as per current guidelines; screening for HPV is not required prior to vaccination and screening for cervical cancer should continue as recommended following vaccination. Observe for syncope for 15 minutes following administration. If seizure-like activity associated with syncope occurs, maintain patient in supine or Trendelenburg position to reestablish adequate cerebral perfusion.

Additional Information Federal law requires that the name of medication, date of administration, the vaccine manufacturer, lot number of vaccine, and the administering person's name, title and address be entered into the patient's permanent medical record. Ideally, administration of vaccine should occur prior to potential HPV exposure.

Comparison of HPV vaccines: Cervarix® and Gardasil® are both vaccines formulated to protect against infection with the human papillomavirus. Both are inactive vaccines which contain proteins HPV16 L1 and HPV 18 L1, the cause of >70% of invasive cervical cancer. The vaccines differ in that Gardasil® also contains HPV 6 L1 and HPV 11 L1 proteins which protect against 75% to 90% of genital warts. The vaccines also differ in their preparation and adjuvants used. The viral proteins in Cervarix® are prepared using *Trichoplusia ni* (insect cells) which are adsorbed on to an aluminum salt which is also combined with a monophosphoryl lipid. The viral proteins in Gardasil® are prepared using *S. cerevisiae* (baker's yeast) which are then adsorbed onto an aluminum salt. Results from a short-term study (measurements obtained 1 month following the third vaccination in the series) have shown that the immune response to HPV 16 and HPV 18 may be greater with Cervarix®; although the clinical significance of this differences is not known, local adverse events may also occur more frequently with this preparation. Both vaccines were effective and results from long-term studies are pending.

Dosage Forms Excipient information presented when available (limited, particularly for generics); consult specific product labeling. [DSC] = Discontinued product

Injection, suspension [preservative free]:

Cervarix®: HPV 16 L1 protein 20 mcg and HPV 18 L1 protein 20 mcg per 0.5 mL (0.5 mL [DSC]) [contains aluminum; manufactured using *Trichoplusia ni* (insect cells)]

Cervarix®: HPV 16 L1 protein 20 mcg and HPV 18 L1 protein 20 mcg per 0.5 mL (0.5 mL) [contains aluminum, natural rubber/natural latex in prefilled syringe; manufactured using *Trichoplusia ni* (insect cells)]

Papillomavirus (Types 6, 11, 16, 18) Vaccine (Human, Recombinant)

(pap ih LO ma VYE rus typs six e LEV en SIX teen AYE teen vak SEEN YU man ree KOM be nant)

Brand Names: U.S. Gardasil®

Brand Names: Canada Gardasil®

Index Terms HPV Vaccine; HPV4; Human Papillomavirus Vaccine; Papillomavirus Vaccine, Recombinant; Quadrivalent Human Papillomavirus Vaccine

Pharmacologic Category Vaccine, Inactivated (Viral)

Additional Appendix Information

Immunization Recommendations *on page 1922*

Use

U.S. labeling:

Females ≥9 years and ≤26 years of age: Prevention of cervical, vulvar, vaginal, and anal cancer caused by HPV types 16 and 18; genital warts caused by HPV types 6 and 11; cervical adenocarcinoma *in situ*, and vulvar, vaginal, cervical, or anal intraepithelial neoplasia caused by HPV types 6, 11, 16, and 18

Males ≥9 years and ≤26 years of age: Prevention of genital warts caused by human papillomavirus (HPV) types 6 and 11; anal cancer caused by HPV types 16 and 18, and anal intraepithelial neoplasia caused by HPV types 6, 11, 16, and 18

Canadian labeling:

Females ≥9 years and ≤26 years of age: Prevention of anal cancer caused by HPV types 16 and 18; anal intraepithelial neoplasia caused by HPV types 6, 11, 16, and 18

Females ≥9 years and ≤45 years of age: Prevention of cervical, vulvar, and vaginal cancer caused by HPV types 16 and 18; genital warts caused by HPV types 6 and 11; cervical adenocarcinoma *in situ*, vulvar, vaginal, or cervical intraepithelial neoplasia caused by HPV types 6, 11, 16, and 18

Males ≥9 years and ≤26 years of age: Prevention of anal cancer caused by HPV types 16 and 18; anal intraepithelial neoplasia caused by HPV types 6, 11, 16, and 18; genital warts caused by HPV types 6 and 11

The Advisory Committee on Immunization Practices (ACIP) recommends routine vaccination for females and males 11-12 years of age; catch-up vaccination is recommended for females 13-26 years of age and males 13-21 years of age. Males 22-26 years may also be vaccinated. The ACIP also recommends routine vaccination for men who have sex with men (MSM) through 26 years of age.

Pregnancy Risk Factor B

Pregnancy Considerations Teratogenic effects were not observed in animal studies. In clinical trials, women who were found to be pregnant before the completion of the 3-dose regimen were instructed to defer any remaining dose until pregnancy resolution. Pregnancies detected within 30 days of vaccination had a higher rate of congenital anomalies (pyloric stenosis, congenital megacolon, congenital hydronephrosis, hip dysplasia, club foot) than the placebo group. Pregnancies with onset beyond 30 days of vaccination had a rate of congenital anomalies consistent with the general population. Overall, the type of teratogenic events were the same as those generally observed for this age group. A registry has been established for women exposed to the HPV vaccine during pregnancy (1-800-986-8999). Administration of the vaccine in pregnancy is not recommended; until additional information is available, the vaccine series (or completion of the series) should be delayed until pregnancy is completed.

Lactation Excretion in breast milk unknown/use caution

Contraindications Hypersensitivity to papillomavirus recombinant vaccine or any component of the formulation

Warnings/Precautions Immediate treatment for anaphylactoid reaction should be available during vaccine use. Patients who develop hypersensitivity after administration should not receive further dosing. There is no evidence that individuals already infected with HPV will be protected; those already infected with 1 or more HPV types were protected from disease in the remaining HPV types. Not for the treatment of active disease; will not protect against diseases not caused by human papillomavirus (HPV) vaccine types 6, 11, 16, and 18. May administer with mild concurrent febrile illness; consider deferring vaccination with serious illness. Immunocompromised patients may have a reduced response to vaccination. In general, household and close contacts of persons with altered immunocompetence may receive all age appropriate vaccines. Administered I.M., therefore use caution in patients at risk for bleeding. The entire 3-dose regimen should be completed for maximum efficacy. Not recommended for use during pregnancy. Syncope may occur following vaccination and may be associated with tonic-clonic movements or other seizure-like activity; observe for 15 minutes following administration. Safety and efficacy in children <9 years of age have not been established. Product may contain yeast. In order to maximize vaccination rates, the ACIP recommends simultaneous administration of all age-appropriate vaccines (live or inactivated) for which a person is eligible at a single clinic visit, unless contraindications exist.

Adverse Reactions All serious adverse reactions must be reported to the U.S. Department of Health and Human Services (DHHS) Vaccine Adverse Event Reporting System (VAERS) 1-800-822-7967 or online at https://vaers.hhs.gov/esub/index. In Canada, adverse reactions may be reported to local provincial/territorial health agencies or to the Vaccine Safety Section at Public Health Agency of Canada (1-866-844-0018).

>10%:

Central nervous system: Headache (12% to 28%), fever (8% to 13%)

Local: Injection site: Pain (61% to 84%), erythema (17% to 25%), swelling (14% to 25%)

1% to 10%:

Central nervous system: Dizziness (1% to 4%), malaise (1%), insomnia (1%)

Gastrointestinal: Nausea (2% to 7%), diarrhea (3% to 4%), vomiting (1% to 2%), toothache (2%)

Local: Injection site: Bruising (3%), pruritus (3%), hematoma (1%)

Neuromuscular & skeletal: Arthralgia (1%), myalgia (≤1%)

Respiratory: Pharyngolaryngeal pain (3%), cough (2%), nasal congestion (1%)

<1% (Limited to important or life-threatening): Acute disseminated encephalomyelitis, alopecia areata, anaphylactic/anaphylactoid reaction, appendicitis, arrhythmia, arthritis, asthma, autoimmune hemolytic anemia and other autoimmune diseases, bronchospasm, cellulitis, cerebrovascular accident, chills, DVT, fatigue, gastroenteritis, Guillain-Barré syndrome, hypersensitivity reaction, hyper-/hypothyroidism, injection site joint movement impairment, ITP, JIA, lymphadenopathy, motor neuron disease, pancreatitis, paralysis, pelvic inflammatory disease, pulmonary embolus, RA, renal failure (acute), seizure, sepsis, syncope (may result in falls with injury or be associated with tonic-clonic movements), transverse myelitis, urticaria, weakness

Drug Interactions

Metabolism/Transport Effects None known.

Avoid Concomitant Use There are no known interactions where it is recommended to avoid concomitant use.

Increased Effect/Toxicity There are no known significant interactions involving an increase in effect.

Decreased Effect

The levels/effects of Papillomavirus (Types 6, 11, 16, 18) Vaccine (Human, Recombinant) may be decreased by: Belimumab; Fingolimod; Immunosuppressants

Stability Store at 2°C to 8°C (36°F to 46°F); do not freeze. Protect from light. May be stored at temperatures ≤25°C (≤77°F) for a total time of ≤72 hours.

Mechanism of Action Contains inactive human papillomavirus (HPV) proteins HPV 6 L1, HPV 11 L1, HPV 16 L1, and HPV 18 L1 which produce neutralizing antibodies to prevent cervical cancer, cervical adenocarcinoma, cervical, vaginal and vulvar neoplasia, and genital warts caused by HPV.

Pharmacodynamics/Kinetics

Onset: Peak seroconversion was observed 1 month following the last dose of vaccine

Duration: Not well defined; at least 5 years

Dosage

U.S. labeling: I.M.: Children ≥9 years and Adults ≤26 years: 0.5 mL followed by 0.5 mL at 2 and 6 months after initial dose

Canadian labeling: I.M. Children ≥9 years and Adults ≤45 years: 0.5 mL followed by 0.5 mL at 2 and 6 months after initial dose

CDC recommended immunization schedule: Administer first dose at age 11-12 years; begin series in females aged 13-26 years or males 13-21 years if not previously vaccinated. Males may also be vaccinated through 26 years of age. Minimum interval between first and second doses is 4 weeks; the minimum interval between first and third doses is 24 weeks. Inadequate doses or doses received following a shorter than recommended dosing interval should be repeated. The HPV vaccine series should be completed with the same product whenever possible (CDC, 2007; CDC, 60[50] 2011).

Administration Shake suspension well before use. Inject the entire dose I.M. into the deltoid region of the upper arm or higher anterolateral thigh area. Observe for syncope for 15 minutes following administration. If the vaccine series is interrupted and only one dose was given, administer the second dose as soon as possible and give the third dose ≥12 weeks later. If the vaccine series is interrupted and the first two doses were given, administer the third dose as soon as possible. The HPV vaccine series should be completed with the same product whenever possible.

For patients at risk of hemorrhage following intramuscular injection, the ACIP recommends "it should be administered intramuscularly if, in the opinion of the physician familiar with the patients bleeding risk, the vaccine can be administered by this route with reasonable safety. If the patient receives antihemophilia or other similar therapy, intramuscular vaccination can be scheduled shortly after such therapy is administered. A fine needle (23 gauge or smaller) can be used for the vaccination and firm pressure applied to the site (without rubbing) for at least 2 minutes. The patient should be instructed concerning the risk of hematoma from the injection." Patients on anticoagulant therapy should be considered to have the same bleeding risks and treated as those with clotting factor disorders (CDC, 2011).

Simultaneous administration of vaccines helps ensure the patients will be fully vaccinated by the appropriate age. Simultaneous administration of vaccines is defined as administering >1 vaccine on the same day at different anatomic sites. Separate vaccines should not be combined in the same syringe unless indicated by product specific labeling. Separate needles and syringes should be used for each injection. The ACIP prefers each dose of a specific vaccine in a series come from the same manufacturer when possible. Adolescents and adults should be vaccinated while seated or lying down. In general, preterm infants should be vaccinated at the same chronological age as full-term infants (CDC, 2011).

Antipyretics have not been shown to prevent febrile seizures. Antipyretics may be used to treat fever or discomfort following vaccination (CDC, 2011). One study reported that routine prophylactic administration of acetaminophen to prevent fever prior to vaccination decreased the immune response of some vaccines; the clinical significance of this reduction in immune response has not been established (Prymula, 2009).

Monitoring Parameters Gynecologic screening exam, papillomavirus test as per current guidelines; screening for HPV is not required prior to vaccination and screening for cervical cancer should continue as recommended following vaccination. Observe for syncope/fainting for ~15 minutes after administration of vaccine. If seizure-like activity associated with syncope occurs, maintain patient in supine or Trendelenburg position to reestablish adequate cerebral perfusion.

Females: Gynecologic screening exam, papillomavirus test; screening for cervical cancer should continue per current guidelines following vaccination

Additional Information Federal law requires that the name of medication, date of administration, the vaccine manufacturer, lot number of vaccine, and the administering person's name, title and address be entered into the patient's permanent medical record. Ideally, administration of vaccine should occur prior to potential HPV exposure. Benefits of vaccine decrease once infected with ≥1 of the HPV vaccine types, although patients are protected from precancerous cervical lesions and external genital lesions caused by other HPV vaccine types.

Comparison of HPV vaccines: Cervarix® and Gardasil® are both vaccines formulated to protect against infection with the human papillomavirus. Both are inactive vaccines which contain proteins HPV16 L1 and HPV 18 L1, the cause of >70% of invasive cervical cancer. The vaccines differ in that Gardasil® also contains HPV 6 L1 and HPV 11 L1 proteins which protect against 75% to 90% of genital warts. The vaccines also differ in their preparation and adjuvants used. The viral proteins in Cervarix® are prepared using *Trichoplusia ni* (insect cells) which are adsorbed on to an aluminum salt which is also combined with a monophosphoryl lipid. The viral proteins in Gardasil® are prepared using *S. cerevisiae* (baker's yeast) which are then adsorbed onto an aluminum salt. Results from a short term study (measurements obtained 1 month following the third vaccination in the series) have shown that the immune response to HPV 16 and HPV 18 may be greater with Cervarix®; although the clinical significance of this differences is not known, local adverse events may also occur more frequently with this preparation. Both vaccines were effective and results from long term studies are pending.

Dosage Forms Excipient information presented when available (limited, particularly for generics); consult specific product labeling.

Injection, suspension [preservative free]:

Gardasil®: HPV 6 L1 protein 20 mcg, HPV 11 L1 protein 40 mcg, HPV 16 L1 protein 40 mcg, and HPV 18 L1 protein 20 mcg per 0.5 mL (0.5 mL) [contains aluminum, polysorbate 80; manufactured using *S. cerevisiae* (baker's yeast)]

◆ **Papillomavirus Vaccine, Recombinant** *see* Papillomavirus (Types 6, 11, 16, 18) Vaccine (Human, Recombinant) *on page* 1294

◆ **Papillomavirus Vaccine, Recombinant** *see* Papillomavirus (Types 16, 18) Vaccine (Human, Recombinant) *on page* 1292

◆ **PAR-101** *see* Fidaxomicin *on page* 710

◆ **Paracetamol** *see* Acetaminophen *on page 27*
◆ **Parafon Forte® (Can)** *see* Chlorzoxazone *on page 351*
◆ **Parafon Forte® DSC** *see* Chlorzoxazone *on page 351*
◆ **Paraplatin** *see* CARBOplatin *on page 287*
◆ **Paraplatin-AQ (Can)** *see* CARBOplatin *on page 287*
◆ **Parathyroid Hormone (1-34)** *see* Teriparatide *on page 1651*
◆ **Parcaine™ [DSC]** *see* Proparacaine *on page 1421*
◆ **Parcopa®** *see* Carbidopa and Levodopa *on page 284*

Paregoric (par e GOR ik)

Index Terms Camphorated Tincture of Opium (error-prone synonym)

Pharmacologic Category Analgesic, Opioid

Use Treatment of diarrhea or relief of pain

Pregnancy Risk Factor B/D (prolonged use or high doses)

Lactation Enters breast milk/use caution

Contraindications Hypersensitivity to opium or any component of the formulation; diarrhea caused by poisoning until the toxic material has been removed; pregnancy (prolonged use or high doses)

Warnings/Precautions May cause CNS depression, which may impair physical or mental abilities; patients must be cautioned about performing tasks which require mental alertness (eg, operating machinery or driving). Effects may be potentiated when used with other sedative drugs or ethanol. Use with caution in patients with respiratory, hepatic or renal dysfunction, adrenal insufficiency, morbid obesity, severe prostatic hyperplasia, urinary stricture, head trauma, thyroid dysfunction, seizure disorder, CNS depression/coma, or history of narcotic abuse. Use with caution in patients with biliary tract dysfunction; acute pancreatitis may cause constriction of sphincter of Oddi. May obscure diagnosis or clinical course of patients with acute abdominal conditions. Opium shares the toxic potential of opiate agonists, and usual precautions of opiate agonist therapy should be observed; some preparations contain sulfites which may cause allergic reactions; infants <3 months of age are more susceptible to respiratory depression, use with caution and generally in reduced doses in this age group; tolerance or drug dependence may result from extended use. Concurrent use of agonist/antagonist analgesics may precipitate withdrawal symptoms and/or reduced analgesic efficacy in patients following prolonged therapy with mu opioid agonists. Abrupt discontinuation following prolonged use may also lead to withdrawal symptoms. Use with caution in the elderly and debilitated patients; may be more sensitive to adverse effects.

Adverse Reactions Frequency not defined.

Cardiovascular: Hypotension, peripheral vasodilation

Central nervous system: CNS depression, dizziness, drowsiness, headache, increased intracranial pressure, insomnia, malaise, mental depression, restlessness

Gastrointestinal: Anorexia, biliary tract spasm, constipation, nausea, stomach cramps, vomiting

Genitourinary: Decreased urination, ureteral spasms, urinary tract spasm

Hepatic: Increased liver function tests

Neuromuscular & skeletal: Weakness

Ocular: Miosis

Respiratory: Respiratory depression

Miscellaneous: Physical and psychological dependence, histamine release

Drug Interactions

Metabolism/Transport Effects None known.

Avoid Concomitant Use There are no known interactions where it is recommended to avoid concomitant use.

Increased Effect/Toxicity

Paregoric may increase the levels/effects of: Alcohol (Ethyl); Alvimopan; CNS Depressants; Desmopressin; Selective Serotonin Reuptake Inhibitors; Thiazide Diuretics

The levels/effects of Paregoric may be increased by: Amphetamines; Antipsychotic Agents (Phenothiazines); Droperidol; HydrOXYzine; Succinylcholine

Decreased Effect

Paregoric may decrease the levels/effects of: Pegvisomant

The levels/effects of Paregoric may be decreased by: Ammonium Chloride; Mixed Agonist / Antagonist Opioids

Ethanol/Nutrition/Herb Interactions Ethanol: May increase CNS depression; monitor for increased effects with coadministration. Caution patients about effects.

Stability Store in light-resistant, tightly-closed container.

Mechanism of Action Increases smooth muscle tone in GI tract, decreases motility and peristalsis, diminishes digestive secretions

Pharmacodynamics/Kinetics In terms of opium:

Metabolism: Hepatic

Excretion: Urine (primarily as morphine glucuronide conjugates and unchanged drug - morphine, codeine, papaverine, etc)

Dosage Oral:

Children: 0.25-0.5 mL/kg 1-4 times/day

Adults: 5-10 mL 1-4 times/day

Additional Information Contains morphine 0.4 mg/mL and alcohol 45%. Do **not** confuse this product with opium tincture which is 25 times **more** potent; each 5 mL of paregoric contains 2 mg morphine equivalent, 0.02 mL anise oil, 20 mg benzoic acid, 20 mg camphor, 0.2 mL glycerin and alcohol; final alcohol content 45%; paregoric also contains papaverine and noscapine; because all of these additives may be harmful to neonates, **a 25-fold dilution of opium tincture** is often preferred for treatment of neonatal abstinence syndrome (opiate withdrawal).

Dosage Forms Excipient information presented when available (limited, particularly for generics); consult specific product labeling.

Liquid, oral: Morphine equivalent 2 mg/5 mL (473 mL) [contains ethanol ≤47.7% and benzoic acid]

Controlled Substance C-III

◆ **Parenteral Nutrition** *see* Total Parenteral Nutrition *on page 1714*

Paricalcitol (pah ri KAL si tole)

Brand Names: U.S. Zemplar®

Brand Names: Canada Zemplar®

Pharmacologic Category Vitamin D Analog

Use

I.V.: Prevention and treatment of secondary hyperparathyroidism associated with stage 5 chronic kidney disease (CKD)

Oral: Prevention and treatment of secondary hyperparathyroidism associated with stage 3 and 4 CKD and stage 5 CKD patients on hemodialysis or peritoneal dialysis

Pregnancy Risk Factor C

Pregnancy Considerations

There are no adequate and well-controlled studies in pregnant women; use during pregnancy only if potential benefit to mother outweighs possible risk to fetus.

Lactation Excretion in breast milk unknown/not recommended

Contraindications Hypersensitivity to paricalcitol or any component of the formulation; patients with evidence of vitamin D toxicity; hypercalcemia

Warnings/Precautions Excessive administration may lead to over suppression of PTH, hypercalcemia, hypercalciuria, hyperphosphatemia and adynamic bone disease. Acute hypercalcemia may increase risk of cardiac arrhythmias and seizures; use caution with cardiac glycosides as digitalis toxicity may be increased. Chronic hypercalcemia may lead to generalized vascular and other soft-tissue calcification. Phosphate and vitamin D (and its derivatives) should be withheld during therapy to avoid hypercalcemia. Risk of hypercalcemia may be increased by concomitant use of calcium-containing supplements and/or medications that increase serum calcium (eg, thiazide diuretics). Avoid regular administration to prevent aluminum overload and toxicity. Dialysate concentration of aluminum should be maintained at <10 mcg/L.

Adverse Reactions

>10%:

Gastrointestinal: Nausea (5% to 13%), diarrhea (7% to 12%)

Miscellaneous: Infection (bacterial, fungal, viral: 3% to 15%)

2% to 10%:

Cardiovascular: Edema (7%), hypertension (7%), hypervolemia (5%), hypotension (5%), palpitation (3%), chest pain (3%), peripheral edema (3%), syncope (3%)

Central nervous system: Pain (8%), dizziness (5% to 7%), chills (5%), insomnia (5%), lightheadedness (5%), vertigo (5%), fever (3% to 5%), headache (3% to 5%), anxiety (3%), depression (3%)

Dermatologic: Rash (6%), bruising (3%), skin ulcer (3%)

Endocrine & metabolic: Dehydration (3%), hypoglycemia (3%)

Gastrointestinal: Vomiting (5% to 8%), GI bleeding (5%), constipation (4% to 5%), abdominal pain (4%), dyspepsia (3%), xerostomia (3%)

Genitourinary: Urinary tract infection (3%)

Neuromuscular & skeletal: Arthritis (5%), weakness (3% to 5%), back pain (4%), leg cramps (3%)

Renal: Uremia (3%)

Respiratory: Pneumonia (5%), rhinitis (5%), oropharyngeal pain (4%), bronchitis (3%), cough (3%), sinusitis (3%)

Miscellaneous: Allergic reaction (6%), flu-like syndrome (5%), peritonitis (5%), sepsis (5%)

<2% (Limited to important or life-threatening): Agitation, anemia, angioedema (including laryngeal edema), arrhythmia, atrial flutter, bleeding time prolonged, breast cancer, cardiac arrest, cerebrovascular accident, chest discomfort, confusional state, conjunctivitis, delirium, dysphagia, dyspnea, erectile dysfunction, gait disturbance, gastritis, gastroesophageal reflux, glaucoma, hepatic enzyme (abnormal), hirsutism, hypercalciuria, hyper-/hypocalcemia, hyper-/hypoparathyroidism, hyperkalemia, hyperphosphatemia, injection site extravasation, injection site pain, intestinal ischemia, lymphadenopathy, myalgia, myoclonus, nasopharyngitis, night sweats, ocular hyperemia, oral edema, orthopnea, paresthesia, pruritus, pulmonary edema, rectal hemorrhage, skin burning sensation, taste perversion (metallic), upper respiratory tract infection, urticaria, vaginal infection, weight loss, wheezing

Drug Interactions

Metabolism/Transport Effects Substrate of CYP3A4 (minor); **Note:** Assignment of Major/Minor substrate status based on clinically relevant drug interaction potential

Avoid Concomitant Use

Avoid concomitant use of Paricalcitol with any of the following: Aluminum Hydroxide; Sucralfate; Vitamin D Analogs

Increased Effect/Toxicity

Paricalcitol may increase the levels/effects of: Aluminum Hydroxide; Cardiac Glycosides; Digoxin; Sucralfate; Vitamin D Analogs

The levels/effects of Paricalcitol may be increased by: Calcium Salts; CYP3A4 Inhibitors (Strong); Danazol; Thiazide Diuretics

Decreased Effect

The levels/effects of Paricalcitol may be decreased by: Bile Acid Sequestrants; Mineral Oil; Orlistat; Tocilizumab

Stability Store at 25°C (77°F); excursions permitted between 15°C to 30°C (59°F to 86°F).

Mechanism of Action Decreased renal conversion of vitamin D to its primary active metabolite (1,25-hydroxyvitamin D) in chronic renal failure leads to reduced activation of vitamin D receptor (VDR), which subsequently removes inhibitory suppression of parathyroid hormone (PTH) release; increased serum PTH (secondary hyperparathyroidism) reduces calcium excretion and enhances bone resorption. Paricalcitol is a synthetic vitamin D analog which binds to and activates the VDR in kidney, parathyroid gland, intestine and bone, thus reducing PTH levels and improving calcium and phosphate homeostasis.

Pharmacodynamics/Kinetics

Distribution: V_d:

Healthy subjects: Oral: 34 L; I.V.: 24 L

Stage 3 and 4 CKD: Oral: 44-46 L

Stage 5 CKD: Oral: 38-49 L; I.V.: 31-35 L

Protein binding: >99%

Metabolism: Hydroxylation and glucuronidation via hepatic and nonhepatic enzymes, including CYP24, CYP3A4, UGT1A4; forms metabolites (at least one active)

Bioavailability: Oral: 72% to 86% in healthy subjects

Half-life elimination:

Healthy subjects: Oral: 4-6 hours; I.V.: 5-7 hours

Stage 3 and 4 CKD: Oral: 14-20 hours

Stage 5 CKD: Oral: 14-20 hours; I.V.: 14-15 hours

Time to peak, plasma: 3 hours: Delayed by food

Excretion: Healthy subjects: Feces (oral: 70%; I.V.: 63%); urine (oral: 18%, I.V.: 19%)

Dosage Note: In stage 3-5 CKD maintain calcium phosphorus product (Ca x P) <55 mg^2/dL^2, reduce or interrupt dosing if recommended Ca x P is exceeded or hypercalcemia is observed (K/DOQI Clinical Practice Guidelines, 2003).

Secondary hyperparathyroidism associated with chronic renal failure (stage 5 CKD):

Children ≥5 years and Adults: I.V.: 0.04-0.1 mcg/kg (2.8-7 mcg) given as a bolus dose no more frequently than every other day at any time during dialysis; dose may be increased by 2-4 mcg every 2-4 weeks; doses as high as 0.24 mcg/kg (16.8 mcg) have been administered safely; the dose of paricalcitol should be adjusted based on serum intact PTH (iPTH) levels, as follows:

Same or increasing iPTH level: Increase paricalcitol dose

iPTH level decreased by <30%: Increase paricalcitol dose

iPTH level decreased by >30% and <60%: Maintain paricalcitol dose

iPTH level decrease by >60%: Decrease paricalcitol dose

iPTH level 1.5-3 times upper limit of normal: Maintain paricalcitol dose

Adults: Oral: Initial dose, in mcg, based on baseline iPTH level divided by 80. Administered 3 times weekly, no more frequently than every other day. **Note:** To reduce the risk of hypercalcemia initiate only after baseline serum calcium has been adjusted to ≤9.5 mg/dL.

Dose titration:

Titration dose (mcg) = Most recent iPTH level (pg/mL) divided by 80

Note: In situations where monitoring of iPTH, calcium, and phosphorus occurs less frequently than once per week, a more modest initial and dose titration rate may be warranted:

Modest titration dose (mcg) = Most recent iPTH level (pg/mL) divided by 100

Dosage adjustment for hypercalcemia or elevated Ca x P: Decrease calculated dose by 2-4 mcg. If further adjustment is required, dose should be reduced or interrupted until these parameters are normalized. If applicable, phosphate binder dosing may also be adjusted or withheld, or switch to a noncalcium-based phosphate binder

Secondary hyperparathyroidism associated with stage 3 and 4 CKD: Adults: Oral: Initial dose based on baseline serum iPTH:

iPTH ≤500 pg/mL: 1 mcg/day or 2 mcg 3 times/week

iPTH >500 pg/mL: 2 mcg/day or 4 mcg 3 times/week

Dosage adjustment based on iPTH level relative to baseline, adjust dose at 2-4 week intervals:

iPTH same or increased: Increase paricalcitol dose by 1 mcg/day or 2 mcg 3 times/week

iPTH decreased by <30%: Increase paricalcitol dose by 1 mcg/day or 2 mcg 3 times/week

iPTH decreased by ≥30% and ≤60%: Maintain paricalcitol dose

iPTH decreased by >60%: Decrease paricalcitol dose by 1 mcg/day* or 2 mcg 3 times/week

iPTH <60 pg/mL: Decrease paricalcitol dose by 1 mcg/day* or 2 mcg 3 times/week

*If patient is taking the lowest dose on a once-daily regimen, but further dose reduction is needed, decrease dose to 1 mcg 3 times/week. If further dose reduction is required, withhold drug as needed and restart at a lower dose. If applicable, calcium-phosphate binder dosing may also be adjusted or withheld, or switch to noncalcium-based binder.

Dosage adjustment in hepatic impairment:

Mild-to-moderate hepatic impairment: No dosage adjustment required

Severe hepatic impairment: Use has not been evaluated

Dietary Considerations May be taken with or without food. Some products may contain coconut or palm kernel oil.

Administration

Oral: May be administered with or without food. With the 3 times/week dosing schedule, doses should not be given more frequently than every other day.

I.V.: Administered as a bolus dose at anytime during dialysis. Doses should not be administered more often than every other day.

Monitoring Parameters

Signs and symptoms of vitamin D intoxication

Serum calcium and phosphorus (closely monitor levels during dosage titration and after initiation of a strong CYP3A4 inhibitor):

I.V.: Twice weekly during initial phase, then at least monthly once dose established

Oral: At least every 2 weeks for 3 months or following dose adjustment, then monthly for 3 months, then every 3 months

Serum or plasma intact PTH (iPTH):

I.V.: Every 3 months

Oral: At least every 2 weeks for 3 months or following dose adjustment, then monthly for 3 months, then every 3 months

Reference Range

Corrected total serum calcium (K/DOQI, 2003): CKD stages 3 and 4: 8.4-10.2 mg/dL (2.1-2.6 mmol/L); CKD stage 5: 8.4-9.5 mg/dL (2.1-2.37 mmol/L); KDIGO guidelines recommend maintaining normal ranges for all stages of CKD (3-5D) (KDIGO, 2009)

Phosphorus (K/DOQI, 2003):

CKD stages 3 and 4: 2.7-4.6 mg/dL (0.87-1.48 mmol/L) (adults); maintain within age-appropriate limits (children)

CKD stage 5 (including those treated with dialysis): 3.5-5.5 mg/dL (1.13-1.78 mmol/L) (children >12 years and adults); 4-6 mg/dL (1.29-1.94 mmol/L) (children 1-12 years)

KDIGO guidelines recommend maintaining normal ranges for CKD stages 3-5 and lowering elevated phosphorus levels toward the normal range for CKD stage 5D (KDIGO, 2009)

Serum calcium-phosphorus product (K/DOQI, 2003): CKD stage 3-5: <55 mg^2/dL^2 (children >12 years and adults); <65 mg^2/dL^2 (children ≤12 years)

PTH: Whole molecule, immunochemiluminometric assay (ICMA): 1.0-5.2 pmol/L; whole molecule, radioimmunoassay (RIA): 10.0-65.0 pg/mL; whole molecule, immunoradiometric, double antibody (IRMA): 1.0-6.0 pmol/L

Target ranges by stage of chronic kidney disease (KDIGO, 2009): CKD stage 3-5: Optimal iPTH is unknown; maintain normal range (assay-dependent); CKD stage 5D: Maintain iPTH within 2-9 times the upper limit of normal for the assay used

Dosage Forms Excipient information presented when available (limited, particularly for generics); consult specific product labeling.

Capsule, soft gelatin, oral:

Zemplar®: 1 mcg, 2 mcg, 4 mcg [contains coconut oil (may have trace amounts), ethanol, palm kernel oil (may have trace amounts)]

Injection, solution:

Zemplar®: 2 mcg/mL (1 mL); 5 mcg/mL (1 mL, 2 mL) [contains ethanol 20%, propylene glycol 30%]

◆ **Pariet® (Can)** *see* RABEprazole *on page 1451*

◆ **Pariprazole** *see* RABEprazole *on page 1451*

◆ **Parlodel®** *see* Bromocriptine *on page 236*

◆ **Parlodel® SnapTabs®** *see* Bromocriptine *on page 236*

◆ **Parnate®** *see* Tranylcypromine *on page 1720*

Paromomycin (par oh moe MYE sin)

Brand Names: Canada Humatin®

Index Terms Paromomycin Sulfate

Pharmacologic Category Amebicide

Use Treatment of acute and chronic intestinal amebiasis; hepatic coma

Unlabeled Use Treatment of cryptosporidiosis

Pregnancy Considerations Paromomycin is poorly absorbed when given orally. Because it does not reach the maternal serum, it would not be expected to adversely affect the fetus. No adverse effects were observed in two infants whose mothers took paromomycin during pregnancy.

Contraindications Hypersensitivity to paromomycin or any component of the formulation; intestinal obstruction

Warnings/Precautions Use with caution in patients with impaired renal function or possible or proven ulcerative bowel lesions. Prolonged use may result in fungal or bacterial superinfection, including *C. difficile*-associated diarrhea (CDAD) and pseudomembranous colitis; CDAD has been observed >2 months postantibiotic treatment.

Adverse Reactions

1% to 10%: Gastrointestinal: Diarrhea, abdominal cramps, nausea, vomiting, heartburn

<1% (Limited to important or life-threatening): Eosinophilia, exanthema, headache, ototoxicity, pruritus, rash, secondary enterocolitis, steatorrhea, vertigo

Drug Interactions

Metabolism/Transport Effects None known.

Avoid Concomitant Use There are no known interactions where it is recommended to avoid concomitant use.

Increased Effect/Toxicity There are no known significant interactions involving an increase in effect.

Decreased Effect There are no known significant interactions involving a decrease in effect.

Ethanol/Nutrition/Herb Interactions Food: Paromomycin may cause malabsorption of xylose, sucrose, and fats.

Mechanism of Action Acts directly on ameba; has antibacterial activity against normal and pathogenic organisms in the GI tract; interferes with bacterial protein synthesis by binding to 30S ribosomal subunits

Pharmacodynamics/Kinetics

Absorption: Poor oral absorption

Excretion: Feces (100% as unchanged drug)

Dosage Oral:

Intestinal amebiasis: Children and Adults: 25-35 mg/kg/day in 3 divided doses for 5-10 days

Dientamoeba fragilis: Children and Adults: 25-30 mg/kg/day in 3 divided doses for 7 days

Cryptosporidium (unlabeled use): Adults with AIDS: 1.5-2.25 g/day in 3-6 divided doses for 10-14 days (occasionally courses of up to 4-8 weeks may be needed)

Tapeworm (fish, dog, bovine, porcine):

Children: 11 mg/kg every 15 minutes for 4 doses

Adults: 1 g every 15 minutes for 4 doses

Hepatic coma: Adults: 4 g/day in 2-4 divided doses for 5-6 days

Dwarf tapeworm: Children and Adults: 45 mg/kg/dose every day for 5-7 days

Dosage Forms Excipient information presented when available (limited, particularly for generics); consult specific product labeling.

Capsule, oral: 250 mg

◆ **Paromomycin Sulfate** *see* Paromomycin *on page 1298*

PARoxetine (pa ROKS e teen)

Brand Names: U.S. Paxil CR®; Paxil®; Pexeva®

Brand Names: Canada Apo-Paroxetine®; CO Paroxetine; Dom-Paroxetine; Mylan-Paroxetine; Novo-Paroxetine; Paxil CR®; Paxil®; PHL-Paroxetine; PMS-Paroxetine; ratio-Paroxetine; Riva-paroxetine; Sandoz-Paroxetine; Teva-Paroxetine

Index Terms Paroxetine Hydrochloride; Paroxetine Mesylate

Pharmacologic Category Antidepressant, Selective Serotonin Reuptake Inhibitor

Additional Appendix Information

Antidepressant Agents *on page 1874*

Selective Serotonin Reuptake Inhibitors (SSRIs) Pharmacokinetics *on page 1897*

Use Treatment of major depressive disorder (MDD); treatment of panic disorder with or without agoraphobia; obsessive-compulsive disorder (OCD); social anxiety disorder (social phobia); generalized anxiety disorder (GAD); posttraumatic stress disorder (PTSD); premenstrual dysphoric disorder (PMDD)

Unlabeled Use May be useful in eating disorders, impulse control disorders; vasomotor symptoms of menopause; treatment of obsessive-compulsive disorder (OCD) in children; treatment of mild dementia-associated agitation in nonpsychotic patients

Pregnancy Risk Factor D

Pregnancy Considerations Due to adverse events observed in human studies, paroxetine is classified as pregnancy category D. Paroxetine crosses the placenta. The risk of cardiovascular and other congenital malformations may be higher with paroxetine than with other antidepressants. Nonteratogenic effects in the newborn following SSRI exposure late in the third trimester include respiratory distress, cyanosis, apnea, seizures, temperature instability, feeding difficulty, vomiting, hypoglycemia, hypo- or hypertonia, hyper-reflexia, jitteriness, irritability, constant crying, and tremor. An increased risk of low birth weight, lower Apgar scores, and blunted behavioral response to pain for a prolonged period after delivery has also been reported. Exposure to SSRIs after the twentieth week of gestation has been associated with persistent pulmonary hypertension of the newborn (PPHN). Adverse effects may be due to toxic effects of the SSRI or drug withdrawal due to discontinuation. The long-term effects of *in utero* SSRI exposure on infant development and behavior are not known.

Due to pregnancy-induced physiologic changes, women who are pregnant may require increased doses of paroxetine to achieve euthymia. Women treated for major depression and who are euthymic prior to pregnancy are more likely to experience a relapse when medication is discontinued as compared to pregnant women who continue taking antidepressant medications. The ACOG recommends that therapy with SSRIs or SNRIs during pregnancy be individualized; treatment of depression during pregnancy should incorporate the clinical expertise of the mental health clinician, obstetrician, primary healthcare provider, and pediatrician. The ACOG also recommends that therapy with paroxetine be avoided during pregnancy if possible and that fetuses exposed in early pregnancy be assessed with a fetal echocardiography. If treatment during pregnancy is required, consider tapering therapy during the third trimester in order to prevent withdrawal symptoms in the infant. If this is done and the woman is considered to be at risk of relapse from her major depressive disorder, the medication can be restarted following delivery, although the dose should be readjusted to that required before pregnancy. Treatment algorithms have been developed by the ACOG and the APA for the management of depression in women prior to conception and during pregnancy (Yonkers, 2009).

Lactation Enters breast milk/use caution (AAP rates "of concern"; AAP 2001 update pending)

Medication Guide Available Yes

Contraindications Hypersensitivity to paroxetine or any component of the formulation; use with or within 14 days of MAO inhibitors intended to treat depression; concurrent use with reversible MAO inhibitors (eg, linezolid, methylene blue); concurrent use with thioridazine or pimozide

Warnings/Precautions Hazardous agent - use appropriate precautions for handling and disposal. **[U.S. Boxed Warning]: Antidepressants increase the risk of suicidal thinking and behavior in children, adolescents, and young adults (18-24 years of age) with major depressive disorder (MDD) and other psychiatric disorders;** consider risk prior to prescribing. Short-term studies did not show an increased risk in patients >24 years of age and showed a decreased risk in patients ≥65 years. Closely monitor patients for clinical worsening, suicidality, or unusual changes in behavior, particularly during the initial 1-2 months of therapy or during periods of dosage adjustments (increases or decreases); the patient's family or caregiver should be instructed to closely observe the patient and communicate condition with healthcare provider. A medication guide concerning the use of antidepressants should be dispensed with each prescription. **Paroxetine is not FDA approved for use in children.**

The possibility of a suicide attempt is inherent in major depression and may persist until remission occurs. Patients treated with antidepressants (for any indication) should be observed for clinical worsening and suicidality, especially during the initial few months of a course of drug therapy, or at times of dose changes, either increases or decreases. Use caution in high-risk patients. Worsening depression and severe abrupt suicidality that are not part of the presenting symptoms may require discontinuation or modification of drug therapy. The patient's family or caregiver should be alerted to monitor patients for the emergence of suicidality and associated behaviors (such as agitation, irritability, hostility, impulsivity, and hypomania) and call healthcare provider.

May worsen psychosis in some patients or precipitate a shift to mania or hypomania in patients with bipolar disorder. Patients presenting with depressive symptoms should be screened for bipolar disorder. Monotherapy in patients with bipolar disorder should be avoided. **Paroxetine is not FDA approved for the treatment of bipolar depression.**

Serotonin syndrome and neuroleptic malignant syndrome (NMS)-like reactions have occurred with serotonin/norepinephrine reuptake inhibitors (SNRIs) and selective serotonin reuptake inhibitors (SSRIs) when used alone, and particularly when used in combination with serotonergic agents (eg, triptans) or antidopaminergic agents (eg, antipsychotics). Concurrent use with MAO inhibitors, including reversible MAO inhibitors (eg, linezolid, methylene blue) is contraindicated. If the administration of linezolid or methylene blue cannot be avoided, paroxetine should be discontinued prior to administration of the reversible MAO inhibitor. Monitor for symptoms of serotonin syndrome/NMS-like reactions for 2 weeks or 24 hours after the last dose of the reversible MAO inhibitor (whichever comes first). Paroxetine may then be resumed 24 hours after the last dose of linezolid or methylene blue.

Paroxetine may increase the risks associated with electroconvulsive therapy. Has a low potential to impair cognitive or motor performance - use caution when operating hazardous machinery or driving. Symptoms of agitation and/or restlessness may occur during initial few weeks of therapy. Low potential for sedation or anticholinergic effects relative to cyclic antidepressants.

Use caution in patients with a previous seizure disorder or condition predisposing to seizures such as brain damage, alcoholism, or concurrent therapy with other drugs which lower the seizure threshold. Use with caution in patients with hepatic dysfunction and in elderly patients. May cause hyponatremia/SIADH (elderly at increased risk); volume depletion (diuretics may increase risk). Use caution with concomitant use of NSAIDs, ASA, or other drugs that affect coagulation; the risk of bleeding may be potentiated. Concurrent use with tamoxifen may decrease the efficacy of tamoxifen; consider an alternative antidepressant with little or no CYP2D6 inhibition when using tamoxifen for the treatment or prevention of breast cancer. Use with caution in patients with renal insufficiency or other concurrent illness (due to limited experience); dose reduction recommended with severe renal impairment. May cause or exacerbate sexual dysfunction. Use caution in patients with narrow-angle glaucoma. Avoid use in the first trimester of pregnancy.

Upon discontinuation of paroxetine therapy, gradually taper dose and monitor for discontinuation symptoms (eg, dizziness, dysphoric mood, irritability, agitation, confusion, paresthesias). If intolerable symptoms occur following a decrease in dosage or upon discontinuation of therapy, then resuming the previous dose with a more gradual taper should be considered.

Adverse Reactions Frequency varies by dose and indication. Adverse reactions reported as a composite of all indications.

>10%:

Central nervous system: Somnolence (15% to 24%), insomnia (11% to 24%), headache (17% to 18%), dizziness (6% to 14%)

Endocrine & metabolic: Libido decreased (3% to 15%)

Gastrointestinal: Nausea (19% to 26%), xerostomia (9% to 18%), constipation (5% to 16%), diarrhea (9% to 12%)

Genitourinary: Ejaculatory disturbances (13% to 28%)

Neuromuscular & skeletal: Weakness (12% to 22%), tremor (4% to 11%)

Miscellaneous: Diaphoresis (5% to 14%)

1% to 10%:

Cardiovascular: Vasodilation (2% to 4%), chest pain (3%), palpitation (2% to 3%), hypertension (≥1%), tachycardia (≥1%)

Central nervous system: Nervousness (4% to 9%), anxiety (5%), agitation (3% to 5%), abnormal dreams (3% to 4%), concentration impaired (3% to 4%), yawning (2% to 4%), depersonalization (≤3%), amnesia (2%), chills (2%), emotional lability (≥1%), vertigo (≥1%), confusion (1%)

Dermatologic: Rash (2% to 3%), pruritus (≥1%)

Endocrine & metabolic: Orgasmic disturbance (2% to 9%), dysmenorrhea (5%)

Gastrointestinal: Appetite decreased (5% to 9%), dyspepsia (2% to 5%), flatulence (4%), abdominal pain (4%), appetite increased (2% to 4%), vomiting (2% to 3%), taste perversion (2%), weight gain (≥1%)

Genitourinary: Genital disorder (male 10%; female 2% to 9%), impotence (2% to 9%), urinary frequency (2% to 3%), urinary tract infection (2%)

Neuromuscular & skeletal: Paresthesia (4%), myalgia (2% to 4%), back pain (3%), myoclonus (2% to 3%), myopathy (2%), myasthenia (1%), arthralgia (≥1%)

Ocular: Blurred vision (4%), abnormal vision (2% to 4%)

Otic: Tinnitus (≥1%)

Respiratory: Respiratory disorder (≤7%), pharyngitis (4%), sinusitis (≤4%), rhinitis (3%)

Miscellaneous: Infection (5% to 6%)

<1%, postmarketing, and/or case reports (limited to important or life-threatening): Acute renal failure, adrenergic syndrome, akinesia, alkaline phosphatase increased, allergic reaction, anaphylaxis, anemias (various), angina pectoris, angioedema, aphasia, aphthous stomatitis, arrhythmias (atrial and ventricular), arthrosis, asthma, behavioral disturbances (various), bilirubinemia, bleeding time increased, blood dyscrasias, bloody diarrhea, bradycardia, bronchitis, bulimia, BUN increased, bundle branch block, cardiospasm, cataract, cellulitis, cerebral ischemia, cerebrovascular accident, cholelithiasis, colitis, congestive heart failure, creatine phosphokinase increased, deafness, dehydration, delirium, diabetes mellitus, drug dependence, dyskinesia, dysphagia, dyspnea, dystonia, ecchymosis, eclampsia, electrolyte abnormalities, emphysema, erythema, exfoliative dermatitis, extrapyramidal syndrome, fecal impactions, fungal dermatitis, gamma globulins increased, gastroenteritis, glaucoma, goiter, Guillain-Barré syndrome, hallucinations, hematemesis, hematoma, hemorrhage, hemoptysis, hepatic necrosis, hepatitis, hypercholesteremia, hyper-/hypoglycemia, hyper-/hypothyroidism, hypotension, ileus, intestinal obstruction, jaundice, ketosis, lactic dehydrogenase increased, liver function tests abnormal, low cardiac output, lung fibrosis, lymphadenopathy, meningitis, MI, migraine, myelitis, myocardial ischemia, neuroleptic malignant syndrome, neuropathy, osteoporosis, pancreatitis, pancytopenia, peptic ulcer, peritonitis, phlebitis, pneumonia, platelet count abnormalities, pulmonary edema, pulmonary embolus, pulmonary hypertension, seizure, sepsis, serotonin syndrome, status epilepticus, suicidal tendencies, syncope, tetany, thrombophlebitis,

thrombosis, tongue edema, torsade de pointes, toxic epidermal necrolysis, vasculitic syndrome

Drug Interactions

Metabolism/Transport Effects Substrate of CYP2D6 (major); **Note:** Assignment of Major/Minor substrate status based on clinically relevant drug interaction potential; **Inhibits** CYP1A2 (weak), CYP2B6 (moderate), CYP2C19 (weak), CYP2C9 (weak), CYP2D6 (strong), CYP3A4 (weak)

Avoid Concomitant Use

Avoid concomitant use of PARoxetine with any of the following: Iobenguane I 123; MAO Inhibitors; Methylene Blue; Pimozide; Tamoxifen; Tryptophan

Increased Effect/Toxicity

PARoxetine may increase the levels/effects of: Alpha-/Beta-Blockers; Anticoagulants; Antidepressants (Serotonin Reuptake Inhibitor/Antagonist); Antiplatelet Agents; Aspirin; Atomoxetine; Beta-Blockers; BusPIRone; CarBAMazepine; CloZAPine; Collagenase (Systemic); CYP2B6 Substrates; CYP2D6 Substrates; Desmopressin; Dextromethorphan; Drotrecogin Alfa (Activated); DULoxetine; Fesoterodine; Galantamine; Ibritumomab; Lithium; Methadone; Methylene Blue; Metoclopramide; Mexiletine; NSAID (COX-2 Inhibitor); NSAID (Nonselective); Pimozide; Propafenone; RisperiDONE; Rivaroxaban; Salicylates; Serotonin Modulators; Tamoxifen; Tetrabenazine; Thrombolytic Agents; Tositumomab and Iodine I 131 Tositumomab; TraMADol; Tricyclic Antidepressants; Vitamin K Antagonists

The levels/effects of PARoxetine may be increased by: Abiraterone Acetate; Alcohol (Ethyl); Analgesics (Opioid); Antipsychotics; Asenapine; BusPIRone; Cimetidine; CNS Depressants; CYP2D6 Inhibitors (Moderate); CYP2D6 Inhibitors (Strong); Dasatinib; Glucosamine; Herbs (Anticoagulant/Antiplatelet Properties); Linezolid; MAO Inhibitors; Metoclopramide; Omega-3-Acid Ethyl Esters; Pentosan Polysulfate Sodium; Pentoxifylline; Pravastatin; Prostacyclin Analogues; TraMADol; Tryptophan; Vitamin E

Decreased Effect

PARoxetine may decrease the levels/effects of: Aprepitant; Fosaprepitant; Iobenguane I 123; Ioflupane I 123

The levels/effects of PARoxetine may be decreased by: Aprepitant; CarBAMazepine; Cyproheptadine; Darunavir; Fosamprenavir; Fosaprepitant; NSAID (Nonselective); Peginterferon Alfa-2b

Ethanol/Nutrition/Herb Interactions

Ethanol: May increase CNS depression; monitor for increased effects with coadministration. Caution patients about effects.

Food: Peak concentration is increased, but bioavailability is not significantly altered by food.

Herb/Nutraceutical: Avoid valerian, St John's wort, SAMe, kava kava.

Stability

Suspension: Store at ≤25°C (≤77°F).

Tablets:

Paxil®: Store at 15°C to 30°C (59°F to 86°F).

Paxil CR®: Store at ≤25°C (≤77°F).

Pexeva®: Store at 25°C (77°F); excursions permitted to 15°C to 30°C (59°F to 86°F).

Mechanism of Action Paroxetine is a selective serotonin reuptake inhibitor, chemically unrelated to tricyclic, tetracyclic, or other antidepressants; presumably, the inhibition of serotonin reuptake from brain synapse stimulated serotonin activity in the brain

Pharmacodynamics/Kinetics

Onset of action: Depression: The onset of action is within a week; however, individual response varies greatly and full response may not be seen until 8-12 weeks after initiation of treatment.

Absorption: Completely absorbed following oral administration

Distribution: V_d: 8.7 L/kg (3-28 L/kg)

Protein binding: 93% to 95%

Metabolism: Extensively hepatic via CYP2D6 enzymes; primary metabolites are formed via oxidation and methylation of parent drug, with subsequent glucuronide/sulfate conjugation; nonlinear pharmacokinetics (via 2D6 saturation) may be seen with higher doses and longer duration of therapy. Metabolites exhibit ~2% potency of parent compound. C_{min} concentrations are 70% to 80% greater in the elderly compared to nonelderly patients; clearance is also decreased.

Half-life elimination: 21 hours (3-65 hours)

Time to peak: Immediate release: 5.2-8.1 hours; controlled release: 6-10 hours

Excretion: Urine (64%, 2% as unchanged drug); feces (36% primarily via bile, <1% as unchanged drug)

Dosage Oral:

Children ≥8 years:

Obsessive-compulsive disorder (unlabeled use): Initial: 10 mg/day; titrate every 7-14 days in 10 mg/day increments as necessary to a maximum 60 mg/day; trials have typically continued for a 10- to 12-week treatment course (Geller, 2004; Rosenberg, 1999)

Social anxiety disorder (unlabeled use): Initial: 2.5-10 mg/day; titrate every ≥7 days in 5-10 mg/day increments to a maximum of 50 mg/day; trials have typically continued for a 16-week treatment course (Mancini, 1999; Wagner, 2004)

Adults:

Major depressive disorder:

Paxil®, Pexeva®: Initial: 20 mg once daily, preferably in the morning; increase if needed by 10 mg/day increments at intervals of at least 1 week; maximum dose: 50 mg/day

Paxil CR®: Initial: 25 mg once daily; increase if needed by 12.5 mg/day increments at intervals of at least 1 week; maximum dose: 62.5 mg/day

Generalized anxiety disorder (Paxil®, Pexeva®): Initial: 20 mg once daily, preferably in the morning (if dose is increased, adjust in increments of 10 mg/day at 1-week intervals); doses of 20-50 mg/day were used in clinical trials, however, no greater benefit was seen with doses >20 mg.

Obsessive-compulsive disorder (Paxil®, Pexeva™): Initial: 20 mg once daily, preferably in the morning; increase if needed by 10 mg/day increments at intervals of at least 1 week; recommended dose: 40 mg/day; range: 20-60 mg/day; maximum dose: 60 mg/day

Panic disorder:

Paxil®, Pexeva®: Initial: 10 mg once daily, preferably in the morning; increase if needed by 10 mg/day increments at intervals of at least 1 week; recommended dose: 40 mg/day; range: 10-60 mg/day; maximum dose: 60 mg/day

Paxil CR®: Initial: 12.5 mg once daily; increase if needed by 12.5 mg/day at intervals of at least 1 week; maximum dose: 75 mg/day

Premenstrual dysphoric disorder (Paxil CR®): Initial: 12.5 mg once daily in the morning; may be increased to 25 mg/day; dosing changes should occur at intervals of at least 1 week. May be given daily throughout the menstrual cycle or limited to the luteal phase.

Post-traumatic stress disorder (PTSD) (Paxil®): Initial: 20 mg once daily, preferably in the morning; increase if needed by 10 mg/day increments at intervals of at least 1 week; range: 20-50 mg. Limited data suggest doses of 40 mg/day were not more efficacious than 20 mg/day.

Social anxiety disorder:
Paxil®: Initial: 20 mg once daily, preferably in the morning; recommended dose: 20 mg/day; range: 20-60 mg/day; doses >20 mg may not have additional benefit
Paxil CR®: Initial: 12.5 mg once daily, preferably in the morning; may be increased by 12.5 mg/day at intervals of at least 1 week; maximum dose: 37.5 mg/day
Vasomotor symptoms of menopause (unlabeled use, Paxil CR®): 12.5-25 mg/day
Elderly:
Paxil®, Pexeva®: Initial: 10 mg/day; increase if needed by 10 mg/day increments at intervals of at least 1 week; maximum dose: 40 mg/day
Paxil CR®: Initial: 12.5 mg/day; increase if needed by 12.5 mg/day increments at intervals of at least 1 week; maximum dose: 50 mg/day

Note: Upon discontinuation of paroxetine therapy, gradually taper dose:
Paxil®, Pexeva®: 10 mg/day at weekly intervals; when 20 mg/day dose is reached, continue for 1 week before treatment is discontinued. Some patients may need to be titrated to 10 mg/day for 1 week before discontinuation.
Paxil CR®: Patients receiving 37.5 mg/day in clinical trials had their dose decreased by 12.5 mg/day to a dose of 25 mg/day and remained at a dose of 25 mg/day for 1 week before treatment was discontinued.

Dosage adjustment in renal impairment: Adults:
Cl_{cr} 30-60 mL/minute: Plasma concentration is 2 times that seen in normal function. There are no dosage adjustments provided in manufacturer's labeling.
Severe impairment (Cl_{cr} <30 mL/minute): Mean plasma concentration is ~4 times that seen in normal function.
Paxil®, Pexeva®: Initial: 10 mg/day; increase if needed by 10 mg/day increments at intervals of at least 1 week; maximum dose: 40 mg/day
Paxil CR®: Initial: 12.5 mg/day; increase if needed by 12.5 mg/day increments at intervals of at least 1 week; maximum dose: 50 mg/day

Dosage adjustment in hepatic impairment: Adults: In hepatic dysfunction, plasma concentration is 2 times that seen in normal function.
Mild-to-moderate impairment: There are no dosage adjustments provided in manufacturer's labeling.
Severe impairment:
Paxil®, Pexeva®: Initial: 10 mg/day; increase if needed by 10 mg/day increments at intervals of at least 1 week; maximum dose: 40 mg/day
Paxil CR®: Initial: 12.5 mg/day; increase if needed by 12.5 mg/day increments at intervals of at least 1 week; maximum dose: 50 mg/day

Dietary Considerations May be taken without regard to meals.

Administration May be administered without regard to meals, preferably in the morning. Do not crush, break, or chew controlled release tablets.

Monitoring Parameters Mental status for depression, suicide ideation (especially at the beginning of therapy or when doses are increased or decreased), anxiety, social functioning, mania, panic attacks; akathisia

Additional Information Paxil CR® incorporates a degradable polymeric matrix (Geomatrix™) to control dissolution rate over a period of 4-5 hours. An enteric coating delays the start of drug release until tablets have left the stomach.

Dosage Forms Excipient information presented when available (limited, particularly for generics); consult specific product labeling.

Suspension, oral, as hydrochloride [strength expressed as base]:
Paxil®: 10 mg/5 mL (250 mL) [contains propylene glycol; orange flavor]
Tablet, oral, as hydrochloride [strength expressed as base]: 10 mg, 20 mg, 30 mg, 40 mg
Paxil®: 10 mg, 20 mg [scored]
Paxil®: 30 mg, 40 mg
Tablet, oral, as mesylate [strength expressed as base]:
Pexeva®: 10 mg
Pexeva®: 20 mg [scored]
Pexeva®: 30 mg, 40 mg
Tablet, controlled release, enteric coated, oral, as hydrochloride [strength expressed as base]: 12.5 mg, 25 mg, 37.5 mg
Paxil CR®: 12.5 mg, 25 mg, 37.5 mg
Tablet, extended release, enteric coated, oral, as hydrochloride [strength expressed as base]: 12.5 mg, 25 mg

- **Paroxetine Hydrochloride** *see* PARoxetine *on page 1299*
- **Paroxetine Mesylate** *see* PARoxetine *on page 1299*
- **Parvolex® (Can)** *see* Acetylcysteine *on page 34*
- **Pataday™** *see* Olopatadine (Ophthalmic) *on page 1239*
- **Patanase®** *see* Olopatadine (Nasal) *on page 1238*
- **Patanol®** *see* Olopatadine (Ophthalmic) *on page 1239*
- **PAT-Galantamine ER (Can)** *see* Galantamine *on page 776*
- **Pathocil® (Can)** *see* Dicloxacillin *on page 499*
- **Pavabid** *see* Papaverine *on page 1292*
- **Pavulon [DSC]** *see* Pancuronium *on page 1287*
- **Paxil®** *see* PARoxetine *on page 1299*
- **Paxil CR®** *see* PARoxetine *on page 1299*

Pazopanib (paz OH pa nib)

Brand Names: U.S. Votrient™
Brand Names: Canada Votrient™
Index Terms GW786034; Pazopanib Hydrochloride
Pharmacologic Category Antineoplastic Agent, Tyrosine Kinase Inhibitor; Vascular Endothelial Growth Factor (VEGF) Inhibitor
Use Treatment of advanced renal cell cancer (RCC)
Unlabeled Use Treatment of advanced, differentiated thyroid cancer; treatment of some histologic types of refractory metastatic soft tissue sarcomas
Pregnancy Risk Factor D
Pregnancy Considerations Adverse effects were observed in animal studies. Based on its mechanism of action, pazopanib would be expected to cause fetal harm if administered to a pregnant woman. Women of childbearing potential should avoid becoming pregnant during treatment.
Lactation Excretion in breast milk unknown/not recommended
Medication Guide Available Yes
Contraindications There are no contraindications listed within the manufacturer's labeling.
Warnings/Precautions **[U.S. Boxed Warning]: Severe and fatal hepatotoxicity (transaminase and bilirubin elevations) has been reported with use; monitor hepatic function; may require dosage interruption, reduction, or discontinuation.** Transaminase elevations usually occur early in the treatment course. Use is not recommended in patients with pre-existing severe hepatic impairment (bilirubin >3 times ULN with any ALT level); dosage reductions is recommended for pre-existing moderate hepatic impairment (bilirubin >1.5-3 times ULN). Patients >60 years of age may be at higher risk for ALT

>3 times ULN. Mild indirect (unconjugated) hyperbilirubinemia may occur in patients with Gilbert's syndrome; for patients with known Gilbert's syndrome (only a mild indirect bilirubin elevation) and ALT >3 times ULN, follow isolated ALT elevation dosage modification recommendations.

Arterial thrombotic events, including angina, transient ischemic attack, MI, and ischemic stroke were observed more frequently in the pazopanib group (versus placebo) in clinical trials; fatalities were observed. Use with caution in patients with a history of or an increased risk for these events. Use in patients with recent arteriothrombotic event (within 6 months) has not been studied and is not recommended. Hemorrhagic events (including fatal) have been reported; use is not recommended in patients with a history of hemoptysis, cerebral hemorrhage or clinically significant gastrointestinal hemorrhage within 6 months (these populations were excluded from clinical trials).

May cause and/or worsen hypertension (hypertensive crisis has been observed); monitor; blood pressure should be controlled prior to treatment initiation; antihypertensive therapy should be used if needed. Hypertension usually occurs early in the treatment course. Dosage reduction may be necessary for persistent hypertension (despite antihypertensive therapy); discontinue for hypertensive crisis, or for severe and persistent hypertension which is refractory to dose reduction and antihypertensive therapy. QT_c prolongation, including torsade de pointes, has been observed; use caution in patients with a history of QT_c prolongation, with medications known to prolong the QT interval, or with pre-existing cardiac disease. Obtain baseline and periodic ECGs; correct electrolyte (potassium, calcium, and magnesium) abnormalities prior to and during treatment.

Gastrointestinal perforation and fistula (including fatal) have been reported; monitor for symptoms of gastrointestinal perforation and fistula. Proteinuria has been reported with use. Obtain baseline and periodic urinalysis. Discontinue for grade 4 proteinuria. Hypothyroidism has been reported with use; monitor thyroid function tests. Vascular endothelial growth factor (VEGF) receptor inhibitors are associated with impaired wound healing. Discontinue treatment at least 7 days prior to scheduled surgery; treatment reinitiation should be guided by clinical judgment. Discontinue if wound dehiscence occurs.

Patients with mild-to-moderate renal impairment (Cl_{cr} ≥30 mL/minute) were included in trials. There are no pharmacokinetic data in patients with severe renal impairment undergoing dialysis (peritoneal and hemodialysis); however, renal impairment is not expected to significantly influence pazopanib pharmacokinetics or exposure. Avoid use with strong CYP3A4 inhibitors or inducers. If pazopanib must be administered concomitantly with a potent enzyme inhibitor, dose reductions are recommended. Use is not recommended in situations where the use of a strong CYP3A4 inducer is required. Pazopanib inhibits UGT1A1 and OATP1B1; pazopanib may increase concentration of drugs eliminated by UGT1A1 and OATP1B1. Concurrent use with other drugs which may prolong QT_c interval may increase the risk of potentially-fatal arrhythmias.

Adverse Reactions

>10%:

- Cardiovascular: Hypertension (40%; grade 3: 4%)
- Central nervous system: Fatigue (19%)
- Dermatologic: Hair color change (38%)
- Endocrine & metabolic: Hyperglycemia (41%), hypophosphatemia (34%), hyponatremia (31%), thyroid-stimulating hormone (TSH) increased (27%), hypomagnesemia (26%), hypoglycemia (17%)
- Gastrointestinal: Diarrhea (52%; grade 3: 3%; grade 4: <1%), lipase increased (4% to 27%), nausea (26%), anorexia (22%), vomiting (21%), abdominal pain (11%)
- Hematologic: Leukopenia (37%), neutropenia (34%; grade 3: 1%; grade 4: <1%), thrombocytopenia (32%; grades 3/4: <1%), lymphocytopenia (31%; grade 3: 4%; grade 4: <1%), hemorrhage (13% to 16%)
- Hepatic: ALT increased (53%; grade 3: 10%; grade 4: 2%), AST increased (53%; grade 3: 7%; grade 4: <1%), bilirubin increased (36%; grade 3: 3%; grade 4: <1%)
- Neuromuscular & skeletal: Weakness (14%)

1% to 10%:

- Cardiovascular: Chest pain (5%), MI/ischemia (2%), facial edema (1%), QT prolongation (1%), transient ischemic event (1%)
- Central nervous system: Headache (10%)
- Dermatologic: Alopecia (8%), rash (8%), palmar-plantar erythrodysesthesia (6%), skin depigmentation (3%)
- Endocrine & metabolic: Hypothyroidism (7%)
- Gastrointestinal: Weight loss (9%), taste alteration (8%), dyspepsia (5%), rectal hemorrhage (1%)
- Renal: Proteinuria (9%), hematuria (4%)
- Respiratory: Epistaxis (2%), hemoptysis (2%)

<1% (Limited to important or life-threatening): Cardiac dysfunction, cerebral hemorrhage, cerebrovascular event, DVT, extrapyramidal symptoms, gastrointestinal fistula, gastrointestinal perforation, hepatotoxicity, hypertensive crisis, intracranial hemorrhage, pancreatitis, torsade de pointes, tumor hemorrhage

Drug Interactions

Metabolism/Transport Effects **Substrate** of CYP1A2 (minor), CYP2C8 (minor), CYP3A4 (major), P-glycoprotein; **Note:** Assignment of Major/Minor substrate status based on clinically relevant drug interaction potential; **Inhibits** CYP2C8 (weak), CYP2D6 (weak), CYP3A4 (weak), SLCO1B1, UGT1A1

Avoid Concomitant Use

Avoid concomitant use of Pazopanib with any of the following: Artemether; BCG; CYP3A4 Inducers (Strong); Dronedarone; Grapefruit Juice; Lumefantrine; Natalizumab; Nilotinib; Pimecrolimus; Pimozide; QUEtiapine; QuiNINE; Tacrolimus (Topical); Tetrabenazine; Thioridazine; Toremifene; Vaccines (Live); Vandetanib; Vemurafenib; Ziprasidone

Increased Effect/Toxicity

Pazopanib may increase the levels/effects of: Dronedarone; Leflunomide; Natalizumab; Pimozide; QTc-Prolonging Agents; QuiNINE; Tetrabenazine; Thioridazine; Toremifene; Vaccines (Live); Vandetanib; Vemurafenib; Vitamin K Antagonists; Ziprasidone

The levels/effects of Pazopanib may be increased by: Alfuzosin; Artemether; Chloroquine; Ciprofloxacin; Ciprofloxacin (Systemic); CYP3A4 Inhibitors (Moderate); CYP3A4 Inhibitors (Strong); Denosumab; Gadobutrol; Grapefruit Juice; Indacaterol; Lapatinib; Lumefantrine; Nilotinib; P-glycoprotein/ABCB1 Inhibitors; Pimecrolimus; QUEtiapine; QuiNINE; Roflumilast; Tacrolimus (Topical); Trastuzumab

Decreased Effect

Pazopanib may decrease the levels/effects of: BCG; Cardiac Glycosides; Coccidioidin Skin Test; Sipuleucel-T; Vaccines (Inactivated); Vaccines (Live); Vitamin K Antagonists

The levels/effects of Pazopanib may be decreased by: CYP3A4 Inducers (Strong); Cyproterone; Deferasirox; Echinacea; P-glycoprotein/ABCB1 Inducers; Tocilizumab

Ethanol/Nutrition/Herb Interactions

Food: Systemic exposure of pazopanib is increased when administered with food (AUC twofold higher with a meal). Avoid grapefruit juice (may increase the levels/effects of pazopanib).

Herb/Nutraceutical: Avoid St John's wort (may increase metabolism and decrease pazopanib concentrations).

Stability Store at room temperature of 25°C (77°F); excursions permitted between 15°C and 30°C (59°F and 86°F).

Mechanism of Action Tyrosine kinase (multikinase) inhibitor; limits tumor growth via inhibition of angiogenesis angiogenesis by inhibiting cell surface vascular endothelial growth factor receptors (VEGFR-1, VEGFR-2, VEGFR-3), platelet-derived growth factor receptors (PDGFR-alpha and -beta), fibroblast growth factor receptor (FGFR-1 and -3), cytokine receptor (cKIT), interleukin-2 receptor inducible T-cell kinase, leukocyte-specific protein tyrosine kinase (Lck), and transmembrane glycoprotein receptor tyrosine kinase (c-Fms)

Pharmacodynamics/Kinetics

Protein binding: >99%

Metabolism: Hepatic; primarily via CYP3A4, minor metabolism via CYP1A2 and CYP2C8

Bioavailability: Rate and extent of bioavailability are increased with food and increased if tablets are crushed (do not crush tablets)

Half-life elimination: ~31 hours

Time to peak, plasma: 2-4 hours

Excretion: Feces (primarily); urine (<4%)

Dosage Oral: Adults:

Renal cell cancer (RCC): 800 mg once daily

Soft tissue sarcoma, refractory/metastatic (unlabeled use): 800 mg once daily until disease progression or unacceptable toxicity (Van Der Graaf, 2011)

Thyroid cancer, advanced differentiated (unlabeled use): 800 mg once daily until disease progression or unacceptable toxicity (Bible, 2010)

Dosage adjustment for toxicity:

Initial dosage reduction: Reduce to 400 mg once daily

Further modification: Adjust dose in 200 mg increments or decrements based on individual tolerance; maximum dose: 800 mg

Proteinuria (grade 4), hypertension (severe, persistent, and refractory to antihypertensives and dose reduction), wound dehiscence: Discontinue treatment

Concomitant CYP3A4 inhibitors/inducers:

CYP3A4 inhibitors: Avoid concomitant strong CYP3A4 inhibitors (may increase pazopanib concentrations). If pazopanib must be administered concomitantly with a potent enzyme inhibitor, reduce pazopanib to 400 mg once daily with careful monitoring; further dosage reductions may be needed if adverse events occur.

CYP3A4 inducers: Avoid concomitant strong CYP3A4 inducers (may decrease pazopanib concentrations); use of pazopanib is not recommended in situations where the use of a strong CYP3A4 inducer is required.

Dosage adjustment in renal impairment: No adjustment necessary (renal impairment is not likely to significantly influence pazopanib pharmacokinetics).

Dosage adjustment in hepatic impairment:

Pre-existing impairment:

Mild (bilirubin <1.5 times ULN or ALT >ULN): No adjustment required (Shibata, 2010)

Moderate (bilirubin 1.5-3 times ULN): Reduce to 200 mg once daily (maximum tolerated dose in moderate hepatic impairment) (Shibata, 2010)

Severe (bilirubin >3 times ULN with any ALT level): Use is not recommended

During treatment:

Isolated ALT elevations 3-8 times ULN: Continue treatment, monitor liver function weekly until ALT returns to grade 1 or baseline

Isolated ALT elevations >8 times ULN: Interrupt treatment until ALT returns to grade 1 or baseline. If therapy benefit is greater than the risk of hepatotoxicity, may reinitiate treatment at ≤400 mg once daily (with liver function monitored weekly for 8 weeks); permanently discontinue if ALT >3 times ULN occur with reinitiation

ALT >3 times ULN concurrently with bilirubin >2 times ULN: Permanently discontinue; monitor until resolution

Gilbert's syndrome with mild indirect bilirubin elevation and ALT >3 times ULN: Refer to isolated ALT elevations dosage recommendations above

Dietary Considerations Take on an empty stomach, 1 hour before or 2 hours after a meal. Avoid grapefruit juice.

Administration Administer on an empty stomach, 1 hour before or 2 hours after a meal. Do not crush tablet. If a dose is missed, do not take if <12 hours until the next dose.

Monitoring Parameters Monitor liver function tests at baseline and at least every 4 weeks for the first 4 months (more frequently if clinically indicated) and periodically thereafter; serum electrolytes (eg, calcium, magnesium, potassium); urinalysis (for proteinuria; baseline and periodic); thyroid function (TSH and T_4 at baseline and TSH every 6-8 weeks during treatment; Appleby, 2011); blood pressure; ECG (baseline and periodic); symptoms of gastrointestinal perforation or fistula

Additional Information Hand-foot skin reaction (Appleby, 2011): Hand-foot skin reaction (HFSR) observed with tyrosine kinase inhibitors (TKIs) is distinct from hand-foot syndrome (palmar-plantar erythrodysesthesia) associated with traditional chemotherapy agents. HFSR due to TKIs is localized with defined hyperkeratotic lesions; symptoms include burning, dysesthesia, paresthesia, or tingling, and generally occur within the first 2-3 weeks of treatment. Pressure and flexor areas may develop blisters (callus-like), dry/cracked skin, edema, desquamation, or hyperkeratosis. The incidence of hand-foot skin reaction (HFSR) is lower with pazopanib (compared to other tyrosine kinase inhibitors). Examine skin at baseline (remove calluses with pedicure prior to treatment) and with each visit; apply an emollient based moisturizer twice daily during treatment. If HSFR develops, consider changing moisturizer to a urea-based product; topical steroids may be utilized for the anti-inflammatory effect; avoid excessive friction or pressure to affected areas and avoid restrictive footwear. Temporary dose reduction or treatment interruption may be necessary.

Dosage Forms Excipient information presented when available (limited, particularly for generics); consult specific product labeling.

Tablet, oral:

Vortrient™: 200 mg

◆ **Pazopanib Hydrochloride** *see* Pazopanib *on page 1302*

◆ **PCA (error-prone abbreviation)** *see* Procainamide *on page 1408*

◆ **PCC** *see* Factor IX Complex (Human) *on page 684*

◆ **PCE®** *see* Erythromycin (Systemic) *on page 617*

◆ **PCEC** *see* Rabies Vaccine *on page 1453*

◆ **PCV** *see* Pneumococcal Conjugate Vaccine (7-Valent) *on page 1365*

◆ **PCV-7** *see* Pneumococcal Conjugate Vaccine (7-Valent) *on page 1365*

◆ **PCV-13** *see* Pneumococcal Conjugate Vaccine (13-Valent) *on page 1366*

◆ **PCV13-CRM(197)** *see* Pneumococcal Conjugate Vaccine (13-Valent) *on page 1366*

◆ **PD-Cof [DSC]** *see* Chlorpheniramine, Phenylephrine, and Dextromethorphan *on page 346*

◆ **PD-Hist-D** *see* Chlorpheniramine and Phenylephrine *on page 345*

◆ **PDX** *see* PRALAtrexate *on page 1387*

- **PediaCare® Children's Allergy [OTC]** *see* DiphenhydrAMINE (Systemic) *on page* 516
- **PediaCare® Children's Decongestant [OTC]** *see* Phenylephrine (Systemic) *on page* 1344
- **PediaCare® Children's NightTime Cough [OTC]** *see* DiphenhydrAMINE (Systemic) *on page* 516
- **PediaCare® Children's Multi-Symptom Cold [OTC]** *see* Dextromethorphan and Phenylephrine *on page* 490
- **Pediacel® (Can)** *see* Diphtheria and Tetanus Toxoids, Acellular Pertussis, Poliovirus and *Haemophilus* b Conjugate Vaccine *on page* 522
- **Pediaderm™ AF** *see* Nystatin (Topical) *on page* 1225
- **Pediaderm™ HC** *see* Hydrocortisone (Topical) *on page* 841
- **Pediaderm™ TA** *see* Triamcinolone (Topical) *on page* 1735
- **Pediapred®** *see* PrednisoLONE (Systemic) *on page* 1396
- **Pedia Relief Cough and Cold [OTC]** *see* Pseudoephedrine and Dextromethorphan *on page* 1431
- **Pedia Relief™ Cough-Cold [OTC]** *see* Chlorpheniramine, Pseudoephedrine, and Dextromethorphan *on page* 347
- **Pediarix®** *see* Diphtheria, Tetanus Toxoids, Acellular Pertussis, Hepatitis B (Recombinant), and Poliovirus (Inactivated) Vaccine *on page* 527
- **Pediatex® TD** *see* Triprolidine and Pseudoephedrine *on page* 1741
- **Pediatric Digoxin CSD (Can)** *see* Digoxin *on page* 503
- **Pediatrix (Can)** *see* Acetaminophen *on page* 27
- **Pediazole® (Can)** *see* Erythromycin and Sulfisoxazole *on page* 620
- **Pedi-Boro® [OTC]** *see* Aluminum Sulfate and Calcium Acetate *on page* 81
- **Pedi-Dri®** *see* Nystatin (Topical) *on page* 1225
- **PedvaxHIB®** *see* *Haemophilus* b Conjugate Vaccine *on page* 815
- **PEG** *see* Polyethylene Glycol 3350 *on page* 1372
- **PEG-L-asparaginase** *see* Pegaspargase *on page* 1306

Pegademase Bovine (peg A de mase BOE vine)

Brand Names: U.S. Adagen®

Brand Names: Canada Adagen®

Pharmacologic Category Enzyme

Use Enzyme replacement therapy for adenosine deaminase (ADA) deficiency in patients with severe combined immunodeficiency disease (SCID) who are not candidates for or who have failed bone marrow transplant

Pregnancy Risk Factor C

Dosage Note: Dose should be individualized based on monitoring of plasma ADA activity levels and dATP content.

Infants and Children: I.M.: Dose given every 7 days, 10 units/kg the first dose, 15 units/kg the second dose, and 20 units/kg the third dose; maintenance dose: 20 units/kg/week is recommended depending on patient's ADA level; maximum single dose: 30 units/kg

Additional Information Complete prescribing information for this medication should be consulted for additional detail.

Dosage Forms Excipient information presented when available (limited, particularly for generics); consult specific product labeling.

Injection, solution [preservative free]:

Adagen®: 250 units/mL (1.5 mL)

Pegaptanib (peg AP ta nib)

Brand Names: U.S. Macugen®

Brand Names: Canada Macugen®

Index Terms EYE001; Pegaptanib Sodium

Pharmacologic Category Ophthalmic Agent; Vascular Endothelial Growth Factor (VEGF) Inhibitor

Use Treatment of neovascular (wet) age-related macular degeneration (AMD)

Pregnancy Risk Factor B

Pregnancy Considerations Teratogenic effects were not reported in animal studies. There are no adequate and well-controlled studies in pregnant women.

Lactation Excretion in breast milk unknown/use caution

Contraindications Hypersensitivity to pegaptanib or any component of the formulation; ocular or periocular infection

Warnings/Precautions Intravitreous injections may be associated with endophthalmitis and retinal detachments. Proper aseptic injection techniques should be used and patients should be instructed to report any signs of infection immediately. Intraocular pressure may increase following injection. Safety and efficacy for administration into both eyes concurrently have not been studied. Safety and efficacy have not been established with hepatic impairment, or in patients requiring hemodialysis. Rare hypersensitivity reactions (including anaphylaxis) have been associated with pegaptanib, occurring within several hours of use; monitor closely. Equipment and appropriate personnel should be available for monitoring and treatment of anaphylaxis. Thromboembolic events (eg, nonfatal stroke/MI, vascular death) have been reported following intravitreal administration of other VEGF inhibitors.

Adverse Reactions

10% to 40%:

Cardiovascular: Hypertension

Ocular: Anterior chamber inflammation, blurred vision, cataract, conjunctival hemorrhage, corneal edema, eye discharge, eye irritation, eye pain, intraocular pressure increased, ocular discomfort, punctate keratitis, visual acuity decreased, visual disturbance, vitreous floaters, vitreous opacities

1% to 10%:

Cardiovascular: Carotid artery occlusion (1% to 5%), cerebrovascular accident (1% to 5%), chest pain (1% to 5%), transient ischemic attack (1% to 5%)

Central nervous system: Dizziness (6% to 10%), headache (6% to 10%), vertigo (1% to 5%)

Dermatologic: Contact dermatitis (1% to 5%)

Endocrine & metabolic: Diabetes mellitus (1% to 5%)

Gastrointestinal: Diarrhea (6% to 10%), nausea (6% to 10%), dyspepsia (1% to 5%), vomiting (1% to 5%)

Genitourinary: Urinary retention (1% to 5%)

Neuromuscular & skeletal: Arthritis (1% to 5%), bone spur (1% to 5%)

Ocular: Blepharitis (6% to 10%), conjunctivitis (6% to 10%), photopsia (6% to 10%), vitreous disorder (6% to 10%), allergic conjunctivitis (1% to 5%), conjunctival edema (1% to 5%), corneal abrasion (1% to 5%), corneal deposits (1% to 5%), corneal epithelium disorder (1% to 5%), endophthalmitis (1% to 5%), eye inflammation (1% to 5%), eye swelling (1% to 5%), eyelid irritation (1% to 5%), meibomianitis (1% to 5%), mydriasis (1% to 5%), periorbital hematoma (1% to 5%), retinal edema (1% to 5%), vitreous hemorrhage (1% to 5%)

Otic: Hearing loss (1% to 5%)

Renal: Urinary tract infection (6% to 10%)

Respiratory: Bronchitis (6% to 10%), pleural effusion (1% to 5%)

Miscellaneous: Contusion (1% to 5%)

<1% (Limited to important or life-threatening): Anaphylaxis, anaphylactoid reaction, angioedema, hypersensitivity, iatrogenic traumatic cataract, endophthalmitis, retinal detachment

Drug Interactions

Metabolism/Transport Effects None known.

Avoid Concomitant Use There are no known interactions where it is recommended to avoid concomitant use.

Increased Effect/Toxicity There are no known significant interactions involving an increase in effect.

Decreased Effect

The levels/effects of Pegaptanib may be decreased by: Pegloticase

Stability Store under refrigeration at 2°C to 8°C (36°F to 46°F); do not freeze. Do not shake vigorously.

Mechanism of Action Pegaptanib is an apatamer, an oligonucleotide covalently bound to polyethylene glycol, which can adopt a three-dimensional shape and bind to vascular endothelial growth factor (VEGF). Pegaptanib binds to extracellular VEGF, inhibiting VEGF from binding to its receptors and thereby suppressing neovascularization and slowing vision loss.

Pharmacodynamics/Kinetics

Absorption: Slow systemic absorption following intravitreous injection

Metabolism: Metabolized by endo- and exonucleases

Half-life elimination: Plasma: 6-14 days

Dosage Intravitreous injection: Adults: AMD: 0.3 mg into affected eye every 6 weeks

Dosage adjustment in renal impairment: Adjustment not required with renal impairment; information not available for patients requiring hemodialysis

Administration For ophthalmic intravitreal injection only. Attach a 30 gauge 1/2 inch needle to the medication syringe. Depress plunger to expel excess air and medication (refer to product labeling for detailed instructions). Adequate anesthesia and a broad spectrum antibiotic should be administered prior to the procedure.

Monitoring Parameters Intraocular pressure (within 30 minutes and 2-7 days after injection); signs of infection/inflammation (for first week following injection); retinal perfusion, endophthalmitis, visual acuity

Dosage Forms Excipient information presented when available (limited, particularly for generics); consult specific product labeling.

Injection, solution [preservative free]:

Macugen®: 0.3 mg/0.09 mL (0.09 mL)

- **Pegaptanib Sodium** *see* Pegaptanib *on page 1305*
- **PEG-ASP** *see* Pegaspargase *on page 1306*
- **PEG-asparaginase** *see* Pegaspargase *on page 1306*

Pegaspargase (peg AS par jase)

Brand Names: U.S. Oncaspar®

Index Terms L-asparaginase with Polyethylene Glycol; PEG-ASP; PEG-asparaginase; PEG-L-asparaginase; PEGLA; Polyethylene Glycol-L-asparaginase

Pharmacologic Category Antineoplastic Agent, Miscellaneous; Enzyme

Use Treatment of acute lymphocytic leukemia (ALL); treatment of ALL with previous hypersensitivity to native L-asparaginase

Pregnancy Risk Factor C

Pregnancy Considerations Reproduction studies have not been conducted with pegaspargase.

Lactation Excretion in breast milk unknown/not recommended

Contraindications History of serious allergic reactions to pegaspargase; history of any of the following with prior L-asparaginase treatment: pancreatitis, serious hemorrhagic events, serious thrombosis

Warnings/Precautions Hazardous agent - use appropriate precautions for handling and disposal. Serious allergic reactions may occur; discontinue in patients with serious allergic reaction. Observe patients for at least 1 hour after administration; immediate treatment for hypersensitivity reactions should be available during administration. Pegaspargase is indicated for use in patients who have had hypersensitivity reactions to native L-asparaginase; however, in one study, 32% of patients with a history of allergic reaction to *E. coli* asparaginase products also experienced allergic reaction to pegaspargase.

Serious thrombotic events, including sagittal sinus thrombosis may occur; discontinue with serious thrombotic event. Pancreatitis may occur; promptly evaluate patients with abdominal pain; discontinue if pancreatitis occurs during treatment. May cause glucose intolerance; irreversible in some cases; use with caution in patients with hyperglycemia, or diabetes. Coagulopathy has been reported; monitor coagulation parameters; severe or symptomatic coagulopathy may require treatment with fresh-frozen plasma; use with caution in patients with underlying coagulopathy. Reversible hepatotoxicity (hyperbilirubinemia and liver enzyme elevation) may occur; use with caution in patients with hepatic dysfunction or concomitant hepatotoxic medications. Use cautiously in patients with previous hematologic complications from asparaginase.

Adverse Reactions

>5%:

Cardiovascular: Edema

Central nervous system: Fever, malaise

Dermatologic: Rash

Gastrointestinal: Nausea, vomiting

Hematologic: Coagulopathy (7%; grades 3/4: 2%)

Hepatic: Transaminases increased (11%; grades 3/4: 3%)

Miscellaneous: Allergic reactions (including bronchospasm, chills, dyspnea, edema, erythema, hypotension, rash, swelling, urticaria; no prior asparaginase hypersensitivity: 1% to 10%; grades 3/4: 2%; prior asparaginase hypersensitivity: 32%; grades 3/4: 8%)

1% to 5%:

Cardiovascular: Hypotension, peripheral edema, tachycardia, thrombosis (4%)

Central nervous system: Chills, CNS thrombosis (2% to 4%; grades 3/4: 3%), CNS hemorrhage (2%), headache, seizure

Dermatologic: Lip edema, urticaria

Endocrine & metabolic: Hyperglycemia (3% to 5%; grades 3/4: ≤5%), hyperuricemia, hypoglycemia, hypoproteinemia

Gastrointestinal: Abdominal pain, anorexia, diarrhea, pancreatitis (1% to 2%; grades 3/4: 2%)

Hematologic: Anticoagulant effect decreased, disseminated intravascular coagulation (DIC), fibrinogen decreased, hemolytic anemia, leukopenia, pancytopenia, thrombocytopenia, thromboplastin increased, myelosuppression

Hepatic: Liver function tests abnormal (grades 3/4: 5%), hyperbilirubinemia (grades 3/4: 2%), jaundice

Local: Injection site hypersensitivity, pain or reaction

Neuromuscular & skeletal: Arthralgia, limb pain, myalgia, paresthesia

Respiratory: Dyspnea

Miscellaneous: Anaphylactic reactions, night sweats

<1% (Limited to important or life-threatening): Abnormal renal function, alopecia, amylase increased, anemia, antithrombin III decreased, ascites, bacteremia, bone pain, bronchospasm, bruising, BUN increased, chest pain, coagulation time increased, colitis, coma, confusion, constipation, cough, creatinine increased, dizziness, DVT, emotional lability, endocarditis, epistaxis, excessive thirst, face edema, fatigue, fatty liver deposits,

gastrointestinal pain, hematuria, hemorrhagic cystitis, hepatomegaly, hyperammonemia, hypertension, hypoalbuminemia, hyponatremia, lipase increased, liver failure, metabolic acidosis, mucositis, petechial rash, proteinuria, prothrombin time increased, purpura, renal failure, sagittal sinus thrombosis, sepsis, septic shock, subacute bacterial endocarditis, superficial venous thrombosis, uric acid nephropathy

Drug Interactions

Metabolism/Transport Effects None known.

Avoid Concomitant Use

Avoid concomitant use of Pegaspargase with any of the following: BCG; Natalizumab; Pimecrolimus; Tacrolimus (Topical); Vaccines (Live)

Increased Effect/Toxicity

Pegaspargase may increase the levels/effects of: Leflunomide; Natalizumab; Vaccines (Live)

The levels/effects of Pegaspargase may be increased by: Denosumab; Pimecrolimus; Roflumilast; Tacrolimus (Topical); Trastuzumab

Decreased Effect

Pegaspargase may decrease the levels/effects of: BCG; Coccidioidin Skin Test; Sipuleucel-T; Vaccines (Inactivated); Vaccines (Live)

The levels/effects of Pegaspargase may be decreased by: Echinacea; Pegloticase

Stability Refrigerate at 2°C to 8°C (36°F to 46°F); do not freeze. Do not use product if it is known to have been frozen. Do not use vial if stored at room temperature for >48 hours. Avoid excessive agitation; do **not** shake. Do not use if cloudy, discolored, or if precipitate is present.

I.V.: Dilute in 100 mL NS or D_5W; solutions for infusion should be refrigerated immediately after aseptic preparation and administered within 24 hours of preparation [Data on file (Enzon Pharmaceuticals, 2009)].

Mechanism of Action Pegaspargase is a modified version of asparaginase. Leukemic cells, especially lymphoblasts, require exogenous asparagine; normal cells can synthesize asparagine. Asparaginase contains L-asparaginase amidohydrolase type EC-2 which inhibits protein synthesis by deaminating asparagine to aspartic acid and ammonia in the plasma and extracellular fluid and therefore deprives tumor cells of the amino acid for protein synthesis. Asparaginase is cycle-specific for the G_1 phase of the cell cycle.

Pharmacodynamics/Kinetics

Onset: Asparagine depletion: I.M.: Within 4 days

Duration: Asparagine depletion: I.M.: ~21 days; I.V. (in asparaginase naive adults): 2-4 weeks

Absorption: I.M.: Slow

Distribution: I.M.: Children: 1.5 L/m^2; I.V.: Adults (asparaginase naive): 2.4 L/m^2

Metabolism: Systemically degraded

Half-life elimination: I.M.: ~5.5-6 days; unaffected by age, renal or hepatic function; half life decreased to 1.8-3.2 days in patients with previous hypersensitivity to native L-asparaginase; I.V.: Adults (asparaginase naive): 7 days

Time to peak: I.M.: 3-4 days

Excretion: Urine (trace amounts)

Dosage Details concerning dosing in combinations regimens should also be consulted.

Children and Adults: I.M., I.V.: 2500 units/m^2 (as part of a combination chemotherapy regimen), do not administer more frequently than every 14 days

Hemodialysis, peritoneal dialysis: Significant drug removal is unlikely based on physiochemical characteristics

Administration Have available appropriate agents for maintenance of an adequate airway and treatment of a hypersensitivity reaction (antihistamine, epinephrine, oxygen, I.V. corticosteroids). Be prepared to treat anaphylaxis at each administration.

I.M.: Must only be administered as a deep intramuscular injection into a large muscle. Do not exceed 2 mL per injection site; use multiple injection sites for I.M. injection volume >2 mL.

I.V.: Administer over 1-2 hours through a running I.V. infusion line; **do not administer I.V. push.**

Monitoring Parameters Vital signs during administration, CBC with differential, platelets, amylase, liver enzymes, fibrinogen, PT, PTT (coagulation parameters [baseline and periodic]), renal function tests, urine glucose, blood glucose; monitor for onset of abdominal pain; observe for allergic reaction (for 1 hour after administration)

Dosage Forms Excipient information presented when available (limited, particularly for generics); consult specific product labeling.

Injection, solution [preservative free]:

Oncaspar®: 750 int. units/mL (5 mL)

◆ **Pegasys®** *see* Peginterferon Alfa-2a *on page 1308*

Pegfilgrastim (peg fil GRA stim)

Brand Names: U.S. Neulasta®

Brand Names: Canada Neulasta®

Index Terms G-CSF (PEG Conjugate); Granulocyte Colony Stimulating Factor (PEG Conjugate); Pegylated G-CSF; SD/01

Pharmacologic Category Colony Stimulating Factor

Use To decrease the incidence of infection, by stimulation of granulocyte production, in patients with nonmyeloid malignancies receiving myelosuppressive therapy associated with a significant risk of febrile neutropenia

Pregnancy Risk Factor C

Pregnancy Considerations Animal studies have demonstrated adverse effects and fetal loss. There are no adequate and well-controlled studies in pregnant women; use only if potential benefit to mother justifies the potential risk to the fetus.

Lactation Excretion in breast milk unknown/use caution

Contraindications Hypersensitivity to pegfilgrastim, filgrastim, or any component of the formulation

Warnings/Precautions Do not use pegfilgrastim in the period 14 days before to 24 hours after administration of cytotoxic chemotherapy because of the potential sensitivity of rapidly dividing myeloid cells to cytotoxic chemotherapy. Benefit has not been demonstrated with regimens under a two-week duration. Administration on the same day as chemotherapy is not recommended (NCCN Myeloid Growth Factor Guidelines, v.1.2011). Pegfilgrastim can potentially act as a growth factor for any tumor type, particularly myeloid malignancies. Caution should be exercised in the usage of pegfilgrastim in any malignancy with myeloid characteristics. Tumors of nonhematopoietic origin may have surface receptors for pegfilgrastim. Pegfilgrastim has not been evaluated with patients receiving radiation therapy, or with chemotherapy associated with delayed myelosuppression (nitrosoureas, mitomycin C). Safety and efficacy have not been evaluated for peripheral blood progenitor cell (PBPC) mobilization.

Allergic-type reactions (anaphylaxis, angioedema, erythema, skin rash, urticaria) have occurred primarily with the initial dose and may recur (possibly delayed) after discontinuation; close follow up for several days and permanent discontinuation are recommended for severe reactions. Rare cases of splenic rupture have been reported; patients must be instructed to report left upper quadrant pain or shoulder tip pain. Acute respiratory distress syndrome (ARDS) has been associated with use; evaluate patients with pulmonary symptoms such as fever, lung infiltrates, or respiratory distress; discontinue or withhold pegfilgrastim if ARDS occurs. May precipitate sickle cell crises in patients with sickle cell disease; carefully ▶

evaluate potential risks and benefits. The packaging (needle cover) contains latex. The 6 mg fixed dose should not be used in infants, children, and adolescents weighing <45 kg.

Adverse Reactions

>10%:

Cardiovascular: Peripheral edema (12%)

Central nervous system: Headache (16%)

Gastrointestinal: Vomiting (13%)

Neuromuscular & skeletal: Bone pain (31% to 57%), myalgia (21%), arthralgia (16%), weakness (13%)

1% to 10%:

Gastrointestinal: Constipation (10%)

Miscellaneous: Antibody formation (1% to 6%)

<1% (Limited to important or life-threatening): Acute respiratory distress syndrome (ARDS), allergic reaction, anaphylaxis, cutaneous vasculitis, erythema, fever, flushing, hyperleukocytosis, hypoxia, injection site reactions (erythema, induration, pain), leukocytosis, rash, sickle cell crisis, splenic rupture, Sweet's syndrome (acute febrile dermatosis), urticaria. Cytopenias resulting from an antibody response to exogenous growth factors have been reported on rare occasions in patients treated with other recombinant growth factors.

Drug Interactions

Metabolism/Transport Effects None known.

Avoid Concomitant Use There are no known interactions where it is recommended to avoid concomitant use.

Increased Effect/Toxicity There are no known significant interactions involving an increase in effect.

Decreased Effect

The levels/effects of Pegfilgrastim may be decreased by: Pegloticase

Stability Store under refrigeration 2°C to 8°C (36°F to 46°F); do not freeze. If inadvertently frozen, allow to thaw in refrigerator; discard if frozen more than one time. Protect from light. Do not shake. Allow to reach room temperature prior to injection. May be kept at room temperature for up to 48 hours.

Mechanism of Action Stimulates the production, maturation, and activation of neutrophils, pegfilgrastim activates neutrophils to increase both their migration and cytotoxicity. Pegfilgrastim has a prolonged duration of effect relative to filgrastim and a reduced renal clearance.

Pharmacodynamics/Kinetics Half-life elimination: SubQ: Adults: 15-80 hours; Children (100 mcg/kg dose): ~20-30 hours (range: up to 68 hours)

Dosage SubQ: **Note:** Do not administer in the period between 14 days before and 24 hours after administration of cytotoxic chemotherapy. According to the NCCN guidelines, efficacy has been demonstrated with every-2-week chemotherapy regimens, however, benefit has not been demonstrated with regimens under a 2-week duration (NCCN Myeloid Growth Factor Guidelines, v.1.2011)

Children (unlabeled dose): 100 mcg/kg (maximum dose: 6 mg) once per chemotherapy cycle, beginning 24-72 hours after completion of chemotherapy

Adolescents >45 kg and Adults: 6 mg once per chemotherapy cycle, beginning 24-72 hours after completion of chemotherapy

Dosage adjustment in renal impairment: No adjustment necessary

Administration Administer subcutaneously. Do not use 6 mg fixed dose in infants, children, or adolescents <45 kg. Engage/activate needle guard following use to prevent accidental needlesticks.

Monitoring Parameters Complete blood count (with differential) and platelet count should be obtained prior to chemotherapy. Leukocytosis (white blood cell counts 100,000/mm^3) has been observed in <1% of patients receiving pegfilgrastim. Monitor platelets and hematocrit regularly. Evaluate fever, pulmonary infiltrates, and respiratory distress; evaluate for left upper abdominal pain, shoulder tip pain, or splenomegaly. Monitor for sickle cell crisis (in patients with sickle cell anemia).

Test Interactions May interfere with bone imaging studies; increased hematopoietic activity of the bone marrow may appear as transient positive bone imaging changes

Dosage Forms Excipient information presented when available (limited, particularly for generics); consult specific product labeling.

Injection, solution [preservative free]:

Neulasta®: 6 mg/0.6 mL (0.6 mL) [contains natural rubber/natural latex in packaging]

◆ **PEG-IFN Alfa-2b** *see* Peginterferon Alfa-2b *on page* 1311

Peginterferon Alfa-2a

(peg in ter FEER on AL fa too aye)

Brand Names: U.S. Pegasys®

Brand Names: Canada Pegasys®

Index Terms Interferon Alfa-2a (PEG Conjugate); Pegylated Interferon Alfa-2a

Pharmacologic Category Interferon

Use Treatment of chronic hepatitis C (CHC), alone or in combination with ribavirin, in patients with compensated liver disease and not previously treated with alfa interferons (includes patients with histological evidence of cirrhosis [Child-Pugh class A] and patients with clinically-stable HIV disease); treatment of patients with HBeAg-positive and HBeAg-negative chronic hepatitis B with compensated liver disease and evidence of viral replication and liver inflammation

Pregnancy Risk Factor C / X in combination with ribavirin

Pregnancy Considerations Reproduction studies with pegylated interferon alfa have not been conducted. Animal studies with nonpegylated interferon alfa-2b have demonstrated abortifacient effects. Disruption of the normal menstrual cycle was also observed in animal studies; therefore, the manufacturer recommends that reliable contraception is used in women of childbearing potential. Alfa interferon is endogenous to normal amniotic fluid. *In vitro* administration studies have reported that when administered to the mother, it does not cross the placenta. Case reports of use in pregnant women are limited. The Perinatal HIV Guidelines Working Group does not recommend that peginterferon-alfa be used during pregnancy. Peginterferon monotherapy should only be used in pregnancy when the potential benefit to the mother justifies the possible risk to the fetus. **[U.S. Boxed Warning]: Combination therapy with ribavirin may cause birth defects; avoid pregnancy in females and female partners of male patients;** combination therapy with ribavirin is contraindicated in pregnancy (refer to Ribavirin monograph); a pregnancy registry has been established for women inadvertently exposed to ribavirin while pregnant (800-593-2214).

Lactation Excretion in breast milk unknown/not recommended

Medication Guide Available Yes

Contraindications Hypersensitivity to polyethylene glycol (PEG), interferon alfa, or any component of the formulation; autoimmune hepatitis; decompensated liver disease in cirrhotic patients (Child-Pugh score >6); decompensated liver disease (Child-Pugh score ≥6, class B and C) in CHC coinfected with HIV; neonates and infants

Warnings/Precautions Hazardous agent: Use appropriate precautions for handling and disposal.

[U.S. Boxed Warning]: May cause or aggravate fatal or life-threatening autoimmune disorders, neuropsychiatric symptoms (including depression and/or suicidal thoughts/behaviors), ischemic and/or infectious

disorders; discontinue treatment for persistent severe or worsening symptoms.

Neuropsychiatric disorders: Severe psychiatric adverse effects (including depression, suicidal ideation, and suicide attempt) may occur in patients with or without a prior history of psychiatric disorder. Avoid use in severe psychiatric disorders; use with extreme caution in patients with a history of depression. Patients who experience dizziness, confusion, somnolence or fatigue should use caution when performing tasks which require mental alertness (eg, operating machinery or driving).

Bone marrow suppression: May cause myelosuppression (including neutropenia, thrombocytopenia, lymphopenia, aplastic anemia). Use caution with baseline neutrophil count <1500/mm^3, platelet count <90,000/mm^3 or hemoglobin <10 g/dL. Discontinue therapy (at least temporarily) if ANC <500/mm^3 or platelet count <25,000/mm^3. Use with caution in patients with an increased risk for severe anemia (eg, spherocytosis, history of GI bleeding).

Hepatic disease: Hepatic decompensation and death have been associated with the use of alpha interferons including Pegasys®, in cirrhotic chronic hepatitis C patients; patients coinfected with HIV and receiving highly active antiretroviral therapy have shown an increased risk. Monitor hepatic function; discontinue if decompensation occurs (Child-Pugh score >6) in monoinfected patients and (Child-Pugh score ≥6, class B and C) in patients coinfected with HIV. In hepatitis B patients, flares (transient and potentially severe increases in serum ALT) may occur during or after treatment; more frequent monitoring of LFTs and a dose reduction are recommended. Discontinue if ALT elevation continues despite dose reduction or if increased bilirubin or hepatic decompensation occur.

Gastrointestinal disorders: Gastrointestinal hemorrhage, ulcerative and hemorrhagic/ischemic colitis have been observed with interferon alfa treatment; may be severe and/or life-threatening; discontinue if symptoms of colitis (eg, abdominal pain, bloody diarrhea, and/or fever) develop. Discontinue therapy if known or suspected pancreatitis develops.

Dermatologic disorders: Serious cutaneous reactions, including vesiculobullous eruptions, Stevens-Johnson syndrome and exfoliative dermatitis, have been reported (rarely) with use, with or without ribavirin therapy; discontinue with signs or symptoms of severe skin reactions.

Ophthalmic disease: Discontinue if new or worsening ophthalmologic disorders occur including retinal hemorrhages, cotton wool spots, retinal detachment (serous), and retinal artery or vein obstruction; visual exams are recommended in these instances, at the initiation of therapy, and periodically during therapy.

Pulmonary disorders: May cause or aggravate dyspnea, pulmonary infiltrates, pneumonia, bronchiolitis obliterans, interstitial pneumonia, and sarcoidosis, resulting in potentially fatal respiratory failure may occur with treatment; may recur upon rechallenge with interferons. Discontinue with unexplained pulmonary infiltrates or evidence of impaired pulmonary function. Use caution in patients with a history of pulmonary disease.

Endocrine disorders: Use with caution in patients with diabetes mellitus; hyper- or hypoglycemia have been reported which may require adjustments in medications. Use with caution in patients with pre-existing thyroid disease; thyroid disorders (hyper- or hypothyroidism) or exacerbations have been reported.

Severe acute hypersensitivity reactions have occurred rarely; prompt discontinuation is advised. Commonly associated with flu-like symptoms, including fever; rule out other causes/infection with persistent or high fever. Serious and severe infections (bacterial, viral and fungal) have been reported with treatment. Use with caution in patients with renal dysfunction (Cl_{cr} <30 mL/minute); monitor for signs/symptoms of toxicity (dosage adjustment required if toxicity occurs). Use with caution in patients with pulmonary dysfunction, prior cardiovascular disease, or autoimmune disease. Use with caution in the elderly. **Due to differences in dosage, patients should not change brands of interferon without the concurrence of their healthcare provider.** Safety and efficacy have not been established in patients who have failed other alpha interferon therapy, have received organ transplants, have been coinfected with HBV **and** HCV or HIV, have been coinfected with HCV **and** HBV or HIV with a CD4$^+$ cell count <100 cells/microL, or been treated for >48 weeks.

[U.S. Boxed Warning]: Combination treatment with ribavirin may cause birth defects and/or fetal mortality (avoid pregnancy in females and female partners of male patients); hemolytic anemia (which may worsen cardiac disease), genotoxicity, mutagenicity, and may possibly be carcinogenic.

Adverse Reactions Note: Percentages are reported for peginterferon alfa-2a in chronic hepatitis C (CHC) patients. Other percentages indicated as "with ribavirin" or "in HIV/CHC" are those which significantly exceed incidence reported for peginterferon monotherapy in CHC patients.

>10%:

- Central nervous system: Headache (54%), fatigue (56%), fever (37%; 41% with ribavirin; 54% in hepatitis B), insomnia (19%; 30% with ribavirin), depression (18%), dizziness (16%), irritability/anxiety/nervousness (19%; 33% with ribavirin), pain (11%)
- Dermatologic: Alopecia (23%; 28% with ribavirin), pruritus (12%; 19% with ribavirin), dermatitis (16% with ribavirin)
- Gastrointestinal: Nausea/vomiting (24%), anorexia (17%; 24% with ribavirin), diarrhea (16%), weight loss (16% in HIV/CHC), abdominal pain (15%)
- Hematologic: Neutropenia (21%; 27% with ribavirin; 40% in HIV/CHC), lymphopenia (14% with ribavirin), anemia (11% with ribavirin; 14% in HIV/CHC)
- Hepatic: ALT increases 5-10 x ULN during treatment (25% to 27% in hepatitis B); ALT increases >10 x ULN during treatment (12% to 18% in hepatitis B); ALT increases 5-10 x ULN after treatment (13% to 16% in hepatitis B); ALT increases >10 x ULN after treatment (7% to 12% in hepatitis B)
- Local: Injection site reaction (22%)
- Neuromuscular & skeletal: Weakness (56%; 65% with ribavirin), myalgia (37%), rigors (35%; 25% to 27% in hepatitis B), arthralgia (28%)
- Respiratory: Dyspnea (13% with ribavirin)

1% to 10%:

- Central nervous system: Concentration impaired (8%), memory impaired (5%), mood alteration (3%; 9% in HIV/CHC)
- Dermatologic: Dermatitis (8%), rash (5%), dry skin (4%; 10% with ribavirin), eczema (1%; 5% with ribavirin)
- Endocrine & metabolic: Hypothyroidism (3% to 4%), hyperthyroidism (≤1%)
- Gastrointestinal: Xerostomia (6%), dyspepsia (<1%; 6% with ribavirin), weight loss (4%; 10% with ribavirin)
- Hematologic: Thrombocytopenia (5%; 8% in HIV/CHC), lymphopenia (3%), anemia (2%)
- Hepatic: Hepatic decompensation (2% in CHC/HIV)
- Neuromuscular & skeletal: Back pain (9%)
- Ocular: Blurred vision (4%)
- Respiratory: Cough (4%; 10% with ribavirin), dyspnea (4%), exertional dyspnea (4% with ribavirin)
- Miscellaneous: Diaphoresis (6%), bacterial infection (3%; 5% in HIV/CHC)

≤1% (Limited to important or life-threatening): Aggression, anaphylaxis, angioedema, angina, aplastic anemia, arrhythmia, autoimmune disorders, bronchiolitis obliterans, bronchoconstriction, cerebral hemorrhage, chest pain, cholangitis, colitis, coma, corneal ulcer, cotton wool spots, dehydration, diabetes mellitus, endocarditis, erythema multiforme major, exertional dyspnea, exfoliative dermatitis, fatty liver, gastrointestinal bleeding, hallucination, hearing impairment, hearing loss, hemoglobin decreased, hematocrit decreased, hepatic dysfunction, hepatic graft rejection, hepatitis B flares, hyper-/hypoglycemia, hypersensitivity reactions, hypertension, influenza, interstitial pneumonitis, macular edema, MI, myositis, optic neuritis, papilledema, pancreatitis, peptic ulcer, peripheral neuropathy, pneumonia, psychiatric disorder, psychosis, pulmonary embolism, pulmonary infiltrates, pure red cell aplasia, renal graft rejection, retinal artery/vein thrombosis, retinal detachment, retinal hemorrhage, retinopathy, rheumatoid arthritis, sarcoidosis, seizures, Stevens-Johnson syndrome, substance overdose, suicidal ideation, suicide, supraventricular arrhythmia, systemic lupus erythematosus, thrombotic thrombocytopenic purpura, triglycerides (increased), urticaria, vesiculobullous eruptions, vision decreased/loss

Drug Interactions

Metabolism/Transport Effects Inhibits CYP1A2 (weak)

Avoid Concomitant Use

Avoid concomitant use of Peginterferon Alfa-2a with any of the following: CloZAPine; Telbivudine

Increased Effect/Toxicity

Peginterferon Alfa-2a may increase the levels/effects of: Aldesleukin; CloZAPine; Methadone; Ribavirin; Telbivudine; Theophylline Derivatives; Zidovudine

Decreased Effect

The levels/effects of Peginterferon Alfa-2a may be decreased by: Pegloticase

Ethanol/Nutrition/Herb Interactions Ethanol: Avoid use in patients with hepatitis C virus.

Stability Store in refrigerator at 2°C to 8°C (36°F to 46°F). Do not freeze or shake. Protect from light. The following stability information has also been reported:

Intact vial: May be stored at room temperature for up to 14 days (Cohen, 2007).

Prefilled syringe: May be stored at room temperature for up to 6 days (Cohen, 2007).

Mechanism of Action Alpha interferons are a family of proteins, produced by nucleated cells that have antiviral, antiproliferative, and immune-regulating activity. There are 16 known subtypes of alpha interferons. Interferons interact with cells through high affinity cell surface receptors. Following activation, multiple effects can be detected including induction of gene transcription. Interferons inhibit cellular growth, alter the state of cellular differentiation, interfere with oncogene expression, alter cell surface antigen expression, increase phagocytic activity of macrophages, and augment cytotoxicity of lymphocytes for target cells.

Pharmacodynamics/Kinetics

Half-life elimination: Terminal: 50-160 hours; increased with renal dysfunction

Time to peak, serum: 72-96 hours

Dosage SubQ: Adults:

Chronic hepatitis C (monoinfection or coinfection with HIV):

Monotherapy: 180 mcg once weekly for 48 weeks

Combination therapy with ribavirin: Recommended dosage: 180 mcg once/week with ribavirin (Copegus®)

Duration of therapy: Monoinfection (based on genotype):

Genotype 1,4: 48 weeks

Genotype 2,3: 24 weeks

Duration of therapy: Coinfection with HIV: 48 weeks

Note: *American Association for the Study of Liver Diseases (AASLD) guidelines recommendation:* Adults with chronic HCV infection (Ghany, 2009): Treatment of choice: Ribavirin plus **peginterferon**; clinical condition and ability of patient to tolerate therapy should be evaluated to determine length and/or likely benefit of therapy. Recommended treatment duration (AASLD guidelines): Genotypes 1,4: 48 weeks; Genotypes 2,3: 24 weeks; Coinfection with HIV: 48 weeks.

Chronic hepatitis B: 180 mcg once weekly for 48 weeks

Dose modifications for adverse reactions/toxicity:

For moderate-to-severe adverse reactions: Initial: 135 mcg/week; may need decreased to 90 mcg/week in some cases

Based on hematologic parameters:

ANC <750/mm^3: 135 mcg/week

ANC <500/mm^3: Suspend therapy until >1000/mm^3, then restart at 90 mcg/week; monitor ANC

Platelet count <50,000/mm^3: 90 mcg/week

Platelet count <25,000/mm^3: Discontinue therapy

Depression (severity based on DSM-IV criteria):

Mild depression: No dosage adjustment required; evaluate once weekly by visit/phone call. If depression remains stable, continue weekly visits. If depression improves, resume normal visit schedule

Moderate depression: Decrease interferon dose to 90-135 mcg once/week; evaluate once weekly with an office visit at least every other week. If depression remains stable, consider psychiatric evaluation and continue with reduced dosing. If symptoms improve and remain stable for 4 weeks, resume normal visit schedule; continue reduced dosing or return to normal dose.

Severe depression: Discontinue interferon permanently. Obtain immediate psychiatric consultation. Discontinue ribavirin if using concurrently.

Dosage adjustment in renal impairment:

Cl_{cr} ≥30 mL/minute: No adjustment required.

Cl_{cr} <30 mL/minute: 135 mcg/week; monitor for toxicity

End-stage renal disease requiring hemodialysis: 135 mcg/week; monitor for toxicity

If severe adverse reactions/toxicity or laboratory abnormalities occur, may decrease dose to 90 mcg/week until reactions abate. If toxicity persists, after dosage adjustment, discontinue therapy. Also refer to dose modifications for adverse reactions/toxicity.

Dosage adjustment in hepatic impairment:

HCV: ALT progressively rising above baseline: Decrease dose to 135 mcg/week. If ALT continues to rise or is accompanied by increased bilirubin or hepatic decompensation, discontinue therapy immediately. Therapy may resume after ALT flare subsides.

HBV:

ALT >5 x ULN: Monitor LFTs more frequently; consider decreasing dose to 135 mcg/week or temporarily discontinuing (may resume after ALT flare subsides).

ALT >10 x ULN: Consider discontinuing.

Dietary Considerations Avoid ethanol use in patients with hepatitis C virus.

Administration SubQ: Administer in the abdomen or thigh. Rotate injection site. Do not use if solution contains particulate matter or is discolored. Discard unused solution. Administration should be done on the same day and at approximately the same time each week.

Monitoring Parameters Clinical studies tested as follows: CBC (including hemoglobin, WBC, and platelets) and chemistries (including liver function tests and uric acid) measured at weeks 1, 2, 4, 6, and 8, and then every 4-6 weeks (more frequently if abnormal); TSH measured every 12 weeks

In addition, the following baseline values were used as entrance criteria:

- Platelet count ≥90,000/mm^3 (as low as 75,000/mm^3 in patients with cirrhosis or transition to cirrhosis)
- ANC ≥1500/mm^3
- Serum creatinine <1.5 times ULN
- TSH and T_4 within normal limits or adequately controlled
- CD4$^+$ cell count ≥200 cells/mcL or CD4$^+$ cell count ≥100 cells/mcL, but <200 cells/mcL and HIV-1 RNA <5000 copies/mL in CHC patients coinfected with HIV
- Hemoglobin ≥12 g/dL for women and ≥13 g/dL for men in CHC monoinfected patients
- Hemoglobin ≥11 g/dL for women and ≥12 g/dL for men in CHC patients coinfected with HIV

Serum HCV RNA levels (pretreatment, 12- and 24 weeks after therapy initiation, 24 weeks after completion of therapy). **Note:** Discontinuation of therapy may be considered after 12 weeks in patients with HCV (genotype 1) who fail to achieve an early virologic response (EVR) (defined as ≥2-log decrease in HCV RNA compared to pretreatment) or after 24 weeks with detectable HCV RNA. Treat patients with HCV (genotypes 2,3) for 24 weeks (if tolerated) and then evaluate HCV RNA levels (Ghany, 2009).

Prior to treatment, pregnancy screening should occur for women of childbearing age who are receiving treatment or who have male partners who are receiving treatment. In combination therapy with ribavirin, pregnancy tests should continue monthly up to 6 months after discontinuation of therapy. Evaluate for depression and other psychiatric symptoms before and during therapy; baseline eye examination and periodically in patients with baseline disorders; baseline echocardiogram in patients with cardiac disease.

Dosage Forms Excipient information presented when available (limited, particularly for generics); consult specific product labeling.

Injection, solution:

- Pegasys®: 180 mcg/mL (1 mL) [contains benzyl alcohol, polysorbate 80; vial]
- Pegasys®: 180 mcg/0.5 mL (0.5 mL) [contains benzyl alcohol, polysorbate 80; prefilled syringe]

Peginterferon Alfa-2b

(peg in ter FEER on AL fa too bee)

Brand Names: U.S. PegIntron®; PegIntron™ Redipen®; Sylatron™

Brand Names: Canada PegIntron®

Index Terms Interferon Alfa-2b (PEG Conjugate); PEG-IFN Alfa-2b; Pegylated Interferon Alfa-2b; Polyethylene Glycol Interferon Alfa-2b; Sylatron™

Pharmacologic Category Interferon

Use

PegIntron®: Treatment of chronic hepatitis C (CHC; in combination with ribavirin) in patients who have compensated liver disease; treatment of chronic hepatitis C (as monotherapy) in adult patients with compensated liver disease who have never received alfa interferons

Sylatron™: Adjuvant treatment of melanoma (with microscopic or gross nodal involvement within 84 days of definitive surgical resection, including lymphadenectomy)

Pregnancy Risk Factor C / X in combination with ribavirin

Pregnancy Considerations Reproduction studies with pegylated interferon alfa have not been conducted. Animal studies with nonpegylated interferon alfa-2b have demonstrated abortifacient effects. Disruption of the normal menstrual cycle was also observed in animal studies; therefore, the manufacturer recommends that reliable contraception is used in women of childbearing potential. Alfa interferon is endogenous to normal amniotic fluid. *In vitro* administration studies have reported that when administered to the mother, it does not cross the placenta. Case reports of use in pregnant women are limited. The Perinatal HIV Guidelines Working Group does not recommend that peginterferon alfa be used during pregnancy. Peginterferon alfa-2b monotherapy should only be used in pregnancy when the potential benefit to the mother justifies the possible risk to the fetus. **[U.S. Boxed Warning]: Combination therapy with ribavirin may cause birth defects and/or fetal mortality; avoid pregnancy in females and female partners of male patients;** combination therapy with ribavirin is contraindicated in pregnancy. Two forms of contraception should be used during combination therapy; patients should have monthly pregnancy tests. A pregnancy registry has been established for women inadvertently exposed to ribavirin while pregnant (800-593-2214).

Lactation Excretion in breast milk unknown/not recommended

Medication Guide Available Yes

Contraindications Hypersensitivity (including urticaria, angioedema, bronchoconstriction, anaphylaxis, Stevens Johnson syndrome and toxic epidermal necrolysis) to peginterferon alfa-2b, interferon alfa-2b, other alfa interferons, or any component of the formulation; autoimmune hepatitis; decompensated liver disease (Child-Pugh score >6, classes B and C)

Combination therapy with peginterferon alfa-2b and ribavirin is also contraindicated in pregnancy, women who may become pregnant, males with pregnant partners; hemoglobinopathies (eg, thalassemia major, sickle-cell anemia); renal dysfunction (Cl_{cr} <50 mL/minute)

Warnings/Precautions Hazardous agent - use appropriate precautions for handling and disposal.

[U.S. Boxed Warnings]: May cause or aggravate severe depression or other neuropsychiatric adverse events (including suicide and suicidal ideation) in patients with and without a history of psychiatric disorder; may be irreversible; discontinue treatment permanently with worsening or persistently severe signs/symptoms of neuropsychiatric disorders (eg, depression, encephalopathy, psychosis). May cause or aggravate fatal or life-threatening autoimmune disorders, infectious disorders, ischemic disorders, and/or hemorrhagic cerebrovascular events; discontinue treatment for persistent severe or worsening symptoms.

Neuropsychiatric disorders: Neuropsychiatric effects may occur in patients with and without a history of psychiatric disorder; addiction relapse, aggression, depression, homicidal ideation and suicidal behavior/ideation have been observed with peginterferon alfa-2b; bipolar disorder, encephalopathy, hallucinations, mania, and psychosis have been observed with other alfa interferons. Onset may be delayed (up to 6 months after discontinuation). Higher doses may be associated with the development of encephalopathy (higher risk in elderly patients). Use with extreme caution in patients with a history of psychiatric disorders, including depression. Monitor all patients for evidence of depression; patients being treated for melanoma should be monitored for depression and psychiatric symptoms every 3 weeks during the first eight weeks of treatment and every 6 months thereafter; discontinue treatment if psychiatric symptoms persist, worsen or if suicidal behavior develops. All patients should continue to be monitored for 6 months after completion of therapy.

Bone marrow suppression: Causes bone marrow suppression, including potentially severe cytopenias; alfa interferons may (rarely) cause aplastic anemia. Use with caution in patients who are chronically immunosuppressed, with low peripheral blood counts or myelosuppression, including concurrent use of myelosuppressive therapy. Use with caution in patients with an increased risk for severe anemia (eg, spherocytosis, history of GI bleeding). Dosage modification may be necessary for hematologic toxicity.

Combination therapy with ribavirin may potentiate the neutropenic effects of alfa interferons. When used in combination with ribavirin, an increased incidence of anemia was observed when using ribavirin weight-based dosing, as compared to flat-dose ribavirin.

Hepatic disease: Use is contraindicated in patients with hepatic decompensation. Discontinue treatment immediately with hepatic decompensation (Child Pugh score >6). Patients with chronic hepatitis C (CHC) with cirrhosis receiving peginterferon alfa-2b are at risk for hepatic decompensation. CHC patients coinfected with human immunodeficiency virus (HIV) are at increased risk for hepatic decompensation when receiving highly active antiretroviral therapy (HAART); monitor closely. A transient increase in ALT (2-5 times above baseline) which is not associated with deterioration of liver function may occur with peginterferon alfa-2b use (for the treatment of chronic hepatitis C); therapy generally may continue with monitoring.

Gastrointestinal disorders: Pancreatitis has been observed with alfa interferon therapy; discontinue therapy if known or suspected pancreatitis develops. Ulcerative or hemorrhagic/ischemic colitis has been observed with alfa interferons; withhold treatment for suspected pancreatitis; discontinue therapy for known pancreatitis. Ulcerative or hemorrhagic/ischemic colitis has been observed with alfa interferons; discontinue therapy if signs of colitis (abdominal pain, bloody diarrhea, fever) develop; symptoms typically resolve within 1-3 weeks.

Autoimmune disorders: Thyroiditis, thrombotic thrombocytopenic purpura, idiopathic thrombocytopenic purpura, rheumatoid arthritis, interstitial nephritis, systemic lupus erythematosus, and psoriasis have been reported with therapy; use with caution in patients with autoimmune disorders.

Cardiovascular disease: Use with caution in patients with cardiovascular disease or a history of cardiovascular disease; hypotension, arrhythmia, bundle branch block, tachycardia, cardiomyopathy, angina pectoris and MI have been observed with treatment. Patients with pre-existing cardiac abnormalities should have baseline ECGs prior to combination treatment with ribavirin; closely monitor patients with a history of MI or arrhythmia. Patients with a history of significant or unstable cardiac disease should not receive combination treatment with ribavirin. Discontinue treatment (permanently) for new-onset ventricular arrhythmia or cardiovascular decompensation.

Endocrine disorders: Diabetes mellitus (including new-onset type I diabetes), hyperglycemia, and thyroid disorders have been reported; discontinue peginterferon alfa-2b if cannot be effectively managed with medication. Use caution in patients with a history of diabetes mellitus, particularly if prone to DKA. Use with caution in patients with thyroid disorders; may cause or aggravate hyper- or hypothyroidism.

Pulmonary disease: May cause or aggravate dyspnea, pulmonary infiltrates, pneumonia, bronchiolitis obliterans, interstitial pneumonitis, pulmonary hypertension, and sarcoidosis which may result in respiratory failure; may recur upon rechallenge with treatment; monitor closely. Use with caution in patients with existing pulmonary disease (eg, chronic obstructive pulmonary disease). Withhold combination therapy with ribavirin for development of pulmonary infiltrate or pulmonary function impairment.

Ophthalmic disorders: Ophthalmologic disorders (including decreased visual acuity, blindness, macular edema, retinal hemorrhages, optic neuritis, papilledema, cotton wool spots, retinal detachment [serous], and retinal artery or vein thrombosis) have occurred with peginterferon alfa-2b and/or with other alfa interferons. Prior to start of therapy, ophthalmic exams are recommended for all patients; patients with diabetic or hypertensive retinopathy should have periodic ophthalmic exams during treatment; a complete eye exam should be done promptly in patients who develop ocular symptoms. Permanently discontinue treatment with new or worsening ophthalmic disorder.

[U.S. Boxed Warning]: Combination treatment with ribavirin may cause birth defects and/or fetal mortality (avoid pregnancy in females and female partners of male patients); hemolytic anemia (which may worsen cardiac disease), genotoxicity, mutagenicity, and may possibly be carcinogenic. Interferon therapy is commonly associated with flu-like symptoms, including fever; rule out other causes/infection with persistent or high fever. Acute hypersensitivity reactions and cutaneous reactions (eg, Stevens-Johnson syndrome, toxic epidermal necrolysis) have been reported (rarely) with alfa interferons; prompt discontinuation is recommended; transient rashes do not require interruption of therapy. Hypertriglyceridemia has been reported with use; discontinue if persistent and severe (triglycerides >1000 mg/dL), particularly if combined with symptoms of pancreatitis. Use with caution in patients with renal impairment (Cl_{cr} <50 mL/minute); monitor closely. For the treatment of chronic hepatitis C, dosage adjustments are recommended with monotherapy in patients with moderate-to-severe impairment; do not use combination therapy with ribavirin in adult patients renal dysfunction (Cl_{cr} <50 mL/minute); discontinue if serum creatinine >2 mg/dL in children. Has not been studied in melanoma patients with renal impairment. Serum creatinine increases have been reported in patients with renal insufficiency. Use with caution in the elderly; the potential adverse effects may be more pronounced in the elderly. Elderly patients generally do not respond to interferon treatment as well as younger patients. Dental/periodontal disorders have been reported with combination therapy; dry mouth may affect teeth and mucous membranes; instruct patients to brush teeth twice daily; encourage regular dental exams.

Combination therapy with ribavirin is preferred over monotherapy for the treatment of chronic hepatitis C (combination therapy provides a better response). Safety and efficacy have not been established in patients who have received organ transplants, are coinfected with HIV or hepatitis B, or received treatment for >1 year. Patients with significant bridging fibrosis or cirrhosis, genotype 1 infection or who have not responded to prior therapy, including previous pegylated interferon treatment are less likely to benefit from combination therapy with peginterferon alfa-2b and ribavirin. Growth velocity (height and weight) was decreased in children on combination treatment with ribavirin, particularly during the first 6 months of treatment. **[U.S. Boxed Warning]: Combination therapy with ribavirin is contraindicated in pregnancy.** Due to differences in dosage, patients should not change brands of interferon.

Adverse Reactions Note: Percentages reported for adults receiving monotherapy unless noted:

>10%:

Central nervous system: Fatigue (52% to 94%), fever (22% to 75%), headache (56% to 70%), chills (≤63%), depression (29% to 59%; may be severe), dizziness (12% to 35%), anxiety/emotional liability/irritability (28%), insomnia (23%), olfactory nerve disorder (≤23%)

Dermatologic: Rash (6% to 36%), alopecia (22% to 34%), pruritus (12%), dry skin (11%)

Gastrointestinal: Anorexia (20% to 69%), nausea (26% to 64%), taste perversion (≤38%), diarrhea (18% to 37%), vomiting (7% to 26%), abdominal pain (15%), weight loss (11%)
Hematologic: Neutropenia (6% to 70%; grade 4: 1%), thrombocytopenia (7% to 20%; grades 3/4: <4%), anemia (6%; in combination with ribavirin: 12% to 47%)
Hepatic: Transaminases increased (10% to 77%), alkaline phosphatase increased (≤23%)
Local: Injection site inflammation/reaction (23% to 62%)
Neuromuscular & skeletal: Myalgia (54% to 68%), weakness (52%), arthralgia (23% to 51%), musculoskeletal pain (28%), rigors (23%), paresthesia (21%)
Miscellaneous: Viral infection (11%)

>1% to 10%:
Cardiovascular: Chest pain (6%), flushing (6%)
Central nervous system: Concentration impaired (10%), malaise (7%), nervousness (4%), agitation (2%), suicidal behavior (ideation/attempt/suicide ≤2%)
Endocrine & metabolic: Hypothyroidism (5%), menstrual disorder (4%), hyperthyroidism (3%)
Gastrointestinal: Dyspepsia (6%), xerostomia (6%), constipation (1%)
Hepatic: GGT increased (8%), hepatomegaly (6%)
Local: Injection site pain (2% to 3%)
Ocular: Conjunctivitis (4%), blurred vision (2%)
Renal: Proteinuria (≤7%)
Respiratory: Pharyngitis (10%), cough (5% to 8%), sinusitis (7%), dyspnea (4% to 6%), rhinitis (2%)
Miscellaneous: Diaphoresis (6%), neutralizing antibodies (2%)

≤1% (Limited to important and life-threatening): Abscess, addiction (drug) relapse, aggressive behavior, anaphylaxis, angina, angioedema, aphthous stomatitis, aplastic anemia, arrhythmia, autoimmune thrombocytopenia (with or without purpura), bacterial infection, blindness, bronchiolitis obliterans, bronchoconstriction, bundle branch block, cardiac arrest, cardiomyopathy, cellulitis, cerebral hemorrhage, cerebral ischemia, colitis, cotton wool spots, cytopenia, diabetes mellitus, diabetic ketoacidosis, drug overdose, emphysema, encephalopathy, erythema multiforme, fungal infection, gastroenteritis, gout, hallucinations, hearing impairment/loss, hemorrhagic colitis, homicidal ideation, hyperglycemia, hyper-/hypotension, hypersensitivity reactions, hypertriglyceridemia, injection site necrosis, interstitial nephritis, interstitial pneumonitis, ischemic colitis, leukopenia, loss of consciousness, lupus-like syndrome, macular edema, memory loss, MI, migraine, myositis, nerve palsy (facial/oculomotor), optic neuritis, palpitation, pancreatitis, papilledema, pericardial effusion, peripheral neuropathy, phototoxicity, pleural effusion, pneumonia, pneumonitis, polyneuropathy, psoriasis, psychosis, pulmonary hypertension, pulmonary infiltrates, pure red cell aplasia, renal failure, renal insufficiency, retinal artery or vein thrombosis, retinal detachment (serous), retinal hemorrhage, retinal ischemia, rhabdomyolysis, rheumatoid arthritis, sarcoidosis, seizure, sepsis, serum creatinine increased, Stevens-Johnson syndrome, supraventricular arrhythmia, systemic lupus erythematosus, tachycardia, thrombotic thrombocytopenic purpura, thyroiditis, toxic epidermal necrolysis, transient ischemic attack, ulcerative colitis, urticaria, vasculitis, vertigo, vision decrease/loss, visual acuity decreased, Vogt-Koyanagi-Harada syndrome

Drug Interactions

Metabolism/Transport Effects Inhibits CYP1A2 (weak)

Avoid Concomitant Use

Avoid concomitant use of Peginterferon Alfa-2b with any of the following: CloZAPine; Telbivudine

Increased Effect/Toxicity

Peginterferon Alfa-2b may increase the levels/effects of: Aldesleukin; CloZAPine; Methadone; Ribavirin; Telbivudine; Theophylline Derivatives; Zidovudine

Decreased Effect

Peginterferon Alfa-2b may decrease the levels/effects of: CYP2C9 Substrates; CYP2D6 Substrates; FLUoxetine

The levels/effects of Peginterferon Alfa-2b may be decreased by: Pegloticase

Ethanol/Nutrition/Herb Interactions Ethanol: Avoid use in patients with hepatitis C virus.

Stability Prior to reconstitution, store Redipen® at 2°C to 8°C (36°F to 46°F). Store intact vials at 25°C (77°F); excursions permitted to 15°C to 30°C (59°F to 86°F). Do not freeze.

Redipen®: Hold cartridge upright and press the two halves together until there is a "click". Gently invert to mix; do not shake. Single-use pen.

Pegintron® (vial): Add 0.7 mL sterile water for injection, USP (supplied single-use diluent) to the vial. Gently swirl. Do not re-enter vial after dose removed.

Sylatron™ (vial): Add 0.7 mL sterile water for injection and swirl gently, resulting in the following concentrations:
296 mcg vial: 40 mcg/0.1 mL
444 mcg vial: 60 mcg/0.1 mL
888 mcg vial: 120 mcg/0.1 mL

Once reconstituted each product should be used immediately or may be stored for ≤24 hours at 2°C to 8°C (36°F to 46°F); do not freeze. Do not shake. Products do not contain preservative.

Mechanism of Action Alpha interferons are a family of proteins, produced by nucleated cells, that have antiviral, antiproliferative, and immune-regulating activity. There are 16 known subtypes of alpha interferons. Interferons interact with cells through high affinity cell surface receptors. Following activation, multiple effects can be detected including induction of gene transcription. Inhibits cellular growth, alters the state of cellular differentiation, interferes with oncogene expression, alters cell surface antigen expression, increases phagocytic activity of macrophages, and augments cytotoxicity of lymphocytes for target cells.

Pharmacodynamics/Kinetics
Bioavailability: Increases with chronic dosing
Half-life elimination: CHC: ~40 hours (range: 22-60 hours); Melanoma: ~43-51 hours
Time to peak: CHC: 15-44 hours
Excretion: Urine (~30%)

Dosage SubQ:

Children ≥3 years: CHC:

Manufacturer labeling: Combination therapy with ribavirin: 60 mcg/m^2 once weekly (in combination with ribavirin 15 mg/kg/day in 2 divided doses); **Note:** Children who reach their 18th birthday during treatment should remain on the pediatric regimen. Treatment duration is 48 weeks for genotype 1, 24 weeks for genotypes 2 and 3. Discontinue combination therapy in patients with HCV (genotype 1) at 12 weeks if HCV-RNA decreases <2 log (compared to pretreatment) or if detectable HCV-RNA at 24 weeks.

American Association for the Study of Liver Diseases (AASLD) guideline recommendations (Ghany, 2009): Children 2-17 years: Treatment of choice: **Peginterferon alfa-2b** 60 mcg/m^2 once weekly in combination with oral ribavirin 15 mg/kg/day for 48 weeks

Adults:

Melanoma: 6 mcg/kg/week for 8 doses, followed by 3 mcg/kg/week for up to 5 years. **Note:** Premedicate with acetaminophen (500-1000 mg orally) 30 minutes prior to the first dose and as needed thereafter.

CHC: Administer dose once weekly; **Note:** Treatment duration is 48 weeks for genotype 1, 24 weeks for genotypes 2 and 3, or 48 weeks for patients who previously failed therapy (regardless of genotype). Discontinue in patients with HCV (genotype 1) after 12 weeks if HCV RNA decreases <2 log (compared to pretreatment) or if detectable HCV RNA at 24 weeks.

Monotherapy: Initial (based on average weekly dose of 1 mcg/kg):
- ≤45 kg: 40 mcg once weekly
- 46-56 kg: 50 mcg once weekly
- 57-72 kg: 64 mcg once weekly
- 73-88 kg: 80 mcg once weekly
- 89-106 kg: 96 mcg once weekly
- 107-136 kg: 120 mcg once weekly
- 137-160 kg: 150 mcg once weekly

Combination therapy with ribavirin: Initial (based on an average weekly dose of 1.5 mcg/kg):
- <40 kg: 50 mcg once weekly (with ribavirin 800 mg/day)
- 40-50 kg: 64 mcg once weekly (with ribavirin 800 mg/day)
- 51-60 kg: 80 mcg once weekly (with ribavirin 800 mg/day)
- 61-65 kg: 96 mcg once weekly (with ribavirin 800 mg/day)
- 66-75 kg: 96 mcg once weekly (with ribavirin 1000 mg/day)
- 76-80 kg: 120 mcg once weekly (with ribavirin 1000 mg/day)
- 81-85 kg: 120 mcg once weekly (with ribavirin 1200 mg/day)
- 86-105 kg: 150 mcg once weekly (with ribavirin 1200 mg/day)
- >105 kg: 1.5 mcg/kg once weekly (with ribavirin 1400 mg/day)

Note: *American Association for the Study of Liver Diseases (AASLD) guidelines recommendation:* Adults with chronic HCV infection: Treatment of choice: Ribavirin plus **peginterferon**; clinical condition and ability of patient to tolerate therapy should be evaluated to determine length and/or likely benefit of therapy. Recommended treatment duration (AASLD guidelines; Ghany, 2009): Genotypes 1,4: 48 weeks; Genotypes 2,3: 24 weeks; Coinfection with HIV: 48 weeks.

Elderly: May require dosage reduction based upon renal dysfunction; however, no established guidelines are available.

Dosage adjustment for toxicity:
Melanoma:

Discontinue for any of the following: Persistent or worsening severe neuropsychiatric disorders (depression, psychosis, encephalopathy), grade 4 nonhematologic toxicity, new or worsening retinopathy, new-onset ventricular arrhythmia or cardiovascular decompensation, evidence of hepatic injury (severe) or hepatic decompensation, development of hyper- or hypothyroidism or diabetes that cannot be effectively managed with medication, or inability to tolerate a dose of 1 mcg/kg/week

Temporarily withhold for any of the following: ANC <500/mm^3, platelets <50,000/mm^3, ECOG performance status (PS) ≥2, nonhematologic toxicity ≥ grade 3. May reinitiate at a reduced dose once ANC ≥500/mm^3, platelets ≥50,000/mm^3, ECOG PS at 0-1, and nonhematologic toxicity completely resolved or improved to grade 1.

Reduced dose schedule, Weeks 1-8:
- First dose reduction (if prior dose 6 mcg/kg/week): 3 mcg/kg/week
- Second dose reduction (if prior dose 3 mcg/kg/week): 2 mcg/kg/week
- Third dose reduction (if prior dose 2 mcg/kg/week): 1 mcg/kg/week
- Discontinue permanently if unable to tolerate 1 mcg/kg/week

Reduced dose schedule, Weeks 9-260:
- First dose reduction (if prior dose 3 mcg/kg/week): 2 mcg/kg/week
- Second dose reduction (if prior dose 2 mcg/kg/week): 1 mcg/kg/week
- Discontinue permanently if unable to tolerate 1 mcg/kg/week

***Chronic hepatitis C:* Dosage adjustment for depression (severity based upon DSM-IV criteria):**

Mild depression: No dosage adjustment required; evaluate once weekly by visit/phone call. If depression remains stable, continue weekly visits. If depression improves, resume normal visit schedule. For worsening depression, see "Moderate depression" or "Severe depression".

Moderate depression:
- Children: Decrease peginterferon alfa-2b dose to 40 mcg/m^2/week, may further decrease to 20 mcg/m^2/week if needed
- Adults:
  - Peginterferon alfa-2b monotherapy: Refer to adult weight-based dosage reduction with monotherapy for depression below
  - Peginterferon alfa-2b combination therapy: Refer to adult weight-based dosage reduction with combination therapy for depression below
- **Note:** Evaluate once weekly (visit or phone) with an office visit at least every other week. If depression remains stable, consider psychiatric evaluation and continue with reduced dosing. If symptoms improve and remain stable for 4 weeks, resume normal visit schedule; continue reduced dosing or return to normal dose. For worsening depression, see "Severe depression".

Severe depression: Discontinue peginterferon alfa-2b and ribavirin permanently. Obtain immediate psychiatric consultation.

***Chronic hepatitis C:* Dosage adjustment in hematologic toxicity:**

Children:
- Hemoglobin decrease ≥2 g/dL in any 4-week period in patients with pre-existing cardiac disease: Monitor and evaluate weekly
- Hemoglobin <10 g/dL: Decrease ribavirin dose to 12 mg/kg/day; may further reduce to 8 mg/kg/day
- WBC <1500/mm^3, neutrophils <750/mm^3, or platelets <70,000/mm^3: Reduce peginterferon alfa-2b dose to 40 mcg/m^2/week; may further reduce to 20 mcg/m^2/week
- Hemoglobin <8.5 g/dL, WBC <1000/mm^3, neutrophils <500/mm^3, or platelets <50,000/mm^3: Permanently discontinue peginterferon alfa-2b and ribavirin

Adults:
- Hemoglobin decrease >2 g/dL in any 4-week period and stable cardiac disease: Decrease peginterferon alfa-2b dose by 50%; decrease ribavirin dose by 200 mg/day. Hemoglobin <12 g/dL after dose reductions: Permanently discontinue both peginterferon alfa-2b and ribavirin
- Hemoglobin <10 g/dL in patients with cardiac disease: Reduce peginterferon alfa-2b dose by 50%; decrease ribavirin dose by 200 mg/day (patients receiving 1400 mg/day should decrease dose by 400 mg/day [ie, first dose reduction to 1000 mg/day]); may further reduce ribavirin dose by additional 200 mg/day if needed

WBC <1500/mm^3, neutrophils <750/mm^3, or platelets <50,000/mm^3:
Peginterferon alfa-2b monotherapy: Refer to adult weight-based dosage reduction monotherapy for hematologic toxicity below
Peginterferon alfa-2b combination therapy: Refer to adult weight-based dosage reduction with combination therapy for hematologic toxicity below
Hemoglobin <8.5 g/dL, WBC <1000/mm^3, neutrophils <500/mm^3, or platelets <25,000/mm^3: Permanently discontinue peginterferon alfa-2b and ribavirin

***Chronic hepatitis C:* Adult weight-based dosage reduction for depression or hematologic toxicity:**
Peginterferon alfa-2b monotherapy: Reduce to average weekly dose of 0.5 mcg/kg as follows:
≤45 kg: 20 mcg once weekly
46-56 kg: 25 mcg once weekly
57-72 kg: 30 mcg once weekly
73-88 kg: 40 mcg once weekly
89-106 kg: 50 mcg once weekly
107-136 kg: 64 mcg once weekly
≥137 kg: 80 mcg once weekly
Peginterferon alfa-2b combination therapy: Initially reduce to average weekly dose of 1 mcg/kg; may further reduce to average weekly dose of 0.5 mcg/kg if needed as follows:
<40 kg: 35 mcg once weekly; may further reduce to 20 mcg once weekly if needed
40-50 kg: 45 mcg once weekly; may further reduce to 25 mcg once weekly if needed
51-60 kg: 50 mcg once weekly; may further reduce to 30 mcg once weekly if needed
61-75 kg: 64 mcg once weekly; may further reduce to 35 mcg once weekly if needed
76-85 kg: 80 mcg once weekly; may further reduce to 45 mcg once weekly if needed
86-104 kg: 96 mcg once weekly; may further reduce to 50 mcg once weekly if needed
105-125 kg: 108 mcg once weekly; may further reduce to 64 mcg once weekly if needed
>125 kg: 135 mcg once weekly; may further reduce to 72 mcg once weekly if needed

Dosage adjustment in renal impairment: Chronic hepatitis C:
Peginterferon alfa-2b monotherapy:
Cl_{cr} 30-50 mL/minute: Reduce dose by 25%
Cl_{cr} 10-29 mL/minute: Reduce dose by 50%
Hemodialysis: Reduce dose by 50%
Discontinue use if renal function declines during treatment.
Peginterferon alfa-2b combination with ribavirin:
Children: Serum creatinine >2 mg/dL: Discontinue treatment
Adults: Cl_{cr} <50 mL/minute: Combination therapy with ribavirin is not recommended

Dosage adjustment in hepatic impairment: Contraindicated in decompensated liver disease

Administration For SubQ administration; rotate injection site; thigh, outer surface of upper arm, and abdomen are preferred injection sites; do not inject near navel or waistline; patients who are thin should only use thigh or upper arm. Do not inject into bruised, infected, irritated, red, or scarred skin. The weekly dose may be administered at bedtime to reduce flu-like symptoms.

Monitoring Parameters Baseline and periodic TSH (for patients being treated for melanoma, obtain baseline within 4 weeks prior to treatment initiation, and then at 3 and 6 months, and every 6 months thereafter during treatment); hematology (including hemoglobin, CBC with differential, platelets); chemistry (including LFTs) testing, renal function, triglycerides. Clinical studies (for combination therapy) tested as follows: CBC (including hemoglobin, WBC, and platelets) and chemistries (including liver function tests and uric acid) measured at weeks 2, 4, 8, and 12, and then every 6 weeks; TSH measured every 12 weeks during treatment.

Serum HCV RNA levels (pretreatment, 12 and 24 weeks after therapy initiation, 24 weeks after completion of therapy). **Note:** Discontinuation of therapy may be considered after 12 weeks in patients with HCV (genotype 1) who fail to achieve an early virologic response (EVR) (defined as ≥2-log decrease in HCV RNA compared to pretreatment) or after 24 weeks with detectable HCV RNA. Treat patients with HCV (genotypes 2,3) for 24 weeks (if tolerated) and then evaluate HCV RNA levels (Ghany, 2009).

Evaluate for depression and other psychiatric symptoms before and after initiation of therapy; patients being treated for melanoma should be monitored for depression and psychiatric symptoms every 3 weeks during the first eight weeks of treatment and every 6 months thereafter; baseline ophthalmic eye examination; periodic ophthalmic exam in patients with diabetic or hypertensive retinopathy; baseline ECG in patients with cardiac disease; serum glucose or Hb A_{1c} (for patients with diabetes mellitus). In combination therapy with ribavirin, pregnancy tests (for women of childbearing age who are receiving treatment or who have male partners who are receiving treatment), continue monthly up to 6 months after discontinuation of therapy.

Reference Range Chronic hepatitis C:
Early viral response (EVR): ≥2 log decrease in HCV RNA after 12 weeks of treatment
End of treatment response (ETR): Absence of detectable HCV RNA at end of the recommended treatment period
Sustained treatment response (STR): Absence of HCV RNA in the serum 6 months following completion of full treatment course

Dosage Forms Excipient information presented when available (limited, particularly for generics); consult specific product labeling.
Injection, powder for reconstitution:
Sylatron™: 296 mcg [contains polysorbate 80, sucrose 59.2 mg; supplied with diluent]
Sylatron™: 444 mcg [contains polysorbate 80, sucrose 59.2 mg; suppled with diluent]
Sylatron™: 888 mcg [contains polysorbate 80, sucrose 59.2 mg; supplied with diluent]
Injection, powder for reconstitution [preservative free]:
PegIntron®: 50 mcg, 80 mcg, 120 mcg, 150 mcg [contains polysorbate 80, sucrose 59.2 mg; supplied with diluent]
PegIntron™ Redipen®: 50 mcg, 80 mcg, 120 mcg, 150 mcg [contains polysorbate 80, sucrose 54 mg; supplied with diluent]

◆ **PegIntron®** *see* Peginterferon Alfa-2b *on page 1311*

◆ **PegIntron™ Redipen®** *see* Peginterferon Alfa-2b *on page 1311*

◆ **PEGLA** *see* Pegaspargase *on page 1306*

Pegloticase (peg LOE ti kase)

Brand Names: U.S. Krystexxa™

Index Terms PEG-Uricase; Pegylated Urate Oxidase; Polyethylene Glycol-Conjugated Uricase; Recombinant Urate Oxidase, Pegylated; Urate Oxidase, Pegylated

Pharmacologic Category Enzyme; Enzyme, Urate-Oxidase (Recombinant)

Use Treatment of chronic gout refractory to conventional therapy

Pregnancy Risk Factor C

Pregnancy Considerations Adequate animal reproduction studies have not been conducted. There are no adequate and well-controlled studies in pregnant women. Use during pregnancy only if the benefit to the mother outweigh the potential risk to the fetus.

Lactation Excretion in breast milk unknown/not recommended

Medication Guide Available Yes

Contraindications Glucose-6-phosphate dehydrogenase (G6PD) deficiency

Warnings/Precautions [U.S. Boxed Warning]: Anaphylaxis and infusion reactions have been reported during and after administration; patients should be closely monitored during infusion and for an appropriate period of time after the infusion. Therapy should be administered in a healthcare facility by skilled medical personnel prepared for the immediate treatment of anaphylaxis. All patients should be premedicated with antihistamines and corticosteroids. Anaphylaxis may occur at any time during treatment (including the initial dose). **Reactions generally occur within 2 hours of administration; however, delayed hypersensitivity reactions have also been reported.** Infusion reactions are varied; symptoms range from chest pain, pruritus/urticaria, or dyspnea to a clinical presentation of anaphylaxis (eg, hemodynamic instability, perioral or lingual edema). If a less severe (nonanaphylactic) infusion reaction occurs, the infusion may be slowed, or stopped and restarted at a slower rate, at the physician's discretion. **Risk of an infusion reaction is increased in patients whose uric acid is >6 mg/dL; therefore, monitor serum uric acid concentrations prior to infusion and consider discontinuing treatment if concentrations exceed 6 mg/dL, particularly in the event of 2 consecutive concentrations >6 mg/dL.**

Therapy with antihyperuricemic agents commonly results in gout flare, particularly upon initiation due to rapid lowering of urate concentrations; gout flare-ups during treatment do not warrant discontinuation of therapy. Gout flare prophylaxis is recommended, using nonsteroidal anti-inflammatory agents (NSAID) or colchicines, unless contraindicated, beginning ≥1 week before initiation of pegloticase and continuing for at least 6 months. Exacerbation of heart failure has been observed in clinical trials; use caution in patients with pre-existing heart failure. Due to the risk for hemolysis and methemoglobinemia, pegloticase is contraindicated in patients with G6PD deficiency. Patients at higher risk for G6PD deficiency (eg, African, Mediterranean) should be screened prior to therapy. Therapy is not appropriate for the treatment of asymptomatic hyperuricemia. Potential for immunogenicity exists with the use of therapeutic proteins. Antipegloticase antibodies and antiPEG antibodies commonly occurred during clinical trials in pegloticase-treated patients. High antipegloticase antibody titers were associated with failure to maintain uric acid normalization and were also associated with a higher incidence of infusion reactions. Due to potential for immunogenicity, closely monitor patients who reinitiate therapy after discontinuing treatment for >4 weeks; patients may be at increased risk for anaphylaxis and infusion reactions.

Adverse Reactions

>10%:

Dermatologic: Bruising (11%), urticaria (11%)

Gastrointestinal: Nausea (12%)

Miscellaneous: Antibody formation (antipegloticase antibodies: 92%; antiPEG antibodies: 42%), gout flare (74% within the first 3 months), infusion reactions (26%)

1% to 10%:

Cardiovascular: Chest pain (6% to 10%)

Dermatologic: Erythema (10%), pruritus (10%)

Gastrointestinal: Constipation (6%), vomiting (5%)

Respiratory: Dyspnea (7%), nasopharyngitis (7%)

Miscellaneous: Anaphylaxis (≤7%)

Frequency not defined: Anemia, diarrhea, headache, muscle spasms, nephrolithiasis

Drug Interactions

Metabolism/Transport Effects None known.

Avoid Concomitant Use There are no known interactions where it is recommended to avoid concomitant use.

Increased Effect/Toxicity There are no known significant interactions involving an increase in effect.

Decreased Effect

Pegloticase may decrease the levels/effects of: Certolizumab Pegol; Pegademase Bovine; Pegaptanib; Pegaspargase; Pegfilgrastim; Peginterferon Alfa-2a; Peginterferon Alfa-2b; Pegvisomant

Stability Prior to use, vials must be stored in the carton to protect from light and kept under refrigeration between 2°C to 8°C (36° to 46°F) at all times. Do **not** shake or freeze.

To prepare solution for administration, withdraw 1 mL (8 mg) and add to a 250 mL bag of NS or 1/2NS; invert bag several times to mix thoroughly (do **not** shake). Do not use vial if particulate matter is present or if solution is discolored (solution should be a clear and colorless). After withdrawal, discard any unused portion of the product remaining in the vial. Diluted solution may be stored up to 4 hours at 2°C to 8°C (36°F to 46°F). Diluted solution is also stable for 4 hours at room temperature of 20°C to 25°C (68°F to 77°F); however, refrigeration is preferred. The diluted solution should be protected from light, not frozen, and used within 4 hours of dilution. Prior to administration, allow the diluted solution to reach room temperature; do not warm to room temperature using any form of artificial heating such as a microwave or warm water bath.

Mechanism of Action Pegloticase is a pegylated recombinant form of urate-oxidase enzyme, also known as uricase (an enzyme normally absent in humans and high primates), which converts uric acid to allantoin (an inactive and water soluble metabolite of uric acid); it does not inhibit the formation of uric acid.

Pharmacodynamics/Kinetics

Onset of action: ~24 hours following the first dose, serum uric acid concentrations decreased

Duration: >300 hours (12.5 days)

Half-life elimination: Median: ~14 days

Dosage Note: Premedicate with antihistamines and corticosteroids. Gout flare prophylaxis with either NSAIDs or colchicine is also recommended, beginning at least 1 week prior to initiation and continuing for at least 6 months.

I.V.: Adults: Refractory gout: 8 mg every 2 weeks

Dosage adjustment in renal impairment: Creatinine clearance did not alter the pharmacokinetics; dosage adjustments are not needed

Administration Administer diluted solution by I.V. infusion over ≥120 minutes via gravity feed or an infusion pump or syringe-type pump. Do **not** administer by I.V. push or bolus. Administer in a healthcare setting by healthcare providers prepared to manage potential anaphylaxis. Monitor closely for infusion reactions during infusion and for an appropriate period of time after the infusion (anaphylaxis has been reported within 2 hours of the infusion). In the event or a less severe infusion reaction, infusion may be slowed, or stopped and restarted at a slower rate, based on the discretion of the physician.

Reference Range

Uric acid, serum: An increase occurs during childhood

Adults:

Males: 3.4-7 mg/dL or slightly more

Females: 2.4-6 mg/dL or slightly more

Values >7 mg/dL are sometimes arbitrarily regarded as hyperuricemia, but there is no sharp line between normals on the one hand, and the serum uric acid of those with clinical gout. Normal ranges cannot be adjusted for purine ingestion, but high purine diet increases uric acid. Uric acid may be increased with body size, exercise, and stress.

Dosage Forms Excipient information presented when available (limited, particularly for generics); consult specific product labeling.

Injection, solution:

Krystexxa™: Uricase protein 8 mg/mL (2 mL)

- **PegLyte® (Can)** *see* Polyethylene Glycol-Electrolyte Solution *on page 1372*
- **PEG-Uricase** *see* Pegloticase *on page 1315*

Pegvisomant (peg VI soe mant)

Brand Names: U.S. Somavert®

Brand Names: Canada Somavert®

Index Terms B2036-PEG

Pharmacologic Category Growth Hormone Receptor Antagonist

Use Treatment of acromegaly in patients resistant to or unable to tolerate other therapies

Pregnancy Risk Factor B

Dosage SubQ: Adults: Initial loading dose: 40 mg; maintenance dose: 10 mg once daily; doses may be adjusted by 5 mg increments in 4- to 6-week intervals based on IGF-I concentrations (maximum maintenance dose: 30 mg/day)

Dosage adjustment in hepatic impairment:

At initiation of therapy:

Normal liver function test (LFT): Initiate therapy; monitor LFT monthly for first 6 months, quarterly for next 6 months, then biannually the following year.

Baseline LFT elevated but ≤3 x ULN: May initiate therapy with monthly evaluation of LFT for 1 year then biannually the following year.

Baseline LFT >3 x ULN: Do not initiate treatment without comprehensive work-up to determine cause; monitor closely if treatment is started.

With ongoing therapy:

LFT ≥3 x but <5 x ULN without signs/symptoms of hepatitis, hepatic injury, or increase in total bilirubin: Continue treatment, but monitor LFT weekly for further increases; perform comprehensive hepatic work-up to rule out alternative cause of hepatic dysfunction

LFT ≥5 x ULN or transaminase ≥3 x ULN associated with any increase in total bilirubin: Discontinue immediately and perform comprehensive hepatic work-up. If LFTs return to normal, may cautiously consider restarting therapy with frequent LFT monitoring.

Signs or symptoms of hepatitis or hepatic injury: Discontinue therapy immediately and perform comprehensive hepatic work-up; discontinue permanently if liver injury is confirmed.

Additional Information Complete prescribing information for this medication should be consulted for additional detail.

Dosage Forms Excipient information presented when available (limited, particularly for generics); consult specific product labeling.

Injection, powder for reconstitution:

Somavert®: 10 mg, 15 mg, 20 mg [supplied with diluent]

- **Pegylated DOXOrubicin Liposomal** *see* DOXOrubicin (Liposomal) *on page 555*
- **Pegylated G-CSF** *see* Pegfilgrastim *on page 1307*
- **Pegylated Interferon Alfa-2a** *see* Peginterferon Alfa-2a *on page 1308*
- **Pegylated Interferon Alfa-2b** *see* Peginterferon Alfa-2b *on page 1311*
- **Pegylated Liposomal DOXOrubicin** *see* DOXOrubicin (Liposomal) *on page 555*
- **Pegylated Urate Oxidase** *see* Pegloticase *on page 1315*
- **PE-Hist-DM [OTC]** *see* Chlorpheniramine, Phenylephrine, and Dextromethorphan *on page 346*

PEMEtrexed (pem e TREKS ed)

Brand Names: U.S. Alimta®

Brand Names: Canada Alimta®

Index Terms LY231514; Pemetrexed Disodium

Pharmacologic Category Antineoplastic Agent, Antimetabolite; Antineoplastic Agent, Antimetabolite (Antifolate)

Use Treatment of unresectable malignant pleural mesothelioma (in combination with cisplatin); treatment of locally advanced or metastatic **non**squamous nonsmall cell lung cancer (NSCLC; as initial treatment in combination with cisplatin, as single-agent maintenance treatment after 4 cycles of initial platinum-based double therapy, and single-agent treatment after prior chemotherapy)

Note: Not indicated for the treatment of **squamous** cell NSCLC

Unlabeled Use Treatment of bladder cancer (metastatic), cervical cancer (recurrent or metastatic), ovarian cancer (recurrent or persistent), thymic malignancies; treatment of malignant pleural mesothelioma (either as a single agent or in combination with carboplatin)

Pregnancy Risk Factor D

Pregnancy Considerations Adverse effects (embryotoxicity, fetotoxicity and teratogenicity) were observed in animal reproduction studies. Based on the mechanism of action, may cause fetal harm if administered to a pregnant woman. Women of childbearing potential should have a negative serum pregnancy test prior to treatment and should use effective contraceptive measures to avoid becoming pregnant during treatment. Irreversible infertility has been reported in males; prior to receiving treatment, males should be counseled on sperm storage. The Canadian labeling recommends that males receiving therapy use effective contraceptive measures and not father a child during, and for up to 6 months after therapy.

Lactation Excretion in breast milk unknown/not recommended

Contraindications Severe hypersensitivity to pemetrexed or any component of the formulation

Canadian labeling (additional contraindications; not in U.S. labeling): Concomitant yellow fever vaccine

Warnings/Precautions Hazardous agent - use appropriate precautions for handling and disposal. Hypersensitivity (including anaphylaxis) has been reported with use. May cause bone marrow suppression (anemia, neutropenia, thrombocytopenia and/or pancytopenia); may require dose reductions in subsequent cycles. Prophylactic folic acid and vitamin B_{12} supplements are necessary to reduce hematologic and gastrointestinal toxicity and infection; initiate supplementation 1 week before the first dose of pemetrexed. Pretreatment with corticosteroids (dexamethasone or equivalent) reduces the incidence and severity of cutaneous reactions. Rarely, Stevens-Johnson syndrome and toxic epidermal necrolysis have been reported. Although the effect of third space fluid is not fully defined, studies have determined pemetrexed concentrations in patients with mild-to-moderate ascites/pleural effusions were similar to concentrations in trials of patients without third space fluid accumulation. Drainage of fluid from ascites/effusions may be considered, but is not likely necessary. Use caution with hepatic dysfunction not due to metastases; may require dose adjustment. Interstitial pneumonitis with respiratory insufficiency has been observed with use; interrupt therapy and evaluate promptly with progressive dyspnea and cough.

The manufacturer does not recommend use in patients with Cl_{cr} <45 mL/minute. Decreased renal function results in increased toxicity. Use caution in patients receiving concurrent nephrotoxins; may result in delayed pemetrexed clearance. NSAIDs may reduce the clearance of pemetrexed. In patients with Cl_{cr} 45-79 mL/minute, interruption of NSAID therapy may be necessary prior to, during, and immediately after pemetrexed therapy. Not indicated for use in patients with squamous cell NSCLC.

Adverse Reactions Note: Reported for single-agent therapy in patients who received folate and B_{12} supplementation.

>10%:

- Central nervous system: Fatigue (25% to 34%; dose-limiting)
- Dermatologic: Rash/desquamation (10% to 14%)
- Gastrointestinal: Nausea (19% to 31%), anorexia (19% to 22%), vomiting (9% to 16%), stomatitis (7% to 15%), diarrhea (5% to 13%)
- Hematologic: Anemia (15% to 19%; grades 3/4: 3% to 4%), leukopenia (6% to 12%; grades 3/4: 2% to 4%), neutropenia (6% to 11%; grades 3/4: 3% to 5%; dose-limiting; nadir: 8-10 days; recovery: 4-8 days after nadir)
- Respiratory: Pharyngitis (15%)

1% to 10%:

- Cardiovascular: Edema (1% to 5%)
- Central nervous system: Fever (1% to 8%)
- Dermatologic: Pruritus (1% to 7%), alopecia (1% to 6%), erythema multiforme (≤5%)
- Gastrointestinal: Constipation (1% to 6%), weight loss (1%), abdominal pain (≤5%)
- Hematologic: Thrombocytopenia (1% to 8%; grades 3/4: 2%; dose-limiting), febrile neutropenia (grades 3/4: 2%)
- Hepatic: ALT increased (8% to 10%; grades 3/4: ≤2%), AST increased (7% to 8%; grades 3/4: ≤1%)
- Neuromuscular & skeletal: Sensory neuropathy (≤9%), motor neuropathy (≤5%)
- Ocular: Conjunctivitis (≤5%), lacrimation increased (≤5%)
- Renal: Creatinine increased/creatinine clearance decreased (1% to 5%)
- Miscellaneous: Allergic reaction/hypersensitivity (≤5%), infection (≤5%), sepsis (1%)

<1% (Limited to important or life-threatening; single-agent or combination therapy): Arrhythmia, chest pain, colitis, dehydration, hypertension, GGT increased, hemolytic anemia, hepatobiliary failure, interstitial pneumonitis, pancytopenia, peripheral ischemia, radiation recall (median onset: 6 days; range: 1-35 days), renal failure, Stevens-Johnson syndrome, supraventricular arrhythmia, thrombosis/embolism, toxic epidermal necrolysis

Drug Interactions

Metabolism/Transport Effects None known.

Avoid Concomitant Use

Avoid concomitant use of PEMEtrexed with any of the following: BCG; CloZAPine; Natalizumab; Pimecrolimus; Tacrolimus (Topical); Vaccines (Live)

Increased Effect/Toxicity

PEMEtrexed may increase the levels/effects of: CloZAPine; Leflunomide; Natalizumab; Vaccines (Live)

The levels/effects of PEMEtrexed may be increased by: Denosumab; NSAID (Nonselective); Pimecrolimus; Roflumilast; Tacrolimus (Topical); Trastuzumab

Decreased Effect

PEMEtrexed may decrease the levels/effects of: BCG; Coccidioidin Skin Test; Sipuleucel-T; Vaccines (Inactivated); Vaccines (Live)

The levels/effects of PEMEtrexed may be decreased by: Echinacea

Ethanol/Nutrition/Herb Interactions Lower ANC nadirs occur in patients with elevated baseline cystathionine or homocysteine concentrations. Levels of these substances can be reduced by folic acid and vitamin B_{12} supplementation.

Stability Store intact vials at room temperature of 25°C (77°F); excursions permitted to 15°C to 30°C (59°F to 86°F). Reconstitute with NS (preservative free); add 4.2 mL to the 100 mg vial and 20 mL to the 500 mg vial, resulting in a 25 mg/mL concentration. Gently swirl. Solution may be colorless to green-yellow. Further dilute in 100 mL NS for infusion; may also dilute in D_5W (Zhang, 2006), although the manufacturer recommends NS. Use appropriate precautions for handling and disposal. Reconstituted solution in NS and infusion solutions (in D_5W or NS) are stable for 24 hours when refrigerated at 2°C to 8°C (36°F to 46°F) or stored at room temperature of 15°C to 30°C (59°F to 86°F). Concentrations at 25 mg/mL are stable in polypropylene syringes for 2 days at room temperature (23°C) (Zhang, 2005).

Mechanism of Action Antifolate; disrupts folate-dependent metabolic processes essential for cell replication. Inhibits thymidylate synthase (TS), dihydrofolate reductase (DHFR), glycinamide ribonucleotide formyltransferase (GARFT), and aminoimidazole carboxamide ribonucleotide formyltransferase (AICARFT), the enzymes involved in folate metabolism and DNA synthesis, resulting in inhibition of purine and thymidine nucleotide and protein synthesis.

Pharmacodynamics/Kinetics

- Duration: V_{dss}: 16.1 L
- Protein binding: ~73% to 81%
- Metabolism: Minimal
- Half-life elimination: Normal renal function: 3.5 hours; Cl_{cr} 40-59 mL/minute: 5.3-5.8 hours
- Excretion: Urine (70% to 90% as unchanged drug)

Dosage Details concerning dosing in combination regimens should also be consulted. **Note:** Start vitamin supplements 1 week before initial pemetrexed dose: Folic acid 350-1000 mcg/day orally (must be taken at least 5 out of 7 days prior to treatment initiation; continue daily during treatment and for 21 days after last pemetrexed dose) and vitamin B_{12} 1000 mcg I.M. during the week prior to treatment initiation and then every 3 cycles. Give dexamethasone 4 mg orally twice daily for 3 days, beginning the day before treatment to minimize cutaneous reactions. New treatment cycles should not begin unless ANC ≥1500/mm³, platelets ≥100,000/mm³, and Cl_{cr} ≥45 mL/minute.

I.V.: Adults:

- Malignant pleural mesothelioma: 500 mg/m² on day 1 of each 21-day cycle (in combination with cisplatin) **or** (unlabeled) in combination with carboplatin (Castagneto, 2008; Ceresoli, 2006) **or** (unlabeled) as single-agent therapy (Jassem, 2008; Taylor, 2008)
- Nonsmall cell lung cancer:
  - *Initial treatment:* 500 mg/m² on day 1 of each 21-day cycle (in combination with cisplatin)
  - *Maintenance or second-line treatment:* 500 mg/m² on day 1 of each 21-day cycle (as a single-agent)
- Bladder cancer (unlabeled use): 500 mg/m² on day 1 of each 21-day cycle (Sweeney, 2006)

Dosage adjustments for toxicities:

Toxicity: Discontinue if patient develops grade 3 or 4 toxicity after two dose reductions or immediately if grade 3 or 4 neurotoxicity develops

Hematologic toxicity: Upon recovery, reinitiate therapy

Nadir ANC <500/mm³ and nadir platelets ≥50,000/mm³: Reduce dose to 75% of previous dose of pemetrexed (and cisplatin)

Nadir platelets <50,000/mm^3 **without bleeding** (regardless of nadir ANC): Reduce dose to 75% of previous dose of pemetrexed (and cisplatin)

Nadir platelets <50,000/mm^3 **with bleeding** (regardless of nadir ANC): Reduce dose to 50% of previous dose of pemetrexed (and cisplatin)

Nonhematologic toxicity ≥grade 3 (excluding neurotoxicity): Withhold treatment until recovery to baseline; upon recovery, reinitiate therapy as follows:

Grade 3 or 4 toxicity (excluding mucositis): Reduce dose to 75% of previous dose of pemetrexed (and cisplatin)

Grade 3 or 4 diarrhea or any diarrhea requiring hospitalization: Reduce dose to 75% of previous dose of pemetrexed (and cisplatin)

Grade 3 or 4 mucositis: Reduce pemetrexed dose to 50% of previous dose (continue cisplatin at 100% of previous dose)

Neurotoxicity:

Grade 0-1: Continue pemetrexed at 100% of previous dose (and cisplatin)

Grade 2: Continue pemetrexed at 100% of previous dose; reduce cisplatin dose to 50% of previous dose

Dosage adjustment in renal impairment: Renal function may be estimated using the Cockcroft-Gault formula (using actual body weight) or glomerular filtration rate (GFR) measured by Tc99m-DPTA serum clearance.

Cl_{cr} ≥45 mL/minute: No dosage adjustment necessary.

Cl_{cr} <45 mL/minute: Use not recommended (an insufficient number of patients have been studied for dosage recommendations).

Concomitant NSAID use with renal dysfunction:

Cl_{cr} ≥80 mL/minute: No dosage adjustment necessary.

Cl_{cr} 45 to 79 mL/minute and NSAIDs with short half-lives (eg, ibuprofen, indomethacin, ketoprofen, ketorolac): Avoid NSAID for 2 days before, the day of, and for 2 days following a dose of pemetrexed

Any creatinine clearance and NSAIDs with long half-lives (eg, nabumetone, naproxen, oxaprozin, piroxicam): Avoid NSAID for 5 days before, the day of, and 2 days following a dose of pemetrexed

Dosage adjustment in hepatic impairment: Grade 3 (5.1-20 times ULN) **or** 4 (>20 times ULN) transaminase elevation during treatment: Reduce pemetrexed dose to 75% of previous dose (and cisplatin)

Dietary Considerations Initiate folic acid supplementation 1 week before first dose of pemetrexed, continue for full course of therapy, and for 21 days after last dose. Institute vitamin B_{12} 1 week before the first dose; administer every 9 weeks thereafter.

Administration I.V.: Infuse over 10 minutes.

Monitoring Parameters CBC with differential and platelets (before each dose; monitor for nadir and recovery); serum creatinine, creatinine clearance, BUN, total bilirubin, ALT, AST (periodic); signs/symptoms of mucositis and diarrhea

Dosage Forms Excipient information presented when available (limited, particularly for generics); consult specific product labeling.

Injection, powder for reconstitution:

Alimta®: 100 mg, 500 mg

◆ **Pemetrexed Disodium** *see* PEMEtrexed *on page* 1317

Pemirolast (pe MIR oh last)

Brand Names: U.S. Alamast®

Brand Names: Canada Alamast®

Pharmacologic Category Mast Cell Stabilizer; Ophthalmic Agent, Miscellaneous

Use Prevention of itching of the eye due to allergic conjunctivitis

Pregnancy Risk Factor C

Dosage Children >3 years and Adults: 1-2 drops instilled in affected eye(s) 4 times/day

Additional Information Complete prescribing information for this medication should be consulted for additional detail.

Dosage Forms Excipient information presented when available (limited, particularly for generics); consult specific product labeling.

Solution, ophthalmic, as potassium [drops]:

Alamast®: 0.1% (10 mL) [contains lauralkonium chloride]

Penciclovir (pen SYE kloe veer)

Brand Names: U.S. Denavir®

Pharmacologic Category Antiviral Agent

Use Topical treatment of recurrent herpes simplex labialis (cold sores)

Pregnancy Risk Factor B

Dosage Children ≥12 years and Adults: Topical: Apply cream at the first sign or symptom of cold sore (eg, tingling, swelling); apply every 2 hours during waking hours for 4 days

Additional Information Complete prescribing information for this medication should be consulted for additional detail.

Dosage Forms Excipient information presented when available (limited, particularly for generics); consult specific product labeling.

Cream, topical:

Denavir®: 1% (1.5 g, 5 g)

PenicillAMINE (pen i SIL a meen)

Brand Names: U.S. Cuprimine®; Depen®

Brand Names: Canada Cuprimine®; Depen®

Index Terms D-3-Mercaptovaline; D-Penicillamine; β,β-Dimethylcysteine

Pharmacologic Category Chelating Agent

Use Treatment of Wilson's disease, cystinuria; adjunctive treatment of rheumatoid arthritis

Unlabeled Use Chelation therapy for the treatment of lead poisoning (third-line agent)

Pregnancy Risk Factor D

Pregnancy Considerations Birth defects, including congenital cutix laxa and associated defects, have been reported in infants following penicillamine exposure during pregnancy. Use for the treatment of rheumatoid arthritis during pregnancy is contraindicated. Use for the treatment of cystinuria only if the possible benefits to the mother outweigh the potential risks to the fetus. Continued treatment of Wilson's disease during pregnancy protects the mother against relapse. Discontinuation has detrimental maternal and fetal effects. Daily dosage should be limited to 750 mg. For planned cesarean section, reduce dose to 250 mg/day for the last 6 weeks of pregnancy, and continue at this dosage until wound healing is complete.

Lactation Excretion in breast milk unknown/contraindicated

Contraindications Hypersensitivity to penicillamine or any component of the formulation; renal insufficiency (in patients with rheumatoid arthritis); patients with previous penicillamine-related aplastic anemia or agranulocytosis; breast-feeding; pregnancy (in patients with rheumatoid arthritis)

Warnings/Precautions Patients with a penicillin allergy may theoretically have cross-sensitivity to penicillamine; however, the possibility has been eliminated now that penicillamine is produced synthetically and no longer contains trace amounts of penicillin. Once instituted for Wilson's disease or cystinuria, continue treatment on a ▶

daily basis; interruptions of even a few days have been followed by hypersensitivity with reinstitution of therapy. Penicillamine has been associated with fatalities due to agranulocytosis, aplastic anemia, thrombocytopenia, Goodpasture's syndrome, and myasthenia gravis. **[U.S. Boxed Warning]: Patients should be warned to report promptly any symptoms suggesting toxicity (fever, sore throat, chills, bruising, or bleeding);** approximately 33% of patients will experience an allergic reaction; toxicity may be dose related, use caution in the elderly. Use caution with other hematopoietic-depressant drugs (eg, gold, immunosuppressants, antimalarials, phenylbutazone); hematologic and renal adverse reactions are similar. Proteinuria or hematuria may develop; monitor for membranous glomerulopathy which can lead to nephrotic syndrome. In rheumatoid arthritis patients, discontinue if gross hematuria or persistent microscopic hematuria develop. Monitor liver function tests periodically due to rare reports of intrahepatic cholestasis or toxic hepatitis. **[U.S. Boxed Warning]: Should be administered under the close supervision of a physician familiar with the toxicity and dosage considerations.**

Lead poisoning: Investigate, identify, and remove sources of lead exposure prior to treatment. Penicillamine is considered to be a third-line agent for the treatment of lead poisoning in children due to the overall toxicity associated with its use; penicillamine should only be used when unacceptable reactions have occurred with edetate CALCIUM disodium and succimer. Primary care providers should consult experts in chemotherapy of lead toxicity before using chelation drug therapy.

Adverse Reactions Frequency not defined, may vary by indication. Adverse effects requiring discontinuation of treatment have been reported in 20% to 30% of patients with Wilson's disease.

Cardiovascular: Vasculitis

Central nervous system: Anxiety, agitation, fever, hyperpyrexia, psychiatric disturbances; worsening neurologic symptoms (10% to 50% patients with Wilson's disease)

Dermatologic: Alopecia, cheilosis, dermatomyositis, exfoliative dermatitis, lichen planus, rash (early and late 5%), pemphigus, pruritus, skin friability increased, toxic epidermal necrolysis, urticaria, wrinkling (excessive), yellow nail syndrome

Endocrine & metabolic: Hypoglycemia, thyroiditis

Gastrointestinal: Anorexia, diarrhea (17%), epigastric pain, gingivostomatitis, glossitis, nausea, oral ulcerations, pancreatitis, peptic ulcer reactivation, taste alteration (12%), vomiting

Hematologic: Eosinophilia, hemolytic anemia, leukocytosis, leukopenia (2% to 5%), monocytosis, red cell aplasia, thrombocytopenia (4% to 5%), thrombotic thrombocytopenia purpura, thrombocytosis

Hepatic: Alkaline phosphatase increased, hepatic failure, intrahepatic cholestasis, toxic hepatitis

Local: Thrombophlebitis, white papules at venipuncture and surgical sites

Neuromuscular & skeletal: Arthralgia, dystonia, myasthenia gravis, muscle weakness, neuropathies, polyarthralgia (migratory, often with objective synovitis), polymyositis

Ocular: Diplopia, extraocular muscle weakness, optic neuritis, ptosis, visual disturbances

Otic: Tinnitus

Renal: Goodpasture's syndrome, hematuria, nephrotic syndrome, proteinuria (6%), renal failure, renal vasculitis

Respiratory: Asthma, interstitial pneumonitis, pulmonary fibrosis, obliterative bronchiolitis

Miscellaneous: Allergic alveolitis, anetoderma, elastosis perforans serpiginosa, lupus-like syndrome, lactic dehydrogenase increased, lymphadenopathy, mammary hyperplasia, positive ANA test

Drug Interactions

Metabolism/Transport Effects None known.

Avoid Concomitant Use There are no known interactions where it is recommended to avoid concomitant use.

Increased Effect/Toxicity There are no known significant interactions involving an increase in effect.

Decreased Effect

PenicillAMINE may decrease the levels/effects of: Digoxin

The levels/effects of PenicillAMINE may be decreased by: Antacids; Iron Salts

Ethanol/Nutrition/Herb Interactions

Ethanol: Avoid or limit ethanol.

Food: Penicillamine serum levels may be decreased if taken with food. Do not administer with milk.

Stability Store in tight, well-closed containers.

Mechanism of Action Chelates with lead, copper, mercury and other heavy metals to form stable, soluble complexes that are excreted in urine; depresses circulating IgM rheumatoid factor, depresses T-cell but not B-cell activity; combines with cystine to form a compound which is more soluble, thus cystine calculi are prevented

Pharmacodynamics/Kinetics

Onset of action: Rheumatoid arthritis: 2-3 months; Wilson's disease: 1-3 months

Absorption: 40% to 70%

Protein binding: 80% to albumin and ceruloplasmin

Metabolism: Hepatic (small amounts metabolized to s-methyl-d-penicillamine)

Half-life elimination: 1.7-7 hours

Time to peak, serum: 1-3 hours

Excretion: Urine (>80% as unchanged drug)

Dosage Oral:

Rheumatoid arthritis:

Children (unlabeled use): Initial: 3 mg/kg/day (≤250 mg/day) for 3 months, then 6 mg/kg/day (≤500 mg/day) in divided doses twice daily for 3 months to a maximum of 10 mg/kg/day in 3-4 divided doses; maximum dose: 750 mg/day

Adults: 125-250 mg/day, may increase dose at 1- to 3-month intervals up to 1-1.5 g/day; maximum in older adults: 750 mg/day

Wilson's disease: **Note:** Decrease dose for surgery and during last trimester of pregnancy

Children (unlabeled): AASLD guidelines: 20 mg/kg/day in 2-3 divided doses, round off to the nearest 250 mg dose

Adults: 750-1500 mg/day in divided doses (dose that results in an initial 24-hour urinary copper excretion >2 mg/day should be continued for ~3 months; maintenance dose defined by amount resulting in <10 mcg serum free copper/dL); maximum dose: 2000 mg/day. **Note:** Therapy in elderly patients should be initiated at low end of dosing range and titrated upward cautiously. AASLD guidelines recommend to increase tolerability, therapy may be initiated at 250-500 mg/day then titrated upward 250 mg every 4-7 days; usual maintenance dose: 750-1000 mg/day in 2 divided doses; maximum: 1000-1500 mg/day in 2-4 divided doses (Roberts, 2008)

Cystinuria: **Note:** Adjust dose to limit cystine excretion to 100-200 mg/day (<100 mg/day with history of stone formation)

Children: 30 mg/kg/day in 4 divided doses

Adults: 1-4 g/day in 4 divided doses; usual dose: 2 g/day

Lead poisoning (unlabeled use): Children: 20-30 mg/kg/day, administered in 3-4 divided doses; initiating treatment at 25% of this dose and gradually increasing to the full dose over 2-3 weeks may minimize adverse reactions. Doses of 15 mg/kg/day may also be effective and have less adverse effects (Shannon, 2000). **Note:** For the treatment of high blood lead concentrations in children, the CDC recommends chelation treatment when blood lead concentrations are >45 mcg/dL (CDC, 2002). Children with blood lead concentrations >70 mcg/dL or symptomatic lead poisoning should be treated with parenteral agents (AAP, 2005).

Dosing adjustment/comments in renal impairment: Cl_{cr} <50 mL/minute: Avoid use

Hemodialysis: Dialyzable; a dosing decrease from 250 mg/day to 250 mg 3 times/week after dialysis has been suggested in the treatment of rheumatoid arthritis.

Dietary Considerations Should be taken at least 1 hour before a meal on an empty stomach. Iron may decrease drug action. Patients with Wilson's disease or cystinuria should receive pyridoxine supplementation 25 mg/day. For Wilson's disease, decrease copper in diet to <1-2 mg/day and omit chocolate, nuts, shellfish, mushrooms, liver, raisins, broccoli, copper-enriched cereal, multivitamins with copper, and molasses. For lead poisoning, decrease calcium in diet. For cystinuria, increase daily fluid intake including 1 pint of fluid prior to bedtime and 1 additional pint during the night.

Administration For patients who cannot swallow, contents of capsules may be administered in 15-30 mL of chilled puréed fruit or fruit juice. Give on an empty stomach (1 hour before meals and at bedtime).

Cystinuria: If administering 4 equal doses is not feasible, administer the larger dose at bedtime.

Rheumatoid arthritis: Doses ≤500 mg/day may be given as a single dose; >500 mg administer in divided doses

Monitoring Parameters Urinalysis, CBC with differential, platelet count, skin, lymph nodes, and body temperature twice weekly during the first month of therapy, then every 2 weeks for 5 months, then monthly; LFTs every 6 months

Cystinuria: Urinary cystine, annual X-ray for renal stones

Lead poisoning: Serum lead concentration (baseline and 7-21 days after completing chelation therapy); hemoglobin or hematocrit, iron status, free erythrocyte protoporphyrin or zinc protoporphyrin; neurodevelopmental changes

Wilson's disease: Serum non-ceruloplasmin bound copper, 24-hour urinary copper excretion, LFTs every 3 months during the first year of treatment; periodic ophthalmic exam

CBC: WBC <3500/mm^3 indicate need to stop therapy immediately; platelet counts <100,000/mm^3 indicate need to stop therapy until numbers of platelets increase

Urinalysis: Monitor for proteinuria and hematuria. A quantitative 24-hour urine protein at 1- to 2-week intervals initially (first 2-3 months) is recommended if proteinuria develops; in patients with rheumatoid arthritis, discontinue or decrease dose with proteinuria >1 g/24 hours, progressively increasing proteinuria or hematuria.

Reference Range Wilson's disease: 24-hour urinary copper excretion: 200-500 mcg (3-8 micromoles)/day

Dosage Forms Excipient information presented when available (limited, particularly for generics); consult specific product labeling.

Capsule, oral:

Cuprimine®: 250 mg

Tablet, oral:

Depen®: 250 mg [scored]

Extemporaneous Preparations A 50 mg/mL oral suspension may be made with capsules. Mix the contents of sixty 250 mg capsules with 3 g carboxymethylcellulose, 150 g sucrose, 300 mg citric acid, and parabens (methylparaben 120 mg, propylparaben 12 mg). Add quantity of propylene glycol sufficient to make 100 mL, then add quantity of purified water sufficient to make 300 mL. Cherry flavor may be added. Label "shake well" and "refrigerate". Stable for 30 days refrigerated.

DeCastro FJ, Jaeger RQ, and Rolfe UT, "An Extemporaneously Prepared Penicillamine Suspension Used to Treat Lead Intoxication," *Hosp Pharm*, 1977, 2:446-8.

Penicillin G Benzathine

(pen i SIL in jee BENZ a theen)

Brand Names: U.S. Bicillin® L-A

Brand Names: Canada Bicillin® L-A

Index Terms Benzathine Benzylpenicillin; Benzathine Penicillin G; Benzylpenicillin Benzathine

Pharmacologic Category Antibiotic, Penicillin

Use Active against some gram-positive organisms, few gram-negative organisms such as *Neisseria gonorrhoeae*, and some anaerobes and spirochetes; used in the treatment of syphilis; used only for the treatment of mild to moderately-severe upper respiratory tract infections caused by organisms susceptible to low concentrations of penicillin G or for prophylaxis of infections caused by these organisms; primary and secondary prevention of rheumatic fever

Pregnancy Risk Factor B

Pregnancy Considerations Adverse events have not been observed in animal studies; therefore, penicillin G is classified as pregnancy category B. Penicillin crosses the placenta and distributes into amniotic fluid. There is no evidence of adverse fetal effects after penicillin use during pregnancy in humans. Penicillin G is the drug of choice for treatment of syphilis during pregnancy.

Lactation Enters breast milk/use caution

Contraindications Hypersensitivity to penicillin(s) or any component of the formulation

Warnings/Precautions Use with caution in patients with impaired renal function, seizure disorder, or history of hypersensitivity to other beta-lactams; CDC and AAP do not currently recommend the use of penicillin G benzathine to treat congenital syphilis or neurosyphilis due to reported treatment failures and lack of published clinical data on its efficacy. Prolonged use may result in fungal or bacterial superinfection, including *C. difficile*-associated diarrhea (CDAD) and pseudomembranous colitis; CDAD has been observed >2 months postantibiotic treatment. **[U.S. Boxed Warning]: Not for intravenous use; cardiopulmonary arrest and death have occurred from inadvertent I.V. administration;** administer by deep I.M. injection only; injection into or near an artery or nerve could result in severe neurovascular damage or permanent neurological damage. Extended duration of therapy or use associated with high serum concentrations may be associated with an increased risk for some adverse reactions.

Adverse Reactions Frequency not defined.

Cardiovascular: Cardiac arrest, cerebral vascular accident, cyanosis, gangrene, hypotension, pallor, palpitations, syncope, tachycardia, vasodilation, vasospasm, vasovagal reaction

Central nervous system: Anxiety, coma, confusion, dizziness, euphoria, fatigue, headache, nervousness, pain, seizure, somnolence

In addition, a syndrome of CNS symptoms has been reported which includes: Severe agitation with confusion, hallucinations (auditory and visual), and fear of death (Hoigne's syndrome); other symptoms include cyanosis, dizziness, palpitations, psychosis, seizures, tachycardia, taste disturbance, tinnitus

Gastrointestinal: Bloody stool, intestinal necrosis, nausea, vomiting

Genitourinary: Impotence, priapism

Hepatic: AST increased

Local: Injection site reactions: Abscess, atrophy, bruising, cellulitis, edema, hemorrhage, inflammation, lump, necrosis, pain, skin ulcer

Neuromuscular & skeletal: Arthritis exacerbation, joint disorder, neurovascular damage, numbness, periostitis, rhabdomyolysis, transverse myelitis, tremor, weakness

Ocular: Blindness, blurred vision

Renal: BUN increased, creatinine increased, hematuria, myoglobinuria, neurogenic bladder, proteinuria, renal failure

Miscellaneous: Diaphoresis, hypersensitivity reactions, Jarisch-Herxheimer reaction, lymphadenopathy, mottling, warmth

Drug Interactions

Metabolism/Transport Effects None known.

Avoid Concomitant Use

Avoid concomitant use of Penicillin G Benzathine with any of the following: BCG

Increased Effect/Toxicity

Penicillin G Benzathine may increase the levels/effects of: Methotrexate; Vitamin K Antagonists

The levels/effects of Penicillin G Benzathine may be increased by: Probenecid

Decreased Effect

Penicillin G Benzathine may decrease the levels/effects of: BCG; Mycophenolate; Typhoid Vaccine

The levels/effects of Penicillin G Benzathine may be decreased by: Fusidic Acid; Tetracycline Derivatives

Stability Refrigerate at 2°C to 8°C (36°F to 46°F); do not freeze. The following stability information has also been reported: May be stored at 25°C (77°F) for 7 days (Cohen, 2007).

Mechanism of Action Interferes with bacterial cell wall synthesis during active multiplication, causing cell wall death and resultant bactericidal activity against susceptible bacteria

Pharmacodynamics/Kinetics

Duration: 1-4 weeks (dose dependent); larger doses result in more sustained levels

Distribution: Highest levels in the kidney; lesser amounts in liver, skin, intestines

Protein Binding: ~60%

Absorption: I.M.: Slow

Time to peak, serum: 12-24 hours

Dosage Note: Administer undiluted injection; higher doses result in more sustained rather than higher levels. Use a penicillin G benzathine-penicillin G procaine combination to achieve early peak levels in acute infections.

Usual dosage range:

Children: I.M.: 25,000-50,000 units/kg as a single dose (maximum: 2.4 million units)

Adults: I.M.: 1.2-2.4 million units as a single dose

Indication-specific dosing:

Infants and Children: I.M.:

Group A streptococcal upper respiratory infection:

Primary prevention of rheumatic fever (Gerber, 2009): ≤27 kg: 600,000 units as a single dose; >27 kg: 1.2 million units as a single dose

Secondary prevention of rheumatic fever (Gerber, 2009): ≤27 kg: 600,000 units every 3-4 weeks; >27 kg: 1.2 million units every 3-4 weeks

Syphilis (CDC, 2010):

Primary, Secondary, Early Latent (<1 year duration): Infants and Children: I.M.: 50,000 units/kg as a single injection (maximum: 2.4 million units)

Late Latent, Latent with unknown duration: Children: I.M.: 50,000 units/kg every week for 3 doses (maximum: 2.4 million units/dose)

Adults: I.M.:

Group A streptococcal upper respiratory infection: 1.2 million units as a single dose

Secondary prevention of glomerulonephritis: 1.2 million units every 4 weeks or 600,000 units twice monthly

Secondary prevention of rheumatic fever: 1.2 million units every 3-4 weeks or 600,000 units twice monthly

Syphilis (CDC, 2010):

Primary, Secondary, Early Latent (<1 year duration): 2.4 million units as a single dose in 2 injection sites

Late Latent, Latent with unknown duration: 2.4 million units in 2 injection sites once weekly for 3 doses

Neurosyphilis: Not indicated as single-drug therapy, but may be given once weekly for 3 weeks following I.V. treatment; refer to Penicillin G (Parenteral/Aqueous) monograph for dosing

Administration Warm to room temperature before administration to lessen the pain associated with injection. Administer by deep I.M. injection in the upper outer quadrant of the buttock; in children <2 years of age, I.M. injections should be made into the midlateral muscle of the thigh, not the gluteal region. Do not inject near an artery or a nerve; permanent neurological damage or gangrene may result. When doses are repeated, rotate the injection site. **Do not administer I.V., intra-arterially, or SubQ.**

Monitoring Parameters Observe for signs and symptoms of anaphylaxis during first dose

Test Interactions Positive Coombs' [direct], false-positive urinary and/or serum proteins; false-positive or negative urinary glucose using Clinitest®

Dosage Forms Excipient information presented when available (limited, particularly for generics); consult specific product labeling.

Injection, suspension:

Bicillin® L-A: 600,000 units/mL (1 mL, 2 mL, 4 mL)

Penicillin G Benzathine and Penicillin G Procaine

(pen i SIL in jee BENZ a theen & pen i SIL in jee PROE kane)

Brand Names: U.S. Bicillin® C-R; Bicillin® C-R 900/300

Index Terms Penicillin G Procaine and Benzathine Combined

Pharmacologic Category Antibiotic, Penicillin

Use May be used in specific situations in the treatment of streptococcal infections; primary prevention of rheumatic fever

Pregnancy Risk Factor B

Dosage

Usual dosage range and indication-specific dosing:

Streptococcal infections:

Children: I.M.:

<14 kg: 600,000 units in a single dose

14-27 kg: 900,000 units to 1.2 million units in a single dose

Children >27 kg and Adults: 2.4 million units in a single dose

Rheumatic fever, primary prevention (Bicillin® C-R 900/300): Children 6 months to 12 years: 1.2 million units as a single dose (Bass, 1976; Gerber, 2009). **Note:** The efficacy of this regimen for heavier patients is unknown.

Additional Information Complete prescribing information for this medication should be consulted for additional detail.

Dosage Forms Excipient information presented when available (limited, particularly for generics); consult specific product labeling. [DSC] = Discontinued product

Injection, suspension [prefilled syringe]:

Bicillin® C-R:

600,000 units: Penicillin G benzathine 300,000 units and penicillin G procaine 300,000 units per 1 mL (1 mL) [DSC]

1,200,000 units: Penicillin G benzathine 600,000 units and penicillin G procaine 600,000 units per 2 mL (2 mL)
2,400,000 units: Penicillin G benzathine 1,200,000 units and penicillin G procaine 1,200,000 units per 4 mL (4 mL) [DSC]
Bicillin® C-R 900/300: 1,200,000 units: Penicillin G benzathine 900,000 units and penicillin G procaine 300,000 units per 2 mL (2 mL)

Penicillin G (Parenteral/Aqueous)

(pen i SIL in jee, pa REN ter al, AYE kwee us)

Brand Names: U.S. Pfizerpen®

Brand Names: Canada Crystapen®

Index Terms Benzylpenicillin Potassium; Benzylpenicillin Sodium; Crystalline Penicillin; Penicillin G Potassium; Penicillin G Sodium

Pharmacologic Category Antibiotic, Penicillin

Additional Appendix Information

Antibiotic Treatment of Adults With Infective Endocarditis *on page 1956*

Use Treatment of infections (including sepsis, pneumonia, pericarditis, endocarditis, meningitis, anthrax) caused by susceptible organisms; active against some gram-positive organisms, generally not *Staphylococcus aureus*; some gram-negative organisms such as *Neisseria gonorrhoeae*, and some anaerobes and spirochetes

Pregnancy Risk Factor B

Pregnancy Considerations Adverse events have not been observed in animal studies; therefore, penicillin G is classified as pregnancy category B. Penicillin crosses the placenta and distributes into amniotic fluid. There is no evidence of adverse fetal effects after penicillin use during pregnancy in humans. Penicillin G is the drug of choice for treatment of syphilis during pregnancy and penicillin G (parenteral/aqueous) is the drug of choice for the prevention of early-onset Group B Streptococcal (GBS) disease in newborns.

Lactation Enters breast milk/compatible

Contraindications Hypersensitivity to penicillin or any component of the formulation

Warnings/Precautions Avoid intra-arterial administration or injection into or near major peripheral nerves or blood vessels since such injections may cause severe and/or permanent neurovascular damage; use with caution in patients with renal impairment (dosage reduction required), concomitant renal and hepatic impairment (further dosage adjustment may be required), pre-existing seizure disorders, or with a history of hypersensitivity to cephalosporins. Prolonged use may result in fungal or bacterial superinfection, including *C. difficile*-associated diarrhea (CDAD) and pseudomembranous colitis; CDAD has been observed >2 months postantibiotic treatment. Serious and occasionally severe or fatal hypersensitivity (anaphylactoid) reactions have been reported in patients on penicillin therapy, especially with a history of beta-lactam hypersensitivity, history of sensitivity to multiple allergens, or previous IgE-mediated reactions (eg, anaphylaxis, angioedema, urticaria). Use with caution in asthmatic patients. Extended duration of therapy or use associated with high serum concentrations may be associated with an increased risk for some adverse reactions. Neonates may have decreased renal clearance of penicillin and require frequent dosage adjustments depending on age. Product contains sodium and potassium; high doses of I.V. therapy may alter serum levels.

Adverse Reactions Frequency not defined.

Central nervous system: Coma (high doses), hyperreflexia (high doses), seizures (high doses)
Dermatologic: Contact dermatitis, rash
Endocrine & metabolic: Electrolyte imbalance (high doses)
Gastrointestinal: Pseudomembranous colitis
Hematologic: Neutropenia, positive Coombs' hemolytic anemia (rare, high doses)
Local: Injection site reaction, phlebitis, thrombophlebitis
Neuromuscular & skeletal: Myoclonus (high doses)
Renal: Acute interstitial nephritis (high doses), renal tubular damage (high doses)
Miscellaneous: Anaphylaxis, hypersensitivity reactions (immediate and delayed), Jarisch-Herxheimer reaction, serum sickness

Drug Interactions

Metabolism/Transport Effects None known.

Avoid Concomitant Use

Avoid concomitant use of Penicillin G (Parenteral/Aqueous) with any of the following: BCG

Increased Effect/Toxicity

Penicillin G (Parenteral/Aqueous) may increase the levels/effects of: Methotrexate; Vitamin K Antagonists

The levels/effects of Penicillin G (Parenteral/Aqueous) may be increased by: Probenecid

Decreased Effect

Penicillin G (Parenteral/Aqueous) may decrease the levels/effects of: BCG; Mycophenolate; Typhoid Vaccine

The levels/effects of Penicillin G (Parenteral/Aqueous) may be decreased by: Fusidic Acid; Tetracycline Derivatives

Stability

Penicillin G potassium powder for injection should be stored below 86°F (30°C). Following reconstitution, solution may be stored for up to 7 days under refrigeration. Premixed bags for infusion should be stored in the freezer (-20°C to -4°F); frozen bags may be thawed at room temperature or in refrigerator. Once thawed, solution is stable for 14 days if stored in refrigerator or for 24 hours when stored at room temperature. Do not refreeze once thawed.

Penicillin G sodium powder for injection should be stored at controlled room temperature. Reconstituted solution may be stored under refrigeration for up to 3 days.

Reconstitution:

Intermittent I.V.: 5 million unit vial: Add 8.2 mL for a final concentration of 500,000 units/mL; add 3.2 mL for a final concentration of 1,000,000 units/mL. Dilute further to 50,000-145,000 units/mL prior to infusion.

Continuous I.V. infusion: 20 million unit vial: Add 11.5 mL for a final concentration of 1,000,000 units/mL. Dilute further in 1-2 L of infusion solution and administer over a 24-hour period.

Mechanism of Action Interferes with bacterial cell wall synthesis during active multiplication, causing cell wall death and resultant bactericidal activity against susceptible bacteria

Pharmacodynamics/Kinetics

Distribution: Poor penetration across blood-brain barrier, despite inflamed meninges
Relative diffusion from blood into CSF: Poor unless meninges inflamed (exceeds usual MICs)
CSF:blood level ratio: Normal meninges: <1%; Inflamed meninges: 2% to 6%
Protein binding: 65%
Metabolism: Hepatic (30%) to penicilloic acid
Half-life elimination:
Neonates: <6 days old: 3.2-3.4 hours; 7-13 days old: 1.2-2.2 hours; >14 days old: 0.9-1.9 hours
Children and Adults: Normal renal function: 30-50 minutes
End-stage renal disease: 3.3-5.1 hours
Time to peak, serum: I.M.: ~30 minutes; I.V.: ~1 hour
Excretion: Urine (58% to 85% as unchanged drug)

Dosage

Usual dosage range:

Infants ≥1 month and Children: I.M., I.V.: 100,000-400,000 units/kg/day in divided doses every 4-6 hours (maximum dose: 24 million units/day)

Adults: I.M., I.V.: 2-30 million units/day in divided doses every 4-6 hours depending on sensitivity of the organism and severity of the infection

Indication-specific dosing:

Infants ≥1 month and Children:

Community-acquired pneumonia (CAP) (IDSA/PIDS, 2011): I.V.: Infants >3 months and Children: **Note:** May consider addition of vancomycin or clindamycin to empiric therapy if community-acquired MRSA suspected. In children ≥5 years, a macrolide antibiotic should be added if atypical pneumonia cannot be ruled out.

Empiric treatment or *S. pneumoniae* (moderate-to-severe; MICs to penicillin ≤2.0 mcg/mL) (preferred): 200,000-250,000 units/kg/day divided every 4-6 hours

Group A *Streptococcus* (moderate-to-severe) (preferred): 100,000-250,000 units/kg/day divided every 4-6 hours

***Meningitis* (gonococcal):** I.V.: 250,000 units/kg/day in 4 divided doses

Moderate infections: I.M., I.V.: 100,000-250,000 units/kg/day in 4 divided doses

Neurosyphilis: I.V.: 200,000-300,000 units/kg/day divided every 4-6 hours for 10-14 days (maximum dose: 24 million units/day)

Severe infections: I.M., I.V.: 250,000-400,000 units/kg/day in divided doses every 4-6 hours (maximum dose: 24 million units/day)

Syphilis (congenital): I.V.:

Infants: 50,000 units/kg every 12 hours for first 7 days of life, then every 8 hours for a total of 10 days (CDC, 2010)

Children: 50,000 units/kg every 4-6 hours for 10 days (CDC, 2010)

Adults:

***Actinomyces* species:** I.V.: 10-20 million units/day in divided doses every 4-6 hours for 4-6 weeks

Clostridium perfringens: I.V.: 24 million units/day in divided doses every 4-6 hours with clindamycin

Corynebacterium diphtheriae: I.V.: 2-3 million units/day in divided doses every 4-6 hours for 10-12 days

Erysipelas: I.V.: 1-2 million units every 4-6 hours

Erysipelothrix: I.V.: 2-4 million units every 4 hours

Fascial space infections: I.V.: 2-4 million units every 4-6 hours with metronidazole

Leptospirosis: I.V.: 1.5 million units every 6 hours for 7 days

Listeria: I.V.: 15-20 million units/day in divided doses every 4-6 hours for 2 weeks (meningitis) or 4 weeks (endocarditis)

Lyme disease (meningitis): I.V.: 20 million units/day in divided doses

Neurosyphilis: I.V.: 18-24 million units/day in divided doses every 4 hours (or by continuous infusion) for 10-14 days (CDC, 2006; CDC, 2009; CDC, 2010)

Streptococcus:

Brain abscess: I.V.: 18-24 million units/day in divided doses every 4 hours with metronidazole

Endocarditis or osteomyelitis: I.V.: 3-4 million units every 4 hours for at least 4 weeks

Pregnancy (prophylaxis GBS): I.V.: 5 million units x 1 dose, then 2.5 million units every 4 hours until delivery (AGOG, 2002; CDC, 2002)

Skin and soft tissue: I.V.: 3-4 million units every 4 hours for 10 days

Toxic shock: I.V.: 24 million units/day in divided doses with clindamycin

Streptococcal pneumonia: I.V.: 2-3 million units every 4 hours

Whipple's disease: I.V.: 2 million units every 4 hours for 2 weeks, followed by oral trimethoprim/sulfamethoxazole or doxycycline for 1 year

Relapse or CNS involvement: 4 million units every 4 hours for 4 weeks

Dosing adjustment in renal impairment:

Uremic patients with Cl_{cr} >10 mL/minute/1.73 m^2: Administer full loading dose followed by 1/2 of the loading dose given every 4-5 hours

Cl_{cr} <10 mL/minute/1.73 m^2: Administer full loading dose followed by 1/2 of the loading dose given every 8-10 hours

Intermittent hemodialysis (IHD) (administer after hemodialysis on dialysis days): Administer normal loading dose followed by either 25% to 50% of normal dose every 4-6 hours **or** 50% to 100% of normal dose every 8-12 hours. For mild-to-moderate infections, administer 0.5-1 million units every 4-6 hours **or** 1-2 million units every 8-12 hours. For neurosyphilis, endocarditis, or serious infections, administer up to 2 million units every 4-6 hours; administer after dialysis on dialysis days **or** supplement with 500,000 units after dialysis (Heintz, 2009). **Note:** Dosing dependent on the assumption of 3 times/week, complete IHD sessions.

Continuous renal replacement therapy (CRRT) (Heintz, 2009; Trotman, 2005): Drug clearance is highly dependent on the method of renal replacement, filter type, and flow rate. Appropriate dosing requires close monitoring of pharmacologic response, signs of adverse reactions due to drug accumulation, as well as drug concentrations in relation to target trough (if appropriate). The following are general recommendations only (based on dialysate flow/ultrafiltration rates of 1-2 L/hour and minimal residual renal function) and should not supersede clinical judgment:

CVVH: Loading dose of 4 million units, followed by 2 million units every 4-6 hours

CVVHD: Loading dose of 4 million units, followed by 2-3 million units every 4-6 hours

CVVHDF: Loading dose of 4 million units, followed by 2-4 million units every 4-6 hours

Dietary Considerations Some products may contain potassium and/or sodium.

Administration

I.M.: Administer I.M. by deep injection in the upper outer quadrant of the buttock

I.V.: **Note:** The 20 million unit dosage form may be administered by continuous I.V. infusion only.

Intermittent I.V.: May be dissolved in small amounts of SWFI, NS, D_5W and administered peripherally as a 50,000-100,000 unit/mL solution. In fluid-restricted patients, 146,000 units/mL in SW results in a maximum recommended osmolality for peripheral infusion. Infuse over 15-30 minutes.

Continuous I.V. infusion: Determine the volume of fluid and rate of its administration required by the patient in a 24-hour period. Add the appropriate daily dosage of penicillin to this fluid. For example, if the daily dose is 10 million units and 2 L of fluid/day is required, add 5 million units to 1 L and adjust the rate of flow so the liter will be infused over 12 hours (83 mL/hour). Repeat steps (5 million units/L at 83 mL/hour) for the remaining 12 hours.

Monitoring Parameters Periodic electrolyte, hepatic, renal, cardiac and hematologic function tests during prolonged/high-dose therapy; observe for signs and symptoms of anaphylaxis during first dose

Test Interactions False-positive or negative urinary glucose determination using Clinitest®; positive Coombs' [direct]; false-positive urinary and/or serum proteins

Additional Information 1 million units is approximately equal to 625 mg.

Dosage Forms Excipient information presented when available (limited, particularly for generics); consult specific product labeling.

Infusion, premixed iso-osmotic dextrose solution, as potassium: 1 million units (50 mL); 2 million units (50 mL); 3 million units (50 mL)

Injection, powder for reconstitution, as potassium: 5 million units, 20 million units

Pfizerpen®: 5 million units, 20 million units [contains potassium 65.6 mg (1.68 mEq) per 1 million units, sodium 6.8 mg (0.3 mEq) per 1 million units]

Injection, powder for reconstitution, as sodium: 5 million units

◆ **Penicillin G Potassium** *see* Penicillin G (Parenteral/Aqueous) *on page* 1323

Penicillin G Procaine (pen i SIL in jee PROE kane)

Brand Names: Canada Pfizerpen-AS®; Wycillin®

Index Terms APPG; Aqueous Procaine Penicillin G; Procaine Benzylpenicillin; Procaine Penicillin G; Wycillin [DSC]

Pharmacologic Category Antibiotic, Penicillin

Use Treatment of moderately-severe infections due to *Treponema pallidum* and other penicillin G-sensitive microorganisms that are susceptible to low, but prolonged serum penicillin concentrations; anthrax due to *Bacillus anthracis* (postexposure) to reduce the incidence or progression of disease following exposure to aerolized *Bacillus anthracis*

Pregnancy Risk Factor B

Pregnancy Considerations Adverse events have not been observed in animal studies; therefore, penicillin G is classified as pregnancy category B. Penicillin crosses the placenta and distributes into amniotic fluid. There is no evidence of adverse fetal effects after penicillin use during pregnancy in humans.

Lactation Enters breast milk/compatible

Contraindications Hypersensitivity to penicillin, procaine, or any component of the formulation

Warnings/Precautions May need to modify dosage in patients with severe renal impairment or seizure disorders; avoid I.V., intravascular, or intra-arterial administration of penicillin G procaine since severe and/or permanent neurovascular damage may occur. Serious and occasionally severe or fatal hypersensitivity (anaphylactoid) reactions have been reported in patients on penicillin therapy, especially with a history of beta-lactam hypersensitivity, history of sensitivity to multiple allergens, or previous IgE-mediated reactions (eg, anaphylaxis, angioedema, urticaria). Use with caution in asthmatic patients. Extended duration of therapy or use associated with high serum concentrations may be associated with an increased risk for some adverse reactions. Prolonged use may result in fungal or bacterial superinfection, including *C. difficile*-associated diarrhea (CDAD) and pseudomembranous colitis; CDAD has been observed >2 months postantibiotic treatment.

Adverse Reactions Frequency not defined.

Cardiovascular: Conduction disturbances, myocardial depression, vasodilation

Central nervous system: CNS stimulation, confusion, drowsiness, myoclonus, seizure

Hematologic: Hemolytic anemia, neutropenia, positive Coombs' reaction

Local: Pain at injection site, sterile abscess at injection site, thrombophlebitis

Renal: Interstitial nephritis

Miscellaneous: Hypersensitivity reactions, Jarisch-Herxheimer reaction, pseudoanaphylactic reactions, serum sickness

Drug Interactions

Metabolism/Transport Effects None known.

Avoid Concomitant Use

Avoid concomitant use of Penicillin G Procaine with any of the following: BCG

Increased Effect/Toxicity

Penicillin G Procaine may increase the levels/effects of: Methotrexate; Vitamin K Antagonists

The levels/effects of Penicillin G Procaine may be increased by: Probenecid

Decreased Effect

Penicillin G Procaine may decrease the levels/effects of: BCG; Mycophenolate; Typhoid Vaccine

The levels/effects of Penicillin G Procaine may be decreased by: Fusidic Acid; Tetracycline Derivatives

Stability Refrigerate

Mechanism of Action Inhibits bacterial cell wall synthesis by binding to one or more of the penicillin-binding proteins (PBPs); which in turn inhibits the final transpeptidation step of peptidoglycan synthesis in bacterial cell walls, thus inhibiting cell wall biosynthesis. Bacteria eventually lyse due to ongoing activity of cell wall autolytic enzymes (autolysins and murein hydrolases) while cell wall assembly is arrested.

Pharmacodynamics/Kinetics

Duration: Therapeutic: 15-24 hours

Absorption: I.M.: Slow

Distribution: Penetration across the blood-brain barrier is poor, despite inflamed meninges

Protein binding: 65%

Metabolism: ~30% hepatically inactivated

Time to peak, serum: 1-4 hours

Excretion: Urine (60% to 90% as unchanged drug)

Clearance: Renal: Delayed in neonates, young infants, and with impaired renal function

Dosage

Usual dosage range:

Infants and Children: I.M.: 25,000-50,000 units/kg/day in divided doses 1-2 times/day (maximum: 4.8 million units/day)

Adults: I.M.: 0.6-4.8 million units/day in divided doses every 12-24 hours

Indication-specific dosing:

Children: I.M.:

Anthrax, inhalational (postexposure prophylaxis): 25,000 units/kg every 12 hours (maximum: 1,200,000 units every 12 hours); see **"Note"** in adult dosing

Syphilis (congenital): 50,000 units/kg/day for 10 days; if more than 1 day of therapy is missed, the entire course should be restarted

Adults: I.M.:

Anthrax:

Inhalational (postexposure prophylaxis): 1,200,000 units every 12 hours

Note: Overall treatment duration should be 60 days. Available safety data suggest continued administration of penicillin G procaine for longer than 2 weeks may incur additional risk for adverse reactions. Clinicians may consider switching to effective alternative treatment for completion of therapy beyond 2 weeks.

Cutaneous (treatment): 600,000-1,200,000 units/day; alternative therapy is recommended in severe cutaneous or other forms of anthrax infection

Endocarditis caused by susceptible viridans *Streptococcus* (when used in conjunction with an aminoglycoside): 1.2 million units every 6 hours for 2-4 weeks

Gonorrhea (uncomplicated): 4.8 million units as a single dose divided in 2 sites given 30 minutes after probenecid 1 g orally

Neurosyphilis: 2.4 million units/day with 500 mg probenecid by mouth 4 times/day for 10-14 days; **Note: Penicillin G aqueous I.V. is the preferred agent**

Whipple's disease: 1.2 million units/day (with streptomycin) for 10-14 days, followed by oral trimethoprim/sulfamethoxazole or doxycycline for 1 year

Hemodialysis: Moderately dialyzable (20% to 50%)

Administration Procaine suspension for deep I.M. injection only; do not inject in gluteal muscle in children <2 years of age; rotate the injection site; avoid I.V., intravascular, or intra-arterial administration of penicillin G procaine since severe and/or permanent neurovascular damage may occur

Monitoring Parameters Periodic renal and hematologic function tests with prolonged therapy; fever, mental status, WBC count

Test Interactions Positive Coombs' [direct], false-positive urinary and/or serum proteins

Dosage Forms Excipient information presented when available (limited, particularly for generics); consult specific product labeling.

Injection, suspension: 600,000 units/mL (1 mL, 2 mL)

◆ **Penicillin G Procaine and Benzathine Combined** *see* Penicillin G Benzathine and Penicillin G Procaine *on page* 1322

◆ **Penicillin G Sodium** *see* Penicillin G (Parenteral/Aqueous) *on page* 1323

Penicillin V Potassium

(pen i SIL in vee poe TASS ee um)

Brand Names: Canada Apo-Pen VK®; Novo-Pen-VK; Nu-Pen-VK

Index Terms Pen VK; Phenoxymethyl Penicillin

Pharmacologic Category Antibiotic, Penicillin

Use Treatment of infections caused by susceptible organisms involving the respiratory tract, otitis media, sinusitis, skin, and urinary tract; prophylaxis in rheumatic fever

Pregnancy Risk Factor B

Pregnancy Considerations Adverse events have not been observed in animal studies; therefore, penicillin V is classified as pregnancy category B. Penicillin crosses the placenta and distributes into amniotic fluid. There is no evidence of adverse fetal effects after penicillin use during pregnancy in humans. Due to pregnancy-induced physiologic changes, some pharmacokinetic parameters of penicillin V may be altered in the second and third trimester. Higher doses or increased dosing frequency may be required.

Lactation Enters breast milk/compatible

Contraindications Hypersensitivity to penicillin or any component of the formulation

Warnings/Precautions Use with caution in patients with severe renal impairment (modify dosage) or history of seizures. Serious and occasionally severe or fatal hypersensitivity (anaphylactoid) reactions have been reported in patients on penicillin therapy, especially with a history of beta-lactam hypersensitivity, history of sensitivity to multiple allergens, or previous IgE-mediated reactions (eg, anaphylaxis, angioedema, urticaria). Use with caution in asthmatic patients. Extended duration of therapy or use associated with high serum concentrations may be associated with an increased risk for some adverse reactions. Prolonged use may result in fungal or bacterial superinfection, including *C. difficile*-associated diarrhea (CDAD) and pseudomembranous colitis; CDAD has been observed >2 months postantibiotic treatment.

Adverse Reactions

>10%: Gastrointestinal: Mild diarrhea, vomiting, nausea, oral candidiasis

<1% (Limited to important or life-threatening): Acute interstitial nephritis, convulsions, hemolytic anemia, positive Coombs' reaction

Drug Interactions

Metabolism/Transport Effects None known.

Avoid Concomitant Use

Avoid concomitant use of Penicillin V Potassium with any of the following: BCG

Increased Effect/Toxicity

Penicillin V Potassium may increase the levels/effects of: Methotrexate; Vitamin K Antagonists

The levels/effects of Penicillin V Potassium may be increased by: Probenecid

Decreased Effect

Penicillin V Potassium may decrease the levels/effects of: BCG; Mycophenolate; Typhoid Vaccine

The levels/effects of Penicillin V Potassium may be decreased by: Fusidic Acid; Tetracycline Derivatives

Ethanol/Nutrition/Herb Interactions Food: Decreases drug absorption rate; decreases drug serum concentration.

Stability Refrigerate suspension after reconstitution; discard after 14 days

Mechanism of Action Inhibits bacterial cell wall synthesis by binding to one or more of the penicillin-binding proteins (PBPs); which in turn inhibits the final transpeptidation step of peptidoglycan synthesis in bacterial cell walls, thus inhibiting cell wall biosynthesis. Bacteria eventually lyse due to ongoing activity of cell wall autolytic enzymes (autolysins and murein hydrolases) while cell wall assembly is arrested.

Pharmacodynamics/Kinetics

Absorption: 60% to 73%

Distribution: Widely distributed to kidneys, liver, skin, tonsils, and into synovial, pleural, and pericardial fluids

Protein binding, plasma: 80%

Half-life elimination: 30 minutes; prolonged with renal impairment

Time to peak, serum: 0.5-1 hour

Excretion: Urine (as unchanged drug and metabolites)

Dosage

Usual dosage range:

Children <12 years: Oral: 25-50 mg/kg/day in divided doses every 6-8 hours (maximum dose: 3 g/day)

Children ≥12 years and Adults: Oral: 125-500 mg every 6-8 hours

Indication-specific dosing:

Infants >3 months and Children: Oral:

Community-acquired pneumonia (CAP) due to group A *Streptococcus*, mild infection or step-down therapy (preferred) (IDSA/PIDS, 2011): 50-75 mg/kg/day in 3-4 divided doses

Children: Oral:

Pharyngitis (streptococcal): 250 mg 2-3 times/day for 10 days

Prophylaxis of pneumococcal infections:

Children <5 years: 125 mg twice daily

Children ≥5 years: 250 mg twice daily

Prophylaxis of recurrent rheumatic fever:

Children <5 years: 125 mg twice daily

Children ≥5 years: 250 mg twice daily

Adults: Oral:

Actinomycosis:

Mild: 2-4 g/day in 4 divided doses for 8 weeks

Surgical: 2-4 g/day in 4 divided doses for 6-12 months (after I.V. penicillin G therapy of 4-6 weeks)

Erysipelas: 500 mg 4 times/day

Periodontal infections: 250-500 mg every 6 hours for 5-7 days

Note: Efficacy of antimicrobial therapy in periapical abscess is questionable; the American Academy of Periodontology recommends use of antibiotic therapy only when systemic symptoms (eg, fever, lymphadenopathy) are present or in immunocompromised patients.

Pharyngitis (streptococcal): 500 mg 3-4 times/day for 10 days

Prophylaxis of pneumococcal or recurrent rheumatic fever infections: 250 mg twice daily

Dosing interval in renal impairment: Cl_{cr} <10 mL/minute: Administer 250 mg every 6 hours

Dietary Considerations Take on an empty stomach 1 hour before or 2 hours after meals.

Administration Administer on an empty stomach to increase oral absorption

Monitoring Parameters Periodic renal and hematologic function tests during prolonged therapy; monitor for signs of anaphylaxis during first dose

Test Interactions False-positive or negative urinary glucose determination using Clinitest®; positive Coombs' [direct]; false-positive urinary and/or serum proteins

Additional Information 0.7 mEq of potassium per 250 mg penicillin V; 250 mg equals 400,000 units of penicillin

Dosage Forms Excipient information presented when available (limited, particularly for generics); consult specific product labeling.

Powder for solution, oral: 125 mg/5 mL (100 mL, 200 mL); 250 mg/5 mL (100 mL, 200 mL)

Tablet, oral: 250 mg, 500 mg

- **Penlac®** *see* Ciclopirox *on page 356*
- **Pentacel®** *see* Diphtheria and Tetanus Toxoids, Acellular Pertussis, Poliovirus and *Haemophilus* b Conjugate Vaccine *on page 522*
- **Pentahydrate** *see* Sodium Thiosulfate *on page 1577*
- **Pentam® 300** *see* Pentamidine *on page 1327*

Pentamidine (pen TAM i deen)

Brand Names: U.S. Nebupent®; Pentam® 300

Index Terms Pentamidine Isethionate

Pharmacologic Category Antifungal Agent; Antiprotozoal

Use

I.M., I.V.: Treatment of pneumonia caused by *Pneumocystis jirovecii* pneumonia (PCP)

Inhalation: Prevention of PCP in high-risk, HIV-infected patients either with a history of PCP or with a CD4+ count ≤200/mm^3

Unlabeled Use Prevention of PCP in nonHIV-infected patients; treatment of African trypanosomiasis, cutaneous leishmaniasis, and amebic meningoencephalitis

Pregnancy Risk Factor C

Pregnancy Considerations Animal reproductive studies were not conducted by the manufacturer; therefore, pentamidine is classified pregnancy category C. In postmarketing studies, pentamidine was embryocidal but not teratogenic when administered to animals. Pentamidine crosses the human placenta. Administration via the aerosolized route may minimize maternal serum concentrations. Concern regarding occupational exposure of pregnant healthcare workers has been discussed in the literature. Pregnant healthcare workers should avoid aerolized exposure if possible. If avoidance is not possible, they should wear a mask and gloves and ensure proper ventilation. Pentamidine may be used in pregnancy for prophylaxis or treatment of PCP if the patient is unable to take first line medications.

Lactation Excretion in breast milk unknown/not recommended

Contraindications Hypersensitivity to pentamidine isethionate or any component of the formulation

Warnings/Precautions Hazardous agent - use appropriate precautions for handling and disposal. Severe hypotension (some fatalities) has been observed (even after a single dose); may occur with either I.V. or I.M administration, although more common with rapid I.V. administration; monitor blood pressure during (and after) infusion. May cause QT prolongation and subsequent torsade de pointes; avoid use in patients with diagnosed or suspected congenital long QT syndrome. Use with caution in patients with pre-existing cardiovascular disease; hyper-/hypotension and arrhythmia, including ventricular tachycardia (eg, torsade de pointes) have been reported.

Use with caution in patients with diabetes mellitus or hypocalcemia; hyper-/hypoglycemia and pancreatic islet cell necrosis with hyperinsulinemia has been reported. Symptoms may occur months after therapy; monitor blood glucose daily on therapy and periodically thereafter. Use with caution in patients with a history of pancreatic disease or elevated amylase/lipase levels; acute pancreatitis (with fatality) has been reported. Discontinue if signs/symptoms of acute pancreatitis occur. Concurrent use with other bone marrow suppressants may increase the risk for myelotoxicity; use with caution in patients with current evidence and/or prior history of hematologic disorders; anemia, leukopenia and/or thrombocytopenia have been reported. Use with caution in patients with hepatic or renal disease. Concurrent use with other nephrotoxic drugs may increase the risk for nephrotoxicity. Avoid concurrent use with other drugs known to prolong QT_c interval. Stevens-Johnson syndrome has been reported with use. Avoid extravasation; may cause tissue ulceration, necrosis, and/or sloughing; if extravasation occurs, treat symptomatically. Assess catheter position before and during infusion.

Aerosolized pentamidine may induce bronchospasm or cough, especially in patients with a smoking or asthma history (an inhaled bronchodilator prior to pentamidine may ameliorate symptoms). Use appropriate precautions to minimize exposure to healthcare personnel; refer to individual institutional policy. Acute PCP may develop despite aerosolized pentamidine prophylaxis. Although rare, extrapulmonary PCP disease may occur and has been associated with aerosolized pentamidine.

Adverse Reactions

Aerosol:

>10%:

Central nervous system: Fatigue (66%), fever (51%), dizziness/lightheadedness (45%)

Gastrointestinal: Appetite decreased (50%)

Respiratory: Cough (1% to 63%), dyspnea (48%), wheezing (32%)

Miscellaneous: Infection (15%)

1% to 10%:

Central nervous system: Headache

Gastrointestinal: Diarrhea, nausea, oral candida, taste alteration

Hematologic: Anemia

Respiratory: Bronchitis, chest pain, pharyngitis, sinusitis, upper respiratory tract infection

Miscellaneous: Herpes infection, influenza, night sweats

Injection:

>10%:

Local: Local reactions at I.M. injection site (11%; includes sterile abscess, necrosis, pain, induration)

Renal: Renal function impaired (29%), creatinine increased (24%)

1% to 10%:
- Cardiovascular: Hypotension (5%)
- Central nervous system: Confusion/hallucinations (2%)
- Dermatologic: Rash (3%)
- Endocrine & metabolic: Hypoglycemia (6%)
- Gastrointestinal: Nausea/anorexia (6%), taste alteration (2%)
- Hematologic: Leukopenia (10%), thrombocytopenia (3%), anemia (1%)
- Hepatic: Liver function tests increased (9%)
- Renal: Azotemia (9%), BUN increased (7%)

Aerosol or injection: <1% (Limited to important or life-threatening): Abdominal pain, allergic reaction, anaphylaxis, anxiety, arthralgia, asthma, blepharitis, blurred vision, bronchitis, bronchospasm, cardiac arrhythmia, central venous line related sepsis, cerebrovascular accident, chest tightness, chills, clotting time prolonged, CMV infection, colitis, confusion, congestion (chest, nasal), conjunctivitis, cough, cryptococcal meningitis, cyanosis, defibrination, depression, dermatitis, desquamation, diabetes mellitus, diabetic ketoacidosis, diarrhea, dizziness, drowsiness, dyspepsia, dyspnea, emotional lability, eosinophilia, erythema, esophagitis, extrapulmonary pneumocystosis, extravasation (tissue ulceration, necrosis, and/or sloughing), facial edema, flank pain, gait unsteady, gagging, gingivitis, headache, hearing loss, hematochezia, hematuria, hemoptysis, hepatic dysfunction, hepatitis, hepatomegaly, histoplasmosis, hyperglycemia, hyperkalemia, hypersalivation, hypertension, hyperventilation, hypesthesia, hypocalcemia, hypomagnesemia, incontinence, insomnia, laryngitis, laryngospasm, leg edema, melena, memory loss, nephritis, nervousness, neuralgia, neuropathy, neutropenia, night sweats, palpitation, pancreatitis, pancytopenia, paranoia, paresthesia, peripheral neuropathy, phlebitis, pleuritis, pneumonitis (eosinophilic or interstitial), pneumothorax, pruritus, rales, renal dysfunction, renal failure, rhinitis, seizure, splenomegaly, Stevens-Johnson syndrome, ST segment abnormal, syncope, syndrome of inappropriate antidiuretic hormone (SIADH), tachycardia, tachypnea, temperature abnormal, torsade de pointes, tremor, vasodilation, vasculitis, ventricular tachycardia, vertigo, vomiting, urticaria, xerostomia

Drug Interactions

Metabolism/Transport Effects Substrate of CYP2C19 (major); **Note:** Assignment of Major/Minor substrate status based on clinically relevant drug interaction potential; **Inhibits** CYP2C19 (weak), CYP2C9 (weak), CYP2D6 (weak), CYP3A4 (weak)

Avoid Concomitant Use

Avoid concomitant use of Pentamidine with any of the following: Artemether; BCG; Dronedarone; Lumefantrine; Nilotinib; Pimozide; QUEtiapine; QuiNINE; Tetrabenazine; Thioridazine; Toremifene; Vandetanib; Vemurafenib; Ziprasidone

Increased Effect/Toxicity

Pentamidine may increase the levels/effects of: Dronedarone; Pimozide; QTc-Prolonging Agents; QuiNINE; Tetrabenazine; Thioridazine; Toremifene; Vandetanib; Vemurafenib; Ziprasidone

The levels/effects of Pentamidine may be increased by: Alfuzosin; Artemether; Chloroquine; Ciprofloxacin; Ciprofloxacin (Systemic); CYP2C19 Inhibitors (Moderate); CYP2C19 Inhibitors (Strong); Gadobutrol; Indacaterol; Lumefantrine; Nilotinib; QUEtiapine; QuiNINE

Decreased Effect

Pentamidine may decrease the levels/effects of: BCG; Typhoid Vaccine

The levels/effects of Pentamidine may be decreased by: CYP2C19 Inducers (Strong)

Ethanol/Nutrition/Herb Interactions Ethanol: Avoid ethanol (may increase CNS depression or aggravate hypoglycemia).

Stability Store intact vials at 20°C to 25°C (68°F to 77°F); protect from light. Do not use sodium chloride for initial reconstitution (sodium chloride will cause precipitation).

Aerosol: Reconstitute with 6 mL SWFI. The manufacturer recommends the use of freshly prepared solutions for inhalation; however, may be stored for up to 48 hours in the vial at room temperature if protected from light. Do not mix with other nebulizer solutions.

Injection: I.M.: Reconstitute with 3 mL SWFI; I.V.: Reconstitute with 3-5 mL SWFI or D_5W; the manufacturer recommends further dilution in 50-250 mL D_5W; however, stability with further dilution in NS has also been documented. Store at room temperature to avoid crystallization. Reconstituted solution is stable for 48 hours in the vial at room temperature and protected from light. Solutions for injection (1-2.5 mg/mL) in D_5W are stable for at least 24 hours at room temperature.

Mechanism of Action Interferes with microbial RNA/DNA, phospholipids and protein synthesis, through inhibition of oxidative phosphorylation and/or interference with incorporation of nucleotides and nucleic acids into RNA and DNA

Pharmacodynamics/Kinetics

Absorption: I.M.: Well absorbed; Inhalation: Limited systemic absorption

Distribution: V_{dss}: I.V.: 286-1356 L; I.M.: 1658-3790 L

Half-life elimination: I.V.: 5-8 hours; I.M.: 7-11 hours; may be prolonged with severe renal impairment

Excretion: Urine (I.V.: ≤12% as unchanged drug)

Dosage

Children:

PCP:

FDA-approved labeling: Children >4 months: Treatment: I.M., I.V.: 4 mg/kg once daily for 14-21 days

CDC recommendation:

Prevention (children ≥5 years): Inhalation: 300 mg/dose monthly via Respirgard® II nebulizer

Treatment: I.V.: 3-4 mg/kg once daily for 21 days

AIDS*info* guidelines (2009):

Prevention: Children ≥5 years: Inhalation: 300 mg/dose monthly via Respirgard® II nebulizer

Treatment: I.V.: 4 mg/kg once daily, if clinical improvement may change to atovaquone after 7-10 days

PCP prevention in pediatric oncology patients (age <5 years, intolerant to trimethoprim-sulfamethoxazole; unlabeled use): 4 mg/kg I.V. once monthly (Kim, 2008; Prasad, 2007)

Cutaneous leishmaniasis (unlabeled use; CDC recommendation): I.M., I.V.: 2-3 mg/kg once daily or every second day for 4-7 doses

Trypanosomiasis (unlabeled use; CDC recommendation): I.M.: 4 mg/kg once daily for 7 days

Adults:

PCP:

FDA-approved labeling:

Prevention: Inhalation: 300 mg every 4 weeks via Respirgard® II nebulizer

Treatment: I.M., I.V.: 4 mg/kg once daily for 14-21 days

CDC recommendation:

Prevention: Inhalation: 300 mg monthly via Respirgard® II nebulizer

Treatment: I.V.: 3-4 mg/kg once daily for 21 days

AIDS*info* guidelines (2009):

Prevention: Inhalation: 300 mg/dose monthly via Respirgard® II nebulizer

Treatment: I.V.: 4 mg/kg once daily, 3 mg/kg may be used by some clinicians

Cutaneous leishmaniasis (unlabeled use; CDC recommendation): I.M., I.V.: 2-3 mg/kg once daily or every second day for 4-7 doses

Trypanosomiasis (unlabeled use; CDC recommendation): I.M.: 4 mg/kg once daily for 7 days

Dosing adjustment in renal impairment: I.V.: The FDA-approved labeling recommends that caution should be used in patients with renal impairment; however, no specific dosage adjustment guidelines are available. The following guidelines have been used by some clinicians (Aronoff, 2007):

Children:

Cl_{cr} >30 mL/minute: No adjustment required

Cl_{cr} 10-30 mL/minute: Administer 4 mg/kg every 36 hours

Cl_{cr} <10 mL/minute and peritoneal dialysis: Administer 4 mg/kg every 48 hours

Hemodialysis: Administer 4 mg/kg every 48 hours, after dialysis on dialysis days

Adults:

Cl_{cr} ≥10 mL/minute: No adjustment required

Cl_{cr} <10 mL/minute: Administer 4 mg/kg every 24-36 hours

Administration Do not use NS to reconstitute.

Inhalation: Deliver via Respirgard® II nebulizer until nebulizer is emptied (30-45 minutes). Administer at a flow rate of 5-7 L/minute from a 40-50 pound-per-square inch (PSI) oxygen or air source. A 40-50 PSI air compressor can be used alternatively, with a set flow rate at 5-7 L/minute or a set pressure of 22-25 PSI. Air compressors <20 PSI should not be used. Use appropriate precautions to minimize exposure to healthcare personnel; refer to individual institutional policy.

I.V.: Infuse slowly over 60-120 minutes. Avoid extravasation; assess catheter position before and during infusion.

I.M.: Administer deep I.M.

Monitoring Parameters Liver function tests, renal function tests, blood glucose, serum potassium and calcium, CBC and platelets; ECG, blood pressure

Dosage Forms Excipient information presented when available (limited, particularly for generics); consult specific product labeling.

Injection, powder for reconstitution, as isethionate:

Pentam® 300: 300 mg

Powder for solution, for nebulization, as isethionate:

Nebupent®: 300 mg

◆ **Pentamidine Isethionate** *see* Pentamidine *on page* 1327

◆ **Pentamycetin® (Can)** *see* Chloramphenicol *on page* 338

◆ **Pentasa®** *see* Mesalamine *on page* 1081

◆ **Pentasodium Colistin Methanesulfonate** *see* Colistimethate *on page* 409

◆ **Pentavalent Human-Bovine Reassortant Rotavirus Vaccine (PRV)** *see* Rotavirus Vaccine *on page* 1526

Pentazocine (pen TAZ oh seen)

Brand Names: U.S. Talwin®

Brand Names: Canada Talwin®

Index Terms Pentazocine Lactate

Pharmacologic Category Analgesic, Opioid; Analgesic, Opioid Partial Agonist

Additional Appendix Information

Beers Criteria - Potentially Inappropriate Medications for Geriatrics *on page* 1973

Opioid Analgesics *on page* 1896

Use Relief of moderate-to-severe pain; has also been used as a sedative prior to surgery and as a supplement to surgical anesthesia

Pregnancy Risk Factor C

Dosage

Preoperative/preanesthetic: Children 1-16 years: I.M.: 0.5 mg/kg

Analgesia:

Children (unlabeled use): I.M.:

5-8 years: 15 mg

9-14 years: 30 mg

Adults:

I.M., SubQ: 30-60 mg every 3-4 hours; do not exceed 60 mg/dose (maximum: 360 mg/day)

I.V.: 30 mg every 3-4 hours; do not exceed 30 mg/dose (maximum: 360 mg/day)

Labor pain: Adults:

I.M.: 30 mg once

I.V.: 20 mg every 2-3 hours as needed (maximum total dose: 60 mg)

Elderly: Elderly patients may be more sensitive to the analgesic and sedating effects. The elderly may also have impaired renal function. If needed, dosing should be started at the lower end of dosing range and adjust dose for renal function.

Dosing adjustment in renal impairment:

Cl_{cr} 10-50 mL/minute: Administer 75% of normal dose

Cl_{cr} <10 mL/minute: Administer 50% of normal dose

Dosing adjustment in hepatic impairment: Reduce dose or avoid use in patients with liver disease

Additional Information Complete prescribing information for this medication should be consulted for additional detail.

Dosage Forms Excipient information presented when available (limited, particularly for generics); consult specific product labeling.

Injection, solution:

Talwin®: 30 mg/mL (1 mL)

Talwin®: 30 mg/mL (10 mL) [contains sodium bisulfite]

Controlled Substance C-IV

◆ **Pentazocine Lactate** *see* Pentazocine *on page* 1329

PENTobarbital (pen toe BAR bi tal)

Brand Names: U.S. Nembutal®

Brand Names: Canada Nembutal® Sodium

Index Terms Pentobarbital Sodium

Pharmacologic Category Anticonvulsant, Barbiturate; Barbiturate

Additional Appendix Information

Status Epilepticus *on page* 2010

Use Sedative/hypnotic; refractory status epilepticus

Unlabeled Use Barbiturate coma in patients with severe brain injury (eg, hemorrhagic stroke, traumatic brain injury) and increased intracranial pressure

Pregnancy Risk Factor D

Pregnancy Considerations Barbiturates can be detected in the placenta, fetal liver and fetal brain. Fetal and maternal blood concentrations may be similar following parenteral administration. An increased incidence of fetal abnormalities may occur following maternal use. When used during the third trimester of pregnancy, withdrawal symptoms may occur in the neonate including seizures and hyperirritability; symptoms may be delayed up to 14 days. Use during labor does not impair uterine activity; however, respiratory depression may occur in the newborn; resuscitation equipment should be available, especially for premature infants.

Lactation Enters breast milk/use caution

Contraindications Hypersensitivity to barbiturates or any component of the formulation; porphyria

Warnings/Precautions May cause hypotension particularly when administered intravenously; use with caution in hemodynamically unstable patients (hypotension or shock). High doses used to induce pentobarbital coma cause hypotension requiring vasopressor therapy. May cause respiratory depression particularly when administered intravenously; use with caution in patients with respiratory disease. Intubation is typically required prior to treatment for status epilepticus or traumatic brain injury. Anticonvulsants should not be discontinued abruptly because of the possibility of increasing seizure frequency; therapy should be withdrawn gradually to minimize the potential of increased seizure frequency, unless safety concerns require a more rapid withdrawal. Do not administer to patients in acute pain; may heighten/worsen sense of pain.

Use with caution in patients with hepatic or renal impairment; reduce dose as appropriate. Do not use in patients with premonitory signs of hepatic coma. Use with caution in patients with a history of drug abuse; potential for drug dependency exists. Tolerance, psychological and physical dependence may occur with prolonged use. Use with caution in patients with depression or suicidal tendencies. Use with caution in the elderly; closely monitor elderly or debilitated patients for impaired cognitive or motor performance; may be inappropriate in this age group due to increased risk for adverse effects and high addiction potential. May cause CNS depression, which may impair physical or mental abilities; patients must be cautioned about performing tasks which require mental alertness (eg, operating machinery or driving). Effects with other sedative drugs or ethanol may be potentiated.

Solution for injection is highly alkaline and extravasation may cause local tissue damage. Intravenous solution may contain propylene glycol (PG). One case report has described a patient who developed lactic acidosis possibly secondary to PG accumulation following a continuous infusion of pentobarbital (Miller, 2008). Consider monitoring for signs of PG toxicity (eg, lactic acidosis, acute renal failure, osmol gap) in patients who require a continuous infusion of pentobarbital.

Adverse Reactions Frequency not defined.

Cardiovascular: Bradycardia, hypotension, syncope

Central nervous system: Abnormal thinking, agitation, anxiety, ataxia, CNS excitation, confusion, depression, dizziness, drowsiness, fever, hallucinations, headache, hyperkinesia, insomnia, nervousness, nightmares, psychiatric disturbances, somnolence

Dermatologic: Angioedema, exfoliative dermatitis, rash

Gastrointestinal: Constipation, nausea, vomiting

Hematologic: Megaloblastic anemia

Hepatic: Hepatotoxicity

Local: Injection site reactions

Respiratory: Apnea (especially with rapid I.V. use), hypoventilation, laryngospasm, respiratory depression

Miscellaneous: Gangrene with inadvertent intra-arterial injection, hypersensitivity reactions

Drug Interactions

Metabolism/Transport Effects **Induces** CYP2A6 (strong), CYP3A4 (strong)

Avoid Concomitant Use

Avoid concomitant use of PENTobarbital with any of the following: Bortezomib; Crizotinib; Dronedarone; Everolimus; Lapatinib; Lurasidone; Nilotinib; Pazopanib; Praziquantel; Ranolazine; Rivaroxaban; Roflumilast; RomiDEPsin; SORAfenib; Ticagrelor; Tolvaptan; Toremifene; Vandetanib

Increased Effect/Toxicity

PENTobarbital may increase the levels/effects of: Alcohol (Ethyl); Clarithromycin; CNS Depressants; Meperidine; QuiNIDine; Selective Serotonin Reuptake Inhibitors; Thiazide Diuretics

The levels/effects of PENTobarbital may be increased by: Carbonic Anhydrase Inhibitors; Chloramphenicol; Clarithromycin; Divalproex; Droperidol; Felbamate; HydrOXYzine; Primidone; Valproic Acid

Decreased Effect

PENTobarbital may decrease the levels/effects of: Acetaminophen; ARIPiprazole; Beta-Blockers; Boceprevir; Bortezomib; Brentuximab Vedotin; Calcium Channel Blockers; Chloramphenicol; Clarithromycin; Contraceptives (Estrogens); Contraceptives (Progestins); Corticosteroids (Systemic); Crizotinib; CycloSPORINE; CycloSPORINE (Systemic); CYP2A6 Substrates; CYP3A4 Substrates; Dasatinib; Disopyramide; Divalproex; Doxycycline; Dronedarone; Etoposide; Etoposide Phosphate; Everolimus; Exemestane; Felbamate; Fosphenytoin; Gefitinib; Griseofulvin; GuanFACINE; Imatinib; Ixabepilone; LamoTRIgine; Lapatinib; Linagliptin; Lurasidone; Maraviroc; Methadone; Nilotinib; Pazopanib; Phenytoin; Praziquantel; Propafenone; QuiNIDine; Ranolazine; Rivaroxaban; Roflumilast; RomiDEPsin; Saxagliptin; SORAfenib; SUNItinib; Tadalafil; Teniposide; Theophylline Derivatives; Ticagrelor; Tolvaptan; Toremifene; Tricyclic Antidepressants; Ulipristal; Valproic Acid; Vandetanib; Vemurafenib; Vitamin K Antagonists; Zuclopenthixol

The levels/effects of PENTobarbital may be decreased by: Ketorolac; Ketorolac (Nasal); Ketorolac (Systemic); Mefloquine; Pyridoxine; Rifamycin Derivatives

Ethanol/Nutrition/Herb Interactions Ethanol: May increase CNS depression; monitor for increased effects with coadministration. Caution patients about effects.

Stability Store at controlled room temperature of 15°C to 30°C (68°F to 77°F); protect from freezing and avoid excessive heat. When mixed with an acidic solution, precipitate may form. Use only clear solution.

Mechanism of Action Barbiturate with sedative, hypnotic, and anticonvulsant properties. Barbiturates depress the sensory cortex, decrease motor activity, alter cerebellar function, and produce drowsiness, sedation, and hypnosis. In high doses, barbiturates exhibit anticonvulsant activity; barbiturates produce dose-dependent respiratory depression; reduce brain metabolism and cerebral blood flow in order to decrease intracranial pressure

Pharmacodynamics/Kinetics

Onset of action: I.M.: 10-15 minutes (Krauss, 2006); I.V.: Almost immediate, within 3-5 minutes (Krauss, 2006)

Duration: I.V.: Variable

Distribution: V_d: Children: 0.8 L/kg (Schaible, 1982); Adults: 1 L/kg (Ehrnebo, 1974)

Protein binding: 45% to 70%

Metabolism: Hepatic via hydroxylation and glucuronidation (Wermeling, 1985)

Half-life elimination: Terminal: Children: 26 ± 16 hours (Schaible, 1982); Adults: Healthy: 22 hours (average; Ehrnebo, 1974); (range: 15-50 hours; dose dependent)

Excretion: Urine

Dosage Note: Adjust dose based on patients age, weight, and condition.

Children:

Hypnotic/sedative:

I.M.: 2-6 mg/kg; maximum: 100 mg/dose

I.V.: 1-6 mg/kg titrated in 1-2 mg/kg increments every 3-5 minutes to desired effect (Krauss, 2006)

Refractory status epilepticus: I.V.: **Note:** Intubation required; adjust dose based on hemodynamics, seizure activity, and EEG. Various regimens available (Abend, 2008; Hanhan, 2001; Holmes, 1999; Kim, 2001):

Loading dose: 5-15 mg/kg given slowly over 1 hour; maintenance infusion: 0.5-5 mg/kg/hour to maintain burst suppression; continue for 12-48 hours of no seizure activity; may taper infusion rate by 0.5 mg/kg/hour every 12 hours

Adults:
Hypnotic/sedative:
I.M.: 150-200 mg
I.V.: Initial: 100 mg; decrease dose for elderly or debilitated patients. If needed, may administer additional increments after at least 1 minute, up to a total dose of 200-500 mg
Barbiturate coma in severe brain injury patients/elevated intracranial pressure (unlabeled use; Bratton, 2007): I.V.: Loading dose: 10 mg/kg given over 30 minutes (or ≤25 mg/minute), followed by 5 mg/kg every hour for 3 doses; monitor blood pressure and respiratory rate. Maintenance infusion: Initial: 1 mg/kg/hour; may increase to 2-4 mg/kg/hour; maintain burst suppression on EEG.
Refractory status epilepticus: I.V.: **Note:** Intubation required; adjust dose based on hemodynamics, seizure activity, and EEG. Various regimens available (Abou Khaled, 2008; Millikan, 2009; Mirski, 2008; Yaffe, 1993):
Loading dose: 10-15 mg/kg (5-10 mg/kg in patients with pre-existing hypotension) administer slowly over 1 hour; initial maintenance infusion: 0.5-1 mg/kg/hour; adjust to maintain burst suppression pattern on EEG; maintenance infusion dose range: 0.5-10 mg/kg/hour
Note: During active seizure activity when increasing maintenance infusion rate, some experts suggest administration of an additional 5 mg/kg bolus given the long half-life of pentobarbital.
Elderly: Not recommended for use in the elderly; decrease dose if use becomes necessary

Dosing adjustment in renal impairment: Reduce dosage in patients with renal dysfunction
Dosing adjustment in hepatic impairment: Reduce dosage in patients with liver dysfunction

Administration Pentobarbital may be administered by deep I.M. or slow I.V. injection.
I.M.: Inject into a large muscle. No more than 5 mL (250 mg) should be injected at any one site because of possible tissue irritation.
I.V.: Do not exceed 50 mg/minute; I.V. push doses may be given undiluted. Parenteral solutions are highly alkaline; avoid extravasation; avoid intra-arterial injection.

Monitoring Parameters Respiratory status (for conscious sedation, includes pulse oximetry), cardiovascular status, CNS status; cardiac monitor and blood pressure monitor required; temperature with high doses (eg, barbiturate coma)

Elevated ICP: Monitor ICP, CPP, EEG

Reference Range
Therapeutic:
Sedation: 1-5 mcg/mL (SI: 4-22 micromole/L)
Coma or intracranial pressure therapy: Target: 30-40 mcg/mL (SI: 132-176 micromole/L) (Bratton, 2007)
Potentially toxic: >10 mcg/mL (SI: >44 micromole/L); dependent on reason for use and patient condition

Dosage Forms Excipient information presented when available (limited, particularly for generics); consult specific product labeling.
Injection, solution, as sodium:
Nembutal®: 50 mg/mL (20 mL, 50 mL) [contains ethanol 10%, propylene glycol 40%]

Controlled Substance C-II

◆ **Pentobarbital Sodium** *see* PENTobarbital *on page 1329*

Pentosan Polysulfate Sodium
(PEN toe san pol i SUL fate SOW dee um)

Brand Names: U.S. Elmiron®
Brand Names: Canada Elmiron®
Index Terms PPS
Pharmacologic Category Analgesic, Urinary
Use Relief of bladder pain or discomfort due to interstitial cystitis
Pregnancy Risk Factor B
Dosage Children ≥16 years and Adults: Oral: 100 mg 3 times/day taken with water 1 hour before or 2 hours after meals

Note: Patients should be evaluated at 3 months and may be continued an additional 3 months if there has been no improvement and if there are no therapy-limiting side effects. **The risks and benefits of continued use beyond 6 months in patients who have not responded is not yet known.**

Additional Information Complete prescribing information for this medication should be consulted for additional detail.

Dosage Forms Excipient information presented when available (limited, particularly for generics); consult specific product labeling.
Capsule, oral:
Elmiron®: 100 mg

Pentostatin (pen toe STAT in)

Brand Names: U.S. Nipent®
Brand Names: Canada Nipent®
Index Terms 2′-Deoxycoformycin; Co-Vidarabine; dCF; Deoxycoformycin; NSC-218321
Pharmacologic Category Antineoplastic Agent, Antibiotic; Antineoplastic Agent, Antimetabolite (Purine Analog)
Use Treatment of hairy cell leukemia
Unlabeled Use Treatment of cutaneous T-cell lymphoma, chronic lymphocytic leukemia (CLL), and acute and chronic graft-versus-host-disease (GVHD)
Pregnancy Risk Factor D
Pregnancy Considerations Animal studies have demonstrated teratogenicity, maternal toxicity, and fetal loss. There are no adequate and well-controlled studies in pregnant women. Women of childbearing potential should be advised to avoid becoming pregnant.
Lactation Excretion in breast milk unknown/not recommended
Contraindications Hypersensitivity to pentostatin or any component of the formulation
Warnings/Precautions Hazardous agent - use appropriate precautions for handling and disposal. **[U.S. Boxed Warnings]: Severe renal, liver, pulmonary and CNS toxicities have occurred with doses higher than recommended; do not exceed the recommended dose. Do not administer concurrently with fludarabine; concomitant use has resulted in serious or fatal pulmonary toxicity.** Bone marrow suppression may occur, primarily early in treatment; if neutropenia persists beyond early cycles, evaluate for disease status. In patients who present with infections prior to treatment, infections should be resolved, if possible, prior to initiation of treatment; treatment should be temporarily withheld for active infections during therapy. Use cautiously in patients with renal dysfunction (the half-life is prolonged); appropriate dosing guidelines in renal insufficiency have not been determined. May cause elevations (reversible) in liver function tests. Withhold treatment for CNS toxicity or severe rash. Fatal pulmonary edema and hypotension have been reported in patients treated with pentostatin in combination with carmustine, etoposide, or high-dose cyclophosphamide as part of a myeloablative regimen for bone marrow transplant. **[U.S. Boxed Warning]: Should be administered under the supervision of an experienced cancer chemotherapy physician.** Safety and efficacy in children have not been established.

Adverse Reactions

>10%:

Central nervous system: Fever (42% to 46%), fatigue (29% to 42%), pain (8% to 20%), chills (11% to 19%), headache (13% to 17%), CNS toxicity (1% to 11%)

Dermatologic: Rash (26% to 43%), pruritus (10% to 21%), skin disorder (4% to 17%)

Gastrointestinal: Nausea/vomiting (22% to 63%), diarrhea (15% to 17%), anorexia (13% to 16%), abdominal pain (4% to 16%), stomatitis (5% to 12%)

Hematologic: Myelosuppression (nadir: 7 days; recovery: 10-14 days), leukopenia (22% to 60%), anemia (8% to 35%), thrombocytopenia (6% to 32%)

Hepatic: Transaminases increased (2% to 19%)

Neuromuscular & skeletal: Myalgia (11% to 19%), weakness (10% to 12%)

Respiratory: Cough (17% to 20%), upper respiratory infection (13% to 16%), rhinitis (10% to 11%), dyspnea (8% to 11%)

Miscellaneous: Infection (7% to 36%), allergic reaction (2% to 11%)

1% to 10%:

Cardiovascular: Chest pain (3% to 10%), facial edema (3% to 10%), hypotension (3% to 10%), peripheral edema (3% to 10%), angina (<3%), arrhythmia (<3%), AV block (<3%), bradycardia (<3%), cardiac arrest (<3%), deep thrombophlebitis (<3%), heart failure (<3%), hypertension (<3%), pericardial effusion (<3%), sinus arrest (<3%), syncope (<3%), tachycardia (<3%), vasculitis (<3%), ventricular extrasystoles (<3%)

Central nervous system: Anxiety (3% to 10%), confusion (3% to 10%), depression (3% to 10%), dizziness (3% to 10%), insomnia (3% to 10%), nervousness (3% to 10%), somnolence (3% to 10%), abnormal dreams/thinking (<3%), amnesia (<3%), ataxia (<3%), emotional lability (<3%), encephalitis (<3%), hallucination (<3%), hostility (<3%), meningism (<3%), neuritis (<3%), neurosis (<3%), seizure (<3%), vertigo (<3%)

Dermatologic: Cellulitis (6%), furunculosis (4%), dry skin (3% to 10%), urticaria (3% to 10%), acne (<3%), alopecia (<3%), eczema (<3%), petechial rash (<3%), photosensitivity (<3%), abscess (2%)

Endocrine & metabolic: Amenorrhea (<3%), hypercalcemia (<3%), hyponatremia (<3%), gout (<3%), libido decreased/loss (<3%)

Gastrointestinal: Dyspepsia (3% to 10%) flatulence (3% to 10%), gingivitis (3% to 10%), constipation (<3%), dysphagia (<3%), glossitis (<3%), ileus (<3%), taste perversion (<3%), oral moniliasis (2%)

Genitourinary: Urinary tract infection (3%), impotence (<3%)

Hematologic: Agranulocytosis (3% to 10%), hemorrhage (3% to 10%), acute leukemia (<3%), aplastic anemia (<3%), hemolytic anemia (<3%)

Local: Phlebitis (<3%)

Neuromuscular & skeletal: Arthralgia (3% to 10%), paresthesia (3% to 10%), arthritis (<3%), dysarthria (<3%), hyperkinesia (<3%), neuralgia (<3%), neuropathy (<3%), paralysis (<3%), twitching (<3%), osteomyelitis (1%)

Ocular: Conjunctivitis (4%), amblyopia (<3%), eyes nonreactive (<3%), lacrimation disorder (<3%), photophobia (<3%), retinopathy (<3%), vision abnormal (<3%), watery eyes (<3%), xerophthalmia (<3%)

Otic: Deafness (<3%), earache (<3%), labyrinthitis (<3%), tinnitus (<3%)

Renal: Creatinine increased (3% to 10%), nephropathy (<3%), renal failure (<3%), renal insufficiency (<3%), renal function abnormal (<3%), renal stone (<3%)

Respiratory: Pharyngitis (8% to 10%), sinusitis (6%), pneumonia (5%), asthma (3% to 10%), bronchitis (3%), bronchospasm (<3%), laryngeal edema (<3%), pulmonary embolus (<3%)

Miscellaneous: Diaphoresis (8% to 10%), herpes zoster (8%), viral infection (≤8%), bacterial infection (5%), herpes simplex (4%), sepsis (3%), flu-like syndrome (<3%)

<1% (Limited to important or life-threatening): Dysuria, fungal infection (skin), hematuria, lethargy, pulmonary edema, pulmonary toxicity (fatal; in combination with fludarabine), uveitis/vision loss

Drug Interactions

Metabolism/Transport Effects None known.

Avoid Concomitant Use

Avoid concomitant use of Pentostatin with any of the following: BCG; CloZAPine; Fludarabine; Natalizumab; Nelarabine; Pegademase Bovine; Pimecrolimus; Tacrolimus (Topical); Vaccines (Live)

Increased Effect/Toxicity

Pentostatin may increase the levels/effects of: CloZAPine; Cyclophosphamide; Fludarabine; Leflunomide; Natalizumab; Vaccines (Live)

The levels/effects of Pentostatin may be increased by: Denosumab; Fludarabine; Pimecrolimus; Roflumilast; Tacrolimus (Topical); Trastuzumab

Decreased Effect

Pentostatin may decrease the levels/effects of: BCG; Coccidioidin Skin Test; Nelarabine; Pegademase Bovine; Sipuleucel-T; Vaccines (Inactivated); Vaccines (Live)

The levels/effects of Pentostatin may be decreased by: Echinacea; Pegademase Bovine

Stability Store intact vials under refrigeration at 2°C to 8°C (36°F to 46°F); reconstituted vials, or further dilutions, are stable at room temperature for 8 hours in D_5W or 48 hours in NS. Reconstitute with 5 mL SWFI to a concentration of 2 mg/mL. The solution may be further diluted in 25-50 mL NS or D_5W for infusion.

Mechanism of Action Pentostatin is a purine antimetabolite that inhibits adenosine deaminase, preventing the deamination of adenosine to inosine. Accumulation of deoxyadenosine (dAdo) and deoxyadenosine 5′-triphosphate (dATP) results in a reduction of purine metabolism and DNA synthesis and cell death.

Pharmacodynamics/Kinetics

Distribution: I.V.: V_d: 36.1 L (20.1 L/m^2); rapidly to body tissues

Protein binding: ~4%

Half-life elimination:

Distribution half-life: 11-85 minutes

Terminal: 3-7 hours

Renal impairment (Cl_{cr} <50 mL/minute): 4-18 hours

Excretion: Urine (~50% to 96%) within 24 hours (30% to 90% as unchanged drug)

Dosage I.V.: Adults (refer to individual protocols):

Hairy cell leukemia: 4 mg/m^2 every 2 weeks

CLL (unlabeled use): 4 mg/m^2 weekly for 3 weeks, then every 2 weeks

Cutaneous T-cell lymphoma (unlabeled use): 3.75-5 mg/m^2 daily for 3 days every 3 weeks

Acute GVHD (unlabeled use): 1.5 mg/m^2 daily for 3 days; may repeat after 2 weeks if needed

Chronic GVHD (unlabeled use): 4 mg/m^2 every 2 weeks for 12 doses; then 4 mg/m^2 every 3-4 weeks (if still improving)

Dosage adjustment in renal impairment: The FDA-approved labeling does not contain renal dosage adjustment guidelines; use with caution in patients with Cl_{cr} <60 mL/minute. Two patients with Cl_{cr} 50-60 mL/minute achieved responses when treated with 2 mg/m^2/dose. The following guidelines have been used by some clinicians:

Kintzel, 1995:

Cl_{cr} 46-60 mL/minute: Administer 70% of dose

Cl_{cr} 31-45 mL/minute: Administer 60% of dose

Cl_{cr} <30 mL/minute: Consider use of alternative drug

Lathia, 2002:

Cl_{cr} 40-59 mL/minute: Administer 3 mg/m^2/dose

Cl_{cr} 20-39 mL/minute: Administer 2 mg/m^2/dose

Administration Administer I.V. 20- to 30-minute infusion or I.V. bolus over 5 minutes. Hydrate with 500-1000 mL fluid prior to infusion and 500 mL after infusion.

Monitoring Parameters CBC with differential, platelet count, liver function, serum uric acid, renal function (creatinine clearance), bone marrow evaluation

Dosage Forms Excipient information presented when available (limited, particularly for generics); consult specific product labeling.

Injection, powder for reconstitution:

Nipent®: 10 mg [contains mannitol]

Injection, powder for reconstitution [preservative free]: 10 mg

◆ **Pentothal® [DSC]** *see* Thiopental *on page 1671*

◆ **Pentothal® (Can)** *see* Thiopental *on page 1671*

Pentoxifylline (pen toks IF i lin)

Brand Names: U.S. TRENtal®

Brand Names: Canada Albert® Pentoxifylline; Apo-Pentoxifylline SR®; Nu-Pentoxifylline SR; ratio-Pentoxifylline; Trental®

Index Terms Oxpentifylline

Pharmacologic Category Blood Viscosity Reducer Agent

Use Treatment of intermittent claudication on the basis of chronic occlusive arterial disease of the limbs; may improve function and symptoms, but not intended to replace more definitive therapy

Unlabeled Use Venous leg ulcers (Jull, 2007)

Pregnancy Risk Factor C

Pregnancy Considerations Teratogenic effects were not observed in animal studies. There are no adequate and well-controlled studies in pregnant women.

Lactation Enters breast milk/not recommended

Contraindications Hypersensitivity to pentoxifylline, xanthines (eg, caffeine, theophylline), or any component of the formulation; recent cerebral and/or retinal hemorrhage

Warnings/Precautions Use with caution in renal impairment; active metabolite may accumulate in renal impairment leading to increased risk of adverse effects. Use caution in the elderly and assess renal function before initiating. Safety and efficacy in pediatric patients have not been established.

Adverse Reactions

1% to 10%: Gastrointestinal: Nausea (2%), vomiting (1%)

<1% (Limited to important or life-threatening): Anaphylactoid reaction, angioedema, angina, anorexia, anxiety, aplastic anemia, arrhythmia, aseptic meningitis, bloating, blurred vision, brittle fingernails, chest pain, cholecystitis, confusion, conjunctivitis, constipation, depression, dyspnea, earache, edema, epistaxis, eructation, fibrinogen decreased (serum), flatus, flu-like syndrome, hallucinations, hepatitis, hypotension, jaundice, laryngitis, leukemia, leukopenia, liver enzymes increased, malaise, nasal congestion, pancytopenia, pruritus, purpura, rash, scotoma, seizure, sialism, sore throat, taste perversion, tachycardia, thrombocytopenia, tremor, urticaria, weight change, xerostomia

Drug Interactions

Metabolism/Transport Effects Inhibits CYP1A2 (weak)

Avoid Concomitant Use

Avoid concomitant use of Pentoxifylline with any of the following: Ketorolac; Ketorolac (Nasal); Ketorolac (Systemic)

Increased Effect/Toxicity

Pentoxifylline may increase the levels/effects of: Antihypertensives; Antiplatelet Agents; Heparin; Heparin (Low Molecular Weight); Theophylline Derivatives; Vitamin K Antagonists

The levels/effects of Pentoxifylline may be increased by: Cimetidine; Ciprofloxacin; Ciprofloxacin (Systemic); Ketorolac; Ketorolac (Nasal); Ketorolac (Systemic)

Decreased Effect There are no known significant interactions involving a decrease in effect.

Ethanol/Nutrition/Herb Interactions Food: Food may decrease rate but not extent of absorption. Pentoxifylline peak serum levels may be decreased if taken with food.

Stability Store between 15°C to 30°C (59°F to 86°F).

Mechanism of Action Reduces blood viscosity via increased leukocyte and erythrocyte deformability and decreased neutrophil adhesion/activation; improves peripheral tissue oxygenation presumably through enhanced blood flow.

Pharmacodynamics/Kinetics

Absorption: Well absorbed

Metabolism: Hepatic to 3-carboxybutyl (M-IV, inactive) and 3-carboxypropyl (M-V, active) and via erythrocytes to 5-hydroxyhexyl (M-I, active); extensive first-pass effect; M-I is further metabolized in the liver

Half-life elimination: Parent drug: 24-48 minutes; Metabolites: 60-96 minutes

Time to peak, serum: 2-4 hours

Excretion: Primarily urine (50% to 80% as M-V, 20% as other metabolites); feces (<4%)

Dosage Oral:

Adults: 400 mg 3 times/day with meals; maximal therapeutic benefit may take 2-4 weeks to develop; recommended to maintain therapy for at least 8 weeks. May reduce to 400 mg twice daily if GI or CNS side effects occur.

Elderly: Dosage adjustment based on creatinine clearance can be considered.

Dosage adjustment in renal impairment: Dosage adjustments are not required by manufacturer; however, consider dosing adjustments based on degree of renal impairment (Paap, 1996):

Moderate renal impairment (Cl_{cr} ~60 mL/minute): 400 mg twice daily

Severe renal impairment (Cl_{cr} ~20 mL/minute): 400 mg once daily; further reduction may be required; Paap suggests 200 mg once daily, but with current products (extended or controlled release; unscored) may require adaptation to 400 mg once every other day

Dietary Considerations May be taken with meals.

Administration Tablets should be swallowed whole; do not chew, break, or crush. May be administered with food.

Test Interactions Decreased calcium (S), magnesium (S); false-positive theophylline levels

Dosage Forms Excipient information presented when available (limited, particularly for generics); consult specific product labeling.

Tablet, controlled release, oral:

TRENtal®: 400 mg

Tablet, extended release, oral: 400 mg

Extemporaneous Preparations A 20 mg/mL oral suspension may be made using tablets. Crush ten 400 mg tablets and reduce to a fine powder. Add a small amount of purified water and mix to a uniform paste; mix while adding purified water to **almost** 200 mL; transfer to a calibrated bottle, rinse mortar with vehicle, and add quantity of vehicle sufficient to make 200 mL. Label "shake well" and "refrigerate". Stable 91 days.

Nahata MC, Pai VB, and Hipple TF, *Pediatric Drug Formulations*, 5th ed, Cincinnati, OH: Harvey Whitney Books Co, 2004.

◆ **Pen VK** *see* Penicillin V Potassium *on page 1326*

◆ **Pepcid®** *see* Famotidine *on page 688*

- **Pepcid® AC [OTC]** *see* Famotidine *on page 688*
- **Pepcid® AC (Can)** *see* Famotidine *on page 688*
- **Pepcid® AC Maximum Strength [OTC]** *see* Famotidine *on page 688*
- **Pepcid® I.V. (Can)** *see* Famotidine *on page 688*
- **Peptic Relief [OTC]** *see* Bismuth *on page 220*
- **Pepto-Bismol® [OTC]** *see* Bismuth *on page 220*
- **Pepto-Bismol® Maximum Strength [OTC]** *see* Bismuth *on page 220*
- **Pepto Relief [OTC]** *see* Bismuth *on page 220*
- **Percocet®** *see* Oxycodone and Acetaminophen *on page 1269*
- **Percocet®-Demi (Can)** *see* Oxycodone and Acetaminophen *on page 1269*
- **Percodan®** *see* Oxycodone and Aspirin *on page 1269*
- **Percogesic® Extra Strength [OTC]** *see* Acetaminophen and Diphenhydramine *on page 31*
- **Perforomist®** *see* Formoterol *on page 754*
- **Periactin** *see* Cyproheptadine *on page 427*
- **Peri-Colace® [OTC]** *see* Docusate and Senna *on page 538*
- **Peridex®** *see* Chlorhexidine Gluconate *on page 341*
- **Peridex® Oral Rinse (Can)** *see* Chlorhexidine Gluconate *on page 341*

Perindopril Erbumine (per IN doe pril er BYOO meen)

Brand Names: U.S. Aceon®

Brand Names: Canada Apo-Perindopril®; Coversyl®

Pharmacologic Category Angiotensin-Converting Enzyme (ACE) Inhibitor

Additional Appendix Information

Angiotensin Agents *on page 1869*

Heart Failure (Systolic) *on page 1991*

Use Treatment of hypertension; reduction of cardiovascular mortality or nonfatal myocardial infarction in patients with stable coronary artery disease

Canadian labeling: Additional use (unlabeled use in U.S.): Treatment of mild-moderate (NYHA I-III) heart failure

Unlabeled Use To delay the progression of nephropathy and reduce risks of cardiovascular events in hypertensive patients with type 1 or 2 diabetes mellitus

Pregnancy Risk Factor D

Pregnancy Considerations Due to adverse events observed in humans, perindopril is considered pregnancy category D. Perindopril crosses the placenta. First trimester exposure to ACE inhibitors may cause major congenital malformations. An increased risk of cardiovascular and/or central nervous system malformations was observed in one study; however, an increased risk of teratogenic events was not observed in other studies. Second and third trimester use of an ACE inhibitor is associated with oligohydramnios. Oligohydramnios due to decreased fetal renal function may lead to fetal limb contractures, craniofacial deformation, and hypoplastic lung development. The use of ACE inhibitors during the second and third trimesters is also associated with anuria, hypotension, renal failure (reversible or irreversible), skull hypoplasia, and death in the fetus/neonate. Chronic maternal hypertension itself is also associated with adverse events in the fetus/infant. ACE inhibitors are not recommended during pregnancy to treat maternal hypertension or heart failure. Those who are planning a pregnancy should be considered for other medication options if an ACE inhibitor is currently prescribed or the ACE inhibitor should be discontinued as soon as possible once pregnancy is detected. The exposed fetus should be monitored for fetal growth, amniotic fluid volume, and organ formation. Infants exposed to an ACE inhibitor *in utero*, especially during the second and third trimester, should be monitored for hyperkalemia, hypotension, and oliguria.

[U.S. Boxed Warning]: Based on human data, ACE inhibitors can cause injury and death to the developing fetus. ACE inhibitors should be discontinued as soon as possible once pregnancy is detected.

Lactation Excretion in breast milk unknown/use caution

Contraindications Hypersensitivity to perindopril, any other ACE inhibitor, or any component of the formulation; angioedema related to previous treatment with an ACE inhibitor

Canadian labeling: Additional contraindications (not in U.S. labeling): History of hereditary/idiopathic angioedema; pregnant women during the second and third trimesters

Warnings/Precautions Anaphylactic reactions may occur rarely with ACE inhibitors. At any time during treatment (especially following first dose), angioedema may occur rarely with ACE inhibitors; it may involve the head and neck (potentially compromising airway) or the intestine (presenting with abdominal pain). African-Americans and patients with idiopathic or hereditary angioedema may be at an increased risk. Prolonged frequent monitoring may be required especially if tongue, glottis, or larynx are involved as they are associated with airway obstruction. Patients with a history of airway surgery may have a higher risk of airway obstruction. Aggressive early and appropriate management is critical. Use in patients with previous angioedema associated with ACE inhibitor therapy is contraindicated. Severe anaphylactoid reactions may be seen during hemodialysis (eg, CVVHD) with high-flux dialysis membranes (eg, AN69), and rarely, during low density lipoprotein apheresis with dextran sulfate cellulose. Rare cases of anaphylactoid reactions have been reported in patients undergoing sensitization treatment with hymenoptera (bee, wasp) venom while receiving ACE inhibitors.

Symptomatic hypotension with or without syncope can occur with ACE inhibitors (usually with the first several doses); effects are most often observed in volume-depleted patients; correct volume depletion prior to initiation; close monitoring of patient is required especially with initial dosing and dosing increases; blood pressure must be lowered at a rate appropriate for the patient's clinical condition. Initiation of therapy in patients with ischemic heart disease or cerebrovascular disease warrants close observation due to the potential consequences posed by falling blood pressure (eg, MI, stroke). Use with caution in hypertrophic cardiomyopathy with outflow tract obstruction, severe aortic stenosis, or before, during, or immediately after major surgery. **[U.S. Boxed Warning]: Based on human data, ACEIs can cause injury and death to the developing fetus when used in the second and third trimesters. ACEIs should be discontinued as soon as possible once pregnancy is detected.**

Hyperkalemia may occur with ACE inhibitors; risk factors include renal dysfunction, diabetes mellitus, concomitant use of potassium-sparing diuretics, potassium supplements, and/or potassium-containing salts. Use cautiously, if at all, with these agents and monitor potassium closely. Cough may occur with ACE inhibitors. Other causes of cough should be considered (eg, pulmonary congestion in patients with heart failure) and excluded prior to discontinuation.

May be associated with deterioration of renal function and/or increases in serum creatinine, particularly in patients with low renal blood flow (eg, renal artery stenosis, heart failure) whose glomerular filtration rate (GFR) is dependent on efferent arteriolar vasoconstriction by angiotensin II; deterioration may result in oliguria, acute renal failure, and progressive azotemia. Small increases in serum creatinine may occur following initiation; consider discontinuation only in patients with progressive and/or significant deterioration in renal function. Use with caution in patients with unstented unilateral/bilateral renal artery stenosis. When unstented bilateral renal artery stenosis is present, use is generally avoided due to the elevated risk of deterioration in renal function unless possible benefits outweigh risks. Concurrent use of angiotensin receptor blockers may increase the risk of clinically-significant adverse events (eg, renal dysfunction, hyperkalemia).

Rare toxicities associated with ACE inhibitors include cholestatic jaundice (which may progress to fulminant hepatic necrosis), agranulocytosis, neutropenia or leukopenia with myeloid hypoplasia. Patients with collagen vascular diseases (especially with concomitant renal impairment) or renal impairment alone may be at increased risk for hematologic toxicity; periodically monitor CBC with differential in these patients.

Adverse Reactions

>10%:

- Central nervous system: Headache (24%)
- Respiratory: Cough (incidence is higher in women, 3:1) (12%)

1% to 10%:

- Cardiovascular: Edema (4%), chest pain (2%), ECG abnormal (2%), palpitation (1%)
- Central nervous system: Dizziness (8%, less than placebo), sleep disorders (3%), depression (2%), fever (2%), nervousness (1%), somnolence (1%)
- Dermatologic: Rash (2%)
- Endocrine & metabolic: Hyperkalemia (1%, less than placebo), triglycerides increased (1%), menstrual disorder (1%)
- Gastrointestinal: Diarrhea (4%), abdominal pain (3%), nausea (2%), vomiting (2%), dyspepsia (2%), flatulence (1%)
- Genitourinary: Urinary tract infection (3%), sexual dysfunction (male 1%)
- Hepatic: ALT increased (2%)
- Neuromuscular & skeletal: Weakness (8%), back pain (6%), lower extremity pain (5%), upper extremity pain (3%), hypertonia (3%), paresthesia (2%), joint pain (1%), myalgia (1%), arthritis (1%), neck pain (1%)
- Renal: Proteinuria (2%)
- Respiratory: Upper respiratory tract infection (9%), sinusitis (5%), rhinitis (5%), pharyngitis (3%)
- Otic: Tinnitus (2%), ear infection (1%)
- Miscellaneous: Viral infection (3%), seasonal allergy (2%)

Note: Some reactions occurred at an i[illegible]% but ≤ placebo.

<1% (Limited to important or life-threatening): Amnesia, anaphylaxis, angioedema, anxiety, AST increased, dyspnea, erythema, fluid retention, gout, leukopenia, migraine, MI, nephrolithiasis, neutropenia, orthostatic hypotension, pruritus, psychosocial disorder, pulmonary fibrosis, purpura, stroke, syncope, urinary retention, vertigo

Additional adverse effects that have been reported with **ACE inhibitors** include agranulocytosis (especially in patients with renal impairment or collagen vascular disease), neutropenia, anemia, bullous pemphigoid, cardiac arrest, eosinophilic pneumonitis, exfoliative dermatitis, falls, hepatic failure, hyponatremia, jaundice, pancreatitis (acute), pancytopenia, pemphigus, psoriasis, thrombocytopenia; decreases in creatinine clearance in some elderly hypertensive patients or those with chronic renal failure, and worsening of renal function in patients with bilateral renal artery stenosis or hypovolemic patients (diuretic therapy). In addition, a syndrome which may include fever, myalgia, arthralgia, interstitial nephritis, vasculitis, rash, eosinophilia and positive ANA, and elevated ESR has been reported with ACE inhibitors.

Drug Interactions

Metabolism/Transport Effects None known.

Avoid Concomitant Use There are no known interactions where it is recommended to avoid concomitant use.

Increased Effect/Toxicity

Perindopril Erbumine may increase the levels/effects of: Allopurinol; Amifostine; Antihypertensives; AzaTHIOprine; CycloSPORINE; CycloSPORINE (Systemic); Ferric Gluconate; Gold Sodium Thiomalate; Hypotensive Agents; Iron Dextran Complex; Lithium; Nonsteroidal Anti-Inflammatory Agents; RiTUXimab; Sodium Phosphates

The levels/effects of Perindopril Erbumine may be increased by: Alfuzosin; Angiotensin II Receptor Blockers; Diazoxide; DPP-IV Inhibitors; Eplerenone; Everolimus; Herbs (Hypotensive Properties); Loop Diuretics; MAO Inhibitors; Pentoxifylline; Phosphodiesterase 5 Inhibitors; Potassium Salts; Potassium-Sparing Diuretics; Prostacyclin Analogues; Sirolimus; Temsirolimus; Thiazide Diuretics; TiZANidine; Tolvaptan; Trimethoprim

Decreased Effect

The levels/effects of Perindopril Erbumine may be decreased by: Antacids; Aprotinin; Herbs (Hypertensive Properties); Icatibant; Lanthanum; Methylphenidate; Nonsteroidal Anti-Inflammatory Agents; Salicylates; Yohimbine

Ethanol/Nutrition/Herb Interactions

- Food: Perindopril active metabolite concentrations may be lowered if taken with food.
- Herb/Nutraceutical: Avoid bayberry, blue cohosh, cayenne, ephedra, ginger, ginseng (American), kola, licorice (may worsen hypertension). Avoid black cohosh, California poppy, coleus, golden seal, hawthorn, mistletoe, periwinkle, quinine, shepherd's purse (may have increased antihypertensive effect).

Stability Store at room temperature of 20°C to 25°C (68°F to 77°F). Protect from moisture.

Mechanism of Action Perindopril is a prodrug for perindoprilat, which acts as a competitive inhibitor of angiotensin-converting enzyme (ACE); prevents conversion of angiotensin I to angiotensin II, a potent vasoconstrictor; results in lower levels of angiotensin II which, in turn, causes an increase in plasma renin activity and a reduction in aldosterone secretion

Pharmacodynamics/Kinetics

- Onset of action: Peak effect: 1-2 hours
- Protein binding: Perindopril: 60%; Perindoprilat: 10% to 20%
- Metabolism: Hepatically hydrolyzed to active metabolite, perindoprilat (~17% to 20% of a dose) and other inactive metabolites
- Bioavailability: Perindopril: 75%; Perindoprilat ~25% (~16% with food)
- Half-life elimination: Parent drug: 1.5-3 hours; Metabolite: Effective: 3-10 hours, Terminal: 30-120 hours
- Time to peak: Chronic therapy: Perindopril: 1 hour; Perindoprilat: 3-7 hours (maximum perindoprilat serum levels are 2-3 times higher and T_{max} is shorter following chronic therapy); CHF: Perindoprilat: 6 hours
- Excretion: Urine (75%, 4% to 12% as unchanged drug)

Dosage Oral:

Adults:

Heart failure (Canadian labeling; unlabeled use in U.S.): Initial: 2 mg once daily; if necessary, may titrate over 2-4 weeks to 4 mg once daily. The American College of Cardiology/ American Heart Association (ACC/AHA) 2009 Heart Failure Guidelines recommend an initial dose of 2 mg once daily with dose titration at 1- to 2-week intervals to a target dose of 8-16 mg once daily.

Hypertension: Initial: 4 mg/day but may be titrated to response; usual range: 4-8 mg/day (may be given in 2 divided doses); increase at 1- to 2-week intervals (maximum: 16 mg/day). **Note:** The Canadian labeling recommended maximum dose is 8 mg/day.

Concomitant therapy with diuretics: To reduce the risk of hypotension, discontinue diuretic, if possible, 2-3 days prior to initiating perindopril. If unable to stop diuretic, initiate perindopril at 2-4 mg/day (given in 1-2 divided doses) and monitor blood pressure closely for the first 2 weeks of therapy, and after any dose adjustment of perindopril or diuretic.

Stable coronary artery disease: Initial: 4 mg once daily for 2 weeks; then increase as tolerated to 8 mg once daily.

Elderly:

Hypertension: >65 years:

U.S. labeling: Initial: 4 mg/day; maintenance: 8 mg/day; experience with doses >8 mg/day is limited; may be given in 1-2 divided doses

Canadian labeling: Initial: 2 mg/day; if necessary may increase dose after 4 weeks to 4 mg/day; then to 8 mg/day (based on renal function); may be given in 1 or 2 divided doses.

ACCF/AHA Expert Consensus recommendations: Consider lower initial doses and titrating to response (Aronow, 2011)

Stable coronary artery disease: >70 years: Initial: 2 mg/day for 1 week; then increase as tolerated to 4 mg/day for 1 week; then increase as tolerated to 8 mg/day.

Dosing adjustment in renal impairment:

U.S. labeling:

Cl_{cr} >30 mL/minute: Initial: 2 mg/day; maintenance dosing not to exceed 8 mg/day.

Cl_{cr} <30 mL/minute: Safety and efficacy not established.

Hemodialysis: Perindopril and its metabolites are dialyzable

Canadian labeling:

Cl_{cr} ≥60 mL/minute: Initial: 4 mg/day; maintenance dosing not to exceed 8 mg/day

Cl_{cr} 30-60 mL/minute: 2 mg/day

Cl_{cr} 15-30 mL/minute: 2 mg every other day

Hemodialysis (Cl_{cr} <15 mL/minute): 2 mg on dialysis days (given after dialysis)

Dosing adjustment in hepatic impairment: No adjustment necessary

Administration Administer prior to a meal.

Monitoring Parameters Blood pressure; serum creatinine and potassium; if patient has collagen vascular disease and/or renal impairment, periodically monitor CBC with differential

Dosage Forms Excipient information presented when available (limited, particularly for generics); consult specific product labeling.

Tablet, oral: 2 mg, 4 mg, 8 mg

Aceon®: 2 mg, 4 mg, 8 mg [scored]

- **periochip®** *see* Chlorhexidine Gluconate *on page 341*
- **PerioGard® [OTC]** *see* Chlorhexidine Gluconate *on page 341*
- **PerioMed™** *see* Fluoride *on page 728*
- **Periostat®** *see* Doxycycline *on page 557*
- **Perlane®** *see* Hyaluronate and Derivatives *on page 831*

Permethrin (per METH rin)

Brand Names: U.S. A200® Lice [OTC]; Nix® Complete Lice Treatment System [OTC]; Nix® Creme Rinse Lice Treatment [OTC]; Nix® Creme Rinse [OTC]; Nix® Lice Control Spray [OTC]; Rid® [OTC]

Brand Names: Canada Kwellada-P™; Nix®

Index Terms Elimite

Pharmacologic Category Antiparasitic Agent, Topical; Pediculocide; Scabicidal Agent

Use Single-application treatment of infestation with *Pediculus humanus capitis* (head louse) and its nits or *Sarcoptes scabiei* (scabies); indicated for prophylactic use during epidemics of lice

Pregnancy Risk Factor B

Dosage Topical:

Head lice: Children >2 months and Adults: After hair has been washed with shampoo, rinsed with water, and towel dried, apply a sufficient volume of topical liquid (lotion or cream rinse) to saturate the hair and scalp. Leave on hair for 10 minutes before rinsing off with water; remove remaining nits; may repeat in 1 week if lice or nits still present.

Scabies: Apply cream from head to toe; leave on for 8-14 hours before washing off with water; for infants, also apply on the hairline, neck, scalp, temple, and forehead; may reapply in 1 week if live mites appear

Additional Information Complete prescribing information for this medication should be consulted for additional detail.

Dosage Forms Excipient information presented when available (limited, particularly for generics); consult specific product labeling.

Cream, topical: 5% (60 g)

Liquid, topical [creme rinse formulation]:

Nix® Complete Lice Treatment System: 1% (1s) [contains isopropyl alcohol 20%]

Nix® Creme Rinse: 1% (60 mL) [contains isopropyl alcohol 20%]

Nix® Creme Rinse Lice Treatment: 1% (60 mL) [contains isopropyl alcohol 20%]

Liquid, topical [for bedding, furniture and garments/spray]:

Nix® Lice Control Spray: 0.25% (150 mL)

Lotion, topical: 1% (60 mL)

Solution, topical [for bedding, furniture and garments/spray]:

A200® Lice: 0.5% (170.1 g)

Rid®: 0.5% (150 mL)

Perphenazine (per FEN a zeen)

Brand Names: Canada Apo-Perphenazine®

Index Terms Trilafon

Pharmacologic Category Antiemetic; Antipsychotic Agent, Typical, Phenothiazine

Additional Appendix Information

Antipsychotic Agents *on page 1880*

Use Treatment of schizophrenia; severe nausea and vomiting

Unlabeled Use Psychosis; psychosis/agitation related to Alzheimer's dementia (risks vs benefits)

Dosage Oral:

Adults:

Schizophrenia:

Nonhospitalized: Initial: 4-8 mg 3 times/day; reduce dose as soon as possible to minimum effective dosage (maximum: 24 mg/day)

Hospitalized: 8-16 mg 2-4 times/day (maximum: 64 mg/day)

Nausea/vomiting: 8-16 mg/day in divided doses; reduce dose as soon as possible to minimum effective dosage (maximum: 24 mg/day)

Elderly: No dosage adjustment provided in manufacturer's labeling; however, initiate dosing at the lower end of the dosing range. Refer to adult dosing.

Dosing adjustment in renal impairment: 0% to 5% removed by hemodialysis (HD); no dosage adjustment provided in manufacturer's labeling.

Dosing adjustment in hepatic impairment: No dosage adjustment provided in manufacturer's labeling.

Additional Information Complete prescribing information for this medication should be consulted for additional detail.

Dosage Forms Excipient information presented when available (limited, particularly for generics); consult specific product labeling.

Tablet, oral: 2 mg, 4 mg, 8 mg, 16 mg

- ◆ **Perphenazine and Amitriptyline Hydrochloride** *see* Amitriptyline and Perphenazine *on page 96*
- ◆ **Persantine®** *see* Dipyridamole *on page 527*
- ◆ **Pertussis, Acellular (Adsorbed)** *see* Diphtheria and Tetanus Toxoids, Acellular Pertussis, Poliovirus and *Haemophilus* b Conjugate Vaccine *on page 522*
- ◆ **Pethidine Hydrochloride** *see* Meperidine *on page 1074*
- ◆ **Pexeva®** *see* PARoxetine *on page 1299*
- ◆ **PF-02341066** *see* Crizotinib *on page 416*
- ◆ **PFA** *see* Foscarnet *on page 760*
- ◆ **Pfizerpen®** *see* Penicillin G (Parenteral/Aqueous) *on page 1323*
- ◆ **Pfizerpen-AS® (Can)** *see* Penicillin G Procaine *on page 1325*
- ◆ **PGE_1** *see* Alprostadil *on page 74*
- ◆ **PGE_2** *see* Dinoprostone *on page 514*
- ◆ **PGI_2** *see* Epoprostenol *on page 604*
- ◆ **PGX** *see* Epoprostenol *on page 604*
- ◆ **Pharmorubicin® (Can)** *see* Epirubicin *on page 597*
- ◆ **Phenabid® [DSC]** *see* Chlorpheniramine and Phenylephrine *on page 345*
- ◆ **Phenadoz®** *see* Promethazine *on page 1416*
- ◆ **Phenazo™ (Can)** *see* Phenazopyridine *on page 1337*

Phenazopyridine (fen az oh PEER i deen)

Brand Names: U.S. AZO Standard® Maximum Strength [OTC]; AZO Standard® [OTC]; Azo-Gesic™ [OTC]; Baridium [OTC]; Pyridium®; ReAzo [OTC]; UTI Relief® [OTC]

Brand Names: Canada Phenazo™

Index Terms Phenazopyridine Hydrochloride; Phenylazo Diamino Pyridine Hydrochloride

Pharmacologic Category Analgesic, Urinary

Use Symptomatic relief of urinary burning, itching, frequency, and urgency in association with urinary tract infection or following urologic procedures

Pregnancy Risk Factor B

Dosage Oral:

Children: 12 mg/kg/day in 3 divided doses administered after meals for 2 days

Adults: 100-200 mg 3 times/day after meals for 2 days when used concomitantly with an antibacterial agent

Dosing interval in renal impairment:

Cl_{cr} 50-80 mL/minute: Administer every 8-16 hours

Cl_{cr} <50 mL/minute: Avoid use

Additional Information Complete prescribing information for this medication should be consulted for additional detail.

Dosage Forms Excipient information presented when available (limited, particularly for generics); consult specific product labeling.

Tablet, oral, as hydrochloride: 100 mg, 200 mg

AZO Standard®: 95 mg [gluten free]

AZO Standard® Maximum Strength: 97.5 mg

AZO Standard® Maximum Strength: 97.5 mg [gluten free]

Azo-Gesic™: 95 mg

Baridium: 97.2 mg

Pyridium®: 100 mg, 200 mg

ReAzo: 95 mg

UTI Relief®: 97.2 mg

◆ **Phenazopyridine Hydrochloride** *see* Phenazopyridine *on page 1337*

Phenelzine (FEN el zeen)

Brand Names: U.S. Nardil®

Brand Names: Canada Nardil®

Index Terms Phenelzine Sulfate

Pharmacologic Category Antidepressant, Monoamine Oxidase Inhibitor

Additional Appendix Information

Antidepressant Agents *on page 1874*

Use Symptomatic treatment of atypical, nonendogenous, or neurotic depression

Pregnancy Risk Factor C

Pregnancy Considerations Safe use during pregnancy has not been established; use only if benefits outweigh the risks.

Lactation Excretion in breast milk unknown/not recommended

Medication Guide Available Yes

Contraindications Hypersensitivity to phenelzine or any component of the formulation; congestive heart failure; pheochromocytoma; abnormal liver function tests or history of hepatic disease; renal disease or severe renal disease/impairment

Concurrent use of sympathomimetics (including amphetamines, cocaine, dopamine, epinephrine, methylphenidate, norepinephrine, or phenylephrine) and related compounds (methyldopa, levodopa, phenylalanine, tryptophan, or tyrosine), ophthalmic $alpha_2$-agonists (apraclonidine, brimonidine), CNS depressants, cyclobenzaprine, dextromethorphan, ethanol, meperidine, bupropion, or buspirone

At least 2 weeks should elapse between the discontinuation of serotoninergic agents (including SNRIs, SSRIs, and tricyclics) and other MAO inhibitors and the initiation of phenelzine. At least 5 weeks should elapse between the discontinuation of fluoxetine and the initiation of phenelzine. In all cases, a sufficient amount of time must be allowed for the clearance of the serotoninergic agent and any active metabolites prior to the initiation of phenelzine.

At least 2 weeks should elapse between the discontinuation of phenelzine and the initiation of the following agents: Serotoninergic agents (including SNRIs, SSRIs, fluoxetine, and tricyclics), bupropion, buspirone, and other antidepressants.

General anesthesia, spinal anesthesia (hypotension may be exaggerated). Use caution with local anesthetics containing sympathomimetic agents. Phenelzine should be discontinued ≥10 days prior to elective surgery.

Foods high in tyramine or dopamine content; foods and/or supplements containing tyrosine, phenylalanine, tryptophan, or caffeine

Warnings/Precautions [U.S. Boxed Warning]: Antidepressants increase the risk of suicidal thinking and behavior in children, adolescents, and young adults (18-24 years of age) with major depressive disorder (MDD) and other psychiatric disorders; consider risk prior to prescribing. Short-term studies did not show an increased risk in patients >24 years of age and showed a decreased risk in patients ≥65 years. Closely monitor for clinical worsening, suicidality, or unusual changes in ▶

behavior; the patient's family or caregiver should be instructed to closely observe the patient and communicate condition with healthcare provider. Such observation would generally include at least weekly face-to-face contact with patients or their family members or caregivers during the first 4 weeks of treatment, then every other week visits for the next 4 weeks, then at 12 weeks, and as clinically indicated beyond 12 weeks. Additional contact by telephone may be appropriate between face-to-face visits. Adults treated with antidepressants should be observed similarly for clinical worsening and suicidality, especially during the initial few months of a course of drug therapy, or at times of dose changes, either increases or decreases. A medication guide should be dispensed with each prescription. Phenelzine is not generally considered a first-line agent for the treatment of depression; phenelzine is typically used in patients who have failed to respond to other treatments. **Phenelzine is not FDA approved for the treatment of depression in children ≤16 years of age.**

The possibility of a suicide attempt is inherent in major depression and may persist until remission occurs. Monitor for worsening of depression or suicidality, especially during initiation of therapy (generally first 1-2 months) or with dose increases or decreases. Worsening depression and severe abrupt suicidality that are not part of the presenting symptoms may require discontinuation or modification of drug therapy. Use caution in high-risk patients during initiation of therapy. Prescriptions should be written for the smallest quantity consistent with good patient care. The patient's family or caregiver should be alerted to monitor patients for the emergence of suicidality and associated behaviors such as anxiety, agitation, panic attacks, insomnia, irritability, hostility, impulsivity, akathisia, hypomania, and mania; patients should be instructed to notify their healthcare provider if any of these symptoms or worsening depression occur.

May worsen psychosis in some patients or precipitate a shift to mania or hypomania in patients with bipolar disorder. Monotherapy in patients with bipolar disorder should be avoided. Patients presenting with depressive symptoms should be screened for bipolar disorder. Phenelzine is not FDA approved for the treatment of bipolar depression.

Sensitization to the effects of insulin may occur; monitor blood glucose closely in patients with diabetes. Use with caution in patients who have glaucoma, or hyperthyroidism. Cases of hypertensive crisis (sometimes fatal) have occurred; symptoms include: severe headache, nausea/vomiting, neck stiffness/soreness, photophobia, and sweating. Monitor blood pressure closely in all patients. Hypertensive crisis may occur with tyramine-, tryptophan-, or dopamine-containing foods. Phentolamine is recommended for the treatment of hypertensive crisis. Do not use with other MAO inhibitors or antidepressants. Do not use within 5 weeks of fluoxetine discontinuation or 2 weeks of other antidepressant discontinuation. Avoid products containing sympathomimetic stimulants or dextromethorphan. Concurrent use with antihypertensive agents may lead to exaggeration of hypotensive effects. May cause orthostatic hypotension; use with caution in patients with hypotension or patients who would not tolerate transient hypotensive episodes (cardiovascular or cerebrovascular disease); effects may be additive with other agents which cause orthostasis. Use with caution in patients at risk of seizures, or in patients receiving other drugs which may lower seizure threshold. Discontinue at least 48 hours prior to myelography. May increase the risks associated with electroconvulsive therapy. Consider discontinuing, when possible, prior to elective surgery. Pyridoxine deficiency has occurred; symptoms include numbness and edema of hands; may respond to supplementation.

Adverse Reactions Frequency not defined.

Cardiovascular: Edema, orthostatic hypotension

Central nervous system: Anxiety (acute), ataxia, coma, delirium, dizziness, drowsiness, euphoria, fatigue, fever, headache, hyper-reflexia, hypersomnia, insomnia, mania, schizophrenia, seizure, twitching

Dermatologic: Pruritus, rash

Endocrine & metabolic: Decreased sexual ability (anorgasmia, ejaculatory disturbances, impotence), hypermetabolic syndrome, hypernatremia

Gastrointestinal: Constipation, weight gain, xerostomia

Genitourinary: Urinary retention

Hematologic: Leukopenia

Hepatic: Jaundice, necrotizing hepatocellular necrosis (rare), transaminases increased

Neuromuscular & skeletal: Myoclonia, paresthesia, tremor, weakness

Ocular: Blurred vision, glaucoma, nystagmus

Respiratory: Edema (glottis)

Miscellaneous: Diaphoresis, Lupus-like syndrome, transient cardiac or respiratory depression (following ECT), withdrawal syndrome (nausea, vomiting, malaise)

Drug Interactions

Metabolism/Transport Effects Inhibits Monoamine Oxidase

Avoid Concomitant Use

Avoid concomitant use of Phenelzine with any of the following: Alpha-/Beta-Agonists (Indirect-Acting); Alpha1-Agonists; Alpha2-Agonists (Ophthalmic); Amphetamines; Anilidopiperidine Opioids; Antidepressants (Serotonin Reuptake Inhibitor/Antagonist); Atomoxetine; Bezafibrate; Buprenorphine; BuPROPion; BusPIRone; CarBAMazepine; Cyclobenzaprine; Dexmethylphenidate; Dextromethorphan; Diethylpropion; HYDROmorphone; Linezolid; Maprotiline; Meperidine; Methyldopa; Methylene Blue; Methylphenidate; Mirtazapine; Oxymorphone; Pizotifen; Selective Serotonin Reuptake Inhibitors; Serotonin 5-HT1D Receptor Agonists; Serotonin/Norepinephrine Reuptake Inhibitors; Tapentadol; Tetrabenazine; Tetrahydrozoline; Tetrahydrozoline (Nasal); Tricyclic Antidepressants; Tryptophan

Increased Effect/Toxicity

Phenelzine may increase the levels/effects of: Alpha-/Beta-Agonists (Direct-Acting); Alpha-/Beta-Agonists (Indirect-Acting); Alpha1-Agonists; Alpha2-Agonists (Ophthalmic); Amphetamines; Anticholinergics; Antidepressants (Serotonin Reuptake Inhibitor/Antagonist); Antihypertensives; Atomoxetine; Beta2-Agonists; Bezafibrate; BuPROPion; Dexmethylphenidate; Dextromethorphan; Diethylpropion; Doxapram; HYDROmorphone; Linezolid; Lithium; Meperidine; Methadone; Methyldopa; Methylene Blue; Methylphenidate; Metoclopramide; Mirtazapine; Orthostatic Hypotension Producing Agents; Pizotifen; Reserpine; Selective Serotonin Reuptake Inhibitors; Serotonin 5-HT1D Receptor Agonists; Serotonin Modulators; Serotonin/Norepinephrine Reuptake Inhibitors; Succinylcholine; Tetrahydrozoline; Tetrahydrozoline (Nasal); Tricyclic Antidepressants

The levels/effects of Phenelzine may be increased by: Altretamine; Anilidopiperidine Opioids; Antipsychotics; Buprenorphine; BusPIRone; CarBAMazepine; COMT Inhibitors; Cyclobenzaprine; Levodopa; MAO Inhibitors; Maprotiline; Oxymorphone; Pramlintide; Tapentadol; Tetrabenazine; TraMADol; Tryptophan

Decreased Effect

Phenelzine may decrease the levels/effects of: Acetylcholinesterase Inhibitors (Central)

The levels/effects of Phenelzine may be decreased by: Acetylcholinesterase Inhibitors (Central)

Ethanol/Nutrition/Herb Interactions

Ethanol: May increase CNS depression; monitor for increased effects with coadministration. Caution patients about effects. Avoid beverages containing tyramine (hearty red wine and beer).

Food: Concurrent ingestion of foods rich in tyramine may cause sudden and severe high blood pressure (hypertensive crisis). Avoid tyramine-containing foods with MAOIs.

Herb/Nutraceutical: Avoid valerian, St John's wort, SAMe, kava kava (may increase risk of serotonin syndrome and/or excessive sedation); Avoid supplements containing caffeine, tyrosine, tryptophan, or phenylalanine. Ingestion of large quantities may increase the risk of severe side effects (eg, hypertensive reactions, serotonin syndrome).

Stability Store at 20°C to 25°C (68°F to 77°F). Protect from heat and light.

Mechanism of Action Thought to act by increasing endogenous concentrations of norepinephrine, dopamine, and serotonin through inhibition of the enzyme (monoamine oxidase) responsible for the breakdown of these neurotransmitters

Pharmacodynamics/Kinetics

Onset of action: Therapeutic: 2-4 weeks; geriatric patients receiving an average of 55 mg/day developed a mean platelet MAO activity inhibition of about 85%.

Duration: May continue to have a therapeutic effect and interactions 2 weeks after discontinuing therapy

Absorption: Well absorbed

Metabolism: Oxidized via monoamine oxidase (primary pathway) and acetylation (minor pathway)

Half-life elimination: 12 hours

Excretion: Urine (73% as metabolites)

Dosage Oral:

Adults: Depression: Initial: 15 mg 3 times/day

Early phase: Increase rapidly, based on patient tolerance, to 60-90 mg/day (may take 4 weeks of 60 mg/day therapy before clinical response)

Maintenance: After maximum benefit is obtained, slowly reduce dose over several weeks; dose may be as low as 15 mg/day to 15 mg every other day

Elderly: Depression: Select dose with caution; generally initiating at the lower end of the dosing range; some clinicians recommend an initial dose of 7.5 mg, with dose increases of 7.5 mg/day every 4-8 days as tolerated to a usual therapeutic dose of 22.5-60 mg/day in older adults (Alexopoulos, 2004).

Dietary Considerations Avoid tyramine-containing foods/beverages. Some examples include aged or matured cheese, air-dried or cured meats (including sausages and salamis), fava or broad bean pods, tap/draft beers, Marmite concentrate, sauerkraut, soy sauce and other soybean condiments. Food's freshness is also an important concern; improperly stored or spoiled food can create an environment where tyramine concentrations may increase.

Monitoring Parameters Blood pressure, heart rate; diet, weight; mood (if depressive symptoms), suicide ideation (especially during the initial months of therapy or when doses are increased or decreased)

Dosage Forms Excipient information presented when available (limited, particularly for generics); consult specific product labeling.

Tablet, oral: 15 mg

Nardil®: 15 mg

◆ **Phenelzine Sulfate** *see* Phenelzine *on page 1337*

◆ **Phenergan®** *see* Promethazine *on page 1416*

◆ **Pheniramine and Naphazoline** *see* Naphazoline and Pheniramine *on page 1177*

PHENobarbital (fee noe BAR bi tal)

Brand Names: Canada PMS-Phenobarbital

Index Terms Luminal Sodium; Phenobarbital Sodium; Phenobarbitone; Phenylethylmalonylurea

Pharmacologic Category Anticonvulsant, Barbiturate; Barbiturate

Additional Appendix Information

Status Epilepticus *on page 2010*

Use Management of generalized tonic-clonic (grand mal), status epilepticus, and partial seizures; sedative/hypnotic

Note: Use to treat insomnia is not recommended (Schutte-Rodin, 2008)

Unlabeled Use Prevention and treatment of neonatal hyperbilirubinemia and lowering of bilirubin in chronic cholestasis; neonatal seizures

Pregnancy Risk Factor B/D (manufacturer dependent)

Pregnancy Considerations Barbiturates can be detected in the placenta, fetal liver, and fetal brain. Fetal and maternal blood concentrations may be similar following parenteral administration. An increased incidence of fetal abnormalities may occur following maternal use. The use of folic acid throughout pregnancy and vitamin K during the last month of pregnancy is recommended; epilepsy itself, number of medications, genetic factors, or a combination of these probably influence the teratogenicity of anticonvulsant therapy. When used during the third trimester of pregnancy, withdrawal symptoms may occur in the neonate, including seizures and hyperirritability; symptoms of withdrawal may be delayed in the neonate up to 14 days after birth. Use during labor does not impair uterine activity; however, respiratory depression may occur in the newborn; resuscitation equipment should be available, especially for premature infants.

Lactation Enters breast milk/use caution (AAP recommends use "with caution"; AAP 2001 update pending)

Contraindications Hypersensitivity to barbiturates or any component of the formulation; marked hepatic impairment; dyspnea or airway obstruction; porphyria (manifest and latent); intra-arterial administration, subcutaneous administration (not recommended); use in patients with a history of sedative/hypnotic addiction is not recommended; nephritic patients (large doses)

Warnings/Precautions Potential for drug dependency exists, abrupt cessation may precipitate withdrawal, including status epilepticus in epileptic patients. Do not administer to patients in acute pain. Use caution in elderly, debilitated, renal or hepatic dysfunction, and pediatric patients. May cause paradoxical responses, including agitation and hyperactivity, particularly in acute pain and pediatric patients. Use with caution in patients with depression or suicidal tendencies, or in patients with a history of drug abuse. Tolerance, psychological and physical dependence may occur with prolonged use. May cause CNS depression, which may impair physical or mental abilities. Effects with other sedative drugs or ethanol may be potentiated. May cause respiratory depression or hypotension, particularly when administered intravenously. Use with caution in hemodynamically unstable patients (hypovolemic shock, CHF) or patients with respiratory disease. Due to its long half-life and risk of dependence, phenobarbital is not recommended as a sedative in the elderly. Use has been associated with cognitive deficits in children. Use with caution in patients with hypoadrenalism. Intra-arterial administration may cause reactions ranging from transient pain to gangrene and is contraindicated. Subcutaneous administration may cause tissue irritation (eg, redness, tenderness, necrosis) and is not recommended. ▶

Adverse Reactions Frequency not defined.

Cardiovascular: Bradycardia, hypotension, syncope

Central nervous system: Agitation, anxiety, ataxia, CNS excitation or depression, confusion, dizziness drowsiness, hallucinations, "hangover" effect, headache, hyperkinesia, impaired judgment, insomnia, lethargy, nervousness, nightmares, somnolence

Dermatologic: Exfoliative dermatitis, rash, Stevens-Johnson syndrome

Gastrointestinal: Nausea, vomiting, constipation

Hematologic: Agranulocytosis, thrombocytopenia, megaloblastic anemia

Local: Pain at injection site, thrombophlebitis with I.V. use

Renal: Oliguria

Respiratory: Laryngospasm, respiratory depression, apnea (especially with rapid I.V. use), hypoventilation

Miscellaneous: Gangrene with inadvertent intra-arterial injection

Drug Interactions

Metabolism/Transport Effects Substrate of CYP2C19 (major), CYP2C9 (minor), CYP2E1 (minor); **Note:** Assignment of Major/Minor substrate status based on clinically relevant drug interaction potential; **Induces** CYP1A2 (strong), CYP2A6 (strong), CYP2B6 (strong), CYP2C8 (strong), CYP2C9 (strong), CYP3A4 (strong)

Avoid Concomitant Use

Avoid concomitant use of PHENobarbital with any of the following: Boceprevir; Bortezomib; Crizotinib; Darunavir; Dronedarone; Etravirine; Everolimus; Lapatinib; Lurasidone; Nilotinib; Pazopanib; Praziquantel; Ranolazine; Rilpivirine; Rivaroxaban; Roflumilast; RomiDEPsin; SORAfenib; Telaprevir; Ticagrelor; Tolvaptan; Toremifene; Vandetanib; Voriconazole

Increased Effect/Toxicity

PHENobarbital may increase the levels/effects of: Alcohol (Ethyl); Clarithromycin; CNS Depressants; Meperidine; Prilocaine; QuiNIDine; Selective Serotonin Reuptake Inhibitors; Thiazide Diuretics

The levels/effects of PHENobarbital may be increased by: Carbonic Anhydrase Inhibitors; Chloramphenicol; Clarithromycin; CYP2C19 Inhibitors (Moderate); CYP2C19 Inhibitors (Strong); Dexmethylphenidate; Divalproex; Droperidol; Felbamate; HydrOXYzine; Methylphenidate; Primidone; QuiNINE; Rufinamide; Telaprevir; Valproic Acid

Decreased Effect

PHENobarbital may decrease the levels/effects of: Acetaminophen; ARIPiprazole; Bendamustine; Beta-Blockers; Boceprevir; Bortezomib; Brentuximab Vedotin; Calcium Channel Blockers; Chloramphenicol; Clarithromycin; Contraceptives (Estrogens); Contraceptives (Progestins); Corticosteroids (Systemic); Crizotinib; CycloSPORINE; CycloSPORINE (Systemic); CYP1A2 Substrates; CYP2A6 Substrates; CYP2B6 Substrates; CYP2C8 Substrates; CYP2C9 Substrates; CYP3A4 Substrates; Darunavir; Dasatinib; Deferasirox; Diclofenac; Disopyramide; Divalproex; Doxycycline; Dronedarone; Etoposide; Etoposide Phosphate; Etravirine; Everolimus; Exemestane; Felbamate; Fosphenytoin; Gefitinib; Griseofulvin; GuanFACINE; Imatinib; Irinotecan; Ixabepilone; Lacosamide; LamoTRIgine; Lapatinib; Linagliptin; Lopinavir; Lurasidone; Maraviroc; Methadone; MetroNIDAZOLE; MetroNIDAZOLE (Systemic); Nilotinib; OXcarbazepine; Pazopanib; Phenytoin; Praziquantel; Propafenone; QuiNIDine; QuiNINE; Ranolazine; Rilpivirine; Rivaroxaban; Roflumilast; RomiDEPsin; Rufinamide; Saxagliptin; SORAfenib; SUNItinib; Tadalafil; Telaprevir; Teniposide; Theophylline Derivatives; Ticagrelor; Tipranavir; Tolvaptan; Toremifene; Treprostinil; Tricyclic Antidepressants; Ulipristal; Valproic Acid; Vandetanib; Vemurafenib; Vitamin K Antagonists; Voriconazole; Zonisamide; Zuclopenthixol

The levels/effects of PHENobarbital may be decreased by: Amphetamines; Cholestyramine Resin; CYP2C19 Inducers (Strong); Cyproterone; Folic Acid; Ketorolac; Ketorolac (Nasal); Ketorolac (Systemic); Leucovorin Calcium-Levoleucovorin; Levomefolate; Mefloquine; Methylfolate; Pyridoxine; Rifamycin Derivatives; Telaprevir; Tipranavir

Ethanol/Nutrition/Herb Interactions

Ethanol: May increase CNS depression; monitor for increased effects with coadministration. Caution patients about effects.

Food: May cause decrease in vitamin D and calcium.

Herb/Nutraceutical: Avoid evening primrose (seizure threshold decreased). Avoid valerian, St John's wort, kava kava, gotu kola (may increase CNS depression).

Stability Protect elixir from light. Not stable in aqueous solutions; use only clear solutions. Do not add to acidic solutions; precipitation may occur.

Mechanism of Action Long-acting barbiturate with sedative, hypnotic, and anticonvulsant properties. Barbiturates depress the sensory cortex, decrease motor activity, alter cerebellar function, and produce drowsiness, sedation, and hypnosis. In high doses, barbiturates exhibit anticonvulsant activity; barbiturates produce dose-dependent respiratory depression.

Pharmacodynamics/Kinetics

Onset of action: Oral: Hypnosis: 20-60 minutes; I.V.: ~5 minutes

Peak effect: I.V.: ~30 minutes

Duration: Oral: 6-10 hours; I.V.: 4-10 hours

Absorption: Oral: 70% to 90%

Protein binding: 20% to 45%; decreased in neonates

Metabolism: Hepatic via hydroxylation and glucuronide conjugation

Half-life elimination: Neonates: 45-500 hours; Infants: 20-133 hours; Children: 37-73 hours; Adults: 53-140 hours

Time to peak, serum: Oral: 1-6 hours

Excretion: Urine (20% to 50% as unchanged drug)

Dosage

Children:

Sedation: Oral: 2 mg/kg 3 times/day

Preoperative sedation: Oral, I.M., I.V.: 1-3 mg/kg 1-1.5 hours before procedure

Adults:

Sedation: Oral, I.M.: 30-120 mg/day in 2-3 divided doses

Preoperative sedation: I.M.: 100-200 mg 1-1.5 hours before procedure

Anticonvulsant: Status epilepticus: **Loading dose:** I.V.:

Infants and Children: 15-20 mg/kg (maximum: 1000 mg/dose, maximum rate ≤30 mg/minute in children <60 kg); may repeat dose after 15 minutes as needed (maximum total dose: 40 mg/kg)

Adults: 10-20 mg/kg (maximum rate ≤60 mg/minute in patients ≥60 kg); may repeat dose in 20-minute intervals as needed (maximum total dose: 30 mg/kg)

Anticonvulsant maintenance dose: Oral, I.V.:

Infants: 5-8 mg/kg/day in 1-2 divided doses

Children:

1-5 years: 6-8 mg/kg/day in 1-2 divided doses

5-12 years: 4-6 mg/kg/day in 1-2 divided doses

Children >12 years and Adults: 1-3 mg/kg/day in divided doses or 50-100 mg 2-3 times/day

Sedative/hypnotic withdrawal (unlabeled use): Initial daily requirement is determined by substituting phenobarbital 30 mg for every 100 mg pentobarbital used during tolerance testing; then daily requirement is decreased by 10% of initial dose

Elderly or debilitated: Initiate at the lowest recommended dose.

Dosing adjustment in renal impairment: Cl_{cr} <10 mL/minute: Administer every 12-16 hours

Hemodialysis: Moderately dialyzable (20% to 50%)

Dosing adjustment in hepatic impairment: Reduce dose in patients with hepatic impairment.

Dietary Considerations Vitamin D: Loss in vitamin D due to malabsorption; increase intake of foods rich in vitamin D. Supplementation of vitamin D and/or calcium may be necessary. Injection may contain sodium.

Administration May be administered I.V., I.M. or orally. Avoid rapid I.V. administration >60 mg/minute in adults and >30 mg/minute in children; intra-arterial injection is contraindicated; avoid subcutaneous administration; parenteral solutions are highly alkaline; avoid extravasation. For I.M. administration, inject deep into muscle. Do not exceed 5 mL per injection site due to potential for tissue irritation

Monitoring Parameters Phenobarbital serum concentrations, mental status, CBC, LFTs, seizure activity

Reference Range

Therapeutic:

Infants and Children: 15-30 mcg/mL (SI: 65-129 micromole/L)

Adults: 20-40 mcg/mL (SI: 86-172 micromole/L)

Toxic: >40 mcg/mL (SI: >172 micromole/L)

Toxic concentration: Slowness, ataxia, nystagmus: 35-80 mcg/mL (SI: 150-344 micromole/L)

Coma with reflexes: 65-117 mcg/mL (SI: 279-502 micromole/L)

Coma without reflexes: >100 mcg/mL (SI: >430 micromole/L)

Test Interactions Assay interference of LDH

Additional Information Injectable solutions contain propylene glycol.

Phenobarbital tablets are also available from some generic manufacturers in strengths that are exactly equivalent to fractional grain strengths: 16.2 mg (1/4 grain), 32.4 mg (1/2 grain), 64.8 mg (1 grain). To avoid medication errors, do not prescribe phenobarbital in grains.

Dosage Forms Excipient information presented when available (limited, particularly for generics); consult specific product labeling.

Elixir, oral: 20 mg/5 mL (5 mL, 7.5 mL, 15 mL, 473 mL)

Injection, solution, as sodium: 65 mg/mL (1 mL); 130 mg/mL (1 mL)

Tablet, oral: 15 mg, 30 mg, 60 mg, 100 mg

Controlled Substance C-IV

Extemporaneous Preparations An alcohol-free 10 mg/mL phenobarbital oral suspension may be made from tablets and one of two different vehicles (a 1:1 mixture of Ora-Plus® and Ora-Sweet® or a 1:1 mixture of Ora-Plus® and Ora-Sweet® SF). Crush ten phenobarbital 60 mg tablets in a glass mortar and reduce to a fine powder. Mix 30 mL of Ora-Plus® and 30 mL of either Ora-Sweet® or Ora-Sweet® SF; stir vigorously. Add 15 mL of the vehicle to the powder and mix to a uniform paste. Transfer the mixture to a 2 ounce amber plastic prescription bottle. Rinse mortar and pestle with 15 mL of the vehicle; transfer to bottle. Repeat, then add quantity of vehicle sufficient to make 60 mL. Label "shake well." May mix dose with chocolate syrup (1:1 volume) immediately before administration to mask the bitter aftertaste. Stable for 115 days when stored in amber plastic prescription bottles at room temperature.

Cober M and Johnson CE, "Stability of an Extemporaneously Prepared Alcohol-Free Phenobarbital Suspension," *Am J Health Syst Pharm*, 2007, 64(6):644-6.

◆ **Phenobarbital, Hyoscyamine, Atropine, and Scopolamine** *see* Hyoscyamine, Atropine, Scopolamine, and Phenobarbital *on page* 855

◆ **Phenobarbital Sodium** *see* PHENobarbital *on page* 1339

◆ **Phenobarbitone** *see* PHENobarbital *on page* 1339

◆ **Phenoptin** *see* Sapropterin *on page* 1536

Phenoxybenzamine (fen oks ee BEN za meen)

Brand Names: U.S. Dibenzyline®

Index Terms Phenoxybenzamine Hydrochloride

Pharmacologic Category $Alpha_1$ Blocker; Antidote

Use Symptomatic management of pheochromocytoma

Unlabeled Use Micturition problems associated with neurogenic bladder, functional outlet obstruction, and partial prostate obstruction; treatment of hypertensive crisis caused by sympathomimetic amines

Pregnancy Risk Factor C

Dosage Oral:

Children (unlabeled use): Initial: 0.25-1 mg/kg/day (maximum: 10 mg); increase slowly to blood pressure control

Adults:

Pheochromocytoma, hypertension: Initial: 10 mg twice daily; increase by 10 mg every other day until optimal blood pressure response is achieved; usual range: 20-40 mg 2-3 times/day. Doses up to 240 mg/day have been reported (Kinney, 2000).

Micturition disorders (unlabeled use): 10-20 mg 1-2 times/day

Additional Information Complete prescribing information for this medication should be consulted for additional detail.

Dosage Forms Excipient information presented when available (limited, particularly for generics); consult specific product labeling.

Capsule, oral, as hydrochloride:

Dibenzyline®: 10 mg

◆ **Phenoxybenzamine Hydrochloride** *see* Phenoxybenzamine *on page* 1341

◆ **Phenoxymethyl Penicillin** *see* Penicillin V Potassium *on page* 1326

Phentermine (FEN ter meen)

Brand Names: U.S. Adipex-P®

Index Terms Phentermine Hydrochloride; Suprenza™

Pharmacologic Category Anorexiant; Sympathomimetic

Use Short-term (few weeks) adjunct therapy in obese patients with an initial body mass index (BMI) ≥30 kg/m^2 or ≥27 kg/m^2 in the presence of other risk factors (eg, diabetes, hyperlipidemia, hypertension); therapy should be used in conjunction with a comprehensive weight management program.

Pregnancy Risk Factor C/X (manufacturer specific)

Pregnancy Considerations Animal reproduction studies have not been conducted. The use of Suprenza™ is contraindicated during pregnancy. The risks of using appetite suppressing drugs in pregnant women are not known and limited information is available about the use of phentermine in pregnancy. Weight loss therapy is generally not recommended for pregnant women. Obese and overweight women should be encouraged to participate in weight reduction programs prior to attempting pregnancy; weight gain during pregnancy should be determined by their prepregnancy BMI and current guidelines.

Lactation Excretion in breast milk unknown/not recommended

Contraindications Hypersensitivity or idiosyncrasy to phentermine or other sympathomimetic amines or any component of the formulation; cardiovascular disease (current or a history of), advanced arteriosclerosis, moderate-to-severe hypertension; hyperthyroidism, glaucoma, agitated states, patients with a history of drug abuse; use during or within 14 days following MAO inhibitor therapy

Suprenza™: Additional contraindications: Pregnancy, breast-feeding

Warnings/Precautions Hazardous agent - use appropriate precautions for handling and disposal. Primary pulmonary hypertension (PPH), a rare and frequently fatal pulmonary disease, has been reported to occur in patients receiving a combination of phentermine and fenfluramine or dexfenfluramine. The possibility of an association between PPH and the use of phentermine alone cannot be ruled out. Discontinue in patients experiencing new-onset dyspnea, chest pain, syncope or lower extremity edema. The use of phentermine has been associated with the development of valvular heart disease. Avoid stimulants in patients with known serious structural cardiac abnormalities, cardiomyopathy, serious heart rhythm abnormalities, or other serious cardiac problems that could increase the risk of sudden death that these conditions alone carry. Caution should be used in patients with mild hypertension and other cardiovascular conditions that might be exacerbated by increases in blood pressure or heart rate.

Use caution with diabetes; antidiabetic agent requirements may be decreased with anorexigens and concomitant dietary restrictions. Stimulants may unmask tics in individuals with coexisting Tourette's syndrome. Use caution with seizure disorders. Phentermine is pharmacologically related to the amphetamines, which have a high abuse potential; prolonged use may lead to dependency. Prescriptions should be written for the smallest quantity consistent with good patient care to minimize possibility of overdose. Amphetamines may impair the ability to engage in potentially hazardous activities. Use caution in patients with renal impairment; use has not been studied; however, an increase in exposure is expected in renal impairment.

May be inappropriate for use in the elderly due to the risk for causing dependence, hypertension, angina, and myocardial infarction (Beers Criteria).

Discontinue if satisfactory weight loss has not occurred within the first 4 weeks of treatment. Tolerance to the anorectic effect usually develops within a few weeks; discontinue use when tolerance develops, do not exceed recommended dosage in an attempt to overcome tolerance. Safety and efficacy have not been established for use with other weight loss medications including SSRIs, over-the-counter, or herbal products.

Adverse Reactions Frequency not defined.

Cardiovascular: Hypertension, ischemic events, palpitation, primary pulmonary hypertension and/or regurgitant cardiac valvular disease, tachycardia

Central nervous system: Dizziness, dysphoria, euphoria, headache, insomnia, overstimulation, psychosis, restlessness

Dermatologic: Urticaria

Endocrine & metabolic: Changes in libido

Gastrointestinal: Constipation, diarrhea, unpleasant taste, xerostomia

Genitourinary: Impotence

Neuromuscular & skeletal: Tremor

Drug Interactions

Metabolism/Transport Effects None known.

Avoid Concomitant Use

Avoid concomitant use of Phentermine with any of the following: Iobenguane I 123; MAO Inhibitors

Increased Effect/Toxicity

Phentermine may increase the levels/effects of: Analgesics (Opioid); Sympathomimetics

The levels/effects of Phentermine may be increased by: Alcohol (Ethyl); Alkalinizing Agents; Antacids; Atomoxetine; Cannabinoids; Carbonic Anhydrase Inhibitors; MAO Inhibitors; Proton Pump Inhibitors; Tricyclic Antidepressants

Decreased Effect

Phentermine may decrease the levels/effects of: Antihistamines; Ethosuximide; Iobenguane I 123; Ioflupane I 123; PHENobarbital; Phenytoin

The levels/effects of Phentermine may be decreased by: Ammonium Chloride; Antipsychotics; Gastrointestinal Acidifying Agents; Lithium; Methenamine

Ethanol/Nutrition/Herb Interactions Ethanol: Concurrent use of phentermine with ethanol may result in adverse effects.

Stability Store at controlled room temperature of 20°C to 25°C (68°F to 77°F).

Mechanism of Action Phentermine is a sympathomimetic amine with pharmacologic properties similar to the amphetamines. The mechanism of action in reducing appetite appears to be secondary to CNS effects, including stimulation of the hypothalamus to release norepinephrine.

Pharmacodynamics/Kinetics

Absorption: Well absorbed

Time to peak: Orally disintegrating tablet: 3-4.4 hours

Excretion: Primarily urine

Dosage Note: Dosing is presented in terms of the salt, phentermine hydrochloride (not as phentermine base).

Oral: Children >16 years and Adults: Obesity:

Capsule, tablet: 15-37.5 mg/day given in 1-2 divided doses. Individualize to achieve adequate response with lowest effective dose.

Orally disintegrating tablet (ODT): One tablet (15 mg or 30 mg) every morning. Individualize to achieve adequate response with lowest effective dose.

Dietary Considerations Capsules, tablets: Should be taken before breakfast or 1-2 hours after breakfast; avoid taking in the late evening. Most effective when combined with a low-calorie diet and behavior modification counseling.

Administration Avoid late evening administration.

Capsules, tablets: Administer before breakfast or 1-2 hours after breakfast. Tablets may be divided in half and dose may be given in 2 divided doses.

Orally disintegrating tablets (Suprenza™): With dry hands, place tablet on the tongue and allow to dissolve, then swallow with or without water. May administer with or without food.

Monitoring Parameters Weight, waist circumference; blood pressure

Reference Range

Adult classification of weight by BMI (kg/m^2):

Underweight: <18.5

Normal: 18.5-24.9

Overweight: 25-29.9

Obese, class I: 30-34.9

Obese, class II: 35-39.9

Extreme obesity (class III): ≥40

Waist circumference: In adults with a BMI of 25-34.9 kg/m^2, high-risk waist circumference is defined as:

Men >102 cm (>40 in)

Women >88 cm (>35 in)

Test Interactions May interfere with urine detection of amphetamines/methamphetamines (false-positive).

Product Availability

Suprenza™: FDA approved June 2011; expected availability is undetermined.

Suprenza™ is an oral disintegrating tablet formulation approved as a short-term adjunct in a comprehensive weight reduction regimen.

Dosage Forms Excipient information presented when available (limited, particularly for generics); consult specific product labeling.

Capsule, oral, as hydrochloride: 15 mg, 30 mg, 37.5 mg
Adipex-P®: 37.5 mg

Tablet, oral, as hydrochloride: 37.5 mg
Adipex-P®: 37.5 mg [scored]

Controlled Substance C-IV

◆ **Phentermine Hydrochloride** *see* Phentermine *on page 1341*

Phentolamine (fen TOLE a meen)

Brand Names: U.S. OraVerse™

Brand Names: Canada Regitine®; Rogitine®

Index Terms Phentolamine Mesylate; Regitine [DSC]

Pharmacologic Category Alpha$_1$ Blocker

Additional Appendix Information

Hypertension *on page 2001*

Use Diagnosis of pheochromocytoma and treatment of hypertension associated with pheochromocytoma or other forms of hypertension caused by excess sympathomimetic amines; treatment of dermal necrosis after extravasation of drugs with alpha-adrenergic effects (ie, dopamine, epinephrine, norepinephrine, phenylephrine)

OraVerse™: Reversal of soft tissue anesthesia and the associated functional deficits resulting from a local dental anesthetic containing a vasoconstrictor

Unlabeled Use Treatment of pralidoxime-induced hypertension

Pregnancy Risk Factor C

Lactation Excretion in breast milk unknown

Contraindications Hypersensitivity to phentolamine or any component of the formulation; renal impairment; coronary or cerebral arteriosclerosis; concurrent use with phosphodiesterase-5 (PDE-5) inhibitors including sildenafil (>25 mg), tadalafil, or vardenafil

OraVerse™: There are no contraindications listed in the manufacturer's labeling.

Warnings/Precautions Myocardial infarction, cerebrovascular spasm, and cerebrovascular occlusion have occurred following administration; use with caution in patients with gastritis or peptic ulcer, tachycardia, or a history of cardiac arrhythmias. Discontinue if symptoms of angina occur or worsen. OraVerse™: Efficacy has not been established in children <6 years of age or <15 kg (33 pounds).

Adverse Reactions Frequency not always defined.

Cardiovascular: Arrhythmia, flushing, hypertension (OraVerse™), hypotension, orthostatic hypotension, tachycardia (OraVerse™ ≤6%), bradycardia (OraVerse™ ≤4%)

Central nervous system: Dizziness, headache (OraVerse™ ≤6%)

Dermatologic: Pruritus (OraVerse™)

Gastrointestinal: Nausea, vomiting, diarrhea

Local: Injection site pain (OraVerse™ 4% to 6%)

Neuromuscular & skeletal: Paresthesia (OraVerse™), weakness

Respiratory: Nasal congestion

Postmarketing and/or case reports: Pulmonary hypertension

Drug Interactions

Metabolism/Transport Effects None known.

Avoid Concomitant Use

Avoid concomitant use of Phentolamine with any of the following: Alpha1-Blockers

Increased Effect/Toxicity

Phentolamine may increase the levels/effects of: Alpha1-Blockers; Amifostine; Antihypertensives; Calcium Channel Blockers; RiTUXimab

The levels/effects of Phentolamine may be increased by: Beta-Blockers; Diazoxide; Herbs (Hypotensive Properties); MAO Inhibitors; Pentoxifylline; Phosphodiesterase 5 Inhibitors; Prostacyclin Analogues

Decreased Effect

The levels/effects of Phentolamine may be decreased by: Herbs (Hypertensive Properties); Methylphenidate; Yohimbine

Stability Reconstituted solution is stable for 48 hours at room temperature and 1 week when refrigerated.

OraVerse™: Store at 20°C to 25°C (68°F to 77°F); excursions permitted between 15°C to 30°C (59°F to 86°F).

Mechanism of Action Competitively blocks alpha-adrenergic receptors to produce brief antagonism of circulating epinephrine and norepinephrine to reduce hypertension caused by alpha effects of these catecholamines; also has a positive inotropic and chronotropic effect on the heart

OraVerse™: Causes vasodilation and increased blood flow in injection area via alpha-adrenergic blockade to accelerate reversal of soft tissue anesthetic

Pharmacodynamics/Kinetics

Onset of action: I.M.: 15-20 minutes; I.V.: Immediate
Peak effect: OraVerse™: 10-20 minutes

Duration: I.M.: 30-45 minutes; I.V.: 15-30 minutes

Metabolism: Hepatic

Half-life elimination: 19 minutes

Excretion: Urine (10% as unchanged drug)

Dosage

Treatment of alpha-adrenergic agonist drug extravasation: SubQ:

Children: Infiltrate area with a small amount (eg, 1 mL given in 0.2 mL aliquots) of a 0.5-1 mg/mL solution (made by diluting 5-10 mg in 10 mL of NS) within 12 hours of extravasation; in general, do not exceed 0.1-0.2 mg/kg or 5 mg total

Adults: Infiltrate area with small amount of solution made by diluting 5-10 mg in 10 mL 0.9% sodium chloride within 12 hours of extravasation; in general, do not exceed 0.1-0.2 mg/kg (5 mg total); typically doses of ≤5 mg are effective; a case using 50 mg for a large extravasation has been reported (Cooper, 1989).

If dose is effective, normal skin color should return to the blanched area within 1 hour

Diagnosis of pheochromocytoma: I.M., I.V.:

Children: 0.05-0.1 mg/kg/dose, maximum single dose: 5 mg

Adults: 5 mg

Surgery for pheochromocytoma: Hypertension: I.M., I.V.:

Children: 0.05-0.1 mg/kg/dose given 1-2 hours before procedure; repeat as needed every 2-4 hours until hypertension is controlled; maximum single dose: 5 mg

Adults: 5 mg given 1-2 hours before procedure and repeated as needed every 2-4 hours

Hypertensive crisis: Adults: 5-20 mg

Treatment of pralidoxime-induced hypertension (unlabeled use): I.V.:

Children: 1 mg

Adults and Elderly: 5 mg

Reversal of soft tissue (lip, tongue) anesthesia (OraVerse™): Infiltration or block technique: Submucosal oral injection:

Children: 15-30 kg: 0.2 mg maximum dose

Children >30 kg and <12 years: 0.4 mg maximum dose

Adults: **Note:** Dose is based upon the number of cartridges of local anesthetic administered. Infiltration or block injection:
- 0.2 mg if one-half cartridge of anesthesia was administered
- 0.4 mg if 1 cartridge of anesthesia was administered
- 0.8 mg if 2 cartridges of anesthesia were administered

Administration

Vasoconstrictor (alpha-adrenergic agonist) extravasation: Infiltrate the area of extravasation with multiple small injections using only 27- or 30-gauge needles and changing the needle between each skin entry. Be careful not to cause so much swelling of the extremity or digit that a compartment syndrome occurs. If infiltration is severe, may also need to consult vascular surgeon.

Pheochromocytoma: Inject each 5 mg over 1 minute.

Monitoring Parameters Blood pressure, heart rate; area of infiltration; monitor patient for orthostasis; assist patient with ambulation

Test Interactions Increased LFTs rarely

Dosage Forms Excipient information presented when available (limited, particularly for generics); consult specific product labeling.

Injection, powder for reconstitution, as mesylate: 5 mg

Injection, solution, as mesylate [preservative free]:

OraVerse™: 0.4 mg/1.7 mL (1.7 mL) [contains edetate disodium; dental cartridge]

◆ **Phentolamine Mesylate** *see* Phentolamine *on page 1343*

◆ **Phenylalanine Mustard** *see* Melphalan *on page 1065*

◆ **Phenylazo Diamino Pyridine Hydrochloride** *see* Phenazopyridine *on page 1337*

Phenylephrine (Systemic) (fen il EF rin)

Brand Names: U.S. LuSonal™ [DSC]; Medi-First® Sinus Decongestant [OTC]; Medi-Phenyl [OTC]; PediaCare® Children's Decongestant [OTC]; Sudafed PE® Children's [OTC]; Sudafed PE® Congestion [OTC]; Sudafed PE™ Nasal Decongestant [OTC]; Sudogest™ PE [OTC]; Triaminic Thin Strips® Children's Cold with Stuffy Nose [OTC]

Index Terms Phenylephrine Hydrochloride

Pharmacologic Category Alpha-Adrenergic Agonist

Additional Appendix Information

Vasoactive Agents, Intravenous *on page 1898*

Use Treatment of hypotension, vascular failure in shock; as a vasoconstrictor in regional analgesia; supraventricular tachycardia (**Note:** Not for routine use in treatment of supraventricular tachycardias); as a decongestant [OTC]

Pregnancy Risk Factor C

Pregnancy Considerations Animal reproduction studies have not been conducted; therefore, the manufacturer classifies phenylephrine as pregnancy category C. Phenylephrine crosses the placenta at term. Maternal use of phenylephrine during the first trimester of pregnancy is not strongly associated with an increased risk of fetal malformations; maternal dose and duration of therapy were not reported in available publications. Phenylephrine is available over-the-counter (OTC) for the symptomatic relief of nasal congestion. Decongestants are not the preferred agents for the treatment of rhinitis during pregnancy. Oral phenylephrine should be avoided during the first trimester of pregnancy; short-term use (<3 days) of intranasal phenylephrine may be beneficial to some patients although its safety during pregnancy has not been studied. Phenylephrine injection is used at delivery for the prevention and/or treatment of maternal hypotension associated with spinal anesthesia in women undergoing cesarean section. Phenylephrine may be associated with a more favorable fetal acid base status than ephedrine; however, overall fetal outcomes appear to be similar. Nausea or vomiting may be less with phenylephrine than ephedrine but is also dependent upon blood pressure control. Phenylephrine may be preferred in the absence of maternal bradycardia.

Lactation Excretion in breast milk unknown/use caution

Contraindications Hypersensitivity to phenylephrine or any component of the formulation; hypertension; ventricular tachycardia

Oral: Use with or within 14 days of MAO inhibitor therapy

Warnings/Precautions Some products contain sulfites which may cause allergic reactions in susceptible individuals. Use with extreme caution in patients taking MAO inhibitors.

Intravenous: Use with caution in the elderly, patients with hyperthyroidism, bradycardia, partial heart block, myocardial disease, or severe CAD. Avoid or use with extreme caution in patients with heart failure or cardiogenic shock; increased systemic vascular resistance may significantly reduce cardiac output. Assure adequate circulatory volume to minimize need for vasoconstrictors. Avoid hypertension; monitor blood pressure closely and adjust infusion rate. Avoid extravasation; infuse into a large vein if possible. Avoid infusion into leg veins. Watch I.V. site closely. If extravasation occurs, infiltrate the area subcutaneously with diluted phentolamine (5-10 mg in 10 mL of saline) with a fine hypodermic needle. **Phentolamine should be administered as soon as possible after extravasation is noted. [U.S. Boxed Warning]: Should be administered by adequately trained individuals familiar with its use.**

Oral: Use caution with asthma, bowel obstruction/narrowing, hyperthyroidism, diabetes mellitus, cardiovascular disease, ischemic heart disease, increased intraocular pressure, prostatic hyperplasia or in the elderly. Notify healthcare provider if symptoms do not improve within 7 days or are accompanied by fever. Discontinue and contact healthcare provider if nervousness, dizziness, or sleeplessness occur.

Adverse Reactions Frequency not defined.

Injection:

Cardiovascular: Arrhythmia (rare), decreased cardiac output, hypertension, pallor, precordial pain or discomfort, reflex bradycardia, severe peripheral and visceral vasoconstriction

Central nervous system: Anxiety, dizziness, excitability, giddiness, headache, insomnia, nervousness, restlessness

Endocrine & metabolic: Metabolic acidosis

Gastrointestinal: Gastric irritation, nausea

Local: I.V.: Extravasation which may lead to necrosis and sloughing of surrounding tissue, blanching of skin

Neuromuscular & skeletal: Paresthesia, pilomotor response, tremor, weakness

Renal: Decreased renal perfusion, reduced urine output

Respiratory: Respiratory distress

Miscellaneous: Hypersensitivity reactions (including rash, urticaria, leukopenia, agranulocytosis, thrombocytopenia)

Oral: Central nervous system: Anxiety, dizziness, excitability, giddiness, headache, insomnia, nervousness, restlessness

Drug Interactions

Metabolism/Transport Effects None known.

Avoid Concomitant Use

Avoid concomitant use of Phenylephrine (Systemic) with any of the following: Ergot Derivatives; Iobenguane I 123; MAO Inhibitors

Increased Effect/Toxicity

Phenylephrine (Systemic) may increase the levels/effects of: Sympathomimetics

The levels/effects of Phenylephrine (Systemic) may be increased by: Atomoxetine; Cannabinoids; Ergot Derivatives; MAO Inhibitors; Tricyclic Antidepressants

Decreased Effect

Phenylephrine (Systemic) may decrease the levels/effects of: Benzylpenicilloyl Polylysine; FentaNYL; Iobenguane I 123

Ethanol/Nutrition/Herb Interactions Herb/Nutraceutical: Avoid ephedra, yohimbe (may cause CNS stimulation).

Stability

Solution for injection: Store vials at controlled room temperature of 15°C to 30°C (59°F to 86°F). Protect from light. Do not use solution if brown or contains a precipitate.

I.V. infusion: Usual concentration: 10 mg in 500 mL NS or D_5W. May also dilute 50 mg in 500 mL NS or 100 mg in 500 mL NS; both concentrations are stable for at least 14 days at room temperature of 25°C (77°F) (Gupta, 2004). Dilution of 1250 mg in 500 mL NS retained potency for at least 24 hours at 22°C (Weber, 1970).

I.V. injection: May dilute with SWFI to a concentration of 1 mg/mL.

Stability in syringes (Kiser, 2007): Concentration of 0.1 mg/mL in NS (polypropylene syringes) is stable for at least 30 days at -20°C (-4°F), 3°C to 5°C (37°F to 41°F), or 23°C to 25°C (73.4°F to 77°F).

Oral: Store at controlled room temperature of 15°C to 25°C (59°F to 77°F). Protect from light.

Mechanism of Action Potent, direct-acting alpha-adrenergic agonist with virtually no beta-adrenergic activity; produces systemic arterial vasoconstriction. Such increases in systemic vascular resistance result in dose dependent increases in systolic and diastolic blood pressure and reductions in heart rate and cardiac output especially in patients with heart failure.

Pharmacodynamics/Kinetics

Onset of action:

Blood pressure increase/vasoconstriction: I.M., SubQ: 10-15 minutes; I.V.: Immediate

Nasal decongestant: Oral: 15-30 minutes (Kollar, 2007)

Duration:

Blood pressure increase/vasoconstriction: I.M.: 1-2 hours; I.V.: ~15-20 minutes; SubQ: 50 minutes

Nasal decongestant: Oral: ≤4 hours (Kollar, 2007)

Absorption: Oral: Rapid and complete (Kanfer, 1993)

Distribution: V_d: Initial: 26-61 L; V_{dss}: 184-543 L (mean: 340 L) (Hengstmann 1982)

Metabolism: Hepatic via oxidative deamination (Oral: 24%; I.V.: 50%); Undergoes sulfation (Oral [mostly within gut wall]: 46%; I.V.: 8%) and some glucuronidation; forms inactive metabolites (Kanfer 1993)

Bioavailability: Oral: ≤38% (Hengstmann, 1982; Kanfer, 1993)

Half-life elimination: Alpha phase: ~5 minutes; Terminal phase: 2-3 hours (Hengstmann, 1982; Kanfer, 1993)

Time to peak: Oral: 0.75-2 hours (Kanfer, 1993)

Excretion: Urine (mostly as inactive metabolites)

Dosage

Hypotension/shock:

Children:

I.V. bolus: 5-20 mcg/kg/dose every 10-15 minutes as needed

I.V. infusion: 0.1-0.5 mcg/kg/minute

Adults:

I.V. bolus: 100-500 mcg/dose every 10-15 minutes as needed (initial dose should not exceed 500 mcg)

I.V. infusion: Initial dose: 100-180 mcg/minute, **or alternatively**, 0.5 mcg/kg/minute; titrate to desired response. Dosing ranges between 0.4-9.1 mcg/kg/minute have been reported when treating septic shock (Gregory, 1991).

Nasal decongestant: Oral:

Children:

4 to <6 years: 2.5 mg every 4 hours as needed for ≤7 days

6 to <12 years: 5 mg every 4 hours as needed for ≤7 days

Children ≥12 years and Adults: 10-20 mg every 4 hours as needed for ≤7 days

Paroxysmal supraventricular tachycardia (**Note:** Not recommended for routine use in treatment of supraventricular tachycardias): I.V.:

Children: 5-10 mcg/kg/dose over 20-30 seconds

Adults: 250-500 mcg/dose over 20-30 seconds

Dietary Considerations Some products may contain phenylalanine and/or sodium.

Administration I.V.: May cause necrosis or sloughing tissue if extravasation occurs during I.V. administration or SubQ administration.

Extravasation management: Use phentolamine as antidote; mix 5-10 mg with 10 mL of NS. Inject a small amount of this dilution subcutaneously into extravasated area. Blanching should reverse immediately. Monitor site. If blanching should recur, additional injections of phentolamine may be needed.

Monitoring Parameters Blood pressure (or mean arterial pressure), heart rate; cardiac output (as appropriate), intravascular volume status, pulmonary capillary wedge pressure (as appropriate); monitor infusion site closely

Dosage Forms Excipient information presented when available (limited, particularly for generics); consult specific product labeling. [DSC] = Discontinued product

Injection, solution, as hydrochloride: 1% [10 mg/mL] (1 mL, 2 mL [DSC], 5 mL, 10 mL)

Liquid, oral, as hydrochloride:

LuSonal™: 7.5 mg/5 mL (473 mL [DSC]) [contains phenylalanine; strawberry flavor]

PediaCare® Children's Decongestant: 2.5 mg/5 mL (118 mL) [contains sodium 14 mg/5 mL, sodium benzoate; raspberry flavor]

Sudafed PE® Children's: 2.5 mg/5 mL (118 mL) [ethanol free, sugar free; contains sodium 14 mg/5 mL, sodium benzoate; raspberry flavor]

Strip, orally disintegrating, oral, as hydrochloride:

Triaminic Thin Strips® Children's Cold with Stuffy Nose: 2.5 mg (14s) [raspberry flavor]

Tablet, oral, as hydrochloride: 10 mg

Medi-First® Sinus Decongestant: 10 mg

Medi-Phenyl: 5 mg

Sudafed PE® Congestion: 10 mg

Sudafed PE™ Nasal Decongestant: 10 mg

Sudogest™ PE: 10 mg

◆ **Phenylephrine and Chlorpheniramine** *see* Chlorpheniramine and Phenylephrine *on page 345*

◆ **Phenylephrine and Cyclopentolate** *see* Cyclopentolate and Phenylephrine *on page 420*

◆ **Phenylephrine and Dextromethorphan** *see* Dextromethorphan and Phenylephrine *on page 490*

◆ **Phenylephrine and Diphenhydramine** *see* Diphenhydramine and Phenylephrine *on page 518*

◆ **Phenylephrine, Chlorpheniramine, and Dextromethorphan** *see* Chlorpheniramine, Phenylephrine, and Dextromethorphan *on page 346*

◆ **Phenylephrine, Chlorpheniramine, and Dihydrocodeine** *see* Dihydrocodeine, Chlorpheniramine, and Phenylephrine *on page 508*

◆ **Phenylephrine, Chlorpheniramine, and Pyrilamine** *see* Chlorpheniramine, Pyrilamine, and Phenylephrine *on page 348*

◆ **Phenylephrine Hydrochloride** *see* Phenylephrine (Systemic) *on page 1344*

- **Phenylephrine Hydrochloride and Diphenhydramine Hydrochloride** *see* Diphenhydramine and Phenylephrine *on page 518*
- **Phenylephrine Hydrochloride and Guaifenesin** *see* Guaifenesin and Phenylephrine *on page 812*
- **Phenylephrine Tannate and Diphenhydramine Tannate** *see* Diphenhydramine and Phenylephrine *on page 518*
- **Phenylethylmalonylurea** *see* PHENobarbital *on page 1339*
- **Phenyl Salicylate, Methenamine, Methylene Blue, Benzoic Acid, and Hyoscyamine** *see* Methenamine, Phenyl Salicylate, Methylene Blue, Benzoic Acid, and Hyoscyamine *on page 1094*
- **Phenyl Salicylate, Methenamine, Methylene Blue, Sodium Biphosphate, and Hyoscyamine** *see* Methenamine, Sodium Biphosphate, Phenyl Salicylate, Methylene Blue, and Hyoscyamine *on page 1094*
- **Phenytek®** *see* Phenytoin *on page 1346*

Phenytoin (FEN i toyn)

Brand Names: U.S. Dilantin-125®; Dilantin®; Phenytek®

Brand Names: Canada Dilantin®

Index Terms Diphenylhydantoin; DPH; Phenytoin Sodium; Phenytoin Sodium, Extended; Phenytoin Sodium, Prompt

Pharmacologic Category Anticonvulsant, Hydantoin

Additional Appendix Information

Anticonvulsant Drugs of Choice *on page 1873*

Status Epilepticus *on page 2010*

Use Management of generalized tonic-clonic (grand mal), complex partial seizures; prevention of seizures following head trauma/neurosurgery

Pregnancy Risk Factor D

Pregnancy Considerations Phenytoin crosses the placenta. Congenital malformations (including a pattern of malformations termed the "fetal hydantoin syndrome" or "fetal anticonvulsant syndrome") have been reported in infants. Isolated cases of malignancies (including neuroblastoma) and coagulation defects in the neonate following delivery have also been reported. Epilepsy itself, the number of medications, genetic factors, or a combination of these probably influence the teratogenicity of anticonvulsant therapy.

Total plasma concentrations of phenytoin are decreased by 56% in the mother during pregnancy; unbound plasma (free) concentrations are decreased by 31%. Because protein binding is decreased, monitoring of unbound plasma concentrations is recommended. Concentrations should be monitored through the 8th week postpartum. The use of folic acid throughout pregnancy and vitamin K during the last month of pregnancy is recommended.

Patients exposed to phenytoin during pregnancy are encouraged to enroll themselves into the AED Pregnancy Registry by calling 1-888-233-2334. Additional information is available at www.aedpregnancyregistry.org.

Lactation Enters breast milk/not recommended (AAP rates "compatible"; AAP 2001 update pending)

Medication Guide Available Yes

Contraindications Hypersensitivity to phenytoin, other hydantoins, or any component of the formulation; pregnancy

Warnings/Precautions Antiepileptics are associated with an increased risk of suicidal behavior/thoughts with use (regardless of indication); patients should be monitored for signs/symptoms of depression, suicidal tendencies, and other unusual behavior changes during therapy and instructed to inform their healthcare provider immediately if symptoms occur.

[U.S. Boxed Warning]: Phenytoin must be administered slowly. Intravenous administration should not exceed 50 mg/minute in adult patients. In neonates, intravenous administration rate should not exceed 1-3 mg/kg/minute (most clinicians use a lower maximum rate of infusion in neonates of 0.5-1 mg/kg/minute). Hypotension may occur with rapid administration. I.V. form may cause skin necrosis at I.V. site; avoid I.V. administration in small veins; may increase frequency of petit mal seizures; use with caution in patients with porphyria; discontinue if rash or lymphadenopathy occurs; a spectrum of hematologic effects have been reported with use (eg, neutropenia, leukopenia, thrombocytopenia, pancytopenia, and anemias); use with caution in patients with hepatic dysfunction, sinus bradycardia, S-A block, or AV block; use with caution in elderly or debilitated patients, or in any condition associated with low serum albumin levels, which will increase the free fraction of phenytoin in the serum and, therefore, the pharmacologic response. Sedation, confusional states, or cerebellar dysfunction (loss of motor coordination) may occur at higher total serum concentrations, or at lower total serum concentrations when the free fraction of phenytoin is increased. Effects with other sedative drugs or ethanol may be potentiated. Abrupt withdrawal may precipitate status epilepticus. Severe reactions, including toxic epidermal necrolysis and Stevens-Johnson syndromes, although rarely reported, have resulted in fatalities; drug should be discontinued if there are any signs of rash. Patients of Asian descent with the variant *HLA-B*1502* may be at an increased risk of developing Stevens-Johnson syndrome and/or toxic epidermal necrolysis.

Adverse Reactions I.V. effects: Hypotension, bradycardia, cardiac arrhythmia, cardiovascular collapse (especially with rapid I.V. use), venous irritation and pain, thrombophlebitis

Effects not related to plasma phenytoin concentrations: Hypertrichosis, gingival hypertrophy, thickening of facial features, carbohydrate intolerance, folic acid deficiency, peripheral neuropathy, vitamin D deficiency, osteomalacia, systemic lupus erythematosus

Concentration-related effects: Nystagmus, blurred vision, diplopia, ataxia, slurred speech, dizziness, drowsiness, lethargy, coma, rash, fever, nausea, vomiting, gum tenderness, confusion, mood changes, folic acid depletion, osteomalacia, hyperglycemia

Related to elevated concentrations:

>20 mcg/mL: Far lateral nystagmus

>30 mcg/mL: 45° lateral gaze nystagmus and ataxia

>40 mcg/mL: Decreased mentation

>100 mcg/mL: Death

Cardiovascular: Hypotension, bradycardia, cardiac arrhythmia, cardiovascular collapse

Central nervous system: Psychiatric changes, slurred speech, dizziness, drowsiness, headache, insomnia

Dermatologic: Rash

Gastrointestinal: Constipation, nausea, vomiting, gingival hyperplasia, enlargement of lips

Hematologic: Leukopenia, thrombocytopenia, agranulocytosis

Hepatic: Hepatitis

Local: Thrombophlebitis

Neuromuscular & skeletal: Tremor, peripheral neuropathy, paresthesia

Ocular: Diplopia, nystagmus, blurred vision

Rarely seen effects: Blood dyscrasias, coarsening of facial features, dyskinesias, hepatitis, hypertrichosis, lymphadenopathy, lymphoma, pseudolymphoma, SLE-like syndrome, Stevens-Johnson syndrome, toxic epidermal necrolysis, venous irritation and pain

Drug Interactions

Metabolism/Transport Effects Substrate of CYP2C19 (major), CYP2C9 (major), CYP3A4 (minor); **Note:** Assignment of Major/Minor substrate status based on clinically relevant drug interaction potential; **Induces** CYP2B6 (strong), CYP2C19 (strong), CYP2C8 (strong), CYP2C9 (strong), CYP3A4 (strong)

Avoid Concomitant Use

Avoid concomitant use of Phenytoin with any of the following: Boceprevir; Bortezomib; Crizotinib; Darunavir; Delavirdine; Dronedarone; Etravirine; Everolimus; Lapatinib; Lurasidone; Nilotinib; Pazopanib; Praziquantel; Ranolazine; Rilpivirine; Rivaroxaban; Roflumilast; RomiDEPsin; SORAfenib; Telaprevir; Ticagrelor; Tolvaptan; Toremifene; Vandetanib

Increased Effect/Toxicity

Phenytoin may increase the levels/effects of: Clarithromycin; CNS Depressants; Fosamprenavir; Lithium; Methotrimeprazine; Prilocaine; Selective Serotonin Reuptake Inhibitors; Vecuronium; Vitamin K Antagonists

The levels/effects of Phenytoin may be increased by: Alcohol (Ethyl); Allopurinol; Amiodarone; Antifungal Agents (Azole Derivatives, Systemic); Benzodiazepines; Calcium Channel Blockers; Capecitabine; CarBAMazepine; Carbonic Anhydrase Inhibitors; CeFAZolin; Chloramphenicol; Cimetidine; Clarithromycin; Conivaptan; CYP2C19 Inhibitors (Moderate); CYP2C19 Inhibitors (Strong); CYP2C9 Inhibitors (Moderate); CYP2C9 Inhibitors (Strong); Delavirdine; Dexmethylphenidate; Disulfiram; Droperidol; Efavirenz; Ethosuximide; Felbamate; Floxuridine; Fluconazole; Fluorouracil; Fluorouracil (Systemic); Fluorouracil (Topical); FLUoxetine; FluvoxaMINE; Halothane; HydrOXYzine; Isoniazid; Methotrimeprazine; Methylphenidate; MetroNIDAZOLE; MetroNIDAZOLE (Systemic); OXcarbazepine; Proton Pump Inhibitors; Rufinamide; Sertraline; Sulfonamide Derivatives; Tacrolimus; Tacrolimus (Systemic); Telaprevir; Ticlopidine; Topiramate; TraZODone; Trimethoprim; Vitamin K Antagonists

Decreased Effect

Phenytoin may decrease the levels/effects of: Acetaminophen; Amiodarone; Antifungal Agents (Azole Derivatives, Systemic); ARIPiprazole; Boceprevir; Bortezomib; Brentuximab Vedotin; Busulfan; CarBAMazepine; Caspofungin; Chloramphenicol; Clarithromycin; CloZAPine; Contraceptives (Estrogens); Contraceptives (Progestins); Crizotinib; CycloSPORINE; CycloSPORINE (Systemic); CYP2B6 Substrates; CYP2C19 Substrates; CYP2C8 Substrates; CYP2C9 Substrates; CYP3A4 Substrates; Darunavir; Dasatinib; Deferasirox; Delavirdine; Diclofenac; Disopyramide; Divalproex; Doxycycline; Dronedarone; Efavirenz; Ethosuximide; Etoposide; Etoposide Phosphate; Etravirine; Everolimus; Exemestane; Felbamate; Flunarizine; Gefitinib; GuanFACINE; HMG-CoA Reductase Inhibitors; Imatinib; Irinotecan; Ixabepilone; Lacosamide; LamoTRIgine; Lapatinib; Levodopa; Linagliptin; Loop Diuretics; Lopinavir; Lurasidone; Maraviroc; Mebendazole; Meperidine; Methadone; MetroNIDAZOLE; MetroNIDAZOLE (Systemic); Metyrapone; Mexiletine; Nilotinib; OXcarbazepine; Pazopanib; Praziquantel; Primidone; QUEtiapine; QuiNIDine; QuiNINE; Ranolazine; Rilpivirine; Ritonavir; Rivaroxaban; Roflumilast; RomiDEPsin; Rufinamide; Saxagliptin; Sertraline; Sirolimus; SORAfenib; SUNItinib; Tacrolimus; Tacrolimus (Systemic); Tadalafil; Telaprevir; Temsirolimus; Teniposide; Theophylline Derivatives; Thyroid Products; Ticagrelor; Tipranavir; Tolvaptan; Topiramate; Toremifene; TraZODone; Treprostinil; Ulipristal; Valproic Acid; Vandetanib; Vecuronium; Vemurafenib; Zonisamide; Zuclopenthixol

The levels/effects of Phenytoin may be decreased by: Alcohol (Ethyl); Amphetamines; Antacids; Barbiturates; CarBAMazepine; Ciprofloxacin; Ciprofloxacin (Systemic); CISplatin; Colesevelam; CYP2C19 Inducers (Strong); CYP2C9 Inducers (Strong); Diazoxide; Divalproex; Folic Acid; Fosamprenavir; Ketorolac; Ketorolac (Nasal); Ketorolac (Systemic); Leucovorin Calcium-Levoleucovorin; Levomefolate; Lopinavir; Mefloquine; Methylfolate; Nelfinavir; Peginterferon Alfa-2b; Pyridoxine; Rifamycin Derivatives; Ritonavir; Telaprevir; Theophylline Derivatives; Tipranavir; Tocilizumab; Valproic Acid; Vigabatrin

Ethanol/Nutrition/Herb Interactions

Ethanol:

Acute use: Avoid or limit ethanol (inhibits metabolism of phenytoin). Ethanol may also increase CNS depression; monitor for increased effects with coadministration. Caution patients about effects.

Chronic use: Avoid or limit ethanol (stimulates metabolism of phenytoin).

Food: Phenytoin serum concentrations may be altered if taken with food. If taken with enteral nutrition, phenytoin serum concentrations may be decreased. Tube feedings decrease bioavailability; hold tube feedings 1-2 hours before and 1-2 hours after phenytoin administration. May decrease calcium, folic acid, and vitamin D levels.

Herb/Nutraceutical: Avoid evening primrose (seizure threshold decreased). Avoid valerian, St John's wort, kava kava, gotu kola (may increase CNS depression).

Stability

Capsule, tablet: Store at controlled room temperature. Protect from light and moisture.

Oral suspension: Store at room temperature of 20°C to 25°C (68°F to 77°F); do not freeze. Protect from light.

Solution for injection: Store at room temperature of 15°C to 30°C (59°F to 86°F). Use only clear solutions free of precipitate and haziness; slightly yellow solutions may be used. Precipitation may occur if solution is refrigerated and may dissolve at room temperature.

Further dilution of the solution for I.V. infusion is controversial and no consensus exists as to the optimal concentration and length of stability. Stability is concentration and pH dependent. Based on limited clinical consensus, NS or LR are recommended diluents. Dilutions of 1-10 mg/mL have been used and should be administered as soon as possible after preparation (some recommend to discard if not used within 4 hours). Do not refrigerate.

Mechanism of Action Stabilizes neuronal membranes and decreases seizure activity by increasing efflux or decreasing influx of sodium ions across cell membranes in the motor cortex during generation of nerve impulses; prolongs effective refractory period and suppresses ventricular pacemaker automaticity, shortens action potential in the heart

Pharmacodynamics/Kinetics

Onset of action: I.V.: ~0.5-1 hour

Absorption: Oral: Slow

Distribution: V_d:

Neonates: Premature: 1-1.2 L/kg; Full-term: 0.8-0.9 L/kg

Infants: 0.7-0.8 L/kg

Children: 0.7 L/kg

Adults: 0.6-0.7 L/kg

Protein binding:

Neonates: ≥80% (≤20% free)

Infants: ≥85% (≤15% free)

Adults: 90% to 95%

Others: Decreased protein binding

Disease states resulting in a decrease in serum albumin concentration: Burns, hepatic cirrhosis, nephrotic syndrome, pregnancy, cystic fibrosis

Disease states resulting in an apparent decrease in affinity of phenytoin for serum albumin: Renal failure, jaundice (severe), other drugs (displacers), hyperbilirubinemia (total bilirubin >15 mg/dL), Cl_{cr} <25 mL/minute (unbound fraction is increased two- to threefold in uremia)

Metabolism: Follows dose-dependent capacity-limited (Michaelis-Menten) pharmacokinetics with increased V_{max} in infants >6 months of age and children versus adults; major metabolite (via oxidation), HPPA, undergoes enterohepatic recirculation

Bioavailability: Form dependent

Half-life elimination: Oral: 22 hours (range: 7-42 hours)

Time to peak, serum (form dependent): Oral: Extended-release capsule: 4-12 hours; Immediate release preparation: 2-3 hours

Excretion: Urine (<5% as unchanged drug); as glucuronides

Clearance: Highly variable, dependent upon intrinsic hepatic function and dose administered; increased clearance and decreased serum concentrations with febrile illness

Dosage Note: Phenytoin base (eg, oral suspension, chewable tablets) contains ~8% more drug than phenytoin sodium (~92 mg base is equivalent to 100 mg phenytoin sodium). Dosage adjustments and closer serum monitoring may be necessary when switching dosage forms.

Status epilepticus: I.V.:

Infants and Children: Loading dose: 15-20 mg/kg in a single or divided dose; maintenance dose: Initial: 5 mg/kg/day in 2 divided doses; usual doses:

6 months to 3 years: 8-10 mg/kg/day

4-6 years: 7.5-9 mg/kg/day

7-9 years: 7-8 mg/kg/day

10-16 years: 6-7 mg/kg/day, some patients may require every 8 hours dosing

Adults: Loading dose: Manufacturer recommends 10-15 mg/kg, however, 15-20 mg/kg is generally recommended; maximum rate: 50 mg/minute; initial maintenance dose: I.V. or Oral: 100 mg every 6-8 hours

Anticonvulsant: Children and Adults: Oral:

Loading dose: 15-20 mg/kg; consider prior phenytoin serum concentrations and/or recent dosing history if available; administer oral loading dose in 3 divided doses given every 2-4 hours to decrease GI adverse effects and to ensure complete oral absorption

Maintenance dose:

Children: Initial maintenance dose: 5 mg/kg/day in 2-3 divided doses; usual maintenance dose range: 4-8 mg/kg/day

Adults: Initial maintenance dose: 300 mg/day in 3 divided doses; may also administer in 1-2 divided doses using extended release formulation; adjust dosage based on individual requirements; usual maintenance dose range: 300-600 mg/day

Dosage adjustment in obesity: Adults: Loading dose: Use adjusted body weight (ABW) correction based on a pharmacokinetic study of phenytoin loading doses in obese patients (Abernethy, 1985). The larger correction factor (ie, 1.33) is due to a doubling of V_d estimated in these obese patients.

ABW = [(Actual body weight – IBW) x 1.33] + IBW

Maximum loading dose: I.V.: 2000 mg (Erstad, 2004)

Maintenance doses should be based on ideal body weight, conventional daily doses with adjustments based upon therapeutic drug monitoring and clinical effectiveness. (Abernethy, 1985; Erstad, 2002; Erstad, 2004)

Neurosurgery (prophylactic): Adults: I.V.: 100-200 mg at ~4-hour intervals during surgery and the immediate postoperative period. **Note:** While the manufacturer recommends I.M. administration, this route should be **avoided** due to severe risk of local tissue destruction and necrosis; use **fos**phenytoin if I.M. administration necessary (Boucher, 1996; Meek, 1999).

Dosing adjustment/comments in renal impairment or hepatic disease: Safe in usual doses in mild liver disease; clearance may be substantially reduced in cirrhosis and plasma level monitoring with dose adjustment advisable. Free phenytoin levels should be monitored closely.

Dietary Considerations

Folic acid: Phenytoin may decrease mucosal uptake of folic acid; to avoid folic acid deficiency and megaloblastic anemia, some clinicians recommend giving patients on anticonvulsants prophylactic doses of folic acid and cyanocobalamin. However, folate supplementation may increase seizures in some patients (dose dependent). Discuss with healthcare provider prior to using any supplements.

Calcium: Hypocalcemia has been reported in patients taking prolonged high-dose therapy with an anticonvulsant. Some clinicians have given an additional 4000 units/week of vitamin D (especially in those receiving poor nutrition and getting no sun exposure) to prevent hypocalcemia.

Vitamin D: Phenytoin interferes with vitamin D metabolism and osteomalacia may result; may need to supplement with vitamin D

Tube feedings: Tube feedings decrease phenytoin absorption. To avoid decreased serum levels with continuous NG feeds, hold feedings for 1-2 hours prior to and 1-2 hours after phenytoin administration, if possible. There is a variety of opinions on how to administer phenytoin with enteral feedings. Be **consistent** throughout therapy.

Injection may contain sodium.

Administration

Oral: Suspension: Shake well prior to use. Absorption is impaired when phenytoin suspension is given concurrently to patients who are receiving continuous nasogastric feedings. A method to resolve this interaction is to divide the daily dose of phenytoin and withhold the administration of nutritional supplements for 1-2 hours before and after each phenytoin dose.

I.M.: **Avoid** this route (manufacturer recommends I.M. administration) due to severe risk of local tissue destruction and necrosis; use **fos**phenytoin if I.M. administration necessary (Boucher, 1996; Meek, 1999).

I.V.: Vesicant. Fosphenytoin may be considered for loading in patients who are in status epilepticus, hemodynamically unstable, or develop hypotension/bradycardia with I.V. administration of phenytoin. Although, phenytoin may be administered by direct I.V. injection, it is preferable that phenytoin be administered via infusion pump either undiluted or diluted in normal saline as an I.V. piggyback (IVPB) to prevent exceeding the maximum infusion rate (monitor closely for extravasation during infusion). The maximum rate of I.V. administration is 50 mg/minute in adults. Highly sensitive patients (eg, elderly, patients with pre-existing cardiovascular conditions) should receive phenytoin more slowly (eg, 20 mg/minute) (Meek, 1999). In neonates, the manufacturer recommends a maximum rate of 1-3 mg/kg/minute; however, a lower maximum rate of 0.5-1 mg/kg/minute is used clinically (Sankar, 2010; Shields, 1989). An in-line 0.22-5 micron

filter is recommended for IVPB solutions due to the high potential for precipitation of the solution. Avoid extravasation. Following I.V. administration, NS should be injected through the same needle or I.V. catheter to prevent irritation.
pH: 10.0-12.3
SubQ: SubQ administration is not recommended because of the possibility of local tissue damage (due to high pH).

Monitoring Parameters CBC, liver function; suicidality (eg, suicidal thoughts, depression, behavioral changes); plasma phenytoin concentrations (if available, free phenytoin concentrations should be obtained in patients with renal impairment and/or hypoalbuminemia; if free phenytoin concentrations are unavailable, the adjusted total concentration may be determined based upon equations in adult patients). Trough concentrations are generally recommended for routine monitoring.

Additional monitoring with I.V. use: Continuous cardiac monitoring (rate, rhythm, blood pressure) and observation during administration recommended; blood pressure and pulse should be monitored every 15 minutes for 1 hour after administration (Meek, 1999); infusion site reactions

Reference Range Timing of serum samples: Because it is slowly absorbed, peak blood levels may occur 4-8 hours after ingestion of an oral dose. The serum half-life varies with the dosage and the drug follows Michaelis-Menten kinetics. The average adult half-life is about 24 hours. Steady-state concentrations are reached in 5-10 days.

Children and Adults: Toxicity is measured clinically, and some patients require levels outside the suggested therapeutic range
Therapeutic range:
Total phenytoin: 10-20 mcg/mL (children and adults), 8-15 mcg/mL (neonates)
Concentrations of 5-10 mcg/mL may be therapeutic for some patients but concentrations <5 mcg/mL are not likely to be effective
50% of patients show decreased frequency of seizures at concentrations >10 mcg/mL
86% of patients show decreased frequency of seizures at concentrations >15 mcg/mL
Add another anticonvulsant if satisfactory therapeutic response is not achieved with a phenytoin concentration of 20 mcg/mL
Free phenytoin: 1-2.5 mcg/mL
Total phenytoin:
Toxic: >30 mcg/mL (SI: <120-200 micromole/L)
Lethal: >100 mcg/mL (SI: >400 micromole/L)

When to draw levels: This is dependent on the disease state being treated and the clinical condition of the patient
Key points:
Slow absorption of extended capsules and prolonged half-life minimize fluctuations between peak and trough concentrations, timing of sampling not crucial
Trough concentrations are generally recommended for routine monitoring. Daily levels are not necessary and may result in incorrect dosage adjustments. If it is determined essential to monitor free phenytoin concentrations, concomitant monitoring of total phenytoin concentrations is not necessary and expensive.
After a loading dose: If rapid therapeutic levels are needed, initial levels may be drawn after 1 hour (I.V. loading dose) or within 24 hours (oral loading dose) to aid in determining maintenance dose or need to reload.
Rapid achievement: Draw within 2-3 days of therapy initiation to ensure that the patient's metabolism is not remarkably different from that which would be predicted by average literature-derived pharmacokinetic parameters; early levels should be used cautiously in design of new dosing regimens
Second concentration: Draw within 6-7 days with subsequent doses of phenytoin adjusted accordingly
If plasma concentrations have not changed over a 3- to 5-day period, monitoring interval may be increased to once weekly in the acute clinical setting
In stable patients requiring long-term therapy, generally monitor levels at 3- to 12-month intervals

Adjustment of serum concentration: See tables.
Note: Although it is ideal to obtain free phenytoin concentrations to assess serum concentrations in patients with hypoalbuminemia or renal failure (Cl_{cr} ≤10 mL/minute), it may not always be possible. If free phenytoin concentrations are unavailable, the following equations may be utilized in adult patients.

Adjustment of Serum Concentration in Adults With Low Serum Albumin

Measured Total Phenytoin Concentration (mcg/mL)	Patient's Serum Albumin (g/dL)			
	3.5	3	2.5	2
	Adjusted Total Phenytoin Concentration (mcg/mL)[1]			
5	6	7	8	10
10	13	14	17	20
15	19	21	25	30

[1]Adjusted concentration = measured total concentration divided by [(0.2 x albumin) + 0.1].

Adjustment of Serum Concentration in Adults With Renal Failure (Cl_{cr} ≤10 mL/min)

Measured Total Phenytoin Concentration (mcg/mL)	Patient's Serum Albumin (g/dL)				
	4	3.5	3	2.5	2
	Adjusted Total Phenytoin Concentration (mcg/mL)[1]				
5	10	11	13	14	17
10	20	22	25	29	33
15	30	33	38	43	50

[1]Adjusted concentration = measured total concentration divided by [(0.1 x albumin) + 0.1].

Dosage Forms Excipient information presented when available (limited, particularly for generics); consult specific product labeling.
Capsule, extended release, oral, as sodium: 100 mg, 200 mg, 300 mg
Dilantin®: 30 mg, 100 mg
Phenytek®: 200 mg, 300 mg
Injection, solution, as sodium: 50 mg/mL (2 mL, 5 mL)
Suspension, oral: 100 mg/4 mL (4 mL); 125 mg/5 mL (120 mL, 237 mL, 240 mL)
Dilantin-125®: 125 mg/5 mL (240 mL) [contains ethanol ≤0.6%, sodium benzoate; orange-vanilla flavor]
Tablet, chewable, oral:
Dilantin®: 50 mg [scored]

◆ **Phenytoin Sodium** *see* Phenytoin *on page 1346*
◆ **Phenytoin Sodium, Extended** *see* Phenytoin *on page 1346*
◆ **Phenytoin Sodium, Prompt** *see* Phenytoin *on page 1346*
◆ **Phillips'® M-O [OTC]** *see* Magnesium Hydroxide and Mineral Oil *on page 1046*
◆ **Phillips'® Laxative Dietary Supplement Cramp-Free [OTC]** *see* Magnesium Oxide *on page 1046*
◆ **Phillips'® Liquid-Gels® [OTC]** *see* Docusate *on page 537*
◆ **Phillips'® Milk of Magnesia [OTC]** *see* Magnesium Hydroxide *on page 1045*

Physostigmine (fye zoe STIG meen)

Index Terms Eserine Salicylate; Physostigmine Salicylate; Physostigmine Sulfate

Pharmacologic Category Acetylcholinesterase Inhibitor

Use Reverse toxic, life-threatening delirium caused by atropine, diphenhydramine, dimenhydrinate, *Atropa belladonna* (deadly nightshade), or jimson weed (*Datura* spp)

Pregnancy Risk Factor C

Lactation Excretion in breast milk unknown

Contraindications Hypersensitivity to physostigmine or any component of the formulation; GI or GU obstruction; asthma; gangrene; diabetes, cardiovascular disease; any vagotonic state; coadministration of choline esters and depolarizing neuromuscular-blocking agents

Warnings/Precautions Hazardous agent - use appropriate precautions for handling and disposal. Patient must have a normal QRS interval, as measured by ECG, in order to receive; use caution in poisoning with agents known to prolong intraventricular conduction. Concomitant administration of choline esters or depolarizing neuromuscular-blocking agents (ie, succinylcholine) are contraindicated. Use with caution in patients with epilepsy, asthma, diabetes, gangrene, cardiovascular disease, bradycardia. Discontinue if excessive salivation or emesis, frequent urination or diarrhea occur. Reduce dosage if excessive sweating or nausea occurs. Administer slowly over 5 minutes to prevent respiratory distress and seizures. Continuous infusions should never be used. Due to the possibility of hypersensitivity or overdose/cholinergic crisis, atropine should be readily available; not intended as a first-line agent for anticholinergic toxicity or Parkinson's disease. Asystole and seizures have been reported when physostigmine was administered to TCA poisoned patients. Physostigmine is not recommended in patients with known or suspected TCA intoxication. Products may contain benzyl alcohol. Products may contain sodium bisulfate.

Adverse Reactions Frequency not defined.

Cardiovascular: Asystole, bradycardia, palpitation

Central nervous system: Hallucinations, nervousness, restlessness, seizure

Gastrointestinal: Diarrhea, nausea, salivation, stomach pain

Genitourinary: Urinary frequency

Neuromuscular & skeletal: Twitching

Ocular: Lacrimation, miosis

Respiratory: Bronchospasm, dyspnea, pulmonary edema, respiratory paralysis

Miscellaneous: Diaphoresis

Drug Interactions

Metabolism/Transport Effects None known.

Avoid Concomitant Use There are no known interactions where it is recommended to avoid concomitant use.

Increased Effect/Toxicity

Physostigmine may increase the levels/effects of: Beta-Blockers; Cholinergic Agonists; Succinylcholine

The levels/effects of Physostigmine may be increased by: Corticosteroids (Systemic)

Decreased Effect

Physostigmine may decrease the levels/effects of: Neuromuscular-Blocking Agents (Nondepolarizing)

The levels/effects of Physostigmine may be decreased by: Dipyridamole

Ethanol/Nutrition/Herb Interactions Herb/Nutraceutical: Ginkgo biloba may enhance the adverse/toxic effect of physostigmine; monitor.

Stability Do not use solution if cloudy or dark brown.

Mechanism of Action Inhibits destruction of acetylcholine by acetylcholinesterase which facilitates transmission of impulses across myoneural junction and prolongs the central and peripheral effects of acetylcholine

Pharmacodynamics/Kinetics

Onset of action: ~5 minutes

Duration: 1-2 hours

Absorption: I.M.: Readily absorbed

Distribution: Crosses blood-brain barrier readily and reverses both central and peripheral anticholinergic effects

Metabolism: Hepatic and via hydrolysis by cholinesterases

Half-life elimination: 15-40 minutes

Dosage Reversal of toxic anticholinergic effects: **Note:** Administer slowly over 5 minutes to prevent respiratory distress and seizures. Continuous infusions of physostigmine should never be used.

Children: **Note:** Reserve for life-threatening situations only: I.V.: 0.01-0.03 mg/kg/dose; may repeat after 5-10 minutes to a maximum total dose of 2 mg or until response occurs or adverse cholinergic effects occur

Adults: I.M., I.V.: 0.5-2 mg to start, repeat every 20 minutes until response occurs or adverse effect occurs; repeat 1-4 mg every 30-60 minutes as life-threatening symptoms recur

Administration Injection: Infuse slowly I.V. over 5 minutes. Too rapid administration can cause bradycardia and hypersalivation leading to respiratory distress and seizures.

Monitoring Parameters ECG, vital signs

Test Interactions Increased aminotransferase [ALT/AST] (S), increased amylase (S)

Dosage Forms Excipient information presented when available (limited, particularly for generics); consult specific product labeling.

Injection, solution, as salicylate: 1 mg/mL (2 mL)

- ◆ **Physostigmine Salicylate** *see* Physostigmine *on page* 1350
- ◆ **Physostigmine Sulfate** *see* Physostigmine *on page* 1350
- ◆ **Phytomenadione** *see* Phytonadione *on page* 1351

Phytonadione (fye toe na DYE one)

Brand Names: U.S. Mephyton®

Brand Names: Canada AquaMEPHYTON®; Konakion; Mephyton®

Index Terms Methylphytyl Napthoquinone; Phylloquinone; Phytomenadione; Vitamin K_1

Pharmacologic Category Vitamin, Fat Soluble

Use Prevention and treatment of hypoprothrombinemia caused by coumarin derivative-induced or other drug-induced vitamin K deficiency, hypoprothrombinemia caused by malabsorption or inability to synthesize vitamin K; hemorrhagic disease of the newborn

Unlabeled Use Treatment of hypoprothrombinemia caused by anticoagulant rodenticides

Pregnancy Risk Factor C

Pregnancy Considerations Animal reproduction studies have not been conducted.

Lactation Enters breast milk/use caution (AAP rates "compatible"; AAP 2001 update pending)

Contraindications Hypersensitivity to phytonadione or any component of the formulation

Warnings/Precautions **[U.S. Boxed Warning]: Severe reactions resembling hypersensitivity (eg, anaphylaxis) reactions have occurred rarely during or immediately after I.V. administration.** Allergic reactions have also occurred with I.M. and SubQ injections; oral administration is the safest. In obstructive jaundice or with biliary fistulas concurrent administration of bile salts is necessary. Manufacturers recommend the SubQ route over other parenteral routes. SubQ is less predictable when compared to the oral route. The American College of Chest Physicians recommends the I.V. route in patients with serious or life-threatening bleeding secondary to warfarin. The I.V. route should be restricted to emergency situations where oral phytonadione cannot be used. Efficacy is delayed regardless of route of administration; patient management may require other treatments in the interim. Administer a dose that will quickly lower the INR into a safe range without causing resistance to warfarin. High phytonadione doses may lead to warfarin resistance for at least one week. Use caution in newborns especially premature infants; hemolysis, jaundice and hyperbilirubinemia have been reported with larger than recommended doses. Some dosage forms contain benzyl alcohol which has been associated with "gasping syndrome" in premature infants. In liver disease, if initial doses do not reverse coagulopathy then higher doses are unlikely to have any effect. Ineffective in hereditary hypoprothrombinemia. Use caution with renal dysfunction (including premature infants). Injectable products may contain aluminum; may result in toxic levels following prolonged administration. Product may contain polysorbate 80.

Adverse Reactions Parenteral administration: Frequency not defined.

Cardiovascular: Cyanosis, flushing, hypotension
Central nervous system: Dizziness
Dermatologic: Scleroderma-like lesions
Endocrine & metabolic: Hyperbilirubinemia (newborn; greater than recommended doses)
Gastrointestinal: Abnormal taste
Local: Injection site reactions
Respiratory: Dyspnea
Miscellaneous: Anaphylactoid reactions, diaphoresis, hypersensitivity reactions

Drug Interactions

Metabolism/Transport Effects None known.

Avoid Concomitant Use There are no known interactions where it is recommended to avoid concomitant use.

Increased Effect/Toxicity There are no known significant interactions involving an increase in effect.

Decreased Effect

Phytonadione may decrease the levels/effects of: Vitamin K Antagonists

The levels/effects of Phytonadione may be decreased by: Mineral Oil; Orlistat

Stability

Injection: Store at 15°C to 30°C (59°F to 86°F). Dilute in preservative-free NS, D_5W, or D_5NS.

Note: Store Hospira product at 20°C to 25°C (68°F to 77°F).

Oral: Store tablets at 15°C to 30°C (59°F to 86°F). Protect from light.

Mechanism of Action Promotes liver synthesis of clotting factors (II, VII, IX, X); however, the exact mechanism as to this stimulation is unknown. Menadiol is a water soluble form of vitamin K; phytonadione has a more rapid and prolonged effect than menadione; menadiol sodium diphosphate (K_4) is half as potent as menadione (K_3).

Pharmacodynamics/Kinetics

Onset of action: Increased coagulation factors: Oral: 6-10 hours; I.V.: 1-2 hours

Peak effect: INR values return to normal: Oral: 24-48 hours; I.V.: 12-14 hours

Absorption: Oral: From intestines in presence of bile; SubQ: Variable

Metabolism: Rapidly hepatic

Excretion: Urine and feces

Dosage Note: According to the manufacturer, SubQ is the preferred parenteral route; I.M. route should be avoided due to the risk of hematoma formation; I.V. route should be restricted for emergency use only. The American College of Chest Physicians recommends the I.V. route in patients with serious or life-threatening bleeding secondary to use of vitamin K antagonists.

Adequate intake:
Children:
1-3 years: 30 mcg/day
4-8 years: 55 mcg/day
9-13 years: 60 mcg/day
14-18 years: 75 mcg/day
Adults: Males: 120 mcg/day; Females: 90 mcg/day

Hemorrhagic disease of the newborn:
Prophylaxis: I.M.: 0.5-1 mg within 1 hour of birth
Treatment: I.M., SubQ: 1 mg/dose/day; higher doses may be necessary if mother has been receiving oral anticoagulants

Hypoprothrombinemia due to drugs (other than coumarin derivatives) or factors limiting absorption or synthesis: Adults: Oral, SubQ, I.M., I.V.: Initial: 2.5-25 mg (rarely up to 50 mg)

Vitamin K deficiency (supratherapeutic INR) secondary to coumarin derivative (Ansell, 2008): Adults:

If INR above therapeutic range to <5 (no significant bleeding and rapid reversal unnecessary): Lower or hold next dose and monitor frequently; when INR approaches desired range, resume dosing with a lower dose.

If INR ≥5 and <9 (no significant bleeding): If no risk factors for bleeding exist, omit next 1 or 2 doses, monitor INR more frequently, and resume with an appropriately adjusted dose when INR in desired range.

Alternatively, if other risk factors for bleeding exist, omit next dose and administer vitamin K orally 1-2.5 mg; resume with an appropriately adjusted dose when INR in desired range.

If INR ≥5 and <9 (no significant bleeding and rapid reversal required for surgery): Administer vitamin K orally ≤5 mg and hold warfarin. Expect INR to be reduced within 24 hours; if INR still elevated, another 1-2 mg of vitamin K orally may be given.

If INR ≥9 (no significant bleeding): Hold warfarin, administer vitamin K orally 2.5-5 mg, expect INR to be reduced within 24-48 hours, monitor INR more frequently and give additional vitamin K at an appropriate dose if necessary. Resume warfarin at an appropriately adjusted dose when INR is in desired range.

If serious bleeding at any INR elevation: Hold warfarin, administer vitamin K 10 mg by slow I.V. infusion and supplement with FFP, PCC, or rFVIIa depending on the urgency of the situation; I.V. Vitamin K may be repeated every 12 hours.

If life-threatening bleeding: Hold warfarin, give FFP, PCC, or rFVIIa supplemented with vitamin K 10 mg slow I.V. infusion; repeat if necessary, depending on INR.

Notes:

If mild-moderate INR elevation without major bleeding occurs, administer vitamin K orally instead of subcutaneously.

Use of high doses of vitamin K (eg, 10-15 mg) may cause warfarin resistance for ≥1 week. During this period of resistance, heparin or low molecular weight heparin may be given until INR responds.

FFP=fresh frozen plasma; PCC=prothrombin complex concentrate; rFVIIa=recombinant factor VIIa

Administration

I.V. administration: Infuse slowly; rate of infusion should not exceed 1 mg/minute (3 mg/m^2/minute in children and infants). The injectable route should be used only if the oral route is not feasible or there is a greater urgency to reverse anticoagulation.

Oral: The parenteral formulation may also be used for small oral doses (eg, 1 mg) or situations in which tablets cannot be swallowed (Crowther, 2000; O'Connor, 1986).

Monitoring Parameters PT, INR

Dosage Forms Excipient information presented when available (limited, particularly for generics); consult specific product labeling.

Injection, aqueous colloidal: 1 mg/0.5 mL (0.5 mL) [contains benzyl alcohol]; 10 mg/mL (1 mL) [contains benzyl alcohol]

Injection, aqueous colloidal [preservative free]: 1 mg/0.5 mL (0.5 mL) [contains polysorbate 80, propylene glycol 10.4 mg/0.5 mL]

Tablet, oral: 100 mcg
Mephyton®: 5 mg [scored]

Extemporaneous Preparations A 1 mg/mL oral suspension may be made with tablets. Crush six 5 mg tablets in a mortar and reduce to a fine powder. Add 5 mL each of water and methylcellulose 1% and mix to a uniform paste. Mix while adding sorbitol in incremental proportions to **almost** 30 mL; transfer to a calibrated bottle, rinse mortar with sorbitol, and add quantity of sorbitol sufficient to make 30 mL. Label "shake well" and "refrigerate". Stable for 3 days.

Nahata MC and Hipple TF, *Pediatric Drug Formulations*, 3rd ed, Cincinnati, OH: Harvey Whitney Books Co, 1997.

Note: The parenteral formulation may also be used for small oral doses (eg, 1 mg) or situations in which tablets cannot be swallowed (Crowther, 2000; O'Connor, 1986).

◆ **Pidorubicin** *see* Epirubicin *on page 597*

◆ **Pidorubicin Hydrochloride** *see* Epirubicin *on page 597*

Pilocarpine (Systemic) (pye loe KAR peen)

Brand Names: U.S. Salagen®

Brand Names: Canada Salagen®

Index Terms Pilocarpine Hydrochloride

Pharmacologic Category Cholinergic Agonist

Use Symptomatic treatment of xerostomia caused by salivary gland hypofunction resulting from radiotherapy for cancer of the head and neck or Sjögren's syndrome

Pregnancy Risk Factor C

Dosage Oral: Adults: Xerostomia:

Following head and neck cancer: 5 mg 3 times/day, titration up to 10 mg 3 times/day may be considered for patients who have not responded adequately; do not exceed 2 tablets/dose

Sjögren's syndrome: 5 mg 4 times/day

Dosage adjustment in hepatic impairment:

Moderate impairment: 5 mg 2 times/day regardless of indication; adjust dose based on response and tolerability

Severe impairment (Child-Pugh score >10): Contraindicated

Additional Information Complete prescribing information for this medication should be consulted for additional detail.

Dosage Forms Excipient information presented when available (limited, particularly for generics); consult specific product labeling.

Tablet, oral, as hydrochloride: 5 mg, 7.5 mg

Salagen®: 5 mg, 7.5 mg

Pilocarpine (Ophthalmic) (pye loe KAR peen)

Brand Names: U.S. Isopto® Carpine; Pilopine HS®

Brand Names: Canada Diocarpine; Isopto® Carpine; Pilopine HS®

Index Terms Pilocarpine Hydrochloride

Pharmacologic Category Ophthalmic Agent, Antiglaucoma; Ophthalmic Agent, Miotic

Use Management of chronic simple glaucoma, chronic and acute angle-closure glaucoma

Unlabeled Use Counter effects of cycloplegics

Pregnancy Risk Factor C

Dosage Ophthalmic: Adults:

Glaucoma:

Solution: Instill 1-2 drops up to 6 times/day; adjust the concentration and frequency as required to control elevated intraocular pressure

Gel: Instill 0.5" ribbon into lower conjunctival sac once daily at bedtime

To counteract the mydriatic effects of sympathomimetic agents (unlabeled use): Solution: Instill 1 drop of a 1% solution in the affected eye

Additional Information Complete prescribing information for this medication should be consulted for additional detail.

Dosage Forms Excipient information presented when available (limited, particularly for generics); consult specific product labeling.

Gel, ophthalmic, as hydrochloride:

Pilopine HS®: 4% (4 g) [contains benzalkonium chloride]

Solution, ophthalmic, as hydrochloride [drops]: 1% (15 mL); 2% (15 mL); 4% (15 mL)

Isopto® Carpine: 1% (15 mL); 2% (15 mL); 4% (15 mL) [contains benzalkonium chloride]

◆ **Pilocarpine Hydrochloride** *see* Pilocarpine (Ophthalmic) *on page 1353*

◆ **Pilocarpine Hydrochloride** *see* Pilocarpine (Systemic) *on page 1353*

◆ **Pilopine HS®** *see* Pilocarpine (Ophthalmic) *on page 1353*

◆ **Pimaricin** *see* Natamycin *on page 1182*

Pimecrolimus (pim e KROE li mus)

Brand Names: U.S. Elidel®

Brand Names: Canada Elidel®

Pharmacologic Category Immunosuppressant Agent; Topical Skin Product

Use Short-term and intermittent long-term treatment of mild-to-moderate atopic dermatitis in patients not responsive to conventional therapy or when conventional therapy is not appropriate

Pregnancy Risk Factor C

Pregnancy Considerations There are no adequate and well-controlled studies in pregnant women; use only if clearly needed.

Lactation Excretion in breast milk unknown/not recommended

Medication Guide Available Yes

Contraindications Hypersensitivity to pimecrolimus or any component of the formulation

Warnings/Precautions [U.S. Boxed Warning]: Topical calcineurin inhibitors have been associated with rare cases of lymphoma and skin malignancy. Avoid use on malignant or premalignant skin conditions (eg, cutaneous T-cell lymphoma). Topical calcineurin agents are considered second-line therapies in the treatment of atopic dermatitis/eczema, and should be limited to use in patients who have failed treatment with other therapies. **[U.S. Boxed Warning]: They should be used for short-term and intermittent treatment using the minimum amount necessary for the control of symptoms should be used.** Application should be limited to involved areas. Diagnosis should be reconfirmed if sign/symptoms do not improve within 6 weeks of treatment. Safety of intermittent use for >1 year has not been established.

May cause local symptoms (eg, burning, soreness, stinging) during first few days of treatment; usually self-resolving. Should not be used in immunocompromised patients. Do not apply to areas of active bacterial or viral infection; infections at the treatment site should be cleared prior to therapy. Patients with atopic dermatitis are predisposed to skin infections, and pimecrolimus therapy has been associated with risk of developing eczema herpeticum, varicella zoster, and herpes simplex. Papilloma/warts have been observed with use; discontinue pimecrolimus until resolution if worsening or do not respond to conventional treatment. Pimecrolimus may be associated with development of lymphadenopathy; possible infectious causes should be investigated. Discontinue use in patients with unknown cause of lymphadenopathy or acute infectious mononucleosis. Not recommended for use in patients with skin disease which may increase the potential for systemic absorption (eg, Netherton's syndrome). Avoid artificial or natural sunlight exposure, even when Elidel® is not on the skin. Safety not established in patients with generalized erythroderma. **[U.S. Boxed Warning]: The use of Elidel® in children <2 years of age is not recommended,** particularly since the effect on immune system development is unknown.

Adverse Reactions

>10%:

Central nervous system: Headache (7% to 25%), fever (1% to 13%)

Local: Burning at application site (2% to 26%; tends to resolve/improve as lesions resolve)

Respiratory: Nasopharyngitis (8% to 27%), cough (2% to 16%), upper respiratory tract infection (4% to 19%), bronchitis (≤11%)

Miscellaneous: Influenza (3% to 13%)

1% to 10%:

Dermatologic: Skin infection (2% to 6%), folliculitis (1% to 6%), impetigo (2% to 4%), skin papilloma (warts) (≤3%), acne (≤2%), herpes simplex dermatitis (≤2%), molluscum contagiosum (≤2%), urticaria (≤1%)

Endocrine & metabolic: Dysmenorrhea (1% to 2%)

Gastrointestinal: Diarrhea (1% to 8%), gastroenteritis (≤7%), abdominal pain (≤4%), constipation (≤4%)

Local: Irritation at application site (≤6%), pruritus at application site (1% to 6%), erythema at application site (≤2%)

Ocular: Eye infection (≤1%)

Otic: Ear infection (1% to 6%), otitis media (1% to 3%)

Respiratory: Pharyngitis (1% to 8%), asthma (1% to 4%), asthma aggravated (≤4%), nasal congestion (1% to 3%), sinusitis (1% to 3%), epistaxis (≤3%), dyspnea (≤2%), pneumonia (≤2%), rhinorrhea (≤2%), wheezing (≤1%)

Miscellaneous: Viral infection (≤7%), tonsillitis (≤6%), hypersensitivity (3% to 5%), herpes simplex infection (≤4%), bacterial infection (1% to 2%)

<1% (Limited to important or life-threatening): Anaphylaxis, angioneurotic edema, eczema herpeticum, facial edema, flushing (ethanol-associated), lymphadenopathy, ocular irritation (following application near eyes), malignancy (basal cell carcinoma, squamous cell carcinoma, malignant melanoma, lymphoma), skin discoloration

Drug Interactions

Metabolism/Transport Effects Substrate of CYP3A4 (minor); **Note:** Assignment of Major/Minor substrate status based on clinically relevant drug interaction potential

Avoid Concomitant Use

Avoid concomitant use of Pimecrolimus with any of the following: Immunosuppressants

Increased Effect/Toxicity

Pimecrolimus may increase the levels/effects of: Immunosuppressants

The levels/effects of Pimecrolimus may be increased by: CYP3A4 Inhibitors (Moderate); CYP3A4 Inhibitors (Strong)

Decreased Effect There are no known significant interactions involving a decrease in effect.

Ethanol/Nutrition/Herb Interactions Ethanol: Avoid ethanol (topical pimecrolimus may increase the potential for experiencing facial flushing following the consumption of alcoholic beverages).

Stability Store at 15°C to 30°C (59°F to 86°F); do not freeze.

Mechanism of Action Penetrates inflamed epidermis to inhibit T cell activation by blocking transcription of proinflammatory cytokine genes such as interleukin-2, interferon gamma (Th1-type), interleukin-4, and interleukin-10 (Th2-type). Pimecrolimus binds to the intracellular protein FKBP-12, inhibiting calcineurin, which blocks cytokine transcription and inhibits T-cell activation. Prevents release of inflammatory cytokines and mediators from mast cells *in vitro* after stimulation by antigen/IgE.

Pharmacodynamics/Kinetics Absorption: Poor when applied to 13% to 62% body surface area in adults for up to a year; detectable blood levels were observed in a higher proportion of children, as compared to adults

Dosage Children ≥2 years and Adults: Topical: Apply thin layer to affected area twice daily; rub in gently and completely. **Note:** Limit application to involved areas. Continue as long as signs and symptoms persist; discontinue if resolution occurs; re-evaluate if symptoms persist >6 weeks.

Administration Do not use with occlusive dressings. Burning at the application site is most common in first few days; improves as atopic dermatitis improves. Limit application to areas of involvement. Continue as long as signs and symptoms persist; discontinue if resolution occurs; re-evaluate if symptoms persist >6 weeks.

Dosage Forms Excipient information presented when available (limited, particularly for generics); consult specific product labeling.

Cream, topical:

Elidel®: 1% (30 g, 60 g, 100 g) [contains benzyl alcohol]

Pimozide (PI moe zide)

Brand Names: U.S. Orap®

Brand Names: Canada Apo-Pimozide®; Orap®; PMS-Pimozide

Pharmacologic Category Antipsychotic Agent, Typical

Additional Appendix Information

Antipsychotic Agents *on page 1880*

Use Suppression of severe motor and phonic tics in patients with Tourette's disorder who have failed to respond satisfactorily to standard treatment

Unlabeled Use Psychosis; reported use in individuals with delusions focused on physical symptoms (ie, preoccupation with parasitic infestation); Huntington's chorea

Pregnancy Risk Factor C

Dosage Oral: **Note:** An ECG should be performed baseline and periodically thereafter, especially during dosage adjustment:

Children ≤12 years: Tourette's disorder: Initial: 0.05 mg/kg preferably once at bedtime; may be increased every third day; usual range: 2-4 mg/day; do not exceed 10 mg/day (0.2 mg/kg/day); maximum dose: 10 mg/day or 0.2 mg/kg/day (whichever is less)

Children >12 years and Adults: Tourette's disorder: Initial: 1-2 mg/day in divided doses, then increase dosage as needed every other day; range is usually 7-10 mg/day, maximum dose: 10 mg/day or 0.2 mg/kg/day (whichever is less)

Dosage adjustment for toxicity:

ECG changes:

Children: QT_c prolongation >0.47 seconds or >25% above baseline: Decrease dose

Adults: QT_c prolongation >0.52 seconds or >25% above baseline: Decrease dose

NMS syndrome: Discontinue (monitor carefully if therapy is reinitiated)

Tardive dyskinesia signs/symptoms: Consider discontinuing.

Additional Information Complete prescribing information for this medication should be consulted for additional detail.

Dosage Forms Excipient information presented when available (limited, particularly for generics); consult specific product labeling.

Tablet, oral:

Orap®: 1 mg, 2 mg [scored]

◆ **Pin-X® [OTC]** *see* Pyrantel Pamoate *on page 1434*

Pindolol (PIN doe lole)

Brand Names: Canada Apo-Pindol®; Dom-Pindolol; Mylan-Pindolol; Novo-Pindol; Nu-Pindol; PMS-Pindolol; Sandoz-Pindolol; Teva-Pindolol; Visken®

Pharmacologic Category Beta Blocker With Intrinsic Sympathomimetic Activity

Additional Appendix Information
Beta-Blockers *on page 1884*

Use Treatment of hypertension, alone or in combination with other agents

Unlabeled Use Potential augmenting agent for antidepressants; ventricular arrhythmias/tachycardia, antipsychotic-induced akathisia, situational anxiety; aggressive behavior associated with dementia

Pregnancy Risk Factor B

Dosage Oral:

Adults:

Hypertension: Initial: 5 mg twice daily, increase as necessary by 10 mg/day every 3-4 weeks (maximum daily dose: 60 mg); usual dose range (JNC 7): 10-40 mg twice daily

Antidepressant augmentation (unlabeled use): 2.5 mg 3 times/day

Elderly: Initial: 5 mg once daily, increase as necessary by 5 mg/day every 3-4 weeks

Dosing adjustment in renal impairment: Use with caution. Clearance significantly decreased in uremic patients. Dosage reduction may be necessary.

Dosage adjustment in hepatic impairment: Use with caution. Elimination half-life in cirrhotic patients may be 10 times as long compared to normal patients. Dosage reduction is necessary in severely impaired.

Additional Information Complete prescribing information for this medication should be consulted for additional detail.

Dosage Forms Excipient information presented when available (limited, particularly for generics); consult specific product labeling.

Tablet, oral: 5 mg, 10 mg

◆ **Pink Bismuth** *see* Bismuth *on page 220*

Pioglitazone (pye oh GLI ta zone)

Brand Names: U.S. Actos®

Brand Names: Canada Accel-Pioglitazone; Actos®; Apo-Pioglitazone®; Ava-Pioglitazone; CO Pioglitazone; Dom-Pioglitazone; JAMP-Pioglitazone; Mint-Pioglitazone; Mylan-Pioglitazone; Novo-Pioglitazone; PHL-Pioglitazone; PMS-Pioglitazone; PRO-Pioglitazone; ratio-Pioglitazone; Sandoz-Pioglitazone; Teva-Pioglitazone; ZYM-Pioglitazone

Pharmacologic Category Antidiabetic Agent, Thiazolidinedione

Additional Appendix Information
Diabetes Mellitus Management, Adults *on page 1983*

Use

Type 2 diabetes mellitus (noninsulin dependent, NIDDM), monotherapy: Adjunct to diet and exercise, to improve glycemic control

Type 2 diabetes mellitus (noninsulin dependent, NIDDM), combination therapy with sulfonylurea, metformin, or insulin: When diet, exercise, and a single agent alone does not result in adequate glycemic control

Pregnancy Risk Factor C

Pregnancy Considerations Pioglitazone is classified as pregnancy category C due to adverse effects observed in animal studies. The use of pioglitazone in pregnant women is limited to very few case reports where pregnancy occurred during treatment for polycystic ovarian syndrome (PCOS); details concerning fetal outcomes are limited. Thiazolidinediones may cause ovulation in anovulatory premenopausal women, increasing the risk of pregnancy; adequate contraception in premenopausal women is recommended. Maternal hyperglycemia can be associated with adverse effects in the fetus, including macrosomia, neonatal hyperglycemia, and hyperbilirubinemia; the risk of congenital malformations is increased when the Hb A_{1c} is above the normal range. Diabetes can also be associated with adverse effects in the mother. Poorly-treated diabetes may cause end-organ damage that may in turn negatively affect obstetric outcomes. Physiologic glucose levels should be maintained prior to and during pregnancy to decrease the risk of adverse events in the mother and the fetus. Until additional safety and efficacy data are obtained, the use of oral agents is generally not recommended as routine management of GDM or type 2 diabetes mellitus during pregnancy. Insulin is the drug of choice for the control of diabetes mellitus during pregnancy.

Lactation Excretion in breast milk unknown/not recommended

Medication Guide Available Yes

Contraindications Hypersensitivity to pioglitazone or any component of the formulation; NYHA Class III/IV heart failure (initiation of therapy)

Canadian labeling: Additional contraindications (not is U.S. labeling): Any stage of heart failure (eg, NYHA Class I, II, III, IV); serious hepatic impairment; pregnancy

Warnings/Precautions [U.S. Boxed Warning]: Thiazolidinediones, including pioglitazone, may cause or exacerbate heart failure; closely monitor for signs and symptoms of heart failure (eg, rapid weight gain, dyspnea, edema), particularly after initiation or dose increases. Not recommended for use in any patient with symptomatic heart failure. In the U.S., initiation of therapy is contraindicated in patients with NYHA class III or IV heart failure. If used in patients with NYHA class II (systolic heart failure), initiate at lowest dosage and monitor closely. In Canada, use in any stage of heart failure (NYHA I, II, III, IV) is contraindicated. Use with caution in patients with edema; may increase plasma volume and/or cause fluid retention. Dose reduction or discontinuation is recommended if heart failure suspected. Dose-related weight gain observed with use; mechanism unknown but likely associated with fluid retention and fat accumulation.

Should not be used in diabetic ketoacidosis. Mechanism requires the presence of insulin; therefore use in type 1 diabetes is not recommended. Use with caution in premenopausal, anovulatory women - may result in a resumption of ovulation, increasing the risk of pregnancy. Use with caution in patients with anemia (may reduce hemoglobin and hematocrit). Increased incidence of bone fractures in females treated with pioglitazone; majority of fractures occurred in the lower limb and distal upper limb.

Use with caution in patients with elevated transaminases (AST or ALT); do not initiate in patients with active liver disease of ALT >2.5 times the upper limit of normal at baseline. During therapy, if ALT >3 times the upper limit of normal, re-evaluate levels promptly and discontinue if elevation persists or if jaundice occurs at any time during use. Idiosyncratic hepatotoxicity has been reported with another thiazolidinedione agent (troglitazone); avoid use in patients who previously experienced jaundice during troglitazone therapy. Monitoring should include periodic determinations of liver function. Use caution with preexisting macular edema or diabetic retinopathy. Postmarketing reports of new-onset or worsening diabetic macular edema with decreased visual acuity has been reported. Safety and efficacy have not been established in children.

Canadian labeling (not in U.S. labeling) states use with insulin **or** as part of triple therapy (pioglitazone in combination with a sulfonylurea and metformin) is not indicated.

Adverse Reactions

>10%:

Cardiovascular: Edema (5%; in combination trials with sulfonlyureas or insulin, the incidence of edema was as high as 15%)

Respiratory: Upper respiratory tract infection (13%)

1% to 10%:

Cardiovascular: Heart failure (requiring hospitalization; up to 6% in patients with prior macrovascular disease)

Central nervous system: Headache (9%), fatigue (4%)

Hematologic: Anemia (≤2%)

Neuromuscular & skeletal: Myalgia (5%)

Respiratory: Sinusitis (6%), pharyngitis (5%)

<1% (Limited to important or life-threatening): Bladder cancer, blurred vision, CPK increased, dyspnea (associated with weight gain and/or edema), fractures (females; usually in distal upper limbs or distal lower limbs), hepatic failure (very rare), hepatitis, macular edema (new onset or worsening), transaminases increased, pulmonary edema, rhabdomyolysis, visual acuity decreased

Frequency not defined: HDL-cholesterol increased, hematocrit/hemoglobin decreased, hypoglycemia (in combination trials with sulfonylureas or insulin), serum triglycerides decreased, weight gain/loss

Drug Interactions

Metabolism/Transport Effects Substrate of CYP2C8 (major), CYP3A4 (minor); **Note:** Assignment of Major/Minor substrate status based on clinically relevant drug interaction potential; **Inhibits** CYP2C19 (weak), CYP2C8 (moderate), CYP2C9 (weak); **Induces** CYP3A4 (weak/moderate)

Avoid Concomitant Use There are no known interactions where it is recommended to avoid concomitant use.

Increased Effect/Toxicity

Pioglitazone may increase the levels/effects of: CYP2C8 Substrates; Hypoglycemic Agents

The levels/effects of Pioglitazone may be increased by: Conivaptan; CYP2C8 Inhibitors (Moderate); CYP2C8 Inhibitors (Strong); Deferasirox; Gemfibrozil; Herbs (Hypoglycemic Properties); Insulin; Pegvisomant; Pregabalin; Trimethoprim

Decreased Effect

Pioglitazone may decrease the levels/effects of: ARIPiprazole; Saxagliptin

The levels/effects of Pioglitazone may be decreased by: Bile Acid Sequestrants; Corticosteroids (Orally Inhaled); Corticosteroids (Systemic); CYP2C8 Inducers (Strong); Luteinizing Hormone-Releasing Hormone Analogs; Rifampin; Somatropin; Thiazide Diuretics; Tocilizumab

Ethanol/Nutrition/Herb Interactions

Ethanol: Caution with ethanol (may cause hypoglycemia).

Food: Peak concentrations are delayed when administered with food, but the extent of absorption is not affected. Pioglitazone may be taken without regard to meals.

Herb/Nutraceutical: Caution with alfalfa, aloe, bilberry, bitter melon, burdock, celery, damiana, fenugreek, garcinia, garlic, ginger, ginseng (American), gymnema, marshmallow, and stinging nettle (may cause hypoglycemia).

Mechanism of Action Thiazolidinedione antidiabetic agent that lowers blood glucose by improving target cell response to insulin, without increasing pancreatic insulin secretion. It has a mechanism of action that is dependent on the presence of insulin for activity. Pioglitazone is a potent and selective agonist for peroxisome proliferator-activated receptor-gamma (PPARgamma). Activation of nuclear PPARgamma receptors influences the production of a number of gene products involved in glucose and lipid metabolism. PPARgamma is abundant in the cells within the renal collecting tubules; fluid retention results from stimulation by thiazolidinediones which increases sodium reabsorption.

Pharmacodynamics/Kinetics

Onset of action: Delayed

Peak effect: Glucose control: Several weeks

Distribution: V_{ss} (apparent): 0.63 L/kg

Protein binding: Pioglitazone >99% and active metabolites >98%; primarily to albumin

Metabolism: Hepatic (99%) via CYP2C8 and 3A4 to both active and inactive metabolites

Half-life elimination: Parent drug: 3-7 hours; Total: 16-24 hours

Time to peak: ~2 hours; delayed with food

Excretion: Urine (15% to 30%) and feces as metabolites

Dosage Oral:

Adults:

Monotherapy: Initial: 15-30 mg once daily; if response is inadequate, the dosage may be increased in increments up to 45 mg once daily; maximum recommended dose: 45 mg once daily

Combination therapy: Maximum recommended dose: 45 mg/day

With sulfonylureas: Initial: 15-30 mg once daily; dose of sulfonylurea should be reduced if the patient reports hypoglycemia

With metformin: Initial: 15-30 mg once daily; it is unlikely that the dose of metformin will need to be reduced due to hypoglycemia

With insulin: Initial: 15-30 mg once daily; dose of insulin should be reduced by 10% to 25% if the patient reports hypoglycemia or if the plasma glucose falls to <100 mg/dL.

Dosage adjustment in patients with CHF (NYHA Class II) in mono- or combination therapy: Initial: 15 mg once daily; may be increased after several months of treatment, with close attention to heart failure symptoms

Elderly: No dosage adjustment is recommended in elderly patients.

Dosage adjustment in renal impairment: No dosage adjustment is required.

Dosage adjustment in hepatic impairment: Clearance is significantly lower in hepatic impairment (Child-Pugh Grade B/C). Therapy should not be initiated if the patient exhibits active liver disease or increased transaminases (>2.5 times ULN) at baseline. During treatment if ALT levels elevate >3 times ULN, the test should be repeated as soon as possible. If ALT levels remain >3 times ULN or if the patient is jaundiced, therapy should be discontinued.

Dietary Considerations Management of type 2 diabetes mellitus (noninsulin dependent, NIDDM) should include diet control. May be taken without regard to meals.

Administration May be administered without regard to meals

Monitoring Parameters Hemoglobin A_{1c}, serum glucose; signs and symptoms of heart failure; liver enzymes prior to initiation and periodically during treatment (per clinician judgment). If the ALT is increased to >2.5 times the upper limit of normal, liver function testing should be performed more frequently until the levels return to normal or pretreatment values. Patients with an elevation in ALT >3 times the upper limit of normal should be rechecked as soon as possible. If the ALT levels remain >3 times the upper limit of normal, therapy with pioglitazone should be discontinued. Routine ophthalmic exams are recommended; patients reporting visual deterioration should have a prompt referral to an ophthalmologist and consideration should be given to discontinuing pioglitazone.

Reference Range Recommendations for glycemic control in adults with diabetes:

Hb A_{1c}: <7%

Preprandial capillary plasma glucose: 70-130 mg/dL

Peak postprandial capillary blood glucose: <180 mg/dL

Dosage Forms Excipient information presented when available (limited, particularly for generics); consult specific product labeling.

Tablet, oral:

Actos®: 15 mg, 30 mg, 45 mg

Pioglitazone and Glimepiride

(pye oh GLI ta zone & GLYE me pye ride)

Brand Names: U.S. Duetact™

Index Terms Glimepiride and Pioglitazone; Glimepiride and Pioglitazone Hydrochloride

Pharmacologic Category Antidiabetic Agent, Sulfonylurea; Antidiabetic Agent, Thiazolidinedione; Hypoglycemic Agent, Oral

Use Management of type 2 diabetes mellitus (noninsulin dependent, NIDDM) as an adjunct to diet and exercise

Pregnancy Risk Factor C

Medication Guide Available Yes

Dosage Oral: Type 2 diabetes mellitus:

Adults: Initial dose should be based on current dose of pioglitazone and/or sulfonylurea.

Patients inadequately controlled on **glimepiride** alone: Initial dose: 30 mg/2 mg or 30 mg/4 mg once daily

Patients inadequately controlled on **pioglitazone** alone: Initial dose: 30 mg/2 mg once daily

Patients with systolic dysfunction (eg, NYHA Class I and II): Initiate only after patient has been safely titrated to 30 mg of pioglitazone. Initial dose: 30 mg/2 mg or 30 mg/4 mg once daily.

Note: No exact dosing relationship exists between glimepiride and other sulfonlyureas. Dosing should be limited to less than or equal to the maximum initial dose of glimepiride (2 mg). When converting patients from other sulfonylureas with longer half-lives (eg, chlorpropamide) to glimepiride, observe patient carefully for 1-2 weeks due to overlapping hypoglycemic effects.

Dosing adjustment: Dosage may be increased up to max dose and formulation strengths available; tablet should not be given more than once daily; see individual agents for frequency of adjustments. Dosage adjustments in patients with systolic dysfunction should be done carefully and patient monitored for symptoms of worsening heart failure.

Maximum dose: Pioglitazone 45 mg/glimepiride 8 mg daily

Elderly: Initial: Glimepiride 1 mg/day prior to initiating Duetact™; dose titration and maintenance dosing should be conservative to avoid hypoglycemia

Dosage adjustment in renal impairment: Cl_{cr} <22 mL/minute: Initial dose should be 1 mg of glimepiride and dosage increments should be based on fasting blood glucose levels

Dosage adjustment in hepatic impairment: Do not initiate treatment with active liver disease or ALT >2.5 times ULN. During treatment, if ALT levels elevate >3 times ULN, the test should be repeated as soon as possible. If ALT levels remain >3 times ULN or if the patient is jaundiced, Duetact™ should be discontinued.

Additional Information Complete prescribing information for this medication should be consulted for additional detail.

Dosage Forms Excipient information presented when available (limited, particularly for generics); consult specific product labeling.

Tablet:

Duetact™:

30 mg/2 mg: Pioglitazone 30 mg and glimepiride 2 mg

30 mg/4 mg: Pioglitazone 30 mg and glimepiride 4 mg

Pioglitazone and Metformin

(pye oh GLI ta zone & met FOR min)

Brand Names: U.S. Actoplus Met®; Actoplus Met® XR

Index Terms Metformin Hydrochloride and Pioglitazone Hydrochloride

Pharmacologic Category Antidiabetic Agent, Biguanide; Antidiabetic Agent, Thiazolidinedione

Use Management of type 2 diabetes mellitus (noninsulin dependent, NIDDM)

Pregnancy Risk Factor C

Medication Guide Available Yes

Dosage Oral: Type 2 diabetes mellitus:

Adults: Initial dose should be based on current dose of pioglitazone and/or metformin; metformin dose may be titrated every 1-2 weeks and pioglitazone dose may be titrated every 2-3 months as necessary to achieve goals

Immediate release tablet: **Note:** Daily doses higher than pioglitazone 15 mg plus metformin 850 mg should be divided. Initial: Pioglitazone 15 mg plus metformin 500 mg **or** pioglitazone 15 mg plus metformin 850 mg tablets once or twice daily. Maximum daily dose: Pioglitazone 45 mg/metformin 2550 mg

Variable release tablet: Pioglitazone 15 mg plus metformin 1000 mg tablet **or** pioglitazone 30 mg plus metformin 1000 mg tablet once daily with evening meal. Maximum daily dose: Pioglitazone 45 mg/metformin 2000 mg

Elderly: The initial and maintenance dosing should be conservative, due to the potential for decreased renal function (monitor). Generally, elderly patients should not be titrated to the maximum; do not use in patients ≥80 years of age unless normal renal function has been established.

Dosage adjustment in renal impairment: Do not use with renal disease or renal dysfunction (serum creatinine ≥1.5 mg/dL in males or ≥1.4 mg/dL in females or abnormal clearance).

Dosage adjustment in hepatic impairment: Do not initiate treatment with active liver disease or ALT >2.5 times ULN. During treatment, if ALT concentrations increase >3 times ULN, the test should be repeated as soon as possible. If ALT concentrations remain >3 times ULN or if the patient is jaundiced, therapy should be discontinued.

Additional Information Complete prescribing information for this medication should be consulted for additional detail.

Dosage Forms Excipient information presented when available (limited, particularly for generics); consult specific product labeling.

Tablet, oral:

Actoplus Met®:

15/500: Pioglitazone 15 mg and metformin hydrochloride 500 mg

15/850: Pioglitazone 15 mg and metformin hydrochloride 850 mg

Tablet, variable release, oral:

Actoplus Met® XR:

15/1000: Pioglitazone 15 mg [immediate release] and metformin hydrochloride 1000 mg [extended release]

30/1000: Pioglitazone 30 mg [immediate release] and metformin hydrochloride 1000 mg [extended release]

Piperacillin (pi PER a sil in)

Brand Names: Canada Piperacillin for Injection, USP
Index Terms Piperacillin Sodium
Pharmacologic Category Antibiotic, Penicillin
Use Treatment of susceptible infections such as septicemia, acute and chronic respiratory tract infections, skin and soft tissue infections, and urinary tract infections due to susceptible strains of *Pseudomonas*, *Proteus*, and *Escherichia coli* and *Enterobacter*; active against some streptococci and some anaerobic bacteria; febrile neutropenia (as part of combination regimen)
Pregnancy Risk Factor B
Dosage
Usual dosage range:
Infants and Children: I.M., I.V.: 200-300 mg/kg/day in divided doses every 4-6 hours
Adults: I.M., I.V.: 2-4 g/dose every 4-6 hours (maximum: 24 g/day)
Indication-specific dosing:
Children: I.M., I.V.:
Cystic fibrosis: 350-500 mg/kg/day in divided doses every 4-6 hours
Adults:
Burn wound sepsis: I.V.: 4 g every 4 hours with vancomycin and amikacin
Cholangitis, acute: I.V.: 4 g every 6 hours
Keratitis *(Pseudomonas)*: Ophthalmic: 6-12 mg/mL every 15-60 minutes around the clock for 24-72 hours, then slow reduction
Malignant otitis externa: I.V.: 4-6 g every 4-6 hours with tobramycin
Moderate infections: I.M., I.V.: 2-3 g/dose every 6-12 hours (maximum: 2 g I.M./site)
Prosthetic joint *(Pseudomonas)*: I.V.: 3 g every 6 hours with aminoglycoside
***Pseudomonas* infections:** I.V.: 4 g every 4 hours
Severe infections: I.M., I.V.: 3-4 g/dose every 4-6 hours (maximum: 24 g/24 hours)
Urinary tract infections: I.V.: 2-3 g/dose every 6-12 hours
Uncomplicated gonorrhea: I.M.: 2 g in a single dose accompanied by 1 g probenecid 30 minutes prior to injection
Dosing adjustment in renal impairment: Adults: I.V.:
Cl_{cr} 20-40 mL/minute: Administer 3-4 g every 8 hours
Cl_{cr} <20 mL/minute: Administer 3-4 g every 12 hours
Moderately dialyzable (20% to 50%)
Continuous arteriovenous or venovenous hemodiafiltration effects: Dose as for Cl_{cr} 10-50 mL/minute
Additional Information Complete prescribing information for this medication should be consulted for additional detail.
Dosage Forms Excipient information presented when available (limited, particularly for generics); consult specific product labeling. [DSC] = Discontinued product
Injection, powder for reconstitution: 2 g [DSC], 3 g [DSC], 4 g [DSC], 40 g [DSC]

Piperacillin and Tazobactam
(pi PER a sil in & ta zoe BAK tam)

Brand Names: U.S. Zosyn®
Brand Names: Canada Piperacillin and Tazobactam for Injection; Tazocin®
Index Terms Piperacillin and Tazobactam Sodium; Piperacillin Sodium and Tazobactam Sodium; Tazobactam and Piperacillin
Pharmacologic Category Antibiotic, Penicillin
Use Treatment of moderate-to-severe infections caused by susceptible organisms, including infections of the lower respiratory tract (community-acquired pneumonia, nosocomial pneumonia); uncomplicated and complicated skin and skin structures (including diabetic foot infections); gynecologic (endometritis, pelvic inflammatory disease); and intra-abdominal infections (appendicitis with rupture/abscess, peritonitis). Tazobactam expands activity of piperacillin to include beta-lactamase producing strains of *S. aureus*, *H. influenzae*, *E. coli*, *Bacteroides* spp, and other gram-positive and gram-negative aerobic and anaerobic bacteria.
Unlabeled Use Treatment of moderate-to-severe infections caused by susceptible organisms, including urinary tract infections, bone and joint infections, septicemia, endocarditis, and cystic fibrosis exacerbations
Pregnancy Risk Factor B
Pregnancy Considerations Adverse events have not been observed in animal studies; therefore, piperacillin/tazobactam is classified as pregnancy category B. Piperacillin and tazobactam both cross the placenta and are found in the fetal serum, placenta, amniotic fluid, and fetal urine. When used during pregnancy, the clearance and volume of distribution of piperacillin/tazobactam are increased; half-life and AUC are decreased.
Lactation Enters breast milk/use caution
Contraindications Hypersensitivity to penicillins, cephalosporins, beta-lactamase inhibitors, or any component of the formulation
Warnings/Precautions Serious and occasionally severe or fatal hypersensitivity (anaphylactic/anaphylactoid) reactions have been reported in patients on penicillin therapy, especially with a history of beta-lactam hypersensitivity, history of sensitivity to multiple allergens, or previous IgE-mediated reactions (eg, anaphylaxis, angioedema, urticaria). Bleeding disorders have been observed, particularly in patients with renal impairment; discontinue if thrombocytopenia or bleeding occurs. Due to sodium load and to the adverse effects of high serum concentrations of penicillins, dosage modification is required in patients with impaired or underdeveloped renal function; use with caution in patients with seizures or in patients with history of beta-lactam allergy; associated with an increased incidence of rash and fever in cystic fibrosis patients. Use may result in fungal or bacterial superinfection, including *C. difficile*-associated diarrhea (CDAD) and pseudomembranous colitis; CDAD has been observed >2 months postantibiotic treatment.
Adverse Reactions
>10%: Gastrointestinal: Diarrhea (7% to 11%)
1% to 10%:
Cardiovascular: Hypertension (2%), chest pain (1%), edema (1%)
Central nervous system: Insomnia (7%), headache (8%), fever (2% to 5%), agitation (2%), pain (2%), anxiety (1% to 2%), dizziness (1% to 2%)
Dermatologic: Rash (4%), pruritus (3%)
Gastrointestinal: Constipation (1% to 8%), nausea (7%), vomiting (3% to 4%), dyspepsia (3%), stool changes (2%), abdominal pain (1% to 2%)
Hepatic: AST increased (1%)
Local: Local reaction (3%), abscess (2%), phlebitis (1%)
Respiratory: Pharyngitis (2%), dyspnea (1%), rhinitis (1%)
Miscellaneous: Moniliasis (2%), sepsis (2%), infection (2%)
<1%, postmarketing, and/or case reports (Limited to important and life-threatening): Agranulocytosis, anaphylaxis/anaphylactoid reaction, anemia, anxiety, arrhythmia, arthralgia, atrial fibrillation, back pain, bradycardia, bronchospasm, *C. difficile*-associated diarrhea (CDAD), candidiasis, cardiac arrest, cardiac failure, cholestatic jaundice, circulatory failure, confusion, convulsions, coughing, depression, diaphoresis, dysuria, epistaxis, erythema multiforme, flatulence, flushing, gastritis, genital pruritus, hallucination, hematuria, hemolytic anemia,

hemorrhage, hepatitis, hiccough, hypoglycemia, hypokalemia, hypotension, ileus, incontinence, inflammation, injection site reaction, interstitial nephritis, leukorrhea, malaise, melena, mesenteric embolism, myalgia, myocardial infarction, oliguria, pancytopenia, photophobia, pulmonary edema, pulmonary embolism, purpura, renal failure, rigors, Stevens-Johnson syndrome, syncope, tachycardia (supraventricular and ventricular), taste perversion, thirst, thrombocytopenia, thrombocytosis, thrombophlebitis, tinnitus, toxic epidermal necrolysis, tremor, ulcerative stomatitis, urinary retention, vaginitis, ventricular fibrillation, vertigo

Drug Interactions

Metabolism/Transport Effects None known.

Avoid Concomitant Use

Avoid concomitant use of Piperacillin and Tazobactam with any of the following: BCG

Increased Effect/Toxicity

Piperacillin and Tazobactam may increase the levels/effects of: Methotrexate; Vitamin K Antagonists

The levels/effects of Piperacillin and Tazobactam may be increased by: Probenecid

Decreased Effect

Piperacillin and Tazobactam may decrease the levels/effects of: Aminoglycosides; BCG; Mycophenolate; Typhoid Vaccine

The levels/effects of Piperacillin and Tazobactam may be decreased by: Fusidic Acid; Tetracycline Derivatives

Stability

Vials: Store at controlled room temperature of 20°C to 25°C (68°F to 77°F). Use single-dose vials immediately after reconstitution (discard unused portions after 24 hours at room temperature and 48 hours if refrigerated). Reconstitute with 5 mL of diluent per 1 g of piperacillin and then further dilute. After reconstitution, vials or solution are stable in NS or D_5W for 24 hours at room temperature and 48 hours (vials) or 7 days (solution) when refrigerated.

Premixed solution: Store frozen at -20°C (-4°F). Thawed solution is stable for 24 hours at room temperature or 14 days under refrigeration; do not refreeze.

Mechanism of Action Piperacillin inhibits bacterial cell wall synthesis by binding to one or more of the penicillin-binding proteins (PBPs); which in turn inhibits the final transpeptidation step of peptidoglycan synthesis in bacterial cell walls, thus inhibiting cell wall biosynthesis. Bacteria eventually lyse due to ongoing activity of cell wall autolytic enzymes (autolysins and murein hydrolases) while cell wall assembly is arrested. Piperacillin exhibits time-dependent killing. Tazobactam inhibits many beta-lactamases, including staphylococcal penicillinase and Richmond-Sykes types 2, 3, 4, and 5, including extended spectrum enzymes; it has only limited activity against class 1 beta-lactamases other than class 1C types.

Pharmacodynamics/Kinetics Both AUC and peak concentrations are dose proportional; hepatic impairment does not affect kinetics

Distribution: Well into lungs, intestinal mucosa, uterus, ovary, fallopian tube, interstitial fluid, gallbladder, and bile; penetration into CSF is low in subjects with noninflamed meninges

Protein binding: Piperacillin and tazobactam: ~30%

Metabolism:

Piperacillin: 6% to 9% to desethyl metabolite (weak activity)

Tazobactam: ~26% to inactive metabolite

Bioavailability:

Piperacillin: I.M.: 71%

Tazobactam: I.M.: 84%

Half-life elimination: Piperacillin and tazobactam: 0.7-1.2 hours (unaffected by dose or duration of infusion)

Time to peak, plasma: Immediately following completion of 30-minute infusion

Excretion: Clearance of both piperacillin and tazobactam are directly proportional to renal function

Piperacillin: Urine (68% as unchanged drug); feces (10% to 20%)

Tazobactam: Urine (80% as unchanged drug; remainder as inactive metabolite)

Dialysis: Hemodialysis removes 30% to 40% of a piperacillin/tazobactam dose; peritoneal dialysis removes 6% of piperacillin and 21% of tazobactam

Dosage Note: Dosing presented is based on traditional infusion method (I.V. infusion over 30 minutes) unless otherwise specified as the extended infusion method (I.V. infusion over 4 hours [unlabeled method]).

Usual dosage range:

Children: I.V.:

2-8 months: 80 mg of piperacillin component/kg every 8 hours

≥9 months and ≤40 kg: 100 mg of piperacillin component/kg every 8 hours

Adults: I.V.: 3.375 g every 6 hours **or** 4.5 g every 6-8 hours; maximum: 18 g/day

Extended infusion method (unlabeled dosing): 3.375-4.5 g I.V. over 4 hours every 8 hours (Kim, 2007; Shea, 2009); an alternative regimen of 4.5 g I.V. over 3 hours every 6 hours has also been described (Kim, 2007)

Indication-specific dosing: I.V.:

Children: **Note:** Dosing based on piperacillin component:

Appendicitis, peritonitis:

2-8 months: 80 mg/kg every 8 hours

≥9 months and ≤40 kg: 100 mg/kg every 8 hours

>40 kg: refer to Adult dosing

Intra-abdominal infection, complicated: 200-300 mg/kg/day divided every 6-8 hours (Solomkin, 2010)

Cystic fibrosis, pseudomonal infections (unlabeled use): 350-450 mg/kg/day in divided doses

Adults:

Diverticulitis, intra-abdominal abscess, peritonitis: I.V.: 3.375 g every 6 hours; **Note:** Some clinicians use 4.5 g every 8 hours for empiric coverage since the % time>MIC is similar between the regimens for most pathogens; however, this regimen is NOT recommended for nosocomial pneumonia or *Pseudomonas* coverage.

Intra-abdominal infection, complicated: I.V.: 3.375 g every 6 hours for 4-7 days (provided source controlled). **Note:** Increase to 3.375 g every 4 hours or 4.5 g every 6 hours if *P. aeruginosa* is suspected. Not recommended for mild-to-moderate, community-acquired intra-abdominal infections due to risk of toxicity and the development of resistant organisms (Solomkin, 2010).

Pneumonia (nosocomial): I.V.: 4.5 g every 6 hours for 7-14 days (when used empirically, combination with an aminoglycoside or antipseudomonal fluoroquinolone is recommended; consider discontinuation of additional agent if *P. aeruginosa* is not isolated)

Severe infections: I.V.: 3.375 g every 6 hours for 7-10 days; **Note:** Some clinicians use 4.5 g every 8 hours for empiric coverage since the %time>MIC is similar between the regimens for most pathogens; however, this regimen is NOT recommended for nosocomial pneumonia or *Pseudomonas* coverage.

Skin and soft tissue infection: I.V.: 3.375 g every 6-8 hours for 7-14 days (when used for necrotizing infection of skin, fascia, or muscle, combination with clindamycin and ciprofloxacin is recommended) (Stevens, 2005)

Dosing interval in renal impairment:

Traditional infusion method (ie, I.V. infusion over 30 minutes): Manufacturer's labeling:

Cl_{cr} >40 mL/minute: No dosage adjustment required

Cl_{cr} 20-40 mL/minute: Administer 2.25 g every 6 hours (3.375 g every 6 hours for nosocomial pneumonia)

Cl_{cr} <20 mL/minute: Administer 2.25 g every 8 hours (2.25 g every 6 hours for nosocomial pneumonia)

Note: Some clinicians suggest adjusting the dose at Cl_{cr} ≤20 mL/minute (rather than Cl_{cr} <40 mL/minute) in patients receiving either traditional or extended-infusion methods, particularly if treating serious gram-negative infections (empirically or definitively) (Patel, 2010).

Extended infusion method (unlabeled dosing): Cl_{cr} ≤20 mL/minute: 3.375 g I.V. over 4 hours every 12 hours (Patel, 2010)

Intermittent hemodialysis (IHD)/peritoneal dialysis (PD): 2.25 g every 12 hours (2.25 g every 8 hours for nosocomial pneumonia). **Note:** Dosing dependent on the assumption of 3 times/week, complete IHD sessions. Administer scheduled doses after hemodialysis on dialysis days; if next regularly scheduled dose is not due right after dialysis session, administer an additional dose of 0.75 g after the dialysis session.

Continuous renal replacement therapy (CRRT) (Heintz, 2009; Trotman, 2005): Drug clearance is highly dependent on the method of renal replacement, filter type, and flow rate. Appropriate dosing requires close monitoring of pharmacologic response, signs of adverse reactions due to drug accumulation, as well as drug concentrations in relation to target trough (if appropriate). The following are general recommendations only (based on dialysate flow/ultrafiltration rates of 1-2 L/hour and minimal residual renal function) and should not supersede clinical judgment (Trotman, 2005):

CVVH: 2.25-3.375 g every 6-8 hours

CVVHD: 2.25-3.375 g every 6 hours

CVVHDF: 3.375 g every 6 hours

Note: Higher dose of 3.375 g should be considered when treating resistant pathogens (especially *Pseudomonas* spp); alternative recommendations suggest dosing of 4.5 g every 8 hours (Valtonen, 2001); regardless of regimen, there is some concern of tazobactam (TAZ) accumulation, given its lower clearance relative to piperacillin (PIP). Some clinicians advocate dosing with PIP to alternate with PIP/TAZ, particularly in CVVH-dependent patients, to lessen this concern.

Dosage adjustment in hepatic impairment: No dosage adjustment necessary.

Dietary Considerations Some products may contain sodium.

Administration Administer by I.V. infusion over 30 minutes. For extended infusion administration (unlabeled dosing), administer over 3-4 hours (Kim 2007; Shea, 2009).

Some penicillins (eg, carbenicillin, ticarcillin, and piperacillin) have been shown to inactivate aminoglycosides *in vitro*. This has been observed to a greater extent with tobramycin and gentamicin, while amikacin has shown greater stability against inactivation. Concurrent use of these agents may pose a risk of reduced antibacterial efficacy *in vivo*, particularly in the setting of profound renal impairment. However, definitive clinical evidence is lacking. If combination penicillin/aminoglycoside therapy is desired in a patient with renal dysfunction, separation of doses (if feasible), and routine monitoring of aminoglycoside levels, CBC, and clinical response should be considered. **Note:** Reformulated Zosyn® containing EDTA (applies only to specific concentrations and diluents and varies by product; consult manufacturer's labeling) has been shown to be compatible *in vitro* for Y-site infusion with amikacin and gentamicin, but not compatible with tobramycin.

Monitoring Parameters Creatinine, BUN, CBC with differential, PT, PTT, serum electrolytes, LFTs, urinalysis; signs of bleeding; monitor for signs of anaphylaxis during first dose

Test Interactions Positive Coombs' [direct] test; false positive reaction for urine glucose using copper-reduction method (Clinitest®); may result in false positive results with the Platelia® *Aspergillus* enzyme immunoassay (EIA)

Some penicillin derivatives may accelerate the degradation of aminoglycosides *in vitro*, leading to a potential underestimation of aminoglycoside serum concentration. **Note:** Reformulated Zosyn® containing EDTA (applies only to specific concentrations and diluents and varies by product; consult manufacturer's labeling) has been shown to be compatible *in vitro* for Y-site infusion with amikacin and gentamicin, but not compatible with tobramycin.

Dosage Forms Excipient information presented when available (limited, particularly for generics); consult specific product labeling.

Note: 8:1 ratio of piperacillin sodium/tazobactam sodium

Infusion [premixed iso-osmotic solution]:

Zosyn®: 2.25 g: Piperacillin 2 g and tazobactam 0.25 g (50 mL) [contains edetate disodium, sodium 128 mg (5.58 mEq)]

Zosyn®: 3.375 g: Piperacillin 3 g and tazobactam 0.375 g (50 mL) [contains edetate disodium, sodium 192 mg (8.38 mEq)]

Zosyn®: 4.5 g: Piperacillin 4 g and tazobactam 0.5 g (100 mL) [contains edetate disodium, sodium 256 mg (11.17 mEq)]

Injection, powder for reconstitution: 2.25 g: Piperacillin 2 g and tazobactam 0.25 g; 3.375 g: Piperacillin 3 g and tazobactam 0.375 g; 4.5 g: Piperacillin 4 g and tazobactam 0.5 g; 40.5 g: Piperacillin 36 g and tazobactam 4.5 g

Zosyn®: 2.25 g: Piperacillin 2 g and tazobactam 0.25 g [contains edetate disodium, sodium 128 mg (5.58 mEq)]

Zosyn®: 3.375 g: Piperacillin 3 g and tazobactam 0.375 g [contains edetate disodium, sodium 192 mg (8.38 mEq)]

Zosyn®: 4.5 g: Piperacillin 4 g and tazobactam 0.5 g [contains edetate disodium, sodium 256 mg (11.17 mEq)]

Zosyn®: 40.5 g: Piperacillin 36 g and tazobactam 4.5 g [contains edetate disodium, sodium 2304 mg (100.4 mEq); bulk pharmacy vial]

◆ **Piperacillin and Tazobactam for Injection (Can)** *see* Piperacillin and Tazobactam *on page 1358*

◆ **Piperacillin and Tazobactam Sodium** *see* Piperacillin and Tazobactam *on page 1358*

◆ **Piperacillin for Injection, USP (Can)** *see* Piperacillin *on page 1358*

◆ **Piperacillin Sodium** *see* Piperacillin *on page 1358*

◆ **Piperacillin Sodium and Tazobactam Sodium** *see* Piperacillin and Tazobactam *on page 1358*

◆ **Piperazine Estrone Sulfate** *see* Estropipate *on page 648*

◆ **Piperonyl Butoxide and Pyrethrins** *see* Pyrethrins and Piperonyl Butoxide *on page 1435*

Pirbuterol (peer BYOO ter ole)

Brand Names: U.S. Maxair® Autohaler®

Index Terms Pirbuterol Acetate

Pharmacologic Category $Beta_2$-Adrenergic Agonist

Additional Appendix Information

Bronchodilators *on page 1886*

Use Prevention and treatment of reversible bronchospasm including asthma

Pregnancy Risk Factor C

Dosage Children ≥12 years and Adults: 2 inhalations every 4-6 hours for prevention; two inhalations at an interval of at least 1-3 minutes, followed by a third inhalation in treatment of bronchospasm, not to exceed 12 inhalations/day

Additional Information Complete prescribing information for this medication should be consulted for additional detail.

Dosage Forms Excipient information presented when available (limited, particularly for generics); consult specific product labeling.

Aerosol, for oral inhalation, as acetate:

Maxair® Autohaler®: 200 mcg/actuation (14 g) [contains chlorofluorocarbon; 400 actuations]

◆ **Pirbuterol Acetate** *see* Pirbuterol *on page 1360*

Piroxicam (peer OKS i kam)

Brand Names: U.S. Feldene®

Brand Names: Canada Apo-Piroxicam®; Dom-Piroxicam; Novo-Pirocam; Nu-Pirox; PMS-Piroxicam

Pharmacologic Category Nonsteroidal Anti-inflammatory Drug (NSAID), Oral

Additional Appendix Information

Beers Criteria – Potentially Inappropriate Medications for Geriatrics *on page 1973*

Use Symptomatic treatment of acute and chronic rheumatoid arthritis and osteoarthritis

Canadian labeling: Additional use (not in U.S. labeling): Symptomatic treatment of ankylosing spondylitis

Pregnancy Risk Factor C

Medication Guide Available Yes

Dosage Oral:

Adults: 10-20 mg/day in 1-2 divided doses (maximum dose: 20 mg/day)

Elderly: Initiate therapy cautiously at low end of dosing range.

Dosing adjustment in renal impairment: Use is contraindicated in severe renal failure (**Note:** Canadian labeling also contraindicates use in patients with deteriorating renal disease).

Mild-to-moderate impairment: U.S. labeling suggests that dosing adjustments may not be required. Canadian labeling suggests that dose reductions may be necessary although the manufacturer labeling does not provide specific dose recommendations.

Dosing adjustment in hepatic impairment: Use is contraindicated in severe hepatic failure. Dose reductions may be necessary with lesser degrees of hepatic impairment although the manufacturer labeling does not provide specific dose recommendations.

Additional Information Complete prescribing information for this medication should be consulted for additional detail.

Dosage Forms Excipient information presented when available (limited, particularly for generics); consult specific product labeling.

Capsule, oral: 10 mg, 20 mg

Feldene®: 10 mg, 20 mg

◆ ***p*-Isobutylhydratropic Acid** *see* Ibuprofen *on page 860*

◆ **Pit** *see* Oxytocin *on page 1272*

Pitavastatin (pi TA va sta tin)

Brand Names: U.S. Livalo®

Index Terms Pitavastatin Calcium

Pharmacologic Category Antilipemic Agent, HMG-CoA Reductase Inhibitor

Additional Appendix Information

Hyperlipidemia Management *on page 1996*

Use Adjunct to dietary therapy to reduce elevations in total cholesterol (TC), LDL-C, apolipoprotein B (Apo B), and triglycerides (TG), and to increase low HDL-C in patients with primary hyperlipidemia and mixed dyslipidemia

Pregnancy Risk Factor X

Dosage Oral: **Note:** Doses should be individualized according to the baseline LDL-cholesterol levels, the recommended goal of therapy, and patient response; adjustments should be made at intervals of 4 weeks.

Adults: Primary hyperlipidemia and mixed dyslipidemia: Initial: 2 mg once daily; may be increased to maximum 4 mg once daily

Dosage adjustment with concomitant medications:

Erythromycin: Pitavastatin dose should not exceed 1 mg once daily

Rifampin: Pitavastatin dose should not exceed 2 mg once daily

Dosing adjustment in renal impairment: Cl_{cr} <60 mL/minute/1.73 m^2 including hemodialysis: Initial: 1 mg once daily; maximum: 2 mg once daily

Dosing adjustment in hepatic impairment: Contraindicated in active liver disease or in patients with unexplained persistent elevations of serum transaminases

Additional Information Complete prescribing information for this medication should be consulted for additional detail.

Dosage Forms Excipient information presented when available (limited, particularly for generics); consult specific product labeling.

Tablet, oral:

Livalo®: 1 mg, 2 mg, 4 mg

◆ **Pitavastatin Calcium** *see* Pitavastatin *on page 1361*

◆ **Pitocin®** *see* Oxytocin *on page 1272*

◆ **Pitressin®** *see* Vasopressin *on page 1775*

◆ **Pitrex (Can)** *see* Tolnaftate *on page 1704*

◆ **PLA** *see* Poly-L-Lactic Acid *on page 1374*

◆ **Plan B** *see* Levonorgestrel *on page 1001*

◆ **Plan B® (Can)** *see* Levonorgestrel *on page 1001*

◆ **Plan B® One Step** *see* Levonorgestrel *on page 1001*

◆ **Plantago Seed** *see* Psyllium *on page 1432*

◆ **Plantain Seed** *see* Psyllium *on page 1432*

◆ **Plaquenil®** *see* Hydroxychloroquine *on page 848*

◆ **Plasbumin®-5** *see* Albumin *on page 51*

◆ **Plasbumin®-25** *see* Albumin *on page 51*

◆ **Platinol** *see* CISplatin *on page 368*

◆ **Platinol-AQ** *see* CISplatin *on page 368*

◆ **Plavix®** *see* Clopidogrel *on page 395*

◆ **Plendil** *see* Felodipine *on page 692*

◆ **Plendil® (Can)** *see* Felodipine *on page 692*

Plerixafor (pler IX a fore)

Brand Names: U.S. Mozobil™

Index Terms AMD3100; LM3100

Pharmacologic Category Hematopoietic Stem Cell Mobilizer

Use Mobilization of hematopoietic stem cells (HSC) for collection and subsequent autologous transplantation (in combination with filgrastim) in patients with non-Hodgkin's lymphoma (NHL) and multiple myeloma (MM)

Pregnancy Risk Factor D

Pregnancy Considerations Adverse effects (including fetal mortality, decreased fetal weights, and teratogenicity) have been reported in animal studies. May cause fetal harm if administered to pregnant women. There are no adequate and well-controlled studies in pregnant women. Women of childbearing potential should use effective contraceptive measures to avoid becoming pregnant during treatment.

Lactation Excretion in breast milk unknown/not recommended

Contraindications There are no contraindications listed within the manufacturer's labeling.

Warnings/Precautions Increases circulating leukocytes when used in conjunction with filgrastim; monitor WBC; use with caution in patients with neutrophil count >50,000/mm^3. Thrombocytopenia has been observed with use; monitor platelet count. Not intended for mobilization in patients with leukemia; may contaminate apheresis product by mobilizing leukemic cells. When used in combination with filgrastim, tumor cells released from marrow could be collected in leukapheresis product; potential effect of tumor cell reinfusion is unknown. Splenomegaly and splenic rupture have been reported (rarely) with filgrastim use; instruct patients to report left upper quadrant pain or scapular/shoulder tip pain; promptly evaluate in any patient who report these symptoms.

Primary route of elimination is urinary; dosage reduction is recommended in patients with moderate-severe renal impairment (Cl_{cr} ≤50 mL/minute). Medications that may reduce renal function or compete for active tubular secretion may increase serum concentrations of plerixafor. Use has not been studied in patients weighing >175% of ideal body weight. Safety and efficacy have not been established in children.

Adverse Reactions Adverse reactions reported with filgrastim combination therapy.

>10%:

- Central nervous system: Fatigue (27%), headache (22%), dizziness (11%)
- Gastrointestinal: Diarrhea (37%), nausea (34%)
- Local: Injection site reactions (34%, including erythema, hematoma, hemorrhage, induration, inflammation, irritation, pain, paresthesia, pruritus, rash, swelling, urticaria)
- Neuromuscular & skeletal: Arthralgia (13%)

5% to 10%:

- Central nervous system: Insomnia (7%)
- Gastrointestinal: Vomiting (10%), flatulence (7%)

<5% (Limited to important or life-threatening): Abdominal discomfort, abdominal distension, abdominal pain, constipation, diaphoresis, dyspepsia, dyspnea, erythema, hypesthesia (oral), hypoxia, leukocytes increased, malaise, musculoskeletal pain, orthostatic hypotension, periorbital swelling, syncope, thrombocytopenia, urticaria, vasovagal reaction, xerostomia

Drug Interactions

Metabolism/Transport Effects None known.

Avoid Concomitant Use There are no known interactions where it is recommended to avoid concomitant use.

Increased Effect/Toxicity There are no known significant interactions involving an increase in effect.

Decreased Effect There are no known significant interactions involving a decrease in effect.

Stability Store at 25°C (77°F); excursions permitted to 15°C to 30°C (59°F to 86°F). The manufacturer recommends discarding unused drug remaining in the vial after use.

Mechanism of Action Reversibly inhibits binding of stromal cell-derived factor-1-alpha (SDF-1α), expressed on bone marrow stromal cells, to the CXC chemokine receptor 4 (CXCR4), resulting in mobilization of hematopoietic stem and progenitor cells from bone marrow into peripheral blood. Plerixafor used in combination with filgrastim results in synergistic increase in CD34+ cell mobilization. Mobilized CD34+ cells are capable of engrafting with extended repopulating capacity.

Pharmacodynamics/Kinetics

Onset of action: Peak CD34+ mobilization: Plerixafor monotherapy: 6-9 hours after administration; Plerixafor + filgrastim: 10-14 hours

Duration: WBC counts return toward baseline at ~24 after administration

Absorption: SubQ: Rapid

Distribution: 0.3 L/kg; primarily to extravascular fluid space

Protein binding: ≤58%

Metabolism: Not metabolized

Half-life elimination: Terminal: 3-6 hours

Time to peak, plasma: SubQ: 30-60 minutes

Excretion: Urine (~70%; as parent drug)

Dosage Note: Dosing is based on actual body weight. Begin plerixafor after patient has received filgrastim 10 mcg/kg once daily for 4 days; plerixafor, filgrastim, and apheresis should be continued daily until sufficient cell collection up to a maximum of 4 days.

SubQ: Adults: HSC mobilization: 0.24 mg/kg once daily ~11 hours prior to apheresis for up to 4 consecutive days; maximum dose: 40 mg/day

Dosage adjustment in renal impairment:

Cl_{cr} >50 mL/minute: No adjustment required

Cl_{cr} ≤50 mL/minute: 0.16 mg/kg; maximum dose: 27 mg/day

Hemodialysis: Insufficient information for dosing recommendation

Administration Administer subcutaneously, ~11 hours prior to initiation of apheresis. In some clinical trials, plerixafor administration began in the evening prior to apheresis. (filgrastim was begun on day 1, plerixafor initiated in the evening on day 4 and apheresis in the morning on day 5; with filgrastim, plerixafor and apheresis then continued daily until sufficient cell collection for autologous transplant.)

Monitoring Parameters CBC with differential and platelets

Dosage Forms Excipient information presented when available (limited, particularly for generics); consult specific product labeling.

Injection, solution [preservative free]:

Mozobil™: 20 mg/mL (1.2 mL)

- ◆ **Pletal®** *see* Cilostazol *on page* 358
- ◆ **Plexion®** *see* Sulfur and Sulfacetamide *on page* 1607
- ◆ **Plexion SCT®** *see* Sulfur and Sulfacetamide *on page* 1607
- ◆ **PLX4032** *see* Vemurafenib *on page* 1778
- ◆ **PMPA** *see* Tenofovir *on page* 1645
- ◆ **PMS-Adenosine (Can)** *see* Adenosine *on page* 46
- ◆ **PMS-Alendronate (Can)** *see* Alendronate *on page* 61
- ◆ **PMS-Alendronate-FC (Can)** *see* Alendronate *on page* 61
- ◆ **PMS-Amantadine (Can)** *see* Amantadine *on page* 82
- ◆ **PMS-Amiodarone (Can)** *see* Amiodarone *on page* 90
- ◆ **PMS-Amitriptyline (Can)** *see* Amitriptyline *on page* 94
- ◆ **PMS-Amlodipine (Can)** *see* AmLODIPine *on page* 97
- ◆ **PMS-Amoxicillin (Can)** *see* Amoxicillin *on page* 103
- ◆ **PMS-Anagrelide (Can)** *see* Anagrelide *on page* 119
- ◆ **PMS-Atenolol (Can)** *see* Atenolol *on page* 161
- ◆ **PMS-Atorvastatin (Can)** *see* Atorvastatin *on page* 165
- ◆ **PMS-Azithromycin (Can)** *see* Azithromycin (Systemic) *on page* 180

◆ **PMS-Venlafaxine XR (Can)** *see* Venlafaxine *on page 1780*
◆ **PMS-Verapamil SR (Can)** *see* Verapamil *on page 1783*
◆ **PMS-Zolmitriptan (Can)** *see* ZOLMitriptan *on page 1824*
◆ **PMS-Zolmitriptan ODT (Can)** *see* ZOLMitriptan *on page 1824*
◆ **PN** *see* Total Parenteral Nutrition *on page 1714*
◆ **PN401** *see* Uridine Triacetate *on page 1750*
◆ **Pneumo 23™ (Can)** *see* Pneumococcal Polysaccharide Vaccine (Polyvalent) *on page 1368*

Pneumococcal Conjugate Vaccine (7-Valent)

(noo moe KOK al KON ju gate vak SEEN, seven vay lent)

Brand Names: U.S. Prevnar®

Brand Names: Canada Prevnar®

Index Terms Diphtheria CRM_{197} Protein; PCV; PCV-7; PCV7; Pneumococcal 7-Valent Conjugate Vaccine

Pharmacologic Category Vaccine, Inactivated (Bacterial)

Additional Appendix Information

Immunization Recommendations *on page 1922*

Use Note: In March 2010, the Advisory Committee on Immunization Practices (ACIP) released recommendations that pneumococcal 13-valent conjugate vaccine (PCV13; Prevnar 13™) replace pneumococcal 7-valent conjugate vaccine (PCV7; Prevnar®) for all doses for immunization of all children 2-59 months of age. Refer to the Pneumococcal Conjugate Vaccine (13-Valent) monograph for additional information.

Immunization of infants and toddlers against *Streptococcus pneumoniae* infection caused by serotypes included in the vaccine

Immunization of infants and toddlers against otitis media caused by serotypes included in the vaccine

The Advisory Committee on Immunization Practices (ACIP) recommends pneumococcal conjugate vaccine (PCV) for routine vaccination of all children 2-59 months and children 60-71 months with underlying medical conditions. PCV13 should be used to complete the vaccination of children who received ≥1 dose of PCV7.

Pregnancy Risk Factor C

Pregnancy Considerations Reproduction studies have not been conducted. This product is indicated for use in infants and toddlers.

Lactation

Excretion in breast milk unknown/not recommended

Contraindications Hypersensitivity to pneumococcal vaccine or any component of the formulation, including diphtheria toxoid

Warnings/Precautions Use caution in latex sensitivity. Children with impaired immune responsiveness may have a reduced response to active immunization. In general, household and close contacts of persons with altered immune competence may receive all age appropriate vaccines. The decision to administer or delay vaccination because of current or recent febrile illness depends on the severity of symptoms and the etiology of the disease. Immunization should be delayed during the course of an acute severe febrile illness; may administer to patients with mild acute illness (with or without fever). Use caution in children with coagulation disorders (including thrombocytopenia) where intramuscular injections should not be used. Epinephrine 1:1000 should be readily available. Use of pneumococcal conjugate vaccine does not replace use of the 23-valent pneumococcal polysaccharide vaccine in children ≥24 months of age with sickle cell disease, asplenia, HIV infection, chronic illness or if immunocompromised. Not to be used to treat pneumococcal infections or to provide immunity against diphtheria. In order to maximize vaccination rates, the ACIP recommends simultaneous administration of all age-appropriate vaccines (live or inactivated) for which a person is eligible at a single clinic visit, unless contraindications exist. Not for I.V. use.

Adverse Reactions All serious adverse reactions must be reported to the U.S. Department of Health and Human Services (DHHS) Vaccine Adverse Event Reporting System (VAERS) 1-800-822-7967 or online at https://vaers.hhs.gov/esub/index. In Canada, adverse reactions may be reported to local provincial/territorial health agencies or to the Vaccine Safety Section at Public Health Agency of Canada (1-866-844-0018).

>10%:

Central nervous system: Fever, irritability, drowsiness, restlessness

Dermatologic: Erythema

Gastrointestinal: Decreased appetite, vomiting, diarrhea

Local: Induration, tenderness, nodule

1% to 10%: Dermatologic: Rash

Postmarketing and/or case reports: Anaphylactic reaction, anaphylactoid reaction, angioneurotic edema, apnea, bronchospasm, crying, dyspnea, erythema multiforme, facial edema, febrile seizure, hypersensitivity reaction, injection site reaction (eg, dermatitis, lymphadenopathy, pruritus, urticaria), shock

Drug Interactions

Metabolism/Transport Effects None known.

Avoid Concomitant Use There are no known interactions where it is recommended to avoid concomitant use.

Increased Effect/Toxicity There are no known significant interactions involving an increase in effect.

Decreased Effect

The levels/effects of Pneumococcal Conjugate Vaccine (7-Valent) may be decreased by: Belimumab; Fingolimod; Immunosuppressants

Stability Store refrigerated at 2°C to 8°C (36°F to 46°F); do not freeze. The following stability information has also been reported: May be stored at room temperature for up to 7 days (Cohen, 2007).

Mechanism of Action Promotes active immunization against invasive disease caused by *S. pneumoniae* capsular serotypes 4, 6B, 9V, 14, 18C, 19F, and 23F, all which are individually conjugated to CRM197 protein

Dosage Note: As of March 10, 2010, the Advisory Committee on Immunization Practices (ACIP) recommended that the use of pneumococcal 13-valent conjugate vaccine (PCV13; Prevnar 13™) replace all doses of pneumococcal 7-valent conjugate vaccine (PCV7; Prevnar®). The manufacturer, Wyeth Pharmaceuticals, intends to phase out the previous Prevnar® product. Refer to the Pneumococcal Conjugate Vaccine (13-Valent) monograph for transitioning from PCV7 to PCV13.

Infants 2-6 months (manufacturer's labeling): I.M.: 0.5 mL at approximately 2-month intervals for 3 consecutive doses, followed by a fourth dose of 0.5 mL at 12-15 months of age; first dose may be given as young as 6 weeks of age, but is typically given at 2 months of age.

Administration Shake well prior to use. Administer I.M. (deltoid muscle for toddlers and young children or lateral midthigh in infants). Do not inject I.V.; avoid intradermal route.

For patients at risk of hemorrhage following intramuscular injection, the ACIP recommends "it should be administered intramuscularly if, in the opinion of the physician familiar with the patients bleeding risk, the vaccine can be administered by this route with reasonable safety. If the patient receives antihemophilia or other similar therapy, intramuscular vaccination can be scheduled shortly after such therapy is administered. A fine needle (23 gauge or smaller) can be used for the vaccination and firm pressure applied to the site (without rubbing) for at least 2 minutes. The patient should be instructed concerning the risk of hematoma from the injection." Patients on anticoagulant therapy should be considered to have the same bleeding risks and treated as those with clotting factor disorders (CDC, 2011).

Antipyretics have not been shown to prevent febrile seizures. Antipyretics may be used to treat fever or discomfort following vaccination (CDC, 2011). One study reported that routine prophylactic administration of acetaminophen to prevent fever prior to vaccination decreased the immune response of some vaccines; the clinical significance of this reduction in immune response has not been established (Prymula, 2009).

Simultaneous administration of vaccines helps ensure the patients will be fully vaccinated by the appropriate age. Simultaneous administration of vaccines is defined as administering >1 vaccine on the same day at different anatomic sites. Separate vaccines should not be combined in the same syringe unless indicated by product specific labeling. Separate needles and syringes should be used for each injection. The ACIP prefers each dose of a specific vaccine in a series come from the same manufacturer when possible. Adolescents and adults should be vaccinated while seated or lying down. In general, preterm infants should be vaccinated at the same chronological age as full-term infants (CDC, 2011).

Monitoring Parameters Monitor for syncope for ≥15 minutes following vaccination.

Additional Information Federal law requires that the name of medication, date of administration, the vaccine manufacturer, lot number of vaccine, and the administering person's name, title and address be entered into the patient's permanent medical record.

Pneumococcal 13-valent conjugate vaccine (PCV13; Prevnar 13™) is the successor to the previously-marketed pneumococcal 7-valent conjugate vaccine (PCV7; Prevnar®). Prevnar 13™ contains an additional 6 serotypes of *Streptococcus pneumoniae*, compared to the 7 serotypes provided in the original Prevnar® formulation.

Dosage Forms Excipient information presented when available (limited, particularly for generics); consult specific product labeling.

Injection, suspension:

Prevnar®: 2 mcg of each capsular saccharide for serotypes 4, 9V, 14, 18C, 19F, and 23F, and 4 mcg of serotype 6B [bound to diphtheria CRM_{197} protein ~20 mcg] per 0.5 mL (0.5 mL) [contains aluminum, natural rubber/natural latex in packaging, and yeast]

Pneumococcal Conjugate Vaccine (13-Valent)

(noo moe KOK al KON ju gate vak SEEN, thur TEEN vay lent)

Brand Names: U.S. Prevnar 13™

Brand Names: Canada Prevnar 13™

Index Terms Diphtheria CRM_{197} Protein; PCV-13; PCV13; PCV13-CRM(197); Pneumococcal 13-Valent Conjugate Vaccine

Pharmacologic Category Vaccine, Inactivated (Bacterial)

Additional Appendix Information

Immunization Recommendations *on page 1922*

Use

Immunization of infants and children against *Streptococcus pneumoniae* infection caused by serotypes included in the vaccine

Immunization of infants and children against otitis media caused by *Streptococcus pneumoniae* serotypes 4, 6B, 9V, 14, 18C, 19F, and 23F

Immunization of adults ≥50 years against pneumococcal pneumonia and invasive disease caused by *Streptococcus pneumoniae* serotypes included in the vaccine

The Advisory Committee on Immunization Practices (ACIP) recommends routine vaccination for the following:

All children age 2-59 months

Children 60-71 months with underlying medical conditions including: Cochlear implants, functional or anatomic asplenia (includes sickle cell disease and other hemoglobinopathies, congenital or acquired asplenia, or splenic dysfunction); immunocompromising conditions (includes HIV infection, congenital immunodeficiencies [excluding chronic granulomatous disease], chronic renal failure, nephrotic syndrome, diseases associated with immunosuppressive or radiation therapy, solid organ transplant); chronic illnesses (cardiac disease, cerebrospinal fluid leaks, diabetes mellitus, pulmonary disease [excluding asthma unless on high dose oral corticosteroids])

Children who received ≥1 dose of PCV7

Children 6-18 years of age at increased risk for invasive pneumococcal disease due to anatomic or functional asplenia (including sickle cell disease), HIV infection or other immunocompromising conditions, cochlear implant, or cerebrospinal fluid leaks (regardless of prior receipt of PCV7 or PPSV23). Routine use is not recommended for healthy children ≥5 years of age.

Pregnancy Risk Factor B

Pregnancy Considerations Animal reproduction studies have not shown adverse fetal effects. Inactivated vaccines have not been shown to cause increased risks to the fetus (CDC, 2011).

Lactation Excretion in breast milk unknown/use caution

Contraindications Hypersensitivity to pneumococcal vaccine or any component of the formulation, including diphtheria toxoid

Warnings/Precautions Immediate treatment (including epinephrine 1:1000) for anaphylactoid and/or hypersensitivity reactions should be available during vaccine use. Use with caution in patients with a history of bleeding disorders (including thrombocytopenia) and/or patients on anticoagulant therapy; bleeding/hematoma may occur from I.M. administration. Use with caution in severely immunocompromised patients (eg, patients receiving chemo/radiation therapy or other immunosuppressive therapy including high dose corticosteroids); may have a reduced response to vaccination. In general, household and close contacts of persons with altered immunocompetence may receive all age appropriate vaccines.

The decision to administer or delay vaccination because of current or recent febrile illness depends on the severity of symptoms and the etiology of the disease. Immunization should be delayed during the course of an acute severe febrile illness; may administer to patients with mild acute illness (with or without fever). In order to maximize vaccination rates, the ACIP recommends simultaneous administration of all age-appropriate vaccines (live or inactivated) for which a person is eligible at a single clinic visit, unless contraindications exist.

Use of pneumococcal conjugate vaccine does not replace use of the 23-valent pneumococcal polysaccharide vaccine in children ≥24 months of age with chronic illness, asplenia, sickle cell disease or are immunocompromised or have HIV infection. Antibody responses were lower in older adults >65 years of age compared to adults 50-59 years of age. Apnea has been reported following I.M. vaccine administration in premature infants; consider risk versus benefit in infants born prematurely. Not to be used to treat pneumococcal infections or to provide immunity against diphtheria.

Adverse Reactions All serious adverse reactions must be reported to the U.S. Department of Health and Human Services (DHHS) Vaccine Adverse Event Reporting System (VAERS) 1-800-822-7967 or online at https://vaers.hhs.gov/esub/index.

>10%:

Central nervous system: Chills, drowsiness, fatigue, fever, headache, insomnia, irritability

Dermatologic: Rash

Gastrointestinal: Appetite decreased

Local: Erythema, limitation of arm motion, pain, swelling, tenderness

Neuromuscular & skeletal: Arthralgia, myalgia

1% to 10%: Gastrointestinal: Diarrhea, vomiting

<1% (Limited to important or life-threatening): Abnormal crying, erythema multiforme, febrile seizures, hypersensitivity reaction (bronchospasm, dyspnea, facial edema), seizure, urticaria, urticaria-like rash

Adverse reactions observed with PCV7 which may also be seen with PCV-13: Anaphylactic reaction, angioneurotic edema, apnea, breath holding, edema, erythema multiforme, hypotonic hyporesponsive episode, injection site reaction (dermatitis, pruritus), lymphadenopathy (localized), shock

Drug Interactions

Metabolism/Transport Effects None known.

Avoid Concomitant Use There are no known interactions where it is recommended to avoid concomitant use.

Increased Effect/Toxicity There are no known significant interactions involving an increase in effect.

Decreased Effect

Pneumococcal Conjugate Vaccine (13-Valent) may decrease the levels/effects of: Influenza Virus Vaccine (Inactivated)

The levels/effects of Pneumococcal Conjugate Vaccine (13-Valent) may be decreased by: Belimumab; Fingolimod; Immunosuppressants; Influenza Virus Vaccine (Inactivated)

Mechanism of Action

Promotes active immunization against invasive disease caused by *S. pneumoniae* capsular serotypes 1, 3, 4, 5, 6A, 6B, 7F, 9V, 14, 18C, 19A, 19F, and 23F, all which are individually conjugated to CRM197 protein

Dosage I.M.:

Infants and Children

Primary immunization: *Infants and Children 6 weeks-59 months:* 0.5 mL/dose for a total of 4 doses. The first dose may be given as young as 6 weeks of age, but is typically given at 2 months of age. The 3 remaining doses are usually given at 4, 6, and 12-15 months of age. The recommended dosing interval is 4-8 weeks. The minimum interval between doses in children <1 year of age is 1 month. The minimum interval between the third and fourth dose is 2 months.

Previously unvaccinated Older Infants and Children:

Children 7-11 months: 0.5 mL for a total of 3 doses; 2 doses at least 4 weeks apart, followed by a third dose after the 1-year birthday (12-15 months), separated from the second dose by at least 2 months

Children 12-23 months: 0.5 mL for a total of 2 doses, separated by at least 2 months

Healthy Children 24-59 months: 0.5 mL as a single dose

Children 24-71 months with an underlying medical condition: ACIP recommendations: 0.5 mL for a total of 2 doses, separated by 2 months

Previously vaccinated with PCV7 and/or PCV13, and with a lapse in vaccine administration (ACIP recommendations):

Children 7-11 months: Previously received 1 or 2 doses: 0.5 mL dose at 7-11 months of age, followed by a second dose ≥2 months later at 12-15 months of age

Children 12-23 months:

Previously received 1 dose <12 months of age: 0.5 mL dose, followed by a second dose ≥2 months later

Previously received 1 dose at ≥12 months of age: 0.5 mL dose ≥2 months after the most recent dose

Previously received 2 or 3 doses before age 12 months: 0.5 mL dose ≥2 months after the most recent dose

Healthy Children 24-59 months with any incomplete schedule: 0.5 mL dose ≥ 2 months after the most recent dose

Children 24-71 months with an underlying medical condition:

Previously received <3 doses: 0.5 mL dose ≥2 months after the most recent dose, followed by a second dose ≥8 weeks later

Previously received 3 doses: 0.5 mL as a single dose ≥2 months after the most recent dose

Previously vaccinated with PCV7 and completed vaccination series of 4 doses (ACIP recommendations):

Children 14-59 months: 0.5 mL as a single supplemental dose ≥2 months after the most recent dose

Children 24-71 months with an underlying medical condition: 0.5 mL as a single supplemental dose ≥2 months after the most recent dose of PCV7 or PPSV23

Previously vaccinated or not previously vaccinated with PCV7 or PPSV23 (ACIP recommendations):

Children 6-18 years at high risk for invasive pneumococcal disease: 0.5 mL as a single dose ≥2 months after the most recent dose

Adults ≥50 years: **Immunization:** 0.5 mL as a single dose. **Note:** Efficacy of PCV13 administered <5 years after PPSV23 is unknown.

Administration Shake well prior to use. Do not use if a homogenous white suspension does not form. Administer I.M. (deltoid muscle for toddlers, young children, and adults or lateral midthigh in infants). Do not inject I.V. or SubQ; avoid intradermal route. Concurrent administration of PCV13 and PPV23 has not been studied and is not recommended (CDC, 2010).

For patients at risk of hemorrhage following intramuscular injection, the ACIP recommends "it should be administered intramuscularly if, in the opinion of the physician familiar with the patients bleeding risk, the vaccine can be administered by this route with reasonable safety. If the patient receives antihemophilia or other similar therapy, intramuscular vaccination can be scheduled shortly after such therapy is administered. A fine needle (23 gauge or smaller) can be used for the vaccination and firm pressure applied to the site (without rubbing) for at least 2 minutes. The patient should be instructed concerning the risk of hematoma from the injection." Patients on anticoagulant therapy should be considered to have the same bleeding risks and treated as those with clotting factor disorders (CDC, 2011).

Antipyretics have not been shown to prevent febrile seizures. Antipyretics may be used to treat fever or discomfort following vaccination (CDC, 2011). One study reported that routine prophylactic administration of acetaminophen to prevent fever prior to vaccination decreased the immune response of some vaccines; the clinical significance of this reduction in immune response has not been established (Prymula, 2009).

Simultaneous administration of vaccines helps ensure the patients will be fully vaccinated by the appropriate age. Simultaneous administration of vaccines is defined as administering >1 vaccine on the same day at different anatomic sites. Separate vaccines should not be combined in the same syringe unless indicated by product specific labeling. Separate needles and syringes should be used for each injection. The ACIP prefers each dose of a specific vaccine in a series come from the same manufacturer when possible. Adolescents and adults should be vaccinated while seated or lying down. In general, preterm infants should be vaccinated at the same chronological age as full-term infants (CDC, 2011).

Additional Information Federal law requires that the name of medication, date of administration, the vaccine manufacturer, lot number of vaccine, and the administering person's name, title and address be entered into the patient's permanent medical record.

Pneumococcal 13-valent conjugate vaccine (PCV13; Prevnar 13™) is the successor to the previously-marketed pneumococcal 7-valent conjugate vaccine (PCV7; Prevnar®). Prevnar 13™ contains an additional 6 serotypes of *Streptococcus pneumoniae*, compared to the 7 serotypes provided in the original Prevnar® formulation.

Dosage Forms Excipient information presented when available (limited, particularly for generics); consult specific product labeling.

Injection, suspension:

Prevnar 13™: 2 mcg of each capsular saccharide for serotypes 1, 3, 4, 5, 6A, 7F, 9V, 14, 18C, 19A, 19F, and 23F, and 4 mcg of serotype 6B [bound to diphtheria CRM_{197} protein ~34 mcg] per 0.5 mL (0.5 mL) [contains aluminum, polysorbate 80, and yeast]

Pneumococcal Polysaccharide Vaccine (Polyvalent)

(noo moe KOK al pol i SAK a ride vak SEEN, pol i VAY lent)

Brand Names: U.S. Pneumovax® 23

Brand Names: Canada Pneumo 23™; Pneumovax® 23

Index Terms 23-Valent Pneumococcal Polysaccharide Vaccine; 23PS; PPSV; PPSV23; PPV23

Pharmacologic Category Vaccine, Inactivated (Bacterial)

Additional Appendix Information

Immunization Recommendations *on page 1922*

Use Immunization against pneumococcal disease caused by serotypes included in the vaccine. Routine vaccination is recommended for persons ≥50 years of age and persons ≥2 years in certain situations.

The Advisory Committee on Immunization Practices (ACIP) recommends routine vaccination for the following:

All immunocompetent patients ≥65 years of age

Patients 2-18 years of age with certain high-risk condition(s):

- Chronic heart disease (particularly cyanotic congenital heart disease and cardiac failure)
- Chronic lung disease (including asthma if treated with high-dose oral corticosteroids)

Patients 2-64 years of age with certain high-risk condition(s):

- Diabetes mellitus
- Cochlear implants
- Cerebrospinal fluid leaks
- Functional or anatomic asplenia (including sickle cell disease and other hemoglobinopathies, splenic dysfunction, or splenectomy)
- Immunocompromising conditions including congenital immunodeficiency (includes B- or T-lymphocyte deficiency, complement deficiencies, and phagocytic disorders [excluding chronic granulomatous disease]); HIV infection; leukemia, lymphoma, Hodgkin's disease, multiple myeloma, generalized malignancy; chronic renal failure, nephrotic syndrome; patients requiring treatment with immunosuppressive therapy, including chemotherapy, long-term systemic corticosteroids, or radiation therapy; patients who have received a solid organ transplant

Patients 19-64 years of age with certain high-risk condition(s):

- Chronic heart disease (including heart failure and cardiomyopathy, and excluding hypertension)
- Chronic lung disease (including COPD, emphysema, and asthma)
- Persons who smoke cigarettes
- Alcoholism
- Chronic liver disease (including cirrhosis)

Routine vaccination is not recommended for Alaska Natives or American Indian persons unless they have underlying conditions which are indications for vaccination; in special situations, vaccination may be recommended when living in an area at increased risk of invasive pneumococcal disease.

Pregnancy Risk Factor C

Pregnancy Considerations Animal reproduction studies have not been conducted. Vaccination should be considered in pregnant women at high risk for infection. Inactivated vaccines have not been shown to cause increased risks to the fetus (CDC, 2011)

Lactation Excretion in breast milk unknown/use caution

Contraindications Hypersensitivity to pneumococcal vaccine or any component of the formulation

Warnings/Precautions Use caution in patients with severely compromised cardiovascular function or pulmonary disease where a systemic reaction may pose a significant risk. May cause relapse in patients with stable idiopathic thrombocytopenia purpura. Epinephrine injection (1:1000) must be immediately available in the case of anaphylaxis.

Patients who will be receiving immunosuppressive therapy (including Hodgkin's disease, cancer chemotherapy, or transplantation) should be vaccinated at least 2 weeks prior to the initiation of therapy. Immune responses may be impaired for several months following intensive immunosuppressive therapy (up to 2 years in Hodgkin's disease patients). Patients who will undergo splenectomy should also be vaccinated 2 weeks prior to surgery, if possible. In general, household and close contacts of persons with altered immunocompetence may receive all age appropriate vaccines. Patients with HIV should be vaccinated as soon as possible (following confirmation of the diagnosis). The decision to administer or delay vaccination because of current or recent febrile illness depends on the severity of symptoms and the etiology of the disease. Immunization should be delayed during the course of an acute febrile illness or other active infection. In order to maximize vaccination rates, the ACIP recommends simultaneous administration of all age-appropriate vaccines (live or inactivated) for which a person is eligible at a single clinic visit, unless contraindications exist. If a person has not received any pneumococcal vaccine or if pneumococcal vaccination status is unknown, PPSV23 should be administered as indicated. Postmarketing reports of adverse effects in the elderly, especially those with comorbidities, have been significant enough to require hospitalization.

Adverse Reactions All serious adverse reactions must be reported to the U.S. Department of Health and Human Services (DHHS) Vaccine Adverse Event Reporting System (VAERS) 1-800-822-7967 or online

at https://vaers.hhs.gov/esub/index. In Canada, adverse reactions may be reported to local provincial/territorial health agencies or to the Vaccine Safety Section at Public Health Agency of Canada (1-866-844-0018).

Frequency not defined.

Central nervous system: Chills, Guillain-Barré syndrome, fever ≤102°F*, fever >102°F, headache, malaise, pain, radiculoneuropathy, seizure (febrile)

Dermatologic: Angioneurotic edema, cellulitis, rash, urticaria

Gastrointestinal: Nausea, vomiting

Hematologic: Hemolytic anemia (in patients with other hematologic disorders), leukocytosis, thrombocytopenia (in patients with stabilized ITP)

Local: Injection site reaction* (erythema, induration, swelling, soreness, warmth); peripheral edema in injected extremity

Neuromuscular & skeletal: Arthralgia, arthritis, limb mobility decreased, myalgia, paresthesia, weakness

Miscellaneous: Anaphylactoid reaction, C-reactive protein increased, lymphadenitis, lymphadenopathy, serum sickness

*Reactions most commonly reported in clinical trials.

Drug Interactions

Metabolism/Transport Effects None known.

Avoid Concomitant Use There are no known interactions where it is recommended to avoid concomitant use.

Increased Effect/Toxicity There are no known significant interactions involving an increase in effect.

Decreased Effect

Pneumococcal Polysaccharide Vaccine (Polyvalent) may decrease the levels/effects of: Zoster Vaccine

The levels/effects of Pneumococcal Polysaccharide Vaccine (Polyvalent) may be decreased by: Belimumab; Fingolimod; Immunosuppressants

Stability Store under refrigeration at 2°C to 8°C (36°F to 46°F).

Mechanism of Action Although there are more than 80 known pneumococcal capsular types, pneumococcal disease is mainly caused by only a few types of pneumococci. Pneumococcal vaccine contains capsular polysaccharides of 23 pneumococcal types of *Streptococcal pneumoniae* which represent at least 85% to 90% of pneumococcal disease isolates in the United States. The 23 capsular pneumococcal vaccine contains purified capsular polysaccharides of pneumococcal types 1, 2, 3, 4, 5, 6B, 7F, 8, 9N, 9V, 10A, 11A, 12F, 14, 15B, 17F, 18C, 19F, 19A, 20, 22F, 23F, and 33F.

Dosage I.M., SubQ:

Children ≥2 years and Adults: 0.5 mL

Children at increased risk of invasive pneumococcal disease: One dose of PPSV23 should be given at ≥2 years of age in children with underlying medical conditions. Immunization with PCV13 (or PCV7) should be completed prior to PPSV23 as recommended. The minimum interval between the last dose of PCV13 (or PCV7) and PPSV23 is 8 weeks (CDC, December 10, 2010).

Revaccination:

Immunocompetent individuals: Revaccination generally not recommended

Children ≥2 years and Adults at highest risk for pneumococcal disease: One revaccination ≥5 years after first dose of PPSV23. Patients at highest risk for infection include those with asplenia or immunocompromising conditions (eg, sickle cell anemia, HIV infection, leukemia, lymphoma, Hodgkin's disease, multiple myeloma, generalized malignancy, chronic renal failure, nephrotic syndrome, solid organ transplant, and patients on immunosuppressive therapy [including corticosteroids]) (CDC, September 3, 2010; CDC, December 10, 2010).

Adults ≥65 years: One revaccination if ≥5 years after first dose of PPSV23 and if <65 years of age at the time of the initial vaccination (CDC, September 3, 2010).

Administration Do not inject I.V.; avoid intradermal administration (may cause severe local reactions); administer SubQ or I.M. (deltoid muscle or lateral midthigh)

For patients at risk of hemorrhage following intramuscular injection, the ACIP recommends "it should be administered intramuscularly if, in the opinion of the physician familiar with the patients bleeding risk, the vaccine can be administered by this route with reasonable safety. If the patient receives antihemophilia or other similar therapy, intramuscular vaccination can be scheduled shortly after such therapy is administered. A fine needle (23 gauge or smaller) can be used for the vaccination and firm pressure applied to the site (without rubbing) for at least 2 minutes. The patient should be instructed concerning the risk of hematoma from the injection." Patients on anticoagulant therapy should be considered to have the same bleeding risks and treated as those with clotting factor disorders (CDC, 2011).

Antipyretics have not been shown to prevent febrile seizures. Antipyretics may be used to treat fever or discomfort following vaccination (CDC, 2011). One study reported that routine prophylactic administration of acetaminophen to prevent fever prior to vaccination decreased the immune response of some vaccines; the clinical significance of this reduction in immune response has not been established (Prymula, 2009).

Simultaneous administration of vaccines helps ensure the patients will be fully vaccinated by the appropriate age. Simultaneous administration of vaccines is defined as administering >1 vaccine on the same day at different anatomic sites. Separate vaccines should not be combined in the same syringe unless indicated by product specific labeling. Separate needles and syringes should be used for each injection. The ACIP prefers each dose of a specific vaccine in a series come from the same manufacturer when possible. Adolescents and adults should be vaccinated while seated or lying down. In general, preterm infants should be vaccinated at the same chronological age as full-term infants (CDC, 2011).

Monitoring Parameters Monitor for syncope for ≥15 minutes following vaccination.

Additional Information Federal law requires that the name of medication, date of administration, the vaccine manufacturer, lot number of vaccine, and the administering person's name, title, and address be entered into the patient's permanent medical record.

Dosage Forms Excipient information presented when available (limited, particularly for generics); consult specific product labeling.

Injection, solution:

Pneumovax® 23: 25 mcg each of 23 capsular polysaccharide isolates/0.5 mL (0.5 mL, 2.5 mL)

◆ **Pneumococcal 7-Valent Conjugate Vaccine** *see* Pneumococcal Conjugate Vaccine (7-Valent) *on page 1365*

◆ **Pneumococcal 13-Valent Conjugate Vaccine** *see* Pneumococcal Conjugate Vaccine (13-Valent) *on page 1366*

◆ **Pneumovax® 23** *see* Pneumococcal Polysaccharide Vaccine (Polyvalent) *on page 1368*

◆ **PNU-140690E** *see* Tipranavir *on page 1691*

◆ **Podactin Cream [OTC]** *see* Miconazole (Topical) *on page 1126*

◆ **Podactin Powder [OTC]** *see* Tolnaftate *on page 1704*

◆ **Podocon-25®** *see* Podophyllum Resin *on page 1370*

◆ **Podofilm® (Can)** *see* Podophyllum Resin *on page 1370*

◆ **Podophyllin** *see* Podophyllum Resin *on page 1370*

Podophyllum Resin (po DOF fil um REZ in)

Brand Names: U.S. Podocon-25®

Brand Names: Canada Podofilm®

Index Terms Mandrake; May Apple; Podophyllin

Pharmacologic Category Keratolytic Agent

Use Topical treatment of soft external genital (venereal) warts (condylomata acuminate); compound benzoin tincture generally is used as the medium for topical application

Dosage Topical: Children and Adults: Condylomata acuminatum: Applied by physician only.

Additional Information Complete prescribing information for this medication should be consulted for additional detail.

Dosage Forms Excipient information presented when available (limited, particularly for generics); consult specific product labeling.

Liquid, topical:

Podocon-25®: 25% (15 mL) [in benzoin tincture]

Polidocanol (pol i DOE kuh nol)

Brand Names: U.S. Asclera™

Pharmacologic Category Sclerosing Agent

Use Treatment of small, uncomplicated varicose veins of the lower extremities

Pregnancy Risk Factor C

Pregnancy Considerations Teratogenic effects were reported in some animal reproductive studies. There are no adequate and well-controlled studies in pregnant women. Polidocanol should not be used in pregnant women.

Lactation Excretion in breast milk is unknown/not recommended

Contraindications Hypersensitivity to polidocanol or any component of the formulation; acute thromboembolic diseases

Warnings/Precautions Severe allergic reactions, including anaphylaxis and fatal anaphylactoid reactions have been reported with polidocanol; more frequent with larger volumes (>3 mL), therefore, dose should be minimized. Observe 15-20 minutes following injection to monitor for hypersensitivity/anaphylactic reaction; emergency resuscitation equipment should be available. Necrosis of the tissue may occur; pain may occur with inadvertent perivascular injection and may be resolved with a local anesthetic (without epinephrine). Severe necrosis, ischemia, or gangrene can occur with accidental intra-arterial injection; consult vascular surgeon immediately.

After injection is complete, apply compression/bandage, and have patient walk for 15-20 minutes.

Adverse Reactions

>10%: Local: Hematoma (42%), irritation (41%), discoloration (38%), pain (24%), pruritus (19%), warmth (16%)

1% to 10%: Local: Neovascularization (8%), injection site thrombosis (6%)

Postmarketing and/or case reports: Allergic dermatitis, anaphylactic shock, angioedema, asthma, cardiac arrest, cerebrovascular accident, circulatory collapse, confusion, deep vein thrombosis, dizziness, dyspnea, hot flush, hypertrichosis, injection site necrosis, loss of consciousness, migraine, nerve injury, palpitation, paresthesia, pulmonary embolism, pyrexia, skin hyperpigmentation, syncope (vasovagal), urticaria, vasculitis

Drug Interactions

Metabolism/Transport Effects None known.

Avoid Concomitant Use There are no known interactions where it is recommended to avoid concomitant use.

Increased Effect/Toxicity There are no known significant interactions involving an increase in effect.

Decreased Effect There are no known significant interactions involving a decrease in effect.

Stability Store at 15°C to 30°C (59°F to 86°F). Each ampul is intended for immediate use.

Mechanism of Action Acts by irritation of the vein intimal endothelium and causes thrombosis formation leading to occlusion of the injected vein

Pharmacodynamics/Kinetics Half-life elimination: 1.5 hours

Dosage I.V.: Adults: Varicose veins:

Reticular veins (1-3 mm diameter): 0.1-0.3 mL of 1% solution per injection (maximum: 10 mL per session); may repeat in 7-14 days

Spider veins (≤1 mm diameter): 0.1-0.3 mL of 0.5% solution per injection (maximum: 10 mL per session); may repeat in 7-14 days

Administration For intravenous use only. Avoid extravasation. After injection, apply compression in the form of a stocking or bandage (maintain for 2-3 days [spider veins] and 5-7 days [reticular veins]). After applying compression, patient should walk for 15-20 minutes and be observed for anaphylactic or allergic reaction.

Monitoring Parameters Monitor patient for anaphylactic or allergic reaction after injection, and for signs/symptoms of DVT or PE.

Dosage Forms Excipient information presented when available (limited, particularly for generics); consult specific product labeling.

Injection, solution [preservative free]:

Asclera™: 0.5% (2 mL); 1% (2 mL) [contains ethanol]

◆ **Polio Vaccine** *see* Poliovirus Vaccine (Inactivated) *on page 1370*

◆ **Poliovirus, Inactivated (IPV)** *see* Diphtheria and Tetanus Toxoids, Acellular Pertussis, and Poliovirus Vaccine *on page 522*

◆ **Poliovirus, Inactivated (IPV)** *see* Diphtheria and Tetanus Toxoids, Acellular Pertussis, Poliovirus and *Haemophilus* b Conjugate Vaccine *on page 522*

Poliovirus Vaccine (Inactivated)

(POE lee oh VYE rus vak SEEN, in ak ti VAY ted)

Brand Names: U.S. IPOL®

Brand Names: Canada Imovax® Polio

Index Terms Enhanced-Potency Inactivated Poliovirus Vaccine; IPV; Polio Vaccine; Salk Vaccine

Pharmacologic Category Vaccine, Inactivated (Viral)

Additional Appendix Information

Immunization Recommendations *on page 1922*

Use Active immunization against poliomyelitis caused by poliovirus types 1, 2 and 3. **Note:** Combination products containing polio vaccine are also available and may be preferred in certain age groups if recipients are likely to be susceptible to the agents contained within each vaccine.

The Advisory Committee on Immunization Practices (ACIP) recommends routine vaccination for the following:

- All children (first dose given at 2 months of age)

Routine immunization of adults in the United States is generally not recommended. Adults with previous wild poliovirus disease, who have never been immunized, or those who are incompletely immunized may receive inactivated poliovirus vaccine if they fall into one of the following categories:

- Travelers to regions or countries where poliomyelitis is endemic or epidemic
- Healthcare workers in close contact with patients who may be excreting poliovirus

- Laboratory workers handling specimens that may contain poliovirus
- Members of communities or specific population groups with diseases caused by wild poliovirus
- Incompletely vaccinated or unvaccinated adults in a household or with other close contact with children receiving oral poliovirus (may be at increased risk of vaccine associated paralytic poliomyelitis)

Pregnancy Risk Factor C

Pregnancy Considerations Animal reproduction studies have not been conducted. Although adverse effects of IPV have not been documented in pregnant women or their fetuses, vaccination of pregnant women should be avoided on theoretical grounds. Pregnant women at increased risk for infection and requiring immediate protection against polio may be administered the vaccine.

Lactation Excretion into breast milk unknown/use caution

Contraindications Hypersensitivity to any component of the vaccine

Warnings/Precautions Patients with prior clinical poliomyelitis, incomplete immunization with oral poliovirus vaccine (OPV), HIV infection, severe combined immunodeficiency, hypogammaglobulinemia, agammaglobulinemia, or altered immunity (due to corticosteroids, alkylating agents, antimetabolites or radiation) may receive inactivated poliovirus vaccine (IPV). In general, household and close contacts of persons with altered immunocompetence may receive all age appropriate vaccines. Immune response may be decreased in patients receiving immune globulin. Vaccination may be deferred with an acute febrile illness; minor illnesses with or without a low-grade fever are not reasons to postpone vaccination. Immediate treatment for anaphylactic/anaphylactoid reaction should be available during vaccine use. In order to maximize vaccination rates, the ACIP recommends simultaneous administration of all age-appropriate vaccines (live or inactivated) for which a person is eligible at a single clinic visit, unless contraindications exist. The use of combination vaccines is generally preferred over separate injections, taking into consideration provider assessment, patient preference, and adverse events.

The injection contains 2-phenoxyethanol, calf serum protein, formaldehyde, neomycin, streptomycin, and polymyxin B; the packaging contains natural latex rubber. Use of the minimum age and minimum intervals during the first 6 months of life should only be done when the vaccine recipient is at risk for imminent exposure to circulating poliovirus (shorter intervals and earlier start dates may lead to lower seroconversion).

Adverse Reactions All serious adverse reactions must be reported to the U.S. Department of Health and Human Services (DHHS) Vaccine Adverse Event Reporting System (VAERS) 1-800-822-7967 or online at https://vaers.hhs.gov/esub/index. In Canada, adverse reactions may be reported to local provincial/territorial health agencies or to the Vaccine Safety Section at Public Health Agency of Canada (1-866-844-0018).

Percentages noted with concomitant administration of DTP or DTaP vaccine and observed within 48 hours of injection.

>10%:

Central nervous system: Irritability (7% to 65%), tiredness (4% to 61%)

Gastrointestinal: Anorexia (1% to 17%)

Local: Injection Site: Tenderness (≤29%), swelling (≤11%)

1% to 10%:

Central nervous system: Fever >39°C (≤4%)

Gastrointestinal: Vomiting (1% to 3%)

Local: Injection site: Erythema (≤3%)

Miscellaneous: Persistent crying (up to 1% reported within 72 hours)

Postmarketing and/or case reports: Guillain-Barré syndrome has been temporally related to another inactivated poliovirus vaccine

Drug Interactions

Metabolism/Transport Effects None known.

Avoid Concomitant Use There are no known interactions where it is recommended to avoid concomitant use.

Increased Effect/Toxicity There are no known significant interactions involving an increase in effect.

Decreased Effect

The levels/effects of Poliovirus Vaccine (Inactivated) may be decreased by: Belimumab; Fingolimod; Immunosuppressants

Stability Store under refrigeration 2°C to 8°C (35°F to 46°F); do not freeze.

Dosage I.M., SubQ:

Children:

Primary immunization: Administer three 0.5 mL doses, at 2, 4, and 6-18 months of age; do not administer more frequently than 4 weeks apart (preferably given more than 8 weeks apart)

Booster dose: 0.5 mL at 4-6 years of age; Minimum interval between booster and previous dose is 6 months. The final (booster) dose should be given at ≥4 years of age, regardless of the number of previous doses. If the final dose is not given at 4-6 years of age, it should be given as soon as feasible.

Note: Use of the minimum age and minimum intervals during the first 6 months of life should only be done when the vaccine recipient is at risk for imminent exposure to circulating poliovirus (shorter intervals and earlier start dates may lead to lower seroconversion).

Adults:

Previously unvaccinated: Two 0.5 mL doses administered at 1- to 2-month intervals, followed by a third dose 6-12 months later. If <3 months, but at least 2 months are available before protection is needed, 3 doses may be administered at least 1 month apart. If administration must be completed within 1-2 months, give 2 doses at least 1 month apart. If <1 month is available, give 1 dose.

Incompletely vaccinated: Adults with at least 1 previous dose of OPV, <3 doses of IPV, or a combination of OPV and IPV equaling <3 doses, administer at least one 0.5 mL dose of IPV. Additional doses to complete the series may be given if time permits.

Completely vaccinated and at increased risk of exposure: One 0.5 mL dose

Administration Do not administer I.V.; for I.M. or SubQ administration. Administer to midlateral aspect of the thigh in infants and small children. Administer in the deltoid area to adults or older children.

Simultaneous administration of vaccines helps ensure the patients will be fully vaccinated by the appropriate age. Simultaneous administration of vaccines is defined as administering >1 vaccine on the same day at different anatomic sites. The use of licensed combination vaccines is generally preferred over separate injections of the equivalent components. Separate vaccines should not be combined in the same syringe unless indicated by product specific labeling. Separate needles and syringes should be used for each injection. The ACIP prefers each dose of a specific vaccine in a series come from the same manufacturer when possible. Adolescents and adults should be vaccinated while seated or lying down. In general, preterm infants should be vaccinated at the same chronological age as full-term infants (CDC, 2011).

Antipyretics have not been shown to prevent febrile seizures. Antipyretics may be used to treat fever or discomfort following vaccination (CDC, 2011). One study reported that routine prophylactic administration of acetaminophen to prevent fever prior to vaccination decreased the immune response of some vaccines; the clinical significance of this reduction in immune response has not been established (Prymula, 2009).

Monitoring Parameters Monitor for syncope for ≥15 minutes following vaccination.

Test Interactions May temporarily suppress tuberculin skin test sensitivity (4-6 weeks)

Additional Information Federal law requires that the name of medication, date of administration, the vaccine manufacturer, lot number of vaccine, and the administering person's name, title, and address be entered into the patient's permanent medical record.

As the global eradication of poliomyelitis continues, the risk for importation of wild-type poliovirus into the United States decreases dramatically. To eliminate the risk for vaccine-associated paralytic poliomyelitis (VAPP), an all-IPV schedule is recommended for routine childhood vaccination in the United States. Oral poliovirus vaccine (OPV), is not commercially available in the United States, but has been stockpiled for use in the following special circumstances:

Mass vaccination campaigns to control outbreaks of paralytic polio

Unvaccinated children who will be traveling within 4 weeks to areas where polio is endemic or epidemic

Children of parents who do not accept the recommended number of vaccine injections; these children may receive OPV only for the third or fourth dose or both. In this situation, healthcare providers should administer OPV only after discussing the risk for VAPP with parents or caregivers.

Currently, the primary risk for paralytic polio in U.S. residents is through travel to countries where polio remains endemic or where polio outbreaks are occurring. Unvaccinated persons traveling to countries that use OPV should be aware of the risk caused by OPV and should consider polio vaccination prior to travel.

Dosage Forms Excipient information presented when available (limited, particularly for generics); consult specific product labeling.

Injection, suspension:

IPOL®: Type 1 poliovirus 40 D-antigen units, type 2 poliovirus 8 D-antigen units, and type 3 poliovirus 32 D-antigen units per 0.5 mL (0.5 mL, 5 mL) [contains 2-phenoxyethanol, formaldehyde, calf serum protein, neomycin (may have trace amounts), streptomycin (may have trace amounts), and polymyxin B (may have trace amounts)]

◆ **Polocaine®** *see* Mepivacaine *on page 1076*

◆ **Polocaine® Dental** *see* Mepivacaine *on page 1076*

◆ **Polocaine® MPF** *see* Mepivacaine *on page 1076*

◆ **Polycin™** *see* Bacitracin and Polymyxin B *on page 186*

◆ **Polycitra** *see* Citric Acid, Sodium Citrate, and Potassium Citrate *on page 372*

◆ **Polycitra K** *see* Potassium Citrate and Citric Acid *on page 1382*

◆ **Poly-Dex™ [DSC]** *see* Neomycin, Polymyxin B, and Dexamethasone *on page 1189*

◆ **Polyethylene Glycol-L-asparaginase** *see* Pegaspargase *on page 1306*

Polyethylene Glycol 3350

(pol i ETH i leen GLY kol 3350)

Brand Names: U.S. Dulcolax Balance® [OTC]; MiraLAX® [OTC]

Index Terms PEG

Pharmacologic Category Laxative, Osmotic

Additional Appendix Information

Laxatives, Classification and Properties *on page 1893*

Use Treatment of occasional constipation in adults

Unlabeled Use Treatment of constipation in children; bowel preparation before colonoscopy

Pregnancy Risk Factor C

Dosage Oral:

Children ≥6 months: Occasional constipation (unlabeled use): 0.5-1.5 g/kg daily (initial dose: 0.5-1 g/kg; titrate to effect); not to exceed 17 g/day; do not use for >2 weeks (Bell, 2004; Loening-Baucke, 2005; Michail, 2004; Voskuijl, 2004)

Adults:

Occasional constipation: 17 g of powder (~1 heaping tablespoon) dissolved in 4-8 ounces of beverage, once daily; do not use for >1 week unless directed by healthcare provider

Bowel preparation before colonoscopy (unlabeled use): Mix 17 g of powder (~1 heaping tablespoon) in 8 ounces of clear liquid and administer the entire mixture every 10 minutes until 2 L are consumed (start within 6 hours after administering 20 mg bisacodyl delayed-release tablets) (Wexner, 2006)

Additional Information Complete prescribing information for this medication should be consulted for additional detail.

Dosage Forms Excipient information presented when available (limited, particularly for generics); consult specific product labeling.

Powder for solution, oral: 17 g/dose (119 g, 238 g, 255 g, 510 g, 527 g); 17 g/packet (14s, 30s)

Dulcolax Balance®: 17 g/dose (119 g, 238 g, 510 g)

MiraLAX®: 17 g/dose (119 g, 238 g, 510 g); 17 g/packet (10s)

◆ **Polyethylene Glycol-Conjugated Uricase** *see* Pegloticase *on page 1315*

Polyethylene Glycol-Electrolyte Solution

(pol i ETH i leen GLY kol ee LEK troe lite soe LOO shun)

Brand Names: U.S. Colyte®; GaviLyte™-C; GaviLyte™-G; GaviLyte™-N; GoLYTELY®; MoviPrep®; NuLYTELY®; TriLyte®

Brand Names: Canada Colyte™; Klean-Prep®; PegLyte®

Index Terms Electrolyte Lavage Solution

Pharmacologic Category Laxative, Osmotic

Use Bowel cleansing prior to GI examination

Unlabeled Use Whole bowel irrigation (WBI) in the following toxic ingestions: Packets of illicit drugs (body packers, body stuffers), potentially toxic sustained-release or enteric-coated agents, substantial amounts of iron (AACT, 2004)

Pregnancy Risk Factor C

Pregnancy Considerations Reproduction studies have not been conducted in animals or in humans.

Lactation Excretion in breast milk unknown/use caution

Medication Guide Available Yes

Contraindications Hypersensitivity to polyethylene glycol or any component of the formulation; ileus, gastrointestinal obstruction, gastric retention, bowel perforation, toxic colitis, toxic megacolon

Warnings/Precautions Seizures associated with electrolyte abnormalities (eg, hyponatremia, hypokalemia) have occurred. Use caution with concomitant administration of medications that alter electrolyte balance or in patients with underlying hyponatremia. Do not add flavorings, unless provided by the manufacturer, as additional ingredients before use; observe unconscious or semiconscious patients with impaired gag reflex or those who are otherwise prone to regurgitation or aspiration during administration; use with caution in patients with severe ulcerative colitis. Evaluate patients with symptoms of bowel obstruction (nausea, vomiting, abdominal pain or distension) prior to use.

MoviPrep®: May be safer to use in patients who cannot tolerate fluid load (eg, heart failure, renal insufficiency, ascites). Use cautiously in patients with G6PD deficiency. Contains phenylalanine.

Adverse Reactions

>10%:

Central nervous system: Malaise (18% to 27%)

Gastrointestinal: Abdominal distension (<60%), anal irritation (<52%), nausea (14% to 47%), abdominal pain (13% to 39%), vomiting (7% to 12%)

Neuromuscular & skeletal: Rigors (34%)

Miscellaneous: Thirst (<47%)

1% to 10%:

Central nervous system: Dizziness (7%), headache (2%)

Gastrointestinal: Dyspepsia (1% to 3%)

Frequency not defined, postmarketing, and/or case reports: Abdominal cramps, abdominal fullness, allergic reactions, anaphylaxis, aspiration, asystole, bloating, chest tightness, dehydration, dermatitis, dyspnea (acute), esophageal perforation, facial edema, fever, flatulence, hypersensitivity reactions, hypokalemia (children), Mallory-Weiss tear, pulmonary edema, rash, rhinorrhea, seizure, shock, throat tightness, upper GI bleeding, urticaria

Drug Interactions

Metabolism/Transport Effects None known.

Avoid Concomitant Use There are no known interactions where it is recommended to avoid concomitant use.

Increased Effect/Toxicity There are no known significant interactions involving an increase in effect.

Decreased Effect There are no known significant interactions involving a decrease in effect.

Stability

CoLyte®, GaviLyte™-C, GaviLyte™-G, GaviLyte™-N, GoLYTELY®, NuLYTELY®, TriLyte®: Store at controlled room temperature of 25°C (77°F) before reconstitution. Use within 48 hours of preparation; refrigerate reconstituted solution; tap water may be used for preparation of the solution; shake container vigorously several times to ensure dissolution of powder.

MoviPrep®: Store at controlled room temperature of 25°C (77°F) before reconstitution. Mix the contents of pouch A and pouch B (one each) in container provided. Add 1 L of lukewarm water; mix the solution until dissolved. Repeat mixing procedure if second liter is needed. Refrigerate reconstituted solution. Use within 24 hours of preparation.

Mechanism of Action Induces catharsis by strong electrolyte and osmotic effects

Pharmacodynamics/Kinetics Onset of effect: Oral: ~1-2 hours

Dosage

Oral:

Children ≥6 months: Bowel cleansing prior to GI exam (GaviLyte™-N, NuLYTELY®, TriLyte®): 25 mL/kg/hour (some studies have used up to 40 mL/kg/hour) for 4-10 hours (until rectal effluent is clear). Maximum total dose: 4 L. **Note:** The solution may be given via nasogastric tube to patients who are unwilling or unable to drink the solution. Patients <2 years should be monitored closely.

Adults: Bowel cleansing prior to GI exam:

CoLyte®, GaviLyte™-C, GaviLyte™-G, GaviLyte™-N, GoLYTELY®, NuLYTELY®, TriLyte®: 240 mL (8 oz) every 10 minutes, until 4 L are consumed or the rectal effluent is clear; rapid drinking of each portion is preferred to drinking small amounts continuously. Ideally, patients should fast for ~3-4 hours prior to administration; absolutely no solid food for at least 2 hours before the solution is given. **Note:** The solution may be given via nasogastric tube to patients who are unwilling or unable to drink the solution.

MoviPrep®: Administer 2 L total with an additional 1 L of clear fluid prior to colonoscopy as follows:

Split dose: Evening before colonoscopy: 240 mL (8 oz) every 15 minutes until 1 L is consumed. Then drink 16 oz of clear liquid. On the morning of the colonoscopy, repeat process with second liter over 1 hour and then drink 16 oz of clear liquid at least 1 hour before the procedure.

Full dose: Evening before colonoscopy (~6 PM): 240 mL (8 oz every 15 minutes) until 1 L is consumed; 90 minutes later (~7:30 PM), repeat dose. Then drink 32 oz of clear liquid.

Nasogastric tube (CoLyte®, GoLYTELY®, NuLYTELY®, TriLyte®):

Bowel cleansing prior to GI exam:

Children ≥6 months: 25 mL/kg/hour until rectal effluent is clear.

Adults: Bowel cleansing prior to GI exam: 20-30 mL/minute (1.2-1.8 L/hour); the first bowel movement should occur ~1 hour after the start of administration.

Toxic ingestion (unlabeled use; AACT, 2004):

Children ≥9 months to 6 years: 500 mL/hour until rectal effluent is clear

Children 6-12 years: 1000 mL/hour until rectal effluent is clear

Adolescents and Adults: 1500-2000 mL/hour until rectal effluent is clear

Note: May take several hours for the rectal effluent to become clear. Duration may be extended if evidence of continued presence of toxins in GI tract (eg, radiographic evidence or ongoing elimination of toxins)

Dietary Considerations

CoLyte®, GaviLyte™-C, GaviLyte™-G, GaviLyte™-N, GoLYTELY®, NuLYTELY®, TriLyte®: Ideally, the patient should fast for ~3-4 hours prior to administration, but in no case should solid food be given for at least 2 hours before the solution is given. Some products contain aspartame which is metabolized to phenylalanine.

MoviPrep®: Patient should not eat solid food from start of solution administration until after colonoscopy. Patient may have clear liquid soup/plain yogurt for dinner; finish at least 1 hour before start of colon prep.

Administration Oral: Rapid drinking of each portion is preferred to drinking small amounts continuously. Do not add flavorings, unless provided by the manufacturer, as additional ingredients before use. Chilled solution often more palatable. Oral medications should not be administered within 1 hour of start of therapy.

Monitoring Parameters Electrolytes, serum glucose, BUN, urine osmolality; children <2 years of age should be monitored for hypoglycemia, dehydration, hypokalemia

Dosage Forms Excipient information presented when available (limited, particularly for generics); consult specific product labeling.

Powder, for solution, oral: PEG 3350 240 g, sodium sulfate 22.72 g, sodium bicarbonate 6.72 g, sodium chloride 5.84 g, and potassium chloride 2.98 g (4000 mL); PEG 3350 236 g, sodium sulfate 22.74 g, sodium bicarbonate 6.74 g, sodium chloride 5.86 g, and potassium chloride 2.97 g (4000 mL); PEG 3350 240 g, sodium bicarbonate 5.72 g, sodium chloride 11.2 g, and potassium chloride 1.48 g (4000 mL)

Colyte®: PEG 3350 240 g, sodium sulfate 22.72 g, sodium bicarbonate 6.72 g, sodium chloride 5.84 g, and potassium chloride 2.98 g (4000 mL) [available with lemon lime, cherry, and orange flavor packets]

GaviLyte™-C: PEG 3350 240 g, sodium sulfate 22.72 g, sodium bicarbonate 6.72 g, sodium chloride 5.84 g, and potassium chloride 2.98 g (4000 mL) [supplied with lemon flavor packet]

GaviLyte™-G: PEG 3350 236 g, sodium sulfate 22.74 g, sodium bicarbonate 6.74 g, sodium chloride 5.86 g, and potassium chloride 2.97 g (4000 mL) [supplied with lemon flavor packet]

GaviLyte™-N: PEG 3350 420 g, sodium bicarbonate 5.72 g, sodium chloride 11.2 g, and potassium chloride 1.48 g (4000 mL) [supplied with lemon flavor packet]

GoLYTELY®:

PEG 3350 236 g, sodium sulfate 22.74 g, sodium bicarbonate 6.74 g, sodium chloride 5.86 g, and potassium chloride 2.97 g (4000 mL) [regular and pineapple flavor]

PEG 3350 227.1 g, sodium sulfate 21.5 g, sodium bicarbonate 6.36 g, sodium chloride 5.53 g, and potassium chloride 2.82 g per packet (1s) [regular flavor; makes 1 gallon of solution after mixing]

MoviPrep®: Pouch A: PEG 3350 100g, sodium sulfate 7.5 g, sodium chloride 2.69 g, potassium chloride 1.015 g; Pouch B: Ascorbic acid 4.7 g, sodium ascorbate 5.9 g (1000 mL) [contains phenylalanine 2.33 mg/treatment; lemon flavor; packaged with 2 of Pouch A and 2 of Pouch B in carton and a disposable reconstitution container]

NuLYTELY®: PEG 3350 420 g, sodium bicarbonate 5.72 g, sodium chloride 11.2 g, and potassium chloride 1.48 g (4000 mL) [cherry, lemon-lime, orange, and pineapple flavors]

TriLyte®: PEG 3350 420 g, sodium bicarbonate 5.72 g, sodium chloride 11.2 g, and potassium chloride 1.48 g (4000 mL) [supplied with flavor packets]

◆ **Polyethylene Glycol Interferon Alfa-2b** *see* Peginterferon Alfa-2b *on page* 1311

◆ **Poly-Iron 150 [OTC]** *see* Polysaccharide-Iron Complex *on page* 1375

Poly-L-Lactic Acid (POL i el LAK tik AS id)

Brand Names: U.S. Sculptra®; Sculptra® Aesthetic

Index Terms New-Fill®; PLA

Pharmacologic Category Cosmetic Agent, Implant

Use Restoration and/or correction of facial lipoatrophy in patients with HIV; correction of shallow to deep nasolabial fold contour deficiencies and other facial wrinkles in immunocompetent patients

Dosage Adults:

Facial wrinkles (Sculptra® Aesthetic): Intradermal: 0.1-0.2 mL per individual injection to a maximum of 2.5 mL per nasolabial fold as a single treatment; may repeat treatment at ≥3 week intervals up to 4 times

Lipoatrophy (Sculptra®): Intradermal or SubQ: ~0.05-0.2 mL per individual injection depending on technique used; ~20 injections may be needed per cheek. Treatment should be individualized. Separate treatments by ≥2 weeks. Typical course involves 3-6 treatments. Supplemental injections may be needed. Do not overfill contour deficiency. For patients with severe facial fat loss, the average treatment requires ~1 vial per cheek area per treatment.

Additional Information Complete prescribing information for this medication should be consulted for additional detail.

Dosage Forms Excipient information presented when available (limited, particularly for generics); consult specific product labeling.

Injection, powder for suspension:

Sculptra®, Sculptra® Aesthetic: Poly-L-lactic acid USP

Polymyxin B (pol i MIKS in bee)

Brand Names: U.S. Poly-Rx [DSC]

Index Terms Polymyxin B Sulfate

Pharmacologic Category Antibiotic, Irrigation; Antibiotic, Miscellaneous

Additional Appendix Information

Prevention of Wound Infection and Sepsis in Surgical Patients *on page* 1954

Use Treatment of acute infections caused by susceptible strains of *Pseudomonas aeruginosa*; used occasionally for gut decontamination; parenteral use of polymyxin B has mainly been replaced by less toxic antibiotics, reserved for life-threatening infections caused by organisms resistant to the preferred drugs (eg, pseudomonal meningitis - intrathecal administration)

Pregnancy Risk Factor B

Pregnancy Considerations [U.S. Boxed Warning]: Safety in pregnant women has not been established. A teratogenic potential has not been identified for polymyxin B, but very limited data is available. Based on the relative toxicity compared to other antibiotics, systemic use in pregnancy cannot be recommended. Due to limited absorption through the maternal skin, limited fetal exposure would be expected after topical polymyxin use.

Lactation Excretion in breast milk unknown/use caution

Contraindications Hypersensitivity to polymyxin B or any component of the formulation; concurrent use of neuromuscular blockers

Warnings/Precautions [U.S. Boxed Warning]: May cause neurotoxicity, nephrotoxicity, and/or neuromuscular blockade and respiratory paralysis; usual risk factors include pre-existing renal impairment, concomitant neuro-/nephrotoxic medications, advanced age and dehydration. Use with caution in patients with impaired renal function (modify dosage); polymyxin B-induced nephrotoxicity may be manifested by albuminuria, cellular casts, and azotemia. Discontinue therapy with decreasing urinary output and increasing BUN; neurotoxic reactions are usually associated with high serum levels, often in patients with renal dysfunction. Avoid concurrent or sequential use of other nephrotoxic and neurotoxic drugs (eg, aminoglycosides). The drug's neurotoxicity can result in respiratory paralysis from neuromuscular blockade, especially when the drug is given soon after anesthesia or muscle relaxants. Polymyxin B sulfate is most toxic when given parenterally; avoid parenteral use whenever possible. Prolonged use may result in fungal or bacterial superinfection, including *C. difficile*-associated diarrhea (CDAD) and pseudomembranous colitis; CDAD has been observed >2 months postantibiotic treatment. **[U.S. Boxed Warnings]: Safety in pregnant women not established; intramuscular/intrathecal administration only to hospitalized patients.**

Adverse Reactions Frequency not defined (limited to important or life-threatening):

Central nervous system: Neurotoxicity (irritability, drowsiness, ataxia, perioral paresthesia, numbness of the extremities, and blurred vision); dizziness

Neuromuscular & skeletal: Neuromuscular blockade

Renal: Nephrotoxicity

Respiratory: Respiratory arrest

Drug Interactions

Metabolism/Transport Effects None known.

Avoid Concomitant Use

Avoid concomitant use of Polymyxin B with any of the following: BCG

Increased Effect/Toxicity

Polymyxin B may increase the levels/effects of: Colistimethate; Neuromuscular-Blocking Agents

The levels/effects of Polymyxin B may be increased by: Capreomycin

Decreased Effect

Polymyxin B may decrease the levels/effects of: BCG

Stability Prior to reconstitution, store at room temperature of 15°C to 30°C (59°F to 86°F). Protect from light. After reconstitution, store under refrigeration at 2°C to 8°C (36°F to 46°F). Discard any unused solution after 72 hours.

Mechanism of Action Binds to phospholipids, alters permeability, and damages the bacterial cytoplasmic membrane permitting leakage of intracellular constituents

Pharmacodynamics/Kinetics

Absorption: Well absorbed from peritoneum; minimal from GI tract (except in neonates) from mucous membranes or intact skin. Clinically insignificant amounts are absorbed following irrigation of an intact urinary bladder; systemic absorption may occur from a denuded bladder. Small amounts are systemically absorbed following ophthalmic installation.

Distribution: Minimal into CSF; V_d: 71-194 mL/kg

Protein binding: 79% to 92% (critically ill patients)

Half-life elimination: 6 hours; 2-3 days with anuria

Time to peak, serum: I.M.: ~2 hours

Excretion: Urine (<1% as unchanged drug)

Dosage

Otic (in combination with other drugs): 1-2 drops, 3-4 times/day; should be used sparingly to avoid accumulation of excess debris

Infants <2 years:

I.M.: Up to 40,000 units/kg/day divided every 6 hours (not routinely recommended due to pain at injection sites)

I.V.: Up to 40,000 units/kg/day divided every 12 hours

Intrathecal: 20,000 units/day for 3-4 days, then 25,000 units every other day for at least 2 weeks after CSF cultures are negative and CSF (glucose) has returned to within normal limits

Children ≥2 years and Adults:

I.M.: 25,000-30,000 units/kg/day divided every 4-6 hours (not routinely recommended due to pain at injection sites)

I.V.: 15,000-25,000 units/kg/day divided every 12 hours

Intrathecal: 50,000 units/day for 3-4 days, then every other day for at least 2 weeks after CSF cultures are negative and CSF (glucose) has returned to within normal limits

Total daily dose should not exceed 2,000,000 units/day

Bladder irrigation: Continuous irrigant or rinse in the urinary bladder for up to 10 days using 20 mg (equal to 200,000 units) added to 1 L of normal saline; usually no more than 1 L of irrigant is used per day unless urine flow rate is high; administration rate is adjusted to patient's urine output

Topical irrigation or topical solution: 500,000 units/L of normal saline; topical irrigation should not exceed 2 million units/day in adults

Gut sterilization: Oral: 15,000-25,000 units/kg/day in divided doses every 6 hours

Clostridium difficile enteritis: Oral: 25,000 units every 6 hours for 10 days

Ophthalmic: A concentration of 0.1% to 0.25% is administered as 1-3 drops every hour, then increasing the interval as response indicates to 1-2 drops 4-6 times/day

Dosing adjustment/interval in renal impairment:

Cl_{cr} 20-50 mL/minute: Administer 75% to 100% of the normal daily dose given in divided doses every 12 hours

Cl_{cr} 5-20 mL/minute: Administer 50% of normal daily dose given in divided doses every 12 hours

Cl_{cr} <5 mL/minute: Administer 15% of normal daily dose given in divided doses every 12 hours

Administration Dissolve 500,000 units in 300-500 mL D_5W for continuous I.V. drip; dissolve 500,000 units in 2 mL water for injection, saline, or 1% procaine solution for I.M. injection; dissolve 500,000 units in 10 mL physiologic solution for intrathecal administration

Extravasation management: Monitor I.V. site closely; extravasation may cause serious injury with possible necrosis and tissue sloughing. Rotate infusion site frequently.

Monitoring Parameters Neurologic symptoms and signs of superinfection; renal function (decreasing urine output and increasing BUN may require discontinuance of therapy)

Reference Range Serum concentrations >5 mcg/mL are toxic in adults

Additional Information 1 mg = 10,000 units

Dosage Forms Excipient information presented when available (limited, particularly for generics); consult specific product labeling. [DSC] = Discontinued product

Injection, powder for reconstitution: 500,000 units

Powder, for prescription compounding [micronized]:

Poly-Rx: 100 million units (13 g [DSC])

- ◆ **Polymyxin B and Bacitracin** *see* Bacitracin and Polymyxin B *on page 186*
- ◆ **Polymyxin B and Neomycin** *see* Neomycin and Polymyxin B *on page 1188*
- ◆ **Polymyxin B and Trimethoprim** *see* Trimethoprim and Polymyxin B *on page 1741*
- ◆ **Polymyxin B, Bacitracin, and Neomycin** *see* Bacitracin, Neomycin, and Polymyxin B *on page 186*
- ◆ **Polymyxin B, Bacitracin, Neomycin, and Hydrocortisone** *see* Bacitracin, Neomycin, Polymyxin B, and Hydrocortisone *on page 187*
- ◆ **Polymyxin B, Neomycin, and Dexamethasone** *see* Neomycin, Polymyxin B, and Dexamethasone *on page 1189*
- ◆ **Polymyxin B, Neomycin, and Gramicidin** *see* Neomycin, Polymyxin B, and Gramicidin *on page 1189*
- ◆ **Polymyxin B, Neomycin, and Hydrocortisone** *see* Neomycin, Polymyxin B, and Hydrocortisone *on page 1190*
- ◆ **Polymyxin B Sulfate** *see* Polymyxin B *on page 1374*
- ◆ **Poly-Rx [DSC]** *see* Polymyxin B *on page 1374*

Polysaccharide-Iron Complex

(pol i SAK a ride-EYE ern KOM pleks)

Brand Names: U.S. Ferrex™ 150 Plus [OTC]; Ferrex™ 150 [OTC]; Niferex® [OTC] [DSC]; Nu-Iron® 150 [OTC]; Poly-Iron 150 [OTC]; ProFe [OTC]

Index Terms Iron-Polysaccharide Complex

Pharmacologic Category Iron Salt

Use Prevention and treatment of iron-deficiency anemias

Dosage

Dietary Reference Intake: Dose is RDA presented as elemental iron unless otherwise noted:

0-6 months: 0.27 mg/day (adequate intake)
7-12 months: 11 mg/day
1-3 years: 7 mg/day
4-8 years: 10 mg/day
9-13 years: 8 mg/day
14-18 years: Males: 11 mg/day; Females: 15 mg/day; Pregnant females: 27 mg/day; Lactating females: 10 mg/day
19-50 years: Males: 8 mg/day; Females: 18 mg/day; Pregnant females: 27 mg/day; Lactating females: 9 mg/day
≥50 years: 8 mg/day

Iron deficiency: Oral:

Children ≥6 years: 50-100 mg/day; may be given in divided doses
Adults: 150-300 mg/day

Additional Information Complete prescribing information for this medication should be consulted for additional detail.

Dosage Forms Excipient information presented when available (limited, particularly for generics); consult specific product labeling. [DSC] = Discontinued product

Capsule, oral: Elemental iron 150 mg [DSC]
Ferrex™ 150: Elemental iron 150 mg [contains tartrazine]
Ferrex™ 150 Plus: Elemental iron 150 mg (50 mg as ferrous asparto glycinate) [contains ascorbic acid 50 mg and succinic acid 50 mg]
Niferex®: Elemental iron 60 mg [DSC]
Nu-Iron® 150: Elemental iron 150 mg
Poly-Iron 150: Elemental iron 150 mg [contains tartrazine]
ProFe: Elemental iron 180 mg

Elixir, oral:
Niferex®: Elemental iron 100 mg/5 mL (236 mL [DSC]) [dye free, sugar free; contains ethanol 10%]

◆ **Polysporin® [OTC]** *see* Bacitracin and Polymyxin B *on page 186*
◆ **Polytrim®** *see* Trimethoprim and Polymyxin B *on page 1741*
◆ **Polytrim™ (Can)** *see* Trimethoprim and Polymyxin B *on page 1741*
◆ **P-OM3** *see* Omega-3-Acid Ethyl Esters *on page 1241*
◆ **Ponstan® (Can)** *see* Mefenamic Acid *on page 1060*
◆ **Ponstel®** *see* Mefenamic Acid *on page 1060*
◆ **Pontocaine® [DSC]** *see* Tetracaine (Topical) *on page 1661*
◆ **Pontocaine® (Can)** *see* Tetracaine (Ophthalmic) *on page 1661*
◆ **Pontocaine® (Can)** *see* Tetracaine (Systemic) *on page 1660*
◆ **Pontocaine® (Can)** *see* Tetracaine (Topical) *on page 1661*

Porfimer (POR fi mer)

Brand Names: U.S. Photofrin®

Brand Names: Canada Photofrin®

Index Terms CL-184116; Dihematoporphyrin Ether; Porfimer Sodium

Pharmacologic Category Antineoplastic Agent, Miscellaneous

Use Palliation in patients with obstructing (partial or complete) esophageal cancer; treatment of microinvasive endobronchial nonsmall cell lung cancer (NSCLC); reduction of obstruction and palliation in patients with obstructing (partial or complete) NSCLC; ablation of high-grade dysplasia in Barrett's esophagus

Canadian labeling (additional use; not in U.S. labeling): Second-line treatment of recurrent, superficial papillary bladder cancer

Unlabeled Use Treatment of actinic keratoses and low-risk basal and squamous cell skin cancers

Pregnancy Risk Factor C

Dosage I.V.: Adults:

Photodynamic therapy in esophageal cancer or endobronchial nonsmall cell lung cancer: 2 mg/kg, followed by endoscopic exposure to the appropriate laser light and debridement; repeat courses must be separated by at least 30 days (delay subsequent treatment for insufficient healing) for a maximum of 3 courses

Photodynamic therapy in Barrett's esophagus dysplasia: 2 mg/kg, followed by endoscopic exposure to the appropriate laser light; repeat courses must be separated by at least 90 days (delay subsequent treatment for insufficient healing) for a maximum of 3 courses

Photodynamic therapy in papillary bladder cancer (Canadian labeling; not in U.S. labeling): 2 mg/kg, followed by cystoscopic exposure to the appropriate laser light. **Note:** Repeat dosing is not recommended due to increased risk of bladder contracture.

Additional Information Complete prescribing information for this medication should be consulted for additional detail.

Dosage Forms Excipient information presented when available (limited, particularly for generics); consult specific product labeling.

Injection, powder for reconstitution, as sodium:
Photofrin®: 75 mg

Dosage Forms: Canada Excipient information presented when available (limited, particularly for generics); consult specific product labeling.

Injection, powder for reconstitution, as sodium:
Photofrin®: 15 mg

◆ **Porfimer Sodium** *see* Porfimer *on page 1376*
◆ **Portia®** *see* Ethinyl Estradiol and Levonorgestrel *on page 656*

Posaconazole (poe sa KON a zole)

Brand Names: U.S. Noxafil®

Brand Names: Canada Posanol™

Index Terms SCH 56592

Pharmacologic Category Antifungal Agent, Oral

Additional Appendix Information

Antifungal Agents *on page 1876*

Use Prophylaxis of invasive *Aspergillus* and *Candida* infections in severely-immunocompromised patients [eg, hematopoietic stem cell transplant (HSCT) recipients with graft-versus-host disease (GVHD) or those with prolonged neutropenia secondary to chemotherapy for hematologic malignancies]; treatment of oropharyngeal candidiasis (including patients refractory to itraconazole and/or fluconazole)

Unlabeled Use Salvage therapy of refractory or relapsed invasive fungal infections; mucormycosis; pulmonary infection (nonimmunosuppressed)

Pregnancy Risk Factor C

Pregnancy Considerations Posaconazole has been shown to be teratogenic in animal studies. There are no adequate and well-controlled studies in pregnant women. Use only if the benefit to the mother justifies potential risk to the fetus.

Lactation Excretion in breast milk unknown/not recommended

Contraindications Hypersensitivity to posaconazole, other azole antifungals, or any component of the formulation; coadministration of cisapride, ergot alkaloids, pimozide, quinidine, simvastatin, or sirolimus

Warnings/Precautions Hepatic dysfunction has occurred, ranging from reversible mild/moderate increases of ALT, AST, alkaline phosphatase, total bilirubin, and/or clinical hepatitis to severe reactions (cholestasis, hepatic failure including death). Consider discontinuation of therapy in patients who develop clinical evidence of liver disease that may be secondary to posaconazole. Use caution in patients with an increased risk of arrhythmia (long QT syndrome, concurrent QT_c-prolonging drugs, hypokalemia). Correct electrolyte abnormalities (eg, potassium, magnesium, and calcium) before initiating therapy. Concurrent use with cyclosporine or tacrolimus may significantly increase cyclosporine/tacrolimus concentrations and may result in rare serious adverse events (eg, nephrotoxicity, leukoencephalopathy, and death); dose reduction and close monitoring are recommended with initiation of posaconazole therapy. Concurrent use with midazolam may increase midazolam concentrations and potentiate midazolam-related adverse effects.

Use caution in hypersensitivity with other azole antifungal agents; cross-reaction may occur, but has not been established. Consider alternative therapy or closely monitor for breakthrough fungal infections in patients receiving drugs that decrease absorption or increase the metabolism of posaconazole or in any patient unable to eat or tolerate an oral liquid nutritional supplement. Use caution in severe renal impairment or GI disturbances; monitor for breakthrough fungal infections.

Adverse Reactions Note: Percentages reflect data from use in comparator trials with multiple concomitant conditions and medications; some adverse reactions may be due to underlying condition(s).

>10%:
- Cardiovascular: Hypertension (18%), edema (9% to 15%), hypotension (14%), tachycardia (12%)
- Central nervous system: Fever (6% to 45%), headache (8% to 28%), fatigue (3% to 17%), insomnia (1% to 17%), dizziness (11%), pain (1% to 11%)
- Endocrine & metabolic: Hypokalemia (≤30%), hypomagnesemia (18%), dehydration (1% to 11%), hyperglycemia (11%)
- Gastrointestinal: Diarrhea (10% to 42%), nausea (9% to 38%), vomiting (7% to 29%), abdominal pain (5% to 27%), constipation (21%), anorexia (2% to 19%), mucositis (17%), weight loss (1% to 14%), oral candidiasis (1% to 12%)
- Hematologic: Thrombocytopenia (29%), anemia (2% to 25%), neutropenia (4% to 23%), neutropenic fever (20%)
- Hepatic: ALT increased (6% to 17%)
- Neuromuscular & skeletal: Rigors (≤20%), musculoskeletal pain (16%), weakness (2% to 13%), arthralgia (11%)
- Respiratory: Cough (3% to 25%), dyspnea (1% to 20%), epistaxis (14%), pharyngitis (12%)
- Miscellaneous: Bacteremia (18%), herpes simplex (3% to 15%), CMV infection (14%)

1% to 10%:
- Central nervous system: Anxiety (9%)
- Endocrine & metabolic: Hypocalcemia (9%)
- Gastrointestinal: Dyspepsia (10%)
- Genitourinary: Vaginal hemorrhage (10%)
- Hepatic: Hyperbilirubinemia (7% to 10%), AST increased (3% to 4%), alkaline phosphatase increased (1% to 3%)
- Neuromuscular & skeletal: Back pain (10%)
- Respiratory: Pneumonia (3% to 10%), upper respiratory infection (7%)
- Miscellaneous: Diaphoresis (2% to 10%)

<1% (Limited to important or life-threatening): Acute renal failure, adrenal insufficiency, allergic reaction, atrial fibrillation, cholestasis, ejection fraction decreased, hemolytic uremic syndrome, hepatic failure, hepatitis, hepatomegaly, hypersensitivity, jaundice, paresthesia, pulmonary embolus, QT_c prolongation, syncope, thrombotic thrombocytopenic purpura, torsade de pointes

Drug Interactions

Metabolism/Transport Effects Inhibits CYP3A4 (strong)

Avoid Concomitant Use

Avoid concomitant use of Posaconazole with any of the following: Alfuzosin; Cisapride; Conivaptan; Crizotinib; Dofetilide; Dronedarone; Efavirenz; Eplerenone; Ergot Derivatives; Everolimus; Fluticasone (Oral Inhalation); Halofantrine; Lapatinib; Lovastatin; Lurasidone; Nilotinib; Nisoldipine; Pimozide; Proton Pump Inhibitors; QuiNIDine; Ranolazine; Rivaroxaban; RomiDEPsin; Salmeterol; Silodosin; Simvastatin; Sirolimus; Tamsulosin; Ticagrelor; Tolvaptan; Toremifene

Increased Effect/Toxicity

Posaconazole may increase the levels/effects of: Alfentanil; Alfuzosin; Almotriptan; Alosetron; Antineoplastic Agents (Vinca Alkaloids); Aprepitant; ARIPiprazole; Benzodiazepines (metabolized by oxidation); Boceprevir; Bortezomib; Bosentan; Brentuximab Vedotin; Brinzolamide; Budesonide (Nasal); Budesonide (Systemic, Oral Inhalation); BusPIRone; Busulfan; Calcium Channel Blockers; CarBAMazepine; Cardiac Glycosides; Ciclesonide; Cilostazol; Cinacalcet; Cisapride; Colchicine; Conivaptan; Corticosteroids (Orally Inhaled); Corticosteroids (Systemic); Crizotinib; CycloSPORINE; CycloSPORINE (Systemic); CYP3A4 Substrates; Dienogest; DOCEtaxel; Dofetilide; Dronedarone; Dutasteride; Eletriptan; Eplerenone; Ergot Derivatives; Erlotinib; Eszopiclone; Etravirine; Everolimus; FentaNYL; Fesoterodine; Fluticasone (Nasal); Fluticasone (Oral Inhalation); Fosamprenavir; Fosaprepitant; Fosphenytoin; Gefitinib; GlipiZIDE; GuanFACINE; Halofantrine; HMG-CoA Reductase Inhibitors; Iloperidone; Imatinib; Irinotecan; Ixabepilone; Lapatinib; Losartan; Lovastatin; Lumefantrine; Lurasidone; Macrolide Antibiotics; Maraviroc; Methadone; MethylPREDNISolone; Nilotinib; Nisoldipine; Paricalcitol; Pazopanib; Phenytoin; Phosphodiesterase 5 Inhibitors; Pimecrolimus; Pimozide; Propafenone; Protease Inhibitors; QuiNIDine; Ramelteon; Ranolazine; Repaglinide; Rifamycin Derivatives; Rivaroxaban; RomiDEPsin; Ruxolitinib; Salmeterol; Saxagliptin; Sildenafil; Silodosin; Simvastatin; Sirolimus; Solifenacin; SORAfenib; SUNItinib; Tacrolimus; Tacrolimus (Systemic); Tacrolimus (Topical); Tadalafil; Tamsulosin; Telaprevir; Temsirolimus; Ticagrelor; Tolterodine; Tolvaptan; Toremifene; Vardenafil; Vemurafenib; Vilazodone; Vitamin K Antagonists; Ziprasidone; Zolpidem; Zuclopenthixol

The levels/effects of Posaconazole may be increased by: Boceprevir; Etravirine; Grapefruit Juice; Macrolide Antibiotics; Protease Inhibitors; Tacrolimus; Telaprevir

Decreased Effect

Posaconazole may decrease the levels/effects of: Amphotericin B; Prasugrel; Saccharomyces boulardii; Ticagrelor

The levels/effects of Posaconazole may be decreased by: Didanosine; Efavirenz; Etravirine; Fosamprenavir; Fosphenytoin; H2-Antagonists; Metoclopramide; Phenytoin; Proton Pump Inhibitors; Rifamycin Derivatives; Sucralfate

Ethanol/Nutrition/Herb Interactions Food: Bioavailability increased ~3 times when posaconazole is administered with a nonfat meal or an oral liquid nutritional supplement; increased ~4 times when administered with a high-fat meal. Grapefruit juice may decrease the levels/effects of posaconazole; concurrent use should be avoided.

Stability Store at 25°C (77°F); excursions permitted to 15°C to 30°C (59°F to 86°F). Do not freeze.

Mechanism of Action Interferes with fungal cytochrome P450 (latosterol-14α-demethylase) activity, decreasing ergosterol synthesis (principal sterol in fungal cell membrane) and inhibiting fungal cell membrane formation.

Pharmacodynamics/Kinetics

Absorption: Coadministration with food, liquid nutritional supplements, and/or acidic carbonated beverages (eg, ginger ale) increases absorption; fasting states do not provide sufficient absorption to ensure adequate plasma concentrations.

Distribution: V_d: 465-1774 L

Protein binding: >98%; predominantly bound to albumin

Metabolism: Not significantly metabolized; ~15% to 17% undergoes non-CYP-mediated metabolism, primarily via hepatic glucuronidation into metabolites

Half-life elimination: 35 hours (range: 20-66 hours)

Time to peak, plasma: ~3-5 hours

Excretion: Feces 71% to 77% (~66% of the total dose as unchanged drug); urine 13% to 14% (<0.2% of the total dose as unchanged drug)

Dosage Oral:

Children ≥13 years and Adults:

Aspergillosis, invasive:

Prophylaxis: 200 mg 3 times/day; duration of therapy is based is based on recovery from neutropenia or immunosuppression

Salvage treatment of refractory infection (unlabeled use): 200 mg 4 times/day initially; after disease stabilization may decrease frequency to 400 mg 2 times/day (Walsh, 2007). **Note:** Duration of therapy should be a minimum of 6-12 weeks or throughout period of immunosuppression (Walsh, 2008).

Candidal infections:

Prophylaxis: 200 mg 3 times/day; duration of therapy is based on recovery from neutropenia or immunosuppression

Treatment of oropharyngeal infection: Initial: 100 mg 2 times/day for 1 day; maintenance: 100 mg once daily for 13 days

Treatment of refractory oropharyngeal infection: 400 mg 2 times/day; duration of therapy is based on underlying disease and clinical response

Adults:

Mucormycosis (unlabeled use): 800 mg/day in 2 or 4 divided doses; duration of therapy is based on response and risk of relapse due to immunosuppression (Greenburg, 2006)

Cryptococcal infections:

Pulmonary, nonimmunosuppressed (unlabeled use): 400 mg 2 times/day. **Note:** Fluconazole is considered first-line treatment (Perfect, 2010).

Salvage treatment of relapsed infection (unlabeled use): 400 mg 2 times/day (or 200 mg 4 times/day) for 10-12 weeks. **Note:** Salvage treatment should only be started after an appropriate course of an induction regimen (Perfect, 2010).

Dosage adjustment in renal impairment:

Mild-to-moderate renal insufficiency (Cl_{cr} 20-80 mL/minute/1.73 m^2): No adjustment necessary

Severe renal insufficiency (Cl_{cr} <20 mL/minute/1.73 m^2): No adjustment necessary; however, monitor for breakthrough fungal infections due to variability in posaconazole exposure.

Dosage adjustment in hepatic impairment:

Mild-to-severe hepatic insufficiency (Child-Pugh classes A, B, and C): No adjustment necessary

Clinical signs and symptoms of liver disease due to posaconazole: Consider discontinuing therapy

Dietary Considerations Give during or within 20 minutes following a full meal or liquid nutritional supplement; alternatively, posaconazole may be administered with an acidic carbonated beverage (eg, ginger ale). Consider alternative antifungal therapy in patients with inadequate oral intake or severe diarrhea/vomiting; if alternative therapy is not an option, closely monitoring for breakthrough fungal infections. Adequate posaconazole absorption from GI tract and subsequent plasma concentrations are dependent on food for efficacy. Lower average plasma concentrations have been associated with an increased risk of treatment failure.

Administration Oral: Shake well before use. Must be administered during or within 20 minutes following a full meal or an oral liquid nutritional supplement; alternatively, posaconazole may be administered with an acidic carbonated beverage (eg, ginger ale). In patients able to swallow, administer oral suspension using dosing spoon provided by the manufacturer; spoon should be rinsed clean with water after each use and before storage.

Monitoring Parameters Hepatic function (eg, AST/ALT, alkaline phosphatase and bilirubin) prior to initiation and during treatment; renal function; electrolyte disturbances (eg, calcium, magnesium, potassium); CBC

Dosage Forms Excipient information presented when available (limited, particularly for generics); consult specific product labeling.

Suspension, oral:

Noxafil®: 40 mg/mL (123 mL) [contains sodium benzoate; cherry flavor; delivers 105 mL of suspension]

◆ **Posanol™ (Can)** *see* Posaconazole *on page 1376*

Potassium Acetate (poe TASS ee um AS e tate)

Pharmacologic Category Electrolyte Supplement, Parenteral

Use Potassium deficiency; to avoid chloride when high concentration of potassium is needed, source of bicarbonate

Pregnancy Risk Factor C

Contraindications Severe renal impairment; hyperkalemia

Warnings/Precautions Close monitoring of serum potassium concentrations is needed to avoid hyperkalemia. Use with caution in patients with renal impairment, cardiac disease, acid/base disorders, or potassium-altering conditions/disorders. Use with caution in digitalized patients or patients receiving concomitant medications or therapies that increase potassium (eg, ACEIs, potassium-sparing diuretics, potassium containing salt substitutes). Do **NOT** administer undiluted or I.V. push; inappropriate parenteral administration may be fatal. Always administer potassium further diluted; refer to appropriate dilution and administration rate recommendations. Pain and phlebitis may occur during parenteral infusion requiring a decrease in infusion rate or potassium concentration. Potassium acetate solution for injection contains aluminum; use caution with impaired renal function and in premature infants.

Adverse Reactions

1% to 10%:

Cardiovascular: Bradycardia

Endocrine & metabolic: Hyperkalemia

Neuromuscular & skeletal: Weakness

Respiratory: Dyspnea

Local: Local tissue necrosis with extravasation

<1% (Limited to important or life-threatening): Abdominal pain, alkalosis, chest pain, mental confusion, paralysis, paresthesia, phlebitis, throat pain

Drug Interactions

Metabolism/Transport Effects None known.

Avoid Concomitant Use There are no known interactions where it is recommended to avoid concomitant use.

Increased Effect/Toxicity

Potassium Acetate may increase the levels/effects of: ACE Inhibitors; Angiotensin II Receptor Blockers; Potassium-Sparing Diuretics

The levels/effects of Potassium Acetate may be increased by: Eplerenone

Decreased Effect There are no known significant interactions involving a decrease in effect.

Mechanism of Action Potassium is the major cation of intracellular fluid and is essential for the conduction of nerve impulses in heart, brain, and skeletal muscle; contraction of cardiac, skeletal and smooth muscles; maintenance of normal renal function, acid-base balance, carbohydrate metabolism, and gastric secretion

Pharmacodynamics/Kinetics

Distribution: Enters cells via active transport from extracellular fluid

Excretion: Primarily urine; skin and feces (small amounts); most intestinal potassium reabsorbed

Dosage I.V. doses should be incorporated into the patient's maintenance I.V. fluids, intermittent I.V. potassium administration should be reserved for severe depletion situations and requires ECG monitoring; doses listed as mEq of potassium

Children:

Treatment of hypokalemia: I.V.: 2-5 mEq/kg/day

I.V. intermittent infusion (must be diluted prior to administration): 0.5-1 mEq/kg/dose (maximum: 30 mEq/dose) to infuse at 0.3-0.5 mEq/kg/hour (maximum: 1 mEq/kg/hour)

Note: Use caution in premature neonates; potassium acetate for injection contains aluminum.

Adults:

Treatment of hypokalemia: I.V.: 40-100 mEq/day

I.V. intermittent infusion (must be diluted prior to administration): 5-10 mEq/dose (maximum: 40 mEq/dose) to infuse over 2-3 hours (maximum: 40 mEq over 1 hour)

Note: Continuous cardiac monitor recommended for rates >0.5 mEq/hour

Potassium dosage/rate of infusion guidelines:

Serum potassium >2.5 mEq/L: Maximum infusion rate: 10 mEq/hour; maximum concentration: 40 mEq/L; maximum 24-hour dose: 200 mEq

Serum potassium <2.5 mEq/L: Maximum infusion rate: 40 mEq/hour; maximum concentration: 80 mEq/L; maximum 24-hour dose: 400 mEq

Dosage adjustment in renal impairment: Use caution; potassium acetate injection contains aluminum

Administration Potassium must be diluted prior to parenteral administration; maximum recommended concentration (peripheral line): 80 mEq/L; maximum recommended concentration (central line): 150 mEq/L or 15 mEq/100 mL; in severely fluid-restricted patients (with central lines): 200 mEq/L or 20 mEq/100 mL has been used; maximum rate of infusion, see Dosage, I.V. intermittent infusion

Monitoring Parameters Serum potassium, magnesium (to facilitate potassium repletion), and bicarbonate; cardiac monitor (if intermittent infusion or potassium infusion rates 0.5 mEq/kg/hour in children or >10 mEq/hour in adults); to assess adequate replacement, repeat serum potassium level 2-4 hours after dose

Reference Range Note: Reference ranges may vary depending on the laboratory

Serum potassium: 3.5-5.2 mEq/L

Additional Information 1 mEq of acetate is equivalent to the alkalinizing effect of 1 mEq of bicarbonate.

Dosage Forms Excipient information presented when available (limited, particularly for generics); consult specific product labeling. [DSC] = Discontinued product

Injection, solution: 2 mEq/mL (20 mL, 50 mL)

Injection, solution [preservative free]: 2 mEq/mL (20 mL, 100 mL [DSC])

Injection, solution [concentrate, preservative free]: 4 mEq/mL (50 mL)

Potassium Acid Phosphate

(poe TASS ee um AS id FOS fate)

Brand Names: U.S. K-Phos® Original

Pharmacologic Category Urinary Acidifying Agent

Use Acidifies urine and lowers urinary calcium concentration; reduces odor and rash caused by ammoniacal urine; increases the antibacterial activity of methenamine

Pregnancy Risk Factor C

Contraindications Severe renal impairment; hyperkalemia, hyperphosphatemia; infected magnesium ammonium phosphate stones

Warnings/Precautions Use with caution in patients receiving concomitant medications or therapies that increase potassium (eg, ACEI, potassium-sparing diuretics, potassium containing salt substitutes). Use caution in patients with renal insufficiency or severe tissue breakdown (eg, chemotherapy or hemodialysis). May cause GI upset (eg, nausea, vomiting, diarrhea, abdominal pain, discomfort) and lead to GI ulceration, bleeding, perforation and/or obstruction. Close monitoring of serum potassium concentrations is needed to avoid hyperkalemia.

Adverse Reactions

>10%: Gastrointestinal: Diarrhea, nausea, stomach pain, flatulence, vomiting

1% to 10%:

Cardiovascular: Bradycardia

Endocrine & metabolic: Hyperkalemia

Local: Local tissue necrosis with extravasation

Neuromuscular & skeletal: Weakness

Respiratory: Dyspnea

<1% (Limited to important or life-threatening): Arrhythmia, dyspnea, edema, hyperphosphatemia, hypocalcemia, mental confusion, paralysis, paresthesia, tetany

Drug Interactions

Metabolism/Transport Effects None known.

Avoid Concomitant Use There are no known interactions where it is recommended to avoid concomitant use.

Increased Effect/Toxicity

Potassium Acid Phosphate may increase the levels/effects of: ACE Inhibitors; Angiotensin II Receptor Blockers; Potassium-Sparing Diuretics; Salicylates

The levels/effects of Potassium Acid Phosphate may be increased by: Eplerenone

Decreased Effect There are no known significant interactions involving a decrease in effect.

Mechanism of Action The principal intracellular cation; involved in transmission of nerve impulses, muscle contractions, enzyme activity, and glucose utilization

Pharmacodynamics/Kinetics

Absorption: Well absorbed from upper GI tract

Distribution: Enters cells via active transport from extracellular fluid

Excretion: Primarily urine; skin and feces (small amounts); most intestinal potassium reabsorbed

Dosage Adults: Oral: 1000 mg dissolved in 6-8 oz of water 4 times/day with meals and at bedtime; for best results, soak tablets in water for 2-5 minutes, then stir and swallow

Dietary Considerations May be taken with meals.

Monitoring Parameters Serum potassium, phosphorus, calcium; serum salicylates (if taking salicylates)

Reference Range Note: Reference ranges may vary depending on the laboratory

Serum phosphorus: Both low and high ends of the normal range are higher in children than in adults.

Infants: 4.5-7.5 mg/dL (1.45-2.42 mmol/L)

Children: ~4-6 mg/dL (1.29-1.94 mmol/L)

Adults: 2.5-4.5 mg/dL (0.81-1.45 mmol/L)

Urinary pH: 4.6-8.0

Test Interactions Decreased ammonia (B)

Dosage Forms Excipient information presented when available (limited, particularly for generics); consult specific product labeling.

Tablet, oral:

K-Phos® Original: 500 mg [scored; phosphorus 114 mg and potassium 144 mg (3.7 mEq) per tablet]

Potassium Bicarbonate and Potassium Chloride

(poe TASS ee um bye KAR bun ate & poe TASS ee um KLOR ide)

Index Terms K-Lyte/Cl; Potassium Bicarbonate and Potassium Chloride (Effervescent)

Pharmacologic Category Electrolyte Supplement, Oral

Use Treatment or prevention of hypokalemia

Pregnancy Risk Factor C

Dosage Oral:

Children: 1-4 mEq/kg/24 hours in divided doses as required to maintain normal serum potassium

Adults:

Prevention: 16-24 mEq/day in 2-4 divided doses

Treatment: 40-100 mEq/day in 2-4 divided doses

Additional Information Complete prescribing information for this medication should be consulted for additional detail.

Dosage Forms Excipient information presented when available (limited, particularly for generics); consult specific product labeling.

Tablet for solution, oral [effervescent]: Potassium chloride 25 mEq [potassium bicarbonate 0.5 g and potassium chloride 1.5 g]

◆ **Potassium Bicarbonate and Potassium Chloride (Effervescent)** *see* Potassium Bicarbonate and Potassium Chloride *on page* 1380

Potassium Bicarbonate and Potassium Citrate

(poe TASS ee um bye KAR bun ate & poe TASS ee um SIT rate)

Brand Names: U.S. Effer-K®; Klor-Con®/EF

Index Terms Potassium Bicarbonate and Potassium Citrate (Effervescent)

Pharmacologic Category Electrolyte Supplement, Oral

Use Treatment or prevention of hypokalemia

Pregnancy Risk Factor C

Dosage Oral:

Children: 1-4 mEq/kg/24 hours in divided doses as required to maintain normal serum potassium

Adults:

Prevention: 16-24 mEq/day in 2-4 divided doses

Treatment: 40-100 mEq/day in 2-4 divided doses

Additional Information Complete prescribing information for this medication should be consulted for additional detail.

Dosage Forms Excipient information presented when available (limited, particularly for generics); consult specific product labeling.

Tablet for solution, oral [effervescent]:

Effer-K®: Potassium 10 mEq [unflavored and cherry vanilla flavor]

Effer-K®: Potassium 20 mEq [unflavored and orange cream flavor]

Effer-K®: Potassium 25 mEq [unflavored, orange, lemon citrus, and cherry berry flavor]

Klor-Con®/EF: Potassium 25 mEq [sugar free; orange flavor]

◆ **Potassium Bicarbonate and Potassium Citrate (Effervescent)** *see* Potassium Bicarbonate and Potassium Citrate *on page* 1380

Potassium Chloride (poe TASS ee um KLOR ide)

Brand Names: U.S. Epiklor™; Epiklor™/25; K-Tab®; Kaon-CL® 10; Klor-Con®; Klor-Con® 10; Klor-Con® 8; Klor-Con® M10; Klor-Con® M15; Klor-Con® M20; Klor-Con®/25; microK®; microK® 10

Brand Names: Canada Apo-K®; K-10®; K-Dur®; Micro-K Extencaps®; Roychlor®; Slo-Pot; Slow-K®

Index Terms KCl; Kdur

Pharmacologic Category Electrolyte Supplement, Oral; Electrolyte Supplement, Parenteral

Use Treatment or prevention of hypokalemia

Pregnancy Risk Factor C

Pregnancy Considerations Reproduction studies have not been conducted. Potassium supplementation (that does not cause maternal hyperkalemia) would not be expected to cause adverse fetal events.

Lactation Enters breast milk/compatible

Contraindications Hypersensitivity to any component of the formulation; hyperkalemia. In addition, solid oral dosage forms are contraindicated in patients in whom there is a structural, pathological, and/or pharmacologic cause for delay or arrest in passage through the GI tract.

Warnings/Precautions Close monitoring of serum potassium concentrations is needed to avoid hyperkalemia. Use with caution in patients with renal impairment, cardiac disease, acid/base disorders, or potassium-altering conditions/disorders. Use with caution in digitalized patients or patients receiving concomitant medications or therapies that increase potassium (eg, ACEI, potassium-sparing diuretics, potassium containing salt substitutes). Do **NOT** administer undiluted or I.V. push; inappropriate parenteral administration may be fatal. Always administer potassium further diluted; refer to appropriate dilution and administration rate recommendations. Pain and phlebitis may occur during parenteral infusion requiring a decrease in infusion rate or potassium concentration. Avoid administering potassium diluted in dextrose solutions during initial therapy; potential for transient decreases in serum potassium due to intracellular shift of potassium from dextrose-stimulated insulin release. May cause GI upset (eg, nausea, vomiting, diarrhea, abdominal pain, discomfort) and lead to GI ulceration, bleeding, perforation, and/or obstruction. Oral liquid preparations (not solid) should be used in patients with esophageal compression or delayed gastric emptying.

Adverse Reactions Frequency not defined.

Dermatologic: Rash

Endocrine & metabolic: Hyperkalemia

Gastrointestinal: Abdominal pain/discomfort, diarrhea, flatulence, GI bleeding (oral), GI obstruction (oral), GI perforation (oral), nausea, vomiting

Drug Interactions

Metabolism/Transport Effects None known.

Avoid Concomitant Use

Avoid concomitant use of Potassium Chloride with any of the following: Glycopyrrolate

Increased Effect/Toxicity

Potassium Chloride may increase the levels/effects of: ACE Inhibitors; Angiotensin II Receptor Blockers; Potassium-Sparing Diuretics

The levels/effects of Potassium Chloride may be increased by: Anticholinergic Agents; Eplerenone; Glycopyrrolate

Decreased Effect There are no known significant interactions involving a decrease in effect.

Stability

Capsule: MicroK®: Store between 20°C to 25°C (68°F to 77°F).

Powder for oral solution: Klor-Con®: Store at room temperature of 15°C to 30°C (59°F to 86°F).

Solution for injection: Store at room temperature; do not freeze. Use only clear solutions. Use admixtures within 24 hours.

Tablet: K-Tab®: Store below 30°C (86°F).

Mechanism of Action Potassium is the major cation of intracellular fluid and is essential for the conduction of nerve impulses in heart, brain, and skeletal muscle; contraction of cardiac, skeletal and smooth muscles; maintenance of normal renal function, acid-base balance, carbohydrate metabolism, and gastric secretion

Pharmacodynamics/Kinetics

Absorption: Well absorbed from upper GI tract

Distribution: Enters cells via active transport from extracellular fluid

Excretion: Primarily urine; skin and feces (small amounts); most intestinal potassium reabsorbed

Dosage I.V. doses should be incorporated into the patient's maintenance I.V. fluids; intermittent I.V. potassium administration should be reserved for severe depletion situations in patients undergoing ECG monitoring. Doses expressed as mEq of potassium.

Normal daily requirements: Oral, I.V.:

- Children: 1-2 mEq/kg/day
- Adults: 40-80 mEq/day

Prevention of hypokalemia: Oral:

- Children: 1-2 mEq/kg/day in 1-2 divided doses
- Adults: 20-40 mEq/day in 1-2 divided doses

Treatment of hypokalemia: Children:

Oral: 1-2 mEq/kg initially, then as needed based on frequently obtained lab values. If deficits are severe or ongoing losses are great, I.V. route should be considered.

I.V. intermittent infusion: 0.5-1 mEq/kg/dose (maximum dose: 40 mEq). If infusion exceeds 0.5 mEq/kg/hour, physician should be at bedside and patient should have continuous ECG monitoring; repeat as needed based on frequently obtained lab values.

Treatment of hypokalemia: Adults:

Oral:

Asymptomatic, mild hypokalemia: Usual dosage range: 40-100 mEq/day divided in 2-5 doses; generally recommended to limit doses to 20-25 mEq/dose to avoid GI discomfort.

Mild-to-moderate hypokalemia: Some clinicians may administer up to 120-240 mEq/day divided in 3-4 doses; generally recommended to limit doses to 40-60 mEq/dose. If deficits are severe or ongoing losses are great, I.V. route should be considered.

I.V. intermittent infusion: Peripheral or central line: ≤10 mEq/hour; repeat as needed based on frequently obtained lab values; central line infusion and continuous ECG monitoring highly recommended for infusions >10 mEq/hour.

Potassium dosage/rate of infusion general guidelines (per product labeling): **Note:** High variability exists in dosing/infusion rate recommendations; therapy guided by patient condition and specific institutional guidelines.

Serum potassium >2.5 mEq/L: Maximum infusion rate: 10 mEq/hour; maximum concentration: 40 mEq/L; maximum 24-hour dose: 200 mEq

Serum potassium <2 mEq/L and symptomatic (excluding emergency treatment of cardiac arrest): Maximum infusion rate (central line only): 40 mEq/hour in presence of continuous ECG monitoring and frequent lab monitoring; In selected situations, patients may require up to 400 mEq/24 hours.

Dietary Considerations Administer with plenty of fluid to decrease stomach irritation and discomfort. Some dietary sources of potassium include leafy green vegetables (eg, spinach, cabbage), tomatoes, cucumbers, zucchini, fruits (eg, apples, oranges, and bananas), root vegetables (eg, carrots, radishes), beans, and peas.

Administration

Parenteral: Potassium must be diluted prior to parenteral administration. Do not administer I.V. push. In general, the dose, concentration of infusion and rate of administration may be dependent on patient condition and specific institution policy. Some clinicians recommend that the maximum concentration for peripheral infusion is 10 mEq/100 mL and maximum rate of administration for peripheral infusion is 10 mEq/hour. ECG monitoring is recommended for peripheral or central infusions >10 mEq/hour in adults. Concentrations and rates of infusion may be greater with central line administration. Some clinicians recommend that the maximum concentration for central infusion is 20-40 mEq/100 mL and maximum rate of administration for central infusion is 40 mEq/hour.

Oral: Oral dosage forms should be taken with meals and a full glass of water or other liquid to minimize the risk of GI irritation. Prescribing information for the various oral preparations recommend that no more than 20 mEq or 25 mEq should be given as single dose.

Capsule: MicroK®: Swallow whole, do not chew. Capsules may also be opened and contents sprinkled on a spoonful of applesauce or pudding and should be swallowed immediately without chewing.

Powder: Klor-Con®: Dissolve one packet in 4-5 ounces of water or other beverage prior to administration.

Tablet:

K-Tab®, Kaon-Cl®, Klor-Con®: Swallow tablets whole; do not crush, chew, or suck on tablet.

Klor-Con® M: Swallow tablets whole; do not crush, chew, or suck on tablet. Tablet may also be broken in half and each half swallowed separately; the whole tablet may be dissolved in ~4 ounces of water (allow ~2 minutes to dissolve, stir well and drink immediately)

Monitoring Parameters Serum potassium, chloride, magnesium (to facilitate potassium repletion), cardiac monitor (if intermittent infusion or potassium infusion rates 0.5 mEq/kg/hour in children or >10 mEq/hour in adults); to assess adequate replacement, repeat serum potassium level 2-4 hours after dose

Reference Range Note: Reference ranges may vary depending on the laboratory

Serum potassium: 3.5-5.2 mEq/L

Dosage Forms Excipient information presented when available (limited, particularly for generics); consult specific product labeling. [DSC] = Discontinued product

Capsule, extended release, microencapsulated, oral: 8 mEq, 10 mEq
- microK®: 8 mEq [600 mg]
- microK® 10: 10 mEq [750 mg]

Infusion, premixed in 1/2 NS: 20 mEq (1000 mL)

Infusion, premixed in D_{10} 1/4 NS: 5 mEq (250 mL [DSC])

Infusion, premixed in D_5 1/2 NS: 10 mEq (500 mL, 1000 mL); 20 mEq (1000 mL); 30 mEq (1000 mL); 40 mEq (1000 mL)

Infusion, premixed in D_5 1/3 NS: 20 mEq (1000 mL)

Infusion, premixed in D_5 1/4 NS: 5 mEq (250 mL); 10 mEq (500 mL, 1000 mL [DSC]); 20 mEq (1000 mL); 30 mEq (1000 mL [DSC]); 40 mEq (1000 mL)

Infusion, premixed in D_5LR: 20 mEq (1000 mL)

Infusion, premixed in D_5NS: 20 mEq (1000 mL); 40 mEq (1000 mL)

Infusion, premixed in D_5W: 20 mEq (1000 mL); 40 mEq (1000 mL)

Infusion, premixed in NS: 20 mEq (1000 mL); 40 mEq (1000 mL)

Infusion, premixed in water for injection [highly concentrated]: 10 mEq (50 mL, 100 mL); 20 mEq (50 mL, 100 mL); 30 mEq (100 mL); 40 mEq (100 mL)

Injection, solution [concentrate]: 2 mEq/mL (5 mL, 10 mL, 15 mL, 20 mL, 30 mL, 250 mL, 500 mL [DSC])

Injection, solution [concentrate, preservative free]: 2 mEq/mL (5 mL, 10 mL, 15 mL, 20 mL)

Powder for solution, oral:
- Epiklor™: 20 mEq/packet (30s, 100s) [sugar free; orange flavor]
- Epiklor™/25: 25 mEq/packet (30s, 100s) [sugar free; orange flavor]
- Klor-Con®: 20 mEq/packet (30s, 100s) [sugar free; fruit flavor]
- Klor-Con®/25: 25 mEq/packet (30s, 100s) [sugar free; fruit flavor]

Solution, oral: 20 mEq/15 mL (15 mL, 30 mL, 473 mL); 40 mEq/15 mL (15 mL, 473 mL)

Tablet, extended release, oral: 10 mEq

Tablet, extended release, microencapsulated, oral: 8 mEq, 10 mEq, 20 mEq
- Klor-Con® M10: 10 mEq [750 mg]
- Klor-Con® M15: 15 mEq [scored; 1125 mg]
- Klor-Con® M20: 20 mEq [scored; 1500 mg]

Tablet, extended release, wax matrix, oral: 8 mEq, 10 mEq
- K-Tab®: 10 mEq [750 mg]
- Kaon-CL® 10: 10 mEq [750 mg]
- Klor-Con® 8: 8 mEq [600 mg]
- Klor-Con® 10: 10 mEq [750 mg]

Potassium Citrate and Citric Acid

(poe TASS ee um SIT rate & SI trik AS id)

Brand Names: U.S. Cytra-K

Index Terms Citric Acid and Potassium Citrate; Polycitra K

Pharmacologic Category Alkalinizing Agent, Oral

Use Treatment of metabolic acidosis; alkalinizing agent in conditions where long-term maintenance of an alkaline urine is desirable

Pregnancy Risk Factor A

Dosage Urine alkalizing agent:

Children: Solution: 5-15 mL after meals and at bedtime; adjust dose based on urinary pH

Adults:
- Powder: One packet dissolved in water after meals and at bedtime; adjust dose to urinary pH
- Solution: 15-30 mL after meals and at bedtime; adjust dose based on urinary pH

Additional Information Complete prescribing information for this medication should be consulted for additional detail.

Dosage Forms Excipient information presented when available (limited, particularly for generics); consult specific product labeling.

Powder for solution, oral:
- Cytra-K: Potassium citrate monohydrate 3300 mg and citric acid monohydrate 1002 mg per packet (100s) [sugar free; fruit-punch flavor; each packet contains potassium 30 mEq equivalent to bicarbonate 30 mEq]

Solution: Potassium citrate monohydrate 1100 mg and citric acid monohydrate 334 mg per 5 mL (480 mL)
- Cytra-K: Potassium citrate monohydrate 1100 mg and citric acid monohydrate 334 mg per 5 mL (480 mL) [ethanol free, sugar free; contains propylene glycol; cherry flavor; contains potassium 2 mEq/mL equivalent to bicarbonate 2 mEq /mL]

◆ **Potassium Citrate, Citric Acid, and Sodium Citrate** *see* Citric Acid, Sodium Citrate, and Potassium Citrate *on page 372*

Potassium Gluconate

(poe TASS ee um GLOO coe nate)

Pharmacologic Category Electrolyte Supplement, Oral

Use Treatment or prevention of hypokalemia

Pregnancy Risk Factor A

Contraindications Severe renal impairment, untreated Addison's disease, heat cramps, hyperkalemia, severe tissue trauma; solid oral dosage forms are contraindicated in patients in whom there is a structural, pathological, and/or pharmacologic cause for delay or arrest in passage through the GI tract

Warnings/Precautions Use caution in patients with acid/base disorders, cardiovascular disease, potassium-altering conditions/disorders, or renal impairment. Use with caution in patients receiving concomitant medications or therapies that increase potassium (eg, ACEI, potassium-sparing diuretics, potassium containing salt substitutes). Close monitoring of serum potassium concentrations is needed to avoid hyperkalemia. May cause GI upset (eg, nausea, vomiting, diarrhea, abdominal pain, discomfort) and lead to GI ulceration, bleeding, perforation and/or obstruction. Oral liquid preparations (not solid) should be used in patients with esophageal compression or delayed gastric emptying.

Adverse Reactions

>10%: Gastrointestinal: Diarrhea, nausea, stomach pain, flatulence, vomiting (oral)

1% to 10%:
- Cardiovascular: Bradycardia
- Endocrine & metabolic: Hyperkalemia
- Neuromuscular & skeletal: Weakness
- Respiratory: Dyspnea

<1% (Limited to important or life-threatening): Mental confusion, paralysis, paresthesia, phlebitis

Drug Interactions

Metabolism/Transport Effects None known.

Avoid Concomitant Use There are no known interactions where it is recommended to avoid concomitant use.

Increased Effect/Toxicity

Potassium Gluconate may increase the levels/effects of: ACE Inhibitors; Angiotensin II Receptor Blockers; Potassium-Sparing Diuretics

The levels/effects of Potassium Gluconate may be increased by: Eplerenone

Decreased Effect There are no known significant interactions involving a decrease in effect.

Stability Store at room temperature.

Mechanism of Action Potassium is the major cation of intracellular fluid and is essential for the conduction of nerve impulses in heart, brain, and skeletal muscle; contraction of cardiac, skeletal and smooth muscles; maintenance of normal renal function, acid-base balance, carbohydrate metabolism, and gastric secretion

Pharmacodynamics/Kinetics

Absorption: Well absorbed from upper GI tract

Distribution: Enters cells via active transport from extracellular fluid

Excretion: Primarily urine; skin and feces (small amounts); most intestinal potassium reabsorbed

Dosage Oral: **Note:** Doses listed as mEq of potassium (approximately 4.3 mEq potassium/g potassium gluconate, and 1 mEq potassium is equivalent to 39 mg elemental potassium):

Normal daily requirement:
- Children: 2-3 mEq/kg/day
- Adults: 40-80 mEq/day

Prevention of hypokalemia during diuretic therapy:
- Children: 1-2 mEq/kg/day in 1-2 divided doses
- Adults: 16-24 mEq/day in 1-2 divided doses

Treatment of hypokalemia:
- Children: 2-5 mEq/kg/day in 2-4 divided doses
- Adults: 40-100 mEq/day in 2-4 divided doses

Monitoring Parameters Serum potassium and magnesium (to facilitate potassium repletion)

Reference Range Note: Reference ranges may vary depending on the laboratory

Serum potassium: 3.5-5.2 mEq/L

Test Interactions Decreased ammonia (B)

Additional Information 9.4 g potassium gluconate is approximately equal to 40 mEq potassium (4.3 mEq potassium/g potassium gluconate).

Dosage Forms Excipient information presented when available (limited, particularly for generics); consult specific product labeling.

Caplet, oral: 595 mg [equivalent to potassium 99 mg]

Capsule, oral [strength expressed as base]: 99 mg

Tablet, oral: 550 mg [equivalent to potassium 90 mg], 595 mg [equivalent to potassium 99 mg]

Tablet, oral [strength expressed as base]: 99 mg

Tablet, timed release, oral [strength expressed as base]: 95 mg

Potassium Iodide (poe TASS ee um EYE oh dide)

Brand Names: U.S. iOSAT™ [OTC]; SSKI®; ThyroSafe™; Thyroshield™ [OTC]

Index Terms KI

Pharmacologic Category Antithyroid Agent; Expectorant

Use Expectorant for the symptomatic treatment of chronic pulmonary diseases complicated by mucous; block thyroidal uptake of radioactive isotopes of iodine in a radiation emergency

Unlabeled Use Lymphocutaneous and cutaneous sporotrichosis; reduce thyroid vascularity prior to thyroidectomy; management of thyrotoxic crisis; block thyroidal uptake of radioactive isotopes of iodine after therapeutic or diagnostic exposure to radioactive iodine

Pregnancy Risk Factor D

Pregnancy Considerations Iodide crosses the placenta (may cause hypothyroidism and goiter in fetus/newborn). Use as an expectorant during pregnancy is contraindicated by the AAP. Use for protection against thyroid cancer secondary to radioactive iodine exposure is considered acceptable based upon risk:benefit, keeping in mind the dose and duration. Repeat dosing should be avoided if possible.

Lactation Enters breast milk/use caution (AAP rates "compatible"; AAP 2001 update pending)

Contraindications Hypersensitivity to iodine or any component of the formulation; dermatitis herpetiformis; hypocomplementemic vasculitis, nodular thyroid condition with heart disease

Warnings/Precautions Prolonged use can lead to hypothyroidism; cystic fibrosis patients have an exaggerated response; can cause acne flare-ups, can cause dermatitis; use with caution in patients with a history of renal impairment, hyperthyroidism, Addison's disease, cardiac disease, myotonia congenita, tuberculosis, acute bronchitis; use with caution in patients receiving concomitant medications or therapies that increase potassium (eg, ACEI, potassium-sparing diuretics, potassium containing salt substitutes). Potassium iodide must be administered prior to receiving radiopharmaceuticals that require thyroid gland protection.

Adverse Reactions Frequency not defined.

Cardiovascular: Irregular heart beat

Central nervous system: Confusion, tiredness, fever

Dermatologic: Skin rash

Endocrine & metabolic: Goiter, salivary gland swelling/tenderness, thyroid adenoma, swelling of neck/throat, myxedema, lymph node swelling, hyper-/hypothyroidism

Gastrointestinal: Diarrhea, gastrointestinal bleeding, metallic taste, nausea, stomach pain, stomach upset, vomiting

Neuromuscular & skeletal: Joint pain, numbness, tingling, weakness

Miscellaneous: Chronic iodine poisoning (with prolonged treatment/high doses); iodism, hypersensitivity reactions (angioedema, cutaneous and mucosal hemorrhage, serum sickness-like symptoms)

Drug Interactions

Metabolism/Transport Effects None known.

Avoid Concomitant Use

Avoid concomitant use of Potassium Iodide with any of the following: Sodium Iodide I131

Increased Effect/Toxicity

Potassium Iodide may increase the levels/effects of: ACE Inhibitors; Angiotensin II Receptor Blockers; Cardiac Glycosides; Lithium; Potassium-Sparing Diuretics; Theophylline Derivatives

The levels/effects of Potassium Iodide may be increased by: Eplerenone

Decreased Effect

Potassium Iodide may decrease the levels/effects of: Sodium Iodide I131; Vitamin K Antagonists

Stability Store at controlled room temperature of 25°C (77°F); excursions permitted to 15°C to 30°C (59°F to 86°F). Protect from light; keep tightly closed.

SSKI®: If exposed to cold, crystallization may occur. Warm and shake to redissolve. If solution becomes brown/yellow, it should be discarded. May be mixed in water, fruit juice, or milk.

Mechanism of Action Reduces viscosity of mucus by increasing respiratory tract secretions; inhibits secretion of thyroid hormone, fosters colloid accumulation in thyroid follicles. Following radioactive iodine exposure, potassium iodide blocks uptake of radioiodine by the thyroid, reducing the risk of thyroid cancer.

Pharmacodynamics/Kinetics

Onset of action: Hyperthyroidism: 24-48 hours

Peak effect: 10-15 days after continuous therapy

Duration: Radioactive iodine exposure: ~24 hours

Dosage Oral:

Adults: RDA: 150 mcg (iodine)

Expectorant: Adults: SSKI®: 300-600 mg 3-4 times/day

Preparation for thyroidectomy (unlabeled use):

Children: 150-350 mg (3-7 drops **or** 0.15-0.35 mL SSKI®) 3 times/day; administer for 10 days before surgery; if not euthyroid prior to surgery, consider concurrent beta-blockade (eg, propranolol) in the immediate preoperative period to reduce the risk of thyroid storm (Bahn, 2011)

Adults: 50-100 mg (1-2 drops **or** 0.05-0.1 mL SSKI®) 3 times/day; administer for 10 days before surgery; if not euthyroid prior to surgery, consider concurrent beta-blockade (eg, propranolol) in the immediate preoperative period to reduce the risk of thyroid storm (Bahn, 2011)

To reduce risk of thyroid cancer following nuclear accident (Iosat™, ThyroSafe™, ThyroShield™): Dosing should continue until risk of exposure has passed or other measures are implemented:

Children 1 month to 3 years: 32.5 mg once daily

Children 3-18 years: 65 mg once daily

Children >68 kg and Adults (including pregnant/lactating women): 130 mg once daily

Thyroid gland protection during radiopharmaceutical use (unlabeled use):

Note: Begin at 1-48 hours prior to exposure. Continue potassium iodide after radiopharmaceutical administration until risk of exposure has diminished (treatment duration and time of initiation is dependent on the radiopharmaceutical, consult specific protocol).

Children (Giammarile, 2008; Olivier, 2003):

Infants <5 kg: 16 mg once daily

1 month to 3 years or 5-15 kg: 32 mg once daily

3-13 years or 15-50 kg: 65 mg once daily

>13 years or >50 kg: 130 mg once daily

Adults: Tablet: 130 mg once daily or Solution (SSKI®): 4 drops 3 times/day

Thyrotoxic crisis/thyroid storm (unlabeled use): **Note:** Administer at least 1-2 hours after antithyroid drug administration:

Infants: 100 mg (2 drops **or** 0.1 mL SSKI®) 4 times/day (Eyal, 2008)

Children: 250 mg (5 drops **or** 0.25 mL SSKI®) 2-4 times/day (Eyal, 2008)

Adults: 250 mg (5 drops **or** 0.25 mL SSKI®) every 6 hours (Bahn, 2011)

Sporotrichosis (cutaneous, lymphocutaneous; unlabeled use): Adults: Initial: 5 drops (SSKI®) 3 times/day; increase to 40-50 drops (SSKI®) 3 times/day as tolerated until 2-4 weeks after lesions have resolved (usual duration 3-6 months) (Kauffman, 2007)

Dietary Considerations SSKI®: Take with food to decrease gastric irritation.

Administration SSKI®: Dilute in a glassful of water, fruit juice, or milk. Take with food to decrease gastric irritation.

Monitoring Parameters Thyroid function tests, signs/symptoms of hyperthyroidism; thyroid function should be monitored in pregnant women, neonates, and young infants if repeat doses are required following radioactive iodine exposure

Test Interactions May alter thyroid function tests.

Additional Information 10 drops of SSKI® = potassium iodide 500 mg

Dosage Forms Excipient information presented when available (limited, particularly for generics); consult specific product labeling.

Solution, oral:

SSKI®: 1 g/mL (30 mL, 237 mL)

Thyroshield™: 65 mg/mL (30 mL) [black raspberry flavor]

Tablet, oral:

iOSAT™: 130 mg [scored]

ThyroSafe™: 65 mg [scored; equivalent to iodine 50 mg]

Extemporaneous Preparations A 16.25 mg/5 mL oral solution may be made with tablets. Crush one 130 mg tablet and reduce to a fine powder. Add 20 mL of water and mix until powder is dissolved. Add an additional 20 mL of low-fat milk (white or chocolate), orange juice, flat soda, raspberry syrup, or infant formula. Stable for 7 days under refrigeration.

To prepare an 8.125 mg/5 mL oral solution, crush one 65 mg tablet and reduce to a fine powder. Add 20 mL of water and mix until powder is dissolved. Add an additional 20 mL of low-fat milk (white or chocolate), orange juice, flat soda, raspberry syrup, or infant formula. Stable for 7 days under refrigeration.

Potassium Iodide and Iodine

(poe TASS ee um EYE oh dide & EYE oh dine)

Index Terms Iodine and Potassium Iodide; Lugol's Solution; Strong Iodine Solution

Pharmacologic Category Antithyroid Agent

Use Topical antiseptic

Unlabeled Use Reduce thyroid vascularity prior to thyroidectomy and management of thyrotoxic crisis; block thyroidal uptake of radioactive isotopes of iodine in a radiation emergency or after therapeutic/diagnostic use of radioactive iodine

Pregnancy Risk Factor D (potassium iodide)

Pregnancy Considerations Iodide crosses the placenta (may cause hypothyroidism and goiter in fetus/newborn). Use for protection against thyroid cancer secondary to radioactive iodine exposure is considered acceptable based upon risk/benefit, keeping in mind the dose and duration. Repeat dosing should be avoided if possible.

Lactation Enters breast milk/use caution (AAP rates "compatible"; AAP 2001 update pending)

Contraindications Hypersensitivity to iodine or any component of the formulation; iodine-induced goiter; dermatitis herpetiformis; hypocomplementemic vasculitis; nodular thyroid disease with heart disease

Warnings/Precautions Prolonged use can lead to hypothyroidism; cystic fibrosis patients have an exaggerated response; can cause acne flare-ups and/or dermatitis; use with caution in patients with a history of renal impairment, hyperthyroidism, Addison's disease, cardiac disease, myotonia congenita, tuberculosis, acute bronchitis. Use with caution in patients receiving concomitant medications or therapies that increase potassium (eg, ACEI, potassium-sparing diuretics, potassium containing salt substitutes). Potassium iodide and iodine solution must be administered prior to receiving radiopharmaceuticals that require thyroid gland protection.

Adverse Reactions Frequency not defined.

Cardiovascular: Irregular heart beat

Central nervous system: Confusion, tiredness, fever

Dermatologic: Skin rash

Endocrine & metabolic: Goiter, salivary gland swelling/tenderness, thyroid adenoma, swelling of neck/throat, myxedema, lymph node swelling, hyper-/hypothyroidism

Gastrointestinal: Diarrhea, gastrointestinal bleeding, metallic taste, nausea, stomach pain, stomach upset, vomiting

Neuromuscular & skeletal: Numbness, tingling, weakness, joint pain

Miscellaneous: Chronic iodine poisoning (with prolonged treatment/high doses); iodism, hypersensitivity reactions (angioedema, cutaneous and mucosal hemorrhage, serum sickness-like symptoms)

Drug Interactions

Metabolism/Transport Effects None known.

Avoid Concomitant Use

Avoid concomitant use of Potassium Iodide and Iodine with any of the following: Sodium Iodide I131

Increased Effect/Toxicity

Potassium Iodide and Iodine may increase the levels/effects of: ACE Inhibitors; Angiotensin II Receptor Blockers; Cardiac Glycosides; Lithium; Potassium-Sparing Diuretics; Theophylline Derivatives

The levels/effects of Potassium Iodide and Iodine may be increased by: Eplerenone

Decreased Effect

Potassium Iodide and Iodine may decrease the levels/effects of: Sodium Iodide I131; Vitamin K Antagonists

Stability Store at controlled room temperature of 25°C (77°F); excursions permitted to 15°C to 30°C (59°F to 86°F). Protect from light and keep container tightly closed.

Mechanism of Action In hyperthyroidism, iodine temporarily inhibits thyroid hormone synthesis and secretion into the circulation; use also decreases thyroid gland size and vascularity. Serum T_4 and T_3 concentrations can be reduced for several weeks with use but effect will not be maintained.

Following radioactive iodine exposure, potassium iodide blocks uptake of radioiodine by the thyroid, reducing the risk of thyroid cancer.

Pharmacodynamics/Kinetics

Onset of action: Hyperthyroidism: 24-48 hours

Peak effect: 10-15 days after continuous therapy

Dosage Oral:

Children and Adults:

Thyrotoxic crisis (unlabeled use):

Children: 4-8 drops 3 times/day; begin therapy preferably 2 hours following the initial dose of propylthiouracil or alternatively, methimazole (Eyal, 2008)

Adults: 4-8 drops every 6-8 hours; begin administration ≥1 hour following the initial dose of either propylthiouracil or methimazole (Nayak, 2006)

Adults:

RDA: 150 mcg (iodine)

Preparation for thyroidectomy (unlabeled use): 5-7 drops (0.25-0.35 mL) 3 times/day; administer for 10 days before surgery; if not euthyroid prior to surgery, consider concurrent beta-blockade (eg, propranolol) in the immediate preoperative period to reduce the risk of thyroid storm (Bahn, 2011)

Thyroid gland protection during radiopharmaceutical use (unlabeled use): 1 drop/kg/day; (maximum: 40 drops/day or 20 drops twice daily) (Giammarile, 2008); alternatively, 20 drops 3 times/day has also been used (Bexxar® prescribing information, 2005)

Note: Initiate 1-48 hours prior to radiopharmaceutical exposure and continue after radiopharmaceutical administration until risk of exposure has diminished (treatment initiation time and duration is dependent on the radiopharmaceutical agent used, consult specific protocol or labeling.

Monitoring Parameters Thyroid function tests, signs/symptoms of hyperthyroidism; thyroid function should be monitored in pregnant women, neonates, and young infants if repeat doses are required following radioactive iodine exposure

Test Interactions May alter thyroid function tests.

Dosage Forms Excipient information presented when available (limited, particularly for generics); consult specific product labeling.

Solution, oral: Potassium iodide 100 mg/mL and iodine 50 mg/mL (473 mL)

Solution, topical: Potassium iodide 100 mg/mL and iodine 50 mg/mL (8 mL)

Potassium Phosphate (poe TASS ee um FOS fate)

Brand Names: U.S. Neutra-Phos®-K [OTC] [DSC]

Index Terms Phosphate, Potassium

Pharmacologic Category Electrolyte Supplement, Parenteral

Use Treatment and prevention of hypophosphatemia; **Note:** The concomitant amount of potassium must be calculated into the total electrolyte content. For each 1 mmol of phosphate, ~1.5 mEq of potassium will be administered. Therefore, if ordering 30 mmol of potassium phosphate, the patient will receive ~45 mEq of potassium.

Pregnancy Risk Factor C

Pregnancy Considerations Reproduction studies have not been conducted with this product.

Contraindications Hyperphosphatemia, hyperkalemia, hypocalcemia, hypomagnesemia, renal failure (oral product)

Warnings/Precautions Close monitoring of serum potassium concentrations is needed to avoid hyperkalemia. Use with caution in patients with renal insufficiency, cardiac disease, metabolic alkalosis. Use with caution in digitalized patients and patients receiving concomitant potassium-altering therapies. Parenteral potassium may cause pain and phlebitis, requiring a decrease in infusion rate or potassium concentration. Solutions for injection may contain aluminum; toxic levels may occur following prolonged administration in premature neonates or patients with renal impairment.

Adverse Reactions Frequency not defined.

Cardiovascular: Arrhythmia, bradycardia, chest pain, ECG changes, edema, heart block, hypotension

Central nervous system: Listlessness, mental confusion, tetany (with large doses of phosphate)

Endocrine & metabolic: Hyperkalemia

Gastrointestinal: Diarrhea, nausea, stomach pain, vomiting

Genitourinary: Urine output decreased

Local: Phlebitis

Neuromuscular & skeletal: Paralysis, paresthesia, weakness

Renal: Acute renal failure

Respiratory: Dyspnea

Drug Interactions

Metabolism/Transport Effects None known.

Avoid Concomitant Use There are no known interactions where it is recommended to avoid concomitant use.

Increased Effect/Toxicity

Potassium Phosphate may increase the levels/effects of: ACE Inhibitors; Angiotensin II Receptor Blockers; Potassium-Sparing Diuretics

The levels/effects of Potassium Phosphate may be increased by: Bisphosphonate Derivatives; Eplerenone

Decreased Effect There are no known significant interactions involving a decrease in effect.

Ethanol/Nutrition/Herb Interactions Food: Avoid administering with oxalate (berries, nuts, chocolate, beans, celery, tomato) or phytate-containing foods (bran, whole wheat).

Stability Store at room temperature; do not freeze. Use only clear solutions. Up to 10-15 mEq of calcium may be added per liter before precipitate may occur.

Stability of parenteral admixture at room temperature (25°C) is 24 hours.

Phosphate salts may precipitate when mixed with calcium salts. Solubility is improved in amino acid parenteral nutrition solutions. Check with a pharmacist to determine compatibility.

Dosage

I.V.: **Caution: The concomitant amount of potassium must be calculated into the total electrolyte content. For each 1 mmol of phosphate, ~1.5 mEq of potassium will be administered. Therefore, if ordering 30 mmol of potassium phosphate, the patient will receive ~45 mEq of potassium. With orders for I.V. phosphate, there is considerable confusion**

associated with the use of millimoles (mmol) versus milliequivalents (mEq) to express the phosphate requirement. The most reliable method of ordering I.V. phosphate is by millimoles, then specifying the potassium or sodium salt. Doses listed as mmol of phosphate.

Acute treatment of hypophosphatemia: Repletion of severe hypophosphatemia should be done I.V. because large doses of oral phosphate may cause diarrhea and intestinal absorption may be unreliable. Reserve intermittent I.V. infusion for severe depletion situations; may require continuous cardiac monitoring depending on potassium administration rate. Guidelines differ based on degree of illness, need/use of parenteral nutrition, and severity of hypophosphatemia. If potassium >4.0 mEq/L consider phosphate replacement strategy without potassium (eg, sodium phosphates). Patients with severe renal impairment were excluded from phosphate supplement trials. **Note:** 1 mmol phosphate = 31 mg phosphorus; 1 mg phosphorus = 0.032 mmol phosphate.

Children and Adults: **Note:** There are no prospective studies of parenteral phosphate replacement in children. The following weight-based guidelines for adult dosing may be cautiously employed in pediatric patients.

General replacement guidelines (Lentz, 1978):

Low dose, if serum phosphate losses are recent and uncomplicated: 0.08 mmol/kg over 6 hours

Intermediate dose, if serum phosphorus level 0.5-1 mg/dL (0.16-0.32 mmol/L): 0.16-0.24 mmol/kg over 4-6 hours

Note: The initial dose may be increased by 25% to 50% if the patient is symptomatic secondary to hypophosphatemia and lowered by 25% to 50% if the patient is hypercalcemic.

Critically-ill adult patients receiving concurrent enteral/parenteral nutrition (Brown, 2006; Clark, 2006): Note: Round doses to the nearest 7.5 mmol for ease of preparation. If administering with phosphate-containing parenteral nutrition, do not exceed 15 mmol/L within parenteral nutrition. May use adjusted body weight for patients weighing >130% of ideal body weight (and BMI<40 kg/m^2) by using [IBW + 0.25 (ABW-IBW)]:

Low dose, serum phosphorus level 2.3-3 mg/dL (0.74-0.96 mmol/L): 0.16-0.32 mmol/kg over 4-6 hours

Intermediate dose, serum phosphorus level 1.6-2.2 mg/dL (0.51-0.71 mmol/L): 0.32-0.64 mmol/kg over 4-6 hours

High dose, serum phosphorus <1.5 mg/dL (<0.5 mmol/L): 0.64-1 mmol/kg over 8-12 hours

Parenteral nutrition:

Infants and Children: 0.5-2 mmol/kg/24 hours (Mirtallo, 2004 [ASPEN guidelines])

Children >50 kg and Adolescents: 10-40 mmol/24 hours (Mirtallo, 2004 [ASPEN guidelines])

Adults: 10-15 mmol/1000 kcal (Hicks, 2001) **or** 20-40 mmol/24 hours (Mirtallo, 2004 [ASPEN guidelines])

Administration Injection must be diluted in appropriate I.V. solution and volume prior to administration. In general, the dose, concentration of infusion, and rate of administration may be dependent on patient condition and specific institution policy. Must consider administration precautions for phosphate and potassium when prescribing.

For adult patients with severe symptomatic hypophosphatemia (ie, <1.5 mg/dL), may administer at rates up to 15 mmol phosphate/hour (this rate will deliver potassium at 22.5 mEq/hour) (Charron, 2003; Rosen, 1995). Potassium infusion rates >10 mEq/hour should be administered via central line (minimizes burning and phlebitis). ECG monitoring is recommended for potassium infusions >10 mEq/hour in adults or >0.5 mEq/kg/hour in children. In patients with renal dysfunction and/or less severe hypophosphatemia, slower administration rates (eg, over 4-6 hours) or oral repletion is recommended.

Intermittent infusion doses of potassium phosphate are typically prepared in 100-250 mL of NS or D_5W (usual phosphate concentration range: 0.15-0.6 mmol/mL) (Charron, 2003; Rosen, 1995). Suggested maximum concentrations:

Peripheral line administration: 6.7 mmoL potassium phosphate/100 mL (10 mEq potassium/100 mL)

Central line administration: 26.8 mmoL potassium phosphate/100 mL (40 mEq potassium/100 mL)

Monitoring Parameters Serum potassium, calcium, phosphorus, magnesium (to facilitate potassium repletion); cardiac monitor (if intermittent infusion or potassium infusion rates 0.5 mEq/kg/hour in children or >10 mEq/hour in adults); to assess adequate replacement, repeat serum potassium and phosphorus levels 2-4 hours after dose

Reference Range Note: Reference ranges may vary depending on the laboratory

Serum calcium: 8.4-10.2 mg/dL

Serum phosphorus: Both low and high ends of the normal range are higher in children than in adults.

Infants: 4.5-7.5 mg/dL (1.45-2.42 mmol/L)

Children: ~4-6 mg/dL (1.29-1.94 mmol/L)

Adults: 2.5-4.5 mg/dL (0.81-1.45 mmol/L)

Serum potassium: 3.5-5.2 mEq/L

Dosage Forms Excipient information presented when available (limited, particularly for generics); consult specific product labeling. [DSC] = Discontinued product

Injection, solution: Potassium 4.4 mEq and phosphorus 3 mmol per mL (5 mL, 15 mL, 50 mL) [equivalent to potassium 170 mg and elemental phosphorus 93 mg per mL]

Potassium Phosphate and Sodium Phosphate

(poe TASS ee um FOS fate & SOW dee um FOS fate)

Brand Names: U.S. K-Phos® MF; K-Phos® Neutral; K-Phos® No. 2; Phos-NaK; Phospha 250™ Neutral

Index Terms Neutra-Phos; Sodium Phosphate and Potassium Phosphate

Pharmacologic Category Electrolyte Supplement, Oral

Use Treatment of conditions associated with excessive renal phosphate loss or inadequate GI absorption of phosphate; to acidify the urine to lower calcium concentrations; to increase the antibacterial activity of methenamine; reduce odor and rash caused by ammonia in urine

Pregnancy Risk Factor C

Dosage Oral:

Children ≥4 years: Elemental phosphorus 250 mg 4 times/day after meals and at bedtime

Adults: Elemental phosphorus 250-500 mg 4 times/day after meals and at bedtime

Additional Information Complete prescribing information for this medication should be consulted for additional detail.

Dosage Forms Excipient information presented when available (limited, particularly for generics); consult specific product labeling.

Powder for solution, oral:

Phos-NaK: Dibasic potassium phosphate, monobasic potassium phosphate, dibasic sodium phosphate, and monobasic sodium phosphate per packet (100s) [sugar free; equivalent to elemental phosphorus 250 mg (8 mmol), sodium 160 mg (6.9 mEq), and potassium 280 mg (7.1 mEq) per packet; fruit flavor]

Tablet, oral:

K-Phos® MF: Potassium acid phosphate 155 mg and sodium acid phosphate 350 mg [equivalent to elemental phosphorus 125.6 mg (4 mmol), sodium 67 mg (2.9 mEq), and potassium 44.5 mg (1.1 mEq)]

K-Phos® Neutral: Monobasic potassium phosphate 155 mg, dibasic sodium phosphate 852 mg, and monobasic sodium phosphate 130 mg [equivalent to elemental phosphorus 250 mg (8 mmol), sodium 298 mg (13 mEq), and potassium 45 mg (1.1 mEq)]

K-Phos® No. 2: Potassium acid phosphate 305 mg and sodium acid phosphate 700 mg [equivalent to elemental phosphorus 250 mg (8 mmol), sodium 134 mg (5.8 mEq), and potassium 88 mg (2.3 mEq)]

Phospha 250™ Neutral: Monobasic potassium phosphate 155 mg, dibasic sodium phosphate 852 mg, and monobasic sodium phosphate 130 mg [equivalent to elemental phosphorus 250 mg (8 mmol), sodium 298 mg (13 mEq), and potassium 45 mg (1.1 mEq)]

◆ **Potassium Sulfate, Magnesium Sulfate, and Sodium Sulfate** *see* Sodium Sulfate, Potassium Sulfate, and Magnesium Sulfate *on page 1576*
◆ **Potassium Sulfate, Sodium Sulfate, and Magnesium Sulfate** *see* Sodium Sulfate, Potassium Sulfate, and Magnesium Sulfate *on page 1576*
◆ **PPD** *see* Tuberculin Tests *on page 1744*
◆ **PPI-0903** *see* Ceftaroline Fosamil *on page 315*
◆ **PPI-0903M** *see* Ceftaroline Fosamil *on page 315*
◆ **PPS** *see* Pentosan Polysulfate Sodium *on page 1331*
◆ **PPSV** *see* Pneumococcal Polysaccharide Vaccine (Polyvalent) *on page 1368*
◆ **PPSV23** *see* Pneumococcal Polysaccharide Vaccine (Polyvalent) *on page 1368*
◆ **PPV23** *see* Pneumococcal Polysaccharide Vaccine (Polyvalent) *on page 1368*
◆ **Pradax™ (Can)** *see* Dabigatran Etexilate *on page 435*
◆ **Pradaxa®** *see* Dabigatran Etexilate *on page 435*

PRALAtrexate (pral a TREX ate)

Brand Names: U.S. Folotyn®

Index Terms PDX

Pharmacologic Category Antineoplastic Agent, Antimetabolite (Antifolate)

Use Treatment of relapsed or refractory peripheral T-cell lymphoma (PTCL)

Unlabeled Use Treatment of relapsed or refractory cutaneous T-cell lymphoma (CTCL)

Pregnancy Risk Factor D

Pregnancy Considerations Adverse effects were observed in animal studies. May cause fetal harm if administered to a pregnant woman.

Lactation Excretion in breast milk unknown/not recommended

Contraindications There are no contraindications listed within the manufacturer's labeling.

Warnings/Precautions Hazardous agent - use appropriate precautions for handling and disposal. May cause bone marrow suppression (thrombocytopenia, neutropenia and anemia); may require dosage modification. Mucositis, including stomatitis or mucosal inflammation of gastrointestinal and genitourinary tracts, may occur with treatment; may require dosage modification. Prophylactic folic acid and vitamin B_{12} supplements are necessary to reduce hematologic toxicity and treatment-related mucositis. Severe and potentially fatal dermatologic reactions, including skin exfoliation, ulceration, and toxic epidermal necrolysis (TEN) have been reported. Skin reaction may be progressive; severity may increase with continued treatment; may also involve skin and subcutaneous tissues which are affected by lymphoma; monitor all dermatologic reactions closely; withhold or discontinue treatment for severe dermatologic reaction.

Tumor lysis syndrome (TLS) has been reported in patients being treated for lymphoma; monitor closely, if TLS develops, treat for associated complications. Use with caution in patients with moderate-to-severe renal impairment (has not been studied in patients with renal impairment); monitor renal function and for systemic toxicity due to increased exposure. Concurrent use with drugs with substantial renal clearance (eg, NSAIDs, sulfamethoxazole/trimethoprim) may result in delayed pralatrexate clearance. Liver function test abnormalities have been observed with use; monitor liver function; persistent abnormalities may indicate hepatotoxicity and may require dosage modification.

Adverse Reactions

>10%:

Cardiovascular: Edema (30%)

Central nervous system: Fatigue (36%), fever (32%)

Dermatologic: Rash (15%; grades 3/4: 0%), pruritus (14%; grade 3: 2%; grade 4: 0%)

Endocrine & metabolic: Hypokalemia (15%)

Gastrointestinal: Mucositis (70%; grade 3: 17%; grade 4: 4%), nausea (40%), constipation (33%), vomiting (25%), diarrhea (21%), anorexia (15%), abdominal pain (12%)

Hematologic: Thrombocytopenia (41%; grade 3: 14%; grade 4: 19%), anemia (34%; grade 4: 2%), neutropenia (24%; grade 3: 13%; grade 4: 7%), leukopenia (11%; grade 3: 3%; grade 4: 4%)

Hepatic: Transaminases increased (13%; grade 3: 5%; grade 4: 0%)

Neuromuscular & skeletal: Limb pain (12%), back pain (11%)

Respiratory: Cough (28%), epistaxis (26%), dyspnea (19%), pharyngolaryngeal pain (14%)

Miscellaneous: Night sweats (11%), infection

1% to 10%:

Cardiovascular: Tachycardia (10%)

Endocrine & metabolic: Dehydration (serious >3%)

Hematologic: Neutropenic fever (serious >3%)

Neuromuscular & skeletal: Weakness (10%)

Respiratory: Upper respiratory infection (10%)

Miscellaneous: Sepsis (serious >3%)

<1% (Limited to important or life-threatening): Bowel obstruction, cardiopulmonary arrest, lymphopenia, odynophagia, pancytopenia, skin exfoliation, skin ulceration, toxic epidermal necrolysis (TEN), tumor lysis syndrome (TLS)

Drug Interactions

Metabolism/Transport Effects None known.

Avoid Concomitant Use

Avoid concomitant use of PRALAtrexate with any of the following: BCG; Natalizumab; Pimecrolimus; Tacrolimus (Topical); Vaccines (Live)

Increased Effect/Toxicity

PRALAtrexate may increase the levels/effects of: Leflunomide; Natalizumab; Vaccines (Live); Vitamin K Antagonists

The levels/effects of PRALAtrexate may be increased by: Denosumab; Nonsteroidal Anti-Inflammatory Agents; Pimecrolimus; Probenecid; Roflumilast; Salicylates; Sulfamethoxazole; Tacrolimus (Topical); Trastuzumab; Trimethoprim

Decreased Effect

PRALAtrexate may decrease the levels/effects of: BCG; Cardiac Glycosides; Coccidioidin Skin Test; Sapropterin; Sipuleucel-T; Vaccines (Inactivated); Vaccines (Live); Vitamin K Antagonists

The levels/effects of PRALAtrexate may be decreased by: Echinacea

Stability Store intact vials refrigerated at 2°C to 8°C (36°F to 46°F). Store in original carton to protect from light until use. Unopened vials (stored in the original carton) are stable for up to 72 hours at room temperature (discard after 72 hours). Withdraw into syringe for administration; do not dilute. Discard unused portion in the vial. The manufacturer recommends immediate use after placing in syringe. Use appropriate precautions for handling (hazardous agent).

Mechanism of Action Antifolate analog; inhibits DNA, RNA, and protein synthesis by selectively entering cells expressing reduced folate carrier (RFC-1), is polyglutamylated by folylpolyglutamate synthetase (FPGS) and then competes for the DHFR-folate binding site to inhibit dihydrofolate reductase (DHFR)

Pharmacodynamics/Kinetics

Distribution: *S*-diastereomer: 105 L; *R*-diastereomer: 37 L

Protein binding: ~67%

Half-life elimination: 12-18 hours

Excretion: Urine (~34% as unchanged drug)

Dosage Note: Start vitamin supplements before initial pralatrexate dose: Folic acid 1-1.25 mg/day orally beginning within 10 days prior to initiating pralatrexate (continue during treatment and for 30 days after last pralatrexate dose) and vitamin B_{12} 1000 mcg I.M. within 10 weeks prior to treatment and every 8-10 weeks thereafter (after initial dose, B_{12} may be administered on the same day as pralatrexate).

Prior to administering any dose, mucositis should be ≤grade 1, platelets should be ≥100,000/mm^3 for the first dose and ≥50,000/mm^3 for subsequent doses, and absolute neutrophil count (ANC) should be ≥1000/mm^3.

I.V.: Adults:

Peripheral T-cell lymphoma (PTCL), relapsed or refractory: 30 mg/m^2 once weekly for 6 weeks of a 7-week treatment cycle (continue until disease progression or unacceptable toxicity)

Cutaneous T-cell lymphoma (CTCL), relapsed or refractory (unlabeled use): 15 mg/m^2 once weekly for 3 weeks of a 4-week treatment cycle (Horwitz, 2010)

Dosage adjustment for toxicity: Severe or intolerable adverse events may require dose omission, reduction or interruption. Do not make up omitted doses at the end of the cycle; do not re-escalate dose after a reduction due to toxicity.

Hematologic toxicity:

Platelets:

<50,000/mm^3 (for 1-week duration): Omit dose; continue at previous dose if platelets recover within 1 week

<50,000/mm^3 (for 2-week duration): Omit dose; decrease to 20 mg/m^2 if platelets recover within 2 weeks

<50,000/mm^3 (for 3-week duration): Discontinue treatment

ANC:

500-1000/mm^3 without fever (for 1-week duration): Omit dose; continue at previous dose if ANC recovers within 1 week

500-1000/mm^3 with fever **or** ANC <500/mm^3 (for 1-week duration): Omit dose, give filgrastim or sargramostim support; continue at previous dose (with growth factor support) if ANC recovers within 1 week

500-1000/mm^3 with fever **or** ANC <500/mm^3 (recurrent or for 2-week duration): Omit dose and give filgrastim or sargramostim support; decrease to 20 mg/m^2 (with growth factor support) if ANC recovers within 2 weeks

500-1000/mm^3 with fever **or** ANC <500/mm^3 (second recurrence or for 3-week duration): Discontinue treatment

Nonhematologic toxicity: Mucositis (on day of treatment):

Grade 2: Omit dose; continue at previous dose when recovers to ≤grade 1

Grade 3 or recurrent grade 2: Omit dose and decrease to 20 mg/m^2 when recovers to ≤grade 1

Grade 4: Discontinue treatment

Nonhematologic toxicity (other than mucositis):

Grade 3: Omit dose; decrease to 20 mg/m^2 when recovers to ≤grade 2

Grade 4: Discontinue treatment

Dosage adjustment in renal impairment: Moderate-to-severe renal impairment: Use with caution (has not been studied in patients with renal impairment). Monitor for possible systemic toxicity due to increased exposure.

Dosage adjustment in hepatic impairment: Patients with total bilirubin >1.5 mg/dL, AST or ALT >2.5 times the upper limit of normal (ULN), and ALT or AST >5 times ULN if documented hepatic lymphoma involvement were excluded from clinical trials. Persistent abnormalities may indicate hepatotoxicity requiring dosage modification; refer to dosage adjustment for nonhematologic (other than mucositis) toxicity for adjustment recommendations.

Administration Administer I.V. push over 3-5 minutes into the line of a free-flowing normal saline I.V.

Monitoring Parameters CBC with differential (weekly), serum chemistries, including renal and liver function tests (prior to the first and fourth doses in each cycle); mucositis severity (weekly); monitor for signs of tumor lysis syndrome

Dosage Forms Excipient information presented when available (limited, particularly for generics); consult specific product labeling.

Injection, solution [preservative free]:

Folotyn®: 20 mg/mL (1 mL, 2 mL)

Pralidoxime (pra li DOKS eem)

Brand Names: U.S. Protopam®

Index Terms 2-PAM; 2-Pyridine Aldoxime Methochloride; Pralidoxime Chloride

Pharmacologic Category Antidote

Use Treatment of muscle weakness and/or respiratory depression secondary to poisoning due to organophosphate anticholinesterase pesticides and chemicals (eg, nerve agents); control of overdose of anticholinesterase medications used to treat myasthenia gravis (ambenonium, neostigmine, pyridostigmine)

Pregnancy Risk Factor C

Pregnancy Considerations Animal reproduction studies have not been conducted. A case report did not show evidence of adverse events after pralidoxime administration during the second trimester (Kamha, 2005).

Lactation Excretion in breast milk unknown/use caution

Contraindications There are no absolute contraindications listed within the manufacturer's labeling.

Warnings/Precautions Pralidoxime is not indicated for the treatment of poisoning due to phosphorus, inorganic phosphates, organophosphates without anticholinesterase activity, or carbamate pesticides (acetylcholinesterase is weakly, but not permanently, affected by carbamates). Use with caution in patients with myasthenia gravis (may precipitate a myasthenic crisis); dosage modification required in patients with impaired renal function. Clinical symptoms that are consistent with suspected organophosphate poisoning should be treated with antidote immediately; administration should not be delayed for confirmatory laboratory tests. Treatment should include proper evacuation and decontamination procedures as indicated; medical personnel should protect themselves from inadvertent contamination. Antidote administration is intended only for initial management; definitive and more intensive medical care is required following administration. Individuals should not rely solely on antidote for treatment; the concomitant use of atropine will be necessary and other supportive measures (eg, artificial respiration) may still be required.

Adverse Reactions Frequency not defined.

Cardiovascular: Cardiac arrest, hypertension, tachycardia
Central nervous system: Dizziness, drowsiness, headache, seizure
Dermatologic: Rash
Gastrointestinal: Nausea
Hepatic: ALT increased (transient), AST increased (transient)
Local: Pain at injection (I.M. administration)
Neuromuscular & skeletal: CPK increased, fasciculations, muscle rigidity, paralysis, weakness
Ocular: Accommodation impaired, blurred vision, diplopia
Renal: Renal function decreased
Respiratory: Apnea, hyperventilation, laryngospasm

Drug Interactions

Metabolism/Transport Effects None known.

Avoid Concomitant Use There are no known interactions where it is recommended to avoid concomitant use.

Increased Effect/Toxicity There are no known significant interactions involving an increase in effect.

Decreased Effect There are no known significant interactions involving a decrease in effect.

Stability Store at 20°C to 25°C (68°F to 77°F); excursions permitted to 15°C to 30°C (59°F to 86°F).

I.V. administration: Dilute 1 g with 20 mL SWFI (50 mg/mL). The solution should be further diluted with NS to a final concentration of 10-20 mg/mL. If this is not practical or in cases of fluid overload, may prepare and administer as a 50 mg/mL solution.

I.M. administration: Dilute 1 g with 3.3 mL SWFI (300 mg/mL)

Mechanism of Action Reactivates cholinesterase that had been inactivated by phosphorylation due to exposure to organophosphate pesticides and cholinesterase inhibiting nerve agents (eg, terrorism and chemical warfare agents such as sarin) by displacing the enzyme from its receptor sites; removes the phosphoryl group from the active site of the inactivated enzyme

Pharmacodynamics/Kinetics

Distribution: V_{dss}: 0.6-2.7 L/kg; may increase with increasing severity of organophosphate intoxication (~9 L/kg in a severely poisoned pediatric patients; Schexnayder, 1998)
Protein binding: None
Metabolism: Hepatic
Half-life elimination: Apparent: 74-77 minutes; Poisoned patients (I.M., I.V.): 3-4 hours
Time to peak, serum: I.V.: 5-15 minutes; I.M.: ~35 minutes
Excretion: Urine (~80% as metabolites and unchanged drug)

Dosage

I.V.: Use in conjunction with atropine; atropine effects should be established before pralidoxime is administered.

Anticholinesterase poisoning (eg, neostigmine, pyridostigmine): Adults: 1000-2000 mg; followed by increments of 250 mg every 5 minutes as needed

Organophosphate poisoning: **Note:** May be given I.M. or SubQ if I.V. administration is not feasible:

Children ≤16 years: Loading dose: 20-50 mg/kg (maximum: 2000 mg/dose); Maintenance infusion: 10-20 mg/kg/hour; alternatively, a repeat bolus of 20-50 mg/kg (maximum: 2000 mg/dose) may be administered after 1 hour and repeated every 10-12 hours thereafter, as needed

Children >16 years and Adults: Loading dose: 1000-2000 mg; Maintenance: Repeat bolus of 1000-2000 mg after 1 hour and repeated every 10-12 hours thereafter, as needed. Alternatively, administer a loading dose of 30 mg/kg followed by a maintenance infusion of 8 mg/kg/hour (unlabeled dose; Roberts, 2007).

I.M.: Organophosphate poisoning: **Note:** Use in conjunction with atropine; atropine effects should be established before pralidoxime is administered. Consider I.M. or SubQ administration when I.V. administration is not feasible:

Children <40 kg:

Mild symptoms: 15 mg/kg; repeat as needed for persistent mild symptoms every 15 minutes to a maximum total dose of 45 mg/kg; may administer doses in rapid succession if severe symptoms develop

Severe symptoms: 15 mg/kg; repeat twice in rapid succession to deliver a total dose of 45 mg/kg

Persistent symptoms: May repeat the entire series (45 mg/kg) beginning ~1 hour after administration of the last injection

Children ≥40 kg and Adults:

Mild symptoms: 600 mg; repeat as needed for persistent mild symptoms every 15 minutes to a maximum total dose of 1800 mg; may administer doses in rapid succession if severe symptoms develop

Severe symptoms: 600 mg; repeat twice in rapid succession to deliver a total dose of 1800 mg

Persistent symptoms: May repeat the entire series (1800 mg) beginning ~1 hour after administration of the last injection

Elderly: Refer to adult dosing; dosing should be cautious, considering possibility of decreased hepatic, renal, or cardiac function

Dosing adjustment in renal impairment: Dose should be reduced; no specific recommendations are provided by the manufacturer

Administration

I.V.:

Loading dose: Infuse as a 10-20 mg/mL solution over 15-30 minutes. Alternatively, if this is not practical or if pulmonary edema is present and/or fluid restriction is necessary, may administer as a 50 mg/mL solution over ≥5 minutes.

Maintenance dose: Administer as a continuous or intermittent infusion at a rate not to exceed 200 mg/minute.

I.M., SubQ: May administer I.M. or SubQ if I.V. administration is not feasible.

Monitoring Parameters Heart rate, respiratory rate, muscle fasciculations and strength, pulse oximetry; cardiac monitor and blood pressure monitor required for I.V. administration

Dosage Forms Excipient information presented when available (limited, particularly for generics); consult specific product labeling.

Injection, powder for reconstitution, as chloride:
Protopam®: 1 g

Injection, solution, as chloride: 300 mg/mL (2 mL)

◆ **Pralidoxime and Atropine** *see* Atropine and Pralidoxime *on page 172*

◆ **Pralidoxime Chloride** *see* Pralidoxime *on page 1388*

Pramipexole (pra mi PEKS ole)

Brand Names: U.S. Mirapex®; Mirapex® ER®

Brand Names: Canada Apo-Pramipexole®; Ava-Pramipexole; CO Pramipexole; Mirapex®; PMS-Pramipexole; Sandoz-Pramipexole; Teva-Pramipexole

Index Terms Pramipexole Dihydrochloride Monohydrate

Pharmacologic Category Anti-Parkinson's Agent, Dopamine Agonist

Additional Appendix Information

Antiparkinsonian Agents *on page 1879*

Use

Immediate release: Treatment of the signs and symptoms of idiopathic Parkinson's disease; treatment of moderate-to-severe primary Restless Legs Syndrome (RLS)

Extended release: Treatment of the signs and symptoms of idiopathic Parkinson's disease

Unlabeled Use Treatment of depression; treatment of fibromyalgia

Pregnancy Risk Factor C

Pregnancy Considerations Early embryonic loss and postnatal growth inhibition were observed in animal studies. There are no adequate and well-controlled studies in pregnant women.

Lactation Excretion in breast milk unknown/not recommended

Contraindications Hypersensitivity to pramipexole or any component of the formulation

Warnings/Precautions Caution should be taken in patients with renal insufficiency; dose adjustment necessary. May cause or exacerbate dyskinesias; use caution in patients with pre-existing dyskinesias. May cause orthostatic hypotension; Parkinson's disease patients appear to have an impaired capacity to respond to a postural challenge. Use with caution in patients at risk of hypotension or where transient hypotensive episodes would be poorly tolerated. Parkinson's patients being treated with dopaminergic agonists ordinarily require careful monitoring for signs and symptoms of postural hypotension, especially during dose escalation. May cause hallucinations.

Dopamine agonists have been associated with compulsive behaviors and/or loss of impulse control, which has manifested as pathological gambling, libido increases (hypersexuality), and/or binge eating. Causality has not been established, and controversy exists as to whether this phenomenon is related to the underlying disease, prior behaviors/addictions and/or drug therapy. Dose reduction or discontinuation of therapy has been reported to reverse these behaviors in some, but not all cases. Risk for melanoma development is increased in Parkinson's disease patients; drug causation or factors contributing to risk have not been established. Patients should be monitored closely and periodic skin examinations should be performed.

Taper gradually over a period of 1 week when discontinuing therapy; dopaminergic agents have been associated with a syndrome resembling neuroleptic malignant syndrome on abrupt withdrawal or significant dosage reduction after long-term use. Ergot-derived dopamine agonists have been associated with fibrotic complications (eg, retroperitoneal fibrosis, pleural thickening, and pulmonary infiltrates). Although pramipexole is not an ergot, there have been postmarketing reports of possible fibrotic complications with pramipexole; monitor closely for signs and symptoms of fibrosis.

Pramipexole has been associated with somnolence, particularly at higher dosages (>1.5 mg/day). In addition, patients have been reported to fall asleep during activities of daily living, including driving, while taking this medication. Whether these patients exhibited somnolence prior to these events is not clear. Patients should be advised of this issue and factors which may increase risk (sleep disorders, other sedating medications, or concomitant medications which increase pramipexole concentrations) and instructed to report daytime somnolence or sleepiness to the prescriber. Patients should use caution in performing activities which require alertness (driving or operating machinery), and to avoid other medications which may cause CNS depression, including ethanol. Use caution in the elderly as they may be more sensitive to these adverse drug reactions.

Pathologic degenerative changes were observed in the retinas of albino rats during studies with this agent, but were not observed in the retinas of albino mice or in other species. The significance of these data for humans remains uncertain. Augmentation (earlier onset of symptoms in the evening/afternoon, increase and/or spread of symptoms to other extremities) or rebound (shifting of symptoms to early morning hours) may occur in some RLS patients.

Adverse Reactions

Parkinson's disease: Actual frequency may be dependent on dose and/or formulation:

>10%:

Cardiovascular: Postural hypotension (dose related; ≤53%)

Central nervous system: Somnolence (dose related; 9% to 36%), extrapyramidal syndrome (28%), insomnia (4% to 27%), dizziness (2% to 26%), hallucinations (5% to 17%), abnormal dreams (11%), headache (4% to 7%)

Gastrointestinal: Nausea (dose related; 11% to 28%), constipation (dose related; 6% to 14%)

Neuromuscular & skeletal: Dyskinesia (17% to 47%), weakness (1% to 14%)

1% to 10%:

Cardiovascular: Edema (2% to 8%), chest pain (3%)

Central nervous system: Confusion (4% to 10%), dystonia (2% to 8%), fatigue (6%), amnesia (dose related; 4% to 6%), sudden onset of sleep (3% to 6%), vertigo (2% to 4%), hypesthesia (3%), abnormal thinking (2% to 3%), akathisia (2% to 3%), malaise (2% to 3%), paranoia (2%), sleep disorder (1% to 3%), depression (≤2%), delusions (1%), fever (1%), myoclonus (1%)

Endocrine & metabolic: Libido decreased (1%)

Gastrointestinal: Xerostomia (4% to 7%), anorexia (1% to 5%), vomiting (4%), abdominal discomfort/pain (1% to 4%), dyspepsia (3%), appetite increased (2% to 3%), dysphagia (2%), weight loss (2%), salivary hypersecretion (≤2%), diarrhea (1% to 2%)

Genitourinary: Urinary frequency (6%), urinary tract infection (4%), impotence (2%), urinary incontinence (2%)

Neuromuscular & skeletal: Gait abnormalities (7%), hypertonia (7%), muscle spasm (3% to 5%), falls (4%), arthritis (3%), tremor (3%), back pain (2% to 3%), bursitis (2%), muscle twitching (2%), balance abnormalities (≤2%), CPK increased (1%), myasthenia (1%)

Ocular: Accommodation abnormalities (4%), vision abnormalities (3%), diplopia (1%)

Respiratory: Dyspnea (4%), cough (3%), rhinitis (3%), pneumonia (2%)

Postmarketing and/or case reports (limited to important or life-threatening): Blackouts, impulsive/compulsive behaviors (eg, binge eating, hypersexuality, pathological gambling, shopping), libido increased, liver transaminases increased, pruritus, rhabdomyolysis, syncope, weight gain

Restless legs syndrome: Actual frequency may be dependent on dose:

>10%:

Central nervous system: Headache (16%), insomnia (9% to 13%), abnormal dreams (1% to 8%), somnolence (6%)

Gastrointestinal: Nausea (11% to 27%), constipation (4%)

1% to 10%:

Central nervous system: Fatigue (3% to 9%)

Gastrointestinal: Diarrhea (1% to 7%), xerostomia (3%)

Neuromuscular & skeletal: Extremity pain (3% to 7%)

Respiratory: Nasal congestion (≤6%)

Miscellaneous: Influenza (1% to 7%)

Postmarketing and/or case reports (limited to important or life-threatening): Augmentation (~20% but similar to placebo), blackouts, impulsive/compulsive behaviors (eg, binge eating, hypersexuality, pathological gambling, shopping), libido increased, liver transaminases increased, pruritus, rebound, tolerance, syncope, weight gain

Drug Interactions

Metabolism/Transport Effects None known.

Avoid Concomitant Use There are no known interactions where it is recommended to avoid concomitant use.

Increased Effect/Toxicity

Pramipexole may increase the levels/effects of: Alcohol (Ethyl); CNS Depressants; Selective Serotonin Reuptake Inhibitors

The levels/effects of Pramipexole may be increased by: Antipsychotics (Typical); Cimetidine; HydrOXYzine; MAO Inhibitors; Methylphenidate

Decreased Effect

Pramipexole may decrease the levels/effects of: Antipsychotics (Typical)

The levels/effects of Pramipexole may be decreased by: Antipsychotics (Atypical); Metoclopramide

Ethanol/Nutrition/Herb Interactions

Ethanol: May increase CNS depression; monitor for increased effects with coadministration. Caution patients about effects.

Food: Food intake does not affect the extent of drug absorption although the time to maximal plasma concentration is delayed when taken with a meal.

Herb/Nutraceutical: Avoid valerian, St John's wort, SAMe, kava kava (may increase risk of serotonin syndrome and/or excessive sedation).

Stability Store at 25°C (77°F); excursions permitted to 15°C to 30°C (59°F to 86°F). Protect from light and high humidity.

Mechanism of Action Pramipexole is a nonergot dopamine agonist with specificity for the D_2 subfamily dopamine receptor, and has also been shown to bind to D_3 and D_4 receptors. By binding to these receptors, it is thought that pramipexole can stimulate dopamine activity on the nerves of the striatum and substantia nigra.

Pharmacodynamics/Kinetics

Absorption: Rapid

Distribution: V_d: 500 L

Protein binding: ~15%

Metabolism: Negligible (<10%)

Bioavailability: Immediate release: >90%; Extended release (as compared to immediate release): 100%

Half-life elimination: 8.5 hours; Elderly: 12 hours

Time to peak, serum: Immediate release: ~2 hours; Extended release: 6 hours

Excretion: Urine (90% as unchanged drug)

Dosage Oral: Adults:

Immediate release formulation:

Parkinson's disease: Initial: 0.375 mg/day given in 3 divided doses, increase gradually every 5-7 days; range: 1.5-4.5 mg/day

Restless legs syndrome: Initial: 0.125 mg once daily 2-3 hours before bedtime. Dose may be doubled every 4-7 days up to 0.5 mg/day. Maximum dose: 0.5 mg/day (manufacturer's recommendation).

Note: Most patients require <0.5 mg/day, but higher doses have been used (2 mg/day). If augmentation occurs, dose earlier in the day.

Depression (unlabeled use): Initial: 0.25-0.375 mg/day given in 2-3 divided doses with a gradual titration; mean dose: 1.6-1.7 mg/day (Aiken, 2007; Goldberg, 2004)

Fibromyalgia (unlabeled use): Initial: 0.25 mg once daily at bedtime; may be increased weekly by 0.25 mg/day increments up to 4.5 mg/day (Holman, 2005)

Extended release formulation (Mirapex® ER™): Parkinson's disease: Initial: 0.375 mg once daily; increase gradually to 0.75 mg once daily. If necessary, may increase by 0.75 mg/dose not more frequently than every 5-7 days; maximum recommended dose 4.5 mg/day

Converting from immediate release to extended release: May initiate extended release preparation the morning after the last immediate release evening tablet is taken. The total daily dose should remain the same.

Dosage adjustment in renal impairment: Use caution; renally-eliminated

Parkinson's disease: Immediate release formulation:

Cl_{cr} 35-59 mL/minute: Initial: 0.125 mg twice daily (maximum dose: 1.5 mg twice daily)

Cl_{cr} 15-34 mL/minute: Initial: 0.125 mg once daily (maximum dose: 1.5 mg once daily)

Cl_{cr} <15 mL/minute: Not adequately studied

Hemodialysis: Not adequately studied; a negligible amount of pramipexole is removed by dialysis

Parkinson's disease: Extended release formulation:

Cl_{cr} >50 mL/minute: Dosing adjustment not necessary

Cl_{cr} 30-50 mL/minute: Initial: 0.375 mg every other day; may increase to 0.375 mg once daily no sooner than 1 week after initiation. If necessary, may increase by 0.375 mg/dose not more frequently than every 7 days; maximum recommended dose: 2.25 mg/day

Cl_{cr} <30 mL/minute: Not recommended

Hemodialysis: Not recommended; a negligible amount of pramipexole is removed by dialysis

Restless legs syndrome: Immediate release formulation:

Cl_{cr} 20-60 mL/minute: Duration between titration should be increased to 14 days

Cl_{cr} <20 mL/minute: Not adequately studied

Dietary Considerations May be taken with or without food. May be taken with food to decrease nausea.

Administration Doses should be titrated gradually in all patients to avoid the onset of intolerable side effects. The dosage should be increased to achieve a maximum therapeutic effect, balanced against the side effects of dyskinesia, hallucinations, somnolence, and dry mouth. May be administered with or without food; may be administered with food to decrease nausea. Extended release tablets should be swallowed whole and not chewed, crushed, or divided.

Monitoring Parameters Blood pressure, heart rate; body weight changes; CNS depression, fall risk

Dosage Forms Excipient information presented when available (limited, particularly for generics); consult specific product labeling.

Tablet, oral, as dihydrochloride monohydrate: 0.125 mg, 0.25 mg, 0.5 mg, 0.75 mg, 1 mg, 1.5 mg

Mirapex®: 0.125 mg

Mirapex®: 0.25 mg, 0.5 mg [scored]

Mirapex®: 0.75 mg

Mirapex®: 1 mg, 1.5 mg [scored]

Tablet, extended release, oral, as dihydrochloride monohydrate:

Mirapex® ER®: 0.375 mg, 0.75 mg, 1.5 mg, 2.25 mg, 3 mg, 3.75 mg, 4.5 mg

◆ **Pramipexole Dihydrochloride Monohydrate** *see* Pramipexole *on page 1389*

Pramlintide (PRAM lin tide)

Brand Names: U.S. SymlinPen®; Symlin® [DSC]

Index Terms Pramlintide Acetate

Pharmacologic Category Amylinomimetic; Antidiabetic Agent

Additional Appendix Information

Diabetes Mellitus Management, Adults *on page 1983*

Use

Adjunctive treatment with mealtime insulin in type 1 diabetes mellitus (insulin dependent, IDDM) patients who have failed to achieve desired glucose control despite optimal insulin therapy

Adjunctive treatment with mealtime insulin in type 2 diabetes mellitus (noninsulin dependent, NIDDM) patients who have failed to achieve desired glucose control despite optimal insulin therapy, with or without concurrent sulfonylurea and/or metformin

Pregnancy Risk Factor C

Pregnancy Considerations Due to adverse events observed in some animal studies, pramlintide is classified as pregnancy category C. Based on *in vitro* data, pramlintide has a low potential to cross the placenta. Maternal hyperglycemia can be associated with adverse effects in the fetus, including macrosomia, neonatal hyperglycemia, and hyperbilirubinemia; the risk of congenital malformations is increased when the Hb A_{1c} is above the normal range. Diabetes can also be associated with adverse effects in the mother. Poorly-treated diabetes may cause end-organ damage that may in turn negatively affect obstetric outcomes. Physiologic glucose levels should be maintained prior to and during pregnancy to decrease the risk of adverse events in the mother and the fetus. Until additional safety and efficacy data are obtained, the use of pramlintide is generally not recommended in the routine management of diabetes mellitus during pregnancy. Insulin is the drug of choice for the control of diabetes mellitus during pregnancy.

Lactation Excretion in breast milk unknown/use caution

Medication Guide Available Yes

Contraindications Hypersensitivity to pramlintide or any component of the formulation; confirmed diagnosis of gastroparesis; hypoglycemia unawareness

Warnings/Precautions [U.S. Boxed Warning]: Coadministration with insulin may induce severe hypoglycemia (usually within 3 hours following administration); coadministration with insulin therapy is an approved indication but does require an initial dosage reduction of insulin and frequent pre and post blood glucose monitoring to reduce risk of severe hypoglycemia. Concurrent use of other glucose-lowering agents may increase risk of hypoglycemia. Avoid use in patients with poor compliance with their insulin regimen and/or blood glucose monitoring. Do not use in patients with Hb A_{1c} levels >9% or recent, recurrent episodes of hypoglycemia; obtain detailed history of glucose control (eg, Hb A_{1c}, incidence of hypoglycemia, glucose monitoring, and medication compliance) and body weight before initiating therapy. Use caution in patients with visual or dexterity impairment. Use caution when driving or operating heavy machinery until effects on blood sugar are known. Use caution with certain antihypertensive agents (eg, beta-adrenergic blockers) or neuropathic conditions which may mask signs/symptoms of hypoglycemia. Use caution in patients with history of nausea; avoid use in patients with conditions or concurrent medications likely to impair gastric motility (eg, anticholinergics); do not use in patients requiring medication(s) to stimulate gastric emptying.

Adverse Reactions

>10%:

Central nervous system: Headache (5% to 13%)

Gastrointestinal: Nausea (28% to 48%), vomiting (7% to 11%), anorexia (≤17%)

Endocrine & metabolic: Severe hypoglycemia (type 1 diabetes ≤17%)

Miscellaneous: Inflicted injury (8% to 14%)

1% to 10%:

Central nervous system: Fatigue (3% to 7%), dizziness (2% to 6%)

Endocrine & metabolic: Severe hypoglycemia (type 2 diabetes ≤8%)

Gastrointestinal: Abdominal pain (2% to 8%)

Respiratory: Pharyngitis (3% to 5%), cough (2% to 6%)

Neuromuscular & skeletal: Arthralgia (2% to 7%)

Miscellaneous: Allergic reaction (≤6%)

Postmarketing and/or case reports: Injection site reactions

Drug Interactions

Metabolism/Transport Effects None known.

Avoid Concomitant Use There are no known interactions where it is recommended to avoid concomitant use.

Increased Effect/Toxicity

Pramlintide may increase the levels/effects of: Anticholinergics

Decreased Effect There are no known significant interactions involving a decrease in effect.

Ethanol/Nutrition/Herb Interactions

Ethanol: Use caution with ethanol (may increase hypoglycemia).

Herb/Nutraceutical: Use caution with garlic, chromium, gymnema (may increase hypoglycemia).

Stability Store unopened vials at 2°C to 8°C (36°F to 46°F); do not freeze. Opened vials may be kept refrigerated or at room temperature ≤30°C (≤86°F). Discard opened vial after 30 days. Protect from light.

Mechanism of Action Synthetic analog of human amylin cosecreted with insulin by pancreatic beta cells; reduces postprandial glucose increases via the following mechanisms: 1) prolongation of gastric emptying time, 2) reduction of postprandial glucagon secretion, and 3) reduction of caloric intake through centrally-mediated appetite suppression

Pharmacodynamics/Kinetics

Duration: 3 hours

Protein binding: ~60%

Metabolism: Primarily renal to des-lys[1] pramlintide (active metabolite)

Bioavailability: ~30% to 40%

Half-life elimination: ~48 minutes

Time to peak, plasma: 20 minutes

Excretion: Primarily urine

Dosage SubQ: Adults: **Note:** When initiating pramlintide, reduce current insulin dose (including rapidly- and mixed-acting preparations) by 50% to avoid hypoglycemia.

Type 1 diabetes mellitus (insulin dependent, IDDM): Initial: 15 mcg immediately prior to meals; titrate in 15 mcg increments every 3 days (if no significant nausea occurs) to target dose of 30-60 mcg (consider discontinuation if intolerant of 30 mcg dose)

Type 2 diabetes mellitus (noninsulin dependent, NIDDM): Initial: 60 mcg immediately prior to meals; after 3-7 days, increase to 120 mcg prior to meals if no significant nausea occurs (if nausea occurs at 120 mcg dose, reduce to 60 mcg)

If pramlintide is discontinued for any reason, restart therapy with same initial titration protocol.

Dosage adjustment in renal impairment: No dosage adjustment required; not evaluated in dialysis patients

Dietary Considerations Dietary modification based on ADA recommendations is a part of therapy; pramlintide to be administered prior to major meals consisting of ≥250 Kcal or ≥30 g carbohydrates

Administration Do not mix with other insulins; administer subcutaneously into abdominal or thigh areas at sites distinct from concomitant insulin injections (do not administer into arm due to variable absorption); rotate injection sites frequently. Allow solution to reach room temperature before administering; may reduce injection site reactions. For oral medications in which a rapid onset of action is desired, administer 1 hour before, or 2 hours after pramlintide, if possible. When using the pen-injector, do not transfer drug to a syringe; dosing errors could occur.

Monitoring Parameters Prior to initiating therapy: Hb A_{1c}, hypoglycemic history, body weight. During therapy: urine sugar and acetone, pre- and postprandial and bedtime serum glucose, electrolytes, Hb A_{1c}, lipid profile

Dosage Forms Excipient information presented when available (limited, particularly for generics); consult specific product labeling. [DSC] = Discontinued product

Injection, solution, as acetate:

SymlinPen®: 1000 mcg/mL (2.7 mL) [120 pen-injector]

SymlinPen®: 1000 mcg/mL (1.5 mL) [60 pen-injector]

Symlin®: 600 mcg/mL (5 mL [DSC])

◆ **Pramlintide Acetate** *see* Pramlintide *on page* 1391

◆ **Pramosone®** *see* Pramoxine and Hydrocortisone *on page* 1393

◆ **Pramosone E™** *see* Pramoxine and Hydrocortisone *on page* 1393

◆ **Pramox® HC (Can)** *see* Pramoxine and Hydrocortisone *on page* 1393

Pramoxine and Hydrocortisone

(pra MOKS een & hye droe KOR ti sone)

Brand Names: U.S. Analpram E™; Analpram HC®; Epifoam®; Pramosone E™; Pramosone®; ProCort®; Proctofoam® HC; Zypram™

Brand Names: Canada Pramox® HC; Proctofoam™-HC

Index Terms Hydrocortisone and Pramoxine; Pramoxine Hydrochloride and Hydrocortisone Acetate

Pharmacologic Category Anesthetic/Corticosteroid

Use Relief of inflammatory and pruritic manifestations of corticosteroid-responsive dermatoses

Pregnancy Risk Factor C

Dosage Topical/rectal: Apply to affected areas 3-4 times/day. If clinical improvement is not seen within 2-3 weeks after initiating treatment or if condition worsens, product should be discontinued.

Additional Information Complete prescribing information for this medication should be consulted for additional detail.

Dosage Forms Excipient information presented when available (limited, particularly for generics); consult specific product labeling.

Aerosol, foam, rectal:

ProctoFoam® HC: Pramoxine hydrochloride 1% and hydrocortisone acetate 1% (10 g)

Aerosol, foam, topical:

Epifoam®: Pramoxine hydrochloride 1% and hydrocortisone acetate 1% (10 g)

Cream, topical: Pramoxine hydrochloride 1% and hydrocortisone acetate 1% (30 g); pramoxine hydrochloride 1% and hydrocortisone acetate 2.5% (30 g)

Analpram Advanced™ Kit: Pramoxine hydrochloride 1% and hydrocortisone acetate 2.5% (1s) [kit includes Analpram HC® cream (4 g x 30), diosmiplex (Vasculera™) tablets, AloeClean™ wipes, and applicators]

Analpram Advanced™ Kit: Pramoxine hydrochloride 1% and hydrocortisone acetate 2.5% (1s) [kit includes Analpram HC® cream (30 g), diosmiplex (Vasculera™) tablets, AloeClean™ wipes, and applicator]

Analpram E™: Pramoxine hydrochloride 1% and hydrocortisone acetate 2.5% (4 g, 30 g)

Analpram HC®: Pramoxine hydrochloride 1% and hydrocortisone acetate 1% (4 g, 30 g); pramoxine hydrochloride 1% and hydrocortisone acetate 2.5% (4 g, 30 g)

Pramosone®: Pramoxine hydrochloride 1% and hydrocortisone acetate 1% (30 g, 60 g); pramoxine hydrochloride 1% and hydrocortisone acetate 2.5% (30 g, 60 g)

Pramosone E™: Pramoxine hydrochloride 1% and hydrocortisone acetate 2.5% (30 g, 60 g)

ProCort®: Pramoxine hydrochloride 1.15% and hydrocortisone acetate 1.85% (60 g)

Zypram™: Pramoxine hydrochloride 1% and hydrocortisone acetate 2.35% (30 g) [contains benzyl alcohol, propylene glycol]

Lotion, topical:

Analpram-HC®: Pramoxine hydrochloride 1% and hydrocortisone acetate 2.5% (60 mL)

Pramosone®: Pramoxine hydrochloride 1% and hydrocortisone acetate 1% (60 mL, 120 mL, 240 mL); pramoxine hydrochloride 1% and hydrocortisone acetate 2.5% (60 mL, 120 mL)

Ointment, topical:

Pramosone®: Pramoxine hydrochloride 1% and hydrocortisone acetate 1% (30 g); pramoxine hydrochloride 1% and hydrocortisone acetate 2.5% (30 g)

◆ **Pramoxine Hydrochloride and Hydrocortisone Acetate** *see* Pramoxine and Hydrocortisone *on page* 1393

◆ **PrandiMet®** *see* Repaglinide and Metformin *on page* 1474

◆ **Prandin®** *see* Repaglinide *on page* 1472

◆ **Prascion®** *see* Sulfur and Sulfacetamide *on page* 1607

◆ **Prascion® FC** *see* Sulfur and Sulfacetamide *on page* 1607

◆ **Prascion® RA** *see* Sulfur and Sulfacetamide *on page* 1607

Prasugrel (PRA soo grel)

Brand Names: U.S. Effient®

Index Terms CS-747; LY-640315; Prasugrel Hydrochloride

Pharmacologic Category Antiplatelet Agent; Antiplatelet Agent, Thienopyridine

Use Reduces rate of thrombotic cardiovascular events (eg, stent thrombosis) in patients who are to be managed with percutaneous coronary intervention (PCI) for unstable angina, non-ST-segment elevation MI, or ST-elevation MI (STEMI)

Pregnancy Risk Factor B

Medication Guide Available Yes

Dosage Oral:

Adults: Acute coronary syndrome managed with PCI: Loading dose: 60 mg administered promptly (as soon as coronary anatomy is known or before if risk for bleeding is low and need for CABG considered unlikely) and no later than 1 hour after PCI; Maintenance dose: 10 mg once daily (in combination with aspirin 81-325 mg/day). **Note:** In patients weighing <60 kg, the manufacturer suggests to consider decreasing maintenance dose to 5 mg once daily; however, prospective clinical trial data does not exist to support this recommendation and may place some patients at risk of thrombotic complications (eg, stent thrombosis); consider use of full dose while monitoring closely for bleeding complications or administration of an alternative agent (eg, clopidogrel).

Duration of prasugrel (in combination with aspirin) after stent placement: **Premature interruption of therapy may result in stent thrombosis with subsequent fatal and nonfatal MI.** Those with ACS receiving either stent type (bare metal [BMS] or drug-eluting stent [DES]) or those receiving a DES for a non-ACS indication, prasugrel for at least 12 months is recommended. A duration >12 months may be considered in patients with DES placement (Levine, 2011; Wright, 2011). Those receiving a BMS for a non-ACS indication should be given at least 1 month and ideally up to 12 months; if patient is at increased risk of bleeding, give for a minimum of 2 weeks (Levine, 2011).

Elderly: Refer to adult dosing. Patients ≥75 years: Use not recommended; may be considered in high-risk situations (eg, patients with diabetes or history of MI)

Dosing adjustment in renal impairment: No dosage adjustment necessary

Dosing adjustment in hepatic impairment: No dosage adjustment necessary for mild-to-moderate hepatic impairment; use in severe hepatic impairment has not been evaluated

Additional Information Complete prescribing information for this medication should be consulted for additional detail.

Dosage Forms Excipient information presented when available (limited, particularly for generics); consult specific product labeling.

Tablet, oral:

Effient®: 5 mg, 10 mg

◆ **Prasugrel Hydrochloride** *see* Prasugrel *on page 1393*

◆ **Pravachol®** *see* Pravastatin *on page 1394*

Pravastatin (prav a STAT in)

Brand Names: U.S. Pravachol®

Brand Names: Canada Apo-Pravastatin®; CO Pravastatin; Dom-Pravastatin; Mylan-Pravastatin; Novo-Pravastatin; Nu-Pravastatin; PHL-Pravastatin; PMS-Pravastatin; Pravachol®; RAN™-Pravastatin; ratio-Pravastatin; Riva-Pravastatin; Sandoz-Pravastatin; ZYM-Pravastatin

Index Terms Pravastatin Sodium

Pharmacologic Category Antilipemic Agent, HMG-CoA Reductase Inhibitor

Additional Appendix Information

Hyperlipidemia Management *on page 1996*

Use Use with dietary therapy for the following:

Primary prevention of coronary events: In hypercholesterolemic patients without established coronary heart disease to reduce cardiovascular morbidity (myocardial infarction, coronary revascularization procedures) and mortality.

Secondary prevention of cardiovascular events in patients with established coronary heart disease: To slow the progression of coronary atherosclerosis; to reduce cardiovascular morbidity (myocardial infarction, coronary vascular procedures) and to reduce mortality; to reduce the risk of stroke and transient ischemic attacks

Hyperlipidemias: Reduce elevations in total cholesterol, LDL-C, apolipoprotein B, and triglycerides (elevations of 1 or more components are present in Fredrickson type IIa, IIb, III, and IV hyperlipidemias)

Heterozygous familial hypercholesterolemia (HeFH): In pediatric patients, 8-18 years of age, with HeFH having LDL-C ≥190 mg/dL **or** LDL ≥160 mg/dL with positive family history of premature cardiovascular disease (CVD) or 2 or more CVD risk factors in the pediatric patient

Pregnancy Risk Factor X

Pregnancy Considerations Cholesterol biosynthesis may be important in fetal development. Contraindicated in pregnancy. Administer to women of childbearing potential only when conception is highly unlikely and patients have been informed of potential hazards.

Lactation Enters breast milk/contraindicated

Contraindications Hypersensitivity to pravastatin or any component of the formulation; active liver disease; unexplained persistent elevations of serum transaminases; pregnancy; breast-feeding

Warnings/Precautions Secondary causes of hyperlipidemia should be ruled out prior to therapy. Liver function must be monitored by periodic laboratory assessment. Rhabdomyolysis with acute renal failure has occurred. Risk may be increased with concurrent use of other drugs which may cause rhabdomyolysis (including colchicine, gemfibrozil, fibric acid derivatives, or niacin at doses ≥1 g/day). The manufacturer recommends temporary discontinuation for elective major surgery, acute medical or surgical conditions, or in any patient experiencing an acute or serious condition predisposing to renal failure (eg, sepsis, hypotension, trauma, uncontrolled seizures). However, based upon current evidence, HMG-CoA reductase inhibitor therapy should be continued in the perioperative period unless risk outweighs cardioprotective benefit. Use with caution in patients with advanced age, these patients are predisposed to myopathy. Use caution in patients with previous liver disease or heavy ethanol use. Treatment in patients <8 years of age is not recommended.

Adverse Reactions As reported in short-term trials; safety and tolerability with long-term use were similar to placebo

1% to 10%:

Cardiovascular: Chest pain (4%)

Central nervous system: Headache (2% to 6%), fatigue (4%), dizziness (1% to 3%)

Dermatologic: Rash (4%)

Gastrointestinal: Nausea/vomiting (7%), diarrhea (6%), heartburn (3%)

Hepatic: Transaminases increased (>3x normal on two occasions - 1%)

Neuromuscular & skeletal: Myalgia (2%)

Respiratory: Cough (3%)

Miscellaneous: Influenza (2%)

<1% (Limited to important or life-threatening): Allergy, lens opacity, libido change, memory impairment, muscle weakness, neuropathy, paresthesia, taste disturbance, tremor, vertigo

Postmarketing and/or case reports: Anaphylaxis, angioedema, cholestatic jaundice, cirrhosis, cranial nerve dysfunction, dermatomyositis, erythema multiforme, ESR increase, fulminant hepatic necrosis, gynecomastia, hemolytic anemia, hepatitis, hepatoma, lupus erythematosus-like syndrome, myopathy, pancreatitis, peripheral nerve palsy, polymyalgia rheumatica, positive ANA, purpura, rhabdomyolysis, Stevens-Johnson syndrome, vasculitis

Additional class-related events or case reports (not necessarily reported with pravastatin therapy): Angioedema, cataracts, depression, dyspnea, eosinophilia, erectile dysfunction, facial paresis, hypersensitivity reaction, impaired extraocular muscle movement, impotence, interstitial lung disease, leukopenia, malaise, memory loss, ophthalmoplegia, paresthesia, peripheral neuropathy, photosensitivity, psychic disturbance, skin discoloration, thrombocytopenia, thyroid dysfunction, toxic epidermal necrolysis, transaminases increased, vomiting

Drug Interactions

Metabolism/Transport Effects Substrate of CYP3A4 (minor), P-glycoprotein, SLCO1B1; **Note:** Assignment of Major/Minor substrate status based on clinically relevant drug interaction potential; **Inhibits** CYP2C9 (weak), CYP2D6 (weak), CYP3A4 (weak)

Avoid Concomitant Use

Avoid concomitant use of Pravastatin with any of the following: Pimozide; Red Yeast Rice

Increased Effect/Toxicity

Pravastatin may increase the levels/effects of: DAPTOmycin; PARoxetine; Pimozide; Trabectedin; Vitamin K Antagonists

The levels/effects of Pravastatin may be increased by: Antifungal Agents (Azole Derivatives, Systemic); Colchicine; Conivaptan; CycloSPORINE; CycloSPORINE (Systemic); Eltrombopag; Fenofibrate; Fenofibric Acid; Gemfibrozil; Niacin; Niacinamide; P-glycoprotein/ABCB1 Inhibitors; Protease Inhibitors; Red Yeast Rice

Decreased Effect

Pravastatin may decrease the levels/effects of: Lanthanum

The levels/effects of Pravastatin may be decreased by: Antacids; Bile Acid Sequestrants; Efavirenz; Fosphenytoin; P-glycoprotein/ABCB1 Inducers; Phenytoin; Rifamycin Derivatives; Tocilizumab

Ethanol/Nutrition/Herb Interactions

Ethanol: Consumption of large amounts of ethanol may increase the risk of liver damage with HMG-CoA reductase inhibitors.

Food: Red yeast rice contains an estimated 2.4 mg lovastatin per 600 mg rice.

Herb/Nutraceutical: St John's wort may decrease pravastatin levels.

Stability Store at 25°C (77°F); excursions permitted to 15°C to 30°C (59°F to 86°F). Protect from moisture and light.

Mechanism of Action Pravastatin is a competitive inhibitor of 3-hydroxy-3-methylglutaryl coenzyme A (HMG-CoA) reductase, which is the rate-limiting enzyme involved in *de novo* cholesterol synthesis.

Pharmacodynamics/Kinetics

Onset of action: Several days

Peak effect: 4 weeks

Absorption: Rapidly absorbed; average absorption 34%

Protein binding: 50%

Metabolism: Hepatic multiple metabolites; primary metabolite is 3α-hydroxy-iso-pravastatin (2.5% to 10% activity of parent drug)

Bioavailability: 17%

Half-life elimination: 77 hours (including all metabolites); pravastatin: ~2-3 hours (Pan, 1990); 3α-hydroxy-iso-pravastatin: ~1.5 hours (Gustavson, 2005)

Time to peak, serum: 1-1.5 hours

Excretion: Feces (70%); urine (≤20%, 8% as unchanged drug)

Dosage Oral: **Note:** Doses should be individualized according to the baseline LDL-cholesterol levels, the recommended goal of therapy, and patient response; adjustments should be made at intervals of 4 weeks or more; doses may need adjusted based on concomitant medications

Children: HeFH:

8-13 years: 20 mg/day

14-18 years: 40 mg/day

Dosage adjustment for pravastatin based on concomitant cyclosporine: Refer to adult dosing section

Adults: Hyperlipidemias, primary prevention of coronary events, secondary prevention of cardiovascular events: Initial: 40 mg once daily; titrate dosage to response; usual range: 10-80 mg; (maximum dose: 80 mg once daily)

Dosage adjustment for pravastatin based on concomitant cyclosporine: Initial: 10 mg/day, titrate with caution (maximum dose: 20 mg/day)

Elderly: No specific dosage recommendations. Clearance is reduced in the elderly, resulting in an increase in AUC between 25% to 50%. However, substantial accumulation is not expected.

Dosing adjustment in renal impairment: Initial: 10 mg/day

Dosing adjustment in hepatic impairment: Initial: 10 mg/day

Dietary Considerations May be taken without regard to meals. Before initiation of therapy, patients should be placed on a standard cholesterol-lowering diet for 6 weeks and the diet should be continued during drug therapy. Red yeast rice contains an estimated 2.4 mg lovastatin per 600 mg rice.

Administration May be administered without regard to meals.

Monitoring Parameters Obtain baseline LFTs and total cholesterol profile; creatine phosphokinase due to possibility of myopathy. Repeat LFTs prior to elevation of dose. May be measured when clinically indicated and/or periodically thereafter; baseline CPK (recheck CPK in any patient with symptoms suggestive of myopathy). Monitor LDL-C at intervals no less than 4 weeks.

Dosage Forms Excipient information presented when available (limited, particularly for generics); consult specific product labeling.

Tablet, oral, as sodium: 10 mg, 20 mg, 40 mg, 80 mg

Pravachol®: 10 mg, 20 mg, 40 mg, 80 mg

◆ **Pravastatin Sodium** *see* Pravastatin *on page 1394*

◆ **Praxis ASA EC 81 Mg Daily Dose (Can)** *see* Aspirin *on page 154*

Praziquantel (pray zi KWON tel)

Brand Names: U.S. Biltricide®

Brand Names: Canada Biltricide®

Pharmacologic Category Anthelmintic

Use Treatment of all stages of schistosomiasis caused by all *Schistosoma* species; treatment of infection (clonorchiasis and opisthorchiasis) due to liver flukes

Unlabeled Use Cysticercosis and many intestinal tapeworms

Pregnancy Risk Factor B

Pregnancy Considerations Adverse effects have not been observed in animal reproduction studies. There are no adequate and well-controlled studies in pregnant women. Use in pregnant women only if clearly needed.

Lactation Enters breast milk/not recommended

Contraindications Hypersensitivity to praziquantel or any component of the formulation; ocular cysticercosis; concurrent use with strong CYP3A4 inducers, particularly rifampin

Warnings/Precautions Use caution in patients with moderate-to-severe hepatic disease or patients with cardiac abnormalities; patients with cerebral cysticercosis require hospitalization. Use not recommended in patients with a history of seizures or signs of central nervous system involvement (eg, subcutaneous nodules suggestive of cysticercosis); may exacerbate condition. Therapeutic levels of praziquantel may not be achieved with concurrent administration of strong inducers of cytochrome P450 (eg, rifampin); concurrent use is contraindicated. Patients should be instructed to not drive or operate machinery on the day of treatment and the day after treatment.

Adverse Reactions Frequency not defined.

Central nervous system: Dizziness, fever, headache, malaise

Dermatologic: Urticaria (rare)

Gastrointestinal: Abdominal discomfort, nausea

Postmarketing and/or case reports: Allergic reaction, anorexia, arrhythmia, AV block, bloody diarrhea, bradycardia, ectopic rhythms, eosinophilia, hypersensitivity, liver enzymes increased, myalgia, polyserositis, pruritus, seizure, somnolence, ventricular fibrillation, vertigo, vomiting, weakness

Drug Interactions

Metabolism/Transport Effects Substrate of CYP3A4 (major); **Note:** Assignment of Major/Minor substrate status based on clinically relevant drug interaction potential; **Inhibits** CYP2D6 (weak)

Avoid Concomitant Use

Avoid concomitant use of Praziquantel with any of the following: Conivaptan; CYP3A4 Inducers (Strong)

Increased Effect/Toxicity

The levels/effects of Praziquantel may be increased by: Cimetidine; Conivaptan; CYP3A4 Inhibitors (Moderate); CYP3A4 Inhibitors (Strong); Dasatinib; Ketoconazole; Ketoconazole (Systemic)

Decreased Effect

The levels/effects of Praziquantel may be decreased by: Aminoquinolines (Antimalarial); CYP3A4 Inducers (Strong); Deferasirox; Herbs (CYP3A4 Inducers); Tocilizumab

Stability Store below 30°C (86°F).

Mechanism of Action Increases the cell permeability to calcium in schistosomes, causing strong contractions and paralysis of worm musculature leading to detachment of suckers from the blood vessel walls and to dislodgment

Pharmacodynamics/Kinetics

Absorption: Oral: 80%

Protein binding: ~80%

Metabolism: Extensive first-pass effect

Half-life elimination: Parent drug: 0.8-1.5 hours; Metabolites: 4.5 hours

Time to peak, serum: 1-3 hours

Excretion: Urine ~80% (>99% as metabolites)

Dosage Oral: Children ≥4 years and Adults:

Schistosomiasis: 20 mg/kg/dose 3 times/day for 1 day at 4- to 6-hour intervals

Clonorchiasis/opisthorchiasis: 25 mg/kg/dose 3 times/day for 1 day at 4- to 6-hour intervals

Cysticercosis (unlabeled use): 50 mg/kg/day divided every 8 hours for 14 days (Takayanagui, 2004)

Tapeworms (unlabeled use): 5-10 mg/kg as a single dose (25 mg/kg for *Hymenolepis nana*) (Liu, 1996)

Administration Administer tablets with water during meals. Tablets should be promptly swallowed to avoid bitter taste that may cause gagging or vomiting. Tablets may be halved or quartered; do not chew.

Monitoring Parameters Culture urine or feces for ova prior to instituting therapy

Dosage Forms Excipient information presented when available (limited, particularly for generics); consult specific product labeling.

Tablet, oral:

Biltricide®: 600 mg [scored]

Prazosin (PRAZ oh sin)

Brand Names: U.S. Minipress®

Brand Names: Canada Apo-Prazo®; Minipress®; Novo-Prazin; Nu-Prazo; Teva-Prazosin

Index Terms Furazosin; Prazosin Hydrochloride

Pharmacologic Category Alpha$_1$ Blocker

Use Treatment of hypertension

Unlabeled Use Post-traumatic stress disorder (PTSD) related nightmares and sleep disruption; benign prostatic hyperplasia; Raynaud's syndrome

Pregnancy Risk Factor C

Dosage Oral:

Children: Hypertension (unlabeled use): Initial: 0.05-0.1 mg/kg/day in 3 divided doses; maximum: 0.5 mg/kg/day (not to exceed 20 mg) (NHBPEP, Fourth Report)

Adults:

Hypertension: Initial: 1 mg/dose 2-3 times/day; usual maintenance dose: 2-20 mg/day in divided doses 2-3 times/day (JNC 7); maximum daily dose: 20 mg

PTSD-related nightmares and sleep disruption (unlabeled use): Initial: 1 mg at bedtime (Raskind, 2002; Raskind, 2007); titrate as tolerated to 2-15 mg at bedtime (Benedek, 2009)

Raynaud's (unlabeled use): Dosage range: 1-5 mg twice daily (Bakst, 2008)

Benign prostatic hyperplasia (unlabeled use): Initial: 0.5 mg twice daily; titrate as tolerated to 2 mg twice daily (Moran, 2001)

Elderly: Hypertension: Consider lower initial doses and titrate to response (Aronow, 2011)

Additional Information Complete prescribing information for this medication should be consulted for additional detail.

Dosage Forms Excipient information presented when available (limited, particularly for generics); consult specific product labeling.

Capsule, oral, as hydrochloride: 1 mg, 2 mg, 5 mg

Minipress®: 1 mg, 2 mg, 5 mg

- **Prazosin Hydrochloride** *see* Prazosin *on page 1396*
- **Precedex®** *see* Dexmedetomidine *on page 484*
- **Precose®** *see* Acarbose *on page 26*
- **Pred Forte®** *see* PrednisoLONE (Ophthalmic) *on page 1398*
- **Pred-G®** *see* Prednisolone and Gentamicin *on page 1399*
- **Pred Mild®** *see* PrednisoLONE (Ophthalmic) *on page 1398*

Prednicarbate (pred ni KAR bate)

Brand Names: U.S. Dermatop®

Brand Names: Canada Dermatop®

Pharmacologic Category Corticosteroid, Topical

Additional Appendix Information

Corticosteroids *on page 1888*

Use Relief of the inflammatory and pruritic manifestations of corticosteroid-responsive dermatoses (medium potency topical corticosteroid)

Pregnancy Risk Factor C

Dosage Note: Therapy should be discontinued when control is achieved; if no improvement is seen within 2 weeks, reassessment of diagnosis may be necessary.

Cream: Children ≥1 year and Adults: Topical: Apply a thin film to affected area twice daily

Ointment: Children ≥10 year and Adults: Topical: Apply a thin film to affected area twice daily

Additional Information Complete prescribing information for this medication should be consulted for additional detail.

Dosage Forms Excipient information presented when available (limited, particularly for generics); consult specific product labeling.

Cream, topical: 0.1% (15 g, 60 g)

Dermatop®: 0.1% (60 g)

Ointment, topical: 0.1% (15 g, 60 g)

Dermatop®: 0.1% (60 g)

PrednisoLONE (Systemic) (pred NISS oh lone)

Brand Names: U.S. Flo-Pred™; Millipred™; Millipred™ DP; Orapred ODT®; Orapred®; Pediapred®; Veripred™ 20

Brand Names: Canada Hydeltra T.B.A.®; Novo-Prednisolone; Pediapred®

Index Terms Prednisolone Sodium Phosphate

Pharmacologic Category Corticosteroid, Systemic

Additional Appendix Information

Corticosteroids *on page 1888*

Use Treatment of endocrine disorders, rheumatic disorders, collagen diseases, allergic states, respiratory diseases, hematologic disorders, neoplastic diseases, edematous states, and gastrointestinal diseases; resolution of acute exacerbations of multiple sclerosis; management of fulminating or disseminated tuberculosis and trichinosis; acute or chronic solid organ rejection

Pregnancy Risk Factor C/D (Flo-Pred™)

Pregnancy Considerations Adverse events have been observed with corticosteroids in animal reproduction studies. Prednisolone crosses the placenta; prior to reaching the fetus, prednisolone is converted by placental enzymes to prednisone. As a result, the amount of prednisolone reaching the fetus is ~8-10 times lower than the maternal serum concentration (healthy women at term; similar results observed with preterm pregnancies complicated by HELLP syndrome). Human studies have shown an association between first trimester corticosteroid use and oral clefts. Additional adverse events in the fetus/neonate, including low birth weight, have been noted in case reports following large doses of systemic corticosteroids during pregnancy. Women exposed to prednisolone during pregnancy for the treatment of an autoimmune disease may contact the OTIS Autoimmune Diseases Study at 877-311-8972.

Lactation Enters breast milk/use caution (AAP rates "compatible"; AAP 2001 update pending)

Contraindications Hypersensitivity to prednisolone or any component of the formulation; acute superficial herpes simplex keratitis; live or attenuated virus vaccines (with immunosuppressive doses of corticosteroids); systemic fungal infections; varicella

Warnings/Precautions May cause hypercorticism or suppression of hypothalamic-pituitary-adrenal (HPA) axis, particularly in younger children or in patients receiving high doses for prolonged periods. HPA axis suppression may lead to adrenal crisis. Withdrawal and discontinuation of a corticosteroid should be done slowly and carefully. Particular care is required when patients are transferred from systemic corticosteroids to inhaled products due to possible adrenal insufficiency or withdrawal from steroids, including an increase in allergic symptoms. Patients receiving >20 mg per day of prednisone (or equivalent) may be most susceptible. Fatalities have occurred due to adrenal insufficiency in asthmatic patients during and after transfer from systemic corticosteroids to aerosol steroids; aerosol steroids do **not** provide the systemic steroid needed to treat patients having trauma, surgery, or infections.

Acute myopathy has been reported with high dose corticosteroids, usually in patients with neuromuscular transmission disorders; may involve ocular and/or respiratory muscles; monitor creatine kinase; recovery may be delayed. Corticosteroid use may cause psychiatric disturbances, including depression, euphoria, insomnia, mood swings, and personality changes. Pre-existing psychiatric conditions may be exacerbated by corticosteroid use. Prolonged use of corticosteroids may also increase the incidence of secondary infection, mask acute infection (including fungal infections), prolong or exacerbate viral infections, or limit response to vaccines. Exposure to chickenpox should be avoided; corticosteroids should not be used to treat ocular herpes simplex. Corticosteroids should not be used for cerebral malaria or viral hepatitis. Close observation is required in patients with latent tuberculosis and/or TB reactivity; restrict use in active TB (only in conjunction with antituberculosis treatment). Prolonged use of corticosteroids may result in glaucoma; cataract formation may occur. Prolonged treatment with corticosteroids has been associated with the development of Kaposi's sarcoma (case reports); if noted, discontinuation of therapy should be considered.

Use with caution in patients with thyroid disease, hepatic impairment, renal impairment, cardiovascular disease, diabetes, glaucoma, cataracts, myasthenia gravis, patients at risk for osteoporosis, patients at risk for seizures, or GI diseases (diverticulitis, peptic ulcer, ulcerative colitis) due to perforation risk. Use caution following acute MI (corticosteroids have been associated with myocardial rupture). Because of the risk of adverse effects, systemic corticosteroids should be used cautiously in the elderly in the smallest possible effective dose for the shortest duration. Withdraw therapy with gradual tapering of dose. May affect growth velocity; growth should be routinely monitored in pediatric patients.

Adverse Reactions Frequency not defined.

Cardiovascular: Cardiomyopathy, CHF, edema, facial edema, hypertension

Central nervous system: Headache, insomnia, malaise, nervousness, pseudotumor cerebri, psychic disorders, seizure, vertigo

Dermatologic: Bruising, facial erythema, hirsutism, petechiae, skin test reaction suppression, thin fragile skin, urticaria

Endocrine & metabolic: Carbohydrate tolerance decreased, Cushing's syndrome, diabetes mellitus, growth suppression, hyperglycemia, hypernatremia, hypokalemia, hypokalemic alkalosis, menstrual irregularities, negative nitrogen balance, pituitary adrenal axis suppression

Gastrointestinal: Abdominal distention, increased appetite, indigestion, nausea, pancreatitis, peptic ulcer, ulcerative esophagitis, weight gain

Hepatic: LFTs increased (usually reversible)

Neuromuscular & skeletal: Arthralgia, aseptic necrosis (humeral/femoral heads), fractures, muscle mass decreased, muscle weakness, osteoporosis, steroid myopathy, tendon rupture, weakness

Ocular: Cataracts, exophthalmus, eyelid edema, glaucoma, intraocular pressure increased, irritation

Respiratory: Epistaxis

Miscellaneous: Diaphoresis increased, impaired wound healing

Drug Interactions

Metabolism/Transport Effects Substrate of CYP3A4 (minor); **Note:** Assignment of Major/Minor substrate status based on clinically relevant drug interaction potential; **Inhibits** CYP3A4 (weak)

Avoid Concomitant Use

Avoid concomitant use of PrednisoLONE (Systemic) with any of the following: Aldesleukin; BCG; Natalizumab; Pimecrolimus; Pimozide; Tacrolimus (Topical)

Increased Effect/Toxicity

PrednisoLONE (Systemic) may increase the levels/effects of: Acetylcholinesterase Inhibitors; Amphotericin B; CycloSPORINE; CycloSPORINE (Systemic); Deferasirox; Leflunomide; Loop Diuretics; Natalizumab; NSAID (COX-2 Inhibitor); NSAID (Nonselective); Pimozide; Thiazide Diuretics; Vaccines (Live); Warfarin

The levels/effects of PrednisoLONE (Systemic) may be increased by: Antifungal Agents (Azole Derivatives, Systemic); Aprepitant; Calcium Channel Blockers (Nondihydropyridine); Conivaptan; CycloSPORINE; CycloSPORINE (Systemic); Denosumab; Estrogen Derivatives; Fluconazole; Fosaprepitant; Indacaterol; Macrolide Antibiotics; Neuromuscular-Blocking Agents (Nondepolarizing); Pimecrolimus; Quinolone Antibiotics; Roflumilast; Salicylates; Tacrolimus (Topical); Telaprevir; Trastuzumab

Decreased Effect

PrednisoLONE (Systemic) may decrease the levels/effects of: Aldesleukin; Antidiabetic Agents; BCG; Calcitriol; Coccidioidin Skin Test; Corticorelin; CycloSPORINE; CycloSPORINE (Systemic); Isoniazid; Salicylates; Sipuleucel-T; Telaprevir; Vaccines (Inactivated)

The levels/effects of PrednisoLONE (Systemic) may be decreased by: Aminoglutethimide; Antacids; Barbiturates; Bile Acid Sequestrants; Echinacea; Mitotane; Primidone; Rifamycin Derivatives; Tocilizumab

Ethanol/Nutrition/Herb Interactions

Ethanol: Avoid ethanol (may increase gastric mucosal irritation).

Food: Prednisolone interferes with calcium absorption. Limit caffeine.

Herb/Nutraceutical: St John's wort may decrease prednisolone levels. Avoid cat's claw, echinacea (have immunostimulant properties).

Stability

Flo-Pred™: Store at 20°C to 25°C (68°F to 77°F). Flo-Pred™ should be dispensed in the original container (to avoid loss of formulation during transfer).

Millipred™: Store at 20°C to 25°C (68°F to 77°F).

Orapred ODT®: Store at 20°C to 25°C (68°F to 77°F) in blister pack. Protect from moisture.

Orapred®, Veripred™ 20: 2°C to 8°C (36°F to 46°F).

Pediapred®: 4°C to 25°C (39°F to 77°F); may be refrigerated.

Mechanism of Action Decreases inflammation by suppression of migration of polymorphonuclear leukocytes and reversal of increased capillary permeability; suppresses the immune system by reducing activity and volume of the lymphatic system

Pharmacodynamics/Kinetics

Duration: 18-36 hours

Protein binding (concentration dependent): 65% to 91%; decreased in elderly

Metabolism: Primarily hepatic, but also metabolized in most tissues, to inactive compounds

Half-life elimination: 3.6 hours; End-stage renal disease: 3-5 hours

Excretion: Primarily urine (as glucuronides, sulfates, and unconjugated metabolites)

Dosage Dose depends upon condition being treated and response of patient; dosage for infants and children should be based on severity of the disease and response of the patient rather than on strict adherence to dosage indicated by age, weight, or body surface area. Oral dosage expressed in terms of prednisolone base. Consider alternate day therapy for long-term therapy. Discontinuation of long-term therapy requires gradual withdrawal by tapering the dose. Patients undergoing unusual stress while receiving corticosteroids should receive increased doses prior to, during, and after the stressful situation.

Children: Oral:

Acute asthma: 1-2 mg/kg/day in divided doses 1-2 times/day for 3-5 days

Anti-inflammatory or immunosuppressive dose: 0.1-2 mg/kg/day in divided doses 1-4 times/day

Nephrotic syndrome:

Initial (first 3 episodes): 2 mg/kg/day **or** 60 mg/m^2/day (maximum: 80 mg/day) in divided doses 3-4 times/day until urine is protein free for 3 consecutive days (maximum: 28 days); followed by 1-1.5 mg/kg/dose **or** 40 mg/m^2/dose given every other day for 4 weeks

Maintenance (long-term maintenance dose for frequent relapses): 0.5-1 mg/kg/dose given every other day for 3-6 months

Adults: Oral:

Usual range: 5-60 mg/day

Multiple sclerosis: 200 mg/day for 1 week followed by 80 mg every other day for 1 month

Rheumatoid arthritis: Initial: 5-7.5 mg/day; adjust dose as necessary

Elderly: Use lowest effective dose

Dosing adjustment in hyperthyroidism: Prednisolone dose may need to be increased to achieve adequate therapeutic effects

Hemodialysis: Slightly dialyzable (5% to 20%); administer dose posthemodialysis

Peritoneal dialysis: Supplemental dose is not necessary

Dietary Considerations Should be taken after meals or with food or milk to decrease GI effects; increase dietary intake of pyridoxine, vitamin C, vitamin D, folate, calcium, and phosphorus.

Administration Administer oral formulation with food or milk to decrease GI effects.

Flo-Pred™: Administer using the provided calibrated syringe (supplied by manufacturer) to accurately measure the dose. Syringe should be washed prior to next use.

Orapred ODT®: Do not break or use partial tablet. Remove tablet from blister pack just prior to use. May swallow whole or allow to dissolve on tongue.

Monitoring Parameters Blood pressure; blood glucose, electrolytes; intraocular pressure (use >6 weeks); bone mineral density; growth in children

Test Interactions Response to skin tests

Dosage Forms Excipient information presented when available (limited, particularly for generics); consult specific product labeling.

Solution, oral, as base: 15 mg/5 mL (240 mL, 480 mL)

Solution, oral, as sodium phosphate [strength expressed as base]: 5 mg/5 mL (120 mL); 15 mg/5 mL (237 mL, 473 mL)

Millipred™: 10 mg/5 mL (237 mL) [dye free, ethanol free; grape flavor]

Orapred®: 15 mg/5 mL (20 mL, 237 mL) [dye free; contains ethanol 2%, sodium benzoate; grape flavor]

Pediapred®: 5 mg/5 mL (120 mL) [dye free; raspberry flavor]

Veripred™ 20: 20 mg/5 mL (237 mL) [dye free, ethanol free; grape flavor]

Suspension, oral, as acetate [strength expressed as base]:

Flo-Pred™: 15 mg/5 mL (52 mL) [contains propylene glycol; cherry flavor]

Tablet, orally disintegrating, oral, as sodium phosphate [strength expressed as base]:

Orapred ODT®: 10 mg, 15 mg, 30 mg [grape flavor]

PrednisoLONE (Ophthalmic) (pred NISS oh lone)

Brand Names: U.S. Omnipred™; Pred Forte®; Pred Mild®

Brand Names: Canada Diopred®; Ophtho-Tate®; Pred Forte®; Pred Mild®

Index Terms Econopred; Prednisolone Acetate, Ophthalmic; Prednisolone Sodium Phosphate, Ophthalmic

Pharmacologic Category Corticosteroid, Ophthalmic

Use Treatment of palpebral and bulbar conjunctivitis; corneal injury from chemical, radiation, thermal burns, or foreign body penetration; steroid-responsive inflammatory ophthalmic diseases

Pregnancy Risk Factor C

Dosage Ophthalmic suspension/solution: Children and Adults: Instill 1-2 drops in the eye 2-4 times daily

Additional Information Complete prescribing information for this medication should be consulted for additional detail.

Dosage Forms Excipient information presented when available (limited, particularly for generics); consult specific product labeling. [DSC] = Discontinued product

Solution, ophthalmic, as sodium phosphate [drops]: 1% (5 mL [DSC], 10 mL, 15 mL [DSC])

Suspension, ophthalmic, as acetate [drops]: 1% (5 mL, 10 mL, 15 mL)

Omnipred™: 1% (5 mL, 10 mL) [contains benzalkonium chloride]

Pred Forte®: 1% (1 mL, 5 mL, 10 mL, 15 mL) [contains benzalkonium chloride, sodium bisulfite]

Pred Mild®: 0.12% (5 mL, 10 mL) [contains benzalkonium chloride, sodium bisulfite]

◆ **Prednisolone Acetate, Ophthalmic** *see* PrednisoLONE (Ophthalmic) *on page 1398*

Prednisolone and Gentamicin

(pred NIS oh lone & jen ta MYE sin)

Brand Names: U.S. Pred-G®

Index Terms Gentamicin and Prednisolone

Pharmacologic Category Antibiotic/Corticosteroid, Ophthalmic

Use Treatment of steroid responsive inflammatory conditions and superficial ocular infections due to microorganisms susceptible to gentamicin

Pregnancy Risk Factor C

Dosage Ophthalmic: Children and Adults:

Ointment: Apply 1/2 inch ribbon in the conjunctival sac 1-3 times/day

Suspension: 1 drop 2-4 times/day; during the initial 24-48 hours, the dosing frequency may be increased if necessary up to 1 drop every hour

Additional Information Complete prescribing information for this medication should be consulted for additional detail.

Dosage Forms Excipient information presented when available (limited, particularly for generics); consult specific product labeling. [DSC] = Discontinued product

Ointment, ophthalmic:

Pred-G®: Prednisolone acetate 0.6% and gentamicin sulfate 0.3% (3.5 g)

Suspension, ophthalmic:

Pred-G®: Prednisolone acetate 1% and gentamicin sulfate 0.3% (5 mL, 10 mL [DSC]) [contains benzalkonium chloride]

◆ **Prednisolone and Sulfacetamide** *see* Sulfacetamide and Prednisolone *on page 1600*

◆ **Prednisolone Sodium Phosphate** *see* PrednisoLONE (Systemic) *on page 1396*

◆ **Prednisolone Sodium Phosphate, Ophthalmic** *see* PrednisoLONE (Ophthalmic) *on page 1398*

PredniSONE (PRED ni sone)

Brand Names: U.S. PredniSONE Intensol™

Brand Names: Canada Apo-Prednisone®; Novo-Prednisone; Winpred™

Index Terms Deltacortisone; Deltadehydrocortisone

Pharmacologic Category Corticosteroid, Systemic

Additional Appendix Information

Contrast Media Reactions, Premedication for Prophylaxis *on page 1976*

Corticosteroids *on page 1888*

Use Treatment of a variety of diseases, including:

Allergic states (including adjunctive treatment of anaphylaxis)

Autoimmune disorders (including systemic lupus erythematosus [SLE])

Collagen diseases

Dermatologic conditions/diseases

Edematous states (including nephrotic syndrome)

Endocrine disorders

Gastrointestinal diseases

Hematologic disorders (including idiopathic thrombocytopenia purpura [ITP])

Multiple sclerosis exacerbations

Neoplastic diseases

Ophthalmic diseases

Respiratory diseases (including acute asthma exacerbation)

Rheumatic disorders (including rheumatoid arthritis)

Trichinosis with neurologic or myocardial involvement

Tuberculous meningitis

Unlabeled Use Adjunctive therapy for *Pneumocystis jirovecii* (formerly *carinii*) pneumonia (PCP); autoimmune hepatitis; adjunctive therapy for pain management in immunocompetent patients with herpes zoster; tuberculosis (severe, paradoxical reactions); Takayasu arteritis; giant cell arteritis; Grave's ophthalmopathy prophylaxis; subacute thyroiditis; thyrotoxicosis (type II amiodarone-induced)

Pregnancy Considerations Adverse events have been observed with corticosteroids in animal reproduction studies. Prednisone and prednisolone cross the human placenta. In the mother, prednisone is converted to the active metabolite prednisolone by the liver. Prior to reaching the fetus, prednisolone is converted by placental enzymes back to prednisone. As a result, the level of prednisone remaining in the maternal serum and reaching the fetus are similar; however, the amount of prednisolone reaching the fetus is ~8-10 times lower than the maternal serum concentration (healthy women at term). Some studies have shown an association between first trimester prednisone use and oral clefts; adverse events in the fetus/neonate have been noted in case reports following large doses of systemic corticosteroids during pregnancy. Pregnant women exposed to prednisone for antirejection therapy following a transplant may contact the National Transplantation Pregnancy Registry (NTPR) at 215-955-4820. Women exposed to prednisone during pregnancy for the treatment of an autoimmune disease (eg, rheumatoid arthritis) may contact the OTIS Autoimmune Diseases Study at 877-311-8972.

Lactation Enters breast milk/AAP rates "compatible" (AAP 2001 update pending)

Contraindications Hypersensitivity to any component of the formulation; systemic fungal infections; administration of live or live attenuated vaccines with immunosuppressive doses of prednisone

Warnings/Precautions May cause hypercorticism or suppression of hypothalamic-pituitary-adrenal (HPA) axis, particularly in younger children or in patients receiving high doses for prolonged periods. HPA axis suppression may lead to adrenal crisis. Withdrawal and discontinuation of a corticosteroid should be done slowly and carefully. Particular care is required when patients are transferred from systemic corticosteroids to inhaled products due to possible adrenal insufficiency or withdrawal from steroids, including an increase in allergic symptoms. Patients receiving >20 mg per day of prednisone (or equivalent) may be most susceptible. Fatalities have occurred due to adrenal insufficiency in asthmatic patients during and after transfer from systemic corticosteroids to aerosol steroids; aerosol steroids do **not** provide the systemic steroid needed to treat patients having trauma, surgery, or infections.

Acute myopathy has been reported with high dose corticosteroids, usually in patients with neuromuscular transmission disorders; may involve ocular and/or respiratory muscles; monitor creatine kinase; recovery may be delayed. Prolonged use of corticosteroids may increase the incidence of secondary infection, mask acute infection (including fungal infections), prolong or exacerbate viral infections, or limit response to vaccines. Exposure to chickenpox should be avoided. Corticosteroids should not be used to treat ocular herpes simplex or cerebral malaria. Close observation is required in patients with latent tuberculosis and/or TB reactivity; restrict use in active TB (only in conjunction with antituberculosis treatment). Prolonged treatment with corticosteroids has been associated with the development of Kaposi's sarcoma (case reports); if noted, discontinuation of therapy should be considered. Prolonged use may cause posterior subcapsular cataracts, glaucoma (with possible nerve damage) and may increase the risk for ocular infections. Corticosteroid use may cause psychiatric disturbances, including depression, euphoria, insomnia, mood swings, and personality changes. Pre-existing psychiatric conditions may be exacerbated by corticosteroid use.

Use with caution in patients with HF, diabetes, GI diseases (diverticulitis, peptic ulcer, ulcerative colitis; due to risk of perforation), hepatic impairment, myasthenia gravis, MI, patients with or who are at risk for osteoporosis, seizure disorders or thyroid disease. May affect growth velocity; growth should be routinely monitored in pediatric patients.

Prior to use, the dose and duration of treatment should be based on the risk versus benefit for each individual patient. In general, use the smallest effective dose for the shortest duration of time to minimize adverse events. A gradual tapering of dose may be required prior to discontinuing therapy.

Adverse Reactions Frequency not defined.

Cardiovascular: Congestive heart failure (in susceptible patients), hypertension

Central nervous system: Emotional instability, headache, intracranial pressure increased (with papilledema), psychic derangements (including euphoria, insomnia, mood swings, personality changes, severe depression), seizure, vertigo

Dermatologic: Bruising, facial erythema, petechiae, thin fragile skin, urticaria, wound healing impaired

Endocrine & metabolic: Adrenocortical and pituitary unresponsiveness (in times of stress), carbohydrate intolerance, Cushing's syndrome, diabetes mellitus, fluid retention, growth suppression (in children), hypokalemic alkalosis, hypothyroidism enhanced, menstrual irregularities, negative nitrogen balance due to protein catabolism, potassium loss, sodium retention

Gastrointestinal: Abdominal distension, pancreatitis, peptic ulcer (with possible perforation and hemorrhage), ulcerative esophagitis

Hepatic: ALT increased, AST increased, alkaline phosphatase increased

Neuromuscular & skeletal: Aseptic necrosis of femoral and humeral heads, muscle mass loss, muscle weakness, osteoporosis, pathologic fracture of long bones, steroid myopathy, tendon rupture (particularly Achilles tendon), vertebral compression fractures

Ocular: Exophthalmos, glaucoma, intraocular pressure increased, posterior subcapsular cataracts

Miscellaneous: Allergic reactions, anaphylactic reactions, diaphoresis, hypersensitivity reactions, infections, Kaposi's sarcoma

Drug Interactions

Metabolism/Transport Effects Substrate of CYP3A4 (minor); **Note:** Assignment of Major/Minor substrate status based on clinically relevant drug interaction potential; **Induces** CYP2C19 (weak/moderate), CYP3A4 (weak/moderate)

Avoid Concomitant Use

Avoid concomitant use of PredniSONE with any of the following: Aldesleukin; BCG; Natalizumab; Pimecrolimus; Tacrolimus (Topical)

Increased Effect/Toxicity

PredniSONE may increase the levels/effects of: Acetylcholinesterase Inhibitors; Amphotericin B; CycloSPORINE; CycloSPORINE (Systemic); Deferasirox; Leflunomide; Loop Diuretics; Natalizumab; NSAID (COX-2 Inhibitor); NSAID (Nonselective); Thiazide Diuretics; Vaccines (Live); Warfarin

The levels/effects of PredniSONE may be increased by: Antifungal Agents (Azole Derivatives, Systemic); Aprepitant; Calcium Channel Blockers (Nondihydropyridine); Conivaptan; CycloSPORINE; CycloSPORINE (Systemic); Denosumab; Estrogen Derivatives; Fluconazole; Fosaprepitant; Indacaterol; Macrolide Antibiotics; Neuromuscular-Blocking Agents (Nondepolarizing); Pimecrolimus; Quinolone Antibiotics; Ritonavir; Roflumilast; Salicylates; Tacrolimus (Topical); Telaprevir; Trastuzumab

Decreased Effect

PredniSONE may decrease the levels/effects of: Aldesleukin; Antidiabetic Agents; ARIPiprazole; BCG; Calcitriol; Coccidioidin Skin Test; Corticorelin; CycloSPORINE; CycloSPORINE (Systemic); Isoniazid; Salicylates; Sipuleucel-T; Telaprevir; Vaccines (Inactivated)

The levels/effects of PredniSONE may be decreased by: Aminoglutethimide; Antacids; Barbiturates; Bile Acid Sequestrants; Echinacea; Mitotane; Primidone; Rifamycin Derivatives; Somatropin; Tesamorelin; Tocilizumab

Ethanol/Nutrition/Herb Interactions

Ethanol: Avoid ethanol (may increase gastric mucosal irritation)

Food: Prednisone interferes with calcium absorption. Limit caffeine.

Herb/Nutraceutical: St John's wort may decrease prednisone levels. Avoid cat's claw, echinacea (have immunostimulant properties).

Mechanism of Action Decreases inflammation by suppression of migration of polymorphonuclear leukocytes and reversal of increased capillary permeability; suppresses the immune system by reducing activity and volume of the lymphatic system; suppresses adrenal function at high doses. Antitumor effects may be related to inhibition of glucose transport, phosphorylation, or induction of cell death in immature lymphocytes. Antiemetic effects are thought to occur due to blockade of cerebral innervation of the emetic center via inhibition of prostaglandin synthesis.

Pharmacodynamics/Kinetics

Absorption: 50% to 90% (may be altered in IBS or hyperthyroidism)

Protein binding (concentration dependent): 65% to 91%

Metabolism: Hepatically converted from prednisone (inactive) to prednisolone (active); may be impaired with hepatic dysfunction

Half-life elimination: Normal renal function: ~3.5 hours

Excretion: Urine (small portion)

Dosage Oral:

General dosing range: Children and Adults: Initial: 5-60 mg/day: **Note:** Dose depends upon condition being treated and response of patient; dosage for infants and children should be based on severity of the disease and response of the patient rather than on strict adherence to dosage indicated by age, weight, or body surface area. Consider alternate day therapy for long-term therapy. Discontinuation of long-term therapy requires gradual withdrawal by tapering the dose.

Prednisone taper (other regimens also available):
Day 1: 30 mg divided as 10 mg before breakfast, 5 mg at lunch, 5 mg at dinner, 10 mg at bedtime
Day 2: 5 mg at breakfast, 5 mg at lunch, 5 mg at dinner, 10 mg at bedtime
Day 3: 5 mg 4 times/day (with meals and at bedtime)
Day 4: 5 mg 3 times/day (breakfast, lunch, bedtime)
Day 5: 5 mg 2 times/day (breakfast, bedtime)
Day 6: 5 mg before breakfast

Indication-specific dosing:
Children:
Acute asthma (NIH guidelines, 2007):
0-11 years 1-2 mg/kg/day for 3-10 days (maximum: 60 mg/day)
≥12 years: Refer to Adults dosing
Autoimmune hepatitis (unlabeled use; Czaja, 2002): Initial treatment: 2 mg/kg/day for 2 weeks (maximum: 60 mg/day), followed by a taper over 6-8 weeks to a dose of 0.1-0.2 mg/kg/day or 5 mg/day
Nephrotic syndrome (Pediatric Nephrology Panel recommendations [Hogg, 2000]): Initial: 2 mg/kg/day or 60 mg/m^2/day given every day in 1-3 divided doses (maximum: 80 mg/day) until urine is protein free or for 4-6 weeks; followed by maintenance dose: 2 mg/kg/dose or 40 mg/m^2/dose given every other day in the morning; gradually taper and discontinue after 4-6 weeks. **Note:** No definitive treatment guidelines exist. Dosing is dependent on institution protocols and individual response.
PCP pneumonia (AIDS*info* guidelines, 2008): 1 mg/kg twice daily for 5 days, *followed by* 0.5-1 mg/kg twice daily for 5 days, *followed by* 0.5 mg/kg once daily for 11-21 days
Adolescents and Adults:
PCP pneumonia (AIDS*info* guidelines, 2008): Note: Begin within 72 hours of PCP therapy: 40 mg twice daily for 5 days, *followed by* 40 mg once daily for 5 days, *followed by* 20 mg once daily for 11 days or until antimicrobial regimen is completed
Adults:
Acute asthma (NIH guidelines, 2007): 40-60 mg per day for 3-10 days; administer as single or 2 divided doses
Anaphylaxis, adjunctive treatment (Lieberman, 2005): 0.5 mg/kg
Antineoplastic: Usual range: 10 mg/day to 100 mg/m^2/day (depending on indication). **Note:** Details concerning dosing in combination regimens should also be consulted.
Autoimmune hepatitis (unlabeled use; Czaja, 2002): Initial treatment: 60 mg/day for 1 week, *followed by* 40 mg/day for 1 week, *then* 30 mg/day for 2 weeks, *then* 20 mg/day. Half this dose should be given when used in combination with azathioprine
Dermatomyositis/polymyositis: Oral: 1 mg/kg daily (range: 0.5-1.5 mg/kg/day), often in conjunction with steroid-sparing therapies; depending on response/tolerance, consider slow tapering after 2-8 weeks depending on response; taper regimens vary widely, but often involve 5-10 mg decrements per week and may require 6-12 months to reach a low once-daily or every-other-day dose to prevent disease flare (Briemberg, 2003; Hengstman, 2009; Iorizzo, 2008; Wiendl, 2008)
Giant cell arteritis (unlabeled use): Oral: Initial: 40-60 mg/day; typically requires 1-2 years of treatment, but may begin to taper after 2-3 months; alternative dosing of 30-40 mg/day has demonstrated similar efficacy (Hiratzka, 2010)
Graves' ophthalmopathy prophylaxis (unlabeled use): 0.4-0.5 mg/kg/day, starting 1-3 days after radioactive iodine treatment, and continued for 1 month, then gradually taper over 2 months (Bahn, 2011)
Herpes zoster (unlabeled use; Dworkin, 2007): 60 mg/day for 7 days, *followed by* 30 mg/day for 7 days, *then* 15 mg/day for 7 days
Idiopathic thrombocytopenia purpura (American Society of Hematology, 1997): 1-2 mg/kg/day
Rheumatoid arthritis (American College of Rheumatology, 2002): ≤10 mg/day
Subacute thyroiditis (unlabeled use): 40 mg/day for 1-2 weeks; gradually taper over 2-4 weeks or longer depending on clinical response. **Note:** NSAIDs should be considered first-line therapy in such patients (Bahn, 2011).
Systemic lupus erythematosus (American College of Rheumatology, 1999):
Mild SLE: ≤10 mg/day
Refractory or severe organ-threatening disease: 20-60 mg/day
Takayasu arteritis (unlabeled use): Oral: Initial: 40-60 mg/day; taper to lowest effective dose when ESR and CRP levels are normal; usual duration: 1-2 years (Hiratzka, 2010)
Thyrotoxicosis (type II amiodarone-induced; unlabeled use): 40 mg/day for 14-28 days; gradually taper over 2-3 months depending on clinical response (Bahn, 2011)
Tuberculosis, severe, paradoxical reactions (unlabeled use, AIDS*info* guidelines, 2008): 1 mg/kg/day, gradually reduce after 1-2 weeks
Elderly: Use the lowest effective dose

Dosing adjustment in hepatic impairment: Prednisone is inactive and must be metabolized by the liver to prednisolone. This conversion may be impaired in patients with liver disease, however, prednisolone levels are observed to be higher in patients with severe liver failure than in normal patients. Therefore, compensation for the inadequate conversion of prednisone to prednisolone occurs.

Dosing adjustment in hyperthyroidism: Prednisone dose may need to be increased to achieve adequate therapeutic effects

Hemodialysis: Supplemental dose is not necessary
Peritoneal dialysis: Supplemental dose is not necessary

Dietary Considerations Should be taken after meals or with food or milk; may require increased dietary intake of pyridoxine, vitamin C, vitamin D, folate, calcium, and phosphorus; may require decreased dietary intake of sodium

Administration Administer with food to decrease gastrointestinal upset

Monitoring Parameters Blood pressure, blood glucose, electrolytes

Following prolonged use: Bone mass density, growth in children, signs and symptoms of infection, cataract formation, intraocular pressure (use >6 weeks)

Test Interactions Decreased response to skin tests

Additional Information Tapering of corticosteroids after a short course of therapy (<7-10 days) is generally not required unless the disease/inflammatory process is slow to respond. Tapering after prolonged exposure is dependent upon the individual patient, duration of corticosteroid treatments, and size of steroid dose. Recovery of the HPA axis may require several months. Subtle but important HPA axis suppression may be present for as long as several months after a course of as few as 10-14 days duration. Testing of HPA axis (cosyntropin) may be required, and signs/symptoms of adrenal insufficiency should be monitored in patients with a history of use.

Dosage Forms Excipient information presented when available (limited, particularly for generics); consult specific product labeling.

Solution, oral: 1 mg/mL (5 mL, 120 mL, 500 mL)

Solution, oral [concentrate]:

PredniSONE Intensol™: 5 mg/mL (30 mL) [dye free, sugar free; contains ethanol 30%, propylene glycol]

Tablet, oral: 1 mg, 2.5 mg, 5 mg, 10 mg, 20 mg, 50 mg

◆ **PredniSONE Intensol™** *see* PredniSONE *on page 1399*

Pregabalin (pre GAB a lin)

Brand Names: U.S. Lyrica®

Brand Names: Canada Lyrica®

Index Terms CI-1008; S-(+)-3-isobutylgaba

Pharmacologic Category Analgesic, Miscellaneous; Anticonvulsant, Miscellaneous

Additional Appendix Information

Anticonvulsant Drugs of Choice *on page 1873*

Use Management of pain associated with diabetic peripheral neuropathy; management of postherpetic neuralgia; adjunctive therapy for partial-onset seizure disorder in adults; management of fibromyalgia

Pregnancy Risk Factor C

Pregnancy Considerations Increased incidence of fetal abnormalities, particularly skeletal malformations, were observed in animal studies. Male-mediated teratogenicity has been observed in animal studies; implications in humans are not defined. Impaired male and female fertility has been noted in animal studies. There are no adequate and well-controlled studies in pregnant women. Use only when potential benefit to the mother outweighs possible risk to the fetus.

Patients exposed to pregabalin during pregnancy are encouraged to enroll themselves into the AED Pregnancy Registry by calling 1-888-233-2334. Additional information is available at www.aedpregnancyregistry.org.

Lactation Excretion in breast milk unknown/not recommended

Medication Guide Available Yes

Contraindications Hypersensitivity to pregabalin or any component of the formulation

Warnings/Precautions Antiepileptics are associated with an increased risk of suicidal behavior/thoughts with use (regardless of indication); patients should be monitored for signs/symptoms of depression, suicidal tendencies, and other unusual behavior changes during therapy and instructed to inform their healthcare provider immediately if symptoms occur.

Angioedema has been reported; may be life threatening; use with caution in patients with a history of angioedema episodes. Concurrent use with other drugs known to cause angioedema (eg, ACE inhibitors) may increase risk. Hypersensitivity reactions, including skin redness, blistering, hives, rash, dyspnea and wheezing have been reported; discontinue treatment of hypersensitivity occurs. May cause CNS depression and/or dizziness, which may impair physical or mental abilities. Patients must be cautioned about performing tasks which require mental alertness (eg, operating machinery or driving). Effects with other sedative drugs or ethanol may be potentiated. Visual disturbances (blurred vision, decreased acuity and visual field changes) have been associated with pregabalin therapy; patients should be instructed to notify their physician if these effects are noted.

Pregabalin has been associated with increases in CPK and rare cases of rhabdomyolysis. Patients should be instructed to notify their prescriber if unexplained muscle pain, tenderness, or weakness, particularly if fever and/or malaise are associated with these symptoms. Use may be associated with weight gain and peripheral edema; use caution in patients with congestive heart failure, hypertension, or diabetes. Effect on weight gain/edema may be additive to thiazolidinedione antidiabetic agent; particularly in patients with prior cardiovascular disease. May decrease platelet count or prolong PR interval.

Has been noted to be tumorigenic (increased incidence of hemangiosarcoma) in animal studies; significance of these findings in humans is unknown. Pregabalin has been associated with discontinuation symptoms following abrupt cessation, and increases in seizure frequency (when used as an antiepileptic) may occur. Should not be discontinued abruptly; dosage tapering over at least 1 week is recommended. Use caution in renal impairment; dosage adjustment required.

Adverse Reactions Note: Frequency of adverse effects may be influenced by dose or concurrent therapy. In add-on trials in epilepsy, frequency of CNS and adverse effects were higher than those reported in pain management trials. Range noted below is inclusive of all trials.

>10%:

Cardiovascular: Peripheral edema (up to 16%)

Central nervous system: Dizziness (8% to 45%), somnolence (4% to 28%), ataxia (up to 20%), headache (up to 14%)

Gastrointestinal: Weight gain (up to 16%), xerostomia (1% to 15%)

Neuromuscular & skeletal: Tremor (up to 11%)

Ocular: Blurred vision (1% to 12%), diplopia (up to 12%)

Miscellaneous: Infection (up to 14%), accidental injury (2% to 11%)

1% to 10%:

Cardiovascular: Chest pain (up to 4%), edema (up to 6%)

Central nervous system: Neuropathy (up to 9%), thinking abnormal (up to 9%), fatigue (up to 8%), confusion (up to 7%), euphoria (up to 7%), speech disorder (up to 7%), attention disturbance (up to 6%), incoordination (up to 6%), amnesia (up to 6%), pain (up to 5%), memory impaired (up to 4%), vertigo (up to 4%), feeling abnormal (up to 3%), hypoesthesia (up to 3%), anxiety (up to 2%), depression (up to 2%), disorientation (up to 2%), lethargy (up to 2%), fever (≥1%), depersonalization (≥1%), hypertonia (≥1%), stupor (≥1%), nervousness (up to 1%)

Dermatologic: Facial edema (up to 3%), bruising (≥1%), pruritus (≥1%)

Endocrine & metabolic: Fluid retention (up to 3%), hypoglycemia (up to 3%), libido decreased (≥1%)

Gastrointestinal: Constipation (up to 10%), appetite increased (up to 7%), flatulence (up to 3%), vomiting (up to 3%), abdominal distension (up to 2%), abdominal pain (≥1%), gastroenteritis (≥1%)

Genitourinary: Incontinence (up to 2%), anorgasmia (≥1%), impotence (≥1%), urinary frequency (≥1%)

Hematologic: Thrombocytopenia (3%)

Neuromuscular & skeletal: Balance disorder (up to 9%), abnormal gait (up to 8%), weakness (up to 7%), arthralgia (up to 6%), twitching (up to 5%), back pain (up to 4%), muscle spasm (up to 4%), myoclonus (up to 4%), paresthesia (>2%), CPK increased (2%), leg cramps (≥1%), myalgia (≥1%), myasthenia (up to 1%)

Ocular: Visual abnormalities (up to 5%), visual field defect (≥2%), eye disorder (up to 2%), nystagmus (>2%), conjunctivitis (≥1%)

Otic: Otitis media (≥1%), tinnitus (≥1%)

Respiratory: Sinusitis (up to 7%), dyspnea (up to 3%), bronchitis (up to 3%), pharyngolaryngeal pain (up to 3%)

Miscellaneous: Flu-like syndrome (up to 2%), allergic reaction (≥1%)

<1% (Limited to important or life-threatening): Abscess, acute renal failure, addiction (rare), agitation, albuminuria, anaphylactoid reaction, anemia, angioedema, aphasia, aphthous stomatitis, apnea, ascites, atelectasis, blepharitis, blindness, breast enlargement, bronchiolitis, cellulitis, cerebellar syndrome, cervicitis, chills, cholecystitis, cholelithiasis, chondrodystrophy, circumoral paresthesia, cogwheel rigidity, colitis, coma, corneal ulcer, crystalluria (urate), delirium, delusions, diarrhea, dysarthria, dysautonomia, dyskinesia, dysphagia, dystonia, dysuria, encephalopathy, eosinophilia, esophageal ulcer, esophagitis, exfoliative dermatitis, extraocular palsy, extrapyramidal syndrome, gastritis, GI hemorrhage, glomerulitis, glucose tolerance decreased, granuloma, Guillain-Barré syndrome, gynecomastia, hallucinations, heart failure, hematuria, hostility, hyper-/hypokinesia; hypersensitivity (including skin redness, blistering, hives, rash, dyspnea, and wheezing); hypotension, hypotonia, intracranial hypertension, laryngismus, leukopenia, leukorrhea, leukocytosis, lymphadenopathy, manic reaction, melena, myelofibrosis, nausea, nephritis, neuralgia, ocular hemorrhage, oliguria, optic atrophy, pancreatitis, papilledema, paranoid reaction, pelvic pain, periodontal abscess, peripheral neuritis, polycythemia, postural hypotension, prothrombin decreased, psychotic depression, ptosis, pulmonary edema, pulmonary fibrosis, purpura, pyelonephritis, rectal hemorrhage, renal calculus, retinal edema, retinal vascular disorder, retroperitoneal fibrosis, rhabdomyolysis, schizophrenic reaction, shock, skin necrosis, skin ulcer, spasm (generalized), ST depression, Stevens-Johnson syndrome, subcutaneous nodule, suicide, suicide attempt, syncope, thrombocythemia, thrombophlebitis, tongue edema, torticollis, trismus, uveitis, ventricular fibrillation

Drug Interactions

Metabolism/Transport Effects None known.

Avoid Concomitant Use There are no known interactions where it is recommended to avoid concomitant use.

Increased Effect/Toxicity

Pregabalin may increase the levels/effects of: Alcohol (Ethyl); Antidiabetic Agents (Thiazolidinedione); CNS Depressants; Methotrimeprazine; Selective Serotonin Reuptake Inhibitors

The levels/effects of Pregabalin may be increased by: Droperidol; HydrOXYzine; Methotrimeprazine

Decreased Effect

The levels/effects of Pregabalin may be decreased by: Ketorolac; Ketorolac (Nasal); Ketorolac (Systemic); Mefloquine

Ethanol/Nutrition/Herb Interactions

Ethanol: May increase CNS depression; monitor for increased effects with coadministration. Caution patients about effects.

Herb/Nutraceutical: Avoid valerian, St John's wort, kava kava, gotu kola (may increase CNS depression).

Stability Store at 15°C to 30°C (59°F to 86°F).

Mechanism of Action Binds to alpha$_2$-delta subunit of voltage-gated calcium channels within the CNS, inhibiting excitatory neurotransmitter release. Although structurally related to GABA, it does not bind to GABA or benzodiazepine receptors. Exerts antinociceptive and anticonvulsant activity. Decreases symptoms of painful peripheral neuropathies and, as adjunctive therapy in partial seizures, decreases the frequency of seizures.

Pharmacodynamics/Kinetics

Onset of action: Pain management: Effects may be noted as early as the first week of therapy.

Distribution: V_d: 0.5 L/kg

Protein binding: 0%

Metabolism: Negligible

Bioavailability: >90%

Half-life elimination: 6.3 hours

Time to peak, plasma: 1.5 hours (3 hours with food)

Excretion: Urine (90% as unchanged drug; minor metabolites)

Dosage Oral: Adults:

Fibromyalgia: Initial: 150 mg/day in divided doses (75 mg 2 times/day); may be increased to 300 mg/day (150 mg 2 times/day) within 1 week based on tolerability and effect; may be further increased to 450 mg/day (225 mg 2 times/day). Maximum dose: 450 mg/day (dosages up to 600 mg/day were evaluated with no significant additional benefit and an increase in adverse effects)

Neuropathic pain (diabetes-associated): Initial: 150 mg/day in divided doses (50 mg 3 times/day); may be increased within 1 week based on tolerability and effect; maximum dose: 300 mg/day (dosages up to 600 mg/day were evaluated with no significant additional benefit and an increase in adverse effects)

Postherpetic neuralgia: Initial: 150 mg/day in divided doses (75 mg 2 times/day or 50 mg 3 times/day); may be increased to 300 mg/day within 1 week based on tolerability and effect; further titration (to 600 mg/day) after 2-4 weeks may be considered in patients who do not experience sufficient relief of pain provided they are able to tolerate pregabalin. Maximum dose: 600 mg/day

Partial-onset seizures (adjunctive therapy): Initial: 150 mg per day in divided doses (75 mg 2 times/day or 50 mg 3 times/day); may be increased based on tolerability and effect (optimal titration schedule has not been defined). Maximum dose: 600 mg/day

Discontinuing therapy: Pregabalin should not be abruptly discontinued; taper dosage over at least 1 week

Dosage adjustment in renal impairment: Renal function may be estimated using the Cockcroft-Gault formula. Then determine recommended dosage regimen based on the indication-specific total daily dose for normal renal function (Cl_{cr} ≥60 mL/minute). For example, if the indication-specific daily dose is 450 mg/day for normal renal function, the daily dose should be reduced to 225 mg/day (in 2-3 divided doses) for a creatinine clearance of 30-60 mL/minute (see table).

Pregabalin Renal Impairment Dosing

Cl_{cr} (mL/minute)	Total Pregabalin Daily Dose (mg/day)				Dosing Frequency
≥60 (normal renal function)	150	300	450	600	2-3 divided doses
30-60	75	150	225	300	2-3 divided doses
15-30	25-50	75	100-150	150	1-2 divided doses
<15	25	25-50	50-75	75	Single daily dose

Posthemodialysis supplementary dosage (as a single additional dose):
25 mg/day schedule: Single supplementary dose of 25 mg **or** 50 mg
25-50 mg/day schedule: Single supplementary dose of 50 mg **or** 75 mg
50-75 mg/day schedule: Single supplementary dose of 75 mg **or** 100 mg
75 mg/day schedule: Single supplementary dose of 100 mg **or** 150 mg

Dietary Considerations May be taken with or without food.

Administration May be administered with or without food.

Monitoring Parameters Measures of efficacy (pain intensity/seizure frequency); degree of sedation; symptoms of myopathy or ocular disturbance; weight gain/edema; CPK; skin integrity (in patients with diabetes); suicidality (eg, suicidal thoughts, depression, behavioral changes)

Product Availability Lyrica® oral solution: FDA approved December 2009; anticipated availability is currently undetermined

Dosage Forms Excipient information presented when available (limited, particularly for generics); consult specific product labeling.

Capsule, oral:

Lyrica®: 25 mg, 50 mg, 75 mg, 100 mg, 150 mg, 200 mg, 225 mg, 300 mg

Controlled Substance C-V

- **Pregnenedione** *see* Progesterone *on page 1414*
- **Pregnyl®** *see* Chorionic Gonadotropin (Human) *on page 352*
- **Premarin®** *see* Estrogens (Conjugated/Equine, Systemic) *on page 641*
- **Premarin®** *see* Estrogens (Conjugated/Equine, Topical) *on page 643*
- **Premjact®** *see* Lidocaine (Topical) *on page 1009*
- **Preparation H® Hydrocortisone [OTC]** *see* Hydrocortisone (Topical) *on page 841*
- **Prepidil®** *see* Dinoprostone *on page 514*
- **Pressyn® (Can)** *see* Vasopressin *on page 1775*
- **Pressyn® AR (Can)** *see* Vasopressin *on page 1775*
- **Pretz® [OTC]** *see* Sodium Chloride *on page 1567*
- **Prevacid®** *see* Lansoprazole *on page 972*
- **Prevacid® 24 HR [OTC]** *see* Lansoprazole *on page 972*
- **Prevacid® FasTab (Can)** *see* Lansoprazole *on page 972*
- **Prevacid® SoluTab™** *see* Lansoprazole *on page 972*
- **Prevalite®** *see* Cholestyramine Resin *on page 351*
- **Prevex® B (Can)** *see* Betamethasone *on page 208*
- **Prevex® HC (Can)** *see* Hydrocortisone (Topical) *on page 841*
- **PreviDent®** *see* Fluoride *on page 728*
- **PreviDent® 5000 Booster** *see* Fluoride *on page 728*
- **PreviDent® 5000 Dry Mouth** *see* Fluoride *on page 728*
- **PreviDent® 5000 Plus®** *see* Fluoride *on page 728*
- **PreviDent® 5000 Sensitive** *see* Fluoride *on page 728*
- **Prevnar®** *see* Pneumococcal Conjugate Vaccine (7-Valent) *on page 1365*
- **Prevnar 13™** *see* Pneumococcal Conjugate Vaccine (13-Valent) *on page 1366*
- **Prevpac®** *see* Lansoprazole, Amoxicillin, and Clarithromycin *on page 975*
- **Prezista®** *see* Darunavir *on page 451*
- **Prialt®** *see* Ziconotide *on page 1813*
- **Priftin®** *see* Rifapentine *on page 1487*
- **Prilocaine and Lidocaine** *see* Lidocaine and Prilocaine *on page 1010*
- **PriLOSEC®** *see* Omeprazole *on page 1241*
- **PriLOSEC OTC® [OTC]** *see* Omeprazole *on page 1241*
- **Primaclone** *see* Primidone *on page 1405*
- **Primacor® (Can)** *see* Milrinone *on page 1136*

Primaquine (PRIM a kween)

Index Terms Primaquine Phosphate; Prymaccone

Pharmacologic Category Aminoquinoline (Antimalarial)

Use Prevention of relapse of *P. vivax* malaria

Unlabeled Use Prevention of relapse of *P. ovale* malaria; prevention of malaria; treatment of uncomplicated *P. vivax* and *P. ovale* malaria; treatment of *Pneumocystis jirovecii* pneumonia (PCP); prevention of malaria

Lactation Excretion in breast milk unknown

Contraindications Use in acutely-ill patients who have a tendency to develop granulocytopenia (eg, rheumatoid arthritis, SLE); concurrent use with other medications causing hemolytic anemia or myeloid bone marrow suppression; concurrent use with or recent use of quinacrine

Warnings/Precautions Use with caution in patients with G6PD deficiency (hemolytic anemia may occur), NADH methemoglobin reductase deficiency (methemoglobinemia may occur); do not exceed recommended dosage and duration. Moderate-to-severe hemolytic reactions may occur in individuals with G6PD deficiency and personal or familial history of favism. Geographic regions with a high prevalence of G6PD deficiency (eg, Africa, southern Europe, Mediterranean region, Middle East, southeast Asia, Oceania) are associated with a higher incidence of hemolytic anemia. Promptly discontinue with signs of hemolytic anemia (darkening of urine, marked fall in hemoglobin or erythrocyte count). The CDC recommends screening for G6PD deficiency prior to therapy initiation. Anemia, methemoglobinemia, and leukopenia have been associated with primaquine use; monitor during treatment. **[U.S. Boxed Warning]: Should be prescribed only by physicians familiar with its use.**

Adverse Reactions Frequency not defined.

Cardiovascular: Arrhythmias (rare)

Central nervous system: Headache

Dermatologic: Pruritus

Gastrointestinal: Abdominal cramps, dyspepsia, nausea, vomiting

Hematologic: Agranulocytosis, anemia, hemolytic anemia (in patients with G6PD deficiency), leukopenia, leukocytosis, methemoglobinemia (in NADH-methemoglobin reductase-deficient individuals)

Ocular: Interference with visual accommodation

Drug Interactions

Metabolism/Transport Effects Substrate of CYP3A4 (major); **Note:** Assignment of Major/Minor substrate status based on clinically relevant drug interaction potential; **Inhibits** CYP1A2 (strong), CYP2D6 (weak), CYP3A4 (weak); **Induces** CYP1A2 (weak/moderate)

Avoid Concomitant Use

Avoid concomitant use of Primaquine with any of the following: Artemether; Lumefantrine; Mefloquine; Pimozide

Increased Effect/Toxicity

Primaquine may increase the levels/effects of: Antipsychotic Agents (Phenothiazines); Bendamustine; Beta-Blockers; Cardiac Glycosides; CYP1A2 Substrates; Dapsone; Dapsone (Systemic); Dapsone (Topical); Lumefantrine; Mefloquine; Pimozide; Prilocaine

The levels/effects of Primaquine may be increased by: Artemether; Conivaptan; Dapsone; Dapsone (Systemic); Mefloquine

Decreased Effect

Primaquine may decrease the levels/effects of: Anthelmintics

The levels/effects of Primaquine may be decreased by: CYP3A4 Inducers (Strong); Deferasirox; Herbs (CYP3A4 Inducers); Tocilizumab

Ethanol/Nutrition/Herb Interactions Ethanol: Avoid ethanol (due to GI irritation).

Mechanism of Action Eliminates the primary tissue exoerythrocytic forms of *P. falciparum*; disrupts mitochondria and binds to DNA

Pharmacodynamics/Kinetics

Absorption: Well absorbed

Metabolism: Hepatic to carboxyprimaquine (active)

Half-life elimination: 3.7-9.6 hours

Time to peak, serum: 1-2 hours

Excretion: Urine (small amounts as unchanged drug)

Dosage Oral: Dosage expressed as mg of base (15 mg base = 26.3 mg primaquine phosphate). **Note:** The CDC requires screening for G6PD deficiency prior to initiating treatment with primaquine.

Malaria:

Treatment or prevention of relapse of *P. vivax* malaria:

Adults: 30 mg once daily for 14 days

Treatment of uncomplicated *P. vivax* and *P. ovale* malaria (unlabeled use):

Children: 0.5 mg /kg (maximum: 30 mg/day) daily for 14 days with chloroquine or hydroxychloroquine (CDC, 2009)

Adults: 30 mg once daily for 14 days with chloroquine or hydroxychloroquine; alternative regimen (for mild G6PD deficiency or as an alternative to daily regimen): 45 mg once weekly for 8 weeks (use only after consultation with an infectious disease/tropical medicine expert) (CDC, 2009)

Chemoprophylaxis (unlabeled use):

Children: 0.5 mg/kg once daily (maximum dose: 30 mg/day); start 1-2 days prior to travel and continue for 7 days after departure from malaria-endemic area (CDC, 2012)

Adults: 30 mg once daily; start 1-2 days prior to travel and continue for 7 days after departure from malaria-endemic area (CDC, 2012)

Presumptive antirelapse therapy for *P. vivax* and *P. ovale* malaria (unlabeled use):

Children: 0.5 mg/kg (maximum dose: 30 mg/day) once daily for 14 days after departure from malaria-endemic area (CDC, 2012)

Adults: 30 mg once daily for 14 days after departure from malaria-endemic area (CDC, 2012)

***Pneumocystis jirovecii* pneumonia treatment (unlabeled use):** CDC recommendation (as alternative):

Children: 0.3 mg/kg once daily for 21 days (in combination with clindamycin)

Adults: 30 mg once daily for 21 days (in combination with clindamycin)

Administration Take with meals to decrease adverse GI effects. Drug has a bitter taste.

Monitoring Parameters Periodic CBC, visual color check of urine, glucose, electrolytes; if hemolysis suspected, monitor CBC, haptoglobin, peripheral smear, urinalysis dipstick for occult blood, G6PD deficiency screening (prior to initiating treatment; CDC recommendation)

Dosage Forms Excipient information presented when available (limited, particularly for generics); consult specific product labeling.

Tablet, oral, as phosphate: 26.3 mg [15 mg base]

Extemporaneous Preparations A 6 mg base/5 mL oral suspension may be made using tablets. Crush ten 15 mg base tablets and reduce to a fine powder. In small amounts, add a total of 10 mL Carboxymethylcellulose 1.5% and mix to a uniform paste; mix while adding Simple Syrup, NF to **almost** 125 mL; transfer to a calibrated bottle, rinse mortar with vehicle, and add quantity of vehicle sufficient to make 125 mL. Label "shake well" and "refrigerate". Stable 7 days.

Nahata MC, Pai VB, and Hipple TF, *Pediatric Drug Formulations*, 5th ed, Cincinnati, OH: Harvey Whitney Books Co, 2004.

- **Primaquine Phosphate** *see* Primaquine *on page 1404*
- **Primatene® Mist [OTC] [DSC]** *see* EPINEPHrine (Systemic, Oral Inhalation) *on page 594*
- **Primaxin® I.M. [DSC]** *see* Imipenem and Cilastatin *on page 875*
- **Primaxin® I.V.** *see* Imipenem and Cilastatin *on page 875*
- **Primaxin® I.V. Infusion (Can)** *see* Imipenem and Cilastatin *on page 875*

Primidone (PRI mi done)

Brand Names: U.S. Mysoline®

Brand Names: Canada Apo-Primidone®

Index Terms Desoxyphenobarbital; Primaclone

Pharmacologic Category Anticonvulsant, Miscellaneous; Barbiturate

Use Management of grand mal, psychomotor, and focal seizures

Unlabeled Use Benign familial tremor (essential tremor)

Pregnancy Considerations Primidone and its metabolites (PEMA, phenobarbital, and p-hydroxyphenobarbital) cross the placenta; neonatal serum concentrations at birth are similar to those in the mother. Withdrawal symptoms may occur in the neonate and may be delayed due to the long half-life of primidone and its metabolites. Use may be associated with birth defects and adverse events; the use of folic acid throughout pregnancy and vitamin K during the last month of pregnancy is recommended. Epilepsy itself, number of medications, genetic factors, or a combination of these probably influence the teratogenicity of anticonvulsant therapy.

Patients exposed to primidone during pregnancy are encouraged to enroll themselves into the NAAED Pregnancy Registry by calling 1-888-233-2334. Additional information is available at www.aedpregnancyregistry.org.

Lactation Enters breast milk/not recommended (AAP recommends use "with caution"; AAP 2001 update pending)

Medication Guide Available Yes

Contraindications Hypersensitivity to phenobarbital; porphyria

Warnings/Precautions Antiepileptics are associated with an increased risk of suicidal behavior/thoughts with use (regardless of indication); patients should be monitored for signs/symptoms of depression, suicidal tendencies, and other unusual behavior changes during therapy and instructed to inform their healthcare provider immediately if symptoms occur.

Use with caution in patients with renal or hepatic impairment, pulmonary insufficiency; abrupt withdrawal may precipitate status epilepticus. Potential for drug dependency exists. Do not administer to patients in acute pain. Use caution in elderly, debilitated, or pediatric patients - may cause paradoxical responses. May cause CNS depression, which may impair physical or mental abilities. Patients must cautioned about performing tasks which require mental alertness (eg, operating machinery or driving). Effects with other sedative drugs or ethanol may be potentiated. Use with caution in patients with depression or suicidal tendencies, or in patients with a history of drug abuse. Tolerance or psychological and physical dependence may occur with prolonged use. Primidone's metabolite, phenobarbital, has been associated with cognitive deficits in children. Use with caution in patients with hypoadrenalism.

Adverse Reactions Frequency not defined.

Central nervous system: Ataxia, drowsiness, emotional disturbances, fatigue, hyperirritability, suicidal ideation, vertigo

Dermatologic: Morbilliform skin eruptions

Gastrointestinal: Anorexia, nausea, vomiting

Genitourinary: Impotence

Hematologic: Agranulocytosis, granulocytopenia, megaloblastic anemia (idiosyncratic), red cell aplasia/hypoplasia

Ocular: Diplopia, nystagmus

Drug Interactions

Metabolism/Transport Effects Induces CYP1A2 (strong), CYP2B6 (strong), CYP2C8 (strong), CYP2C9 (strong), CYP3A4 (strong)

Avoid Concomitant Use

Avoid concomitant use of Primidone with any of the following: Boceprevir; Bortezomib; Crizotinib; Dienogest; Dronedarone; Everolimus; Lapatinib; Lurasidone; Nilotinib; Nisoldipine; Pazopanib; Praziquantel; Ranolazine; Rilpivirine; Rivaroxaban; Roflumilast; RomiDEPsin; SORAfenib; Ticagrelor; Tolvaptan; Toremifene; Vandetanib

Increased Effect/Toxicity

Primidone may increase the levels/effects of: Alcohol (Ethyl); Barbiturates; Clarithromycin; CNS Depressants; Methotrimeprazine; Selective Serotonin Reuptake Inhibitors

The levels/effects of Primidone may be increased by: Carbonic Anhydrase Inhibitors; Clarithromycin; Dexmethylphenidate; Divalproex; Droperidol; Felbamate; HydrOXYzine; Methotrimeprazine; Methylphenidate; Valproic Acid

Decreased Effect

Primidone may decrease the levels/effects of: ARIPiprazole; Bendamustine; Boceprevir; Bortezomib; Brentuximab Vedotin; Clarithromycin; Corticosteroids (Systemic); Crizotinib; CYP1A2 Substrates; CYP2B6 Substrates; CYP2C8 Substrates; CYP2C9 Substrates; CYP3A4 Substrates; Dasatinib; Diclofenac; Dienogest; Divalproex; Dronedarone; Everolimus; Exemestane; Felbamate; Gefitinib; GuanFACINE; Imatinib; Ixabepilone; LamoTRIgine; Lapatinib; Linagliptin; Lurasidone; Maraviroc; NIFEdipine; Nilotinib; Nisoldipine; Pazopanib; Praziquantel; QuiNIDine; Ranolazine; Rilpivirine; Rivaroxaban; Roflumilast; RomiDEPsin; Rufinamide; Saxagliptin; SORAfenib; SUNItinib; Tadalafil; Ticagrelor; Tolvaptan; Toremifene; Treprostinil; Ulipristal; Valproic Acid; Vandetanib; Vemurafenib; Zuclopenthixol

The levels/effects of Primidone may be decreased by: Carbonic Anhydrase Inhibitors; Folic Acid; Fosphenytoin; Ketorolac; Ketorolac (Nasal); Ketorolac (Systemic); Leucovorin Calcium-Levoleucovorin; Levomefolate; Mefloquine; Methylfolate; Phenytoin

Ethanol/Nutrition/Herb Interactions

Ethanol: May increase CNS depression; monitor for increased effects with coadministration. Caution patients about effects.

Food: Protein-deficient diets increase duration of action of primidone.

Herb/Nutraceutical: Avoid valerian, St John's wort, kava kava, gotu kola (may increase CNS depression).

Stability Store at 20°C to 25°C (68°F to 77°F).

Mechanism of Action Decreases neuron excitability, raises seizure threshold similar to phenobarbital; primidone has two active metabolites, phenobarbital and phenylethylmalonamide (PEMA); PEMA may enhance the activity of phenobarbital

Pharmacodynamics/Kinetics

Absorption: 60% to 80%

Distribution: Adults: V_d: 0.6 L/kg

Protein binding: 30%

Metabolism: Hepatic to phenobarbital (active) by oxidation and to phenylethylmalonamide (PEMA; active) by scission of the heterocyclic ring

Half-life elimination (age dependent): Primidone: Mean: 5-15 hours (variable); PEMA: 16 hours (variable)

Time to peak, serum: ~3 hours (variable)

Excretion: Urine (40% as unchanged drug; the remainder is unconjugated PEMA, phenobarbital and its metabolites)

Dosage Oral:

Seizure disorders:

Children <8 years: Initial: Days 1-3: 50 mg/day given at bedtime; days 4-6: 50 mg twice daily; days 7-9: 100 mg twice daily; usual dose: 375-750 mg/day in 3-4 divided doses (10-25 mg/kg/day)

Children ≥8 years and Adults: Days 1-3: 100-125 mg/day at bedtime; days 4-6: 100-125 twice daily; days 7-9: 100-125 mg 3 times daily; usual dose: 750-1500 mg/day in divided doses 3-4 times/day with maximum dosage of 2 g/day

Patients already receiving other anticonvulsants: Initial: 100-125 mg at bedtime; gradually increase to maintenance dose as other drug is gradually decreased, continue until desired level obtained or other drug completely withdrawn. If goal is monotherapy, conversion should be completed over ≥2 weeks.

Essential tremor (unlabeled use): Adults: Initial 12.5-25 mg/day at bedtime; titrate up to 250 mg/day in 1-2 divided doses; doses up to 750 mg/day may be beneficial

Dosing interval in renal impairment: Adults (Aronoff, 2007): **Note:** Avoid in renal failure if possible; due to active metabolites with long half-lives and complex kinetics:

Cl_{cr} ≥50 mL/minute: Administer every 12 hours

Cl_{cr} 10-50 mL/minute: Administer every 12-24 hours

Cl_{cr} <10 mL/minute: Administer every 24 hours

Hemodialysis: Administer dose postdialysis

Dietary Considerations Folic acid: Low erythrocyte and CSF folate concentrations. Megaloblastic anemia has been reported. To avoid folic acid deficiency and megaloblastic anemia, some clinicians recommend giving patients on anticonvulsants prophylactic doses of folic acid and cyanocobalamin.

Monitoring Parameters Serum primidone and phenobarbital concentration, neurological status. Due to CNS effects, monitor closely when initiating drug in elderly. Monitor CBC and sequential multiple analysis-12 (SMA-12) at 6-month intervals to compare with baseline obtained at start of therapy. Monitor for suicidality (eg, suicidal thoughts, depression, behavioral changes). Since elderly metabolize phenobarbital at a slower rate than younger adults, it is suggested to measure both primidone and phenobarbital levels together.

Reference Range Therapeutic: Children <5 years: 7-10 mcg/mL (SI: 32-46 micromole/L); Adults: 5-12 mcg/mL (SI: 23-55 micromole/L); toxic effects rarely present with levels <10 mcg/mL (SI: 46 micromole/L) if phenobarbital concentrations are low. Dosage of primidone is adjusted with reference mostly to the phenobarbital level; Toxic: >15 mcg/mL (SI: >69 micromole/L)

Dosage Forms Excipient information presented when available (limited, particularly for generics); consult specific product labeling.

Tablet, oral: 50 mg, 250 mg

Mysoline®: 50 mg, 250 mg [scored]

Dosage Forms: Canada Excipient information presented when available (limited, particularly for generics); consult specific product labeling.

Tablet, oral:

Apo-Primidone®: 125 mg, 250 mg

◆ **Primlev™** *see* Oxycodone and Acetaminophen *on page 1269*

◆ **Primsol®** *see* Trimethoprim *on page 1740*

◆ **Prinivil®** *see* Lisinopril *on page 1020*

◆ **Prinzide®** *see* Lisinopril and Hydrochlorothiazide *on page 1023*

◆ **Priorix™ (Can)** *see* Measles, Mumps, and Rubella Virus Vaccine *on page 1054*

◆ **Priorix-Tetra™ (Can)** *see* Measles, Mumps, Rubella, and Varicella Virus Vaccine *on page 1055*

◆ **PrismaSol** *see* Electrolyte Solution, Renal Replacement *on page 578*

◆ **Pristinamycin** *see* Quinupristin and Dalfopristin *on page 1450*

◆ **Pristiq®** *see* Desvenlafaxine *on page 479*
◆ **Privigen®** *see* Immune Globulin *on page 880*
◆ **Privine® [OTC]** *see* Naphazoline (Nasal) *on page 1176*
◆ **ProAir® HFA** *see* Albuterol *on page 52*
◆ **ProAmatine** *see* Midodrine *on page 1130*
◆ **PRO-Amiodarone (Can)** *see* Amiodarone *on page 90*
◆ **PRO-Azithromycin (Can)** *see* Azithromycin (Systemic) *on page 180*

Probenecid (proe BEN e sid)

Brand Names: Canada Benuryl™
Index Terms Benemid [DSC]
Pharmacologic Category Uricosuric Agent
Use Treatment of hyperuricemia associated with gout or gouty arthritis; prolongation and elevation of beta-lactam plasma levels (eg, uncomplicated gonococcal infection)
Unlabeled Use Prolongation and elevation of beta-lactam plasma levels (eg, neurosyphilis, pelvic inflammatory disease)
Pregnancy Considerations Probenecid crosses the placenta; adverse fetal events have not been reported.
Lactation Enters breast milk; based on a single case report, very small amounts of probenecid have been detected in breast milk
Contraindications Hypersensitivity to probenecid or any component of the formulation; small- or large-dose aspirin therapy; blood dyscrasias; uric acid kidney stones; children <2 years of age; initiation during an acute gout attack
Warnings/Precautions Use with caution in patients with peptic ulcer. Salicylates may diminish the therapeutic effect of probenecid. This effect may be more pronounced with high, chronic doses, however, the manufacturer recommends the use of an alternative analgesic even in place of small doses of aspirin. Use of probenecid with penicillin in patients with renal insufficiency is not recommended. Probenecid monotherapy may not be effective in patients with a creatinine clearance <30 mL/minute. Probenecid may increase the serum concentration of methotrexate. Avoid concomitant use of probenecid and methotrexate if possible. If used together, consider lower methotrexate doses and monitor for methotrexate toxicity. May cause exacerbation of acute gouty attack. If hypersensitivity reaction or anaphylaxis occurs, discontinue medication. Use caution in patients with G6PD deficiency; may increase risk for hemolytic anemia.
Adverse Reactions Frequency not defined.
Cardiovascular: Flushing
Central nervous system: Dizziness, fever, headache
Dermatologic: Alopecia, dermatitis, pruritus, rash
Gastrointestinal: Anorexia, dyspepsia, gastroesophageal reflux, nausea, sore gums, vomiting
Genitourinary: Hematuria, polyuria
Hematologic: Anemia, aplastic anemia, hemolytic anemia (in G6PD deficiency), leukopenia
Hepatic: Hepatic necrosis
Neuromuscular & skeletal: Costovertebral pain, gouty arthritis (acute)
Renal: Nephrotic syndrome, renal colic
Miscellaneous: Anaphylaxis, hypersensitivity
Drug Interactions
Metabolism/Transport Effects Inhibits CYP2C19 (weak)
Avoid Concomitant Use
Avoid concomitant use of Probenecid with any of the following: Doripenem; Ketorolac; Ketorolac (Nasal); Ketorolac (Systemic); Meropenem
Increased Effect/Toxicity
Probenecid may increase the levels/effects of: Acetaminophen; Cefotaxime; Cephalosporins; Dapsone; Dapsone (Systemic); Doripenem; Ertapenem; Ganciclovir-Valganciclovir; Gemifloxacin; Imipenem; Ketoprofen; Ketorolac; Ketorolac (Nasal); Ketorolac (Systemic); Loop Diuretics; LORazepam; Meropenem; Methotrexate; Mycophenolate; Nitrofurantoin; Nonsteroidal Anti-Inflammatory Agents; Oseltamivir; Penicillins; PRALAtrexate; Quinolone Antibiotics; Sodium Benzoate; Sodium Phenylacetate; Theophylline Derivatives; Zidovudine
Decreased Effect
Probenecid may decrease the levels/effects of: Loop Diuretics
The levels/effects of Probenecid may be decreased by: Salicylates
Stability Store at 20°C to 25°C (68°F to 77°F). Protect from light.
Mechanism of Action Competitively inhibits the reabsorption of uric acid at the proximal convoluted tubule, thereby promoting its excretion and reducing serum uric acid levels; increases plasma levels of weak organic acids (penicillins, cephalosporins, or other beta-lactam antibiotics) by competitively inhibiting their renal tubular secretion
Pharmacodynamics/Kinetics
Onset of action: Effect on penicillin levels: 2 hours
Absorption: Rapid and complete
Metabolism: Hepatic
Half-life elimination (dose dependent): Normal renal function: 6-12 hours
Time to peak, serum: 2-4 hours
Excretion: Urine
Dosage Oral:
Children:
<2 years: Contraindicated
2-14 years: Prolong penicillin serum levels: Initial: 25 mg/kg, then 40 mg/kg/day in 4 divided doses (maximum: 500 mg/dose)
Gonorrhea: >50 kg: Refer to adult dosing.
Adults:
Hyperuricemia with gout: 250 mg twice daily for 1 week; may increase to 500 mg twice daily; if needed, may increase to a maximum of 2 g/day (increase dosage in 500 mg increments every 4 weeks). If serum uric acid levels are within normal limits and gout attacks have been absent for 6 months, daily dosage may be reduced by 500 mg every 6 months.
Prolong penicillin serum levels: 500 mg 4 times/day. **Note:** Dosing per manufacturer, see indication-specific dosing.
Gonorrhea, uncomplicated infections of cervix, urethra, and rectum: Oral: 1 g once with cefoxitin 2 g I.M. (CDC, 2010)
Pelvic inflammatory disease (unlabeled use): Oral: 1 g once with cefoxitin 2 g I.M. plus doxycycline (CDC, 2010)
Neurosyphilis (unlabeled use): Oral: 500 mg 4 times/day with procaine penicillin 2.4 million units/day I.M for 10-14 days (CDC, 2010). **Note:** Penicillin G aqueous I.V. is the preferred agent.
Dosing adjustment in renal impairment: Cl_{cr} <30 mL/minute: Avoid use
Dietary Considerations Drug may cause GI upset; take with food if GI upset. Drink plenty of fluids.
Administration Administer with food or antacids to minimize GI effects.
Monitoring Parameters Uric acid, renal function, CBC
Reference Range
Uric acid, serum: An increase occurs during childhood
Adults:
Males: 3.4-7 mg/dL or slightly more
Females: 2.4-6 mg/dL or slightly more
Target: <6 mg/dL

Values >7 mg/dL are sometimes arbitrarily regarded as hyperuricemia, but there is no sharp line between normals and the serum uric acid of those with clinical gout. Normal ranges cannot be adjusted for purine ingestion, but high-purine diet increases uric acid. Uric acid may be increased with body size, exercise, and stress.

Test Interactions False-positive glucosuria with Clinitest®, a falsely high determination of theophylline has occurred and the renal excretion of phenolsulfonphthalein 17-ketosteroids and bromsulfophthalein (BSP) may be inhibited

Additional Information Avoid fluctuation in uric acid (increase or decrease); may precipitate gout attack. The manufacturer recommends the use of sodium bicarbonate (3-7.5 g daily) or potassium citrate (7.5 g daily) is suggested until serum uric acid normalizes and tophaceous deposits disappear.

Dosage Forms Excipient information presented when available (limited, particularly for generics); consult specific product labeling.

Tablet, oral: 500 mg

- **Probenecid and Colchicine** *see* Colchicine and Probenecid *on page 408*
- **PRO-Bicalutamide (Can)** *see* Bicalutamide *on page 217*
- **PRO-Bisoprolol (Can)** *see* Bisoprolol *on page 220*

Procainamide (pro KANE a mide)

Brand Names: Canada Apo-Procainamide®; Procainamide Hydrochloride Injection, USP; Procan SR®

Index Terms PCA (error-prone abbreviation); Procainamide Hydrochloride; Procaine Amide Hydrochloride; Procanbid; Pronestyl

Pharmacologic Category Antiarrhythmic Agent, Class Ia

Use

Intravenous: Treatment of life-threatening ventricular arrhythmias

Oral (Canadian labeling; not available in U.S.): Treatment of supraventricular arrhythmias. **Note:** In the treatment of atrial fibrillation, use only when preferred treatment is ineffective or cannot be used. Use in paroxysmal atrial tachycardia when reflex stimulation or other measures are ineffective.

Unlabeled Use

Paroxysmal supraventricular tachycardia (PSVT); prevent recurrence of ventricular tachycardia; symptomatic premature ventricular contractions

ACLS guidelines: I.V.: Treatment of the following arrhythmias in patients with preserved left ventricular function: Stable monomorphic VT; pre-excited atrial fibrillation; stable wide complex regular tachycardia (likely VT)

PALS guidelines: I.V.: Tachycardia with pulses and poor perfusion (probable SVT [unresponsive to vagal maneuvers and adenosine or synchronized cardioversion]; probable VT [unresponsive to synchronized cardioversion or adenosine])

Pregnancy Risk Factor C

Pregnancy Considerations Animal reproduction studies have not been conducted. Procainamide crosses the placenta; procainamide and its active metabolite (N-acetyl procainamide) can be detected in the cord blood and neonatal serum.

Lactation Enters breast milk/not recommended (AAP rates "compatible"; AAP 2001 update pending)

Contraindications Hypersensitivity to procainamide, procaine, other ester-type local anesthetics, or any component of the formulation; complete heart block; second-degree AV block or various types of hemiblock (without a functional artificial pacemaker); SLE; torsade de pointes

Warnings/Precautions Monitor and adjust dose to prevent QT_c prolongation. Watch for proarrhythmic effects. Avoid use in patients with QT prolongation (ACLS, 2010). May precipitate or exacerbate HF due to negative inotropic actions; use with caution or avoid (ACLS, 2010) in patients with HF. Correct electrolyte disturbances, especially hypokalemia or hypomagnesemia, prior to use and throughout therapy. Reduce dosage in renal impairment. May increase ventricular response rate in patients with atrial fibrillation or flutter; control AV conduction before initiating. Correct hypokalemia before initiating therapy; hypokalemia may worsen toxicity. Reduce dose if first-degree heart block occurs. Use caution with concurrent use of other antiarrhythmics; may exacerbate or increase the risk of conduction disturbances. Avoid concurrent use with other drugs known to prolong QT_c interval. Avoid use in myasthenia gravis (may worsen condition). Use caution and dose cautiously; renal clearance of procainamide/NAPA declines in patients ≥50 years of age (independent of creatinine clearance reductions) and in the presence of concomitant renal impairment. This product contains sodium metabisulfite which may cause allergic-type reactions, including anaphylactic symptoms and life-threatening asthmatic episodes in susceptible people; this is seen more frequently in asthmatics.

[U.S. Boxed Warning]: Potentially fatal blood dyscrasias (eg, agranulocytosis) have occurred with therapeutic doses; weekly monitoring is recommended during the first 3 months of therapy and periodically thereafter. Discontinue procainamide if this occurs.

[U.S. Boxed Warning]: Long-term administration leads to the development of a positive antinuclear antibody (ANA) test in 50% of patients which may result in a drug-induced lupus erythematosus-like syndrome (in 20% to 30% of patients); discontinue procainamide with rising ANA titers or with SLE symptoms and choose an alternative agent.

[U.S. Boxed Warning] In the Cardiac Arrhythmia Suppression Trial (CAST), recent (>6 days but <2 years ago) myocardial infarction patients with asymptomatic, non-life-threatening ventricular arrhythmias did not benefit and may have been harmed by attempts to suppress the arrhythmia with flecainide or encainide. An increased mortality or nonfatal cardiac arrest rate (7.7%) was seen in the active treatment group compared with patients in the placebo group (3%). The applicability of the CAST results to other populations is unknown. Procainamide should be reserved for patients with life-threatening ventricular arrhythmias.

Adverse Reactions

>1%:

Cardiovascular: Hypotension (I.V. up to 5%)

Dermatologic: Rash

Gastrointestinal: Diarrhea (oral: 3% to 4%), nausea (oral: 3% to 4%), taste disorder (oral: 3% to 4%), vomiting (oral: 3% to 4%)

Miscellaneous: Positive ANA (≤50%), SLE-like syndrome (≤30%, increased incidence with long-term therapy or slow acetylators; syndrome may include abdominal pain, arthralgia, arthritis, chills, fever, hepatomegaly, myalgia, pericarditis, pleural effusion, pulmonary infiltrates, rash)

<1% (Limited to important or life-threatening): Agranulocytosis, alkaline phosphatase increased, angioedema, anorexia, aplastic anemia, arrhythmia exacerbated, arthralgia, asystole, bone marrow suppression, cerebellar ataxia, confusion, demyelinating polyradiculoneuropathy, disorientation, dizziness, drug fever, fever, first degree heart block, flushing, granulomatous hepatitis, hallucinations, hemolytic anemia, hepatic failure, hyperbilirubinemia, hypoplastic anemia, intrahepatic cholestasis, leukopenia, lightheadedness, maculopapular rash, mania, mental depression, myasthenia gravis worsened,

myocardial contractility depressed, myocarditis, myopathy, neuromuscular blockade, neutropenia, pancreatitis, pancytopenia, paradoxical increase in ventricular rate in atrial fibrillation/flutter, peripheral/polyneuropathy, pleural effusion, positive Coombs' test, proarrhythmia, pseudo-obstruction, psychosis, pulmonary embolism, QT_c-interval prolongation, pruritus, rash, respiratory failure due to myopathy, second-degree heart block, tachycardia, thrombocytopenia, torsade de pointes, transaminases increased, urticaria, vasculitis, ventricular fibrillation, weakness

Drug Interactions

Metabolism/Transport Effects **Substrate** of CYP2D6 (major); **Note:** Assignment of Major/Minor substrate status based on clinically relevant drug interaction potential

Avoid Concomitant Use

Avoid concomitant use of Procainamide with any of the following: Artemether; Dronedarone; Lumefantrine; Nilotinib; Pimozide; QUEtiapine; QuiNINE; Tetrabenazine; Thioridazine; Toremifene; Vandetanib; Vemurafenib; Ziprasidone

Increased Effect/Toxicity

Procainamide may increase the levels/effects of: Dronedarone; Neuromuscular-Blocking Agents; Pimozide; QTc-Prolonging Agents; QuiNINE; Tetrabenazine; Thioridazine; Toremifene; Vandetanib; Vemurafenib; Ziprasidone

The levels/effects of Procainamide may be increased by: Abiraterone Acetate; Alfuzosin; Amiodarone; Artemether; Chloroquine; Cimetidine; Ciprofloxacin; Ciprofloxacin (Systemic); CYP2D6 Inhibitors (Moderate); CYP2D6 Inhibitors (Strong); Darunavir; Eribulin; Fingolimod; Gadobutrol; Indacaterol; Lumefantrine; Lurasidone; Nilotinib; QUEtiapine; QuiNINE; Ranitidine; Trimethoprim

Decreased Effect

The levels/effects of Procainamide may be decreased by: Peginterferon Alfa-2b

Ethanol/Nutrition/Herb Interactions

Ethanol: Avoid ethanol (acute ethanol administration reduces procainamide serum concentrations).

Herb/Nutraceutical: Avoid ephedra (may worsen arrhythmia).

Stability Store undiluted vials at room temperature of 15°C to 30°C (59°F to 86°F). The solution is initially colorless but may turn slightly yellow on standing. Injection of air into the vial causes solution to darken. Discard solutions darker than light amber. Color formation may occur upon refrigeration.

Maximum concentration (loading dose only): 20 mg/mL

Maximum admixture concentration: 8 mg/mL

Usual admixture concentration: 1 g/250 mL NS/D_5W or 1 g/500 mL NS/D_5W

When admixed in NS or D_5W to a final concentration of 2-4 mg/mL, solution is stable at room temperature for 24 hours and for 7 days under refrigeration.

Some information indicates that procainamide may be subject to greater decomposition in D_5W unless the admixture is refrigerated or the pH is adjusted. Procainamide is believed to form an association complex with dextrose - the bioavailability of procainamide in this complex is not known and the complex formation is reversible (Raymond, 1988).

Mechanism of Action Decreases myocardial excitability and conduction velocity and may depress myocardial contractility, by increasing the electrical stimulation threshold of ventricle, His-Purkinje system and through direct cardiac effects

Pharmacodynamics/Kinetics

Onset of action: I.M. 10-30 minutes

Distribution: V_d: Children: 2.2 L/kg; Adults: 2 L/kg; decreased with congestive heart failure or shock

Protein binding: 15% to 20%

Metabolism: Hepatic via acetylation to produce N-acetyl procainamide (NAPA) (active metabolite)

Half-life elimination:

Procainamide (hepatic acetylator, phenotype, cardiac and renal function dependent): Children: 1.7 hours; Adults: 2.5-4.7 hours; Anephric: 11 hours

NAPA (dependent upon renal function): Children: 6 hours; Adults: 6-8 hours; Anephric: 42 hours

Time to peak, serum: I.M.: 15-60 minutes

Excretion: Urine (30% to 60% unchanged procainamide; 6% to 52% as NAPA); feces (<5% unchanged procainamide. **Note:** >80% of formed NAPA is renally eliminated in contrast to procainamide which is ~50% renally eliminated (Gibson, 1977).

Dosage Must be titrated to patient's response

Children:

I.M.: 20-30 mg/kg/day divided every 4-6 hours; maximum: 4 g/day

I.V.:

Load: 3-6 mg/kg/dose over 5 minutes not to exceed 100 mg/dose; may repeat every 5-10 minutes to maximum of 15 mg/kg/load

Maintenance as continuous I.V. infusion: 20-80 mcg/kg/minute; maximum: 2 g/24 hours

Possible VT (PALS, 2010): I.V.; I.O.: 15 mg/kg over 30-60 minutes

Adults:

I.M.: 50 mg/kg/day divided every 3-6 hours **or** 0.5-1 g every 4-8 hours (Koch-Weser, 1971)

I.V.:

Loading dose: 15-18 mg/kg administered as slow infusion over 25-30 minutes **or** 100 mg/dose at a rate not to exceed 50 mg/minute repeated every 5 minutes as needed to a total dose of 1 g.

Hemodynamically stable monomorphic VT or pre-excited atrial fibrillation (ACLS, 2010): Loading dose: Infuse 20-50 mg/minute **or** 100 mg every 5 minutes until arrhythmia controlled, hypotension occurs, QRS complex widens by 50% of its original width, or total of 17 mg/kg is given. Follow with a continuous infusion of 1-4 mg/minute. **Note:** Not recommended for use in ongoing ventricular fibrillation (VF) or pulseless ventricular tachycardia (VT) due to prolonged administration time and uncertain efficacy.

Maintenance dose: 1-4 mg/minute by continuous infusion. Maintenance infusions should be reduced by one-third in patients with moderate renal or cardiac impairment and by two-thirds in patients with severe renal or cardiac impairment.

Oral (not available in the U.S.; Canadian labeling): Sustained release formulation (Procan SR®): Maintenance: 50 mg/kg/24 hours given in divided doses every 6 hours

Suggested Procan SR® maintenance dose:

<55 kg: 500 mg every 6 hours

55-91 kg: 750 mg every 6 hours

>91 kg: 1000 mg every 6 hours

Elderly: Initiate doses at lower end of dosage range.

Dosing interval in renal impairment:

Oral:

Cl_{cr} 10-50 mL/minute: Administer every 6-12 hours.

Cl_{cr} <10 mL/minute: Administer every 8-24 hours.

I.V.:

Loading dose: Reduce dose to 12 mg/kg in severe renal impairment.

Maintenance infusion: Reduce dose by one-third in patients with mild renal impairment. Reduce dose by two-thirds in patients with severe renal impairment.

Dialysis:

Procainamide: Moderately hemodialyzable (20% to 50%): Monitor procainamide/N-acetylprocainamide (NAPA) concentrations; supplementation may be necessary.

NAPA: Not dialyzable (0% to 5%)

Procainamide/NAPA: Not peritoneal dialyzable (0% to 5%)

Procainamide/NAPA: Replace according to blood concentration monitoring during continuous arteriovenous or venovenous hemofiltration.

Dosing adjustment in hepatic impairment: Reduce dose by 50%.

Administration

Oral: Do **not** crush or chew sustained release drug products (not available in the U.S.).

I.V.: Must dilute prior to I.V. administration. Loading dose: Maximum rate: 50 mg/minute

Monitoring Parameters ECG, blood pressure, renal function; with prolonged use monitor CBC with differential, platelet count; procainamide and NAPA blood concentrations in patients with hepatic impairment, renal impairment, or receiving constant infusion >3 mg/minute for longer than 24 hours; ANA titers

Reference Range

Timing of serum samples: Draw 6-12 hours after I.V. infusion has started; half-life is 2.5-5 hours

Therapeutic concentrations: Procainamide: 4-10 mcg/mL; NAPA 15-25 mcg/mL; Combined: 10-30 mcg/mL

Toxic concentration: Procainamide: >10-12 mcg/mL

Test Interactions In the presence of propranolol or supra-pharmacologic concentrations of lidocaine or meprobamate, tests which depend on fluorescence to measure procainamide/NAPA concentrations may be affected.

Dosage Forms Excipient information presented when available (limited, particularly for generics); consult specific product labeling.

Injection, solution, as hydrochloride: 100 mg/mL (10 mL); 500 mg/mL (2 mL)

Dosage Forms: Canada Excipient information presented when available (limited, particularly for generics); consult specific product labeling.

Tablet, sustained release, oral, as hydrochloride:

Procan SR®: 250 mg, 500 mg, 750 mg

◆ **Procainamide Hydrochloride** *see* Procainamide *on page 1408*

◆ **Procainamide Hydrochloride Injection, USP (Can)** *see* Procainamide *on page 1408*

◆ **Procaine Amide Hydrochloride** *see* Procainamide *on page 1408*

◆ **Procaine Benzylpenicillin** *see* Penicillin G Procaine *on page 1325*

◆ **Procaine Penicillin G** *see* Penicillin G Procaine *on page 1325*

◆ **PRO-Calcitonin (Can)** *see* Calcitonin *on page 262*

◆ **Procanbid** *see* Procainamide *on page 1408*

◆ **Procan SR® (Can)** *see* Procainamide *on page 1408*

Procarbazine (proe KAR ba zeen)

Brand Names: U.S. Matulane®

Brand Names: Canada Matulane®; Natulan®

Index Terms Benzmethyzin; N-Methylhydrazine; Procarbazine Hydrochloride

Pharmacologic Category Antineoplastic Agent, Alkylating Agent

Use Treatment of Hodgkin's disease

Unlabeled Use Treatment of non-Hodgkin's lymphoma, brain tumors

Pregnancy Risk Factor D

Pregnancy Considerations Animal studies have demonstrated teratogenic effects. There are no adequate and well-controlled studies in pregnant women. There are, however, case reports of fetal malformations in the offspring of pregnant women exposed to procarbazine as part of a combination chemotherapy regimen. Women of childbearing potential should avoid becoming pregnant during treatment.

Lactation Excretion in breast milk unknown/not recommended

Contraindications Hypersensitivity to procarbazine or any component of the formulation; pre-existing bone marrow aplasia; ethanol ingestion; pregnancy

Warnings/Precautions Hazardous agent - use appropriate precautions for handling and disposal. Use with caution in patients with pre-existing renal or hepatic impairment. Procarbazine possesses MAO inhibitor activity and has potential for severe drug and food interactions; follow MAO-I diet. Avoid ethanol consumption, may cause disulfiram-like reaction. May cause hemolysis and/or presence of Heinz inclusion bodies in erythrocytes. Bone marrow depression may occur 2-8 weeks after treatment initiation. Allow ≥1 month interval between radiation therapy or myelosuppressive chemotherapy and initiation of treatment. Withhold treatment for CNS toxicity, leukopenia (WBC <4000/mm^3), thrombocytopenia (platelets <100,000/mm^3), hypersensitivity, stomatitis, diarrhea, or hemorrhage. Procarbazine is a carcinogen which may cause acute leukemia. May cause infertility. **[U.S. Boxed Warning]: Should be administered under the supervision of an experienced cancer chemotherapy physician.**

Adverse Reactions Most frequencies not defined.

Cardiovascular: Edema, flushing, hypotension, syncope, tachycardia

Central nervous system: Apprehension, ataxia, chills, coma, confusion, depression, dizziness, drowsiness, fatigue, fever, hallucination, headache, insomnia, lethargy, nervousness, nightmares, pain, seizure, slurred speech

Dermatologic: Alopecia, dermatitis, hyperpigmentation, petechiae, pruritus, purpura, rash, urticaria

Endocrine & metabolic: Gynecomastia (in prepubertal and early pubertal males)

Hematologic: Eosinophilia; hemolysis (in patients with G6PD deficiency); hemolytic anemia; myelosuppression (leukopenia, anemia, thrombocytopenia); pancytopenia

Gastrointestinal: Abdominal pain, anorexia, constipation, diarrhea, dysphagia, hematemesis, melena; nausea and vomiting ([60% to 90%], increasing the dose in a stepwise fashion over several days may minimize); stomatitis, xerostomia

Genitourinary: Azoospermia (reported with combination chemotherapy), hematuria, nocturia, polyuria, reproductive dysfunction (>10%)

Hepatic: Hepatic dysfunction, jaundice

Neuromuscular & skeletal: Arthralgia, falling, foot drop, myalgia, neuropathy, paresthesia, reflex diminished, tremor, unsteadiness, weakness

Ocular: Diplopia, inability to focus, nystagmus, papilledema, photophobia, retinal hemorrhage

Otic: Hearing loss

Respiratory: Cough, epistaxis, hemoptysis, hoarseness, pleural effusion, pneumonitis, pulmonary toxicity (<1%)

Miscellaneous: Allergic reaction, diaphoresis, herpes, infection, secondary malignancies (2% to 15%; reported with combination therapy)

Drug Interactions

Metabolism/Transport Effects Inhibits Monoamine Oxidase

Avoid Concomitant Use

Avoid concomitant use of Procarbazine with any of the following: Alpha-/Beta-Agonists (Indirect-Acting); Alpha1-Agonists; Alpha2-Agonists (Ophthalmic); Amphetamines; Anilidopiperidine Opioids; Antidepressants (Serotonin Reuptake Inhibitor/Antagonist); Atomoxetine; BCG; Bezafibrate; Buprenorphine; BuPROPion; BusPIRone;

CarBAMazepine; CloZAPine; Cyclobenzaprine; Dexmethylphenidate; Dextromethorphan; Diethylpropion; HYDROmorphone; Linezolid; Maprotiline; Meperidine; Methyldopa; Methylene Blue; Methylphenidate; Mirtazapine; Natalizumab; Oxymorphone; Pimecrolimus; Pizotifen; Selective Serotonin Reuptake Inhibitors; Serotonin 5-HT1D Receptor Agonists; Serotonin/Norepinephrine Reuptake Inhibitors; Tacrolimus (Topical); Tapentadol; Tetrabenazine; Tetrahydrozoline; Tetrahydrozoline (Nasal); Tricyclic Antidepressants; Tryptophan; Vaccines (Live)

Increased Effect/Toxicity

Procarbazine may increase the levels/effects of: Alpha-/Beta-Agonists (Direct-Acting); Alpha-/Beta-Agonists (Indirect-Acting); Alpha1-Agonists; Alpha2-Agonists (Ophthalmic); Amphetamines; Antidepressants (Serotonin Reuptake Inhibitor/Antagonist); Antihypertensives; Atomoxetine; Beta2-Agonists; Bezafibrate; BuPROPion; CloZAPine; Dexmethylphenidate; Dextromethorphan; Diethylpropion; Doxapram; HYDROmorphone; Leflunomide; Linezolid; Lithium; Meperidine; Methadone; Methyldopa; Methylene Blue; Methylphenidate; Metoclopramide; Mirtazapine; Natalizumab; Orthostatic Hypotension Producing Agents; Pizotifen; Reserpine; Selective Serotonin Reuptake Inhibitors; Serotonin 5-HT1D Receptor Agonists; Serotonin Modulators; Serotonin/Norepinephrine Reuptake Inhibitors; Tetrahydrozoline; Tetrahydrozoline (Nasal); Tricyclic Antidepressants; Vaccines (Live); Vitamin K Antagonists

The levels/effects of Procarbazine may be increased by: Altretamine; Anilidopiperidine Opioids; Antipsychotics; Buprenorphine; BusPIRone; CarBAMazepine; COMT Inhibitors; Cyclobenzaprine; Denosumab; Levodopa; MAO Inhibitors; Maprotiline; Oxymorphone; Pimecrolimus; Roflumilast; Tacrolimus (Topical); Tapentadol; Tetrabenazine; TraMADol; Trastuzumab; Tryptophan

Decreased Effect

Procarbazine may decrease the levels/effects of: BCG; Cardiac Glycosides; Coccidioidin Skin Test; Sipuleucel-T; Vaccines (Inactivated); Vaccines (Live); Vitamin K Antagonists

The levels/effects of Procarbazine may be decreased by: Echinacea

Ethanol/Nutrition/Herb Interactions

Ethanol: May enhance the adverse/toxic effects of procarbazine; concurrent use not recommended.

Food: Concurrent ingestion of foods rich in tyramine may cause sudden and severe high blood pressure (hypertensive crisis). Avoid tyramine-containing foods with MAO-Is. Food's freshness is also an important concern; improperly stored or spoiled food can create an environment where tyramine concentrations may increase.

Herb/Nutraceuticals: Avoid supplements containing caffeine, tyrosine, tryptophan, or phenylalanine. Ingestion of large quantities may increase the risk of severe side effects (eg, hypertensive reactions, serotonin syndrome).

Stability Protect from light.

Mechanism of Action Mechanism of action is not clear, methylating of nucleic acids; inhibits DNA, RNA, and protein synthesis; may damage DNA directly and suppresses mitosis; metabolic activation required by host

Pharmacodynamics/Kinetics

Absorption: Rapid and complete

Distribution: Crosses blood-brain barrier; equilibrates between plasma and CSF

Metabolism: Hepatic and renal

Half-life elimination: 1 hour

Time to peak, plasma: 1 hour

Excretion: Urine and respiratory tract (<5% as unchanged drug, 70% as metabolites)

Dosage Refer to individual protocols. Manufacturer states that the dose is based on patient's ideal weight if the patient is obese or has abnormal fluid retention. Other studies suggest that ideal body weight may not be necessary. Oral (may be given as a single daily dose or in 2-3 divided doses):

Children:

BMT aplastic anemia conditioning regimen (unlabeled use): 12.5 mg/kg/day every other day for 4 doses

Hodgkin's disease: MOPP/IC-MOPP regimens: 100 mg/m^2/day for 14 days and repeated every 4 weeks

Neuroblastoma and medulloblastoma (unlabeled use): Doses as high as 100-200 mg/m^2/day once daily have been used

Adults: Initial: 2-4 mg/kg/day in single or divided doses for 7 days then increase dose to 4-6 mg/kg/day until response is obtained or leukocyte count decreased <4000/mm^3 or the platelet count decreased <100,000/mm^3; maintenance: 1-2 mg/kg/day

Dosing in renal impairment: The FDA-approved labeling does not contain dosing adjustment guidelines; use with caution; may result in increased toxicity.

Dosing in hepatic impairment: The FDA-approved labeling does not contain dosing adjustment guidelines; use with caution; may result in increased toxicity. The following guidelines have been used by some clinicians:

Floyd, 2006:

Transaminases 1.6-6 times ULN: Administer 75% of dose

Transaminases >6 times ULN: Use clinical judgment

Serum bilirubin >5 mg/dL or transaminases >3 times ULN: Avoid use

King, 2001: Serum bilirubin >5 mg/dL or transaminases >180 units/L: Avoid use

Dietary Considerations Avoid tyramine-containing foods/beverages. Some examples include aged or matured cheese, air-dried or cured meats (including sausages and salamis), fava or broad bean pods, tap/draft beers, Marmite concentrate, sauerkraut, soy sauce and other soybean condiments.

Administration May be given as a single daily dose or in 2-3 divided doses.

Monitoring Parameters CBC with differential, platelet and reticulocyte count, urinalysis, liver function test, renal function test.

Dosage Forms Excipient information presented when available (limited, particularly for generics); consult specific product labeling.

Capsule, oral, as hydrochloride:

Matulane®: 50 mg

Extemporaneous Preparations Hazardous agent: Use appropriate precautions for handling and disposal.

A 10 mg/mL oral suspension may be prepared using capsules, glycerin, and strawberry syrup. Empty the contents of ten 50 mg capsules into a mortar. Add 2 mL glycerin and mix to a thick uniform paste. Add 10 mL strawberry syrup in incremental proportions; mix until uniform. Transfer the mixture to an amber glass bottle and rinse mortar with small amounts of strawberry syrup; add rinses to the bottle in sufficient quantity to make 50 mL. Label "shake well" and "protect from light". Stable for 7 days at room temperature.

Matulane® data on file, Sigma Tau Pharmaceuticals, Inc.

◆ **Procarbazine Hydrochloride** *see* Procarbazine *on page 1410*

◆ **Procardia®** *see* NIFEdipine *on page 1202*

◆ **Procardia XL®** *see* NIFEdipine *on page 1202*

◆ **PRO-Cefadroxil (Can)** *see* Cefadroxil *on page 301*

◆ **PRO-Cefuroxime (Can)** *see* Cefuroxime *on page 322*

◆ **ProCentra®** *see* Dextroamphetamine *on page 487*

◆ **Procetofene** *see* Fenofibrate *on page 693*

Prochlorperazine (proe klor PER a zeen)

Brand Names: U.S. Compro®

Brand Names: Canada Apo-Prochlorperazine®; Nu-Prochlor; Stemetil®

Index Terms Chlormeprazine; Compazine; Prochlorperazine Edisylate; Prochlorperazine Maleate

Pharmacologic Category Antiemetic; Antipsychotic Agent, Typical, Phenothiazine

Use Management of nausea and vomiting; psychotic disorders, including schizophrenia and anxiety

Unlabeled Use Behavioral syndromes in dementia; psychosis/agitation related to Alzheimer's dementia

Pregnancy Considerations Jaundice or hyper-/hyporeflexia have been reported in newborn infants following maternal use of phenothiazines. Antipsychotic use during the third trimester of pregnancy has a risk for abnormal muscle movements (extrapyramidal symptoms [EPS]) and withdrawal symptoms in newborns following delivery. Symptoms in the newborn may include agitation, feeding disorder, hypertonia, hypotonia, respiratory distress, somnolence, and tremor; these effects may be self-limiting or require hospitalization.

Lactation Excretion in breast milk unknown/use caution

Contraindications Hypersensitivity to prochlorperazine or any component of the formulation (cross-reactivity between phenothiazines may occur); severe CNS depression; coma; pediatric surgery; Reye's syndrome; should not be used in children <2 years of age or <9 kg

Warnings/Precautions [U.S. Boxed Warning]: Elderly patients with dementia-related psychosis treated with antipsychotics are at an increased risk of death compared to placebo. Most deaths appeared to be either cardiovascular (eg, heart failure, sudden death) or infectious (eg, pneumonia) in nature. Prochlorperazine is not approved for the treatment of dementia-related psychosis.

Leukopenia, neutropenia, and agranulocytosis (sometimes fatal) have been reported in clinical trials and postmarketing reports with antipsychotic use; presence of risk factors (eg, pre-existing low WBC or history of drug-induced leuko-/neutropenia) should prompt periodic blood count assessment. Discontinue therapy at first signs of blood dyscrasias or if absolute neutrophil count <1000/mm^3.

May be sedating; use with caution in disorders where CNS depression is a feature. May obscure intestinal obstruction or brain tumor. May impair physical or mental abilities. Effects with other sedative drugs or ethanol may be potentiated. Use with caution in Parkinson's disease; hemodynamic instability; predisposition to seizures; subcortical brain damage; and in severe cardiac, hepatic, or renal disease. May alter temperature regulation or mask toxicity of other drugs. Use caution with exposure to heat. May alter cardiac conduction. May cause orthostatic hypotension. Hypotension may occur following administration, particularly when parenteral form is used or in high dosages. Antipsychotic use has been associated with esophageal dysmotility and aspiration; use with caution in patients at risk of pneumonia (ie, Alzheimer's disease).

May cause pigmentary retinopathy, and lenticular and corneal deposits, particularly with prolonged therapy. Use associated with increased prolactin levels; clinical significance of hyperprolactinemia in patients with breast cancer or other prolactin-dependent tumors is unknown.

Phenothiazines may cause anticholinergic effects; therefore, they should be used with caution in patients with decreased gastrointestinal motility, urinary retention, BPH, xerostomia, or visual problems. Conditions which also may be exacerbated by cholinergic blockade include narrow-angle glaucoma and worsening of myasthenia gravis. May cause extrapyramidal symptoms (EPS), including pseudoparkinsonism, acute dystonic reactions, akathisia, and tardive dyskinesia. Risk of dystonia (and possibly other EPS) may be greater with increased doses, use of conventional antipsychotics, males, and younger patients. Use caution in the elderly. Children with acute illness or dehydration are more susceptible to neuromuscular reactions; use cautiously. May be associated with neuroleptic malignant syndrome (NMS). Injection contains benzyl alcohol which has been associated with "gasping syndrome" in neonates.

Adverse Reactions Reported with prochlorperazine or other phenothiazines. Frequency not defined.

Cardiovascular: Cardiac arrest, hypotension, peripheral edema, Q-wave distortions, T-wave distortions

Central nervous system: Agitation, catatonia, cerebral edema, cough reflex suppressed, dizziness, drowsiness, fever (mild - I.M.), headache, hyperactivity, hyperpyrexia, impairment of temperature regulation, insomnia, neuroleptic malignant syndrome (NMS), paradoxical excitement, restlessness, seizure

Dermatologic: Angioedema, contact dermatitis, discoloration of skin (blue-gray), epithelial keratopathy, erythema, eczema, exfoliative dermatitis (injectable), itching, photosensitivity, rash, skin pigmentation, urticaria

Endocrine & metabolic: Amenorrhea, breast enlargement, galactorrhea, gynecomastia, glucosuria, hyper-/hypoglycemia, lactation, libido (changes in), menstrual irregularity, SIADH

Gastrointestinal: Appetite increased, atonic colon, constipation, ileus, nausea, weight gain, xerostomia

Genitourinary: Ejaculating dysfunction, ejaculatory disturbances, impotence, incontinence, polyuria, priapism, urinary retention, urination difficulty

Hematologic: Agranulocytosis, aplastic anemia, eosinophilia, hemolytic anemia, leukopenia, pancytopenia, thrombocytopenic purpura

Hepatic: Biliary stasis, cholestatic jaundice, hepatotoxicity

Neuromuscular & skeletal: Dystonias (torticollis, opisthotonos, carpopedal spasm, trismus, oculogyric crisis, protrusion of tongue); extrapyramidal symptoms (pseudoparkinsonism, akathisia, dystonias, tardive dyskinesia); SLE-like syndrome, tremor

Ocular: blurred vision, cornea and lens changes, lenticular/corneal deposits, miosis, mydriasis, pigmentary retinopathy

Respiratory: Asthma, laryngeal edema, nasal congestion

Miscellaneous: Allergic reactions, diaphoresis

Drug Interactions

Metabolism/Transport Effects None known.

Avoid Concomitant Use

Avoid concomitant use of Prochlorperazine with any of the following: Dofetilide; Metoclopramide

Increased Effect/Toxicity

Prochlorperazine may increase the levels/effects of: Alcohol (Ethyl); Analgesics (Opioid); Anticholinergics; Antidepressants (Serotonin Reuptake Inhibitor/Antagonist); Anti-Parkinson's Agents (Dopamine Agonist); Beta-Blockers; CNS Depressants; Dofetilide; Methotrimeprazine; Methylphenidate; Porfimer; Serotonin Modulators

The levels/effects of Prochlorperazine may be increased by: Acetylcholinesterase Inhibitors (Central); Antidepressants (Serotonin Reuptake Inhibitor/Antagonist); Antimalarial Agents; Beta-Blockers; Deferoxamine; Droperidol; HydrOXYzine; Lithium formulations; Methotrimeprazine; Methylphenidate; Metoclopramide; Pramlintide; Tetrabenazine

Decreased Effect

Prochlorperazine may decrease the levels/effects of: Amphetamines; Quinagolide

The levels/effects of Prochlorperazine may be decreased by: Antacids; Anti-Parkinson's Agents (Dopamine Agonist); Lithium formulations

Ethanol/Nutrition/Herb Interactions

Ethanol: May increase CNS depression; monitor for increased effects with coadministration. Caution patients about effects.

Food: Limit caffeine.

Herb/Nutraceutical: Avoid dong quai, St John's wort (may also cause photosensitization). Avoid kava kava, gotu kola, valerian, St John's wort (may increase CNS depression).

Stability

Injection: Store at <30°C (<86°F); do not freeze. Protect from light. Clear or slightly yellow solutions may be used.

I.V. infusion: Injection may be diluted in 50-100 mL NS or D_5W.

Suppository, tablet: Store at 15°C to 30°C (59°F to 86°F). Protect from light.

Mechanism of Action Prochlorperazine is a piperazine phenothiazine antipsychotic which blocks postsynaptic mesolimbic dopaminergic D_1 and D_2 receptors in the brain, including the chemoreceptor trigger zone; exhibits a strong alpha-adrenergic and anticholinergic blocking effect and depresses the release of hypothalamic and hypophyseal hormones; believed to depress the reticular activating system, thus affecting basal metabolism, body temperature, wakefulness, vasomotor tone and emesis

Pharmacodynamics/Kinetics

Onset of action: Oral: 30-40 minutes; I.M.: 10-20 minutes; Rectal: ~60 minutes

Peak antiemetic effect: I.V.: 30-60 minutes

Duration: Rectal: 12 hours; Oral: 3-4 hours; I.M., I.V.: Adults: 4-6 hours; I.M.: Children: 12 hours

Distribution: V_d: 1400-1548 L; crosses placenta; enters breast milk

Metabolism: Primarily hepatic; N-desmethyl prochlorperazine (major active metabolite)

Bioavailability: Oral: 12.5%

Half-life elimination: Oral: 6-10 hours (single dose), 14-22 hours (repeated dosing); I.V.: 6-10 hours

Dosage

Antiemetic: Children (therapy >1 day usually not required): **Note:** Not recommended for use in children <9 kg or <2 years:

Oral, rectal: >9 kg: 0.4 mg/kg/24 hours in 3-4 divided doses; **or**

9-13 kg: 2.5 mg every 12-24 hours as needed; maximum: 7.5 mg/day

13.1-17 kg: 2.5 mg every 8-12 hours as needed; maximum: 10 mg/day

17.1-37 kg: 2.5 mg every 8 hours or 5 mg every 12 hours as needed; maximum: 15 mg/day

I.M.: 0.13 mg/kg/dose; change to oral as soon as possible

Antiemetic: Adults:

Oral (tablet): 5-10 mg 3-4 times/day; usual maximum: 40 mg/day; larger doses may rarely be required

I.M. (deep): 5-10 mg every 3-4 hours; usual maximum: 40 mg/day

I.V.: 2.5-10 mg; maximum: 10 mg/dose or 40 mg/day; may repeat dose every 3-4 hours as needed

Rectal: 25 mg twice daily

Surgical nausea/vomiting: Adults: **Note:** Should not exceed 40 mg/day

I.M.: 5-10 mg 1-2 hours before induction or to control symptoms during or after surgery; may repeat once if necessary

I.V. (administer slow IVP <5 mg/minute): 5-10 mg 15-30 minutes before induction or to control symptoms during or after surgery; may repeat once if necessary

Rectal (unlabeled use): 25 mg

Antipsychotic:

Children 2-12 years (not recommended in children <9 kg or <2 years):

Oral, rectal: 2.5 mg 2-3 times/day; do not give more than 10 mg the first day; increase dosage as needed to maximum daily dose of 20 mg for 2-5 years and 25 mg for 6-12 years

I.M.: 0.13 mg/kg/dose; change to oral as soon as possible

Adults:

Oral: 5-10 mg 3-4 times/day; titrate dose slowly every 2-3 days; doses up to 150 mg/day may be required in some patients for treatment of severe disturbances

I.M.: Initial: 10-20 mg; if necessary repeat initial dose every 1-4 hours to gain control; more than 3-4 doses are rarely needed. If parenteral administration is still required; give 10-20 mg every 4-6 hours; change to oral as soon as possible.

Nonpsychotic anxiety: Oral (tablet): Adults: Usual dose: 15-20 mg/day in divided doses; do not give doses >20 mg/day or for longer than 12 weeks

Elderly: Behavioral symptoms associated with dementia (unlabeled use): Initial: 2.5-5 mg 1-2 times/day; increase dose at 4- to 7-day intervals by 2.5-5 mg/day; increase dosing intervals (twice daily, 3 times/day, etc) as necessary to control response or side effects; maximum daily dose should probably not exceed 75 mg in elderly; gradual increases (titration) may prevent some side effects or decrease their severity

Dietary Considerations Increase dietary intake of riboflavin; should be administered with food or water. Rectal suppositories may contain coconut and palm oil.

Administration May be administered orally, I.M., or I.V.

I.M.: Inject by deep IM into outer quadrant of buttocks.

I.V.: Administer slow I.V. at a rate not exceeding 5 mg/minute. To reduce the risk of hypotension, patients receiving I.V. prochlorperazine must remain lying down and be observed for at least 30 minutes following administration.

Monitoring Parameters Vital signs; lipid profile, fasting blood glucose/Hgb A_{1c}; BMI; mental status, abnormal involuntary movement scale (AIMS); periodic ophthalmic exams (if chronically used); extrapyramidal symptoms (EPS)

Test Interactions False-positives for phenylketonuria, pregnancy, urinary amylase, uroporphyrins, urobilinogen

Additional Information Not recommended as an antipsychotic due to inferior efficacy compared to other phenothiazines.

Dosage Forms Excipient information presented when available (limited, particularly for generics); consult specific product labeling.

Injection, solution, as edisylate [strength expressed as base]: 5 mg/mL (2 mL, 10 mL)

Suppository, rectal: 25 mg (12s)

Compro®: 25 mg (12s) [contains coconut oil, palm oil]

Tablet, oral, as maleate [strength expressed as base]: 5 mg, 10 mg

◆ **Prochlorperazine Edisylate** *see* Prochlorperazine *on page 1412*

◆ **Prochlorperazine Maleate** *see* Prochlorperazine *on page 1412*

◆ **PRO-Ciprofloxacin (Can)** *see* Ciprofloxacin (Systemic) *on page 362*

◆ **PRO-Clonazepam (Can)** *see* ClonazePAM *on page 390*

◆ **ProCort®** *see* Pramoxine and Hydrocortisone *on page 1393*

◆ **Procrit®** *see* Epoetin Alfa *on page 601*

- ◆ **Proctocort®** *see* Hydrocortisone (Topical) *on page 841*
- ◆ **ProctoCream®-HC** *see* Hydrocortisone (Topical) *on page 841*
- ◆ **Proctofene** *see* Fenofibrate *on page 693*
- ◆ **ProctoFoam® HC** *see* Pramoxine and Hydrocortisone *on page 1393*
- ◆ **Proctofoam™-HC (Can)** *see* Pramoxine and Hydrocortisone *on page 1393*
- ◆ **Procto-Pak™** *see* Hydrocortisone (Topical) *on page 841*
- ◆ **Proctosol-HC®** *see* Hydrocortisone (Topical) *on page 841*
- ◆ **Proctozone-HC 2.5%™** *see* Hydrocortisone (Topical) *on page 841*
- ◆ **Procytox® (Can)** *see* Cyclophosphamide *on page 421*
- ◆ **PRO-Diclo-Rapide (Can)** *see* Diclofenac (Systemic) *on page 495*
- ◆ **PRO-Enalapril (Can)** *see* Enalapril *on page 584*
- ◆ **ProFe [OTC]** *see* Polysaccharide-Iron Complex *on page 1375*
- ◆ **PRO-Feno-Super (Can)** *see* Fenofibrate *on page 693*
- ◆ **Profilnine® SD** *see* Factor IX Complex (Human) *on page 684*
- ◆ **Proflavanol C™ (Can)** *see* Ascorbic Acid *on page 149*
- ◆ **PRO-Fluconazole (Can)** *see* Fluconazole *on page 718*
- ◆ **PRO-Fluoxetine (Can)** *see* FLUoxetine *on page 731*
- ◆ **PRO-Gabapentin (Can)** *see* Gabapentin *on page 773*

Progesterone (proe JES ter one)

Brand Names: U.S. Crinone®; Endometrin®; First™-Progesterone VGS 100; First™-Progesterone VGS 200; First™-Progesterone VGS 25; First™-Progesterone VGS 400; First™-Progesterone VGS 50; Prometrium®

Brand Names: Canada Crinone®; Prometrium®

Index Terms Pregnenedione; Progestin

Pharmacologic Category Progestin

Use

Oral: Prevention of endometrial hyperplasia in nonhysterectomized, postmenopausal women who are receiving conjugated estrogen tablets; secondary amenorrhea

I.M.: Amenorrhea; abnormal uterine bleeding due to hormonal imbalance

Intravaginal gel: Part of assisted reproductive technology (ART) for infertile women with progesterone deficiency; secondary amenorrhea

Vaginal tablet: Part of ART for infertile women with progesterone deficiency

Pregnancy Risk Factor B (Prometrium®, per manufacturer); none established for vaginal gel, vaginal tablet, or injection

Pregnancy Considerations Adverse events were not observed following oral administration in animal reproduction studies. There is an increased risk of minor birth defects in children whose mothers take progesterones during the first 4 months of pregnancy. Hypospadias has been reported in male and mild masculinization of the external genitalia has been reported in female babies exposed during the first trimester. Cleft lip, cleft palate, congenital heart disease, patent ductus arteriosus, ventricular septal defect, intrauterine death, and spontaneous abortion have been noted in case reports following use of oral progesterone during pregnancy. High doses of progesterone would be expected to impair fertility. According to the American College of Obstetricians and Gynecologists, additional studies are needed to evaluate the use of progesterone to reduce the risk of preterm birth. If needed, use should be restricted to women with history of previous spontaneous abortion at <37 weeks. The vaginal gel and tablet are indicated for use in ART. The oral capsules are contraindicated for use during pregnancy.

Lactation Enters breast milk/use caution (AAP rates "compatible"; AAP 2001 update pending)

Contraindications Hypersensitivity to progesterone or any component of the formulation; undiagnosed abnormal vaginal bleeding; history of or current thrombophlebitis or venous thromboembolic disorders (including DVT, PE); history of, active or recent (within 1 year) arterial thromboembolic disease (eg, stroke, MI); history of or known or suspected carcinoma of the breast or genital organs; hepatic dysfunction or disease; missed abortion or ectopic pregnancy; diagnostic test for pregnancy; capsules are also contraindicated for use during pregnancy

Warnings/Precautions [U.S. Boxed Warning]: Progestins used in combination with estrogen should not be used to prevent cardiovascular disease. Use caution with cardiovascular disease or dysfunction. Progestins used in combination with estrogen may increase the risks of hypertension, myocardial infarction (MI), stroke, pulmonary emboli (PE), and deep vein thrombosis; incidence of these effects was shown to be significantly increased in postmenopausal women using CEE in combination with MPA. Similar risk should be assumed with other progestins.

[U.S. Boxed Warning]: The risk of dementia may be increased in postmenopausal women; progestins used in combination with estrogen should not be used to prevent dementia. Increased incidence was observed in women ≥65 years of age taking CEE alone or in combination with MPA.

[U.S. Boxed Warning]: An increased risk of invasive breast cancer was observed in postmenopausal women using conjugated equine estrogens (CEE) in combination with medroxyprogesterone acetate (MPA). An increase in abnormal mammograms has also been reported with estrogen and progestin therapy

Unopposed estrogens may increase the risk of endometrial carcinoma in postmenopausal women with an intact uterus. Risk appears to be associated with long-term use. The use of a progestin should be considered when administering estrogens to postmenopausal women with an intact uterus. Adequate diagnostic measures, including endometrial sampling (if indicated), should be performed to rule out malignancy in all cases of undiagnosed abnormal vaginal bleeding. Postmenopausal estrogen therapy and combined estrogen/progesterone therapy may increase the risk of ovarian cancer; however, the absolute risk to an individual woman is small. Although results from various studies are not consistent, risk does not appear to be significantly associated with the duration, route, or dose of therapy. In one study, the risk decreased after 2 years following discontinuation of therapy.

Discontinue pending examination in cases of sudden partial or complete vision loss, sudden onset of proptosis, diplopia, or migraine; discontinue permanently if papilledema or retinal vascular lesions are observed on examination. Use with caution in patients with diseases that may be exacerbated by fluid retention, including asthma, epilepsy, migraine, diabetes or renal dysfunction. Use caution with history of depression. Patients should be warned that progesterone might cause transient dizziness or drowsiness during initial therapy. Whenever possible, progestins in combination with estrogens should be discontinued at least 4-6 weeks prior to surgeries associated with an increased risk of thromboembolism or during periods of prolonged immobilization. Progestins used in combination with estrogen should be used for shortest duration possible consistent with treatment goals. Conduct periodic risk: benefit assessments.

Products may contain palm oil, peanut oil, sesame oil, or benzyl alcohol. Not for use prior to menarche.

Adverse Reactions

Injection (I.M.):

Cardiovascular: Cerebral edema, cerebral thrombosis, edema

Central nervous system: Depression, fever, insomnia, somnolence

Dermatologic: Acne, allergic rash (rare), alopecia, hirsutism, pruritus, rash, urticaria

Endocrine & metabolic: Amenorrhea, breakthrough bleeding, breast tenderness, galactorrhea, menstrual flow changes, spotting

Gastrointestinal: Nausea, weight gain/loss

Genitourinary: Cervical erosion changes, cervical secretion changes

Hepatic: Cholestatic jaundice

Local: Injection site: Irritation, pain, redness

Ocular: Optic neuritis, retinal thrombosis

Respiratory: Pulmonary embolism

Miscellaneous: Anaphylactoid reactions

Oral capsule (percentages reported when used in combination with or cycled with conjugated estrogens):

>10%:

Central nervous system: Headache (16% to 31%), dizziness (15% to 24%), depression (19%)

Endocrine & metabolic: Breast tenderness (27%), breast pain (6% to 16%)

Gastrointestinal: Abdominal pain (10% to 20%), abdominal bloating (8% to 12%)

Genitourinary: Urinary problems (11%)

Neuromuscular & skeletal: Joint pain (20%), musculoskeletal pain (12%)

Miscellaneous: Viral infection (12%)

5% to 10%:

Cardiovascular: Chest pain (7%)

Central nervous system: Fatigue (8%), irritability (8%), worry (8%)

Gastrointestinal: Nausea/vomiting (8%), diarrhea (7% to 8%)

Genitourinary: Vaginal discharge (10%)

Respiratory: Cough (8%)

<5%: Breast biopsy, breast cancer, cholecystectomy, constipation

Postmarketing and/or case reports: Aggression, alopecia, anaphylactic reaction, arthralgia, asthma, blurred vision, choking, cholestasis, cholestatic hepatitis, circulatory collapse, confusion, consciousness depressed/loss, convulsion, depersonalization, diplopia, disorientation, drunk feeling, dysarthria, dysphagia, dyspnea, endometrial carcinoma, facial edema, feeling abnormal, gait abnormal, hepatic enzymes increased, hepatic failure, hepatic necrosis, hepatitis, hyperglycemia, hyper-/hypotension, hypersensitivity, jaundice, liver function tests increased, menorrhagia, menstrual disorder, metrorrhagia, muscle cramps, ovarian cyst, pancreatitis (acute), paresthesia, pruritus, sedation, slurred speech, stupor, suicidal ideation, syncope, tachycardia, throat tightness, TIA, tinnitus, tongue swelling, urticaria, vertigo, visual disturbance, walking difficulty, weight gain/loss

Vaginal gel (percentages reported with ART); also refer to oral capsule reactions listing for additional effects noted with progesterone:

>10%:

Central nervous system: Somnolence (27%), headache (13% to 17%), nervousness (16%), depression (11%)

Endocrine & metabolic: Breast enlargement (40%), breast pain (13%), libido decreased (11%)

Gastrointestinal: Constipation (27%), nausea (7% to 22%), cramps (15%), abdominal pain (12%)

Genitourinary: Perineal pain (17%), nocturia (13%)

5% to 10%:

Central nervous system: Pain (8%), dizziness (5%)

Gastrointestinal: Diarrhea (8%), bloating (7%), vomiting (5%)

Genitourinary: Vaginal discharge (7%), dyspareunia (6%), genital moniliasis (5%), genital pruritus (5%)

Neuromuscular & skeletal: Arthralgia (8%)

Vaginal tablet (percentages reported with ART); also refer to oral capsule reactions listing for additional effects noted with progesterone:

>10%:

Gastrointestinal: Abdominal pain (12%)

Miscellaneous: Post-oocyte retrieval pain (25% to 28%)

1% to 10%:

Central nervous system: Headache (3% to 4%), fatigue (2% to 3%)

Endocrine & metabolic: Ovarian hyperstimulation syndrome (7%)

Gastrointestinal: Nausea (7% to 8%), abdominal distension (4%), constipation (2% to 3%), vomiting (2% to 3%)

Genitourinary: Uterine spasm (3% to 4%), vaginal bleeding (3%), urinary tract infection (1% to 2%)

<1%: Burning, discomfort, itching, peripheral edema, urticaria, vaginal irritation

Drug Interactions

Metabolism/Transport Effects Substrate of CYP1A2 (minor), CYP2A6 (minor), CYP2C19 (major), CYP2C9 (minor), CYP2D6 (minor), CYP3A4 (major); **Note:** Assignment of Major/Minor substrate status based on clinically relevant drug interaction potential; **Inhibits** CYP2C19 (weak), CYP2C9 (weak), CYP3A4 (weak), P-glycoprotein

Avoid Concomitant Use

Avoid concomitant use of Progesterone with any of the following: Pimozide; Silodosin; Topotecan

Increased Effect/Toxicity

Progesterone may increase the levels/effects of: Colchicine; Dabigatran Etexilate; Everolimus; P-glycoprotein/ABCB1 Substrates; Pimozide; Rivaroxaban; Silodosin; Topotecan

The levels/effects of Progesterone may be increased by: Conivaptan; Herbs (Progestogenic Properties)

Decreased Effect

The levels/effects of Progesterone may be decreased by: Aminoglutethimide; CYP2C19 Inducers (Strong); CYP3A4 Inducers (Strong); Cyproterone; Deferasirox; Herbs (CYP3A4 Inducers); Peginterferon Alfa-2b; Tocilizumab

Ethanol/Nutrition/Herb Interactions

Food: Food increases oral bioavailability.

Herb/Nutraceutical: St John's wort may decrease progesterone levels. Herbs with progestogenic properties may enhance the adverse/toxic effects of progestin; example herbs include bloodroot, chasteberry, damiana, oregano, yucca.

Stability Store at controlled room temperature. Protect capsules from excessive moisture.

Mechanism of Action Natural steroid hormone that induces secretory changes in the endometrium, promotes mammary gland development, relaxes uterine smooth muscle, blocks follicular maturation and ovulation, and maintains pregnancy. When used as part of an ART program in the luteal phase, progesterone supports embryo implantation.

Pharmacodynamics/Kinetics

Absorption: Vaginal gel: Prolonged

Absorption half-life: 25-50 hours

Protein binding: Albumin (50% to 54%) and cortisol-binding protein (43% to 48%)

Metabolism: Hepatic to metabolites

Half-life elimination: Vaginal gel: 5-20 minutes

Time to peak: Oral: Within 3 hours; I.M.: ~8 hours; Vaginal tablet: ~17-24 hours

Excretion: Urine, bile, feces

Dosage Adults:

I.M.: Females:

Amenorrhea: 5-10 mg/day for 6-8 consecutive days

Functional uterine bleeding: 5-10 mg/day for 6 doses

Oral: Females:

Prevention of endometrial hyperplasia (in postmenopausal women with a uterus who are receiving daily conjugated estrogen tablets): 200 mg as a single daily dose every evening for 12 days sequentially per 28-day cycle

Amenorrhea: 400 mg every evening for 10 days

Intravaginal gel: Females:

ART in women who require progesterone supplementation: 90 mg (8% gel) once daily; if pregnancy occurs, may continue treatment for up to 10-12 weeks

ART in women with partial or complete ovarian failure: 90 mg (8% gel) intravaginally twice daily; if pregnancy occurs, may continue up to 10-12 weeks

Secondary amenorrhea: 45 mg (4% gel) intravaginally every other day for up to 6 doses; women who fail to respond may be increased to 90 mg (8% gel) every other day for up to 6 doses

Intravaginal tablet: Females: ART: 100 mg 2-3 times daily starting at oocyte retrieval and continuing for up to 10 weeks.

Administration

I.M.: Administer deep I.M. only

Intravaginal:

Vaginal gel: (A small amount of gel will remain in the applicator following insertion): Administer into the vagina directly from sealed applicator. Remove applicator from wrapper; holding applicator by thickest end, shake down to move contents to thin end; while holding applicator by flat section of thick end, twist off tab; gently insert into vagina and squeeze thick end of applicator.

For use at altitudes above 2500 feet: Remove applicator from wrapper; hold applicator on both sides of bubble in the thick end; using a lancet, make a single puncture in the bubble to relieve air pressure; holding applicator by thickest end, shake down to move contents to thin end; while holding applicator by flat section of thick end, twist off tab; gently insert into vagina and squeeze thick end of applicator.

Vaginal tablet: Insert tablet in vagina using disposable applicator provided.

Oral capsule: For patients who experience difficulty swallowing the capsules, taking with a full glass of water in the standing position may be beneficial.

Monitoring Parameters Routine physical examination that includes blood pressure and Papanicolaou smear, breast exam, mammogram. Adequate diagnostic measures, including endometrial sampling, if indicated, should be performed to rule out malignancy in all cases of undiagnosed abnormal vaginal bleeding. Signs and symptoms of thromboembolic disorders, vision changes

Test Interactions Thyroid function, metyrapone, liver function, coagulation tests, endocrine function tests

Dosage Forms Excipient information presented when available (limited, particularly for generics); consult specific product labeling.

Capsule, oral:

Prometrium®: 100 mg, 200 mg [contains peanut oil]

Gel, vaginal:

Crinone®: 4% (1.45 g) [contains palm oil; 45 mg/dose]

Crinone®: 8% (1.45 g) [contains palm oil; 90 mg/dose]

Injection, oil: 50 mg/mL (10 mL)

Suppository, vaginal [compounding kit]:

First™-Progesterone VGS 25: 25 mg (30s)

First™-Progesterone VGS 50: 50 mg (30s)

First™-Progesterone VGS 100: 100 mg (30s)

First™-Progesterone VGS 200: 200 mg (30s)

First™-Progesterone VGS 400: 400 mg (30s)

Tablet, vaginal:

Endometrin®: 100 mg

◆ **Progestin** *see* Progesterone *on page 1414*
◆ **PRO-Glyburide (Can)** *see* GlyBURIDE *on page 799*
◆ **Proglycem®** *see* Diazoxide *on page 495*
◆ **Prograf®** *see* Tacrolimus (Systemic) *on page 1615*
◆ **Proguanil and Atovaquone** *see* Atovaquone and Proguanil *on page 168*
◆ **Proguanil Hydrochloride and Atovaquone** *see* Atovaquone and Proguanil *on page 168*
◆ **PRO-Hydroxyquine (Can)** *see* Hydroxychloroquine *on page 848*
◆ **PRO-Indapamide (Can)** *see* Indapamide *on page 886*
◆ **Pro-Indo (Can)** *see* Indomethacin *on page 890*
◆ **PRO-ISMN (Can)** *see* Isosorbide Mononitrate *on page 938*
◆ **Proleukin®** *see* Aldesleukin *on page 55*
◆ **PRO-Levetiracetam (Can)** *see* LevETIRAcetam *on page 994*
◆ **PRO-Levocarb (Can)** *see* Carbidopa and Levodopa *on page 284*
◆ **Prolia®** *see* Denosumab *on page 471*
◆ **PRO-Lisinopril (Can)** *see* Lisinopril *on page 1020*
◆ **PRO-Lorazepam (Can)** *see* LORazepam *on page 1032*
◆ **PRO-Lovastatin (Can)** *see* Lovastatin *on page 1038*
◆ **Promacet** *see* Butalbital and Acetaminophen *on page 255*
◆ **Promacta®** *see* Eltrombopag *on page 579*
◆ **PRO-Metformin (Can)** *see* MetFORMIN *on page 1086*

Promethazine (proe METH a zeen)

Brand Names: U.S. Phenadoz®; Phenergan®; Promethegan™

Brand Names: Canada Bioniche Promethazine; Histantil; Phenergan®; PMS-Promethazine

Index Terms Promethazine Hydrochloride

Pharmacologic Category Antiemetic; Histamine H_1 Antagonist; Histamine H_1 Antagonist, First Generation; Phenothiazine Derivative

Additional Appendix Information

Beers Criteria − Potentially Inappropriate Medications for Geriatrics *on page 1973*

Use Symptomatic treatment of various allergic conditions; antiemetic; motion sickness; sedative; adjunct to postoperative analgesia and anesthesia

Pregnancy Risk Factor C

Pregnancy Considerations Teratogenic effects were not observed in animal studies. There are no adequate and well-controlled studies in pregnant women. Crosses the placenta. Use during pregnancy only if benefits outweigh risk. May be used alone or as an adjunct to narcotic analgesics during labor.

Lactation Excretion in breast milk unknown/not recommended

Contraindications Hypersensitivity to promethazine or any component of the formulation (cross-reactivity between phenothiazines may occur); coma; treatment of lower respiratory tract symptoms, including asthma; children <2 years of age; intra-arterial or subcutaneous administration

Warnings/Precautions [U.S. Boxed Warning]: Respiratory fatalities have been reported in children <2 years of age. Contraindicated in children <2 years of age. In children ≥2 years, use the lowest possible dose; other drugs with respiratory depressant effects should be avoided.

[U.S. Boxed Warning]: Promethazine injection can cause severe tissue injury (including gangrene) regardless of the route of administration. Tissue irritation and damage may result from perivascular extravasation, unintentional intra-arterial administration, and intraneuronal or perineuronal infiltration. In addition to gangrene, adverse events reported include tissue necrosis, abscesses, burning, pain, erythema, edema, paralysis, severe spasm of distal vessels, phlebitis, thrombophlebitis, venous thrombosis, sensory loss, paralysis, and palsies. Surgical intervention including fasciotomy, skin graft, and/or amputation have been necessary in some cases. The preferred route of administration is by deep intramuscular (I.M.) injection. Subcutaneous administration is contraindicated. Discontinue intravenous injection immediately with onset of pain and evaluate for arterial injection or perivascular extravasation. Although there is no proven successful management of unintentional intra-arterial injection or perivascular extravasation, sympathetic block and heparinization have been used in the acute management of unintentional intra-arterial injection based on results from animal studies.

May be sedating; use with caution in disorders where CNS depression is a feature. May impair physical or mental abilities; patients must be cautioned about performing tasks which require mental alertness. Use with caution in hemodynamic instability; bone marrow suppression; subcortical brain damage; and in severe cardiac, hepatic or respiratory disease. Avoid use in Reye's syndrome. May lower seizure threshold; use caution in persons with seizure disorders or in persons using narcotics or local anesthetics which may also affect seizure threshold. May alter temperature regulation or mask toxicity of other drugs due to antiemetic effects. May alter cardiac conduction (life-threatening arrhythmias have occurred with therapeutic doses of phenothiazines). May cause orthostatic hypotension; use with caution in patients at risk of hypotension or where transient hypotensive episodes would be poorly tolerated (cardiovascular disease or cerebrovascular disease).

Phenothiazines may cause anticholinergic effects; therefore, they should be used with caution in patients with decreased gastrointestinal motility, GI or GU obstruction, urinary retention, BPH, xerostomia, or visual problems. Conditions which also may be exacerbated by cholinergic blockade include narrow-angle glaucoma (screening is recommended) and worsening of myasthenia gravis. Use with caution in Parkinson's disease. May cause extrapyramidal symptoms, including pseudoparkinsonism, acute dystonic reactions, akathisia, and tardive dyskinesia. May be associated with neuroleptic malignant syndrome (NMS). May cause photosensitivity. May be inappropriate for use in the elderly due to potent anticholinergic effects (Beers Criteria). Injection may contain sodium metabisulfite.

Adverse Reactions Frequency not defined.

Cardiovascular: Bradycardia, hyper-/hypotension, nonspecific QT changes, postural hypotension, tachycardia

Central nervous system: Agitation akathisia, catatonic states, confusion, delirium, disorientation, dizziness, drowsiness, dystonias, euphoria, excitation, extrapyramidal symptoms, faintness, fatigue, hallucinations, hysteria, insomnia, lassitude, pseudoparkinsonism, tardive dyskinesia, nervousness, neuroleptic malignant syndrome, nightmares, sedation, seizure, somnolence

Dermatologic: Angioneurotic edema, dermatitis, photosensitivity, skin pigmentation (slate gray), urticaria

Endocrine & metabolic: Amenorrhea, breast engorgement, gynecomastia, hyperglycemia, lactation

Gastrointestinal: Constipation, nausea, vomiting, xerostomia

Genitourinary: Ejaculatory disorder, impotence, urinary retention

Hematologic: Agranulocytosis, leukopenia, thrombocytopenia, thrombocytopenic purpura

Hepatic: Jaundice

Local: Abscess, distal vessel spasm, gangrene, injection site reactions (burning, edema, erythema, pain), palsies, paralysis, phlebitis, sensory loss, thrombophlebitis, tissue necrosis, venous thrombosis

Neuromuscular & skeletal: Incoordination, tremor

Ocular: Blurred vision, corneal and lenticular changes, diplopia, epithelial keratopathy, pigmentary retinopathy

Otic: Tinnitus

Respiratory: Apnea, asthma, nasal congestion, respiratory depression

Drug Interactions

Metabolism/Transport Effects Substrate of CYP2B6 (major), CYP2D6 (major); **Note:** Assignment of Major/Minor substrate status based on clinically relevant drug interaction potential; **Inhibits** CYP2D6 (weak)

Avoid Concomitant Use

Avoid concomitant use of Promethazine with any of the following: Metoclopramide

Increased Effect/Toxicity

Promethazine may increase the levels/effects of: Anticholinergics; Metoclopramide; Serotonin Modulators

The levels/effects of Promethazine may be increased by: Abiraterone Acetate; Antipsychotics; CYP2B6 Inhibitors (Moderate); CYP2B6 Inhibitors (Strong); CYP2D6 Inhibitors (Moderate); CYP2D6 Inhibitors (Strong); Darunavir; MAO Inhibitors; Metoclopramide; Pramlintide; Quazepam

Decreased Effect

Promethazine may decrease the levels/effects of: Acetylcholinesterase Inhibitors (Central)

The levels/effects of Promethazine may be decreased by: Acetylcholinesterase Inhibitors (Central); CYP2B6 Inducers (Strong); Peginterferon Alfa-2b

Ethanol/Nutrition/Herb Interactions

Ethanol: Avoid ethanol (may increase CNS depression).

Herb/Nutraceutical: Avoid valerian, St John's wort, kava kava, gotu kola (may increase CNS depression).

Stability

Injection: Prior to dilution, store at 20°C to 25°C (68°F to 77°F). Protect from light. Solutions in NS or D_5W are stable for 24 hours at room temperature.

Oral solution: Store at 15°C to 25°C (59°F to 77°F). Protect from light.

Suppositories: Store refrigerated at 2°C to 8°C (36°F to 46°F).

Tablets: Store at 20°C to 25°C (68°F to 77°F). Protect from light.

Mechanism of Action Phenothiazine derivative; blocks postsynaptic mesolimbic dopaminergic receptors in the brain; exhibits a strong alpha-adrenergic blocking effect and depresses the release of hypothalamic and hypophyseal hormones; competes with histamine for the H_1-receptor; muscarinic-blocking effect may be responsible for antiemetic activity; reduces stimuli to the brainstem reticular system

Pharmacodynamics/Kinetics
Onset of action: Oral, I.M.: ~20 minutes; I.V.: ~5 minutes
Peak effect: C_{max}: ~9 ng/mL (suppository); ~19 ng/mL (syrup)
Duration: Usually 4-6 hours (up to 12 hours)
Absorption:
I.M.: Bioavailability may be greater than with oral or rectal administration
Oral: Rapid and complete; large first pass effect limits systemic bioavailability
Distribution: V_d: 970 L
Protein binding: 93%
Metabolism: Hepatic; primarily oxidation; forms metabolites
Half-life elimination: 9-16 hours
Time to maximum serum concentration: ~4.5 hours (syrup); ~7-9 hours (suppositories)
Excretion: Primarily urine and feces (as inactive metabolites)

Dosage
Children ≥2 years:
Allergic conditions: Oral, rectal: 0.1 mg/kg/dose (maximum: 12.5 mg) every 6 hours during the day and 0.5 mg/kg/dose (maximum: 25 mg) at bedtime as needed
Antiemetic: Oral, I.M., I.V., rectal: 0.25-1 mg/kg 4-6 times/day as needed (maximum: 25 mg/dose)
Motion sickness: Oral, rectal: 0.5 mg/kg/dose 30 minutes to 1 hour before departure, then every 12 hours as needed (maximum dose: 25 mg twice daily)
Preoperative analgesia/hypnotic adjunct: I.M., I.V.: 1.1 mg/kg in combination with an analgesic or hypnotic (at reduced doses) and an atropine-like agent. **Note:** Dose should not exceed half of suggested adult dose.
Sedation: Oral, I.M., I.V., rectal: 0.5-1 mg/kg/dose every 6 hours as needed (maximum: 50 mg/dose)
Adults:
Allergic conditions (including allergic reactions to blood or plasma):
Oral, rectal: 25 mg at bedtime **or** 12.5 mg before meals and at bedtime (range: 6.25-12.5 mg 3 times/day)
I.M., I.V.: 25 mg, may repeat in 2 hours when necessary; switch to oral route as soon as feasible
Antiemetic: Oral, I.M., I.V., rectal: 12.5-25 mg every 4-6 hours as needed
Motion sickness: Oral, rectal: 25 mg 30-60 minutes before departure, then every 12 hours as needed
Obstetrics (labor) as adjunct to analgesia: I.M., I.V.: Early labor: 50 mg; Established labor: 25-75 mg; may repeat every 4 hours for up to 2 additional doses (maximum: 100 mg/day while in labor). **Note:** Dosage of concomitant analgesic should be reduced.
Pre-/postoperative analgesia/hypnotic adjunct: I.M., I.V.: 25-50 mg in combination with analgesic or hypnotic (at reduced dosage)
Sedation: Oral, I.M., I.V., rectal: 12.5-50 mg/dose

Dietary Considerations Increase dietary intake of riboflavin.

Administration Formulations available for oral, rectal, I.M./I.V.; not for SubQ or intra-arterial administration. Administer I.M. into deep muscle (preferred route of administration). I.V. administration is **not** the preferred route; severe tissue damage may occur. Solution for injection should be administered in a maximum concentration of 25 mg/mL (more dilute solutions are recommended). Administer via running I.V. line at port farthest from patient's vein, or through a large bore vein (not hand or wrist). Consider administering over 10-15 minutes (maximum: 25 mg/minute). Discontinue immediately if burning or pain occurs with administration.

Monitoring Parameters Relief of symptoms, mental status; signs and symptoms of tissue injury (burning or pain at injection site, phlebitis, edema) with I.V. administration

Test Interactions May interfere with urine detection of amphetamine/methamphetamine (false-positive); alters the flare response in intradermal allergen tests; hCG-based pregnancy tests may result in false-negatives or false-positives

Dosage Forms Excipient information presented when available (limited, particularly for generics); consult specific product labeling.
Injection, solution, as hydrochloride: 25 mg/mL (1 mL); 50 mg/mL (1 mL)
Phenergan®: 25 mg/mL (1 mL); 50 mg/mL (1 mL) [contains edetate disodium, sodium metabisulfite]
Suppository, rectal, as hydrochloride: 12.5 mg (12s); 25 mg (12s)
Phenadoz®: 12.5 mg (12s); 25 mg (12s)
Promethegan™: 12.5 mg (12s); 25 mg (12s); 50 mg (12s)
Syrup, oral, as hydrochloride: 6.25 mg/5 mL (118 mL, 473 mL)
Tablet, oral, as hydrochloride: 12.5 mg, 25 mg, 50 mg

Promethazine and Codeine
(proe METH a zeen & KOE deen)

Index Terms Codeine and Promethazine

Pharmacologic Category Alpha/Beta Agonist; Analgesic, Opioid; Histamine H_1 Antagonist; Histamine H_1 Antagonist, First Generation; Phenothiazine Derivative

Use Temporary relief of coughs and upper respiratory symptoms associated with allergy or the common cold

Pregnancy Risk Factor C

Dosage Oral:
Children:
<6 years: **Note:** Use of promethazine/codeine combination is contraindicated in children <6 years of age
6-11 years: 2.5-5 mL every 4-6 hours (maximum: 30 mL/24 hours)
Children ≥12 years and Adults: 5 mL every 4-6 hours (maximum: 30 mL/24 hours)
Elderly: Use with caution; consider decreased dose
Dosage adjustment in renal/hepatic impairment: Use with caution; consider decreased dose

Additional Information Complete prescribing information for this medication should be consulted for additional detail.

Dosage Forms Excipient information presented when available (limited, particularly for generics); consult specific product labeling.
Syrup: Promethazine hydrochloride 6.25 mg and codeine phosphate 10 mg per 5 mL (5 mL, 118 mL, 473 mL)

Controlled Substance C-V

Promethazine and Dextromethorphan
(proe METH a zeen & deks troe meth OR fan)

Index Terms Dextromethorphan and Promethazine

Pharmacologic Category Antitussive; Histamine H_1 Antagonist; Histamine H_1 Antagonist, First Generation; Phenothiazine Derivative

Use Temporary relief of coughs and upper respiratory symptoms associated with allergy or the common cold

Pregnancy Risk Factor C

Dosage Oral:
Children:
<2 years: Use of promethazine is contraindicated
2-6 years: 1.25-2.5 mL every 4-6 hours up to 10 mL in 24 hours
6-12 years: 2.5-5 mL every 4-6 hours up to 20 mL in 24 hours
Adults: 5 mL every 4-6 hours up to 30 mL in 24 hours

Additional Information Complete prescribing information for this medication should be consulted for additional detail.

Dosage Forms Excipient information presented when available (limited, particularly for generics); consult specific product labeling.

Syrup: Promethazine hydrochloride 6.25 mg and dextromethorphan hydrobromide 15 mg per 5 mL (120 mL, 480 mL) [contains alcohol 7%]

◆ **Promethazine Hydrochloride** *see* Promethazine *on page 1416*

◆ **Promethegan™** *see* Promethazine *on page 1416*

◆ **Prometrium®** *see* Progesterone *on page 1414*

◆ **PRO-Mirtazapine (Can)** *see* Mirtazapine *on page 1140*

◆ **PRO-Naproxen EC (Can)** *see* Naproxen *on page 1177*

◆ **Pronestyl** *see* Procainamide *on page 1408*

◆ **Pronto® Complete Lice Removal System [OTC]** *see* Pyrethrins and Piperonyl Butoxide *on page 1435*

◆ **Pronto® Lice Control (Can)** *see* Pyrethrins and Piperonyl Butoxide *on page 1435*

◆ **Pronto® Plus Lice Killing Mousse Plus Vitamin E [OTC]** *see* Pyrethrins and Piperonyl Butoxide *on page 1435*

◆ **Pronto® Plus Lice Killing Mousse Shampoo Plus Natural Extracts and Oils [OTC]** *see* Pyrethrins and Piperonyl Butoxide *on page 1435*

◆ **Pronto® Plus Warm Oil Treatment and Conditioner [OTC]** *see* Pyrethrins and Piperonyl Butoxide *on page 1435*

Propafenone (pro PAF en one)

Brand Names: U.S. Rythmol®; Rythmol® SR

Brand Names: Canada Apo-Propafenone®; Mylan-Propafenone; PMS-Propafenone; Rythmol® Gen-Propafenone

Index Terms Propafenone Hydrochloride

Pharmacologic Category Antiarrhythmic Agent, Class Ic

Use Treatment of life-threatening ventricular arrhythmias; treatment of paroxysmal atrial fibrillation/flutter (PAF) or paroxysmal supraventricular tachycardia (PSVT) in patients with disabling symptoms and without structural heart disease

Extended release capsule: Prolong the time to recurrence of symptomatic atrial fibrillation in patients without structural heart disease

Unlabeled Use Cardioversion of recent-onset atrial fibrillation (single dose); supraventricular tachycardia in patients with Wolff-Parkinson-White syndrome

Pregnancy Risk Factor C

Pregnancy Considerations There are no adequate and well-controlled studies in pregnant women; use only if potential benefit to the mother justifies potential risk to the fetus.

Lactation Enters breast milk/not recommended

Contraindications Hypersensitivity to propafenone or any component of the formulation; sinoatrial, AV, and intraventricular disorders of impulse generation and/or conduction (except in patients with a functioning artificial pacemaker); sinus bradycardia; cardiogenic shock; uncompensated cardiac failure; hypotension; bronchospastic disorders or severe obstructive pulmonary disease; uncorrected electrolyte abnormalities; concurrent use of ritonavir

Warnings/Precautions **[U.S. Boxed Warning]: In the Cardiac Arrhythmia Suppression Trial (CAST), recent (>6 days but <2 years ago) myocardial infarction patients with asymptomatic, non-life-threatening ventricular arrhythmias did not benefit and may have been harmed by attempts to suppress the arrhythmia with flecainide or encainide.** An increased mortality or nonfatal cardiac arrest rate (7.7%) was seen in the active treatment group compared with patients in the placebo group (3%). The applicability of the CAST results to other populations is unknown. Antiarrhythmic agents should be reserved for patients with life-threatening ventricular arrhythmias. Monitor for proarrhythmic events. May prolong QT_c interval; use caution with other QT_c-prolonging drugs. Hold Class Ia or Class III antiarrhythmics for at least five half-lives prior to starting propafenone Slows atrioventricular conduction, potentially leading to first degree AV block; degree of PR interval prolongation and increased QRS duration are dose and concentration related. Avoid in patients with conduction disturbances (unless functioning pacemaker present).

May alter pacing and sensing thresholds of artificial pacemakers. The use of propafenone is not recommended in patients with obstructive lung disease (eg, COPD) (Fuster, 2006). Use in patients with bronchospastic disease or severe obstructive lung disease is contraindicated.

Avoid use in patients with heart failure; similar agents have been shown to increase mortality in this population; may precipitate or exacerbate condition. Correct electrolyte disturbances, especially hypokalemia or hypomagnesemia, prior to use and throughout therapy. Administer cautiously in significant hepatic or renal dysfunction. Use with caution in patients with myasthenia gravis; may exacerbate condition. Avoid the concurrent use of a CYP2D6 inhibitor and CYP3A4 inhibitor; may result in an increased risk of proarrhythmia or exaggerated beta-adrenergic blocking activity Agranulocytosis has been reported; generally occurring within the first 2 months of therapy. Upon therapy discontinuation, WBC usually normalized by 14 days. Positive ANA titers have been reported. Titers have decreased with and without propafenone discontinuation. Positive titers have not usually been associated with clinical symptoms, although at least one case of drug induced lupus erythematosus has been reported. Consider therapy discontinuation in symptomatic patients with positive ANA titers.

Adverse Reactions

1% to 10%:

Cardiovascular: New or worsened arrhythmia (proarrhythmic effect) (2% to 10%), angina (2% to 5%), CHF (1% to 4%), ventricular tachycardia (1% to 3%), palpitation (1% to 3%), AV block (first-degree) (1% to 3%), syncope (1% to 2%), increased QRS interval (1% to 2%), chest pain (1% to 2%), PVCs (1% to 2%), bradycardia (1% to 2%), edema (0% to 1%), bundle branch block (0% to 1%), atrial fibrillation (1%), hypotension (0% to 1%), intraventricular conduction delay (0% to 1%)

Central nervous system: Dizziness (4% to 15%), fatigue (2% to 6%), headache (2% to 5%), ataxia (0% to 2%), insomnia (0% to 2%), anxiety (1% to 2%), drowsiness (1%)

Dermatologic: Rash (1% to 3%)

Gastrointestinal: Nausea/vomiting (2% to 11%), unusual taste (3% to 23%), constipation (2% to 7%), dyspepsia (1% to 3%), diarrhea (1% to 3%), xerostomia (1% to 2%), anorexia (1% to 2%), abdominal pain (1% to 2%), flatulence (0% to 1%)

Neuromuscular & skeletal: Tremor (0% to 1%), arthralgia (0% to 1%), weakness (1% to 2%)

Ocular: Blurred vision (1% to 6%)

Respiratory: Dyspnea (2% to 5%)

Miscellaneous: Diaphoresis (1%)

<1% (Limited to important or life-threatening): Agranulocytosis, alopecia, amnesia, anemia, apnea, AV block (second or third degree), AV dissociation, cardiac arrest, cholestasis (0.1%), coma, confusion, CHF, depression, granulocytopenia, hepatitis (0.03%), hyperglycemia,

impotence, increased bleeding time, leukopenia, lupus erythematosus, mania, memory loss, nephrotic syndrome, paresthesia, peripheral neuropathy, pruritus, psychosis, purpura, renal failure, seizure (0.3%), SIADH, sinus node dysfunction, thrombocytopenia, tinnitus, vertigo

Drug Interactions

Metabolism/Transport Effects **Substrate** of CYP1A2 (minor), CYP2D6 (major), CYP3A4 (minor); **Note:** Assignment of Major/Minor substrate status based on clinically relevant drug interaction potential; **Inhibits** CYP1A2 (weak), CYP2D6 (weak)

Avoid Concomitant Use

Avoid concomitant use of Propafenone with any of the following: Amiodarone; Artemether; Dronedarone; Lumefantrine; Nilotinib; Pimozide; QUEtiapine; QuiNIDine; QuiNINE; Ritonavir; Saquinavir; Tetrabenazine; Thioridazine; Tipranavir; Toremifene; Vandetanib; Vemurafenib; Ziprasidone

Increased Effect/Toxicity

Propafenone may increase the levels/effects of: Beta-Blockers; Cardiac Glycosides; CYP2D6 Inhibitors (Moderate); Dronedarone; Pimozide; Propranolol; QTc-Prolonging Agents; QuiNINE; Tetrabenazine; Theophylline Derivatives; Thioridazine; Toremifene; Vandetanib; Vemurafenib; Venlafaxine; Vitamin K Antagonists; Ziprasidone

The levels/effects of Propafenone may be increased by: Abiraterone Acetate; Alfuzosin; Amiodarone; Artemether; Boceprevir; Chloroquine; Cimetidine; Ciprofloxacin; Ciprofloxacin (Systemic); CYP2D6 Inhibitors (Strong); CYP3A4 Inhibitors (Moderate); CYP3A4 Inhibitors (Strong); FLUoxetine; FluvoxaMINE; Gadobutrol; Indacaterol; Lumefantrine; Nilotinib; PARoxetine; QUEtiapine; QuiNIDine; QuiNINE; Ritonavir; Saquinavir; Telaprevir; Tipranavir

Decreased Effect

The levels/effects of Propafenone may be decreased by: Barbiturates; Cyproterone; Etravirine; Orlistat; Peginterferon Alfa-2b; Rifamycin Derivatives; Tocilizumab

Ethanol/Nutrition/Herb Interactions

Food: Propafenone serum concentrations may be increased if taken with food.

Herb/Nutraceutical: St John's wort may decrease propafenone levels. Avoid ephedra (may worsen arrhythmia).

Stability Store at 25°C (77°F); excursions permitted to 15°C to 30°C (59°F to 86°F).

Mechanism of Action Propafenone is a class 1c antiarrhythmic agent which possesses local anesthetic properties, blocks the fast inward sodium current, and slows the rate of increase of the action potential. Prolongs conduction and refractoriness in all areas of the myocardium, with a slightly more pronounced effect on intraventricular conduction; it prolongs effective refractory period, reduces spontaneous automaticity and exhibits some beta-blockade activity.

Pharmacodynamics/Kinetics

Absorption: Well absorbed

Distribution; V_d: Adults: 252 L

Protein binding: 95% to alpha$_1$-acid glycoprotein

Metabolism: Hepatic via CYP2D6, CYP3A4 and CYP1A2 to two active metabolites (5-hydroxypropafenone and N-depropylpropafenone) then ultimately to glucuronide or sulfate conjugates. Two genetically determined metabolism groups exist (extensive and poor metabolizers); 10% of Caucasians are poor metabolizers. Exhibits nonlinear pharmacokinetics; when dose is increased from 300-900 mg/day, serum concentrations increase tenfold; this nonlinearity is thought to be due to saturable first-pass effect.

Bioavailability: Immediate release (IR): 150 mg: 3.4%; 300 mg: 10.6%; relative bioavailability of extended release (ER) capsule is less than IR tablet; the bioavailability of an ER capsule regimen of 325 mg twice-daily regimen approximates an IR tablet regimen of 150 mg 3 times/day.

Half-life elimination: Extensive metabolizers: 2-10 hours; Poor metabolizers: 10-32 hours

Time to peak, serum: IR: 3.5 hours; ER: 3-8 hours

Excretion: Urine (<1% unchanged; remainder as glucuronide or sulfate conjugates); feces

Dosage Oral: Adults: **Note:** Patients who exhibit significant widening of QRS complex or second- or third-degree AV block may need dose reduction.

Atrial fibrillation (to prevent recurrence): Extended release capsule: Initial: 225 mg every 12 hours; dosage increase may be made at a minimum of 5-day intervals; may increase to 325 mg every 12 hours; if further increase is necessary, may increase to 425 mg every 12 hours

Paroxysmal atrial fibrillation/flutter, paroxysmal supraventricular tachycardia, ventricular arrhythmias: Immediate release tablet: Initial: 150 mg every 8 hours; dosage increase may be made at minimum of 3- to 4-day intervals, may increase to 225 mg every 8 hours; if further increase is necessary, may increase to 300 mg every 8 hours

Atrial fibrillation, pharmacologic cardioversion (unlabeled use): **Note:** To prevent rapid AV conduction, start an AV nodal-blocking agent (eg, beta-blocker, nondihydropyridine calcium channel blocker) prior to pharmacologic cardioversion. Effect occurs between 2-6 hours after administration.

Immediate release tablet: 600 mg as single dose (Fuster, 2006)

Dosing adjustment in renal impairment: No dosage adjustments provided in manufacturer's labeling; however, 50% of propafenone metabolites (active) are excreted in the urine; use with caution in renal impairment

Dosing adjustment in hepatic impairment:

Immediate release tablet: Reduce dose by 70% to 80% in patients with hepatic impairment

Extended release capsule: Specific dosage adjustments are not provided in manufacturer's labeling; however, dosage reduction should be considered as drug undergoes hepatic metabolism.

Dietary Considerations Capsule: May be taken without regard to meals.

Administration Capsules should be swallowed whole; do not crush or chew; may be taken without regard to meals.

Monitoring Parameters ECG, blood pressure, pulse (particularly at initiation of therapy)

Dosage Forms Excipient information presented when available (limited, particularly for generics); consult specific product labeling. [DSC] = Discontinued product

Capsule, extended release, oral, as hydrochloride: 225 mg, 325 mg, 425 mg

Rythmol® SR: 225 mg, 325 mg, 425 mg [contains soy lecithin]

Tablet, oral, as hydrochloride: 150 mg, 225 mg, 300 mg

Rythmol®: 150 mg, 225 mg, 300 mg [DSC] [scored]

◆ **Propafenone Hydrochloride** *see* Propafenone *on page 1419*

Propantheline (proe PAN the leen)

Index Terms Propantheline Bromide

Pharmacologic Category Anticholinergic Agent

Additional Appendix Information
Beers Criteria - Potentially Inappropriate Medications for Geriatrics *on page 1973*
Use Adjunctive treatment of peptic ulcer
Unlabeled Use Decreased salivation and drooling
Pregnancy Risk Factor C
Dosage Oral:
Antisecretory (unlabeled use):
Children: 1-2 mg/kg/day in 3-4 divided doses
Adults: 15 mg 3 times/day before meals or food and 30 mg at bedtime
Elderly: 7.5 mg 3 times/day before meals and at bedtime
Antispasmodic:
Children: 2-3 mg/kg/day in divided doses every 4-6 hours and at bedtime
Adults: 15 mg 3 times/day before meals or food and 30 mg at bedtime
Additional Information Complete prescribing information for this medication should be consulted for additional detail.
Dosage Forms Excipient information presented when available (limited, particularly for generics); consult specific product labeling.
Tablet, oral, as bromide: 15 mg

◆ **Propantheline Bromide** *see* Propantheline *on page 1420*

Proparacaine (proe PAR a kane)

Brand Names: U.S. Alcaine®; Parcaine™ [DSC]
Brand Names: Canada Alcaine®; Diocaine®
Index Terms Proparacaine Hydrochloride; Proxymetacaine
Pharmacologic Category Local Anesthetic, Ophthalmic
Use Anesthesia for tonometry, gonioscopy; suture removal from cornea; removal of corneal foreign body; cataract extraction, glaucoma surgery; short operative procedure involving the cornea and conjunctiva
Pregnancy Risk Factor C
Dosage Children and Adults:
Ophthalmic surgery: Instill 1 drop of 0.5% solution in eye every 5-10 minutes for 5-7 doses
Tonometry, gonioscopy, suture removal: Instill 1-2 drops of 0.5% solution in eye just prior to procedure
Additional Information Complete prescribing information for this medication should be consulted for additional detail.
Dosage Forms Excipient information presented when available (limited, particularly for generics); consult specific product labeling. [DSC] = Discontinued product
Solution, ophthalmic, as hydrochloride [drops]: 0.5% (15 mL)
Alcaine®: 0.5% (15 mL) [contains benzalkonium chloride]
Parcaine™: 0.5% (15 mL [DSC]) [contains benzalkonium chloride]

Proparacaine and Fluorescein
(proe PAR a kane & FLURE e seen)

Brand Names: U.S. Flucaine
Index Terms Fluorescein and Proparacaine
Pharmacologic Category Diagnostic Agent; Local Anesthetic
Use Anesthesia for tonometry, gonioscopy; suture removal from cornea; removal of corneal foreign body; cataract extraction, glaucoma surgery
Pregnancy Risk Factor C
Dosage
Ophthalmic surgery: Children and Adults: Instill 1 drop in each eye every 5-10 minutes for 5-7 doses
Tonometry, gonioscopy, suture removal: Adults: Instill 1-2 drops in each eye just prior to procedure
Additional Information Complete prescribing information for this medication should be consulted for additional detail.
Dosage Forms Excipient information presented when available (limited, particularly for generics); consult specific product labeling. [DSC] = Discontinued product
Solution, ophthalmic: Proparacaine hydrochloride 0.5% and fluorescein sodium 0.25% (5 mL)
Flucaine: Proparacaine hydrochloride 0.5% and fluorescein sodium 0.25% (5 mL)

◆ **Proparacaine Hydrochloride** *see* Proparacaine *on page 1421*
◆ **Propecia®** *see* Finasteride *on page 713*
◆ **Propine® (Can)** *see* Dipivefrin *on page 527*
◆ **PRO-Pioglitazone (Can)** *see* Pioglitazone *on page 1355*

Propofol (PROE po fole)

Brand Names: U.S. Diprivan®
Brand Names: Canada Diprivan®
Pharmacologic Category General Anesthetic
Additional Appendix Information
Status Epilepticus *on page 2010*
Use Induction of anesthesia in patients ≥3 years of age; maintenance of anesthesia in patients >2 months of age; in adults, for monitored anesthesia care sedation during procedures; sedation in intubated, mechanically-ventilated ICU patients
Unlabeled Use Postoperative antiemetic; refractory delirium tremens (case reports)
Pregnancy Risk Factor B
Pregnancy Considerations Propofol should only be used in pregnancy if clearly needed. Propofol is not recommended for obstetrics, including cesarean section deliveries. Propofol crosses the placenta and may be associated with neonatal CNS and respiratory depression.
Lactation Enters breast milk/not recommended
Contraindications Hypersensitivity to propofol or any component of the formulation; hypersensitivity to eggs, egg products, soybeans, or soy products; when general anesthesia or sedation is contraindicated
Warnings/Precautions May rarely cause hypersensitivity, anaphylaxis, anaphylactoid reactions, angioedema, bronchospasm, and erythema; medications for the treatment of hypersensitivity reactions should be available for immediate use. The major cardiovascular effect of propofol is hypotension especially if patient is hypovolemic or if bolus dosing is used; use with caution in patients who are hemodynamically unstable, hypovolemic, or have abnormally low vascular tone (eg, sepsis). Use requires careful patient monitoring, should only be used by experienced personnel who are not actively engaged in the procedure or surgery. If used in a nonintubated and/or nonmechanically-ventilated patient, qualified personnel and appropriate equipment for rapid institution of respiratory and/or cardiovascular support must be immediately available. Use to induce moderate (conscious) sedation in patients warrants monitoring equivalent to that seen with deep anesthesia.

Use a lower induction dose, a slower maintenance rate of administration, and avoid rapidly administered boluses in the elderly, debilitated, or ASA-PS (American Society of Anesthesiologists - Physical Status) 3/4 patients to reduce the incidence of unwanted cardiorespiratory depressive events. Use caution in patients with severe cardiac disease (ejection fraction <50%) or respiratory disease; may have more profound adverse cardiovascular responses to propofol. Use caution in patients with a history of epilepsy or seizures; seizure may occur during recovery phase. Use caution in patients with increased intracranial pressure or impaired cerebral circulation; substantial decreases in mean arterial pressure and subsequent decreases in cerebral perfusion pressure may occur; consider continuous infusion or administer as a slow bolus.

Propofol-related infusion syndrome is a serious side effect with a high mortality rate characterized by dysrhythmia (eg, bradycardia or tachycardia), heart failure, hyperkalemia, lipemia, metabolic acidosis, and/or rhabdomyolysis or myoglobinuria with subsequent renal failure. Risk factors include poor oxygen delivery, sepsis, serious cerebral injury, and the administration of high doses of propofol (usually doses >83 mcg/kg/minute or >5 mg/kg/hour for >48 hours), but has also been reported following large dose, short term infusions during surgical anesthesia. The onset of the syndrome is rapid, occurring within 4 days of initiation. Alternate sedative therapy should be considered for patients with escalating doses of vasopressors or inotropes, when cardiac failure occurs during high-dose propofol infusion, when metabolic acidosis is observed, or in whom lengthy and/or high-dose sedation is needed.

Because propofol is formulated within a 10% fat emulsion, hypertriglyceridemia is an expected side effect. Patients who develop hypertriglyceridemia (eg, >500 mg/dL) are at risk of developing pancreatitis. An alternative sedative agent should be employed if significant hypertriglyceridemia occurs. Use with caution in patients with preexisting pancreatitis; use of propofol may exacerbate this condition. Use caution in patients with preexisting hyperlipidemia as evidenced by increased serum triglyceride levels or serum turbidity. Transient local pain may occur during I.V. injection; perioperative myoclonia has occurred. Propofol should only be used in pregnancy if clearly needed. Not recommended for use in obstetrics, including cesarean section deliveries. Safety and efficacy in pediatric intensive care unit patients have not been established. Concurrent use of fentanyl and propofol in pediatric patients may result in bradycardia.

Concomitant use may lead to increased sedative or anesthetic effects of propofol, more pronounced decreases in systolic, diastolic, and mean arterial pressures and cardiac output. Lower doses of propofol may be needed. In addition, fentanyl may cause serious bradycardia when used with propofol in pediatric patients. Alfentanil use with propofol has precipitated seizure activity in patients without any history of epilepsy. Discontinue opioids and paralytic agents prior to weaning. Avoid abrupt discontinuation prior to weaning or daily wake up assessments. Abrupt discontinuation can result in rapid awakening, anxiety, agitation, and resistance to mechanical ventilation; wean the infusion rate so the patient awakens slowly. Propofol lacks analgesic properties; pain management requires specific use of analgesic agents, at effective dosages, propofol must be titrated separately from the analgesic agent.

Propofol vials and prefilled syringes have the potential to support the growth of various microorganisms despite product additives intended to suppress microbial growth. To limit the potential for contamination, recommendations in product labeling for handling and administering propofol should be strictly adhered to. Some formulations may contain edetate disodium which may lead to decreased zinc levels in patients with prolonged therapy (>5 days) or a predisposition to zinc deficiency (eg, burns, diarrhea, or sepsis). A holiday from propofol infusion should take place after 5 days of therapy to allow for evaluation and necessary replacement of zinc. Some formulations may contain sulfites. Some products may contain benzyl alcohol; benzyl alcohol has been associated with the "gasping syndrome" in neonates and low-birth-weight infants.

Adverse Reactions

>10%:

Cardiovascular: Hypotension (children 17%; adults 3% to 26%)

Central nervous system: Movement (children 17%; adults 3% to 10%)

Local: Injection site burning, stinging, or pain (children 10%; adults 18%)

Respiratory: Apnea lasting 30-60 seconds (children 10%; adults 24%), apnea lasting >60 seconds (children 5%; adults 12%)

1% to 10%:

Cardiovascular: Hypertension (children 8%), arrhythmia (1% to 3%), bradycardia (1% to 3%), cardiac output decreased (1% to 3%; concurrent opioid use increases incidence), tachycardia (1% to 3%)

Dermatologic: Pruritus (1% to 3%), rash (children 5%; adults 1% to 3%)

Endocrine & metabolic: Hypertriglyceridemia (3% to 10%)

Respiratory: Respiratory acidosis during weaning (3% to 10%)

<1% (Limited to important or life-threatening): Agitation, amblyopia, anaphylaxis, anaphylactoid reaction, anticholinergic syndrome, asystole, atrial arrhythmia, bigeminy, cardiac arrest, chills, cough, dizziness, delirium, discoloration (green [urine, hair, or nailbeds]), extremity pain, fever, flushing, hemorrhage, hypersalivation, hypertonia, hypomagnesemia, hypoxia, infusion site reactions (including pain, swelling, blisters and/or tissue necrosis following accidental extravasation); laryngospasm, leukocytosis, lung function decreased, myalgia, myoclonia (rarely including convulsions and opisthotonos), nausea, pancreatitis, paresthesia, phlebitis, postoperative unconsciousness with or without increase in muscle tone, premature atrial contractions, premature ventricular contractions, pulmonary edema, propofol-related infusion syndrome, rhabdomyolysis, somnolence, syncope, thrombosis, urine cloudy, vision abnormality, wheezing

Drug Interactions

Metabolism/Transport Effects **Substrate** of CYP1A2 (minor), CYP2A6 (minor), CYP2B6 (major), CYP2C19 (minor), CYP2C9 (minor), CYP2D6 (minor), CYP2E1 (minor), CYP3A4 (minor); **Note:** Assignment of Major/Minor substrate status based on clinically relevant drug interaction potential; **Inhibits** CYP1A2 (weak), CYP2C9 (weak), CYP2D6 (weak), CYP2E1 (weak), CYP3A4 (weak)

Avoid Concomitant Use

Avoid concomitant use of Propofol with any of the following: Pimozide

Increased Effect/Toxicity

Propofol may increase the levels/effects of: Midazolam; Pimozide; Ropivacaine

The levels/effects of Propofol may be increased by: Alfentanil; Conivaptan; CYP2B6 Inhibitors (Moderate); CYP2B6 Inhibitors (Strong); Midazolam; Quazepam

Decreased Effect

The levels/effects of Propofol may be decreased by: Cyproterone; Peginterferon Alfa-2b; Tocilizumab

Ethanol/Nutrition/Herb Interactions Food: Edetate disodium, an ingredient of propofol emulsion, may lead to decreased zinc levels in patients on prolonged therapy (>5 days) or those predisposed to deficiency (burns, diarrhea, and/or major sepsis).

Stability Store between 4°C to 22°C (40°F to 72°F); refrigeration is not required. Do not freeze. If transferred to a syringe or other container prior to administration, use within 6 hours. If used directly from vial/prefilled syringe, use within 12 hours. Shake well before use. Do not use if there is evidence of separation of phases of emulsion.

Does not need to be diluted; however, propofol may be further diluted in 5% dextrose in water to a concentration of ≥2 mg/mL and is stable for 8 hours at room temperature.

Mechanism of Action Propofol is a short-acting, lipophilic intravenous general anesthetic. The drug is unrelated to any of the currently used barbiturate, opioid, benzodiazepine, arylcyclohexylamine, or imidazole intravenous anesthetic agents. Propofol causes global CNS depression, presumably through it's agonist actions on $GABA_A$ receptors, and perhaps also involving reduced glutamatergic activity through NMDA receptor blockade.

Pharmacodynamics/Kinetics

Onset of action: Anesthetic: Bolus infusion (dose dependent): 9-51 seconds (average 30 seconds)

Duration (dose and rate dependent): 3-10 minutes

Distribution: V_d: 2-10 L/kg; after a 10-day infusion, V_d approaches 60 L/kg; decreased in the elderly

Protein binding: 97% to 99%

Metabolism: Hepatic to water-soluble sulfate and glucuronide conjugates (~50%)

Half-life elimination: Biphasic: Initial: 40 minutes; Terminal: 4-7 hours (after 10-day infusion, may be up to 1-3 days)

Excretion: Urine (~88% as metabolites, 40% as glucuronide metabolite); feces (<2%)

Dosage Dosage must be individualized based on total body weight and titrated to the desired clinical effect; wait at least 3-5 minutes between dosage adjustments to clinically assess drug effects; smaller doses are required when used with narcotics; the following are general dosing guidelines:

General anesthesia: Note: Increase dose in patients with chronic alcoholism (Fassoulaki, 1993); decrease dose with acutely intoxicated (alcoholic) patients.

Induction: I.V.:

Children (healthy) 3-16 years, ASA-PS 1 or 2: 2.5-3.5 mg/kg over 20-30 seconds; use a lower dose for children ASA-PS 3 or 4

Adults (healthy), ASA-PS 1 or 2, <55 years: 2-2.5 mg/kg (~40 mg every 10 seconds until onset of induction)

Elderly, debilitated, or ASA-PS 3 or 4: 1-1.5 mg/kg (~20 mg every 10 seconds until onset of induction)

Maintenance: I.V. infusion:

Children (healthy) 2 months to 16 years, ASA-PS 1 or 2: 125-300 mcg/kg/minute (or 7.5-18 mg/kg/**hour**); after 30 minutes, if clinical signs of light anesthesia are absent, decrease the infusion rate. Children ≤5 years may require larger infusion rates compared to older children.

Adults (healthy), ASA-PS 1 or 2, <55 years: Initial: 100-200 mcg/kg/minute (or 6-12 mg/kg/**hour**) for 10-15 minutes; usual maintenance infusion rate: 50-100 mcg/kg/minute (or 3-6 mg/kg/**hour**) to optimize recovery time

Elderly, debilitated, ASA-PS 3 or 4: 50-100 mcg/kg/minute (or 3-6 mg/kg/**hour**)

Maintenance: I.V. intermittent bolus: Adults (healthy), ASA-PS 1 or 2, <55 years: 25-50 mg increments as needed

Monitored anesthesia care sedation:

Adults (healthy), ASA-PS 1 or 2, <55 years: Slow I.V. infusion: 100-150 mcg/kg/minute (or 6-9 mg/kg/**hour**) for 3-5 minutes **or** slow injection: 0.5 mg/kg over 3-5 minutes followed by I.V. infusion of 25-75 mcg/kg/minute (or 1.5-4.5 mg/kg/**hour**) **or** incremental bolus doses: 10 mg or 20 mg

Elderly, debilitated, or ASA-PS 3 or 4 patients: Use 80% of healthy adult dose

ICU sedation in intubated mechanically-ventilated patients: Avoid rapid bolus injection; individualize dose and titrate to response. Adults: Continuous infusion: Initial: 5 mcg/kg/minute (or 0.3 mg/kg/**hour**); increase by 5-10 mcg/kg/minute (or 0.3-0.6 mg/kg/**hour**) every 5-10 minutes until desired sedation level is achieved; usual maintenance (Jacobi, 2002): 5-80 mcg/kg/minute (or 0.3-4.8 mg/kg/**hour**); reduce dose after adequate sedation established and adjust to response (eg, evaluate frequently to use minimum dose for sedation). Daily interruption with retitration is recommended to minimize prolonged sedative effects (Jacobi, 2002).

Postoperative nausea and vomiting (PONV), rescue therapy (unlabeled use; Gan, 2007; Unlugenc, 2004): Adults: I.V.: 20 mg, may be repeated

Refractory status epilepticus (unlabeled use): Adults: 1-2 mg/kg bolus (optional), then 33-167 mcg/kg/minute (or 2-10 mg/kg/**hour**) (Claassen, 2002; Kälviäinen, 2007; Meierkord, 2010; Rossetti, 2004); titrate to desired effect (eg, burst suppression on EEG). **Note:** Doses >83 mcg/kg/minute (or >5 mg/kg/**hour**) may increase the risk of hypotension and propofol-related infusion syndrome (PRIS) especially if used for >48 hours; consider alternative therapies to avoid the risk of PRIS in longer term propofol infusions.

Dosing adjustment in renal impairment: No dosage adjustment necessary.

Dosing adjustment in hepatic impairment: No dosage adjustment necessary.

Dietary Considerations Propofol is formulated in an oil-in-water emulsion. If on parenteral nutrition, may need to adjust the amount of lipid infused. Propofol emulsion contains 1.1 kcal/mL. Soybean fat emulsion is used as a vehicle for propofol. Formulations also contain egg phosphatide and glycerol.

Administration Strict aseptic technique must be maintained in handling although a preservative has been added. Do not use if contamination is suspected. Do not administer through the same I.V. catheter with blood or plasma. Tubing and any unused portions of propofol vials should be discarded after 12 hours.

To reduce pain associated with injection, use larger veins of forearm or antecubital fossa; lidocaine I.V. (1 mL of a 1% solution) may also be used prior to administration or it may be added to propofol immediately before administration in a quantity not to exceed 20 mg lidocaine per 200 mg propofol. Do not use filter <5 micron for administration.

Monitoring Parameters Cardiac monitor, blood pressure, oxygen saturation (during monitored anesthesia care sedation), arterial blood gas (with prolonged infusions). With prolonged infusions (eg, ICU sedation), monitor for metabolic acidosis, hyperkalemia, rhabdomyolysis or elevated CPK, hepatomegaly, and progression of cardiac and renal failure.

ICU sedation: Assess and adjust sedation according to scoring system; assess CNS function daily. Serum triglyceride levels should be obtained prior to initiation of therapy and every 3-7 days thereafter, especially if receiving for >48 hours with doses exceeding 50 mcg/kg/minute (Devlin, 2005); use intravenous port opposite propofol infusion or temporarily suspend infusion and flush port prior to blood draw.

Diprivan®: Monitor zinc levels in patients predisposed to deficiency (burns, diarrhea, major sepsis) or after 5 days of treatment.

Dosage Forms Excipient information presented when available (limited, particularly for generics); consult specific product labeling.

Injection, emulsion: 10 mg/mL (20 mL, 50 mL, 100 mL)

Diprivan®: 10 mg/mL (20 mL, 50 mL, 100 mL) [contains edetate disodium, egg lecithin, soybean oil]

Propranolol (proe PRAN oh lole)

Brand Names: U.S. Inderal® LA; InnoPran XL®

Brand Names: Canada Apo-Propranolol®; Dom-Propranolol; Inderal®; Inderal® LA; Novo-Pranol; Nu-Propranolol; PMS-Propranolol; Propranolol Hydrochloride Injection, USP; Teva-Propranolol

Index Terms Propranolol Hydrochloride

Pharmacologic Category Antianginal Agent; Antiarrhythmic Agent, Class II; Beta-Adrenergic Blocker, Nonselective

Additional Appendix Information

Beta-Blockers *on page 1884*

Use Management of hypertension; angina pectoris; pheochromocytoma; essential tremor; supraventricular arrhythmias (such as atrial fibrillation and flutter, AV nodal reentrant tachycardias), ventricular tachycardias (catecholamine-induced arrhythmias, digoxin toxicity); prevention of myocardial infarction; migraine headache prophylaxis; symptomatic treatment of hypertrophic subaortic stenosis (hypertrophic obstructive cardiomyopathy)

Unlabeled Use Tremor due to Parkinson's disease; aggressive behavior (not recommended for dementia-associated aggression), anxiety, schizophrenia; antipsychotic-induced akathisia; primary and secondary prophylaxis of variceal hemorrhage; acute panic; thyrotoxicosis; tetralogy of Fallot (TOF) hypercyanotic spells

Pregnancy Risk Factor C

Pregnancy Considerations Adverse events have been observed in some animal reproduction studies; therefore, the manufacturer classifies propranolol as pregnancy category C. Propranolol crosses the placenta and is measurable in the newborn serum following maternal use during pregnancy. In a cohort study, an increased risk of cardiovascular defects was observed following maternal use of beta-blockers during pregnancy. Intrauterine growth restriction (IUGR), small placentas, as well as fetal/neonatal bradycardia, hypoglycemia, and/or respiratory depression have been observed following *in utero* exposure to beta-blockers as a class. Adequate facilities for monitoring infants at birth should be available. Untreated chronic maternal hypertension and pre-eclampsia are also associated with adverse events in the fetus, infant, and mother. The peak maternal serum concentrations of propranolol and the active metabolite 4-hydroxypropranolol do not change during pregnancy; peak serum concentrations of naphthoxylactic acid are lower in the third trimester when compared to postpartum. Propranolol is recommended for use in the management of thyrotoxicosis in pregnancy. Propranolol has been evaluated for the treatment of hypertension in pregnancy, but other agents may be more appropriate for use. Propranolol has also been used in the management of hypertrophic obstructive cardiomyopathy in pregnancy and has been studied for use as an adjunctive agent in the management of dysfunctional labor (dystocia).

Lactation Enters breast milk/use caution (AAP rates "compatible"; AAP 2001 update pending)

Contraindications Hypersensitivity to propranolol, beta-blockers, or any component of the formulation; uncompensated congestive heart failure (unless the failure is due to tachyarrhythmias being treated with propranolol), cardiogenic shock, severe sinus bradycardia or heart block greater than first-degree (except in patients with a functioning artificial pacemaker), severe hyperactive airway disease (asthma or COPD)

Warnings/Precautions Consider pre-existing conditions such as sick sinus syndrome before initiating. Administer cautiously in compensated heart failure and monitor for a worsening of the condition (efficacy of propranolol in HF has not been demonstrated). **[U.S. Boxed Warning]: Beta-blocker therapy should not be withdrawn abruptly (particularly in patients with CAD), but gradually tapered to avoid acute tachycardia, hypertension, and/or ischemia.** Chronic beta-blocker therapy should not be routinely withdrawn prior to major surgery. May precipitate or aggravate symptoms of arterial insufficiency in patients with PVD and Raynaud's disease; use with caution and monitor for progression of arterial obstruction. Bradycardia may be observed more frequently in elderly patients (>65 years of age); dosage reductions may be necessary. Use caution with concurrent use of digoxin, verapamil, or diltiazem; bradycardia or heart block can occur. Avoid concurrent I.V. use of both agents. Use with caution in patients receiving inhaled anesthetic agents known to depress myocardial contractility.

Use cautiously in patients with diabetes because it can mask prominent hypoglycemic symptoms. May mask signs of hyperthyroidism (eg, tachycardia); if hyperthyroidism is suspected, carefully manage and monitor; abrupt withdrawal may exacerbate symptoms of hyperthyroidism or precipitate thyroid storm. May alter thyroid-function tests. Use with caution in myasthenia gravis or psychiatric disease (may cause CNS depression). Use cautiously in renal and hepatic dysfunction; dosage adjustment required in hepatic impairment. In general, patients with bronchospastic disease should not receive beta-blockers; if used at all, should be used cautiously with close monitoring. Adequate alpha-blockade is required prior to use of any beta-blocker for patients with untreated pheochromocytoma. May induce or exacerbate psoriasis. Use caution with history of severe anaphylaxis to allergens; patients taking beta-blockers may become more sensitive to repeated challenges. Treatment of anaphylaxis (eg, epinephrine) in patients taking beta-blockers may be ineffective or promote undesirable effects.

Adverse Reactions Frequency not defined.

Cardiovascular: Angina, arterial insufficiency, AV conduction disturbance increased, bradycardia, cardiogenic shock, CHF, hypotension, impaired myocardial contractility, mesenteric arterial thrombosis (rare), Raynaud's syndrome, syncope

Central nervous system: Amnesia, catatonia, cognitive dysfunction, confusion, depression, dizziness, emotional lability, fatigue, hallucinations, hypersomnolence, insomnia, lethargy, lightheadedness, psychosis, vertigo, vivid dreams

Dermatologic: Alopecia, contact dermatitis, cutaneous ulcers, eczematous eruptions, erythema multiforme, exfoliative dermatitis, hyperkeratosis, nail changes, oculomucocutaneous reactions, pruritus, psoriasiform eruptions, rash, Stevens-Johnson syndrome, toxic epidermal necrolysis, ulcers, ulcerative lichenoid, urticaria

Endocrine & metabolic: Hyper-/hypoglycemia, hyperkalemia, hyperlipidemia

Gastrointestinal: Anorexia, cramping, constipation, diarrhea, ischemic colitis, nausea, stomach discomfort, vomiting

Genitourinary: Impotence, interstitial nephritis (rare), oliguria (rare), Peyronie's disease, proteinuria (rare)

Hematologic: Agranulocytosis, nonthrombocytopenic purpura, thrombocytopenia, thrombocytopenic purpura

Hepatic: Alkaline phosphatase increased, transaminases increased

Neuromuscular & skeletal: Arthropathy, carpal tunnel syndrome (rare), myotonus, paresthesia, polyarthritis, weakness

Ocular: Hyperemia of the conjunctiva, mydriasis, visual acuity decreased, visual disturbances, xerophthalmia

Renal: BUN increased

Respiratory: Bronchospasm, dyspnea, laryngospasm, pharyngitis, pulmonary edema, respiratory distress, wheezing

Miscellaneous: Anaphylactic/anaphylactoid allergic reaction, cold extremities, lupus-like syndrome (rare)

Drug Interactions

Metabolism/Transport Effects **Substrate** of CYP1A2 (major), CYP2C19 (minor), CYP2D6 (major), CYP3A4 (minor); **Note:** Assignment of Major/Minor substrate status based on clinically relevant drug interaction potential; **Inhibits** CYP1A2 (weak), CYP2D6 (weak), P-glycoprotein

Avoid Concomitant Use

Avoid concomitant use of Propranolol with any of the following: Beta2-Agonists; Floctafenine; Methacholine; Silodosin; Topotecan

Increased Effect/Toxicity

Propranolol may increase the levels/effects of: Alpha-/Beta-Agonists (Direct-Acting); Alpha1-Blockers; Alpha2-Agonists; Amifostine; Antihypertensives; Antipsychotic Agents (Phenothiazines); Bupivacaine; Cardiac Glycosides; Cholinergic Agonists; Colchicine; Dabigatran Etexilate; Everolimus; Fingolimod; Hypotensive Agents; Insulin; Lidocaine; Lidocaine (Systemic); Lidocaine (Topical); Mepivacaine; Methacholine; Midodrine; P-glycoprotein/ABCB1 Substrates; RiTUXimab; Rivaroxaban; Rizatriptan; Silodosin; Sulfonylureas; Topotecan; ZOLMitriptan

The levels/effects of Propranolol may be increased by: Abiraterone Acetate; Acetylcholinesterase Inhibitors; Alcohol (Ethyl); Aminoquinolines (Antimalarial); Amiodarone; Anilidopiperidine Opioids; Antipsychotic Agents (Phenothiazines); Calcium Channel Blockers (Dihydropyridine); Calcium Channel Blockers (Nondihydropyridine); Conivaptan; CYP1A2 Inhibitors (Moderate); CYP1A2 Inhibitors (Strong); CYP2D6 Inhibitors (Moderate); CYP2D6 Inhibitors (Strong); Darunavir; Deferasirox; Diazoxide; Dipyridamole; Disopyramide; Dronedarone; Floctafenine; FluvoxaMINE; Herbs (Hypotensive Properties); Lacidipine; MAO Inhibitors; Pentoxifylline; Phosphodiesterase 5 Inhibitors; Propafenone; Prostacyclin Analogues; QuiNIDine; Reserpine; Selective Serotonin Reuptake Inhibitors; Zileuton

Decreased Effect

Propranolol may decrease the levels/effects of: Beta2-Agonists; Lacidipine; Theophylline Derivatives

The levels/effects of Propranolol may be decreased by: Alcohol (Ethyl); Barbiturates; Bile Acid Sequestrants; CYP1A2 Inducers (Strong); Cyproterone; Herbs (Hypertensive Properties); Methylphenidate; Nonsteroidal Anti-Inflammatory Agents; Peginterferon Alfa-2b; Rifamycin Derivatives; Tocilizumab; Yohimbine

Ethanol/Nutrition/Herb Interactions

Ethanol: Ethanol may increase or decrease plasma levels of propranolol. Reports are variable and have shown both enhanced as well as inhibited hepatic metabolism (of propranolol). Caution advised with consumption of alcohol and monitor for heart rate and/or blood pressure changes.

Food: Propranolol serum levels may be increased if taken with food. Protein-rich foods may increase bioavailability; a change in diet from high carbohydrate/low protein to low carbohydrate/high protein may result in increased oral clearance.

Cigarette: Smoking may decrease plasma levels of propranolol by increasing metabolism.

Herb/Nutraceutical: Avoid dong quai if using for hypertension (has estrogenic activity). Avoid bayberry, blue cohosh, cayenne, ephedra, ginger, ginseng (American), gotu kola, licorice, yohimbe (may worsen hypertension). Avoid black cohosh, california poppy, coleus, garlic, golden seal, hawthorn, mistletoe, periwinkle, quinine, shepherd's purse (have antihypertensive activity, may cause hypotension).

Stability

Injection: Store at 20°C to 25°C (68°F to 77°F); protect from freezing or excessive heat. Once diluted, propranolol is stable for 24 hours at room temperature in D_5W or NS. Protect from light. Solution has a maximum stability at pH of 3 and decomposes rapidly in alkaline pH.

Capsule, tablet: Store at 20°C to 25°C (68°F to 77°F); protect from freezing or excessive heat. Protect from light and moisture.

Mechanism of Action Nonselective beta-adrenergic blocker (class II antiarrhythmic); competitively blocks response to $beta_1$- and $beta_2$-adrenergic stimulation which results in decreases in heart rate, myocardial contractility, blood pressure, and myocardial oxygen demand. Nonselective beta-adrenergic blockers (propranolol, nadolol) reduce portal pressure by producing splanchnic vasoconstriction ($beta_2$ effect) thereby reducing portal blood flow.

Pharmacodynamics/Kinetics

Onset of action: Beta-blockade: Oral: 1-2 hours

Duration: Immediate release: 6-12 hours; Extended-release formulations: ~24-27 hours

Absorption: Oral: Rapid and complete

Distribution: V_d: 4 L/kg in adults

Protein binding: Newborns: 68%; Adults: ~90% (S-isomer primarily to $alpha_1$-acid glycoprotein; R-isomer primarily to albumin)

Metabolism: Hepatic via CYP2D6, and CYP1A2 to 4-hydroxypropranolol (active) and inactive compounds; extensive first-pass effect

Bioavailability: ~25% reaches systemic circulation due to high first-pass metabolism; protein-rich foods increase bioavailability by ~50%

Half-life elimination: Neonates and Infants: Possible increased half-life; Children: 3.9-6.4 hours; Adults: Immediate release formulation: 3-6 hours; Extended-release formulations: 8-10 hours

Time to peak: Immediate release: 1-4 hours; Extended-release formulations: ~6-14 hours

Excretion: Metabolites are excreted primarily in urine (96% to 99%); <1% excreted in urine as unchanged drug

Dosage

Akathisia (unlabeled use): Oral: Adults: 30-120 mg/day in 2-3 divided doses

Essential tremor: Oral: Adults: 40 mg twice daily initially; maintenance doses: Usually 120-320 mg/day

Hypertension:

Oral:

Children (unlabeled use): Initial: 0.5-1 mg/kg/day in divided doses every 6-12 hours; increase gradually every 5-7 days; maximum: 16 mg/kg/24 hours

Adults: Initial: 40 mg twice daily; increase dosage every 3-7 days; usual dose: 120-240 mg divided in 2-3 doses/day; maximum daily dose: 640 mg; usual dosage range (JNC 7): 40-160 mg/day in 2 divided doses

Extended release formulations:

Inderal® LA: Initial: 80 mg once daily; usual maintenance: 120-160 mg once daily; maximum daily dose: 640 mg; usual dosage range (JNC 7): 60-180 mg/day once daily

InnoPran XL®: Initial: 80 mg once daily at bedtime; if initial response is inadequate, may be increased at 2-3 week intervals to a maximum dose of 120 mg

Elderly: Consider lower initial doses and titrate to response (Aronow, 2011)

Hypertrophic subaortic stenosis: Oral: Adults: 20-40 mg 3-4 times/day

Inderal® LA: 80-160 mg once daily

Migraine headache prophylaxis: Oral:

Children (unlabeled use): Initial: 2-4 mg/kg/day **or**

≤35 kg: 10-20 mg 3 times/day

>35 kg: 20-40 mg 3 times/day

Adults: Initial: 80 mg/day divided every 6-8 hours; increase by 20-40 mg/dose every 3-4 weeks to a maximum of 160-240 mg/day given in divided doses every 6-8 hours; if satisfactory response not achieved within 6 weeks of starting therapy, drug should be withdrawn gradually over several weeks

Inderal® LA: Initial: 80 mg once daily; effective dose range: 160-240 mg once daily

Post-MI mortality reduction: Oral: Adults: Initial: 40 mg 3 times/day; usual dosage range: 180-240 mg/day in 3-4 divided doses

Pheochromocytoma: Oral: Adults: 30-60 mg/day in divided doses

Stable angina: Oral: Adults: 80-320 mg/day in doses divided 2-4 times/day

Inderal® LA: Initial: 80 mg once daily; maximum dose: 320 mg once daily

Tachyarrhythmias:

Oral:

Children (unlabeled use): Initial: 0.5-1 mg/kg/day in divided doses every 6-8 hours; titrate dosage upward every 3-7 days; usual dose: 2-6 mg/kg/day; higher doses may be needed; do not exceed 16 mg/kg/day or 60 mg/day

Adults: 10-30 mg/dose every 6-8 hours

Elderly: Initial: 10 mg twice daily; increase dosage every 3-7 days; usual dosage range: 10-320 mg given in 2 divided doses

I.V.:

Children (unlabeled use): 0.01-0.1 mg/kg/dose slow IVP over 10 minutes; maximum dose: 1 mg for infants; 3 mg for children

Adults: 1-3 mg/dose slow IVP; repeat every 2-5 minutes up to a total of 5 mg; titrate initial dose to desired response

or

0.5-1 mg over 1 minute; may repeat, if necessary, up to a total maximum dose of 0.1 mg/kg (ACLS guidelines, 2010)

Note: Once response achieved or maximum dose administered, additional doses should not be given for at least 4 hours.

Elderly: Use caution; initiate at lower end of the dosing range.

Hypercyanotic spells (TOF) (unlabeled use): Children:

Oral: Palliation: Initial: 1 mg/kg/day every 6 hours; if ineffective, may increase dose after 1 week by 1 mg/kg/day to a maximum of 5 mg/kg/day; if patient becomes refractory, may increase slowly to a maximum of 10-15 mg/kg/day. Allow 24 hours between dosing changes.

I.V.: 0.01-0.2 mg/kg/dose infused over 10 minutes; maximum dose: 5 mg

Thyroid storm (unlabeled use):

Children: 0.5 mg/kg/dose every 4-8 hours; titrate to effective dose (Eyal, 2008)

Adults:

Oral: 60-80 mg every 4 hours; may consider the use of an intravenous shorter-acting beta-blocker (ie, esmolol) (Bahn, 2011)

I.V.: 0.5-1 mg administered over 10 minutes every 3 hours (Gardner, 2011)

Thyrotoxicosis (unlabeled use): Oral:

Children: 10-40 mg every 6 hours; titrate to effective dose (Eyal, 2008)

Adolescents and Adults: Oral: 10-40 mg/dose every 6-8 hours; may also consider administering extended or sustained release formulations (Bahn, 2011)

Variceal hemorrhage prophylaxis (unlabeled use; Garcia-Tsao, 2007): Oral: Adults:

Primary prophylaxis: Initial: 20 mg twice daily; adjust to maximal tolerated dose. **Note:** Risk factors for hemorrhage include Child-Pugh class B/C or variceal red wale markings on endoscopy.

Secondary prophylaxis: Initial: 20 mg twice daily; adjust to maximal tolerated dose

Dosing adjustment in renal impairment:

Not dialyzable (0% to 5%); supplemental dose is not necessary.

Peritoneal dialysis effects: Supplemental dose is not necessary.

Dosing adjustment in hepatic disease: Marked slowing of heart rate may occur in chronic liver disease with conventional doses; low initial dose and regular heart rate monitoring

Dietary Considerations Tablets (immediate release) should be taken on an empty stomach; capsules (extended release) may be taken with or without food, but should always be taken consistently (with food or on an empty stomach)

Administration I.V. dose is much smaller than oral dose. When administered acutely for cardiac treatment, monitor ECG and blood pressure. May administer by rapid infusion (I.V. push) at a rate of 1 mg/minute or by slow infusion over ~30 minutes. Necessary monitoring for surgical patients who are unable to take oral beta-blockers (prolonged ileus) has not been defined. Some institutions require monitoring of baseline and postinfusion heart rate and blood pressure when a patient's response to beta-blockade has not been characterized (ie, the patient's initial dose or following a change in dose). Consult individual institutional policies and procedures. Do not crush long-acting oral forms.

Monitoring Parameters Acute cardiac treatment: Monitor ECG, heart rate, and blood pressure with I.V. administration; heart rate and blood pressure with oral administration

Reference Range Therapeutic: 50-100 ng/mL (SI: 190-390 nmol/L) at end of dose interval

Dosage Forms Excipient information presented when available (limited, particularly for generics); consult specific product labeling.

Capsule, extended release, oral, as hydrochloride: 60 mg, 80 mg, 120 mg, 160 mg

InnoPran XL®: 80 mg, 120 mg

Capsule, sustained release, oral, as hydrochloride:

Inderal® LA: 60 mg, 80 mg, 120 mg, 160 mg

Injection, solution, as hydrochloride: 1 mg/mL (1 mL)

Injection, solution, as hydrochloride [preservative free]: 1 mg/mL (1 mL)

Solution, oral, as hydrochloride: 4 mg/mL (500 mL); 8 mg/mL (500 mL)

Tablet, oral, as hydrochloride: 10 mg, 20 mg, 40 mg, 60 mg, 80 mg

◆ **Propranolol Hydrochloride** *see* Propranolol *on page 1424*

◆ **Propranolol Hydrochloride Injection, USP (Can)** *see* Propranolol *on page 1424*

◆ **Proprinal® [OTC]** *see* Ibuprofen *on page 860*

◆ **Proprinal® Cold and Sinus [OTC]** *see* Pseudoephedrine and Ibuprofen *on page 1432*

◆ **Propylene Glycol Diacetate, Acetic Acid, and Hydrocortisone** *see* Acetic Acid, Propylene Glycol Diacetate, and Hydrocortisone *on page 33*

◆ **2-Propylpentanoic Acid** *see* Valproic Acid *on page 1757*

Propylthiouracil (proe pil thye oh YOOR a sil)

Brand Names: Canada Propyl-Thyracil®

Index Terms PTU (error-prone abbreviation)

Pharmacologic Category Antithyroid Agent; Thioamide

Use Adjunctive therapy in patients intolerant of methimazole to ameliorate hyperthyroidism symptoms in preparation for surgical treatment or radioactive iodine therapy; treatment of hyperthyroidism in patients intolerant of methimazole and not candidates for surgical/radiotherapy

Unlabeled Use Management of Graves' disease, thyrotoxic crisis, or thyroid storm

Pregnancy Risk Factor D

Pregnancy Considerations Studies in pregnant women have demonstrated a risk to the fetus. Propylthiouracil has been found to readily cross the placenta. Teratogenic effects have not been observed. Nonteratogenic adverse effects, including fetal and neonatal hypothyroidism, goiter, and hyperthyroidism, have been observed following maternal propylthiouracil use. The transfer of thyroid-stimulating immunoglobulins can stimulate the fetal thyroid *in utero* and transiently after delivery and may increase the risk of fetal or neonatal hyperthyroidism.

The pharmacokinetics of propylthiouracil are not significantly changed during pregnancy; however, the severity of hyperthyroidism may fluctuate throughout pregnancy. Doses of propylthiouracil may be decreased as pregnancy progresses and discontinued weeks to months prior to delivery. Possible exacerbation of hyperthyroidism after delivery may require the reinitiation of antithyroid therapy.

Uncontrolled maternal hyperthyroidism may result in adverse neonatal outcomes (eg, prematurity, low birth weight) and adverse maternal outcomes (eg, pre-eclampsia, congestive heart failure, stillbirth, and abortion). To prevent adverse fetal and maternal events, normal maternal thyroid function should be maintained prior to conception and throughout pregnancy. Antithyroid treatment is recommended for the control of hyperthyroidism during pregnancy. Propylthiouracil is considered first-line therapy, especially during the first trimester. Due to an increased risk of liver toxicity, use of methimazole may be preferred during the second and third trimesters. Propylthiouracil, along with other medications, is used for the treatment of thyroid storm in pregnant women; alternative therapy is recommended if oral administration is not possible.

Lactation Enters breast milk/AAP rates "compatible" (AAP 2001 update pending)

Medication Guide Available Yes

Contraindications Hypersensitivity to propylthiouracil or any component of the formulation

Warnings/Precautions [U.S. Boxed Warning]: Severe liver injury (some fatal) and acute liver failure (some cases requiring transplantation) have been reported. Patients should be counseled to recognize and report symptoms suggestive of hepatic dysfunction (especially in first 6 months of treatment), which should prompt immediate discontinuation. Routine liver function test monitoring may not reduce risk due to unpredictable and rapid onset.

Has been associated with significant bone marrow depression. The most severe manifestation is agranulocytosis (commonly within first 3 months of therapy). Aplastic anemia, thrombocytopenia, and leukopenia may also occur. Use with caution in patients receiving other drugs known to cause myelosuppression particularly agranulocytosis. Discontinue if significant bone marrow suppression occurs, particularly agranulocytosis or aplastic anemia.

Rare hypersensitivity reactions have been reported, including the development of ANCA-positive vasculitis, drug fever, interstitial pneumonitis, exfoliative dermatitis, glomerulonephritis, leukocytoclastic vasculitis, and a lupus-like syndrome; prompt discontinuation is warranted in patients who develop symptoms consistent with a form of autoimmunity or other hypersensitivity during therapy. May cause hypoprothrombinemia and bleeding.

Adverse Reactions Frequency not defined.

Cardiovascular: Periarteritis, vasculitis (ANCA-positive, cutaneous, leukocytoclastic)

Central nervous system: Drowsiness, drug fever, fever, headache, neuritis, vertigo

Dermatologic: Alopecia, erythema nodosum, exfoliative dermatitis, pruritus, skin pigmentation, skin rash, skin ulcers, urticaria

Endocrine & metabolic: Goiter, weight gain

Gastrointestinal: Constipation, loss of taste, nausea, sialoadenopathy, splenomegaly, stomach pain, taste perversion, vomiting

Hematologic: Agranulocytosis, aplastic anemia, bleeding, granulopenia, hypoprothrombinemia, leukopenia, thrombocytopenia

Hepatic: Acute liver failure, cholestatic jaundice, hepatitis

Neuromuscular & skeletal: Arthralgia, myalgia, paresthesia

Renal: Acute renal failure, glomerulonephritis, nephritis

Respiratory: Alveolar hemorrhage, interstitial pneumonitis

Miscellaneous: Lymphadenopathy, SLE-like syndrome

Drug Interactions

Metabolism/Transport Effects None known.

Avoid Concomitant Use

Avoid concomitant use of Propylthiouracil with any of the following: CloZAPine; Sodium Iodide I131

Increased Effect/Toxicity

Propylthiouracil may increase the levels/effects of: Cardiac Glycosides; CloZAPine; Theophylline Derivatives

Decreased Effect

Propylthiouracil may decrease the levels/effects of: Sodium Iodide I131; Vitamin K Antagonists

Ethanol/Nutrition/Herb Interactions Food: Propylthiouracil serum levels may be altered if taken with food.

Stability Store at 25°C (77°F); excursions permitted to 15°C to 30°C (59°F to 86°F).

Mechanism of Action Inhibits the synthesis of thyroid hormones by blocking the oxidation of iodine in the thyroid gland; blocks synthesis of thyroxine and triiodothyronine

Pharmacodynamics/Kinetics

Duration: 12-24 hours

Distribution: Concentrated in the thyroid gland

Protein binding: 80% to 85%

Metabolism: Hepatic

Bioavailability: 53% to 88%

Half-life elimination: ~1 hour

Time to peak, serum: 1-2 hours

Excretion: Urine (35%; primarily as metabolites)

Dosage Oral: Administer in equally divided doses every 8 hours. Adjust dosage to maintain T_3, T_4, and TSH levels in normal range; elevated T_3 may be sole indicator of inadequate treatment. Elevated TSH indicates excessive antithyroid treatment.

Children: Initial: 5-7 mg/kg/day **or** 150-200 mg/m^2/day in divided doses every 8 hours

or

Manufacturer's recommendations:

6-10 years: 50-150 mg/day

>10 years: 150-300 mg/day

Adults:

Hyperthyroidism: Initial: 300 mg/day in 3 divided doses; 400 mg/day in patients with severe hyperthyroidism and/or very large goiters; an occasional patient will require 600-900 mg/day; usual maintenance: 100-150 mg/day

Graves' disease (unlabeled use): Initial: 50-150 mg (depending on severity) 3 times daily to restore euthyroidism; maintenance: 50 mg 2-3 times daily for a total of 12-18 months, then tapered or discontinued if TSH is normal at that time (Bahn, 2011)

Thyrotoxic crisis/thyroid storm (unlabeled use): **Note:** Recommendations vary widely and have not been evaluated in comparative trials. Typical dosing is 800-1200 mg/day given as 200-300 mg every 4-6 hours; some clinicians advocate an initial loading dose of 600-1000 mg. After initial response, dose may be reduced gradually to a maintenance dosage (100-600 mg/day in divided doses) (Goldberg, 2003; Nayak, 2006). The American Thyroid Association and the American Association of Clinical Endocrinologists recommend 500-1000 mg loading dose followed by 250 mg every 4 hours (Bahn, 2011).

Duration of therapy: Clinical improvement generally occurs in 1-3 months, after which dosage reduction may be employed (to prevent hypothyroidism), with discontinuation considered after 12-18 months of therapy. Thyroid function should be monitored every 2 months thereafter for 6 months until remission is confirmed, followed by annual evaluations (Cooper, 2005).

Dosing adjustment in renal impairment: Adjustment is not necessary.

Dietary Considerations Take at the same time in relation to meals each day, either always with meals or always between meals.

Administration Administer at the same time in relation to meals each day, either always with meals or always between meals.

Monitoring Parameters CBC with differential, prothrombin time, liver function tests (bilirubin, alkaline phosphatase, transaminases), and thyroid function tests (TSH, T_3, T_4) every 4-6 weeks until euthyroid; periodic blood counts are recommended for chronic therapy

Reference Range Normal laboratory values:

Total T_4: 5-12 mcg/dL

Serum T_3: 90-185 ng/dL

Free thyroxine index (FT_4 I): 6-10.5

TSH: 0.5-4.0 microunits/mL

Additional Information Preferred over methimazole in thyroid storm due to inhibition of peripheral conversion as well as synthesis of thyroid hormone.

Graves' hyperthyroidism: Elevated T_3 may be the sole indicator of inadequate treatment. Elevated TSH indicates excessive antithyroid treatment. Monitoring of TSH is a poor indicator of treatment effectiveness, as levels may remain suppressed for months, despite euthyroid state (Cooper, 2005).

A potency ratio of methimazole to propylthiouracil of at least 20-30:1 is recommended when changing from one drug to another (eg, 300 mg of propylthiouracil would be roughly equivalent to 10-15 mg of methimazole) (Bahn, 2011).

Dosage Forms Excipient information presented when available (limited, particularly for generics); consult specific product labeling.

Tablet, oral: 50 mg

Extemporaneous Preparations A 5 mg/mL oral suspension may be made with tablets and a 1:1 mixture of Ora-Plus® and Ora-Sweet®. Crush twenty 50 mg propylthiouracil tablets in a mortar and reduce to a fine powder. Add small portions of vehicle and mix to a uniform paste; mix while adding vehicle in incremental proportions to **almost** 200 mL; transfer to a calibrated bottle, rinse mortar with vehicle, and add quantity of vehicle sufficient to make 200 mL. Label "shake well" and "refrigerate". Stable for 91 days refrigerated (preferred) and 70 days at room temperature.

Nahata MC, Pai VB, and Hipple TF, *Pediatric Drug Formulations*, 5th ed, Cincinnati, OH: Harvey Whitney Books Co, 2004.

- ◆ **Propyl-Thyracil® (Can)** *see* Propylthiouracil *on page* 1426
- ◆ **2-Propylvaleric Acid** *see* Valproic Acid *on page* 1757
- ◆ **ProQuad®** *see* Measles, Mumps, Rubella, and Varicella Virus Vaccine *on page* 1055
- ◆ **PRO-Quetiapine (Can)** *see* QUEtiapine *on page* 1440
- ◆ **PRO-Rabeprazole (Can)** *see* RABEprazole *on page* 1451
- ◆ **PRO-Risperidone (Can)** *see* RisperiDONE *on page* 1496
- ◆ **Proscar®** *see* Finasteride *on page* 713
- ◆ **Prosed®/DS** *see* Methenamine, Phenyl Salicylate, Methylene Blue, Benzoic Acid, and Hyoscyamine *on page* 1094
- ◆ **ProSom** *see* Estazolam *on page* 627
- ◆ **PRO-Sotalol (Can)** *see* Sotalol *on page* 1586
- ◆ **Prostacyclin** *see* Epoprostenol *on page* 604
- ◆ **Prostacyclin PGI_2** *see* Iloprost *on page* 870
- ◆ **Prostaglandin E_1** *see* Alprostadil *on page* 74
- ◆ **Prostaglandin E_2** *see* Dinoprostone *on page* 514
- ◆ **Prostaglandin F_2** *see* Carboprost Tromethamine *on page* 290
- ◆ **Prostate Cancer Vaccine, Cell-Based** *see* Sipuleucel-T *on page* 1557
- ◆ **Prostigmin®** *see* Neostigmine *on page* 1190
- ◆ **Prostin E2®** *see* Dinoprostone *on page* 514
- ◆ **Prostin E_2® (Can)** *see* Dinoprostone *on page* 514
- ◆ **Prostin® VR (Can)** *see* Alprostadil *on page* 74
- ◆ **Prostin VR Pediatric®** *see* Alprostadil *on page* 74

Protamine (PROE ta meen)

Index Terms Protamine Sulfate

Pharmacologic Category Antidote

Use Treatment of heparin overdosage; neutralize heparin during surgery or dialysis procedures

Unlabeled Use Treatment of low molecular weight heparin (LMWH) overdose

Pregnancy Risk Factor C

Lactation Excretion in breast milk unknown

Contraindications Hypersensitivity to protamine or any component of the formulation

Warnings/Precautions May not be totally effective in some patients following cardiac surgery despite adequate doses. May cause hypersensitivity reaction in patients (have epinephrine 1:1000 and resuscitation equipment available). **[U.S. Boxed Warning]: Hypotension, cardiovascular collapse, noncardiogenic pulmonary edema, pulmonary vasoconstriction, and pulmonary hypertension may occur. Risk factors for such events include: use of high doses or overdose, repeated doses, previous protamine administration (including protamine-containing drugs), fish allergy, vasectomy, severe left ventricular dysfunction, abnormal preoperative pulmonary hemodynamics.** Too rapid administration can cause severe hypotensive and anaphylactoid-like reactions. Heparin rebound associated with anticoagulation and bleeding has been reported to occur occasionally; symptoms typically occur 8-9 hours after protamine administration, but may occur as long as 18 hours later.

Adverse Reactions Frequency not defined.

Cardiovascular: Sudden fall in blood pressure, bradycardia, flushing, hypotension

Central nervous system: Lassitude

Gastrointestinal: Nausea, vomiting

Hematologic: Hemorrhage

Respiratory: Dyspnea, pulmonary hypertension

Miscellaneous: Hypersensitivity reactions

Drug Interactions

Metabolism/Transport Effects None known.

Avoid Concomitant Use There are no known interactions where it is recommended to avoid concomitant use.

Increased Effect/Toxicity There are no known significant interactions involving an increase in effect.

Decreased Effect There are no known significant interactions involving a decrease in effect.

Stability Refrigerate; do not freeze. Stable for at least 2 weeks at room temperature. Preservative-free formulation does not require refrigeration. Reconstitute vial with 5 mL sterile water. If using protamine in neonates, reconstitute with preservative-free sterile water for injection; resulting solution equals 10 mg/mL.

Mechanism of Action Combines with strongly acidic heparin to form a stable complex (salt) neutralizing the anticoagulant activity of both drugs

Pharmacodynamics/Kinetics Onset of action: I.V.: Heparin neutralization: ~5 minutes

Dosage

Heparin neutralization: I.V.: Protamine dosage is determined by the dosage of heparin; 1 mg of protamine neutralizes 90 USP units of heparin (lung) and 115 USP units of heparin (intestinal); maximum dose: 50 mg

Heparin overdosage, following intravenous administration: I.V.: Since blood heparin concentrations decrease rapidly **after** administration, adjust the protamine dosage depending upon the duration of time since heparin administration as follows: See table.

Time Elapsed	Dose of Protamine (mg) to Neutralize 100 units of Heparin
Immediate	1-1.5
30-60 min	0.5-0.75
>2 h	0.25-0.375

Heparin overdosage, following SubQ injection: I.V.: 1-1.5 mg protamine per 100 units heparin; this may be done by a portion of the dose (eg, 25-50 mg) given slowly I.V. followed by the remaining portion as a continuous infusion over 8-16 hours (the expected absorption time of the SubQ heparin dose)

LMWH overdose (unlabeled use): **Note:** Antifactor Xa activity never completely neutralized (maximum: ~60% to 75%)

Enoxaparin: 1 mg protamine for each mg of enoxaparin (1 mg of enoxaparin is equal to 100 int. units of anti-Xa activity); if PTT prolonged 2-4 hours after first dose, consider additional dose of 0.5 mg for each mg of enoxaparin.

Dalteparin or tinzaparin: 1 mg protamine for each 100 anti-Xa int. units of dalteparin or tinzaparin; if PTT prolonged 2-4 hours after first dose, consider additional dose of 0.5 mg for each 100 anti-Xa int. units of dalteparin or tinzaparin.

Note: Excessive protamine doses may worsen bleeding potential.

Administration For I.V. use only; **incompatible** with cephalosporins and penicillins; administer slow IVP (50 mg over 10 minutes); rapid I.V. infusion causes hypotension; resulting solution equals 10 mg/mL; inject without further dilution over 1-3 minutes; maximum of 50 mg in any 10-minute period

Monitoring Parameters Coagulation test, aPTT or ACT, cardiac monitor and blood pressure monitor required during administration

Dosage Forms Excipient information presented when available (limited, particularly for generics); consult specific product labeling.

Injection, solution, as sulfate [preservative free]: 10 mg/mL (5 mL, 25 mL)

- **Protamine Sulfate** *see* Protamine *on page 1428*
- **Protease, Lipase, and Amylase** *see* Pancrelipase *on page 1285*
- **Protein C** *see* Protein C Concentrate (Human) *on page 1429*
- **Protein C (Activated), Human, Recombinant** *see* Drotrecogin Alfa (Activated) *on page 564*
- **Protein-Bound Paclitaxel** *see* PACLitaxel (Protein Bound) *on page 1275*

Protein C Concentrate (Human)

(PROE teen cee KON suhn trate HYU man)

Brand Names: U.S. Ceprotin

Index Terms Protein C

Pharmacologic Category Anticoagulant

Use Replacement therapy for severe congenital protein C deficiency for the prevention and/or treatment of venous thromboembolism and purpura fulminans

Pregnancy Risk Factor C

Dosage Patient variables (including age, clinical condition, and plasma levels of protein C) will influence dosing and duration of therapy. Individualize dosing based on protein C activity and patient pharmacokinetic profile. Dosing is dependent on the severity of protein C deficiency, age of patient, clinical condition, and patient's level of protein C. The frequency, duration, and dose should be individualized.

I.V.: Children and Adults: Severe congenital protein C deficiency:

Acute episode/short-term prophylaxis: Initial dose: 100-120 int. units/kg (for determination of recovery and half-life)

Subsequent 3 doses: 60-80 int. units/kg every 6 hours (adjust to maintain peak protein C activity of 100%)

Maintenance dose: 45-60 int. units/kg every 6 or 12 hours (adjust to maintain recommended maintenance trough protein C activity levels >25%)

Long-term prophylaxis: Maintenance dose: 45-60 int. units/kg every 12 hours (recommended maintenance trough protein C activity levels >25%)

Note: Maintain target peak protein C activity of 100% during acute episodes and short-term prophylaxis. Maintain trough levels of protein C activity >25%. Higher peak levels of protein C may be necessary in prophylactic therapy of patients at increased risk for thrombosis (eg, infection, trauma, surgical intervention).

Additional Information Complete prescribing information for this medication should be consulted for additional detail.

Dosage Forms Excipient information presented when available (limited, particularly for generics); consult specific product labeling.

Injection, powder for reconstitution [preservative free]:

Ceprotin: ~500 int. units, ~1000 int. units [contains albumin (human), heparin (may have trace amounts), mouse protein (may have trace amounts), sodium; actual potency is printed on the vial label; supplied with diluent]

- **Prothrombin Complex Concentrate** *see* Factor IX Complex (Human) *on page 684*
- **Protonix®** *see* Pantoprazole *on page 1289*
- **Protonix® I.V.** *see* Pantoprazole *on page 1289*
- **Protopam®** *see* Pralidoxime *on page 1388*
- **Protopic®** *see* Tacrolimus (Topical) *on page 1619*
- **PRO-Topiramate (Can)** *see* Topiramate *on page 1706*
- **Pro-Triazide (Can)** *see* Hydrochlorothiazide and Triamterene *on page 836*

Protriptyline (proe TRIP ti leen)

Brand Names: U.S. Vivactil®

Index Terms Protriptyline Hydrochloride

Pharmacologic Category Antidepressant, Tricyclic (Secondary Amine)

Additional Appendix Information

Antidepressant Agents *on page 1874*

Use Treatment of depression

Medication Guide Available Yes

Dosage Oral:

Adolescents: 15-20 mg/day

Adults: 15-60 mg/day in 3-4 divided doses

Elderly: Initial: 5-10 mg/day; increase every 3-7 days by 5-10 mg; usual dose: 15-20 mg/day

Additional Information Complete prescribing information for this medication should be consulted for additional detail.

Dosage Forms Excipient information presented when available (limited, particularly for generics); consult specific product labeling.

Tablet, oral, as hydrochloride: 5 mg, 10 mg

Vivactil®: 5 mg, 10 mg

◆ **Protriptyline Hydrochloride** *see* Protriptyline *on page 1430*
◆ **PRO-Valacyclovir (Can)** *see* ValACYclovir *on page 1753*
◆ **Provenge®** *see* Sipuleucel-T *on page 1557*
◆ **Proventil® HFA** *see* Albuterol *on page 52*
◆ **Provera®** *see* MedroxyPROGESTERone *on page 1058*
◆ **Provera-Pak (Can)** *see* MedroxyPROGESTERone *on page 1058*
◆ **PRO-Verapamil SR (Can)** *see* Verapamil *on page 1783*
◆ **Provigil®** *see* Modafinil *on page 1147*
◆ **Provisc®** *see* Hyaluronate and Derivatives *on page 831*
◆ **Provocholine®** *see* Methacholine *on page 1088*
◆ **Proxymetacaine** *see* Proparacaine *on page 1421*
◆ **PROzac®** *see* FLUoxetine *on page 731*
◆ **Prozac® (Can)** *see* FLUoxetine *on page 731*
◆ **PROzac® Weekly™** *see* FLUoxetine *on page 731*
◆ **PRP-OMP** *see Haemophilus* b Conjugate Vaccine *on page 815*
◆ **PRP-T** *see Haemophilus* b Conjugate Vaccine *on page 815*
◆ **Prudoxin™** *see* Doxepin (Topical) *on page 552*
◆ **Prussian Blue** *see* Ferric Hexacyanoferrate *on page 705*
◆ **Prymaccone** *see* Primaquine *on page 1404*
◆ **23PS** *see* Pneumococcal Polysaccharide Vaccine (Polyvalent) *on page 1368*
◆ **PS-341** *see* Bortezomib *on page 228*

Pseudoephedrine (soo doe e FED rin)

Brand Names: U.S. Children's Nasal Decongestant [OTC]; Contac® Cold + Flu Maximum Strength Non-Drowsy [OTC]; Genaphed™ [OTC] [DSC]; Oranyl [OTC]; Silfedrine Children's [OTC]; Sudafed® 12 Hour [OTC]; Sudafed® 24 Hour [OTC]; Sudafed® Children's [OTC]; Sudafed® Maximum Strength Nasal Decongestant [OTC]; Sudo-Tab® [OTC]; SudoGest 12 Hour [OTC]; SudoGest Children's [OTC]; SudoGest [OTC]

Brand Names: Canada Balminil Decongestant; Benylin® D for Infants; Contac® Cold 12 Hour Relief Non Drowsy; Drixoral® ND; Eltor®; PMS-Pseudoephedrine; Pseudofrin; Robidrine®; Sudafed® Decongestant

Index Terms *d*-Isoephedrine Hydrochloride; Pseudoephedrine Hydrochloride; Pseudoephedrine Sulfate; Sudafed

Pharmacologic Category Alpha/Beta Agonist

Use Temporary symptomatic relief of nasal congestion due to common cold, upper respiratory allergies, and sinusitis; also promotes nasal or sinus drainage

Pregnancy Considerations Use of pseudoephedrine during the first trimester may be associated with a possible risk of gastroschisis, small intestinal atresia, and hemifacial microsomia due to pseudoephedrine's vasoconstrictive effects; additional studies are needed to define the magnitude of risk. Single doses of pseudoephedrine were not found to adversely affect the fetus during the third trimester of pregnancy (limited data); however, fetal tachycardia was noted in a case report following maternal use of an extended release product for multiple days. Decongestants are not the preferred agents for the treatment of rhinitis during pregnancy. Oral pseudoephedrine should be avoided during the first trimester.

Lactation Enters breast milk (AAP rates "compatible"; AAP 2001 update pending)

Contraindications Hypersensitivity to pseudoephedrine or any component of the formulation; with or within 14 days of MAO inhibitor therapy

Warnings/Precautions Use with caution in the elderly; may be more sensitive to adverse effects; administer with caution to patients with hypertension, hyperthyroidism, diabetes mellitus, cardiovascular disease, ischemic heart disease, increased intraocular pressure, prostatic hyperplasia, seizure disorders, or renal impairment. When used for self-medication (OTC), notify healthcare provider if symptoms do not improve within 7 days or are accompanied by fever. Discontinue and contact healthcare provider if nervousness, dizziness, or sleeplessness occur. Some products may contain sodium. Not for OTC use in children <4 years of age.

Adverse Reactions Frequency not defined.

Cardiovascular: Arrhythmia, hypotension, palpitation, tachycardia

Central nervous system: Chills, confusion, coordination impaired, dizziness, drowsiness, excitability, fatigue, hallucination, headache, insomnia, nervousness, neuritis, restlessness, seizure, transient stimulation, vertigo

Dermatologic: Photosensitivity, rash, urticaria

Gastrointestinal: Anorexia, constipation, diarrhea, dry throat, ischemic colitis, nausea, vomiting, xerostomia

Genitourinary: Difficult urination, dysuria, polyuria, urinary retention

Hematologic: Agranulocytosis, hemolytic anemia, thrombocytopenia

Neuromuscular & skeletal: Tremor, weakness

Ocular: Blurred vision, diplopia

Otic: Tinnitus

Respiratory: Chest/throat tightness, dry nose, dyspnea, nasal congestion, thickening of bronchial secretions, wheezing

Miscellaneous: Anaphylaxis, diaphoresis

Drug Interactions

Metabolism/Transport Effects None known.

Avoid Concomitant Use

Avoid concomitant use of Pseudoephedrine with any of the following: Ergot Derivatives; Iobenguane I 123; MAO Inhibitors

Increased Effect/Toxicity

Pseudoephedrine may increase the levels/effects of: Bromocriptine; Sympathomimetics

The levels/effects of Pseudoephedrine may be increased by: Antacids; Atomoxetine; Cannabinoids; Carbonic Anhydrase Inhibitors; Ergot Derivatives; MAO Inhibitors; Serotonin/Norepinephrine Reuptake Inhibitors

Decreased Effect

Pseudoephedrine may decrease the levels/effects of: Benzylpenicilloyl Polylysine; FentaNYL; Iobenguane I 123

The levels/effects of Pseudoephedrine may be decreased by: Spironolactone

Ethanol/Nutrition/Herb Interactions

Food: Onset of effect may be delayed if pseudoephedrine is taken with food.

Herb/Nutraceutical: Avoid ephedra, yohimbe (may cause hypertension).

Mechanism of Action Directly stimulates alpha-adrenergic receptors of respiratory mucosa causing vasoconstriction; directly stimulates beta-adrenergic receptors causing bronchial relaxation, increased heart rate and contractility

Pharmacodynamics/Kinetics

Onset of action: Decongestant: Oral: 30 minutes (Chua 1989)

Peak effect: Decongestant: Oral: ~1-2 hours (Chua, 1989)

Duration: Immediate release tablet: 3-8 hours (Chua 1989)

Absorption: Rapid (Simons 1996)

Distribution: Children: ~2.5 L/kg (Simons 1996); Adults: 2.64-3.51 L/kg (Kanfer 1993)

Metabolism: Undergoes n-demethylation to norpseudoephedrine (active) (Chua 1989, Kanfer 1993); Hepatic (<1%) (Kanfer 1993)

Half-life elimination: Varies by urine pH and flow rate; alkaline urine decreases renal elimination of pseudoephedrine (Kanfer 1993)

Children: ~3 hours (urine pH ~6.5) (Simons 1996)

Adults: 9-16 hours (pH 8); 3-6 hours (pH 5) (Chua 1989)

Time to peak:

Children (immediate release) ~2 hours (Simons 1996)

Adults (immediate release): 1-3 hours (dose dependent) (Kanfer 1993)

Excretion: Urine (43% to 96% as unchanged drug, 1% to 6% as active norpseudoephedrine); dependent on urine pH and flow rate; alkaline urine decreases renal elimination of pseudoephedrine (Kanfer 1993)

Dosage Oral: General dosing guidelines:

Children:

4-5 years: 15 mg every 4-6 hours: maximum 60 mg/24 hours

6-12 years: 30 mg every 4-6 hours; maximum: 120 mg/24 hours

Children >12 years and Adults: Immediate release: 60 mg every 4-6 hours; Extended release: 120 mg every 12 hours **or** 240 mg every 24 hours; maximum: 240 mg/24 hours

Dosing adjustment in renal impairment: Consider reducing dose

Dietary Considerations Some products may contain sodium. May be taken with or without food.

Administration Do not crush extended release drug product, swallow whole. May administer with or without food. Sudafed® 24 Hour tablet may not completely dissolve and appear in stool

Test Interactions Interferes with urine detection of amphetamine (false-positive)

Dosage Forms Excipient information presented when available (limited, particularly for generics); consult specific product labeling. [DSC] = Discontinued product

Caplet, oral:

Contac® Cold + Flu Maximum Strength Non-Drowsy: Acetaminophen 500 mg and phenylephrine hydrochloride 5 mg

Caplet, extended release, oral, as hydrochloride:

Sudafed® 12 Hour: 120 mg

Liquid, oral, as hydrochloride: 30 mg/5 mL (473 mL)

Children's Nasal Decongestant: 30 mg/5 mL (118 mL) [contains sodium benzoate; raspberry flavor]

Silfedrine Children's: 15 mg/5 mL (118 mL, 237 mL) [ethanol free, sugar free; grape flavor]

Sudafed® Children's: 15 mg/5 mL (118 mL) [ethanol free, sugar free; contains menthol, sodium 5 mg/5 mL, sodium benzoate; grape flavor]

Syrup, oral, as hydrochloride: 30 mg/5 mL (118 mL)

SudoGest Children's: 15 mg/5 mL (118 mL) [ethanol free, sugar free; contains sodium 5 mg/5 mL, sodium benzoate; grape flavor]

Tablet, oral, as hydrochloride: 30 mg

Genaphed™: 30 mg [DSC]

Oranyl: 30 mg [sugar free]

Sudafed® Maximum Strength Nasal Decongestant: 30 mg [contains sodium benzoate]

Sudo-Tab®: 30 mg [contains sodium benzoate]

SudoGest: 30 mg

SudoGest: 60 mg [scored]

Tablet, extended release, oral, as hydrochloride:

Sudafed® 24 Hour: 240 mg

SudoGest 12 Hour: 120 mg

- ◆ **Pseudoephedrine and Acetaminophen** *see* Acetaminophen and Pseudoephedrine *on page 31*
- ◆ **Pseudoephedrine and Carbetapentane** *see* Carbetapentane and Pseudoephedrine *on page 283*
- ◆ **Pseudoephedrine and Chlorpheniramine** *see* Chlorpheniramine and Pseudoephedrine *on page 346*
- ◆ **Pseudoephedrine and Desloratadine** *see* Desloratadine and Pseudoephedrine *on page 476*

Pseudoephedrine and Dextromethorphan

(soo doe e FED rin & deks troe meth OR fan)

Brand Names: U.S. Pedia Relief Cough and Cold [OTC]; Sudafed® Children's Cold & Cough [OTC]

Brand Names: Canada Balminil DM D; Benylin® DM-D; Koffex DM-D; Novahistex® DM Decongestant; Novahistine® DM Decongestant; Robitussin® Childrens Cough & Cold

Index Terms Dextromethorphan and Pseudoephedrine

Pharmacologic Category Antitussive/Decongestant

Use Temporary symptomatic relief of nasal congestion and cough due to common cold, hay fever, upper respiratory allergies

Dosage Relief of nasal congestion and cough: Oral:

General dosing guidelines base on pseudoephedrine component:

Children 2-6 years: 15 mg every 4-6 hours (maximum: 60 mg/24 hours)

Children 6-12 years: 30 mg every 4-6 hours (maximum: 120 mg/24 hours)

Children ≥12 years and Adults: 60 mg every 4-6 hours (maximum: 240 mg/24 hours)

Product-specific dosing:

Children 2-6 years (Sudafed® Children's Cold & Cough): 5 mL every 4 hours (maximum: 20 mL/24 hours)

Children 6-12 years (Sudafed® Children's Cold & Cough): 10 mL every 4 hours (maximum: 40 mL/24 hours)

Children ≥12 years and Adults (Sudafed® Children's Cold & Cough): 20 mL every 4 hours (maximum: 80 mL/24 hours)

Additional Information Complete prescribing information for this medication should be consulted for additional detail.

Dosage Forms Excipient information presented when available (limited, particularly for generics); consult specific product labeling.

Liquid:

Sudafed® Children's Cold & Cough: Pseudoephedrine hydrochloride 15 mg and dextromethorphan hydrobromide 5 mg per 5 mL (120 mL) [alcohol free, sugar free; contains sodium benzoate; cherry berry flavor]

Syrup:

Pedia Relief Cough and Cold: Pseudoephedrine hydrochloride 15 mg and dextromethorphan hydrobromide 7.5 mg per 5 mL (120 mL) [cherry flavor]

◆ **Pseudoephedrine and Fexofenadine** *see* Fexofenadine and Pseudoephedrine *on page 709*

◆ **Pseudoephedrine and Guaifenesin** *see* Guaifenesin and Pseudoephedrine *on page 813*

Pseudoephedrine and Ibuprofen

(soo doe e FED rin & eye byoo PROE fen)

Brand Names: U.S. Advil® Cold & Sinus [OTC]; Proprinal® Cold and Sinus [OTC]

Brand Names: Canada Advil® Cold & Sinus; Advil® Cold & Sinus Daytime; Children's Advil® Cold; Sudafed® Sinus Advance

Index Terms Ibuprofen and Pseudoephedrine

Pharmacologic Category Decongestant/Analgesic

Use For temporary relief of cold, sinus, and flu symptoms (including nasal congestion, sinus pressure, headache, minor body aches and pains, and fever)

Pregnancy Risk Factor Ibuprofen: B/D (3rd trimester)

Dosage OTC labeling: Oral: Children ≥12 years and Adults: Ibuprofen 200 mg and pseudoephedrine 30 mg per dose: One dose every 4-6 hours as needed; may increase to 2 doses if necessary (maximum: 6 doses/24 hours). Contact healthcare provider if symptoms have not improved within 7 days when treating cold symptoms or within 3 days when treating fever.

Additional Information Complete prescribing information for this medication should be consulted for additional detail.

Dosage Forms Excipient information presented when available (limited, particularly for generics); consult specific product labeling.

Caplet:

Advil® Cold & Sinus, Proprinal® Cold and Sinus: Pseudoephedrine hydrochloride 30 mg and ibuprofen 200 mg

Capsule, liquid filled:

Advil® Cold & Sinus: Pseudoephedrine hydrochloride 30 mg and ibuprofen 200 mg [solubilized ibuprofen as free acid and potassium salt; contains potassium 20 mg/capsule and coconut oil]

◆ **Pseudoephedrine and Loratadine** *see* Loratadine and Pseudoephedrine *on page 1032*

Pseudoephedrine and Methscopolamine

(soo doe e FED rin & meth skoe POL a meen)

Brand Names: U.S. AlleRx™-D [DSC]

Index Terms Methscopolamine and Pseudoephedrine; Pseudoephedrine hydrochloride and Methscopolamine Nitrate

Pharmacologic Category Decongestant/Anticholingeric Combination

Use Relief of symptoms of allergic rhinitis, vasomotor rhinitis, sinusitis, and the common cold

Pregnancy Risk Factor C

Dosage Oral: Children ≥12 years and Adults (Allerx™-D): One tablet every 12 hours (maximum: 2 tablets/24 hours)

Additional Information Complete prescribing information for this medication should be consulted for additional detail.

Dosage Forms Excipient information presented when available (limited, particularly for generics); consult specific product labeling. [DSC] = Discontinued product

Tablet:

AlleRx™-D [DSC]: Pseudoephedrine hydrochloride 120 mg and methscopolamine nitrate 2.5 mg

◆ **Pseudoephedrine and Triprolidine** *see* Triprolidine and Pseudoephedrine *on page 1741*

◆ **Pseudoephedrine, Chlorpheniramine, and Dextromethorphan** *see* Chlorpheniramine, Pseudoephedrine, and Dextromethorphan *on page 347*

◆ **Pseudoephedrine, Dextromethorphan, and Guaifenesin** *see* Guaifenesin, Pseudoephedrine, and Dextromethorphan *on page 814*

◆ **Pseudoephedrine, Guaifenesin, and Codeine** *see* Guaifenesin, Pseudoephedrine, and Codeine *on page 813*

◆ **Pseudoephedrine Hydrochloride** *see* Pseudoephedrine *on page 1430*

◆ **Pseudoephedrine Hydrochloride and Acetaminophen** *see* Acetaminophen and Pseudoephedrine *on page 31*

◆ **Pseudoephedrine Hydrochloride and Acrivastine** *see* Acrivastine and Pseudoephedrine *on page 39*

◆ **Pseudoephedrine hydrochloride and Methscopolamine Nitrate** *see* Pseudoephedrine and Methscopolamine *on page 1432*

◆ **Pseudoephedrine Sulfate** *see* Pseudoephedrine *on page 1430*

◆ **Pseudofrin (Can)** *see* Pseudoephedrine *on page 1430*

◆ **Pseudomonic Acid A** *see* Mupirocin *on page 1161*

Psyllium (SIL i yum)

Brand Names: U.S. Bulk-K [OTC]; Fiberall® [OTC]; Fibro-Lax [OTC]; Fibro-XL [OTC]; Genfiber™ [OTC] [DSC]; Hydrocil® Instant [OTC]; Konsyl-D™ [OTC]; Konsyl® Easy Mix™ [OTC]; Konsyl® Orange [OTC]; Konsyl® Original [OTC]; Konsyl® [OTC]; Metamucil® Plus Calcium [OTC]; Metamucil® Smooth Texture [OTC]; Metamucil® [OTC]; Natural Fiber Therapy Smooth Texture [OTC]; Natural Fiber Therapy [OTC]; Reguloid [OTC]

Brand Names: Canada Metamucil®

Index Terms Plantago Seed; Plantain Seed; Psyllium Husk; Psyllium Hydrophilic Mucilloid

Pharmacologic Category Antidiarrheal; Fiber Supplement; Laxative, Bulk-Producing

Additional Appendix Information

Laxatives, Classification and Properties *on page 1893*

Use OTC labeling: Dietary fiber supplement; treatment of occasional constipation; reduce risk of coronary heart disease (CHD)

Unlabeled Use Treatment of diarrhea, chronic constipation, irritable bowel syndrome, inflammatory bowel disease, colon cancer, or diabetes

Contraindications Hypersensitivity to psyllium or any component of the formulation; fecal impaction; GI obstruction

Warnings/Precautions Use with caution in patients with esophageal strictures, ulcers, stenosis, intestinal adhesions, or difficulty swallowing. Use with caution in the elderly; may have insufficient fluid intake which may predispose them to fecal impaction and bowel obstruction. Products must be taken with at least 8 ounces of fluid in order to prevent choking. To reduce the risk of CHD, the soluble fiber from psyllium should be used in conjunction with a diet low in saturated fat and cholesterol. Some products may contain calcium, potassium, sodium, soy lecithin, or phenylalanine.

When used for self-medication (OTC), do not use in the presence of abdominal pain, nausea, or vomiting. Notify healthcare provider in case of sudden changes of bowel habits which last >2 weeks or in case of rectal bleeding. Not for self-treatment of constipation lasting >1 week

Adverse Reactions Frequency not defined.

Gastrointestinal: Abdominal cramps, constipation, diarrhea, esophageal or bowel obstruction

Respiratory: Bronchospasm

Miscellaneous: Anaphylaxis upon inhalation in susceptible individuals, rhinoconjunctivitis

Drug Interactions

Metabolism/Transport Effects None known.

Avoid Concomitant Use There are no known interactions where it is recommended to avoid concomitant use.

Increased Effect/Toxicity There are no known significant interactions involving an increase in effect.

Decreased Effect There are no known significant interactions involving a decrease in effect.

Mechanism of Action Psyllium is a soluble fiber. It absorbs water in the intestine to form a viscous liquid which promotes peristalsis and reduces transit time.

Pharmacodynamics/Kinetics

Onset of action: Relief of constipation: 12-72 hours

Absorption: None; small amounts of grain extracts present in the preparation have been reportedly absorbed following colonic hydrolysis

Dosage Oral: General dosing guidelines; consult specific product labeling.

Adequate intake for total fiber: Note: The definition of "fiber" varies; however, the soluble fiber in psyllium is only one type of fiber which makes up the daily recommended intake of total fiber.

Children 1-3 years: 19 g/day

Children 4-8 years: 25 g/day

Children 9-13 years: Males: 31 g/day; Females: 26 g/day

Children 14-18 years: Males: 38 g/day; Females: 26 g/day

Adults 19-50 years: Males: 38 g/day; Females: 25 g/day

Adults ≥51 years: Males: 30 g/day; Females: 21 g/day

Pregnancy: 28 g/day

Lactation: 29 g/day

Constipation:

Children 6-11 years: Psyllium: 1.25-15 g per day in divided doses

Children ≥12 years and Adults: Psyllium: 2.5-30 g per day in divided doses

Reduce risk of CHD: Children ≥12 years and Adults: Soluble fiber ≥7 g (psyllium seed husk ≥10.2 g) per day

Dietary Considerations Products should be taken with at least 8 ounces of fluids. Some products may contain phenylalanine, potassium, sodium, as well as additional ingredients. Check individual product information for caloric and nutritional value.

When used to reduce the risk of CHD, the amount of **soluble fiber** from psyllium should be ≥7 g/day and it should be used in conjunction with a diet low in saturated fat and cholesterol.

Administration Inhalation of psyllium dust may cause sensitivity to psyllium (eg, runny nose, watery eyes, wheezing). Drink at least 8 ounces of liquid with each dose. Powder must be mixed in a glass of water or juice. Capsules should be swallowed one at a time. When more than one dose is required, they should be divided throughout the day. Separate dose by at least 2 hours from other drug therapies.

Dosage Forms Excipient information presented when available (limited, particularly for generics); consult specific product labeling. [DSC] = Discontinued product

Capsule, oral: 500 mg

Fibro-XL: 0.675 g [sugar free; provides dietary fiber 3.8 g and soluble fiber 3 g per 7 capsules]

Genfiber™: 0.52 g [DSC] [provides dietary fiber 3 g and soluble fiber 2 g per 6 capsules]

Konsyl®: 0.52 g [sugar free; contains calcium 8 mg/capsule, potassium <11 mg/capsule, sodium 1 mg/capsule; provides dietary fiber 3 g and soluble fiber 2 g per 5 capsules]

Metamucil®: 0.52 g [contains potassium 5 mg/capsule; provides dietary fiber 3 g and soluble fiber 2.1 g per 6 capsules]

Metamucil® Plus Calcium: 0.52 g [contains calcium 60 mg/capsule, potassium 6 mg/capsule; provides dietary fiber 3 g and soluble fiber 2.1 g per 5 capsules]

Reguloid: 0.52 g [provides dietary fiber 3 g and soluble fiber 2 g per 6 capsules]

Powder, oral: (454 g)

Bulk-K: (392 g)

Fiberall®: (454 g) [sugar free; contains phenylalanine; orange flavor; psyllium is in combination with other fiber sources; also contains vitamins and minerals]

Fibro-Lax: (140 g, 392 g)

Genfiber™: (397 g [DSC]) [contains sodium; natural flavor]

Genfiber™: (397 g [DSC]) [contains sodium; orange flavor]

Hydrocil® Instant: (300 g) [sugar free]

Hydrocil® Instant: 3.5 g/packet (30s, 500s) [sugar free; provides dietary fiber 3 g and soluble fiber 2.4 g per packet]

Konsyl-D™: (325 g, 397 g, 500 g) [contains calcium, dextrose, potassium, sodium]

Konsyl-D™: 3.4 g/packet (100s, 500s) [contains calcium 6 mg/packet, dextrose 3.1 g/packet, potassium 31 mg/packet, sodium 3 mg/packet; provides dietary fiber 3 g and soluble fiber 2 g per packet]

Konsyl® Easy Mix™: (250 g) [sugar free; contains calcium, potassium, sodium]

Konsyl® Easy Mix™: 6 g/packet (500s) [sugar free; contains calcium 10 mg/packet, potassium 55 mg/packet, sodium 5 mg/packet; provides dietary fiber 5 g and soluble fiber 3 g per packet]

Konsyl® Orange: (538 g) [contains calcium, potassium, sodium, sucrose; orange flavor]

Konsyl® Orange: 3.4 g/packet (30s) [contains calcium 6 mg/packet, potassium 31 mg/packet, sodium 3 mg/packet, sucrose 8 g/packet; orange flavor; provides dietary fiber 3 g and soluble fiber 2 g per packet]

Konsyl® Orange: (425 g) [sugar free; contains calcium, phenylalanine, potassium, sodium; orange flavor]

Konsyl® Original: (300 g, 450 g) [sugar free; contains calcium, potassium, sodium]

Konsyl® Original: 6 g/packet (30s, 100s, 500s) [sugar free; contains calcium 10 mg/packet, potassium 55 mg/packet, sodium 5 mg/packet; provides dietary fiber 5 g and soluble fiber 3 g per packet]

Metamucil®: (390 g, 570 g, 870 g) [contains potassium, sodium; unflavored]

Metamucil®: (570 g, 870 g, 1254 g) [contains potassium, sodium; orange flavor]

Metamucil® Smooth Texture: (609 g, 912 g, 1368 g) [contains potassium, sodium; orange flavor]

Metamucil® Smooth Texture: 3.4 g/packet (30s) [contains potassium 30 mg/packet, sodium 5 mg/packet; orange flavor; provides dietary fiber 3 g and soluble fiber ~2 g per packet]
Metamucil® Smooth Texture: (283 g, 425 g, 660 g) [sugar free; contains phenylalanine, potassium, sodium; berry burst flavor]
Metamucil® Smooth Texture: (173 g, 300 g, 450 g, 660 g, 1020 g) [sugar free; contains phenylalanine, potassium, sodium; orange flavor]
Metamucil® Smooth Texture: (288 g, 432 g, 684 g) [sugar free; contains phenylalanine, potassium, sodium; pink lemonade flavor]
Metamucil® Smooth Texture: (300 g, 450 g, 690 g) [sugar free; contains potassium, sodium; unflavored]
Metamucil® Smooth Texture: 3.4 g/packet (30s) [sugar free; contains phenylalanine 16 mg/packet, potassium 30 mg/packet, sodium 5 mg/packet; berry burst flavor; provides dietary fiber 3 g and soluble fiber ~2 g per packet]
Metamucil® Smooth Texture: 3.4 g/packet (30s) [sugar free; contains phenylalanine 25 mg/packet, potassium 30 mg/packet, sodium 5 mg/packet; orange flavor; provides dietary fiber 3 g and soluble fiber ~2 g per packet]
Natural Fiber Therapy: (390 g, 539 g) [natural flavor]
Natural Fiber Therapy: (390 g, 539 g) [contains sodium; orange flavor]
Natural Fiber Therapy Smooth Texture: (300 g) [sugar free; orange flavor]
Reguloid: (369 g, 540 g) [contains sodium; orange flavor]
Reguloid: (369 g, 540 g) [contains sodium; regular flavor]
Reguloid: (284 g, 426 g) [sugar free; contains phenylalanine, sodium; orange flavor]
Reguloid: (284 g, 426 g) [sugar free; contains phenylalanine, sodium; regular flavor]

Wafer, oral:
Metamucil®: 3.4 g/2 wafers (24s) [contains potassium 60 mg/2 wafers, sodium 20 mg/2 wafers, soya lecithin; apple flavor; provides dietary fiber 6 g and soluble fiber 3 g per 2 wafers]
Metamucil®: 3.4 g/2 wafers (24s) [contains potassium 60 mg/2 wafers, sodium 20 mg/2 wafers, soya lecithin; cinnamon-spice flavor; provides dietary fiber 6 g and soluble fiber 3 g per 2 wafers]

- **Psyllium Husk** *see* Psyllium *on page 1432*
- **Psyllium Hydrophilic Mucilloid** *see* Psyllium *on page 1432*
- **Pteroylglutamic Acid** *see* Folic Acid *on page 748*
- **PTG** *see* Teniposide *on page 1644*
- **PTU (error-prone abbreviation)** *see* Propylthiouracil *on page 1426*
- **Pulmicort® (Can)** *see* Budesonide (Systemic) *on page 237*
- **Pulmicort Flexhaler®** *see* Budesonide (Systemic) *on page 237*
- **Pulmicort Respules®** *see* Budesonide (Systemic) *on page 237*
- **Pulmophylline (Can)** *see* Theophylline *on page 1667*
- **Pulmozyme®** *see* Dornase Alfa *on page 547*
- **Puregon® (Can)** *see* Follitropin Beta *on page 750*
- **Purified Chick Embryo Cell** *see* Rabies Vaccine *on page 1453*
- **Purinethol®** *see* Mercaptopurine *on page 1077*

Pyrantel Pamoate (pi RAN tel PAM oh ate)

Brand Names: U.S. Pin-X® [OTC]; Reese's Pinworm Medicine [OTC]
Brand Names: Canada Combantrin™
Pharmacologic Category Anthelmintic
Use Treatment of pinworms (*Enterobius vermicularis*) and roundworms (*Ascaris lumbricoides*)
Unlabeled Use Treatment of whipworms (*Trichuris trichiura*) and hookworms (*Ancylostoma duodenale*)
Pregnancy Risk Factor C
Contraindications Hypersensitivity to pyrantel pamoate or any component of the formulation
Warnings/Precautions Use with caution in patients with liver impairment, anemia, malnutrition, or pregnancy. Since pinworm infections are easily spread to others, treat all family members in close contact with the patient.
Adverse Reactions Frequency not defined.
Central nervous system: Dizziness, drowsiness, insomnia, headache
Dermatologic: Rash
Gastrointestinal: Abdominal cramps, anorexia, diarrhea, nausea, tenesmus, vomiting
Hepatic: Liver enzymes increased
Neuromuscular & skeletal: Weakness

Drug Interactions
Metabolism/Transport Effects None known.
Avoid Concomitant Use There are no known interactions where it is recommended to avoid concomitant use.
Increased Effect/Toxicity There are no known significant interactions involving an increase in effect.
Decreased Effect
The levels/effects of Pyrantel Pamoate may be decreased by: Aminoquinolines (Antimalarial)

Stability Protect from light.
Mechanism of Action Causes the release of acetylcholine and inhibits cholinesterase; acts as a depolarizing neuromuscular blocker, paralyzing the helminths
Pharmacodynamics/Kinetics
Absorption: Oral: Poor
Metabolism: Partially hepatic
Time to peak, serum: 1-3 hours
Excretion: Feces (50% as unchanged drug); urine (7% as unchanged drug)

Dosage Children and Adults (purgation is not required prior to use): Oral: **Note:** Dose is expressed as pyrantel base:
Roundworm, pinworm, or trichostrongyliasis: 11 mg/kg administered as a single dose; maximum dose: 1 g. (**Note:** For pinworm infection, dosage should be repeated in 2 weeks and all family members should be treated).
Hookworm (unlabeled use): 11 mg/kg administered once daily for 3 days

Administration May be mixed with milk or fruit juice.
Monitoring Parameters Stool for presence of eggs, worms, and occult blood, serum AST and ALT
Dosage Forms Excipient information presented when available (limited, particularly for generics); consult specific product labeling.
Suspension, oral, as pamoate:
Pin-X®: 144 mg/mL (30 mL, 60 mL) [sugar free; contains sodium benzoate; caramel flavor; equivalent to pyrantel base 50 mg/mL]
Reese's Pinworm Medicine: 144 mg/mL (30 mL, 60 mL, 240 mL) [equivalent to pyrantel base 50 mg/mL]
Tablet, chewable, oral, as pamoate:
Pin-X®: 720.5 mg [scored; contains aspartame; equivalent to pyrantel base 250 mg]

Pyrazinamide (peer a ZIN a mide)

Brand Names: Canada Tebrazid™
Index Terms Pyrazinoic Acid Amide
Pharmacologic Category Antitubercular Agent
Use Adjunctive treatment of tuberculosis in combination with other antituberculosis agents
Pregnancy Risk Factor C

Pregnancy Considerations Teratogenic effects have not been observed in animal reproduction studies. Due to the risk of tuberculosis to the fetus, treatment is recommended when the probability of maternal disease is moderate to high. Although not recommended as the initial treatment regimen, the use of pyrazinamide during pregnancy is recommended by The World Health Organization (Blumberg, 2003).

Lactation Enters breast milk/use caution

Contraindications Hypersensitivity to pyrazinamide or any component of the formulation; acute gout; severe hepatic damage

Warnings/Precautions Use with caution in patients with a history of alcoholism, renal failure, chronic gout, diabetes mellitus, or porphyria. Dose-related hepatotoxicity ranging from transient ALT/AST elevations to jaundice, hepatitis and/or liver atrophy (rare) has occurred. Use with caution in patients receiving concurrent medications associated with hepatotoxicity (particularly with rifampin).

Adverse Reactions

1% to 10%:

Central nervous system: Malaise

Gastrointestinal: Anorexia, nausea, vomiting

Neuromuscular & skeletal: Arthralgia, myalgia

<1% (Limited to important or life-threatening): Acne, angioedema (rare), anticoagulant effect, dysuria, fever, gout, hepatotoxicity, interstitial nephritis, itching, photosensitivity, porphyria, rash, sideroblastic anemia, thrombocytopenia, urticaria

Drug Interactions

Metabolism/Transport Effects None known.

Avoid Concomitant Use There are no known interactions where it is recommended to avoid concomitant use.

Increased Effect/Toxicity

Pyrazinamide may increase the levels/effects of: CycloSPORINE (Systemic); Rifampin

Decreased Effect

Pyrazinamide may decrease the levels/effects of: CycloSPORINE

Stability Store at controlled room temperature of 15°C to 30°C (59°F to 86°F).

Mechanism of Action Converted to pyrazinoic acid in susceptible strains of *Mycobacterium* which lowers the pH of the environment; exact mechanism of action has not been elucidated

Pharmacodynamics/Kinetics Bacteriostatic or bactericidal depending on drug's concentration at infection site

Absorption: Well absorbed

Distribution: Widely into body tissues and fluids including liver, lung, and CSF

Relative diffusion from blood into CSF: Adequate with or without inflammation (exceeds usual MICs)

CSF:blood level ratio: Inflamed meninges: 100%

Protein binding: 50%

Metabolism: Hepatic

Half-life elimination: 9-10 hours

Time to peak, serum: Within 2 hours

Excretion: Urine (4% as unchanged drug)

Dosage Oral: Treatment of tuberculosis:

Note: Used as part of a multidrug regimen. Treatment regimens consist of an initial 2-month phase, followed by a continuation phase of 4 or 7 additional months; pyrazinamide is administered in the initial phase of treatment.

Children:

HIV negative (CDC, 2003):

Daily therapy: 15-30 mg/kg/day (maximum: 2 g/day)

Twice weekly directly observed therapy (DOT): 50 mg/kg/dose (maximum: 2 g/dose)

HIV-exposed/-infected: Daily therapy: 20-40 mg/kg/dose once daily (maximum: 2 g/day) (CDC, 2009)

Adults: Suggested dosing based on lean body weight (Blumberg, 2003; CDC, 2003):

Daily therapy:

40-55 kg: 1000 mg

56-75 kg: 1500 mg

76-90 kg: 2000 mg (maximum dose regardless of weight)

Twice weekly directly observed therapy (DOT):

40-55 kg: 2000 mg

56-75 kg: 3000 mg

76-90 kg: 4000 mg (maximum dose regardless of weight)

Three times/week DOT:

40-55 kg: 1500 mg

56-75 kg: 2500 mg

76-90 kg: 3000 mg (maximum dose regardless of weight)

Dosing adjustment in renal impairment: Adults: Cl_{cr} <30 mL/minute or receiving hemodialysis: Treatment of TB: 25-35 mg/kg/dose 3 times per week administered after dialysis (Blumberg, 2003; CDC, 2003)

Monitoring Parameters Periodic liver function tests, serum uric acid, sputum culture, chest x-ray 2-3 months into treatment and at completion

Test Interactions Reacts with Acetest® and Ketostix® to produce pinkish-brown color

Dosage Forms Excipient information presented when available (limited, particularly for generics); consult specific product labeling.

Tablet, oral: 500 mg

Extemporaneous Preparations A 100 mg/mL oral suspension may be made with tablets. Crush two-hundred pyrazinamide 500 mg tablets and mix with a suspension containing 500 mL methylcellulose 1% and 500 mL simple syrup. Add to this a suspension containing one-hundred forty crushed pyrazinamide tablets in 350 mL methylcellulose 1% and 350 mL simple syrup to make 1.7 L suspension. Label "shake well" and "refrigerate". Stable for 60 days refrigerated (preferred) and 45 days at room temperature.

Nahata MC, Morosco RS, and Peritre SP, "Stability of Pyrazinamide in Two Suspensions," *Am J Health Syst Pharm*, 1995, 52(14):1558-60.

◆ **Pyrazinoic Acid Amide** *see* Pyrazinamide *on page 1434*

Pyrethrins and Piperonyl Butoxide

(pye RE thrins & pi PER oh nil byo TOKS ide)

Brand Names: U.S. A-200® Lice Treatment Kit [OTC]; A-200® Maximum Strength [OTC]; Licide® [OTC]; Pronto® Complete Lice Removal System [OTC]; Pronto® Plus Lice Killing Mousse Plus Vitamin E [OTC]; Pronto® Plus Lice Killing Mousse Shampoo Plus Natural Extracts and Oils [OTC]; Pronto® Plus Warm Oil Treatment and Conditioner [OTC]; RID® Maximum Strength [OTC]

Brand Names: Canada Pronto® Lice Control; R & C™ II; R & C™ Shampoo/Conditioner; RID® Mousse

Index Terms Piperonyl Butoxide and Pyrethrins

Pharmacologic Category Antiparasitic Agent, Topical; Pediculocide; Shampoo, Pediculocide

Use Treatment of *Pediculus humanus* infestations (head lice, body lice, pubic lice, and their eggs)

Pregnancy Risk Factor C

Dosage Application of pyrethrins: Topical products:

Apply enough solution to completely wet infested area, including hair

Allow to remain on area for 10 minutes

Wash and rinse with large amounts of warm water.

Use fine-toothed comb to remove lice and eggs from hair

Shampoo hair to restore body and luster

Treatment may be repeated if necessary once in a 24-hour period

Repeat treatment in 7-10 days to kill newly hatched lice

Note: Keep out of eyes when rinsing hair; protect eyes with a wash cloth or towel

Additional Information Complete prescribing information for this medication should be consulted for additional detail.

Dosage Forms Excipient information presented when available (limited, particularly for generics); consult specific product labeling.

Kit:

A-200® Lice Treatment Kit:

Shampoo: Pyrethrins 0.33% and piperonyl butoxide 4% (120 mL)

Solution [spray; for bedding; not for human or animal use]: Permethrin 0.5% (180 mL)

[packaged with nit removal comb]

Pronto® Complete Lice Removal System:

Shampoo: Pyrethrins 0.33% and piperonyl butoxide 4% (60 mL)

Solution, topical: Benzalkonium chloride 0.1% (60 mL) [lice egg remover antiseptic]

[packaged with household furniture spray and nit removal comb]

Oil, topical:

Pronto® Plus Warm Oil Treatment and Conditioner: Pyrethrins 0.33% and piperonyl butoxide 4% (36 mL) [fruity herbal scent; packaged with nit removal comb]

Shampoo:

A-200® Maximum Strength: Pyrethrins 0.33% and piperonyl butoxide 4% (60 mL, 120 mL) [contains benzyl alcohol; packaged with nit removal comb]

Licide®: Pyrethrins 0.33% and piperonyl butoxide 4% (120 mL) [packaged with nit removal comb; also available in a kit containing shampoo, household spray, and nit removal comb]

Pronto® Plus Lice Killing Mousse Shampoo Plus Natural Extracts and Oils: Pyrethrins 0.33% and piperonyl butoxide 4% (60 mL) [packaged with nit removal comb]

Pronto® Plus Lice Killing Mousse Shampoo Plus Vitamin E: Pyrethrins 0.33% and piperonyl butoxide 4% (120 mL) [blue mousse shampoo; contains vitamin E; packaged with nit removal comb]

RID® Maximum Strength: Pyrethrins 0.33% and piperonyl butoxide 4% (60 mL, 120 mL, 180 mL, 240 mL) [packaged with nit removal comb; also available in a kit containing shampoo, gel, and furniture spray]

◆ **Pyri-500 [OTC]** *see* Pyridoxine *on page 1437*

◆ **Pyrichlor PE™** *see* Chlorpheniramine, Pyrilamine, and Phenylephrine *on page 348*

◆ **2-Pyridine Aldoxime Methochloride** *see* Pralidoxime *on page 1388*

◆ **Pyridium®** *see* Phenazopyridine *on page 1337*

Pyridostigmine (peer id oh STIG meen)

Brand Names: U.S. Mestinon®; Mestinon® Timespan®; Regonol®

Brand Names: Canada Mestinon®; Mestinon®-SR

Index Terms Pyridostigmine Bromide

Pharmacologic Category Acetylcholinesterase Inhibitor

Use Symptomatic treatment of myasthenia gravis; antagonism of nondepolarizing neuromuscular blockers

Military use: Pretreatment for Soman nerve gas exposure

Pregnancy Risk Factor B

Pregnancy Considerations Safety has not been established for use during pregnancy. The potential benefit to the mother should outweigh the potential risk to the fetus. When pyridostigmine is needed in myasthenic mothers, giving dose parenterally 1 hour before completion of the second stage of labor may facilitate delivery and protect the neonate during the immediate postnatal state.

Lactation Enters breast milk/compatible

Contraindications Hypersensitivity to pyridostigmine, bromides, or any component of the formulation; GI or GU obstruction

Warnings/Precautions Use with caution in patients with epilepsy, bradycardia, hyperthyroidism, cardiac arrhythmias, or peptic ulcer; use with extreme caution in patients with asthma or bronchospastic disease; adequate facilities should be available for cardiopulmonary resuscitation when testing and adjusting dose for myasthenia gravis; have atropine and epinephrine ready to treat hypersensitivity reactions; overdosage may result in cholinergic crisis, this must be distinguished from myasthenic crisis; anticholinesterase insensitivity can develop for brief or prolonged periods. Regonol® injection contains 1% benzyl alcohol as the preservative (not intended for use in newborns). **[U.S. Boxed Warning]: Regonol® injection must be administered by trained personnel.**

Adverse Reactions Frequency not defined.

Cardiovascular: Arrhythmias (especially bradycardia), AV block, cardiac arrest, decreased carbon monoxide, flushing, hypotension, nodal rhythm, nonspecific ECG changes, syncope, tachycardia

Central nervous system: Convulsions, dizziness, drowsiness, dysphonia, headache, loss of consciousness

Dermatologic: Skin rash, thrombophlebitis (I.V.), urticaria

Gastrointestinal: Abdominal pain, diarrhea, dysphagia, flatulence, hyperperistalsis, nausea, salivation, stomach cramps, vomiting

Genitourinary: Urinary urgency

Neuromuscular & skeletal: Arthralgia, dysarthria, fasciculations, muscle cramps, myalgia, spasms, weakness

Ocular: Amblyopia, lacrimation, small pupils

Respiratory: Bronchial secretions increased, bronchiolar constriction, bronchospasm, dyspnea, laryngospasm, respiratory arrest, respiratory depression, respiratory muscle paralysis

Miscellaneous: Allergic reactions, anaphylaxis, diaphoresis increased

Drug Interactions

Metabolism/Transport Effects None known.

Avoid Concomitant Use There are no known interactions where it is recommended to avoid concomitant use.

Increased Effect/Toxicity

Pyridostigmine may increase the levels/effects of: Beta-Blockers; Cholinergic Agonists; Succinylcholine

The levels/effects of Pyridostigmine may be increased by: Corticosteroids (Systemic)

Decreased Effect

Pyridostigmine may decrease the levels/effects of: Neuromuscular-Blocking Agents (Nondepolarizing)

The levels/effects of Pyridostigmine may be decreased by: Dipyridamole; Methocarbamol

Stability

Injection: Protect from light.

Tablet:

30 mg: Store under refrigeration at 2°C to 8°C (36°F to 46°F). Protect from light. Stable at room temperature for up to 3 months.

Mestinon®: Store at 25°C (77°F). Protect from moisture.

Mechanism of Action Inhibits destruction of acetylcholine by acetylcholinesterase which facilitates transmission of impulses across myoneural junction

Pharmacodynamics/Kinetics

Onset of action: Oral, I.M.: 15-30 minutes; I.V. injection: 2-5 minutes

Duration: Oral: Up to 6-8 hours (due to slow absorption); I.V.: 2-3 hours

Absorption: Oral: Very poor

Distribution: 19 ± 12 L

Metabolism: Hepatic

Bioavailability: 10% to 20%
Half-life elimination: 1-2 hours; Renal failure: ≤6 hours
Excretion: Urine (80% to 90% as unchanged drug)

Dosage

Myasthenia gravis:

Oral:

Children: 7 mg/kg/24 hours divided into 5-6 doses

Adults: Highly individualized dosing ranges: 60-1500 mg/day, usually 600 mg/day divided into 5-6 doses, spaced to provide maximum relief

Sustained release formulation: Highly individualized dosing ranges: 180-540 mg once or twice daily (doses separated by at least 6 hours); **Note:** Most clinicians reserve sustained release dosage form for bedtime dose only.

I.M., slow I.V. push:

Children: 0.05-0.15 mg/kg/dose

Adults: To supplement oral dosage pre- and postoperatively during labor and postpartum, during myasthenic crisis, or when oral therapy is impractical: ~1/30th of oral dose; observe patient closely for cholinergic reactions

or

I.V. infusion: Initial: 2 mg/hour with gradual titration in increments of 0.5-1 mg/hour, up to a maximum rate of 4 mg/hour

Reversal of nondepolarizing muscle relaxants: **Note:** Atropine sulfate (0.6-1.2 mg) I.V. immediately prior to pyridostigmine to minimize side effects: I.V.:

Children: Dosing range: 0.1-0.25 mg/kg/dose*

Adults: 0.1-0.25 mg/kg/dose; 10-20 mg is usually sufficient*

*Full recovery usually occurs ≤15 minutes, but ≥30 minutes may be required

Pretreatment for Soman nerve gas exposure (military use): Oral: Adults: 30 mg every 8 hours beginning several hours prior to exposure; discontinue at first sign of nerve agent exposure, then begin atropine and pralidoxime

Dosage adjustment in renal dysfunction: Lower dosages may be required due to prolonged elimination; no specific recommendations have been published

Administration Do **not** crush sustained release tablet.

Monitoring Parameters Observe for cholinergic reactions, particularly when administered I.V.

Test Interactions Increased aminotransferase [ALT/AST] (S), increased amylase (S)

Dosage Forms Excipient information presented when available (limited, particularly for generics); consult specific product labeling.

Injection, solution, as bromide:

Regonol®: 5 mg/mL (2 mL) [contains benzyl alcohol]

Syrup, oral, as bromide:

Mestinon®: 60 mg/5 mL (480 mL) [contains ethanol 5%, sodium benzoate; raspberry flavor]

Tablet, oral, as bromide: 60 mg

Mestinon®: 60 mg [scored]

Tablet, sustained release, oral, as bromide:

Mestinon® Timespan®: 180 mg [scored]

◆ **Pyridostigmine Bromide** *see* Pyridostigmine *on page 1436*

Pyridoxine (peer i DOKS een)

Brand Names: U.S. Aminoxin® [OTC]; Pyri-500 [OTC]

Index Terms B6; B_6; Pyridoxine Hydrochloride; Vitamin B_6

Pharmacologic Category Vitamin, Water Soluble

Use Prevention and treatment of vitamin B_6 deficiency, pyridoxine-dependent seizures in infants

Unlabeled Use Treatment and prophylaxis of neurological toxicities (ie, seizures, coma) associated with isoniazid, hydrazine, and Gyromitrin-containing mushroom (false morel) overdose/toxicity

Pregnancy Risk Factor A

Pregnancy Considerations Crosses the placenta; available evidence suggests safe use during pregnancy

Lactation Enters breast milk/compatible (AAP rates "compatible"; AAP 2001 update pending)

Contraindications Hypersensitivity to pyridoxine or any component of the formulation

Warnings/Precautions Severe, permanent peripheral neuropathies have been reported; neurotoxicity is more common with long-term administration of large doses (>2 g/day). Dependence and withdrawal may occur with doses >200 mg/day. Single vitamin deficiency is rare; evaluate for other deficiencies. Some parenteral products contain aluminum; use caution in patients with impaired renal function and neonates. Guidelines suggest that at least 8-24 g be stocked. This is enough to treat 1 patient weighing 100 kg for an initial 8- to 24-hour period. In areas where tuberculosis is common, hospitals should consider stocking 24 g. This is enough to treat 1 patient for 24 hours (Dart, 2009).

Adverse Reactions Frequency not defined.

Central nervous system: Headache, seizure (following very large I.V. doses), somnolence

Endocrine & metabolic: Acidosis, folic acid decreased

Gastrointestinal: Nausea

Hepatic: AST increased

Neuromuscular & skeletal: Neuropathy, paresthesia

Miscellaneous: Allergic reactions

Drug Interactions

Metabolism/Transport Effects None known.

Avoid Concomitant Use There are no known interactions where it is recommended to avoid concomitant use.

Increased Effect/Toxicity There are no known significant interactions involving an increase in effect.

Decreased Effect

Pyridoxine may decrease the levels/effects of: Altretamine; Barbiturates; Fosphenytoin; Levodopa; Phenytoin

Stability Store at 20°C to 25°C (68°F to 77°F). Protect from light.

Mechanism of Action Precursor to pyridoxal, which functions in the metabolism of proteins, carbohydrates, and fats; pyridoxal also aids in the release of liver and muscle-stored glycogen and in the synthesis of GABA (within the central nervous system) and heme

Pharmacodynamics/Kinetics

Absorption: Enteral, parenteral: Well absorbed

Metabolism: Hepatic to 4-pyridoxic acid (active form) and other metabolites

Half-life elimination: Biologic: 15-20 days

Excretion: Urine

Dosage

Recommended daily allowance (RDA):

Children:

1-3 years: 0.9 mg

4-6 years: 1.3 mg

7-10 years: 1.6 mg

Adults:

Males: 1.7-2 mg

Females: 1.4-1.6 mg

Pyridoxine-dependent Infants:

Oral: 2-100 mg/day

I.M., I.V., SubQ: 10-100 mg

Dietary deficiency: Oral:

Children: 5-25 mg/24 hours for 3 weeks, then 1.5-2.5 mg/day in multiple vitamin product

Adults: 10-20 mg/day for 3 weeks

Drug-induced neuritis (eg, isoniazid, hydralazine, penicillamine, cycloserine): Oral:
Children:
Treatment: 10-50 mg/24 hours
Prophylaxis: 1-2 mg/kg/24 hours
Adults:
Treatment: 100-200 mg/24 hours
Prophylaxis: 25-100 mg/24 hours

Treatment of isoniazid-induced seizures and/or coma (unlabeled use): I.V.:
Children:
Acute ingestion of known amount: Initial: A total dose of pyridoxine equal to the amount of isoniazid ingested (maximum dose: 70 mg/kg, up to 5 g); administer at a rate of 0.5-1 g/minute until seizures stop or the maximum initial dose has been administered; may repeat every 5-10 minutes as needed to control persistent seizure activity and/or CNS toxicity. If seizures stop prior to the administration of the calculated initial dose, infuse the remaining pyridoxine over 4-6 hours (Howland, 2006; Morrow, 2006).
Acute ingestion of unknown amount: Initial: 70 mg/kg (maximum dose: 5 g); administer at a rate of 0.5-1 g/minute; may repeat every 5-10 minutes as needed to control persistent seizure activity and/or CNS toxicity (Howland, 2006; Morrow, 2006; Santucci, 1999)
Adults:
Acute ingestion of known amount: Initial: A total dose of pyridoxine equal to the amount of isoniazid ingested (maximum dose: 5 g); administer at a rate of 0.5-1 g/minute until seizures stop or the maximum initial dose has been administered; may repeat every 5-10 minutes as needed to control persistent seizure activity and/or CNS toxicity. If seizures stop prior to the administration of the calculated initial dose, infuse the remaining pyridoxine over 4-6 hours (Howland, 2006; Morrow, 2006).
Acute ingestion of unknown amount: Initial: 5 g; administer at a rate of 0.5-1 g/minute; may repeat every 5-10 minutes as needed to control persistent seizure activity and/or CNS toxicity (Howland, 2006; Morrow, 2006)

Prevention of isoniazid-induced seizures and/or coma (unlabeled use): I.V.: Children and Adults: Asymptomatic patients who present within 2 hours of ingesting a potentially toxic amount of isoniazid should receive a prophylactic dose of pyridoxine (Boyer, 2006). Dosing recommendations are the same as for the treatment of symptomatic patients.

Treatment of acute hydrazine toxicity (unlabeled use): I.V.: Adults: A total dose of 25 mg/kg should be given over 15-30 minutes

Treatment of seizures from acute Gyromitrin-containing mushroom toxicity (unlabeled use; Diaz, 2005): I.V.: Children and Adults: 25 mg/kg over 15-30 minutes; repeat dose as needed to control seizures

Administration Burning may occur at the injection site after I.M. or SubQ administration; seizures have occurred following I.V. administration of very large doses.

Isoniazid toxicity (unlabeled use): Initial doses should be administered at a rate of 0.5-1 g/minute. If the parenteral formulation is not available, anecdotal reports suggest that pyridoxine tablets may be crushed and made into a slurry and given at the same dose orally or via nasogastric (NG) tube (Boyer, 2006). Oral administration is not recommended for acutely poisoned patients with seizure activity.

Monitoring Parameters For treatment of isoniazid, hydrazine, or Gyromitrin-containing mushroom toxicity: Anion gap, arterial blood gases, electrolytes, neurological exam, seizure activity

Reference Range Over 50 ng/mL (SI: 243 nmol/L) (varies considerably with method). A broad range is ~25-80 ng/mL (SI: 122-389 nmol/L). HPLC method for pyridoxal phosphate has normal range of 3.5-18 ng/mL (SI: 17-88 nmol/L).

Test Interactions False positive urobilinogen spot test using Ehrlich's reagent

Dosage Forms Excipient information presented when available (limited, particularly for generics); consult specific product labeling.
Capsule, oral, as hydrochloride: 50 mg, 250 mg
Aminoxin®: 20 mg
Injection, solution, as hydrochloride: 100 mg/mL (1 mL)
Liquid, oral, as hydrochloride: 200 mg/5 mL (120 mL)
Tablet, oral, as hydrochloride: 25 mg, 50 mg, 100 mg, 250 mg, 500 mg
Tablet, sustained release, oral, as hydrochloride:
Pyri-500: 500 mg

Extemporaneous Preparations A 1 mg/mL oral solution may be made using pyridoxine injection. Withdraw 100 mg (1 mL of a 100 mg/mL injection) from a vial with a needle and syringe; add to 99 mL simple syrup in an amber bottle. Label "refrigerate". Stable for 30 days refrigerated.

Nahata MC, Pai VB, and Hipple TF, *Pediatric Drug Formulations*, 5th ed, Cincinnati, OH: Harvey Whitney Books Co, 2004.

◆ **Pyridoxine, Folic Acid, and Cyanocobalamin** *see* Folic Acid, Cyanocobalamin, and Pyridoxine *on page 749*
◆ **Pyridoxine Hydrochloride** *see* Pyridoxine *on page 1437*
◆ **Pyrilamine, Chlorpheniramine, and Phenylephrine** *see* Chlorpheniramine, Pyrilamine, and Phenylephrine *on page 348*

Pyrimethamine (peer i METH a meen)

Brand Names: U.S. Daraprim®
Brand Names: Canada Daraprim®
Pharmacologic Category Antimalarial Agent
Use Prophylaxis of malaria due to susceptible strains of plasmodia; used in conjunction with a sulfonamide for the treatment of uncomplicated malaria due to susceptible strains of plasmodia (alternative agent; not preferred therapy); synergistic combination with sulfonamide in treatment of toxoplasmosis
Pregnancy Risk Factor C
Pregnancy Considerations Teratogenic effects have been observed in animal reproduction studies. If administered during pregnancy (ie, for toxoplasmosis), supplementation of folate is strongly recommended. Pregnancy should be avoided during therapy.
Lactation Enters breast milk/not recommended (AAP rates "compatible"; AAP 2001 update pending)
Contraindications Hypersensitivity to pyrimethamine or any component of the formulation; megaloblastic anemia secondary to folate deficiency
Warnings/Precautions When used for more than 3-4 days, it may be advisable to administer leucovorin calcium to prevent hematologic complications; monitor CBC and platelet counts every 2 weeks; use with caution in patients with impaired renal or hepatic function or with possible G6PD. Use caution in patients with seizure disorders or possible folate deficiency (eg, malabsorption syndrome, pregnancy, alcoholism).
Adverse Reactions Frequency not defined.
Cardiovascular: Arrhythmias (large doses)
Dermatologic: Erythema multiforme, rash, Stevens-Johnson syndrome, toxic epidermal necrolysis
Gastrointestinal: Anorexia, atrophic glossitis, vomiting
Hematologic: Leukopenia, megaloblastic anemia, pancytopenia, pulmonary eosinophilia, thrombocytopenia
Genitourinary: Hematuria
Miscellaneous: Anaphylaxis

Drug Interactions

Metabolism/Transport Effects Inhibits CYP2C9 (moderate), CYP2D6 (moderate)

Avoid Concomitant Use

Avoid concomitant use of Pyrimethamine with any of the following: Artemether; Lumefantrine

Increased Effect/Toxicity

Pyrimethamine may increase the levels/effects of: Antipsychotic Agents (Phenothiazines); Carvedilol; CYP2C9 Substrates; CYP2D6 Substrates; Dapsone; Dapsone (Systemic); Dapsone (Topical); Fesoterodine; Lumefantrine; Nebivolol; Tamoxifen

The levels/effects of Pyrimethamine may be increased by: Artemether; Dapsone; Dapsone (Systemic); Propafenone

Decreased Effect

Pyrimethamine may decrease the levels/effects of: Codeine; TraMADol

The levels/effects of Pyrimethamine may be decreased by: Methylfolate

Stability Store at 15°C to 25°C (59°F to 77°F). Protect from light.

Mechanism of Action Inhibits parasitic dihydrofolate reductase, resulting in inhibition of vital tetrahydrofolic acid synthesis

Pharmacodynamics/Kinetics

Onset of action: ~1 hour

Absorption: Well absorbed

Distribution: Widely, mainly in blood cells, kidneys, lungs, liver, and spleen; crosses into CSF

Protein binding: 80% to 87%

Metabolism: Hepatic

Half-life elimination: 80-95 hours

Time to peak, serum: 1.5-8 hours

Excretion: Urine (20% to 30% as unchanged drug)

Dosage Oral:

Isosporiasis (*Isospora belli* infection) in HIV-positive patients (unlabeled use; CDC, 2009): Adults:

Treatment (alternative to trimethoprim-sulfamethoxazole): 50-75 mg once daily in combination with leucovorin calcium

Chronic maintenance (secondary prophylaxis): 25 mg once daily in combination with leucovorin calcium

Malaria chemoprophylaxis: Begin prophylaxis before entering endemic area: **Note:** Current CDC recommendations for malaria prophylaxis do not include the use of pyrimethamine; resistance to pyrimethamine is prevalent worldwide.

Manufacturer's labeling:

Children <4 years: 6.25 mg once weekly

Children 4-10 years: 12.5 mg once weekly

Children >10 years and Adults: 25 mg once weekly

Malaria treatment (non- *falciparum* malaria; use in conjunction with a sulfonamide [eg, sulfadoxine]): Note: Current CDC recommendations for the malaria treatment do not include the use of pyrimethamine; resistance to pyrimethamine is prevalent worldwide.

Manufacturer's labeling:

Children 4-10 years: 25 mg daily for 2 days; following clinical cure, administer a once weekly chemoprophylaxis regimen for ≥10 weeks

Children >10 years and Adults: 25 mg daily for 2 days; following clinical cure, administer a once weekly chemoprophylaxis regimen for ≥10 weeks

Note: Pyrimethamine use alone is **not** recommended; if circumstances arise where it must be used alone in semi-immune patients, give adults 50 mg daily for 2 days (children receive 25 mg daily for 2 days), then (following clinical cure) administer a once-weekly chemoprophylaxis regimen for ≥10 weeks.

***Pneumocystis jirovecii* pneumonia (PCP) in HIV-positive patients (unlabeled use; CDC, 2009):** Adults:

Prophylaxis (alternative to trimethoprim-sulfamethoxazole): 50 mg once weekly in combination with dapsone and leucovorin calcium; **or** 25 mg once daily with atovaquone in combination with oral leucovorin calcium

Chronic maintenance (secondary prophylaxis; alternative to trimethoprim-sulfamethoxazole): 50-75 mg once weekly in combination with dapsone and leucovorin calcium; **or** 25 mg once daily with atovaquone in combination with leucovorin calcium

Toxoplasmosis treatment: *Manufacturer's labeling:*

Children: Loading dose: 1 mg/kg/day divided into 2 equal daily doses for 2-4 days, then may decrease dose to 0.5 mg/kg/day divided into 2 doses for 4 weeks; use with a sulfonamide in combination with leucovorin calcium

Adults: 50-75 mg/day for 1-3 weeks depending on patient's tolerance and response, then may reduce dose by 50% and continue for 4-5 weeks; use with a sulfonamide in combination with leucovorin calcium

Toxoplasmosis prophylaxis and treatment in HIV-positive patients (unlabeled; CDC, 2009):

Prophylaxis for first episode of Toxoplasma gondii:

Children ≥1 month of age: 1 mg/kg/day (or 15 mg/m^2) once daily (maximum: 25 mg), with dapsone or atovaquone in combination with leucovorin calcium

Adolescents and Adults (alternative to trimethoprim sulfamethoxazole): 50 mg or 75 mg once weekly with dapsone in combination with leucovorin calcium; **or** 25 mg once daily with atovaquone in combination with leucovorin calcium

Prophylaxis to prevent recurrence of Toxoplasma gondii:

Children ≥1 month of age: 1 mg/kg/day (or 15 mg/m^2) once daily (maximum: 25 mg) given with sulfadiazine (or atovaquone or clindamycin) in combination with leucovorin calcium

Adolescents and Adults: 25-50 mg once daily with sulfadiazine in combination with leucovorin calcium (preferred); **or** 25-50 mg once daily with clindamycin in combination with leucovorin calcium; **or** 25 mg once daily with atovaquone in combination with leucovorin calcium

Treatment of congenital toxoplasmosis: Infants and Children: Loading dose: 2 mg/kg/day once daily for 2 days, then 1 mg/kg/day once daily for 2-6 months, followed by 1 mg/kg administered 3 times weekly, with sulfadiazine or clindamycin in combination with leucovorin calcium (treatment duration: 12 months)

Treatment of acquired toxoplasmosis: Infants and Children: Acute induction: Loading dose: 2 mg/kg once daily (maximum: 50 mg/day) for 3 days, then 1 mg/kg/day once daily (maximum: 25 mg/day), with sulfadiazine or clindamycin in combination with leucovorin calcium (treatment duration: ≥6 weeks)

Treatment of Toxoplasma gondii encephalitis: Adolescents and Adults: 200 mg as a single dose, followed by 50 mg (<60 kg) or 75 mg (≥60 kg) daily, with sulfadiazine in combination with leucovorin calcium for at least 6 weeks (preferred); **or** 200 mg as a single dose, followed by 50 mg (<60 kg) or 75 mg (≥60 kg) daily, with clindamycin, atovaquone, or azithromycin in combination with leucovorin calcium

Dietary Considerations Take with meals to minimize GI distress.

Administration Administer with meals to minimize GI distress.

Monitoring Parameters CBC, including platelet counts

Dosage Forms Excipient information presented when available (limited, particularly for generics); consult specific product labeling.

Tablet, oral:

Daraprim®: 25 mg [scored]

Extemporaneous Preparations A 2 mg/mL oral suspension may be made with tablets and a 1:1 mixture of Simple Syrup, NF and methylcellulose 1%. Crush forty 25 mg tablets in a mortar and reduce to a fine powder. Add small portions of vehicle and mix to a uniform paste; mix while adding vehicle in incremental proportions to **almost** 500 mL; transfer to a calibrated bottle, rinse mortar with vehicle, and add quantity of vehicle sufficient to make 500 mL. Label "shake well" and "refrigerate". Stable for 91 days.

Nahata MC, Pai VB, and Hipple TF, *Pediatric Drug Formulations*, 5th ed, Cincinnati, OH: Harvey Whitney Books Co, 2004.

◆ **Pyrimethamine and Sulfadoxine** *see* Sulfadoxine and Pyrimethamine *on page 1601*

◆ **QAB149** *see* Indacaterol *on page 885*

◆ **Qinghao Derivative** *see* Artesunate *on page 148*

◆ **Qinghaosu Derivative** *see* Artesunate *on page 148*

◆ **Q-Pantoprazole (Can)** *see* Pantoprazole *on page 1289*

◆ **Quadrivalent Human Papillomavirus Vaccine** *see* Papillomavirus (Types 6, 11, 16, 18) Vaccine (Human, Recombinant) *on page 1294*

◆ **Qualaquin®** *see* QuiNINE *on page 1448*

◆ **Quasense®** *see* Ethinyl Estradiol and Levonorgestrel *on page 656*

◆ **Quaternium-18 Bentonite** *see* Bentoquatam *on page 201*

Quazepam (KWAZ e pam)

Brand Names: U.S. Doral®
Brand Names: Canada Doral®
Pharmacologic Category Benzodiazepine
Additional Appendix Information

Beers Criteria – Potentially Inappropriate Medications for Geriatrics *on page 1973*

Benzodiazepines *on page 1882*

Use Treatment of insomnia
Pregnancy Risk Factor X
Medication Guide Available Yes
Dosage

Adults: Oral: Initial: 15 mg at bedtime; in some patients, the dose may be reduced to 7.5 mg after a few nights

Elderly: Dosing should be cautious; begin at lower end of dosing range (ie, 7.5 mg)

Dosing adjustment in renal impairment: Use caution; monitor for signs of excessive sedation or impaired coordination

Dosing adjustment in hepatic impairment: Use caution; monitor for signs of excessive sedation or impaired coordination

Additional Information Complete prescribing information for this medication should be consulted for additional detail.

Dosage Forms Excipient information presented when available (limited, particularly for generics); consult specific product labeling.

Tablet, oral:

Doral®: 15 mg

Controlled Substance C-IV

◆ **Quelicin®** *see* Succinylcholine *on page 1596*

◆ **Questran®** *see* Cholestyramine Resin *on page 351*

◆ **Questran® Light** *see* Cholestyramine Resin *on page 351*

◆ **Questran® Light Sugar Free (Can)** *see* Cholestyramine Resin *on page 351*

QUEtiapine (kwe TYE a peen)

Brand Names: U.S. SEROquel XR®; SEROquel®
Brand Names: Canada Apo-Quetiapine®; CO Quetiapine; Dom-Quetiapine; JAMP-Quetiapine; Mylan-Quetiapine; PHL-Quetiapine; PMS-Quetiapine; PRO-Quetiapine; ratio-Quetiapine; Riva-Quetiapine; Sandoz-Quetiapine; Seroquel XR®; Seroquel®; Teva-Quetiapine
Index Terms Quetiapine Fumarate
Pharmacologic Category Antipsychotic Agent, Atypical
Additional Appendix Information

Antipsychotic Agents *on page 1880*

Use Treatment of schizophrenia; treatment of acute manic or mixed episodes associated with bipolar I disorder (as monotherapy or in combination with lithium or divalproex); maintenance treatment of bipolar I disorder (in combination with lithium or divalproex); treatment of acute depressive episodes associated with bipolar disorder; adjunctive treatment of major depressive disorder
Unlabeled Use Autism; delirium in the critically-ill patient; psychosis/agitation related to Alzheimer's dementia
Pregnancy Risk Factor C
Pregnancy Considerations Quetiapine was embryo and fetal toxic, but not teratogenic in animal reproduction studies. Congenital malformations have not been observed in humans (based on limited data). The long term effects of *in utero* exposure on infant development and behavior are not known. Antipsychotic use during the third trimester of pregnancy has a risk for abnormal muscle movements (extrapyramidal symptoms [EPS]) and withdrawal symptoms in newborns following delivery. Symptoms in the newborn may include agitation, feeding disorder, hypertonia, hypotonia, respiratory distress, somnolence, and tremor; these effects may be self-limiting or require hospitalization. Treatment algorithms have been developed by the ACOG and the APA for the management of depression in women prior to conception and during pregnancy. Healthcare providers are encouraged to enroll women 18-45 years of age exposed to quetiapine during pregnancy in the Atypical Antipsychotics Pregnancy Registry (1-866-961-2388).
Lactation Enters breast milk/not recommended
Medication Guide Available Yes
Contraindications There are no contraindications listed in manufacturers labeling.

Canadian labeling: Hypersensitivity to quetiapine or any component of the formulation

Warnings/Precautions [U.S. Boxed Warning]: Antidepressants increase the risk of suicidal thinking and behavior in children, adolescents, and young adults (18-24 years of age) with major depressive disorder (MDD) and other psychiatric disorders; consider risk prior to prescribing. Short-term studies did not show an increased risk in patients >24 years of age and showed a decreased risk in patients ≥65 years. Closely monitor all patients for clinical worsening, suicidality, or unusual changes in behavior; particularly during the initial 1-2 months of therapy or during periods of dosage adjustments (increased or decreases); the patient's family or caregiver should be instructed to closely observe the patient and communicate condition with healthcare provider. A medication guide concerning the use of antidepressants should be dispensed with each prescription.

[U.S. Boxed Warning]: Elderly patients with dementia-related psychosis treated with antipsychotics are at an increased risk of death compared to placebo. Most deaths appeared to be either cardiovascular (eg, heart failure, sudden death) or infectious (eg, pneumonia) in nature. Quetiapine is not approved for the treatment of dementia-related psychosis.

Leukopenia, neutropenia, and agranulocytosis (sometimes fatal) have been reported in clinical trials and postmarketing reports with antipsychotic use; presence of risk factors (eg, pre-existing low WBC or history of drug-induced leuko-/neutropenia) should prompt periodic blood count assessment. Discontinue therapy at first signs of blood dyscrasias or if absolute neutrophil count <1000/mm^3.

May be sedating, use with caution in disorders where CNS depression is a feature. Use with caution in Parkinson's disease. May induce orthostatic hypotension associated with dizziness, tachycardia, and, in some cases, syncope, especially during the initial dose titration period. Should be used with particular caution in patients with known cardiovascular disease (history of MI or ischemic heart disease, heart failure, or conduction abnormalities), cerebrovascular disease, or conditions that predispose to hypotension. Use has been associated with QT prolongation; postmarketing reports have occurred in patients with concomitant illness, quetiapine overdose, or who were receiving concomitant therapy known to affect QT interval or cause electrolyte imbalance. Esophageal dysmotility and aspiration have been associated with antipsychotic use; use with caution in patients at risk of aspiration pneumonia (eg, Alzheimer's disease). May cause dose-related decreases in thyroid levels, including cases requiring thyroid replacement therapy. Development of cataracts has been observed in animal studies; lens changes have been observed in humans during long-term treatment. Lens examination on initiation of therapy and every 6 months thereafter is recommended.

Due to anticholinergic effects, use with caution in patients with decreased gastrointestinal motility, urinary retention, BPH, xerostomia, visual problems, and narrow-angle glaucoma. Relative to other antipsychotics, quetiapine has a moderate potency of cholinergic blockade. May cause extrapyramidal symptoms (EPS), pseudoparkinsonism, and/or tardive dyskinesia. Risk of dystonia (and probably other EPS) may be greater with increased doses, use of conventional antipsychotics, males, and younger patients. Impaired core body temperature regulation may occur; caution with strenuous exercise, heat exposure, dehydration, and concomitant medication possessing anticholinergic effects. Neuroleptic malignant syndrome (NMS) is a potentially fatal symptom complex that has been reported in association with administration of antipsychotic drugs. Clinical manifestations of NMS are hyperpyrexia, muscle rigidity, altered mental status, and evidence of autonomic instability (irregular pulse or blood pressure, tachycardia, diaphoresis, and cardiac dysrhythmia). Management of NMS should include immediate discontinuation of antipsychotic drugs and other drugs not essential to concurrent therapy, intensive symptomatic treatment and medication monitoring, and treatment of any concomitant medical problems for which specific treatment are available.

Use caution in patients with a history of seizures. May cause decreases in total free thyroxine, elevations of liver enzymes, cholesterol levels, and/or triglyceride increases. Rare cases of priapism have been reported. May increase prolactin levels; clinical significance of hyperprolactinemia in patients with breast cancer or other prolactin-dependent tumors is unknown.

May cause hyperglycemia; in some cases may be extreme and associated with ketoacidosis, hyperosmolar coma, or death. Use with caution in patients with diabetes or other disorders of glucose regulation; monitor for worsening of glucose control. Significant weight gain has been observed with antipsychotic therapy; incidence varies with product. Monitor waist circumference and BMI. Patients using immediate release tablets may be switched to extended release tablets at the same total daily dose taken once daily. Dosage adjustments may be necessary based on response and tolerability. May cause withdrawal symptoms (rare) with abrupt cessation; gradually taper dose during discontinuation.

Adverse Reactions Actual frequency may be dependent upon dose and/or indication. Unless otherwise noted, frequency of adverse effects is reported for adult patients; spectrum and incidence of adverse effects similar in children (with significant exceptions noted).

>10%:

Cardiovascular: Diastolic blood pressure increased (children and adolescents, 41%), systolic blood pressure increased (children and adolescents, 15%)

Central nervous system: Somnolence (18% to 57%), headache (7% to 21%), agitation (5% to 20%), dizziness (1% to 18%), fatigue (3% to 14%), extrapyramidal symptoms (1% to 13%)

Endocrine & metabolic: Triglycerides increased (≥200 mg/dL, 8% to 22%), HDL cholesterol decreased (≤40 mg/dL, 6% to 19%), total cholesterol increased (≥240 mg/dL, 7% to 18%), LDL cholesterol increased (≥160 mg/dL, 4% to 17%), hyperglycemia (≥200 mg/dL post glucose challenge or fasting glucose ≥126 mg/dL, 2% to 12%)

Gastrointestinal: Xerostomia (9% to 44%), weight gain (dose related; 3% to 23%), appetite increased (2% to 12%), constipation (6% to 11%)

1% to 10%:

Cardiovascular: Orthostatic hypotension (2% to 7%; children and adolescents <1%), tachycardia (1% to 6%), syncope (<5%), palpitation (4%), peripheral edema (4%), hypotension (3%), hypertension (1% to 2%)

Central nervous system: Insomnia (9%), akathisia (≤8%), pain (1% to 7%), dystonia (≤6%), lethargy (1% to 5%), tardive dyskinesia (<5%), anxiety (2% to 4%), irritability (1% to 4%), parkinsonism (≤4%), abnormal dreams (2% to 3%), depression (1% to 3%), hypersomnia (1% to 3%), abnormal thinking (2%), ataxia (2%), attention disturbance (2%), coordination impaired (2%), disorientation (2%), hypoesthesia (2%), mental impairment (2%), migraine (2%), sluggishness (2%), vertigo (2%), confusion (1% to 2%), restlessness (1% to 2%), fever (1% to 2%), chills (1%)

Dermatologic: Rash (4%), hyperhidrosis (2%)

Endocrine & metabolic: Hyperprolactinemia (4%), libido decreased (≤2%), hypothyroidism (≤2%), female lactation (1%)

Gastrointestinal: Nausea (7% to 8%), abdominal pain (dose related; 4% to 7%), dyspepsia (dose related; 2% to 7%), vomiting (1% to 6%), drooling (<5%), gastroenteritis (2% to 4%), toothache (2% to 3%), appetite decreased (2%), dysphagia (2%), flatulence (2%), GERD (2%), anorexia (≥1%), abnormal taste (1%), abdominal distension (≤1%)

Genitourinary: Pollakiuria (2%), urinary tract infection (2%), impotence (1%)

Hematologic: Neutropenia (≤2%), leukopenia (≥1%), hemorrhage (1%)

Hepatic: Transaminases increased (1% to 6%), GGT increased (1%)

Neuromuscular & skeletal: Weakness (2% to 10%), tremor (2% to 8%), back pain (3% to 5%), dysarthria (1% to 5%), hypertonia (4%), twitching (4%), dyskinesia (≤4%), arthralgia (1% to 4%), paresthesia (3%), muscle spasm (1% to 3%), limb pain (2%), myalgia (2%), neck pain (2%), neck rigidity (1%)

Ocular: Blurred vision (1% to 4%), amblyopia (2% to 3%)

Otic: Ear pain (1% to 2%)

Respiratory: Pharyngitis (4% to 6%), nasal congestion (5%), rhinitis (3% to 4%), upper respiratory tract infection (2% to 3%), sinus congestion (2%), sinus headache (2%), sinusitis (2%), cough (3%), dyspnea (≥1%), dry throat (1%)

Miscellaneous: Diaphoresis (2%), restless legs syndrome (2%), flu-like syndrome (1% to 2%), lymphadenopathy (1%)

<1% (Limited to important or life-threatening): Acute renal failure, agranulocytosis, alkaline phosphatase increased, amnesia, anaphylactic reaction, anaphylaxis, anemia, angina, asthma, atrial arrhythmia, AV block, bradycardia, bundle branch block, cardiomyopathy, cataract formation, cerebral ischemia, cerebrovascular accident, HF, CPK increased, creatinine increased, dehydration, diabetes mellitus, dysuria, eosinophilia, epistaxis, exfoliative dermatitis, galactorrhea, hallucinations, hematemesis, hypersensitivity, hypoglycemia, hypokalemia, hyponatremia, intestinal obstruction, involuntary movements, leukocytosis, myocarditis, neuroleptic malignant syndrome, nightmares, palpitation, pancreatitis, pneumonia, priapism, QRS duration increased, QT prolongation, rectal bleeding, rhabdomyolysis, seizure, SIADH, Stevens-Johnson syndrome, ST segment elevation, suicidal ideation, suicide attempt, thrombocytopenia, tinnitus, T-wave abnormal, T-wave inversion, urinary retention

Drug Interactions

Metabolism/Transport Effects Substrate of CYP2D6 (minor), CYP3A4 (major); **Note:** Assignment of Major/Minor substrate status based on clinically relevant drug interaction potential

Avoid Concomitant Use

Avoid concomitant use of QUEtiapine with any of the following: Artemether; Conivaptan; Dronedarone; Lumefantrine; Metoclopramide; Nilotinib; Pimozide; QTc-Prolonging Agents; QuiNINE; Tetrabenazine; Thioridazine; Toremifene; Vandetanib; Vemurafenib; Ziprasidone

Increased Effect/Toxicity

QUEtiapine may increase the levels/effects of: Alcohol (Ethyl); Anticholinergics; CNS Depressants; Dronedarone; Methylphenidate; Pimozide; QTc-Prolonging Agents; QuiNINE; Serotonin Modulators; Tetrabenazine; Thioridazine; Toremifene; Vandetanib; Vemurafenib; Ziprasidone

The levels/effects of QUEtiapine may be increased by: Acetylcholinesterase Inhibitors (Central); Alfuzosin; Artemether; Chloroquine; Ciprofloxacin; Ciprofloxacin (Systemic); Conivaptan; CYP3A4 Inhibitors (Moderate); CYP3A4 Inhibitors (Strong); Gadobutrol; HydrOXYzine; Indacaterol; Lithium formulations; Lumefantrine; Methylphenidate; Metoclopramide; Nilotinib; Pramlintide; QuiNINE; Tetrabenazine

Decreased Effect

QUEtiapine may decrease the levels/effects of: Amphetamines; Anti-Parkinson's Agents (Dopamine Agonist); Quinagolide

The levels/effects of QUEtiapine may be decreased by: CYP3A4 Inducers (Strong); Deferasirox; Fosphenytoin; Lithium formulations; Peginterferon Alfa-2b; Phenytoin; Tocilizumab

Ethanol/Nutrition/Herb Interactions

Ethanol: May increase CNS depression; monitor for increased effects with coadministration. Caution patients about effects.

Food: In healthy volunteers, administration of quetiapine (immediate release) with food resulted in an increase in the peak serum concentration and AUC by 25% and 15%, respectively, compared to the fasting state. Administration of the extended release formulation with a high-fat meal (~800-1000 calories) resulted in an increase in peak serum concentration by 44% to 52% and AUC by 20% to 22% for the 50 mg and 300 mg tablets; administration with a light meal (≤300 calories) had no significant effect on the C_{max} or AUC.

Herb/Nutraceutical: St John's wort may decrease quetiapine levels. Avoid valerian, St John's wort, kava kava, gotu kola (may increase CNS depression).

Stability Store at controlled room temperature of 25°C (77°F); excursions permitted to 15°C to 30°C (59°F to 86°F).

Mechanism of Action Quetiapine is a dibenzothiazepine atypical antipsychotic. It has been proposed that this drug's antipsychotic activity is mediated through a combination of dopamine type 2 (D_2) and serotonin type 2 ($5\text{-}HT_2$) antagonism. It is an antagonist at multiple neurotransmitter receptors in the brain: Serotonin $5\text{-}HT_{1A}$ and $5\text{-}HT_2$, dopamine D_1 and D_2, histamine H_1, and adrenergic $alpha_1$- and $alpha_2$- receptors; but appears to have no appreciable affinity at cholinergic muscarinic and benzodiazepine receptors. Norquetiapine, an active metabolite, differs from its parent molecule by exhibiting high affinity for muscarinic M1 receptors.

Antagonism at receptors other than dopamine and $5\text{-}HT_2$ with similar receptor affinities may explain some of the other effects of quetiapine. The drug's antagonism of histamine H_1-receptors may explain the somnolence observed. The drug's antagonism of adrenergic $alpha_1$-receptors may explain the orthostatic hypotension observed.

Pharmacodynamics/Kinetics

Absorption: Rapidly absorbed following oral administration

Distribution: V_d: 6-14 L/kg

Protein binding, plasma: 83%

Metabolism: Primarily hepatic; via CYP3A4; forms the metabolite N-desalkyl quetiapine (active) and two inactive metabolites

Bioavailability: 100% (relative to oral solution)

Half-life elimination:

Mean: Terminal: Quetiapine: ~6 hours; Extended release: ~7 hours

Metabolite: N-desalkyl quetiapine: 9-12 hours

Time to peak, plasma: Immediate release: 1.5 hours; Extended release: 6 hours

Excretion: Urine (73% as metabolites, <1% of total dose as unchanged drug); feces (20%)

Dosage Oral:

Children ≥10 years: **Note:** Total daily doses may also be divided into 3 doses per day.

Bipolar disorder:

Mania: Immediate release tablet: Initial: 25 mg twice daily on day 1; increase to 50 mg twice daily on day 2, further increasing by 100 mg/day each day until a target dose of 400 mg/day is reached on day 5. May increase up to 600 mg/day at increments ≤100 mg/day; however, no additional benefit seen with 600 mg/day. Usual dosage range: 400-600 mg/day.

Maintenance therapy: Immediate release tablet: Continue therapy at lowest dose needed to maintain remission; periodically assess maintenance treatment needs.

Autism (unlabeled use): 100-350 mg/day (1.6-5.2 mg/kg/day) (Martin, 1999)

Adolescents ≥13 years: **Note:** Total daily doses may also be divided into 3 doses per day: Schizophrenia: Immediate release tablet: Initial: 25 mg twice daily on day 1; increase to 50 mg twice daily on day 2, further increasing by 100 mg/day each day until a target dose of 400 mg/day is reached on day 5. May increase up to 800 mg/day at increments ≤100 mg/day; however, no additional benefit seen with 800 mg/day. Usual dosage range: 400-800 mg/day; periodically assess maintenance treatment needs.

Adults:

Bipolar disorder:

Depression:

Immediate release tablet: Initial: 50 mg once daily the first day; increase to 100 mg once daily on day 2, further increasing by 100 mg/day each day until a target dose of 300 mg once daily is reached by day 4. Further increases up to 600 mg once daily by day 8 have been evaluated in clinical trials, but no additional antidepressant efficacy was noted.

Extended release tablet: Initial: 50 mg/day the first day; increase to 100 mg on day 2, further increasing by 100 mg/day each day until a target dose of 300 mg/day is reached by day 4.

Mania:

Immediate release tablet: Initial: 50 mg twice daily on day 1, increase dose in increments of 100 mg/day to 200 mg twice daily on day 4; may increase to a target dose of 800 mg/day by day 6 at increments ≤200 mg/day. Usual dosage range: 400-800 mg/day.

Extended release tablet: Initial: 300 mg on day 1; increase to 600 mg on day 2 and adjust dose to 400-800 mg once daily on day 3, depending on response and tolerance.

Maintenance therapy: Immediate release tablet: 200-400 mg twice daily with lithium or divalproex; **Note:** Average time of stabilization was 15 weeks in clinical trials.

Major depressive disorder (adjunct to antidepressants): Extended release tablet: Initial: 50 mg once daily; may be increased to 150 mg on day 3. Usual dosage range: 150-300 mg/day

Schizophrenia/psychoses:

Immediate release tablet: Initial: 25 mg twice daily; followed by increases in the total daily dose on the second and third day in increments of 25-50 mg divided 2-3 times/day, if tolerated, to a target dose of 300-400 mg/day in 2-3 divided doses by day 4. Make further adjustments as needed at intervals of at least 2 days in adjustments of 25-50 mg divided twice daily. Usual maintenance range: 300-800 mg/day.

Extended release tablet: Initial: 300 mg once daily; increase in increments of up to 300 mg/day (in intervals of ≥1 day). Usual maintenance range: 400-800 mg/day.

Note: Dose reductions should be attempted periodically to establish lowest effective dose in patients with psychosis. Patients being restarted after 1 week of no drug need to be titrated as above.

ICU delirium: Initial: 50 mg twice daily; may increase as necessary on a daily basis in increments of 50 mg twice daily to a maximum dose of 400 mg/day (Devlin, 2010)

Elderly: 40% lower mean oral clearance of quetiapine in adults >65 years of age; higher plasma levels expected and, therefore, dosage adjustment may be needed; elderly patients usually require 50-200 mg/day of immediate release tablets or 50 mg/day of extended release tablets with a slower titration schedule. Increase immediate release dose by 25-50 mg/day or extended release dose by 50 mg/day to effective dose, based on clinical response and tolerability. If initiated with immediate release tablets, patient may transition to extended release formulation (at equivalent total daily dose) when effective dose has been reached. See **"Note"** in adult dosing.

Psychosis/agitation related to Alzheimer's dementia (unlabeled use): Initial: 12.5-50 mg/day; if necessary, gradually increase as tolerated not to exceed 200-300 mg/day (Rabins, 2007)

Dosing comments in renal insufficiency: 25% lower mean oral clearance of quetiapine than normal subjects; however, plasma concentrations similar to normal subjects receiving the same dose; no dosage adjustment required

Dosing comments in hepatic insufficiency: 30% lower mean oral clearance of quetiapine than normal subjects; higher plasma levels expected in hepatically impaired subjects; dosage adjustment may be needed

Immediate release tablet: Initial: 25 mg/day, increase dose by 25-50 mg/day to effective dose, based on clinical response and tolerability to patient. If initiated with immediate-release formulation, patient may transition to extended-release formulation (at equivalent total daily dose) when effective dose has been reached.

Extended release tablet: Initial: 50 mg/day; increase dose by 50 mg/day to effective dose, based on clinical response and tolerability to patient.

Dietary Considerations Immediate-release tablet may be taken without regard to meals. Extended release tablet should be taken without food or with a light meal (≤300 calories).

Administration

Oral:

Immediate release tablet: May be administered with or without food.

Extended release tablet: Administer without food or with a light meal (≤300 calories), preferably in the evening. Swallow tablet whole; do not break, crush, or chew.

Nasogastric/enteral tube (unlabeled route): Hold tube feeds for 30 minutes before administration; flush with 25 mL of sterile water. Crush dose using immediate-release formulation, mix in 10 mL water and administer via NG/enteral tube; follow with a 50 mL flush of sterile water (Devlin, 2010).

Monitoring Parameters Vital signs; fasting lipid profile and fasting blood glucose/Hgb A_{1c} (prior to treatment, at 3 months, then annually); CBC frequently during first few months of therapy in patients with pre-existing low WBC or a history of drug-induced leukopenia/neutropenia; BMI, personal/family history of obesity, waist circumference; mental status, abnormal involuntary movement scale (AIMS). Weight should be assessed prior to treatment, at 4 weeks, 8 weeks, 12 weeks, and then at quarterly intervals. Consider titrating to a different antipsychotic agent for a weight gain ≥5% of the initial weight. Patients should have eyes checked for cataracts every 6 months while on this medication. Observe for new or worsening depression, anxiety, irritability, aggression, or other symptoms of unusual behavior, mood, or suicide ideation (especially at the beginning of therapy or when doses are increased or decreased).

Test Interactions May interfere with urine detection of methadone (false-positives); may cause false-positive serum TCA screen

Dosage Forms Excipient information presented when available (limited, particularly for generics); consult specific product labeling.

Tablet, oral:

SEROquel®: 25 mg, 50 mg, 100 mg, 200 mg, 300 mg, 400 mg

Tablet, extended release, oral:

SEROquel XR®: 50 mg, 150 mg, 200 mg, 300 mg, 400 mg

Dosage Forms: Canada Excipient information presented when available (limited, particularly for generics); consult specific product labeling.

Tablet:

Seroquel®: 25 mg, 50 mg, 100 mg, 200 mg, 300 mg, 400 mg

Tablet, extended release:

Seroquel XR®: 50 mg, 150 mg, 200 mg, 300 mg, 400 mg

◆ **Quetiapine Fumarate** *see* QUEtiapine *on page 1440*

◆ **Quinalbarbitone Sodium** *see* Secobarbital *on page 1543*

Quinapril (KWIN a pril)

Brand Names: U.S. Accupril®

Brand Names: Canada Accupril®

Index Terms Quinapril Hydrochloride

Pharmacologic Category Angiotensin-Converting Enzyme (ACE) Inhibitor

Additional Appendix Information

Angiotensin Agents *on page 1869*

Heart Failure (Systolic) *on page 1991*

Use Treatment of hypertension; treatment of heart failure

Unlabeled Use Treatment of left ventricular dysfunction after myocardial infarction; pediatric hypertension; to delay the progression of nephropathy and reduce risks of cardiovascular events in hypertensive patients with type 1 or 2 diabetes mellitus

Pregnancy Risk Factor C (1st trimester); D (2nd and 3rd trimesters)

Pregnancy Considerations Due to adverse events observed in some animal studies, quinapril is considered pregnancy category C during the first trimester. Based on human data, quinapril is considered pregnancy category D if used during the second and third trimesters (per the manufacturer; however, one study suggests that fetal injury may occur at anytime during pregnancy). Quinapril crosses the placenta. First trimester exposure to ACE inhibitors may cause major congenital malformations. An increased risk of cardiovascular and/or central nervous system malformations was observed in one study; however, an increased risk of teratogenic events was not observed in other studies. Second and third trimester use of an ACE inhibitor is associated with oligohydramnios. Oligohydramnios due to decreased fetal renal function may lead to fetal limb contractures, craniofacial deformation, and hypoplastic lung development. The use of ACE inhibitors during the second and third trimesters is also associated with anuria, hypotension, renal failure (reversible or irreversible), skull hypoplasia, and death in the fetus/neonate. Chronic maternal hypertension itself is also associated with adverse events in the fetus/infant. ACE inhibitors are not recommended during pregnancy to treat maternal hypertension or heart failure. Those who are planning a pregnancy should be considered for other medication options if an ACE inhibitor is currently prescribed or the ACE inhibitor should be discontinued as soon as possible once pregnancy is detected. The exposed fetus should be monitored for fetal growth, amniotic fluid volume, and organ formation. Infants exposed to an ACE inhibitor *in utero*, especially during the second and third trimester, should be monitored for hyperkalemia, hypotension, and oliguria.

[U.S. Boxed Warning]: Based on human data, ACE inhibitors can cause injury and death to the developing fetus when used in the second and third trimesters. ACE inhibitors should be discontinued as soon as possible once pregnancy is detected.

Lactation Enters breast milk/use caution

Contraindications Hypersensitivity to quinapril or any component of the formulation; angioedema related to previous treatment with an ACE inhibitor

Warnings/Precautions Anaphylactic reactions may occur rarely with ACE inhibitors. At any time during treatment (especially following first dose) angioedema may occur rarely with ACE inhibitors; it may involve the head and neck (potentially compromising airway) or the intestine (presenting with abdominal pain). African-Americans and patients with idiopathic or hereditary angioedema may be at an increased risk. Prolonged frequent monitoring may be required especially if tongue, glottis, or larynx are involved as they are associated with airway obstruction. Patients with a history of airway surgery may have a higher risk of airway obstruction. Aggressive early and appropriate management is critical. Use in patients with previous angioedema associated with ACE inhibitor therapy is contraindicated. Severe anaphylactoid reactions may be seen during hemodialysis (eg, CVVHD) with high-flux dialysis membranes (eg, AN69), and rarely, during low density lipoprotein apheresis with dextran sulfate cellulose. Rare cases of anaphylactoid reactions have been reported in patients undergoing sensitization treatment with hymenoptera (bee, wasp) venom while receiving ACE inhibitors.

Symptomatic hypotension with or without syncope can occur with ACE inhibitors (usually with the first several doses); effects are most often observed in volume-depleted patients; close monitoring of patient is required especially with initial dosing and dosing increases; blood pressure must be lowered at a rate appropriate for the patient's clinical condition. Initiation of therapy in patients with ischemic heart disease or cerebrovascular disease warrants close observation due to the potential consequences posed by falling blood pressure (eg, MI, stroke). Use with caution in hypertrophic cardiomyopathy with outflow tract obstruction, severe aortic stenosis, or before, during, or immediately after major surgery. **[U.S. Boxed Warning]: Based on human data, ACEIs can cause injury and death to the developing fetus when used in the second and third trimesters. ACEIs should be discontinued as soon as possible once pregnancy is detected.**

Hyperkalemia may occur with ACE inhibitors; risk factors include renal dysfunction, diabetes mellitus, concomitant use of potassium-sparing diuretics, potassium supplements, and/or potassium-containing salts. Use cautiously, if at all, with these agents and monitor potassium closely. Cough may occur with ACE inhibitors. Other causes of cough should be considered (eg, pulmonary congestion in patients with heart failure) and excluded prior to discontinuation.

May be associated with deterioration of renal function and/or increases in serum creatinine, particularly in patients with low renal blood flow (eg, renal artery stenosis, heart failure) whose glomerular filtration rate (GFR) is dependent on efferent arteriolar vasoconstriction by angiotensin II; deterioration may result in oliguria, acute renal failure, and progressive azotemia. Small increases in serum creatinine may occur following initiation; consider discontinuation only in patients with progressive and/or significant deterioration in renal function. Use with caution in patients with unstented unilateral/bilateral renal artery stenosis. When unstented bilateral renal artery stenosis is present, use is generally avoided due to the elevated risk of deterioration in renal function unless possible benefits outweigh risks. Concurrent use of angiotensin receptor blockers may increase the risk of clinically-significant adverse events (eg, renal dysfunction, hyperkalemia).

Rare toxicities associated with ACE inhibitors include cholestatic jaundice (which may progress to fulminant hepatic necrosis), agranulocytosis, neutropenia, or leukopenia with myeloid hypoplasia. Patients with collagen vascular diseases (especially with concomitant renal impairment) or renal impairment alone may be at increased risk for hematologic toxicity; periodically monitor CBC with differential in these patients.

Adverse Reactions Note: Frequency ranges include data from hypertension and heart failure trials. Higher rates of adverse reactions have generally been noted in patients with CHF. However, the frequency of adverse effects associated with placebo is also increased in this population.

1% to 10%:

Cardiovascular: Hypotension (3%), chest pain (2%), first-dose hypotension (up to 3%)

Central nervous system: Dizziness (4% to 8%), headache (2% to 6%), fatigue (3%)

Dermatologic: Rash (1%)

Endocrine & metabolic: Hyperkalemia (2%)

Gastrointestinal: Vomiting/nausea (1% to 2%), diarrhea (1.7%)

Neuromuscular & skeletal: Myalgias (2% to 5%), back pain (1%)

Renal: BUN/serum creatinine increased (2%, transient elevations may occur with a higher frequency), worsening of renal function (in patients with bilateral renal artery stenosis or hypovolemia)

Respiratory: Upper respiratory symptoms, cough (2% to 4%; up to 13% in some studies), dyspnea (2%)

<1% (Limited to important or life-threatening): Acute renal failure, agranulocytosis, alopecia, amblyopia, anaphylactoid reaction, angina, angioedema, arrhythmia, arthralgia, depression, dermatopolymyositis, edema, eosinophilic pneumonitis, exfoliative dermatitis, hemolytic anemia, hepatitis, hyperkalemia, hypertensive crisis, impotence, insomnia, MI, orthostatic hypotension, pancreatitis, paresthesia, pemphigus, photosensitivity, pruritus, shock, somnolence, stroke, syncope, thrombocytopenia, vertigo

A syndrome which may include fever, myalgia, arthralgia, interstitial nephritis, vasculitis, rash, eosinophilia and positive ANA, and elevated ESR has been reported with ACE inhibitors. In addition, pancreatitis, hepatic necrosis, neutropenia, and/or agranulocytosis (particularly in patients with collagen-vascular disease or renal impairment) have been associated with many ACE inhibitors.

Drug Interactions

Metabolism/Transport Effects None known.

Avoid Concomitant Use There are no known interactions where it is recommended to avoid concomitant use.

Increased Effect/Toxicity

Quinapril may increase the levels/effects of: Allopurinol; Amifostine; Antihypertensives; AzaTHIOprine; CycloSPORINE; CycloSPORINE (Systemic); Ferric Gluconate; Gold Sodium Thiomalate; Hypotensive Agents; Iron Dextran Complex; Lithium; Nonsteroidal Anti-Inflammatory Agents; RiTUXimab; Sodium Phosphates

The levels/effects of Quinapril may be increased by: Alfuzosin; Angiotensin II Receptor Blockers; Diazoxide; DPP-IV Inhibitors; Eplerenone; Everolimus; Herbs (Hypotensive Properties); Loop Diuretics; MAO Inhibitors; Pentoxifylline; Phosphodiesterase 5 Inhibitors; Potassium Salts; Potassium-Sparing Diuretics; Prostacyclin Analogues; Sirolimus; Temsirolimus; Thiazide Diuretics; TiZANidine; Tolvaptan; Trimethoprim

Decreased Effect

Quinapril may decrease the levels/effects of: Quinolone Antibiotics; Tetracycline Derivatives

The levels/effects of Quinapril may be decreased by: Antacids; Aprotinin; Herbs (Hypertensive Properties); Icatibant; Lanthanum; Methylphenidate; Nonsteroidal Anti-Inflammatory Agents; Salicylates; Yohimbine

Ethanol/Nutrition/Herb Interactions Herb/Nutraceutical: Avoid bayberry, blue cohosh, cayenne, ephedra, ginger, ginseng (American), kola, licorice (may worsen hypertension). Avoid black cohosh, California poppy, coleus, golden seal, hawthorn, mistletoe, periwinkle, quinine, shepherd's purse (may have increased antihypertensive effect).

Stability Store at room temperature. To prepare solution for oral administration, mix prior to administration and use within 10 minutes.

Mechanism of Action Competitive inhibitor of angiotensin-converting enzyme (ACE); prevents conversion of angiotensin I to angiotensin II, a potent vasoconstrictor; results in lower levels of angiotensin II which causes an increase in plasma renin activity and a reduction in aldosterone secretion; a CNS mechanism may also be involved in hypotensive effect as angiotensin II increases adrenergic outflow from CNS; vasoactive kallikreins may be decreased in conversion to active hormones by ACE inhibitors, thus reducing blood pressure

Pharmacodynamics/Kinetics

Onset of action: 1 hour

Duration: 24 hours

Absorption: Quinapril: ≥60%

Protein binding: Quinapril: 97%; Quinaprilat: 97%

Metabolism: Rapidly hydrolyzed to quinaprilat, the active metabolite

Half-life elimination: Quinapril: 0.8 hours; Quinaprilat: 3 hours; increases as Cl_{cr} decreases

Time to peak, serum: Quinapril: 1 hour; Quinaprilat: ~2 hours

Excretion: Urine (50% to 60% primarily as quinaprilat)

Dosage Oral:

Children (unlabeled use): Hypertension: Initial 5-10 mg once daily; maximum: 80 mg/day

Adults:

Heart failure: Initial: 5 mg once or twice daily, titrated at weekly intervals to 20-40 mg daily in 2 divided doses; target dose (heart failure): 20 mg twice daily (ACC/AHA 2009 Heart Failure Guidelines)

Hypertension: Initial: 10-20 mg once daily, adjust according to blood pressure response at peak and trough blood levels; initial dose may be reduced to 5 mg in patients receiving diuretic therapy if the diuretic is continued; usual dose range (JNC 7): 10-40 mg once daily

Elderly: Initial: 2.5-5 mg/day; increase dosage at increments of 2.5-5 mg at 1- to 2-week intervals.

Dosing adjustment in renal impairment: Lower initial doses should be used; after initial dose (if tolerated), administer initial dose twice daily; may be increased at weekly intervals to optimal response:

Heart failure: Initial:

Cl_{cr} >30 mL/minute: Administer 5 mg/day

Cl_{cr} 10-30 mL/minute: Administer 2.5 mg/day

Hypertension: Initial:

Cl_{cr} >60 mL/minute: Administer 10 mg/day

Cl_{cr} 30-60 mL/minute: Administer 5 mg/day

Cl_{cr} 10-30 mL/minute: Administer 2.5 mg/day

Dosing comments in hepatic impairment: In patients with alcoholic cirrhosis, hydrolysis of quinapril to quinaprilat is impaired; however, the subsequent elimination of quinaprilat is unaltered.

Monitoring Parameters Blood pressure; serum creatinine and potassium; if patient has collagen vascular disease and/or renal impairment, periodically monitor CBC with differential

Dosage Forms Excipient information presented when available (limited, particularly for generics); consult specific product labeling.

Tablet, oral: 5 mg, 10 mg, 20 mg, 40 mg

Accupril®: 5 mg, 10 mg, 20 mg [scored]

Accupril®: 40 mg

◆ **Quinapril Hydrochloride** *see* Quinapril *on page 1444*

◆ **Quinate® (Can)** *see* QuiNIDine *on page 1446*

QuiNIDine (KWIN i deen)

Brand Names: Canada Apo-Quinidine®; BioQuin® Durules™; Novo-Quinidin; Quinate®

Index Terms Quinidine Gluconate; Quinidine Polygalacturonate; Quinidine Sulfate

Pharmacologic Category Antiarrhythmic Agent, Class Ia; Antimalarial Agent

Use

Quinidine gluconate and sulfate salts: Conversion and prevention of relapse into atrial fibrillation and/or flutter; suppression of ventricular arrhythmias. **Note:** Due to proarrhythmic effects, use should be reserved for life-threatening arrhythmias. Moreover, the use of quinidine has largely been replaced by more effective/safer antiarrhythmic agents and/or nonpharmacologic therapies (eg, radiofrequency ablation).

Quinidine gluconate (I.V. formulation): Conversion of atrial fibrillation/flutter and ventricular tachycardia. **Note:** The use of I.V. quinidine gluconate for these indications has been replaced by more effective/safer antiarrhythmic agents (eg, amiodarone and procainamide).

Quinidine gluconate (I.V. formulation) and quinidine sulfate: Treatment of malaria (*Plasmodium falciparum*)

Unlabeled Use Paroxysmal supraventricular tachycardia, paroxysmal AV junctional rhythm, and symptomatic atrial or ventricular premature contractions; short QT syndrome; Brugada syndrome

Pregnancy Risk Factor C

Pregnancy Considerations Animal reproduction studies have not been conducted. Quinidine crosses the placenta and can be detected in the amniotic fluid, cord blood, and neonatal serum. Quinidine is indicated for use in the treatment of severe malaria infection in pregnant women (CDC, 2011; Smereck, 2011) and has also been used to treat arrhythmias in pregnancy when other agents are ineffective (European Society of Cardiology, 2003).

Lactation Enters breast milk/not recommended (AAP rates "compatible"; AAP 2001 update pending)

Contraindications Hypersensitivity to quinidine or any component of the formulation; thrombocytopenia; thrombocytopenic purpura; myasthenia gravis; heart block greater than first degree; idioventricular conduction delays (except in patients with a functioning artificial pacemaker); those adversely affected by anticholinergic activity; concurrent use of quinolone antibiotics which prolong QT interval, cisapride, amprenavir, or ritonavir

Warnings/Precautions Watch for proarrhythmic effects; may cause QT prolongation and subsequent torsade de pointes. Monitor and adjust dose to prevent QT_c prolongation. Avoid use in patients with diagnosed or suspected congenital long QT syndrome. Correct hypokalemia before initiating therapy. Hypokalemia may worsen toxicity. **[U.S. Boxed Warning]: Antiarrhythmic drugs have not been shown to enhance survival in non-life-threatening ventricular arrhythmias and may increase mortality; the risk is greatest with structural heart disease. Quinidine may increase mortality in treatment of atrial fibrillation/flutter.** May precipitate or exacerbate HF. Reduce dosage in hepatic impairment. Use may cause digoxin-induced toxicity (adjust digoxin's dose). Use caution with concurrent use of other antiarrhythmics. Hypersensitivity reactions can occur. Can unmask sick sinus syndrome (causes bradycardia); use with caution in patients with heart block. Has been associated with severe hepatotoxic reactions, including granulomatous hepatitis. Hemolysis may occur in patients with G6PD (glucose-6-phosphate dehydrogenase) deficiency. Different salt products are not interchangeable.

Adverse Reactions

Frequency not defined: Hypotension, syncope

>10%:

Cardiovascular: QT_c prolongation (modest prolongation is common, however, excessive prolongation is rare and indicates toxicity)

Central nervous system: Lightheadedness (15%)

Gastrointestinal: Diarrhea (35%), upper GI distress, bitter taste, diarrhea, anorexia, nausea, vomiting, stomach cramping (22%)

1% to 10%:

Cardiovascular: Angina (6%), palpitation (7%), new or worsened arrhythmia (proarrhythmic effect)

Central nervous system: Syncope (1% to 8%), headache (7%), fatigue (7%), sleep disturbance (3%), tremor (2%), nervousness (2%), incoordination (1%)

Dermatologic: Rash (5%)

Neuromuscular & skeletal: Weakness (5%)

Ocular: Blurred vision

Otic: Tinnitus

Respiratory: Wheezing

<1% (Limited to important or life-threatening): Abnormal pigmentation, acute psychotic reactions, agranulocytosis, angioedema, arthralgia, bronchospasm, cerebral hypoperfusion (possibly resulting in ataxia, apprehension, and seizure), cholestasis, confusion, delirium, depression, drug-induced lupus-like syndrome, eczematous dermatitis, esophagitis, exacerbated bradycardia (in sick sinus syndrome), exfoliative rash, fever, flushing, granulomatous hepatitis, hallucinations, heart block, hemolytic anemia, hepatotoxic reaction (rare), hearing impaired, CPK increased, lichen planus, livedo reticularis, lymphadenopathy, melanin pigmentation of the hard palate, myalgia, mydriasis, nephropathy, optic neuritis, pancytopenia, paradoxical increase in ventricular rate during atrial fibrillation/flutter, photosensitivity, pneumonitis, pruritus, psoriaform rash, QT_c prolongation (excessive), respiratory depression, sicca syndrome, tachycardia, thrombocytopenia, thrombocytopenic purpura, torsade de pointes, urticaria, uveitis, vascular collapse, vasculitis, ventricular fibrillation, ventricular tachycardia, vertigo, visual field loss

Note: Cinchonism, a syndrome which may include tinnitus, high-frequency hearing loss, deafness, vertigo, blurred vision, diplopia, photophobia, headache, confusion, and delirium has been associated with quinidine use. Usually associated with chronic toxicity, this syndrome has also been described after brief exposure to a moderate dose in sensitive patients. Vomiting and diarrhea may also occur as isolated reactions to therapeutic quinidine levels.

Drug Interactions

Metabolism/Transport Effects Substrate of CYP2C9 (minor), CYP2E1 (minor), CYP3A4 (major), P-glycoprotein; **Note:** Assignment of Major/Minor substrate status based on clinically relevant drug interaction potential; **Inhibits** CYP2C9 (weak), CYP2D6 (strong), CYP3A4 (weak), P-glycoprotein

Avoid Concomitant Use

Avoid concomitant use of QuiNIDine with any of the following: Antifungal Agents (Azole Derivatives, Systemic); Artemether; Conivaptan; Crizotinib; Dronedarone; Lumefantrine; Mefloquine; Nilotinib; Pimozide; Propafenone; Protease Inhibitors; QUEtiapine; QuiNINE; Silodosin; Tetrabenazine; Thioridazine; Topotecan; Toremifene; Vandetanib; Vemurafenib; Ziprasidone

Increased Effect/Toxicity

QuiNIDine may increase the levels/effects of: Atomoxetine; Beta-Blockers; Calcium Channel Blockers (Dihydropyridine); Cardiac Glycosides; Colchicine; CYP2D6 Substrates; Dabigatran Etexilate; Dextromethorphan; Dronedarone; Everolimus; Fesoterodine; Haloperidol;

Mefloquine; Neuromuscular-Blocking Agents; P-glycoprotein/ABCB1 Substrates; Pimozide; Propafenone; QTc-Prolonging Agents; QuiNINE; Rivaroxaban; Silodosin; Tetrabenazine; Thioridazine; Topotecan; Toremifene; Tricyclic Antidepressants; Vandetanib; Vemurafenib; Verapamil; Vitamin K Antagonists; Ziprasidone

The levels/effects of QuiNIDine may be increased by: Alfuzosin; Amiodarone; Antacids; Antifungal Agents (Azole Derivatives, Systemic); Artemether; Barbiturates; Boceprevir; Calcium Channel Blockers (Dihydropyridine); Carbonic Anhydrase Inhibitors; Chloroquine; Cimetidine; Ciprofloxacin; Ciprofloxacin (Systemic); Conivaptan; Crizotinib; CYP3A4 Inhibitors (Moderate); CYP3A4 Inhibitors (Strong); Diltiazem; Eribulin; Fingolimod; Fluconazole; Gadobutrol; Haloperidol; Indacaterol; Lumefantrine; Lurasidone; Macrolide Antibiotics; Nilotinib; P-glycoprotein/ABCB1 Inhibitors; Protease Inhibitors; QUEtiapine; QuiNINE; Reserpine; Selective Serotonin Reuptake Inhibitors; Telaprevir; Tricyclic Antidepressants; Verapamil

Decreased Effect

QuiNIDine may decrease the levels/effects of: Codeine; Dihydrocodeine; Hydrocodone; TraMADol

The levels/effects of QuiNIDine may be decreased by: Barbiturates; Calcium Channel Blockers (Dihydropyridine); CYP3A4 Inducers (Strong); Cyproterone; Deferasirox; Etravirine; Fosphenytoin; Kaolin; P-glycoprotein/ABCB1 Inducers; Phenytoin; Potassium-Sparing Diuretics; Primidone; Rifamycin Derivatives; Sucralfate; Tocilizumab

Ethanol/Nutrition/Herb Interactions

Food: Dietary salt intake may alter the rate and extent of quinidine absorption. A decrease in dietary salt may lead to an increase in quinidine serum concentrations. Avoid changes in dietary salt intake. Quinidine serum levels may be increased if taken with food. Food has a variable effect on absorption of sustained release formulation. The rate of absorption of quinidine may be decreased following the ingestion of grapefruit juice. In addition, CYP3A4 metabolism of quinidine may be reduced by grapefruit juice. Grapefruit juice should be avoided. Excessive intake of fruit juices or vitamin C may decrease urine pH and result in increased clearance of quinidine with decreased serum concentration. Alkaline foods may result in increased quinidine serum concentrations.

Herb/Nutraceutical: St John's wort may decrease quinidine levels. Avoid ephedra (may worsen arrhythmia).

Stability

Solution for injection: Store at room temperature of 25°C (77°F).

Tablets: Store at controlled room temperature of 20°C to 25°C (68°F to 77°F). Protect from light.

Mechanism of Action Class Ia antiarrhythmic agent; depresses phase O of the action potential; decreases myocardial excitability and conduction velocity, and myocardial contractility by decreasing sodium influx during depolarization and potassium efflux in repolarization; also reduces calcium transport across cell membrane

Pharmacodynamics/Kinetics

Distribution: V_d: Adults: 2-3 L/kg, decreased with congestive heart failure (0.5 L/kg), malaria; increased with cirrhosis

Protein binding: Newborns: 50% to 70%; Adults: 80% to 88%

Binds mainly to alpha$_1$-acid glycoprotein and to a lesser extent albumin; protein-binding changes may occur in periods of stress due to increased alpha$_1$-acid glycoprotein concentrations (eg, acute myocardial infarction) or in certain disease states due to decreased alpha$_1$-acid glycoprotein concentrations (eg, cirrhosis,hyperthyroidism, malnutrition)

Metabolism: Extensively hepatic (50% to 90%) to inactive compounds

Bioavailability: Sulfate: ~70% with wide variability between patients (45% to 100%); Gluconate: 70% to 80%

Half-life elimination, plasma: Children: 3-4 hours; Adults: 6-8 hours; prolonged with elderly, cirrhosis, and congestive heart failure

Time to peak, serum: Sulfate: 2 hours; Gluconate: 3-6 hours

Excretion: Urine (15% to 25% as unchanged drug)

Dosage Note: Dosage expressed in terms of the salt: 267 mg of quinidine gluconate = 200 mg of quinidine sulfate.

Antiarrhythmic: Adults: Oral:

Immediate release formulations: Quinidine sulfate: Initial: 200-400 mg/dose every 6 hours the dose may be increased cautiously to desired effect

Extended release formulations:

Quinidine sulfate: Initial: 300 mg every 8-12 hours; the dose may be increased cautiously to desired effect

Quinidine gluconate: Initial: 324 mg every 8-12 hours; the dose may be increased cautiously to desired effect

Severe malaria, treatment: Children and Adults: I.V. (quinidine gluconate): 10 mg/kg infused over 60-120 minutes followed by 0.02 mg/kg/minute continuous infusion for ≥24 hours; alternatively, may administer 24 mg/kg loading dose over 4 hours, followed by 12 mg/kg over 4 hours every 8 hours (beginning 8 hours after initiation of the loading dose); complete treatment with oral quinine once parasite density <1% and patient can receive oral medication; total duration of treatment (quinidine/quinine): 3 days (Africa or South America) or 7 days (Southeast Asia); use in combination with doxycycline, tetracycline or clindamycin (CDC malaria guidelines, 2009). **Note:** Close monitoring, including telemetry, required.

Dosing adjustment in renal impairment: The FDA-approved labeling recommends that caution should be used in patients with renal impairment; however, no specific dosage adjustment guidelines are available. The following guidelines have been used by some clinicians (Aronoff, 2007): Oral:

Cl_{cr} ≥10 mL/minute: No adjustment required.

Cl_{cr} <10 mL/minute: Administer 75% of normal dose.

Hemodialysis: Dose following hemodialysis

Peritoneal dialysis: Supplemental dose is not necessary

CRRT: No dosage adjustment required; monitor serum concentrations

Dosing adjustment/comments in hepatic impairment: Use caution; hepatic impairment decreases clearance; dosage adjustments are not provided in the manufacturers' labeling although toxicity may occur if the dose is not appropriately adjusted.

Dietary Considerations Administer with food or milk to decrease gastrointestinal irritation. Avoid changes in dietary salt intake.

Administration Administer around-the-clock to promote less variation in peak and trough serum levels

Oral: Do not crush, chew, or break sustained release dosage forms. Some preparations of quinidine gluconate extended release tablets may be split in half to facilitate dosage titration; tablets are not scored.

Parenteral: Minimize use of PVC tubing to enhance bioavailability; shorter tubing lengths are recommended by the manufacturer

Monitoring Parameters Cardiac monitor required during I.V. administration; CBC, liver and renal function tests, should be routinely performed during long-term administration

Reference Range Therapeutic: 2-5 mcg/mL (SI: 6.2-15.4 micromole/L). Patient-dependent therapeutic response occurs at levels of 3-6 mcg/mL (SI: 9.2-18.5 micromole/L). Optimal therapeutic level is method dependent; >6 mcg/mL (SI: >18 micromole/L).

Dosage Forms Excipient information presented when available (limited, particularly for generics); consult specific product labeling.

Injection, solution, as gluconate: 80 mg/mL (10 mL) [equivalent to quinidine base 50 mg/mL]

Tablet, oral, as sulfate: 200 mg, 300 mg

Tablet, extended release, oral, as gluconate: 324 mg [equivalent to quinidine base 202 mg]

Tablet, extended release, oral, as sulfate: 300 mg [equivalent to quinidine base 249 mg]

Extemporaneous Preparations A 10 mg/mL oral liquid preparation may be made with tablets and one of three different vehicles (cherry syrup, a 1:1 mixture of Ora-Sweet® and Ora-Plus®, or a 1:1 mixture of Ora-Sweet® SF and Ora-Plus®). Crush six 200 mg tablets in a mortar and reduce to a fine powder. Add 15 mL of the chosen vehicle and mix to a uniform paste; mix while adding vehicle in incremental proportions to **almost** 120 mL; transfer to a calibrated bottle, rinse mortar with vehicle, and add quantity of vehicle sufficient to make 120 mL. Label "shake well" and "protect from light". Stable for 60 days when stored in amber plastic prescription bottles in the dark at room temperature or refrigerated.

Allen LV and Erickson MA, "Stability of Bethanechol Chloride, Pyrazinamide, Quinidine Sulfate, Rifampin, and Tetracycline in Extemporaneously Compounded Oral Liquids," *Am J Health Syst Pharm*, 1998, 55(17):1804-9.

◆ **Quinidine and Dextromethorphan** *see* Dextromethorphan and Quinidine *on page 490*

◆ **Quinidine Gluconate** *see* QuiNIDine *on page 1446*

◆ **Quinidine Polygalacturonate** *see* QuiNIDine *on page 1446*

◆ **Quinidine Sulfate** *see* QuiNIDine *on page 1446*

QuiNINE (KWYE nine)

Brand Names: U.S. Qualaquin®

Brand Names: Canada Apo-Quinine®; Novo-Quinine; Quinine-Odan

Index Terms Quinine Sulfate

Pharmacologic Category Antimalarial Agent

Use In conjunction with other antimalarial agents, treatment of uncomplicated chloroquine-resistant *P. falciparum* malaria

Unlabeled Use Treatment of *Babesia microti* infection in conjunction with clindamycin; treatment of uncomplicated chloroquine-resistant *P. vivax* malaria (in conjunction with other antimalarial agents)

Pregnancy Risk Factor C

Pregnancy Considerations Teratogenic effects have been reported in some animal studies. Quinine crosses the human placenta. Cord plasma to maternal plasma quinine ratios have been reported as 0.18-0.46 and should not be considered therapeutic to the infant. Teratogenic effects, optic nerve hypoplasia, and deafness have been reported in the infant following maternal use of very high doses; however, therapeutic doses used for malaria are generally considered safe. Quinine may also cause significant hypoglycemia when used during pregnancy. Malaria infection in pregnant women may be more severe than in nonpregnant women. Because *P. falciparum* malaria can cause maternal death and fetal loss, pregnant women traveling to malaria-endemic areas must use personal protection against mosquito bites. Quinine may be used for the treatment of malaria in pregnant women; consult current CDC guidelines. Pregnant women should be advised not to travel to areas of *P. falciparum* resistance to chloroquine.

Lactation Enters breast milk/use caution (AAP rate "compatible"; AAP 2001 update pending)

Medication Guide Available Yes

Contraindications Hypersensitivity to quinine or any component of the formulation; hypersensitivity to mefloquine or quinidine (cross sensitivity reported); history of potential hypersensitivity reactions (including black water fever, thrombotic thrombocytopenia purpura [TTP], hemolytic uremic syndrome [HUS], or thrombocytopenia) associated with prior quinine use; prolonged QT interval; myasthenia gravis; optic neuritis; G6PD deficiency

Warnings/Precautions [U.S. Boxed Warning]: Quinine is not recommended for the prevention/treatment of nocturnal leg cramps due to the potential for severe and/or life-threatening side effects (eg, cardiac arrhythmias, thrombocytopenia, HUS/TTP, severe hypersensitivity reactions). These risks, as well as the absence of clinical effectiveness, do not justify its use in the unapproved/unlabeled prevention and/or treatment of leg cramps.

Quinine may cause QT interval prolongation, with maximum increase corresponding to maximum plasma concentration. Use caution with medications or clinical conditions which may further prolong the QT interval or cause cardiac arrhythmias. Use caution with atrial fibrillation or flutter, renal or hepatic impairment. Quinine interacts with many medications due to its hepatic metabolism; use caution with other medications metabolized via the CYP3A4 isoenzyme system. Severe hypersensitivity reactions (eg, Stevens-Johnson syndrome, anaphylactic shock) have occurred; discontinue following any signs of sensitivity. Other events (including acute interstitial nephritis, neutropenia, and granulomatous hepatitis) may also be attributed to hypersensitivity reactions. Immune-mediated thrombocytopenia, including life-threatening cases and hemolytic uremic syndrome/thrombotic thrombocytopenic purpura (HUS/TTP), has occurred with use. Chronic renal failure associated with TTP has also been reported. Thrombocytopenia generally resolves within a week upon discontinuation. Re-exposure may result in increased severity of thrombocytopenia and faster onset.

Use may cause significant hypoglycemia due to quinine-induced insulin release. Use with caution in patients with hepatic impairment. Use with caution in patients with renal impairment; dosage adjustment recommended. Quinine should not be used for the prevention of malaria or in the treatment of complicated or severe *P. falciparum* malaria (oral antimalarial agents are not appropriate for initial therapy of severe malaria).

Adverse Reactions

Frequency not defined.

Cardiovascular: Atrial fibrillation, atrioventricular block, bradycardia, cardiac arrest, chest pain, hypotension, irregular rhythm, nodal escape beats, palpitation, postural hypotension, QT prolongation, syncope, tachycardia, torsade de pointes, unifocal premature ventricular contractions, U waves, vasodilation, ventricular fibrillation, ventricular tachycardia

Central nervous system: Aphasia, ataxia, chills, coma, confusion, disorientation, dizziness, dystonic reaction, fever, flushing, headache, mental status altered, restlessness, seizure, suicide, vertigo

Dermatologic: Acral necrosis, allergic contact dermatitis, bullous dermatitis, bruising, cutaneous rash (urticaria, papular, scarlatinal), cutaneous vasculitis, exfoliative dermatitis, erythema multiforme, petechiae, photosensitivity, pruritus, Stevens-Johnson syndrome, toxic epidermal necrolysis

Endocrine & metabolic: Hypoglycemia

Gastrointestinal: Abdominal pain, anorexia, diarrhea, esophagitis, gastric irritation, nausea, vomiting
Hematologic: Agranulocytosis, aplastic anemia, coagulopathy, disseminated intravascular coagulation, hemolytic anemia, hemolytic uremic syndrome, hemorrhage, hypoprothrombinemia, idiopathic thrombocytopenic purpura, leukopenia, neutropenia, pancytopenia, thrombocytopenia, thrombotic thrombocytopenic purpura
Hepatic: Granulomatous hepatitis, hepatitis, jaundice, liver function test abnormalities
Neuromuscular & skeletal: Myalgia, tremor, weakness
Ocular: Blindness, blurred vision (with or without scotomata), color vision disturbance, diminished visual fields, diplopia, night blindness, optic neuritis, photophobia, pupillary dilation, vision loss (sudden)
Otic: Deafness, hearing impaired, tinnitus
Renal: Acute interstitial nephritis, hemoglobinuria, renal failure, renal impairment
Respiratory: Asthma, dyspnea, pulmonary edema
Miscellaneous: Black water fever, diaphoresis, hypersensitivity reaction, lupus anticoagulant, lupus-like syndrome

Drug Interactions

Metabolism/Transport Effects Substrate of CYP1A2 (minor), CYP2C19 (minor), CYP3A4 (major), P-glycoprotein; **Note:** Assignment of Major/Minor substrate status based on clinically relevant drug interaction potential; **Inhibits** CYP2C8 (moderate), CYP2C9 (moderate), CYP2D6 (moderate), CYP3A4 (weak), P-glycoprotein

Avoid Concomitant Use

Avoid concomitant use of QuiNINE with any of the following: Antacids; Artemether; Conivaptan; Halofantrine; Lumefantrine; Macrolide Antibiotics; Mefloquine; Neuromuscular-Blocking Agents; QTc-Prolonging Agents; Rifampin; Ritonavir; Silodosin; Topotecan

Increased Effect/Toxicity

QuiNINE may increase the levels/effects of: Antihypertensives; Antipsychotic Agents (Phenothiazines); CarBAMazepine; Cardiac Glycosides; Colchicine; CYP2C8 Substrates; CYP2C9 Substrates; CYP2D6 Substrates; Dabigatran Etexilate; Dapsone; Dapsone (Systemic); Dapsone (Topical); Everolimus; Fesoterodine; Halofantrine; Herbs (Hypotensive Properties); HMG-CoA Reductase Inhibitors; Lumefantrine; Mefloquine; Nebivolol; Neuromuscular-Blocking Agents; P-glycoprotein/ABCB1 Substrates; PHENobarbital; Prilocaine; QTc-Prolonging Agents; Ritonavir; Rivaroxaban; Silodosin; Theophylline Derivatives; Topotecan; Vitamin K Antagonists

The levels/effects of QuiNINE may be increased by: Alkalinizing Agents; Artemether; Cimetidine; Conivaptan; CYP3A4 Inhibitors (Moderate); CYP3A4 Inhibitors (Strong); Dapsone; Dapsone (Systemic); Macrolide Antibiotics; Mefloquine; P-glycoprotein/ABCB1 Inhibitors; QTc-Prolonging Agents; Ritonavir

Decreased Effect

QuiNINE may decrease the levels/effects of: Codeine; TraMADol

The levels/effects of QuiNINE may be decreased by: Antacids; CarBAMazepine; CYP3A4 Inducers (Strong); Cyproterone; Deferasirox; Fosphenytoin; P-glycoprotein/ABCB1 Inducers; PHENobarbital; Phenytoin; Rifampin; Tocilizumab

Ethanol/Nutrition/Herb Interactions Herb/Nutraceutical: St John's wort may decrease quinine levels. Black cohosh, California poppy, coleus, golden seal, hawthorn, mistletoe, periwinkle, and shepherd's purse may cause excessive decreases in blood pressure.

Stability Store at 20°C to 25°C (68°F to 77°F).

Mechanism of Action Depresses oxygen uptake and carbohydrate metabolism; intercalates into DNA, disrupting the parasite's replication and transcription; cardiovascular effects similar to quinidine

Pharmacodynamics/Kinetics

Absorption: Readily, mainly from upper small intestine
Distribution: Children: ~0.9 L/kg (subjects with malaria); Adults: 2.5-7.1 L/kg (varies with severity of infection)
Intraerythrocytic levels are ~30% to 50% of the plasma concentration; distributes poorly to the CSF (~2% to 7% of plasma concentration)
Protein binding: 69% to 92% in healthy subjects; 78% to 95% with malaria
Metabolism: Hepatic via CYP450 enzymes, primarily CYP3A4; forms metabolites; major metabolite, 3-hydroxyquinine, is less active than parent
Bioavailability: 76% to 88% in healthy subjects; increased with malaria
Half-life elimination:
Children: ~3 hours in healthy subjects; ~12 hours with malaria
Healthy adults: 10-13 hours
Healthy elderly subjects: 18 hours
Time to peak, serum:
Children: 2 hours in healthy subjects; 4 hours with malaria
Adults: 2-4 hours in healthy subjects; 1-11 hours with malaria
Excretion: Urine (<20% as unchanged drug)

Dosage Note: Actual duration of quinine treatment for malaria may be dependent upon the geographic region or pathogen. Dosage expressed in terms of the salt; 1 capsule Qualaquin® = 324 mg of quinine sulfate = 269 mg of base.

Children: Oral:
Treatment of uncomplicated chloroquine-resistant *P. falciparum* malaria (CDC guidelines): 30 mg/kg/day in divided doses every 8 hours for 3-7 days. Tetracycline, doxycycline, or clindamycin (consider risk versus benefit of using tetracycline or doxycycline in children <8 years) should also be given.
Treatment of uncomplicated chloroquine-resistant *P. vivax* malaria (unlabeled use; CDC guidelines): 30 mg/kg/day in divided doses every 8 hours for 3-7 days. Tetracycline or doxycycline (consider risk versus benefit of using tetracycline or doxycycline in children <8 years) plus primaquine should also be given.
Babesiosis (unlabeled use): 30 mg/kg/day divided every 8 hours for 7-10 days with clindamycin
Adults: Oral:
Treatment of uncomplicated chloroquine-resistant *P. falciparum* malaria (CDC guidelines): 648 mg every 8 hours for 3-7 days. Tetracycline, doxycycline, or clindamycin should also be given.
Treatment of uncomplicated chloroquine-resistant *P. vivax* malaria (unlabeled use; CDC guidelines): 648 mg every 8 hours for 3-7 days. Tetracycline or doxycycline plus primaquine should also be given.
Babesiosis (unlabeled use): 650 mg every 8 hours for 7-10 days with clindamycin

Dosing interval/adjustment in renal impairment:
Cl_{cr} 10-50 mL/minute: Administer every 8-12 hours
Cl_{cr} <10 mL/minute: Administer every 24 hours
Severe chronic renal failure not on dialysis: Initial dose: 648 mg followed by 324 mg every 12 hours
Dialysis: Administer dose after dialysis. **Note:** Clearance of ~6.5% achieved with 1 hour of hemodialysis.
Peritoneal dialysis: Dose as for Cl_{cr} <10 mL/minute
Continuous arteriovenous or hemodialysis: Dose as for Cl_{cr} 10-50 mL/minute

Dosing adjustment in hepatic impairment:
Mild-to-moderate impairment: No dosing adjustment required; monitor closely
Severe impairment (Child-Pugh class C): Data not available

Dietary Considerations Take with food to decrease incidence of gastric upset.

Administration Avoid use of aluminum- or magnesium-containing antacids because of drug absorption problems. Swallow dose whole to avoid bitter taste. May be administered with food.

Monitoring Parameters Monitor CBC with platelet count, liver function tests, blood glucose, ophthalmologic examination

Test Interactions May interfere with urine detection of opioids (false-positive); positive Coombs' [direct]; false elevation of urinary steroids (when assayed by Zimmerman method) and catecholamines

Dosage Forms Excipient information presented when available (limited, particularly for generics); consult specific product labeling.

Capsule, oral, as sulfate:

Qualaquin®: 324 mg

◆ **Quinine-Odan (Can)** *see* QuiNINE *on page 1448*

◆ **Quinine Sulfate** *see* QuiNINE *on page 1448*

◆ **Quinnostik** *see* Urea *on page 1749*

◆ **Quinol** *see* Hydroquinone *on page 846*

Quinupristin and Dalfopristin

(kwi NYOO pris tin & dal FOE pris tin)

Brand Names: U.S. Synercid®

Brand Names: Canada Synercid®

Index Terms Dalfopristin and Quinupristin; Pristinamycin; RP-59500

Pharmacologic Category Antibiotic, Streptogramin

Additional Appendix Information

Antibiotic Treatment of Adults With Infective Endocarditis *on page 1956*

Use Treatment of complicated skin and skin structure infections caused by methicillin-susceptible *Staphylococcus aureus* or *Streptococcus pyogenes*

Pregnancy Risk Factor B

Pregnancy Considerations Because adverse effects were not observed in animal reproduction studies, quinupristin/dalfopristin is classified pregnancy category B. There are no adequate and well-controlled studies of quinupristin/dalfopristin in pregnant women.

Lactation Excretion in breast milk unknown/use caution

Contraindications Hypersensitivity to quinupristin, dalfopristin, pristinamycin, or virginiamycin, or any component of the formulation

Warnings/Precautions Use with caution in patients with hepatic or renal dysfunction. May cause pain and phlebitis when infused through a peripheral line (not relieved by hydrocortisone or diphenhydramine). Prolonged use may result in fungal or bacterial superinfection, including *C. difficile*-associated diarrhea (CDAD) and pseudomembranous colitis; CDAD has been observed >2 months post-antibiotic treatment. May cause arthralgias, myalgias, and hyperbilirubinemia. May inhibit the metabolism of many drugs metabolized by CYP3A4. Concurrent therapy with cisapride (which may prolong QT_c interval and lead to arrhythmias) should be avoided.

Adverse Reactions

>10%:

Hepatic: Hyperbilirubinemia (3% to 35%)

Local: Local pain (40% to 44%), inflammation at infusion site (38% to 42%), local edema (17% to 18%), infusion site reaction (12% to 13%)

Neuromuscular & skeletal: Arthralgia (up to 47%), myalgia (up to 47%)

1% to 10%:

Central nervous system: Pain (2% to 3%), headache (2%)

Dermatologic: Rash (3%), pruritus (2%)

Endocrine & metabolic: Hyperglycemia (1%)

Gastrointestinal: Nausea (3% to 5%), vomiting (3% to 4%), diarrhea (3%)

Hematologic: Anemia (3%)

Hepatic: GGT increased (2%), LDH increased (3%)

Local: Thrombophlebitis (2%)

Neuromuscular & skeletal: CPK increased (2%)

<1% (Limited to important or life-threatening): Allergic reaction, anaphylactoid reaction, angina, apnea, arrhythmia, cardiac arrest, coagulation disorder, dysautonomia, dyspnea, encephalopathy, gout, hematuria, hemolytic anemia, hepatitis, hyperkalemia, hypotension, maculopapular rash, mesenteric artery occlusion, myasthenia, neuropathy, pancreatitis, pancytopenia, paraplegia, paresthesia, pericarditis, pleural effusion, pseudomembranous colitis, respiratory distress, seizure, shock, stomatitis, syncope, thrombocytopenia, urticaria

Drug Interactions

Avoid Concomitant Use

Avoid concomitant use of Quinupristin and Dalfopristin with any of the following: Pimozide

Increased Effect/Toxicity

Quinupristin and Dalfopristin may increase the levels/effects of: CycloSPORINE; CycloSPORINE (Systemic); Pimozide

Decreased Effect There are no known significant interactions involving a decrease in effect.

Stability Store unopened vials under refrigeration at 2°C to 8°C (36°F to 46°F). The following stability information has also been reported: May be stored at room temperature for up to 7 days (Cohen, 2007).

Reconstitute single dose vial with 5 mL of 5% dextrose in water or sterile water for injection. Swirl gently to dissolve; do not shake (to limit foam formation). The reconstituted solution should be diluted within 30 minutes. Stability of the diluted solution prior to the infusion is established as 5 hours at room temperature or 54 hours if refrigerated at 2°C to 8°C (36°F to 46°F). Reconstituted solution should be added to at least 250 mL of 5% dextrose in water for peripheral administration (increase to 500 mL or 750 mL if necessary to limit venous irritation). An infusion volume of 100 mL may be used for central line infusions. Do not freeze solution.

Mechanism of Action Quinupristin/dalfopristin inhibits bacterial protein synthesis by binding to different sites on the 50S bacterial ribosomal subunit thereby inhibiting protein synthesis

Pharmacodynamics/Kinetics

Distribution: Quinupristin: 0.45 L/kg; Dalfopristin: 0.24 L/kg

Metabolism: To active metabolites via nonenzymatic reactions

Half-life elimination: Quinupristin: 0.85 hour; Dalfopristin: 0.7 hour (mean elimination half-lives, including metabolites: 3 and 1 hours, respectively)

Excretion: Feces (75% to 77% as unchanged drug and metabolites); urine (15% to 19%)

Dosage I.V.: Children ≥12 years and Adults: Complicated skin and skin structure infection: 7.5 mg/kg every 12 hours for at least 7 days

Dosage adjustment in renal impairment: No adjustment required in renal failure, hemodialysis, or peritoneal dialysis

Dosage adjustment in hepatic impairment: Pharmacokinetic data suggest dosage adjustment may be necessary; however, specific recommendations have not been proposed

Elderly: No dosage adjustment is required

Administration Line should be flushed with 5% dextrose in water prior to and following administration. Infusion should be completed over 60 minutes (toxicity may be increased with shorter infusion). If severe venous irritation occurs following peripheral administration of quinupristin/dalfopristin diluted in 250 mL 5% dextrose in water, consideration should be given to increasing the infusion volume to 500 mL or 750 mL, changing the infusion site, or infusing by a peripherally-inserted central catheter (PICC) or a central venous catheter.

Monitoring Parameters Culture and sensitivity

Dosage Forms Excipient information presented when available (limited, particularly for generics); consult specific product labeling.

Injection, powder for reconstitution:

Synercid®: 500 mg: Quinupristin 150 mg and dalfopristin 350 mg

- ◆ **Quixin®** *see* Levofloxacin (Ophthalmic) *on page 1000*
- ◆ **QVAR®** *see* Beclomethasone (Systemic) *on page 192*
- ◆ **R & C™ II (Can)** *see* Pyrethrins and Piperonyl Butoxide *on page 1435*
- ◆ **R & C™ Shampoo/Conditioner (Can)** *see* Pyrethrins and Piperonyl Butoxide *on page 1435*
- ◆ **R-1569** *see* Tocilizumab *on page 1700*
- ◆ **RabAvert®** *see* Rabies Vaccine *on page 1453*

RABEprazole (ra BEP ra zole)

Brand Names: U.S. AcipHex®

Brand Names: Canada Pariet®; PMS-Rabeprazole EC; PRO-Rabeprazole; Rabeprazole EC; RAN™-Rabeprazole; Riva-Rabeprazole EC; Sandoz-Rabeprazole; Teva-Rabeprazole EC

Index Terms Pariprazole

Pharmacologic Category Proton Pump Inhibitor; Substituted Benzimidazole

Use Short-term (4-8 weeks) treatment and maintenance of erosive or ulcerative gastroesophageal reflux disease (GERD); symptomatic GERD; short-term (up to 4 weeks) treatment of duodenal ulcers; long-term treatment of pathological hypersecretory conditions, including Zollinger-Ellison syndrome; *H. pylori* eradication (in combination therapy)

Canadian labeling: Additional uses (not in U.S. labeling): Treatment of nonerosive reflux disease (NERD); treatment of gastric ulcers

Unlabeled Use Maintenance of duodenal ulcer

Pregnancy Risk Factor B

Pregnancy Considerations Not shown to be teratogenic in animal studies, however, adequate and well-controlled studies have not been done in humans; use during pregnancy only if clearly needed

Lactation Excretion in breast milk unknown/not recommended

Contraindications Hypersensitivity to rabeprazole, substituted benzimidazoles (ie, esomeprazole, lansoprazole, omeprazole, pantoprazole), or any component of the formulation

Warnings/Precautions Use of proton pump inhibitors (PPIs) may increase the risk of gastrointestinal infections (eg, *Salmonella, Campylobacter*). Use caution in severe hepatic impairment. Relief of symptoms with rabeprazole does not preclude the presence of a gastric malignancy. Decreased *H. pylori* eradication rates have been observed with short-term (≤7 days) combination therapy. The American College of Gastroenterology recommends 10-14 days of therapy (triple or quadruple) for eradication of *H. pylori* (Chey, 2007).

PPIs may diminish the therapeutic effect of clopidogrel, thought to be due to reduced formation of the active metabolite of clopidogrel. The manufacturer of clopidogrel recommends either avoidance of omeprazole or use of a PPI with less potent CYP2C19 inhibition (eg, pantoprazole); given the potency of CYP2C19 inhibitory activity, avoidance of rabeprazole would appear prudent. Others have recommended the continued use of PPIs, regardless of the degree of inhibition, in patients with a history of GI bleeding or multiple risk factors for GI bleeding who are also receiving clopidogrel since no evidence has established clinically meaningful differences in outcome; however, a clinically-significant interaction cannot be excluded in those who are poor metabolizers of clopidogrel (Abraham, 2010; Levine, 2011).

Increased incidence of osteoporosis-related bone fractures of the hip, spine, or wrist may occur with PPI therapy. Patients on high-dose (multiple daily doses) or long-term therapy (≥1 year) should be monitored. Use the lowest effective dose for the shortest duration of time, use vitamin D and calcium supplementation, and follow appropriate guidelines to reduce risk of fractures in patients at risk.

Hypomagnesemia, reported rarely, usually with prolonged PPI use of >3 months (most cases >1 year of therapy); may be symptomatic or asymptomatic; severe cases may cause tetany, seizures, and cardiac arrhythmias. Consider obtaining serum magnesium concentrations prior to beginning long-term therapy, especially if taking concomitant digoxin, diuretics, or other drugs known to cause hypomagnesemia; and periodically thereafter. Hypomagnesemia may be corrected by magnesium supplementation, although discontinuation of rabeprazole may be necessary; magnesium levels typically return to normal within 1 week of stopping.

Adverse Reactions

1% to 10%:

Central nervous system: Pain (3%), headache (2% to 5%)

Gastrointestinal: Diarrhea (3%), flatulence (3%), constipation (2%), nausea (2%)

Respiratory: Pharyngitis (3%)

Miscellaneous: Infection (2%)

<1% (Limited to important or life-threatening): Abdomen enlarged, abdominal pain, abnormal stools, abnormal vision, agitation, agranulocytosis, albuminuria, allergic reaction, alopecia, amblyopia, anaphylaxis, anemia, angina pectoris, angioedema, anorexia, apnea, arrhythmia, arthralgia, arthritis, ascites, asthma, bloody diarrhea, bone pain, bradycardia, breast enlargement, bullous and other drug eruptions of skin, bundle branch block, bursitis, cataract, cellulitis, cerebral hemorrhage, chest pain substernal, cholangitis, cholecystitis, cholelithiasis, colitis, coma, constipation, contact dermatitis, convulsions, corneal opacity, CPK increased, cystitis, deafness, delirium, depression, diaphoresis, diabetes mellitus, diplopia, disorientation, dizziness, duodenitis, dysmenorrhea, dyspepsia, dysphagia, dyspnea, dysuria, edema, electrocardiogram abnormal, embolus, epistaxis, erythema multiforme, esophageal stenosis, esophagitis, extrapyramidal syndrome, eye hemorrhage, facial edema, fever, flatulence, fracture, fungal dermatitis, gastritis, gastroenteritis, gastrointestinal hemorrhage, gingivitis, glaucoma, glossitis, gout, gynecomastia, hematuria, hemolytic anemia, hepatic encephalopathy, hepatic cirrhosis, hepatic enzymes increased, hepatitis, hepatoma, hernia, hyperammonemia, hypercholesteremia, hyperglycemia, hyperkinesia, hyperlipemia, hypertension, hyper-/hypothyroidism, hypertonia, hypokalemia, hypomagnesemia, hyponatremia, hypoxia, impotence, injection site hemorrhage/pain/reaction, insomnia, interstitial nephritis, interstitial pneumonia, jaundice, kidney calculus, leukocytosis, leukopenia, leukorrhea, liver fatty deposit,

lymphadenopathy, malaise, melena, menorrhagia, metrorrhagia, MI, migraine, myalgia, nausea, neck rigidity, nervousness, neuralgia, neuropathy, neutropenia, orchitis, osteoporosis-related fracture, palpitation, pancreatitis, pancytopenia, paresthesia, peripheral edema, photosensitivity, polycystic kidney, polyuria, proctitis, pruritus, PSA increased, psoriasis, pulmonary embolus, QT_c prolongation, rash, rectal hemorrhage, retinal degeneration, rhabdomyolysis, salivary gland enlargement, sinus bradycardia, skin discoloration, somnolence, Stevens-Johnson syndrome, stomatitis, strabismus, sudden death, supraventricular tachycardia, syncope, tachycardia, taste abnormal, thrombocytopenia, thrombophlebitis, thrombosis, thirst (rare) tinnitus, toxic epidermal necrolysis, tremor, TSH increased, ulcerative colitis, urinary incontinence, urticaria, vasodilation, ventricular arrhythmias, vertigo, vomiting, weakness, weight gain/loss, xerostomia

Drug Interactions

Metabolism/Transport Effects Substrate of CYP2C19 (major), CYP3A4 (major); **Note:** Assignment of Major/Minor substrate status based on clinically relevant drug interaction potential; **Inhibits** CYP2C19 (moderate), CYP2C8 (moderate), CYP2D6 (weak), CYP3A4 (weak)

Avoid Concomitant Use

Avoid concomitant use of RABEprazole with any of the following: Delavirdine; Erlotinib; Nelfinavir; Pimozide; Posaconazole; Rilpivirine

Increased Effect/Toxicity

RABEprazole may increase the levels/effects of: Amphetamines; Citalopram; CYP2C19 Substrates; CYP2C8 Substrates; Dexmethylphenidate; Methotrexate; Methylphenidate; Pimozide; Raltegravir; Saquinavir; Tacrolimus; Tacrolimus (Systemic); Voriconazole

The levels/effects of RABEprazole may be increased by: Conivaptan; Fluconazole; Ketoconazole; Ketoconazole (Systemic)

Decreased Effect

RABEprazole may decrease the levels/effects of: Atazanavir; Bisphosphonate Derivatives; Cefditoren; Clopidogrel; Dabigatran Etexilate; Dasatinib; Delavirdine; Erlotinib; Gefitinib; Indinavir; Iron Salts; Itraconazole; Ketoconazole; Ketoconazole (Systemic); Mesalamine; Mycophenolate; Nelfinavir; Posaconazole; Rilpivirine

The levels/effects of RABEprazole may be decreased by: CYP2C19 Inducers (Strong); CYP3A4 Inducers (Strong); Deferasirox; Herbs (CYP3A4 Inducers); Tipranavir; Tocilizumab

Ethanol/Nutrition/Herb Interactions

Ethanol: Avoid ethanol (may cause gastric mucosal irritation).

Food: High-fat meals may delay absorption, but C_{max} and AUC are not altered.

Herb/Nutraceutical: St John's wort may increase the metabolism and thus decrease the levels/effects of rabeprazole.

Stability Store at 25°C (77°F). Protect from moisture.

Mechanism of Action Potent proton pump inhibitor; suppresses gastric acid secretion by inhibiting the parietal cell H+/K+ ATP pump

Pharmacodynamics/Kinetics

Onset of action: Within 1 hour

Duration: 24 hours

Absorption: Oral: Well absorbed within 1 hour

Protein binding, serum: ~96%

Metabolism: Hepatic via CYP3A and 2C19 to inactive metabolites

Bioavailability: Oral: ~52%

Half-life elimination (dose dependent): 1-2 hours

Time to peak, plasma: 2-5 hours

Excretion: Urine (90% primarily as thioether carboxylic acid metabolites); remainder in feces

Dosage Oral:

Children ≥12 years: *U.S. labeling:* Short-term treatment of GERD: 20 mg once daily for ≤8 weeks

Adults >18 years and Elderly:

Erosive/ulcerative GERD: Treatment: 20 mg once daily for 4-8 weeks; if inadequate response, may repeat up to an additional 8 weeks; maintenance: 20 mg once daily

Canadian labeling: 20 mg once daily for 4 weeks; if inadequate response, may repeat for an additional 4 weeks (lack of symptom control after 4 weeks warrants further evaluation); maintenance: 10 mg once daily (maximum: 20 mg once daily)

Symptomatic GERD: Treatment: 20 mg once daily for 4 weeks; if inadequate response, may repeat for an additional 4 weeks

Canadian labeling: 10 mg once daily (maximum: 20 mg once daily) for 4 weeks; lack of symptom control after 4 weeks warrants further evaluation

Duodenal ulcer: 20 mg/day before breakfast for 4 weeks; additional therapy may be required for some patients

Gastric ulcers (*Canadian labeling*): 20 mg once daily up to 6 weeks; additional therapy may be required for some patients

Helicobacter pylori eradication:

Manufacturer labeling: 20 mg twice daily administered with amoxicillin 1000 mg *and* clarithromycin 500 mg twice daily for 7 days

American College of Gastroenterology guidelines (Chey, 2007):

Nonpenicillin allergy: 20 mg twice daily administered with amoxicillin 1000 mg *and* clarithromycin 500 mg twice daily for 10-14 days

Penicillin allergy: 20 mg twice daily administered with clarithromycin 500 mg *and* metronidazole 500 mg twice daily for 10-14 days **or** 20 mg once or twice daily administered with bismuth subsalicylate 525 mg *and* metronidazole 250 mg *plus* tetracycline 500 mg 4 times/day for 10-14 days

Hypersecretory conditions: 60 mg once daily; dose may need to be adjusted as necessary. Doses as high as 100 mg once daily and 60 mg twice daily have been used, and continued as long as necessary (up to 1 year in some patients).

NERD (*Canadian labeling*): Treatment: 10 mg (maximum: 20 mg once daily) for 4 weeks; lack of symptom control after 4 weeks warrants further evaluation

Dosage adjustment in renal impairment: No dosage adjustment required

Dosage adjustment in hepatic impairment:

Mild-to-moderate: Elimination decreased; no dosage adjustment required

Severe: Use caution

Dietary Considerations May be taken without regard to meals; best if taken before breakfast.

Administration May be administered without regard to meals; best if taken before breakfast. Do not crush, split, or chew tablet. May be administered with an antacid.

Dosage Forms Excipient information presented when available (limited, particularly for generics); consult specific product labeling.

Tablet, delayed release, enteric coated, oral, as sodium:

AcipHex®: 20 mg

Dosage Forms: Canada Excipient information presented when available (limited, particularly for generics); consult specific product labeling.

Tablet, delayed release, enteric coated, as sodium:

Pariet®: 10 mg, 20 mg

◆ **Rabeprazole EC (Can)** *see* RABEprazole *on page* 1451

Rabies Immune Globulin (Human)

(RAY beez i MYUN GLOB yoo lin, HYU man)

Brand Names: U.S. HyperRAB™ S/D; Imogam® Rabies-HT

Brand Names: Canada HyperRAB™ S/D; Imogam® Rabies Pasteurized

Index Terms HRIG; RIG

Pharmacologic Category Blood Product Derivative; Immune Globulin

Use Part of postexposure prophylaxis of persons with rabies exposure. Provides passive immunity until active immunity with rabies vaccine is established. Not for use in persons with a history of pre-exposure vaccination, history of postexposure prophylaxis, or previous vaccination with rabies vaccine and documentation of antibody response.

Pregnancy Risk Factor C

Pregnancy Considerations Reproduction studies have not been conducted. Pregnancy is not a contraindication to postexposure prophylaxis.

Contraindications There are no contraindications listed within the FDA-approved manufacturer's labeling.

Warnings/Precautions Hypersensitivity and anaphylactic reactions can occur; immediate treatment (including epinephrine 1:1000) should be available. Use with caution in patients with isolated immunoglobulin A deficiency or a history of systemic hypersensitivity to human immunoglobulins. Use with caution in patients with thrombocytopenia or coagulation disorders; I.M. injections may be contraindicated. Product of human plasma; may potentially contain infectious agents which could transmit disease. Screening of donors, as well as testing and/or inactivation or removal of certain viruses, reduces the risk. Infections thought to be transmitted by this product should be reported to the manufacturer. Not for intravenous administration.

Adverse Reactions Frequency not defined.

Central nervous system: Fever (mild), headache, malaise

Dermatologic: Angioneurotic edema, rash

Local: Injection site: Pain, stiffness, soreness, tenderness

Renal: Nephrotic syndrome

Miscellaneous: Anaphylaxis

Drug Interactions

Metabolism/Transport Effects None known.

Avoid Concomitant Use There are no known interactions where it is recommended to avoid concomitant use.

Increased Effect/Toxicity There are no known significant interactions involving an increase in effect.

Decreased Effect

Rabies Immune Globulin (Human) may decrease the levels/effects of: Vaccines (Live)

Stability Store between 2°C to 8°C (36°F to 46°F); do not freeze. Discard product exposed to freezing. The following stability information has also been reported for HyperRAB™ S/D: May be exposed to room temperature for a cumulative 7 days (Cohen, 2007).

Mechanism of Action Rabies immune globulin is a solution of globulins dried from the plasma or serum of selected adult human donors who have been immunized with rabies vaccine and have developed high titers of rabies antibody. It generally contains 10% to 18% of protein of which not less than 80% is monomeric immunoglobulin G.

Dosage Children and Adults: Postexposure prophylaxis: Local wound infiltration: 20 units/kg in a single dose, RIG should always be administered as part of rabies vaccine regimen. If anatomically feasible, the full rabies immune globulin dose should be infiltrated around and into the wound(s); remaining volume should be administered I.M. at a site distant from the vaccine administration site. If rabies vaccine was initiated without rabies immune globulin, rabies immune globulin may be administered through the seventh day after the administration of the first dose of the vaccine. Administration of RIG is not recommended after the seventh day post vaccine since an antibody response to the vaccine is expected during this time period.

Note: Not for use in persons with a history of pre-exposure vaccination, history of postexposure prophylaxis, or previous vaccination with rabies vaccine and documentation of antibody response.

Administration Do not administer I.V.

Postexposure wound infiltration: If anatomically feasible, the full rabies immune globulin dose should be infiltrated around and into the wound(s); remaining volume should be administered I.M. in the deltoid muscle of the upper arm or lateral thigh muscle. The gluteal area should be avoided to reduce the risk of sciatic nerve damage. Do not administer rabies vaccine in the same syringe or at the same administration site as RIG.

Measles-containing vaccines should be given ≥4 months after rabies immune globulin.

Dosage Forms Excipient information presented when available (limited, particularly for generics); consult specific product labeling.

Injection, solution [preservative free]:

HyperRAB™ S/D: 150 int. units/mL (2 mL, 10 mL) [solvent/detergent treated]

Imogam® Rabies-HT: 150 int. units/mL (2 mL, 10 mL) [heat treated]

Rabies Vaccine (RAY beez vak SEEN)

Brand Names: U.S. Imovax® Rabies; RabAvert®

Brand Names: Canada Imovax® Rabies; RabAvert®

Index Terms HDCV; Human Diploid Cell Cultures Rabies Vaccine; PCEC; Purified Chick Embryo Cell

Pharmacologic Category Vaccine, Inactivated (Viral)

Use Pre-exposure and postexposure vaccination against rabies

The Advisory Committee on Immunization Practices (ACIP) recommends a primary course of prophylactic immunization (pre-exposure vaccination) for the following:

- Persons with continuous risk of infection, including rabies research laboratory and biologics production workers
- Persons with frequent risk of infection in areas where rabies is enzootic, including rabies diagnostic laboratory workers, cavers, veterinarians and their staff, and animal control and wildlife workers; persons who frequently handle bats
- Persons with infrequent risk of infection, including veterinarians and animal control staff with terrestrial animals in areas where rabies infection is rare, veterinary students, and travelers visiting areas where rabies is enzootic and immediate access to medical care and biologicals is limited

The ACIP recommends the use of postexposure vaccination for a particular person be assessed by the severity and likelihood versus the actual risk of acquiring rabies. Consideration should include the type of exposure, epidemiology of rabies in the area, species of the animal, circumstances of the incident, and the availability of the exposing animal for observation or rabies testing. Postexposure vaccination is used in both previously vaccinated and previously unvaccinated individuals.

Pregnancy Risk Factor C

Pregnancy Considerations Animal reproduction studies have not been conducted. Pregnancy is not a contraindication to postexposure prophylaxis. Pre-exposure prophylaxis during pregnancy may also be considered if risk of rabies is great.

Lactation Excretion in breast milk unknown

Contraindications

Pre-exposure prophylaxis: Hypersensitivity to rabies vaccine or any component of the formulation

Postexposure prophylaxis: There are no contraindications listed within the FDA-approved manufacturer's labeling.

Warnings/Precautions Rabies vaccine should not be used in persons with a confirmed diagnosis of rabies; use after the onset of symptoms may be detrimental. Postexposure vaccination may begin regardless of the length of time from documented or likely exposure, as long as clinical signs of rabies are not present. Immediate treatment (including epinephrine 1:1000) for anaphylactoid and/or hypersensitivity reactions should be available during vaccine use. Once postexposure prophylaxis has begun, administration should generally not be interrupted or discontinued due to local or mild adverse events. Continuation of vaccination following severe systemic reactions should consider the persons risk of developing rabies. Report serious reactions to the State Health Department or the manufacturer/distributor. An immune complex reaction is possible 2-21 days following booster doses of HDCV. Symptoms may include arthralgia, arthritis, angioedema, fever, generalized urticaria, malaise, nausea, and vomiting. Use with caution in severely immunocompromised patients (eg, patients receiving chemo/radiation therapy or other immunosuppressive therapy [including high-dose corticosteroids]); may have a reduced response to vaccination. Withhold nonessential immunosuppressive agents during postexposure prophylaxis; if possible postpone pre-exposure prophylaxis until the immunocompromising condition is resolved. Persons with altered immunocompetence should receive the five-dose postexposure vaccine regimen. In general, household and close contacts of persons with altered immunocompetence may receive all age appropriate vaccines. Imovax® Rabies contains albumin and neomycin. RabAvert® contains amphotericin B, bovine gelatin, chicken protein, chlortetracycline, and neomycin. For I. M. administration only.

Adverse Reactions All serious adverse reactions must be reported to the U.S. Department of Health and Human Services (DHHS) Vaccine Adverse Event Reporting System (VAERS) 1-800-822-7967 or online at https://vaers.hhs.gov/esub/index. In Canada, adverse reactions may be reported to local provincial/territorial health agencies or to the Vaccine Safety Section at Public Health Agency of Canada (1-866-844-0018).

>10%:

- Central nervous system: Dizziness, headache, malaise
- Gastrointestinal: Abdominal pain, nausea
- Local: Erythema, itching, pain, swelling
- Neuromuscular & skeletal: Myalgia
- Miscellaneous: Lymphadenopathy

Uncommon, frequency not defined, postmarketing, and/or case reports:

- Cardiovascular: Circulatory reactions, edema, palpitation
- Central nervous system: Chills, fatigue, fever >38°C (100°F), Guillain-Barré syndrome, encephalitis, meningitis, multiple sclerosis, myelitis, neuroparalysis, vertigo
- Dermatologic: Pruritus, urticaria, urticaria pigmentosa
- Endocrine & metabolic: Hot flashes
- Local: Limb swelling (extensive)
- Neuromuscular & skeletal: Limb pain, monoarthritis, paralysis (transient), paresthesias (transient)
- Ocular: Retrobulbar neuritis, visual disturbances
- Respiratory: Bronchospasm
- Miscellaneous: Allergic reactions, anaphylaxis, hypersensitivity reactions, swollen lymph nodes

Drug Interactions

Metabolism/Transport Effects None known.

Avoid Concomitant Use There are no known interactions where it is recommended to avoid concomitant use.

Increased Effect/Toxicity There are no known significant interactions involving an increase in effect.

Decreased Effect

The levels/effects of Rabies Vaccine may be decreased by: Belimumab; Chloroquine; Fingolimod; Immunosuppressants

Stability Prior to reconstitution, store under refrigeration at 2°C to 8°C (36°F to 46°F); do not freeze. Protect from light. Reconstitute with provided diluent; gently swirl to dissolve. Use immediately after reconstitution.

Imovax®: Suspension will appear pink to red

RabAvert®: Suspension will appear clear to slightly opaque

Mechanism of Action Rabies vaccine is an inactivated virus vaccine which promotes immunity by inducing an active immune response. The production of specific antibodies requires about 7-10 days to develop. Rabies immune globulin or antirabies serum, equine (ARS) is given in conjunction with rabies vaccine to provide immune protection until an antibody response can occur.

Pharmacodynamics/Kinetics

Onset of action: I.M.: Rabies antibody: ~7-10 days

Peak effect: ~30-60 days

Duration: ≥1 year

Dosage

Pre-exposure vaccination: I.M: A total of 3 doses, 1 mL each, on days 0, 7, and 21-28. **Note:** Prolonging the interval between doses does not interfere with immunity achieved after the concluding dose of the basic series.

Postexposure vaccination: All postexposure treatment should begin with immediate cleansing of the wound with soap and water

Persons not previously immunized as above: I.M.: 5 doses (1 mL each) on days 0, 3, 7, 14, 28. In addition, patients should also receive rabies immune globulin with the first dose (day 0). **Note:** A regimen of 4 doses (1 mL each) on days 0, 3, 7, 14 may be used in persons who are not immunosuppressed (ACIP recommendations, 2010).

Persons who have previously received postexposure prophylaxis with rabies vaccine, received a recommended I.M. pre-exposure series of rabies vaccine or have a previously documented rabies antibody titer considered adequate: I.M.: Two doses (1 mL each) on days 0 and 3; do not administer rabies immune globulin

Booster (for persons with continuous or frequent risk of infection): 1 mL I.M. based on antibody titers

Administration For I.M. administration only; this rabies vaccine product must not be administered intradermally; in adults and children, administer I.M. injections in the deltoid muscle, not the gluteal; for younger children, use the outer aspect of the thigh. Postexposure prophylaxis should begin with immediate cleansing of wounds with soap and water; if available, a virucidal agent (eg povidone-iodine solution) should be used to irrigate the wounds.

For patients at risk of hemorrhage following intramuscular injection, the ACIP recommends "it should be administered intramuscularly if, in the opinion of the physician familiar with the patients bleeding risk, the vaccine can be administered by this route with reasonable safety. If the patient receives antihemophilia or other similar therapy, intramuscular vaccination can be scheduled shortly after such therapy is administered. A fine needle (23 gauge or smaller) can be used for the vaccination and firm pressure applied to the site (without rubbing) for at least 2 minutes. The patient should be instructed concerning the risk of hematoma from the injection." Patients on anticoagulant therapy should be considered to have the same bleeding risks and treated as those with clotting factor disorders (CDC, 2011).

Simultaneous administration of vaccines helps ensure the patients will be fully vaccinated by the appropriate age. Simultaneous administration of vaccines is defined as administering >1 vaccine on the same day at different anatomic sites. The use of licensed combination vaccines is generally preferred over separate injections of the equivalent components. Separate vaccines should not be combined in the same syringe unless indicated by product specific labeling. Separate needles and syringes should be used for each injection. The ACIP prefers each dose of a specific vaccine in a series come from the same manufacturer when possible. Adolescents and adults should be vaccinated while seated or lying down. In general, preterm infants should be vaccinated at the same chronological age as full-term infants (CDC, 2011).

Antipyretics have not been shown to prevent febrile seizures. Antipyretics may be used to treat fever or discomfort following vaccination (CDC, 2011). One study reported that routine prophylactic administration of acetaminophen to prevent fever prior to vaccination decreased the immune response of some vaccines; the clinical significance of this reduction in immune response has not been established (Prymula, 2009).

Monitoring Parameters Monitor for syncope for ≥15 minutes following vaccination.

Antibody response to vaccination is not recommended for otherwise healthy persons who complete the pre-exposure or postexposure regimen. Serologic testing to determine if the antibody titer is at an acceptable level is required for the following persons (booster vaccination recommended if titer is below the acceptable level):

Persons with continuous risk of infection: Serologic testing every 6 months

Persons with frequent risk of infection: Serologic testing every 2 years

Persons who are immunocompromised: Serologic testing after completion of pre-exposure or postexposure prophylaxis series

Monitoring of antibody response to vaccination is not recommended for otherwise healthy persons who complete the pre-exposure or postexposure regimen.

Reference Range Adequate adaptive immune response: antibody titers of 0.5 int. units/mL [WHO] or complete virus neutralization at a 1:5 serum dilution by the rapid fluorescent focus inhibition test (RFFIT) [ACIP]

Additional Information Federal law requires that the name of medication, date of administration, the vaccine manufacturer, lot number of vaccine, and the administering person's name, title, and address be entered into the patient's permanent medical record.

Dosage Forms Excipient information presented when available (limited, particularly for generics); consult specific product labeling.

Injection, powder for reconstitution [preservative free]:

Imovax® Rabies: ≥ 2.5 int. units [contains albumin (human), neomycin (may have trace amounts); HDCV; grown in human diploid cell culture]

RabAvert®: ≥ 2.5 int. units [contains albumin (human), amphotericin B (may have trace amounts), bovine gelatin, chicken egg protein, chlortetracycline (may have trace amounts), neomycin (may have trace amounts); PCEC; grown in chicken fibroblast culture]

◆ **Racemic Epinephrine** *see* EPINEPHrine (Systemic, Oral Inhalation) *on page 594*

◆ **Racepinephrine** *see* EPINEPHrine (Systemic, Oral Inhalation) *on page 594*

◆ **RAD001** *see* Everolimus *on page 673*

◆ **Radiogardase®** *see* Ferric Hexacyanoferrate *on page 705*

◆ **rAHF** *see* Antihemophilic Factor (Recombinant) *on page 127*

◆ **R-albuterol** *see* Levalbuterol *on page 992*

◆ **Ralivia™ ER (Can)** *see* TraMADol *on page 1715*

Raloxifene (ral OKS i feen)

Brand Names: U.S. Evista®

Brand Names: Canada Apo-Raloxifene®; Evista®; Novo-Raloxifene; Teva-Raloxifene

Index Terms Keoxifene Hydrochloride; Raloxifene Hydrochloride

Pharmacologic Category Selective Estrogen Receptor Modulator (SERM)

Use Prevention and treatment of osteoporosis in postmenopausal women; risk reduction for invasive breast cancer in postmenopausal women with osteoporosis and in postmenopausal women with high risk for invasive breast cancer

Pregnancy Risk Factor X

Pregnancy Considerations Animal studies have demonstrated teratogenicity and fetal loss. There are no adequate and well-controlled studies in pregnant women. Raloxifene should not be used by women who are or may become pregnant.

Lactation Excretion in breast milk unknown/contraindicated

Medication Guide Available Yes

Contraindications History of or current venous thromboembolic disorders (including DVT, PE, and retinal vein thrombosis); pregnancy or women who could become pregnant; breast-feeding

Warnings/Precautions Hazardous agent - use appropriate precautions for handling and disposal. **[U.S. Boxed Warning]: May increase the risk for DVT or PE; use contraindicated in patients with history of or current venous thromboembolic disorders.** Use with caution in patients at high risk for venous thromboembolism; the risk for DVT and PE are higher in the first 4 months of treatment. Discontinue at least 72 hours prior to and during prolonged immobilization (postoperative recovery or prolonged bedrest). **[U.S. Boxed Warning]: The risk of death due to stroke may be increased in women with coronary heart disease or in women at risk for coronary events;** use with caution in patients with cardiovascular disease. Not be used for the prevention of cardiovascular disease. Use caution with moderate-to-severe renal dysfunction, hepatic impairment, unexplained uterine bleeding, and in women with a history of elevated triglycerides in response to treatment with oral estrogens (or estrogen/progestin). Safety with concomitant estrogen therapy has not been established. Safety and efficacy in premenopausal women or men have not been established. Not indicated for treatment of invasive breast cancer, to reduce the risk of recurrence of invasive breast cancer or to reduce the risk of noninvasive breast cancer. The efficacy (for breast cancer risk reduction) in women with inherited BRCA1 and BRCA1 mutations has not been established.

Adverse Reactions Note: Raloxifene has been associated with increased risk of thromboembolism (DVT, PE) and superficial thrombophlebitis; risk is similar to reported risk of HRT

>10%:

Cardiovascular: Peripheral edema (3% to 14%)

Endocrine & metabolic: Hot flashes (8% to 29%)

Neuromuscular & skeletal: Arthralgia (11% to 16%), leg cramps/muscle spasm (6% to 12%)

Miscellaneous: Flu syndrome (14% to 15%), infection (11%)

1% to 10%:

Cardiovascular: Chest pain (3%), venous thromboembolism (1% to 2%)

Central nervous system: Insomnia (6%)

Dermatologic: Rash (6%)

Endocrine & metabolic: Breast pain (4%)

Gastrointestinal: Weight gain (9%), abdominal pain (7%), vomiting (5%), flatulence (2% to 3%), cholelithiasis (≤3%), gastroenteritis (≤3%)

Genitourinary: Vaginal bleeding (6%), leukorrhea (3%), urinary tract disorder (3%), uterine disorder (3%), vaginal hemorrhage (3%), endometrial disorder (≤3%)

Neuromuscular & skeletal: Myalgia (8%), tendon disorder (4%)

Respiratory: Bronchitis (10%), sinusitis (10%), pharyngitis (8%), pneumonia (3%), laryngitis (≤2%)

Miscellaneous: Diaphoresis (3%)

<1% (Limited to important or life-threatening): Apolipoprotein A-1 increased, apolipoprotein B decreased, death related to VTE, fibrinogen decreased, hypertriglyceridemia (in women with a history of increased triglycerides in response to oral estrogens), intermittent claudication, LDL cholesterol decreased, lipoprotein decreased, retinal vein occlusion, stroke related to VTE, superficial thrombophlebitis, total serum cholesterol decreased

Drug Interactions

Metabolism/Transport Effects None known.

Avoid Concomitant Use There are no known interactions where it is recommended to avoid concomitant use.

Increased Effect/Toxicity There are no known significant interactions involving an increase in effect.

Decreased Effect

Raloxifene may decrease the levels/effects of: Levothyroxine

The levels/effects of Raloxifene may be decreased by: Bile Acid Sequestrants

Ethanol/Nutrition/Herb Interactions Ethanol: Avoid ethanol (may increase risk of osteoporosis).

Stability Store at controlled room temperature of 20°C to 25°C (68°F to 77°F); excursions permitted to 15°C to 30°C (59°F to 86°F).

Mechanism of Action A selective estrogen receptor modulator (SERM), meaning that it affects some of the same receptors that estrogen does, but not all, and in some instances, it antagonizes or blocks estrogen; it acts like estrogen to prevent bone loss and has the potential to block some estrogen effects in the breast and uterine tissues. Raloxifene decreases bone resorption, increasing bone mineral density and decreasing fracture incidence.

Pharmacodynamics/Kinetics

Onset of action: 8 weeks

Absorption: Rapid; ~60%

Distribution: 2348 L/kg

Protein binding: >95% to albumin and α-glycoprotein; does not bind to sex-hormone-binding globulin

Metabolism: Hepatic, extensive first-pass effect; metabolized to glucuronide conjugates

Bioavailability: ~2%

Half-life elimination: 28-33 hours

Excretion: Primarily feces; urine (<0.2% as unchanged drug; <6% as glucuronide conjugates)

Dosage Adults: Females: Oral:

Osteoporosis: 60 mg once daily

Invasive breast cancer risk reduction: 60 mg once daily for 5 years per ASCO guidelines (Visvanathan, 2009)

Dosage adjustment in renal impairment: Moderate-to-severe impairment: Use caution; safety and efficacy have not been established.

Dosage adjustment in hepatic impairment: Mild impairment (Child-Pugh class A): Plasma concentrations were higher and correlated with total bilirubin. Safety and efficacy in hepatic insufficiency have not been established.

Dietary Considerations May be taken without regard to meals. Osteoporosis prevention or treatment: Ensure adequate calcium and vitamin D intake; postmenopausal women should consume ~1500 mg/day of elemental calcium and 400-800 int. units/day of vitamin D.

Administration May be administered without regard to meals.

Monitoring Parameters Bone mineral density (BMD), lipid profile; adequate diagnostic measures, including endometrial sampling, if indicated, should be performed to rule out malignancy in all cases of undiagnosed abnormal vaginal bleeding

Additional Information The decrease in estrogen-related adverse effects with the selective estrogen-receptor modulators in general and raloxifene in particular should improve compliance and decrease the incidence of cardiovascular events and fractures while not increasing breast cancer.

Oncology Comment: The American Society of Clinical Oncology (ASCO) guidelines for breast cancer risk reduction (Visvanathan, 2009) recommend raloxifene (for 5 years) as an option to reduce the risk of ER-positive invasive breast cancer in postmenopausal women with a 5-year projected risk (based on NCI trial model) of ≥1.66%, or with lobular carcinoma *in situ*. Raloxifene should not be used in premenopausal women. Women with osteoporosis may use raloxifene beyond 5 years of treatment. According to the NCCN breast cancer risk reduction guidelines (v.2.2009), raloxifene is only recommended for postmenopausal women (≥35 years of age), and is equivalent to tamoxifen although, raloxifene has a better adverse event profile; however, tamoxifen is superior in reducing the risk on noninvasive breast cancer.

Dosage Forms Excipient information presented when available (limited, particularly for generics); consult specific product labeling.

Tablet, oral, as hydrochloride:

Evista®: 60 mg

◆ **Raloxifene Hydrochloride** *see* Raloxifene *on page 1455*

Raltegravir (ral TEG ra vir)

Brand Names: U.S. Isentress®

Brand Names: Canada Isentress®

Index Terms MK-0518

Pharmacologic Category Antiretroviral Agent, Integrase Inhibitor

Additional Appendix Information

Perinatal HIV Guidelines *on page 1946*

Use Treatment of HIV-1 infection in combination with other antiretroviral agents

Pregnancy Risk Factor C

Pregnancy Considerations Adverse events were observed in some animal reproduction studies. Raltegravir crosses the placenta and can be detected in neonatal serum after delivery. Standard doses appear to be appropriate in pregnant women. The DHHS Perinatal HIV Guidelines note that available data are insufficient to recommend use in pregnancy.

Regardless of CD4 count or HIV RNA copy number, all HIV-infected pregnant women should receive a combination antepartum antiretroviral (ARV) drug regimen; this includes women who require therapy for their own health, as well as women who do not yet require therapy for their own health. ARV therapy should be started as soon as possible if required for the woman's health or immediately after the first trimester if not needed for the mothers health (although earlier initiation may be considered). Long-term follow-up is recommended for all infants exposed to ARV medications.

Healthcare providers are encouraged to enroll pregnant women exposed to antiretroviral medications in the Antiretroviral Pregnancy Registry (1-800-258-4263 or www.-APRegistry.com). Healthcare providers caring for HIV-infected women and their infants may contact the National Perinatal HIV Hotline (888-448-8765) for clinical consultation (DHHS [perinatal], 2011).

Lactation Excretion in breast milk unknown/contraindicated

Contraindications There are no contraindications listed in the manufacturer's labeling.

Canadian labeling: Hypersensitivity to raltegravir or any other component of the formulation

Warnings/Precautions Patients may develop immune reconstitution syndrome resulting in the occurrence of an inflammatory response to an indolent or residual opportunistic infection; further evaluation and treatment may be required. Severe, life-threatening or fatal cases of Stevens-Johnson syndrome and toxic epidermal necrolysis have been reported. Hypersensitivity reactions (rash [may occur with fever, fatigue, malaise, conjunctivitis, or other constitutional symptoms], organ dysfunction and/or hepatic failure) have also been reported. Discontinue immediately if a severe skin reaction or hypersensitivity symptoms develop. Monitor liver transaminases and start supportive therapy. Myopathy and rhabdomyolysis have been reported; use caution in patients with risk factors for CK elevations and/or skeletal muscle abnormalities. Use caution with medications known to induce (eg, rifampin) or inhibit (eg, atazanavir) UGT1A1 glucuronidation, as serum levels/therapeutic effects may be reduced or increased, respectively. Avoid use as a boosted PI replacement in antiretroviral experienced patients with documented resistance to nucleoside reverse transcriptase inhibitors.

Adverse Reactions

>10%: Endocrine & metabolic: Total cholesterol increased (grade 2: 16%; grade 3: 6%)

2% to 10%:

Cardiovascular: Hypertension (≤3%)

Central nervous system: Fatigue (<2% to 8%), dizziness (≤4%), insomnia (4%), headache (≥2%)

Dermatologic: Rash (≤5%), pruritus (≤3%), folliculitis (≤2%)

Endocrine & metabolic: LDL-cholesterol increased (grade 2: 9%; grade 3: 4%), glucose increased (126-250 mg/dL: 8%; 251-500 mg/dL: 2%), hypertriglyceridemia (grade 3: 4%)

Gastrointestinal: Abdominal pain (≤5%), lipase increased (1.6-3 x ULN: 4%), amylase increased (1.6-2 x ULN: 2%; 2.1-5 x ULN: 3%), gastroenteritis (≤3%), nausea (≥2%), constipation (≤2%)

Hepatic: AST increased (2.6-5 x ULN: 3% to 9%), hyperbilirubinemia (1.6-2.5 x ULN: 4% to 5%), ALT increased (5.1-10 x ULN: <1% to 3%), alkaline phosphatase increased (2.6-5 x ULN: <1% to 2%)

Neuromuscular & skeletal: Weakness (≥2%), creatine kinase increased (grade 4: 2%)

Renal: Creatinine increased (1.4-1.8 x ULN: 3%)

Respiratory: Nasopharyngitis (≤6%), cough (≤5%), influenza (≤3%)

Miscellaneous: Lymphadenopathy (≤3%), anogenital warts (≤2%)

Frequency <2% or not defined: Abnormal dreams, absolute neutrophil count decreased, acneiform dermatitis, allodynia, anemia, anxiety, appetite increased, arthralgia, back pain, cellulitis, central obesity, cerebellar ataxia, chest discomfort, chills, depression, diabetes mellitus, drug rash with eosinophilia and systemic symptoms (DRESS), dry skin, dyspepsia, dyslipidemia, epistaxis, erectile dysfunction, erythema, extremity pain, facial wasting, flatulence, fever, gastritis, GERD, glossitis, gynecomastia, hepatic failure, hepatitis, hepatomegaly, herpes simplex, herpes zoster, hyperhidrosis, hyperlactacidemia, hypersensitivity, insomnia, irritability, lipodystrophy, macrocytic anemia, maculopapular rash, MI, muscle atrophy, muscle spasms, myalgia, myopathy, myositis, nephrolithiasis, nephropathy, nephrotic syndrome, neuropathy, night sweats, nocturia, palpitation, paranoia, paresthesia, platelets decreased, pollakiuria, prurigo, renal failure, renal tubular necrosis, rhabdomyolysis, somnolence, Stevens-Johnson syndrome, suicidal ideation/behavior, thrombocytopenia, vertigo, ventricular extrasystoles, visual disturbance, vomiting, weight changes

Drug Interactions

Metabolism/Transport Effects None known.

Avoid Concomitant Use There are no known interactions where it is recommended to avoid concomitant use.

Increased Effect/Toxicity

The levels/effects of Raltegravir may be increased by: Proton Pump Inhibitors

Decreased Effect

Raltegravir may decrease the levels/effects of: Fosamprenavir

The levels/effects of Raltegravir may be decreased by: Efavirenz; Fosamprenavir; Rifampin; Tipranavir

Ethanol/Nutrition/Herb Interactions

Food: High-fat meal increased AUC by 19%, but raltegravir was administered without regard to meals in clinical trials.

Herb/Nutraceutical: Avoid St John's wort (may decrease the levels/effects of raltegravir).

Stability Store at room temperature of 20°C to 25°C (68°F to 77°F); excursions permitted to 15°C to 30°C (59°F to 86°F).

Mechanism of Action Incorporation of viral DNA into the host cell's genome is required to produce a self-replicating provirus and propagation of infectious virion particles. The viral cDNA strand produced by reverse transcriptase is subsequently processed and inserted into the human genome by the enzyme HIV-1 integrase (encoded by the pol gene of HIV). Raltegravir inhibits the catalytic activity of integrase, thus preventing integration of the proviral gene into human DNA.

Pharmacodynamics/Kinetics

Absorption: AUC increased ~19% with high-fat meal

Protein binding: ~83%

Metabolism: Primarily hepatic glucuronidation mediated by UGT1A1

Half-life elimination: ~9 hours

Time to peak, plasma: ~3 hours

Excretion: Feces (~51%, as unchanged drug); urine (~32%; 9% as unchanged drug)

Dosage Oral: Adolescents ≥16 years and Adults: 400 mg twice daily. **Note:** Recommended as a first-line therapy with tenofovir/emtricitabine in antiretroviral naïve patients (Lennox, 2009; DHHS, 2011).

Dosage adjustment for rifampin coadministration: 800 mg twice daily

Dosage adjustment in renal impairment: Severe renal impairment: No dosage adjustment required

Dosage adjustment in hepatic impairment:

Mild-to-moderate hepatic impairment: No dosage adjustment required

Severe impairment: No data available

Dietary Considerations May be taken without regard to meals.

Administration May be administered without regard to meals.

Monitoring Parameters Viral load, CD4 count, lipid profile

Product Availability Isentress® chewable tablets (25 mg, 100 mg): FDA approved December 2011; availability anticipated mid-2012

Dosage Forms Excipient information presented when available (limited, particularly for generics); consult specific product labeling.

Tablet, oral:

Isentress®: 400 mg

Ramelteon (ra MEL tee on)

Brand Names: U.S. Rozerem®

Index Terms TAK-375

Pharmacologic Category Hypnotic, Nonbenzodiazepine

Use Treatment of insomnia characterized by difficulty with sleep onset

Pregnancy Risk Factor C

Pregnancy Considerations Animal studies have demonstrated teratogenic effects. May cause disturbances of reproductive hormonal regulation (eg, disruption of menses or decreased libido). There are no adequate and well-controlled studies in pregnant women.

Lactation Excretion in breast milk unknown/use caution

Medication Guide Available Yes

Contraindications History of angioedema with previous ramelteon therapy (do not rechallenge); concurrent use with fluvoxamine

Warnings/Precautions Symptomatic treatment of insomnia should be initiated only after careful evaluation of potential causes of sleep disturbance. Failure of sleep disturbance to resolve after a reasonable period of treatment may indicate psychiatric and/or medical illness. Because of the rapid onset of action, administer immediately prior to bedtime or after the patient has gone to bed and is having difficulty falling asleep. Hypnotics/sedatives have been associated with abnormal thinking and behavior changes including decreased inhibition, aggression, bizarre behavior, agitation, hallucinations, and depersonalization. These changes may occur unpredictably and may indicate previously unrecognized psychiatric disorders; evaluate appropriately. Postmarketing studies have indicated that the use of hypnotic/sedative agents (including ramelteon) for sleep has been associated with hypersensitivity reactions including anaphylaxis as well as angioedema. Do not rechallenge patients who have developed angioedema with ramelteon therapy. An increased risk for hazardous sleep-related activities such as sleep-driving; cooking and eating food, and making phone calls while asleep have also been noted. Use caution with preexisting depression or other psychiatric conditions. Caution when using with other CNS depressants; avoid engaging in hazardous activities or activities requiring mental alertness. Not recommended for use in patients with severe sleep apnea or COPD. Use caution with moderate hepatic impairment; not recommended in patients with severe impairment. May cause disturbances of hormonal regulation. Use caution when administered concomitantly with strong CYP1A2 inhibitors.

Adverse Reactions

1% to 10%:

Central nervous system: Dizziness (4% to 5%), somnolence (3% to 5%), fatigue (3% to 4%), insomnia worsened (3%), depression (2%)

Endocrine & metabolic: Serum cortisol decreased (1%)

Gastrointestinal: Nausea (3%), taste perversion (2%)

Neuromuscular & skeletal: Myalgia (2%), arthralgia (2%)

Respiratory: Upper respiratory infection (3%)

Miscellaneous: Influenza (1%)

Postmarketing and/or case reports: Anaphylaxis, angioedema, complex sleep-related behavior (sleep-driving, cooking or eating food, making phone calls), prolactin levels increased, testosterone levels decreased

Drug Interactions

Metabolism/Transport Effects Substrate of CYP1A2 (major), CYP2C19 (minor), CYP3A4 (minor); **Note:** Assignment of Major/Minor substrate status based on clinically relevant drug interaction potential

Avoid Concomitant Use

Avoid concomitant use of Ramelteon with any of the following: FluvoxaMINE

Increased Effect/Toxicity

Ramelteon may increase the levels/effects of: Alcohol (Ethyl); CNS Depressants; Methotrimeprazine; Selective Serotonin Reuptake Inhibitors

The levels/effects of Ramelteon may be increased by: Abiraterone Acetate; Antifungal Agents (Azole Derivatives, Systemic); Conivaptan; CYP1A2 Inhibitors (Moderate); CYP1A2 Inhibitors (Strong); Deferasirox; Droperidol; Fluconazole; FluvoxaMINE; HydrOXYzine; Methotrimeprazine

Decreased Effect

The levels/effects of Ramelteon may be decreased by: Cyproterone; Rifamycin Derivatives; Tocilizumab

Ethanol/Nutrition/Herb Interactions

Ethanol: May increase CNS depression; monitor for increased effects with coadministration. Caution patients about effects.

Food: Taking with high-fat meal delays T_{max} and increases AUC (~31%).

Herb/Nutraceutical: Avoid valerian, St John's wort, kava kava, gotu kola (may increase CNS depression).

Stability Store at 25°C (77°F); excursions permitted to 15°C to 30°C (59°F to 86°F). Protect from moisture.

Mechanism of Action Potent, selective agonist of melatonin receptors MT_1 and MT_2 (with little affinity for MT_3) within the suprachiasmic nucleus of the hypothalamus, an area responsible for determination of circadian rhythms and synchronization of the sleep-wake cycle. Agonism of MT_1 is thought to preferentially induce sleepiness, while MT_2 receptor activation preferentially influences regulation of circadian rhythms. Ramelteon is eightfold more selective for MT_1 than MT_2 and exhibits nearly sixfold higher affinity for MT_1 than melatonin, presumably allowing for enhanced effects on sleep induction.

Pharmacodynamics/Kinetics

Onset of action: 30 minutes

Absorption: Rapid; high-fat meal delays T_{max} and increases AUC (~31%)

Distribution: 74 L

Protein binding: ~82%

Metabolism: Extensive first-pass effect; oxidative metabolism primarily through CYP1A2 and to a lesser extent through CYP2C and CYP3A4; forms active metabolite (M-II)

Bioavailability: Absolute: 1.8%

Half-life elimination: Ramelteon: 1-2.6 hours; M-II: 2-5 hours

Time to peak, plasma: Median: 0.5-1.5 hours

Excretion: Primarily as metabolites: Urine (84%); feces (4%)

Dosage Oral: Adults: One 8 mg tablet within 30 minutes of bedtime

Dosage adjustment in renal impairment: No dosage adjustment required

Dosage adjustment in hepatic impairment: No adjustment required for mild-to-moderate impairment; use caution. Not recommended with severe impairment.

Dietary Considerations Do not take with high-fat meal.

Administration Do not administer with a high-fat meal. Swallow tablet whole; do not break.

Dosage Forms Excipient information presented when available (limited, particularly for generics); consult specific product labeling.

Tablet, oral:

Rozerem®: 8 mg

Ramipril (RA mi pril)

Brand Names: U.S. Altace®

Brand Names: Canada Altace®; Apo-Ramipril®; Ava-Ramipril; CO Ramipril; Dom-Ramipril; JAMP-Ramipril; Mylan-Ramipril; PHL-Ramipril; PMS-Ramipril; RAN™-Ramipril; ratio-Ramipril; Sandoz-Ramipril; Teva-Ramipril

Pharmacologic Category Angiotensin-Converting Enzyme (ACE) Inhibitor

Additional Appendix Information

Angiotensin Agents *on page 1869*

Heart Failure (Systolic) *on page 1991*

Use Treatment of hypertension, alone or in combination with thiazide diuretics; treatment of left ventricular dysfunction after MI; to reduce risk of MI, stroke, and death in patients at increased risk for these events

Unlabeled Use Treatment of heart failure; to delay the progression of nephropathy and reduce risks of cardiovascular events in hypertensive patients with type 1 or 2 diabetes mellitus

Pregnancy Risk Factor C (1st trimester); D (2nd and 3rd trimesters)

Pregnancy Considerations Due to adverse events observed in some animal studies, ramipril is considered pregnancy category C during the first trimester. Based on human data, ramipril is considered pregnancy category D if used during the second and third trimesters (per the manufacturer; however, one study suggests that fetal injury may occur at anytime during pregnancy). Ramipril crosses the placenta. First trimester exposure to ACE inhibitors may cause major congenital malformations. An increased risk of cardiovascular and/or central nervous system malformations was observed in one study; however, an increased risk of teratogenic events was not observed in other studies. Second and third trimester use of an ACE inhibitor is associated with oligohydramnios. Oligohydramnios due to decreased fetal renal function may lead to fetal limb contractures, craniofacial deformation, and hypoplastic lung development. The use of ACE inhibitors during the second and third trimesters is also associated with anuria, hypotension, renal failure (reversible or irreversible), skull hypoplasia, and death in the fetus/neonate. Chronic maternal hypertension itself is also associated with adverse events in the fetus/infant. ACE inhibitors are not recommended during pregnancy to treat maternal hypertension or heart failure. Those who are planning a pregnancy should be considered for other medication options if an ACE inhibitor is currently prescribed or the ACE inhibitor should be discontinued as soon as possible once pregnancy is detected. The exposed fetus should be monitored for fetal growth, amniotic fluid volume, and organ formation. Infants exposed to an ACE inhibitor *in utero*, especially during the second and third trimester, should be monitored for hyperkalemia, hypotension, and oliguria.

[U.S. Boxed Warning]: Based on human data, ACE inhibitors can cause injury and death to the developing fetus when used in the second and third trimesters. ACE inhibitors should be discontinued as soon as possible once pregnancy is detected.

Lactation Excretion in breast milk unknown/not recommended

Contraindications Hypersensitivity to ramipril or any component of the formulation; prior hypersensitivity (including angioedema) to ACE inhibitors

Warnings/Precautions Anaphylactic reactions may occur rarely with ACE inhibitors. At any time during treatment (especially following first dose) angioedema may occur rarely with ACE inhibitors; it may involve the head and neck (potentially compromising airway) or the intestine (presenting with abdominal pain). African-Americans and patients with idiopathic or hereditary angioedema may be at an increased risk. Prolonged frequent monitoring may be required especially if tongue, glottis, or larynx are involved as they are associated with airway obstruction. Patients with a history of airway surgery may have a higher risk of airway obstruction. Aggressive early and appropriate management is critical. Use in patients with previous angioedema associated with ACE inhibitor therapy is contraindicated. Severe anaphylactoid reactions may be seen during hemodialysis (eg, CVVHD) with high-flux dialysis membranes (eg, AN69), and rarely, during low density lipoprotein apheresis with dextran sulfate cellulose. Rare cases of anaphylactoid reactions have been reported in patients undergoing sensitization treatment with hymenoptera (bee, wasp) venom while receiving ACE inhibitors.

Symptomatic hypotension with or without syncope can occur with ACE inhibitors (usually with the first several doses); effects are most often observed in volume-depleted patients; close monitoring of patient is required especially with initial dosing and dosing increases; blood pressure must be lowered at a rate appropriate for the patient's clinical condition. Initiation of therapy in patients with ischemic heart disease or cerebrovascular disease warrants close observation due to the potential consequences posed by falling blood pressure (eg, MI, stroke). Use with caution in hypertrophic cardiomyopathy with outflow tract obstruction, severe aortic stenosis, or before, during, or immediately after major surgery. **[U.S. Boxed Warning]: Based on human data, ACEIs can cause injury and death to the developing fetus when used in the second and third trimesters. ACEIs should be discontinued as soon as possible once pregnancy is detected.**

Hyperkalemia may occur with ACE inhibitors; risk factors include renal dysfunction, diabetes mellitus, concomitant use of potassium-sparing diuretics, potassium supplements, and/or potassium containing salts. Use cautiously, if at all, with these agents and monitor potassium closely. Cough may occur with ACE inhibitors. Other causes of cough should be considered (eg, pulmonary congestion in patients with heart failure) and excluded prior to discontinuation.

May be associated with deterioration of renal function and/or increases in serum creatinine, particularly in patients with low renal blood flow (eg, renal artery stenosis, heart failure) whose glomerular filtration rate (GFR) is dependent on efferent arteriolar vasoconstriction by angiotensin II; deterioration may result in oliguria, acute renal failure, and progressive azotemia. Small increases in serum creatinine may occur following initiation; consider discontinuation only in patients with progressive and/or significant deterioration in renal function. Use with caution in patients with unstented unilateral/bilateral renal artery stenosis. When unstented bilateral renal artery stenosis is present, use is generally avoided due to the elevated risk of deterioration in renal function unless possible benefits outweigh risks. Concurrent use of angiotensin receptor blockers may increase the risk of clinically-significant adverse events (eg, renal dysfunction, hyperkalemia). Concurrent use with telmisartan is not recommended.

Rare toxicities associated with ACE inhibitors include cholestatic jaundice (which may progress to fulminant hepatic necrosis), agranulocytosis, neutropenia, or leukopenia with myeloid hypoplasia. Patients with collagen vascular diseases (especially with concomitant renal impairment) or renal impairment alone may be at increased risk for hematologic toxicity; periodically monitor CBC with differential in these patients.

Adverse Reactions Note: Frequency ranges include data from hypertension and heart failure trials. Higher rates of adverse reactions have generally been noted in patients with CHF. However, the frequency of adverse effects associated with placebo is also increased in this population.

>10%: Respiratory: Cough increased (7% to 12%)

1% to 10%:

Cardiovascular: Hypotension (11%), angina (up to 3%), postural hypotension (2%), syncope (up to 2%)

Central nervous system: Headache (1% to 5%), dizziness (2% to 4%), fatigue (2%), vertigo (up to 2%)

Endocrine & metabolic: Hyperkalemia (1% to 10%)

Gastrointestinal: Nausea/vomiting (1% to 2%)

Neuromuscular & skeletal: Chest pain (noncardiac) (1%)

Renal: Renal dysfunction (1%), serum creatinine increased (1% to 2%), BUN increased (<1% to 3%); transient increases of creatinine and/or BUN may occur more frequently

Respiratory: Cough (estimated 1% to 10%)

<1% (Limited to important or life-threatening): Agitation, agranulocytosis, amnesia, anaphylactoid reaction, angioedema, arrhythmia, bone marrow depression, convulsions, depression, dysphagia, dyspnea, edema, eosinophilia, erythema multiforme, hearing loss, hemolytic anemia, hepatitis, hypersensitivity reactions (urticaria, rash, fever), impotence, insomnia, myalgia, MI, neuropathy, onycholysis, pancreatitis, pancytopenia, paresthesia, pemphigoid, pemphigus, photosensitivity, proteinuria, somnolence, Stevens-Johnson syndrome, symptomatic hypotension, thrombocytopenia, toxic epidermal necrolysis

Worsening of renal function may occur in patients with bilateral renal artery stenosis or in hypovolemia. In addition, a syndrome which may include fever, myalgia, arthralgia, interstitial nephritis, vasculitis, rash, eosinophilia and positive ANA, and elevated ESR has been reported with ACE inhibitors. Risk of pancreatitis and/or agranulocytosis may be increased in patients with collagen vascular disease or renal impairment.

Drug Interactions

Metabolism/Transport Effects None known.

Avoid Concomitant Use There are no known interactions where it is recommended to avoid concomitant use.

Increased Effect/Toxicity

Ramipril may increase the levels/effects of: Allopurinol; Amifostine; Antihypertensives; AzaTHIOprine; CycloSPORINE; CycloSPORINE (Systemic); Ferric Gluconate; Gold Sodium Thiomalate; Hypotensive Agents; Iron Dextran Complex; Lithium; Nonsteroidal Anti-Inflammatory Agents; RiTUXimab; Sodium Phosphates

The levels/effects of Ramipril may be increased by: Alfuzosin; Angiotensin II Receptor Blockers; Diazoxide; DPP-IV Inhibitors; Eplerenone; Everolimus; Herbs (Hypotensive Properties); Loop Diuretics; MAO Inhibitors; Pentoxifylline; Phosphodiesterase 5 Inhibitors; Potassium Salts; Potassium-Sparing Diuretics; Prostacyclin Analogues; Sirolimus; Telmisartan; Temsirolimus; Thiazide Diuretics; TiZANidine; Tolvaptan; Trimethoprim

Decreased Effect

The levels/effects of Ramipril may be decreased by: Aprotinin; Herbs (Hypertensive Properties); Icatibant; Lanthanum; Methylphenidate; Nonsteroidal Anti-Inflammatory Agents; Salicylates; Yohimbine

Ethanol/Nutrition/Herb Interactions Herb/Nutraceutical: Avoid bayberry, blue cohosh, cayenne, ephedra, ginger, ginseng (American), kola, licorice (may worsen hypertension). Avoid black cohosh, California poppy, coleus, golden seal, hawthorn, mistletoe, periwinkle, quinine, shepherd's purse (may have increased antihypertensive effect).

Stability Store at controlled room temperature.

Mechanism of Action Ramipril is an ACE inhibitor which prevents the formation of angiotensin II from angiotensin I and exhibits pharmacologic effects that are similar to captopril. Ramipril must undergo enzymatic saponification by esterases in the liver to its biologically active metabolite, ramiprilat. The pharmacodynamic effects of ramipril result from the high-affinity, competitive, reversible binding of ramiprilat to angiotensin-converting enzyme, thus preventing the formation of the potent vasoconstrictor angiotensin II. This isomerized enzyme-inhibitor complex has a slow rate of dissociation, which results in high potency and a long duration of action; a CNS mechanism may also be involved in the hypotensive effect as angiotensin II increases adrenergic outflow from CNS; vasoactive kallikreins may be decreased in conversion to active hormones by ACE inhibitors, thus reducing blood pressure

Pharmacodynamics/Kinetics

Onset of action: 1-2 hours

Duration: 24 hours

Absorption: Well absorbed (50% to 60%)

Distribution: Plasma levels decline in a triphasic fashion; rapid decline is a distribution phase to peripheral compartment, plasma protein and tissue ACE (half-life: 2-4 hours); second phase is an apparent elimination phase representing the clearance of free ramiprilat (half-life: 9-18 hours); and final phase is the terminal elimination phase representing the equilibrium phase between tissue binding and dissociation

Protein binding: Ramipril: 73%; Ramiprilat: 56%

Metabolism: Hepatic to the active form, ramiprilat

Bioavailability: Ramipril: 28%; Ramiprilat: 44%

Half-life elimination: Ramiprilat: Effective: 13-17 hours; Terminal: >50 hours

Time to peak, serum: Ramipril: ~1 hour; Ramiprilat: 2-4 hours

Excretion: Urine (60%) and feces (40%) as parent drug and metabolites

Dosage Oral:

Adults:

Heart failure (unlabeled use): Initial: 1.25-2.5 mg once daily; target dose: 10 mg once daily (ACC/AHA 2009 Heart Failure Guidelines)

Hypertension: 2.5-5 mg once daily, maximum: 20 mg/day

LV dysfunction postmyocardial infarction: Initial: 2.5 mg twice daily titrated upward, if possible, to 5 mg twice daily

Reduction in risk of MI, stroke, and death from cardiovascular causes: Initial: 2.5 mg once daily for 1 week, then 5 mg once daily for the next 3 weeks, then increase as tolerated to 10 mg once daily (may be given as divided dose)

Elderly: Adjust for renal function for elderly since glomerular filtration rates are decreased; may see exaggerated hypotensive effects if renal clearance is not considered. In the management of hypertension, consider lower initial doses and titrate to response (Aronow, 2011).

Note: The dose of any concomitant diuretic should be reduced. If the diuretic cannot be discontinued, initiate therapy with 1.25 mg. After the initial dose, the patient should be monitored carefully until blood pressure has stabilized.

Dosing adjustment in renal impairment:

Cl_{cr} <40 mL/minute: Administer 25% of normal dose.

Renal failure and heart failure: Administer 1.25 mg once daily, increasing to 1.25 mg twice daily up to 2.5 mg twice daily as tolerated.

Renal failure and hypertension: Administer 1.25 mg once daily, titrated upward as possible; maximum daily dose 5 mg

Administration Capsule is usually swallowed whole, but contents may be mixed in water, apple juice, or applesauce.

Monitoring Parameters Blood pressure; serum creatinine and potassium; if patient has collagen vascular disease and/or renal impairment, periodically monitor CBC with differential

Test Interactions Positive Coombs' [direct]; may cause false-positive results in urine acetone determinations using sodium nitroprusside reagent

Dosage Forms Excipient information presented when available (limited, particularly for generics); consult specific product labeling.

Capsule, oral: 1.25 mg, 2.5 mg, 5 mg, 10 mg

Altace®: 1.25 mg, 2.5 mg, 5 mg, 10 mg

- ◆ **RAN™-Amlodipine (Can)** *see* AmLODIPine *on page 97*
- ◆ **RAN™-Atenolol (Can)** *see* Atenolol *on page 161*
- ◆ **RAN™-Atorvastatin (Can)** *see* Atorvastatin *on page 165*
- ◆ **RAN™-Carvedilol (Can)** *see* Carvedilol *on page 295*
- ◆ **RAN™-Cefprozil (Can)** *see* Cefprozil *on page 314*
- ◆ **RAN™-Ciprofloxacin (Can)** *see* Ciprofloxacin (Systemic) *on page 362*
- ◆ **RAN™-Citalo (Can)** *see* Citalopram *on page 370*
- ◆ **RAN™-Clarithromycin (Can)** *see* Clarithromycin *on page 374*
- ◆ **RAN™-Enalapril (Can)** *see* Enalapril *on page 584*
- ◆ **Ranexa®** *see* Ranolazine *on page 1464*
- ◆ **RAN™-Fentanyl Matrix Patch (Can)** *see* FentaNYL *on page 697*
- ◆ **RAN™-Fentanyl Transdermal System (Can)** *see* FentaNYL *on page 697*
- ◆ **RAN™-Fosinopril (Can)** *see* Fosinopril *on page 763*
- ◆ **RAN™-Gabapentin (Can)** *see* Gabapentin *on page 773*

Ranibizumab (ra ni BIZ oo mab)

Brand Names: U.S. Lucentis®

Brand Names: Canada Lucentis®

Index Terms rhuFabV2

Pharmacologic Category Monoclonal Antibody; Ophthalmic Agent; Vascular Endothelial Growth Factor (VEGF) Inhibitor

Use Treatment of neovascular (wet) age-related macular degeneration (AMD); treatment of macular edema following retinal vein occlusion (RVO)

Canadian labeling: Additional use (not in in U.S. labeling): Treatment of visual impairment associated with diabetic macular edema (DME)

Pregnancy Risk Factor C

Pregnancy Considerations Animal reproduction studies have not been conducted. Use during pregnancy only if clearly needed. Canadian labeling recommends that women of childbearing potential use effective contraception during therapy.

Lactation Excretion in breast milk unknown/use caution

Contraindications Hypersensitivity to ranibizumab or any component of the formulation; ocular or periocular infection

Canadian labeling: Additional contraindications (not in U.S. labeling): Active intraocular inflammation

Warnings/Precautions Intravitreous injections may be associated with endophthalmitis and retinal detachments. Proper aseptic injection techniques should be used and patients should be instructed to report any signs of infection immediately. Intraocular pressure may increase following injection. Intravitreal injections of ranibizumab may induce temporary visual disturbances that impair the ability to drive or operate machinery. Affected patients should be advised to abstain from driving or using machinery until resolution of disturbances. Use for >24 months has not been evaluated.

Risk of thromboembolic events, particularly stroke, may be increased following intravitreal administration of VEGF inhibitors. Use caution in patients with known risk factors (eg, history of stroke, TIA). Rare hypersensitivity reactions (including anaphylaxis) have been associated with another VEGF inhibitor, pegaptanib, occurring within several hours of use; monitor closely. Equipment and appropriate personnel should be available for monitoring and treatment of anaphylaxis.

Adverse Reactions Note: Rates of ocular adverse reactions reported for control group when percentages overlapped with treatment group.

As reported with AMD or RVO:

>10%:

Central nervous system: Headache (3% to 12%)

Neuromuscular & skeletal: Arthralgia (2% to 11%)

Ocular: Conjunctival hemorrhage (48% to 74%; control: 37% to 60%), eye pain (17% to 35%; control 12% to 30%), vitreous floaters (7% to 27%), intraocular pressure increased (7% to 24%), blurred vision/visual disturbance (5% to 18%), intraocular inflammation (1% to 18%; control 3% to 8%), blepharitis (≤12%), maculopathy (6% to 11%; control 6% to 9%), ocular hyperemia (5% to 11%; control 3% to 8%)

Note: Cataract, dry eye, eye irritation, foreign body sensation, lacrimation increased, pruritus, and vitreous detachment occurred in >10% of patients, but also occurred in similar percentages to the control; visual acuity blurred/decreased occurred more often in the control.

Respiratory: Nasopharyngitis (5% to 16%), bronchitis (≤11%)

1% to 10%:

Cardiovascular: Atrial fibrillation (1% to 5%), arterial thromboembolic events (4%; stroke ≤3%)

Gastrointestinal: Nausea (1% to 9%), viral gastroenteritis (1% to 4%)

Hematologic: Anemia (1% to 8%; control up to 7%)

Ocular: Retinal disorder (2% to 10%), retinal degeneration (1% to 8%), posterior capsule opacification (≤7%), injection site hemorrhage (≤5%)

Note: Conjunctival hyperemia and ocular discomfort occurred in 1% to 10% of patients, but also occurred in similar percentages to the control; retinal exudates occurred more often in the control.

Respiratory: Cough (2% to 9%), upper respiratory tract infection (≤9%), sinusitis (3% to 8%), chronic obstructive pulmonary disease (COPD) (≤6%), dyspnea (≤4%)

Miscellaneous: Ranibizumab antibodies (1% to 8%), influenza (3% to 7%)

As reported with DME:

>10%: Ocular: Intraocular pressure increased (≤28%), conjunctival hemorrhage (7% to 26%), vitreous floaters (2% to 14%)

1% to 10%:

Cardiovascular: Arrhythmia (2% to 4%), arterial thromboembolic events (≤4%), hypertension exacerbated (≤2%)

Gastrointestinal: Nausea (≤2%)

Local: Facial pain (≤2%)

Ocular: Conjunctival hyperemia (2% to 7%), foreign body sensation (4%), lacrimation increased (2% to 6%), eye irritation (2%to 6%), eye pruritus (4%), endophthalmitis (2% to 4%), vision blurred (2% to 4%), vitreous hemorrhage (2% to 4%), ocular hyperemia (1% to 4%), visual impairment (3%), eye discharge (2%), allergic blepharitis (≤2%), conjunctival edema (≤2%), corneal disorder (≤2%), eyelid edema (≤2%), eyelid erythema (≤2%), hypopyon (≤2%), lenticular opacities (≤2%), retinal artery occlusion (≤2%), retinal disorder (≤2%), retinal exudates (≤2%), ulcerative keratitis (≤2%)

All indications: <1% (Limited to important or life-threatening): Anterior chamber inflammation, anxiety, back pain, corneal edema, corneal epithelium defect, corneal erosion, coronary artery occlusion, dizziness, endophthalmitis, eyelid pain, hypoglycemia, iatrogenic traumatic cataracts, influenza, intestinal obstruction, lid margin discharge, maculopathy, photophobia, retinal tear, rhegmatogenous retinal detachments, rhinorrhea, subscapular cataract, urticaria, visual acuity decreased

Drug Interactions

Metabolism/Transport Effects None known.

Avoid Concomitant Use There are no known interactions where it is recommended to avoid concomitant use.

Increased Effect/Toxicity There are no known significant interactions involving an increase in effect.

Decreased Effect There are no known significant interactions involving a decrease in effect.

Stability Store in original carton under refrigeration at 2°C to 8°C (36°F to 46°F); protect from light. Do not freeze.

Mechanism of Action Ranibizumab is a recombinant humanized monoclonal antibody fragment which binds to and inhibits human vascular endothelial growth factor A (VEGF-A). Ranibizumab inhibits VEGF from binding to its receptors and thereby suppressing neovascularization and slowing vision loss.

Pharmacodynamics/Kinetics

Absorption: Low levels are detected in the serum following intravitreal injection

Half-life elimination: Vitreous: ~9 days

Dosage Intravitreal: Adults:

Age-related macular degeneration (AMD):

U.S. labeling: 0.5 mg (0.05 mL) once a month. Frequency may be reduced after the first 4 injections to once every 3 months if monthly injections are not feasible.

Canadian labeling: 0.5 mg (0.05 mL) once a month. Frequency may be reduced after the first 3 injections to once every 3 months if monthly injections are not feasible.

Note: Every-3-month dosing regimen has reportedly resulted in a ~5 letter (1 line) loss of visual acuity over 9 months, as compared to monthly dosing.

Macular edema following retinal vein occlusion (RVO): 0.5 mg (0.05 mL) once a month. **Note:** Canadian labeling recommends continuing therapy until achievement of stable visual acuity for 3 consecutive months; upon discontinuation, may resume monthly therapy with loss of visual acuity.

Visual impairment associated with diabetic macular edema (DME): *Canadian labeling (not in U.S. labeling):* 0.5 mg (0.05 mL) once a month until achievement of stable visual acuity for 3 consecutive months. Upon discontinuation, may resume monthly therapy with loss of visual acuity.

Dosage adjustment in renal impairment: Dose adjustment not expected

Dosage adjustment in hepatic impairment: Dose adjustment not expected

Administration For ophthalmic intravitreal injection only. Remove contents from vial using a 5 micron 19-gauge filter needle attached to a tuberculin syringe. Discard filter needle and replace with a sterile 30 gauge 1/2 inch needle for injection (do not use filter needle for intravitreal injection). Adequate anesthesia and a broad-spectrum antimicrobial agent should be administered prior to the procedure. Canadian labeling recommends administering ranibizumab at least 30 minutes after laser photocoagulation therapy when administered on the same day.

Monitoring Parameters Intraocular pressure (within 30 minutes and between 2-7 days following administration); signs of infection/inflammation (for first week following injection); retinal perfusion, endophthalmitis; visual acuity

Dosage Forms Excipient information presented when available (limited, particularly for generics); consult specific product labeling.

Injection, solution [preservative free]:

Lucentis®: 10 mg/mL (0.2 mL)

Dosage Forms: Canada Excipient information presented when available (limited, particularly for generics); consult specific product labeling.

Injection, solution [preservative free]:

Lucentis®: 10 mg/mL (0.3 mL)

◆ **RAN™-Imipenem-Cilastatin (Can)** *see* Imipenem and Cilastatin *on page 875*

◆ **Ran™-Irbesartan HCTZ (Can)** *see* Irbesartan and Hydrochlorothiazide *on page 926*

Ranitidine (ra NI ti deen)

Brand Names: U.S. Zantac 150® [OTC]; Zantac 75® [OTC]; Zantac®; Zantac® EFFERdose®

Brand Names: Canada Acid Reducer; Apo-Ranitidine®; CO Ranitidine; Dom-Ranitidine; Myl-Ranitidine; Mylan-Ranitidine; Nu-Ranit; PHL-Ranitidine; PMS-Ranitidine; Ranitidine Injection, USP; RAN™-Ranitidine; ratio-Ranitidine; Riva-Ranitidine; Sandoz-Ranitidine; ScheinPharm Ranitidine; Teva-Ranitidine; Zantac 75®; Zantac Maximum Strength Non-Prescription; Zantac®

Index Terms Ranitidine Hydrochloride

Pharmacologic Category Histamine H_2 Antagonist

Use

Zantac®: Short-term and maintenance therapy of duodenal ulcer, gastric ulcer, gastroesophageal reflux disease (GERD), active benign ulcer, erosive esophagitis, and pathological hypersecretory conditions; as part of a multidrug regimen for *H. pylori* eradication to reduce the risk of duodenal ulcer recurrence

Zantac 75® [OTC]: Relief of heartburn, acid indigestion, and sour stomach

Unlabeled Use Recurrent postoperative ulcer, upper GI bleeding, prevention of acid-aspiration pneumonitis during surgery, and prevention of stress-induced ulcers

Pregnancy Risk Factor B

Pregnancy Considerations Adverse events were not observed in animal studies; therefore, ranitidine is classified as pregnancy category B. Ranitidine crosses the placenta. An increased risk of congenital malformations or adverse events in the newborn has generally not been observed following maternal use of ranitidine during pregnancy. Histamine H_2 antagonists have been evaluated for the treatment of gastroesophageal reflux disease (GERD) as well as gastric and duodenal ulcers during pregnancy. If needed, ranitidine is the agent of choice. Histamine H_2 antagonists may be used for aspiration prophylaxis prior to cesarean delivery.

Lactation Enters breast milk/use caution

Contraindications Hypersensitivity to ranitidine or any component of the formulation

Warnings/Precautions Ranitidine has been associated with confusional states (rare). Use with caution in patients with hepatic impairment; use with caution in renal impairment, dosage modification required. Avoid use in patients with history of acute porphyria (may precipitate attacks); long-term therapy may be associated with vitamin B_{12} deficiency. Symptoms of GI distress may be associated with a variety of conditions; symptomatic response to H_2 antagonists does not rule out the potential for significant pathology (eg, malignancy). EFFERdose® formulation contains phenylalanine.

Adverse Reactions Frequency not defined.

Cardiovascular: Asystole, atrioventricular block, bradycardia (with rapid I.V. administration), premature ventricular beats, tachycardia, vasculitis

Central nervous system: Agitation, dizziness, depression, hallucinations, headache, insomnia, malaise, mental confusion, somnolence, vertigo

Dermatologic: Alopecia, erythema multiforme, rash

Endocrine & metabolic: Prolactin levels increased

Gastrointestinal: Abdominal discomfort/pain, constipation, diarrhea, nausea, pancreatitis, vomiting

Hematologic: Acquired immune hemolytic anemia, acute porphyritic attack, agranulocytosis, aplastic anemia, granulocytopenia, leukopenia, pancytopenia, thrombocytopenia

Hepatic: Cholestatic hepatitis, hepatic failure, hepatitis, jaundice

Local: Transient pain, burning or itching at the injection site

Neuromuscular & skeletal: Arthralgia, involuntary motor disturbance, myalgia

Ocular: Blurred vision

Renal: Acute interstitial nephritis, serum creatinine increased

Respiratory: Pneumonia (causal relationship not established)

Miscellaneous: Anaphylaxis, angioneurotic edema, hypersensitivity reactions (eg, bronchospasm, fever, eosinophilia)

Drug Interactions

Metabolism/Transport Effects Substrate of CYP1A2 (minor), CYP2C19 (minor), CYP2D6 (minor), P-glycoprotein; **Note:** Assignment of Major/Minor substrate status based on clinically relevant drug interaction potential; **Inhibits** CYP1A2 (weak), CYP2D6 (weak)

Avoid Concomitant Use

Avoid concomitant use of Ranitidine with any of the following: Delavirdine

Increased Effect/Toxicity

Ranitidine may increase the levels/effects of: Dexmethylphenidate; Methylphenidate; Procainamide; Saquinavir; Sulfonylureas; Varenicline; Warfarin

The levels/effects of Ranitidine may be increased by: P-glycoprotein/ABCB1 Inhibitors

Decreased Effect

Ranitidine may decrease the levels/effects of: Atazanavir; Cefditoren; Cefpodoxime; Cefuroxime; Dasatinib; Delavirdine; Erlotinib; Fosamprenavir; Gefitinib; Indinavir; Iron Salts; Itraconazole; Ketoconazole; Ketoconazole (Systemic); Mesalamine; Nelfinavir; Posaconazole; Prasugrel; Rilpivirine

The levels/effects of Ranitidine may be decreased by: Cyproterone; Peginterferon Alfa-2b; P-glycoprotein/ABCB1 Inducers

Ethanol/Nutrition/Herb Interactions

Ethanol: Avoid ethanol (may cause gastric mucosal irritation).

Food: Does not interfere with absorption of ranitidine.

Stability

Injection: Vials: Store between 4°C to 25°C (39°F to 77°F); excursion permitted to 30°C (86°F). Protect from light. Solution is a clear, colorless to yellow solution; slight darkening does not affect potency.

Premixed bag: Store between 2°C to 25°C (36°F to 77°F). Protect from light.

EFFERdose® formulations: Store between 2°C to 30°C (36°F to 86°F).

Syrup: Store between 4°C to 25°C (39°F to 77°F). Protect from light.

Tablet: Store in dry place, between 15°C to 30°C (59°F to 86°F). Protect from light.

Vials can be mixed with NS or D_5W; solutions are stable for 48 hours at room temperature.

Intermittent bolus injection, continuous infusion: Dilute to maximum of 2.5 mg/mL.

Intermittent infusion: Dilute to maximum of 0.5 mg/mL.

Mechanism of Action Competitive inhibition of histamine at H_2-receptors of the gastric parietal cells, which inhibits gastric acid secretion, gastric volume, and hydrogen ion concentration are reduced. Does not affect pepsin secretion, pentagastrin-stimulated intrinsic factor secretion, or serum gastrin.

Pharmacodynamics/Kinetics

Absorption: Oral: 50%

Distribution: Normal renal function: V_d: ~1.4 L/kg; Cl_{cr} 25-35 mL/minute: 1.76 L/kg minimally penetrates the blood-brain barrier

Protein binding: 15%

Metabolism: Hepatic to N-oxide, S-oxide, and N-desmethyl metabolites

Bioavailability: Oral: 48% to 50%; I.M.: 90% to 100%

Half-life elimination:

- Oral: Normal renal function: 2.5-3 hours; Cl_{cr} 25-35 mL/minute: 4.8 hours
- I.V.: Normal renal function: 2-2.5 hours

Time to peak, serum: Oral: 2-3 hours; I.M.: ≤15 minutes

Excretion: Urine: Oral: 30%, I.V.: 70% (as unchanged drug); feces (as metabolites)

Dosage

Children 1 month to 16 years:

- Duodenal and gastric ulcer:
  - Oral:
    - Treatment: 4-8 mg/kg/day divided twice daily; maximum: 300 mg/day
    - Maintenance: 2-4 mg/kg/day once daily; maximum: 150 mg/day
  - I.V.: 2-4 mg/kg/day divided every 6-8 hours; maximum: 200 mg/day
- GERD and erosive esophagitis:
  - Oral: 5-10 mg/kg/day divided twice daily; maximum: GERD: 300 mg/day, erosive esophagitis: 600 mg/day
  - I.V. (unlabeled): 2-4 mg/kg/day divided every 6-8 hours; maximum: 200 mg/day **or as an alternative**
    - Continuous infusion: Initial: 1 mg/kg/dose for one dose followed by infusion of 0.08-0.17 mg/kg/hour or 2-4 mg/kg/day

Children ≥12 years: Prevention of heartburn: Oral: Zantac 75® [OTC]: 75 mg 30-60 minutes before eating food or drinking beverages which cause heartburn; maximum: 150 mg/24 hours; do not use for more than 14 days

Adults:

- Duodenal ulcer: Oral: Treatment: 150 mg twice daily, or 300 mg once daily after the evening meal or at bedtime; maintenance: 150 mg once daily at bedtime
- *Helicobacter pylori* eradication: 150 mg twice daily; requires combination therapy
- Pathological hypersecretory conditions:
  - Oral: 150 mg twice daily; adjust dose or frequency as clinically indicated; doses of up to 6 g/day have been used
  - I.V.: Continuous infusion for Zollinger-Ellison: Initial: 1 mg/kg/hour; measure gastric acid output at 4 hours, if >10 mEq or if patient is symptomatic, increase dose in increments of 0.5 mg/kg/hour; doses of up to 2.5 mg/kg/hour (or 220 mg/hour) have been used
- Gastric ulcer, benign: Oral: 150 mg twice daily; maintenance: 150 mg once daily at bedtime
- GERD: Oral: 150 mg twice daily
- Erosive esophagitis: Oral: Treatment: 150 mg 4 times/day; maintenance: 150 mg twice daily

Prevention of heartburn: Oral: Zantac 75® [OTC]: 75 mg 30-60 minutes before eating food or drinking beverages which cause heartburn; maximum: 150 mg in 24 hours; do not use for more than 14 days

Patients not able to take oral medication:

I.M.: 50 mg every 6-8 hours

I.V.: Intermittent bolus or infusion: 50 mg every 6-8 hours

Continuous I.V. infusion: 6.25 mg/hour

Elderly: Ulcer healing rates and incidence of adverse effects are similar in the elderly, when compared to younger patients; dosing adjustments not necessary based on age alone

Dosing adjustment in renal impairment: Adults: Cl_{cr} <50 mL/minute:

Oral: 150 mg every 24 hours; adjust dose cautiously if needed

I.V.: 50 mg every 18-24 hours; adjust dose cautiously if needed

Hemodialysis: Adjust dosing schedule so that dose coincides with the end of hemodialysis

Dosing adjustment/comments in hepatic disease: Patients with hepatic impairment may have minor changes in ranitidine half-life, distribution, clearance, and bioavailability; dosing adjustments not necessary, monitor

Dietary Considerations Some products may contain phenylalanine and/or sodium. Oral dosage forms may be taken with or without food.

Administration

Ranitidine injection may be administered I.M. or I.V.:

I.M.: Injection is administered undiluted

I.V.: Must be diluted; may be administered I.V. push, intermittent I.V. infusion, or continuous I.V. infusion

I.V. push: Ranitidine (usually 50 mg) should be diluted to a total of 20 mL (or a concentration not exceeding 2.5 mg/mL) with NS or D_5W and administered over at least 5 minutes or a maximum rate of 10 mg/minute

Intermittent I.V. infusion: Dilute to a maximum concentration of 0.5 mg/mL; administer over 15-20 minutes

Continuous I.V. infusion: Dilute to a maximum concentration of 2.5 mg/mL. Titrate dosage based on gastric pH.

EFFERdose®: Should not be chewed, swallowed whole, or dissolved on tongue: 25 mg tablet: Dissolve in at least 5 mL of water; wait until completely dissolved before administering

Monitoring Parameters AST, ALT, serum creatinine; when used to prevent stress-related GI bleeding, measure the intragastric pH and try to maintain pH >4; signs and symptoms of peptic ulcer disease, occult blood with GI bleeding, monitor renal function to correct dose

Test Interactions False-positive urine protein using Multistix®; gastric acid secretion test; skin test allergen extracts. May also interfere with urine detection of amphetamine/methamphetamine (false-positive).

Dosage Forms Excipient information presented when available (limited, particularly for generics); consult specific product labeling.

Capsule, oral: 150 mg, 300 mg

Infusion, premixed in 1/2 NS [preservative free]:

Zantac®: 50 mg (50 mL)

Injection, solution: 25 mg/mL (2 mL, 6 mL, 40 mL)

Zantac®: 25 mg/mL (2 mL, 6 mL, 40 mL)

Syrup, oral: 15 mg/mL (5 mL, 10 mL, 120 mL, 473 mL, 474 mL, 480 mL)

Zantac®: 15 mg/mL (480 mL) [contains ethanol 7.5%; peppermint flavor]

Tablet, oral: 75 mg, 150 mg, 300 mg

Zantac 150®: 150 mg

Zantac 150®: 150 mg [cool mint flavor]

Zantac 75®: 75 mg

Zantac 75®: 75 mg [sugar free]

Zantac®: 150 mg, 300 mg

Tablet for solution, oral [effervescent]:

Zantac® EFFERdose®: 25 mg [contains phenylalanine 2.81 mg/tablet, sodium 1.33 mEq/tablet, sodium benzoate]

◆ **Ranitidine Hydrochloride** *see* Ranitidine *on page 1462*

◆ **Ranitidine Injection, USP (Can)** *see* Ranitidine *on page 1462*

◆ **RAN™-Lisinopril (Can)** *see* Lisinopril *on page 1020*

◆ **RAN™-Lovastatin (Can)** *see* Lovastatin *on page 1038*

◆ **RAN™-Metformin (Can)** *see* MetFORMIN *on page 1086*

Ranolazine (ra NOE la zeen)

Brand Names: U.S. Ranexa®

Pharmacologic Category Antianginal Agent; Cardiovascular Agent, Miscellaneous

Use Treatment of chronic angina

Pregnancy Risk Factor C

Pregnancy Considerations Adverse effects were observed in animal studies. There are no adequate and well-controlled studies in pregnant women.

Lactation Excretion in breast milk unknown/not recommended

Contraindications Hepatic cirrhosis; concurrent strong CYP3A inhibitors; concurrent CYP3A inducers

Warnings/Precautions Ranolazine does not relieve acute angina attacks. Has been shown to prolong QT interval in a dose/plasma concentration-related manner; assess risk versus benefit of use in patients with potential for prolonged QT including a family history. Hepatically-impaired patients may have a more significant increase in QT interval. Use is contraindicated in patients with cirrhosis (Child-Pugh class ≥A). Use caution in patients ≥75 years of age; they may experience more adverse events. Use caution and monitor blood pressure in patients with renal dysfunction; has not been evaluated in patients requiring dialysis.

Ranolazine is a substrate for and a moderate inhibitor of P-glycoprotein. Inhibitors of P-glycoprotein may increase serum concentrations of ranolazine. Ranolazine may increase serum concentrations of substrates for P-glycoprotein (eg, digoxin). Ranolazine is primarily metabolized by CYP3A; use is contraindicated with inducers and strong inhibitors of CYP3A. Ranolazine has potential to prolong the QT-interval; use caution when administered concomitantly with QT-prolonging drugs. Use caution when administering ranolazine to patients with a history of malignant neoplasms or adenomatous polyps.

Adverse Reactions

>0.5% to 10%:

Cardiovascular: Bradycardia (≤4%), hypotension (≤4%), orthostatic hypotension (≤4%), palpitation (≤4%), peripheral edema (≤4%), QT_c prolongation (>500 msec: ≤1%)

Central nervous system: Headache (≤6%), dizziness (1% to 6%), confusion (≤4%), vasovagal attacks (≤4%), vertigo (≤4%)

Dermatologic: Hyperhidrosis (≤4%)

Gastrointestinal: Constipation (≤9%), abdominal pain (≤4%), anorexia (≤4%), dyspepsia (≤4%), nausea (≤4%; dose related), vomiting (≤4%), xerostomia (≤4%)

Neuromuscular: Weakness (≤4%)

Ocular: Blurred vision (≤4%)

Otic: Tinnitus (≤4%)

Renal: Hematuria (≤4%)
Respiratory: Dyspnea (≤4%)
≤0.5% (Limited to important or life-threatening): Angioedema, blood pressure increased, blood urea nitrogen increased, eosinophilia, hallucination, hemoglobin A_{1c} decreased, hypoesthesia, leukopenia, pancytopenia, paresthesia, pruritus, pulmonary fibrosis, rash, renal failure, serum creatinine increased, thrombocytopenia, T-wave amplitude decreased, T-wave changes (notched), torsade de pointes (case report [Morrow, 2007]), tremor

Drug Interactions

Metabolism/Transport Effects Substrate of CYP2D6 (minor), CYP3A4 (major), P-glycoprotein; **Note:** Assignment of Major/Minor substrate status based on clinically relevant drug interaction potential; **Inhibits** CYP2D6 (weak), CYP3A4 (weak), P-glycoprotein

Avoid Concomitant Use

Avoid concomitant use of Ranolazine with any of the following: Antifungal Agents (Azole Derivatives, Systemic); Artemether; CYP3A4 Inducers (Strong); CYP3A4 Inhibitors (Strong); Dronedarone; Lumefantrine; Nilotinib; Pimozide; QUEtiapine; QuiNINE; Rifampin; Silodosin; St Johns Wort; Tetrabenazine; Thioridazine; Topotecan; Toremifene; Vandetanib; Vemurafenib; Ziprasidone

Increased Effect/Toxicity

Ranolazine may increase the levels/effects of: Colchicine; Dabigatran Etexilate; Digoxin; Dronedarone; Everolimus; P-glycoprotein/ABCB1 Substrates; Pimozide; QTc-Prolonging Agents; QuiNINE; Rivaroxaban; Silodosin; Simvastatin; Tacrolimus; Tacrolimus (Systemic); Tetrabenazine; Thioridazine; Topotecan; Toremifene; Vandetanib; Vemurafenib; Ziprasidone

The levels/effects of Ranolazine may be increased by: Alfuzosin; Antifungal Agents (Azole Derivatives, Systemic); Artemether; Calcium Channel Blockers (Nondihydropyridine); Chloroquine; Ciprofloxacin; Ciprofloxacin (Systemic); CYP3A4 Inhibitors (Moderate); CYP3A4 Inhibitors (Strong); Gadobutrol; Indacaterol; Lumefantrine; Nilotinib; P-glycoprotein/ABCB1 Inhibitors; QUEtiapine; QuiNINE

Decreased Effect

The levels/effects of Ranolazine may be decreased by: CYP3A4 Inducers (Strong); Deferasirox; Peginterferon Alfa-2b; P-glycoprotein/ABCB1 Inducers; Rifampin; St Johns Wort; Tocilizumab

Ethanol/Nutrition/Herb Interactions Food: Limit the use of grapefruit, grapefruit juice, or grapefruit-containing products; if use is significant and consistent, the dose of ranolazine should be limited to 500 mg twice daily.

Stability Store at 25°C (77°F); excursions permitted to 15°C to 30°C (59°F to 86°F).

Mechanism of Action Ranolazine exerts antianginal and anti-ischemic effects without changing hemodynamic parameters (heart rate or blood pressure). At therapeutic levels, ranolazine inhibits the late phase of the inward sodium channel (late I_{Na}) in ischemic cardiac myocytes during cardiac repolarization reducing intracellular sodium concentrations and thereby reducing calcium influx via Na^+-Ca^{2+} exchange. Decreased intracellular calcium reduces ventricular tension and myocardial oxygen consumption. It is thought that ranolazine produces myocardial relaxation and reduces anginal symptoms through this mechanism although this is uncertain. At higher concentrations, ranolazine inhibits the rapid delayed rectifier potassium current (I_{Kr}) thus prolonging the ventricular action potential duration and subsequent prolongation of the QT interval.

Pharmacodynamics/Kinetics

Absorption: Highly variable; ranolazine is a substrate of P-glycoprotein; concurrent use of P-glycoprotein inhibitors may increase absorption
Protein binding: ~62%
Metabolism: Hepatic via CYP3A (major) and 2D6 (minor); gut
Bioavailability: 35% to 55%
Half-life elimination: Ranolazine: Terminal: 7 hours; Metabolites (activity undefined): 6-22 hours
Time to peak, plasma: 2-5 hours
Excretion: Primarily urine (75% mostly as metabolites); feces (25% mostly as metabolites); in feces and urine, <5% to 7% excreted unchanged

Dosage Oral: Chronic angina:

Adults: Initial: 500 mg twice daily; maximum recommended dose: 1000 mg twice daily

Elderly: Select dose cautiously, starting at the lower end of the dosing range

Dosage adjustment for ranolazine with concomitant medications:

Diltiazem, erythromycin, verapamil, and other moderate CYP3A inhibitors: Ranolazine dose should not exceed 500 mg twice daily

P-glycoprotein inhibitors (eg, cyclosporine): Titrate ranolazine based on clinical response

Dosage adjustment for concomitant medications with ranolazine: *Simvastatin:* Simvastatin dose should not exceed 20 mg/day

Dosage adjustment in renal impairment: There is no dosage adjustments provided in manufacturer's labeling. However, plasma ranolazine levels increased ~50% in patients with varying degrees of renal dysfunction. Patients with severe renal dysfunction had an increase in mean diastolic blood pressure of 10-15 mm Hg. Ranolazine has not been evaluated in patients requiring dialysis.

Dosage adjustment in hepatic impairment: Use is contraindicated with any degree of hepatic cirrhosis.

Dietary Considerations May be taken without regard to meals. Limit the use of grapefuit juice.

Administration May be taken with or without meals. Swallow tablet whole; do not crush, break, or chew.

Monitoring Parameters Baseline and follow up ECG to evaluate QT interval; blood pressure in patients with renal dysfunction; correct and maintain serum potassium in normal limits

Dosage Forms Excipient information presented when available (limited, particularly for generics); consult specific product labeling.

Tablet, extended release, oral:
Ranexa®: 500 mg, 1000 mg

◆ **RAN™-Ondansetron (Can)** *see* Ondansetron *on page 1246*
◆ **RAN™-Pantoprazole (Can)** *see* Pantoprazole *on page 1289*
◆ **RAN™-Pravastatin (Can)** *see* Pravastatin *on page 1394*
◆ **RAN™-Rabeprazole (Can)** *see* RABEprazole *on page 1451*
◆ **RAN™-Ramipril (Can)** *see* Ramipril *on page 1459*
◆ **RAN™-Ranitidine (Can)** *see* Ranitidine *on page 1462*
◆ **RAN™-Risperidone (Can)** *see* RisperiDONE *on page 1496*
◆ **RAN™-Ropinirole (Can)** *see* ROPINIRole *on page 1517*
◆ **RAN™-Simvastatin (Can)** *see* Simvastatin *on page 1555*
◆ **RAN™-Tamsulosin (Can)** *see* Tamsulosin *on page 1626*
◆ **Ran-Valsartan (Can)** *see* Valsartan *on page 1761*
◆ **Rapaflo®** *see* Silodosin *on page 1554*
◆ **Rapamune®** *see* Sirolimus *on page 1557*
◆ **Rapamycin** *see* Sirolimus *on page 1557*

Rasagiline (ra SA ji leen)

Brand Names: U.S. Azilect®

Index Terms AGN 1135; Rasagiline Mesylate; TVP-1012

Pharmacologic Category Anti-Parkinson's Agent, MAO Type B Inhibitor

Additional Appendix Information

Antiparkinsonian Agents *on page 1879*

Use Treatment of idiopathic Parkinson's disease (initial monotherapy or as adjunct to levodopa)

Pregnancy Risk Factor C

Pregnancy Considerations Animal studies have documented decreased offspring survival and birth weight. An increased incidence of teratogenic effects, embryo-fetal deaths, and cardiovascular abnormalities were also noted with rasagiline in combination with levodopa/carbidopa. There are no adequate and well-controlled studies in pregnant women.

Lactation Excretion in breast milk unknown/use caution

Contraindications Concomitant use of cyclobenzaprine, dextromethorphan, methadone, propoxyphene, St John's wort, or tramadol; concomitant use of meperidine or an MAO inhibitor (including selective MAO-B inhibitors) within 14 days of rasagiline

Warnings/Precautions Hazardous agent - use appropriate precautions for handling and disposal.

Cardiovascular system: May cause orthostatic hypotension, particularly in combination with levodopa; use with caution in patients with hypotension or patients who would not tolerate transient hypotensive episodes (cardiovascular or cerebrovascular disease); orthostasis is usually most problematic during first 2 months of therapy and tends to abate thereafter. Due to the potential for hemodynamic instability, patients should not undergo elective surgery requiring general anesthesia and should avoid local anesthesia containing sympathomimetic vasoconstrictors within 14 days of discontinuing rasagiline. If surgery is required, benzodiazepines, mivacurium, fentanyl, morphine or codeine may be used cautiously. In patients taking recommended doses of rasagiline, dietary restriction of most tyramine-containing products is not necessary; however, certain foods (eg, aged cheeses) may contain high amounts (>150 mg) of tyramine and could lead to hypertensive crisis. Avoid concomitant use with foods high in tyramine.

Central nervous system: Serotonin syndrome (SS)/neuroleptic malignant syndrome (NMS)-like reactions may occur rarely, particularly when used at doses exceeding recommendations or when used in combination with an antidepressant (eg, SSRI, SNRI, TCA). May cause hallucinations; signs of severe CNS toxicity (some fatal), including hyperpyrexia, hyperthermia, rigidity, altered mental status, seizure and coma have been reported with selective and nonselective MAO inhibitor use in combination with antidepressants. Do not use within 5 weeks of fluoxetine discontinuation; do not initiate tricyclic, SSRI, or SNRI therapy within 2 weeks of discontinuing rasagiline. Addition to levodopa therapy may result in exacerbation of dyskinesias, requiring a reduction in levodopa dosage.

Dermatologic: Risk of melanoma may be increased with rasagiline, although increased risk has been associated with Parkinson's disease itself; patients should have regular and frequent skin examinations.

Organ dysfunction: Use caution in mild hepatic impairment; dose reduction recommended. Do not use with moderate-to-severe hepatic impairment.

Adverse Reactions Unless otherwise noted, the following adverse reactions are as reported for monotherapy. Spectrum of adverse events was generally similar with adjunctive (levodopa) therapy, though the incidence tended to be higher.

>10%:

Cardiovascular: Postural hypotension (6% to 13% adjunct therapy, dose dependent)

Central nervous system: Dyskinesia (18% adjunct therapy), headache (14%)

Gastrointestinal: Nausea (10% to 12% adjunct therapy)

1% to 10%:

Cardiovascular: Angina, bundle branch block, chest pain, syncope

Central nervous system: Depression (5%), hallucinations (4% to 5% adjunct therapy), fever (3%), malaise (2%), vertigo (2%), anxiety, dizziness

Dermatologic: Bruising (2%), alopecia, skin carcinoma, vesiculobullous rash

Endocrine & metabolic: Impotence, libido decreased

Gastrointestinal: Constipation (4% to 9% adjunct therapy), weight loss (2% to 9% adjunct therapy; dose dependent), dyspepsia (7%), xerostomia (2% to 6% adjunct therapy; dose dependent), gastroenteritis (3%), anorexia, diarrhea, gastrointestinal hemorrhage, vomiting

Genitourinary: Hematuria, urinary incontinence

Hematologic: Leukopenia

Hepatic: Liver function tests increased

Neuromuscular & skeletal: Arthralgia (7%), neck pain (2%), arthritis (2%), paresthesia (2%), abnormal gait, hyperkinesias, hypertonia, neuropathy, tremor, weakness

Ocular: Conjunctivitis (3%)

Renal: Albuminuria

Respiratory: Rhinitis (3%), asthma, cough increased

Miscellaneous: Fall (5%), flu-like syndrome (5%), allergic reaction

<1%, postmarketing, and/or case reports (limited to important or life-threatening): Acute kidney failure, aphasia, apnea, atrial arrhythmia, AV block, bigeminy, blepharitis, blindness, bone necrosis, cerebral hemorrhage, cerebral ischemia, circumoral paresthesia, deafness, deep thrombophlebitis, delirium, diplopia, dysautonomia, dysesthesia, emphysema, esophageal ulcer, exfoliative dermatitis, facial paralysis, glaucoma, gynecomastia, heart failure, hematemesis, hemiplegia, hemorrhage (various locations), hostility, hypersexuality, hypertension, hypocalcemia, impulse control symptoms, interstitial pneumonia, intestinal obstruction, intestinal perforation, intestinal stenosis, jaundice, keratitis, kidney calculus, large intestine perforation, laryngismus, larynx edema, leukoderma, leukorrhea, libido increased, lung fibrosis, macrocytic anemia, manic depressive reaction, mania, megacolon, menstrual abnormalities, MI, muscle atrophy, myelitis, neuralgia, neuritis, neurosis, nocturia, paranoid reaction, parosmia, pathological gambling, personality disorder, pleural effusion, pneumothorax, polyuria, psychosis, psychotic depression, ptosis, purpura, retinal degeneration, retinal detachment, seizure, stomach ulcer, strabismus, stupor, thrombocythemia, thrombosis, tongue edema, urinary disorders, vaginal moniliasis, ventricular fibrillation, ventricular tachycardia, vestibular disorder, visual field defect

Drug Interactions

Metabolism/Transport Effects Substrate of CYP1A2 (major); **Note:** Assignment of Major/Minor substrate status based on clinically relevant drug interaction potential; **Inhibits** Monoamine Oxidase

Avoid Concomitant Use

Avoid concomitant use of Rasagiline with any of the following: Alpha-/Beta-Agonists (Indirect-Acting); Alpha1-Agonists; Alpha2-Agonists (Ophthalmic); Amphetamines; Anilidopiperidine Opioids; Antidepressants (Serotonin Reuptake Inhibitor/Antagonist); Atomoxetine; Bezafibrate; Buprenorphine; BuPROPion; BusPIRone; CarBAMazepine; Cyclobenzaprine; Dexmethylphenidate; Dextromethorphan; Diethylpropion; HYDROmorphone; Linezolid; Maprotiline; Meperidine; Methyldopa; Methylene Blue; Methylphenidate; Mirtazapine; Oxymorphone; Pizotifen; Selective Serotonin Reuptake Inhibitors; Serotonin 5-HT1D Receptor Agonists; Serotonin/Norepinephrine Reuptake Inhibitors; Tapentadol; Tetrabenazine; Tetrahydrozoline; Tetrahydrozoline (Nasal); Tricyclic Antidepressants; Tryptophan

Increased Effect/Toxicity

Rasagiline may increase the levels/effects of: Alpha-/Beta-Agonists (Direct-Acting); Alpha-/Beta-Agonists (Indirect-Acting); Alpha1-Agonists; Alpha2-Agonists (Ophthalmic); Amphetamines; Antidepressants (Serotonin Reuptake Inhibitor/Antagonist); Antihypertensives; Atomoxetine; Beta2-Agonists; Bezafibrate; BuPROPion; Dexmethylphenidate; Dextromethorphan; Diethylpropion; Doxapram; HYDROmorphone; Linezolid; Lithium; Meperidine; Methadone; Methyldopa; Methylene Blue; Methylphenidate; Metoclopramide; Mirtazapine; Orthostatic Hypotension Producing Agents; Pizotifen; Reserpine; Selective Serotonin Reuptake Inhibitors; Serotonin 5-HT1D Receptor Agonists; Serotonin Modulators; Serotonin/Norepinephrine Reuptake Inhibitors; Tetrahydrozoline; Tetrahydrozoline (Nasal); Tricyclic Antidepressants

The levels/effects of Rasagiline may be increased by: Abiraterone Acetate; Altretamine; Anilidopiperidine Opioids; Antipsychotics; Buprenorphine; BusPIRone; CarBAMazepine; COMT Inhibitors; Cyclobenzaprine; CYP1A2 Inhibitors (Moderate); CYP1A2 Inhibitors (Strong); Deferasirox; Levodopa; MAO Inhibitors; Maprotiline; Oxymorphone; Tapentadol; Tetrabenazine; TraMADol; Tryptophan

Decreased Effect

The levels/effects of Rasagiline may be decreased by: CYP1A2 Inducers (Strong); Cyproterone

Ethanol/Nutrition/Herb Interactions

Ethanol: Avoid ethanol.

Food: Concurrent ingestion of foods rich in tyramine may cause sudden and severe high blood pressure (hypertensive crisis). Avoid foods (such as aged cheeses) containing high amounts (>150 mg) of tyramine.

Herb/Nutraceutical: Avoid valerian, St John's wort, SAMe, kava kava (may increase risk of serotonin syndrome and/or excessive sedation); Avoid supplements containing caffeine, tyrosine, tryptophan, or phenylalanine. Ingestion of large quantities may increase the risk of severe side effects (eg, hypertensive reactions, serotonin syndrome).

Stability Store at 25°C (77°F); excursions permitted to 15°C to 30°C (59°F to 86°F).

Mechanism of Action Potent, irreversible and selective inhibitor of brain monoamine oxidase (MAO) type B, which plays a major role in the catabolism of dopamine. Inhibition of dopamine depletion in the striatal region of the brain reduces the symptomatic motor deficits of Parkinson's disease. There is also experimental evidence of rasagiline conferring neuroprotective effects (antioxidant, antiapoptotic), which may delay onset of symptoms and progression of neuronal deterioration.

Pharmacodynamics/Kinetics

Onset of action: Therapeutic: Within 1 hour

Duration: ~1 week (irreversible inhibition); may require ~14-40 days for complete restoration of (brain) MAO-B activity

Absorption: Rapid

Protein binding: 88% to 94%, primarily to albumin

Metabolism: Hepatic N-dealkylation and/or hydroxylation via CYP1A2 to multiple inactive metabolites (nonamphetamine derivatives)

Distribution: V_{dss}: 87 L

Bioavailability: ~36%

Half-life elimination: ~1.3-3 hours (no correlation with biologic effect due to irreversible inhibition)

Time to peak, plasma: ~1 hour

Excretion: Urine (62%, <1% of total dose as unchanged drug); feces (7%)

Dosage Oral: Adults: Parkinson's disease:

Monotherapy: 1 mg once daily

Adjunctive therapy with levodopa: Initial: 0.5 mg once daily; may increase to 1 mg once daily based on response and tolerability

Note: When added to existing levodopa therapy, a dose reduction of levodopa may be required to avoid exacerbation of dyskinesias; typical dose reductions of ~9% to 13% were employed in clinical trials

Dose reduction with concomitant ciprofloxacin or other CYP1A2 inhibitors: 0.5 mg once daily

Dosage adjustment in renal impairment:

Mild-to-moderate impairment: No adjustment necessary

Severe impairment: Not studied

Dosage adjustment in hepatic impairment:

Mild impairment (Child-Pugh ≤6): 0.5 mg once daily

Moderate-to-severe impairment: Not recommended

Dietary Considerations May be taken without regard to meals. Avoid products containing high amounts of tyramine (>150 mg), such as aged cheeses (eg, Stilton cheese). Restriction of tyramine-containing products with lower amounts (<150 mg) of tyramine is not necessary in patients taking recommended doses. Some examples of tyramine-containing products include aged or matured cheese, air-dried or cured meats (including sausages and salamis), fava or broad bean pods, tap/draft beers, Marmite concentrate, sauerkraut, soy sauce and other soybean condiments. Food's freshness is also an important concern; improperly stored or spoiled food can create an environment where tyramine concentrations may increase.

Administration Administer without regard to meals.

Monitoring Parameters Blood pressure; symptoms of parkinsonism; general mood and behavior (increased anxiety, or presence of mania or agitation); skin examination for presence of melanoma (higher incidence in Parkinson's patients- drug causation not established)

Additional Information When adding rasagiline to levodopa/carbidopa, the dose of the latter can usually be decreased. Studies are investigating the use of rasagiline in early Parkinson's disease to slow the progression of the disease.

Dosage Forms Excipient information presented when available (limited, particularly for generics); consult specific product labeling.

Tablet, oral:

Azilect®: 0.5 mg, 1 mg

◆ **Rasagiline Mesylate** *see* Rasagiline *on page 1466*

Rasburicase (ras BYOOR i kayse)

Brand Names: U.S. Elitek®

Brand Names: Canada Fasturtec®

Index Terms Recombinant Urate Oxidase; Urate Oxidase

Pharmacologic Category Enzyme; Enzyme, Urate-Oxidase (Recombinant)

Use Initial management of uric acid levels in patients with leukemia, lymphoma, and solid tumor malignancies receiving chemotherapy expected to result in tumor lysis and elevation of plasma uric acid

Pregnancy Risk Factor C

Pregnancy Considerations Adverse effects were observed in animal studies. There are no adequate and well-controlled studies in pregnant women. Use during pregnancy only if the benefit to the mother outweighs the potential risk to the fetus.

Lactation Excretion in breast milk unknown/not recommended

Contraindications History of anaphylaxis or severe hypersensitivity to rasburicase or any component of the formulation; history of hemolytic reaction or methemoglobinemia associated with rasburicase; glucose-6-phosphatase dehydrogenase (G6PD) deficiency

Warnings/Precautions **[U.S. Boxed Warning]: Severe hypersensitivity reactions (including anaphylaxis) have been reported; immediately and permanently discontinue in patients developing serious hypersensitivity reaction;** reactions may occur at any time during treatment, including the initial dose. Signs and symptoms of hypersensitivity may include bronshospasm, chest pain/tightness, dyspnea, hypotension, hypoxia, shock, or urticaria. **[U.S. Boxed Warning]: Due to the risk for hemolysis (<1%), rasburicase is contraindicated in patients with G6PD deficiency; discontinue immediately and permanently in any patient developing hemolysis. Patients at higher risk for G6PD deficiency (eg, African, Mediterranean, or Southeast Asian descent) should be screened prior to therapy;** severe hemolytic reactions occurred within 2-4 days of rasburicase initiation. **[U.S. Boxed Warning]: Methemoglobinemia has been reported (<1%). Discontinue immediately and permanently in any patient developing methemoglobinemia;** initiate appropriate treatment (eg, transfusion, methylene blue) if methemoglobinemia occurs.

[U.S. Boxed Warning]: Enzymatic degradation of uric acid in blood samples will occur if left at room temperature, which may interfere with serum uric acid measurements; specific guidelines for the collection of plasma uric acid samples must be followed, including collection in pre-chilled tubes with heparin anticoagulant, immediate ice water bath immersion and assay within 4 hours. Patients at risk for tumor lysis syndrome should receive appropriate I.V. hydration as part of uric acid management; however, alkalinization (with sodium bicarbonate) concurrently with rasburicase is not recommended (Coiffier, 2008). Rasburicase is immunogenic and can elicit an antibody response; administration of more than one course is not recommended.

Adverse Reactions

>10%:

- Cardiovascular: Peripheral edema (≤50%), fluid overload (≤12%)
- Central nervous system: Fever (46%; serious: 5%), headache (26%), anxiety (≤24%)
- Dermatologic: Rash (13%; serious: 1%)
- Endocrine & metabolic: Hypophosphatemia (≤17%)
- Gastrointestinal: Vomiting (50%), nausea (27%), abdominal pain (20%), constipation (20%), diarrhea (20%), mucositis (15%; serious: 2%)
- Hepatic: Hyperbilirubinemia (≤16%), ALT increased (≤11%)
- Respiratory: Pharyngolaryngeal pain (≤14%)
- Miscellaneous: Antibody formation (healthy volunteers: 61% to 64%; patients with malignancies: 11%), sepsis (≤12%; serious: 3% to 5%)

1% to 10%:

- Cardiovascular: Ischemic coronary disorder, supraventricular arrhythmia
- Endocrine & metabolic: Hyperphosphatemia (≤10%)
- Gastrointestinal: Abdominal/gastrointestinal infection
- Hematologic: Neutropenic fever (serious: 4%), neutropenia (serious: 2%)
- Respiratory: Respiratory distress (serious: 3%), pulmonary hemorrhage, respiratory failure
- Miscellaneous: Hypersensitivity (≤4%)

<1% (Limited to important or life-threatening): Acute renal failure, anaphylaxis, arrhythmia, cardiac arrest, cardiac failure, cellulitis, cerebrovascular disorder, chest pain, cyanosis, dehydration, hemolysis, hemorrhage, hot flashes, ileus, infection, intestinal obstruction, liver enzymes increased, methemoglobinemia, MI, pancytopenia, paresthesia, pneumonia, pulmonary edema, pulmonary hypertension, retinal hemorrhage, rigors, seizure, thrombosis, thrombophlebitis

Drug Interactions

Metabolism/Transport Effects None known.

Avoid Concomitant Use There are no known interactions where it is recommended to avoid concomitant use.

Increased Effect/Toxicity There are no known significant interactions involving an increase in effect.

Decreased Effect There are no known significant interactions involving a decrease in effect.

Stability Prior to reconstitution, store with diluent at 2°C to 8°C (36°F to 46°F); do not freeze. Protect from light. Reconstitute with provided diluent (use 1 mL diluent for the 1.5 mg vial and 5 mL diluent for the 7.5 mg vial). Mix by gently swirling; do **not** shake or vortex. Discard if discolored or containing particulate matter. Total dose should be further diluted in NS to a final volume of 50 mL. Reconstituted and final solution may be stored up to 24 hours at 2°C to 8°C (36°F to 46°F). Discard unused product.

Mechanism of Action Rasburicase is a recombinant urate-oxidase enzyme, which converts uric acid to allantoin (an inactive and soluble metabolite of uric acid); it does not inhibit the formation of uric acid.

Pharmacodynamics/Kinetics

- Onset: Uric acid levels decrease within 4 hours of initial administration
- Distribution: Children: 110-127 mL/kg; Adults: 76-138 mL/kg
- Half-life elimination: ~16-23 hours

Dosage I.V.: Hyperuricemia associated with malignancy:

Children: 0.2 mg/kg once daily for up to 5 days (manufacturer-recommended dose) **or**

Alternate dosing (unlabeled; Coiffier, 2008): 0.05-0.2 mg/kg once daily for 1-7 days (average of 2-3 days) with the duration of treatment dependent on plasma uric acid levels and clinical judgment (patients with significant tumor burden may require an increase to twice daily); the following dose levels are recommended based on risk of tumor lysis syndrome (TLS):

- High risk: 0.2 mg/kg once daily (duration is based on plasma uric acid levels)
- Intermediate risk: 0.15 mg/kg once daily (duration is based on plasma uric acid levels); may consider managing initially with a single dose
- Low risk: 0.1 mg/kg once daily (duration is based on clinical judgment); a dose of 0.05 mg/kg was used effectively in one trial

Single-dose rasburicase (unlabeled use; based on limited data): 0.15 mg/kg; additional doses may be needed based on serum uric acid levels (Liu, 2005)

Adults: 0.2 mg/kg once daily for up to 5 days (manufacturer-recommended dose) **or**

Alternate dosing (unlabeled; Coiffier, 2008): 0.05-0.2 mg/kg once daily for 1-7 days (average of 2-3 days) with the duration of treatment dependent on plasma uric acid levels and clinical judgment (patients with significant tumor burden may require an increase to twice daily); the following dose levels are recommended based on risk of tumor lysis syndrome (TLS):

High risk: 0.2 mg/kg once daily (duration is based on plasma uric acid levels)

Intermediate risk: 0.15 mg/kg once daily (duration is based on plasma uric acid levels)

Low risk: 0.1 mg/kg once daily (duration is based on clinical judgment); a dose of 0.05 mg/kg was used effectively in one trial

Single-dose rasburicase (unlabeled use; based on limited data): 0.15 mg/kg (Campara, 2009; Liu, 2005) **or** 3-7.5 mg as a single dose (Hutcherson, 2006; McDonnell, 2006; Reeves, 2008; Trifilio, 2006); repeat doses (1.5-6 mg) may be needed based on serum uric acid levels

Administration I.V. infusion over 30 minutes; do **not** administer as a bolus infusion. Do **not** filter during infusion. If not possible to administer through a separate line, I.V. line should be flushed with at least 15 mL saline prior to and following rasburicase infusion. May begin chemotherapy 4 hours after the initiation of reasburicase (Coiffier, 2008).

Monitoring Parameters Plasma uric acid levels (4 hours after rasburicase administration, then every 6-8 hours until TLS resolution), CBC, G6PD deficiency screening (in patients at high risk for deficiency); monitor for hypersensitivity

Test Interactions Specific handling procedures must be followed to prevent the degradation of uric acid in plasma samples. Blood must be collected in prechilled tubes containing heparin anticoagulant. Samples must then be **immediately** immersed in an ice water bath. Prepare samples by centrifugation in a precooled centrifuge (4°C). Samples must be kept in ice water bath and analyzed within 4 hours of collection.

Dosage Forms Excipient information presented when available (limited, particularly for generics); consult specific product labeling.

Injection, powder for reconstitution:

Elitek®: 1.5 mg, 7.5 mg [supplied with diluent]

- ◆ **Rasilez® (Can)** *see* Aliskiren *on page 66*
- ◆ **Rasilez HCT (Can)** *see* Aliskiren and Hydrochlorothiazide *on page 67*
- ◆ **rATG** *see* Antithymocyte Globulin (Rabbit) *on page 133*
- ◆ **ratio-Aclavulanate (Can)** *see* Amoxicillin and Clavulanate *on page 105*
- ◆ **ratio-Acyclovir (Can)** *see* Acyclovir (Systemic) *on page 39*
- ◆ **ratio-Alendronate (Can)** *see* Alendronate *on page 61*
- ◆ **ratio-Amiodarone (Can)** *see* Amiodarone *on page 90*
- ◆ **ratio-Amlodipine (Can)** *see* AmLODIPine *on page 97*
- ◆ **ratio-Atenolol (Can)** *see* Atenolol *on page 161*
- ◆ **ratio-Atorvastatin (Can)** *see* Atorvastatin *on page 165*
- ◆ **ratio-Azithromycin (Can)** *see* Azithromycin (Systemic) *on page 180*
- ◆ **ratio-Baclofen (Can)** *see* Baclofen *on page 187*
- ◆ **ratio-Bicalutamide (Can)** *see* Bicalutamide *on page 217*
- ◆ **ratio-Brimonidine (Can)** *see* Brimonidine *on page 235*
- ◆ **ratio-Bupropion SR (Can)** *see* BuPROPion *on page 247*
- ◆ **ratio-Buspirone (Can)** *see* BusPIRone *on page 250*
- ◆ **ratio-Carvedilol (Can)** *see* Carvedilol *on page 295*
- ◆ **ratio-Cefuroxime (Can)** *see* Cefuroxime *on page 322*
- ◆ **ratio-Ciprofloxacin (Can)** *see* Ciprofloxacin (Systemic) *on page 362*
- ◆ **ratio-Citalopram (Can)** *see* Citalopram *on page 370*
- ◆ **ratio-Clarithromycin (Can)** *see* Clarithromycin *on page 374*
- ◆ **ratio-Clindamycin (Can)** *see* Clindamycin (Systemic) *on page 378*
- ◆ **ratio-Clobetasol (Can)** *see* Clobetasol *on page 384*
- ◆ **ratio-Codeine (Can)** *see* Codeine *on page 403*
- ◆ **ratio-Cyclobenzaprine (Can)** *see* Cyclobenzaprine *on page 419*
- ◆ **ratio-Diltiazem CD (Can)** *see* Diltiazem *on page 510*
- ◆ **ratio-Ectosone (Can)** *see* Betamethasone *on page 208*
- ◆ **ratio-Emtec (Can)** *see* Acetaminophen and Codeine *on page 30*
- ◆ **ratio-Enalapril (Can)** *see* Enalapril *on page 584*
- ◆ **ratio-Fenofibrate MC (Can)** *see* Fenofibrate *on page 693*
- ◆ **ratio-Fentanyl (Can)** *see* FentaNYL *on page 697*
- ◆ **ratio-Finasteride (Can)** *see* Finasteride *on page 713*
- ◆ **ratio-Fluoxetine (Can)** *see* FLUoxetine *on page 731*
- ◆ **ratio-Fluticasone (Can)** *see* Fluticasone (Nasal) *on page 741*
- ◆ **ratio-Gabapentin (Can)** *see* Gabapentin *on page 773*
- ◆ **ratio-Glimepiride (Can)** *see* Glimepiride *on page 793*
- ◆ **ratio-Glyburide (Can)** *see* GlyBURIDE *on page 799*
- ◆ **ratio-Indomethacin (Can)** *see* Indomethacin *on page 890*
- ◆ **ratio-Ipra-Sal (Can)** *see* Albuterol *on page 52*
- ◆ **ratio-Ipra Sal UDV (Can)** *see* Ipratropium and Albuterol *on page 924*
- ◆ **ratio-Irbesartan (Can)** *see* Irbesartan *on page 925*
- ◆ **ratio-Irbesartan HCTZ (Can)** *see* Irbesartan and Hydrochlorothiazide *on page 926*
- ◆ **ratio-Ketorolac (Can)** *see* Ketorolac (Ophthalmic) *on page 959*
- ◆ **ratio-Lamotrigine (Can)** *see* LamoTRIgine *on page 967*
- ◆ **ratio-Lenoltec (Can)** *see* Acetaminophen and Codeine *on page 30*
- ◆ **ratio-Lisinopril (Can)** *see* Lisinopril *on page 1020*
- ◆ **ratio-Lisinopril P (Can)** *see* Lisinopril *on page 1020*
- ◆ **ratio-Lisinopril Z (Can)** *see* Lisinopril *on page 1020*
- ◆ **ratio-Lovastatin (Can)** *see* Lovastatin *on page 1038*
- ◆ **ratio-Meloxicam (Can)** *see* Meloxicam *on page 1063*
- ◆ **ratio-Memantine (Can)** *see* Memantine *on page 1068*
- ◆ **ratio-Metformin (Can)** *see* MetFORMIN *on page 1086*
- ◆ **ratio-Methotrexate (Can)** *see* Methotrexate *on page 1098*
- ◆ **ratio-Methylphenidate (Can)** *see* Methylphenidate *on page 1107*
- ◆ **ratio-Minocycline (Can)** *see* Minocycline *on page 1137*
- ◆ **ratio-Mirtazapine (Can)** *see* Mirtazapine *on page 1140*
- ◆ **ratio-Mometasone (Can)** *see* Mometasone (Topical) *on page 1151*
- ◆ **ratio-Morphine (Can)** *see* Morphine (Systemic) *on page 1153*
- ◆ **ratio-Morphine SR (Can)** *see* Morphine (Systemic) *on page 1153*
- ◆ **ratio-Omeprazole (Can)** *see* Omeprazole *on page 1241*

◆ **Remicade®** *see* InFLIXimab *on page 893*

Remifentanil (rem i FEN ta nil)

Brand Names: U.S. Ultiva®

Brand Names: Canada Ultiva®

Index Terms GI87084B

Pharmacologic Category Analgesic, Opioid; Anilidopiperidine Opioid

Use Analgesic for use during the induction and maintenance of general anesthesia; for continued analgesia into the immediate postoperative period; analgesic component of monitored anesthesia

Unlabeled Use Management of pain in mechanically-ventilated patients

Pregnancy Risk Factor C

Pregnancy Considerations Remifentanil has been shown to cross the placenta. Neonatal respiratory depression and sedation may occur.

Lactation Excretion in breast milk unknown/use caution

Contraindications Not for intrathecal or epidural administration, due to the presence of glycine in the formulation; hypersensitivity to remifentanil, fentanyl, or fentanyl analogs, or any component of the formulation

Warnings/Precautions Remifentanil is not recommended as the sole agent in general anesthesia, because the loss of consciousness cannot be assured and due to the high incidence of apnea, hypotension, tachycardia and muscle rigidity; it should be administered by individuals specifically trained in the use of anesthetic agents and should not be used in diagnostic or therapeutic procedures outside the monitored anesthesia setting; resuscitative and intubation equipment should be readily available. May cause hypotension; use with caution in patients with hypovolemia, cardiovascular disease (including acute MI), or drugs which may exaggerate hypotensive effects (including phenothiazines or general anesthetics). Shares the toxic potentials of opiate agonists, and precautions of opiate agonist therapy should be observed. In patients <55 years of age, intraoperative awareness has been reported when used with propofol rates of ≤75 mcg/kg/minute.

Use with caution when administering to patients with bradycardia. Inject slowly over 3-5 minutes; rapid I.V. infusion may result in skeletal muscle and chest wall rigidity, impaired ventilation, or respiratory distress/arrest; nondepolarizing skeletal muscle relaxant may be required. Interruption of an infusion will result in offset of effects within 5-10 minutes; the discontinuation of remifentanil infusion should be preceded by the establishment of adequate postoperative analgesia orders, especially for patients in whom postoperative pain is anticipated. Use caution in the morbidly obese. Safety and efficacy for postoperative analgesic or monitored anesthesia care have not been established in children.

Adverse Reactions

>10%: Gastrointestinal: Nausea, vomiting

1% to 10%:

- Cardiovascular: Bradycardia (dose dependent), hypertension, hypotension (dose dependent), tachycardia
- Central nervous system: Agitation, dizziness, fever, headache
- Dermatologic: Pruritus
- Neuromuscular & skeletal: Muscle rigidity (dose dependent)
- Ocular: Visual disturbances
- Respiratory: Apnea, hypoxia, respiratory depression
- Miscellaneous: Postoperative pain, shivering

<1% (Limited to important or life-threatening): Anaphylactic/anaphylactoid reactions, anemia, anxiety, arrhythmia, asystole, bronchospasm, confusion, constipation, CPK-MB increased, diarrhea, dysphagia, electrolyte disorders, hallucinations, heart block, pleural effusion, prolonged emergence from anesthesia, pulmonary edema, syncope, thrombocytopenia, xerostomia

Drug Interactions

Metabolism/Transport Effects None known.

Avoid Concomitant Use

Avoid concomitant use of Remifentanil with any of the following: MAO Inhibitors

Increased Effect/Toxicity

Remifentanil may increase the levels/effects of: Alcohol (Ethyl); Alvimopan; Beta-Blockers; Calcium Channel Blockers (Nondihydropyridine); CNS Depressants; Desmopressin; MAO Inhibitors; Selective Serotonin Reuptake Inhibitors; Thiazide Diuretics

The levels/effects of Remifentanil may be increased by: Amphetamines; Antipsychotic Agents (Phenothiazines); Droperidol; HydrOXYzine; Succinylcholine

Decreased Effect

Remifentanil may decrease the levels/effects of: Pegvisomant

The levels/effects of Remifentanil may be decreased by: Ammonium Chloride; Mixed Agonist / Antagonist Opioids

Stability Prior to reconstitution, store at 2°C to 25°C (36°F to 77°F). Prepare solution by adding 1 mL of diluent per 1 mg of remifentanil. Shake well. Further dilute to a final concentration of 20, 25, 50, or 250 mcg/mL. Stable for 24 hours at room temperature after reconstitution and further dilution to concentrations of 20-250 mcg/mL (4 hours if diluted with LR).

Mechanism of Action Binds with stereospecific mu-opioid receptors at many sites within the CNS, increases pain threshold, alters pain reception, inhibits ascending pain pathways

Pharmacodynamics/Kinetics

Onset of action: I.V.: 1-3 minutes

Distribution: V_d: 100 mL/kg; increased in children

Protein binding: ~70% (primarily $alpha_1$ acid glycoprotein)

Metabolism: Rapid via blood and tissue esterases

Half-life elimination (dose dependent): Terminal: 10-20 minutes; effective: 3-10 minutes

Excretion: Urine

Dosage I.V. continuous infusion: Dose should be based on ideal body weight (IBW) in obese patients (>30% over IBW).

Children Birth to 2 months: Maintenance of anesthesia with nitrous oxide (70%): 0.4 mcg/kg/minute (range: 0.4-1 mcg/kg/minute); supplemental bolus dose of 1 mcg/kg may be administered, smaller bolus dose may be required with potent inhalation agents, potent neuraxial anesthesia, significant comorbidities, significant fluid shifts, or without atropine pretreatment. Clearance in neonates is highly variable; dose should be carefully titrated.

Children 1-12 years: Maintenance of anesthesia with halothane, sevoflurane, or isoflurane: 0.25 mcg/kg/minute (range: 0.05-1.3 mcg/kg/minute); supplemental bolus dose of 1 mcg/kg may be administered every 2-5 minutes. Consider increasing concomitant anesthetics with infusion rate >1 mcg/kg/minute. Infusion rate can be titrated upward in increments up to 50% or titrated downward in decrements of 25% to 50%. May titrate every 2-5 minutes.

Adults:

Induction of anesthesia: 0.5-1 mcg/kg/minute; if endotracheal intubation is to occur in <8 minutes, an initial dose of 1 mcg/kg may be given over 30-60 seconds

Coronary bypass surgery: 1 mcg/kg/minute

Maintenance of anesthesia: **Note:** Supplemental bolus dose of 1 mcg/kg may be administered every 2-5 minutes. Consider increasing concomitant anesthetics with infusion rate >1 mcg/kg/minute. Infusion rate can be titrated upward in increments of 25% to 100% or downward in decrements of 25% to 50%. May titrate every 2-5 minutes.

With nitrous oxide (66%): 0.4 mcg/kg/minute (range: 0.1-2 mcg/kg/minute)

With isoflurane: 0.25 mcg/kg/minute (range: 0.05-2 mcg/kg/minute)

With propofol: 0.25 mcg/kg/minute (range: 0.05-2 mcg/kg/minute)

Coronary bypass surgery: 1 mcg/kg/minute (range: 0.125-4 mcg/kg/minute); supplemental dose: 0.5-1 mcg/kg

Continuation as an analgesic in immediate postoperative period: 0.1 mcg/kg/minute (range: 0.025-0.2 mcg/kg/minute). Infusion rate may be adjusted every 5 minutes in increments of 0.025 mcg/kg/minute. Bolus doses are not recommended. Infusion rates >0.2 mcg/kg/minute are associated with respiratory depression.

Coronary bypass surgery, continuation as an analgesic into the ICU: 1 mcg/kg/minute (range: 0.05-1 mcg/kg/minute)

Analgesic component of monitored anesthesia care: **Note:** Supplemental oxygen is recommended:

Single I.V. dose given 90 seconds prior to local anesthetic:

Remifentanil alone: 1 mcg/kg over 30-60 seconds

With midazolam: 0.5 mcg/kg over 30-60 seconds

Continuous infusion beginning 5 minutes prior to local anesthetic:

Remifentanil alone: 0.1 mcg/kg minute

With midazolam: 0.05 mcg/kg/minute

Continuous infusion given after local anesthetic:

Remifentanil alone: 0.05 mcg/kg/minute (range: 0.025-0.2 mcg/kg/minute)

With midazolam: 0.025 mcg/kg/minute (range: 0.025-0.2 mcg/kg/minute)

Note: Following local or anesthetic block, infusion rate should be decreased to 0.05 mcg/kg/minute; rate adjustments of 0.025 mcg/kg/minute may be done at 5-minute intervals

Critically-ill patients (unlabeled dose): Continuous infusion: 0.01-0.25 mcg/kg/minute (**or** 0.6-15 mcg/kg/**hour**) (Jacobi, 2002)

Elderly: Elderly patients have an increased sensitivity to effect of remifentanil; doses should be decreased by 50% and titrated.

Administration An infusion device should be used to administer continuous infusions. During the maintenance of general anesthesia, I.V. boluses may be administered over 30-60 seconds. Injections should be given into I.V. tubing close to the venous cannula; tubing should be cleared after treatment to prevent residual effects when other fluids are administered through the same I.V. line.

Monitoring Parameters Respiratory and cardiovascular status, blood pressure, heart rate

Additional Information Ultra short-acting narcotic that is unique compared to other short-acting narcotics. This agent is not considered suitable as the sole agent for induction; remifentanil should be used in combination with other induction agents. Bolus doses are not recommended for sedation cases and in treatment of postoperative pain due to risk of respiratory depression and muscle rigidity. Due to remifentanil's short duration of action, when postoperative pain is anticipated, discontinuation of an infusion of remifentanil should be preceded by an adequate postoperative analgesic (ie, fentanyl, morphine).

Dosage Forms Excipient information presented when available (limited, particularly for generics); consult specific product labeling.

Injection, powder for reconstitution:

Ultiva®: 1 mg, 2 mg, 5 mg [contains glycine 15 mg]

Controlled Substance C-II

- **Reminyl® (Can)** *see* Galantamine *on page 776*
- **Reminyl® ER (Can)** *see* Galantamine *on page 776*
- **Remodulin®** *see* Treprostinil *on page 1727*
- **Renagel®** *see* Sevelamer *on page 1550*
- **Renal Replacement Solution** *see* Electrolyte Solution, Renal Replacement *on page 578*
- **Renedil® (Can)** *see* Felodipine *on page 692*
- **Renova®** *see* Tretinoin (Topical) *on page 1731*
- **Renvela®** *see* Sevelamer *on page 1550*
- **Reopro®** *see* Abciximab *on page 22*
- **ReoPro® (Can)** *see* Abciximab *on page 22*

Repaglinide (re PAG li nide)

Brand Names: U.S. Prandin®

Brand Names: Canada GlucoNorm®; Prandin®

Pharmacologic Category Antidiabetic Agent, Meglitinide Derivative

Additional Appendix Information

Diabetes Mellitus Management, Adults *on page 1983*

Use Management of type 2 diabetes mellitus (noninsulin dependent, NIDDM) as an adjunct to diet and exercise; may be used in combination with metformin or thiazolidinediones

Pregnancy Risk Factor C

Pregnancy Considerations Adverse events have been observed in some animal studies; therefore, repaglinide is classified as pregnancy category C. Information describing the effects of repaglinide on pregnancy outcomes is limited. Maternal hyperglycemia can be associated with adverse effects in the fetus, including macrosomia, neonatal hyperglycemia, and hyperbilirubinemia; the risk of congenital malformations is increased when the Hb A_{1c} is above the normal range. Diabetes can also be associated with adverse effects in the mother. Poorly-treated diabetes may cause end-organ damage that may in turn negatively affect obstetric outcomes. Physiologic glucose levels should be maintained prior to and during pregnancy to decrease the risk of adverse events in the mother and the fetus. Until additional safety and efficacy data are obtained, the use of oral agents is generally not recommended as routine management of GDM or type 2 diabetes mellitus during pregnancy. Insulin is the drug of choice for the control of diabetes mellitus during pregnancy.

Lactation Excretion in breast milk unknown/not recommended

Contraindications Hypersensitivity to repaglinide or any component of the formulation; diabetic ketoacidosis, with or without coma; type 1 diabetes (insulin dependent, IDDM); concurrent gemfibrozil therapy

Warnings/Precautions Use with caution in patients with hepatic impairment. Use caution in severe renal dysfunction, elderly, malnourished, or patients with adrenal/pituitary dysfunction; may be more susceptible to glucose-lowering effects. May cause hypoglycemia; appropriate patient selection, dosage, and patient education are important to avoid hypoglycemic episodes. It may be necessary to discontinue repaglinide and administer insulin if the patient is exposed to stress (fever, trauma, infection, surgery). Theoretically, repaglinide may increase cardiovascular events as observed in some studies using sulfonylureas, but there are no long-term studies assessing this concern. Not indicated for use in combination with NPH insulin as there have been case reports of myocardial ischemia; further evaluation required to assess the safety of this combination.

Adverse Reactions

>10%:

Central nervous system: Headache (9% to 11%)
Endocrine & metabolic: Hypoglycemia (16% to 31%)
Respiratory: Upper respiratory tract infection (10% to 16%)

1% to 10%:

Cardiovascular: Ischemia (4%), chest pain (2% to 3%)
Gastrointestinal: Diarrhea (4% to 5%), constipation (2% to 3%)
Genitourinary: Urinary tract infection (2% to 3%)
Neuromuscular & skeletal: Back pain (5% to 6%), arthralgia (3% to 6%)
Respiratory: Sinusitis (3% to 6%), bronchitis (2% to 6%)
Miscellaneous: Allergy (1% to 2%)

<1% (Limited to important or life-threatening): Anaphylactoid reaction, arrhythmia, hemolytic anemia, hepatic dysfunction (severe), hepatitis, hypertension, leukopenia, MI, pancreatitis, Stevens-Johnson syndrome, thrombocytopenia, visual disturbances (transient)

Drug Interactions

Metabolism/Transport Effects Substrate of CYP2C8 (major), CYP3A4 (major), SLCO1B1; **Note:** Assignment of Major/Minor substrate status based on clinically relevant drug interaction potential

Avoid Concomitant Use

Avoid concomitant use of Repaglinide with any of the following: Conivaptan; Gemfibrozil

Increased Effect/Toxicity

Repaglinide may increase the levels/effects of: Hypoglycemic Agents

The levels/effects of Repaglinide may be increased by: Antifungal Agents (Azole Derivatives, Systemic); Conivaptan; CycloSPORINE; CycloSPORINE (Systemic); CYP2C8 Inhibitors (Moderate); CYP2C8 Inhibitors (Strong); CYP3A4 Inhibitors (Moderate); CYP3A4 Inhibitors (Strong); Dasatinib; Deferasirox; Eltrombopag; Gemfibrozil; Herbs (Hypoglycemic Properties); Macrolide Antibiotics; Pegvisomant; Trimethoprim

Decreased Effect

The levels/effects of Repaglinide may be decreased by: Corticosteroids (Orally Inhaled); Corticosteroids (Systemic); CYP2C8 Inducers (Strong); CYP3A4 Inducers (Strong); Deferasirox; Herbs (CYP3A4 Inducers); Luteinizing Hormone-Releasing Hormone Analogs; Rifamycin Derivatives; Somatropin; Thiazide Diuretics; Tocilizumab

Ethanol/Nutrition/Herb Interactions

Ethanol: Avoid ethanol; may increase risk of hypoglycemia.

Food: When given with food, the AUC of repaglinide is decreased.

Herb/Nutraceutical: Avoid alfalfa, aloe, bilberry, bitter melon, burdock, celery, damiana, fenugreek, garcinia, garlic, ginger, ginseng (American), gymnema, marshmallow, and stinging nettle (may enhance the hypoglycemic effects of antidiabetic agents). St John's wort may decrease the levels/effect of repaglinide.

Stability Do not store above 25°C (77°F). Protect from moisture.

Mechanism of Action Nonsulfonylurea hypoglycemic agent which blocks ATP-dependent potassium channels, depolarizing the membrane and facilitating calcium entry through calcium channels. Increased intracellular calcium stimulates insulin release from the pancreatic beta cells. Repaglinide-induced insulin release is glucose-dependent.

Pharmacodynamics/Kinetics

Onset of action: Single dose: Increased insulin levels: ~15-60 minutes
Duration: 4-6 hours
Absorption: Rapid and complete
Distribution: V_d: 31 L
Protein binding, plasma: >98% to albumin
Metabolism: Hepatic via CYP3A4 and CYP2C8 isoenzymes and glucuronidation to inactive metabolites
Bioavailability: ~56%
Half-life elimination: ~1 hour
Time to peak, plasma: ~1 hour
Excretion: Feces (~90%, <2% as unchanged drug); Urine (~8%, 0.1% as unchanged drug)

Dosage Oral: Adults:

Initial: For patients not previously treated or whose Hb A_{1c} is <8%, the starting dose is 0.5 mg before each meal. For patients previously treated with blood glucose-lowering agents whose Hb A_{1c} is ≥8%, the initial dose is 1 or 2 mg before each meal.

Dose adjustment: Determine dosing adjustments by blood glucose response, usually fasting blood glucose. Double the preprandial dose up to 4 mg until satisfactory blood glucose response is achieved. At least 1 week should elapse to assess response after each dose adjustment.

Dose range: 0.5-4 mg taken with meals. Repaglinide may be dosed preprandially 2, 3, or 4 times/day in response to changes in the patient's meal pattern. Maximum recommended daily dose: 16 mg.

Patients receiving other oral hypoglycemic agents: When repaglinide is used to replace therapy with other oral hypoglycemic agents, it may be started the day after the final dose is given. Observe patients carefully for hypoglycemia because of potential overlapping of drug effects. When transferred from longer half-life sulfonylureas (eg, chlorpropamide), close monitoring may be indicated for up to ≥1 week.

Combination therapy: If repaglinide monotherapy does not result in adequate glycemic control, metformin or a thiazolidinedione may be added. Or, if metformin or thiazolidinedione therapy does not provide adequate control, repaglinide may be added. The starting dose and dose adjustments for combination therapy are the same as repaglinide monotherapy. Carefully adjust the dose of each drug to determine the minimal dose required to achieve the desired pharmacologic effect. Failure to do so could result in an increase in the incidence of hypoglycemic episodes. Use appropriate monitoring of FPG and Hb A_{1c} measurements to ensure that the patient is not subjected to excessive drug exposure or increased probability of secondary drug failure. If glucose is not achieved after a suitable trial of combination therapy, consider discontinuing these drugs and using insulin.

Dosing adjustment in renal impairment:

Cl_{cr} 40-80 mL/minute (mild-to-moderate renal dysfunction): Initial dosage adjustment does not appear to be necessary.

Cl_{cr} 20-40 mL/minute (severe renal impairment): Initial: 0.5 mg with meals; titrate carefully.

Cl_{cr} <20 mL/minute: Not studied.

Hemodialysis: Not studied

Dosing adjustment in hepatic impairment: Use conservative initial and maintenance doses. Use longer intervals between dosage adjustments.

Dietary Considerations Take repaglinide 15-30 minutes before meals. Individualized medical nutrition therapy (MNT) based on ADA recommendations is an integral part of therapy. May cause hypoglycemia. Must be able to recognize symptoms of hypoglycemia (palpitations, tachycardia, sweaty palms, diaphoresis, lightheadedness).

Administration Administer 15 minutes before meals; however, time may vary from immediately preceding a meal to as long as 30 minutes before a meal. If the patient misses a meal or is unable to take anything by mouth, repaglinide should not be administered to avoid hypoglycemia. Patients consuming extra meals should be instructed to add a dose for the extra meal.

Monitoring Parameters Monitor fasting blood glucose (periodically) and glycosylated hemoglobin (Hb A_{1c}) levels (every 3 months) with a goal of decreasing these levels towards the normal range. During dose adjustment, fasting glucose can be used to determine response.

Reference Range Recommendations for glycemic control in adults with diabetes mellitus (ADA, 2010):

Hb A_{1c}: <7%

Preprandial capillary plasma glucose: 70-130 mg/dL

Peak postprandial capillary blood glucose: <180 mg/dL

Dosage Forms Excipient information presented when available (limited, particularly for generics); consult specific product labeling.

Tablet, oral:

Prandin®: 0.5 mg, 1 mg, 2 mg

Repaglinide and Metformin

(re PAG li nide & met FOR min)

Brand Names: U.S. PrandiMet®

Index Terms Metformin and Repaglinide; Repaglinide and Metformin Hydrochloride

Pharmacologic Category Antidiabetic Agent, Biguanide; Antidiabetic Agent, Meglitinide Derivative; Hypoglycemic Agent, Oral

Use Management of type 2 diabetes mellitus (noninsulin dependent, NIDDM), as an adjunct to diet and exercise, in patients currently receiving or not adequately controlled on metformin and/or a meglitinide

Pregnancy Risk Factor C

Dosage Oral: Adults: Type 2 diabetes mellitus: **Note:** Daily doses should be divided and given 2-3 times daily with meals (maximum single dose: 4 mg/dose [repaglinide], 1000 mg/dose [metformin]; maximum daily dose: 10 mg/day [repaglinide], 2500 mg/day [metformin])

Patients currently taking repaglinide and metformin: Initial doses should be based on (but not exceeding) the patient's current doses of repaglinide and metformin; titrate as needed to the maximum daily dose to achieve targeted glycemic control

Patients inadequately controlled on metformin alone: Initial dose: repaglinide 1 mg/ metformin 500 mg twice daily with meals. Titrate slowly to reduce the risk of repaglinide-induced hypoglycemia.

Patients inadequately controlled on a meglitinide alone: Initial dose: metformin 500 mg twice daily plus repaglinide at a dose similar to (but not exceeding) the patient's current dose. Titrate slowly to reduce the risk of metformin-induced gastrointestinal adverse effects.

Dosing adjustment in renal impairment: Do not use in renal impairment; metformin use is contraindicated in patients with renal impairment (serum creatinine ≥1.5 mg/dL in males or ≥1.4 mg/dL in females)

Dosing adjustment in hepatic impairment: Avoid use in patients with impaired liver function

Additional Information Complete prescribing information for this medication should be consulted for additional detail.

Dosage Forms Excipient information presented when available (limited, particularly for generics); consult specific product labeling.

Tablet:

PrandiMet®:

1/500: Repaglinide 1 mg and metformin hydrochloride 500 mg

2/500: Repaglinide 2 mg and metformin hydrochloride 500 mg

◆ **Repaglinide and Metformin Hydrochloride** *see* Repaglinide and Metformin *on page 1474*

◆ **Repan®** *see* Butalbital, Acetaminophen, and Caffeine *on page 255*

◆ **Reprexain™** *see* Hydrocodone and Ibuprofen *on page 838*

◆ **Repronex®** *see* Menotropins *on page 1073*

◆ **Requa® Activated Charcoal [OTC]** *see* Charcoal, Activated *on page 335*

◆ **Requip®** *see* ROPINIRole *on page 1517*

◆ **Requip® XL™** *see* ROPINIRole *on page 1517*

◆ **Rescon DM [OTC]** *see* Chlorpheniramine, Pseudoephedrine, and Dextromethorphan *on page 347*

◆ **Rescon GG [OTC]** *see* Guaifenesin and Phenylephrine *on page 812*

◆ **Rescriptor®** *see* Delavirdine *on page 467*

Reserpine

(re SER peen)

Pharmacologic Category Central Monoamine-Depleting Agent; Rauwolfia Alkaloid

Additional Appendix Information

Beers Criteria – Potentially Inappropriate Medications for Geriatrics *on page 1973*

Hypertension *on page 2001*

Use Management of mild-to-moderate hypertension; treatment of agitated psychotic states (schizophrenia)

Unlabeled Use Management of tardive dyskinesia

Pregnancy Risk Factor C

Dosage Note: When used for management of hypertension, full antihypertensive effects may take as long as 3 weeks.

Oral:

Children: Hypertension: 0.01-0.02 mg/kg/24 hours divided every 12 hours; maximum dose: 0.25 mg/day (not recommended in children)

Adults:

Hypertension:

Manufacturer's labeling: Initial: 0.5 mg/day for 1-2 weeks; maintenance: 0.1-0.25 mg/day

Note: Clinically, the need for a "loading" period (as recommended by the manufacturer) is not well supported, and alternative dosing is preferred.

Alternative dosing (unlabeled): Initial: 0.1 mg once daily; adjust as necessary based on response.

Usual dose range (JNC 7): 0.05-0.25 mg once daily; 0.1 mg every other day may be given to achieve 0.05 mg once daily

Schizophrenia (labeled use) or tardive dyskinesia (unlabeled use): Dosing recommendations vary; initial dose recommendations generally range from 0.05-0.25 mg (although manufacturer recommends 0.5 mg once daily initially in schizophrenia). May be increased in increments of 0.1-0.25 mg; maximum dose in tardive dyskinesia: 5 mg/day.

Elderly: Initial: 0.05 mg once daily, increasing by 0.05 mg every week as necessary (Beers Criteria: Avoid doses >0.25 mg daily)

Dosing adjustment in renal impairment: Cl_{cr} <10 mL/minute: Avoid use

Dialysis: Not removed by hemo or peritoneal dialysis; supplemental dose is not necessary

Additional Information Complete prescribing information for this medication should be consulted for additional detail.

Dosage Forms Excipient information presented when available (limited, particularly for generics); consult specific product labeling.

Tablet, oral: 0.1 mg, 0.25 mg

- **Resistant Dextrin** *see* Wheat Dextrin *on page 1805*
- **Resistant Maltodextrin** *see* Wheat Dextrin *on page 1805*
- **Resource® GlutaSolve® [OTC]** *see* Glutamine *on page 799*
- **Respa®-BR [DSC]** *see* Brompheniramine *on page 237*
- **Respaire®-30 [DSC]** *see* Guaifenesin and Pseudoephedrine *on page 813*
- **Restasis®** *see* CycloSPORINE (Ophthalmic) *on page 427*
- **Restoril™** *see* Temazepam *on page 1638*
- **Restylane®** *see* Hyaluronate and Derivatives *on page 831*

Retapamulin (re te PAM ue lin)

Brand Names: U.S. Altabax™

Pharmacologic Category Antibiotic, Pleuromutilin; Antibiotic, Topical

Use Treatment of impetigo caused by susceptible strains of *S. pyogenes* or methicillin-susceptible *S. aureus*

Pregnancy Risk Factor B

Dosage Topical: Impetigo:

Children ≥9 months: Apply to affected area twice daily for 5 days. Total treatment area should not exceed 2% of total body surface area.

Adults: Apply to affected area twice daily for 5 days. Total treatment area should not exceed 100 cm^2 total body surface area.

Additional Information Complete prescribing information for this medication should be consulted for additional detail.

Dosage Forms Excipient information presented when available (limited, particularly for generics); consult specific product labeling. [DSC] = Discontinued product

Ointment, topical:

Altabax™: 1% (5 g [DSC], 10 g [DSC], 15 g)

- **Retavase® (Can)** *see* Reteplase *on page 1475*
- **Retavase® Half-Kit** *see* Reteplase *on page 1475*
- **Retavase® Kit** *see* Reteplase *on page 1475*

Reteplase (RE ta plase)

Brand Names: U.S. Retavase® Half-Kit; Retavase® Kit

Brand Names: Canada Retavase®

Index Terms r-PA; Recombinant Plasminogen Activator

Pharmacologic Category Thrombolytic Agent

Use Management of ST-elevation myocardial infarction (STEMI); improvement of ventricular function; reduction of the incidence of CHF and the reduction of mortality following AMI

Recommended criteria for treatment: STEMI: Chest pain ≥20 minutes duration, onset of chest pain within 12 hours of treatment (or within prior 12-24 hours in patients with continuing ischemic symptoms), and ST-segment elevation >0.1 mV in at least two contiguous precordial leads or two adjacent limb leads on ECG or new or presumably new left bundle branch block (LBBB)

Pregnancy Risk Factor C

Pregnancy Considerations Adverse events have been observed in some animal reproduction studies. The risk of bleeding may be increased in pregnant women.

Lactation Excretion in breast milk unknown/use caution

Contraindications Hypersensitivity to reteplase or any component of the formulation; active internal bleeding; history of cerebrovascular accident; recent intracranial or intraspinal surgery or trauma; intracranial neoplasm, arteriovenous malformations, or aneurysm; known bleeding diathesis; severe uncontrolled hypertension

Warnings/Precautions Concurrent heparin anticoagulation can contribute to bleeding; careful attention to all potential bleeding sites. I.M. injections and nonessential handling of the patient should be avoided. Venipunctures should be performed carefully and only when necessary. If arterial puncture is necessary, use an upper extremity vessel that can be manually compressed. If serious bleeding occurs then the infusion of anistreplase and heparin should be stopped.

For the following conditions the risk of bleeding is higher with use of reteplase and should be weighed against the benefits of therapy: recent major surgery (eg, CABG, obstetrical delivery, organ biopsy, previous puncture of noncompressible vessels), cerebrovascular disease, recent gastrointestinal or genitourinary bleeding, recent trauma including CPR, hypertension (systolic BP >180 mm Hg and/or diastolic BP >110 mm Hg), high likelihood of left heart thrombus (eg, mitral stenosis with atrial fibrillation), acute pericarditis, subacute bacterial endocarditis, hemostatic defects including ones caused by severe renal or hepatic dysfunction, significant hepatic dysfunction, pregnancy, diabetic hemorrhagic retinopathy or other hemorrhagic ophthalmic conditions, septic thrombophlebitis or occluded AV cannula at seriously infected site, advanced age (eg, >75 years), patients receiving oral anticoagulants, any other condition in which bleeding constitutes a significant hazard or would be particularly difficult to manage because of location.

Coronary thrombolysis may result in reperfusion arrhythmias. Follow standard MI management. Rare anaphylactic reactions can occur. Safety and efficacy in pediatric patients have not been established.

Adverse Reactions Bleeding is the most frequent adverse effect associated with reteplase. Heparin and aspirin have been administered concurrently with reteplase in clinical trials. The incidence of adverse events is a reflection of these combined therapies, and are comparable with comparison thrombolytics.

>10%: Local: Injection site bleeding (4.6% to 48.6%)

1% to 10%:

Gastrointestinal: Bleeding (1.8% to 9.0%)

Genitourinary: Bleeding (0.9% to 9.5%)

Hematologic: Anemia (0.9% to 2.6%)

<1% (Limited to important or life-threatening): Allergic/anaphylactoid reactions, cholesterol embolization, intracranial hemorrhage (0.8%)

Other adverse effects noted are frequently associated with MI (and therefore may or may not be attributable to Retavase®) and include arrhythmia, arrest, cardiac reinfarction, cardiogenic shock, embolism, hypotension, pericarditis, pulmonary edema, tamponade, thrombosis

Drug Interactions

Metabolism/Transport Effects None known.

Avoid Concomitant Use There are no known interactions where it is recommended to avoid concomitant use.

Increased Effect/Toxicity

Reteplase may increase the levels/effects of: Anticoagulants; Drotrecogin Alfa (Activated)

The levels/effects of Reteplase may be increased by: Antiplatelet Agents; Herbs (Anticoagulant/Antiplatelet Properties); Nonsteroidal Anti-Inflammatory Agents; Salicylates

Decreased Effect

The levels/effects of Reteplase may be decreased by: Aprotinin

Stability Dosage kits should be stored at 2°C to 25°C (36°F to 77°F) and remain sealed until use in order to protect from light. Reteplase should be reconstituted using the diluent, syringe, needle, and dispensing pin provided with each kit.

Mechanism of Action Reteplase is a nonglycosylated form of tPA produced by recombinant DNA technology using *E. coli*; it initiates local fibrinolysis by binding to fibrin in a thrombus (clot) and converts entrapped plasminogen to plasmin

Pharmacodynamics/Kinetics

Onset of action: Thrombolysis: 30-90 minutes

Half-life elimination: 13-16 minutes

Excretion: Feces and urine

Clearance: Plasma: 250-450 mL/minute

Dosage

Children: Not recommended

Adults: 10 units I.V. over 2 minutes, followed by a second dose 30 minutes later of 10 units I.V. over 2 minutes; withhold second dose if serious bleeding or anaphylaxis occurs

Note: All patients should receive 162-325 mg of chewable nonenteric coated aspirin as soon as possible and then daily. Administer concurrently with heparin 60 units/kg bolus (maximum: 4000 units) followed by continuous infusion of 12 units/kg/hour (maximum: 1000 units/hour) and adjust to aPTT target of 50-70 seconds (or 1.5-2 times the upper limit of control).

Administration Reteplase should be reconstituted using the diluent, syringe, needle and dispensing pin provided with each kit and the each reconstituted dose should be administered I.V. over 2 minutes; no other medication should be added to the injection solution

Monitoring Parameters Monitor for signs of bleeding (hematuria, GI bleeding, gingival bleeding); CBC, PTT; ECG monitoring

Dosage Forms Excipient information presented when available (limited, particularly for generics); consult specific product labeling.

Injection, powder for reconstitution [preservative free]:

Retavase® Half-Kit: 10.4 units [contains polysorbate 80, sucrose 364 mg/vial; equivalent to reteplase 18.1 mg; one Reteplase® vial; supplied with diluent]

Retavase® Kit: 10.4 units [contains polysorbate 80, sucrose 364 mg/vial; equivalent to reteplase 18.1 mg; two Retavase® vials; supplied with diluents]

- ◆ **Retin-A®** *see* Tretinoin (Topical) *on page* 1731
- ◆ **Retin-A Micro®** *see* Tretinoin (Topical) *on page* 1731
- ◆ **Retinoic Acid** *see* Tretinoin (Topical) *on page* 1731
- ◆ **Retinova® (Can)** *see* Tretinoin (Topical) *on page* 1731
- ◆ **Retrovir®** *see* Zidovudine *on page* 1814
- ◆ **Retrovir® (AZT™) (Can)** *see* Zidovudine *on page* 1814
- ◆ **Revatio®** *see* Sildenafil *on page* 1552
- ◆ **ReVia®** *see* Naltrexone *on page* 1174
- ◆ **RevitaDERM® 40** *see* Urea *on page* 1749
- ◆ **Revitalose C-1000® (Can)** *see* Ascorbic Acid *on page* 149
- ◆ **Revlimid®** *see* Lenalidomide *on page* 981
- ◆ **Revolade®** *see* Eltrombopag *on page* 579
- ◆ **Revolade™ (Can)** *see* Eltrombopag *on page* 579
- ◆ **Revonto™** *see* Dantrolene *on page* 443
- ◆ **Reyataz®** *see* Atazanavir *on page* 158
- ◆ **rFSH-alpha** *see* Follitropin Alfa *on page* 750
- ◆ **rFSH-beta** *see* Follitropin Beta *on page* 750
- ◆ **rFVIIa** *see* Factor VIIa (Recombinant) *on page* 681
- ◆ **RG7204** *see* Vemurafenib *on page* 1778
- ◆ **R-Gene® 10** *see* Arginine *on page* 142
- ◆ **rhAPC** *see* Drotrecogin Alfa (Activated) *on page* 564
- ◆ **rhAT** *see* Antithrombin *on page* 130
- ◆ **rhATIII** *see* Antithrombin *on page* 130
- ◆ **r-hCG** *see* Chorionic Gonadotropin (Recombinant) *on page* 353
- ◆ **rhDNase** *see* Dornase Alfa *on page* 547
- ◆ **Rheumatrex®** *see* Methotrexate *on page* 1098
- ◆ **rhFSH-alpha** *see* Follitropin Alfa *on page* 750
- ◆ **rhFSH-beta** *see* Follitropin Beta *on page* 750
- ◆ **rhGAA** *see* Alglucosidase Alfa *on page* 65
- ◆ **r-h α-GAL** *see* Agalsidase Beta *on page* 49
- ◆ **RhIG** *see* Rh_o(D) Immune Globulin *on page* 1476
- ◆ **rhIL-11** *see* Oprelvekin *on page* 1249
- ◆ **Rhinalar® (Can)** *see* Flunisolide (Nasal) *on page* 726
- ◆ **Rhinaris® [OTC]** *see* Sodium Chloride *on page* 1567
- ◆ **Rhinaris-CS Anti-Allergic Nasal Mist (Can)** *see* Cromolyn (Nasal) *on page* 418
- ◆ **Rhinocort Aqua®** *see* Budesonide (Nasal) *on page* 240
- ◆ **Rhinocort® Aqua™ (Can)** *see* Budesonide (Nasal) *on page* 240
- ◆ **Rhinocort® Turbuhaler® (Can)** *see* Budesonide (Nasal) *on page* 240
- ◆ **r-Hirudin** *see* Desirudin *on page* 475
- ◆ **rhKGF** *see* Palifermin *on page* 1276
- ◆ **r-hLH** *see* Lutropin Alfa *on page* 1043
- ◆ **Rho(D) Immune Globulin (Human)** *see* Rh_o(D) Immune Globulin *on page* 1476
- ◆ **Rho®-Clonazepam (Can)** *see* ClonazePAM *on page* 390

Rh_o(D) Immune Globulin

(ar aych oh (dee) i MYUN GLOB yoo lin)

Brand Names: U.S. HyperRHO™ S/D Full Dose; HyperRHO™ S/D Mini-Dose; MICRhoGAM® UF Plus; RhoGAM® UF Plus; Rhophylac®; WinRho® SDF

Brand Names: Canada WinRho® SDF

Index Terms RhIG; Rho(D) Immune Globulin (Human); RhoIGIV; RhoIVIM

Pharmacologic Category Blood Product Derivative; Immune Globulin

Use

Suppression of Rh isoimmunization: Use in the following situations when an Rh_o(D)-negative individual is exposed to Rh_o(D)-positive blood: During delivery of an Rh_o(D)-positive infant; abortion; amniocentesis; chorionic villus sampling; ruptured tubal pregnancy; abdominal trauma; hydatidiform mole; transplacental hemorrhage. Used when the mother is Rh_o(D)-negative, the father of the child is either Rh_o(D)-positive or Rh_o(D)-unknown, or the baby is either Rh_o(D)-positive or Rh_o(D)-unknown.

Transfusion: Suppression of Rh isoimmunization in Rh_o(D)-negative individuals transfused with Rh_o(D) antigen-positive RBCs or blood components containing Rh_o(D) antigen-positive RBCs

Treatment of idiopathic thrombocytopenic purpura (ITP): Used intravenously in the following nonsplenectomized $Rh_o(D)$-positive individuals: Children with acute or chronic ITP, adults with chronic ITP, and children and adults with ITP secondary to HIV infection

Pregnancy Risk Factor C

Pregnancy Considerations Animal studies have not been conducted. Available evidence suggests that $Rh_o(D)$ immune globulin administration during pregnancy does not harm the fetus or affect future pregnancies.

Lactation Does not enter breast milk

Contraindications Hypersensitivity to immune globulins or any component of the formulation; prior sensitization to $Rh_o(D)$

WinRho® SDF product labeling: Patients with autoimmune hemolytic anemia; patients with pre-existing hemolysis or at high risk for hemolysis; IgA-deficient patients with antibodies against IgA; suppression of isoimmunization in infants

WinRho® SDF Canadian labeling: Additional contraindications (not in U.S. labeling):

Rh immunization prophylaxis: $Rh_o(D)$-negative women who are not pregnant or have had a recent delivery or abortion and who are Rh sensitized

Treatment of ITP: Patients who are $Rh_o(D)$-negative or have had splenectomy, ITP secondary to conditions including leukemia, lymphoma, or active infections with Epstein-Barr virus (EBV) or hepatits C virus (HCV), elderly with comorbidities predisposing to acute hemolytic reaction (AHR), evidence of autoimmune hemolytic anemia (Evan's syndrome), systemic lupus erythematosus (SLE) or antiphospholipid antibody syndrome

Warnings/Precautions [U.S. Boxed Warning]: May cause IVH in patients treated for immune thrombocytopenic purpura (WinRho® SDF product labeling). Rare but serious signs and symptoms (eg, back pain, shaking, chills, fever, discolored urine; onset within 4 hours of infusion) of intravascular hemolysis (IVH) have been reported in postmarketing experience in patients treated for ITP and may result in clinically-compromising anemia and multiorgan system failure including acute respiratory distress syndrome. Acute renal insufficiency and disseminated intravascular coagulation (DIC) have also been reported. ITP patients should be advised of the signs and symptoms of IVH and instructed to report them immediately.

Product of human plasma; may potentially contain infectious agents which could transmit disease. Screening of donors, as well as testing and/or inactivation or removal of certain viruses, reduces the risk. Infections thought to be transmitted by this product should be reported to the manufacturer. Not for replacement therapy in immune globulin deficiency syndromes. Pulmonary edema may occur following IVIG treatment in patients being treated for ITP. Symptoms are usually present within 1-6 hours after administration; monitor patients for pulmonary reactions. Use caution with IgA deficiency, may contain trace amounts of IgA; patients who are IgA deficient may have the potential for developing IgA antibodies, anaphylactic reactions may occur. Administer I.M. injections with caution in patients with thrombocytopenia or coagulation disorders. Some products may contain maltose, which may result in falsely-elevated blood glucose readings. Use caution with renal dysfunction. Thrombotic events have been reported with administration of intravenous immune globulins (IVIG); use with caution in patients with a history of atherosclerosis or cardiovascular and/or thrombotic risk factors or patients with known/suspected hyperviscosity. Consider a baseline assessment of blood viscosity in patients at risk for hyperviscosity.

Administer at the minimum practical infusion rate in patients with renal impairment or in patients at risk for thrombotic events. Monitor for signs and symptoms of transfusion-related acute lung injury.

ITP: Do not administer I.M. or SubQ for the treatment of ITP; administer dose I.V. only. Safety and efficacy not established in $Rh_o(D)$ negative, non-ITP thrombocytopenia, or splenectomized patients. When using WinRho® SDF, decrease dose with hemoglobin <10 g/dL; use with extreme caution if hemoglobin <8 g/dL. Safety and efficacy have not been established for Rhophylac® in patients with anemia.

$Rh_o(D)$ suppression: For use in the mother; do not administer to the neonate.

Adverse Reactions Frequency not defined.

Cardiovascular: Hyper-/hypotension, pallor, vasodilation

Central nervous system: Chills, dizziness, fever, headache, malaise, somnolence

Dermatologic: Pruritus, rash

Gastrointestinal: Abdominal pain, diarrhea, nausea, vomiting

Hematologic: Haptoglobin decreased, hemoglobin decreased (patients with ITP), intravascular hemolysis (patients with ITP)

Hepatic: Bilirubin increased, LDH increased

Local: Injection site reaction: Discomfort, induration, mild pain, redness, swelling

Neuromuscular & skeletal: Arthralgia, back pain, hyperkinesia, myalgia, weakness

Renal: Acute renal insufficiency

Miscellaneous: Anaphylaxis, diaphoresis, infusion-related reactions, positive anti-C antibody test (transient), shivering

Postmarketing and/or case reports: Anemia (clinically-compromising), anuria, ARDS, cardiac arrest, cardiac failure, chest pain, chromaturia, DIC, edema, erythema, fatigue, hematuria, hemoglobinemia, hemoglobinuria (transient in patients with ITP), hyperhidrosis, hypersensitivity, injection site irritation, jaundice, myocardial infarction, muscle spasm, nausea, pain in extremities, renal failure, renal impairment, tachycardia, transfusion-related acute lung injury

Drug Interactions

Metabolism/Transport Effects None known.

Avoid Concomitant Use There are no known interactions where it is recommended to avoid concomitant use.

Increased Effect/Toxicity There are no known significant interactions involving an increase in effect.

Decreased Effect

Rho(D) Immune Globulin may decrease the levels/effects of: Vaccines (Live)

Stability Store at 2°C to 8°C (35°F to 46°F); do not freeze.

RhoGAM® UF Plus, MICRhoGAM® UF Plus: May be stored at 25°C (77°F) for up to 10 days (data on file [Ortho Clinical Diagnostics, 2011]). However, the manufacturer recommends storage under refrigeration. Room temperature stability information should only be utilized in situations where the drug has been inadvertently exposed to prolonged room temperature.

HyperRHO™ SD may be stored at 25°C (77°F) for ~2 weeks (data on file [Talecris Biotherapeutics, 2011]). However, the manufacturer recommends storage under refrigeration. Room temperature stability information should only be utilized in situations where the drug has been inadvertently exposed to prolonged room temperature.

Rhophylac®: Protect from light.

WinRho® SDF: After reconstitution, store at room temperature for no longer than 12 hours. Do not shake or freeze.

Mechanism of Action

Rh suppression: Prevents isoimmunization by suppressing the immune response and antibody formation by $Rh_o(D)$ negative individuals to $Rh_o(D)$ positive red blood cells.

ITP: Not completely characterized; $Rh_o(D)$ immune globulin is thought to form anti-D-coated red blood cell complexes which bind to macrophage Fc receptors within the spleen; blocking or saturating the spleens ability to clear antibody-coated cells, including platelets. In this manner, platelets are spared from destruction.

Pharmacodynamics/Kinetics

Onset of platelet increase: ITP: Platelets should rise within 1-2 days

Peak effect: In 7-14 days

Duration: Suppression of Rh isoimmunization: ~12 weeks; Treatment of ITP: 30 days (variable)

Distribution: V_d: I.M.: 8.59 L

Bioavailability: I.M.: Rhophylac®: 69%

Half-life elimination: ~24-30 days

Time to peak, plasma: I.M.: 5-10 days; I.V. (WinRho® SDF): ≤2 hours

Dosage

ITP: Children and Adults:

Rhophylac®: I.V.: 50 mcg/kg

WinRho® SDF: I.V.:

Initial: 50 mcg/kg as a single injection, or can be given as a divided dose on separate days. If hemoglobin is <10 g/dL: Dose should be reduced to 25-40 mcg/kg.

Subsequent dosing: 25-60 mcg/kg can be used if required to increase platelet count

Maintenance dosing if patient **did respond** to initial dosing: 25-60 mcg/kg based on platelet count and hemoglobin concentration

Maintenance dosing if patient **did not respond** to initial dosing:

Hemoglobin <8 g/dL: Alternative treatment should be used

Hemoglobin 8-10 g/dL: Redose between 25-40 mcg/kg

Hemoglobin >10 g/dL: Redose between 50-60 mcg/kg

Rh_o (D) suppression: Adults: **Note:** One "full dose" (300 mcg) provides enough antibody to prevent Rh sensitization if the volume of RBC entering the circulation is ≤15 mL. When >15 mL is suspected, a fetal red cell count should be performed to determine the appropriate dose.

Pregnancy:

Antepartum prophylaxis: In general, dose is given at 28 weeks. If given early in pregnancy, administer every 12 weeks to ensure adequate levels of passively acquired anti-Rh

HyperRHO™ S/D Full Dose, RhoGAM®: I.M.: 300 mcg

Rhophylac®, WinRho® SDF: I.M., I.V.: 300 mcg

Postpartum prophylaxis: In general, dose is administered as soon as possible after delivery, preferably within 72 hours. Can be given up to 28 days following delivery

HyperRHO™ S/D Full Dose, RhoGAM®: I.M.: 300 mcg

Rhophylac®: I.M., I.V.: 300 mcg

WinRho® SDF: I.M., I.V.: 120 mcg

Threatened abortion, any time during pregnancy (with continuation of pregnancy):

HyperRHO™ S/D Full Dose, RhoGAM®: I.M.: 300 mcg; administer as soon as possible

Rhophylac®, WinRho® SDF: I.M., I.V.: 300 mcg; administer as soon as possible

Abortion, miscarriage, termination of ectopic pregnancy:

RhoGAM®: I.M.: ≥13 weeks gestation: 300 mcg.

HyperRHO™ S/D Mini Dose, MICRhoGAM®: <13 weeks gestation: I.M.: 50 mcg

Rhophylac®: I.M., I.V.: 300 mcg

WinRho® SDF: I.M., I.V.: After 34 weeks gestation: 120 mcg; administer immediately or within 72 hours

Amniocentesis, chorionic villus sampling:

HyperRHO™ S/D Full Dose, RhoGAM®: I.M.: At 15-18 weeks gestation or during the 3rd trimester: 300 mcg. If dose is given between 13-18 weeks, repeat at 26-28 weeks and within 72 hours of delivery.

Rhophylac®: I.M., I.V.: 300 mcg

WinRho® SDF: I.M., I.V.: Before 34 weeks gestation: 300 mcg; administer immediately, repeat dose every 12 weeks during pregnancy; After 34 weeks gestation: 120 mcg, administered immediately or within 72 hours

Excessive fetomaternal hemorrhage (>15 mL): Rhophylac®: I.M., I.V.: 300 mcg within 72 hours plus 20 mcg/mL fetal RBCs in excess of 15 mL if excess transplacental bleeding is quantified **or** 300 mcg/dose if bleeding cannot be quantified

Abdominal trauma, manipulation:

HyperRHO™ S/D Full Dose, RhoGAM®: I.M.: 2nd or 3rd trimester: 300 mcg. If dose is given between 13-18 weeks, repeat at 26-28 weeks and within 72 hours of delivery

Rhophylac®: I.M., I.V.: 300 mcg within 72 hours

WinRho® SDF: I.M./I.V.: After 34 weeks gestation: 120 mcg; administer immediately or within 72 hours

Transfusion:

Children and Adults: WinRho® SDF: Administer within 72 hours after exposure of incompatible blood transfusions or massive fetal hemorrhage.

I.V.: Calculate dose as follows; administer 600 mcg every 8 hours until the total dose is administered:

Exposure to $Rh_o(D)$ positive whole blood: 9 mcg/mL blood

Exposure to $Rh_o(D)$ positive red blood cells: 18 mcg/mL cells

I.M.: Calculate dose as follows; administer 1200 mcg every 12 hours until the total dose is administered:

Exposure to $Rh_o(D)$ positive whole blood: 12 mcg/mL blood

Exposure to $Rh_o(D)$ positive red blood cells: 24 mcg/mL cells

Adults:

HyperRHO™ S/D Full Dose, RhoGAM®: I.M.: Multiply the volume of Rh positive whole blood administered by the hematocrit of the donor unit to equal the volume of RBCs transfused. The volume of RBCs is then divided by 15 mL, providing the number of 300 mcg doses (vials/syringes) to administer. If the dose calculated results in a fraction, round up to the next higher whole 300 mcg dose (vial/syringe).

Rhophylac®: I.M., I.V.: 20 mcg/2 mL transfused blood or 20 mcg/mL erythrocyte concentrate

Elderly: Patients >65 years of age with a concurrent comorbid condition (eg, infection, malignancy, autoimmune disorders) may be at increased risk of developing acute hemolytic reactions. Fatal outcomes associated with IVH have occurred most frequently in those >65 years. Careful consideration should be used when selecting dosage for elderly patients due to a higher probability of decreased hepatic, renal, or cardiac function; consider starting at lower doses.

Dosage adjustment in renal impairment: I.V. infusion: Use caution; may require infusion rate reduction or discontinuation.

Administration The total volume can be administered in divided doses at different sites at one time or may be divided and given at intervals, provided the total dosage is given within 72 hours of the fetomaternal hemorrhage or transfusion.

I.M.: Administer into the deltoid muscle of the upper arm or anterolateral aspect of the upper thigh; avoid gluteal region due to risk of sciatic nerve injury. If large doses (>5 mL) are needed, administration in divided doses at different sites is recommended. **Note:** Do not administer I.M. Rh_o(D) immune globulin for ITP.

I.V.:

Rhophylac®: ITP: Infuse at 2 mL per 15-60 seconds

WinRho® SDF: Infuse over at least 3-5 minutes; do not administer with other medications

Note: If preparing dose using liquid formulation, withdraw the entire contents of the vial to ensure accurate calculation of the dosage requirement.

Monitoring Parameters Signs and symptoms of intravascular hemolysis (IVH), anemia, renal insufficiency, back pain, shaking, chills, discolored urine, or hematuria; observe patient for side effects for 8 hours following administration

Patients with suspected IVH: CBC, haptoglobin, plasma hemoglobin, urine dipstick, BUN, serum creatinine, liver function tests, DIC-specific tests (D-dimer, fibrin degradation products [FDP] or fibrin split products [FSP]) for differential diagnosis. In patients at increased risk of developing acute renal failure, periodically monitor renal function and urine output. Clinical response may be determined by monitoring platelets, red blood cell (RBC) counts, hemoglobin, and reticulocyte levels.

ITP: Check blood type, CBC, reticulocyte count, DAT, urine dipstick before initiating treatment with WinRho® SDF, repeat urine dipstick at 2 and 4 hours after administration and prior to end of the 8-hour monitoring period.

Test Interactions Some infants born to women given Rh_o(D) antepartum have a weakly positive Coombs' test at birth. Fetal-maternal hemorrhage may cause false blood-typing result in the mother; when there is any doubt to the patients' Rh type, Rh_o(D) immune globulin should be administered. WinRho® SDF liquid contains maltose; may result in falsely elevated blood glucose levels with dehydrogenase pyrroloquinolinequinone or glucose-dye-oxidoreductase testing methods. WinRho® SDF contains trace amounts of anti-A, B, C and E; may alter Coombs' tests following administration.

Additional Information A "full dose" of Rh_o(D) immune globulin has previously been referred to as a 300 mcg dose. It is not the actual anti-D content. Although dosing has traditionally been expressed in mcg, potency is listed in int. units (1 mcg = 5 int. units). ITP patients requiring transfusions should be transfused with Rho-negative blood cells to avoid exacerbating hemolysis; platelet products may contain red blood cells; caution should be exercised if platelets are from Rh_o-positive donors.

Dosage Forms Excipient information presented when available (limited, particularly for generics); consult specific product labeling.

Injection, solution [preservative free]:

HyperRHO™ S/D Full Dose: ≥300 mcg/mL (1 mL) [solvent/detergent treated; ≥1500 int. units; for I.M. use only]

HyperRHO™ S/D Mini-Dose: ≥50 mcg/0.17 mL (0.17 mL) [solvent/detergent treated; ≥250 int. units; for I.M. use only]

MICRhoGAM® UF Plus: ~50 mcg/0.75 mL (0.75 mL) [contains polysorbate 80; 250 int. units; for I.M. use only; volume is expressed as an approximate value]

RhoGAM® UF Plus: ~300 mcg/0.75 mL (0.75 mL) [contains polysorbate 80; 1500 int. units; for I.M. use only; volume is expressed as an approximate value]

Rhophylac®: ≥300 mcg/2 mL (2 mL) [contains albumin (human); 1500 int. units; for I.M. or I.V. use]

WinRho® SDF: 3000 mcg/~13 mL (13 mL) [contains maltose, polysorbate 80; 15,000 int. units; for I.M. or I.V. use; volume is expressed as an approximate value]

WinRho® SDF: 300 mcg/~1.3 mL (1.3 mL) [contains maltose, polysorbate 80; 1500 int. units; for I.M. or I.V. use; volume is expressed as an approximate value]

WinRho® SDF: 500 mcg/~2.2 mL (2.2 mL) [contains maltose, polysorbate 80; 2500 int. units; for I.M. or I.V. use; volume is expressed as an approximate value]

WinRho® SDF: 1000 mcg/~4.4 mL (4.4 mL) [contains maltose, polysorbate 80; 5000 int. units; for I.M. or I.V. use; volume is expressed as an approximate value]

- ◆ **RhoGAM® UF Plus** *see* Rh_o(D) Immune Globulin *on page 1476*
- ◆ **RhoIGIV** *see* Rh_o(D) Immune Globulin *on page 1476*
- ◆ **RhoIVIM** *see* Rh_o(D) Immune Globulin *on page 1476*
- ◆ **Rho®-Loperamine (Can)** *see* Loperamide *on page 1026*
- ◆ **Rho®-Nitro Pump Spray (Can)** *see* Nitroglycerin *on page 1212*
- ◆ **Rhophylac®** *see* Rh_o(D) Immune Globulin *on page 1476*
- ◆ **Rhotral (Can)** *see* Acebutolol *on page 27*
- ◆ **Rhoxal-cyclosporine (Can)** *see* CycloSPORINE (Systemic) *on page 422*
- ◆ **Rhoxal-fluvoxamine (Can)** *see* FluvoxaMINE *on page 746*
- ◆ **Rhoxal-glimepiride (Can)** *see* Glimepiride *on page 793*
- ◆ **Rhoxal-loperamide (Can)** *see* Loperamide *on page 1026*
- ◆ **Rhoxal-nabumetone (Can)** *see* Nabumetone *on page 1167*
- ◆ **Rhoxal-orphendrine (Can)** *see* Orphenadrine *on page 1252*
- ◆ **Rhoxal-pamidronate (Can)** *see* Pamidronate *on page 1282*
- ◆ **Rhoxal-sotalol (Can)** *see* Sotalol *on page 1586*
- ◆ **Rhoxal-valproic (Can)** *see* Valproic Acid *on page 1757*
- ◆ **rhPTH(1-34)** *see* Teriparatide *on page 1651*
- ◆ **Rh-TSH** *see* Thyrotropin Alfa *on page 1677*
- ◆ **rHuEPO** *see* Epoetin Alfa *on page 601*
- ◆ **rhuFabV2** *see* Ranibizumab *on page 1461*
- ◆ **rhuGM-CSF** *see* Sargramostim *on page 1538*
- ◆ **rhu Keratinocyte Growth Factor** *see* Palifermin *on page 1276*
- ◆ **rHu-KGF** *see* Palifermin *on page 1276*
- ◆ **rhuMAb-E25** *see* Omalizumab *on page 1240*
- ◆ **rHuMAb-EGFr** *see* Panitumumab *on page 1288*
- ◆ **rhuMAb HER2** *see* Trastuzumab *on page 1722*
- ◆ **rhuMAb-VEGF** *see* Bevacizumab *on page 212*
- ◆ **RiaSTAP®** *see* Fibrinogen Concentrate (Human) *on page 710*
- ◆ **Ribasphere®** *see* Ribavirin *on page 1479*
- ◆ **Ribasphere® RibaPak®** *see* Ribavirin *on page 1479*

Ribavirin (rye ba VYE rin)

Brand Names: U.S. Copegus®; Rebetol®; Ribasphere®; Ribasphere® RibaPak®; Virazole®

Brand Names: Canada Virazole®

Index Terms RTCA; Tribavirin

Pharmacologic Category Antiviral Agent

Use

Inhalation: Treatment of hospitalized infants and young children with respiratory syncytial virus (RSV) infections; specially indicated for treatment of severe lower respiratory tract RSV infections in patients with an underlying compromising condition (prematurity, cardiopulmonary disease, or immunosuppression)

Oral capsule:

In combination with interferon alfa-2b (Intron® A) injection for the treatment of chronic hepatitis C in patients with compensated liver disease who have relapsed after alpha interferon therapy or were previously untreated with alpha interferons

In combination with peginterferon alfa-2b (PEG-Intron®) injection for the treatment of chronic hepatitis C in patients with compensated liver disease who were previously untreated with alpha interferons

Oral solution: In combination with interferon alfa 2b (Intron® A) injection for the treatment of chronic hepatitis C in patients with compensated liver disease who were previously untreated with alpha interferons or patients who have relapsed after alpha interferon therapy

Oral tablet: In combination with peginterferon alfa-2a (Pegasys®) injection for the treatment of chronic hepatitis C in patients with compensated liver disease who were previously untreated with alpha interferons (includes patients with histological evidence of cirrhosis [Child-Pugh class A] and patients with clinically-stable HIV disease)

Unlabeled Use

Inhalation: Treatment for RSV in adult hematopoietic stem cell or heart/lung transplant recipients

Used in other viral infections including influenza A and B and adenovirus

Pregnancy Risk Factor X

Pregnancy Considerations **[U.S. Boxed Warning]: Significant teratogenic effects have been observed in all animal studies** at ~0.01 times the maximum recommended daily human dose. Use is contraindicated in pregnancy. Negative pregnancy test is required before initiation and monthly thereafter. Avoid pregnancy in female patients and female partners of male patients during therapy by using two effective forms of contraception; continue contraceptive measures for at least 6 months after completion of therapy. If patient or female partner becomes pregnant during treatment, she should be counseled about potential risks of exposure. If pregnancy occurs during use or within 6 months after treatment, report to the ribavirin pregnancy registry (800-593-2214).

Lactation Excretion in breast milk unknown/not recommended

Medication Guide Available Yes

Contraindications Hypersensitivity to ribavirin or any component of the formulation; women of childbearing age who will not use contraception reliably; pregnancy

Additional contraindications for oral formulation: Male partners of pregnant women; hemoglobinopathies (eg, thalassemia major, sickle cell anemia); patients with autoimmune hepatitis; ribavirin tablets are contraindicated in patients with hepatic decompensation (Child-Pugh class B and C); concomitant use of didanosine

Additional contraindication for Ribasphere® capsules and Rebetrol® capsules/solution: Patients with a Cl_{cr} <50 mL/minute

Refer to individual monographs for Interferon Alfa-2b (Intron® A) and Peginterferon Alfa-2a (Pegasys®) for additional contraindication information.

Warnings/Precautions Oral: **[U.S. Boxed Warning]: Significant teratogenic effects have been observed in all animal studies.** A negative pregnancy test is required before initiation and monthly thereafter. Avoid pregnancy in female patients and female partners of male patients, during therapy, and for at least 6 months after treatment; two forms of contraception should be used. Safety and efficacy have not been established in patients who have failed other alfa interferon therapy, received organ transplants, or been coinfected with hepatitis B or HIV (Copegus® may be used in HIV coinfected patients unless CD4+ cell count is <100 cells/microL). Oral products should not be used for HIV infection, adenovirus, RSV, or influenza infections.

[U.S. Boxed Warning]: Monotherapy not effective for chronic hepatitis C infection. Severe psychiatric events have occurred including depression and suicidal behavior during combination therapy. Avoid use in patients with a psychiatric history; discontinue if severe psychiatric symptoms occur. Acute hypersensitivity reactions (eg, anaphylaxis, angioedema, bronchoconstriction, and urticaria) have been observed (rarely) with ribavirin and alfa interferon combination therapy. Severe cutaneous reactions, including Stevens-Johnson syndrome and exfoliative dermatitis have been reported (rarely) with ribavirin and alfa interferon combination therapy; discontinue with signs or symptoms of severe skin reactions. Use with caution in patients with renal impairment; dosage adjustment or discontinuation may be required. Elderly patients are more susceptible to adverse effects; use caution.

[U.S. Boxed Warning]: Hemolytic anemia is the primary toxicity of oral therapy; usually occurring within 1-2 weeks of therapy initiation; observed in ~10% to 13% of patients when alfa interferons were combined with ribavirin. Assess cardiac disease before initiation. Anemia may worsen underlying cardiac disease; avoid use in patients with significant/unstable cardiac disease. If deterioration in cardiovascular status occurs, discontinue therapy. Patients with renal dysfunction and/or those >50 years of age should be carefully assessed for development of anemia. Pancytopenia and bone marrow suppression have been reported with the combination of ribavirin, interferon, and azathioprine. Use caution in pulmonary disease; pulmonary symptoms have been associated with administration. Discontinue therapy if evidence of hepatic decompensation (Child-Pugh score ≥6) is observed. Use caution in patients with sarcoidosis (exacerbation reported). Dental and periodontal disorders have been reported with ribavirin and interferon therapy; patients should be instructed to brush teeth twice daily and have regular dental exams. Serious ophthalmologic disorders have occurred with combination therapy. All patients require an eye exam at baseline; those with pre-existing ophthalmologic disorders (eg, diabetic or hypertensive retinopathy) require periodic follow up. In combination with peginterferon alfa-2b, ribavirin may cause a reduction in growth velocity in pediatric patients during treatment and for about 6 months post-treatment.

Inhalation: **[U.S. Boxed Warning]: Use with caution in patients requiring assisted ventilation because precipitation of the drug in the respiratory equipment may interfere with safe and effective patient ventilation; sudden deterioration of respiratory function has been observed;** monitor carefully in patients with COPD and asthma for deterioration of respiratory function. Ribavirin is potentially mutagenic, tumor-promoting, and gonadotoxic. Although anemia has not been reported with inhalation therapy, consider monitoring for anemia 1-2 weeks post-treatment. Pregnant healthcare workers may consider unnecessary occupational exposure; ribavirin has been detected in healthcare workers' urine. Healthcare professionals or family members who are pregnant (or may become pregnant) should be counseled about potential risks of exposure and counseled about risk reduction strategies. Hazardous agent - use appropriate precautions for handling and disposal.

Adverse Reactions

Inhalation:

1% to 10%:

Central nervous system: Fatigue, headache, insomnia
Gastrointestinal: Nausea, anorexia
Hematologic: Anemia

<1%: Hypotension, cardiac arrest, digitalis toxicity, conjunctivitis, mild bronchospasm, worsening of respiratory function, apnea

Note: Incidence of adverse effects (approximate) in healthcare workers: Headache (51%); conjunctivitis (32%); rhinitis, nausea, rash, dizziness, pharyngitis, and lacrimation (10% to 20%); bronchospasm and/or chest pain (case reports in individuals with underlying airway disease)

Oral (all adverse reactions are documented while receiving combination therapy with alfa interferons; percentages as reported in adults); asterisked (*) percentages are those similar to interferon therapy alone:

>10%:

Central nervous system: Fatigue (60% to 70%)*, headache (43% to 66%)*, fever (32% to 55%)*, insomnia (26% to 41%), depression (20% to 36%)*, irritability (23% to 33%), dizziness (14% to 26%), impaired concentration (10% to 21%)*, emotional lability (7% to 12%)*

Dermatologic: Alopecia (27% to 36%), pruritus (13% to 29%), rash (5% to 28%), dry skin (10% to 24%), dermatitis (≤16%)

Endocrine and metabolic: Hyperuricemia (33% to 38%)

Gastrointestinal: Nausea (25% to 47%), anorexia (21% to 32%), weight decrease (10% to 29%), vomiting (9% to 25%)*, diarrhea (10% to 22%), dyspepsia (6% to 16%), abdominal pain (8% to 13%), xerostomia (≤12%), RUQ pain (≤12%)

Hematologic: Leukopenia (6% to 45%), neutropenia (8% to 42%; grade 4: 2% to 11%; 40% with HIV coinfection), hemoglobin decreased (11% to 35%), anemia (11% to 17%), thrombocytopenia (<1% to 15%), lymphopenia (12% to 14%), hemolytic anemia (10% to 13%)

Hepatic: Bilirubin increase (10% to 32%)

Neuromuscular & skeletal: Myalgia (40% to 64%)*, rigors (25% to 48%), arthralgia (22% to 34%)*, musculoskeletal pain (19% to 28%)

Respiratory: Dyspnea (13% to 26%), cough (7% to 23%), pharyngitis (≤13%), sinusitis (≤12%)*

Miscellaneous: Flu-like syndrome (13% to 18%)*, viral infection (≤12%), diaphoresis (≤11%)

1% to 10%:

Cardiovascular: Chest pain (5% to 9%)*, flushing (≤4%)

Central nervous system: Pain (≤10%), mood alteration (≤6%; 9% with HIV coinfection), agitation (5% to 8%), nervousness (6%)*, memory impairment (≤6%), malaise (≤6%), suicidal ideation (adolescents: 2%; adults: 1%)

Dermatologic: Eczema (4% to 5%)

Endocrine & metabolic: Menstrual disorder (≤7%), hypothyroidism (≤5%)

Gastrointestinal: Taste perversion (4% to 9%), constipation (5%)

Hepatic: Hepatomegaly (4%), transaminases increased (1% to 3%), hepatic decompensation (2% with HIV coinfection)

Neuromuscular & skeletal: Weakness (9% to 10%), back pain (5%)

Ocular: Blurred vision (≤6%), conjunctivitis (≤5%)

Respiratory: Rhinitis (≤8%), exertional dyspnea (≤7%)

Miscellaneous: Fungal infection (≤6%), bacterial infection (3% to 5%)

<1% (Limited to important or life-threatening): Aggression, angina, anxiety, aplastic anemia, arrhythmia; autoimmune disorders (systemic lupus erythematosus, rheumatoid arthritis, sarcoidosis); bone marrow suppression, cerebral hemorrhage, cholangitis, colitis, coma, corneal ulcer, dehydration, diabetes mellitus, drug abuse relapse/overdose, exfoliative dermatitis, fatty liver, hearing impairment/loss, gastrointestinal bleeding, gout, hallucination, hepatic dysfunction, hyper-/hypothyroidism, hypersensitivity (including anaphylaxis, angioedema, bronchoconstriction, and urticaria), macular edema, myositis, optic neuritis, papilledema, pancreatitis, peptic ulcer, peripheral neuropathy, pneumonitis, psychosis, psychotic disorder, pulmonary dysfunction, pulmonary embolism, pulmonary infiltrates, pure red cell aplasia, retinal artery/vein thrombosis, retinal detachment, retinal hemorrhage, retinopathy, sarcoidosis exacerbation; skin reactions (erythema multiforme, exfoliative dermatitis, urticaria, vesiculobullous eruptions); Stevens-Johnson syndrome, suicide, thrombotic thrombocytopenic purpura, thyroid function test abnormalities; transplant rejection (kidney, liver); vision loss

Note: Incidence of anorexia, headache, fever, suicidal ideation, and vomiting are higher in children.

Drug Interactions

Metabolism/Transport Effects None known.

Avoid Concomitant Use

Avoid concomitant use of Ribavirin with any of the following: Didanosine

Increased Effect/Toxicity

Ribavirin may increase the levels/effects of: AzaTHIOprine; Didanosine; Reverse Transcriptase Inhibitors (Nucleoside)

The levels/effects of Ribavirin may be increased by: Interferons (Alfa); Zidovudine

Decreased Effect

Ribavirin may decrease the levels/effects of: Influenza Virus Vaccine (Live/Attenuated)

Ethanol/Nutrition/Herb Interactions Food: Oral: High-fat meal increases the AUC and C_{max}.

Stability

Inhalation: Store vials in a dry place at 15°C to 30°C (59°F to 86°F). Do not use any water containing an antimicrobial agent to reconstitute drug. Reconstituted solution is stable for 24 hours at room temperature. Should not be mixed with other aerosolized medication.

Oral: Store at controlled room temperature of 25°C (77°F). Solution may also be refrigerated at 2°C to 8°C (36°F to 46°F).

Mechanism of Action Inhibits replication of RNA and DNA viruses; inhibits influenza virus RNA polymerase activity and inhibits the initiation and elongation of RNA fragments resulting in inhibition of viral protein synthesis

Pharmacodynamics/Kinetics

Absorption: Inhalation: Systemic; dependent upon respiratory factors and method of drug delivery; maximal absorption occurs with the use of aerosol generator via endotracheal tube; highest concentrations in respiratory tract and erythrocytes

Distribution: Oral capsule: Single dose: V_d: 2825 L; distribution significantly prolonged in the erythrocyte (16-40 days), which can be used as a marker for intracellular metabolism

Protein binding: Oral: None

Metabolism: Hepatically and intracellularly (forms active metabolites); may be necessary for drug action

Bioavailability: Oral: 64%

Half-life elimination, plasma:

Children: Inhalation: 6.5-11 hours

Adults: Oral:

Capsule, single dose (Rebetol®, Ribasphere®): 24 hours in healthy adults, 44 hours with chronic hepatitis C infection (increases to ~298 hours at steady state)

Tablet, single dose (Copegus®): ~120-170 hours

Time to peak, serum: Inhalation: At end of inhalation period; Oral capsule: Multiple doses: 3 hours; Tablet: 2 hours

Excretion: Inhalation: Urine (40% as unchanged drug and metabolites); Oral capsule: Urine (61%), feces (12%)

Dosage

Infants and Children: Aerosol inhalation: RSV infection: Use with Viratek® small particle aerosol generator (SPAG-2) at a concentration of 20 mg/mL (6 g reconstituted with 300 mL of sterile water without preservatives). Continuous aerosol administration: 12-18 hours/day for 3 days, up to 7 days in length

Children ≥3 years: Oral capsule or solution (Rebetol®): Chronic hepatitis C (in combination with interferon alfa-2b): **Note:** Oral solution should be used in children 3-5 years of age, children ≤25 kg, or those unable to swallow capsules. Recommended therapy duration (manufacturer labeling): Genotype 1: 48 weeks; genotypes 2,3: 24 weeks

Capsule/solution: 15 mg/kg/day in 2 divided doses (morning and evening)

Capsule dosing recommendations:

25-36 kg: 400 mg/day (200 mg morning and evening)

37-49 kg: 600 mg/day (200 mg in the morning and 400 mg in the evening)

50-61 kg: 800 mg/day (400 mg in the morning and evening)

>61 kg: Refer to adult dosing

Note: *American Association for the Study of Liver Diseases (AASLD) guidelines recommendation:* Children 2-17 years with chronic HCV infection (Ghany, 2009): Treatment of choice: Ribavirin 15 mg/kg daily in combination with SubQ peginterferon alfa-2b 60 mcg/m^2 once weekly for 48 weeks

Adults:

Oral capsule (Rebetol®, Ribasphere®):

Chronic hepatitis C (in combination with interferon alfa-2b):

≤75 kg: 400 mg in the morning, then 600 mg in the evening

>75 kg: 600 mg in the morning, then 600 mg in the evening

Chronic hepatitis C (in combination with peginterferon alfa-2b): 400 mg twice daily

Tablet (Copegus®): Chronic hepatitis C (in combination with peginterferon alfa-2a):

Monoinfection, genotype 1,4:

<75 kg: 1000 mg/day in 2 divided doses for 48 weeks

≥75 kg: 1200 mg/day in 2 divided doses for 48 weeks

Monoinfection, genotype 2,3: 800 mg/day in 2 divided doses for 24 weeks

Coinfection with HIV: 800 mg/day in 2 divided doses for 48 weeks (regardless of genotype)

Note: *American Association for the Study of Liver Diseases (AASLD) guidelines recommendation:* Adults with chronic HCV infection (Ghany, 2009): Treatment of choice: Ribavirin plus **peginterferon**; clinical condition and ability of patient to tolerate therapy should be evaluated to determine length and/or likely benefit of therapy. Recommended treatment duration (AASLD guidelines): Genotypes 1,4: 48 weeks; Genotypes 2,3: 24 weeks; Coinfection with HIV: 48 weeks.

Aerosol inhalation: RSV Infection in hematopoietic cell or heart/lung transplant recipients (unlabeled use): 2 g (over 2 hours) every 8 hours

Note: Heart/lung transplant recipients also received IVIG, methylprednisolone and palivizumab. Dosage and protocol may be institution specific. (Boeckh, 2007; Chemaly, 2006; Liu, 2010).

Dosage adjustment for toxicity: Oral: Capsule, solution, tablet:

Patient **without** cardiac history:

Hemoglobin <10 g/dL:

Children: Decrease dose to 7.5 mg/kg/day

Adults: Decrease dose to 600 mg/day

Hemoglobin <8.5 g/dL: Children and Adults: Permanently discontinue treatment

Patient **with** cardiac history:

Hemoglobin has decreased ≥2 g/dL during any 4-week period of treatment:

Children: Decrease dose to 7.5 mg/kg/day

Adults: Decrease dose to 600 mg/day

Hemoglobin <12 g/dL after 4 weeks of reduced dose: Children and Adults: Permanently discontinue treatment

Dosage adjustment in renal impairment: Oral:

Rebetol® capsules/solution, Ribasphere® capsules:

Cl_{cr} ≥50 mL/minute: No dosage adjustments are recommended

Cl_{cr} <50 mL/minute: Use is contraindicated

Ribasphere® tablets:

Cl_{cr} ≥50 mL/minute: No dosage adjustments are recommended

Cl_{cr} <50 mL/minute: Use is not recommended

Copegus® tablets:

Cl_{cr} >50 mL/minute: No dosage adjustments are recommended

Cl_{cr} 30-50 mL/minute: Alternate 200 mg and 400 mg every other day

Cl_{cr} <30 mL/minute: 200 mg once daily

ESRD requiring hemodialysis: 200 mg once daily

Dosage adjustment in hepatic impairment: Hepatic decompensation (Child-Pugh class B and C): Use of ribavirin tablets is contraindicated.

Dietary Considerations When used in combination with interferon alfa-2b, capsules and solution may be taken with or without food, but always in a consistent manner in regard to food intake (ie, always take with food or always take on an empty stomach). When used in combination with peginterferon alfa-2b, capsules should be taken with food. Tablets should be taken with food.

Administration

Inhalation: Ribavirin should be administered in well-ventilated rooms (at least 6 air changes/hour). In mechanically-ventilated patients, ribavirin can potentially be deposited in the ventilator delivery system depending on temperature, humidity, and electrostatic forces; this deposition can lead to malfunction or obstruction of the expiratory valve, resulting in inadvertently high positive end-expiratory pressures. The use of one-way valves in the inspiratory lines, a breathing circuit filter in the expiratory line, and frequent monitoring and filter replacement have been effective in preventing these problems. Solutions in SPAG-2 unit should be discarded at least every 24 hours and when the liquid level is low before adding newly reconstituted solution. Should not be mixed with other aerosolized medication.

Oral: Administer concurrently with interferon alfa injection. Capsule should not be opened, crushed, chewed, or broken. Capsules are not for use in children <5 years of age. Use oral solution for children 3-5 years, those ≤25 kg, or those who cannot swallow capsules.

Capsule, in combination with interferon alfa-2b: May be administered with or without food, but always in a consistent manner in regard to food intake.

Capsule, in combination with peginterferon alfa-2b: Administer with food.

Solution, in combination with interferon alfa-2b: May be administered with or without food, but always in a consistent manner in regard to food intake.

Tablet: Should be administered with food.

Monitoring Parameters

Inhalation: Respiratory function, hemoglobin, reticulocyte count, CBC with differential, I & O

Oral: Clinical studies tested as follows: CBC (including hemoglobin, WBC, and platelets) and chemistries (including liver function tests and uric acid) measured at weeks 1, 2, 4, 6, and 8, and then every 4 weeks; TSH measured every 12 weeks

Baseline values used in clinical trials:

Platelet count ≥90,000/mm^3 (75,000/mm^3 for cirrhosis or 70,000/mm^3 for coinfection with HIV)

ANC ≥1500/mm^3

Hemoglobin ≥12 g/dL for women and ≥13 g/dL for men (11 g/dL for HIV coinfected women and 12 g/dL for HIV coinfected men)

TSH and T_4 within normal limits or adequately controlled

$CD4^+$ cell count ≥200 cells/microL or $CD4^+$ cell count 100-200 cells/microL and HIV-1 RNA <5000 copies/mL for coinfection with HIV

Serum HCV RNA (pretreatment, week 12 and week 24, and 24 weeks after completion of therapy). **Note:** Discontinuation of therapy may be considered after 12 weeks in patients with HCV (genotypes 1,4) who fail to achieve an early virologic response (EVR) (defined as ≥2-log decrease in HCV RNA compared to pretreatment) or after 24 weeks with detectable HCV RNA. Treat patients with HCV (genotypes 2,3) for 24 weeks (if tolerated) and then evaluate HCV RNA levels (Ghany, 2009).

Pretreatment and monthly pregnancy test up to 6 months following discontinuation of therapy for women of childbearing age; pretreatment ECG in patients with preexisting cardiac disease; dental exams; ophthalmic exam pretreatment (all patients) and periodically for those with pre-existing ophthalmologic disorders. In pediatric patients, monitor growth closely during and after treatment.

Reference Range

Rapid virological response (RVR): Absence of detectable HCV RNA after 4 weeks of treatment

Early viral response (EVR): ≥2-log decrease in HCV RNA after 12 weeks of treatment

End of treatment response (ETR): Absence of detectable HCV RNA at end of the recommended treatment period

Sustained treatment response (STR): Absence of HCV RNA in the serum 6 months following completion of full treatment course

Dosage Forms Excipient information presented when available (limited, particularly for generics); consult specific product labeling.

Capsule, oral: 200 mg

Rebetol®: 200 mg

Ribasphere®: 200 mg

Combination package, oral [dose-pack/each package contains]:

Ribasphere® RibaPak®: Tablet: 400 mg (7s) [medium blue tablets] and Tablet: 600 mg (7s) [dark blue tablets] (14s, 56s)

Powder for solution, for nebulization:

Virazole®: 6 g [reconstituted product contains ribavirin 20 mg/mL]

Solution, oral:

Rebetol®: 40 mg/mL (100 mL) [contains propylene glycol, sodium benzoate; bubblegum flavor]

Tablet, oral: 200 mg

Copegus®: 200 mg

Ribasphere®: 200 mg, 400 mg, 600 mg

Tablet, oral [dose-pack]:

Ribasphere® RibaPak®: 400 mg [14s]

Ribasphere® RibaPak®: 400 mg [56s]

Ribasphere® RibaPak®: 600 mg [14s]

Ribasphere® RibaPak®: 600 mg [56s]

◆ **Ribavirin and Interferon Alfa-2b Combination Pack** *see* Interferon Alfa-2b and Ribavirin *on page 915*

◆ **Ribo-100 [OTC]** *see* Riboflavin *on page 1483*

Riboflavin (RYE boe flay vin)

Brand Names: U.S. Ribo-100 [OTC]

Index Terms Lactoflavin; Vitamin B_2; Vitamin G

Pharmacologic Category Vitamin, Water Soluble

Use Prevention of riboflavin deficiency and treatment of ariboflavinosis

Pregnancy Risk Factor A/C (dose exceeding RDA recommendation)

Dosage Oral:

Riboflavin deficiency:

Children: 2.5-10 mg/day in divided doses

Adults: 5-30 mg/day in divided doses

Recommended daily allowance:

Children: 0.4-1.8 mg

Adults: 1.2-1.7 mg

Additional Information Complete prescribing information for this medication should be consulted for additional detail.

Dosage Forms Excipient information presented when available (limited, particularly for generics); consult specific product labeling.

Tablet, oral: 25 mg, 50 mg, 100 mg

Ribo-100: 100 mg

◆ **Rid® [OTC]** *see* Permethrin *on page 1336*

◆ **Rid-A-Pain Dental [OTC]** *see* Benzocaine *on page 202*

◆ **Ridaura®** *see* Auranofin *on page 173*

◆ **RID® Maximum Strength [OTC]** *see* Pyrethrins and Piperonyl Butoxide *on page 1435*

◆ **RID® Mousse (Can)** *see* Pyrethrins and Piperonyl Butoxide *on page 1435*

Rifabutin (rif a BYOO tin)

Brand Names: U.S. Mycobutin®

Brand Names: Canada Mycobutin®

Index Terms Ansamycin

Pharmacologic Category Antibiotic, Miscellaneous; Antitubercular Agent

Use Prevention of disseminated *Mycobacterium avium* complex (MAC) in patients with advanced HIV infection

Unlabeled Use Utilized in multidrug regimens for treatment of MAC; alternative to rifampin as prophylaxis for latent tuberculosis infection (LTBI) or part of multidrug regimen for treatment active tuberculosis infection

Pregnancy Risk Factor B

Lactation Excretion in breast milk unknown/not recommended

Contraindications Hypersensitivity to rifabutin, any other rifamycins, or any component of the formulation

Warnings/Precautions Rifabutin must not be administered for MAC prophylaxis to patients with active tuberculosis since its use may lead to the development of tuberculosis that is resistant to both rifabutin and rifampin. May be associated with neutropenia and/or thrombocytopenia (rarely). Dosage reduction recommended in severe impairment (Cl_{cr} <30 mL/minute). Prolonged use may result in fungal or bacterial superinfection, including *C. difficile*-associated diarrhea (CDAD) and pseudomembranous colitis; CDAD has been observed >2 months postantibiotic treatment. May cause brown/orange discoloration of urine, feces, saliva, sweat, tears, and skin. Remove soft contact lenses during therapy since permanent staining may occur.

Adverse Reactions

>10%:

Dermatologic: Rash (11%)

Genitourinary: Discoloration of urine (30%)

Hematologic: Neutropenia (25%), leukopenia (17%)

1% to 10%:

Central nervous system: Headache (3%), fever (2%)

Gastrointestinal: Nausea (3% to 6%), abdominal pain (4%), dyspepsia (3%), eructation (3%), taste perversion (3%), vomiting (3%), flatulence (2%)

Hematologic: Thrombocytopenia (5%)

Hepatic: ALT increased (7% to 9%; incidence less than placebo), AST increased (7% to 9%; incidence less than placebo)

Neuromuscular & skeletal: Myalgia (2%)

<1% (Limited to important or life-threatening): Aphasia, arthralgia, chest pain, confusion, dyspnea, flu-like syndrome, hepatitis, hemolysis, myositis, parasthesia, seizures, skin discoloration, T-wave abnormalities, uveitis

Drug Interactions

Metabolism/Transport Effects Substrate of CYP1A2 (minor), CYP3A4 (major); **Note:** Assignment of Major/Minor substrate status based on clinically relevant drug interaction potential; **Induces** CYP3A4 (strong)

Avoid Concomitant Use

Avoid concomitant use of Rifabutin with any of the following: BCG; Boceprevir; Bortezomib; Crizotinib; Dronedarone; Everolimus; Lapatinib; Lurasidone; Mycophenolate; Nilotinib; Pazopanib; Praziquantel; Ranolazine; Rilpivirine; Rivaroxaban; Roflumilast; RomiDEPsin; SORAfenib; Telaprevir; Ticagrelor; Tolvaptan; Toremifene; Vandetanib; Voriconazole

Increased Effect/Toxicity

Rifabutin may increase the levels/effects of: Clopidogrel; Darunavir; Fosamprenavir; Isoniazid; Lopinavir; Pitavastatin

The levels/effects of Rifabutin may be increased by: Antifungal Agents (Azole Derivatives, Systemic); Atazanavir; Boceprevir; Conivaptan; Darunavir; Delavirdine; Fluconazole; Fosamprenavir; Indinavir; Lopinavir; Macrolide Antibiotics; Nelfinavir; Nevirapine; Ritonavir; Saquinavir; Telaprevir; Tipranavir; Voriconazole

Decreased Effect

Rifabutin may decrease the levels/effects of: Alfentanil; Amiodarone; Angiotensin II Receptor Blockers; Antiemetics (5HT3 Antagonists); Antifungal Agents (Azole Derivatives, Systemic); Aprepitant; ARIPiprazole; Atovaquone; Barbiturates; BCG; Benzodiazepines (metabolized by oxidation); Boceprevir; Bortezomib; Brentuximab Vedotin; BusPIRone; Calcium Channel Blockers; Contraceptives (Estrogens); Contraceptives (Progestins); Corticosteroids (Systemic); Crizotinib; CycloSPORINE; CycloSPORINE (Systemic); CYP3A4 Substrates; Dapsone; Dapsone (Systemic); Dasatinib; Delavirdine; Disopyramide; Dronedarone; Efavirenz; Etravirine; Everolimus; Exemestane; FentaNYL; Fluconazole; Fosphenytoin; Gefitinib; GuanFACINE; HMG-CoA Reductase Inhibitors; Imatinib; Indinavir; Ixabepilone; Lapatinib; Linagliptin; Lurasidone; Maraviroc; Morphine (Systemic); Morphine Sulfate; Mycophenolate; Nelfinavir; Nevirapine; Nilotinib; Pazopanib; Phenytoin; Praziquantel; Propafenone; QuiNIDine; Ramelteon; Ranolazine; Repaglinide; Rilpivirine; Rivaroxaban; Roflumilast; RomiDEPsin; Saxagliptin; SORAfenib; SUNItinib; Tacrolimus; Tacrolimus (Systemic); Tadalafil; Tamoxifen; Telaprevir; Temsirolimus; Terbinafine (Systemic); Ticagrelor; Tolvaptan; Toremifene; Typhoid Vaccine; Ulipristal; Vandetanib; Vemurafenib; Vitamin K Antagonists; Voriconazole; Zaleplon; Zolpidem; Zuclopenthixol

The levels/effects of Rifabutin may be decreased by: CYP3A4 Inducers (Strong); Cyproterone; Deferasirox; Efavirenz; Herbs (CYP3A4 Inducers); Nevirapine; Tocilizumab

Ethanol/Nutrition/Herb Interactions Food: High-fat meal may decrease the rate but not the extent of absorption.

Stability Store at 25°C (77°F); excursions permitted to 15°C to 30°C (59°F to 86°F).

Mechanism of Action Inhibits DNA-dependent RNA polymerase at the beta subunit which prevents chain initiation

Pharmacodynamics/Kinetics

Absorption: Readily, 53%

Distribution: V_d: 9.32 L/kg; distributes to body tissues including the lungs, liver, spleen, eyes, and kidneys

Protein binding: 85%

Metabolism: To 5 metabolites; predominantly 25-O-desacetyl-rifabutin (antimicrobial activity equivalent to parent drug; serum AUC 10% of parent drug) and 31-hydroxy-rifabutin (serum AUC 7% of parent drug)

Bioavailability: Absolute: HIV: 20%

Half-life elimination: Terminal: 45 hours (range: 16-69 hours)

Time to peak, serum: 2-4 hours

Excretion: Urine (53% as metabolites); feces (30%)

Dosage Oral:

Infants and Children:

Prophylaxis for recurrence of *Mycobacterium avium* complex (MAC) in HIV-exposed/-infected patients (unlabeled use; CDC, 2009): 5 mg/kg (maximum dose: 300 mg) once daily as an optional add-on to primary therapy of clarithromycin and ethambutol

Treatment of active TB (as alternative to rifampin) in HIV-exposed/-infected patients (unlabeled use; CDC, 2009): 10-20 mg/kg (maximum dose: 300 mg) once daily or intermittently 2-3 times weekly

Treatment of severe MAC in HIV-exposed/-infected patients (unlabeled use; CDC, 2009): 10-20 mg/kg (maximum dose: 300 mg) once daily, in addition to primary therapy of clarithromycin and ethambutol

Children ≥6 years: Prophylaxis for first episode of MAC in HIV-exposed/-infected patients (unlabeled use; CDC, 2009): 300 mg once daily

Adolescents and Adults:

Disseminated MAC in advanced HIV infection:

Prophylaxis: 300 mg once daily or 150 mg twice daily to reduce gastrointestinal upset

Treatment (unlabeled use; AIDS*info* guidelines): 300 mg once daily as an optional add-on to primary therapy of clarithromycin and ethambutol

Tuberculosis (unlabeled use as alternative to rifampin; AIDS*info* guidelines):

Prophylaxis of LTBI: 300 mg once daily for 4 months

Treatment of active TB: 300 mg once daily or intermittently 2-3 times weekly as part of multidrug regimen

Dosage adjustment for concurrent nelfinavir, amprenavir, indinavir: Reduce rifabutin dose to 150 mg/day; no change in dose if administered twice weekly

Dosage adjustment for concurrent efavirenz (no concomitant protease inhibitor): Increase rifabutin dose to 450-600 mg daily, or 600 mg 3 times/week

Dosage adjustment in renal impairment: Cl_{cr} <30 mL/minute: Reduce dose by 50%

Dietary Considerations May be taken with meals.

Administration May be taken with meals to minimize nausea or vomiting.

Monitoring Parameters Periodic liver function tests, CBC with differential, platelet count

Dosage Forms Excipient information presented when available (limited, particularly for generics); consult specific product labeling.

Capsule, oral:

Mycobutin®: 150 mg

Extemporaneous Preparations A 20 mg/mL rifabutin oral suspension may be made with capsules and a 1:1 mixture of Ora-Sweet® and Ora-Plus®. Empty the the powder from eight 150 mg rifabutin capsules into a glass mortar; add 20 mL of vehicle and mix to a uniform paste. Mix while adding vehicle in incremental proportions to **almost** 60 mL; transfer to a calibrated bottle, rinse mortar with vehicle, and add quantity of vehicle sufficient to make 60 mL. Label "shake well". Stable for 12 weeks at 4°C, 25°C, 30°C, and 40°C.

Haslam JL, Egodage KL, Chen Y, et al, "Stability of Rifabutin in Two Extemporaneously Compounded Oral Liquids," *Am J Health Syst Pharm*, 1999, 56(4):333-6.

◆ **Rifadin®** *see* Rifampin *on page 1485*

◆ **Rifampicin** *see* Rifampin *on page 1485*

Rifampin (rif AM pin)

Brand Names: U.S. Rifadin®

Brand Names: Canada Rifadin®; Rofact™

Index Terms Rifampicin

Pharmacologic Category Antibiotic, Miscellaneous; Antitubercular Agent

Additional Appendix Information

Antibiotic Treatment of Adults With Infective Endocarditis *on page 1956*

Use Management of active tuberculosis in combination with other agents; elimination of meningococci from the nasopharynx in asymptomatic carriers

Unlabeled Use Prophylaxis of *Haemophilus influenzae* type b infection; *Legionella* pneumonia; used in combination with other anti-infectives in the treatment of staphylococcal infections; treatment of *M. leprae* infections

Pregnancy Risk Factor C

Pregnancy Considerations Teratogenic effects have been reported in animal studies. Rifampin crosses the human placenta. Due to the risk of tuberculosis to the fetus, treatment is recommended when the probability of maternal disease is moderate to high. Postnatal hemorrhages have been reported in the infant and mother with isoniazid administration during the last few weeks of pregnancy.

Lactation Enters breast milk/not recommended (AAP rates "compatible"; AAP 2001 update pending)

Contraindications Hypersensitivity to rifampin, any rifamycins, or any component of the formulation; concurrent use of amprenavir, saquinavir/ritonavir (possibly other protease inhibitors)

Warnings/Precautions Use with caution and modify dosage in patients with liver impairment; observe for hyperbilirubinemia; discontinue therapy if this in conjunction with clinical symptoms or any signs of significant hepatocellular damage develop. Use with caution in patients receiving concurrent medications associated with hepatotoxicity. Use with caution in patients with a history of alcoholism (even if ethanol consumption is discontinued during therapy). Since rifampin since rifampin has enzyme-inducing properties, porphyria exacerbation is possible; use with caution in patients with porphyria; do not use for meningococcal disease, only for short-term treatment of asymptomatic carrier states

Regimens of >600 mg once or twice weekly have been associated with a high incidence of adverse reactions including a flu-like syndrome, hypersensitivity, thrombocytopenia, leukopenia, and anemia. Urine, feces, saliva, sweat, tears, and CSF may be discolored to red/orange; remove soft contact lenses during therapy since permanent staining may occur. Do not administer I.V. form via I.M. or SubQ routes; restart infusion at another site if extravasation occurs. Prolonged use may result in fungal or bacterial superinfection, including *C. difficile*-associated diarrhea (CDAD) and pseudomembranous colitis; CDAD has been observed >2 months postantibiotic treatment. Monitor for compliance in patients on intermittent therapy.

Adverse Reactions

1% to 10%:

Dermatologic: Rash (1% to 5%)

Gastrointestinal (1% to 2%): Anorexia, cramps, diarrhea, epigastric distress, flatulence, heartburn, nausea, pseudomembranous colitis, pancreatitis, vomiting

Hepatic: LFTs increased (up to 14%)

Frequency not defined:

Cardiovascular: Edema, flushing

Central nervous system: Ataxia, behavioral changes, concentration impaired, confusion, dizziness, drowsiness, fatigue, fever, headache, numbness, psychosis

Dermatologic: Pemphigoid reaction, pruritus, urticaria

Endocrine & metabolic: Adrenal insufficiency, menstrual disorders

Hematologic: Agranulocytosis (rare), DIC, eosinophilia, hemoglobin decreased, hemolysis, hemolytic anemia, leukopenia, thrombocytopenia (especially with high-dose therapy)

Hepatic: Hepatitis (rare), jaundice

Neuromuscular & skeletal: Myalgia, osteomalacia, weakness

Ocular: Exudative conjunctivitis, visual changes

Renal: Acute renal failure, BUN increased, hemoglobinuria, hematuria, interstitial nephritis, uric acid increased

Miscellaneous: Flu-like syndrome

Drug Interactions

Metabolism/Transport Effects Substrate of P-glycoprotein, SLCO1B1; **Induces** CYP1A2 (strong), CYP2A6 (strong), CYP2B6 (strong), CYP2C19 (strong), CYP2C8 (strong), CYP2C9 (strong), CYP3A4 (strong), P-glycoprotein

Avoid Concomitant Use

Avoid concomitant use of Rifampin with any of the following: Atazanavir; BCG; Boceprevir; Bortezomib; Dabigatran Etexilate; Darunavir; Esomeprazole; Etravirine; Fosamprenavir; Indinavir; Lopinavir; Lurasidone; Mycophenolate; Nelfinavir; Omeprazole; Praziquantel; QuiNINE; Ranolazine; Rilpivirine; Ritonavir; Roflumilast; Saquinavir; SORAfenib; Telaprevir; Ticagrelor; Tipranavir; Toremifene; Voriconazole

Increased Effect/Toxicity

Rifampin may increase the levels/effects of: Clopidogrel; Isoniazid; Leflunomide; Lopinavir; Pitavastatin; Saquinavir

The levels/effects of Rifampin may be increased by: Antifungal Agents (Azole Derivatives, Systemic); Delavirdine; Eltrombopag; Fluconazole; Macrolide Antibiotics; P-glycoprotein/ABCB1 Inhibitors; Pyrazinamide; Voriconazole

Decreased Effect

Rifampin may decrease the levels/effects of: Alfentanil; Amiodarone; Angiotensin II Receptor Blockers; Antidiabetic Agents (Thiazolidinedione); Antiemetics (5HT3 Antagonists); Antifungal Agents (Azole Derivatives, Systemic); Aprepitant; ARIPiprazole; Atazanavir; Atovaquone; Barbiturates; BCG; Bendamustine; Benzodiazepines (metabolized by oxidation); Beta-Blockers; Boceprevir; Bortezomib; Brentuximab Vedotin; BusPIRone; Calcium Channel Blockers; Caspofungin; Chloramphenicol; Contraceptives (Estrogens); Contraceptives (Progestins); Corticosteroids (Systemic); CycloSPORINE; CycloSPORINE (Systemic); CYP1A2 Substrates; CYP2A6 Substrates; CYP2B6 Substrates; ▶

CYP2C19 Substrates; CYP2C8 Substrates; CYP2C9 Substrates; CYP3A4 Substrates; Dabigatran Etexilate; Dapsone; Dapsone (Systemic); Darunavir; Dasatinib; Deferasirox; Delavirdine; Diclofenac; Disopyramide; Divalproex; Efavirenz; Erlotinib; Esomeprazole; Etravirine; Exemestane; FentaNYL; Fexofenadine; Fluconazole; Fosamprenavir; Fosaprepitant; Fosphenytoin; Gefitinib; GuanFACINE; HMG-CoA Reductase Inhibitors; Imatinib; Indinavir; Ixabepilone; LamoTRIgine; Linagliptin; Lopinavir; Lurasidone; Maraviroc; Methadone; Morphine (Systemic); Morphine Sulfate; Mycophenolate; Nelfinavir; Nevirapine; Omeprazole; OxyCODONE; P-glycoprotein/ABCB1 Substrates; Phenytoin; Prasugrel; Praziquantel; Propafenone; QuiNIDine; QuiNINE; Raltegravir; Ramelteon; Ranolazine; Repaglinide; Rilpivirine; Ritonavir; Roflumilast; Saquinavir; Sirolimus; SORAfenib; Sulfonylureas; Tacrolimus; Tacrolimus (Systemic); Tadalafil; Tamoxifen; Telaprevir; Temsirolimus; Terbinafine; Terbinafine (Systemic); Thyroid Products; Ticagrelor; Tipranavir; Toremifene; Treprostinil; Typhoid Vaccine; Ulipristal; Valproic Acid; Vitamin K Antagonists; Voriconazole; Zaleplon; Zidovudine; Zolpidem; Zuclopenthixol

The levels/effects of Rifampin may be decreased by: P-glycoprotein/ABCB1 Inducers

Ethanol/Nutrition/Herb Interactions

Ethanol: Avoid ethanol (may increase risk of hepatotoxicity).

Food: Food decreases the extent of absorption; rifampin concentrations may be decreased if taken with food.

Herb/Nutraceutical: St John's wort may decrease rifampin levels.

Stability Rifampin powder is reddish brown. Intact vials should be stored at room temperature and protected from excessive heat and light. Reconstitute powder for injection with SWFI. Prior to injection, dilute in appropriate volume of compatible diluent (eg, 100 mL D_5W). Reconstituted vials are stable for 24 hours at room temperature.

Stability of parenteral admixture at room temperature (25°C) is 4 hours for D_5W and 24 hours for NS.

Mechanism of Action Inhibits bacterial RNA synthesis by binding to the beta subunit of DNA-dependent RNA polymerase, blocking RNA transcription

Pharmacodynamics/Kinetics

Duration: ≤24 hours

Absorption: Oral: Well absorbed; food may delay or slightly reduce peak

Distribution: Highly lipophilic; crosses blood-brain barrier well

Relative diffusion from blood into CSF: Adequate with or without inflammation (exceeds usual MICs)

CSF:blood level ratio: Inflamed meninges: 25%

Protein binding: 80%

Metabolism: Hepatic; undergoes enterohepatic recirculation

Half-life elimination: 3-4 hours; prolonged with hepatic impairment; End-stage renal disease: 1.8-11 hours

Time to peak, serum: Oral: 2-4 hours

Excretion: Feces (60% to 65%) and urine (~30%) as unchanged drug

Dosage

Usual dosage ranges: Oral, I.V.:

Infants and Children: 10-20 mg/kg/day as a single dose or in 2 divided doses; maximum: 600 mg/day

Adults: 600 mg once or twice daily

Indication-specific dosing: Oral, I.V.:

Endocarditis, prosthetic valve due to MRSA (unlabeled use): Adults: 300 mg every 8 hours for at least 6 weeks (combine with vancomycin for the entire duration of therapy and gentamicin for the first 2 weeks) (Liu, 2011)

***H. influenzae* prophylaxis (unlabeled use):**

Infants and Children: 20 mg/kg/day every 24 hours for 4 days, not to exceed 600 mg/dose

Adults: 600 mg every 24 hours for 4 days

Leprosy (unlabeled use): Adults:

Multibacillary: 600 mg once monthly for 24 months in combination with ofloxacin and minocycline

Paucibacillary: 600 mg once monthly for 6 months in combination with dapsone

Single lesion: 600 mg as a single dose in combination with ofloxacin 400 mg and minocycline 100 mg

Meningitis *(Pneumococcus* or *Staphylococcus)* (unlabeled use): Adults: 600 mg once daily

Note: Recommended only for organisms known to be rifampin-susceptible and highly penicillin- or cephalosporin-resistant. May be used in place of or in addition to vancomycin when dexamethasone therapy employed.

Meningococcal meningitis prophylaxis (unlabeled use):

Infants <1 month: 10 mg/kg/day in divided doses every 12 hours for 2 days

Infants ≥1 month and Children: 20 mg/kg/day in divided doses every 12 hours for 2 days (maximum: 600 mg/dose)

Adults: 600 mg every 12 hours for 2 days

Nasal carriers of *Staphylococcus aureus* (unlabeled use): Note: Must use in combination with at least one other systemic antistaphylococcal antibiotic. Not recommended as first-line drug for decolonization; evidence is weak for use in patients with recurrent infections (Liu, 2011).

Children: 15 mg/kg/day divided every 12 hours for 5-10 days in combination with other antibiotics

Adults: 600 mg/day for 5-10 days in combination with other antibiotics

Nontuberculous mycobacterium *(M. kansasii)* (unlabeled use): Adults: 10 mg/kg/day (maximum: 600 mg/day) for duration to include 12 months of culture-negative sputum; typically used in combination with ethambutol and isoniazid

***Staphylococcus aureus* infections, adjunctive therapy (unlabeled use):** Adults: 600 mg once daily or 300-450 mg every 12 hours with other antibiotics. **Note:** Must be used in combination with another antistaphylococcal antibiotic to avoid rapid development of resistance (Liu, 2011).

Tuberculosis, active: Note: A four-drug regimen (isoniazid, rifampin, pyrazinamide, and ethambutol) is preferred for the initial, empiric treatment of TB. When the drug susceptibility results are available, the regimen should be altered as appropriate.

Infants and Children <12 years:

Daily therapy: 10-20 mg/kg/day usually as a single dose (maximum: 600 mg/day)

Twice weekly directly observed therapy (DOT): 10-20 mg/kg (maximum: 600 mg)

Adults:

Daily therapy: 10 mg/kg/day (maximum: 600 mg/day)

Twice weekly directly observed therapy (DOT): 10 mg/kg (maximum: 600 mg); 3 times/week: 10 mg/kg (maximum: 600 mg)

Tuberculosis, latent infection (LTBI): As an alternative to isoniazid:

Children: 10-20 mg/kg/day (maximum: 600 mg/day) for 6 months

Adults: 10 mg/kg/day (maximum: 600 mg/day) for 4 months. **Note:** Combination with pyrazinamide should not generally be offered (*MMWR*, Aug 8, 2003).

Dosing adjustment in renal impairment: No dosage adjustment required in renal impairment.

Poorly dialyzed; no supplemental dose or dosage adjustment necessary, including patients on intermittent hemodialysis, peritoneal dialysis, or continuous renal replacement therapy (eg, CVVHD).

Dosing adjustment in hepatic impairment: Dose reductions may be necessary to reduce hepatotoxicity

Dietary Considerations Rifampin should be taken on an empty stomach.

Administration

I.V.: Administer I.V. preparation by slow I.V. infusion over 30 minutes to 3 hours at a final concentration not to exceed 6 mg/mL.

Oral: Administer on an empty stomach (ie, 1 hour prior to, or 2 hours after meals or antacids) to increase total absorption. The compounded oral suspension must be shaken well before using. May mix contents of capsule with applesauce or jelly.

Monitoring Parameters Periodic (baseline and every 2-4 weeks during therapy) monitoring of liver function (AST, ALT, bilirubin), CBC, mental status, sputum culture, chest x-ray 2-3 months into treatment

Test Interactions May interfere with urine detection of opiates (false-positive); positive Coombs' reaction [direct], rifampin inhibits standard assay's ability to measure serum folate and B_{12}; transient increase in LFTs and decreased biliary excretion of contrast media

Dosage Forms Excipient information presented when available (limited, particularly for generics); consult specific product labeling.

Capsule, oral: 150 mg, 300 mg

Rifadin®: 150 mg, 300 mg

Injection, powder for reconstitution: 600 mg

Rifadin®: 600 mg

Extemporaneous Preparations A rifampin 1% w/v suspension (10 mg/mL) may be made with capsules and one of four syrups (Syrup NF, simple syrup, Syrpalta® syrup, or raspberry syrup). Empty the contents of four 300 mg capsules or eight 150 mg capsules onto a piece of weighing paper. If necessary, crush contents to produce a fine powder. Transfer powder to a 4-ounce amber glass or plastic prescription bottle. Rinse paper and spatula with 20 mL of chosen syrup and add the rinse to bottle; shake vigorously. Add 100 mL syrup to the bottle and shake vigorously. Label "shake well". Stable for 4 weeks at room temperature or refrigerated.

A 25 mg/mL oral suspension may be made with capsules and cherry syrup concentrate diluted 1:4 with simple syrup, NF. Empty the contents of ten 300 mg capsules into a mortar and reduce to a fine powder. Add 20 mL of the vehicle and mix to a uniform paste; mix while adding the vehicle in incremental proportions to **almost** 120 mL; transfer to a calibrated bottle, rinse mortar with vehicle, and add quantity of vehicle sufficient to make 120 mL. Label "shake well" and "refrigerate". Stable for 28 days refrigerated (preferred) or at room temperature.

Nahata MC, Pai VB, and Hipple TF, *Pediatric Drug Formulations*, 5th ed, Cincinnati, OH: Harvey Whitney Books Co, 2004.

Rifapentine (rif a PEN teen)

Brand Names: U.S. Priftin®

Brand Names: Canada Priftin®

Pharmacologic Category Antitubercular Agent

Use Treatment of pulmonary tuberculosis; rifapentine must always be used in conjunction with at least one other antituberculosis drug to which the isolate is susceptible; it may also be necessary to add a third agent (either streptomycin or ethambutol) until susceptibility is known.

Pregnancy Risk Factor C

Pregnancy Considerations Has been shown to be teratogenic in rats and rabbits. Rat offspring showed cleft palates, right aortic arch, and delayed ossification and increased number of ribs. Rabbits displayed ovarian agenesis, pes varus, arhinia, microphthalmia, and irregularities of the ossified facial tissues. Rat studies also show decreased fetal weight, increased number of stillborns, and decreased gestational survival. There are no adequate and well-controlled studies in pregnant women. Rifapentine should be used during pregnancy only if the potential benefits justifies the potential risk to the fetus.

Lactation Excretion in breast milk unknown/contraindicated

Contraindications Hypersensitivity to rifapentine, rifampin, rifabutin, any rifamycin analog, or any component of the formulation

Warnings/Precautions Patients with abnormal liver tests and/or liver disease should only be given rifapentine when absolutely necessary and under strict medical supervision. Monitoring of liver function tests should be carried out prior to therapy and then every 2-4 weeks during therapy if signs of liver disease occur or worsen, rifapentine should be discontinued. All patients treated with rifapentine should have baseline measurements of liver function tests and enzymes, bilirubin, and a complete blood count. Patients should be seen monthly and specifically questioned regarding symptoms associated with adverse reactions. Routine laboratory monitoring in people with normal baseline measurements is generally not necessary. Use with caution in patients with porphyria; exacerbation is possible.

Rifapentine may produce a red-orange discoloration of body tissues/fluids including skin, teeth, tongue, urine, feces, saliva, sputum, tears, sweat, and cerebral spinal fluid. Contact lenses may become permanently stained. Prolonged use may result in fungal or bacterial superinfection, including *C. difficile*-associated diarrhea (CDAD) and pseudomembranous colitis; CDAD has been observed >2 months postantibiotic treatment. Experience in treating TB in HIV-infected patients is limited. Compliance with dosing regimen is absolutely necessary for successful drug therapy.

Adverse Reactions

>10%: Endocrine & metabolic: Hyperuricemia (most likely due to pyrazinamide from initiation phase combination therapy)

1% to 10%:

Cardiovascular: Hypertension

Central nervous system: Headache, dizziness

Dermatologic: Rash, pruritus, acne

Gastrointestinal: Anorexia, nausea, vomiting, dyspepsia, diarrhea

Genitourinary: Pyuria, proteinuria, hematuria, urinary casts

Hematologic: Neutropenia, lymphopenia, anemia, leukopenia, thrombocytosis

Hepatic: ALT increased, AST increased

Neuromuscular & skeletal: Arthralgia, pain

Respiratory: Hemoptysis

<1% (Limited to important or life-threatening): Aggressive reaction, arthrosis, gout, hepatitis, hyperkalemia, pancreatitis, purpura, thrombocytopenia

Drug Interactions

Metabolism/Transport Effects Induces CYP2C8 (strong), CYP2C9 (strong), CYP3A4 (strong)

Avoid Concomitant Use

Avoid concomitant use of Rifapentine with any of the following: Bortezomib; Crizotinib; Dronedarone; Etravirine; Everolimus; Lapatinib; Lurasidone; Mycophenolate; Nilotinib; Pazopanib; Praziquantel; Ranolazine; Rilpivirine; Rivaroxaban; Roflumilast; RomiDEPsin; SORAfenib; Ticagrelor; Tolvaptan; Toremifene; Vandetanib; Voriconazole

Increased Effect/Toxicity

Rifapentine may increase the levels/effects of: Clarithromycin; Clopidogrel; Isoniazid; Pitavastatin

The levels/effects of Rifapentine may be increased by: Antifungal Agents (Azole Derivatives, Systemic); Clarithromycin; Delavirdine; Fluconazole; Voriconazole

Decreased Effect

Rifapentine may decrease the levels/effects of: Alfentanil; Amiodarone; Angiotensin II Receptor Blockers; Antiemetics (5HT3 Antagonists); Antifungal Agents (Azole Derivatives, Systemic); Aprepitant; ARIPiprazole; Atovaquone; Barbiturates; Benzodiazepines (metabolized by oxidation); Beta-Blockers; Boceprevir; Bortezomib; Brentuximab Vedotin; BusPIRone; Calcium Channel Blockers; Clarithromycin; Contraceptives (Estrogens); Contraceptives (Progestins); Corticosteroids (Systemic); Crizotinib; CycloSPORINE; CycloSPORINE (Systemic); CYP2C8 Substrates; CYP2C9 Substrates; CYP3A4 Substrates; Dapsone; Dapsone (Systemic); Dasatinib; Delavirdine; Diclofenac; Disopyramide; Dronedarone; Etravirine; Everolimus; Exemestane; FentaNYL; Fluconazole; Fosphenytoin; Gefitinib; GuanFACINE; HMG-CoA Reductase Inhibitors; Imatinib; Ixabepilone; Lapatinib; Linagliptin; Lurasidone; Maraviroc; Methadone; Morphine (Systemic); Morphine Sulfate; Mycophenolate; Nilotinib; Pazopanib; Phenytoin; Praziquantel; Propafenone; QuiNIDine; Ramelteon; Ranolazine; Repaglinide; Rilpivirine; Rivaroxaban; Roflumilast; RomiDEPsin; Saxagliptin; SORAfenib; SUNItinib; Tacrolimus; Tacrolimus (Systemic); Tadalafil; Tamoxifen; Temsirolimus; Terbinafine (Systemic); Ticagrelor; Tolvaptan; Toremifene; Treprostinil; Ulipristal; Vandetanib; Vemurafenib; Vitamin K Antagonists; Voriconazole; Zaleplon; Zidovudine; Zolpidem; Zuclopenthixol

Ethanol/Nutrition/Herb Interactions Food: Food increases AUC and maximum serum concentration by 43% and 44% respectively as compared to fasting conditions.

Stability Store at room temperature (15°C to 30°C; 59°F to 86°F). Protect from excessive heat and humidity.

Mechanism of Action Inhibits DNA-dependent RNA polymerase in susceptible strains of *Mycobacterium tuberculosis* (but not in mammalian cells). Rifapentine is bactericidal against both intracellular and extracellular MTB organisms. MTB resistant to other rifamycins including rifampin are likely to be resistant to rifapentine. Cross-resistance does not appear between rifapentine and other nonrifamycin antimycobacterial agents.

Pharmacodynamics/Kinetics

Absorption: Food increases AUC and C_{max} by 43% and 44% respectively.

Distribution: V_d: ~70.2 L; rifapentine and metabolite accumulate in human monocyte-derived macrophages with intracellular/extracellular ratios of 24:1 and 7:1 respectively

Protein binding: Rifapentine and 25-desacetyl metabolite: 97.7% and 93.2%, primarily to albumin

Metabolism: Hepatic; hydrolyzed by an esterase and esterase enzyme to form the active metabolite 25-desacetyl rifapentine

Bioavailability: ~70%

Half-life elimination: Rifapentine: 14-17 hours; 25-desacetyl rifapentine: 13 hours

Time to peak, serum: 5-6 hours

Excretion: Urine (17% primarily as metabolites)

Dosage

Children: No dosing information available

Adults: **Rifapentine should not be used alone**; initial phase should include a 3- to 4-drug regimen

Intensive phase (initial 2 months) of short-term therapy: 600 mg (four 150 mg tablets) given twice weekly (with an interval of not less than 72 hours between doses); following the intensive phase, treatment should continue with rifapentine 600 mg once weekly for 4 months in combination with INH or appropriate agent for susceptible organisms

Dosing adjustment in renal or hepatic impairment: Unknown

Monitoring Parameters Patients with pre-existing hepatic problems should have liver function tests monitored every 2-4 weeks during therapy

Test Interactions Rifampin has been shown to inhibit standard microbiological assays for serum folate and vitamin B_{12}; this should be considered for rifapentine; therefore, alternative assay methods should be considered.

Additional Information Rifapentine has only been studied in patients with tuberculosis receiving a 6-month short-course intensive regimen approval. Outcomes have been based on 6-month follow-up treatment observed in clinical trial 008 as a surrogate for the 2-year follow-up generally accepted as evidence for efficacy in the treatment of pulmonary tuberculosis.

Dosage Forms Excipient information presented when available (limited, particularly for generics); consult specific product labeling.

Tablet, oral:

Priftin®: 150 mg

Rifaximin (rif AX i min)

Brand Names: U.S. Xifaxan®

Pharmacologic Category Antibiotic, Miscellaneous

Use Treatment of travelers' diarrhea caused by noninvasive strains of *E. coli*; reduction in the risk of overt hepatic encephalopathy (HE) recurrence

Unlabeled Use Treatment of hepatic encephalopathy; alternative treatment for *Clostridium difficile*-associated diarrhea (CDAD)

Pregnancy Risk Factor C

Pregnancy Considerations Adverse events have been observed in animal reproduction studies; therefore, the manufacturer classifies rifaximin as pregnancy category C. Due to the limited oral absorption of rifaximin in patients with normal hepatic function, exposure to the fetus is expected to be extremely low.

Lactation Excretion in breast milk unknown/not recommended

Contraindications Hypersensitivity to rifaximin, other rifamycin antibiotics, or any component of the formulation

Warnings/Precautions Efficacy has not been established for the treatment of diarrhea due to pathogens other than *E. coli*, including *C. jejuni*, *Shigella* and *Salmonella*. Consider alternative therapy if symptoms persist or worsen after 24-48 hours of treatment. Not for treatment of systemic infections; <1% is absorbed orally. Prolonged use may result in fungal or bacterial superinfection, including *C. difficile*-associated diarrhea (CDAD) and pseudomembranous colitis; CDAD has been observed >2 months postantibiotic treatment. Use caution in severe hepatic impairment (Child-Pugh class C); efficacy for prevention of encephalopathy has not been established in patients with a Model for End-Stage Liver Disease (MELD) score >25.

Adverse Reactions Note: Frequency of adverse events generally higher following treatment for hepatic encephalopathy (HE). Percentages are presented for HE unless otherwise stated.

>10%:

Cardiovascular: Peripheral edema (15%)

Central nervous system: Dizziness (13%), fatigue (12%)

Hepatic: Ascites (11%)

Gastrointestinal: Nausea (14%)

2% to 10%:

Cardiovascular: Chest pain (>2% to 5%), edema (>2% to 5%), hypotension (>2% to 5%)

Central nervous system: Headache (travelers' diarrhea 10%), depression (7%), fever (6%), amnesia (>2% to 5%), attention disturbance (>2% to 5%), confusion (>2% to 5%), hypoesthesia (>2% to 5%), pain (>2% to 5%), tremor (>2% to 5%), vertigo (>2% to 5%)

Dermatological: Pruritus (9%), rash (5%), cellulitis (>2% to 5%)

Endocrine and metabolism: Hyper-/hypoglycemia (>2% to 5%), hyperkalemia (>2% to 5%), hyponatremia (>2% to 5%)

Gastrointestinal: Abdominal pain (>2% to 9%), abdominal tenderness (>2% to 5%), anorexia (>2% to 5%), dehydration (>2% to 5%), esophageal varices (>2% to 5%), weight gain (>2% to 5%), xerostomia (>2% to 5%)

Hematologic: Anemia (8%)

Neuromuscular & skeletal: Muscle spasms (9%), arthralgia (6%), myalgia (>2% to 5%)

Respiratory: Nasopharyngitis (7%), dyspnea (6%), epistaxis(>2% to 5%), pneumonia (>2% to 5%), rhinitis (>2% to 5%), upper respiratory tract infection (>2% to 5%)

Miscellaneous: Influenza-like illness (>2% to 5%)

All indications: <2% (Limited to important or life-threatening): Abnormal dreams, allergic dermatitis, anaphylaxis, angioneurotic edema, AST increased, choluria, CDAD, dry lips, dysuria, ear pain, exfoliative dermatitis, flushing, gingival disorder, hematuria, hot flashes, hypersensitivity reactions, lymphocytosis, migraine, monocytosis, motion sickness, nasal irritation, nasopharyngitis, neck pain, neutropenia, pharyngitis, pharyngolaryngeal pain, polyuria, proteinuria, sunburn, syncope, taste loss, tinnitus, urticaria, weakness, weight loss

Drug Interactions

Metabolism/Transport Effects None known.

Avoid Concomitant Use

Avoid concomitant use of Rifaximin with any of the following: BCG

Increased Effect/Toxicity There are no known significant interactions involving an increase in effect.

Decreased Effect

Rifaximin may decrease the levels/effects of: BCG

Stability Store at controlled room temperature of 20°C to 25°C (68°F to 77°F).

Mechanism of Action Rifaximin inhibits bacterial RNA synthesis by binding to bacterial DNA-dependent RNA polymerase.

Pharmacodynamics/Kinetics

Absorption: Oral: Travelers' diarrhea: Low; Increased in prevention of hepatic encephalopathy with Child-Pugh class C having a greater exposure than A

Protein binding: Healthy subjects: ~68%; Hepatic impairment: 62%

Half-life elimination: ~2-5 hours

Time to peak: Hepatic encephalopathy prevention: ~1 hour

Excretion: Feces (~97% as unchanged drug); urine (<1%)

Dosage Oral:

Children ≥12 years and Adults: Travelers' diarrhea: 200 mg 3 times/day for 3 days

Adults:

Hepatic encephalopathy:

Reduction of overt hepatic encephalopathy recurrence: 550 mg 2 times/day. **Note:** Supporting clinical trial evaluated efficacy over 6-month treatment period.

Treatment of hepatic encephalopathy (unlabeled use): 400 mg every 8 hours for 5-10 days (Mas, 2003)

Clostridium difficile-associated diarrhea (unlabeled use): 200-400 mg 2-3 times/day for 14 days (Johnson, 2007)

Dosage adjustment in renal impairment: Not studied; no dosing recommendation available

Dosage adjustment in hepatic impairment: No adjustment necessary, but use with caution in severe impairment (Child-Pugh class C) as systemic absorption does occur and pharmacokinetic parameters are highly variable

Dietary Considerations May be taken with or without food.

Administration May be administered with or without food.

Monitoring Parameters Temperature, blood in stool, change in symptoms; monitor changes in mental status in hepatic encephalopathy

Dosage Forms Excipient information presented when available (limited, particularly for generics); consult specific product labeling.

Tablet, oral:

Xifaxan®: 200 mg, 550 mg

Extemporaneous Preparations A 20 mg/mL oral suspension may be made using tablets. Crush six 200 mg tablets and reduce to a fine powder. Add 30 mL of a 1:1 mixture of Ora-Sweet® and Ora-Plus® or a 1:1 mixture of Ora-Sweet® SF and Ora-Plus®; mix well while adding the vehicle in geometric proportions to **almost** 60 mL; transfer to a calibrated bottle, rinse mortar with vehicle, and add quantity of vehicle sufficient to make 60 mL. Label "shake well". Stable 60 days at room temperature.

Cober MP, Johnson CE, Lee J, et al, "Stability of Extemporaneously Prepared Rifaximin Oral Suspensions," *Am J Health Syst Pharm*, 2010, 67(4):287-89.

- **rIFN beta-1a** *see* Interferon Beta-1a *on page 916*
- **rIFN beta-1b** *see* Interferon Beta-1b *on page 918*
- **RIG** *see* Rabies Immune Globulin (Human) *on page 1453*

Rilonacept (ri LON a sept)

Brand Names: U.S. Arcalyst™

Pharmacologic Category Interleukin-1 Inhibitor

Use Treatment of cryopyrin-associated periodic syndromes (CAPS) including familial cold autoinflammatory syndrome (FCAS) and Muckle-Wells syndrome (MWS)

Pregnancy Risk Factor C

Pregnancy Considerations Animal studies have demonstrated teratogenic effects and fetal loss. There are no adequate and well-controlled studies in pregnant women. Use during pregnancy only if potential benefit to the mother outweighs potential risk to the fetus.

Lactation Excretion in breast milk unknown/use caution

Contraindications There are no contraindications listed in the manufacturer's labeling.

Warnings/Precautions May cause rare hypersensitivity, anaphylaxis, or anaphylactoid reactions; medications for the treatment of hypersensitivity reactions should be available for immediate use. Caution should be exercised when considering use in patients with a history of new/recurrent infections, with conditions that predispose them to infections, or with latent or localized infections. Therapy should not be initiated in patients with active or chronic infections. Use may impair defenses against malignancies; impact on the development and course of malignancies is not fully defined. Use may increase total cholesterol, HDL, LDL, and triglycerides; periodic assessment of lipid profile should occur. Tumor necrosis factor (TNF)-blocking agents should not be used in combination with rilonacept; risk of serious infection is increased. Immunizations should be up to date including pneumococcal and influenza vaccines before initiating therapy. Live vaccines should not be given concurrently. Administration of inactivated (killed) vaccines while on therapy may not be effective. Use with caution in the elderly due to the potential higher risk for infections. Safety and efficacy has not been established in patients <12 years of age.

Adverse Reactions
>10%:
Local: Injection site reactions (48%; majority mild-moderate; typically lasting 1-2 days; characterized by erythema, bruising, dermatitis, inflammation, pain, pruritus, swelling, urticaria, vesicles, warmth, and hemorrhage)
Respiratory: Upper respiratory tract infection (26%)
Miscellaneous: Infection (48% during winter months; 18% during summer months), antibody formation to rilonacept (35%)
1% to 10%:
Central nervous system: Hypoesthesia (9%)
Respiratory: Cough (9%), sinusitis (9%)
<1% (Limited to important or life-threatening): HDL cholesterol increased, LDL cholesterol increased, neutropenia (transient), triglycerides increased, total cholesterol increased

Drug Interactions

Metabolism/Transport Effects None known.

Avoid Concomitant Use

Avoid concomitant use of Rilonacept with any of the following: Anti-TNF Agents; BCG; Canakinumab; Natalizumab; Pimecrolimus; Tacrolimus (Topical); Vaccines (Live)

Increased Effect/Toxicity

Rilonacept may increase the levels/effects of: Canakinumab; Leflunomide; Natalizumab; Vaccines (Live)

The levels/effects of Rilonacept may be increased by: Anti-TNF Agents; Denosumab; Pimecrolimus; Roflumilast; Tacrolimus (Topical); Trastuzumab

Decreased Effect

Rilonacept may decrease the levels/effects of: BCG; Coccidioidin Skin Test; Sipuleucel-T; Vaccines (Inactivated); Vaccines (Live)

The levels/effects of Rilonacept may be decreased by: Echinacea

Stability Store powder in refrigerator at 2°C to 8°C (36°F to 46°F); do not freeze. Do not shake. Protect from light. Reconstitute rilonacept 220 mg powder for injection with SWFI 2.3 mL; do not use bacteriostatic water containing benzyl alcohol or parabens. After reconstituting with SWFI, gently shake the vial for 1 minute, then allow solution to sit for 1 minute. Each reconstituted vial allows for withdrawal of 2 mL (160 mg) for SubQ administration. After reconstitution, may be stored at controlled room temperature. Protect from light. Use within 3 hours of reconstitution.

Mechanism of Action Cryopyrin-associated periodic syndromes (CAPS) refers to rare genetic syndromes caused by mutations in the nucleotide-binding domain, leucine rich family (NLR), pyrin domain containing 3 (NLRP-3) gene or the cold-induced autoinflammatory syndrome-1 (CIAS1) gene. Cryopyrin, a protein encoded by this gene, regulates interleukin-1 beta (IL-1β) activation. Deficiency of cryopyrin results in excessive inflammation. Rilonacept reduces inflammation by binding to IL-1β (some binding of IL-1α and IL-1 receptor antagonist) and preventing interaction with cell surface receptors.

Pharmacodynamics/Kinetics Onset of action: Steady state reached by 6 weeks

Dosage SubQ: Cryopyrin-associated periodic syndromes:
Children ≥12 years: Loading dose 4.4 mg/kg (maximum dose: 320 mg) given as 1-2 separate injections (maximum: 2 mL/injection) on the same day, followed by 2.2 mg/kg (maximum dose: 160 mg) once weekly. **Note:** Do not administer more frequently than once weekly.
Adults: Loading dose 320 mg given as 2 separate injections (160 mg each) on the same day at 2 different sites, followed a week later by 160 mg, then once weekly. **Note:** Do not administer more frequently than once weekly.

Administration SubQ: Rotate injection sites (thigh, abdomen, upper arm); injections should never be made at sites that are bruised, red, tender, or hard

Monitoring Parameters CBC with differential, lipid profile, C-reactive protein (CRP), serum amyloid A; signs of infection

Dosage Forms Excipient information presented when available (limited, particularly for generics); consult specific product labeling.
Injection, powder for reconstitution:
Arcalyst™: 220 mg

Rilpivirine (ril pi VIR een)

Brand Names: U.S. Edurant™

Brand Names: Canada Edurant™

Index Terms TMC278

Pharmacologic Category Antiretroviral Agent, Reverse Transcriptase Inhibitor (Non-nucleoside)

Use Treatment of HIV-1 infections in combination with at least two other antiretroviral agents

Pregnancy Risk Factor B

Pregnancy Considerations No evidence of fetal toxicity has been noted in animal reproduction studies. Available data in pregnant women are insufficient and the DHHS Perinatal HIV Guidelines do not recommend use unless other alternatives are not available. Hypersensitivity reactions (including hepatic toxicity and rash) are more common in women on NNRTI therapy; it is not known if pregnancy increases this risk.

Regardless of CD4 count or HIV RNA copy number, all HIV-infected pregnant women should receive a combination antepartum antiretroviral (ARV) drug regimen; this includes women who require therapy for their own health, as well as women who do not yet require therapy for their own health. ARV therapy should be started as soon as possible if required for the woman's health or immediately after the first trimester if not needed for the mother's health (although earlier initiation may be considered). Long-term follow-up is recommended for all infants exposed to ARV medications.

Healthcare providers are encouraged to enroll pregnant women exposed to antiretroviral medications in the Antiretroviral Pregnancy Registry (1-800-258-4263 or www.APRegistry.com). Healthcare providers caring for HIV-infected women and their infants may contact the National Perinatal HIV Hotline (888-448-8765) for clinical consultation (DHHS [perinatal], 2011).

Lactation Excretion in breast milk unknown/contraindicated

Contraindications Concurrent use of carbamazepine, dexamethasone (>1 dose), oxcarbazepine, phenobarbital, phenytoin, proton pump inhibitors (PPIs), rifabutin, rifampin, rifapentine, or St John's wort

Warnings/Precautions Not for use in treatment-experienced patients. May cause depressive disorders (depression, depressed mood, dysphoria, mood changes, negative thoughts, suicide attempts, or suicidal ideation); monitor for changes and need for intervention. May cause redistribution of fat (eg, buffalo hump, peripheral wasting with increased abdominal girth, cushingoid appearance). Patients may develop immune reconstitution syndrome resulting in the occurrence of an inflammatory response to an indolent or residual opportunistic infection; further evaluation and treatment may be required.

Use with caution in patients taking major CYP3A4 (see Drug Interactions) inducers or drugs that increase gastric pH. Use caution with drugs known to prolong the QT_c interval.

Adverse Reactions

2% to 10%:

Central nervous system: Depressive disorders (depression, depressed mood, dysphoria, mood changes, negative thoughts, suicide attempts, suicidal ideation) (4% to 8%; grades 3/4: 1%), headache (3%), insomnia (3%)

Dermatologic: Rash (3%)

Endocrine & metabolic: Cholesterol increased (200-300 mg/dL: 19%; >300 mg/dL: <1%), LDL increased (130-190 mg/dL: 17%; >191 mg/dL: <1%), triglycerides increased (500-750 mg/dL: 2%; >750 mg/dL: <1%)

Hepatic: ALT increased (≤5 x ULN: 19%; >5 x ULN: <1%), AST increased (≤5 x ULN: 15%; >5 x ULN: ~2%), bilirubin increased (≤2.5 x ULN: 7%; >2.5 x ULN: <1%)

Renal: Creatinine increased (≤1.8 x ULN: ~5%)

<2% (Limited to important or life-threatening): Abdominal discomfort/pain, abnormal dreams, anxiety, appetite decreased, cholecystitis, cholelithiasis, diarrhea, dizziness, fatigue, glomerulonephritis (membranous and mesangioproliferative), nausea, somnolence, sleep disorders, vomiting

Drug Interactions

Metabolism/Transport Effects Substrate of CYP3A4 (major); **Note:** Assignment of Major/Minor substrate status based on clinically relevant drug interaction potential

Avoid Concomitant Use

Avoid concomitant use of Rilpivirine with any of the following: CarBAMazepine; Conivaptan; Dexamethasone; Dexamethasone (Systemic); Etravirine; Fosphenytoin; OXcarbazepine; PHENobarbital; Phenytoin; Primidone; Proton Pump Inhibitors; Reverse Transcriptase Inhibitors (Non-Nucleoside); Rifamycin Derivatives; St Johns Wort

Increased Effect/Toxicity

Rilpivirine may increase the levels/effects of: Etravirine; PACLitaxel

The levels/effects of Rilpivirine may be increased by: Conivaptan; CYP3A4 Inhibitors (Moderate); CYP3A4 Inhibitors (Strong); Darunavir; Dasatinib; Ketoconazole; Ketoconazole (Systemic); Lopinavir; Reverse Transcriptase Inhibitors (Non-Nucleoside)

Decreased Effect

Rilpivirine may decrease the levels/effects of: Dexamethasone; Didanosine; Etravirine; Ketoconazole; Ketoconazole (Systemic); Methadone

The levels/effects of Rilpivirine may be decreased by: Antacids; CarBAMazepine; CYP3A4 Inducers (Strong); Deferasirox; Dexamethasone (Systemic); Didanosine; Fosphenytoin; H2-Antagonists; OXcarbazepine; PHENobarbital; Phenytoin; Primidone; Proton Pump Inhibitors; Reverse Transcriptase Inhibitors (Non-Nucleoside); Rifamycin Derivatives; St Johns Wort; Tocilizumab

Ethanol/Nutrition/Herb Interactions

Food: Absorption increased by ~40% when taken with a normal to high-caloric meal. Administration with a protein supplement drink alone does not increase absorption.

Herb/Nutraceutical: St John's wort (*Hypericum perforatum*) may decrease the levels/effects of rilpivirine; do not coadminister.

Stability Store at 25°C (77°F); excursions permitted to 15°C to 30°C (59°F to 86°F). Keep in original container; protect from light.

Mechanism of Action As a non-nucleoside reverse transcriptase inhibitor, rilpivirine has activity against HIV-1 by binding to reverse transcriptase. It consequently blocks the RNA-dependent and DNA-dependent DNA polymerase activities, including HIV-1 replication. It does not require intracellular phosphorylation for antiviral activity.

Pharmacodynamics/Kinetics

Absorption: Increased 40% with a meal (normal-to-high calorie)

Protein binding: 99.7% (primarily albumin)

Metabolism: Hepatic, primarily by CYP3A4

Half-life elimination: ~50 hours

Time to peak, plasma: 4-5 hours

Excretion: Feces (85%, ~25% as unchanged drug); urine (~6%; <1% as unchanged drug)

Dosage Oral: Adults: 25 mg once daily

Dosage adjustment in renal impairment:

Mild-to-moderate renal impairment: No dosage adjustment necessary

Severe or end-stage renal impairment: No dosage adjustment necessary (DHHS, 2011)

Hemodialysis/peritoneal dialysis: Due to extensive protein binding, significant removal by hemodialysis or peritoneal dialysis is unlikely.

Dosage adjustment in hepatic impairment:

Mild-to-moderate impairment (Child-Pugh class A, B): No dosage adjustment necessary

Severe impairment (Child-Pugh class C): No dosage adjustment provided in the manufacturer's labeling (has not been studied); DHHS HIV guidelines also have no dosage recommendation (DHHS, 2011).

Dietary Considerations Take with a normal- to high-calorie meal. Taking with a protein supplement drink alone does not increase absorption.

Administration Administer with a normal- to high-calorie meal. Taking with a protein supplement drink alone does not increase absorption.

Monitoring Parameters Cholesterol, triglycerides, hepatic transaminases; signs of skin rash, signs and symptoms of infection

Additional Information Rilpivirine has been shown in several studies to be noninferior to efavirenz in treatment-naive HIV-1 patients. Patients with increased HIV-1 viral loads at treatment initiation (HIV-1 RNA >100,000 copies/mL) are more likely to develop treatment failure. These patients also are more likely to develop rilpivirine-resistance and NNRTI class cross-resistance. Rilpivirine resistance patterns are very similar to those of etravirine (including cross resistance with single substitutions at K101P, Y181I, and Y181V) (Aziin, 2010).

Dosage Forms Excipient information presented when available (limited, particularly for generics); consult specific product labeling.

Tablet, oral:

Edurant™: 25 mg

◆ **Rilpivirine, Emtricitabine, and Tenofovir** *see* Emtricitabine, Rilpivirine, and Tenofovir *on page 583*

◆ **Rilutek®** *see* Riluzole *on page 1491*

Riluzole (RIL yoo zole)

Brand Names: U.S. Rilutek®

Brand Names: Canada Rilutek®

Index Terms 2-Amino-6-Trifluoromethoxy-benzothiazole; RP-54274

Pharmacologic Category Glutamate Inhibitor

Use Treatment of amyotrophic lateral sclerosis (ALS); riluzole can extend survival or time to tracheostomy

Pregnancy Risk Factor C

Pregnancy Considerations Impaired fertility, decreased implantation, increased intrauterine death, and adverse effects on offspring growth and viability were observed in animal studies. There are no adequate or well-controlled studies in pregnant women.

Lactation Excretion in breast milk unknown/not recommended

Contraindications Severe hypersensitivity reactions to riluzole or any component of the formulation

Warnings/Precautions Among 4000 patients given riluzole for ALS, there were 3 cases of marked neutropenia (ANC <500/mm^3), all seen within the first 2 months of treatment. Interstitial lung disease (primarily hypersensitivity pneumonitis) has occurred, requires prompt evaluation and possible discontinuation. Use with caution in patients with concomitant renal insufficiency. Use with caution in patients with current evidence or history of abnormal liver function; do not administer if baseline liver function tests are elevated. May cause elevations in transaminases (usually transient). May cause elevations in transaminases (usually transient) within first 3 months of therapy; discontinue if ALT levels are ≥5 times upper limit of normal or if jaundice develops. The elderly or female patients may have decreased clearance of riluzole; use with caution. May cause dizziness or somnolence; caution should be used performing tasks which require alertness (operating machinery or driving).

Adverse Reactions

>10%:

Gastrointestinal: Nausea (16%)

Neuromuscular & skeletal: Weakness (19%)

1% to 10%:

Cardiovascular: Hypertension (5%), peripheral edema (3%), tachycardia (3%)

Central nervous system: Dizziness (4%), somnolence (2%), vertigo (2%), malaise (1%)

Dermatologic: Pruritus (4%), eczema (2%), exfoliative dermatitis (1%)

Gastrointestinal: Abdominal pain (5%), vomiting (4%), flatulence (3%), oral moniliasis (1%), stomatitis (1%), tooth caries (1%)

Genitourinary: Urinary tract infection (3%), dysuria (1%)

Hepatic: Liver function tests increased (8% >3 x ULN; 2% >5 x ULN)

Neuromuscular & skeletal: Arthralgia (4%), paresthesia (circumoral; 2%), tremor (1%)

Respiratory: Lung function decreased (10%), cough increased (3%)

<1% (Limited to important or life-threatening): Alkaline phosphatase increased, amblyopia, anaphylactoid reaction, anaphylaxis, angioedema, aplastic anemia, arthrosis, asthma, ataxia, bone necrosis, bradycardia, bundle branch block, cataract, cerebral hemorrhage, deafness, dementia, diabetes mellitus, diabetes insipidus, edema, erythema multiforme, extrapyramidal syndrome, facial paralysis, gastrointestinal hemorrhage, gastrointestinal ulcer, GGT increased, glaucoma, hallucination, heart failure, hematemesis, hematuria, hemoptysis, hepatitis, hypercalcemia, hypokalemia, hypokinesia, hyponatremia, hypotension, hypersensitivity pneumonitis, interstitial lung disease, jaundice, LDH increased, leukocytosis, leukopenia, lymphadenopathy, mania, myoclonus, neutropenia, osteoporosis, pancreatitis, peripheral neuritis, pleural effusion, pseudomembranous colitis, purpura, respiratory acidosis, seizure, subarachnoid hemorrhage, thrombosis, urinary retention, urticaria, uterine hemorrhage, ventricular fibrillation, ventricular tachycardia

Drug Interactions

Metabolism/Transport Effects **Substrate** of CYP1A2 (major); **Note:** Assignment of Major/Minor substrate status based on clinically relevant drug interaction potential

Avoid Concomitant Use There are no known interactions where it is recommended to avoid concomitant use.

Increased Effect/Toxicity There are no known significant interactions involving an increase in effect.

Decreased Effect

The levels/effects of Riluzole may be decreased by: CYP1A2 Inducers (Strong); Cyproterone

Ethanol/Nutrition/Herb Interactions

Ethanol: Avoid ethanol (due to CNS depression and possible risk of liver toxicity).

Food: A high-fat meal decreases absorption of riluzole (decreasing AUC by 20% and peak blood levels by 45%). Charbroiled food may increase riluzole elimination.

Stability Store at 20°C to 25°C (68°F to 77°F). Protect from bright light.

Mechanism of Action Mechanism of action is not known. Pharmacologic properties include inhibitory effect on glutamate release, inactivation of voltage-dependent sodium channels; and ability to interfere with intracellular events that follow transmitter binding at excitatory amino acid receptors

Pharmacodynamics/Kinetics

Absorption: ~90%; high-fat meal decreases AUC by 20% and peak blood levels by 45%

Protein binding, plasma: 96%, primarily to albumin and lipoproteins

Metabolism: Extensively hepatic to six major and a number of minor metabolites via CYP1A2 dependent hydroxylation and glucuronidation

Bioavailability: Oral: Absolute: ~60%

Half-life elimination: 12 hours

Excretion: Urine (90%; 85% as metabolites, 2% as unchanged drug) and feces (5%) within 7 days

Dosage Adults: Oral: 50 mg every 12 hours; no increased benefit can be expected from higher daily doses, but adverse events are increased

Dosage adjustment in smoking: Cigarette smoking is known to induce CYP1A2; patients who smoke cigarettes would be expected to eliminate riluzole faster. There is no information, however, on the effect of, or need for, dosage adjustment in these patients.

Dosage adjustment in renal impairment: No specific dosage adjustments recommended by manufacturer; use caution.

Dosage adjustment in hepatic impairment: No specific dosage adjustments recommended by manufacturer; use caution.

Dietary Considerations Take at least 1 hour before or 2 hours after a meal.

Administration Administer at the same time each day, at least 1 hour before or 2 hours after a meal.

Monitoring Parameters Monitor serum aminotransferases including ALT levels before and during therapy. Evaluate serum ALT levels every month during the first 3 months of therapy, every 3 months during the remainder of the first year and periodically thereafter. Evaluate ALT levels more frequently in patients who develop elevations. Maximum increases in serum ALT usually occurred within 3 months after the start of therapy and were usually transient when <5 times ULN (upper limits of normal). Discontinue therapy if ALT levels are ≥5 times upper limit of normal or if jaundice develops.

In trials, if ALT levels were <5 times ULN, treatment continued and ALT levels usually returned to below 2 times ULN within 2-6 months. There is no experience with continued treatment of ALS patients once ALT values exceed 5 times ULN.

Dosage Forms Excipient information presented when available (limited, particularly for generics); consult specific product labeling.

Tablet, oral:

Rilutek®: 50 mg

RimabotulinumtoxinB

(rime uh BOT yoo lin num TOKS in bee)

Brand Names: U.S. Myobloc®

Index Terms Botulinum Toxin Type B

Pharmacologic Category Neuromuscular Blocker Agent, Toxin

Use Treatment of cervical dystonia (spasmodic torticollis)

Unlabeled Use Treatment of cervical dystonia in patients who have developed resistance to onabotulinumtoxinA or abobotulinumtoxinA

Pregnancy Risk Factor C (manufacturer)

Medication Guide Available Yes

Dosage

Children: Not established in pediatric patients

Adults: Cervical dystonia: I.M.: Initial: 2500-5000 units divided among the affected muscles in patients **previously treated** with botulinum toxin; initial dose in **previously untreated** patients should be lower. Subsequent dosing should be optimized according to patient's response.

Elderly: No dosage adjustments required, but limited experience in patients ≥75 years old

Dosage adjustment in renal impairment: No specific adjustment recommended

Dosage adjustment in hepatic impairment: No specific adjustment recommended

Additional Information Complete prescribing information for this medication should be consulted for additional detail.

Dosage Forms Excipient information presented when available (limited, particularly for generics); consult specific product labeling.

Injection, solution [preservative free]:

Myobloc®: 5000 units/mL (0.5 mL, 1 mL, 2 mL) [contains albumin (human)]

Rimantadine (ri MAN ta deen)

Brand Names: U.S. Flumadine®

Brand Names: Canada Flumadine®

Index Terms Rimantadine Hydrochloride

Pharmacologic Category Antiviral Agent; Antiviral Agent, Adamantane

Use Prophylaxis (adults and children >1 year of age) and treatment (adults) of influenza A viral infection (per manufacturer labeling; also refer to current ACIP guidelines for recommendations during current flu season)

Note: In certain circumstances, the ACIP recommends use of rimantadine in combination with oseltamivir for the treatment or prophylaxis of influenza A infection when resistance to oseltamivir is suspected.

Pregnancy Risk Factor C

Pregnancy Considerations Animal data suggest embryotoxicity, maternal toxicity, and offspring mortality at doses 7-11 times the recommended human dose. There are no adequate and well-controlled studies in pregnant women.

Influenza infection may be more severe in pregnant women. Untreated influenza infection is associated with an increased risk of adverse events to the fetus and an increased risk of complications or death to the mother. Oseltamivir and zanamivir are currently recommended for the treatment or prophylaxis influenza in pregnant women and women up to 2 weeks postpartum. Appropriate antiviral agents are currently recommended as an adjunct to vaccination and should not be used as a substitute for vaccination in pregnant women (consult current CDC guidelines).

Healthcare providers are encouraged to refer women exposed to influenza vaccine, or who have taken an antiviral medication during pregnancy to the Vaccines and Medications in Pregnancy Surveillance System (VAMPSS) by contacting The Organization of Teratology Information Specialists (OTIS) at (877) 311-8972.

Lactation Excretion in breast milk unknown/ not recommended

Contraindications Hypersensitivity to drugs of the adamantine class, including rimantadine and amantadine, or any component of the formulation

Warnings/Precautions Use with caution in patients with renal and hepatic dysfunction; avoid use, if possible, in patients with uncontrolled psychosis or severe psychoneurosis. An increase in seizure incidence may occur in patients with seizure disorders; discontinue drug if seizures occur; resistance may develop during treatment; viruses exhibit cross-resistance between amantadine and rimantadine. Due to increased resistance, the ACIP has recommended that rimantadine and amantadine no longer be used for the treatment or prophylaxis of influenza A in the United States until susceptibility has been re-established; consult current guidelines. Rimantadine is not effective in the prevention or treatment of influenza B virus infections. The elderly are at higher risk for CNS (eg, dizziness, headache, weakness) and gastrointestinal (eg, nausea/vomiting, abdominal pain) adverse events; dosage adjustment is recommended in elderly patients >65 years of age.

Adverse Reactions

1% to 10%:

Central nervous system: Insomnia (2% to 3%), concentration impaired (≤2%), dizziness (1% to 2%), nervousness (1% to 2%), fatigue (1%), headache (1%)

Gastrointestinal: Nausea (3%), anorexia (2%), vomiting (2%), xerostomia (2%), abdominal pain (1%)

Neuromuscular & skeletal: Weakness (1%)

<1% (Limited to important or life-threatening): Agitation, ataxia, bronchospasm, cardiac failure, confusion, convulsions, depression, diarrhea, dyspnea, euphoria, gait abnormality, hallucinations, heart block, hyperkinesias, hypertension, lactation, palpitation, parosmia, pedal edema, rash, syncope, tachycardia, taste alteration, tremor

Drug Interactions

Metabolism/Transport Effects None known.

Avoid Concomitant Use There are no known interactions where it is recommended to avoid concomitant use.

Increased Effect/Toxicity

The levels/effects of Rimantadine may be increased by: MAO Inhibitors

Decreased Effect

Rimantadine may decrease the levels/effects of: Influenza Virus Vaccine (Live/Attenuated)

Ethanol/Nutrition/Herb Interactions Food: Food does not affect rate or extent of absorption

Stability Store at 25°C (77°F); excursions permitted to 15°C to 30°C (59°F to 86°F).

Mechanism of Action Exerts its inhibitory effect on three antigenic subtypes of influenza A virus (H1N1, H2N2, H3N2) early in the viral replicative cycle, possibly inhibiting the uncoating process; it has no activity against influenza B virus and is two- to eightfold more active than amantadine

Pharmacodynamics/Kinetics

Onset of action: Antiviral activity: No data exist establishing a correlation between plasma concentration and antiviral effect

Protein Binding: ~40%, primarily to albumin

Metabolism: Extensively hepatic

Half-life elimination: 25.4 hours; prolonged in elderly, severe liver and severe renal impairment

Time to peak: 6 hours

Excretion: Urine (<25% as unchanged drug)

Clearance: Hemodialysis does not contribute to clearance

Dosage Oral:
Prophylaxis:
Children
1-9 years: 5 mg/kg/day in 1-2 divided doses; maximum: 150 mg/day
≥10 years and <40 kg: 5 mg/kg/day in 2 divided doses (CDC, 2011)
Children ≥10 years (and ≥40 kg) and Adults: 100 mg twice daily
Elderly: 100 mg daily in the elderly (≥65 years), including elderly nursing home patients
Note: Prophylaxis (institutional outbreak): In order to control outbreaks in institutions, if influenza A virus subtyping is unavailable and oseltamivir resistant viruses are circulating, rimantadine may be used in combination with oseltamivir if zanamivir cannot be used. Treatment should continue for ≥2 weeks and until ~10 days after illness onset in the last patient (CDC, 2011; Harper 2009).
Treatment:
Children ≥17 years and Adults: 100 mg twice daily
Elderly: 100 mg daily in the elderly (≥ 65 years) or nursing home patients

Dosage adjustment in renal impairment:
Cl_{cr} ≥30 mL/minute: Dose adjustment not required
Cl_{cr} <30 mL/minute: 100 mg daily
Dosage adjustment in hepatic impairment: Severe dysfunction: 100 mg daily
Administration Initiation of rimantadine within 48 hours of the onset of influenza A illness halves the duration of illness and significantly reduces the duration of viral shedding and increased peripheral airways resistance; continue therapy for 5-7 days after symptoms begin; discontinue as soon as clinically warranted to reduce the emergence of antiviral drug resistant viruses
Monitoring Parameters Monitor for CNS or GI effects in elderly or patients with renal or hepatic impairment
Dosage Forms Excipient information presented when available (limited, particularly for generics); consult specific product labeling.
Tablet, oral, as hydrochloride: 100 mg
Flumadine®: 100 mg
Extemporaneous Preparations Rimantadine 10 mg/mL
Suspension:
To prepare suspension, 10 mL of Ora-Sweet® will be required for every 100 mg tablet of rimantadine. (Do not prepare more than a 14-day supply).
- Calculate the total dose needed (daily dose x number of days = mg of rimantadine needed) and round the final mg of rimantadine needed up to the next 100 mg (eg, 750 mg would be 800 mg, or eight 100 mg tablets).
- Calculate the total volume of Ora-Sweet® by taking the rounded mg of rimantadine and dividing by 10 mg/mL (eg, 800 mg divided by 10 mg/mL = 80 mL).
- Grind required number of tablets in mortar and triturate to a fine powder. Slowly add 1/3 of the total volume of Ora-Sweet® to the mortar and triturate until a uniform suspension is achieved.
- Transfer to an amber glass or PET plastic bottle. Slowly add another 1/3 of the total volume of Ora-Sweet® to the mortar, rinsing the mortar, then transferring the contents into the bottle. Repeat using the final 1/3 of Ora-Sweet®. Add additional vehicle to bottle, if needed, to achieve the total calculated volume.
- Shake well to ensure homogeneous suspension. Some inert ingredients in the tablet may be insoluble.
- Label: Shake gently prior to each use.
- Suspension is stable for 14 days when stored at room temperature (25°C/77°F).

◆ **Rimantadine Hydrochloride** *see* Rimantadine *on page 1493*

Rimexolone (ri MEKS oh lone)

Brand Names: U.S. Vexol®
Brand Names: Canada Vexol®
Pharmacologic Category Corticosteroid, Ophthalmic
Use Treatment of inflammation after ocular surgery and the treatment of anterior uveitis
Pregnancy Risk Factor C
Dosage Ophthalmic: Adults:
Anti-inflammatory: Instill 1-2 drops in conjunctival sac of affected eye 4 times/day beginning 24 hours after surgery and continuing through the first 2 weeks of the postoperative period
Anterior uveitis: Instill 1-2 drops in conjunctival sac of affected eye every hour during waking hours for the first week, then 1 drop every 2 hours during waking hours of the second week, and then taper until uveitis is resolved
Additional Information Complete prescribing information for this medication should be consulted for additional detail.
Dosage Forms Excipient information presented when available (limited, particularly for generics); consult specific product labeling.
Suspension, ophthalmic [drops]:
Vexol®: 1% (5 mL, 10 mL) [contains benzalkonium chloride]

◆ **Riomet®** *see* MetFORMIN *on page 1086*

◆ **Riopan Plus** *see* Magaldrate and Simethicone *on page 1043*

Risedronate (ris ED roe nate)

Brand Names: U.S. Actonel®; Atelvia™
Brand Names: Canada Actonel®; Actonel® DR; Apo-Risedronate®; Dom-Risedronate; Novo-Risedronate; PMS-Risedronate; ratio-Risedronate; Riva-Risedronate; Sandoz-Risedronate; Teva-Risedronate
Index Terms Risedronate Sodium
Pharmacologic Category Bisphosphonate Derivative
Use
Actonel®: Treatment of Paget's disease of the bone; treatment and prevention of glucocorticoid-induced osteoporosis; treatment and prevention of osteoporosis in postmenopausal women; treatment of osteoporosis in men
Atelvia™: Treatment of osteoporosis in postmenopausal women
Pregnancy Risk Factor C
Pregnancy Considerations Teratogenic and nonteratogenic embryo/fetal effects have been reported in animal studies. There are no adequate and well-controlled studies in pregnant women. Bisphosphonates are incorporated into the bone matrix and gradually released over time. Theoretically, there may be a risk of fetal harm when pregnancy follows the completion of therapy. Based on limited case reports with pamidronate, serum calcium levels in the newborn may be altered if administered during pregnancy.
Lactation Excretion in breast milk unknown/not recommended
Medication Guide Available Yes
Contraindications Hypersensitivity to risedronate, bisphosphonates, or any component of the formulation; hypocalcemia; inability to stand or sit upright for at least 30 minutes; abnormalities of the esophagus which delay esophageal emptying, such as stricture or achalasia
Warnings/Precautions Bisphosphonates may cause upper gastrointestinal disorders such as dysphagia, esophagitis, esophageal ulcer, and gastric ulcer; risk increases in patients unable to comply with dosing

instructions. Use with caution in patients with dysphagia, esophageal disease, gastritis, duodenitis, or ulcers (may worsen underlying condition). Discontinue if new or worsening symptoms occur. Use caution in patients with renal impairment (not recommended in patients with a Cl_{cr} <30 mL/minute). Hypocalcemia must be corrected before therapy initiation with risedronate. Ensure adequate calcium and vitamin D intake, especially for patients with Paget's disease in whom the pretreatment rate of bone turnover may be greatly elevated.

Bisphosphonate therapy has been associated with osteonecrosis, primarily of the jaw. Risk factors for osteonecrosis of the jaw (ONJ) include invasive dental procedures (eg, tooth extraction, dental implants, boney surgery); a diagnosis of cancer, with concomitant chemotherapy or corticosteroids; poor oral hygiene, ill-fitting dentures; and comorbid disorders (anemia, coagulopathy, infection, preexisting dental disease). Most reported cases occurred after I.V. bisphosphonate therapy; however, cases have been reported following oral therapy. A dental exam and preventative dentistry should be performed prior to placing patients with risk factors on chronic bisphosphonate therapy. The manufacturer's labeling states that discontinuing bisphosphonates in patients requiring invasive dental procedures may reduce the risk of ONJ. However, other experts suggest that there is no evidence that discontinuing therapy reduces the risk of developing ONJ (Assael, 2009). The benefit/risk must be assessed by the treating physician and/or dentist/surgeon prior to any invasive dental procedure. Patients developing ONJ while on bisphosphonates should receive care by an oral surgeon.

Atypical femur fractures have been reported in patients receiving bisphosphonates for treatment/prevention of osteoporosis. The fractures include subtrochanteric femur (bone just below the hip joint) and diaphyseal femur (long segment of the thigh bone). Some patients experience prodromal pain weeks or months before the fracture occurs. It is unclear if bisphosphonate therapy is the cause for these fractures, although the majority have been reported in patients taking bisphosphonates. Patients receiving long-term (>3-5 years) therapy may be at an increased risk. Discontinue bisphosphonate therapy in patients who develop a femoral shaft fracture.

Infrequently, severe (and occasionally debilitating) bone, joint, and/or muscle pain have been reported during bisphosphonate treatment. The onset of pain ranged from a single day to several months. Consider discontinuing therapy in patients who experience severe symptoms; symptoms usually resolve upon discontinuation. Some patients experienced recurrence when rechallenged with same drug or another bisphosphonate; avoid use in patients with a history of these symptoms in association with bisphosphonate therapy.

When using for glucocorticoid-induced osteoporosis, evaluate sex steroid hormonal status prior to treatment initiation; consider appropriate hormone replacement if necessary. Not approved for use in pediatric patients with osteogenesis imperfecta due to lack of efficacy in reducing the risk of fracture.

Adverse Reactions Frequency may vary with product, dose, and indication.

>10%:

- Cardiovascular: Hypertension (11%)
- Central nervous system: Headache (3% to 18%)
- Dermatologic: Rash (8% to 12%)
- Endocrine & metabolic: Serum PTH levels increased (transient; <30%)
- Gastrointestinal: Diarrhea (5% to 20%), nausea (4% to 13%), constipation (3% to 13%), abdominal pain (2% to 12%), dyspepsia (4% to 11%)
- Genitourinary: Urinary tract infection (11%)
- Neuromuscular & skeletal: Arthralgia (7% to 33%), back pain (6% to 28%)
- Miscellaneous: Infection (≤31%)

1% to 10%:

- Cardiovascular: Peripheral edema (8%), chest pain (5% to 7%), arrhythmia (2%)
- Central nervous system: Depression (7%), dizziness (3% to 7%)
- Endocrine & metabolic: Hypocalcemia (≤5%), hypophosphatemia (<3%)
- Gastrointestinal: Vomiting (2% to 5%), gastritis (3%), duodenitis (≤1%), glossitis (≤1%)
- Genitourinary: Prostatic hyperplasia (5%; benign), nephrolithiasis (3%)
- Neuromuscular & skeletal: Joint disorder (7%), myalgia (2% to 7%), neck pain (5%), muscle spasm (1% to 2%)
- Ocular: Cataract (7%)
- Respiratory: Bronchitis (3% to 10%), pharyngitis (6%), rhinitis (6%), dyspnea (4%)
- Miscellaneous: Flu-like syndrome (10%), acute phase reaction (≤8%; includes fever, influenza-like illness)

<1% (Limited to important or life-threatening): Diaphyseal femur fracture, dysphagia, esophageal cancer, esophageal ulcer, esophagitis, gastric ulcer, hypersensitivity reaction, musculoskeletal pain (rarely severe or incapacitating), osteonecrosis (primarily of the jaw), subtrochanteric femur fracture

Drug Interactions

Metabolism/Transport Effects None known.

Avoid Concomitant Use There are no known interactions where it is recommended to avoid concomitant use.

Increased Effect/Toxicity

Risedronate may increase the levels/effects of: Deferasirox; Phosphate Supplements

The levels/effects of Risedronate may be increased by: Aminoglycosides; Nonsteroidal Anti-Inflammatory Agents

Decreased Effect

The levels/effects of Risedronate may be decreased by: Antacids; Calcium Salts; Iron Salts; Magnesium Salts; Proton Pump Inhibitors

Ethanol/Nutrition/Herb Interactions

Ethanol: Avoid ethanol (may increase risk of osteoporosis).

Food: Food reduces absorption (similar to other bisphosphonates); mean oral bioavailability is decreased when given with food.

Stability Store at room temperature of 20°C to 25°C (68°F to 77°F).

Mechanism of Action A bisphosphonate which inhibits bone resorption via actions on osteoclasts or on osteoclast precursors; decreases the rate of bone resorption, leading to an indirect increase in bone mineral density. In Paget's disease, characterized by disordered resorption and formation of bone, inhibition of resorption leads to an indirect decrease in bone formation; but the newly-formed bone has a more normal architecture.

Pharmacodynamics/Kinetics

Onset of action: May require weeks

Absorption: Rapid

Distribution: V_d: 13.8 L/kg

Protein binding: ~24%

Metabolism: None

Bioavailability: Poor, ~0.54% to 0.75%

Half-life elimination: Initial: 1.5 hours; Terminal: 480-561 hours

Time to peak, serum: 1-3 hours

Excretion: Urine (up to 85%); feces (as unabsorbed drug)

Dosage Oral: Adults: **Note:** Patients should receive supplemental calcium and vitamin D if dietary intake is inadequate.

Immediate release tablet:
Paget's disease of bone: 30 mg once daily for 2 months
Retreatment may be considered (following post-treatment observation of at least 2 months) if relapse occurs, or if treatment fails to normalize serum alkaline phosphatase. For retreatment, the dose and duration of therapy are the same as for initial treatment. No data are available on more than one course of retreatment.
Osteoporosis (postmenopausal) prevention and treatment: 5 mg once daily **or** 35 mg once weekly **or** 150 mg once a month
Osteoporosis (males) treatment: 35 mg once weekly
Osteoporosis (glucocorticoid-induced) prevention and treatment: 5 mg once daily
Delayed release tablet: Osteoporosis (postmenopausal) treatment: 35 mg once weekly

Dosage adjustment in renal impairment:
Cl_{cr} ≥30 mL/minute: No adjustment required
Cl_{cr} <30 mL/minute: **Not** recommended for use
Dosage adjustment in hepatic impairment: No studies performed in hepatic impairment; no dosage adjustment necessary due to lack of hepatic metabolism

Dietary Considerations Ensure adequate calcium and vitamin D intake. Take immediate release tablet with at least 6 oz of **plain water** (not mineral water) ≥30 minutes before the first food or drink of the day other than water. Take delayed release tablet with at least 4 ounces of **plain water** immediately **after** breakfast.

Administration Note: Avoid administration of oral calcium supplements, antacids, magnesium supplements/laxatives, and iron preparations within 30 minutes of risedronate administration.
Immediate release tablet: Risedronate immediate release tablets must be taken on an empty stomach with a full glass (6-8 oz) of **plain water** (not mineral water) at least 30 minutes before any food, drink, or other medications orally to avoid interference with absorption. Patient must remain sitting upright or standing for at least 30 minutes after taking (to reduce esophageal irritation). Tablet should be swallowed whole; do not crush or chew.
Delayed release tablet: Risedronate delayed release tablets must be taken with at least 4 oz of **plain water** (not mineral water) immediately after breakfast. Patient must remain sitting upright or standing for at least 30 minutes after taking (to reduce esophageal irritation). Tablet should be swallowed whole; do not cut, split, crush, or chew.

Monitoring Parameters
Osteoporosis: Bone mineral density as measured by central dual-energy x-ray absorptiometry (DXA) of the hip or spine prior to initiation of therapy and at least every 2 years thereafter (6-12 months post-baseline if combined glucocorticoid and risedronate treatment, then every 2 years thereafter); annual measurements of height and weight, assessment of chronic back pain; serum calcium and 25(OH)D; consider measuring biochemical markers of bone turnover
Paget's disease: Alkaline phosphatase; pain; serum calcium and 25(OH)D

Test Interactions Bisphosphonates may interfere with diagnostic imaging agents such as technetium-99m-diphosphonate in bone scans.

Dosage Forms Excipient information presented when available (limited, particularly for generics); consult specific product labeling.
Tablet, oral, as sodium:
Actonel®: 5 mg, 30 mg, 35 mg, 150 mg
Tablet, delayed release, oral, as sodium:
Atelvia™: 35 mg

◆ **Risedronate Sodium** *see* Risedronate *on page* 1494
◆ **RisperDAL®** *see* RisperiDONE *on page* 1496
◆ **Risperdal® (Can)** *see* RisperiDONE *on page* 1496
◆ **Risperdal M-Tab** *see* RisperiDONE *on page* 1496
◆ **RisperDAL® M-Tab®** *see* RisperiDONE *on page* 1496
◆ **Risperdal® M-Tab® (Can)** *see* RisperiDONE *on page* 1496
◆ **RisperDAL® Consta®** *see* RisperiDONE *on page* 1496
◆ **Risperdal® Consta® (Can)** *see* RisperiDONE *on page* 1496

RisperiDONE (ris PER i done)

Brand Names: U.S. RisperDAL®; RisperDAL® Consta®; RisperDAL® M-Tab®

Brand Names: Canada Apo-Risperidone®; Ava-Risperidone; CO Risperidone; Dom-Risperidone; JAMP-Risperidone; Mint-Risperidon; Mylan-Risperidone; Novo-Risperidone; PHL-Risperidone; PMS-Risperidone; PMS-Risperidone ODT; PRO-Risperidone; RAN™-Risperidone; ratio-Risperidone; Risperdal®; Risperdal® Consta®; Risperdal® M-Tab®; Riva-Risperidone; Sandoz-Risperidone

Index Terms Risperdal M-Tab

Pharmacologic Category Antimanic Agent; Antipsychotic Agent, Atypical

Additional Appendix Information
Antipsychotic Agents *on page* 1880

Use
Oral: Treatment of schizophrenia; treatment of acute mania or mixed episodes associated with bipolar I disorder (as monotherapy in children or adults, or in combination with lithium or valproate in adults); treatment of irritability/aggression associated with autistic disorder
Injection: Treatment of schizophrenia; maintenance treatment of bipolar I disorder in adults as monotherapy or in combination with lithium or valproate

Unlabeled Use Treatment of Tourette's syndrome; psychosis/agitation related to Alzheimer's dementia; post-traumatic stress disorder (PTSD)

Pregnancy Risk Factor C

Pregnancy Considerations Animal studies indicate an increase in fetal mortality. Reversible EPS symptoms were noted in neonates following use of risperidone during the last trimester. Agenesis of the corpus callosum has also been noted in one case report of an infant exposed *in utero*. Antipsychotic use during the third trimester of pregnancy has a risk for abnormal muscle movements (extrapyramidal symptoms [EPS]) and withdrawal symptoms in newborns following delivery. Symptoms in the newborn may include agitation, feeding disorder, hypertonia, hypotonia, respiratory distress, somnolence, and tremor; these effects may be self-limiting or require hospitalization. There are no adequate and well-controlled studies in pregnant women. When using Risperdal® Consta®, patients should notify healthcare provider if they become or intend to become pregnant during therapy or within 12 weeks of last injection. Risperidone may cause hyperprolactinemia, which may decrease reproductive function in both males and females. Healthcare providers are encouraged to enroll women 18-45 years of age exposed to risperidone during pregnancy in the Atypical Antipsychotics Pregnancy Registry (1-866-961-2388).

Lactation Enters breast milk/not recommended

Contraindications Hypersensitivity to risperidone or any component of the formulation

Warnings/Precautions Hazardous agent - use appropriate precautions for handling and disposal. **[U.S. Boxed Warning]: Elderly patients with dementia-related psychosis treated with antipsychotics are at an increased risk of death compared to placebo.** Most deaths appeared to be either cardiovascular (eg, heart failure, sudden death) or infectious (eg, pneumonia) in nature. In addition, an increased incidence of cerebrovascular effects (eg, transient ischemic attack, cerebrovascular accidents) has been reported in studies of placebo-controlled trials of risperidone in elderly patients with dementia-related psychosis. Risperidone is not approved for the treatment of dementia-related psychosis.

Leukopenia, neutropenia, and agranulocytosis (sometimes fatal) have been reported in clinical trials and postmarketing reports with antipsychotic use; presence of risk factors (eg, pre-existing low WBC or history of drug-induced leuko-/neutropenia) should prompt periodic blood count assessment. Discontinue therapy at first signs of blood dyscrasias or if absolute neutrophil count <1000/mm^3.

Low to moderately sedating, use with caution in disorders where CNS depression is a feature. Use with caution in Parkinson's disease. Caution in patients with predisposition to seizures. Use with caution in renal or hepatic dysfunction; dose reduction recommended. Esophageal dysmotility and aspiration have been associated with antipsychotic use; use with caution in patients at risk of aspiration pneumonia (ie, Alzheimer's disease). Use is associated with increased prolactin levels; clinical significance of hyperprolactinemia in patients with breast cancer or other prolactin-dependent tumors is unknown. May alter temperature regulation. May mask toxicity of other drugs or conditions (eg intestinal obstruction, Reyes syndrome, brain tumor) due to antiemetic effects. Neutropenia has been reported with antipsychotic use, including fatal cases of agranulocytosis. Pre-existing myelosuppression (disease or drug-induced) increases risk and these patients should have frequent CBC monitoring; decreased blood counts in absence of other causative factors should prompt discontinuation of therapy.

Use with caution in patients with cardiovascular diseases (eg, heart failure, history of myocardial infarction or ischemia, cerebrovascular disease, conduction abnormalities). May cause orthostatic hypotension; use with caution in patients at risk of this effect (eg, concurrent medication use which may predispose to hypotension/bradycardia or presence of hypovolemia) or in those who would not tolerate transient hypotensive episodes. May alter cardiac conduction (low risk relative to other neuroleptics); life-threatening arrhythmias have occurred with therapeutic doses of neuroleptics.

May cause anticholinergic effects (confusion, agitation, constipation, xerostomia, blurred vision, urinary retention); therefore, they should be used with caution in patients with decreased gastrointestinal motility, urinary retention, BPH, xerostomia, or visual problems (including narrow-angle glaucoma). Relative to other neuroleptics, risperidone has a low potency of cholinergic blockade.

May cause extrapyramidal symptoms (EPS), including pseudoparkinsonism, acute dystonic reactions, akathisia, and tardive dyskinesia (risk of these reactions is low relative to other neuroleptics, and is dose dependent). Risk of dystonia (and probably other EPS) may be greater with increased doses, use of conventional antipsychotics, males, and younger patients. Risk of neuroleptic malignant syndrome (NMS) may be increased in patients with Parkinson's disease or Lewy body dementia; monitor for symptoms of confusion, obtundation, postural instability and extrapyramidal symptoms. May cause hyperglycemia; in some cases may be extreme and associated with ketoacidosis, hyperosmolar coma, or death. Use with caution in patients with diabetes or other disorders of glucose regulation; monitor for worsening of glucose control. Significant weight gain has been observed with antipsychotic therapy; incidence varies with product. Monitor waist circumference and BMI. Rare cases of priapism have been reported.

The possibility of a suicide attempt is inherent in psychotic illness or bipolar disorder; use caution in high-risk patients during initiation of therapy. Prescriptions should be written for the smallest quantity consistent with good patient care. Long-term effects on growth or sexual maturation have not been evaluated. Vehicle used in injectable (polylactide-co-glycolide microspheres) has rarely been associated with retinal artery occlusion in patients with abnormal arteriovenous anastomosis.

Adverse Reactions The frequency of adverse effects is reported as absolute percentages and is not based upon net frequencies as compared to placebo. Actual frequency may be dependent upon dose and/or indication. Events are reported from placebo-controlled studies. Unless otherwise noted, frequency of adverse effects is reported for the oral formulation in adults.

>10%:

- Central nervous system: Somnolence (children 12% to 67%; adults 5% to 14%; I.M. injection 5% to 6%), fatigue (children 18% to 42%; adults 1% to 3%), headache (I.M. injection 15% to 21%), fever (children 20%; adults 1% to 2%), dystonia (children 9% to 18%; adults 5% to 11%), anxiety (children ≤16%; adults 2% to 16%), dizziness (children 7% to 16%; adults 4% to 10%), Parkinsonism (children 2% to 16%; adults 12% to 20%)
- Dermatologic: Rash (children ≤11%; adults 2% to 4%)
- Gastrointestinal: Appetite increased (children 4% to 49%), weight gain (≥7% kg increase from baseline: children 33%; adults 9% to 21%), vomiting (children 10% to 25%), salivation increased (children ≤22%; adults 1% to 3%), constipation (children 21%; adults 8% to 9%), abdominal pain (children 15% to 18%; adults 3% to 4%), nausea (children 8% to 16%; adults 4% to 9%), dyspepsia (children 5% to 16%; adults 4% to 10%), xerostomia (children 13%; adults ≤4%)
- Genitourinary: Urinary incontinence (children 5% to 22%; adults <2%)
- Neuromuscular & skeletal: Tremor (adults 6%; children 10% to 12%)
- Respiratory: Rhinitis (children 13% to 36%; adults 7% to 11%), upper respiratory infection (children 34%; adults 2% to 3%), cough (children 34%; adults 3%)

1% to 10%:

- Cardiovascular: Tachycardia (children ≤7%; adults 1% to 5%), hypertension (I.M. injection 3%), chest pain (1% to 3%), creatine phosphokinase increased (≤2%), postural hypotension (≤2%), arrhythmia (≤1%), edema (≤1%), hypotension (≤1%), syncope (≤1%)
- Central nervous system: Akathisia (children ≤10%; adults 5% to 9%), automatism (children 7%), confusion (children 5%)
- Dermatologic: Seborrhea (up to 2%), acne (1%)
- Endocrine & metabolic: Lactation nonpuerperal (children 2% to 5%; adults 1%), ejaculation failure (≤1%)
- Gastrointestinal: Diarrhea (children 7% to 8%; adults ≤3%), anorexia (children 8%; adults ≤2%), toothache (I.M. injection 1% to 3%)
- Genitourinary: Urinary tract infection (≤3%)
- Hematologic: Neutropenia (I.M. injection <2%), anemia (I.M. injection <2%; oral ≤1%)
- Hepatic: Transaminases increased (I.M. injection ≥1%; oral 1%)
- Neuromuscular & skeletal: Dyskinesia (children 7%; adults 1%), arthralgia (2% to 3%), back pain (2% to 3%), myalgia (≤2%), weakness (1%)
- Ocular: Abnormal vision (children 4% to 7%; adults 1% to 3%), blurred vision (I.M. injection 2% to 3%)
- Otic: Earache (1%)
- Respiratory: Dyspnea (children 2% to 5%; adults 2%), epistaxis (≤2%)

≤1% (Limited to important or life-threatening): Agranulocytosis, allergic reaction, amnesia, anaphylactic reaction, anemias (oral formulations), angina pectoris, angioedema, antidiuretic hormone disorder, aphasia, apnea, ascites, aspiration, atrial fibrillation, AV block, bronchospasm, cachexia, catatonic reaction, cerebrovascular accident, cerebrovascular disorder, cholecystitis, cholelithiasis, cholestatic hepatitis, cholesterol increased, cholinergic syndrome, coma, dehydration, delirium, depression, diabetes mellitus, diabetic ketoacidosis, diverticulitis, dysgeusia, dysphagia, esophagitis, esophageal dysmotility, fecal incontinence, flu-like syndrome, gastroenteritis, hematemesis, hematuria, hemorrhage, hepatic failure, hepatocellular damage, hyper-/hypoglycemia, hyperphosphatemia, hypertriglyceridemia, hyperuricemia, hypokalemia, hyponatremia, hypoproteinemia, intestinal obstruction, jaundice, leukocytosis, leukopenia, leukorrhea, lymphadenopathy, mastitis, menstrual irregularities, migraine, myocardial infarction, myocarditis, palpitation, pancreatitis, Pelger-Huët anomaly, pituitary adenomas, pneumonia, precocious puberty, premature atrial contractions, priapism, pulmonary embolism, QT_c prolongation, RBC disorders, renal insufficiency, retinal artery occlusion (I.M. formulation), rigors, sarcoidosis, skin exfoliation, skin ulceration, ST depression, stomatitis, stridor, stroke, superficial phlebitis, synostosis, T wave inversions, thrombocytopenia, thrombophlebitis, thrombotic thrombocytopenic purpura, tinnitus, tongue edema, tongue paralysis, torticollis, transient ischemic attack, urinary retention, urticaria, ventricular extrasystoles, ventricular tachycardia, water intoxication, withdrawal syndrome, xerophthalmia

Drug Interactions

Metabolism/Transport Effects **Substrate** of CYP2D6 (major), CYP3A4 (minor); **Note:** Assignment of Major/Minor substrate status based on clinically relevant drug interaction potential; **Inhibits** CYP2D6 (weak), CYP3A4 (weak)

Avoid Concomitant Use

Avoid concomitant use of RisperiDONE with any of the following: Artemether; Dronedarone; Lumefantrine; Metoclopramide; Nilotinib; Pimozide; QUEtiapine; QuiNINE; Tetrabenazine; Thioridazine; Toremifene; Vandetanib; Vemurafenib; Ziprasidone

Increased Effect/Toxicity

RisperiDONE may increase the levels/effects of: Alcohol (Ethyl); Anticholinergics; CNS Depressants; Dronedarone; Methylphenidate; Paliperidone; Pimozide; QTc-Prolonging Agents; QuiNINE; Serotonin Modulators; Tetrabenazine; Thioridazine; Toremifene; Vandetanib; Vemurafenib; Ziprasidone

The levels/effects of RisperiDONE may be increased by: Abiraterone Acetate; Acetylcholinesterase Inhibitors (Central); Alfuzosin; Artemether; Chloroquine; Ciprofloxacin; Ciprofloxacin (Systemic); Conivaptan; CYP2D6 Inhibitors (Moderate); CYP2D6 Inhibitors (Strong); Darunavir; Divalproex; Gadobutrol; HydrOXYzine; Indacaterol; Lithium formulations; Loop Diuretics; Lumefantrine; Methylphenidate; Metoclopramide; Nilotinib; Pramlintide; QUEtiapine; QuiNINE; Selective Serotonin Reuptake Inhibitors; Tetrabenazine; Valproic Acid; Verapamil

Decreased Effect

RisperiDONE may decrease the levels/effects of: Amphetamines; Anti-Parkinson's Agents (Dopamine Agonist); Quinagolide

The levels/effects of RisperiDONE may be decreased by: CarBAMazepine; Lithium formulations; Peginterferon Alfa-2b; Tocilizumab

Ethanol/Nutrition/Herb Interactions

Ethanol: May increase CNS depression; monitor for increased effects with coadministration. Caution patients about effects.

Herb/Nutraceutical: Avoid kava kava, gotu kola, valerian, St John's wort (may increase CNS depression).

Stability

Injection: Risperdal® Consta®: Store in refrigerator at 2°C to 8°C (36°F to 46°F) and protect from light. May be stored at room temperature of 25°C (77°F) for up to 7 days prior to administration. Bring to room temperature prior to reconstitution. Reconstitute with provided diluent only. Shake vigorously to mix; will form thick, milky suspension. Following reconstitution, store at room temperature and use within 6 hours. Suspension settles in ~2 minutes; shake vigorously to resuspend prior to administration.

Oral solution, tablet: Store at 15°C to 25°C (59°F to 77°F). Protect from light and moisture. Keep orally-disintegrating tablets sealed in foil pouch until ready to use. Do not freeze solution.

Mechanism of Action Risperidone is a benzisoxazole atypical antipsychotic with mixed serotonin-dopamine antagonist activity that binds to 5-HT_2-receptors in the CNS and in the periphery with a very high affinity; binds to dopamine-D_2 receptors with less affinity. The binding affinity to the dopamine-D_2 receptor is 20 times lower than the 5-HT_2 affinity. The addition of serotonin antagonism to dopamine antagonism (classic neuroleptic mechanism) is thought to improve negative symptoms of psychoses and reduce the incidence of extrapyramidal side effects. $Alpha_1$, $alpha_2$ adrenergic, and histaminergic receptors are also antagonized with high affinity. Risperidone has low to moderate affinity for 5-HT_{1C}, 5-HT_{1D}, and 5-HT_{1A} receptors, weak affinity for D_1 and no affinity for muscarinics or $beta_1$ and $beta_2$ receptors

Pharmacodynamics/Kinetics

Absorption:

Oral: Rapid and well absorbed; food does not affect rate or extent

Injection: <1% absorbed initially; main release occurs at ~3 weeks and is maintained from 4-6 weeks

Distribution: V_d: 1-2 L/kg

Protein binding, plasma: Risperidone 90%; 9-hydroxyrisperidone: 77%

Metabolism: Extensively hepatic via CYP2D6 to 9-hydroxyrisperidone (similar pharmacological activity as risperidone); *N*-dealkylation is a second minor pathway

Bioavailability: Oral: 70%; Tablet (relative to solution): 94%; orally-disintegrating tablets and oral solution are bioequivalent to tablets

Half-life elimination: Active moiety (risperidone and its active metabolite 9-hydroxyrisperidone)

Oral: 20 hours (mean)

Extensive metabolizers: Risperidone: 3 hours; 9-hydroxyrisperidone: 21 hours

Poor metabolizers: Risperidone: 20 hours; 9-hydroxyrisperidone: 30 hours

Injection: 3-6 days; related to microsphere erosion and subsequent absorption of risperidone

Time to peak, plasma: Oral: Risperidone: Within 1 hour; 9-hydroxyrisperidone: Extensive metabolizers: 3 hours; Poor metabolizers: 17 hours

Excretion: Urine (70%); feces (14%)

Dosage Note: When reinitiating treatment after discontinuation, the initial titration schedule should be followed.

Oral:

Children ≥5 years and Adolescents: Autism:

<15 kg: Use with caution; specific dosing recommendations not available

<20 kg: Initial: 0.25 mg/day; may increase dose to 0.5 mg/day after ≥4 days, maintain dose for ≥14 days. In patients not achieving sufficient clinical response, may increase dose by 0.25 mg/day in ≥2-week intervals. Therapeutic effect reached plateau at 1 mg/day in clinical trials. Following clinical response, consider gradually lowering dose. May be administered once daily or in divided doses twice daily.

≥20 kg: Initial: 0.5 mg/day; may increase dose to 1 mg/day after ≥4 days, maintain dose for ≥14 days. In patients not achieving sufficient clinical response, may increase dose by 0.5 mg/day in ≥2-week intervals. Therapeutic effect reached plateau at 2.5 mg/day (3 mg/day in children >45 kg) in clinical trials. Following clinical response, consider gradually lowering dose. May be administered once daily or in divided doses twice daily.

Children and Adolescents:

Schizophrenia: Adolescents 13-17 years: Initial: 0.5 mg once daily; dose may be adjusted in increments of 0.5-1 mg/day at intervals ≥24 hours to a dose of 3 mg/day. Doses ranging from 1-6 mg/day have been evaluated, however, doses >3 mg/day do not confer additional benefit and are associated with increased adverse events.

Bipolar mania: Children and Adolescents 10-17 years: Initial: 0.5 mg once daily; dose may be adjusted in increments of 0.5-1 mg/day at intervals ≥24 hours to a dose of 2.5 mg/day. Doses ranging from 0.5-6 mg/day have been evaluated, however doses >2.5 mg/day do not confer additional benefit and are associated with increased adverse events.

Maintenance: No dosing recommendation available for treatment >3 weeks duration

Adolescents and Adults: Tourette's syndrome (unlabeled use): Initial: 0.25 mg once daily for 2 days, then 0.25 mg twice daily for 3 days, then 0.5 mg twice daily for 2 days; titrate slowly thereafter in increments/decrements ≤0.5 mg twice daily and at intervals ≥3 days; maximum dose: 6 mg/day (Dion, 2002)

Adults:

Schizophrenia:

Initial: 2 mg/day in 1-2 divided doses; may be increased by 1-2 mg/day at intervals ≥24 hours to a recommended dosage range of 4-8 mg/day; may be given as a single daily dose once maintenance dose is achieved; daily dosages >6 mg do not appear to confer any additional benefit, and the incidence of extrapyramidal symptoms is higher than with lower doses. Further dose adjustments should be made in increments/decrements of 1-2 mg/day on a weekly basis. Dose range studied in clinical trials: 4-16 mg/day.

Maintenance: Recommended dosage range: 2-8 mg/day

Bipolar mania:

Initial: 2-3 mg once daily; if needed, adjust dose by 1 mg/day in intervals ≥24 hours; dosing range: 1-6 mg/day

Maintenance: No dosing recommendation available for treatment >3 weeks duration.

Post-traumatic stress disorder (PTSD) (unlabeled use): 0.5-8 mg/day (Bandelow, 2008; Benedek, 2009)

Elderly:

Initial: 0.5 mg twice daily; titration should progress slowly in increments of no more than 0.5 mg twice daily; increases to dosages >1.5 mg twice daily should occur at intervals of ≥1 week.

Note: Additional monitoring of renal function and orthostatic blood pressure may be warranted. If once-a-day dosing in the elderly or debilitated patient is considered, a twice daily regimen should be used to titrate to the target dose, and this dose should be maintained for 2-3 days prior to attempts to switch to a once-daily regimen.

Psychosis/agitation related to Alzheimer's dementia (unlabeled use): Initial: 0.25-1 mg/day; if necessary, gradually increase as tolerated not to exceed 1.5-2 mg/day; doses >1 mg/day are associated with higher rates of extrapyramidal symptoms (Rabins, 2007)

I.M.: **Note:** Oral risperidone (or other antipsychotic) should be administered with the initial injection of Risperdal® Consta® and continued for 3 weeks (then discontinued) to maintain adequate therapeutic plasma concentrations prior to main release phase of risperidone from injection site. When switching from depot administration to a short-acting formulation, administer short-acting agent in place of the next regularly-scheduled depot injection.

Adults: Schizophrenia, bipolar I maintenance (Risperdal® Consta®): Initial: 25 mg every 2 weeks; if unresponsive, some may benefit from larger doses (37.5-50 mg); maximum dose: 50 mg every 2 weeks. Dosage adjustments should not be made more frequently than every 4 weeks. A lower initial dose of 12.5 mg may be appropriate in some patients (eg, demonstrated poor tolerability to other psychotropic medications).

Elderly (Risperdal® Consta®): 25 mg every 2 weeks; a lower initial dose of 12.5 mg may be appropriate in some patients

Dosing adjustment in renal impairment:

Oral: Starting dose of 0.5 mg twice daily; titration should progress slowly in increments of no more than 0.5 mg twice daily; increases to dosages >1.5 mg twice daily should occur at intervals of ≥1 week. Clearance of the active moiety is decreased by 60% in patients with moderate-to-severe renal disease compared to healthy subjects.

I.M.: Initiate with **oral** dosing (0.5 mg twice daily for 1 week then 2 mg/day for 1 week); if tolerated, begin 25 mg **I.M.** every 2 weeks; continue oral dosing for 3 weeks after the first I.M. injection. An initial I.M. dose of 12.5 mg may also be considered.

Dosing adjustment in hepatic impairment:

Oral: Starting dose of 0.5 mg twice daily; titration should progress slowly in increments of no more than 0.5 mg twice daily; increases to dosages >1.5 mg twice daily should occur at intervals of ≥1 week. The mean free fraction of risperidone in plasma was increased by 35% in patients with hepatic impairment compared to healthy subjects.

I.M.: Initiate with **oral** dosing (0.5 mg twice daily for 1 week then 2 mg/day for 1 week); if tolerated, begin 25 mg **I.M.** every 2 weeks; continue oral dosing for 3 weeks after the first I.M. injection. An initial I.M. dose of 12.5 mg may also be considered.

Dietary Considerations May be taken without regard to meals. Some products may contain phenylalanine.

Administration

Oral: May be administered without regard to meals.

Oral solution can be administered directly from the provided pipette or may be mixed with water, coffee, orange juice, or low-fat milk, but is **not compatible** with cola or tea.

In children or adolescents experiencing somnolence, half the daily dose may be administered twice daily **or** the once-daily dose may be administered at bedtime.

Risperdal® M-Tab® should not be removed from blister pack until administered. Using dry hands, place immediately on tongue. Tablet will dissolve within seconds, and may be swallowed with or without liquid. Do not split or chew.

I.M.: Risperdal® Consta® should be administered into either the deltoid muscle or the upper outer quadrant of the gluteal area. Avoid inadvertent injection into vasculature. Injection should alternate between the two arms or buttocks. Do not combine two different dosage strengths into one single administration. Do not substitute any components of the dose-pack; administer with needle provided (1-inch needle for deltoid administration or 2-inch needle for gluteal administration).

Monitoring Parameters Vital signs; fasting lipid profile and fasting blood glucose/Hgb A_{1c} (prior to treatment, at 3 months, then annually); CBC; BMI, personal/family history of obesity, waist circumference; blood pressure; mental status, abnormal involuntary movement scale (AIMS), extrapyramidal symptoms; orthostatic blood pressure changes for 3-5 days after starting or increasing dose. Weight should be assessed prior to treatment, at 4 weeks, 8 weeks, 12 weeks, and then at quarterly intervals. Consider titrating to a different antipsychotic agent for a weight gain ≥5% of the initial weight.

Additional Information Risperdal® Consta® is an injectable formulation of risperidone using the extended release Medisorb® drug-delivery system; small polymeric microspheres degrade slowly, releasing the medication at a controlled rate.

Dosage Forms Excipient information presented when available (limited, particularly for generics); consult specific product labeling.

Injection, microspheres for reconstitution, extended release:
RisperDAL® Consta®: 12.5 mg, 25 mg, 37.5 mg, 50 mg [contains polylactide-co-glycolide; supplied in a dose-pack containing vial with active ingredient in microsphere formulation, prefilled syringe with diluent, needle-free vial access device, and 2 safety needles (a 21 G UTW 1-inch and a 20 G TW 2-inch)]

Solution, oral: 1 mg/mL (30 mL)
RisperDAL®: 1 mg/mL (30 mL) [contains benzoic acid]

Tablet, oral: 0.25 mg, 0.5 mg, 1 mg, 2 mg, 3 mg, 4 mg
RisperDAL®: 0.25 mg, 0.5 mg
RisperDAL®: 1 mg [scored]
RisperDAL®: 2 mg, 3 mg, 4 mg

Tablet, orally disintegrating, oral: 0.25 mg, 0.5 mg, 1 mg, 2 mg, 3 mg, 4 mg
RisperDAL® M-Tab®: 0.5 mg [contains phenylalanine 0.14 mg/tablet]
RisperDAL® M-Tab®: 1 mg [contains phenylalanine 0.28 mg/tablet]
RisperDAL® M-Tab®: 2 mg [contains phenylalanine 0.42 mg/tablet]
RisperDAL® M-Tab®: 3 mg [contains phenylalanine 0.63 mg/tablet]
RisperDAL® M-Tab®: 4 mg [contains phenylalanine 0.84 mg/tablet]

◆ **Ritalin®** *see* Methylphenidate *on page 1107*
◆ **Ritalin LA®** *see* Methylphenidate *on page 1107*
◆ **Ritalin-SR®** *see* Methylphenidate *on page 1107*
◆ **Ritalin® SR (Can)** *see* Methylphenidate *on page 1107*

Ritonavir (ri TOE na veer)

Brand Names: U.S. Norvir®

Brand Names: Canada Norvir®; Norvir® SEC

Pharmacologic Category Antiretroviral Agent, Protease Inhibitor

Additional Appendix Information

Management of Healthcare Worker Exposures to HBV, HCV, and HIV *on page 1935*

Perinatal HIV Guidelines *on page 1946*

Use Treatment of HIV infection; should always be used as part of a multidrug regimen (at least three antiretroviral agents); may be used as a pharmacokinetic "booster" for other protease inhibitors

Pregnancy Risk Factor B

Pregnancy Considerations Adverse events were observed in animal reproduction studies only with doses which were also maternally toxic. Ritonavir crosses the placenta in minimal amounts; no increased risk of overall birth defects has been observed following first trimester exposure according to data collected by the antiretroviral pregnancy registry. Early studies have shown lower plasma levels during pregnancy compared to postpartum. The DHHS Perinatal HIV Guidelines consider ritonavir to be an alternative protease inhibitor (PI) for use during pregnancy to be used only as a booster for other PIs. A small increased risk of preterm birth has been associated with maternal use of protease inhibitor-based combination antiretroviral (ARV) therapy during pregnancy; however, the benefits of use generally outweigh this risk and PIs should not be withheld if otherwise recommended. Hyperglycemia, new onset of diabetes mellitus, or diabetic ketoacidosis have been reported with protease inhibitors; it is not clear if pregnancy increases this risk.

Regardless of CD4 count or HIV RNA copy number, all HIV-infected pregnant women should receive a combination antepartum ARV drug regimen; this includes women who require therapy for their own health, as well as women who do not yet require therapy for their own health. ARV therapy should be started as soon as possible if required for the woman's health or immediately after the first trimester if not needed for the mothers health (although earlier initiation may be considered). Long-term follow-up is recommended for all infants exposed to ARV medications.

Healthcare providers are encouraged to enroll pregnant women exposed to antiretroviral medications in the Antiretroviral Pregnancy Registry (1-800-258-4263 or www.APRegistry.com). Healthcare providers caring for HIV-infected women and their infants may contact the National Perinatal HIV Hotline (888-448-8765) for clinical consultation (DHHS [perinatal], 2011).

Lactation Excretion in breast milk unknown/not recommended

Contraindications Hypersensitivity to ritonavir or any component of the formulation; concurrent alfuzosin, amiodarone, bepridil, cisapride, dihydroergotamine, ergonovine, ergotamine, flecainide, lovastatin, methylergonovine, midazolam (oral), pimozide, propafenone, quinidine, sildenafil (when used for the treatment of pulmonary arterial hypertension [eg, Revatio®]), simvastatin, St John's wort, triazolam, and voriconazole (when ritonavir ≥800 mg/day)

Warnings/Precautions [U.S. Boxed Warning]: Ritonavir may interact with many medications, resulting in potentially serious and/or life-threatening adverse events. Use with caution in patients taking strong CYP3A4 inhibitors, moderate or strong CYP3A4 inducers and major CYP3A4 substrates (see Drug Interactions); consider alternative agents that avoid or lessen the potential for CYP-mediated interactions. Concomitant use with fluticasone, salmeterol, or high-dose or long-term use of meperidine is not recommended. Do not coadminister colchicine in patient with renal or hepatic impairment

Pancreatitis has been observed; use with caution in patients with increased triglycerides; monitor serum lipase and amylase and for gastrointestinal symptoms. Increases in total cholesterol and triglycerides have been reported; screening should be done prior to therapy and periodically throughout treatment.

Protease inhibitors have been associated with a variety of hypersensitivity events (some severe), including rash, anaphylaxis (rare), angioedema, bronchospasm, erythema multiforme, toxic epidermal necrolysis, and/or Stevens-Johnson syndrome (rare). It is generally recommended to discontinue treatment if severe rash or moderate symptoms accompanied by other systemic symptoms occur. Use with caution in patients with cardiomyopathy, ischemic heart disease, pre-existing conduction abnormalities, or structural heart disease; may be at increased risk of conduction abnormalities (eg, second- or third-degree AV block). Ritonavir has been associated with AV block due to prolongation of PR interval; use caution with drugs that prolong the PR interval. Use with caution in patients with hemophilia A or B; increased bleeding during protease inhibitor therapy has been reported. Changes in glucose tolerance, hyperglycemia, exacerbation of diabetes, DKA, and new-onset diabetes mellitus have been reported in patients receiving protease inhibitors. May be associated with fat redistribution (buffalo hump, increased abdominal girth, breast engorgement, facial atrophy, and dyslipidemia). Immune reconstitution syndrome may develop resulting in the occurrence of an inflammatory response to an indolent or residual opportunistic infection; further evaluation and treatment may be required. May cause hepatitis or exacerbate pre-existing hepatic dysfunction; use with caution in patients with hepatitis B or C and in hepatic disease. Norvir® tablets are **not** bioequivalent to Norvir® capsules. Gastrointestinal side effects (eg, nausea, vomiting, abdominal pain, diarrhea) or paresthesias may be more common when patients are switching from the capsule to the tablet formulation due to a higher C_{max} (26% increase) observed with the tablet formulation compared to the capsule. These side effects should decrease as therapy is continued. Safety and efficacy have not been established in children <1 month of age.

Adverse Reactions Percentages as reported for combined experiences in both treatment-naive and experienced adults:

>10%:

Endocrine & metabolic: Hypercholesterolemia (>240 mg/dL: 37% to 45%), triglycerides increased (>800 mg/dL: 17% to 34%; >1500 mg/dL: 1% to 13%)

Gastrointestinal: Nausea (26% to 30%), diarrhea (15% to 23%), vomiting (14% to 17%), taste perversion (7% to 11%)

Hepatic: GGT increased (5% to 20%)

Neuromuscular & skeletal: Weakness (10% to 15%), creatine phosphokinase increased (9% to 12%)

2% to 10%:

Cardiovascular: Vasodilation (2%), syncope (1% to 2%)

Central nervous system: Headache (6% to 7%), fever (1% to 5%), dizziness (3% to 4%), insomnia (2% to 3%), somnolence (2% to 3%), depression (2%), anxiety (up to 2%), malaise (1% to 2%)

Dermatologic: Rash (up to 4%)

Endocrine & metabolic: Uric acid increased (up to 4%)

Gastrointestinal: Abdominal pain (6% to 8%), anorexia (2% to 8%), dyspepsia (up to 6%), local throat irritation (2% to 3%), flatulence (1% to 2%)

Hepatic: Transaminases increased (6% to 10%)

Neuromuscular & skeletal: Paresthesia (3% to 7%), arthralgia (up to 2%), myalgia (2%)

Respiratory: Pharyngitis (≤1% to 3%)

Miscellaneous: Diaphoresis (2% to 3%)

<2% (Limited to important or life-threatening): Abnormal vision. acute myeloblastic leukemia, adrenal cortex insufficiency, adrenal suppression, anaphylaxis, allergic reaction, amnesia, anemia, angioedema, aphasia, asthma, atrioventricular block (first, second, or third degree), bleeding increased (in patients with hemophilia A or B), bronchospasm, cachexia, cerebral ischemia, cerebral venous thrombosis, chest pain, cholestatic jaundice, coma, Cushing's syndrome, dehydration, dementia, depersonalization, diabetes mellitus, dyspnea, edema, esophageal ulcer, gastroenteritis, gastrointestinal hemorrhage, hallucinations, hepatic coma, hepatitis, hepatomegaly, hepatosplenomegaly, hyper-/hypotension, hypercholesteremia, hypothermia, hypoventilation, ileus, interstitial pneumonia, kidney failure, larynx edema, leukopenia, lymphadenopathy, lymphocytosis, manic reaction, MI, myeloproliferative disorder, neuropathy, orthostatic hypotension,palpitation, pancreatitis, paralysis, postural hypotension, pseudomembranous colitis, QT prolongation, rectal hemorrhage, redistribution of body fat,right bundle branch block, seizure, skin melanoma, Stevens-Johnson syndrome, subdural hematoma, syncope, tachycardia, thrombocytopenia, tongue edema, torsade de pointes, toxic epidermal necrolysis, ulcerative colitis, urticaria, vasospasm

Drug Interactions

Metabolism/Transport Effects **Substrate** of CYP1A2 (minor), CYP2B6 (minor), CYP2D6 (minor), CYP3A4 (major), P-glycoprotein; **Note:** Assignment of Major/Minor substrate status based on clinically relevant drug interaction potential; **Inhibits** CYP2C19 (weak), CYP2C8 (strong), CYP2C9 (weak), CYP2D6 (strong), CYP2E1 (weak), CYP3A4 (strong), P-glycoprotein; **Induces** CYP1A2 (weak/moderate), CYP2C9 (weak/moderate), CYP3A4 (weak/moderate)

Avoid Concomitant Use

Avoid concomitant use of Ritonavir with any of the following: Alfuzosin; Amiodarone; Cisapride; Conivaptan; Crizotinib; Disulfiram; Dronedarone; Eplerenone; Ergot Derivatives; Etravirine; Everolimus; Flecainide; Fluticasone (Nasal); Fluticasone (Oral Inhalation); Halofantrine; Lapatinib; Lovastatin; Lurasidone; Midazolam; Nilotinib; Nisoldipine; Pimozide; Propafenone; QuiNIDine; QuiNINE; Ranolazine; Rifampin; Rivaroxaban; RomiDEPsin; Salmeterol; Silodosin; Simvastatin; St Johns Wort; Tamsulosin; Thioridazine; Ticagrelor; Tolvaptan; Topotecan; Toremifene; Triazolam; Voriconazole

Increased Effect/Toxicity

Ritonavir may increase the levels/effects of: Alfuzosin; Almotriptan; Alosetron; ALPRAZolam; Amiodarone; Antifungal Agents (Azole Derivatives, Systemic); ARIPiprazole; Atomoxetine; Bortezomib; Bosentan; Brentuximab Vedotin; Brinzolamide; Budesonide (Nasal); Budesonide (Systemic, Oral Inhalation); Calcium Channel Blockers (Dihydropyridine); Calcium Channel Blockers (Nondihydropyridine); CarBAMazepine; Ciclesonide; Cisapride; Clarithromycin; Clorazepate; Colchicine; Conivaptan; Corticosteroids (Orally Inhaled); Crizotinib; CycloSPORINE; CycloSPORINE (Systemic); CYP2C8 Substrates; CYP2D6 Substrates; CYP3A4 Substrates; Dabigatran Etexilate; Diazepam; Dienogest; Digoxin; Dronabinol; Dronedarone; Dutasteride; Enfuvirtide; Eplerenone; Ergot Derivatives; Estazolam; Everolimus; FentaNYL; Fesoterodine; Flecainide; Flurazepam; Fluticasone (Nasal); Fluticasone (Oral Inhalation); Fusidic Acid; GuanFACINE; Halofantrine; HMG-CoA Reductase Inhibitors; Iloperidone; Ixabepilone; Lapatinib; Linagliptin; Lovastatin; Lumefantrine; Lurasidone; Maraviroc; Meperidine; MethylPREDNISolone; Midazolam; Nebivolol; Nefazodone; Nilotinib; Nisoldipine; Paricalcitol; Pazopanib; P-glycoprotein/ABCB1 Substrates; Pimecrolimus; Pimozide; PrednisoLONE; PredniSONE; Propafenone; Protease Inhibitors; QuiNIDine; QuiNINE; Ranolazine; Rifabutin; Rivaroxaban; RomiDEPsin; Ruxolitinib; Salmeterol; Saxagliptin; Sildenafil; Silodosin; Simvastatin; Sirolimus; SORAfenib; Tacrolimus; Tacrolimus (Systemic); Tacrolimus (Topical); Tadalafil; Tamsulosin; Telaprevir; Temsirolimus; Tenofovir; Tetrabenazine; Thioridazine; Ticagrelor; Tolterodine; Tolvaptan; Topotecan; Toremifene; TraZODone; Treprostinil; Triazolam; Tricyclic Antidepressants; Vardenafil; Vemurafenib; Vilazodone; VinBLAStine; VinCRIStine; Zuclopenthixol

The levels/effects of Ritonavir may be increased by: Antifungal Agents (Azole Derivatives, Systemic); Clarithromycin; CycloSPORINE; CycloSPORINE (Systemic); Delavirdine; Disulfiram; Efavirenz; Enfuvirtide; Fusidic Acid; MetroNIDAZOLE (Topical); P-glycoprotein/ABCB1 Inhibitors; QuiNINE

Decreased Effect

Ritonavir may decrease the levels/effects of: Abacavir; ARIPiprazole; Atovaquone; BuPROPion; Clarithromycin; Codeine; Contraceptives (Estrogens); Deferasirox; Delavirdine; Divalproex; Etravirine; Fosphenytoin; LamoTRIgine; Meperidine; Methadone; Phenytoin; Prasugrel; Telaprevir; Theophylline Derivatives; Ticagrelor; TraMADol; Valproic Acid; Voriconazole; Warfarin; Zidovudine

The levels/effects of Ritonavir may be decreased by: Antacids; CarBAMazepine; CYP3A4 Inducers (Strong); Cyproterone; Efavirenz; Fosphenytoin; Garlic; Peginterferon Alfa-2b; P-glycoprotein/ABCB1 Inducers; Phenytoin; Rifampin; St Johns Wort; Tenofovir; Tocilizumab

Ethanol/Nutrition/Herb Interactions

Food: Food enhances absorption.

Herb/Nutraceutical: St John's wort may decrease ritonavir serum levels. Avoid use.

Stability

Capsule: Store under refrigeration at 2°C to 8°C (36°F to 46°F); may be left out at room temperature of <25°C (<77°F) if used within 30 days. Protect from light. Avoid exposure to excessive heat.

Solution: Store at room temperature at 20°C to 25°C (68°F to 77°F); do not refrigerate. Avoid exposure to excessive heat.

Tablet: Store at room temperature at 20°C to 25°C (68°F to 77°F); excursions permitted to 15°C to 30°C (59°F to 86°F); avoid exposure to excessive heat. Exposure to high humidity outside of the original container (or a USP equivalent container) for >2 weeks is not recommended.

Mechanism of Action Binds to the site of HIV-1 protease activity and inhibits cleavage of viral Gag-Pol polyprotein precursors into individual functional proteins required for infectious HIV. This results in the formation of immature, noninfectious viral particles.

Pharmacodynamics/Kinetics

Absorption: Variable; increased with food; In the fed state, mean C_{max} of the tablet formulation increased by 26% compared to the capsule.

Distribution: High concentrations in serum and lymph nodes; V_d: 0.16-0.66 L/kg

Protein binding: 98% to 99%

Metabolism: Hepatic via CYP3A4 and 2D6; five metabolites, low concentration of an active metabolite (M-2) achieved in plasma (oxidative)

Half-life elimination: 3-5 hours

Time to peak, plasma: Oral solution: 2 hours (fasted); 4 hours (nonfasted)

Excretion: Urine (~11%, ~4% as unchanged drug); feces (~86%, ~34% as unchanged drug)

Dosage Note: Norvir® tablets are **not** bioequivalent to Norvir® capsules. Gastrointestinal side effects or paresthesias may be more common initially when patients are switching from the capsule to the tablet formulation.

Treatment of HIV infection: Oral:

Children >1 month: 350-400 mg/m² twice daily (maximum dose: 600 mg twice daily). Initiate dose at 250 mg/m² twice daily; titrate dose upward every 2-3 days by 50 mg/m² twice daily.

Adults (not recommended as the primary protease inhibitor in any regimen [DHHS, 2011]): 600 mg twice daily; dose escalation tends to avoid nausea that many patients experience upon initiation of full dosing. Escalate the dose as follows: 300 mg twice daily for 1 day, then increase by 100 mg twice daily every 2-3 days to recommended dosage of 600 mg twice daily

Pharmacokinetic "booster" in combination with other protease inhibitors: 100-400 mg/day

Note: Recommended as the "booster" component in the following regimens in treatment-naive patients: Atazanavir and tenofovir/emtricitabine, or darunavir and tenofovir/emtricitabine (DHHS, 2011). In patients without evidence of PI resistance, once-daily booster-dosing of 100 mg ritonavir may be preferred to 200 mg/day due to less gastrointestinal and metabolic adverse events. Refer to individual protease inhibitor monographs; specific dosage recommendations often require adjustment of both agents.

Dosage adjustments for concomitant therapy: Adults:

Coadministration with bosentan:

Coadministration of bosentan in patients currently receiving ritonavir: For patients receiving ritonavir for at least 10 days, begin with bosentan 62.5 mg once daily or every other day based on tolerability

Coadministration of ritonavir in patients currently receiving bosentan: Discontinue bosentan 36 hours prior to the initiation of ritonavir. After at least 10 days of ritonavir, resume bosentan 62.5 mg once daily or every other day based on tolerability.

Coadministration with colchicine:

Familial Mediterranean fever (FMF): Maximum colchicine dose: 0.6 mg/day (0.3 mg twice daily)

Gout prophylaxis:

If original colchicine dose is 0.6 mg twice daily, adjust dose to 0.3 mg once daily

If original colchicine dose is 0.6 mg once daily, adjust dose to 0.3 mg every other day

Gout flare treatment: Initial: Colchicine 0.6 mg, followed in 1 hour by a single dose of 0.3 mg; do not repeat for at least 3 days

Coadministration with phosphodiesterase-5 enzyme (PDE-5) inhibitor:

Pulmonary arterial hypertension: Ritonavir coadministered with tadalafil:

Patient receiving ritonavir for at least 1 week: Initiate tadalafil at 20 mg once daily; increase to 40 mg once daily based on individual tolerability

Patient receiving tadalafil when initiating ritonavir: Stop tadalafil at least 24 hours prior to starting ritonavir. After at least 1 week following the initiation of ritonavir, resume tadalafil at 20 mg once daily; increase to 40 mg once daily based on individual tolerability.

Erectile dysfunction: Ritonavir coadministered with:

Sildenafil (Viagra®): Maximum sildenafil dose: 25 mg in a 48-hour period

Tadalafil (Cialis®): Maximum tadalafil dose: 10 mg in a 72-hour period

Vardenafil: Maximum vardenafil dose: 2.5 mg in a 72-hour period

Dosing adjustment in renal impairment: None necessary

Dosing adjustment in hepatic impairment: No adjustment required in mild or moderate impairment; however, careful monitoring is required in moderate hepatic impairment (levels may be decreased); caution advised with severe impairment (no data available)

Dietary Considerations Should be taken with food. Oral solution contains 43% ethanol by volume.

Administration Administer capsules or oral solution with or without food (DHHS, 2011). Food improves tolerability. Liquid formulations usually have an unpleasant taste. Consider mixing it with chocolate milk or a liquid nutritional supplement. Whenever possible, administer oral solution with calibrated dosing syringe. Shake liquid well before use. Tablets should be administered with food and swallowed whole; do not chew, break, or crush.

Monitoring Parameters Triglycerides, cholesterol, CBC, LFTs, CPK, uric acid, basic HIV monitoring, viral load, CD4 count, glucose, serum amylase and lipase

Additional Information Potential compliance problems, frequency of administration and adverse effects should be discussed with patients before initiating therapy to help prevent the emergence of resistance.

Tipranavir with "boosted" ritonavir is not a recommended regimen due to inferior virilogic efficacy; do not use (DHHS, 2011).

Dosage Forms Excipient information presented when available (limited, particularly for generics); consult specific product labeling.

Capsule, soft gelatin, oral:
  Norvir®: 100 mg [contains ethanol, polyoxyl 35 castor oil]
Solution, oral:
  Norvir®: 80 mg/mL (240 mL) [contains ethanol, polyoxyl 35 castor oil, propylene glycol; peppermint-caramel flavor]
Tablet, oral:
  Norvir®: 100 mg

◆ **Ritonavir and Lopinavir** *see* Lopinavir and Ritonavir *on page 1028*

◆ **Rituxan®** *see* RiTUXimab *on page 1503*

RiTUXimab (ri TUK si mab)

Brand Names: U.S. Rituxan®

Brand Names: Canada Rituxan®

Index Terms Anti-CD20 Monoclonal Antibody; C2B8 Monoclonal Antibody; IDEC-C2B8

Pharmacologic Category Antineoplastic Agent, Monoclonal Antibody; Monoclonal Antibody

Use

Treatment of CD20-positive non-Hodgkin's lymphomas (NHL):
  Relapsed or refractory, low-grade or follicular B-cell NHL (as a single agent)
  Follicular B-cell NHL, previously untreated (in combination with first-line chemotherapy, and as single-agent maintenance therapy if response to first-line rituximab with chemotherapy)
  Nonprogressing, low-grade B-cell NHL (as a single agent after first-line CVP treatment)
  Diffuse large B-cell NHL, previously untreated (in combination with CHOP chemotherapy [or other anthracycline-based regimen])
Treatment of CD20-positive chronic lymphocytic leukemia (CLL) (in combination with fludarabine and cyclophosphamide)
Treatment of moderately- to severely-active rheumatoid arthritis (in combination with methotrexate) in adult patients with inadequate response to one or more TNF antagonists
Treatment of Wegener's granulomatosis (WG) (in combination with glucocorticoids)
Treatment of microscopic polyangiitis (MPA) (in combination with glucocorticoids)

Unlabeled Use Treatment of Burkitt's lymphoma, central nervous system lymphoma, Hodgkin's lymphoma (lymphocyte predominant); mucosal associated lymphoid tissue (MALT) lymphoma (gastric and nongastric), splenic marginal zone lymphoma; Waldenström's macroglobulinemia (WM); post-transplant lymphoproliferative disorder (PTLD); autoimmune hemolytic anemia (AIHA) in children; chronic immune thrombocytopenic purpura (ITP); refractory pemphigus vulgaris; treatment of steroid-refractory chronic graft-versus-host disease (GVHD)

Pregnancy Risk Factor C

Pregnancy Considerations Animal studies have demonstrated adverse effects including decreased (reversible) B-cells and immunosuppression. IgG molecules are known to cross the placenta (rituximab is an engineered IgG molecule) and rituximab has been detected in the serum of infants exposed in utero. B-Cell lymphocytopenia lasting <6 months may occur in exposed infants. Retrospective case reports of inadvertent pregnancy during rituximab treatment (often combined with concomitant teratogenic therapies) describe premature births, and infant hematologic abnormalities and infections; no specific pattern of birth defects has been observed (limited data). Effective contraception should be used during and for 12 months following treatment. Healthcare providers are encouraged to enroll women with rheumatoid arthritis exposed to rituximab during pregnancy in the OTIS AutoImmune Diseases Study by contacting the Organization of Teratology Information Specialists (877-311-8972).

Lactation Excretion in breast milk unknown/not recommended

Medication Guide Available Yes

Contraindications There are no contraindications listed in the FDA-approved manufacturer's labeling.

Canadian labeling (not in U.S. labeling): Type 1 hypersensitivity or anaphylactic reaction to murine proteins, Chinese Hamster Ovary (CHO) cell proteins, or any component of the formulation; patients who have or have had progressive multifocal leukoencephalopathy (PML)

Warnings/Precautions **[U.S. Boxed Warning]: Severe (occasionally fatal) infusion-related reactions have been reported, usually with the first infusion; fatalities have been reported within 24 hours of infusion; monitor closely during infusion; discontinue with grades 3 or 4 infusion reactions.** Reactions usually occur within 30-120 minutes and may include hypotension, angioedema, bronchospasm, hypoxia, urticaria, and in more severe cases pulmonary infiltrates, acute respiratory distress syndrome, myocardial infarction, ventricular fibrillation, cardiogenic shock and/or anaphylaxis. Risk factors associated with fatal outcomes include chronic lymphocytic leukemia, female gender, mantle cell lymphoma, or pulmonary infiltrates. Closely monitor patients with a history of prior cardiopulmonary reactions or with pre-existing cardiac or pulmonary conditions and patients with high numbers of circulating malignant cells (>25,000/mm^3). Prior to infusion, premedicate patients with acetaminophen and an antihistamine (and methylprednisolone for patients with RA). Discontinue infusion for severe reactions; treatment is symptomatic. Medications for the treatment of hypersensitivity reactions (eg, bronchodilators, epinephrine, antihistamines, corticosteroids) should be available for immediate use. Discontinue infusion for serious or life-threatening cardiac arrhythmias; subsequent doses should include cardiac monitoring during and after the infusion. Mild-to-moderate infusion-related reactions (eg, chills, fever, rigors) occur frequently and are typically managed through slowing or interrupting the infusion. Infusion may be resumed at a 50% infusion rate reduction upon resolution of symptoms. Due to the potential for hypotension, consider withholding antihypertensives 12 hours prior to treatment.

[U.S. Boxed Warning]: Progressive multifocal leukoencephalopathy (PML) due to JC virus infection has been reported with rituximab use; may be fatal. Cases were reported in patients with hematologic malignancies receiving rituximab either with combination chemotherapy, or with hematopoietic stem cell transplant. Cases were also reported in patients receiving rituximab for autoimmune diseases who had received prior or concurrent immunosuppressant therapy. Onset may be delayed, although most cases were diagnosed within 12 months of the last rituximab dose. A retrospective analysis of patients (n=57) diagnosed with PML following rituximab therapy, found a median of 16 months (following rituximab initiation), 5.5 months (following last rituximab dose), and 6 rituximab doses preceded PML diagnosis. Clinical findings included confusion/disorientation, motor weakness/hemiparesis, altered vision/speech, and poor motor coordination with symptoms progressing over weeks to months (Carson, 2009). Promptly evaluate any patient presenting with neurological changes; consider neurology consultation, brain MRI and lumbar puncture for suspected PML. Discontinue rituximab in patients who develop PML; consider reduction/discontinuation of concurrent chemotherapy or immunosuppressants. Avoid use if severe active infection is present. Serious and potentially fatal bacterial, fungal, and either new or reactivated viral infections may occur during treatment, and up to 1 year after completing rituximab. Associated new or reactivated viral infections have included cytomegalovirus, herpes simplex virus, parvovirus B19, varicella zoster virus, West Nile virus, and hepatitis B and C. Rarely, reactivation of hepatitis B (with fulminant hepatitis, hepatic failure, and death) has been reported in association with rituximab; median time to hepatitis diagnosis was ~4 months after initiation of therapy and 1 month following last dose; screen high-risk patients prior to therapy initiation; monitor for several months following completion of therapy. Discontinue rituximab (and concomitant chemotherapy) in patients who develop viral hepatitis and initiate antiviral therapy. Discontinue rituximab in patients who develop other serious infections and initiate appropriate anti-infective treatment.

[U.S. Boxed Warning]: Tumor lysis syndrome leading to acute renal failure requiring dialysis may occur 12-24 hours following the first dose when used as a single agent in the treatment of NHL. Hyperkalemia, hypocalcemia, hyperuricemia, and/or hyperphosphatemia may occur. Administer prophylaxis (allopurinol, hydration) in patients at high risk (high numbers of circulating malignant cells ≥25,000/mm^3 or high tumor burden). May cause fatal renal toxicity in patients with hematologic malignancies. Patients who received combination therapy with cisplatin and rituximab for NHL experienced renal toxicity during clinical trials; this combination is not an approved treatment regimen. Monitor for signs of renal failure; discontinue rituximab with increasing serum creatinine or oliguria. Correct electrolyte abnormalities; monitor hydration status.

[U.S. Boxed Warning]: Severe and sometimes fatal mucocutaneous reactions (lichenoid dermatitis, paraneoplastic pemphigus, Stevens-Johnson syndrome, toxic epidermal necrolysis and vesiculobullous dermatitis) have been reported, occurring from 1-13 weeks following exposure. Discontinue in patients experiencing severe mucocutaneous skin reactions; the safety of re-exposure following mucocutaneous reactions has not been evaluated. Use caution with pre-existing cardiac or pulmonary disease, or prior cardiopulmonary events. Rheumatoid arthritis patients are at increased risk for cardiovascular events; monitor closely during and after each infusion. Elderly patients are at higher risk for cardiac (supraventricular arrhythmia) and pulmonary adverse events (pneumonia, pneumonitis). Abdominal pain, bowel obstruction, and perforation (rarely fatal) have been reported with an average onset of symptoms of ~6 days (range: 1-77 days); complaints of abdominal pain should be evaluated, especially if early in the treatment course. Live vaccines should not be given concurrently with rituximab; there is no data available concerning secondary transmission of live vaccines with or following rituximab treatment. RA patients should be brought up to date with nonlive immunizations (following current guidelines) at least 4 weeks before initiating therapy; evaluate risks of therapy delay versus benefit (of nonlive vaccines) for NHL patients. Safety and efficacy of rituximab in combination with biologic agents or disease-modifying antirheumatic drugs (DMARD) other than methotrexate have not been established. Rituximab is not recommended for use in RA patients who have not had prior inadequate response to TNF antagonists. Safety and efficacy of retreatment for RA have not been established. The safety of concomitant immunosuppressants other than corticosteroids has not been evaluated in patients with Wegener's granulomatosis (WG) or microscopic polyangiitis (MPA) after rituximab-induced B-cell depletion. There are only limited data on subsequent courses of rituximab for WG or MPA; safety and efficacy of retreatment has not been established.

Adverse Reactions Note: Patients treated with rituximab for rheumatoid arthritis (RA) may experience fewer adverse reactions.

>10%:

Cardiovascular: Peripheral edema (8% to 16%), hypertension (6% to 12%)

Central nervous system: Fever (5% to 53%), fatigue (13% to 39%), chills (3% to 33%), headache (17% to 19%), insomnia (≤14%), pain (12%)

Dermatologic: Rash (10% to 17%; grades 3/4: 1%), pruritus (5% to 17%), angioedema (11%; grades 3/4: 1%)

Gastrointestinal: Nausea (8% to 23%), diarrhea (10% to 17%), abdominal pain (2% to 14%), weight gain (11%)

Hematologic: Cytopenias (grades 3/4: ≤48%; may be prolonged), lymphopenia (48%; grades 3/4: 40%; median duration 14 days), anemia (8% to 35%; grades 3/4: 3%), leukopenia (NHL: 14%; grades 3/4: 4%; CLL: grades 3/4: 23%; WG/MPA: 10%), neutropenia (NHL: 14%; grades 3/4: 4% to 6%; median duration 13 days; CLL: grades 3/4: 30% to 49%), neutropenic fever (CLL: grades 3/4: 9% to 15%), thrombocytopenia (12%; grades 3/4: 2% to 11%)

Hepatic: ALT increased (≤13%)

Neuromuscular & skeletal: Neuropathy (≤30%), weakness (2% to 26%), muscle spasm (≤17%), arthralgia (6% to 13%)

Respiratory: Cough (13%), rhinitis (3% to 12%), epistaxis (≤11%)

Miscellaneous: Infusion-related reactions (lymphoma: first dose 77%; decreases with subsequent infusions; may include angioedema, bronchospasm, chills, dizziness, fever, headache, hyper-/hypotension, myalgia, nausea, pruritus, rash, rigors, urticaria, and vomiting; reactions reported are lower [first infusion: 32%] in RA; CLL: 59%; grades 3/4: 7% to 9%; WG/MPA: 12%); infection (19% to 62%; grades 3/4: 4%; bacterial: 19%; viral 10%; fungal: 1%), human antichimeric antibody (HACA) positive (1% to 23%), night sweats (15%)

1% to 10%:

Cardiovascular: Hypotension (10%; grades 3/4: 2%), flushing (5%)

Central nervous system: Dizziness (10%), anxiety (2% to 5%), migraine (RA: 2%)

Dermatologic: Urticaria (2% to 8%)

Endocrine & metabolic: Hyperglycemia (9%)

Gastrointestinal: Vomiting (10%), dyspepsia (RA: 3%)

Neuromuscular & skeletal: Back pain (10%), myalgia (10%), paresthesia (2%)

Respiratory: Dyspnea (≤10%), throat irritation (2% to 9%), bronchospasm (8%), dyspnea (7%), upper respiratory tract infection (RA: 7%), sinusitis (6%)

Miscellaneous: LDH increased (7%)

Postmarketing and/or case reports: Acute renal failure, anaphylactoid reaction/anaphylaxis, angina, aplastic anemia, ARDS, arrhythmia, bowel obstruction/perforation, bronchiolitis obliterans, cardiac failure, cardiogenic shock, encephalomyelitis, fatal infusion-related reactions, fulminant hepatitis, gastrointestinal perforation, hemolytic anemia, hepatic failure, hepatitis, hepatitis B reactivation, hyperviscosity syndrome (in Waldenström's macroglobulinemia), hypogammaglobulinemia, hypoxia, interstitial pneumonitis, laryngeal edema, lichenoid dermatitis, lupus-like syndrome, marrow hypoplasia, MI, mucositis, mucocutaneous reaction, neutropenia (late-onset occurring >40 days after last dose), optic neuritis, pancytopenia (prolonged), paraneoplastic pemphigus (uncommon), pleuritis, pneumonia, pneumonitis, polyarticular arthritis, polymyositis, posterior reversible encephalopathy syndrome (PRES), progressive multifocal leukoencephalopathy (PML), pure red cell aplasia, renal toxicity, reversible posterior leukoencephalopathy syndrome (RPLS), serum sickness, Stevens-Johnson syndrome, supraventricular arrhythmia, systemic vasculitis, toxic epidermal necrolysis, tuberculosis reactivation, tumor lysis syndrome, uveitis, vasculitis with rash, ventricular fibrillation, ventricular tachycardia, vesiculobullous dermatitis, viral reactivation (includes JC virus, cytomegalovirus, herpes simplex virus, parvovirus B19, varicella zoster virus, West Nile virus, and hepatitis C), wheezing

Drug Interactions

Metabolism/Transport Effects None known.

Avoid Concomitant Use

Avoid concomitant use of RiTUXimab with any of the following: BCG; Belimumab; Certolizumab Pegol; CloZAPine; Natalizumab; Pimecrolimus; Tacrolimus (Topical); Vaccines (Live)

Increased Effect/Toxicity

RiTUXimab may increase the levels/effects of: Belimumab; Certolizumab Pegol; CloZAPine; Hypoglycemic Agents; Leflunomide; Natalizumab; Vaccines (Live)

The levels/effects of RiTUXimab may be increased by: Abciximab; Antihypertensives; Denosumab; Herbs (Hypoglycemic Properties); Pimecrolimus; Roflumilast; Tacrolimus (Topical); Trastuzumab

Decreased Effect

RiTUXimab may decrease the levels/effects of: BCG; Coccidioidin Skin Test; Sipuleucel-T; Vaccines (Inactivated); Vaccines (Live)

The levels/effects of RiTUXimab may be decreased by: Echinacea

Ethanol/Nutrition/Herb Interactions Herb/Nutraceutical: Avoid echinacea (may diminish the therapeutic effect of immunosuppressants). Avoid hypoglycemic herbs, including alfalfa, aloe, bilberry, bitter melon, burdock, celery, damiana, fenugreek, garcinia, garlic, ginger, ginseng (American), gymnema, marshmallow, and stinging nettle (may enhance the hypoglycemic effect of rituximab).

Stability Store vials under refrigeration at 2°C to 8°C (36°F to 46°F); do not freeze. Do not shake. Protect vials from direct sunlight.

Withdraw the necessary amount of rituximab and dilute to a final concentration of 1-4 mg/mL with 0.9% sodium chloride or 5% dextrose in water. Gently invert the bag to mix the solution; do not shake. Solutions for infusion are stable at 2°C to 8°C (36°F to 46°F) for 24 hours and at room temperature for an additional 24 hours.

Mechanism of Action Rituximab is a monoclonal antibody directed against the CD20 antigen on B-lymphocytes. CD20 regulates cell cycle initiation; and, possibly, functions as a calcium channel. Rituximab binds to the antigen on the cell surface, activating complement-dependent B-cell cytotoxicity; and to human Fc receptors, mediating cell killing through an antibody-dependent cellular toxicity. B-cells are believed to play a role in the development and progression of rheumatoid arthritis. Signs and symptoms of RA are reduced by targeting B-cells and the progression of structural damage is delayed.

Pharmacodynamics/Kinetics

Duration: Detectable in serum 3-6 months after completion of treatment; B-cell recovery begins ~6 months following completion of treatment; median B-cell levels return to normal by 12 months following completion of treatment

Absorption: I.V.: Immediate and results in a rapid and sustained depletion of circulating and tissue-based B cells

Distribution: RA: 3.1 L; WG/MPA: 4.5 L

Half-life elimination:

CLL: Median terminal half-life: 32 days (range: 14-62 days)

NHL: Median terminal half-life: 22 days (range: 6-52 days)

RA: Mean terminal half-life: 18 days (range: 5-78 days)

WG/MPA: 23 days (range: 9-49 days)

Excretion: Uncertain; may undergo phagocytosis and catabolism in the reticuloendothelial system (RES)

Dosage Note: Details concerning dosing in combination regimens should also be consulted. Pretreatment with acetaminophen and an antihistamine is recommended for all indications. For oncology uses, a uricostatic agent (eg, allopurinol) and aggressive hydration is recommended for patients at risk for tumor lysis syndrome (high tumor burden or lymphocytes >25,000/mm^3). In patients with CLL, *Pneumocystis jirovecii* pneumonia (PCP) and anti-herpetic viral prophylaxis is recommended during treatment (and for up to 12 months following treatment). In patients with WG and MPA, PCP prophylaxis is recommended during and for 6 months after rituximab treatment. For patients with RA, premedication with methylprednisolone 100 mg I.V. (or equivalent) is recommended 30 minutes prior to each dose.

Children: I.V. infusion:

AIHA (unlabeled use): 375 mg/m^2 once weekly for 2-4 doses (Zecca, 2003)

Chronic ITP (unlabeled use): 375 mg/m^2 once weekly for 4 doses (Parodi, 2009; Wang, 2005)

Adults: I.V. infusion:

CLL: 375 mg/m^2 on the day prior to fludarabine/cyclophosphamide in cycle 1, then 500 mg/m^2 on day 1 (every 28 days) of cycles 2-6

NHL (relapsed/refractory, low-grade or follicular CD20-positive, B-cell): 375 mg/m^2 once weekly for 4 or 8 doses

Retreatment following disease progression: 375 mg/m^2 once weekly for 4 doses

NHL (diffuse large B-cell): 375 mg/m^2 given on day 1 of each chemotherapy cycle for up to 8 doses

NHL (follicular, CD20-positive, B-cell, previously untreated): 375 mg/m^2 given on day 1 of each chemotherapy cycle for up to 8 doses

Maintenance therapy (as a single agent, in patients with partial or complete response to rituximab plus chemotherapy; begin 8 weeks after completion of combination chemotherapy): 375 mg/m^2 every 8 weeks for 12 doses

NHL (nonprogressing, low-grade, CD20-positive, B-cell, after first line CVP): 375 mg/m^2 once weekly for 4 doses every 6 months for up to 4 cycles (initiate after 6-8 cycles of chemotherapy are completed)

NHL: Combination therapy with ibritumomab: 250 mg/m^2 I.V. day 1; repeat in 7-9 days with ibritumomab (also see Ibritumomab monograph)

Canadian labeling: NHL, low grade or follicular:

Initial: 375 mg/m^2 once weekly for 4 doses (as a single agent) or 375 mg/m^2 on day 1 of each 21-day cycle for 8 cycles (in combination with CVP chemotherapy)

Maintenance (responding to induction therapy): 375 mg/m^2 every 3 months until disease progression or up to a maximum of 2 years

Rheumatoid arthritis: 1000 mg on days 1 and 15 in combination with methotrexate; subsequent courses may be administered every 24 weeks (based on clinical evaluation), if necessary may be repeated no sooner than every 16 weeks

Wegener's granulomatosis (WG): 375 mg/m^2 once weekly for 4 doses (in combination with methylprednisolone I.V. for 1-3 days followed by daily prednisone)

Microscopic polyangiitis (MPA): 375 mg/m^2 once weekly for 4 doses (in combination with methylprednisolone I.V. for 1-3 days followed by daily prednisone)

Chronic GVHD, refractory (unlabeled use): 375 mg/m^2 once weekly for 4 doses (Cutler, 2006)

Chronic ITP (unlabeled use): 375 mg/m^2 once weekly for 4 doses (Arnold, 2007; Godeau, 2008)

Hodgkin's lymphoma (unlabeled use): 375 mg/m^2 once weekly for 4 weeks (Ekstrand, 2003; Schulz, 2008)

Pemphigus vulgaris, refractory (unlabeled use): 375 mg/m^2 once weekly of weeks 1, 2, and 3 of a 4-week cycle, repeat for 1 additional cycle, then 1 dose per month for 4 months (total of 10 doses in 6 months) (Ahmed, 2006)

Post-transplant lymphoproliferative disorder (unlabeled use): 375 mg/m^2 once weekly for 4 doses (Choquet, 2006)

Waldenström's macroglobulinemia (unlabeled use): 375 mg/m^2 once weekly for 4 doses (Dimopoulos, 2002)

Administration Do **not** administer I.V. push or bolus.

I.V.: Initial infusion: Start rate of 50 mg/hour; if there is no reaction, increase the rate by 50 mg/hour increments every 30 minutes, to a maximum rate of 400 mg/hour.

Subsequent infusions: If patient did not tolerate initial infusion follow initial infusion guidelines. If patient tolerated initial infusion, start at 100 mg/hour; if there is no reaction, increase the rate by 100 mg/hour increments every 30 minutes, to a maximum rate of 400 mg/hour.

Note: If a reaction occurs, slow or stop the infusion. If the reaction abates, restart infusion at 50% of the previous rate.

In patients with NHL who are receiving a corticosteroid as part of their combination chemotherapy regimen and after tolerance has been established at the recommended infusion rate in cycle 1, a rapid infusion rate has been used beginning with cycle 2. The daily corticosteroid, acetaminophen, and diphenhydramine are administered prior to treatment, then the rituximab dose is administered over 90 minutes, with 20% of the dose administered in the first 30 minutes and the remaining 80% is given over 60 minutes (Sehn, 2007).

Monitoring Parameters CBC with differential and platelets (obtain at weekly to monthly intervals and more frequently in patients with cytopenias, or at 2-4 month intervals in rheumatoid arthritis patients, WG and MPA), peripheral CD20$^+$ cells; HAMA/HACA titers (high levels may increase the risk of allergic reactions); renal function, fluid balance; vital signs; monitor for infusion reactions, cardiac monitoring during and after infusion in rheumatoid arthritis patients and in patients with pre-existing cardiac disease or if arrhythmias develop during or after subsequent infusions

Screen for hepatitis B in high-risk patients prior to initiation of rituximab therapy (the NCCN NHL guidelines recommend screening **all** NHL patients prior to therapy). In addition, carriers and patients with evidence of recovery from prior hepatitis B infection should be monitored closely for clinical and laboratory signs of HBV infection during therapy and for up to a year following completion of treatment. High-risk patients should be screened for hepatitis C (per NCCN guidelines).

Complaints of abdominal pain, especially early in the course of treatment, should prompt a thorough diagnostic evaluation and appropriate treatment. Signs or symptoms of progressive multifocal leukoencephalopathy (focal neurologic deficits, which may present as hemiparesis, visual field deficits, cognitive impairment, aphasia, ataxia, and/or cranial nerve deficits). If PML is suspected, obtain brain MRI scan and lumbar puncture.

Dosage Forms Excipient information presented when available (limited, particularly for generics); consult specific product labeling.

Injection, solution [preservative free]:

Rituxan®: 10 mg/mL (10 mL, 50 mL) [contains polysorbate 80]

◆ **Riva-Alendronate (Can)** *see* Alendronate *on page 61*

◆ **Riva-Amiodarone (Can)** *see* Amiodarone *on page 90*

◆ **Riva-Amlodipine (Can)** *see* AmLODIPine *on page 97*

◆ **Riva-Atenolol (Can)** *see* Atenolol *on page 161*

◆ **Riva-Azithromycin (Can)** *see* Azithromycin (Systemic) *on page 180*

◆ **Riva-Baclofen (Can)** *see* Baclofen *on page 187*

◆ **Riva-Buspirone (Can)** *see* BusPIRone *on page 250*

◆ **Riva-Ciprofloxacin (Can)** *see* Ciprofloxacin (Systemic) *on page 362*

◆ **Riva-Citalopram (Can)** *see* Citalopram *on page 370*

◆ **Riva-Clarithromycin (Can)** *see* Clarithromycin *on page 374*

◆ **Riva-Clindamycin (Can)** *see* Clindamycin (Systemic) *on page 378*

◆ **Riva-Cycloprine (Can)** *see* Cyclobenzaprine *on page 419*

◆ **Riva-Dicyclomine (Can)** *see* Dicyclomine *on page 499*

◆ **Riva-Enalapril (Can)** *see* Enalapril *on page 584*

◆ **Riva-Fenofibrate Micro (Can)** *see* Fenofibrate *on page 693*

◆ **Riva-Fluconazole (Can)** *see* Fluconazole *on page 718*

◆ **Riva-Fluoxetine (Can)** *see* FLUoxetine *on page 731*

◆ **Riva-Fluvox (Can)** *see* FluvoxaMINE *on page 746*

◆ **Riva-Fosinopril (Can)** *see* Fosinopril *on page 763*

◆ **Riva-Gabapentin (Can)** *see* Gabapentin *on page 773*

◆ **Riva-Glyburide (Can)** *see* GlyBURIDE *on page 799*

◆ **Riva-Hydroxyzine (Can)** *see* HydrOXYzine *on page 853*

◆ **Riva-Indapamide (Can)** *see* Indapamide *on page 886*

◆ **Riva-Lisinopril (Can)** *see* Lisinopril *on page 1020*

◆ **Riva-Loperamide (Can)** *see* Loperamide *on page 1026*

◆ **Riva-Lovastatin (Can)** *see* Lovastatin *on page 1038*

◆ **Riva-Memantine (Can)** *see* Memantine *on page 1068*

◆ **Riva-Metformin (Can)** *see* MetFORMIN *on page 1086*

◆ **Riva-Metoprolol (Can)** *see* Metoprolol *on page 1117*

◆ **Riva-Minocycline (Can)** *see* Minocycline *on page 1137*

◆ **Riva-Mirtazapine (Can)** *see* Mirtazapine *on page 1140*

◆ **Riva-Naproxen (Can)** *see* Naproxen *on page 1177*

◆ **Riva-Naproxen Sodium (Can)** *see* Naproxen *on page 1177*

◆ **Riva-Naproxen Sodium DS (Can)** *see* Naproxen *on page 1177*

◆ **Rivanase AQ (Can)** *see* Beclomethasone (Nasal) *on page 194*

◆ **Riva-Norfloxacin (Can)** *see* Norfloxacin *on page 1219*

◆ **Riva-Olanzapine (Can)** *see* OLANZapine *on page 1233*

◆ **Riva-Olanzapine ODT (Can)** *see* OLANZapine *on page 1233*

- ◆ **Riva-Oxazepam (Can)** *see* Oxazepam *on page 1261*
- ◆ **Riva-Oxybutynin (Can)** *see* Oxybutynin *on page 1264*
- ◆ **Riva-Pantoprazole (Can)** *see* Pantoprazole *on page 1289*
- ◆ **Riva-paroxetine (Can)** *see* PARoxetine *on page 1299*
- ◆ **Riva-Pravastatin (Can)** *see* Pravastatin *on page 1394*
- ◆ **Riva-Quetiapine (Can)** *see* QUEtiapine *on page 1440*
- ◆ **Riva-Rabeprazole EC (Can)** *see* RABEprazole *on page 1451*
- ◆ **Riva-Ranitidine (Can)** *see* Ranitidine *on page 1462*
- ◆ **Riva-Risedronate (Can)** *see* Risedronate *on page 1494*
- ◆ **Riva-Risperidone (Can)** *see* RisperiDONE *on page 1496*

Rivaroxaban (riv a ROX a ban)

Brand Names: U.S. Xarelto®
Brand Names: Canada Xarelto®
Index Terms BAY 59-7939
Pharmacologic Category Factor Xa Inhibitor
Use Postoperative thromboprophylaxis in patients who have undergone hip or knee replacement surgery; prevention of stroke and systemic embolism in patients with nonvalvular atrial fibrillation
Pregnancy Risk Factor C
Pregnancy Considerations Postimplantation pregnancy loss, increased fetal toxicity, and maternal hemorrhagic complications have been observed in animal studies. There are no adequate and well-controlled studies in pregnant women. Use with caution during pregnancy; may increase the risk of pregnancy related hemorrhage. Clinicians should note that the anticoagulant effect cannot be easily monitored or readily reversed. Prompt clinical evaluation is warranted with any unexplained decrease in hemoglobin, hematocrit or blood pressure, or fetal distress. Use during pregnancy is contraindicated in the Canadian labeling.
Lactation Excretion in breast milk unknown/not recommended
Medication Guide Available Yes
Contraindications Hypersensitivity to rivaroxaban or any component of the formulation; active pathological bleeding

Canadian labeling: Additional contraindications (not in U.S. labeling): Hepatic disease (including Child-Pugh classes B and C) associated with coagulopathy and clinically relevant bleeding risk; clinically significant active bleeding, including hemorrhagic manifestations and bleeding diathesis; lesions at increased risk of clinically significant bleeding (eg, hemorrhagic or ischemic cerebral infarction) within previous 6 months; spontaneous hemostasis impairment; concomitant systemic treatment with strong CYP3A4 and P-glycoprotein (P-gp) inhibitors; pregnancy; lactation

Warnings/Precautions Most common complication is bleeding; major hemorrhages (eg, intracranial, GI, retinal, epidural hematoma, adrenal bleeding) have been reported. Certain patients are at increased risk of bleeding; risk factors include bacterial endocarditis, congenital or acquired bleeding disorders, thrombocytopenia, recent puncture of large vessels or organ biopsy, stroke, intracerebral surgery, or other neuraxial procedure, severe uncontrolled hypertension, renal impairment, recent major surgery, recent major bleeding (intracranial, GI, intraocular, or pulmonary), concomitant use of drugs that affect hemostasis. Monitor for signs and symptoms of bleeding. Prompt clinical evaluation is warranted with any unexplained decrease in hemoglobin or blood pressure. Avoid use with direct thrombin inhibitors (eg, bivalirudin), unfractionated heparin or heparin derivatives, low molecular weight heparins (eg, enoxaparin), aspirin, coumarin derivatives, and sulfinpyrazone. NSAIDs and other platelet aggregation inhibitors (eg, clopidogrel) should be used cautiously.

[U.S. Boxed Warning]: Spinal or epidural hematomas, including subsequent paralysis, may occur with neuraxial anesthesia (epidural or spinal anesthesia) or spinal puncture in patients who are anticoagulated; the risk is increased with concomitant administration of other drugs that affect hemostasis (eg, NSAIDS, platelet inhibitors, other anticoagulants), in patients with a history of traumatic or repeated epidural or spinal punctures, or a history of spinal deformity or surgery. In patients who receive both rivaroxaban and neuraxial anesthesia, avoid removal of epidural catheter for at least 18 hours following last rivaroxaban dose; avoid rivaroxaban administration for at least 6 hours following epidural catheter removal; if traumatic puncture occurs, avoid rivaroxaban administration for at least 24 hours. Monitor for signs of neurologic impairment (eg, numbness/weakness of legs, bowel/bladder dysfunction); prompt diagnosis and treatment are necessary.

[U.S. Boxed Warning]: An increased risk of stroke was noted upon discontinuation of rivaroxaban in clinical trials of patients with atrial fibrillation; consider the addition of alternative anticoagulant therapy when discontinuing rivaroxaban for reasons other than bleeding.

Avoid use in patients with moderate-to-severe hepatic impairment (Child-Pugh classes B and C) or in patients with any hepatic disease associated with coagulopathy; use in this patient population is contraindicated in the Canadian labeling. Use with caution in patients with moderate renal impairment (Cl_{cr} 30-49 mL/minute) when used for postoperative thromboprophylaxis including patients receiving concomitant drug therapy that may increase rivaroxaban systemic exposure and those with deteriorating renal function. Monitor for any signs or symptoms of blood loss. Avoid use in severe renal impairment (postoperative thromboprophylaxis: Cl_{cr} <30 mL/minute; nonvalvular atrial fibrillation: Cl_{cr} <15 mL/minute); discontinue use in patients who develop acute renal failure.

Concomitant use with combined P-gp and strong CYP3A4 inducers should be avoided. Concomitant use with combined P-gp and strong CYP3A4 inhibitors should be avoided; concurrent use is contraindicated in the Canadian labeling. In patients with renal impairment, concomitant use of rivaroxaban with combined P-gp and weak or moderate CYP3A4 inhibitors should only occur if the potential benefit outweighs the risk of bleeding. Formulation contains lactose; use is not recommended in patients with lactose or galactose intolerance (eg, Lapp lactase deficiency, glucose-galactose malabsorption).

Discontinue rivaroxaban at least 24 hours prior to surgery/invasive procedures; reinitiate when adequate hemostasis has been achieved unless oral therapy cannot be administered then consider administration of a parenteral anticoagulant.

Adverse Reactions

1% to 10%:
- Central nervous system: Syncope (1%)
- Dermatologic: Pruritus (2%), blister (1%)
- Gastrointestinal: Nausea (1%)
- Hematologic: Bleeding (DVT prophylaxis: 6% [major: <1%]; atrial fibrillation: 21% [major: 6%]), thrombocytopenia (<100,000/mm^3 or <50% baseline: 3%), anemia (1%)

Hepatic: GGT increased (>3 times ULN: 7%), ALT increased (>3 times ULN: 3%), AST increased (>3 times ULN: 3%), bilirubin increase (>1.5 times ULN: 3%)

Local: Wound secretion (3%)

Neuromuscular & skeletal: Extremity pain (2%), muscle spasm (1%)

<1% (Limited to important or life-threatening): Abdominal pain, agranulocytosis, alkaline phosphatase increased, allergic dermatitis, amylase increased, anaphylactic shock, anaphylaxis, BUN increased, cholestasis, cytolytic hepatitis, constipation, creatinine increased, diarrhea, dizziness, dyspepsia, dysuria, ecchymosis, fatigue, fever, headache, hematoma (epidural, subdural) hematuria, hemiparesis, hemorrhage (cerebral, retroperitoneal), hypersensitivity, hypotension, jaundice, LDH increased, lipase increased, pain, peripheral edema, rash, Stevens-Johnson syndrome, tachycardia, thrombocythemia, urticaria, vomiting, weakness, xerostomia

Drug Interactions

Metabolism/Transport Effects Substrate of CYP3A4 (major), P-glycoprotein; **Note:** Assignment of Major/Minor substrate status based on clinically relevant drug interaction potential

Avoid Concomitant Use

Avoid concomitant use of Rivaroxaban with any of the following: Anticoagulants; CYP3A4 Inducers (Strong); CYP3A4 Inhibitors (Strong); St Johns Wort

Increased Effect/Toxicity

Rivaroxaban may increase the levels/effects of: Collagenase (Systemic); Deferasirox; Ibritumomab; Tositumomab and Iodine I 131 Tositumomab

The levels/effects of Rivaroxaban may be increased by: Anticoagulants; Antiplatelet Agents; Azithromycin; Clarithromycin; CYP3A4 Inhibitors (Strong); Dasatinib; Diltiazem; Erythromycin; Erythromycin (Systemic); Herbs (Anticoagulant/Antiplatelet Properties); Nonsteroidal Anti-Inflammatory Agents; Pentosan Polysulfate Sodium; P-glycoprotein/ABCB1 Inhibitors; Prostacyclin Analogues; Salicylates; Thrombolytic Agents; Verapamil

Decreased Effect

The levels/effects of Rivaroxaban may be decreased by: CYP3A4 Inducers (Strong); Deferasirox; P-glycoprotein/ABCB1 Inducers; St Johns Wort; Tocilizumab

Ethanol/Nutrition/Herb Interactions

Food: Grapefruit juice may increase levels/effects of rivaroxaban; use caution.

Herb/Nutraceutical: Avoid concomitant use of St John's wort if possible (may decrease levels/effects of rivaroxaban; use with caution and consider dosage adjustment of rivaroxaban if concomitant use cannot be avoided).

Stability Store at 25°C (77°F); excursions permitted to 15°C to 30°C (59°F to 86°F).

Mechanism of Action Inhibits platelet activation and fibrin clot formation via direct, selective and reversible inhibition of factor Xa (FXa) in both the intrinsic and extrinsic coagulation pathways. FXa, as part of the prothrombinase complex consisting also of factor Va, calcium ions, factor II and phospholipid, catalyzes the conversion of prothrombin to thrombin. Thrombin both activates platelets and catalyzes the conversion of fibrinogen to fibrin.

Pharmacodynamics/Kinetics

Absorption: Rapid

Distribution: V_{dss}: ~50 L

Protein binding: ~92% to 95% (primarily to albumin)

Metabolism: Hepatic via CYP3A4/5 and CYP2J2

Bioavailability: Absolute bioavailability: 10 mg dose: ~80% to 100%; 20 mg dose: ~66% (fasting; increased with food)

Half-life elimination: Terminal: 5-9 hours; Elderly: 11-13 hours

Time to peak, plasma: 2-4 hours

Excretion: Urine (66% primarily via active tubular secretion [36% as unchanged drug; 30% as inactive metabolites]); feces (28% [7% as unchanged drug; 21% as inactive metabolites])

Dosage Oral:

Adults:

Nonvalvular atrial fibrillation (to prevent stroke and systemic embolism): 20 mg once daily

Conversion from warfarin: Discontinue warfarin and initiate rivaroxaban as soon as INR falls below 3.0

Conversion to warfarin: Initiate warfarin and a parenteral anticoagulant 24 hours after discontinuation of rivaroxaban (manufacturer recommended approach; other approaches to conversion may be acceptable). **Note:** Rivaroxaban affects INR; therefore, initial INR measurements after initiating warfarin may be unreliable.

Conversion from continuous infusion unfractionated heparin: Initiate rivaroxaban at the time of heparin discontinuation

Conversion to continuous infusion unfractionated heparin: Initiate continuous infusion unfractionated heparin 24 hours after discontinuation of rivaroxaban

Conversion from anticoagulants (other than warfarin and continuous infusion unfractionated heparin): Discontinue current anticoagulant and initiate rivaroxaban ≤2 hours prior to the next regularly scheduled evening dose of the discontinued anticoagulant.

Conversion to other anticoagulants (other than warfarin): Initiate the anticoagulant 24 hours after discontinuation of rivaroxaban

Postoperative thromboprophylaxis: **Note:** Initiate therapy after hemostasis has been established, 6-10 hours postoperatively.

Knee replacement: 10 mg once daily; recommended total duration of therapy: 12-14 days

Hip replacement: 10 mg once daily; total duration of therapy: 35 days

Elderly: Refer to adult dosing.

Dosing adjustment in renal impairment:

Nonvalvular atrial fibrillation:

Cl_{cr} >50 mL/minute: No dosage adjustment necessary

Cl_{cr} 15-50 mL/minute: 15 mg once daily

Cl_{cr} <15 mL/minute: Avoid use

ESRD requiring hemodialysis: Avoid use

Postoperative thromboprophylaxis:

Cl_{cr} >50 mL/minute: No dosage adjustment necessary

Cl_{cr} 30-50 mL/minute: No dosage adjustment provided in manufacturer's labeling; use with caution

Cl_{cr} <30 mL/minute: Avoid use

ESRD requiring hemodialysis: Avoid use.

Dosing adjustment in hepatic impairment:

Mild hepatic impairment: No dosage adjustment provided in manufacturer's labeling. Limited data indicates pharmacokinetics and pharmacodynamic response were similar to healthy subjects.

Moderate-to-severe hepatic impairment (Child-Pugh classes B and C) and patients with any hepatic disease associated with coagulopathy: Avoid use. **Note:** The Canadian labeling contraindicates use in these patient populations.

Administration Administer doses ≥15 mg/day with food; dose of 10 mg/day may be administered without regard to meals.

A decrease in the AUC and C_{max} (29% and 56%, respectively) was observed when rivaroxaban was delivered to the proximal small intestine; further decreases may be seen with delivery to the distal small intestine or ascending colon. Avoid administering via a feeding tube that delivers the rivaroxaban directly into the small intestine or ascending colon.

Monitoring Parameters Prothrombin time (PT), CBC with differential, renal function, hepatic function; **Note:** In major clinical trials, monitoring of aPTT, PT/INR, or antifactor Xa levels did not occur. However, certain patient populations (eg, renal insufficiency, hepatic impairment, low body weight, extreme obesity) may require monitoring of the PT time which correlates well with rivaroxaban concentrations (Abrams, 2009; Kubitza, 2005).

Test Interactions Prolongs activated partial thromboplastin time (aPTT), HepTest®, and Russell viper venom time

Dosage Forms Excipient information presented when available (limited, particularly for generics); consult specific product labeling.

Tablet, oral:

Xarelto®: 10 mg, 15 mg, 20 mg

◆ **Riva-Sertraline (Can)** *see* Sertraline *on page 1548*

◆ **Riva-Simvastatin (Can)** *see* Simvastatin *on page 1555*

◆ **Rivasol (Can)** *see* Zinc Sulfate *on page 1818*

◆ **Rivasone (Can)** *see* Betamethasone *on page 208*

◆ **Riva-Sotalol (Can)** *see* Sotalol *on page 1586*

Rivastigmine (ri va STIG meen)

Brand Names: U.S. Exelon®

Brand Names: Canada Exelon®; Mylan-Rivastigmine; Novo-Rivastigmine; PMS-Rivastigmine; ratio-Rivastigmine; Sandoz-Rivastigmine

Index Terms ENA 713; Rivastigmine Tartrate; SDZ ENA 713

Pharmacologic Category Acetylcholinesterase Inhibitor (Central)

Use Treatment of mild-to-moderate dementia associated with Alzheimer's disease or Parkinson's disease

Unlabeled Use Severe dementia associated with Alzheimer's disease; Lewy body dementia

Pregnancy Risk Factor B

Pregnancy Considerations Teratogenic effects were not observed in animal studies. There are no adequate and well-controlled studies in pregnant women. Should be used only if the benefit outweighs the potential risk to the fetus.

Lactation Excretion in breast milk unknown/use caution

Contraindications Hypersensitivity to rivastigmine, other carbamate derivatives (eg, neostigmine, pyridostigmine, physostigmine), or any component of the formulation

Warnings/Precautions Significant nausea, vomiting, anorexia, and weight loss are associated with use; occurs more frequently in women and during the titration phase. Nausea and/or vomiting may be severe, particularly at doses higher than recommended. Monitor weight during therapy. Therapy should be initiated at lowest dose and titrated; if treatment is interrupted for more than several days, reinstate at the lowest daily dose. Cholinesterase inhibitors may have vagotonic effects which may cause bradycardia and/or heart block with or without a history of cardiac disease. Alzheimer's treatment guidelines consider bradycardia to be a relative contraindication for use of centrally-active cholinesterase inhibitors. Post-market cases of overdose (including a few fatalities) have been reported in association with medication errors/improper use of rivastigmine transdermal patches. No more than 1 patch should be applied daily and existing patch must be removed prior to applying new patch.

Use caution in patients with a history of peptic ulcer disease or concurrent NSAID use. Use caution in patients undergoing anesthesia who will receive succinylcholine-type muscle relaxation, patients with sick-sinus syndrome, bradycardia or supraventricular conduction conditions, urinary obstruction, seizure disorders, or pulmonary conditions such as asthma or COPD. Use caution in patients with low body weight (<50 kg) due to increased risk of adverse reactions.

Adverse Reactions Note: Many concentration-related effects are reported at a lower frequency by transdermal route.

>10%:

Central nervous system: Dizziness (2% to 21%), headache (3% to 17%)

Gastrointestinal: Nausea (7% to 47%), vomiting (6% to 31%), diarrhea (5% to 19%), anorexia (3% to 17%), abdominal pain (1% to 13%)

1% to 10%:

Cardiovascular: Syncope (3%), hypertension (3%)

Central nervous system: Fatigue (2% to 9%), insomnia (1% to 9%), confusion (8%), depression (4% to 6%), anxiety (2% to 5%), malaise (5%), somnolence (4% to 5%), hallucinations (4%), aggressiveness (3%), parkinsonism symptoms worsening (2% to 3%), vertigo (≤2%)

Gastrointestinal: Dyspepsia (9%), constipation (5%), flatulence (4%), weight loss (3% to 8%), eructation (2%), dehydration (2%)

Genitourinary: Urinary tract infection (1% to 7%)

Neuromuscular & skeletal: Weakness (2% to 6%), tremor (1%; up to 10% in Parkinson's patients)

Respiratory: Rhinitis (4%)

Miscellaneous: Diaphoresis (4%), flu-like syndrome (3%)

<1% (Limited to important or life-threatening symptoms; reactions may be at a similar frequency to placebo): Abnormal hepatic function, acute renal failure, albuminuria, allergy, anemia, angina, aphasia, apnea, apraxia, ataxia, atrial fibrillation, AV block, bradycardia, bronchospasm, bundle branch block, cachexia, cardiac arrest, cardiac failure, chest pain, cholecystitis, diplopia, diverticulitis, dysphagia, dyspnea, dysphonia, edema, esophagitis, extrasystoles, fecal incontinence, gastritis, gastroesophageal reflux, GGT increased, glaucoma, hematuria, hot flashes, hyper-/hypoglycemia, hypercholesterolemia, hyper-/hypokinesia, hypertonia, hypokalemia, hyponatremia, hypotension (including postural), hypothermia, hypothyroidism, intestinal obstruction, intracranial hemorrhage, mastitis, MI, migraine, neuralgia, palpitation, pancreatitis, paresthesia, periorbital or facial edema, peripheral ischemia, peripheral neuropathy, pneumonia, pruritus, psychiatric disorders (eg, delirium, depersonalization, psychosis, emotional lability, suicidal ideation or tendencies), rash, respiratory depression, retinopathy, rigors, salivation, seizure, severe vomiting with esophageal rupture (following inappropriate reinitiation of dose), sick-sinus syndrome, Stevens-Johnson syndrome, sudden cardiac death, supraventricular tachycardia, thrombocytopenia, thrombophlebitis, thrombosis, transient ischemic attack, ulcerative stomatitis, urinary incontinence, urticaria, vasovagal syncope

Drug Interactions

Metabolism/Transport Effects None known.

Avoid Concomitant Use There are no known interactions where it is recommended to avoid concomitant use.

Increased Effect/Toxicity

Rivastigmine may increase the levels/effects of: Antipsychotics; Beta-Blockers; Cholinergic Agonists; Succinylcholine

The levels/effects of Rivastigmine may be increased by: Corticosteroids (Systemic)

Decreased Effect

Rivastigmine may decrease the levels/effects of: Anticholinergics; Neuromuscular-Blocking Agents (Nondepolarizing)

The levels/effects of Rivastigmine may be decreased by: Anticholinergics; Dipyridamole

Ethanol/Nutrition/Herb Interactions

Smoking: Nicotine increases the clearance of rivastigmine by 23%.

Ethanol: Avoid ethanol (due to risk of sedation; may increase GI irritation).

Food: Food delays absorption by 90 minutes, lowers C_{max} by 30% and increases AUC by 30%.

Herb/Nutraceutical: Avoid ginkgo biloba (may increase cholinergic effects).

Stability

Oral: Store at 15°C to 30°C (59°F to 86°F); do not freeze. Store solution in an upright position.

Transdermal patch: Store at 15°C to 30°C (59°F to 86°F). Patches should be kept in sealed pouch until use.

Mechanism of Action A deficiency of cortical acetylcholine is thought to account for some of the symptoms of Alzheimer's disease and the dementia of Parkinson's disease; rivastigmine increases acetylcholine in the central nervous system through reversible inhibition of its hydrolysis by cholinesterase

Pharmacodynamics/Kinetics

Duration: Anticholinesterase activity (CSF): ~10 hours (6 mg oral dose)

Absorption: Oral: Fasting: Rapid and complete within 1 hour

Distribution: V_d: 1.8-2.7 L/kg; penetrates blood-brain barrier (CSF levels are ~40% of plasma levels following oral administration)

Protein binding: 40%

Metabolism: Extensively via cholinesterase-mediated hydrolysis in the brain; metabolite undergoes N-demethylation and/or sulfate conjugation hepatically; CYP minimally involved; linear kinetics at 3 mg twice daily, but nonlinear at higher doses

Bioavailability: Oral: 36% to 40%

Half-life elimination: Oral: 1.5 hours; Transdermal patch: 3 hours (after removal)

Time to peak: Oral: 1 hour; Transdermal patch: 10-16 hours following first dose

Excretion: Urine (97% as metabolites); feces (0.4%)

Dosage Adults:

Oral: **Note:** Exelon® oral solution and capsules are bioequivalent.

Mild-to-moderate Alzheimer's dementia: Initial: 1.5 mg twice daily; may increase by 3 mg/day (1.5 mg/dose) every 2 weeks based on tolerability (maximum recommended dose: 6 mg twice daily)

Note: If GI adverse events occur, discontinue treatment for several doses then restart at the same or next lower dosage level; antiemetics have been used to control GI symptoms. If treatment is interrupted for longer than several days, restart the treatment at the lowest dose and titrate as previously described.

Mild-to-moderate Parkinson's-related dementia: Initial: 1.5 mg twice daily; may increase by 3 mg/day (1.5 mg/dose) every 4 weeks based on tolerability (maximum recommended dose: 6 mg twice daily)

Transdermal patch: Mild-to-moderate Alzheimer's- or Parkinson's-related dementia:

Initial: 4.6 mg/24 hours; if well tolerated, may be increased (after at least 4 weeks) to 9.5 mg/24 hours (recommended effective dose)

Maintenance: 9.5 mg/24 hours (maximum dose: 9.5 mg/24 hours)

Note: If intolerance is noted (nausea, vomiting), patch should be removed and treatment interrupted for several days and restarted at the same or lower dosage. If interrupted for more than several days, reinitiate at lowest dosage and increase to maintenance dose after 4 weeks.

Conversion from oral therapy: If oral daily dose <6 mg, switch to 4.6 mg/24 hours patch; if oral daily dose 6-12 mg, switch to 9.5 mg/24 hours patch. Apply patch on the next day following last oral dose.

Elderly: Following oral administration, clearance is significantly lower in patients >60 years of age, but dosage adjustments are not recommended. Age was not associated with exposure in patients treated transdermally. Titrate dose to individual's tolerance.

Dosage adjustment in renal impairment: Dosage adjustments are not recommended; however, titrate the dose to the individual's tolerance.

Dosage adjustment in hepatic impairment: Clearance is significantly reduced in mild to moderately impaired patients. Although dosage adjustments are not recommended, use lowest possible dose and titrate according to individual's tolerance. Consider intervals of >2 weeks between dosage adjustments.

Dietary Considerations Capsules should be taken with meals.

Administration

Oral: Should be administered with meals (breakfast or dinner). Capsule should be swallowed whole. Liquid form is available for patients who cannot swallow capsules (can be swallowed directly from syringe or mixed with water, soda, or cold fruit juice). Stir well and drink within 4 hours of mixing.

Topical: Apply transdermal patch to upper or lower back (alternatively, may apply to upper arm or chest). Avoid reapplication to same spot of skin for 14 days (may rotate sections of back, for example). Do not apply to red, irritated, or broken skin. Avoid areas of recent application of lotion or powder. After removal, fold patch to press adhesive surfaces together, and discard. Avoid eye contact; wash hands after handling patch. Replace patch every 24 hours. Avoid exposing the patch to external sources of heat (eg, sauna, excessive light) for prolonged periods of time. No more than 1 patch should be applied daily and existing patch must be removed prior to applying new patch.

Monitoring Parameters Cognitive function at periodic intervals, symptoms of GI intolerance, weight

Dosage Forms Excipient information presented when available (limited, particularly for generics); consult specific product labeling.

Capsule, oral: 1.5 mg, 3 mg, 4.5 mg, 6 mg

Exelon®: 1.5 mg, 3 mg, 4.5 mg, 6 mg

Patch, transdermal:

Exelon®: 4.6 mg/24 hours (30s) [5 cm^2; contains rivastigmine 9 mg]

Exelon®: 9.5 mg/24 hours (30s) [10 cm^2; contains rivastigmine 18 mg]

Solution, oral:

Exelon®: 2 mg/mL (120 mL) [contains sodium benzoate]

◆ **Rivastigmine Tartrate** *see* Rivastigmine *on page 1509*

◆ **Riva-Sumatriptan (Can)** *see* SUMAtriptan *on page 1609*

◆ **Riva-Terbinafine (Can)** *see* Terbinafine (Systemic) *on page 1648*

◆ **Riva-Valacyclovir (Can)** *see* ValACYclovir *on page 1753*

◆ **Riva-Venlafaxine XR (Can)** *see* Venlafaxine *on page 1780*

◆ **Riva-Verapamil SR (Can)** *see* Verapamil *on page 1783*

◆ **Riva-Zide (Can)** *see* Hydrochlorothiazide and Triamterene *on page 836*

◆ **Rivotril® (Can)** *see* ClonazePAM *on page 390*

Rizatriptan (rye za TRIP tan)

Brand Names: U.S. Maxalt-MLT®; Maxalt®

Brand Names: Canada Maxalt RPD™; Maxalt™

Index Terms MK462

Pharmacologic Category Antimigraine Agent; Serotonin $5\text{-}HT_{1B,\ 1D}$ Receptor Agonist

Additional Appendix Information

Antimigraine Drugs: 5-HT_1 Receptor Agonists *on page 1878*

Use Acute treatment of migraine with or without aura

Pregnancy Risk Factor C

Pregnancy Considerations There are no adequate and well-controlled studies using rizatriptan in pregnant women. Use only if potential benefit to the mother outweighs the potential risk to the fetus. A pregnancy registry has been established to monitor outcomes of women exposed to rizatriptan during pregnancy (800-986-8999). In some animal studies, administration was associated with decreased weight gain, developmental toxicity and increased mortality in the offspring. Teratogenic effects were not observed.

Lactation Excretion in breast milk unknown/use caution

Contraindications Hypersensitivity to rizatriptan or any component of the formulation; documented ischemic heart disease or Prinzmetal's angina; uncontrolled hypertension; basilar or hemiplegic migraine; during or within 2 weeks of MAO inhibitors; during or within 24 hours of treatment with another 5-HT_1 agonist, or an ergot-containing or ergot-type medication (eg, methysergide, dihydroergotamine)

Warnings/Precautions Only indicated for treatment of acute migraine; if a patient does not respond to the first dose, the diagnosis of migraine should be reconsidered. Coronary artery vasospasm, transient ischemia, myocardial infarction, ventricular tachycardia/fibrillation, cardiac arrest, and death have been reported with 5-HT_1 agonist administration. Patients who experience sensations of chest pain/pressure/tightness or symptoms suggestive of angina following dosing should be evaluated for coronary artery disease or Prinzmetal's angina before receiving additional doses; if dosing is resumed and similar symptoms recur, monitor with ECG. Should not be given to patients who have risk factors for CAD (eg, hypertension, hypercholesterolemia, smoker, obesity, diabetes, strong family history of CAD, menopause, male >40 years of age) without adequate cardiac evaluation. Patients with suspected CAD should have cardiovascular evaluation to rule out CAD before considering use; if cardiovascular evaluation is "satisfactory," first dose should be given in the healthcare provider's office (consider ECG monitoring). Periodic evaluation of cardiovascular status should be done in all patients. Significant elevation in blood pressure, including hypertensive crisis, has also been reported on rare occasions in patients with and without a history of hypertension. Cerebral/subarachnoid hemorrhage, stroke, peripheral vascular ischemia, and colonic ischemia have been reported with 5-HT_1 agonist administration.

Use with caution in elderly or patients with hepatic or renal impairment (including dialysis patients). Symptoms of agitation, confusion, hallucinations, hyper-reflexia, myoclonus, shivering, and tachycardia may occur with concomitant proserotonergic drugs (eg, SSRIs/SNRIs or triptans) or agents which reduce rizatriptan's metabolism. Concurrent use of serotonin precursors (eg, tryptophan) is not recommended. If concomitant administration with SSRIs is warranted, monitor closely, especially at initiation and with dose increases. Maxalt-MLT® tablets contain phenylalanine.

Adverse Reactions

>10%:

Central nervous system: Fatigue (adults 7% to 30%, dose related; children >1%)

Gastrointestinal: Xerostomia (<5% to 13%)

1% to 10%:

Cardiovascular: Chest pain (<2% to 5%), flushing (>1%), palpitation (>1%), systolic/diastolic blood pressure increases (5-10 mm Hg)

Central nervous system: Dizziness (9%), somnolence (8%), headache (≤2%), euphoria (>1%), hypoesthesia (>1%), drowsiness

Dermatologic: Skin flushing

Endocrine & metabolic: Growth hormone increased (mild), hot flashes

Gastrointestinal: Nausea (3%), diarrhea (>1%), vomiting (>1%), abdominal pain

Neuromuscular & skeletal: Weakness (4% to 7%), paresthesia (3% to 4%); myalgia (3%); neck, throat, and jaw pain/tightness/pressure (≤2%), tremor (>1%)

Respiratory: Dyspnea (>1%)

Miscellaneous: Feeling of heaviness (<1% to 2%)

<1% (Limited to important or life-threatening): Akinesia, anaphylaxis/anaphylactoid reactions, angina, angioedema, arrhythmia, bradycardia, bradykinesia, confusion, hallucinations (children), hypertensive crisis, memory impairment, mental activity decreased, MI, myocardial ischemia, neurological/psychiatric abnormalities, pruritus, seizures, stroke, syncope, tachycardia, tinnitus, toxic epidermal necrolysis, vasospasm, vertigo, wheezing

Drug Interactions

Metabolism/Transport Effects None known.

Avoid Concomitant Use

Avoid concomitant use of Rizatriptan with any of the following: Ergot Derivatives; MAO Inhibitors

Increased Effect/Toxicity

Rizatriptan may increase the levels/effects of: Ergot Derivatives; Metoclopramide; Serotonin Modulators

The levels/effects of Rizatriptan may be increased by: Antipsychotics; Ergot Derivatives; MAO Inhibitors; Propranolol

Decreased Effect There are no known significant interactions involving a decrease in effect.

Ethanol/Nutrition/Herb Interactions Food: Food delays absorption.

Stability Store in blister pack until administration.

Mechanism of Action Selective agonist for serotonin (5-HT_{1B} and 5-HT_{1D}receptors) in cranial arteries; causes vasoconstriction and reduces sterile inflammation associated with antidromic neuronal transmission correlating with relief of migraine

Pharmacodynamics/Kinetics

Onset of action: ~30 minutes

Duration: 14-16 hours

Protein binding: 14%

Metabolism: Via monoamine oxidase-A; first-pass effect

Bioavailability: 40% to 50%

Half-life elimination: 2-3 hours

Time to peak: 1-1.5 hours

Excretion: Urine (82%, 8% to 16% as unchanged drug); feces (12%)

Dosage Note: In patients with risk factors for coronary artery disease, following adequate evaluation to establish the absence of coronary artery disease, the initial dose should be administered in a setting where response may be evaluated (physician's office or similarly staffed setting). ECG monitoring may be considered.

Oral: 5-10 mg, repeat after 2 hours if significant relief is not attained; maximum: 30 mg in a 24-hour period (use 5 mg dose in patients receiving propranolol with a maximum of 15 mg in 24 hours)

Note: For orally-disintegrating tablets (Maxalt-MLT®): Patient should be instructed to place tablet on tongue and allow to dissolve. Dissolved tablet will be swallowed with saliva.

Dietary Considerations Some products may contain phenylalanine.

Monitoring Parameters Headache severity, signs/symptoms suggestive of angina; consider monitoring blood pressure, heart rate, and/or ECG with first dose in patients with likelihood of unrecognized coronary disease, such as patients with significant hypertension, hypercholesterolemia, obese patients, patients with diabetes, smokers with other risk factors or strong family history of coronary artery disease

Dosage Forms Excipient information presented when available (limited, particularly for generics); consult specific product labeling.

Tablet, oral:

Maxalt®: 5 mg, 10 mg

Tablet, orally disintegrating, oral:

Maxalt-MLT®: 5 mg [contains phenylalanine 1.05 mg/tablet; peppermint flavor]

Maxalt-MLT®: 10 mg [contains phenylalanine 2.1 mg/tablet; peppermint flavor]

- ◆ **rLFN-α2** *see* Interferon Alfa-2b *on page* 912
- ◆ **R-modafinil** *see* Armodafinil *on page* 145
- ◆ **Ro 5488** *see* Tretinoin (Systemic) *on page* 1729
- ◆ **RO5185426** *see* Vemurafenib *on page* 1778
- ◆ **RoActemra®** *see* Tocilizumab *on page* 1700
- ◆ **Robafen [OTC]** *see* GuaiFENesin *on page* 809
- ◆ **Robafen AC** *see* Guaifenesin and Codeine *on page* 810
- ◆ **Robafen DM [OTC]** *see* Guaifenesin and Dextromethorphan *on page* 810
- ◆ **Robafen DM Clear [OTC]** *see* Guaifenesin and Dextromethorphan *on page* 810
- ◆ **Robaxin®** *see* Methocarbamol *on page* 1096
- ◆ **Robaxin®-750** *see* Methocarbamol *on page* 1096
- ◆ **Robidrine® (Can)** *see* Pseudoephedrine *on page* 1430
- ◆ **Robinul®** *see* Glycopyrrolate *on page* 802
- ◆ **Robinul® Forte** *see* Glycopyrrolate *on page* 802
- ◆ **Robitussin® (Can)** *see* GuaiFENesin *on page* 809
- ◆ **Robitussin AC** *see* Guaifenesin and Codeine *on page* 810
- ◆ **Robitussin® Childrens Cough & Cold (Can)** *see* Pseudoephedrine and Dextromethorphan *on page* 1431
- ◆ **Robitussin® Children's Cough & Cold Long-Acting [OTC]** *see* Dextromethorphan and Chlorpheniramine *on page* 489
- ◆ **Robitussin® Cough & Chest Congestion DM [OTC] [DSC]** *see* Guaifenesin and Dextromethorphan *on page* 810
- ◆ **Robitussin® Cough & Chest Congestion DM Max [OTC] [DSC]** *see* Guaifenesin and Dextromethorphan *on page* 810
- ◆ **Robitussin® Cough & Chest Congestion Sugar-Free DM [OTC] [DSC]** *see* Guaifenesin and Dextromethorphan *on page* 810
- ◆ **Robitussin® Cough & Cold Long-Acting [OTC] [DSC]** *see* Dextromethorphan and Chlorpheniramine *on page* 489
- ◆ **Robitussin® DM (Can)** *see* Guaifenesin and Dextromethorphan *on page* 810
- ◆ **Robitussin® Night Time Cough & Cold [OTC] [DSC]** *see* Diphenhydramine and Phenylephrine *on page* 518
- ◆ **Robitussin® Peak Cold Cough + Chest Congestion DM [OTC]** *see* Guaifenesin and Dextromethorphan *on page* 810
- ◆ **Robitussin® Peak Cold Maximum Strength Cough + Chest Congestion DM [OTC]** *see* Guaifenesin and Dextromethorphan *on page* 810
- ◆ **Robitussin® Peak Cold Sugar-Free Cough + Chest Congestion DM [OTC]** *see* Guaifenesin and Dextromethorphan *on page* 810
- ◆ **Rocaltrol®** *see* Calcitriol *on page* 263
- ◆ **Rocephin®** *see* CefTRIAXone *on page* 318

Rocuronium (roe kyoor OH nee um)

Brand Names: U.S. Zemuron®

Brand Names: Canada Rocuronium Bromide Injection; Zemuron®

Index Terms ORG 9426; Rocuronium Bromide

Pharmacologic Category Neuromuscular Blocker Agent, Nondepolarizing

Use Facilitate both rapid sequence and routine endotracheal intubation and to relax skeletal muscles during surgery; to facilitate mechanical ventilation in ICU patients

Pregnancy Risk Factor C

Pregnancy Considerations Teratogenic effects were not observed in animal studies. Rocuronium crosses the placenta; umbilical venous plasma levels are ~18% of the maternal concentration. The manufacturer does not recommend use for rapid sequence induction during cesarean section.

Lactation Excretion in breast milk unknown/use caution

Contraindications Hypersensitivity to rocuronium, other neuromuscular-blocking agents, or any component of the formulation

Warnings/Precautions Use with caution in patients with cardiovascular disease and pulmonary disease; ventilation must be supported during neuromuscular blockade; certain clinical conditions may result in potentiation or antagonism of neuromuscular blockade:

Potentiation: Electrolyte abnormalities, severe hyponatremia, severe hypocalcemia, severe hypokalemia, hypermagnesemia, cachexia, neuromuscular diseases, metabolic acidosis, metabolic alkalosis, Eaton-Lambert syndrome, and myasthenia gravis

Antagonism: Respiratory alkalosis, hypercalcemia, demyelinating lesions, peripheral neuropathies, denervation, infection, and muscle trauma

Use with caution in patients with hepatic impairment; clinical duration may be prolonged. Resistance may occur in burn patients (>30% of body) for period of 5-70 days postinjury or in immobilized patients. Cross-sensitivity with other neuromuscular-blocking agents may occur; use caution in patients with previous anaphylactic reactions to other neuromuscular blockers. Use with caution in patients with pulmonary hypertension or valvular heart disease. Use caution in the elderly. Should be administered by adequately trained individuals familiar with its use. Use appropriate anesthesia, pain control, and sedation. In patients requiring long-term administration in the ICU, use of a peripheral nerve stimulator to monitor drug effects is strongly recommended. Additional doses of rocuronium or any other neuromuscular-blocking agent should be avoided unless definite excessive response to nerve stimulation is present.

Some patients may experience prolonged recovery of neuromuscular function after administration (especially after prolonged use). Patients should be adequately recovered prior to extubation. Other factors associated with prolonged recovery should be considered (eg, corticosteroid use, patient condition). In addition to prolonging recovery from neuromuscular blockade, concomitant use with corticosteroids has been associated with development of acute quadriplegic myopathy syndrome (AQMS). Current guidelines recommend neuromuscular blockers be discontinued as soon as possible in patients receiving corticosteroids or interrupted daily until necessary to restart them based on clinical condition (Murray, 2002).

Numerous drugs either *antagonize* (eg, acetylcholinesterase inhibitors) or *potentiate* (eg, calcium channel blockers, certain antimicrobials, inhalation anesthetics) the effects of neuromuscular blockade; use with caution in patients receiving these agents. Immediate treatment (including epinephrine 1:1000) for anaphylactoid and/or hypersensitivity reactions should be available during use. Not recommended by the manufacturer for rapid sequence intubation in pediatric patients; however, it has been used successfully in clinical trials for this indication.

Adverse Reactions

>1%: Cardiovascular: Hypertension (≤2%), hypotension (transient; ≤2%)

<1% (Limited to important or life-threatening): Abnormal ECG, anaphylactoid reaction, anaphylaxis, arrhythmia, bronchospasm, injection site edema, hiccups, pruritus, nausea, pulmonary vascular resistance (increased), rash, rhonchi, shock, tachycardia, vomiting, wheezing

Drug Interactions

Metabolism/Transport Effects None known.

Avoid Concomitant Use

Avoid concomitant use of Rocuronium with any of the following: QuiNINE

Increased Effect/Toxicity

Rocuronium may increase the levels/effects of: Cardiac Glycosides; Corticosteroids (Systemic); OnabotulinumtoxinA; RimabotulinumtoxinB

The levels/effects of Rocuronium may be increased by: AbobotulinumtoxinA; Aminoglycosides; Calcium Channel Blockers; Capreomycin; Colistimethate; Inhalational Anesthetics; Ketorolac; Ketorolac (Nasal); Ketorolac (Systemic); Lincosamide Antibiotics; Lithium; Loop Diuretics; Magnesium Salts; Polymyxin B; Procainamide; QuiNIDine; QuiNINE; Spironolactone; Tetracycline Derivatives; Vancomycin

Decreased Effect

The levels/effects of Rocuronium may be decreased by: Acetylcholinesterase Inhibitors; Loop Diuretics

Stability Store unopened/undiluted vials under refrigeration at 2°C to 8°C (36°F to 46°F); do not freeze. When stored at room temperature, it is stable for 60 days; once opened, use within 30 days. Dilutions up to 5 mg/mL in 0.9% sodium chloride, dextrose 5% in water, 5% dextrose in sodium chloride 0.9%, or lactated Ringer's are stable for up to 24 hours at room temperature.

Mechanism of Action Blocks acetylcholine from binding to receptors on motor endplate inhibiting depolarization

Pharmacodynamics/Kinetics

Onset of action: Good intubation conditions within 1-2 minutes (depending on dose administered); maximum neuromuscular blockade within 4 minutes

Duration: ~30 minutes (with standard doses, increases with higher doses and inhalational anesthetic agents; patient age dependent)

Distribution: V_d: ~0.25 L/kg

Protein binding: ~30%

Metabolism: Minimally hepatic; 17-desacetylrocuronium (5% to 10% activity of parent drug)

Half-life elimination: 60-70 minutes

Excretion: Feces (50%); urine (30%)

Dosage Dose to effect; doses will vary due to interpatient variability. Dosing also dependent on anesthetic technique and age of patient.

Infants 28 days to 3 months and Children ≥3 months: **Note:** In general, onset is shortened and duration is prolonged as dose increases. Duration is shortest in children >2 to ≤11 years and longest in neonates and infants.

Rapid sequence intubation (unlabeled use): I.V.: 0.9 mg/kg or 1.2 mg/kg. Not recommended, per the manufacturer, for rapid sequence intubation in pediatric patients; however, it has been used successfully in clinical trials for this indication in children >1 year of age (Cheng, 2002; Fuchs-Buder, 1996; Mazurek, 1998; Naguib, 1997).

Tracheal intubation: I.V.: 0.45 mg/kg or 0.6 mg/kg

Maintenance for continued surgical relaxation: I.V.: 0.075-0.15 mg/kg; redosing interval is guided by monitoring with a peripheral nerve stimulator **or** 7-12 **mcg**/kg/minute as a continuous infusion; use lower end of the continuous infusion dosing range for neonates and infants up to age 28 days and the upper end for children >2 to ≤11 years of age

Adults:

Rapid sequence intubation: I.V.: 0.6-1.2 mg/kg

Tracheal intubation: I.V.: **Note:** May use ideal body weight (IBW) for morbidly obese (BMI >40 kg/m^2) adult patients (Leykin, 2004); onset time may be slightly delayed using IBW. The manufacturer recommends dosing based on actual body weight in all obese patients.

Initial: 0.45-0.6 mg/kg; administration of 0.3 mg/kg may also provide optimal conditions for tracheal intubation (Barclay, 1997)

Maintenance for continued surgical relaxation: 0.1-0.2 mg/kg; repeat as needed **or** a continuous infusion of 8-12 **mcg**/kg/minute only after recovery of neuromuscular function is evident; infusion rates have ranged from 4-16 **mcg**/kg/minute

Note: Inhaled anesthetic agents prolong the duration of action of rocuronium. Use lower end of the dosing range; redosing interval guided by monitoring with a peripheral nerve stimulator.

Preinduction defasciculating dose: I.V.: 0.03-0.06 mg/kg given 1.5-3 minutes before administration of succinylcholine (Harvey, 1998; Martin, 1998)

ICU paralysis (eg, facilitate mechanical ventilation) in selected adequately sedated patients (Murray, 2002; Rudis, 1996; Sparr, 1997): Initial bolus dose: 0.6-1 mg/kg, then a continuous I.V. infusion of 8-12 **mcg**/kg/minute; monitor depth of blockade every 2-3 hours initially until stable dose, then every 8-12 hours; adjust rate of administration by 10% increments according to peripheral nerve stimulation response or desired clinical response

Note: When possible, minimize depth and duration of paralysis. Stopping the infusion for some time until forced to restart based on patient condition is recommended to reduce post-paralytic complications (eg, acute quadriplegic myopathy syndrome [AQMS]) (Murray, 2002).

Intermittent dosing has also been described with an initial loading dose of 50 mg followed by 25 mg given when peripheral nerve stimulation returns (Sparr, 1997).

Dosing adjustment in renal impairment: No adjustments required; duration of neuromuscular blockade may vary in patients with renal impairment.

Dosing adjustment in hepatic impairment: Reductions may be necessary in patients with liver disease; duration of neuromuscular blockade may be prolonged due to increased volume of distribution. When rapid sequence intubation is required in adult patients with ascites, a dose on the higher end of the dosage range may be necessary to achieve adequate neuromuscular blockade.

Administration Administer I.V. only; may be administered undiluted as a bolus injection or via a continuous infusion using an infusion pump

Monitoring Parameters Peripheral nerve stimulator measuring twitch response, heart rate, blood pressure, assisted ventilation status

Additional Information Rocuronium is classified as an intermediate-duration neuromuscular-blocking agent. Do not mix in the same syringe with barbiturates. Rocuronium does not relieve pain or produce sedation.

Dosage Forms Excipient information presented when available (limited, particularly for generics); consult specific product labeling.

Injection, solution, as bromide: 10 mg/mL (5 mL, 10 mL)
 Zemuron®: 10 mg/mL (5 mL, 10 mL)
Injection, solution, as bromide [preservative free]: 10 mg/mL (5 mL, 10 mL)

◆ **Rocuronium Bromide** *see* Rocuronium *on page 1512*

◆ **Rocuronium Bromide Injection (Can)** *see* Rocuronium *on page 1512*

◆ **Rofact™ (Can)** *see* Rifampin *on page 1485*

Roflumilast (roe FLUE mi last)

Brand Names: U.S. Daliresp®
Brand Names: Canada Daxas™
Pharmacologic Category Phosphodiesterase-4 Enzyme Inhibitor
Use Adjunct to bronchodilator therapy in the maintenance treatment of severe chronic obstructive pulmonary disease (COPD) associated with chronic bronchitis
Pregnancy Risk Factor C
Pregnancy Considerations Animal studies have demonstrated reproductive toxicity (incomplete ossification, post-implantive losses) at doses greater than the human recommended dose. There are no adequate and well controlled studies in pregnant women. Avoid use during pregnancy.
Medication Guide Available Yes
Contraindications Moderate or severe hepatic impairment (Child-Pugh class B or C)

Canadian labeling: Additional contraindication (not in U.S. labeling): Hypersensitivity to roflumilast or any component of the formulation

Warnings/Precautions Not indicated for relieving acute bronchospasms or for use as monotherapy of COPD; use only as adjunctive therapy to bronchodilator therapy. Neuropsychiatric effects (eg, anxiety, depression) have been reported with use; rarely, suicidal behavior/ ideation and completed suicide were reported. Avoid use in patients with a history of depression with suicidal behavior/ideations; instruct patients/caregivers to report psychiatric symptoms and consider discontinuation of therapy in such patients. Systemic exposure may be increased in patients with mild hepatic impairment; use in moderate-to-severe impairment is contraindicated.

May cause weight loss and/or diarrhea (sometimes severe); weight loss usually observed within 6 months of initiating therapy and diarrhea within 4 weeks. Instruct patients to monitor weight regularly. Avoid initiation of therapy or discontinue therapy with unexplained/pronounced weight loss.

Adverse Reactions
2% to 10%:
 Central nervous system: Headache (4%), dizziness (2%), insomnia (2%)
 Gastrointestinal: Gastrointestinal: Diarrhea (10%), weight loss (8%; 7%: >10% loss), nausea (5%), appetite decreased (2%)
 Neuromuscular & skeletal: Back pain (3%)
 Miscellaneous: Influenza (3%)
<2% (Limited to important or life-threatening): Abdominal pain, anemia, arthralgia, arthritis, AST increased, atrial fibrillation depression, epistaxis, gastritis, GERD, GGT increased, gynecomastia, hematochezia, hypersensitivity, LDH increased, lung cancer, malaise, muscle spasm, muscle weakness, myalgia, pancreatitis, paresthesia, prostate cancer, rash, renal failure, respiratory tract infection, rhinitis, sinusitis, suicidal ideation/behavior, suicide completed, supraventricular arrhythmia, taste abnormal, tremor, urinary tract infection, urticaria, vertigo, vomiting

Drug Interactions
Metabolism/Transport Effects **Substrate** of CYP1A2 (minor), CYP3A4 (major); **Note:** Assignment of Major/ Minor substrate status based on clinically relevant drug interaction potential
Avoid Concomitant Use
Avoid concomitant use of Roflumilast with any of the following: CYP3A4 Inducers (Strong); Rifampin
Increased Effect/Toxicity
Roflumilast may increase the levels/effects of: Immunosuppressants

The levels/effects of Roflumilast may be increased by: Cimetidine; Ciprofloxacin; Conivaptan; FluvoxaMINE
Decreased Effect
The levels/effects of Roflumilast may be decreased by: CYP3A4 Inducers (Strong); Cyproterone; Deferasirox; Herbs (CYP3A4 Inducers); Rifampin

Stability Store at 20°C to 25°C (68°F to 77°F), excursions permitted from 15°C to 30°C (59°F to 86°F).
Mechanism of Action Roflumilast and its active N-oxide metabolite selectively inhibit phosphodiesterase-4 (PDE4) leading to an accumulation of cyclic AMP (cAMP) within inflammatory and structural cells important in the pathogenesis of COPD. Anti-inflammatory effects include suppression of cytokine release and inhibition of lung infiltration by neutrophils and other leukocytes. Pulmonary remodeling and mucociliary malfunction are also attenuated.
Pharmacodynamics/Kinetics
Distribution: V_d: 2.9 L/kg
Protein binding: 99%; N-oxide metabolite: 97%
Metabolism: Hepatic via CYP3A4 and CYP1A2 to active N-oxide metabolite; also undergoes conjugation
Bioavailability: ~80%
Half-life elimination: 17 hours; N-oxide metabolite: 30 hours
Time to peak: ~1 hour (delayed by food); N-oxide metabolite: ~8 hours
Excretion: Urine (~70% as metabolites)
Dosage Oral: Adults: COPD: 500 mcg once daily
Dosage adjustment in renal impairment: No dosage adjustment is recommended.
Dosage adjustment in hepatic impairment:
 Mild impairment (Child-Pugh class A): No dosage adjustment is recommended. Use with caution; 500 mcg once daily dose has not been evaluated in mild impairment.
 Moderate-to-severe impairment (Child-Pugh class B or C): Use is contraindicated.
Dietary Considerations May be given with or without food.
Administration Administer without regard to meals.
Monitoring Parameters Measure weight regularly during therapy
Dosage Forms Excipient information presented when available (limited, particularly for generics); consult specific product labeling.
Tablet, oral:
 Daliresp®: 500 mcg
Dosage Forms: Canada Excipient information presented when available (limited, particularly for generics); consult specific product labeling.
Tablet, oral:
 Daxas™: 500 mcg

◆ **Rogaine® (Can)** *see* Minoxidil (Topical) *on page 1139*

◆ **Rogaine® Extra Strength for Men [OTC]** *see* Minoxidil (Topical) *on page 1139*

RomiDEPsin (roe mi DEP sin)

Brand Names: U.S. Istodax®

Index Terms Depsipeptide; FK228; FR901228

Pharmacologic Category Antineoplastic Agent, Histone Deacetylase Inhibitor

Use Treatment of refractory cutaneous T-cell lymphoma (CTCL) and refractory peripheral T-cell lymphoma (PTCL)

Pregnancy Risk Factor D

Pregnancy Considerations Adverse events were observed in animal reproduction studies. Based on the mechanism of action, romidepsin may cause fetal harm if administered during pregnancy.

Lactation Excretion in breast milk unknown/not recommended

Contraindications There are no contraindications listed within the manufacturer's labeling.

Warnings/Precautions Hazardous agent - use appropriate precautions for handling and disposal. Anemia, leukopenia, neutropenia, lymphopenia and thrombocytopenia may occur; may require dosage modification; monitor blood counts during treatment. Serious infections (occasionally fatal), including pneumonia and sepsis have occurred during or within 30 days of treatment; the risk of life-threatening infection is increased in patients who have received prior intensive or extensive chemotherapy. QT_c prolongation has been observed; use caution in patients with a history of QT_c prolongation, congenital long QT syndrome, with medications known to prolong the QT interval, or with pre-existing cardiac disease. Obtain baseline and periodic ECG (12-lead); monitor and correct electrolyte (potassium, magnesium, and calcium) abnormalities prior to and during treatment. T-wave and ST-segment changes have also been reported. Use with caution in patients with moderate-to-severe hepatic impairment or end-stage renal disease. Avoid use with strong CYP3A4 inhibitors or inducers. Use with caution with moderate CYP3A4 inhibitors and P-glycoprotein inhibitors. Tumor lysis syndrome (TLS) has been observed; closely monitor patients with advanced disease and/or with a high tumor burden; if TLS occurs, initiate appropriate treatment.

Adverse Reactions

>10%:

Cardiovascular: ST-T wave changes (2% to 63%), hypotension (7% to 23%)

Central nervous system: Fatigue (53% to 77%), fever (20% to 47%), headache (15% to 34%), chills (11% to 17%)

Dermatologic: Pruritus (7% to 31%), dermatitis/exfoliative dermatitis (4% to 27%)

Endocrine & metabolic: Hypocalcemia (4% to 52%), hyperglycemia (2% to 51%), hypoalbuminemia (3% to 48%), hyperuricemia (≤33%), hypomagnesemia (22% to 28%), hypermagnesemia (≤27%), hypophosphatemia (≤27%), hypokalemia (6% to 20%), hyponatremia (≤20%)

Gastrointestinal: Nausea (56% to 86%; grades 3/4: 2% to 6%), anorexia (23% to 54%), vomiting (34% to 52%; grades 3/4: ≤10%), taste alteration (15% to 40%), constipation (12% to 40%), diarrhea (20% to 36%), weight loss (10% to 15%), abdominal pain (13% to 14%)

Hematologic: Anemia (19% to 72%; grades 3/4: 3% to 28%), thrombocytopenia (17% to 72%; grades 3/4: ≤36%), neutropenia (11% to 66%; grades 3/4: 4% to 47%), lymphopenia (4% to 57%; grades 3/4: ≤37%), leukopenia (4% to 55%; grades 3/4: ≤45%)

Hepatic: AST increased (3% to 28%), ALT increased (3% to 22%)

Neuromuscular & skeletal: Weakness (53% to 77%)

Respiratory: Cough (18% to 21%), dyspnea (13% to 21%)

Miscellaneous: Infection (46% to 54%; grades 3/4: 11% to 33%)

1% to 10%:

Cardiovascular: Peripheral edema (6% to 10%), tachycardia (≤10%), chest pain, DVT, edema, QT prolongation, supraventricular arrhythmia, syncope, ventricular arrhythmia

Dermatologic: Cellulitis

Endocrine & metabolic: Dehydration

Gastrointestinal: Stomatitis (6% to 10%)

Hematologic: Neutropenic fever

Hepatic: Hyperbilirubinemia

Respiratory: Hypoxia, pneumonia, pneumonitis, pulmonary embolism

Miscellaneous: Central line infection, hypersensitivity, sepsis, tumor lysis syndrome (1% to 2%)

<1% (Limited to important or life-threatening): Acute renal failure, acute respiratory distress syndrome, atrial fibrillation, bacteremia, candida infection, cardiopulmonary failure, cardiogenic shock, Epstein-Barr virus reactivation, multiorgan failure, septic shock

Drug Interactions

Metabolism/Transport Effects Substrate of CYP3A4 (major), P-glycoprotein; **Note:** Assignment of Major/Minor substrate status based on clinically relevant drug interaction potential

Avoid Concomitant Use

Avoid concomitant use of RomiDEPsin with any of the following: Artemether; CYP3A4 Inducers (Strong); CYP3A4 Inhibitors (Strong); Dronedarone; Lumefantrine; Nilotinib; Pimozide; QUEtiapine; QuiNINE; Tetrabenazine; Thioridazine; Toremifene; Vandetanib; Vemurafenib; Ziprasidone

Increased Effect/Toxicity

RomiDEPsin may increase the levels/effects of: Dronedarone; Pimozide; QTc-Prolonging Agents; QuiNINE; Tetrabenazine; Thioridazine; Toremifene; Vandetanib; Vemurafenib; Warfarin; Ziprasidone

The levels/effects of RomiDEPsin may be increased by: Alfuzosin; Artemether; Chloroquine; Ciprofloxacin; Ciprofloxacin (Systemic); CYP3A4 Inhibitors (Moderate); CYP3A4 Inhibitors (Strong); Gadobutrol; Indacaterol; Lumefantrine; Nilotinib; P-glycoprotein/ABCB1 Inhibitors; QUEtiapine; QuiNINE

Decreased Effect

The levels/effects of RomiDEPsin may be decreased by: CYP3A4 Inducers (Strong); Deferasirox; P-glycoprotein/ABCB1 Inducers; Tocilizumab

Ethanol/Nutrition/Herb Interactions

Food: Avoid grapefruit juice (may increase the levels/effects of romidepsin).

Herb/Nutraceutical: Avoid St John's wort (may increase metabolism and decrease romidepsin concentrations).

Stability Store intact vials at room temperature of 20°C to 25°C (68°F to 77°F); excursions permitted between 15°C and 30°C (59°F and 86°F). Use appropriate precautions for handling and disposal. Reconstitute each 10 mg vial with 2 mL of supplied diluent to a reconstituted concentration of 5 mg/mL; swirl until dissolved. The reconstituted solution is stable for 8 hours at room temperature. Further dilute in 500 mL normal saline; compatible with polyvinyl chloride (PVC), ethylene vinyl acetate (EVA), polyethylene (PE) and glass infusion containers. Solutions diluted for infusion are stable for 24 hours at room temperature; however, the manufacturer recommends use as soon as possible after dilution.

Mechanism of Action Histone deacetylase inhibitor; catalyzes acetyl group removal from protein lysine residues (including histone and transcription factors). Inhibition of histone deacetylase results in accumulation of acetyl groups, leading to alterations in chromatin structure and transcription factor activation causing termination of cell growth (induces arrest in cell cycle at G_1 and G_2/M phases) leading to cell death.

Pharmacodynamics/Kinetics

Protein binding: 92% to 94%; primarily to α_1-acid glycoprotein

Metabolism: Hepatic, primarily via CYP3A4, minor metabolism from CYP3A5, 1A1, 2B6, and 2C19

Half-life elimination: ~3 hours

Dosage I.V.: Adults:

Cutaneous T-cell lymphoma: 14 mg/m^2 days 1, 8, and 15 of a 28-day treatment cycle; repeat cycle as long as benefit continues and treatment is tolerated

Peripheral T-cell lymphoma: 14 mg/m^2 days 1, 8, and 15 of a 28-day treatment cycle; repeat cycle as long as benefit continues and treatment is tolerated

Dosage adjustment for toxicity:

Nonhematologic toxicity (excluding alopecia):

Grade 2 or 3: Delay treatment until toxicity returns to ≤grade 1 or baseline, may restart at 14 mg/m^2

Grade 4 or recurrent grade 3 toxicity: Delay treatment until toxicity returns to ≤grade 1 or baseline, permanently reduce dose to 10 mg/m^2

Recurrent grade 3 or 4 toxicity despite dosage reduction: Discontinue treatment

Hematologic toxicity:

Grade 3 or 4 neutropenia or thrombocytopenia: Delay treatment until ANC ≥1500/mm^3 and/or platelets ≥75,000/mm^3 or baseline, may restart at 14 mg/m^2

Grade 4 febrile neutropenia or thrombocytopenia requiring platelet transfusion: Delay treatment until toxicity returns to ≤grade 1 or baseline, permanently reduce dose to 10 mg/m^2

Dosage adjustment in renal impairment: The pharmacokinetics of romidepsin are unaffected by mild, moderate, or severe renal impairment (based on pharmacokinetic analysis). Use with caution in patients with end-stage renal disease (has not been studied).

Dosage adjustment in hepatic impairment: Mild hepatic impairment does not significantly influence the pharmacokinetics of romidepsin. The effect of moderate or severe impairment is unknown; use with caution.

Dietary Considerations Avoid grapefruit juice.

Administration Infuse over 4 hours. Antiemetics to prevent nausea and vomiting were used in clinical trials (Piekarz, 2009; Piekarz, 2011).

Monitoring Parameters Serum electrolytes (baseline and periodic; especially potassium and magnesium); CBC with differential and platelets, ECG (baseline and periodic; in patients with significant cardiovascular disease, congenital long QT syndrome, and in patients taking QT-prolonging medications); signs/symptoms of infection or tumor lysis syndrome

Dosage Forms Excipient information presented when available (limited, particularly for generics); consult specific product labeling.

Injection, powder for reconstitution:

Istodax®: 10 mg [contains dehydrated ethanol (in diluent), propylene glycol (in diluent); supplied with diluent]

RomiPLOStim (roe mi PLOE stim)

Brand Names: U.S. Nplate®

Brand Names: Canada Nplate®

Index Terms AMG 531

Pharmacologic Category Colony Stimulating Factor; Thrombopoietic Agent

Use Treatment of thrombocytopenia in patients with chronic immune (idiopathic) thrombocytopenia purpura (ITP) who have had insufficient response to corticosteroids, immune globulin, or splenectomy

Note: Should be used only when the degree of thrombocytopenia and clinical condition increase the risk for bleeding; should not be used in attempt to normalize platelet counts; **not** indicated for the treatment of thrombocytopenia due to myelodysplastic syndrome.

Pregnancy Risk Factor C

Pregnancy Considerations Adverse effects were observed in animal reproduction studies. There are no adequate and well-controlled studies in pregnant women. Use during pregnancy only if the potential benefit to the mother outweighs the potential risk to the fetus. The Nplate® pregnancy registry has been established to monitor outcomes of women exposed to romiplostim during pregnancy (1-800-772-6436).

Lactation Excretion in breast milk unknown/ not recommended.

Medication Guide Available Yes

Contraindications There are no contraindications listed within the manufacturer's labeling.

Warnings/Precautions May increase the risk for bone marrow reticulin formation or progression. In patients where reticulin formation occurred, doses were ≥5 mcg/kg. A baseline peripheral blood smear is recommended prior to treatment to establish baseline level of cellular morphologic abnormalities, then monthly (after stable dose achieved) for new or worsening abnormalities (teardrop or nucleated RBC, immature WBCs) or cytopenias. Progression to marrow fibrosis with cytopenias was not observed in clinical trials, although the risk has not been excluded. Onset of new or worsening cellular abnormalities or cytopenias may warrant therapy discontinuation and subsequent bone marrow biopsy. Thromboembolism or thrombotic complications may occur with increased platelets; maintain appropriate platelet levels with dosage adjustments; portal vein thrombosis has been reported in patients with chronic liver disease; use with caution in patients with a history of cerebrovascular disease. Progression of underlying myelodysplastic syndrome (MDS) to acute myeloid leukemia (AML) has been observed in MDS clinical trials (not indicated for the treatment of thrombocytopenia due to MDS). An increase in the percentage of circulating myeloblasts in peripheral blood smears was also noted (both in patients who progressed to AML and in those who did not); blast cells decreased to baseline after discontinuation in some patients.

Inadequate platelet response may be due to neutralizing antibodies (to romiplostim or TPO) or bone marrow fibrosis. Indicated only when the degree of thrombocytopenia and clinical conditions increase the risk for bleeding; use the lowest dose necessary to achieve and maintain platelet count ≥50,000/mm^3. Do not use to normalize platelet counts. Discontinue if platelet count does not respond to a level to avoid clinically important bleeding after 4 weeks at the maximum recommended dose. May be used in combination with other therapies for ITP, including corticosteroids, danazol, azathioprine, immune globulin, or Rho(D) immune globulin. Reduce dose or discontinue ITP medications when platelet count ≥50,000/mm^3.

Upon discontinuation of therapy, thrombocytopenia may worsen. Severity may be greater than pretreatment level. Risk of bleeding is increased, particularly in patients receiving anticoagulants or antiplatelet agents; monitor closely. Rebound thrombocytopenia generally resolves within 14 days.

Use with caution in patients with hepatic and renal impairment (has not been studied).

Adverse Reactions

>10%:

Central nervous system: Headache (35%), dizziness (17%), insomnia (16%)

Gastrointestinal: Abdominal pain (11%)

Hematologic: Circulating myeloblasts increased (MDS patients: 17%)

Neuromuscular & skeletal: Arthralgia (26%), myalgia (14%), limb pain (13%)

1% to 10%:

Gastrointestinal: Dyspepsia (7%)

Hematologic: Rebound thrombocytopenia (7%), AML (MDS patients: 4% to 6%), bone marrow reticulin formation/deposition (4%)

Neuromuscular & skeletal: Shoulder pain (8%), paresthesia (6%)

Miscellaneous: Antibody formation (romiplostim 6%; TPO 4%)

<1% (Limited to important or life-threatening): Erythromelalgia, marrow fibrosis with collagen, thromboembolism, thrombotic complications

Drug Interactions

Metabolism/Transport Effects None known.

Avoid Concomitant Use There are no known interactions where it is recommended to avoid concomitant use.

Increased Effect/Toxicity There are no known significant interactions involving an increase in effect.

Decreased Effect There are no known significant interactions involving a decrease in effect.

Stability Store intact vials refrigerated at 2°C to 8°C (36°F to 46°F); do not freeze. Protect from light. Store in original carton until use. Reconstitute with preservative free SWFI (add 0.72 mL to 250 mcg vial or 1.2 mL to 500 mcg vial) to a final concentration of 500 mcg/mL. Gently invert vial and swirl; do not shake. Usually dissolves within 2 minutes. Reconstituted solution may be stored at room temperature of 25°C (77°F) or refrigerated at 2°C to 8°C (36°F to 46°F) for up to 24 hours prior to administration. Protect reconstituted solution from light; discard any unused portion.

Mechanism of Action Thrombopoietin (TPO) peptide mimetic which increases platelet counts in ITP by binding to and activating the human TPO receptor.

Pharmacodynamics/Kinetics

Onset of action: Platelet count increase: SubQ: 4-9 days; Peak platelet count increase: Days 12-16

Duration: Platelet counts return to baseline by day 28

Absorption: SubQ: Slow

Half-life elimination: Median: 3.5 days (range: 1-34 days)

Time to peak, plasma: SubQ: Median: 14 hours (range: 7-50 hours)

Dosage Note: Initial dose is based on actual body weight. Use the lowest dose sufficient to maintain platelet count ≥50,000/mm^3 as necessary to reduce the risk of bleeding. Discontinue if platelet count does not respond to a level that avoids clinically important bleeding after 4 weeks at the maximum recommended dose.

SubQ: Adults: Chronic ITP: Initial: 1 mcg/kg once weekly; adjust dose by 1 mcg/kg/week to achieve platelet count ≥50,000/mm^3 and to reduce the risk of bleeding; Maximum: 10 mcg/kg/week (median dose needed to achieve response in clinical trials: 2 mcg/kg)

Dosage adjustment recommendations:

Platelet count <50,000/mm^3: Increase dose by 1 mcg/kg

Platelet count >200,000/mm^3 for 2 consecutive weeks: Reduce dose by 1 mcg/kg

Platelet count >400,000/mm^3: Withhold dose; assess platelet count weekly; when platelet count <200,000/mm^3, resume with the dose reduced by 1 mcg/kg

Dosage adjustment in renal impairment: No dosage adjustment provided in manufacturer's labeling (has not been studied)

Dosage adjustment in hepatic impairment: No dosage adjustment provided in manufacturer's labeling (has not been studied)

Dietary Considerations Some products may contain sucrose.

Administration Administer SubQ. Administration volume may be small; use appropriate syringe (with graduations to 0.01 mL) for administration.

Monitoring Parameters CBC with differential and platelets (baseline, during treatment [weekly until platelet response stable for at least 4 weeks then monthly] and weekly for at least 2 weeks following completion of treatment)

Evaluate for neutralizing antibodies in patients with inadequate response (blood samples may be submitted to Amgen for assay [1-800-772-6436]).

Reference Range Target platelet count of 50,000-200,000/mm^3; platelet life span: 8-11 days

Additional Information Restricted access to Nplate® was previously a REMS requirement via the Nplate® NEXUS (Network of Experts Understanding and Supporting Nplate® and Patients) program. Patients, prescribers, and pharmacies were required to be enrolled in this program. However, the FDA eliminated this REMS requirement in December 2011. There is currently no restricted access to obtaining Nplate®.

Dosage Forms Excipient information presented when available (limited, particularly for generics); consult specific product labeling.

Injection, powder for reconstitution:

Nplate®: 250 mcg [contains sucrose 15 mg/vial]

Nplate®: 500 mcg [contains sucrose 25 mg/vial]

ROPINIRole (roe PIN i role)

Brand Names: U.S. Requip®; Requip® XL™

Brand Names: Canada CO Ropinirole; JAMP-Ropinirole; PMS-Ropinirole; RAN™-Ropinirole; Requip®

Index Terms Ropinirole Hydrochloride

Pharmacologic Category Anti-Parkinson's Agent, Dopamine Agonist

Additional Appendix Information

Antiparkinsonian Agents *on page 1879*

Use Treatment of idiopathic Parkinson's disease; in patients with early Parkinson's disease who were not receiving concomitant levodopa therapy as well as in patients with advanced disease on concomitant levodopa; treatment of moderate-to-severe primary Restless Legs Syndrome (RLS)

Pregnancy Risk Factor C

Pregnancy Considerations Teratogenic effects have been observed in animal studies. There are no adequate and well-controlled studies in pregnant women; use only if potential benefit outweighs the risk to the fetus.

Lactation Excretion in breast milk unknown/not recommended

Contraindications Hypersensitivity to ropinirole or any component of the formulation

Warnings/Precautions Syncope, sometimes associated with bradycardia, was observed in association with ropinirole in both early Parkinson's disease (without levodopa) patients and advanced Parkinson's disease (with levodopa) patients. Dopamine agonists appear to impair the systemic regulation of blood pressure resulting in postural hypotension, especially during dose escalation. Parkinson's disease patients appear to have an impaired capacity to respond to a postural challenge; use with caution in patients at risk of hypotension (ie, those receiving antihypertensive or antiarrhythmic drugs) or where transient hypotensive episodes would be poorly tolerated (cardiovascular disease or cerebrovascular disease). Parkinson's patients being treated with dopaminergic agonists ordinarily require careful monitoring for signs and symptoms of postural hypotension, especially during dose escalation, and should be informed of this risk.

May cause hallucinations (dose dependent); risk may be increased in the elderly. Use with caution in patients with pre-existing dyskinesia, hepatic or severe renal dysfunction (use in patients with severe renal impairment and who are not undergoing regular hemodialysis is not recommended in the Canadian labeling). Avoid use in patients with a major psychotic disorder; may exacerbate psychosis.

Patients treated with ropinirole have reported falling asleep while engaging in activities of daily living; this has been reported to occur without significant warning signs. Monitor for daytime somnolence or pre-existing sleep disorder; caution with concomitant sedating medication; discontinue if significant daytime sleepiness or episodes of falling asleep occur. Patients must be cautioned about performing tasks which require mental alertness (eg, operating machinery or driving). Use with caution in patients receiving other CNS depressants or psychoactive agents. Effects with other sedative drugs or ethanol may be potentiated.

Dopamine agonists have been associated with compulsive behaviors and/or loss of impulse control, which has manifested as pathological gambling, libido increases (hypersexuality), and/or binge eating. Causality has not been established, and controversy exists as to whether this phenomenon is related to the underlying disease, prior behaviors/addictions and/or drug therapy. Dose reduction or discontinuation of therapy has been reported to reverse these behaviors in some, but not all cases. Risk for melanoma development is increased in Parkinson's disease patients; drug causation or factors contributing to risk have not been established. Patients should be monitored closely and periodic skin examinations should be performed.

Some patients treated for RLS may experience worsening of symptoms in the early morning hours (rebound) or an increase and/or spread of daytime symptoms (augmentation); clinical management of these phenomena has not been evaluated in controlled clinical trials. Pathologic degenerative changes were observed in the retinas of albino rats during studies with this agent, but were not observed in the retinas of albino mice or in other species. The significance of these data for humans remains uncertain.

Other dopaminergic agents have been associated with a syndrome resembling neuroleptic malignant syndrome on withdrawal or significant dosage reduction after long-term use. Risk of fibrotic complications (eg, pleural effusion/fibrosis, interstitial lung disease) and melanoma has been reported in patients receiving ropinirole; drug causation has not been established.

Adverse Reactions

Data inclusive of trials in early Parkinson's disease (without levodopa) and Restless Legs Syndrome:

>10%:

Cardiovascular: Syncope (1% to 12%)

Central nervous system: Somnolence (11% to 40%), dizziness (6% to 40%), fatigue (8% to 11%)

Gastrointestinal: Nausea (immediate release: 40% to 60%; extended release: 19%), vomiting (11% to 12%)

Miscellaneous: Viral infection (11%)

1% to 10%:

Cardiovascular: Dependent/leg edema (2% to 7%), orthostasis (1% to 6%), hypertension (5%), chest pain (4%), flushing (3%), palpitation (3%), peripheral ischemia (2% to 3%), atrial fibrillation (2%), extrasystoles (2%), hypotension (2%), tachycardia (2%)

Central nervous system: Pain (3% to 8%), headache (extended release: 6%), confusion (5%), hallucinations (up to 5%; dose related), hypoesthesia (4%), amnesia (3%), malaise (3%), yawning (3%), concentration impaired (2%), vertigo (2%)

Dermatologic: Hyperhidrosis (3%)

Gastrointestinal: Dyspepsia (4% to 10%), abdominal pain (3% to 7%), constipation (≥5%), xerostomia (3% to 5%), diarrhea (5%), anorexia (4%), flatulence (3%)

Genitourinary: Urinary tract infection (5%), impotence (3%)

Hepatic: Alkaline phosphatase increased (3%)

Neuromuscular & skeletal: Weakness (6%), arthralgia (4%), muscle cramps (3%), paresthesia (3%), hyperkinesia (2%)

Ocular: Abnormal vision (6%), xerophthalmia (2%)

Respiratory: Pharyngitis (6% to 9%), rhinitis (4%), sinusitis (4%), bronchitis (3%), dyspnea (3%), influenza (3%), cough (3%), nasal congestion (2%)

Miscellaneous: Diaphoresis increased (3% to 6%)

Advanced Parkinson's disease (with levodopa):

>10%:

Central nervous system: Dizziness (immediate release: 26%; extended-release: 8%), somnolence (immediate release: 20%, extended release: 7%), headache (17%)

Gastrointestinal: Nausea (immediate release: 30%; extended-release: 11%)

Neuromuscular & skeletal: Dyskinesias (immediate release: 34%; extended-release: 13%; dose related)

1% to 10%:

Cardiovascular: Hypotension (2% to 5%; including orthostatic), peripheral edema (4%), syncope (3%), hypertension (3%; dose related)

Central nervous system: Hallucinations (7% to 10%; dose related), confusion (9%), anxiety (2% to 6%), amnesia (5%), nervousness (5%), pain (5%), vertigo (4%), abnormal dreaming (3%), paresis (3%), aggravated parkinsonism, insomnia

Gastrointestinal: Abdominal pain (6% to 9%), vomiting (7%), constipation (4% to 6%), diarrhea (3% to 5%), xerostomia (2% to 5%), dysphagia (2%), flatulence (2%), salivation increased (2%), weight loss (2%)

Genitourinary: Urinary tract infection (6%), pyuria (2%), urinary incontinence (2%)

Hematologic: Anemia (2%)

Neuromuscular & skeletal: Falls (2% to 10%; dose related), arthralgia (7%), tremor (6%), hypokinesia (5%), paresthesia (5%), arthritis (3%), back pain (3%)

Ocular: Diplopia (2%)

Respiratory: Upper respiratory tract infection (9%), dyspnea (3%)

Miscellaneous: Injury, diaphoresis increased (7%), viral infection, increased drug level (7%)

Other adverse effects (all phase 2/3 trials for Parkinson's disease and Restless Leg Syndrome):

≥1%: Asthma, BUN increased, depression, gastroenteritis, gastrointestinal reflux, irritability, migraine, muscle spasm, myalgia, neck pain, neuralgia, osteoarthritis, pharyngolaryngeal pain, rash, rigors, sleep disorder, tendonitis

<1% (Limited to important or life-threatening): Abnormal coordination, acidosis, agitation, aneurysm, angina, aphasia, behavioral disorders, bradycardia, bundle branch block, cardiac arrest, cardiac failure, cardiac valvulopathy, cardiomegaly, cellulitis, cholecystitis, cholelithiasis, choreoathetosis, colitis, coma, conjunctival hemorrhage, dehydration, delusion, delirium, diabetes mellitus, diverticulitis, Dupuytren's contracture, dysphonia, electrolyte disturbances, eosinophilia, extrapyramidal symptoms, gangrene, gastrointestinal hemorrhage, gastrointestinal ulceration, glaucoma, goiter, gynecomastia, hematuria, hemiparesis, hemiplegia, hepatitis (ischemic), hyperbilirubinemia, hypercholesterolemia, hyper-/hypothyroidism, hyper-/hypotonia, hypoglycemia, hyponatremia, hyperphosphatemia, hypersensitivity reactions (angioedema, pruritus), hyperuricemia, impulsive/compulsive behaviors (eg, pathological gambling, hypersexuality, binge eating), infections (bacterial, viral, or fungal); interstitial lung disease, intestinal obstruction, leukocytosis, leukopenia, limb embolism, liver enzymes increased, lymphadenopathy, lymphedema, lymphocytosis, lymphopenia, menstrual abnormalities, mitral insufficiency, MI, neoplasms (various), pancreatitis, paralysis, paranoia, peripheral neuropathy, photosensitivity, pleural effusion, pleural fibrosis, proteinuria, psychiatric disorders, pulmonary edema, pulmonary embolism, renal calculus, renal failure (acute), seizure, sepsis, SIADH, skin disorders, stomatitis, stupor, subarachnoid hemorrhage, suicide attempt, SVT, thrombocytopenia, thrombosis, tinnitus, tongue edema, torticollis, urticaria, vagina/uterine hemorrhage, ventricular tachycardia, visual disturbances

Drug Interactions

Metabolism/Transport Effects Substrate of CYP1A2 (major), CYP3A4 (minor); **Note:** Assignment of Major/Minor substrate status based on clinically relevant drug interaction potential; **Inhibits** CYP1A2 (weak), CYP2D6 (weak)

Avoid Concomitant Use There are no known interactions where it is recommended to avoid concomitant use.

Increased Effect/Toxicity

The levels/effects of ROPINIRole may be increased by: Abiraterone Acetate; Antipsychotics (Typical); Ciprofloxacin; Ciprofloxacin (Systemic); Conivaptan; CYP1A2 Inhibitors (Moderate); CYP1A2 Inhibitors (Strong); Deferasirox; Estrogen Derivatives; MAO Inhibitors; Methylphenidate

Decreased Effect

ROPINIRole may decrease the levels/effects of: Antipsychotics (Typical)

The levels/effects of ROPINIRole may be decreased by: Antipsychotics (Atypical); CYP1A2 Inducers (Strong); Cyproterone; Metoclopramide; Tocilizumab

Ethanol/Nutrition/Herb Interactions

Ethanol: Avoid ethanol (may increase CNS depression).

Herb/Nutraceutical: Avoid kava kava, gotu kola, valerian, St John's wort (may increase CNS depression).

Stability Store at controlled room temperature of 20°C to 25°C (68°F to 77°F). Protect from light.

Mechanism of Action Ropinirole has a high relative *in vitro* specificity and full intrinsic activity at the D_2 and D_3 dopamine receptor subtypes, binding with higher affinity to D_3 than to D_2 or D_4 receptor subtypes; relevance of D_3 receptor binding in Parkinson's disease is unknown. Ropinirole has moderate *in vitro* affinity for opioid receptors. Ropinirole and its metabolites have negligible *in vitro* affinity for dopamine D_1, 5-HT_1, 5-HT_2, benzodiazepine, GABA, muscarinic, alpha$_1$-, alpha$_2$-, and beta-adrenoreceptors. Although precise mechanism of action of ropinirole is unknown, it is believed to be due to stimulation of postsynaptic dopamine D_2-type receptors within the caudate putamen in the brain. Ropinirole caused decreases in systolic and diastolic blood pressure at doses >0.25 mg. The mechanism of ropinirole-induced postural hypotension is believed to be due to D_2-mediated blunting of the noradrenergic response to standing and subsequent decrease in peripheral vascular resistance.

Pharmacodynamics/Kinetics

Absorption: Not affected by food

Distribution: V_d: 525 L

Protein binding: 40%

Metabolism: Extensively hepatic via CYP1A2 to inactive metabolites; first-pass effect

Bioavailability: Absolute: 45% to 55%

Half-life elimination: ~6 hours

Time to peak: Immediate release: ~1-2 hours; Extended release: 6-10 hours; T_{max} increased by 2.5-3 hours when drug taken with food

Excretion: Urine (<10% as unchanged drug, 60% as metabolites)

Clearance: Reduced by 15% to 30% in patients >65 years of age

Dosage Oral: Adults:

Parkinson's disease:

Immediate release tablet: The dosage should be increased to achieve a maximum therapeutic effect, balanced against the principal side effects of nausea, dizziness, somnolence and dyskinesia. Recommended starting dose is 0.25 mg 3 times/day; based on individual patient response, the dosage should be titrated with weekly increments as described below:

- Week 1: 0.25 mg 3 times/day; total daily dose: 0.75 mg
- Week 2: 0.5 mg 3 times/day; total daily dose: 1.5 mg
- Week 3: 0.75 mg 3 times/day; total daily dose: 2.25 mg
- Week 4: 1 mg 3 times/day; total daily dose: 3 mg

Note: After week 4, if necessary, daily dosage may be increased by 1.5 mg/day on a weekly basis up to a dose of 9 mg/day, and then by up to 3 mg/day weekly to a total of 24 mg/day

Parkinson's disease discontinuation taper: Ropinirole should be gradually tapered over 7 days as follows: reduce frequency of administration from 3 times daily to twice daily for 4 days, then reduce to once daily for remaining 3 days.

Extended release tablet: Initial: 2 mg once daily for 1-2 weeks, followed by increases of 2 mg/day at weekly or longer intervals based on therapeutic response and tolerability (maximum: 24 mg/day); **Note:** When discontinuing gradually taper over 7 days.

Restless legs syndrome: Immediate release tablets: Initial: 0.25 mg once daily 1-3 hours before bedtime. Dose may be increased after 2 days to 0.5 mg daily, and after 7 days to 1 mg daily. Dose may be further titrated upward in 0.5 mg increments every week until reaching a daily dose of 3 mg during week 6. If symptoms persist or reappear, the daily dose may be increased to a maximum of 4 mg beginning week 7.

Note: Doses up to 4 mg per day may be discontinued without tapering.

Converting from ropinirole immediate release tablets to ropinirole extended-release tablets: Choose a once daily extended-release dose that most closely matches current immediate-release daily dose.

Elderly: Clearance is reduced; however, no dosage adjustment necessary. Titrate dose to clinical response. Refer to adult dosing.

Dosage adjustment in renal impairment:
Moderate renal impairment (Cl_{cr} 30-50 mL/minute): No adjustment needed
Severe renal impairment (Cl_{cr} <30 mL/minute): Use with caution; has not been studied in this patient population. **Note:** The Canadian labeling recommends to avoid use in patients with severe renal impairment and who are not undergoing regular hemodialysis.
Hemodialysis: Canadian labeling (not in U.S. labeling): Initial: 0.25 mg 3 times daily; may titrate dose upward based on tolerability and efficacy (maximum dose: 18 mg/day); postdialysis supplemental doses are not required

Dosage adjustment in hepatic impairment: Titrate with caution; has not been studied.

Dietary Considerations May be taken without regard to meals; taking with food may reduce nausea.

Administration May be administered without regard to meals; taking with food may reduce nausea. Swallow extended-release tablet whole; do not crush, split, or chew.

Monitoring Parameters
Blood pressure (orthostatic); daytime alertness

Additional Information If therapy with a drug known to be a potent inhibitor of CYP1A2 is stopped or started during treatment with ropinirole, adjustment of ropinirole dose may be required. Ropinirole binds to melanin-containing tissues (ie, eyes, skin) in pigmented rats. After a single dose, long-term retention of drug was demonstrated, with a half-life in the eye of 20 days; not known if ropinirole accumulates in these tissues over time.

Dosage Forms Excipient information presented when available (limited, particularly for generics); consult specific product labeling.
Tablet, oral: 0.25 mg, 0.5 mg, 1 mg, 2 mg, 3 mg, 4 mg, 5 mg
Requip®: 0.25 mg, 0.5 mg, 1 mg, 2 mg, 3 mg, 4 mg, 5 mg
Tablet, extended release, oral:
Requip® XL™: 2 mg, 4 mg, 6 mg, 8 mg, 12 mg

◆ **Ropinirole Hydrochloride** *see* ROPINIRole *on page 1517*

Ropivacaine (roe PIV a kane)

Brand Names: U.S. Naropin®
Brand Names: Canada Naropin®
Index Terms Ropivacaine Hydrochloride
Pharmacologic Category Local Anesthetic
Use Local anesthetic for use in surgery, postoperative pain management, and obstetrical procedures when local or regional anesthesia is needed
Pregnancy Risk Factor B
Pregnancy Considerations Teratogenic events were not observed in animal studies. When used for epidural block during labor and delivery, systemically absorbed ropivacaine may cross the placenta, resulting in varying degrees of fetal or neonatal effects (eg, CNS or cardiovascular depression). Fetal or neonatal adverse events include fetal bradycardia (12%), neonatal jaundice (8%), low Apgar scores (3%), fetal distress (2%), neonatal respiratory disorder (3%). Maternal hypotension may also result from systemic absorption. In cases of hypotension, position pregnant woman in left lateral decubitus position to prevent aortocaval compression by the gravid uterus. Epidural anesthesia may prolong the second stage of labor.
Lactation Excretion in breast milk unknown/use caution
Contraindications Hypersensitivity to ropivacaine, amide-type local anesthetics (eg, bupivacaine, mepivacaine, lidocaine), or any component of the formulation

Warnings/Precautions Careful and constant monitoring of the patient's state of consciousness should be done following each local anesthetic injection; at such times, restlessness, anxiety, tinnitus, dizziness, blurred vision, tremors, depression, or drowsiness may be early warning signs of CNS toxicity. Treatment is primarily symptomatic and supportive. Intravascular injections should be avoided. Continuous intra-articular infusion of local anesthetics after arthroscopic or other surgical procedures is **not** an approved use; chondrolysis (primarily in the shoulder joint) has occurred following infusion, with some cases requiring arthroplasty or shoulder replacement. Local anesthetics have been associated with rare occurrences of sudden respiratory arrest, seizures, and cardiac arrest. When administering this agent, have ready access to drugs and equipment for resuscitation. Use with caution in patients with liver disease, cardiovascular disease, neurological or psychiatric disorders, and in the elderly or debilitated; these patients may be at greater risk for toxicity. Cardiovascular adverse events (bradycardia, hypotension) may be age-related (more common in patients >61 years of age). Use caution in patients on type III antiarrhythmics (eg, amiodarone); consider ECG monitoring since cardiac effects may be additive. Use cautiously in hypotension, hypovolemia, or heart block. Ropivacaine is not recommended for use in emergency situations where rapid administration is necessary. Safety and efficacy have not been established in pediatric patients.

Adverse Reactions
>10%:
Cardiovascular: Hypotension (dose-related and age-related: 32% to 69%), bradycardia (6% to 20%)
Gastrointestinal: Nausea (11% to 29%), vomiting (7% to 14%)
Neuromuscular & skeletal: Back pain (7% to 16%)
1% to 10%:
Cardiovascular: Hypertension, tachycardia, chest pain (1% to 5%)
Central nervous system: Fever (3% to 9%), headache (5% to 8%), dizziness (3%), chills (2% to 3%), anxiety (1%), lightheadedness
Dermatologic: Pruritus (1% to 5%)
Endocrine & metabolic: Hypokalemia
Genitourinary: Urinary retention (1% to 5%), urinary tract infection (1% to 5%)
Hematologic: Anemia (6%)
Neuromuscular & skeletal: Paresthesia (2% to 6%), hypoesthesia, rigors, circumoral paresthesia
Renal: Oliguria
Respiratory: Dyspnea
Miscellaneous: Shivering
<1% (Limited to important or life-threatening): Accidental I.V. injection (0.2%), angioedema, allergic reaction, apnea (usually associated with epidural block in head/neck region), bronchospasm, cardiac arrest, cardiovascular collapse, chondrolysis (continuous intra-articular administration), dyskinesia, hallucination, hyperthermia, laryngeal edema, myocardial depression, MI, rash, seizure, syncope, tinnitus, urticaria, ventricular arrhythmia

Drug Interactions
Metabolism/Transport Effects **Substrate** of CYP1A2 (major), CYP2B6 (minor), CYP2D6 (minor), CYP3A4 (minor); **Note:** Assignment of Major/Minor substrate status based on clinically relevant drug interaction potential
Avoid Concomitant Use There are no known interactions where it is recommended to avoid concomitant use.
Increased Effect/Toxicity
The levels/effects of Ropivacaine may be increased by: Abiraterone Acetate; Ciprofloxacin; Ciprofloxacin (Systemic); Conivaptan; CYP1A2 Inhibitors (Moderate); CYP1A2 Inhibitors (Strong); Deferasirox; FluvoxaMINE; Fospropofol; Propofol

Decreased Effect

The levels/effects of Ropivacaine may be decreased by: Cyproterone; Peginterferon Alfa-2b; Tocilizumab

Stability Store at 20°C to 25°C (68°F to 77°F). Infusions should be discarded after 24 hours.

Mechanism of Action Blocks both the initiation and conduction of nerve impulses by decreasing the neuronal membrane's permeability to sodium ions, which results in inhibition of depolarization with resultant blockade of conduction

Pharmacodynamics/Kinetics

Onset of action: Anesthesia (route dependent): 3-15 minutes

Duration (dose and route dependent): 3-15 hours

Metabolism: Hepatic, via CYP1A2 to metabolites

Half-life elimination: Epidural: 5-7 hours; I.V.: Terminal: 111 ± 62 minutes (Lee, 1989)

Excretion: Urine (86% as metabolites)

Dosage Dose varies with procedure, onset and depth of anesthesia desired, vascularity of tissues, duration of anesthesia, and condition of patient: Adults:

Surgical anesthesia:
- Lumbar epidural: 15-30 mL of 0.5% to 1% solution
- Lumbar epidural block for cesarean section:
  - 20-30 mL dose of 0.5% solution
  - 15-20 mL dose of 0.75% solution
- Thoracic epidural block: 5-15 mL dose of 0.5% or 0.75% solution
- Major nerve block:
  - 35-50 mL dose of 0.5% solution (175-250 mg)
  - 10-40 mL dose of 0.75% solution (75-300 mg)
- Field block: 1-40 mL dose of 0.5% solution (5-200 mg)

Labor pain management: Lumbar epidural: Initial: 10-20 mL 0.2% solution; continuous infusion dose: 6-14 mL/hour of 0.2% solution with incremental injections of 10-15 mL/hour of 0.2% solution

Postoperative pain management:
- Peripheral nerve block: Continuous infusion dose: 5-10 mL/hour of 0.2% solution (Bagry, 2008; Klein, 2000)
- Lumbar or thoracic epidural: Continuous infusion dose: 6-14 mL/hour of 0.2% solution
- Infiltration/minor nerve block:
  - 1-100 mL dose of 0.2% solution
  - 1-40 mL dose of 0.5% solution

Administration Administered via local infiltration, epidural block and epidural infusion, or intermittent bolus

Monitoring Parameters Heart rate, blood pressure, ECG monitoring (if used with antiarrhythmics)

Dosage Forms Excipient information presented when available (limited, particularly for generics); consult specific product labeling.

Injection, solution, as hydrochloride [preservative free]:
- Naropin®: 2 mg/mL (10 mL, 20 mL, 100 mL, 200 mL); 5 mg/mL (20 mL, 30 mL, 100 mL, 200 mL); 7.5 mg/mL (20 mL); 10 mg/mL (10 mL, 20 mL)

◆ **Ropivacaine Hydrochloride** *see* Ropivacaine *on page 1520*

◆ **Rosanil®** *see* Sulfur and Sulfacetamide *on page 1607*

◆ **Rosasol® (Can)** *see* MetroNIDAZOLE (Topical) *on page 1122*

Rosiglitazone (roh si GLI ta zone)

Brand Names: U.S. Avandia®

Brand Names: Canada Avandia®

Pharmacologic Category Antidiabetic Agent, Thiazolidinedione

Additional Appendix Information

Diabetes Mellitus Management, Adults *on page 1983*

Use Type 2 diabetes mellitus (noninsulin dependent, NIDDM):

Monotherapy: Improve glycemic control as an adjunct to diet and exercise

Note: Canadian labeling approves use as monotherapy only when metformin is contraindicated or not tolerated.

Combination therapy: **Note:** Use when diet, exercise, and a single agent do not result in adequate glycemic control.
- U.S. labeling: In combination with a sulfonylurea, metformin, or sulfonylurea plus metformin
- Canadian labeling: In combination with metformin; in combination with a sulfonylurea only when metformin use is contraindicated or not tolerated

Pregnancy Risk Factor C

Pregnancy Considerations Rosiglitazone is classified as pregnancy category C due to adverse effects observed in initial animal studies. Rosiglitazone has been found to cross the placenta during the first trimester of pregnancy. Inadvertent use early in pregnancy has not shown adverse fetal effects although in the majority of cases, the medication was stopped as soon as pregnancy was detected. Thiazolidinediones may cause ovulation in anovulatory premenopausal women, increasing the risk of pregnancy; adequate contraception in premenopausal women is recommended. Maternal hyperglycemia can be associated with adverse effects in the fetus, including macrosomia, neonatal hyperglycemia, and hyperbilirubinemia; the risk of congenital malformations is increased when the Hb A_{1c} is above the normal range. Diabetes can also be associated with adverse effects in the mother. Poorly-treated diabetes may cause end-organ damage that may in turn negatively affect obstetric outcomes. Physiologic glucose levels should be maintained prior to and during pregnancy to decrease the risk of adverse events in the mother and the fetus. Until additional safety and efficacy data are obtained, the use of oral agents is generally not recommended as routine management of GDM or type 2 diabetes mellitus during pregnancy. Insulin is the drug of choice for the control of diabetes mellitus during pregnancy.

Lactation Excretion in breast milk unknown/not recommended

Prescribing and Access Restrictions Health Canada requires written informed consent for new and current patients receiving rosiglitazone.

Medication Guide Available Yes

Contraindications NYHA Class III/IV heart failure (initiation of therapy)

Canadian labeling: Hypersensitivity to rosiglitazone or any component of the formulation; any stage of heart failure (eg, NYHA Class I, II, III, IV); serious hepatic impairment; pregnancy

Warnings/Precautions [U.S. Boxed Warning]: Thiazolidinediones, including rosiglitazone, may cause or exacerbate congestive heart failure; closely monitor for signs/symptoms of congestive heart failure (eg, rapid weight gain, dyspnea, edema), particularly after initiation or dose increases. Not recommended for use in any patient with symptomatic heart failure. In the U.S., initiation of therapy is contraindicated in patients with NYHA class III or IV heart failure; in Canada use is contraindicated in patients with any stage of heart failure (NYHA Class I, II, III, IV). Use with caution in patients with edema; may increase plasma volume and/or cause fluid retention, leading to heart failure. Dose-related weight gain observed with use; mechanism unknown but likely associated with fluid retention and fat accumulation. Use may also be associated with an increased risk of angina and MI. Use caution in patients at risk for cardiovascular events and monitor closely. Discontinue if any deterioration in cardiac status occurs.

Should not be used in diabetic ketoacidosis. Mechanism requires the presence of insulin; therefore, use in type 1 diabetes (insulin dependent, IDDM) is not recommended. Combination therapy with other hypoglycemic agents may increase risk for hypoglycemic events; dose reduction with the concomitant agent may be warranted. Concomitant use with nitrates is not recommended due to increased risk of myocardial ischemia. Avoid use with insulin due to an increased risk of edema, congestive heart failure, and myocardial ischemic events.

Use with caution in patients with elevated transaminases (AST or ALT); do not initiate in patients with active liver disease or ALT >2.5 times ULN at baseline; evaluate patients with ALT ≤2.5 times ULN at baseline or during therapy for cause of enzyme elevation; during therapy, if ALT >3 times ULN, reevaluate levels promptly and discontinue if elevation persists or if jaundice occurs at any time during use. Idiosyncratic hepatotoxicity has been reported with another thiazolidinedione agent (troglitazone); avoid use in patients who previously experienced jaundice during troglitazone therapy. Monitoring should include periodic determinations of liver function. Increased incidence of bone fractures in females treated with rosiglitazone observed during analysis of long-term trial; majority of fractures occurred in the upper arm, hand, and foot (differing from the hip or spine fractures usually associated with postmenopausal osteoporosis). May decrease hemoglobin/hematocrit and/or WBC count (slight); effects may be related to increased plasma volume and/or dose related; use with caution in patients with anemia.

Rosiglitazone has been associated with new onset and/or worsening of macular edema in patients with diabetes. Rosiglitazone should be used with caution in patients with a pre-existing macular edema or diabetic retinopathy. Discontinuation of rosiglitazone should be considered in any patient who reports visual deterioration. In addition, ophthalmological consultation should be initiated in these patients. Use with caution in premenopausal, anovulatory women; may result in resumption of ovulation, increasing the risk of pregnancy. Safety and efficacy in pediatric patients have not been established.

Additional Canadian warnings (not included in U.S. labeling): If glycemic control is inadequate, rosiglitazone may be added to metformin or a sulfonylurea (if metformin use is contraindicated or not tolerated); use of triple therapy (rosiglitazone in combination with both metformin and a sulfonylurea) is not indicated due to increased risks of heart failure and fluid retention.

Adverse Reactions Note: The rate of certain adverse reactions (eg, anemia, edema, hypoglycemia) may be higher with some combination therapies.

>10%: Endocrine & metabolic: HDL-cholesterol increased, LDL-cholesterol increased, total cholesterol increased, weight gain

1% to 10%:

Cardiovascular: Edema (5%), hypertension (4%); heart failure/CHF (up to 2% to 3% in patients receiving insulin; incidence likely higher in patients with preexisting HF; myocardial ischemia (3%; incidence likely higher in patients with preexisting CAD)

Central nervous system: Headache (6%)

Endocrine & metabolic: Hypoglycemia (1% to 3%; combination therapy with insulin: 12% to 14%)

Gastrointestinal: Diarrhea (3%)

Hematologic: Anemia (2%)

Neuromuscular & skeletal: Fractures (up to 9%; incidence greater in females; usually upper arm, hand, or foot), arthralgia (5%), back pain (4% to 5%)

Respiratory: Upper respiratory tract infection (4% to 10%), nasopharyngitis (6%)

Miscellaneous: Injury (8%)

<1% (Limited to important or life-threatening): Anaphylaxis, angina, angioedema, bilirubin increased, blurred vision, cardiac arrest, dyspnea, coronary artery disease, coronary thrombosis, hematocrit decreased, hemoglobin decreased, hepatic failure, hepatitis, HDL-cholesterol decreased, jaundice (reversible), macular edema, MI, pleural effusion, pruritus, pulmonary edema, rash, Stevens-Johnson syndrome, thrombocytopenia, transaminases increased, urticaria, visual acuity decreased, weight gain (rapid, excessive; usually due to fluid accumulation), WBC count decreased

Note: Rare cases of hepatocellular injury have been reported in men in their 60s within 2-3 weeks after initiation of rosiglitazone therapy. LFTs in these patients revealed severe hepatocellular injury which responded with rapid improvement of liver function and resolution of symptoms upon discontinuation of rosiglitazone. Patients were also receiving other potentially hepatotoxic medications (Al-Salman, 2000; Freid, 2000).

Drug Interactions

Metabolism/Transport Effects Substrate of CYP2C8 (major), CYP2C9 (minor); **Note:** Assignment of Major/Minor substrate status based on clinically relevant drug interaction potential; **Inhibits** CYP2C19 (weak), CYP2C8 (moderate), CYP2C9 (weak)

Avoid Concomitant Use There are no known interactions where it is recommended to avoid concomitant use.

Increased Effect/Toxicity

Rosiglitazone may increase the levels/effects of: CYP2C8 Substrates; Hypoglycemic Agents

The levels/effects of Rosiglitazone may be increased by: CYP2C8 Inhibitors (Moderate); CYP2C8 Inhibitors (Strong); Deferasirox; Gemfibrozil; Herbs (Hypoglycemic Properties); Insulin; Pegvisomant; Pregabalin; Trimethoprim; Vasodilators (Organic Nitrates)

Decreased Effect

The levels/effects of Rosiglitazone may be decreased by: Bile Acid Sequestrants; Corticosteroids (Orally Inhaled); Corticosteroids (Systemic); CYP2C8 Inducers (Strong); Luteinizing Hormone-Releasing Hormone Analogs; Rifampin; Somatropin; Thiazide Diuretics

Ethanol/Nutrition/Herb Interactions

Ethanol: Avoid ethanol (may cause hypoglycemia).

Food: Peak concentrations are lower by 28% and delayed when administered with food, but these effects are not believed to be clinically significant.

Herb/Nutraceutical: Avoid alfalfa, aloe, bilberry, bitter melon, burdock, celery, damiana, fenugreek, garcinia, garlic, ginger, ginseng (American), gymnema, marshmallow, stinging nettle (may cause hypoglycemia).

Stability Store at 15°C to 30°C (59°F to 86°F). Protect from light.

Mechanism of Action Thiazolidinedione antidiabetic agent that lowers blood glucose by improving target cell response to insulin, without increasing pancreatic insulin secretion. It has a mechanism of action that is dependent on the presence of insulin for activity. Rosiglitazone is an agonist for peroxisome proliferator-activated receptor-gamma (PPARgamma). Activation of nuclear PPAR-gamma receptors influences the production of a number of gene products involved in glucose and lipid metabolism. PPARgamma is abundant in the cells within the renal collecting tubules; fluid retention results from stimulation by thiazolidinediones which increases sodium reabsorption.

Pharmacodynamics/Kinetics

Onset of action: Delayed; Maximum effect: Up to 12 weeks

Distribution: V_{dss} (apparent): 17.6 L

Protein binding: 99.8%; primarily albumin

Metabolism: Hepatic (99%) via CYP2C8; minor metabolism via CYP2C9
Bioavailability: 99%
Half-life elimination: 3-4 hours
Time to peak, plasma: 1 hour; delayed with food
Excretion: Urine (~64%) and feces (~23%) as metabolites

Dosage Oral:

Adults: **Note:** All patients should be initiated at the lowest recommended dose.

Monotherapy: Initial: 4 mg daily as a single daily dose or in divided doses twice daily. If response is inadequate after 8-12 weeks of treatment, the dosage may be increased to 8 mg daily as a single daily dose or in divided doses twice daily. In clinical trials, the 4 mg twice-daily regimen resulted in the greatest reduction in fasting plasma glucose and Hb A_{1c}.

Combination therapy: When adding rosiglitazone to existing therapy, continue current dose(s) of previous agents:

U.S. labeling: With sulfonylureas or metformin (or sulfonylurea plus metformin): Initial: 4 mg daily as a single daily dose or in divided doses twice daily. If response is inadequate after 8-12 weeks of treatment, the dosage may be increased to 8 mg daily as a single daily dose or in divided doses twice daily. Reduce dose of sulfonylurea if hypoglycemia occurs. It is unlikely that the dose of metformin will need to be reduced due to hypoglycemia.

Canadian labeling:

With metformin: Initial: 4 mg daily as a single daily dose or in divided doses twice daily. If response is inadequate after 8-12 weeks of treatment, the dosage may be increased to 8 mg daily as a single daily dose or in divided doses twice daily.

With a sulfonylurea: 4 mg daily as a single daily dose or in divided doses twice daily. Dose should not exceed 4 mg daily when using in combination with a sulfonylurea. Reduce dose of sulfonylurea if hypoglycemia occurs.

Elderly: No dosage adjustment is recommended

Dosage adjustment in renal impairment: No dosage adjustment is required

Dosage comment in hepatic impairment: Clearance is significantly lower in hepatic impairment. Therapy should not be initiated if the patient exhibits active liver disease or increased transaminases (ALT >2.5 times the upper limit of normal) at baseline.

Dietary Considerations Management of type 2 diabetes mellitus (noninsulin dependent, NIDDM) should include diet control. May be taken without regard to meals.

Administration May be administered without regard to meals.

Monitoring Parameters Hemoglobin A_{1c}, fasting serum glucose; signs and symptoms of fluid retention or heart failure; liver enzymes (prior to initiation of therapy, then periodically thereafter); ophthalmic exams. Evaluate patients with ALT ≤2.5 times ULN at baseline or during therapy for cause of enzyme elevation. Patients with an elevation in ALT >3 times ULN should be rechecked as soon as possible. If the ALT levels remain >3 times ULN, therapy with rosiglitazone should be discontinued.

Reference Range Recommendations for glycemic control in adults with diabetes:

Hb A_{1c}: <7%
Preprandial capillary plasma glucose: 70-130 mg/dL
Peak postprandial capillary blood glucose: <180 mg/dL

Dosage Forms Excipient information presented when available (limited, particularly for generics); consult specific product labeling.

Tablet, oral:
Avandia®: 2 mg, 4 mg, 8 mg

Rosiglitazone and Glimepiride
(roh si GLI ta zone & GLYE me pye ride)

Brand Names: U.S. Avandaryl®
Brand Names: Canada Avandaryl®
Index Terms Glimepiride and Rosiglitazone Maleate
Pharmacologic Category Antidiabetic Agent, Sulfonylurea; Antidiabetic Agent, Thiazolidinedione
Use Management of type 2 diabetes mellitus (noninsulin dependent, NIDDM) as an adjunct to diet and exercise
Pregnancy Risk Factor C
Prescribing and Access Restrictions Health Canada requires written informed consent for new and current patients receiving rosiglitazone
Medication Guide Available Yes

Dosage Oral: Adults: Type 2 diabetes mellitus:

Initial: Rosiglitazone 4 mg and glimepiride 1 mg once daily **or** rosiglitazone 4 mg and glimepiride 2 mg once daily (for patients previously treated with sulfonylurea or thiazolidinedione monotherapy)

Patients switching from combination rosiglitazone and glimepiride as separate tablets: Use current dose

Titration:

Dose adjustment in patients previously on sulfonylurea monotherapy: May take 2 weeks to observe decreased blood glucose and 2-3 months to see full effects of rosiglitazone component. If not adequately controlled after 8-12 weeks, increase daily dose of rosiglitazone component.

Dose adjustment in patients previously on thiazolidinedione monotherapy: If not adequately controlled after 1-2 weeks, increase daily dose of glimepiride component in ≤2 mg increments in 1-2 week intervals.

Maximum dose:

U.S. labeling: Rosiglitazone 8 mg and glimepiride 4 mg once daily

Canadian labeling: Rosiglitazone 4 mg and glimepiride 4 mg once daily

Elderly: Rosiglitazone 4 mg and glimepiride 1 mg once daily; carefully titrate dose.

Dosage adjustment in renal impairment: Rosiglitazone 4 mg and glimepiride 1 mg once daily; carefully titrate dose.

Dosage adjustment in hepatic impairment: Rosiglitazone 4 mg and glimepiride 1 mg once daily; carefully titrate dose.

ALT ≤2.5 times ULN: Use with caution
ALT >2.5 times ULN: Do not initiate therapy
ALT >3 times ULN or jaundice: Discontinue

Additional Information Complete prescribing information for this medication should be consulted for additional detail.

Dosage Forms Excipient information presented when available (limited, particularly for generics); consult specific product labeling.

Tablet:
Avandaryl® 4 mg/1 mg: Rosiglitazone maleate 4 mg and glimepiride 1 mg
Avandaryl® 4 mg/2 mg: Rosiglitazone maleate 4 mg and glimepiride 2 mg
Avandaryl® 4 mg/4 mg: Rosiglitazone maleate 4 mg and glimepiride 4 mg
Avandaryl® 8 mg/2 mg: Rosiglitazone maleate 8 mg and glimepiride 2 mg
Avandaryl® 8 mg/4 mg: Rosiglitazone maleate 8 mg and glimepiride 4 mg

Rosiglitazone and Metformin
(roh si GLI ta zone & met FOR min)

Brand Names: U.S. Avandamet®

Brand Names: Canada Avandamet®

Index Terms Metformin and Rosiglitazone; Metformin Hydrochloride and Rosiglitazone Maleate; Rosiglitazone Maleate and Metformin Hydrochloride

Pharmacologic Category Antidiabetic Agent, Biguanide; Antidiabetic Agent, Thiazolidinedione

Use Management of type 2 diabetes mellitus (noninsulin dependent, NIDDM) as an adjunct to diet and exercise in patients where dual rosiglitazone and metformin therapy is appropriate

Pregnancy Risk Factor C

Prescribing and Access Restrictions Health Canada requires written informed consent for new and current patients receiving rosiglitazone.

Medication Guide Available Yes

Dosage Oral:

Adults: Type 2 diabetes mellitus: Daily dose should be divided and given with meals:

First-line therapy (drug-naive patients): Initial: Rosiglitazone 2 mg and metformin 500 mg once or twice daily; may increase by 2 mg/500 mg per day after 4 weeks to a maximum of 8 mg/2000 mg per day.

Second-line therapy:

Patients inadequately controlled on **metformin alone**: Initial dose: Rosiglitazone 4 mg/day plus current dose of metformin

Patients inadequately controlled on **rosiglitazone alone**: Initial dose: Metformin 1000 mg/day plus current dose of rosiglitazone

Note: When switching from combination rosiglitazone and metformin as separate tablets: Use current dose

Dose adjustment: Doses may be increased as increments of rosiglitazone 4 mg and/or metformin 500 mg, up to the maximum dose; doses should be titrated gradually.

After a change in the metformin dosage, titration can be done after 1-2 weeks

After a change in the rosiglitazone dosage, titration can be done after 8-12 weeks

Maximum dose: Rosiglitazone 8 mg/metformin 2000 mg daily

Elderly: The initial and maintenance dosing should be conservative, due to the potential for decreased renal function (monitor). Generally, elderly patients should not be titrated to the maximum; do not use in patients ≥80 years unless normal renal function has been established.

Dosage adjustment in renal impairment: Do not use with renal disease or renal dysfunction (serum creatinine ≥1.5 mg/dL in males or ≥1.4 mg/dL in females or abnormal clearance)

Dosage adjustment in hepatic impairment: Do not initiate therapy with active liver disease or ALT >2.5 times the upper limit of normal

Additional Information Complete prescribing information for this medication should be consulted for additional detail.

Dosage Forms Excipient information presented when available (limited, particularly for generics); consult specific product labeling.

Tablet:

Avandamet®: 2/500: Rosiglitazone 2 mg and metformin hydrochloride 500 mg

Avandamet®: 4/500: Rosiglitazone 4 mg and metformin hydrochloride 500 mg

Avandamet®: 2/1000: Rosiglitazone 2 mg and metformin hydrochloride 1000 mg

Avandamet®: 4/1000: Rosiglitazone 4 mg and metformin hydrochloride 1000 mg

◆ **Rosiglitazone Maleate and Metformin Hydrochloride** *see* Rosiglitazone and Metformin *on page 1523*

◆ **Rosone (Can)** *see* Betamethasone *on page 208*

◆ **Rosula®** *see* Sulfur and Sulfacetamide *on page 1607*

◆ **Rosula® Clarifying** *see* Sulfur and Sulfacetamide *on page 1607*

◆ **Rosula® NS** *see* Sulfacetamide (Topical) *on page 1599*

Rosuvastatin (roe soo va STAT in)

Brand Names: U.S. Crestor®

Brand Names: Canada Crestor®

Index Terms Rosuvastatin Calcium

Pharmacologic Category Antilipemic Agent, HMG-CoA Reductase Inhibitor

Additional Appendix Information

Hyperlipidemia Management *on page 1996*

Use

Treatment of dyslipidemias:

Used with dietary therapy for hyperlipidemias to reduce elevations in total cholesterol (TC), LDL-C, apolipoprotein B, nonHDL-C, and triglycerides (TG) in patients with primary hypercholesterolemia (elevations of 1 or more components are present in Fredrickson type IIa, IIb, and IV hyperlipidemias); increase HDL-C; treatment of primary dysbetalipoproteinemia (Fredrickson type III hyperlipidemia); treatment of homozygous familial hypercholesterolemia (FH); to slow progression of atherosclerosis as an adjunct to diet to lower TC and LDL-C

Heterozygous familial hypercholesterolemia (HeFH): In adolescent patients (10-17 years of age, females >1 year postmenarche) with HeFH having LDL-C >190 mg/dL or LDL >160 mg/dL with positive family history of premature cardiovascular disease (CVD), or ≥2 other CVD risk factors.

Primary prevention of cardiovascular disease: To reduce the risk of stroke, myocardial infarction, or arterial revascularization procedures in patients without clinically evident coronary heart disease or lipid abnormalities but with all of the following: 1) an increased risk of cardiovascular disease based on age ≥50 years old in men and ≥60 years old in women, 2) hsCRP ≥2 mg/L, and 3) the presence of at least one additional cardiovascular disease risk factor such as hypertension, low HDL-C, smoking, or a family history of premature coronary heart disease.

Secondary prevention of cardiovascular disease: To slow progression of atherosclerosis

Pregnancy Risk Factor X

Pregnancy Considerations Cholesterol biosynthesis may be important in fetal development. Contraindicated in pregnancy. Administer to women of childbearing potential only when conception is highly unlikely and patients have been informed of potential hazards.

Lactation Excretion in breast milk unknown/contraindicated

Contraindications Hypersensitivity to rosuvastatin or any component of the formulation; active liver disease; unexplained persistent elevations of serum transaminases (>3 times ULN); pregnancy; breast-feeding

Canadian labeling: Additional contraindications (not in U.S. labeling): Concomitant administration of cyclosporine; use of 40 mg dose in Asian patients, patients with predisposing risk factors for myopathy/rhabdomyolysis (eg, hereditary muscle disorders, history of myotoxicity with other HMC-CoA reductase inhibitors, concomitant use with fibrates or niacin, severe hepatic impairment, severe renal impairment [Cl_{cr} <30 mL/minute/1.73 m^2], hypothyroidism, alcohol abuse)

Warnings/Precautions Secondary causes of hyperlipidemia should be ruled out prior to therapy. Rosuvastatin has not been studied when the primary lipid abnormality is chylomicron elevation (Fredrickson types I and V). Liver function must be monitored by periodic laboratory assessment. Use with caution in patients who consume large amounts of ethanol or have a history of liver disease. Use is contraindicated with active liver disease or unexplained transaminase elevations; may cause hepatic dysfunction. Rhabdomyolysis with acute renal failure has occurred. Hematuria (microscopic) and proteinuria have been observed; more commonly reported in patients receiving rosuvastatin 40 mg daily. Typically, transient and not associated with a decrease in renal function. Consider dosage reduction if unexplained hematuria and proteinuria persists. Discontinue in any patient in which CPK levels are markedly elevated (>10 times ULN) or if myopathy is suspected/diagnosed. An increased incidence of rosuvastatin-associated myopathy has been reported during concomitant therapy with fibric acid derivatives, niacin, cyclosporine, and lopinavir/ritonavir, and in certain subgroups of the Asian population; dosage adjustment should be considered for patients of Asian descent. The Canadian labeling contraindicates concomitant use of rosuvastatin with cyclosporine and the use of rosuvastatin 40 mg/day in Asian patients and/or patients receiving fibrates or niacin. Use with caution with concurrent protease inhibitor/ritonavir combinations. Atazanavir/ritonavir and lopinavir/ritonavir significantly increase rosuvastatin serum concentration; limit dose of rosuvastatin to 10 mg/day. Monitor closely if used with other drugs associated with myopathy (eg, colchicine). Risk is also elevated at higher dosages of rosuvastatin. Patients should be instructed to report unexplained muscle pain, tenderness, or weakness, particularly if associated with fever and/or malaise. Use caution in patients predisposed to myopathy (eg, renal failure, advanced age, inadequately treated hypothyroidism). The manufacturer recommends temporary discontinuation for elective major surgery, acute medical or surgical conditions, or in any patient experiencing an acute or serious condition predisposing to renal failure (eg, sepsis, hypotension, trauma, uncontrolled seizures). However, based upon current evidence, HMG-CoA reductase inhibitor therapy should be continued in the perioperative period unless risk outweighs cardioprotective benefit. In the JUPITER study, small increases in hemoglobin (Hb) A1c (mean HbA1c increased by ~0.1%) and physician-reported diabetes was significantly higher in the rosuvastatin group compared to placebo (Ridker, 2008). Overall, evidence supporting an association with diabetes risk is lacking. Because the clear benefits on cardiovascular disease risk outweigh any potential detrimental effects on glucose metabolism, the use of HMG-CoA reductase inhibitors in patients with diabetes continues to be recommended (ADA, 2011).

Adverse Reactions

>10%: Neuromuscular & skeletal: Myalgia (3% to 13%)

2% to 10%:

- Central nervous system: Headache (6%), dizziness (4%)
- Gastrointestinal: Nausea (3%), abdominal pain (2%), constipation (2%)
- Hepatic: ALT increased (2%; >3 times ULN)
- Neuromuscular & skeletal: Arthralgia (4% to 10%), CPK increased (3%; >10 x ULN: Children 3%), weakness (3%)

<2%, postmarketing, and/or case reports: Alkaline phosphatase increased, AST increased, bilirubin increased, depression, GGT increased, gynecomastia, hematuria (microscopic), hepatic failure, hepatitis, hyperglycemia, hypersensitivity reactions (including angioedema, pruritus, rash, urticaria), insomnia, jaundice, memory deficits, myoglobinuria, myositis, myopathy, nightmares, pancreatitis, proteinuria (dose related), renal failure, rhabdomyolysis, thyroid function test abnormalities

Adverse reactions reported with other HMG-CoA reductase inhibitors (not necessarily reported with rosuvastatin therapy) include a hypersensitivity syndrome (symptoms may include anaphylaxis, angioedema, arthralgia, erythema multiforme, eosinophilia, hemolytic anemia, interstitial lung disease, lupus syndrome, photosensitivity, polymyalgia rheumatica, positive ANA, purpura, Stevens-Johnson syndrome, toxic epidermal necrolysis, urticaria, vasculitis)

Drug Interactions

Metabolism/Transport Effects Substrate of CYP2C9 (minor), CYP3A4 (minor), SLCO1B1; **Note:** Assignment of Major/Minor substrate status based on clinically relevant drug interaction potential

Avoid Concomitant Use

Avoid concomitant use of Rosuvastatin with any of the following: Red Yeast Rice

Increased Effect/Toxicity

Rosuvastatin may increase the levels/effects of: DAPTOmycin; Trabectedin; Vitamin K Antagonists

The levels/effects of Rosuvastatin may be increased by: Amiodarone; Colchicine; Conivaptan; CycloSPORINE; CycloSPORINE (Systemic); Eltrombopag; Fenofibrate; Fenofibric Acid; Gemfibrozil; Niacin; Niacinamide; Protease Inhibitors; Red Yeast Rice

Decreased Effect

Rosuvastatin may decrease the levels/effects of: Lanthanum

The levels/effects of Rosuvastatin may be decreased by: Antacids; Tocilizumab

Ethanol/Nutrition/Herb Interactions

Ethanol: Avoid excessive ethanol consumption (due to potential hepatic effects).

Food: Red yeast rice contains an estimated 2.4 mg lovastatin per 600 mg rice.

Stability Store between 20°C and 25°C (68°F to 77°F). Protect from moisture.

Mechanism of Action Inhibitor of 3-hydroxy-3-methylglutaryl coenzyme A (HMG-CoA) reductase, the rate-limiting enzyme in cholesterol synthesis (reduces the production of mevalonic acid from HMG-CoA); this then results in a compensatory increase in the expression of LDL receptors on hepatocyte membranes and a stimulation of LDL catabolism

Pharmacodynamics/Kinetics

Onset of action: Within 1 week; maximal at 4 weeks

Distribution: V_d: 134 L

Protein binding: 88%

Metabolism: Hepatic (10%), via CYP2C9 (1 active metabolite identified: N-desmethyl rosuvastatin, one-sixth to one-half the HMG-CoA reductase activity of the parent compound)

Bioavailability: 20% (high first-pass extraction by liver)

Asian patients have been noted to have increased bioavailability.

Half-life elimination: 19 hours

Time to peak, plasma: 3-5 hours

Excretion: Feces (90%), primarily as unchanged drug

Dosage Oral: **Note:** Doses should be individualized according to the baseline LDL-cholesterol levels, the recommended goal of therapy, and patient response; adjustments should be made at intervals of 4 weeks or more

Children 10-17 years (females >1 year postmenarche): HeFH:

U.S. labeling: 5-20 mg once daily; maximum: 20 mg/day

Dosage adjustment for rosuvastatin with concomitant cyclosporine, atazanavir/ritonavir or lopinavir/ritonavir: Refer to drug-specific dosing in adult dosing section

Canadian labeling: 5-10 mg once daily; maximum: 10 mg/day

Adults:

Hyperlipidemia, mixed dyslipidemia, hypertriglyceridemia, primary dysbetalipoproteinemia, slowing progression of atherosclerosis:

Initial dose:

General dosing: 10 mg once daily; 20 mg once daily may be used in patients with severe hyperlipidemia (LDL >190 mg/dL) and aggressive lipid targets

Conservative dosing: Patients requiring less aggressive treatment or predisposed to myopathy (including patients of Asian descent): 5 mg once daily

Titration: After 2 weeks, may be increased by 5-10 mg once daily; dosing range: 5-40 mg/day (maximum dose: 40 mg once daily)

Note: The 40 mg dose should be reserved for patients who have not achieved goal cholesterol levels on a dose of 20 mg/day, including patients switched from another HMG-CoA reductase inhibitor.

Homozygous familial hypercholesterolemia (FH): Initial: 20 mg once daily (maximum dose: 40 mg/day)

Dosage adjustment with concomitant medications:

U.S. labeling:

Cyclosporine: Rosuvastatin dose should not exceed 5 mg/day

Gemfibrozil: Avoid concurrent use; if unable to avoid concurrent use, rosuvastatin dose should not exceed 10 mg/day

Atazanavir/ritonavir or lopinavir/ritonavir: Rosuvastatin dose should not exceed 10 mg/day

Canadian labeling:

Cyclosporine: Concomitant use is contraindicated

Gemfibrozil: Rosuvastatin dose should not exceed 20 mg/day

Dosage adjustment for hematuria and/or persistent, unexplained proteinuria while on 40 mg/day: Reduce dose and evaluate causes

Dosage adjustment in renal impairment:

Mild-to-moderate impairment: No dosage adjustment required.

Cl_{cr} <30 mL/minute/1.73 m^2: Initial: 5 mg/day; do not exceed 10 mg once daily

Dosage adjustment in hepatic impairment:

U.S. labeling: Active hepatic disease, including unexplained persistent transaminase elevations: Use is contraindicated

Canadian labeling:

Active hepatic disease or unexplained persistent transaminase >3 x ULN: Use is contraindicated

Mild-to-moderate impairment: No dosage adjustment required

Severe impairment: Initial: 5 mg/day; do not exceed 20 mg once daily

Dietary Considerations May be taken with or without food. Red yeast rice contains an estimated 2.4 mg lovastatin per 600 mg rice.

Administration May be administered with or without food. May be taken at any time of the day.

Monitoring Parameters Total cholesterol, LDL, and HDL cholesterol within 2-4 weeks of treatment initiation or dose change; liver function tests should be determined at baseline (prior to initiation), 3 months following initiation, 3 months after any increase in dose, and periodically thereafter (eg, semiannually); baseline CPK (recheck CPK in any patient with symptoms suggestive of myopathy). Monitor LDL-C at intervals no less than 4 weeks.

Dosage Forms Excipient information presented when available (limited, particularly for generics); consult specific product labeling.

Tablet, oral:

Crestor®: 5 mg, 10 mg, 20 mg, 40 mg

◆ **Rosuvastatin Calcium** *see* Rosuvastatin *on page 1524*

◆ **Rotarix®** *see* Rotavirus Vaccine *on page 1526*

◆ **RotaTeq®** *see* Rotavirus Vaccine *on page 1526*

Rotavirus Vaccine (ROE ta vye rus vak SEEN)

Brand Names: U.S. Rotarix®; RotaTeq®

Brand Names: Canada Rotarix®; RotaTeq®

Index Terms Human Rotavirus Vaccine, Attenuated (HRV); Pentavalent Human-Bovine Reassortant Rotavirus Vaccine (PRV); Rotavirus Vaccine, Pentavalent; RV1 (Rotarix®); RV5 (RotaTeq®)

Pharmacologic Category Vaccine, Live (Viral)

Additional Appendix Information

Immunization Recommendations *on page 1922*

Use Prevention of rotavirus gastroenteritis in infants and children

The Advisory Committee on Immunization Practices (ACIP) recommends routine vaccination of all infants.

Pregnancy Risk Factor C

Pregnancy Considerations Reproduction studies have not been conducted. Not indicated for use in women of reproductive age. Infants living in households with pregnant women may be vaccinated.

Contraindications Hypersensitivity to rotavirus vaccine or any component of the formulation; use in infants with severe combined immunodeficiency disease (SCID); infants with a history of intussusception

Rotarix®: Additional contraindication: Contraindicated with a history of an uncorrected congenital malformation of the GI tract

Warnings/Precautions Information is not available for use in postexposure prophylaxis. May consider deferring administration in patients with moderate or severe acute illness (with or without fever); may administer to patients with mild acute illness (with or without fever). Use caution with history of GI disorders, acute GI illness, chronic diarrhea, failure to thrive, congenital abdominal disorders, abdominal surgery, and intussusception. Vaccine may be used with controlled gastroesophageal reflux disease. Consider delaying administration to infants with acute diarrhea or vomiting. Intussusception was observed with a previously licensed rotavirus vaccine; an increased risk in intussusception was not observed in clinical trials with current vaccines; however, cases have been noted in postmarketing reports. Preliminary postmarketing data has found an increased risk of intussusception following the first dose of Rotarix® vaccine in a study conducted in Mexico. Based on an interim analysis, the relative risk of intussusception within 31 days of first vaccination is 1.8 (99% CI 1-3.1); most cases occurred within the first 7 days. Rotarix® is contraindicated with a history of an uncorrected congenital malformation of the GI tract; RotaTeq® and Rotarix® are contraindicated with a history of intussusception.

Virus from live virus vaccines may be transmitted to nonvaccinated contacts; use caution in presence immunocompromised family members. The ACIP recommends vaccination of infants living in households with persons who are immunocompromised. Safety and efficacy have not been established for use in immunocompromised infants (including blood dyscrasias, leukemia, lymphoma, malignant neoplasms affecting bone marrow or lymphatic system), infants on immunosuppressants (including high-dose corticosteroids; may be administered with topical corticosteroids or inhaled steroids), or infants with primary and acquired immunodeficiencies (including HIV/AIDS, cellular immune deficiencies, hypogammaglobulinemic and dysgammaglobulinemic states). The ACIP recommendations support vaccination of HIV-exposed or infected infants, since the diagnosis of infection may not be made prior to the first dose of the vaccine and also because strains of rotavirus vaccine are considerably attenuated.

Immediate treatment (including epinephrine 1:1000) for anaphylactoid and/or hypersensitivity reactions should be available during vaccine use. Some packaging may contain natural latex/natural rubber. Not intended for use in adults. In order to maximize vaccination rates, the ACIP recommends simultaneous administration of all age-appropriate vaccines (live or inactivated) for which a person is eligible at a single clinic visit, unless contraindications exist.

Adverse Reactions All serious adverse reactions must be reported to the U.S. Department of Health and Human Services (DHHS) Vaccine Adverse Event Reporting System (VAERS) 1-800-822-7967 or online at https://vaers.hhs.gov/esub/index.

Note: Ranges reported; actual percentage may vary between products.

>10%:

Central nervous system: Fever ≥38.1°C (17% to 43%; equal to or less than placebo), fussiness/irritability (3% to 52%)

Gastrointestinal: Diarrhea (4% to 24%), vomiting (3% to 15%)

Otic: Otitis media (15%)

1% to 10%:

Gastrointestinal: Flatulence (2%)

Respiratory: Nasopharyngitis (7%), bronchospasm (1%)

<1% (Limited to important or life-threatening): Gastroenteritis with severe diarrhea and prolonged vaccine viral shedding in infants with SCID, hematochezia, idiopathic thrombocytopenic purpura, intussusception, Kawasaki disease, seizure, transmission of vaccine virus from recipient to nonvaccinated contacts, urticaria

Drug Interactions

Metabolism/Transport Effects None known.

Avoid Concomitant Use

Avoid concomitant use of Rotavirus Vaccine with any of the following: Belimumab; Fingolimod; Immunosuppressants

Increased Effect/Toxicity

The levels/effects of Rotavirus Vaccine may be increased by: AzaTHIOprine; Belimumab; Corticosteroids (Systemic); Fingolimod; Hydroxychloroquine; Immunosuppressants; Leflunomide; Mercaptopurine; Methotrexate

Decreased Effect

Rotavirus Vaccine may decrease the levels/effects of: Tuberculin Tests

The levels/effects of Rotavirus Vaccine may be decreased by: Fingolimod; Immune Globulins; Immunosuppressants

Stability

Rotarix®: Prior to reconstitution, store powder under refrigeration at 2°C to 8°C (36°F to 46°F); diluent may be stored at room temperature 20°C to 25°C (68°F to 77°F). Protect from light; discard if frozen. Reconstitute only with provided diluent and transfer adapter. Shake to form suspension. Following reconstitution, may be refrigerated or stored at room temperature for up to 24 hours. Discard if frozen.

RotaTeq®: Store and transport under refrigeration at 2°C to 8°C (36°F to 46°F). Use as soon as possible once removed from refrigerator. Protect from light.

Mechanism of Action A live vaccine; replicates in the small intestine and promotes active immunity to rotavirus gastroenteritis. Rotarix® is specifically indicated for prevention of rotavirus gastroenteritis caused by serotypes G1, G3, G4, and G9 and RotaTeq® is specifically indicated for prevention of rotavirus gastroenteritis caused by serotypes G1, G2, G3, and G4. However, vaccines may provide immunity to other serotypes.

Pharmacodynamics/Kinetics Note: There is no established relationship between antibody response and protection against gastroenteritis.

Seroconversion:

Rotarix®: Antirotavirus IgA antibodies were noted 1-2 months following completion of the 2-dose series in 77% to 87% of infants.

RotaTeq®: A threefold increase in antirotavirus IgA was noted following completion of the 3-dose regimen in 93% to 100% of infants.

Duration: Following administration of rotavirus vaccine, efficacy of protecting against any grade of rotavirus gastroenteritis through two seasons was 70% to 79%

Dosage Oral:

Manufacturer's labeling:

Infants 6-24 weeks of age: Rotarix®: A total of two 1 mL doses, the first dose given at 6 weeks of age. The first and second dose should be separated by ≥4 weeks. The 2-dose series should be completed by 24 weeks of age.

Infants 6-32 weeks: RotaTeq®: A total of three 2 mL doses, the first dose given at 6-12 weeks of age, followed by subsequent doses at 4- to 10-week intervals. Administer all doses by 32 weeks of age.

ACIP recommendations: The first dose can be given at 6-14 weeks of age. The series should not be started in infants ≥15 weeks. The final dose in the series should be administered by 8 months 0 days of age. The minimum interval between doses is 4 weeks. RotaTeq® should be given in 3 doses administered at 2-, 4-, and 6 months of age. Rotarix® should be given in 2 doses administered at 2- and 4 months of age. For infants inadvertently administered rotavirus vaccine at ≥15 weeks of age, the vaccine series may be completed according to schedule. The ACIP recommendations for vaccination recommend completing the vaccine series with the same product whenever possible. If continuing with same product will cause vaccination to be deferred, or if product used previously is unknown, vaccination should be completed with the product available. If RotaTeq® was used in any previous doses, or if the specific product used was unknown, a total of 3 doses should be given. Infants who have had rotavirus gastroenteritis before getting the full course of vaccine should still initiate or complete the recommended schedule; initial infection provides only partial immunity.

Dietary Considerations Do not mix or dilute vaccine. May be administered before or after food, milk, or breast milk.

Administration

Rotarix®: Using oral applicator, administer contents into infant's inner cheek. Dispose of applicator and vaccine vial in biologic waste container.

RotaTeq®: Gently squeeze dose from ready-to-use dosing tube into infant's inner cheek. After use, dispose of the empty tube and cap in a biologic waste container.

Note: A single dose of the rotavirus vaccine should not be readministered to an infant who regurgitates, spits out, or vomits the vaccine during administration. Any remaining dose(s) should be administered on schedule (CDC, 2009).

Simultaneous administration of vaccines helps ensure the patients will be fully vaccinated by the appropriate age. Simultaneous administration of vaccines is defined as administering >1 vaccine on the same day at different anatomic sites. Separate vaccines should not be combined in the same syringe unless indicated by product specific labeling. The ACIP prefers each dose of a specific vaccine in a series come from the same manufacturer when possible. In general, preterm infants should be vaccinated at the same chronological age as full-term infants (CDC, 2011).

Antipyretics have not been shown to prevent febrile seizures. Antipyretics may be used to treat fever or discomfort following vaccination (CDC, 2011). One study reported that routine prophylactic administration of acetaminophen to prevent fever prior to vaccination decreased the immune response of some vaccines; the clinical significance of this reduction in immune response has not been established (Prymula, 2009).

Test Interactions Tuberculin tests: Rotavirus vaccine may diminish the diagnostic effect of tuberculin tests.

Additional Information Federal law requires that the name of medication, date of administration, the vaccine manufacturer, lot number of vaccine, and the administering person's name, title and address be entered into the patient's permanent medical record.

Dosage Forms Excipient information presented when available (limited, particularly for generics); consult specific product labeling.

Powder, for suspension, oral [preservative free; human derived]:

Rotarix®: G1P[8] ≥10^6 $CCID_{50}$ per 1 mL [contains sorbitol, sucrose; supplied with diluent which may contain natural rubber/natural latex in packaging]

Suspension, oral [preservative free; bovine and human derived]:

RotaTeq®: G1 ≥2.2 x 10^6 infectious units, G2 ≥2.8 x 10^6 infectious units, G3 ≥2.2 x 10^6 infectious units, G4 ≥2 x 10^6 infectious units, and P1A [8] ≥2.3 x 10^6 infectious units per 2 mL (2 mL)

◆ **Rotavirus Vaccine, Pentavalent** *see* Rotavirus Vaccine *on page 1526*

◆ **Rowasa®** *see* Mesalamine *on page 1081*

◆ **Roxanol** *see* Morphine (Systemic) *on page 1153*

◆ **Roxicet™** *see* Oxycodone and Acetaminophen *on page 1269*

◆ **Roxicet™ 5/500** *see* Oxycodone and Acetaminophen *on page 1269*

◆ **Roxicodone®** *see* OxyCODONE *on page 1266*

◆ **Roychlor® (Can)** *see* Potassium Chloride *on page 1380*

◆ **Rozerem®** *see* Ramelteon *on page 1458*

◆ **RP-6976** *see* DOCEtaxel *on page 534*

◆ **RP-54274** *see* Riluzole *on page 1491*

◆ **RP-59500** *see* Quinupristin and Dalfopristin *on page 1450*

◆ **r-PA** *see* Reteplase *on page 1475*

◆ **rPDGF-BB** *see* Becaplermin *on page 192*

◆ **RPR-116258A** *see* Cabazitaxel *on page 257*

◆ **(R,R)-Formoterol L-Tartrate** *see* Arformoterol *on page 139*

◆ **RS-25259** *see* Palonosetron *on page 1281*

◆ **RS-25259-197** *see* Palonosetron *on page 1281*

◆ **R-Tanna** *see* Chlorpheniramine and Phenylephrine *on page 345*

◆ **R-Tanna Pediatric** *see* Chlorpheniramine and Phenylephrine *on page 345*

◆ **RTCA** *see* Ribavirin *on page 1479*

◆ **RU 0211** *see* Lubiprostone *on page 1040*

◆ **RU-486** *see* Mifepristone *on page 1131*

◆ **RU-23908** *see* Nilutamide *on page 1205*

◆ **RU-38486** *see* Mifepristone *on page 1131*

◆ **Rubella, Measles and Mumps Vaccines** *see* Measles, Mumps, and Rubella Virus Vaccine *on page 1054*

◆ **Rubella, Varicella, Measles, and Mumps Vaccine** *see* Measles, Mumps, Rubella, and Varicella Virus Vaccine *on page 1055*

◆ **Rubidomycin Hydrochloride** *see* DAUNOrubicin (Conventional) *on page 457*

◆ **RUF 331** *see* Rufinamide *on page 1528*

Rufinamide (roo FIN a mide)

Brand Names: U.S. Banzel®

Brand Names: Canada Banzel™

Index Terms CGP 33101; E 2080; RUF 331; Xilep

Pharmacologic Category Anticonvulsant, Triazole Derivative

Use Adjunctive therapy in the treatment of generalized seizures of Lennox-Gastaut syndrome

Pregnancy Risk Factor C

Pregnancy Considerations Adverse effects were seen in animal studies. There are no adequate and well-controlled studies in pregnant women; use during pregnancy only if clearly needed. Hormonal contraceptives may be less effective with concurrent rufinamide use; additional forms of nonhormonal contraceptives should be used.

Patients exposed to rufinamide during pregnancy are encouraged to enroll themselves into the AED Pregnancy Registry by calling 1-888-233-2334. Additional information is available at www.aedpregnancyregistry.org.

Lactation Excretion in breast milk unknown/not recommended

Medication Guide Available Yes

Contraindications Patients with familial short QT syndrome

Canadian labeling: Additional contraindications (not in U.S. labeling): Family history of short QT syndrome; presence or history of short QT interval; hypersensitivity to rufinamide, triazole derivatives, or any component of the formulation

Warnings/Precautions Has been associated with shortening of the QT interval. Use caution in patients receiving concurrent medications that shorten the QT interval. Contraindicated in patients with familial short-QT syndrome (Canadian labeling also contraindicates use in patients with a family history of short QT syndrome or presence or history of short QT interval). Use has been associated with CNS-related adverse events, most significant of these were cognitive symptoms (including somnolence or fatigue) and coordination abnormalities (including ataxia, dizziness, and gait disturbances). Caution patients about performing tasks which require mental alertness (eg, operating machinery or driving). Effects with other sedative drugs or ethanol may be potentiated. Potentially serious, sometimes fatal, multiorgan hypersensitivity reactions have been reported with some antiepileptic drugs, including rufinamide; monitor for signs and symptoms of possible disparate manifestations associated with lymphatic, hepatic, renal, and/or hematologic organ systems; gradual discontinuation and conversion to alternate therapy may be required. Closely monitor any patient who develops a rash; instruct patients to report any rash associated with fever.

Antiepileptics are associated with an increased risk of suicidal behavior/thoughts with use (regardless of indication); patients should be monitored for signs/symptoms of depression, suicidal tendencies, and other unusual behavior changes during therapy and instructed to inform their healthcare provider immediately if symptoms occur. Use with caution in patients with mild-to-moderate hepatic impairment; use in not recommended in patients with severe hepatic impairment. Concurrent use with hormonal contraceptives may lead to contraceptive failure. Anticonvulsants should not be discontinued abruptly because of the possibility of increasing seizure frequency; therapy should be withdrawn gradually to minimize the potential of increased seizure frequency, unless safety concerns require a more rapid withdrawal. Reducing dose by ~25% every two days was effective in trials.

Adverse Reactions

>10%:

Cardiovascular: QT shortening (46% to 65%; dose related)

Central nervous system: Headache (16% to 27%), somnolence (11% to 24%), dizziness (3% to 19%), fatigue (9% to 16%)

Gastrointestinal: Vomiting (5% to 17%), nausea (7% to 12%)

1% to 10%:

Central nervous system: Ataxia (4% to 5%), seizure (children 5%), status epilepticus (≤4%), aggression (children 3%), anxiety (adults 3%), attention disturbance (children 3%), hyperactivity (children 3%), vertigo (adults 3%)

Dermatologic: Rash (children 4%), pruritus (children 3%)

Gastrointestinal: Appetite decreased (≥1% to 5%), abdominal pain (3%), constipation (adults 3%), dyspepsia (adults 3%), appetite increased (≥1%)

Hematologic: Leukopenia (≤4%), anemia (≥1%)

Neuromuscular & skeletal: Tremor (adults 6%), back pain (adults 3%), gait disturbance (1% to 3%)

Ocular: Diplopia (4% to 9%), blurred vision (adults 6%), nystagmus (adults 6%)

Otic: Otitis media (children 3%)

Renal: Pollakiuria (≥1%)

Respiratory: Nasopharyngitis (children 5%), bronchitis (children 3%), sinusitis (children 3%)

Miscellaneous: Influenza (children 5%)

<1% (Limited to important or life-threatening): Atrioventricular block (first degree), bundle branch block (right), dysuria, enuresis, hematuria; hypersensitivity (multiorgan; includes eosinophilia, facial edema, fever, hepatitis [severe], LFTs increased, rash, stupor, urticaria); incontinence, iron-deficiency anemia, lymphadenopathy, nephrolithiasis, neutropenia, nocturia, polyuria, thrombocytopenia, urinary incontinence

Drug Interactions

Metabolism/Transport Effects Inhibits CYP2E1 (weak); **Induces** CYP3A4 (weak/moderate)

Avoid Concomitant Use There are no known interactions where it is recommended to avoid concomitant use.

Increased Effect/Toxicity

Rufinamide may increase the levels/effects of: Fosphenytoin; PHENobarbital; Phenytoin

The levels/effects of Rufinamide may be increased by: Divalproex; Valproic Acid

Decreased Effect

Rufinamide may decrease the levels/effects of: ARIPiprazole; CarBAMazepine; Ethinyl Estradiol; Norethindrone; Saxagliptin

The levels/effects of Rufinamide may be decreased by: CarBAMazepine; Fosphenytoin; PHENobarbital; Phenytoin; Primidone

Ethanol/Nutrition/Herb Interactions

Ethanol: Avoid ethanol (may increase CNS depression).

Food: Food increases the absorption of rufinamide.

Herb/Nutraceutical: Avoid evening primrose (seizure threshold decreased).

Stability Store at 25°C (77°F); excursions permitted to 15°C to 30°C (59°F to 86°F). Protect tablets from moisture. The cap to the oral suspension bottle fits over the adapter.

Mechanism of Action A triazole-derivative antiepileptic whose exact mechanism is unknown. *In vitro*, it prolongs the inactive state of the sodium channels, thereby limiting repetitive firing of sodium-dependent action potentials mediating anticonvulsant effects.

Pharmacodynamics/Kinetics

Absorption: Slow; extensive ≥85%; increased with food

Distribution: V_d: ~50 L

Protein binding: 34%, primarily to albumin

Metabolism: Extensively via carboxylesterase-mediated hydrolysis of the carboxylamide group to CGP 47292 (inactive metabolite); weak inhibitor of CYP2E1 and weak inducer of CYP3A4

Bioavailability: Extent decreased with increased dose; oral tablets and oral suspension are bioequivalent

Half-life elimination: ~6-10 hours

Time to peak, plasma: 4-6 hours

Excretion: Urine (85%, ~66% as CGP 47292, <2% as unchanged drug)

Dosage Oral: Lennox-Gastaut (adjunctive):

U.S. labeling:

Children ≥4 years: Initial: 10 mg/kg/day in 2 equally divided doses; increase dose by ~10 mg/kg every other day to a target dose of 45 mg/kg/day **or** 3200 mg/day (whichever is lower) in 2 equally divided doses

Adults: Initial: 400-800 mg/day in 2 equally divided doses; increase dose by 400-800 mg/day every other day to a maximum dose of 3200 mg/day in 2 equally divided doses

Canadian labeling: Children ≥4 years and Adults:

<30 kg: Initial: 100 mg twice daily; increase dose by 5 mg/kg/day every 2 weeks until satisfactory control (maximum dose: 1300 mg/day)

≥30 kg: Initial: 200 mg twice daily; increase dose by 5 mg/kg/day every 2 weeks until satisfactory control (maximum dose: 30-50 kg: 1800 mg/day; 50.1-70 kg: 2400 mg/day; ≥70.1 kg: 3200 mg/day). **Note:** Dose was increased as frequently as every other day in clinical trials.

Dosage adjustment for concomitant medications: Valproate:

U.S. labeling: Initial rufinamide dose should be <10 mg/kg/day (children) or 400 mg/day (adults)

Canadian labeling: Initial rufinamide dose should be less than the initial daily recommended dosage; however, a specific dosage recommendation is not included in the manufacturer's labeling.

Dosage adjustment in renal impairment: Cl_{cr} <30 mL/minute: No dosage adjustment needed

Hemodialysis: No specific guidelines available; consider dosage adjustment for loss of drug

Dosage adjustment in hepatic impairment:

Mild-to-moderate impairment: Use caution

Severe impairment: Use in severe impairment has not been studied and is not recommended

Dietary Considerations Take with food.

Administration Administer with food. Tablets may be swallowed whole, split in half, or crushed. Oral suspension should be administered using the provided adapter and oral syringe; shake well before every administration.

Monitoring Parameters Seizure (frequency and duration); serum levels of concurrent anticonvulsants; suicidality (eg, suicidal thoughts, depression, behavioral changes)

Dosage Forms Excipient information presented when available (limited, particularly for generics); consult specific product labeling.

Suspension, oral:

Banzel®: 40 mg/mL (460 mL) [dye free, gluten free, lactose free; contains propylene glycol; orange flavor]

Tablet, oral:

Banzel®: 200 mg, 400 mg [scored]

Dosage Forms: Canada Excipient information presented when available (limited, particularly for generics); consult specific product labeling.

Tablet, oral:

Banzel™: 100 mg [scored]

Extemporaneous Preparations A 40 mg/mL oral suspension may be made using tablets. Crush twelve 400 mg tablets (or twenty-four 200 mg tablets) and reduce to a fine powder. Add 60 mL of Ora-Plus® in incremental proportions until a smooth suspension is obtained; then mix well while adding 60 mL of Ora-Sweet® or Ora-Sweet® SF; transfer to a calibrated bottle. Label "shake well". Stable 90 days at room temperature.

Hutchinson DJ, Liou Y, Best R, et al, "Stability of Extemporaneously Prepared Rufinamide Oral Suspensions," *Ann Pharmacother*, 2010, 44(3):462-5.

◆ **Ru-Hist Forte [DSC]** *see* Chlorpheniramine, Pyrilamine, and Phenylephrine *on page 348*

◆ **Rulox [OTC]** *see* Aluminum Hydroxide, Magnesium Hydroxide, and Simethicone *on page 80*

Ruxolitinib (rux oh LI ti nib)

Brand Names: U.S. Jakafi™

Index Terms INCB 18424; INCB018424; Jakafi™; Ruxolitinib Phosphate

Pharmacologic Category Antineoplastic Agent, Janus Associated Kinase Inhibitor; Antineoplastic Agent, Tyrosine Kinase Inhibitor; Janus Associated Kinase Inhibitor

Use Treatment of intermediate or high-risk myelofibrosis, including primary myelofibrosis, post-polycythemia vera (post-PV) myelofibrosis and post-essential thrombocythemia (post-ET) myelofibrosis

Pregnancy Risk Factor C

Pregnancy Considerations Increased resorptions (late) and reduced fetal weights were observed in animal reproduction studies. Use during human pregnancy only if the potential treatment benefits outweigh risks.

Lactation Excretion in breast milk unknown/ not recommended

Prescribing and Access Restrictions Available through specialty/network pharmacies. Further information may be obtained from the manufacturer, Incyte, at 1-855-452-5234 or at www.Jakafi.com.

Contraindications There are no contraindications listed within the manufacturer's labeling.

Warnings/Precautions Hematologic toxicity, including thrombocytopenia, anemia and neutropenia may occur; may require dosage modification; monitor complete blood counts. Patients with baseline platelets <200,000/mm^3 are more likely to develop thrombocytopenia during treatment. Thrombocytopenia is generally reversible with treatment interruption or dose reduction; platelet transfusions may be administered during treatment if clinically indicated. Anemia may require blood transfusion; may consider dose modification. Neutropenia (ANC <500/mm^3) is generally reversible and managed by treatment interruption.

Assess for risk of developing serious bacterial, mycobacterial, fungal or viral infection; monitor for infections during treatment. Active serious infections should be resolved prior to treatment initiation. Prompt treatment is recommended if symptoms of herpes zoster infection develop. May require initial dosage reduction for hepatic impairment; avoid use if platelets <100,000/mm^3 and with hepatic impairment (any degree). May require initial dosage reduction for renal impairment; avoid use if platelets <100,000/mm^3 and with moderate-to-severe renal impairment or in patients with ESRD not requiring dialysis. Ruxolitinib is not removed by dialysis, however, some active metabolites may be removed. On dialysis days, patients are advised to take their dose following dialysis sessions. Reduced initial doses are recommended with concomitant use of strong CYP3A4 inhibitors (eg, clarithromycin, conivaptin, itraconazole, ketoconazole, nefazodone, posaconazole, protease inhibitors, telithromycin, voriconazole, grapefruit juice); if platelets <100,000/mm^3, avoid concomitant use with strong CYP3A4 inhibitors. No adjustment is recommended with concomitant use of mild or moderate CYP3A4 inhibitors or with CYP3A4 inducers (monitor closely for efficacy and titrate dose appropriately). Discontinue treatment after 6 months if no reduction in spleen size or no improvement in symptoms. Gradually taper off if discontinuing for reasons other than thrombocytopenia. Within ~1 week after discontinuation, symptoms of myelofibrosis generally return to pretreatment levels. Acute relapse of myelofibrosis symptoms, splenomegaly, worsening cytopenias, hemodynamic compensation, and septic shock-like syndrome have been reported with treatment discontinuation (Tefferi, 2011); gradually taper off if discontinuing for reasons other than thrombocytopenia.

Adverse Reactions

>10%:

Central nervous system: Dizziness (18%), headache (15%)

Dermatologic: Bruising (23%)

Endocrine& metabolic: Cholesterol increased (17%; grade 2: <1%)

Hematologic: Anemia (96%; grade 3: 34%; grade 4: 11%), thrombocytopenia (70%; grade 3: 9%; grade 4: 4%), neutropenia (19%; grade 3: 5%; grade 4: 2%)

Hepatic: ALT increased (25%; grades 2/3: 2%), AST increased (17%; grade 2: <1%)

1% to 10%:

Gastrointestinal: Weight gain (7%), flatulence (5%)

Genitourinary: Urinary tract infection (9%)

Miscellaneous: Herpes zoster infection (2%)

<1% (Limited to important or life-threatening): Anxiety, cardiac murmur, diarrhea, dyspnea, edema, epistaxis, fatigue, fever, insomnia, limb pain, musculoskeletal pain, nausea, peripheral edema, peripheral neuropathy, weakness, withdrawal syndrome (acute relapse of myelofibrosis symptoms, splenomegaly, worsening cytopenias, hemodynamic compensation, and septic shock-like syndrome)

Drug Interactions

Metabolism/Transport Effects Substrate of CYP3A4 (major); **Note:** Assignment of Major/Minor substrate status based on clinically relevant drug interaction potential

Avoid Concomitant Use

Avoid concomitant use of Ruxolitinib with any of the following: BCG; CloZAPine; Natalizumab; Pimecrolimus; Tacrolimus (Topical); Vaccines (Live)

Increased Effect/Toxicity

Ruxolitinib may increase the levels/effects of: CloZAPine; Leflunomide; Natalizumab; Vaccines (Live)

The levels/effects of Ruxolitinib may be increased by: CYP3A4 Inhibitors (Moderate); CYP3A4 Inhibitors (Strong); Dasatinib; Denosumab; Grapefruit Juice; Pimecrolimus; Roflumilast; Tacrolimus (Topical); Trastuzumab

Decreased Effect

Ruxolitinib may decrease the levels/effects of: BCG; Coccidioidin Skin Test; Sipuleucel-T; Vaccines (Inactivated); Vaccines (Live)

The levels/effects of Ruxolitinib may be decreased by: CYP3A4 Inducers (Strong); Deferasirox; Echinacea; Herbs (CYP3A4 Inducers); Tocilizumab

Ethanol/Nutrition/Herb Interactions Food: Avoid grapefruit juice (may increase the effects of ruxolitinib).

Stability Store at room temperature of 20°C to 25°C (68°F to 77°F); excursions permitted to 15°C to 30°C (59°F to 86°F).

Mechanism of Action Kinase inhibitor which selectively inhibits Janus Associated Kinases (JAKs), JAK1 and JAK2. JAK1 and JAK2 mediate signaling of cytokine and growth factors responsible for hematopoiesis and immune function; JAK mediated signaling involves recruitment of STATs (signal transducers and activators of transcription) to cytokine receptors which leads to modulation of gene expression. In myelofibrosis, JAK1/2 activity is dysregulated; ruxolitinib modulates the affected JAK1/2 activity.

Pharmacodynamics/Kinetics

Absorption: Rapid

Distribution: V_d: 53-65 L

Protein binding: ~97%; primarily to albumin

Metabolism: Hepatic, primarily via CYP3A4; forms active metabolites responsible for 20% to 50% of activity

Half-life elimination: Ruxolitinib: 2.8-3 hours (hepatic impairment: 5 hours); Ruxolitinib + metabolites: ~6 hours

Time to peak: Within 1-2 hours

Excretion: Urine (74%, <1% as unchanged drug); feces (22%, <1% as unchanged drug)

Dosage Oral: Adults: Myelofibrosis: Initial dose (based on platelet count, titrate dose thereafter based on efficacy and safety):

Platelets >200,000/mm^3: 20 mg twice daily

Platelets 100,000-200,000/mm^3: 15 mg twice daily

Dosage modification based on response: For insufficient response (with adequate platelet and neutrophil counts), may increase the dose in 5 mg twice daily increments to a maximum dose of 25 mg twice daily. Do not increase during initial 4 weeks and no more frequently than every 2 weeks. Discontinue treatment after 6 months if no reduction in spleen size or no improvement in symptoms. When discontinuing for reasons other than thrombocytopenia, gradually taper by ~5 mg twice daily per week.

Dose increases may be considered if meet all of the following situations:

- Failure to achieve either a 50% reduction (from baseline) in palpable spleen length or a 35% reduction (from baseline) in spleen volume (measured by CT or MRI)
- Platelet count >125,000/mm^3 at 4 weeks (and never <100,000/mm^3)
- Absolute neutrophil count (ANC) >750/mm^3

Dosage modification for treatment interruption: Platelets <50,000/mm^3: Interrupt treatment; upon platelet recovery (to >50,000/mm^3), dosing may be restarted or increased based on the following platelet levels and **maximum allowable doses** (when restarting, begin with a dose that is at least 5 mg twice daily below the dose at treatment interruption):

Platelets ≥125,000/mm^3: 20 mg twice daily

Platelets 100,000 to <125,000/mm^3: 15 mg twice daily

Platelets 75,000 to <100,000/mm^3: 10 mg twice daily for at least 2 weeks; may increase to 15 mg twice daily if stable

Platelets 50,000 to <75,000/mm^3: 5 mg twice daily for at least 2 weeks; may increase to 10 mg twice daily if stable

Platelets <50,000/mm^3: Continue to withhold treatment

Note: Long-term maintenance at 5 mg twice daily has not demonstrated responses; limit use of the dose level to patients where the benefits outweigh risks

Dosage reduction for thrombocytopenia:

Platelet Count	Dose at Time of Thrombocytopenia				
	25 mg twice/day	20 mg twice/day	15 mg twice/day	10 mg twice/day	5 mg twice/day
	New Dose	New Dose	New Dose	New Dose	New Dose
100,000 to <125,000/mm^3	20 mg twice/day	15 mg twice/day	No change	No change	No change
75,000 to <100,000/mm^3	10 mg twice/day	10 mg twice/day	10 mg twice/day	No change	No change
50,000 to <75,000/mm^3	5 mg twice/day	5 mg twice/day	5 mg twice/day	5 mg twice/day	No change
<50,000/mm^3	Hold dose	Hold dose	Hold dose	Hold dose	Hold dose

Note: Long-term maintenance at 5 mg twice daily has not demonstrated responses; limit use of the dose level to patients where the benefits outweigh risks

Dosage adjustment with concomitant strong CYP3A4 inhibitors: Initial dose: 10 mg twice daily (if platelet count ≥100,000/mm^3); additional dose adjustments should be made with careful monitoring. Avoid concomitant use if platelet count <100,000/mm^3.

Dosage adjustment in renal impairment:

Cl_{cr} 15-59 mL/minute and platelets 100,000-150,000/mm^3: Initial dose: 10 mg twice daily; additional dose adjustments should be made with careful monitoring

Cl_{cr} 15-59 mL/minute and platelets <100,000/mm^3: Avoid use

End-stage renal disease (ESRD) on dialysis and platelets 100,000-200,000/mm^3: Initial dose: 15 mg; administer subsequent doses after dialysis on dialysis days. Additional dose adjustments should be made with careful monitoring.

ESRD on dialysis and platelets >200,000/mm^3: Initial dose: 20 mg; administer subsequent doses after dialysis on dialysis days. Additional dose adjustments should be made with careful monitoring.

ESRD not requiring dialysis: Avoid use

Dosage adjustment in hepatic impairment:

Hepatic impairment and platelets 100,000-150,000/mm^3: Initial dose: 10 mg twice daily; additional dose adjustments should be made with careful monitoring

Hepatic impairment and platelets <100,000/mm^3: Avoid use

Dietary Considerations May be taken with or without food. Avoid grapefruit juice (may increase the effects of ruxolitinib).

Administration May be administered orally with or without food. If a dose is missed, return to the usual dosing schedule and do **not** administer an additional dose.

If unable to ingest tablets, may administer through a nasogastric (NG) tube (≥8 Fr): Suspend tablet in ~40 mL water and stir for ~10 minutes and administer (within 6 hours after dispersion) with appropriate syringe; rinse NG tube with ~75 mL water (effect of enteral tube feeding on ruxolitinib exposure has not been evaluated)

Monitoring Parameters CBC (baseline, every 2-4 weeks until dose stabilized, then as clinically indicated), renal function, hepatic function

Dosage Forms Excipient information presented when available (limited, particularly for generics); consult specific product labeling.

Tablet, oral:

Jakafi™: 5 mg, 10 mg, 15 mg, 20 mg, 25 mg

Extemporaneous Preparations A suspension for nasogastric administration may be prepared with tablets. Place one tablet into ~40 mL water; stir for approximately 10 minutes. Administer within 6 hour after preparation.

Jakafi™ prescribing information November, 2011. Incyte Corporation, Wilmington, DE.

◆ **Ruxolitinib Phosphate** *see* Ruxolitinib *on page 1530*
◆ **RV1 (Rotarix®)** *see* Rotavirus Vaccine *on page 1526*
◆ **RV5 (RotaTeq®)** *see* Rotavirus Vaccine *on page 1526*
◆ **Rybix™ ODT** *see* TraMADol *on page 1715*
◆ **Rylosol (Can)** *see* Sotalol *on page 1586*
◆ **Rynatan® [DSC]** *see* Chlorpheniramine and Phenylephrine *on page 345*
◆ **Rynatan® Pediatric [DSC]** *see* Chlorpheniramine and Phenylephrine *on page 345*
◆ **Rythmodan® (Can)** *see* Disopyramide *on page 529*
◆ **Rythmodan®-LA (Can)** *see* Disopyramide *on page 529*
◆ **Rythmol®** *see* Propafenone *on page 1419*
◆ **Rythmol® Gen-Propafenone (Can)** *see* Propafenone *on page 1419*
◆ **Rythmol® SR** *see* Propafenone *on page 1419*
◆ **Ryzolt™** *see* TraMADol *on page 1715*
◆ **S2® [OTC]** *see* EPINEPHrine (Systemic, Oral Inhalation) *on page 594*
◆ **S-(+)-3-isobutylgaba** *see* Pregabalin *on page 1402*
◆ **S-4661** *see* Doripenem *on page 545*
◆ **Sabril®** *see* Vigabatrin *on page 1787*

Sacrosidase (sak ROE si dase)

Brand Names: U.S. Sucraid®
Brand Names: Canada Sucraid®
Pharmacologic Category Enzyme, Gastrointestinal
Use Orphan drug: Oral replacement therapy in sucrase deficiency, as seen in congenital sucrase-isomaltase deficiency (CSID)
Pregnancy Risk Factor C
Prescribing and Access Restrictions Sucraid® is not available in retail pharmacies or via mail-order pharmacies. To obtain the product, please refer to http://www.qolmed.com/sucraid.htm or call 1-866-740-2743.
Dosage Oral:
Infants ≥5 months and Children <15 kg: 8500 int. units (1 mL) per meal or snack
Children >15 kg and Adults: 17,000 int. units (2 mL) per meal or snack
Doses should be diluted with 2-4 oz of water, milk, or formula with each meal or snack. Approximately one-half of the dose may be taken before, and the remainder of a dose taken at the completion of each meal or snack.
Additional Information Complete prescribing information for this medication should be consulted for additional detail.
Dosage Forms Excipient information presented when available (limited, particularly for generics); consult specific product labeling.
Solution, oral:
Sucraid®: 8500 int. units/mL (118 mL)

◆ **Safetussin® CD [OTC]** *see* Dextromethorphan and Phenylephrine *on page 490*
◆ **Safe Tussin® DM [OTC]** *see* Guaifenesin and Dextromethorphan *on page 810*
◆ **Safyral™** *see* Ethinyl Estradiol, Drospirenone, and Levomefolate *on page 664*
◆ **SAHA** *see* Vorinostat *on page 1800*
◆ **Saizen®** *see* Somatropin *on page 1579*
◆ **Salagen®** *see* Pilocarpine (Systemic) *on page 1353*
◆ **Salazopyrin® (Can)** *see* SulfaSALAzine *on page 1605*
◆ **Salazopyrin En-Tabs® (Can)** *see* SulfaSALAzine *on page 1605*
◆ **Salbutamol** *see* Albuterol *on page 52*
◆ **Salbutamol and Ipratropium** *see* Ipratropium and Albuterol *on page 924*
◆ **Salbutamol Sulphate** *see* Albuterol *on page 52*
◆ **Salflex® (Can)** *see* Salsalate *on page 1534*
◆ **Salicylazosulfapyridine** *see* SulfaSALAzine *on page 1605*
◆ **Salicylsalicylic Acid** *see* Salsalate *on page 1534*
◆ **Saline** *see* Sodium Chloride *on page 1567*
◆ **Saline Mist [OTC]** *see* Sodium Chloride *on page 1567*
◆ **Salk Vaccine** *see* Poliovirus Vaccine (Inactivated) *on page 1370*

Salmeterol (sal ME te role)

Brand Names: U.S. Serevent® Diskus®
Brand Names: Canada Serevent® Diskhaler® Disk; Serevent® Diskus®
Index Terms Salmeterol Xinafoate
Pharmacologic Category $Beta_2$-Adrenergic Agonist; $Beta_2$-Adrenergic Agonist, Long-Acting
Additional Appendix Information
Bronchodilators *on page 1886*
Use Maintenance treatment of asthma and prevention of bronchospasm (as concomitant therapy) in patients with reversible obstructive airway disease, including patients with symptoms of nocturnal asthma; prevention of exercise-induced bronchospasm (monotherapy may be indicated in patients without persistent asthma); maintenance treatment of bronchospasm associated with COPD
Pregnancy Risk Factor C
Pregnancy Considerations Animal studies have demonstrated (dose-dependent) teratogenicity. There are no adequate and well-controlled studies in pregnant women. Beta-agonists may interfere with uterine contractility if administered during labor. Use only if clearly needed.
Lactation Enters breast milk/use caution
Medication Guide Available Yes
Contraindications Hypersensitivity to salmeterol or any component of the formulation (milk proteins); monotherapy in the treatment of asthma (ie, use without a concomitant long-term asthma control medication, such as an inhaled corticosteroid); status asthmaticus or other acute episodes of asthma or COPD
Warnings/Precautions
Asthma treatment: [U.S. Boxed Warning]: Long-acting $beta_2$-agonists (LABAs) increase the risk of asthma-related deaths. Salmeterol should only be used in asthma patients as adjuvant therapy in patients who are currently receiving but are not adequately controlled on a long-term asthma control medication (ie, an inhaled corticosteroid). Monotherapy with an LABA is contraindicated in the treatment of asthma. In a large, randomized, placebo-controlled U.S. clinical trial (SMART, 2006), salmeterol was associated with an increase in asthma-related deaths (when added to usual asthma therapy); risk is considered a class effect among all LABAs. Data are not available to determine if the addition of an inhaled corticosteroid lessens this increased risk of death associated with LABA use. Assess patients at regular intervals once asthma control is maintained on combination therapy to determine if step-down therapy is appropriate and the LABA can be discontinued (without loss of asthma control), and the patient can be maintained

on an inhaled corticosteroid. LABAs are not appropriate in patients whose asthma is adequately controlled on low- or medium-dose inhaled corticosteroids. Do **not** use for acute bronchospasm. Short-acting beta$_2$-agonist (eg, albuterol) should be used for acute symptoms and symptoms occurring between treatments. Do **not** initiate in patients with significantly worsening or acutely deteriorating asthma; reports of severe (sometimes fatal) respiratory events have been reported when salmeterol has been initiated in this situation. Corticosteroids should not be stopped or reduced when salmeterol is initiated. During initiation, watch for signs of worsening asthma. Patients must be instructed to use short-acting beta$_2$-agonists (eg, albuterol) for acute asthmatic or COPD symptoms and to seek medical attention in cases where acute symptoms are not relieved or a previous level of response is diminished. The need to increase frequency of use of short-acting beta$_2$-agonist may indicate deterioration of asthma, and treatment must not be delayed. Because LABAs may disguise poorly controlled persistent asthma, frequent or chronic use of LABAs for exercise-induced bronchospasm is discouraged by the NIH Asthma Guidelines (NIH, 2007). Salmeterol should not be used more than twice daily; do not use with other long-acting beta$_2$-agonists. **[U.S. Boxed Warning]: LABAs may increase the risk of asthma-related hospitalization in pediatric and adolescent patients.** In general, a combination product containing a LABA and an inhaled corticosteroid is preferred in patients <18 years of age to ensure compliance.

COPD treatment: Appropriate use: Do **not** use for acute episodes of COPD. Do **not** initiate in patients with significantly worsening or acutely deteriorating COPD. Data are not available to determine if LABA use increases the risk of death in patients with COPD.

Concurrent diseases: Use caution in patients with cardiovascular disease (eg, arrhythmia, hypertension, or HF), seizure disorders, diabetes, hyperthyroidism, hepatic impairment, or hypokalemia. Beta-agonists may cause elevation in blood pressure, heart rate, CNS stimulation/excitation, increased risk of arrhythmia, increase serum glucose, or decrease serum potassium.

Adverse events: Immediate hypersensitivity reactions (urticaria, angioedema, rash, bronchospasm) have been reported. There have been reports of laryngeal spasm, irritation, swelling (stridor, choking) with use. Salmeterol should not be used more than twice daily; do not exceed recommended dose; do not use with other long-acting beta$_2$-agonists; serious adverse events have been associated with excessive use of inhaled sympathomimetics. Rarely, paradoxical bronchospasm may occur with use of inhaled bronchodilating agents; this should be distinguished from inadequate response. Use with strong CYP3A4 inhibitors (see Drug Interactions) is not recommended due to potential for an increased risk of cardiovascular events. Powder for oral inhalation contains lactose; very rare anaphylactic reactions have been reported in patients with severe milk protein allergy.

Adverse Reactions

>10%:

Central nervous system: Headache (13% to 17%)

Neuromuscular & skeletal: Pain (1% to 12%)

1% to 10%:

Cardiovascular: Hypertension (4%), edema (1% to 3%), pallor

Central nervous system: Dizziness (4%), sleep disturbance (1% to 3%), fever (1% to 3%), anxiety (1% to 3%), migraine (1% to 3%)

Dermatologic: Rash (1% to 4%), contact dermatitis (1% to 3%), eczema (1% to 3%), urticaria (3%), photodermatitis (1% to 2%)

Endocrine & metabolic: Hyperglycemia (1% to 3%)

Gastrointestinal: Throat irritation (7%), nausea (1% to 3%), dyspepsia (1% to 3%), dental pain (1% to 3%), gastrointestinal infection (1% to 3%), oropharyngeal candidiasis (1% to 3%), xerostomia (1% to 3%)

Hepatic: Liver enzymes increased

Neuromuscular & skeletal: Muscular cramps/spasm (3%), articular rheumatism (1% to 3%), arthralgia (1% to 3%), joint pain (1% to 3%), muscular stiffness (1% to 3%), paresthesia (1% to 3%), rigidity (1% to 3%)

Ocular: Keratitis/conjunctivitis (1% to 3%)

Respiratory: Nasal congestion (4% to 9%), tracheitis/bronchitis (7%), pharyngitis (≤6%), cough (5%), influenza (5%), viral respiratory tract infection (5%), sinusitis (4% to 5%), rhinitis (4% to 5%), asthma (3% to 4%)

<1% (Limited to important or life-threatening): Abdominal pain, agitation, aggression, anaphylactic reaction (some in patients with severe milk allergy [Diskus®]), angioedema, aphonia, arrhythmia, atrial fibrillation, bronchospasm and immediate bronchospasm, cataracts, chest congestion, chest tightness, choking, contusions, Cushing syndrome, Cushingoid features, depression, dysmenorrhea, dyspnea, earache, ecchymoses, edema (facial, oropharyngeal), eosinophilic conditions, glaucoma, growth velocity reduction in children/adolescents, hypercorticism, hypersensitivity reaction (immediate and delayed), hypokalemia, hypothyroidism, intraocular pressure increased, laryngeal spasm/irritation, irregular menstruation, myositis, oropharyngeal irritation, osteoporosis, pallor, paradoxical tracheitis, paranasal sinus pain, PID, restlessness, stridor, supraventricular tachycardia, syncope, tremor, vaginal candidiasis, vaginitis, vulvovaginitis, rare cases of vasculitis (Churg-Strauss syndrome), ventricular tachycardia, weight gain

Drug Interactions

Metabolism/Transport Effects Substrate of CYP3A4 (major); **Note:** Assignment of Major/Minor substrate status based on clinically relevant drug interaction potential

Avoid Concomitant Use

Avoid concomitant use of Salmeterol with any of the following: Beta-Blockers (Nonselective); CYP3A4 Inhibitors (Strong); Iobenguane I 123; Telaprevir

Increased Effect/Toxicity

Salmeterol may increase the levels/effects of: Loop Diuretics; Sympathomimetics; Thiazide Diuretics

The levels/effects of Salmeterol may be increased by: Atomoxetine; Cannabinoids; CYP3A4 Inhibitors (Moderate); CYP3A4 Inhibitors (Strong); Dasatinib; MAO Inhibitors; Telaprevir; Tricyclic Antidepressants

Decreased Effect

Salmeterol may decrease the levels/effects of: Iobenguane I 123

The levels/effects of Salmeterol may be decreased by: Alpha-/Beta-Blockers; Beta-Blockers (Beta1 Selective); Beta-Blockers (Nonselective); Betahistine; Tocilizumab

Stability Inhalation powder: Store at controlled room temperature 20°C to 25°C (68°F to 77°F) in a dry place away from direct heat or sunlight. Stable for 6 weeks after removal from foil pouch.

Mechanism of Action Relaxes bronchial smooth muscle by selective action on beta$_2$-receptors with little effect on heart rate; salmeterol acts locally in the lung.

Pharmacodynamics/Kinetics

Onset of action: Asthma: 30-48 minutes, COPD: 2 hours

Peak effect: Asthma: 3 hours, COPD: 2-5 hours

Duration: 12 hours

Absorption: Systemic: Inhalation: Undetectable to poor

Protein binding: 96%

Metabolism: Hepatic; hydroxylated via CYP3A4

Half-life elimination: 5.5 hours

Time to peak, serum: ~20 minutes

Excretion: Feces (60%); urine (25%)

Dosage Inhalation, powder (50 mcg/inhalation):
Asthma, maintenance and prevention: Children ≥4 years and Adults: One inhalation twice daily (~12 hours apart); maximum: 1 inhalation twice daily. **Note:** For asthma control, long acting $beta_2$-agonists (LABAs) should be used in combination with inhaled corticosteroids and not as monotherapy.
Exercise-induced asthma, prevention: Children ≥4 years and Adults: One inhalation at least 30 minutes prior to exercise; additional doses should not be used for 12 hours; should not be used in individuals already receiving salmeterol twice daily. **Note:** Because LABAs may disguise poorly controlled persistent asthma, frequent or chronic use of LABAs for exercise-induced bronchospasm is discouraged by the NIH Asthma Guidelines (NIH, 2007).
COPD maintenance: Adults: One inhalation twice daily (~12 hours apart); maximum: 1 inhalation twice daily
Dosage adjustment in hepatic impairment: No dosage adjustment required; manufacturer suggests monitoring of patients with hepatic impairment.

Dietary Considerations Some products may contain lactose; very rare anaphylactic reactions have been reported in patients with severe milk protein allergy.

Administration Inhalation: **Not** to be used for the relief of acute attacks. Not for use with a spacer device. Administer with Diskus® in a level, horizontal position. Do not wash mouthpiece; Diskus® should be kept dry. Discard device 6 weeks after removal from foil pouch or when the dose counter reads "0" (whichever comes first).

Monitoring Parameters FEV_1, peak flow, and/or other pulmonary function tests; blood pressure, heart rate; CNS stimulation. Monitor for increased use of short-acting $beta_2$-agonist inhalers; may be marker of a deteriorating asthma condition.

Dosage Forms Excipient information presented when available (limited, particularly for generics); consult specific product labeling.
Powder, for oral inhalation:
Serevent® Diskus®: 50 mcg (28s, 60s) [contains lactose]

Dosage Forms: Canada Excipient information presented when available (limited, particularly for generics); consult specific product labeling.
Powder for oral inhalation:
Serevent® Diskhaler® Disk: Salmeterol xinafoate 50 mcg (60s) [delivers 50 mcg/inhalation; contains lactose]

- ◆ **Salmeterol and Fluticasone** *see* Fluticasone and Salmeterol *on page 741*
- ◆ **Salmeterol Xinafoate** *see* Salmeterol *on page 1532*
- ◆ **Salofalk® (Can)** *see* Mesalamine *on page 1081*
- ◆ **Salofalk® 5-ASA (Can)** *see* Mesalamine *on page 1081*
- ◆ **Salonpas® [OTC]** *see* Methyl Salicylate and Menthol *on page 1113*
- ◆ **Salonpas® Arthritis Pain® [OTC]** *see* Methyl Salicylate and Menthol *on page 1113*
- ◆ **Salonpas® Pain Relief Patch® [OTC]** *see* Methyl Salicylate and Menthol *on page 1113*

Salsalate (SAL sa late)

Brand Names: Canada Amigesic®; Salflex®
Index Terms Disalicylic Acid; Salicylsalicylic Acid
Pharmacologic Category Salicylate
Use Treatment of rheumatoid arthritis, osteoarthritis, and related rheumatic disorders
Pregnancy Risk Factor C
Dosage Oral:
Adults: 3 g/day in 2-3 divided dose
Elderly: May require lower dosage

Additional Information Complete prescribing information for this medication should be consulted for additional detail.

Dosage Forms Excipient information presented when available (limited, particularly for generics); consult specific product labeling.
Tablet, oral: 500 mg, 750 mg

- ◆ **Salt** *see* Sodium Chloride *on page 1567*
- ◆ **Salt Poor Albumin** *see* Albumin *on page 51*
- ◆ **Samsca™** *see* Tolvaptan *on page 1706*
- ◆ **Sanctura®** *see* Trospium *on page 1743*
- ◆ **Sanctura® XR** *see* Trospium *on page 1743*
- ◆ **Sancuso®** *see* Granisetron *on page 807*
- ◆ **SandIMMUNE®** *see* CycloSPORINE (Systemic) *on page 422*
- ◆ **Sandimmune® I.V. (Can)** *see* CycloSPORINE (Systemic) *on page 422*
- ◆ **SandoSTATIN®** *see* Octreotide *on page 1226*
- ◆ **Sandostatin® (Can)** *see* Octreotide *on page 1226*
- ◆ **SandoSTATIN LAR®** *see* Octreotide *on page 1226*
- ◆ **Sandostatin LAR® (Can)** *see* Octreotide *on page 1226*
- ◆ **Sandoz-Acebutolol (Can)** *see* Acebutolol *on page 27*
- ◆ **Sandoz-Alendronate (Can)** *see* Alendronate *on page 61*
- ◆ **Sandoz-Alfuzosin (Can)** *see* Alfuzosin *on page 64*
- ◆ **Sandoz-Amiodarone (Can)** *see* Amiodarone *on page 90*
- ◆ **Sandoz Amlodipine (Can)** *see* AmLODIPine *on page 97*
- ◆ **Sandoz-Anagrelide (Can)** *see* Anagrelide *on page 119*
- ◆ **Sandoz-Atenolol (Can)** *see* Atenolol *on page 161*
- ◆ **Sandoz-Atorvastatin (Can)** *see* Atorvastatin *on page 165*
- ◆ **Sandoz-Azithromycin (Can)** *see* Azithromycin (Systemic) *on page 180*
- ◆ **Sandoz-Betaxolol (Can)** *see* Betaxolol (Systemic) *on page 211*
- ◆ **Sandoz-Bicalutamide (Can)** *see* Bicalutamide *on page 217*
- ◆ **Sandoz-Bisoprolol (Can)** *see* Bisoprolol *on page 220*
- ◆ **Sandoz-Brimonidine (Can)** *see* Brimonidine *on page 235*
- ◆ **Sandoz-Bupropion SR (Can)** *see* BuPROPion *on page 247*
- ◆ **Sandoz-Calcitonin (Can)** *see* Calcitonin *on page 262*
- ◆ **Sandoz-Candesartan (Can)** *see* Candesartan *on page 273*
- ◆ **Sandoz-Carbamazepine (Can)** *see* CarBAMazepine *on page 280*
- ◆ **Sandoz-Cefprozil (Can)** *see* Cefprozil *on page 314*
- ◆ **Sandoz-Ciprofloxacin (Can)** *see* Ciprofloxacin (Systemic) *on page 362*
- ◆ **Sandoz-Citalopram (Can)** *see* Citalopram *on page 370*
- ◆ **Sandoz-Clarithromycin (Can)** *see* Clarithromycin *on page 374*
- ◆ **Sandoz-Clonazepam (Can)** *see* ClonazePAM *on page 390*
- ◆ **Sandoz-Cyclosporine (Can)** *see* CycloSPORINE (Systemic) *on page 422*
- ◆ **Sandoz-Diclofenac (Can)** *see* Diclofenac (Systemic) *on page 495*
- ◆ **Sandoz-Diclofenac Rapide (Can)** *see* Diclofenac (Systemic) *on page 495*
- ◆ **Sandoz-Diclofenac SR (Can)** *see* Diclofenac (Systemic) *on page 495*

- **Sandoz-Zolmitriptan ODT (Can)** *see* ZOLMitriptan *on page 1824*
- **Sans Acne® (Can)** *see* Erythromycin (Topical) *on page 619*
- **Santyl®** *see* Collagenase (Topical) *on page 410*
- **Saphris®** *see* Asenapine *on page 150*

Sapropterin (sap roe TER in)

Brand Names: U.S. Kuvan™

Index Terms 6R-BH4; Phenoptin; Sapropterin Dihydrochloride

Pharmacologic Category Enzyme Cofactor

Use Adjunct to dietary management in the treatment of tetrahydrobiopterin (BH4) responsive phenylketonuria (PKU)

Pregnancy Risk Factor C

Dosage Oral: PKU: Children ≥4 years and Adults: Initial: 10 mg/kg once daily; adjust after 1 month based on blood phenylalanine levels (if phenylalanine levels do not decrease from baseline, increase dose to 20 mg/kg once daily); discontinue if phenylalanine levels do not decrease after 1 month of treatment at 20 mg/kg/day (nonresponder). Maintenance range: 5-20 mg/kg once daily

Additional Information Complete prescribing information for this medication should be consulted for additional detail.

Dosage Forms Excipient information presented when available (limited, particularly for generics); consult specific product labeling.

Tablet, as dihydrochloride:

Kuvan™: 100 mg

- **Sapropterin Dihydrochloride** *see* Sapropterin *on page 1536*

Saquinavir (sa KWIN a veer)

Brand Names: U.S. Invirase®

Brand Names: Canada Invirase®

Index Terms Saquinavir Mesylate; SQV

Pharmacologic Category Antiretroviral Agent, Protease Inhibitor

Additional Appendix Information

Management of Healthcare Worker Exposures to HBV, HCV, and HIV *on page 1935*

Perinatal HIV Guidelines *on page 1946*

Use Treatment of HIV infection; used in combination with at least two other antiretroviral agents

Pregnancy Risk Factor B

Pregnancy Considerations Adverse events were not observed in animal reproduction studies. Saquinavir crosses the human placenta in minimal amounts. Based on limited data, Invirase® 1000 mg (capsules and tablets) administered twice daily with ritonavir 100 mg twice daily provide adequate levels in pregnant women. The DHHS Perinatal HIV Guidelines consider Invirase® capsules and ritonavir to be an alternative combination for use during pregnancy; use without ritonavir is **not** recommended. A small increased risk of preterm birth has been associated with maternal use of protease inhibitor-based combination antiretroviral (ARV) therapy during pregnancy; however, the benefits of use generally outweigh this risk and protease inhibitors (PIs) should not be withheld if otherwise recommended. Hyperglycemia, new onset of diabetes mellitus, or diabetic ketoacidosis have been reported with PIs; it is not clear if pregnancy increases this risk.

Regardless of CD4 count or HIV RNA copy number, all HIV-infected pregnant women should receive a combination antepartum ARV drug regimen; this includes women who require therapy for their own health, as well as women who do not yet require therapy for their own health. ARV therapy should be started as soon as possible if required for the woman's health or immediately after the first trimester if not needed for the mothers health (although earlier initiation may be considered). Long-term follow-up is recommended for all infants exposed to ARV medications.

Healthcare providers are encouraged to enroll pregnant women exposed to antiretroviral medications in the Antiretroviral Pregnancy Registry (1-800-258-4263 or www.APRegistry.com). Healthcare providers caring for HIV-infected women and their infants may contact the National Perinatal HIV Hotline (888-448-8765) for clinical consultation (DHHS [perinatal], 2011).

Lactation Excretion in breast milk unknown/contraindicated

Medication Guide Available Yes

Contraindications Hypersensitivity to saquinavir or any component of the formulation; congenital or acquired QT prolongation, refractory hypokalemia or hypomagnesemia, concomitant use of other medications that both increase saquinavir plasma concentrations and prolong the QT interval; complete AV block (without implanted ventricular pacemaker) or patients at high risk of complete AV block; severe hepatic impairment; coadministration of saquinavir/ritonavir with alfuzosin, amiodarone, bepridil, cisapride, dofetilide, ergot derivatives, flecainide, lidocaine (systemic), lovastatin, midazolam (oral), pimozide, propafenone, quinidine, rifampin, sildenafil (when used for pulmonary artery hypertension [eg, Revatio®]),simvastatin, trazodone, or triazolam

Warnings/Precautions Use caution in patients with hepatic insufficiency. May exacerbate pre-existing hepatic dysfunction; use with caution in patients with hepatitis B or C and in cirrhosis. May be associated with fat redistribution (buffalo hump, increased abdominal girth, breast engorgement, facial atrophy). Use caution in hemophilia. May increase cholesterol and/or triglycerides. Changes in glucose tolerance, hyperglycemia, exacerbation of diabetes, DKA, and new-onset diabetes mellitus have been reported in patients receiving protease inhibitors.

Altered cardiac conduction: Saquinavir/ritonavir prolongs the QT interval, potentially leading to torsade de pointes, and prolongs the PR interval, potentially leading to heart block. An ECG should be performed for all patients prior to starting saquinavir/ritonavir therapy; do not initiate therapy in patients with a baseline QT interval >450 msec. If baseline QT interval <450 msec, may initiate therapy but a subsequent ECG is recommended after ~3-4 days of therapy. If subsequent QT interval is >480 msec or is prolonged over baseline by >20 msec, therapy should be discontinued. Patients who may be at increased risk for QT- or PR-interval prolongation include those with heart failure, bradyarrhythmias, hepatic impairment, electrolyte abnormalities, ischemic heart disease, cardiomyopathy, structural heart disease, or those with pre-existing cardiac conduction abnormalities; ECG monitoring is recommended for these patients.

Use with caution in patients taking strong CYP3A4 inhibitors, moderate or strong CYP3A4 inducers and major CYP3A4 substrates (see Drug Interactions); consider alternative agents that avoid or lessen the potential for CYP-mediated interactions. St John's wort, lovastatin, and simvastatin should not be used concurrently with saquinavir/ritonavir. A listing of medications that should not be used is available with each bottle and patients should be provided with this information. Do not coadminister colchicine in patient with renal or hepatic impairment; avoid concurrent use with salmeterol. Patients may develop immune reconstitution syndrome resulting in the occurrence of an inflammatory response to an indolent or residual opportunistic infection; further evaluation and treatment may be required. Invirase® may be used only if combined with ritonavir. Safety and efficacy have not been established in children ≤16 years of age.

Adverse Reactions

Incidence data shown for saquinavir soft gel capsule formulation (no longer available) in combination with ritonavir.

10%: Gastrointestinal: Nausea (11%)

1% to 10%:

Cardiovascular: Chest pain

Central nervous system: Fatigue (6%), fever (3%), anxiety, depression, headache, insomnia, pain

Dermatologic: Pruritus (3%), rash (3%), dry lips/skin (2%), eczema (2%), verruca

Endocrine & metabolic: Lipodystrophy (5%), hyperglycemia (3%), hypoglycemia, hyperkalemia, libido disorder, serum amylase increased

Gastrointestinal: Diarrhea (8%), vomiting (7%), abdominal pain (6%), constipation (2%), abdominal discomfort, appetite decreased, buccal mucosa ulceration, dyspepsia, flatulence, taste alteration

Hepatic: AST increased, ALT increased, bilirubin increased

Neuromuscular & skeletal: Back pain (2%), CPK increased, paresthesia, weakness

Renal: Creatinine kinase increased

Respiratory: Pneumonia (5%), bronchitis (3%), sinusitis (3%)

Miscellaneous: Influenza (3%)

Incidence not currently defined (limited to significant reactions; reported for hard or soft gel capsule with/without ritonavir)

Cardiovascular: Cyanosis, heart valve disorder (including murmur), hyper-/hypotension, peripheral vasoconstriction, prolonged QT interval, prolonged PR interval, syncope, thrombophlebitis

Central nervous system: Agitation, amnesia, ataxia, confusion, hallucination, hyper-/hyporeflexia, myelopolyradiculoneuritis, neuropathies, poliomyelitis, progressive multifocal encephalopathy, psychosis, seizures, somnolence, speech disorder, suicide attempt

Dermatologic: Alopecia, bullous eruption, dermatitis, erythema, maculopapular rash, photosensitivity, Stevens-Johnson syndrome, skin ulceration, urticaria

Endocrine & metabolic: Dehydration, diabetes, electrolyte changes, TSH increased

Gastrointestinal: Ascites, colic, dysphagia, esophagitis, bloody stools, gastritis, intestinal obstruction, hemorrhage (rectal), pancreatitis, stomatitis

Genitourinary: impotence, prostate enlarged, hematuria, UTI

Hematologic; Acute myeloblastic leukemia, anemia (including hemolytic), leukopenia, neutropenia, pancytopenia, splenomegaly, thrombocytopenia

Hepatic: Alkaline phosphatase increased, GGT increased, hepatitis, hepatomegaly, hepatosplenomegaly, jaundice, liver disease exacerbation

Neuromuscular & skeletal: Arthritis, LDH increased

Ocular: Blepharitis, visual disturbance

Otic: Otitis, hearing decreased, tinnitus

Renal: Nephrolithiasis, renal calculus

Respiratory: Dyspnea, hemoptysis, pharyngitis, upper respiratory tract infection

Miscellaneous: Infections (bacterial, fungal, viral)

Postmarketing and/or case reports: AV block (second or third degree), torsade de pointes

Drug Interactions

Metabolism/Transport Effects Substrate of CYP2D6 (minor), CYP3A4 (major), P-glycoprotein; **Note:** Assignment of Major/Minor substrate status based on clinically relevant drug interaction potential; **Inhibits** CYP2C19 (weak), CYP2C9 (weak), CYP2D6 (weak), CYP3A4 (strong), P-glycoprotein

Avoid Concomitant Use

Avoid concomitant use of Saquinavir with any of the following: Alfuzosin; Amiodarone; Artemether; Bepridil [Off Market]; Cisapride; Conivaptan; Crizotinib; Darunavir; Dofetilide; Dronedarone; Eplerenone; Ergot Derivatives; Everolimus; Flecainide; Fluticasone (Oral Inhalation); Halofantrine; Lapatinib; Lidocaine (Systemic); Lovastatin; Lumefantrine; Lurasidone; Midazolam; Nilotinib; Nisoldipine; Pimozide; Propafenone; QUEtiapine; QuiNIDine; QuiNINE; Ranolazine; Rifampin; Rivaroxaban; RomiDEPsin; Salmeterol; Silodosin; Simvastatin; St Johns Wort; Tamsulosin; Tetrabenazine; Thioridazine; Ticagrelor; Tolvaptan; Topotecan; Toremifene; TraZODone; Triazolam; Vandetanib; Vemurafenib; Ziprasidone

Increased Effect/Toxicity

Saquinavir may increase the levels/effects of: Alfuzosin; Almotriptan; Alosetron; ALPRAZolam; Amiodarone; Antifungal Agents (Azole Derivatives, Systemic); ARIPiprazole; Bepridil [Off Market]; Bortezomib; Brentuximab Vedotin; Brinzolamide; Budesonide (Nasal); Budesonide (Systemic, Oral Inhalation); Calcium Channel Blockers (Dihydropyridine); Calcium Channel Blockers (Nondihydropyridine); CarBAMazepine; Ciclesonide; Cisapride; Clarithromycin; Clorazepate; Colchicine; Conivaptan; Corticosteroids (Orally Inhaled); Crizotinib; CycloSPORINE; CycloSPORINE (Systemic); CYP3A4 Substrates; Dabigatran Etexilate; Diazepam; Dienogest; Digoxin; Dofetilide; Dronedarone; Dutasteride; Enfuvirtide; Eplerenone; Ergot Derivatives; Everolimus; FentaNYL; Fesoterodine; Flecainide; Flurazepam; Fluticasone (Nasal); Fluticasone (Oral Inhalation); Fusidic Acid; GuanFACINE; Halofantrine; HMG-CoA Reductase Inhibitors; Iloperidone; Ixabepilone; Lapatinib; Lidocaine (Systemic); Lovastatin; Lumefantrine; Lurasidone; Maraviroc; Meperidine; MethylPREDNISolone; Midazolam; Nefazodone; Nilotinib; Nisoldipine; Paricalcitol; Pazopanib; P-glycoprotein/ABCB1 Substrates; Pimecrolimus; Pimozide; Propafenone; Protease Inhibitors; QTc-Prolonging Agents; QuiNIDine; QuiNINE; Ranolazine; Rifabutin; Rivaroxaban; RomiDEPsin; Ruxolitinib; Salmeterol; Saxagliptin; Sildenafil; Silodosin; Simvastatin; Sirolimus; SORAfenib; Tacrolimus; Tacrolimus (Systemic); Tacrolimus (Topical); Tadalafil; Tamsulosin; Temsirolimus; Tetrabenazine; Thioridazine; Ticagrelor; Tolterodine; Tolvaptan; Topotecan; Toremifene; TraZODone; Triazolam; Tricyclic Antidepressants; Vandetanib; Vardenafil; Vemurafenib; Vilazodone; Warfarin; Ziprasidone; Zuclopenthixol

The levels/effects of Saquinavir may be increased by: Alfuzosin; Antifungal Agents (Azole Derivatives, Systemic); Artemether; Bepridil [Off Market]; Chloroquine; Ciprofloxacin; Ciprofloxacin (Systemic); Clarithromycin; CycloSPORINE; CycloSPORINE (Systemic); Delavirdine; Efavirenz; Enfuvirtide; Etravirine; Fusidic Acid; Gadobutrol; H2-Antagonists; Indacaterol; Lumefantrine; Nilotinib; P-glycoprotein/ABCB1 Inhibitors; Proton Pump Inhibitors; QUEtiapine; QuiNINE; Rifampin

Decreased Effect

Saquinavir may decrease the levels/effects of: Abacavir; Clarithromycin; Contraceptives (Estrogens); Darunavir; Delavirdine; Divalproex; Etravirine; Meperidine; Methadone; Prasugrel; Theophylline Derivatives; Ticagrelor; Valproic Acid; Zidovudine

The levels/effects of Saquinavir may be decreased by: Antacids; CarBAMazepine; CYP3A4 Inducers (Strong); Deferasirox; Efavirenz; Garlic; Nevirapine; Peginterferon Alfa-2b; P-glycoprotein/ABCB1 Inducers; Rifampin; St Johns Wort; Tocilizumab

Ethanol/Nutrition/Herb Interactions
Food: A high-fat meal maximizes bioavailability. Saquinavir levels may increase if taken with grapefruit juice.
Herb/Nutraceutical: Saquinavir serum concentrations may be decreased by St John's wort; avoid concurrent use. Garlic capsules may decrease saquinavir serum concentrations; avoid use if saquinavir is the only protease inhibitor.

Stability Invirase®: Store at room temperature.

Mechanism of Action Binds to the site of HIV-1 protease activity and inhibits cleavage of viral Gag-Pol polyprotein precursors into individual functional proteins required for infectious HIV. This results in the formation of immature, noninfectious viral particles.

Pharmacodynamics/Kinetics
Absorption: Poor; increased with high fat meal; Fortovase® has improved absorption over Invirase®
Distribution: V_d: 700 L; does not distribute into CSF
Protein binding, plasma: ~98%
Metabolism: Extensively hepatic via CYP3A4; extensive first-pass effect
Bioavailability: Invirase®: ~4%
Excretion: Feces (81% to 88%), urine (1% to 3%) within 5 days

Dosage Note: ECG should be done prior to starting therapy; do not initiate therapy if pretreatment QT interval >450 msec. Saquinavir should not be used in "unboosted regimens."
Oral: Children >16 years and Adults: 1000 mg (five 200 mg capsules or two 500 mg tablets) twice daily given in combination with ritonavir 100 mg twice daily. This combination should be given together and within 2 hours after a full meal in combination with a nucleoside analog.

Dosage adjustments when administered in combination therapy: Saquinavir: 1000 mg twice daily administered with lopinavir 400 mg/ritonavir 100 mg (Kaletra™) twice daily; no additional ritonavir is necessary

Dosage adjustments for concomitant therapy: Adults:
Coadministration with bosentan:
Coadministration of bosentan in patients currently receiving saquinavir/ritonavir: For patients receiving saquinavir/ritonavir for at least 10 days, begin with bosentan 62.5 mg once daily or every other day based on tolerability
Coadministration of saquinavir/ritonavir in patients currently receiving bosentan: Discontinue bosentan 36 hours prior to the initiation of saquinavir/ritonavir. After at least 10 days of saquinavir/ritonavir, resume bosentan 62.5 mg once daily or every other day based on tolerability.
Coadministration with colchicine:
Familial Mediterranean fever (FMF): Maximum colchicine dose: 0.6 mg/day (0.3 mg twice daily)
Gout prophylaxis:
If original colchicine dose is 0.6 mg twice daily, adjust dose to 0.3 mg once daily
If original colchicine dose is 0.6 mg once daily, adjust dose to 0.3 mg every other day
Gout flare treatment: Initial: Colchicine 0.6 mg, followed in 1 hour by a single dose of 0.3 mg; do not repeat for at least 3 days
Coadministration with phosphodiesterase-5 enzyme (PDE-5) inhibitor:
Pulmonary arterial hypertension: Saquinavir/ritonavir coadministered with tadalafil:
Patient receiving saquinavir/ritonavir for at least 1 week: Initiate tadalafil at 20 mg once daily; increase to 40 mg once daily based on individual tolerability
Patient receiving tadalafil when initiating saquinavir/ritonavir: Stop tadalafil at least 24 hours prior to starting saquinavir/ritonavir. After at least 1 week following the initiation of saquinavir/ritonavir, resume tadalafil at 20 mg once daily; increase to 40 mg once daily based on individual tolerability.
Erectile dysfunction: Saquinavir/ritonavir coadministered with:
Sildenafil: Maximum sildenafil dose: 25 mg in a 48-hour period
Tadalafil: Maximum tadalafil dose: 10 mg in a 72-hour period
Vardenafil: Maximum vardenafil dose: 2.5 mg in a 72-hour period

Elderly: Clinical studies did not include sufficient numbers of patients ≥65 years of age; use caution due to increased frequency of organ dysfunction

Dietary Considerations Take within 2 hours of a meal. Invirase® capsules contain lactose (not expected to induce symptoms of intolerance).

Administration Administer within 2 hours after a full meal. When used with ritonavir, saquinavir and ritonavir should be administered at the same time.

Monitoring Parameters Monitor ECG (prior to therapy and after 3-4 days of therapy); serum potassium and magnesium levels, triglycerides and cholesterol (prior to initiation and periodically during therapy); viral load, CD4 count; glucose

Dosage Forms Excipient information presented when available (limited, particularly for generics); consult specific product labeling.
Capsule, oral:
Invirase®: 200 mg [contains lactose 63.3 mg/capsule]
Tablet, oral:
Invirase®: 500 mg

◆ **Saquinavir Mesylate** *see* Saquinavir *on page 1536*

◆ **Sarafem®** *see* FLUoxetine *on page 731*

Sargramostim (sar GRAM oh stim)

Brand Names: U.S. Leukine®
Brand Names: Canada Leukine®
Index Terms GM-CSF; Granulocyte-Macrophage Colony Stimulating Factor; NSC-613795; rhuGM-CSF
Pharmacologic Category Colony Stimulating Factor
Use
Acute myelogenous leukemia (AML) following induction chemotherapy in older adults (≥55 years of age) to shorten time to neutrophil recovery and to reduce the incidence of severe and life-threatening infections and infections resulting in death
Bone marrow transplant (allogeneic or autologous) failure or engraftment delay
Myeloid reconstitution after allogeneic bone marrow transplantation
Myeloid reconstitution after autologous bone marrow transplantation: Non-Hodgkin's lymphoma (NHL), acute lymphoblastic leukemia (ALL), Hodgkin's lymphoma
Peripheral stem cell transplantation: Mobilization and myeloid reconstitution following autologous peripheral stem cell transplantation

Pregnancy Risk Factor C

Pregnancy Considerations Clinical effects to the fetus: Animal reproduction studies have not been conducted. It is not known whether sargramostim can cause fetal harm when administered to a pregnant woman or can affect reproductive capability. Sargramostim should be given to a pregnant woman only if clearly needed.

Lactation Excretion in breast milk unknown/use caution

Contraindications Hypersensitivity to sargramostim, yeast-derived products, or any component of the formulation; concurrent (24 hours preceding/following) myelosuppressive chemotherapy or radiation therapy; patients with excessive (≥10%) leukemic myeloid blasts in bone marrow or peripheral blood

Warnings/Precautions Simultaneous administration, or administration 24 hours preceding/following cytotoxic chemotherapy or radiotherapy is not recommended. Use with caution in patients with pre-existing cardiac problems or HF; supraventricular arrhythmias have been reported in patients with history of arrhythmias. Edema, capillary leak syndrome, pleural and/or pericardial effusion have been reported; use with caution in patients with pre-existing fluid retention; may worsen. Use with caution in patients with hepatic or renal impairment; monitor hepatic and/or renal function in patients with history of hepatic or renal dysfunction. Elevations in bilirubin, transaminases, and serum creatinine have been observed with use. Dyspnea may occur; monitor respiratory symptoms during and following infusion; use with caution in patients with hypoxia or pulmonary infiltrates.

With rapid increase in blood counts (ANC >20,000/mm^3, WBC >50,000/mm^3, or platelets >500,000/mm^3); decrease dose by 50% or discontinue drug (counts will fall to normal within 3-7 days after discontinuing drug). May potentially act as a growth factor for any tumor type, particularly myeloid malignancies; caution should be exercised when using in any malignancy with myeloid characteristics; tumors of nonhematopoietic origin may have surface receptors for sargramostim. Discontinue use if disease progression occurs during treatment.

There is a "first-dose effect" (refer to Adverse Reactions for details) which is seen (rarely) with the first dose of a cycle and does not usually occur with subsequent doses within that cycle. Anaphylaxis or other serious allergic reactions have been reported; discontinue immediately if occur. Solution contains benzyl alcohol; do not use in premature infants or neonates.

Adverse Reactions

>10%:

- Cardiovascular: Hypertension (34%), pericardial effusion (4% to 25%), edema (13% to 25%), chest pain (15%), peripheral edema (11%), tachycardia (11%)
- Central nervous system: Fever (81%), malaise (57%), headache (26%), chills (25%), anxiety (11%), insomnia (11%)
- Dermatologic: Rash (44%), pruritus (23%)
- Endocrine & metabolic: Hyperglycemia (25%), hypercholesterolemia (17%), hypomagnesemia (15%)
- Gastrointestinal: Diarrhea (≤89%), nausea (58% to 70%), vomiting (46% to 70%), abdominal pain (38%), weight loss (37%), anorexia (13%), hematemesis (13%), dysphagia (11%), gastrointestinal hemorrhage (11%)
- Genitourinary: Urinary tract disorder (14%)
- Hepatic: Hyperbilirubinemia (30%)
- Neuromuscular & skeletal: Weakness (66%), bone pain (21%), arthralgia (11% to 21%) myalgia (18%)
- Ocular: Eye hemorrhage (11%)
- Renal: BUN increased (23%), serum creatinine increased (15%)
- Respiratory: Pharyngitis (23%), epistaxis (17%), dyspnea (15%)

1% to 10%: Respiratory: Pleural effusion (1%)

<1% (Limited to important or life-threatening): Allergic reaction, anaphylaxis, arrhythmia, capillary leak syndrome, constipation, dizziness, eosinophilia; first-dose effect (syndrome with respiratory distress, hypoxia, flushing, hypotension, syncope, and/or tachycardia occurring with the first dose of a treatment cycle); injection site reaction, lethargy, leukocytosis, liver function abnormalities (transient), pain, pericarditis, prothrombin time prolonged, rigors, sore throat, supraventricular arrhythmia (transient), thrombocytosis, thrombophlebitis, thrombosis

Drug Interactions

Metabolism/Transport Effects None known.

Avoid Concomitant Use There are no known interactions where it is recommended to avoid concomitant use.

Increased Effect/Toxicity

Sargramostim may increase the levels/effects of: Bleomycin

Decreased Effect There are no known significant interactions involving a decrease in effect.

Stability Store at 2°C to 8°C (36°F to 46°F); do not freeze. Do not shake.

Solution for injection: May be stored for up to 20 days at 2°C to 8°C (36°F to 46°F) once the vial has been entered. Discard remaining solution after 20 days.

Powder for injection: May be reconstituted with preservative free SWFI or bacteriostatic water for injection (with benzyl alcohol 0.9%). Preparations made with SWFI should be administered as soon as possible, and discarded within 6 hours of reconstitution. Preparations made with bacteriostatic water may be stored for up to 20 days at 2°C to 8°C (36°F to 46°F). Gently swirl to reconstitute; do not shake.

Sargramostim may also be further diluted in 25-50 mL NS to a concentration ≥10 mcg/mL for I.V. infusion administration; preparations diluted with NS are stable for 48 hours at room temperature and refrigeration.

If the final concentration of sargramostim is <10 mcg/mL, 1 mg of human albumin/1 mL of NS (eg, 1 mL of 5% human albumin/50 mL of NS) should be added.

Mechanism of Action Stimulates proliferation, differentiation and functional activity of neutrophils, eosinophils, monocytes, and macrophages, as indicated.

Pharmacodynamics/Kinetics

Onset of action: Increase in WBC: 7-14 days

Duration: WBCs return to baseline within 1 week of discontinuing drug

Half-life elimination: I.V.: 60 minutes; SubQ: 2.7 hours

Time to peak, serum: SubQ: 1-3 hours

Dosage

Children (unlabeled use) and Adults: I.V. infusion over ≥2 hours or SubQ: **Rounding the dose to the nearest vial size enhances patient convenience and reduces costs without clinical detriment**

Myeloid reconstitution after allogeneic or autologous bone marrow transplant: I.V.: 250 mcg/m^2/day (over 2 hours), begin 2-4 hours after the marrow infusion and ≥24 hours after chemotherapy or radiotherapy, when the post marrow infusion ANC is <500 cells/mm^3, and continue until ANC >1500 cells/mm^3 for 3 consecutive days

If a severe adverse reaction occurs, reduce dose by 50% or temporarily discontinue the dose until the reaction abates

If blast cells appear or progression of the underlying disease occurs, discontinue treatment

If ANC >20,000 cells/mm^3, interrupt treatment or reduce the dose by 50%

Neutrophil recovery following chemotherapy in AML: I.V.: 250 mcg/m^2/day (over 4 hours) starting approximately on day 11 or 4 days following the completion of induction chemotherapy, if day 10 bone marrow is hypoplastic with <5% blasts

If a second cycle of chemotherapy is necessary, administer ~4 days after the completion of chemotherapy if the bone marrow is hypoplastic with <5% blasts

Continue sargramostim until ANC is >1500 cells/mm^3 for 3 consecutive days or a maximum of 42 days

Discontinue sargramostim immediately if leukemic regrowth occurs

If a severe adverse reaction occurs, reduce the dose by 50% or temporarily discontinue the dose until the reaction abates

If ANC >20,000 cells/mm^3, interrupt treatment or reduce the dose by 50%

Mobilization of peripheral blood progenitor cells: I.V., SubQ: 250 mcg/m^2/day I.V. over 24 hours or SubQ once daily

Continue the same dose through the period of PBPC collection

The optimal schedule for PBPC collection has not been established (usually begun by day 5 and performed daily until protocol specified targets are achieved)

If WBC >50,000 cells/mm^3, reduce the dose by 50%

If adequate numbers of progenitor cells are not collected, consider other mobilization therapy

Postperipheral blood progenitor cell transplantation: I.V., SubQ: 250 mcg/m^2/day I.V. over 24 hours or SubQ once daily beginning immediately following infusion of progenitor cells and continuing until ANC is >1500 cells/mm^3 for 3 consecutive days is attained

BMT failure or engraftment delay: I.V.: 250 mcg/m^2/day over 2 hours for 14 days

May be repeated after 7 days off therapy if engraftment has not occurred

If engraftment still has not occurred, a third course of 500 mcg/m^2/day for 14 days may be tried after another 7 days off therapy; if there is still no improvement, it is unlikely that further dose escalation will be beneficial

If a severe adverse reaction occurs, reduce the dose by 50% or temporarily discontinue the dose until the reaction abates

If blast cells appear or disease progression occurs, discontinue treatment

If ANC >20,000 cells/mm^3, interrupt treatment or reduce the dose by 50%

Administration Can premedicate with analgesics and antipyretics (eg, acetaminophen) to control adverse events (eg, fever, chills, myalgia, etc); control bone pain with non-narcotic analgesics. Sargramostim is administered as a subcutaneous injection or intravenous infusion; intravenous infusion should be over 2-24 hours; continuous infusions may be more effective than short infusion or bolus injection. An in-line membrane filter should **NOT** be used for intravenous administration. When administering GM-CSF subcutaneously, rotate injection sites.

Monitoring Parameters Vital signs, hydration status, weight, CBC with differential twice weekly during therapy, renal/liver function tests at least biweekly during therapy (in patients displaying renal or hepatic dysfunction prior to initiation of treatment), pulmonary function

Reference Range Excessive leukocytosis: ANC >20,000/mm^3 or WBC >50,000 cells/mm^3

Test Interactions May interfere with bone imaging studies; increased hematopoietic activity of the bone marrow may appear as transient positive bone imaging changes

Additional Information Reimbursement Hotline (Leukine®): 1-800-321-4669

Dosage Forms Excipient information presented when available (limited, particularly for generics); consult specific product labeling.

Injection, powder for reconstitution:

Leukine®: 250 mcg [contains sucrose 10 mg/mL]

Injection, solution:

Leukine®: 500 mcg/mL (1 mL) [contains benzyl alcohol, sucrose 10 mg/mL]

◆ **Sarna® HC (Can)** *see* Hydrocortisone (Topical) *on page 841*

◆ **Savella®** *see* Milnacipran *on page 1134*

Saxagliptin (sax a GLIP tin)

Brand Names: U.S. Onglyza™

Brand Names: Canada Onglyza™

Index Terms BMS-477118

Pharmacologic Category Antidiabetic Agent, Dipeptidyl Peptidase IV (DPP-IV) Inhibitor

Additional Appendix Information

Diabetes Mellitus Management, Adults *on page 1983*

Use Treatment of type 2 diabetes mellitus (noninsulin dependent, NIDDM) as an adjunct to diet and exercise as monotherapy or in combination therapy with other antidiabetic agents to improve glycemic control

Pregnancy Risk Factor B

Pregnancy Considerations Teratogenic effects were not observed in animal studies. However, there are no adequate and well-controlled studies in pregnant women.

Lactation Excretion in breast milk unknown/use caution

Medication Guide Available Yes

Contraindications Hypersensitivity to saxagliptin or any component of the formulation.

Warnings/Precautions Use with caution in patients with moderate-to-severe renal dysfunction, end-stage renal disease (ESRD) requiring hemodialysis, and in patients taking strong CYP3A4/5 inhibitors (eg, atazanavir, clarithromycin, indinavir, itraconazole, nefazodone, nelfinavir, ritonavir, saquinavir, telithromycin [also see Drug Interactions]); dosing adjustment required. Use caution when used in conjunction with insulin secretagogues (eg, sulfonylureas); risk of hypoglycemia is increased. Monitor blood glucose closely; dosage adjustments of the insulin secretagogue may be necessary. Rare hypersensitivity reactions, including anaphylaxis, angioedema, and/or exfoliative dermatologic reactions have been reported; discontinue if signs/symptoms of severe hypersensitivity reactions occur. Cases of acute pancreatitis have been reported; discontinue immediately if suspected.

Adverse Reactions Note: Frequencies and adverse reactions reported with monotherapy unless otherwise noted.

1% to 10%:

Cardiovascular: Peripheral edema (≤4%; incidence increased in conjunction with thiazolidinediones: ≤8%)

Central nervous system: Headache (7%)

Endocrine & metabolic: Hypoglycemia (≤6%; incidence increased in conjunction with insulin secretagogues: ≤15%)

Gastrointestinal: Abdominal pain (2%), gastroenteritis (2%), vomiting (2%)

Genitourinary: Urinary tract infection (7%)

Hematologic: Lymphopenia (≤2%; dose related)

Respiratory: Sinusitis (3%)

Miscellaneous: Hypersensitivity reactions (2%; including urticaria and facial edema)

<1% (Limited to important or life-threatening): Angioedema, anaphylaxis, creatinine increased, creatine phosphokinase increased, exfoliative skin reactions, idiopathic thrombocytopenic purpura, pancreatitis (acute), rash

Drug Interactions

Metabolism/Transport Effects Substrate of CYP3A4 (major), P-glycoprotein; **Note:** Assignment of Major/Minor substrate status based on clinically relevant drug interaction potential

Avoid Concomitant Use There are no known interactions where it is recommended to avoid concomitant use.

Increased Effect/Toxicity

Saxagliptin may increase the levels/effects of: ACE Inhibitors; Hypoglycemic Agents

The levels/effects of Saxagliptin may be increased by: CYP3A4 Inhibitors (Moderate); CYP3A4 Inhibitors (Strong); Dasatinib; Herbs (Hypoglycemic Properties); Pegvisomant; P-glycoprotein/ABCB1 Inhibitors

Decreased Effect

The levels/effects of Saxagliptin may be decreased by: Corticosteroids (Orally Inhaled); Corticosteroids (Systemic); CYP3A4 Inducers; Luteinizing Hormone-Releasing Hormone Analogs; P-glycoprotein/ABCB1 Inducers; Somatropin; Thiazide Diuretics; Tocilizumab

Stability Store at 20°C to 25°C (68°F to 77°F); excursions permitted between 15°C to 30°C (59°F to 86°F).

Mechanism of Action Saxagliptin inhibits dipeptidyl peptidase IV (DPP-IV) enzyme resulting in prolonged active incretin levels. Incretin hormones (eg, glucagon-like peptide-1 [GLP-1] and glucose-dependent insulinotropic polypeptide [GIP]) regulate glucose homeostasis by increasing insulin synthesis and release from pancreatic beta cells and decreasing glucagon secretion from pancreatic alpha cells. Decreased glucagon secretion results in decreased hepatic glucose production. Under normal physiologic circumstances, incretin hormones are released by the intestine throughout the day and levels are increased in response to a meal; incretin hormones are rapidly inactivated by the DPP-IV enzyme.

Pharmacodynamics/Kinetics

Duration: 24 hours

Protein binding: Negligible

Metabolism: Hepatic via CYP3A4/5 to 5-hydroxy saxagliptin (active; ~50% potency of the parent compound)

Half-life elimination: Saxagliptin: 2.5 hours; 5-hydroxy saxagliptin: 3.1 hours

Time to peak, plasma: Saxagliptin: 2 hours; 5-hydroxy saxagliptin: 4 hours

Excretion: Urine (75%, 24% of the total dose as saxagliptin, 36% of the total dose as 5-hydroxy saxagliptin); feces (22%)

Dosage Oral: Adults: Type 2 diabetes: 2.5-5 mg once daily

Concomitant use with strong CYP3A4/5 inhibitors: 2.5 mg once daily

Concomitant use with insulin secretagogues: Reduced dose of the insulin secretagogue (eg, sulfonylurea) may be needed

Dosage adjustment in renal impairment:

Note: Renal function may be estimated using the Cockcroft-Gault formula or the MDRD formula for dosage adjustment purposes.

Cl_{cr} >50 mL/minute: No dosage adjustment necessary

Cl_{cr} ≤50 mL/minute: 2.5 mg once daily

ESRD requiring hemodialysis: 2.5 mg once daily; administer postdialysis

Peritoneal dialysis: Not studied

Dosage adjustment in hepatic impairment: No dosage adjustment necessary

Dietary Considerations May be taken without regard to meals.

Administration May be administered without regard to meals.

Monitoring Parameters Plasma glucose, Hb A_{1c}, renal function

Reference Range Recommendations for glycemic control in adults with diabetes mellitus (ADA, 2010):

Hb A_{1c}: <7%

Preprandial capillary plasma glucose: 70-130 mg/dL

Peak postprandial capillary blood glucose: <180 mg/dL

Dosage Forms Excipient information presented when available (limited, particularly for generics); consult specific product labeling.

Tablet, oral:

Onglyza™: 2.5 mg, 5 mg

Saxagliptin and Metformin

(sax a GLIP tin & met FOR min)

Brand Names: U.S. Kombiglyze™ XR

Index Terms Metformin and Saxagliptin; Metformin Hydrochloride and Saxagliptin; Saxagliptin and Metformin Hydrochloride

Pharmacologic Category Antidiabetic Agent, Biguanide; Antidiabetic Agent, Dipeptidyl Peptidase IV (DPP-IV) Inhibitor

Use Management of type 2 diabetes mellitus (noninsulin dependent, NIDDM) as an adjunct to diet and exercise when treatment with both saxagliptin and metformin is appropriate

Pregnancy Risk Factor B

Medication Guide Available Yes

Dosage Oral: Type 2 diabetes mellitus: **Note:** Patients receiving concomitant insulin secretagogues (eg, sulfonylureas) may require dosage adjustments of these agents.

Adults: Initial doses should be based on current dose of saxagliptin and metformin; daily doses should be given once daily with the evening meal. Maximum: Saxagliptin 5 mg/metformin 2000 mg daily

Patients inadequately controlled on metformin alone: Initial dose: Saxagliptin 2.5-5 mg/day plus current dose of metformin. **Note:** Patients who require saxagliptin 2.5 mg (eg, dose adjusted for concomitant use of strong CYP3A4/5 inhibitors) and metformin >1000 mg should not be switched to the combination product.

Patients inadequately controlled on saxagliptin alone: Initial dose: Metformin 500 mg/day plus saxagliptin 5 mg/day. **Note:** Metformin-naïve patients currently receiving saxagliptin 2.5 mg daily (eg, dose adjusted for concomitant use of strong CYP3A4/5 inhibitors) should not be switched to the combination product.

Concomitant use with strong CYP3A4/5 inhibitors: Maximum: Saxagliptin 2.5 mg/metformin 1000 mg daily

Elderly: The initial and maintenance dosing should be conservative, due to the potential for decreased renal function (monitor). Do not use in patients ≥80 years of age unless normal renal function has been established.

Dosage adjustment in renal impairment: Do not use in patients with renal disease or renal dysfunction (serum creatinine ≥1.5 mg/dL [≥136 micromole/L] in males or ≥1.4 mg/dL [≥124 micromole/L] in females or abnormal clearance).

Dosage adjustment in hepatic impairment: Avoid metformin; liver disease is a risk factor for the development of lactic acidosis during metformin therapy.

Additional Information Complete prescribing information for this medication should be consulted for additional detail.

Dosage Forms Excipient information presented when available (limited, particularly for generics); consult specific product labeling.

Tablet, variable release, oral:

Kombiglyze™ XR 2.5/1000: Saxagliptin 2.5 mg [immediate release] and metformin hydrochloride 1000 mg [extended release]

Kombiglyze™ XR 5/500: Saxagliptin 5 mg [immediate release] and metformin hydrochloride 500 mg [extended release]

Kombiglyze™ XR 5/1000: Saxagliptin 5 mg [immediate release] and metformin hydrochloride 1000 mg [extended release]

◆ **Saxagliptin and Metformin Hydrochloride** *see* Saxagliptin and Metformin *on page* 1541

◆ **SB-265805** *see* Gemifloxacin *on page* 786

◆ **SB-497115** *see* Eltrombopag *on page* 579

◆ **SB-497115-GR** *see* Eltrombopag *on page* 579

Scopolamine (Systemic) (skoe POL a mee)

Brand Names: U.S. Scopace™ [DSC]; Transderm Scōp®

Brand Names: Canada Buscopan®; Transderm-V®

Index Terms Hyoscine Butylbromide; Scopolamine Base; Scopolamine Butylbromide; Scopolamine Hydrobromide

Pharmacologic Category Anticholinergic Agent

Use

Scopolamine base: Transdermal: Prevention of nausea/vomiting associated with motion sickness and recovery from anesthesia and surgery

Scopolamine hydrobromide:

Injection: Preoperative medication to produce amnesia, sedation, tranquilization, antiemetic effects, and decrease salivary and respiratory secretions

Oral: Symptomatic treatment of postencephalitic parkinsonism and paralysis agitans; in spastic states; inhibits excessive motility and hypertonus of the gastrointestinal tract in such conditions as the irritable colon syndrome, mild dysentery, diverticulitis, pylorospasm, and cardiospasm

Scopolamine butylbromide [not available in the U.S.]: Oral/injection: Treatment of smooth muscle spasm of the genitourinary or gastrointestinal tract; injection may also be used to prior to radiological/diagnostic procedures to prevent spasm

Unlabeled Use Scopolamine base: Transdermal: Breakthrough treatment of nausea and vomiting associated with chemotherapy

Pregnancy Risk Factor C

Pregnancy Considerations Teratogenic effects were not observed in animal studies; embryotoxic events were observed in some studies. Scopolamine crosses the placenta; may cause respiratory depression and/or neonatal hemorrhage when used during pregnancy. Transdermal scopolamine has been used as an adjunct to epidural anesthesia for cesarean delivery without adverse CNS effects on the newborn. Except when used prior to cesarean section, use during pregnancy only if the benefit to the mother outweighs the potential risk to the fetus.

Lactation Enters breast milk/use caution (AAP rates "compatible"; AAP 2001 update pending)

Contraindications Hypersensitivity to scopolamine, other belladonna alkaloids, or any component of the formulation; narrow-angle glaucoma; acute hemorrhage; paralytic ileus; tachycardia secondary to cardiac insufficiency; myasthenia gravis

Tablet formulations are also contraindicated in patients with prostatic hyperplasia, pyloric obstruction, or patients with an idiosyncrasy to anticholinergic drugs.

Injectable formulations are also contraindicated in patients with chronic lung disease (repeated administration).

Warnings/Precautions Use with caution in patients with coronary artery disease, tachyarrhythmias, heart failure, or hypertension; evaluate tachycardia prior to administration. Use with caution with hepatic or renal impairment; adverse CNS effects occur more often in these patients. Use injectable and transdermal products with caution in patients with prostatic hyperplasia (nonobstructive) or urinary retention; oral products are contraindicated. Discontinue if patient reports unusual visual disturbances or pain within the eye. Use caution in hiatal hernia, reflux esophagitis, and ulcerative colitis. Use with caution in patients with a history of seizure or psychosis; may exacerbate these conditions. Patients with idiosyncratic reaction to anticholinergics, including scopolamine, may experience disorientation, delirium and/or marked somnolence; may be accompanied by dilated pupils, rapid pulse and xerostomia. May cause CNS depression, which may impair physical or mental abilities; patients must be cautioned about performing tasks which require mental alertness (eg, operating machinery or driving).

Transdermal patch may contain conducting metal (eg, aluminum); remove patch prior to MRI. Scopolamine (hyoscine) hydrobromide should not be interchanged with scopolamine butylbromide formulations; dosages are not equivalent.

Use with caution in infants and children since they may be more susceptible to adverse effects of scopolamine. Safety and efficacy have not been established for the use of transdermal and oral scopolamine in children.

Adverse Reactions Frequency not defined.

Cardiovascular: Flushing, orthostatic hypotension, palpitation, tachycardia, ventricular fibrillation

Central nervous system: Acute toxic psychosis (rare), agitation (rare), ataxia, confusion, delusion (rare), disorientation, dizziness, drowsiness, fatigue, hallucination (rare), headache, loss of memory, paranoid behavior (rare), restlessness

Dermatologic: Dry skin, erythema, photosensitivity increased, rash

Endocrine & metabolic: Decreased flow of breast milk, thirst

Gastrointestinal: Bloated feeling, constipation, dry throat, dysphagia, nausea, vomiting, xerostomia

Genitourinary: Dysuria, urinary retention

Local: Irritation at injection site

Neuromuscular & skeletal: Tremor, weakness

Ocular: Accommodation impaired, blurred vision, cycloplegia, dryness, glaucoma (narrow-angle), increased intraocular pain, itching, photophobia, pupil dilation

Respiratory: Dry nose

Miscellaneous: Diaphoresis decreased, heat intolerance

Drug Interactions

Metabolism/Transport Effects None known.

Avoid Concomitant Use There are no known interactions where it is recommended to avoid concomitant use.

Increased Effect/Toxicity

Scopolamine (Systemic) may increase the levels/effects of: AbobotulinumtoxinA; Alcohol (Ethyl); Anticholinergics; Cannabinoids; CNS Depressants; Methotrimeprazine; OnabotulinumtoxinA; Potassium Chloride; RimabotulinumtoxinB; Selective Serotonin Reuptake Inhibitors

The levels/effects of Scopolamine (Systemic) may be increased by: Droperidol; HydrOXYzine; Methotrimeprazine; Pramlintide

Decreased Effect

Scopolamine (Systemic) may decrease the levels/effects of: Acetylcholinesterase Inhibitors (Central); Secretin

The levels/effects of Scopolamine (Systemic) may be decreased by: Acetylcholinesterase Inhibitors (Central)

Ethanol/Nutrition/Herb Interactions Ethanol: May increase CNS depression; monitor for increased effects with coadministration. Caution patients about effects.

Stability

Injection: Store at room temperature of 15°C to 30°C (58°F to 86°F). Protect from light.

Hydrobromide injection: Avoid acid solutions, hydrolysis occurs at pH <3.

Butylbromide injection: Stable in D_5W, NS, $D_{10}W$, and LR for up to 8 hours.

Tablet: Store at room temperature of 15°C to 30°C (58°F to 86°F).

Transdermal system: Store at 20°C to 25°C (68°F to 77°F).

Mechanism of Action Blocks the action of acetylcholine at parasympathetic sites in smooth muscle, secretory glands and the CNS; increases cardiac output, dries secretions, antagonizes histamine and serotonin

Pharmacodynamics/Kinetics

Onset of action: Oral, I.M.: 0.5-1 hour; I.V.: 10 minutes

Peak effect: 20-60 minutes; may take 3-7 days for full recovery; transdermal: 24 hours

Duration: Oral, I.M.: 4-6 hours; I.V.: 2 hours

Absorption: Tertiary salts (hydrobromide) are well absorbed; quaternary salts (butylbromide) are poorly absorbed (local concentrations in the GI tract following oral dosing may be high)

Metabolism: Hepatic

Half-life elimination: Hyoscine-N-butylbromide: 4.8 hours; Scopolamine: 9.5 hours

Excretion: Urine (<10%, as parent drug and metabolites)

Dosage Note: Scopolamine (hyoscine) hydrobromide should not be interchanged with scopolamine butylbromide formulations. Dosages are not equivalent.

Scopolamine base: Transdermal patch: Adults:

Preoperative: Apply 1 patch to hairless area behind ear the night before surgery or 1 hour prior to cesarean section (apply no sooner than 1 hour before surgery to minimize newborn exposure); remove 24 hours after surgery

Motion sickness: Apply 1 patch behind the ear at least 4 hours prior to exposure and every 3 days as needed; effective if applied as soon as 2-3 hours before anticipated need, best if 12 hours before

Chemotherapy-induced nausea and vomiting, breakthrough (unlabeled use): Apply 1 patch every 72 hours (NCCN Antiemesis guidelines v.1.2012)

Scopolamine hydrobromide:

Antiemetic: SubQ:

Children: 0.006 mg/kg

Adults: 0.6-1 mg

Preoperative: I.M., I.V., SubQ:

Children 6 months to 3 years: 0.1-0.15 mg

Children 3-6 years: 0.2-0.3 mg

Adults: 0.3-0.65 mg

Sedation, tranquilization: I.M., I.V., SubQ: Adults: 0.6 mg 3-4 times/day

Parkinsonism, spasticity, motion sickness: Adults: Oral: 0.4-0.8 mg. May repeat every 8-12 hours as needed; the dosage may be cautiously increased in parkinsonism and spastic states. For motion sickness, administration at least 1 hour before exposure is recommended.

Scopolamine butylbromide: Gastrointestinal/genitourinary spasm (Buscopan® [CAN]; not available in the U.S.): Adults:

Oral: 10-20 mg daily (1-2 tablets); maximum: 6 tablets/day

I.M., I.V., SubQ: 10-20 mg; maximum: 100 mg/day. Intramuscular injections should be administered 10-15 minutes prior to radiological/diagnostic procedures.

Administration

I.M.: **Butylbromide:** Intramuscular injections should be administered 10-15 minutes prior to radiological/diagnostic procedures.

I.V.:

Hydrobromide: Dilute with an equal volume of sterile water and administer by direct I.V.; inject over 2-3 minutes

Butylbromide: No dilution is necessary prior to injection; inject at a rate of 1 mL/minute

Transdermal: Topical patch is programmed to deliver 1 mg over 3 days. Once applied, do not remove the patch for 3 full days. Apply to hairless area of skin behind the ear. Wash hands before and after applying the disc to avoid drug contact with eyes.

Monitoring Parameters Body temperature, heart rate, urinary output, intraocular pressure

Test Interactions Interferes with gastric secretion test

Dosage Forms Excipient information presented when available (limited, particularly for generics); consult specific product labeling. [DSC] = Discontinued product

Injection, solution, as hydrobromide: 0.4 mg/mL (1 mL)

Patch, transdermal:

Transderm Scōp®: 1.5 mg (4s, 10s, 24s) [contains metal; releases ~1 mg over 72 hours]

Tablet, soluble, oral, as hydrobromide:

Scopace™: 0.4 mg [DSC]

Dosage Forms: Canada Excipient information presented when available (limited, particularly for generics); consult specific product labeling.

Injection, solution, as hyoscine-N-butylbromide:

Buscopan®: 20 mg/mL [not available in U.S.]

Tablet, as hyoscine-N-butylbromide:

Buscopan®: 10 mg

- **Scopolamine Base** *see* Scopolamine (Systemic) *on page* 1542
- **Scopolamine Butylbromide** *see* Scopolamine (Systemic) *on page* 1542
- **Scopolamine Hydrobromide** *see* Scopolamine (Systemic) *on page* 1542
- **Scopolamine, Hyoscyamine, Atropine, and Phenobarbital** *see* Hyoscyamine, Atropine, Scopolamine, and Phenobarbital *on page* 855
- **Scorpion Antivenin** *see* *Centruroides* Immune $F(ab')_2$ (Equine) *on page* 326
- **Scorpion Antivenom** *see* *Centruroides* Immune $F(ab')_2$ (Equine) *on page* 326
- **Scot-Tussin® DM Maximum Strength [OTC]** *see* Dextromethorphan and Chlorpheniramine *on page* 489
- **Scot-Tussin® Expectorant [OTC]** *see* GuaiFENesin *on page* 809
- **Scot-Tussin® Senior [OTC]** *see* Guaifenesin and Dextromethorphan *on page* 810
- **Sculptra®** *see* Poly-L-Lactic Acid *on page* 1374
- **Sculptra® Aesthetic** *see* Poly-L-Lactic Acid *on page* 1374
- **SD/01** *see* Pegfilgrastim *on page* 1307
- **SDX-105** *see* Bendamustine *on page* 199
- **SDZ ENA 713** *see* Rivastigmine *on page* 1509
- **Se-100 [OTC]** *see* Selenium *on page* 1547
- **Seasonale®** *see* Ethinyl Estradiol and Levonorgestrel *on page* 656
- **Seasonique®** *see* Ethinyl Estradiol and Levonorgestrel *on page* 656
- **SE Aspartate [OTC]** *see* Selenium *on page* 1547
- **Seb-Prev™** *see* Sulfacetamide (Topical) *on page* 1599

Secobarbital (see koe BAR bi tal)

Brand Names: U.S. Seconal®

Index Terms Quinalbarbitone Sodium; Secobarbital Sodium

Pharmacologic Category Barbiturate

Use Preanesthetic agent; short-term treatment of insomnia

Pregnancy Risk Factor D

Dosage Oral:

Children:

Preoperative sedation: 2-6 mg/kg (maximum dose: 100 mg/dose) 1-2 hours before procedure

Sedation: 6 mg/kg/day divided every 8 hours

Adults:

Hypnotic: Usual: 100 mg/dose at bedtime; range: 100-200 mg/dose

Preoperative sedation: 100-300 mg 1-2 hours before procedure

Additional Information Complete prescribing information for this medication should be consulted for additional detail.

Dosage Forms Excipient information presented when available (limited, particularly for generics); consult specific product labeling.

Capsule, oral, as sodium:

Seconal®: 100 mg

Controlled Substance C-II

- **Secobarbital Sodium** *see* Secobarbital *on page 1543*
- **Seconal®** *see* Secobarbital *on page 1543*
- **Sectral®** *see* Acebutolol *on page 27*
- **Secura® Antifungal Extra Thick [OTC]** *see* Miconazole (Topical) *on page 1126*
- **Secura® Antifungal Greaseless [OTC]** *see* Miconazole (Topical) *on page 1126*
- **Sedapap®** *see* Butalbital and Acetaminophen *on page 255*
- **Selax® (Can)** *see* Docusate *on page 537*
- **Select™ 1/35 (Can)** *see* Ethinyl Estradiol and Norethindrone *on page 660*

Selegiline (se LE ji leen)

Brand Names: U.S. Eldepryl®; Emsam®; Zelapar®

Brand Names: Canada Apo-Selegiline®; Gen-Selegiline; Mylan-Selegiline; Novo-Selegiline; Nu-Selegiline

Index Terms Deprenyl; L-Deprenyl; Selegiline Hydrochloride

Pharmacologic Category Anti-Parkinson's Agent, MAO Type B Inhibitor; Antidepressant, Monoamine Oxidase Inhibitor

Additional Appendix Information

Antidepressant Agents *on page 1874*

Antiparkinsonian Agents *on page 1879*

Use Adjunct in the management of parkinsonian patients in which levodopa/carbidopa therapy is deteriorating (oral products); treatment of major depressive disorder (transdermal product)

Unlabeled Use Early Parkinson's disease; attention-deficit/hyperactivity disorder (ADHD)

Pregnancy Risk Factor C

Pregnancy Considerations Teratogenic and adverse behavioral events were noted in animal studies. There are no adequate and well-controlled studies in pregnant women.

Lactation Excretion in breast milk unknown/use caution

Medication Guide Available Yes

Contraindications Hypersensitivity to selegiline or any component of the formulation; concomitant use of meperidine

Orally disintegrating tablet: Additional contraindications: Concomitant use of dextromethorphan, methadone, propoxyphene, tramadol, oral selegiline, other MAO inhibitors

Transdermal: Additional contraindications: Pheochromocytoma; concomitant use of bupropion, selective or dual serotonin reuptake inhibitors (including SSRIs and SNRIs), tricyclic antidepressants, tramadol, propoxyphene, methadone, dextromethorphan, St. John's wort, mirtazapine, cyclobenzaprine, oral selegiline and other MAO inhibitors; carbamazepine, and oxcarbazepine; elective surgery requiring general anesthesia, local anesthesia containing sympathomimetic vasoconstrictors; sympathomimetics (and related compounds); foods high in tyramine content; supplements containing tyrosine, phenylalanine, tryptophan, or caffeine

Warnings/Precautions

Oral: MAO-B selective inhibition should not pose a problem with tyramine-containing products as long as the typical oral doses are employed, however, rare reactions have been reported. Increased risk of nonselective MAO inhibition occurs with oral capsule/tablet doses >10 mg/day or orally disintegrating tablet doses >2.5 mg/day. Use of oral selegiline with tricyclic antidepressants and SSRIs has also been associated with rare reactions and should generally be avoided. Addition to levodopa therapy may result in exacerbation of levodopa adverse effects, requiring a reduction in levodopa dosage. Dopaminergic agents used for Parkinson's disease or restless legs syndrome have been associated with compulsive behaviors and/or loss of impulse control, which has manifested as pathological gambling, libido increases (hypersexuality), and/or binge eating. Causality has not been established, and controversy exists as to whether this phenomenon is related to the underlying disease, prior behaviors/addictions and/or drug therapy. Dose reduction or discontinuation of therapy has been reported to reverse these behaviors in some, but not all cases. Use caution in patients with hepatic or renal impairment. Incidence of orthostatic hypotension may be increased in older adults and when titrating to the 2.5 mg dosage in patients taking the orally disintegrating tablet. Risk for melanoma development is increased in Parkinson's disease patients; drug causation or factors contributing to risk have not been established. Patients should be monitored closely and periodic skin examinations should be performed. Orally disintegrating tablet may cause oral mucosa edema, irritation, pain, ulceration and/or swallowing pain. Do not use orally disintegrating tablet concurrently with other selegiline products; wait at least 14 days from discontinuation before initiating treatment with another selegiline dosage form. Some products may contain phenylalanine.

Transdermal: Nonselective MAO inhibition occurs with transdermal delivery and is necessary for antidepressant efficacy. Hypertensive crisis as a result of ingesting tyramine-rich foods is always a concern with nonselective MAO inhibition. Although transdermal delivery minimizes inhibition of MAO-A in the gut, there is limited data with higher transdermal doses; dietary modifications are recommended with doses >6 mg/24 hours.

Transdermal patch: May cause orthostatic hypotension; use with caution in patients at risk of this effect or in those who would not tolerate transient hypotensive episodes (cerebrovascular disease, cardiovascular disease, hypovolemia, or concurrent medication use which may predispose to hypotension/bradycardia). Discontinue transdermal product at least 10 days prior to elective surgery. May contain conducting metal (eg, aluminum); remove patch prior to MRI. Avoid exposure of application site and surrounding area to direct external heat sources.

Transdermal: **[U.S. Boxed Warning]: Antidepressants increase the risk of suicidal thinking and behavior in children, adolescents, and young adults (18-24 years of age) with major depressive disorder (MDD) and other psychiatric disorders;** consider risk prior to prescribing. Short-term studies did not show an increased risk in patients >24 years of age and showed a decreased risk in patients ≥65 years. Closely monitor patients for worsening of depression, suicidality and/or associated behaviors, particularly during the initial 1-2 months of therapy or during periods of dosage adjustments (increases or decreases); the patient's family or caregiver should be instructed to closely observe the patient and communicate condition with healthcare provider. A medication guide concerning the use of antidepressants should be dispensed with each prescription. **Transdermal selegiline is not FDA approved for use in children <12 years of age.**

Transdermal: The possibility of a suicide attempt is inherit in major depression and may persist until remission occurs. Patients treated with antidepressants (for any indication) should be observed for clinical worsening and suicidality, especially during the initial few months of a course of drug therapy, or at times of dose changes, either increases or decreases. Use caution in high-risk patients. Worsening depression and severe abrupt suicidality that are not part of the presenting symptoms may require discontinuation or modification of drug therapy. Use caution in high-risk patients during initiation of therapy. The patient's family or caregiver should be alerted to monitor patients for the emergence of suicidality and associated behaviors (such as agitation, irritability, hostility, and hypomania) and call healthcare provider.

Transdermal selegiline may worsen psychosis in some patients or precipitate a shift to mania or hypomania in patients with bipolar disorder. Monotherapy in patients with bipolar disorder should be avoided. Patients presenting with depressive symptoms should be screened for bipolar disorder. **Selegiline is not FDA approved for the treatment of bipolar depression.**

Adverse Reactions Unless otherwise noted, the percentage of adverse events is reported for the transdermal patch (**Note:** ODT = orally disintegrating tablet, Oral = capsule/tablet)

>10%:

Central nervous system: Headache (18%; ODT 7%; oral 4%), insomnia (12%; ODT 7%), dizziness (oral 14%; ODT 11%)

Gastrointestinal: Nausea (oral 20%; ODT 11%)

Local: Application site reaction (24%)

1% to 10%:

Cardiovascular: Hypotension (including postural 3% to 10%), palpitation (oral 2%), chest pain (≥1%; ODT 2%), hypertension (≥1%; ODT 3%), peripheral edema (≥1%)

Central nervous system: Pain (ODT 8%; oral 2%), hallucinations (oral 6%; ODT 4%), confusion (oral 6%; ODT 4%), vivid dreams (oral 4%), ataxia (ODT 3%), somnolence (ODT 3%), lethargy (oral 2%), agitation (≥1%), amnesia (≥1%), paresthesia (≥1%), thinking abnormal (≥1%), depression (<1%; ODT 2%)

Dermatologic: Rash (4%), bruising (≥1%; ODT 2%), pruritus (≥1%), acne (≥1%)

Endocrine & metabolic: Weight loss (5%; oral 2%), hypokalemia (ODT 2%), sexual side effects (≤1%)

Gastrointestinal: Diarrhea (9%; ODT 2%; oral 2%), xerostomia (8%; oral 6%; ODT 4%), stomatitis (ODT 5%), abdominal pain (oral 8%), dyspepsia (4%; ODT 5%), dysphagia (ODT 2%), dental caries (ODT 2%), constipation (≥1%; ODT 4%), flatulence (≥1%; ODT 2%), anorexia (≥1%), gastroenteritis (≥1%), taste perversion (≥1%; ODT 2%), vomiting (≥1%; ODT 3%)

Genitourinary: Urinary retention (oral 2%), dysmenorrhea (≥1%), metrorrhagia (≥1%), UTI (≥1%), urinary frequency (≥1%)

Neuromuscular & skeletal: Dyskinesia (ODT 6%), back pain (ODT 5%; oral 2%), ataxia (<1%; ODT 3%), leg cramps (ODT 3%; oral 2%), myalgia (≥1%; ODT 3%), neck pain (≥1%), tremor (<1%; ODT 3%)

Otic: Tinnitus (≥1%)

Respiratory: Rhinitis (ODT 7%), pharyngitis (3%; ODT 4%), sinusitis (3%), cough (≥1%), bronchitis (≥1%), dyspnea (<1%; ODT 3%)

Miscellaneous: Diaphoresis (≥1%)

Oral and/or transdermal patch: <1% or frequency not defined (limited to important or life-threatening): Abnormal liver function tests, alkaline phosphatase increased, appetite increased, arrhythmia, asthma, ataxia, atrial fibrillation, bacterial infection, behavior/mood changes, bilirubinemia, bradycardia, bradykinesia, breast neoplasm (female), breast pain, chorea, circumoral paresthesia, colitis, dehydration, delusions, depersonalization, depression, emotional lability, epistaxis, eructation, euphoria, face edema, fever, fungal infection, gastritis, generalized spasm, glossitis, heat stroke, hematuria (female), hernia, hostility, hypercholesterolemia, hyperesthesia, hyperglycemia, hyperkinesias, hypertonia, hypoglycemic reaction, hyponatremia, impulsive/compulsive behaviors (eg, pathological gambling, hypersexuality, binge eating), kidney calculus (female), lactate dehydrogenase increased, laryngismus, leukocytosis, leukopenia, libido increased, loss of balance, lymphadenopathy, maculopapular rash, manic reaction, melena, MI, migraine, moniliasis, myasthenia, myoclonus, neoplasia, neurosis, osteoporosis, otitis external, palpitation, paranoid reaction, parasitic infection, parosmia, pelvic pain, periodontal abscess, peripheral vascular disorder, pneumonia, polyuria (female), prostatic hyperplasia, rectal hemorrhage, salivation increased, skin hypertrophy, skin benign neoplasm, suicide attempt, syncope, tachycardia, tenosynovitis, tongue edema, twitching, urinary retention, urinary urgency (male and female), urination impaired (male), urticaria, vaginal hemorrhage, vaginal moniliasis, vaginitis, vasodilatation, vertigo, vesiculobullous rash, viral infection, visual field defect

Drug Interactions

Metabolism/Transport Effects Substrate of CYP1A2 (minor), CYP2A6 (minor), CYP2B6 (major), CYP2C8 (minor), CYP2D6 (minor), CYP3A4 (minor); **Note:** Assignment of Major/Minor substrate status based on clinically relevant drug interaction potential; **Inhibits** CYP1A2 (weak), CYP2A6 (weak), CYP2C19 (weak), CYP2D6 (weak), CYP2E1 (weak), CYP3A4 (weak), Monoamine Oxidase

Avoid Concomitant Use

Avoid concomitant use of Selegiline with any of the following: Alpha-/Beta-Agonists (Indirect-Acting); Alpha1-Agonists; Alpha2-Agonists (Ophthalmic); Amphetamines; Anilidopiperidine Opioids; Antidepressants (Serotonin Reuptake Inhibitor/Antagonist); Atomoxetine; Bezafibrate; Buprenorphine; BuPROPion; BusPIRone; CarBAMazepine; Cyclobenzaprine; Dexmethylphenidate; Dextromethorphan; Diethylpropion; HYDROmorphone; Linezolid; Maprotiline; Meperidine; Methyldopa; Methylene Blue; Methylphenidate; Mirtazapine; OXcarbazepine; Oxymorphone; Pizotifen; Selective Serotonin Reuptake Inhibitors; Serotonin 5-HT1D Receptor Agonists; Serotonin/Norepinephrine Reuptake Inhibitors; Tapentadol; Tetrabenazine; Tetrahydrozoline; Tetrahydrozoline (Nasal); Tricyclic Antidepressants; Tryptophan

Increased Effect/Toxicity

Selegiline may increase the levels/effects of: Alpha-/Beta-Agonists (Direct-Acting); Alpha-/Beta-Agonists (Indirect-Acting); Alpha1-Agonists; Alpha2-Agonists (Ophthalmic); Amphetamines; Antidepressants (Serotonin Reuptake Inhibitor/Antagonist); Antihypertensives; Atomoxetine; Beta2-Agonists; Bezafibrate; BuPROPion; Dexmethylphenidate; Dextromethorphan; Diethylpropion; Doxapram; HYDROmorphone; Linezolid; Lithium; Meperidine; Methadone; Methyldopa; Methylene Blue; Methylphenidate; Metoclopramide; Mirtazapine; Orthostatic Hypotension Producing Agents; Pizotifen; Reserpine; Selective Serotonin Reuptake Inhibitors; Serotonin 5-HT1D Receptor Agonists; Serotonin Modulators; Serotonin/Norepinephrine Reuptake Inhibitors; Tetrahydrozoline; Tetrahydrozoline (Nasal); Tricyclic Antidepressants

The levels/effects of Selegiline may be increased by: Altretamine; Anilidopiperidine Opioids; Antipsychotics; Buprenorphine; BusPIRone; CarBAMazepine; COMT Inhibitors; Conivaptan; Contraceptives (Estrogens); Contraceptives (Progestins); Cyclobenzaprine; CYP2B6 Inhibitors (Moderate); CYP2B6 Inhibitors (Strong); Levodopa; MAO Inhibitors; Maprotiline; OXcarbazepine; Oxymorphone; Quazepam; Tapentadol; Tetrabenazine; TraMADol; Tryptophan

Decreased Effect

Selegiline may decrease the levels/effects of: Ioflupane I 123

The levels/effects of Selegiline may be decreased by: CYP2B6 Inducers (Strong); Cyproterone; Peginterferon Alfa-2b; Tocilizumab

Ethanol/Nutrition/Herb Interactions

Ethanol: Avoid ethanol (based on CNS depressant effects and potential tyramine content)

Food: Concurrent ingestion of foods rich in tyramine may cause sudden and severe high blood pressure (hypertensive crisis). Avoid or limit tyramine-containing foods with MAO-Is (product and/or dose-dependent).

Herb/Nutraceuticals: Avoid valerian, St John's wort, SAMe, kava kava. Avoid supplements containing caffeine, tryptophan, or phenylalanine. Ingestion of large quantities may increase the risk of severe side effects (eg, hypertensive reactions, serotonin syndrome).

Stability

Capsule, tablet, transdermal: Store at 20°C to 25°C (68°F to 77°F). Store patch in sealed pouch and apply immediately after removal.

Orally disintegrating tablet: Store at controlled room temperature 25°C (77°F); excursions permitted to 15°C to 30°C (59°F to 86°F). Use within 3 months of opening pouch and immediately after opening individual blister.

Mechanism of Action Potent, irreversible inhibitor of monoamine oxidase (MAO). Plasma concentrations achieved via administration of oral dosage forms in recommended doses confer selective inhibition of MAO type B, which plays a major role in the metabolism of dopamine; selegiline may also increase dopaminergic activity by interfering with dopamine reuptake at the synapse. When administered transdermally in recommended doses, selegiline achieves higher blood levels and effectively inhibits both MAO-A and MAO-B, which blocks catabolism of other centrally-active biogenic amine neurotransmitters.

Pharmacodynamics/Kinetics

Onset of action: Therapeutic: Oral: Within 1 hour

Duration: Oral: 24-72 hours

Absorption:

- Orally disintegrating tablet: Rapid; greater bioavailability than capsule/tablet
- Transdermal: 25% to 30% (of total selegiline content) over 24 hours

Protein binding: ~90%

Metabolism: Hepatic, primarily via CYP2B6 to active (N-desmethylselegiline, amphetamine, methamphetamine) and inactive metabolites

Half-life elimination: Oral: 10 hours; Transdermal: 18-25 hours

Excretion: Urine (primarily metabolites); feces

Dosage

Capsule/tablet:

- Children and Adolescents: ADHD (unlabeled use): Oral: 5-15 mg/day (Jankovic, 1993)
- Adults: Parkinson's disease: 5 mg twice daily with breakfast and lunch
- Elderly: Parkinson's disease: ≤5 mg/day (when combined with levodopa) is recommended by some clinicians to decrease the enhanced dopaminergic side effects (Olanow, 2001)

Orally disintegrating tablet (Zelapar®): Adults: Parkinson's disease: Initial 1.25 mg daily for at least 6 weeks; may increase to 2.5 mg daily based on clinical response (maximum: 2.5 mg daily)

Transdermal (Emsam®): Depression:

- Adults: Initial: 6 mg/24 hours once daily; may titrate based on clinical response in increments of 3 mg/day every 2 weeks up to a maximum of 12 mg/24 hours
- Elderly: 6 mg/24 hours

Dosage adjustment in renal impairment:

- Oral: Use caution, has not been studied.
- Transdermal: No adjustment required in patients with mild-to-moderate renal impairment.

Dosage adjustment in hepatic impairment:

- Oral: Use caution, has not been studied.
- Transdermal: No adjustment required in patients with mild-to-moderate hepatic impairment.

Dietary Considerations Avoid or limit tyramine-containing foods/beverages (product and/or dose-dependent). Some examples include aged or matured cheese, air-dried or cured meats (including sausages and salamis), fava or broad bean pods, tap/draft beers, Marmite concentrate, sauerkraut, soy sauce and other soybean condiments. Food's freshness is also an important concern; improperly stored or spoiled food can create an environment where tyramine concentrations may increase.

Emsam® 9 mg/24 hours or 12 mg/24 hours: Avoid tyramine-rich foods or beverages beginning the first day of treatment or for 2 weeks after discontinuation or dose reduction to 6 mg/24 hours.

Zelapar®: Do not take with food or liquid.

Some products may contain phenylalanine.

Administration

Oral: Orally disintegrating tablet (Zelapar®): Take in morning before breakfast; place on top of tongue and allow to dissolve. Avoid food or liquid 5 minutes before and after administration.

Topical: Transdermal (Emsam®): Apply to clean, dry, intact skin to the upper torso (below the neck and above the waist), upper thigh, or outer surface of the upper arm. Avoid exposure of application site to external heat source, which may increase the amount of drug absorbed. Apply at the same time each day and rotate application sites. Wash hands with soap and water after handling. Avoid touching the sticky side of the patch.

Monitoring Parameters Blood pressure; symptoms of parkinsonism; general mood and behavior (increased anxiety, presence of mania or agitation); suicidal ideation (especially at the beginning of therapy or when doses are increased or decreased)

Test Interactions May interfere with urine detection of amphetamine/methamphetamine (false-positive).

Additional Information When adding selegiline to levodopa/carbidopa, the dose of the latter can usually be decreased.

Dosage Forms Excipient information presented when available (limited, particularly for generics); consult specific product labeling.
Capsule, oral, as hydrochloride: 5 mg
Eldepryl®: 5 mg
Patch, transdermal:
Emsam®: 6 mg/24 hours (30s) [20 cm^2, total selegiline 20 mg]
Emsam®: 9 mg/24 hours (30s) [30 cm^2, total selegiline 30 mg]
Emsam®: 12 mg/24 hours (30s) [40 cm^2, total selegiline 40 mg]
Tablet, oral, as hydrochloride: 5 mg
Tablet, orally disintegrating, oral, as hydrochloride:
Zelapar®: 1.25 mg [contains phenylalanine 1.25 mg/tablet; grapefruit flavor]

◆ **Selegiline Hydrochloride** *see* Selegiline *on page 1544*
◆ **Selenicaps** *see* Selenium *on page 1547*
◆ **Selenimin** *see* Selenium *on page 1547*

Selenium (se LEE nee um)

Brand Names: U.S. SE Aspartate [OTC]; Se-100 [OTC]; Selenicaps; Selenimin
Pharmacologic Category Trace Element, Parenteral
Use Trace metal supplement
Pregnancy Risk Factor C
Dosage I.V. in TPN solutions:
Children: 3 mcg/kg/day
Adults:
Metabolically stable: 20-40 mcg/day
Deficiency from prolonged TPN support: 100 mcg/day for 24 and 31 days
Additional Information Complete prescribing information for this medication should be consulted for additional detail.
Dosage Forms Excipient information presented when available (limited, particularly for generics); consult specific product labeling.
Capsule, oral: 200 mcg
Se-100: 100 mcg
Selenicaps: 200 mcg [gluten free, sugar free]
Injection, solution: 40 mcg/mL (10 mL)
Tablet, oral: 50 mcg, 100 mcg, 200 mcg
SE Aspartate: 50 mcg
Selenimin: 50 mcg [contains calcium 115 mg/tablet]
Selenimin: 125 mcg, 200 mcg [gluten free, sugar free]
Tablet, timed release, oral: 200 mcg

Selenium Sulfide (se LEE nee um SUL fide)

Brand Names: U.S. Dandrex; Head & Shoulders® Clinical Strength [OTC]; Selseb® [DSC]; Selsun blue® 2-in-1 [OTC]; Selsun blue® Medicated [OTC]; Selsun blue® Moisturizing [OTC]; Selsun blue® Normal to Oily [OTC]; Tersi
Brand Names: Canada Versel®
Pharmacologic Category Topical Skin Product
Use Treatment of itching and flaking of the scalp associated with dandruff, to control scalp seborrheic dermatitis; treatment of tinea versicolor
Pregnancy Risk Factor C
Dosage Topical: Adults:
Dandruff, seborrhea: Massage 5-10 mL of shampoo into wet scalp, leave on scalp 2-3 minutes, rinse thoroughly. Usually 2 applications each week for 2 weeks will provide control. After this, may repeat at less frequent intervals (eg, once weekly, every 2-4 weeks). Rub foam into affected skin twice daily.
Tinea versicolor: Apply the 2.5% lotion to affected area and lather with small amounts of water; leave on skin for 10 minutes, then rinse thoroughly; apply every day for 7 days; rub foam into affected skin twice daily
Additional Information Complete prescribing information for this medication should be consulted for additional detail.
Dosage Forms Excipient information presented when available (limited, particularly for generics); consult specific product labeling. [DSC] = Discontinued product
Aerosol, foam, topical:
Tersi: 2.25% (70 g)
Lotion, topical: 2.5% (120 mL)
Shampoo, topical: 1% (210 mL)
Dandrex: 1% (236 mL)
Head & Shoulders® Clinical Strength: 1% (420 mL)
Selseb®: 2.25% (180 mL [DSC])
Selsun blue® Medicated: 1% (120 mL, 207 mL, 325 mL) [contains menthol]
Selsun blue® Moisturizing: 1% (207 mL, 325 mL) [contains aloe, moisturizers]
Selsun blue® Normal to Oily: 1% (207 mL, 325 mL)
Shampoo, topical [with conditioner]:
Selsun blue® 2-in-1: 1% (207 mL, 325 mL)

◆ **Selfemra® [DSC]** *see* FLUoxetine *on page 731*
◆ **Selseb® [DSC]** *see* Selenium Sulfide *on page 1547*
◆ **Selsun blue® 2-in-1 [OTC]** *see* Selenium Sulfide *on page 1547*
◆ **Selsun blue® Medicated [OTC]** *see* Selenium Sulfide *on page 1547*
◆ **Selsun blue® Moisturizing [OTC]** *see* Selenium Sulfide *on page 1547*
◆ **Selsun blue® Normal to Oily [OTC]** *see* Selenium Sulfide *on page 1547*
◆ **Selzentry®** *see* Maraviroc *on page 1052*
◆ **Semprex®-D** *see* Acrivastine and Pseudoephedrine *on page 39*
◆ **Senexon-S [OTC]** *see* Docusate and Senna *on page 538*
◆ **Senna and Docusate** *see* Docusate and Senna *on page 538*
◆ **Senna Plus [OTC]** *see* Docusate and Senna *on page 538*
◆ **Senna-S** *see* Docusate and Senna *on page 538*
◆ **Senokot-S® [OTC]** *see* Docusate and Senna *on page 538*
◆ **SenoSol™-SS [OTC]** *see* Docusate and Senna *on page 538*
◆ **Sensipar®** *see* Cinacalcet *on page 360*
◆ **Sensorcaine®** *see* Bupivacaine *on page 242*
◆ **Sensorcaine®-MPF** *see* Bupivacaine *on page 242*
◆ **Sensorcaine®-MPF Spinal** *see* Bupivacaine *on page 242*
◆ **Sepasoothe® [OTC]** *see* Benzocaine *on page 202*
◆ **Septa-Amlodipine (Can)** *see* AmLODIPine *on page 97*
◆ **Septa-Atenolol (Can)** *see* Atenolol *on page 161*
◆ **Septa-Citalopram (Can)** *see* Citalopram *on page 370*
◆ **Septra® [DSC]** *see* Sulfamethoxazole and Trimethoprim *on page 1602*
◆ **Septra® DS** *see* Sulfamethoxazole and Trimethoprim *on page 1602*
◆ **Septra® Injection (Can)** *see* Sulfamethoxazole and Trimethoprim *on page 1602*
◆ **Serax** *see* Oxazepam *on page 1261*

- **Serevent® Diskhaler® Disk (Can)** *see* Salmeterol *on page 1532*
- **Serevent® Diskus®** *see* Salmeterol *on page 1532*
- **Serophene®** *see* ClomiPHENE *on page 387*
- **SEROquel®** *see* QUEtiapine *on page 1440*
- **Seroquel® (Can)** *see* QUEtiapine *on page 1440*
- **SEROquel XR®** *see* QUEtiapine *on page 1440*
- **Seroquel XR® (Can)** *see* QUEtiapine *on page 1440*
- **Serostim®** *see* Somatropin *on page 1579*

Sertaconazole (ser ta KOE na zole)

Brand Names: U.S. Ertaczo®

Index Terms Sertaconazole Nitrate

Pharmacologic Category Antifungal Agent, Topical

Use Topical treatment of tinea pedis (athlete's foot)

Pregnancy Risk Factor C

Dosage Topical: Children ≥12 years and Adults: Apply between toes and to surrounding healthy skin twice daily for 4 weeks

Additional Information Complete prescribing information for this medication should be consulted for additional detail.

Dosage Forms Excipient information presented when available (limited, particularly for generics); consult specific product labeling.

Cream, topical, as nitrate:

Ertaczo®: 2% (30 g, 60 g)

- **Sertaconazole Nitrate** *see* Sertaconazole *on page 1548*

Sertraline (SER tra leen)

Brand Names: U.S. Zoloft®

Brand Names: Canada Apo-Sertraline®; CO Sertraline; Dom-Sertraline; GD-Sertraline; Mylan-Sertraline; Nu-Sertraline; PHL-Sertraline; PMS-Sertraline; ratio-Sertraline; Riva-Sertraline; Sandoz-Sertraline; Teva-Sertraline; Zoloft®

Index Terms Sertraline Hydrochloride

Pharmacologic Category Antidepressant, Selective Serotonin Reuptake Inhibitor

Additional Appendix Information

Antidepressant Agents *on page 1874*

Selective Serotonin Reuptake Inhibitors (SSRIs) Pharmacokinetics *on page 1897*

Use Treatment of major depression; obsessive-compulsive disorder (OCD); panic disorder; post-traumatic stress disorder (PTSD); premenstrual dysphoric disorder (PMDD); social anxiety disorder

Unlabeled Use Eating disorders; generalized anxiety disorder (GAD); impulse control disorders; treatment of mild dementia-associated agitation in nonpsychotic patients

Pregnancy Risk Factor C

Pregnancy Considerations Due to adverse effects observed in animal studies, sertraline is classified as pregnancy category C. Sertraline crosses the human placenta. Nonteratogenic effects in the newborn following SSRI exposure late in the third trimester include respiratory distress, cyanosis, apnea, seizures, temperature instability, feeding difficulty, vomiting, hypoglycemia, hypo- or hypertonia, hyper-reflexia, jitteriness, irritability, constant crying, and tremor. An increased risk of low birth weight, lower Apgar scores, and blunted behavioral response to pain for a prolonged period after delivery has also been reported. Exposure to SSRIs after the twentieth week of gestation has been associated with persistent pulmonary hypertension of the newborn (PPHN). Adverse effects may be due to toxic effects of the SSRI or drug discontinuation. The long-term effects of *in utero* SSRI exposure on infant development and behavior are not known.

Due to pregnancy-induced physiologic changes, women who are pregnant may require increased doses of sertraline to achieve euthymia. Women treated for major depression and who are euthymic prior to pregnancy are more likely to experience a relapse when medication is discontinued as compared to pregnant women who continue taking antidepressant medications. The ACOG recommends that therapy with SSRIs or SNRIs during pregnancy be individualized; treatment of depression during pregnancy should incorporate the clinical expertise of the mental health clinician, obstetrician, primary healthcare provider, and pediatrician. If treatment during pregnancy is required, consider tapering therapy during the third trimester in order to prevent withdrawal symptoms in the infant. If this is done and the woman is considered to be at risk of relapse from her major depressive disorder, the medication can be restarted following delivery, although the dose should be readjusted to that required before pregnancy. Treatment algorithms have been developed by the ACOG and the APA for the management of depression in women prior to conception and during pregnancy (Yonkers, 2009).

Lactation Enters breast milk/use caution (AAP rates "of concern"; AAP 2001 update pending)

Medication Guide Available Yes

Contraindications Hypersensitivity to sertraline or any component of the formulation; use of MAO inhibitors within 14 days; concurrent use of pimozide; concurrent use of sertraline oral concentrate with disulfiram

Warnings/Precautions [U.S. Boxed Warning]: Antidepressants increase the risk of suicidal thinking and behavior in children, adolescents, and young adults (18-24 years of age) with major depressive disorder (MDD) and other psychiatric disorders; consider risk prior to prescribing. Short-term studies did not show an increased risk in patients >24 years of age and showed a decreased risk in patients ≥65 years. Closely monitor patients for clinical worsening, suicidality, or unusual changes in behavior, particularly during the initial 1-2 months of therapy or during periods of dosage adjustments (increases or decreases); the patient's family or caregiver should be instructed to closely observe the patient and communicate condition with healthcare provider. A medication guide concerning the use of antidepressants should be dispensed with each prescription. **Sertraline is not FDA approved for use in children with major depressive disorder (MDD). However, it is approved for the treatment of obsessive-compulsive disorder (OCD) in children ≥6 years of age.**

The possibility of a suicide attempt is inherent in major depression and may persist until remission occurs. Use caution in high-risk patients. Worsening depression and severe abrupt suicidality that are not part of the presenting symptoms may require discontinuation or modification of drug therapy. The patient's family or caregiver should be alerted to monitor patients for the emergence of suicidality and associated behaviors (such as agitation, irritability, hostility, impulsivity, and hypomania) and call healthcare provider.

May worsen psychosis in some patients or precipitate a shift to mania or hypomania in patients with bipolar disorder. Patients presenting with depressive symptoms should be screened for bipolar disorder. Monotherapy in patients with bipolar disorder should be avoided. **Sertraline is not FDA approved for the treatment of bipolar depression.**

Serotonin syndrome and neuroleptic malignant syndrome (NMS)-like reactions have occurred with serotonin/norepinephrine reuptake inhibitors (SNRIs) and selective serotonin reuptake inhibitors (SSRIs) when used alone, and particularly when used in combination with serotonergic agents (eg, triptans) or antidopaminergic agents (eg, antipsychotics). Concurrent use with MAO inhibitors is contraindicated. Has a very low potential to impair cognitive or motor performance. However, caution patients regarding activities requiring alertness until response to sertraline is known. Does not appear to potentiate the effects of alcohol, however, ethanol use is not advised.

Use caution in patients with a previous seizure disorder or condition predisposing to seizures such as brain damage, alcoholism, or concurrent therapy with other drugs which lower the seizure threshold. May increase the risks associated with electroconvulsive therapy. Use with caution in patients with hepatic or renal dysfunction and in elderly patients. May cause hyponatremia/SIADH (elderly at increased risk); volume depletion (diuretics may increase risk). Use with caution in patients with renal insufficiency or other concurrent illness (due to limited experience). Sertraline acts as a mild uricosuric; use with caution in patients at risk of uric acid nephropathy. Use caution with concomitant use of NSAIDs, ASA, or other drugs that affect coagulation; the risk of bleeding may be potentiated. Use with caution in patients where weight loss is undesirable. May cause or exacerbate sexual dysfunction.

Use oral concentrate formulation with caution in patients with latex sensitivity; dropper dispenser contains dry natural rubber. Monitor growth in pediatric patients. Discontinuation symptoms (eg, dysphoric mood, irritability, agitation, confusion, anxiety, insomnia, hypomania) may occur upon abrupt discontinuation. Taper dose when discontinuing therapy.

Adverse Reactions

>10%:

Central nervous system: Dizziness, fatigue, headache, insomnia, somnolence

Endocrine & metabolic: Libido decreased

Gastrointestinal: Anorexia, diarrhea, nausea, xerostomia

Genitourinary: Ejaculatory disturbances

Neuromuscular & skeletal: Tremors

Miscellaneous: Diaphoresis

1% to 10%:

Cardiovascular: Chest pain, palpitation

Central nervous system: Agitation, anxiety, hypoesthesia, malaise, nervousness, pain

Dermatologic: Rash

Endocrine & metabolic: Impotence

Gastrointestinal: Appetite increased, constipation, dyspepsia, flatulence, vomiting, weight gain

Neuromuscular & skeletal: Back pain, hypertonia, myalgia, paresthesia, weakness

Ocular: Visual difficulty, abnormal vision

Otic: Tinnitus

Respiratory: Rhinitis

Miscellaneous: Yawning

<1% (Limited to important or life-threatening): Abdominal pain, acute renal failure, agranulocytosis, allergic reaction, anaphylactoid reaction, angioedema, aplastic anemia, atrial arrhythmia, AV block, bilirubin increased, blindness, bradycardia, cataract, dystonia, extrapyramidal symptoms, galactorrhea, gum hyperplasia, gynecomastia, hallucinations, hepatic failure, hepatitis, hepatomegaly, hyperglycemia, hyperprolactinemia, hypothyroidism, jaundice, leukopenia, lupus-like syndrome, micturition disorders, neuroleptic malignant syndrome, oculogyric crisis, serotonin syndrome, SIADH, Stevens-Johnson syndrome (and other severe dermatologic reactions), optic neuritis, pancreatitis (rare), photosensitivity, priapism, psychosis, PT/INR increased, pulmonary hypertension, QT_c prolongation, serum sickness, thrombocytopenia, torsade de pointes, transaminases increased, vasculitis, ventricular tachycardia

Additional adverse reactions reported in pediatric patients (frequency >2%): Aggressiveness, epistaxis, hyperkinesia, purpura, sinusitis, urinary incontinence

Drug Interactions

Metabolism/Transport Effects **Substrate** of CYP2B6 (minor), CYP2C19 (minor), CYP2C9 (minor), CYP2D6 (major), CYP3A4 (minor); **Note:** Assignment of Major/Minor substrate status based on clinically relevant drug interaction potential; **Inhibits** CYP1A2 (weak), CYP2B6 (moderate), CYP2C19 (moderate), CYP2C8 (weak), CYP2C9 (weak), CYP2D6 (moderate), CYP3A4 (moderate)

Avoid Concomitant Use

Avoid concomitant use of Sertraline with any of the following: Clopidogrel; Disulfiram; Iobenguane I 123; MAO Inhibitors; Methylene Blue; Pimozide; Tolvaptan; Tryptophan

Increased Effect/Toxicity

Sertraline may increase the levels/effects of: Alpha-/Beta-Blockers; Anticoagulants; Antidepressants (Serotonin Reuptake Inhibitor/Antagonist); Antiplatelet Agents; Aspirin; Beta-Blockers; Budesonide (Systemic, Oral Inhalation); BusPIRone; CarBAMazepine; CloZAPine; Colchicine; Collagenase (Systemic); CYP2B6 Substrates; CYP2C19 Substrates; CYP2D6 Substrates; CYP3A4 Substrates; Desmopressin; Dextromethorphan; Drotrecogin Alfa (Activated); Eplerenone; Everolimus; Fesoterodine; Fosphenytoin; Galantamine; Halofantrine; Ibritumomab; Lithium; Methadone; Methylene Blue; Metoclopramide; NSAID (COX-2 Inhibitor); NSAID (Nonselective); Phenytoin; Pimecrolimus; Pimozide; Ranolazine; RisperiDONE; Rivaroxaban; Salicylates; Salmeterol; Saxagliptin; Serotonin Modulators; Tamoxifen; Thrombolytic Agents; Tolvaptan; Tositumomab and Iodine I 131 Tositumomab; TraMADol; Tricyclic Antidepressants; Vitamin K Antagonists

The levels/effects of Sertraline may be increased by: Abiraterone Acetate; Alcohol (Ethyl); Analgesics (Opioid); Antipsychotics; BusPIRone; Cimetidine; CNS Depressants; Conivaptan; CYP2D6 Inhibitors (Moderate); CYP2D6 Inhibitors (Strong); Dasatinib; Disulfiram; Glucosamine; Herbs (Anticoagulant/Antiplatelet Properties); Linezolid; Macrolide Antibiotics; MAO Inhibitors; Metoclopramide; Omega-3-Acid Ethyl Esters; Pentosan Polysulfate Sodium; Pentoxifylline; Prostacyclin Analogues; TraMADol; Tryptophan; Vitamin E

Decreased Effect

Sertraline may decrease the levels/effects of: Clopidogrel; Iobenguane I 123; Ioflupane I 123

The levels/effects of Sertraline may be decreased by: CarBAMazepine; Cyproheptadine; Darunavir; Efavirenz; Fosphenytoin; NSAID (Nonselective); Peginterferon Alfa-2b; Phenytoin; Tocilizumab

Ethanol/Nutrition/Herb Interactions

Ethanol: May increase CNS depression; monitor for increased effects with coadministration. Caution patients about effects.

Food: Sertraline average peak serum levels may be increased if taken with food.

Herb/Nutraceutical: Avoid valerian, St John's wort, kava kava, gotu kola (may increase CNS depression).

Stability Tablets and oral solution should be stored at controlled room temperature of 15°C to 30°C (59°F to 86°F).

Mechanism of Action Antidepressant with selective inhibitory effects on presynaptic serotonin (5-HT) reuptake and only very weak effects on norepinephrine and dopamine neuronal uptake. *In vitro* studies demonstrate no significant affinity for adrenergic, cholinergic, GABA, dopaminergic, histaminergic, serotonergic, or benzodiazepine receptors.

Pharmacodynamics/Kinetics

Onset of action: Depression: The onset of action is within a week, however, individual response varies greatly and full response may not be seen until 8-12 weeks after initiation of treatment.

Absorption: Slow

Protein binding: 98%

Metabolism: Hepatic; may involve CYP2C19 and CYP2D6; extensive first pass metabolism; forms metabolite N-desmethylsertraline

Bioavailability: Bioavailability of tablets and solution are equivalent

Half-life elimination: Sertraline: 26 hours; N-desmethylsertraline: 66 hours (range: 62-104 hours)

Time to peak, plasma: Sertraline: 4.5-8.4 hours

Excretion: Urine and feces

Dosage Oral:

Children and Adolescents: Obsessive-compulsive disorder:

6-12 years: Initial: 25 mg once daily

13-17 years: Initial: 50 mg once daily

Note: May increase daily dose, at intervals of not less than 1 week, to a maximum of 200 mg/day. If somnolence is noted, give at bedtime.

Adults:

Depression/obsessive-compulsive disorder: Oral: Initial: 50 mg/day (see **"Note"** above)

Panic disorder, post-traumatic stress disorder, social anxiety disorder: Initial: 25 mg once daily; increase to 50 mg once daily after 1 week; maximum dose: 200 mg/day

Premenstrual dysphoric disorder: 50 mg/day either daily throughout menstrual cycle **or** limited to the luteal phase of menstrual cycle, depending on physician assessment. Patients not responding to 50 mg/day may benefit from dose increases (50 mg increments per menstrual cycle) up to 150 mg/day when dosing throughout menstrual cycle **or** up to 100 mg day when dosing during luteal phase only. If a 100 mg/day dose has been established with luteal phase dosing, a 50 mg/day titration step for 3 days should be utilized at the beginning of each luteal phase dosing period.

Elderly: Depression/obsessive-compulsive disorder: Start treatment with 25 mg/day in the morning and increase by 25 mg/day increments every 2-3 days if tolerated to 50-100 mg/day; additional increases may be necessary; maximum dose: 200 mg/day. **Note:** Patients with Alzheimer's dementia-related depression may require a lower starting dosage of 12.5 mg/day, with titration intervals of 1-2 weeks, up to 150-200 mg/day maximum.

Dosage adjustment/comment in renal impairment: Multiple-dose pharmacokinetics are unaffected by renal impairment.

Hemodialysis: Not removed by hemodialysis

Dosage adjustment/comment in hepatic impairment: Sertraline is extensively metabolized by the liver; caution should be used in patients with hepatic impairment; a lower dose or less frequent dosing should be used.

Administration Oral concentrate: Must be diluted before use. Immediately before administration, use the dropper provided to measure the required amount of concentrate; mix with 4 ounces (1/2 cup) of water, ginger ale, lemon/lime soda, lemonade, or orange juice **only**. Do not mix with any other liquids than these. The dose should be taken immediately after mixing; do not mix in advance. A slight haze may appear after mixing; this is normal. **Note:** Use with caution in patients with latex sensitivity; dropper dispenser contains dry natural rubber.

Monitoring Parameters Monitor nutritional intake and weight; mental status for depression, suicide ideation (especially at the beginning of therapy or when doses are increased or decreased), anxiety, social functioning, mania, panic attacks; akathisia; growth in pediatric patients

Test Interactions Increased (minor) serum triglycerides, LFTs; decreased serum uric acid; may interfere with urine detection of benzodiazepines (false-positive)

Additional Information Buspirone (15-60 mg/day) may be useful in treatment of sexual dysfunction during treatment with a selective serotonin reuptake inhibitor. May exacerbate tics in Tourette's syndrome.

Dosage Forms Excipient information presented when available (limited, particularly for generics); consult specific product labeling.

Solution, oral [concentrate]: 20 mg/mL (60 mL)

Zoloft®: 20 mg/mL (60 mL) [contains ethanol 12%, menthol, natural rubber/natural latex in packaging]

Tablet, oral: 25 mg, 50 mg, 100 mg

Zoloft®: 25 mg, 50 mg, 100 mg [scored]

- **Sertraline Hydrochloride** *see* Sertraline *on page 1548*
- **Serzone** *see* Nefazodone *on page 1184*

Sevelamer (se VEL a mer)

Brand Names: U.S. Renagel®; Renvela®

Brand Names: Canada Renagel®

Index Terms Sevelamer Carbonate; Sevelamer Hydrochloride

Pharmacologic Category Phosphate Binder

Use Reduction or control of serum phosphorous in patients with chronic kidney disease on hemodialysis

Pregnancy Risk Factor C

Pregnancy Considerations Animal studies have shown reduced or irregular ossification of fetal bones. Because sevelamer may cause a reduction in the absorption of some vitamins, it should be used with caution in pregnant women.

Lactation Excretion in breast milk unknown/use caution (not absorbed systemically but may alter maternal nutrition)

Contraindications Bowel obstruction

Warnings/Precautions Use with caution in patients with gastrointestinal disorders including dysphagia, swallowing disorders, severe gastrointestinal motility disorders (including constipation), or major gastrointestinal surgery. May cause reductions in vitamin D, E, K, or folic acid absorption. May bind to some drugs in the gastrointestinal tract and decrease their absorption; when changes in absorption of oral medications may have significant clinical consequences (such as antiarrhythmic and antiseizure medications), these medications should be taken at least 1 hour before or 3 hours after a dose of sevelamer. Tablets should not be taken apart or chewed; broken or crushed tablets will rapidly expand in water/saliva and may be a choking hazard.

Adverse Reactions

>10%: Gastrointestinal: Vomiting (22%), nausea (20%), diarrhea (19%), dyspepsia (16%)

1% to 10%:

Endocrine & metabolic: Hypercalcemia (5% to 7%)

Gastrointestinal: Abdominal pain (9%), flatulence (8%), constipation (8%)

Miscellaneous: Peritonitis (peritoneal dialysis: 8%)

Postmarketing and/or case reports: Fecal impaction, ileus (rare), intestinal obstruction (rare), intestinal perforation (rare), pruritus, rash

Drug Interactions

Metabolism/Transport Effects None known.

Avoid Concomitant Use There are no known interactions where it is recommended to avoid concomitant use.

Increased Effect/Toxicity There are no known significant interactions involving an increase in effect.

Decreased Effect

Sevelamer may decrease the levels/effects of: Calcitriol; Levothyroxine; Mycophenolate; Quinolone Antibiotics

Stability Store at controlled room temperature of 25°C (77°F); excursions permitted to 15°C to 30°C (59°F to 86°F). Protect from moisture.

Mechanism of Action Sevelamer (a polymeric compound) binds phosphate within the intestinal lumen, limiting absorption and decreasing serum phosphate concentrations without altering calcium, aluminum, or bicarbonate concentrations.

Pharmacodynamics/Kinetics

Absorption: Not systemically absorbed

Excretion: Feces

Dosage Oral: **Note:** The dosing of sevelamer carbonate and sevelamer hydrochloride are similar; when switching from one product to another, the same dose (on a mg per mg basis) should be utilized.

Children (unlabeled use): In a pilot study of 17 pediatric patients aged 11.8 ± 3.7 years on hemodialysis (n=3) or peritoneal dialysis (n=14), initial doses of 121 ± 50 mg/kg/day (4.5 ± 5 g/day) were used. Doses were adjusted based on the serum phosphorus with final doses of 163 ± 46 mg/kg (6.7 ± 2.4 g/day) without any adverse effects (Mahdavi, 2003). In a study of 18 patients aged 0.9-18 years with chronic kidney disease, a mean dose of 140 ± 86 mg/kg/day (5.38 ± 3.24 g/day) resulted in good phosphorus control with minimal adverse effects. Initial doses were based on prior phosphate-binder dose and were adjusted based on the serum phosphorus (Pieper, 2006).

Adults: Patients not taking a phosphate binder: 800-1600 mg 3 times/day with meals; the initial dose may be based on serum phosphorous levels:

>5.5 mg/dL to <7.5 mg/dL: 800 mg 3 times/day

≥7.5 mg/dL to <9.0 mg/dL: 1200-1600 mg 3 times/day

≥9.0 mg/dL: 1600 mg 3 times/day

Maintenance dose adjustment based on serum phosphorous concentration (goal range of 3.5-5.5 mg/dL; maximum dose studied was equivalent to 13 g/day [sevelamer hydrochloride] or 14 g/day [sevelamer carbonate]):

>5.5 mg/dL: Increase by 400-800 mg per meal at 2-week intervals

3.5-5.5 mg/dL: Maintain current dose

<3.5 mg/dL: Decrease by 400-800 mg per meal

Dosage adjustment when switching between phosphate-binder products: 667 mg of calcium acetate is equivalent to ~800 mg sevelamer (carbonate or hydrochloride)

Conversion based on dose per meal:

Calcium acetate 667 mg: Convert to 800 mg Renagel® / Renvela®

Calcium acetate 1334 mg: Convert to 1600 mg Renagel® 800 mg/ Renvela® **or** 1200 mg Renagel® 400 mg

Calcium acetate 2001 mg: Convert to 2400 mg Renagel® 800 mg / Renvela® **or** 2000 mg Renagel® 400 mg

Dietary Considerations Take with meals. Reduced levels of folic acid, and vitamins D, E, and K may occur; most hemodialysis patients in clinical trials received vitamin supplementation.

Administration Must be administered with meals.

Powder for oral suspension: Mix powder with water prior to administration. The 0.8 g packet should be mixed with 30 mL of water and the 2.4 g packet should be mixed with 60 mL of water (multiple packets may be mixed together using the appropriate amount of water). Stir vigorously to suspend mixture just prior to drinking; powder does not dissolve. Drink within 30 minutes of preparing and resuspend just prior to drinking.

Tablets: Swallow whole; do not crush, chew, or break

Monitoring Parameters

Serum chemistries, including bicarbonate and chloride

Serum calcium and phosphorus: Frequency of measurement may be dependent upon the presence and magnitude of abnormalities, the rate of progression of CKD, and the use of treatments for CKD-mineral and bone disorders (KDIGO, 2009):

CKD stage 3: Every 6-12 months

CKD stage 4: Every 3-6 months

CKD stage 5 and 5D: Every 1-3 months

Periodic 24-hour urinary calcium and phosphorus; magnesium; alkaline phosphatase every 12 months or more frequently in the presence of elevated PTH; creatinine, BUN, albumin; intact parathyroid hormone (iPTH) every 3-12 months depending on CKD severity

Reference Range

Corrected total serum calcium (K/DOQI, 2003): CKD stages 3 and 4: 8.4-10.2 mg/dL (2.1-2.6 mmol/L); CKD stage 5: 8.4-9.5 mg/dL (2.1-2.37 mmol/L); KDIGO guidelines recommend maintaining normal ranges for all stages of CKD (3-5D) (KDIGO, 2009)

Phosphorus (K/DOQI, 2003):

CKD stages 3 and 4: 2.7-4.6 mg/dL (0.87-1.48 mmol/L) (adults); maintain within age-appropriate limits (children)

CKD stage 5 (including those treated with dialysis): 3.5-5.5 mg/dL (1.13-1.78 mmol/L) (children >12 years and adults); 4-6 mg/dL (1.29-1.94 mmol/L) (children 1-12 years)

KDIGO guidelines recommend maintaining normal ranges for CKD stages 3-5 and lowering elevated phosphorus levels toward the normal range for CKD stage 5D (KDIGO, 2009)

Serum calcium-phosphorus product (K/DOQI, 2003): CKD stage 3-5: <55 mg^2/dL^2 (children >12 years and adults); <65 mg2/dL2 (children ≤12 years)

PTH: Whole molecule, immunochemiluminometric assay (ICMA): 1.0-5.2 pmol/L; whole molecule, radioimmunoassay (RIA): 10.0-65.0 pg/mL; whole molecule, immunoradiometric, double antibody (IRMA): 1.0-6.0 pmol/L

Target ranges by stage of chronic kidney disease (KDIGO, 2009): CKD stage 3-5: Optimal iPTH is unknown; maintain normal range (assay-dependent); CKD stage 5D: Maintain iPTH within 2-9 times the upper limit of normal for the assay used

Dosage Forms Excipient information presented when available (limited, particularly for generics); consult specific product labeling.

Powder for suspension, oral, as carbonate:

Renvela®: 0.8 g/packet (90s); 2.4 g/packet (90s) [contains propylene glycol; citrus-cream flavor]

Tablet, oral, as carbonate:

Renvela®: 800 mg

Tablet, oral, as hydrochloride:

Renagel®: 400 mg, 800 mg

◆ **Sevelamer Carbonate** *see* Sevelamer *on page 1550*

◆ **Sevelamer Hydrochloride** *see* Sevelamer *on page 1550*

◆ **sfRowasa™** *see* Mesalamine *on page 1081*

◆ **SGN-35** *see* Brentuximab Vedotin *on page 234*

◆ **Shingles Vaccine** *see* Zoster Vaccine *on page 1830*

◆ **Shohl's Solution (Modified)** *see* Sodium Citrate and Citric Acid *on page 1570*

◆ **Sig-Enalapril (Can)** *see* Enalapril *on page 584*

◆ **Silace [OTC]** *see* Docusate *on page 537*

◆ **Siladryl Allergy [OTC]** *see* DiphenhydrAMINE (Systemic) *on page 516*

◆ **Silafed [OTC]** *see* Triprolidine and Pseudoephedrine *on page 1741*

- **Silapap Children's [OTC]** *see* Acetaminophen *on page 27*
- **Silapap Infant's [OTC]** *see* Acetaminophen *on page 27*
- **Sildec PE [DSC]** *see* Chlorpheniramine and Phenylephrine *on page 345*
- **Sildec PE-DM [DSC]** *see* Chlorpheniramine, Phenylephrine, and Dextromethorphan *on page 346*

Sildenafil (sil DEN a fil)

Brand Names: U.S. Revatio®; Viagra®

Brand Names: Canada ratio-Sildenafil R; Revatio®; Viagra®

Index Terms Sildenafil Citrate; UK92480

Pharmacologic Category Phosphodiesterase-5 Enzyme Inhibitor

Use

Revatio®: Treatment of pulmonary arterial hypertension (PAH) (WHO Group I) to improve exercise ability and delay clinical worsening

Viagra®: Treatment of erectile dysfunction (ED)

Unlabeled Use PAH in children; pulmonary hypertension (WHO Group II, III, and IV); persistent pulmonary hypertension after recent left ventricular assist device placement

Pregnancy Risk Factor B

Pregnancy Considerations Teratogenic effects were not observed in animal studies. There are no adequate and well-controlled studies in pregnant women. Less than 0.001% appears in the semen.

Lactation Excretion in breast milk unknown/use caution

Contraindications Hypersensitivity to sildenafil or any component of the formulation; concurrent use (regularly/intermittently) of organic nitrates in any form (eg, nitroglycerin, isosorbide dinitrate); concurrent use with a protease inhibitor regimen when sildenafil used for pulmonary artery hypertension (eg, Revatio®)

Warnings/Precautions Decreases in blood pressure may occur due to vasodilator effects; use with caution in patients with left ventricular outflow obstruction (aortic stenosis or hypertrophic obstructive cardiomyopathy); may be more sensitive to hypotensive actions. Concurrent use with alpha-adrenergic antagonist therapy or substantial ethanol consumption may cause symptomatic hypotension; patients should be hemodynamically stable prior to initiating therapy at the lowest possible dose. Use with caution in patients with hypotension (<90/50 mm Hg); uncontrolled hypertension (>170/110 mm Hg); life-threatening arrhythmias, stroke or MI within the last 6 months; cardiac failure or coronary artery disease causing unstable angina; safety and efficacy have not been studied in these patients. There is a degree of cardiac risk associated with sexual activity; therefore, physicians should consider the cardiovascular status of their patients prior to initiating any treatment for erectile dysfunction. If pulmonary edema occurs when treating pulmonary arterial hypertension (PAH), consider the possibility of pulmonary veno-occlusive disease (PVOD); continued use is not recommended in patient with PVOD.

Sildenafil should be used with caution in patients with anatomical deformation of the penis (angulation, cavernosal fibrosis, or Peyronie's disease) and in patients who have conditions which may predispose them to priapism (sickle cell anemia, multiple myeloma, leukemia). All patients should be instructed to seek medical attention if erection persists >4 hours.

Vision loss may occur rarely and be a sign of nonarteritic anterior ischemic optic neuropathy (NAION). Risk may be increased with history of vision loss. Other risk factors for NAION include low cup-to-disc ratio ("crowded disc"), coronary artery disease, diabetes, hypertension, hyperlipidemia, smoking, and age >50 years. May cause dose-related impairment of color discrimination. Use caution in patients with retinitis pigmentosa; a minority have genetic disorders of retinal phosphodiesterases (no safety information available). Sudden decrease or loss of hearing has been reported rarely; hearing changes may be accompanied by tinnitus and dizziness. A direct relationship between therapy and vision or hearing loss has not been determined.

The potential underlying causes of erectile dysfunction should be evaluated prior to treatment. The safety and efficacy of sildenafil with other treatments for erectile dysfunction have not been established; use is not recommended. Efficacy with concurrent bosentan therapy has not been evaluated; use with caution. Use with caution in patients taking strong CYP3A4 inhibitors or alpha-blockers. Concomitant use with all forms of nitrates is contraindicated. If nitrate administration is medically necessary, it is not known when nitrates can be safely administered following the use of sildenafil (per manufacturer); the ACC/AHA 2007 guidelines supports administration of nitrates only if 24 hours have elapsed.

Avoid abrupt discontinuation, especially if used as monotherapy in PAH as exacerbation may occur. Use caution in patients with bleeding disorders or with active peptic ulcer disease; safety and efficacy have not been established. Efficacy has not be established for treatment of pulmonary hypertension associated with sickle cell disease. Use with caution in the elderly, or patients with renal or hepatic dysfunction; dose adjustment may be needed.

Adverse Reactions Based upon normal doses for either indication or route. (Adverse effects such as flushing, diarrhea, myalgia, and visual disturbances may be increased with doses >100 mg/24 hours.)

>10%:

Central nervous system: Headache (16% to 46%)

Gastrointestinal: Dyspepsia (7% to 17%; dose related)

2% to 10%:

Cardiovascular: Flushing (10%)

Central nervous system: Insomnia (≤7%), pyrexia (6%), dizziness (2%)

Dermatologic: Erythema (6%), rash (2%)

Gastrointestinal: Diarrhea (3% to 9%), gastritis (≤3%)

Genitourinary: Urinary tract infection (3%)

Hepatic: LFTs increased

Neuromuscular & skeletal: Myalgia (≤7%), paresthesia (≤3%)

Ocular: Abnormal vision (color changes, blurred vision, or increased sensitivity to light 3% to 11%; dose related)

Respiratory: Epistaxis (9% to 13%), dyspnea exacerbated (≤7%), nasal congestion (4%), rhinitis (4%), sinusitis (3%)

<2% (Limited to important or life-threatening): Allergic reaction, amnesia (transient global), anemia, angina pectoris, anorgasmia, asthma, AV block, cardiac arrest, cardiomyopathy, cataract, cerebral thrombosis, cerebrovascular hemorrhage, colitis, cystitis, depression, dysphagia, edema, exfoliative dermatitis, eye hemorrhage, gout, hearing decreased, hearing loss, heart failure, hematuria, hemorrhage, hyper-/hypoglycemia, hypernatremia, hyper-/hypotension, hyperuricemia, intracerebral hemorrhage, intraocular pressure increased, leukopenia, migraine, myocardial ischemia, MI, myasthenia, mydriasis, neuralgia, nonarteritic ischemic optic neuropathy (NAION), palpitation, postural hypotension, priapism, pulmonary hemorrhage, rectal hemorrhage, retinal vascular disease or bleeding, seizure, shock, sickle cell crisis (vaso-occlusive crisis in patients with pulmonary hypertension associated with sickle cell disease), stomatitis, subarachnoid hemorrhage, syncope, tachycardia, tendon rupture, TIA, urinary incontinence, ventricular arrhythmia,

vertigo, visual field loss, vitreous detachment/traction, vomiting

Drug Interactions

Metabolism/Transport Effects Substrate of CYP1A2 (minor), CYP2C19 (minor), CYP2C9 (minor), CYP2D6 (minor), CYP2E1 (minor), CYP3A4 (major); **Note:** Assignment of Major/Minor substrate status based on clinically relevant drug interaction potential; **Inhibits** CYP2C9 (weak), CYP3A4 (weak)

Avoid Concomitant Use

Avoid concomitant use of Sildenafil with any of the following: Amyl Nitrite; Boceprevir; Phosphodiesterase 5 Inhibitors; Pimozide; Telaprevir; Vasodilators (Organic Nitrates)

Increased Effect/Toxicity

Sildenafil may increase the levels/effects of: Alpha1-Blockers; Amyl Nitrite; Antihypertensives; Bosentan; HMG-CoA Reductase Inhibitors; Phosphodiesterase 5 Inhibitors; Pimozide; Vasodilators (Organic Nitrates)

The levels/effects of Sildenafil may be increased by: Antifungal Agents (Azole Derivatives, Systemic); Boceprevir; CYP3A4 Inhibitors (Moderate); CYP3A4 Inhibitors (Strong); Dasatinib; Erythromycin; Protease Inhibitors; Sapropterin; Telaprevir

Decreased Effect

The levels/effects of Sildenafil may be decreased by: Bosentan; CYP3A4 Inducers (Strong); Cyproterone; Deferasirox; Etravirine; Herbs (CYP3A4 Inducers); Peginterferon Alfa-2b; Tocilizumab

Ethanol/Nutrition/Herb Interactions

Food: Amount and rate of absorption of sildenafil is reduced when taken with a high-fat meal. Serum concentrations/toxicity may be increased with grapefruit juice; avoid concurrent use.

Herb/Nutraceutical: St John's wort may decrease sildenafil levels.

Stability Store at controlled room temperature of 25°C (77°F); excursions permitted to 15°C to 30°C (59°F to 86°F).

Mechanism of Action

Erectile dysfunction: Does not directly cause penile erections, but affects the response to sexual stimulation. The physiologic mechanism of erection of the penis involves release of nitric oxide (NO) in the corpus cavernosum during sexual stimulation. NO then activates the enzyme guanylate cyclase, which results in increased levels of cyclic guanosine monophosphate (cGMP), producing smooth muscle relaxation and inflow of blood to the corpus cavernosum. Sildenafil enhances the effect of NO by inhibiting phosphodiesterase type 5 (PDE-5), which is responsible for degradation of cGMP in the corpus cavernosum; when sexual stimulation causes local release of NO, inhibition of PDE-5 by sildenafil causes increased levels of cGMP in the corpus cavernosum, resulting in smooth muscle relaxation and inflow of blood to the corpus cavernosum; at recommended doses, it has no effect in the absence of sexual stimulation.

Pulmonary arterial hypertension (PAH): Inhibits phosphodiesterase type 5 (PDE-5) in smooth muscle of pulmonary vasculature where PDE-5 is responsible for the degradation of cyclic guanosine monophosphate (cGMP). Increased cGMP concentration results in pulmonary vasculature relaxation; vasodilation in the pulmonary bed and the systemic circulation (to a lesser degree) may occur.

Pharmacodynamics/Kinetics

Onset of action: ~60 minutes

Duration: 2-4 hours

Absorption: Rapid; slower with a high-fat meal

Distribution: V_{dss}: 105 L

Protein binding, plasma: ~96%

Metabolism: Hepatic via CYP3A4 (major) and CYP2C9 (minor route); forms N-desmethyl metabolite (active)

Bioavailability: 40% (25% to 63%)

Half-life elimination: ~4 hours; the elderly and those with severe renal impairment have reduced clearance of sildenafil and its active N-desmethyl metabolite

Time to peak: 30-120 minutes; delayed by 60 minutes with a high-fat meal

Excretion: Feces (~80%); urine (~13%)

Dosage

I.V.: Adults: Pulmonary arterial hypertension (PAH) (Revatio®): 10 mg 3 times/day

Oral:

Children ≥1 month: PAH (unlabeled use): 0.25-2 mg/kg/dose every 4-6 hours. Most reports used 0.5 mg/kg/dose and titrated up to 2 mg/kg/dose

Adults:

Erectile dysfunction (Viagra®): Usual dose: 50 mg once daily 1 hour (range: 30 minutes to 4 hours) before sexual activity; dosing range: 25-100 mg once daily

PAH (Revatio®): 20 mg 3 times/day, taken 4-6 hours apart

Note: A delay in clinical worsening was observed in a short-term trial in which most patients achieved a target dose of 80 mg 3 times daily (unlabeled dose). The patients had an incremental dosage escalation while on a stable epoprostenol regimen (Simonneau, 2008).

Elderly >65 years: Use with caution

Revatio®: Refer to adult dosing.

Viagra®: Starting dose of 25 mg should be considered.

Dosage considerations for patients stable on alpha-blockers: Viagra®: Initial 25 mg

Dosage adjustment for concomitant use of potent CYP34A inhibitors:

Revatio®:

Erythromycin: No dosage adjustment

Itraconazole, ketoconazole: Not recommended

Viagra®:

Erythromycin, itraconazole, ketoconazole: Starting dose of 25 mg should be considered

Protease inhibitors: Maximum sildenafil dose: 25 mg every 48 hours

Dosage adjustment in renal impairment:

Revatio®: Dose adjustment not necessary

Viagra®: Cl_{cr} <30 mL/minute: Starting dose of 25 mg should be considered

Dosage adjustment in hepatic impairment:

Revatio®: Child-Pugh class A and B: Dose adjustment not necessary; not studied in severe impairment (Child-Pugh class C)

Viagra®: Child-Pugh class A and B: Starting dose of 25 mg should be considered; not studied in severe impairment (Child-Pugh class C)

Dietary Considerations Avoid grapefruit juice.

Administration

Revatio®: Administer tablets without regard to meals at least 4-6 hours apart. Administer injection as an I.V. bolus.

Viagra®: Administer orally 30 minutes to 4 hours before sexual activity

Additional Information Sildenafil is ~10 times more selective for PDE-5 as compared to PDE6. This enzyme is found in the retina and is involved in phototransduction. At higher plasma levels, interference with PDE6 is believed to be the basis for changes in color vision noted in some patients.

Dosage Forms Excipient information presented when available (limited, particularly for generics); consult specific product labeling.
Injection, solution:
Revatio®: 0.8 mg/mL (12.5 mL)
Tablet, oral:
Revatio®: 20 mg
Viagra®: 25 mg, 50 mg, 100 mg

Extemporaneous Preparations A 2.5 mg/mL sildenafil citrate oral suspension may be made with tablets and either a 1:1 mixture of methylcellulose 1% and simple syrup NF or a 1:1 mixture of Ora-Sweet® and Ora-Plus®. Crush thirty sildenafil 25 mg tablets (Viagra®) in a mortar and reduce to a fine powder. Add small portions of chosen vehicle and mix to a uniform paste; mix while adding vehicle in incremental proportions to **almost** 300 mL; transfer to a graduated cylinder, rinse mortar with vehicle, and add quantity of vehicle sufficient to make 300 mL. Store in amber plastic bottles and label "shake well". Stable for 90 days at room temperature or refrigerated.

Nahata MC, Morosco RS, and Brady MT, "Extemporaneous Sildenafil Citrate Oral Suspensions for the Treatment of Pulmonary Hypertension in Children," *Am J Health-Syst Pharm*, 2006, 63(3):254-7.

◆ **Sildenafil Citrate** *see* Sildenafil *on page 1552*

◆ **Silenor®** *see* Doxepin (Systemic) *on page 550*

◆ **Silexin [OTC]** *see* Guaifenesin and Dextromethorphan *on page 810*

◆ **Silfedrine Children's [OTC]** *see* Pseudoephedrine *on page 1430*

Silodosin (SI lo doe sin)

Brand Names: U.S. Rapaflo®
Index Terms KMD 3213
Pharmacologic Category Alpha$_1$ Blocker
Use Treatment of signs and symptoms of benign prostatic hyperplasia (BPH)
Pregnancy Risk Factor B
Dosage Oral: Adults: BPH: 8 mg once daily with a meal
Dosage adjustment in renal impairment:
Cl_{cr} >50 mL/minute: No adjustment needed
Cl_{cr} 30-50 mL/minute: 4 mg once daily
Cl_{cr} <30 mL/minute: Use is contraindicated
Dosage adjustment in hepatic impairment:
Mild-to-moderate impairment (Child-Pugh classes A and B): No adjustment needed
Severe impairment (Child-Pugh class C): Use is contraindicated
Additional Information Complete prescribing information for this medication should be consulted for additional detail.
Dosage Forms Excipient information presented when available (limited, particularly for generics); consult specific product labeling.
Capsule, oral:
Rapaflo®: 4 mg, 8 mg

◆ **Silphen [OTC]** *see* DiphenhydrAMINE (Systemic) *on page 516*

◆ **Siltussin DM [OTC]** *see* Guaifenesin and Dextromethorphan *on page 810*

◆ **Siltussin DM DAS [OTC]** *see* Guaifenesin and Dextromethorphan *on page 810*

◆ **Siltussin SA [OTC]** *see* GuaiFENesin *on page 809*

◆ **Silvadene®** *see* Silver Sulfadiazine *on page 1554*

Silver Nitrate (SIL ver NYE trate)

Index Terms $AgNO_3$
Pharmacologic Category Antibiotic, Topical; Cauterizing Agent, Topical; Topical Skin Product, Antibacterial
Use Cauterization of wounds and sluggish ulcers, removal of granulation tissue and warts; aseptic prophylaxis of burns
Pregnancy Risk Factor C
Dosage Children and Adults:
Sticks: Apply to mucous membranes and other moist skin surfaces only on area to be treated 2-3 times/week for 2-3 weeks
Topical solution: Apply a cotton applicator dipped in solution on the affected area 2-3 times/week for 2-3 weeks
Additional Information Complete prescribing information for this medication should be consulted for additional detail.
Dosage Forms Excipient information presented when available (limited, particularly for generics); consult specific product labeling.
Applicator sticks, topical: Silver nitrate 75% and potassium nitrate 25% (6", 12", 18")
Solution, topical: 0.5% (960 mL); 10% (30 mL); 25% (30 mL); 50% (30 mL)

Silver Sulfadiazine (SIL ver sul fa DYE a zeen)

Brand Names: U.S. Silvadene®; SSD AF®; SSD®; Thermazene®
Brand Names: Canada Flamazine®
Pharmacologic Category Antibiotic, Topical
Use Prevention and treatment of infection in second and third degree burns
Pregnancy Risk Factor B
Dosage Children and Adults: Topical: Apply once or twice daily with a sterile-gloved hand; apply to a thickness of 1/16"; burned area should be covered with cream at all times
Additional Information Complete prescribing information for this medication should be consulted for additional detail.
Dosage Forms Excipient information presented when available (limited, particularly for generics); consult specific product labeling.
Cream, topical: 1% (20 g, 25 g, 50 g, 85 g, 400 g)
Silvadene®: 1% (20 g, 50 g, 85 g, 400 g, 1000 g)
SSD AF®: 1% (50 g, 400 g)
SSD®: 1% (25 g, 50 g, 85 g, 400 g)
Thermazene®: 1% (20 g, 50 g, 85 g, 400 g, 1000 g)

◆ **Simethicone, Aluminum Hydroxide, and Magnesium Hydroxide** *see* Aluminum Hydroxide, Magnesium Hydroxide, and Simethicone *on page 80*

◆ **Simethicone and Loperamide Hydrochloride** *see* Loperamide and Simethicone *on page 1027*

◆ **Simethicone and Magaldrate** *see* Magaldrate and Simethicone *on page 1043*

◆ **Simply Saline® [OTC]** *see* Sodium Chloride *on page 1567*

◆ **Simply Saline® Baby [OTC]** *see* Sodium Chloride *on page 1567*

◆ **Simply Saline® Nasal Moist® [OTC]** *see* Sodium Chloride *on page 1567*

◆ **Simply Sleep® [OTC]** *see* DiphenhydrAMINE (Systemic) *on page 516*

◆ **Simply Sleep® (Can)** *see* DiphenhydrAMINE (Systemic) *on page 516*

◆ **Simponi®** *see* Golimumab *on page 803*

◆ **Simuc-DM [DSC]** *see* Guaifenesin and Dextromethorphan *on page 810*

◆ **Simulect®** *see* Basiliximab *on page 190*

Simvastatin (sim va STAT in)

Brand Names: U.S. Zocor®

Brand Names: Canada Apo-Simvastatin®; CO Simvastatin; Dom-Simvastatin; JAMP-Simvastatin; Mylan-Simvastatin; Nu-Simvastatin; PHL-Simvastatin; PMS-Simvastatin; RAN™-Simvastatin; ratio-Simvastatin; Riva-Simvastatin; Sandoz-Simvastatin; Taro-Simvastatin; Teva-Simvastatin; Zocor®; ZYM-Simvastatin

Pharmacologic Category Antilipemic Agent, HMG-CoA Reductase Inhibitor

Additional Appendix Information

Hyperlipidemia Management *on page 1996*

Use Used with dietary therapy for the following:

Secondary prevention of cardiovascular events in hypercholesterolemic patients with established coronary heart disease (CHD) or at high risk for CHD: To reduce cardiovascular morbidity (myocardial infarction, coronary/noncoronary revascularization procedures) and mortality; to reduce the risk of stroke

Hyperlipidemias: To reduce elevations in total cholesterol (total-C), LDL-C, apolipoprotein B, triglycerides, and VLDL-C, and to increase HDL-C in patients with primary hypercholesterolemia (elevations of 1 or more components are present in Fredrickson type IIa, IIb, III, and IV hyperlipidemias); treatment of homozygous familial hypercholesterolemia

Heterozygous familial hypercholesterolemia (HeFH): In adolescent patients (10-17 years of age, females >1 year postmenarche) with HeFH having LDL-C ≥190 mg/dL **or** LDL-C ≥160 mg/dL with positive family history of premature cardiovascular disease (CVD), or 2 or more CVD risk factors in the adolescent patient

Pregnancy Risk Factor X

Pregnancy Considerations Cholesterol biosynthesis may be important in fetal development. Contraindicated in pregnancy. Administer to women of childbearing potential only when conception is highly unlikely and patients have been informed of potential hazards. If pregnancy occurs during treatment, discontinue simvastatin immediately.

Lactation Excretion in breast milk unknown/contraindicated

Contraindications Hypersensitivity to simvastatin or any component of the formulation; active liver disease; unexplained persistent elevations of serum transaminases; pregnancy; breast-feeding; concomitant use of strong CYP3A4 inhibitors (eg, clarithromycin, erythromycin, HIV protease inhibitors, itraconazole, ketoconazole, nefazodone, posaconazole, telithromycin), cyclosporine, danazol, and gemfibrozil

Warnings/Precautions Secondary causes of hyperlipidemia should be ruled out prior to therapy. Liver function must be monitored by laboratory assessment. Rhabdomyolysis with acute renal failure has occurred. Risk is dose-related and is increased with high doses (80 mg), concurrent use of lipid-lowering agents which may cause rhabdomyolysis (gemfibrozil, other fibric acid derivatives, or niacin at doses ≥1 g/day) or moderate-to-strong CYP3A4 inhibitors (including amiodarone, cyclosporine, grapefruit juice in large quantities, or verapamil), age ≥65 years, female gender, uncontrolled hypothyroidism, and renal dysfunction. If concurrent use of a contraindicated interacting medication is unavoidable, treatment with simvastatin should be suspended during use or consider the use of an alternative HMG-CoA reductase inhibitor void of CYP3A4 metabolism. Monitor closely if used with other drugs associated with myopathy (eg, colchicine). Weigh the risk versus benefit when combining any of these drugs with simvastatin. The manufacturer recommends temporary discontinuation for elective major surgery, acute medical or surgical conditions, or in any patient experiencing an acute or serious condition predisposing to renal failure (eg, sepsis, hypotension, trauma, uncontrolled seizures). However, based upon current evidence, HMG-CoA reductase inhibitor therapy should be continued in the perioperative period unless risk outweighs cardioprotective benefit. Use with caution in patients who consume large amounts of ethanol or have a history of liver disease. Use with caution in patients with severe renal impairment; initial dosage adjustment is necessary; monitor closely. Use is contraindicated with active liver disease and with unexplained transaminase elevations. Concomitant use of high-dose simvastatin (80 mg) and niacin ≥1 g/day may increase risk of myopathy in Chinese patients.

Adverse Reactions

1% to 10%:

Cardiovascular: Atrial fibrillation (6%; placebo 5%), edema (3%; placebo 2%)

Central nervous system: Headache (3% to 7%), vertigo (5%)

Dermatologic: Eczema (5%)

Gastrointestinal: Abdominal pain (7%), constipation (2% to 7%), gastritis (5%), nausea (5%)

Hepatic: Transaminases increased (>3 x ULN; 1%)

Neuromuscular & skeletal: CPK increased (>3 x normal; 5%), myalgia (4%)

Respiratory: Upper respiratory infections (9%), bronchitis (7%)

<1% (Limited to important or life-threatening): Alkaline phosphatase increased, alopecia, anaphylaxis, anemia, angioedema, arthralgia, arthritis, chills, depression, dermatomyositis, diarrhea, dizziness, dryness of skin/mucous membranes, dyspepsia, dyspnea, eosinophilia, erythema multiforme, ESR increased, fever, flatulence, flushing, GGT increased, hemolytic anemia, hepatic failure, hepatitis, hypersensitivity reaction, jaundice, leukopenia, malaise, memory loss, muscle cramps, nail changes, nodules, pancreatitis, paresthesia, peripheral neuropathy, photosensitivity, polymyalgia rheumatica, positive ANA, pruritus, purpura, rash, rhabdomyolysis, skin discoloration, Stevens-Johnson syndrome, systemic lupus erythematosus-like syndrome, thrombocytopenia, toxic epidermal necrolysis, urticaria, vasculitis, vomiting, weakness

Additional class-related events or case reports (not necessarily reported with simvastatin therapy): Alteration in taste, anorexia, anxiety, bilirubin increased, cataracts, cholestatic jaundice, cirrhosis, decreased libido, depression, erectile dysfunction/impotence, facial paresis, fatty liver, fulminant hepatic necrosis, gynecomastia, hepatoma, hyperbilirubinemia, impaired extraocular muscle movement, increased CPK (>10 x normal), interstitial lung disease, ophthalmoplegia, peripheral nerve palsy, psychic disturbance, renal failure (secondary to rhabdomyolysis), thyroid dysfunction, tremor, vertigo

Drug Interactions

Metabolism/Transport Effects **Substrate** of CYP3A4 (major), SLCO1B1; **Note:** Assignment of Major/Minor substrate status based on clinically relevant drug interaction potential; **Inhibits** CYP2C8 (weak), CYP2C9 (weak), CYP2D6 (weak)

Avoid Concomitant Use

Avoid concomitant use of Simvastatin with any of the following: Boceprevir; CYP3A4 Inhibitors (Strong); Erythromycin; Gemfibrozil; Protease Inhibitors; Red Yeast Rice; Telaprevir

Increased Effect/Toxicity

Simvastatin may increase the levels/effects of: DAPTOmycin; Diltiazem; Trabectedin; Vitamin K Antagonists

The levels/effects of Simvastatin may be increased by: Amiodarone; AmLODIPine; Antifungal Agents (Azole Derivatives, Systemic); Boceprevir; Colchicine; CycloSPORINE; CycloSPORINE (Systemic); CYP3A4 Inhibitors (Moderate); CYP3A4 Inhibitors (Strong); Cyproterone; Danazol; Dasatinib; Diltiazem; Dronedarone; Eltrombopag; Erythromycin; Fenofibrate; Fenofibric Acid; Fluconazole; Fusidic Acid; Gemfibrozil; Grapefruit Juice; Green Tea; Imatinib; Macrolide Antibiotics; Niacin; Niacinamide; Protease Inhibitors; QuiNINE; Ranolazine; Red Yeast Rice; Sildenafil; Telaprevir; Ticagrelor; Verapamil

Decreased Effect

Simvastatin may decrease the levels/effects of: Lanthanum

The levels/effects of Simvastatin may be decreased by: Antacids; Bosentan; CYP3A4 Inducers (Strong); Deferasirox; Efavirenz; Etravirine; Fosphenytoin; Phenytoin; Rifamycin Derivatives; St Johns Wort; Tocilizumab

Ethanol/Nutrition/Herb Interactions

Ethanol: Avoid excessive ethanol consumption (due to potential hepatic effects).

Food: Simvastatin serum concentration may be increased when taken with grapefruit juice; avoid concurrent intake of large quantities (>1 quart/day). Red yeast rice contains an estimated 2.4 mg lovastatin per 600 mg rice.

Herb/Nutraceutical: St John's wort may decrease simvastatin levels.

Stability Tablets should be stored in tightly-closed containers at temperatures between 5°C to 30°C (41°F to 86°F).

Mechanism of Action Simvastatin is a methylated derivative of lovastatin that acts by competitively inhibiting 3-hydroxy-3-methylglutaryl-coenzyme A (HMG-CoA) reductase, the enzyme that catalyzes the rate-limiting step in cholesterol biosynthesis

Pharmacodynamics/Kinetics

Onset of action: >3 days

Peak effect: 2 weeks

Absorption: 85%

Protein binding: ~95%

Metabolism: Hepatic via CYP3A4; extensive first-pass effect

Bioavailability: <5%

Half-life elimination: Unknown

Time to peak: 1.3-2.4 hours

Excretion: Feces (60%); urine (13%)

Dosage Oral: **Note:** Doses should be individualized according to the baseline LDL-cholesterol levels, the recommended goal of therapy, and the patient's response; adjustments should be made at intervals of 4 weeks or more; doses may need adjusted based on concomitant medications

Children 10-17 years (females >1 year postmenarche): HeFH: 10 mg once daily in the evening; range: 10-40 mg/day (maximum: 40 mg/day)

Dosage adjustment for simvastatin with concomitant amiodarone, amlodipine, diltiazem, ranolazine, or verapamil: Refer to drug-specific dosing in adult dosing section

Adults:

Note: Dosing limitation: Simvastatin 80 mg is limited to patients that have been taking this dose for >12 consecutive months without evidence of myopathy and are not currently taking or beginning to take a simvastatin dose-limiting or contraindicated interacting medication. If patient is unable to achieve low-density lipoprotein cholesterol (LDL-C) goal using the 40 mg dose of simvastatin, increasing to 80 mg dose is not recommended. Instead, switch patient to an alternative LDL-C-lowering treatment providing greater LDL-C reduction.

Homozygous familial hypercholesterolemia: 40 mg once daily in the evening

Prevention of cardiovascular events, hyperlipidemias: 10-20 mg once daily in the evening; range: 5-40 mg/day

Patients requiring only moderate reduction of LDL-C may be started at 5-10 mg once daily in the evening; adjust to achieve recommended LDL-C goal

Patients requiring reduction of >40% of LDL-C may be started at 40 mg once daily in the evening; adjust to achieve recommended LDL-C goal

Patients with CHD or at high risk for cardiovascular events (patients with diabetes, PVD, history of stroke or other cerebrovascular disease): Dosing should be started at 40 mg once daily in the evening; start simultaneously with diet therapy.

Dosage adjustment with concomitant medications: Note: Patients currently tolerating and requiring a dose of simvastatin 80 mg who require initiation of an interacting drug with a dose cap for simvastatin should be switched to an alternative statin with less potential for drug-drug interaction.

Amiodarone, amlodipine, or ranolazine: Simvastatin dose should **not** exceed 20 mg/day

Diltiazem or verapamil: Simvastatin dose should **not** exceed 10 mg/day

Dosage adjustment in Chinese patients on niacin doses ≥1 g/day: Use caution with simvastatin doses exceeding 20 mg/day; because of an increased risk of myopathy, do not administer simvastatin 80 mg concurrently.

Dosing adjustment in renal impairment:

Manufacturer's recommendations:

Mild-to-moderate renal impairment: No dosage adjustment necessary; simvastatin does not undergo significant renal excretion

Severe renal impairment: Cl_{cr} <30 mL/minute: Initial: 5 mg/day with close monitoring

Alternative recommendation: No dosage adjustment necessary for any degree of renal impairment (Aronoff, 2007)

Dietary Considerations May be taken without regard to meals. Red yeast rice contains an estimated 2.4 mg lovastatin per 600 mg rice.

Administration May be administered without regard to meals. Administer in the evening for maximal efficacy.

Monitoring Parameters Serum cholesterol (total and fractionated); baseline CPK (recheck CPK in any patient with symptoms suggestive of myopathy)

Obtain liver function tests prior to initiation and thereafter when clinically indicated. Patients with elevated transaminase levels should have a second (confirmatory) test and frequent monitoring until values normalize. Discontinue if increase in ALT/AST is persistently >3 times ULN. Monitor LDL-C at intervals no less than 4 weeks.

Dosage Forms Excipient information presented when available (limited, particularly for generics); consult specific product labeling.

Tablet, oral: 5 mg, 10 mg, 20 mg, 40 mg, 80 mg

Zocor®: 5 mg, 10 mg, 20 mg, 40 mg, 80 mg

◆ **Simvastatin and Ezetimibe** *see* Ezetimibe and Simvastatin *on page* 681

◆ **Simvastatin and Sitagliptin** *see* Sitagliptin and Simvastatin *on page* 1562

◆ **Sina-12X® [DSC]** *see* Guaifenesin and Phenylephrine *on page* 812

◆ **Sinemet®** *see* Carbidopa and Levodopa *on page* 284

◆ **Sinemet® CR** *see* Carbidopa and Levodopa *on page* 284

◆ **Sinequan® (Can)** *see* Doxepin (Systemic) *on page* 550

- **Singulair®** *see* Montelukast *on page 1152*
- **Sinutab® Non Drowsy (Can)** *see* Acetaminophen and Pseudoephedrine *on page 31*

Sipuleucel-T (si pu LOO sel tee)

Brand Names: U.S. Provenge®

Index Terms APC8015; Prostate Cancer Vaccine, Cell-Based

Pharmacologic Category Cellular Immunotherapy, Autologous

Use Treatment of metastatic hormone-refractory prostate cancer in patients who are asymptomatic or minimally symptomatic

Prescribing and Access Restrictions Patients may currently receive Sipuleucel-T at one of the ~50 sites that participated in the clinical trials until the program is expanded to additional sites. Physicians must go through an inservice and register to prescribe the treatment; patients must also complete an enrollment form. Information on registration and enrollment is available at 1-877-336-3736.

Dosage Note: Premedicate with oral acetaminophen 650 mg and an antihistamine (eg, diphenhydramine 50 mg) ~30 minutes prior to infusion. For autologous use only.

I.V.: Adults: Prostate cancer, metastatic: Each dose contains ≥50 million autologous CD54+ cells (obtained through leukapheresis) activated with PAP-GM-CSF; administer doses at ~2 week intervals for a total of 3 doses

Dosage adjustment for toxicity: Acute infusion reaction: Interrupt or slow infusion rate (depending on the severity of infusion reaction); may require acetaminophen, I.V. H_1 and/or H_2 antagonists, or low-dose meperidine to manage acute symptoms.

Additional Information Complete prescribing information for this medication should be consulted for additional detail.

Dosage Forms Excipient information presented when available (limited, particularly for generics); consult specific product labeling.

Infusion, premixed in LR [preservative free]:

Provenge®: ≥50 million autologous $CD54^+$ cells activated with PAP-GM-CSF (250 mL)

- **Sirdalud®** *see* TiZANidine *on page 1695*

Sirolimus (sir OH li mus)

Brand Names: U.S. Rapamune®

Brand Names: Canada Rapamune®

Index Terms Rapamycin

Pharmacologic Category Immunosuppressant Agent; mTOR Kinase Inhibitor

Use Prophylaxis of organ rejection in patients receiving renal transplants

Unlabeled Use Prophylaxis of organ rejection in heart transplant recipients; prevention acute graft-versus-host disease (GVHD) in allogeneic stem cell transplantation; treatment of refractory acute or chronic GVHD; treatment of soft tissue sarcoma (chordoma, angiomyolipoma, or lymphangioleiomyomatosis)

Pregnancy Risk Factor C

Pregnancy Considerations Animal studies have demonstrated embryotoxicity and fetotoxicity, as evidenced by increased mortality, reduced fetal weights and delayed ossification. There are no adequate and well-controlled studies in pregnant women. Effective contraception must be initiated before therapy with sirolimus and continued for 12 weeks after discontinuation.

The National Transplantation Pregnancy Registry (NTPR, Temple University) is a registry for pregnant women taking immunosuppressants following any solid organ transplant. The NTPR encourages reporting of all immunosuppressant exposures during pregnancy in transplant recipients at 877-955-6877.

Lactation Excretion in breast milk unknown/not recommended

Medication Guide Available Yes

Contraindications Hypersensitivity to sirolimus or any component of the formulation

Warnings/Precautions Hazardous agent - use appropriate precautions for handling and disposal. **[U.S. Boxed Warning]: Immunosuppressive agents, including sirolimus, increase the risk of infection and may be associated with the development of lymphoma.** Immune suppression may also increase the risk of opportunistic infections (including activation of latent viral infections including BK virus-associated nephropathy), fatal infections, and sepsis. Prophylactic treatment for *Pneumocystis jirovecii* pneumonia (PCP) should be administered for 1 year post-transplant; prophylaxis for cytomegalovirus (CMV) should be taken for 3 months post-transplant in patients at risk for CMV. Progressive multifocal leukoencephalopathy (PML), an opportunistic CNS infection caused by reactivation of the JC virus, has been reported in patients receiving immunosuppressive therapy, including sirolimus. Clinical findings of PML include apathy, ataxia, cognitive deficiency, confusion, and hemiparesis; promptly evaluate any patient presenting with neurological changes; consider decreasing the degree of immunosuppression with consideration to the risk of organ rejection in transplant patients.

[U.S. Boxed Warning]: Sirolimus is not recommended for use in liver or lung transplantation. Bronchial anastomotic dehiscence cases have been reported in lung transplant patients when sirolimus was used as part of an immunosuppressive regimen; most of these reactions were fatal. Studies indicate an association with an increase risk of hepatic artery thrombosis (HAT), graft failure, and increased mortality (with evidence of infection) in liver transplant patients when sirolimus is used in combination with cyclosporine and/or tacrolimus. Most cases of HAT occurred within 30 days of transplant.

In renal transplant patients, *de novo* use without cyclosporine has been associated with higher rates of acute rejection. Sirolimus should be used in combination with cyclosporine (and corticosteroids) initially. Cyclosporine may be withdrawn in low-to-moderate immunologic risk patients after 2-4 months, in conjunction with an increase in sirolimus dosage. In high immunologic risk patients, use in combination with cyclosporine and corticosteroids is recommended for the first year. Safety and efficacy of combination therapy with cyclosporine in high immunologic risk patients has not been studied beyond 12 months of treatment; adjustment of immunosuppressive therapy beyond 12 months should be considered based on clinical judgement. Monitor renal function closely when combined with cyclosporine; consider dosage adjustment or discontinue in patients with increasing serum creatinine.

May increase serum creatinine and decrease GFR. Use caution when used concurrently with medications which may alter renal function. May delay recovery of renal function in patients with delayed allograft function. Increased urinary protein excretion has been observed when converting renal transplant patients from calcineurin inhibitors to sirolimus during maintenance therapy. A higher level of proteinuria prior to sirolimus conversion correlates with a higher degree of proteinuria after conversion. In some patients, proteinuria may reach nephrotic levels; nephrotic syndrome (new onset) has been reported. Increased risk of BK viral-associated nephropathy which may impair renal function and cause graft loss; consider decreasing immunosuppressive burden if evidence of deteriorating renal function.

Use caution with hepatic impairment; a reduction in the maintenance dose is recommended. Has been associated with an increased risk of fluid accumulation and lymphocele; peripheral edema, lymphedema, ascites, and pleural and pericardial effusions (including significant effusions and tamponade) were reported; use with caution in patients in whom fluid accumulation may be poorly tolerated, such as in cardiovascular disease (heart failure or hypertension) and pulmonary disease. Cases of interstitial lung disease (eg, pneumonitis, bronchiolitis obliterans organizing pneumonia [BOOP], pulmonary fibrosis) have been observed; risk may be increased with higher trough levels. Avoid concurrent use of strong CYP3A4 and/or P-glycoprotein (P-gp) inhibitors (eg, clarithromycin, erythromycin, telithromycin, itraconazole, ketoconazole, voriconazole) and strong inducers of CYP3A4 and/or P-gp (eg, rifampin, rifabutin). Concurrent use with a calcineurin inhibitor (cyclosporine, tacrolimus) may increase the risk of calcineurin inhibitor-induced hemolytic uremic syndrome/thrombotic thrombocytopenic purpura/thrombotic microangiopathy (HUS/TTP/TMA).

Hypersensitivity reactions, including anaphylactic/anaphylactoid reactions, angioedema, exfoliative dermatitis, and hypersensitivity vasculitis have been reported. Concurrent use with other drugs known to cause angioedema (eg, ACE inhibitors) may increase risk. Immunosuppressant therapy is associated with an increased risk of skin cancer; limit sun and ultraviolet light exposure; use appropriate sun protection. May increase serum lipids (cholesterol and triglycerides); use with caution in patients with hyperlipidemia. May be associated with wound dehiscence and impaired healing; use caution in the perioperative period. Patients with a body mass index (BMI) >30 kg/m^2 are at increased risk for abnormal wound healing.

Sirolimus tablets and oral solution are not bioequivalent, due to differences in absorption. Clinical equivalence was seen using 2 mg tablet and 2 mg solution. It is not known if higher doses are also clinically equivalent. Monitor sirolimus levels if changes in dosage forms are made. **[U.S. Boxed Warning]: Should only be used by physicians experienced in immunosuppressive therapy and management of transplant patients. Adequate laboratory and supportive medical resources must be readily available.** Sirolimus concentrations are dependent on the assay method (eg, chromatographic and immunoassay) used; assay methods are not interchangeable. Variations in methods to determine sirolimus whole blood concentrations, as well as interlaboratory variations, may result in improper dosage adjustments, which may lead to subtherapeutic or toxic levels. Determine the assay method used to assure consistency (or accommodations if changes occur), and for monitoring purposes, be aware of alterations to assay method or reference range. The manufacturer recommends high performance liquid chromatography (HPLC) as the reference standard to determine sirolimus trough concentrations.

Adverse Reactions Incidence of many adverse effects is dose related.

>20%:

Cardiovascular: Peripheral edema (54% to 58%), hypertension (45% to 49%), edema (18% to 20%)

Central nervous system: Headache (34%), pain (29% to 33%), insomnia (13% to 22%)

Dermatologic: Acne (22%)

Endocrine & metabolic: Hypertriglyceridemia (45% to 57%), hypercholesterolemia (43% to 46%)

Gastrointestinal: Constipation (36% to 38%), abdominal pain (29% to 36%), diarrhea (25% to 36%), nausea (25% to 31%)

Genitourinary: Urinary tract infection (26% to 33%)

Hematologic: Anemia (23% to 33%), thrombocytopenia (14% to 30%)

Neuromuscular & skeletal: Arthralgia (25% to 31%)

Renal: Serum creatinine increased (39% to 40%)

3% to 20%:

Cardiovascular: Atrial fibrillation, CHF, DVT, facial edema, hypervolemia, hypotension, palpitation, peripheral vascular disorder, postural hypotension, syncope, tachycardia, thrombosis, vasodilation

Central nervous system: Anxiety, chills, confusion, depression, dizziness, emotional lability, hypoesthesia, malaise, neuropathy, somnolence

Dermatologic: Rash (10% to 20%), skin carcinoma (up to 3%; includes basal cell carcinoma, squamous cell carcinoma, melanoma), cellulitis, dermal ulcer, dermatitis (fungal), ecchymosis, hirsutism, pruritus, skin hypertrophy, wound healing abnormal

Endocrine & metabolic: Acidosis, Cushing's syndrome, dehydration, diabetes mellitus, glycosuria, hypercalcemia, hyperglycemia, hyperphosphatemia, hypocalcemia, hypoglycemia, hypomagnesemia, hyponatremia

Gastrointestinal: Abdomen enlarged, anorexia, dysphagia, eructation, esophagitis, flatulence, gastritis, gastroenteritis, gingival hyperplasia, gingivitis, ileus, mouth ulceration, oral moniliasis, stomatitis, weight loss

Genitourinary: Impotence, pelvic pain, scrotal edema, testis disorder

Hematologic: Hemolytic-uremic syndrome, hemorrhage, leukopenia, leukocytosis, polycythemia, TTP

Hepatic: Abnormal liver function tests, alkaline phosphatase increased, LDH increased

Local: Thrombophlebitis

Neuromuscular & skeletal: Arthrosis, bone necrosis, CPK increased, hyper-/hypotonia, leg cramps, myalgia, osteoporosis, paresthesia, tetany

Ocular: Abnormal vision, cataract, conjunctivitis

Otic: Ear pain, otitis media, tinnitus

Renal: Albuminuria, bladder pain, BUN increased, dysuria, hematuria, hydronephrosis, kidney pain, nephropathy (toxic), nocturia, oliguria, pyelonephritis, pyuria, tubular necrosis, urinary frequency, urinary incontinence, urinary retention

Respiratory: Asthma, atelectasis, bronchitis, cough, epistaxis, hypoxia, lung edema, pleural effusion, pneumonia, pulmonary embolism, rhinitis, sinusitis

Miscellaneous: Lymphoproliferative disease/lymphoma (1% to 3%), abscess, diaphoresis, flu-like syndrome, hernia, herpesvirus infection, infection (including opportunistic), lymphadenopathy, lymphocele, peritonitis, sepsis

<3% (Limited to important or life-threatening): ALT increased, alveolar proteinosis, anaphylactoid reaction, anaphylaxis, anastomotic disruption, angioedema, ascites, AST increased, azoospermia, BK virus-associated nephropathy, *Clostridium difficile* colitis, cytomegalovirus, Epstein-Barr virus, exfoliative dermatitis, fascial dehiscence, focal segmental glomerulosclerosis, hepatic necrosis, hepatotoxicity, hypersensitivity reaction, hypersensitivity vasculitis, hypophosphatemia, incisional hernia; interstitial lung disease (dose-related; includes pneumonitis, pulmonary fibrosis, and bronchiolitis obliterans organizing pneumonia [BOOP] with no identified infectious etiology); joint disorders, lymphedema, myocardial infarction, mycobacterial infection, nephropathy, nephropathy (BK viral-induced), nephrotic syndrome, neutropenia, pancreatitis, pancytopenia, pericardial effusion, *Pneumocystis* pneumonia, progressive multifocal leukoencephalopathy (PML), proteinuria, pulmonary hemorrhage, reversible posterior leukoencephalopathy

syndrome (RPLS), tamponade, tuberculosis, wound dehiscence

Note: Hepatic artery thrombosis (HAT) and graft failure have been reported in liver transplant patients (not an approved use); bronchial anastomotic dehiscence has been reported in lung transplant patients (not an approved use)

Drug Interactions

Metabolism/Transport Effects **Substrate** of CYP3A4 (major), P-glycoprotein; **Note:** Assignment of Major/Minor substrate status based on clinically relevant drug interaction potential; **Inhibits** CYP3A4 (weak)

Avoid Concomitant Use

Avoid concomitant use of Sirolimus with any of the following: BCG; CloZAPine; Conivaptan; Crizotinib; Natalizumab; Pimecrolimus; Pimozide; Posaconazole; Tacrolimus (Systemic); Tacrolimus (Topical); Vaccines (Live); Voriconazole

Increased Effect/Toxicity

Sirolimus may increase the levels/effects of: ACE Inhibitors; CloZAPine; CycloSPORINE; CycloSPORINE (Systemic); Hypoglycemic Agents; Leflunomide; Natalizumab; Pimozide; Tacrolimus; Tacrolimus (Systemic); Tacrolimus (Topical); Vaccines (Live)

The levels/effects of Sirolimus may be increased by: Conivaptan; Crizotinib; CycloSPORINE; CycloSPORINE (Systemic); CYP3A4 Inhibitors (Moderate); CYP3A4 Inhibitors (Strong); Dasatinib; Denosumab; Fluconazole; Herbs (Hypoglycemic Properties); Itraconazole; Ketoconazole; Ketoconazole (Systemic); Macrolide Antibiotics; P-glycoprotein/ABCB1 Inhibitors; Pimecrolimus; Posaconazole; Protease Inhibitors; Roflumilast; Tacrolimus; Tacrolimus (Systemic); Tacrolimus (Topical); Telaprevir; Trastuzumab; Voriconazole

Decreased Effect

Sirolimus may decrease the levels/effects of: BCG; Coccidioidin Skin Test; Sipuleucel-T; Tacrolimus; Tacrolimus (Systemic); Vaccines (Inactivated); Vaccines (Live)

The levels/effects of Sirolimus may be decreased by: CYP3A4 Inducers (Strong); Deferasirox; Echinacea; Efavirenz; Fosphenytoin; P-glycoprotein/ABCB1 Inducers; Phenytoin; Rifampin; Tocilizumab

Ethanol/Nutrition/Herb Interactions

Food: Avoid grapefruit juice; may decrease clearance of sirolimus. Ingestion with high-fat meals decreases peak concentrations but increases AUC by 23% to 35%. Sirolimus should be taken consistently (either with or without food) to minimize variability.

Herb/Nutraceutical: St John's wort may decrease sirolimus levels; avoid concurrent use. Avoid cat's claw, echinacea (have immunostimulant properties; consider therapy modifications). Herbs with hypoglycemic properties may increase the risk of sirolimus-induced hypoglycemia; includes alfalfa, aloe, bilberry, bitter melon, burdock, celery, damiana, fenugreek, garcinia, garlic, ginger, ginseng (American), gymnema, marshmallow, stinging nettle.

Stability

Oral solution: Store under refrigeration, 2°C to 8°C (36°F to 46°F). Protect from light. A slight haze may develop in refrigerated solutions, but the quality of the product is not affected. After opening, solution should be used in 1 month. If necessary, may be stored at temperatures up to 25°C (77°F) for ≤15 days after opening. Product may be stored in amber syringe for a maximum of 24 hours (at room temperature or refrigerated). Discard syringe after single use. Solution should be used immediately following dilution.

Tablet: Store at room temperature of 20°C to 25°C (68°F to 77°F). Protect from light.

Mechanism of Action Sirolimus inhibits T-lymphocyte activation and proliferation in response to antigenic and cytokine stimulation and inhibits antibody production. Its mechanism differs from other immunosuppressants. Sirolimus binds to FKBP-12, an intracellular protein, to form an immunosuppressive complex which inhibits the regulatory kinase, mTOR (mammalian target of rapamycin). This inhibition suppresses cytokine mediated T-cell proliferation, halting progression from the G1 to the S phase of the cell cycle. It inhibits acute rejection of allografts and prolongs graft survival.

Pharmacodynamics/Kinetics

Absorption: Rapid

Distribution: 12 L/kg (range: 4-20 L/kg)

Protein binding: ~92%, primarily to albumin

Metabolism: Extensive; in intestinal wall via P-glycoprotein and hepatic via CYP3A4; to 7 major metabolites

Bioavailability: Oral solution: 14%; Oral tablet: 18%

Half-life elimination: Mean: 62 hours (range: 46-78 hours); extended in hepatic impairment (Child-Pugh class A or B) to 113 hours

Time to peak: Oral solution: 1-3 hours; Tablet: 1-6 hours

Excretion: Feces (91% due to P-glycoprotein-mediated efflux into gut lumen); urine (2%)

Dosage Oral:

Low-to-moderate immunologic risk renal transplant patients: Children ≥13 years and Adults: Dosing by body weight:

<40 kg: Loading dose: 3 mg/m^2 on day 1, followed by maintenance dosing of 1 mg/m^2 once daily

≥40 kg: Loading dose: 6 mg on day 1; maintenance: 2 mg once daily

High immunologic risk renal transplant patients: Adults: Loading dose: Up to 15 mg on day 1; maintenance: 5 mg/day; obtain trough concentration between days 5-7 and adjust accordingly. Continue concurrent cyclosporine/sirolimus therapy for 1 year following transplantation. Further adjustment of the regimen must be based on clinical status.

Dosage adjustment: Sirolimus dosages should be adjusted to maintain trough concentrations within desired range based on risk and concomitant therapy. Maximum daily dose: 40 mg. Dosage should be adjusted at intervals of 7-14 days to account for the long half-life of sirolimus. In general, dose proportionality may be assumed. New sirolimus dose **equals** current dose **multiplied by** (target concentration **divided by** current concentration). **Note:** If large dose increase is required, consider loading dose calculated as:

Loading dose **equals** (new maintenance dose **minus** current maintenance dose) **multiplied by** 3

Maximum dose in 1 day: 40 mg; if required dose is >40 mg (due to loading dose), divide loading dose over 2 days. Whole blood concentrations should not be used as the sole basis for dosage adjustment (monitor clinical signs/symptoms, tissue biopsy, and laboratory parameters).

Maintenance therapy after withdrawal of cyclosporine: Cyclosporine withdrawal is not recommended in high immunological risk patients. Following 2-4 months of combined therapy, withdrawal of cyclosporine may be considered in low-to-moderate immunologic risk patients. Cyclosporine should be discontinued over 4-8 weeks, and a necessary increase in the dosage of sirolimus (up to fourfold) should be anticipated due to removal of metabolic inhibition by cyclosporine and to maintain adequate immunosuppressive effects. Dose-adjusted trough target concentrations are typically 16-24 ng/mL for the first year post-transplant and 12-20 ng/mL thereafter (measured by chromatographic methodology).

GVHD prophylaxis (unlabeled use): 12 mg loading dose on day -3, followed by 4 mg daily (target trough level: 3-12 ng/mL); taper off after 6-9 months (Armand, 2008; Cutler, 2007)

Treatment of refractory acute GVHD (unlabeled use): 4-5 mg/m^2 for 14 days (no loading dose) (Benito, 2001)

Treatment of chronic GVHD (unlabeled use): 6 mg loading dose, followed by 2 mg daily (target trough level: 7-12 ng/mL) for 6-9 months (Couriel, 2005)

Dosage adjustment in renal impairment: No dosage adjustment (in loading or maintenance dose) is necessary in renal impairment. However, adjustment of regimen (including discontinuation of therapy) should be considered when used concurrently with cyclosporine and elevated or increasing serum creatinine is noted.

Dosage adjustment in hepatic impairment:

Loading dose: No adjustment required

Maintenance dose:

Mild-to-moderate hepatic impairment: reduce maintenance dose by ~33%

Severe hepatic impairment: reduce maintenance dose by ~50%

Dietary Considerations Take consistently (with or without food) to minimize variability of absorption.

Administration Initial dose should be administered as soon as possible after transplant. Sirolimus should be taken 4 hours after oral cyclosporine (Neoral® or Gengraf®). Should be administered consistently (with or without food).

Solution: Mix (by stirring vigorously) with at least 2 ounces of water or orange juice. No other liquids should be used for dilution. Patient should drink diluted solution immediately. The cup should then be refilled with an additional 4 ounces of water or orange juice, stirred vigorously, and the patient should drink the contents at once.

Tablet: Do not crush, split, or chew.

Monitoring Parameters Monitor LFTs and CBC during treatment. Monitor sirolimus levels in all patients (especially in pediatric patients, patients ≥13 years of age weighing <40 kg, patients with hepatic impairment, or on concurrent potent inhibitors or inducers of CYP3A4 or P-gp, and/or if cyclosporine dosing is markedly reduced or discontinued), and when changing dosage forms of sirolimus. Also monitor serum cholesterol and triglycerides, blood pressure, serum creatinine, and urinary protein. Serum drug concentrations should be determined 3-4 days after loading doses and 7-14 days after dosage adjustments; however, these concentrations should not be used as the sole basis for dosage adjustment, especially during withdrawal of cyclosporine (monitor clinical signs/symptoms, tissue biopsy, and laboratory parameters). **Note:** Concentrations and ranges are dependent on and will vary with assay methodology (chromatographic or immunoassay); assay methods are not interchangeable.

Reference Range Note: Sirolimus concentrations are dependent on the assay method (eg, chromatographic and immunoassay) used; assay methods are not interchangeable. Determine the assay method used to assure consistency (or accommodations if changes occur) and for monitoring purposes, be aware of alterations to assay method or reference range.

Serum trough concentration goals for renal transplantation (based on HPLC methods):

Concomitant cyclosporine: 4-12 ng/mL

Low-to-moderate immunologic risk (after cyclosporine withdrawal): 16-24 ng/mL for the first year after transplant; after 1 year: 12-20 ng/mL

High immunologic risk (with cyclosporine): 10-15 ng/mL

Note: Trough concentrations vary based on clinical context and use of additional immunosuppressants. The following represents typical ranges.

When combined with tacrolimus and mycophenolate mofetil (MMF) without steroids: 6-8 ng/mL

As a substitute for tacrolimus (starting 4-8 weeks post-transplant), in combination with MMF and steroids: 8-12 ng/mL

Following conversion from tacrolimus to sirolimus >6 months post-transplant due to chronic allograft nephropathy: 4-6 ng/mL

Serum trough concentrations for GVHD prophylaxis in allogeneic stem cell transplant: 3-12 ng/mL (Armand, 2008; Cutler, 2007)

Additional Information Sirolimus tablets and oral solution are not bioequivalent, due to differences in absorption. Clinical equivalence was seen using 2 mg tablet and 2 mg solution. It is not known if higher doses are also clinically equivalent. Monitor sirolimus levels if changes in dosage forms are made.

Sirolimus solution may cause irritation if administered undiluted.

High-risk renal transplant patients are defined (per the manufacturer's labeling) as African-American transplant recipients and/or repeat renal transplant recipients who lost a previous allograft based on an immunologic process and/or patients with high PRA (panel-reactive antibodies; peak PRA level >80%). Individual transplant centers may have differences in their definitions. For example, some centers would consider a PRA >50% to be at higher risk of rejection.

Dosage Forms Excipient information presented when available (limited, particularly for generics); consult specific product labeling.

Solution, oral:

Rapamune®: 1 mg/mL (60 mL) [contains ethanol 1.5%-2.5%, propylene glycol, soy]

Tablet, oral:

Rapamune®: 0.5 mg, 1 mg, 2 mg

SitaGLIPtin (sit a GLIP tin)

Brand Names: U.S. Januvia®

Brand Names: Canada Januvia®

Index Terms MK-0431; Sitagliptin Phosphate

Pharmacologic Category Antidiabetic Agent, Dipeptidyl Peptidase IV (DPP-IV) Inhibitor

Additional Appendix Information

Diabetes Mellitus Management, Adults *on page 1983*

Use Management of type 2 diabetes mellitus (noninsulin dependent, NIDDM) as an adjunct to diet and exercise as monotherapy or in combination therapy with other antidiabetic agents

Pregnancy Risk Factor B

Pregnancy Considerations Adverse events have not been observed in animal reproduction studies; therefore, sitagliptan is classified as pregnancy category B. There are no adequate and well controlled studies in pregnant women. Maternal hyperglycemia can be associated with adverse effects in the fetus, including macrosomia, neonatal hyperglycemia, and hyperbilirubinemia; the risk of congenital malformations is increased when the Hb A_{1c} is above the normal range. Diabetes can also be associated with adverse effects in the mother. Poorly-treated diabetes may cause end-organ damage that may in turn negatively affect obstetric outcomes. Physiologic glucose levels should be maintained prior to and during pregnancy to decrease the risk of adverse events in the mother and the fetus. Until additional safety and efficacy data are obtained, the use of oral agents is generally not recommended as routine management of GDM or type 2 diabetes mellitus during pregnancy. Insulin is the drug of choice for the control of diabetes mellitus during pregnancy. Health professionals are encouraged to report any prenatal exposure to sitagliptin by contacting Merck's pregnancy registry (1-800-986-8999).

Lactation Excretion in breast milk unknown/use caution

Medication Guide Available Yes

Contraindications Serious hypersensitivity (eg, anaphylaxis, angioedema) to sitagliptan or any component of the formulation

Warnings/Precautions Avoid use in type 1 diabetes mellitus (insulin dependent, IDDM) and diabetic ketoacidosis (DKA) due to lack of efficacy in these populations. Use caution when used in conjunction with insulin or insulin secretagogues; risk of hypoglycemia is increased. Monitor blood glucose closely; dosage adjustments of insulin or insulin secretagogues may be necessary. Use with caution in patients with moderate-to-severe renal dysfunction and end-stage renal disease (ESRD) requiring hemodialysis or peritoneal dialysis; dosing adjustment required. Safety and efficacy have not been established in severe hepatic dysfunction.

Rare hypersensitivity reactions, including anaphylaxis, angioedema, and/or severe dermatologic reactions (such as Stevens-Johnson syndrome), have been reported in postmarketing surveillance; discontinue if signs/symptoms of hypersensitivity reactions occur. Cases of acute pancreatitis (including hemorrhagic and necrotizing with some fatalities) have been reported with use; monitor for signs/symptoms of pancreatitis. Discontinue use immediately if pancreatitis is suspected and initiate appropriate management. Use with caution in patients with a history of pancreatitis (not known if this population is at greater risk).

Clinical trials included only a limited number of patients with heart failure (HF). No specific recommendations regarding this population are provided in the approved U.S. labeling (Canadian labeling recommends against use in this population). Diabetes self-management education (DSME) is essential to maximize the effectiveness of therapy.

Adverse Reactions As reported with monotherapy:

1% to 10%:

- Cardiovascular: Peripheral edema (2%)
- Endocrine & metabolic: Hypoglycemia (1%)
- Gastrointestinal: Diarrhea (4%), constipation (3%), nausea (2%)
- Neuromuscular & skeletal: Osteoarthritis (1%)
- Respiratory: Nasopharyngitis (5%), pharyngitis (1%), upper respiratory tract infection (viral; 1%)

<1% (Limited to important or life-threatening): Abdominal discomfort/pain/tenderness, acute renal failure (possibly requiring dialysis), anaphylaxis, anemia, angioedema, anxiety, appetite decreased, bundle branch block, coordination abnormal, cough, cutaneous vasculitis, depression, dizziness, dry skin, dysmenorrhea, dyspepsia, erectile dysfunction, erythema, exanthema, exfoliative dermatitis, facial edema, fever, flatulence, gastritis (*Helicobacter*), GERD, hepatic steatosis, hyperhidrosis, hyper-/hypotension, hypersensitivity, liver enzymes increased, malaise, migraine, muscle tightness, orthostasis, pain, palpitation, pancreatitis (acute cases including hemorrhagic or necrotizing forms with some fatalities), peripheral neuropathy, pruritus, rash (including macular), renal function decreased, retching, rosacea, salivation increased, serum creatinine increased, somnolence, Stevens-Johnson syndrome, uric acid increased, urticaria, white blood cells increased

Drug Interactions

Metabolism/Transport Effects **Substrate** of P-glycoprotein

Avoid Concomitant Use There are no known interactions where it is recommended to avoid concomitant use.

Increased Effect/Toxicity

SitaGLIPtin may increase the levels/effects of: ACE Inhibitors; Digoxin; Hypoglycemic Agents

The levels/effects of SitaGLIPtin may be increased by: Herbs (Hypoglycemic Properties); Pegvisomant; P-glycoprotein/ABCB1 Inhibitors

Decreased Effect

The levels/effects of SitaGLIPtin may be decreased by: Corticosteroids (Orally Inhaled); Corticosteroids (Systemic); Luteinizing Hormone-Releasing Hormone Analogs; P-glycoprotein/ABCB1 Inducers; Somatropin; Thiazide Diuretics

Stability Store at 20°C to 25°C (68°F to 77°F); excursions permitted to 15°C to 30°C (59°F to 86°F).

Mechanism of Action Sitagliptin inhibits dipeptidyl peptidase IV (DPP-IV) enzyme resulting in prolonged active incretin levels. Incretin hormones (eg, glucagon-like peptide-1 [GLP-1] and glucose-dependent insulinotropic polypeptide [GIP]) regulate glucose homeostasis by increasing insulin synthesis and release from pancreatic beta cells and decreasing glucagon secretion from pancreatic alpha cells. Decreased glucagon secretion results in decreased hepatic glucose production. Under normal physiologic circumstances, incretin hormones are released by the intestine throughout the day and levels are increased in response to a meal; incretin hormones are rapidly inactivated by the DPP-IV enzyme.

Pharmacodynamics/Kinetics

Absorption: Rapid

Distribution: ~198 L

Protein binding: 38%

Metabolism: Not extensively metabolized; minor metabolism via CYP3A4 and 2C8 to metabolites (inactive) suggested by *in vitro* studies

Bioavailability: ~87%

Half-life elimination: 12 hours

Time to peak, plasma: 1-4 hours

Excretion: Urine 87% (79% as unchanged drug, 16% as metabolites); feces 13%

Dosage Oral: Adults: Type 2 diabetes: 100 mg once daily

Concomitant use with insulin and/or insulin secretagogues (eg, sulfonylureas): Reduced dose of insulin and/or insulin secretagogues may be needed.

Dosage adjustment in renal impairment:

Cl_{cr} ≥50 mL/minute: No adjustment required

Cl_{cr} ≥30 to <50 mL/minute: 50 mg once daily

S_{cr}: Males: >1.7 to ≤3.0 mg/dL; Females: >1.5 to ≤2.5 mg/dL: 50 mg once daily

Cl_{cr}<30 mL/minute: 25 mg once daily

S_{cr}: Males: >3.0 mg/dL; Females: >2.5 mg/dL: 25 mg once daily

ESRD requiring hemodialysis or peritoneal dialysis: 25 mg once daily; administered without regard to timing of hemodialysis

Dosage adjustment in hepatic impairment:

Mild-to-moderate impairment (Child-Pugh score 7-9): No dosage adjustment required

Severe impairment (Child-Pugh score >9): Not studied

Dietary Considerations May be taken with or without food. Individualized medical nutrition therapy (MNT) based on ADA recommendations is an integral part of therapy.

Administration May be administered with or without food.

Monitoring Parameters Hb A_{1c}, serum glucose; renal function prior to initiation and periodically during treatment

Reference Range Recommendations for glycemic control in adults with diabetes:

Hb A_{1c}: <7%

Preprandial capillary plasma glucose: 70-130 mg/dL

Peak postprandial capillary blood glucose: <180 mg/dL

Dosage Forms Excipient information presented when available (limited, particularly for generics); consult specific product labeling.

Tablet, oral:

Januvia®: 25 mg, 50 mg, 100 mg

Sitagliptin and Metformin
(sit a GLIP tin & met FOR min)

Brand Names: U.S. Janumet®
Brand Names: Canada Janumet®
Index Terms Metformin and Sitagliptin; Sitagliptin Phosphate and Metformin Hydrochloride
Pharmacologic Category Antidiabetic Agent, Biguanide; Antidiabetic Agent, Dipeptidyl Peptidase IV (DPP-IV) Inhibitor; Hypoglycemic Agent, Oral
Use Management of type 2 diabetes mellitus (noninsulin dependent, NIDDM) as an adjunct to diet and exercise in patients not adequately controlled on metformin or sitagliptin monotherapy
Pregnancy Risk Factor B
Medication Guide Available Yes
Dosage Oral: Type 2 diabetes mellitus: **Note:** Patients receiving concomitant insulin and/or insulin secretagogues (eg, sulfonylureas) may require dosage adjustments of these agents.

Adults: Initial doses should be based on current dose of sitagliptin and metformin; daily doses should be divided and given twice daily with meals. Maximum: Sitagliptin 100 mg/metformin 2000 mg daily

Patients inadequately controlled on metformin alone: Initial dose: Sitagliptin 100 mg/day plus current dose of metformin. **Note:** The U.S. labeling recommends that patients currently receiving metformin 850 mg twice daily receive an initial dose of sitagliptin 50 mg and metformin 1000 mg twice daily

Patients inadequately controlled on sitagliptin alone: Initial dose: Metformin 1000 mg/day plus sitagliptin 100 mg/day. **Note:** Patients currently receiving a renally adjusted dose of sitagliptin should not be switched to combination product.

Dosing adjustment: Metformin component may be gradually increased up to the maximum dose. Maximum dose: Sitagliptin 100 mg/metformin 2000 mg daily

Elderly: The initial and maintenance dosing should be conservative, due to the potential for decreased renal function (monitor). Do not use in patients ≥80 years of age unless normal renal function has been established.

Dosage adjustment in renal impairment: Do not use with renal disease or renal dysfunction (serum creatinine ≥1.5 mg/dL [≥136 micromole/L] in males or ≥1.4 mg/dL [≥124 micromole/L] in females or abnormal clearance).

Dosage adjustment in hepatic impairment: Avoid metformin; liver disease is a risk factor for the development of lactic acidosis during metformin therapy.

Additional Information Complete prescribing information for this medication should be consulted for additional detail.

Dosage Forms Excipient information presented when available (limited, particularly for generics); consult specific product labeling.

Tablet, oral:
- Janumet® 50/500: Sitagliptin 50 mg and metformin hydrochloride 500 mg
- Janumet® 50/1000: Sitagliptin 50 mg and metformin hydrochloride 1000 mg

Dosage Forms: Canada Excipient information presented when available (limited, particularly for generics); consult specific product labeling.

Tablet, oral:
- Janumet® 50/850: Sitagliptin 50 mg and metformin hydrochloride 850 mg

Sitagliptin and Simvastatin
(sit a GLIP tin & sim va STAT in)

Brand Names: U.S. Juvisync™
Index Terms Simvastatin and Sitagliptin; Sitagliptin Phosphate and Simvastatin
Pharmacologic Category Antidiabetic Agent, Dipeptidyl Peptidase IV (DPP-IV) Inhibitor; Antilipemic Agent, HMG-CoA Reductase Inhibitor
Use For use when treatment with both sitagliptin and simvastatin is appropriate:

Sitagliptin: Management of type 2 diabetes mellitus (noninsulin dependent, NIDDM) as an adjunct to diet and exercise as monotherapy or in combination therapy with other antidiabetic agents

Simvastatin: Used with dietary therapy for the following:

Secondary prevention of cardiovascular events in hypercholesterolemic patients with established coronary heart disease (CHD) or at high risk for CHD: To reduce cardiovascular morbidity (myocardial infarction, coronary/noncoronary revascularization procedures) and mortality; to reduce the risk of stroke

Hyperlipidemias: To reduce elevations in total cholesterol (total-C), LDL-C, apolipoprotein B, triglycerides, and VLDL-C, and to increase HDL-C in patients with primary hypercholesterolemia (elevations of 1 or more components are present in Fredrickson type IIa, IIb, III, and IV hyperlipidemias); treatment of homozygous familial hypercholesterolemia

Pregnancy Risk Factor X
Medication Guide Available Yes
Dosage Oral: Adults: Hyperlipidemia and type 2 diabetes: Initial dose: Sitagliptin 100 mg and simvastatin 40 mg once daily. **Note:** Patients already taking simvastatin <40 mg/day (with or without sitagliptin 100 mg daily) can be converted to the comparable equivalent of the combination product. Dose adjustments should be made at intervals of ≥4 weeks.

Concomitant use with insulin and/or insulin secretagogues (eg, sulfonylureas): Reduced dose of insulin and/or insulin secretagogues may be needed.

Dosage adjustment for simvastatin with concomitant medications:

Diltiazem or verapamil: Simvastatin dose should **not** exceed 10 mg/day

Amiodarone, amlodipine, or ranolazine: Simvastatin dose should **not** exceed 20 mg/day

Dosage adjustment for simvastatin in Chinese patients on niacin doses ≥1 g/day: Use caution with simvastatin doses of 40 mg/day because of an increased risk of myopathy

Dosage adjustment in renal impairment: Note: Renal function may be estimated using Cockcroft-Gault formula for dosage adjustment purposes.

Cl_{cr} ≥50 mL/minute: No dosage adjustment necessary
Cl_{cr} <50 mL/minute: Use is not recommended
End-stage renal disease (ESRD): Use is not recommended

Dosage adjustment in hepatic impairment: Use is contraindicated

Additional Information Complete prescribing information for this medication should be consulted for additional detail.

Dosage Forms Excipient information presented when available (limited, particularly for generics); consult specific product labeling.

Tablet, oral:
- Juvisync™ 100/10: Sitagliptin 100 mg and simvastatin 10 mg
- Juvisync™ 100/20: Sitagliptin 100 mg and simvastatin 20 mg
- Juvisync™ 100/40: Sitagliptin 100 mg and simvastatin 40 mg

◆ **Sitagliptin Phosphate** *see* SitaGLIPtin *on page* 1560

- ◆ **Sitagliptin Phosphate and Metformin Hydrochloride** *see* Sitagliptin and Metformin *on page 1562*
- ◆ **Sitagliptin Phosphate and Simvastatin** *see* Sitagliptin and Simvastatin *on page 1562*
- ◆ **Skeeter Stik® [OTC]** *see* Benzocaine *on page 202*
- ◆ **Skelaxin®** *see* Metaxalone *on page 1085*
- ◆ **Skelid®** *see* Tiludronate *on page 1685*
- ◆ **SKF 104864** *see* Topotecan *on page 1709*
- ◆ **SKF 104864-A** *see* Topotecan *on page 1709*
- ◆ **Sleep-ettes D [OTC]** *see* DiphenhydrAMINE (Systemic) *on page 516*
- ◆ **Sleepinal® [OTC]** *see* DiphenhydrAMINE (Systemic) *on page 516*
- ◆ **Sleep-Tabs [OTC]** *see* DiphenhydrAMINE (Systemic) *on page 516*
- ◆ **S-leucovorin** *see* LEVOleucovorin *on page 1000*
- ◆ **6S-leucovorin** *see* LEVOleucovorin *on page 1000*
- ◆ **Slo-Niacin® [OTC]** *see* Niacin *on page 1195*
- ◆ **Slo-Pot (Can)** *see* Potassium Chloride *on page 1380*
- ◆ **Slow FE® [OTC]** *see* Ferrous Sulfate *on page 706*
- ◆ **Slow-K® (Can)** *see* Potassium Chloride *on page 1380*
- ◆ **Slow-Mag® [OTC]** *see* Magnesium Chloride *on page 1044*
- ◆ **Slow Release [OTC]** *see* Ferrous Sulfate *on page 706*
- ◆ **SM-13496** *see* Lurasidone *on page 1041*

Smallpox Vaccine (SMAL poks vak SEEN)

Brand Names: U.S. ACAM2000®

Index Terms Live Smallpox Vaccine; Vaccinia Vaccine

Pharmacologic Category Vaccine, Live (Viral)

Use Active immunization against vaccinia virus, the causative agent of smallpox in persons determined to be at risk for smallpox infection.

The Advisory Committee on Immunization Practices (ACIP) recommends routine vaccination for the following:

- Laboratory workers at risk of exposure from cultures or contaminated animals which may be a source of vaccinia or related Orthopoxviruses capable of causing infections in humans (monkeypox, cowpox, or variola).
- Consideration may also be given for vaccination of healthcare workers having contact with clinical specimens, contaminated material, or patients receiving vaccinia or recombinant vaccinia viruses.

In a Pre-Event Vaccination Program, the ACIP recommends vaccination for the following:

- Persons designated by authorities to investigate smallpox cases with the likelihood of direct patient contact
- Persons responsible for administering smallpox vaccine

In the event of an intentional release of smallpox virus, the ACIP recommends vaccination for the following:

- Persons exposed to the initial release of the virus
- Persons who had close contact with a confirmed or suspected smallpox patient at any time from the onset of the patient's fever until all scabs have separated
- Healthcare providers involved in evaluation, care, or transport of confirmed or suspected smallpox patients
- Laboratory personnel involved in processing specimens of confirmed or suspected smallpox patients
- Persons likely to have increased contact with infectious materials from smallpox patients

Pregnancy Risk Factor D

Pregnancy Considerations **[U.S. Boxed Warning]: Pregnant women are at increased risk for severe adverse reactions.** Animal reproduction studies have not been conducted with this vaccine. Vaccinia vaccine has not been associated with the development of congenital malformations. On rare occasions, vaccination has been reported to cause fetal infection. Fetal vaccina infection is associated with stillbirth or neonatal mortality. Vaccination of pregnant women is not recommended in a pre-event setting. Pregnancy should be avoided for at least 4 weeks following vaccination. Healthcare providers may enroll pregnant women who were inadvertently vaccinated during pregnancy (or who were a close contact of a vaccinee within 4 weeks of vaccination) in the CDC pregnancy registry by calling 404-639-8253 or 877-554-4625. Military cases should be reported to the Department of Defense.

Lactation Excretion in breast milk unknown/not recommended

Prescribing and Access Restrictions ACAM2000® is deemed to have an approved REMS program. The smallpox vaccine is not available for general public use. All supplies are currently owned by the federal government for inclusion in the Strategic National Stockpile. In October 2002, the FDA approved the licensing of the stockpile of smallpox vaccine. This approval allows the vaccine to be distributed and administered in the event of a smallpox attack. The bulk of current supplies have been designated for use by the U.S. military. Additionally, laboratory workers who may be at risk of exposure may require vaccination. Bioterrorism experts have proposed immunization of first responders (including police, fire, and emergency workers), but these plans may not be implemented until additional stocks of vaccine are licensed.

Medication Guide Available Yes

Contraindications Manufacturer labeling: Severe immune deficiency (eg, persons undergoing bone marrow transplant, individuals with primary or acquired immunodeficiency requiring isolation). There are very few absolute contraindications regarding vaccination of individuals at high-risk for exposure to smallpox. The decision to vaccinate must be based on a careful analysis of potential benefits and possible risks.

ACIP contraindications in a pre-event vaccination program: Hypersensitivity to the vaccine or any component of the formulation; history or presence of atopic dermatitis, eczema or other acute, chronic or exfoliative skin conditions (or persons with household contacts with these conditions); immunosuppression (or persons with household contacts who are immunosuppressed); pregnant or breast-feeding women (or household contacts of pregnant women); children <1 year of age

According to ACIP, persons exposed to smallpox virus in an emergency situation have no contraindications to vaccination.

Warnings/Precautions **[U.S. Boxed Warning]: Acute myocarditis and/or pericarditis, encephalitis, encephalomyelitis, and encephalopathy have been observed following vaccination. [U.S. Boxed Warning]: Progressive vaccinia, general vaccinia, and severe vaccinial skin infections have been observed following vaccination. [U.S. Boxed Warning]: Severe skin and systemic reactions, including Stevens-Johnson syndrome, have also occurred. [U.S. Boxed Warning]: Patients with congenital or acquired immune deficiency disorders (including those on immunosuppressive medications), patients with or with a history of cardiovascular disease, patients with eye diseases treated with topical steroids, infants <12 months of age, and pregnant women may be at an increased risk for severe adverse reactions** and should not be vaccinated in nonemergency situations. **[U.S. Boxed Warning]: Following vaccination, eczema vaccinatum has been reported. Patients with eczema, a history of eczema, or other acute or chronic exfoliative skin conditions may be at an increased risk for severe skin infections;** these patients should not be vaccinated in nonemergency situations. **[U.S. Boxed Warning]: The risk of vaccination complications must be weighed against the risk of experiencing a potentially fatal smallpox infection.** Patients at greatest risk for adverse reactions from the vaccine are also at increased risk for death from smallpox infection. **[U.S. Boxed Warning]: Live vaccinia virus may be transmitted to close contacts of the vaccinee; risks for the close contact are the same as those receiving the vaccine.**

For percutaneous administration only. Vaccination is given by scarification (multiple punctures into superficial layers of the skin) only. **Not for I.M., I.V., or SubQ injection.** Some dosage forms may contain neomycin, polymyxin B, and/or human albumin. Virus may be cultured from vaccination sites until scab separates from lesion. Individuals should be instructed to avoid contact with patients at high risk of transmission/adverse effects, including pregnant or breast-feeding women and patients with eczema or immunodeficiency during this time. Patients should be advised not to donate blood or organs for 21-30 days; contacts who have inadvertently contracted vaccinia should avoid donating blood for 14 days. Appropriate precautions should be used for the handling and disposal of vaccine and all supplies. Per the ACIP, vaccine is contraindicated for use in infants <12 months of age (nonemergency situation) and use is not recommended in pediatric patients <18 years of age (nonemergency situations). Safety and efficacy has not been established in patients ≥65 years of age. In order to maximize vaccination rates, the ACIP recommends simultaneous administration of all age-appropriate vaccines (live or inactivated) for which a person is eligible at a single clinic visit, unless contraindications exist.

Adverse Reactions All serious adverse reactions must be reported to the U.S. Department of Health and Human Services (DHHS) Vaccine Adverse Event Reporting System (VAERS) 1-800-822-7967 or online at https://vaers.hhs.gov/esub/index. In addition, clinicians may enroll patients with adverse reactions in the CDC Registry at 877-554-4625. Serious adverse reactions to ACAM2000® may also be reported to the manufacturer, Acambis Inc, at 866-440-9440.

>10%:
- Central nervous system: Headache (32% to 51%), fatigue (34% to 48%), malaise (28% to 37%)
- Dermatologic: Erythema (18% to 24%); rash (6% to 11% erythematous, folliculitis, papulovesicular, urticarial, nonspecific)
- Gastrointestinal: Nausea (10% to 19%), diarrhea (12% to 16%)
- Local: Injection site: Pruritus (82% to 92%), erythema (61% to 74%), pain (37% to 67%), edema (28% to 48%)
- Neuromuscular & skeletal: Myalgia (27% to 46%), rigors (12% to 21%)
- Miscellaneous: Lymph node pain (19% to 57%), feeling hot (20% to 32%), exercise tolerance decreased (8% to 11%)

1% to 10%:
- Gastrointestinal: Constipation (6%), vomiting (3% to 5%)
- Neuromuscular & skeletal: Arthralgia, back pain
- Respiratory: Dyspnea (3% to 4%)
- Miscellaneous: Lymphadenopathy (6% to 8%)

Frequency not defined: Abdominal pain, Bell's palsy, blindness, cardiomyopathy (nonischemic/dilated), contact dermatitis, corneal scarring, death, dizziness, eczema vaccinatum, encephalitis, encephalomyelitis, encephalopathy, erythema multiforme, fever, generalized vaccinia, Guillain-Barré syndrome, hypersensitivity reactions; inadvertent inoculation at other sites (including autoinoculation to eyelid, face, genitalia, lips, mouth, nose, rectum); ischemic heart disease, keratitis, meningitis, myelitis, myocarditis, myopericarditis (asymptomatic or symptomatic), ocular vaccinia, paresthesia, pericarditis, photophobia, progressive vaccinia, secondary pyogenic infection, seizure, Stevens-Johnson syndrome, toothache, vaccinial skin infection, vertigo

Drug Interactions

Metabolism/Transport Effects None known.

Avoid Concomitant Use

Avoid concomitant use of Smallpox Vaccine with any of the following: Belimumab; Fingolimod; Immunosuppressants

Increased Effect/Toxicity

Smallpox Vaccine may increase the levels/effects of: Varicella Virus Vaccine

The levels/effects of Smallpox Vaccine may be increased by: AzaTHIOprine; Belimumab; Corticosteroids (Systemic); Fingolimod; Hydroxychloroquine; Immunosuppressants; Leflunomide; Mercaptopurine; Methotrexate

Decreased Effect

Smallpox Vaccine may decrease the levels/effects of: Tuberculin Tests

The levels/effects of Smallpox Vaccine may be decreased by: Fingolimod; Immune Globulins; Immunosuppressants

Stability Prior to reconstitution, store frozen at -15°C to -25°C (5°F to -13°F); may also be stored at 2°C to 8°C (36°F to 46°F) for up to 18 months. Bring to room temperature prior to reconstitution. Using the syringe provided, inject 0.3 mL of provided diluent into the vaccine vial. Swirl gently until the solution becomes a slightly hazy, colorless to straw-colored liquid free from particulate matter; avoid contact between the solution and the rubber stopper. Following reconstitution, stable for 6 to 8 hours at room temperature of 20°C to 25°C (68°F to 77°F) or for up to 30 days when refrigerated at 2°C to 8°C (36°F to 46°F). The provided diluent should be stored at room temperature of 15°C to 30°C (59°F to 86°F).

Mechanism of Action Vaccinia virus is similar to the variola (smallpox) virus. By inducing a localized infection with vaccinia virus, immunity to both vaccinia and smallpox is achieved. Vaccination results in viral replication, production of neutralizing antibodies, immunity, and cellular hypersensitivity.

Pharmacodynamics/Kinetics Onset of action: Neutralizing antibodies appear 15-20 days after vaccination.

Dosage Percutaneous: Not for I.M., I.V., or SubQ injection: Vaccination by scarification (multiple-puncture technique) only: **Note:** A trace of blood should appear at vaccination site after 15-20 seconds; if no trace of blood is visible, an additional 3 insertions should be made using the same needle, without reinserting the needle into the vaccine bottle.

Children ≥12 months (in emergency conditions only) and Adults (ACAM2000®):

Primary vaccination and revaccination: Use a single drop of vaccine suspension and 15 needle punctures (using the same bifurcated needle) into the superficial skin

Note: According to the manufacturer, revaccination is recommended every 3 years for patients at a continued high risk for smallpox infection. The ACIP recommends routine nonemergency revaccination every 3-10 years, depending on type of exposure. Additional information can be obtained from the Department of Defense and the CDC.

Dosage adjustment in renal impairment: No dosage adjustment required

Administration Vaccination should only be performed by healthcare providers trained in the safe and efficacious administration of the smallpox vaccine via the percutaneous route. Using a bifurcated needle, 1 drop of vaccine is introduced into the superficial layers of the skin using a multiple-puncture technique. The skin over the insertion of the deltoid muscle is the preferred site for vaccination.

A single-use bifurcated needle should be dipped carefully into the reconstituted vaccine (following removal of rubber stopper). Visually confirm that the needle picks up a drop of vaccine solution. Deposit the drop of vaccine onto clean, dry skin at the vaccination site. If alcohol is used to clean the skin, allow site to dry completely prior to administration to prevent the inactivation of the vaccine by the alcohol. Holding the bifurcated needle perpendicular to the skin, punctures are to be made rapidly within a diameter of about 5 mm into the superficial skin of the vaccination site. The puncture strokes should be vigorous enough to allow a trace of blood to appear after approximately 15-20 seconds. Wipe off any remaining vaccine with dry sterile gauze. Dispose of all materials in a biohazard waste container. All materials must be burned, boiled, or autoclaved. If no evidence of vaccine take is apparent after 7 days, the individual may be vaccinated again.

To prevent transmission of the virus, avoid scratching the vaccination site and cover with gauze; cover gauze with a semipermeable barrier or clothing. Ointment or salves should not be applied to the vaccination site. Good handwashing prevents inadvertent inoculation. Vaccinees should change bandages away from others and launder their own linens separately to prevent transmission.

Simultaneous administration of vaccines helps ensure the patients will be fully vaccinated by the appropriate age. Simultaneous administration of vaccines is defined as administering >1 vaccine on the same day at different anatomic sites. Separate vaccines should not be combined in the same syringe unless indicated by product specific labeling. Separate needles and syringes should be used for each injection. The ACIP prefers each dose of a specific vaccine in a series come from the same manufacturer when possible. Adolescents and adults should be vaccinated while seated or lying down. In general, preterm infants should be vaccinated at the same chronological age as full-term infants (CDC, 2011).

Antipyretics have not been shown to prevent febrile seizures. Antipyretics may be used to treat fever or discomfort following vaccination (CDC, 2011). One study reported that routine prophylactic administration of acetaminophen to prevent fever prior to vaccination decreased the immune response of some vaccines; the clinical significance of this reduction in immune response has not been established (Prymula, 2009).

Monitoring Parameters

Primary vaccines: Monitor vaccination site; inspect after 6-8 days. Evidence of a major reaction (vesicular or pustular lesion or an area of palpable induration surrounding a central lesion) confirms success of vaccination. An equivocal reaction (all responses other than a major reaction) requires revaccination in patients undergoing primary vaccination only (preferably with another vial or vaccine lot, if available). Consult CDC or state or local health department if response to a second vaccination from a different vial or lot is equivocal.

Revaccination: Successful vaccination is confirmed when a major cutaneous reaction is observed 6-8 days post-vaccination. Prior vaccinations may reduce the cutaneous response and does not necessarily indicate a vaccination failure. A revaccinated individual without a cutaneous response does not require revaccination.

Test Interactions Rapid plasma regain (RPR) test: Smallpox vaccine may induce false-positive RPR test for syphilis; confirm positive RPR test using a more specific test (eg, FTA assay).

Tuberculin skin (PPD) and blood tests: Smallpox vaccine may diminish the diagnostic utility of tuberculin skin (PPD) and blood tests; avoid skin test for ≥1 month after vaccine to prevent false-negative results.

Additional Information Initial reaction of the vaccine includes formation of a papule (2-5 days following vaccination). The papule forms a vesicle on day 5 or day 6, which becomes pustular, with surrounding erythema and induration. The maximal area of erythema usually occurs between day 8 and day 10, and crusting of the lesion normally occurs between day 14 and day 21. Formation of a major cutaneous reaction in patients undergoing primary vaccination by day 6-8 is indicative of successful acquisition of protective immunity. In patients previously vaccinated, the major cutaneous reaction typically seen by day 6-8 may be modified and/or reduced; a lack of cutaneous response does not indicate vaccination failure and revaccination is not required in these patients. At the peak of the reaction, systemic symptoms (fever, malaise) and lymphadenopathy may occur. All materials used in vaccination must be burned, boiled, or autoclaved. Vaccination can decrease the rate of severe or fatal smallpox if administered during the first 4 days of exposure. If vaccination failure occurs, revaccination should be attempted using a different vial or vaccine lot. If the second vaccination (from a different vial or lot) also fails, contact the Centers for Disease Control and Prevention (CDC) at 404-639-3670 and/or the state or local health department prior to administering any additional vaccine. Vaccinia immune globulin (VIG) is available from the CDC for the treatment of severe adverse reactions.

If vaccination failure occurs, revaccination should be attempted using a different vial or vaccine lot. If the second vaccination (from a different vial or lot) also fails, contact the Centers for Disease Control and Prevention (CDC) at 404-639-3670 and/or the state or local health department prior to administering any additional vaccine.

Vaccinia immune globulin (VIG) is available from the CDC for the treatment of severe adverse reactions.

Dosage Forms Excipient information presented when available (limited, particularly for generics); consult specific product labeling. [DSC] = Discontinued product

Injection, powder for reconstitution [purified monkey cell source]:

ACAM2000®: 1-5 x 10^8 plaque-forming units per mL [contains polymyxin B, neomycin (trace amounts) and human albumin; packed with diluent, tuberculin syringes for reconstitution, and 100 bifurcated needles for administration]

- ◆ **SMX-TMP** *see* Sulfamethoxazole and Trimethoprim *on page 1602*
- ◆ **SMZ-TMP** *see* Sulfamethoxazole and Trimethoprim *on page 1602*
- ◆ **(+)-(*S*)-*N*-Methyl-γ-(1-naphthyloxy)-2-thiophenepropylamine Hydrochloride** *see* DULoxetine *on page 565*
- ◆ **Sodium 2-Mercaptoethane Sulfonate** *see* Mesna *on page 1083*
- ◆ **Sodium 4-Hydroxybutyrate** *see* Sodium Oxybate *on page 1572*
- ◆ **Sodium *L*-Triiodothyronine** *see* Liothyronine *on page 1016*

Sodium Acetate (SOW dee um AS e tate)

Pharmacologic Category Electrolyte Supplement, Parenteral

Use Sodium source in large volume I.V. fluids to prevent or correct hyponatremia in patients with restricted intake; used to counter acidosis through conversion to bicarbonate

Pregnancy Risk Factor C

Contraindications Alkalosis, hypocalcemia, low sodium diets, edema, cirrhosis

Warnings/Precautions Avoid extravasation, use with caution in patients with edema, heart failure, severe hepatic failure, or renal impairment. Use with caution in patients with acid/base alterations; contains acetate, monitor closely during acid/base correction. Close monitoring of serum sodium concentrations is needed to avoid hypernatremia. Solution for injection contains aluminum; use with caution in patients with impaired renal function and in premature infants.

Adverse Reactions 1% to 10%:

Cardiovascular: Thrombosis, hypervolemia

Dermatologic: Chemical cellulitis at injection site (extravasation)

Endocrine & metabolic: Hypernatremia, dilution of serum electrolytes, overhydration, hypokalemia, metabolic alkalosis, hypocalcemia

Gastrointestinal: Gastric distension, flatulence

Local: Phlebitis

Respiratory: Pulmonary edema

Miscellaneous: Congestive conditions

Drug Interactions

Metabolism/Transport Effects None known.

Avoid Concomitant Use There are no known interactions where it is recommended to avoid concomitant use.

Increased Effect/Toxicity There are no known significant interactions involving an increase in effect.

Decreased Effect There are no known significant interactions involving a decrease in effect.

Stability Protect from light, heat, and freezing.

Dosage Sodium acetate is metabolized to bicarbonate on an equimolar basis outside the liver; administer in large volume I.V. fluids as a sodium source. Refer to Sodium Bicarbonate monograph.

Maintenance electrolyte requirements of sodium in parenteral nutrition solutions:

Daily requirements: 3-4 mEq/kg/24 hours or 25-40 mEq/1000 kcal/24 hours

Maximum: 100-150 mEq/24 hours

Dietary Considerations Sodium acetate anhydrous (2 mEq/mL): 1 mL = 164 mg sodium acetate anhydrous = 2 mEq of sodium (46 mg) and acetate (118 mg)

Administration Must be diluted prior to I.V. administration; infusion hypertonic solutions (>154 mEq/L) via a central line; maximum rate of administration: 1 mEq/kg/hour

Dosage Forms Excipient information presented when available (limited, particularly for generics); consult specific product labeling.

Injection, solution, as anhydrous [concentrate, preservative free]: 2 mEq/mL (20 mL, 50 mL, 100 mL); 4 mEq/mL (50 mL, 100 mL)

◆ **Sodium Acid Carbonate** *see* Sodium Bicarbonate *on page 1566*

◆ **Sodium Acid Phosphate and Methenamine** *see* Methenamine and Sodium Acid Phosphate *on page 1094*

◆ **Sodium Artesunate** *see* Artesunate *on page 148*

◆ **Sodium Benzoate and Caffeine** *see* Caffeine *on page 259*

◆ **Sodium Benzoate and Sodium Phenylacetate** *see* Sodium Phenylacetate and Sodium Benzoate *on page 1572*

Sodium Bicarbonate (SOW dee um bye KAR bun ate)

Brand Names: U.S. Brioschi® [OTC]; Neut®

Index Terms Baking Soda; $NaHCO_3$; Sodium Acid Carbonate; Sodium Hydrogen Carbonate

Pharmacologic Category Alkalinizing Agent; Antacid; Electrolyte Supplement, Oral; Electrolyte Supplement, Parenteral

Additional Appendix Information

Contrast Media Reactions, Premedication for Prophylaxis *on page 1976*

Use Management of metabolic acidosis; gastric hyperacidity; as an alkalinization agent for the urine; treatment of hyperkalemia; management of overdose of certain drugs, including tricyclic antidepressants and aspirin

Unlabeled Use Prevention of contrast-induced nephropathy (CIN)

Pregnancy Risk Factor C

Lactation Enters breast milk/compatible

Contraindications Alkalosis, hypernatremia, severe pulmonary edema, hypocalcemia, unknown abdominal pain

Warnings/Precautions Rapid administration in neonates and children <2 years of age has led to hypernatremia, decreased CSF pressure and intracranial hemorrhage. **Use of I.V. $NaHCO_3$ should be reserved for documented metabolic acidosis and for hyperkalemia-induced cardiac arrest.** Routine use in cardiac arrest is not recommended. Avoid extravasation, tissue necrosis can occur due to the hypertonicity of $NaHCO_3$. May cause sodium retention especially if renal function is impaired; not to be used in treatment of peptic ulcer; use with caution in patients with HF, edema, cirrhosis, or renal failure. Not the antacid of choice for the elderly because of sodium content and potential for systemic alkalosis.

Adverse Reactions Frequency not defined.

Cardiovascular: Cerebral hemorrhage, CHF (aggravated), edema

Central nervous system: Tetany

Gastrointestinal: Belching, flatulence (with oral), gastric distension

Endocrine & metabolic: Hypernatremia, hyperosmolality, hypocalcemia, hypokalemia, increased affinity of hemoglobin for oxygen-reduced pH in myocardial tissue necrosis when extravasated, intracranial acidosis, metabolic alkalosis, milk-alkali syndrome (especially with renal dysfunction)

Respiratory: Pulmonary edema

Drug Interactions

Metabolism/Transport Effects None known.

Avoid Concomitant Use There are no known interactions where it is recommended to avoid concomitant use.

Increased Effect/Toxicity

Sodium Bicarbonate may increase the levels/effects of: Alpha-/Beta-Agonists; Amphetamines; Calcium Polystyrene Sulfonate; Dexmethylphenidate; Flecainide; Memantine; Methylphenidate; QuiNIDine; QuiNINE

The levels/effects of Sodium Bicarbonate may be increased by: AcetaZOLAMIDE

Decreased Effect

Sodium Bicarbonate may decrease the levels/effects of: ACE Inhibitors; Anticonvulsants (Hydantoin); Antipsychotic Agents (Phenothiazines); Atazanavir; Bisacodyl; Cefditoren; Cefpodoxime; Cefuroxime; Chloroquine; Corticosteroids (Oral); Dabigatran Etexilate; Dasatinib; Delavirdine; Erlotinib; Flecainide; Gabapentin; HMG-CoA Reductase Inhibitors; Iron Salts; Isoniazid; Itraconazole; Ketoconazole; Ketoconazole (Systemic); Lithium; Mesalamine; Methenamine; PenicillAMINE; Phosphate Supplements; Protease Inhibitors; Rilpivirine; Tetracycline Derivatives; Trientine

Ethanol/Nutrition/Herb Interactions Herb/Nutraceutical: Concurrent doses with iron may decrease iron absorption.

Stability Store injection at room temperature; do not freeze. Protect from heat. Use only clear solutions.

Prevention of contrast-induced nephropathy (unlabeled use): Remove 154 mL from 1000 mL bag of D_5W; replace with 154 mL of 8.4% sodium bicarbonate; resultant concentration is 154 mEq/L (Merten, 2004); more practically, institutions may remove 150 mL from 1000 mL bag of D_5W and replace with 150 mL of 8.4% sodium bicarbonate; resultant concentration is 150 mEq/L

Mechanism of Action Dissociates to provide bicarbonate ion which neutralizes hydrogen ion concentration and raises blood and urinary pH

Pharmacodynamics/Kinetics

Onset of action: Oral: Rapid; I.V.: 15 minutes

Duration: Oral: 8-10 minutes; I.V.: 1-2 hours

Absorption: Oral: Well absorbed

Excretion: Urine (<1%)

Dosage

Cardiac arrest (ACLS, 2010; PALS, 2010): **Routine use of $NaHCO_3$ is not recommended.** May be considered in the setting of prolonged cardiac arrest only after adequate alveolar ventilation has been established and effective cardiac compressions. **Note:** In some cardiac arrest situations (eg, metabolic acidosis, hyperkalemia, or tricyclic antidepressant overdose), sodium bicarbonate may be beneficial.

Infants and Children: I.V., I.O.: 1 mEq/kg/dose; repeat doses should be guided by arterial blood gases; children <2 years of age should receive 4.2% (0.5 mEq/mL) solution. **Note:** If I.O. route is used for administration and is subsequently used to obtain blood samples for acid-base analysis, results will be inaccurate.

Adults: I.V.: Initial: 1 mEq/kg/dose; repeat doses should be guided by arterial blood gases

Metabolic acidosis: Infants, Children, and Adults: Dosage should be based on the following formula if blood gases and pH measurements are available:

HCO_3^-(mEq) = 0.5 x weight (kg) x [24 - serum HCO_3^- (mEq/L)] **or** HCO_3^-(mEq) = 0.5 x weight (kg) x [desired increase in serum HCO_3^-(mEq/L)]

Administer 1/2 dose initially, then remaining 1/2 dose over the next 24 hours; monitor pH, serum HCO_3^-, and clinical status. **Note:** These equations provide an estimated replacement dose. The underlying cause and degree of acidosis may result in the need for larger or smaller replacement doses. In most cases, the initial goal of therapy is to target a pH of ~7.2 and a plasma bicarbonate level of ~10 mEq/L to prevent overalkalinization.

Note: If acid-base status is not available: Dose for older Children and Adults: 2-5 mEq/kg I.V. infusion over 4-8 hours; subsequent doses should be based on patient's acid-base status

Chronic renal failure: Oral: Initiate when plasma HCO_3^- <15 mEq/L

Children: 1-3 mEq/kg/day

Adults: Start with 20-36 mEq/day in divided doses, titrate to bicarbonate level of 18-20 mEq/L

Hyperkalemia (ACLS, 2010): Adults: I.V.: 50 mEq over 5 minutes (as appropriate, consider methods of enhancing potassium removal/excretion)

Renal tubular acidosis: Oral:

Distal:

Children: 2-3 mEq/kg/day

Adults: 0.5-2 mEq/kg/day in 4-5 divided doses

Proximal: Children and Adults: Initial: 5-10 mEq/kg/day; maintenance: Increase as required to maintain serum bicarbonate in the normal range

Urine alkalinization: Oral:

Children: 1-10 mEq (84-840 mg)/kg/day in divided doses every 4-6 hours; dose should be titrated to desired urinary pH

Adults: Initial: 48 mEq (4 g), then 12-24 mEq (1-2 g) every 4 hours; dose should be titrated to desired urinary pH; doses up to 16 g/day (200 mEq) in patients <60 years and 8 g (100 mEq) in patients >60 years

Antacid: Adults: Oral: 325 mg to 2 g 1-4 times/day

Prevention of contrast-induced nephropathy (unlabeled use): Adults: I.V. infusion: 154 mEq/L sodium bicarbonate in D_5W solution: 3 mL/kg/hour for 1 hour immediately before contrast injection, then 1mL/kg/hour during contrast exposure and for 6 hours after procedure

To prepare solution, remove 154 mL from 1000 mL bag of D_5W; replace with 154 mL of 8.4% sodium bicarbonate; resultant concentration is 154 mEq/L (Merten, 2004); more practically, institutions may remove 150 mL from 1000 mL bag of D_5W and replace with 150 mL of 8.4% sodium bicarbonate; resultant concentration is 150 mEq/L

Dietary Considerations Some products may contain sodium. Oral product should be taken 1-3 hours after meals.

Administration For I.V. administration to infants, use the 0.5 mEq/mL solution or dilute the 1 mEq/mL solution 1:1 with **sterile water**; for direct I.V. infusion in emergencies, administer slowly (maximum rate in infants: 10 mEq/minute); for infusion, dilute to a maximum concentration of 0.5 mEq/mL in dextrose solution and infuse over 2 hours (maximum rate of administration: 1 mEq/kg/hour)

Oral product should be administered 1-3 hours after meals.

Dosage Forms Excipient information presented when available (limited, particularly for generics); consult specific product labeling. [DSC] = Discontinued product

Granules for solution, oral [effervescent]:

Brioschi®: 2.69 g/capful (120 g, 240 g) [contains sodium 770 mg/capful; lemon flavor]

Brioschi®: 2.69 g/packet (12s) [contains sodium 770 mg/packet; lemon flavor]

Infusion, premixed in water for injection: 5% (500 mL [DSC]) [5.95 mEq/10 mL]

Injection, solution: 4.2% (10 mL) [5 mEq/10 mL]; 7.5% (50 mL [DSC]) [8.92 mEq/10 mL]; 8.4% (50 mL, 250 mL [DSC], 500 mL [DSC]) [10 mEq/10 mL]

Neut®: 4% (5 mL) [contains edetate disodium; 2.4 mEq/5 mL]

Injection, solution [preservative free]: 4.2% (5 mL) [5 mEq/10 mL]; 7.5% (50 mL) [8.92 mEq/10 mL]; 8.4% (10 mL, 50 mL) [10 mEq/10 mL]

Powder, oral: USP: 100% (120 g, 480 g)

Tablet, oral: 325 mg [3.8 mEq], 650 mg [7.6 mEq]

- ◆ **Sodium Bicarbonate and Omeprazole** *see* Omeprazole and Sodium Bicarbonate *on page 1244*
- ◆ **Sodium Biphosphate, Methenamine, Methylene Blue, Phenyl Salicylate, and Hyoscyamine** *see* Methenamine, Sodium Biphosphate, Phenyl Salicylate, Methylene Blue, and Hyoscyamine *on page 1094*

Sodium Chloride (SOW dee um KLOR ide)

Brand Names: U.S. 4-Way® Saline Moisturizing Mist [OTC]; Altachlore [OTC]; Altamist [OTC]; Ayr® Allergy Sinus [OTC]; Ayr® Baby Saline [OTC]; Ayr® Saline No-Drip [OTC]; Ayr® Saline [OTC]; Breathe Free® [OTC]; Deep Sea [OTC]; Entsol® [OTC]; HuMist® for Kids [OTC]; HuMist® [OTC]; HyperSal®; Little Noses® Saline [OTC]; Little Noses® Sterile Saline Nasal Mist [OTC]; Little Noses® Stuffy Nose Kit [OTC]; Muro 128® [OTC]; Na-Zone® [OTC]; Nasal Moist® Saline [OTC]; Nasal Spray [OTC] [DSC]; NāSal™ [OTC]; Ocean® for Kids [OTC]; Ocean® [OTC]; Pretz® [OTC]; Rhinaris® [OTC]; Saline Mist [OTC]; Simply Saline® Baby [OTC]; Simply Saline® Nasal Moist® [OTC]; Simply Saline® [OTC]; Syrex; Wound Wash Saline™ [OTC]

Index Terms Hypertonic Saline; NaCl; Normal Saline; Saline; Salt

Pharmacologic Category Electrolyte Supplement, Parenteral; Genitourinary Irrigant; Irrigant; Lubricant, Ocular; Sodium Salt

Additional Appendix Information
Contrast Media Reactions, Premedication for Prophylaxis *on page 1976*

Use
Parenteral: Restores sodium ion in patients with restricted oral intake (especially hyponatremia states or low salt syndrome).
Concentrated sodium chloride: Additive for parenteral fluid therapy
Hypertonic sodium chloride: For severe hyponatremia and hypochloremia
Hypotonic sodium chloride: Hydrating solution
Normal saline: Restores water/sodium losses
Ophthalmic: Reduces corneal edema
Inhalation: Restores moisture to pulmonary system; loosens and thins congestion caused by colds or allergies; diluent for bronchodilator solutions that require dilution before inhalation
Intranasal: Restores moisture to nasal membranes
Irrigation: Wound cleansing, irrigation, and flushing

Unlabeled Use Parenteral: Hypertonic saline: Refractory elevated intracranial pressure (ICP) due to various etiologies (eg, subarachnoid hemorrhage, neoplasm); transtentorial herniation syndrome; traumatic brain injury with elevated ICP. **Note:** May be used in patients in whom mannitol may not be recommended (eg, renal failure).

Pregnancy Risk Factor C

Contraindications Hypersensitivity to sodium chloride or any component of the formulation; hypertonic uterus, hypernatremia, fluid retention

Warnings/Precautions Use with caution in patients with HF, renal insufficiency, liver cirrhosis, hypertension, edema; sodium toxicity is almost exclusively related to how fast a sodium deficit is corrected; both rate and magnitude are extremely important; do not use bacteriostatic sodium chloride in newborns since benzyl alcohol preservatives have been associated with toxicity. Administration of low sodium or sodium-free I.V. solutions may result in significant hyponatremia or water intoxication in pediatric patients; monitor serum sodium concentration. Wound Wash Saline™ is for single-patient use only.

Irrigants: For external use only; not for parenteral use. Do not use during electrosurgical procedures. Irrigating fluids may be absorbed into systemic circulation; monitor for fluid or solute overload.

Adverse Reactions Frequency not defined.
Cardiovascular: Congestive heart failure, transient hypotension (especially with administration of 23.4% NaCl)
Central nervous system: Central pontine myelinolysis (due to rapid correction of hyponatremia)
Endocrine & metabolic: Dilution of serum electrolytes, extravasation, hypernatremia, hypervolemia, hypokalemia, overhydration
Local: Thrombosis, phlebitis, extravasation
Respiratory: Pulmonary edema

Drug Interactions

Metabolism/Transport Effects None known.

Avoid Concomitant Use
Avoid concomitant use of Sodium Chloride with any of the following: Tolvaptan

Increased Effect/Toxicity
Sodium Chloride may increase the levels/effects of: Tolvaptan

Decreased Effect
Sodium Chloride may decrease the levels/effects of: Lithium

Stability Store injection at room temperature; do not freeze. Protect from heat. Use only clear solutions.

Mechanism of Action Principal extracellular cation; functions in fluid and electrolyte balance, osmotic pressure control, and water distribution

Pharmacodynamics/Kinetics
Absorption: Oral: Rapid
Distribution: Widely distributed
Excretion: Primarily urine; also sweat, tears, saliva

Dosage
Children: I.V.: Hypertonic solutions (>0.9%) should only be used for the initial treatment of acute serious symptomatic hyponatremia or increased intracranial pressure in the setting of traumatic brain injury.
Maintenance: 3-4 mEq/kg/day; maximum: 100-150 mEq/day; dosage varies widely depending on clinical condition
Replacement: Determined by laboratory determinations mEq
Sodium deficiency (mEq/kg) = [% dehydration (L/kg)/100 x 70 (mEq/L)] + [0.6 (L/kg) x (140 - serum sodium) (mEq/L)]
Increased intracranial pressure (unlabeled use): Hypertonic saline (3%): 0.1-1 mL/kg/hour continuous infusion titrated to maintain ICP <20 mm Hg (Addleson, 2003)
Children ≥2 years and Adults:
Intranasal: 2-3 sprays in each nostril as needed
Irrigation: Spray affected area
Children and Adults: Inhalation: Bronchodilator diluent: 1-3 sprays (1-3 mL) to dilute bronchodilator solution in nebulizer prior to administration
Adults:
Refractory elevated ICP due to various etiologies (eg, subarachnoid hemorrhage, trauma, neoplasm), transtentorial herniation syndromes (unlabeled use): I.V.: Hypertonic saline: 23.4% (30-60 mL) given over 2-20 minutes administered via central venous access only (Koenig, 2008; Suarez, 1998; Ware, 2005)
Subarachnoid hemorrhage with hyponatremia (ie, ≤135 mEq/L) to enhance cerebral perfusion (unlabeled use): I.V.: Hypertonic saline: 3% sodium chloride/acetate (50:50 mixture) 100-200 mL/hour administered via central venous catheter; titrate to clinical response up to a maximum serum sodium between 150-160 mEq/L (achieved at a rate of 0.5-1 mEq/L/hour) (Suarez, 1999)
Traumatic brain injury with elevated ICP (unlabeled use): I.V.: Hypertonic saline: **Note:** Optimal dose has not been established; due to insufficient evidence, the Brain Trauma Foundation guidelines (Bratton, 2007) do not make specific recommendations on the use of hypertonic saline for the treatment of traumatic intracranial hypertension. Clinical trials are small; few are prospective. **Some concentrations may not be commercially available; administer via central venous catheter;** protocols include:
3%: 300 mL administered over 20 minutes when ICP values exceed 20 mm Hg (Huang, 2006)
7.2%: 1.5 mL/kg administered over 15 minutes when ICP values exceed 15 mm Hg (Munar, 2000)
7.5%: 2 mL/kg administered over 20 minutes when ICP values exceed 25 mm Hg (Vialet, 2003)
23.4%: 30 mL administered over 2 minutes (Ware, 2005) **or** over >30 minutes when ICP values exceed 20 mm Hg (Kerwin, 2009)
GU irrigant: 1-3 L/day by intermittent irrigation
Replacement I.V.: Determined by laboratory determinations mEq
Hyponatremia: Sodium deficiency (mEq/kg) = [% dehydration (L/kg)/100 x 70 (mEq/L)] + [0.6 (L/kg) x (140 - serum sodium) (mEq/L)]
To correct acute, serious hyponatremia: mEq sodium = [desired sodium (mEq/L) - actual sodium (mEq/L)] x [0.6 x wt (kg)]; for acute correction use 125 mEq/L as the desired serum sodium; acutely correct serum sodium in 5 mEq/L/dose increments; more gradual correction in increments of 10 mEq/L/day is indicated in the asymptomatic patient

Chloride maintenance electrolyte requirement in parenteral nutrition: 2-4 mEq/kg/24 hours or 25-40 mEq/1000 kcals/24 hours; maximum: 100-150 mEq/24 hours
Sodium maintenance electrolyte requirement in parenteral nutrition: 3-4 mEq/kg/24 hours or 25-40 mEq/1000 kcals/24 hours; maximum: 100-150 mEq/24 hours.

Approximate Deficits of Water and Electrolytes in Moderately Severe Dehydration[1]

Condition	Water (mL/kg)	Sodium (mEq/kg)
Fasting and thirsting	100-120	5-7
Diarrhea		
isonatremic	100-120	8-10
hypernatremic	100-120	2-4
hyponatremic	100-120	10-12
Pyloric stenosis	100-120	8-10
Diabetic acidosis	100-120	9-10

[1]A **negative** deficit indicates total body **excess** prior to treatment.

Adapted from Behrman RE, Kleigman RM, Nelson WE, et al, eds, *Nelson Textbook of Pediatrics*, 14th ed, WB Saunders Co, 1992.

Ophthalmic:
Ointment: Apply once daily or more often
Solution: Instill 1-2 drops into affected eye(s) every 3-4 hours

Administration
Irrigation solution: Do not warm >66°C (150°F); not for I.V. use. Wound Wash Saline™: Before use, expel a short stream into air to clear nozzle.
I.V.: ≥3% solutions: Administration through a central line is recommended due to high osmolarity and tonicity

Monitoring Parameters Serum sodium, potassium, chloride, and bicarbonate concentrations; I & O, weight

Reference Range Serum/plasma sodium concentration:
Neonates:
Full-term: 133-142 mEq/L
Premature: 132-140 mEq/L
Children ≥2 months to Adults: 135-145 mEq/L

Dosage Forms Excipient information presented when available (limited, particularly for generics); consult specific product labeling. [DSC] = Discontinued product
Aerosol, spray, intranasal [preservative free]:
Entsol®: 3% (100 mL) [chlorofluorocarbon free]
Little Noses® Sterile Saline Nasal Mist: 0.9% (50 mL) [ethanol free]
Gel, intranasal:
Ayr® Saline: < 0.5% (14 g) [contains aloe, soybean oil]
Entsol®: 3% (20 g) [contains aloe, benzalkonium chloride, vitamin E]
Rhinaris®: 0.2% (28.4 g) [contains benzalkonium chloride]
Simply Saline® Nasal Moist®: 0.65% (30 g) [contains aloe]
Gel, intranasal [spray]:
Ayr® Saline No-Drip: < 0.5% (22 mL) [contains benzalkonium chloride, benzyl alcohol, soybean oil]
Injection, solution: 0.45% (50 mL, 100 mL, 250 mL, 500 mL, 1000 mL); 0.9% (25 mL, 50 mL, 100 mL, 150 mL, 250 mL, 500 mL, 1000 mL); 3% (500 mL); 5% (500 mL)
Injection, solution [preservative free]: 0.9% (2 mL, 3 mL, 5 mL, 10 mL, 20 mL, 50 mL, 100 mL)
Injection, solution [I.V. flush]: 0.9% (10 mL)
Injection, solution [I.V. flush, preservative free]: 0.9% (1 mL, 2 mL, 2.5 mL, 3 mL, 5 mL, 10 mL, 50 mL, 125 mL)
Syrex: 0.9% (2.5 mL, 3 mL, 5 mL, 10 mL)
Injection, solution [bacteriostatic]: 0.9% (10 mL, 20 mL, 30 mL)
Injection, solution [concentrate]: 14.6% (20 mL, 40 mL); 23.4% (100 mL, 250 mL)
Injection, solution [concentrate, preservative free]: 14.6% (20 mL, 40 mL); 23.4% (30 mL, 100 mL, 200 mL)
Ointment, ophthalmic: 5% (3.5 g)
Altachlore: 5% (3.5 g)
Ointment, ophthalmic [preservative free]:
Muro 128®: 5% (3.5 g)
Powder for solution, intranasal [preservative free]:
Entsol®: 3% (10s)
Powder for solution, intranasal [concentrate, preservative free]:
Pretz®: 1 teaspoon/dose (360 g) [with yerba santa]
Solution, for blood processing [not for injection]: 0.9% (3000 mL)
Solution, for inhalation [preservative free]: 0.9% (3 mL, 5 mL, 15 mL); 3% (15 mL); 10% (15 mL)
Solution, for irrigation: 0.45% (2000 mL [DSC]); 0.9% (250 mL, 500 mL, 1000 mL, 1500 mL, 2000 mL, 3000 mL, 4000 mL, 5000 mL)
Solution, for irrigation [preservative free]: 0.9% (250 mL, 500 mL, 1000 mL, 1500 mL, 2000 mL, 3000 mL)
Solution, for irrigation [slush solution]: 0.9% (1000 mL)
Solution, for nebulization [preservative free]: 7% (4 mL)
HyperSal®: 3.5% (4 mL); 7% (4 mL)
Solution, intranasal [preservative free]:
Simply Saline®: 3% (44 mL)
Solution, intranasal [buffered/spray, preservative free]:
Pretz®: 0.75% (20 mL) [chlorofluorocarbon free; with yerba santa]
Solution, intranasal [drops]:
Ayr® Saline: 0.65% (50 mL) [ethanol free; contains benzalkonium chloride]
Solution, intranasal [drops/mist/spray]:
HuMist®: 0.65% (45 mL) [ethanol free]
HuMist® for Kids: 0.65% (30 mL) [ethanol free; bubblegum flavor]
Ocean®: 0.65% (45 mL, 473 mL) [gluten free; contains benzalkonium chloride, benzyl alcohol]
Ocean® for Kids: 0.65% (37.5 mL) [ethanol free; contains benzalkonium chloride]
Solution, intranasal [drops/spray]:
Ayr® Baby Saline: 0.65% (30 mL) [ethanol free; contains benzalkonium chloride]
Little Noses® Saline: 0.65% (30 mL) [contains benzalkonium chloride]
Little Noses® Stuffy Nose Kit: 0.65% (15 mL) [contains benzalkonium chloride]
Solution, intranasal [irrigation]:
Pretz®: 0.75% (960 mL) [contains benzalkonium chloride, sodium benzoate; with yerba santa]
Solution, intranasal [isotonic, buffered/spray]:
Pretz®: 0.75% (50 mL) [contains benzalkonium chloride, sodium benzoate; with yerba santa]
Solution, intranasal [mist]:
4-Way® Saline Moisturizing Mist: 0.74% (29.6 mL) [ethanol free; contains benzalkonium chloride, menthol]
Ayr® Allergy Sinus: 2.65% (50 mL)
Ayr® Saline: 0.65% (50 mL) [ethanol free; contains benzalkonium chloride]
Entsol®: 3% (30 mL) [contains benzalkonium chloride]
Rhinaris®: 0.2% (30 mL) [contains benzalkonium chloride]
Saline Mist: 0.65% (45 mL) [contains benzalkonium chloride]
Solution, intranasal [mist, preservative free]:
Simply Saline®: 0.9% (44 mL, 90 mL)
Simply Saline® Baby: 0.9% (45 mL)
Solution, intranasal [nasal wash, preservative free]:
Entsol®: 3% (240 mL)

Solution, intranasal [spray]: 0.65% (45 mL, 88 mL)
- Altamist: 0.65% (60 mL) [contains benzalkonium chloride]
- Breathe Free®: 0.65% (44.3 mL) [contains benzalkonium chloride]
- Deep Sea: 0.65% (45 mL) [contains benzalkonium chloride, benzyl alcohol]
- Na-Zone®: 0.65% (60 mL) [contains benzalkonium chloride]
- Nasal Moist® Saline: 0.65% (45 mL)
- Nasal Spray: 0.65% (45 mL [DSC]) [contains benzalkonium chloride, benzyl alcohol]
- NāSal™: 0.65% (30 mL) [ethanol free; contains benzalkonium chloride, thimerosal]

Solution, ophthalmic [drops]: 5% (15 mL)
- Altachlore: 5% (15 mL, 30 mL)
- Muro 128®: 2% (15 mL); 5% (15 mL, 30 mL)

Solution, topical [preservative free]:
- Wound Wash Saline™: 0.9% (90 mL, 210 mL)

Swab, intranasal:
- Ayr® Saline: < 0.5% (20s) [contains aloe, soybean oil]

Tablet, oral: 1 g

Tablet for solution, topical: 1000 mg

Sodium Chondroitin Sulfate and Sodium Hyaluronate

(SOW de um kon DROY tin SUL fate & SOW de um hye al yoor ON ate)

Brand Names: U.S. DisCoVisc®; Viscoat®

Index Terms Chondroitin Sulfate and Sodium Hyaluronate; Sodium Hyaluronate and Chondroitin Sulfate

Pharmacologic Category Ophthalmic Agent, Viscoelastic

Use Ophthalmic surgical aid in the anterior segment during cataract extraction and intraocular lens implantation

Pregnancy Risk Factor C

Dosage Ophthalmic: Adults: Carefully introduce (using a 27-gauge cannula) into anterior chamber during surgery

Additional Information Complete prescribing information for this medication should be consulted for additional detail.

Dosage Forms Excipient information presented when available (limited, particularly for generics); consult specific product labeling.

Injection, solution, intraocular:
- DisCoVisc®: Sodium chondroitin sulfate ≤4% and sodium hyaluronate ≤1.7% (1 mL) [provided in a kit which also contains 27-gauge cannula and cannula locking ring]
- Viscoat®: Sodium chondroitin sulfate ≤4% and sodium hyaluronate ≤3% (0.5 mL, 0.75 mL) [packaged with 27-gauge cannula and cannula locking ring]

Sodium Citrate and Citric Acid

(SOW dee um SIT rate & SI trik AS id)

Brand Names: U.S. Cytra-2; Oracit®; Shohl's Solution (Modified)

Brand Names: Canada PMS-Dicitrate

Index Terms Bicitra; Citric Acid and Sodium Citrate; Modified Shohl's Solution

Pharmacologic Category Alkalinizing Agent, Oral

Use Treatment of metabolic acidosis; alkalinizing agent in conditions where long-term maintenance of an alkaline urine is desirable

Pregnancy Risk Factor Not established

Dosage Oral: Systemic alkalization:

Infants and Children: 2-3 mEq/kg/day in divided doses 3-4 times/day **or** 5-15 mL with water after meals and at bedtime

Adults: 10-30 mL with water after meals and at bedtime

Additional Information Complete prescribing information for this medication should be consulted for additional detail.

Dosage Forms Excipient information presented when available (limited, particularly for generics); consult specific product labeling. **Note:** Contains sodium 1 mEq/mL and is equivalent to bicarbonate 1 mEq/mL

Solution, oral: Sodium citrate 500 mg and citric acid 334 mg per 5 mL (480 mL)
- Cytra-2: Sodium citrate 500 mg and citric acid 334 mg per 5 mL (480 mL) [alcohol free, dye free, sugar free; contains propylene glycol and sodium benzoate; grape flavor]
- Oracit®: Sodium citrate 490 mg and citric acid 640 mg per 5 mL (15 mL, 30 mL, 500 mL, 3840 mL)
- Shohl's Solution (Modified): Sodium citrate 500 mg and citric acid 300 mg per 5 mL (480 mL) [contains alcohol]

◆ **Sodium Citrate, Citric Acid, and Potassium Citrate** *see* Citric Acid, Sodium Citrate, and Potassium Citrate *on page* 372

◆ **Sodium Diuril®** *see* Chlorothiazide *on page* 344

◆ **Sodium Edecrin®** *see* Ethacrynic Acid *on page* 651

◆ **Sodium Etidronate** *see* Etidronate *on page* 666

◆ **Sodium Ferric Gluconate** *see* Ferric Gluconate *on page* 705

◆ **Sodium Fluorescein** *see* Fluorescein *on page* 727

◆ **Sodium Fluoride** *see* Fluoride *on page* 728

◆ **Sodium Hyaluronate** *see* Hyaluronate and Derivatives *on page* 831

◆ **Sodium Hyaluronate and Chondroitin Sulfate** *see* Sodium Chondroitin Sulfate and Sodium Hyaluronate *on page* 1570

◆ **Sodium Hydrogen Carbonate** *see* Sodium Bicarbonate *on page* 1566

Sodium Hypochlorite Solution

(SOW dee um hye poe KLOR ite soe LOO shun)

Brand Names: U.S. Dakin's Solution; Di-Dak-Sol

Index Terms Modified Dakin's Solution

Pharmacologic Category Disinfectant, Antibacterial (Topical)

Use Treatment of athlete's foot (0.5%); wound irrigation (0.5%); disinfection of utensils and equipment (5%)

Pregnancy Risk Factor C

Dosage Topical via irrigation: Children and Adults:

Lightly-to-moderately exudative wounds: Apply once daily

Highly exudative or contaminated wounds: Apply twice daily.

Additional Information Complete prescribing information for this medication should be consulted for additional detail.

Dosage Forms Excipient information presented when available (limited, particularly for generics); consult specific product labeling.

Solution, topical:
- Dakin's Solution: 0.125% (473 mL); 0.25% (473 mL); 0.5% (473 mL)
- Di-Dak-Sol: 0.0125% (473 mL)

◆ **Sodium Hyposulfate** *see* Sodium Thiosulfate *on page* 1577

◆ **Sodium Nafcillin** *see* Nafcillin *on page* 1170

Sodium Nitrite and Sodium Thiosulfate

(SOW dee um NYE trite & SOW dee um thye oh SUL fate)

Brand Names: U.S. Nithiodote™

Index Terms Sodium Thiosulfate and Sodium Nitrite

Pharmacologic Category Antidote

Use Acute, life-threatening cyanide poisoning

Pregnancy Risk Factor C

Pregnancy Considerations Teratogenic effects were not observed in animal reproduction studies of sodium nitrite or sodium thiosulfate. Embryotoxic and nonteratogenic effects were observed in animal reproduction studies of sodium nitrite. Methemoglobin reductase is lower in the fetus compared to adults and may result in adverse effects due to nitrite-induced prenatal hypoxia. There are no adequate and well-controlled studies of Nithiodote™ in pregnant women; use in pregnant women only if the benefit to the mother outweighs the potential risk to the fetus.

Lactation Excretion in breast milk unknown/use caution

Contraindications There are no contraindications listed within the manufacturer's labeling.

Warnings/Precautions [U.S. Boxed Warning]: Sodium nitrite may cause methemoglobin formation and hypotension resulting in diminished oxygen carrying capacity; serious adverse effects may occur at doses less than the recommended therapeutic dose. Monitor for adequate perfusion and oxygenation; ensure patient is euvolemic. Use with caution in patients where the diagnosis of cyanide poisoning is uncertain, patients with pre-existing diminished oxygen or cardiovascular reserve (eg, smoke inhalation victims, anemia, substantial blood loss, and cardiac or respiratory compromise), in patients at greater risk for developing methemoglobinemia (eg, congenital methemoglobin reductase deficiency), and in patients who may be susceptible to injury from vasodilation. Use with caution with concomitant medications known to cause methemoglobinemia (eg, nitroglycerin). Collection of pretreatment blood cyanide concentrations does not preclude administration and should not delay administration in the emergency management of highly suspected or confirmed cyanide toxicity. Monitor patients for return of symptoms for 24-48 hours. Use nitrites cautiously in patients with cyanide poisoning related to smoke inhalation because methemoglobinemia and carboxyhemoglobinemia may worsen oxygen-carrying capacity. Consider consultation with a poison control center at 1-800-222-1222.

Concurrent use of antihypertensives, diuretics, and phosphodiesterase-5 enzyme (PDE5) inhibitors should be done with caution. Patients with anemia will form more methemoglobin; dosage reduction in proportion to oxygen carrying capacity is recommended. Patients with G6PD deficiency are at an increased risk for hemolytic crisis following sodium nitrite administration; monitor for an acute drop in hematocrit. The presence of sulfite hypersensitivity should not preclude the use of this medication.

Methemoglobin reductase, which is responsible for converting methemoglobin back to hemoglobin, has reduced activity in pediatric patients. In addition, infants and young children have some proportion of fetal hemoglobin which forms methemoglobin more readily than adult hemoglobin. Therefore, pediatric patients (eg, neonates and infants <6 months of age) are more susceptible to excessive nitrite-induced methemoglobinemia.

Adverse Reactions Frequency not defined.

Sodium nitrite:

Cardiovascular: Arrhythmias, cyanosis, flushing, hypotension, palpitation, tachycardia, syncope

Central nervous system: Anxiety, coma, confusion, dizziness, fatigue, headache, lightheadedness, seizure

Dermatologic: Urticaria

Endocrine & metabolic: Acidosis

Gastrointestinal: Abdominal pain, nausea, vomiting

Hematologic: Methemoglobinemia

Local: Injection site tingling

Neuromuscular & skeletal: Numbness, paresthesia, weakness

Ocular: Blurred vision

Respiratory: Dyspnea, tachypnea

Miscellaneous: Diaphoresis

Sodium thiosulfate:

Cardiovascular: Hypotension

Central nervous system: Disorientation, headache

Gastrointestinal: Nausea, salty taste, vomiting

Hematologic: Bleeding time prolonged

Miscellaneous: Warmth

Drug Interactions

Metabolism/Transport Effects None known.

Avoid Concomitant Use There are no known interactions where it is recommended to avoid concomitant use.

Increased Effect/Toxicity

Sodium Nitrite and Sodium Thiosulfate may increase the levels/effects of: Prilocaine

Decreased Effect There are no known significant interactions involving a decrease in effect.

Stability Store at 20°C to 25°C (68°F to 77°F); excursions permitted to 15°C to 30°C (59°F to 86°F); do not freeze. Protect from direct light.

Mechanism of Action

Sodium thiosulfate serves as a sulfur donor to increase endogenous rhondanese-catalyzed thiocyanate (much less toxic than cyanide) formation.

Sodium nitrite promotes formation of methemoglobin which competes with cytochrome oxidase for the cyanide ion. Cyanide combines with methemoglobin to form cyanomethemoglobin and frees the cytochrome oxidase, allowing aerobic metabolism to continue.

Pharmacodynamics/Kinetics

Sodium nitrite:

Onset: Peak effect: Methemoglobinemia: 30-60 minutes

Duration: Methemoglobinemia: ~55 minutes

Metabolism: To ammonia and other metabolites

Excretion: Urine (~40% as unchanged drug)

Sodium thiosulfate:

Half-life elimination: ~3 hours; renal impairment: ≤9 days

Excretion: Urine (~20% to 50% as unchanged drug)

Dosage I.V.:

Sodium nitrite:

Children: 6 mg/kg (0.2 mL/kg or 6-8 mL/m^2 of a 3% solution); maximum dose: 300 mg (10 mL of a 3% solution); may repeat at one-half the original dose if symptoms of cyanide toxicity return

Adults: 300 mg (10 mL of a 3% solution); may repeat at one-half the original dose if symptoms of cyanide toxicity return

Alternatively, patients who are unable to tolerate significant methemoglobinemia (ie, patients with comorbidities that compromise oxygen delivery, such as heart disease, lung disease, etc), dosing may be based on hemoglobin levels (when rapid bedside testing is available) to prevent fatal methemoglobinemia; see table (Berlin, 1970):

Hemoglobin Level (g/dL)	Dose of 3% Sodium Nitrite Solution
7	0.19 mL/kg
8	0.22 mL/kg
9	0.25 mL/kg
10	0.27 mL/kg
11	0.3 mL/kg
12	0.33 mL/kg
13	0.36 mL/kg
14	0.39 mL/kg

Sodium thiosulfate:

Children: 7 g/m^2 or 250 mg/kg (1 mL/kg or 28-40 mL/m^2 of a 25% solution); maximum dose: 12.5 g (50 mL of a 25% solution); may repeat at one-half the original dose if symptoms of cyanide toxicity return

Adults: 12.5 g (50 mL of a 25% solution); may repeat at one-half the original dose if symptoms of cyanide toxicity return

Note: Monitor the patient for 24-48 hours; if symptoms return, repeat both sodium nitrite and sodium thiosulfate at one-half the original doses.

Administration Administer via slow I.V. injection as soon as possible after diagnosis of acute, life-threatening cyanide poisoning. Administer sodium nitrite first over ≥5 minutes (2.5-5 mL/minute), followed immediately by the administration sodium thiosulfate over 10-20 minutes. Decrease rate of infusion in the event of significant hypotension, nausea, or vomiting.

Monitoring Parameters Monitor for at least 24-48 hours after administration; blood pressure and heart rate during and after infusion; hemoglobin/hematocrit; co-oximetry; serum lactate levels; venous-arterial PO_2 gradient; serum methemoglobin and oxyhemoglobin. Pretreatment cyanide levels may be useful diagnostically.

Dosage Forms Excipient information presented when available (limited, particularly for generics); consult specific product labeling.

Injection, solution [combination package]:

Nithiodote™: Sodium nitrite 300 mg/10 mL (10 mL) and sodium thiosulfate 12.5 g/50 mL (50 mL)

◆ **Sodium Nitroferricyanide** *see* Nitroprusside *on page 1214*

◆ **Sodium Nitroprusside** *see* Nitroprusside *on page 1214*

Sodium Oxybate (SOW dee um ox i BATE)

Brand Names: U.S. Xyrem®

Brand Names: Canada Xyrem®

Index Terms 4-Hydroxybutyrate; Gamma Hydroxybutyric Acid; GHB; Oxybate; Sodium 4-Hydroxybutyrate

Pharmacologic Category Central Nervous System Depressant

Additional Appendix Information

Patient Information for Disposal of Unused Medications *on page 2026*

Use Treatment of cataplexy and daytime sleepiness in patients with narcolepsy

Pregnancy Risk Factor B

Prescribing and Access Restrictions Sodium oxybate is deemed to have an approved REMS program. As a requirement of the REMS program, access to this medication is restricted. Sodium oxybate oral solution will be available only to prescribers enrolled in the Xyrem® Patient Success Program® and dispensed to the patient through the designated centralized pharmacy (1-866-997-3688). Prior to dispensing the first prescription, prescribers will be sent educational materials to be reviewed with the patient and enrollment forms for the postmarketing surveillance program. Patients must be seen at least every 3 months; prescriptions can be written for a maximum of 3 months (the first prescription may only be written for a 1-month supply).

Medication Guide Available Yes

Dosage Oral:

Children ≥16 years and Adults: Narcolepsy: Initial: 4.5 g/day, in 2 equal doses; first dose to be given at bedtime after the patient is in bed, and second dose to be given 2.5-4 hours later. Dose may be increased or adjusted in 2-week intervals; average dose: 6-9 g/day (maximum: 9 g/day)

Elderly: Safety and efficacy have not been studied in patients >65 years.

Dosage adjustment in renal impairment: Adjustment not necessary; consider sodium content

Dosage adjustment in hepatic impairment: Decrease starting dose to half and titrate doses carefully in patients with liver dysfunction. Elimination half-life significantly longer in patients with Child's class C liver dysfunction.

Additional Information Complete prescribing information for this medication should be consulted for additional detail.

Dosage Forms Excipient information presented when available (limited, particularly for generics); consult specific product labeling.

Solution, oral:

Xyrem®: 500 mg/mL (180 mL) [contains sodium 91 mg/mL]

Controlled Substance C-I (illicit use); C-III (medical use)

Sodium Phenylacetate and Sodium Benzoate

(SOW dee um fen il AS e tate & SOW dee um BENZ oh ate)

Brand Names: U.S. Ammonul®

Index Terms NAPA and NABZ; Sodium Benzoate and Sodium Phenylacetate

Pharmacologic Category Antidote; Urea Cycle Disorder (UCD) Treatment Agent

Use Adjunct to treatment of acute hyperammonemia and encephalopathy in patients with urea cycle disorders involving partial or complete deficiencies of carbamyl-phosphate synthetase (CPS), ornithine transcarbamoylase (OTC), argininosuccinate lysase (ASL), or argininosuccinate synthetase (ASS); for use with hemodialysis in acute neonatal hyperammonemic coma, moderate-to-severe hyperammonemic encephalopathy and hyperammonemia which fails to respond to initial therapy

Pregnancy Risk Factor C

Dosage Administer as a loading dose over 90-120 minutes, followed by an equivalent maintenance infusion given over 24 hours. Dosage based on weight and specific enzyme deficiency; therapy should continue until ammonia levels are in normal range. Repeat loading doses are not recommended due to the prolonged plasma levels.

Children ≤20 kg:

CPS and OTC deficiency: Ammonul® 2.5 mL/kg and arginine 10% 2 mL/kg (provides sodium phenylacetate 250 mg/kg, sodium benzoate 250 mg/kg, and arginine hydrochloride 200 mg/kg).

ASS and ASL deficiency: Ammonul® 2.5 mL/kg and arginine 10% 6 mL/kg (provides sodium phenylacetate 250 mg/kg, sodium benzoate 250 mg/kg, and arginine hydrochloride 600 mg/kg)

Note: Pending a specific diagnosis in infants, the bolus and maintenance dose of arginine should be 6 mL/kg. If ASS or ASL are excluded as diagnostic possibilities, reduce dose of arginine to 2 mL/kg/day.

Children >20 kg and Adults:

CPS and OTC deficiency: Ammonul® 55 mL/m^2 and arginine 10% 2 mL/kg (provides sodium phenylacetate 5.5 g/m^2, sodium benzoate 5.5 g/m^2, and arginine hydrochloride 200 mg/kg)

ASS and ASL deficiency: Ammonul® 55 mL/m^2 and arginine 10% 6 mL/kg (provides sodium phenylacetate 5.5 g/m^2, sodium benzoate 5.5 g/m^2, and arginine hydrochloride 600 mg/kg)

Dosage adjustment in renal impairment: Use with caution; monitor closely

Dialysis: Ammonia clearance is ~10 times greater with hemodialysis than by peritoneal dialysis or hemofiltration. Exchange transfusion is ineffective.

Dosage adjustment in hepatic impairment: Use with caution

Additional Information Complete prescribing information for this medication should be consulted for additional detail.

Dosage Forms Excipient information presented when available (limited, particularly for generics); consult specific product labeling.

Injection, solution [concentrate]:

Ammonul®: Sodium phenylacetate 100 mg and sodium benzoate 100 mg per 1 mL (50 mL)

Sodium Phenylbutyrate

(SOW dee um fen il BYOO ti rate)

Brand Names: U.S. Buphenyl®

Index Terms Ammonapse

Pharmacologic Category Urea Cycle Disorder (UCD) Treatment Agent

Use Adjunctive therapy in the chronic management of patients with urea cycle disorder involving deficiencies of carbamoylphosphate synthetase, ornithine transcarbamylase, or argininosuccinic acid synthetase

Pregnancy Risk Factor C

Dosage Oral: Management of urea cycle disorders:

Children <20 kg: Powder: 450-600 mg/kg/day, administered in equally divided amounts with each meal or feeding, 3-6 times daily (maximum dose: 20 g/day)

Children ≥20 kg and Adults: Powder or tablet: 9.9-13 g/m^2/day, administered in equally divided amounts with each meal or feeding, 3-6 times daily (maximum dose: 20 g/day)

Additional Information Complete prescribing information for this medication should be consulted for additional detail.

Dosage Forms Excipient information presented when available (limited, particularly for generics); consult specific product labeling.

Powder for solution, oral:

Buphenyl®: (250 g) [contains sodium 125 mg/g]

Tablet, oral:

Buphenyl®: 500 mg [contains sodium 62 mg/tablet]

◆ **Sodium Phosphate and Potassium Phosphate** *see* Potassium Phosphate and Sodium Phosphate *on page 1386*

Sodium Phosphates (SOW dee um FOS fates)

Brand Names: U.S. Fleet® Enema Extra® [OTC]; Fleet® Enema [OTC]; Fleet® Pedia-Lax™ Enema [OTC]; LaCrosse Complete [OTC]; OsmoPrep®; Visicol®

Brand Names: Canada Fleet Enema®

Index Terms Phosphates, Sodium

Pharmacologic Category Cathartic; Electrolyte Supplement, Parenteral; Laxative, Bowel Evacuant

Additional Appendix Information

Laxatives, Classification and Properties *on page 1893*

Use

Oral solution, rectal: Short-term treatment of constipation

Oral tablets (OsmoPrep®, Visicol®): Bowel cleansing prior to colonoscopy

I.V.: Source of phosphate in large volume I.V. fluids and parenteral nutrition; treatment and prevention of hypophosphatemia

Pregnancy Risk Factor C

Pregnancy Considerations Reproduction studies have not been conducted with these products. Use with caution in pregnant women.

Lactation Use caution in nursing women.

Medication Guide Available Yes

Contraindications Hypersensitivity to sodium phosphate salts or any component of the formulation; additional contraindications vary by product:

Enema: Ascites, clinically significant renal impairment, heart failure, imperforate anus, known or suspected GI obstruction, megacolon (congenital or acquired)

Intravenous preparation: Diseases with hyperphosphatemia, hypocalcemia, or hypernatremia

Oral preparation: Acute phosphate nephropathy (biopsy proven), bowel obstruction, congenital megacolon, toxic megacolon

Warnings/Precautions [U.S. Boxed Warning]: Acute phosphate nephropathy has been reported (rarely) with use of oral products as a colon cleanser prior to colonoscopy. Some cases have resulted in permanent renal impairment (some requiring dialysis). Risk factors for acute phosphate nephropathy may include increased age (>55 years of age), pre-existing renal dysfunction, bowel obstruction, active colitis, or dehydration, and the use of medicines that affect renal perfusion or function (eg, ACE inhibitors, angiotensin receptor blockers, diuretics, and possibly NSAIDs), although some cases have been reported in patients without apparent risk factors. Other preventive measures may include avoid exceeding maximum recommended doses and concurrent use of other laxatives containing sodium phosphate; encourage patients to adequately hydrate before, during, and after use; obtain baseline and postprocedure labs in patients at risk; consider hospitalization and intravenous hydration during bowel cleansing for patients unable to hydrate themselves (eg, frail patients).

Use with caution in patients with impaired renal dysfunction, pre-existing electrolyte imbalances, risk of electrolyte disturbance (hypocalcemia, hyperphosphatemia, hypernatremia), or dehydration. If using as a bowel evacuant, correct electrolyte abnormalities before administration. Use caution in patients with unstable angina, history of myocardial infarction arrhythmia, cardiomyopathy; use caution in patients with or at risk for arrhythmias (eg, cardiomyopathy, prolonged QT interval, history of uncontrolled arrhythmias, recent MI) or with concurrent use of other QT-prolonging medications; pre-/postdose ECGs should be considered in high-risk patients.

Use caution in inflammatory bowel disease; may induce colonic aphthous ulceration. Use caution in patients with any of the following: Bowel obstruction (including pseudo) or perforation, gastric retention or hypomotility, ileus, severe, chronic constipation, colitis, gastric bypass or bariatric surgery.

Use with caution in patients with a history of seizures and those at higher risk of seizures. Inadequate fluid intake may lead to dehydration. Use with caution in debilitated patients; consider each patient's ability to hydrate properly. Use with caution in geriatric patients. Laxatives and purgatives have the potential for abuse by bulimia nervosa patients. Other oral medications may not be well absorbed when given during bowel evacuation because of rapid intestinal peristalsis. Solutions for injection may contain aluminum; toxic levels may occur following prolonged administration in premature neonates or patients with renal impairment. Enemas and oral solution are available in pediatric and adult sizes; prescribe by "volume" not by "bottle."

Visicol®: Use caution with history of swallowing difficulties or esophageal narrowing. Tablet particles may be seen in the stool.

Adverse Reactions Frequency not defined.

Cardiovascular: Edema, hypotension

Central nervous system: Dizziness, headache

Endocrine & metabolic: Calcium phosphate precipitation, hypernatremia, hyperphosphatemia, hypocalcemia

Gastrointestinal: Abdominal bloating, abdominal pain, diarrhea, mucosal bleeding, nausea, superficial mucosal ulcerations, vomiting

Renal: Acute renal failure

Postmarketing and/or case reports: Acute phosphate nephropathy, anaphylaxis, arrhythmia, atrial fibrillation (following severe vomiting [tablet formulation]), BUN increased, creatinine increased, nephrocalcinosis (oral solution), pruritus, rash, renal tubular necrosis, swelling (face, lips, tongue), urticaria, seizure

Drug Interactions

Metabolism/Transport Effects None known.

Avoid Concomitant Use There are no known interactions where it is recommended to avoid concomitant use.

Increased Effect/Toxicity

Sodium Phosphates may increase the levels/effects of: Nonsteroidal Anti-Inflammatory Agents

The levels/effects of Sodium Phosphates may be increased by: ACE Inhibitors; Angiotensin II Receptor Blockers; Bisphosphonate Derivatives; Diuretics; Tricyclic Antidepressants

Decreased Effect

The levels/effects of Sodium Phosphates may be decreased by: Antacids; Calcium Salts; Iron Salts; Magnesium Salts; Sucralfate

Stability Store at 15°C to 30°C (59°F to 86°F).

Mechanism of Action As a laxative, exerts osmotic effect in the small intestine by drawing water into the lumen of the gut, producing distention and promoting peristalsis and evacuation of the bowel; phosphorous participates in bone deposition, calcium metabolism, utilization of B complex vitamins, and as a buffer in acid-base equilibrium

Pharmacodynamics/Kinetics

Onset of action: Cathartic: 3-6 hours; Rectal: 2-5 minutes

Absorption: Oral: ~1% to 20%

Excretion: Urine

Dosage Caution: With orders for I.V. phosphate, there is considerable confusion associated with the use of millimoles (mmol) versus milliequivalents (mEq) to express the phosphate requirement. The most reliable method of ordering I.V. phosphate is by millimoles, then specifying the potassium or sodium salt. Intravenous doses listed as mmol of phosphate.

Acute treatment of hypophosphatemia: I.V.: It is difficult to provide concrete guidelines for the treatment of severe hypophosphatemia because the extent of total body deficits and response to therapy are difficult to predict. Aggressive doses of phosphate may result in a transient serum elevation followed by redistribution into intracellular compartments or bone tissue. It is recommended that repletion of severe hypophosphatemia be done I.V. because large doses of oral phosphate may cause diarrhea and intestinal absorption may be unreliable. Intermittent I.V. infusion should be reserved for severe depletion situations; requires continuous cardiac monitoring. Guidelines differ based on degree of illness, need/use of TPN, and severity of hypophosphatemia. If hypokalemia exists (some clinicians recommend threshold of <4 mmol/L), consider phosphate replacement strategy with potassium (eg, potassium phosphates). Obese patients and/or severe renal impairment were excluded from phosphate supplement trials.

Children and Adults: There are no prospective studies of parenteral phosphate replacement in children. The following weight-based guidelines for adult dosing may be cautiously employed in pediatric patients. **Note:** 1 mmol phosphate = 31 mg phosphorus; 1 mg phosphorus = 0.032 mmol phosphate

General replacement guidelines (Lentz, 1978):

Low dose, serum phosphorus losses are recent and uncomplicated: 0.08 mmol/kg over 6 hours

Intermediate dose, serum phosphorus level 0.5-1 mg/dL (0.16-0.32 mmol/L): 0.16-0.24 mmol/kg over 6 hours

Note: The initial dose may be increased by 25% to 50% if the patient is symptomatic secondary to hypophosphatemia and lowered by 25% to 50% if the patient is hypercalcemic.

Critically-ill adult patients receiving concurrent enteral/parenteral nutrition (Brown, 2006; Clark, 1995): **Note:** Round doses to the nearest 7.5 mmol for ease of preparation. If administering with phosphate-containing parenteral nutrition, do not exceed 15 mmol/L within parenteral nutrition. May use adjusted body weight for patients weighing >130% of ideal body weight (and BMI <40 kg/m^2) by using [IBW + 0.25 (ABW-IBW)]:

Low dose, serum phosphorus level 2.3-3 mg/dL (0.74-0.96 mmol/L): 0.16-0.32 mmol/kg over 4-6 hours

Intermediate dose, serum phosphorus level 1.6-2.2 mg/dL (0.51-0.71 mmol/L): 0.32-0.64 mmol/kg over 4-6 hours

High dose, serum phosphorus <1.5 mg/dL (<0.5 mmol/L): 0.64-1 mmol/kg over 8-12 hours

Parenteral nutrition: I.V.:

Infants and Children: 0.5-2 mmol/kg/24 hours (Mirtallo, 2004 [ASPEN guidelines])

Children >50 kg and Adolescents: 10-40 mmol/24 hours (Mirtallo, 2004 [ASPEN guidelines])

Adults: 10-15 mmol/1000 kcal (Hicks, 2001) **or** 20-40 mmol/24 hours (Mirtallo, 2004 [ASPEN guidelines])

Laxative (Fleet®): Rectal:

Children 2-4 years: One-half contents of one 2.25 oz pediatric enema

Children 5-11 years: Contents of one 2.25 oz pediatric enema

Children ≥12 years and Adults: Contents of one 4.5 oz enema as a single dose

Laxative: Oral solution:

Children 5-9 years: 7.5 mL as a single dose; maximum single daily dose: 7.5 mL

Children 10-11 years: 15 mL as a single dose; maximum single daily dose: 15 mL

Children ≥12 years and Adults: 15 mL as a single dose; maximum single daily dose: 45 mL

Bowel cleansing prior to colonoscopy: Oral tablets:

Adults: **Note:** Do not use additional agents, especially sodium phosphate products.

Visicol®: A total of 40 tablets divided as follows:

Evening before colonoscopy: 3 tablets every 15 minutes for 6 doses, then 2 additional tablets in 15 minutes (total of 20 tablets)

3-5 hours prior to colonoscopy: 3 tablets every 15 minutes for 6 doses, then 2 additional tablets in 15 minutes (total of 20 tablets)

OsmoPrep®: A total of 32 tablets divided as follows:

Evening before colonoscopy: 4 tablets every 15 minutes for 5 doses (total of 20 tablets)

3-5 hours prior to colonoscopy: 4 tablets every 15 minutes for 3 doses (total of 12 tablets)

Elderly: Use with caution due to increased risk of renal impairment in the elderly

Dosage adjustment in renal impairment: Use with caution; ionized inorganic phosphate is excreted by the kidneys; oral solution is contraindicated in patients with kidney disease

Dosage adjustment in hepatic impairment: Not expected to be metabolized in the liver

Dietary Considerations Should be taken on an empty stomach with water; a clear liquid diet should be used for 12 hours prior to tablet administration. Some products may contain phenylalanine and/or sodium.

Administration

Intermittent I.V. infusion; do **not** administer I.V. push. Must be diluted prior to parenteral administration. In general, the dose, concentration of infusion, and rate of administration may be dependent on patient condition and specific institution policy. Intermittent infusion doses are typically prepared in 100-250 mL of NS or D_5W (usual concentration range: 0.15-0.6 mmol/mL). For adult patients with severe symptomatic hypophosphatemia (ie, <1.5 mg/dL), may administer at rates up to 15 mmol/hour (Rosen, 1995; Charron, 2003). In patients with renal dysfunction and/or less severe hypophosphatemia, slower administration rates (eg, over 4-6 hours) or oral repletion is recommended.

Bowel cleansing: Have patient drink ~8 ounces of water with each dose of sodium phosphate (total of 2 quarts/64 ounces); have patient rehydrate before and after colonoscopy

Constipation: Take on an empty stomach; dilute dose with 8 ounces cool water, then follow dose with 8 ounces water; **do not repeat dose within 24 hours**

Monitoring Parameters

I.V.: Serum calcium, sodium and phosphorus levels; renal function; after I.V. phosphate repletion, repeat serum phosphorus level should be checked 2-4 hours later

Oral: Bowel cleansing: Baseline and postprocedure labs (electrolytes, calcium, phosphorus, BUN, creatinine) in patients at risk for acute renal nephropathy, seizure, or who have a history of electrolyte abnormality; ECG in patients with risks for prolonged QT or arrhythmias. Ensure euvolemia before initiating bowel preparation.

Reference Range Note: Reference ranges may vary depending on the laboratory

Serum calcium: 8.4-10.2 mg/dL

Serum phosphorus: Both low and high ends of the normal range are higher in children than in adults.

Infants: 4.5-7.5 mg/dL (1.45-2.42 mmol/L)

Children: ~4.0-6.0 mg/dL (1.29-1.94 mmol/L)

Adults: 2.5-4.5 mg/dL (0.81-1.45 mmol/L)

Additional Information Phosphate salts may precipitate when mixed with calcium salts; solubility is improved in amino acid parenteral nutrition solutions; check with a pharmacist to determine compatibility.

Dosage Forms Excipient information presented when available (limited, particularly for generics); consult specific product labeling.

Injection, solution [concentrate; preservative free]: Phosphorus 3 mmol and sodium 4 mEq per 1 mL (5 mL, 15 mL, 50 mL) [equivalent to phosphorus 93 mg and sodium 92 mg per 1 mL; source of electrolytes; monobasic and dibasic sodium phosphate]

Solution, oral: Monobasic sodium phosphate monohydrate 2.4 g and dibasic sodium phosphate heptahydrate 0.9 g per 5 mL [sugar free; contains sodium 556 mg/5 mL, sodium benzoate; ginger-lemon flavor] (45 mL)

Solution, rectal [enema]: Monobasic sodium phosphate monohydrate 19 g and dibasic sodium phosphate heptahydrate 7 g per 118 mL delivered dose (133 mL)

Fleet® Enema: Monobasic sodium phosphate monohydrate 19 g and dibasic sodium phosphate heptahydrate 7 g per 118 mL delivered dose (133 mL) [contains sodium 4.4 g/118 mL]

Fleet® Enema Extra®: Monobasic sodium phosphate monohydrate 19 g and dibasic sodium phosphate heptahydrate 7 g per 197 mL delivered dose (230 mL) [contains sodium 4.4 g/197 mL]

Fleet® Pedia-Lax™ Enema: Monobasic sodium phosphate monohydrate 9.5 g and dibasic sodium phosphate heptahydrate 3.5 g per 59 mL delivered dose (66 mL) [contains sodium 2.2 g/59 mL]

LaCrosse Complete: Monobasic sodium phosphate monohydrate 19 g and dibasic sodium phosphate heptahydrate 7 g per 118 mL delivered dose (133 mL) [contains sodium 4.4 g/118 mL]

Tablet, oral [scored]:

OsmoPrep®, Visicol®: Monobasic sodium phosphate monohydrate 1.102 g and dibasic sodium phosphate anhydrous 0.398 g [sodium phosphate 1.5 g per tablet; gluten free]

Sodium Polystyrene Sulfonate

(SOW dee um pol ee STYE reen SUL fon ate)

Brand Names: U.S. Kalexate; Kayexalate®; Kionex®; SPS®

Brand Names: Canada Kayexalate®; PMS-Sodium Polystyrene Sulfonate

Pharmacologic Category Antidote

Use Treatment of hyperkalemia

Pregnancy Risk Factor C

Pregnancy Considerations Animal reproductive studies have not been conducted. There are no adequate and well-controlled studies in pregnant women. Use during pregnancy only if benefits outweigh the risks.

Lactation Excretion in breast milk unknown/use caution

Contraindications Hypersensitivity to sodium polystyrene sulfonate or any component of the formulation; hypokalemia; obstructive bowel disease; neonates with reduced gut motility (postoperatively or drug-induced); oral administration in neonates

Additional contraindications: Sodium polystyrene sulfonate suspension (**with** sorbitol): Rectal administration in neonates (particularly in premature infants); any postoperative patient until normal bowel function resumes

Warnings/Precautions Intestinal necrosis (including fatalities) and other serious gastrointestinal events (eg, bleeding, ischemic colitis, perforation) have been reported, especially when administered with sorbitol. Increased risk may be associated with a history of intestinal disease or surgery, hypovolemia, prematurity, and renal insufficiency or failure; use with sorbitol is not recommended. Avoid use in any postoperative patient until normal bowel function resumes or in patients at risk for constipation or impaction; discontinue use if constipation occurs. Oral or rectal administration of sorbitol-containing sodium polystyrene sulfonate suspensions is contraindicated in neonates (particularly with prematurity). Use with caution in patients with severe HF, hypertension, or edema; sodium load may exacerbate condition. Effective lowering of serum potassium from sodium polystyrene sulfonate may take hours to days after administration; consider alternative measures (eg, dialysis) or concomitant therapy (eg, I.V. sodium bicarbonate) in situations where rapid correction of severe hyperkalemia is required. Severe hypokalemia may occur; frequent monitoring of serum potassium is recommended within each 24-hour period; ECG monitoring may be appropriate in select patients. In addition to serum potassium-lowering effects, cation-exchange resins may also affect other cation concentrations possibly resulting in decreased serum magnesium and calcium. Large oral doses may cause fecal impaction (especially in elderly).

Concomitant administration of oral sodium polystyrene sulfonate with nonabsorbable cation-donating antacids or laxatives (eg, magnesium hydroxide) may result in systemic alkalosis and may diminish ability to reduce serum potassium concentrations; use with such agents is not recommended. In addition, intestinal obstruction has been reported with concomitant administration of aluminum hydroxide due to concretion formation. Enema will reduce the serum potassium faster than oral administration, but the oral route will result in a greater reduction over several hours. Oral administration in neonates and use in neonates with reduced gut motility (postoperatively or drug-induced) is contraindicated. Oral or rectal administration of sorbitol-containing sodium polystyrene sulfonate suspensions in neonates (particularly with prematurity) is also contraindicated due to propylene glycol content and risk of intestinal necrosis and digestive hemorrhage. Use sodium polystyrene sulfonate (**without** sorbitol) with caution in premature or low-birth-weight infants. Use with caution in children when administering rectally; excessive dosage or inadequate dilution may result in fecal impaction.

Adverse Reactions

Frequency not defined:

Endocrine & metabolic: Hypernatremia, hypocalcemia, hypokalemia, hypomagnesemia, sodium retention

Gastrointestinal: Anorexia, constipation, diarrhea, fecal impaction, intestinal necrosis (rare), intestinal obstruction (due to concretions in association with aluminum hydroxide), nausea, vomiting

<1% (Limited to important or life-threatening): Acute bronchitis (rare; associated with inhalation of particles), concretions, gastrointestinal bleeding, gastrointestinal ulceration, intestinal perforation, ischemic colitis

Drug Interactions

Metabolism/Transport Effects None known.

Avoid Concomitant Use

Avoid concomitant use of Sodium Polystyrene Sulfonate with any of the following: Laxatives; Meloxicam; Sorbitol

Increased Effect/Toxicity

Sodium Polystyrene Sulfonate may increase the levels/effects of: Aluminum Hydroxide; Digoxin

The levels/effects of Sodium Polystyrene Sulfonate may be increased by: Antacids; Laxatives; Meloxicam; Sorbitol

Decreased Effect

Sodium Polystyrene Sulfonate may decrease the levels/effects of: Lithium; Thyroid Products

Stability Store at 25°C (77°F); excursions permitted to 15°C to 30°C (59°F to 86°F). Store repackaged product in refrigerator and use within 14 days. Freshly prepared suspensions should be used within 24 hours. Do not heat resin suspension.

Mechanism of Action Removes potassium by exchanging sodium ions for potassium ions in the intestine (especially the large intestine) before the resin is passed from the body; exchange capacity is 1 mEq/g *in vivo*, and *in vitro* capacity is 3.1 mEq/g, therefore, a wide range of exchange capacity exists such that close monitoring of serum electrolytes is necessary

Pharmacodynamics/Kinetics

Onset of action: 2-24 hours

Absorption: None

Excretion: Completely feces (primarily as potassium polystyrene sulfonate)

Dosage

Children: Hyperkalemia:

Oral: 1 g/kg/dose every 6 hours

Rectal: 1 g/kg/dose every 2-6 hours (In small children and infants, employ lower doses by using the practical exchange ratio of 1 mEq K^+/g of resin as the basis for calculation)

Adults: Hyperkalemia:

Oral: 15 g 1-4 times/day

Rectal: 30-50 g every 6 hours

Dietary Considerations Do **not** mix in orange juice or in any fruit juice known to contain potassium. Some products may contain sodium.

Administration

Oral: Shake suspension well prior to administration. Administer orally (or via NG tube) as a suspension. **Do not mix in orange juice.** Chilling the oral mixture will increase palatability.

Powder for suspension: For each 1 g of the powdered resin, add 3-4 mL of water or syrup (amount of fluid usually ranges from 20-100 mL)

Rectal: Enema route is less effective than oral administration. Administer cleansing enema first. Each dose of the powder for suspension should be suspended in 100 mL of aqueous vehicle and administered as a warm emulsion (body temperature). The commercially available suspension should also be warmed to body temperature. During administration, the solution should be agitated gently. Retain enema in colon for at least 30-60 minutes and for several hours, if possible. Once retention time is complete, irrigate colon with a non-sodium-containing solution to remove resin.

Monitoring Parameters Serum electrolytes (potassium, sodium, calcium, magnesium); ECG in select patients

Reference Range Serum potassium: Adults: 3.5-5.2 mEq/L

Additional Information 1 g of resin binds approximately 1 mEq of potassium

Historically, sorbitol was often recommended as a cathartic agent to be administered with sodium polystyrene sulfonate (SPS) to prevent SPS-induced fecal impaction. However, SPS, particularly when used with sorbitol, has been associated with cases of intestinal necrosis and other serious GI adverse events. Due to the concern that sorbitol may increase the risk of intestinal necrosis, concomitant use of sorbitol is no longer recommended.

Sodium polystyrene sulfonate is commercially available in a liquid suspension containing 33% sorbitol (~20 grams sorbitol per 60 mL suspension).

Dosage Forms Excipient information presented when available (limited, particularly for generics); consult specific product labeling.

Powder for suspension, oral/rectal: (454 g)

Kalexate: (454 g) [contains sodium 100 mg (4.1 mEq)/g]

Kayexalate®: (454 g) [contains sodium 100 mg (4.1 mEq)/g]

Kionex®: (454 g) [contains sodium 100 mg (4.1 mEq)/g]

Suspension, oral/rectal:

Kionex®: 15 g/60 mL (60 mL, 480 mL) [contains ethanol 0.2%, propylene glycol, sodium 1500 mg (65 mEq)/60 mL, sorbitol; raspberry flavor]

SPS®: 15 g/60 mL (60 mL, 120 mL, 473 mL) [contains ethanol 0.3%, propylene glycol, sodium 1500 mg (65 mEq)/60 mL, sorbitol; cherry flavor]

◆ **Sodium Sulamyd (Can)** *see* Sulfacetamide (Ophthalmic) *on page 1599*

◆ **Sodium Sulfacetamide** *see* Sulfacetamide (Ophthalmic) *on page 1599*

◆ **Sodium Sulfacetamide** *see* Sulfacetamide (Topical) *on page 1599*

◆ **Sodium Sulfacetamide and Sulfur** *see* Sulfur and Sulfacetamide *on page 1607*

◆ **Sodium Sulfate, Magnesium Sulfate, and Potassium Sulfate** *see* Sodium Sulfate, Potassium Sulfate, and Magnesium Sulfate *on page 1576*

Sodium Sulfate, Potassium Sulfate, and Magnesium Sulfate

(SOW dee um SUL fate, poe TASS ee um SUL fate, & mag NEE zhum SUL fate)

Brand Names: U.S. Suprep® Bowel Prep Kit

Index Terms Magnesium Sulfate, Potassium Sulfate, and Sodium Sulfate; Magnesium Sulfate, Sodium Sulfate, and Potassium Sulfate; Potassium Sulfate, Magnesium Sulfate, and Sodium Sulfate; Potassium Sulfate, Sodium Sulfate, and Magnesium Sulfate; Sodium Sulfate, Magnesium Sulfate, and Potassium Sulfate

Pharmacologic Category Laxative, Osmotic

Use Bowel cleansing prior to GI examination

Pregnancy Risk Factor C

Medication Guide Available Yes

Dosage Oral: Adults: Bowel cleansing prior to GI exam:

Split-dose regimen: Total volume of liquid consumed over the course of treatment: 2880 mL (96 oz)

Evening before colonoscopy: Drink the entire contents of 1 bottle, diluted to a final volume of 480 mL (16 oz). Then drink 2 additional containers of water each (filled to the 16-ounce line) over the next hour, for an additional volume of 960 mL (32 oz).

Morning of the colonoscopy (10-12 hours after the evening dose): Repeat entire process with the second bottle: Drink entire contents of second bottle diluted to a final volume of 480 mL (16 oz); then drink 2 additional containers of water (each filled to the 16-ounce line) over the next hour, for an additional volume of 960 mL (32 oz). Complete at least 1 hour before the procedure.

Additional Information Complete prescribing information for this medication should be consulted for additional detail.

Dosage Forms Excipient information presented when available (limited, particularly for generics); consult specific product labeling. [DSC] = Discontinued product

Solution, oral:

Suprep® Bowel Prep Kit: Sodium sulfate 17.5 g, potassium sulfate 3.13 g, and magnesuim sulfate 1.6 g per 180 mL (180 mL) [contains sodium benzoate]

Sodium Tetradecyl (SOW dee um tetra DEK il)

Brand Names: U.S. Sotradecol®

Brand Names: Canada Trombovar®

Index Terms Sodium Tetradecyl Sulfate

Pharmacologic Category Sclerosing Agent

Use Treatment of small, uncomplicated varicose veins of the lower extremities

Pregnancy Risk Factor C

Dosage I.V.: Test dose: 0.5 mL given several hours prior to administration of larger dose; 0.5-2 mL (preferred maximum: 1 mL) in each vein, maximum: 10 mL per treatment session; 3% solution reserved for large varices

Additional Information Complete prescribing information for this medication should be consulted for additional detail.

Dosage Forms Excipient information presented when available (limited, particularly for generics); consult specific product labeling.

Injection, solution, as sulfate:

Sotradecol®: 1% (2 mL); 3% (2 mL) [contains benzyl alcohol]

◆ **Sodium Tetradecyl Sulfate** *see* Sodium Tetradecyl *on page 1577*

Sodium Thiosulfate (SOW dee um thye oh SUL fate)

Brand Names: U.S. Versiclear™

Index Terms Disodium Thiosulfate Pentahydrate; Pentahydrate; Sodium Hyposulfate; Sodium Thiosulphate; Thiosulfuric Acid Disodium Salt

Pharmacologic Category Antidote

Use

Parenteral: Used alone or with sodium nitrite or amyl nitrite in cyanide poisoning; reduce the risk of nephrotoxicity associated with cisplatin therapy; treatment of cyanide poisoning due to nitroprusside

Topical: Treatment of tinea versicolor

Unlabeled Use Management of I.V. extravasation

Pregnancy Risk Factor C

Pregnancy Considerations Safety has not been established in pregnant women. Use only when potential benefit to the mother outweighs the possible risk to the fetus.

Contraindications Hypersensitivity to sodium thiosulfate or any component of the formulation

Warnings/Precautions Safety in pregnancy has not been established; discontinue topical use if irritation or sensitivity occurs; rapid I.V. infusion has caused transient hypotension and ECG changes in dogs; can increase risk of thiocyanate intoxication; use caution with renal impairment.

Fire victims may present with both cyanide and carbon monoxide poisoning. Collection of pretreatment blood cyanide concentrations does not preclude administration and should not delay administration in the emergency management of highly suspected or confirmed cyanide toxicity. Patients receiving treatment for acute cyanide toxicity must be monitored for return of symptoms for 24-48 hours.

Adverse Reactions Frequency not defined

Cardiovascular: Hypotension (infusion rate-dependent)

Dermatologic: Contact dermatitis, local irritation

Gastrointestinal: Nausea, vomiting

Miscellaneous: Hypersensitivity reactions

Drug Interactions

Metabolism/Transport Effects None known.

Avoid Concomitant Use There are no known interactions where it is recommended to avoid concomitant use.

Increased Effect/Toxicity There are no known significant interactions involving an increase in effect.

Decreased Effect There are no known significant interactions involving a decrease in effect.

Stability Store at 15°C to 30°C (59°F to 86°F); stable diluted in NS, D_5W, or $D_5{}^1/_2NS$ at concentrations of 1.5% and 9.76% sodium thiosulfate for 24 hours (Redkar, 1986)

Mechanism of Action

Cyanide toxicity: Accelerates the clearance of cyanide via the rhodanase-catalyzed detoxification of cyanide to thiocyanate (much less toxic than cyanide). The accelerated action of rhodanase is a result of the exogenous sulfur provided by sodium thiosulfate.

Cisplatin toxicity: Complexes with cisplatin to form a compound that is nontoxic to either normal or cancerous cells

Pharmacodynamics/Kinetics

Absorption: Oral: Poor

Distribution: Extracellular fluid

Half-life elimination: 0.65 hour

Excretion: Urine (28.5% as unchanged drug)

Dosage

Cyanide poisoning: I.V.: **Note:** Death from cyanide poisoning may occur rapidly, do not delay antidote administration in the event of highly suspected or confirmed cyanide poisoning; usually given in conjunction with amyl nitrite and sodium nitrite

Children: 7 g/m^2 (maximum dose: 12.5 g) given over 10 minutes; may repeat at $^1/_2$ the original dose if symptoms return

Adults: 12.5 g given over 10 minutes; may repeat at $^1/_2$ the original dose if symptoms return

Cisplatin rescue should be given before or during cisplatin administration: I.V. infusion (in sterile water): 12 g/m^2 over 6 hours or 9 g/m^2 I.V. push followed by 1.2 g/m^2 continuous infusion for 6 hours

Tinea versicolor: Children and Adults: Topical: 20% to 25% solution: Apply a thin layer to affected areas twice daily

Drug extravasation (unlabeled use): Children and Adults: SubQ: 1/6 M (~4%) solution: Inject into the affected area; various volumes have also been suggested for direct injection into existing I.V. line; however, the optimal volume and efficacy of such practices have not been thoroughly evaluated. **Note:** Use only for large cisplatin infiltrates (>20 mL) and cisplatin concentrations >0.5 mg/mL.

Administration

I.V.: Inject slowly, over at least 10 minutes; rapid administration may cause hypotension.

Topical: Do not apply to or near eyes.

Monitoring Parameters Monitor for signs of thiocyanate toxicity; monitor for hypotension and hypersensitivity reactions

Dosage Forms Excipient information presented when available (limited, particularly for generics); consult specific product labeling.

Injection, solution [preservative free]: 100 mg/mL (10 mL); 250 mg/mL (50 mL)

Lotion, topical:

Versiclear™: Sodium thiosulfate 25% and salicylic acid 1% (120 mL)

- **Sodium Thiosulfate and Sodium Nitrite** *see* Sodium Nitrite and Sodium Thiosulfate *on page 1570*
- **Sodium Thiosulphate** *see* Sodium Thiosulfate *on page 1577*
- **Soflax™ (Can)** *see* Docusate *on page 537*
- **Solaquin® (Can)** *see* Hydroquinone *on page 846*
- **Solaquin Forte® (Can)** *see* Hydroquinone *on page 846*
- **Solarcaine® cool aloe Burn Relief [OTC]** *see* Lidocaine (Topical) *on page 1009*
- **Solia® [DSC]** *see* Ethinyl Estradiol and Desogestrel *on page 653*

Solifenacin (sol i FEN a sin)

Brand Names: U.S. VESIcare®

Index Terms Solifenacin Succinate; YM905

Pharmacologic Category Anticholinergic Agent

Use Treatment of overactive bladder with symptoms of urinary frequency, urgency, or urge incontinence

Pregnancy Risk Factor C

Pregnancy Considerations Decreased fetal weight, increased incidence of cleft palate, and delayed physical development were observed in some animal studies. There are no adequate or well-controlled studies in pregnant women. Use during pregnancy only if the benefit to the mother outweighs the potential risk to the fetus.

Lactation Excretion in breast milk unknown/not recommended

Contraindications Hypersensitivity to solifenacin or any component of the formulation; urinary retention; gastric retention; uncontrolled narrow-angle glaucoma.

Warnings/Precautions Cases of angioedema involving the face, lips, tongue, and/or larynx have been reported. Immediately discontinue if tongue, hypopharynx, or larynx are involved. May cause drowsiness and/or blurred vision, which may impair physical or mental abilities; patients must be cautioned about performing tasks which require mental alertness (eg, operating machinery or driving). Heat prostration may occur in the presence of increased environmental temperature; use caution in hot weather and/or exercise. Use with caution in patients with bladder outflow obstruction, gastrointestinal obstructive disorders, and decreased gastrointestinal motility. Use with caution in patients with a known history of QT prolongation or other risk factors for QT prolongation (eg, concomitant use of medications known to prolong QT interval and/or electrolyte abnormalities); the risk for QT prolongation is dose-related. Use with caution in patients with controlled (treated) narrow-angle glaucoma; use is contraindicated with uncontrolled narrow-angle glaucoma. Dosage adjustment is required for patients with severe renal impairment (Cl_{cr} <30 mL/minute) or moderate (Child-Pugh class B) hepatic impairment; use is not recommended with severe hepatic impairment (Child-Pugh class C). Patients on potent CYP3A4 inhibitors require the lower dose of solifenacin.

Adverse Reactions

>10%: Gastrointestinal: Xerostomia (11% to 28%; dose-related), constipation (5% to 13%; dose-related)

1% to 10%:

Cardiovascular: Edema (≤1%), hypertension (≤1%)

Central nervous system: Headache (3% to 6%), fatigue (1% to 2%), depression (≤1%)

Gastrointestinal: Dyspepsia (1% to 4%), nausea (2% to 3%), upper abdominal pain (1% to 2%)

Genitourinary: Urinary tract infection (3% to 5%), urinary retention (≤1%)

Ocular: Blurred vision (4% to 5%), dry eyes (≤2%)

Respiratory: Cough (≤1%)

Miscellaneous: Influenza (≤2%)

<1% (Limited to important or life-threatening): Angioneurotic edema with airway obstruction, confusion, fecal impaction, gastrointestinal obstruction, hallucination, hypersensitivity, pruritus, QT_c prolongation, rash, torsade de pointes, urticaria

Drug Interactions

Metabolism/Transport Effects Substrate of CYP3A4 (major); **Note:** Assignment of Major/Minor substrate status based on clinically relevant drug interaction potential

Avoid Concomitant Use

Avoid concomitant use of Solifenacin with any of the following: Conivaptan

Increased Effect/Toxicity

Solifenacin may increase the levels/effects of: AbobotulinumtoxinA; Anticholinergics; Cannabinoids; OnabotulinumtoxinA; Potassium Chloride; RimabotulinumtoxinB

The levels/effects of Solifenacin may be increased by: Antifungal Agents (Azole Derivatives, Systemic); Conivaptan; CYP3A4 Inhibitors (Moderate); CYP3A4 Inhibitors (Strong); Dasatinib; Pramlintide

Decreased Effect

Solifenacin may decrease the levels/effects of: Acetylcholinesterase Inhibitors (Central); Secretin

The levels/effects of Solifenacin may be decreased by: Acetylcholinesterase Inhibitors (Central); CYP3A4 Inducers (Strong); Deferasirox; Herbs (CYP3A4 Inducers); Tocilizumab

Ethanol/Nutrition/Herb Interactions

Food: Grapefruit juice may increase the serum level effects of solifenacin.

Herb/Nutraceutical: St John's wort (*Hypericum*) may decrease the levels/effects of solifenacin.

Stability Store at controlled room temperature of 25°C (77°F); excursions permitted to 15°C to 30°C (59°F to 86°F).

Mechanism of Action Inhibits muscarinic receptors resulting in decreased urinary bladder contraction, increased residual urine volume, and decreased detrusor muscle pressure.

Pharmacodynamics/Kinetics

Distribution: V_d: 600 L

Protein binding: ~98% bound primarily to alpha$_1$-acid glycoprotein

Metabolism: Extensively hepatic; via N-oxidation and 4 R-hydroxylation, forms 1 active and 3 inactive metabolites; primary pathway for elimination is via CYP3A4

Bioavailability: ~90%
Half-life elimination: 45-68 hours following chronic dosing; prolonged in severe renal (Cl_{cr} <30 mL/minute) or moderate hepatic (Child-Pugh class B) impairment
Time to peak, plasma: 3-8 hours
Excretion: Urine 69% (<15% as unchanged drug); feces 23%

Dosage Oral: Adults: 5 mg once daily; if tolerated, may increase to 10 mg once daily
Dosage adjustment with concomitant CYP3A4 inhibitors: Maximum solifenacin dose: 5 mg/day

Dosage adjustment in renal impairment: Use with caution in reduced renal function
Cl_{cr} <30 mL/minute: Maximum dose: 5 mg/day

Dosage adjustment in hepatic impairment: Use with caution in reduced hepatic function
Moderate (Child-Pugh class B): Maximum dose: 5 mg/day
Severe (Child-Pugh class C): Use is not recommended

Dietary Considerations May be taken without regard to meals.

Administration Swallow tablet whole; administer with liquids; may be administered without regard to meals.

Monitoring Parameters Anticholinergic effects (eg, fixed and dilated pupils, blurred vision, tremors, or dry skin); creatinine clearance (prior to treatment for dosing adjustment); liver function

Dosage Forms Excipient information presented when available (limited, particularly for generics); consult specific product labeling.
Tablet, oral, as succinate:
VESIcare®: 5 mg, 10 mg

◆ **Solifenacin Succinate** *see* Solifenacin *on page* 1578
◆ **Soliris®** *see* Eculizumab *on page* 570
◆ **Solodyn®** *see* Minocycline *on page* 1137
◆ **Soluble Fluorescein** *see* Fluorescein *on page* 727
◆ **Solu-CORTEF®** *see* Hydrocortisone (Systemic) *on page* 839
◆ **Solu-Cortef® (Can)** *see* Hydrocortisone (Systemic) *on page* 839
◆ **Solumedrol** *see* MethylPREDNISolone *on page* 1110
◆ **Solu-MEDROL®** *see* MethylPREDNISolone *on page* 1110
◆ **Solu-Medrol® (Can)** *see* MethylPREDNISolone *on page* 1110
◆ **Solzira** *see* Gabapentin Enacarbil *on page* 775
◆ **Soma®** *see* Carisoprodol *on page* 291
◆ **Soma® Compound** *see* Carisoprodol and Aspirin *on page* 292
◆ **Soma Compound w/Codeine** *see* Carisoprodol, Aspirin, and Codeine *on page* 292

Somatropin (soe ma TROE pin)

Brand Names: U.S. Genotropin Miniquick®; Genotropin®; Humatrope®; Norditropin FlexPro®; Norditropin® NordiFlex®; Norditropin® [DSC]; Nutropin AQ Pen®; Nutropin AQ®; Nutropin AQ® NuSpin™; Nutropin®; Omnitrope®; Saizen®; Serostim®; Tev-Tropin®; Zorbtive®

Brand Names: Canada Humatrope®; Nutropin®; Nutropin® AQ; Omnitrope®; Saizen®; Serostim®

Index Terms Growth Hormone, Human; hGH; Human Growth Hormone

Pharmacologic Category Growth Hormone

Use
Children:
Treatment of growth failure due to inadequate endogenous growth hormone secretion (Genotropin®, Humatrope®, Norditropin®, Nutropin®, Nutropin AQ®, Omnitrope®, Saizen®, Tev-Tropin®)
Treatment of short stature associated with Turner syndrome (Genotropin®, Humatrope®, Norditropin®, Nutropin®, Nutropin AQ®, Omnitrope®)
Treatment of Prader-Willi syndrome (Genotropin®, Omnitrope®)
Treatment of growth failure associated with chronic renal insufficiency (CRI) up until the time of renal transplantation (Nutropin®, Nutropin AQ®)
Treatment of growth failure in children born small for gestational age who fail to manifest catch-up growth by 2 years of age (Genotropin®, Omnitrope®) or by 2-4 years of age (Humatrope®, Norditropin®)
Treatment of idiopathic short stature (nongrowth hormone-deficient short stature) defined by height standard deviation score (SDS) ≤-2.25 and growth rate not likely to attain normal adult height (Genotropin®, Humatrope®, Nutropin®, Nutropin AQ®, Omnitrope®)
Treatment of short stature or growth failure associated with short stature homeobox gene (SHOX) deficiency (Humatrope®)
Treatment of short stature associated with Noonan syndrome (Norditropin®)
Adults:
HIV patients with wasting or cachexia with concomitant antiviral therapy (Serostim®)
Replacement of endogenous growth hormone in patients with adult growth hormone deficiency who meet both of the following criteria (Genotropin®, Humatrope®, Norditropin®, Nutropin®, Nutropin AQ®, Omnitrope®, Saizen®):
Biochemical diagnosis of adult growth hormone deficiency by means of a subnormal response to a standard growth hormone stimulation test (peak growth hormone ≤5 mcg/L). Confirmatory testing may not be required in patients with congenital/genetic growth hormone deficiency or multiple pituitary hormone deficiencies due to organic diseases.
and
Adult-onset: Patients who have adult growth hormone deficiency whether alone or with multiple hormone deficiencies (hypopituitarism) as a result of pituitary disease, hypothalamic disease, surgery, radiation therapy, or trauma
or
Childhood-onset: Patients who were growth hormone deficient during childhood, confirmed as an adult before replacement therapy is initiated
Treatment of short-bowel syndrome (Zorbtive®)

Unlabeled Use Pediatric HIV patients with wasting/cachexia (Serostim®); HIV-associated adipose redistribution syndrome (HARS) (Serostim®)

Pregnancy Risk Factor B/C (depending upon manufacturer)

Pregnancy Considerations Teratogenic effects were not observed in animal studies. Reproduction studies have not been conducted with all agents. During normal pregnancy, maternal production of endogenous growth hormone decreases as placental growth hormone production increases. Data with somatropin use during pregnancy is limited.

Lactation Excretion in breast milk unknown/use caution

Contraindications Hypersensitivity to growth hormone or any component of the formulation; growth promotion in pediatric patients with closed epiphyses; progression or recurrence of any underlying intracranial lesion or actively growing intracranial tumor; acute critical illness due to complications following open heart or abdominal surgery;

multiple accidental trauma or acute respiratory failure; evidence of active malignancy; active proliferative or severe nonproliferative diabetic retinopathy; use in patients with Prader-Willi syndrome **without** growth hormone deficiency (except Genotropin®) or in patients with Prader-Willi syndrome **with** growth hormone deficiency who are severely obese, have a history of upper airway obstruction or sleep apnea, or have severe respiratory impairment

Warnings/Precautions Initiation of somatropin is contraindicated with acute critical illness due to complications following open heart or abdominal surgery, multiple accidental trauma, or acute respiratory failure; mortality may be increased. The safety of continuing somatropin in patients who develop these illnesses during therapy has not been established; use with caution. Use in contraindicated with active malignancy; monitor patients with pre-existing tumors or growth failure secondary to an intracranial lesion for recurrence or progression of underlying disease; discontinue therapy with evidence of recurrence. An increased risk of second neoplasm has been reported in childhood cancer survivors treated with somatropin; the most common second neoplasms were meningiomas in patients treated with radiation to the head for their first neoplasm. Monitor patients for any malignant transformation of skin lesions.

Somatropin may decrease insulin sensitivity; use with caution in patients with diabetes or with risk factors for impaired glucose tolerance. Adjustment of antidiabetic medications may be necessary. Pancreatitis has been rarely reported; incidence in children (especially girls) with Turner syndrome may be greater than adults. Monitor for hypersensitivity reactions. Patients with hypoadrenalism may require increased dosages of glucocorticoids (especially cortisone acetate and prednisone) due to somatropin-mediated inhibition of 11 beta-hydroxysteroid dehydrogenase type 1; undiagnosed central hypoadrenalism may be unmasked. Excessive glucocorticoid therapy may inhibit the growth promoting effects of somatropin in children; monitor and adjust glucocorticoids carefully. Untreated/undiagnosed hypothyroidism may decrease response to therapy; monitor thyroid function test periodically and initiate/adjust thyroid replacement therapy as needed. Closely monitor other hormonal replacement treatments in patients with hypopituitarism. Obese patients may experience an increased incidence of adverse events when using a weight-based dosing regimen. Intracranial hypertension (IH) with headache, nausea, papilledema, visual changes, and/or vomiting has been reported with somatropin; funduscopic examination prior to initiation of therapy and periodically thereafter is recommended. Treatment should be discontinued in patients who develop papilledema; resuming treatment at a lower dose may be considered once IH-associated signs and symptoms have resolved. Patients with Turner syndrome, chronic renal failure and Prader-Willi syndrome may be at increased risk for IH. Progression of scoliosis may occur in children experiencing rapid growth. Patients with growth hormone deficiency may develop slipped capital epiphyses more frequently, evaluate any child with new onset of a limp or with complaints of hip or knee pain. Patients with Turner syndrome are at increased risk for otitis media and other ear/hearing disorders, cardiovascular disorders (including stroke, aortic aneurysm, hypertension), and thyroid disease, monitor carefully. Fluid retention may occur frequently in adults during use; manifestations of fluid retention (eg, edema, arthralgia, myalgia, nerve compression syndromes/paresthesias) are generally transient and dose dependent. Products may contain benzyl alcohol or m-cresol. When administering to newborns, reconstitute with sterile water or saline for injection. Not for I.V. injection.

Fatalities have been reported in pediatric patients with Prader-Willi syndrome following the use of growth hormone. The reported fatalities occurred in patients with one or more risk factors, including severe obesity, sleep apnea, respiratory impairment, or unidentified respiratory infection; male patients with one or more of these factors may be at greater risk. Treatment interruption is recommended in patients who show signs of upper airway obstruction, including the onset of, or increased, snoring. In addition, evaluation of and/or monitoring for sleep apnea and respiratory infections are recommended.

Patients with HIV infection should be maintained on antiretroviral therapy to prevent the potential increase in viral replication.

Elderly patients may be more sensitive to the actions of somatropin; consider lower starting doses. Safety and efficacy have not been established for the treatment of Noonan syndrome in children with significant cardiac disease. Children with epiphyseal closure who are treated for adult GHD need reassessment of therapy and dose. Administration site rotation is necessary to prevent tissue atrophy.

Adverse Reactions

Growth hormone deficiency: Adverse reactions reported with growth hormone deficiency vary greatly by age. Generally, percentages are less in pediatric patients than adults, and many of the reactions reported in adults are dose related. Percentages reported also vary by product. Below is a listing by age group; events reported more commonly overall are noted with an asterisk (*).

Children: Antibodies development, arthralgia, benign intracranial hypertension, edema, eosinophilia, glycosuria, Hb A_{1c} increased, headache, hematoma, hematuria, hyperglycemia (mild), hypertriglyceridemia, hypoglycemia, hypothyroidism, injection site reaction, intracranial tumor, leg pain, lipoatrophy, leukemia, meningioma, muscle pain, papilledema, pseudotumor cerebri, psoriasis exacerbation, rash, scoliosis progression, seizure, slipped capital femoral epiphysis, weakness

Adults: Acne, ALT increased, AST increased, arthralgia*, back pain, bronchitis, carpal tunnel syndrome, chest pain, cough, depression, diabetes mellitus (type 2), diaphoresis, dizziness, edema*, fatigue, flu-like syndrome*, gastritis, glucose intolerance, glucosuria, headache*, hyperglycemia (mild), hypertension, hypoesthesia, hypothyroidism, infection, insomnia, insulin resistance, joint disorder, leg edema, muscle pain, myalgia*, nausea, pain in extremities, paresthesia*, peripheral edema*, pharyngitis, retinopathy, rhinitis, skeletal pain*, stiffness in extremities, surgical procedure, upper respiratory tract infection, weakness

Additional/postmarketing reactions observed with growth hormone deficiency: Gynecomastia, increased growth of pre-existing nevi, pancreatitis

HARS: Serostim®: Limited to >10%: Edema (peripheral) (19% to 45%), arthralgia (28% to 37%), pain (extremity) (5% to 19%), hypoesthesia (9% to 15%), headache (4% to 14%), blood glucose increased (4% to 14%), paresthesia (11% to 13%), myalgia (3% to 13%)

Idiopathic short stature: Percentages reported using Humatrope® versus placebo: Myalgia (24%), scoliosis (19%), otitis media (16%), arthralgia (11%), arthrosis (11%), hyperlipidemia (8%), gynecomastia (5%), hip pain (3%), hypertension (3%). Additional adverse reactions listed as reported using other products from ISS NCGS Cohort (frequencies <1%): Aggressiveness, benign intracranial hypertension, diabetes, edema, hair loss, headache, injection site reaction

Prader-Willi syndrome: Genotropin® (frequency not defined): Aggressiveness, arthralgia, edema, hair loss, headache, benign intracranial hypertension, myalgia; fatalities associated with use in this population have been reported

Turner syndrome: Percentages reported using Humatrope® compared to untreated patients. Additional adverse reactions reported from other products, frequency not specified: Surgical procedures (45%), otitis media (43%), ear disorders (18%), joint pain, respiratory illness, urinary tract infection

HIV patients with wasting or cachexia: Serostim® (limited to ≥5%): Musculoskeletal disorders (arthralgia, arthrosis, myalgia: 78%), peripheral edema (26%), headache (13%), nausea (9%), paresthesia (8%), edema (6%), gynecomastia (6%), hypoesthesia (5%)

Short-bowel syndrome: Zorbtive® (limited to >10%): Peripheral edema (69% to 81%), facial edema (44% to 50%), arthralgia (31% to 44%), nausea (13% to 31%), injection site pain (up to 31%), flatulence (25%), injection site reaction (19% to 25%), abdominal pain (13% to 25%), vomiting (19%), pain (6% to 19%), chest pain (up to 19%), dehydration (up to 19%), infection (up to 19%), rhinitis (up to 19%), hearing symptoms (13%), dizziness (6% to 13%), rash (6% to 13%), diaphoresis (up to 13%), generalized edema (up to 13%), malaise (up to 13%), moniliasis (up to 13%), myalgia (up to 13%)

SHOX deficiency: Humatrope®: Arthralgia (11%), gynecomastia (8%), excessive cutaneous nevi (7%), scoliosis (4%)

Small for gestational age: Genotropin®, Humatrope® (frequency not defined): Mild, transient hyperglycemia; benign intracranial hypertension (rare); central precocious puberty; jaw prominence (rare); aggravation of pre-existing scoliosis (rare); injection site reactions; progression of pigmented nevi; carpal tunnel syndrome (rare) diabetes mellitus (rare); otitis media; headache; slipped capital femoral epiphysis

Drug Interactions

Metabolism/Transport Effects None known.

Avoid Concomitant Use There are no known interactions where it is recommended to avoid concomitant use.

Increased Effect/Toxicity There are no known significant interactions involving an increase in effect.

Decreased Effect

Somatropin may decrease the levels/effects of: Antidiabetic Agents; Cortisone; PredniSONE

The levels/effects of Somatropin may be decreased by: Estrogen Derivatives

Stability

Genotropin®: Store at 2°C to 8°C (36°F to 46°F); do not freeze. Protect from light. Reconstitute with diluent provided. Following reconstitution of 5.8 mg and 13.8 mg cartridge, store under refrigeration and use within 21 days.

Genotropin® Miniquick®: Store in refrigerator prior to dispensing, but may be stored ≤25°C (77°F) for up to 3 months after dispensing. Reconstitute with diluent provided. Consult the instructions provided with the reconstitution device. Once reconstituted, solution must be refrigerated and used within 24 hours. Discard unused portion.

Humatrope®:

Vial: Before and after reconstitution, store at 2°C to 8°C (36°F to 46°F); do not freeze. When reconstituted with provided diluent or bacteriostatic water for injection, use within 14 days. When reconstituted with sterile water for injection, use within 24 hours and discard unused portion. Reconstitute 5 mg vial with 1.5-5 mL diluent provided; swirl gently, do not shake.

Cartridge: Before and after reconstitution, store at 2°C to 8°C (36°F to 46°F); do not freeze. Consult HumatroPen™ User Guide for complete instructions for reconstitution. **Dilute with solution provided with cartridges ONLY; do not use diluent provided with vials.** Following reconstitution with provided diluent, stable for 28 days under refrigeration.

Norditropin®: Store at 2°C to 8°C (36°F to 46°F); do not freeze. Avoid direct light.

Cartridge: When refrigerated, must be used within 4 weeks once inserted into pen. Orange cartridges (5 mg/1.5 mL) may also be stored up to 3 weeks at ≤25°C (77°F).

Prefilled pen: When refrigerated, must be used within 4 weeks once inserted into pen. Orange and blue cartridges may also be stored up to 3 weeks at ≤25°C (77°F).

Nutropin®: Before and after reconstitution, store at 2°C to 8°C (36°F to 46°F); do not freeze.

Nutropin® vial: Reconstitute with bacteriostatic water for injection. Swirl gently, do not shake. Use reconstituted vials within 14 days. When reconstituted with sterile water for injection, use immediately and discard unused portion.

Nutropin® AQ formulations: Use within 28 days following initial use.

Omnitrope®:

Powder for injection: Prior to reconstitution, store under refrigeration at 2°C to 8°C (36°F to 46°F); do not freeze. Protect from light. Reconstitute with provided diluent. Swirl gently; do not shake. Following reconstitution with the provided diluents, the 5.8 mg vial may be stored under refrigeration for up to 3 weeks. Store vial in carton to protect from light.

Solution: Prior to use, store under refrigeration at 2°C to 8°C (36°F to 46°F). Once the cartridge is loaded into the pen delivery system, store under refrigeration for up to 21 days after first use.

Saizen®: Prior to reconstitution, store at room temperature 15°C to 30°C (59°F to 86°F). Following reconstitution with bacteriostatic water for injection, reconstituted solution should be refrigerated and used within 14 days. When reconstituted with sterile water for injection, use immediately and discard unused portion. The Saizen® easy click cartridge, when reconstituted with the provided bacteriostatic water, should be stored under refrigeration and used within 21 days.

5 mg vial: Reconstitute with 1-3 mL bacteriostatic water for injection or sterile water for injection. Gently swirl; do not shake.

8.8 mg vial: Reconstitute with 2-3 mL bacteriostatic water for injection or sterile water for injection. Gently swirl; do not shake.

Serostim®: Prior to reconstitution, store at room temperature 15°C to 30°C (59°F to 86°F). Reconstitute with sterile water for injection. When reconstituted with sterile water for injection, use immediately and discard unused portion.

Tev-Tropin®: Prior to reconstitution, store at 2°C to 8°C (36°F to 46°F). Reconstitute with 1-5 mL of diluent provided. Gently swirl; do not shake. May use preservative free NS for use in newborns. Following reconstitution with bacteriostatic NS, solution should be refrigerated and used within 14 days. Some cloudiness may occur; do not use if cloudiness persists after warming to room temperature.

Zorbtive®: Store unopened vials and diluent at room temperature of 15°C to 30°C (59°F to 86°F). Store reconstituted vial under refrigeration at 2°C to 8°C (36°F to 46°F) for up to 14 days; do not freeze.

8.8 mg vial: Reconstitute with 1-2 mL bacteriostatic water for injection. Swirl gently.

Mechanism of Action Somatropin is a purified polypeptide hormones of recombinant DNA origin; somatropin contains the identical sequence of amino acids found in human growth hormone; human growth hormone assists growth of linear bone, skeletal muscle, and organs by stimulating chondrocyte proliferation and differentiation, lipolysis, protein synthesis, and hepatic glucose output; stimulates erythropoietin which increases red blood cell mass; exerts both insulin-like and diabetogenic effects; enhances the transmucosal transport of water, electrolytes, and nutrients across the gut

Pharmacodynamics/Kinetics

Duration: Maintains supraphysiologic levels for 18-20 hours

Absorption: I.M., SubQ: Well absorbed

Distribution: ~1 L/kg

Metabolism: Hepatic and renal (~90%)

Bioavailability: SubQ: ~70% to 90%; **Note:** Variable; product-dependent

Half-life elimination: Preparation and route of administration dependent; SubQ: ~2-4 hours

Excretion: Urine (small amount)

Dosage

Children (individualize dose):

Chronic renal insufficiency (CRI): Nutropin®, Nutropin® AQ: SubQ: Weekly dosage: 0.35 mg/kg divided into daily injections; continue until the time of renal transplantation

Dosage recommendations in patients treated for CRI who require dialysis:

Hemodialysis: Administer dose at night prior to bedtime or at least 3-4 hours after hemodialysis to prevent hematoma formation from heparin

CCPD: Administer dose in the morning following dialysis

CAPD: Administer dose in the evening at the time of overnight exchange

Growth hormone deficiency:

Genotropin®, Omnitrope®: SubQ: Weekly dosage: 0.16-0.24 mg/kg divided into equal doses 6-7 days per week

Humatrope®: SubQ: Weekly dosage: 0.18-0.3 mg/kg divided into equal doses 6-7 days per week

Norditropin®: SubQ: 0.024-0.034 mg/kg/day, 6-7 days per week

Nutropin®, Nutropin® AQ: SubQ: Weekly dosage: 0.3 mg/kg divided into equal daily doses; pubertal patients: ≤0.7 mg/kg divided into equal daily doses

Tev-Tropin®: SubQ: Up to 0.1 mg/kg/dose administered 3 days per week

Saizen®: I.M., SubQ: Weekly dosage: 0.18 mg/kg divided into equal daily doses **or** as 0.06 mg/kg/dose administered 3 days per week **or** as 0.03 mg/kg/dose administered 6 days per week

Note: Therapy should be discontinued when patient has reached satisfactory adult height, when epiphyses have fused, or when the patient ceases to respond. Growth of 5 cm/year or more is expected, if growth rate does not exceed 2.5 cm in a 6-month period, double the dose for the next 6 months; if there is still no satisfactory response, discontinue therapy

HIV patients with wasting or cachexia (unlabeled use): Serostim®: SubQ: Limited data; doses of 0.04 mg/kg/day were reported in five children, 6-17 years of age; doses of 0.07 mg/kg/day were reported in six children, 8-14 years of age

Idiopathic short stature:

Genotropin®, Omnitrope®: SubQ: Weekly dosage: 0.47 mg/kg divided into equal doses 6-7 days per week

Humatrope®: SubQ: Weekly dosage: 0.37 mg/kg divided into equal doses 6-7 days per week

Nutropin®, Nutropin AQ®: SubQ: Weekly dosage: Up to 0.3 mg/kg divided into equal daily doses

Noonan syndrome: Norditropin®: SubQ: Up to 0.066 mg/kg/day

Prader-Willi syndrome: Genotropin®, Omnitrope®: SubQ: Weekly dosage: 0.24 mg/kg divided into equal doses 6-7 days per week

SHOX deficiency: Humatrope®: SubQ: Weekly dosage: 0.35 mg/kg divided into equal doses 6-7 days per week

Small for gestational age:

Genotropin®, Omnitrope®: SubQ: Weekly dosage: 0.48 mg/kg divided into equal doses 6-7 days per week

Humatrope®: SubQ: Weekly dosage: 0.47 mg/kg divided into equal doses 6-7 days per week

Norditropin®: SubQ: Up to 0.067 mg/kg/day

Alternate dosing (small for gestational age): In older/early pubertal children or children with very short stature, consider initiating therapy at higher doses (0.067 mg/kg/day) and then consider reducing the dose (0.033 mg/kg/day) if substantial catch-up growth observed. In younger children (<4 years) with less severe short stature, consider initiating therapy with lower doses (0.033 mg/kg/day) and then titrating the dose upwards as needed.

Turner syndrome:

Genotropin®, Omnitrope®: SubQ: Weekly dosage: 0.33 mg/kg divided into equal doses 6-7 days per week

Humatrope®: SubQ: Weekly dosage: 0.375 mg/kg divided into equal doses 6-7 days per week

Norditropin®: SubQ: Up to 0.067 mg/kg/day

Nutropin®, Nutropin® AQ: SubQ: Weekly dosage: ≤0.375 mg/kg divided into equal doses 3-7 days per week

Adults:

Growth hormone deficiency: Adjust dose based on individual requirements: To minimize adverse events in older or overweight patients, reduced dosages may be necessary. During therapy, dosage should be decreased if required by the occurrence of side effects or excessive IGF-I levels.

Weight-based dosing:

Norditropin®: SubQ: Initial dose ≤0.004 mg/kg/day; after 6 weeks of therapy, may increase dose up to 0.016 mg/kg/day

Nutropin®, Nutropin® AQ: SubQ: ≤0.006 mg/kg/day; dose may be increased up to a maximum of 0.025 mg/kg/day in patients <35 years of age, or up to a maximum of 0.0125 mg/kg/day in patients ≥35 years of age

Humatrope®: SubQ: ≤0.006 mg/kg/day; dose may be increased up to a maximum of 0.0125 mg/kg/day

Genotropin®, Omnitrope®: SubQ: Weekly dosage: ≤0.04 mg/kg divided into equal doses 6-7 days per week; dose may be increased at 4- to 8-week intervals to a maximum of 0.08 mg/kg/week

Saizen®: SubQ: ≤0.005 mg/kg/day; dose may be increased to not more than 0.01 mg/kg/day after 4 weeks

Nonweight-based dosing: SubQ: Initial: 0.2 mg/day (range: 0.15-0.3 mg/day); may increase every 1-2 months by 0.1-0.2 mg/day based on response and/or serum IGF-I levels

Dosage adjustment with estrogen supplementation (growth hormone deficiency): Larger doses of somatropin may be needed for women taking oral estrogen replacement products; dosing not affected by topical products

HARS (unlabeled use): Serostim®: SubQ: Induction: 4 mg once daily at bedtime for 12 weeks; Maintenance: 2 mg or 4 mg every other day at bedtime for 12-24 weeks. **Note:** Every-other-day dosing during induction has also been studied. Although a greater response was seen with daily dosing, it was associated with an increased incidence of adverse events.

HIV patients with wasting or cachexia: Serostim®: SubQ: 0.1 mg/kg once daily at bedtime (maximum: 6 mg/day). Alternately, patients at risk for side effects may be started at 0.1 mg/kg every other day. Patients who continue to lose weight after 12 weeks should be re-evaluated for opportunistic infections or other clinical events; rotate injection sites to avoid lipodystrophy

Adjust dose if needed to manage side effects.

Daily dose based on body weight:
- <35 kg: 0.1 mg/kg
- 35-45 kg: 4 mg
- 45-55 kg: 5 mg
- >55 kg: 6 mg

Short-bowel syndrome (Zorbtive®): SubQ: 0.1 mg/kg once daily for 4 weeks (maximum: 8 mg/day)

Fluid retention (moderate) or arthralgias: Treat symptomatically or reduce dose by 50%

Severe toxicity: Discontinue therapy for up to 5 days; when symptoms resolve, restart at 50% of dose. If severe toxicity recurs or does not disappear within 5 days after discontinuation, permanently discontinue treatment.

Elderly: Patients ≥65 years of age may be more sensitive to the action of growth hormone and more prone to adverse effects; in general, dosing should be cautious, beginning at low end of dosing range

Dosage adjustment in renal impairment Reports indicate patients with chronic renal failure tend to have decreased clearance; specific dosing suggestions not available

Dosage adjustment in hepatic impairment: Clearance may be reduced in patients with severe hepatic dysfunction; specific dosing suggestions not available

Dietary Considerations

Prader-Willi syndrome: All patients should have effective weight control (use is contraindicated in severely-obese patients).

Short-bowel syndrome: Intravenous parenteral nutrition requirements may need reassessment as gastrointestinal absorption improves.

Administration Do not shake; administer SubQ or I.M. (not all products are approved for I.M. administration). Rotate administration sites to avoid tissue atrophy. When administering to newborns, do not reconstitute with a diluent that contains benzyl alcohol; sterile water for injection may be used as an alternative.

Norditropin® cartridge must be administered using the corresponding color-coded NordiPen® injection pen.

Omnitrope®: Solution in the cartridges must be administered using the Omnitrope® pen; when installing a new cartridge, prime pen prior to first use.

Humatrope®: When administering for growth hormone deficiency, SubQ route is preferred

Tev-Tropin®: SubQ injections of solutions >1 mL not recommended.

Monitoring Parameters Growth curve, Tanner staging (children), periodic thyroid function tests, bone age (annually), periodical urine testing for glucose, somatomedin C (IGF-I) levels; funduscopic examinations at initiation of therapy and periodically during treatment; serum phosphorus, alkaline phosphatase and parathyroid hormone. If growth deceleration is observed in children treated for growth hormone deficiency, and not due to other causes, evaluate for presence of antibody formation. Periodic blood glucose monitoring; strict blood glucose monitoring in patients with diabetes. Progression or recurrence of pre-existing tumors or malignant transformation of skin lesions. **Note:** Practice guidelines recommend monitoring for efficacy and adverse effects every 1-2 months during dose titration and semiannually, thereafter (TES, 2006).

CRI: Progression of renal osteodystrophy

Prader-Willi syndrome: Monitor for sleep apnea, respiratory infections, snoring (onset of or increased)

Turner syndrome: Ear disorders including otitis media; cardiovascular disorders

Noonan syndrome: Prior to use, verify short stature syndrome.

Dosage Forms Excipient information presented when available (limited, particularly for generics); consult specific product labeling. [DSC] = Discontinued product

Injection, powder for reconstitution [rDNA origin]:
- Genotropin®: 5.8 mg [delivers 5 mg/mL; supplied with diluent]
- Genotropin®: 13.8 mg [delivers 12 mg/mL; supplied with diluent]
- Humatrope®: 5 mg, 6 mg, 12 mg, 24 mg [supplied with diluent]
- Nutropin®: 5 mg, 10 mg [contains benzyl alcohol (in diluent)]
- Omnitrope®: 5.8 mg [contains benzyl alcohol (in diluent)]
- Saizen®: 5 mg [contains benzyl alcohol (in diluent), sucrose 34.2 mg]
- Saizen®: 8.8 mg [contains benzyl alcohol (in diluent), sucrose 60.2 mg]
- Saizen®: 8.8 mg [contains sucrose 60.2 mg; supplied with diluent]
- Serostim®: 4 mg [contains benzyl alcohol (in diluent), sucrose 27.3 mg]
- Serostim®: 5 mg [contains sucrose 34.2 mg; supplied with diluent]
- Serostim®: 6 mg [contains sucrose 41 mg; supplied with diluent]
- Tev-Tropin®: 5 mg [contains benzyl alcohol (in diluent)]
- Zorbtive®: 8.8 mg [contains benzyl alcohol (in diluent), sucrose 60.19 mg]

Injection, powder for reconstitution [rDNA origin, preservative free]:
- Genotropin Miniquick®: 0.2 mg, 0.4 mg, 0.6 mg, 0.8 mg, 1 mg, 1.2 mg, 1.4 mg, 1.6 mg, 1.8 mg, 2 mg [delivers 0.25 mL; supplied with diluent]

Injection, solution [rDNA origin]:
- Norditropin FlexPro®: 5 mg/1.5 mL (1.5 mL); 10 mg/1.5 mL (1.5 mL); 15 mg/1.5 mL (1.5 mL) [prefilled pen]
- Norditropin®: 5 mg/1.5 mL (1.5 mL [DSC]); 15 mg/1.5 mL (1.5 mL [DSC]) [cartridge]
- Norditropin® NordiFlex®: 5 mg/1.5 mL (1.5 mL [DSC]); 10 mg/1.5 mL (1.5 mL [DSC]); 15 mg/1.5 mL (1.5 mL [DSC]); 30 mg/3 mL (3 mL) [prefilled pen]
- Nutropin AQ Pen®: 10 mg/2 mL (2 mL); 20 mg/2 mL (2 mL) [cartridge]
- Nutropin AQ®: 10 mg/2 mL (2 mL) [vial]
- Nutropin AQ® NuSpin™: 5 mg/2 mL (2 mL); 10 mg/2 mL (2 mL); 20 mg/2 mL (2 mL) [prefilled pen]
- Omnitrope®: 5 mg/1.5 mL (1.5 mL) [contains benzyl alcohol; cartridge]
- Omnitrope®: 10 mg/1.5 mL (1.5 mL) [cartridge]

◆ **Somatuline® Autogel® (Can)** *see* Lanreotide *on page 972*

◆ **Somatuline® Depot** *see* Lanreotide *on page 972*

◆ **Somavert®** *see* Pegvisomant *on page 1317*

◆ **Sominex® [OTC]** *see* DiphenhydrAMINE (Systemic) *on page 516*

◆ **Sominex® (Can)** *see* DiphenhydrAMINE (Systemic) *on page 516*

◆ **Sominex® Maximum Strength [OTC]** *see* DiphenhydrAMINE (Systemic) *on page 516*

- **Somnote®** *see* Chloral Hydrate *on page 336*
- **Som Pam (Can)** *see* Flurazepam *on page 737*
- **Sonata®** *see* Zaleplon *on page 1809*

SORAfenib (sor AF e nib)

Brand Names: U.S. NexAVAR®

Brand Names: Canada Nexavar®

Index Terms BAY 43-9006; Sorafenib Tosylate

Pharmacologic Category Antineoplastic Agent, Tyrosine Kinase Inhibitor; Vascular Endothelial Growth Factor (VEGF) Inhibitor

Use Treatment of advanced renal cell cancer (RCC); treatment of unresectable hepatocellular cancer (HCC)

Unlabeled Use Treatment of advanced thyroid cancer, recurrent or metastatic angiosarcoma, resistant gastrointestinal stromal tumor (GIST)

Pregnancy Risk Factor D

Pregnancy Considerations Animal studies have demonstrated teratogenicity and fetal loss. There are no adequate and well-controlled studies in pregnant women. Based on its mechanism of action and because sorafenib inhibits angiogenesis, a critical component of fetal development, adverse effects on pregnancy would be expected. Women of childbearing potential should be advised to avoid pregnancy. Men and women of reproductive potential should use effective birth control during treatment and for at least 2 weeks after treatment is discontinued.

Lactation Excretion in breast milk unknown/not recommended

Contraindications Hypersensitivity to sorafenib or any component of the formulation; use in combination with carboplatin and paclitaxel in patients with squamous cell lung cancer

Warnings/Precautions Hazardous agent - use appropriate precautions for handling and disposal. May cause hypertension (generally mild-to-moderate), especially in the first 6 weeks of treatment; monitor; use caution in patients with underlying or poorly-controlled hypertension; consider discontinuing (temporary or permanent) in patients who develop severe or persistent hypertension while on appropriate antihypertensive therapy. May cause cardiac ischemia or infarction; consider discontinuing (temporarily or permanently) in patients who develop these; use in patients with unstable coronary artery disease or recent myocardial infarction has not been studied. QT prolongation has been observed; may increase the risk for ventricular arrhythmia. Avoid use in patients with congenital long QT syndrome; use with caution and monitor closely in patients with heart failure, bradyarrhythmias, concurrent medications know to prolong the QT interval, and electrolyte (calcium, magnesium, potassium) imbalances.

Serious bleeding events may occur (consider permanently discontinuing if serious); monitor PT/INR in patients on warfarin therapy. May complicate wound healing; temporarily withhold treatment for patients undergoing major surgical procedures (the appropriate timing for reinitiation after surgical procedures has not been determined). Gastrointestinal perforation has been reported (rare); monitor patients for signs/symptoms (abdominal pain, constipation, or vomiting); discontinue treatment if gastrointestinal perforation occurs. Avoid concurrent use with strong CYP3A4 inducers (eg, carbamazepine, dexamethasone, phenobarbital, phenytoin, rifampin, St John's wort); may decrease sorafenib levels/effects. Use caution when administering sorafenib with compounds that are metabolized predominantly via UGT1A1 (eg, irinotecan). Use in combination with carboplatin and paclitaxel in patients with squamous cell lung cancer is contraindicated.

Hand-foot skin reaction and rash are the most common adverse events and typically appear within the first 6 weeks of treatment; usually managed with topical treatment, treatment delays, and/or dose reductions. Consider permanently discontinuing with severe or persistent dermatological toxicities. The risk for hand-foot syndrome increased with cumulative doses of sorafenib. The incidence of hand-foot syndrome is also increased in patients treated with sorafenib plus bevacizumab in comparison to those treated with sorafenib monotherapy. Sorafenib levels in patients with mild-to-moderate hepatic impairment (Child-Pugh classes A and B) were similar to levels observed in patients without hepatic impairment; has not been studied in patients with severe hepatic impairment. In a small study of Asian patients with advanced HCC, sorafenib demonstrated efficacy with adequate tolerability in a hepatitis B-endemic area (Yau, 2009). There have been reports of sorafenib-induced hepatitis, including hepatic failure and death.

Adverse Reactions

>10%:

Cardiovascular: Hypertension (9% to 17%; grade 3: 3% to 4%; grade 4: <1%; onset: ~3 weeks)

Central nervous system: Fatigue (37% to 46%), sensory neuropathy (≤13%), pain (11%)

Dermatologic: Rash/desquamation (19% to 40%; grade 3: ≤1%), hand-foot syndrome (21% to 30%; grade 3: 6% to 8%), alopecia (14% to 27%), pruritus (14% to 19%), dry skin (10% to 11%), erythema

Endocrine & metabolic: Hypoalbuminemia (≤59%), hypophosphatemia (35% to 45%; grade 3: 11% to 13%; grade 4: <1%)

Gastrointestinal: Diarrhea (43% to 55%; grade 3: 2% to 10%; grade 4: <1%), lipase increased (40% to 41% [usually transient]), amylase increased (30% to 34% [usually transient]), abdominal pain (11% to 31%), weight loss (10% to 30%), anorexia (16% to 29%), nausea (23% to 24%), vomiting (15% to 16%), constipation (14% to 15%)

Hematologic: Lymphopenia (23% to 47%; grades 3/4: ≤13%), thrombocytopenia (12% to 46%; grades 3/4: 1% to 4%), INR increased (≤42%), neutropenia (≤18%; grades 3/4: ≤5%), hemorrhage (15% to 18%; grade 3: 2% to 3%; grade 4: ≤2%), leukopenia

Hepatic: Liver dysfunction (≤11%; grade 3: 2%; grade 4: 1%)

Neuromuscular & skeletal: Muscle pain, weakness

Respiratory: Dyspnea (≤14%), cough (≤13%)

1% to 10%:

Cardiovascular: Cardiac ischemia/infarction (≤3%), heart failure (2%; congestive), flushing

Central nervous system: Headache (≤10%), depression, fever

Dermatologic: Acne, exfoliative dermatitis

Gastrointestinal: Appetite decreased, dyspepsia, dysphagia, esophageal varices bleeding (2%), glossodynia, mucositis, stomatitis, xerostomia

Genitourinary: Erectile dysfunction

Hematologic: Anemia

Hepatic: Transaminases increased (transient)

Neuromuscular & skeletal: Joint pain (≤10%), arthralgia, myalgia

Renal: Renal failure

Respiratory: Hoarseness

Miscellaneous: Flu-like syndrome

<1% (Limited to important or life-threatening): Acute renal failure, alkaline phosphatase increased, anaphylactic reaction, angioedema, aortic dissection, arrhythmia, bilirubin increased, bone pain, cardiac failure, cerebral hemorrhage, cholangitis, cholecystitis, dehydration, eczema, epistaxis, erythema multiforme, folliculitis, gastritis, gastrointestinal hemorrhage, gastrointestinal perforation, gastrointestinal reflux, gynecomastia, hepatic failure,

hepatitis, hypersensitivity (skin reaction, urticaria), hypertensive crisis, hyper-/hypothyroidism, hyponatremia, infection, interstitial lung disease (acute respiratory distress, interstitial pneumonia, lung inflammation, pneumonitis, pulmonitis, radiation pneumonitis), jaundice, MI, mouth pain, muscle wasting, myocardial ischemia, nephrotic syndrome, pancreatitis, pleural effusion, preeclampsia-like syndrome (reversible hypertension and proteinuria), QT prolongation, respiratory hemorrhage, reversible posterior leukoencephalopathy syndrome (RPLS), rhinorrhea, skin cancer (squamous cell/keratoacanthomas), Stevens-Johnson syndrome, thromboembolism, tinnitus, toxic epidermal necrolysis (TEN), transient ischemic attack, tumor lysis syndrome, tumor pain, voice alteration

Drug Interactions

Metabolism/Transport Effects **Substrate** of CYP3A4 (minor), UGT1A9; **Note:** Assignment of Major/Minor substrate status based on clinically relevant drug interaction potential; **Inhibits** CYP2B6 (moderate), CYP2C8 (strong), CYP2C9 (moderate), UGT1A1, UGT1A9

Avoid Concomitant Use

Avoid concomitant use of SORAfenib with any of the following: BCG; CARBOplatin; CloZAPine; CYP3A4 Inducers (Strong); Natalizumab; PACLitaxel; Pimecrolimus; St Johns Wort; Tacrolimus (Topical); Vaccines (Live)

Increased Effect/Toxicity

SORAfenib may increase the levels/effects of: Acetaminophen; CARBOplatin; Carvedilol; CloZAPine; CYP2B6 Substrates; CYP2C8 Substrates; CYP2C9 Substrates; DOCEtaxel; DOXOrubicin; Fluorouracil; Fluorouracil (Systemic); Fluorouracil (Topical); Irinotecan; Leflunomide; Natalizumab; PACLitaxel; Treprostinil; Vaccines (Live); Vitamin K Antagonists; Warfarin

The levels/effects of SORAfenib may be increased by: Acetaminophen; Bevacizumab; CYP3A4 Inhibitors (Strong); Denosumab; Pimecrolimus; Roflumilast; Tacrolimus (Topical); Trastuzumab

Decreased Effect

SORAfenib may decrease the levels/effects of: BCG; Cardiac Glycosides; Coccidioidin Skin Test; Dacarbazine; Fluorouracil; Fluorouracil (Systemic); Fluorouracil (Topical); Sipuleucel-T; Vaccines (Inactivated); Vaccines (Live); Vitamin K Antagonists

The levels/effects of SORAfenib may be decreased by: CYP3A4 Inducers (Strong); Echinacea; Herbs (CYP3A4 Inducers); Neomycin; St Johns Wort; Tocilizumab

Ethanol/Nutrition/Herb Interactions

Food: Bioavailability is decreased 29% with a high-fat meal (bioavailability is similar to fasting state when administered with a moderate-fat meal).

Herb/Nutraceutical: Avoid St John's wort (may decrease the levels/effects of sorafenib).

Stability Store at room temperature of 25°C (77°F); excursions permitted to 15°C and 30°C (59°F and 86°F). Protect from moisture.

Mechanism of Action Multikinase inhibitor; inhibits tumor growth and angiogenesis by inhibiting intracellular Raf kinases (CRAF, BRAF, and mutant BRAF), and cell surface kinase receptors (VEGFR-1, VEGFR-2, VEGFR-3, PDGFR-beta, cKIT, FLT-3, and RET)

Pharmacodynamics/Kinetics

Protein binding: 99.5%

Metabolism: Hepatic, via CYP3A4 (primarily oxidated to the pyridine N-oxide; active, minor) and UGT1A9 (glucuronidation)

Bioavailability: 38% to 49%; reduced when administered with a high-fat meal

Half-life elimination: 25-48 hours

Time to peak, plasma: ~3 hours

Excretion: Feces (77%, 51% of dose as unchanged drug); urine (19%, as metabolites)

Dosage Oral: Adults:

Advanced renal cell carcinoma: 400 mg twice daily; continue until no longer clinically benefiting or until unacceptable toxicity

Hepatocellular cancer: 400 mg twice daily; continue until no longer clinically benefiting or until unacceptable toxicity

Angiosarcoma (unlabeled use): 400 mg twice daily (Maki, 2009)

GIST (unlabeled use): 400 mg twice daily (Wiebe, 2008)

Thyroid cancer (unlabeled use): 400 mg twice daily (Gupta-Abramson, 2008)

Dosage adjustment for concomitant CYP3A4 inducers: Avoid the concomitant use of a strong CYP3A4 inducer (eg, carbamazepine, dexamethasone, phenobarbital, phenytoin, rifampin, St John's wort) with sorafenib.

Dosage adjustment for toxicity: Temporary interruption and/or dosage reduction may be necessary for management of adverse drug reactions. The dose may be reduced to 400 mg once daily and then further reduced to 400 mg every other day.

Dose modification for severe/persistent hypertension (despite antihypertensive therapy) or cardiac ischemia/infarction: Consider temporarily or permanently discontinuing treatment.

Dose modification for gastrointestinal perforation: Permanently discontinue treatment.

Dose modification for hemorrhage requiring medical intervention: Consider permanently discontinuing treatment.

Dose modification for skin toxicity:

- Grade 1 (numbness, dysesthesia, paresthesia, tingling, painless swelling, erythema, or discomfort of the hands or feet which do not disrupt normal activities): Continue sorafenib and consider symptomatic treatment with topical therapy.
- Grade 2 (painful erythema and swelling of the hands or feet and/or discomfort affecting normal activities):
  - 1st occurrence: Continue sorafenib and consider symptomatic treatment with topical therapy. **Note:** If no improvement within 7 days, see dosing for 2nd or 3rd occurrence.
  - 2nd or 3rd occurrence (or no improvement after 7 days of 1st occurrence): Hold treatment until resolves to grade 0-1; resume treatment with dose reduced by one dose level (400 mg daily or 400 mg every other day)
  - 4th occurrence: Discontinue treatment
- Grade 3 (moist desquamation, ulceration, blistering, or severe pain of the hands or feet or severe discomfort that prevents working or performing daily activities):
  - 1st or 2nd occurrence: Hold treatment until resolves to grade 0-1; resume treatment with dose reduced by one dose level (400 mg daily or 400 mg every other day)
  - 3rd occurrence: Discontinue treatment

Dosage adjustment in renal impairment:

Manufacturer's recommendations: No dosage adjustment necessary for mild, moderate, or severe renal impairment (not dependent on dialysis); has not been studied in dialysis patients.

Alternate recommendations: Safety and pharmacokinetics were studied in varying degrees of renal dysfunction with the following empiric dose levels recommended based on patient tolerance (Miller, 2009):

Mild renal dysfunction (Cl_{cr} 40-59 mL/minute): 400 mg twice daily

Moderate renal dysfunction (Cl_{cr} 20-39 mL/minute): 200 mg twice daily

Severe renal dysfunction (Cl_{cr} <20 mL/minute): Data inadequate to define dose

Hemodialysis (any Cl_{cr}): 200 mg once daily

Dosage adjustment in hepatic impairment:

Manufacturer's recommendations: No adjustment is required for mild (Child-Pugh class A) to moderate (Child-Pugh class B) hepatic impairment; not studied in severe hepatic impairment (Child-Pugh class C).

Alternate recommendations: Safety and pharmacokinetics were studied in varying degrees of hepatic dysfunction with the following empiric dose levels recommended based on patient tolerance (Miller, 2009):

Mild hepatic dysfunction (bilirubin >1 to ≤1.5 times ULN and/or AST >ULN): 400 mg twice daily

Moderate hepatic dysfunction (bilirubin >1.5 to ≤3 times ULN; any AST): 200 mg twice daily

Severe hepatic dysfunction:

Bilirubin >3-10 x ULN (any AST): 200 mg every 3 days was **not** tolerated

Albumin <2.5 g/dL (any bilirubin and any AST): 200 mg once daily

Dietary Considerations Take without food (1 hour before or 2 hours after eating).

Administration Administer on an empty stomach (1 hour before or 2 hours after eating).

Monitoring Parameters CBC with differential, electrolytes, phosphorus, lipase and amylase levels; thyroid function; blood pressure (baseline, weekly for the first 6 weeks, then periodic); monitor for hand-foot syndrome

Additional Information Hand-foot skin reaction (HFSR) management (Lacouture, 2008): The following treatments may be used in addition to the recommended dosage modifications. Prior to treatment initiation, a pedicure is recommended to remove hyperkeratotic areas/calluses, which may predispose to HFSR; avoid vigorous exercise/activities which may stress hands or feet. During therapy, patients should reduce exposure to hot water (may exacerbate hand-foot symptoms); avoid constrictive footwear and excessive skin friction. Patients may also wear thick cotton gloves or socks and should wear shoes with padded insoles. Grade 1 HFSR may be relieved with moisturizing creams, cotton gloves and socks (at night) and/or keratolytic creams such as urea (20% to 40%) or salicylic acid (6%). Apply topical steroid (eg, clobetasol ointment) twice daily to erythematous areas of Grade 2 HFSR; topical anesthetics (eg, lidocaine 2%) and then systemic analgesics (if appropriate) may be used for pain control. Resolution of acute erythema may result in keratotic areas which may be softened with keratolytic agents.

Dosage Forms Excipient information presented when available (limited, particularly for generics); consult specific product labeling.

Tablet, oral:

NexAVAR®: 200 mg

Extemporaneous Preparations Hazardous agent: Use appropriate precautions for handling and disposal.

An oral suspension may be prepared with tablets. Place two 200 mg tablets into a glass containing 60 mL (2 oz) water; let stand 5 minutes before stirring. Stir until tablets are completely disintegrated, forming a uniform suspension. Administer within 1 hour after preparation. Stir suspension again immediately before administration. To ensure the full dose is administered, rinse glass several times with a total of 180 mL (6 oz) water and administer residue. **Note:** Brown tablet coating may initially form a thin film but has no effect on the dosing accuracy.

Nexavar® data on file, Bayer Healthcare Pharmaceuticals.

◆ **Sorafenib Tosylate** *see* SORAfenib *on page 1584*

Sorbitol (SOR bi tole)

Pharmacologic Category Genitourinary Irrigant; Laxative, Osmotic

Additional Appendix Information

Laxatives, Classification and Properties *on page 1893*

Use Genitourinary irrigant in transurethral prostatic resection or other transurethral resection or other transurethral surgical procedures; diuretic; humectant; sweetening agent; hyperosmotic laxative; facilitate the passage of sodium polystyrene sulfonate through the intestinal tract

Pregnancy Risk Factor C

Dosage Hyperosmotic laxative (as single dose, at infrequent intervals):

Children 2-11 years:

Oral: 2 mL/kg (as 70% solution)

Rectal enema: 30-60 mL as 25% to 30% solution

Children >12 years and Adults:

Oral: 30-150 mL (as 70% solution)

Rectal enema: 120 mL as 25% to 30% solution

Adjunct to sodium polystyrene sulfonate: 15 mL as 70% solution orally until diarrhea occurs (10-20 mL/2 hours) or 20-100 mL as an oral vehicle for the sodium polystyrene sulfonate resin

When administered with charcoal:

Oral:

Children: 4.3 mL/kg of 35% sorbitol with 1 g/kg of activated charcoal

Adults: 4.3 mL/kg of 70% sorbitol with 1 g/kg of activated charcoal every 4 hours until first stool containing charcoal is passed

Topical: 3% to 3.3% as transurethral surgical procedure irrigation

Additional Information Complete prescribing information for this medication should be consulted for additional detail.

Dosage Forms Excipient information presented when available (limited, particularly for generics); consult specific product labeling.

Solution, genitourinary irrigation [preservative free]: 3% (3000 mL); 3.3% (2000 mL, 4000 mL)

Solution, oral: 70% (30 mL, 473 mL, 480 mL, 3840 mL)

◆ **Sore Throat Relief [OTC]** *see* Benzocaine *on page 202*

◆ **Soriatane®** *see* Acitretin *on page 37*

◆ **Sorine®** *see* Sotalol *on page 1586*

Sotalol (SOE ta lole)

Brand Names: U.S. Betapace AF®; Betapace®; Sorine®

Brand Names: Canada Apo-Sotalol®; CO Sotalol; Dom-Sotalol; Med-Sotalol; Mylan-Sotalol; Novo-Sotalol; Nu-Sotalol; PHL-Sotalol; PMS-Sotalol; PRO-Sotalol; ratio-Sotalol; Rhoxal-sotalol; Riva-Sotalol; Rylosol; Sandoz-Sotalol; ZYM-Sotalol

Index Terms Sotalol Hydrochloride

Pharmacologic Category Antiarrhythmic Agent, Class II; Antiarrhythmic Agent, Class III; Beta-Adrenergic Blocker, Nonselective

Additional Appendix Information

Beta-Blockers *on page 1884*

Use Treatment of documented ventricular arrhythmias (ie, sustained ventricular tachycardia), that in the judgment of the physician are life-threatening; maintenance of normal sinus rhythm in patients with symptomatic atrial fibrillation and atrial flutter who are currently in sinus rhythm. Manufacturer states substitutions should not be made for Betapace AF® since Betapace AF® is distributed with a patient package insert specific for atrial fibrillation/flutter.

Injection: Substitution for oral sotalol in those who are unable to take sotalol orally

Unlabeled Use Fetal tachycardia; alternative antiarrhythmic for the treatment of atrial fibrillation in patients with hypertrophic cardiomyopathy (HCM)

Pregnancy Risk Factor B

Pregnancy Considerations Adverse events were not observed in the initial animal reproduction studies; therefore, the manufacturer classifies sotalol as pregnancy category B. Sotalol crosses the placenta and is found in amniotic fluid. In a cohort study, an increased risk of cardiovascular defects was observed following maternal use of beta-blockers during pregnancy. Intrauterine growth restriction (IUGR), small placentas, as well as fetal/neonatal bradycardia, hypoglycemia, and/or respiratory depression have been observed following *in utero* exposure to beta-blockers as a class. Adequate facilities for monitoring infants at birth should be available. Untreated chronic maternal hypertension and pre-eclampsia are also associated with adverse events in the fetus, infant, and mother; however, sotalol is currently not recommended for the initial treatment of hypertension in pregnancy. Because sotalol crosses the placenta in concentrations similar to the maternal serum, it has been used for the treatment of fetal atrial flutter or fetal supraventricular tachycardia without hydrops. The clearance of sotalol is increased during the third trimester of pregnancy, but other pharmacokinetic parameters do not significantly differ from nonpregnant values.

Lactation Enters breast milk/consider risk:benefit (AAP rates "compatible"; AAP 2001 update pending)

Contraindications Hypersensitivity to sotalol or any component of the formulation; bronchial asthma; sinus bradycardia; second- or third-degree AV block (unless a functioning pacemaker is present); congenital or acquired long QT syndromes; cardiogenic shock; uncontrolled heart failure

Additional contraindications: Betapace AF® and the injectable formulation: Baseline QT_c interval >450 msec; bronchospastic conditions; Cl_{cr} <40 mL/minute; serum potassium <4 mEq/L; sick sinus syndrome

Warnings/Precautions [U.S. Boxed Warning] Manufacturer recommends initiation (or reinitiation) and doses increased in a hospital setting with continuous monitoring and staff familiar with the recognition and treatment of life-threatening arrhythmias. Some experts will initiate therapy on an outpatient basis in a patient without heart disease or bradycardia, who has a baseline uncorrected QT interval <450 msec, and normal serum potassium and magnesium levels; close ECG monitoring during this time is necessary. ACC/AHA guidelines for management of atrial fibrillation also recommend that for outpatient initiation the patient not have risk factors predisposing to drug-induced ventricular proarrhythmia (Fuster, 2006). Dosage should be adjusted gradually with 3 days between dosing increments to achieve steady-state concentrations, and to allow time to monitor QT intervals. **[U.S. Boxed Warning]: Adjust dosing interval based on creatinine clearance to decrease risk of proarrhythmia; QT interval prolongation is directly related to sotalol concentration.** Creatinine clearance must be calculated with dose initiation and dose increases. Use cautiously in the renally-impaired (dosage adjustment required). Betapace AF® and the injectable formulation are contraindicated in patients with Cl_{cr} <40 mL/minute.

[U.S. Boxed Warning]: Sotalol injection: Sotalol can cause life-threatening ventricular tachycardia associated with QT-interval prolongation (ie, torsade de pointes). Do not initiate if baseline QTc interval is >450 msec. If QT_c exceeds 500 msec during therapy, reduce the dose, prolong the infusion duration, or discontinue use. If while on oral sotalol therapy baseline QT_c interval is >500 msec, use I.V. sotalol with particular caution; serious consideration should be given to reducing the dose or discontinuing I.V. sotalol when QT_c exceeds 520 msec. QT_c prolongation is directly related to the concentration of sotalol; reduced creatinine clearance, female gender, and large doses increase the risk of QT_c prolongation and subsequent torsade de pointes. Monitor and adjust dose to prevent QT_c prolongation. Concurrent use with other QT_c-prolonging drugs (including Class I and Class III antiarrhythmics) and use within 3 months of discontinuing amiodarone is generally not recommended. To reduce the chance of excessive QT_c-prolongation, withhold QT_c-prolonging drugs for at least 3 half-lives (or 3 months for amiodarone) before initiating sotalol.

Correct electrolyte imbalances before initiating (especially hypokalemia and hypomagnesemia). Consider pre-existing conditions such as sick sinus syndrome before initiating. Conduction abnormalities can occur particularly sinus bradycardia. Use cautiously within the first 2 weeks post-MI especially in patients with markedly impaired ventricular function (experience limited). Administer cautiously in compensated heart failure and monitor for a worsening of the condition. May precipitate or aggravate symptoms of arterial insufficiency in patients with PVD and Raynaud's disease; use with caution and monitor for progression of arterial obstruction. Bradycardia may be observed more frequently in elderly patients (>65 years of age); dosage reductions may be necessary. Beta-blocker therapy should not be withdrawn abruptly (particularly in patients with CAD), but gradually tapered to avoid acute tachycardia, hypertension, and/or ischemia. Chronic beta-blocker therapy should not be routinely withdrawn prior to major surgery. Use caution with concurrent use of digoxin, verapamil, or diltiazem; bradycardia or heart block can occur. Use with caution in patients receiving inhaled anesthetic agents known to depress myocardial contractility. Use cautiously in diabetics because it can mask prominent hypoglycemic symptoms. Use with caution in patients with bronchospastic disease, myasthenia gravis or psychiatric disease. Adequate alpha-blockade is required prior to use of any beta-blocker for patients with untreated pheochromocytoma. May mask signs of hyperthyroidism (eg, tachycardia); if hyperthyroidism is suspected, carefully manage and monitor; abrupt withdrawal may exacerbate symptoms of hyperthyroidism or precipitate thyroid storm. Use caution with history of severe anaphylaxis to allergens; patients taking beta-blockers may become more sensitive to repeated challenges. Treatment of anaphylaxis (eg, epinephrine) in patients taking beta-blockers may be ineffective or promote undesirable effects.

[U.S. Boxed Warning]: Betapace® should not be substituted for Betapace® AF; Betapace® AF is distributed with an educational insert specifically for patients with atrial fibrillation/flutter.

Adverse Reactions Note: No clinical experience with I.V. sotalol; however, since exposure is similar between I.V. and oral sotalol, adverse reactions are expected to be similar.

>10%:

- Cardiovascular: Bradycardia (13% to 16%), chest pain (3% to 16%), palpitation (14%)
- Central nervous system: Fatigue (20%), dizziness (20%), lightheadedness (12%)
- Neuromuscular & skeletal: Weakness (13%)
- Respiratory: Dyspnea (21%)

1% to 10%:

- Cardiovascular: Edema (8%), abnormal ECG (7%), hypotension (6%), proarrhythmia (5%), syncope (5%), CHF (5%), torsade de pointes (dose related; 1% to 4%), peripheral vascular disorders (3%), ventricular tachycardia worsened (1%), QT_c interval prolongation (dose related)
- Central nervous system: Headache (8%), sleep problems (8%), mental confusion (6%), anxiety (4%), depression (4%)
- Dermatologic: Itching/rash (5%)

Endocrine & metabolic: Sexual ability decreased (3%)
Gastrointestinal: Nausea/vomiting (10%), diarrhea (7%), stomach discomfort (3% to 6%), flatulence (2%)
Genitourinary: Impotence (2%)
Hematologic: Bleeding (2%)
Neuromuscular & skeletal: Extremity pain (7%), paresthesia (4%), back pain (3%)
Ocular: Visual problems (5%)
Respiratory: Upper respiratory problems (5% to 8%), asthma (2%)

<1% (Limited to important or life-threatening): Alopecia, bronchiolitis obliterans with organized pneumonia (BOOP), cold extremities, diaphoresis, eosinophilia, leukocytoclastic vasculitis, leukopenia, paralysis, phlebitis, photosensitivity reaction, pruritus, pulmonary edema, Raynaud's phenomenon, red crusted skin, retroperitoneal fibrosis, serum transaminases increased, skin necrosis after extravasation, thrombocytopenia, vertigo

Drug Interactions

Metabolism/Transport Effects None known.

Avoid Concomitant Use

Avoid concomitant use of Sotalol with any of the following: Artemether; Beta2-Agonists; Dronedarone; Floctafenine; Lumefantrine; Methacholine; Nilotinib; Pimozide; QUEtiapine; QuiNINE; Tetrabenazine; Thioridazine; Toremifene; Vandetanib; Vemurafenib; Ziprasidone

Increased Effect/Toxicity

Sotalol may increase the levels/effects of: Alpha-/Beta-Agonists (Direct-Acting); Alpha1-Blockers; Alpha2-Agonists; Amifostine; Antihypertensives; Antipsychotic Agents (Phenothiazines); Bupivacaine; Cardiac Glycosides; Cholinergic Agonists; Dronedarone; Fingolimod; Hypotensive Agents; Insulin; Lidocaine; Lidocaine (Systemic); Lidocaine (Topical); Mepivacaine; Methacholine; Midodrine; Pimozide; QTc-Prolonging Agents; QuiNINE; RiTUXimab; Sulfonylureas; Tetrabenazine; Thioridazine; Toremifene; Vandetanib; Vemurafenib; Ziprasidone

The levels/effects of Sotalol may be increased by: Acetylcholinesterase Inhibitors; Alfuzosin; Aminoquinolines (Antimalarial); Amiodarone; Anilidopiperidine Opioids; Antipsychotic Agents (Phenothiazines); Artemether; Calcium Channel Blockers (Dihydropyridine); Calcium Channel Blockers (Nondihydropyridine); Chloroquine; Ciprofloxacin; Ciprofloxacin (Systemic); Diazoxide; Dipyridamole; Disopyramide; Dronedarone; Eribulin; Fingolimod; Floctafenine; Gadobutrol; Herbs (Hypotensive Properties); Indacaterol; Lidocaine (Topical); Lumefantrine; MAO Inhibitors; Nilotinib; Pentoxifylline; Phosphodiesterase 5 Inhibitors; Propafenone; Prostacyclin Analogues; QUEtiapine; QuiNIDine; QuiNINE; Reserpine

Decreased Effect

Sotalol may decrease the levels/effects of: Beta2-Agonists; Theophylline Derivatives

The levels/effects of Sotalol may be decreased by: Barbiturates; Herbs (Hypertensive Properties); Methylphenidate; Nonsteroidal Anti-Inflammatory Agents; Rifamycin Derivatives; Yohimbine

Ethanol/Nutrition/Herb Interactions

Food: Sotalol peak serum concentrations may be decreased if taken with food.

Herb/Nutraceutical: Avoid ephedra (may worsen arrhythmia).

Stability Store at 25°C (77°F); excursions permitted to 15°C to 30°C (59°F to 86°F). To prepare sotalol infusion, see manufacturer's prescribing information.

Mechanism of Action

Beta-blocker which contains both beta-adrenoreceptor-blocking (Vaughan Williams Class II) and cardiac action potential duration prolongation (Vaughan Williams Class III) properties

Class II effects: Increased sinus cycle length, slowed heart rate, decreased AV nodal conduction, and increased AV nodal refractoriness Sotalol has both $beta_1$- and $beta_2$-receptor blocking activity. The beta-blocking effect of sotalol is a noncardioselective (half maximal at about 80 mg/day and maximal at doses of 320-640 mg/day). Significant beta-blockade occurs at oral doses as low as 25 mg/day.

Class III effects: Prolongation of the atrial and ventricular monophasic action potentials, and effective refractory prolongation of atrial muscle, ventricular muscle, and atrioventricular accessory pathways in both the antegrade and retrograde directions. Sotalol is a racemic mixture of *d*- and *l*-sotalol; both isomers have similar Class III antiarrhythmic effects while the *l*-isomer is responsible for virtually all of the beta-blocking activity. The Class III effects are seen only at oral doses ≥160 mg/day

Pharmacodynamics/Kinetics

Onset of action: Oral: Rapid, 1-2 hours; when administered I.V. for ongoing VT over 5 minutes, onset of action is ~5-10 minutes (Ho, 1994)

Duration: 8-16 hours

Absorption: Oral: Decreased 20% to 30% by meals compared to fasting

Distribution: V_d: 1.2-2.4 L/kg

Protein binding: None

Metabolism: None

Bioavailability: Oral: 90% to 100%

Half-life elimination: 12 hours; Children: 9.5 hours; terminal half-life decreases with age <2 years (time to steady state may be ≥1 week in neonates); increases with renal dysfunction

Time to peak, serum: Oral: 2.5-4 hours

Excretion: Urine (as unchanged drug)

Dosage Baseline QT_c interval and creatinine clearance must be determined prior to initiation. Sotalol should be initiated and doses increased in a hospital with facilities for cardiac rhythm monitoring and assessment. Proarrhythmic events can occur after initiation of therapy and with each upward dosage adjustment.

Children: Oral: The safety and efficacy of sotalol in children have not been established

Note: Dosing per manufacturer, based on pediatric pharmacokinetic data; wait at least 36 hours between dosage adjustments to allow monitoring of QT intervals

≤2 years: Dosage should be adjusted (decreased) by plotting of the child's age on a logarithmic scale; see graph on next page or refer to manufacturer's package labeling.

Sotalol Age Factor Nomogram for Patients ≤2 Years of Age

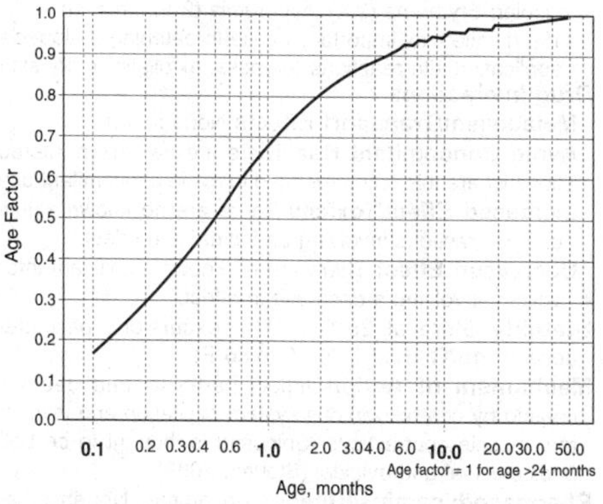

Adapted from U.S. Food and Drug Administration. http://www.fda.gov/cder/foi/label/2001/2115s3lbl.PDF

>2 years: Initial: 90 mg/m²/day in 3 divided doses; may be incrementally increased to a maximum of 180 mg/m²/day

Adults:

I.V.: **Note:** The effects of the initial I.V. dose must be monitored and the dose titrated either upward or downward, if needed, based on clinical effect, QT_c interval, or adverse reactions.

Symptomatic atrial fibrillation/flutter, ventricular arrhythmias: Substitution for oral sotalol: *Initial dose:* 75 mg infused over 5 hours twice daily

Dose adjustment: If the frequency of relapse does not reduce and excessive QT_c prolongation does not occur, may increase to 112.5 mg twice daily. For ventricular arrhythmias, may increase dose every 3 days in increments of 75 mg/day.

Dose range for symptomatic atrial fibrillation/flutter: Usual therapeutic dose: 112.5 mg twice daily; maximum dose: 150 mg twice daily

Dose range for ventricular arrhythmias: Usual therapeutic dose: 75-150 mg twice daily; maximum dose: 300 mg twice daily.

Hemodynamically stable monomorphic VT, ongoing (unlabeled use): 1.5 mg/kg over 5 minutes (ACLS, 2010); **Note:** Clinical trial employed standard dose of 100 mg (Ho, 1994).

Conversion from oral sotalol to I.V. sotalol:

80 mg oral equivalent to 75 mg I.V.
120 mg oral equivalent to 112.5 mg I.V.
160 mg oral equivalent to 150 mg I.V.

Oral:

Ventricular arrhythmias (Betapace®, Sorine®):

Initial: 80 mg twice daily

Dose may be increased gradually to 240-320 mg/day; allow 3 days between dosing increments in order to attain steady-state plasma concentrations and to allow monitoring of QT intervals

Most patients respond to a total daily dose of 160-320 mg/day in 2-3 divided doses.

Some patients, with life-threatening refractory ventricular arrhythmias, may require doses as high as 480-640 mg/day; however, these doses should only be prescribed when the potential benefit outweighs the increased of adverse events.

Atrial fibrillation or atrial flutter (Betapace AF®): Initial: 80 mg twice daily. If the frequency of relapse does not reduce and excessive QT_c prolongation does not occur after 3 days, the dose may be increased to 120 mg twice daily; may further increase to 160 mg twice daily if response is inadequate and QT_c prolongation is not excessive.

Elderly: Age does not significantly alter the pharmacokinetics of sotalol, but impaired renal function in elderly patients can increase the terminal half-life, resulting in increased drug accumulation

Dosage adjustment for toxicity:

QT_c ≥500 msec during initiation period:

Betapace AF®: Reduce dose or discontinue sotalol

Injectable formulation: Reduce dose, decrease infusion rate, or discontinue sotalol

QT_c ≥520 msec (or JT interval ≥430 msec if the QRS >100 msec) during maintenance therapy (Betapace AF®, injectable formulation): Reduce dose and carefully monitor QT_c until <520 msec. If QT_c interval ≥520 msec on the lowest maintenance dose, discontinue sotalol.

QT_c ≥550 msec (Betapace®, Sorine®): Reduce dose or discontinue sotalol.

Dosage adjustment in renal impairment: Adults: Impaired renal function can increase the terminal half-life, resulting in increased drug accumulation. Sotalol (Betapace AF®, injectable formulation) is contraindicated per the manufacturers for treatment of atrial fibrillation/flutter in patients with a Cl_{cr} <40 mL/minute.

Ventricular arrhythmias (Betapace®, Sorine®):

Cl_{cr} >60 mL/minute: Administer every 12 hours
Cl_{cr} 30-60 mL/minute: Administer every 24 hours
Cl_{cr} 10-29 mL/minute: Administer every 36-48 hours
Cl_{cr} <10 mL/minute: Individualize dose

Atrial fibrillation/flutter (Betapace AF®):

Cl_{cr} >60 mL/minute: Administer every 12 hours
Cl_{cr} 40-60 mL/minute: Administer every 24 hours
Cl_{cr} <40 mL/minute: Use is contraindicated

Note: The manufacturer of the injectable formulation recommends adjustment similar to that used for Betapace AF®. However, the injectable formulation may be used for either indication.

Dialysis: Hemodialysis would be expected to reduce sotalol plasma concentrations because sotalol is not bound to plasma proteins and does not undergo extensive metabolism; administer dose postdialysis or administer supplemental 80 mg dose; peritoneal dialysis does not remove sotalol; supplemental dose is not necessary

Dietary Considerations May be taken without regard to meals.

Administration

Oral: Administer without regard to meals.

I.V.:

Substitution for oral: Administer over 5 hours.

Hemodynamically stable monomorphic VT: Administer I.V. push over 5 minutes; use with caution due to increased risk of adverse events (eg, bradycardia, hypotension, torsade de pointes) (ACLS, 2010)

Monitoring Parameters Serum creatinine, magnesium, potassium; heart rate, blood pressure; ECG (eg, QT_c interval, PR interval). If baseline QT_c >450 msec (or JT interval >330 msec if QRS over 100 msec), sotalol is contraindicated.

For oral use (Betapace AF®) during initiation period, monitor QT_c interval 2-4 hours after each dose. If QT_c interval ≥500 msec, discontinue use; if QT_c interval <500 msec after 3 days (after fifth or sixth dose if patient receiving once-daily dosing), patient may be discharged on current regimen. Monitor QT_c interval periodically thereafter.

For I.V. use, measure QT_c interval after completion of each infusion.

Test Interactions May falsely increase urinary metanephrine values when fluorimetric or photometric methods are used; does not interact with HPLC assay with solid phase extraction for determination of urinary catecholamines

Additional Information Pharmacokinetics in children are more relevant for BSA than age.

Dosage Forms Excipient information presented when available (limited, particularly for generics); consult specific product labeling.

Injection, solution, as hydrochloride [preservative free]: 15 mg/mL (10 mL)

Tablet, oral, as hydrochloride: 80 mg [atrial fibrillation], 80 mg, 120 mg [atrial fibrillation], 120 mg, 160 mg [atrial fibrillation], 160 mg, 240 mg

Betapace AF®: 80 mg, 120 mg, 160 mg [scored; atrial fibrillation]

Betapace®: 80 mg, 120 mg, 160 mg, 240 mg [scored]

Sorine®: 80 mg, 120 mg, 160 mg, 240 mg [scored]

Extemporaneous Preparations A 5 mg/mL sotalol hydrochloride syrup may be made with Betapace® or Betapace AF® tablets and Simple Syrup containing sodium benzoate 0.1% (Syrup, NF). Place 120 mL Syrup, NF in a 6-ounce amber plastic (polyethylene terephthalate) prescription bottle; add five Betapace® or Betapace AF® 120 mg tablets and shake the bottle to wet the tablets. Allow tablets to hydrate for at least 2 hours, then shake intermittently over ≥2 hours until the tablets are completely disintegrated; a dispersion of fine particles (water-insoluble inactive ingredients) in syrup should be obtained. **Note:** To simplify the disintegration process, tablets can hydrate overnight; tablets may also be crushed, carefully transferred into the bottle and shaken well until a dispersion of fine particles in syrup is obtained. Label "shake well". Stable for 3 months at controlled room temperature (15°C to 30°C [59°F to 86°F]) and ambient humidity.

Betapace® prescribing information, Bayer HealthCare Pharmaceuticals Inc, Wayne, NJ, 2007.

Betapace AF® prescribing information, Bayer HealthCare Pharmaceuticals Inc, Wayne, NJ, 2009.

◆ **Sotalol Hydrochloride** *see* Sotalol *on page* 1586

◆ **Sotradecol®** *see* Sodium Tetradecyl *on page* 1577

◆ **Sotret®** *see* ISOtretinoin *on page* 939

◆ **SPA** *see* Albumin *on page* 51

◆ **SPD417** *see* CarBAMazepine *on page* 280

◆ **Spectracef®** *see* Cefditoren *on page* 305

◆ **SPI 0211** *see* Lubiprostone *on page* 1040

Spinosad (SPIN oh sad)

Brand Names: U.S. Natroba™

Index Terms NatrOVA

Pharmacologic Category Antiparasitic Agent, Topical; Pediculocide

Use Topical treatment of head lice (*Pediculosis capitis*) infestation in adults and children ≥4 years of age

Unlabeled Use Topical treatment of head lice (*Pediculosis capitis*) infestation in children ≥6 months and <4 years of age

Pregnancy Risk Factor B

Pregnancy Considerations Teratogenic effects were not observed in animal reproduction studies. Human studies did not assess the absorption of benzyl alcohol, an ingredient in the product.

Lactation Use caution

Contraindications There are no contraindications listed in the manufacturer's labeling

Warnings/Precautions For topical use on scalp and scalp hair only; avoid contact with eyes. Wash hands after application. The suspension contains benzyl alcohol and is not recommended for use in children <6 months of age.

Adverse Reactions

1% to 10%:

Dermatologic: Application site erythema (3%), application site irritation (1%), skin irritation

Ocular: Erythema (2%), hyperemia (2%), irritation

<1% (Limited to important or life-threatening): Alopecia, application site reactions (dryness, exfoliation), dry skin

Drug Interactions

Metabolism/Transport Effects None known.

Avoid Concomitant Use There are no known interactions where it is recommended to avoid concomitant use.

Increased Effect/Toxicity There are no known significant interactions involving an increase in effect.

Decreased Effect There are no known significant interactions involving a decrease in effect.

Stability Store at 25°C (77°F); excursions permitted between 15°C to 30°C (59°F to 86°F).

Mechanism of Action Insect paralysis and death is caused by central nervous system excitation and involuntary muscle contractions. Spinosad is thought to be both pediculocidal and ovicidal (Stough, 2009).

Pharmacodynamics/Kinetics Absorption: Not absorbed topically (not detectable in a pediatric patient plasma sampling study); absorption of the benzyl alcohol was not analyzed in this study.

Dosage Topical:

Children ≥6 months to <4 years (unlabeled use): Head lice: Apply to dry scalp; may repeat in 7 days if needed (Stough, 2009)

Children ≥4 years and Adults: Head lice: Apply sufficient amount to cover dry scalp and completely cover dry hair; 120 mL may be necessary depending on the length of hair. If live lice are seen 7 days after first treatment, repeat with second application.

Administration Topical suspension. For external use only. Shake bottle well. Apply to dry scalp and rub gently until the scalp is thoroughly moistened, then apply to dry hair; completely covering scalp and hair. Leave on for 10 minutes (start timing treatment after the scalp and hair have been completely covered). The hair should then be rinsed thoroughly with warm water. Shampoo may be used immediately after the product is completely rinsed off. If live lice are seen 7 days after the first treatment, repeat with second application. Avoid contact with the eyes. Nit combing is not required, although a fine-tooth comb may be used to remove treated lice and nits.

Spinosad should be a portion of a whole lice removal program, which should include washing or dry cleaning all clothing, hats, bedding and towels recently worn or used by the patient and washing combs, brushes and hair accessories in hot water.

Monitoring Parameters Monitor scalp for lice

Dosage Forms Excipient information presented when available (limited, particularly for generics); consult specific product labeling.

Suspension, topical:

Natroba™: 0.9% (120 mL) [contains benzyl alcohol, isopropyl alcohol]

◆ **Spiriva® (Can)** *see* Tiotropium *on page* 1690

◆ **Spiriva® HandiHaler®** *see* Tiotropium *on page* 1690

Spironolactone (speer on oh LAK tone)

Brand Names: U.S. Aldactone®

Brand Names: Canada Aldactone®; Novo-Spiroton; Teva-Spironolactone

Pharmacologic Category Diuretic, Potassium-Sparing; Selective Aldosterone Blocker

Additional Appendix Information
Heart Failure (Systolic) *on page 1991*

Use Management of edema associated with excessive aldosterone excretion; hypertension; primary hyperaldosteronism; hypokalemia; cirrhosis of liver accompanied by edema or ascites; nephrotic syndrome; severe heart failure (NYHA class III-IV) to increase survival and reduce hospitalization when added to standard therapy

Unlabeled Use Female acne (adjunctive therapy); hirsutism; hypertension (pediatric); diuretic (pediatric)

Pregnancy Risk Factor C

Pregnancy Considerations Teratogenic effects were not observed in animal studies; however, doses used were less than or equal to equivalent doses in humans. The antiandrogen effects of spironolactone have been shown to cause feminization of the male fetus in animal studies. Two case reports did not demonstrate this effect in humans however, the authors caution that adequate data is lacking. Use of diuretics during normal pregnancies is not appropriate; use may be considered when edema is due to pathologic causes (as in the nonpregnant patient); monitor.

Lactation Enters breast milk/not recommended (AAP rates "compatible"; AAP 2001 update pending)

Contraindications Anuria; acute renal insufficiency; significant impairment of renal excretory function; hyperkalemia

Warnings/Precautions Monitor serum potassium closely in patients being treated for heart failure. Avoid potassium supplements, potassium-containing salt substitutes, a diet rich in potassium, or other drugs that can cause hyperkalemia. Excess amounts can lead to profound diuresis with fluid and electrolyte loss; close medical supervision and dose evaluation are required. Watch for and correct electrolyte disturbances; adjust dose to avoid dehydration. In cirrhosis, avoid electrolyte and acid/base imbalances that might lead to hepatic encephalopathy. Gynecomastia is related to dose and duration of therapy. Discontinue use prior to adrenal vein catheterization. When evaluating a heart failure patient for spironolactone treatment, creatinine should be ≤2.5 mg/dL in men or ≤2 mg/dL in women and potassium <5 mEq/L. Discontinue or interrupt therapy if serum potassium >5 mEq/L or serum creatinine >4 mg/dL. **[U.S. Boxed Warning]: Shown to be a tumorigen in chronic toxicity animal studies. Avoid unnecessary use.**

Adverse Reactions Frequency not defined.

Cardiovascular: Vasculitis

Central nervous system: Ataxia, confusion, drowsiness, fever, headache, lethargy

Dermatologic: Drug Rash with Eosinophilia and Systemic Symptoms (DRESS), maculopapular or erythematous cutaneous eruptions, Stevens-Johnson syndrome, toxic epidermal necrolysis, urticaria

Endocrine & metabolic: Amenorrhea, gynecomastia, hyperkalemia, impotence, irregular menses, postmenopausal bleeding

Gastrointestinal: Cramps, diarrhea, gastritis, gastric bleeding, nausea, ulceration, vomiting

Hematologic: Agranulocytosis

Hepatic: Cholestatic/hepatocellular toxicity

Renal: BUN increased, renal dysfunction, renal failure

Miscellaneous: Anaphylactic reaction, breast cancer

Drug Interactions

Metabolism/Transport Effects None known.

Avoid Concomitant Use

Avoid concomitant use of Spironolactone with any of the following: CycloSPORINE; CycloSPORINE (Systemic); Tacrolimus; Tacrolimus (Systemic)

Increased Effect/Toxicity

Spironolactone may increase the levels/effects of: ACE Inhibitors; Amifostine; Ammonium Chloride; Antihypertensives; Cardiac Glycosides; CycloSPORINE; CycloSPORINE (Systemic); Digoxin; Hypotensive Agents; Neuromuscular-Blocking Agents (Nondepolarizing); RiTUXimab; Sodium Phosphates; Tacrolimus; Tacrolimus (Systemic)

The levels/effects of Spironolactone may be increased by: Alfuzosin; Angiotensin II Receptor Blockers; Diazoxide; Drospirenone; Eplerenone; Herbs (Hypotensive Properties); MAO Inhibitors; Nitrofurantoin; Nonsteroidal Anti-Inflammatory Agents; Pentoxifylline; Phosphodiesterase 5 Inhibitors; Potassium Salts; Prostacyclin Analogues; Tolvaptan; Trimethoprim

Decreased Effect

Spironolactone may decrease the levels/effects of: Alpha-/Beta-Agonists; Cardiac Glycosides; Mitotane; QuiNIDine

The levels/effects of Spironolactone may be decreased by: Herbs (Hypertensive Properties); Methylphenidate; Nonsteroidal Anti-Inflammatory Agents; Yohimbine

Ethanol/Nutrition/Herb Interactions

Ethanol: Increases risk of orthostasis.

Food: Food increases absorption.

Herb/Nutraceutical: Avoid natural licorice (due to mineralocorticoid activity)

Stability Store below 25°C (77°F).

Mechanism of Action Competes with aldosterone for receptor sites in the distal renal tubules, increasing sodium chloride and water excretion while conserving potassium and hydrogen ions; may block the effect of aldosterone on arteriolar smooth muscle as well

Pharmacodynamics/Kinetics

Duration: 2-3 days

Protein binding: 91% to 98%

Metabolism: Hepatic to multiple metabolites, including active metabolites canrenone and 7-alpha-spirolactone

Half-life elimination: Spironolactone: 78-84 minutes; Canrenone: 10-23 hours; 7-alpha-spirolactone: 7-20 hours

Time to peak, serum: 3-4 hours (primarily as the active metabolite)

Excretion: Urine and feces

Dosage Oral:

Children:

Diuretic, hypertension (unlabeled use): Children 1-17 years: Initial: 1 mg/kg/day divided every 12-24 hours (maximum dose: 3.3 mg/kg/day, up to 100 mg/day)

Diagnosis of primary aldosteronism (unlabeled use): 125-375 mg/m^2/day in divided doses

Adults:

Edema: 25-200 mg/day in 1-2 divided doses

Hypokalemia: 25-100 mg daily

Hypertension (JNC 7): 25-50 mg/day in 1-2 divided doses

Diagnosis of primary aldosteronism: Long test: 400 mg daily for 3-4 weeks; short test: 400 mg daily for 4 days; maintenance until surgical correction: 100-400 mg/day in 1-2 divided doses

Heart failure, severe (NYHA class III-IV; with ACE inhibitor and a loop diuretic ± digoxin): 12.5-25 mg/day; maximum daily dose: 50 mg. If 25 mg once daily not tolerated, reduce to 25 mg every other day was the lowest maintenance dose possible.

Note: If potassium >5 mEq/L or serum creatinine >4 mg/dL, discontinue or interrupt therapy.

Acne in women (unlabeled use): 25-200 mg once daily

Hirsutism in women (unlabeled use): 50-200 mg/day in 1-2 divided doses (Koulouri, 2008; Martin, 2008)

Elderly: Indication specific: Initial: 12.5-50 mg/day in 1-2 divided doses, increasing by 25-50 mg every 5 days as needed; adjust for renal impairment

Dosing interval in renal impairment: Heart failure:
Cl_{cr} 31-50 mL/minute: Decrease initial dose to 12.5 mg once daily
Cl_{cr} <30 mL/minute: Not recommended

Dietary Considerations Should be taken with food to decrease gastrointestinal irritation and to increase absorption. Excessive potassium intake (eg, salt substitutes, low-salt foods, bananas, nuts) should be avoided.

Monitoring Parameters Blood pressure, serum electrolytes (potassium, sodium), renal function, I & O ratios and daily weight throughout therapy

HF: Potassium levels and renal function should be checked in 3 days and 1 week after initiation or increase in dose, then every 2-4 weeks for 3 months, then quarterly for a year, then every 6 months thereafter.

Test Interactions May cause false elevation in serum digoxin concentrations measured by RIA

Additional Information Maximum diuretic effect may be delayed 2-3 days and maximum hypertensive effects may be delayed 2-3 weeks.

Dosage Forms Excipient information presented when available (limited, particularly for generics); consult specific product labeling.

Tablet, oral: 25 mg, 50 mg, 100 mg
Aldactone®: 25 mg
Aldactone®: 50 mg, 100 mg [scored]

Extemporaneous Preparations A 1 mg/mL oral suspension may be made with tablets. Crush ten 25 mg tablets in a mortar and reduce to a fine powder. Add a small amount of purified water and soak for 5 minutes; add 50 mL 1.5% carboxymethylcellulose, 100 mL syrup NF, and mix to a uniform paste; mix while adding purified water in incremental proportions to **almost** 250 mL; transfer to a calibrated bottle, rinse mortar with purified water, and add quantity of purified water sufficient to make 250 mL. Label "shake well". Stable for 3 months at room temperature or refrigerated (Nahata, 1993).

A 2.5 mg/mL oral suspension may be made with tablets. Crush twelve 25 mg tablets in a mortar and reduce to a fine powder. Add small portions of distilled water or glycerin and mix to a uniform paste; mix while adding cherry syrup to **almost** 120 mL; transfer to a calibrated bottle, rinse mortar with cherry syrup, and add quantity of cherry syrup sufficient to make 120 mL. Label "shake well" and "refrigerate". This method may also be used with twenty-four 25 mg tablets for a 5 mg/mL oral suspension. Both concentrations are stable for 28 days refrigerated (Mathur, 1989).

A 25 mg/mL oral suspension may be made with tablets and either a 1:1 mixture of Ora-Sweet® and Ora-Plus® or a 1:1 mixture of Ora-Sweet® SF and Ora-Plus®. Crush one-hundred-twenty 25 mg tablets in a mortar and reduce to a fine powder. Add small portions of chosen vehicle and mix to a uniform paste; mix while adding vehicle in incremental proportions to **almost** 120 mL; transfer to a calibrated bottle, rinse mortar with vehicle, and add quantity of vehicle sufficient to make 120 mL. Store in amber bottles; label "shake well" and "refrigerate". Stable for 60 days refrigerated (Allen, 1996).

Allen LV Jr and Erickson MA 3rd, "Stability of Ketoconazole, Metolazone, Metronidazole, Procainamide Hydrochloride, and Spironolactone in Extemporaneously Compounded Oral Liquids," *Am J Health Syst Pharm*, 1996, 53(17):2073-8.
Mathur LK and Wickman A, "Stability of Extemporaneously Compounded Spironolactone Suspensions," *Am J Hosp Pharm*, 1989, 46(10):2040-2.
Nahata MC, Morosco RS, and Hipple TF, "Stability of Spironolactone in an Extemporaneously Prepared Suspension at Two Temperatures," *Ann Pharmacother*, 1993, 27(10):1198-9.

◆ **SPM 927** *see* Lacosamide *on page* 963
◆ **Sporanox®** *see* Itraconazole *on page* 941
◆ **SPP100** *see* Aliskiren *on page* 66
◆ **Sprintec®** *see* Ethinyl Estradiol and Norgestimate *on page* 663
◆ **Sprix®** *see* Ketorolac (Nasal) *on page* 958
◆ **Sprycel®** *see* Dasatinib *on page* 454
◆ **SPS®** *see* Sodium Polystyrene Sulfonate *on page* 1575
◆ **SQV** *see* Saquinavir *on page* 1536
◆ **SR-89** *see* Strontium-89 *on page* 1595
◆ **SR33589** *see* Dronedarone *on page* 562
◆ **Sronyx®** *see* Ethinyl Estradiol and Levonorgestrel *on page* 656
◆ **SS734** *see* Besifloxacin *on page* 207
◆ **SSD®** *see* Silver Sulfadiazine *on page* 1554
◆ **SSD AF®** *see* Silver Sulfadiazine *on page* 1554
◆ **SSKI®** *see* Potassium Iodide *on page* 1383
◆ **Stadol** *see* Butorphanol *on page* 256
◆ **Stagesic™** *see* Hydrocodone and Acetaminophen *on page* 837
◆ **Stalevo®** *see* Levodopa, Carbidopa, and Entacapone *on page* 996
◆ **StanGard® Perio** *see* Fluoride *on page* 728
◆ **Stannous Fluoride** *see* Fluoride *on page* 728
◆ **Starlix®** *see* Nateglinide *on page* 1182
◆ **Statex® (Can)** *see* Morphine (Systemic) *on page* 1153

Stavudine (STAV yoo deen)

Brand Names: U.S. Zerit®
Brand Names: Canada Zerit®
Index Terms d4T
Pharmacologic Category Antiretroviral Agent, Reverse Transcriptase Inhibitor (Nucleoside)
Additional Appendix Information
Management of Healthcare Worker Exposures to HBV, HCV, and HIV *on page* 1935
Perinatal HIV Guidelines *on page* 1946

Use Treatment of HIV infection in combination with other antiretroviral agents

Pregnancy Risk Factor C

Pregnancy Considerations Adverse events were observed in some animal reproduction studies. Stavudine crosses the placenta. No increased risk of overall birth defects has been observed following first trimester exposure according to data collected by the antiretroviral pregnancy registry. Cases of lactic acidosis/hepatic steatosis syndrome related to mitochondrial toxicity have been reported in pregnant women with prolonged use of nucleoside analogues. It is not known if pregnancy itself potentiates this known side effect; however, women may be at increased risk of lactic acidosis and liver damage. In addition, these adverse events are similar to other rare but life-threatening syndromes which occur during pregnancy (eg, HELLP syndrome). Combination treatment with didanosine may also contribute to the risk of lactic acidosis, and should be considered only if benefit outweighs risk. Hepatic enzymes and electrolytes should be monitored in women receiving nucleoside analogues and clinicians should watch for early signs of the syndrome. In addition, mitochondrial dysfunction may develop in infants following *in utero* exposure. Pharmacokinetics of stavudine are not significantly altered during pregnancy; dose adjustments are not needed. The DHHS Perinatal HIV Guidelines consider stavudine to be an alternative NRTI in dual nucleoside combination regimens; do not use with zidovudine. Due to the reports of lactic acidosis, maternal, and neonatal mortality, didanosine and stavudine should **not** be used in combination during pregnancy; use with didanosine only if no alternatives are available.

Regardless of CD4 count or HIV RNA copy number, all HIV-infected pregnant women should receive a combination antepartum antiretroviral (ARV) drug regimen; this includes women who require therapy for their own health, as well as women who do not yet require therapy for their own health. ARV therapy should be started as soon as possible if required for the woman's health or immediately after the first trimester if not needed for the mother's health (although earlier initiation may be considered). Long-term follow-up is recommended for all infants exposed to ARV medications.

Healthcare providers are encouraged to enroll pregnant women exposed to antiretroviral medications in the Antiretroviral Pregnancy Registry (1-800-258-4263 or www.-APRegistry.com). Healthcare providers caring for HIV-infected women and their infants may contact the National Perinatal HIV Hotline (888-448-8765) for clinical consultation (DHHS [perinatal], 2011).

Lactation Excretion in breast milk unknown/contraindicated

Medication Guide Available Yes

Contraindications Hypersensitivity to stavudine or any component of the formulation

Warnings/Precautions Use with caution in patients who demonstrate previous hypersensitivity to zidovudine, didanosine, zalcitabine, pre-existing bone marrow suppression, renal insufficiency (dosage adjustment recommended), hepatic impairment, or peripheral neuropathy. Peripheral neuropathy may be a treatment-limiting side effect; consider permanent discontinuation. Zidovudine should not be used in combination with stavudine. **[U.S. Boxed Warning]: Lactic acidosis and severe hepatomegaly with steatosis have been reported with stavudine use, including fatal cases;** combination therapy with didanosine may increase risk; use with caution in patients with risk factors for liver disease (although acidosis has occurred in patients without known risk factors, risk may be increased with female gender, obesity, pregnancy, or prolonged exposure). Suspend treatment in any patient who develops clinical or laboratory findings suggestive of lactic acidosis or hepatotoxicity. Mortality of 50% associated in some case series, notably with serum lactate >10 mmol/L (DHHS, 2011). Severe motor weakness (resembling Guillain-Barré syndrome) has been reported (including fatal cases, usually in association with lactic acidosis); manufacturer recommends discontinuation if motor weakness develops (with or without lactic acidosis). May cause redistribution of fat (eg, buffalo hump, peripheral wasting with increased abdominal girth, cushingoid appearance). Patients may develop immune reconstitution syndrome resulting in the occurrence of an inflammatory response to an indolent or residual opportunistic infection; further evaluation and treatment may be required. **[U.S. Boxed Warning]: Pancreatitis (including some fatal cases) has occurred during combination therapy with didanosine.** Suspend stavudine and didanosine combination therapy, and any other agents toxic to the pancreas, in patients with suspected pancreatitis. If pancreatitis diagnosis confirmed, use extreme caution if reinitiating stavudine; monitor closely and do not use didanosine in regimen. Use with caution in combination with interferon alfa with or without ribavirin in HIV/HBV coinfected patients; monitor closely for hepatic decompensation, anemia, or neutropenia; dose reduction or discontinuation of interferon and/or ribavirin may be required if toxicity evident. Combination therapy with didanosine or hydroxyurea may increase risk of hepatotoxicity, pancreatitis, or severe peripheral neuropathy; avoid stavudine or hydroxyurea combination.

Adverse Reactions Adverse reactions reported below represent experience with combination therapy with other nucleoside analogues and protease inhibitors.

>10%:

- Central nervous system: Headache (25% to 46%)
- Dermatologic: Rash (18% to 30%)
- Gastrointestinal: Nausea (43% to 53%; less than comparator group), vomiting (18% to 30%; less than comparator group), diarrhea (34% to 45%)
- Hepatic: Hyperbilirubinemia (65% to 68%; grade 3/4: 7% to 16%), AST increased (42% to 53%; grade 3/4: 5% to 7%), ALT increased (40% to 50%; grade 3/4: 6% to 8%), GGT increased (15% to 28%; grade 3/4: 2% to 5%)
- Neuromuscular & skeletal: Peripheral neuropathy (8% to 21%)
- Miscellaneous: Amylase increased (21% to 31%; grade 3/4: 4% to 8%), lipase increased (~27%; grade 3/4: 5% to 6%)

Postmarketing and/or case reports: Abdominal pain, allergic reaction, anemia, anorexia, chills, diabetes mellitus, fever, hepatic failure, hepatitis, hepatomegaly (with steatosis; some fatal), hyperglycemia, hyperlactatemia (symptomatic), hyperlipidemia, immune reconstitution syndrome, insomnia, insulin resistance, lactic acidosis (some fatal), leukopenia, macrocytosis, myalgia, neuromuscular weakness (severe-resembling Guillain-Barré), neutropenia, pancreatitis (some fatal), redistribution/accumulation/atrophy of body fat, thrombocytopenia

Drug Interactions

Metabolism/Transport Effects None known.

Avoid Concomitant Use

Avoid concomitant use of Stavudine with any of the following: Hydroxyurea; Zidovudine

Increased Effect/Toxicity

Stavudine may increase the levels/effects of: Didanosine; Hydroxyurea

The levels/effects of Stavudine may be increased by: Hydroxyurea; Ribavirin

Decreased Effect

The levels/effects of Stavudine may be decreased by: DOXOrubicin; DOXOrubicin (Liposomal); Zidovudine

Stability Capsules and powder for reconstitution may be stored at controlled room temperature of 25°C (77°F). Reconstitute powder for oral suspension with 202 mL of purified water as specified on the bottle. Shake vigorously until suspended. Final suspension will be 1 mg/mL (200 mL). Reconstituted oral solution should be stored in refrigerator at 2°C to 8°C (36°F to 46°F) and is stable for 30 days.

Mechanism of Action Stavudine is a thymidine analog which interferes with HIV viral DNA dependent DNA polymerase resulting in inhibition of viral replication; nucleoside reverse transcriptase inhibitor

Pharmacodynamics/Kinetics

Distribution: V_d: 46 L

Metabolism: Undergoes intracellular phosphorylation to an active metabolite (stavudine triphosphate)

Bioavailability: Children: 76.9%; Adults: 86.4%

Half-life elimination: HIV-infected Children: 0.96 hours, HIV-infected Adults: 1.6 hours

Time to peak, serum: 1 hour

Excretion: Urine 95% (74% as unchanged drug); feces 3% (62% as unchanged drug)

Dosage Oral:

Newborns (Birth to 13 days): 0.5 mg/kg every 12 hours

Children:

- ≥14 days and <30 kg: 1 mg/kg every 12 hours
- ≥30 kg: Refer to adult dosing

Adults:

- <60 kg: 30 mg every 12 hours
- ≥60 kg: 40 mg every 12 hours

Note: The World Health Organization recommends 30 mg every 12 hours in all adult and adolescent patients regardless of body weight (DHHS, 2011).

Dosing adjustment in renal impairment:

Children: Specific recommendations not available. Reduction in dose or increase in dosing interval should be considered.

Adults:

Cl_{cr} >50 mL/minute:
<60 kg: 30 mg every 12 hours
≥60 kg: 40 mg every 12 hours

Cl_{cr} 26-50 mL/minute:
<60 kg: 15 mg every 12 hours
≥60 kg: 20 mg every 12 hours

Cl_{cr} 10-25 mL/minute, hemodialysis (administer dose after hemodialysis on day of dialysis):
<60 kg: 15 mg every 24 hours
≥60 kg: 20 mg every 24 hours

Elderly: Older patients should be closely monitored for signs and symptoms of peripheral neuropathy; dosage should be carefully adjusted to renal function

Dietary Considerations May be taken without regard to meals. Some products may contain sucrose.

Administration May be administered without regard to meals. Oral solution should be shaken vigorously prior to use.

Monitoring Parameters Monitor liver function tests and renal function tests; signs and symptoms of peripheral neuropathy; monitor viral load and CD4 count

Additional Information Potential compliance problems, frequency of administration and adverse effects should be discussed with patients before initiating therapy to help prevent the emergence of resistance. Concomitant use of stavudine and lamivudine is discouraged; additive toxicities include life-threatening lactic acidosis and pancreatitis; concomitant stavudine with zidovudine, or stavudine with didanosine use should be avoided (DHHS, 2011).

Dosage Forms Excipient information presented when available (limited, particularly for generics); consult specific product labeling.

Capsule, oral: 15 mg, 20 mg, 30 mg, 40 mg
Zerit®: 15 mg, 20 mg, 30 mg, 40 mg

Powder for solution, oral:
Zerit®: 1 mg/mL (200 mL) [dye free; contains sucrose 50 mg/mL; fruit flavor]

- **Stavzor™** *see* Valproic Acid *on page* 1757
- **Staxyn™** *see* Vardenafil *on page* 1769
- **Stelara™** *see* Ustekinumab *on page* 1751
- **Stemetil® (Can)** *see* Prochlorperazine *on page* 1412
- **Sterile Talc** *see* Talc (Sterile) *on page* 1624
- **Sterile Talc Powder™** *see* Talc (Sterile) *on page* 1624
- **Sterile Vancomycin Hydrochloride, USP (Can)** *see* Vancomycin *on page* 1763
- **STI-571** *see* Imatinib *on page* 870
- **Stieprox® (Can)** *see* Ciclopirox *on page* 356
- **Stieva-A (Can)** *see* Tretinoin (Topical) *on page* 1731
- **Stimate®** *see* Desmopressin *on page* 476
- **Sting-Kill® [OTC]** *see* Benzocaine *on page* 202
- **St Joseph® Adult Aspirin [OTC]** *see* Aspirin *on page* 154
- **Stop®** *see* Fluoride *on page* 728
- **Strattera®** *see* Atomoxetine *on page* 163

Streptomycin (strep toe MYE sin)

Index Terms Streptomycin Sulfate

Pharmacologic Category Antibiotic, Aminoglycoside; Antitubercular Agent

Use Part of combination therapy of active tuberculosis; used in combination with other agents for treatment of streptococcal or enterococcal endocarditis, mycobacterial infections, plague, tularemia, and brucellosis

Pregnancy Risk Factor D

Pregnancy Considerations Streptomycin crosses the placenta. Many case reports of hearing impairment in children exposed *in utero* have been published. Impairment has ranged from mild hearing loss to bilateral deafness. Because of several reports of total irreversible bilateral congenital deafness in children whose mothers received streptomycin during pregnancy, the manufacturer classifies streptomycin as pregnancy risk factor D.

Lactation Enters breast milk/not recommended (AAP rates "compatible"; AAP 2001 update pending)

Contraindications Hypersensitivity to streptomycin or any component of the formulation; pregnancy

Warnings/Precautions [U.S. Boxed Warning]: May cause neurotoxicity, nephrotoxicity, and/or neuromuscular blockade and respiratory paralysis; usual risk factors include pre-existing renal impairment, concomitant neuro-/nephrotoxic medications, advanced age and dehydration. The drug's neurotoxicity can result in respiratory paralysis from neuromuscular blockade, especially when the drug is given soon after anesthesia or muscle relaxants. Use with caution in patients with pre-existing vertigo, tinnitus, hearing loss, neuromuscular disorders, or renal impairment; modify dosage in patients with renal impairment; ototoxicity is directly proportional to the amount of drug given and the duration of treatment; tinnitus or vertigo are indications of vestibular injury and impending bilateral irreversible damage; renal damage is usually reversible. **[U.S. Boxed Warning]: Parenteral form should be used only where appropriate audiometric and laboratory testing facilities are available.** Prolonged use may result in fungal or bacterial superinfection, including *C. difficile*-associated diarrhea (CDAD) and pseudomembranous colitis; CDAD has been observed >2 months postantibiotic treatment.

Adverse Reactions Frequency not defined.

Cardiovascular: Hypotension
Central nervous system: Neurotoxicity, drowsiness, headache, drug fever, paresthesia
Dermatologic: Skin rash
Gastrointestinal: Nausea, vomiting
Hematologic: Eosinophilia, anemia
Neuromuscular & skeletal: Arthralgia, weakness, tremor
Otic: Ototoxicity (auditory), ototoxicity (vestibular)
Renal: Nephrotoxicity
Respiratory: Difficulty in breathing

Drug Interactions

Metabolism/Transport Effects None known.

Avoid Concomitant Use

Avoid concomitant use of Streptomycin with any of the following: BCG; Gallium Nitrate

Increased Effect/Toxicity

Streptomycin may increase the levels/effects of: AbobotulinumtoxinA; Bisphosphonate Derivatives; CARBOplatin; Colistimethate; CycloSPORINE; CycloSPORINE (Systemic); Gallium Nitrate; Neuromuscular-Blocking Agents; OnabotulinumtoxinA; RimabotulinumtoxinB

The levels/effects of Streptomycin may be increased by: Amphotericin B; Capreomycin; Cephalosporins (2nd Generation); Cephalosporins (3rd Generation); Cephalosporins (4th Generation); CISplatin; Loop Diuretics; Nonsteroidal Anti-Inflammatory Agents; Vancomycin

Decreased Effect

Streptomycin may decrease the levels/effects of: BCG; Typhoid Vaccine

The levels/effects of Streptomycin may be decreased by: Penicillins

Stability Depending upon manufacturer, reconstituted solution remains stable for 2-4 weeks when refrigerated. Exposure to light causes darkening of solution without apparent loss of potency.

Mechanism of Action Inhibits bacterial protein synthesis by binding directly to the 30S ribosomal subunits causing faulty peptide sequence to form in the protein chain

Pharmacodynamics/Kinetics

Absorption: Oral: Poorly absorbed; I.M.: Well absorbed

Distribution: To extracellular fluid including serum, abscesses, ascitic, pericardial, pleural, synovial, lymphatic, and peritoneal fluids; poorly distributed into CSF

Protein binding: 34%

Half-life elimination: Newborns: 4-10 hours; Adults: 2-4.7 hours, prolonged with renal impairment

Time to peak: I.M.: Within 1 hour

Excretion: Urine (90% as unchanged drug); feces, saliva, sweat, and tears (<1%)

Dosage Note: For I.M. administration; I.V. use is not recommended

Usual dosage range:

Children: 20-40 mg/kg/day (maximum: 1 g)

Adults: 15-30 mg/kg/day or 1-2 g/day

Indication-specific dosing:

Children: **Tuberculosis:** I.M.:

Daily therapy: 20-40 mg/kg/day (maximum: 1 g/day)

Directly observed therapy (DOT): Twice weekly: 25-30 mg/kg (maximum: 1.5 g)

Directly observed therapy DOT: 3 times/week: 25-30 mg/kg (maximum: 1.5 g)

Adults: I.M.:

Brucellosis: 1 g/day for 14-21 days (with doxycycline, 100 mg twice daily for 6 weeks)

Endocarditis:

Enterococcal: 1 g every 12 hours for 2 weeks, 500 mg every 12 hours for 4 weeks in combination with penicillin

Streptococcal: 1 g every 12 hours for 1 week, 500 mg every 12 hours for 1 week

***Mycobacterium avium* complex:** Adjunct therapy (with macrolide, rifamycin, and ethambutol): 15 mg/kg 3 times/week for first 2-3 months for severe disease

Plague: 15 mg/kg (or 1 g) every 12 hours until the patient is afebrile for at least 3 days

Tuberculosis:

Daily therapy: 15 mg/kg/day (maximum: 1 g)

Directly observed therapy (DOT): Twice weekly: 25-30 mg/kg (maximum: 1.5 g)

Directly observed therapy DOT: 3 times/week: 25-30 mg/kg (maximum: 1.5 g)

Tularemia: 10-15 mg/kg every 12 hours (maximum: 2 g/day) for 7-10 days or until patient is afebrile for 5-7 days

Elderly: I.M.: 10 mg/kg/day, not to exceed 750 mg/day; dosing interval should be adjusted for renal function; some authors suggest not to give more than 5 days/week or give as 20-25 mg/kg/dose twice weekly

Dosing interval in renal impairment:

Cl_{cr} 10-50 mL/minute: Administer every 24-72 hours

Cl_{cr} <10 mL/minute: Administer every 72-96 hours

Removed by hemo- and peritoneal dialysis: Administer dose postdialysis

Administration Inject deep I.M. into large muscle mass; I.V. administration is not recommended; has been administered intravenously over 30-60 minutes.

Monitoring Parameters Hearing (audiogram), BUN, creatinine; serum concentration of the drug should be monitored in all patients; eighth cranial nerve damage is usually preceded by high-pitched tinnitus, roaring noises, sense of fullness in ears, or impaired hearing and may persist for weeks after drug is discontinued

Reference Range Therapeutic: Peak: 20-30 mcg/mL; Trough: <5 mcg/mL; Toxic: Peak: >50 mcg/mL; Trough: >10 mcg/mL

Test Interactions False-positive urine glucose with Benedict's solution or Clinitest®; penicillin may decrease aminoglycoside serum concentrations *in vitro*

Dosage Forms Excipient information presented when available (limited, particularly for generics); consult specific product labeling.

Injection, powder for reconstitution: 1 g

- **Streptomycin Sulfate** *see* Streptomycin *on page 1594*
- **Striant®** *see* Testosterone *on page 1654*
- **Strifon Forte® (Can)** *see* Chlorzoxazone *on page 351*
- **Stromectol®** *see* Ivermectin *on page 944*
- **Strong Iodine Solution** *see* Potassium Iodide and Iodine *on page 1384*
- **Strontium-89 Chloride** *see* Strontium-89 *on page 1595*

Strontium-89 (STRON shee um atey nine)

Brand Names: U.S. Metastron®

Brand Names: Canada Metastron®

Index Terms SR-89; Sr89; Strontium Chloride SR 89; Strontium-89 Chloride

Pharmacologic Category Radiopharmaceutical

Use Relief of bone pain in patients with skeletal metastases

Pregnancy Risk Factor D

Dosage Note: Measure dose by a suitable radioactivity calibration system immediately prior to administration.

I.V.: Adults: Bone pain due to skeletal metastases: 148 megabecquerel (4 millicurie) **or** 1.5-2.2 megabecquerel (40-60 microcurie)/kg; repeat doses are generally not recommended at intervals <90 days

Additional Information Complete prescribing information for this medication should be consulted for additional detail.

Dosage Forms Excipient information presented when available (limited, particularly for generics); consult specific product labeling.

Injection, solution, as chloride [preservative free]:

Metastron®: 1 mCi/mL (4 mL) [37 megabecquerel per mL]

- **Strontium Chloride SR 89** *see* Strontium-89 *on page 1595*
- **SU011248** *see* SUNItinib *on page 1612*
- **Suberoylanilide Hydroxamic Acid** *see* Vorinostat *on page 1800*
- **Sublinox™ (Can)** *see* Zolpidem *on page 1826*
- **Suboxone®** *see* Buprenorphine and Naloxone *on page 246*
- **Subsys®** *see* FentaNYL *on page 697*
- **Subutex® [DSC]** *see* Buprenorphine *on page 244*
- **Subutex® (Can)** *see* Buprenorphine *on page 244*

Succimer (SUKS si mer)

Brand Names: U.S. Chemet®

Brand Names: Canada Chemet®

Index Terms DMSA

Pharmacologic Category Antidote

Use Treatment of lead poisoning in children with serum lead levels >45 mcg/dL

Unlabeled Use

Treatment of lead poisoning in symptomatic adults

Pregnancy Risk Factor C

Pregnancy Considerations Adverse events were observed in animal reproduction studies. Following maternal occupational exposure, lead crosses the placenta in amounts related to maternal plasma levels. Possible outcomes of maternal lead exposure >10 mcg/dL includes spontaneous abortion, postnatal developmental delay, and reduced birth weight. Chelation therapy during pregnancy is for maternal benefit only and should be limited to the treatment of severe, symptomatic lead poisoning.

Lactation Excretion in breast milk unknown/not recommended

Contraindications Hypersensitivity to succimer or any component of the formulation

Warnings/Precautions Remove sources of lead exposure prior to treatment. Consult experts before using chelation drug therapy for lead removal. Succimer should not be used to treat encephalopathy associated with lead toxicity. Caution in patients with renal or hepatic impairment; adequate hydration should be maintained during therapy. Succimer is dialyzable, however, the lead chelates are not. Rebounding serum lead levels may occur after treatment.

Adverse Reactions Note: Percentages as reported in pediatric patients unless otherwise noted.

>10%: Gastrointestinal: Appetite decreased, diarrhea, hemorrhoid symptoms, metallic taste, loose stools, nausea, vomiting

1% to 10%:

Cardiovascular: Arrhythmia (adults 2%)

Central nervous system: Chills, dizziness, drowsiness, fatigue, fever, headache, sleepiness

Dermatologic: Rash (including papular rash, herpetic rash and mucocutaneous eruptions); pruritus

Endocrine & metabolic: Cholesterol increased

Gastrointestinal: Abdominal cramps, mucosal irritation, sore throat

Genitourinary: Proteinuria (adults), urine output decreased (adults), voiding difficulty (adults)

Hepatic: Alkaline phosphatase increased, ALT increased, AST increased

Neuromuscular & skeletal: Back pain, flank pain, leg pain (adults), neuropathy, paresthesia, rib pain

Ocular: Cloudy film in eye, watery eyes

Otic: Otitis media, plugged ears

Respiratory: Cough, nasal congestion, rhinorrhea

Miscellaneous: Flu-like syndrome, moniliasis

<1% (Limited to important or life-threatening): Allergic reactions (especially with retreatment), eosinophilia, neutropenia (causal relationship not established)

Drug Interactions

Metabolism/Transport Effects None known.

Avoid Concomitant Use There are no known interactions where it is recommended to avoid concomitant use.

Increased Effect/Toxicity There are no known significant interactions involving an increase in effect.

Decreased Effect There are no known significant interactions involving a decrease in effect.

Stability Store between 15°C to 25°C (59°F to 77°F); avoid excessive heat.

Mechanism of Action Succimer is an analog of dimercaprol. It forms water soluble chelates with heavy metals which are subsequently excreted renally. Succimer binds heavy metals; however, the chemical form of these chelates is not known.

Pharmacodynamics/Kinetics

Absorption: Rapid but incomplete

Protein binding: Highly bound to albumin

Metabolism: Rapidly and extensively to mixed succimer cysteine disulfides

Half-life elimination: 2 days

Time to peak, serum: ~1-2 hours

Excretion: Urine (~25%) with peak urinary excretion between 2-4 hours (90% as mixed succimer-cysteine disulfide conjugates, 10% as unchanged drug); feces (as unabsorbed drug)

Dosage Note: For the treatment of high blood lead levels in children, the CDC recommends chelation treatment when blood lead levels are >45 mcg/dL (CDC, 2002). Children with blood lead levels >70 mcg/dL or symptomatic lead poisoning should be treated with parenteral agents (AAP, 2005). In adults, available guidelines recommend chelation therapy with blood lead levels >50 mcg/dL and significant symptoms; chelation therapy may also be indicated with blood lead levels ≥100 mcg/dL and/or symptoms. (Kosnett, 2007).

Children: Oral: 10 mg/kg/dose (or 350 mg/m^2/dose) every 8 hours for 5 days followed by 10 mg/kg/dose (or 350 mg/m^2/dose) every 12 hours for 14 days. Maximum: 500 mg/dose. For children <5 years of age, dose should be based on mg/m^2; dosing by mg/kg may be suboptimal.

Adults (mild symptoms or blood lead levels 70-100 mg/dL; unlabeled use): 10 mg/kg/dose (or 350 mg/m^2/dose) every 8 hours for 5 days, followed by 10 mg/kg/dose (or 350 mg/m^2/dose) every 12 hours for 14 days; Maximum: 500 mg/dose

Note: Treatment courses may be repeated, but 2-week intervals between courses is generally recommended.

Dosing adjustment in renal/hepatic impairment: Administer with caution and monitor closely

Administration Capsule can be separated and contents sprinkled on a small amount of soft food, or the contents placed on a spoon and administered followed by fruit drink.

Monitoring Parameters Blood lead levels (baseline and 7-21 days after completing chelation therapy); serum aminotransferase, CBC with differential, platelets (baseline, and weekly during treatment); hemoglobin or hematocrit, iron status, free erythrocyte protoporphyrin or zinc protoporphyrin; neurodevelopmental changes

Test Interactions False-positive ketones (U) using nitroprusside methods, falsely decreased serum CPK; falsely decreased uric acid measurement

Dosage Forms Excipient information presented when available (limited, particularly for generics); consult specific product labeling.

Capsule, oral:

Chemet®: 100 mg

Succinylcholine (suks in il KOE leen)

Brand Names: U.S. Anectine®; Quelicin®

Brand Names: Canada Quelicin®

Index Terms Succinylcholine Chloride; Suxamethonium Chloride

Pharmacologic Category Neuromuscular Blocker Agent, Depolarizing

Use To facilitate both rapid sequence and routine endotracheal intubation and to relax skeletal muscles during surgery

Note: Does not relieve pain or produce sedation

Unlabeled Use To reduce the intensity of muscle contractions of electroconvulsive therapy (ECT)

Pregnancy Risk Factor C

Pregnancy Considerations Reproduction studies have not been conducted. Small amounts cross the placenta. Sensitivity to succinylcholine may be increased due to a ~24% decrease in plasma cholinesterase activity during pregnancy and several days postpartum.

Lactation Excretion in breast milk unknown/use caution

Contraindications Hypersensitivity to succinylcholine or any component of the formulation; personal or familial history of malignant hyperthermia; myopathies associated with elevated serum creatine phosphokinase (CPK)

values; acute phase of injury following major burns, multiple trauma, extensive denervation of skeletal muscle or upper motor neuron injury

Warnings/Precautions [U.S. Boxed Warning]: Use caution in children and adolescents. Acute rhabdomyolysis with hyperkalemia, ventricular arrhythmias and cardiac arrest have been reported (rarely) in children with undiagnosed skeletal muscle myopathy. Use in children should be reserved for emergency intubation or where immediate airway control is necessary. Use with caution in patients with pre-existing hyperkalemia, extensive or severe burns; severe hyperkalemia may develop in patients with chronic abdominal infections, burn injuries, children with skeletal muscle myopathy, subarachnoid hemorrhage, or conditions which cause degeneration of the nervous system. Alkalosis, hypercalcemia, demyelinating lesions, peripheral neuropathies, denervation, infection, muscle trauma, and diabetes mellitus may result in antagonism of neuromuscular blockade. Electrolyte abnormalities, severe hyponatremia, severe hypocalcemia, severe hypokalemia, hypermagnesemia, neuromuscular diseases, acidosis, acute intermittent porphyria, Eaton-Lambert syndrome, myasthenia gravis, renal failure, and hepatic failure may result in potentiation of neuromuscular blockade. May increase vagal tone.

Succinylcholine is metabolized by plasma cholinesterase; use with caution (if at all) in patients suspected of being homozygous for the atypical plasma cholinesterase gene.

Use with caution in patients with extensive or severe burns; risk of hyperkalemia is increased following injury. May increase intraocular pressure; use caution with narrow angle glaucoma or penetrating eye injuries. Risk of bradycardia may be increased with second dose and may occur more in children. Use may be associated with acute onset of malignant hyperthermia; risk may be increased with concomitant administration of volatile anesthetics. Use with caution in the elderly; effects and duration are more variable.

Maintenance of an adequate airway and respiratory support is critical. Should be administered by adequately trained individuals familiar with its use.

Adverse Reactions Frequency not defined.

Cardiovascular: Arrhythmias, bradycardia (higher with second dose, more frequent in children), cardiac arrest, hyper-/hypotension, tachycardia

Dermatologic: Rash

Endocrine & metabolic: Hyperkalemia

Gastrointestinal: Salivation (excessive)

Neuromuscular & skeletal: Jaw rigidity, muscle fasciculation, postoperative muscle pain, rhabdomyolysis (with possible myoglobinuric acute renal failure)

Ocular: Intraocular pressure increased

Renal: Acute renal failure (secondary to rhabdomyolysis)

Respiratory: Apnea, respiratory depression (prolonged)

Miscellaneous: Anaphylaxis, malignant hyperthermia

Postmarketing and/or case reports: Acute quadriplegic myopathy syndrome (prolonged use), myositis ossificans (prolonged use)

Drug Interactions

Metabolism/Transport Effects None known.

Avoid Concomitant Use

Avoid concomitant use of Succinylcholine with any of the following: QuiNINE

Increased Effect/Toxicity

Succinylcholine may increase the levels/effects of: Analgesics (Opioid); Cardiac Glycosides; OnabotulinumtoxinA; RimabotulinumtoxinB

The levels/effects of Succinylcholine may be increased by: AbobotulinumtoxinA; Acetylcholinesterase Inhibitors; Aminoglycosides; Capreomycin; Colistimethate; Cyclophosphamide; Echothiophate Iodide; Lincosamide Antibiotics; Lithium; Loop Diuretics; Magnesium Salts; Phenelzine; Polymyxin B; Procainamide; QuiNIDine; QuiNINE; Tetracycline Derivatives; Vancomycin

Decreased Effect

The levels/effects of Succinylcholine may be decreased by: Loop Diuretics

Stability Manufacturer recommends refrigeration at 2°C to 8°C (36°F to 46°F) and may be stored at room temperature for 14 days; however, additional testing has demonstrated stability for ≤6 months unrefrigerated (25°C) (Ross, 1988; Roy, 2008). May dilute to a final concentration of 1-2 mg/mL. Do not mix with alkaline solutions (pH >8.5). Stability in polypropylene syringes (20 mg/mL) at room temperature (25°C) is 45 days (Storms, 2003). Stability of parenteral admixture (1-2 mg/mL) at refrigeration temperature (4°C) is 24 hours in D_5W or NS.

Mechanism of Action Acts similar to acetylcholine, produces depolarization of the motor endplate at the myoneural junction which causes sustained flaccid skeletal muscle paralysis produced by state of accommodation that develops in adjacent excitable muscle membranes

Pharmacodynamics/Kinetics

Onset of action: I.M.: 2-3 minutes; I.V.: Complete muscular relaxation: 30-60 seconds

Duration: I.M.: 10-30 minutes; I.V.: 4-6 minutes with single administration

Metabolism: Rapidly hydrolyzed by plasma pseudocholinesterase

Excretion: Urine

Dosage I.M., I.V.: Dose to effect; doses will vary due to interpatient variability; use total body weight for obese patients (Bentley, 1982; Brunette, 2004; Rose, 2000). Use carefully and/or consider dose reduction in patients with reduced plasma cholinesterase activity due to genetic abnormalities of plasma cholinesterase or when associated with other conditions (eg, pregnancy, severe liver disease, renal disease); prolonged neuromuscular blockade may occur.

I.M.: Children and Adults: Up to 3-4 mg/kg, total dose should not exceed 150 mg

I.V.:

Smaller Children: Intermittent: Initial: 2 mg/kg/dose; maintenance: 0.3-0.6 mg/kg/dose every 5-10 minutes as needed

Older Children and Adolescents: Intermittent: Initial: 1 mg/kg/dose; maintenance: 0.3-0.6 mg/kg every 5-10 minutes as needed

Adults:

Intubation: 0.6 mg/kg (range: 0.3-1.1 mg/kg)

Rapid sequence intubation: 1-1.5 mg/kg (Sluga, 2005; Weiss, 1997)

Note: Initial dose of succinylcholine must be increased when nondepolarizing agent pretreatment used because of the antagonism between succinylcholine and nondepolarizing neuromuscular-blocking agents.

Dosing adjustment in renal impairment: Use carefully and/or consider dose reduction; prolonged neuromuscular blockade may occur if reduced plasma cholinesterase activity coexists.

Dosing adjustment in hepatic impairment: Use carefully and/or consider dose reduction; prolonged neuromuscular blockade may occur if reduced plasma cholinesterase activity coexists.

Administration May be administered by rapid I.V. injection without further dilution. I.M. injections should be made deeply, preferably high into deltoid muscle; use only when I.V. access is not available.

Monitoring Parameters Monitor cardiac, blood pressure, and oxygenation during administration; temperature, serum potassium and calcium, assisted ventilator status; neuromuscular function with a peripheral nerve stimulator

Dosage Forms Excipient information presented when available (limited, particularly for generics); consult specific product labeling.

Injection, solution, as chloride:
Anectine®: 20 mg/mL (10 mL)
Quelicin®: 20 mg/mL (10 mL)
Injection, solution, as chloride [preservative free]:
Quelicin®: 100 mg/mL (10 mL)

- **Succinylcholine Chloride** *see* Succinylcholine *on page 1596*
- **Suclor™ [DSC]** *see* Chlorpheniramine and Pseudoephedrine *on page 346*
- **Sucraid®** *see* Sacrosidase *on page 1532*

Sucralfate (soo KRAL fate)

Brand Names: U.S. Carafate®

Brand Names: Canada Apo-Sucralfate; Dom-Sucralfate; Novo-Sucralate; Nu-Sucralate; PMS-Sucralate; Sucralfate-1; Sulcrate®; Sulcrate® Suspension Plus; Teva-Sucralfate

Index Terms Aluminum Sucrose Sulfate, Basic

Pharmacologic Category Gastrointestinal Agent, Miscellaneous

Use Short-term (≤8 weeks) management of duodenal ulcers; maintenance therapy for duodenal ulcers

Unlabeled Use Gastric ulcers; suspension may be used topically for treatment of stomatitis due to cancer chemotherapy and other causes of esophageal and gastric erosions; GERD, esophagitis; treatment of NSAID mucosal damage; prevention of stress ulcers; postsclerotherapy for esophageal variceal bleeding

Pregnancy Risk Factor B

Dosage Oral:

Children (unlabeled use): Doses of 40-80 mg/kg/day divided every 6 hours have been used
Stomatitis (unlabeled use): 5-10 mL (1 g/10 mL suspension), swish and spit or swish and swallow 4 times/day

Adults:
Stress ulcer (unlabeled use):
Prophylaxis: 1 g 4 times/day
Treatment: 1 g every 4 hours
Duodenal ulcer:
Treatment: 1 g 4 times/day on an empty stomach and at bedtime for 4-8 weeks, or alternatively 2 g twice daily; treatment is recommended for 4-8 weeks in adults
Maintenance: Prophylaxis: 1 g twice daily
Stomatitis (unlabeled use): 10 mL (1 g/10 mL suspension), swish and spit or swish and swallow 4 times/day

Dosage comment in renal impairment: Aluminum salt is minimally absorbed (<5%), however, may accumulate in renal failure

Additional Information Complete prescribing information for this medication should be consulted for additional detail.

Dosage Forms Excipient information presented when available (limited, particularly for generics); consult specific product labeling.

Suspension, oral: 1 g/10 mL (10 mL)
Carafate®: 1 g/10 mL (420 mL)
Tablet, oral: 1 g
Carafate®: 1 g [scored]

- **Sucralfate-1 (Can)** *see* Sucralfate *on page 1598*
- **Sucrets® Children's [OTC]** *see* Dyclonine *on page 568*
- **Sucrets® Maximum Strength [OTC]** *see* Dyclonine *on page 568*
- **Sucrets® Regular Strength [OTC]** *see* Dyclonine *on page 568*
- **Sudafed** *see* Pseudoephedrine *on page 1430*
- **Sudafed® 12 Hour [OTC]** *see* Pseudoephedrine *on page 1430*
- **Sudafed® 24 Hour [OTC]** *see* Pseudoephedrine *on page 1430*
- **Sudafed® Children's [OTC]** *see* Pseudoephedrine *on page 1430*
- **Sudafed® Children's Cold & Cough [OTC]** *see* Pseudoephedrine and Dextromethorphan *on page 1431*
- **Sudafed® Decongestant (Can)** *see* Pseudoephedrine *on page 1430*
- **Sudafed® Head Cold and Sinus Extra Strength (Can)** *see* Acetaminophen and Pseudoephedrine *on page 31*
- **Sudafed® Maximum Strength Nasal Decongestant [OTC]** *see* Pseudoephedrine *on page 1430*
- **Sudafed PE® Children's [OTC]** *see* Phenylephrine (Systemic) *on page 1344*
- **Sudafed PE® Children's Cold & Cough [OTC]** *see* Dextromethorphan and Phenylephrine *on page 490*
- **Sudafed PE® Congestion [OTC]** *see* Phenylephrine (Systemic) *on page 1344*
- **Sudafed PE™ Nasal Decongestant [OTC]** *see* Phenylephrine (Systemic) *on page 1344*
- **Sudafed PE® Non-Drying Sinus [OTC]** *see* Guaifenesin and Phenylephrine *on page 812*
- **Sudafed PE® Sinus + Allergy [OTC]** *see* Chlorpheniramine and Phenylephrine *on page 345*
- **Sudafed® Sinus Advance (Can)** *see* Pseudoephedrine and Ibuprofen *on page 1432*
- **SudaHist® [DSC]** *see* Chlorpheniramine and Pseudoephedrine *on page 346*
- **SudaTex-G [OTC]** *see* Guaifenesin and Pseudoephedrine *on page 813*
- **SudoGest [OTC]** *see* Pseudoephedrine *on page 1430*
- **SudoGest 12 Hour [OTC]** *see* Pseudoephedrine *on page 1430*
- **SudoGest Children's [OTC]** *see* Pseudoephedrine *on page 1430*
- **Sudogest™ PE [OTC]** *see* Phenylephrine (Systemic) *on page 1344*
- **Sudo-Tab® [OTC]** *see* Pseudoephedrine *on page 1430*
- **Sufenta®** *see* SUFentanil *on page 1598*

SUFentanil (soo FEN ta nil)

Brand Names: U.S. Sufenta®

Brand Names: Canada Sufentanil Citrate Injection, USP; Sufenta®

Index Terms Sufentanil Citrate

Pharmacologic Category Analgesic, Opioid; Anilidopiperidine Opioid; General Anesthetic

Use Analgesic supplement in maintenance of general anesthesia; epidural analgesic in conjunction with a local anesthetic

Pregnancy Risk Factor C

Dosage

I.V.:
Children 2-12 years: Induction: 10-25 mcg/kg (10-15 mcg/kg most common dose) with 100% O_2; Maintenance: Up to 1-2 mcg/kg total dose

Adults: Dose should be based on body weight. **Note:** In obese patients (eg, >20% above ideal body weight), use lean body weight to determine dosage.

Surgical analgesia (surgery 1-2 hours long): Total dose: 1-2 mcg/kg; ≥75% of dose administered prior to intubation; administered with N_2O/O_2; Maintenance: 5-20 mcg as needed. Total dose should not exceed 1 mcg/kg/hour of expected surgical time.

Epidural: Adults: Analgesia: Labor and delivery: 10-15 mcg with 10 mL bupivacaine 0.125% with/without epinephrine. May repeat at ≥1-hour interval for 2 additional doses.

Additional Information Complete prescribing information for this medication should be consulted for additional detail.

Dosage Forms Excipient information presented when available (limited, particularly for generics); consult specific product labeling.

Injection, solution [preservative free]: 50 mcg/mL (1 mL, 2 mL, 5 mL)

Sufenta®: 50 mcg/mL (1 mL, 2 mL, 5 mL)

Controlled Substance C-II

- **Sufentanil Citrate** *see* SUFentanil *on page 1598*
- **Sufentanil Citrate Injection, USP (Can)** *see* SUFentanil *on page 1598*
- **Sulamyd** *see* Sulfacetamide (Ophthalmic) *on page 1599*
- **Sulamyd** *see* Sulfacetamide (Topical) *on page 1599*
- **Sular®** *see* Nisoldipine *on page 1208*
- **Sulbactam and Ampicillin** *see* Ampicillin and Sulbactam *on page 117*

Sulconazole (sul KON a zole)

Brand Names: U.S. Exelderm®

Brand Names: Canada Exelderm®

Index Terms Sulconazole Nitrate

Pharmacologic Category Antifungal Agent, Topical

Use Treatment of superficial fungal infections of the skin, including tinea cruris (jock itch), tinea corporis (ringworm), tinea versicolor, and tinea pedis (athlete's foot, cream only)

Pregnancy Risk Factor C

Dosage Adults: Topical: Apply a small amount to the affected area and gently massage once or twice daily (tinea pedis apply twice daily) for 3 weeks (tinea cruris, tinea corporis, tinea versicolor) to 4 weeks (tinea pedis).

Additional Information Complete prescribing information for this medication should be consulted for additional detail.

Dosage Forms Excipient information presented when available (limited, particularly for generics); consult specific product labeling.

Cream, topical, as nitrate:

Exelderm®: 1% (15 g, 30 g, 60 g)

Solution, topical, as nitrate:

Exelderm®: 1% (30 mL)

- **Sulconazole Nitrate** *see* Sulconazole *on page 1599*
- **Sulcrate® (Can)** *see* Sucralfate *on page 1598*
- **Sulcrate® Suspension Plus (Can)** *see* Sucralfate *on page 1598*

Sulfacetamide (Ophthalmic) (sul fa SEE ta mide)

Brand Names: U.S. Bleph®-10; Sulfamide

Brand Names: Canada AK Sulf Liq; Bleph 10 DPS; Diosulf™; PMS-Sulfacetamide; Sodium Sulamyd

Index Terms Sodium Sulfacetamide; Sulamyd

Pharmacologic Category Antibiotic, Ophthalmic

Use Treatment and prophylaxis of conjunctivitis due to susceptible organisms; corneal ulcers; adjunctive treatment with systemic sulfonamides for therapy of trachoma

Pregnancy Risk Factor C

Dosage Children >2 months and Adults: Ophthalmic: Solution: Instill 1-2 drops several times daily up to every 2-3 hours in lower conjunctival sac during waking hours and less frequently at night; increase dosing interval as condition responds. Usual duration of treatment: 7-10 days

Trachoma: Instill 2 drops into the conjunctival sac every 2 hours; must be used in conjunction with systemic therapy

Additional Information Complete prescribing information for this medication should be consulted for additional detail.

Dosage Forms Excipient information presented when available (limited, particularly for generics); consult specific product labeling.

Solution, ophthalmic, as sodium [drops]: 10% (15 mL)

Bleph®-10: 10% (5 mL) [contains benzalkonium chloride]

Sulfamide: 10% (15 mL)

Sulfacetamide (Topical) (sul fa SEE ta mide)

Brand Names: U.S. Carmol® Scalp Treatment; Klaron®; Ovace®; Ovace® Plus; Rosula® NS; Seb-Prev™

Brand Names: Canada Sulfacet-R

Index Terms Sodium Sulfacetamide; Sulamyd; Sulfacetamide Sodium

Pharmacologic Category Acne Products; Antibiotic, Sulfonamide Derivative; Topical Skin Product, Acne

Use Scaling dermatosis (seborrheic); bacterial infections of the skin; acne vulgaris

Pregnancy Risk Factor C

Dosage Topical: Children >12 years and Adults:

Acne: Apply thin film to affected area twice daily

Seborrheic dermatitis: Apply at bedtime and allow to remain overnight; in severe cases, may apply twice daily. Duration of therapy is usually 8-10 applications; dosing interval may be increased as eruption subsides. Applications once or twice weekly, or every other week may be used to prevent eruptions.

Secondary cutaneous bacterial infections: Apply 2-4 times/day until infection clears

Additional Information Complete prescribing information for this medication should be consulted for additional detail.

Dosage Forms Excipient information presented when available (limited, particularly for generics); consult specific product labeling. [DSC] = Discontinued product

Aerosol, foam, topical, as sodium:

Ovace®: 10% (70 g [DSC])

Cream, topical, as sodium:

Seb-Prev™: 10% (30 g [DSC], 60 g [DSC]) [contains benzyl alcohol]

Gel, topical, as sodium:

Seb-Prev™: 10% (30 g [DSC], 60 g [DSC])

Gel, topical, as sodium [emulsion-based/wash]:

Ovace® Plus: 10% (355 mL)

Lotion, topical, as sodium: 10% (118 mL)

Carmol® Scalp Treatment: 10% (85 g) [contains urea 10%]

Klaron®: 10% (118 mL) [contains sodium metabisulfite]

Lotion, topical, as sodium [wash]: 10% (177 mL, 354.8 mL)

Ovace®: 10% (180 mL [DSC], 355 mL, 360 mL [DSC])

Pad, topical, as sodium: 10% (30s)

Rosula® NS: 10% (30s) [contains urea 10%]

Soap, topical, as sodium [wash]:

Seb-Prev™: 10% (170 mL, 340 mL)

Suspension, topical, as sodium: 10% (118 mL)

Sulfacetamide and Prednisolone

(sul fa SEE ta mide & pred NIS oh lone)

Brand Names: U.S. Blephamide®

Brand Names: Canada AK Cide Oph; Blephamide®; Dioptimyd®

Index Terms Prednisolone and Sulfacetamide

Pharmacologic Category Antibiotic/Corticosteroid, Ophthalmic

Use Steroid-responsive inflammatory ocular conditions in which a corticosteroid is indicated and where infection is present or there is a risk of infection

Pregnancy Risk Factor C

Dosage Ophthalmic:

Children ≥6 years and Adults:

Ointment: Apply ~1/2 inch ribbon to lower conjunctival sac 3-4 times/day and 1-2 times at night

Solution: Instill 2 drops every 4 hours

Suspension: Instill 2 drops every 4 hours during the day and at bedtime

Additional Information Complete prescribing information for this medication should be consulted for additional detail.

Dosage Forms Excipient information presented when available (limited, particularly for generics); consult specific product labeling.

Ointment, ophthalmic:

Blephamide®: Sulfacetamide sodium 10% and prednisolone acetate 0.2% (3.5 g)

Solution, ophthalmic [drops]: Sulfacetamide sodium 10% and prednisolone sodium phosphate 0.25% (5 mL, 10 mL)

Suspension, ophthalmic [drops]:

Blephamide®: Sulfacetamide sodium 10% and prednisolone acetate 0.2% (5 mL, 10 mL) [contains benzalkonium chloride]

◆ **Sulfacetamide and Sulfur** *see* Sulfur and Sulfacetamide *on page 1607*

◆ **Sulfacetamide Sodium** *see* Sulfacetamide (Topical) *on page 1599*

◆ **Sulfacet-R®** *see* Sulfur and Sulfacetamide *on page 1607*

◆ **Sulfacet-R (Can)** *see* Sulfacetamide (Topical) *on page 1599*

SulfADIAZINE

(sul fa DYE a zeen)

Pharmacologic Category Antibiotic, Sulfonamide Derivative

Use Treatment of the following conditions (per product labeling): Chancroid, trachoma, inclusion conjunctivitis, nocardiosis, urinary tract infections, toxoplasmosis encephalitis, malaria, meningococcal meningitis, acute otitis media, rheumatic fever (prophylaxis), meningitis (adjunctive)

Refer to current guidelines for appropriate use.

Pregnancy Risk Factor C

Pregnancy Considerations Adverse events have been observed in animal reproduction studies; therefore, the manufacturer classifies sulfadiazine as pregnancy category C. Sulfadiazine crosses the placenta. Available studies and case reports have failed to show an increased risk for congenital malformations after use. Sulfadiazine is indicated for use in children <2 months of age for the treatment of congenital toxoplasmosis and may be used in pregnancy for the maternal treatment of *Toxoplasmic gondii* encephalitis and as an alternative agent for the secondary prevention of rheumatic fever. Because of the theoretical increased risk for hyperbilirubinemia and kernicterus, sulfadiazine is contraindicated by the manufacturer for use near term. Neonatal healthcare providers should be informed if maternal sulfonamide therapy is used near the time of delivery.

Lactation Enters breast milk/contraindicated

Contraindications Hypersensitivity to any sulfa drug or any component of the formulation; children <2 months of age unless indicated for the treatment of congenital toxoplasmosis; pregnancy (at term); breast-feeding

Warnings/Precautions Fatalities associated with severe reactions including agranulocytosis, aplastic anemia and other blood dyscrasias, hepatic necrosis, Stevens-Johnson syndrome, and toxic epidermal necrolysis have occurred; discontinue use at first sign of rash or signs of serious adverse reactions. Use with caution in patients with allergies or asthma.

Chemical similarities are present among sulfonamides, sulfonylureas, carbonic anhydrase inhibitors, thiazides, and loop diuretics (except ethacrynic acid). Use in patients with sulfonamide allergy is specifically contraindicated in product labeling; however, a risk of cross-reaction exists in patients with allergy to any of these compounds; avoid use when previous reaction has been severe.

Prolonged use may result in fungal or bacterial superinfection, including *C. difficile*-associated diarrhea (CDAD) and pseudomembranous colitis; CDAD has been observed >2 months postantibiotic treatment. Use with caution in patients with G6PD deficiency; hemolysis may occur. Use with caution in patients with hepatic impairment. Use with caution in patients with renal impairment; dosage modification required. Maintain adequate hydration to prevent crystalluria. Not for the treatment of group A beta-hemolytic streptococcal infections.

Adverse Reactions Frequency not defined.

Cardiovascular: Allergic myocarditis, periarteritis nodosa

Central nervous system: Ataxia, chills, convulsions, depression, fever, hallucinations, headache, insomnia, vertigo

Dermatologic: Epidermal necrolysis, erythema multiforme, exfoliative dermatitis, photosensitivity, pruritus, purpura, rash, skin eruptions, Stevens-Johnson syndrome, urticaria

Endocrine & metabolic: Hypoglycemia, thyroid function disturbance

Gastrointestinal: Abdominal pain, anorexia, diarrhea, nausea, pancreatitis, stomatitis, vomiting

Genitourinary: Crystalluria, stone formation, toxic nephrosis with oliguria and anuria

Hematologic: Agranulocytopenia, aplastic anemia, hemolytic anemia, hypoprothrombinemia, leukopenia, methemoglobinemia, thrombocytopenia

Hepatic: Hepatitis

Neuromuscular & skeletal: Arthralgia, peripheral neuritis

Ocular: Conjunctival/scleral injection, periorbital edema

Otic: Tinnitus

Renal: Diuresis

Miscellaneous: Anaphylactoid reactions, lupus erythematosus, serum sickness-like reactions

Drug Interactions

Metabolism/Transport Effects Substrate of CYP2C9 (major), CYP2E1 (minor), CYP3A4 (minor); **Note:** Assignment of Major/Minor substrate status based on clinically relevant drug interaction potential; **Inhibits** CYP2C9 (strong)

Avoid Concomitant Use

Avoid concomitant use of SulfADIAZINE with any of the following: BCG; Methenamine; Potassium P-Aminobenzoate; Procaine

Increased Effect/Toxicity

SulfADIAZINE may increase the levels/effects of: Carvedilol; CycloSPORINE; CycloSPORINE (Systemic); CYP2C9 Substrates; Diclofenac; Fosphenytoin;

Methotrexate; Phenytoin; Porfimer; Prilocaine; Sulfonylureas; Vitamin K Antagonists

The levels/effects of SulfADIAZINE may be increased by: Conivaptan; CYP2C9 Inhibitors (Moderate); CYP2C9 Inhibitors (Strong); Methenamine

Decreased Effect

SulfADIAZINE may decrease the levels/effects of: BCG; CycloSPORINE; CycloSPORINE (Systemic); Typhoid Vaccine

The levels/effects of SulfADIAZINE may be decreased by: CYP2C9 Inducers (Strong); Cyproterone; Peginterferon Alfa-2b; Potassium P-Aminobenzoate; Procaine; Tocilizumab

Ethanol/Nutrition/Herb Interactions

Food: Avoid large quantities of vitamin C or acidifying agents (cranberry juice) to prevent crystalluria.

Herb/Nutraceutical: Avoid dong quai, St John's wort (may also cause photosensitization).

Stability Store at controlled room temperature of 20°C to 25°C (68°F to 77°F). Protect from light.

Mechanism of Action Interferes with bacterial growth by inhibiting bacterial folic acid synthesis through competitive antagonism of PABA

Pharmacodynamics/Kinetics

Absorption: Well absorbed

Distribution: Throughout body tissues and fluids including pleural, peritoneal, synovial, and ocular fluids; throughout total body water; readily diffused into CSF

Protein binding: 38% to 48%

Metabolism: Via N-acetylation

Half-life elimination: 10 hours

Time to peak: Within 3-6 hours

Excretion: Urine (43% to 60% as unchanged drug, 15% to 40% as metabolites)

Dosage Oral:

General dosing guidelines:

Children >2 months of age: Initial: 75 mg/kg; Maintenance: 150 mg/kg/day in 4-6 divided doses (maximum: 6 g/24 hours)

Adults: 2-4 g/day in 3-6 divided doses

Rheumatic fever prophylaxis: Children and Adults:

<30 kg: 0.5 g/day

≥30 kg: 1 g/day

Toxoplasmosis (HIV-exposed/-positive patients) (CDC, 2009):

Congenital toxoplasmosis: Infants: 100 mg/kg/day in divided doses every 12 hours for 12 months in combination with pyrimethamine plus leucovorin calcium

Acquired toxoplasmosis: Infants and Children:

Acute induction therapy: 25-50 mg/kg/dose given 4 times/day (maximum: 1-1.5 g/dose) in combination with pyrimethamine and leucovorin calcium. Continue acute induction therapy for ≥6 weeks, then follow with chronic suppressive therapy.

Prophylaxis to prevent recurrence (prior to encephalitis): 85-120 mg/kg/day divided every 6-12 hours (maximum: 2-4 g/day) in combination with pyrimethamine plus leucovorin calcium

Toxoplasma gondii encephalitis: Adolescents and Adults:

Acute therapy (duration of therapy: ≥6 weeks): 1000 mg (<60 kg) or 1500 mg (≥60 kg) every 6 hours in combination with pyrimethamine plus leucovorin calcium (preferred) **or** alternatively, may give 1000-1500 mg every 6 hours in combination with atovaquone

Prophylaxis to prevent recurrence: 2000-4000 mg/day in 2-4 divided doses in combination with pyrimethamine and leucovorin calcium (preferred) **or** alternatively, may give 2000-4000 mg/day in 2-4 divided doses in combination with atovaquone

Dietary Considerations Supplemental leucovorin calcium should be administered to reverse symptoms or prevent problems due to folic acid deficiency.

Administration Administer with at least 8 ounces of water and around-the-clock to promote less variation in peak and trough serum levels. Oral sodium bicarbonate may be used to alkalinize the urine of patients unable to maintain adequate fluid intake (in order to prevent crystalluria, azotemia, oliguria) (Lerner, 1996).

Monitoring Parameters Perform culture and sensitivity testing prior to initiating therapy; frequent CBC and urinalysis during therapy; signs of serious blood disorders (sore throat, fever, pallor, purpura, jaundice); CD4+ count in HIV-exposed/-positive patients treated for toxoplasmosis; sulfonamide blood concentrations may be monitored for severe infections (target: 12-15 mg/100 mL)

Dosage Forms Excipient information presented when available (limited, particularly for generics); consult specific product labeling.

Tablet, oral: 500 mg

Extemporaneous Preparations A 200 mg/mL oral suspension may be made with sulfadiazine powder and sterile water. Place 50 g sulfadiazine powder in a glass mortar. Add small portions of sterile water and mix to a uniform paste; mix while incrementally adding sterile water to **almost** 250 mL; transfer to a calibrated bottle, rinse mortar with sterile water, and add sufficient quantity of sterile water to make 250 mL. Label "shake well" and "refrigerate". Stable for 3 days refrigerated. **Note:** Suspension may also be prepared by crushing one-hundred 500 mg tablets; however, it is stable for only 2 days.

Pathmanathan U, Halgrain D, Chiadmi F, et al, "Stability of Sulfadiazine Oral Liquids Prepared From Tablets and Powder," *J Pharm Pharm Sci*, 2004, 7(1):84-7.

Sulfadoxine and Pyrimethamine

(sul fa DOKS een & peer i METH a meen)

Brand Names: U.S. Fansidar® [DSC]

Index Terms Pyrimethamine and Sulfadoxine

Pharmacologic Category Antimalarial Agent

Use Treatment of *Plasmodium falciparum* malaria in patients in whom chloroquine resistance is suspected; malaria prophylaxis for travelers to areas where chloroquine-resistant malaria is endemic

Pregnancy Risk Factor C/D (at term)

Dosage Children and Adults: Oral:

Treatment of acute attack of malaria: A single dose of the following number of Fansidar® tablets is used in sequence with quinine or alone:

2-11 months: 1/4 tablet

1-3 years: 1/2 tablet

4-8 years: 1 tablet

9-14 years: 2 tablets

>14 years: 3 tablets

Malaria prophylaxis: A single dose should be carried for self-treatment in the event of febrile illness when medical attention is not immediately available:

2-11 months: 1/4 tablet

1-3 years: 1/2 tablet

4-8 years: 1 tablet

9-14 years: 2 tablets

>14 years and Adults: 3 tablets

Additional Information Complete prescribing information for this medication should be consulted for additional detail.

Dosage Forms Excipient information presented when available (limited, particularly for generics); consult specific product labeling. [DSC] = Discontinued product

Tablet:

Fansidar®: Sulfadoxine 500 mg and pyrimethamine 25 mg [DSC]

Sulfamethoxazole and Trimethoprim

(sul fa meth OKS a zole & trye METH oh prim)

Brand Names: U.S. Bactrim™; Bactrim™ DS; Septra® DS; Septra® [DSC]

Brand Names: Canada Apo-Sulfatrim®; Apo-Sulfatrim® DS; Apo-Sulfatrim® Pediatric; Novo-Trimel; Novo-Trimel D.S.; Nu-Cotrimox; Septra® Injection

Index Terms Co-Trimoxazole; SMX-TMP; SMZ-TMP; Sulfatrim; TMP-SMX; TMP-SMZ; Trimethoprim and Sulfamethoxazole

Pharmacologic Category Antibiotic, Miscellaneous; Antibiotic, Sulfonamide Derivative

Additional Appendix Information

Prevention of Wound Infection and Sepsis in Surgical Patients *on page 1954*

Use

Oral treatment of urinary tract infections due to *E. coli*, *Klebsiella* and *Enterobacter* sp, *M. morganii*, *P. mirabilis* and *P. vulgaris*; acute otitis media in children; acute exacerbations of chronic bronchitis in adults due to susceptible strains of *H. influenzae* or *S. pneumoniae*; treatment and prophylaxis of *Pneumocystis jirovecii* pneumonia (PCP); traveler's diarrhea due to enterotoxigenic *E. coli*; treatment of enteritis caused by *Shigella flexneri* or *Shigella sonnei*

I.V. treatment of severe or complicated infections when oral therapy is not feasible, for documented PCP, empiric treatment of PCP in immune compromised patients; treatment of documented or suspected shigellosis, typhoid fever, or other infections caused by susceptible bacteria

Unlabeled Use Cholera and *Salmonella*-type infections and nocardiosis; chronic prostatitis; as prophylaxis in neutropenic patients with *P. jirovecii* infections, in leukemia patients, and in patients following renal transplantation, to decrease incidence of PCP; treatment of *Cyclospora* infection, typhoid fever, *Nocardia asteroides* infection; prophylaxis against urinary tract infection; alternative treatment for MRSA infections

Pregnancy Risk Factor C

Pregnancy Considerations Adverse events have been observed in animal reproduction studies; therefore, the manufacturer classifies TMP-SMX as pregnancy category C. TMP-SMX crosses the placenta and distributes to amniotic fluid. Due to trimethoprim's potential effect on folic acid metabolism, TMP-SMX should only be used during pregnancy if the benefit justifies the potential risk. The use of dihydrofolate reductase inhibitors, including trimethoprim, during pregnancy may increase the risk of congenital anomalies including cardiovascular defects, oral clefts, urinary tract anomalies, and neural tube defects. Folic acid supplementation may decrease this risk. A few case reports have described additional congenital anomalies after TMP-SMX exposure, but none of these have proven causality. Most studies and case reports have failed to show an increased risk for congenital malformations after use of TMP-SMX. Per the manufacturer, TMP-SMX is contraindicated in late pregnancy because sulfonamides pass the placenta and may cause kernicterus in the newborn, but this has not been observed specifically with SMX. Neonatal healthcare providers should be informed if maternal sulfonamide therapy is used near the time of delivery. TMP-SMX may be used in pregnancy for prophylaxis or treatment of *Pneumocystis jirovecii* pneumonia (PCP), the prophylaxis of *Toxoplasmic gondii* encephalitis (TE), and may prevent fetal loss in patients with Q fever (*Coxiella burnetii*). The pharmacokinetics of TMP-SMX are similar to nonpregnant values in early pregnancy.

Lactation Enters breast milk/contraindicated (AAP rates "compatible"; AAP 2001 update pending)

Contraindications Hypersensitivity to any sulfa drug, trimethoprim, or any component of the formulation; megaloblastic anemia due to folate deficiency; infants <2 months of age; marked hepatic damage or severe renal disease (if patient not monitored); pregnancy (at term); breast-feeding

Warnings/Precautions Use with caution in patients with G6PD deficiency, impaired renal or hepatic function or potential folate deficiency (malnourished, chronic anticonvulsant therapy, or elderly); maintain adequate hydration to prevent crystalluria; adjust dosage in patients with renal impairment. Injection vehicle contains benzyl alcohol and sodium metabisulfite.

Chemical similarities are present among sulfonamides, sulfonylureas, carbonic anhydrase inhibitors, thiazides, and loop diuretics (except ethacrynic acid). Use in patients with sulfonamide allergy is specifically contraindicated in product labeling, however, a risk of cross-reaction exists in patients with allergy to any of these compounds; avoid use when previous reaction has been severe.

Fatalities associated with severe reactions including Stevens-Johnson syndrome, toxic epidermal necrolysis, hepatic necrosis, agranulocytosis, aplastic anemia, and other blood dyscrasias; discontinue use at first sign of rash or serious adverse reactions. Elderly patients appear at greater risk for more severe adverse reactions. May cause hypoglycemia, particularly in malnourished, or patients with renal or hepatic impairment. Use with caution in patients with porphyria or thyroid dysfunction. Slow acetylators may be more prone to adverse reactions. Caution in patients with allergies or asthma. May cause hyperkalemia (associated with high doses of trimethoprim). Incidence of adverse effects appears to be increased in patients with AIDS. Prolonged use may result in fungal or bacterial superinfection, including *C. difficile*-associated diarrhea (CDAD) and pseudomembranous colitis; CDAD has been observed >2 months postantibiotic treatment.

Adverse Reactions The most common adverse reactions include gastrointestinal upset (nausea, vomiting, anorexia) and dermatologic reactions (rash or urticaria). Rare, life-threatening reactions have been associated with co-trimoxazole, including severe dermatologic reactions, blood dyscrasias, and hepatotoxic reactions. Most other reactions listed are rare, however, frequency cannot be accurately estimated.

Cardiovascular: Allergic myocarditis

Central nervous system: Apathy, aseptic meningitis, ataxia, chills, depression, fatigue, fever, hallucinations, headache, insomnia, kernicterus (in neonates), nervousness, peripheral neuritis, seizure, vertigo

Dermatologic: Photosensitivity, pruritus, rash, skin eruptions, urticaria; rare reactions include erythema multiforme, exfoliative dermatitis, Henoch-Schönlein purpura, Stevens-Johnson syndrome, and toxic epidermal necrolysis

Endocrine & metabolic: Hyperkalemia (generally at high dosages), hypoglycemia (rare), hyponatremia

Gastrointestinal: Abdominal pain, anorexia, diarrhea, glottitis, nausea, pancreatitis, pseudomembranous colitis, stomatitis, vomiting

Hematologic: Agranulocytosis, aplastic anemia, eosinophilia, hemolysis (with G6PD deficiency), hemolytic anemia, hypoprothrombinemia, leukopenia, megaloblastic anemia, methemoglobinemia, neutropenia, thrombocytopenia

Hepatic: Hepatotoxicity (including hepatitis, cholestasis, and hepatic necrosis), hyperbilirubinemia, transaminases increased

Neuromuscular & skeletal: Arthralgia, myalgia, rhabdomyolysis, weakness

Otic: Tinnitus

Renal: BUN increased, crystalluria, diuresis (rare), interstitial nephritis, nephrotoxicity (in association with cyclosporine), renal failure, serum creatinine increased, toxic nephrosis (with anuria and oliguria)

Respiratory: Cough, dyspnea, pulmonary infiltrates

Miscellaneous: Allergic reaction, anaphylaxis, angioedema, periarteritis nodosa (rare), serum sickness, systemic lupus erythematosus (rare)

Drug Interactions

Metabolism/Transport Effects Refer to individual components.

Avoid Concomitant Use

Avoid concomitant use of Sulfamethoxazole and Trimethoprim with any of the following: BCG; Dofetilide; Methenamine; Potassium P-Aminobenzoate; Procaine

Increased Effect/Toxicity

Sulfamethoxazole and Trimethoprim may increase the levels/effects of: ACE Inhibitors; Amantadine; Angiotensin II Receptor Blockers; Antidiabetic Agents (Thiazolidinedione); AzaTHIOprine; Carvedilol; CycloSPORINE; CycloSPORINE (Systemic); CYP2C8 Substrates; CYP2C9 Substrates; Dapsone; Dapsone (Systemic); Dapsone (Topical); Dofetilide; Eplerenone; Fosphenytoin; LamiVUDine; Memantine; Mercaptopurine; Methotrexate; Phenytoin; Porfimer; PRALAtrexate; Prilocaine; Procainamide; Repaglinide; Spironolactone; Sulfonylureas; Varenicline; Vitamin K Antagonists

The levels/effects of Sulfamethoxazole and Trimethoprim may be increased by: Amantadine; Conivaptan; CYP2C9 Inhibitors (Moderate); CYP2C9 Inhibitors (Strong); Dapsone; Dapsone (Systemic); Memantine; Methenamine

Decreased Effect

Sulfamethoxazole and Trimethoprim may decrease the levels/effects of: BCG; CycloSPORINE; CycloSPORINE (Systemic); Typhoid Vaccine

The levels/effects of Sulfamethoxazole and Trimethoprim may be decreased by: CYP2C9 Inducers (Strong); CYP3A4 Inducers (Strong); Deferasirox; Herbs (CYP3A4 Inducers); Leucovorin Calcium-Levoleucovorin; Peginterferon Alfa-2b; Potassium P-Aminobenzoate; Procaine; Tocilizumab

Ethanol/Nutrition/Herb Interactions Herb/Nutraceutical: Avoid dong quai; St John's wort (may diminish effects and also cause photosensitization).

Stability

Injection: Store at room temperature; do not refrigerate. Less soluble in more alkaline pH. Protect from light. Solution must be diluted prior to administration. Following dilution, store at room temperature; do not refrigerate. Manufacturer recommended dilutions and stability of parenteral admixture at room temperature (25°C):

5 mL/125 mL D_5W; stable for 6 hours.

5 mL/100 mL D_5W; stable for 4 hours.

5 mL/75 mL D_5W; stable for 2 hours.

Studies have also confirmed limited stability in NS; detailed references should be consulted.

Suspension, tablet: Store at controlled room temperature of 15°C to 25°C (59°F to 77°F). Protect from light.

Mechanism of Action Sulfamethoxazole interferes with bacterial folic acid synthesis and growth via inhibition of dihydrofolic acid formation from para-aminobenzoic acid; trimethoprim inhibits dihydrofolic acid reduction to tetrahydrofolate resulting in sequential inhibition of enzymes of the folic acid pathway

Pharmacodynamics/Kinetics

Absorption: Oral: Almost completely, 90% to 100%

Protein binding: SMX: 68%, TMP: 45%

Metabolism: SMX: N-acetylated and glucuronidated; TMP: Metabolized to oxide and hydroxylated metabolites

Half-life elimination: SMX: 9 hours, TMP: 6-17 hours; both are prolonged in renal failure

Time to peak, serum: Within 1-4 hours

Excretion: Both are excreted in urine as metabolites and unchanged drug

Effects of aging on the pharmacokinetics of both agents has been variable; increase in half-life and decreases in clearance have been associated with reduced creatinine clearance

Dosage Dosage recommendations are based on the trimethoprim component. Double-strength tablets are equivalent to sulfamethoxazole 800 mg and trimethoprim 160 mg.

Usual dosage ranges:

Children >2 months: Manufacturer's labeling:

Mild-to-moderate infections: Oral: 8 mg TMP/kg/day in divided doses every 12 hours

Serious infection:

Oral: 15-20 mg TMP/kg/day in divided doses every 6 hours

I.V.: 8-12 mg TMP/kg/day in divided doses every 6-12 hours

Adults:

Oral: 1-2 double-strength tablets (sulfamethoxazole 800 mg; trimethoprim 160 mg) every 12-24 hours

I.V.: 8-20 mg TMP/kg/day divided every 6-12 hours

Indication-specific dosing:

Children >2 months:

Acute otitis media: Oral: 8 mg TMP/kg/day in divided doses every 12 hours for 10 days. **Note:** Recommended by the American Academy of Pediatrics as an alternative agent in penicillin-allergic patients at a dose of 6-10 mg TMP/kg/day (AOM guidelines, 2004).

Cyclosporiasis (unlabeled use): Oral, I.V.: 5 mg TMP/kg twice daily for 7-10 days (*Red Book*, 2009)

Pneumocystis jirovecii:

Treatment: Oral, I.V.: 15-20 mg TMP/kg/day in divided doses every 6-8 hours for 21 days

Prophylaxis: Oral, 150 mg TMP/m^2/day in divided doses every 12 hours and administered for 3 days/week on consecutive or alternate days; an alternative dosing regimen allows for same dose to be administered in 2 divided doses daily (maximum: trimethoprim 320 mg and sulfamethoxazole 1600 mg daily) (CDC, 2009)

Shigellosis:

Oral: 8 mg TMP/kg/day in divided doses every 12 hours for 5 days

I.V.: 8-10 mg TMP/kg/day in divided doses every 6, 8, or 12 hours for up to 5 days

Skin/soft tissue infection due to community-acquired MRSA (unlabeled use): Oral: 4-6 mg TMP/kg/dose every 12 hours for 5-10 days (Liu, 2011); **Note:** If beta-hemolytic *Streptococcus* spp are also suspected, a beta-lactam antibiotic should be added to the regimen (Liu, 2011)

Toxoplasmosis primary prophylaxis in HIV-exposed/infected patients (unlabeled use; CDC, 2009): Oral: 150 mg TMP/m^2/day in 2 divided doses (preferred) or 150 mg TMP/m^2/day in a single dose 3 times/week on consecutive days; or 150 mg TMP/m^2/day in 2 divided doses 3 times/week on alternate days

Urinary tract infection:

Treatment:

Oral: 8 mg TMP/kg/day in divided doses every 12 hours

I.V.: 8-10 mg TMP/kg/day in divided doses every 6, 8, or 12 hours for up to 14 days with serious infections

Prophylaxis: Oral: 2 mg TMP/kg/dose daily or 5 mg TMP/kg/dose twice weekly

Adults:

Chronic bronchitis (acute): Oral: One double-strength tablet every 12 hours for 10-14 days

Cyclosporiasis (unlabeled use): Oral, I.V.: 160 mg TMP twice daily for 7-10 days. **Note:** AIDS patients: Oral: One double-strength tablet 2-4 times/day for 10 days, then 1 double-strength tablet 3 times/week for 10 weeks (Pape, 1994; Verdier, 2000)

Granuloma inguinale (donovanosis) (unlabeled use): Oral: One double-strength tablet every 12 hours for at least 3 weeks and until lesions have healed (CDC, 2010)

Isosporiasis (*Isospora belli* infection) in HIV-positive patients (unlabeled use; CDC, 2009):
- Treatment: Oral, I.V.: 160 mg TMP 4 times/day for 10 days **or** 160 mg TMP 2 times/day for 7-10 days. May increase dose and/or duration up to 3-4 weeks if symptoms worsen or persist
- Secondary prophylaxis (in patients with CD4+ count <200 /microL): Oral: 160 mg TMP 3 times/week (preferred) **or** alternatively, 160 mg TMP daily **or** 320 mg TMP 3 times/week

Meningitis (bacterial): I.V.: 10-20 mg TMP/kg/day in divided doses every 6-12 hours

Nocardia (unlabeled use): Oral, I.V.:
- Cutaneous infections: 5-10 mg TMP/kg/day in 2-4 divided doses
- Severe infections (pulmonary/cerebral): 15 mg TMP/kg/day in 2-4 divided doses for 3-4 weeks, then 10 mg TMP/kg/day in 2-4 divided doses. Treatment duration is controversial; an average of 7 months has been reported.
- **Note:** Therapy for severe infection may be initiated I.V. and converted to oral therapy (frequently converted to approximate dosages of oral solid dosage forms: 2 DS tablets every 8-12 hours). Although not widely available, sulfonamide levels should be considered in patients with questionable absorption, at risk for dose-related toxicity, or those with poor therapeutic response.

Osteomyelitis due to MRSA (unlabeled use): Oral, I.V.: 3.5-4 mg TMP/kg/dose every 8-12 hours for a minimum of 8 weeks with rifampin 600 mg once daily (Liu, 2011)

***Pneumocystis jirovecii* pneumonia (PCP):** Oral: Manufacturer's labeling:
- Prophylaxis: 160 mg TMP daily
- Treatment: 15-20 mg TMP/kg/day divided every 6 hours for 14-21 days

***Pneumocystis jirovecii* pneumonia (PCP) prophylaxis and treatment in HIV-positive patients (CDC, 2009):**
- **Note:** Sulfamethoxazole and trimethoprim is the preferred regimen for this indication.
- Prophylaxis: Oral: 80-160 mg TMP daily **or** alternatively, 160 mg TMP 3 times/week
- Treatment:
  - Mild-to-moderate: Oral: 15-20 mg TMP/kg/day in 3 divided doses for 21 days **or** alternatively, 320 mg TMP 3 times/day for 21 days
  - Moderate-to-severe: Oral, I.V.: 15-20 mg TMP/kg/day in 3-4 divided doses for 21 days

Sepsis: I.V.: 20 TMP/kg/day divided every 6 hours

Septic arthritis due to MRSA (unlabeled use): Oral, I.V.: 3.5-4 mg TMP/kg/dose every 8-12 hours for 3-4 weeks (some experts combine with rifampin) (Liu, 2011)

Shigellosis:
- Oral: One double-strength tablet every 12 hours for 5 days
- I.V.: 8-10 mg TMP/kg/day in divided doses every 6, 8, or 12 hours for up to 5 days

Skin/soft tissue infection due to community-acquired MRSA (unlabeled use): Oral: 1-2 double-strength tablets every 12 hours for 5-10 days (Liu, 2011); **Note:** If beta-hemolytic *Streptococcus* spp are also suspected, a beta-lactam antibiotic should be added to the regimen (Liu, 2011)

***Stenotrophomonas maltophilia* (ventilator-associated pneumonia):** I.V.: Most clinicians have utilized 12-15 mg TMP/kg/day for the treatment of VAP caused by *Stenotrophomonas maltophilia*. Higher doses (up to 20 mg TMP/kg/day) have been mentioned for treatment of severe infection in patients with normal renal function (Looney, 2009; Vartivarian, 1989; Wood, 2010)

***Toxoplasma gondii* encephalitis (unlabeled use; CDC, 2009):** Oral:
- Primary prophylaxis: Oral: 160 mg TMP daily (preferred) **or** 160 mg TMP 3 times/week **or** 80 mg TMP daily
- Treatment (alternative to sulfadiazine, pyrimethamine and leucovorin calcium): Oral, I.V.: 5 mg/kg TMP twice daily

Travelers' diarrhea: Oral: One double-strength tablet every 12 hours for 5 days

Urinary tract infection:
- Oral: One double-strength tablet every 12 hours
  - Duration of therapy: Uncomplicated: 3-5 days; Complicated: 7-10 days
  - Pyelonephritis: 14 days
  - Prostatitis: Acute: 2 weeks; Chronic: 2-3 months
- I.V.: 8-10 mg TMP/kg/day in divided doses every 6, 8, or 12 hours for up to 14 days with severe infections

Dosing adjustment in renal impairment: Oral, I.V.:

Manufacturer's recommendation: Children and Adults:
- Cl_{cr} >30 mL/minute: No dosage adjustment required
- Cl_{cr} 15-30 mL/minute: Administer 50% of recommended dose
- Cl_{cr} <15 mL/minute: Use is not recommended

Alternate recommendations:
- Cl_{cr} 15-30 mL/minute:
  - Treatment: Administer full daily dose (divided every 12 hours) for 24-48 hours, then decrease daily dose by 50% and administer every 24 hours (**Note:** For serious infections including *Pneumocystis jirovecii* pneumonia (PCP), full daily dose is given in divided doses every 6-8 hours for 2 days, followed by reduction to 50% daily dose divided every 12 hours) (Nahata, 1995).
  - PCP prophylaxis: One-half single-strength tablet (40 mg trimethoprim) daily **or** 1 single-strength tablet (80 mg trimethoprim) daily or 3 times weekly (Masur, 2002).
- Cl_{cr} <15 mL/minute:
  - Treatment: Administer full daily dose every 48 hours (Nahata, 1995)
  - PCP prophylaxis: One-half single-strength tablet (40 mg trimethoprim) daily **or** 1 single-strength tablet (80 mg trimethoprim) 3 times weekly (Masur, 2002). While the guidelines do acknowledge the alternative of giving 1 single-strength tablet daily, this may be inadvisable in the uremic/ESRD patient.

Intermittent Hemodialysis (IHD) (administer after hemodialysis on dialysis days):
- Treatment: Full daily dose before dialysis and 50% dose after dialysis (Nahata, 1995)
- Children: GFR <10 mL/minute/1.73 m^2: Not recommended, but if required 5-10 mg TMP/kg every 24 hours (Aronoff, 2007)
- PCP prophylaxis: One single-strength tablet (80 mg trimethoprim) after each dialysis session (Masur, 2002)
- **Note:** Dosing dependent on the assumption of 3 times/week, complete IHD sessions.

Peritoneal dialysis (PD):
- Use Cl_{cr} <15 mL/minute dosing recommendations. Not significantly removed by PD; supplemental dosing is not required (Aronoff, 2007):
- Exit-site and tunnel infections: Oral: One single-strength tablet daily (Li, 2010)

Peritonitis: Oral: One double-strength tablet twice daily (Li, 2010)

Children: GFR <10 mL/minute/1.73 m^2: Not recommended, but if required 5-10 mg TMP/kg every 24 hours. Intraperitoneal: Loading dose: TMP-SMX 320/1600 mg/L; Maintenance: TMP-SMX 80/400 mg/L (Aronoff, 2007; Warady, 2000)

Continuous renal replacement therapy (CRRT) (Heintz, 2009; Trotman, 2005): Drug clearance is highly dependent on the method of renal replacement, filter type, and flow rate. Appropriate dosing requires close monitoring of pharmacologic response, signs of adverse reactions due to drug accumulation, as well as drug concentrations in relation to target trough (if appropriate). The following are general recommendations only (based on dialysate flow/ultrafiltration rates of 1-2 L/hour and minimal residual renal function) and should not supersede clinical judgment:

CVVH/CVVHD/CVVHDF: 2.5-7.5 mg/kg of TMP every 12 hours. **Note:** Dosing regimen dependent on clinical indication. Critically-ill patients with *P. jirovecii* pneumonia receiving CVVHDF may require up to 10 mg/kg every 12 hours (Heintz, 2009).

Dietary Considerations Should be taken with 8 oz of water. May be taken without regard to meals.

Administration

I.V.: Infuse over 60-90 minutes, must dilute well before giving (ie, 1:15 to 1:25, which equates to 5 mL of drug solution diluted in 75-125 mL base solution); not for I.M. injection

Oral: Administer without regard to meals. Administer with at least 8 ounces of water.

Monitoring Parameters Perform culture and sensitivity testing prior to initiating therapy; CBC, serum potassium, creatinine, BUN

Test Interactions Increased creatinine (Jaffé alkaline picrate reaction); increased serum methotrexate by dihydrofolate reductase method

Dosage Forms Excipient information presented when available (limited, particularly for generics); consult specific product labeling. **Note:** The 5:1 ratio (SMX:TMP) remains constant in all dosage forms. [DSC] = Discontinued products

Injection, solution: Sulfamethoxazole 80 mg and trimethoprim 16 mg per mL (5 mL, 10 mL, 30 mL) [contains benzyl alcohol, ethanol 12.2%, propylene glycol 400 mg/mL, sodium metabisulfite]

Suspension, oral: Sulfamethoxazole 200 mg and trimethoprim 40 mg per 5 mL (480 mL)

Tablet: Sulfamethoxazole 400 mg and trimethoprim 80 mg

Bactrim™: Sulfamethoxazole 400 mg and trimethoprim 80 mg

Septra®: Sulfamethoxazole 400 mg and trimethoprim 80 mg [DSC]

Tablet, double-strength: Sulfamethoxazole 800 mg and trimethoprim 160 mg

Bactrim™ DS: Sulfamethoxazole 800 mg and trimethoprim 160 mg

Septra® DS: Sulfamethoxazole 800 mg and trimethoprim 160 mg

◆ **Sulfamide** *see* Sulfacetamide (Ophthalmic) *on page 1599*

◆ **Sulfamylon®** *see* Mafenide *on page 1043*

Sulfanilamide (sul fa NIL a mide)

Brand Names: U.S. AVC™

Index Terms p-amino-benzenesulfonamide

Pharmacologic Category Antifungal Agent, Vaginal

Use Treatment of vulvovaginitis caused by *Candida albicans*

Pregnancy Risk Factor C

Pregnancy Considerations Adverse events have been observed in animal reproduction studies with sulfonamides, including sulfanilamide. Sulfonamides cross the placenta and distribute to amniotic fluid. The fetal concentration is 50% to 90% of that measured in the maternal blood. Because of the theoretical increased risk for hyperbilirubinemia and kernicterus, neonatal healthcare providers should be informed if maternal sulfonamide therapy is used near the time of delivery.

Lactation Enters breast milk/not recommended

Contraindications Hypersensitivity to sulfanilamide or any component of the formulation

Warnings/Precautions Severe reactions, including agranulocytosis, aplastic anemia, and other blood dyscrasias, have occurred with sulfonamides (regardless of route). Severe dermatologic reactions, including Stevens-Johnson syndrome and toxic epidermal necrolysis, have occurred with sulfonamides (regardless of route). Fatalities associated with fulminant hepatic necrosis have occurred with sulfonamides (regardless of route). Chemical similarities are present among sulfonamides, sulfonylureas, carbonic anhydrase inhibitors, thiazides, and loop diuretics (except ethacrynic acid). Use in patients with sulfonamide allergy is specifically contraindicated in product labeling; however, a risk of cross-reaction exists in patients with allergy to any of these compounds; avoid use when previous reaction has been severe.

Topical antifungal agents or oral fluconazole are generally considered to be the preferred treatment for uncomplicated vulvovaginal candidiasis (Reef, 1993; Pappas, 2009; Sobel, 2007). Sulfanilamide is not recognized as a preferred or as an alternative agent for the treatment of uncomplicated vulvovaginitis candidiasis in the available literature.

Adverse Reactions <1% (Limited to important or life-threatening): Local: Sensitivity reactions (burning, discomfort)

Drug Interactions

Metabolism/Transport Effects None known.

Avoid Concomitant Use There are no known interactions where it is recommended to avoid concomitant use.

Increased Effect/Toxicity There are no known significant interactions involving an increase in effect.

Decreased Effect There are no known significant interactions involving a decrease in effect.

Mechanism of Action Interferes with microbial folic acid synthesis and growth via inhibition of para-aminiobenzoic acid metabolism; exerts a bacteriostatic action

Dosage Intravaginal: Adults: Females: Insert one applicatorful intravaginally once or twice daily; treatment should continue for a period of 30 days

Dosage Forms Excipient information presented when available (limited, particularly for generics); consult specific product labeling.

Cream, vaginal:

AVC™: 15% (120 g) [~6 g/applicator]

SulfaSALAzine (sul fa SAL a zeen)

Brand Names: U.S. Azulfidine EN-tabs®; Azulfidine®

Brand Names: Canada Alti-Sulfasalazine; Salazopyrin En-Tabs®; Salazopyrin®

Index Terms Salicylazosulfapyridine

Pharmacologic Category 5-Aminosalicylic Acid Derivative

Use Treatment of mild-to-moderate ulcerative colitis or as adjunctive therapy in severe ulcerative colitis; enteric coated tablets are also used for rheumatoid arthritis (including juvenile idiopathic arthritis [JIA]) in patients who inadequately respond to analgesics and NSAIDs

Unlabeled Use Ankylosing spondylitis, Crohn's disease, psoriasis, psoriatic arthritis

Pregnancy Risk Factor B

Pregnancy Considerations Adverse events have not been observed in animal reproduction studies. Sulfasalazine and sulfapyridine cross the placenta; a potential for kernicterus in the newborn exists. Agranulocytosis was noted in an infant following maternal use of sulfasalazine during pregnancy. Based on available data, an increase in fetal malformations has not been observed following maternal use of sulfasalazine for the treatment of inflammatory bowel disease or ulcerative colitis.

Lactation Enters breast milk/use caution (AAP recommends use "with caution"; AAP 2001 update pending)

Contraindications Hypersensitivity to sulfasalazine, sulfa drugs, salicylates, or any component of the formulation; porphyria; GI or GU obstruction

Warnings/Precautions Use with extreme caution in patients with renal impairment, impaired hepatic function or blood dyscrasias. Use caution in patients with severe allergies or asthma, or G6PD deficiency; may cause folate deficiency (consider providing 1 mg/day folate supplement). Deaths from irreversible neuromuscular or central nervous system changes, fibrosing alveolitis, agranulocytosis, aplastic anemia, and other blood dyscrasias have been reported. In males, oligospermia (rare) has been reported. Chemical similarities are present among sulfonamides, sulfonylureas, carbonic anhydrase inhibitors, thiazides, and loop diuretics (except ethacrynic acid). Nausea, vomiting, and abdominal discomfort commonly occur; titration of dose and/or using the enteric coated formulation may decrease GI adverse effects. Use in patients with sulfonamide allergy is specifically contraindicated in product labeling, however, a risk of cross-reaction exists in patients with allergy to any of these compounds; avoid use when previous reaction has been severe. Slow acetylators may be more prone to adverse reactions.

Adverse Reactions

>10%:

- Central nervous system: Headache
- Dermatologic: Rash
- Gastrointestinal: Anorexia, dyspepsia, gastric distress, nausea, vomiting
- Genitourinary: Oligospermia (reversible)

1% to 10%:

- Cardiovascular: Cyanosis
- Central nervous system: Dizziness, fever
- Dermatologic: Pruritus, urticaria
- Gastrointestinal: Abdominal pain, stomatitis
- Hematologic: Heinz body anemia, hemolytic anemia, leukopenia, thrombocytopenia
- Hepatic: Liver function tests abnormal

<1% (limited to important or life-threatening; includes reactions reported with mesalamine or other sulfonamides): Agranulocytosis, alopecia, anaphylaxis, aplastic anemia, arthralgia, ataxia, cholestatic jaundice, cirrhosis, crystalluria, depression, diarrhea, drowsiness, drug rash with eosinophilia and systemic symptoms (DRESS), eosinophilia, epidermal necrolysis, exfoliative dermatitis, fibrosing alveolitis, fulminant hepatitis, Guillain-Barré syndrome, hallucinations, hearing loss, hemolytic-uremic syndrome, hematuria, hepatic failure, hepatic necrosis, hepatitis, hypoglycemia, hypoprothrombinemia, insomnia, interstitial lung disease, interstitial nephritis, jaundice, Kawasaki-like syndrome (single case report), lupus-like syndrome, megaloblastic anemia, meningitis, methemoglobinemia, myelitis, myelodysplastic syndrome, myocarditis (allergic), nephropathy (acute), nephrotic syndrome, neutropenia (congenital), neutropenic enterocolitis, pancreatitis, pericarditis, periorbital edema, peripheral neuropathy, photosensitization, pleuritis, pneumonitis, polyarteritis nodosa, proteinuria, purpura, rhabdomyolysis, seizure, serum sickness-like reactions, skin discoloration, Stevens-Johnson syndrome, thyroid function disturbance, tinnitus, urine discoloration, vasculitis, vertigo

Drug Interactions

Metabolism/Transport Effects None known.

Avoid Concomitant Use There are no known interactions where it is recommended to avoid concomitant use.

Increased Effect/Toxicity

SulfaSALAzine may increase the levels/effects of: Heparin; Heparin (Low Molecular Weight); Methotrexate; Prilocaine; Thiopurine Analogs; Varicella Virus-Containing Vaccines

Decreased Effect

SulfaSALAzine may decrease the levels/effects of: Cardiac Glycosides; Methylfolate

Ethanol/Nutrition/Herb Interactions

Food: May impair folate absorption.

Herb/Nutraceutical: Avoid dong quai, St John's wort (may also cause photosensitization)

Stability Store at 25°C (77°F); excursions permitted to 15°C to 30°C (59°F to 86°F).

Mechanism of Action Acts locally in the colon to decrease the inflammatory response and systemically interferes with secretion by inhibiting prostaglandin synthesis

Pharmacodynamics/Kinetics

Absorption: ≤15% as unchanged drug from small intestine

Distribution: Small amounts enter feces

Metabolism: Via colonic intestinal flora to sulfapyridine and 5-aminosalicylic acid (5-ASA). Following absorption, sulfapyridine undergoes acetylation to form AcSP and ring hydroxylation while 5-ASA undergoes N-acetylation (non-acetylation phenotype dependent process); rate of metabolism via acetylation dependent on acetylation phenotype

Bioavailability: Sulfasalazine: <15%; sulfapyridine: ~60%; 5-aminosalicylic acid: ~10% to 30%

Half-life elimination: 5.7-10 hours (prolonged in elderly); sulfapyridine half-life prolonged in slow acetylators (14.8 hours)

Time to peak: Sulfasalazine: 3-12 hours (mean: 6 hours); metabolites: ~10 hours

Excretion: Primarily urine (as unchanged drug, components, and acetylated metabolites)

Dosage Oral:

Children ≥6 years:

- Ulcerative colitis: Initial: 40-60 mg/kg/day in 3-6 divided doses; maintenance dose: 30 mg/kg/day in 4 divided doses
- Juvenile idiopathic arthritis (JIA): Enteric coated tablet: 30-50 mg/kg/day in 2 divided doses; Initial: Begin with 1/4 to 1/3 of expected maintenance dose; increase weekly; maximum: 2 g/day typically

Adults:

- Ulcerative colitis:
  - Initial: 3-4 g/day in evenly divided doses at ≤8-hour intervals. **Note:** American College of Gastroenterology guideline recommendations: Titrate to 4-6 g/day in 4 divided doses (Kornbluth, 2010).
  - Maintenance dose: 2 g/day in evenly divided doses at ≤8-hour intervals; may initiate therapy with 1-2 g/day to reduce GI intolerance
- Rheumatoid arthritis: Enteric coated tablet: Initial: 0.5-1 g/day; increase weekly to maintenance dose of 2 g/day in 2 divided doses; maximum: 3 g/day (if response to 2 g/day is inadequate after 12 weeks of treatment)

Dosing interval in renal impairment: Use not recommended; weigh risk vs benefit

Dosing adjustment in hepatic impairment: Use not recommended; weigh risk vs benefit

Dietary Considerations Since sulfasalazine impairs folate absorption, consider providing 1 mg/day folate supplement.

Administration GI intolerance is common during the first few days of therapy (administer with meals). Do not crush enteric coated tablets.

Monitoring Parameters CBC with differential and liver function tests (prior to therapy, then every other week for first 3 months of therapy, followed by every month for the second 3 months, then once every 3 months thereafter); periodic urinalysis and renal function tests; stool frequency; signs of infection

Dosage Forms Excipient information presented when available (limited, particularly for generics); consult specific product labeling.

Tablet, oral: 500 mg

Azulfidine®: 500 mg [scored]

Tablet, delayed release, enteric coated, oral: 500 mg

Azulfidine EN-tabs®: 500 mg

Extemporaneous Preparations A 100 mg/mL oral suspension may be made with tablets. Place twenty 500 mg tablets in a mortar and add a small amount of a 1:1 mixture of Ora-Sweet® and Ora-Plus® to cover the tablets. Let soak for 20-30 minutes. Crush the tablets and mix to a uniform paste; mix while adding the vehicle in equal proportions to **almost** 100 mL; transfer to a calibrated bottle, rinse mortar with vehicle, and add sufficient quantity of vehicle to make 100 mL. Label "shake well". Stable 91 days under refrigeration or at room temperature.

Lingertat-Walsh K, Walker SE, Law S, et al, "Stability of Sulfasalazine Oral Suspension," *Can J Hosp Pharm*, 2006, 59(4):194-200.

◆ **Sulfatol®** *see* Sulfur and Sulfacetamide *on page 1607*

◆ **Sulfatol C™** *see* Sulfur and Sulfacetamide *on page 1607*

◆ **Sulfatol®-M [DSC]** *see* Sulfur and Sulfacetamide *on page 1607*

◆ **Sulfatol SS™** *see* Sulfur and Sulfacetamide *on page 1607*

◆ **Sulfatrim** *see* Sulfamethoxazole and Trimethoprim *on page 1602*

◆ **Sulfisoxazole and Erythromycin** *see* Erythromycin and Sulfisoxazole *on page 620*

Sulfur and Sulfacetamide

(SUL fur & sul fa SEE ta mide)

Brand Names: U.S. AVAR™; AVAR™ LS; AVAR™-e; AVAR™-e Green [DSC]; AVAR™-e LS; BP Cleansing Wash; BP10-1; Clarifoam™ EF; Clenia™; Plexion SCT®; Plexion®; Prascion®; Prascion® FC; Prascion® RA; Rosanil®; Rosula®; Rosula® Clarifying; Sulfacet-R®; Sulfatol C™; Sulfatol SS™; Sulfatol®; Sulfatol®-M [DSC]; Sumaxin™

Brand Names: Canada Sulfacet-R®

Index Terms Sodium Sulfacetamide and Sulfur; Sulfacetamide and Sulfur; Sulfur and Sulfacetamide Sodium

Pharmacologic Category Acne Products; Antibiotic, Sulfonamide Derivative; Antiseborrheic Agent, Topical; Topical Skin Product, Acne

Use Aid in the treatment of acne vulgaris, acne rosacea, and seborrheic dermatitis

Pregnancy Risk Factor C

Dosage Topical: Children ≥12 years and Adults: Apply in a thin film 1-3 times/day. Cleansing products should be used 1-2 times/day.

Dosage adjustment in renal impairment: Use is contraindicated.

Additional Information Complete prescribing information for this medication should be consulted for additional detail.

Dosage Forms Excipient information presented when available (limited, particularly for generics); consult specific product labeling. [DSC] = Discontinued product

Aerosol, foam, topical:

Clarifoam™ EF: Sulfur 5% and sulfacetamide sodium 10% (60 g)

Cleanser, topical: Sulfur 5% and sulfacetamide sodium 10% (170 g, 340 g)

AVAR™: Sulfur 5% and sulfacetamide sodium 10% (227 g) [contains benzyl alcohol]

AVAR™ LS: Sulfur 2% and sulfacetamide sodium 10% (227 g) [contains benzyl alcohol]

Plexion®: Sulfur 5% and sulfacetamide sodium 10% (170 g, 340 g)

Prascion®: Sulfur 5% and sulfacetamide sodium 10% (170 g, 340 g)

Rosanil®: Sulfur 5% and sulfacetamide sodium 10% (170 g, 390 g)

Rosula®: Sulfur 5% and sulfacetamide sodium 10% (355 mL) [contains urea 10%]

Cleanser, topical [emulsion-based]:

Sulfatol®: Sulfur 5% and sulfacetamide sodium 10% (355 mL) [contains urea 10%]

Cream, topical:

AVAR™-e: Sulfur 5% and sulfacetamide sodium 10% (45 g) [contains benzyl alcohol]

AVAR™-e Green: Sulfur 5% and sulfacetamide sodium 10% (45 g) [contains benzyl alcohol; color corrective cream] [DSC]

AVAR™-e LS: Sulfur 2% and sulfacetamide sodium 10% (45 g) [contains benzyl alcohol]

Clenia™: Sulfur 5% and sulfacetamide sodium 10% (28 g)

Plexion SCT®: Sulfur 5% and sulfacetamide sodium 10% (120 g) [contains benzyl alcohol]

Prascion® RA: Sulfur 5% and sulfacetamide sodium 10% (45 g) [contains benzyl alcohol and sunscreen]

Sulfatol C™: Sulfur 5% and sulfacetamide sodium 10% (28 g) [contains benzyl alcohol]

Sulfatol SS™: Sulfur 5% and sulfacetamide sodium 10% (45 g) [contains benzyl alcohol and sunscreen]

Gel, topical: Sulfur 5% and sulfacetamide sodium 10% (45 mL)

AVAR™: Sulfur 5% and sulfacetamide sodium 10% (45 g) [contains benzyl alcohol] [DSC]

Rosula®: Sulfur 5% and sulfacetamide sodium 10% (45 mL) [contains urea 10% and benzyl alcohol]

Gel, topical [emulsion-based]:

Sulfatol®: Sulfur 5% and sulfacetamide sodium 10% (45 mL) [contains urea 10%]

Lotion, topical: Sulfur 5% and sulfacetamide sodium 10% (25 g, 30 g, 45 g, 60 g)

Sulfacet-R®: Sulfur 5% and sulfacetamide sodium 10% (25 g) [contains sodium metabisulfite; tint formulation]

Sulfatol-M®: Sulfur 5% and sulfacetamide sodium 10% (25 g) [contains sodium metabisulfite; tint formulation] [DSC]

Sulfatol-M®: Sulfur 5% and sulfacetamide sodium 10% (25 g) [contains sodium metabisulfite; tint-free formulation] [DSC]

Pad, topical [cleansing cloth]:

Plexion®: Sulfur 5% and sulfacetamide sodium 10% (30s, 60s) [contains aloe vera]

Prascion® FC: Sulfur 5% and sulfacetamide sodium 10% (30s, 60s)

Sumaxin™: Sulfur 4% and sulfacetamide sodium 10% (60s) [contains aloe]

Suspension, topical: Sulfur 5% and sulfacetamide sodium 10% (30 g)

Wash, topical: Sulfur 5% and sulfacetamide sodium 10% (170 g, 340 g)
BP10-1: Sulfur 1% and sulfacetamide sodium 10% (170 g)
BP Cleansing Wash: Sulfur 5% and sulfacetamide sodium 10% (480 mL) [contains urea]
Clenia™: Sulfur 5% and sulfacetamide sodium 10% (170 g, 340 g)
Wash, topical [emulsion-based]:
Rosula® Clarifying: Sulfur 4% and sulfacetamide sodium 10% (473 mL) [contains urea 10%]

◆ **Sulfur and Sulfacetamide Sodium** *see* Sulfur and Sulfacetamide *on page 1607*

Sulindac (SUL in dak)

Brand Names: U.S. Clinoril®

Brand Names: Canada Apo-Sulin®; Novo-Sundac; Nu-Sulindac; Nu-Sundac; Teva-Sulindac

Pharmacologic Category Nonsteroidal Anti-inflammatory Drug (NSAID), Oral

Use Management of inflammatory diseases including osteoarthritis, rheumatoid arthritis, acute gouty arthritis, ankylosing spondylitis, acute painful shoulder (bursitis/tendonitis)

Unlabeled Use Management of preterm labor

Pregnancy Risk Factor C

Pregnancy Considerations Adverse events were not observed in the initial animal reproduction studies; therefore, the manufacturer classifies sulindac as pregnancy category C. Sulindac and the sulfide metabolite have been found to cross the placenta. NSAID exposure during the first trimester is not strongly associated with congenital malformations; however, cardiovascular anomalies and cleft palate have been observed following NSAID exposure in some studies. The use of an NSAID in the first trimester may be associated with an increased risk of miscarriage. Nonteratogenic effects have been observed following NSAID administration during the third trimester including myocardial degenerative changes, prenatal constriction of the ductus arteriosus, failure of the ductus arteriosus to close postnatally, and fetal tricuspid regurgitation; renal dysfunction or failure, oligohydramnios; gastrointestinal bleeding or perforation, increased risk of necrotizing enterocolitis; intracranial bleeding, platelet dysfunction with resultant bleeding; or pulmonary hypertension. Because they may cause premature closure of the ductus arteriosus, use of NSAIDs late in pregnancy should be avoided (use after 31-32 weeks gestation is not recommended by some clinicians). Sulindac has been used in the management of preterm labor. The chronic use of NSAIDs in women of reproductive age may be associated with infertility that is reversible upon discontinuation of the medication. A registry is available for pregnant women exposed to autoimmune medications including sulindac. For additional information contact the Organization of Teratology Information Specialists, OTIS Autoimmune Diseases Study, at (877) 311-8972.

Lactation Excretion in breast milk unknown/not recommended

Medication Guide Available Yes

Contraindications Hypersensitivity or allergic-type reactions to sulindac, aspirin, other NSAIDs, or any component of the formulation; perioperative pain in the setting of coronary artery bypass graft (CABG) surgery

Warnings/Precautions [U.S. Boxed Warning]: NSAIDs are associated with an increased risk of adverse cardiovascular thrombotic events, including MI and stroke. Use caution with fluid retention. Avoid use in heart failure. Concurrent administration of ibuprofen, and potentially other nonselective NSAIDs, may interfere with aspirin's cardioprotective effect. May cause new-onset hypertension or worsening of existing hypertension. NSAID use may compromise existing renal function; dose-dependent decreases in prostaglandin synthesis may result from NSAID use, reducing renal blood flow which may cause renal decompensation. NSAID use may increase the risk for hyperkalemia. Patients with impaired renal function, dehydration, heart failure, liver dysfunction, those taking diuretics, and ACE inhibitors, and the elderly are at greater risk of renal toxicity and hyperkalemia. Rehydrate patient before starting therapy; monitor renal function closely. Not recommended for use in patients with advanced renal disease. Long-term NSAID use may result in renal papillary necrosis. Use caution in patients with renal lithiasis; sulindac metabolites have been reported as components of renal stones. Maintain adequate hydration in patients with a history of renal stones. Use with caution in patients with decreased hepatic function. May require dosage adjustment in hepatic dysfunction; sulfide and sulfone metabolites may accumulate. The elderly are at increased risk for adverse effects.

[U.S. Boxed Warning]: Use is contraindicated for treatment of perioperative pain in the setting of coronary artery bypass graft (CABG) surgery. Risk of MI and stroke may be increased with use following CABG surgery.

[U.S. Boxed Warning]: NSAIDs may increase risk of gastrointestinal irritation, inflammation, ulceration, bleeding, and perforation. Use the lowest effective dose for the shortest duration of time, consistent with individual patient goals, to reduce risk of cardiovascular or GI adverse events. When used concomitantly with ≤325 mg of aspirin, a substantial increase in the risk of gastrointestinal complications (eg, ulcer) occurs; concomitant gastroprotective therapy (eg, proton pump inhibitors) is recommended (Bhatt, 2008). Pancreatitis has been reported; discontinue with suspected pancreatitis.

NSAIDS may cause drowsiness, dizziness, blurred vision and other neurologic effects which may impair physical or mental abilities; patients must be cautioned about performing tasks which require mental alertness (eg, operating machinery or driving). Discontinue use with blurred or diminished vision and perform ophthalmologic exam. Monitor vision with long-term therapy.

Platelet adhesion and aggregation may be decreased, may prolong bleeding time; patients with coagulation disorders or who are receiving anticoagulants should be monitored closely. Anemia may occur; patients on long-term NSAID therapy should be monitored for anemia. Rarely, NSAID use may cause severe blood dyscrasias (eg, agranulocytosis, aplastic anemia, thrombocytopenia). NSAIDs may cause serious skin adverse events including exfoliative dermatitis, Stevens-Johnson syndrome (SJS) and toxic epidermal necrolysis (TEN); discontinue use at first sign of skin rash or hypersensitivity. Anaphylactoid reactions may occur. Do not use in patients who experience bronchospasm, asthma, rhinitis, or urticaria with NSAID or aspirin therapy. Use caution in other forms of asthma. May increase the risk of aseptic meningitis, especially in patients with systemic lupus erythematosus (SLE) and mixed connective tissue disorders.

Withhold for at least 4-6 half-lives prior to surgical or dental procedures.

Adverse Reactions

1% to 10%:
Cardiovascular: Edema (1% to 3%)
Central nervous system: Dizziness (3% to 9%), headache (3% to 9%), nervousness (1% to 3%)
Dermatologic: Rash (3% to 9%), pruritus (1% to 3%)

Gastrointestinal: GI pain (10%), constipation (3% to 9%), diarrhea (3% to 9%), dyspepsia (3% to 9%), nausea (3% to 9%), abdominal cramps (1% to 3%), anorexia (1% to 3%), flatulence (1% to 3%), vomiting (1% to 3%)

Otic: Tinnitus (1% to 3%)

<1% (Limited to important or life-threatening): Agranulocytosis, ageusia, alopecia, anaphylaxis, angioneurotic edema, aplastic anemia, arrhythmia, aseptic meningitis, bitter taste, blurred vision, bone marrow depression, bronchial spasm, bruising, CHF, cholestasis, colitis, conjunctivitis, crystalluria, depression, dry mucous membranes, dyspnea, dysuria, epistaxis, erythema multiforme, exfoliative dermatitis, fever, gastritis, GI bleeding, GI perforation, glossitis, gynecomastia, hearing decreased, hematuria, hemolytic anemia, hepatitis, hepatic failure, hyperglycemia, hyperkalemia, hypersensitivity reaction, hypersensitivity syndrome (includes chills, diaphoresis, fever, flushing), hypersensitivity vasculitis, hypertension, insomnia, intestinal stricture, interstitial nephritis, jaundice, leukopenia, liver function abnormal, metallic taste, necrotizing fascitis, nephrotic syndrome, neuritis, neutropenia, palpitation, pancreatitis, paresthesia, peptic ulcer, photosensitivity, proteinuria, psychosis, purpura, renal calculi, renal failure, renal impairment, retinal disturbances, seizure, somnolence, Stevens-Johnson syndrome, stomatitis, syncope, thrombocytopenia, toxic epidermal necrolysis, urine discoloration, urticaria, vaginal bleeding, vertigo, visual disturbance, weakness

Drug Interactions

Metabolism/Transport Effects None known.

Avoid Concomitant Use

Avoid concomitant use of Sulindac with any of the following: Floctafenine; Ketorolac; Ketorolac (Nasal); Ketorolac (Systemic)

Increased Effect/Toxicity

Sulindac may increase the levels/effects of: Aminoglycosides; Anticoagulants; Antiplatelet Agents; Bisphosphonate Derivatives; Collagenase (Systemic); CycloSPORINE; CycloSPORINE (Systemic); Deferasirox; Desmopressin; Digoxin; Drotrecogin Alfa (Activated); Eplerenone; Haloperidol; Ibritumomab; Methotrexate; Nonsteroidal Anti-Inflammatory Agents; PEMEtrexed; Porfimer; Potassium-Sparing Diuretics; PRALAtrexate; Quinolone Antibiotics; Rivaroxaban; Salicylates; Thrombolytic Agents; Tositumomab and Iodine I 131 Tositumomab; Vancomycin; Vitamin K Antagonists

The levels/effects of Sulindac may be increased by: ACE Inhibitors; Angiotensin II Receptor Blockers; Antidepressants (Tricyclic, Tertiary Amine); Corticosteroids (Systemic); CycloSPORINE; CycloSPORINE (Systemic); Dasatinib; Dimethyl Sulfoxide; Floctafenine; Glucosamine; Herbs (Anticoagulant/Antiplatelet Properties); Ketorolac; Ketorolac (Nasal); Ketorolac (Systemic); Nonsteroidal Anti-Inflammatory Agents; Omega-3-Acid Ethyl Esters; Pentosan Polysulfate Sodium; Pentoxifylline; Probenecid; Prostacyclin Analogues; Selective Serotonin Reuptake Inhibitors; Serotonin/Norepinephrine Reuptake Inhibitors; Sodium Phosphates; Treprostinil; Vitamin E

Decreased Effect

Sulindac may decrease the levels/effects of: ACE Inhibitors; Angiotensin II Receptor Blockers; Antiplatelet Agents; Beta-Blockers; Eplerenone; HydrALAZINE; Loop Diuretics; Potassium-Sparing Diuretics; Salicylates; Selective Serotonin Reuptake Inhibitors; Thiazide Diuretics

The levels/effects of Sulindac may be decreased by: Bile Acid Sequestrants; Nonsteroidal Anti-Inflammatory Agents; Salicylates

Ethanol/Nutrition/Herb Interactions

Ethanol: Avoid ethanol (may enhance gastric mucosal irritation).

Herb/Nutraceutical: Avoid alfalfa, anise, bilberry, bladderwrack, bromelain, cat's claw, celery, chamomile, coleus, cordyceps, dong quai, evening primrose, fenugreek, feverfew, garlic, ginger, ginkgo biloba, ginseng (American, Panax, Siberian), grapeseed, green tea, guggul, horse chestnut seed, horseradish, licorice, prickly ash, red clover, reishi, SAMe (S-adenosylmethionine), sweet clover, turmeric, white willow (all have additional antiplatelet activity).

Stability Store at room temperature of 15°C to 30°C (59°F to 86°F).

Mechanism of Action Reversibly inhibits cyclooxygenase-1 and 2 (COX-1 and 2) enzymes, which results in decreased formation of prostaglandin precursors; has antipyretic, analgesic, and anti-inflammatory properties

Other proposed mechanisms not fully elucidated (and possibly contributing to the anti-inflammatory effect to varying degrees), include inhibiting chemotaxis, altering lymphocyte activity, inhibiting neutrophil aggregation/activation, and decreasing proinflammatory cytokine levels.

Pharmacodynamics/Kinetics

Absorption: 90%

Distribution: Crosses blood-brain barrier (brain concentrations <4% of plasma concentrations)

Protein binding: Sulindac: 93%, sulfone metabolite: 95%, sulfide metabolite: 98%; primarily to albumin

Metabolism: Hepatic; prodrug metabolized to sulfide metabolite (active) for therapeutic effects and to sulfone metabolites (inactive); parent and inactive sulfone metabolite undergo extensive enterohepatic recirculation

Half-life elimination: Sulindac: ~8 hours; Sulfide metabolite: ~16 hours

Time to peak: Sulindac: 3-4 hours; Sulfide and sulfone metabolites: 5-6 hours

Excretion: Urine (~50%, primarily as inactive metabolites, <1% as active metabolite); feces (~25%, primarily as metabolites)

Dosage Oral:

Children: Dose not established

Adults: **Note:** Maximum daily dose: 400 mg

Osteoarthritis, rheumatoid arthritis, ankylosing spondylitis: 150 mg twice daily

Acute painful shoulder (bursitis/tendonitis): 200 mg twice daily; usual treatment: 7-14 days

Acute gouty arthritis: 200 mg twice daily; usual treatment: 7 days

Dosing adjustment in renal impairment: Not recommended with advanced renal impairment; if required, decrease dose and monitor closely

Dosing adjustment in hepatic impairment: Dose reduction is necessary; discontinue if abnormal liver function tests occur

Dietary Considerations Drug may cause GI upset, bleeding, ulceration, perforation; take with food or milk to minimize GI upset.

Administration Should be administered with food or milk.

Monitoring Parameters Liver enzymes, BUN, serum creatinine, CBC, blood pressure; signs and symptoms of GI bleeding; ophthalmic exam (if ocular complaints develop during treatment)

Test Interactions Increased chloride (S), increased sodium (S), increased bleeding time

Dosage Forms Excipient information presented when available (limited, particularly for generics); consult specific product labeling.

Tablet, oral: 150 mg, 200 mg

Clinoril®: 200 mg [scored]

SUMAtriptan (soo ma TRIP tan)

Brand Names: U.S. Alsuma™; Imitrex®; Sumavel™ DosePro™

Brand Names: Canada Apo-Sumatriptan®; Ava-Sumatriptan; CO Sumatriptan; Dom-Sumatriptan; Imitrex®; Imitrex® DF; Imitrex® Injection; Imitrex® Nasal Spray; Mylan-Sumatriptan; PHL-Sumatriptan; PMS-Sumatriptan; Riva-Sumatriptan; Sandoz-Sumatriptan; Sumatriptan Injection; Sumatriptan Sun Injection; Sumatryx; Teva-Sumatriptan; Teva-Sumatriptan DF

Index Terms Sumatriptan Succinate

Pharmacologic Category Antimigraine Agent; Serotonin 5-$HT_{1B, 1D}$ Receptor Agonist

Additional Appendix Information

Antimigraine Drugs: 5-HT_1 Receptor Agonists *on page 1878*

Use

Intranasal, Oral, SubQ: Acute treatment of migraine with or without aura

SubQ: Acute treatment of cluster headache episodes

Pregnancy Risk Factor C

Pregnancy Considerations There are no adequate and well-controlled studies using sumatriptan in pregnant women. Use only if potential benefit to the mother outweighs the potential risk to the fetus. A pregnancy registry has been established to monitor outcomes of women exposed to sumatriptan during pregnancy (800-336-2176). Preliminary data from the registry do not suggest a greater risk of birth defects than the general population and so far a specific pattern of malformations has not been identified. However, sample sizes are small and studies are ongoing. In some (but not all) animal studies, administration was associated with embryolethality, fetal malformations and pup mortality.

Lactation Enters breast milk/use caution (AAP rates "compatible"; AAP 2001 update pending)

Contraindications Hypersensitivity to sumatriptan or any component of the formulation; patients with ischemic heart disease or signs or symptoms of ischemic heart disease (including Prinzmetal's angina, angina pectoris, myocardial infarction, silent myocardial ischemia); cerebrovascular syndromes (including strokes, transient ischemic attacks); peripheral vascular disease (including ischemic bowel disease); uncontrolled hypertension; use within 24 hours of ergotamine derivatives; use within 24 hours of another 5-HT_1 agonist; concurrent administration or within 2 weeks of discontinuing an MAO type A inhibitors (oral and nasal sumatriptan only; see Warnings/Precautions); management of hemiplegic or basilar migraine; severe hepatic impairment (oral and nasal sumatriptan, and injectable Imitrex® only); not for I.V. administration

Warnings/Precautions Sumatriptan is only indicated for the acute treatment of migraine or cluster headache (product dependent); not indicated for migraine prophylaxis, or for the treatment of hemiplegic or basilar migraine. If a patient does not respond to the first dose, the diagnosis of migraine or cluster headache should be reconsidered; rule out underlying neurologic disease in patients with atypical headache and in patients with no prior history of migraine or cluster headache. Cardiac events (coronary artery vasospasm, transient ischemia, myocardial infarction, ventricular tachycardia/fibrillation, cardiac arrest and death), cerebral/subarachnoid hemorrhage, and stroke have been reported with 5-HT_1 agonist administration. Patients who experience sensations of chest pain/pressure/tightness or symptoms suggestive of angina following dosing should be evaluated for coronary artery disease or Prinzmetal's angina before receiving additional doses; if dosing is resumed and similar symptoms recur, monitor with ECG. Do not give to patients with risk factors for CAD until a cardiovascular evaluation has been performed; if evaluation is satisfactory, the healthcare provider should administer the first dose (consider ECG monitoring) and cardiovascular status should be periodically evaluated.

Significant elevation in blood pressure, including hypertensive crisis, has also been reported on rare occasions in patients with and without a history of hypertension; use is contraindicated in patients with uncontrolled hypertension. Vasospasm-related reactions have been reported other than coronary artery vasospasm. Peripheral vascular ischemia and colonic ischemia with abdominal pain and bloody diarrhea have occurred. Transient and permanent blindness and significant partial vision loss have been very rarely reported. Use with caution in patients with a history of seizure disorder or in patients with a lowered seizure threshold. Use the oral formulation with caution (and with dosage limitations) in patients with hepatic impairment where treatment is necessary and advisable. Presystemic clearance of orally administered sumatriptan is reduced in hepatic impairment, leading to increased plasma concentrations; dosage reduction of the oral product is recommended. Non-oral routes of administration (nasal, subcutaneous formulations) do not undergo similar hepatic first-pass metabolism and are not expected to result in significantly altered pharmacokinetics in patients with hepatic impairment. Use of the oral, nasal, or Imitrex® injectable is contraindicated in severe hepatic impairment.

Symptoms of agitation, confusion, hallucinations, hyperreflexia, myoclonus, shivering, and tachycardia (serotonin syndrome) may occur with concomitant proserotonergic drugs (ie, SSRIs/SNRIs or triptans) or agents which reduce sumatriptan's metabolism. Concurrent use of serotonin precursors (eg, tryptophan) is not recommended. If concomitant administration with SSRIs is warranted, monitor closely, especially at initiation and with dose increases. Concurrent use with an MAO inhibitor may result in increased sumatriptan concentrations and increased risk for dose-related adverse effects (eg, serotonin syndrome); use with oral or nasal sumatriptan is contraindicated. Although generally not recommended, if concomitant use of MAO inhibitors with injectable sumatriptan is deemed necessary, careful monitoring and appropriate dosage adjustments are required. I.V. administration is contraindicated due to the potential to cause coronary vasospasm. Not recommended for use in elderly patients; older adults are at a higher risk for coronary artery disease and may be more likely to have reduced hepatic function.

Adverse Reactions

Injection:

>10%:

Central nervous system: Dizziness (12%), warm/hot sensation (11%)

Local: Injection site reaction (≤86%; includes bleeding, bruising, edema, and erythema)

Neuromuscular & skeletal: Paresthesia (5% to 14%)

1% to 10%:

Cardiovascular: Chest discomfort/tightness/pressure (2% to 5%)

Central nervous system: Burning sensation (7%), feeling of heaviness (7%), flushing (7%), pressure sensation (7%), feeling of tightness (5%), drowsiness (3%), feeling strange (2%), headache (2%), tight feeling in head (2%), anxiety (1%), cold sensation (1%), malaise/fatigue (1%)

Gastrointestinal: Nausea/vomiting (4%), abdominal discomfort (1%), dysphagia (1%)

Neuromuscular & skeletal: Neck pain/stiffness (5%), numbness (5%), weakness (5%), jaw discomfort (2%), myalgia (2%), muscle cramps (1%)

Ocular: Vision alterations (1%)

Respiratory: Throat discomfort (3%), nasal disorder/discomfort (2%), bronchospasm (1%)

Miscellaneous: Diaphoresis (2%)

Nasal spray:

>10%: Gastrointestinal: Bad taste (13% to 24%), nausea (11% to 13%), vomiting (11% to 13%)

1% to 10%:
- Central nervous system: Dizziness (1% to 2%)
- Respiratory: Nasal disorder/discomfort (2% to 4%), throat discomfort (1% to 2%)

Tablet:

1% to 10%:
- Cardiovascular: Chest pain/tightness/heaviness/pressure (1% to 2%), palpitation (1%), syncope (1%)
- Central nervous system: Burning (1%), dizziness (>1%), drowsiness (>1%), malaise/fatigue (2% to 3%), headache (>1%), nonspecified pain (1% to 2%, placebo 1%), vertigo (<1% to 2%), migraine (>1%), sleepiness (>1%)
- Gastrointestinal: Diarrhea (1%), nausea (>1%), vomiting (>1%), hyposalivation (>1%)
- Hematologic: Hemolytic anemia (1%)
- Neuromuscular & skeletal: Neck, throat, and jaw pain/tightness/pressure (2% to 3%), paresthesia (3% to 5%), myalgia (1%), numbness (1%)
- Otic: Ear hemorrhage (1%), hearing loss (1%), sensitivity to noise (1%), tinnitus (1%)
- Renal: Hematuria (1%)
- Respiratory: Allergic rhinitis (1%), dyspnea (1%), nasal inflammation (1%), nose/throat hemorrhage (1%), sinusitis (1%), upper respiratory inflammation (1%)
- Miscellaneous: Hypersensitivity reactions (1%), nonspecified pressure/tightness/heaviness (1% to 3%, placebo 2%); warm/cold sensation (2% to 3%, placebo 2%)

Route unspecified: <1%: Postmarketing and uncontrolled studies (limited to important or life-threatening): Abdominal aortic aneurysm, abnormal/elevated liver function tests, accommodation disorders, acute renal failure, anaphylactoid reaction, anaphylaxis, anemia, angioneurotic edema, arrhythmia, atrial fibrillation, bronchospasm, cardiomyopathy, cerebral ischemia, cerebrovascular accident, colonic ischemia, coronary artery vasospasm, cyanosis, deafness, ECG changes, hallucinations, heart block, hematuria, hemolytic anemia, hypersensitivity reactions, hyper-/hypotension, hypertensive crises, intestinal obstruction, intracranial pressure increased, ischemic colitis, MI, nose/throat hemorrhage, optic neuropathy (ischemic), pancytopenia, paresthesia, phlebitis, photosensitivity, Prinzmetal's angina, pulmonary embolism, Raynaud syndrome, retinal artery occlusion, retinal vein thrombosis, seizures, serotonin syndrome, shock, subarachnoid hemorrhage, syncope, temporal arteritis, thrombocytopenia, thrombophlebitis, thrombosis, transaminases increased, transient myocardial ischemia, TSH increased, vasculitis, ventricular fibrillation, ventricular tachycardia, vision loss

Drug Interactions

Metabolism/Transport Effects None known.

Avoid Concomitant Use

Avoid concomitant use of SUMAtriptan with any of the following: Ergot Derivatives; MAO Inhibitors

Increased Effect/Toxicity

SUMAtriptan may increase the levels/effects of: Ergot Derivatives; Metoclopramide; Serotonin Modulators

The levels/effects of SUMAtriptan may be increased by: Antipsychotics; Ergot Derivatives; MAO Inhibitors

Decreased Effect There are no known significant interactions involving a decrease in effect.

Stability

Alsuma™: Store at 25°C (77°F); excursions permitted between 15°C and 30°C (59°F and 86°F); do not refrigerate. Protect from light.

Imitrex® injectable, tablet, nasal spray: Store at 2°C to 30°C (36°F to 86°F). Protect from light.

Sumavel™ DosePro™: Store at 20°C to 25°C (68°F to 77°F); excursions permitted between 15°C and 30°C (59°F and 86°F); do not freeze.

Mechanism of Action Selective agonist for serotonin (5-HT_{1B} and 5-HT_{1D} receptors) in cranial arteries; causes vasoconstriction and reduces neurogenic inflammation associated with antidromic neuronal transmission correlating with relief of migraine

Pharmacodynamics/Kinetics

Onset of action: Oral: ~30 minutes; Nasal: ~15-30 minutes; SubQ: ~10 minutes

Distribution: V_d: 2.4 L/kg

Protein binding: 14% to 21%

Metabolism: Hepatic, primarily via MAO-A isoenzyme; extensive first-pass metabolism following oral administration

Bioavailability: Nasal: 17% (compared to SubQ); Oral: 15%; SubQ: 97% ± 16%

Half-life elimination: ~2-2.5 hours

Time to peak, serum: Oral: 2-2.5 hours; SubQ: 12 minutes (range: 4-20 minutes)

Excretion:
- Nasal spray: Urine (42% of total dose as indole acetic acid metabolite; 3% of total dose as unchanged drug)
- Oral: Urine (~60% of total dose, mostly as indole acetic acid metabolite; 3% of total dose as unchanged drug); feces (~40%)
- SubQ: Urine (38% of total dose as indole acetic acid metabolite; 22% of total dose as unchanged drug)

Dosage

Adults:

Oral: A single dose of 25 mg, 50 mg, or 100 mg (taken with fluids). If a satisfactory response has not been obtained at 2 hours, a second dose may be administered. Results from clinical trials show that initial doses of 50 mg and 100 mg are more effective than doses of 25 mg, and that 100 mg doses do not provide a greater effect than 50 mg and may have increased incidence of side effects. Although doses of up to 300 mg/day have been studied, the total daily dose should not exceed 200 mg. The safety of treating an average of >4 headaches in a 30-day period have not been established.

Intranasal: A single dose of 5 mg, 10 mg, or 20 mg administered in one nostril. A 10 mg dose may be achieved by administering a single 5 mg dose in each nostril. If headache returns, the dose may be repeated once after 2 hours, not to exceed a total daily dose of 40 mg. In clinical trials, a greater number of patients responded to initial doses of 20 mg versus 5 or 10 mg. The safety of treating an average of >4 headaches in a 30-day period has not been established.

SubQ: Initial: Up to 6 mg; may repeat if needed ≥1 hour after initial dose (maximum: Two 6 mg injections per 24-hour period). However, controlled clinical trials have failed to document a benefit with administration of a second 6 mg dose in nonresponders.

Elderly: Use is not recommended (due to increased potential for adverse effects).

Dosage adjustment in renal impairment: No dosage adjustments are recommended.

Dosage adjustment in hepatic impairment:

Mild-to-moderate hepatic impairment:
- Oral: Bioavailability of oral sumatriptan is increased with liver disease. If treatment is needed, do not exceed single doses of 50 mg.
- Nasal spray: Has not been studied in patients with hepatic impairment, however, because the spray does not undergo first-pass metabolism, levels would not be expected to be altered.
- Subcutaneous: Has been studied and pharmacokinetics were not altered in patients with hepatic impairment compared to healthy patients.

Severe hepatic impairment: Oral, nasal, and subcutaneous (limited to Imitrex® injection, per prescribing information) formulations are contraindicated with severe hepatic impairment.

Administration Should be administered as soon as symptoms appear.

Intranasal: Each nasal spray unit is preloaded with 1 dose; **do not** test the spray unit before use; remove unit from plastic pack when ready to use; while sitting down, gently blow nose to clear nasal passages; keep head upright and close one nostril gently with index finger; hold container with other hand, with thumb supporting bottom and index and middle fingers on either side of nozzle; insert nozzle into nostril about 1/2 inch; close mouth; take a breath through nose while releasing spray into nostril by pressing firmly on blue plunger; remove nozzle from nostril; keep head level for 10-20 seconds and gently breathe in through nose and out through mouth; **do not breathe deeply**

SubQ: Not for I.M. or I.V. use. Needle penetrates 1/4 inch of skin; use in areas of the body with adequate skin and subcutaneous thickness. Alsuma™ is a prefilled single-use autoinjector device.

Needleless administration (Sumavel™ DosePro™): Administer to the abdomen (>2 inches from the navel) or thigh; not for I.M. or I.V. administration. Do not administer to other areas of the body (eg, arm). Device is for single use only, discard after use; do not use if the tip of the device is tilted or broken.

Dosage Forms Excipient information presented when available (limited, particularly for generics); consult specific product labeling.

Injection, solution, as succinate [strength expressed as base]: 4 mg/0.5 mL (0.5 mL); 6 mg/0.5 mL (0.5 mL)

Alsuma™: 6 mg/0.5 mL (0.5 mL) [autoinjector]

Imitrex®: 4 mg/0.5 mL (0.5 mL); 6 mg/0.5 mL (0.5 mL) [cartridge]

Imitrex®: 6 mg/0.5 mL (0.5 mL) [vial]

Sumavel™ DosePro™: 6 mg/0.5 mL (0.5 mL) [needleless autoinjector]

Injection, solution, as succinate [strength expressed as base, preservative free]: 6 mg/0.5 mL (0.5 mL)

Solution, intranasal [spray]: 5 mg/0.1 mL (6s); 20 mg/0.1 mL (6s)

Imitrex®: 5 mg/0.1 mL (6s); 20 mg/0.1 mL (6s)

Tablet, oral, as succinate [strength expressed as base]: 25 mg, 50 mg, 100 mg

Imitrex®: 25 mg, 50 mg, 100 mg

Extemporaneous Preparations A 5 mg/mL oral liquid preparation made from tablets and one of three different vehicles (Ora-Sweet®, Ora-Sweet® SF, or Syrpalta® syrups). **Note:** Ora-Plus® Suspending Vehicle is used with Ora-Sweet® or Ora-Sweet® SF to facilitate dispersion of the tablets (Ora-Plus® is not necessary if Syrpalta® is the vehicle). Crush nine 100 mg tablets in a mortar and reduce to a fine powder. Add 40 mL of Ora-Plus® in 5 mL increments and mix thoroughly between each addition; rinse mortar and pestle 5 times with 10 mL of Ora-Plus®, pouring into bottle each time, and add quantity of appropriate syrup (Ora-Sweet® or Ora-Sweet® SF) sufficient to make 180 mL. Store in amber glass bottles in the dark; label "shake well", "refrigerate", and "protect from light". Stable for 21 days refrigerated.

Fish DN, Beall HD, Goodwin SD, et al, "Stability of Sumatriptan Succinate in Extemporaneously Prepared Oral Liquids," *Am J Health Syst Pharm*, 1997, 54(14):1619-22.

Sumatriptan and Naproxen

(soo ma TRIP tan & na PROKS en)

Brand Names: U.S. Treximet™

Index Terms Naproxen and Sumatriptan; Naproxen Sodium and Sumatriptan; Naproxen Sodium and Sumatriptan Succinate; Sumatriptan Succinate and Naproxen; Sumatriptan Succinate and Naproxen Sodium

Pharmacologic Category Antimigraine Agent; Nonsteroidal Anti-inflammatory Drug (NSAID), Oral; Serotonin 5-$HT_{1B, 1D}$ Receptor Agonist

Use Acute treatment of migraine with or without aura

Pregnancy Risk Factor C

Medication Guide Available Yes

Dosage Oral: Adults: 1 tablet (sumatriptan 85 mg and naproxen 500 mg). If a satisfactory response has not been obtained at 2 hours, a second dose may be administered (maximum: 2 tablets/24 hours). **Note:** The safety of treating an average of >5 migraine headaches in a 30-day period has not been established.

Dosage adjustment in renal impairment:

Cl_{cr} ≥30 mL/minute Dosage adjustment not necessary

Cl_{cr} <30 mL/minute: Use not recommended

Dosage adjustment in hepatic impairment: Mild-to-severe impairment: Use is contraindicated by the manufacturer

Additional Information Complete prescribing information for this medication should be consulted for additional detail.

Dosage Forms Excipient information presented when available (limited, particularly for generics); consult specific product labeling.

Tablet:

Treximet™ 85/500: Sumatriptan 85 mg and naproxen sodium 500 mg [contains sodium 61.2 mg/tablet (~2.7 mEq/tablet)]

◆ **Sumatriptan Injection (Can)** *see* SUMAtriptan *on page 1609*

◆ **Sumatriptan Succinate** *see* SUMAtriptan *on page 1609*

◆ **Sumatriptan Succinate and Naproxen** *see* Sumatriptan and Naproxen *on page 1612*

◆ **Sumatriptan Succinate and Naproxen Sodium** *see* Sumatriptan and Naproxen *on page 1612*

◆ **Sumatriptan Sun Injection (Can)** *see* SUMAtriptan *on page 1609*

◆ **Sumatryx (Can)** *see* SUMAtriptan *on page 1609*

◆ **Sumavel™ DosePro™** *see* SUMAtriptan *on page 1609*

◆ **Sumaxin™** *see* Sulfur and Sulfacetamide *on page 1607*

SUNItinib

(su NIT e nib)

Brand Names: U.S. Sutent®

Brand Names: Canada Sutent®

Index Terms SU011248; SU11248; Sunitinib Malate

Pharmacologic Category Antineoplastic Agent, Tyrosine Kinase Inhibitor; Vascular Endothelial Growth Factor (VEGF) Inhibitor

Use Treatment of gastrointestinal stromal tumor (GIST) intolerant to or with disease progression on imatinib; treatment of advanced renal cell cancer (RCC); treatment of advanced, metastatic or unresectable pancreatic neuroendocrine tumors (PNET)

Unlabeled Use Treatment of advanced thyroid cancer; treatment of non-GIST soft tissue sarcomas

Pregnancy Risk Factor D

Pregnancy Considerations Animal studies have demonstrated teratogenicity, embryotoxicity, and fetal loss. There are no adequate and well-controlled studies in pregnant women. Because sunitinib inhibits angiogenesis, a critical component of fetal development, adverse effects on pregnancy would be expected. Women of childbearing potential should be advised to avoid pregnancy if receiving sunitinib.

Lactation Excretion in breast milk unknown/not recommended

Medication Guide Available Yes

Contraindications There are no contraindications listed within the FDA-approved manufacturer's labeling.

Canadian labeling: Hypersensitivity to sunitinib or any component of the formulation; pregnancy

Warnings/Precautions Hazardous agent - use appropriate precautions for handling and disposal. **[U.S. Boxed Warning]: Hepatotoxicity, which may be severe and/or result in fatal liver failure, has been observed in clinical trials and in postmarketing surveillance.** Signs of liver failure include jaundice, elevated transaminases, and/or hyperbilirubinemia, in conjunction with encephalopathy, coagulopathy and/or renal failure. Monitor liver function tests at baseline, with each treatment cycle and if clinically indicated. Withhold treatment for grade 3 or 4 hepatotoxicity; discontinue if hepatotoxicity does not resolve. Do not reinitiate in patients with severe changes in liver function tests or other signs/symptoms of liver failure. Sunitinib has not been studied in patients with ALT or AST >2.5 times ULN (or >5 times ULN if due to liver metastases).

May cause a decrease in left ventricular ejection fraction (LVEF), including grade 3 reductions; consider obtaining LVEF evaluation prior to treatment. Mean onset of symptomatic heart failure (HF) is 22 days from treatment initiation. Interrupt therapy or decrease dose with LVEF <50% or >20% reduction from baseline. Discontinue with clinical signs and symptoms of HF. Cardiovascular events (some fatal), including symptomatic HF, myocardial disorders and cardiomyopathy have been reported with use. QT_c prolongation and torsade de pointes have been observed (dose dependent); a baseline and periodic ECG should be obtained; correct electrolyte abnormalities prior to treatment and monitor and correct potassium, calcium and magnesium levels during therapy; use caution in patients with a history of QT_c prolongation, with medications known to prolong the QT_c interval, or patients with pre-existing (relevant) cardiac disease, bradycardia, or electrolyte imbalance. Use with caution in patients with cardiac dysfunction; monitor for clinical signs/symptoms of HF, obtain baseline and periodic LVEF evaluation patients with MI, bypass grafts, symptomatic HF, vascular diseases (including CVA and TIA), and PE were excluded from clinical trials. May cause hypertension; monitor and control with antihypertensives if needed; interrupt therapy until hypertension is controlled for severe hypertension. Use caution and closely monitor in patients with underlying or poorly-controlled hypertension. Use with caution in patients concurrently taking strong CYP3A4 inhibitors (may increase sunitinib levels; eg, ketoconazole) or inducers (may decrease sunitinib levels; eg, rifampin); dosage adjustments of sunitinib may be required.

Hemorrhagic events have been reported including epistaxis, rectal, gingival, upper GI, urinary tract, genital, brain, wound bleeding, tumor-related, and hemoptysis/pulmonary hemorrhage; may be serious and/or fatal. Proteinuria and (rare) cases of nephrotic syndrome have been reported; discontinue treatment in patients with nephrotic syndrome. Microangiopathic hemolytic anemia (MAHA) and dose-limiting hypertension have been reported when sunitinib has been used in combination with bevacizumab. Impaired wound healing has been reported with sunitinib; temporarily withhold treatment for patients undergoing major surgical procedures; the optimal time to resume treatment after a procedure has not been determined. Serious and fatal gastrointestinal complications, including gastrointestinal perforation, have occurred (rarely). Pancreatitis has been observed in RCC patients; discontinue sunitinib if symptoms are present. Hypothyroidism may occur; the risk for hypothyroidism appears to increase with therapy duration; hyperthyroidism, sometimes followed by hypothyroidism has also been reported; monitor thyroid function at baseline and if symptomatic. Adrenal function abnormalities have been reported; monitor for adrenal insufficiency for patients with stress such as trauma, severe infection, or undergoing surgery. May cause skin and/or hair depigmentation or discoloration. Reversible posterior leukoencephalopathy syndrome (RPLS) has been reported (rarely); symptoms include confusion, headache, hypertension, lethargy, seizure, blindness and/or other vision, or neurologic disturbances; interrupt treatment and begin hypertension management. Dosing schedules vary by indication; some treatment regimens are continuous daily dosing; other treatment schedules are daily dosing for 4 weeks of a 6-week cycle (4 weeks on, 2 weeks off).

Adverse Reactions

>10%:

Cardiovascular: Hypertension (15% to 34%; grade 3: 4% to 13%), peripheral edema (24%), LVEF decreased (11% to 16%; grades 3/4: 1% to 3%), heart failure (≤15%), chest pain (13%)

Central nervous system: Fatigue (33% to 62%), headache (≤23%), fever (≤22%), insomnia (15% to 18%), chills (14%), depression (11%), dizziness (11%)

Dermatologic: Skin discoloration (25% to 30%), rash (14% to 29%), hand-foot syndrome (14% to 29%; grades 3/4: 4% to 8%), hair color changes (7% to 29%), dry skin (≤23%), alopecia (5% to 14%), erythema (12%), pruritus (12%)

Endocrine & metabolic: Hyperglycemia (23% to 71%), hyperuricemia (≤46%), hypocalcemia (34% to 42%), hypoalbuminemia (28% to 41%), hypophosphatemia (≤36%), hyponatremia (≤29%), hypoglycemia (17% to 22%), hypokalemia (12% to 21%), hypomagnesemia (≤19%), hyperkalemia (≤18%), hypothyroidism (4% to 16%; grades 3/4: ≤2%), hypercalcemia (13%), hypernatremia (10% to 13%)

Gastrointestinal: Diarrhea (40% to 66%), nausea (24% to 58%), lipase increased (17% to 56%), anorexia (33% to 48%), mucositis/stomatitis (29% to 48%), taste perversion (21% to 47%), abdominal pain (39%), vomiting (16% to 39%), amylase increased (17% to 35%), dyspepsia (15% to 34%), constipation (20% to 23%), weight loss (16%), flatulence (14%), oral pain (6% to 14%), xerostomia (13%), GERD/reflux (12%), glossodynia (11%)

Hematologic: Anemia (26% to 79%; grades 3/4: ≤8%), leukopenia (78%; grades 3/4: 8%), neutropenia (53% to 77%; grades 3/4: 10% to 17%), lymphopenia (38% to 68%; grades 3/4: ≤18%), thrombocytopenia (38% to 68%; grades 3/4: 5% to 9%), hemorrhage/bleeding (18% to 37%)

Hepatic: AST increased (39% to 72%; grades 3/4: 2% to 5%), alkaline phosphatase increased (24% to 63%; grades 3/4: 2% to 10%), ALT increased (39% to 61%; grades 3/4: 2% to 4%), hyperbilirubinemia (10% to 37%; grades 3/4 ≤1%)

Neuromuscular & skeletal: Creatine kinase increased (49%), limb pain (14% to 40%), weakness (22% to 34%), arthralgia (15% to 30%), back pain (≤28%), myalgia (14%)

Renal: Creatinine increased (12% to 70%)

Respiratory: Cough (27%), dyspnea (26%), epistaxis (21%), nasopharyngitis (14%), upper respiratory tract infection (11%)

1% to 10%:

Cardiovascular: Venous thrombotic events (1% to 3%), DVT (2% to 3%)

Gastrointestinal: Hemorrhoids (10%), pancreatitis (1%)

Respiratory: Pulmonary embolism (2%)

Miscellaneous: Flu-like syndrome (5%)

<1% (Limited to important or life-threatening): Acute renal failure, adrenal dysfunction, angioedema, aortic dissection, arterio thrombotic events, atrial flutter,

cardiomyopathy, cerebral infarction, cerebrovascular accident, coma, epistaxis, febrile neutropenia, fistula formation, gastrointestinal perforation, glomerular sclerosis (segmental), hepatic failure, hepatotoxicity, hypersensitivity, hyperthyroidism, infection, macrocytosis, microangiopathic hemolytic anemia (when used in combination with bevacizumab), MI, myocardial disorders, myopathy, nephrotic syndrome, neutropenic infection, pneumonitis (recall), preeclampsia-like syndrome (proteinuria and reversible hypertension), proteinuria, pulmonary hemorrhage, QT_c prolongation, renal impairment, reversible posterior leukoencephalopathy syndrome (RPLS), rhabdomyolysis, seizure, thrombotic microangiopathy, torsade de pointes, transient ischemic attack, tumor hemorrhage, tumor necrosis, ventricular arrhythmia, wound healing complications

Drug Interactions

Metabolism/Transport Effects Substrate of CYP3A4 (major); **Note:** Assignment of Major/Minor substrate status based on clinically relevant drug interaction potential; **Inhibits** BCRP, P-glycoprotein

Avoid Concomitant Use

Avoid concomitant use of SUNItinib with any of the following: Artemether; BCG; Bevacizumab; Conivaptan; Dronedarone; Lumefantrine; Natalizumab; Nilotinib; Pimecrolimus; Pimozide; QUEtiapine; QuiNINE; Silodosin; St Johns Wort; Tacrolimus (Topical); Temsirolimus; Tetrabenazine; Thioridazine; Topotecan; Toremifene; Vaccines (Live); Vandetanib; Vemurafenib; Ziprasidone

Increased Effect/Toxicity

SUNItinib may increase the levels/effects of: Bevacizumab; Colchicine; Dabigatran Etexilate; Dronedarone; Everolimus; Leflunomide; Natalizumab; P-glycoprotein/ABCB1 Substrates; Pimozide; QTc-Prolonging Agents; QuiNINE; Rivaroxaban; Silodosin; Tetrabenazine; Thioridazine; Topotecan; Toremifene; Vaccines (Live); Vandetanib; Vemurafenib; Vitamin K Antagonists; Ziprasidone

The levels/effects of SUNItinib may be increased by: Alfuzosin; Antifungal Agents (Azole Derivatives, Systemic); Artemether; Bevacizumab; Chloroquine; Ciprofloxacin; Ciprofloxacin (Systemic); Conivaptan; CYP3A4 Inhibitors (Moderate); CYP3A4 Inhibitors (Strong); Denosumab; Gadobutrol; Indacaterol; Lumefantrine; Nilotinib; Pimecrolimus; QUEtiapine; QuiNINE; Roflumilast; Tacrolimus (Topical); Temsirolimus; Trastuzumab

Decreased Effect

SUNItinib may decrease the levels/effects of: BCG; Cardiac Glycosides; Coccidioidin Skin Test; Sipuleucel-T; Vaccines (Inactivated); Vaccines (Live); Vitamin K Antagonists

The levels/effects of SUNItinib may be decreased by: CYP3A4 Inducers (Strong); Deferasirox; Echinacea; St Johns Wort; Tocilizumab

Ethanol/Nutrition/Herb Interactions

Food: Grapefruit juice may increase the levels/effects of sunitinib. Food has no effect on the bioavailability of sunitinib.

Herb/Nutraceutical: Avoid St John's wort (may increase metabolism and decrease sunitinib concentrations).

Stability Store at room temperature of 25°C (77°F); excursions permitted to 15°C to 30°C (59°F to 86°F).

Mechanism of Action Exhibits antitumor and antiangiogenic properties by inhibiting multiple receptor tyrosine kinases, including platelet-derived growth factors (PDGFRα and PDGFRβ), vascular endothelial growth factors (VEGFR1, VEGFR2, and VEGFR3), FMS-like tyrosine kinase-3 (FLT3), colony-stimulating factor type 1 (CSF-1R), and glial cell-line-derived neurotrophic factor receptor (RET).

Pharmacodynamics/Kinetics

Distribution: V_d/F: 2230 L

Protein binding: Sunitinib: 95%; SU12662: 90%

Metabolism: Hepatic; primarily metabolized by CYP3A4 to the N-desethyl metabolite SU12662 (active)

Half-life elimination: Terminal: Sunitinib: 40-60 hours; SU12662: 80-110 hours

Time to peak, plasma: 6-12 hours

Excretion: Feces (61%); urine (16%)

Dosage Oral: Adults: **Note:** Dosage modifications should be done in increments or decrements of 12.5 mg; individualize based on safety and tolerability.

Gastrointestinal stromal tumor (GIST): 50 mg once daily for 4 weeks of a 6-week treatment cycle (4 weeks on, 2 weeks off)

GIST unlabeled dosing: 37.5 mg once daily, continuous daily dosing (George, 2009, *EJC*)

Pancreatic neuroendocrine tumors, advanced (PNET): 37.5 mg once daily, continuous daily dosing (maximum daily dose used in clinical trials: 50 mg)

Renal cell cancer, advanced (RCC): 50 mg once daily for 4 weeks of a 6-week treatment cycle (4 weeks on, 2 weeks off)

Soft tissue sarcoma, non-GIST (unlabeled use): 37.5 mg once daily, continuous daily dosing (George, 2009, *JCO*)

Thyroid cancer, refractory (unlabeled use): 50 mg once daily for 4 weeks of a 6-week treatment cycle (4 weeks on, 2 weeks off) (Cohen, 2008; Ravaud, 2008)

Dosage adjustment with concurrent CYP3A4 inhibitor: Avoid concomitant administration with strong CYP3A4 inhibitors (eg, clarithromycin, erythromycin, itraconazole, ketoconazole, nefazodone, protease inhibitors, telithromycin, voriconazole); if concomitant administration with a strong CYP3A4 inhibitor cannot be avoided, consider a dose reduction to a minimum of 37.5 mg/day (GIST, RCC) or 25 mg/day (PNET).

Dosage adjustment with concurrent CYP3A4 inducer: Avoid concomitant administration with strong CYP3A4 inducers (eg, carbamazepine, dexamethasone, phenobarbital, phenytoin, rifampin, St John's wort); if concomitant administration with a strong CYP3A4 inducer cannot be avoided, consider a dosage increase (with careful monitoring) to a maximum of 87.5 mg/day (GIST, RCC) or 62.5 mg/day (PNET).

Dosage adjustment for toxicity: Dosage modifications should be done in increments or decrements of 12.5 mg; individualize based on safety and tolerability.

Cardiac toxicity:

Ejection fraction <50% and >20% below baseline without evidence of CHF: Interrupt treatment and/or reduce dose

LV dysfunction with CHF clinical manifestations: Discontinue treatment

Hepatotoxicity: Hepatic adverse events ≥ grade 3 or 4: Withhold treatment; discontinue if hepatotoxicity does not resolve. Do not reinitiate in patients with severe changes in liver function tests or other signs/symptoms of liver failure.

Severe hypertension: Temporarily interrupt treatment until hypertension is controlled

Nephrotic syndrome or pancreatitis: Discontinue treatment

Reversible posterior leukoencephalopathy (RPLS) or thrombotic microangiopathy: Temporarily withhold treatment; after resolution, may resume with discretion.

Dosage adjustment in renal impairment:

Mild, moderate, or severe impairment: No initial adjustment required; subsequent adjustments may be needed based on safety and tolerance.

ESRD on hemodialysis: No initial adjustment required; subsequent dosage **increases** (up to 2 fold) may be required due to reduced (47%) exposure

Dosage adjustment in hepatic impairment: No adjustment is necessary with mild-to-moderate (Child-Pugh class A or B) hepatic impairment; not studied in patients with severe (Child-Pugh class C) hepatic impairment. Studies excluded patients with ALT or AST >2.5 x ULN, or if due to liver metastases, ALT or AST >5 x ULN.

Dietary Considerations May be taken with or without food. Avoid grapefruit juice.

Administration May be administered with or without food.

Monitoring Parameters LVEF, baseline (and periodic with cardiac risk factors), ECG (12-lead; baseline and periodic), blood pressure, adrenal function, CBC with differential and platelets (prior to each treatment cycle), liver function tests (baseline, with each cycle and if clinically indicated), serum chemistries including magnesium, phosphate, and potassium (prior to each treatment cycle), thyroid function (baseline; then if symptomatic), urinalysis (for proteinuria development or worsening)

Additional Information Hand-foot skin reaction (HFSR) management (Lacouture, 2008): The following treatments may be used in addition to the recommended dosage modifications. Prior to treatment initiation, a pedicure is recommended to remove hyperkeratotic areas/calluses, which may predispose to HFSR; avoid vigorous exercise/activities which may stress hands or feet. During therapy, patients should reduce exposure to hot water (may exacerbate hand-foot symptoms); avoid constrictive footwear and excessive skin friction. Patients may also wear thick cotton gloves or socks and should wear shoes with padded insoles. Grade 1 HFSR may be relieved with moisturizing creams, cotton gloves and socks (at night) and/or keratolytic creams such as urea (20% to 40%) or salicylic acid (6%). Apply topical steroid (eg, clobetasol ointment) twice daily to erythematous areas of Grade 2 HFSR; topical anesthetics (eg, lidocaine 2%) and then systemic analgesics (if appropriate) may be used for pain control. Resolution of acute erythema may result in keratotic areas which may be softened with keratolytic agents.

Dosage Forms Excipient information presented when available (limited, particularly for generics); consult specific product labeling.

Capsule, oral:

Sutent®: 12.5 mg, 25 mg, 50 mg

Extemporaneous Preparations Hazardous agent: Use appropriate precautions for handling and disposal.

A 10 mg/mL sunitinib oral suspension may be made with capsules and a 1:1 mixture of Ora-Sweet® and Ora-Plus®. Empty the contents of three 50 mg sunitinib capsules into a mortar; add small portions of vehicle and mix to a uniform paste. Mix while adding vehicle in incremental proportions to 15 mL. Transfer to amber plastic bottle and label "shake well". This suspension maintains an average concentration of 96% to 106% (of the original concentration) at room temperature or refrigerated for up to 60 days in plastic amber prescription bottles.

Navid F, Christensen R, Minkin P, et al, "Stability of Sunitinib in Oral Suspension," *Ann Pharmacother*, 2008, 42(7):962-6.

- **Sunitinib Malate** *see* SUNItinib *on page 1612*
- **Supartz®** *see* Hyaluronate and Derivatives *on page 831*
- **Super Calcium 600 [OTC]** *see* Calcium Carbonate *on page 266*
- **Supeudol® (Can)** *see* OxyCODONE *on page 1266*
- **Suplasyn® (Can)** *see* Hyaluronate and Derivatives *on page 831*
- **Supprelin® LA** *see* Histrelin *on page 830*
- **Suprax®** *see* Cefixime *on page 307*
- **Suprenza™** *see* Phentermine *on page 1341*
- **Suprep® Bowel Prep Kit** *see* Sodium Sulfate, Potassium Sulfate, and Magnesium Sulfate *on page 1576*
- **Survanta®** *see* Beractant *on page 206*
- **Sustiva®** *see* Efavirenz *on page 575*
- **Sutent®** *see* SUNItinib *on page 1612*
- **Su-Tuss DM [DSC]** *see* Guaifenesin and Dextromethorphan *on page 810*
- **Suxamethonium Chloride** *see* Succinylcholine *on page 1596*
- **Sween Cream® [OTC]** *see* Vitamin A and Vitamin D *on page 1796*
- **Syeda™** *see* Ethinyl Estradiol and Drospirenone *on page 654*
- **Sylatron™** *see* Peginterferon Alfa-2b *on page 1311*
- **Sylatron™** *see* Peginterferon Alfa-2b *on page 1311*
- **Symax® DuoTab** *see* Hyoscyamine *on page 854*
- **Symax® FasTab** *see* Hyoscyamine *on page 854*
- **Symax® SL** *see* Hyoscyamine *on page 854*
- **Symax® SR** *see* Hyoscyamine *on page 854*
- **Symbicort®** *see* Budesonide and Formoterol *on page 240*
- **Symlin® [DSC]** *see* Pramlintide *on page 1391*
- **SymlinPen®** *see* Pramlintide *on page 1391*
- **Symmetrel** *see* Amantadine *on page 82*
- **Symmetrel® (Can)** *see* Amantadine *on page 82*
- **Sympt-X [OTC]** *see* Glutamine *on page 799*
- **Sympt-X G.I. [OTC]** *see* Glutamine *on page 799*
- **Synacthen** *see* Cosyntropin *on page 415*
- **Synagis®** *see* Palivizumab *on page 1280*
- **Synalar® (Can)** *see* Fluocinolone (Topical) *on page 726*
- **Synalgos®-DC** *see* Dihydrocodeine, Aspirin, and Caffeine *on page 508*
- **Synarel®** *see* Nafarelin *on page 1170*
- **Synera™** *see* Lidocaine and Tetracaine *on page 1011*
- **Synercid®** *see* Quinupristin and Dalfopristin *on page 1450*
- **Synphasic® (Can)** *see* Ethinyl Estradiol and Norethindrone *on page 660*
- **Synthroid®** *see* Levothyroxine *on page 1004*
- **Synvisc®** *see* Hyaluronate and Derivatives *on page 831*
- **Synvisc-One®** *see* Hyaluronate and Derivatives *on page 831*
- **Syprine®** *see* Trientine *on page 1736*
- **Syrex** *see* Sodium Chloride *on page 1567*
- **T_3 Sodium (error-prone abbreviation)** *see* Liothyronine *on page 1016*
- **T_3/T_4 Liotrix** *see* Liotrix *on page 1017*
- **T_4** *see* Levothyroxine *on page 1004*
- **T-20** *see* Enfuvirtide *on page 587*
- **T-91825** *see* Ceftaroline Fosamil *on page 315*
- **Tabloid®** *see* Thioguanine *on page 1670*
- **Taclonex®** *see* Calcipotriene and Betamethasone *on page 261*
- **Taclonex Scalp®** *see* Calcipotriene and Betamethasone *on page 261*

Tacrolimus (Systemic) (ta KROE li mus)

Brand Names: U.S. Prograf®

Brand Names: Canada Advagraf®; Prograf®

Index Terms FK506

Pharmacologic Category Calcineurin Inhibitor; Immunosuppressant Agent

Use
Prograf®:
U.S. labeling: Prevention of organ rejection in heart, kidney, or liver transplant recipients
Canadian labeling: Prevention of organ rejection in heart, kidney, or liver transplant recipients; treatment of refractory rejection in kidney or liver transplant recipients; treatment of active rheumatoid arthritis in adult patients nonresponsive to disease-modifying antirheumatic drug (DMARD) therapy or when DMARD therapy is inappropriate
Advagraf® (Canadian availability; not available in U.S.): Prevention of organ rejection in kidney transplant recipients

Unlabeled Use Prevention of organ rejection in lung, small bowel transplant recipients; prevention and treatment of graft-versus-host disease (GVHD) in allogenic hematopoietic stem cell transplantation

Pregnancy Risk Factor C

Pregnancy Considerations Adverse events were observed in animal reproduction studies. Tacrolimus crosses the human placenta and is measurable in the cord blood, amniotic fluid, and newborn serum. Tacrolimus concentrations in the placenta may be higher than the maternal serum. No consistent pattern of congenital anomalies has been observed. Transient neonatal hyperkalemia and renal dysfunction have been reported.

The National Transplantation Pregnancy Registry (NTPR, Temple University) is a registry for pregnant women taking immunosuppressants following any solid organ transplant. The NTPR encourages reporting of all immunosuppressant exposures during pregnancy in transplant recipients at 877-955-6877.

Lactation Enters breast milk/not recommended

Medication Guide Available Yes

Contraindications Hypersensitivity to tacrolimus or any component of the formulation

Warnings/Precautions Hazardous agent - use appropriate precautions for handling and disposal. **[U.S. Boxed Warning]: Risk of developing infections (including bacterial, viral [including CMV], fungal, and protozoal infections [including opportunistic infections]) is increased.** Latent viral infections may be activated, including BK virus (associated with polyoma virus-associated nephropathy [PVAN]) and JC virus (associated with progressive multifocal leukoencephalopathy [PML]); may result in serious adverse effects. The risk of CMV disease is increased for patients who are CMV-seronegative prior to transplant and receive a graft from a CMV-seropositive donor. Consider reduction in immunosuppression if PVAN, PML, CMV viremia and/or CMV disease occurs. **[U.S. Boxed Warning]: Immunosuppressive therapy may result in the development of lymphoma and other malignancies (predominantly skin malignancies).** The risk for new-onset diabetes and insulin-dependent post-transplant diabetes mellitus (PTDM) is increased with tacrolimus use after transplantation, including in patients without pretransplant history of diabetes mellitus; insulin dependence may be reversible; increased risk in African-American and Hispanic kidney transplant patients. Nephrotoxicity has has been reported, especially with higher doses; to avoid excess nephrotoxicity do not administer simultaneously with other nephrotoxic drugs (eg sirolimus, cyclosporine). Neurotoxicity may occur especially when used in high doses; tremor headache, coma and delirium have been reported and are associated with serum concentrations. Seizures may also occur. Posterior reversible encephalopathy syndrome (PRES) may also occur; symptoms (altered mental status, headache, hypertension, seizures, and visual disturbances) are reversible with dose reduction or discontinuation of therapy; stabilize blood pressure and reduce dose with suspected or confirmed PRES diagnosis.

Pure red cell aplasia (PRCA) has been reported in patients receiving tacrolimus. Use with caution in patients with risk factors for PRCA including parvovirus B19 infection, underlying disease, or use of concomitant medications associated with PRCA (eg, mycophenolate). Discontinuation of therapy should be considered with diagnosis of PRCA. Monitoring of serum concentrations (trough for oral therapy) is essential to prevent organ rejection and reduce drug-related toxicity. A period of ≥24 hours should elapse between discontinuation of cyclosporine and the initiation of tacrolimus. Delay initiation further with persistently elevated tacrolimus/cyclosporine levels. Use caution in renal or hepatic dysfunction, dosing adjustments may be required. Delay initiation of therapy in kidney transplant patients if postoperative oliguria occurs; begin therapy no sooner than 6 hours and within 24 hours post-transplant, but may be delayed until renal function has recovered. Use may be associated with the development of hypertension (common); hyperkalemia has been reported; avoid use of potassium-sparing diuretics. Myocardial hypertrophy has been reported (rare). Concurrent use with strong CYP3A4 inhibitors (eg, ritonavir, ketoconazole, itraconazole, voriconazole, clarithromycin) or inducers (eg, rifampin, rifabutin) is not recommended without close monitoring of tacrolimus trough concentrations.

Each mL of injection contains polyoxyl 60 hydrogenated castor oil (HCO-60) (200 mg) and dehydrated alcohol USP 80% v/v. Anaphylaxis has been reported with the injection, use should be reserved for those patients not able to take oral medications. Patients should not be immunized with live vaccines during or shortly after treatment and should avoid close contact with recently vaccinated (live vaccine) individuals. Oral formulations contain lactose; the Canadian labeling does not recommend use of these products in patients who may be lactose intolerant (eg, Lapp lactase deficiency, glucose-galactose malabsorption, galactose intolerance). **[U.S. Boxed Warning]: Should be administered under the supervision of a physician experienced in immunosuppressive therapy and organ transplantation in a facility appropriate for monitoring and managing therapy.**

Adverse Reactions As reported for kidney, liver, and heart transplantation:

≥15%:
Cardiovascular: Hypertension (13% to 62%), edema (peripheral 11% to 36%), chest pain (19%), edema (18%), pericardial effusion (heart transplant 15%)
Central nervous system: Headache (24% to 64%), insomnia (30% to 64%), pain (24% to 63%), fever (19% to 48%), postprocedural pain (kidney transplant 29%), dizziness (19%)
Dermatologic: Pruritus (15% to 36%), rash (10% to 24%)
Endocrine & metabolic: New-onset diabetes after transplant (75% kidney transplant), hypophosphatemia (28% to 49%), hypomagnesemia (16% to 48%), hyperglycemia (21% to 47%), hyperkalemia (13% to 45%), hyperlipemia (10% to 31%), hypokalemia (13% to 29%), diabetes mellitus (24% to 26%), post-transplant diabetes mellitus (heart transplant 13% to 22%; kidney transplant 20%; liver transplant 11% to 18%)
Gastrointestinal: Diarrhea (25% to 72%), abdominal pain (29% to 59%), nausea (32% to 46%), constipation (23% to 36%), anorexia (7% to 34%), vomiting (14% to 29%), dyspepsia (18% to 28%)
Genitourinary: Urinary tract infection (16% to 34%)
Hematologic: Anemia (5% to 50%), leukopenia (13% to 48%), leukocytosis (8% to 32%), thrombocytopenia (14% to 24%)
Hepatic: Liver function tests abnormal (6% to 36%), ascites (7% to 27%)

Local: Incision site complication (kidney transplant 28%)
Neuromuscular & skeletal: Tremor (15% to 56%; heart transplant 15%), weakness (11% to 52%), paresthesia (17% to 40%), back pain (17% to 30%), arthralgia (25%)
Renal: Abnormal kidney function (36% to 56%), creatinine increased (23% to 45%), BUN increased (12% to 30%), oliguria (18% to 19%)
Respiratory: Atelectasis (5% to 28%), pleural effusion (30% to 36%), dyspnea (5% to 29%), cough increased (18%), bronchitis (17%)
Miscellaneous: Infection (24% to 45%), CMV infection (heart transplant 32%), graft dysfunction (kidney transplant 24%)

<15%:
Cardiovascular: Abnormal ECG (QRS or ST segment abnormal), arrhythmia, atrial fibrillation, atrial flutter, bradycardia, cardiopulmonary failure, deep thrombophlebitis, heart failure, heart rate decreased, hemorrhage, hemorrhagic stroke, hypervolemia, hypotension, peripheral vascular disorder, phlebitis, postural hypotension, syncope, tachycardia, thrombosis, vasodilation
Central nervous system: Abnormal dreams, abnormal thinking, agitation, amnesia, anxiety, chills, confusion, depression, emotional lability, encephalopathy, flaccid paralysis, hallucinations, mood elevated, nervousness, psychosis, quadriparesis, seizure, somnolence, vertigo
Dermatologic: Acne, alopecia, bruising, cellulitis, exfoliative dermatitis, fungal dermatitis, hirsutism, photosensitivity reaction, skin discoloration, skin disorder, skin neoplasm, skin ulcer, wound healing impaired
Endocrine & metabolic: Acidosis, alkalosis, bicarbonate decreased, Cushing's syndrome, dehydration, gout, hypercholesterolemia, hyper-/hypocalcemia, hyponatremia, hyperphosphatemia, hyperuricemia, hypoproteinemia, serum iron decreased
Gastrointestinal: Appetite increased, cramps, duodenitis, dysphagia, enlarged abdomen, esophagitis (including ulcerative), flatulence, gastritis, gastroesophagitis, GI perforation/hemorrhage, ileus, oral moniliasis, pancreatic pseudocyst, rectal disorder, stomatitis, weight gain
Genitourinary: Bladder spasm, cystitis, dysuria, nocturia, urge incontinence, urinary frequency, urinary incontinence, urinary retention, vaginitis
Hematologic: Coagulation disorder, decreased prothrombin, hypochromic anemia, polycythemia
Hepatic: Alkaline phosphatase increased, bilirubinemia, cholangitis, cholestatic jaundice, GGT increased, hepatitis (including granulomatous), jaundice, LDH increased, liver damage
Local: Phlebitis
Neuromuscular & skeletal: Hypertonia, incoordination, joint disorder, leg cramps, monoparesis, myalgia, myasthenia, myoclonus, nerve compression, neuropathy, osteoporosis, quadriparesis
Ocular: Abnormal vision, amblyopia
Otic: Ear pain, otitis media, tinnitus
Renal: Acute renal failure, albuminuria, BK nephropathy, hematuria, hydronephrosis, renal tubular necrosis, toxic nephropathy
Respiratory: Asthma, emphysema, lung disorder, lung function decreased, pharyngitis, pneumonia, pneumothorax, pulmonary edema, respiratory disorder, rhinitis, sinusitis, voice alteration
Miscellaneous: Abscess, abnormal healing, allergic reaction, crying, diaphoresis, flu-like syndrome, generalized spasm, hernia, herpes simplex, hiccups, peritonitis, sepsis, writing impaired

Postmarketing and/or case reports (limited to important or life-threatening): Anaphylaxis, anaphylactoid reaction, angioedema, ARDS, atrial flutter, basal cell carcinoma, bile duct stenosis, blindness, cardiac arrest, cerebral infarction, cerebrovascular accident, deafness, delirium, DIC, hemiparesis, hemolytic-uremic syndrome, hemorrhagic cystitis, hepatic necrosis, hepatotoxicity, interstitial lung disease, leukoencephalopathy, lymphoproliferative disorder (related to EBV), malignant melanoma, myocardial hypertrophy (associated with ventricular dysfunction; reversible upon discontinuation), MI, neutropenia, osteomyelitis, pancreatitis (hemorrhagic and necrotizing), pancytopenia, posterior reversible encephalopathy syndrome (PRES), progressive multifocal leukoencephalopathy (PML), quadriplegia, QT_c prolongation, respiratory failure, septicemia, squamous cell carcinoma, Stevens-Johnson syndrome, toxic epidermal necrolysis, thrombocytopenic purpura, torsade de pointes, TTP, veno-occlusive hepatic disease, venous thrombosis, ventricular fibrillation

Note: Calcineurin inhibitor-induced hemolytic uremic syndrome/thrombotic thrombocytopenic purpura/thrombotic microangiopathy (HUS/TTP/TMA) have been reported (with concurrent sirolimus).

Drug Interactions

Metabolism/Transport Effects **Substrate** of CYP3A4 (major), P-glycoprotein; **Note:** Assignment of Major/Minor substrate status based on clinically relevant drug interaction potential; **Inhibits** CYP3A4 (weak), P-glycoprotein

Avoid Concomitant Use

Avoid concomitant use of Tacrolimus (Systemic) with any of the following: Artemether; BCG; Conivaptan; Crizotinib; CycloSPORINE (Systemic); Dronedarone; Eplerenone; Grapefruit Juice; Lumefantrine; Natalizumab; Nilotinib; Pimecrolimus; Pimozide; Potassium-Sparing Diuretics; QUEtiapine; QuiNINE; Silodosin; Sirolimus; Tacrolimus (Topical); Temsirolimus; Tetrabenazine; Thioridazine; Topotecan; Toremifene; Vaccines (Live); Vandetanib; Vemurafenib; Ziprasidone

Increased Effect/Toxicity

Tacrolimus (Systemic) may increase the levels/effects of: Colchicine; CycloSPORINE (Systemic); Dabigatran Etexilate; Dronedarone; Everolimus; Fosphenytoin; Leflunomide; Natalizumab; P-glycoprotein/ABCB1 Substrates; Phenytoin; Pimozide; QTc-Prolonging Agents; QuiNINE; Rivaroxaban; Silodosin; Sirolimus; Temsirolimus; Tetrabenazine; Thioridazine; Topotecan; Toremifene; Vaccines (Live); Vandetanib; Vemurafenib; Ziprasidone

The levels/effects of Tacrolimus (Systemic) may be increased by: Alfuzosin; Antidepressants (Serotonin Reuptake Inhibitor/Antagonist); Artemether; Calcium Channel Blockers (Dihydropyridine); Calcium Channel Blockers (Nondihydropyridine); Chloramphenicol; Chloroquine; Ciprofloxacin; Ciprofloxacin (Systemic); Clotrimazole; Clotrimazole (Oral); Conivaptan; Crizotinib; CycloSPORINE (Systemic); CYP3A4 Inhibitors (Moderate); CYP3A4 Inhibitors (Strong); Danazol; Denosumab; Eplerenone; Fluconazole; Gadobutrol; Grapefruit Juice; Indacaterol; Itraconazole; Ketoconazole; Ketoconazole (Systemic); Lumefantrine; Macrolide Antibiotics; MetroNIDAZOLE; MetroNIDAZOLE (Systemic); Nilotinib; P-glycoprotein/ABCB1 Inhibitors; Pimecrolimus; Posaconazole; Potassium-Sparing Diuretics; Protease Inhibitors; Proton Pump Inhibitors; QUEtiapine; QuiNINE; Ranolazine; Roflumilast; Sirolimus; Tacrolimus (Topical); Telaprevir; Temsirolimus; Trastuzumab; Voriconazole

Decreased Effect

Tacrolimus (Systemic) may decrease the levels/effects of: BCG; Coccidioidin Skin Test; Sipuleucel-T; Vaccines (Inactivated); Vaccines (Live)

The levels/effects of Tacrolimus (Systemic) may be decreased by: Caspofungin; Cinacalcet; CYP3A4 Inducers (Strong); Deferasirox; Echinacea; Efavirenz; Fosphenytoin; P-glycoprotein/ABCB1 Inducers;

Phenytoin; Rifamycin Derivatives; Sirolimus; St Johns Wort; Temsirolimus; Tocilizumab

Ethanol/Nutrition/Herb Interactions

Food: Decreases rate and extent of absorption. High-fat meals have most pronounced effect (37% decrease in AUC, 77% decrease in C_{max}). Grapefruit juice, CYP3A4 inhibitor, may increase serum level and/or toxicity of tacrolimus; avoid concurrent use.

Herb/Nutraceutical: St John's wort: May reduce tacrolimus serum concentrations (avoid concurrent use).

Stability

Injection: Prior to dilution, store at 5°C to 25°C (41°F to 77°F). Following dilution, stable for 24 hours in D_5W or NS in glass or polyethylene containers. Dilute with 5% dextrose injection or 0.9% sodium chloride injection to a final concentration between 0.004 mg/mL and 0.02 mg/mL.

Capsules: Store at room temperature of 25°C (77°F); excursions permitted to 15°C to 30°C (59°F to 86°F).

Mechanism of Action Suppresses cellular immunity (inhibits T-lymphocyte activation), by binding to an intracellular protein, FKBP-12 and complexes with calcineurin dependent proteins to inhibit calcineurin phosphatase activity

Pharmacodynamics/Kinetics

Absorption: Better in resected patients with a closed stoma; unlike cyclosporine, clamping of the T-tube in liver transplant patients does not alter trough concentrations or AUC; Oral: Incomplete and variable; the rate and extent of absorption is affected by food and may be most pronounced with a high-fat meal. Oral absorption may be variable in stem cell transplant patients with mucositis due to the conditioning regimen.

Distribution: V_d: Children: 0.5-4.7 L/kg; Adults: 0.55-2.47 L/kg

Protein binding: ~99% primarily to albumin and alpha$_1$-acid glycoprotein glycoprotein

Metabolism: Extensively hepatic via CYP3A4 to eight possible metabolites (major metabolite, 31-demethyl tacrolimus, shows same activity as tacrolimus *in vitro*)

Bioavailability: Oral: Children: 7% to 55%, Adults: 7% to 32%; Absolute: Unknown

Half-life elimination: Variable, 23-46 hours in healthy volunteers; 2.1-36 hours in transplant patients

Time to peak: 0.5-6 hours

Excretion: Feces (~93%); urine (<1% as unchanged drug)

Dosage

Oral:

Prevention of organ rejection in transplant recipients: The initial dose of tacrolimus should begin no sooner than 6 hours after liver and heart transplant and within 24 hours of kidney transplant (but may be delayed until renal function has recovered). Adjunctive therapy with corticosteroids is recommended early post-transplant. I.V. route should only be used in patients not able to take oral medications and continued only until oral medication can be tolerated; anaphylaxis has been reported with I.V. administration. If switching from I.V. to oral, the oral dose should be started 8-12 hours after stopping the infusion.

Children: Patients without pre-existing renal or hepatic dysfunction have required (and tolerated) higher doses than adults to achieve similar blood concentrations. It is recommended that therapy be initiated at the ***high end*** of the recommended adult I.V. and oral dosing ranges; dosage adjustments may be required.

Liver transplant: Initial dose: 0.15-0.20 mg/kg/day in 2 divided doses, given every 12 hours

Adults:

Heart transplant: Initial dose: 0.075 mg/kg/day in 2 divided doses, given every 12 hours. Use in combination with azathioprine or mycophenolate mofetil is recommended.

Kidney transplant:

U.S. labeling: Initial dose: 0.2 mg/kg/day in combination with azathioprine **or** 0.1 mg/kg/day in combination with mycophenolate mofetil. Administer in 2 divided doses, given every 12 hours; African-American patients may require larger doses to maintain trough concentration.

Canadian labeling:

Prograf®: Initial: 0.2-0.3 mg/kg/day in 2 divided doses, given every 12 hours in combination with corticosteroids and other immunosuppressive agents.

Advagraf®: Initial: 0.15-0.2 mg/kg/day. Administer once daily in combination with corticosteroids and mycophenolate mofetil (MMF) in *de novo* kidney transplant recipients. Antibody induction therapy should also be used.

Conversion from Prograf® to Advagraf®: Initiate Advagraf® therapy using previously established total daily dose of Prograf®. Administer once daily.

Liver transplant: Initial dose: 0.1-0.15 mg/kg/day in 2 divided doses, given every 12 hours

Prevention of graft-versus-host disease (unlabeled use): Children and Adults: Convert from I.V. to oral dose (1:4 ratio): Multiply total daily I.V. dose times 4 and administer in 2 divided oral doses per day, every 12 hours (Uberti, 1999; Yanik, 2000).

Rheumatoid arthritis: Canadian labeling (not in U.S. labeling): Adults: 3 mg once daily; carefully monitor serum creatinine during therapy

Treatment of graft-versus-host disease (unlabeled use): Adults: 0.06 mg/kg twice daily (Furlong, 2000; Przepiorka, 1999)

I.V.:

Prevention of organ rejection in transplant recipients: The initial dose of tacrolimus should begin no sooner than 6 hours after liver and heart transplant and within 24 hours of kidney transplant (but may be delayed until renal function has recovered). Adjunctive therapy with corticosteroids is recommended early post-transplant. I.V. route should only be used in patients not able to take oral medications and continued only until oral medication can be tolerated; anaphylaxis has been reported with I.V. administration. If switching from I.V. to oral, the oral dose should be started 8-12 hours after stopping the infusion.

Children: It is recommended that therapy be initiated at the ***high end*** of the dosing range.

Liver transplant: Initial dose: 0.03-0.05 mg/kg/day as a continuous infusion

Adults: It is recommended that therapy be initiated at the ***lower end*** of the dosing range.

Heart transplant: Initial dose: 0.01 mg/kg/day as a continuous infusion. Use in combination with azathioprine or mycophenolate mofetil is recommended.

Kidney transplant: Initial dose: 0.03-0.05 mg/kg/day as a continuous infusion. Use in combination with azathioprine or mycophenolate mofetil is recommended.

Liver transplant: Initial dose: 0.03-0.05 mg/kg/day as a continuous infusion.

Prevention of graft-versus-host disease (unlabeled use): Children and Adults: Initial: 0.03 mg/kg/day (based on lean body weight) as continuous infusion. Treatment should begin at least 24 hours prior to stem cell infusion and continued only until oral medication can be tolerated (Przepiorka, 1999; Yanik, 2000).

Treatment of graft-versus-host disease (unlabeled use): Adults: Initial: 0.03 mg/kg/day (based on lean body weight) as continuous infusion (Furlong, 2000; Przepiorka, 1999)

Dosing adjustment in renal impairment: Systemic therapy: Evidence suggests that lower doses should be used; patients should receive doses at the lowest value of the recommended I.V. and oral dosing ranges; further reductions in dose below these ranges may be required.

Kidney transplant: Tacrolimus therapy in patients with postoperative oliguria should begin no sooner than 6 hours and within 24 hours post-transplant, but may be delayed until renal function has recovered.

Hemodialysis: Not removed by hemodialysis; supplemental dose is not necessary.

Peritoneal dialysis: Significant drug removal is unlikely based on physiochemical characteristics.

Dosing adjustment in hepatic impairment: Systemic therapy: Use of tacrolimus in liver transplant recipients experiencing post-transplant hepatic impairment may be associated with increased risk of developing renal insufficiency related to high whole blood levels of tacrolimus. The presence of moderate-to-severe hepatic dysfunction (serum bilirubin >2 mg/dL; Child-Pugh score ≥10) appears to affect the metabolism of tacrolimus. The half-life of the drug was prolonged and the clearance reduced after I.V. administration. The bioavailability of tacrolimus was also increased after oral administration. The higher plasma concentrations as determined by ELISA, in patients with severe hepatic dysfunction are probably due to the accumulation of metabolites of lower activity. These patients should be monitored closely and dosage adjustments should be considered. Some evidence indicates that lower doses could be used in these patients.

Dietary Considerations Capsule: Administer with or without food; be consistent with timing and composition of meals, food decreases bioavailability. Avoid grapefruit juice.

Administration

I.V.: If I.V. administration is necessary, administer by continuous infusion only. Do not use PVC tubing when administering diluted solutions. Tacrolimus is usually intended to be administered as a continuous infusion over 24 hours. Do not mix with solutions with a pH ≥9 (eg, acyclovir or ganciclovir) due to chemical degradation of tacrolimus (use different ports in multilumen lines). Do not alter dose with concurrent T-tube clamping. Adsorption of the drug to PVC tubing may become clinically significant with low concentrations.

Oral: Administer with or without food; be consistent with timing and composition of meals if GI intolerance occurs and administration with food becomes necessary (per manufacturer). If dosed once daily, administer in the morning. If dosed twice daily, doses should be 12 hours apart. If the morning and evening doses differ, the larger dose (differences are never >0.5-1 mg) should be given in the morning. If dosed 3 times/day, separate doses by 8 hours.

Advagraf®: Canadian labeling recommends that missed doses may be taken up to 14 hours after scheduled time; if >14 hours, resume at next regularly scheduled time.

Monitoring Parameters Renal function, hepatic function, serum electrolytes (especially potassium), glucose and blood pressure, measure 3 times/week for first few weeks, then gradually decrease frequency as patient stabilizes. Whole blood concentrations should be used for monitoring (trough for oral therapy). Signs/symptoms of anaphylactic reactions during infusion should also be monitored. Patients should be monitored during the first 30 minutes of the infusion, and frequently thereafter.

Tacrolimus serum levels may be falsely elevated in infected liver transplant patients due to interference from β-galactosidase antibodies.

Reference Range

Heart transplant: Typical whole blood trough concentrations:

- Months 1-3: 10-20 ng/mL
- Months ≥4: 5-15 ng/mL

Kidney transplant: Whole blood trough concentrations:

- In combination with azathioprine:
  - Months 1-3: 7-20 ng/mL
  - Months 4-12: 5-15 ng/mL
- In combination with mycophenolate mofetil/IL-2 receptor antagonist (eg, daclizumab): Months 1-2: 4-11 ng/mL

Liver transplant: Whole blood trough concentrations: Months 1-12: 5-20 ng/mL

Prevention of graft-versus-host disease (unlabeled use): 10-20 ng/mL (Uberti, 1999) although some institutions use a lower limit of 5 ng/mL and an upper limit of 15 ng/mL (Przepiorka, 1999; Yanik, 2000)

Dosage Forms Excipient information presented when available (limited, particularly for generics); consult specific product labeling.

Capsule, oral: 0.5 mg, 1 mg, 5 mg

Prograf®: 0.5 mg, 1 mg, 5 mg

Injection, solution:

Prograf®: 5 mg/mL (1 mL) [contains dehydrated ethanol 80%, polyoxyl 60 hydrogenated castor oil]

Dosage Forms: Canada Excipient information presented when available (limited, particularly for generics); consult specific product labeling.

Capsule, oral:

Advagraf®: 0.5 mg, 1 mg, 3 mg, 5 mg

Extemporaneous Preparations Hazardous agent: Use appropriate precautions for handling and disposal.

A 0.5 mg/mL tacrolimus oral suspension may be made with capsules and a 1:1 mixture of Ora-Plus® and Simple Syrup, N.F. Mix the contents of six 5 mg tacrolimus capsules with quantity of vehicle sufficient to make 60 mL. Store in glass or plastic amber prescription bottles; label "shake well". Stable for 56 days at room temperature (Esquivel, 1996; Foster, 1996).

A 1 mg/mL tacrolimus oral suspension may be made with capsules, sterile water, Ora-Plus®, and Ora-Sweet®. Pour the contents of six 5 mg capsules into a plastic amber prescription bottle. Add ~5 mL of sterile water and agitate bottle until drug disperses into a slurry. Add equal parts Ora-Plus® and Ora-Sweet® in sufficient quantity to make 30 mL. Store in plastic amber prescription bottles; label "shake well". Stable for 4 months at room temperature (Elefante, 2006).

Elefante A, Muindi J, West K, et al, "Long-Term Stability of a Patient-Convenient 1 mg/mL Suspension of Tacrolimus for Accurate Maintenance of Stable Therapeutic Levels," *Bone Marrow Transplant*, 2006, 37(8):781-4.

Esquivel C, So S, McDiarmid S, Andrews W, and Colombani PM, "Suggested Guidelines for the Use of Tacrolimus in Pediatric Liver Transplant Patients," *Transplantation*, 1996, 61(5):847-8.

Foster JA, Jacobson PA, Johnson CE, et al, "Stability of Tacrolimus in an Extemporaneously Compounded Oral Liquid (Abstract of Meeting Presentation)," *American Society of Health-System Pharmacists Annual Meeting*, 1996, 53:P-52(E).

Tacrolimus (Topical) (ta KROE li mus)

Brand Names: U.S. Protopic®

Brand Names: Canada Protopic®

Pharmacologic Category Calcineurin Inhibitor; Topical Skin Product

Use Moderate-to-severe atopic dermatitis in immunocompetent patients not responsive to conventional therapy or when conventional therapy is not appropriate

Canadian labeling: Additional use (not in U.S. labeling): Maintenance therapy to prevent flares and extend flare-free intervals in patients with moderate-to-severe atopic dermatitis who are responsive to initial therapy and experiencing ≥5 flares per year

Pregnancy Risk Factor C

Pregnancy Considerations Adverse events were observed in animal reproduction studies. Tacrolimus crosses the human placenta and is measurable in the cord blood, amniotic fluid, and newborn serum following systemic use. Refer to the Tacrolimus (Systemic) monograph for additional information.

Lactation Enters breast milk/not recommended

Medication Guide Available Yes

Contraindications Hypersensitivity to tacrolimus or any component of the formulation

Warnings/Precautions [U.S. Boxed Warning]: Topical calcineurin inhibitors have been associated with rare cases of malignancy (including skin and lymphoma); therefore, it should be limited to short-term and intermittent treatment using the minimum amount necessary for the control of symptoms and only on involved areas. Use in children <2 years of age is not recommended, children ages 2-15 should only use the 0.03% ointment. Avoid use on malignant or premalignant skin conditions (eg cutaneous T-cell lymphoma). Should not be used in immunocompromised patients. Do not apply to areas of active bacterial or viral infection; infections at the treatment site should be cleared prior to therapy. Topical calcineurin agents are considered second-line therapies in the treatment of atopic dermatitis/eczema, and should be limited to use in patients who have failed treatment with other therapies. Patients with atopic dermatitis are predisposed to skin infections, and tacrolimus therapy has been associated with risk of developing eczema herpeticum, varicella zoster, and herpes simplex. If atopic dermatitis is not improved in <6 weeks, re-evaluate to confirm diagnosis. May be associated with development of lymphadenopathy; possible infectious causes should be investigated. Discontinue use in patients with unknown cause of lymphadenopathy or acute infectious mononucleosis. Acute renal failure has been observed (rarely) with topical use. Not recommended for use in patients with skin disease which may increase systemic absorption (eg, Netherton's syndrome). Minimize sunlight exposure during treatment. Safety not established in patients with generalized erythroderma. Safety of intermittent use for >1 year has not been established, particularly since the effect on immune system development is unknown. Should not be used in immunocompromised patients; safety and efficacy have not been evaluated.

Adverse Reactions As reported in children and adults, unless otherwise noted:

>10%:

- Central nervous system: Headache (5% to 20%), fever (1% to 21%)
- Dermatologic: Skin burning (43% to 58%; tends to improve as lesions resolve), pruritus (41% to 46%), erythema (12% to 28%)
- Respiratory: Increased cough (children 18%)
- Miscellaneous: Flu-like syndrome (23% to 31%), allergic reaction (4% to 12%)

1% to 10%:

- Cardiovascular: Peripheral edema (adults 3% to 4%)
- Central nervous system: Hyperesthesia (adults 3% to 7%), pain (1% to 2%)
- Dermatologic: Skin tingling (2% to 8%), acne (adults 4% to 7%), localized flushing (following ethanol consumption; adults 3% to 7%), folliculitis (2% to 6%), urticaria (1% to 6%), rash (2% to 5%), pustular rash (2% to 4%), vesiculobullous rash (children 4%), contact dermatitis (3% to 4%), cyst (adults 1% to 3%), eczema herpeticum (1% to 2%), fungal dermatitis (adults 1% to 2%), sunburn (adults 1% to 2%), alopecia (adults 1%), dry skin (children 1%)
- Endocrine & metabolic: Dysmenorrhea (adult females 4%)
- Gastrointestinal: Diarrhea (3% to 5%), dyspepsia (adults 1% to 4%), abdominal pain (children 3%), vomiting (adults 1%), gastroenteritis (adults 2%), nausea (children 1%)
- Neuromuscular & skeletal: Paresthesia (adults 3%), myalgia (adults 2% to 3%), weakness (adults 2% to 3%), arthralgia (adults 1% to 3%), back pain (adults 2%)
- Ocular: Conjunctivitis (2% adults)
- Otic: Otitis media (12% children)
- Respiratory: Rhinitis (6% children), sinusitis (2% to 4% adults), bronchitis (2% adults), pneumonia (1% adults)
- Miscellaneous: Varicella/herpes zoster (1% to 5%), lymphadenopathy (3% children)

<1% (Limited to important or life-threatening): Acute renal failure, anaphylaxis, anaphylactoid reaction, anemia, basal cell carcinoma, chest pain, hypercholesterolemia, malignant melanoma, osteomyelitis, photosensitivity reaction, seizure, septicemia, skin discoloration, squamous cell carcinoma

Drug Interactions

Metabolism/Transport Effects Substrate of CYP3A4 (minor), P-glycoprotein; **Note:** Assignment of Major/Minor substrate status based on clinically relevant drug interaction potential

Avoid Concomitant Use

Avoid concomitant use of Tacrolimus (Topical) with any of the following: Immunosuppressants

Increased Effect/Toxicity

Tacrolimus (Topical) may increase the levels/effects of: Alcohol (Ethyl); CycloSPORINE; CycloSPORINE (Systemic); Immunosuppressants; Sirolimus; Temsirolimus

The levels/effects of Tacrolimus (Topical) may be increased by: Antidepressants (Serotonin Reuptake Inhibitor/Antagonist); Antifungal Agents (Azole Derivatives, Systemic); Calcium Channel Blockers (Nondihydropyridine); Conivaptan; CycloSPORINE; CycloSPORINE (Systemic); Danazol; Fluconazole; Grapefruit Juice; Macrolide Antibiotics; Protease Inhibitors; Sirolimus; Temsirolimus

Decreased Effect There are no known significant interactions involving a decrease in effect.

Ethanol/Nutrition/Herb Interactions Ethanol: Localized flushing (redness, warm sensation) may occur at application site of topical tacrolimus following ethanol consumption.

Stability Store at room temperature of 25°C (77°F); excursions permitted to 15°C to 30°C (59°F to 86°F).

Mechanism of Action Suppresses cellular immunity (inhibits T-lymphocyte activation), by binding to an intracellular protein, FKBP-12 and complexes with calcineurin dependent proteins to inhibit calcineurin phosphatase activity

Pharmacodynamics/Kinetics

Absorption: Minimally absorbed; serum concentrations range from undetectable to 20 ng/mL (~2 ng/mL in majority of adult patients studied)

Bioavailability: ~0.5%

Dosage Topical: Atopic dermatitis (moderate-to-severe):

Treatment:

Children ≥2-15 years: Apply thin layer of 0.03% ointment to affected area twice daily; rub in gently and completely. Discontinue use when symptoms have cleared. If no improvement within 6 weeks, patients should be re-examined to confirm diagnosis.

Children >15 years and Adults: Apply thin layer of 0.03% or 0.1% ointment to affected area twice daily; rub in gently and completely. Discontinue use when symptoms have cleared. If no improvement within 6 weeks, patients should be re-examined to confirm diagnosis.

Maintenance therapy (Canadian labeling; not in U.S. labeling):

Children ≥2-15 years: Apply one application (thin layer of 0.03% ointment) to areas usually affected twice a week, allowing 2-3 days between applications (eg, one application on Monday and Thursday). Reevaluate after 12 months. Safety of maintenance therapy >12 months has not been established.

Children >15 years and Adults: Apply one application (thin layer of 0.03% or 0.1% ointment) to areas usually affected twice a week, allowing 2-3 days between applications (eg, one application on Monday and Thursday). Reevaluate after 12 months. Safety of maintenance therapy >12 months has not been established.

Note: Patients experiencing flares should resume twice daily treatment.

Administration Do not use with occlusive dressings. Burning at the application site is most common in first few days; improves as atopic dermatitis improves. Limit application to involved areas. Continue as long as signs and symptoms persist; discontinue if resolution occurs; reevaluate if symptoms persist >6 weeks.

Dosage Forms Excipient information presented when available (limited, particularly for generics); consult specific product labeling.

Ointment, topical:

Protopic®: 0.03% (30 g, 60 g, 100 g); 0.1% (30 g, 60 g, 100 g)

◆ **Tactuo™ (Can)** *see* Adapalene and Benzoyl Peroxide *on page 44*

Tadalafil (tah DA la fil)

Brand Names: U.S. Adcirca®; Cialis®

Brand Names: Canada Adcirca®; Cialis®

Index Terms GF196960

Pharmacologic Category Phosphodiesterase-5 Enzyme Inhibitor

Use

Adcirca®: Treatment of pulmonary arterial hypertension (PAH) (WHO Group I) to improve exercise ability

Cialis®: Treatment of erectile dysfunction (ED); treatment of signs and symptoms of benign prostatic hyperplasia (BPH)

Pregnancy Risk Factor B

Pregnancy Considerations Teratogenic events were not reported in animal reproduction studies. Postnatal development and pup survival was decreased at some doses. There are no adequate and well-controlled studies in pregnant women. Less than 0.0005% is found in the semen of healthy males.

Lactation Excretion in breast milk unknown/use caution

Contraindications Known serious hypersensitivity to tadalafil or any component of the formulation; concurrent use (regularly/intermittently) of organic nitrates in any form (eg, nitroglycerin, isosorbide dinitrate)

Warnings/Precautions There is a degree of cardiac risk associated with sexual activity; therefore, physicians should consider the cardiovascular status of their patients prior to initiation. Use is not recommended in patients with hypotension (<90/50 mm Hg), uncontrolled hypertension (>170/100 mm Hg), NYHA class II-IV heart failure within the last 6 months, uncontrolled arrhythmias, stroke within the last 6 months, MI within the last 3 months, unstable angina or angina during sexual intercourse; safety and efficacy have not been evaluated in these patients. Safety and efficacy in PAH have not been evaluated in patients with clinically significant aortic and/or mitral valve disease, life-threatening arrhythmias, hypotension (<90/50 mm Hg), uncontrolled hypertension, significant left ventricular dysfunction, pericardial constriction, restrictive or congestive cardiomyopathy, symptomatic coronary artery disease. Use caution in patients with left ventricular outflow obstruction (eg, aortic stenosis, hypertrophic obstructive cardiomyopathy); may be more sensitive to vasodilator effects.

Patients experiencing anginal chest pain after tadalafil administration should seek immediate medical attention. Concomitant use (regularly/intermittently) with all forms of nitrates is contraindicated. When used for BPH, erectile dysfunction, or PAH and nitrate administration is medically necessary following use, at least 48 hours should elapse after the tadalafil dose and nitrate administration. When used for PAH, per the manufacturer, nitrate may be administered within 48 hours of tadalafil. For both situations, administration of nitrates should only be done under close medical supervision with hemodynamic monitoring.

Concurrent use with alpha-adrenergic antagonist therapy or substantial alcohol consumption may cause symptomatic hypotension; patients should be hemodynamically stable prior to initiating tadalafil therapy at the lowest possible dose. When used for BPH or erectile dysfunction, use caution in patients receiving strong CYP3A4 inhibitors. When used for PAH, avoid use in patients taking strong CYP3A4 inducers/inhibitors. Use in patients receiving or about to receive ritonavir requires dosage adjustment or interruption of therapy, respectively. Canadian labeling does not recommend use of tadalafil in patients with PAH who are also receiving protease inhibitors.

Pulmonary vasodilators may exacerbate the cardiovascular status in patients with pulmonary veno-occlusive disease (PVOD); use is not recommended. In patients with unrecognized PVOD, signs of pulmonary edema should prompt investigation into this diagnosis. Use with caution in patients with mild-to-moderate hepatic impairment; dosage adjustment/limitation is needed. Use is not recommended in patients with severe hepatic impairment or cirrhosis. Use with caution in patients with renal impairment; dosage adjustment/limitation is needed. Safety and efficacy with other tadalafil brands or other PDE-5 inhibitors (ie, sildenafil and vardenafil) have not been established. Patients should be informed not to take with other tadalafil brands or other PDE-5 inhibitors. Use caution in patients with bleeding disorders or peptic ulcer disease due to effect on platelets (bleeding).

When used to treat BPH or erectile dysfunction, potential underlying causes of BPH or erectile dysfunction should be evaluated prior to treatment. Use with caution in patients with anatomical deformation of the penis (angulation, cavernosal fibrosis, or Peyronie's disease), or who have conditions which may predispose them to priapism (sickle cell anemia, multiple myeloma, leukemia). Instruct patients to seek immediate medical attention if erection persists >4 hours. Safety and efficacy with other tadalafil brands or other PDE-5 inhibitors (ie, sildenafil and vardenafil) have not been established. Patients should be informed not to take with other tadalafil brands or other PDE-5 inhibitors. The safety and efficacy of tadalafil with other treatments for erectile dysfunction have not been studied and are, therefore, not recommended as combination therapy.

Rare cases of nonarteritic anterior ischemic optic neuropathy (NAION) have been reported; risk may be increased with history of vision loss or NAION in one eye. Other risk factors for NAION include heart disease, diabetes, hypertension, smoking, age >50 years, or history of certain eye problems. Sudden decrease or loss of hearing has been reported rarely; hearing changes may be accompanied by tinnitus and dizziness. A direct relationship between therapy and vision or hearing loss has not been determined. Instruct patients to seek medical assistance for sudden loss of vision in one or both eyes, sudden decrease in hearing, or sudden loss of hearing.

Patients with genetic retinal disorders (eg, retinitis pigmentosa) were not evaluated in clinical trials; use is not recommended. Use with caution in the elderly.

Adverse Reactions Based upon usual doses for either indication. For erectile dysfunction, similar adverse events are reported with once-daily versus intermittent dosing, but are generally lower than with doses used intermittently.

>10%:

Cardiovascular: Flushing (1% to 13%; dose related)

Central nervous system: Headache (3% to 42%; dose related)

Gastrointestinal: Dyspepsia (1% to 13%), nausea (10% to 11%)

Neuromuscular & skeletal: Myalgia (1% to 14%; dose related), back pain (2% to 12%), extremity pain (1% to 11%)

Respiratory: Respiratory tract infection (3% to 13%), nasopharyngitis (2% to 13%)

2% to 10%:

Cardiovascular: Hypertension (1% to 3%)

Gastrointestinal: Gastroenteritis (viral; 3% to 5%), GERD (1% to 3%), abdominal pain (1% to 2%), diarrhea (1% to 2%)

Genitourinary: Urinary tract infection (≤2%)

Respiratory: Nasal congestion (≤9%), cough (2% to 4%), bronchitis (≤2%)

Miscellaneous: Flu-like syndrome (2% to 5%)

<2% (Limited to important or life-threatening): Amnesia (transient global), angina pectoris, arthralgia, blurred vision, chest pain, color vision decreased, conjunctival hyperemia, conjunctivitis, diaphoresis, dizziness, dysphagia, dyspnea, epistaxis, esophagitis, exfoliative dermatitis, eye pain, eyelid swelling, facial edema, fatigue, gastritis, GGTP increased, hearing decreased, hearing loss, hepatic enzymes increased, hypoesthesia, hypotension, insomnia, lacrimation, migraine, MI, neck pain, nonarteritic ischemic optic neuropathy (NAION), pain, palpitation, paresthesia, pharyngitis, postural hypotension, priapism, pruritus, rash, retinal artery occlusion, retinal vein occlusion, seizure, somnolence, spontaneous penile erection, Stevens-Johnson syndrome, stroke, sudden cardiac death, syncope, tachycardia, tinnitus, urticaria, vertigo, visual field loss, vomiting, weakness, xerostomia

Drug Interactions

Metabolism/Transport Effects Substrate of CYP3A4 (major); **Note:** Assignment of Major/Minor substrate status based on clinically relevant drug interaction potential

Avoid Concomitant Use

Avoid concomitant use of Tadalafil with any of the following: Amyl Nitrite; Boceprevir; Phosphodiesterase 5 Inhibitors; Telaprevir; Vasodilators (Organic Nitrates)

Increased Effect/Toxicity

Tadalafil may increase the levels/effects of: Alpha1-Blockers; Amyl Nitrite; Antihypertensives; Bosentan; Phosphodiesterase 5 Inhibitors; Vasodilators (Organic Nitrates)

The levels/effects of Tadalafil may be increased by: Antifungal Agents (Azole Derivatives, Systemic); Boceprevir; CYP3A4 Inhibitors (Moderate); CYP3A4 Inhibitors (Strong); Dasatinib; Ritonavir; Sapropterin; Telaprevir

Decreased Effect

The levels/effects of Tadalafil may be decreased by: Bosentan; CYP3A4 Inducers (Strong); Etravirine; Tocilizumab

Ethanol/Nutrition/Herb Interactions

Ethanol: Substantial consumption of ethanol may increase the risk of hypotension and orthostasis. Lower ethanol consumption has not been associated with significant changes in blood pressure or increase in orthostatic symptoms.

Food: Rate and extent of absorption are not affected by food. Grapefruit juice may increase serum levels/toxicity of tadalafil. Use tadalafil with caution in patients who regularly consume grapefruit juice. In general, use of grapefruit juice should be limited or avoided; the manufacturer does not give specific recommendations.

Herb/Nutraceutical: St John's wort: Use caution with concomitant use.

Stability Store at 25°C (77°F); excursions permitted to 15°C to 30°C (59°F to 86°F).

Mechanism of Action

BPH: Exact mechanism unknown; effects likely due to PDE-5 mediated reduction in smooth muscle and endothelial cell proliferation, decreased nerve activity, and increased smooth muscle relaxation and tissue perfusion of the prostate and bladder

Erectile dysfunction: Does not directly cause penile erections, but affects the response to sexual stimulation. The physiologic mechanism of erection of the penis involves release of nitric oxide (NO) in the corpus cavernosum during sexual stimulation. NO then activates the enzyme guanylate cyclase, which results in increased levels of cyclic guanosine monophosphate (cGMP), producing smooth muscle relaxation and inflow of blood to the corpus cavernosum. Tadalafil enhances the effect of NO by inhibiting phosphodiesterase type 5 (PDE-5), which is responsible for degradation of cGMP in the corpus cavernosum; when sexual stimulation causes local release of NO, inhibition of PDE-5 by tadalafil causes increased levels of cGMP in the corpus cavernosum, resulting in smooth muscle relaxation and inflow of blood to the corpus cavernosum. At recommended doses, it has no effect in the absence of sexual stimulation.

PAH: Inhibits phosphodiesterase type 5 (PDE-5) in smooth muscle of pulmonary vasculature where PDE-5 is responsible for the degradation of cyclic guanosine monophosphate (cGMP). Increased cGMP concentration results in pulmonary vasculature relaxation; vasodilation in the pulmonary bed and the systemic circulation (to a lesser degree) may occur.

Pharmacodynamics/Kinetics

Onset of action: Within 1 hour

Peak effect (pulmonary artery vasodilation): 75-90 minutes (Ghofrani, 2004)

Duration: Erectile dysfunction: Up to 36 hours

Distribution: V_d: 63-77 L

Protein binding: 94%

Metabolism: Hepatic, via CYP3A4 to metabolites (inactive)

Half-life elimination: 15-17.5 hours; Pulmonary hypertension (not receiving bosentan): 35 hours

Time to peak, plasma: ~2-4 hours (range: 30 minutes to 8 hours)

Excretion: Feces (~61%, predominantly as metabolites); urine (~36%, predominantly as metabolites)

Dosage Oral: Adults:

Benign prostatic hyperplasia (with or without concomitant erectile dysfunction) (Cialis®): 5 mg once daily

Dosing adjustment with concomitant medications:

CYP3A4 inhibitors (strong): 2.5 mg once daily; maximum: 2.5 mg once daily

Erectile dysfunction (Cialis®):

As-needed dosing: 10 mg (U.S. labeling) or 20 mg (Canadian labeling) at least 30 minutes prior to anticipated sexual activity (dosing range: 5-20 mg); to be given as one single dose and not given more than once daily. **Note:** Erectile function may be improved for up to 36 hours following a single dose; adjust dose.

Once-daily dosing: 2.5 mg once daily (U.S. labeling) or 5 mg once daily (Canadian labeling) to be given at approximately the same time daily without regard to timing of sexual activity. Dose may be adjusted based on tolerability (dosage range: 2.5-5 mg/day).

Dosing adjustment with concomitant medications:

U.S. labeling: $Alpha_1$-blockers: If stabilized on either alpha-blockers or tadalafil therapy, initiate new therapy with the other agent at the lowest possible dose.

Canadian labeling: Nonselective alpha-blockers (eg, doxazosin): *As-needed dosing:* 10 mg at least 30 minutes prior to anticipated sexual activity

CYP3A4 inhibitors (strong):

As-needed dosing:

U.S. labeling: Maximum: 10 mg, not to be given more frequently than every 72 hours

Canadian labeling: 10 mg, not to be given more frequently than every 48 hours (maximum 3 doses/week); may increase to 20 mg if lower dose is tolerated but ineffective. Discontinue use if 10 mg dose is not tolerated.

Once-daily dosing:

U.S. labeling: 2.5 mg once daily; maximum: 2.5 mg once daily

Canadian labeling: 2.5-5 mg once daily

Pulmonary arterial hypertension (Adcirca®): 40 mg once daily

Dosing adjustment with concomitant medications:

Coadministration with protease inhibitor regimen:

Concurrent use with atazanavir/ritonavir, darunavir/ritonavir, fosamprenavir, ritonavir, saquinavir/ritonavir, tipranavir/ritonavir:

Coadministration of tadalafil in patients currently receiving one of these protease inhibitor regimens for at least 1 week: Initiate tadalafil at 20 mg once daily; increase to 40 mg once daily based on individual tolerability.

Coadministration of one of these protease inhibitor regimens in patients currently receiving tadalafil: Discontinue tadalafil at least 24 hours prior to the initiation of the protease inhibitor regimen. After at least 1 week of the protease inhibitor regimen, resume tadalafil at 20 mg once daily; increase to 40 mg once daily based on individual tolerability.

Concurrent use with indinavir or nelfinavir:

Patient receiving indinavir/nelfinavir when initiating tadalafil: Initiate tadalafil at 20 mg once daily; increase to 40 mg once daily based on individual tolerability

Patient receiving tadalafil when initiating indinavir/nelfinavir: Adjust tadalafil to 20 mg once daily; increase to 40 mg once daily based on individual tolerability

Elderly: No dose adjustment for patients >65 years of age in the absence of renal or hepatic impairment

Dosage adjustment in renal impairment:

Benign prostatic hyperplasia (with or without concomitant erectile dysfunction) (Cialis®):

Cl_{cr} ≥51 mL/minute: No dosage adjustment necessary

Cl_{cr} 30-50 mL/minute: Initial: 2.5 mg once daily; maximum: 5 mg once daily

Cl_{cr} <30 mL/minute: Use not recommended

ESRD requiring hemodialysis: Use not recommended

Erectile dysfunction (Cialis®):

As-needed use:

U.S. labeling:

Cl_{cr} ≥51 mL/minute: No dosage adjustment necessary

Cl_{cr} 30-50 mL/minute: Initial: 5 mg once daily; maximum: 10 mg (not to be given more frequently than every 48 hours)

Cl_{cr} <30 mL/minute: Maximum: 5 mg (not to be given more frequently than every 72 hours)

ESRD requiring hemodialysis: Maximum: 5 mg (not to be given more frequently than every 72 hours)

Canadian labeling:

Cl_{cr} >80 mL/minute: No dosage adjustment necessary

Cl_{cr} ≥31-80 mL/minute: 10 mg, not to be given more frequently than every 48 hours (maximum 3 doses/week); may increase to 20 mg if lower dose is tolerated but ineffective. Discontinue use if 10 mg dose is not tolerated.

Cl_{cr} <30 mL/minute: Use with extreme caution; has not been adequately studied

ESRD requiring hemodialysis: Use with extreme caution; has not been adequately studied

Once-daily use:

Cl_{cr} ≥31 mL/minute: No dosage adjustment necessary

Cl_{cr} <30 mL/minute: Use not recommended

ESRD requiring hemodialysis: Use not recommended

Pulmonary arterial hypertension (Adcirca®):

Cl_{cr} >80 mL/minute: No dosage adjustment necessary

Cl_{cr} 31-80 mL/minute: Initial: 20 mg once daily; increase to 40 mg once daily based on individual tolerability

Cl_{cr} ≤30 mL/minute: Avoid use due to increased tadalafil exposure, limited clinical experience, and lack of ability to influence clearance by dialysis.

Dosage adjustment in hepatic impairment:

Benign prostatic hyperplasia (with or without concomitant erectile dysfunction) (Cialis®):

Mild-to-moderate impairment (Child-Pugh class A or B): Use with caution

Severe impairment (Child-Pugh class C): Use is not recommended

Erectile dysfunction (Cialis®):

As-needed use:

U.S. labeling:

Mild-to-moderate impairment (Child-Pugh class A or B): Use with caution; dose should not exceed 10 mg once daily

Severe impairment (Child-Pugh class C): Use is not recommended

Canadian labeling:

Mild-to-moderate impairment (Child-Pugh class A or B): 10 mg, not to be given more frequently than every 48 hours (maximum 3 doses/week); may increase to 20 mg if lower dose is tolerated but ineffective. Discontinue use if 10 mg dose is not tolerated.

Severe impairment (Child-Pugh class C): Use with extreme caution; has not been adequately studied

Once-daily use:

U.S. labeling:

Mild-to-moderate impairment (Child-Pugh class A or B): Use with caution

Severe impairment (Child-Pugh class C): Use is not recommended

Canadian labeling:

Mild-to-moderate impairment (Child-Pugh class A or B): No dosage adjustment necessary

Severe impairment (Child-Pugh class C): Use with extreme caution; has not been adequately studied

Pulmonary arterial hypertension (Adcirca®):

Mild-to-moderate impairment (Child-Pugh class A or B): Use with caution; consider initial dose of 20 mg once daily

Severe impairment (Child-Pugh class C): Avoid use; has not been studied in patients with severe hepatic cirrhosis.

Dietary Considerations May be taken with or without food.

Administration May be administered with or without food.

Adcirca®: Administer daily dose all at once; dividing doses throughout the day is not advised.

Cialis®: When used on an as-needed basis, should be taken at least 30 minutes prior to sexual activity. When used on a once-daily basis, should be taken at the same time each day, without regard to timing of sexual activity.

Monitoring Parameters Blood pressure, response and adverse effects; urine flow, PSA

Dosage Forms Excipient information presented when available (limited, particularly for generics); consult specific product labeling.

Tablet, oral:

Adcirca®: 20 mg

Cialis®: 2.5 mg, 5 mg, 10 mg, 20 mg

- ◆ **Tagamet® HB (Can)** *see* Cimetidine *on page 359*
- ◆ **Tagamet HB 200® [OTC]** *see* Cimetidine *on page 359*
- ◆ **TAK-375** *see* Ramelteon *on page 1458*
- ◆ **TAK-390MR** *see* Dexlansoprazole *on page 483*
- ◆ **TAK-599** *see* Ceftaroline Fosamil *on page 315*
- ◆ **Talc** *see* Talc (Sterile) *on page 1624*
- ◆ **Talc for Pleurodesis** *see* Talc (Sterile) *on page 1624*

Talc (Sterile) (talk STARE il)

Brand Names: U.S. Sclerosol®; Sterile Talc Powder™

Index Terms Intrapleural Talc; Sterile Talc; Talc; Talc for Pleurodesis

Pharmacologic Category Sclerosing Agent

Use Prevention of recurrence of malignant pleural effusion in symptomatic patients

Pregnancy Risk Factor B

Dosage Adults: Pleural effusion:

Intrapleural aerosol: 4-8 g (1-2 cans) as a single dose

Intrapleural instillation: 5 g

Additional Information Complete prescribing information for this medication should be consulted for additional detail.

Dosage Forms Excipient information presented when available (limited, particularly for generics); consult specific product labeling.

Aerosol, powder, intrapleural:

Sclerosol®: 4 g (4 g) [contains chlorofluorocarbon]

Powder, intrapleural:

Sterile Talc Powder™: USP: 100% (5 g)

- ◆ **Talwin®** *see* Pentazocine *on page 1329*
- ◆ **Tambocor™** *see* Flecainide *on page 716*
- ◆ **Tamiflu®** *see* Oseltamivir *on page 1253*

Tamoxifen (ta MOKS i fen)

Brand Names: Canada Apo-Tamox®; Mylan-Tamoxifen; Nolvadex®-D; PMS-Tamoxifen; Teva-Tamoxifen

Index Terms ICI-46474; Nolvadex; Tamoxifen Citras; Tamoxifen Citrate

Pharmacologic Category Antineoplastic Agent, Estrogen Receptor Antagonist; Selective Estrogen Receptor Modulator (SERM)

Use Treatment of metastatic (female and male) breast cancer; adjuvant treatment of breast cancer after primary treatment with surgery and radiation; reduce risk of invasive breast cancer in women with ductal carcinoma *in situ* (DCIS) after surgery and radiation; reduce the incidence of breast cancer in women at high risk

Unlabeled Use Treatment of mastalgia, gynecomastia, ovarian cancer, endometrial cancer, uterine sarcoma, and desmoid tumors; risk reduction in women with Paget's disease of the breast (with DCIS or without associated cancer); induction of ovulation; treatment of precocious puberty in females, secondary to McCune-Albright syndrome

Pregnancy Risk Factor D

Pregnancy Considerations Animal studies have demonstrated fetal adverse effects and fetal loss. There have been reports of vaginal bleeding, birth defects and fetal loss in pregnant women. Tamoxifen use during pregnancy may have a potential long term risk to the fetus of a DES-like syndrome. For sexually-active women of childbearing age, initiate during menstruation (negative β-hCG immediately prior to initiation in women with irregular cycles). Tamoxifen may induce ovulation. Barrier or nonhormonal contraceptives are recommended. Pregnancy should be avoided during treatment and for 2 months after treatment has been discontinued.

Lactation Excretion in breast milk unknown/not recommended

Medication Guide Available Yes

Contraindications Hypersensitivity to tamoxifen or any component of the formulation; concurrent warfarin therapy or history of deep vein thrombosis or pulmonary embolism (when tamoxifen is used for cancer risk reduction in women at high risk for breast cancer and in women with DCIS)

Warnings/Precautions Hazardous agent - use appropriate precautions for handling and disposal. **[U.S. Boxed Warning]: Serious and life-threatening events (including stroke, pulmonary emboli, and uterine malignancy) have occurred at an incidence greater than placebo during use for breast cancer risk reduction in women at high-risk for breast cancer and in women with DCIS;** these events are rare, but require consideration in risk: benefit evaluation. An increased incidence of thromboembolic events, including DVT and pulmonary embolism, has been associated with use for breast cancer; risk is increased with concomitant chemotherapy; use with caution in individuals with a history of thromboembolic events. Thrombocytopenia and/or leukopenia may occur; neutropenia and pancytopenia have been reported rarely. Although the relationship to tamoxifen therapy is uncertain, rare hemorrhagic episodes have occurred in patients with significant thrombocytopenia. Use with caution in patients with hyperlipidemias; infrequent postmarketing cases of hyperlipidemias have been reported. Decreased visual acuity, retinal vein thrombosis, retinopathy, corneal changes, color perception changes, and increased incidence of cataracts (and the need for cataract surgery), have been reported. Hypercalcemia has occurred in patients with bone metastasis, usually within a few weeks of therapy initiation; institute appropriate hypercalcemia management; discontinue if severe. Local disease flare and increased bone and tumor pain may occur in patients with metastatic breast cancer; may be associated with (good) tumor response.

Tamoxifen is associated with a high potential for drug interactions, including CYP- and Pgp-mediated interactions. Decreased efficacy and an increased risk of breast cancer recurrence has been reported with concurrent moderate or strong CYP2D6 inhibitors (Aubert, 2009; Dezentje, 2009). Concomitant use with select SSRIs may result in decreased tamoxifen efficacy. Strong CYP2D6 inhibitors (eg, fluoxetine, paroxetine) and moderate CYP2D6 inhibitors (eg, sertraline) are reported to interfere with transformation to the active metabolite endoxifen. Weak CYP2D6 inhibitors (eg, venlafaxine, citalopram) have minimal effect on the conversion to endoxifen (Jin, 2005; NCCN Breast Cancer Risk Reduction Guidelines v.2.2010); escitalopram is also a weak CYP2D6 inhibitor. Lower plasma concentrations of endoxifen (active metabolite) have been observed in patients associated with reduced CYP2D6 activity (Jin, 2005) and may be associated with reduced efficacy. In a retrospective analysis of breast cancer patients taking tamoxifen and SSRIs, concomitant use of paroxetine and tamoxifen was associated with an increased risk of death due to breast cancer (Kelly, 2010).

Tamoxifen use may be associated with changes in bone mineral density (BMD) and the effects may be dependent upon menstrual status. In postmenopausal women, tamoxifen use is associated with a protective effect on bone mineral density (BMD), preventing loss of BMD which lasts over the 5-year treatment period. In premenopausal women, a decline (from baseline) in BMD mineral density has been observed in women who continued to menstruate; may be associated with an increased risk of fractures. Liver abnormalities such as cholestasis, fatty liver, hepatitis, and hepatic necrosis have occurred. Hepatocellular carcinomas have been reported in some studies; relationship to treatment is unclear. Tamoxifen is associated with an increased incidence of uterine or endometrial cancers. Endometrial hyperplasia, polyps, endometriosis, uterine fibroids, and ovarian cysts have occurred. Monitor and promptly evaluate any report of abnormal vaginal bleeding. Amenorrhea and menstrual irregularities have been reported with tamoxifen use.

Adverse Reactions

>10%:

Cardiovascular: Vasodilation (41%), flushing (33%), hypertension (11%), peripheral edema (11%)

Central nervous system: Mood changes (12% to 18%), pain (3% to 16%), depression (2% to 12%)

Dermatologic: Skin changes (6% to 19%), rash (13%)

Endocrine & metabolic: Hot flashes (3% to 80%), fluid retention (32%), altered menses (13% to 25%), amenorrhea (16%)

Gastrointestinal: Nausea (5% to 26%), weight loss (23%), vomiting (12%)

Genitourinary: Vaginal discharge (13% to 55%), vaginal bleeding (2% to 23%)

Neuromuscular & skeletal: Weakness (18%), arthritis (14%), arthralgia (11%)

Respiratory: Pharyngitis (14%)

Miscellaneous: Lymphedema (11%)

1% to 10%:

Cardiovascular: Chest pain (5%), venous thrombotic events (5%), edema (4%), cardiovascular ischemia (3%), angina (2%), deep venous thrombus (≤2%), MI (1%)

Central nervous system: Insomnia (9%), dizziness (8%), headache (8%), anxiety (6%), fatigue (4%)

Dermatologic: Alopecia (≤5%)

Endocrine & metabolic: Oligomenorrhea (9%), breast pain (6%), menstrual disorder (6%), breast neoplasm (5%), hypercholesterolemia (4%)

Gastrointestinal: Abdominal pain (9%), weight gain (9%), constipation (4% to 8%), diarrhea (7%), dyspepsia (6%), throat irritation (oral solution 5%), abdominal cramps (1%), anorexia (1%)

Genitourinary: Urinary tract infection (10%), leukorrhea (9%), vaginal hemorrhage (6%), vaginitis (5%), vulvovaginitis (5%), ovarian cyst (3%)

Hematologic: Thrombocytopenia (≤10%), anemia (5%)

Hepatic: AST increased (5%), serum bilirubin increased (2%)

Neuromuscular & skeletal: Back pain (10%), bone pain (6% to 10%), osteoporosis (7%), fracture (7%), arthrosis (5%), joint disorder (5%), myalgia (5%), paresthesia (5%), musculoskeletal pain (3%)

Ocular: Cataract (7%)

Renal: Serum creatinine increased (≤2%)

Respiratory: Cough (4% to 9%), dyspnea (8%), bronchitis (5%), sinusitis (5%)

Miscellaneous: Infection/sepsis (≤9%), diaphoresis (6%), flu-like syndrome (6%), cyst (5%), neoplasm (5%), allergic reaction (3%)

<1 or frequency not defined (limited to important or life-threatening): Angioedema, bullous pemphigoid, cholestasis, corneal changes, endometrial cancer, endometrial hyperplasia, endometrial polyps, endometriosis, erythema multiforme, fatty liver, hepatic necrosis, hepatitis, hypercalcemia, hyperlipidemia, hypersensitivity reactions, hypertriglyceridemia, impotence (males), interstitial pneumonitis, loss of libido (males), pancreatitis, phlebitis, pruritus vulvae, pulmonary embolism, retinal vein thrombosis, retinopathy, second primary tumors, Stevens-Johnson syndrome, stroke; tumor pain and local disease flare (including increase in lesion size and erythema) during treatment of metastatic breast cancer (generally resolves with continuation); uterine fibroids, vaginal dryness, visual color perception changes

Drug Interactions

Metabolism/Transport Effects Substrate of CYP2A6 (minor), CYP2B6 (minor), CYP2C9 (major), CYP2D6 (major), CYP2E1 (minor), CYP3A4 (major); **Note:** Assignment of Major/Minor substrate status based on clinically relevant drug interaction potential; **Inhibits** CYP2B6 (weak), CYP2C8 (moderate), CYP2C9 (weak), CYP3A4 (weak), P-glycoprotein

Avoid Concomitant Use

Avoid concomitant use of Tamoxifen with any of the following: Conivaptan; CYP2D6 Inhibitors (Strong); Pimozide; Silodosin; Topotecan; Vitamin K Antagonists

Increased Effect/Toxicity

Tamoxifen may increase the levels/effects of: Colchicine; CYP2C8 Substrates; Dabigatran Etexilate; Everolimus; P-glycoprotein/ABCB1 Substrates; Pimozide; Rivaroxaban; Silodosin; Topotecan; Vitamin K Antagonists

The levels/effects of Tamoxifen may be increased by: Abiraterone Acetate; Conivaptan; CYP2C9 Inhibitors (Moderate); CYP2C9 Inhibitors (Strong); CYP2D6 Inhibitors (Moderate); CYP2D6 Inhibitors (Strong); CYP3A4 Inhibitors (Moderate); CYP3A4 Inhibitors (Strong); Darunavir; Dasatinib

Decreased Effect

Tamoxifen may decrease the levels/effects of: Anastrozole; Letrozole

The levels/effects of Tamoxifen may be decreased by: Aminoglutethimide; CYP2C9 Inducers (Strong); CYP3A4 Inducers (Strong); Cyproterone; Deferasirox; Herbs (CYP3A4 Inducers); Peginterferon Alfa-2b; Rifamycin Derivatives; Tocilizumab

Ethanol/Nutrition/Herb Interactions

Food: Avoid grapefruit juice (may decrease the metabolism of tamoxifen).

Herb/Nutraceutical: Avoid black cohosh, dong quai in estrogen-dependent tumors. Avoid St John's wort (may decrease levels/effects of tamoxifen).

Stability Store at room temperature of 20°C to 25°C (68°F to 77°F). Protect from light.

Mechanism of Action Competitively binds to estrogen receptors on tumors and other tissue targets, producing a nuclear complex that decreases DNA synthesis and inhibits estrogen effects; nonsteroidal agent with potent antiestrogenic properties which compete with estrogen for binding sites in breast and other tissues; cells accumulate in the G_0 and G_1 phases; therefore, tamoxifen is cytostatic rather than cytocidal.

Pharmacodynamics/Kinetics

Absorption: Well absorbed

Distribution: High concentrations found in uterus, endometrial and breast tissue

Protein binding: 99%

Metabolism: Hepatic; via CYP2D6 to 4-hydroxytamoxifen and via CYP3A4/5 to N-desmethyl-tamoxifen. Each is then further metabolized into endoxifen (4-hydroxy-tamoxifen via CYP3A4/5 and N-desmethyl-tamoxifen via CYP2D6); both 4-hydroxy-tamoxifen and endoxifen are 30- to 100-fold more potent than tamoxifen

Half-life elimination: Tamoxifen: ~5-7 days; N-desmethyl tamoxifen: ~14 days

Time to peak, serum: ~5 hours

Excretion: Feces (26% to 51%); urine (9% to 13%)

Dosage Oral: **Note:** For the treatment of breast cancer, patients receiving both tamoxifen and chemotherapy, should receive treatment sequentially, with tamoxifen following completion of chemotherapy.

Children: Females: Precocious puberty and McCune-Albright syndrome (unlabeled use): A dose of 20 mg/day has been reported in patients 2-10 years of age; safety and efficacy have not been established for treatment of longer than 1 year duration (Eugster, 2003)

Adults:

Breast cancer treatment:

Adjuvant therapy (females): 20 mg once daily for 5 years

Metastatic (males and females): 20-40 mg/day (doses >20 mg should be given in 2 divided doses). **Note:** Although the FDA-approved labeling recommends dosing up to 40 mg/day, clinical benefit has not been demonstrated with doses above 20 mg/day (Bratherton, 1984).

Premenopausal women: Duration of treatment is 5 years (NCCN Breast Cancer guidelines v.1.2011)

Postmenopausal women: Duration of tamoxifen treatment is 2-3 years followed by an aromatase inhibitor (AI) to complete 5 years; if contraindications or intolerant to AI, may take tamoxifen for the full 5 years **or** extended therapy: 4.5-6 years of tamoxifen followed by 5 years of an AI (NCCN Breast Cancer guidelines v.1.2011)

DCIS (females), to reduce the risk for invasive breast cancer: 20 mg once daily for 5 years

Breast cancer risk reduction (pre- and postmenopausal high-risk females): 20 mg once daily for 5 years

Induction of ovulation (unlabeled use): 20 mg once daily (range: 20-80 mg once daily) for 5 days (Steiner, 2005)

Paget's disease of the breast (risk reduction; with DCIS or without associated cancer): 20 mg once daily for 5 years (NCCN Breast Cancer Guidelines, v.1.2011)

Dosage adjustment for DVT, pulmonary embolism, cerebrovascular accident, or prolonged immobilization: Discontinue tamoxifen (NCCN Breast Cancer Risk Reduction Guidelines, v.2.2010)

Dietary Considerations May be taken with or without food. Avoid grapefruit and grapefruit juice.

Administration Administer orally with or without food.

Monitoring Parameters CBC with platelets, serum calcium, LFTs; triglycerides and cholesterol (in patients with pre-existing hyperlipidemias); INR and PT (in patients on vitamin K antagonists); abnormal vaginal bleeding; breast and gynecologic exams (baseline and routine), mammogram (baseline and routine); signs/symptoms of DVT (leg swelling, tenderness) or PE (shortness of breath); ophthalmic exam (if vision problem or cataracts); bone mineral density (premenopausal women)

Test Interactions T_4 elevations (which may be explained by increases in thyroid-binding globulin) have been reported; not accompanied by clinical hyperthyroidism

Additional Information Estrogen receptor status may predict if adjuvant treatment with tamoxifen is of benefit. In metastatic breast cancer, patients with estrogen receptor positive tumors are more likely to benefit from tamoxifen treatment. With tamoxifen use to reduce the incidence of breast cancer in high risk-women, high risk is defined as women ≥35 years of age with a 5 year NCI Gail model predicted risk of breast cancer ≥1.67%.

Oncology Comment: The American Society of Clinical Oncology (ASCO) guidelines for adjuvant endocrine therapy in postmenopausal women with HR-positive breast cancer (Burstein, 2010) recommend considering aromatase inhibitor (AI) therapy at some point in the treatment course (primary, sequentially, or extended). Optimal duration at this time is not known; however, treatment with an AI should not exceed 5 years in primary and extended therapies, and 2-3 years if followed by tamoxifen in sequential therapy (total of 5 years). If initial therapy with AI has been discontinued before the 5 years, consideration should be taken to receive tamoxifen for a total of 5 years. The optimal time to switch to an AI is also not known; but data supports switching after 2-3 years of tamoxifen (sequential) or after 5 years of tamoxifen (extended). If patient becomes intolerant or has poor adherence, consideration should be made to switch to another AI or initiate tamoxifen.

The adjuvant endocrine therapy of choice is tamoxifen for men with breast cancer and for pre- or perimenopausal women at diagnosis. CYP2D6 genotyping is not recommended, however, due to the potential for drug-drug interactions use caution and consider avoiding concomitant therapy with tamoxifen and known CYP2D6 inhibitors.

Dosage Forms Excipient information presented when available (limited, particularly for generics); consult specific product labeling.

Tablet, oral: 10 mg, 20 mg

Extemporaneous Preparations Hazardous agent: Use appropriate precautions for handling and disposal.

A 0.5 mg/mL oral suspension may be prepared with tablets. Place two 10 mg tablets into 40 mL purified water and let stand ~2-5 minutes. Stir until tablets are completely disintegrated (dispersion time for each 10 mg tablet is ~2-5 minutes). Administer immediately after preparation. To ensure the full dose is administered, rinse glass several times with water and administer residue.

Lam MS, "Extemporaneous Compounding of Oral Liquid Dosage Formulations and Alternative Drug Delivery Methods for Anticancer Drugs," *Pharmacotherapy*, 2011, 31(2):164-92.

◆ **Tamoxifen Citras** *see* Tamoxifen *on page 1624*

◆ **Tamoxifen Citrate** *see* Tamoxifen *on page 1624*

Tamsulosin (tam SOO loe sin)

Brand Names: U.S. Flomax®

Brand Names: Canada Ava-Tamsulosin CR; Flomax® CR; JAMP-Tamsulosin; Mylan-Tamsulosin; RAN™-Tamsulosin; ratio-Tamsulosin; Sandoz-Tamsulosin; Sandoz-Tamsulosin CR; Teva-Tamsulosin

Index Terms Tamsulosin Hydrochloride

Pharmacologic Category Alpha$_1$ Blocker

Use Treatment of signs and symptoms of benign prostatic hyperplasia (BPH)

Unlabeled Use Symptomatic treatment of bladder outlet obstruction or dysfunction; facilitation of expulsion of ureteral stones

Pregnancy Risk Factor B

Pregnancy Considerations Teratogenic effects were not observed in animal studies.

Contraindications Hypersensitivity to tamsulosin or any component of the formulation

Warnings/Precautions Not intended for use as an antihypertensive drug. May cause significant orthostatic hypotension and syncope, especially with first dose; anticipate a similar effect if therapy is interrupted for a few days, if dosage is rapidly increased, or if another antihypertensive drug (particularly vasodilators) or a PDE-5 inhibitor (eg, sildenafil, tadalafil, vardenafil) is introduced. "First-dose" orthostatic hypotension may occur 4-8 hours after dosing; may be dose related. Patients should be cautioned about performing hazardous tasks when starting new therapy or adjusting dosage upward. Discontinue if symptoms of angina occur or worsen. Rule out prostatic carcinoma before beginning therapy with tamsulosin. Intraoperative floppy iris syndrome has been observed in cataract surgery patients who were on or were previously treated with alpha$_1$-blockers; causality has not been established and there appears to be no benefit in discontinuing alpha-blocker therapy prior to surgery; instruct patients to inform ophthalmologist of tamsulosin use when considering eye surgery. Priapism has been associated with use (rarely). Rarely, patients with a sulfa allergy have also developed an allergic reaction to tamsulosin; avoid use when previous reaction has been severe.

Adverse Reactions

>10%:

- Cardiovascular: Orthostatic hypotension (6 % to 19%)
- Central nervous system: Headache (19% to 21%), dizziness (15% to 17%)
- Genitourinary: Abnormal ejaculation (8% to 18%)
- Respiratory: Rhinitis (13% to 18%)
- Miscellaneous: Infection (9% to 11%)

1% to 10%:

- Cardiovascular: Chest pain (4%)
- Central nervous system: Somnolence (3% to 4%), insomnia (1% to 2%), vertigo (≤1%)
- Endocrine & metabolic: Libido decreased (1% to 2%)
- Gastrointestinal: Diarrhea (4% to 6%), nausea (3% to 4%), gum pain, toothache
- Neuromuscular & skeletal: Weakness (8% to 9%), back pain (7% to 8%)
- Ocular: Blurred vision (≤2%)
- Respiratory: Pharyngitis (5% to 6%), cough (3% to 5%), sinusitis (2% to 4%)

<1% (Limited to important or life-threatening): Allergic reactions (angioedema, pruritus, rash, urticaria, respiratory symptoms); constipation, hypotension, intraoperative floppy iris syndrome, lightheadedness, orthostasis (symptomatic), palpitation, priapism, skin desquamation, syncope, vomiting

Drug Interactions

Metabolism/Transport Effects Substrate of CYP2D6 (minor), CYP3A4 (major); **Note:** Assignment of Major/Minor substrate status based on clinically relevant drug interaction potential

Avoid Concomitant Use

Avoid concomitant use of Tamsulosin with any of the following: Alpha1-Blockers; CYP3A4 Inhibitors (Strong)

Increased Effect/Toxicity

Tamsulosin may increase the levels/effects of: Alpha1-Blockers; Calcium Channel Blockers

The levels/effects of Tamsulosin may be increased by: Beta-Blockers; CYP3A4 Inhibitors (Moderate); CYP3A4 Inhibitors (Strong); Dasatinib; MAO Inhibitors; Phosphodiesterase 5 Inhibitors

Decreased Effect

The levels/effects of Tamsulosin may be decreased by: CYP3A4 Inducers (Strong); Deferasirox; Herbs (CYP3A4 Inducers); Peginterferon Alfa-2b; Tocilizumab

Ethanol/Nutrition/Herb Interactions

Food: Fasting increases bioavailability by 30% and peak concentration 40% to 70%.

Herb/Nutraceutical: St John's wort: May decrease the levels/effects of tamsulosin. Avoid herbs with hypotensive properties (black cohosh, California poppy, coleus, golden seal, hawthorn, mistletoe, periwinkle, quinine, Shepherd's purse); may enhance the hypotensive effect of tamsulosin. Avoid saw palmetto (due to limited experience with this combination).

Stability Store at room temperature of 25°C (77°F); excursions permitted to 15°C to 30°C (59°F to 86°F).

Mechanism of Action Tamsulosin is an antagonist of alpha$_{1A}$-adrenoreceptors in the prostate. Smooth muscle tone in the prostate is mediated by alpha$_{1A}$-adrenoreceptors; blocking them leads to relaxation of smooth muscle in the bladder neck and prostate causing an improvement of urine flow and decreased symptoms of BPH. Approximately 75% of the alpha$_1$-receptors in the prostate are of the alpha$_{1A}$ subtype.

Pharmacodynamics/Kinetics

- Absorption: >90%
- Distribution: V_d: 16 L
- Protein binding: 94% to 99%, primarily to alpha$_1$ acid glycoprotein (AAG)
- Metabolism: Hepatic (extensive) via CYP3A4 and 2D6; metabolites undergo extensive conjugation to glucuronide or sulfate
- Bioavailability: Fasting: 30% increase
- Steady-state: By the fifth day of once-daily dosing
- Half-life elimination: Healthy volunteers: 9-13 hours; Target population: 14-15 hours
- Time to peak: Fasting: 4-5 hours; With food: 6-7 hours
- Excretion: Urine (76%, <10% as unchanged drug); feces (21%)

Dosage Oral: Adults:

Benign prostatic hyperplasia (BPH): 0.4 mg once daily ~30 minutes after the same meal each day; dose may be increased after 2-4 weeks to 0.8 mg once daily in patients who fail to respond. If therapy is interrupted for several days, restart with 0.4 mg once daily.

Bladder outlet obstruction symptoms (unlabeled use): 0.4 mg once daily (Rossi, 2001)

Ureteral stones, expulsion (unlabeled use): 0.4 mg once daily, discontinue after successful expulsion (average time to expulsion was 1-2 weeks) (Agrawal, 2009; Ahmed, 2010). **Note:** Patients with stones >10 mm were excluded from studies.

Dosage adjustment in renal impairment:

Cl_{cr} ≥10 mL/minute: No adjustment needed

Cl_{cr} <10 mL/minute: Not studied

Dosage adjustment in hepatic impairment:

Mild-to-moderate impairment: No adjustment needed

Severe impairment: Not studied

Dietary Considerations Take once daily, 30 minutes after the same meal each day.

Administration Administer 30 minutes after the same meal each day. Capsules should be swallowed whole; do not crush, chew, or open.

Dosage Forms Excipient information presented when available (limited, particularly for generics); consult specific product labeling.

Capsule, oral, as hydrochloride: 0.4 mg

Flomax®: 0.4 mg

Tablet, oral, as hydrochloride: 0.4 mg

◆ **Tamsulosin and Dutasteride** *see* Dutasteride and Tamsulosin *on page 568*

◆ **Tamsulosin Hydrochloride** *see* Tamsulosin *on page 1626*

◆ **Tamsulosin Hydrochloride and Dutasteride** *see* Dutasteride and Tamsulosin *on page 568*

◆ **Tanac® [OTC]** *see* Benzocaine *on page 202*
◆ **TanaCof-XR [DSC]** *see* Brompheniramine *on page 237*
◆ **Tanafed DMX™** *see* Chlorpheniramine, Pseudoephedrine, and Dextromethorphan *on page 347*
◆ **Tanta-Orciprenaline® (Can)** *see* Metaproterenol *on page 1085*
◆ **TAP-144** *see* Leuprolide *on page 989*
◆ **Tapazole®** *see* Methimazole *on page 1095*

Tapentadol (ta PEN ta dol)

Brand Names: U.S. Nucynta®; Nucynta® ER
Brand Names: Canada Nucynta™ CR
Index Terms CG5503; Tapentadol Hydrochloride
Pharmacologic Category Analgesic, Opioid
Use

Immediate release formulation: Relief of moderate-to-severe acute pain

Long acting formulation: Relief of moderate-to-severe chronic pain when continuous, around-the-clock analgesia is necessary for an extended period of time

Pregnancy Risk Factor C

Pregnancy Considerations Embryo-fetal toxicity, including malformations, was observed in animal studies only at doses that were maternally toxic. There are no adequate and well-controlled studies in pregnant women. Not recommended for use during labor and delivery. Neonates exposed to tapentadol *in utero* should be monitored for respiratory depression.

Lactation Excretion in breast milk unknown/not recommended

Medication Guide Available Yes

Contraindications Hypersensitivity to tapentadol or any component of the formulation; impaired pulmonary function (severe respiratory depression, acute or severe asthma or hypercapnia) in unmonitored settings or in absence of resuscitative equipment or ventilatory support; paralytic ileus; use of MAO inhibitors within 14 days

Canadian labeling: Additional contraindications (not in U.S. labeling): Hypersensitivity to opioids; any disease/condition that affects bowel transit (eg, ileus of any type, strictures); severe renal impairment (Cl_{cr} <30 mL/minute); severe hepatic impairment (Child-Pugh class C); mild, intermittent, or short-duration pain that can be managed with alternative pain medication; management of perioperative pain; acute alcoholism, delirium tremens, and seizure disorders; severe CNS depression, increased cerebrospinal or intracranial pressure or head injury; pregnancy; breast-feeding; use during labor/delivery

Warnings/Precautions Extended release tablets: **[U.S. Boxed Warning]: Use of alcohol or alcohol-containing medications should be avoided;** concomitant use with alcohol may increase tapentadol systemic exposure which may lead to possible fatal overdose. **[U.S. Boxed warning]: NOT intended for use as an as-needed analgesic; NOT intended for the management of acute or postoperative pain;** approved for the treatment of chronic pain only (not an as-needed basis). **[U.S. Boxed Warning]: Extended-release tablets must be swallowed whole and should NOT be split, crushed, broken, chewed or dissolved. [U.S. Boxed Warning]: Healthcare provider should be alert to problems of abuse, misuse, and diversion.** May cause severe hypotension; use with caution in patients with risk factors (eg. hypovolemia, concomitant use of other hypotensive agents).

Use with caution in patients with respiratory disease or respiratory compromise (eg, asthma, chronic obstructive pulmonary disease [COPD], cor pulmonale, sleep apnea, severe obesity, kyphoscoliosis, hypoxia, hypercapnia); critical respiratory depression may occur, even at therapeutic dosages. May cause CNS depression, which may impair physical or mental abilities; patients must be cautioned about performing tasks which require mental alertness (eg, operating machinery or driving). Use with caution in patients with CNS depression or coma. Effects may be potentiated when used with other sedative drugs or ethanol. Use with caution in patients with adrenal insufficiency, hypothyroidism or prostatic hyperplasia/urinary stricture.

Serotonin syndrome (SS) may occur with serotonin/norepinephrine reuptake inhibitors (SNRIs), including tapentadol. Signs of SS may include agitation, tachycardia, hyperthermia, nausea, and vomiting. Avoid use with serotonergic agents such as TCAs, triptans, venlafaxine, trazodone, lithium, sibutramine, meperidine, dextromethorphan, St John's wort, SNRIs, and SSRIs; concomitant use has been associated with the development of serotonin syndrome. Contraindicated with MAO inhibitor use within 14 days.

Use caution in patients with biliary tract dysfunction or acute pancreatitis; opioids may cause spasm of the sphincter of Oddi. Opioid use may obscure diagnosis or clinical course of patients with acute abdominal conditions. Use with extreme caution in patients with head injury, intracranial lesions, or elevated intracranial pressure (ICP); exaggerated elevation of ICP may occur. Serum concentrations are increased in hepatic impairment; use with caution in patients with moderate hepatic impairment (dosage adjustment required). Not recommended for use in severe hepatic impairment (not studied). Use with caution in patients with mild-to-moderate renal impairment (no dosage adjustment recommended). Not recommended for use in severe renal impairment (not studied). Use caution in patients with a history of seizures or conditions predisposing patients to seizures; patients with a history of seizures were excluded in clinical trials of tapentadol. Tramadol, an analgesic with similar pharmacologic properties to tapentadol, has been associated with seizures, particularly in patients with predisposing factors.

Prolonged use increases risk of abuse, addiction, and withdrawal symptoms. An opioid-containing regimen should be tailored to each patient's needs with respect to degree of tolerance for opioids (naïve versus chronic user), age, weight, and medical condition. Healthcare provider should be alert to problems of abuse, misuse, and diversion. Abrupt discontinuation may lead to withdrawal symptoms. Symptoms may be decreased by tapering prior to discontinuation. Use opioids with caution in elderly; consider decreasing initial dose. Use caution in debilitated patients; there is a greater potential for critical respiratory depression, even at therapeutic dosages.

During dosage adjustments, the Canadian labeling recommends that immediate release tramadol may be used as rescue medication (maximum dose: 400 mg/day) and that fentanyl should not be used as rescue medication.

Adverse Reactions

Immediate release:

>10%:

Central nervous system: Dizziness (24%), somnolence (15%)

Gastrointestinal: Nausea (30%), vomiting (18%), constipation (8%)

≤1% to 10%:

Central nervous system: Fatigue (3%), insomnia (2%), anxiety (1%), confusion (1%), dreams abnormal (1%), lethargy (1%), attention disturbances (<1%), headache (<1%)

Dermatologic: Pruritus (3% to 5%), hyperhidrosis (3%), rash (1%)

Endocrine & metabolic: Hot flushes (1%)

Gastrointestinal: Xerostomia (4%), appetite decreased (2%), dyspepsia (2%)
Genitourinary: Urinary tract infection (1%)
Neuromuscular & skeletal: Arthralgia (1%), tremor (1%)
Respiratory: Nasopharyngitis (1%), upper respiratory tract infection (1%), dyspnea (<1%)

Extended release:
>10%:
Central nervous system: Dizziness (17%), headache (15%), somnolence (12%)
Gastrointestinal: Nausea (21%), constipation (17%), vomiting (8%)
1% to 10%:
Central nervous system: Fatigue (9%), insomnia (4%), anxiety (2%), lethargy (2%), vertigo (2%), attention disturbances (1%), chills (1%), depression/depressed mood (1%)
Dermatologic: Hyperhidrosis (5%), pruritus (5%), rash (1%)
Endocrine & metabolic: Hot flushes (2%)
Gastrointestinal: Xerostomia (7%), dyspepsia (3%), appetite decreased (2%)
Genitourinary: Erectile dysfunction (1%)
Neuromuscular & skeletal: Weakness (2%), tremor (1%)
Ocular: Vision blurred (1%)
Respiratory: Dyspnea (1%)

Immediate and/or extended release: <1%, postmarketing, and/or case reports: Abdominal discomfort, agitation, ALT increased, angioedema, AST increased, ataxia, blood pressure decreased, consciousness decreased, diarrhea, disorientation, drunk feeling, dysarthria, edema, euphoria, gastric emptying impaired, GGT increased, hallucination, heart rate increased/decreased, heaviness sensation, hypersensitivity, hyper-/hypotension, hypoesthesia, involuntary muscle contractions, memory impairment, nervousness, oxygen saturation decreased, paresthesia, pharyngolaryngeal pain, pollakiuria, presyncope, respiratory depression, sedation, seizure, serotonin syndrome, syncope, thinking abnormal, urinary hesitation, visual disturbance, weakness, withdrawal syndrome

Drug Interactions

Metabolism/Transport Effects **Substrate** of CYP2C9 (minor), CYP2D6 (minor); **Note:** Assignment of Major/Minor substrate status based on clinically relevant drug interaction potential

Avoid Concomitant Use

Avoid concomitant use of Tapentadol with any of the following: Alcohol (Ethyl); MAO Inhibitors

Increased Effect/Toxicity

Tapentadol may increase the levels/effects of: Alvimopan; CNS Depressants; Desmopressin; MAO Inhibitors; Metoclopramide; Selective Serotonin Reuptake Inhibitors; Serotonin Modulators; Thiazide Diuretics

The levels/effects of Tapentadol may be increased by: Alcohol (Ethyl); Amphetamines; Antipsychotic Agents (Phenothiazines); Antipsychotics; HydrOXYzine; Succinylcholine

Decreased Effect

Tapentadol may decrease the levels/effects of: Pegvisomant

The levels/effects of Tapentadol may be decreased by: Ammonium Chloride; Mixed Agonist / Antagonist Opioids; Peginterferon Alfa-2b

Ethanol/Nutrition/Herb Interactions

Ethanol: May increase CNS depression; monitor for increased effects with coadministration. Caution patients about effects. Bioavailability of extended release tablets may be increased by alcohol; combined use should be avoided.

Food: When administered after a high fat/calorie meal, the AUC and C_{max} increased by 25% and 16%, respectively; may administer without regard to meals.

Herb/Nutraceutical: Avoid St John's wort (may increase CNS depression and risk of serotonin syndrome).

Stability Store at room temperature up to 25°C (77°F); excursions permitted to 15°C to 30°C (59°F to 86°F). Protect from moisture.

Mechanism of Action Binds to μ-opiate receptors in the CNS causing inhibition of ascending pain pathways, altering the perception of and response to pain; also inhibits the reuptake of norepinephrine, which also modifies the ascending pain pathway

Pharmacodynamics/Kinetics

Absorption: Rapid and complete
Distribution: V_d: I.V.: 442-638 L
Protein binding: ~20%
Metabolism: Extensive metabolism, including first pass metabolism; metabolized primarily via phase 2 glucuronidation to glucuronides (major metabolite: tapentadol-O-glucuronide); minimal phase 1 oxidative metabolism; also metabolized to a lesser degree by CYP2C9, CYP2C19, and CYP2D6; all metabolites pharmacologically inactive
Bioavailability: ~32%
Half-life elimination: Immediate release: ~4 hours; Long acting formulations: ~5-6 hours
Time to peak, plasma: Immediate release: 1.25 hours; Long acting formulations: 3-6 hours
Excretion: Urine (99%: 70% conjugated metabolites; 3% unchanged drug)

Dosage Oral: **Note:** Dose and dosage intervals should be individualized according to pain severity with respect to patient's previous experience with similar opioid analgesics. To reduce the risk of withdrawal symptoms, it is recommended to taper the dose when discontinuing therapy.

Adults:

Acute moderate-severe pain: *U.S. labeling (immediate release):* Day 1: 50-100 mg every 4-6 hours as needed; may administer a second dose ≥1 hour after the initial dose (maximum dose on first day: 700 mg/day); Day 2 and subsequent dosing: 50-100 mg every 4-6 hours as needed (maximum: 600 mg/day)

Chronic moderate-severe pain:

U.S. labeling (extended release):

Opioid naive: Initial: 50 mg twice daily (recommended interval: ~12 hours); titrate in increments of 50 mg no more frequently than twice daily every 3 days to effective dose (therapeutic range: 100-250 mg twice daily) (maximum dose: 500 mg/day)

Opioid experienced: Initial: 50 mg titrated to an effective dose; titrate in increments of 50 mg no more frequently than twice daily every 3 days (therapeutic range: 100-250 mg twice daily) (maximum dose: 500 mg/day). **Note:** No adequate data on converting patients from other opioids to tapentadol extended release.

Conversion from Nucynta® immediate release to extended release: Convert using same total daily dose but divide into two equal doses and administer twice daily (recommended interval: ~12 hours) (maximum dose: 500 mg/day).

Canadian labeling (controlled release):

Opioid naive: Initial: 50 mg twice daily (recommended interval: ~12 hours); titrate to effective dose (therapeutic range: 100-250 mg twice daily)

Opioid experienced (**Note:** Decrease initial dose by 50% when switching from other opioid analgesics): Titrate in increments of 50 mg twice daily every 3 days to recommended dosing range of 100-250 mg twice daily (maximum dose should not exceed 500 mg/day)

Elderly: Initial: Consider initiating at lower range of dosing. Refer to adult dosing.

Dosage adjustment in renal impairment:
Mild-moderate renal impairment: No adjustment necessary
Severe renal impairment: Not recommended (not studied); use is contraindicated in the Canadian labeling
Dosage adjustment in hepatic impairment:
Mild hepatic impairment: No adjustment necessary
Moderate hepatic impairment:
U.S. labeling:
Immediate release: Initial: 50 mg every 8 hours or longer (maximum: 3 doses/24 hours). Further treatment for maintenance of analgesia may be achieved by either shortening or lengthening the dosing interval.
Extended release: Initial: 50 mg every 24 hours; maximum: 100 mg once daily
Canadian labeling (controlled release): Initial: 50 mg every 24 hours; titrate dose cautiously; manufacturer labeling does not provide specific recommendations.
Severe hepatic impairment: Not recommended (not studied); use is contraindicated in the Canadian labeling

Dietary Considerations May be taken without regard to meals.

Administration Administer orally with or without food. Long acting formulations must be swallowed whole and should **not** be split, crushed, broken, chewed, or dissolved.

Dosage Forms Excipient information presented when available (limited, particularly for generics); consult specific product labeling.
Tablet, oral:
Nucynta®: 50 mg, 75 mg, 100 mg
Tablet, extended release, oral:
Nucynta® ER: 50 mg, 100 mg, 150 mg, 200 mg, 250 mg

Dosage Forms: Canada Excipient information presented when available (limited, particularly for generics); consult specific product labeling.
Tablet, controlled release, oral, as hydrochloride:
Nucynta™ CR: 50 mg, 100 mg, 150 mg, 200 mg, 250 mg

Controlled Substance C-II

◆ **Tapentadol Hydrochloride** *see* Tapentadol *on page 1628*
◆ **Tarceva®** *see* Erlotinib *on page 612*
◆ **Targretin®** *see* Bexarotene (Systemic) *on page 215*
◆ **Targretin®** *see* Bexarotene (Topical) *on page 216*
◆ **Tarka®** *see* Trandolapril and Verapamil *on page 1718*
◆ **Taro-Carbamazepine Chewable (Can)** *see* CarBAMazepine *on page 280*
◆ **Taro-Ciprofloxacin (Can)** *see* Ciprofloxacin (Systemic) *on page 362*
◆ **Taro-Clindamycin (Can)** *see* Clindamycin (Topical) *on page 381*
◆ **Taro-Clobetasol (Can)** *see* Clobetasol *on page 384*
◆ **Taro-Desoximetasone (Can)** *see* Desoximetasone *on page 479*
◆ **Taro-Enalapril (Can)** *see* Enalapril *on page 584*
◆ **Taro-Fluconazole (Can)** *see* Fluconazole *on page 718*
◆ **Taro-Mometasone (Can)** *see* Mometasone (Topical) *on page 1151*
◆ **Taro-Simvastatin (Can)** *see* Simvastatin *on page 1555*
◆ **Taro-Sone (Can)** *see* Betamethasone *on page 208*
◆ **Taro-Warfarin (Can)** *see* Warfarin *on page 1802*
◆ **Tasigna®** *see* Nilotinib *on page 1205*
◆ **Tasmar®** *see* Tolcapone *on page 1702*
◆ **Tavist® Allergy [OTC]** *see* Clemastine *on page 377*
◆ **Tavist® ND Allergy [OTC]** *see* Loratadine *on page 1031*
◆ **Taxol** *see* PACLitaxel *on page 1273*
◆ **Taxol® (Can)** *see* PACLitaxel *on page 1273*
◆ **Taxotere®** *see* DOCEtaxel *on page 534*

Tazarotene (taz AR oh teen)

Brand Names: U.S. Avage®; Tazorac®
Brand Names: Canada Tazorac®
Pharmacologic Category Acne Products; Keratolytic Agent; Topical Skin Product, Acne
Use Topical treatment of facial acne vulgaris; topical treatment of stable plaque psoriasis; mitigation (palliation) of facial skin wrinkling, facial mottled hyper-/hypopigmentation, and benign facial lentigines
Pregnancy Risk Factor X
Dosage Topical: **Note:** In patients experiencing excessive pruritus, burning, skin redness, or peeling, discontinue until integrity of the skin is restored, or reduce dosing to an interval the patient is able to tolerate.
Children ≥12 years and Adults:
Acne: Tazorac® cream/gel 0.1%: Apply a thin film (2 mg/cm^2) to affected area once daily
Psoriasis: Tazorac® gel: Initial: 0.05%: Apply once daily to psoriatic lesions using enough (2 mg/cm^2) to cover only the lesion with a thin film to no more than 20% of body surface area. May increase strength to 0.1% if tolerated and necessary.
Children ≥17 years and Adults: Palliation of fine facial wrinkles, facial mottled hyper-/hypopigmentation, benign facial lentigines: Avage™: Apply a pea-sized amount once daily
Adults: Psoriasis: Tazorac® cream: Initial: 0.05%: Apply once daily to psoriatic lesions using enough (2 mg/cm^2) to cover only the lesion with a thin film. May increase strength to 0.1% if tolerated and necessary.

Additional Information Complete prescribing information for this medication should be consulted for additional detail.

Dosage Forms Excipient information presented when available (limited, particularly for generics); consult specific product labeling.
Cream, topical:
Avage®: 0.1% (30 g) [contains benzyl alcohol]
Tazorac®: 0.05% (30 g, 60 g); 0.1% (30 g, 60 g) [contains benzyl alcohol]
Gel, topical:
Tazorac®: 0.05% (30 g, 100 g); 0.1% (30 g, 100 g) [contains benzyl alcohol]

◆ **Tazicef®** *see* CefTAZidime *on page 315*
◆ **Tazobactam and Piperacillin** *see* Piperacillin and Tazobactam *on page 1358*
◆ **Tazocin® (Can)** *see* Piperacillin and Tazobactam *on page 1358*
◆ **Tazorac®** *see* Tazarotene *on page 1630*
◆ **Taztia XT®** *see* Diltiazem *on page 510*
◆ **TBC** *see* Trypsin, Balsam Peru, and Castor Oil *on page 1744*
◆ **TB Skin Test** *see* Tuberculin Tests *on page 1744*
◆ **3TC** *see* LamiVUDine *on page 965*
◆ **3TC® (Can)** *see* LamiVUDine *on page 965*
◆ **3TC, Abacavir, and Zidovudine** *see* Abacavir, Lamivudine, and Zidovudine *on page 20*
◆ **T-Cell Growth Factor** *see* Aldesleukin *on page 55*
◆ **TCGF** *see* Aldesleukin *on page 55*
◆ **TCN** *see* Tetracycline *on page 1661*
◆ **Td** *see* Diphtheria and Tetanus Toxoid *on page 520*
◆ **TD-6424** *see* Telavancin *on page 1633*

Telaprevir (tel A pre vir)

Brand Names: U.S. Incivek™

Brand Names: Canada Incivek™

Index Terms LY570310; MP-424; MP424; VRT111950; VX-950; VX950

Pharmacologic Category Antiviral Agent; Protease Inhibitor

Use Treatment of genotype 1 chronic hepatitis C (in combination with peginterferon alfa and ribavirin) in adult patients with compensated liver disease (including cirrhosis) who are treatment naive or who have received previous interferon-based treatment, including null or partial responders, and treatment relapsers.

Pregnancy Risk Factor B / X (in combination with ribavirin)

Pregnancy Considerations Adverse events were not observed in telaprevir animal developmental studies; however, telaprevir must not be used as monotherapy (must be used in combination with peginterferon alfa and ribavirin). Significant ribavirin teratogenic effects have been observed in all animal studies at ~0.01 times the maximum recommended daily human dose. Use of ribavirin is contraindicated in pregnancy. In addition, animal studies with interferons have demonstrated abortifacient effects. Negative pregnancy test is required before initiation and monthly thereafter. Hormonal contraceptive measures may not be effective in patients taking telaprevir or for 2 weeks after discontinuing therapy. Avoid pregnancy in female patients and female partners of male patients during therapy by using two effective nonhormonal forms of contraception; continue contraceptive measures for at least 6 months after completion of therapy. If patient or female partner becomes pregnant during treatment, she should be counseled about potential risks of exposure. If pregnancy occurs during use or within 6 months after treatment, report to the ribavirin pregnancy registry (800-593-2214).

Lactation Excretion in breast milk unknown/not recommended

Medication Guide Available Yes

Contraindications Hypersensitivity to telaprevir or any component of the formulation; pregnancy; male partners of pregnant women

Coadministration with CYP 3A4 highly dependent substrates (alfuzosin, atorvastatin, cisapride, ergot derivatives, lovastatin, midazolam [oral], pimozide, sildenafil/tadalafil [when used for treatment of pulmonary arterial hypertension], simvastatin, triazolam), or strong CYP 3A4 inducers (rifampin, St John's wort)

Canadian labeling: Additional contraindications (not in U.S. labeling): Coadministration with amiodarone, eletriptan, flecainide, propafenone, quinidine, terfenadine, vardenafil

Also refer to Peginterferon Alfa and Ribavirin monographs for individual product contraindications.

Warnings/Precautions Avoid pregnancy in female patients and female partners of male patients, during therapy, and for at least 6 months after treatment; two forms of nonhormonal contraception should be used. Safety and efficacy have not been established in patients who have uncompensated cirrhosis, received organ transplants, or been coinfected with hepatitis B or HIV, or who have failed to respond to other NS3/4A inhibitors. Monotherapy is not effective for chronic hepatitis C infection.

Anemia has been reported with peginterferon alfa and ribavirin; addition of telaprevir is associated with further hemoglobin decreases. Low hemoglobin levels were measured during the first 4 weeks of treatment, and the lowest at the end of telaprevir treatment (week 12). Dose modifications of ribavirin were needed more often in patients also taking telaprevir. Assess complete blood count (CBC) pretreatment and at weeks 2, 4, 8, and 12, and when clinically indicated. May require ribavirin dose reduction, interruption or discontinuation of treatment. Do not reduce telaprevir dose. If ribavirin is discontinued, telaprevir must also be discontinued. Do not restart telaprevir if ribavirin therapy is reinitiated. Mild-to-severe skin reactions, including DRESS (drug rash with eosinophilia with systemic symptoms [fever, facial edema, hepatitis or nephritis with or without eosinophilia]) and Stevens-Johnson syndrome (SJS) have been reported; discontinue telaprevir combination therapy immediately if patient develops DRESS or SJS. Severe rashes (other than DRESS, SJS) are generalized, bullous, vesicular or ulcerative; may also have an eczematous appearance. Discontinue telaprevir (may continue peginterferon alfa and ribavirin) for severe rash or for mild-to-moderate rash that progresses or leads to systemic involvement; if no improvement in rash within 1 week of stopping telaprevir, interruption or discontinuation of peginterferon alfa and/or ribavirin should be considered (or sooner if clinically indicated). May use oral antihistamines/topical corticosteroids for rash treatment; do not use systemic corticosteroids. Do not restart telaprevir if discontinued due to any rash severity. High potential for CYP3A-mediated interactions. Hormonal contraceptives may not be effective in patients taking telaprevir or for two weeks after discontinuing therapy. Not recommended in moderate or severe hepatic impairment (Child-Pugh class B or C) or decompensated hepatic disease.

Adverse Reactions

>10%:

Central nervous system: Fatigue (56%)

Dermatologic: Rash (56%), pruritus (47%)

Endocrine and Metabolic: Hyperuricemia (<12.1 mg/dL: 66%; ≥12.1 mg/dL: 7%)

Gastrointestinal: Nausea (39%), diarrhea (26%), vomiting (13%), hemorrhoids (12%), anorectal discomfort (11%)

Hematologic: Anemia (36%), lymphopenia (15%)

Hepatic: Hyperbilirubinemia (<2.6 x ULN: 37%; ≥2.6 x ULN: 4%)

1% to 10%:

Gastrointestinal: Abnormal taste (10%), anal pruritus (6%)

Hematologic: Thrombocytopenia (3%)

Drug Interactions

Metabolism/Transport Effects Substrate of CYP3A4 (major), P-glycoprotein; **Note:** Assignment of Major/Minor substrate status based on clinically relevant drug interaction potential; **Inhibits** CYP3A4 (strong), P-glycoprotein

Avoid Concomitant Use

Avoid concomitant use of Telaprevir with any of the following: Alfuzosin; Atorvastatin; CarBAMazepine; Cisapride; Conivaptan; Crizotinib; Darunavir; Dronedarone; Eplerenone; Ergot Derivatives; Everolimus; Fluticasone (Oral Inhalation); Fosamprenavir; Fosphenytoin; Halofantrine; Lapatinib; Lopinavir; Lovastatin; Lurasidone; Midazolam; Nilotinib; Nisoldipine; PHENobarbital; Phenytoin; Pimozide; Ranolazine; Rifabutin; Rifampin; Rivaroxaban; RomiDEPsin; Salmeterol; Sildenafil; Silodosin; Simvastatin; St Johns Wort; Tadalafil; Tamsulosin; Ticagrelor; Tolvaptan; Topotecan; Toremifene; Triazolam

Increased Effect/Toxicity

Telaprevir may increase the levels/effects of: Alfuzosin; Almotriptan; Alosetron; ALPRAZolam; Amiodarone; ARIPiprazole; Atazanavir; Atorvastatin; Bepridil [Off Market]; Bortezomib; Bosentan; Brentuximab Vedotin; Brinzolamide; Budesonide (Nasal); Budesonide (Systemic, Oral Inhalation); CarBAMazepine; Ciclesonide; Cisapride; Clarithromycin; Colchicine; Conivaptan; Corticosteroids; Corticosteroids (Orally Inhaled); Corticosteroids (Systemic); Crizotinib; CycloSPORINE; CycloSPORINE (Systemic); CYP3A4 Substrates; Dabigatran Etexilate; Desipramine; Dienogest; Digoxin; Dronedarone; Dutasteride; Eplerenone; Ergot Derivatives; Erythromycin; Everolimus; FentaNYL; Fesoterodine; Flecainide; Fluticasone (Nasal); Fluticasone (Oral Inhalation); Fosphenytoin; GuanFACINE; Halofantrine; Iloperidone; Itraconazole; Ixabepilone; Ketoconazole; Ketoconazole (Systemic); Lapatinib; Lidocaine; Lidocaine (Systemic); Lovastatin; Lumefantrine; Lurasidone; Maraviroc; MethylPREDNISolone; Midazolam; Nilotinib; Nisoldipine; Paricalcitol; Pazopanib; P-glycoprotein/ABCB1 Substrates; PHENobarbital; Phenytoin; Pimecrolimus; Pimozide; Posaconazole; Propafenone; QuiNIDine; Ranolazine; Rifabutin; Rivaroxaban; RomiDEPsin; Ruxolitinib; Salmeterol; Saxagliptin; Sildenafil; Silodosin; Simvastatin; Sirolimus; SORAfenib; Tacrolimus; Tacrolimus (Systemic); Tadalafil; Tamsulosin; Telithromycin; Tenofovir; Ticagrelor; Tolterodine; Tolvaptan; Topotecan; Toremifene; TraZODone; Triazolam; Vardenafil; Vemurafenib; Vilazodone; Voriconazole; Warfarin; Zuclopenthixol

The levels/effects of Telaprevir may be increased by: Clarithromycin; CYP3A4 Inhibitors (Moderate); CYP3A4 Inhibitors (Strong); Dasatinib; Erythromycin; Itraconazole; Ketoconazole; Ketoconazole (Systemic); P-glycoprotein/ABCB1 Inhibitors; Posaconazole; Ritonavir; Telithromycin; Voriconazole

Decreased Effect

Telaprevir may decrease the levels/effects of: Contraceptives (Estrogens); Contraceptives (Progestins); Darunavir; Efavirenz; Escitalopram; Fosamprenavir; Fosphenytoin; Methadone; PHENobarbital; Phenytoin; Prasugrel; Ticagrelor; Voriconazole; Warfarin; Zolpidem

The levels/effects of Telaprevir may be decreased by: Atazanavir; Bosentan; CarBAMazepine; Corticosteroids; Corticosteroids (Systemic); CYP3A4 Inducers (Strong); Darunavir; Deferasirox; Efavirenz; Fosamprenavir; Fosphenytoin; Lopinavir; P-glycoprotein/ABCB1 Inducers; PHENobarbital; Phenytoin; Rifabutin; Rifampin; Ritonavir; St Johns Wort; Tocilizumab

Stability Store at 25°C (77°F); excursions permitted to 15°C to 30°C (59°F to 86°F). Keep container tightly closed. Opened bottle must be used within 28 days.

Mechanism of Action Binds reversibly to nonstructural protein 3 (NS 3) serine protease and inhibits replication of the hepatitis C virus. Considered a direct-acting antiviral treatment for HCV, also called a specifically targeted antiviral therapy for HCV (STAT-C).

Pharmacodynamics/Kinetics

Absorption: Food (not low fat) enhances absorption

Distribution: V_d: ~252 L

Protein binding: 59% to 76%

Metabolism: Primarily hepatic to less active (30x) and inactive metabolites. Some oxidative CYP3A4 metabolism.

Half-life elimination: Plasma: Adults: ~4-5 hours (single dose); steady state: ~9-11 hours

Time to peak, serum: 4-5 hours

Excretion: Feces (82%); urine (1%)

Dosage Oral: Adults: 750 mg 3 times/day (in combination with peginterferon alfa and ribavirin)

Treatment-naive or prior relapse patients: **Note:** Relapse includes patients with an undetectable HCV-RNA upon completion of treatment (non-telaprevir based regimen) but with detectable HCV-RNA during the follow up period.

Weeks 1-12: Triple therapy: Telaprevir 750 mg 3 times/day in combination with peginterferon alfa and ribavirin

Weeks 13-23 (based on HCV-RNA results at weeks 4 and 12):

HCV-RNA **undetectable** (level less than ~10-15 int. units/mL) at both weeks 4 and 12 (eRVR): Dual therapy: Peginterferon alfa and ribavirin only (through week 24)

HCV-RNA **detectable** (level greater than ~10-15 int. units/mL but ≤1000 int. units/mL) at week 4 and/or week 12: Dual therapy: Peginterferon alfa and ribavirin only (through week 48 discussed below)

HCV-RNA **detectable** (level >1000 int. units/mL) at week 4 or week 12 (treatment futility): Discontinue telaprevir, peginterferon alfa and ribavirin at week 12

Weeks ≥24 (based on HCV-RNA results at week 24):

HCV-RNA **detectable** (level greater than ~10-15 int. units/mL but ≤1000 int. units/mL) at week 4 and/or week 12: Peginterferon alfa with concomitant ribavirin only (through week 48)

HCV-RNA **detectable** (level greater than ~10-15 int. units/mL) at week 24 (treatment futility): Discontinue peginterferon alfa and concomitant ribavirin

Treatment naïve patients with cirrhosis, compensated:

Weeks 1-12: Triple therapy: Telaprevir 750 mg 3 times/day in combination with peginterferon alfa and ribavirin

Weeks 13-24 (based on HCV-RNA results at weeks 4 and 12):

HCV-RNA **undetectable** at both weeks 4 and 12 (eRVR): Dual therapy: Peginterferon alfa and ribavirin only (through week 48 discussed below)

HCV-RNA **detectable** (level greater than ~10-15 int. units/mL but ≤1000 int. units/mL) at week 4 and/or week 12: Dual therapy: Peginterferon alfa and ribavirin only (through week 48 discussed below)

HCV-RNA **detectable** (level >1000 int. units/mL) at week 4 or week 12 (treatment futility): Discontinue telaprevir, peginterferon alfa and ribavirin at week 12

Weeks ≥ 24 (based on HCV-RNA results at week 24):

HCV-RNA **undetectable** at week 24: Peginterferon alfa with concomitant ribavirin only (through week 48)

HCV-RNA **detectable** (level greater than ~10-15 int. units/mL) at week 24 (treatment futility): Discontinue peginterferon alfa and ribavirin

Previously-treated patients (partial response or null responders): **Note:** Previously treated does not include prior treatment with telaprevir. Partial response includes patients with a >2-$\log_{10}$ HCV-RNA decrease by week 12 but a nonsustained virologic response thereafter. Null response includes patients with a <2-$\log_{10}$ HCV-RNA decrease at week 12.

Weeks 1-12: Triple therapy: Telaprevir 750 mg 3 times/day with peginterferon alfa and ribavirin

Weeks 13-48 (based on HCV-RNA results at weeks 4 and 12):

HCV-RNA **undetectable** (level less than ~10-15 int. units/mL) or detectable (level ≤1000 int. units/mL) at both weeks 4 and 12: Dual therapy: Peginterferon alfa and ribavirin only (through week 48)

HCV-RNA **detectable** (level >1000 int. units/mL) at week 4 or week 12: Discontinue telaprevir, peginterferon alfa, and ribavirin at week 12
HCV-RNA **detectable** (level greater than ~10-15 int. units/mL) at week 24: Discontinue peginterferon alfa and concomitant ribavirin

Dosage adjustment in renal impairment:
Telaprevir: No adjustment required. Not studied in patients with Cl_{cr} ≤50 mL/minute or in hemodialysis.
Peginterferon Alfa and Ribavirin: Refer to individual monographs.

Dosage adjustment in hepatic impairment: Telaprevir:
Mild impairment (Child-Pugh class A): No adjustment required
Moderate or severe impairment (Child-Pugh class B or C): Not studied
Peginterferon Alfa and Ribavirin: Refer to individual monographs.

Dietary Considerations Take with a meal (not low fat).

Administration Administer with a meal (not low fat). Doses should be taken approximately every 7-9 hours. Administer concurrently with peginterferon alfa and ribavirin.

Monitoring Parameters
CBC with differential, serum electrolytes, TSH, bilirubin, liver enzymes, and uric acid at baseline and weeks 2, 4, 8 and 12, then periodically (and when clinically indicated)
Serum HCV-RNA at baseline, weeks 4, 8, 12 and 24, end of treatment, during treatment follow up, and when clinically indicated
Pretreatment and monthly pregnancy test up to 6 months following discontinuation of therapy for women of child-bearing age

Reference Range
Treatment futility: HCV-RNA ≥1000 int. units/mL at treatment week 4 or 12 or confirmed, detectable HCV-RNA at treatment week 24
Rapid virologic response (RVR): Absence of detectable HCV-RNA after 4 weeks of treatment
Extended rapid virologic response (eRVR): Absence of detectable HCV-RNA after 4 and 12 weeks of treatment
Early virologic response (EVR): Absence of detectable HCV-RNA after 12 weeks of treatment
Sustained virologic response (SVR): Absence of HCV-RNA in the serum 6 months following completion of full treatment course

Additional Information In clinical studies of treatment-naive patients, a sustained virologic response (SVR) of ~75% (~65% in African-Americans) was observed with peginterferon alfa, ribavirin, and telaprevir versus 44% with peginterferon and ribavirin alone. Adherence to 3-times-day dosing is needed; resistance is increased and efficacy is affected when dosed every 12 hours.

Dosage Forms Excipient information presented when available (limited, particularly for generics); consult specific product labeling.
Tablet, oral:
Incivek™: 375 mg

Telavancin (tel a VAN sin)

Brand Names: U.S. Vibativ™

Index Terms TD-6424; Telavancin Hydrochloride

Pharmacologic Category Glycopeptide

Use Treatment of complicated skin and skin structure infections caused by susceptible gram-positive organisms including methicillin-susceptible or -resistant *Staphylococcus aureus*, vancomycin-susceptible *Enterococcus faecalis*, and *Streptococcus pyogenes*, *Streptococcus agalactiae*, or *Streptococcus anginosus* group

Pregnancy Risk Factor C

Pregnancy Considerations Animal studies noted decreased fetal weight and increased deaths. There are no adequate or well-controlled studies in pregnant women. Use is not recommended during pregnancy unless the potential benefit outweighs the risk to the fetus.

Pregnant women should be registered with the Vibativ™ Pregnancy Registry by calling 1-888-658-4228.

Lactation Excretion in breast milk unknown/use caution

Medication Guide Available Yes

Contraindications There are no contraindications listed within the manufacturers labeling.

Warnings/Precautions [U.S. Boxed Warning]: Based on animal data, adverse developmental outcomes have been observed. Prior to use, women of child-bearing potential should have a serum pregnancy test. Use of telavancin is not recommended during pregnancy unless the potential benefit outweighs the risk to the fetus. May prolong QT_c interval; avoid use in patients with a history of QT_c prolongation, uncompensated heart failure, severe left ventricular hypertrophy, or concurrent administration of other medications known to prolong the QT interval (including Class Ia and Class III antiarrhythmics, cisapride, erythromycin, antipsychotics, and tricyclic antidepressants). Clinical studies indicate mean maximal QT_c prolongation of 12-15 msec at the end of 10 mg/kg infusion. Use with caution in patients with renal impairment or those receiving other nephrotoxic drugs; dosage modification required and efficacy may be reduced in patients with Cl_{cr} ≤50 mL/minute. May cause nephrotoxicity; usual risk factors include pre-existing renal impairment, concomitant nephrotoxic medications, advanced age, and dehydration. Monitor renal function prior to, during, and following therapy. Contains solubilizer cyclodextrin (hydroxypropyl-beta-cyclodextrin) which may accumulate in patients with renal dysfunction. Prolonged use may result in fungal or bacterial superinfection, including *C. difficile*-associated diarrhea (CDAD) and pseudomembranous colitis; CDAD has been observed >2 months postantibiotic treatment.

May interfere with tests used to monitor coagulation (eg, prothrombin time, INR, activated partial thromboplastin time, activated clotting time, coagulation based factor Xa tests) when samples drawn ≤18 hours after drug administration. Blood samples should be collected as close to the next dose of telavancin as possible. Rapid I.V. administration may result in flushing, rash, urticaria, and/or pruritus; slowing or stopping the infusion may alleviate these symptoms. In the elderly, lower doses are often required secondary to age-related decreases in renal function.

Adverse Reactions
>10%:
Central nervous system: Insomnia (13%), psychiatric disorder (12%), headache (11%)
Gastrointestinal: Metallic/soapy taste (33%), nausea (27%), vomiting (14%)
Genitourinary: Foamy urine (13%)
1% to 10%:
Central nervous system: Dizziness (6%)
Dermatologic: Pruritus (3% to 6%), rash (4%)
Endocrine & metabolic: Hypokalemia (7%)
Gastrointestinal: Diarrhea (7%), appetite decreased (3%), abdominal pain (2%)
Hematologic: Thrombocytopenia (7%)
Local: Infusion site pain (4%), infusion site erythema (3%)
Neuromuscular & skeletal: Paresthesia (5%), rigors (4%)
Renal: Serum creatinine increased (8%), microalbuminuria (7%)
Respiratory: Dyspnea (8%)
<1% (Limited to important or life-threatening): *C. difficile*-associated diarrhea, hearing loss (transient), QT_c interval prolongation

Drug Interactions

Metabolism/Transport Effects None known.

Avoid Concomitant Use

Avoid concomitant use of Telavancin with any of the following: Artemether; BCG; Dronedarone; Lumefantrine; Nilotinib; Pimozide; QUEtiapine; QuiNINE; Tetrabenazine; Thioridazine; Toremifene; Vandetanib; Vemurafenib; Ziprasidone

Increased Effect/Toxicity

Telavancin may increase the levels/effects of: Dronedarone; Pimozide; QTc-Prolonging Agents; QuiNINE; Tetrabenazine; Thioridazine; Toremifene; Vandetanib; Vemurafenib; Ziprasidone

The levels/effects of Telavancin may be increased by: Alfuzosin; Artemether; Chloroquine; Ciprofloxacin; Ciprofloxacin (Systemic); Gadobutrol; Indacaterol; Lumefantrine; Nilotinib; QUEtiapine; QuiNINE

Decreased Effect

Telavancin may decrease the levels/effects of: BCG; Typhoid Vaccine

Stability Store at 2°C to 8°C (35°F to 46°F); excursions permitted up to 25°C (77°F); avoid excess heat. **Note:** Vials contain no bacteriostatic agent.

Reconstitute 250 mg vial with 15 mL of D_5W, NS, or SWFI to yield 15 mg/mL (total volume of ~17 mL). Reconstitute 750 mg vial with 45 mL of of D_5W, NS, or SWFI to yield 15 mg/mL (total volume of ~50 mL). Reconstitution may take 2-20 minutes. Discard vial if vacuum did not pull the diluent into the vial. Prior to administration, dilute dose in 100-250 mL D_5W, LR, or NS to a final concentration of 0.6-8 mg/mL.

Reconstituted solution in the vial or admixed in either D_5W, NS, or SWFI are stable at room temperature for 4 hours or under refrigeration for 72 hours. Total time in vial **plus** time in infusion bag should not exceed 4 hours at room temperature or 72 hours if refrigerated at 2°C to 8°C (35°F to 46°F).

Mechanism of Action Exerts concentration-dependent bactericidal activity; inhibits bacterial cell wall synthesis by blocking polymerization and cross-linking of peptidoglycan by binding to D-Ala-D-Ala portion of cell wall. Unlike vancomycin, additional mechanism involves disruption of membrane potential and changes cell permeability due to presence of lipophilic side chain moiety.

Pharmacodynamics/Kinetics

Distribution: V_{ss}: 0.13 L/kg

Protein binding: ~90%; primarily to albumin

Half-life elimination: 6.6-9.6 hours

Excretion: Urine (~76%); feces (<1%)

Dosage I.V.: Adults: Complicated skin and skin structure Infection: 10 mg/kg every 24 hours for 1-2 weeks

Dosing adjustment in renal impairment: ***Note:*** *Renal function may be estimated using the Cockcroft-Gault formula for dosage adjustment purposes.*

Cl_{cr} 30-50 mL/minute: 7.5 mg/kg every 24 hours

Cl_{cr} 10 to <30 mL/minute: 10 mg/kg every 48 hours

Cl_{cr} <10 mL/minute and hemodialysis patients: Dosage adjustment recommendations are not available; use caution or avoid.

Dosing adjustment in hepatic impairment:

Mild-to-moderate hepatic impairment: no dosage adjustment necessary

Severe hepatic impairment: Has not been evaluated

Administration Administer I.V. over 60 minutes. Other medications should not be infused simultaneously through the same I.V. line. When the same intravenous line is used for sequential infusion of other medications, flush line with D_5W, LR, or NS before and after infusing telavancin.

Red-man syndrome may occur if the infusion is too rapid. It is not an allergic reaction, but may be characterized by hypotension and/or a maculopapular rash appearing on the face, neck, trunk, and/or upper extremities. If this should occur, discontinuing or slowing the infusion rate may eliminate these reactions.

Monitoring Parameters Renal function, pregnancy test

Test Interactions Interferes with the following coagulation assessments (causes artificially increased clotting times): PT, INR, aPTT, ACT, Xa; interferes with urine protein via qualitative dipstick and quantitative dye methods

Dosage Forms Excipient information presented when available (limited, particularly for generics); consult specific product labeling.

Injection, powder for reconstitution:

Vibativ™: 250 mg, 750 mg [contains cyclodextrin]

◆ **Telavancin Hydrochloride** *see* Telavancin *on page 1633*

Telithromycin (tel ith roe MYE sin)

Brand Names: U.S. Ketek®

Brand Names: Canada Ketek®

Index Terms HMR 3647

Pharmacologic Category Antibiotic, Ketolide

Use Treatment of community-acquired pneumonia (mild-to-moderate) caused by susceptible strains of *Streptococcus pneumoniae* (including multidrug-resistant isolates), *Haemophilus influenzae*, *Chlamydophila pneumoniae*, *Moraxella catarrhalis*, and *Mycoplasma pneumoniae*

Pregnancy Risk Factor C

Pregnancy Considerations Because adverse effects were observed in some animal studies, telithromycin is classified pregnancy category C. There are no adequate and well-controlled studies of telithromycin in pregnant women.

Lactation Excretion in breast milk unknown/use caution

Medication Guide Available Yes

Contraindications Hypersensitivity to telithromycin, macrolide antibiotics, or any component of the formulation; myasthenia gravis; history of hepatitis and/or jaundice associated with telithromycin or other macrolide antibiotic use; concurrent use of cisapride or pimozide

Warnings/Precautions Acute hepatic failure and severe liver injury, including hepatitis and hepatic necrosis (leading to some fatalities) have been reported, in some cases after only a few doses; if signs/symptoms of hepatitis or liver damage occur, discontinue therapy and initiate liver function tests. **[U.S. Boxed Warning]: Life-threatening (including fatal) respiratory failure has occurred in patients with myasthenia gravis;** use in these patients is contraindicated. May prolong QT_c interval, leading to a risk of ventricular arrhythmias; closely-related antibiotics have been associated with malignant ventricular arrhythmias and torsade de pointes. Avoid in patients with prolongation of QTc interval due to congenital causes, history of long QT syndrome, uncorrected electrolyte disturbances (hypokalemia or hypomagnesemia), significant bradycardia (<50 bpm), or concurrent therapy with QT_c-prolonging drugs (eg, class Ia and class III antiarrhythmics). Avoid use in patients with a prior history of confirmed cardiogenic syncope or ventricular arrhythmias while receiving macrolide antibiotics or other QT_c-prolonging drugs. May cause severe visual disturbances (eg, changes in accommodation ability, diplopia, blurred vision). May cause loss of consciousness (possibly vagal-related); caution patients that these events may interfere with ability to operate machinery or drive, and to use caution until effects are known. Use caution in renal impairment; severe impairment (Cl_{cr} <30 mL/minute) requires dosage adjustment. Pseudomembranous colitis has been reported. Safety and efficacy not established in pediatric patients <13 years of age per Canadian approved labeling and <18 years of age per U.S. approved labeling.

Adverse Reactions

>10%: Gastrointestinal: Diarrhea (10% to 11%)

2% to 10%:

Central nervous system: Headache (2% to 6%), dizziness (3% to 4%)

Gastrointestinal: Nausea (7% to 8%), vomiting (2% to 3%), loose stools (2%), dysgeusia (2%)

≥0.2% to <2%:

Central nervous system: Fatigue, insomnia, somnolence, vertigo

Dermatologic: Rash

Gastrointestinal: Abdominal distension, abdominal pain, anorexia, constipation, dyspepsia, flatulence, gastritis, gastroenteritis, GI upset, glossitis, stomatitis, watery stools, xerostomia

Genitourinary: Vaginal candidiasis, vaginitis

Hematologic: Platelets increased

Hepatic: Transaminases increased

Ocular: Blurred vision, accommodation delayed, diplopia

Miscellaneous: Candidiasis, diaphoresis increased

<0.2% (Limited to important or life-threatening): Acute repiratory failure, alkaline phosphatase increased, allergic reaction, anaphylaxis, angioedema, anxiety, arrhythmia, bilirubin increased, bradycardia, edema (facial), eosinophilia, erythema multiforme, flushing, hepatitis, hepatitis, hepatocellular injury (including necrosis), hypotension, jaundice, liver failure, loss of consciousness (may be vagal-related), muscle cramps, myasthenia gravis exacerbation (rare), palpitation, pancreatitis, paresthesia, pruritus, pseudomembranous colitis, QT_c prolongation, syncope, torsade de pointes

Drug Interactions

Metabolism/Transport Effects **Substrate** of CYP1A2 (minor), CYP3A4 (major); **Note:** Assignment of Major/Minor substrate status based on clinically relevant drug interaction potential; **Inhibits** CYP2D6 (weak), CYP3A4 (strong)

Avoid Concomitant Use

Avoid concomitant use of Telithromycin with any of the following: Alfuzosin; Artemether; BCG; Cisapride; Conivaptan; Crizotinib; Disopyramide; Dronedarone; Eplerenone; Everolimus; Fluticasone (Oral Inhalation); Halofantrine; Lapatinib; Lovastatin; Lumefantrine; Lurasidone; Nilotinib; Nisoldipine; Pimozide; QUEtiapine; QuiNINE; Ranolazine; Rivaroxaban; RomiDEPsin; Salmeterol; Silodosin; Simvastatin; Tamsulosin; Terfenadine; Tetrabenazine; Thioridazine; Ticagrelor; Tolvaptan; Toremifene; Vandetanib; Vemurafenib; Ziprasidone

Increased Effect/Toxicity

Telithromycin may increase the levels/effects of: Alfentanil; Alfuzosin; Almotriptan; Alosetron; Antifungal Agents (Azole Derivatives, Systemic); Antineoplastic Agents (Vinca Alkaloids); ARIPiprazole; Benzodiazepines (metabolized by oxidation); Bortezomib; Brentuximab Vedotin; Brinzolamide; Budesonide (Nasal); Budesonide (Systemic, Oral Inhalation); BusPIRone; Calcium Channel Blockers; CarBAMazepine; Cardiac Glycosides; Ciclesonide; Cilostazol; Cisapride; CloZAPine; Colchicine; Conivaptan; Corticosteroids (Orally Inhaled); Corticosteroids (Systemic); Crizotinib; CycloSPORINE; CycloSPORINE (Systemic); CYP3A4 Substrates; Dienogest; Disopyramide; Dronedarone; Dutasteride; Eletriptan; Eplerenone; Ergot Derivatives; Everolimus; FentaNYL; Fesoterodine; Fluticasone (Nasal); Fluticasone (Oral Inhalation); GuanFACINE; Halofantrine; HMG-CoA Reductase Inhibitors; Iloperidone; Ixabepilone; Lapatinib; Lovastatin; Lumefantrine; Lurasidone; Maraviroc; MethylPREDNISolone; Nilotinib; Nisoldipine; Paricalcitol; Pazopanib; Pimecrolimus; Pimozide; Propafenone; QTc-Prolonging Agents; QuiNIDine; QuiNINE; Ranolazine; Repaglinide; Rifamycin Derivatives; Rivaroxaban; RomiDEPsin; Ruxolitinib; Salmeterol; Saxagliptin; Selective Serotonin Reuptake Inhibitors; Sildenafil; Silodosin; Simvastatin; Sirolimus; SORAfenib; Tacrolimus; Tacrolimus (Systemic); Tacrolimus (Topical); Tadalafil; Tamsulosin; Telaprevir; Temsirolimus; Terfenadine; Tetrabenazine; Thioridazine; Ticagrelor; Tolterodine; Tolvaptan; Toremifene; Vandetanib; Vardenafil; Vemurafenib; Verapamil; Vilazodone; Vitamin K Antagonists; Ziprasidone; Zopiclone; Zuclopenthixol

The levels/effects of Telithromycin may be increased by: Alfuzosin; Antifungal Agents (Azole Derivatives, Systemic); Artemether; Chloroquine; Ciprofloxacin; Ciprofloxacin (Systemic); CYP3A4 Inhibitors (Moderate); CYP3A4 Inhibitors (Strong); Gadobutrol; Indacaterol; Lumefantrine; Nilotinib; QUEtiapine; QuiNINE; Telaprevir

Decreased Effect

Telithromycin may decrease the levels/effects of: BCG; Clopidogrel; Prasugrel; Ticagrelor; Typhoid Vaccine

The levels/effects of Telithromycin may be decreased by: CYP3A4 Inducers (Strong); Cyproterone; Deferasirox; Etravirine; Herbs (CYP3A4 Inducers); Tocilizumab

Ethanol/Nutrition/Herb Interactions Herb/nutraceutical: St John's wort: May decrease the levels/effects of telithromycin.

Stability Store at 15°C to 30°C (59°F to 86°F).

Mechanism of Action Inhibits bacterial protein synthesis by binding to two sites on the 50S ribosomal subunit. Telithromycin has also been demonstrated to alter secretion of IL-1alpha and TNF-alpha; the clinical significance of this immunomodulatory effect has not been evaluated.

Pharmacodynamics/Kinetics

Absorption: Rapid

Distribution: 2.9 L/kg

Protein binding: 60% to 70%; primarily to albumin

Metabolism: Hepatic, via CYP3A4 (50%) and non-CYP-mediated pathways

Bioavailability: 57% (significant first-pass metabolism)

Half-life elimination: 10 hours

Time to peak, plasma: 1 hour

Excretion: Urine (13% unchanged drug, remainder as metabolites); feces (7%)

Dosage Oral:

Children ≥13 years and Adults: Tonsillitis/pharyngitis (unlabeled use; Canadian indication): 800 mg once daily for 5 days

Adults: Community-acquired pneumonia: 800 mg once daily for 7-10 days

Dosage adjustment in renal impairment:

U.S. product labeling: Cl_{cr} <30 mL/minute, including dialysis: 600 mg once daily; when renal impairment is accompanied by hepatic impairment, reduce dosage to 400 mg once daily

Canadian product labeling: Cl_{cr} <30 mL/minute: Reduce dose to 400 mg once daily

Hemodialysis: Administer following dialysis

Dosage adjustment in hepatic impairment: No adjustment recommended, unless concurrent severe renal impairment is present

Dietary Considerations May be taken with or without food.

Administration May be administered with or without food.

Monitoring Parameters Liver function tests; signs/symptoms of liver failure (eg, jaundice, fatigue, malaise, anorexia, nausea, bilirubinemia, acholic stools, liver tenderness, hepatomegaly); visual acuity

Dosage Forms Excipient information presented when available (limited, particularly for generics); consult specific product labeling.

Tablet, oral:

Ketek®: 300 mg, 400 mg

Dosage Forms: Canada Excipient information presented when available (limited, particularly for generics); consult specific product labeling.

Tablet:

Ketek®: 400 mg

Telmisartan (tel mi SAR tan)

Brand Names: U.S. Micardis®

Brand Names: Canada Micardis®

Pharmacologic Category Angiotensin II Receptor Blocker

Additional Appendix Information

Angiotensin Agents *on page 1869*

Use Treatment of hypertension (may be used alone or in combination with other antihypertensive agents); cardiovascular risk reduction in patients ≥55 years of age unable to take ACE inhibitors and who are at high risk of major cardiovascular events (eg, MI, stroke, death)

Pregnancy Risk Factor C (1st trimester); D (2nd and 3rd trimesters)

Pregnancy Considerations Medications which act on the renin-angiotensin system are reported to have the following fetal/neonatal effects: Hypotension, neonatal skull hypoplasia, anuria, renal failure, and death; oligohydramnios is also reported. These effects are reported to occur with exposure during the second and third trimesters. There are no adequate and well-controlled studies in pregnant women. **[U.S. Boxed Warning]: Based on human data, drugs that act on the angiotensin system can cause injury and death to the developing fetus when used in the second and third trimesters. Angiotensin receptor blockers should be discontinued as soon as possible once pregnancy is detected.**

Lactation Excretion in breast milk unknown/not recommended

Contraindications There are no contraindications listed in manufacturer's labeling.

Canadian labeling: Hypersensitivity to telmisartan or any component of the formulation; second and third trimesters of pregnancy; breast-feeding; fructose intolerance

Warnings/Precautions [U.S. Boxed Warning]: Based on human data, drugs that act on the angiotensin system can cause injury and death to the developing fetus when used in the second and third trimesters. Angiotensin receptor blockers should be discontinued as soon as possible once pregnancy is detected. May cause hyperkalemia; avoid potassium supplementation unless specifically required by healthcare provider. Avoid use or use a smaller dose in patients who are volume depleted; correct depletion first. May be associated with deterioration of renal function and/or increases in serum creatinine, particularly in patients with low renal blood flow (eg, renal artery stenosis, heart failure) whose glomerular filtration rate (GFR) is dependent on efferent arteriolar vasoconstriction by angiotensin II. Use with caution in unstented unilateral/bilateral renal artery stenosis. When unstented bilateral renal artery stenosis is present, use is generally avoided due to the elevated risk of deterioration in renal function unless possible benefits outweigh risks. Use with caution with pre-existing renal insufficiency; significant aortic/mitral stenosis. Concurrent use of ACE inhibitors may increase the risk of clinically-significant adverse events (eg, renal dysfunction, hyperkalemia). Concurrent use with ramipril is not recommended. Use with caution in patients who have biliary obstructive disorders or hepatic dysfunction. Product contains sorbitol. The Canadian labeling (not in U.S. labeling) contraindicates use in fructose intolerant patients.

Adverse Reactions May be associated with worsening of renal function in patients dependent on renin-angiotensin-aldosterone system.

1% to 10%:

Cardiovascular: Intermittent claudication (7%; placebo 6%), chest pain (≥1%), hypertension (≥1%), peripheral edema (≥1%)

Central nervous system: Dizziness (≥1%), fatigue (≥1%), headache (≥1%), pain (≥1%)

Dermatologic: Skin ulcer (3%; placebo 2%)

Gastrointestinal: Diarrhea (3%), abdominal pain (≥1%), dyspepsia (≥1%), nausea (≥1%)

Genitourinary: Urinary tract infection (≥1%)

Neuromuscular & skeletal: Back pain (3%), myalgia (≥1%)

Respiratory: Upper respiratory infection (7%), sinusitis (3%), cough (≥1%), pharyngitis (1%)

<1% (Limited to important or life-threatening): Abnormal ECG, abnormal vision, abscess, allergic reaction, anemia, angina, angioedema, angioneurotic edema, anxiety, arthralgia, arthritis, asthma, atrial fibrillation, bradycardia, bronchitis, BUN increased, cerebrovascular disorder, CHF, conjunctivitis, constipation, cramps, creatinine kinase increased, cystitis, depression, dermatitis, diabetes mellitus, diaphoresis, dyspnea, earache, eczema, edema, enteritis, epistaxis, eosinophilia, erectile dysfunction, erythema, facial edema, fever, flatulence, flushing, frequent urination, fungal infection, gastroenteritis, gout, hemoglobin decreased, hemorrhoids, hepatic dysfunction, hypercholesterolemia, hyperkalemia, hypersensitivity, hypotension, impotence, insomnia, liver enzymes increased, malaise, MI, migraine, muscle cramps, neoplasm, nervousness, orthostatic hypotension (more frequent in dialysis patients), otitis media, palpitation, paresthesia, pruritus, renal dysfunction, renal failure, rhabdomyolysis, rash, reflux, rhinitis, serum creatinine increased, somnolence, syncope, tachycardia, tendon pain, tendonitis, tenosynovitis, thrombocytopenia, tinnitus, toothache, uric acid increased, urticaria, vertigo, vomiting, weakness, xerostomia

Drug Interactions

Metabolism/Transport Effects Inhibits CYP2C19 (weak)

Avoid Concomitant Use There are no known interactions where it is recommended to avoid concomitant use.

Increased Effect/Toxicity

Telmisartan may increase the levels/effects of: ACE Inhibitors; Amifostine; Antihypertensives; Cardiac Glycosides; Hypotensive Agents; Lithium; Nonsteroidal Anti-Inflammatory Agents; Potassium-Sparing Diuretics; Ramipril; RiTUXimab; Sodium Phosphates

The levels/effects of Telmisartan may be increased by: Alfuzosin; Diazoxide; Eplerenone; Herbs (Hypotensive Properties); MAO Inhibitors; Pentoxifylline; Phosphodiesterase 5 Inhibitors; Potassium Salts; Prostacyclin Analogues; Tolvaptan; Trimethoprim

Decreased Effect

The levels/effects of Telmisartan may be decreased by: Herbs (Hypertensive Properties); Methylphenidate; Nonsteroidal Anti-Inflammatory Agents; Yohimbine

Ethanol/Nutrition/Herb Interactions Herb/Nutraceutical: Avoid herbs with hypertensive properties (bayberry, blue cohosh, cayenne, ephedra, ginger, ginseng [American], kola, licorice); may diminish the antihypertensive effect of telmisartan. Avoid herbs with hypotensive properties (black cohosh, California poppy, coleus, golden seal, hawthorn, mistletoe, periwinkle, quinine, shepherd's purse); may enhance the hypotensive effect of telmisartan.

Stability Store at 25°C (77°F); excursions between 15°C to 30°C (59°F to 86°F) permitted. Protect from moisture and do not remove from blister pack until immediately before use.

Mechanism of Action Angiotensin II acts as a vasoconstrictor. In addition to causing direct vasoconstriction, angiotensin II also stimulates the release of aldosterone. Once aldosterone is released, sodium as well as water are reabsorbed. The end result is an elevation in blood pressure. Telmisartan is a nonpeptide AT1 angiotensin II receptor antagonist. This binding prevents angiotensin II from binding to the receptor thereby blocking the vasoconstriction and the aldosterone secreting effects of angiotensin II.

Pharmacodynamics/Kinetics Orally active, not a prodrug

Onset of action: 1-2 hours

Duration: Up to 24 hours

Distribution: V_d: 500 L

Protein binding: >99.5%; primarily to albumin and $alpha_1$-acid glycoprotein

Metabolism: Hepatic via conjugation to inactive metabolites; not metabolized via CYP

Bioavailability (dose dependent): 42% to 58%; Hepatic impairment: Approaches 100%

Half-life elimination: Terminal: 24 hours

Time to peak, plasma: 0.5-1 hours

Excretion: Feces (97%)

Clearance: Total body: 800 mL/minute

Dosage Oral:

Adults:

Hypertension: Initial: 40 mg once daily; usual maintenance dose range: 20-80 mg/day. Patients with volume depletion should be initiated on the lower dosage with close supervision.

Cardiovascular risk reduction: Initial: 80 mg once daily. **Note:** It is unknown whether doses <80 mg/day are associated with a reduction in risk of cardiovascular morbidity or mortality.

Elderly:

Hypertension: Initial: 20 mg/day; usual maintenance dose range: 20-80 mg/day

Cardiovascular risk reduction: Initial 80 mg once daily

Dosage adjustment in renal impairment: No adjustment required; hemodialysis patients are more susceptible to orthostatic hypotension

Dosage adjustment in hepatic impairment: Initiate therapy with low dose; titrate slowly and monitor closely.

Canadian labeling: Recommended initial dose: 40 mg/day

Dietary Considerations May be taken without regard to meals. Product contains sorbitol.

Administration May be administered without regard to meals.

Monitoring Parameters Blood pressure; electrolytes, serum creatinine, BUN

Dosage Forms Excipient information presented when available (limited, particularly for generics); consult specific product labeling.

Tablet, oral:

Micardis®: 20 mg

Micardis®: 40 mg, 80 mg [scored]

Telmisartan and Amlodipine

(tel mi SAR tan & am LOE di peen)

Brand Names: U.S. Twynsta®

Brand Names: Canada Twynsta®

Index Terms Amlodipine and Telmisartan; Amlodipine Besylate and Telmisartan

Pharmacologic Category Angiotensin II Receptor Blocker; Antianginal Agent; Calcium Channel Blocker; Calcium Channel Blocker, Dihydropyridine

Use Treatment of hypertension, including initial treatment in patients who will require multiple antihypertensives for adequate control

Pregnancy Risk Factor C (1st trimester); D (2nd and 3rd trimesters)

Dosage Oral: Adults: Dose is individualized; combination product may be substituted for individual components in patients currently maintained on both agents separately or in patients not adequately controlled with monotherapy (using one of the agents or an agent within the same antihypertensive class). May also be used as initial therapy in patients who are likely to need >1 antihypertensive to control blood pressure. **Note:** Use as initial therapy is not an approved indication in the Canadian labeling.

Hypertension:

Initial therapy (antihypertensive naive): Telmisartan 40 mg/amlodipine 5 mg once daily; dose may be increased after 2 weeks of therapy. Patients requiring larger blood pressure reductions may be started on telmisartan 80 mg/amlodipine 5 mg once daily. Maximum recommended dose: Telmisartan 80 mg/day, amlodipine 10 mg/day

Add-on/replacement therapy: Telmisartan 40-80 mg and amlodipine 5-10 mg once daily depending upon previous doses, current control, and goals of therapy; dose may be titrated after 2 weeks of therapy. Maximum recommended dose: Telmisartan 80 mg/day; amlodipine 10 mg/day

Elderly: Not recommended for initial therapy in patients ≥75 years of age. For add-on/replacement therapy, initiate amlodipine therapy at 2.5 mg once daily and titrate slowly. **Note:** Use of individual agents may be necessary if the appropriate combination dose is not available.

Dosage adjustment in renal impairment:

Mild-to-moderate impairment: No dosage adjustments are recommended.

Severe impairment: No dosage adjustments are recommended; titrate slowly

Dosage adjustment in hepatic impairment: Not recommended for initial therapy. For add-on/replacement therapy, initiate amlodipine at 2.5 mg once daily with low-dose telmisartan and titrate slowly; **Note:** Use of individual agents is necessary as the appropriate combination dose is not available. Upon titration to therapeutic dose, may initiate combination dose if available. Canadian labeling contraindicates use in severe hepatic impairment or with biliary obstructive disorders.

Additional Information Complete prescribing information for this medication should be consulted for additional detail.

Dosage Forms Excipient information presented when available (limited, particularly for generics); consult specific product labeling.

Tablet, oral:

Twynsta® 40/5: Telmisartan 40 mg and amlodipine 5 mg

Twynsta® 40/10: Telmisartan 40 mg and amlodipine 10 mg

Twynsta® 80/5: Telmisartan 80 mg and amlodipine 5 mg

Twynsta® 80/10: Telmisartan 80 mg and amlodipine 10 mg

Telmisartan and Hydrochlorothiazide

(tel mi SAR tan & hye droe klor oh THYE a zide)

Brand Names: U.S. Micardis® HCT

Brand Names: Canada Micardis® Plus

Index Terms Hydrochlorothiazide and Telmisartan

Pharmacologic Category Angiotensin II Receptor Blocker; Diuretic, Thiazide

Use Treatment of hypertension; combination product should not be used for initial therapy

Pregnancy Risk Factor C (1st trimester); D (2nd and 3rd trimesters)

Dosage Adults: Oral: Replacement therapy: Combination product can be substituted for individual titrated agents. Initiation of combination therapy when monotherapy has failed to achieve desired effects:

Patients currently on telmisartan: Initial dose if blood pressure is not currently controlled on monotherapy of 80 mg telmisartan: Telmisartan 80 mg/hydrochlorothiazide 12.5 mg once daily; may titrate up to telmisartan 160 mg/hydrochlorothiazide 25 mg if needed

Patients currently on hydrochlorothiazide: Initial dose if blood pressure is not currently controlled on monotherapy of 25 mg once daily: Telmisartan 80 mg/hydrochlorothiazide 12.5 mg once daily or telmisartan 80 mg/hydrochlorothiazide 25 mg once daily; may titrate up to telmisartan 160 mg/hydrochlorothiazide 25 mg if blood pressure remains uncontrolled after 2-4 weeks of therapy. Patients who develop hypokalemia while on hydrochlorothiazide 25 mg may be switched to telmisartan 80 mg/hydrochlorothiazide 12.5 mg.

Dosage adjustment in renal impairment:

Cl_{cr} >30 mL/minute: No dosage adjustment necessary

Cl_{cr} ≤30 mL/minute: Not recommended

Dosage adjustment in hepatic impairment:

Mild-to-moderate hepatic impairment or biliary obstructive disorders: Initial: Telmisartan 40 mg/hydrochlorothiazide 12.5 mg

Severe hepatic impairment: Not recommended

Additional Information Complete prescribing information for this medication should be consulted for additional detail.

Dosage Forms Excipient information presented when available (limited, particularly for generics); consult specific product labeling.

Tablet, oral:

Micardis® HCT:

40/12.5: Telmisartan 40 mg and hydrochlorothiazide 12.5 mg

80/12.5: Telmisartan 80 mg and hydrochlorothiazide 12.5 mg

80/25: Telmisartan 80 mg and hydrochlorothiazide 25 mg

Dosage Forms: Canada Excipient information presented when available (limited, particularly for generics); consult specific product labeling.

Tablet, oral:

Micardis® Plus: 80/25: Telmisartan 80 mg and hydrochlorothiazide 25 mg

◆ **Telzir® (Can)** *see* Fosamprenavir *on page 756*

Temazepam (te MAZ e pam)

Brand Names: U.S. Restoril™

Brand Names: Canada Apo-Temazepam®; CO Temazepam; Dom-Temazepam; Gen-Temazepam; Novo-Temazepam; Nu-Temazepam; PHL-Temazepam; PMS-Temazepam; ratio-Temazepam; Restoril™

Pharmacologic Category Hypnotic, Benzodiazepine

Additional Appendix Information

Beers Criteria - Potentially Inappropriate Medications for Geriatrics *on page 1973*

Benzodiazepines *on page 1882*

Use Short-term treatment of insomnia

Unlabeled Use Treatment of anxiety

Pregnancy Risk Factor X

Medication Guide Available Yes

Dosage Oral:

Adults: Usual dose: 15-30 mg at bedtime; some patients may respond to 7.5 mg in transient insomnia

Elderly or debilitated patients: Initial: 7.5 mg at bedtime

Additional Information Complete prescribing information for this medication should be consulted for additional detail.

Dosage Forms Excipient information presented when available (limited, particularly for generics); consult specific product labeling.

Capsule, oral: 7.5 mg, 15 mg, 22.5 mg, 30 mg

Restoril™: 7.5 mg, 15 mg, 22.5 mg, 30 mg

Controlled Substance C-IV

◆ **Temodal® (Can)** *see* Temozolomide *on page 1638*

◆ **Temodar®** *see* Temozolomide *on page 1638*

◆ **Temovate®** *see* Clobetasol *on page 384*

◆ **Temovate E®** *see* Clobetasol *on page 384*

Temozolomide (te moe ZOE loe mide)

Brand Names: U.S. Temodar®

Brand Names: Canada Temodal®

Index Terms SCH 52365; TMZ

Pharmacologic Category Antineoplastic Agent, Alkylating Agent (Triazene)

Use Treatment of newly-diagnosed glioblastoma multiforme (initially in combination with radiotherapy, then as maintenance treatment); treatment of refractory anaplastic astrocytoma

Canadian labeling (not an approved indication in the U.S.): Treatment of recurrent or progressive glioblastoma multiforme

Unlabeled Use Treatment of recurrent glioblastoma multiforme, low-grade astrocytoma, low-grade oligodendroglioma, anaplastic oligodendroglioma, metastatic CNS lesions, refractory primary CNS lymphoma, advanced or metastatic melanoma, cutaneous T-cell lymphomas (mycosis fungoides [MF] and Sézary syndrome [SS]), advanced neuroendocrine tumors (carcinoid or islet cell), Ewing's sarcoma (recurrent or progressive), soft tissue sarcomas (extremity/retroperitoneal/intra-abdominal or hemangiopericytoma/solitary fibrous tumor), treatment of pediatric neuroblastoma

Pregnancy Risk Factor D

Pregnancy Considerations May cause fetal harm when administered to pregnant women. Animal studies, at doses less than used in humans, resulted in numerous birth defects. Testicular toxicity was demonstrated in animal studies using smaller doses than recommended for cancer treatment. There are no adequate and well-controlled studies in pregnant women. Male and female patients should avoid pregnancy while receiving drug.

Lactation Excretion in breast milk unknown/not recommended

Contraindications Hypersensitivity (eg, allergic reaction, anaphylaxis, urticaria, Stevens-Johnson syndrome, toxic epidermal necrolysis) to temozolomide or any component of the formulation; hypersensitivity to dacarbazine (both drugs are metabolized to MTIC)

Canadian labeling: Additional contraindications (not in U.S. labeling): Not recommended in patients with severe myelosuppression

Warnings/Precautions Hazardous agent - use appropriate precautions for handling and disposal. *Pneumocystis jirovecii* pneumonia (PCP) may occur; risk is increased in those receiving steroids or longer dosing regimens; PCP prophylaxis is required in patients receiving radiotherapy in combination with the 42-day temozolomide regimen. Myelosuppression may occur; an increased incidence has been reported in geriatric and female patients. Prolonged pancytopenia resulting in aplastic anemia has been reported; concurrent use of temozolomide with medications associated with aplastic anemia (eg, carbamazepine, co-trimoxazole, phenytoin) may obscure assessment for development of aplastic anemia. Rare cases of myelodysplastic syndrome and secondary malignancies, including acute myeloid leukemia have been reported. Use caution in patients with severe hepatic or renal impairment; has not been studied in dialysis patients.

Increased MGMT (O-6-methylguanine-DNA methyltransferase) activity/levels within tumor tissue is associated with temozolomide resistance. Glioblastoma patients with decreased levels (due to methylated MGMT promoter) may be more likely to benefit from the combination of radiation therapy and temozolomide (Hegi, 2008; Stupp, 2009). Determination of MGMT status may be predictive for response to alkylating agents.

Adverse Reactions Note: With CNS malignancies, it may be difficult to distinguish between CNS adverse events caused by temozolomide versus the effects of progressive disease.

>10%:

Cardiovascular: Peripheral edema (11%)

Central nervous system: Fatigue (34% to 61%), headache (23% to 41%), seizure (6% to 23%), hemiparesis (18%), fever (13%), dizziness (5% to 12%), coordination abnormality (11%)

Dermatologic: Alopecia (55%), rash (8% to 13%)

Gastrointestinal: Nausea (49% to 53%; grades 3/4: 1% to 10%), vomiting (29% to 42%; grades 3/4: 2% to 6%), constipation (22% to 33%), anorexia (9% to 27%), diarrhea (10% to 16%)

Hematologic: Lymphopenia (grades 3/4: 55%), thrombocytopenia (grades 3/4: adults: 4% to 19%; children: 25%), neutropenia (grades 3/4: adults: 8% to 14%; children: 20%), leukopenia (grades 3/4: 11%)

Neuromuscular & skeletal: Weakness (7% to 13%)

Miscellaneous: Viral infection (11%)

1% to 10%:

Central nervous system: Amnesia (10%), insomnia (4% to 10%), somnolence (9%), ataxia (8%), paresis (8%), anxiety (7%), memory impairment (7%), depression (6%), confusion (5%)

Dermatologic: Pruritus (5% to 8%), dry skin (5%), radiation injury (2% maintenance phase after radiotherapy), erythema (1%)

Endocrine & metabolic: Hypercorticism (8%), breast pain (females 6%)

Gastrointestinal: Stomatitis (9%), abdominal pain (5% to 9%), dysphagia (7%), taste perversion (5%), weight gain (5%)

Genitourinary: Incontinence (8%), urinary tract infection (8%), urinary frequency (6%)

Hematologic: Anemia (grades 3/4: 4%)

Neuromuscular & skeletal: Paresthesia (9%), back pain (8%), abnormal gait (6%), arthralgia (6%), myalgia (5%)

Ocular: Blurred vision (5% to 8%), diplopia (5%), vision abnormality (visual deficit/vision changes 5%)

Respiratory: Pharyngitis (8%), upper respiratory tract infection (8%), cough (5% to 8%), sinusitis (6%), dyspnea (5%)

Miscellaneous: Allergic reaction (≤3%)

<1% (Limited to important or life-threatening): Alkaline phosphatase increased, alveolitis, anaphylaxis, aplastic anemia, cholestasis, emotional lability, erythema multiforme, febrile neutropenia, flu-like syndrome, hallucination, hematoma, hemorrhage, hepatitis, hepatotoxicity, herpes simplex, herpes zoster, hyperbilirubinemia, hyperglycemia, hypokalemia, injection site reactions (erythema, irritation, pain, pruritus, swelling, warmth), interstitial pneumonia/pneumonitis, myelodysplastic syndrome, opportunistic infection (eg, PCP), oral candidiasis, pancytopenia (may be prolonged), peripheral neuropathy, petechiae, pneumonitis, pulmonary fibrosis, secondary malignancies (including myeloid leukemia), Stevens-Johnson syndrome, toxic epidermal necrolysis, transaminases increased

Drug Interactions

Metabolism/Transport Effects None known.

Avoid Concomitant Use

Avoid concomitant use of Temozolomide with any of the following: BCG; CloZAPine; Natalizumab; Pimecrolimus; Tacrolimus (Topical); Vaccines (Live)

Increased Effect/Toxicity

Temozolomide may increase the levels/effects of: CloZAPine; Leflunomide; Natalizumab; Vaccines (Live)

The levels/effects of Temozolomide may be increased by: Denosumab; Divalproex; Pimecrolimus; Roflumilast; Tacrolimus (Topical); Trastuzumab; Valproic Acid

Decreased Effect

Temozolomide may decrease the levels/effects of: BCG; Coccidioidin Skin Test; Sipuleucel-T; Vaccines (Inactivated); Vaccines (Live)

The levels/effects of Temozolomide may be decreased by: Echinacea

Ethanol/Nutrition/Herb Interactions Food: Food reduces rate and extent of absorption.

Stability

Injection: Store intact vials refrigerated at 2°C to 8°C (36°F to 46°F). Bring to room temperature prior to reconstitution. Reconstitute each 100 mg vial with 41 mL sterile water for injection to a final concentration of 2.5 mg/mL. Swirl gently; do not shake. Place dose without further dilution into a 250 mL empty sterile infusion bag. Reconstituted vials may be stored for up to 14 hours at room temperature of 25°C (77°F); infusion must be completed within 14 hours of reconstitution. Use appropriate precautions for handling and disposal.

Capsule: Store at room temperature of 25°C (77°F); excursions permitted to 15°C to 30°C (59°F to 86°F).

Mechanism of Action Like dacarbazine, temozolomide (a prodrug) is rapidly and nonenzymatically converted to the active alkylating metabolite MTIC [(methyl-triazene-1-yl)-imidazole-4-carboxamide]. Unlike dacarbazine, however, this conversion is spontaneous, nonenzymatic, and occurs under physiologic conditions in all tissues to which it distributes. The cytotoxic effects of MTIC are manifested through alkylation of DNA at the O^6, N^7 guanine positions.

Pharmacodynamics/Kinetics

Absorption: Oral: Rapid and complete

Distribution: V_d: Parent drug: 0.4 L/kg; penetrates blood-brain barrier; CSF levels are ~35% to 39% of plasma levels

Protein binding: 15%

Metabolism: Prodrug, hydrolyzed to the active form, MTIC; MTIC is eventually eliminated as CO_2 and 5-aminoimidazole-4-carboxamide (AIC), a natural constituent in urine; CYP isoenzymes play only a minor role in metabolism (of temozolomide and MTIC)

Bioavailability: Oral: 100% (on a mg-per-mg basis, I.V. temozolomide, infused over 90 minutes, is bioequivalent to an oral dose)

Half-life elimination: Mean: Parent drug: 1.8 hours

Time to peak: Oral: Empty stomach: 1 hour; with food (high-fat meal): 2.25 hours

Excretion: Urine (~38%; parent drug 6%); feces <1%

Dosage

Children:

Ewing's sarcoma, recurrent or progressive (unlabeled use): Oral: Refer to adult dosing.

Neuroblastoma, relapsed or refractory (unlabeled use): Oral: 100 mg/m^2/dose days 1-5 days every 21 days (in combination with irinotecan) for up to 6 cycles (Bagatell, 2011)

Adults:

Anaplastic astrocytoma (refractory): Oral, I.V.: Initial dose: 150 mg/m^2/day for 5 days; repeat every 28 days. Subsequent doses of 100-200 mg/m^2/day for 5 days per treatment cycle; based upon hematologic tolerance.

Dosage modification for toxicity:

ANC <1000/mm^3 or platelets <50,000/mm^3 on day 22 or day 29 (day 1 of next cycle): Postpone therapy until ANC >1500/mm^3 and platelets >100,000/mm^3; reduce dose by 50 mg/m^2/day for subsequent cycle

ANC 1000-1500/mm^3 or platelets 50,000-100,000/mm^3 on day 22 or day 29 (day 1 of next cycle): Postpone therapy until ANC >1500/mm^3 and platelets >100,000/mm^3; maintain initial dose

ANC ≥1500/mm^3 and platelets ≥100,000/mm^3 on day 22 or day 29 (day 1 of next cycle): Increase dose to or maintain dose at 200 mg/m^2/day for 5 days for subsequent cycle

Glioblastoma multiforme (newly diagnosed, high-grade glioma): Oral, I.V.:

Concomitant phase: 75 mg/m^2/day for 42 days with focal radiotherapy (60 Gy administered in 30 fractions). **Note:** PCP prophylaxis is required during concomitant phase and should continue in patients who develop lymphocytopenia until lymphocyte recovery to ≤grade 1. Obtain weekly CBC.

Continue at 75 mg/m^2/day throughout the 42-day concomitant phase (up to 49 days) as long as ANC ≥1500/mm^3, platelet count ≥100,000/mm^3, and nonhematologic toxicity ≤grade 1 (excludes alopecia, nausea/vomiting)

Dosage modification for toxicity:

ANC ≥500/mm^3 but <1500/mm^3 **or** platelet count ≥10,000/mm^3 but <100,000/mm^3 **or** grade 2 nonhematologic toxicity (excludes alopecia, nausea/vomiting): Interrupt therapy

ANC <500/mm^3 **or** platelet count <10,000/mm^3 **or** grade 3/4 nonhematologic toxicity (excludes alopecia, nausea/vomiting): Discontinue therapy

Maintenance phase (consists of 6 treatment cycles): Begin 4 weeks after concomitant phase completion. **Note:** Each subsequent cycle is 28 days (consisting of 5 days of drug treatment followed by 23 days without treatment). Draw CBC within 48 hours of day 22; hold next cycle and do weekly CBC until ANC >1500/mm^3 and platelet count >100,000/mm^3; dosing modification should be based on lowest blood counts and worst nonhematologic toxicity during the previous cycle.

Cycle 1: 150 mg/m^2/day for 5 days; repeat every 28 days

Cycles 2-6: May increase to 200 mg/m^2/day for 5 days every 28 days (if ANC ≥1500/mm^3, platelets ≥100,000/mm^3 and nonhematologic toxicities for cycle 1 are ≤grade 2 [excludes alopecia, nausea/vomiting]); **Note:** If dose was not escalated at the onset of cycle 2, do not increase for cycles 3-6)

Dosage modification (during maintenance phase) for toxicity:

ANC <1000/mm^3, platelet count <50,000/mm^3, or grade 3 nonhematologic toxicity (excludes for alopecia, nausea/vomiting) during previous cycle: Decrease dose by 1 dose level (by 50 mg/m^2/day for 5 days), unless dose has already been lowered to 100 mg/m^2/day, then discontinue therapy.

If dose reduction <100 mg/m^2/day is required or grade 4 nonhematologic toxicity (excludes for alopecia, nausea/vomiting), or if the same grade 3 nonhematologic toxicity occurs after dose reduction: Discontinue therapy

Glioblastoma multiforme (recurrent glioma): *Canadian labeling (unlabeled use in the U.S.):* 200 mg/m^2/day for 5 days every 28 days; if previously treated with chemotherapy, initiate at 150 mg/m^2/day for 5 days every 28 days and increase to 200 mg/m^2/day for 5 days every 28 days with cycle 2 if no hematologic toxicity (Brada, 2001; Yung, 2000)

Ewing's sarcoma, recurrent or progressive (unlabeled use): Oral: 100 mg/m^2/dose days 1-5 every 21 days (in combination with irinotecan) (Casey, 2009)

Melanoma, advanced or metastatic (unlabeled use): Oral: 200 mg/m^2/day for 5 days every 28 days (for up to 12 cycles). For subsequent cycles reduce dose to 75% of the original dose for grade 3/4 hematologic toxicity and reduce the dose to 50% of the original dose for grade 3/4 nonhematologic toxicity (Middleton, 2000).

Neuroendocrine tumors, advanced (unlabeled use): Oral: 150 mg/m^2/day for 7 days every 14 days in combination with thalidomide (Kulke, 2006)

Primary CNS lymphoma, refractory (unlabeled use): Oral: 150 mg/m^2/day for 5 days every 28 days, initially in combination with rituximab, followed by temozolomide monotherapy: 150 mg/m^2/day for 5 days every 28 days (Wong, 2004) **or** 150 mg/m^2/day for 7 days every 14 days, initially in combination with rituximab, followed by temozolomide monotherapy: 150 mg/m^2/day for 5 days every 28 days (Enting, 2004)

Soft tissue sarcoma (unlabeled use): Oral: 75 mg/m^2/day for 6 weeks (Garcia del Muro, 2005)

Elderly: Refer to adult dosing. **Note:** Patients ≥70 years of age in the anaplastic astrocytoma study had a higher incidence of grade 4 neutropenia and thrombocytopenia in the first cycle of therapy than patients <70 years of age.

Dosage adjustment in renal impairment: Oral:

Cl_{cr} ≥36 mL/minute/m^2: No effect on temozolomide clearance was demonstrated.

Severe renal impairment (Cl_{cr} <36 mL/minute/m^2): Use with caution.

Dialysis patients: Use has not been studied

Dosage adjustment in hepatic impairment: Severe hepatic impairment: Use with caution

Dietary Considerations The incidence of nausea/vomiting is decreased when taken on an empty stomach. Take capsules consistently either with food or without food (absorption is affected by food).

Administration Standard antiemetics may be administered if needed.

Oral: Swallow capsules whole with a glass of water. Absorption is affected by food. Administer consistently either with food or without food (was administered in studies under fasting and nonfasting conditions). May administer on an empty stomach or at bedtime to reduce nausea and vomiting. Do not repeat if vomiting occurs after dose is administered; wait until the next scheduled dose. Do not open or chew capsules; avoid contact with skin if capsules are accidentally opened or damaged.

I.V.: Infuse over 90 minutes. Flush line before and after administration. May be administered through the same I.V. line as sodium chloride 0.9%; do not administer other medications through the same I.V. line.

Monitoring Parameters CBC with differential and platelets (prior to each cycle; weekly during glioma concomitant phase treatment; at or within 48 hours of day 22 and weekly until ANC >1500/mm^3 for glioma maintenance and astrocytoma treatment)

Dosage Forms Excipient information presented when available (limited, particularly for generics); consult specific product labeling.

Capsule, oral:

Temodar®: 5 mg, 20 mg, 100 mg, 140 mg, 180 mg, 250 mg

Injection, powder for reconstitution:

Temodar®: 100 mg [contains polysorbate 80]

Extemporaneous Preparations Hazardous agent: Use appropriate precautions for handling and disposal.

A 10 mg/mL temozolomide oral suspension may be compounded in a vertical flow hood. Mix the contents of ten 100 mg capsules and 500 mg of povidone K-30 powder in a glass mortar; add 25 mg anhydrous citric acid dissolved in 1.5 mL purified water and mix to a uniform paste; mix while adding 50 mL Ora-Plus® in incremental proportions. Transfer to an amber plastic bottle, rinse mortar 4 times with small portions of either Ora-Sweet® or Ora-Sweet® SF, and add quantity of Ora-Sweet® or Ora-Sweet® SF sufficient to make 100 mL. Store in plastic amber prescription bottles; label "shake well" and "refrigerate"; include the beyond-use date. Stable for 7 days at room temperature or 60 days refrigerated (preferred).

Trissel LA, Yanping Z, and Koontz SE, "Temozolomide Stability in Extemporaneously Compounded Oral Suspension," *Int J Pharm Compound*, 2006, 10(5):396-9.

◆ **Tempra® (Can)** *see* Acetaminophen *on page* 27

Temsirolimus (tem sir OH li mus)

Brand Names: U.S. Torisel®

Brand Names: Canada Torisel®

Index Terms CCI-779

Pharmacologic Category Antineoplastic Agent, mTOR Kinase Inhibitor

Use Treatment of advanced renal cell cancer (RCC)

Pregnancy Risk Factor D

Pregnancy Considerations Embryotoxicity and fetotoxicity (as evidenced by increased mortality, reduced fetal weights, and delayed ossification) occurred in animal studies at oral doses lower than the usual human dose. There are no adequate and well-controlled studies in pregnant women. Women of childbearing potential should be advised to avoid pregnancy. Men and women should use effective birth control during temsirolimus treatment, and continue for 3 months after temsirolimus discontinuation.

Lactation Excretion in breast milk unknown/not recommended

Contraindications Bilirubin >1.5 times the upper limit of normal (ULN)

Canadian labeling: Additional contraindications (not in U.S. labeling): History of anaphylaxis after exposure to temsirolimus, sirolimus, or any component of the formulation

Warnings/Precautions Hazardous agent - use appropriate precautions for handling and disposal.

Hypersensitivity/infusion reactions (eg, anaphylaxis, apnea, dyspnea, flushing, loss of consciousness, hypotension, and/or chest pain) have been reported. Infusion reaction may occur during the initial infusion (early in infusion) or with subsequent infusions. Premedicate with an antihistamine (H_1 antagonist) prior to infusion; monitor throughout infusion (appropriate supportive care should be available); interrupt infusion for hypersensitivity reaction and observe patient for 30-60 minutes. With discretion, treatment may be resumed at a slower infusion rate; administer an H_1 antagonist (if not given as premedication) and/or an H_2 antagonist ~30 minutes prior to resuming infusion. For severe infusion reactions, asses risk versus benefit of continued treatment. Use with caution in patients with hypersensitivity temsirolimus, sirolimus (a metabolite), or polysorbate 80. Angioneurotic edema has been reported; concurrent use with other drugs known to cause angioedema (eg, ACE inhibitors) may increase risk.

Temsirolimus is predominantly cleared by the liver; use with caution and reduce dose in patients with mild hepatic impairment (bilirubin >1-1.5 x ULN or AST >ULN with bilirubin ≤ULN). Toxicities were increased in patients with baseline bilirubin >1.5 x ULN. Use is contraindicated in patients with moderate-to-severe hepatic impairment (bilirubin >1.5 x ULN).

Avoid concomitant use with strong CYP3A4 inhibitors and strong CYP3A4 inducers (see Drug Interactions); consider alternative agents that avoid or lessen the potential for CYP-mediated interactions. Patients should not be immunized with live, viral vaccines during or shortly after treatment and should avoid close contact with recently vaccinated (live vaccine) individuals. Patients who are receiving anticoagulant therapy or those with CNS tumors/metastases may be at increased risk for developing intracerebral bleeding. Combination therapy with temsirolimus and sunitinib has resulted in dose-limiting toxicities, including grade 3 or 4 rash, gout, and/or cellulitis.

Increases in serum glucose commonly occur during treatment; initiation or alteration of insulin and/or oral hypoglycemic therapy may be required; monitor serum glucose before and during treatment; use with caution in patients with diabetes. Use with caution in patients with hyperlipidemia; may increase serum lipids (cholesterol and triglycerides); initiation or dosage adjustment of of antihyperlipidemic agents may be required; monitor cholesterol/triglyceride panel. Treatment may result in immunosuppression, may increase risk of opportunistic infections and/or sepsis. Interstitial lung disease (ILD), sometimes fatal, has been reported; symptoms include dyspnea, cough, hypoxia, and/or fever, although asymptomatic or mild cases may present; promptly evaluate worsening respiratory symptoms; may require corticosteroids, antibiotic therapy, and/or treatment discontinuation; baseline chest radiographic assessment (CT scan or xray) is recommended. Cases of bowel perforation (fatal) have occurred (usually presenting with abdominal pain, bloody stools, diarrhea, fever, or metabolic acidosis); promptly evaluate any new or worsening abdominal pain or bloody stools. Temsirolimus may be associated with impaired wound healing; use caution in the perioperative period. Cases of acute renal failure with rapid progression have been reported (unrelated to disease progression), including cases unresponsive to dialysis.

Adverse Reactions

>10%:

Cardiovascular: Edema (35%), peripheral edema (27%), chest pain (16%)

Central nervous system: Pain (28%), fever (24%), headache (15%), insomnia (12%)

Dermatologic: Rash (47%), pruritus (19%), nail disorder/thinning (14%), dry skin (11%)

Endocrine & metabolic: Hyperglycemia (26% to 89%; grades 3/4: 16%), hypercholesterolemia (24% to 87%; grades 3/4: 2%), hypertriglyceridemia (83%; grades 3/4: 44%), hypophosphatemia (49%; grades 3/4: 18%), hyperlipidemia (27%), hypokalemia (21%; grades 3/4: 5%)

Gastrointestinal: Mucositis (41%), nausea (37%), anorexia (32%), diarrhea (27%), abdominal pain (21%), constipation (20%), stomatitis (20%), taste disturbance (20%), vomiting (19%), weight loss (19%)

Genitourinary: Urinary tract infection (15%)

Hematologic: Anemia (45% to 94%; grades 3/4: 20%), lymphopenia (53%; grades 3/4: 16%), thrombocytopenia (14% to 40%; grades 3/4: 1%; dose-limiting toxicity), leukopenia (6% to 32%; grades 3/4: 1%), neutropenia (7% to 19%; grades 3/4: 3% to 5%)
Hepatic: Alkaline phosphatase increased (68%; grades 3/4: 3%), AST increased (8% to 38%; grades 3/4: 1% to 2%)
Neuromuscular & skeletal: Weakness (51%), back pain (20%), arthralgia (18%)
Renal: Creatinine increased (14% to 57%; grades 3/4: 3%)
Respiratory: Dyspnea (28%), cough (26%), epistaxis (12%), pharyngitis (12%)
Miscellaneous: Infection (20% to 27%; includes abscess, bronchitis, cellulitis, herpes simplex, herpes zoster)

1% to 10%:
Cardiovascular: Hypertension, thrombophlebitis, venous thromboembolism (includes DVT and PE)
Central nervous system: Chills, depression
Dermatologic: Acne, wound healing impaired
Gastrointestinal: Bowel perforation
Hepatic: Hyperbilirubinemia
Neuromuscular & skeletal: Myalgia
Ocular: Conjunctivitis
Respiratory: Interstitial lung disease (ILD), pneumonia, rhinitis, upper respiratory tract infection
Miscellaneous: Allergic/hypersensitivity/infusion reaction (includes anaphylaxis, apnea, chest pain, dyspnea, flushing, hypotension, loss of consciousness)

<1% (Limited to important or life-threatening): Acute renal failure, angioneurotic edema, glucose intolerance, infusion site extravasation (with pain, swelling, warmth, erythema), pericardial effusion, pleural effusion, pneumonitis, reflex sympathetic dystrophy, rhabdomyolysis, seizure, Stevens-Johnson syndrome

Drug Interactions

Metabolism/Transport Effects **Substrate** of CYP3A4 (major), P-glycoprotein; **Note:** Assignment of Major/Minor substrate status based on clinically relevant drug interaction potential; **Inhibits** CYP2D6 (weak), CYP3A4 (weak)

Avoid Concomitant Use

Avoid concomitant use of Temsirolimus with any of the following: BCG; CloZAPine; Conivaptan; Natalizumab; Pimecrolimus; Pimozide; SUNItinib; Tacrolimus; Tacrolimus (Systemic); Tacrolimus (Topical); Vaccines (Live)

Increased Effect/Toxicity

Temsirolimus may increase the levels/effects of: ACE Inhibitors; CloZAPine; CycloSPORINE; CycloSPORINE (Systemic); Hypoglycemic Agents; Leflunomide; Natalizumab; Pimozide; SUNItinib; Tacrolimus; Tacrolimus (Systemic); Tacrolimus (Topical); Vaccines (Live)

The levels/effects of Temsirolimus may be increased by: Conivaptan; CYP3A4 Inhibitors (Moderate); CYP3A4 Inhibitors (Strong); Dasatinib; Denosumab; Fluconazole; Herbs (Hypoglycemic Properties); Itraconazole; Ketoconazole; Ketoconazole (Systemic); Macrolide Antibiotics; P-glycoprotein/ABCB1 Inhibitors; Pimecrolimus; Posaconazole; Protease Inhibitors; Roflumilast; Tacrolimus; Tacrolimus (Systemic); Tacrolimus (Topical); Trastuzumab

Decreased Effect

Temsirolimus may decrease the levels/effects of: BCG; Coccidioidin Skin Test; Sipuleucel-T; Tacrolimus; Tacrolimus (Systemic); Vaccines (Inactivated); Vaccines (Live)

The levels/effects of Temsirolimus may be decreased by: CarBAMazepine; CYP3A4 Inducers (Strong); Deferasirox; Echinacea; Fosphenytoin; P-glycoprotein/ABCB1 Inducers; Phenytoin; Rifamycin Derivatives; Tocilizumab

Ethanol/Nutrition/Herb Interactions Herb/Nutraceutical: St John's wort may decrease sirolimus (the active metabolite of temsirolimus) levels; avoid concurrent use. Herbs with hypoglycemic properties may increase the risk of temsirolimus-induced hypoglycemia; includes alfalfa, aloe, bilberry, bitter melon, burdock, celery, damiana, fenugreek, garcinia, garlic, ginger, ginseng (American), gymnema, marshmallow, stinging nettle. Avoid grapefruit and grapefruit juice (may increase the levels/effects of sirolimus).

Stability Store intact vials refrigerated at 2°C to 8°C (36°F to 46°F). Protect from light during storage, preparation, and handling. Preparation requires a two-step dilution process (do not add undiluted temsirolimus to aqueous solution; addition to aqueous solution prior to step 1 will result in precipitation). *Step 1:* Total amount in undiluted vial is 30 mg/1.2 mL (25 mg/mL concentration); contains overfill. Vials should initially be diluted with 1.8 mL of provided diluent to a concentration of 10 mg/mL. Once diluted with provided diluent, mix by inverting vial. Diluted solution in the vial (10 mg/mL) is stable for 24 hours at room temperature. *Step 2:* After allowing air bubbles to subside, the intended dose should be withdrawn from the 10 mg/mL diluted vial (ie, 2.5 mL for a 25 mg dose) and further diluted in 250 mL of NS in a non-DEHP/non-PVC container (glass, polyolefin, or polypropylene). Mix by inverting bottle or bag; avoid excessive shaking (may result in foaming). Solutions diluted for infusion (in NS) must be infused within 6 hours of preparation. Use appropriate precautions for handling and disposal.

Mechanism of Action Temsirolimus and its active metabolite, sirolimus, are targeted inhibitors of mTOR (mammalian target of rapamycin) kinase activity. Temsirolimus (and sirolimus) bind to FKBP-12, an intracellular protein, to form a complex which inhibits mTOR signaling, halting the cell cycle at the G1 phase in tumor cells. In renal cell carcinoma, mTOR inhibition also exhibits anti-angiogenesis activity by reducing levels of HIF-1 and HIF-2 alpha (hypoxia inducible factors) and vascular endothelial growth factor (VEGF).

Pharmacodynamics/Kinetics

Distribution: V_{dss}: 172 L
Metabolism: Hepatic; via CYP3A4 to sirolimus (primary active metabolite) and 4 minor metabolites
Half-life elimination: Temsirolimus: ~17 hours; Sirolimus: ~55 hours
Time to peak, plasma: Temsirolimus: At end of infusion; Sirolimus: 0.5-2 hours after temsirolimus infusion
Excretion: Feces (78%); urine (<5%)

Dosage **Note:** For infusion reaction prophylaxis, premedicate with an H_1 antagonist (eg, diphenhydramine 25-50 mg I.V.) 30 minutes prior to infusion.

I.V.: Adults: Renal cell cancer (RCC), advanced: 25 mg once weekly; continue until disease progression or unacceptable toxicity

Dosage adjustment for concomitant CYP3A4 inhibitors/inducers:

CYP3A4 inhibitors: Avoid concomitant administration with strong CYP3A4 inhibitors (eg, clarithromycin, itraconazole, ketoconazole, nefazodone, protease inhibitors, telithromycin, voriconazole); if concomitant administration with a strong CYP3A4 inhibitor cannot be avoided, consider a dose reduction to 12.5 mg/week. When a strong CYP3A4 inhibitor is discontinued; allow ~1 week to elapse prior to adjusting the temsirolimus upward to the dose used prior to initiation of the CYP3A4 inhibitor.

CYP3A4 inducers: Avoid concomitant administration with strong CYP3A4 inducers (eg, carbamazepine, dexamethasone, phenobarbital, phenytoin, rifampin, St John's wort); if concomitant administration with a strong CYP3A4 inducer cannot be avoided, consider adjusting temsirolimus dose up to 50 mg/week. If the strong CYP3A4 enzyme inducer is discontinued, reduce the temsirolimus to the dose used prior to initiation of the CYP3A4 inducer.

Dosage adjustment for toxicity:

Hematologic toxicity: ANC <1000/mm^3 or platelets <75,000/mm^3: Withhold treatment until resolves and reinitiate treatment with a 5 mg/week dose reduction; minimum dose: 15 mg/week if adjustment for toxicity is needed.

Nonhematologic toxicity: Any toxicity ≥grade 3: Withhold treatment until resolves to ≤grade 2; reinitiate treatment with a 5 mg/week dose reduction; minimum dose: 15 mg/week if adjustment for toxicity is needed.

Infusion/hypersensitivity reaction: Interrupt infusion and observe for 30-60 minutes; treatment may be resumed with discretion at a slower infusion rate (up to 60 minutes); administer an H_1 antagonist (if not given as premedication) and/or an H_2 antagonist 30 minutes prior to resuming infusion.

Interstitial lung disease: Consider withholding treatment for clinically significant respiratory symptoms until after recovery of symptoms or radiographic improvement.

Dosage adjustment in renal impairment: No adjustments are recommended (renal impairment is not expected to significantly impact exposure). Has not been studied in hemodialysis patients.

Dosage adjustment in hepatic impairment:

Mild hepatic impairment (bilirubin >1-1.5 x ULN or AST >ULN with bilirubin ≤ULN): Reduce dose to 15 mg once weekly

Moderate-to-severe hepatic impairment (bilirubin >1.5 x ULN): Use is contraindicated

Dietary Considerations Avoid grapefruit juice (may increase the levels of the major metabolite, sirolimus).

Administration Infuse over 30-60 minutes via an infusion pump (preferred). Use polyethylene-lined non-DEHP administration tubing. Administer through an inline polyethersulfone filter ≤5 micron; if set does not contain an inline filter, a polyethersulfone end filter (0.2-5 micron) should be added (do not use both an inline and an end filter). Premedicate with an H_1 antagonist (eg, diphenhydramine 25-50 mg I.V.) ~30 minutes prior to infusion. Monitor during infusion; interrupt infusion for hypersensitivity/infusion reaction; monitor for 30-60 minutes; may reinitiate at a reduced infusion rate (over 60 minutes) with discretion, 30 minutes after administration of a histamine H_1 antagonist and/or a histamine H_2 antagonist (eg, famotidine or ranitidine). Administration should be completed within 6 hours of admixture.

Monitoring Parameters CBC with differential and platelets (weekly), serum chemistries including glucose (baseline and every other week), serum cholesterol and triglycerides (baseline and periodic), liver function (baseline and periodic), renal function tests (baseline and periodic)

Monitor for infusion reactions; infection; symptoms of ILD (or radiographic changes), symptoms of hyperglycemia (excessive thirst, polyuria)

Dosage Forms Excipient information presented when available (limited, particularly for generics); consult specific product labeling.

Injection, solution [concentrate]:

Torisel®: 25 mg/mL (1.2 mL) [contains dehydrated ethanol, dehydrated ethanol (in diluent), polyethylene glycol 400, polysorbate 80 (in diluent), propylene glycol; supplied with diluent]

◆ **Tenar™ PSE [DSC]** *see* Guaifenesin and Pseudoephedrine *on page 813*

Tenecteplase (ten EK te plase)

Brand Names: U.S. TNKase®

Brand Names: Canada TNKase®

Pharmacologic Category Thrombolytic Agent

Use Thrombolytic agent used in the management of ST-elevation myocardial infarction (STEMI) for the lysis of thrombi in the coronary vasculature to restore perfusion and reduce mortality.

Recommended criteria for treatment: STEMI: Chest pain ≥20 minutes duration, onset of chest pain within 12 hours of treatment (or within prior 12-24 hours in patients with continuing ischemic symptoms), and S-T segment elevation >0.1 mV in at least two contiguous precordial leads or two adjacent limb leads on ECG or new or presumably new left bundle branch block (LBBB)

Unlabeled Use Acute MI - combination regimen of tenecteplase (unlabeled dose), abciximab, and heparin (unlabeled dose)

Pregnancy Risk Factor C

Pregnancy Considerations Administer to pregnant women only if the potential benefits justify the risk to the fetus.

Lactation Use caution

Contraindications Hypersensitivity to tenecteplase or any component of the formulation; active internal bleeding; history of stroke; intracranial/intraspinal surgery or trauma within 2 months; intracranial neoplasm; arteriovenous malformation or aneurysm; bleeding diathesis; severe uncontrolled hypertension

Warnings/Precautions Stop antiplatelet agents and heparin if serious bleeding occurs. Avoid I.M. injections and nonessential handling of the patient for a few hours after administration. Monitor for bleeding complications. Venipunctures should be performed carefully and only when necessary. If arterial puncture is necessary, then use an upper extremity that can be easily compressed manually. For the following conditions, the risk of bleeding is higher with use of tenecteplase and should be weighed against the benefits: Recent major surgery, cerebrovascular disease, recent GI or GU bleed, recent trauma, uncontrolled hypertension (systolic BP ≥180 mm Hg and/or diastolic BP ≥110 mm Hg), suspected left heart thrombus, acute pericarditis, subacute bacterial endocarditis, hemostatic defects, severe hepatic dysfunction, pregnancy, hemorrhagic diabetic retinopathy or other hemorrhagic ophthalmic conditions, septic thrombophlebitis or occluded arteriovenous cannula at seriously infected site, advanced age (see Dosage, Elderly), anticoagulants, recent administration of GP IIb/IIIa inhibitors. Coronary thrombolysis may result in reperfusion arrhythmias. Caution with readministration of tenecteplase. Safety and efficacy have not been established in pediatric patients. Cholesterol embolism has rarely been reported.

Adverse Reactions As with all drugs which may affect hemostasis, bleeding is the major adverse effect associated with tenecteplase. Hemorrhage may occur at virtually any site. Risk is dependent on multiple variables, including the dosage administered, concurrent use of multiple agents which alter hemostasis, and patient predisposition. Rapid lysis of coronary artery thrombi by thrombolytic agents may be associated with reperfusion-related arterial and/or ventricular arrhythmia.

>10%:

Local: Hematoma (12% minor)

Hematologic: Bleeding (22% minor: ASSENT-2 trial)

1% to 10%:

Central nervous system: Stroke (2%)

Gastrointestinal: GI hemorrhage (1% major, 2% minor), epistaxis (2% minor)

Genitourinary: GU bleeding (4% minor)

Hematologic: Bleeding (5% major; ASSENT-2 trial)
Local: Bleeding at catheter puncture site (4% minor), hematoma (2% major)
Respiratory: Pharyngeal (3% minor)

The incidence of stroke and bleeding increase with age above 65 years.

<1% (Limited to important or life-threatening): Anaphylaxis, angioedema, bleeding at catheter puncture site (<1% major), cholesterol embolism (clinical features may include livedo reticularis, "purple toe" syndrome, acute renal failure, gangrenous digits, hypertension, pancreatitis, MI, cerebral infarction, spinal cord infarction, retinal artery occlusion, bowel infarction, rhabdomyolysis), GU bleeding (<1% major), intracranial hemorrhage (0.9%), laryngeal edema, rash, respiratory tract bleeding, retroperitoneal bleeding, urticaria

Additional cardiovascular events associated with use in MI: Arrhythmias, AV block, cardiac arrest, cardiac tamponade, cardiogenic shock, electromechanical dissociation, embolism, fever, heart failure, hypotension, mitral regurgitation, myocardial reinfarction, myocardial rupture, nausea, pericardial effusion, pericarditis, pulmonary edema, recurrent myocardial ischemia, thrombosis, vomiting

Drug Interactions

Metabolism/Transport Effects None known.

Avoid Concomitant Use There are no known interactions where it is recommended to avoid concomitant use.

Increased Effect/Toxicity

Tenecteplase may increase the levels/effects of: Anticoagulants; Drotrecogin Alfa (Activated)

The levels/effects of Tenecteplase may be increased by: Antiplatelet Agents; Herbs (Anticoagulant/Antiplatelet Properties); Nonsteroidal Anti-Inflammatory Agents; Salicylates

Decreased Effect

The levels/effects of Tenecteplase may be decreased by: Aprotinin

Stability Store at room temperature not to exceed 30°C (86°F) or under refrigeration 2°C to 8°C (36°F to 46°F). Tenecteplase should be reconstituted using the supplied 10 mL syringe with TwinPak™ Dual Cannula Device and 10 mL sterile water for injection. If reconstituted and not used immediately, store in refrigerator and use within 8 hours.

Mechanism of Action Initiates fibrinolysis by binding to fibrin and converting plasminogen to plasmin.

Pharmacodynamics/Kinetics

Distribution: V_d is weight related and approximates plasma volume
Metabolism: Primarily hepatic
Half-life elimination: 90-130 minutes
Excretion: Clearance: Plasma: 99-119 mL/minute

Dosage I.V.:

Adult: Recommended total dose should not exceed 50 mg and is based on patient's weight; administer as a bolus over 5 seconds

If patient's weight:
- <60 kg, dose: 30 mg
- ≥60 to <70 kg, dose: 35 mg
- ≥70 to <80 kg, dose: 40 mg
- ≥80 to <90 kg, dose: 45 mg
- ≥90 kg, dose: 50 mg

Note: All patients should receive 162-325 mg of chewable nonenteric coated aspirin as soon as possible and then daily. Administer concurrently with heparin 60 units/kg bolus (maximum: 4000 units) followed by continuous infusion of 12 units/kg/hour (maximum: 1000 units/hour) and adjust to aPTT target of 50-70 seconds (or 1.5-2 times the upper limit of control).

Elderly: Although dosage adjustments are not recommended, the elderly have a higher incidence of morbidity and mortality with the use of tenecteplase. The 30-day mortality in the ASSENT-2 trial was 2.5% for patients <65 years, 8.5% for patients 65-74 years, and 16.2% for patients ≥75 years. The intracranial hemorrhage rate was 0.4% for patients <65, 1.6% for patients 65-74 years, and 1.7% for patients ≥75 years. The risks and benefits of use should be weighted carefully in the elderly.

Combination regimen (unlabeled): Half-dose tenecteplase (15-25 mg based on weight) and abciximab 0.25 mg/kg bolus then 0.125 mcg/kg/minute (maximum: 10 mcg/minute) for 12 hours with heparin dosing as follows: Concurrent bolus of 40 units/kg (maximum: 3000 units), then 7 units/kg/hour (maximum: 800 units/hour) as continuous infusion. Adjust to aPTT target of 50-70 seconds.

Note: The 2004 ACC/AHA guidelines for the management of patients with STEMI suggests that abciximab and half-dose reteplase or tenecteplase may be considered for prevention of reinfarction in patients with anterior MI, who are <75 years of age and have no risk factors for bleeding. However, more recently the American College of Chest Physicians recommends against the combination of half-dose reteplase or tenecteplase and standard-dose abciximab (with low dose unfractionated heparin) in any patient with STEMI due to the lack of mortality benefit and the risk of major bleeding (Goodman, 2008).

Dosage adjustment in renal impairment: No formal recommendations for renal impairment

Dosage adjustment in hepatic impairment: Severe hepatic failure is a relative contraindication. Recommendations were not made for mild-to-moderate hepatic impairment.

Administration Tenecteplase should be reconstituted using the supplied 10 mL syringe with TwinPak™ dual cannula device and 10 mL sterile water for injection. Do not shake when reconstituting. Slight foaming is normal and will dissipate if left standing for several minutes. The reconstituted solution is 5 mg/mL. Any unused solution should be discarded. Tenecteplase is **incompatible** with dextrose solutions. Dextrose-containing lines must be flushed with a saline solution before and after administration. Administer as a single I.V. bolus over 5 seconds. Avoid I.M. injections and nonessential handling of patient.

Monitoring Parameters CBC, aPTT, signs and symptoms of bleeding, ECG monitoring

Dosage Forms Excipient information presented when available (limited, particularly for generics); consult specific product labeling.

Injection, powder for reconstitution [recombinant]:
TNKase®: 50 mg

◆ **Tenex®** *see* GuanFACINE *on page 814*

Teniposide (ten i POE side)

Brand Names: U.S. Vumon®

Brand Names: Canada Vumon®

Index Terms EPT; PTG; VM-26

Pharmacologic Category Antineoplastic Agent, Podophyllotoxin Derivative

Use Treatment of refractory childhood acute lymphoblastic leukemia (ALL) in combination with other chemotherapy

Unlabeled Use Treatment of refractory acute lymphoblastic leukemia (ALL) in adults

Pregnancy Risk Factor D

Dosage I.V.: **Note:** Patients with Down syndrome and leukemia may be more sensitive to the myelosuppressive effects; administer the first course at half the usual dose and adjust dose in subsequent cycles upward based on degree of toxicities (myelosuppression and mucositis) in the previous course(s).

Children: Acute lymphoblastic leukemia (ALL; combination chemotherapy): 165 mg/m^2 twice weekly for 8-9 doses **or** 250 mg/m^2 weekly for 4-8 weeks **or** (unlabeled dosing) 165 mg/m^2/dose days 1 and 2 of weeks 3, 13, and 23 (Lauer, 2001)

Adults: ALL consolidation treatment (unlabeled use; combination chemotherapy): 165 mg/m^2/dose days 1, 4, 8, and 11 of alternating consolidation cycles (Linker, 1991)

Dosage adjustment in renal impairment: Data is insufficient, but dose adjustments may be necessary in patient with significant renal impairment.

Dosage adjustment in hepatic impairment: Data is insufficient, but dose adjustments may be necessary in patient with significant hepatic impairment.

Additional Information Complete prescribing information for this medication should be consulted for additional detail.

Dosage Forms Excipient information presented when available (limited, particularly for generics); consult specific product labeling.

Injection, solution:

Vumon®: 10 mg/mL (5 mL) [contains benzyl alcohol, dehydrated ethanol 42.7%, polyoxyethylated castor oil]

Tenofovir (te NOE fo veer)

Brand Names: U.S. Viread®

Brand Names: Canada Viread®

Index Terms PMPA; TDF; Tenofovir Disoproxil Fumarate

Pharmacologic Category Antiretroviral Agent, Reverse Transcriptase Inhibitor (Nucleotide)

Additional Appendix Information

Management of Healthcare Worker Exposures to HBV, HCV, and HIV *on page 1935*

Perinatal HIV Guidelines *on page 1946*

Use Management of HIV infections in combination with at least two other antiretroviral agents; treatment of chronic hepatitis B virus (HBV) in patients with compensated or decompensated liver disease

Pregnancy Risk Factor B

Pregnancy Considerations Adverse events were not observed in rat and rabbit reproduction studies. Decreased fetal growth and reduced fetal bone porosity were observed in monkeys. Clinical studies in children have shown bone demineralization with chronic use. Tenofovir crosses the human placenta. No increased risk of overall birth defects has been observed following first trimester exposure according to data collected by the antiretroviral pregnancy registry. Limited data indicate decreased maternal bioavailability during the third trimester. Cases of lactic acidosis/hepatic steatosis syndrome related to mitochondrial toxicity have been reported in pregnant women with prolonged use of nucleoside analogues. It is not known if pregnancy itself potentiates this known side effect; however, women may be at increased risk of lactic acidosis and liver damage. In addition, these adverse events are similar to other rare but life-threatening syndromes which occur during pregnancy (eg HELLP syndrome). Hepatic enzymes and electrolytes should be monitored in women receiving nucleoside analogues and clinicians should watch for early signs of the syndrome. In addition, mitochondrial dysfunction may develop in infants following *in utero* exposure. Renal function should also be monitored. The DHHS Perinatal HIV Guidelines consider tenofovir to be an alternative NRTI in dual nucleoside combination regimens. The DHHS Perinatal HIV Guidelines consider emtricitabine plus tenofovir, or lamivudine plus tenofovir as recommended dual NRTI/NtRTI backbones for HIV/HBV coinfected pregnant women. Hepatitis B flare may occur if tenofovir is discontinued postpartum.

Regardless of CD4 count or HIV RNA copy number, all HIV-infected pregnant women should receive a combination antepartum antiretroviral (ARV) drug regimen; this includes women who require therapy for their own health, as well as women who do not yet require therapy for their own health. ARV therapy should be started as soon as possible if required for the woman's health or immediately after the first trimester if not needed for the mother's health (although earlier initiation may be considered). Long-term follow-up is recommended for all infants exposed to ARV medications.

Healthcare providers are encouraged to enroll pregnant women exposed to antiretroviral medications in the Antiretroviral Pregnancy Registry (1-800-258-4263 or www.-APRegistry.com). Healthcare providers caring for HIV-infected women and their infants may contact the National Perinatal HIV Hotline (888-448-8765) for clinical consultation (DHHS [perinatal], 2011).

Lactation Enters breast milk/contraindicated

Contraindications There are no contraindications listed within the FDA-approved labeling.

Warnings/Precautions [U.S Boxed Warning]: Lactic acidosis and severe hepatomegaly with steatosis have been reported with tenofovir and other nucleoside analogues, including fatal cases; use with caution in patients with risk factors for liver disease (risk may be increased in obese patients or prolonged exposure) and suspend treatment in any patient who develops clinical or laboratory findings suggestive of lactic acidosis (transaminase elevation may/may not accompany hepatomegaly and steatosis). May cause redistribution of fat (eg, buffalo hump, peripheral wasting with increased abdominal girth, cushingoid appearance). Immune reconstitution syndrome may develop resulting in the occurrence of an inflammatory response to an indolent or residual opportunistic infection; further evaluation and treatment may be required. Use caution in hepatic impairment; no dosage adjustment is required; limited studies indicate the pharmacokinetics of tenofovir are not altered in hepatic dysfunction. Limited data supporting treatment of chronic hepatitis B in patients with decompensated liver disease; observe for increased adverse reactions, including renal dysfunction.

May cause osteomalacia; increased biochemical markers of bone metabolism, serum parathyroid hormone levels, and 1,25 vitamin D levels have been noted with tenofovir use. A 5% to 7% loss of bone mineral density (BMD) has been reported in some patients. BMD monitoring should be considered in patients with a history of bone fracture or risk factors for osteopenia or bone loss. Bone effects in tenofovir-treated HIV adolescents were similar to adults; long-term bone health and fracture risk unknown.

Do not use as monotherapy in treatment of HIV. Treatment of HIV in patients with unrecognized/untreated HBV may lead to rapid HBV resistance. Patients should be tested for presence of chronic hepatitis B infection prior to initiation of therapy.

Use caution in renal impairment. Calculate creatinine clearance prior to initiation of therapy and monitor renal function (including recalculation of creatinine clearance and serum phosphorus) during therapy. Dosage adjustment required in patients with Cl_{cr} <50 mL/minute. May cause acute renal failure or Fanconi syndrome; use caution with other nephrotoxic agents (especially those which compete for active tubular secretion), patients with low body weight, or concurrent medications which increase tenofovir levels. Use caution in the elderly; dosage adjustment based on renal function may be required.

[U.S. Boxed Warning]: If treating HBV, acute exacerbation of hepatitis B may occur upon discontinuation.

Monitor liver function closely for several months after discontinuing treatment; reinitiation of antihepatitis B therapy may be required. Treatment of HBV in patients with unrecognized/untreated HIV may lead to HIV resistance; patients should be tested for presence of HIV infection prior to initiating therapy. Do not use as monotherapy in treatment of HIV. Treatment of HIV in patients with unrecognized/untreated HBV may lead to rapid HBV resistance. Patients should be tested for presence of chronic hepatitis B prior to initiation of therapy. Use with caution in patients taking strong CYP3A4 inhibitors, moderate or strong CYP3A4 inducers and major CYP3A4 substrates (see Drug Interactions); consider alternative agents that avoid or lessen the potential for CYP-mediated interactions. Do not use concurrently with adefovir or tenofovir combination products.

Adverse Reactions Frequencies listed are treatment-emergent adverse effects noted at higher frequency than in the placebo group or comparator group. Only adverse events from treatment-naive studies which varied significantly were noted (eg, rash event). Patients treated for chronic hepatitis B had similar reactions and frequencies.

>10%:

Central nervous system: Insomnia (3% to 4%; decompensated liver disease 18%), pain (7% to 13%), dizziness (3%; treatment naïve 8%; decompensated liver disease 13%), depression (4% to 8%; treatment naïve 9% to 11%), fever (2% to 4%; treatment naïve 8%; decompensated liver disease 11%)

Dermatologic: Rash event (includes maculopapular, pustular, or vesiculobullous rash, pruritus or urticaria 5% to 7%; treatment naïve 18%)

Endocrine & metabolic: Triglycerides increased (grades 3/4: 11%; treatment naïve 4%)

Gastrointestinal: Abdominal pain (4% to 7%; decompensated liver disease 22%), nausea (8% to 11%; decompensated liver disease 20%), diarrhea (11% to 16%), vomiting (4% to 7%; decompensated liver disease 13%)

Neuromuscular & skeletal: Creatine kinase increased (9% to 12%), weakness (7% to 11%)

1% to 10%:

Cardiovascular: Chest pain (3%)

Central nervous system: Fatigue (9%), headache (5% to 8%), anxiety (6%)

Endocrine & metabolic: Hyperglycemia (grades 3/4: 3%)

Gastrointestinal: Serum amylase increased (grades 3/4: 4% to 7%; treatment naïve 8% to 9%), anorexia (3% to 4%), dyspepsia (3% to 4%), flatulence (3% to 4%), weight loss (2% to 4%)

Genitourinary: Hematuria (grades 3/4: 3% to 7%)

Hematologic: Neutropenia (1% to 3%)

Hepatic: Transaminases increased (2% to 5%), alkaline phosphatase increased (1%)

Neuromuscular & skeletal: Back pain (3% to 4%; treatment naive 9%), peripheral neuropathy (3% to 5%), myalgia (3% to 4%)

Renal: Serum creatinine increased (decompensated liver disease 9%), renal failure (decompensated liver disease 7%), glycosuria (grades 3/4: 3%)

Respiratory: Upper respiratory tract infection (8%), sinusitis (8%), nasopharyngitis (5%), pneumonia (2% to 3%; treatment naive 5%)

Miscellaneous: Diaphoresis (3%)

Postmarketing and/or case reports: Acute tubular necrosis, allergic reaction, angioedema, bone mineral density decreased, dyspnea, Fanconi syndrome, hepatic steatosis, hepatitis, hypokalemia, hypophosphatemia, immune reconstitution syndrome, interstitial nephritis, lactic acidosis, muscle weakness, myopathy, nephrogenic diabetes insipidus, nephrotoxicity, osteomalacia, pancreatitis, polyuria, proteinuria, proximal renal tubulopathy, renal insufficiency, renal myopathy, rhabdomyolysis

Drug Interactions

Metabolism/Transport Effects Inhibits CYP1A2 (weak)

Avoid Concomitant Use

Avoid concomitant use of Tenofovir with any of the following: Adefovir; Didanosine

Increased Effect/Toxicity

Tenofovir may increase the levels/effects of: Adefovir; Didanosine; Ganciclovir-Valganciclovir

The levels/effects of Tenofovir may be increased by: Acyclovir-Valacyclovir; Adefovir; Atazanavir; Ganciclovir-Valganciclovir; Lopinavir; Protease Inhibitors; Telaprevir

Decreased Effect

Tenofovir may decrease the levels/effects of: Atazanavir; Didanosine; Protease Inhibitors

The levels/effects of Tenofovir may be decreased by: Adefovir

Ethanol/Nutrition/Herb Interactions Food: Fatty meals may increase the bioavailability of tenofovir. Tenofovir may be taken with or without food.

Stability Store at 25°C (77°F); excursions permitted to 15°C to 30°C (59°F to 86°F).

Mechanism of Action Tenofovir disoproxil fumarate (TDF) is an analog of adenosine 5'-monophosphate; it interferes with the HIV viral RNA dependent DNA polymerase resulting in inhibition of viral replication. TDF is first converted intracellularly by hydrolysis to tenofovir and subsequently phosphorylated to the active tenofovir diphosphate; nucleotide reverse transcriptase inhibitor. Tenofovir inhibits replication of HBV by inhibiting HBV polymerase.

Pharmacodynamics/Kinetics

Distribution: V_d: 1.2-1.3 L/kg

Protein binding: <7% to serum proteins

Metabolism: Tenofovir disoproxil fumarate (TDF) is converted intracellularly by hydrolysis (by non-CYP enzymes) to tenofovir, then phosphorylated to the active tenofovir diphosphate

Bioavailability: ~25% (fasting); increases ~40% with high-fat meal

Half-life elimination: ~17 hours

Time to peak, serum: Fasting: 36-84 minutes; With food: 96-144 minutes

Excretion: Urine (70% to 80%) via filtration and active secretion, primarily as unchanged tenofovir

Dosage Oral: **Note:** Concurrent use with adefovir and/or tenofovir combination products should be avoided.

Children ≥12 years and ≥35 kg and Adults: HIV infection: 300 mg once daily (in combination with other antiretrovirals)

Adults: Hepatitis B infection: 300 mg once daily; **Note:** Tenofovir is recommended for first-line treatment of HBV (Lok, 2009)

Treatment duration (AASLD practice guidelines, 2009):

Note: Patients not achieving <2 log decrease in serum HBV DNA after at least 6 months of therapy should either receive additional treatment or be switched to an alternative therapy (Lok, 2009).

Hepatitis Be antigen (HBeAg) positive chronic hepatitis: Treat ≥1 year until HBeAg seroconversion and undetectable serum HBV DNA; continue therapy for ≥6 months after HBeAg seroconversion

HBeAg negative chronic hepatitis: Treat >1 year until hepatitis B surface antigen (HBsAg) clearance

Decompensated liver disease: Lifelong treatment is recommended

Dosage adjustment in renal impairment: Adults:
Cl_{cr} ≥50 mL/minute: No adjustment necessary
Cl_{cr} 30-49 mL/minute: 300 mg every 48 hours
Cl_{cr} 10-29 mL/minute: 300 mg every 72-96 hours
Cl_{cr} <10 mL/minute without hemodialysis: No recommendation available.

Hemodialysis: 300 mg following dialysis every 7 days or after a total of ~12 hours of dialysis (usually once weekly assuming 3 dialysis sessions lasting about 4 hours each)

Dosage adjustment in hepatic impairment: No dosage adjustment required.

Dietary Considerations May be taken without regard to meals. Consider calcium and vitamin D supplementation in patients with history of bone fracture or osteopenia.

Administration May be administered without regard to meals.

Monitoring Parameters

Patients with HIV: CBC with differential, reticulocyte count, creatine kinase, CD4 count, HIV RNA plasma levels, renal and hepatic function tests, bone density (long-term), serum phosphorus; testing for HBV is recommended prior to the initiation of antiretroviral therapy

Patients with HBV: HIV status (prior to initiation of therapy); bone density (long-term), serum phosphorus; serum creatinine (prior to initiation and as clinically indicated therapy; HBV DNA (every 3-6 months during therapy); HBeAg and anti-HBe; LFTs every 3 months during therapy and for several months following discontinuation of tenofovir; signs/symptoms of HBV relapse/exacerbation following discontinuation of therapy

Patients with HIV and HBV coinfection should be monitored for several months following tenofovir discontinuation.

Additional Information Approval was based on two clinical trials involving patients who were previously treated with antiretrovirals with continued evidence of HIV replication despite therapy. The risk:benefit ratio for untreated patients has not been established (studies currently ongoing), however, patients who received tenofovir showed significant decreases in HIV replication as compared to continuation of standard therapy.

A high rate of early virologic nonresponse was observed when abacavir, lamivudine, and tenofovir were used as the initial regimen in treatment-naive patients. A high rate of early virologic nonresponse was also observed when didanosine, lamivudine, and tenofovir were used as the initial regimen in treatment-naive patients. Use of either of these combinations is not recommended; patients currently on either of these regimens should be closely monitored for modification of therapy. Early virologic failure was also observed with tenofovir and didanosine delayed release capsules, plus either efavirenz or nevirapine; use caution in treatment-naive patients with high baseline viral loads.

Dosage Forms Excipient information presented when available (limited, particularly for generics); consult specific product labeling.

Tablet, oral, as disoproxil fumarate:
Viread®: 300 mg [equivalent to 245 mg tenofovir disoproxil]

- ◆ **Tenofovir and Emtricitabine** *see* Emtricitabine and Tenofovir *on page 583*
- ◆ **Tenofovir Disoproxil Fumarate** *see* Tenofovir *on page 1645*
- ◆ **Tenofovir Disoproxil Fumarate, Efavirenz, and Emtricitabine** *see* Efavirenz, Emtricitabine, and Tenofovir *on page 577*
- ◆ **Tenofovir Disoproxil Fumarate, Rilpivirine, and Emtricitabine** *see* Emtricitabine, Rilpivirine, and Tenofovir *on page 583*
- ◆ **Tenofovir, Emtricitabine, and Rilpivirine** *see* Emtricitabine, Rilpivirine, and Tenofovir *on page 583*
- ◆ **Tenormin®** *see* Atenolol *on page 161*
- ◆ **Tensilon® (Can)** *see* Edrophonium *on page 573*
- ◆ **Tenuate® (Can)** *see* Diethylpropion *on page 502*
- ◆ **Tenuate® Dospan® (Can)** *see* Diethylpropion *on page 502*
- ◆ **Terazol® (Can)** *see* Terconazole *on page 1651*
- ◆ **Terazol® 3** *see* Terconazole *on page 1651*
- ◆ **Terazol® 7** *see* Terconazole *on page 1651*

Terazosin (ter AY zoe sin)

Brand Names: Canada Apo-Terazosin®; Dom-Terazosin; Hytrin®; Nu-Terazosin; PHL-Terazosin; PMS-Terazosin; ratio-Terazosin; Teva-Terazosin

Index Terms Hytrin

Pharmacologic Category $Alpha_1$ Blocker

Use Management of mild-to-moderate hypertension; alone or in combination with other agents such as diuretics or beta-blockers; benign prostate hyperplasia (BPH)

Unlabeled Use Pediatric hypertension

Pregnancy Risk Factor C

Pregnancy Considerations Teratogenic effects have not been observed in animal studies. Decreased fetal weight and increased risk of fetal mortality were noted in some animal reproduction studies. There are no adequate and well-controlled studies in pregnant women. Use only if benefit outweighs risk.

Lactation Excretion in breast milk unknown/use caution

Contraindications Hypersensitivity to terazosin or any component of the formulation

Warnings/Precautions Can cause significant orthostatic hypotension and syncope, especially with first dose; anticipate a similar effect if therapy is interrupted for a few days, if dosage is rapidly increased, or if another antihypertensive drug (particularly vasodilators) or a PDE-5 inhibitor is introduced. Discontinue if symptoms of angina occur or worsen. Patients should be cautioned about performing hazardous tasks when starting new therapy or adjusting dosage upward. Prostate cancer should be ruled out before starting for BPH. Intraoperative floppy iris syndrome has been observed in cataract surgery patients who were on or were previously treated with $alpha_1$-blockers. Causality has not been established and there appears to be no benefit in discontinuing alpha-blocker therapy prior to surgery. Priapism has been associated with use (rarely).

Adverse Reactions

>10%:
Central nervous system: Dizziness (9% to 19%)
Neuromuscular & skeletal: Muscle weakness (7% to 11%)

1% to 10%:
Cardiovascular: Peripheral edema (1% to 6%), orthostatic hypotension (1% to 4%), palpitation (≤4%), tachycardia (≤2%), syncope (≤1%
Central nervous system: Somnolence (4% to 5%), vertigo (1%)
Gastrointestinal: Nausea (2% to 4%)
Genitourinary: Impotence (≤2%), libido decreased (≤1%)
Neuromuscular & skeletal: Extremity pain (≤4%), paresthesia (≤3%), back pain (≤2%)
Ocular: Blurred vision (≤2%)
Respiratory: Nasal congestion (2% to 6%), dyspnea (2% to 3%), sinusitis (≤3%)

<1% (Limited to important or life-threatening): Abdominal pain, abnormal vision, allergic reactions, anaphylaxis, anxiety, arrhythmia, arthralgia, arthritis, atrial fibrillation, bronchitis, chest pain, conjunctivitis, constipation, cough, diaphoresis, diarrhea, dyspepsia, epistaxis, facial edema,

fever, flatulence, flu-like syndrome, gout, insomnia, intraoperative floppy iris syndrome (IFIS), joint disorder, myalgia, neck pain, pharyngitis, polyuria, priapism, pruritus, rash, rhinitis, shoulder pain, thrombocytopenia, tinnitus, urinary incontinence, urinary tract infection, vasodilation, vomiting, xerostomia

Drug Interactions

Metabolism/Transport Effects None known.

Avoid Concomitant Use

Avoid concomitant use of Terazosin with any of the following: Alpha1-Blockers

Increased Effect/Toxicity

Terazosin may increase the levels/effects of: Alpha1-Blockers; Amifostine; Antihypertensives; Calcium Channel Blockers; Hypotensive Agents; RiTUXimab

The levels/effects of Terazosin may be increased by: Beta-Blockers; Diazoxide; Herbs (Hypotensive Properties); MAO Inhibitors; Pentoxifylline; Phosphodiesterase 5 Inhibitors; Prostacyclin Analogues

Decreased Effect

The levels/effects of Terazosin may be decreased by: Herbs (Hypertensive Properties); Methylphenidate; Yohimbine

Ethanol/Nutrition/Herb Interactions Herb/Nutraceutical: Avoid dong quai if using for hypertension (has estrogenic activity). Avoid ephedra, yohimbe, ginseng (may worsen hypertension). Avoid saw palmetto. Avoid garlic (may have increased antihypertensive effect).

Stability Store below 30°C (86°F).

Mechanism of Action $Alpha_1$-specific blocking agent with minimal $alpha_2$ effects; this allows peripheral postsynaptic blockade, with the resultant decrease in arterial tone, while preserving the negative feedback loop which is mediated by the peripheral presynaptic $alpha_2$-receptors; terazosin relaxes the smooth muscle of the bladder neck, thus reducing bladder outlet obstruction

Pharmacodynamics/Kinetics

Onset of action: 1-2 hours

Absorption: Rapid and complete

Protein binding: 90% to 95%

Metabolism: Hepatic; minimal first-pass

Half-life elimination: ~12 hours

Time to peak, serum: ~1 hour

Excretion: Feces (~60%, ~20% as unchanged drug); urine (~40%, ~10% as unchanged drug)

Dosage Oral: **Note:** If drug is discontinued for greater than several days, consider beginning with initial dose and retitrate as needed.

Hypertension:

Children (unlabeled use): Initial: 1 mg once daily; gradually increase dose as necessary, up to maximum of 20 mg/day

Adults: Initial: 1 mg at bedtime; slowly increase dose to achieve desired blood pressure, up to 20 mg/day; usual dose range (JNC 7): 1-20 mg once daily. **Note:** Dosage may be given on a twice daily regimen if response is diminished at 24 hours and hypotension is observed at 2-4 hours following a dose.

Elderly: Consider lower initial doses (eg, immediate release: 0.5 mg once daily) and titrate to response (Aronow, 2011)

Benign prostatic hyperplasia: Adults: Initial: 1 mg at bedtime; thereafter, titrate upwards, if needed, over several weeks, balancing therapeutic benefit with terazosin-induced postural hypotension; most patients require 10 mg day; if no response after 4-6 weeks of 10 mg/day, may increase to 20 mg/day

Dosage adjustment with concurrent medication:

Concurrent use with a diuretic or other antihypertensive agent (especially verapamil): Dosage reduction may be needed when adding

Concurrent use with PDE-5 inhibitors: Initiate PDE-5 inhibitor therapy at the lowest dose due to additive orthostatic and blood pressure lowering effects

Dietary Considerations May be taken without regard to meals at the same time each day.

Administration Administer without regard to meals at the same time each day.

Monitoring Parameters Standing and sitting/supine blood pressure, especially following the initial dose at 2-4 hours following the dose and thereafter at the trough point to ensure adequate control throughout the dosing interval; urinary symptoms

Dosage Forms Excipient information presented when available (limited, particularly for generics); consult specific product labeling.

Capsule, oral: 1 mg, 2 mg, 5 mg, 10 mg

Terbinafine (Systemic) (TER bin a feen)

Brand Names: U.S. LamISIL®; Terbinex™

Brand Names: Canada Apo-Terbinafine®; Auro-Terbinafine; CO Terbinafine; Dom-Terbinafine; JAMP-Terbinafine; Lamisil®; Mylan-Terbinafine; Nu-Terbinafine; PHL-Terbinafine; PMS-Terbinafine; Riva-Terbinafine; Sandoz-Terbinafine; Teva-Terbinafine

Index Terms Terbinafine Hydrochloride

Pharmacologic Category Antifungal Agent, Oral

Additional Appendix Information

Antifungal Agents *on page 1876*

Use Active against most strains of *Trichophyton mentagrophytes*, *Trichophyton rubrum*; may be effective for infections of *Microsporum gypseum* and *M. nanum*, *Trichophyton verrucosum*, *Epidermophyton floccosum*, *Candida albicans*, and *Scopulariopsis brevicaulis*

Onychomycosis of the toenail or fingernail due to susceptible dermatophytes; treatment of tinea capitis

Pregnancy Risk Factor B

Pregnancy Considerations Adverse events were not observed in animal reproduction studies. Avoid use in pregnancy since treatment of onychomycosis is postponable.

Lactation Enters breast milk/not recommended

Contraindications Hypersensitivity to terbinafine or any component of the formulation

Warnings/Precautions While rare, the following complications have been reported and may require discontinuation of therapy: Changes in the ocular lens and retina, pancytopenia, neutropenia, Stevens-Johnson syndrome, toxic epidermal necrolysis. Precipitation or exacerbation of cutaneous or systemic lupus erythematosus has been observed; discontinue if signs and/or symptoms develop. Rare cases of hepatic failure, including fatal cases, have been reported following treatment of onychomycosis. Not recommended for use in patients with active or chronic liver disease. Discontinue if symptoms or signs of hepatobiliary dysfunction or cholestatic hepatitis develop. Products are not recommended for use with pre-existing liver or renal disease (Cl_{cr} ≤50 mL/minute). Use caution in patients sensitive to allylamine antifungals (eg, naftifine, butenafine); cross sensitivity to terbinafine may exist.

Adverse Reactions Adverse events listed for tablets unless otherwise specified. Granules were studied in patients 4-12 years of age.

>10%: Central nervous system: Headache (13%; granules 7%)

1% to 10%:

Central nervous system: Fever (granules 7%)

Dermatologic: Rash (6%; granules 2%), pruritus (3%; granules 1%), urticaria (1%)

Gastrointestinal: Diarrhea (6%; granules 3%), vomiting (<1%; granules 5%), dyspepsia (4%), nausea (3%; granules 2%), taste disturbance (3%), abdominal pain (2%; granules 2% to 4%), toothache (granules 1%)
Hepatic: Liver enzyme abnormalities (3%)
Respiratory: Nasopharyngitis (granules 10%), cough (granules 6%), nasal congestion (granules 2%), pharyngeal pain (granules 2%), rhinorrhea (granules 2%)
<1%, postmarketing, and/or case reports (Limited to important or life-threatening): Angioedema, agranulocytosis, allergic reactions, alopecia, anaphylaxis, depression, fatigue, generalized exanthematous pustulosis (acute), hepatic failure, loss of smell, neutropenia (severe), ocular lens and retina changes, pancreatitis (acute), pancytopenia, photosensitivity, precipitation/exacerbation of cutaneous and systemic lupus erythematosus, psoriasiform eruption, psoriasis exacerbation, rhabdomyolysis, Stevens-Johnson syndrome, thrombocytopenia, toxic epidermal necrolysis, vasculitis, visual field acuity decreased, visual field defects

Drug Interactions

Metabolism/Transport Effects Substrate of CYP1A2 (minor), CYP2C19 (minor), CYP2C9 (minor), CYP3A4 (minor); **Note:** Assignment of Major/Minor substrate status based on clinically relevant drug interaction potential; **Inhibits** CYP2D6 (strong); **Induces** CYP3A4 (weak/moderate)

Avoid Concomitant Use

Avoid concomitant use of Terbinafine (Systemic) with any of the following: Pimozide; Tamoxifen; Thioridazine

Increased Effect/Toxicity

Terbinafine (Systemic) may increase the levels/effects of: Atomoxetine; CYP2D6 Substrates; Fesoterodine; Iloperidone; Nebivolol; Pimozide; Propafenone; Tamoxifen; Tetrabenazine; Thioridazine; Tricyclic Antidepressants

The levels/effects of Terbinafine (Systemic) may be increased by: Conivaptan

Decreased Effect

Terbinafine (Systemic) may decrease the levels/effects of: ARIPiprazole; Codeine; CycloSPORINE; Iloperidone; Saccharomyces boulardii; Saxagliptin; TraMADol

The levels/effects of Terbinafine (Systemic) may be decreased by: Cyproterone; Rifamycin Derivatives; Tocilizumab

Stability

Granules: Store at controlled room temperature of 15°C to 30°C (59°F to 86°F).
Tablet: Store below 25°C (77°F). Protect from light.

Mechanism of Action Synthetic allylamine derivative which inhibits squalene epoxidase, a key enzyme in sterol biosynthesis in fungi. This results in a deficiency in ergosterol within the fungal cell wall and results in fungal cell death.

Pharmacodynamics/Kinetics

Absorption: Children and Adults: >70%
Distribution: V_d: 1000 L; distributed to sebum and skin predominantly
Protein binding: Children and Adults: Plasma: >99%
Metabolism: Hepatic; no active metabolites; first-pass effect; little effect on CYP
Bioavailability: 40%; Children 36% to 64%
Half-life elimination: Terminal half-life: 200-400 hours; very slow release of drug from skin and adipose tissues occurs; effective half-life: ~36 hours; Children 27-31 hours
Time to peak, plasma: Children and Adults: 1-2 hours
Excretion: Urine (70% to 75%; Children 70%)

Dosage Oral:

Granules: Tinea capitis: Children ≥4 years:
<25 kg: 125 mg once daily for 6 weeks
25-35 kg: 187.5 mg once daily for 6 weeks
>35 kg: 250 mg once daily for 6 weeks

Tablet: Onychomycosis:
Children (unlabeled use):
10-20 kg: 62.5 mg once daily for 6 weeks (fingernails) **or** 12 weeks (toenails)
20-40 kg: 125 mg once daily for 6 weeks (fingernails) **or** 12 weeks (toenails)
>40 kg: 250 mg once daily for 6 weeks (fingernails) **or** 12 weeks (toenails)
Adults:
Superficial mycoses: Fingernail: 250 mg/day for up to 6 weeks; toenail: 250 mg/day for 12 weeks; doses may be given in 2 divided doses
Systemic mycosis (unlabeled use): 250-500 mg/day for up to 16 months

Dosing adjustment in renal impairment: Cl_{cr} <50 mL/minute: Clearance decreased by ~50%; oral administration is not recommended

Dosing adjustment in hepatic impairment: Clearance is decreased by ~50% with hepatic cirrhosis; oral administration is not recommended

Administration Tablets may be administered without regard to meals. Granules should be sprinkled on a spoonful of nonacidic food (eg, mashed potatoes); swallow granules without chewing.

Monitoring Parameters AST/ALT prior to initiation, repeat if used >6 weeks; CBC

Additional Information Due to potential toxicity, the manufacturer recommends confirmation of diagnosis testing of nail specimens prior to treatment of onychomycosis. Patients should not be considered therapeutic failures until they have been symptom-free for 2-4 weeks off following a course of treatment; GI complaints usually subside with continued administration.

A meta-analysis of efficacy studies for toenail infections revealed that weighted average mycological cure rates for continuous therapy were 36.7% (griseofulvin), 54.7% (itraconazole), and 77% (terbinafine). Cure rate for 4-month pulse therapy for itraconazole and terbinafine were 73.3% and 80%. Additionally, the final outcome measure of final costs per cured infections for continuous therapy was significantly lower for terbinafine.

Dosage Forms Excipient information presented when available (limited, particularly for generics); consult specific product labeling.

Granules, oral:
LamISIL®: 125 mg/packet (14s, 42s); 187.5 mg/packet (14s, 42s)
Tablet, oral: 250 mg
LamISIL®: 250 mg
Terbinex™: 250 mg [kit includes Terbinex™ tablets (42s) and Eco-Formula™ nail enhancer]

Extemporaneous Preparations A 25 mg/mL oral suspension may be made using tablets. Crush twenty 250 mg tablets and reduce to a fine powder. Add small amount of a 1:1 mixture of Ora-Sweet® and Ora-Plus® and mix to a uniform paste; mix while adding the vehicle in geometric proportions to **almost** 200 mL; transfer to a calibrated bottle, rinse mortar with vehicle, and add quantity of vehicle sufficient to make 200 mL. Label "shake well" and "refrigerate". Stable 42 days.

Nahata MC, Pai VB, and Hipple TF, *Pediatric Drug Formulations*, 5th ed, Cincinnati, OH: Harvey Whitney Books Co, 2004.

Terbinafine (Topical) (TER bin a feen)

Brand Names: U.S. LamISIL AT® [OTC]
Brand Names: Canada Lamisil®
Index Terms Terbinafine Hydrochloride
Pharmacologic Category Antifungal Agent, Topical

Use Antifungal for the treatment of tinea pedis (athlete's foot), tinea cruris (jock itch), and tinea corporis (ringworm) [OTC/prescription formulations]; tinea versicolor [prescription formulations]

Dosage Topical:

Cream, gel, solution: Children ≥12 years and Adults:

Athlete's foot (tinea pedis): Apply to affected area once daily for at least 1 week, not to exceed 4 weeks [OTC/Canadian/prescription formulations]

Cutaneous candidiasis: Apply to affected area once or twice daily for 7-14 days

Ringworm (tinea corporis) and jock itch (tinea cruris): Apply cream to affected area once daily for at least 1 week, not to exceed 4 weeks; apply gel or solution once daily for 7 days [OTC formulations]

Cream, solution: Adults: Tinea versicolor: Apply to affected area once or twice daily for 2 weeks [Canadian/prescription formulation]

Additional Information Complete prescribing information for this medication should be consulted for additional detail.

Dosage Forms Excipient information presented when available (limited, particularly for generics); consult specific product labeling. [DSC] = Discontinued product

Cream, topical, as hydrochloride: 1% (12 g [DSC], 15 g, 24 g [DSC], 30 g)

LamISIL AT®: 1% (12 g, 15 g, 24 g, 30 g, 36 g) [contains benzyl alcohol]

Gel, topical:

LamISIL AT®: 1% (6 g, 12 g) [contains benzyl alcohol]

Solution, topical, as hydrochloride [spray]:

LamISIL AT®: 1% (30 mL) [contains ethanol]

Dosage Forms: Canada Excipient information presented when available (limited, particularly for generics); consult specific product labeling.

Cream, topical, as hydrochloride: 1% (12 g, 24 g)

Lamisil®: 1% (15 g, 30 g)

Solution, topical, as hydrochloride [spray]:

Lamisil®: 1% (30 mL)

◆ **Terbinafine Hydrochloride** *see* Terbinafine (Systemic) *on page 1648*

◆ **Terbinafine Hydrochloride** *see* Terbinafine (Topical) *on page 1649*

◆ **Terbinex™** *see* Terbinafine (Systemic) *on page 1648*

Terbutaline (ter BYOO ta leen)

Brand Names: Canada Bricanyl®

Index Terms Brethaire [DSC]; Brethine; Bricanyl [DSC]

Pharmacologic Category $Beta_2$-Adrenergic Agonist

Additional Appendix Information

Bronchodilators *on page 1886*

Use Bronchodilator in reversible airway obstruction and bronchial asthma

Unlabeled Use Injection: Tocolytic agent (short-term [≤72 hours] prevention or management of preterm labor

Pregnancy Risk Factor B

Lactation Enters breast milk/compatible

Contraindications Hypersensitivity to terbutaline or any component of the formulation; cardiac arrhythmias associated with tachycardia; tachycardia caused by digitalis intoxication

Injection: Additional contraindications: Prolonged (>72 hours) prevention or management of preterm labor

Oral: Additional contraindications: Prevention or treatment of preterm labor

Warnings/Precautions When used for tocolysis, terbutaline causes tachycardia, transient hyperglycemia, hypokalemia, cardiac arrhythmias, pulmonary edema and myocardial ischemia in the mother and increased fetal heart rate and neonatal hypoglycemia as a result of maternal administration. Injectable terbutaline has not been approved for and should not be used for prolonged tocolysis (beyond 48-72 hours). Oral terbutaline should not be used in preterm labor.

Use caution in patients with cardiovascular disease (arrhythmia or hypertension or HF), convulsive disorders, diabetes, glaucoma, hyperthyroidism, or hypokalemia. Beta-agonists may cause elevation in blood pressure, heart rate, and result in CNS stimulation/excitation. $Beta_2$-agonists may increase risk of arrhythmia, increase serum glucose, or decrease serum potassium.

When used as a bronchodilator, optimize anti-inflammatory treatment before initiating maintenance treatment with terbutaline. Do not use as a component of chronic therapy without an anti-inflammatory agent. Only the mildest form of asthma (Step 1 and/or exercise-induced) would not require concurrent use based upon asthma guidelines. Patient must be instructed to seek medical attention in cases where acute symptoms are not relieved or a previous level of response is diminished. The need to increase frequency of use may indicate deterioration of asthma, and treatment must not be delayed.

Immediate hypersensitivity reactions (urticaria, angioedema, rash, bronchospasm) have been reported. Do not exceed recommended dose; serious adverse events including fatalities, have been associated with excessive use of inhaled sympathomimetics. Rarely, paradoxical bronchospasm may occur with use of inhaled bronchodilating agents; this should be distinguished from inadequate response.

Adverse Reactions

>10%:

Central nervous system: Nervousness, restlessness

Endocrine & metabolic: Serum glucose increased, serum potassium decreased

Neuromuscular & skeletal: Trembling

1% to 10%:

Cardiovascular: Tachycardia, hypertension, pounding heartbeat

Central nervous system: Dizziness, lightheadedness, drowsiness, headache, insomnia

Gastrointestinal: Dry mouth, nausea, vomiting, bad taste in mouth

Neuromuscular & skeletal: Muscle cramps, weakness

Miscellaneous: Diaphoresis

<1% (Limited to important or life-threatening): Arrhythmia, cardiac arrest (preterm labor), chest pain, hyperglycemia (preterm labor), hypokalemia (preterm labor), hypotension (preterm labor), paradoxical bronchospasm, myocardial infarction (preterm labor), myocardial ischemia (preterm labor), pulmonary edema (preterm labor)

Drug Interactions

Metabolism/Transport Effects None known.

Avoid Concomitant Use

Avoid concomitant use of Terbutaline with any of the following: Beta-Blockers (Nonselective); Iobenguane I 123

Increased Effect/Toxicity

Terbutaline may increase the levels/effects of: Loop Diuretics; Sympathomimetics; Thiazide Diuretics

The levels/effects of Terbutaline may be increased by: Atomoxetine; Cannabinoids; MAO Inhibitors; Tricyclic Antidepressants

Decreased Effect

Terbutaline may decrease the levels/effects of: Iobenguane I 123

The levels/effects of Terbutaline may be decreased by: Alpha-/Beta-Blockers; Beta-Blockers (Beta1 Selective); Beta-Blockers (Nonselective); Betahistine

Ethanol/Nutrition/Herb Interactions Herb/Nutraceutical: Avoid ephedra, yohimbe (may cause CNS stimulation).

Stability Store injection at room temperature; do not freeze. Protect from heat and light. Use only clear solutions. Store powder for inhalation (Bricanyl® Turbuhaler [CAN]) at room temperature between 15°C and 30°C (58°F and 86°F).

Mechanism of Action Relaxes bronchial and uterine smooth muscle by action on beta$_2$-receptors with less effect on heart rate

Pharmacodynamics/Kinetics

Onset of action: Oral: 30-45 minutes; SubQ: 6-15 minutes
Protein binding: 25%
Metabolism: Hepatic to inactive sulfate conjugates
Bioavailability: SubQ doses are more bioavailable than oral
Half-life elimination: 11-16 hours
Excretion: Urine

Dosage

Children <12 years: Bronchoconstriction:
- Oral: Initial: 0.05 mg/kg/dose 3 times/day, increased gradually as required; maximum: 0.15 mg/kg/dose 3-4 times/day or a total of 5 mg/24 hours
- SubQ: 0.005-0.01 mg/kg/dose to a maximum of 0.4 mg/dose every 15-20 minutes for 3 doses; may repeat every 2-6 hours as needed

Children ≥6 years and Adults: Bronchospasm (acute): Inhalation (Bricanyl® [CAN] MDI: 500 mcg/puff, *not labeled for use in the U.S.*): One puff as needed; may repeat with 1 inhalation (after 5 minutes); more than 6 inhalations should not be necessary in any 24 hour period. **Note:** If a previously effective dosage regimen fails to provide the usual relief, or the effects of a dose last for >3 hours, medical advice should be sought immediately; this is a sign of seriously worsening asthma that requires reassessment of therapy.

Children >12 years and Adults: Bronchoconstriction:
- Oral:
  - 12-15 years: 2.5 mg every 6 hours 3 times/day; not to exceed 7.5 mg in 24 hours
  - >15 years: 5 mg/dose every 6 hours 3 times/day; if side effects occur, reduce dose to 2.5 mg every 6 hours; not to exceed 15 mg in 24 hours
- SubQ:
  - Manufacturer's labeling: 0.25 mg/dose; may repeat in 15-30 minutes (maximum: 0.5 mg/4-hour period)
  - Unlabeled dose: 0.25 mg/dose; may repeat every 20 minutes for 3 doses (maximum: 0.75 mg/1-hour period) (NIH Guidelines, 2007)

Adults: Premature labor (acute; short-term [≤72 hours] tocolysis; unlabeled use):
- I.V.: 2.5-5 mcg/minute; increased gradually every 20-30 minutes by 2.5-5 mcg/minute; effective maximum dosages from 17.5-30 mcg/minute have been used with caution. Duration of infusion is at least 12 hours (Travis, 1993).
- SubQ: 0.25 mg every 20 minutes to 3 hours; hold for pulse >120 beats per minute. Terbutaline has not been approved for and should not be used for prolonged tocolysis (beyond 48-72 hours) (ACOG, 2003).

Dosing adjustment/comments in renal impairment:
- Cl_{cr} 10-50 mL/minute: Administer at 50% of normal dose
- Cl_{cr} <10 mL/minute: Avoid use

Administration

I.V.: Use infusion pump.
Oral: Administer around-the-clock to promote less variation in peak and trough serum levels

Monitoring Parameters Serum potassium, glucose; intake/output; heart rate, blood pressure, respiratory rate; chest pain, shortness of breath; monitor for signs and symptoms of pulmonary edema (when used as a tocolytic); monitor FEV$_1$, peak flow, and/or other pulmonary function tests (when used as bronchodilator)

Dosage Forms Excipient information presented when available (limited, particularly for generics); consult specific product labeling.

Injection, solution, as sulfate: 1 mg/mL (1 mL)
Tablet, oral, as sulfate: 2.5 mg, 5 mg

Dosage Forms: Canada Excipient information presented when available (limited, particularly for generics); consult specific product labeling.

Powder for oral inhalation:
- Bricanyl® Turbuhaler: 500 mcg/actuation [50 or 200 metered actuations]

Extemporaneous Preparations A 1 mg/mL oral suspension may be made with tablets. Crush twenty-four 5 mg tablets in a mortar and reduce to a fine powder. Add 5 mL purified water USP and mix to a uniform paste; mix while adding simple syrup, NF in incremental proportions to **almost** 120 mL; transfer to a calibrated bottle, rinse mortar with vehicle, and add quantity of simple syrup, NF sufficient to make 120 mL. Label "shake well" and "refrigerate". Stable for 30 days.

Nahata MC, Pai VB, and Hipple TF, *Pediatric Drug Formulations*, 5th ed, Cincinnati, OH: Harvey Whitney Books Co, 2004.

Terconazole (ter KONE a zole)

Brand Names: U.S. Terazol® 3; Terazol® 7; Zazole™ [DSC]

Brand Names: Canada Terazol®

Index Terms Triaconazole

Pharmacologic Category Antifungal Agent, Vaginal

Use Local treatment of vulvovaginal candidiasis

Pregnancy Risk Factor C

Dosage Intravaginal: Adults: Females:
- Terazol® 3, Zazole™ (0.8%) vaginal cream: Insert 1 applicatorful intravaginally at bedtime for 3 consecutive days
- Terazol® 7, Zazole™ (0.4%) vaginal cream: Insert 1 applicatorful intravaginally at bedtime for 7 consecutive days
- Terazol® 3 vaginal suppository: Insert 1 suppository intravaginally at bedtime for 3 consecutive days

Additional Information Complete prescribing information for this medication should be consulted for additional detail.

Dosage Forms Excipient information presented when available (limited, particularly for generics); consult specific product labeling. [DSC] = Discontinued product

Cream, vaginal: 0.4% (45 g); 0.8% (20 g)
- Terazol® 7: 0.4% (45 g)
- Terazol® 3: 0.8% (20 g)
- Zazole™: 0.4% (45 g [DSC]); 0.8% (20 g [DSC])

Suppository, vaginal: 80 mg (3s)
- Terazol® 3: 80 mg (3s) [contains coconut oil (may have trace amounts), palm kernel oil (may have trace amounts)]

◆ **Terfluzine (Can)** *see* Trifluoperazine *on page* *1736*

Teriparatide (ter i PAR a tide)

Brand Names: U.S. Forteo®

Brand Names: Canada Forteo®

Index Terms Parathyroid Hormone (1-34); Recombinant Human Parathyroid Hormone (1-34); rhPTH(1-34)

Pharmacologic Category Parathyroid Hormone Analog

Use Treatment of osteoporosis in postmenopausal women at high risk of fracture; treatment of primary or hypogonadal osteoporosis in men at high risk of fracture; treatment of glucocorticoid-induced osteoporosis in men and women at high risk for fracture

Pregnancy Risk Factor C

Pregnancy Considerations Adverse events were observed in animal studies; the effect on human fetal development has not been studied. Teriparatide is not indicated for use in pregnant or premenopausal women.

Lactation Excretion in breast milk unknown/not recommended

Medication Guide Available Yes

Contraindications Hypersensitivity to teriparatide or any component of the formulation

Canadian labeling: Additional contraindications (not in U.S. labeling): Pre-existing hypercalcemia; severe renal impairment; metabolic bone diseases other than primary osteoporosis (including hyperparathyroidism and Paget's disease of the bone); unexplained elevations of alkaline phosphatase; prior external beam or implant radiation therapy involving the skeleton; bone metastases or history of skeletal malignancies; pregnancy; breast-feeding mothers; pediatric patients or young adults with open epiphysis

Warnings/Precautions [U.S. Boxed Warning]: In animal studies, teriparatide has been associated with an increase in osteosarcoma; risk was dependent on both dose and duration. Avoid use in patients with an increased risk of osteosarcoma (including Paget's disease, prior radiation, unexplained elevation of alkaline phosphatase, or in patients with open epiphyses). Do not use in patients with a history of skeletal metastases, hyperparathyroidism, or pre-existing hypercalcemia. Not for use in patients with metabolic bone disease other than osteoporosis. Use caution in patients with active or recent urolithiasis. Use caution in patients at risk of orthostasis (including concurrent antihypertensive therapy), or in patients who may not tolerate transient hypotension (cardiovascular or cerebrovascular disease). Use caution in patients with cardiac, renal or hepatic impairment (limited data available concerning safety and efficacy). Use in severe renal impairment is contraindicated in the Canadian labeling. Use of teriparatide for longer than 2 years is not recommended. Not approved for use in pediatric patients.

Adverse Reactions

>10%: Endocrine & metabolic: Hypercalcemia (transient increases noted 4-6 hours postdose [women 11%; men 6%])

1% to 10%:

Cardiovascular: Orthostatic hypotension (5%; transient), chest pain (3%), syncope (3%)

Central nervous system: Dizziness (8%), insomnia (4% to 5%), anxiety (≤4%), depression (4%), vertigo (4%)

Dermatologic: Rash (5%)

Endocrine & metabolic: Hyperuricemia (3%)

Gastrointestinal: Nausea (9% to 14%), gastritis (≤7%), dyspepsia (5%), vomiting (3%)

Neuromuscular & skeletal: Arthralgia (10%), weakness (9%), leg cramps (3%)

Respiratory: Rhinitis (10%), pharyngitis (6%), dyspnea (4% to 6%), pneumonia (4% to 6%)

Miscellaneous: Antibodies to teriparatide (3% of women in long-term treatment; hypersensitivity reactions or decreased efficacy were not associated in preclinical trials), herpes zoster (≤3%)

Postmarketing and/or case reports: Acute dyspnea, allergic reactions, edema (facial/oral), hypercalcemia >13 mg/dL, injection site reactions (bruising, pain, swelling), muscle spasm, osteosarcoma, urticaria

Drug Interactions

Metabolism/Transport Effects None known.

Avoid Concomitant Use There are no known interactions where it is recommended to avoid concomitant use.

Increased Effect/Toxicity There are no known significant interactions involving an increase in effect.

Decreased Effect There are no known significant interactions involving a decrease in effect.

Ethanol/Nutrition/Herb Interactions

Ethanol: Excessive intake may increase risk of osteoporosis.

Herb/Nutraceutical: Ensure adequate calcium and vitamin D intake.

Stability Store at 2°C to 8°C (36°F to 46°F); do not freeze. Protect from light. Discard pen 28 days after first injection. Do not use if solution is cloudy, colored or contains solid particles.

Mechanism of Action Teriparatide is a recombinant formulation of endogenous parathyroid hormone (PTH), containing a 34-amino-acid sequence which is identical to the N-terminal portion of this hormone. The pharmacologic activity of teriparatide, which is similar to the physiologic activity of PTH, includes stimulating osteoblast function, increasing gastrointestinal calcium absorption, and increasing renal tubular reabsorption of calcium. Treatment with teriparatide results in increased bone mineral density, bone mass, and strength. In postmenopausal women, teriparatide has been shown to decrease osteoporosis-related fractures.

Pharmacodynamics/Kinetics

Distribution: V_d: ~0.12 L/kg

Metabolism: Hepatic (nonspecific proteolysis)

Bioavailability: 95%

Half-life elimination: I.V.: 5 minutes; SubQ: ~1 hour

Time to peak, serum: ~30 minutes

Excretion: Urine (as metabolites)

Dosage SubQ: Adults: 20 mcg once daily; **Note:** Initial administration should occur under circumstances in which the patient may sit or lie down, in the event of orthostasis.

Dosage adjustment in renal impairment: No dosage adjustment required. Bioavailability and half-life increase with Cl_{cr} <30 mL/minute. Use in severe renal impairment is contraindicated in the Canadian labeling.

Administration Administer by subcutaneous injection into the thigh or abdominal wall. Initial administration should occur under circumstances in which the patient may sit or lie down, in the event of orthostasis. **Note:** The 3 mL prefilled pen (Canadian availability; not available in U.S.) must be primed prior to each dose.

Monitoring Parameters Serum calcium, serum phosphorus, uric acid; blood pressure; bone mineral density

Test Interactions Transiently increases serum calcium; maximal effect 4-6 hours postdose; generally returns to baseline ~16 hours postdose

Additional Information Teriparatide was formerly marketed as a diagnostic agent (Perithar™); that agent was withdrawn from the market in 1997. Teriparatide (Forteo®) is manufactured through recombinant DNA technology using a strain of *E. coli*.

Patients are encouraged to enroll in the Forteo® Patient Registry which is designed to monitor the potential risk of osteosarcoma and teriparatide treatment. Enrollment information may be found at www.forteoregistry.rti.org or by calling 1-866-382-6813.

Dosage Forms Excipient information presented when available (limited, particularly for generics); consult specific product labeling.

Injection, solution:

Forteo®: 250 mcg/mL (2.4 mL) [delivers teriparatide 20 mcg/dose]

Dosage Forms: Canada Excipient information presented when available (limited, particularly for generics); consult specific product labeling.

Injection, solution:

Forteo®: 250 mcg/mL (3 mL) [delivers teriparatide 20 mcg/dose]

◆ **Tersi** *see* Selenium Sulfide *on page* 1547

Tesamorelin (tes a moe REL in)

Brand Names: U.S. Egrifta™

Index Terms Tesamorelin Acetate; TH9507

Pharmacologic Category Growth Hormone Releasing Factor

Use Reduction of excess abdominal fat in HIV-infected patients with lipodystrophy

Pregnancy Risk Factor X

Pregnancy Considerations Adverse effects were noted in animal reproduction studies. During pregnancy, there is an increased deposition of visceral adipose tissue due to metabolic and hormonal changes. Tesamorelin decreases the deposition of visceral fat and could potentially cause harm to the unborn fetus. Therefore, use during pregnancy is contraindicated.

Lactation Excretion in breast milk unknown/not recommended

Prescribing and Access Restrictions In order to prescribe Egrifta™, healthcare providers must call the Axis Center at 1-877-714-2947. Egrifta™ is only available through specialty pharmacy distribution.

Contraindications Hypersensitivity to tesamorelin, mannitol, or any component of the formulation; disruption of hypothalamic-pituitary-axis due to hypophysectomy, hypopituitarism, pituitary tumor/surgery, head irradiation or head trauma; active malignancy (newly diagnosed or recurrent); pregnancy

Warnings/Precautions Hypersensitivity reactions (eg, pruritus, erythema, flushing, urticaria, rash) may occur. If hypersensitivity is suspected; discontinue and instruct patient to seek immediate medical attention. Tesamorelin use may result in peripheral edema manifested by increased skin turgor and musculoskeletal discomfort. Injection site reactions (including erythema, pruritus, pain, irritation, and bruising) may occur; incidence decreases with treatment continued beyond 26 weeks; rotating the site of injection to different areas of the abdomen may reduce incidence of reactions. Tesamorelin may increase risk of development of diabetes due to glucose intolerance; evaluate glucose status prior to treatment initiation; monitor periodically for glucose metabolism changes. Patients with diabetes should be monitored for the development or worsening of retinopathy due to increased IGF-1 levels.

HIV-positive patients are at an increased risk for development of malignancies. Due to increased IGF-1 levels, use may be associated with a reactivation of malignancies in patients with a history of malignancies. Use is contraindicated in patients with active malignancies; treatment for malignancy should be completed prior to initiation of tesamorelin. IGF-1 levels should be monitored during treatment; consider discontinuing with persistent IGF-1 elevations (eg, >3 standard deviation scores). Growth hormone is associated with an increased risk of mortality in patients with acute critical illness due to complications following open heart surgery, abdominal surgery, trauma, or acute respiratory failure; consider discontinuing in critically ill patients. Should not be used in children due to risk of excess growth (gigantism) when epiphyses are open and is not indicated for weight loss management in non-HIV infected patients

Adverse Reactions Note: The incidence of adverse reactions generally decreases with treatment continued beyond 26 weeks.

>10%:

Local: Injection site reactions (6% to 25%; includes erythema [1% to 9%], pruritus [2% to 8%], pain [4%], irritation [3%], hemorrhage [2%], swelling [2%], urticaria [2%], rash [1%])

Neuromuscular & skeletal: Arthralgia (13%)

1% to 10%:

Cardiovascular: Peripheral edema (2% to 6%), hypertension (1% to 2%), chest pain (1%), palpitation (1%)

Central nervous system: Hypoesthesia (2% to 4%), depression (2%), pain (2%), insomnia (1%)

Dermatologic: Rash (4%), pruritus (1% to 2%), urticaria (1%)

Endocrine & metabolic: Hb A_{1c} increased (5%), hot flush (1%), hyperglycemia

Gastrointestinal: Nausea (4%), vomiting (2% to 3%), dyspepsia (2%), abdominal pain (1%)

Neuromuscular & skeletal: Pain in extremity (3% to 6%), myalgia (1% to 6%), paresthesia (2% to 5%), carpal tunnel syndrome (2%), creatine phosphokinase increased (2%), muscle stiffness (2%), musculoskeletal pain (2%), joint stiffness (2%), peripheral neuropathy (2%), joint swelling (1%), muscle spasm (1%), muscle strain (1%)

Miscellaneous: Hypersensitivity reactions (1% to 4%), night sweats (1%)

<1% (Limited to important or life-threatening): Anemia, abdominal abscess, basal cell carcinoma, bipolar II disorder, cellulitis, cerebellar syndrome, chorioretinopathy, coronary artery arteriosclerosis, dehydration, diarrhea, fracture, heart failure (congestive), mental status changes, pneumonia, rectal cancer, sepsis, small intestinal obstruction, spontaneous abortion, trigeminal neuralgia, upper respiratory tract infection, viral bronchitis

Drug Interactions

Metabolism/Transport Effects None known.

Avoid Concomitant Use There are no known interactions where it is recommended to avoid concomitant use.

Increased Effect/Toxicity There are no known significant interactions involving an increase in effect.

Decreased Effect

Tesamorelin may decrease the levels/effects of: Cortisone; PredniSONE

Stability Store refrigerated at 2°C to 8°C (36°F to 46°F). Protect from light and store in original container until time of use. Store diluent, (sterile water for injection USP), syringes, and needles at room temperature at 20°C to 25°C (68°F to 77°F). Use reconstituted solution immediately after prepared; do not refrigerate or freeze. Discard if not used immediately.

Mechanism of Action Tesamorelin binds to pituitary growth hormone-releasing factor (GRF) receptors and stimulates the secretion of endogenous growth hormone which has anabolic and lipolytic properties. Growth hormone exerts its effects by interacting with receptors on target cells such as osteoblasts, myocytes, hepatocytes, and adipocytes to promote the reduction of total fat mass. These effects are primarily mediated by IGF-1 produced in the liver and in peripheral tissues.

Pharmacodynamics/Kinetics

Distribution: V_d: Healthy adults: 9.4 ± 3.1 L/kg; HIV-infected patients: 10.5 ± 6.1 L/kg

Bioavailability: SubQ: Healthy adults: <4%

Half-life elimination: Healthy adults: 26 minutes; HIV-infected patients: 38 minutes

Time to peak: 9 minutes

Dosage SubQ: Adults: HIV-associated lipodystrophy: 2 mg once daily

Dosing adjustment for toxicity: Discontinue if symptoms of hypersensitivity occur.

Administration SubQ: The abdomen is the preferred site of administration; site should be rotated within the abdomen. Avoid injection into scar tissue, bruises, or the navel. The reconstituted solution should be visually inspected for particulate matter and discoloration; do not administer if solution is not clear, colorless and free of particulate matter. **Note:** Syringes and needles are single-use only and should not be shared between patients.

Monitoring Parameters Serum IGF-1 levels should be monitored at baseline and during therapy due to the potential increased risk of malignancy from sustained elevation of IGF-1 levels.

Dosage Forms Excipient information presented when available (limited, particularly for generics); consult specific product labeling.

Injection, powder for reconstitution:
Egrifta™: 1 mg [contains mannitol]

- **Tesamorelin Acetate** *see* Tesamorelin *on page 1653*
- **TESPA** *see* Thiotepa *on page 1674*
- **Tessalon®** *see* Benzonatate *on page 205*
- **Tessalon Perles** *see* Benzonatate *on page 205*
- **Testim®** *see* Testosterone *on page 1654*
- **Testopel®** *see* Testosterone *on page 1654*

Testosterone (tes TOS ter one)

Brand Names: U.S. Androderm®; AndroGel®; Axiron®; Delatestryl®; Depo®-Testosterone; First®-Testosterone; First®-Testosterone MC; Fortesta™; Striant®; Testim®; Testopel®

Brand Names: Canada Andriol®; Androderm®; AndroGel®; Andropository; Delatestryl®; Depotest® 100; Everone® 200; PMS-Testosterone; Testim®

Index Terms Axiron®; Testosterone Cypionate; Testosterone Enanthate

Pharmacologic Category Androgen

Use

Injection: Androgen replacement therapy in the treatment of delayed male puberty; male hypogonadism (primary or hypogonadotropic); inoperable metastatic female breast cancer (enanthate only)

Pellet: Androgen replacement therapy in the treatment of delayed male puberty; male hypogonadism (primary or hypogonadotropic)

Buccal system, topical gel, topical solution, transdermal system: Male hypogonadism (primary or hypogonadotropic)

Capsule (not available in U.S.): Conditions associated with a deficiency or absence of endogenous testosterone

Unlabeled Use Androgen deficiency in men with AIDS wasting; postmenopausal women (short-term use in select cases)

Pregnancy Risk Factor X

Pregnancy Considerations Testosterone may cause adverse effects, including masculinization of the female fetus, if used during pregnancy. Females who are or may become pregnant should also avoid skin-to-skin contact to areas where testosterone has been applied topically on another person.

Lactation Enters breast milk/contraindicated

Medication Guide Available Yes

Contraindications Hypersensitivity to testosterone or any component of the formulation; males with known or suspected carcinoma of the breast or prostate; specific products are contraindicated in women

Depo®-Testosterone: Also contraindicated in serious hepatic, renal, or cardiac disease

Warnings/Precautions When used to treat delayed male puberty, perform radiographic examination of the hand and wrist every 6 months to determine the rate of bone maturation. May cause hypercalcemia in patients with prolonged immobilization or cancer. May accelerate bone maturation without producing compensating gain in linear growth. Has both androgenic and anabolic activity, the anabolic action may enhance hypoglycemia. May alter serum cholesterol; use caution with history of MI or coronary artery disease. Use caution in elderly patients or patients with other demographic factors which may increase the risk of prostatic carcinoma; careful monitoring is required. Urethral obstruction may develop in patients with BPH; treatment should be discontinued if this should occur (use lower dose if restarted). Withhold treatment pending urological evaluation in patients with palpable prostate nodule or induration, PSA >4 ng/mL, or PSA >3 ng/mL in men at high risk of prostate cancer (Bhasin, 2010). Use with caution in patients with conditions influenced by edema (eg, cardiovascular disease, migraine, seizure disorder, renal or hepatic impairment) or medications that enhance edema formation (eg, corticosteroids); testosterone may cause fluid retention. May cause gynecomastia. Large doses may suppress spermatogenesis. During treatment for metastatic breast cancer, women should be monitored for signs of virilization; discontinue if mild virilization is present to prevent irreversible symptoms.

Prolonged use of high doses of androgens has been associated with serious hepatic effects (peliosis hepatis, hepatic neoplasms, cholestatic hepatitis, jaundice). May potentiate sleep apnea in some male patients (obesity or chronic lung disease). May increase hematocrit requiring dose adjustment or discontinuation; monitor.

[U.S. Boxed Warning]: Virilization in children has been reported following contact with unwashed or unclothed application sites of men using topical testosterone. Patients should strictly adhere to instructions for use in order to prevent secondary exposure. Virilization of female sexual partners has also been reported with male use of topical testosterone. Symptoms of virilization generally regress following removal of exposure; however, in some children, enlarged genitalia and bone age did not fully return to age appropriate normal. Signs of inappropriate virilization in women or children following secondary exposure to topical testosterone should be brought to the attention of a healthcare provider. Axiron® and Fortesta™ are not interchangeable with other topical testosterone products; AndroGel® 1% and AndroGel® 1.62% are not interchangeable. Transdermal patch may contain conducting metal (eg, aluminum); remove patch prior to MRI. Gels, solution, transdermal, and buccal system have not been evaluated in males <18 years of age; safety and efficacy of injection have not been established in males <12 years of age. Some testosterone products may be chemically synthesized from soy. Some products may contain benzyl alcohol. Use of Axiron® in males with BMI >35 kg/m^2 has not been established.

Adverse Reactions Frequency not always defined.

Cardiovascular: Deep venous thrombosis, edema, hypertension, vasodilation

Central nervous system: Abnormal dreams, aggressive behavior, anger, amnesia, anxiety, blood pressure increased/decreased, chills, depression, dizziness, emotional lability, excitation, fatigue, headache, hostility, insomnia, malaise, memory loss, mood swings, nervousness, seizure, sleep apnea, sleeplessness

Dermatologic: Acne, alopecia, contact dermatitis, dry skin, erythema, folliculitis, hair discoloration, hirsutism (increase in pubic hair growth), pruritus, rash, seborrhea

Endocrine & metabolic: Breast pain/soreness, gonadotropin secretion decreased, growth acceleration, gynecomastia, hot flashes, hypercalcemia, hyperchloremia, hypercholesterolemia, hyper-/hypoglycemia, hyper-/hypokalemia, hyperlipidemia, hypernatremia, inorganic phosphate retention, libido changes, menstrual problems (including amenorrhea), virilism, water retention

Gastrointestinal: Appetite increased, diarrhea, gastroesophageal reflux, GI bleeding, GI irritation, nausea, taste disorder, vomiting, weight gain

Following buccal administration (most common): Bitter taste, gum edema, gum or mouth irritation, gum pain, gum tenderness, taste perversion

Genitourinary: Bladder irritability, impotence, oligospermia, penile erections (spontaneous), priapism, prostatic carcinoma, prostatic hyperplasia, prostatitis, PSA increased, testicular atrophy, urination impaired

Hepatic: Bilirubin increased, cholestatic hepatitis, cholestatic jaundice, hepatic dysfunction, hepatic necrosis, hepatocellular neoplasms, liver function test changes, peliosis hepatis

Hematologic: Anemia, bleeding, hematocrit/hemoglobin increased, leukopenia, polycythemia, suppression of clotting factors

Local: Application site reaction (gel, solution), injection site inflammation/pain

Transdermal system: Pruritus at application site (17% to 37%), burn-like blisters under system (12%), erythema at application site (≤7%), vesicles at application site (6%), allergic contact dermatitis to system (4%), burning at application site (3%), induration at application site (3%), exfoliation at application site (<3%)

Neuromuscular & skeletal: Back pain, hemarthrosis, hyperkinesias, paresthesia, weakness

Ocular: Lacrimation increased

Renal: Creatinine increased, hematuria, polyuria

Respiratory: Dyspnea, nasopharyngitis

Miscellaneous: Anaphylactoid reactions, diaphoresis, hypersensitivity reactions, smell disorder

Postmarketing and/or case reports: Injection: Cough, coughing fits, respiratory distress; migraine; virilization of children following secondary exposure to topical gel (advanced bone age, aggressive behavior, enlargement of clitoris requiring surgery, enlargement of penis, erections increased, libido increased, pubic hair development); vitreous detachment

Drug Interactions

Metabolism/Transport Effects Substrate of CYP2B6 (minor), CYP2C19 (minor), CYP2C9 (minor), CYP3A4 (minor); **Note:** Assignment of Major/Minor substrate status based on clinically relevant drug interaction potential

Avoid Concomitant Use There are no known interactions where it is recommended to avoid concomitant use.

Increased Effect/Toxicity

Testosterone may increase the levels/effects of: CycloSPORINE; CycloSPORINE (Systemic); Vitamin K Antagonists

The levels/effects of Testosterone may be increased by: Conivaptan

Decreased Effect

The levels/effects of Testosterone may be decreased by: Tocilizumab

Ethanol/Nutrition/Herb Interactions Herb/Nutraceutical: St John's wort may decrease testosterone levels.

Stability

Androderm®: Store at room temperature. Do not store outside of pouch. Excessive heat may cause system to burst.

AndroGel® 1%, AndroGel® 1.62%, Axiron®, Delatestryl®, Striant®, Testim®: Store at room temperature.

Depo® Testosterone: Store at room temperature. Protect from light.

Fortesta™: Store at room temperature; do not freeze

Testopel®: Store in a cool location.

Mechanism of Action Principal endogenous androgen responsible for promoting the growth and development of the male sex organs and maintaining secondary sex characteristics in androgen-deficient males

Pharmacodynamics/Kinetics

Duration (route and ester dependent): I.M.: Cypionate and enanthate esters have longest duration, ≤2-4 weeks; gel: 24-48 hours

Absorption: Transdermal gel: ~10% of applied dose

Protein binding: 98%; bound to sex hormone-binding globulin (40%) and albumin

Metabolism: Hepatic; forms metabolites, including dihydrotestosterone (DHT) and estradiol (both active)

Half-life elimination: Variable: 10-100 minutes

Excretion: Urine (90%); feces (6%)

Dosage

Adolescents and Adults: Males:

I.M.:

Primary hypogonadism or hypogonadotropic hypogonadism: Testosterone enanthate or testosterone cypionate: 50-400 mg every 2-4 weeks (FDA-approved dosing range); 75-100 mg/week or 150-200 mg every 2 weeks (Bhasin, 2010)

Delayed puberty: Testosterone enanthate: 50-200 mg every 2-4 weeks for a limited duration

Pellet (for subcutaneous implantation): Delayed puberty, primary hypogonadism or hypogonadotropic hypogonadism: 150-450 mg every 3-6 months

Adults:

I.M.: Females: Inoperable metastatic breast cancer: Testosterone enanthate: 200-400 mg every 2-4 weeks

Oral: Males: Conditions associated with a deficiency or absence of endogenous testosterone: Capsule (Andriol®; not available in U.S.): Initial: 120-160 mg/day in 2 divided doses for 2-3 weeks; adjust according to individual response; usual maintenance dose: 40-120 mg/day (in divided doses)

Topical: Primary male hypogonadism **or** hypogonadotropic hypogonadism:

Buccal: 30 mg twice daily (every 12 hours) applied to the gum region above the incisor tooth

Gel: Apply to clean, dry, intact skin. **Do not apply testosterone gel to the genitals.**

AndroGel® 1%, Testim®: 5 g (to deliver 50 mg of testosterone with 5 mg systemically absorbed) applied once daily (preferably in the morning) to the shoulder and upper arms. AndroGel® 1% may also be applied to the abdomen. Dosage may be increased to a maximum of 10 g (100 mg).

Dose adjustment based on testosterone levels:

Less than normal range: Increase dose from 5 g to 7.5 g to 10 g

Greater than normal range: Decrease dose. Discontinue if consistently above normal at 5 g/day

AndroGel® 1.62%: 40.5 mg applied once daily in the morning to the shoulder and upper arms. Dosage may be increased to a maximum of 81 mg.

Dose adjustment based on testosterone levels:

>750 ng/dL: Decrease dose by 20.25 mg/day

≥350 ng/dL to ≤750 ng/dL: Maintain current dose

<350 ng/dL: Increase dose by 20.25 mg/day

Fortesta™: 40 mg once daily in the morning. Apply to the thighs. Dosing range: 10-70 mg/day

Dose adjustment based on serum testosterone levels:

≥2500 ng/dL: Decrease dose by 20 mg/day

≥1250 to <2500 ng/dL: Decrease dose by 10 mg/day

≥500 and <1250 ng/dL: Maintain current dose

<500 ng/dL: Increase dose by 10 mg/day

Solution: Axiron®: 60 mg once daily. (Dosage range 30-120 mg/day). Apply to the axilla at the same time each morning; do not apply to other parts of the body. Apply to clean, dry, intact skin. **Do not apply testosterone solution to the genitals.**

Dose adjustment based on serum testosterone levels:

>1050 ng/dL: Decrease 60 mg/day dose to 30 mg/day; if levels >1050 ng/dL persist after dose reduction discontinue therapy

<300 ng/dL: Increase 60 mg/day dose to 90 mg/day, or increase 90 mg/day dose to 120 mg/day

Transdermal system (Androderm®): **Note:** Patches are available in 2 mg, 2.5 mg, 4 mg, and 5 mg strengths. Initial dose is either 4 mg/day or 5 mg/day and dose adjustment varies as follows:

Initial: 4 mg/day (as one 4 mg/day patch; do **not** use two 2 mg/day patches)

Dose adjustment based on testosterone levels:

>930 ng/dL: Decrease dose to 2 mg/day

400-930 ng/dL: Continue 4 mg/day

<400 ng/dL: Increase dose to 6 mg/day (as one 4 mg/day and one 2 mg/day patch)

Initial: 5 mg/day (as one 5 mg/day or two 2.5 mg/day patches)

Dose adjustment based on testosterone levels:

>1030 ng/dL: Decrease dose to 2.5 mg/day

300-1030 ng/dL: Continue 5 mg/day

<300 ng/dL: Increase dose to 7.5 mg/day (as one 5 mg/day and one 2.5 mg/day patch)

Dosing conversion: If needed, patients may be switched from the 2.5 mg/day, 5 mg/day, and 7.5 mg/day patches as follows. Patch change should occur at their next scheduled dosing. Measure early morning testosterone concentrations ~2 weeks after switching therapy:

From 2.5 mg/day patch to 2 mg/day patch

From 5 mg/day patch to 4 mg/day patch

From 7.5 mg/day patch to 6 mg/day patch (one 2 mg/day and one 4 mg/day patch)

Dosing adjustment in renal impairment: No dosage adjustment provided in manufacturer's labeling (has not been studied). Use with caution; may enhance edema formation.

Dosing adjustment in hepatic impairment: No dosage adjustment provided in manufacturer's labeling (has not been studied). Use with caution; may enhance edema formation.

Dietary Considerations Testosterone USP may be synthesized from soy. Food and beverages have not been found to interfere with buccal system; ensure system is in place following eating, drinking, or brushing teeth.

Administration

I.M.: Warm to room temperature; shaking vial will help redissolve crystals that have formed after storage. Administer by deep I.M. injection into the upper outer quadrant of the gluteus maximus.

Oral, buccal application (Striant®): One mucoadhesive for buccal application (buccal system) should be applied to a comfortable area above the incisor tooth. Apply flat side of system to gum. Rotate to alternate sides of mouth with each application. Hold buccal system firmly in place for 30 seconds to ensure adhesion. The buccal system should adhere to gum for 12 hours. If the buccal system falls out, replace with a new system. If the system falls out within 4 hours of next dose, the new buccal system should remain in place until the time of the following scheduled dose. System will soften and mold to shape of gum as it absorbs moisture from mouth. Do not chew or swallow the buccal system. The buccal system will not dissolve; gently remove by sliding downwards from gum; avoid scratching gum.

Oral, capsule (Andriol®; not available in the U.S.): Should be administered with meals. Should be swallowed whole; do not crush or chew.

Transdermal patch (Androderm®): Apply patch to clean, dry area of skin on the back, abdomen, upper arms, or thigh. Do not apply to bony areas or parts of the body that are subject to prolonged pressure while sleeping or sitting. **Do not apply to the scrotum.** Avoid showering, washing the site, or swimming for 3 hours after application. Following patch removal, mild skin irritation may be treated with OTC hydrocortisone cream. A small amount of triamcinolone acetonide 0.1% cream may be applied under the system to decrease irritation; do not use ointment. Patch should be applied nightly. Rotate administration sites, allowing 7 days between applying to the same site.

Topical gel and solution: Apply to clean, dry, intact skin. Application sites should be allowed to dry for a few minutes prior to dressing. Hands should be washed with soap and water after application. **Do not apply testosterone gel or solution to the genitals.** Alcohol-based gels and solutions are flammable; avoid fire or smoking until dry. Testosterone may be transferred to another person following skin-to-skin contact with the application site. Strict adherence to application instructions is needed in order to decrease secondary exposure. Thoroughly wash hands after application and cover application site with clothing (ie, shirt) once gel or solution has dried, or clean application site thoroughly with soap and water prior to contact in order to minimize transfer. In addition to skin-to-skin contact, secondary exposure has also been reported following exposure to secondary items (eg, towel, shirt, sheets). If secondary exposure occurs, the other person should thoroughly wash the skin with soap and water as soon as possible.

AndroGel® 1%, AndroGel® 1.62%, Testim®: Apply (preferably in the morning) to clean, dry, intact skin of the shoulder and upper arms. AndroGel® 1% may also be applied to the abdomen; do not apply AndroGel® 1.62% or Testim® to the abdomen. Area of application should be limited to what will be covered by a short sleeve t-shirt. Apply at the same time each day. Upon opening the packet(s), the entire contents should be squeezed into the palm of the hand and immediately applied to the application site(s). Alternatively, a portion may be squeezed onto palm of hand and applied, repeating the process until entire packet has been applied. Application site should not be washed for ≥2 hours following application of AndroGel® 1.62% or Testim®, or >5 hours for AndroGel® 1%.

AndroGel® 1% multidose pump: Prime pump 3 times (and discard this portion of product) prior to initial use. Each actuation delivers 1.25 g of gel (4 actuations = 5 g; 6 actuations = 7.5 g; 8 actuations = 10 g); each actuation may be applied individually or all at the same time.

AndroGel® 1.62% multidose pump: Prime pump 3 times (and discard this portion of product) prior to initial use. Each actuation delivers 20.25 mg of gel (2 actuations = 40.5 mg; 3 actuations = 60.75 mg; 4 actuations = 81 mg); each actuation may be applied individually or all at the same time.

Axiron®: Apply using the applicator to the axilla at the same time each morning. Do not apply to other parts of the body (eg, abdomen, genitals, shoulders, upper arms). Avoid washing the site or swimming for 2 hours after application. Prior to first use, prime the applicator pump by depressing it 3 times (discard this portion of the product). After priming, position the nozzle over the applicator cup and depress pump fully one time; ensure liquid enters cup. Each pump actuation delivers testosterone 30 mg. No more than 30 mg (one pump) should be added to the cup at one time. The total dose should be divided between axilla (example, 30 mg/day: apply to one axilla only; 60 mg/day: apply 30 mg to each axilla; 90 mg/day: apply 30 mg to each axilla, allow to dry, then apply an additional 30 mg to one axilla; etc). To apply dose, keep applicator upright and wipe into the axilla; if solution runs or drips, use cup to wipe. Do not rub into skin with fingers or hand. If more than one 30 mg dose is needed, repeat process. Apply roll-on or stick antiperspirants or deodorants prior to testosterone. Once application site is dry, cover with clothing. After use, rinse applicator under running water and pat dry with a tissue. The application site and dose of this product are not interchangeable with other topical testosterone products.

Fortesta™: Apply to skin of front and inner thighs. Do not apply to other parts of the body. Use one finger to rub gel evenly onto skin of each thigh. Avoid showering, washing the site, or swimming for 2 hours after application. Prior to first dose, prime the pump by holding canister upright and fully depressing the pump 8 times (discard this portion of the product). Each pump actuation delivers testosterone 10 mg. The total dose should be divided between thighs (example, 10 mg/day: apply 10 mg to one thigh only; 20 mg/day: apply 10 mg to each thigh; 30 mg/day: apply 20 mg to one thigh and 10 mg to the other thigh; etc). Once application site is dry, cover with clothing. The application site and dose of this product are not interchangeable with other topical testosterone products.

Monitoring Parameters Periodic liver function tests, cholesterol, hemoglobin and hematocrit (prior to therapy, at 3-6 months, then annually); radiologic examination of wrist and hand every 6 months (when using in prepubertal children). Withhold initial treatment with hematocrit >50%, hyperviscosity, untreated obstructive sleep apnea, or uncontrolled severe heart failure. Monitor urine and serum calcium and signs of virilization in women treated for breast cancer. Serum glucose (may be decreased by testosterone, monitor patients with diabetes). Evaluate males for response to treatment and adverse events 3-6 months after initiation and then annually.

Bone mineral density: Monitor after 1-2 years of therapy in hypogonadal men with osteoporosis or low trauma fracture (Bhasin, 2010)

PSA: In men >40 years of age with baseline PSA >0.6 ng/mL, PSA and prostate exam (prior to therapy, at 3-6 months, then as based on current guidelines). Withhold treatment pending urological evaluation in patients with palpable prostate nodule or induration or PSA >4 ng/mL or if PSA >3 ng/mL in men at high risk of prostate cancer (Bhasin, 2010).

Do not treat with severe untreated BPH with IPSS symptom score >19.

Serum testosterone: After initial dose titration (if applicable), monitor 3-6 months after initiating treatment, then annually.

Injection: Measure midway between injections. Adjust dose or frequency if testosterone concentration is <400 ng/dL or >700 ng/dL (Bhasin, 2010).

AndroGel® 1%, Testim®: Morning serum testosterone levels ~14 days after start of therapy or dose adjustments

AndroGel® 1.62%: Morning serum testosterone levels after 14 and 28 days of starting therapy or dose adjustments and periodically thereafter

Androderm®: Morning serum testosterone levels (following application the previous evening) ~14 days after start of therapy or dose adjustments

Axiron®: Serum testosterone levels can be measured 2-8 hours after application and after 14 days of starting therapy or dose adjustments

Fortesta™: Serum testosterone levels can be measured 2 hours after application and after 14 and 35 days of starting therapy or dose adjustments

Striant®: Application area of gums; total serum testosterone 4-12 weeks after initiating treatment, prior to morning dose

Testopel®: Measure at the end of the dosing interval (Bhasin, 2010)

Reference Range

Total testosterone, males:

12-13 years: <800 ng/dL
14 years: <1200 ng/dL
15-16 years: 100-1200ng/dL
17-18 years: 300-1200 ng/dL
19-40 years: 300-950 ng/dL
>40 years: 240-950 ng/dL

Free testosterone, males: 9-30 ng/dL

Test Interactions Testosterone may decrease thyroxine-binding globulin, resulting in decreased total T_4; free thyroid hormone levels are not changed.

Dosage Forms Excipient information presented when available (limited, particularly for generics); consult specific product labeling. [DSC] = Discontinued product

Cream, topical [compounding kit]:
First®-Testosterone MC: 2% (60 g) [contains benzyl alcohol, sesame oil]

Gel, topical:
AndroGel®: 1% [5 g gel/packet] (30s); 1% [2.5 g gel/packet] (30s); 1% [1.25 g gel/actuation] (75 g) [contains ethanol 67%; may be chemically synthesized from soy]
AndroGel®: 1.62% [1.25 g gel/actuation] (75 g) [contains ethanol]
Fortesta™: 10 mg/actuation (60 g) [contains ethanol; 0.5 g gel/actuation; 120 metered actuations]
Testim®: 1% [5 g gel/tube] (30s) [contains ethanol 74%; may be chemically synthesized from soy]

Implant, subcutaneous:
Testopel®: 75 mg (10s, 24s, 100s)

Injection, oil, as cypionate: 100 mg/mL (10 mL); 200 mg/mL (1 mL, 10 mL)
Depo®-Testosterone: 100 mg/mL (10 mL); 200 mg/mL (1 mL, 10 mL) [contains benzyl alcohol, benzyl benzoate, cottonseed oil]

Injection, oil, as enanthate: 200 mg/mL (5 mL)
Delatestryl®: 200 mg/mL (5 mL) [contains chlorobutanol, sesame oil]

Mucoadhesive, for buccal application [buccal system]:
Striant®: 30 mg (60s) [may be chemically synthesized from soy]

Ointment, topical [compounding kit]:
First®-Testosterone: 2% (60 g) [contains benzyl alcohol, sesame oil]

Patch, transdermal:
Androderm®: 2 mg/24 hours (60s); 2.5 mg/24 hours (60s [DSC]); 4 mg/24 hours (30s); 5 mg/24 hours (30s [DSC]) [contains ethanol, metal]

Powder, for prescription compounding [micronized]: USP: 100% (5 g, 25 g)

Powder, for prescription compounding, as propionate: USP: 100% (5 g, 25 g)

Solution, topical:
Axiron®: 30 mg/actuation (110 mL) [contains ethanol, isopropyl alcohol; 60 metered actuations]

Dosage Forms: Canada Excipient information presented when available (limited, particularly for generics); consult specific product labeling.

Capsule, gelatin, as undecanoate:
Andriol™: 40 mg (10s)

Controlled Substance C-III

◆ **Testosterone Cypionate** *see* Testosterone *on page 1654*

◆ **Testosterone Enanthate** *see* Testosterone *on page 1654*

◆ **Testred®** *see* MethylTESTOSTERone *on page 1114*

◆ **Tetanus and Diphtheria Toxoid** *see* Diphtheria and Tetanus Toxoid *on page 520*

Tetanus Immune Globulin (Human)

(TET a nus i MYUN GLOB yoo lin HYU man)

Brand Names: U.S. HyperTET™ S/D
Brand Names: Canada HyperTET™ S/D
Index Terms TIG
Pharmacologic Category Immune Globulin

Use Prophylaxis against tetanus following injury in patients where immunization status is not known or uncertain

The Advisory Committee on Immunization Practices (ACIP) recommends passive immunization with TIG for the following:

- Persons with a wound that is not clean or minor and in whom contraindications to a tetanus-toxoid containing vaccine exist and they have not completed a primary series of tetanus toxoid immunization.
- Persons who are wounded in bombings or similar mass casualty events who have penetrating injuries or non-intact skin exposure and who cannot confirm receipt of a tetanus booster within the previous 5 years. In case of shortage, use should be reserved for persons ≥60 years of age.

Pregnancy Risk Factor C

Pregnancy Considerations Animal reproduction studies have not been conducted. Tetanus immune globulin and a tetanus toxoid containing vaccine are recommended by the ACIP as part of the standard wound management to prevent tetanus in pregnant women.

Warnings/Precautions Hypersensitivity and anaphylactic reactions can occur; immediate treatment (including epinephrine 1:1000) should be available. Use caution in patients with isolated immunoglobulin A deficiency or a history of systemic hypersensitivity to human immunoglobulins. Use with caution in patients with thrombocytopenia or coagulation disorders; I.M. injections may be contraindicated. Product of human plasma; may potentially contain infectious agents which could transmit disease. Screening of donors, as well as testing and/or inactivation or removal of certain viruses, reduces the risk. Infections thought to be transmitted by this product should be reported to the manufacturer. Skin testing should not be performed as local irritation can occur and be misinterpreted as a positive reaction. Not for intravenous administration.

Adverse Reactions Frequency not defined.

Central nervous system: Temperature increased
Dermatologic: Angioneurotic edema (rare)
Local: Injection site: Pain, soreness, tenderness
Renal: Nephritic syndrome (rare)
Miscellaneous: Anaphylactic shock (rare)

Drug Interactions

Metabolism/Transport Effects None known.

Avoid Concomitant Use There are no known interactions where it is recommended to avoid concomitant use.

Increased Effect/Toxicity There are no known significant interactions involving an increase in effect.

Decreased Effect

Tetanus Immune Globulin (Human) may decrease the levels/effects of: Vaccines (Live)

Stability Store at 2°C to 8°C (26°F to 46°F). Do not use if frozen. The following stability information has also been reported for HyperTET™ S/D: May be exposed to room temperature for a cumulative 7 days (Cohen, 2007).

Mechanism of Action Passive immunity toward tetanus

Pharmacodynamics/Kinetics Absorption: Well absorbed

Dosage I.M.:

Prophylaxis of tetanus:

Children <7 years: 4 units/kg; some recommend administering 250 units to small children

Children ≥7 years and Adults: 250 units

Tetanus prophylaxis in wound management: Children and Adults: Tetanus prophylaxis in patients with wounds should consider if the wound is clean or contaminated, the immunization status of the patient, proper use of tetanus toxoid and/or tetanus immune globulin (TIG), wound cleaning, and (if required) surgical debridement and the proper use of antibiotics. Patients with an uncertain or incomplete tetanus immunization status should have additional follow up to ensure a series is completed. Patients with a history of Arthus reaction following a previous dose of a tetanus toxoid-containing vaccine should not receive a tetanus toxoid-containing vaccine until >10 years after the most recent dose even if they have a wound that is neither clean nor minor. See table.

Tetanus Prophylaxis in Wound Management

History of Tetanus Immunization Doses	Clean, Minor Wounds		All Other Wounds[1]	
	Tetanus Toxoid[2]	TIG	Tetanus Toxoid[2]	TIG
Uncertain or <3 doses	Yes	No	Yes	Yes
3 or more doses	No[3]	No	No[4]	No

[1]Such as, but not limited to, wounds contaminated with dirt, feces, soil, and saliva; puncture wounds; wounds from crushing, tears, burns, and frostbite.

[2]Tetanus toxoid in this chart refers to a tetanus toxoid-containing vaccine. For children <7 years of age, DTaP (DT, if pertussis vaccine contraindicated) is preferred to tetanus toxoid alone. For children ≥7 years and Adults, Td preferred to tetanus toxoid alone; Tdap may be preferred if the patient has not previously been vaccinated with Tdap.

[3]Yes, if ≥10 years since last dose.

[4]Yes, if ≥5 years since last dose.

Adapted from CDC "Yellow Book" (*Health Information for International Travel 2010*), "Routine Vaccine-Preventable Diseases, Tetanus" (available at http://www.cdc.gov/yellowbook) and *MMWR* 2006, 55 (RR-17).

Abbreviations: **DT** = Diphtheria and Tetanus Toxoids (formulation for age ≤6 years); **DTaP** = Diphtheria and Tetanus Toxoids, and Acellular Pertussis (formulation for age ≤6 years; Daptacel®, Infanrix®, Tripedia®); **Td** = Diphtheria and Tetanus Toxoids (formulation for age ≥7 years; Decavac®); **TT**= Tetanus toxoid (adsorbed [formulation for age ≥7 years]); **Tdap** = Diphtheria and Tetanus Toxoids, and Acellular Pertussis (Adacel® or Boostrix® [formulations for age ≥7 years]); **TIG** = Tetanus Immune Globulin

Treatment of tetanus: Children and Adults: 500-6000 units. Infiltration of part of the dose around the wound is recommended.

Administration Do not administer I.V.; I.M. use only. Administer in the anterolateral aspects of the upper thigh or the deltoid muscle of the upper arm. Avoid gluteal region due to risk of injury to sciatic nerve; if gluteal region is used, administer only in the upper outer quadrant. If tetanus vaccine and tetanus immune globulin are administered simultaneously, separate sites should be used for each injection. When used for the treatment of tetanus, infiltration of part of the dose around the wound is recommended.

Additional Information Tetanus immune globulin (TIG) must not contain <50 units/mL. Protein makes up 10% to 18% of TIG preparations. The great majority of this (≥90%) is IgG. TIG has almost no color or odor and it is a sterile, nonpyrogenic, concentrated preparation of immunoglobulins that has been derived from the plasma of adults hyperimmunized with tetanus toxoid. The pooled material from which the immunoglobulin is derived may be from fewer than 1000 donors. This plasma has been shown to be free of hepatitis B surface antigen.

Dosage Forms Excipient information presented when available (limited, particularly for generics); consult specific product labeling.

Injection, solution [preservative free]:

HyperTET™ S/D: 250 units/mL (~1 mL)

◆ **Tetanus Toxoid** *see* Diphtheria and Tetanus Toxoids, Acellular Pertussis, Poliovirus and *Haemophilus* b Conjugate Vaccine *on page* 522

Tetanus Toxoid (Adsorbed)

(TET a nus TOKS oyd, ad SORBED)

Index Terms TT

Pharmacologic Category Vaccine, Inactivated (Bacterial)

Additional Appendix Information

Immunization Recommendations *on page 1922*

Use Active immunization against tetanus when combination antigen preparations are not indicated; tetanus prophylaxis in wound management. **Note:** Tetanus and diphtheria toxoids for adult use (Td) is the preferred immunizing agent for most adults and for children after their seventh birthday. Young children should receive trivalent DTaP (diphtheria/tetanus/acellular pertussis) as part of their childhood immunization program, unless pertussis is contraindicated, then DT is warranted.

Pregnancy Risk Factor C

Pregnancy Considerations Animal studies have not been conducted. Inactivated bacterial vaccines have not been shown to cause increased risks to the fetus (CDC, 2011). The ACIP recommends vaccination in previously unvaccinated women or in women with an incomplete vaccination series, whose child may be born in unhygienic conditions. Tetanus immune globulin and a tetanus toxoid-containing vaccine are recommended by the ACIP as part of the standard wound management to prevent tetanus in pregnant women. Vaccination using Td is preferred.

Lactation Excretion in breast milk unknown/use caution

Contraindications Hypersensitivity to tetanus toxoid or any component of the formulation

Warnings/Precautions Avoid injection into a blood vessel; allergic reactions may occur; epinephrine 1:1000 must be available. Patients who are immunocompromised may have reduced response; may be used in patients with HIV infection. In general, household and close contacts of persons with altered immunocompetence may receive all age appropriate vaccines. May defer elective immunization during febrile illness or acute infection. In patients with a history of severe local reaction (Arthus-type) following previous dose, do not give further routine or emergency doses of tetanus and diphtheria toxoids for 10 years. Use caution in patients on anticoagulants, with thrombocytopenia, or bleeding disorders (bleeding may occur following intramuscular injection). Use with caution if Guillain-Barré syndrome occurred within 6 weeks of prior tetanus toxoid. Contains thimerosal. This product is not indicated for use in children <7 years of age. In order to maximize vaccination rates, the ACIP recommends simultaneous administration of all age-appropriate vaccines (live or inactivated) for which a person is eligible at a single clinic visit, unless contraindications exist. The use of combination vaccines is generally preferred over separate injections, taking into consideration provider assessment, patient preference, and adverse events. When using combination vaccines, the minimum age for administration is the oldest minimum age for any individual component; the minimum interval between dosing is the greatest minimum interval between any individual component.

Adverse Reactions All serious adverse reactions must be reported to the U.S. Department of Health and Human Services (DHHS) Vaccine Adverse Event Reporting System (VAERS) 1-800-822-7967 or online at https://vaers.hhs.gov/esub/index.

Frequency not defined.

Cardiovascular: Hypotension

Central nervous system: Brachial neuritis, fever, malaise, pain

Gastrointestinal: Nausea

Local: Edema, induration (with or without tenderness), rash, redness, urticaria, warmth

Neuromuscular: Arthralgia, Guillain-Barré syndrome

Miscellaneous: Anaphylactic reaction, Arthus-type hypersensitivity reaction

Drug Interactions

Metabolism/Transport Effects None known.

Avoid Concomitant Use There are no known interactions where it is recommended to avoid concomitant use.

Increased Effect/Toxicity There are no known significant interactions involving an increase in effect.

Decreased Effect

The levels/effects of Tetanus Toxoid (Adsorbed) may be decreased by: Belimumab; Fingolimod; Immunosuppressants

Stability Store at 2°C to 8°C (26°F to 46°F); do not freeze.

Mechanism of Action Tetanus toxoid preparations contain the toxin produced by virulent tetanus bacilli (detoxified growth products of *Clostridium tetani*). The toxin has been modified by treatment with formaldehyde so that it has lost toxicity but still retains ability to act as antigen and produce active immunity; the aluminum salt, a mineral adjuvant, delays the rate of absorption and prolongs and enhances its properties; duration ~10 years.

Pharmacodynamics/Kinetics Duration: Primary immunization: ~10 years

Dosage Note: In most patients, Td is the recommended product for primary immunization, booster doses, and tetanus immunization in wound management (refer to Diphtheria and Tetanus Toxoid monograph).

Children ≥7 years and Adults: I.M.:

Primary immunization: 0.5 mL; repeat 0.5 mL at 4-8 weeks after first dose and at 6-12 months after second dose

Routine booster dose: Recommended every 10 years

Tetanus prophylaxis in wound management: Tetanus prophylaxis in patients with wounds should consider if the wound is clean or contaminated, the immunization status of the patient, proper use of tetanus toxoid and/or tetanus immune globulin (TIG), wound cleaning, and (if required) surgical debridement and the proper use of antibiotics. Patients with an uncertain or incomplete tetanus immunization status should have additional follow up to ensure a series is completed. Patients with a history of Arthus reaction following a previous dose of a tetanus toxoid-containing vaccine should not receive a tetanus toxoid-containing vaccine until >10 years after the most recent dose even if they have a wound that is neither clean nor minor. See table.

Tetanus Prophylaxis in Wound Management

History of Tetanus Immunization Doses	Clean, Minor Wounds		All Other Wounds[1]	
	Tetanus Toxoid[2]	TIG	Tetanus Toxoid[2]	TIG
Uncertain or <3 doses	Yes	No	Yes	Yes
3 or more doses	No[3]	No	No[4]	No

[1]Such as, but not limited to, wounds contaminated with dirt, feces, soil, and saliva; puncture wounds; wounds from crushing, tears, burns, and frostbite.

[2]Tetanus toxoid in this chart refers to a tetanus toxoid-containing vaccine. For children <7 years of age, DTaP (DT, if pertussis vaccine contraindicated) is preferred to tetanus toxoid alone. For children ≥7 years and Adults, Td preferred to tetanus toxoid alone; Tdap may be preferred if the patient has not previously been vaccinated with Tdap.

[3]Yes, if ≥10 years since last dose.

[4]Yes, if ≥5 years since last dose.

Adapted from CDC "Yellow Book" (*Health Information for International Travel 2010*), "Routine Vaccine-Preventable Diseases, Tetanus" (available at http://www.cdc.gov/yellowbook) and *MMWR* 2006, 55 (RR-17).

Abbreviations: **DT** = Diphtheria and Tetanus Toxoids (formulation for age ≤6 years); **DTaP** = Diphtheria and Tetanus Toxoids, and Acellular Pertussis (formulation for age ≤6 years; Daptacel®, Infanrix®, Tripedia®); **Td** = Diphtheria and Tetanus Toxoids (formulation for age ≥7 years; Decavac®); **TT**= Tetanus toxoid (adsorbed [formulation for age ≥7 years]); **Tdap** = Diphtheria and Tetanus Toxoids, and Acellular Pertussis (Adacel® or Boostrix® [formulations for age ≥7 years]); **TIG** = Tetanus Immune Globulin

Administration Inject intramuscularly in the area of the vastus lateralis (midthigh laterally) or deltoid. Do not inject into gluteal area. Shake well prior to withdrawing dose; do not use if product does not form a suspension.

For patients at risk of hemorrhage following intramuscular injection, the ACIP recommends "it should be administered intramuscularly if, in the opinion of the physician familiar with the patients bleeding risk, the vaccine can be administered by this route with reasonable safety. If the patient receives antihemophilia or other similar therapy, intramuscular vaccination can be scheduled shortly after such therapy is administered. A fine needle (23 gauge or smaller) can be used for the vaccination and firm pressure applied to the site (without rubbing) for at least 2 minutes. The patient should be instructed concerning the risk of hematoma from the injection." Patients on anticoagulant therapy should be considered to have the same bleeding risks and treated as those with clotting factor disorders (CDC, 2011).

Simultaneous administration of vaccines helps ensure the patients will be fully vaccinated by the appropriate age. Simultaneous administration of vaccines is defined as administering >1 vaccine on the same day at different anatomic sites. The use of licensed combination vaccines is generally preferred over separate injections of the equivalent components. Separate vaccines should not be combined in the same syringe unless indicated by product specific labeling. Separate needles and syringes should be used for each injection. The ACIP prefers each dose of a specific vaccine in a series come from the same manufacturer when possible. Adolescents and adults should be vaccinated while seated or lying down. In general, preterm infants should be vaccinated at the same chronological age as full-term infants (CDC, 2011).

Antipyretics have not been shown to prevent febrile seizures. Antipyretics may be used to treat fever or discomfort following vaccination (CDC, 2011). One study reported that routine prophylactic administration of acetaminophen to prevent fever prior to vaccination decreased the immune response of some vaccines; the clinical significance of this reduction in immune response has not been established (Prymula, 2009).

Additional Information Federal law requires that the name of medication, date of administration, the vaccine manufacturer, lot number of vaccine, and the administering person's name, title and address be entered into the patient's permanent medical record.

Dosage Forms Excipient information presented when available (limited, particularly for generics); consult specific product labeling.

Injection, suspension: 5 Lf units/0.5 mL (0.5 mL) [contains aluminum and thimerosal (may have trace amounts)]

◆ **Tetanus Toxoid, Reduced Diphtheria Toxoid, and Acellular Pertussis, Adsorbed** *see* Diphtheria and Tetanus Toxoids, and Acellular Pertussis Vaccine *on page 523*

◆ **Tetcaine** *see* Tetracaine (Ophthalmic) *on page 1661*

Tetrabenazine (tet ra BEN a zeen)

Brand Names: U.S. Xenazine®

Brand Names: Canada Nitoman™

Pharmacologic Category Central Monoamine-Depleting Agent

Use Treatment of chorea associated with Huntington's disease

Canadian labeling: Treatment of hyperkinetic movement disorders, including Huntington's chorea, hemiballismus, senile chorea, Tourette syndrome, and tardive dyskinesia

Pregnancy Risk Factor C

Prescribing and Access Restrictions Xenazine® is available only through specialty pharmacies. For more information regarding the procurement of Xenazine®, healthcare providers, patients, and caregivers may contact the Xenazine® Information Center (XIC) at 1-888-882-6013 or at:

Healthcare providers: http://www.xenazineusa.com/HCP/PrescribingXenazine/Default.aspx

Patients and caregivers: http://www.xenazineusa.com/AboutXenazine/Getting-Your-Prescription.aspx

Medication Guide Available Yes

Dosage Oral: Dose should be individualized; titrate slowly

Chorea associated with Huntington's disease: Adults:

Initial: 12.5 mg once daily, may increase to 12.5 mg twice daily after 1 week

Maintenance: May be increased by 12.5 mg/day at weekly intervals; doses >37.5 mg/day should be divided into 3 doses (maximum single dose: 25 mg)

Patients requiring doses >50 mg/day: Genotype for CYP2D6:

Extensive/intermediate metabolizers: Maximum: 100 mg/day; 37.5 mg/dose

Poor metabolizers: Maximum: 50 mg/day; 25 mg/dose

Concomitant use with strong CYP2D6 inhibitors (eg, fluoxetine, paroxetine, quinidine): Dose of tetrabenazine should be reduced by 50% in patients receiving strong CYP2D6 inhibitors, follow dosing for poor CYP2D6 metabolizers. Use caution when adding a CYP2D6 inhibitor to patients already taking tetrabenazine.

Note: If treatment is interrupted for >5 days, retitration is recommended. If treatment is interrupted for <5 days resume at previous maintenance dose.

Canadian labeling: Hyperkinetic movement disorders:

Adults: Initial: 12.5 mg twice daily (may be given 3 times/day); may be increased by 12.5 mg/day every 3-5 days; should be titrated slowly to maximal tolerated and effective dose (dose is individualized)

Usual maximum tolerated dosage: 25 mg 3 times/day; maximum recommended dose: 200 mg/day

Note: If there is no improvement at the maximum tolerated dose after 7 days, improvement is unlikely; discontinuation should be considered.

Elderly and/or debilitated patients: Consider initiation at lower doses; must be titrated slowly to individualize dosage

Dosage adjustment for toxicity: For toxicity/adverse reaction, including akathisia, restlessness, parkinsonism, insomnia, depression, suicidality, anxiety, sedation (intolerable): Suspend upward dosage titration and reduce dose; consider discontinuing if adverse reaction does not resolve (may be discontinued without tapering).

Dosage adjustment in hepatic impairment: Use is contraindicated

Additional Information Complete prescribing information for this medication should be consulted for additional detail.

Dosage Forms Excipient information presented when available (limited, particularly for generics); consult specific product labeling.

Tablet, oral:

Xenazine®: 12.5 mg

Xenazine®: 25 mg [scored]

Dosage Forms: Canada Excipient information presented when available (limited, particularly for generics); consult specific product labeling.

Tablet:

Nitoman™: 25 mg

Tetracaine (Systemic) (TET ra kane)

Brand Names: Canada Pontocaine®

Index Terms Amethocaine Hydrochloride; Tetracaine Hydrochloride
Pharmacologic Category Local Anesthetic
Use Spinal anesthesia
Pregnancy Risk Factor C
Dosage Injection: Adults: Spinal anesthesia: **Note:** Dosage varies with the anesthetic procedure, the degree of anesthesia required, and the individual patient response; it is administered by subarachnoid injection for spinal anesthesia.
Perineal anesthesia: 5 mg
Perineal and lower extremities: 10 mg
Anesthesia extending up to costal margin: 15 mg; doses up to 20 mg may be given, but are reserved for exceptional cases
Low spinal anesthesia (saddle block): 2-5 mg
Additional Information Complete prescribing information for this medication should be consulted for additional detail.
Dosage Forms Excipient information presented when available (limited, particularly for generics); consult specific product labeling.
Injection, solution, as hydrochloride [preservative free]: 1% [10 mg/mL] (2 mL)

Tetracaine (Ophthalmic) (TET ra kane)

Brand Names: U.S. Altacaine; Tetcaine; TetraVisc™; TetraVisc™ FORTE
Brand Names: Canada Pontocaine®
Index Terms Amethocaine Hydrochloride; Tetracaine Hydrochloride
Pharmacologic Category Local Anesthetic
Use Local anesthesia for various ophthalmic procedures of short duration (eg, tonometry, gonioscopy); minor ophthalmic surgical procedures (eg, removal of corneal foreign bodies, suture removal); and for various diagnostic purposes (eg, conjunctival scrapings)
Pregnancy Risk Factor C
Dosage Ophthalmic: Adults:
Short-term (nonsurgical procedures) anesthesia: Instill 1-2 drops into affected eye just prior to evaluation
Minor surgical procedures: Instill 1-2 drops into affected eye every 5-10 minutes for up to 3 doses
Prolonged surgical procedures: Instill 1-2 drops into affected eye every 5-10 minutes for up to 5 doses
Additional Information Complete prescribing information for this medication should be consulted for additional detail.
Dosage Forms Excipient information presented when available (limited, particularly for generics); consult specific product labeling.
Solution, ophthalmic, as hydrochloride [drops]: 0.5% [5 mg/mL] (2 mL, 15 mL)
Altacaine: 0.5% [5 mg/mL] (15 mL, 30 mL) [contains chlorobutanol]
Tetcaine: 0.5% [5 mg/mL] (15 mL)
TetraVisc™: 0.5% [5 mg/mL) (0.6 mL, 5 mL) [contains benzalkonium chloride]
TetraVisc™ FORTE: 0.5% [5 mg/mL] (0.6 mL, 5 mL) [contains benzalkonium chloride]

Tetracaine (Topical) (TET ra kane)

Brand Names: U.S. Pontocaine® [DSC]
Brand Names: Canada Ametop™; Pontocaine®
Index Terms Amethocaine Hydrochloride; Tetracaine Hydrochloride
Pharmacologic Category Local Anesthetic
Use Applied to nose and throat for diagnostic procedures
Pregnancy Risk Factor C
Dosage Adults: Topical mucous membranes (rhinolaryngology): Used as a 0.25% or 0.5% solution by direct application or nebulization; total dose should not exceed 20 mg
Additional Information Complete prescribing information for this medication should be consulted for additional detail.
Dosage Forms Excipient information presented when available (limited, particularly for generics); consult specific product labeling. [DSC] = Discontinued product
Solution, topical, as hydrochloride [for rhinolaryngology]:
Pontocaine®: 2% [20 mg/mL] (30 mL [DSC], 118 mL [DSC])

◆ **Tetracaine and Lidocaine** *see* Lidocaine and Tetracaine *on page 1011*
◆ **Tetracaine, Benzocaine, and Butamben** *see* Benzocaine, Butamben, and Tetracaine *on page 204*
◆ **Tetracaine Hydrochloride** *see* Tetracaine (Ophthalmic) *on page 1661*
◆ **Tetracaine Hydrochloride** *see* Tetracaine (Systemic) *on page 1660*
◆ **Tetracaine Hydrochloride** *see* Tetracaine (Topical) *on page 1661*
◆ **Tetracosactide** *see* Cosyntropin *on page 415*

Tetracycline (tet ra SYE kleen)

Brand Names: Canada Apo-Tetra®; Nu-Tetra
Index Terms Achromycin; TCN; Tetracycline Hydrochloride
Pharmacologic Category Antibiotic, Tetracycline Derivative
Use Treatment of susceptible bacterial infections of both gram-positive and gram-negative organisms; also infections due to *Mycoplasma*, *Chlamydia*, and *Rickettsia*; indicated for acne, exacerbations of chronic bronchitis, and treatment of gonorrhea and syphilis in patients who are allergic to penicillin; as part of a multidrug regimen for *H. pylori* eradication to reduce the risk of duodenal ulcer recurrence
Unlabeled Use Treatment of periodontitis associated with presence of *Actinobacillus actinomycetemcomitans* (AA)
Pregnancy Risk Factor D
Pregnancy Considerations Tetracyclines cross the placenta, enter fetal circulation, and may cause permanent discoloration of teeth if used during the second or third trimester. Maternal hepatic toxicity has been associated with the use of tetracycline during pregnancy, especially in patients with azotemia or pyelonephritis. Because use during pregnancy may cause fetal harm, tetracycline is classified as pregnancy category D.
Lactation Enters breast milk/not recommended (AAP rates "compatible"; AAP 2001 update pending)
Contraindications Hypersensitivity to tetracycline or any component of the formulation; children <8 years of age; pregnancy
Warnings/Precautions Use with caution in patients with renal or hepatic impairment (eg, elderly); dosage modification required in patients with renal impairment since it may increase BUN as an antianabolic agent. Hepatotoxicity has been reported rarely; risk may be increased in patients with pre-existing hepatic or renal impairment. Pseudotumor cerebri has been reported with tetracycline use (usually resolves with discontinuation); outdated drug can cause nephropathy; use protective measure to avoid photosensitivity. Prolonged use may result in fungal or bacterial superinfection, including *C. difficile*-associated diarrhea (CDAD) and pseudomembranous colitis; CDAD has been observed >2 months postantibiotic treatment. May cause tissue hyperpigmentation, enamel hypoplasia,

or permanent tooth discoloration; use of tetracyclines should be avoided during tooth development (children <8 years of age) unless other drugs are not likely to be effective or are contraindicated. Do not use during pregnancy. In addition to affecting tooth development, tetracycline use has been associated with retardation of skeletal development and reduced bone growth.

Adverse Reactions Frequency not defined.

Cardiovascular: Pericarditis

Central nervous system: Bulging fontanels in infants, increased intracranial pressure, paresthesia, pseudotumor cerebri

Dermatologic: Exfoliative dermatitis, photosensitivity, pigmentation of nails, pruritus

Gastrointestinal: Abdominal cramps, anorexia, antibiotic-associated pseudomembranous colitis, diarrhea, discoloration of teeth and enamel hypoplasia (young children), esophagitis, nausea, pancreatitis, staphylococcal enterocolitis, vomiting

Hematologic: Thrombophlebitis

Hepatic: Hepatotoxicity

Renal: Acute renal failure, azotemia, renal damage

Miscellaneous: Anaphylaxis, candidal superinfection, hypersensitivity reactions, superinfection

Drug Interactions

Metabolism/Transport Effects Substrate of CYP3A4 (major); **Note:** Assignment of Major/Minor substrate status based on clinically relevant drug interaction potential; **Inhibits** CYP3A4 (moderate)

Avoid Concomitant Use

Avoid concomitant use of Tetracycline with any of the following: BCG; Pimozide; Retinoic Acid Derivatives; Tolvaptan

Increased Effect/Toxicity

Tetracycline may increase the levels/effects of: ARIPiprazole; Budesonide (Systemic, Oral Inhalation); Colchicine; CYP3A4 Substrates; Eplerenone; Everolimus; FentaNYL; Halofantrine; Lurasidone; Neuromuscular-Blocking Agents; Pimecrolimus; Pimozide; Porfimer; Propafenone; Ranolazine; Retinoic Acid Derivatives; Salmeterol; Saxagliptin; Tolvaptan; Vilazodone; Vitamin K Antagonists; Zuclopenthixol

The levels/effects of Tetracycline may be increased by: Conivaptan

Decreased Effect

Tetracycline may decrease the levels/effects of: Atovaquone; BCG; Penicillins; Typhoid Vaccine

The levels/effects of Tetracycline may be decreased by: Antacids; Bile Acid Sequestrants; Bismuth; Bismuth Subsalicylate; Calcium Salts; CYP3A4 Inducers (Strong); Deferasirox; Herbs (CYP3A4 Inducers); Iron Salts; Lanthanum; Magnesium Salts; Quinapril; Sucralfate; Tocilizumab; Zinc Salts

Ethanol/Nutrition/Herb Interactions

Food: Serum concentrations may be decreased if taken with dairy products.

Herb/Nutraceutical: Avoid dong quai, St John's wort (may also cause photosensitization).

Stability Outdated tetracyclines have caused a Fanconi-like syndrome. Protect oral dosage forms from light.

Mechanism of Action Inhibits bacterial protein synthesis by binding with the 30S and possibly the 50S ribosomal subunit(s) of susceptible bacteria; may also cause alterations in the cytoplasmic membrane

Pharmacodynamics/Kinetics

Absorption: Oral: 75%

Distribution: Small amount appears in bile

Relative diffusion from blood into CSF: Good only with inflammation (exceeds usual MICs)

CSF:blood level ratio: Inflamed meninges: 25%

Protein binding: ~65%

Half-life elimination: Normal renal function: 8-11 hours; End-stage renal disease: 57-108 hours

Time to peak, serum: Oral: 2-4 hours

Excretion: Urine (60% as unchanged drug); feces (as active form)

Dosage

Usual dosage range:

Children >8 years: Oral: 25-50 mg/kg/day in divided doses every 6 hours

Adults: Oral: 250-500 mg/dose every 6 hours

Indication-specific dosing:

Children ≥8 years: Oral:

Malaria, severe, treatment (unlabeled use): 25 mg/kg/day in divided doses every 6 hours (maximum dose: 250 mg every 6 hours) for 7 days with quinidine gluconate. **Note:** Quinidine gluconate duration is region specific; consult CDC for current recommendations (CDC, 2009).

Malaria, uncomplicated, treatment (unlabeled use): 25 mg/kg/day in divided doses every 6 hours (maximum dose: 250 mg every 6 hours) for 7 days with quinine sulfate. **Note:** Quinine sulfate duration is region specific; consult CDC for current recommendations (CDC, 2009).

Adults: Oral:

Acne: 250-500 twice daily

Chronic bronchitis, acute exacerbation: 500 mg 4 times/day

Erlichiosis: 500 mg 4 times/day for 7-14 days

Malaria, severe, treatment (unlabeled use): Oral: 250 mg 4 times/day for 7 days with quinidine gluconate. **Note:** Quinidine gluconate duration is region specific; consult CDC for current recommendations (CDC, 2009).

Malaria, uncomplicated, treatment (unlabeled use): Oral: 250 mg 4 times/day for 7 days with quinine sulfate. **Note:** Quinine sulfate duration is region specific; consult CDC for current recommendations (CDC, 2009).

Peptic ulcer disease: Eradication of *Helicobacter pylori*: 500 mg 2-4 times/day depending on regimen; requires combination therapy with at least one other antibiotic and an acid-suppressing agent (proton pump inhibitor or H_2 blocker)

Periodontitis (unlabeled use): 250 mg every 6 hours until improvement (usually 10 days)

Vibrio cholerae: 500 mg 4 times/day for 3 days

Dosing interval in renal impairment:

Cl_{cr} 50-80 mL/minute: Administer every 8-12 hours

Cl_{cr} 10-50 mL/minute: Administer every 12-24 hours

Cl_{cr} <10 mL/minute: Administer every 24 hours

Dialysis: Slightly dialyzable (5% to 20%) via hemo- and peritoneal dialysis or via continuous arteriovenous or venovenous hemofiltration; no supplemental dosage necessary

Dosing adjustment in hepatic impairment: Use caution; no dosing adjustment required

Dietary Considerations Take on an empty stomach (ie, 1 hour prior to, or 2 hours after meals). Take at least 1-2 hours prior to, or 4 hours after antacid.

Administration Should be administered on an empty stomach (ie, 1 hour prior to, or 2 hours after meals) to increase total absorption. Administer at least 1-2 hours prior to, or 4 hours after antacid because aluminum and magnesium cations may chelate with tetracycline and reduce its total absorption.

Monitoring Parameters Renal, hepatic, and hematologic function test, temperature, WBC, cultures and sensitivity, appetite, mental status

Test Interactions False-negative urine glucose with Clinistix®

Dosage Forms Excipient information presented when available (limited, particularly for generics); consult specific product labeling.

Capsule, oral, as hydrochloride: 250 mg, 500 mg

Extemporaneous Preparations A 25 mg/mL oral suspension may be made using capsules. Empty the contents of six 500 mg capsules into mortar. Add a small amount (~20 mL) of a 1:1 mixture of Ora-Sweet® and Ora-Plus® and mix to a uniform paste; mix while adding the vehicle in geometric proportions to **almost** 120 mL; transfer to a calibrated bottle, rinse mortar with vehicle, and add quantity of vehicle sufficient to make 120 mL. Label "shake well" and "refrigerate". Stable 28 days refrigerated.

Nahata MC, Pai VB, and Hipple TF, *Pediatric Drug Formulations*, 5th ed, Cincinnati, OH: Harvey Whitney Books Co, 2004.

- ◆ **Tetracycline Hydrochloride** *see* Tetracycline *on page 1661*
- ◆ **Tetrahydrocannabinol** *see* Dronabinol *on page 561*
- ◆ **Tetraiodothyronine and Triiodothyronine** *see* Thyroid, Desiccated *on page 1676*
- ◆ **2,2,2-tetramine** *see* Trientine *on page 1736*

Tetrastarch (TET ra starch)

Brand Names: U.S. Voluven®
Brand Names: Canada Voluven®
Index Terms HES; HES 130/0.4; Hydroxyethyl Starch
Pharmacologic Category Plasma Volume Expander, Colloid
Use Blood volume expander used in treatment and prevention of hypovolemia
Pregnancy Risk Factor C
Dosage I.V. infusion: Plasma volume expansion: **Note:** With severe dehydration, administer crystalloid first. Daily dose and rate of infusion dependent on amount of blood lost, on maintenance or restoration of hemodynamics, and on amount of hemodilution. Titrate to individual colloid needs, hemodynamics, and hydration status.

Infants and Children <2 years:

Manufacturer labeling: Average dose: 7-25 mL/kg

Unlabeled dosing: 10 mL/kg/dose (range: 7-50 mL/kg) individualized to patient colloid needs based on intraoperative hemodynamic and hydration status (Chong Sung, 2006; Hanart, 2009; Lochbühler, 2003; Osthaus, 2008; Sumpelman, 2008; Witt, 2008).

Children 2-12 years (unlabeled dosing): 10 mL/kg/dose (maximum dose: 50 mL/kg/day) individualized to patient colloid needs based on intraoperative hemodynamic and hydration status (Chong Sung, 2006; Hanart, 2009; Osthaus, 2008; Sumpelman, 2008, Witt, 2008).

Children >12 years: Administer up to 50 mL/kg/day (or up to 3500 mL in a 70 kg patient); may administer repetitively over several days.

Adults: Administer up to 50 mL/kg/day (or up to 3500 mL in a 70 kg patient); may administer repetitively over several days

Dosage adjustment in renal impairment: Contraindicated in oliguric/anuric renal failure unrelated to hypovolemia or patients receiving hemodialysis

Dosage adjustment in hepatic impairment: Use with caution in severe impairment

Additional Information Complete prescribing information for this medication should be consulted for additional detail.

Dosage Forms Excipient information presented when available (limited, particularly for generics); consult specific product labeling.

Infusion, premixed in NS:

Voluven®: 6% (500 mL)

- ◆ **TetraVisc™** *see* Tetracaine (Ophthalmic) *on page 1661*
- ◆ **TetraVisc™ FORTE** *see* Tetracaine (Ophthalmic) *on page 1661*
- ◆ **Teva-Acebutolol (Can)** *see* Acebutolol *on page 27*
- ◆ **Teva-Acyclovir (Can)** *see* Acyclovir (Systemic) *on page 39*
- ◆ **Teva-Alendronate (Can)** *see* Alendronate *on page 61*
- ◆ **Teva-Alfuzosin PR (Can)** *see* Alfuzosin *on page 64*
- ◆ **Teva-Alprazolam (Can)** *see* ALPRAZolam *on page 72*
- ◆ **Teva-Amiodarone (Can)** *see* Amiodarone *on page 90*
- ◆ **Teva-Amlodipine (Can)** *see* AmLODIPine *on page 97*
- ◆ **Teva-Atenolol (Can)** *see* Atenolol *on page 161*
- ◆ **Teva-Azathioprine (Can)** *see* AzaTHIOprine *on page 176*
- ◆ **Teva-Captopril (Can)** *see* Captopril *on page 277*
- ◆ **Teva-Carbamazepine (Can)** *see* CarBAMazepine *on page 280*
- ◆ **Teva-Citalopram (Can)** *see* Citalopram *on page 370*
- ◆ **Teva-Clindamycin (Can)** *see* Clindamycin (Systemic) *on page 378*
- ◆ **Teva-Diltiazem (Can)** *see* Diltiazem *on page 510*
- ◆ **Teva-Diltiazem CD (Can)** *see* Diltiazem *on page 510*
- ◆ **Teva-Diltiazem HCL ER Capsules (Can)** *see* Diltiazem *on page 510*
- ◆ **Teva-Enalapril (Can)** *see* Enalapril *on page 584*
- ◆ **Teva-Finasteride (Can)** *see* Finasteride *on page 713*
- ◆ **Teva-Fluoxetine (Can)** *see* FLUoxetine *on page 731*
- ◆ **Teva-Flutamide (Can)** *see* Flutamide *on page 738*
- ◆ **Teva-Fosinopril (Can)** *see* Fosinopril *on page 763*
- ◆ **Teva-Gabapentin (Can)** *see* Gabapentin *on page 773*
- ◆ **Teva-Glyburide (Can)** *see* GlyBURIDE *on page 799*
- ◆ **Teva-Irbesartan (Can)** *see* Irbesartan *on page 925*
- ◆ **Teva-Irbesartan HCTZ (Can)** *see* Irbesartan and Hydrochlorothiazide *on page 926*
- ◆ **Teva-Lamotrigine (Can)** *see* LamoTRIgine *on page 967*
- ◆ **Teva-Lansoprazole (Can)** *see* Lansoprazole *on page 972*
- ◆ **Teva-Lisinopril/Hctz (Type P) (Can)** *see* Lisinopril and Hydrochlorothiazide *on page 1023*
- ◆ **Teva-Lisinopril/Hctz (Type Z) (Can)** *see* Lisinopril and Hydrochlorothiazide *on page 1023*
- ◆ **Teva-Lisinopril (Type P) (Can)** *see* Lisinopril *on page 1020*
- ◆ **Teva-Lisinopril (Type Z) (Can)** *see* Lisinopril *on page 1020*
- ◆ **Teva-Maprotiline (Can)** *see* Maprotiline *on page 1052*
- ◆ **Teva-Medroxyprogesterone (Can)** *see* MedroxyPROGESTERone *on page 1058*
- ◆ **Teva-Meloxicam (Can)** *see* Meloxicam *on page 1063*
- ◆ **Teva-Metoprolol (Can)** *see* Metoprolol *on page 1117*
- ◆ **Teva-Montelukast (Can)** *see* Montelukast *on page 1152*
- ◆ **Teva-Morphine SR (Can)** *see* Morphine (Systemic) *on page 1153*
- ◆ **Teva-Nadolol (Can)** *see* Nadolol *on page 1169*
- ◆ **Teva-Naproxen (Can)** *see* Naproxen *on page 1177*
- ◆ **Teva-Naproxen EC (Can)** *see* Naproxen *on page 1177*
- ◆ **Teva-Naproxen Sodium (Can)** *see* Naproxen *on page 1177*
- ◆ **Teva-Naproxen Sodium DS (Can)** *see* Naproxen *on page 1177*
- ◆ **Teva-Naproxen SR (Can)** *see* Naproxen *on page 1177*

- ◆ **Teva-Nitrofurantoin (Can)** *see* Nitrofurantoin *on page 1210*
- ◆ **Teva-Olanzapine (Can)** *see* OLANZapine *on page 1233*
- ◆ **Teva-Olanzapine OD (Can)** *see* OLANZapine *on page 1233*
- ◆ **Teva-Ondansetron (Can)** *see* Ondansetron *on page 1246*
- ◆ **Teva-Pantoprazole (Can)** *see* Pantoprazole *on page 1289*
- ◆ **Teva-Paroxetine (Can)** *see* PARoxetine *on page 1299*
- ◆ **Teva-Pindolol (Can)** *see* Pindolol *on page 1355*
- ◆ **Teva-Pioglitazone (Can)** *see* Pioglitazone *on page 1355*
- ◆ **Teva-Pramipexole (Can)** *see* Pramipexole *on page 1389*
- ◆ **Teva-Prazosin (Can)** *see* Prazosin *on page 1396*
- ◆ **Teva-Propranolol (Can)** *see* Propranolol *on page 1424*
- ◆ **Teva-Quetiapine (Can)** *see* QUEtiapine *on page 1440*
- ◆ **Teva-Rabeprazole EC (Can)** *see* RABEprazole *on page 1451*
- ◆ **Teva-Raloxifene (Can)** *see* Raloxifene *on page 1455*
- ◆ **Teva-Ramipril (Can)** *see* Ramipril *on page 1459*
- ◆ **Teva-Ranitidine (Can)** *see* Ranitidine *on page 1462*
- ◆ **Teva-Risedronate (Can)** *see* Risedronate *on page 1494*
- ◆ **Teva-Sertraline (Can)** *see* Sertraline *on page 1548*
- ◆ **Teva-Simvastatin (Can)** *see* Simvastatin *on page 1555*
- ◆ **Teva-Spironolactone (Can)** *see* Spironolactone *on page 1590*
- ◆ **Teva-Sucralfate (Can)** *see* Sucralfate *on page 1598*
- ◆ **Teva-Sulindac (Can)** *see* Sulindac *on page 1608*
- ◆ **Teva-Sumatriptan (Can)** *see* SUMAtriptan *on page 1609*
- ◆ **Teva-Sumatriptan DF (Can)** *see* SUMAtriptan *on page 1609*
- ◆ **Teva-Tamoxifen (Can)** *see* Tamoxifen *on page 1624*
- ◆ **Teva-Tamsulosin (Can)** *see* Tamsulosin *on page 1626*
- ◆ **Teva-Terazosin (Can)** *see* Terazosin *on page 1647*
- ◆ **Teva-Terbinafine (Can)** *see* Terbinafine (Systemic) *on page 1648*
- ◆ **Teva-Theophylline SR (Can)** *see* Theophylline *on page 1667*
- ◆ **Teva-Ticlopidine (Can)** *see* Ticlopidine *on page 1682*
- ◆ **Teva-Timolol (Can)** *see* Timolol (Systemic) *on page 1686*
- ◆ **Teva-Trazodone (Can)** *see* TraZODone *on page 1725*
- ◆ **Teva-Triamterene HCTZ (Can)** *see* Hydrochlorothiazide and Triamterene *on page 836*
- ◆ **Teva-Valsartan (Can)** *see* Valsartan *on page 1761*
- ◆ **Teva-Valsartan HCTZ (Can)** *see* Valsartan and Hydrochlorothiazide *on page 1763*
- ◆ **Teva-Venlafaxine XR (Can)** *see* Venlafaxine *on page 1780*
- ◆ **Teva-Zolmitriptan (Can)** *see* ZOLMitriptan *on page 1824*
- ◆ **Teva-Zolmitriptan OD (Can)** *see* ZOLMitriptan *on page 1824*
- ◆ **Teveten®** *see* Eprosartan *on page 607*
- ◆ **Teveten® HCT** *see* Eprosartan and Hydrochlorothiazide *on page 608*
- ◆ **Teveten® Plus (Can)** *see* Eprosartan and Hydrochlorothiazide *on page 608*
- ◆ **Tev-Tropin®** *see* Somatropin *on page 1579*
- ◆ **Texacort™** *see* Hydrocortisone (Topical) *on page 841*
- ◆ **TG** *see* Thioguanine *on page 1670*
- ◆ **6-TG (error-prone abbreviation)** *see* Thioguanine *on page 1670*
- ◆ **TH9507** *see* Tesamorelin *on page 1653*

Thalidomide (tha LI doe mide)

Brand Names: U.S. Thalomid®

Brand Names: Canada Thalomid®

Pharmacologic Category Angiogenesis Inhibitor; Immunomodulator, Systemic; Tumor Necrosis Factor (TNF) Blocking Agent

Use Treatment of newly-diagnosed multiple myeloma; treatment and maintenance of cutaneous manifestations of erythema nodosum leprosum (ENL)

Unlabeled Use Treatment of refractory Crohn's disease; treatment of chronic graft-versus-host disease (GVHD) in hematopoietic stem cell transplantation; AIDS-related aphthous stomatitis; Waldenström's macroglobulinemia; maintenance therapy of multiple myeloma (following autologous stem cell transplant)

Pregnancy Risk Factor X

Pregnancy Considerations [U.S. Boxed Warning]: Thalidomide is a known teratogen; either abstinence or 2 forms of effective contraception must be used for at least 4 weeks before initiating therapy, during therapy, and for 4 weeks following discontinuation of thalidomide for women of childbearing potential. Distribution is restricted; physicians, pharmacists, and patients must be registered with the S.T.E.P.S.® program. Women of childbearing potential should be treated only if they are able to comply with the conditions of the S.T.E.P.S.® program. Embryotoxic with limb defects noted from the 27th to 40th gestational day of exposure; all cases of phocomelia occur from the 27th to 42nd gestational day; fetal cardiac, gastrointestinal, bone, external ear, eye, and genitourinary tract abnormalities have also been described. Mortality at or shortly after birth has also been reported. A negative pregnancy test (sensitivity of at least 50 mIU/mL) within 24 hours prior to beginning therapy, weekly during the first 4 weeks, and every 4 weeks (every 2 weeks for women with irregular menstrual cycles) thereafter is required for women of childbearing potential. Males (even those vasectomized) must use a latex condom during any sexual contact with women of childbearing age. Risk to the fetus from semen of male patients is unknown. The parent or legal guardian for patients between 12 and 18 years of age must agree to ensure compliance with the required guidelines. Thalidomide must be immediately discontinued and the patient referred to a reproductive toxicity specialist if pregnancy occurs during treatment. Any suspected fetal exposure to thalidomide must be reported to the FDA via the MedWatch program (1-800-FDA-1088) and to Celgene Corporation (1-888-423-5436). In Canada, thalidomide is available only through a restricted-distribution program called RevAid® (1-888-738-2431).

Lactation Excretion in breast milk unknown/not recommended

Prescribing and Access Restrictions U.S.: As a requirement of the REMS program, access to this medication is restricted. Thalidomide is approved for marketing only under a special distribution program. This program, called the "System for Thalidomide Education and Prescribing Safety" (STEPS® 1-888-423-5436), has been approved by the FDA. Prescribers and pharmacists must be registered with the program. No more than a 4-week supply should be dispensed. Blister packs should be dispensed intact (do not repackage capsules). Prescriptions must be filled within 7 days. Subsequent prescriptions may be filled only if fewer than 7 days of therapy remain on the previous prescription. A new prescription is required for further dispensing (a telephone prescription may not be accepted.) Pregnancy testing is required for females of childbearing potential.

Canada: Access to thalidomide is restricted through a controlled distribution program called RevAid®. Only physicians and pharmacists enrolled in this program are authorized to prescribe or dispense thalidomide. Patients must be enrolled in the program by their physicians. Further information is available by calling 1-888-738-2431.

Medication Guide Available Yes

Contraindications Hypersensitivity to thalidomide or any component of the formulation; patient unable to comply with STEPS® program (including males); women of childbearing potential unless alternative therapies are inappropriate and adequate precautions are taken to avoid pregnancy; pregnancy

Canadian labeling: Additional contraindications (not in U.S. labeling): Hypersensitivity to lenalidomide; breast-feeding

Warnings/Precautions Hazardous agent - use appropriate precautions for handling and disposal. **[U.S. Boxed Warning]: Thalidomide should only be prescribed to patients (male and female) who can understand and comply with the conditions of the S.T.E.P.S.® program. Distribution is restricted; physicians, pharmacists, and patients must be registered with the S.T.E.P.S.® program. [U.S. Boxed Warning]: Thalidomide is a known teratogen; effective contraception must be used for at least 4 weeks before initiating therapy, during therapy, and for 4 weeks following discontinuation of thalidomide for women of childbearing potential.** Use caution with drugs which may decrease the efficacy of hormonal contraceptives.

[U.S. Boxed Warning]: Thrombotic events have been reported, generally in patients with other risk factors for thrombosis (neoplastic disease, inflammatory disease, or concurrent therapy with combination chemotherapy. Use in combination with dexamethasone is associated with increased risk for deep vein thrombosis (DVT) and pulmonary embolism (PE), monitor for signs and symptoms of thromboembolism; patients at risk may benefit from prophylactic anticoagulation or aspirin. The NCCN multiple myeloma guidelines (v.1.2011) recommend anticoagulant prophylaxis with thalidomide-based therapy. Anticoagulant prophylaxis should be individualized and selected based on the venous thromboembolism risk of the combination treatment regimen, using the safest and easiest to administer (Palumbo, 2008). The Canadian labeling recommends anticoagulant prophylaxis for at least the first 5 months of thalidomide-based therapy.

May cause sedation; patients must be warned to use caution when performing tasks which require alertness. Use caution in patients with neurological disorders or constipation. Thalidomide has been associated with the development of peripheral neuropathy, which may be irreversible; generally occurs following chronic use (over months), but may occur with short-term use; use caution with other medications which may cause peripheral neuropathy. Consider immediate discontinuation (if clinically appropriate) in patients who develop neuropathy. May cause seizures; use caution in patients with a history of seizures, concurrent therapy with drugs which alter seizure threshold, or conditions which predispose to seizures. May cause neutropenia; discontinue therapy if absolute neutrophil count decreases to <750/mm^3. Use caution in patients with HIV infection; has been associated with increased viral loads. May cause orthostasis and/or bradycardia; use with caution in patients with cardiovascular disease or in patients who would not tolerate transient hypotensive episodes. Hypersensitivity, Stevens-Johnson syndrome (SJS) and toxic epidermal necrolysis (TEN) have been reported; withhold therapy and evaluate with skin rashes; permanently discontinue if rash is exfoliative, purpuric, bullous or if SJS or TEN is suspected.

Adverse Reactions

>10%:

- Cardiovascular: Edema (57%), thrombosis/embolism (23%; grade 3: 13%, grade 4: 9%), hypotension (16%)
- Central nervous system: Fatigue (79%; grade 3: 14%, grade 4: 3%), somnolence (36% to 38%), dizziness (4% to 20%), sensory neuropathy (54%), confusion (28%), anxiety/agitation (9% to 26%), fever (19% to 23%), motor neuropathy (22%), headache (13% to 19%)
- Dermatologic: Rash/desquamation (21% to 30%; grade 3: 4%), dry skin (21%), maculopapular rash (4% to 19%), acne (3% to 11%)
- Endocrine & metabolic: Hypocalcemia (72%)
- Gastrointestinal: Constipation (3% to 55%), nausea (4% to 28%), anorexia (3% to 28%), weight loss (23%), weight gain (22%), diarrhea (4% to 19%), oral moniliasis (4% to 11%)
- Hematologic: Leukopenia (17% to 35%), neutropenia (31%), anemia (6% to 13%), lymphadenopathy (6% to 13%)
- Hepatic: AST increased (3% to 25%), bilirubin increased (14%)
- Neuromuscular & skeletal: Muscle weakness (40%), tremor (4% to 26%), weakness (6% to 22%), myalgia (17%), paresthesia (6% to 16%), arthralgia (13%)
- Renal: Hematuria (11%)
- Respiratory: Dyspnea (42%)
- Miscellaneous: Diaphoresis (13%)

1% to 10%:

- Cardiovascular: Peripheral edema (3% to 8%), facial edema (4%)
- Central nervous system: Insomnia (9%), nervousness (3% to 9%), malaise (8%), vertigo (8%), pain (3% to 8%)
- Dermatologic: Dermatitis (fungal 4% to 9%), pruritus (3% to 8%), nail disorder (3% to 4%)
- Endocrine & metabolic: Hyperlipemia (6% to 9%)
- Gastrointestinal: Xerostomia (8% to 9%), flatulence (8%), tooth pain (4%)
- Genitourinary: Impotence (3% to 8%)
- Hepatic: LFTs abnormal (9%)
- Neuromuscular & skeletal: Neuropathy (8%), back pain (4% to 6%), neck pain (4%), neck rigidity (4%)
- Renal: Albuminuria (3% to 8%)
- Respiratory: Pharyngitis (4% to 8%), rhinitis (4%), sinusitis (3% to 8%)
- Miscellaneous: Infection (6% to 8%)

Postmarketing and/or case reports (limited to important or life-threatening): Acute renal failure, alkaline phosphatase increased, ALT increased, amenorrhea, aphthous stomatitis, arrhythmia, atrial fibrillation, bile duct obstruction, bradycardia, BUN increased, CML, creatinine clearance decreased, creatinine increased, deafness, depression, diplopia, ECG abnormalities, eosinophilia, erythema multiforme, erythema nodosum, erythroleukemia, febrile neutropenia, foot drop, galactorrhea, granulocytopenia, gynecomastia, hepatomegaly, Hodgkin's disease, hypercalcemia, hyper-/hypokalemia, hypersensitivity, hypertension, hyper-/hypothyroidism, hyperuricemia, hypomagnesemia, hyponatremia, hypoproteinemia, intestinal obstruction, intestinal perforation, interstitial pneumonitis, LDH increased, leukocytosis, lymphedema, lymphopenia, myxedema, nystagmus, oliguria, orthostatic hypotension, pancytopenia, petechiae, peripheral neuritis, pleural effusion, prothrombin time changes, psychosis, pulmonary embolus, pulmonary hypertension, purpura, Raynaud's syndrome, seizure, status epilepticus, Stevens-Johnson syndrome, stomach ulcer, suicide attempt, syncope, tachycardia, thrombocytopenia, toxic epidermal necrolysis, tumor lysis syndrome

Drug Interactions

Metabolism/Transport Effects None known.

Avoid Concomitant Use

Avoid concomitant use of Thalidomide with any of the following: Abatacept; Anakinra; BCG; Canakinumab; Certolizumab Pegol; CloZAPine; Natalizumab; Pimecrolimus; Rilonacept; Tacrolimus (Topical); Vaccines (Live)

Increased Effect/Toxicity

Thalidomide may increase the levels/effects of: Abatacept; Alcohol (Ethyl); Anakinra; Canakinumab; Certolizumab Pegol; CloZAPine; CNS Depressants; Leflunomide; Methotrimeprazine; Natalizumab; Pamidronate; Rilonacept; Selective Serotonin Reuptake Inhibitors; Vaccines (Live); Zoledronic Acid

The levels/effects of Thalidomide may be increased by: Denosumab; Dexamethasone; Dexamethasone (Systemic); Droperidol; HydrOXYzine; Methotrimeprazine; Pimecrolimus; Roflumilast; Tacrolimus (Topical); Trastuzumab

Decreased Effect

Thalidomide may decrease the levels/effects of: BCG; Coccidioidin Skin Test; Sipuleucel-T; Vaccines (Inactivated); Vaccines (Live)

The levels/effects of Thalidomide may be decreased by: Echinacea

Ethanol/Nutrition/Herb Interactions

Ethanol: May increase CNS depression; monitor for increased effects with coadministration. Caution patients about effects.

Herb/Nutraceutical: Avoid cat's claw and echinacea (have immunostimulant properties; consider therapy modifications).

Stability Store at 25°C (77°F); excursions permitted to 15°C to 30°C (59°F to 86°F). Protect from light. Keep in original package.

Mechanism of Action Immunomodulatory and antiangiogenic characteristics; immunologic effects may vary based on conditions; may suppress excessive tumor necrosis factor-alpha production in patients with ENL, yet may increase plasma tumor necrosis factor-alpha levels in HIV-positive patients. In multiple myeloma, thalidomide is associated with an increase in natural killer cells and increased levels of interleukin-2 and interferon gamma. Other proposed mechanisms of action include suppression of angiogenesis, prevention of free-radical-mediated DNA damage, increased cell mediated cytotoxic effects, and altered expression of cellular adhesion molecules.

Pharmacodynamics/Kinetics

Protein binding: 55% to 66%

Metabolism: Nonenzymatic hydrolysis in plasma; forms multiple metabolites

Bioavailability: Capsule: 90%

Half-life elimination: 5-7 hours

Time to peak, plasma: 3-6 hours

Excretion: Urine (<1% as unchanged drug)

Dosage Oral:

Children ≥3 years: Chronic graft-versus-host disease (refractory), treatment (unlabeled second-line use; limited data): 3 mg/kg 4 times/day (dose adjusted to goal thalidomide concentration of ≥5 mcg/mL 2 hours postdose) (Vogelsang, 1992) **or** Initial: 3-6 mg/kg/day in 2-4 divided doses; target dose 12 mg/kg/day; Maximum daily dose: 800 mg (Rovelli, 1998)

Children ≥12 years and Adults: Cutaneous ENL: Initial: 100-300 mg once daily

Adjustments to initial dose:

Patients weighing <50 kg: Initiate at lower end of the dosing range

Severe cutaneous reaction or patients previously requiring high dose may be initiated at 400 mg/day; doses may be divided, but taken 1 hour after meals

Duration and tapering/maintenance:

Maintenance: Dosing should continue until active reaction subsides (usually at least 2 weeks), then tapered in 50 mg decrements every 2-4 weeks

Patients who flare during tapering or with a history of requiring prolonged maintenance should be maintained on the minimum dosage necessary to control the reaction. Efforts to taper should be repeated every 3-6 months, in decrements of 50 mg every 2-4 weeks.

Adults:

Multiple myeloma: **Note:** Details concerning dosing for multiple myeloma with combination regimens should also be consulted.

200 mg once daily at bedtime (in combination with dexamethasone 40 mg daily on days 1-4, 9-12, and 17-20 of a 28-day treatment cycle)

In combination with melphalan and prednisone (unlabeled combination in U.S.): 200-400 mg once daily (Facon, 2007) **or** 100 mg once daily (Palumbo, 2008)

Canadian labeling: Adults ≥65 years: 200 mg once daily (in combination with melphalan and prednisone)

AIDS-related aphthous stomatitis (unlabeled use): 200 mg once daily at bedtime for up to 8 weeks, if no response, then 200 mg twice daily for 4 weeks (Jacobson, 1997)

Chronic graft-versus-host disease (refractory), treatment (unlabeled second-line use; optimum dose not determined): Initial: 100 mg at bedtime, with dose escalation up to 400 mg/day in 3-4 divided doses (Wolff, 2010) **or** Initial: 50-100 mg 3 times/day; maximum dose: 600-1200 mg/day (Kulkarni, 2003) **or** 200 mg 4 times/day (dose adjusted to goal thalidomide concentration of ≥5 mcg/mL 2 hours postdose) (Vogelsang, 1992) **or** 100-300 mg 4 times/day (Parker, 1995)

Crohn's disease, refractory (unlabeled use): 50-100 mg/day at bedtime (Vasiliauskas, 1999) **or** 200-300 mg/day at bedtime (Ehrenpreis, 1999)

Multiple myeloma, maintenance (following autologous stem cell transplant; unlabeled use): 200 mg/day starting 3-6 months after transplant; continue until disease progression or unacceptable toxicity (Brinker, 2006) **or** 100 mg/day starting 42-60 days following transplant; increase to 200 mg/day after 2 weeks if tolerated; continue for up to 12 months (in combination with prednisolone) (Spencer, 2009)

Waldenström's macroglobulinemia (unlabeled use): 200 mg/day for up to 52 weeks (in combination with rituximab) (Treon, 2008)

Dosing adjustment for toxicity:

ANC ≤750/mm^3: Withhold treatment if clinically appropriate

Multiple myeloma:

U.S. labeling: Constipation, oversedation, peripheral neuropathy: Temporarily withhold or continue with a reduced dose

Canadian labeling:

ANC <1500/mm^3: Withhold melphalan and prednisone for 1 week; resume melphalan and prednisone after 1 week if ANC >1500/mm^3 **or** if ANC 1000-1500/mm^3 reduce melphalan dose by 50% **or** if ANC <1000/mm^3 adjust chemotherapy dose based on clinical status of patient.

Constipation, oversedation: Temporarily withhold thalidomide treatment or continue with a reduced dose

Peripheral neuropathy, Grade 1 (paresthesia, weakness and/or loss of reflexes) without loss of function): Evaluate patient and consider dose reduction with worsening of symptoms; symptom improvement may not follow dose reduction, however.

Peripheral neuropathy, Grade 2 (interferes with function but not with daily activities), Grade 3 (interferes with daily activities), or Grade 4 (disabling neuropathy): Discontinue thalidomide treatment

Thromboembolic events: Withhold therapy and initiate standard anticoagulant treatment; may resume thalidomide therapy at original dose following stabilization of patient and resolution of thromboembolic event; maintain anticoagulant treatment for duration of thalidomide therapy

Dosing adjustment in renal impairment: No adjustment is required for patients with renal impairment and on dialysis (per manufacturer). In a study of 6 patients with end-stage renal disease on dialysis, although clearance was increased by dialysis, a supplemental dose was not needed (Eriksson, 2003).

Multiple myeloma: An evaluation of 29 newly-diagnosed myeloma patients with renal failure (serum creatinine ≥2 mg/dL) treated with thalidomide and dexamethasone (some also received cyclophosphamide) found that toxicities and efficacy were similar to patients with normal renal function (Seol, 2010). A study evaluating induction therapy with thalidomide and dexamethasone in 31 newly-diagnosed myeloma patients with renal failure (Cl_{cr} <50 mL/minute), including 16 patients with severe renal impairment (Cl_{cr} <30 mL/minute) and 7 patients on chronic hemodialysis found that toxicities were similar to patients without renal impairment and that thalidomide and dexamethasone could be administered safely (Tosi, 2009).

Dosing adjustment in hepatic impairment: Thalidomide does not appear to undergo significant hepatic metabolism; the pharmacokinetics of thalidomide have not been studied in patients with liver dysfunction (per manufacturer).

Dietary Considerations Should be taken at least 1 hour after the evening meal.

Administration Administer orally with water, preferably at bedtime once daily on an empty stomach, at least 1 hour after the evening meal. Doses >400 mg/day may be given in 2-3 divided doses. For missed doses, if <12 hours patient may receive dose; if >12 hours wait till next dose due.

Avoid extensive handling of capsules; capsules should remain in blister pack until ingestion. If exposed to the powder content from broken capsules or body fluids from patients receiving thalidomide, the exposed area should be washed with soap and water.

Monitoring Parameters CBC with differential, platelets; signs of neuropathy monthly for the first 3 months, then periodically during treatment; consider monitoring of sensory nerve application potential amplitudes (at baseline and every 6 months) to detect asymptomatic neuropathy. Monitor for signs and symptoms of thromboembolism (shortness of breath, chest pain, arm/leg swelling). In HIV-seropositive patients: viral load after 1 and 3 months, then every 3 months. Pregnancy testing (sensitivity of at least 50 mIU/mL) is required within 24 hours prior to initiation of therapy, weekly during the first 4 weeks, then every 4 weeks in women with regular menstrual cycles or every 2 weeks in women with irregular menstrual cycles.

Reference Range Graft-vs-host disease: Therapeutic plasma thalidomide levels are 5-8 mcg/mL, although it has been suggested that lower plasma levels (0.5-1.5 mcg/mL) may be therapeutic; peak serum thalidomide level after a 200 mg dose: 1.8 mcg/mL

Dosage Forms Excipient information presented when available (limited, particularly for generics); consult specific product labeling.

Capsule, oral:

Thalomid®: 50 mg, 100 mg, 150 mg, 200 mg

- ◆ **Thalitone®** *see* Chlorthalidone *on page 350*
- ◆ **Thalomid®** *see* Thalidomide *on page 1664*
- ◆ **THAM®** *see* Tromethamine *on page 1742*
- ◆ **THC** *see* Dronabinol *on page 561*
- ◆ **Theo-24®** *see* Theophylline *on page 1667*
- ◆ **Theo ER (Can)** *see* Theophylline *on page 1667*
- ◆ **Theolair (Can)** *see* Theophylline *on page 1667*

Theophylline (thee OFF i lin)

Brand Names: U.S. Elixophyllin® Elixir; Theo-24®

Brand Names: Canada Apo-Theo LA®; Novo-Theophyl SR; PMS-Theophylline; Pulmophylline; ratio-Theo-Bronc; Teva-Theophylline SR; Theo ER; Theolair; Uniphyl

Index Terms Theophylline Anhydrous

Pharmacologic Category Theophylline Derivative

Additional Appendix Information

Asthma *on page 1967*

Use Treatment of symptoms and reversible airway obstruction due to chronic asthma, or other chronic lung diseases

Note: The Global Initiative for Asthma Guidelines (2009) and the National Heart, Lung and Blood Institute Guidelines (2007) do not recommend oral theophylline as a long-term control medication for asthma in children ≤5 years of age; use has been shown to be effective as an add-on (but not preferred) agent in older children and adults with severe asthma treated with inhaled or oral glucocorticoids. The guidelines do not recommend theophylline for the treatment of exacerbations of asthma.

The Global Initiative for Chronic Obstructive Lung Disease Guidelines (2009) suggest that while higher doses of slow release formulations of theophylline have been proven to be effective for use in COPD, it is not a preferred agent due to its potential for toxicity.

Pregnancy Risk Factor C

Pregnancy Considerations Teratogenic effects were observed in animal reproduction studies. Theophylline crosses the placenta; adverse effects may be seen in the newborn. Use is generally safe when used at the recommended doses (serum concentrations 5-12 mcg/mL) however maternal adverse events may be increased and efficacy may be decreased in pregnant women. Theophylline metabolism may change during pregnancy; the half-life is similar to that observed in otherwise healthy, nonsmoking adults with asthma during the first and second trimesters (~8.7 hours), but may increase to 13 hours (range: 8-18 hours) during the third trimester. The volume of distribution is also increased during the third trimester. Monitor serum levels. The recommendations for the use of theophylline in pregnant women with asthma are similar to those used in nonpregnant adults (National Heart, Lung, and Blood Institute Guidelines, 2004).

Lactation Enters breast milk/compatible (AAP rates "compatible"; AAP 2001 update pending)

Contraindications Hypersensitivity to theophylline or any component of the formulation; premixed injection may contain corn-derived dextrose and its use is contraindicated in patients with allergy to corn-related products

Warnings/Precautions If a patient develops signs and symptoms of theophylline toxicity (eg, persistent, repetitive vomiting), a serum theophylline level should be measured and subsequent doses held. Serum theophylline monitoring may be lessened as lower therapeutic ranges are established. More intense monitoring may be required during acute illness or when interacting drugs are introduced into the regimen. Use with caution in patients with peptic ulcer, hyperthyroidism, seizure disorders, and patients with tachyarrhythmias (eg, sinus tachycardia, atrial fibrillation); use may exacerbate these conditions. ▶

Theophylline clearance may be decreased in patients with acute pulmonary edema, congestive heart failure, cor-pulmonale, fever, hepatic disease, acute hepatitis, cirrhosis, hypothyroidism, sepsis with multiorgan failure, and shock; clearance may also be decreased in neonates, infants <3 months of age with decreased renal function, children <1 year of age, the elderly >60 years, and patients following cessation of smoking.

Adverse Reactions Frequency not defined. Adverse events observed at therapeutic serum levels:

Cardiovascular: Flutter, tachycardia

Central nervous system: Headache, hyperactivity (children), insomnia, restlessness, seizures

Endocrine & metabolic: Hypercalcemia (with concomitant hyperthyroid disease)

Gastrointestinal: Nausea, reflux or ulcer aggravation, vomiting

Genitourinary: Difficulty urinating (elderly males with prostatism)

Neuromuscular & skeletal: Tremor

Renal: Diuresis (transient)

Drug Interactions

Metabolism/Transport Effects Substrate of CYP1A2 (major), CYP2C9 (minor), CYP2D6 (minor), CYP2E1 (major), CYP3A4 (major); **Note:** Assignment of Major/Minor substrate status based on clinically relevant drug interaction potential; **Inhibits** CYP1A2 (weak)

Avoid Concomitant Use

Avoid concomitant use of Theophylline with any of the following: Conivaptan; Deferasirox; Iobenguane I 123

Increased Effect/Toxicity

Theophylline may increase the levels/effects of: Formoterol; Indacaterol; Pancuronium; Sympathomimetics

The levels/effects of Theophylline may be increased by: Abiraterone Acetate; Allopurinol; Antithyroid Agents; Atomoxetine; Cannabinoids; Cimetidine; Conivaptan; Contraceptives (Estrogens); CYP1A2 Inhibitors (Moderate); CYP1A2 Inhibitors (Strong); CYP3A4 Inhibitors (Moderate); CYP3A4 Inhibitors (Strong); Dasatinib; Deferasirox; Disulfiram; Febuxostat; FluvoxaMINE; Interferons; Isoniazid; Linezolid; Macrolide Antibiotics; Methotrexate; Mexiletine; Pentoxifylline; Propafenone; QuiNINE; Quinolone Antibiotics; Thiabendazole; Ticlopidine; Zafirlukast; Zileuton

Decreased Effect

Theophylline may decrease the levels/effects of: Adenosine; Benzodiazepines; CarBAMazepine; Fosphenytoin; Iobenguane I 123; Lithium; Pancuronium; Phenytoin; Regadenoson; Zafirlukast

The levels/effects of Theophylline may be decreased by: Aminoglutethimide; Barbiturates; Beta-Blockers (Beta1 Selective); Beta-Blockers (Nonselective); CarBAMazepine; CYP1A2 Inducers (Strong); CYP3A4 Inducers (Strong); Cyproterone; Fosphenytoin; Herbs (CYP3A4 Inducers); Isoproterenol; Phenytoin; Protease Inhibitors; Thyroid Products; Tocilizumab

Ethanol/Nutrition/Herb Interactions Food: Food does not appreciably affect the absorption of liquid, fast-release products, and most sustained release products; however, food may induce a sudden release (dose-dumping) of once-daily sustained release products resulting in an increase in serum drug levels and potential toxicity. Avoid excessive amounts of caffeine. Avoid extremes of dietary protein and carbohydrate intake. Changes in diet may affect the elimination of theophylline; charbroiled foods may increase elimination, reducing half-life by 50%.

Stability Tablet, premixed infusion, solution: Store at controlled room temperature of 25°C (77°F).

Mechanism of Action Causes bronchodilatation, diuresis, CNS and cardiac stimulation, and gastric acid secretion by blocking phosphodiesterase which increases tissue concentrations of cyclic adenine monophosphate (cAMP) which in turn promotes catecholamine stimulation of lipolysis, glycogenolysis, and gluconeogenesis and induces release of epinephrine from adrenal medulla cells

Pharmacodynamics/Kinetics

Absorption: Oral: Dosage form dependent

Distribution: 0.45 L/kg (range: 0.3-0.7 L/kg) based on ideal body weight; distributes poorly into body fat; V_d may increase in premature neonates, patients with hepatic cirrhosis, acidemia (uncorrected), the elderly

Metabolism: Children >1 year and Adults: Hepatic; involves CYP1A2, 2E1 and 3A4; forms active metabolites (caffeine and 3-methylxanthine)

Protein binding: 40%, primarily to albumin

Half-life elimination: Highly variable and dependent upon age, liver function, cardiac function, lung disease, and smoking history

- Premature infants, postnatal age 3-15 days: 30 hours (range: 17-43 hours)
- Premature infants, postnatal age 25-57 days: 20 hours (range: 9.4-30.6 hours)
- Children 6-17 years: 3.7 hours (range: 1.5-5.9 hours)
- Adults 16-60 years with asthma, nonsmoking, otherwise healthy: 8.7 hours (range: 6.1-12.8 hours)

Time to peak, serum:

- Oral: Liquid: 1 hour
- I.V.: Within 30 minutes

Excretion: Urine

- Neonates: 50% as unchanged theophylline
- Children >3 months and Adults: ~10% as unchanged theophylline

Dosage Doses should be individualized based on steady-state serum concentrations and ideal body weight.

Acute symptoms: Loading dose: Children and Adults: Oral, I.V.:

Asthma exacerbations: While theophylline may be considered for relief of asthma symptoms, the role of treating exacerbations is not supported by current practice.

COPD treatment: Theophylline is currently considered second-line intravenous therapy in the emergency department or hospital setting when there is inadequate or insufficient response to short acting bronchodilators (Global Initiative for COPD Guidelines, 2009).

If no theophylline received within the previous 24 hours: 4.6 mg/kg loading dose (~5.8 mg/kg hydrous aminophylline) I.V. or 5 mg/kg orally. Loading dose intended to achieve a serum level of approximately 10 mcg/mL; loading doses should be given intravenously (preferred) or with a rapidly absorbed oral product (not an extended-release product). **Note:** On the average, for every 1 mg/kg theophylline given, blood levels will rise 2 mcg/mL.

If theophylline has been administered in the previous 24 hours: A loading dose is not recommended without obtaining a serum theophylline concentration. The loading dose should be calculated as follows:

Dose = (desired serum theophylline concentration - measured serum theophylline concentration) (V_d)

Acute symptoms: Maintenance dose: Children and Adults: I.V.: **Note:** To achieve a target concentration of 10 mcg/mL unless otherwise noted. Lower initial doses may be required in patients with reduced theophylline clearance. Dosage should be adjusted according to serum level measurements during the first 12- to 24-hour period.

Infants 6-52 weeks: mg/kg/hour = (0.008) (age in weeks) + 0.21

Children 1-9 years: 0.8 mg/kg/hour

Children 9-12 years: 0.7 mg/kg/hour

Adolescents 12-16 years (cigarette or marijuana smokers): 0.7 mg/kg/hour

Adolescents 12-16 years (nonsmokers): 0.5 mg/kg/hour; maximum 900 mg/day unless serum levels indicate need for larger dose

Adults 16-60 years (otherwise healthy, nonsmokers): 0.4 mg/kg/hour; maximum 900 mg/day unless serum levels indicate need for larger dose

Adults >60 years: 0.3 mg/kg/hour; maximum 400 mg/day unless serum levels indicate need for larger dose

Treatment of chronic conditions: With newer guidelines suggesting lower therapeutic theophylline ranges, it is unlikely that doses larger than >10 mg/kg/day will be required in children ≥1 year or adults.

Oral solution:

Infants <1 year: **Note:** Doses should be adjusted to maintain the peak steady state serum concentrations. The time to reach steady state will vary based on age and the presence of risk factors which may affect theophylline clearance.

Full-term Infants and Infants <26 weeks: Total daily dose (mg)= [(0.2 x age in weeks) +5] x (weight in kg); divide dose into 3 equal amounts and administer at 8-hour intervals

Full-term Infants and Infants ≥26 weeks and <52 weeks: Total daily dose (mg) = [(0.2 x age in weeks) +5] x (weight in kg); divide dose into 4 equal amounts and administer at 6-hour intervals

Children ≥1 year and <45 kg: Initial dose: 10-14 mg/kg/day (maximum 300 mg/day) administered in divided doses every 4-6 hours; Maintenance: Up to 20 mg/kg/day (maximum: 600 mg/day)

Children >45 kg and Adults: Initial dose: 300 mg/day administered in divided doses every 6-8 hours; Maintenance: 400-600 mg/day (maximum: 600 mg/day)

Oral extended release formulations:

Children ≥1 year and <45 kg: Initial: 10-14 mg/kg once daily (maximum 300 mg/day); Maintenance up to 20 mg/kg/day (maximum: 600 mg/day)

Children >45 kg and Adults: Initial dose: 300-400 mg once daily; Maintenance: 400-600 mg once daily (maximum: 600 mg/day)

Dosage adjustment after serum theophylline measurement: Asthma: Within normal limits: Children: 5-10 mcg/mL; Adults: 5-15 mcg/mL: Maintain dosage if tolerated. Recheck serum theophylline concentration at 24-hour intervals (for acute I.V. dosing) or at 6- to 12-month intervals (for oral dosing). Finer adjustments in dosage may be needed for some patients. If levels ≥15 mcg/mL, consider 10% dose reduction to improve safety margin.

Note: Recheck serum theophylline levels after 3 days when using oral dosing, or after 12 hours (children) or 24 hours (adults) when dosing intravenously. Patients maintained with oral therapy may be reassessed at 6- to 12-month intervals.

Dietary Considerations Should be taken with water 1 hour before or 2 hours after meals. Premixed injection may contain corn-derived dextrose and its use is contraindicated in patients with allergy to corn-related products.

Administration

I.V.: Administer loading dose over 30 minutes; follow with a continuous infusion as appropriate

Oral: Long-acting preparations should be taken with a full glass of water, swallowed whole, or cut in half if scored. Do **not** crush. Extended release capsule forms may be opened and the contents sprinkled on soft foods; do **not** chew beads.

Monitoring Parameters Monitor heart rate, CNS effects (insomnia, irritability); respiratory rate (COPD patients often have resting controlled respiratory rates in low 20s); arterial or capillary blood gases (if applicable)

Theophylline levels: Serum theophylline levels should be monitored prior to making dose increases; in the presence of signs or symptoms of toxicity; or when a new illness, worsening of a present illness, or medication changes occur that may change theophylline clearance

I.V. loading dose: Measure serum concentrations 30 minutes after the end of an I.V. loading dose

I.V. infusion: Measure serum concentrations one half-life after starting a continuous infusion, then every 12-24 hours

Reference Range Therapeutic levels: Asthma:

Children: 5-10 mcg/mL

Adults: 5-15 mcg/mL

Test Interactions Plasma glucose, uric acid, free fatty acids, total cholesterol, HDL, HDL/LDL ratio, and urinary free cortisol excretion may be increased by theophylline. Theophylline may decrease triiodothyronine.

Dosage Forms Excipient information presented when available (limited, particularly for generics); consult specific product labeling. [DSC] = Discontinued product

Capsule, extended release, oral:

Theo-24®: 100 mg, 200 mg, 300 mg, 400 mg [24 hours]

Infusion, premixed in D_5W: 400 mg (250 mL [DSC], 500 mL); 800 mg (500 mL)

Solution, oral: 80 mg/15 mL (15 mL, 473 mL)

Elixophyllin® Elixir: 80 mg/15 mL (473 mL) [contains ethanol 20%; mixed fruit flavor]

Tablet, extended release, oral: 100 mg, 200 mg, 300 mg, 400 mg, 450 mg, 600 mg

Extemporaneous Preparations Note: An alcohol-containing commercial oral solution is available (80 mg/15mL).

A 5 mg/mL oral suspension may be made with tablets. Crush one 300 mg extended release tablet in a mortar and reduce to a fine powder. Add small portions of a 1:1 mixture of Ora-Sweet® and Ora-Plus® and mix to a uniform paste; mix while adding the vehicle in equal proportions to **almost** 60 mL; transfer to a calibrated bottle, rinse mortar with vehicle, and add sufficient quantity of vehicle to make 60 mL. Label "shake well". Stable for 90 days at room temperature.

Johnson CE, VanDeKoppel S, and Myers E, "Stability of Anhydrous Theophylline in Extemporaneously Prepared Alcohol-Free Oral Suspensions," *Am J Health-Syst Pharm*, 2005, 62(23):2518-20.

◆ **Theophylline Anhydrous** *see* Theophylline *on page 1667*

◆ **TheraCys®** *see* BCG *on page 191*

◆ **Theraflu® Thin Strips® Multi Symptom [OTC]** *see* DiphenhydrAMINE (Systemic) *on page 516*

◆ **Thera-Gesic® [OTC]** *see* Methyl Salicylate and Menthol *on page 1113*

◆ **Thera-Gesic® Plus [OTC]** *see* Methyl Salicylate and Menthol *on page 1113*

◆ **Thermazene®** *see* Silver Sulfadiazine *on page 1554*

◆ **Thiamazole** *see* Methimazole *on page 1095*

◆ **Thiamin** *see* Thiamine *on page 1669*

Thiamine (THYE a min)

Brand Names: Canada Betaxin®

Index Terms Aneurine Hydrochloride; Thiamin; Thiamine Hydrochloride; Thiaminium Chloride Hydrochloride; Vitamin B_1

Pharmacologic Category Vitamin, Water Soluble

Use Treatment of thiamine deficiency including beriberi, Wernicke's encephalopathy, Korsakoff's syndrome, neuritis associated with pregnancy, or in alcoholic patients; dietary supplement

Pregnancy Risk Factor A

Dosage

Adequate Intake:

0-6 months: 0.2 mg/day

7-12 months: 0.3 mg/day

Recommended daily intake:
1-3 years: 0.5 mg
4-8 years: 0.6 mg
9-13 years: 0.9 mg
14-18 years: Females: 1 mg; Males: 1.2 mg
≥19 years: Females: 1.1 mg; Males: 1.2 mg
Pregnancy, lactation: 1.4 mg

Parenteral nutrition supplementation:
Infants: 1.2 mg/day
Adults: 6 mg/day; may be increased to 25-50 mg/day with history of alcohol abuse

Thiamine deficiency (beriberi):
Children: 10-25 mg/dose I.M. or I.V. daily (if critically ill), or 10-50 mg/dose orally every day for 2 weeks, then 5-10 mg/dose orally daily for 1 month
Adults: 5-30 mg/dose I.M. or I.V. 3 times/day (if critically ill); then orally 5-30 mg/day in single or divided doses 3 times/day for 1 month

Alcohol withdrawal syndrome: Adults: 100 mg/day I.M. or I.V. for several days, followed by 50-100 mg/day orally

Wernicke's encephalopathy: Adults: Treatment (manufacturer labeling): Initial: 100 mg I.V., then 50-100 mg/day I.M. or I.V. until consuming a regular, balanced diet. However, larger doses may be required based on failure of lower doses to produce clinical improvement in some patients.

Alternate dosage: The Royal College of Physicians (U.K.) has recommended the use of higher doses of thiamine (in combination with other B vitamins, ascorbic acid, potassium, phosphate, and magnesium) for the management of Wernicke's encephalopathy (Thomson, 2002):
Prophylaxis: 250 mg I.V. once daily for 3-5 days
Treatment: Initial: 500 mg I.V. 3 times/day for 3 days. If response to thiamine after 3 days, continue with 250 mg I.M. or I.V. once daily for an additional 5 days or until clinical improvement.

Additional Information Complete prescribing information for this medication should be consulted for additional detail.

Dosage Forms Excipient information presented when available (limited, particularly for generics); consult specific product labeling.
Injection, solution, as hydrochloride: 100 mg/mL (2 mL)
Tablet, oral, as hydrochloride: 50 mg, 100 mg, 250 mg, 500 mg

- **Thiamine Hydrochloride** *see* Thiamine *on page 1669*
- **Thiaminium Chloride Hydrochloride** *see* Thiamine *on page 1669*

Thioguanine (thye oh GWAH neen)

Brand Names: U.S. Tabloid®
Brand Names: Canada Lanvis®
Index Terms 2-Amino-6-Mercaptopurine; 6-TG (error-prone abbreviation); 6-Thioguanine (error-prone abbreviation); TG; Tioguanine
Pharmacologic Category Antineoplastic Agent, Antimetabolite (Purine Analog)
Use Treatment of acute myelogenous (nonlymphocytic) leukemia (AML)
Unlabeled Use Treatment of pediatric acute lymphoblastic leukemia (ALL)
Pregnancy Risk Factor D
Pregnancy Considerations Animal studies have demonstrated adverse effects. There are no adequate and well-controlled studies in pregnant women. May cause fetal harm if administered during pregnancy. Women of child-bearing potential should avoid becoming pregnant during treatment.
Lactation Excretion in breast milk unknown/not recommended
Contraindications Prior resistance to thioguanine (or mercaptopurine)

Canadian labeling: Additional contraindications (not in US labeling): Hypersensitivity to thioguanine or any component of the formulation

Warnings/Precautions Hazardous agent - use appropriate precautions for handling and disposal.

Not recommended for maintenance therapy or long-term continuous treatment; long-term continuous therapy or maintenance treatment is associated with a high risk for hepatotoxicity, hepatic sinusoidal obstruction syndrome (SOS; formerly called veno-occlusive disease), or portal hypertension; monitor liver function carefully for liver toxicity and discontinue in patients with evidence of hepatic SOS (eg, hyperbilirubinemia, hepatomegaly [tender], and weight gain due to ascites and fluid retention) or portal hypertension (eg, splenomegaly, thrombocytopenia, esophageal varices); hepatotoxicity with or without transaminase elevations may occur; pathologic findings of hepatotoxicity include hepatoportal sclerosis, nodular regenerative hyperplasia, peliosis hepatitis, and periportal fibrosis.

Myelosuppression (anemia, leukopenia, and/or thrombocytopenia) is a common dose-related toxicity (may be delayed); monitor for infection (due to leukopenia) or bleeding(due to thrombocytopenia); withhold treatment with abnormally significant drop in blood counts. Patients with genetic enzyme deficiency of thiopurine methyltransferase (TPMT) or who are receiving drugs which inhibit this enzyme (mesalazine, olsalazine, sulfasalazine) may be highly sensitive to myelosuppressive effects and may require substantial dose reductions.

Hyperuricemia occurs commonly with treatment; institute adequate hydration and prophylactic allopurinol. Thioguanine is potentially carcinogenic. Cross resistance with mercaptopurine generally occurs. Avoid vaccination with live vaccines during treatment.

Adverse Reactions Frequency not defined.
Endocrine & metabolic: Fluid retention, hyperuricemia (common)
Gastrointestinal: Anorexia, intestinal necrosis, intestinal perforation, nausea, splenomegaly, stomatitis, vomiting, weight gain
Hematologic: Anemia (may be delayed), bleeding, granulocytopenia, leukopenia (common; may be delayed), marrow hypoplasia, pancytopenia, thrombocytopenia (common; may be delayed)
Hepatic: Ascites, esophageal varices, hepatic necrosis (centrilobular), hepatic sinusoidal obstruction syndrome (SOS; veno-occlusive disease), hepatitis, hepatomegaly [tender], hepatoportal sclerosis, hepatotoxicity, hyperbilirubinemia, jaundice, LFTs increased, nodular regenerative hyperplasia, peliosis hepatitis, periportal fibrosis, portal hypertension
Miscellaneous: Infection

Drug Interactions
Metabolism/Transport Effects None known.
Avoid Concomitant Use
Avoid concomitant use of Thioguanine with any of the following: BCG; CloZAPine; Natalizumab; Pimecrolimus; Tacrolimus (Topical); Vaccines (Live)
Increased Effect/Toxicity
Thioguanine may increase the levels/effects of: CloZAPine; Leflunomide; Natalizumab; Vaccines (Live)
The levels/effects of Thioguanine may be increased by: 5-ASA Derivatives; Denosumab; Pimecrolimus; Roflumilast; Tacrolimus (Topical); Trastuzumab

Decreased Effect

Thioguanine may decrease the levels/effects of: BCG; Coccidioidin Skin Test; Sipuleucel-T; Vaccines (Inactivated); Vaccines (Live)

The levels/effects of Thioguanine may be decreased by: Echinacea

Ethanol/Nutrition/Herb Interactions Ethanol: Avoid; may increase the risk for hepatotoxicity.

Stability Store tablet at room temperature at 15°C to 25°C (59°F to 77°F). Protect from moisture.

Mechanism of Action Purine analog that is incorporated into DNA and RNA resulting in the blockage of synthesis and metabolism of purine nucleotides

Pharmacodynamics/Kinetics

Absorption: ~30% (range: 14% to 46%; highly variable)

Distribution: Does not reach therapeutic concentrations in the CSF

Metabolism: Hepatic; rapidly and extensively via thiopurine methyltransferase (TPMT) to 2-amino-6-methylthioguanine (MTG; active) and inactive compounds

Half-life elimination: Terminal: 5-9 hours

Time to peak, serum: Within 8 hours; predominantly metabolite(s)

Dosage

Oral: Children: Pediatric ALL (unlabeled use; combination therapy): Delayed intensification treatment phase: 60 mg/m^2/day for 14 days (Lange, 2002; Nachman, 1998)

Dosing comments in renal impairment: Children: No adjustment required (Aronoff, 2007).

Dosing comments in hepatic impairment: Deterioration in transaminases, alkaline phosphatase or bilirubin, toxic hepatitis, biliary stasis, clinical jaundice, evidence of hepatic sinusoidal obstruction syndrome (veno-occlusive disease), or evidence of portal hypertension: Discontinue treatment.

Administration Administer orally; total daily dose can be given at one time.

Monitoring Parameters CBC with differential and platelet count; liver function tests (weekly when beginning therapy then monthly, more frequently in patients with liver disease or concurrent hepatotoxic drugs); serum uric acid; some laboratories offer testing for TPMT deficiency

Hepatotoxicity may present with signs of portal hypertension (splenomegaly, esophageal varices, thrombocytopenia) or sinusoidal obstruction syndrome (veno-occlusive disease; fluid retention, ascites, hepatomegaly with tenderness, or hyperbilirubinemia)

Dosage Forms Excipient information presented when available (limited, particularly for generics); consult specific product labeling.

Tablet, oral:

Tabloid®: 40 mg [scored]

Extemporaneous Preparations Hazardous agent: Use appropriate precautions for handling and disposal.

A 20 mg/mL oral suspension may be made with tablets, methylcellulose 1%, and simple syrup NF. Crush fifteen 40 mg tablets in a mortar and reduce to a fine powder. Add 10 mL methylcellulose 1% in incremental proportions and mix to a uniform paste. Transfer to a graduated cylinder, rinse mortar with simple syrup, and add quantity of simple syrup sufficient to make 30 mL. Label "shake well" and "refrigerate". Stable for 84 days refrigerated (preferred) or at room temperature.

Dressman JB and Poust RI, "Stability of Allopurinol and Five Antineoplastics in Suspension," *Am J Hosp Pharm*, 1983, 40(4):616-8.

Nahata MC, Pai VB, and Hipple TF, *Pediatric Drug Formulations*, 5th ed, Cincinnati, OH: Harvey Whitney Books Co, 2004.

◆ **6-Thioguanine (error-prone abbreviation)** *see* Thioguanine *on page 1670*

Thiopental (thye oh PEN tal)

Brand Names: U.S. Pentothal® [DSC]

Brand Names: Canada Pentothal®

Index Terms Thiopental Sodium

Pharmacologic Category Anticonvulsant, Barbiturate; Barbiturate; General Anesthetic

Use Induction of anesthesia; control of convulsive states; treatment of elevated intracranial pressure

Pregnancy Risk Factor C

Contraindications Hypersensitivity to thiopental, barbiturates, or any component of the formulation; status asthmaticus; severe cardiovascular disease; porphyria (variegate or acute intermittent); should not be administered by intra-arterial injection

Warnings/Precautions Laryngospasm or bronchospasms may occur; use with extreme caution in patients with reactive airway diseases (asthma or COPD). Use with caution when the hypnotic may be prolonged or potentiated (excessive premedication, Addison's disease, hepatic or renal dysfunction, myxedema, increased blood urea, severe anemia, or myasthenia gravis). Potential for drug dependency exists, abrupt cessation may precipitate withdrawal, including status epilepticus in epileptic patients. Do not administer to patients in acute pain. Use caution in patients with unstable aneurysms, cardiovascular disease, renal impairment, or hepatic disease. Use caution in elderly, debilitated, or pediatric patients. May cause paradoxical responses, including agitation and hyperactivity, particularly in acute pain and pediatric patients. Effects with other sedative drugs or ethanol may be potentiated. May cause respiratory depression or hypotension. Use with caution in hemodynamically unstable patients (hypotension or shock) or patients with respiratory disease. Repeated dosing or continuous infusions may cause cumulative effects. Administer only by I.V. route.

Adverse Reactions Frequency not defined.

Cardiovascular: Bradycardia, hypotension, syncope

Central nervous system: Drowsiness, lethargy, CNS excitation or depression, impaired judgment, "hangover" effect, confusion, somnolence, agitation, hyperkinesia, ataxia, nervousness, headache, insomnia, nightmares, hallucinations, anxiety, dizziness, shivering

Dermatologic: Rash, exfoliative dermatitis, Stevens-Johnson syndrome

Gastrointestinal: Nausea, vomiting, constipation

Hematologic: Agranulocytosis, thrombocytopenia, megaloblastic anemia, immune hemolytic anemia (rare)

Local: Pain at injection site, thrombophlebitis with I.V. use

Renal: Oliguria

Respiratory: Laryngospasm, respiratory depression, apnea (especially with rapid I.V. use), hypoventilation, sneezing, cough, bronchospasm

Miscellaneous: Gangrene with inadvertent intra-arterial injection, anaphylaxis, anaphylactic reactions

Drug Interactions

Metabolism/Transport Effects None known.

Avoid Concomitant Use There are no known interactions where it is recommended to avoid concomitant use.

Increased Effect/Toxicity

Thiopental may increase the levels/effects of: Alcohol (Ethyl); CNS Depressants; Meperidine; QuiNIDine; Selective Serotonin Reuptake Inhibitors; Thiazide Diuretics

The levels/effects of Thiopental may be increased by: Carbonic Anhydrase Inhibitors; Chloramphenicol; Divalproex; Droperidol; Felbamate; HydrOXYzine; Primidone; Valproic Acid

Decreased Effect

Thiopental may decrease the levels/effects of: Acetaminophen; Beta-Blockers; Calcium Channel Blockers; Chloramphenicol; Contraceptives (Estrogens); Contraceptives (Progestins); Corticosteroids (Systemic); CycloSPORINE; CycloSPORINE (Systemic); Disopyramide; Divalproex; Doxycycline; Etoposide; Etoposide Phosphate; Felbamate; Fosphenytoin; LamoTRIgine; Methadone; Phenytoin; Propafenone; QuiNIDine; Teniposide; Theophylline Derivatives; Tricyclic Antidepressants; Valproic Acid; Vitamin K Antagonists

The levels/effects of Thiopental may be decreased by: Ketorolac; Ketorolac (Nasal); Ketorolac (Systemic); Mefloquine; Pyridoxine; Rifamycin Derivatives

Stability Reconstituted solutions remain stable for 3 days at room temperature and 7 days when refrigerated.

Mechanism of Action Short-acting barbiturate with sedative, hypnotic, and anticonvulsant properties. Barbiturates depress the sensory cortex, decrease motor activity, alter cerebellar function, and produce drowsiness, sedation, and hypnosis. In high doses, barbiturates exhibit anticonvulsant activity; barbiturates produce dose-dependent respiratory depression.

Pharmacodynamics/Kinetics

Onset of action: Anesthetic: I.V.: 30-60 seconds
Duration: 5-30 minutes
Distribution: V_d: ~1.6 L/kg
Protein binding: 72% to 86%
Metabolism: Hepatic, primarily to inactive metabolites but pentobarbital is also formed
Half-life elimination: 3-11.5 hours; decreased in children

Dosage I.V.:

Induction anesthesia:
- Infants: 5-8 mg/kg
- Children 1-12 years: 5-6 mg/kg
- Adults: 3-5 mg/kg

Maintenance anesthesia:
- Children: 1 mg/kg as needed
- Adults: 25-100 mg as needed

Increased intracranial pressure: Children and Adults: 1.5-5 mg/kg/dose; repeat as needed to control intracranial pressure

Seizures:
- Children: 2-3 mg/kg/dose; repeat as needed
- Adults: 75-250 mg/dose; repeat as needed

Dosing adjustment in renal impairment: Cl_{cr} <10 mL/minute: Administer at 75% of normal dose

Note: Accumulation may occur with chronic dosing due to lipid solubility; prolonged recovery may result from redistribution of thiopental from fat stores

Dietary Considerations Some products may contain sodium.

Administration Administer slowly over 20-30 seconds. Rapid I.V. injection may cause hypotension or decreased cardiac output; avoid extravasation, necrosis may occur. Check I.V. catheter placement prior to administration. If inadvertent intra-arterial administration occurs, treat with a local anesthetic (eg, lidocaine 1%, 5 mL) and/or papaverine (20-40 mg), preferably through the catheter used for the thiopental injection.

Monitoring Parameters Respiratory rate, heart rate, blood pressure

Reference Range Therapeutic: Hypnotic: 1-5 mcg/mL (SI: 4.1-20.7 micromole/L); Coma: 30-100 mcg/mL (SI: 124-413 micromole/L); Anesthesia: 7-130 mcg/mL (SI: 29-536 micromole/L); Toxic: >10 mcg/mL (SI: >41 micromole/L)

Additional Information Thiopental switches from linear to nonlinear pharmacokinetics following prolonged continuous infusions.

Dosage Forms Excipient information presented when available (limited, particularly for generics); consult specific product labeling. [DSC] = Discontinued product

Injection, powder for reconstitution, as sodium:
Pentothal®: 250 mg [DSC], 400 mg [DSC], 500 mg [DSC], 1 g [DSC] [contains sodium 105 mg/g]

Controlled Substance C-III

◆ **Thiopental Sodium** *see* Thiopental *on page* 1671
◆ **Thiophosphoramide** *see* Thiotepa *on page* 1674
◆ **Thioplex** *see* Thiotepa *on page* 1674

Thioridazine (thye oh RID a zeen)

Index Terms Mellaril; Thioridazine Hydrochloride

Pharmacologic Category Antipsychotic Agent, Typical, Phenothiazine

Additional Appendix Information

Antipsychotic Agents *on page* 1880
Beers Criteria – Potentially Inappropriate Medications for Geriatrics *on page* 1973

Use Management of schizophrenic patients who fail to respond adequately to treatment with other antipsychotic drugs, either because of insufficient effectiveness or the inability to achieve an effective dose due to intolerable adverse effects from those medications

Unlabeled Use Behavior problems (children); severe psychoses (children); schizophrenia/psychoses (children); depressive disorders/dementia (children and adults); behavioral symptoms associated with dementia (elderly); psychosis/agitation related to Alzheimer's dementia

Pregnancy Risk Factor C

Pregnancy Considerations Jaundice or hyper-/hyporeflexia have been reported in newborn infants following maternal use of phenothiazines. Antipsychotic use during the third trimester of pregnancy has a risk for abnormal muscle movements (extrapyramidal symptoms [EPS]) and withdrawal symptoms in newborns following delivery. Symptoms in the newborn may include agitation, feeding disorder, hypertonia, hypotonia, respiratory distress, somnolence, and tremor; these effects may be self-limiting or require hospitalization.

Contraindications Severe CNS depression; severe hyper-/hypotensive heart disease; coma; in combination with other drugs that are known to prolong the QT_c interval and/or CYP2D6 inhibitors; in patients with congenital long QT syndrome or a history of cardiac arrhythmias; concurrent use with medications that inhibit the metabolism of thioridazine (fluoxetine, paroxetine, fluvoxamine, propranolol, pindolol); patients known to have genetic defect leading to reduced levels of activity of CYP2D6

Warnings/Precautions [U.S. Boxed Warning]: Thioridazine has dose-related effects on ventricular repolarization leading to QT_c prolongation, a potentially life-threatening effect. Therefore, it should be reserved for patients with schizophrenia who have failed to respond to adequate levels of other antipsychotic drugs. Due to potential for QT_c prolongation; use contraindicated with concomitant CYP2D6 inhibitors and/or concomitant use with other agents that prolong the QT_c interval. May cause orthostatic hypotension; use with caution in patients at risk of this effect or those who would tolerate transient hypotensive episodes (cerebrovascular disease, cardiovascular disease, or other medications which may predispose). **[U.S. Boxed Warning]: Elderly patients with dementia-related psychosis treated with antipsychotics are at an increased risk of death compared to placebo.** Most deaths appeared to be either cardiovascular (eg, heart failure, sudden death) or infectious (eg, pneumonia) in nature. Thioridazine is not approved for the treatment of dementia-related psychosis.

Leukopenia, neutropenia, and agranulocytosis (sometimes fatal) have been reported in clinical trials and postmarketing reports with antipsychotic use; presence of risk factors (eg, pre-existing low WBC or history of drug-induced leuko-/neutropenia) should prompt periodic blood count assessment. Discontinue therapy at first signs of blood dyscrasias or if absolute neutrophil count <1000/mm^3.

Highly sedating, use with caution in disorders where CNS depression is a feature. Use with caution in Parkinson's disease. Use caution in patients with hemodynamic instability; predisposition to seizures; subcortical brain damage; severe cardiac, hepatic, or renal disease. Esophageal dysmotility and aspiration have been associated with antipsychotic use; use with caution in patients at risk of pneumonia (ie, Alzheimer's disease). Use associated with increased prolactin levels; clinical significance of hyperprolactinemia in patients with breast cancer or other prolactin-dependent tumors is unknown. May alter temperature regulation or mask toxicity of other drugs due to antiemetic effects.

Phenothiazines may cause anticholinergic effects (confusion, agitation, constipation, xerostomia, blurred vision, urinary retention); therefore, they should be used with caution in patients with decreased gastrointestinal motility, urinary retention, BPH, xerostomia, or visual problems. Conditions which also may be exacerbated by cholinergic blockade include narrow-angle glaucoma and worsening of myasthenia gravis. Relative to other neuroleptics, thioridazine has a high potency of cholinergic blockade.

May cause extrapyramidal symptoms (EPS), including pseudoparkinsonism, acute dystonic reactions, akathisia, and tardive dyskinesia. Risk of dystonia (and possibly other EPS) may be greater with increased doses, use of conventional antipsychotics, males, and younger patients. May be inappropriate for use in the elderly due to risk of CNS and EPS adverse effects (Beers Criteria). May be associated with neuroleptic malignant syndrome (NMS). May cause pigmentary retinopathy, and lenticular and corneal deposits, particularly with prolonged therapy.

Adverse Reactions Frequency not defined.

Cardiovascular: Hypotension, orthostatic hypotension, peripheral edema, ECG changes

Central nervous system: EPS (pseudoparkinsonism, akathisia, dystonias, tardive dyskinesia), dizziness, drowsiness, neuroleptic malignant syndrome (NMS), impairment of temperature regulation, lowering of seizure threshold

Dermatologic: Increased sensitivity to sun, rash, discoloration of skin (blue-gray)

Endocrine & metabolic: Changes in menstrual cycle, libido (changes in), breast pain, galactorrhea, amenorrhea

Gastrointestinal: Constipation, weight gain, nausea, vomiting, stomach pain, xerostomia, diarrhea

Genitourinary: Difficulty in urination, ejaculatory disturbances, urinary retention, priapism

Hematologic: Agranulocytosis, leukopenia

Hepatic: Cholestatic jaundice, hepatotoxicity

Neuromuscular & skeletal: Tremor, seizure

Ocular: Pigmentary retinopathy, blurred vision, cornea and lens changes

Respiratory: Nasal congestion

Drug Interactions

Metabolism/Transport Effects Substrate of CYP2C19 (minor), CYP2D6 (major); **Note:** Assignment of Major/Minor substrate status based on clinically relevant drug interaction potential; **Inhibits** CYP1A2 (weak), CYP2C9 (weak), CYP2D6 (strong), CYP2E1 (weak)

Avoid Concomitant Use

Avoid concomitant use of Thioridazine with any of the following: Artemether; CYP2D6 Inhibitors; Dronedarone; FluvoxaMINE; Lumefantrine; Metoclopramide; Moclobemide; Nilotinib; Pimozide; QTc-Prolonging Agents; QUEtiapine; QuiNINE; Tamoxifen; Tetrabenazine; Toremifene; Vandetanib; Vemurafenib; Ziprasidone

Increased Effect/Toxicity

Thioridazine may increase the levels/effects of: Alcohol (Ethyl); Analgesics (Opioid); Anticholinergics; Antidepressants (Serotonin Reuptake Inhibitor/Antagonist); Anti-Parkinson's Agents (Dopamine Agonist); Atomoxetine; Beta-Blockers; CNS Depressants; CYP2D6 Substrates; Dronedarone; Fesoterodine; Methylphenidate; Pimozide; Porfimer; QTc-Prolonging Agents; QuiNINE; Serotonin Modulators; Tamoxifen; Tetrabenazine; Toremifene; Vandetanib; Vemurafenib; Ziprasidone

The levels/effects of Thioridazine may be increased by: Abiraterone Acetate; Acetylcholinesterase Inhibitors (Central); Alfuzosin; Antidepressants (Serotonin Reuptake Inhibitor/Antagonist); Antimalarial Agents; Artemether; Beta-Blockers; Chloroquine; Ciprofloxacin; Ciprofloxacin (Systemic); CYP2D6 Inhibitors; Darunavir; FluvoxaMINE; Gadobutrol; HydrOXYzine; Indacaterol; Lithium formulations; Lumefantrine; Methylphenidate; Metoclopramide; Moclobemide; Nilotinib; Pramlintide; QTc-Prolonging Agents; QUEtiapine; QuiNINE; Tetrabenazine

Decreased Effect

Thioridazine may decrease the levels/effects of: Amphetamines; Quinagolide

The levels/effects of Thioridazine may be decreased by: Antacids; Anti-Parkinson's Agents (Dopamine Agonist); Lithium formulations; Peginterferon Alfa-2b

Ethanol/Nutrition/Herb Interactions

Ethanol: May increase CNS depression; monitor for increased effects with coadministration. Caution patients about effects.

Herb/Nutraceutical: Avoid kava kava, valerian, St John's wort, gotu kola (may increase CNS depression). Avoid dong quai, St John's wort (may also cause photosensitization).

Stability Protect from light.

Mechanism of Action Thioridazine is a piperidine phenothiazine which blocks postsynaptic mesolimbic dopaminergic receptors in the brain; exhibits a strong alpha-adrenergic blocking effect and depresses the release of hypothalamic and hypophyseal hormones

Pharmacodynamics/Kinetics

Duration: 4-5 days

Half-life elimination: 21-25 hours

Time to peak, serum: ~1 hour

Dosage Oral:

Children >2-12 years (unlabeled use): Range: 0.5-3 mg/kg/day in 2-3 divided doses; usual: 1 mg/kg/day; maximum: 3 mg/kg/day

Behavior problems (unlabeled use): Initial: 10 mg 2-3 times/day, increase gradually

Severe psychoses (unlabeled use): Initial: 25 mg 2-3 times/day, increase gradually

Children >12 years (unlabeled use) and Adults:

Schizophrenia/psychoses: Initial: 50-100 mg 3 times/day with gradual increments as needed and tolerated; maximum: 800 mg/day in 2-4 divided doses

Depressive disorders/dementia (unlabeled use): Initial: 25 mg 3 times/day; maintenance dose: 20-200 mg/day

Elderly: Behavioral symptoms associated with dementia (unlabeled use): Oral: Initial: 10-25 mg 1-2 times/day; increase at 4- to 7-day intervals by 10-25 mg/day; increase dose intervals (once daily, twice daily, etc) as necessary to control response or side effects. Maximum daily dose: 400 mg; gradual increases (titration) may prevent some side effects or decrease their severity.

Hemodialysis: Not dialyzable (0% to 5%)

Administration Do not take antacid within 2 hours of taking drug.

Monitoring Parameters Baseline and periodic ECG; vital signs; serum potassium, lipid profile, fasting blood glucose and Hgb A_{1c}; BMI; mental status, abnormal involuntary movement scale (AIMS); periodic eye exam; do not initiate if QT_c >450 msec

Reference Range Toxic: >1 mg/mL; lethal: 2-8 mg/dL

Test Interactions False-positives for phenylketonuria, urinary amylase, uroporphyrins, urobilinogen; may interfere with urine detection of methadone and PCP (false-positives)

Dosage Forms Excipient information presented when available (limited, particularly for generics); consult specific product labeling.

Tablet, oral, as hydrochloride: 10 mg, 25 mg, 50 mg, 100 mg

◆ **Thioridazine Hydrochloride** *see* Thioridazine *on page 1672*

◆ **Thiosulfuric Acid Disodium Salt** *see* Sodium Thiosulfate *on page 1577*

Thiotepa (thye oh TEP a)

Index Terms TESPA; Thiophosphoramide; Thioplex; Triethylenethiophosphoramide; TSPA

Pharmacologic Category Antineoplastic Agent, Alkylating Agent

Use Treatment of superficial papillary bladder cancer; palliative treatment of adenocarcinoma of breast or ovary; controlling intracavitary effusions caused by metastatic tumors

Unlabeled Use Intrathecal treatment of leptomeningeal metastases

Pregnancy Risk Factor D

Pregnancy Considerations Animal studies have demonstrated teratogenicity and fetal loss. There are no adequate and well-controlled studies in pregnant women. May cause harm if administered during pregnancy. Effective contraception is recommended for men and women of childbearing potential.

Lactation Excretion in breast milk unknown/not recommended

Contraindications Hypersensitivity to thiotepa or any component of the formulation

Note: May be contraindicated in certain circumstances of hepatic, renal, and/or bone marrow failure; evaluate on an individual basis as lower dose treatment (with close monitoring) may still be appropriate if the potential benefit outweighs the risks

Warnings/Precautions Hazardous agent - use appropriate precautions for handling and disposal. Myelosuppression is common; monitor for infection or bleeding. Myelosuppression has also been reported with intravesicular administration (due to systemic absorption). Potentially teratogenic, mutagenic, and carcinogenic; myelodysplastic syndrome and acute myeloid leukemia (AML) have been reported. Reduce dosage and use extreme caution in patients with hepatic, renal, or bone marrow damage. Use may be contraindicated with impairment/damage and should be limited to cases where benefit outweighs risk.

When used for intrathecal administration, should not be prepared during the preparation of any other agents; after preparation, store intrathecal medications in an isolated location or container clearly marked with a label identifying as "intrathecal" use only; delivery of intrathecal medications to the patient should only be with other medications intended for administration into the central nervous system (Jacobson, 2009).

Adverse Reactions

Frequency not defined:

Central nervous system: Chills, dizziness, fatigue, fever, headache

Dermatologic: Alopecia, contact dermatitis, depigmentation (with topical treatment), dermatitis, rash, urticaria

Endocrine & metabolic: Amenorrhea, spermatogenesis inhibition

Gastrointestinal: Abdominal pain, anorexia, nausea, vomiting

Genitourinary: Dysuria, urinary retention

Hematologic: Anemia, bleeding, leukopenia, thrombocytopenia

Local: Injection site pain

Neuromuscular & skeletal: Weakness

Ocular: Blurred vision, conjunctivitis

Renal: Hematuria

Respiratory: Asthma, epistaxis, laryngeal edema, wheezing

Miscellaneous: Allergic reaction, anaphylactic shock, infection

Infrequent, postmarketing, and/or case reports: Acute myeloid leukemia (AML), chemical cystitis (bladder instillation), hemorrhagic cystitis (bladder instillation), myelodysplastic syndrome

Drug Interactions

Metabolism/Transport Effects Inhibits CYP2B6 (strong)

Avoid Concomitant Use

Avoid concomitant use of Thiotepa with any of the following: BCG; CloZAPine; Natalizumab; Pimecrolimus; Tacrolimus (Topical); Vaccines (Live)

Increased Effect/Toxicity

Thiotepa may increase the levels/effects of: CloZAPine; CYP2B6 Substrates; Leflunomide; Natalizumab; Vaccines (Live)

The levels/effects of Thiotepa may be increased by: Denosumab; Pimecrolimus; Roflumilast; Tacrolimus (Topical); Trastuzumab

Decreased Effect

Thiotepa may decrease the levels/effects of: BCG; Coccidioidin Skin Test; Sipuleucel-T; Vaccines (Inactivated); Vaccines (Live)

The levels/effects of Thiotepa may be decreased by: Echinacea

Ethanol/Nutrition/Herb Interactions

Ethanol: Avoid ethanol (due to GI irritation).

Herb/Nutraceutical: Avoid black cohosh, dong quai in estrogen-dependent tumors.

Stability Store intact vials under refrigeration (2°C to 8°C). Protect from light. Reconstitute each 15 mg vial with 1.5 mL SWFI to a concentration of 10 mg/mL. Reconstituted solutions (10 mg/mL) are stable for up to 28 days under refrigeration (4°C to 8°C) or 7 days at room temperature (25°C), although the manufacturer recommends use within 8 hours when reconstituted solutions are stored under refrigeration. Should be further diluted in 0.9% sodium chloride injection for I.V. use. Solutions further diluted (for I.V. use) in NS to 1 mg/mL are stable for 24 hours and to 3 mg/mL are stable for 48 hours at room temperature, although the manufacturer recommends immediate use. Filter through a 0.22 micron filter (polysulfone membrane [eg, Sterile Aerodisc®] or triton-free cellulose mixed ester [eg, Millex®-GS]) prior to administration; do not use solutions which precipitate or remain opaque after filtering. Use appropriate precautions for handling and disposal.

Intrathecal: Dilute to a concentration of 1-5 mg/mL in preservative-free NS. Intrathecal medications should not be prepared during the preparation of any other agents. After preparation, store intrathecal medications in an isolated location or container clearly marked with a label identifying as "intrathecal" use only.

Intravesicular: Dilute in 30-60 mL NS.

Mechanism of Action Alkylating agent that reacts with DNA phosphate groups to produce cross-linking of DNA strands leading to inhibition of DNA, RNA, and protein synthesis; mechanism of action has not been explored as thoroughly as the other alkylating agents, it is presumed that the aziridine rings open and react as nitrogen mustard; reactivity is enhanced at a lower pH

Pharmacodynamics/Kinetics

Absorption: Intracavitary instillation: Unreliable (10% to 100%) through bladder mucosa

Metabolism: Extensively hepatic; major metabolite (active): TEPA

Half-life elimination: Terminal (dose-dependent clearance): ~2 hours

Excretion: Urine (as metabolites and unchanged drug)

Dosage

Children: HSCT for CNS malignancy (unlabeled use; combination chemotherapy): I.V.: 300 mg/m^2/day for 3 days beginning 8 days prior to transplant (Gilheeney, 2010) **or** 300 mg/m^2/day for 3 days beginning 5 days prior to transplant (Dunkel, 2010; Grodman, 2009)

Adults:

Bladder cancer: Intravesical: 60 mg in 30-60 mL NS retained for 2 hours once weekly for 4 weeks

Ovarian, breast cancer: I.V.: 0.3-0.4 mg/kg by rapid I.V. administration every 1-4 weeks

Effusions: Intracavitary: 0.6-0.8 mg/kg

Leptomeningeal metastases (unlabeled use): Intrathecal: 10 mg twice a week for 4 weeks, then (if CSF cytology is negative) weekly for 4 weeks, then monthly for 4 doses (NCCN CNS cancer guidelines v.1.2010)

HSCT for CNS malignancy (unlabeled use; combination chemotherapy): I.V.: 250 mg/m^2/day for 3 days beginning 9 days prior to transplant (Soussain, 2008) **or** 150 mg/m^2/dose every 12 hours for 6 doses, followed by stem cell reinfusion 96 hours after completion of thiotepa (Abrey, 2006)

Dosage adjustment for hematologic toxicity: I.V.:

WBC ≤3000/mm^3: Discontinue treatment

Platelets ≤150,000/mm^3: Discontinue treatment

Note: Use may be contraindicated with pre-existing marrow damage and should be limited to cases where benefit outweighs risk.

Dosing adjustment in renal impairment: Use with extreme caution, reduced dose may be warranted. Use may be contraindicated with existing renal impairment and should be limited to cases where benefit outweighs risk.

Dosing adjustment in hepatic impairment: Use with extreme caution, reduced dose may be warranted. Use may be contraindicated with existing hepatic impairment and should be limited to cases where benefit outweighs risk.

Administration

I.V.: Administer as a rapid injection. Infusion times may be longer for high-dose (unlabeled use) treatment; refer to specific protocols

Intravesical instillation: Instill directly into the bladder and retain for 2 hours; patient should be repositioned every 15-30 minutes for maximal exposure

Monitoring Parameters CBC with differential and platelet count (monitor weekly during treatment and for at least 3 weeks after treatment); renal and liver function tests; uric acid, urinalysis

Dosage Forms Excipient information presented when available (limited, particularly for generics); consult specific product labeling.

Injection, powder for reconstitution: 15 mg

Thiothixene (thye oh THIKS een)

Brand Names: U.S. Navane® [DSC]

Brand Names: Canada Navane®

Index Terms Tiotixene

Pharmacologic Category Antipsychotic Agent, Typical

Additional Appendix Information

Antipsychotic Agents *on page 1880*

Use Management of schizophrenia

Unlabeled Use Psychotic disorders (children); rapid tranquilization of the agitated patient (children); nonpsychotic patient, dementia behavior (elderly); psychosis/agitation related to Alzheimer's dementia

Pregnancy Considerations Antipsychotic use during the third trimester of pregnancy has a risk for abnormal muscle movements (extrapyramidal symptoms [EPS]) and withdrawal symptoms in newborns following delivery. Symptoms in the newborn may include agitation, feeding disorder, hypertonia, hypotonia, respiratory distress, somnolence, and tremor; these effects may be self-limiting or require hospitalization.

Contraindications Hypersensitivity to thiothixene or any component of the formulation; severe CNS depression; circulatory collapse; blood dyscrasias; coma

Warnings/Precautions [U.S. Boxed Warning]: Elderly patients with dementia-related psychosis treated with antipsychotics are at an increased risk of death compared to placebo. Most deaths appeared to be either cardiovascular (eg, heart failure, sudden death) or infectious (eg, pneumonia) in nature. Thiothixene is not approved for the treatment of dementia-related psychosis.

May alter cardiac conduction; life-threatening arrhythmias have occurred with therapeutic doses of antipsychotics. Avoid use in patients with underlying QT prolongation, in those taking medicines that prolong the QT interval, or cause polymorphic ventricular tachycardia; monitor ECG closely for dose-related QT effects.

Leukopenia, neutropenia, and agranulocytosis (sometimes fatal) have been reported in clinical trials and postmarketing reports with antipsychotic use; presence of risk factors (eg, pre-existing low WBC or history of drug-induced leuko-/neutropenia) should prompt periodic blood count assessment. Discontinue therapy at first signs of blood dyscrasias or if absolute neutrophil count <1000/mm^3.

Antipsychotic use has been associated with esophageal dysmotility and aspiration; use with caution in patients at risk of pneumonia (ie, Alzheimer's disease). May cause extrapyramidal symptoms (EPS), including pseudoparkinsonism, acute dystonic reactions, akathisia, and tardive dyskinesia. Risk of dystonia (and possibly other EPS) may be greater with increased doses, use of conventional antipsychotics, males, and younger patients. Use may be associated with NMS; monitor for mental status changes, fever, muscle rigidity, and/or autonomic instability. May cause orthostatic hypotension; use with caution in patients at risk of this effect or in those who would not tolerate transient hypotensive episodes (cerebrovascular disease, cardiovascular disease, hypovolemia, or concurrent medication use which may predispose to hypotension/bradycardia). May rarely cause pigmentary retinopathy and lenticular pigmentation. Impaired core body temperature regulation may occur; caution with strenuous exercise, heat exposure, dehydration, and concomitant medication possessing anticholinergic effects.

May be sedating, use with caution in disorders where CNS depression is a feature; patients must be cautioned about performing tasks which require mental alertness (eg, operating machinery or driving). Effects may be potentiated when used with other sedative drugs or ethanol. May cause anticholinergic effects (constipation, xerostomia, blurred vision, urinary retention); use with caution in patients with decreased gastrointestinal motility, paralytic ileus, urinary retention, BPH, xerostomia, or visual problems. Relative to other neuroleptics, thiothixene has a low potency of cholinergic blockade. May mask toxicity of other drugs or conditions (eg, intestinal obstruction, Reye's syndrome, brain tumor) due to antiemetic effects. Use is associated with increased prolactin levels; clinical significance of hyperprolactinemia in patients with breast cancer or other prolactin-dependent tumors is unknown.

Use with caution in patients with severe cardiovascular disease, narrow-angle glaucoma, hepatic impairment, myasthenia gravis, Parkinson's disease, renal impairment, or seizure disorder. Use with caution in the elderly.

Adverse Reactions Frequency not defined.

Cardiovascular: Hypotension, nonspecific ECG changes, syncope, tachycardia

Central nervous system: Agitation, dizziness, drowsiness, extrapyramidal symptoms (akathisia, dystonias, lightheadedness, pseudoparkinsonism, tardive dyskinesia), insomnia restlessness

Dermatologic: Discoloration of skin (blue-gray), photosensitivity, pruritus, rash, urticaria

Endocrine & metabolic: Amenorrhea, breast pain, libido (changes in), changes in menstrual cycle, galactorrhea, gynecomastia, hyper-/hypoglycemia, hyperprolactinemia, lactation

Gastrointestinal: Constipation, nausea, salivation increased, stomach pain, vomiting, weight gain, xerostomia

Genitourinary: Difficulty in urination, ejaculatory disturbances, impotence

Hematologic: Leukocytes, leukopenia

Neuromuscular & skeletal: Tremors

Ocular: Blurred vision, pigmentary retinopathy

Respiratory: Nasal congestion

Miscellaneous: Diaphoresis

Drug Interactions

Metabolism/Transport Effects Substrate of CYP1A2 (major); **Note:** Assignment of Major/Minor substrate status based on clinically relevant drug interaction potential; **Inhibits** CYP2D6 (weak)

Avoid Concomitant Use

Avoid concomitant use of Thiothixene with any of the following: Artemether; Dronedarone; Lumefantrine; Metoclopramide; Nilotinib; Pimozide; QUEtiapine; QuiNINE; Tetrabenazine; Thioridazine; Toremifene; Vandetanib; Vemurafenib; Ziprasidone

Increased Effect/Toxicity

Thiothixene may increase the levels/effects of: Alcohol (Ethyl); Anticholinergics; Anti-Parkinson's Agents (Dopamine Agonist); CNS Depressants; Dronedarone; Methylphenidate; Pimozide; QTc-Prolonging Agents; QuiNINE; Serotonin Modulators; Tetrabenazine; Thioridazine; Toremifene; Vandetanib; Vemurafenib; Ziprasidone

The levels/effects of Thiothixene may be increased by: Abiraterone Acetate; Acetylcholinesterase Inhibitors (Central); Alfuzosin; Artemether; Chloroquine; Ciprofloxacin; Ciprofloxacin (Systemic); CYP1A2 Inhibitors (Moderate); CYP1A2 Inhibitors (Strong); Deferasirox; Gadobutrol; HydrOXYzine; Indacaterol; Lithium formulations; Lumefantrine; Methylphenidate; Metoclopramide; Nilotinib; Pramlintide; QUEtiapine; QuiNINE; Tetrabenazine

Decreased Effect

Thiothixene may decrease the levels/effects of: Amphetamines; Quinagolide

The levels/effects of Thiothixene may be decreased by: Anti-Parkinson's Agents (Dopamine Agonist); CYP1A2 Inducers (Strong); Cyproterone; Lithium formulations

Ethanol/Nutrition/Herb Interactions

Ethanol: May increase CNS depression; monitor for increased effects with coadministration. Caution patients about effects.

Herb/Nutraceutical: Avoid kava kava, valerian, St John's wort, gotu kola (may increase CNS depression).

Mechanism of Action Thiothixene is a thioxanthene antipsychotic which elicits antipsychotic activity by postsynaptic blockade of CNS dopamine receptors resulting in inhibition of dopamine-mediated effects; also has alpha-adrenergic blocking activity

Pharmacodynamics/Kinetics

Metabolism: Extensively hepatic

Half-life elimination: >24 hours with chronic use

Dosage Oral:

Children <12 years (unlabeled use): Schizophrenia/psychoses: 0.25 mg/kg/24 hours in divided doses (dose not well established; use not recommended)

Children >12 years (unlabeled use) and Adults:

Mild-to-moderate psychosis: 2 mg 3 times/day, up to 20-30 mg/day; more severe psychosis: Initial: 5 mg 2 times/day, may increase gradually, if necessary; maximum: 60 mg/day

Rapid tranquilization of the agitated patient (administered every 30-60 minutes): 5-10 mg; average total dose for tranquilization: 15-30 mg

Elderly: Nonpsychotic patient, dementia behavior (unlabeled use): Initial: 1-2 mg 1-2 times/day; increase dose at 4- to 7-day intervals by 1-2 mg/day. Increase dosing intervals (bid, tid, etc) as necessary to control response or side effects; maximum daily dose: 30 mg. Gradual increases in dose may prevent some side effects or decrease their severity.

Hemodialysis: Not dialyzable (0% to 5%)

Monitoring Parameters Vital signs; lipid profile, fasting blood glucose/Hgb A_{1c}; BMI; mental status, abnormal involuntary movement scale (AIMS), extrapyramidal symptoms (EPS)

Test Interactions May cause false-positive pregnancy test

Dosage Forms Excipient information presented when available (limited, particularly for generics); consult specific product labeling. [DSC] = Discontinued product

Capsule, oral: 1 mg, 2 mg, 5 mg, 10 mg

Navane®: 2 mg [DSC], 10 mg [DSC], 20 mg [DSC]

◆ **Thonzonium, Neomycin, Colistin, and Hydrocortisone** *see* Neomycin, Colistin, Hydrocortisone, and Thonzonium *on page* 1189

◆ **Thorazine** *see* ChlorproMAZINE *on page* 348

◆ **Thorets [OTC]** *see* Benzocaine *on page* 202

◆ **Thrive™ [OTC]** *see* Nicotine *on page* 1200

◆ **Thrombate III®** *see* Antithrombin *on page* 130

◆ **Thymocyte Stimulating Factor** *see* Aldesleukin *on page* 55

◆ **Thymoglobulin®** *see* Antithymocyte Globulin (Rabbit) *on page* 133

◆ **Thyrogen®** *see* Thyrotropin Alfa *on page* 1677

Thyroid, Desiccated (THYE roid DES i kay tid)

Brand Names: U.S. Armour® Thyroid; Nature-Throid™; Westhroid™

Index Terms Desiccated Thyroid; Levothyroxine and Liothyronine; Tetraiodothyronine and Triiodothyronine; Thyroid Extract; Thyroid USP

Pharmacologic Category Thyroid Product

Use Replacement or supplemental therapy in hypothyroidism; pituitary TSH suppressants (thyroid nodules, thyroiditis, multinodular goiter, thyroid cancer)

Pregnancy Risk Factor A

Dosage Oral: **Note:** The American Association of Clinical Endocrinologists does not recommend the use of desiccated thyroid for thyroid replacement therapy for hypothyroidism (Baskin, 2002).

Children: See table.

Recommended Pediatric Dosage for Congenital Hypothyroidism

Age	Daily Dose (mg)	Daily Dose/kg (mg)
0-6 mo	15-30	4.8-6
6-12 mo	30-45	3.6-4.8
1-5 y	45-60	3-3.6
6-12 y	60-90	2.4-3
>12 y	>90	1.2-1.8

Adults: Initial: 15-30 mg; increase with 15 mg increments every 2-3 weeks; use 15 mg in patients with cardiovascular disease or long-standing myxedema. Maintenance dose: Usually 60-120 mg/day; monitor TSH and clinical symptoms.

Additional Information Complete prescribing information for this medication should be consulted for additional detail.

Dosage Forms Excipient information presented when available (limited, particularly for generics); consult specific product labeling. [DSC] = Discontinued product

Tablet, oral: 30 mg [DSC], 60 mg [DSC], 120 mg [DSC]

Armour® Thyroid: 15 mg, 30 mg, 60 mg, 90 mg, 120 mg

Armour® Thyroid: 180 mg [scored]

Armour® Thyroid: 240 mg

Armour® Thyroid: 300 mg [scored]

Nature-Throid™: 16.25 mg, 32.5 mg, 65 mg, 130 mg, 195 mg

Westhroid™: 32.5 mg, 65 mg, 130 mg

◆ **Thyroid Extract** *see* Thyroid, Desiccated *on page* 1676

◆ **Thyroid USP** *see* Thyroid, Desiccated *on page* 1676

◆ **Thyrolar®** *see* Liotrix *on page* 1017

◆ **ThyroSafe™** *see* Potassium Iodide *on page* 1383

◆ **Thyroshield™ [OTC]** *see* Potassium Iodide *on page* 1383

Thyrotropin Alfa (thye roe TROH pin AL fa)

Brand Names: U.S. Thyrogen®

Brand Names: Canada Thyrogen®

Index Terms Human Thyroid Stimulating Hormone; Recombinant Human Thyrotropin; Rh-TSH; Thyrotropin Alpha; TSH

Pharmacologic Category Diagnostic Agent

Use As an adjunctive diagnostic tool for serum thyroglobulin (Tg) testing; adjunctive treatment for radioiodine ablation of thyroid tissue remnants after total or near-total thyroidectomy in patients with well-differentiated thyroid cancer without evidence of metastatic disease

Potential clinical uses include: Patients with an undetectable Tg on thyroid hormone suppressive therapy to exclude the diagnosis of residual or recurrent thyroid cancer, patients requiring serum Tg testing and radioiodine imaging who are unwilling to undergo thyroid hormone withdrawal testing and whose treating physician believes that use of a less sensitive test is justified, patients who are either unable to mount an adequate endogenous TSH response to thyroid hormone withdrawal or in whom withdrawal is medically contraindicated, and patients without evidence of metastatic disease to ablate thyroid remnants (in combination with radioiodine [I^{131}]) following near-total thyroidectomy.

Pregnancy Risk Factor C

Dosage I.M.: Children >16 years and Adults: Radioiodine imaging or ablation: 0.9 mg, followed 24 hours later by a second 0.9 mg dose

For radioiodine imaging or remnant ablation, radioiodine administration should be given 24 hours following the second thyrotropin injection. Diagnostic scanning should be performed 48 hours after radioiodine administration (72 hours after the second thyrotropin injection). Post-therapy scanning may be delayed (additional days) to allow decline of background activity.

For serum Tg testing, serum Tg should be obtained 72 hours after final injection of thyrotropin.

Additional Information Complete prescribing information for this medication should be consulted for additional detail.

Dosage Forms Excipient information presented when available (limited, particularly for generics); consult specific product labeling.

Injection, powder for reconstitution:

Thyrogen®: 1.1 mg

◆ **Thyrotropin Alpha** *see* Thyrotropin Alfa *on page* 1677

◆ **Tiacumicin B** *see* Fidaxomicin *on page* 710

TiaGABine (tye AG a been)

Brand Names: U.S. Gabitril®

Index Terms Tiagabine Hydrochloride

Pharmacologic Category Anticonvulsant, Miscellaneous

Use Adjunctive therapy in adults and children ≥12 years of age in the treatment of partial seizures

Pregnancy Risk Factor C

Pregnancy Considerations Patients exposed to tiagabine during pregnancy are encouraged to enroll themselves into the AED Pregnancy Registry by calling 1-888-233-2334. Additional information is available at www.aedpregnancyregistry.org.

Lactation Enters breast milk/not recommended

Medication Guide Available Yes

Contraindications Hypersensitivity to tiagabine or any component of the formulation

Warnings/Precautions Antiepileptics are associated with an increased risk of suicidal behavior/thoughts with use (regardless of indication); patients should be monitored for signs/symptoms of depression, suicidal tendencies, and other unusual behavior changes during therapy and instructed to inform their healthcare provider immediately if symptoms occur. New-onset seizures and status epilepticus have been associated with tiagabine use when taken for unlabeled indications. Often these seizures have occurred shortly after the initiation of treatment or shortly after a dosage increase. Seizures have also occurred with very low doses or after several months of therapy. In most cases, patients were using concomitant medications (eg, antidepressants, antipsychotics, stimulants, narcotics). In these instances, the discontinuation of tiagabine, followed by an evaluation for an underlying seizure disorder, is suggested. Use for unapproved indications, however, has not been proven to be safe or effective and is not recommended. When tiagabine is used as an adjunct in partial seizures (an FDA-approved indication), it should not be abruptly discontinued because of the possibility of increasing seizure frequency, unless safety concerns require a more rapid withdrawal. Rarely, nonconvulsive status epilepticus has been reported following abrupt discontinuation or dosage reduction.

Use with caution in patients with hepatic impairment. Experience in patients not receiving enzyme-inducing drugs has been limited; caution should be used in treating any patient who is not receiving one of these medications (decreased dose and slower titration may be required). Weakness, sedation, and confusion may occur with tiagabine use. Patients must be cautioned about performing tasks which require mental alertness (eg, operating machinery or driving). Effects with other sedative drugs or ethanol may be potentiated. May cause serious rash, including Stevens-Johnson syndrome.

Adverse Reactions

>10%:

Central nervous system: Concentration decreased, dizziness, nervousness, somnolence

Gastrointestinal: Nausea

Neuromuscular & skeletal: Weakness, tremor

1% to 10%:

Cardiovascular: Chest pain, edema, hypertension, palpitation, peripheral edema, syncope, tachycardia, vasodilation

Central nervous system: Agitation, ataxia, chills, confusion, difficulty with memory, confusion, depersonalization, depression, euphoria, hallucination, hostility, insomnia, malaise, migraine, paranoid reaction, personality disorder, speech disorder

Dermatologic: Alopecia, bruising, dry skin, pruritus, rash

Gastrointestinal: Abdominal pain, diarrhea, gingivitis, increased appetite, mouth ulceration, stomatitis, vomiting, weight gain/loss

Neuromuscular & skeletal: Abnormal gait, arthralgia, dysarthria, hyper-/hypokinesia, hyper-/hypotonia, myasthenia, myalgia, myoclonus, neck pain, paresthesia, reflexes decreased, stupor, twitching, vertigo

Ocular: Abnormal vision, amblyopia, nystagmus

Otic: Ear pain, hearing impairment, otitis media, tinnitus

Respiratory: Bronchitis, cough, dyspnea, epistaxis, pneumonia

Miscellaneous: Allergic reaction, cyst, diaphoresis, flu-like syndrome, lymphadenopathy

<1% (Limited to important or life-threatening): Abortion, abscess, anemia, angina, apnea, asthma, blepharitis, blindness, cellulitis, cerebral ischemia, cholelithiasis, CNS neoplasm, coma, deafness, dehydration, dysphagia, dystonia, electrocardiogram abnormal, encephalopathy, hemorrhage, erythrocytes abnormal, leukopenia, fecal incontinence, herpes simplex/zoster, glossitis, goiter, hematuria, hemoptysis, hepatomegaly, hypercholesteremia, hyper-/hypoglycemia, hyperlipemia, hypokalemia, hyponatremia, hypotension, hypothyroidism, impotence, kidney failure, liver function tests abnormal, MI, neoplasm, peripheral vascular disorder, paralysis, photophobia, psychosis, petechia, photosensitivity, seizure (when used for unlabeled uses), sepsis, spasm, suicide attempt, thrombocytopenia, thrombophlebitis, urinary retention, urinary urgency, urticaria, visual field defect

Drug Interactions

Metabolism/Transport Effects Substrate of CYP3A4 (major); **Note:** Assignment of Major/Minor substrate status based on clinically relevant drug interaction potential

Avoid Concomitant Use

Avoid concomitant use of TiaGABine with any of the following: Conivaptan

Increased Effect/Toxicity

TiaGABine may increase the levels/effects of: Alcohol (Ethyl); CNS Depressants; Methotrimeprazine; Selective Serotonin Reuptake Inhibitors

The levels/effects of TiaGABine may be increased by: Conivaptan; CYP3A4 Inhibitors (Moderate); CYP3A4 Inhibitors (Strong); Dasatinib; Droperidol; HydrOXYzine; Methotrimeprazine

Decreased Effect

The levels/effects of TiaGABine may be decreased by: CYP3A4 Inducers (Strong); Deferasirox; Herbs (CYP3A4 Inducers); Ketorolac; Ketorolac (Nasal); Ketorolac (Systemic); Mefloquine; Tocilizumab

Ethanol/Nutrition/Herb Interactions

Ethanol: May increase CNS depression; monitor for increased effects with coadministration. Caution patients about effects.

Food: Food reduces the rate but not the extent of absorption.

Herb/Nutraceutical: St John's wort may decrease tiagabine levels. Avoid valerian, St John's wort, kava kava, gotu kola (may increase CNS depression).

Mechanism of Action The exact mechanism by which tiagabine exerts antiseizure activity is not definitively known; however, *in vitro* experiments demonstrate that it enhances the activity of gamma aminobutyric acid (GABA), the major neuroinhibitory transmitter in the nervous system; it is thought that binding to the GABA uptake carrier inhibits the uptake of GABA into presynaptic neurons, allowing an increased amount of GABA to be available to postsynaptic neurons; based on *in vitro* studies, tiagabine does not inhibit the uptake of dopamine, norepinephrine, serotonin, glutamate, or choline

Pharmacodynamics/Kinetics

Absorption: Rapid (45 minutes); prolonged with food

Protein binding: 96%, primarily to albumin and α_1-acid glycoprotein

Metabolism: Hepatic via CYP (primarily 3A4)

Bioavailability: Oral: Absolute: 90%

Half-life elimination: 2-5 hours when administered with enzyme inducers; 7-9 hours when administered without enzyme inducers

Time to peak, plasma: 45 minutes

Excretion: Feces (63%); urine (25%); 2% as unchanged drug; primarily as metabolites

Dosage Oral (administer with food):

Patients receiving enzyme-inducing AED regimens:

Children 12-18 years: 4 mg once daily for 1 week; may increase to 8 mg daily in 2 divided doses for 1 week; then may increase by 4-8 mg weekly to response or up to 32 mg daily in 2-4 divided doses

Adults: 4 mg once daily for 1 week; may increase by 4-8 mg weekly to response or up to 56 mg daily in 2-4 divided doses; usual maintenance: 32-56 mg/day

Patients **not** receiving enzyme-inducing AED regimens: The estimated plasma concentrations of tiagabine in patients not taking enzyme-inducing medications is twice that of patients receiving enzyme-inducing AEDs. Lower doses are required; slower titration may be necessary.

Dietary Considerations Take with food.

Monitoring Parameters A reduction in seizure frequency is indicative of therapeutic response to tiagabine in patients with partial seizures; complete blood counts, renal function tests, liver function tests, and routine blood chemistry should be monitored periodically during therapy; suicidality (eg, suicidal thoughts, depression, behavioral changes)

Reference Range Maximal plasma level after a 24 mg/dose: 552 ng/mL

Additional Information Animal studies suggest that tiagabine may bind to retina and uvea; however, no treatment-related ophthalmoscopic changes were seen long-term; periodic monitoring may be considered.

Dosage Forms Excipient information presented when available (limited, particularly for generics); consult specific product labeling.

Tablet, oral, as hydrochloride:

Gabitril®: 2 mg, 4 mg, 12 mg, 16 mg

Extemporaneous Preparations A 1 mg/mL tiagabine hydrochloride oral suspension may be made with tablets and a 1:1 mixture of Ora-Sweet® and Ora-Plus®. Crush ten 12 mg tablets in a mortar and reduce to a fine powder. Add small portions of the vehicle and mix to a uniform paste; mix while adding the vehicle in incremental proportions to **almost** 120 mL; transfer to a graduated cylinder; rinse mortar with vehicle, and add quantity of vehicle sufficient to make 120 mL. Label "shake well" and "refrigerate". Store in amber plastic prescription bottles; stable for 70 days at room temperature or 91 days refrigerated (preferred).

A 1 mg/mL oral suspension may be made with tablets and a 6:1 mixture of simple syrup, NF and methylcellulose 1%. Crush ten 12 mg tablets in a mortar and reduce to a fine powder. Add 17 mL of methylcellulose 1% gel and mix to a uniform paste; mix while adding simple syrup, NF in incremental proportions to **almost** 120 mL; transfer to a graduated cylinder, rinse mortar with syrup, and add quantity of syrup sufficient to make 120 mL. Label "shake well" and "refrigerate". Store in amber plastic prescription bottles; stable for 42 days at room temperature or 91 days refrigerated (preferred).

Nahata MC, Pai VB, and Hipple TF, *Pediatric Drug Formulations*, 5th ed, Cincinnati, OH: Harvey Whitney Books Co, 2004.

◆ **Tiagabine Hydrochloride** *see* TiaGABine *on page 1677*
◆ **Tiamol® (Can)** *see* Fluocinonide *on page 727*
◆ **Tiazac®** *see* Diltiazem *on page 510*
◆ **Tiazac® XC (Can)** *see* Diltiazem *on page 510*

Ticagrelor (tye KA grel or)

Brand Names: U.S. Brilinta™
Brand Names: Canada Brilinta™
Index Terms AZD6140
Pharmacologic Category Antiplatelet Agent; Antiplatelet Agent, Cyclopentyltriazolopyrimidine
Use Used in conjunction with aspirin for secondary prevention of thrombotic events in patients with unstable angina, non-ST-elevation myocardial infarction (NSTEMI), or ST-elevation myocardial infarction (STEMI) managed medically or with percutaneous coronary intervention (PCI) and/or coronary artery bypass graft (CABG)
Pregnancy Risk Factor C
Pregnancy Considerations Fetal mortality and/or abnormalities were observed in animal studies at doses greater than maximum recommended human doses. There are no adequate and well-controlled studies in pregnant women. Use only if potential benefits outweigh potential risk to fetus. The Canadian labeling recommends women of child-bearing potential use appropriate contraceptive measures.
Medication Guide Available Yes
Contraindications Active pathological bleeding (eg, peptic ulcer or intracranial hemorrhage); history of intracranial hemorrhage; hepatic impairment

Canadian labeling: Additional contraindications (not in U.S. labeling): Hypersensitivity to ticagrelor or any component of the formulation; moderate hepatic impairment; concomitant use of strong CYP3A4 inhibitors (eg, ketoconazole, clarithromycin, ritonavir, atazanavir, nefazodone)

Warnings/Precautions [U.S. Boxed Warning]: Ticagrelor increases the risk of bleeding including significant and sometimes fatal bleeding. Use is contraindicated in patients with active pathological bleeding and presence or history of intracranial hemorrhage. Additional risk factors for bleeding include propensity to bleed (eg, recent trauma or surgery, recent or recurrent GI bleeding, active PUD, moderate-to-severe hepatic impairment), CABG or other surgical procedure, concomitant use of medications that increase risk of bleeding (eg, warfarin, NSAIDs), and advanced age. Bleeding should be suspected if patient becomes hypotensive after undergoing recent coronary angiography, PCI, CABG, or other surgical procedure even if overt signs of bleeding do not exist. **Where possible, manage bleeding without discontinuing ticagrelor as the risk of cardiovascular events is increased upon discontinuation.** If discontinuation of ticagrelor is necessary, resume as soon as possible after the bleeding source is identified and controlled. Hemostatic benefits of platelet transfusions are not known; may inhibit transfused platelets. Premature discontinuation of therapy may increase the risk of cardiac events (eg, stent thrombosis with subsequent fatal or nonfatal MI). Duration of therapy, in general, is determined by the type of stent placed (bare metal or drug eluting) and whether an ACS event was ongoing at the time of placement. Use with caution in patients who are at an increased risk of bradycardia (eg, second- or third-degree AV block, sick sinus syndrome) or taking other bradycardic-inducing agents (eg, beta blockers, nondihydropyridine calcium channel blockers). Ventricular pauses ≥3 seconds were noted more frequently with ticagrelor than with clopidogrel in a substudy of the Platelet Inhibition and Patient Outcomes (PLATO) trial. Dyspnea (often mild-to-moderate and transient) was observed more frequently in patients receiving ticagrelor than clopidogrel during clinical trials. Ticagrelor-related dyspnea does not require specific treatment nor does it warrant therapy interruption (Canadian labeling recommends discontinuing therapy in patients unable to tolerate ticagrelor related dyspnea0.

[U.S. Boxed Warning]: Maintenance doses of aspirin greater than 100 mg/day reduce the efficacy of ticagrelor and should be avoided. Use of higher maintenance doses of aspirin (ie, >100 mg/day) was associated with relatively unfavorable outcomes for ticagrelor versus clopidogrel in the PLATO trial (Gaglia, 2011; Wallentin, 2009). Canadian labeling recommends a maximum maintenance aspirin dose of 150 mg/day.

[U.S. Boxed Warning]: Avoid initiation of ticagrelor when urgent CABG surgery is planned; when possible discontinue use at least 5 days before any surgery. Discontinue 5 days before elective surgery (except in patients with cardiac stents that have not completed their full course of dual antiplatelet therapy; patient-specific situations need to be discussed with cardiologist). When urgent CABG is necessary, the ACCF/AHA CABG guidelines recommend discontinuation for at least 24 hours prior to surgery (Hillis, 2011).

Use is contraindicated in patients with severe hepatic impairment (Canadian labeling also contraindicates use in moderate-to-severe hepatic impairment). Use with caution in patients with renal impairment, a history of hyperuricemia or gouty arthritis. Canadian labeling does not recommend use in patients with uric acid nephropathy. Avoid concomitant use with strong CYP3A4 inhibitors (eg, ketoconazole, ritonavir, nefazodone) or strong CYP3A4 inducers (eg, rifampin, carbamazepine, dexamethasone, phenobarbital, phenytoin). Canadian labeling contraindicates use with strong CYP3A4 inhibitors.

Adverse Reactions Note: As with all drugs which may affect hemostasis, bleeding is associated with ticagrelor. Hemorrhage may occur at virtually any site. Risk is dependent on multiple variables, including the concurrent use of multiple agents which alter hemostasis and patient susceptibility.

Frequencies as reported in PLATO trial versus clopidogrel:

>10%: Respiratory: Dyspnea (≤14%)

1% to 10%:

Cardiovascular: Ventricular pauses (6%; 2% after 1 month of therapy), atrial fibrillation (4%), hypertension (4%), angina (3%), hypotension (3%), bradycardia (1% to 3%), cardiac failure (2%), peripheral edema (2%), ventricular tachycardia (2%), palpitation (1%), syncope (1%), ventricular extrasystoles (1%), ventricular fibrillation (1%)

Central nervous system: Headache (7%), dizziness (5%), fatigue (3%), fever (3%), anxiety (2%), insomnia (2%), vertigo (2%), depression (1%)

Dermatologic: Bruising (2% to 4%), rash (2%), pruritus (1%), subcutaneous or dermal bleeding

Endocrine & metabolic: Hypokalemia (2%), diabetes mellitus (1%), dyslipidemia (1%), hypercholesterolemia (1%)

Gastrointestinal: Diarrhea (4%), nausea (4%), vomiting (3%), abdominal pain (2%), constipation (2%), dyspepsia (2%), GI hemorrhage

Genitourinary: Urinary tract infection (2%), urinary tract bleeding

Hematologic: Major bleeding (12%; composite of major fatal/life threatening and other major bleeding events), minor bleeding (~5%), anemia (2%), hematoma (2%), postprocedural hemorrhage (2%)

Local: Puncture site hematoma (2%)

Neuromuscular & skeletal: Back pain (4%), noncardiac chest pain (4%), extremity pain (2%), arthralgia (2%), musculoskeletal pain (2%), weakness (2%), myalgia (1%)

Renal: Creatinine increased (7%; mechanism undetermined), hematuria (2%), renal failure (1%)

Respiratory: Epistaxis (6%), cough (5%), nasopharyngitis (2%), bronchitis (1%), pneumonia (1%)

<1% (Limited to important or life-threatening): Confusion, conjunctival hemorrhage, gastritis, gout, gynecomastia, hemarthrosis, hemoptysis, intracranial hemorrhage (including fatalities), intraocular hemorrhage, paresthesia, retinal hemorrhage, retroperitoneal hemorrhage

Drug Interactions

Metabolism/Transport Effects Substrate of CYP3A4 (major); **Note:** Assignment of Major/Minor substrate status based on clinically relevant drug interaction potential; **Inhibits** CYP2B6 (weak), CYP2C9 (moderate), CYP2D6 (weak)

Avoid Concomitant Use

Avoid concomitant use of Ticagrelor with any of the following: CYP3A4 Inducers (Strong); CYP3A4 Inhibitors (Strong)

Increased Effect/Toxicity

Ticagrelor may increase the levels/effects of: Anticoagulants; Antiplatelet Agents; Carvedilol; Collagenase (Systemic); CYP2C9 Substrates; Digoxin; Drotrecogin Alfa (Activated); Ibritumomab; Lovastatin; Rivaroxaban; Salicylates; Simvastatin; Thrombolytic Agents; Tositumomab and Iodine I 131 Tositumomab

The levels/effects of Ticagrelor may be increased by: Aspirin; CYP3A4 Inhibitors (Strong); Dasatinib; Glucosamine; Herbs (Anticoagulant/Antiplatelet Properties); Nonsteroidal Anti-Inflammatory Agents; Omega-3-Acid Ethyl Esters; Pentosan Polysulfate Sodium; Pentoxifylline; Prostacyclin Analogues; Vitamin E

Decreased Effect

The levels/effects of Ticagrelor may be decreased by: Aspirin; CYP3A4 Inducers (Strong); CYP3A4 Inhibitors (Strong); Deferasirox; Herbs (CYP3A4 Inducers); Nonsteroidal Anti-Inflammatory Agents; Tocilizumab

Stability Store in the original container at 25°C (77°F); excursions permitted to 15°C to 30°C (59°F to 86°F).

Mechanism of Action Reversibly and noncompetitively binds the adenosine diphosphate (ADP) $P2Y_{12}$ receptor on the platelet surface which prevents ADP-mediated activation of the GPIIb/IIIa receptor complex thereby reducing platelet aggregation. Due to the reversible antagonism of the $P2Y_{12}$ receptor, recovery of platelet function is likely to depend on serum concentrations of ticagrelor and its active metabolite.

Pharmacodynamics/Kinetics

Onset of inhibition of platelet aggregation (IPA): 180 mg loading dose: ~41% within 30 minutes (similar to clopidogrel 600 mg at 8 hours)

Peak effect: Time to maximal IPA: 180 mg loading dose: IPA ~88% at 2 hours post administration

Duration of IPA: 180 mg loading dose: 87% to 89% maintained from 2-8 hours; 24 hours after the last maintenance dose, IPA is 58% (similar to maintenance clopidogrel)

Time after discontinuation when IPA is 30%: ~56 hours; IPA 10%: ~110 hours (Gurbel, 2009). Mean IPA observed with ticagrelor at 3 days post-discontinuation was comparable to that observed with clopidogrel at 5 days post discontinuation.

Absorption: Rapid

Distribution: 88 L

Protein binding: >99% (parent drug and active metabolite)

Metabolism: Hepatic via CYP3A4/5 to active metabolite (AR-C124910XX)

Bioavailability: ~36% (range: 30% to 42%)

Half-life elimination: Parent drug: ~7 hours; active metabolite: ~9 hours

Time to peak: Parent drug: ~1.5 hours; active metabolite (AR-C124910XX): ~2.5 hours

Excretion: Feces (58%); urine (26%); actual amount of parent drug and active metabolite excreted in urine was <1% of total dose administered

Dosage Oral: Adults:

Acute coronary syndrome: Unstable angina, non-ST-segment elevation myocardial infarction (NSTEMI), ST-segment elevation myocardial infarction (STEMI): Initial: 180 mg loading dose (with a loading dose of aspirin [eg, 325 mg] if not already receiving); Maintenance: 90 mg twice daily; initiated 12 hours after initial loading dose (with low-dose aspirin 75-100 mg/day). **Note:** Canadian labeling recommends a maintenance aspirin dose of 75-150 mg/day. Safety and efficacy of therapy beyond 12 months has not been established.

Duration of ticagrelor (in combination with aspirin) after stent placement: **Premature interruption of therapy may result in stent thrombosis with subsequent fatal and nonfatal MI.** Those with ACS receiving either stent type (bare metal [BMS] or drug-eluting stent [DES]) or those receiving a DES for a non-ACS indication, ticagrelor for at least 12 months is recommended. A duration >12 months may be considered in patients with DES placement. Those receiving a BMS for a non-ACS indication should be given at least 1 month and ideally up to 12 months; if patient is at increased risk of bleeding, give for a minimum of 2 weeks (Levine, 2011).

Conversion from clopidogrel to ticagrelor: Initiate ticagrelor 90 mg twice daily beginning 24 hours after clopidogrel dose (loading or maintenance). **Note:** Conversion to ticagrelor results in an absolute inhibition of platelet aggregation (IPA) increase of 26.4%.

Dosage adjustment in renal impairment: No dosage adjustments are recommended

Hemodialysis: Use caution; drug is thought to be nondialyzable

Dosage adjustment in hepatic impairment:

Mild hepatic impairment: No dosage adjustments are recommended

Moderate hepatic impairment: Use has not been studied; however, undergoes hepatic metabolism; use caution. The manufacturer labeling does not provide specific dosing recommendations. Use is contraindicated in the Canadian labeling.

Severe hepatic impairment: Use is contraindicated.

Dietary Considerations May be taken without regard to meals.

Administration May be administered without regard to meals. Missed doses should be taken at their next regularly scheduled time.

Monitoring Parameters Signs of bleeding; hemoglobin and hematocrit periodically; renal function; uric acid levels (patients with gout or at risk of hyperuricemia); signs/symptoms of dyspnea

Additional Information Unlike thienopyridines (eg, clopidogrel, prasugrel) which are prodrugs and require metabolic transformation to their active metabolites for their activity, ticagrelor and its active metabolite both exhibit antiplatelet activity by reversibly and noncompetitively binding to the adenosine diphosphate (ADP) $P2Y_{12}$ receptor on the platelet surface. Due to the reversible antagonism of the $P2Y_{12}$ receptor, recovery of platelet function is faster than with use of irreversible $P2Y_{12}$ receptor antagonists such as clopidogrel or prasugrel.

Dosage Forms Excipient information presented when available (limited, particularly for generics); consult specific product labeling.

Tablet, oral:

Brilinta™: 90 mg

Dosage Forms: Canada Excipient information presented when available (limited, particularly for generics); consult specific product labeling.

Tablet, oral:

Brilinta®: 90 mg

Ticarcillin and Clavulanate Potassium

(tye kar SIL in & klav yoo LAN ate poe TASS ee um)

Brand Names: U.S. Timentin®

Brand Names: Canada Timentin®

Index Terms Ticarcillin and Clavulanic Acid

Pharmacologic Category Antibiotic, Penicillin

Use Treatment of lower respiratory tract, urinary tract, skin and skin structures, bone and joint, gynecologic (endometritis) and intra-abdominal (peritonitis) infections, and septicemia caused by susceptible organisms. Clavulanate expands activity of ticarcillin to include beta-lactamase producing strains of *S. aureus*, *H. influenzae*, *Bacteroides* species, and some other gram-negative bacilli

Pregnancy Risk Factor B

Pregnancy Considerations Adverse events were not observed in animal reproduction studies; therefore, ticarcillin/clavulanate is classified as pregnancy category B. Ticarcillin and clavulanate cross the placenta. Human experience with the penicillins during pregnancy has shown no evidence of adverse effects to the fetus. Ticarcillin/clavulanate is approved for the treatment of postpartum gynecologic infections, including endometritis, caused by susceptible organisms.

Lactation Enters breast milk/use caution

Contraindications Hypersensitivity to ticarcillin, clavulanate, any penicillin, or any component of the formulation

Warnings/Precautions Use with caution and modify dosage in patients with renal impairment; serious and occasionally severe or fatal hypersensitivity (anaphylactoid) reactions have been reported in patients on penicillin therapy (especially with a history of beta-lactam hypersensitivity and/or a history of sensitivity to multiple allergens); use with caution in patients with seizures and in patients with HF due to high sodium load. Particularly in patients with renal impairment, bleeding disorders have been observed; discontinue if thrombocytopenia or bleeding occurs. Prolonged use may result in fungal or bacterial superinfection, including *C. difficile*-associated diarrhea (CDAD) and pseudomembranous colitis; CDAD has been observed >2 months postantibiotic treatment.

Adverse Reactions Frequency not defined.

Central nervous system: Confusion, drowsiness, fever, headache, Jarisch-Herxheimer reaction, seizure

Dermatologic: Erythema multiforme, pruritus, rash, Stevens-Johnson syndrome, toxic epidermal necrolysis, urticaria

Endocrine & metabolic: Electrolyte imbalance

Gastrointestinal: *Clostridium difficile* colitis, diarrhea, nausea, vomiting

Hematologic: Bleeding, eosinophilia, hemolytic anemia, leukopenia, neutropenia, positive Coombs' reaction, prothrombin time prolonged, thrombocytopenia

Hepatic: Hepatotoxicity, jaundice

Local: Injection site reaction (pain, burning, induration); thrombophlebitis

Neuromuscular & skeletal: Myoclonus

Renal: BUN increased, interstitial nephritis (acute), serum creatinine increased

Miscellaneous: Anaphylaxis, hypersensitivity reactions

Drug Interactions

Metabolism/Transport Effects None known.

Avoid Concomitant Use

Avoid concomitant use of Ticarcillin and Clavulanate Potassium with any of the following: BCG

Increased Effect/Toxicity

Ticarcillin and Clavulanate Potassium may increase the levels/effects of: Methotrexate; Vitamin K Antagonists

The levels/effects of Ticarcillin and Clavulanate Potassium may be increased by: Probenecid

Decreased Effect

Ticarcillin and Clavulanate Potassium may decrease the levels/effects of: Aminoglycosides; BCG; Mycophenolate; Typhoid Vaccine

The levels/effects of Ticarcillin and Clavulanate Potassium may be decreased by: Fusidic Acid; Tetracycline Derivatives

Stability

Vials: Store intact vials at <24°C (<75°F). Reconstituted solution is stable for 6 hours at room temperature and 72 hours when refrigerated. I.V. infusion in NS or LR is stable for 24 hours at room temperature, 7 days when refrigerated, or 30 days when frozen. I.V. infusion in D_5W solution is stable for 24 hours at room temperature, 3 days when refrigerated, or 7 days when frozen. After freezing, thawed solution is stable for 8 hours at room temperature. Darkening of drug indicates loss of potency of clavulanate potassium.

Premixed solution: Store frozen at ≤-20°C (-4°F). Thawed solution is stable for 24 hours at room temperature or 7 days under refrigeration; do not refreeze.

Mechanism of Action Inhibits bacterial cell wall synthesis by binding to one or more of the penicillin-binding proteins (PBPs); which in turn inhibits the final transpeptidation step of peptidoglycan synthesis in bacterial cell walls, thus inhibiting cell wall biosynthesis. Bacteria eventually lyse due to ongoing activity of cell wall autolytic enzymes (autolysins and murein hydrolases) while cell wall assembly is arrested.

Pharmacodynamics/Kinetics

Absorption: Ticarcillin: Not absorbed orally

Protein binding: Ticarcillin: ~45%; Clavulanic acid: ~25%

Metabolism: Clavulanic acid: Hepatic

Half-life elimination: Ticarcillin: 1.1 hours; Clavulanic acid: 1.1 hours

Excretion: Ticarcillin: Urine (60% to 70%); Clavulanic acid: Urine (35% to 45% as unchanged drug)

Clearance: Clavulanic acid does not affect clearance of ticarcillin

Dosage Note: Timentin® (ticarcillin/clavulanate) is a combination product; each 3.1 g dosage form contains 3 g ticarcillin disodium and 0.1 g clavulanic acid.

Usual dosage range:

Children and Adults <60 kg: I.V.: 200-300 mg of ticarcillin component/kg/day in divided doses every 4-6 hours

Children ≥60 kg and Adults: I.V.: 3.1 g (ticarcillin 3 g plus clavulanic acid 0.1 g) every 4-6 hours (maximum: 24 g of ticarcillin component/day)

Indication-specific dosing:

Children: I.V.:

Bite wounds (animal): 200 mg of ticarcillin component/kg/day in divided doses

Neutropenic fever: 75 mg of ticarcillin component/kg every 6 hours (maximum: 3.1 g/dose)

Pneumonia (nosocomial): 300 mg of ticarcillin component/kg/day in 4 divided doses (maximum: 18-24 g of ticarcillin component/day)

Children ≥60 kg and Adults: I.V.:

Amnionitis, cholangitis, diverticulitis, endometritis, epididymo-orchitis, mastoiditis, orbital cellulitis, peritonitis, pneumonia (aspiration): 3.1 g every 6 hours

Intra-abdominal infection, complicated, community-acquired, mild-to-moderate: 3.1 g every 6 hours for 4-7 days (provided source controlled)

Liver abscess, parafascial space infections, septic thrombophlebitis: 3.1 g every 4 hours

***Pseudomonas* infections:** 3.1 g every 4 hours

Urinary tract infections: 3.1 g every 6-8 hours

Dosing adjustment in renal impairment: Loading dose: I.V.: 3.1 g one dose, followed by maintenance dose based on creatinine clearance:

Cl_{cr} 30-60 mL/minute: Administer 2 g of ticarcillin component every 4 hours or 3.1 g every 8 hours

Cl_{cr} 10-30 mL/minute: Administer 2 g of ticarcillin component every 8 hours or 3.1 g every 12 hours

Cl_{cr} <10 mL/minute: Administer 2 g of ticarcillin component every 12 hours

Cl_{cr} <10 mL/minute with concomitant hepatic dysfunction: 2 g of ticarcillin component every 24 hours

Intermittent hemodialysis (IHD) (administer after hemodialysis on dialysis days): Dialyzable (20% to 50%): 2 g of ticarcillin component every 12 hours; supplemented with 3.1 g (ticarcillin/clavulanate) after each dialysis session. Alternatively, administer 2 g every 8 hours without a supplemental dose for deep-seated infections (Heintz, 2009). **Note:** Dosing dependent on the assumption of 3 times/week, complete IHD sessions.

Peritoneal dialysis (PD): 3.1 g every 12 hours

Continuous renal replacement therapy (CRRT) (Heintz, 2009; Trotman, 2005): Drug clearance is highly dependent on the method of renal replacement, filter type, and flow rate. Appropriate dosing requires close monitoring of pharmacologic response, signs of adverse reactions due to drug accumulation, as well as drug concentrations in relation to target trough (if appropriate). The following are general recommendations only (based on dialysate flow/ultrafiltration rates of 1-2 L/hour and minimal residual renal function) and should not supersede clinical judgment:

CVVH: Loading dose of 3.1g followed by 2 g every 6-8 hours

CVVHD: Loading dose of 3.1 g followed by 3.1 g every 6-8 hours

CVVHDF: Loading dose of 3.1 g followed by 3.1 g every 6 hours

Note: Do not administer in intervals exceeding every 8 hours. Clavulanate component is hepatically eliminated; extending the dosing interval beyond 8 hours may result in loss of beta-lactamase inhibition.

Dosing adjustment in hepatic dysfunction: With concomitant renal dysfunction (Cl_{cr} <10 mL/minute): 2 g of ticarcillin component every 24 hours

Dietary Considerations Some products may contain potassium and/or sodium.

Administration Infuse over 30 minutes.

Some penicillins (eg, carbenicillin, ticarcillin, and piperacillin) have been shown to inactivate aminoglycosides *in vitro*. This has been observed to a greater extent with tobramycin and gentamicin, while amikacin has shown greater stability against inactivation. Concurrent use of these agents may pose a risk of reduced antibacterial efficacy *in vivo*, particularly in the setting of profound renal impairment. However, definitive clinical evidence is lacking. If combination penicillin/aminoglycoside therapy is desired in a patient with renal dysfunction, separation of doses (if feasible), and routine monitoring of aminoglycoside levels, CBC, and clinical response should be considered.

Monitoring Parameters Observe for signs and symptoms of anaphylaxis during first dose; serum electrolytes, bleeding time, and periodic tests of renal, hepatic, and hematologic function

Test Interactions Positive Coombs' test, false-positive urinary proteins

Some penicillin derivatives may accelerate the degradation of aminoglycosides *in vitro*, leading to a potential underestimation of aminoglycoside serum concentration.

Dosage Forms Excipient information presented when available (limited, particularly for generics); consult specific product labeling.

Infusion [premixed, frozen]: Ticarcillin 3 g and clavulanic acid 0.1 g (100 mL) [contains sodium 4.51 mEq and potassium 0.15 mEq per g]

Injection, powder for reconstitution: Ticarcillin 3 g and clavulanic acid 0.1 g (3.1 g, 31 g) [contains sodium 4.51 mEq and potassium 0.15 mEq per g]

◆ **Ticarcillin and Clavulanic Acid** *see* Ticarcillin and Clavulanate Potassium *on page 1681*

◆ **TICE® BCG** *see* BCG *on page 191*

Ticlopidine (tye KLOE pi deen)

Brand Names: Canada Apo-Ticlopidine®; Dom-Ticlopidine; Gen-Ticlopidine; Mylan-Ticlopidine; Novo-Ticlopidine; Nu-Ticlopidine; PMS-Ticlopidine; Sandoz-Ticlopidine; Teva-Ticlopidine

Index Terms Ticlopidine Hydrochloride

Pharmacologic Category Antiplatelet Agent; Antiplatelet Agent, Thienopyridine

Additional Appendix Information

Beers Criteria – Potentially Inappropriate Medications for Geriatrics *on page 1973*

Use Platelet aggregation inhibitor that reduces the risk of thrombotic stroke in patients who have had a stroke or stroke precursors. **Note:** Due to its association with life-threatening hematologic disorders, ticlopidine should be reserved for patients who are intolerant to aspirin, or who have failed aspirin therapy. Adjunctive therapy (with aspirin) following successful coronary stent implantation to reduce the incidence of subacute stent thrombosis.

Unlabeled Use Protection of aortocoronary bypass grafts, diabetic microangiopathy, ischemic heart disease, prevention of postoperative DVT, reduction of graft loss following renal transplant

Pregnancy Risk Factor B

Pregnancy Considerations Teratogenic effects have not been observed in animal reproduction studies; a case report has demonstrated the safe use of ticlopidine in pregnant women (Ueno, 2001).

Lactation Excretion in breast milk unknown/not recommended

Contraindications Hypersensitivity to ticlopidine or any component of the formulation; active pathological bleeding such as peptic ulcer disease (PUD) or intracranial hemorrhage; severe liver dysfunction; hematopoietic disorders (neutropenia, thrombocytopenia, a past history of TTP or aplastic anemia)

Warnings/Precautions Use with caution in patients who may be at risk of increased bleeding (eg, PUD, trauma, or surgery). Consider discontinuing 10-14 days before elective surgery (except in patients with cardiac stents that have not completed their full course of dual antiplatelet therapy; patient-specific situations need to be discussed with cardiologist; AHA/ACC/SCAI/ACS/ADA Science Advisory provides recommendations). Use caution in concurrent treatment with anticoagulants (eg, heparin, warfarin) or other antiplatelet drugs; bleeding risk is increased.

Because of structural similarities, cross-reactivity is possible among the thienopyridines (clopidogrel, prasugrel, and ticlopidine); use with caution or avoid in patients with previous thienopyridine hypersensitivity. Use of ticlopidine is contraindicated in patients with hypersensitivity to ticlopidine.

Use with caution in patients with mild-to-moderate hepatic impairment; use is contraindicated with severe hepatic impairment. Use with caution in patients with moderate-to-severe renal impairment (experience is limited); bleeding times may be significantly prolonged and the risk of hematologic adverse effects (eg, neutropenia) may be increased. **[U.S. Boxed Warning]: May cause life-threatening hematologic reactions, including neutropenia, agranulocytosis, thrombotic thrombocytopenia purpura (TTP), and aplastic anemia.** Routine monitoring is required (see Monitoring Parameters). Monitor for signs and symptoms of neutropenia including WBC count. Discontinue if the absolute neutrophil count falls to <1200/mm^3 or if the platelet count falls to <80,000/mm^3. Not recommended for use in the elderly as this medication has been shown to be no better than aspirin as an antiplatelet agent and may have more significant adverse effects (Beers Criteria).

Adverse Reactions As with all drugs which may affect hemostasis, bleeding is associated with ticlopidine. Hemorrhage may occur at virtually any site. Risk is dependent on multiple variables, including the use of multiple agents which alter hemostasis and patient susceptibility.

>10%:

- Endocrine & metabolic: Total cholesterol increased (increases of ~8% to 10% within 1 month of therapy), triglycerides increased
- Gastrointestinal: Diarrhea (13%)

1% to 10%:

- Central nervous system: Dizziness (1%)
- Dermatologic: Rash (5%), purpura (2%), pruritus (1%)
- Gastrointestinal: Nausea (7%), dyspepsia (7%), gastrointestinal pain (4%), vomiting (2%), flatulence (2%), anorexia (1%)
- Hematologic: Neutropenia (2%)
- Hepatic: Alkaline phosphatase increased (>2 x upper limit of normal; 8%), abnormal liver function test (1%)

<1% (Limited to important or life-threatening): Agranulocytosis, anaphylaxis, angioedema, aplastic anemia, arthropathy, bilirubin increased, bone marrow suppression, bronchiolitis obliterans-organized pneumonia, chronic diarrhea, conjunctival bleeding, eosinophilia, erythema multiforme, erythema nodosum, exfoliative dermatitis, gastrointestinal bleeding, hematuria, hemolytic anemia, hepatic necrosis, hepatitis, hyponatremia, intracranial bleeding (rare), jaundice, maculopapular rash, menorrhagia, myositis, nephrotic syndrome, pancytopenia, peptic ulcer, peripheral neuropathy, pneumonitis (allergic), positive ANA, renal failure, sepsis, serum creatinine increased, serum sickness, Stevens-Johnson syndrome, systemic lupus erythematosus, thrombocytopenia (immune), thrombocytosis, thrombotic thrombocytopenic purpura, urticaria, vasculitis

Drug Interactions

Metabolism/Transport Effects Substrate of CYP3A4 (major); **Note:** Assignment of Major/Minor substrate status based on clinically relevant drug interaction potential; **Inhibits** CYP1A2 (weak), CYP2B6 (moderate), CYP2C19 (strong), CYP2C9 (weak), CYP2D6 (moderate), CYP2E1 (weak), CYP3A4 (weak)

Avoid Concomitant Use

Avoid concomitant use of Ticlopidine with any of the following: Clopidogrel; Pimozide; Thioridazine

Increased Effect/Toxicity

Ticlopidine may increase the levels/effects of: Anticoagulants; Antiplatelet Agents; Citalopram; Collagenase (Systemic); CYP2B6 Substrates; CYP2C19 Substrates; CYP2D6 Substrates; Drotrecogin Alfa (Activated); Fesoterodine; Fosphenytoin; Ibritumomab; Nebivolol; Phenytoin; Pimozide; Rivaroxaban; Salicylates; Tamoxifen; Theophylline Derivatives; Thioridazine; Thrombolytic Agents; Tositumomab and Iodine I 131 Tositumomab

The levels/effects of Ticlopidine may be increased by: Conivaptan; Dasatinib; Glucosamine; Herbs (Anticoagulant/Antiplatelet Properties); Nonsteroidal Anti-Inflammatory Agents; Omega-3-Acid Ethyl Esters; Pentosan Polysulfate Sodium; Pentoxifylline; Propafenone; Prostacyclin Analogues; Vitamin E

Decreased Effect

Ticlopidine may decrease the levels/effects of: Clopidogrel; Codeine; TraMADol

The levels/effects of Ticlopidine may be decreased by: CYP3A4 Inducers (Strong); Deferasirox; Herbs (CYP3A4 Inducers); Nonsteroidal Anti-Inflammatory Agents; Tocilizumab

Ethanol/Nutrition/Herb Interactions

Food: Ticlopidine bioavailability may be increased (20%) if taken with food. High-fat meals increase absorption, antacids decrease absorption.

Herb/Nutraceutical: Avoid alfalfa, anise, bilberry, bladderwrack, bromelain, cat's claw, chamomile, coleus, cordyceps, dong quai, evening primrose oil, fenugreek, feverfew, garlic, ginger, ginkgo biloba, ginseng (American), ginseng (Panax), ginseng (Siberian), grape seed, green tea, guggul, horse chestnut seed, horseradish, licorice, prickly ash, red clover, reishi, SAMe (S-adenosylmethionine), sweet clover, turmeric, white willow (all have additional antiplatelet activity).

Mechanism of Action Ticlopidine requires *in vivo* biotransformation to an unidentified active metabolite. This active metabolite irreversibly blocks the P2Y12 component of ADP receptors, which prevents activation of the GPIIb/IIIa receptor complex, thereby reducing platelet aggregation. Platelets blocked by ticlopidine are affected for the remainder of their lifespan.

Pharmacodynamics/Kinetics

Onset of action: ~6 hours

Peak effect: 3-5 days; serum levels do not correlate with clinical antiplatelet activity

Absorption: Well absorbed

Protein binding: Parent drug: 98%; <15% bound to alpha$_1$-acid glycoprotein

Metabolism: Extensively hepatic; has at least 1 active metabolite

Half-life elimination: 13 hours

Time to peak, serum: ~2 hours
Excretion: Urine (60%); feces (23%)

Dosage Oral: Adults:

Stroke prevention: 250 mg twice daily

Coronary artery stenting (initiate after successful implantation): 250 mg twice daily (in combination with antiplatelet doses of aspirin) for up to 30 days

Unstable angina, non-ST-segment elevation myocardial infarction (UA/NSTEMI) undergoing percutaneous coronary intervention (PCI) in patients unable to receive clopidogrel (unlabeled dosing): Initial: 500 mg loading dose given at least 6 hours prior to PCI, followed by 250 mg twice daily (in combination with aspirin 75-325 mg once daily). Duration of therapy dependent upon type of stent implanted during PCI.

Note: *Coronary artery stents:* Duration of ticlopidine (clopidogrel preferred) in combination with aspirin: According to the ACC/AHA/SCAI guidelines, ideally 12 months following drug-eluting stent (DES) placement in patients not at high risk for bleeding; at a minimum, 1, 3, and 6 months for bare metal (BMS), sirolimus-eluting, and paclitaxel-eluting stents, respectively, for uninterrupted therapy (Smith, 2005). The 2008 *Chest* guidelines recommend for patients who undergo PCI and receive a BMS (with ongoing ACS) or a DES (with or without ongoing ACS) that ticlopidine (clopidogrel preferred) be continued for at least 12 months. In patients receiving a BMS without ongoing ACS, ticlopidine (or clopidogrel) may be continued for at least 1 month. In patients receiving a DES, therapy with ticlopidine (or clopidogrel) beyond 12 months may be considered in patients without bleeding or tolerability issues (Becker, 2008). Premature interruption of therapy may result in stent thrombosis with subsequent fatal and nonfatal myocardial infarction.

Dosage adjument in renal impairment: No adjustment is necessary

Dosage adjustment in hepatic impairment: No specific guidelines for patients with hepatic impairment; use with caution. Use is contraindicated with severe renal impairment.

Dietary Considerations Should be taken with food to reduce stomach upset.

Administration Administer with food.

Monitoring Parameters Signs of bleeding; CBC with differential every 2 weeks starting the second week through the third month of treatment; more frequent monitoring is recommended for patients whose absolute neutrophil counts have been consistently declining or are 30% less than baseline values. The peak incidence of TTP occurs between 3-4 weeks, the peak incidence of neutropenia occurs at approximately 4-6 weeks, and the incidence of aplastic anemia peaks after 4-8 weeks of therapy. Few cases have been reported after 3 months of treatment. Liver function tests (alkaline phosphatase and transaminases) should be performed in the first 4 months of therapy if liver dysfunction is suspected.

Dosage Forms Excipient information presented when available (limited, particularly for generics); consult specific product labeling.

Tablet, oral, as hydrochloride: 250 mg

◆ **Ticlopidine Hydrochloride** *see* Ticlopidine *on page 1682*

◆ **TIG** *see* Tetanus Immune Globulin (Human) *on page 1657*

◆ **Tigan®** *see* Trimethobenzamide *on page 1739*

Tigecycline (tye ge SYE kleen)

Brand Names: U.S. Tygacil®
Brand Names: Canada Tygacil®

Index Terms GAR-936

Pharmacologic Category Antibiotic, Glycylcycline

Use Treatment of complicated skin and skin structure infections caused by susceptible organisms, including methicillin-resistant *Staphylococcus aureus* and vancomycin-sensitive *Enterococcus faecalis*; complicated intra-abdominal infections (cIAI); community-acquired pneumonia

Pregnancy Risk Factor D

Pregnancy Considerations Because adverse effects were observed in animals and because of the potential for permanent tooth discoloration, tigecycline is classified pregnancy category D. Tigecycline frequently causes nausea and vomiting and, therefore, may not be ideal for use in a patient with pregnancy-related nausea.

Lactation Excretion in breast milk unknown/use caution

Contraindications Hypersensitivity to tigecycline or any component of the formulation

Warnings/Precautions In Phase 3 and 4 clinical trials, an increase in all-cause mortality was observed in patients treated with tigecycline compared to those treated with comparator antibiotics; cause has not been established. In general, deaths were the result of worsening infection, complications of infection, or underlying comorbidity. May cause life-threatening anaphylaxis/anaphylactoid reactions. Due to structural similarity with tetracyclines, use caution in patients with prior hypersensitivity and/or severe adverse reactions associated with tetracycline use. Due to structural similarities with tetracyclines, may be associated with photosensitivity, pseudotumor cerebri, pancreatitis, and antianabolic effects (including increased BUN, azotemia, acidosis, and hyperphosphatemia) observed with this class. Acute pancreatitis (including fatalities) has been reported, including patients without known risk factors; discontinue use when suspected. May cause fetal harm if used during pregnancy; patients should be advised of potential risks associated with use. Permanent discoloration of the teeth may occur if used during tooth development (fetal stage through children up to 8 years of age).

Use caution in hepatic impairment; dosage adjustment recommended in severe hepatic impairment. Abnormal liver function tests (increased total bilirubin, prothrombin time, transaminases) have been reported. Isolated cases of significant hepatic dysfunction and hepatic failure have occurred. Closely monitor for worsening hepatic function in patients that develop abnormal liver function tests during therapy. Adverse hepatic effects may occur after drug discontinuation.

Prolonged use may result in fungal or bacterial superinfection, including *C. difficile*-associated diarrhea (CDAD) and pseudomembranous colitis; CDAD has been observed >2 months postantibiotic treatment. Use with caution if using as monotherapy for patients with intestinal perforation (in the small sample of available cases, septic shock occurred more frequently than patients treated with imipenem/cilastatin comparator). Demonstrated inferior efficacy (versus comparator antibiotic), including lower cure rates and increased mortality in the subgroup of patients with VAP (particularly those with VAP and concurrent bacteremia at baseline).

Adverse Reactions Note: Frequencies relative to placebo are not available; some frequencies are lower than those experienced with comparator drugs.

>10%: Gastrointestinal: Nausea (26%; severe: 1%), vomiting (18%; severe: 1%), diarrhea (12%)

2% to 10%:
Central nervous system: Headache (6%), dizziness (3%)
Dermatologic: Rash (3%)
Endocrine & metabolic: Hypoproteinemia (5%)
Gastrointestinal: Abdominal pain (6%), dyspepsia (2%)
Hematologic: Anemia (4%)

Hepatic: ALT increased (5%), AST increased (4%), alkaline phosphatase increased (4%), amylase increased (3%), bilirubin increased (2%)
Local: Phlebitis (3%)
Neuromuscular & skeletal: Weakness (3%)
Renal: BUN increased (3%)
Miscellaneous: Infection (8%), abnormal healing (4%), abscess (3%)

<2% (Limited to important or life-threatening): Abnormal stools, anaphylaxis/anaphylactoid reactions, anorexia, aPTT prolonged, chills, creatinine increased, eosinophilia, hepatic cholestasis, hypocalcemia, hypoglycemia, hyponatremia, injection site edema, injection site inflammation, injection site pain, injection site phlebitis, injection site reaction, jaundice, leukorrhea, pancreatitis (acute), pruritus, PT prolonged, septic shock, taste perversion, thrombocytopenia, thrombophlebitis, vaginal moniliasis, vaginitis

Drug Interactions

Metabolism/Transport Effects None known.

Avoid Concomitant Use There are no known interactions where it is recommended to avoid concomitant use.

Increased Effect/Toxicity

Tigecycline may increase the levels/effects of: Warfarin

Decreased Effect There are no known significant interactions involving a decrease in effect.

Stability Prior to reconstitution, store at 20°C to 25°C (68°F to 77°F); excursions permitted to 15°C to 30°C (59°F to 86°F). Add 5.3 mL NS, D_5W, or LR to each 50 mg vial. Swirl gently to dissolve. Resulting solution is 10 mg/mL. Reconstituted solution must be further diluted to allow I.V. administration. Transfer to 100 mL I.V. bag for infusion (final concentration should not exceed 1 mg/mL). Reconstituted solution may be stored at room temperature for up to 6 hours or up to 24 hours if further diluted in a compatible I.V. solution. Alternatively, may be stored refrigerated at 2°C to 8°C (36°F to 46°F) for up to 48 hours following immediate transfer of the reconstituted solution into NS or D_5W. Reconstituted solution should be yellow-orange; discard if not this color.

Mechanism of Action A glycylcycline antibiotic that binds to the 30S ribosomal subunit of susceptible bacteria, thereby, inhibiting protein synthesis. Generally considered bacteriostatic; however, bactericidal activity has been demonstrated against isolates of *S. pneumoniae* and *L. pneumophila*. Tigecycline is a derivative of minocycline (9-t-butylglycylamido minocycline), and while not classified as a tetracycline, it may share some class-associated adverse effects. Tigecycline has demonstrated activity against a variety of gram-positive and -negative bacterial pathogens including methicillin-resistant staphylococci.

Pharmacodynamics/Kinetics Note: Systemic clearance is reduced by 55% and half-life increased by 43% in severe hepatic impairment.

Distribution: V_d: 7-9 L/kg; extensive tissue distribution
Protein binding: 71% to 89%
Metabolism: Hepatic, via glucuronidation, N-acetylation, and epimerization to several metabolites, each <10% of the dose
Half-life elimination: Single dose: 27 hours; following multiple doses: 42 hours
Excretion: Feces (59%, primarily as unchanged drug); urine (33%, with 22% of the total dose as unchanged drug)

Dosage I.V.: Adults: **Note:** Duration of therapy dependent on severity/site of infection and clinical status and response to therapy.

Intra-abdominal infections, complicated (cIAI): Initial: 100 mg as a single dose; Maintenance dose: 50 mg every 12 hours for 5-14 days; **Note:** 2010 IDSA guidelines recommend a treatment duration of 4-7 days (provided source controlled) for community-acquired, mild-to-moderate IAI

Pneumonia, community-acquired: Initial: 100 mg as a single dose; Maintenance dose: 50 mg every 12 hours for 7-14 days

Skin/skin structure infections, complicated: Initial: 100 mg as a single dose; Maintenance dose: 50 mg every 12 hours for 5-14 days

Dosage adjustment in renal impairment: No dosage adjustment required in renal impairment.

Poorly dialyzed; no supplemental dose or dosage adjustment necessary, including patients on intermittent hemodialysis, peritoneal dialysis, or continuous renal replacement therapy (eg, CVVHD).

Dosage adjustment in hepatic impairment:

Mild-to-moderate hepatic impairment (Child-Pugh classes A and B): No dosage adjustment required
Severe hepatic impairment (Child-Pugh class C): Initial: 100 mg single dose; Maintenance: 25 mg every 12 hours

Administration Infuse over 30-60 minutes through dedicated line or via Y-site

Dosage Forms Excipient information presented when available (limited, particularly for generics); consult specific product labeling.

Injection, powder for reconstitution:
Tygacil®: 50 mg [contains lactose 100 mg]

- **Tikosyn®** *see* Dofetilide *on page 539*
- **Tilia™ Fe** *see* Ethinyl Estradiol and Norethindrone *on page 660*

Tiludronate (tye LOO droe nate)

Brand Names: U.S. Skelid®

Index Terms Tiludronate Disodium

Pharmacologic Category Bisphosphonate Derivative

Use Treatment of Paget's disease of the bone (osteitis deformans) in patients who have a level of serum alkaline phosphatase (SAP) at least twice the upper limit of normal, or who are symptomatic, or who are at risk for future complications of their disease

Pregnancy Risk Factor C

Pregnancy Considerations Teratogenic and nonteratogenic embryo/fetal effects have been reported in animal studies. There are no adequate and well-controlled studies in pregnant women. Bisphosphonates are incorporated into the bone matrix and gradually released over time. Theoretically, there may be a risk of fetal harm when pregnancy follows the completion of therapy. Based on limited case reports with pamidronate, serum calcium levels in the newborn may be altered if bisphosphonates are administered during pregnancy.

Lactation Excretion in breast milk unknown/use caution

Contraindications Hypersensitivity to tiludronate, bisphosphonates, or any component of the formulation; inability to stand or sit upright for at least 30 minutes

Warnings/Precautions Not recommended in patients with severe renal impairment (Cl_{cr} <30 mL/minute). Use with caution in patients with active upper GI problems (eg, dysphagia, symptomatic esophageal diseases, gastritis, duodenitis, ulcers); discontinue use if new or worsening symptoms develop.

Osteonecrosis of the jaw (ONJ) has been reported in patients receiving bisphosphonates. Risk factors include invasive dental procedures (eg, tooth extraction, dental implants, boney surgery); a diagnosis of cancer, with concomitant chemotherapy or corticosteroids; poor oral hygiene, ill-fitting dentures; and comorbid disorders (anemia, coagulopathy, infection, pre-existing dental disease). Most reported cases occurred after I.V. bisphosphonate therapy; however, cases have been reported following oral therapy. A dental exam and preventative dentistry should be performed prior to placing patients with risk factors on chronic bisphosphonate therapy. The manufacturer's labeling states that discontinuing bisphosphonates in patients requiring invasive dental procedures may reduce the risk of ONJ. However, other experts suggest that there is no evidence that discontinuing therapy reduces the risk of developing ONJ (Assael, 2009). The benefit/risk must be assessed by the treating physician and/or dentist/surgeon prior to any invasive dental procedure. Patients developing ONJ while on bisphosphonates should receive care by an oral surgeon.

Infrequently, severe (and occasionally debilitating) bone, joint, and/or muscle pain have been reported during bisphosphonate treatment. The onset of pain ranged from a single day to several months. Consider discontinuing therapy in patients who experience severe symptoms; symptoms usually resolve upon discontinuation. Some patients experienced recurrence when rechallenged with same drug or another bisphosphonate; avoid use in patients with a history of these symptoms in association with bisphosphonate therapy.

Adverse Reactions

1% to 10%:

Cardiovascular: Chest pain (3%), edema (3%), peripheral edema (3%), flushing, hypertension, syncope

Central nervous system: Anxiety, fatigue, insomnia, nervousness, somnolence, vertigo

Dermatologic: Rash (3%), skin disorder (3%), pruritus

Endocrine & metabolic: Hyperparathyroidism (3%)

Gastrointestinal: Nausea (9%), diarrhea (9%), dyspepsia (5%), vomiting (4%), flatulence (3%), abdominal pain, anorexia, constipation, gastritis, xerostomia

Genitourinary: Urinary tract infection

Neuromuscular & skeletal: Paresthesia (4%), arthrosis (3%), fractures, muscle spasm, weakness

Ocular: Cataract (3%), conjunctivitis (3%), glaucoma (3%)

Respiratory: Rhinitis (5%), sinusitis (5%), pharyngitis (3%), bronchitis

Miscellaneous: Accidental injury (4%), infection (3%), diaphoresis

<1% (Limited to important or life-threatening): Musculoskeletal pain (sometimes severe and/or incapacitating), osteonecrosis (primarily of the jaw), Stevens-Johnson syndrome

Drug Interactions

Metabolism/Transport Effects None known.

Avoid Concomitant Use There are no known interactions where it is recommended to avoid concomitant use.

Increased Effect/Toxicity

Tiludronate may increase the levels/effects of: Deferasirox; Phosphate Supplements

The levels/effects of Tiludronate may be increased by: Aminoglycosides; Indomethacin; Nonsteroidal Anti-Inflammatory Agents

Decreased Effect

The levels/effects of Tiludronate may be decreased by: Antacids; Aspirin; Calcium Salts; Iron Salts; Magnesium Salts; Proton Pump Inhibitors

Ethanol/Nutrition/Herb Interactions Food: In single-dose studies, the bioavailability of tiludronate was reduced by 90% when an oral dose was administered with, or 2 hours after, a standard breakfast compared to the same dose administered after an overnight fast and 4 hours before a standard breakfast.

Stability Store at 25°C (77°F); excursions permitted to 15°C to 30°C (59°F to 86°F). Do not remove tablets from foil strips until they are to be used.

Mechanism of Action Inhibition of normal and abnormal bone resorption. Inhibits osteoclasts through at least two mechanisms: disruption of the cytoskeletal ring structure, possibly by inhibition of protein-tyrosine-phosphatase, thus leading to the detachment of osteoclasts from the bone surface area and the inhibition of the osteoclast proton pump.

Pharmacodynamics/Kinetics

Onset of action: Delayed, may require several weeks

Absorption: Rapid

Distribution: Widely to bone and soft tissue

Protein binding: ~90%, primarily to albumin

Metabolism: Little, if any

Bioavailability: ~6% (range: 2% to 11%); reduced by 90% when given with food

Half-life elimination: Healthy volunteers: Single dose: 50 hours; Cl_{cr} 11-18 mL/minute: 205 hours; Pagetic patients: Repeated dosing: 150 hours

Time to peak, plasma: Within 2 hours

Excretion: Urine (~60%, as tiludronic acid within 13 days)

Dosage Oral: Adults: 400 mg (2 tablets of tiludronic acid) daily for a period of 3 months; allow an interval of 3 months to assess response

Dosing adjustment in renal impairment: Cl_{cr} <30 mL/minute: **Not recommended**

Dosing adjustment in hepatic impairment: Adjustment is not necessary

Dietary Considerations Do not take within 2 hours of food. Ensure adequate intake of vitamin D and calcium supplements during treatment.

Administration Administer as a single oral dose, take with 6-8 oz of plain water. Should not be taken with beverages containing minerals (eg, mineral water), food, or with other medications (may reduce absorption). Do not take within 2 hours of food. Take calcium or mineral supplements at least 2 hours before or after tiludronate. Take aluminum- or magnesium-containing antacids at least 2 hours after taking tiludronate. Patients should be instructed to stay upright (not to lie down) for at least 30 minutes and until after first food of the day (to reduce esophageal irritation).

Monitoring Parameters Alkaline phosphatase; pain; serum calcium and 25(OH)D

Test Interactions Bisphosphonates may interfere with diagnostic imaging agents such as technetium-99m-diphosphonate in bone scans.

Dosage Forms Excipient information presented when available (limited, particularly for generics); consult specific product labeling.

Tablet, oral, as tiludronic acid:

Skelid®: 200 mg [equivalent tiludronate disodium 240 mg]

◆ **Tiludronate Disodium** *see* Tiludronate *on page* 1685

◆ **Tim-AK (Can)** *see* Timolol (Ophthalmic) *on page* 1687

◆ **Time-C® [OTC]** *see* Ascorbic Acid *on page* 149

◆ **Timentin®** *see* Ticarcillin and Clavulanate Potassium *on page* 1681

Timolol (Systemic) (TIM oh lol)

Brand Names: Canada Apo-Timol®; Nu-Timolol; Teva-Timolol

Index Terms Timolol Maleate

Pharmacologic Category Beta-Adrenergic Blocker, Nonselective

Additional Appendix Information

Beta-Blockers *on page* 1884

Use Treatment of hypertension and angina; to reduce mortality following myocardial infarction; prophylaxis of migraine

Pregnancy Risk Factor C

Dosage Oral: Adults:

Hypertension: Initial: 10 mg twice daily, increase gradually every 7 days, usual dosage: 20-40 mg/day in 2 divided doses; maximum: 60 mg/day

Prevention of myocardial infarction: 10 mg twice daily initiated within 1-4 weeks after infarction

Migraine headache: Initial: 10 mg twice daily, increase to maximum of 30 mg/day

Additional Information Complete prescribing information for this medication should be consulted for additional detail.

Dosage Forms Excipient information presented when available (limited, particularly for generics); consult specific product labeling.

Tablet, oral, as maleate: 5 mg, 10 mg, 20 mg

Timolol (Ophthalmic) (TIM oh lol)

Brand Names: U.S. Betimol®; Istalol®; Timolol GFS; Timoptic-XE®; Timoptic®; Timoptic® in OcuDose®

Brand Names: Canada Apo-Timop®; Dom-Timolol; Mylan-Timolol; Novo-Timol; PMS-Timolol; Sandoz-Timolol; Tim-AK; Timolol Maleate-EX; Timoptic-XE®; Timoptic®

Index Terms Timolol Hemihydrate; Timolol Maleate

Pharmacologic Category Beta-Adrenergic Blocker, Nonselective; Ophthalmic Agent, Antiglaucoma

Use Treatment of elevated intraocular pressure such as glaucoma or ocular hypertension

Pregnancy Risk Factor C

Pregnancy Considerations Adverse events were not observed in animal reproduction studies; therefore, the manufacturer classifies timolol ophthalmic as pregnancy category C. Timolol crosses the placenta. Decreased fetal heart rate has been observed following maternal use of oral and ophthalmic timolol during pregnancy. In a cohort study, an increased risk of cardiovascular defects was observed following maternal use of beta-blockers during pregnancy. Intrauterine growth restriction (IUGR), small placentas, as well as fetal/neonatal bradycardia, hypoglycemia, and/or respiratory depression have been observed following *in utero* exposure to beta-blockers as a class. Adequate facilities for monitoring infants at birth should be available. Untreated chronic maternal hypertension and pre-eclampsia are also associated with adverse events in the fetus, infant, and mother. If timolol is required for the treatment of glaucoma during pregnancy, the minimum effective dose should be used in combination with punctual occlusion to decrease exposure to the fetus. Also refer to the Timolol (Systemic) monograph for additional information.

Lactation Enters breast milk/ consider risk:benefit (AAP rates "compatible"; AAP 2001 update pending)

Contraindications Hypersensitivity to timolol or any component of the formulation; sinus bradycardia; sinus node dysfunction; heart block greater than first degree (except in patients with a functioning artificial pacemaker); cardiogenic shock; uncompensated cardiac failure; bronchospastic disease

Warnings/Precautions Consider pre-existing conditions such as sick sinus syndrome before initiating. Use with caution in patients with compensated heart failure and monitor for a worsening of the condition. Use with caution in patients on concurrent digoxin, verapamil, or diltiazem; bradycardia or heart block can occur. Concomitant use with other topical beta-blockers should be avoided; monitor for increased effects (systemic or intraocular) with concomitant use of a systemic beta-blocker. Use with caution in patients receiving inhaled anesthetic agents known to depress myocardial contractility. In general, patients with bronchospastic disease should not receive beta-blockers; if used at all, should be used cautiously with close monitoring. Use with caution in patients with diabetes mellitus; may potentiate hypoglycemia and/or mask signs and symptoms. Can precipitate or aggravate symptoms of arterial insufficiency in patients with PVD and Raynaud's disease. Use with caution and monitor for progression of arterial obstruction. May mask signs of hyperthyroidism (eg, tachycardia); if hyperthyroidism is suspected, carefully manage and monitor; abrupt withdrawal may exacerbate symptoms of hyperthyroidism or precipitate thyroid storm. Use caution with history of severe anaphylaxis to allergens; patients taking beta-blockers may become more sensitive to repeated challenges. Treatment of anaphylaxis (eg, epinephrine) in patients taking beta-blockers may be ineffective or promote undesirable effects.

Should not be used alone in angle-closure glaucoma (has no effect on pupillary constriction). Multidose vials have been associated with development of bacterial keratitis; avoid contamination. Beta-blockade and/or other suppressive therapy have been associated with choroidal detachment following filtration procedures. Some products contain benzalkonium chloride which may be absorbed by soft contact lenses; remove lens prior to administration and wait 15 minutes before reinserting.

Adverse Reactions

>10%: Ocular: Burning, stinging

Frequency not defined:

Cardiovascular: Angina pectoris, arrhythmia, bradycardia, cardiac arrest, cardiac failure, cerebral ischemia, cerebral vascular accident, edema, heart block, hypertension, hypotension, palpitation, Raynaud's phenomenon

Central nervous system: Anxiety, confusion, depression, disorientation, dizziness, hallucinations, headache, insomnia, memory loss, nervousness, nightmares, somnolence

Dermatologic: Alopecia, angioedema, pseudopemphigoid, psoriasiform rash, psoriasis exacerbation, rash, urticaria

Endocrine & metabolic: Hypoglycemia masked, libido decreased

Gastrointestinal: Anorexia, diarrhea, dyspepsia, nausea, xerostomia

Genitourinary: Impotence, retoperitoneal fibrosis

Hematologic: Claudication

Neuromuscular & skeletal: Myasthenia gravis exacerbation, paresthesia

Ocular: Blepharitis, blurred vision, cataract, choroidal detachment (following filtration surgery), conjunctival injection, conjunctivitis, corneal sensitivity decreased, cystoid macular edema, diplopia, dry eyes, foreign body sensation, hyperemia, itching, keratitis, ocular discharge, ocular pain, ptosis, tearing, visual acuity decreased refractive changes, visual disturbances

Otic: Tinnitus

Respiratory: Bronchospasm, cough, dyspnea, nasal congestion, pulmonary edema, respiratory failure

Miscellaneous: Allergic reactions, cold hands/feet, Peyronie's disease, systemic lupus erythematosus

Drug Interactions

Metabolism/Transport Effects Substrate of CYP2D6 (major); **Note:** Assignment of Major/Minor substrate status based on clinically relevant drug interaction potential; **Inhibits** CYP2D6 (weak)

Avoid Concomitant Use

Avoid concomitant use of Timolol (Ophthalmic) with any of the following: Beta2-Agonists; Floctafenine; Methacholine

Increased Effect/Toxicity

Timolol (Ophthalmic) may increase the levels/effects of: Alpha-/Beta-Agonists (Direct-Acting); Alpha1-Blockers; Alpha2-Agonists; Amifostine; Antihypertensives; Antipsychotic Agents (Phenothiazines); Bupivacaine; Cardiac Glycosides; Cholinergic Agonists; Fingolimod; Hypotensive Agents; Insulin; Lidocaine; Lidocaine (Systemic); Lidocaine (Topical); Mepivacaine; Methacholine; Midodrine; RiTUXimab; Sulfonylureas

The levels/effects of Timolol (Ophthalmic) may be increased by: Abiraterone Acetate; Acetylcholinesterase Inhibitors; Aminoquinolines (Antimalarial); Amiodarone; Anilidopiperidine Opioids; Antipsychotic Agents (Phenothiazines); Calcium Channel Blockers (Dihydropyridine); Calcium Channel Blockers (Nondihydropyridine); CYP2D6 Inhibitors (Moderate); CYP2D6 Inhibitors (Strong); Darunavir; Diazoxide; Dipyridamole; Disopyramide; Dronedarone; Floctafenine; Herbs (Hypotensive Properties); MAO Inhibitors; Pentoxifylline; Phosphodiesterase 5 Inhibitors; Propafenone; Prostacyclin Analogues; QuiNIDine; Reserpine; Selective Serotonin Reuptake Inhibitors

Decreased Effect

Timolol (Ophthalmic) may decrease the levels/effects of: Beta2-Agonists; Theophylline Derivatives

The levels/effects of Timolol (Ophthalmic) may be decreased by: Barbiturates; Herbs (Hypertensive Properties); Methylphenidate; Nonsteroidal Anti-Inflammatory Agents; Rifamycin Derivatives; Yohimbine

Stability Drops: Store at room temperature of 15°C to 25°C (59°F to 77°F); do not freeze. Protect from light.

Timolol GFS: Store at 2°C to 25°C (36°F to 77°F). Protect from light.

Timoptic® in OcuDose®: Store in the protective foil wrap and use within 1 month after opening foil package.

Mechanism of Action Blocks both $beta_1$- and $beta_2$-adrenergic receptors, reduces intraocular pressure by reducing aqueous humor production or possibly outflow; reduces blood pressure by blocking adrenergic receptors and decreasing sympathetic outflow, produces a negative chronotropic and inotropic activity through an unknown mechanism

Pharmacodynamics/Kinetics

Onset of action: Intraocular pressure reduction: 30 minutes

Peak effect: 1-2 hours

Duration: 24 hours

Absorption: Timolol is measurable in the serum following ophthalmic use

Dosage Ophthalmic:

Children and Adults:

Solution: Initial: Instill 1 drop (0.25% solution) into affected eye(s) twice daily; increase to 0.5% solution if response not adequate; decrease to 1 drop/day if controlled; do not exceed 1 drop twice daily of 0.5% solution

Gel-forming solution (Timolol GFS, Timoptic-XE®): Instill 1 drop (either 0.25% or 0.5% solution) once daily

Adults: Solution (Istalol®): Instill 1 drop (0.5% solution) once daily in the morning

Administration Administer other topically-applied ophthalmic medications at least 10 minutes before Timoptic-XE®; wash hands before use; invert closed bottle and shake once before use; remove cap carefully so that tip does not touch anything; hold bottle between thumb and index finger; use index finger of other hand to pull down the lower eyelid to form a pocket for the eye drop and tilt head back; place the dispenser tip close to the eye and gently squeeze the bottle to administer 1 drop; remove pressure after a single drop has been released; **do not allow the dispenser tip to touch the eye**; replace cap and store bottle in an upright position in a clean area; do **not** enlarge hole of dispenser; do **not** wash tip with water, soap, or any other cleaner. Some solutions contain benzalkonium chloride; wait at least 10 minutes after instilling solution before inserting soft contact lenses.

Dosage Forms Excipient information presented when available (limited, particularly for generics); consult specific product labeling.

Gel forming solution, ophthalmic, as maleate [strength expressed as base, drops]: 0.25% (5 mL); 0.5% (5 mL)

Timolol GFS: 0.25% (5 mL); 0.5% (5 mL)

Timoptic-XE®: 0.25% (5 mL); 0.5% (5 mL)

Solution, ophthalmic, as hemihydrate [strength expressed as base, drops]:

Betimol®: 0.25% (5 mL); 0.5% (5 mL, 10 mL, 15 mL) [contains benzalkonium chloride]

Solution, ophthalmic, as maleate [drops]: 0.25% (5 mL, 10 mL, 15 mL); 0.5% (5 mL, 10 mL, 15 mL)

Solution, ophthalmic, as maleate [strength expressed as base, drops]: 0.25% (5 mL, 10 mL, 15 mL); 0.5% (5 mL, 10 mL, 15 mL)

Istalol®: 0.5% (2.5 mL, 5 mL) [contains benzalkonium chloride]

Timoptic®: 0.25% (5 mL); 0.5% (5 mL, 10 mL) [contains benzalkonium chloride]

Solution, ophthalmic, as maleate [strength expressed as base, drops, preservative free]:

Timoptic® in OcuDose®: 0.25% (0.2 mL); 0.5% (0.2 mL)

◆ **Timolol and Brimonidine** *see* Brimonidine and Timolol *on page 236*

◆ **Timolol and Dorzolamide** *see* Dorzolamide and Timolol *on page 548*

◆ **Timolol GFS** *see* Timolol (Ophthalmic) *on page 1687*

◆ **Timolol Hemihydrate** *see* Timolol (Ophthalmic) *on page 1687*

◆ **Timolol Maleate** *see* Timolol (Ophthalmic) *on page 1687*

◆ **Timolol Maleate** *see* Timolol (Systemic) *on page 1686*

◆ **Timolol Maleate-EX (Can)** *see* Timolol (Ophthalmic) *on page 1687*

◆ **Timoptic®** *see* Timolol (Ophthalmic) *on page 1687*

◆ **Timoptic® in OcuDose®** *see* Timolol (Ophthalmic) *on page 1687*

◆ **Timoptic-XE®** *see* Timolol (Ophthalmic) *on page 1687*

◆ **Tinactin® Antifungal [OTC]** *see* Tolnaftate *on page 1704*

◆ **Tinactin® Antifungal Deodorant [OTC]** *see* Tolnaftate *on page 1704*

◆ **Tinactin® Antifungal Jock Itch [OTC]** *see* Tolnaftate *on page 1704*

◆ **Tinaderm [OTC]** *see* Tolnaftate *on page 1704*

◆ **Tincture of Opium** *see* Opium Tincture *on page 1249*

◆ **Ting® Cream [OTC]** *see* Tolnaftate *on page 1704*

◆ **Ting® Spray Liquid [OTC]** *see* Tolnaftate *on page 1704*

◆ **Ting® Spray Powder [OTC]** *see* Miconazole (Topical) *on page 1126*

Tinzaparin (tin ZA pa rin)

Brand Names: U.S. Innohep® [DSC]

Brand Names: Canada Innohep®

Index Terms Tinzaparin Sodium

Pharmacologic Category Low Molecular Weight Heparin

Use Treatment of acute symptomatic deep vein thrombosis, with or without pulmonary embolism, in conjunction with warfarin sodium

Unlabeled Use Prophylaxis of deep vein thrombosis following hip or knee replacement surgery, and general surgery

Pregnancy Risk Factor B

Pregnancy Considerations Teratogenic events were not observed in animal studies. Tinzaparin does not cross the human placenta. A pharmacokinetic study in pregnant women found no dose adjustment was needed during pregnancy. Pregnancy may increase the risk of thromboembolism; risk may be further increased with certain pre-existing conditions. As with all anticoagulants, bleeding is the major adverse effect of tinzaparin. Vaginal bleeding was reported in ~10% of pregnant patients during tinzaparin therapy. Contains benzyl alcohol; use with caution in pregnant women.

Lactation Excretion in breast milk unknown/use caution

Contraindications Hypersensitivity to tinzaparin sodium, heparin, or any component of the formulation; active major bleeding; heparin-induced thrombocytopenia (current or history of)

Warnings/Precautions [U.S. Boxed Warning]: Spinal or epidural hematomas, including subsequent paralysis, may occur with recent or anticipated neuraxial anesthesia (epidural or spinal) or spinal puncture in patients anticoagulated with LMWH or heparinoids. Consider risk versus benefit prior to spinal procedures; risk is increased by the use of concomitant agents which may alter hemostasis, the use of indwelling epidural catheters for analgesia, a history of spinal deformity or spinal surgery, as well as traumatic or repeated epidural or spinal punctures. Patient should be observed closely for signs and symptoms of neurological impairment. Not to be used interchangeably (unit for unit) with heparin or any other low molecular weight heparins.

Monitor patient closely for signs or symptoms of bleeding. Certain patients are at increased risk of bleeding. Risk factors include bacterial endocarditis; congenital or acquired bleeding disorders; active ulcerative or angiodysplastic GI diseases; severe uncontrolled hypertension; history of hemorrhagic stroke; use shortly after brain, spinal, or ophthalmologic surgery; patients treated concomitantly with platelet inhibitors; recent GI bleeding; thrombocytopenia or platelet defects; severe liver disease; hypertensive or diabetic retinopathy; or in patients undergoing invasive procedures. Monitor platelet count closely. Rare cases of thrombocytopenia have occurred. Manufacturer recommends discontinuation of therapy if platelets are <100,000/mm^3. Rare cases of thrombocytopenia with thrombosis have occurred.

Reduced tinzaparin clearance was observed in patients with moderate-to-severe renal impairment; use with caution or avoid use in patients with renal insufficiency. The 2008 *Chest* guidelines recommend that patients with Cl_{cr} <30 mL/minute be treated with unfractionated heparin instead of LMWH (Hirsh, 2008). Use with caution in the elderly (delayed elimination may occur). Use in patients ≥70 years of age with renal insufficiency (Cl_{cr} ≤30 mL/minute or ≥75 years of age and Cl_{cr} ≤60 mL/minute) has been associated with an increased risk of death compared to use of unfractionated heparin; consider alternative treatments in these patients.

Heparin can cause hyperkalemia by suppressing aldosterone production; similar reactions could occur with LMWHs. Monitor for hyperkalemia which most commonly occurs in patients with risk factors for the development of hyperkalemia (eg, renal dysfunction, concomitant use of potassium-sparing diuretics or potassium supplements, hematoma in body tissues). For subcutaneous use only; do not administer intramuscularly or intravenously. Clinical experience is limited in patients with BMI >40 kg/m^2. Derived from porcine intestinal mucosa. Contains benzyl alcohol and sodium metabisulfite.

Adverse Reactions As with all anticoagulants, bleeding is the major adverse effect of tinzaparin. Hemorrhage may occur at virtually any site. Risk is dependent on multiple variables.

>10%:

- Hepatic: ALT increased (13%)
- Local: Injection site hematoma (16%)

1% to 10%:

- Cardiovascular: Angina pectoris, chest pain (2%), hyper-/hypotension, tachycardia
- Central nervous system: Confusion, dizziness, fever (2%), headache (2%), insomnia, pain (2%)
- Dermatologic: Bullous eruption, pruritus, rash (1%), skin disorder
- Gastrointestinal: Constipation (1%), dyspepsia, flatulence, nausea (2%), nonspecified gastrointestinal disorder, vomiting (1%)
- Genitourinary: Dysuria, urinary retention, urinary tract infection (4%)
- Hematologic: Anemia, hematoma, hemorrhage (2%), thrombocytopenia (1%)
- Hepatic: AST increased (9%)
- Local: Thrombophlebitis (deep)
- Neuromuscular & skeletal: Back pain (2%)
- Renal: Hematuria (1%)
- Respiratory: Dyspnea (1%), epistaxis (2%), pneumonia, pulmonary embolism (2%), respiratory disorder
- Miscellaneous: Impaired healing, infection, unclassified reactions

<1% (Limited to important or life-threatening): Abscess, acute febrile reaction, agranulocytosis, allergic purpura, allergic reaction, angioedema, anaphylactoid reaction, anorectal bleeding, cardiac arrhythmia, cellulitis, cerebral hemorrhage, cholestatic hepatitis, coronary thrombosis, dependent edema, epidermal necrolysis, erythematous gastrointestinal hemorrhage, granulocytopenia, hemarthrosis, hematemesis, hemoptysis, injection site bleeding, intracranial hemorrhage, ischemic necrosis, melena, MI, necrosis, neoplasm, ocular hemorrhage, pancytopenia, peripheral ischemia, priapism, purpura, rash, retroperitoneal/intra-abdominal bleeding, severe thrombocytopenia, skin necrosis, spinal epidural hematoma, Stevens-Johnson syndrome, thromboembolism, urticaria, vaginal hemorrhage, wound hematoma

Drug Interactions

Metabolism/Transport Effects None known.

Avoid Concomitant Use

Avoid concomitant use of Tinzaparin with any of the following: Rivaroxaban

Increased Effect/Toxicity

Tinzaparin may increase the levels/effects of: Anticoagulants; Collagenase (Systemic); Deferasirox; Drotrecogin Alfa (Activated); Ibritumomab; Rivaroxaban; Tositumomab and Iodine I 131 Tositumomab

The levels/effects of Tinzaparin may be increased by: 5-ASA Derivatives; Antiplatelet Agents; Dasatinib; Herbs (Anticoagulant/Antiplatelet Properties); Nonsteroidal Anti-Inflammatory Agents; Pentosan Polysulfate Sodium; Pentoxifylline; Prostacyclin Analogues; Salicylates; Thrombolytic Agents

Decreased Effect There are no known significant interactions involving a decrease in effect.

Stability Store at 15°C to 30°C (59°F to 86°F).

Mechanism of Action Standard heparin consists of components with molecular weights ranging from 4000-30,000 daltons with a mean of 16,000 daltons. Heparin acts as an anticoagulant by enhancing the inhibition rate of clotting proteases by antithrombin III, impairing normal hemostasis and inhibition of factor Xa. Low molecular weight heparins have a small effect on the activated partial thromboplastin time and strongly inhibit factor Xa. The primary inhibitory activity of tinzaparin is through antithrombin. Tinzaparin is derived from porcine heparin that undergoes controlled enzymatic depolymerization. The average molecular weight of tinzaparin ranges between 5500 and 7500 daltons which is distributed as <2000 daltons (<10%), 2000-8000 daltons (60% to 72%), and >8000 daltons (22% to 36%). The anti-Xa activity is approximately 100 int. units/mg.

Pharmacodynamics/Kinetics
Onset of action: 2-3 hours
Distribution: 3-5 L
Half-life elimination: 3-4 hours
Metabolism: Partially metabolized by desulphation and depolymerization
Bioavailability: 87%
Time to peak: 4-5 hours
Excretion: Urine

Dosage Note: Each 100 int. units of anti-Xa activity is equal to 1 mg of tinzaparin.

SubQ: **Note:** A pharmacokinetic study confirmed that weight-based dosing (single doses of 75 or 175 units/kg) using actual body weight in heavy/obese patients between 100 and 165 kg led to achievement of similar anti-Xa activity levels compared to normal-weight patients (Hainer, 2002). However, there is limited clinical experience in patients with a BMI >40 kg/m^2.

Adults:

DVT (with or without PE) treatment: 175 anti-Xa int. units/kg once daily. The 2008 *Chest* guidelines recommend starting warfarin on the first treatment day and continuing tinzaparin until INR is between 2 and 3 (usually 5-7 days). Administer tinzaparin for at least 5 days and until INR ≥2 for at least 24 hours (Hirsh, 2008).

DVT prophylaxis (unlabeled use):

Hip replacement surgery: 75 anti-Xa int. units/kg once daily, with initial dose given 18-24 hours after surgery for up to 14 days **or** 4500 anti-Xa int. units once daily, with initial dose given 12 hours prior to surgery and continued for up to 15 days (Hull, 1993; Planes, 1999)

Knee replacement surgery: 75 anti-Xa int. units/kg once daily, with initial dose given 18-24 hours after surgery and continued for up to 14 days (Hull, 1993)

General surgery: 3500 anti-Xa int. units once daily, with initial dose given 2 hours prior to surgery and continued for 7-10 days (Leizorovicz, 1991)

Elderly: No significant differences in safety or response were seen when used in patients ≥65 years of age. However, increased sensitivity to tinzaparin in elderly patients may be possible due to a decline in renal function. Increased all-cause mortality noted in patients ≥70 years of age with Cl_{cr} ≤30 mL/minute or ≥75 years of age and Cl_{cr} ≤60 mL/minute; consider alternative treatments in these patients.

Dosage adjustment in renal impairment:

Cl_{cr} ≤50 mL/minute: Use with caution; clearance is decreased

Cl_{cr} <30 mL/minute: Per manufacturer's labeling, use with caution. The 2008 *Chest* guidelines recommend avoiding use (in patients requiring therapeutic anticoagulation); if used, consider monitoring anti-Xa levels (Hirsh, 2008).

Dosage adjustment in hepatic impairment: No specific dosage adjustment has been recommended.

Administration Patient should be lying down or sitting. Administer by deep SubQ injection, alternating between the left and right anterolateral and left and right posterolateral abdominal wall. Vary site daily. The entire needle should be introduced into the skin fold formed by the thumb and forefinger. Hold the skin fold until injection is complete. To minimize bruising, do not rub the injection site.

Monitoring Parameters CBC including platelet count and hematocrit or hemoglobin, and stool for occult blood; the monitoring of PT and/or aPTT is not of clinical value. Patients receiving both warfarin and tinzaparin should have their INR drawn just prior to the next scheduled dose of tinzaparin.

According to 2008 *Chest* guidelines, routine monitoring of anti-Xa levels is generally not recommended; however, anti-Xa levels may be beneficial in certain patients (eg, obese patients, patients with severe renal insufficiency receiving therapeutic doses, and possibly pregnant women receiving therapeutic doses; Hirsh, 2008)

Dosage Forms Excipient information presented when available (limited, particularly for generics); consult specific product labeling. [DSC] = Discontinued product

Injection, solution, as sodium:

Innohep®: 20,000 anti-Xa int. units/mL (2 mL [DSC]) [contains benzyl alcohol, sodium metabisulfite]

◆ **Tinzaparin Sodium** *see* Tinzaparin *on page 1688*

◆ **Tioguanine** *see* Thioguanine *on page 1670*

◆ **Tiotixene** *see* Thiothixene *on page 1675*

Tiotropium (ty oh TRO pee um)

Brand Names: U.S. Spiriva® HandiHaler®

Brand Names: Canada Spiriva®

Index Terms Tiotropium Bromide Monohydrate

Pharmacologic Category Anticholinergic Agent

Use Maintenance treatment of bronchospasm associated with COPD (including bronchitis and emphysema); reduction of COPD exacerbations

Pregnancy Risk Factor C

Pregnancy Considerations Adverse events (fetal loss, decreased birth weights, delayed sexual maturation) were observed in some animal studies. There are no adequate and well-controlled studies in pregnant women. Use only when expected benefit to mother outweighs potential risk to the fetus.

Lactation Excretion in breast milk unknown/use caution

Contraindications Hypersensitivity to tiotropium or ipratropium, or any component of the formulation (contains lactose)

Warnings/Precautions Rarely, paradoxical bronchospasm may occur with use of inhaled bronchodilating agents; discontinue use and consider other therapy if bronchospasm occurs.

Not indicated for the initial (rescue) treatment of acute episodes of bronchospasm. Use with caution in patients with myasthenia gravis, narrow-angle glaucoma, prostatic hyperplasia, moderate-severe renal impairment (Cl_{cr} ≤50 mL/minute), or bladder neck obstruction; avoid inadvertent instillation of powder into the eyes. Immediate hypersensitivity reactions may occur; discontinue immediately if signs/symptoms occur. Use with caution in patients with a history of hypersensitivity to atropine.

The contents of Spiriva® capsules are for inhalation only via the HandiHaler® device. There have been reports of incorrect administration (swallowing of the capsules). Capsule for oral inhalation contains lactose; use with caution in patients with severe milk protein allergy.

Adverse Reactions

>10%:

Gastrointestinal: Xerostomia (5% to 16%)

Respiratory: Upper respiratory tract infection (41%), pharyngitis (9% to 13%), sinusitis (7% to 11%)

1% to 10%:

Cardiovascular: Chest pain (1% to 7%), edema (dependent, 5%)

Central nervous system: Headache (6%), insomnia (4%), depression (1% to 4%), dysphonia (1% to 3%)

Dermatologic: Rash (4%)

Endocrine & metabolic: Hypercholesterolemia (1% to 3%), hyperglycemia (1% to 3%)

Gastrointestinal: Dyspepsia (6%), abdominal pain (5%), constipation (4% to 5%), vomiting (4%), gastroesophageal reflux (1% to 3%), stomatitis (including ulcerative; 1% to 3%)
Genitourinary: Urinary tract infection (7%)
Neuromuscular & skeletal: Arthralgia (4%), myalgia (4%), arthritis (≥3%), leg pain (1% to 3%), paresthesia (1% to 3%), skeletal pain (1% to 3%)
Ocular: Cataract (1% to 3%)
Respiratory: Rhinitis (6%), epistaxis (4%), cough (≥3%), laryngitis (1% to 3%)
Miscellaneous: Infection (4%), moniliasis (4%), flu-like syndrome (≥3%), allergic reaction (1% to 3%), herpes zoster (1% to 3%)

<1% (Limited to important or life-threatening): Angioedema; application site irritation (glossitis, mouth ulceration, pharyngolaryngeal pain); atrial fibrillation, blurred vision, candidiasis (oral), dizziness, dehydration, dry skin, dysphagia, gingivitis, glaucoma, hoarseness, hypersensitivity reactions, ileus (paralytic), intestinal obstruction, intraocular pressure increased, joint swelling, palpitation, paradoxical bronchospasm, pruritus, pupil dilation (if powder comes in contact with eyes), skin infection, skin ulcer, supraventricular tachycardia, tachycardia, throat irritation, urinary difficulty, urinary retention, urticaria

Drug Interactions

Metabolism/Transport Effects **Substrate** of CYP2D6 (minor), CYP3A4 (minor); **Note:** Assignment of Major/Minor substrate status based on clinically relevant drug interaction potential

Avoid Concomitant Use There are no known interactions where it is recommended to avoid concomitant use.

Increased Effect/Toxicity

Tiotropium may increase the levels/effects of: AbobotulinumtoxinA; Anticholinergics; Cannabinoids; OnabotulinumtoxinA; Potassium Chloride; RimabotulinumtoxinB

The levels/effects of Tiotropium may be increased by: Conivaptan; Pramlintide

Decreased Effect

Tiotropium may decrease the levels/effects of: Acetylcholinesterase Inhibitors (Central); Secretin

The levels/effects of Tiotropium may be decreased by: Acetylcholinesterase Inhibitors (Central); Peginterferon Alfa-2b; Tocilizumab

Stability Store at 25°C (77°F); excursions permitted to 15°C to 30°C (59°F to 86°F). Avoid excessive temperatures and moisture. Do not store capsules in HandiHaler® device. Capsules should be stored in the blister pack and only removed immediately before use. Once protective foil is peeled back and/or removed the capsule should be used immediately; if capsule is not used immediately it should be discarded.

Mechanism of Action Competitively and reversibly inhibits the action of acetylcholine at type 3 muscarinic (M_3) receptors in bronchial smooth muscle causing bronchodilation

Pharmacodynamics/Kinetics

Absorption: Poorly absorbed from GI tract, systemic absorption may occur from lung
Distribution: V_d: 32 L/kg
Protein binding: 72%
Metabolism: Hepatic (minimal), via CYP2D6 and CYP3A4
Bioavailability: Following inhalation, 19.5%; oral solution: 2% to 3%
Half-life elimination: 5-6 days
Time to peak, plasma: 5 minutes (following inhalation)
Excretion: Urine (14% of an inhaled dose); feces (primarily nonabsorbed drug)

Dosage Oral inhalation: Adults: Contents of 1 capsule (18 mcg) inhaled once daily using HandiHaler® device. **Note:** To ensure drug delivery the contents of each capsule should be inhaled twice.

Dosage adjustment in renal impairment: Plasma concentrations may increase in renal impairment. Use caution in moderate-to-severe impairment (Cl_{cr} ≤50 mL/minute); although no dosage adjustment is required, monitor closely.

Administration Administer once daily at the same time each day. Remove capsule from foil blister immediately before use. Capsule should not be swallowed. Place capsule in the capsule-chamber in the base of the HandiHaler® Inhaler. Must only use the HandiHaler® Inhaler. Close mouthpiece until a click is heard, leaving dustcap open. Exhale fully. Do not exhale into inhaler. Tilt head slightly back and inhale (rapidly, steadily and deeply); the capsule vibration may be heard within the device. Hold breath as long as possible. If any powder remains in capsule, exhale and inhale again. Repeat until capsule is empty. Throw away empty capsule; do not leave in inhaler. Do not use a spacer with the HandiHaler® Inhaler. Do not use HandiHaler® device for other medications. Always keep capsules and inhaler dry.

Delivery of dose: Instruct patient to place mouthpiece gently between teeth, closing lips around inhaler. Instruct patient to inhale deeply and hold breath for 5-10 seconds. The amount of drug delivered is small, and the individual will not sense the medication as it is inhaled. Remove mouthpiece prior to exhalation. Patient should not breathe out through the mouthpiece.

Monitoring Parameters FEV_1, peak flow (or other pulmonary function studies)

Dosage Forms Excipient information presented when available (limited, particularly for generics); consult specific product labeling.

Powder, for oral inhalation [capsule]:
Spiriva® HandiHaler®: 18 mcg/capsule (5s, 30s, 90s) [contains lactose]

◆ **Tiotropium Bromide Monohydrate** *see* Tiotropium *on page 1690*

Tipranavir (tip RA na veer)

Brand Names: U.S. Aptivus®
Brand Names: Canada Aptivus®
Index Terms PNU-140690E; TPV
Pharmacologic Category Antiretroviral Agent, Protease Inhibitor

Additional Appendix Information

Perinatal HIV Guidelines *on page 1946*

Use Treatment of HIV-1 infections in combination with ritonavir and other antiretroviral agents; limited to highly treatment-experienced or multiprotease inhibitor-resistant patients.

Pregnancy Risk Factor C

Pregnancy Considerations Teratogenic effects were not observed in animal reproduction studies; fetotoxity was observed with some doses. It is not known if tipranavir crosses the human placenta. The DHHS Perinatal HIV Guidelines note there are insufficient data to recommend use during pregnancy; however, if used, tipranavir must be given with low-dose ritonavir boosting. A small increased risk of preterm birth has been associated with maternal use of protease inhibitor-based combination antiretroviral (ARV) therapy during pregnancy; however, the benefits of use generally outweigh this risk and protease inhibitors (PIs) should not be withheld if otherwise recommended. Hyperglycemia, new onset of diabetes mellitus, or diabetic ketoacidosis have been reported with PIs; it is not clear if pregnancy increases this risk.

Regardless of CD4 count or HIV RNA copy number, all HIV-infected pregnant women should receive a combination antepartum ARV drug regimen; this includes women who require therapy for their own health, as well as women who do not yet require therapy for their own health. ARV therapy should be started as soon as possible if required for the woman's health or immediately after the first trimester if not needed for the mothers health (although earlier initiation may be considered). Long-term follow-up is recommended for all infants exposed to ARV medications.

Healthcare providers are encouraged to enroll pregnant women exposed to antiretroviral medications in the Antiretroviral Pregnancy Registry (1-800-258-4263 or www.-APRegistry.com). Healthcare providers caring for HIV-infected women and their infants may contact the National Perinatal HIV Hotline (888-448-8765) for clinical consultation (DHHS [perinatal], 2011).

Women receiving estrogen (as hormonal contraception or replacement therapy) may have an increased incidence of rash.

Lactation Excretion in breast milk unknown/contraindicated

Contraindications Concurrent therapy of tipranavir/ritonavir with alfuzosin, amiodarone, bepridil, cisapride, ergot derivatives (eg, dihydroergotamine, ergonovine, ergotamine, methylergonovine), flecainide, lovastatin, midazolam (oral), pimozide, propafenone, quinidine, rifampin, sildenafil (for pulmonary arterial hypertension [eg, Revatio®]), simvastatin, St John's wort, and triazolam; moderate-to-severe hepatic impairment (Child-Pugh class B or C)

Warnings/Precautions Coadministration with ritonavir is required. **[U.S. Boxed Warning]: In combination with ritonavir, may cause hepatitis (including fatalities) and/or exacerbate pre-existing hepatic dysfunction (causal relationship not established); patients with chronic hepatitis B or C are at increased risk.** Monitor patients closely; discontinue use if signs or symptoms of toxicity occur or if asymptomatic AST/ALT elevations >10 times upper limit of normal or AST/ALT elevations >5-10 times upper limit of normal concurrently with total bilirubin >2.5 times the upper limit of normal occur. Use with caution in patients with mild hepatic impairment; contraindicated in moderate-to-severe impairment. May be associated with fat redistribution (buffalo hump, increased abdominal girth, breast engorgement, facial atrophy). Use caution in hemophilia. May increase cholesterol and/or triglycerides; hypertriglyceridemia may increase risk of pancreatitis. May cause hyperglycemia. Use with caution in patients with sulfonamide allergy. Protease inhibitors have been associated with a variety of hypersensitivity events (some severe), including rash, anaphylaxis (rare), angioedema, bronchospasm, erythema multiforme, and/or Stevens-Johnson syndrome (rare). It is generally recommended to discontinue treatment if severe rash or moderate symptoms accompanied by other systemic symptoms occur. Immune reconstitution syndrome, including inflammatory responses to indolent infections, has been associated with antiretroviral therapy; additional evaluation and treatment may be required.

[U.S. Boxed Warning]: Tipranavir in combination with ritonavir has been associated with rare reports of fatal and nonfatal intracranial hemorrhage; causal relationship not established. Events often occurred in patients with medical conditions (eg, CNS lesions, head trauma, recent neurosurgery, coagulopathy, alcohol abuse) or concurrent therapy which may have influenced these events. Tipranavir may inhibit platelet aggregation. Use with caution in patients who may be at risk for increased bleeding (trauma, surgery or other medical conditions) or in patients receiving concurrent medications which may increase the risk of bleeding, including antiplatelet agents and anticoagulants.

Use with caution in patients taking strong CYP3A4 inhibitors and moderate CYP3A4 inducers. Concomitant use with selected major CYP3A4 substrates and strong CYP3A4 inducers is contraindicated (see Drug Interactions); consider alternative agents that avoid or lessen the potential for CYP-mediated interactions. Do not coadminister colchicine in patient with renal or hepatic impairment; avoid concurrent use with salmeterol. Coadministration with anticoagulants or antiplatelet agents may increase the risk of bleeding. Women receiving estrogen (as hormonal contraception or replacement therapy) have an increased incidence of rash. Alternative forms of contraception may be needed. Do not coadminister with etravirine. Oral solution formulation contains vitamin E; additional vitamin E supplements should be avoided. Safety and efficacy have not been established in children <2 years of age.

Adverse Reactions

>10%:

Dermatologic: Rash (children 21%; adults 3% to 10%)

Endocrine & metabolic: Hypertriglyceridemia (>400 mg/dL: 61%), hypercholesterolemia (>300 mg/dL: 22%)

Gastrointestinal: Diarrhea (15%)

Hepatic: Transaminases increased (>2.5 x ULN: 26% to 32%; grade 3/4: 10% to 20%)

Neuromuscular & skeletal: CPK increased (grade 3/4: children 11%)

2% to 10%:

Central nervous system: Fever (6% to 8%), fatigue (6%), headache (5%)

Endocrine & metabolic: Dehydration (2%)

Gastrointestinal: Nausea (5% to 9%), amylase increased (grade 3: 6% to 8%), vomiting (6%), abdominal pain (4%), diarrhea (children 4%), weight loss (3%)

Hematologic: Bleeding (children 8%), WBC decreased (grades 3: 5%), anemia (3%), neutropenia (2%)

Hepatic: ALT increased (2%, grades 3/4: 10%), AST increased (grades 3/4: 6%), GGT increased (2%)

Neuromuscular & skeletal: Myalgia (2%)

Respiratory: Cough (children 6%), dyspnea (2%), epistaxis (children 4%)

<2% (Limited to important or life-threatening): Abdominal distension, anorexia, appetite decreased, diabetes mellitus, dizziness, dyspepsia, exanthem, facial wasting, flatulence, flu-like syndrome, gastroesophageal reflux, hepatic failure, hepatic steatosis, hepatitis, hyperbilirubinemia, hyperglycemia, hypersensitivity, immune reconstitution syndrome, insomnia, intracranial hemorrhage, lipase increased, lipoatrophy, lipodystrophy (acquired), lipohypertrophy, malaise, mitochondrial toxicity, muscle cramp, neuropathy (peripheral), pancreatitis, pruritus, renal insufficiency, sleep disorder, somnolence, thrombocytopenia

Drug Interactions

Metabolism/Transport Effects Substrate of CYP3A4 (major); **Note:** Assignment of Major/Minor substrate status based on clinically relevant drug interaction potential; **Inhibits** CYP2D6 (strong); **Induces** P-glycoprotein

Avoid Concomitant Use

Avoid concomitant use of Tipranavir with any of the following: Alfuzosin; Amiodarone; Bepridil [Off Market]; Cisapride; Dabigatran Etexilate; Ergot Derivatives; Etravirine; Flecainide; Lovastatin; Midazolam; Pimozide; Propafenone; QuiNIDine; Rifampin; Simvastatin; St Johns Wort; Tamoxifen; Thioridazine; Triazolam

Increased Effect/Toxicity

Tipranavir may increase the levels/effects of: Alfuzosin; ALPRAZolam; Amiodarone; Antifungal Agents (Azole Derivatives, Systemic); Atomoxetine; Bepridil [Off Market]; Calcium Channel Blockers (Dihydropyridine); Calcium Channel Blockers (Nondihydropyridine); CarBAMazepine; Cisapride; Clarithromycin;

CycloSPORINE; CycloSPORINE (Systemic); CYP2D6 Substrates; Digoxin; Enfuvirtide; Eplerenone; Ergot Derivatives; Fesoterodine; Flecainide; Fusidic Acid; HMG-CoA Reductase Inhibitors; Iloperidone; Lovastatin; Meperidine; Midazolam; Nebivolol; Nefazodone; Pimozide; Propafenone; Protease Inhibitors; QuiNIDine; Rifabutin; Sildenafil; Simvastatin; Sirolimus; Tacrolimus; Tacrolimus (Systemic); Tacrolimus (Topical); Tamoxifen; Temsirolimus; Tenofovir; Tetrabenazine; Thioridazine; TraZODone; Triazolam; Tricyclic Antidepressants; Vardenafil; Vitamin E

The levels/effects of Tipranavir may be increased by: Antifungal Agents (Azole Derivatives, Systemic); Clarithromycin; Conivaptan; CycloSPORINE; CycloSPORINE (Systemic); Delavirdine; Disulfiram; Efavirenz; Enfuvirtide; Estrogen Derivatives; Fusidic Acid; MetroNIDAZOLE; MetroNIDAZOLE (Systemic); MetroNIDAZOLE (Topical)

Decreased Effect

Tipranavir may decrease the levels/effects of: Abacavir; Clarithromycin; Codeine; Contraceptives (Estrogens); Dabigatran Etexilate; Delavirdine; Didanosine; Divalproex; Estrogen Derivatives; Etravirine; Fosphenytoin; Iloperidone; Linagliptin; Meperidine; Methadone; P-glycoprotein/ABCB1 Substrates; PHENobarbital; Phenytoin; Proton Pump Inhibitors; Raltegravir; Theophylline Derivatives; TraMADol; Valproic Acid; Zidovudine

The levels/effects of Tipranavir may be decreased by: Antacids; CarBAMazepine; CYP3A4 Inducers (Strong); Deferasirox; Efavirenz; Fosphenytoin; Garlic; PHENobarbital; Phenytoin; Rifampin; St Johns Wort; Tenofovir; Tocilizumab

Ethanol/Nutrition/Herb Interactions

Ethanol: Capsules contain dehydrated alcohol 7% w/w (0.1 g per capsule)

Herb/Nutraceutical: St Johns wort may decrease the levels/effects of tipranavir/ritonavir; concurrent use is contraindicated. Vitamin E (high dose) may increase the risk of bleeding.

Stability

Capsule: Prior to opening bottle, store under refrigeration at 2°C to 8°C (36°F to 46°F). After bottle is opened, may be stored at controlled room temperature of 25°C (77°F) for up to 60 days.

Oral solution: Store at 15°C to 30°C (59°F to 86°F). After bottle is open, use within 60 days. Do not refrigerate or freeze oral solution.

Mechanism of Action Binds to the site of HIV-1 protease activity and inhibits cleavage of viral Gag-Pol polyprotein precursors into individual functional proteins required for infectious HIV. This results in the formation of immature, noninfectious viral particles.

Pharmacodynamics/Kinetics

Absorption: Incomplete (percentage not established)

Distribution: V_d: 7.7-10 L

Protein binding: >99% (albumin, alpha$_1$-acid glycoprotein)

Metabolism: Hepatic, via CYP3A4 (minimal when coadministered with ritonavir)

Bioavailability: Not established

Half-life elimination: Children 2-<6 years of age: ~8 hours, 6-<12 years of age: ~7 hours, 12-18 years: ~5 hours; Adults: 6 hours

Time to peak, plasma: 3 hours

Excretion: Feces (82%); urine (4%); primarily as unchanged drug (when coadministered with ritonavir)

Dosage Oral:

Children ≥2 years: 14 mg/kg or 375 mg/m^2 (maximum: 500 mg/dose) twice daily. **Note:** Coadministration with ritonavir (6 mg/kg or 150 mg/m^2 [maximum: 200 mg/dose] twice daily) is required.

If intolerance or toxicity develops and virus is not resistant to multiple protease inhibitors: May decrease dose to 12 mg/kg or 290 mg/m^2 twice daily. **Note:** Coadministration with ritonavir (5 mg/kg or 115 mg/m^2 twice daily) is required.

Adults: 500 mg twice daily; **Note:** Coadministration with ritonavir (200 mg twice daily) is required.

Dosage adjustments for concomitant therapy: Adults:

Coadministration with bosentan:

Coadministration of bosentan in patients currently receiving tipranavir/ritonavir: For patients receiving tipranavir/ritonavir for at least 10 days, begin with bosentan 62.5 mg once daily or every other day based on tolerability

Coadministration of tipranavir/ritonavir in patients currently receiving bosentan: Discontinue bosentan 36 hours prior to the initiation of tipranavir/ritonavir. After at least 10 days of tipranavir/ritonavir, resume bosentan 62.5 mg once daily or every other day based on tolerability.

Coadministration with colchicine:

Familial Mediterranean fever (FMF): Maximum colchicine dose: 0.6 mg/day (0.3 mg twice daily)

Gout prophylaxis:

If original colchicine dose is 0.6 mg twice daily, adjust dose to 0.3 mg once daily

If original colchicine dose is 0.6 mg once daily, adjust dose to 0.3 mg every other day

Gout flare treatment: Initial: Colchicine 0.6 mg, followed in 1 hour by a single dose of 0.3 mg; do not repeat for at least 3 days

Coadministration with phosphodiesterase-5 enzyme (PDE-5) inhibitor:

Pulmonary arterial hypertension: Tipranavir/ritonavir coadministered with tadalafil:

Patient receiving tipranavir/ritonavir for at least 1 week: Initiate tadalafil at 20 mg once daily; increase to 40 mg once daily based on individual tolerability

Patient receiving tadalafil when initiating tipranavir/ritonavir: Stop tadalafil at least 24 hours prior to starting tipranavir/ritonavir. After at least 1 week following the initiation of tipranavir/ritonavir, resume tadalafil at 20 mg once daily; increase to 40 mg once daily based on individual tolerability.

Erectile dysfunction: Tipranavir/ritonavir coadministered with:

Sildenafil (Viagra®): Maximum sildenafil dose: 25 mg in a 48-hour period

Tadalafil (Cialis®): Maximum tadalafil dose: 10 mg in a 72-hour period

Vardenafil: Maximum vardenafil dose: 2.5 mg in a 72-hour period

Dosage adjustment in renal impairment: No adjustment required

Dosage adjustment in hepatic impairment:

Mild impairment (Child-Pugh class A): No adjustment required

Moderate-to-severe impairment (Child-Pugh class B or C): Concurrent use is contraindicated

Dietary Considerations Capsule contains dehydrated ethanol. Oral solution formulation contains vitamin E; additional vitamin E supplements should be avoided.

Administration Coadministration with ritonavir is required. Administer with ritonavir capsules or solution without regard to meals; administer with ritonavir tablets with meals.

Monitoring Parameters Viral load, CD4, serum glucose, liver function tests, bilirubin

Dosage Forms Excipient information presented when available (limited, particularly for generics); consult specific product labeling.

Capsule, soft gelatin, oral:

Aptivus®: 250 mg [contains dehydrated ethanol 7%/capsule]

Solution, oral:

Aptivus®: 100 mg/mL (95 mL) [contains propylene glycol, vitamin E; buttermint-butter toffee flavor]

Tirofiban (tye roe FYE ban)

Brand Names: U.S. Aggrastat®

Brand Names: Canada Aggrastat®

Index Terms MK383; Tirofiban Hydrochloride

Pharmacologic Category Antiplatelet Agent, Glycoprotein IIb/IIIa Inhibitor

Use Treatment of acute coronary syndrome (ie, unstable angina/non-ST-elevation myocardial infarction [UA/NSTEMI]) in combination with heparin

Unlabeled Use To support PCI (administered at the time of PCI) for ST-elevation myocardial infarction (STEMI), UA/NSTEMI, and stable ischemic heart disease (ie, elective PCI)

Pregnancy Risk Factor B

Lactation Excretion in breast milk unknown/contraindicated

Contraindications Hypersensitivity to tirofiban or any component of the formulation; active internal bleeding or a history of bleeding diathesis within the previous 30 days; history of intracranial hemorrhage, intracranial neoplasm, arteriovenous malformation, or aneurysm; history of thrombocytopenia following prior exposure; history of CVA within 30 days or any history of hemorrhagic stroke; major surgical procedure or severe physical trauma within the previous month; history, symptoms, or findings suggestive of aortic dissection; severe hypertension (systolic BP >180 mm Hg and/or diastolic BP >110 mm Hg); concomitant use of another parenteral GP IIb/IIIa inhibitor; acute pericarditis

Warnings/Precautions Bleeding is the most common complication encountered during this therapy; most major bleeding occurs at the arterial access site for cardiac catheterization. Caution in patients with platelets <150,000/mm^3; patients with hemorrhagic retinopathy; chronic dialysis patients; when used in combination with other drugs impacting on coagulation. Prior to pulling the sheath, heparin should be discontinued for 3-4 hours and ACT <180 seconds or aPTT <45 seconds. Use standard compression techniques after sheath removal. Watch the site closely afterwards for further bleeding. Sheath hemostasis should be achieved at least 4 hours before hospital discharge. Other trauma and vascular punctures should be minimized. Avoid obtaining vascular access through a noncompressible site (eg, subclavian or jugular vein). Discontinue at least 2-4 hours prior to coronary artery bypass graft surgery (Hillis, 2011). Patients with severe renal insufficiency require dosage reduction.

Adverse Reactions Bleeding is the major drug-related adverse effect. Patients received background treatment with aspirin and heparin. Major bleeding was reported in 1.4% to 2.2%; minor bleeding in 10.5% to 12%; transfusion was required in 4% to 4.3%.

>1% (nonbleeding adverse events):

Cardiovascular: Coronary artery dissection (5%), bradycardia (4%), edema (2%)

Central nervous system: Dizziness (3%), vasovagal reaction (2%), fever (>1%), headache (>1%)

Gastrointestinal: Nausea (>1%)

Genitourinary: Pelvic pain (6%)

Hematologic: Thrombocytopenia: <90,000/mm^3 (1.5%), <50,000/mm^3 (0.3%)

Neuromuscular & skeletal: Leg pain (3%)

Miscellaneous: Diaphoresis (2%)

<1% (Limited to important or life-threatening): Acutely decreased platelets in association with fever, anaphylaxis, GI bleeding (0.1% to 0.2%), GU bleeding (up to 0.1%), hemopericardium, intracranial bleeding (up to 0.1%), pulmonary alveolar hemorrhage, rash, retroperitoneal bleeding (up to 0.6%), severe (<10,000/mm^3) thrombocytopenia (rare), spinal-epidural hematoma

Drug Interactions

Metabolism/Transport Effects None known.

Avoid Concomitant Use There are no known interactions where it is recommended to avoid concomitant use.

Increased Effect/Toxicity

Tirofiban may increase the levels/effects of: Anticoagulants; Antiplatelet Agents; Collagenase (Systemic); Drotrecogin Alfa (Activated); Ibritumomab; Rivaroxaban; Salicylates; Thrombolytic Agents; Tositumomab and Iodine I 131 Tositumomab

The levels/effects of Tirofiban may be increased by: Dasatinib; Glucosamine; Herbs (Anticoagulant/Antiplatelet Properties); Nonsteroidal Anti-Inflammatory Agents; Omega-3-Acid Ethyl Esters; Pentosan Polysulfate Sodium; Pentoxifylline; Prostacyclin Analogues; Vitamin E

Decreased Effect

The levels/effects of Tirofiban may be decreased by: Nonsteroidal Anti-Inflammatory Agents

Stability Store at 25°C (77°F); do not freeze. Protect from light during storage.

Mechanism of Action A reversible antagonist of fibrinogen binding to the GP IIb/IIIa receptor, the major platelet surface receptor involved in platelet aggregation. When administered intravenously, it inhibits *ex vivo* platelet aggregation in a dose- and concentration-dependent manner. When given according to the recommended regimen, >90% inhibition is attained by the end of the 30-minute infusion. Platelet aggregation inhibition is reversible following cessation of the infusion.

Pharmacodynamics/Kinetics

Distribution: 35% unbound

Metabolism: Minimally hepatic

Half-life elimination: 2 hours

Excretion: Urine (65%) and feces (25%) primarily as unchanged drug

Clearance: Elderly: Reduced by 19% to 26%

Dosage Adults: I.V.:

Unstable angina/non-ST-elevation myocardial infarction (UA/NSTEMI): Initial rate of 0.4 mcg/kg/minute for 30 minutes and then continued at 0.1 mcg/kg/minute; dosing should be continued through angiography and for 12-24 hours after angioplasty or atherectomy.

Percutaneous coronary intervention (PCI) (unlabeled use): Loading dose: 25 mcg/kg over 3 minutes at the time of PCI; Maintenance infusion: 0.15 mcg/kg/minute continued for up to 18-24 hours (Levine, 2011; Valgimigli, 2008; Van't Hof, 2008)

Dosing adjustment in severe renal impairment: Cl_{cr} <30 mL/minute: Reduce dose to 50% of normal rate.

Administration Intended for intravenous delivery using sterile equipment and technique. Do not add other drugs or remove solution directly from the bag with a syringe. Do not use plastic containers in series connections; such use can result in air embolism by drawing air from the first container if it is empty of solution. Discard unused solution 24 hours following the start of infusion. May be administered through the same catheter as heparin. Tirofiban injection must be diluted to a concentration of 50 mcg/mL (premixed solution does not require dilution). For unstable angina/non-ST-elevation MI (UA/NSTEMI), infuse loading dose over 30 minutes, followed by continuous infusion. When used during percutaneous coronary intervention (PCI), may administer loading dose over 3 minutes, followed by continuous infusion.

Monitoring Parameters Platelet count. Hemoglobin and hematocrit should be monitored prior to treatment, within 6 hours following loading infusion, and at least daily thereafter during therapy. Platelet count may need to be monitored earlier in patients who received prior glycoprotein IIb/IIa antagonists. Persistent reductions of platelet counts <90,000/mm^3 may require interruption or discontinuation of infusion. Because tirofiban requires concurrent heparin therapy, aPTT levels should also be followed. Monitor vital signs and laboratory results prior to, during, and after therapy. Assess infusion insertion site during and after therapy (every 15 minutes or as institutional policy). Observe and teach patient bleeding precautions (avoid invasive procedures and activities that could result in injury). Monitor closely for signs of unusual or excessive bleeding (eg, CNS changes, blood in urine, stool, or vomitus, unusual bruising or bleeding). Breast-feeding is contraindicated.

Dosage Forms Excipient information presented when available (limited, particularly for generics); consult specific product labeling. [DSC] = Discontinued product

Infusion, premixed in NS [preservative free]:

Aggrastat®: 50 mcg/mL (100 mL [DSC], 250 mL)

- ◆ **Tirofiban Hydrochloride** *see* Tirofiban *on page 1694*
- ◆ **Tirosint®** *see* Levothyroxine *on page 1004*
- ◆ **Titralac™ [OTC]** *see* Calcium Carbonate *on page 266*
- ◆ **Ti-U-Lac® H (Can)** *see* Urea and Hydrocortisone *on page 1750*
- ◆ **TIV** *see* Influenza Virus Vaccine (Inactivated) *on page 897*

TiZANidine (tye ZAN i deen)

Brand Names: U.S. Zanaflex Capsules®; Zanaflex®

Brand Names: Canada Apo-Tizanidine®; Gen-Tizanidine; Mylan-Tizanidine; Zanaflex®

Index Terms Sirdalud®

Pharmacologic Category Alpha$_2$-Adrenergic Agonist

Use Skeletal muscle relaxant used for treatment of muscle spasticity

Unlabeled Use Tension headaches, low back pain, and trigeminal neuralgia

Pregnancy Risk Factor C

Pregnancy Considerations Adverse events were observed in some animal reproduction studies.

Lactation Excretion in breast milk unknown

Contraindications Hypersensitivity to tizanidine or any component of the formulation; concomitant therapy with ciprofloxacin or fluvoxamine (potent CYP1A2 inhibitors)

Warnings/Precautions Significant hypotension (possibly with bradycardia or orthostatic hypotension) and sedation may occur; use caution in patients with cardiac disease or those at risk for severe hypotensive or sedative effects. Should not be used with other alpha$_2$-adrenergic agonists. Avoid concomitant administration with CYP1A2 inhibitors; increased tizanidine levels/effects (severe hypotension and sedation) may occur. These effects may also be increased with concomitant administration with other CNS depressants and/or antihypertensives; use caution. Elderly patients are at risk due to decreased clearance, particulary in elderly patients with renal insufficiency (Cl_{cr} <25 mL/minute) compared to healthy elderly subjects; this may lead to an increased risk of adverse effects and/or a longer duration of effects. Use caution in any patient with renal impairment; reduced initial doses recommended in patient with Cl_{cr} <25 mL/minute. Use with extreme caution or avoid in hepatic impairment due to extensive hepatic metabolism and potential hepatotoxicity; AST/ALT elevations (≥2 times baseline) and rarely hepatic failure have occurred; monitoring recommended.

Use has been associated with visual hallucinations or delusions, generally in first 6 weeks of therapy; use caution in patients with psychiatric disorders. Withdrawal resulting in rebound hypertension, tachycardia, and hypertonia may occur upon discontinuation; doses should be decreased slowly, particularly in patients receiving high doses for prolonged periods. Pharmacokinetics and bioequivalence between capsules and tablets altered by nonfasting vs fasting conditions. Limited data exists for chronic use of single doses >8 mg and multiple doses >24 mg/day.

Adverse Reactions Frequency percentages below reported during multiple-dose studies, unless specified otherwise.

>10%:

Cardiovascular: Hypotension (single-dose study with doses ≥8 mg: 16% to 33%)

Central nervous system: Somnolence (48%), dizziness (16%)

Gastrointestinal: Xerostomia (49%)

Neuromuscular & skeletal: Weakness (41%)

1% to 10%:

Cardiovascular: Bradycardia (single-dose study with doses ≥8 mg: 2% to 10%)

Central nervous system: Nervousness (3%), speech disorder (3%), visual hallucinations/delusions (3%; generally occurring in first 6 weeks of therapy), anxiety (1%), depression (1%), fever (1%)

Dermatologic: Rash (1%), skin ulcer (1%)

Gastrointestinal: Constipation (4%), vomiting (3%), abdominal pain (1%), diarrhea (1%), dyspepsia (1%)

Genitourinary: UTI (10%), urinary frequency (3%)

Hepatic: Liver enzymes increased (3% to 5%)

Neuromuscular & skeletal: Dyskinesia (3%), back pain (1%), myasthenia (1%), paresthesia (1%)

Ocular: Blurred vision (3%)

Respiratory: Pharyngitis (3%), rhinitis (3%)

Miscellaneous: Infection (6%), flu-like syndrome (3%), diaphoresis (1%)

<1%, frequency not defined, and postmarketing experience (limited to important or life-threatening): Adrenal insufficiency, allergic reaction, anemia, angina, arrhythmia, carcinoma, cholelithiasis, deafness, dementia, dyslipidemia, gastrointestinal hemorrhage, glaucoma, heart failure, hepatomegaly, hemiplegia, hepatic failure, hepatitis, hepatoma, hyperglycemia, hypokalemia, hyponatremia, hypoproteinemia, hypothyroidism, intestinal obstruction, jaundice, leukopenia, leukocytosis, MI, migraine, neuralgia, optic neuritis, palpitation, paralysis, postural hypotension, psychotic-like symptoms, pulmonary embolus, purpura, respiratory acidosis, retinal hemorrhage, seizure, sepsis, suicide attempt, syncope, thrombocythemia, thrombocytopenia, ventricular extrasystoles, ventricular tachycardia, vertigo

Drug Interactions

Metabolism/Transport Effects **Substrate** of CYP1A2 (major); **Note:** Assignment of Major/Minor substrate status based on clinically relevant drug interaction potential

Avoid Concomitant Use

Avoid concomitant use of TiZANidine with any of the following: Ciprofloxacin; Ciprofloxacin (Systemic); FluvoxaMINE; Iobenguane I 123

Increased Effect/Toxicity

TiZANidine may increase the levels/effects of: ACE Inhibitors; Alcohol (Ethyl); CNS Depressants; Hypotensive Agents; Lisinopril; Methotrimeprazine; Selective Serotonin Reuptake Inhibitors

The levels/effects of TiZANidine may be increased by: Abiraterone Acetate; Beta-Blockers; Ciprofloxacin; Ciprofloxacin (Systemic); Contraceptives (Estrogens); CYP1A2 Inhibitors (Moderate); CYP1A2 Inhibitors (Strong); Deferasirox; Droperidol; FluvoxaMINE; HydrOXYzine; MAO Inhibitors; Methotrimeprazine

Decreased Effect

TiZANidine may decrease the levels/effects of: Iobenguane I 123

The levels/effects of TiZANidine may be decreased by: Antidepressants (Alpha2-Antagonist); Cyproterone; Serotonin/Norepinephrine Reuptake Inhibitors; Tricyclic Antidepressants

Ethanol/Nutrition/Herb Interactions

Ethanol: May increase CNS depression; monitor for increased effects with coadministration. Caution patients about effects.

Food: The tablet and capsule dosage forms are not bioequivalent when administered with food. Food increases both the time to peak concentration and the extent of absorption for both the tablet and capsule. However, maximal concentrations of tizanidine achieved when administered with food were increased by 30% for the tablet, but decreased by 20% for the capsule. Under fed conditions, the capsule is approximately 80% bioavailable relative to the tablet.

Herb/Nutraceutical: Avoid valerian, St John's wort, kava kava, gotu kola (may increase CNS depression). Avoid black cohosh, California poppy, coleus, golden seal, hawthorn, mistletoe, periwinkle, quinine, shepherd's purse (may increase hypotensive effects).

Stability Store at 25°C (77°F); excursions permitted to 15°C to 30°C (59°F to 86°F).

Mechanism of Action An alpha$_2$-adrenergic agonist agent which decreases excitatory input to alpha motor neurons; an imidazole derivative chemically-related to clonidine, which acts as a centrally acting muscle relaxant with alpha$_2$-adrenergic agonist properties; acts on the level of the spinal cord

Pharmacodynamics/Kinetics

Duration: 3-6 hours

Absorption: Tablets and capsules are bioequivalent under fasting conditions, but not under nonfasting conditions.

Tablets administered with food: Peak plasma concentration is increased by ~30%; time to peak increased by 25 minutes; extent of absorption increased by ~30%.

Capsules administered with food: Peak plasma concentration decreased by 20%; time to peak increased by 2-3 hours; extent of absorption increased by ~10%.

Capsules opened and sprinkled on applesauce are not bioequivalent to administration of intact capsules under fasting conditions. Peak plasma concentration and AUC are increased by 15% to 20%.

Distribution: 2.4 L/kg

Protein binding: ~30%

Metabolism: Extensively hepatic via CYP1A2 to inactive metabolites

Bioavailability: ~40% (extensive first-pass metabolism)

Half-life elimination: 2.5 hours

Time to peak, serum:

Fasting state: Capsule, tablet: 1 hour

Fed state: Capsule: 3-4 hours, Tablet: 1.5 hours

Excretion: Urine (60%); feces (20%)

Dosage

Adults: 2-4 mg 3 times/day

Usual initial dose: 4 mg, may increase by 2-4 mg as needed for satisfactory reduction of muscle tone every 6-8 hours to a maximum of 3 doses in any 24-hour period

Maximum: 36 mg/day

Elderly: No specific dosing guidelines exist; clearance is decreased; dose cautiously

Dosing adjustment in renal impairment: Cl_{cr} <25 mL/minute: Use with caution; clearance reduced >50%. During initial dose titration, use reduced doses. If higher doses necessary, increase dose instead of increasing dosing frequency.

Dosing adjustment in hepatic impairment: Avoid use in hepatic impairment; if used, lowest possible dose should be used initially with close monitoring for adverse effects (eg, hypotension).

Dietary Considerations Administration with food compared to administration in the fasting state results in clinically-significant differences in absorption and other pharmacokinetic parameters. Patients should be consistent and should not switch administration of the tablets or the capsules between the fasting and nonfasting state. In addition, switching between the capsules and the tablets in the fed state will also result in significant differences. Opening capsule contents to sprinkle on applesauce compared to swallowing intact capsules whole will also result in significant absorption differences. Patients should be consistent with regards to administration.

Administration Capsules may be opened and contents sprinkled on food; however, extent of absorption is increased up to 20% relative to administration of the capsule under fasted conditions.

Monitoring Parameters Monitor liver function (aminotransferases) at baseline, 1, 3, 6 months and periodically thereafter; blood pressure; renal function

Dosage Forms Excipient information presented when available (limited, particularly for generics); consult specific product labeling.

Capsule, oral:

Zanaflex Capsules®: 2 mg, 4 mg, 6 mg

Tablet, oral: 2 mg, 4 mg

Zanaflex®: 4 mg [scored]

- ◆ **TMC-114** *see* Darunavir *on page 451*
- ◆ **TMC125** *see* Etravirine *on page 673*
- ◆ **TMC278** *see* Rilpivirine *on page 1490*
- ◆ **TMP** *see* Trimethoprim *on page 1740*
- ◆ **TMP-SMX** *see* Sulfamethoxazole and Trimethoprim *on page 1602*
- ◆ **TMP-SMZ** *see* Sulfamethoxazole and Trimethoprim *on page 1602*
- ◆ **TMX-67** *see* Febuxostat *on page 690*
- ◆ **TMZ** *see* Temozolomide *on page 1638*
- ◆ **TNKase®** *see* Tenecteplase *on page 1643*
- ◆ **TOBI®** *see* Tobramycin (Systemic, Oral Inhalation) *on page 1696*
- ◆ **TOBI® Podhaler® (Can)** *see* Tobramycin (Systemic, Oral Inhalation) *on page 1696*
- ◆ **TobraDex®** *see* Tobramycin and Dexamethasone *on page 1700*
- ◆ **Tobradex® (Can)** *see* Tobramycin and Dexamethasone *on page 1700*
- ◆ **TobraDex® ST** *see* Tobramycin and Dexamethasone *on page 1700*

Tobramycin (Systemic, Oral Inhalation)

(toe bra MYE sin)

Brand Names: U.S. TOBI®

Brand Names: Canada TOBI®; TOBI® Podhaler®; Tobramycin Injection, USP

Index Terms Tobramycin Sulfate

Pharmacologic Category Antibiotic, Aminoglycoside

Additional Appendix Information

Prevention of Wound Infection and Sepsis in Surgical Patients *on page 1954*

Use Treatment of documented or suspected infections caused by susceptible gram-negative bacilli, including *Pseudomonas aeruginosa*. Tobramycin solution for inhalation and powder for inhalation (Canadian availability; not available in the U.S.) are indicated for the management of cystic fibrosis patients (>6 years of age) with *Pseudomonas aeruginosa*.

Pregnancy Risk Factor D

Pregnancy Considerations [U.S. Boxed Warning]: Aminoglycosides may cause fetal harm if administered to a pregnant woman. There are several reports of total irreversible bilateral congenital deafness in children whose mothers received another aminoglycoside (streptomycin) during pregnancy; therefore, tobramycin is classified as pregnancy category D. Tobramycin crosses the placenta and produces detectable serum levels in the fetus. Although serious side effects to the fetus have not been reported following maternal use of tobramycin, a potential for harm exists.

Due to pregnancy-induced physiologic changes, some pharmacokinetic parameters of tobramycin may be altered. Pregnant women have an average-to-larger volume of distribution which may result in lower serum peak levels than for the same dose in nonpregnant women. Serum half-life is also shorter.

Lactation Enters breast milk/not recommended

Contraindications Hypersensitivity to tobramycin, other aminoglycosides, or any component of the formulation; pregnancy

Warnings/Precautions [U.S. Boxed Warning]: Aminoglycosides may cause neurotoxicity and/or nephrotoxicity; usual risk factors include pre-existing renal impairment, concomitant neuro-/nephrotoxic medications, advanced age, and dehydration. Ototoxicity may be directly proportional to the amount of drug given and the duration of treatment; tinnitus or vertigo are indications of vestibular injury and impending hearing loss; renal damage is usually reversible. May cause neuromuscular blockade and respiratory paralysis, especially when given soon after anesthesia or muscle relaxants.

Not intended for long-term therapy due to toxic hazards associated with extended administration; use caution in pre-existing renal insufficiency, vestibular or cochlear impairment, myasthenia gravis, hypocalcemia, and conditions which depress neuromuscular transmission. Dosage modification required in patients with impaired renal function. Prolonged use may result in fungal or bacterial superinfection, including *C. difficile*-associated diarrhea (CDAD) and pseudomembranous colitis; CDAD has been observed >2 months postantibiotic treatment. Solution may contain sodium metabisulfate; use caution in patients with sulfite allergy.

Adverse Reactions

Injection: Frequency not defined:

- Central nervous system: Confusion, disorientation, dizziness, fever, headache, lethargy, vertigo
- Dermatologic: Exfoliative dermatitis, itching, rash, urticaria
- Endocrine & metabolic: Serum calcium, magnesium, potassium, and/or sodium decreased
- Gastrointestinal: Diarrhea, nausea, vomiting
- Hematologic: Anemia, eosinophilia, granulocytopenia, leukocytosis, leukopenia, thrombocytopenia
- Hepatic: ALT increased, AST increased, bilirubin increased, LDH increased
- Local: Pain at the injection site
- Otic: Hearing loss, tinnitus, ototoxicity (auditory), ototoxicity (vestibular), roaring in the ears
- Renal: BUN increased, cylindruria, serum creatinine increased, oliguria, proteinuria

Inhalation (as reported for solution for inhalation unless otherwise noted):

>10%:

- Gastrointestinal: Sputum discoloration (21%)
- Respiratory: Cough (22% [powder for inhalation]), voice alteration (13%)

1% to 10%:

- Cardiovascular: Chest discomfort (3% [powder for inhalation])
- Central nervous system: Malaise (6%), pyrexia (1% [powder for inhalation])
- Gastrointestinal: Abnormal taste (5% [powder for inhalation]), xerostomia (2% [powder for inhalation])
- Otic: Tinnitus (3%)
- Respiratory: Dyspnea (4% [powder for inhalation]), oropharyngeal pain (4% [powder for inhalation]), throat irritation (3% [powder for inhalation]), FEV decreased (2% [powder for inhalation]), pulmonary function decreased (2% [powder for inhalation]), bronchospasm (1% [powder for inhalation]), upper respiratory tract infection (1% [powder for inhalation])

<1% (Limited to important or life-threatening): Aphonia, bronchial secretions increased, deafness, diarrhea, exercise tolerance decreased, hearing loss, hypersensitivity (allergic reactions), hypoesthesia (oral), lower respiratory tract infection, musculoskeletal chest pain, nasal congestion, obstructive airway disorder, oral candidiasis, pneumonitis, pruritus, pulmonary congestion, rales, rash, respiratory sounds abnormal, serum glucose increased, urticaria, vital capacity decreased

Drug Interactions

Metabolism/Transport Effects None known.

Avoid Concomitant Use

Avoid concomitant use of Tobramycin (Systemic, Oral Inhalation) with any of the following: BCG; Gallium Nitrate

Increased Effect/Toxicity

Tobramycin (Systemic, Oral Inhalation) may increase the levels/effects of: AbobotulinumtoxinA; Bisphosphonate Derivatives; CARBOplatin; Colistimethate; CycloSPORINE; CycloSPORINE (Systemic); Gallium Nitrate; Neuromuscular-Blocking Agents; OnabotulinumtoxinA; RimabotulinumtoxinB

The levels/effects of Tobramycin (Systemic, Oral Inhalation) may be increased by: Amphotericin B; Capreomycin; Cephalosporins (2nd Generation); Cephalosporins (3rd Generation); Cephalosporins (4th Generation); CISplatin; Loop Diuretics; Nonsteroidal Anti-Inflammatory Agents; Vancomycin

Decreased Effect

Tobramycin (Systemic, Oral Inhalation) may decrease the levels/effects of: BCG; Typhoid Vaccine

The levels/effects of Tobramycin (Systemic, Oral Inhalation) may be decreased by: Penicillins

Stability

Injection: Stable at room temperature both as the clear, colorless solution and as the dry powder. Reconstituted solutions remain stable for 24 hours at room temperature and 96 hours when refrigerated. Dilute in 50-100 mL NS, D_5W for I.V. infusion.

Powder, for inhalation (TOBI® Podhaler®) [Canadian availability; not available in the U.S.]: Store in original package at 15°C to 30°C (59°F to 86°F). Protect from moisture.

Solution, for inhalation (TOBI®): Store under refrigeration at 2°C to 8°C (36°F to 46°F). May be stored in foil pouch at room temperature of 25°C (77°F) for up to 28 days. Avoid intense light. Solution may darken over time; however, do not use if cloudy or contains particles.

Mechanism of Action Interferes with bacterial protein synthesis by binding to 30S and 50S ribosomal subunits, resulting in a defective bacterial cell membrane

Pharmacodynamics/Kinetics

Absorption:

Oral: Poorly absorbed

I.M.: Rapid and complete

Inhalation: Peak serum concentrations:

Solution for inhalation: ~1 mcg/mL following a 300 mg dose

Powder for inhalation: ~1 mcg/mL (range: 0.49-1.55 mcg/mL) following a 112 mg dose

Distribution: V_d: 0.2-0.3 L/kg; Pediatrics: 0.2-0.7 L/kg; to extracellular fluid, including serum, abscesses, ascitic, pericardial, pleural, synovial, lymphatic, and peritoneal fluids; poor penetration into CSF, eye, bone, prostate

Inhalation: Tobramycin remains concentrated primarily in the airways

Protein binding: <30%

Half-life elimination:

Neonates: ≤1200 g: 11 hours; >1200 g: 2-9 hours

Adults: 2-3 hours; directly dependent upon glomerular filtration rate

Adults with impaired renal function: 5-70 hours

Time to peak, serum: I.M.: 30-60 minutes; I.V.: ~30 minutes

Excretion: Normal renal function: Urine (~90% to 95%) within 24 hours

Dosage Note: Dosage individualization is **critical** because of the low therapeutic index.

Use of ideal body weight (IBW) for determining the mg/kg/dose appears to be more accurate than dosing on the basis of total body weight (TBW). In morbid obesity, dosage requirement may best be estimated using a dosing weight of IBW + 0.4 (TBW - IBW).

Initial and periodic plasma drug levels (eg, peak and trough with conventional dosing) should be determined, particularly in critically-ill patients with serious infections or in disease states known to significantly alter aminoglycoside pharmacokinetics (eg, cystic fibrosis, burns, or major surgery).

Usual dosage range:

Infants and Children <5 years: I.M., I.V.: 2.5 mg/kg/dose every 8 hours

Children ≥5 years: I.M., I.V.: 2-2.5 mg/kg/dose every 8 hours

Note: Higher individual doses and/or more frequent intervals (eg, every 6 hours) may be required in selected clinical situations (cystic fibrosis) or serum levels document the need.

Children ≥6 years and Adults: Inhalation:

TOBI®: 300 mg every 12 hours (do not administer doses <6 hours apart); administer in repeated cycles of 28 days on drug followed by 28 days off drug.

TOBI® Podhaler® (Canadian availability; not available in the U.S.): 112 mg (4 x 28 mg capsules) every 12 hours (do not administer doses <6 hours apart); administer in repeated cycles of 28 days on drug followed by 28 days off drug.

Adults: I.M., I.V.:

Conventional: 1-2.5 mg/kg/dose every 8-12 hours; to ensure adequate peak concentrations early in therapy, higher initial dosage may be considered in selected patients when extracellular water is increased (edema, septic shock, postsurgical, and/or trauma)

Once-daily: 4-7 mg/kg/dose once daily; some clinicians recommend this approach for all patients with normal renal function; this dose is at least as efficacious with similar, if not less, toxicity than conventional dosing.

Indication-specific dosing:

Children:

CNS shunt infection: Intrathecal (unlabeled route): Refer to adult dosing

Cystic fibrosis:

I.M., I.V.: 2.5-3.3 mg/kg every 6-8 hours; **Note:** Some patients may require larger or more frequent doses if serum levels document the need (eg, cystic fibrosis or febrile granulocytopenic patients).

Inhalation: Children ≥6 years: Refer to adult dosing.

Adults:

I.M., I.V.:

Brucellosis: 240 mg (I.M.) daily or 5 mg/kg (I.V.) daily for 7 days; either regimen recommended in combination with doxycycline

Cholangitis: 4-6 mg/kg once daily with ampicillin

Diverticulitis, complicated: 1.5-2 mg/kg every 8 hours (with ampicillin and metronidazole)

Infective endocarditis or synergy (for gram-positive infections): I.M., I.V.: 1 mg/kg every 8 hours (with ampicillin)

Meningitis *(Enterococcus or Pseudomonas aeruginosa)*: I.V.: Loading dose: 2 mg/kg, then 1.7 mg/kg/dose every 8 hours (administered with another bactericidal drug)

Pelvic inflammatory disease: Loading dose: 2 mg/kg, then 1.5 mg/kg every 8 hours **or** 4.5 mg/kg once daily

Plague *(Yersinia pestis)*: Treatment: 5 mg/kg/day, followed by postexposure prophylaxis with doxycycline

Pneumonia, hospital- or ventilator-associated: 7 mg/kg/day (with antipseudomonal beta-lactam or carbapenem)

Prophylaxis against endocarditis (dental, oral, upper respiratory procedures, GI/GU procedures): 1.5 mg/kg with ampicillin (50 mg/kg) 30 minutes prior to procedure. **Note:** AHA guidelines now recommend prophylaxis only in patients undergoing invasive procedures and in whom underlying cardiac conditions may predispose to a higher risk of adverse outcomes should infection occur. As of April 2007, routine prophylaxis no longer recommended by the AHA.

Tularemia: 5 mg/kg/day divided every 8 hours for 1-2 weeks

Urinary tract infection: 1.5 mg/kg/dose every 8 hours

Inhalation: **Cystic fibrosis:**

TOBI®: 300 mg every 12 hours (do not administer doses <6 hours apart); administer in repeated cycles of 28 days on drug followed by 28 days off drug.

TOBI® Podhaler® (Canadian availability; not available in the U.S.): 112 mg (4 x 28 mg capsules) every 12 hours (do not administer doses <6 hours apart); administer in repeated cycles of 28 days on drug followed by 28 days off drug.

Intrathecal (unlabeled route): **CNS shunt infection:** 5-20 mg/day (Tunkel, 2004)

Dosing interval in renal impairment: I.M., I.V.:

Conventional dosing:

Cl_{cr} ≥60 mL/minute: Administer every 8 hours

Cl_{cr} 40-60 mL/minute: Administer every 12 hours

Cl_{cr} 20-40 mL/minute: Administer every 24 hours

Cl_{cr} 10-20 mL/minute: Administer every 48 hours

Cl_{cr} <10 mL/minute: Administer every 72 hours

High-dose therapy: Interval may be extended (eg, every 48 hours) in patients with moderate renal impairment (Cl_{cr} 30-59 mL/minute) and/or adjusted based on serum level determinations.

Intermittent hemodialysis (IHD) (administer after hemodialysis on dialysis days) (Heintz, 2009): Dialyzable (25% to 70%; variable; dependent on filter, duration, and type of HD): I.V.:

Loading dose of 2-3 mg/kg, followed by:

Mild UTI or synergy: I.V.: 1 mg/kg every 48-72 hours; consider redosing for pre-HD or post-HD concentrations <1mg/L

Moderate-to-severe UTI: I.V. 1-1.5 mg/kg every 48-72 hours; consider redosing for pre-HD concentrations <1.5-2 mg/L or post-HD concentrations <1 mg/L

Systemic gram-negative infection: I.V.: 1.5-2 mg/kg every 48-72 hours; consider redosing for pre-HD concentrations <3-5 mg/L or post-HD concentrations <2 mg/L

Note: Dosing dependent on the assumption of 3 times/week, complete IHD sessions.

Peritoneal dialysis (PD):

Administration via peritoneal dialysis (PD) fluid:

Gram-negative infection: 4-8 mg/L (4-8 mcg/mL) of PD fluid

Gram-positive infection (ie, synergy): 3-4 mg/L (3-4 mcg/mL) of PD fluid

Administration IVPB/I.M.: Dose as for Cl_{cr} <10 mL/minute and follow levels

Continuous renal replacement therapy (CRRT) (Heintz, 2009; Trotman, 2005): Drug clearance is highly dependent on the method of renal replacement, filter type, and flow rate. Appropriate dosing requires close monitoring of pharmacologic response, signs of adverse reactions due to drug accumulation, as well as drug concentrations in relation to target trough (if appropriate). The following are general recommendations only (based on dialysate flow/ultrafiltration rates of 1-2 L/hour and minimal residual renal function) and should not supersede clinical judgment:

CVVH/CVVHD/CVVHDF: I.V.: Loading dose of 2-3 mg/kg, followed by:

Mild UTI or synergy: I.V. 1 mg/kg every 24-36 hours (redose when concentration <1 mg/L)

Moderate-severe UTI: I.V.: 1-1.5 mg/kg every 24-36 hours (redose when concentration <1.5-2 mg/L)

Systemic gram-negative infection: I.V.: 1.5-2.5 mg/kg every 24-48 hours (redose when concentration <3-5 mg/L)

Dosing adjustment/comments in hepatic disease: No dosage adjustment necessary in hepatic impairment; monitor plasma concentrations as appropriate.

Dietary Considerations May require supplementation of calcium, magnesium, potassium.

Administration

I.V.: Infuse over 30-60 minutes. Flush with saline before and after administration.

Inhalation:

TOBI®: To be inhaled over ~15 minutes using a handheld nebulizer (PARI-LC PLUS™). If multiple different nebulizer treatments are required, administer bronchodilator first, followed by chest physiotherapy, any other nebulized medications, and then TOBI® last. Do not mix with other nebulizer medications.

TOBI® Podhaler® (Canadian availability; not available in the U.S.): Capsules should be administered by oral inhalation via Podhaler® device following manufacturer recommendations for use and handling. Capsules should not be swallowed. Patients requiring bronchodilator therapy should administer the bronchodilator 15-90 minutes prior to TOBI® Podhaler®. The sequence of chest physiotherapy and additional inhaled therapies is at the discretion of the healthcare provider however TOBI® Podhaler® should always be administered last.

Some penicillins (eg, carbenicillin, ticarcillin, and piperacillin) have been shown to inactivate aminoglycosides *in vitro*. This has been observed to a greater extent with tobramycin and gentamicin, while amikacin has shown greater stability against inactivation. Concurrent use of these agents may pose a risk of reduced antibacterial efficacy *in vivo*, particularly in the setting of profound renal impairment. However, definitive clinical evidence is lacking. If combination penicillin/aminoglycoside therapy is desired in a patient with renal dysfunction, separation of doses (if feasible), and routine monitoring of aminoglycoside levels, CBC, and clinical response should be considered.

Monitoring Parameters Urinalysis, urine output, BUN, serum creatinine, peak and trough plasma tobramycin levels; be alert to ototoxicity; hearing should be tested before and during treatment

Some penicillin derivatives may accelerate the degradation of aminoglycosides *in vitro*. This may be clinically-significant for certain penicillin (ticarcillin, piperacillin, carbenicillin) and aminoglycoside (gentamicin, tobramycin) combination therapy in patients with significant renal impairment. Close monitoring of aminoglycoside levels is warranted.

Reference Range

Timing of serum samples: Draw peak 30 minutes after 30-minute infusion has been completed or 1 hour following I.M. injection or beginning of infusion; draw trough immediately before next dose

Therapeutic levels:

Peak:

Serious infections: 6-8 mcg/mL (SI: 12-17 micromole/L)

Life-threatening infections: 8-10 mcg/mL (SI: 17-21 micromole/L)

Urinary tract infections: 4-6 mcg/mL (SI: 7-12 micromole/L)

Synergy against gram-positive organisms: 3-5 mcg/mL

Trough:

Serious infections: 0.5-1 mcg/mL

Life-threatening infections: 1-2 mcg/mL

The American Thoracic Society (ATS) recommends trough levels of <1 mcg/mL for patients with hospital-acquired pneumonia.

Monitor serum creatinine and urine output; obtain drug levels after the third dose unless otherwise directed

Inhalation: Serum levels are ~1 mcg/mL one hour following a 300 mg dose in patients with normal renal function.

Test Interactions Some penicillin derivatives may accelerate the degradation of aminoglycosides *in vitro*, leading to a potential underestimation of aminoglycoside serum concentration.

Additional Information Once-daily dosing: Higher peak serum drug concentration to MIC ratios, demonstrated aminoglycoside postantibiotic effect, decreased renal cortex drug uptake, and improved cost-time efficiency are supportive reasons for the use of once daily dosing regimens for aminoglycosides. Current research indicates these regimens to be as effective for non-life-threatening infections, with no higher incidence of nephrotoxicity, than those requiring multiple daily doses. Doses are determined by calculating the entire day's dose via usual multiple dose calculation techniques and administering this quantity as a single dose. Doses are then adjusted to maintain mean serum concentrations above the MIC(s) of the causative organism(s). (Example: 2.5-5 mg/kg as a single dose; expected Cp_{max}: 10-20 mcg/mL and Cp_{min}: <1 mcg/mL). Further research is needed for universal recommendation in all patient populations and gram-negative disease; exceptions may include those with known high clearance (eg, children, patients with cystic fibrosis, or burns who may require shorter dosage intervals) and patients with renal function impairment for whom longer than conventional dosage intervals are usually required.

Dosage Forms Excipient information presented when available (limited, particularly for generics); consult specific product labeling. [DSC] = Discontinued product

Infusion, premixed in NS: 60 mg (50 mL [DSC]); 80 mg (100 mL)

Injection, powder for reconstitution: 1.2 g

Injection, solution: 10 mg/mL (2 mL); 40 mg/mL (2 mL, 30 mL, 50 mL)

Solution, for nebulization [preservative free]:

TOBI®: 300 mg/5 mL (56s)

Dosage Forms: Canada Excipient information presented when available (limited, particularly for generics); consult specific product labeling.

Powder, for oral inhalation [capsule]:

TOBI® Podhaler®: 28 mg/capsule (224s)

Tobramycin (Ophthalmic) (toe bra MYE sin)

Brand Names: U.S. AK-Tob™; Tobrex®

Brand Names: Canada PMS-Tobramycin; Sandoz-Tobramycin; Tobrex®

Index Terms Tobramycin Sulfate

Pharmacologic Category Antibiotic, Aminoglycoside; Antibiotic, Ophthalmic

Use Treatment of superficial ophthalmic infections caused by susceptible bacteria

Pregnancy Risk Factor B

Dosage Ophthalmic: Children ≥2 months and Adults:

Ointment: Instill 1/2" (1.25 cm) 2-3 times/day; for severe infections, apply every 3-4 hours

Solution: Instill 1-2 drops every 2-4 hours; for severe infections, instill up to 2 drops every hour until improved, then reduce to less frequent intervals

Additional Information Complete prescribing information for this medication should be consulted for additional detail.

Dosage Forms Excipient information presented when available (limited, particularly for generics); consult specific product labeling.

Ointment, ophthalmic:

Tobrex®: 0.3% (3.5 g) [contains chlorobutanol]

Solution, ophthalmic [drops]: 0.3% (5 mL)

AK-Tob™: 0.3% (5 mL) [contains benzalkonium chloride]

Tobrex®: 0.3% (5 mL) [contains benzalkonium chloride]

Tobramycin and Dexamethasone
(toe bra MYE sin & deks a METH a sone)

Brand Names: U.S. TobraDex®; TobraDex® ST

Brand Names: Canada Tobradex®

Index Terms Dexamethasone and Tobramycin

Pharmacologic Category Antibiotic/Corticosteroid, Ophthalmic

Use Treatment of external ocular infection caused by susceptible gram-negative bacteria and steroid responsive inflammatory conditions of the palpebral and bulbar conjunctiva, cornea, and anterior segment of the globe

Pregnancy Risk Factor C

Dosage Ophthalmic: Children ≥2 years and Adults: Ocular infection/inflammation:

Ointment: Apply a small amount (~1/2-inch ribbon of ointment) up to 3-4 times/day

Suspension: Instill 1-2 drops every 4-6 hours; may be increased to 1-2 drops every 2 hours for the first 24-48 hours, then reduce to less frequent intervals

Additional Information Complete prescribing information for this medication should be consulted for additional detail.

Dosage Forms Excipient information presented when available (limited, particularly for generics); consult specific product labeling.

Ointment, ophthalmic:

TobraDex®: Tobramycin 0.3% and dexamethasone 0.1% (3.5 g) [contains chlorobutanol]

Suspension, ophthalmic: Tobramycin 0.3% and dexamethasone 0.1% (2.5 mL, 5 mL, 10 mL)

TobraDex®: Tobramycin 0.3% and dexamethasone 0.1% (2.5 mL, 5 mL, 10 mL) [contains benzalkonium chloride]

TobraDex® ST: Tobramycin 0.3% and dexamethasone 0.05% (5 mL) [contains benzalkonium chloride]

◆ **Tobramycin and Loteprednol Etabonate** *see* Loteprednol and Tobramycin *on page 1038*

◆ **Tobramycin Injection, USP (Can)** *see* Tobramycin (Systemic, Oral Inhalation) *on page 1696*

◆ **Tobramycin Sulfate** *see* Tobramycin (Ophthalmic) *on page 1700*

◆ **Tobramycin Sulfate** *see* Tobramycin (Systemic, Oral Inhalation) *on page 1696*

◆ **Tobrex®** *see* Tobramycin (Ophthalmic) *on page 1700*

Tocilizumab (toe si LIZ oo mab)

Brand Names: U.S. Actemra®

Brand Names: Canada Actemra®

Index Terms Atlizumab; MRA; R-1569; RoActemra®

Pharmacologic Category Antirheumatic, Disease Modifying; Interleukin-6 Receptor Antagonist

Use Treatment of moderately- to severely-active rheumatoid arthritis in adult patients who have had an inadequate response to one or more TNF antagonists (as monotherapy or in combination with nonbiological disease-modifying antirheumatic drugs [DMARDs]); treatment of active systemic juvenile idiopathic arthritis (SJIA) (as monotherapy or in combination with methotrexate)

Pregnancy Risk Factor C

Pregnancy Considerations No evidence of impaired fertility, teratogenic, or dysmorphogenic effects in animal models; an increased incidence of abortion and embryo-fetal death has been observed in animal models. There are no adequate and well-controlled studies in pregnant women. Use during pregnancy only if clearly needed. A pregnancy registry has been established to monitor outcomes of women exposed to tocilizumab during pregnancy (877-311-8972).

Lactation Excretion in breast milk unknown/not recommended

Medication Guide Available Yes

Contraindications Hypersensitivity to tocilizumab or any component of the formulation

Warnings/Precautions [U.S. Boxed Warning]: Serious and potentially fatal infections (including tuberculosis, invasive fungal, bacterial, viral, protozoal, and other opportunistic infections) have been reported in patients receiving tocilizumab. Most of the serious infections have occurred in patients on concomitant immunosuppressive therapy. Do not administer tocilizumab to a patient with an active infection, including localized infection. Caution should be exercised when considering use in patients with chronic or recurrent infections, previous exposure to tuberculosis, previous residence or travel in an area of endemic tuberculosis or mycoses, or predisposition to infection. Patients should be closely monitored for signs and symptoms of infection during and after treatment. If a patient develops a serious infection, therapy should be discontinued. **[U.S. Boxed Warning]: Tuberculosis (disseminated or extrapulmonary) has been reported in patients receiving tocilizumab; both reactivation of latent infection and new infections have been reported.** Patients should be evaluated for latent tuberculosis infection with a tuberculin skin test prior to starting therapy. Treatment of latent tuberculosis should be initiated before therapy is used. Some patients who test negative prior to therapy may develop active infection; monitor for signs and symptoms of tuberculosis in all patients. Rare reactivation of herpes zoster has been reported. Patients should be brought up to date with all immunizations before initiating therapy. Live vaccines should not be given concurrently; there is no data available concerning secondary transmission of infection from live vaccines in patients receiving therapy.

Impact on the development and course of malignancies is not fully defined, however, malignancies were observed in clinical trials. Use with caution in patients with pre-existing or recent onset CNS demyelinating disorders; rare cases of CNS demyelinating disorders (eg, multiple sclerosis) have occurred. All patients should be monitored for signs and symptoms of demyelinating disorders. May cause hypersensitivity, anaphylaxis, or anaphylactoid reactions; permanently discontinue treatment in patients who develop a hypersensitivity reaction to tocilizumab. Medications for the treatment of hypersensitivity reactions should be available for immediate use. Use is not recommended in patients with active hepatic disease or hepatic impairment; use with caution in patients at increased risk for gastrointestinal perforation.

Use may cause increases in total cholesterol, triglycerides, LDL and HDL cholesterol; hyperlipidemia should be managed according to current guidelines. Therapy should not be initiated in patients with an ANC <2000/mm^3, platelet count <100,000/mm^3, or ALT/AST >1.5 times the upper limit of normal (ULN); discontinue treatment in patients who develop an ANC <500/mm^3, platelet count <50,000/mm^3, or ALT/AST >5 x ULN.

Due to higher incidence of serious infections, concomitant use with other biological DMARDs (eg, TNF blockers, IL-1 receptor blockers, anti-CD20 monoclonal antibodies, selective costimulation modulators) should be avoided. Cautious use is recommended in elderly patients due to an increased incidence of serious infections.

Adverse Reactions Incidence as reported for monotherapy, except where noted. Combination therapy refers to use in rheumatoid arthritis with nonbiological DMARDs or use in SJIA in trials where most patients (~70%) were taking methotrexate at baseline.

>10%: Hepatic: ALT increased (≤36%; grades 3/4: <1%), AST increased (≤22%; grades 3/4: <1%)

1% to 10%:

Cardiovascular: Hypertension (1% to 6%), peripheral edema (<2%)

Central nervous system: Headache (1% to 7%), dizziness (3%)

Dermatologic: Rash (2%), skin reaction (combination therapy; 1% [includes pruritus, urticaria])

Endocrine & metabolic: LDL cholesterol increased (>1.5-2 x ULN; combination therapy; children 2%), total cholesterol increased (>1.5-2 x ULN; combination therapy; children 2%), hypothyroidism (<2%)

Gastrointestinal: Diarrhea (children ≤5%), abdominal pain (2%), mouth ulceration (2%), gastric ulcer (<2%), stomatitis (<2%), weight gain (<2%), gastritis (1%)

Hematologic: Neutropenia (combination therapy; grade 3: 2% to 7%; grade 4: <1%), thrombocytopenia (combination therapy; 1% to 2%), leukopenia (<2%)

Hepatic: Bilirubin increased (<2%)

Local: Infusion-related reactions (combination therapy; 4% to 16%)

Ocular: Conjunctivitis (<2%)

Renal: Nephrolithiasis (<2%)

Respiratory: Upper respiratory tract infection (7%), nasopharyngitis (7%), bronchitis (3%), cough (<2%), dyspnea (<2%)

Miscellaneous: Anti-tocilizumab antibody formation (2%), herpes simplex (<2%)

<1% (Limited to important or life-threatening): Anaphylactic/anaphylactoid reaction, angioedema, aspergillosis, bacterial arthritis, candidiasis, cellulitis, chronic inflammatory demyelinating polyneuropathy, cryptococcus, diverticulitis, Epstein-Barr virus reactivation, gastroenteritis, gastrointestinal perforation, HDL cholesterol increased, herpes zoster, hypertriglyceridemia, malignancy (including breast and colon cancer), multiple sclerosis, otitis media, pneumonia, pneumonitis (allergic), pneumocystosis, sepsis, tuberculosis, urinary tract infection, varicella

Drug Interactions

Metabolism/Transport Effects None known.

Avoid Concomitant Use

Avoid concomitant use of Tocilizumab with any of the following: BCG; Belimumab; Natalizumab; Pimecrolimus; Tacrolimus (Topical); Vaccines (Live)

Increased Effect/Toxicity

Tocilizumab may increase the levels/effects of: Belimumab; Leflunomide; Natalizumab; Vaccines (Live)

The levels/effects of Tocilizumab may be increased by: Abciximab; Denosumab; Pimecrolimus; Roflumilast; Tacrolimus (Topical); Trastuzumab

Decreased Effect

Tocilizumab may decrease the levels/effects of: BCG; Coccidioidin Skin Test; CYP3A4 Substrates; Sipuleucel-T; Vaccines (Inactivated); Vaccines (Live)

The levels/effects of Tocilizumab may be decreased by: Echinacea

Stability Store unopened vials at 2°C to 8°C (36°F to 46°F); do not freeze. Protect from light. Prior to administration, dilute to 50 mL (children <30 kg) or 100 mL (children ≥30 kg and adults) using 0.9% sodium chloride. Diluted solutions may be stored under refrigeration or at room temperature for up to 24 hours and are compatible with polypropylene, polyethylene (PE), polyvinyl chloride (PVC), and glass infusion containers.

Mechanism of Action Antagonist of the interleukin-6 (IL-6) receptor. Endogenous IL-6 is induced by inflammatory stimuli and mediates a variety of immunological responses. Inhibition of IL-6 receptors by tocilizumab leads to a reduction in cytokine and acute phase reactant production.

Pharmacodynamics/Kinetics

Distribution: V_{dss}: Children: 2.54 L; Adults: 6.4 L

Half life elimination: Terminal, single dose: 6.3 days (concentration-dependent; may be increased up to 23 days [children] or 13 days [adults] at steady state)

Dosage I.V.:

Children ≥2 years: Systemic juvenile idiopathic arthritis (SJIA): **Note:** Dose adjustment should not be made based solely on a single-visit body weight measurement due to fluctuations in body weight.

<30 kg: 12 mg/kg every 2 weeks

≥30 kg: 8 mg/kg every 2 weeks

Adults: Rheumatoid arthritis: Initial: 4 mg/kg every 4 weeks; may be increased to 8 mg/kg based on clinical response (maximum: 800 mg per infusion)

Dosage adjustment for toxicity:

Rheumatoid arthritis (RA):

Liver enzyme abnormalities:

>1 to 3 x ULN: For persistent increases in this range, reduce tocilizumab dose to 4 mg/kg or interrupt therapy until ALT/AST have normalized; adjust concomitant DMARDs as appropriate

>3 to 5 x ULN: Discontinue tocilizumab until ALT/AST <3 x ULN, then resume tocilizumab at 4 mg/kg. For persistent increases in this range, discontinue therapy.

>5 x ULN: Discontinue therapy

Low absolute neutrophil counts (ANC):

ANC >1000 cells/mm^3: Maintain dose.

ANC 500-1000 cells/mm^3: Interrupt therapy; when ANC >1000 cells/mm^3, resume tocilizumab at 4 mg/kg. May increase to 8 mg/kg as clinically appropriate.

ANC <500 cells/mm^3: Discontinue therapy

Low platelet counts:
Platelets 50,000-100,000 cells/mm^3: Interrupt therapy; when platelet count is >100,000 cells/mm^3, resume tocilizumab at 4 mg/kg; may increase to 8 mg/kg as clinically appropriate
Platelets <50,000 cells/mm^3: Discontinue therapy

Systemic juvenile idiopathic arthritis (SJIA): Dose reductions have not been studied; however, dose interruptions are recommended for liver enzyme abnormalities, low neutrophil counts, and low platelets similar to recommendations provided for rheumatoid arthritis patients. In addition, consider interrupting or discontinuing concomitant methotrexate and/or other medications.

Dosage adjustment for renal impairment:
Mild renal impairment: No dosage adjustment required
Moderate-to-severe renal impairment: Limited experience; no specific dosage adjustment recommended by the manufacturer

Dosage adjustment for hepatic impairment: Not recommended for use in patients with active hepatic disease or hepatic impairment

Administration I.V.: Allow diluted solution to reach room temperature prior to administration; infuse over 60 minutes using a dedicated I.V. line. Do not infuse other agents through same I.V. line. Do not administer I.V. push or I.V. bolus. Do not use if opaque particles or discoloration is visible.

Monitoring Parameters Signs and symptoms of infection (prior to and during therapy); latent TB screening prior to therapy initiation; CBC with differential (prior to and every 2-4 weeks [SJIA] or 4-8 weeks [RA] during therapy); ALT/AST (prior to and every 2-4 weeks [SJIA] or 4-8 weeks [RA] during therapy); additional liver function tests (eg, bilirubin) as clinically indicated; lipid panel (prior to, at 4-8 weeks following initiation, and every ~6 months during therapy); signs and symptoms of CNS demyelinating disorders

Dosage Forms Excipient information presented when available (limited, particularly for generics); consult specific product labeling.
Injection, solution [preservative free]:
Actemra®: 20 mg/mL (4 mL, 10 mL, 20 mL) [contains polysorbate 80, sucrose 50 mg/mL]

◆ **Today® [OTC]** *see* Nonoxynol 9 *on page 1216*
◆ **Tofranil®** *see* Imipramine *on page 877*
◆ **Tofranil-PM®** *see* Imipramine *on page 877*

TOLAZamide (tole AZ a mide)

Brand Names: Canada Tolinase®
Pharmacologic Category Antidiabetic Agent, Sulfonylurea
Additional Appendix Information
Diabetes Mellitus Management, Adults *on page 1983*
Use Adjunct to diet for the management of mild-to-moderately severe, stable, type 2 diabetes mellitus (noninsulin dependent, NIDDM)
Pregnancy Risk Factor C
Dosage Oral: Adults: Doses >500 mg/day should be given in 2 divided doses:
Initial: 100-250 mg/day with breakfast or the first main meal of the day
Fasting blood sugar <200 mg/dL: 100 mg/day
Fasting blood sugar >200 mg/dL: 250 mg/day
Patient is malnourished, underweight, elderly, or not eating properly: 100 mg/day
Adjust dose in increments of 100-250 mg/day at weekly intervals to response; maximum daily dose: 1 g (doses >1 g/day are not likely to improve control)

Conversion from insulin to tolazamide:
<20 units day = 100 mg/day
21-<40 units/day = 250 mg/day
≥40 units/day = 250 mg/day and 50% of insulin dose

Dosing adjustment in renal impairment: Conservative initial and maintenance doses are recommended because tolazamide is metabolized to active metabolites, which are eliminated in the urine

Dosing comments in hepatic impairment: Conservative initial and maintenance doses and careful monitoring of blood glucose are recommended

Additional Information Complete prescribing information for this medication should be consulted for additional detail.

Dosage Forms Excipient information presented when available (limited, particularly for generics); consult specific product labeling.
Tablet, oral: 250 mg, 500 mg

TOLBUTamide (tole BYOO ta mide)

Brand Names: Canada Apo-Tolbutamide®
Index Terms Orinase; Tolbutamide Sodium
Pharmacologic Category Antidiabetic Agent, Sulfonylurea
Additional Appendix Information
Diabetes Mellitus Management, Adults *on page 1983*
Use Adjunct to diet for the management of type 2 diabetes mellitus (noninsulin dependent, NIDDM)
Pregnancy Risk Factor C
Dosage Oral: **Note:** Divided doses may improve gastrointestinal tolerance.
Adults: Initial: 1-2 g/day as a single dose in the morning or in divided doses throughout the day. Maintenance dose: 0.25-3 g/day; however, a maintenance dose >2 g/day is seldom required.
Elderly: Initial: 250 mg 1-3 times/day; usual: 500-2000 mg; maximum: 3 g/day

Dosing adjustment in renal impairment: Adjustment is not necessary
Hemodialysis: Not dialyzable (0% to 5%)

Dosing adjustment in hepatic impairment: Reduction of dose may be necessary in patients with impaired liver function

Additional Information Complete prescribing information for this medication should be consulted for additional detail.

Dosage Forms Excipient information presented when available (limited, particularly for generics); consult specific product labeling.
Tablet, oral: 500 mg

◆ **Tolbutamide Sodium** *see* TOLBUTamide *on page 1702*

Tolcapone (TOLE ka pone)

Brand Names: U.S. Tasmar®
Pharmacologic Category Anti-Parkinson's Agent, COMT Inhibitor
Additional Appendix Information
Antiparkinsonian Agents *on page 1879*
Use Adjunct to levodopa and carbidopa for the treatment of signs and symptoms of idiopathic Parkinson's disease in patients with motor fluctuations not responsive to other therapies
Pregnancy Risk Factor C
Pregnancy Considerations Tolcapone may be teratogenic based on animal studies. There are no adequate and well-controlled studies in pregnant women. Use only if benefit outweighs risk.

Lactation Excretion in breast milk unknown/not recommended

Prescribing and Access Restrictions A patient signed consent form acknowledging the risks of hepatic injury should be obtained by the treating physician.

Contraindications Hypersensitivity to tolcapone or any component of the formulation; history of liver disease or tolcapone-induced hepatocellular injury; nontraumatic rhabdomyolysis or hyperpyrexia and confusion

Warnings/Precautions [U.S. Boxed Warning]: Due to reports of fatal liver injury associated with use of this drug, the manufacturer is advising that tolcapone be reserved for patients who are experiencing inadequate symptom control or who are not appropriate candidates for other available treatments. Patients must provide written consent acknowledging the risks of hepatic injury. Liver disease should be excluded prior to initiation; laboratory monitoring is recommended. Discontinue if signs and/or symptoms of hepatic injury are noted (eg, transaminases >2 times upper limit of normal) or if clinical improvement is not evident after 3 weeks of therapy. Use with caution in patients with pre-existing dyskinesias; exacerbation of pre-existing dyskinesia and severe rhabdomyolysis has been reported. Levodopa dosage reduction may be required, particularly in patients with levodopa dosages >600 mg daily or with moderate-to-severe dyskinesia prior to initiation.

May cause orthostatic hypotension and syncope; Parkinson's disease patients appear to have an impaired capacity to respond to a postural challenge; use with caution in patients at risk of hypotension (such as those receiving antihypertensive drugs) or where transient hypotensive episodes would be poorly tolerated (cardiovascular disease or cerebrovascular disease). Parkinson's patients being treated with dopaminergic agonists ordinarily require careful monitoring for signs and symptoms of postural hypotension, especially during dose escalation, and should be informed of this risk. May cause hallucinations, which may improve with reduction in levodopa therapy. Use with caution in patients with lower gastrointestinal disease or an increased risk of dehydration; tolcapone has been associated with delayed development of diarrhea (onset after 2-12 weeks).

Tolcapone, in conjunction with other drug therapy that alters brain biogenic amine concentrations (eg, MAO inhibitors, SSRIs), has been associated with a syndrome resembling neuroleptic malignant syndrome (hyperpyrexia and confusion - some fatal) on abrupt withdrawal or dosage reduction. Concomitant use of tolcapone and nonselective MAO inhibitors should be avoided. Selegiline is a selective MAO type B inhibitor (when given orally at ≤10 mg/day) and can be taken with tolcapone. Dopaminergic agents have been associated with compulsive behaviors and/or loss of impulse control, which has manifested as pathological gambling, libido increases (hypersexuality), and/or binge eating. Causality has not been established, and controversy exists as to whether this phenomenon is related to the underlying disease, prior behaviors/addictions and/or drug therapy. Dose reduction or discontinuation of therapy has been reported to reverse these behaviors in some, but not all cases. Risk for melanoma development is increased in Parkinson's disease patients; drug causation or factors contributing to risk have not been established. Patients should be monitored closely and periodic skin examinations should be performed. Dopaminergic agents from the ergot class have also been associated with fibrotic complications, such as retroperitoneal fibrosis, pulmonary infiltrates or effusion and pleural thickening. It is unknown whether non-ergot, pro-dopaminergic agents like tolcapone confer this risk. Use caution in patients with hepatic impairment or severe renal impairment.

Adverse Reactions

>10%:

Cardiovascular: Orthostatic hypotension (17%)

Central nervous system: Somnolence (14% to 32%), sleep disorder (24% to 25%), hallucinations (8% to 24%), excessive dreaming (16% to 21%), dizziness (6% to 13%), headache (10% to 11%), confusion (10% to 11%)

Gastrointestinal: Nausea (28% to 50%), diarrhea (16% to 34%; approximately 3% to 4% severe), anorexia (19% to 23%)

Neuromuscular & skeletal: Dyskinesia (42% to 51%), dystonia (19% to 22%), muscle cramps (17% to 18%)

1% to 10%:

Cardiovascular: Syncope (4% to 5%), chest pain (1% to 3%), hypotension (2%), palpitation

Central nervous system: Fatigue (3% to 7%), loss of balance (2% to 3%), agitation (1%), euphoria (1%), hyperactivity (1%), malaise (1%), panic reaction (1%), irritability (1%), mental deficiency (1%), fever (1%), depression, hypoesthesia, tremor, speech disorder, vertigo, emotional lability, hyperkinesia

Dermatologic: Alopecia (1%), bleeding (1%), tumor (1%), rash

Gastrointestinal: Vomiting (8% to 10%), constipation (6% to 8%), xerostomia (5% to 6%), abdominal pain (5% to 6%), dyspepsia (3% to 4%), flatulence (2% to 4%)

Genitourinary: UTI (5%), hematuria (4% to 5%), urine discoloration (2% to 3%), urination disorder (1% to 2%), uterine tumor (1%), incontinence, impotence

Hepatic: Transaminases increased (1% to 3%; 3 times ULN, usually with first 6 months of therapy)

Neuromuscular & skeletal: Paresthesia (1% to 3%), hyper-/hypokinesia (1% to 3%), arthritis (1% to 2%), neck pain (2%), stiffness (2%), myalgia, rhabdomyolysis

Ocular: Cataract (1%), eye inflammation (1%)

Otic: Tinnitus

Respiratory: Upper respiratory infection (5% to 7%), dyspnea (3%), sinus congestion (1% to 2%), bronchitis, pharyngitis

Miscellaneous: Diaphoresis (4% to 7%), influenza (3% to 4%), burning (1% to 2%), flank pain, injury, infection

<1% (Limited to important or life-threatening): Abnormal stools, abscess, allergic reaction, amnesia, anemia, antisocial reaction, apathy, apnea, arteriosclerosis, arthrosis, asthma, bladder calculus, breast neoplasm, carcinoma, cardiovascular disorder, cellulitis, cerebral ischemia, cerebrovascular accident, chills, cholecystitis, cholelithiasis, choreoathetosis, colitis, cough increased, death, dehydration, delirium, delusions, diabetes mellitus, diplopia, duodenal ulcer, dysphagia, dysuria, ear pain, eczema, edema, encephalopathy, epistaxis, erythema multiforme, esophagitis, extrapyramidal syndrome, eye hemorrhage, eye pain, facial edema, furunculosis, gastroenteritis, gastrointestinal carcinoma, gastrointestinal hemorrhage, glaucoma, hemiplegia, hernia, herpes simplex, herpes zoster, hiccup, hostility, hypercholesteremia, hyperventilation, hypoxia, infection (bacterial), infection (fungal), joint disorder, kidney calculus, lacrimation disorder, laryngitis, leukemia, libido changes, lung edema, manic reaction, meningitis, mouth ulceration, myoclonus, neoplasm, nervousness, neuralgia, neuropathy, nocturia, oliguria, otitis media, ovarian carcinoma, pain, paranoid reaction, parosmia, pericardial effusion, polyuria, prostatic carcinoma, prostatic disorder, pruritus, psychosis, rectal disorder, rhinitis, salivation increased, seborrhea, skin discoloration, skin disorder, stomach atony, surgical procedure, tenosynovitis, thinking abnormal, thirst, thrombocytopenia, thrombosis, tongue disorder, twitching, urinary retention, urinary tract disorder, urticaria, uterine atony, uterine disorder, uterine hemorrhage, vaginitis, viral infection

Drug Interactions

Metabolism/Transport Effects **Inhibits** COMT, CYP2C9 (weak)

Avoid Concomitant Use There are no known interactions where it is recommended to avoid concomitant use.

Increased Effect/Toxicity

Tolcapone may increase the levels/effects of: Alcohol (Ethyl); CNS Depressants; COMT Substrates; MAO Inhibitors; Methotrimeprazine; Selective Serotonin Reuptake Inhibitors

The levels/effects of Tolcapone may be increased by: Droperidol; HydrOXYzine; MAO Inhibitors; Methotrimeprazine

Decreased Effect There are no known significant interactions involving a decrease in effect.

Ethanol/Nutrition/Herb Interactions

Ethanol: May increase CNS depression; monitor for increased effects with coadministration. Caution patients about effects.

Food: Tolcapone, taken with food within 1 hour before or 2 hours after the dose, decreases bioavailability by 10% to 20%.

Avoid valerian, St John's wort, kava kava, gotu kola (may increase CNS depression).

Stability Store at 20°C to 25°C (68°F to 77°F).

Mechanism of Action Tolcapone is a selective and reversible inhibitor of catechol-o-methyltransferase (COMT). In the presence of a decarboxylase inhibitor (eg, carbidopa), COMT is the major degradation pathway for levodopa. Inhibition of COMT leads to more sustained plasma levels of levodopa and enhanced central dopaminergic activity.

Pharmacodynamics/Kinetics

Absorption: Rapid

Distribution: 9 L

Protein binding: >99.0%

Metabolism: Hepatic, via glucuronidation, to inactive metabolite (>99%)

Bioavailability: 65%

Half-life elimination: 2-3 hours

Time to peak: ~2 hours

Excretion: Urine (60% as metabolites, 0.5% as unchanged drug); feces (40%)

Dosage Note: If clinical improvement is not observed after 3 weeks of therapy (regardless of dose), tolcapone treatment should be discontinued.

Oral: Adults: Initial: 100 mg 3 times/day; may increase as tolerated to 200 mg 3 times/day. **Note:** Levodopa dose may need to be decreased upon initiation of tolcapone (average reduction in clinical trials was 30%). As many as 70% of patients receiving levodopa doses >600 mg daily required levodopa dosage reduction in clinical trials. Patients with moderate-to-severe dyskinesia prior to initiation are also more likely to require dosage reduction.

Dosage adjustment in renal impairment: No adjustment necessary for mild-moderate impairment. Use caution with severe impairment; no safety information available in patients with Cl_{cr} <25 mL/minute.

Dosage adjustment in hepatic impairment: Do not use. Discontinue immediately if signs/symptoms of hepatic impairment develop.

Dietary Considerations May be taken without regard to meals.

Administration May be administered without regard to meals. In clinical studies, the first dose of the day was administered with carbidopa/levodopa, and the subsequent doses were administered 6 hours and 12 hours later.

Monitoring Parameters Blood pressure, symptoms of Parkinson's disease, liver enzymes at baseline and then every 2-4 weeks for the first 6 months of therapy; thereafter, periodic monitoring should be conducted as deemed clinically relevant. If the dose is increased to 200 mg 3 times/day, reinitiate LFT monitoring every 2-4 weeks for 6 months, and then resume periodic monitoring. Discontinue therapy if the ALT or AST exceeds 2 times ULN or if the clinical signs and symptoms suggest the onset of liver failure.

Dosage Forms Excipient information presented when available (limited, particularly for generics); consult specific product labeling. [DSC] = Discontinued product

Tablet, oral:

Tasmar®: 100 mg, 200 mg [DSC]

◆ **Tolectin** *see* Tolmetin *on page 1704*

◆ **Tolinase® (Can)** *see* TOLAZamide *on page 1702*

Tolmetin (TOLE met in)

Index Terms Tolectin; Tolmetin Sodium

Pharmacologic Category Nonsteroidal Anti-inflammatory Drug (NSAID), Oral

Use Treatment of rheumatoid arthritis and osteoarthritis, juvenile idiopathic arthritis (JIA)

Pregnancy Risk Factor C

Medication Guide Available Yes

Dosage Oral:

Children ≥2 years:

Juvenile idiopathic arthritis (JIA): Initial: 20 mg/kg/day in 3-4 divided doses, then 15-30 mg/kg/day in 3-4 divided doses (maximum dose: 30 mg/kg/day)

Analgesic (unlabeled use): 5-7 mg/kg/dose every 6-8 hours

Adults: RA, osteoarthritis: 400 mg 3 times/day; usual dose: 600 mg to 1.8 g/day; maximum: 1.8 g/day

Additional Information Complete prescribing information for this medication should be consulted for additional detail.

Dosage Forms Excipient information presented when available (limited, particularly for generics); consult specific product labeling.

Capsule, oral: 400 mg

Tablet, oral: 200 mg, 600 mg

◆ **Tolmetin Sodium** *see* Tolmetin *on page 1704*

Tolnaftate (tole NAF tate)

Brand Names: U.S. Blis-To-Sol® [OTC]; Mycocide® NS [OTC]; Podactin Powder [OTC]; Tinactin® Antifungal Deodorant [OTC]; Tinactin® Antifungal Jock Itch [OTC]; Tinactin® Antifungal [OTC]; Tinaderm [OTC]; Ting® Cream [OTC]; Ting® Spray Liquid [OTC]

Brand Names: Canada Pitrex

Pharmacologic Category Antifungal Agent, Topical

Use Treatment of tinea pedis, tinea cruris, tinea corporis

Pregnancy Risk Factor C

Dosage Children ≥2 years and Adults: Topical: Wash and dry affected area; spray aerosol or apply 1-3 drops of solution or a small amount of cream, or powder and rub into the affected areas 2 times/day

Note: May use for up to 4 weeks for tinea pedis or tinea corporis, and up to 2 weeks for tinea cruris

Additional Information Complete prescribing information for this medication should be consulted for additional detail.

Dosage Forms Excipient information presented when available (limited, particularly for generics); consult specific product labeling.

Aerosol, powder, topical:
- Tinactin® Antifungal: 1% (133 g) [contains ethanol 11% v/v, talc]
- Tinactin® Antifungal Deodorant: 1% (133 g) [contains ethanol 11% v/v, talc]
- Tinactin® Antifungal Jock Itch: 1% (133 g) [contains ethanol 11% v/v, talc]

Aerosol, spray, topical:
- Tinactin® Antifungal: 1% (150 g) [contains ethanol 29% v/v]
- Ting® Spray Liquid: 1% (128 g) [contains ethanol 41% w/w]

Cream, topical: 1% (15 g, 30 g, 114 g)
- Tinactin® Antifungal: 1% (15 g, 30 g)
- Tinactin® Antifungal Jock Itch: 1% (15 g)
- Ting® Cream: 1% (15 g)

Liquid, topical:
- Blis-To-Sol®: 1% (30 mL, 55 mL)

Liquid, topical [spray]:
- Tinactin® Antifungal: 1% (59 mL) [contains ethanol 70% v/v]

Powder, topical: 1% (45 g)
- Podactin Powder: 1% (60 g)
- Tinactin® Antifungal: 1% (108 g)

Solution, topical:
- Mycocide® NS: 1% (30 mL)
- Tinaderm: 1% (10 mL)

◆ **Toloxin® (Can)** *see* Digoxin *on page 503*

Tolterodine (tole TER oh deen)

Brand Names: U.S. Detrol®; Detrol® LA

Brand Names: Canada Detrol®; Detrol® LA; Unidet®

Index Terms Tolterodine Tartrate

Pharmacologic Category Anticholinergic Agent

Use Treatment of patients with an overactive bladder with symptoms of urinary frequency, urgency, or urge incontinence

Pregnancy Risk Factor C

Pregnancy Considerations Teratogenic effects were observed in some animal studies. There are no adequate and well-controlled studies in pregnant women. Use during pregnancy only if the potential benefit to the mother outweighs the possible risk to the fetus.

Lactation Excretion in breast milk unknown/not recommended

Contraindications Hypersensitivity to tolterodine or fesoterodine (both are metabolized to 5-hydroxymethyl tolterodine) or any component of the formulation; urinary retention; gastric retention; uncontrolled narrow-angle glaucoma

Warnings/Precautions Cases of angioedema have been reported with oral tolterodine; some cases have occurred after a single dose. Discontinue immediately if develops. May cause drowsiness and/or blurred vision, which may impair physical or mental abilities; patients must be cautioned about performing tasks which require mental alertness (eg, operating machinery or driving). Use with caution in patients with bladder flow obstruction, may increase the risk of urinary retention. Use with caution in patients with gastrointestinal obstructive disorders (ie, pyloric stenosis), may increase the risk of gastric retention. Use with caution in patients with myasthenia gravis and controlled (treated) narrow-angle glaucoma; metabolized in the liver and excreted in the urine and feces, dosage adjustment is required for patients with renal or hepatic impairment. Tolterodine has been associated with QT_c prolongation at high (supratherapeutic) doses. The manufacturer recommends caution in patients with congenital prolonged QT or in patients receiving concurrent therapy with QT_c-prolonging drugs (class Ia or III antiarrhythmics). However, the mean change in QT_c even at supratherapeutic dosages was less than 15 msec. Individuals who are CYP2D6 poor metabolizers or in the presence of inhibitors of CYP2D6 and CYP3A4 may be more likely to exhibit prolongation. Dosage adjustment is recommended in patients receiving CYP3A4 inhibitors (a lower dose of tolterodine is recommended).

Adverse Reactions As reported with immediate release tablet, unless otherwise specified

>10%: Gastrointestinal: Dry mouth (35%; extended release capsules 23%)

1% to 10%:
- Cardiovascular: Chest pain (2%)
- Central nervous system: Headache (7%; extended release capsules 6%), somnolence (3%; extended release capsules 3%), fatigue (4%; extended release capsules 2%), dizziness (5%; extended release capsules 2%), anxiety (extended release capsules 1%)
- Dermatologic: Dry skin (1%)
- Gastrointestinal: Abdominal pain (5%; extended release capsules 4%), constipation (7%; extended release capsules 6%), dyspepsia (4%; extended release capsules 3%), diarrhea (4%), weight gain (1%)
- Genitourinary: Dysuria (2%; extended release capsules 1%)
- Neuromuscular & skeletal: Arthralgia (2%)
- Ocular: Abnormal vision (2%; extended release capsules 1%), dry eyes (3%; extended release capsules 3%)
- Respiratory: Bronchitis (2%), sinusitis (extended release capsules 2%)
- Miscellaneous: Flu-like syndrome (3%), infection (1%)

<1% (Limited to important or life-threatening): Anaphylaxis, angioedema, confusion, dementia aggravated, disorientation, hallucinations, memory impairment, palpitation, peripheral edema, QT_c prolongation, tachycardia

Drug Interactions

Metabolism/Transport Effects Substrate of CYP2C19 (minor), CYP2C9 (minor), CYP2D6 (major), CYP3A4 (major); **Note:** Assignment of Major/Minor substrate status based on clinically relevant drug interaction potential

Avoid Concomitant Use There are no known interactions where it is recommended to avoid concomitant use.

Increased Effect/Toxicity

Tolterodine may increase the levels/effects of: AbobotulinumtoxinA; Anticholinergics; Cannabinoids; OnabotulinumtoxinA; Potassium Chloride; RimabotulinumtoxinB; Warfarin

The levels/effects of Tolterodine may be increased by: Abiraterone Acetate; Antifungal Agents (Azole Derivatives, Systemic); CYP2D6 Inhibitors (Moderate); CYP2D6 Inhibitors (Strong); CYP3A4 Inhibitors (Moderate); CYP3A4 Inhibitors (Strong); Dasatinib; Fluconazole; Pramlintide; VinBLAStine

Decreased Effect

Tolterodine may decrease the levels/effects of: Acetylcholinesterase Inhibitors (Central); Secretin

The levels/effects of Tolterodine may be decreased by: Acetylcholinesterase Inhibitors (Central); CYP3A4 Inducers (Strong); Deferasirox; Herbs (CYP3A4 Inducers); Peginterferon Alfa-2b; Tocilizumab

Ethanol/Nutrition/Herb Interactions

Food: Increases bioavailability (~53% increase) of tolterodine tablets (dose adjustment not necessary); does not affect the pharmacokinetics of tolterodine extended release capsules. As a CYP3A4 inhibitor, grapefruit juice may increase the serum level and/or toxicity of tolterodine, but unlikely secondary to high oral bioavailability.

Herb/Nutraceutical: St John's wort (*Hypericum*) appears to induce CYP3A enzymes.

Stability Store at 25°C (77°F); excursions permitted to 15°C to 30°C (59°F to 86°F). Protect from light.

Mechanism of Action Tolterodine is a competitive antagonist of muscarinic receptors. In animal models, tolterodine demonstrates selectivity for urinary bladder receptors over salivary receptors. Urinary bladder contraction is mediated by muscarinic receptors. Tolterodine increases residual urine volume and decreases detrusor muscle pressure.

Pharmacodynamics/Kinetics

Absorption: Immediate release tablet: Rapid; ≥77%

Distribution: I.V.: V_d: 113 ± 27 L

Protein binding: >96% (primarily to alpha$_1$-acid glycoprotein)

Metabolism: Extensively hepatic, primarily via CYP2D6 to 5-hydroxymethyltolterodine (active) and 3A4 usually (minor pathway). In patients with a genetic deficiency of CYP2D6, metabolism via 3A4 predominates.

Bioavailability: Immediate release tablet: Increased 53% with food

Half-life elimination:

Immediate release tablet: Extensive metabolizers: ~2 hours; Poor metabolizers: ~10 hours

Extended release capsule: Extensive metabolizers: ~7 hours; Poor metabolizers: ~18 hours

Time to peak: Immediate release tablet: 1-2 hours; Extended release tablet: 2-6 hours

Excretion: Urine (77%); feces (17%); primarily as metabolites (<1% unchanged drug) of which the active 5-hydroxymethyl metabolite accounts for 5% to 14% (<1% in poor metabolizers); as unchanged drug (<1%; <2.5% in poor metabolizers)

Dosage

Oral: Adults: Treatment of overactive bladder:

Immediate release tablet: 2 mg twice daily; the dose may be lowered to 1 mg twice daily based on individual response and tolerability

Dosing adjustment in patients concurrently taking CYP3A4 inhibitors: 1 mg twice daily

Extended release capsule: 4 mg once a day; dose may be lowered to 2 mg daily based on individual response and tolerability

Dosing adjustment in patients concurrently taking CYP3A4 inhibitors: 2 mg daily

Elderly: Safety and efficacy in patients >64 years was found to be similar to that in younger patients; no dosage adjustment is needed based on age

Dosing adjustment in renal impairment: Use with caution (studies conducted in patients with Cl_{cr} 10-30 mL/minute):

Immediate release tablet: 1 mg twice daily

Extended release capsule: 2 mg daily

Dosing adjustment in hepatic impairment:

Immediate release tablet: 1 mg twice daily

Extended release capsule: 2 mg daily

Administration Extended release capsule: Swallow whole; do not crush, chew, or open

Monitoring Parameters Renal function (BUN, creatinine); hepatic function

Dosage Forms Excipient information presented when available (limited, particularly for generics); consult specific product labeling.

Capsule, extended release, oral, as tartrate:

Detrol® LA: 2 mg, 4 mg

Tablet, oral, as tartrate:

Detrol®: 1 mg, 2 mg

◆ **Tolterodine Tartrate** *see* Tolterodine *on page* 1705

Tolvaptan (tol VAP tan)

Brand Names: U.S. Samsca™

Brand Names: Canada Samsca™

Index Terms OPC-41061

Pharmacologic Category Vasopressin Antagonist

Use Treatment of clinically significant hypervolemic or euvolemic hyponatremia (associated with heart failure, cirrhosis, or SIADH) with either a serum sodium <125 mEq/L or less marked hyponatremia that is symptomatic and resistant to fluid restriction

Pregnancy Risk Factor C

Medication Guide Available Yes

Dosage Oral: Adults: Hyponatremia: Initial: 15 mg once daily; after at least 24 hours, may increase to 30 mg once daily to a maximum of 60 mg once daily titrating at 24-hour intervals to desired serum sodium concentration

Additional Information Complete prescribing information for this medication should be consulted for additional detail.

Dosage Forms Excipient information presented when available (limited, particularly for generics); consult specific product labeling.

Tablet, oral:

Samsca™: 15 mg, 30 mg

Dosage Forms: Canada Excipient information presented when available (limited, particularly for generics); consult specific product labeling.

Tablet, oral:

Samsca™: 15 mg, 30 mg, 60 mg

◆ **Tomoxetine** *see* Atomoxetine *on page* 163

◆ **Topactin (Can)** *see* Fluocinonide *on page* 727

◆ **Topamax®** *see* Topiramate *on page* 1706

◆ **TopCare® Junior Strength [OTC]** *see* Ibuprofen *on page* 860

◆ **TopCare® Pain Relief PM [OTC]** *see* Acetaminophen and Diphenhydramine *on page* 31

◆ **Topicaine® [OTC]** *see* Lidocaine (Topical) *on page* 1009

◆ **Topicort®** *see* Desoximetasone *on page* 479

◆ **Topicort® LP** *see* Desoximetasone *on page* 479

◆ **Topilene® (Can)** *see* Betamethasone *on page* 208

Topiramate (toe PYRE a mate)

Brand Names: U.S. Topamax®

Brand Names: Canada Apo-Topiramate®; CO Topiramate; Dom-Topiramate; Mint-Topiramate; Mylan-Topiramate; Novo-Topiramate; PHL-Topiramate; PMS-Topiramate; PRO-Topiramate; ratio-Topiramate; Sandoz-Topiramate; Topamax®; ZYM-Topiramate

Pharmacologic Category Anticonvulsant, Miscellaneous

Additional Appendix Information

Anticonvulsant Drugs of Choice *on page* 1873

Use Monotherapy or adjunctive therapy for partial onset seizures and primary generalized tonic-clonic seizures; adjunctive treatment of seizures associated with Lennox-Gastaut syndrome; prophylaxis of migraine headache

Unlabeled Use Diabetic neuropathy, infantile spasms, neuropathic pain; prophylaxis of cluster headache

Pregnancy Risk Factor D

Pregnancy Considerations Topiramate was found to be teratogenic in animal studies. Based on limited data, topiramate was found to cross the placenta. An increase risk of oral clefts (cleft lip and/or palate) has been observed following first trimester exposure. Data, from the North American Antiepileptic Drug (NAAED) Pregnancy Registry, reported that the prevalence of oral clefts was 1.4% for infants exposed to topiramate during the first trimester of pregnancy, versus 0.38% to 0.55% for infants exposed to other antiepileptic drugs and 0.07% with no exposure. Hypospadias and other congenital anomalies have also been reported. Although not evaluated during pregnancy, metabolic acidosis may be induced by topiramate. In general, metabolic acidosis during pregnancy may result in adverse effects and fetal death. Maternal serum concentrations may decrease during the second and third trimesters of pregnancy therefore therapeutic drug monitoring should be considered in pregnant women who require therapy.

Patients exposed to topiramate during pregnancy are encouraged to enroll themselves into the AED Pregnancy Registry by calling 1-888-233-2334. Additional information is available at www.aedpregnancyregistry.org.

Lactation Enters breast milk/use caution

Medication Guide Available Yes

Contraindications There are no contraindications listed in the manufacturers' labeling.

Canadian labeling (not in U.S. labeling): Hypersensitivity to topiramate or any component of the formulation or container; pregnancy and women in childbearing years not using effective contraception (migraine prophylaxis only)

Warnings/Precautions Antiepileptics are associated with an increased risk of suicidal behavior/thoughts with use (regardless of indication); patients should be monitored for signs/symptoms of depression, suicidal tendencies, and other unusual behavior changes during therapy and instructed to inform their healthcare provider immediately if symptoms occur. Use with caution in patients with hepatic, respiratory, or renal impairment. Topiramate may decrease serum bicarbonate concentrations (up to 67% of patients); treatment-emergent metabolic acidosis is less common. Risk may be increased in patients with a predisposing condition (organ dysfunction, ketogenic diet, or concurrent treatment with other drugs which may cause acidosis). Metabolic acidosis may occur at dosages as low as 50 mg/day. Monitor serum bicarbonate as well as potential complications of chronic acidosis (nephrolithiasis, osteomalacia, and reduced growth rates in children). Kidney stones have been reported in both children and adults; the risk of kidney stones is about 2-4 times that of the untreated population; the risk of this event may be reduced by increasing fluid intake.

Cognitive dysfunction, psychiatric disturbances (mood disorders), and sedation (somnolence or fatigue) may occur with topiramate use; incidence may be related to rapid titration and higher doses. Patients must be cautioned about performing tasks which require mental alertness (eg, operating machinery or driving). Topiramate may also cause paresthesia, dizziness, and ataxia. Topiramate has been associated with acute myopia and secondary angle-closure glaucoma in adults and children, typically within 1 month of initiation; discontinue in patients with acute onset of decreased visual acuity or ocular pain. Hyperammonemia with or without encephalopathy may occur with or without concomitant valproate administration; valproic acid dose-dependency was observed in limited pediatric studies; use with caution in patients with inborn errors of metabolism or decreased hepatic mitochondrial activity. Hypothermia (core body temperature <35°C [95°F]) has been reported with concomitant use of topiramate and valproic acid; may occur with or without associated hyperammonemia and may develop after topiramate initiation or dosage increase; discontinuation of topiramate or valproic acid may be necessary. Topiramate may be associated (rarely) with severe oligohydrosis and hyperthermia, most frequently in children; use caution and monitor closely during strenuous exercise, during exposure to high environmental temperature, or in patients receiving receiving other carbonic anhydrase inhibitors and drugs with anticholinergic activity. Concurrent use of topiramate and hydrochlorothiazide may increase the risk for hypokalemia; monitor potassium closely.

Avoid abrupt withdrawal of topiramate therapy, it should be withdrawn/tapered slowly to minimize the potential of increased seizure frequency. Doses were also gradually withdrawn in migraine prophylaxis studies. Effects with other sedative drugs or ethanol may be potentiated. Safety and efficacy have not been established in children <2 years of age for treatment of seizures. In pediatric patients, weight loss may occur most often early in therapy; in clinical trials of at least 1 year, the majority of patients with weight loss had a resumption of weight gain within the study period. Safety and efficacy have not been established in children for migraine prophylaxis.

Adverse Reactions Adverse events are reported for placebo-controlled trials of adjunctive therapy in adult and pediatric patients. Unless otherwise noted, the percentages refer to incidence in epilepsy trials. **Note:** A wide range of dosages were studied; incidence of adverse events was frequently lower in the pediatric population studied.

>10%:

Central nervous system: Somnolence (15% to 29%), dizziness (4% to 25%; dose dependent), fatigue (9% to 16%; dose-dependent), nervousness (9% to 18%), ataxia (6% to 16%), psychomotor slowing (3% to 13%; dose dependent), speech problems (2% to 13%), memory difficulties (2% to 12%), behavior problems (children 11%), confusion (4% to 11%)

Endocrine & metabolic: Serum bicarbonate decreased (dose related: 7% to 67%; marked reductions [to <17 mEq/L] 1% to 11%)

Gastrointestinal: Anorexia (4% to 24%; dose dependent), nausea (6% to 10%; migraine trial: 9% to 14%)

Neuromuscular & skeletal: Paresthesia (1% to 11%; migraine trial: 35% to 51%)

Ocular: Abnormal vision (2% to 13%)

Respiratory: Upper respiratory infection (migraine trial: 12% to 14%)

Miscellaneous: Injury (14%)

1% to 10%:

Cardiovascular: Chest pain (2% to 4%), edema (2%), hypertension (1% to 2%), bradycardia (1%), pallor (1%), syncope (1%)

Central nervous system: Difficulty concentrating (5% to 10%), aggressive reactions (2% to 9%), depression (5% to 9%; dose dependent, insomnia (4% to 8%), mood problems (≤6%), abnormal coordination (4%), agitation (3%), cognitive problems (3%), emotional lability (3%), anxiety (2% to 3%; dose dependent), hypoesthesia (2%; migraine trial: 6% to 8%), stupor (2%), vertigo (2%), fever (migraine trial: 1% to 2%), apathy (1%), hallucination (1%), neurosis (1%), psychosis (1%), seizure (1%), suicide attempt (1%)

Dermatologic: Pruritus (migraine trial: 2% to 4%), skin disorder (2% to 3%), alopecia (2%), dermatitis (2%), hypertrichosis (2%), rash erythematous (1% to 2%), eczema (1%), seborrhea (1%), skin discoloration (1%)

Endocrine & metabolic: Breast pain (4%), hot flashes (1% to 2%), libido decreased (<1% to 2%), menstrual irregularities (1% to 2%), hypoglycemia (1%), metabolic acidosis (hyperchloremia, nonanion gap)

Gastrointestinal: Weight loss (4% to 9%), dyspepsia (2% to 7%), abdominal pain (5% to 6%), salivation increased (6%), constipation (4% to 5%), gastroenteritis (2% to 3%), vomiting (migraine trial: 1% to 3%), diarrhea (2%; migraine trial: 9% to 11%), dysgeusia (2%; migraine trial: 8% to 15%), xerostomia (2%), loss of taste (migraine trial: ≤2%), appetite increased (1%), dysphagia (1%), fecal incontinence (1%), flatulence (1%),

GERD (1%), gingivitis (1%), glossitis (1%), gum hyperplasia (1%), weight gain (1%)

Genitourinary: Incontinence (2% to 4%), UTI (2%), premature ejaculation (migraine trial: ≤3%), cystitis (2%), leukorrhea (2%), impotence (1%), nocturia (1%)

Hematologic: Purpura (8%), leukopenia (2%), anemia (1%), hematoma (1%), prothrombin time increased (1%), thrombocytopenia (1%)

Neuromuscular & skeletal: Tremor (3% to 9%), gait abnormal (3% to 8%), arthralgia (migraine trial: 1% to 7%), weakness (6%), hyperkinesia (5%), back pain (1% to 5%), involuntary muscle contractions (2%; migraine trial: 2% to 4%), leg cramps (2%), leg pain (2%), myalgia (2%), hyporeflexia (2%), rigors (1%), skeletal pain (1%)

Ocular: Diplopia (1% to 10%), nystagmus (10%), conjunctivitis (1%), lacrimation abnormal (1%), myopia (1%)

Otic: Hearing decreased (2%), tinnitus (2%), otitis media (migraine trial: 1% to 2%)

Renal: Hematuria (2%), renal calculus (migraine trial ≤2%)

Respiratory: Rhinitis (4% to 7%), pharyngitis (6%), sinusitis (5%; migraine trial: 6% to 10%), pneumonia (5%), epistaxis (2% to 4%), cough (migraine trial: 2% to 4%), bronchitis (migraine trial: 3%), dyspnea (migraine trial: 1% to 3%)

Miscellaneous: Viral infection (2% to 7%: migraine trial: 3% to 4%), flu-like syndrome (3%), allergy (2%), infection (2%), thirst (2%), body odor (1%), diaphoresis (1%), moniliasis (1%)

<1% (Limited to important or life-threatening): Angina, apraxia, AV block, bone marrow depression, deep vein thrombosis, dehydration, delirium, delusion, diabetes mellitus, dyskinesia, eosinophilia, erythema multiforme, euphoria, granulocytopenia, hepatic failure, hepatitis, hyperammonemia/encephalopathy (with or without valproate therapy), hyperesthesia, hyperthermia (severe), hypokalemia, hypotension, lymphadenopathy, lymphopenia, maculopathy, manic reaction, neuropathy, oligohydrosis, pancreatitis, pancytopenia, paranoid reaction, pemphigus, photosensitivity, pulmonary embolism, renal tubular acidosis, Stevens-Johnson syndrome, suicidal behavior, suicide, suicidal ideation, syndrome of acute myopia/secondary angle-closure glaucoma, tongue edema, toxic epidermal necrolysis

Drug Interactions

Metabolism/Transport Effects Inhibits CYP2C19 (weak); **Induces** CYP3A4 (weak/moderate)

Avoid Concomitant Use

Avoid concomitant use of Topiramate with any of the following: Carbonic Anhydrase Inhibitors

Increased Effect/Toxicity

Topiramate may increase the levels/effects of: Alcohol (Ethyl); Alpha-/Beta-Agonists; Amphetamines; Anticonvulsants (Barbiturate); Anticonvulsants (Hydantoin); CarBAMazepine; Carbonic Anhydrase Inhibitors; CNS Depressants; Flecainide; Fosphenytoin; Lithium; Memantine; Methotrimeprazine; Phenytoin; Primidone; QuiNIDine; Selective Serotonin Reuptake Inhibitors; Valproic Acid

The levels/effects of Topiramate may be increased by: Divalproex; Droperidol; HydrOXYzine; Methotrimeprazine; Salicylates; Thiazide Diuretics

Decreased Effect

Topiramate may decrease the levels/effects of: ARIPiprazole; Contraceptives (Estrogens); Contraceptives (Progestins); Lithium; Methenamine; Primidone; Saxagliptin

The levels/effects of Topiramate may be decreased by: CarBAMazepine; Fosphenytoin; Ketorolac; Ketorolac (Nasal); Ketorolac (Systemic); Mefloquine; Phenytoin

Ethanol/Nutrition/Herb Interactions

Ethanol: May increase CNS depression; monitor for increased effects with coadministration. Caution patients about effects.

Food: Ketogenic diet may increase the possibility of acidosis and/or kidney stones.

Herb/Nutraceutical: Avoid evening primrose (seizure threshold decreased).

Stability Store at room temperature of 15°C to 30°C (59°F to 86°F). Protect from moisture.

Mechanism of Action Anticonvulsant activity may be due to a combination of potential mechanisms: Blocks neuronal voltage-dependent sodium channels, enhances GABA(A) activity, antagonizes AMPA/kainate glutamate receptors, and weakly inhibits carbonic anhydrase.

Pharmacodynamics/Kinetics

Absorption: Good, rapid; unaffected by food

Protein binding: 15% to 41% (inversely related to plasma concentrations)

Metabolism: Hepatic via P450 enzymes

Bioavailability: ~80%

Half-life elimination: Mean: Adults: Normal renal function: 21 hours; shorter in pediatric patients; clearance is 50% higher in pediatric patients; Elderly: ~24 hours

Time to peak, serum: ~1-4 hours

Excretion: Urine (~70% to 80% as unchanged drug)

Dialyzable: Significantly hemodialyzed; dialysis clearance: 120 mL/minute (4-6 times higher than in adults with normal renal function); supplemental doses may be required

Dosage Oral: **Note:** Do not abruptly discontinue therapy; taper dosage gradually to prevent rebound effects. (In clinical trials, adult doses were withdrawn by decreasing in weekly intervals of 50-100 mg/day gradually over 2-8 weeks for seizure treatment, and by decreasing in weekly intervals by 25-50 mg/day for migraine prophylaxis.)

Epilepsy, monotherapy:

Children 2-9 years: Partial onset seizure and primary generalized tonic-clonic seizure:

Initial: 25 mg once daily (in evening); may increase to 25 mg twice daily in week 2; thereafter, may increase by 25-50 mg/day at weekly intervals over 5-7 weeks up to the following minimum recommended maintenance dose:

≤11 kg: 150 mg/day in 2 divided doses
12-22 kg: 200 mg/day in 2 divided doses
23-31 kg: 200 mg/day in 2 divided doses
32-38 kg: 250 mg/day in 2 divided doses
≥39 kg: 250 mg/day in 2 divided doses

Maximum maintenance dose: If additional seizure control is needed and therapy is tolerated, may further increase by 25-50 mg/day at weekly intervals up to the following maximum recommended maintenance dose:

≤11 kg: 250 mg/day in 2 divided doses
12-22 kg: 300 mg/day in 2 divided doses
23-31 kg: 350 mg/day in 2 divided doses
32-38 kg: 350 mg/day in 2 divided doses
≥39 kg: 400 mg/day in 2 divided doses

Children ≥10 years and Adults: Partial onset seizure and primary generalized tonic-clonic seizure: Initial: 25 mg twice daily; may increase weekly by 50 mg/day up to 100 mg twice daily (week 4 dose); thereafter, may further increase weekly by 100 mg/day up to the recommended maximum of 200 mg twice daily.

Canadian labeling: Children ≥6 years and Adults: Initial: 25 mg once daily (in evening); may increase to 25 mg twice daily in weeks 2 or 3, and up to 50 mg twice daily by weeks 3 or 4; may further increase weekly in increments of 50 mg/day up to recommended maximum of 200 mg twice daily.

Epilepsy, adjunctive therapy:

Children 2-16 years:

Partial onset seizure or seizure associated with Lennox-Gastaut syndrome: Initial: 25 mg (1-3 mg/kg/day) once daily (in evening); may increase every 1-2 weeks in increments of 1-3 mg/kg/day up to the recommended maximum of 5-9 mg/kg/day in 2 divided doses

Primary generalized tonic-clonic seizure: Use initial dose listed above for partial onset seizures, but use slower initial titration rate; titrate to the recommended maintenance dose of 6 mg/kg/day by the end of 8 weeks

Canadian labeling: Initial: 25 mg (1-3 mg/kg/day) once daily (in evening); may increase every 1-2 weeks in increments of 1-3 mg/kg/day up to the recommended maximum of 5-9 mg/kg/day in 2 divided doses

Adolescents ≥17 years and Adults:

Partial onset seizure: Initial: 25 mg once or twice daily for 1 week; may increase weekly by 25-50 mg/day until response; usual maintenance dose: 100-200 mg twice daily. Doses >1600 mg/day have not been studied.

Primary generalized tonic-clonic seizure: Use initial dose as listed above for partial onset seizures, but use slower initial titration rate; titrate upwards to recommended dose by the end of 8 weeks; usual maintenance dose: 200 mg twice daily. Doses >1600 mg/day have not been studied.

Canadian labeling: Initial: 25 mg once or twice daily; may increase weekly by 50 mg/day up to the recommended dose of 100-200 mg twice daily (maximum recommended dose: 800 mg/day; doses >400 mg/day have shown no additional benefit)

Migraine prophylaxis: Adults: Initial: 25 mg once daily (in evening); may increase weekly by 25 mg/day, up to the recommended dose of 100 mg/day given in 2 divided doses. Doses >100 mg/day have shown no additional benefit.

Cluster headache prophylaxis (unlabeled use): Adults: Initial: 25 mg/day, titrated at weekly intervals in 25 mg increments, up to 200 mg/day (Pascual, 2007)

Diabetic neuropathy (unlabeled use): Adults: Initial: 25 mg/day, titrated at weekly intervals in 25-50 mg increments to target dose of 400 mg daily in 2 divided doses (Raskin, 2004; Thienel, 2004)

Dosing adjustment in renal impairment: Cl_{cr} <70 mL/minute/1.73 m^2: Administer 50% dose and titrate more slowly

Hemodialysis: Supplemental dose may be needed during hemodialysis

Dosing adjustment in hepatic impairment: Clearance may be reduced; however the manufacturer's labeling provides no specific dosing recommendations

Administration Oral: May be administered without regard to meals

Capsule sprinkles: May be swallowed whole or opened to sprinkle the contents on a small amount (~1 teaspoon) of soft food (drug/food mixture should not be chewed; swallow immediately).

Tablet: Because of bitter taste, tablets should not be broken or chewed.

Monitoring Parameters Seizure frequency, hydration status; electrolytes (recommended monitoring includes serum bicarbonate at baseline and periodically during treatment), serum creatinine; monitor for symptoms of acute acidosis and complications of long-term acidosis (nephrolithiasis, osteomalacia, and reduced growth rates in children); ammonia level in patients with unexplained lethargy, vomiting, or mental status changes; intraocular pressure, symptoms of secondary angle closure glaucoma; suicidality (eg, suicidal thoughts, depression, behavioral changes)

Additional Information May be associated with weight loss in some patients

Dosage Forms Excipient information presented when available (limited, particularly for generics); consult specific product labeling.

Capsule, sprinkle, oral: 15 mg, 25 mg

Topamax®: 15 mg, 25 mg

Tablet, oral: 25 mg, 50 mg, 100 mg, 200 mg

Topamax®: 25 mg, 50 mg, 100 mg, 200 mg

Extemporaneous Preparations A 6 mg/mL topiramate oral suspension may be made with tablets and one of two different vehicles (a 1:1 mixture of Ora-Sweet® and Ora-Plus®, or a mixture of Simple Syrup, NF and methylcellulose 1% with parabens). Crush six 100 mg tablets in a mortar and reduce to a fine powder. Add a small amount of methylcellulose gel and mix to a uniform paste (**Note:** Use a small amount of methylcellulose gel when using the 1:1 Ora-Sweet® and Ora-Plus® mixture as the vehicle; use 10 mL methylcellulose 1% with parabens when using Simple Syrup, NF as the vehicle); mix while adding the chosen vehicle in incremental proportions to **almost** 100 mL; transfer to a graduated cylinder; rinse mortar with vehicle, and add quantity of vehicle sufficient to make 100 mL. Store in plastic prescription bottles; label "shake well" and "refrigerate". Stable for 90 days refrigerated (preferred) or at room temperature.

Nahata MC, Pai VB, and Hipple TF, *Pediatric Drug Formulations*, 5th ed, Cincinnati, OH: Harvey Whitney Books Co, 2004.

◆ **Topisone® (Can)** *see* Betamethasone *on page* 208

◆ **Toposar®** *see* Etoposide *on page* 669

Topotecan (toe poe TEE kan)

Brand Names: U.S. Hycamtin®

Brand Names: Canada Hycamtin®; Topotecan For Injection

Index Terms Hycamptamine; SKF 104864; SKF 104864-A; Topotecan Hydrochloride

Pharmacologic Category Antineoplastic Agent, Camptothecin; Antineoplastic Agent, Natural Source (Plant) Derivative; Antineoplastic Agent, Topoisomerase I Inhibitor

Use Treatment of metastatic ovarian cancer, relapsed or refractory small cell lung cancer, recurrent or resistant (stage IVB) cervical cancer (in combination with cisplatin)

Unlabeled Use Treatment of central nervous system lesions (metastatic from lung cancer), central nervous system lymphoma (primary), Ewing's sarcoma, rhabdomyosarcoma (pediatrics), neuroblastoma (pediatrics)

Pregnancy Risk Factor D

Pregnancy Considerations Animal studies found reduced fetal body weight, eye, brain, skull, and vertebrae malformations. May cause fetal harm in pregnant women. Use during pregnancy is contraindicated.

Lactation Excretion in breast milk unknown/contraindicated

Contraindications Hypersensitivity to topotecan or any component of the formulation; severe bone marrow depression; pregnancy; breast-feeding

Canadian labeling: Additional contraindications (not in U.S. labeling): Severe renal impairment (Cl_{cr} <20 mL/minute)

Warnings/Precautions Hazardous agent - use appropriate precautions for handling and disposal. **[U.S. Boxed Warning]: May cause neutropenia, which may be severe or lead to infection or fatalities. Monitor blood counts frequently. Do NOT administer to patients with baseline neutrophils <1500/mm³ and platelets <100,000/mm³.** The dose-limiting toxicity is bone marrow suppression (primarily neutropenia); may also cause thrombocytopenia and anemia. Neutropenia is not cumulative overtime. In a clinical study comparing I.V. to oral topotecan, G-CSF support was administered in a higher percentage of patients receiving oral topotecan (Eckerd, 2007). Topotecan-induced neutropenia may lead to neutropenic colitis (including fatalities); should be considered in patients presenting with neutropenia, fever and abdominal pain.

Diarrhea has been reported with oral topotecan; may be severe (requiring hospitalization); incidence may be higher in the elderly; educate patients on early recognition and proper management, including diet changes, increase in fluid intake, antidiarrheals, and antibiotics. Interstitial lung disease (ILD) (with fatalities) has been reported; discontinue use in patients with confirmed ILD; risk factors for ILD include a history of ILD, pulmonary fibrosis, lung cancer, thoracic radiation, and the use of colony-stimulating factors or medication with pulmonary toxicity; monitor pulmonary symptoms (cough, fever, dyspnea, and/or hypoxia) and discontinue if ILD is diagnosed. Use caution in renal impairment; may require dose adjustment (use in severe renal impairment is contraindicated in the Canadian labeling).

Adverse Reactions

>10%:

Central nervous system: Fatigue (6% to 29%), fever (5% to 28%), pain (5% to 23%), headache (18%)

Dermatologic: Alopecia (10% to 49%), rash (16%)

Gastrointestinal: Nausea (8% to 64%), vomiting (10% to 45%), diarrhea (6% to 32%; Oral: grade 3: 4%; grade 4: ≤1%; onset: 9 days), constipation (5% to 29%), abdominal pain (5% to 22%), anorexia (7% to 19%), stomatitis (18%)

Hematologic: Anemia (89% to 98%; grade 4: 7% to 37%; nadir: 15 days), neutropenia (83% to 97%; grade 4: 32% to 80%; nadir 12-15 days; duration: 7 days), leukopenia (86% to 97%; grade 4: 15% to 32%), thrombocytopenia (69% to 81%; grade 4: 6% to 27%; nadir: 15 days; duration: 3-5 days), neutropenic fever/sepsis (2% to 43%)

Neuromuscular & skeletal: Weakness (3% to 25%)

Respiratory: Dyspnea (6% to 22%), cough (15%)

1% to 10%:

Gastrointestinal: Obstruction (5%)

Hepatic: Liver enzymes increased (transient; 8%; grades 3/4: 4%), bilirubin increased (grades 3/4: <2%)

Neuromuscular & skeletal: Paresthesia (7%)

Respiratory: Pneumonia (8%)

Miscellaneous: Sepsis (grades 3/4: 5%)

<1% (Limited to important or life-threatening): Allergic reactions, anaphylactoid reactions, angioedema, bleeding (severe, associated with thrombocytopenia), dermatitis (severe), extravasation (inadvertent), interstitial lung disease (ILD), neutropenic colitis, pancytopenia, pruritus (severe)

Drug Interactions

Metabolism/Transport Effects None known.

Avoid Concomitant Use

Avoid concomitant use of Topotecan with any of the following: BCG; CloZAPine; Natalizumab; P-glycoprotein/ABCB1 Inhibitors; Pimecrolimus; Tacrolimus (Topical); Vaccines (Live)

Increased Effect/Toxicity

Topotecan may increase the levels/effects of: CloZAPine; Leflunomide; Natalizumab; Vaccines (Live)

The levels/effects of Topotecan may be increased by: BCRP/ABCG2 Inhibitors; Denosumab; Filgrastim; P-glycoprotein/ABCB1 Inhibitors; Pimecrolimus; Platinum Derivatives; Roflumilast; Tacrolimus (Topical); Trastuzumab

Decreased Effect

Topotecan may decrease the levels/effects of: BCG; Coccidioidin Skin Test; Sipuleucel-T; Vaccines (Inactivated); Vaccines (Live)

The levels/effects of Topotecan may be decreased by: Echinacea

Ethanol/Nutrition/Herb Interactions Ethanol: Avoid ethanol (due to GI irritation).

Stability

I.V.:

Solution for injection: Store intact vials at 2°C to 8°C (36°F to 45°F). Protect from light. Single-use vials should be discarded after initial vial entry; solutions for infusion are stable for 24 hours at room temperature after dilution in at least 50 mL D_5W or NS.

Lyophilized powder: Store intact vials at room temperature of 20°C to 25°C (68°F to 77°F). Protect from light. Reconstitute with 4 mL SWFI. This solution is stable for up to 28 days at room temperature of 20°C to 25°C (68°F to 77°F), although the manufacturer recommends use immediately after reconstitution. Further dilute in 50-100 mL D_5W or NS. This solution is stable for 24 hours at room temperature (manufacturer recommendation) or up to 7 days under refrigeration (Craig, 1997).

Oral: Store at 2°C to 8°C (36°F to 46°F). Protect from light.

Mechanism of Action Binds to topoisomerase I and stabilizes the cleavable complex so that religation of the cleaved DNA strand cannot occur. This results in the accumulation of cleavable complexes and single-strand DNA breaks. Topotecan acts in S phase of the cell cycle.

Pharmacodynamics/Kinetics

Absorption: Oral: Rapid

Distribution: V_{dss} of the lactone is high (mean: 87.3 L/mm^2; range: 25.6-186 L/mm^2), suggesting wide distribution and/or tissue sequestering

Protein binding: ~35%

Metabolism: Undergoes a rapid, pH-dependent hydrolysis of the lactone ring to yield a relatively inactive hydroxy acid in plasma; metabolized in the liver to N-demethylated metabolite

Bioavailability: Oral: ~40%

Half-life elimination: I.V.: 2-3 hours; renal impairment: 5 hours; Oral: 3-6 hours

Time to peak, plasma: Oral: 1-2 hours; delayed with high-fat meal (3-4 hours)

Excretion:

I.V.: Urine (51%; 3% as N-desmethyl topotecan); feces (18%; 2% as N-desmethyl topotecan)

Oral: Urine (20%; 2% as N-desmethyl topotecan); feces (33%; <2% as N-desmethyl topotecan)

Dosage Adults (details concerning dosing in combination regimens should also be consulted): **Note:** Baseline neutrophil count should be ≥1500/mm^3 and platelets should be ≥100,000/mm^3 prior to treatment; for retreatment, neutrophil count should be >1000/mm^3; platelets >100,000/mm^3 and hemoglobin ≥9 g/dL:

Small cell lung cancer:

IVPB: 1.5 mg/m^2/day for 5 days; repeated every 21 days, minimum of 4 cycles recommended in the absence of tumor progression

Oral: 2.3 mg/m^2/day for 5 days; repeated every 21 days (round dose to the nearest 0.25 mg); if patient vomits after dose is administered, do not give a replacement dose.

Metastatic ovarian cancer: IVPB: 1.5 mg/m^2/day for 5 days; repeated every 21 days, minimum of 4 cycles recommended in the absence of tumor progression

Cervical cancer: IVPB: 0.75 mg/m^2/day for 3 days (followed by cisplatin 50 mg/m^2 on day 1 only, [with hydration]); repeated every 21 days

Dosage adjustment for toxicity:

I.V.:

Ovarian and small cell lung cancer: Dosage adjustment for hematological effects: Severe neutropenia (<500/mm^3) or platelet count <25,000/mm^3: Reduce dose to 1.25 mg/m^2/day for subsequent cycles (may consider G-CSF support [beginning on day 6] prior to instituting dose reduction for severe neutropenia). **Note:** The Canadian labeling states that the dose may be further reduced to 1 mg/m^2/day if necessary.

Cervical cancer (cisplatin may also require dosage adjustment): Severe febrile neutropenia (<500/mm^3 with temperature of 38°C) or platelet count <25,000/mm^3: Reduce topotecan to 0.6 mg/m^2/day for subsequent cycles (may consider G-CSF support [beginning on day 4] prior to instituting dose reduction for neutropenic fever.

For neutropenic fever despite G-CSF use, reduce dose to 0.45 mg/m^2/day for subsequent cycles.

Oral:

Small cell lung cancer: Severe neutropenia (neutrophils <500/mm^3 associated with fever or infection or lasting >7 days) or prolonged neutropenia (neutrophils ≥500/mm^3 to ≤1000/mm^3 lasting beyond day 21) or platelets <25,000/mm^3 or grades 3/4 diarrhea: Reduce dose to 1.9 mg/m^2/day for subsequent cycles (may consider same dosage reduction for grade 2 diarrhea if clinically indicated).

Dosing adjustment in renal impairment:

Manufacturer's labeling recommends the following dosage adjustment:

I.V.:

Cl_{cr} ≥40 mL/minute: No dosage adjustment required

Cl_{cr} 20-39 mL/minute: Reduce to 0.75 mg/m^2/dose

Cl_{cr} <20 mL/minute: Insufficient data available for dosing recommendation (contraindicated in the Canadian labeling)

Note: For topotecan in combination with cisplatin for cervical cancer, do not initiate treatment in patients with serum creatinine >1.5 mg/dL; consider discontinuing treatment in patients with serum creatinine >1.5 mg/dL in subsequent cycles.

Oral:

Cl_{cr} ≥50 mL/minute: No dosage adjustment required

Cl_{cr} 30-49 mL/minute: Reduce dose to 1.8 mg/m^2/day

Cl_{cr} <30 mL/minute: Insufficient data available for dosing recommendation

The following guidelines have been used by some clinicians:

Aronoff, 2007: *I.V.:*

Children:

Cl_{cr} 30-50 mL/minute: Administer 75% of dose

Cl_{cr} 10-29 mL/minute: Administer 50% of dose or reduce by 0.75 mg/m^2/dose

Cl_{cr} <10 mL/minute: Administer 25% of dose

Hemodialysis: 0.75 mg/m^2

Continuous renal replacement therapy (CRRT): Administer 50% of dose or reduce by 0.75 mg/m^2/dose

Adults:

Cl_{cr} >50 mL/minute: Administer 75% of dose

Cl_{cr} 10-50 mL/minute: Administer 50% of dose

Cl_{cr} <10 mL/minute: Administer 25% of dose

Hemodialysis: Avoid use

Continuous ambulatory peritoneal dialysis (CAPD): Avoid use

Continuous renal replacement therapy (CRRT): 0.75 mg/m^2

Kintzel, 1995: *I.V.:*

Cl_{cr} 46-60 mL/minute: Administer 80% of dose

Cl_{cr} 31-45 mL/minute: Administer 75% of dose

Cl_{cr} <30 mL/minute: Administer 70% of dose

Dosing adjustment in hepatic impairment: Manufacturer's labeling recommends the following:

I.V.: Bilirubin 1.7-15 mg/dL: No adjustment necessary (the half-life is increased slightly; usual doses are generally tolerated)

Oral: Bilirubin >1.5 mg/dL: No adjustment necessary

Dietary Considerations May be taken without regard to meals.

Administration

I.V.: Administer IVPB over 30 minutes. For combination chemotherapy with cisplatin, administer pretreatment hydration.

Oral: Administer without regard to meals. Swallow whole; do not crush, chew, or divide capsule. If vomiting occurs after dose, do not take replacement dose.

Monitoring Parameters CBC with differential and platelet count, renal function tests, bilirubin; monitor for symptoms of interstitial lung disease

Test Interactions None known

Dosage Forms Excipient information presented when available (limited, particularly for generics); consult specific product labeling.

Capsule, oral:

Hycamtin®: 0.25 mg, 1 mg

Injection, powder for reconstitution: 4 mg

Hycamtin®: 4 mg

Injection, solution [concentrate]: 1 mg/mL (4 mL)

◆ **Topotecan For Injection (Can)** *see* Topotecan *on page 1709*

◆ **Topotecan Hydrochloride** *see* Topotecan *on page 1709*

◆ **Toprol-XL®** *see* Metoprolol *on page 1117*

◆ **Topsyn® (Can)** *see* Fluocinonide *on page 727*

◆ **Toradol** *see* Ketorolac (Systemic) *on page 956*

◆ **Toradol® (Can)** *see* Ketorolac (Systemic) *on page 956*

◆ **Toradol® IM (Can)** *see* Ketorolac (Systemic) *on page 956*

Toremifene (tore EM i feen)

Brand Names: U.S. Fareston®

Brand Names: Canada Fareston®

Index Terms FC1157a; Toremifene Citrate

Pharmacologic Category Antineoplastic Agent, Estrogen Receptor Antagonist; Selective Estrogen Receptor Modulator (SERM)

Use Treatment of metastatic breast cancer in postmenopausal women with estrogen receptor positive or estrogen receptor status unknown

Unlabeled Use Treatment of soft tissue sarcoma (desmoid tumors)

Pregnancy Risk Factor D

Pregnancy Considerations Animal studies have demonstrated embryotoxicity and fetal adverse effects. There are no adequate and well-controlled studies in pregnant women. Only approved for use in postmenopausal women. May cause fetal harm if administered during pregnancy.

Lactation Excretion in breast milk unknown/not recommended

Contraindications Hypersensitivity to toremifene or any component of the formulation; long QT syndrome (congenital or acquired QT prolongation), uncorrected hypokalemia, uncorrected hypomagnesemia

Warnings/Precautions Hazardous agent - use appropriate precautions for handling and disposal.

[U.S. Boxed Warning]: May prolong the QT interval; QT_c prolongation is dose-dependent and concentration dependent. Torsade de pointes, syncope, seizure and/or sudden death may occur. Use is contraindicated in patients with congenital or acquired long QT syndrome, uncorrected hypokalemia, or uncorrected hypomagnesemia. Avoid use with other medications known to prolong the QT interval and with strong CYP3A4 inhibitors. Use with caution in patients with heart failure, hepatic impairment, or electrolyte abnormalities. Monitor electrolytes; correct hypokalemia and hypomagnesemia prior to treatment. Obtain ECG at baseline and as clinically indicated in patients at risk for QT prolongation

Hypercalcemia and tumor flare have been reported during the first weeks of treatment in some breast cancer patients with bone metastases; monitor closely for hypocalcemia. Institute appropriate measures if hypercalcemia occurs, and if severe, discontinue treatment. Tumor flare consists of diffuse musculoskeletal pain and erythema with initial increased size of tumor lesions that later regress; is often accompanied by hypercalcemia. Tumor flare does not imply treatment failure or represent tumor progression. Drugs that decrease renal calcium excretion (eg, thiazide diuretics) may increase the risk of hypercalcemia in patients receiving toremifene. Leukopenia and thrombocytopenia have been reported rarely; monitor leukocyte and platelet counts. Endometrial hyperplasia has been reported; some patients have developed endometrial cancer, although a role of toremifene in endometrial cancer development has not been established. Avoid long-term use in patients with pre-existing endometrial hyperplasia. Use with caution in patients with hepatic failure. Avoid use in patients with a history of thromboembolic disease.

Adverse Reactions

>10%:

Endocrine & metabolic: Hot flashes (35%)
Gastrointestinal: Nausea (14%)
Genitourinary: Vaginal discharge (13%)
Hepatic: Alkaline phosphatase increased (8% to 19%), AST increased (5% to 19%)
Miscellaneous: Diaphoresis (20%)

1% to 10%:

Cardiovascular: Edema (5%), arrhythmia (≤2%), CVA/TIA (≤2%), thrombosis (≤2%), cardiac failure (≤1%), MI (≤1%)
Central nervous system: Dizziness (9%)
Endocrine & metabolic: Hypercalcemia (≤3%)
Gastrointestinal: Vomiting (4%)
Genitourinary: Vaginal bleeding (2%)
Hepatic: Bilirubin increased (1% to 2%)
Local: Thrombophlebitis (≤2%)
Ocular: Cataracts (≤10%), xerophthalmia (≤9%), visual field abnormal (≤4%), corneal keratopathy (≤2%), glaucoma (≤2%), vision abnormal/diplopia (≤2%)
Respiratory: Pulmonary embolism (≤2%)

<1% (Limited to important or life-threatening): Alopecia, angina, ataxia, blurred vision, corneal opacity (reversible), corneal verticulata, depression, dermatitis, dyspnea, endometrial cancer, endometrial hyperplasia, hepatitis (toxic), incoordination, ischemic attack, jaundice, lethargy, leukopenia, paresis, pruritus, QT prolongation, rigors, skin discoloration, thrombocytopenia, tremor, tumor flare, vertigo, weakness

Drug Interactions

Metabolism/Transport Effects Substrate of CYP1A2 (minor), CYP3A4 (major); **Note:** Assignment of Major/Minor substrate status based on clinically relevant drug interaction potential

Avoid Concomitant Use

Avoid concomitant use of Toremifene with any of the following: Artemether; CYP3A4 Inducers (Strong); CYP3A4 Inhibitors (Strong); Dronedarone; Lumefantrine; Nilotinib; Pimozide; QTc-Prolonging Agents; QUEtiapine; QuiNINE; Tetrabenazine; Thioridazine; Vandetanib; Vemurafenib; Ziprasidone

Increased Effect/Toxicity

Toremifene may increase the levels/effects of: Dronedarone; Pimozide; QTc-Prolonging Agents; QuiNINE; Tetrabenazine; Thioridazine; Vandetanib; Vemurafenib; Vitamin K Antagonists; Ziprasidone

The levels/effects of Toremifene may be increased by: Alfuzosin; Artemether; Chloroquine; Ciprofloxacin; Ciprofloxacin (Systemic); CYP3A4 Inhibitors (Strong); Gadobutrol; Indacaterol; Lumefantrine; Nilotinib; QTc-Prolonging Agents; QUEtiapine; QuiNINE; Thiazide Diuretics

Decreased Effect

The levels/effects of Toremifene may be decreased by: CYP3A4 Inducers (Strong); Cyproterone; Deferasirox; Herbs (CYP3A4 Inducers); Tocilizumab

Ethanol/Nutrition/Herb Interactions

Food: Avoid grapefruit juice (may increase toremifene levels).
Herb/Nutraceutical: Avoid St John's wort (may decrease toremifene levels).

Stability Store at 25°C (77°F); excursions permitted to 15°C to 30°C (59°F to 86°F); protect from heat. Protect from light.

Mechanism of Action Nonsteroidal, triphenylethylene derivative with potent antiestrogenic properties (also has estrogenic effects). Competitively binds to estrogen receptors on tumors and other tissue targets, producing a nuclear complex that decreases DNA synthesis and inhibits estrogen effects. Competes with estrogen for binding sites in breast and other tissues; cells accumulate in the G_0 and G_1 phases; therefore, toremifene is cytostatic rather than cytocidal.

Pharmacodynamics/Kinetics

Absorption: Well absorbed
Distribution: V_d: 580 L (range: 457-958 L)
Protein binding, plasma: >99.5%, primarily to albumin
Metabolism: Extensively hepatic, principally by CYP3A4 to N-demethyltoremifene (a weak antiestrogen)
Bioavailability: Not affected by food
Half-life elimination: Toremifene: ~5 days; N-demethyltoremifene: 6 days
Time to peak, serum: ≤3 hours
Excretion: Primarily feces; urine (10%) during a 1-week period

Dosage Oral: Adults: Metastatic breast cancer (postmenopausal): 60 mg once daily, continue until disease progression

Dietary Considerations May be taken with or without food. Avoid grapefruit juice.

Administration Administer orally, as a single daily dose, with or without food.

Monitoring Parameters CBC with differential, electrolytes (calcium, magnesium, and potassium), hepatic function. Obtain ECG in patients at risk for QT prolongation. In patients with bone metastases, monitor closely for hypercalcemia during the first few weeks of treatment.

Dosage Forms Excipient information presented when available (limited, particularly for generics); consult specific product labeling.

Tablet, oral:
Fareston®: 60 mg

◆ **Toremifene Citrate** *see* Toremifene *on page 1711*

◆ **Torisel®** *see* Temsirolimus *on page 1641*

Torsemide (TORE se mide)

Brand Names: U.S. Demadex®
Pharmacologic Category Diuretic, Loop

Additional Appendix Information
Heart Failure (Systolic) *on page 1991*

Use Management of edema associated with heart failure and hepatic or renal disease (including chronic renal failure); treatment of hypertension

Pregnancy Risk Factor B

Pregnancy Considerations A decrease in fetal weight, an increase in fetal resorption, and delayed fetal ossification has occurred in animal studies.

Lactation Excretion in breast milk unknown/use caution

Contraindications Hypersensitivity to torsemide, any component of the formulation, or any sulfonylurea; anuria

Warnings/Precautions Loop diuretics are potent diuretics; excess amounts can lead to profound diuresis with fluid and electrolyte loss; close medical supervision and dose evaluation are required. Potassium supplementation and/or use of potassium-sparing diuretics may be necessary to prevent hypokalemia. Use with caution in patients with cirrhosis; avoid sudden changes in fluid and electrolyte balance and acid/base status which may lead to hepatic encephalopathy. Administration with an aldosterone antagonist or potassium-sparing diuretic may provide additional diuretic efficacy and maintain normokalemia. Coadministration of antihypertensives may increase the risk of hypotension.

Monitor fluid status and renal function in an attempt to prevent oliguria, azotemia, and reversible increases in BUN and creatinine; close medical supervision of aggressive diuresis required. Ototoxicity has been demonstrated following oral administration of torsemide and following rapid I.V. administration of other loop diuretics. Other possible risk factors may include use in renal impairment, excessive doses, and concurrent use of other ototoxins (eg, aminoglycosides).

Chemical similarities are present among sulfonamides, sulfonylureas, carbonic anhydrase inhibitors, thiazides, and loop diuretics (except ethacrynic acid). Use in patients with sulfonylurea allergy is specifically contraindicated in product labeling; a risk of cross-reaction exists in patients with allergy to any of these compounds; avoid use when previous reaction has been severe. Discontinue if signs of hypersensitivity are noted.

Adverse Reactions

1% to 10%:
- Cardiovascular: ECG abnormality (2%), chest pain (1%)
- Central nervous system: Nervousness (1%)
- Gastrointestinal: Constipation (2%), diarrhea (2%), dyspepsia (2%), nausea (2%), sore throat (2%)
- Genitourinary: Excessive urination (7%)
- Neuromuscular & skeletal: Arthralgia (2%), myalgia (2%), weakness (2%)
- Respiratory: Rhinitis (3%), cough (2%)

<1% (Limited to important or life-threatening): Angioedema, arthritis, atrial fibrillation, esophageal hemorrhage, GI hemorrhage, hyperglycemia, hypernatremia, hyperuricemia, hypokalemia, hypotension, hypovolemia, impotence, leukopenia, rash, rectal bleeding, shunt thrombosis, Stevens-Johnson syndrome, syncope, thirst, thrombocytopenia, toxic epidermal necrolysis, ventricular tachycardia, vomiting

Drug Interactions

Metabolism/Transport Effects Substrate of CYP2C8 (minor), CYP2C9 (major), SLCO1B1; **Note:** Assignment of Major/Minor substrate status based on clinically relevant drug interaction potential; **Inhibits** CYP2C19 (weak)

Avoid Concomitant Use There are no known interactions where it is recommended to avoid concomitant use.

Increased Effect/Toxicity

Torsemide may increase the levels/effects of: ACE Inhibitors; Allopurinol; Amifostine; Aminoglycosides; Antihypertensives; Cardiac Glycosides; CISplatin; Dofetilide; Hypotensive Agents; Lithium; Methotrexate; Neuromuscular-Blocking Agents; RisperiDONE; RiTUXimab; Salicylates; Sodium Phosphates; Warfarin

The levels/effects of Torsemide may be increased by: Alfuzosin; Beta2-Agonists; Corticosteroids (Orally Inhaled); Corticosteroids (Systemic); CycloSPORINE (Systemic); CYP2C9 Inhibitors (Moderate); CYP2C9 Inhibitors (Strong); Diazoxide; Eltrombopag; Herbs (Hypotensive Properties); Licorice; MAO Inhibitors; Methotrexate; Pentoxifylline; Phosphodiesterase 5 Inhibitors; Probenecid; Prostacyclin Analogues

Decreased Effect

Torsemide may decrease the levels/effects of: Lithium; Neuromuscular-Blocking Agents

The levels/effects of Torsemide may be decreased by: Bile Acid Sequestrants; CYP2C9 Inducers (Strong); Fosphenytoin; Herbs (Hypertensive Properties); Methotrexate; Methylphenidate; Nonsteroidal Anti-Inflammatory Agents; Peginterferon Alfa-2b; Phenytoin; Probenecid; Salicylates; Yohimbine

Ethanol/Nutrition/Herb Interactions Herb/Nutraceutical: Avoid herbs with *hypertensive* properties (bayberry, blue cohosh, cayenne, ephedra, ginger, ginseng [American], kola, licorice); may diminish the antihypertensive effect of torsemide. Avoid herbs with *hypotensive* properties (black cohosh, California poppy, coleus, golden seal, hawthorn, mistletoe, periwinkle, quinine, shepherd's purse); may enhance the hypotensive effect of torsemide.

Stability

I.V.: Store at 15°C to 30°C (59°F to 86°F). If torsemide is to be administered via continuous infusion, stability has been demonstrated through 24 hours at room temperature in plastic containers for the following fluids and concentrations:
- 200 mg torsemide (10 mg/mL) added to 250 mL D_5W, 250 mL NS or 500 mL 0.45% sodium chloride
- 50 mg torsemide (10 mg/mL) added to 500 mL D_5W, 500 mL NS, or 500 mL 0.45% sodium chloride

Tablets: Store at 15°C to 30°C (59°F to 86°F).

Mechanism of Action Inhibits reabsorption of sodium and chloride in the ascending loop of Henle and distal renal tubule, interfering with the chloride-binding cotransport system, thus causing increased excretion of water, sodium, chloride, magnesium, and calcium; does not alter GFR, renal plasma flow, or acid-base balance

Pharmacodynamics/Kinetics

Onset of action: Diuresis: Oral: Within 1hour
Peak effect: Diuresis: Oral: 1-2 hours; Antihypertensive: Oral: 4-6 weeks (up to 12 weeks)
Duration: Diuresis: Oral: ~6-8 hours
Absorption: Oral: Rapid
Distribution: V_d: 12-15 L; Cirrhosis: Approximately doubled
Protein binding: >99%
Metabolism: Hepatic (~80%) via CYP
Bioavailability: ~80%
Half-life elimination: ~3.5 hours; Cirrhosis: 7-8 hours
Time to peak, plasma: Oral: 1 hour; delayed ~30 minutes when administered with food
Excretion: Urine (~20% as unchanged drug)

Dosage Adults: **Note:** I.V. and oral dosing are equivalent.

Edema:

Chronic renal failure: Oral, I.V.: Initial: 20 mg once daily; may increase gradually by doubling dose until the desired diuretic response is obtained (maximum recommended daily dose: 200 mg)

Heart failure:

Oral: Initial: 10-20 mg once daily; may increase gradually by doubling dose until the desired diuretic response is obtained. **Note:** ACC/AHA 2009 guidelines for heart failure maximum daily dose: 200 mg (Hunt, 2009)

I.V.: Initial: 10-20 mg; may repeat every 2 hours with double the dose as needed. **Note:** ACC/AHA 2009 guidelines for heart failure recommend maximum single dose: 100-200 mg (Hunt, 2009)

Continuous I.V. infusion (unlabeled dose): Initial: 20 mg I.V. load, then 5-20 mg/hour (Hunt, 2009)

Hepatic cirrhosis: Oral: Initial: 5-10 mg once daily; may increase gradually by doubling dose until the desired diuretic response is obtained (maximum recommended single dose: 40 mg). **Note:** Administer with an aldosterone antagonist or a potassium-sparing diuretic.

Hypertension: Oral: Initial: 5 mg once daily; may increase to 10 mg once daily after 4-6 weeks if adequate antihypertensive response is not apparent; if still not effective, an additional antihypertensive agent may be added. Usual dosage range (JNC 7): 2.5-10 mg once daily. **Note:** Thiazide-type diuretics are preferred in the treatment of hypertension (Chobanian, 2003)

Dietary Considerations May be taken without regard to meals; however, food slows the rate and reduces the extent of absorption and may reduce diuretic efficacy (Bard, 2004). May require increased intake of potassium-rich foods.

Administration

I.V.: Administer over ≥2 minutes; reserve I.V. administration for situations which require rapid onset of action

Oral: Administer without regard to meals; patients may be switched from the I.V. form to the oral (and vice-versa) with no change in dose

Monitoring Parameters Renal function, electrolytes, and fluid status (weight and I & O), blood pressure

Additional Information 10-20 mg torsemide is approximately equivalent to furosemide 40 mg or bumetanide 1 mg.

Dosage Forms Excipient information presented when available (limited, particularly for generics); consult specific product labeling.

Injection, solution: 10 mg/mL (2 mL, 5 mL)

Tablet, oral: 5 mg, 10 mg, 20 mg, 100 mg

Demadex®: 5 mg, 10 mg, 20 mg, 100 mg [scored]

◆ **Tositumomab I-131** *see* Tositumomab and Iodine I 131 Tositumomab *on page 1714*

Tositumomab and Iodine I 131 Tositumomab

(toe si TYOO mo mab & EYE oh dyne eye one THUR tee one toe si TYOO mo mab)

Brand Names: U.S. Bexxar®

Index Terms 131 I Anti-B1 Antibody; 131 I-Anti-B1 Monoclonal Antibody; Anti-CD20-Murine Monoclonal Antibody I-131; Iodine I 131 Tositumomab and Tositumomab; Tositumomab I-131

Pharmacologic Category Antineoplastic Agent, Monoclonal Antibody; Radiopharmaceutical

Use Treatment of relapsed or refractory CD20 positive, low-grade, follicular, or transformed non-Hodgkin's lymphoma (NHL)

Unlabeled Use First-line treatment of follicular NHL

Pregnancy Risk Factor X

Dosage I.V.: Adults: NHL: Dosing consists of four components administered in 2 steps. Refer to manufacturer's labeling for additional details. Thyroid protective agents (SSKI, Lugol's solution or potassium iodide) should be administered beginning at least 24 hours prior to step 1. Premedicate with acetaminophen 650 mg and diphenhydramine 50 mg orally prior to step 1 and step 2.

Step 1: Dosimetric step (Day 0):

Tositumomab 450 mg in NS 50 mL administered over 60 minutes

Iodine I 131 tositumomab (containing I-131 5 mCi and tositumomab 35 mg) in NS 30 mL administered over 20 minutes

Note: Whole body dosimetry and biodistribution should be determined on Day 0; days 2, 3, or 4; and day 6 or 7 prior to administration of Step 2. If biodistribution is not acceptable, do not administer the therapeutic step. On day 6 or 7, calculate the patient specific activity of iodine I 131 tositumomab to deliver 75 cGy TBD or 65 cGy TBD (in mCi).

Step 2: Therapeutic step (one dose administered 7-14 days after step 1):

Tositumomab 450 mg in NS 50 mL administered over 60 minutes

Iodine I 131 tositumomab:

Platelets ≥150,000/mm^3: Iodine I 131 calculated to deliver 75 cGy total body irradiation and tositumomab 35 mg over 20 minutes

Platelets ≥100,000/mm^3 and <150,000/mm^3: Iodine I 131 calculated to deliver 65 cGy total body irradiation and tositumomab 35 mg over 20 minutes

Dosage adjustment for toxicity: Infusion-related toxicity (with tositumomab or iodine I-131 tositumomab):

Mild-to-moderate: Reduce infusion rate by 50%

Severe: Interrupt infusion; after complete resolution, resume with infusion rate reduced by 50%

Additional Information Complete prescribing information for this medication should be consulted for additional detail.

Dosage Forms Excipient information presented when available (limited, particularly for generics); consult specific product labeling.

Note: Not all components are shipped from the same facility. When ordering, ensure that all will arrive on the same day.

Kit [dosimetric package]: Tositumomab 225 mg/16.1 mL [2 vials], tositumomab 35 mg/2.5 mL [1 vial], and iodine I 131 tositumomab 0.1 mg/mL and 0.61mCi/mL (20 mL) [1 vial]

Kit [therapeutic package]: Tositumomab 225 mg/16.1 mL [2 vials], tositumomab 35 mg/2.5 mL [1 vial], and iodine I 131 tositumomab 1.1 mg/mL and 5.6 mCi/mL (20 mL) [1 or 2 vials]

Total Parenteral Nutrition

(TOE tal par EN ter al noo TRISH un)

Index Terms Hyperal; Hyperalimentation; Parenteral Nutrition; PN; TPN

Pharmacologic Category Caloric Agent; Intravenous Nutritional Therapy

Use Infusion of nutrient solutions into the bloodstream to support nutritional needs during a time when patient is unable to absorb nutrients via the gastrointestinal tract, cannot take adequate nutrition orally or enterally, or have had (or are expected to have) inadequate oral intake for 7-14 days.

Dosage PN is a highly-individualized therapy. The following general guidelines may be used in the estimation of needs. Electrolytes, vitamins, and trace minerals should be added to TPN mixtures based on patients individualized needs.

Children: I.V.: **Note:** Give within 5-7 days if unable to meet needs orally or with enteral nutrition:

Total calories:

<6 months: 85-105 kcal/kg/day

6-12 months: 80-100 kcal/kg/day

1-7 years: 75-90 kcal/kg/day

7-12 years: 50-75 kcal/kg/day

12-18 years: 30-50 kcal/kg/day

Fluid:
2-10 kg: 100 mL/kg
>10-20 kg: 1000 mL for 10 kg plus 50 mL/kg for each kg >10
>20 kg: 1500 mL for 10 kg plus 20 mL/kg for each kg >20
Carbohydrate (dextrose): 40% to 50% of caloric intake
<1 year: Initial: 6-8 mg/kg/minute; goal: 10-14 mg/kg/minute
1-10 years: Initial: 10% to 12.5%; daily increase: 5% increments (maximum: 15 mg/kg/minute)
>10 years: Initial: 10% to 15%; daily increase: 5% increments (maximum: 8.5 mg/kg/minute)
Protein (amino acids):
1-12 months: Initial: 2-3 g/kg/day; daily increase: 1 g/kg/day (maximum: 3 g/kg/day)
1-10 years: Initial: 1-2 g/kg/day; daily increase: 1 g/kg/day (maximum: 2-2.5 g/kg/day)
>10 years: Initial: 0.8-1.5 g/kg/day; daily increase: 1 g/kg/day (maximum: 1.5-2 g/kg/day)
Fat: Initial: 1 g/kg/day; daily increase: 1 g/kg/day (maximum: 3 g/kg/day); **Note:** Monitor triglycerides while receiving intralipids.

Adults: I.V.:
Total calories: Calculate using Harris-Benedict equation or based on stress level as indicated below:
Harris-Benedict Equation (BEE):
Females: 655.1 + [(9.56 x W) + (1.85 x H) - (4.68 x A)]
Males: 66.47 + [(13.75 x W) + (5 x H) - (6.76 x A)]
Then multiply BEE x (activity factor) x (stress factor)
W = weight in kg; H = height in cm; A = age in years
Activity factor = 1.2 sedentary, 1.3 normal activity, 1.4 active, 1.5 very active
Stress factor = 1.5 for trauma, stressed, or surgical patients and underweight (to promote weight gain); 2.0 for severe burn patients
Stress level:
Normal/mild stress level: 20-25 kcal/kg/day
Moderate stress level: 25-30 kcal/kg/day
Severe stress level: 30-40 kcal/kg/day
Pregnant women in second or third trimester: Add an additional 300 kcal/day
Fluid: mL/day = 30-40 mL/kg
Carbohydrate (dextrose):
5 g/kg/day or 3.5 mg/kg/minute (maximum rate: 4-7 mg/kg/minute)
Minimum recommended amount: 400 calories/day or 100 g/day
Protein (amino acids):
Maintenance: 0.8-1 g/kg/day
Normal/mild stress level: 1-1.2 g/kg/day
Moderate stress level: 1.2-1.5 g/kg/day
Severe stress level: 1.5-2 g/kg/day
Burn patients (severe): Increase protein until significant wound healing achieved
Solid organ transplant: Perioperative: 1.5-2 g/kg/day
Renal failure:
Acute (severely malnourished or hypercatabolic): 1.5-1.8 g/kg/day
Chronic, with dialysis: 1.2-1.3 g/kg/day
Chronic, without dialysis: 0.6-0.8 g/kg/day
Continuous hemofiltration: ≥1 g/kg/day
Hepatic failure:
Acute management when other treatments have failed:
With encephalopathy: 0.6-1 g/kg/day
Without encephalopathy: 1-1.5 g/kg/day
Chronic encephalopathy: Use branch chain amino acid enriched diets only if unresponsive to pharmacotherapy
Pregnant women in second or third trimester: Add an additional 10-14 g/day

Fat:
Initial: 20% to 40 % of total calories (maximum: 60% of total calories or 2.5 g/kg/day); **Note:** Monitor triglycerides while receiving intralipids.
Safe for use in pregnancy
I.V. lipids are safe in adults with pancreatitis if triglyceride levels <400 mg/dL

Additional Information Complete prescribing information for this medication should be consulted for additional detail.

Dosage Forms Excipient information presented when available (limited, particularly for generics); consult specific product labeling. TPN is usually compounded from optimal combinations of macronutrients (water, protein, dextrose, and lipids) and micronutrients (electrolytes, trace elements, and vitamins) to meet the specific nutritional requirements of a patient. Individual hospitals may have designated standard TPN formulas. There are a few commercially-available amino acids with electrolytes solutions; however, these products may not meet an individual's specific nutrition requirements.
See Fat Emulsion on page 690 monograph for additional information.

◆ **Totect®** *see* Dexrazoxane *on page* 486
◆ **Toviaz™** *see* Fesoterodine *on page* 707
◆ **tPA** *see* Alteplase *on page* 76
◆ **TPN** *see* Total Parenteral Nutrition *on page* 1714
◆ **TPV** *see* Tipranavir *on page* 1691
◆ **tRA** *see* Tretinoin (Systemic) *on page* 1729
◆ **Tracleer®** *see* Bosentan *on page* 230
◆ **Tradjenta™** *see* Linagliptin *on page* 1012
◆ **Trajenta** *see* Linagliptin *on page* 1012
◆ **Trajenta™ (Can)** *see* Linagliptin *on page* 1012
◆ **Tramacet (Can)** *see* Acetaminophen and Tramadol *on page* 32

TraMADol (TRA ma dole)

Brand Names: U.S. ConZip™; Rybix™ ODT; Ryzolt™; Ultram®; Ultram® ER

Brand Names: Canada Ralivia™ ER; Tridural™; Zytram® XL

Index Terms Tramadol Hydrochloride

Pharmacologic Category Analgesic, Opioid

Use Relief of moderate to moderately-severe pain
Extended release formulations are indicated for patients requiring around-the-clock management of moderate to moderately-severe pain for an extended period of time

Pregnancy Risk Factor C

Pregnancy Considerations Adverse events were observed in animal studies. Tramadol has been shown to cross the human placenta when administered during labor. Postmarketing reports following tramadol use during pregnancy include neonatal seizures, withdrawal syndrome, fetal death, and stillbirth. Not recommended for use during labor and delivery.

Lactation Enters breast milk/not recommended

Contraindications Hypersensitivity to tramadol, opioids, or any component of the formulation
Additional contraindications for Ultram®, Rybix™ ODT, and Ultram® ER: Any situation where opioids are contraindicated, including acute intoxication with alcohol, hypnotics, centrally-acting analgesics, opioids, or psychotropic drugs
Additional contraindications for ConZip™, Ryzolt™: Severe/acute bronchial asthma, hypercapnia, or significant respiratory depression in the absence of appropriately monitored setting and/or resuscitative equipment

Canadian product labeling:

Tramadol is contraindicated during or within 14 days following MAO inhibitor therapy

Extended release formulations (Ralivia™ ER [CAN], Tridural™[CAN], and Zytram® XL [CAN]): Additional contraindications: Severe (Cl_{cr} <30 mL/minute) renal dysfunction, severe (Child-Pugh class C) hepatic dysfunction

Warnings/Precautions Rare but serious anaphylactoid reactions (including fatalities) often following initial dosing have been reported. Pruritus, hives, bronchospasm, angioedema, toxic epidermal necrolysis (TEN) and Stevens-Johnson syndrome also have been reported with use. Previous anaphylactoid reactions to opioids may increase risks for similar reactions to tramadol. Caution patients to swallow extended release tablets whole. Rapid release and absorption of tramadol from extended release tablets that are broken, crushed, or chewed may lead to a potentially lethal overdose. May cause CNS depression, which may impair physical or mental abilities; patients must be cautioned about performing tasks which require mental alertness (eg, operating machinery or driving). May cause CNS depression and/or respiratory depression, particularly when combined with other CNS depressants. Use with caution and reduce dosage when administered to patients receiving other CNS depressants. An increased risk of seizures may occur in patients receiving serotonin reuptake inhibitors (SSRIs or anorectics), tricyclic antidepressants or other cyclic compounds (including cyclobenzaprine, promethazine), neuroleptics, drugs which may lower seizure threshold, or drugs which impair metabolism of tramadol (ie, CYP2D6 and 3A4 inhibitors). Patients with a history of seizures, or with a risk of seizures (head trauma, metabolic disorders, CNS infection, or malignancy, or during ethanol/drug withdrawal) are also at increased risk. Avoid use, if possible, with serotonergic agents such as TCAs, MAO inhibitors (use with extreme caution; contraindicated in Canadian product labeling), triptans, venlafaxine, trazodone, lithium, sibutramine, meperidine, dextromethorphan, St John's wort, SNRIs, and SSRIs; use caution with drugs which impair metabolism of tramadol (ie, CYP2D6 and 3A4 inhibitors); concomitant may increase the risk of serotonin syndrome.

Elderly (particularly >75 years of age), debilitated patients and patients with chronic respiratory disorders may be at greater risk of adverse events. Use with caution in patients with increased intracranial pressure or head injury. Avoid use in patients who are suicidal or addiction prone; use with caution in patients taking tranquilizers and/or antidepressants, or those with an emotional disturbance including depression. Healthcare provider should be alert to problems of abuse, misuse, and diversion. Use caution in heavy alcohol users. Use caution in treatment of acute abdominal conditions; may mask pain. Use tramadol with caution and reduce dosage in patients with liver disease or renal dysfunction. Avoid using extended release tablets in severe hepatic impairment. Do not use Ryzolt™ in any degree of hepatic impairment. Tolerance or drug dependence may result from extended use (withdrawal symptoms have been reported); abrupt discontinuation should be avoided. Tapering of dose at the time of discontinuation limits the risk of withdrawal symptoms. Some products may contain phenylalanine.

Adverse Reactions

>10%:

Cardiovascular: Flushing (8% to 16%)

Central nervous system: Dizziness (10% to 33%), headache (4% to 32%), somnolence (7% to 25%), insomnia (2% to 11%)

Dermatologic: Pruritus (3% to 12%)

Gastrointestinal: Constipation (9% to 46%), nausea (15% to 40%), vomiting (5% to 17%), dyspepsia (1% to 13%)

Neuromuscular & skeletal: Weakness (4% to 12%)

1% to 10%:

Cardiovascular: Postural hypotension (2% to 5%), chest pain (1% to <5%), hypertension (1% to <5%), peripheral edema (1% to <5%), vasodilation (1% to <5%)

Central nervous system: Agitation (1% to <5%), anxiety (1% to <5%), apathy (1% to <5%), chills (1% to <5%), confusion (1% to <5%), coordination impaired (1% to <5%), depersonalization (1% to <5%), depression (1% to <5%), euphoria (1% to <5%), fever (1% to <5%), hypoesthesia (1% to <5%), lethargy (1% to <5%), nervousness (1% to <5%), pain (1% to <5%), pyrexia (1% to <5%), restlessness (1% to <5%), malaise (<1% to <5%), fatigue (2%), vertigo (2%)

Dermatologic: Dermatitis (1% to <5%), rash (1% to <5%)

Endocrine & metabolic: Hot flashes (2% to 9%), hyperglycemia (1% to <5%), menopausal symptoms (1% to <5%)

Gastrointestinal: Diarrhea (5% to 10%), xerostomia (3% to 13%), anorexia (1% to 6%), abdominal pain (1% to <5%), appetite decreased (1% to <5%), weight loss (1% to <5%), flatulence (<1% to <5%)

Genitourinary: Pelvic pain (1% to <5%), prostatic disorder (1% to <5%), urine abnormalities (1% to <5%), urinary tract infection (1% to <5%), urinary frequency (<1% to <5%), urinary retention (<1% to <5%)

Neuromuscular & skeletal: Arthralgia (1% to 5%), back pain (1% to <5%), creatine phosphokinase increased (1% to <5%), myalgia (1% to <5%), hypertonia (1% to <5%), neck pain (1% to <5%), rigors (1% to <5%), paresthesia (1% to <5%), tremor (1% to <5%)

Ocular: Blurred vision (1% to <5%), miosis (1% to <5%)

Respiratory: Bronchitis (1% to <5%), congestion (nasal/sinus) (1% to <5%), cough (1% to <5%), dyspnea (1% to <5%), nasopharyngitis (1% to <5%), pharyngitis (1% to <5%), rhinitis (1% to <5%), rhinorrhea (1% to <5%), sinusitis (1% to <5%), sneezing (1% to <5%), sore throat (1% to <5%), upper respiratory infection (1% to <5%)

Miscellaneous: Diaphoresis (2% to 9%), flu-like syndrome (1% to < 5%), withdrawal syndrome (1% to <5%), shivering (<1% to <5%)

<1% (Limited to important or life-threatening): Abnormal gait, allergic reaction, amnesia, anaphylactoid reactions, anaphylaxis, anemia, angioedema, appendicitis, ALT increased/decreased, AST increased/decreased, bradycardia, bronchospasm, BUN increased, cataracts, cellulitis, cholecystitis, cholelithiasis, clamminess, cognitive dysfunction, concentration difficulty, creatinine increased, deafness, disorientation, diverticulitis, dreams abnormal, dysphagia, dysuria, ear infection, ECG abnormalities, edema, fecal impaction, gastroenteritis, gastrointestinal bleeding, GGT increased, gout, hallucination, hematuria, hemoglobin decreased, hepatitis, hypotension, hypersensitivity, irritability, joint stiffness, libido decreased, liver enzymes increased, liver failure, menstrual disorder, MI, migraine, muscle cramps, muscle spasms, muscle twitching, myocardial ischemia, night sweats, orthostatic hypotension, palpitation, pancreatitis, peripheral edema, peripheral ischemia, pneumonia, proteinuria, pulmonary edema, pulmonary embolism, sedation, seizure, serotonin syndrome, sleep disorder, speech disorder, Stevens-Johnson syndrome, stomatitis, suicidal tendency, syncope, taste perversion, tachycardia, thrombocytopenia, tinnitus, toxic epidermal necrolysis, urticaria, vesicles, visual disturbance

A withdrawal syndrome may include anxiety, diarrhea, hallucinations (rare), nausea, pain, piloerection, rigors, sweating, and tremor. Uncommon discontinuation symptoms may include severe anxiety, panic attacks, or paresthesia.

Drug Interactions

Metabolism/Transport Effects **Substrate** of CYP2B6 (minor), CYP2D6 (major), CYP3A4 (major); **Note:** Assignment of Major/Minor substrate status based on clinically relevant drug interaction potential

Avoid Concomitant Use

Avoid concomitant use of TraMADol with any of the following: Conivaptan

Increased Effect/Toxicity

TraMADol may increase the levels/effects of: Alcohol (Ethyl); Alvimopan; CNS Depressants; Desmopressin; MAO Inhibitors; Metoclopramide; Selective Serotonin Reuptake Inhibitors; Serotonin Modulators; Thiazide Diuretics; Vitamin K Antagonists

The levels/effects of TraMADol may be increased by: Amphetamines; Antipsychotic Agents (Phenothiazines); Antipsychotics; Conivaptan; CYP3A4 Inhibitors (Moderate); CYP3A4 Inhibitors (Strong); Dasatinib; HydrOXYzine; Selective Serotonin Reuptake Inhibitors; Succinylcholine; Tricyclic Antidepressants

Decreased Effect

TraMADol may decrease the levels/effects of: Pegvisomant

The levels/effects of TraMADol may be decreased by: Ammonium Chloride; CYP2D6 Inhibitors (Moderate); CYP2D6 Inhibitors (Strong); CYP3A4 Inducers (Strong); Deferasirox; Mixed Agonist / Antagonist Opioids; Tocilizumab

Ethanol/Nutrition/Herb Interactions

Ethanol: May increase CNS depression; monitor for increased effects with coadministration. Caution patients about effects.

Food:

Immediate release tablet: Rate and extent of absorption were not significantly affected.

Extended release:

ConZip™: Rate and extent of absorption were unaffected.

Ryzolt™: Increased C_{max}; no effect on AUC.

Ultram® ER: High-fat meal reduced C_{max} and AUC, and increased T_{max} by 3 hours.

Orally disintegrating tablet: Food delays the time to peak serum concentration by 30 minutes; extent of absorption was not significantly affected.

Herb/Nutraceutical: Avoid valerian, St John's wort, kava kava, gotu kola (may increase CNS depression).

Stability Store at 25°C (77°F); excursions permitted to 15°C to 30°C (59°F to 86°F).

Mechanism of Action Tramadol and its active metabolite (M1) binds to µ-opiate receptors in the CNS causing inhibition of ascending pain pathways, altering the perception of and response to pain; also inhibits the reuptake of norepinephrine and serotonin, which also modifies the ascending pain pathway

Pharmacodynamics/Kinetics

Onset of action: Immediate release: ~1 hour

Duration: 9 hours

Absorption: Immediate release formulation: Rapid and complete; Extended release formulation: Delayed

Distribution: V_d: 2.5-3 L/kg

Protein binding, plasma: ~20%

Metabolism: Extensively hepatic via demethylation (mediated by CYP3A4 and CYP2B6), glucuronidation, and sulfation; has pharmacologically active metabolite formed by CYP2D6 (M1; O-desmethyl tramadol)

Bioavailability: Immediate release: 75%; Extended release: Ultram® ER: 85% to 90% (as compared to immediate release), Zytram® XL, Tridural™: 70%, Ryzolt™: ~95% (as compared to immediate release)

Half-life elimination: Tramadol: ~6-8 hours; Active metabolite: 7-9 hours; prolonged in elderly, hepatic or renal impairment; Zytram® XL: ~16 hours; Ralivia™ ER, Ryzolt™, Tridural™: ~5-9 hours

Time to peak: Immediate release: ~2 hours; Extended release: ConZip™: ~10-12 hours, Ryzolt™: ~4 hours, Tridural™: ~4 hours, Ultram® ER: ~12 hours

Excretion: Urine (30% as unchanged drug; 60% as metabolites)

Dosage Oral: Moderate-to-severe pain:

Children ≥17 years and Adults:

Immediate release: 50-100 mg every 4-6 hours (not to exceed 400 mg/day).For patients not requiring rapid onset of effect, tolerability may be improved by starting dose at 25 mg/day and titrating dose by 25 mg every 3 days, until reaching 25 mg 4 times/day. The total daily dose may then be increased by 50 mg every 3 days as tolerated, to reach dose of 50 mg 4 times/day. After titration, 50-100 mg may be given every 4-6 hours as needed up to a maximum 400 mg/day.

Orally-disintegrating tablet (Rybix™ ODT): 50-100 mg every 4-6 hours (not to exceed 400 mg/day); for patients not requiring rapid onset of effect, tolerability may be improved by starting dose at 50 mg/day and titrating dose by 50 mg every 3 days, until reaching 50 mg 4 times/day. After titration, 50-100 mg may be given every 4-6 hours as needed up to a maximum 400 mg/day.

Adults: Extended release:

ConZip™, Ultram® ER:

Patients not currently on immediate-release: 100 mg once daily; titrate every 5 days (maximum: 300 mg/day)

Patients currently on immediate-release: Calculate 24-hour immediate release total dose and initiate total extended release daily dose (round dose to the next lowest 100 mg increment); titrate as tolerated to desired effect (maximum: 300 mg/day)

Ryzolt™:

Patients not currently on immediate-release: 100 mg once daily; titrate every 2-3 days by 100 mg/day increments; usual daily dose: 200-300 mg/day (maximum: 300 mg/day)

Patients currently on immediate-release: Calculate 24 hour immediate release total dose and initiate total extended release daily dose (round dose to the next lowest 100 mg increment); titrate as tolerated to desired effect (maximum: 300 mg/day)

Ralivia™ ER (Canadian labeling, not available in U.S.): 100 mg once daily; titrate every 5 days as needed based on clinical response and severity of pain (maximum: 300 mg/day)

Tridural™ (Canadian labeling, not available in U.S.): 100 mg once daily; titrate by 100 mg/day every 2 days as needed based on clinical response and severity of pain (maximum: 300 mg/day)

Zytram® XL (Canadian labeling, not available in U.S.): 150 mg once daily; if pain relief is not achieved may titrate by increasing dosage incrementally, with sufficient time to evaluate effect of increased dosage; generally not more often than every 7 days (maximum: 400 mg/day)

Elderly >65 years: Use caution and initiate at the lower end of the dosing range

Elderly >75 years:

Immediate release: Do not exceed 300 mg/day; see dosing adjustments for renal and hepatic impairment.

Extended release: Use with great caution. See adult, renal, and hepatic dosing.

Dosing adjustment in renal impairment:
Immediate release: Cl_{cr} <30 mL/minute: Administer 50-100 mg dose every 12 hours (maximum: 200 mg/day)
Extended release: Should not be used in patients with Cl_{cr} <30 mL/minute
Dosing adjustment in hepatic impairment:
Immediate release: Cirrhosis: Recommended dose: 50 mg every 12 hours
Extended release: Should not be used in patients with severe (Child-Pugh class C) hepatic dysfunction; Ryzolt™ should not be used in any degree of hepatic impairment

Dietary Considerations Some products may contain phenylalanine.

Administration
Immediate release: Administer without regard to meals.
Extended release: Swallow whole; do not crush, chew, or split.
ConZip™, Zytram® XL (Canadian labeling, not available in U.S.): May administer without regard to meals.
Ultram® ER, Ralivia™ ER (Canadian labeling, not available in U.S.), Tridural™ (Canadian labeling, not available in U.S.): May administer without regard to meals, but administer in a consistent manner of either with or without meals.
Orally-disintegrating tablet: Remove from foil blister by peeling back (do not push tablet through the foil). Place tablet on tongue and allow to dissolve (may take ~1 minute); water is not needed, but may be administered with water. Do not chew, break, or split tablet.

Monitoring Parameters Pain relief, respiratory rate, blood pressure, and pulse; signs of tolerance, abuse, or suicidal ideation

Reference Range 100-300 ng/mL; however, serum level monitoring is not required

Test Interactions May interfere with urine detection of PCP (false-positive).

Dosage Forms Excipient information presented when available (limited, particularly for generics); consult specific product labeling.
Capsule, variable release, oral, as hydrochloride:
ConZip™: 100 mg [25 mg (immediate release) and 75 mg (extended release)]
ConZip™: 200 mg [50 mg (immediate release) and 150 mg (extended release)]
ConZip™: 300 mg [50 mg (immediate release) and 250 mg (extended release)]
Tablet, oral, as hydrochloride: 50 mg
Ultram®: 50 mg [scored]
Tablet, extended release, oral, as hydrochloride: 100 mg, 200 mg, 300 mg
Ryzolt™: 100 mg, 200 mg, 300 mg
Ultram® ER: 100 mg, 200 mg, 300 mg
Tablet, orally disintegrating, oral, as hydrochloride:
Rybix™ ODT: 50 mg [contains aspartame; mint flavor]

Dosage Forms: Canada Excipient information presented when available (limited, particularly for generics); consult specific product labeling.
Tablet, extended release, as hydrochloride
Ralivia™ ER: 100 mg, 200 mg, 300 mg
Tridural™: 100 mg, 200 mg, 300 mg
Zytram® XL: 75 mg, 150 mg, 200 mg, 300 mg, 400 mg

Extemporaneous Preparations A 5 mg/mL oral suspension may be made with tablets and either Ora-Sweet® SF or a mixture of 30 mL Ora-Plus® and 30 mL strawberry syrup. Crush six 50 mg tramadol tablets in a mortar and reduce to a fine powder. Add small portions of the chosen vehicle and mix to a uniform paste; mix while adding vehicle in incremental proportions to **almost** 60 mL; transfer to a calibrated bottle, rinse mortar with vehicle, and add quantity of vehicle sufficient to make 60 mL. Label "shake well before use". Stable for 90 days refrigerated or at room temperature.

Wagner DS, Johnson CE, Cichon-Hensley BK, et al, "Stability of Oral Liquid Preparations of Tramadol in Strawberry Syrup and a Sugar-Free Vehicle," *Am J Health Syst Pharm*, 2003, 60(12):1268-70.

◆ **Tramadol Hydrochloride** *see* TraMADol *on page 1715*
◆ **Tramadol Hydrochloride and Acetaminophen** *see* Acetaminophen and Tramadol *on page 32*
◆ **Trandate®** *see* Labetalol *on page 960*

Trandolapril (tran DOE la pril)

Brand Names: U.S. Mavik®
Brand Names: Canada Mavik®
Pharmacologic Category Angiotensin-Converting Enzyme (ACE) Inhibitor
Additional Appendix Information
Angiotensin Agents *on page 1869*
Heart Failure (Systolic) *on page 1991*

Use Treatment of hypertension alone or in combination with other antihypertensive agents; treatment of heart failure (HF) or left ventricular (LV) dysfunction after myocardial infarction (MI)

Unlabeled Use To delay the progression of nephropathy and reduce risks of cardiovascular events in hypertensive patients with type 1 or 2 diabetes mellitus

Pregnancy Risk Factor C (1st trimester); D (2nd and 3rd trimesters)

Dosage Adults: Oral:
Hypertension: Initial dose in patients not receiving a diuretic: 1 mg once daily (2 mg/day in black patients). Adjust dosage at intervals of ≥1 week according to blood pressure response; most patients require 2-4 mg/day. There is little experience with doses >8 mg/day. Patients inadequately treated with once daily dosing at 4 mg may be treated with twice daily dosing. If blood pressure is not adequately controlled with trandolapril monotherapy, a diuretic may be added.
Usual dose range (JNC 7): 1-4 mg once daily
Post-MI heart failure or LV dysfunction: Initial: 1 mg once daily; titrate (as tolerated) towards target dose of 4 mg/day. If 4 mg dose is not tolerated, patients may continue therapy with the greatest tolerated dose.

Dosing adjustment in renal impairment: Cl_{cr} <30 mL/minute: Recommended starting dose: 0.5 mg once daily
Dosing adjustment in hepatic impairment: Cirrhosis: Recommended starting dose: 0.5 mg once daily

Additional Information Complete prescribing information for this medication should be consulted for additional detail.

Dosage Forms Excipient information presented when available (limited, particularly for generics); consult specific product labeling.
Tablet, oral: 1 mg, 2 mg, 4 mg
Mavik®: 1 mg [scored]
Mavik®: 2 mg, 4 mg

Trandolapril and Verapamil
(tran DOE la pril & ver AP a mil)

Brand Names: U.S. Tarka®
Brand Names: Canada Tarka®
Index Terms Verapamil and Trandolapril
Pharmacologic Category Angiotensin-Converting Enzyme (ACE) Inhibitor; Calcium Channel Blocker
Use Treatment of hypertension; however, not indicated for initial treatment of hypertension
Pregnancy Risk Factor C/D (2nd and 3rd trimesters)

Dosage Dose is individualized

Additional Information Complete prescribing information for this medication should be consulted for additional detail.

Dosage Forms Excipient information presented when available (limited, particularly for generics); consult specific product labeling.

Tablet, variable release: Trandolapril 2 mg [immediate release] and verapamil hydrochloride 180 mg [sustained release]; Trandolapril 2 mg [immediate release] and verapamil hydrochloride 240 mg [sustained release]; Trandolapril 4 mg [immediate release] and verapamil hydrochloride 240 mg [sustained release]

Tarka®:

1/240: Trandolapril 1 mg [immediate release] and verapamil hydrochloride 240 mg [sustained release]

2/180: Trandolapril 2 mg [immediate release] and verapamil hydrochloride 180 mg [sustained release]

2/240: Trandolapril 2 mg [immediate release] and verapamil hydrochloride 240 mg [sustained release]

4/240: Trandolapril 4 mg [immediate release] and verapamil hydrochloride 240 mg [sustained release]

Tranexamic Acid (tran eks AM ik AS id)

Brand Names: U.S. Cyklokapron®; Lysteda™

Brand Names: Canada Cyklokapron®; Tranexamic Acid Injection BP

Pharmacologic Category Antifibrinolytic Agent; Antihemophilic Agent; Hemostatic Agent; Lysine Analog

Use

Solution for injection: Short-term use (2-8 days) in hemophilia patients to reduce or prevent hemorrhage and reduce need for replacement therapy during and following tooth extraction

Tablet: Treatment of cyclic heavy menstrual bleeding

Unlabeled Use Trauma-associated hemorrhage; treatment of traumatic hyphema; topical treatment (mouth rinse) of bleeding associated with dental procedures in patients on oral anticoagulant therapy; prevention of perioperative bleeding associated with cardiac surgery; prevention of bleeding associated with craniosynostosis surgery, extracorporeal membrane oxygenation (ECMO), orthognathic surgery, spinal surgery (eg, spinal fusion), total knee replacement surgery, or transurethral prostatectomy; reduction of blood loss associated with cesarean delivery; hereditary angioedema (long-term prophylaxis)

Pregnancy Risk Factor B

Dosage

Oral:

Children: Hereditary angioedema (HAE) (unlabeled use):

Long-term prophylaxis: 20-40 mg/kg/day in 2-3 divided doses (maximum dose: 3000 mg/day) (Farkas, 2007) **or** 50 mg/kg/day (or 1000-2000 mg/day; depending on age and size of patient); may consider alternate-day regimen or twice-weekly regimen when frequency of attacks reduces; diarrhea may be a dose-limiting side effect (Gompels, 2005)

Short-term prophylaxis: 20-40 mg/kg/day in 2-3 divided doses (maximum dose: 3000 mg/day) (Farkas, 2007) **or** 500 mg 4 times/day (Gompels, 2005). **Note:** For short-term prophylaxis (eg, dental work), initiate 2-5 days before and continue for 2 days after the procedure (Bowen, 2004; Gompels, 2005).

Children and Adults: Traumatic hyphema (unlabeled use): 25 mg/kg administered 3 times/day for 5-7 days (Rahmani, 1999; Vangsted, 1983; Varnek, 1980). **Note:** This same regimen may also be used for secondary hemorrhage after an initial traumatic hyphema event.

Adults:

Hereditary angioedema (HAE) (unlabeled use):

Long-term prophylaxis: 1000-1500 mg 2-3 times daily; reduce to 500 mg/dose once or twice daily when frequency of attacks reduces (Gompels, 2005; Levy, 2010) **or** 25 mg/kg/dose administered 2-3 times daily (Bowen, 2004)

Short-term prophylaxis (eg, for dental work): 75 mg/kg/day divided 2-3 times daily for 5 days before and 2 days after the event (Bowen, 2004) **or** 1000 mg 4 times/day for 48 hours before and after procedure (Gompels, 2005)

Treatment of acute HAE attack: 25 mg/kg/dose (maximum single dose: 1000 mg) every 3-4 hours (maximum: 75 mg/kg/day) (Bowen, 2004) **or** 1000 mg 4 times/day for 48 hours (Gompels, 2005)

Menorrhagia: 1300 mg 3 times/day (3900 mg/day) for up to 5 days during monthly menstruation

Prevention of dental procedure bleeding in patients on oral anticoagulant therapy (unlabeled use): Oral rinse: 4.8% solution: Hold 10 mL in mouth and rinse for 2 minutes then spit out. Repeat 4 times/day for 2 days after procedure. **Note:** Patient should not eat or drink for 1 hour after using oral rinse (Carter, 2003).

Transurethral prostatectomy, blood loss reduction (unlabeled use): 2000 mg 3 times/day on the operative and first postoperative day (Rannikko, 2004)

I.V.:

Children:

Prevention of perioperative bleeding associated with cardiac surgery (unlabeled use): 10 mg/kg given over 30 minutes prior to incision, 10 mg/kg while on cardiopulmonary bypass, and 10 mg/kg administered after protamine reversal (Chauhan, 2004; Chauhan, 2004)

or

Loading dose of 100 mg/kg over 15 minutes prior to incision, followed by 10 mg/kg/hour infusion (continued until ICU transport); add 100 mg/kg to pump reservoir when cardiopulmonary bypass initiated (Reid, 1997)

Prevention of perioperative bleeding associated with craniosynostosis surgery (unlabeled use): Loading dose of 50 mg/kg over 15 minutes prior to incision, followed by 5 mg/kg/hour (Goobie, 2011) **or** 15 mg/kg over 15 minutes prior to incision, followed by 10 mg/kg/hour until skin closure (Dadure, 2011)

Children and Adolescents:

Prevention of perioperative bleeding associated with spinal surgery (eg, spinal fusion) (unlabeled use): 10 mg/kg given over 15 minutes prior to incision followed by 1 mg/kg/hour for the remainder of the surgery; discontinue at time of wound closure (Neilipovitz, 2001; Verma, 2010)

or

100 mg/kg over 15 minutes prior to incision followed by 10 mg/kg/hour until skin closure (Sethna, 2005)

or

30 mg/kg over 20 minutes prior to incision followed by 1 mg/kg/hour during surgery and for 5 hours postoperatively (Elwatidy, 2008)

Children and Adults: Tooth extraction in patients with hemophilia (in combination with appropriate factor replacement therapy): 10 mg/kg immediately before surgery, then 10 mg/kg/dose 3-4 times/day; may be used for 2-8 days

Adults:

Elective cesarean section, blood loss reduction (unlabeled use): 1000 mg over 5 minutes at least 10 minutes prior to skin incision (Gungorduk, 2011)

Hereditary angioedema (HAE), treatment of acute attack (unlabeled use): 25 mg/kg/dose (maximum single dose: 1000 mg) every 3-4 hours (maximum: 75 mg/kg/day) (Bowen, 2004) **or** 1000 mg 4 times/day for 48 hours (Gompels, 2005)

Orthognathic surgery, blood loss reduction (unlabeled use): 20 mg/kg over 15 minutes prior to incision (Choi, 2009)

Prevention of perioperative bleeding associated with cardiac surgery (unlabeled use): Loading dose of 30 mg/kg over 30 minutes (total loading dose includes a test dose administered over the first 10 minutes followed by the remainder of dose) prior to incision, followed by 16 mg/kg/hour until sternal closure; add an additional 2 mg/kg to cardiopulmonary bypass circuit (Fergusson, 2008)

or

Loading dose of 10 mg/kg over 20 minutes prior to incision followed by 2 mg/kg/hour continued for 2 hours after transfer to ICU; add a prime dose of 50 mg for a 2.5 L cardiopulmonary bypass circuit; maintenance infusion adjusted for renal insufficiency (Nuttall, 2008)

or

Loading dose of 10-15 mg/kg over 10-15 minutes, followed by 1-1.5 mg/kg/hour. The authors suggest adding 2–2.5 mg/kg to cardiopulmonary bypass circuit; however, amounts have varied widely in clinical trials (Gravlee, 2008).

Prevention of perioperative bleeding associated with spinal surgery (eg, spinal fusion) (unlabeled use): 2000 mg over 20 minutes prior to incision followed by 100 mg/hour during surgery and for 5 hours postoperatively (Elwatidy, 2008) **or** 10 mg/kg prior to incision followed by 1 mg/kg/hour for the remainder of the surgery; discontinue at time of wound closure (Wong, 2008)

Total knee replacement surgery, blood loss reduction (unlabeled use): 10 mg/kg over 30 minutes before inflation of tourniquet and 3 hours after first dose (Camarasa, 2006)

or

10 mg/kg over 10 minutes before inflation of tourniquet with a second dose (10 mg/kg) administered immediately after tourniquet release (Lozano, 2008)

or

10 mg/kg administered 30 minutes before deflation of tourniquet followed by 1 mg/kg/hour beginning at the end of the operation and continuing for 6 hours postoperatively (Alvarez, 2008)

Trauma-associated hemorrhage (unlabeled use): Loading dose: 1000 mg over 10 minutes, followed by 1000 mg over the next 8 hours. **Note:** Clinical trial included patients with significant hemorrhage (SBP <90 mm Hg, heart rate >110 bpm, or both) or those at risk of significant hemorrhage. Treatment began within 8 hours of injury (CRASH-2 Trial Collaborators, 2010).

Dosing adjustment/interval in renal impairment:

I.V. formulation:

Tooth extraction in patients with hemophilia:

Serum creatinine 1.36-2.83 mg/dL: Maintenance dose of 10 mg/kg/dose twice daily

Serum creatinine 2.83-5.66 mg/dL: Maintenance dose of 10 mg/kg/dose once daily

Serum creatinine >5.66 mg/dL: Maintenance dose of 10 mg/kg/dose every 48 hours **or** 5 mg/kg/dose once daily

Cardiac surgery (the following dose adjustments have been recommended [Nuttall, 2008]):

Serum creatinine 1.6-3.3 mg/dL: Reduce maintenance infusion to 1.5 mg/kg/hour (based on a 25% reduction from 2 mg/kg/hour)

Serum creatinine 3.3-6.6 mg/dL: Reduce maintenance infusion to 1 mg/kg/hour (based on a 50% reduction from 2 mg/kg/hour)

Serum creatinine >6.6 mg/dL: Reduce maintenance infusion to 0.5 mg/kg/hour (based on a 75% reduction from 2 mg/kg/hour)

Oral formulation: *Heavy menstrual bleeding:*

Serum creatinine >1.4-2.8 mg/dL: 1300 mg twice daily (2600 mg/day) for up to 5 days

Serum creatinine 2.9-5.7 mg/dL: 1300 mg once daily for up to 5 days

Serum creatinine >5.7 mg/dL: 650 mg once daily for up to 5 days

Additional Information Complete prescribing information for this medication should be consulted for additional detail.

Dosage Forms Excipient information presented when available (limited, particularly for generics); consult specific product labeling.

Injection, solution: 100 mg/mL (10 mL)

Cyklokapron®: 100 mg/mL (10 mL)

Tablet, oral:

Lysteda™: 650 mg

- **Tranexamic Acid Injection BP (Can)** *see* Tranexamic Acid *on page 1719*
- **Transamine Sulphate** *see* Tranylcypromine *on page 1720*
- **Transderm-V® (Can)** *see* Scopolamine (Systemic) *on page 1542*
- **Transderm-Nitro® (Can)** *see* Nitroglycerin *on page 1212*
- **Transderm Scōp®** *see* Scopolamine (Systemic) *on page 1542*
- ***trans*-Retinoic Acid** *see* Tretinoin (Systemic) *on page 1729*
- ***trans*-Retinoic Acid** *see* Tretinoin (Topical) *on page 1731*
- ***trans* Vitamin A Acid** *see* Tretinoin (Systemic) *on page 1729*
- **Tranxene T-Tab** *see* Clorazepate *on page 398*
- **Tranxene® T-Tab®** *see* Clorazepate *on page 398*

Tranylcypromine (tran il SIP roe meen)

Brand Names: U.S. Parnate®

Brand Names: Canada Parnate®

Index Terms Transamine Sulphate; Tranylcypromine Sulfate

Pharmacologic Category Antidepressant, Monoamine Oxidase Inhibitor

Additional Appendix Information

Antidepressant Agents *on page 1874*

Use Treatment of major depressive episode without melancholia

Lactation Enters breast milk/not recommended

Medication Guide Available Yes

Contraindications

Cardiovascular disease (including hypertension); cerebrovascular defect; history of headache; history of hepatic disease or abnormal liver function tests; pheochromocytoma

Concurrent use of antihistamines, antihypertensives, antiparkinson drugs, bupropion, buspirone, caffeine (excessive use), CNS depressants (including ethanol and narcotics), dextromethorphan, diuretics, elective surgery requiring general anesthesia (discontinue tranylcypromine ≥10 days prior to elective surgery), local vasoconstrictors, meperidine, MAO inhibitors or dibenzazepine derivatives (eg, amitriptyline, clomipramine, desipramine, imipramine, nortriptyline, protriptyline, doxepin, carbamazepine, cyclobenzaprine, amoxapine, maprotiline, trimipramine), SSRIs or SNRIs, spinal anesthesia (hypotension may be exaggerated), sympathomimetics (including amphetamines, cocaine, phenylephrine, pseudoephedrine) or related compounds (methyldopa, reserpine, levodopa, tryptophan), or foods high in tyramine content

Bupropion: At least 14 days should elapse between MAO inhibitor discontinuation and bupropion initiation.

Buspirone: At least 10 days should elapse between tranylcypromine discontinuation and buspirone initiation.

MAO inhibitors or dibenzazepine derivatives: At least 1-2 weeks should elapse between the use of another MAO inhibitor or dibenzazepine derivative and tranylcypromine use.

Meperidine: At least 2-3 weeks should elapse between MAO inhibitor discontinuation and meperidine use.

SSRIs or SNRIs: At least 2 weeks should elapse between the discontinuation of sertraline or paroxetine and the initiation of tranylcypromine. At least 5 weeks should elapse between the discontinuation of fluoxetine and the initiation of tranylcypromine. At least 1 week should elapse between discontinuation of a SNRI and the initiation of tranylcypromine. At least 2 weeks should elapse between the discontinuation of tranylcypromine and the initiation of SNRIs and SSRIs.

Warnings/Precautions Risk of suicide: [U.S. Boxed Warning]: Antidepressants increase the risk of suicidal thinking and behavior in children, adolescents, and young adults (18-24 years of age) with major depressive disorder (MDD) and other psychiatric disorders; consider risk prior to prescribing. Short-term studies did not show an increased risk in patients >24 years of age and showed a decreased risk inpatients >65 years. Closely monitor for clinical worsening, suicidality, or unusual changes in behavior such as anxiety, agitation, panic attacks, insomnia, irritability, hostility, impulsivity, akathisia, hypomania, and mania. The patient's family or caregiver should be instructed to closely observe the patient and communicate condition with healthcare provider. Such observation would generally include at least weekly face-to-face contact with patients or their family members or caregivers during the first 4 weeks of treatment, then every other week visits for the next 4 weeks, then at 12 weeks, and as clinically indicated beyond 12 weeks. Additional contact by telephone may be appropriate between face-to-face visits. A medication guide should be dispensed with each prescription. **Tranylcypromine is not FDA approved for treatment of children and adolescents.**

All patients treated with antidepressants should be observed similarly for clinical worsening and suicidality, especially during the initial few months of a course of drug therapy, or at times of dose changes, either increases or decreases. The possibility of a suicide attempt is inherent in major depression and may persist until remission occurs. Worsening depression and severe abrupt suicidality that are not part of the presenting symptoms may require discontinuation or modification of drug therapy. Use caution in high-risk patients during initiation of therapy. Prescriptions should be written for the smallest quantity consistent with good patient care.

Hypertensive crisis may occur with foods/supplements high in tyramine, tryptophan, phenylalanine, or tyrosine content; treatment with phentolamine is recommended for hypertensive crisis. Use with caution in patients who have glaucoma, hyperthyroidism, diabetes or hypotension. May cause orthostatic hypotension (especially at dosages >30 mg/day). Use with caution in patients at risk of seizures, or in patients receiving other drugs which may lower seizure threshold. Use with caution in patients with a history of drug abuse or acute alcoholism; potential for drug dependency exists especially in patients using excessive doses. Discontinue at least 48 hours prior to myelography. May increase the risks associated with electroconvulsive therapy. Consider discontinuing, when possible, prior to elective surgery. Use with caution in patients with renal impairment. Do not use with other MAO inhibitors or antidepressants. Avoid products containing sympathomimetic stimulants or dextromethorphan. Concurrent use with antihypertensive agents may lead to exaggeration of hypotensive effects. Tranylcypromine is not generally considered a first-line agent for the treatment of depression; tranylcypromine is typically used in patients who have failed to respond to other treatments. May worsen psychosis in some patients or precipitate a shift to mania or hypomania in patients with bipolar disorder. **Tranylcypromine is not FDA approved for the treatment of bipolar depression.**

Adverse Reactions

Frequency not defined:

Cardiovascular: Edema, orthostatic hypotension, palpitation, tachycardia

Central nervous system: Agitation, anxiety, chills, dizziness, drowsiness, headache, insomnia, mania, restlessness

Dermatologic: Alopecia (rare), rash (rare), urticaria

Endocrine & metabolic: Sexual dysfunction (anorgasmia, ejaculatory disturbances, impotence); SIADH

Gastrointestinal: Abdominal pain, anorexia, constipation, diarrhea, nausea, xerostomia

Genitourinary: Urinary retention

Hematologic: Agranulocytosis, anemia, leukopenia, thrombocytopenia

Hepatic: Hepatitis (rare)

Neuromuscular & skeletal: Muscle spasm, myoclonus, numbness, paresthesia, tremor, weakness

Ocular: Blurred vision

Otic: Tinnitus

Miscellaneous: Diaphoresis

Postmarketing and/or case reports: Akinesia, ataxia, confusion, cystic acne, disorientation, memory loss, mouth fissures, polyuria, scleroderma (localized), urinary incontinence, urticaria, withdrawal symptoms

Drug Interactions

Metabolism/Transport Effects Inhibits CYP1A2 (moderate), CYP2A6 (strong), CYP2C19 (moderate), CYP2C8 (weak), CYP2C9 (weak), CYP2D6 (moderate), CYP2E1 (weak), CYP3A4 (weak), Monoamine Oxidase

Avoid Concomitant Use

Avoid concomitant use of Tranylcypromine with any of the following: Alpha-/Beta-Agonists (Indirect-Acting); Alpha1-Agonists; Alpha2-Agonists (Ophthalmic); Amphetamines; Anilidopiperidine Opioids; Antidepressants (Serotonin Reuptake Inhibitor/Antagonist); Atomoxetine; Bezafibrate; Buprenorphine; BuPROPion; BusPIRone; CarBAMazepine; Clopidogrel; Cyclobenzaprine; Dexmethylphenidate; Dextromethorphan; Diethylpropion; HYDROmorphone; Linezolid; Maprotiline; Meperidine; Methyldopa; Methylene Blue; Methylphenidate; Mirtazapine; Oxymorphone; Pizotifen; Selective Serotonin Reuptake Inhibitors; Serotonin 5-HT1D Receptor Agonists; Serotonin/Norepinephrine Reuptake Inhibitors; Tapentadol; Tetrabenazine; Tetrahydrozoline; Tetrahydrozoline (Nasal); Tricyclic Antidepressants; Tryptophan

Increased Effect/Toxicity

Tranylcypromine may increase the levels/effects of: Alpha-/Beta-Agonists (Direct-Acting); Alpha-/Beta-Agonists (Indirect-Acting); Alpha1-Agonists; Alpha2-Agonists (Ophthalmic); Amphetamines; Anticholinergics;

Antidepressants (Serotonin Reuptake Inhibitor/Antagonist); Antihypertensives; Atomoxetine; Beta2-Agonists; Bezafibrate; BuPROPion; CYP1A2 Substrates; CYP2A6 Substrates; CYP2C19 Substrates; CYP2D6 Substrates; Dexmethylphenidate; Dextromethorphan; Diethylpropion; Doxapram; Fesoterodine; HYDROmorphone; Linezolid; Lithium; Meperidine; Methadone; Methyldopa; Methylene Blue; Methylphenidate; Metoclopramide; Mirtazapine; Orthostatic Hypotension Producing Agents; Pizotifen; Reserpine; Selective Serotonin Reuptake Inhibitors; Serotonin 5-HT1D Receptor Agonists; Serotonin Modulators; Serotonin/Norepinephrine Reuptake Inhibitors; Tamoxifen; Tetrahydrozoline; Tetrahydrozoline (Nasal); Tricyclic Antidepressants

The levels/effects of Tranylcypromine may be increased by: Altretamine; Anilidopiperidine Opioids; Antipsychotics; Buprenorphine; BusPIRone; CarBAMazepine; COMT Inhibitors; Cyclobenzaprine; Levodopa; MAO Inhibitors; Maprotiline; Oxymorphone; Pramlintide; Propafenone; Tapentadol; Tetrabenazine; TraMADol; Tryptophan

Decreased Effect

Tranylcypromine may decrease the levels/effects of: Acetylcholinesterase Inhibitors (Central); Clopidogrel; Codeine

The levels/effects of Tranylcypromine may be decreased by: Acetylcholinesterase Inhibitors (Central)

Ethanol/Nutrition/Herb Interactions

Ethanol: May increase CNS depression; monitor for increased effects with coadministration. Caution patients about effects. Avoid beverages containing tyramine (hearty red wine and beer).

Food: Concurrent ingestion of foods rich in tyramine may cause sudden and severe high blood pressure (hypertensive crisis). Avoid tyramine-containing foods with MAOIs.

Herb/Nutraceutical: Avoid valerian, St John's wort, SAMe, kava kava (may increase risk of serotonin syndrome and/or excessive sedation); Avoid supplements containing caffeine, tyrosine, tryptophan, or phenylalanine. Ingestion of large quantities may increase the risk of severe side effects (eg, hypertensive reactions, serotonin syndrome).

Stability Store at room temperature of 15°C to 30°C (59°F to 86°F).

Mechanism of Action Tranylcypromine is a nonhydrazine monoamine oxidase inhibitor. It increases endogenous concentrations of epinephrine, norepinephrine, dopamine, and serotonin through inhibition of the enzyme (monoamine oxidase) responsible for the breakdown of these neurotransmitters.

Pharmacodynamics/Kinetics

Onset of action: Therapeutic: 2 days to 3 weeks continued dosing

Duration: MAO inhibition may persist for up to 10 days following discontinuation

Half-life elimination: 90-190 minutes

Time to peak, serum: ~2 hours

Excretion: Urine

Dosage Adults: Oral: Usual effective dose: 30 mg/day in divided doses; if symptoms don't improve after 2 weeks, increase by 10 mg increments at 1- to 3-week intervals; maximum: 60 mg/day

Transitioning from another MAO inhibitor or dibenzazepine derivative (eg, TCAs, carbamazepine, cyclobenzaprine) to tranylcypromine therapy: Allow at least 1 medication-free week, then initiate tranylcypromine at 50% of usual starting dose for at least 1 week

Dietary Considerations Avoid tyramine-containing foods/beverages. Some examples include aged or matured cheese, air-dried or cured meats (including sausages and salamis), fava or broad bean pods, tap/draft beers, Marmite concentrate, sauerkraut, soy sauce and other soybean condiments. Food's freshness is also an important concern; improperly stored or spoiled food can create an environment where tyramine concentrations may increase.

Monitoring Parameters Blood glucose; blood pressure, mental status, suicide ideation (especially at the beginning of therapy or when doses are increased or decreased)

Additional Information Tranylcypromine has a more rapid onset of therapeutic effect than other MAO inhibitors, but causes more severe hypertensive reactions.

Dosage Forms Excipient information presented when available (limited, particularly for generics); consult specific product labeling.

Tablet, oral: 10 mg

Parnate®: 10 mg

◆ **Tranylcypromine Sulfate** *see* Tranylcypromine *on page 1720*

Trastuzumab (tras TU zoo mab)

Brand Names: U.S. Herceptin®

Brand Names: Canada Herceptin®

Index Terms anti-c-erB-2; anti-ERB-2; MOAB HER2; rhuMAb HER2

Pharmacologic Category Antineoplastic Agent, Monoclonal Antibody; Monoclonal Antibody

Use Treatment (adjuvant) of HER-2 overexpressing breast cancer; treatment of HER-2 overexpressing metastatic breast cancer; treatment of HER-2 overexpressing metastatic gastric or gastroesophageal junction adenocarcinoma (in patients who have not received prior treatment)

Pregnancy Risk Factor D

Pregnancy Considerations Reproductive studies in cynomolgus monkeys showed no evidence of impaired fertility or fetal harm. Trastuzumab inhibits HER2 protein, which has a role in embryonic development. There are no adequate and well-controlled studies in pregnant women. Effective contraception is recommended during and for 6 months after treatment for women of childbearing potential. **[U.S. Boxed Warning]: Trastuzumab exposure during pregnancy may result in oligohydramnios and oligohydramnios sequence (pulmonary hypoplasia, skeletal malformations and neonatal death).** Oligohydramnios (reversible in some cases) has been reported with trastuzumab use alone or with combination chemotherapy. If trastuzumab exposure occurs during pregnancy, monitor for oligohydramnios. Women exposed to trastuzumab during pregnancy are encouraged to enroll in MotHER (the Herceptin Pregnancy Registry; 1-800-690-6720).

The National Comprehensive Cancer Network (NCCN) breast cancer guidelines (v.3.2010) consider pregnancy a contraindication to trastuzumab treatment and recommend administering trastuzumab (if indicated) in the postpartum period.

Lactation Excretion in breast milk unknown/not recommended

Contraindications There are no contraindications listed within the manufacturer's labeling.

Canadian labeling: Hypersensitivity to trastuzumab, Chinese hamster ovary (CHO) cell proteins, or any component of the formulation

Warnings/Precautions Hazardous agent - use appropriate precautions for handling and disposal. **[U.S. Boxed Warning]: Trastuzumab is associated with symptomatic and asymptomatic reductions in left ventricular ejection fraction (LVEF) and heart failure (HF); the incidence is highest in patients receiving trastuzumab with an anthracycline-containing chemotherapy**

regimen. Evaluate LVEF in all patients prior to and during treatment; discontinue for cardiomyopathy. Extreme caution should be used in patients with preexisting cardiac disease or dysfunction. Prior or concurrent exposure to anthracyclines or radiation therapy significantly increases the risk of cardiomyopathy; other potential risk factors include advanced age, high or low body mass index, smoking, diabetes, and hyper/hypothyroidism. Discontinuation should be strongly considered in patients who develop a clinically significant reduction in LVEF during therapy; treatment with HF medications (eg, ACE inhibitors, beta-blockers) should be initiated. Withhold treatment for ≥16% decrease from pretreatment levels or LVEF below normal limits and ≥10% decrease from baseline (see Dosage adjustment for cardiotoxicity). Cardiomyopathy due to trastuzumab is generally reversible over a period of 1-3 months after discontinuation. Trastuzumab is also associated with arrhythmias, hypertension, mural thrombus formation, stroke, and even cardiac death.

[U.S. Boxed Warning]: Serious adverse events, including hypersensitivity reaction (anaphylaxis), infusion reactions (including fatalities), and pulmonary events (including acute respiratory distress syndrome [ARDS]) have been associated with trastuzumab. Discontinue for anaphylaxis, angioedema, ARDS or interstitial pneumonitis. Most of these events occur with the first infusion; pulmonary events may occur during or within 24 hours of the first infusion; delayed reactions have occurred. Interrupt infusion for dyspnea or significant hypotension; monitor until symptoms resolve. Infusion reactions may consist of fever and chills, and may also include nausea, vomiting, pain, headache dizziness, dyspnea, hypotension, rash and weakness. Retreatment of patients who experienced severe hypersensitivity reactions has been attempted (with premedication). Some patients tolerated retreatment, while others experienced a second severe reaction. When used in combination with myelosuppressive chemotherapy, trastuzumab may increase the incidence of neutropenia (moderate-to-severe) and febrile neutropenia; the incidence of anemia may be higher when trastuzumab is added to chemotherapy. Rare cases of nephrotic syndrome with evidence of glomerulopathy have been reported, with an onset of 4-18 months from trastuzumab initiation; complications may include volume overload and HF. The incidence of renal impairment was increased in metastatic gastric cancer patients when trastuzumab is added to chemotherapy.

May cause serious pulmonary toxicity (dyspnea, hypoxia, interstitial pneumonitis, pulmonary infiltrates, pleural effusion, noncardiogenic pulmonary edema, pulmonary insufficiency, acute respiratory distress syndrome, and/or pulmonary fibrosis); use caution in patients with pre-existing pulmonary disease or patients with extensive pulmonary tumor involvement. **[U.S. Boxed Warning]: Trastuzumab exposure during pregnancy may result in oligohydramnios and oligohydramnios sequence (pulmonary hypoplasia, skeletal malformations and neonatal death).** Effective contraception is recommended during and for 6 months after treatment for women of childbearing potential.

Adverse Reactions Note: Percentages reported with single-agent therapy.

>10%:

Cardiovascular: LVEF decreased (4% to 22%)

Central nervous system: Pain (47%), fever (6% to 36%), chills (5% to 32%), headache (10% to 26%), insomnia (14%), dizziness (4% to 13%)

Dermatologic: Rash (4% to 18%)

Gastrointestinal: Nausea (6% to 33%), diarrhea (7% to 25%), vomiting (4% to 23%), abdominal pain (2% to 22%), anorexia (14%)

Neuromuscular & skeletal: Weakness (4% to 42%), back pain (5% to 22%)

Respiratory: Cough (5% to 26%), dyspnea (3% to 22%), rhinitis (2% to 14%), pharyngitis (12%)

Miscellaneous: Infusion reaction (21% to 40%, chills and fever most common; severe: 1%), infection (20%)

1% to 10%:

Cardiovascular: Peripheral edema (5% to 10%), edema (8%), HF (2% to 7%; severe: <1%), tachycardia (5%), hypertension (4%), arrhythmia (3%), palpitation (3%)

Central nervous system: Depression (6%)

Dermatologic: Acne (2%), nail disorder (2%), pruritus (2%)

Gastrointestinal: Constipation (2%), dyspepsia (2%)

Genitourinary: Urinary tract infection (3% to 5%)

Hematologic: Anemia (4%), leukopenia (3%)

Neuromuscular & skeletal: Paresthesia (2% to 9%), bone pain (3% to 7%), arthralgia (6% to 8%), myalgia (4%), muscle spasm (3%), peripheral neuritis (2%), neuropathy (1%)

Respiratory: Sinusitis (2% to 9%), nasopharyngitis (8%), upper respiratory infection (3%), epistaxis (2%), pharyngolaryngeal pain (2%)

Miscellaneous: Flu-like syndrome (2% to 10%), accidental injury (6%), influenza (4%), allergic reaction (3%), herpes simplex (2%)

<1% (Limited to important or life-threatening; as a single-agent or with combination chemotherapy): Acute respiratory distress syndrome (ARDS), amblyopia, anaphylaxis, anaphylactoid reaction, angioedema, apnea, ascites, asthma, ataxia, bone necrosis, bronchospasm, cardiac arrest, cardiomyopathy, cellulitis, coagulopathy, colitis, confusion, deafness, esophageal ulcer, gastroenteritis, glomerulonephritis (membraneous, focal and fibrillary), glomerulopathy, glomerulosclerosis, hematemesis, hemorrhage, hemorrhagic cystitis, hepatic failure, hepatitis, herpes zoster, hydrocephalus, hydronephrosis, hypercalcemia, hypersensitivity, hypotension, hypothyroidism, hypoxia, ileus, intestinal obstruction, interstitial pneumonitis, laryngitis, leukemia (acute), lymphangitis, mania, mural thrombosis, myopathy, nephrotic syndrome, neutropenia, oligohydramnios, pancreatitis, pancytopenia, paroxysmal nocturnal dyspnea, pathological fracture, pericardial effusion, pleural effusion, pneumonitis, pneumothorax, pulmonary edema (noncardiogenic), pulmonary fibrosis, pulmonary hypertension, pulmonary infiltrate, pyelonephritis, radiation injury, renal failure, respiratory distress, respiratory failure, seizure, sepsis, shock, skin ulcers, stroke, syncope, stomatitis, thyroiditis (autoimmune), vascular thrombosis, ventricular dysfunction, volume overload

Drug Interactions

Metabolism/Transport Effects None known.

Avoid Concomitant Use

Avoid concomitant use of Trastuzumab with any of the following: Belimumab

Increased Effect/Toxicity

Trastuzumab may increase the levels/effects of: Antineoplastic Agents (Anthracycline, Systemic); Belimumab; Immunosuppressants

The levels/effects of Trastuzumab may be increased by: Abciximab; PACLitaxel

Decreased Effect

Trastuzumab may decrease the levels/effects of: PACLitaxel

Stability Prior to reconstitution, store intact vials under refrigeration at 2°C to 8°C (36°F to 46°F). Reconstitute each vial with 20 mL of bacteriostatic sterile water for injection (SWFI) to a concentration of 21 mg/mL. Swirl gently; do not shake. Allow vial to rest for ~5 minutes. Following reconstitution with bacteriostatic SWFI, the solution in the vial is stable refrigerated for 28 days from the date of reconstitution; do not freeze. If the patient has a known hypersensitivity to benzyl alcohol, trastuzumab may be reconstituted with sterile water for injection without preservatives, which must be used immediately.

Further dilute the appropriate volume for the trastuzumab dose in 250 mL NS prior to administration. Gently invert bag to mix. The solution for infusion is stable for 24 hours refrigerated; do not freeze.

Mechanism of Action Trastuzumab is a monoclonal antibody which binds to the extracellular domain of the human epidermal growth factor receptor 2 protein (HER-2); it mediates antibody-dependent cellular cytotoxicity by inhibiting proliferation of cells which overexpress HER-2 protein.

Pharmacodynamics/Kinetics

Distribution: V_d: 44 mL/kg; not likely to cross the (intact) blood-brain barrier (due to the large molecule size)

Half-life elimination: Weekly dosing: Mean: 6 days (range: 1-32 days); every 3 week regimen: Mean: 16 days (range: 11-23 days)

Dosage Adults: I.V. infusion: Details concerning dosing in combination regimens should also be consulted.

Note: Missed dose recommendation (Canadian labeling, 2010): If a dose is missed by ≤1 week, the usual maintenance dose (based on patient's schedule) should be administered as soon as possible (do not wait until the next planned cycle); if a dose is missed by >1 week, then a loading dose (4 mg/kg if patient receives trastuzumab weekly; 8 mg/kg if on an every-3-week schedule) should be administered, followed by the usual maintenance dose and schedule.

Breast cancer, adjuvant treatment:

With concurrent paclitaxel or docetaxel:

Initial loading dose: 4 mg/kg infused over 90 minutes

Maintenance dose: 2 mg/kg infused over 30 minutes weekly for total of 12 weeks, followed 1 week later (when concurrent chemotherapy completed) by 6 mg/kg infused over 30-90 minutes every 3 weeks for total therapy duration of 52 weeks

With concurrent docetaxel/carboplatin:

Initial loading dose: 4 mg/kg infused over 90 minutes

Maintenance dose: 2 mg/kg infused over 30 minutes weekly for total of 18 weeks, followed 1 week later (when concurrent chemotherapy completed) by 6 mg/kg infused over 30-90 minutes every 3 weeks for total therapy duration of 52 weeks

Following completion of anthracycline-based chemotherapy:

Initial loading dose: 8 mg/kg infused over 90 minutes

Maintenance dose: 6 mg/kg infused over 30-90 minutes every 3 weeks for total therapy duration of 52 weeks

Breast cancer, metastatic (either as a single agent or in combination with paclitaxel):

Initial loading dose: 4 mg/kg infused over 90 minutes

Maintenance dose: 2 mg/kg infused over 30 minutes weekly until disease progression

Gastric cancer, metastatic (in combination with cisplatin and either capecitabine or fluorouracil for 6 cycles followed by trastuzumab monotherapy; Bang, 2010; Van Cutsem, 2009):

Initial loading dose: 8 mg/kg infused over 90 minutes

Maintenance dose: 6 mg/kg infused over 30-90 minutes every 3 weeks until disease progression

Dosage adjustment for toxicity:

Cardiotoxicity: LVEF ≥16% decrease from baseline within normal limits or LVEF below normal limits and ≥10% decrease from baseline: Withhold treatment for at least 4 weeks and repeat LVEF every 4 weeks. May resume trastuzumab treatment if LVEF returns to normal limits within 4-8 weeks and remains at ≤15% decrease from baseline value. Discontinue permanently for persistent (>8 weeks) LVEF decline or for >3 incidents of treatment interruptions for cardiomyopathy.

Infusion-related events:

Mild-moderate infusion reactions: Decrease infusion rate

Dyspnea, clinically significant hypotension: Interrupt infusion

Severe or life-threatening infusion reactions: Discontinue

Dosing adjustment in renal impairment: Data suggest that the disposition of trastuzumab is not altered based on serum creatinine (up to 2 mg/dL)

Administration Administered by I.V. infusion; loading doses are infused over 90 minutes; maintenance doses may be infused over 30 minutes if tolerated. Do not administer with D_5W. **Do not administer I.V. push or by rapid bolus.** Treatment with acetaminophen, diphenhydramine, and/or meperidine is usually effective for managing infusion-related events.

Monitoring Parameters Assessment for HER2 overexpression and HER2 gene amplification by validated immunohistochemistry (IHC) or fluorescence *in situ* hybridization (FISH) methodology (pretherapy); test should be specific for cancer type (breast vs gastric cancer). Monitor vital signs during infusion; signs and symptoms of cardiac dysfunction; LVEF (baseline, every 3 months during treatment, upon therapy completion and if component of adjuvant therapy, every 6 months for at least 2 years; if treatment is withheld for significant LVEF dysfunction, monitor LVEF at 4-week intervals); signs and symptoms of infusion reaction; if patient is pregnant, monitor amniotic fluid volume

Dosage Forms Excipient information presented when available (limited, particularly for generics); consult specific product labeling.

Injection, powder for reconstitution:

Herceptin®: 440 mg [contains benzyl alcohol (in diluent)]

◆ **Trasylol® (Can)** *see* Aprotinin *on page* 139

◆ **Trav-L-Tabs® [OTC]** *see* Meclizine *on page* 1057

◆ **Travatan Z®** *see* Travoprost *on page* 1724

Travoprost (TRA voe prost)

Brand Names: U.S. Travatan Z®

Brand Names: Canada Travatan Z®

Pharmacologic Category Ophthalmic Agent, Antiglaucoma; Prostaglandin, Ophthalmic

Use Reduction of elevated intraocular pressure in patients with open-angle glaucoma or ocular hypertension who are intolerant of the other IOP-lowering medications or insufficiently responsive (failed to achieve target IOP determined after multiple measurements over time) to another IOP-lowering medication

Pregnancy Risk Factor C

Dosage Ophthalmic: Adults: Glaucoma (open angle) or ocular hypertension: Instill 1 drop into affected eye(s) once daily in the evening; do not exceed once-daily dosing (may decrease IOP-lowering effect). If used with other topical ophthalmic agents, separate administration by at least 5 minutes.

Additional Information Complete prescribing information for this medication should be consulted for additional detail.

Dosage Forms Excipient information presented when available (limited, particularly for generics); consult specific product labeling.

Solution, ophthalmic [drops]:

Travatan Z®: 0.004% (2.5 mL, 5 mL)

TraZODone (TRAZ oh done)

Brand Names: U.S. Oleptro™

Brand Names: Canada Apo-Trazodone D®; Apo-Trazodone®; Dom-Trazodone; Mylan-Trazodone; Novo-Trazodone; Nu-Trazodone; Nu-Trazodone D; Oleptro™; PHL-Trazodone; PMS-Trazodone; ratio-Trazodone; Teva-Trazodone; Trazorel®; ZYM-Trazodone

Index Terms Desyrel; Trazodone Hydrochloride

Pharmacologic Category Antidepressant, Serotonin Reuptake Inhibitor/Antagonist

Additional Appendix Information

Antidepressant Agents *on page 1874*

Use Treatment of major depressive disorder

Unlabeled Use Potential augmenting agent for antidepressants, hypnotic

Pregnancy Risk Factor C

Pregnancy Considerations Trazodone is classified as pregnancy category C due to adverse effects observed in animal studies. When trazodone is taken during pregnancy, an increased risk of major malformations has not been observed in the small number of pregnancies studied. The long-term effects on neurobehavior have not been evaluated.

Women treated for major depression and who are euthymic prior to pregnancy are more likely to experience a relapse when medication is discontinued as compared to pregnant women who continue taking antidepressant medications. Therapy during pregnancy should be individualized; treatment of depression during pregnancy should incorporate the clinical expertise of the mental health clinician, obstetrician, primary healthcare provider, and pediatrician. If treatment during pregnancy is required, consider tapering therapy during the third trimester to prevent potential withdrawal symptoms in the infant. If this is done and the woman is considered to be at risk of relapse from her major depressive disorder, the medication can be restarted following delivery. Treatment algorithms have been developed by the ACOG and the APA for the management of depression in women prior to conception and during pregnancy (Yonkers, 2009).

Lactation Enters breast milk/use caution (AAP rates "of concern"; AAP 2001 update pending)

Medication Guide Available Yes

Contraindications Hypersensitivity to trazodone or any component of the formulation

Warnings/Precautions [U.S. Boxed Warning]: Antidepressants increase the risk of suicidal thinking and behavior in children, adolescents, and young adults (18-24 years of age) with major depressive disorder (MDD) and other psychiatric disorders; consider risk prior to prescribing. Short-term studies did not show an increased risk in patients >24 years of age and showed a decreased risk in patients ≥65 years of age. Closely monitor for clinical worsening, suicidality, or unusual changes in behavior; the patient's family or caregiver should be instructed to closely observe the patient and communicate condition with healthcare provider. A medication guide should be dispensed with each prescription. **Trazodone is not FDA approved for use in children.**

The possibility of a suicide attempt is inherent in major depression and may persist until remission occurs. Monitor for worsening of depression or suicidality, especially during initiation of therapy (generally first 1-2 months) or with dose increases or decreases. Use caution in high-risk patients. Worsening depression and severe abrupt suicidality that are not part of the presenting symptoms may require discontinuation or modification of drug therapy. The patient's family or caregiver should be alerted to monitor patients for the emergence of suicidality and associated behaviors (such as agitation, irritability, hostility, impulsivity, and hypomania) and call healthcare provider.

May worsen psychosis in some patients or precipitate a shift to mania or hypomania in patients with bipolar disorder. Patients presenting with depressive symptoms should be screened for bipolar disorder. Monotherapy in patients with bipolar disorder should be avoided. **Trazodone is not FDA approved for the treatment of bipolar depression.**

Priapism, including cases resulting in permanent dysfunction, has occurred with the use of trazodone. Instruct patient to seek medical assistance for erection lasting >4 hours; use with caution in patients who have conditions which may predispose them to priapism (eg, sickle cell anemia, multiple myeloma, leukemia). Not recommended for use in a patient during the acute recovery phase of MI. The risks of sedation, postural hypotension, and/or syncope are high relative to other antidepressants. Trazodone frequently causes sedation, which may result in impaired performance of tasks requiring alertness (eg, operating machinery or driving). Sedative effects may be additive with other CNS depressants and ethanol.

Use with caution in patients with a history of cardiovascular disease (including previous MI, stroke, tachycardia, or conduction abnormalities). Although the risk of conduction abnormalities with this agent is low relative to other antidepressants, QT prolongation (with or without torsade de pointes), ventricular tachycardia, and other arrhythmias have been observed with the use of trazodone (reports limited to immediate-release formulation); use with caution in patients with pre-existing cardiac disease. Concurrent use of CYP3A4 inhibitors may increase the risk of QT prolongation and/or proarrhythmia. Concurrent use with other drugs known to prolong QT_c interval is not recommended. May impair platelet aggregation resulting in increased risk of bleeding events (eg, epistaxis, life threatening bleeding), particularly if used concomitantly with aspirin, NSAIDs, warfarin or other anticoagulants. Trazodone should be initiated with caution in patients who are receiving concurrent or recent therapy with a MAO inhibitor. Oleptro™: Avoid use in combination with or within 14 days of an MAO inhibitor.

Serotonin syndrome (SS)/neuroleptic malignant syndrome (NMS)-like reactions may occur with trazodone when used alone, particularly if used with other serotonergic agents (eg, serotonin/norepinephrine reuptake inhibitors [SNRIs], selective serotonin reuptake inhibitors [SSRIs], or triptans), drugs that impair serotonin metabolism (eg, MAO inhibitors), or antidopaminergic agents (eg, antipsychotics). If concurrent use is clinically warranted, carefully observe patient during treatment initiation and dose increases. Do not use concurrently with serotonin precursors (eg, tryptophan).

May cause SIADH and hyponatremia, predominantly in the elderly; volume depletion and/or concurrent use of diuretics likely increases risk. Use with caution in patients taking antihypertensives; may increase the risk of hypotension or syncope. Use with caution in patients taking strong CYP3A4 inhibitors and moderate or strong CYP3A4 inducers; monitor or consider alternative agents that avoid or lessen the potential for CYP-mediated interactions.

Therapy should not be abruptly discontinued in patients receiving high doses for prolonged periods; gradually reduce dosage prior to complete discontinuation to avoid withdrawal symptoms (eg, anxiety, agitation, sleep disturbance). Use caution in patients with a previous seizure disorder or condition predisposing to seizures such as brain damage, alcoholism, or concurrent therapy with other drugs which lower the seizure threshold. Use with caution in patients with hepatic or renal dysfunction and in elderly patients.

Adverse Reactions

>10%:

Central nervous system: Sedation (≤46%), headache (10% to 33%), dizziness (20% to 28%), fatigue (6% to 15%)

Gastrointestinal: Xerostomia (15% to 34%), nausea (10% to 21%)

Ocular: Blurred vision (5% to 15%)

1% to 10%:

Cardiovascular: Edema (3% to 7%), hypotension (≤7%), syncope (≤5%), hypertension (1% to 2%)

Central nervous system: Confusion (5% to 6%), incoordination (2% to 5%), concentration decreased (1% to 3%), disorientation (≤2%), memory impairment (≤1%), agitation, migraine

Endocrine & metabolic: Libido decreased (1% to 2%)

Gastrointestinal: Diarrhea (5% to 9%), constipation (7% to 8%), abdominal pain, abnormal taste, flatulence, vomiting, weight gain/loss

Genitourinary: Ejaculation disorder (2%), urinary urgency

Neuromuscular & skeletal: Back pain (≤5%), tremor (1% to 5%), paresthesia (≤1%), myalgia

Ocular: Visual disturbance

Respiratory: Nasal congestion (3% to 6%), dyspnea

Miscellaneous: Night sweats

<1% (Limited to important or life-threatening): Abnormal dreams, abnormal orgasm, acne, akathisia, allergic reactions, alopecia, amylase increased, anemia, anxiety, aphasia, apnea, appetite increased, arrhythmia, ataxia, atrial fibrillation, bladder pain, bradycardia, breast enlargement/engorgement, cardiac arrest, cardiospasm, cerebrovascular accident, chest pain, CHF, chills, cholestasis, clitorism, conduction block, diplopia, early menses, erectile dysfunction, extrapyramidal symptoms, eye pain, flushing, gait disturbance, hallucination, hearing loss (partial), hematuria, hemolytic anemia, hepatitis, hirsutism, hyperbilirubinemia, hyperhidrosis, hypersalivation, hypersensitivity, hypoesthesia, hypomania, impaired speech, impotence, insomnia, jaundice, lactation, leukocytosis, leukonychia, libido increased, liver enzyme alteration, methemoglobinemia, MI, muscle twitching, orthostatic hypotension, palpitation, paranoia, photophobia, photosensitivity reaction, priapism, pruritus, psoriasis, psychosis, QT prolongation, rash, reflux esophagitis, retrograde ejaculation, salivation increased, seizure, SIADH, speech impairment, stupor, tachycardia, tardive dyskinesia, tinnitus, torsade de pointes, urinary frequency increased, urinary retention, urinary incontinence, urticaria, vasodilation, ventricular ectopy, ventricular tachycardia, vertigo, dry eyes, weakness

Drug Interactions

Metabolism/Transport Effects Substrate of CYP2D6 (minor), CYP3A4 (major); **Note:** Assignment of Major/Minor substrate status based on clinically relevant drug interaction potential; **Inhibits** CYP3A4 (weak); **Induces** P-glycoprotein

Avoid Concomitant Use

Avoid concomitant use of TraZODone with any of the following: Conivaptan; Dabigatran Etexilate; MAO Inhibitors; Methylene Blue; Saquinavir

Increased Effect/Toxicity

TraZODone may increase the levels/effects of: Antipsychotic Agents (Phenothiazines); Fosphenytoin; Methylene Blue; Metoclopramide; Phenytoin; Serotonin Modulators

The levels/effects of TraZODone may be increased by: Antipsychotic Agents (Phenothiazines); Antipsychotics; BusPIRone; Conivaptan; CYP3A4 Inhibitors (Moderate); CYP3A4 Inhibitors (Strong); Dasatinib; Linezolid; MAO Inhibitors; Protease Inhibitors; Saquinavir; Selective Serotonin Reuptake Inhibitors; Telaprevir; Venlafaxine

Decreased Effect

TraZODone may decrease the levels/effects of: Dabigatran Etexilate; Linagliptin; P-glycoprotein/ABCB1 Substrates

The levels/effects of TraZODone may be decreased by: CYP3A4 Inducers (Strong); Deferasirox; Fosphenytoin; Peginterferon Alfa-2b; Phenytoin; Tocilizumab

Ethanol/Nutrition/Herb Interactions

Ethanol: May increase CNS depression; monitor for increased effects with coadministration. Caution patients about effects.

Food: Time to peak serum levels may be increased if immediate release trazodone is taken with food.

Herb/Nutraceutical: Avoid valerian, St John's wort, SAMe, kava kava (may increase risk of serotonin syndrome and/or excessive sedation).

Stability

Immediate release tablet: Store at room temperature; avoid temperatures >40°C (>104°F). Protect from light.

Extended release tablet: Store at room temperature of 15ºC to 30ºC (59ºF to 86ºF). Protect from light.

Mechanism of Action Inhibits reuptake of serotonin, causes adrenoreceptor subsensitivity, and induces significant changes in 5-HT presynaptic receptor adrenoreceptors. Trazodone also significantly blocks histamine (H_1) and alpha$_1$-adrenergic receptors.

Pharmacodynamics/Kinetics

Onset of action: Therapeutic (antidepressant): Up to 6 weeks; sleep aid: 1-3 hours

Absorption: Well absorbed; Extended release: C_{max} increases ~86% when taken shortly after ingestion of a high-fat meal compared to fasting conditions

Protein binding: 85% to 95%

Metabolism: Hepatic via CYP3A4 (extensive) to an active metabolite (mCPP)

Half-life elimination: 7-10 hours

Time to peak, serum:

Immediate release: 30-100 minutes; delayed with food (up to 2.5 hours)

Extended release: 9 hours; not significantly affected by food

Excretion: Primarily urine (<1% excreted unchanged); secondarily feces

Dosage Oral: Therapeutic effects may take up to 6 weeks to occur; therapy is normally maintained for 6-12 months after optimum response is reached to prevent recurrence of depression

Children 6-12 years: Depression (unlabeled use): Initial: 1.5-2 mg/kg/day in divided doses; increase gradually every 3-4 days as needed; maximum: 6 mg/kg/day in 3 divided doses

Adolescents: Depression (unlabeled use): Initial: 25-50 mg/day; increase to 100-150 mg/day in divided doses

Adults:

Depression: Initial: 150 mg/day in 3 divided doses (may increase by 50 mg/day every 3-7 days); maximum dose: 600 mg/day

Extended release formulation: Initial: 150 mg once daily at bedtime (may increase by 75 mg/day every 3 days); maximum dose: 375 mg/day; once adequate response obtained, gradually reduce with adjustment based on therapeutic response

Note: Therapeutic effects may take up to 6 weeks. Therapy is normally maintained for 6-12 months after optimum response is reached to prevent recurrence of depression.

Sedation/hypnotic (unlabeled use): 25-50 mg at bedtime (often in combination with daytime SSRIs); may increase up to 200 mg at bedtime

Elderly: 25-50 mg at bedtime with 25-50 mg/day dose increase every 3 days for inpatients and weekly for outpatients, if tolerated; usual dose: 75-150 mg/day

Administration

Immediate release tablet: Dosing after meals may decrease lightheadedness and postural hypotension

Extended release tablet: Take on an empty stomach; swallow whole or as a half tablet without food. Tablet may be broken along the score line, but do not crush or chew.

Monitoring Parameters Baseline liver function prior to and periodically during therapy; suicide ideation (especially at the beginning of therapy or when doses are increased or decreased)

Reference Range

Plasma levels do not always correlate with clinical effectiveness

Therapeutic: 0.5-2.5 mcg/mL

Potentially toxic: >2.5 mcg/mL

Toxic: >4 mcg/mL

Test Interactions May interfere with urine detection of amphetamine/methamphetamine (false-positive).

Dosage Forms Excipient information presented when available (limited, particularly for generics); consult specific product labeling.

Tablet, oral, as hydrochloride: 50 mg, 100 mg, 150 mg, 300 mg

Tablet, extended release, oral, as hydrochloride:
Oleptro™: 150 mg, 300 mg [scored]

◆ **Trazodone Hydrochloride** *see* TraZODone *on page 1725*

◆ **Trazorel® (Can)** *see* TraZODone *on page 1725*

◆ **Treanda®** *see* Bendamustine *on page 199*

◆ **Trelstar®** *see* Triptorelin *on page 1742*

◆ **TRENtal®** *see* Pentoxifylline *on page 1333*

◆ **Trental® (Can)** *see* Pentoxifylline *on page 1333*

Treprostinil (tre PROST in il)

Brand Names: U.S. Remodulin®; Tyvaso™

Brand Names: Canada Remodulin®

Index Terms Treprostinil Sodium

Pharmacologic Category Prostacyclin; Prostaglandin; Vasodilator

Use

Injection: Treatment of pulmonary arterial hypertension (PAH) (WHO Group I) in patients with NYHA Class II-IV symptoms to decrease exercise-associated symptoms; to diminish clinical deterioration when transitioning from epoprostenol (I.V.)

Inhalation: Treatment of pulmonary arterial hypertension (PAH) (WHO Group I) in patients with NYHA Class III symptoms to improve exercise ability. **Note:** Nearly all controlled clinical trial experience has been with concomitant bosentan or sildenafil.

Pregnancy Risk Factor B

Pregnancy Considerations Some skeletal malformations and maternal toxicity noted in animal studies. There are no adequate and well-controlled studies in pregnant women. Use with caution and only if clearly needed.

Lactation Excretion in breast milk unknown/use caution

Contraindications There are no contraindications listed in the FDA-approved labeling.

Warnings/Precautions May produce symptomatic hypotension; use with caution in patients with low systemic arterial blood pressure. Abrupt withdrawal/large dosage reductions may worsen symptoms of PAH. If a SubQ or I.V. infusion is restarted within a few hours of discontinuation, the same dose rate may be used. Interruptions for longer periods may require retitration. Regardless of administration route (inhalation, I.V., or SubQ), treatment interruptions should be avoided. Immediate access to medication, back-up inhalation device, or pump and infusion sets is essential to prevent treatment interruptions. Chronic continuous I.V. infusion of treprostinil via a chronic indwelling central venous catheter has been associated with serious blood stream infections. This method of administration should be reserved for patients who are intolerant of the SubQ route or in whom the benefit outweighs the potential risks. Treprostinil should only be used by clinicians experienced in the treatment of PAH. Prior to initiation, patients should be carefully evaluated for ability to administer treprostinil, either as an I.V./SubQ infusion or inhalation, and care for the infusion system/inhalation device. Initiation of infusion must occur in a setting where adequate personnel and equipment necessary for hemodynamic monitoring and emergency treatment is available. Use with caution in patients with hepatic impairment; dose reduction is recommended for the initial dose (I.V./SubQ) in patients with mild-to-moderate hepatic insufficiency; titrate dose slowly in patients with hepatic insufficiency; has not been studied in severe hepatic impairment. Has not been studied in renal impairment; use with caution in renal impairment; titrate dose slowly in patients with renal insufficiency. Use with caution in patients ≥65 years of age. Inhalation: Safety and efficacy have not been established in patients with underlying pulmonary disease (eg, asthma, COPD). Patients with acute pulmonary infections should be monitored closely for exacerbation or reduced efficacy. Treprostinil inhibits platelet aggregation, increasing the risk of bleeding; use with caution in patients receiving concurrent anticoagulant/antiplatelet therapy.

Adverse Reactions

>10%:

Cardiovascular: Flushing (11%; inhalation: 15%)

Central nervous system: Headache (27% to 41%)

Dermatologic: Rash (14%)

Gastrointestinal: Diarrhea (25%), nausea (19% to 22%)

Local: Infusion site pain (SubQ: 85%; may improve after several months of therapy), infusion site reaction (SubQ: 83%)

Neuromuscular & skeletal: Jaw pain (13%)

Respiratory: Cough (inhalation: 54%), throat irritation/pharyngolaryngeal pain (inhalation: 25%)

1% to 10%:

Cardiovascular: Edema (9%), syncope (inhalation: 6%), hypotension (4%)

Central nervous system: Dizziness (9%)

Dermatologic: Pruritus (8%)

Respiratory: Epistaxis (inhalation), hemoptysis, pneumonia, wheezing (inhalation)

<1% (Limited to important or life-threatening): Anxiety, arm swelling, bone pain, cellulitis, central venous catheter-related line infections, central venous catheter-related sepsis, hematoma, pain, paresthesia, restlessness, thrombocytopenia, thrombophlebitis

Drug Interactions

Metabolism/Transport Effects Substrate of CYP2C8 (minor); **Note:** Assignment of Major/Minor substrate status based on clinically relevant drug interaction potential

Avoid Concomitant Use There are no known interactions where it is recommended to avoid concomitant use.

Increased Effect/Toxicity

Treprostinil may increase the levels/effects of: Anticoagulants; Antihypertensives; Antiplatelet Agents; Nonsteroidal Anti-Inflammatory Agents; Salicylates

The levels/effects of Treprostinil may be increased by: CYP2C8 Inhibitors (Strong)

Decreased Effect

The levels/effects of Treprostinil may be decreased by: CYP2C8 Inducers (Strong)

Stability Injection solution: Store vials at 25°C (77°F); excursions permitted to 15°C to 30°C (59°F to 86°F). Contents of a vial should not be used past 30 days after initial needle access into the vial. For SubQ infusion, **product should not be diluted prior to use**; contents of a single-reservoir syringe of treprostinil can be administered up to 72 hours at 37°C. For I.V. infusion, dilute in SWFI, NS, or Flolan® sterile diluent to a final volume of either 50 mL or 100 mL (dependent on system reservoir and calculated dose). Stability for up to 48 hours at 37°C has been shown for concentrations as low as 4000 ng/mL.

Solution for inhalation: Store ampules in foil packs at 25°C (77°F); excursions permitted to 15°C to 30°C (59°F to 89°F). Protect from light. Once foil pack is opened, ampules should be used within 7 days. Following transfer of solution to inhalation device, solution should remain in device for no more than 24 hours; discard unused portion.

Mechanism of Action Treprostinil is a direct vasodilator of both pulmonary and systemic arterial vascular beds; also inhibits platelet aggregation.

Pharmacodynamics/Kinetics

Absorption: SubQ: Rapidly and completely

Distribution: 14 L/70 kg ideal body weight

Protein binding: 91%

Metabolism: Hepatic (primarily by CYP2C8); forms 5 inactive metabolites (HU1-HU5)

Bioavailability: Inhalation: 64% to 72% (dose-dependent); SubQ: 100%

Half-life elimination: Terminal: ~4 hours

Excretion: Urine (79%; 4% as unchanged drug, 64% as metabolites); feces (13%)

Dosage Pulmonary arterial hypertension (PAH):

Children: SubQ; I.V. infusion: Limited experience in patients ≤16 years of age.

Adults:

Inhalation: **Note:** Prior to initiation, patients should be carefully evaluated for ability to administer treprostinil and care for the inhalation system and accessories required for administration. Immediate access to a back-up inhalation device, accessories, and medication is essential to prevent treatment interruptions.

Initial: 18 mcg (or 3 inhalations) every 4 hours 4 times/day; if 3 inhalations are not tolerated, reduce to 1-2 inhalations, then increase to 3 inhalations as tolerated

Maintenance: If tolerated, increase dose by an additional 3 inhalations at approximately 1- to 2-week intervals; target dose and maximum dose: 54 mcg (or 9 inhalations) 4 times/day

SubQ (preferred) or I.V. infusion: **Note:** Prior to initiation, patients should be carefully evaluated for ability to administer treprostinil and care for the infusion system outside of inpatient setting. Immediate access to a back-up pump, infusion sets, and medication is essential to prevent treatment interruptions.

New to prostacyclin therapy: Initial: 1.25 ng/kg/minute; if dose cannot be tolerated due to systemic effects, reduce to 0.625 ng/kg/minute. Increase dose in increments of 1.25 ng/kg/minute per week for first 4 weeks, followed by increments of 2.5 ng/kg/minute per week for remainder of therapy. Limited experience with doses >40 ng/kg/minute. **Note:** Dose must be carefully and individually titrated (symptom improvement with minimal adverse effects). Avoid abrupt withdrawal. If infusion is restarted within a few hours of discontinuation, the same dose rate may be used. Interruptions for longer periods may require retitration.

Transitioning from epoprostenol (see table): **Note:** Transition should occur in a hospital setting to follow response (eg, walking distance, sign/symptoms of disease progression). May take 24-48 hours to transition. Transition is accomplished by initiating the infusion of treprostinil, and increasing it while simultaneously reducing the dose of intravenous epoprostenol. During transition, increases in PAH symptoms should be first treated with an increase in treprostinil dose. Occurrence of prostacyclin associated side effects should be treated by decreasing the dose of epoprostenol.

Transitioning From I.V. Epoprostenol to SubQ (Preferred) or I.V. Treprostinil

Step	Epoprostenol Dose	Treprostinil Dose
1	Maintain current dose	Initiate at 10% initial epoprostenol dose
2	Decrease to 80% initial dose	Increase to 30% initial epoprostenol dose
3	Decrease to 60% initial dose	Increase to 50% initial epoprostenol dose
4	Decrease to 40% initial dose	Increase to 70% initial epoprostenol dose
5	Decrease to 20% initial dose	Increase to 90% initial epoprostenol dose
6	Decrease to 5% initial dose	Increase to 110% initial epoprostenol dose
7	Discontinue epoprostenol	Maintain current dose plus additional 5% to 10% as needed

Elderly: Refer to adult dosing. Limited experience in patients ≥65 years; use caution.

Dosage adjustment in renal impairment: Titrate slowly in patients with renal impairment

Dosage adjustment in hepatic impairment:

Mild-to-moderate: Use with caution and titrate slowly in patients with hepatic impairment

SubQ; I.V. infusion: Initial: 0.625 ng/kg/minute (ideal body weight)

Severe: Has not been studied in patients with severe hepatic impairment

Administration Regardless of administration route (inhalation, I.V., or SubQ), treatment interruptions or rapid large dosage reductions should be avoided. Immediate access to medication, a back-up inhalation device, or pump and infusion sets is essential to prevent treatment interruptions.

Inhalation: Do not mix with other medications. For inhalation only via the Tyvaso™ Inhalation System; consists of the Optineb-ir Model ON-100/7 (an ultrasonic, pulsed-delivery device) and accessories. Prior to the first treatment session of each day, transfer the entire contents of one ampule into the medicine chamber; one ampule contains sufficient volume of medication for all 4 treatment sessions in a single day. Between each session, the device should be capped and stored upright with the remaining medication inside. At the end of each day, the medicine chamber and any remaining medication must be discarded. Avoid contact of solution with eyes or skin; wash hands after handling.

I.V. infusion: I.V. use is recommended when SubQ infusion is not tolerated or when the benefit outweighs the potential risks of an indwelling central venous catheter. Solution must be diluted in SWFI, NS, or Flolan® sterile diluent prior to use and administered by continuous infusion using a central indwelling catheter and infusion pump. The ambulatory infusion pump should be small and lightweight; have occlusion/no delivery, low battery, programming error, and motor malfunction alarms; have ± 6% accuracy of the programmed rate; and be positive pressure driven. The reservoir should be made of polyvinyl chloride, polypropylene, or glass. Peripheral infusion may be used temporarily until central line is established.

SubQ infusion (preferred): Administer undiluted via continuous SubQ infusion using an appropriately-designed infusion pump. The ambulatory infusion pump should be small and lightweight; be able to adjust infusion rates in ~0.002 mL/hour increments; have occlusion/no delivery, low battery, programming error, and motor malfunction alarms; have ± 6% accuracy of the programmed rate; and be positive pressure driven. The reservoir should be made of polyvinyl chloride, polypropylene, or glass. Infusion site reactions may be helped by moving the infusion site every 3 days, local application of topical hot and cold packs, topical or oral analgesics. Injection site pain and erythema may improve after several months of treprostinil therapy.

Monitoring Parameters BP, dyspnea, fatigue, activity tolerance, symptoms of excessive dose (eg, headache, nausea, vomiting)

Dosage Forms Excipient information presented when available (limited, particularly for generics); consult specific product labeling.

Injection, solution:

Remodulin®: 1 mg/mL (20 mL); 2.5 mg/mL (20 mL); 5 mg/mL (20 mL) [contains sodium chloride 5.3 mg/mL]

Remodulin®: 10 mg/mL (20 mL) [contains sodium chloride 4 mg/mL]

Solution, for oral inhalation:

Tyvaso™: 0.6 mg/mL (2.9 mL) [delivers ~6 mcg/inhalation]

◆ **Treprostinil Sodium** *see* Treprostinil *on page 1727*

◆ **Tretin-X™** *see* Tretinoin (Topical) *on page 1731*

◆ **Tretinoin and Clindamycin** *see* Clindamycin and Tretinoin *on page 382*

◆ **Tretinoin, Fluocinolone Acetonide, and Hydroquinone** *see* Fluocinolone, Hydroquinone, and Tretinoin *on page 727*

Tretinoin (Systemic) (TRET i noyn, sis TEM ik)

Brand Names: Canada Vesanoid®

Index Terms *trans* Vitamin A Acid; *trans*-Retinoic Acid; All-*trans* Retinoic Acid; All-*trans* Vitamin A Acid; ATRA; Ro 5488; tRA; Tretinoinum; Vesanoid

Pharmacologic Category Antineoplastic Agent, Miscellaneous; Retinoic Acid Derivative

Use Induction of remission in patients with acute promyelocytic leukemia (APL), French American British (FAB) classification M3 (including the M3 variant) characterized by t(15;17) translocation and/or PML/RARα gene presence

Unlabeled Use Post consolidation and maintenance therapy in APL; combination therapy (with arsenic trioxide) for remission induction in APL

Pregnancy Risk Factor D

Pregnancy Considerations **[U.S. Boxed Warning]: High risk of teratogenicity; if treatment with tretinoin is required in women of childbearing potential, two reliable forms of contraception should be used during and for 1 month after treatment.** Within 1 week prior to starting therapy, serum or urine pregnancy test (sensitivity 50 mIU/mL) should be collected. If possible, delay therapy until results are available. Repeat pregnancy testing and contraception counseling monthly throughout the period of treatment. An increase in fetal resorptions and a decrease in live fetuses were observed in all animal studies; teratogenic effects have also been observed. Use in humans is limited, however, major fetal abnormalities and spontaneous abortions have been reported with other retinoids. If the clinical condition of a patient presenting with APL during pregnancy warrants immediate treatment, tretinoin use should be avoided in the first trimester; treatment with tretinoin may be considered in the second and third trimester with careful fetal cardiac monitoring.

Lactation Excretion in breast milk unknown/not recommended

Contraindications Hypersensitivity to tretinoin, other retinoids, parabens, or any component of the formulation

Warnings/Precautions Hazardous agent - use appropriate precautions for handling and disposal.

[U.S. Boxed Warning]: About 25% of patients with APL treated with tretinoin have experienced APL differentiation syndrome (formerly called retinoic-acid-APL [RA-APL] syndrome), which is characterized by fever, dyspnea, acute respiratory distress, weight gain, radiographic pulmonary infiltrates and pleural or pericardial effusions, edema, and hepatic, renal, and/or multiorgan failure. DS usually occurs during the first month of treatment, with some cases reported following the first dose. DS has been observed with or without concomitant leukocytosis and has occasionally been accompanied by impaired myocardial contractility and episodic hypotension; endotracheal intubation and mechanical ventilation have been required in some cases due to progressive hypoxemia, and several patients have expired with multiorgan failure. About one-half of DS cases are severe, which is associated with increased mortality. Management has not been defined, although high-dose steroids given at the first suspicion appear to reduce morbidity and mortality. Regardless of the leukocyte count, at the first signs suggestive of DS, immediately initiate steroid therapy with dexamethasone 10 mg I.V. every 12 hours for 3-5 days; taper off over 2 weeks. Most patients do not require termination of tretinoin therapy during treatment of DS.

[U.S. Boxed Warning]: During treatment, ~40% of patients will develop rapidly evolving leukocytosis. A high WBC at diagnosis increases the risk for further leukocytosis and may be associated with a higher risk of life-threatening complications. If signs and symptoms of the APL-DS syndrome are present together with leukocytosis, initiate treatment with high-dose steroids immediately. Consider adding full-dose chemotherapy (including an anthracycline, if not contraindicated) to the tretinoin therapy on day 1 or 2 for patients presenting with a WBC count of $>5 \times 10^9$/L. Consider adding chemotherapy immediately in patients who presented with a WBC count of $<5 \times 10^9$/L, yet the WBC count reaches $\geq 6 \times 10^9$/L by day 5, or $\geq 10 \times 10^9$/L by day 10, or $\geq 15 \times 10^9$/L by day 28.

[U.S. Boxed Warning]: High risk of teratogenicity; if treatment with tretinoin is required in women of childbearing potential, two reliable forms of contraception should be used during and for 1 month after treatment. Repeat pregnancy testing and contraception counseling monthly throughout the period of treatment. If possible, initiation of treatment with tretinoin should be delayed until negative pregnancy test result is confirmed.

Retinoids have been associated with pseudotumor cerebri (benign intracranial hypertension), especially in children. Concurrent use of other drugs associated with this effect (eg, tetracyclines) may increase risk. Early signs and symptoms include papilledema, headache, nausea, vomiting, visual disturbances, intracranial noises, or pulsate tinnitus.

Up to 60% of patients experienced hypercholesterolemia or hypertriglyceridemia, which were reversible upon completion of treatment. Venous thrombosis and MI have been reported in patient without risk factors for thrombosis or MI;

the risk for thrombosis (arterial and venous) is increased during the first month of treatment. Use with caution with antifibrinolytic agents; thrombotic complications have been reported (rarely) with concomitant use. Elevated liver function test results occur in 50% to 60% of patients during treatment. Carefully monitor liver function test results during treatment and give consideration to a temporary withdrawal of tretinoin if test results reach >5 times the upper limit of normal. Most liver function test abnormalities will resolve without interruption of treatment or after therapy completion. May cause headache, malaise, and/or dizziness; caution patients about performing tasks which require mental alertness (eg, operating machinery or driving). Patients with APL are at high risk and can have severe adverse reactions to tretinoin. **[U.S. Boxed Warning]: Should be administered under the supervision of an experienced cancer chemotherapy physician.** Tretinoin treatment for APL should be initiated early, discontinue if pending cytogenetic analysis does not confirm APL by t(15;17) translocation or the presence of the PML/RARα fusion protein (caused by translocation of the promyelocytic [PML] gene on chromosome 15 and retinoic acid receptor [RAR] alpha gene on chromosome 17).

Adverse Reactions Most patients will experience drug-related toxicity, especially headache, fever, weakness, and fatigue. These are seldom permanent or irreversible and do not typically require therapy interruption.

>10%:

Cardiovascular: Peripheral edema (52%), chest discomfort (32%), edema (29%), arrhythmias (23%), flushing (23%), hypotension (14%), hypertension (11%)

Central nervous system: Headache (86%), fever (83%), malaise (66%), pain (37%), dizziness (20%), anxiety (17%), depression (14%), insomnia (14%), confusion (11%)

Dermatologic: Skin/mucous membrane dryness (77%), rash (54%), pruritus (20%), alopecia (14%), skin changes (14%)

Endocrine & metabolic: Hypercholesterolemia and/or hypertriglyceridemia (≤60%)

Gastrointestinal: Nausea/vomiting (57%), GI hemorrhage (34%), abdominal pain (31%), mucositis (26%), diarrhea (23%), weight gain (23%), anorexia (17%), constipation (17%), weight loss (17%), dyspepsia (14%), abdominal distention (11%)

Hematologic: Hemorrhage (60%), leukocytosis (40%), disseminated intravascular coagulation (DIC) (26%)

Hepatic: Liver function tests increased (50% to 60%)

Local: Phlebitis (11%)

Neuromuscular & skeletal: Bone pain (77%), paresthesia (17%), myalgia (14%)

Ocular: Ocular disorder (17%), visual disturbances (17%)

Otic: Earache/ear fullness (23%)

Renal: Renal insufficiency (11%)

Respiratory: Upper respiratory tract disorders (63%), dyspnea (60%), respiratory insufficiency (26%), pleural effusion (20%), expiratory wheezing (14%), pneumonia (14%), rales (14%)

Miscellaneous: Shivering (63%), infections (58%), retinoic acid-acute promyelocytic leukemia syndrome differentiation syndrome (≤25%), diaphoresis (20%)

1% to 10%:

Cardiovascular: Cerebral hemorrhage (9%), cardiac failure (6%), facial edema (6%), pallor (6%), cardiac arrest (3%), cardiomyopathy (3%), heart enlarged (3%), heart murmur (3%), ischemia (3%), MI (3%), myocarditis (3%), pericarditis (3%), stroke (3%)

Central nervous system: Agitation (9%), intracranial hypertension (9%), hallucination (6%), aphasia (3%), cerebellar edema (3%), CNS depression (3%), coma (3%), dementia (3%), encephalopathy (3%), facial paralysis (3%), forgetfulness (3%), hypotaxia (3%), hypothermia (3%), light reflex absent (3%), seizure (3%), slow speech (3%), somnolence (3%), spinal cord disorder (3%), unconsciousness (3%)

Dermatologic: Cellulitis (8%)

Endocrine & metabolic: Fluid imbalance (6%), acidosis (3%)

Gastrointestinal: Hepatosplenomegaly (9%), ulcer (3%)

Genitourinary: Dysuria (9%), micturition frequency (3%), prostate enlarged (3%)

Hepatic: Ascites (3%), hepatitis (3%)

Neuromuscular & skeletal: Flank pain (9%), abnormal gait (3%), asterixis (3%), bone inflammation (3%), dysarthria (3%), hemiplegia (3%), hyporeflexia (3%), leg weakness (3%), tremor (3%)

Ocular: Visual acuity change (6%), agnosia (3%), visual field deficit (3%)

Otic: Hearing loss (6%)

Renal: Acute renal failure (3%), renal tubular necrosis (3%)

Respiratory: Lower respiratory tract disorders (9%), pulmonary infiltration (6%), bronchial asthma (3%), larynx edema (3%), pulmonary hypertension (3%)

Miscellaneous: Lymph disorder (6%)

<1% (Limited to important or life-threatening): Arterial thrombosis, basophilia, erythema nodosum, genital ulceration, hypercalcemia, hyperhistaminemia, irreversible hearing loss, myositis, organomegaly, pancreatitis, pseudotumor cerebri, renal infarct, Sweet's syndrome, thrombocytosis, vasculitis (skin), venous thrombosis

Drug Interactions

Metabolism/Transport Effects Substrate of CYP2A6 (minor), CYP2B6 (minor), CYP2C8 (major), CYP2C9 (minor); **Note:** Assignment of Major/Minor substrate status based on clinically relevant drug interaction potential; **Inhibits** CYP2C9 (weak); **Induces** CYP2E1 (weak/moderate)

Avoid Concomitant Use

Avoid concomitant use of Tretinoin (Systemic) with any of the following: BCG; Natalizumab; Pimecrolimus; Tacrolimus (Topical); Tetracycline Derivatives; Vaccines (Live); Vitamin A

Increased Effect/Toxicity

Tretinoin (Systemic) may increase the levels/effects of: Antifibrinolytic Agents; Leflunomide; Natalizumab; Porfimer; Vaccines (Live); Vitamin A

The levels/effects of Tretinoin (Systemic) may be increased by: CYP2C8 Inhibitors (Moderate); CYP2C8 Inhibitors (Strong); Deferasirox; Denosumab; Pimecrolimus; Roflumilast; Tacrolimus (Topical); Tetracycline Derivatives; Trastuzumab

Decreased Effect

Tretinoin (Systemic) may decrease the levels/effects of: BCG; Coccidioidin Skin Test; Contraceptives (Estrogens); Contraceptives (Progestins); Sipuleucel-T; Vaccines (Inactivated); Vaccines (Live)

The levels/effects of Tretinoin (Systemic) may be decreased by: CYP2C8 Inducers (Strong); Echinacea

Ethanol/Nutrition/Herb Interactions

Ethanol: Avoid ethanol (may increase CNS depression).

Food: Absorption of retinoids has been shown to be enhanced when taken with food.

Herb/Nutraceutical: St John's wort may decrease tretinoin levels. Avoid dong quai, St John's wort (may also cause photosensitization). Avoid additional vitamin A supplementation; may lead to vitamin A toxicity.

Stability Store capsule at 15°C to 30°C (59°F to 86°F). Protect from light.

Mechanism of Action Tretinoin appears to bind one or more nuclear receptors and decreases proliferation and induces differentiation of APL cells; initially produces maturation of primitive promyelocytes and repopulates the marrow and peripheral blood with normal hematopoietic cells to achieve complete remission

Pharmacodynamics/Kinetics

Absorption: Well absorbed

Protein binding: >95%, predominantly to albumin

Metabolism: Hepatic via CYP; primary metabolite: 4-oxo-all-*trans*-retinoic acid; displays autometabolism

Half-life elimination: Terminal: Parent drug: 0.5-2 hours

Time to peak, serum: 1-2 hours

Excretion: Urine (63%); feces (30%)

Dosage Details concerning dosing in combination regimens should also be consulted. **Note:** Induction treatment of APL with tretinoin should be initiated early; discontinue if pending cytogenetic analysis does not confirm t(15;17) translocation or the presence of the PML/RARα fusion protein.

Oral: Children and Adults: APL:

Remission induction: 45 mg/m^2/day in 2 equally divided doses until documentation of complete remission (CR); discontinue 30 days after CR or after 90 days of treatment, whichever occurs first

Remission induction (in combination with an anthracycline; unlabeled use):

Children: 25 mg/m^2/day in 2 equally divided doses until complete remission or 90 days (Ortega, 2005)

Adults: 45 mg/m^2/day in 2 equally divided doses until complete remission or 90 days (Sanz, 2004; Sanz, 2008)

Consolidation therapy, intermediate- and high-risk patients (unlabeled use):

Children: 25 mg/m^2/day in 2 equally divided doses for 15 days each month for 3 months (Ortega, 2005)

Adults: 45 mg/m^2/day in 2 equally divided doses for 15 days each month for 3 months (Sanz, 2004)

Maintenance therapy, intermediate- and high-risk patients (unlabeled use):

Children: 25 mg/m^2/day in 2 equally divided doses for 15 days every 3 months for 2 years (Ortega, 2005)

Adults: 45 mg/m^2/day in 2 equally divided doses for 15 days every 3 months for 2 years (Sanz, 2004)

Dosage adjustment for toxicity:

APL differentiation syndrome: Initiate dexamethasone 10 mg I.V. every 12 hours for 3-5 days; consider interrupting tretinoin until resolution of hypoxia

Liver function tests >5 times the upper limit of normal: Consider temporarily withholding treatment

Dietary Considerations The absorption of retinoids (as a class) is enhanced when taken with food. Capsule contains soybean oil.

Administration Administer orally with a meal; do not crush capsules.

Although the manufacturer does not recommend the use of the capsule contents to extemporaneously prepare tretinoin suspension, there are limited case reports of use in patients who are unable to swallow the capsules whole. In a patient with a nasogastric (NG) tube, tretinoin capsules were cut open, with partial aspiration of the contents into a glass syringe, the residual capsule contents were mixed with soy bean oil and aspirated into the same syringe and administered (Shaw, 1995). Tretinoin capsules have also been mixed with sterile water (~20 mL) and heated in a water bath (37°C) to melt the capsules and create an oily suspension for NG tube administration (Bargetzi, 1996). Tretinoin has also been administered sublingually by squeezing the capsule contents beneath the tongue (Kueh, 1999). Low plasma concentrations have been reported when tretinoin has been administered through a feeding tube, although patient-specific impaired absorption or a lack of excipient (eg, soybean oil) may have been a contributing factor (Takitani, 2004).

Monitoring Parameters Bone marrow cytology to confirm t(15;17) translocation or the presence of the PML/RARα fusion protein (do not withhold treatment initiation for results); monitor CBC with differential, coagulation profile, liver function test results, and triglyceride and cholesterol levels frequently; monitor closely for signs of APL differentiation syndrome (eg, monitor volume status, pulmonary status, temperature, respiration)

Dosage Forms Excipient information presented when available (limited, particularly for generics); consult specific product labeling.

Capsule, oral: 10 mg

Extemporaneous Preparations Hazardous agent: Use appropriate precautions for handling and disposal.

Although the manufacturer does not recommend the use of the capsule contents to extemporaneously prepare a suspension of tretinoin (due to reports of low plasma levels) (Vesanoid® data on file), there are limited case reports of use in patients who are unable to swallow the capsules whole. In a patient with a nasogastric (NG) tube, tretinoin capsules were cut open, with partial aspiration of the contents aspirated into a glass syringe. The residual capsule contents were mixed with soybean oil, aspirated into the syringe, and administered (Shaw, 1995). Tretinoin capsules have also been mixed with sterile water (~20 mL) and heated in a water bath to melt the capsules and create an oily suspension for NG tube administration (Bargetzi, 1996). Tretinoin has also been administered sublingually by squeezing the capsule contents beneath the tongue (Kueh, 1999).

Bargetzi MJ, Tichelli A, Gratwohl A, et al, "Oral All-Transretinoic Acid Administration in Intubated Patients With Acute Promyelocytic Leukemia," *Schweiz Med Wochenschr*, 1996, 126(45):1944-5.

Kueh YK, Liew PP, Ho PC, et al, "Sublingual Administration of All-*Trans*-Retinoic Acid to a Comatose Patient With Acute Promyelocytic Leukemia," *Ann Pharmacother*, 1999, 33(4):503-5.

Shaw PJ, Atkins MC, Nath CE, et al, "ATRA Administration in the Critically Ill Patient," *Leukemia*, 1995, 9(7):1288.

Vesanoid® data on file, Roche Pharmaceuticals

Tretinoin (Topical) (TRET i noyn, TOP i kal)

Brand Names: U.S. Atralin™; Avita®; Refissa™; Renova®; Retin-A Micro®; Retin-A®; Tretin-X™

Brand Names: Canada Rejuva-A®; Renova®; Retin-A Micro®; Retin-A®; Retinova®; Stieva-A

Index Terms *trans*-Retinoic Acid; Retinoic Acid; Vitamin A Acid

Pharmacologic Category Acne Products; Retinoic Acid Derivative; Topical Skin Product, Acne

Use Treatment of acne vulgaris; photodamaged skin; palliation of fine wrinkles, mottled hyperpigmentation, and tactile roughness of facial skin as part of a comprehensive skin care and sun avoidance program

Unlabeled Use Some skin cancers

Pregnancy Risk Factor C

Pregnancy Considerations Oral tretinoin is teratogenic and fetotoxic in rats at doses 1000 and 500 times the topical human dose, respectively. Tretinoin does not appear to be teratogenic when used topically since it is rapidly metabolized by the skin; however, there are rare reports of fetal defects. Use for acne only if benefit to mother outweighs potential risk to fetus. During pregnancy, do not use for palliation of fine wrinkles, mottled hyperpigmentation, and tactile roughness of facial skin.

Lactation Enters breast milk/compatible

Contraindications Hypersensitivity to tretinoin or any component of the formulation; sunburn

Warnings/Precautions Use with caution in patients with eczema; avoid excessive exposure to sunlight and sunlamps; avoid contact with abraded skin, sunburned skin, mucous membranes, eyes, mouth, angles of the nose. Treatment can increase skin sensitivity to weather extremes of wind or cold. Also, concomitant topical medications (eg, medicated or abrasive soaps, cleansers, or cosmetics with a strong drying effect) should be used with caution due to increased skin irritation. Palliation of fine wrinkles, mottled hyperpigmentation, and tactile roughness of facial skin: Do not use the 0.05% cream for longer than 48 weeks or the 0.02% cream for longer than 52 weeks. Not for use on moderate- to heavily-pigmented skin. Gel is flammable; do not expose to high temperatures or flame. Safety and efficacy have not been established in children <12 years of age.

Adverse Reactions

>10%: Dermatologic: Excessive dryness, erythema, scaling of the skin, pruritus

1% to 10%:

Dermatologic: Hyperpigmentation or hypopigmentation, photosensitivity, initial acne flare-up

Local: Edema, blistering, stinging

Drug Interactions

Metabolism/Transport Effects None known.

Avoid Concomitant Use There are no known interactions where it is recommended to avoid concomitant use.

Increased Effect/Toxicity

Tretinoin (Topical) may increase the levels/effects of: Porfimer

Decreased Effect

Tretinoin (Topical) may decrease the levels/effects of: Contraceptives (Progestins)

Ethanol/Nutrition/Herb Interactions

Food: Avoid excessive intake of vitamin A (cod liver oil, halibut fish oil).

Herb/Nutraceutical: Avoid dong quai, St John's wort (may also cause photosensitization). Avoid excessive amounts of vitamin A supplements.

Stability Store at 25°C (77°F). Gel is flammable; keep away from heat and flame.

Mechanism of Action Keratinocytes in the sebaceous follicle become less adherent which allows for easy removal; inhibits microcomedone formation and eliminates lesions already present

Pharmacodynamics/Kinetics

Absorption: Minimal

Metabolism: Hepatic for the small amount absorbed

Excretion: Urine and feces

Dosage Topical:

Children >12 years and Adults: Acne vulgaris: Begin therapy with a weaker formulation of tretinoin (0.025% cream, 0.04% microsphere gel, or 0.01% gel) and increase the concentration as tolerated; apply once daily to acne lesions before retiring or on alternate days; if stinging or irritation develop, decrease frequency of application

Adults ≥18: Palliation of fine wrinkles, mottled hyperpigmentation, and tactile roughness of facial skin: Pea-sized amount of the 0.02% or 0.05% cream applied to entire face once daily in the evening

Elderly: Use of the 0.02% cream in patients 65-71 years of age showed similar improvement in fine wrinkles as seen in patients <65 years. Safety and efficacy of the 0.02% cream have not been established in patients >71 years of age. Safety and efficacy of the 0.05% cream have not been established in patients >50 years of age.

Administration Palliation of fine wrinkles, mottled hyperpigmentation, and tactile roughness of facial skin: Cream: Prior to application, gently wash face with a mild soap. Pat dry. Wait 20-30 minutes to apply cream. Avoid eyes, ears, nostrils, and mouth.

Dosage Forms Excipient information presented when available (limited, particularly for generics); consult specific product labeling.

Cream, topical: 0.025% (20 g, 45 g); 0.05% (20 g, 45 g); 0.1% (20 g, 45 g)

Avita®: 0.025% (20 g, 45 g)

Refissa™: 0.05% (40 g)

Renova®: 0.02% (40 g, 44 g, 60 g) [contains benzyl alcohol]

Retin-A®: 0.025% (20 g, 45 g); 0.05% (20 g, 45 g); 0.1% (20 g, 45 g)

Tretin-X™: 0.025% (35 g) [kit includes cleanser and moisturizer]

Tretin-X™: 0.0375% (35 g)

Tretin-X™: 0.05% (35 g); 0.1% (35 g) [kit includes cleanser and moisturizer]

Gel, topical: 0.01% (15 g, 45 g); 0.025% (15 g, 45 g)

Atralin™: 0.05% (45 g) [contains benzyl alcohol, fish collagen]

Avita®: 0.025% (20 g, 45 g) [contains ethanol 83%]

Retin-A®: 0.01% (15 g, 45 g); 0.025% (15 g, 45 g) [contains ethanol 90% w/w]

Tretin-X™: 0.01% (35 g); 0.025% (35 g) [contains ethanol 90% w/w; kit includes cleanser and moisturizer]

Gel, topical [microsphere gel]:

Retin-A Micro®: 0.04% (20 g, 45 g, 50 g); 0.1% (20 g, 45 g, 50 g) [contains benzyl alcohol]

◆ **Tretinoinum** *see* Tretinoin (Systemic) *on page* [illegible]

◆ **Trexall™** *see* Methotrexate *on page 1098*

◆ **Treximet™** *see* Sumatriptan and Naproxen *on page 1612*

◆ **Triacetyluridine** *see* Uridine Triacetate *on page 1750*

◆ **Triaconazole** *see* Terconazole *on page 1651*

◆ **Triaderm (Can)** *see* Triamcinolone (Topical) *on page 1735*

Triamcinolone (Systemic) (trye am SIN oh lone)

Brand Names: U.S. Aristospan®; Kenalog®-10; Kenalog®-40

Brand Names: Canada Aristospan®

Index Terms Triamcinolone Acetonide, Parenteral; Triamcinolone Hexacetonide

Pharmacologic Category Corticosteroid, Systemic

Additional Appendix Information

Corticosteroids *on page 1888*

Use

Intra-articular (soft tissue): Acute gouty arthritis, acute/subacute bursitis, acute tenosynovitis, epicondylitis, rheumatoid arthritis, synovitis of osteoarthritis

Intralesional: Alopecia areata, discoid lupus erythematosus, keloids, granuloma annulare lesions (localized hypertrophic, infiltrated, or inflammatory), lichen planus plaques, lichen simplex chronicus plaques, psoriatic plaques, necrobiosis lipoidica diabeticorum, cystic tumors of aponeurosis or tendon (ganglia)

Systemic: Adrenocortical insufficiency, dermatologic diseases, endocrine disorders, gastrointestinal diseases, hematologic and neoplastic disorders, nervous system disorders, nephrotic syndrome, rheumatic disorders, allergic states, respiratory diseases, systemic lupus erythematosus (SLE), and other diseases requiring anti-inflammatory or immunosuppressive effects

Pregnancy Risk Factor C

Pregnancy Considerations Triamcinolone was shown to be teratogenic in animal reproduction studies. Some studies have shown an association between first trimester corticosteroid use and oral clefts; adverse events in the fetus/neonate have been noted in case reports following large doses of systemic corticosteroids during pregnancy.

Lactation Excretion in breast milk unknown/use caution

Contraindications Hypersensitivity to triamcinolone or any component of the formulation; systemic fungal infections; cerebral malaria; idiopathic thrombocytopenic purpura (I.M. injection)

Warnings/Precautions May cause hypercorticism or suppression of hypothalamic-pituitary-adrenal (HPA) axis, particularly in younger children or in patients receiving high doses for prolonged periods. HPA axis suppression may lead to adrenal crisis. Withdrawal and discontinuation of a corticosteroid should be done slowly and carefully.

Acute myopathy has been reported with high-dose corticosteroids, usually in patients with neuromuscular transmission disorders; may involve ocular and/or respiratory muscles; monitor creatine kinase; recovery may be delayed. Corticosteroid use may cause psychiatric disturbances, including depression, euphoria, insomnia, mood swings, and personality changes. Pre-existing psychiatric conditions may be exacerbated by corticosteroid use. Prolonged use of corticosteroids may also increase the incidence of secondary infection, mask acute infection (including fungal infections), prolong or exacerbate viral infections, or limit response to vaccines. Exposure to chickenpox should be avoided; corticosteroids should not be used to treat ocular herpes simplex. Corticosteroids should not be used for cerebral malaria or viral hepatitis. Close observation is required in patients with latent tuberculosis and/or TB reactivity; restrict use in active TB (only in conjunction with antituberculosis treatment). Use with caution in patients with threadworm infection; may cause serious hyperinfection. Prolonged treatment with corticosteroids has been associated with the development of Kaposi's sarcoma (case reports); if noted, discontinuation of therapy should be considered. Avoid use in head injury patients.

Use with caution in patients with thyroid disease, hepatic impairment, renal impairment, cardiovascular disease, diabetes, myasthenia gravis, patients at risk for osteoporosis, patients at risk for seizures, or GI diseases (diverticulitis, peptic ulcer, ulcerative colitis) due to perforation risk. Avoid use in head injury patients. Use caution following acute MI (corticosteroids have been associated with myocardial rupture). Because of the risk of adverse effects, systemic corticosteroids should be used cautiously in the elderly in the smallest possible effective dose for the shortest duration. Patients should not be immunized with live, viral vaccines while receiving immunosuppressive doses of corticosteroids. The ability to respond to dead viral vaccines is unknown.

Withdraw therapy with gradual tapering of dose. There have been reports of systemic corticosteroid withdrawal symptoms (eg, joint/muscle pain, lassitude, depression) when withdrawing oral inhalation therapy. Injection suspension contains benzyl alcohol; benzyl alcohol has been associated with the "gasping syndrome" in neonates and low-birth-weight infants. Administer products only via recommended route (depending on product used). Do **not** administer any triamcinolone product via the epidural or intrathecal route; serious adverse events, including fatalities, have been reported.

Adverse Reactions Frequency not defined; reactions reported with corticosteroid therapy in general:

Cardiovascular: Arrhythmia, bradycardia, cardiac arrest, cardiac enlargement, CHF, circulatory collapse, edema, hypertension, hypertrophic cardiomyopathy (premature infants), myocardial rupture (following recent MI), syncope, tachycardia, thromboembolism, vasculitis

Central nervous system: Arachnoiditis (I.T.), depression, emotional instability, euphoria, headache, insomnia, intracranial pressure increased, malaise, meningitis (I.T.), mood changes, neuritis, neuropathy, personality change, pseudotumor cerebri (with discontinuation), seizure, spinal cord infarction, stroke, vertigo

Dermatologic: Abscess (sterile), acne, allergic dermatitis, angioedema, atrophy (cutaneous/subcutaneous), bruising, dry skin, erythema, hair thinning, hirsutism, hyper-/hypopigmentation, hypertrichosis, impaired wound healing, lupus erythematosus-like lesions, petechiae, purpura, rash, skin test suppression, striae, thin skin

Endocrine & metabolic: Carbohydrate intolerance, Cushingoid state, diabetes mellitus, fluid retention, glucose intolerance, growth suppression (children), hypokalemia, hypokalemic alkalosis, menstrual irregularities, negative nitrogen balance, sodium retention, sperm motility altered

Gastrointestinal: Abdominal distention, appetite increased, GI hemorrhage, GI perforation, nausea, pancreatitis, peptic ulcer, ulcerative esophagitis, weight gain

Hepatic: Hepatomegaly, liver function tests increased

Local: Thrombophlebitis

Neuromuscular & skeletal: Aseptic necrosis of femoral and humeral heads, calcinosis, Charcot-like arthropathy, fractures, joint tissue damage, muscle mass loss, myopathy, osteoporosis, parasthesia, paraplegia, quadriplegia, tendon rupture, vertebral compression fractures, weakness

Ocular: Cataracts, cortical blindness, exophthalmos, glaucoma, ocular pressure increased, papilledema

Renal: Glycosuria

Respiratory: Pulmonary edema

Miscellaneous: Abnormal fat deposits, anaphylactoid reaction, anaphylaxis, diaphoresis, hiccups, infection, moon face

Drug Interactions

Metabolism/Transport Effects None known.

Avoid Concomitant Use

Avoid concomitant use of Triamcinolone (Systemic) with any of the following: Aldesleukin; BCG; Natalizumab; Pimecrolimus; Tacrolimus (Topical)

Increased Effect/Toxicity

Triamcinolone (Systemic) may increase the levels/effects of: Acetylcholinesterase Inhibitors; Amphotericin B; Deferasirox; Leflunomide; Loop Diuretics; Natalizumab; NSAID (COX-2 Inhibitor); NSAID (Nonselective); Thiazide Diuretics; Vaccines (Live); Warfarin

The levels/effects of Triamcinolone (Systemic) may be increased by: Antifungal Agents (Azole Derivatives, Systemic); Aprepitant; Calcium Channel Blockers (Nondihydropyridine); Denosumab; Estrogen Derivatives; Fluconazole; Fosaprepitant; Indacaterol; Macrolide Antibiotics; Neuromuscular-Blocking Agents (Nondepolarizing); Pimecrolimus; Quinolone Antibiotics; Roflumilast; Salicylates; Tacrolimus (Topical); Telaprevir; Trastuzumab

Decreased Effect

Triamcinolone (Systemic) may decrease the levels/effects of: Aldesleukin; Antidiabetic Agents; BCG; Calcitriol; Coccidioidin Skin Test; Corticorelin; Isoniazid; Salicylates; Sipuleucel-T; Telaprevir; Vaccines (Inactivated)

The levels/effects of Triamcinolone (Systemic) may be decreased by: Aminoglutethimide; Barbiturates; Echinacea; Mitotane; Primidone; Rifamycin Derivatives

Stability Injection, suspension:

Acetonide injectable suspension: Kenalog®: Store at 20°C to 25°C (68°F to 77°F); avoid freezing. Protect from light.

Hexacetonide injectable suspension: Store at 20°C to 25°C (68°F to 77°F); avoid freezing. Protect from light. Avoid diluents containing parabens, phenol, or other preservatives (may cause flocculation). Diluted suspension stable up to 1 week. Suspension for intralesional use may be diluted with D_5NS, $D_{10}NS$, NS, or SWFI to a 1:1,

1:2, or 1:4 concentration. Solutions for intra-articular use, may be diluted with lidocaine 1% or 2%.

Mechanism of Action Decreases inflammation by suppression of migration of polymorphonuclear leukocytes and reversal of increased capillary permeability; suppresses the immune system by reducing activity and volume of the lymphatic system; suppresses adrenal function at high doses

Pharmacodynamics/Kinetics

Distribution: V_d: 99.5 L

Protein binding: ~68%

Half-life elimination: Biologic: 18-36 hours

Time to peak: I.M.: 8-10 hours

Excretion: Urine (~40%); feces (~60%)

Dosage The lowest possible dose should be used to control the condition; when dose reduction is possible, the dose should be reduced gradually.

Injection:

Acetonide:

Intra-articular, intrabursal, tendon sheaths: Adults: Initial: Smaller joints: 2.5-5 mg, larger joints: 5-15 mg; may require up to 10 mg for small joints and up to 40 mg for large joints; maximum dose/treatment (several joints at one time): 20-80 mg

Intradermal: Adults: Initial: 1 mg

I.M.: Range: 2.5-100 mg/day

Children: Initial: 0.11-1.6 mg/kg/day in 3-4 divided doses

Children 6-12 years: Initial: 40 mg

Children >12 years and Adults: Initial: 60 mg

Hay fever/pollen asthma: 40-100 mg as a single injection/season

Multiple sclerosis (acute exacerbation): 160 mg daily for 1 week, followed by 64 mg every other day for 1 month

Hexacetonide: Adults:

Intralesional, sublesional: Up to 0.5 mg/square inch of affected skin; range: 2-48 mg/day

Intra-articular: Average dose: 2-20 mg; smaller joints: 2-6 mg; larger joints: 10-20 mg. Frequency of injection into a single joint is every 3-4 weeks as necessary; to avoid possible joint destruction use as infrequently as possible.

Triamcinolone Dosing

	Acetonide	Hexacetonide
Intrasynovial	5-40 mg	
Intralesional	1-30 mg (usually 1 mg per injection site); 10 mg/mL suspension usually used	Up to 0.5 mg/sq inch affected area
Sublesional	1-30 mg	
Systemic I.M.	2.5-60 mg/dose (usual adult dose: 60 mg; may repeat with 20-100 mg dose when symptoms recur)	
Intra-articular	2.5-40 mg	2-20 mg average
large joints	5-15 mg	10-20 mg
small joints	2.5-5 mg	2-6 mg
Tendon sheaths	2.5-10 mg	
Intradermal	1 mg/site	

Dietary Considerations Ensure adequate intake of calcium and vitamins (or consider supplementation) in patients on medium-to-high doses of systemic corticosteroids.

Administration Shake well before use to ensure suspension is uniform. Inspect visually to ensure no clumping; administer immediately after withdrawal so settling does not occur in the syringe. Do **not** administer any product I.V. or via the epidural or intrathecal route.

Aristospan® (20 mg/mL concentration): For intra-articular and soft tissue administration only; a ≥23-gauge needle is preferred.

Aristospan® (5 mg/mL concentration): For intralesional or sublesional administration only; a ≥23-gauge needle is preferred.

Kenalog®-10 injection: For intra-articular or intralesional administration only. When administered intralesionally, inject directly into the lesion (ie, intradermally or subcutaneously). Tuberculin syringes with a 23- to 25-gauge needle are preferable for intralesional injections.

Kenalog®-40 injection: For intra-articular, soft tissue or I.M. administration. When administered I.M., inject deep into the gluteal muscle using a minimum needle length of 1½ inches for adults. Obese patients may require a longer needle. Alternate sites for subsequent injections.

Dosage Forms Excipient information presented when available (limited, particularly for generics); consult specific product labeling.

Injection, suspension, as acetonide:

Kenalog®-10: 10 mg/mL (5 mL) [contains benzyl alcohol, polysorbate 80; **not** for I.V., I.M., intraocular, epidural, or intrathecal use]

Kenalog®-40: 40 mg/mL (1 mL, 5 mL, 10 mL) [contains benzyl alcohol, polysorbate 80; **not** for I.V., intradermal, intraocular, epidural, or intrathecal use]

Injection, suspension, as hexacetonide:

Aristospan®: 5 mg/mL (5 mL); 20 mg/mL (1 mL, 5 mL) [contains benzyl alcohol, polysorbate 80; **not** for I.V. use]

Triamcinolone (Nasal) (trye am SIN oh lone)

Brand Names: U.S. Nasacort® AQ

Brand Names: Canada Nasacort® AQ; Trinasal®

Index Terms Triamcinolone acetonide

Pharmacologic Category Corticosteroid, Nasal

Use Management of seasonal and perennial allergic rhinitis

Pregnancy Risk Factor C

Dosage Intranasal: Perennial allergic rhinitis, seasonal allergic rhinitis:

Nasal spray:

Children 2-5 years: 110 mcg/day as 1 spray in each nostril once daily (maximum: 110 mcg/day)

Children 6-11 years: Initial: 110 mcg/day as 1 spray in each nostril once daily; may increase to 220 mcg/day as 2 sprays in each nostril if response not adequate; once symptoms controlled may reduce to 110 mcg/day

Children ≥12 years and Adults: 220 mcg/day as 2 sprays in each nostril once daily; once symptoms controlled reduce to 110 mcg/day

Nasal inhaler:

Children 6-11 years: Initial: 220 mcg/day as 2 sprays in each nostril once daily

Children ≥12 years and Adults: Initial: 220 mcg/day as 2 sprays in each nostril once daily; may increase dose to 440 mcg/day (given once daily or divided and given 2 or 4 times/day)

Additional Information Complete prescribing information for this medication should be consulted for additional detail.

Dosage Forms Excipient information presented when available (limited, particularly for generics); consult specific product labeling.

Suspension, intranasal, as acetonide [spray]: 55 mcg/inhalation (16.5 g)

Nasacort® AQ: 55 mcg/inhalation (16.5 g) [chlorofluorocarbon free; contains benzalkonium chloride; 120 actuations]

Triamcinolone (Ophthalmic)

(trye am SIN oh lone)

Brand Names: U.S. Triesence™
Index Terms Triamcinolone acetonide
Pharmacologic Category Corticosteroid, Ophthalmic
Additional Appendix Information
Corticosteroids *on page 1888*
Use
Intavitreal: Treatment of sympathetic ophthalmia, temporal arteritis, uveitis, ocular inflammatory conditions unresponsive to topical corticosteroids
Triesence™: Visualization during vitrectomy
Pregnancy Risk Factor D
Dosage Ophthalmic injection: Intravitreal: Children and Adults:
Ocular disease: Initial: 4 mg as a single dose; additional doses may be given as needed over the course of treatment
Visualization during vitrectomy (Triesence™): 1-4 mg
Additional Information Complete prescribing information for this medication should be consulted for additional detail.
Dosage Forms Excipient information presented when available (limited, particularly for generics); consult specific product labeling.
Injection, suspension, ophthalmic, as acetonide:
Triesence™: 40 mg/mL (1 mL) [contains polysorbate 80; not for I.V. use]

Triamcinolone (Topical) (trye am SIN oh lone)

Brand Names: U.S. Kenalog®; Oralone®; Pediaderm™ TA; Trianex™; Triderm®; Zytopic™
Brand Names: Canada Kenalog®; Oracort; Triaderm
Pharmacologic Category Corticosteroid, Topical
Additional Appendix Information
Corticosteroids *on page 1888*
Use
Oral topical: Adjunctive treatment and temporary relief of symptoms associated with oral inflammatory lesions and ulcerative lesions resulting from trauma
Topical: Inflammatory dermatoses responsive to steroids
Pregnancy Risk Factor C
Dosage
Oral topical: Oral inflammatory lesions/ulcers: Press a small dab (about 1/4 inch) to the lesion until a thin film develops. A larger quantity may be required for coverage of some lesions. For optimal results use only enough to coat the lesion with a thin film; do not rub in.

Topical:
Cream, Ointment:
0.025% or 0.05%: Apply thin film to affected areas 2-4 times/day
0.1% or 0.5%: Apply thin film to affected areas 2-3 times/day
Spray: Apply to affected area 3-4 times/day
Additional Information Complete prescribing information for this medication should be consulted for additional detail.
Dosage Forms Excipient information presented when available (limited, particularly for generics); consult specific product labeling.
Aerosol, spray, topical, as acetonide:
Kenalog®: 0.2 mg/2-second spray (63 g, 100 g) [contains dehydrated ethanol 10.3%]
Cream, topical, as acetonide: 0.025% (15 g, 80 g, 454 g); 0.1% (15 g, 30 g, 80 g, 454 g); 0.5% (15 g)
Triderm®: 0.1% (30 g, 85 g)
Cream, topical, as acetonide [kit]:
Pediaderm™ TA: 0.1% (30 g) [packaged with protective emollient]
Zytopic™: 0.1% (85 g) [packaged with cleanser and moisturizer]
Lotion, topical, as acetonide: 0.025% (60 mL); 0.1% (60 mL)
Ointment, topical, as acetonide: 0.025% (15 g, 80 g, 454 g); 0.05% (430 g); 0.1% (15 g, 80 g, 454 g); 0.5% (15 g)
Trianex™: 0.05% (17 g, 85 g)
Paste, oral topical, as acetonide: 0.1% (5 g)
Oralone®: 0.1% (5 g)

- ◆ **Triamcinolone acetonide** *see* Triamcinolone (Nasal) *on page 1734*
- ◆ **Triamcinolone acetonide** *see* Triamcinolone (Ophthalmic) *on page 1735*
- ◆ **Triamcinolone Acetonide, Parenteral** *see* Triamcinolone (Systemic) *on page 1732*
- ◆ **Triamcinolone and Nystatin** *see* Nystatin and Triamcinolone *on page 1226*
- ◆ **Triamcinolone Hexacetonide** *see* Triamcinolone (Systemic) *on page 1732*
- ◆ **Triaminic® Children's Chest & Nasal Congestion [OTC]** *see* Guaifenesin and Phenylephrine *on page 812*
- ◆ **Triaminic™ Children's Fever Reducer Pain Reliever [OTC]** *see* Acetaminophen *on page 27*
- ◆ **Triaminic® Children's Night Time Cold & Cough [OTC]** *see* Diphenhydramine and Phenylephrine *on page 518*
- ◆ **Triaminic® Children's Softchews® Cough & Runny Nose [OTC]** *see* Dextromethorphan and Chlorpheniramine *on page 489*
- ◆ **Triaminic® Children's Thin Strips® Night Time Cold & Cough [OTC]** *see* Diphenhydramine and Phenylephrine *on page 518*
- ◆ **Triaminic® Cold & Allergy (Can)** *see* Chlorpheniramine and Pseudoephedrine *on page 346*
- ◆ **Triaminic® Cold and Allergy [OTC]** *see* Chlorpheniramine and Phenylephrine *on page 345*
- ◆ **Triaminic® Day Time Cold & Cough [OTC]** *see* Dextromethorphan and Phenylephrine *on page 490*
- ◆ **Triaminic Thin Strips® Children's Cold with Stuffy Nose [OTC]** *see* Phenylephrine (Systemic) *on page 1344*
- ◆ **Triaminic Thin Strips® Children's Cough & Runny Nose [OTC]** *see* DiphenhydrAMINE (Systemic) *on page 516*
- ◆ **Triaminic Thin Strips® Children's Day Time Cold & Cough [OTC]** *see* Dextromethorphan and Phenylephrine *on page 490*

Triamterene (trye AM ter een)

Brand Names: U.S. Dyrenium®
Pharmacologic Category Diuretic, Potassium-Sparing
Use Alone or in combination with other diuretics in treatment of edema and hypertension; decreases potassium excretion caused by kaliuretic diuretics
Pregnancy Risk Factor C
Dosage Oral:
Children (unlabeled use): Hypertension: Initial: 1-2 mg/kg/day in 2 divided doses; maximum: 3-4 mg/kg/day, up to 300 mg/day
Adults: Hypertension, edema: 100-300 mg/day in 1-2 divided doses; maximum dose: 300 mg/day; usual dosage range (JNC 7): 50-100 mg/day

Elderly: Hypertension: Consider lower initial doses and titrate to response (Aronow, 2011)

Dosing comments in renal impairment: Cl_{cr} <10 mL/minute: Avoid use.

Dosing adjustment in hepatic impairment: Dose reduction is recommended in patients with cirrhosis.

Additional Information Complete prescribing information for this medication should be consulted for additional detail.

Dosage Forms Excipient information presented when available (limited, particularly for generics); consult specific product labeling.

Capsule, oral:

Dyrenium®: 50 mg, 100 mg

- **Triamterene and Hydrochlorothiazide** *see* Hydrochlorothiazide and Triamterene *on page 836*
- **Trianex™** *see* Triamcinolone (Topical) *on page 1735*
- **Triatec-8 (Can)** *see* Acetaminophen and Codeine *on page 30*
- **Triatec-8 Strong (Can)** *see* Acetaminophen and Codeine *on page 30*
- **Triatec-30 (Can)** *see* Acetaminophen and Codeine *on page 30*

Triazolam (trye AY zoe lam)

Brand Names: U.S. Halcion®

Brand Names: Canada Apo-Triazo®; Gen-Triazolam; Halcion®; Mylan-Triazolam

Pharmacologic Category Hypnotic, Benzodiazepine

Additional Appendix Information

Beers Criteria – Potentially Inappropriate Medications for Geriatrics *on page 1973*

Benzodiazepines *on page 1882*

Use Short-term treatment of insomnia

Unlabeled Use Treatment of anxiety before dental procedures

Pregnancy Risk Factor X

Medication Guide Available Yes

Dosage Oral (onset of action is rapid, patient should be in bed when taking medication):

Children <18 years: Dosage not established

Adults:

Insomnia (short-term): 0.125-0.25 mg at bedtime (maximum dose: 0.5 mg/day)

Preprocedure sedation (unlabeled use): 0.25 mg taken the evening before oral surgery; or 0.25 mg 1 hour before procedure

Elderly: Insomnia (short-term use): Initial: 0.125 mg at bedtime; maximum dose: 0.25 mg/day

Dosing adjustment/comments in hepatic impairment: Reduce dose or avoid use in cirrhosis

Additional Information Complete prescribing information for this medication should be consulted for additional detail.

Dosage Forms Excipient information presented when available (limited, particularly for generics); consult specific product labeling.

Tablet, oral: 0.125 mg, 0.25 mg

Halcion®: 0.25 mg [scored]

Controlled Substance C-IV

- **Tri-B® [OTC]** *see* Folic Acid, Cyanocobalamin, and Pyridoxine *on page 749*
- **Tribavirin** *see* Ribavirin *on page 1479*
- **Tribenzor™** *see* Olmesartan, Amlodipine, and Hydrochlorothiazide *on page 1238*
- **Tri-Buffered Aspirin [OTC]** *see* Aspirin *on page 154*
- **Tricardio B** *see* Folic Acid, Cyanocobalamin, and Pyridoxine *on page 749*
- **Trichloroacetaldehyde Monohydrate** *see* Chloral Hydrate *on page 336*
- **Tricitrates** *see* Citric Acid, Sodium Citrate, and Potassium Citrate *on page 372*
- **Tricode® GF** *see* Guaifenesin, Pseudoephedrine, and Codeine *on page 813*
- **TriCor®** *see* Fenofibrate *on page 693*
- **Tricosal** *see* Choline Magnesium Trisalicylate *on page 351*
- **Tri-Cyclen® (Can)** *see* Ethinyl Estradiol and Norgestimate *on page 663*
- **Tri-Cyclen® Lo (Can)** *see* Ethinyl Estradiol and Norgestimate *on page 663*
- **Triderm®** *see* Triamcinolone (Topical) *on page 1735*
- **Tridil** *see* Nitroglycerin *on page 1212*
- **Tridural™ (Can)** *see* TraMADol *on page 1715*
- **Trien** *see* Trientine *on page 1736*

Trientine (TRYE en teen)

Brand Names: U.S. Syprine®

Brand Names: Canada Syprine®

Index Terms 2,2,2-tetramine; Trien; Trientine Hydrochloride; Triethylene Tetramine Dihydrochloride

Pharmacologic Category Chelating Agent

Use Treatment of Wilson's disease in patients intolerant to penicillamine

Pregnancy Risk Factor C

Dosage Oral:

Children <12 years: 500-750 mg/day in divided doses 2-4 times/day; maximum: 1.5 g/day. AASLD practice guidelines suggest 20 mg/kg/day rounded off to the nearest 250 mg, given in 2-3 divided doses (Roberts, 2008).

Children ≥12 years and Adults: 750-1250 mg/day in divided doses 2-4 times/day; maximum dose: 2 g/day. AASLD practice guidelines suggest typical doses of 750-1500 mg/day in 2-3 divided doses with maintenance therapy of 750-1000 mg/day (Roberts, 2008).

Additional Information Complete prescribing information for this medication should be consulted for additional detail.

Dosage Forms Excipient information presented when available (limited, particularly for generics); consult specific product labeling.

Capsule, oral, as hydrochloride:

Syprine®: 250 mg

- **Trientine Hydrochloride** *see* Trientine *on page 1736*
- **Triesence™** *see* Triamcinolone (Ophthalmic) *on page 1735*
- **Triethylene Tetramine Dihydrochloride** *see* Trientine *on page 1736*
- **Triethylenethiophosphoramide** *see* Thiotepa *on page 1674*

Trifluoperazine (trye floo oh PER a zeen)

Brand Names: Canada Apo-Trifluoperazine®; Novo-Trifluzine; PMS-Trifluoperazine; Terfluzine

Index Terms Trifluoperazine Hydrochloride

Pharmacologic Category Antipsychotic Agent, Typical, Phenothiazine

Additional Appendix Information

Antipsychotic Agents *on page 1880*

Use Treatment of schizophrenia; short-term treatment of generalized nonpsychotic anxiety

Unlabeled Use Management of psychotic disorders; behavioral symptoms associated with dementia behavior (elderly); psychosis/agitation related to Alzheimer's dementia

Pregnancy Considerations Adverse events were not observed in animal reproduction studies, except when using doses that were also maternally toxic. Jaundice or hyper-/hyporeflexia have been reported in newborn infants following maternal use of phenothiazines. Antipsychotic use during the third trimester of pregnancy has a risk for abnormal muscle movements (extrapyramidal symptoms [EPS]) and withdrawal symptoms in newborns following delivery. Symptoms in the newborn may include agitation, feeding disorder, hypertonia, hypotonia, respiratory distress, somnolence, and tremor; these effects may be self-limiting or require hospitalization.

Lactation Enters breast milk/not recommended (AAP rates "of concern"; AAP 2001 update pending)

Contraindications Hypersensitivity to trifluoperazine or any component of the formulation (cross-reactivity between phenothiazines may occur); severe CNS depression; bone marrow suppression; blood dyscrasias; severe hepatic disease; coma

Warnings/Precautions [U.S. Boxed Warning]: Elderly patients with dementia-related psychosis treated with antipsychotics are at an increased risk of death compared to placebo. Most deaths appeared to be either cardiovascular (eg, heart failure, sudden death) or infectious (eg, pneumonia) in nature. Trifluoperazine is not approved for the treatment of dementia-related psychosis.

Leukopenia, neutropenia, and agranulocytosis (sometimes fatal) have been reported in clinical trials and postmarketing reports with antipsychotic use; presence of risk factors (eg, pre-existing low WBC or history of drug-induced leuko-/neutropenia) should prompt periodic blood count assessment. Discontinue therapy at first signs of blood dyscrasias or if absolute neutrophil count <1000/mm^3.

May be sedating, use with caution in disorders where CNS depression is a feature. Use with caution in Parkinson's disease. Caution in patients with hemodynamic instability; predisposition to seizures; subcortical brain damage; severe cardiac or renal disease. Liver damage and jaundice of the cholestatic type of hepatitis have been reported with use; use is contraindicated in patients with pre-existing hepatic disease. Esophageal dysmotility and aspiration have been associated with antipsychotic use - use with caution in patients at risk of pneumonia (ie, Alzheimer's disease). Use associated with increased prolactin levels; clinical significance of hyperprolactinemia in patients with breast cancer or other prolactin-dependent tumors is unknown. May alter temperature regulation or mask toxicity of other drugs due to antiemetic effects. May alter cardiac conduction - life-threatening arrhythmias have occurred with therapeutic doses of phenothiazines. May cause orthostatic hypotension - use with caution in patients at risk of this effect or those who would tolerate transient hypotensive episodes (cerebrovascular disease, cardiovascular disease or other medications which may predispose).

Due to anticholinergic effects, should be used with caution in patients with decreased gastrointestinal motility, urinary retention, BPH, xerostomia, visual problems, narrow-angle glaucoma, and myasthenia gravis. Relative to other antipsychotics, trifluoperazine has a low potency of cholinergic blockade.

May cause extrapyramidal symptoms (EPS), including pseudoparkinsonism, acute dystonic reactions, akathisia, and tardive dyskinesia. Risk of dystonia (and possibly other EPS) may be greater with increased doses, use of conventional antipsychotics, males, and younger patients. Use caution in the elderly. May be associated with neuroleptic malignant syndrome (NMS) or pigmentary retinopathy.

Adverse Reactions Frequency not defined.

Cardiovascular: Cardiac arrest, hypotension, orthostatic hypotension

Central nervous system: Dizziness; extrapyramidal symptoms (akathisia, dystonias, pseudoparkinsonism, tardive dyskinesia); headache, impairment of temperature regulation, lowering of seizure threshold, neuroleptic malignant syndrome (NMS)

Dermatologic: Discoloration of skin (blue-gray), increased sensitivity to sun, photosensitivity, rash

Endocrine & metabolic: Breast pain, galactorrhea, gynecomastia, hyperglycemia, hypoglycemia, lactation, libido (changes in), menstrual cycle (changes in)

Gastrointestinal: Constipation, nausea, stomach pain, vomiting, weight gain, xerostomia

Genitourinary: Difficulty in urination, ejaculatory disturbances, priapism, urinary retention

Hematologic: Agranulocytosis, aplastic anemia, eosinophilia, hemolytic anemia, leukopenia, pancytopenia, thrombocytopenic purpura

Hepatic: Cholestatic jaundice, hepatotoxicity

Neuromuscular & skeletal: Tremor

Ocular: Cornea and lens changes, pigmentary retinopathy

Respiratory: Nasal congestion

Drug Interactions

Metabolism/Transport Effects Substrate of CYP1A2 (major); **Note:** Assignment of Major/Minor substrate status based on clinically relevant drug interaction potential

Avoid Concomitant Use

Avoid concomitant use of Trifluoperazine with any of the following: Metoclopramide

Increased Effect/Toxicity

Trifluoperazine may increase the levels/effects of: Alcohol (Ethyl); Analgesics (Opioid); Anticholinergics; Antidepressants (Serotonin Reuptake Inhibitor/Antagonist); Anti-Parkinson's Agents (Dopamine Agonist); Beta-Blockers; CNS Depressants; Methotrimeprazine; Methylphenidate; Porfimer; Serotonin Modulators

The levels/effects of Trifluoperazine may be increased by: Abiraterone Acetate; Acetylcholinesterase Inhibitors (Central); Antidepressants (Serotonin Reuptake Inhibitor/Antagonist); Antimalarial Agents; Beta-Blockers; CYP1A2 Inhibitors (Moderate); CYP1A2 Inhibitors (Strong); Deferasirox; Droperidol; HydrOXYzine; Lithium formulations; Methotrimeprazine; Methylphenidate; Metoclopramide; Pramlintide; Tetrabenazine

Decreased Effect

Trifluoperazine may decrease the levels/effects of: Amphetamines; Quinagolide

The levels/effects of Trifluoperazine may be decreased by: Antacids; Anti-Parkinson's Agents (Dopamine Agonist); CYP1A2 Inducers (Strong); Cyproterone; Lithium formulations

Ethanol/Nutrition/Herb Interactions

Ethanol: May increase CNS depression; monitor for increased effects with coadministration. Caution patients about effects.

Herb/Nutraceutical: Avoid kava kava, gotu kola, valerian, St John's wort (may increase CNS depression). Avoid dong quai, St John's wort (may also cause photosensitization).

Mechanism of Action Trifluoperazine is a piperazine phenothiazine antipsychotic which blocks postsynaptic mesolimbic dopaminergic receptors in the brain; exhibits alpha-adrenergic blocking effect and depresses the release of hypothalamic and hypophyseal hormones

Pharmacodynamics/Kinetics

Metabolism: Extensively hepatic

Half-life elimination: >24 hours with chronic use

Dosage Oral:
Children 6-12 years: Schizophrenia/psychoses: Hospitalized or well-supervised patients: Initial: 1 mg 1-2 times/day, gradually increase until symptoms are controlled or adverse effects become troublesome; maximum: 15 mg/day
Adults:
Schizophrenia/psychoses:
Outpatients: 1-2 mg twice daily
Hospitalized or well-supervised patients: Initial: 2-5 mg twice daily with optimum response in the 15-20 mg/day range; do not exceed 40 mg/day
Nonpsychotic anxiety: 1-2 mg twice daily; maximum: 6 mg/day; therapy for anxiety should not exceed 12 weeks; do not exceed 6 mg/day for longer than 12 weeks when treating anxiety; agitation, jitteriness, or insomnia may be confused with original neurotic or psychotic symptoms
Elderly:
Schizophrenia/psychoses: Refer to adult dosing. Dose selection should start at the low end of the dosage range and titration must be gradual.
Behavioral symptoms associated with dementia behavior (unlabeled use): Initial: 0.5-1 mg 1-2 times/day; increase dose at 4- to 7-day intervals by 0.5-1 mg/day; increase dosing intervals (bid, tid, etc) as necessary to control response or side effects. Maximum daily dose: 40 mg. Gradual increases (titration) may prevent some side effects or decrease their severity.
Hemodialysis: Not dialyzable (0% to 5%)

Dietary Considerations May be taken with food to decrease GI distress.

Monitoring Parameters Vital signs; lipid profile, fasting blood glucose/Hgb A_{1c}; BMI; mental status, abnormal involuntary movement scale (AIMS)

Reference Range Therapeutic response and blood levels have not been established

Test Interactions False-positive for phenylketonuria

Additional Information Do not exceed 6 mg/day for longer than 12 weeks when treating anxiety. Agitation, jitteriness, or insomnia may be confused with original neurotic or psychotic symptoms.

Dosage Forms Excipient information presented when available (limited, particularly for generics); consult specific product labeling.
Tablet, oral: 1 mg, 2 mg, 5 mg, 10 mg

◆ **Trifluoperazine Hydrochloride** *see* Trifluoperazine *on page 1736*

◆ **Trifluorothymidine** *see* Trifluridine *on page 1738*

Trifluridine (trye FLURE i deen)

Brand Names: U.S. Viroptic®

Brand Names: Canada Sandoz-Trifluridine; Viroptic®

Index Terms F_3T; Trifluorothymidine

Pharmacologic Category Antiviral Agent, Ophthalmic

Use Treatment of primary keratoconjunctivitis and recurrent epithelial keratitis caused by herpes simplex virus types I and II

Pregnancy Risk Factor C

Dosage Adults: Instill 1 drop into affected eye every 2 hours while awake, to a maximum of 9 drops/day, until re-epithelialization of corneal ulcer occurs; then use 1 drop every 4 hours for another 7 days; do **not** exceed 21 days of treatment; if improvement has not taken place in 7-14 days, consider another form of therapy

Additional Information Complete prescribing information for this medication should be consulted for additional detail.

Dosage Forms Excipient information presented when available (limited, particularly for generics); consult specific product labeling.
Solution, ophthalmic [drops]: 1% (7.5 mL)
Viroptic®: 1% (7.5 mL)

◆ **Triglide®** *see* Fenofibrate *on page 693*

◆ **Trihexyphen (Can)** *see* Trihexyphenidyl *on page 1738*

Trihexyphenidyl (trye heks ee FEN i dil)

Brand Names: Canada PMS-Trihexyphenidyl; Trihexyphen; Trihexyphenidyl

Index Terms Artane; Benzhexol Hydrochloride; Trihexyphenidyl Hydrochloride

Pharmacologic Category Anti-Parkinson's Agent, Anticholinergic; Anticholinergic Agent

Additional Appendix Information
Antiparkinsonian Agents *on page 1879*

Use Adjunctive treatment of Parkinson's disease; treatment of drug-induced extrapyramidal symptoms

Lactation Excretion in breast milk unknown/use caution

Contraindications There are no contraindications listed within the manufacturer's labeling.

Warnings/Precautions Use with caution in hot weather or during exercise, especially when administered concomitantly with other atropine-like drugs to chronically-ill patients, alcoholics, patients with CNS disease, or persons doing manual labor in a hot environment. Use with caution in patients with cardiovascular disease (including hypertension), glaucoma, prostatic hyperplasia or any tendency toward urinary retention, liver or kidney disorders, and obstructive disease of the GI tract. May exacerbate mental symptoms when used to treat extrapyramidal symptoms. When given in large doses or to susceptible patients, may cause weakness. May impair physical or mental abilities; patients must be cautioned about performing tasks which require mental alertness (eg, operating machinery or driving). Does not improve symptoms of tardive dyskinesias. Elderly patients require strict dosage regulation.

Adverse Reactions Frequency not defined.
Cardiovascular: Tachycardia
Central nervous system: Agitation, confusion, delusions, dizziness, drowsiness, euphoria, hallucinations, headache, nervousness, paranoia, psychiatric disturbances
Dermatologic: Rash
Gastrointestinal: Constipation, dilatation of colon, ileus, nausea, parotitis, vomiting, xerostomia
Genitourinary: Urinary retention
Neuromuscular & skeletal: Weakness
Ocular: Blurred vision, glaucoma, intraocular pressure increased, mydriasis

Drug Interactions

Metabolism/Transport Effects None known.

Avoid Concomitant Use There are no known interactions where it is recommended to avoid concomitant use.

Increased Effect/Toxicity
Trihexyphenidyl may increase the levels/effects of: AbobotulinumtoxinA; Anticholinergics; Cannabinoids; OnabotulinumtoxinA; Potassium Chloride; RimabotulinumtoxinB

The levels/effects of Trihexyphenidyl may be increased by: Pramlintide

Decreased Effect
Trihexyphenidyl may decrease the levels/effects of: Acetylcholinesterase Inhibitors (Central); Secretin

The levels/effects of Trihexyphenidyl may be decreased by: Acetylcholinesterase Inhibitors (Central)

Ethanol/Nutrition/Herb Interactions Ethanol: Avoid ethanol (may increase CNS depression).

Stability Store at 20°C to 25°C (68°F to 77°F).

Mechanism of Action Exerts a direct inhibitory effect on the parasympathetic nervous system. It also has a relaxing effect on smooth musculature; exerted both directly on the muscle itself and indirectly through parasympathetic nervous system (inhibitory effect)

Pharmacodynamics/Kinetics

Metabolism: Hydroxylation of the alicyclic groups

Half-life elimination: 33 hours

Time to peak, serum: 1.3 hours

Excretion: Urine and bile

Dosage Oral:

Adults:

Parkinson's disease: Initial: 1 mg/day, increase by 2 mg increments at intervals of 3-5 days; usual dose: 6-10 mg/day in 3-4 divided doses; doses of 12-15 mg/day may be required

Drug-induced EPS: Initial: 1 mg/day; increase as necessary to usual range: 5-15 mg/day in 3-4 divided doses

Use in combination with levodopa: Usual range: 3-6 mg/day in divided doses

Elderly: Parkinson's disease: Refer to adult dosing. **Note:** Conservative initial doses and gradual titration is especially important in patients >60 years of age.

Dietary Considerations May be taken before or after meals; tolerated best if given with food.

Administration May be administered before or after meals; tolerated best if given in 3 daily doses and with food. High doses (>10 mg/day) may be divided into 4 doses, at meal times and at bedtime.

Monitoring Parameters IOP monitoring and gonioscopic evaluations should be performed periodically

Additional Information Incidence and severity of side effects are dose related. Patients may be switched to sustained-action capsules when stabilized on conventional dosage forms.

Dosage Forms Excipient information presented when available (limited, particularly for generics); consult specific product labeling.

Elixir, oral, as hydrochloride: 2 mg/5 mL (473 mL)

Tablet, oral, as hydrochloride: 2 mg, 5 mg

- ◆ **Trihexyphenidyl Hydrochloride** *see* Trihexyphenidyl *on page 1738*
- ◆ **TriHIBit® [DSC]** *see* Diphtheria and Tetanus Toxoids, Acellular Pertussis, and *Haemophilus influenzae* b Conjugate Vaccine *on page 522*
- ◆ **Trilafon** *see* Perphenazine *on page 1336*
- ◆ **Tri-Legest™ Fe** *see* Ethinyl Estradiol and Norethindrone *on page 660*
- ◆ **Trileptal®** *see* OXcarbazepine *on page 1262*
- ◆ **TriLipix®** *see* Fenofibric Acid *on page 695*
- ◆ **Trilisate** *see* Choline Magnesium Trisalicylate *on page 351*
- ◆ **Tri-Luma®** *see* Fluocinolone, Hydroquinone, and Tretinoin *on page 727*
- ◆ **TriLyte®** *see* Polyethylene Glycol-Electrolyte Solution *on page 1372*

Trimethobenzamide (trye meth oh BEN za mide)

Brand Names: U.S. Tigan®

Brand Names: Canada Tigan®

Index Terms Trimethobenzamide Hydrochloride

Pharmacologic Category Antiemetic

Additional Appendix Information

Beers Criteria – Potentially Inappropriate Medications for Geriatrics *on page 1973*

Use Treatment of postoperative nausea and vomiting; treatment of nausea associated with gastroenteritis

Pregnancy Considerations Teratogenic effects were not observed in animal studies. Safety and efficacy have not been established in pregnant patients. Trimethobenzamide has been used to treat nausea and vomiting of pregnancy.

Lactation Excretion in breast milk unknown

Contraindications Hypersensitivity to trimethobenzamide or any component of the formulation; injection contraindicated in children

Warnings/Precautions May mask emesis due to Reye's syndrome or mimic CNS effects of Reye's syndrome in patients with emesis of other etiologies. Antiemetic effects may mask toxicity of other drugs or conditions (eg, intestinal obstruction). May cause drowsiness; patient should avoid tasks requiring alertness (eg, driving, operating machinery). May cause extrapyramidal symptoms (EPS) which may be confused with CNS symptoms of primary disease responsible for emesis. May be inappropriate for use in the elderly due to the risk of EPS adverse effects combined with lower efficacy, as compared to other antiemetics (Beers Criteria). Risk of CNS adverse effects (eg, coma, EPS, seizure) may be increased in patients with acute febrile illness, dehydration, electrolyte imbalance, encephalitis, or gastroenteritis; use caution. Allergic-type skin reactions have been reported with use; discontinue with signs of sensitization. Trimethobenzamide clearance is predominantly renal; dosage reductions may be recommended in patient with renal impairment. Use capsule formulation with caution in children; antiemetics are not recommended for uncomplicated vomiting in children, limit antiemetic use to prolonged vomiting of known etiology. Use of injection is contraindicated in children.

Adverse Reactions Frequency not defined.

Cardiovascular: Hypotension (I.V. administration)

Central nervous system: Coma, depression, disorientation, dizziness, drowsiness, EPS, headache, Parkinson-like symptoms, seizure

Dermatologic: Allergic-type skin reactions

Gastrointestinal: Diarrhea

Hematologic: Blood dyscrasias

Hepatic: Jaundice

Local: Injection site burning, pain, redness, stinging, or swelling

Neuromuscular & skeletal: Muscle cramps, opisthotonos

Ocular: Blurred vision

Miscellaneous: Hypersensitivity reactions

Drug Interactions

Metabolism/Transport Effects None known.

Avoid Concomitant Use There are no known interactions where it is recommended to avoid concomitant use.

Increased Effect/Toxicity

Trimethobenzamide may increase the levels/effects of: AbobotulinumtoxinA; Anticholinergics; Cannabinoids; OnabotulinumtoxinA; Potassium Chloride; RimabotulinumtoxinB

The levels/effects of Trimethobenzamide may be increased by: Pramlintide

Decreased Effect

Trimethobenzamide may decrease the levels/effects of: Acetylcholinesterase Inhibitors (Central); Secretin

The levels/effects of Trimethobenzamide may be decreased by: Acetylcholinesterase Inhibitors (Central)

Ethanol/Nutrition/Herb Interactions Ethanol: Concomitant use should be avoided (sedative effects may be additive).

Stability Store capsules and injection solution at room temperature of 25°C (77°F); excursions permitted to 15°C to 30°C (59°F to 86°F).

Mechanism of Action Acts centrally to inhibit the medullary chemoreceptor trigger zone by blocking emetic impulses to the vomiting center

Pharmacodynamics/Kinetics
Onset of action: Antiemetic: Oral: 10-40 minutes; I.M.: 15-35 minutes
Duration: 3-4 hours
Metabolism: Via oxidation, forms metabolite trimethobenzamide N-oxide
Bioavailability: Oral: 60% to 100%
Half-life elimination: 7-9 hours
Time to peak: Oral: ~45 minutes; I.M.: ~30 minutes
Excretion: Urine (30% to 50%, as unchanged drug)

Dosage
Children >40 kg: Oral: 300 mg 3-4 times/day
Adults:
Oral: 300 mg 3-4 times/day
I.M.: 200 mg 3-4 times/day
Postoperative nausea and vomiting (PONV): I.M.: 200 mg, followed 1 hour later by a second 200 mg dose
Elderly: Refer to adult dosing. Consider dosage reduction or increasing dosing interval in elderly patients with renal impairment (specific adjustment guidelines are not provided in the manufacturer's labeling).

Dosage adjustment in renal impairment: Cl_{cr} ≤70 mL/minute: Consider dosage reduction or increasing dosing interval (specific adjustment guidelines are not provided in the manufacturer's labeling)

Administration
Injection: Administer I.M. only; not for I.V. administration. Inject deep into upper outer quadrant of gluteal muscle.
Capsule: Administer capsule orally without regard to meals.

Monitoring Parameters Renal function (at baseline)

Dosage Forms Excipient information presented when available (limited, particularly for generics); consult specific product labeling. [DSC] = Discontinued product
Capsule, oral, as hydrochloride: 300 mg
Tigan®: 300 mg
Injection, solution, as hydrochloride: 100 mg/mL (2 mL [DSC])
Tigan®: 100 mg/mL (20 mL)
Injection, solution, as hydrochloride [preservative free]:
Tigan®: 100 mg/mL (2 mL)

◆ **Trimethobenzamide Hydrochloride** *see* Trimethobenzamide *on page 1739*

Trimethoprim (trye METH oh prim)

Brand Names: U.S. Primsol®
Brand Names: Canada Apo-Trimethoprim®
Index Terms TMP
Pharmacologic Category Antibiotic, Miscellaneous
Use Treatment of urinary tract infections due to susceptible strains of *E. coli*, *P. mirabilis*, *K. pneumoniae*, *Enterobacter* spp and coagulase-negative *Staphylococcus* including *S. saprophyticus*; acute otitis media due to susceptible strains of *S. pneumoniae* and *H. influenzae* in children
Unlabeled Use Alternative agent for *Pneumocystis jirovecii* pneumonia (in combination with dapsone)
Pregnancy Risk Factor C
Pregnancy Considerations Because adverse effects have been observed in animals, trimethoprim is classified pregnancy category C. Trimethoprim crosses the placenta and can be detected in the fetal serum and amniotic fluid. Due to trimethoprim's potential effect on folic acid metabolism, TMP should only be used during pregnancy if the benefit justifies the potential risk. The use of dihydrofolate reductase inhibitors, including trimethoprim, during pregnancy may increase the risk of congenital anomalies including cardiovascular defects, oral clefts, urinary tract anomalies, and neural tube defects. Folic acid supplementation may decrease this risk. The majority of studies evaluating the effects of trimethoprim administration in pregnancy have been conducted with sulfamethoxazole/trimethoprim. Trimethoprim in combination with sulfamethoxazole is used in pregnancy for various indications (see the Sulfamethoxazole and Trimethoprim monograph for details).
Lactation Enters breast milk/use caution
Contraindications Hypersensitivity to trimethoprim or any component of the formulation; megaloblastic anemia due to folate deficiency
Warnings/Precautions Use with caution in patients with impaired renal or hepatic function or with possible folate deficiency. Prolonged use may result in fungal or bacterial superinfection, including *C. difficile*-associated diarrhea (CDAD) and pseudomembranous colitis; CDAD has been observed >2 months postantibiotic treatment.
Adverse Reactions Frequency not defined.
Central nervous system: Aseptic meningitis (rare), fever
Dermatologic: Maculopapular rash (3% to 7% at 200 mg/day; incidence higher with larger daily doses), erythema multiforme (rare), exfoliative dermatitis (rare), pruritus (common), phototoxic skin eruptions, Stevens-Johnson syndrome (rare), toxic epidermal necrolysis (rare)
Endocrine & metabolic: Hyperkalemia, hyponatremia
Gastrointestinal: Epigastric distress, glossitis, nausea, vomiting
Hematologic: Leukopenia, megaloblastic anemia, methemoglobinemia, neutropenia, thrombocytopenia
Hepatic: Cholestatic jaundice (rare), liver enzymes increased
Renal: BUN and creatinine increased
Miscellaneous: Anaphylaxis, hypersensitivity reactions

Drug Interactions
Metabolism/Transport Effects Substrate of CYP2C9 (major), CYP3A4 (major); **Note:** Assignment of Major/Minor substrate status based on clinically relevant drug interaction potential; **Inhibits** CYP2C8 (moderate), CYP2C9 (moderate)

Avoid Concomitant Use
Avoid concomitant use of Trimethoprim with any of the following: BCG; Dofetilide

Increased Effect/Toxicity
Trimethoprim may increase the levels/effects of: ACE Inhibitors; Amantadine; Angiotensin II Receptor Blockers; Antidiabetic Agents (Thiazolidinedione); AzaTHIOprine; Carvedilol; CYP2C8 Substrates; CYP2C9 Substrates; Dapsone; Dapsone (Systemic); Dapsone (Topical); Dofetilide; Eplerenone; Fosphenytoin; LamiVUDine; Memantine; Mercaptopurine; Methotrexate; Phenytoin; PRALAtrexate; Procainamide; Repaglinide; Spironolactone; Varenicline

The levels/effects of Trimethoprim may be increased by: Amantadine; Conivaptan; CYP2C9 Inhibitors (Moderate); CYP2C9 Inhibitors (Strong); Dapsone; Dapsone (Systemic); Memantine

Decreased Effect
Trimethoprim may decrease the levels/effects of: BCG; Typhoid Vaccine

The levels/effects of Trimethoprim may be decreased by: CYP2C9 Inducers (Strong); CYP3A4 Inducers (Strong); Deferasirox; Herbs (CYP3A4 Inducers); Leucovorin Calcium-Levoleucovorin; Peginterferon Alfa-2b; Tocilizumab

Stability
Solution: Store between 15°C to 25°C (59°F to 77°F). Protect from light.
Tablets: Store at 20°C to 25°C (68°F to 77°F). Protect from light.

Mechanism of Action Inhibits folic acid reduction to tetrahydrofolate, and thereby inhibits microbial growth

Pharmacodynamics/Kinetics
Absorption: Readily and extensive
Distribution: Widely into body tissues and fluids (middle ear, prostate, bile, aqueous humor, CSF)
Protein binding: 42% to 46%
Metabolism: Partially hepatic
Half-life elimination: 8-14 hours; prolonged with renal impairment
Time to peak, serum: 1-4 hours
Excretion: Urine (60% to 80%) as unchanged drug

Dosage Oral:
Children:
Susceptible infections: Children ≥2 months: 4-6 mg/kg/day in divided doses every 12 hours (dosing for UTI in Schleiss, 2007); **Note:** AAP guidelines on treatment of UTI recommend 6-12 mg trimethoprim/kg/day (in combination with sulfamethoxazole) in 2 divided doses (AAP, 1999)
Acute otitis media: Children ≥6 months: 10 mg/kg/day in divided doses every 12 hours for 10 days
Adults:
***Pneumocystis jirovecii* pneumonia, mild-to-moderate (unlabeled use) (CDC, 2009):** 15 mg/kg/day in 3 divided doses in combination with dapsone
Susceptible infections: 100 mg every 12 hours or 200 mg every 24 hours for 10 days
Urinary tract infection, uncomplicated (unlabeled duration):
Treatment: 100 mg every 12 hours for 3 days (Gupta, 2011)
Prophylaxis: 100 mg once daily (Kodner, 2010)

Dosing interval in renal impairment:
Cl_{cr} 15-30 mL/minute: Administer 50 mg every 12 hours
Cl_{cr} <15 mL/minute: Not recommended
Hemodialysis: Moderately dialyzable (20% to 50%)

Dietary Considerations May cause folic acid deficiency, supplements may be needed. Should be taken with milk or food.

Administration Administer with milk or food.

Monitoring Parameters Periodic CBC and serum potassium during long-term therapy

Reference Range Therapeutic: Peak: 5-15 mg/L; Trough: 2-8 mg/L

Test Interactions May falsely increase creatinine determination measured by the Jaffé alkaline picrate assay; may interfere with determination of serum methotrexate when measured by methods that use a bacterial dihydrofolate reductase as the binding protein (eg, the competitive binding protein technique); does **not** interfere with RIA for methotrexate

Dosage Forms Excipient information presented when available (limited, particularly for generics); consult specific product labeling.
Solution, oral:
Primsol®: 50 mg (base)/5 mL (473 mL) [dye free, ethanol free; contains propylene glycol, sodium benzoate; bubblegum flavor]
Tablet, oral: 100 mg

Extemporaneous Preparations Note: Commercial oral solution is available (10 mg/mL [dye free, ethanol free; contains propylene glycol, sodium benzoate; bubblegum flavor])

A 10 mg/mL oral suspension may be made with tablets. Crush ten 100 mg tablets in a mortar and reduce to a fine powder. Add 20 mL of a 1:1 mixture of Simple Syrup, NF, and Methylcellulose 1% and mix to a uniform paste; mix while adding the vehicle in incremental proportions to **almost** 100 mL; transfer to a calibrated bottle, rinse mortar with vehicle, and add quantity of vehicle sufficient to make 100 mL. Label "shake well" and "refrigerate". Stable for 91 days.

Nahata MC, Pai VB, and Hipple TF, *Pediatric Drug Formulations*, 5th ed, Cincinnati, OH: Harvey Whitney Books Co, 2004.

Trimethoprim and Polymyxin B

(trye METH oh prim & pol i MIKS in bee)

Brand Names: U.S. Polytrim®
Brand Names: Canada PMS-Polytrimethoprim; Polytrim™
Index Terms Polymyxin B and Trimethoprim
Pharmacologic Category Antibiotic, Ophthalmic
Use Treatment of surface ocular bacterial conjunctivitis and blepharoconjunctivitis
Pregnancy Risk Factor C
Dosage Ophthalmic:
Children ≥2 months and Adults: Instill 1 drop in affected eye(s) every 3 hours (maximum: 6 doses per day) for 7-10 days
Elderly: No overall differences observed between elderly and other adults
Additional Information Complete prescribing information for this medication should be consulted for additional detail.
Dosage Forms Excipient information presented when available (limited, particularly for generics); consult specific product labeling.
Solution, ophthalmic: Trimethoprim 1 mg and polymyxin B sulfate 10,000 units per 1 mL (10 mL)
Polytrim®: Trimethoprim 1 mg and polymyxin B sulfate 10,000 units per 1 mL (10 mL) [contains benzalkonium chloride]

- **Trimethoprim and Sulfamethoxazole** *see* Sulfamethoxazole and Trimethoprim *on page* 1602
- **Trinasal® (Can)** *see* Triamcinolone (Nasal) *on page* 1734
- **TriNessa®** *see* Ethinyl Estradiol and Norgestimate *on page* 663
- **Trinipatch® (Can)** *see* Nitroglycerin *on page* 1212
- **Tri-Norinyl®** *see* Ethinyl Estradiol and Norethindrone *on page* 660
- **Triostat®** *see* Liothyronine *on page* 1016
- **Tripedia® [DSC]** *see* Diphtheria and Tetanus Toxoids, and Acellular Pertussis Vaccine *on page* 523
- **Triphasil® (Can)** *see* Ethinyl Estradiol and Levonorgestrel *on page* 656
- **Triple Antibiotic** *see* Bacitracin, Neomycin, and Polymyxin B *on page* 186
- **Triplex™ AD [DSC]** *see* Chlorpheniramine, Pyrilamine, and Phenylephrine *on page* 348
- **Tripohist™ D** *see* Triprolidine and Pseudoephedrine *on page* 1741

Triprolidine and Pseudoephedrine

(trye PROE li deen & soo doe e FED rin)

Brand Names: U.S. Allerfrim [OTC]; Aprodine [OTC]; Genac™ [OTC] [DSC]; Pediatex® TD; Silafed [OTC]; Tripohist™ D
Brand Names: Canada Actifed®
Index Terms Pseudoephedrine and Triprolidine
Pharmacologic Category Alkylamine Derivative; Alpha/Beta Agonist; Decongestant; Histamine H_1 Antagonist; Histamine H_1 Antagonist, First Generation
Use Temporary relief of nasal congestion, decongest sinus openings, running nose, sneezing, itching of nose or throat and itchy, watery eyes due to common cold, hay fever, or other upper respiratory allergies

Pregnancy Risk Factor C

Dosage Oral:

Liquid:

Children:

6-12 years:

Pediatex® TD: 1.33 mL every 6 hours (maximum: 4 doses/24 hours)

Tripohist™ D: 2.5-5 mL every 4-6 hours (maximum pseudoephedrine: 120 mg/24 hours)

Children ≥12 years and Adults:

Pediatex® TD: 2.67 mL every 6 hours (maximum: 4 doses/24 hours)

Tripohist™ D: 5-10 mL every 4-6 hours (maximum pseudoephedrine: 240 mg/24 hours)

Syrup (Allerfrim, Aprodine):

Children 6-12 years: 5 mL every 4-6 hours; do not exceed 4 doses in 24 hours

Children >12 years and Adults: 10 mL every 4-6 hours; do not exceed 4 doses in 24 hours

Tablet (Aprodine):

Children 6-12 years: 1/2 tablet every 4-6 hours; do not exceed 4 doses in 24 hours

Children >12 years and Adults: One tablet every 4-6 hours; do not exceed 4 doses in 24 hours

Additional Information Complete prescribing information for this medication should be consulted for additional detail.

Dosage Forms Excipient information presented when available (limited, particularly for generics); consult specific product labeling. [DSC] = Discontinued product

Liquid, oral:

Pediatex® TD: Triprolidine hydrochloride 0.938 mg and pseudoephedrine hydrochloride 10 mg per 1 mL (30 mL) [cotton candy flavor]

Tripohist™ D: Triprolidine hydrochloride 1.25 mg and pseudoephedrine hydrochloride 45 mg per 5 mL (473 mL) [ethanol free, sugar free; contains sodium benzoate; blueberry flavor]

Syrup, oral: Triprolidine hydrochloride 1.25 mg and pseudoephedrine hydrochloride 30 mg per 5 mL (120 mL) [DSC]

Allerfrim: Triprolidine hydrochloride 1.25 mg and pseudoephedrine hydrochloride 30 mg per 5 mL (118 mL [DSC], 473 mL [DSC]) [contains sodium benzoate]

Aprodine: Triprolidine hydrochloride 1.25 mg and pseudoephedrine hydrochloride 30 mg per 5 mL (120 mL)

Silafed: Triprolidine hydrochloride 1.25 mg and pseudoephedrine hydrochloride 30 mg per 5 mL (120 mL, 240 mL)

Tablet, oral:

Allerfrim, Aprodine, Genac™ [DSC]: Triprolidine hydrochloride 2.5 mg and pseudoephedrine hydrochloride 60 mg

◆ **TripTone® [OTC]** *see* DimenhyDRINATE *on page 513*

Triptorelin (trip toe REL in)

Brand Names: U.S. Trelstar®

Brand Names: Canada Trelstar®

Index Terms AY-25650; CL-118,532; D-Trp(6)-LHRH; Detryptoreline; Triptorelin Pamoate; Tryptoreline

Pharmacologic Category Gonadotropin Releasing Hormone Agonist

Use Palliative treatment of advanced prostate cancer

Unlabeled Use Treatment of endometriosis, *in vitro* fertilization, precocious puberty, uterine sarcoma

Pregnancy Risk Factor X

Dosage I.M.: Adults: Prostate cancer:

3.75 mg once every 4 weeks **or**

11.25 mg once every 12 weeks **or**

22.5 mg once every 24 weeks

Additional Information Complete prescribing information for this medication should be consulted for additional detail.

Dosage Forms Excipient information presented when available (limited, particularly for generics); consult specific product labeling.

Injection, powder for reconstitution:

Trelstar®: 3.75 mg, 11.25 mg, 22.5 mg [contains polylactide-co-glycolide, polysorbate 80]

◆ **Triptorelin Pamoate** *see* Triptorelin *on page 1742*

◆ **Triquilar® (Can)** *see* Ethinyl Estradiol and Levonorgestrel *on page 656*

◆ **Tris Buffer** *see* Tromethamine *on page 1742*

◆ **Trisenox®** *see* Arsenic Trioxide *on page 146*

◆ **Tris(hydroxymethyl)aminomethane** *see* Tromethamine *on page 1742*

◆ **Tri-Sprintec®** *see* Ethinyl Estradiol and Norgestimate *on page 663*

◆ **Trivagizole-3® (Can)** *see* Clotrimazole (Topical) *on page 399*

◆ **Trivalent Inactivated Influenza Vaccine** *see* Influenza Virus Vaccine (Inactivated) *on page 897*

◆ **Trivora®** *see* Ethinyl Estradiol and Levonorgestrel *on page 656*

◆ **Trizivir®** *see* Abacavir, Lamivudine, and Zidovudine *on page 20*

◆ **Trocaine® [OTC]** *see* Benzocaine *on page 202*

◆ **Trombovar® (Can)** *see* Sodium Tetradecyl *on page 1577*

Tromethamine (troe METH a meen)

Brand Names: U.S. THAM®

Index Terms Tris Buffer; Tris(hydroxymethyl)aminomethane

Pharmacologic Category Alkalinizing Agent, Parenteral

Use Correction of metabolic acidosis associated with cardiac bypass surgery or cardiac arrest; to correct excess acidity of stored blood that is preserved with acid citrate dextrose (ACD); indicated in infants needing alkalinization after receiving maximum sodium bicarbonate (8-10 mEq/kg/24 hours)

Pregnancy Risk Factor C

Dosage

Infants: Metabolic acidosis associated with RDS: Initial: Approximately 1 mL/kg for each pH unit below 7.4; additional doses determined by changes in PaO_2, pH, and pCO_2; **Note:** Although THAM® solution does not raise pCO_2 when treating metabolic acidosis with concurrent respiratory acidosis, bicarbonate may be preferred because the osmotic effects of THAM® are greater.

Adults: Dose depends on buffer base deficit; when deficit is known: tromethamine (mL of 0.3 M solution) = body weight (kg) x base deficit (mEq/L) x 1.1

Metabolic acidosis with cardiac arrest:

I.V.: 3.6-10.8 g (111-333 mL); additional amounts may be required to control acidosis after arrest reversed

Open chest: Intraventricular: 2-6 g (62-185 mL). **Note:** Do not inject into cardiac muscle

Acidosis associated with cardiac bypass surgery: Average dose: 9 mL/kg (2.7 mEq/kg); 500 mL is adequate for most adults; maximum dose: 500 mg/kg in ≤1 hour

Excess acidity of acid citrate dextrose (ACD) blood in coronary artery surgery: 15-77 mL of 0.3 molar solution added to each 500 mL of blood

Dosing comments in renal impairment: Use with caution; monitor for toxicity

Additional Information Complete prescribing information for this medication should be consulted for additional detail.

Dosage Forms Excipient information presented when available (limited, particularly for generics); consult specific product labeling.

Injection, solution:

THAM®: 18 g (500 mL) [0.3 molar]

◆ **Tropicacyl®** *see* Tropicamide *on page 1743*

Tropicamide (troe PIK a mide)

Brand Names: U.S. Mydral™ [DSC]; Mydriacyl®; Tropicacyl®

Brand Names: Canada Diotrope®; Mydriacyl®

Index Terms Bistropamide

Pharmacologic Category Ophthalmic Agent, Mydriatic

Use Short-acting mydriatic used in diagnostic procedures; as well as preoperatively and postoperatively; treatment of some cases of acute iritis, iridocyclitis, and keratitis

Pregnancy Risk Factor C

Dosage Ophthalmic: Children and Adults (individuals with heavily pigmented eyes may require larger doses):

Cycloplegia: Instill 1-2 drops (1%); may repeat in 5 minutes

Exam must be performed within 30 minutes after the repeat dose; if the patient is not examined within 20-30 minutes, instill an additional drop

Mydriasis: Instill 1-2 drops (0.5%) 15-20 minutes before exam; may repeat every 30 minutes as needed

Additional Information Complete prescribing information for this medication should be consulted for additional detail.

Dosage Forms Excipient information presented when available (limited, particularly for generics); consult specific product labeling. [DSC] = Discontinued product

Solution, ophthalmic [drops]: 0.5% (15 mL); 1% (2 mL, 3 mL, 15 mL)

Mydral™: 0.5% (15 mL [DSC]); 1% (15 mL [DSC]) [contains benzalkonium chloride]

Mydriacyl®: 1% (3 mL, 15 mL) [contains benzalkonium chloride]

Tropicacyl®: 0.5% (15 mL); 1% (15 mL) [contains benzalkonium chloride]

◆ **Trosec (Can)** *see* Trospium *on page 1743*

Trospium (TROSE pee um)

Brand Names: U.S. Sanctura®; Sanctura® XR

Brand Names: Canada Sanctura® XR; Trosec

Index Terms Trospium Chloride

Pharmacologic Category Anticholinergic Agent

Use Treatment of overactive bladder with symptoms of urgency, incontinence, and urinary frequency

Pregnancy Risk Factor C

Pregnancy Considerations Adverse events were observed in animal studies. There are no adequate or well-controlled studies in pregnant women; use only if clearly needed.

Lactation Excretion in breast milk unknown/use caution

Contraindications Hypersensitivity to trospium or any component of the formulation; urinary retention; gastric retention; uncontrolled narrow-angle glaucoma

Warnings/Precautions Cases of angioedema involving the face, lips, tongue, and/or larynx have been reported. Immediately discontinue if tongue, hypopharynx, or larynx are involved. May cause drowsiness and/or blurred vision, which may impair physical or mental abilities; patients must be cautioned about performing tasks which require mental alertness (eg, operating machinery or driving). May occur in the presence of increased environmental temperature; use caution in hot weather and/or exercise. Use with caution in patients with bladder flow obstruction, may increase the risk of urinary retention. Use with caution in patients with gastrointestinal obstructive disorders (eg, pyloric stenosis); may increase the risk of gastric retention. Use caution in patients with decreased GI motility (eg, myasthenia gravis, ulcerative colitis). Avoid use of extended release formulation in severe renal impairment (Cl_{cr} <30 mL/minute). Use immediate release formulation with caution in renal dysfunction; dosage adjustment is required. Ethanol should not be ingested within 2 hours of the administration of the extended release formulation. Concurrent ethanol use may increase the incidence of drowsiness. Active tubular secretion (ATS) is a route of elimination; use caution with other medications that are eliminated by ATS (eg, procainamide, pancuronium, vancomycin, morphine, metformin, and tenofovir). Use with extreme caution in patients with controlled (treated) narrow-angle glaucoma. Use caution in patients with moderate or severe hepatic dysfunction. Use caution in Alzheimer's patients. Use caution in the elderly (≥65 years of age); increased anticholinergic side effects are seen.

Adverse Reactions

>10%: Gastrointestinal: Xerostomia (9% to 22%)

1% to 10%:

Cardiovascular: Tachycardia

Central nervous system: Headache (4% to 7%), fatigue (2%)

Dermatologic: Dry skin

Gastrointestinal: Constipation (9% to 10%), abdominal pain (1% to 3%), dyspepsia (1% to 2%), flatulence (1% to 2%), nausea (1%), abdominal distention (<2%), taste abnormal, vomiting

Genitourinary: Urinary tract infection (1% to 7%), urinary retention (≤1%)

Ocular: Dry eyes (1% to 2%), blurred vision (1%)

Respiratory: Nasopharyngitis (3%), nasal dryness (1%)

Miscellaneous: Influenza (2%)

<1% (Limited to important or life-threatening): Anaphylaxis, angioedema, back pain, chest pain, delirium, feces hard, gastritis, hallucinations, hypertensive crisis, palpitation, rash, rhabdomyolysis, somnolence, Stevens-Johnson syndrome, supraventricular tachycardia, syncope, T-wave inversion

Drug Interactions

Metabolism/Transport Effects None known.

Avoid Concomitant Use There are no known interactions where it is recommended to avoid concomitant use.

Increased Effect/Toxicity

Trospium may increase the levels/effects of: AbobotulinumtoxinA; Anticholinergics; Cannabinoids; OnabotulinumtoxinA; Potassium Chloride; RimabotulinumtoxinB

The levels/effects of Trospium may be increased by: Alcohol (Ethyl); Pramlintide

Decreased Effect

Trospium may decrease the levels/effects of: Acetylcholinesterase Inhibitors (Central); Secretin

The levels/effects of Trospium may be decreased by: Acetylcholinesterase Inhibitors (Central); MetFORMIN

Ethanol/Nutrition/Herb Interactions

Ethanol: Avoid use since ethanol may enhance the sedative effects of trospium. Ethanol should not be ingested within 2 hours of the administration of the trospium extended release formulation.

Food: Administration with a fatty meal reduces the absorption and bioavailability of trospium.

Stability Store at 20°C to 25°C (68°F to 77°F).

Mechanism of Action Trospium antagonizes the effects of acetylcholine on muscarinic receptors in cholinergically innervated organs. It reduces the smooth muscle tone of the bladder.

Pharmacodynamics/Kinetics

Absorption: <10%; decreased with food

Distribution: V_d: 395 - >600 L, primarily in plasma

Protein binding: 48% to 85% *in vitro*

Metabolism: Hypothesized to be via esterase hydrolysis and conjugation; forms metabolites

Bioavailability: Immediate release formulation: ~10% (range: 4% to 16%)

Half-life elimination: Immediate release formulation: 20 hours

Severe renal insufficiency (Cl_{cr} <30 mL/minute): ~33 hours; extended release formulation: ~35 hours

Time to peak, plasma: 5-6 hours

Excretion: Feces (85%); urine (~6%; mostly as unchanged drug) primarily via active tubular secretion

Dosage Oral:

Adults: Immediate release formulation: 20 mg twice daily; extended release formulation: 60 mg once daily

Elderly ≥75 years: Immediate release formulation: Consider initial dose of 20 mg once daily (based on tolerability) at bedtime

Dosage adjustment in renal impairment: Cl_{cr} ≤30 mL/minute: Immediate release formulation: 20 mg once daily at bedtime; Extended release formulation: Use not recommended

Dietary Considerations Give 1 hour prior to meals or on an empty stomach.

Administration Administer 1 hour prior to meals or an empty stomach. Administer extended release capsules in the morning with a full glass of water.

Dosage Forms Excipient information presented when available (limited, particularly for generics); consult specific product labeling.

Capsule, extended release, oral, as chloride:

Sanctura® XR: 60 mg

Tablet, oral, as chloride: 20 mg

Sanctura®: 20 mg

◆ **Trospium Chloride** *see* Trospium *on page 1743*

◆ **Trusopt®** *see* Dorzolamide *on page 547*

◆ **Truvada®** *see* Emtricitabine and Tenofovir *on page 583*

Trypsin, Balsam Peru, and Castor Oil

(TRIP sin, BAL sam pe RUE, & KAS tor oyl)

Brand Names: U.S. Granulex®; Optase™; TBC; Vasolex™; Xenaderm®

Index Terms Balsam Peru, Castor Oil, and Trypsin; Castor Oil, Trypsin, and Balsam Peru

Pharmacologic Category Protectant, Topical

Use Treatment of decubitus ulcers, varicose ulcers, debridement of eschar, dehiscent wounds and sunburn; promote wound healing; reduce odor from necrotic wounds

Dosage Topical: Apply a minimum of twice daily or as often as necessary

Additional Information Complete prescribing information for this medication should be consulted for additional detail.

Dosage Forms Excipient information presented when available (limited, particularly for generics); consult specific product labeling.

Aerosol, spray, topical:

Granulex®: Trypsin 0.12 mg, balsam Peru 87 mg, and castor oil 788 mg per gram (60 g, 120 g)

TBC: Trypsin 0.1 mg, balsam Peru 72.5 mg, and castor oil 650 mg per 0.82 mL (60 g, 120 g)

Gel, topical:

Optase™: Trypsin 0.12 mg, balsam Peru 87 mg, and castor oil 788 mg per gram (95 g)

Ointment, topical:

Vasolex™: Trypsin 90 USP units, balsam Peru 87 mg, and castor oil 788 mg per gram (5 g, 30 g, 60 g)

Xenaderm®: Trypsin 90 USP units, balsam Peru 87 mg, and castor oil 788 mg per gram (30 g, 60 g)

◆ **Tryptoreline** *see* Triptorelin *on page 1742*

◆ **TSH** *see* Thyrotropin Alfa *on page 1677*

◆ **TSPA** *see* Thiotepa *on page 1674*

◆ **TST** *see* Tuberculin Tests *on page 1744*

◆ **TT** *see* Tetanus Toxoid (Adsorbed) *on page 1658*

◆ **Tuberculin Purified Protein Derivative** *see* Tuberculin Tests *on page 1744*

◆ **Tuberculin Skin Test** *see* Tuberculin Tests *on page 1744*

Tuberculin Tests (too BER kyoo lin tests)

Brand Names: U.S. Aplisol®; Tubersol®

Index Terms Mantoux; PPD; TB Skin Test; TST; Tuberculin Purified Protein Derivative; Tuberculin Skin Test

Pharmacologic Category Diagnostic Agent

Use Skin test in diagnosis of tuberculosis

Pregnancy Risk Factor C

Pregnancy Considerations Reproduction studies have not been conducted. Pregnancy is not a contraindication to testing.

Contraindications Hypersensitivity to tuberculin purified protein derivative (PPD) or any component of the formulation; previous severe reaction to tuberculin PPD skin test (TST)

Warnings/Precautions Patients with a previous severe reaction to TST (vesiculation, ulceration, necrosis) at the injection site should not receive tuberculin PPD again. Do not administer to persons with documented tuberculosis or a clear history of treatment for tuberculosis; persons with extensive burns or eczema. Skin testing may be deferred with major viral infections or live-virus vaccination within 1 month. Tuberculous or other bacterial infections, viral infection, live virus vaccination, malignancy, immunosuppressive agents, and conditions which impair immune response may cause a decreased response to test. Very young children (<6 weeks of age) may also have an absent or delayed response. For intradermal administration only; do not administer I.V., I.M., or SubQ. Epinephrine (1:1000) should be available to treat possible allergic reactions.

Adverse Reactions Suspected adverse reactions should be reported to the Food and Drug Administration (FDA) MedWatch Program at 1-800-332-1088

Frequency not defined:

Dermatologic: Rash

Local: Injection site reactions: Bleeding, bruising, discomfort, erythematous reaction, hematoma, necrosis, pain, pruritus, redness, scarring, ulceration, vesiculation

Miscellaneous: Anaphylaxis

Drug Interactions

Metabolism/Transport Effects None known.

Avoid Concomitant Use There are no known interactions where it is recommended to avoid concomitant use.

Increased Effect/Toxicity There are no known significant interactions involving an increase in effect.

Decreased Effect

The levels/effects of Tuberculin Tests may be decreased by: Vaccines (Live)

Stability Aplisol®, Tubersol®: Store under refrigeration at 2°C to 8°C (36°F to 46°F); do not freeze. Protect from light. Opened vials should be discarded after 30 days.

Mechanism of Action Tuberculosis results in individuals becoming sensitized to certain antigenic components of the *M. tuberculosis* organism. Culture extracts called tuberculins are contained in tuberculin skin test preparations. Upon intracutaneous injection of these culture extracts, a classic delayed (cellular) hypersensitivity reaction occurs. This reaction is characteristic of a delayed course (peak occurs >24 hours after injection, induration of the skin secondary to cell infiltration, and occasional vesiculation and necrosis). Delayed hypersensitivity reactions to tuberculin may indicate infection with a variety of nontuberculosis mycobacteria, or vaccination with the live attenuated mycobacterial strain of *M. bovis* vaccine, BCG, in addition to previous natural infection with *M. tuberculosis*.

Pharmacodynamics/Kinetics

Onset of action: Delayed hypersensitivity reactions: 5-6 hours

Peak effect: 48-72 hours

Duration: Reactions subside over a few days

Dosage Children and Adults: Intradermal: 0.1 mL

TST interpretation: Criteria for positive TST read at 48-72 hours (see "Note" for healthcare workers):

Induration ≥5 mm: Persons with HIV infection (or risk factors for HIV infection, but unknown status), recent close contact to person with known active TB, persons with chest x-ray consistent with healed TB, persons who are immunosuppressed

Induration ≥10 mm: Persons with clinical conditions which increase risk of TB infection, recent immigrants, I.V. drug users, residents and employees of high-risk settings, children <4 years of age

Induration ≥15 mm: Persons who do not meet any of the above criteria (no risk factors for TB)

Note: A two-step test is recommended when testing will be performed at regular intervals (eg, for healthcare workers). If the first test is negative, a second TST should be administered 1-3 weeks after the first test was read.

TST interpretation (CDC guidelines) in a healthcare setting:

Baseline test: ≥10 mm is positive (either first or second step)

Serial testing without known exposure: Increase of ≥10 mm is positive

Known exposure:

≥5 mm is positive in patients with baseline of 0 mm

≥10 mm is positive in patients with negative baseline or previous screening result of ≥0mm

Read test at 48-72 hours following placement. Test results with 0 mm induration or measured induration less than the defined cutoff point are considered to signify absence of infection with *M. tuberculosis*. Test results should be documented in millimeters even if classified as negative. Erythema and redness of skin are not indicative of a positive test result.

Administration For intradermal administration only. Administer to upper third of forearm (palm up) ≥2 inches from elbow, wrist, or other injection site. If neither arm can be used, may administer to back of shoulder. Administer using inch 1/4 to 1/2 inch 27-gauge needle or finer tuberculin syringe. Should form wheal (6-10 mm in diameter) as liquid is injected which will remain ~10 minutes. Avoid pressure or bandage at injection site. Document date and time of injection, person placing TST, location of injection site, and lot number of solution.

Monitoring Parameters Monitor for immediate hypersensitivity reactions for ~15 minutes following injection.

Test Interactions False-positive reactions may occur with BCG vaccination or previous mycobacteria (nonTB) infection (previous BCG vaccination is not a contraindication to testing). False-negative reactions may occur with impaired cell mediated immunity.

Additional Information Situations where risk of tuberculosis infection may be increased are with contacts of recently-diagnosed persons with active disease, contact with immigrants from countries where tuberculosis is still common, or reactivation with impaired immunity (HIV infection, diabetes, renal failure, immunosuppressant use, pulmonary silicosis). Healthcare workers, staff of correctional facilities, and travelers at high risk of exposure should have routine testing. Patients with HIV infection should be tested as soon as possible following diagnosis.

The date of administration, the product manufacturer, and lot number of product must be entered into the patient's permanent medical record. Results should be recorded in millimeters (even if 0), not "negative" or "positive".

Dosage Forms Excipient information presented when available (limited, particularly for generics); consult specific product labeling.

Injection, solution:

Aplisol®: 5 TU/0.1 mL (1 mL, 5 mL) [contains polysorbate 80]

Tubersol®: 5 TU/0.1 mL (1 mL, 5 mL) [contains polysorbate 80]

- **Tubersol®** *see* Tuberculin Tests *on page 1744*
- **Tums® [OTC]** *see* Calcium Carbonate *on page 266*
- **Tums® Chews Extra Strength (Can)** *see* Calcium Carbonate *on page 266*
- **Tums® E-X [OTC]** *see* Calcium Carbonate *on page 266*
- **Tums Extra Strength (Can)** *see* Calcium Carbonate *on page 266*
- **Tums® Extra Strength Sugar Free [OTC]** *see* Calcium Carbonate *on page 266*
- **Tums® Quickpak [OTC]** *see* Calcium Carbonate *on page 266*
- **Tums® Regular Strength (Can)** *see* Calcium Carbonate *on page 266*
- **Tums® Smoothies™ [OTC]** *see* Calcium Carbonate *on page 266*
- **Tums Smoothies (Can)** *see* Calcium Carbonate *on page 266*
- **Tums® Ultra [OTC]** *see* Calcium Carbonate *on page 266*
- **Tums® Ultra Strength (Can)** *see* Calcium Carbonate *on page 266*
- **Tusscough DHC™** *see* Dihydrocodeine, Chlorpheniramine, and Phenylephrine *on page 508*
- **Tussi-Bid® [OTC] [DSC]** *see* Guaifenesin and Dextromethorphan *on page 810*
- **TussiCaps®** *see* Hydrocodone and Chlorpheniramine *on page 838*
- **Tussigon®** *see* Hydrocodone and Homatropine *on page 838*
- **Tussionex®** *see* Hydrocodone and Chlorpheniramine *on page 838*
- **TVP-1012** *see* Rasagiline *on page 1466*
- **Twelve Resin-K [OTC]** *see* Cyanocobalamin *on page 418*
- **Twilite® [OTC]** *see* DiphenhydrAMINE (Systemic) *on page 516*
- **Twinject®** *see* EPINEPHrine (Systemic, Oral Inhalation) *on page 594*
- **Twinrix®** *see* Hepatitis A and Hepatitis B Recombinant Vaccine *on page 824*
- **Twinrix® Junior (Can)** *see* Hepatitis A and Hepatitis B Recombinant Vaccine *on page 824*
- **Twynsta®** *see* Telmisartan and Amlodipine *on page 1637*
- **Ty21a Vaccine** *see* Typhoid Vaccine *on page 1746*
- **Tygacil®** *see* Tigecycline *on page 1684*
- **Tykerb®** *see* Lapatinib *on page 975*
- **Tylenol® [OTC]** *see* Acetaminophen *on page 27*
- **Tylenol® (Can)** *see* Acetaminophen *on page 27*

- **Tylenol #2** *see* Acetaminophen and Codeine *on page 30*
- **Tylenol #3** *see* Acetaminophen and Codeine *on page 30*
- **Tylenol® 8 Hour [OTC]** *see* Acetaminophen *on page 27*
- **Tylenol® Arthritis Pain Extended Relief [OTC]** *see* Acetaminophen *on page 27*
- **Tylenol® Children's [OTC]** *see* Acetaminophen *on page 27*
- **Tylenol® Children's Meltaways [OTC]** *see* Acetaminophen *on page 27*
- **Tylenol Codeine** *see* Acetaminophen and Codeine *on page 30*
- **Tylenol® Decongestant (Can)** *see* Acetaminophen and Pseudoephedrine *on page 31*
- **Tylenol Elixir with Codeine (Can)** *see* Acetaminophen and Codeine *on page 30*
- **Tylenol® Extra Strength [OTC]** *see* Acetaminophen *on page 27*
- **Tylenol® Infant's Concentrated [OTC]** *see* Acetaminophen *on page 27*
- **Tylenol® Jr. Meltaways [OTC]** *see* Acetaminophen *on page 27*
- **Tylenol No. 1 (Can)** *see* Acetaminophen and Codeine *on page 30*
- **Tylenol No. 1 Forte (Can)** *see* Acetaminophen and Codeine *on page 30*
- **Tylenol No. 2 with Codeine (Can)** *see* Acetaminophen and Codeine *on page 30*
- **Tylenol No. 3 with Codeine (Can)** *see* Acetaminophen and Codeine *on page 30*
- **Tylenol No. 4 with Codeine (Can)** *see* Acetaminophen and Codeine *on page 30*
- **Tylenol® PM [OTC]** *see* Acetaminophen and Diphenhydramine *on page 31*
- **Tylenol® Severe Allergy [OTC]** *see* Acetaminophen and Diphenhydramine *on page 31*
- **Tylenol® Sinus (Can)** *see* Acetaminophen and Pseudoephedrine *on page 31*
- **Tylenol® with Codeine No. 3** *see* Acetaminophen and Codeine *on page 30*
- **Tylenol® with Codeine No. 4** *see* Acetaminophen and Codeine *on page 30*
- **Tylox®** *see* Oxycodone and Acetaminophen *on page 1269*
- **Typherix® (Can)** *see* Typhoid Vaccine *on page 1746*
- **Typhim Vi®** *see* Typhoid Vaccine *on page 1746*

Typhoid Vaccine (TYE foid vak SEEN)

Brand Names: U.S. Typhim Vi®; Vivotif®

Brand Names: Canada Typherix®; Typhim Vi®; Vivotif®

Index Terms Ty21a Vaccine; Typhoid Vaccine Live Oral Ty21a; Vi Vaccine

Pharmacologic Category Vaccine, Inactivated (Bacterial); Vaccine, Live (Bacterial)

Use Active immunization against typhoid fever caused by *Salmonella typhi*

Not for routine vaccination. In the United States and Canada, use should be limited to:

- Travelers to areas with a prolonged risk of exposure to *S. typhi*
- Persons with intimate exposure to a *S. typhi* carrier
- Laboratory technicians with exposure to *S. typhi*
- Travelers with achlorhydria or hypochlorhydria (Canadian recommendation)

Pregnancy Risk Factor C

Pregnancy Considerations Reproduction studies have not been conducted. The manufacturer of the Typhim Vi® injection suggests delaying vaccination until the 2nd or 3rd trimester if possible. Untreated typhoid fever may lead to miscarriage or vertical intrauterine transmission causing neonatal typhoid (rare).

Lactation Excretion in breast milk unknown/use caution

Contraindications Hypersensitivity to any component of the vaccine. In addition, the oral vaccine is contraindicated with congenital or acquired immunodeficient state, acute febrile illness

Warnings/Precautions Not all recipients of typhoid vaccine will be fully protected against typhoid fever. Travelers should take all necessary precautions to avoid contact or ingestion of potentially contaminated food or water sources. Should not be used to treat typhoid fever.

Injection: Administer at least 2 weeks prior to expected exposure. Vaccination may be deferred during acute infection or febrile illness. Immune response may be decreased in those receiving immunosuppressive therapy or are otherwise immunocompromised. In general, household and close contacts of persons with altered immunocompetence may receive all age appropriate vaccines. Use caution with coagulation disorders (including thrombocytopenia) where intramuscular injections should not be used. Epinephrine 1:1000 should be readily available.

Oral: Full immunization schedule should be completed at least 1 week prior to expected exposure. The complete immunization schedule must be followed to achieve optimum immune response. Do not administer during acute GI illness; vaccination may be deferred with persistent diarrhea or vomiting.

In order to maximize vaccination rates, the ACIP recommends simultaneous administration of all age-appropriate vaccines (live or inactivated) for which a person is eligible at a single clinic visit, unless contraindications exist.

Adverse Reactions In the U.S., all serious adverse reactions must be reported to the Department of Health and Human Services (DHHS) Vaccine Adverse Event Reporting System (VAERS) 1-800-822-7967 or online at https://vaers.hhs.gov/esub/index. In Canada, adverse reactions may be reported to local provincial/territorial health agencies or to the Vaccine Safety Section at Public Health Agency of Canada (1-866-844-0018).

Oral:

1% to 10%:

Central nervous system: Headache (5%), fever (3%)

Dermatologic: Rash (1%)

Gastrointestinal: Abdominal pain (6%), nausea (6%), diarrhea (3%), vomiting (2%)

Postmarketing and/or case reports: Anaphylactic reaction, demyelinating disease, myalgia, pain, RA, urticaria, sepsis, weakness

Injection (incidence may vary based on age and/or product used):

>10%:

Central nervous system: Fever (undefined; 2% to 32%), malaise (4% to 24%), headache (16% to 20%)

Local: Injection site: Tenderness (97% to 98%), pain (27% to 41%), soreness (up to 16%), induration (5% to 15%)

Neuromuscular & skeletal: General aches (1% to 13%)

1% to 10%:

Central nervous system: Fever ≥100°F (2%), >102°F (2%)

Dermatologic: Pruritus (up to 8%)

Gastrointestinal: Nausea (up to 8%), vomiting (2%)

Local: Injection site: Erythema (up to 5%), swelling (up to 4%)

Neuromuscular & skeletal: Myalgia (3% to 7%)

Postmarketing and/or case reports: Abdominal pain, allergic reactions, anaphylaxis, arthralgia, cervical pain, diarrhea, dizziness, flu-like syndrome, Guillain-Barré syndrome, hypotension, injection site inflammation (including angioedema and urticaria), loss of consciousness, lymphadenopathy, malaise, perforated jejunum, rash, serum sickness, tremor, urticaria, vasodilation, weakness

Drug Interactions

Metabolism/Transport Effects None known.

Avoid Concomitant Use

Avoid concomitant use of Typhoid Vaccine with any of the following: Belimumab; Fingolimod; Immunosuppressants

Increased Effect/Toxicity

The levels/effects of Typhoid Vaccine may be increased by: AzaTHIOprine; Belimumab; Corticosteroids (Systemic); Fingolimod; Hydroxychloroquine; Immunosuppressants; Leflunomide; Mercaptopurine; Methotrexate

Decreased Effect

Typhoid Vaccine may decrease the levels/effects of: Tuberculin Tests

The levels/effects of Typhoid Vaccine may be decreased by: Antibiotics; Fingolimod; Immune Globulins; Immunosuppressants

Ethanol/Nutrition/Herb Interactions Ethanol: Avoid alcohol within 2 hours of taking the capsule; may disrupt the enteric coating

Stability

Typherix®: Store between 2°C to 8°C (35°F to 46°F); do not freeze. Discard if vaccine has been frozen. Protect from light.

Typhim Vi®: Store between 2°C to 8°C (35°F to 46°F); do not freeze.

Vivotif®: Store between 2°C to 8°C (35°F to 46°F).

Mechanism of Action Virulent strains of *Salmonella typhi* cause disease by penetrating the intestinal mucosa and entering the systemic circulation via the lymphatic vasculature. One possible mechanism of conferring immunity may be the provocation of a local immune response in the intestinal tract induced by oral ingesting of a live strain with subsequent aborted infection. The ability of *Salmonella typhi* to produce clinical disease (and to elicit an immune response) is dependent on the bacteria having a complete lipopolysaccharide. The live attenuate Ty21a strain lacks the enzyme UDP-4-galactose epimerase so that lipopolysaccharide is only synthesized under conditions that induce bacterial autolysis. Thus, the strain remains avirulent despite the production of sufficient lipopolysaccharide to evoke a protective immune response. Despite low levels of lipopolysaccharide synthesis, cells lyse before gaining a virulent phenotype due to the intracellular accumulation of metabolic intermediates.

Pharmacodynamics/Kinetics

Onset of action: Immunity to *Salmonella typhi*: Oral: ~1 week

Duration: Immunity: Oral: ~4-7 years; Parenteral: Typhim Vi®: >17-21 months, Typherix®: ~3 years

Dosage Immunization:

Oral: Children ≥6 years and Adults:

Primary immunization: One capsule on alternate days (day 1, 3, 5, and 7) for a total of 4 doses; all doses should be complete at least 1 week prior to potential exposure

Booster immunization (with repeated or continued exposure to typhoid fever):

U.S. labeling: Repeat full course of primary immunization every 5 years

Canadian labeling: Repeat full course of primary immunization every 7 years

I.M.: Children ≥2 years and Adults: 0.5 mL given at least 2 weeks prior to expected exposure

Reimmunization:

Typhim Vi®: 0.5 mL; optimal schedule has not been established; a single dose every 2 years is currently recommended for repeated or continued exposure

Typherix® (Canadian labeling; not available in U.S.): 0.5 mL every 3 years

Administration

Injection: Typhim Vi® and Typherix® may be given I.M. and are indicated for children ≥2 years of age; administer as a single 0.5 mL (25 mcg) injection in deltoid muscle. **Do not administer Typhim Vi® or Typherix® intravascularly. Note:** For patients at risk of hemorrhage following intramuscular injection, the ACIP recommends "it should be administered intramuscularly if, in the opinion of the physician familiar with the patients bleeding risk, the vaccine can be administered by this route with reasonable safety. If the patient receives antihemophilia or other similar therapy, intramuscular vaccination can be scheduled shortly after such therapy is administered. A fine needle (23 gauge or smaller) can be used for the vaccination and firm pressure applied to the site (without rubbing) for at least 2 minutes. The patient should be instructed concerning the risk of hematoma from the injection." Patients on anticoagulant therapy should be considered to have the same bleeding risks and treated as those with clotting factor disorders (CDC, 2011).

Oral: Swallow capsule whole soon after placing into mouth; do not chew or open capsule. Capsule should be taken with a cold or lukewarm beverage (≤37°C/98.6°F). Take 1 hour prior to a meal. Avoid alcohol 1 hour before or 2 hours after administration.

Simultaneous administration of vaccines helps ensure patients will be fully vaccinated by the appropriate age. Simultaneous administration of vaccines is defined as administering >1 vaccine on the same day at different anatomic sites. The ACIP prefers each dose of a specific vaccine in a series come from the same manufacturer when possible. Adolescents and adults should be vaccinated while seated or lying down. In general, preterm infants should be vaccinated at the same chronological age as full-term infants (CDC, 2011).

Antipyretics have not been shown to prevent febrile seizures. Antipyretics may be used to treat fever or discomfort following vaccination (CDC, 2011). One study reported that routine prophylactic administration of acetaminophen to prevent fever prior to vaccination decreased the immune response of some vaccines; the clinical significance of this reduction in immune response has not been established (Prymula, 2009).

Monitoring Parameters Monitor for syncope for ≥15 minutes following vaccination

Additional Information Federal law requires that the name of medication, date of administration, the vaccine manufacturer, lot number of vaccine, and the administering person's name, title, and address be entered into the patient's permanent medical record.

Dosage Forms Excipient information presented when available (limited, particularly for generics); consult specific product labeling.

Capsule, enteric coated [live]:

Vivotif®: Viable *S. typhi* Ty21a 2-6.8 x 10^9 colony-forming units and nonviable *S. typhi* Ty21a 5-50 x 10^9 bacterial cells [contains lactose 100-180 mg/capsule and sucrose 26-130 mg/capsule]

Injection, solution [inactivated]:

Typhim Vi®: Purified Vi capsular polysaccharide 25 mcg/0.5 mL (0.5 mL, 10 mL) [derived from *S. typhi* Ty2 strain]

Dosage Forms: Canada Excipient information presented when available (limited, particularly for generics); consult specific product labeling.

Injection, solution:

Typherix®: Vi capsular polysaccharide 25 mcg/0.5 mL (0.5 mL) [derived from *S. typhi* Ty2 strain]

- ◆ **Typhoid Vaccine Live Oral Ty21a** *see* Typhoid Vaccine *on page 1746*
- ◆ **Tysabri®** *see* Natalizumab *on page 1181*
- ◆ **Tyvaso™** *see* Treprostinil *on page 1727*
- ◆ **506U78** *see* Nelarabine *on page 1184*
- ◆ **U-90152S** *see* Delavirdine *on page 467*
- ◆ **UCB-P071** *see* Cetirizine *on page 330*
- ◆ **U-Cort®** *see* Hydrocortisone (Topical) *on page 841*
- ◆ **UK-88,525** *see* Darifenacin *on page 450*
- ◆ **UK-427,857** *see* Maraviroc *on page 1052*
- ◆ **UK92480** *see* Sildenafil *on page 1552*
- ◆ **UK109496** *see* Voriconazole *on page 1797*
- ◆ **U-Kera E™ [DSC]** *see* Urea *on page 1749*
- ◆ **Ulcidine (Can)** *see* Famotidine *on page 688*
- ◆ **Ulesfia®** *see* Benzyl Alcohol *on page 206*

Ulipristal (ue li PRIS tal)

Brand Names: U.S. ella®

Index Terms CDB-2914; Ulipristal Acetate

Pharmacologic Category Contraceptive; Progestin Receptor Modulator

Use Emergency contraception following unprotected intercourse or possible contraceptive failure

Pregnancy Risk Factor X

Pregnancy Considerations Embryofetal loss was observed following administration of ulipristal to pregnant rats and rabbits during the period of organogenesis at doses that were 1/3 and 1/2 the human dose (based on BSA), respectively. Teratogenic effects were not observed in surviving fetuses. Pregnancy terminations were also observed in pregnant monkeys following administration of ulipristal during the first trimester in doses ~3 times the human dose (based on BSA). Exclude pregnancy prior to therapy; not indicated for terminating an existing pregnancy. A rapid return of fertility is expected following use for emergency contraception; routine contraceptive measures should be initiated or continued following use to ensure ongoing prevention of pregnancy. Barrier contraception is recommended immediately following emergency contraception and throughout the same menstrual cycle; efficacy of hormonal contraceptives may be decreased.

Lactation Excretion unknown/not recommended

Contraindications Known or suspected pregnancy

Warnings/Precautions Exclude pregnancy prior to therapy via history, physical exam or pregnancy testing; not indicated for terminating an existing pregnancy. Not intended for routine contraception. Barrier contraception is recommended immediately following emergency contraception and throughout the same menstrual cycle; efficacy of hormonal contraception may be decreased. Repeated use within the same menstrual cycle is not recommended. Menstrual bleeding patterns may be altered (cycle length may be delayed or shortened by a few days) but returns to normal in subsequent cycles. Intermenstrual bleeding (spotting) has also been observed. The possibility of pregnancy should be considered if menstruation is delayed for >7 days of the expected menstrual period. A history of ectopic pregnancy is not a contraindication to use in emergency contraception. The possibility of ectopic pregnancy should be considered in patients with abdominal pain after administration of ulipristal. Safety and efficacy have not been established for use in hepatic or renal impairment. Not for use prior to menarche or in postmenopausal women. Does not protect against HIV infection or other sexually-transmitted diseases.

Adverse Reactions

>10%:

Central nervous system: Headache (18% to 19%)

Endocrine & metabolic: Menstruation occurring ≥7 days later than expected (19%), dysmenorrhea (7% to 13%)

Gastrointestinal: Abdominal pain (8% to 15%), nausea (12% to 13%)

1% to 10%:

Central nervous system: Fatigue (6%), dizziness (5%)

Endocrine & metabolic: Intermenstrual bleeding (9%), menstruation occurring ≥7 days earlier than expected (7%)

Postmarketing and/or case reports: Acne

Drug Interactions

Metabolism/Transport Effects Substrate of CYP3A4 (major); **Note:** Assignment of Major/Minor substrate status based on clinically relevant drug interaction potential

Avoid Concomitant Use There are no known interactions where it is recommended to avoid concomitant use.

Increased Effect/Toxicity

The levels/effects of Ulipristal may be increased by: Conivaptan

Decreased Effect

The levels/effects of Ulipristal may be decreased by: CYP3A4 Inducers (Strong); Deferasirox; Herbs (CYP3A4 Inducers); Tocilizumab

Ethanol/Nutrition/Herb Interactions Herb/Nutraceutical: St John's wort (an enzyme inducer) may decrease serum levels of ulipristal.

Stability Store at 20°C to 25°C (68°F to 77°F). Protect from light.

Mechanism of Action Prevents progestin from binding to the progesterone receptor. Ulipristal postpones follicular rupture when administered prior to ovulation, thereby inhibiting or delaying ovulation. May also alter the normal endometrium, impairing implantation.

Pharmacodynamics/Kinetics

Protein binding: Ulipristal: >94% to plasma proteins including albumin, alpha$_1$-acid glycoprotein, and high-density lipoprotein

Metabolism: Hepatic via CYP3A4; forms monodemethylated metabolite (active) and inactive metabolites

Half-life elimination: Ulipristal: ~32 hours; Monodemethylated metabolite: ~27 hours

Time to peak, serum: 1 hour (ulipristal and monodemethylated metabolite)

Dosage Oral: Emergency contraception:

Children: Not for use prior to menarche

Adults: One tablet (30 mg) as soon as possible, but within 120 hours (5 days) of unprotected intercourse or contraceptive failure

Elderly: Not indicated for use in postmenopausal women

Dietary Considerations May be taken with or without food.

Administration Oral: Administer with or without food at anytime during menstrual cycle. If vomiting occurs within 3 hours of administration, consider repeating dose.

Monitoring Parameters Evaluate for pregnancy or ectopic pregnancy if menses is delayed for ≥1 week following emergency contraception, or if lower abdominal pain (3-5 weeks after administration) or persistent irregular bleeding develops.

Dosage Forms Excipient information presented when available (limited, particularly for generics); consult specific product labeling.

Tablet, oral, as acetate:

ella®: 30 mg

◆ **Ulipristal Acetate** *see* Ulipristal *on page 1748*

Urea (yoor EE a)

Brand Names: U.S. Aqua Care® [OTC]; Aquaphilic® with Carbamide [OTC]; BP 50%; Carmol® 10 [OTC]; Carmol® 20 [OTC]; Carmol® 40; Carmol® Deep Cleansing [OTC]; DPM™ [OTC]; Gordon's® Urea [OTC]; Gormel® Ten [OTC]; Gormel® [OTC]; Hydro 35™; Hydro 40™; Kerafoam®; Kerafoam® 42; Keralac™; Keralac™ Nailstik; Keratol 40™ [DSC]; Kerol™; Kerol™ AD; Kerol™ Redi-Cloths; Kerol™ ZX; Lanaphilic® with Urea [OTC]; Nutraplus® [OTC]; Quinnostik; Rea Lo® 30 [OTC]; Rea Lo® 40; Remeven™; RevitaDERM® 40; U-Kera E™ [DSC]; Ultra Mide 25® [OTC]; Umecta PD™; Umecta®; Umecta® Nail Film; Uramaxin®; Uramaxin® GT; Ureacin-10® [OTC]; Ureacin-20® [OTC]; X-Viate™

Brand Names: Canada UltraMide 25™; Uremol®; Urisec®

Index Terms Carbamide

Pharmacologic Category Diuretic, Osmotic; Keratolytic Agent; Topical Skin Product

Use Keratolytic agent to soften nails or skin; OTC: Moisturizer for dry, rough skin

Pregnancy Risk Factor B/C (manufacturer specific)

Dosage Topical: Adults: Hyperkeratotic conditions, dry skin: Apply 1-3 times/day

Additional Information Complete prescribing information for this medication should be consulted for additional detail.

Dosage Forms Excipient information presented when available (limited, particularly for generics); consult specific product labeling. [DSC] = Discontinued product

Aerosol, foam, topical:
- Hydro 35™: 35% (150 g) [contains lactic acid]
- Hydro 40™: 40% (150 g)
- Kerafoam® 42: 42% (60 g, 100 g)
- Kerafoam®: 30% (60 g, 100 g)
- Umecta®: 40% (113.4 g) [contains soy]
- Uramaxin®: 20% (100 g)

Cloth, topical:
- Kerol™ Redi-Cloths: 42% (30s) [contains lactic acid, vitamin E, zinc]

Cream, topical: 40% (28 g, 30 g, 85 g, 199 g, 210 g); 45% (255 g); 50% (142 g, 255 g)
- Aqua Care®: 10% (71 g) [contains benzyl alcohol]
- Carmol® 20: 20% (90 g)
- Carmol® 40: 40% (28 g, 85 g, 199 g)
- DPM™: 20% (118 g) [contains menthol, peppermint oil]
- Gordon's® Urea: 40% (30 g)
- Gormel®: 20% (75 g, 120 g, 454 g, 2270 g)
- Keralac™: 50% (142 g, 255 g) [contains lactic acid, vitamin E, zinc]
- Keratol 40™: 40% (30 g [DSC], 90 g [DSC], 210 g [DSC])
- Nutraplus®: 10% (90 g, 454 g)
- Rea Lo® 30: 30% (60 g, 240 g)
- Rea Lo® 40: 40% (60 g, 240 g)
- Remeven™: 50% (142 g, 255 g) [contains lactic acid, vitamin E, zinc]
- RevitaDERM® 40: 40% (112 g) [contains aloe]
- U-Kera E™: 40% (28 g [DSC])
- Uramaxin®: 45% (255 g) [contains menthol]
- Ureacin-20®: 20% (113 g) [contains lactic acid]
- X-Viate™: 40% (29 g, 85 g, 199 g)

Emulsion, topical: 50% (284 g, 300 g)
- BP 50%: 50% (300 g)
- Kerol™: 50% (284 g) [contains lactic acid, vitamin E, zinc]
- Kerol™ AD: 45% (240 mL) [contains lactic acid, vitamin E, zinc]
- Umecta PD™: 40% (198.5 g) [contains soy; contains sodium hyaluronate 0.3%]
- Umecta®: 40% (114 g, 227 g)

Gel, topical: 40% (15 mL); 45% (28 mL); 50% (18 mL)
- Carmol® 40: 40% (15 mL)
- Keralac™: 50% (18 mL) [contains lactic acid, zinc]
- Keratol 40™: 40% (15 mL [DSC])
- Uramaxin®: 45% (28 mL) [contains menthol]
- Uramaxin® GT: 45% (20 mL) [contains menthol]
- X-Viate™: 40% (15 mL)

Lotion, topical: 35% (207 mL, 325 mL); 40% (237 mL)
- Aqua Care®: 10% (240 mL) [contains lactic acid]
- Carmol® 10: 10% (180 mL)
- Carmol® 40: 40% (237 mL)
- Gormel® Ten: 20% (240 mL)
- Keralac™: 35% (207 mL, 325 mL) [contains lactic acid, vitamin E, zinc]
- Keratol 40™: 40% (240 mL [DSC])
- Nutraplus®: 10% (240 mL, 480 mL)
- Ultra Mide 25®: 25% (120 mL [DSC], 236 mL, 240 mL)
- Uramaxin®: 45% (480 mL) [contains menthol]
- Ureacin-10®: 10% (237 mL) [contains lactic acid]
- X-Viate™: 40% (237 mL)

Ointment, topical: 50% (45 g)
Aquaphilic® with Carbamide: 10% (180 g, 454 g); 20% (454 g) [contains lactic acid]
Keralac™: 50% (45 g) [contains lactic acid, vitamin E, zinc]
Lanaphilic® with Urea: 10% (454 g); 20% (454 g) [contains lactic acid]
Shampoo, topical:
Carmol® Deep Cleansing: 10% (240 mL)
Solution, topical: 50% (2.4 mL, 12 mL)
Keralac™ Nailstik: 50% (2.4 mL) [contains lactic acid, zinc]
Kerol™ ZX: 50% (12 mL) [contains lactic acid, vitamin E, zinc]
Quinnostik: 50% (2.4 mL) [contains lactic acid, zinc; part of RINNOVI Nail System]
Suspension, topical: 40% (18 mL); 50% (284 g)
Kerol™: 50% (284 g) [contains lactic acid, salicylic acid, vitamin E]
Umecta PD™: 40% (255.1 g) [contains soy; contains sodium hyaluronate 0.3%]
Umecta®: 40% (283 g)
Umecta® Nail Film: 40% (3 mL, 18 mL)

Urea and Hydrocortisone
(yoor EE a & hye droe KOR ti sone)

Brand Names: U.S. Carmol-HC®
Brand Names: Canada Ti-U-Lac® H; Uremol® HC
Index Terms Hydrocortisone and Urea
Pharmacologic Category Corticosteroid, Topical
Use Inflammation of corticosteroid-responsive dermatoses
Pregnancy Risk Factor C
Dosage Topical: Children and Adults: Steroid-responsive dermatoses: Apply thin film and rub in well 2-4 times/day. Therapy should be discontinued when control is achieved; if no improvement is seen, reassessment of diagnosis may be necessary.
Additional Information Complete prescribing information for this medication should be consulted for additional detail.
Dosage Forms Excipient information presented when available (limited, particularly for generics); consult specific product labeling.
Cream, topical:
Carmol-HC®: Urea 10% and hydrocortisone acetate 1% (28 g) [in water soluble vanishing cream base]

- **Ureacin-10® [OTC]** *see* Urea *on page 1749*
- **Ureacin-20® [OTC]** *see* Urea *on page 1749*
- **Urea Peroxide** *see* Carbamide Peroxide *on page 283*
- **Urecholine®** *see* Bethanechol *on page 211*
- **Urelle®** *see* Methenamine, Sodium Biphosphate, Phenyl Salicylate, Methylene Blue, and Hyoscyamine *on page 1094*
- **Uremol® (Can)** *see* Urea *on page 1749*
- **Uremol® HC (Can)** *see* Urea and Hydrocortisone *on page 1750*
- **Urex** *see* Methenamine *on page 1093*
- **Uribel™** *see* Methenamine, Sodium Biphosphate, Phenyl Salicylate, Methylene Blue, and Hyoscyamine *on page 1094*

Uridine Triacetate (URE i deen trye AS e tate)

Index Terms PN401; Triacetyluridine; Vistonuridine
Pharmacologic Category Antidote
Unlabeled Use Antidote for fluorouracil overdose or overexposure
Prescribing and Access Restrictions Uridine triacetate (formerly called vistonuridine) is supplied for emergency use under a single-patient Investigational New Drug (IND) provision. Procurement information is available from Wellstat Therapeutics at 1-443-831-5626.
Dosage Oral: Adults: Fluorouracil overdose (unlabeled use): 10 g every 6 hours for 20 doses beginning as soon as possible (8 hours to 4 days) after fluorouracil overdose (von Borstel, 2009)
Additional Information Complete prescribing information for this medication should be consulted for additional detail.

- **Urisec® (Can)** *see* Urea *on page 1749*
- **Urispas** *see* FlavoxATE *on page 716*
- **Urispas® (Can)** *see* FlavoxATE *on page 716*

Urofollitropin (yoor oh fol li TROE pin)

Brand Names: U.S. Bravelle®
Brand Names: Canada Bravelle®; Fertinorm® H.P.
Index Terms Follicle-Stimulating Hormone, Human; FSH; hFSH
Pharmacologic Category Gonadotropin; Ovulation Stimulator
Use Ovulation induction in patients who previously received pituitary suppression; development of multiple follicles with Assisted Reproductive Technologies (ART)
Pregnancy Risk Factor X
Dosage Note: Dose should be individualized. Use the lowest dose consistent with the expectation of good results. Over the course of treatment, doses may vary depending on individual patient response.
Adults: Females:
Ovulation induction: I.M., SubQ: Initial: 150 int. units daily for the first 5 days of treatment. Dose adjustments ≤75-150 int. units can be made every ≥2 days; maximum daily dose: 450 int. units; treatment >12 days is not recommended. If response to follitropin is appropriate, hCG is given 1 day following the last dose. Withhold hCG if serum estradiol is >2000 pg/mL, if the ovaries are abnormally enlarged, or if abdominal pain occurs.
ART: SubQ: 225 int. units daily for the first 5 days; dose may be adjusted based on patient response, but adjustments should not be made more frequently than once every 2 days; maximum adjustment: 75-150 int. units; maximum daily dose: 450 int. units; maximum duration of treatment: 12 days. When a sufficient number of follicles of adequate size are present, the final maturation of the follicles is induced by administering hCG. Withhold hCG in cases where the ovaries are abnormally enlarged on the last day of therapy.
Additional Information Complete prescribing information for this medication should be consulted for additional detail.
Dosage Forms Excipient information presented when available (limited, particularly for generics); consult specific product labeling.
Injection, powder for reconstitution [human origin]:
Bravelle®: 75 int. units [contains lactose 23 mg]

- **Uro-Mag® [OTC]** *see* Magnesium Oxide *on page 1046*
- **Uromax® (Can)** *see* Oxybutynin *on page 1264*
- **Uromitexan (Can)** *see* Mesna *on page 1083*
- **Uroqid-Acid® No. 2** *see* Methenamine and Sodium Acid Phosphate *on page 1094*
- **Uroxatral®** *see* Alfuzosin *on page 64*
- **Urso® (Can)** *see* Ursodiol *on page 1751*
- **Urso 250®** *see* Ursodiol *on page 1751*

◆ **Ursodeoxycholic Acid** *see* Ursodiol *on page 1751*

Ursodiol (ur soe DYE ol)

Brand Names: U.S. Actigall®; Urso 250®; Urso Forte®

Brand Names: Canada Dom-Ursodiol C; PHL-Ursodiol C; PMS-Ursodiol C; Urso®; Urso® DS

Index Terms Ursodeoxycholic Acid

Pharmacologic Category Gallstone Dissolution Agent

Use

Actigall®: Gallbladder stone dissolution; prevention of gallstones in obese patients experiencing rapid weight loss

Urso®, Urso Forte®: Primary biliary cirrhosis

Pregnancy Risk Factor B

Dosage Oral: Adults:

Gallstone dissolution (Actigall®): 8-10 mg/kg/day in 2-3 divided doses; use beyond 24 months is not established

Gallstone prevention (Actigall®): 300 mg twice daily

Primary biliary cirrhosis (Urso®, Urso Forte®): 13-15 mg/kg/day in 2-4 divided doses (with food)

Additional Information Complete prescribing information for this medication should be consulted for additional detail.

Dosage Forms Excipient information presented when available (limited, particularly for generics); consult specific product labeling.

Capsule, oral: 300 mg

Actigall®: 300 mg

Tablet, oral: 250 mg, 500 mg

Urso 250®: 250 mg

Urso Forte®: 500 mg [scored]

◆ **Urso® DS (Can)** *see* Ursodiol *on page 1751*

◆ **Urso Forte®** *see* Ursodiol *on page 1751*

Ustekinumab (yoo stek in YOO mab)

Brand Names: U.S. Stelara™

Brand Names: Canada Stelara™

Index Terms CNTO 1275

Pharmacologic Category Antipsoriatic Agent; Interleukin-12 Inhibitor; Interleukin-23 Inhibitor; Monoclonal Antibody

Use Treatment of moderate-to-severe plaque psoriasis

Pregnancy Risk Factor B

Pregnancy Considerations Reproduction studies have not been conducted in pregnant women. Use during pregnancy only if clearly needed.

Lactation Excretion in breast milk unknown/use caution

Medication Guide Available Yes

Contraindications There are no contraindications listed within the manufacturer's labeling.

Canadian labeling (not in U.S. labeling): Hypersensitivity to ustekinumab or any component of the formulation; severe infections such as sepsis, tuberculosis and opportunistic infections

Warnings/Precautions May increase the risk for malignancy although the impact on the development and course of malignancies is not fully defined. In clinical trials, the incidence of malignancy associated with therapy was comparable to that of the general population. Use with caution in patients with prior malignancy (use not studied in this population).

Infrequent, but serious bacterial, fungal, and viral infections have been observed with use. Avoid use in patients with clinically important active infection. Caution should be exercised when considering use in patients with a history of new/recurrent infections, with conditions that predispose them to infections (eg, diabetes or residence/travel from areas of endemic mycoses), or with chronic, latent, or localized infections. Patients who develop a new infection while undergoing treatment should be monitored closely. If a patient develops a serious infection, therapy should be discontinued or withheld until successful resolution of infection.

Avoid use in patients with active tuberculosis (TB). Patients should be evaluated for latent tuberculosis infection with a tuberculin skin test prior to starting therapy. Treatment of latent TB should be initiated before ustekinumab therapy is used.

Antibody formation to ustekinumab has been observed with therapy and has been associated with decreased serum levels and therapeutic response in some patients. Discontinue immediately with signs/symptoms of hypersensitivity reaction and treat appropriately as indicated. Use in combination with other immunosuppressive drugs or phototherapy has not been studied. Patients should be brought up to date with all immunizations before initiating therapy. **Live vaccines should not be given concurrently;** inactivated or nonlive vaccines may be given concurrently. BCG vaccines should not be given 1 year prior to, during, or 1 year following treatment. Patients >100 kg may require higher dose to achieve adequate serum levels. Use in hepatic or renal impairment has not been studied.

The packaging may contain latex. Product may contain polysorbate 80.

Adverse Reactions

>10%: Miscellaneous: Infection (27% to 61%)

1% to 10%:

Central nervous system: Headache (5%), fatigue (3%), dizziness (1% to 2%), depression (1%)

Dermatologic: Pruritus (1% to 2%), rash (<2%), urticaria (<2%)

Local: Injection site erythema (1% to 2%)

Neuromuscular & skeletal: Back pain (1% to 2%)

Respiratory: Pharyngolaryngeal pain (1% to 2%)

Miscellaneous: Antibody formation (3% to 5%)

<1% (Limited to important or life-threatening): Angina, bacterial infection, cellulitis, dactylitis, diverticulitis, fungal infection, gastroenteritis, herpes zoster, hypertension; injection site reactions (bruising, hemorrhage, induration, irritation, pain, pruritus, swelling); malignancy (breast, colon, head and neck, kidney, prostate, thyroid); MI, nephrolithiasis, osteomyelitis, pneumonia, reversible posterior leukoencephalopathy syndrome, stroke, urinary tract infection, viral infection

Drug Interactions

Metabolism/Transport Effects None known.

Avoid Concomitant Use

Avoid concomitant use of Ustekinumab with any of the following: BCG; Belimumab; Natalizumab; Pimecrolimus; Tacrolimus (Topical); Vaccines (Live)

Increased Effect/Toxicity

Ustekinumab may increase the levels/effects of: Belimumab; Leflunomide; Natalizumab; Vaccines (Live)

The levels/effects of Ustekinumab may be increased by: Abciximab; Denosumab; Pimecrolimus; Roflumilast; Tacrolimus (Topical); Trastuzumab

Decreased Effect

Ustekinumab may decrease the levels/effects of: BCG; Coccidioidin Skin Test; Sipuleucel-T; Vaccines (Inactivated); Vaccines (Live)

The levels/effects of Ustekinumab may be decreased by: Echinacea

Stability Store vials refrigerated at 2°C to 8°C (36°F to 46°F); do not freeze. Do not shake. Protect from light; store in original container. Discard any unused portion.

Mechanism of Action Ustekinumab is a human monoclonal antibody that binds to and interferes with the proinflammatory cytokines, interleukin (IL)-12 and IL-23. Biological effects of IL-12 and IL-23 include natural killer (NK) cell activation, CD4+ T-cell differentiation and activation. Ustekinumab also interferes with the expression of monocyte chemotactic protein-1 (MCP-1), tumor necrosis factor-alpha (TNF-α), interferon-inducible protein-10 (IP-10), and interleukin-8 (IL-8). Significant clinical improvement in psoriasis patients is seen in association with reduction of these proinflammatory signalers.

Pharmacodynamics/Kinetics

Distribution: V_d (terminal elimination phase): 0.096-0.264 L/kg

Bioavailability: Absolute bioavailability: SubQ: ~57%

Half-life elimination: 10-126 days

Time to peak, plasma: 7-13.5 days

Dosage SubQ: Adults: Plaque psoriasis:

Initial and maintenance: **Note:** Following an interruption in therapy, retreatment may be initiated at the initial dosing interval. Consider therapy discontinuation in any patient failing to demonstrate a response after 12 weeks of therapy.

≤100 kg: 45 mg at 0- and 4 weeks, and then every 12 weeks thereafter

>100 kg: 45 mg or 90 mg at 0- and 4 weeks, and then every 12 weeks thereafter

Per Canadian labeling, if response inadequate on every 12 week therapy, may increase to every 8 weeks.

Dosing adjustment in renal impairment: Use has not been studied in renal dysfunction

Dosing adjustment in hepatic impairment: Use has not been studied in hepatic dysfunction

Administration Do not use if cloudy or discolored. Administer by subcutaneous injection into the top of the thigh, abdomen, upper arms, or buttocks. Rotate sites. Avoid areas of skin where psoriasis is present.

Monitoring Parameters Place and read PPD prior to initiating therapy; monitor for signs/symptoms of infection; CBC; Ustekinumab-antibody formation

Dosage Forms Excipient information presented when available (limited, particularly for generics); consult specific product labeling.

Injection, solution [preservative free]:

Stelara™: 45 mg/0.5 mL (0.5 mL) [contains natural rubber/natural latex in packaging, polysorbate 80, sucrose 38 mg/syringe]

Stelara™: 90 mg/mL (1 mL) [contains natural rubber/natural latex in packaging, polysorbate 80, sucrose 76 mg/syringe]

Dosage Forms: Canada Excipient information presented when available (limited, particularly for generics); consult specific product labeling.

Injection, solution [preservative free]:

Stelara™: 45 mg/0.5 mL (0.5 mL)

◆ **Uta®** *see* Methenamine, Sodium Biphosphate, Phenyl Salicylate, Methylene Blue, and Hyoscyamine *on page 1094*

◆ **UTI Relief® [OTC]** *see* Phenazopyridine *on page 1337*

◆ **Utradol™ (Can)** *see* Etodolac *on page 666*

◆ **Uvadex®** *see* Methoxsalen (Systemic) *on page 1102*

Vaccinia Immune Globulin (Intravenous)

(vax IN ee a i MYUN GLOB yoo lin IN tra VEE nus)

Brand Names: U.S. CNJ-016®

Index Terms VIGIV

Pharmacologic Category Blood Product Derivative; Immune Globulin

Use Treatment of infectious complications of smallpox (vaccinia virus) vaccination, such as eczema vaccinatum, progressive vaccinia, and severe generalized vaccinia; treatment of vaccinia infections in individuals with concurrent skin conditions or accidental virus exposure to eyes (except vaccinia keratitis), mouth, or other areas where viral infection would pose significant risk

CDC guidelines for use:

Use is recommended for:

- Inadvertent inoculation (considering severity, toxicity of affected person, and pain)
- Eczema vaccinatum
- Generalized vaccinia (severe form or if underlying illness is present)
- Progressive vaccinia

Use may be considered for:

- Severe ocular complications except isolated keratitis

Use is not recommended for:

- Inadvertent inoculation that is not severe
- Mild or limited generalized vaccinia
- Nonspecific rashes, erythema multiforme, or Stevens-Johnson syndrome
- Postvaccinial encephalitis or encephalomyelitis

Pregnancy Risk Factor C

Pregnancy Considerations Animal reproduction studies have not been conducted. Immune globulins cross the placenta in increased amounts after 30 weeks gestation. There are no adequate and well-controlled studies in pregnant women. Vaccinia immune globulin is currently not recommended for use in persons with contraindications to smallpox vaccine; inadvertent exposure to smallpox vaccine in high risk populations (eg pregnant women) should be reported to the CDC so that standardized treatment may be provided.

Lactation Excretion in breast milk unknown/use caution

Prescribing and Access Restrictions Vaccinia immune globulin is not available for general public use. All supplies are currently owned by the federal government for inclusion in the Strategic National Stockpile. The CDC Smallpox Adverse Events Clinical Consultation team will coordinate shipment. The State Health Department should be contacted first concerning severe or unexpected adverse events from smallpox vaccination.

Contraindications Hypersensitivity to immune globulin or any component of the formulation; isolated vaccinia keratitis; selective IgA deficiency

Warnings/Precautions Vaccinia immune globulin is currently not recommended for use in persons with contraindications to smallpox vaccine; inadvertent exposure to smallpox vaccine in high risk populations should be reported to the CDC so that standardized treatment may be provided.

Hypersensitivity and anaphylactic reactions can occur; immediate treatment (including epinephrine 1:1000) should be available. Contains trace amounts of IgA; use caution in IgA-deficient patients. Aseptic meningitis syndrome (AMS) has been reported with intravenous immune globulin administration (rare); may occur with high doses (≥2 g/kg). Intravenous immune globulin has been associated with antiglobulin hemolysis; monitor for signs of hemolytic anemia. Monitor for transfusion-related acute lung injury (TRALI); noncardiogenic pulmonary edema has been reported with intravenous immune globulin use. TRALI is characterized by severe respiratory distress, pulmonary edema, hypoxemia, and fever in the presence of normal left ventricular function. Usually occurs within 1-6 hours after infusion.

Acute renal dysfunction (increased serum creatinine, oliguria, acute renal failure) can rarely occur; usually within 7 days of use (more likely with products stabilized with sucrose). Use with caution in the elderly, patients with renal disease, diabetes mellitus, volume depletion, sepsis, paraproteinemia, and nephrotoxic medications due to risk of renal dysfunction. In patients at risk of renal dysfunction, the rate of infusion and concentration of solution should be minimized. discontinue if renal function deteriorates. Patients should not be volume depleted prior to therapy. Thrombotic events have been reported with administration of intravenous immune globulin; use with caution in patients with cardiovascular risk factors. Product of human plasma; may potentially contain infectious agents which could transmit disease. Screening of donors, as well as testing and/or inactivation or removal of certain viruses, reduces the risk. Infections thought to be transmitted by this product should be reported to the manufacturer. Product may contain maltose. **[U.S. Boxed Warning]: Maltose in vaccinia immune globulin can interact with glucose monitoring systems and test strips.** Falsely-elevated blood glucose readings may result in unnecessary insulin use and life-threatening hypoglycemia. Glucose specific monitoring systems and test strips are recommended. For intravenous administration only.

Adverse Reactions Note: Actual frequency varies by dose and rate of infusion

Cardiovascular: Peripheral edema

Central nervous system: Cold or hot feeling, dizziness, fatigue, headache, pain, pallor, pyrexia

Dermatologic: Erythema

Gastrointestinal: Appetite decreased, nausea, vomiting

Local: Injection site reaction

Neuromuscular & skeletal: Back pain, paraesthesia, muscle spasm, rigors, tremor, weakness

Miscellaneous: Diaphoresis

Postmarketing and/or case reports: Abdominal pain, anaphylaxis, apnea, acute respiratory distress syndrome, arthralgia, aseptic meningitis, blood pressure changes, bronchospasm, bullous dermatitis, cardiac arrest, chills, coma, Coombs' test positive, cyanosis, diarrhea, dyspnea, epidermolysis, erythema multiforme, flushing, hemolysis, hepatic dysfunction, hypersensitivity reactions, hypoxemia, hypotension, intravascular hemolysis, leukopenia, loss of consciousness, lung injury (transfusion associated), malaise, myalgia, osmotic nephropathy, pancytopenia, proximal tubular nephropathy, pulmonary edema, renal dysfunction/failure (acute), seizure, Stevens-Johnson syndrome, syncope, tachycardia, thrombocytopenia, thromboembolism, transfusion-related acute lung injury (TRALI), urticaria, vascular collapse, wheezing

Drug Interactions

Metabolism/Transport Effects None known.

Avoid Concomitant Use There are no known interactions where it is recommended to avoid concomitant use.

Increased Effect/Toxicity There are no known significant interactions involving an increase in effect.

Decreased Effect

Vaccinia Immune Globulin (Intravenous) may decrease the levels/effects of: Vaccines (Live)

Stability Store between 2°C and 8°C (36°F to 46°F); may also be frozen. If frozen, use within 60 days of thawing at 2°C and 8°C. Infusion should begin within 4 hours after entering vial.

Mechanism of Action Antibodies obtained from pooled human plasma of individuals immunized with the smallpox vaccine provide passive immunity

Pharmacodynamics/Kinetics

Distribution: V_d: 6630 L

Half-life elimination: 30 days (range 13-67 days)

Time to peak, plasma: ≤2 hours

Dosage I.V.: **Note:** Vaccinia immune globulin is currently not recommended for use in persons with contraindications to smallpox vaccine; inadvertent exposure to smallpox vaccine in high-risk populations should be reported to the CDC so that standardized treatment may be provided.

Adults: 6000 units/kg; may repeat dose based on severity of symptoms and response to treatment (specific data are lacking); 9000 units/kg may be considered if patient does not respond to initial dose. Doses up to 24,000 unit/kg were tolerated in healthy volunteers.

Dosage adjustment in renal impairment: Use caution. In patients at risk of renal dysfunction, the rate of infusion and concentration of solution should be minimized; discontinue if renal function deteriorates.

Administration Do not shake; avoid foaming. For intravenous use only. Predilution is not recommended. If dedicated line is not available, flush with NS prior to administration of VIGIV. Do not exceed recommended rates of infusion.

Patients ≥50 kg: Infuse at ≤2 mL/minute; Patients <50 kg: Infuse at ≤0.04 mL/kg/minute. Maximum assessed rate of infusion: 4 mL/minute. Decrease rate of infusion in patients who develop minor adverse reactions (eg, flushing) and in patients with risk factors for thrombosis/thromboembolism and/or renal insufficiency.

Monitoring Parameters Renal function and urine output (at baseline and at appropriate intervals). Baseline assessment of blood viscosity in patients at risk for hyperviscosity. During infusion, monitor patient for signs of infusion-related reactions, including (but not limited to) flushing, fever, chills, respiratory distress, blood pressure or heart rate changes. Transfusion-related lung injury (typically 1-6 hours after infusion) and hemolysis have been reported with infusion.

Test Interactions [U.S. Boxed Warning]: Maltose in vaccinia immune globulin can interact with glucose monitoring systems and test strips. CNJ-016® contains maltose. Falsely-elevated blood glucose levels may occur when glucose monitoring devices and test strips utilizing the glucose dehydrogenase pyrroloquinolinequinone (GDH-PQQ) based methods are used. Glucose monitoring devices and test strips which utilize the glucose-specific method are recommended.

Positive direct Coombs' test due to transitory increase of antibodies.

Dosage Forms Excipient information presented when available (limited, particularly for generics); consult specific product labeling.

Injection, solution [preservative free; solvent-detergent treated]:

CNJ-016®: ≥50,000 units/15 mL (15 mL) [contains maltose 10% and polysorbate 80 0.03%]

◆ **Vaccinia Vaccine** *see* Smallpox Vaccine *on page 1563*

◆ **Vagifem®** *see* Estradiol (Topical) *on page 632*

◆ **Vagifem® 10 (Can)** *see* Estradiol (Topical) *on page 632*

ValACYclovir (val ay SYE kloe veer)

Brand Names: U.S. Valtrex®

Brand Names: Canada Apo-Valacyclovir®; Mylan-Valacyclovir; PHL-Valacyclovir; PMS-Valacyclovir; PRO-Valacyclovir; Riva-Valacyclovir; Valtrex®

Index Terms Valacyclovir Hydrochloride

Pharmacologic Category Antiviral Agent; Antiviral Agent, Oral

Use Treatment of herpes zoster (shingles) in immunocompetent patients; treatment of first-episode and recurrent genital herpes; suppression of recurrent genital herpes and reduction of heterosexual transmission of genital herpes in immunocompetent patients; suppression of genital herpes in HIV-infected individuals; treatment of herpes labialis (cold sores); chickenpox in immunocompetent children

Unlabeled Use Prophylaxis of cancer-related HSV, VZV, and CMV infections; treatment of cancer-related HSV, VZV infection

Pregnancy Risk Factor B

Pregnancy Considerations Teratogenic events were not observed in animal studies. Data from a pregnancy registry has shown no increased rate of birth defects than that of the general population; however, the registry is small and use during pregnancy is only warranted if the potential benefit to the mother justifies the risk of the fetus.

Lactation Enters breast milk/use caution

Contraindications Hypersensitivity to valacyclovir, acyclovir, or any component of the formulation

Warnings/Precautions Thrombotic thrombocytopenic purpura/hemolytic uremic syndrome has occurred in immunocompromised patients (at doses of 8 g/day). Safety and efficacy have not been established for treatment/suppression of recurrent genital herpes or disseminated herpes in patients with profound immunosuppression (eg, advanced HIV with CD4 <100 cells/mm^3). CNS adverse effects (including agitation, hallucinations, confusion, delirium, seizures, and encephalopathy) have been reported. Use caution in patients with renal impairment, the elderly, and/or those receiving nephrotoxic agents. Acute renal failure has been observed in patients with renal dysfunction; dose adjustment may be required. Decreased precipitation in renal tubules may occur leading to urinary precipitation; adequately hydrate patient. For cold sores, treatment should begin at with earliest symptom (tingling, itching, burning). For genital herpes, treatment should begin as soon as possible after the first signs and symptoms (within 72 hours of onset of first diagnosis or within 24 hours of onset of recurrent episodes). For herpes zoster, treatment should begin within 72 hours of onset of rash. For chickenpox, treatment should begin with earliest sign or symptom. Use with caution in the elderly; CNS effects have been reported. Safety and efficacy have not been established in patients <2 years of age.

Adverse Reactions

>10%:

- Central nervous system: Headache (13% to 38%)
- Gastrointestinal: Nausea (5% to 15%), abdominal pain (1% to 11%)
- Hematologic: Neutropenia (≤18%)
- Hepatic: ALT increased (≤14%), AST increased (2% to 16%)
- Respiratory: Nasopharyngitis (≤16%)

1% to 10%:

- Central nervous system: Fatigue (≤8%), depression (≤7%), fever (children 4%), dizziness (2% to 4%)
- Dermatologic: Rash (≤8%)
- Endocrine: Dysmenorrhea (≤1% to 8%), dehydration (children 2%)
- Gastrointestinal: Vomiting (<1% to 6%), diarrhea (children 5%; adults <1%)
- Hematologic: Thrombocytopenia (≤3%)
- Hepatic: Alkaline phosphatase increased (≤4%)
- Neuromuscular & skeletal: Arthralgia (<1 to 6%)
- Respiratory: Rhinorrhea (children 2%)
- Miscellaneous: Herpes simplex (children 2%)

<1% (Limited to important or life-threatening): Acute hypersensitivity reactions (angioedema, anaphylaxis, dyspnea, pruritus, rash, urticaria); aggression, agitation, alopecia, anemia, aplastic anemia, ataxia, creatinine increased, coma, confusion, consciousness decreased, delirium, dysarthria, encephalopathy, erythema multiforme, facial edema, hallucinations (auditory and visual), hemolytic uremic syndrome (HUS), hepatitis, hypertension, leukocytoclastic vasculitis, leukopenia, mania, photosensitivity reaction, psychosis, renal failure, renal pain, seizure, tachycardia, thrombotic thrombocytopenic purpura (TTP), tremor, urinary precipitation, visual disturbances

Drug Interactions

Metabolism/Transport Effects None known.

Avoid Concomitant Use

Avoid concomitant use of ValACYclovir with any of the following: Zoster Vaccine

Increased Effect/Toxicity

ValACYclovir may increase the levels/effects of: Mycophenolate; Tenofovir; Zidovudine

The levels/effects of ValACYclovir may be increased by: Mycophenolate

Decreased Effect

ValACYclovir may decrease the levels/effects of: Zoster Vaccine

Stability Store at 15°C to 25°C (59°F to 77°F).

Mechanism of Action Valacyclovir is rapidly and nearly completely converted to acyclovir by intestinal and hepatic metabolism. Acyclovir is converted to acyclovir monophosphate by virus-specific thymidine kinase then further converted to acyclovir triphosphate by other cellular enzymes. Acyclovir triphosphate inhibits DNA synthesis and viral replication by competing with deoxyguanosine triphosphate for viral DNA polymerase and being incorporated into viral DNA.

Pharmacodynamics/Kinetics

Absorption: Rapid

Distribution: Acyclovir is widely distributed throughout the body including brain, kidney, lungs, liver, spleen, muscle, uterus, vagina, and CSF

Protein binding: ~14% to 18%

Metabolism: Hepatic; valacyclovir is rapidly and nearly completely converted to acyclovir and L-valine by first-pass effect; acyclovir is hepatically metabolized to a very small extent by aldehyde oxidase and by alcohol and aldehyde dehydrogenase (inactive metabolites)

Bioavailability: ~55% once converted to acyclovir

Half-life elimination: Normal renal function: Adults: Acyclovir: 2.5-3.3 hours, Valacyclovir: ~30 minutes; End-stage renal disease: Acyclovir: 14-20 hours; During hemodialysis: 4 hours

Excretion: Urine, primarily as acyclovir (89%); **Note:** Following oral administration of radiolabeled valacyclovir, 46% of the label is eliminated in the feces (corresponding to nonabsorbed drug), while 47% of the radiolabel is eliminated in the urine.

Dosage Oral:

Children 2 to <18 years: Chickenpox: 20 mg/kg/dose 3 times/day for 5 days (maximum: 1 g 3 times/day)

Children ≥12 and Adults: Herpes labialis (cold sores): 2 g twice daily for 1 day (separate doses by ~12 hours)

Adults:

- CMV prophylaxis in allogeneic HSCT recipients (unlabeled use): 2 g 4 times/day
- Herpes zoster (shingles): 1 g 3 times/day for 7 days
- HSV, VZV in cancer patients (unlabeled use): Prophylaxis: 500 mg 2-3 times/day; Treatment: 1 g 3 times/day
- Genital herpes:
  - Initial episode: 1 g twice daily for 10 days
  - Recurrent episode: 500 mg twice daily for 3 days
  - Reduction of transmission: 500 mg once daily (source partner)
  - Suppressive therapy:
    - Immunocompetent patients: 1000 mg once daily (500 mg once daily in patients with <9 recurrences per year)
    - HIV-infected patients (CD4 ≥100 cells/mm^3): 500 mg twice daily

Dosing adjustment in renal impairment:
Herpes zoster: Adults:
Cl_{cr} 30-49 mL/minute: 1 g every 12 hours
Cl_{cr} 10-29 mL/minute: 1 g every 24 hours
Cl_{cr} <10 mL/minute: 500 mg every 24 hours
Genital herpes: Adults:
Initial episode:
Cl_{cr} 10-29 mL/minute: 1 g every 24 hours
Cl_{cr} <10 mL/minute: 500 mg every 24 hours
Recurrent episode: Cl_{cr} <29 mL/minute: 500 mg every 24 hours
Suppressive therapy: Cl_{cr} <29 mL/minute:
For usual dose of 1 g every 24 hours, decrease dose to 500 mg every 24 hours
For usual dose of 500 mg every 24 hours, decrease dose to 500 mg every 48 hours
HIV-infected patients: 500 mg every 24 hours
Herpes labialis: Adolescents and Adults:
Cl_{cr} 30-49 mL/minute: 1 g every 12 hours for 2 doses
Cl_{cr} 10-29 mL/minute: 500 mg every 12 hours for 2 doses
Cl_{cr} <10 mL/minute: 500 mg as a single dose
Hemodialysis: Dialyzable (~33% removed during 4-hour session); administer dose postdialysis
Chronic ambulatory peritoneal dialysis/continuous arteriovenous hemofiltration dialysis: Pharmacokinetic parameters are similar to those in patients with ESRD; supplemental dose not needed following dialysis

Dosing adjustment in hepatic impairment: No adjustment required.

Dietary Considerations May be taken with or without food.

Administration If GI upset occurs, administer with meals.

Monitoring Parameters Urinalysis, BUN, serum creatinine, liver enzymes, and CBC

Dosage Forms Excipient information presented when available (limited, particularly for generics); consult specific product labeling.
Caplet, oral: 500 mg, 1 g
Valtrex®: 500 mg
Valtrex®: 1 g [scored]
Tablet, oral: 500 mg, 1 g

Extemporaneous Preparations A 50 mg/mL oral suspension may be made with caplets and either Ora-Sweet® or Ora-Sweet SF®. Crush eighteen 500 mg caplets in a mortar and reduce to a fine powder. Add 5 mL portions of chosen vehicle (40 mL total) and mix to a uniform paste; transfer to a 180 mL calibrated amber glass bottle, rinse mortar with 10 mL of vehicle 5 times, and add quantity of vehicle sufficient to make 180 mL. Label "shake well" and "refrigerate". Stable for 21 days refrigerated.

Fish DN, Vidaurri VA, and Deeter RG, "Stability of Valacyclovir Hydrochloride in Extemporaneously Prepared Oral Liquids," *Am J Health Syst Pharm*, 1999, 56(19):1957-60.

◆ **Valacyclovir Hydrochloride** *see* ValACYclovir *on page 1753*

◆ **Valcyte®** *see* ValGANciclovir *on page 1755*

◆ **23-Valent Pneumococcal Polysaccharide Vaccine** *see* Pneumococcal Polysaccharide Vaccine (Polyvalent) *on page 1368*

ValGANciclovir (val gan SYE kloh veer)

Brand Names: U.S. Valcyte®
Brand Names: Canada Valcyte®
Index Terms Valganciclovir Hydrochloride
Pharmacologic Category Antiviral Agent

Use Treatment of cytomegalovirus (CMV) retinitis in patients with acquired immunodeficiency syndrome (AIDS); prevention of CMV disease in high-risk patients (donor CMV positive/recipient CMV negative) undergoing kidney, heart, or kidney/pancreas transplantation

Pregnancy Risk Factor C

Pregnancy Considerations Valganciclovir is converted to ganciclovir and shares its reproductive toxicity. **[U.S. Boxed Warning]: Ganciclovir may be teratogenic and cause aspermatogenesis.** Based on animal data, temporary or permanent impairment of fertility may occur in males and females. Ganciclovir is also teratogenic in animals. Females should use effective contraception during treatment and for 30 days after; males should use barrier contraception during treatment and for 90 days after.

Lactation Excretion in breast milk unknown/not recommended

Contraindications Hypersensitivity to valganciclovir, ganciclovir, or any component of the formulation

Warnings/Precautions Hazardous agent - use appropriate precautions for handling and disposal. **[U.S. Boxed Warning]: May cause dose- or therapy-limiting granulocytopenia, anemia, and/or thrombocytopenia;** do not use in patients with an absolute neutrophil count <500/mm^3, platelet count <25,000/mm^3, or hemoglobin <8 g/dL. Use with caution in patients with impaired renal function (dose adjustment required). Acute renal failure (ARF) may occur; ensure adequate hydration and use with caution in patients receiving concomitant nephrotoxic agents. Elderly patients with or without pre-existing renal impairment may develop ARF; use with caution and adjust dose as needed. **[U.S. Boxed Warning]: Ganciclovir may be teratogenic, carcinogenic, and cause aspermatogenesis.** Due to its teratogenic potential, contraceptive precautions for female and male patients need to be followed during and for at least 90 days after therapy with the drug. Fertility may be temporarily or permanently impaired in males and females. Due to differences in bioavailability, valganciclovir tablets cannot be substituted for ganciclovir capsules on a one-to-one basis. The preferred dosage form for pediatric patients is the oral solution; however, valganciclovir tablets may used so long as the calculated dose is within 10% of the available tablet strength (450 mg). Not indicated for use in liver transplant patients (higher incidence of tissue-invasive CMV relative to oral ganciclovir was observed in trials). Use of valganciclovir for the treatment of congenital CMV disease has not been evaluated.

Adverse Reactions
>10%:
Cardiovascular: Hypertension (12% to 18%)
Central nervous system: Fever (9% to 31%), headache (6% to 22%), insomnia (6% to 20%)
Gastrointestinal: Diarrhea (16% to 41%), nausea (8% to 30%), vomiting (3% to 21%), abdominal pain (15%), constipation
Hematologic: Anemia (≤31%), thrombocytopenia (≤22%), neutropenia (3% to 19%)
Neuromuscular & skeletal: Tremor (12% to 28%)
Ocular: Retinal detachment (15%)
Renal: Serum creatinine increased (S_{cr} >1.5-2.5 mg/dL: 12% to 50%; S_{cr} >2.5: 3% to 17%)
Respiratory: Cough, upper respiratory tract infection
5% to 10%: Central nervous system: Peripheral neuropathy (9%), paresthesia (8%)
<5%:
Cardiovascular: Edema, hypotension, peripheral edema
Central nervous system: Agitation, confusion, depression, dizziness, fatigue, hallucination, pain, psychosis, seizure
Dermatologic: Acne, dermatitis, pruritus

Endocrine & metabolic: Dehydration, hyperglycemia, hyper-/hypokalemia, hypocalcemia, hypomagnesemia, hypophosphatemia
Gastrointestinal: Abdominal distention/pain, appetite (decreased), dyspepsia
Genitourinary: Urinary tract infection
Hematologic: Aplastic anemia, bleeding (potentially life-threatening due to thrombocytopenia), bone marrow depression, pancytopenia
Hepatic: Ascites
Neuromuscular & skeletal: Arthralgia, back pain, limb pain, muscle cramps, weakness
Renal: Creatinine clearance (decreased), dysuria, renal impairment
Respiratory: Dyspnea, nasopharyngitis, pharyngitis, pleural effusion, rhinorrhea
Miscellaneous: Allergic reaction, local and systemic infection (including sepsis)

<1% (Limited to important or life-threatening): Valganciclovir is expected to share the toxicities which may occur at a low incidence or due to idiosyncratic reactions which have been associated with ganciclovir

Drug Interactions

Metabolism/Transport Effects None known.

Avoid Concomitant Use

Avoid concomitant use of ValGANciclovir with any of the following: Imipenem

Increased Effect/Toxicity

ValGANciclovir may increase the levels/effects of: Imipenem; Mycophenolate; Reverse Transcriptase Inhibitors (Nucleoside); Tenofovir

The levels/effects of ValGANciclovir may be increased by: Mycophenolate; Probenecid; Tenofovir

Decreased Effect There are no known significant interactions involving a decrease in effect.

Ethanol/Nutrition/Herb Interactions Food: Coadministration with a high-fat meal increased AUC by 30%.

Stability

Oral solution: Store dry powder at 25°C (77°F); excursions permitted to 15°C to 30°C (59°F to 86°F). Prior to dispensing, prepare the oral solution by adding 91 mL of purified water to the bottle; shake well. Store oral solution under refrigeration at 2°C to 8°C (36°F to 46°F); do not freeze. Discard any unused medication after 49 days. A reconstituted 100 mL bottle will only provide 88 mL of solution for administration.

Tablet: Store at 25°C (77°F); excursions permitted to 15°C to 30°C (59°F to 86°F).

Mechanism of Action Valganciclovir is rapidly converted to ganciclovir in the body. The bioavailability of ganciclovir from valganciclovir is increased 10-fold compared to oral ganciclovir. A dose of 900 mg achieved systemic exposure of ganciclovir comparable to that achieved with the recommended doses of intravenous ganciclovir of 5 mg/kg. Ganciclovir is phosphorylated to a substrate which competitively inhibits the binding of deoxyguanosine triphosphate to DNA polymerase resulting in inhibition of viral DNA synthesis.

Pharmacodynamics/Kinetics

Absorption: Well absorbed; high-fat meal increases AUC by 30%
Distribution: V_{dss}: Ganciclovir: 0.7 L/kg; widely to all tissue including CSF and ocular tissue
Protein binding: Ganciclovir: 1% to 2%
Metabolism: Converted to ganciclovir by intestinal mucosal cells and hepatocytes
Bioavailability: With food: 60%
Half-life elimination: Ganciclovir: 4.08 hours; prolonged with renal impairment; Severe renal impairment: Up to 68 hours
Time to peak: Ganciclovir: 1-3 hours
Excretion: Urine (primarily as ganciclovir)

Dosage Oral:

Children 4 months to 16 years: Prevention of CMV disease following kidney or heart transplantation: Dose (mg) = 7 x body surface area x creatinine clearance* once daily beginning within 10 days of transplantation; continue therapy until 100 days post-transplantation. Doses should be rounded to the nearest 25 mg increment; maximum dose: 900 mg/day.

*Cl_{cr} (mL/minute/1.73 m^2) = [k x Height (cm)] divided by serum creatinine (mg/dL)

Note: If the calculated Cl_{cr} is >150 mL/minute/1.73 m^2, then a maximum value of 150 mL/minute/1.73 m^2 should be used to calculate the dose.

Note: Calculated using *modified* Schwartz formula where k is as follows:
Patients <2 years: k = 0.45
Girls 2-16 years: k = 0.55
Boys 2 to <13 years: k = 0.55
Boys 13-16 years: k = 0.7

Children >16 years and Adults:

CMV retinitis:
Induction: 900 mg twice daily for 21 days
Maintenance: Following induction treatment, or for patients with inactive CMV retinitis who require maintenance therapy: 900 mg once daily

Prevention of CMV disease following transplantation: 900 mg once daily beginning within 10 days of transplantation; continue therapy until 100 days (heart or kidney-pancreas transplant) or 200 days (kidney transplant) post-transplantation

Dosage adjustment in renal impairment:

Children 4 months to 16 years: No additional dosage adjustments required; calculation for all patients adjusts for renal function.

Children >16 years and Adults:

Induction dose:
Cl_{cr} 40-59 mL/minute: 450 mg twice daily
Cl_{cr} 25-39 mL/minute: 450 mg once daily
Cl_{cr} 10-24 mL/minute: 450 mg every 2 days

Maintenance dose:
Cl_{cr} 40-59 mL/minute: 450 mg once daily
Cl_{cr} 25-39 mL/minute: 450 mg every 2 days
Cl_{cr} 10-24 mL/minute: 450 mg twice weekly

Note: Valganciclovir is not recommended in patients receiving hemodialysis. For patients on hemodialysis (Cl_{cr} <10 mL/minute), it is recommended that ganciclovir be used (dose adjusted as specified for ganciclovir).

Dosage adjustment in hepatic impairment: Use has not been studied

Dietary Considerations Should be taken with meals.

Administration Valganciclovir should be taken with meals. The preferred dosage form for pediatric patients is the oral solution; however, valganciclovir tablets may used so long as the calculated dose is within 10% of the available tablet strength (450 mg).

Due to the carcinogenic and mutagenic potential, avoid direct contact with broken or crushed tablets, powder for oral solution, and oral solution. Consideration should be given to handling and disposal according to guidelines issued for antineoplastic drugs. However, there is no consensus on the need for these precautions.

Monitoring Parameters Retinal exam (at least every 4-6 weeks), CBC, platelet counts, serum creatinine

Dosage Forms Excipient information presented when available (limited, particularly for generics); consult specific product labeling.

Powder for solution, oral:
Valcyte®: 50 mg/mL (100 mL) [contains sodium benzoate; tutti frutti flavor]

Tablet, oral [strength expressed as base]:
Valcyte®: 450 mg

Extemporaneous Preparations Hazardous agent: Use appropriate precautions for handling and disposal.

Note: Commercial preparation is available (50 mg/mL)

A 60 mg/mL oral suspension may be with tablets and a 1:1 mixture of Ora-Sweet® and Ora-Plus®. Crush sixteen 450 mg tablets and reduce to a fine powder. Add 1 mL portions of chosen vehicle (10 mL total) and mix to a uniform paste; mix while adding the vehicle in incremental proportions to **almost** 120 mL; transfer to a calibrated amber glass bottle, rinse mortar with vehicle, and add quantity of vehicle sufficient to make 120 mL. Label "shake well" and "refrigerate". Stable for 35 days refrigerated.

Henkin CC, Griener JC, and Ten Eick AP, "Stability of Valganciclovir in Extemporaneously Compounded Liquid Formulations," *Am J Health Syst Pharm*, 2003, 60(7):687-90.

◆ **Valganciclovir Hydrochloride** *see* ValGANciclovir *on page 1755*

◆ **Valisone® Scalp Lotion (Can)** *see* Betamethasone *on page 208*

◆ **Valium®** *see* Diazepam *on page 492*

◆ **Valorin [OTC]** *see* Acetaminophen *on page 27*

◆ **Valorin Extra [OTC]** *see* Acetaminophen *on page 27*

◆ **Valproate Semisodium** *see* Divalproex *on page 530*

◆ **Valproate Semisodium** *see* Valproic Acid *on page 1757*

◆ **Valproate Sodium** *see* Valproic Acid *on page 1757*

Valproic Acid (val PROE ik AS id)

Brand Names: U.S. Depacon®; Depakene®; Stavzor™

Brand Names: Canada Apo-Valproic®; Depakene®; Epival® I.V.; Mylan-Valproic; PHL-Valproic Acid; PHL-Valproic Acid E.C.; PMS-Valproic Acid; PMS-Valproic Acid E.C.; ratio-Valproic; ratio-Valproic ECC; Rhoxal-valproic; Sandoz-Valproic

Index Terms 2-Propylpentanoic Acid; 2-Propylvaleric Acid; Dipropylacetic Acid; DPA; Valproate Semisodium; Valproate Sodium

Pharmacologic Category Anticonvulsant, Miscellaneous; Antimanic Agent; Histone Deacetylase Inhibitor

Additional Appendix Information

Anticonvulsant Drugs of Choice *on page 1873*

Use Monotherapy and adjunctive therapy in the treatment of patients with complex partial seizures; monotherapy and adjunctive therapy of simple and complex absence seizures; adjunctive therapy in patients with multiple seizure types that include absence seizures

Stavzor™: Mania associated with bipolar disorder; migraine prophylaxis

Unlabeled Use Status epilepticus, diabetic neuropathy

Pregnancy Risk Factor D

Pregnancy Considerations [U.S. Boxed Warning]: May cause teratogenic effects such as neural tube defects (eg, spina bifida). Teratogenic effects have been reported in animals and humans. Valproic acid crosses the placenta. Neural tube, cardiac, facial (characteristic pattern of dysmorphic facial features), skeletal, multiple other defects reported. Epilepsy itself, number of medications, genetic factors, or a combination of these probably influence the teratogenicity of anticonvulsant therapy. Information from the North American Antiepileptic Drug Pregnancy Registry notes a fourfold increase in congenital malformations with exposure to valproic acid monotherapy during the 1st trimester of pregnancy when compared to monotherapy with other antiepileptic drugs (AED). The risk of neural tube defects is ~1% to 2% (general population risk estimated to be 0.14% to 0.2%). The effect of folic acid supplementation to decrease this risk is unknown, however, folic acid supplementation is recommended for all women contemplating pregnancy. An information sheet describing the teratogenic potential is available from the manufacturer.

Nonteratogenic effects have also been reported. Afibrinogenemia leading to fatal hemorrhage and hepatotoxicity have been noted in case reports of infants following *in utero* exposure to valproic acid. Developmental delay, autism and/or autism spectrum disorder have also been reported. In a prospective cohort study conducted in the U.S. and the United Kingdom, a lower Differential Ability Scale ([D.A.S.]; a battery of tests which measure cognitive development in children) score was observed in children 3 years of age with prenatal exposure to valproate compared to children with prenatal exposure to other antiepileptics (lamotrigine, carbamazepine, or phenytoin). Use in women of childbearing potential requires that benefits of use in mother be weighed against the potential risk to fetus, especially when used for conditions not associated with permanent injury or risk of death (eg, migraine).

Patients exposed to valproic acid during pregnancy are encouraged to enroll themselves into the AED Pregnancy Registry by calling 1-888-233-2334. Additional information is available at www.aedpregnancyregistry.org.

Lactation Enters breast milk/not recommended (AAP considers "compatible"; AAP 2001 update pending)

Contraindications Hypersensitivity to valproic acid, derivatives, or any component of the formulation; hepatic disease or significant impairment; urea cycle disorders

Warnings/Precautions [U.S. Boxed Warning]: Hepatic failure resulting in fatalities has occurred in patients; children <2 years of age are at considerable risk. Other risk factors include organic brain disease, mental retardation with severe seizure disorders, congenital metabolic disorders, and patients on multiple anticonvulsants. Hepatotoxicity has usually been reported within 6 months of therapy initiation. Monitor patients closely for appearance of malaise, weakness, facial edema, anorexia, jaundice, and vomiting; discontinue immediately with signs/symptom of significant or suspected impairment. Liver function tests should be performed at baseline and at regular intervals after initiation of therapy, especially within the first 6 months. Hepatic dysfunction may progress despite discontinuing treatment. Should only be used as monotherapy in children <2 years of age and patients at high risk for hepatotoxicity. Contraindicated with severe impairment.

[U.S. Boxed Warning]: Cases of life-threatening pancreatitis, occurring at the start of therapy or following years of use, have been reported in adults and children. Some cases have been hemorrhagic with rapid progression of initial symptoms to death. Promptly evaluate symptoms of abdominal pain, nausea, vomiting, and/or anorexia; should generally be discontinued if pancreatitis is diagnosed.

[U.S. Boxed Warning]: May cause teratogenic effects such as neural tube defects (eg, spina bifida). Use in women of childbearing potential requires that benefits of use in mother be weighed against the potential risk to fetus, especially when used for conditions not associated with permanent injury or risk of death (eg, migraine).

May cause severe thrombocytopenia, inhibition of platelet aggregation, and bleeding. Tremors may indicate overdosage; use with caution in patients receiving other anticonvulsants. Hypersensitivity reactions affecting multiple organs have been reported in association with valproic acid use; may include dermatologic and/or hematologic changes (eosinophilia, neutropenia, thrombocytopenia) or symptoms of organ dysfunction.

Hyperammonemia and/or encephalopathy, sometimes fatal, have been reported following the initiation of valproic acid therapy and may be present with normal transaminase levels. Ammonia levels should be measured in patients who develop unexplained lethargy and vomiting, changes in mental status, or in patients who present with hypothermia (unintentional drop in core body temperature to <35°C/95°F). Discontinue therapy if ammonia levels are increased and evaluate for possible urea cycle disorder (UCD); contraindicated in patients with UCD. Evaluation of UCD should be considered for the following patients prior to the start of therapy: History of unexplained encephalopathy or coma; encephalopathy associated with protein load; pregnancy or postpartum encephalopathy; unexplained mental retardation; history of elevated plasma ammonia or glutamine; history of cyclical vomiting and lethargy; episodic extreme irritability, ataxia; low BUN or protein avoidance; family history of UCD or unexplained infant deaths (particularly male); or signs or symptoms of UCD (hyperammonemia, encephalopathy, respiratory alkalosis). Hypothermia has been reported with valproic acid therapy; may or may not be associated with hyperammonemia; may also occur with concomitant topiramate therapy.

In vitro studies have suggested valproic acid stimulates the replication of HIV and CMV viruses under experimental conditions. The clinical consequence of this is unknown, but should be considered when monitoring affected patients.

Antiepileptics are associated with an increased risk of suicidal behavior/thoughts with use (regardless of indication); patients should be monitored for signs/symptoms of depression, suicidal tendencies, and other unusual behavior changes during therapy and instructed to inform their healthcare provider immediately if symptoms occur.

Use of Depacon® injection is not recommended for post-traumatic seizure prophylaxis following acute head trauma. Anticonvulsants should not be discontinued abruptly because of the possibility of increasing seizure frequency; valproic acid should be withdrawn gradually to minimize the potential of increased seizure frequency, unless safety concerns require a more rapid withdrawal. Concomitant use with carbapenem antibiotics may reduce valproic acid levels to subtherapeutic levels; monitor levels frequently and consider alternate therapy if levels drop significantly or lack of seizure control occurs. Concomitant use with clonazepam may induce absence status. Patients treated for bipolar disorder should be monitored closely for clinical worsening or suicidality; prescriptions should be written for the smallest quantity consistent with good patient care.

CNS depression may occur with valproic acid use. Patients must be cautioned about performing tasks which require mental alertness (operating machinery or driving). Effects with other sedative drugs or ethanol may be potentiated. Use with caution in the elderly.

Adverse Reactions

>10%:

- Central nervous system: Headache (≤31%), somnolence (≤30%), dizziness (12% to 25%), insomnia (>1% to 15%), nervousness (>1% to 11%), pain (1% to 11%)
- Dermatologic: Alopecia (>1% to 24%)
- Gastrointestinal: Nausea (15% to 48%), vomiting (7% to 27%), diarrhea (7% to 23%), abdominal pain (7% to 23%), dyspepsia (7% to 23%), anorexia (>1% to 12%)
- Hematologic: Thrombocytopenia (1% to 24%; dose related)
- Neuromuscular & skeletal: Tremor (≤57%), weakness (6% to 27%)
- Ocular: Diplopia (>1% to 16%), amblyopia/blurred vision (≤12%)
- Miscellaneous: Infection (≤20%), flu-like syndrome (12%)

1% to 10%:

- Cardiovascular: Peripheral edema (>1% to 8%), chest pain (>1% to <5%), edema (>1% to <5%), facial edema (>1% to <5%), hypertension (>1% to <5%), hypotension (>1% to <5%), palpitation (>1% to <5%), postural hypotension (>1% to <5%), tachycardia (>1% to <5%), vasodilation (>1% to <5%), arrhythmia
- Central nervous system: Ataxia (>1% to 8%), amnesia (>1% to 7%), emotional lability (>1% to 6%), fever (>1% to 6%), abnormal thinking (≤6%), depression (>1% to 5%), abnormal dreams (>1% to <5%), agitation (>1% to <5%), anxiety (>1% to <5%), catatonia (>1% to <5%), chills (>1% to <5%), confusion (>1% to <5%), coordination abnormal (>1% to <5%), hallucination (>1% to <5%), malaise (>1% to <5%), personality disorder (>1% to <5%), speech disorder (>1% to <5%), tardive dyskinesia (>1% to <5%), vertigo (>1% to <5%), euphoria (1%), hypoesthesia (1%)
- Dermatologic: Rash (>1% to 6%), bruising (>1% to 5%), discoid lupus erythematosus (>1% to <5%), dry skin (>1% to <5%), furunculosis (>1% to <5%), petechia (>1% to <5%), pruritus (>1% to <5), seborrhea (>1% to <5%)
- Endocrine & metabolic: Amenorrhea (>1% to <5%), dysmenorrhea (>1% to <5%), metrorrhagia (>1% to <5%), hypoproteinemia
- Gastrointestinal: Weight gain (4% to 9%), weight loss (6%), appetite increased (≤6%), constipation (>1% to 5%), xerostomia (>1% to 5%), eructation (>1% to <5%), fecal incontinence (>1% to <5%), flatulence (>1% to <5%), gastroenteritis (>1% to <5%), glossitis (>1% to <5%), hematemesis (>1% to <5%), pancreatitis (>1% to <5%), periodontal abscess (>1% to <5%), stomatitis (>1% to <5%), taste perversion (>1% to <5%), dysphagia, gum hemorrhage, mouth ulceration
- Genitourinary: Cystitis (>1% to 5%), dysuria (>1% to 5%), urinary frequency (>1% to <5%), urinary incontinence (>1% to <5%), vaginal hemorrhage (>1% to 5%), vaginitis (>1% to <5%)
- Hepatic: ALT increased (>1% to <5%), AST increased (>1% to <5%)
- Local: Injection site pain (3%), injection site reaction (2%), injection site inflammation (1%)
- Neuromuscular & skeletal: Back pain (≤8%), abnormal gait (>1% to <5%), arthralgia (>1% to <5%), arthrosis (>1% to <5%), dysarthria (>1% to <5%), hypertonia (>1% to <5%), hypokinesia (>1% to <5%), leg cramps (>1% to <5%), myalgia (>1% to <5%), myasthenia (>1% to <5%), neck pain (>1% to <5%), neck rigidity (>1% to <5%), paresthesia (>1% to <5%), reflex increased (>1% to <5%), twitching (>1% to <5%)
- Ocular: Nystagmus (1% to 8%), dry eyes (>1% to 5%), eye pain (>1% to 5%), abnormal vision (>1% to <5%), conjunctivitis (>1% to <5%)
- Otic: Tinnitus (1% to 7%), ear pain (>1% to 5%), deafness (>1% to <5%), otitis media (>1% to <5%)
- Respiratory: Pharyngitis (2% to 8%), bronchitis (5%), rhinitis (>1% to 5%), dyspnea (1% to 5%), cough (>1% to <5%), epistaxis (>1% to <5%), pneumonia (>1% to <5%), sinusitis (>1% to <5%)
- Miscellaneous: Diaphoresis (1%), hiccups

<1% (Limited to important and/or life-threatening): Aggression, agranulocytosis, allergic reaction, anaphylaxis, anemia, aplastic anemia, asterixis, behavioral deterioration, bilirubin increased, bleeding time altered, bone marrow suppression, bone pain, bradycardia, breast enlargement, cutaneous vasculitis, carnitine decreased, cerebral atrophy (reversible), coma (rare), dementia, encephalopathy (rare), enuresis, eosinophilia, erythema multiforme, Fanconi-like syndrome (rare, in children), galactorrhea, hematoma formation, hemorrhage, hepatic failure, hepatotoxicity, hostility, hyperactivity, hyperammonemia, hyperammonemic encephalopathy (in patients with

UCD), hyperglycinemia, hypersensitivity reactions (severe, with multiorgan dysfunction), hypofibrinogenemia, hyponatremia, hypothermia, inappropriate ADH secretion, intermittent porphyria, LDH increased, leukopenia, lupus, lymphocytosis, macrocytosis, menstrual irregularities, pancytopenia, parkinsonism, parotid gland swelling, photosensitivity, platelet aggregation inhibited, polycystic ovary disease (rare), psychosis, seeing "spots before the eyes," Stevens-Johnson syndrome, suicidal behavior/ideation, thyroid function tests abnormal, toxic epidermal necrolysis (rare), urinary tract infection

Drug Interactions

Metabolism/Transport Effects Substrate of CYP2A6 (minor), CYP2B6 (minor), CYP2C19 (minor), CYP2C9 (minor), CYP2E1 (minor); **Note:** Assignment of Major/Minor substrate status based on clinically relevant drug interaction potential; **Inhibits** CYP2C9 (weak); **Induces** CYP2A6 (weak/moderate)

Avoid Concomitant Use There are no known interactions where it is recommended to avoid concomitant use.

Increased Effect/Toxicity

Valproic Acid may increase the levels/effects of: Barbiturates; Ethosuximide; LamoTRIgine; LORazepam; Paliperidone; Primidone; RisperiDONE; Rufinamide; Temozolomide; Tricyclic Antidepressants; Vorinostat; Zidovudine

The levels/effects of Valproic Acid may be increased by: ChlorproMAZINE; Felbamate; GuanFACINE; Salicylates; Topiramate

Decreased Effect

Valproic Acid may decrease the levels/effects of: CarBAMazepine; Fosphenytoin; OXcarbazepine; Phenytoin

The levels/effects of Valproic Acid may be decreased by: Barbiturates; CarBAMazepine; Carbapenems; Cyproterone; Ethosuximide; Fosphenytoin; Methylfolate; Phenytoin; Primidone; Protease Inhibitors; Rifampin

Ethanol/Nutrition/Herb Interactions

Ethanol: Avoid ethanol (may increase CNS depression).

Food: Food may delay but does not affect the extent of absorption. Valproic acid serum concentrations may be decreased if taken with food. Milk has no effect on absorption.

Herb/Nutraceutical: Avoid evening primrose (seizure threshold decreased).

Stability

Depakene® solution: Store below 30°C (86°F).

Stavzor™: Store at controlled room temperature of 25°C (77°F).

Depakene® capsule: Store at controlled room temperature of 15°C to 25°C (59°F to 77°F).

Depacon®: Store vial at room temperature of 15°C to 30°C (59°F to 86°F). Injection should be diluted in 50 mL of a compatible diluent. Stable in D_5W, NS, and LR for at least 24 hours when stored in glass or PVC.

Mechanism of Action Causes increased availability of gamma-aminobutyric acid (GABA), an inhibitory neurotransmitter, to brain neurons or may enhance the action of GABA or mimic its action at postsynaptic receptor sites

Pharmacodynamics/Kinetics

Distribution: Total valproate: 11 L/1.73 m^2; free valproate 92 L/1.73 m^2

Protein binding (dose dependent): 80% to 90%; decreased in the elderly and with hepatic or renal dysfunction

Metabolism: Extensively hepatic via glucuronide conjugation and mitochondrial beta-oxidation. The relationship between dose and total valproate concentration is nonlinear; concentration does not increase proportionally with the dose, but increases to a lesser extent due to saturable plasma protein binding. The kinetics of unbound drug are linear.

Half-life elimination (increased in neonates and with liver disease): Children >2 months: 7-13 hours; Adults: 9-16 hours

Time to peak, serum: Stavzor™: 2 hours

Excretion: Urine (30% to 50% as glucuronide conjugate, 3% as unchanged drug)

Dosage

Seizure disorders: **Note:** Administer doses >250 mg/day in divided doses.

Oral:

Simple and complex absence seizures: Children and Adults: Initial: 15 mg/kg/day; increase by 5-10 mg/kg/day at weekly intervals until therapeutic levels are achieved; maximum: 60 mg/kg/day. Larger maintenance doses may be required in younger children.

Complex partial seizures: Children ≥10 years and Adults: Initial: 10-15 mg/kg/day; increase by 5-10 mg/kg/day at weekly intervals until therapeutic levels are achieved; maximum: 60 mg/kg/day. Larger maintenance doses may be required in younger children.

Note: Regular release and delayed release formulations are usually given in 2-4 divided doses/day.

I.V.: Administer as a 60-minute infusion (≤20 mg/minute) with the same frequency as oral products; switch patient to oral products as soon as possible. Rapid infusions ≤45 mg/kg over 5-10 minutes (1.5-6 mg/kg/minute) were generally well tolerated in a clinical trial.

Rectal (unlabeled): Dilute syrup 1:1 with water for use as a retention enema; loading dose: 17-20 mg/kg one time; maintenance: 10-15 mg/kg/dose every 8 hours

Status epilepticus (unlabeled use): Adults:

Loading dose: I.V.: 15-45 mg/kg administered at ≤6 mg/kg/minute.

Maintenance dose: I.V. infusion: 1-4 mg/kg/hour; titrate dose as needed based upon patient response and evaluation of drug-drug interactions

Mania (Stavzor™): Adults: Oral: Initial: 750 mg/day in divided doses; dose should be adjusted as rapidly as possible to desired clinical effect; maximum recommended dosage: 60 mg/kg/day

Migraine prophylaxis (Stavzor™): Children ≥12 years: Oral: 250 mg twice daily; adjust dose based on patient response, up to 1000 mg/day

Diabetic neuropathy (unlabeled use): Adults: Oral: 500-1200 mg/day (Bril, 2011)

Elderly: Elimination is decreased in the elderly. Studies of elderly patients with dementia show a high incidence of somnolence. In some patients, this was associated with weight loss. Starting doses should be lower and increases should be slow, with careful monitoring of nutritional intake and dehydration. Safety and efficacy for use in patients >65 years have not been studied for migraine prophylaxis.

Dosing adjustment in renal impairment: A 27% reduction in clearance of unbound valproate is seen in patients with Cl_{cr} <10 mL/minute. Hemodialysis reduces valproate concentrations by 20%, therefore no dose adjustment is needed in patients with renal failure. Protein binding is reduced, monitoring only total valproate concentrations may be misleading.

Dosing adjustment/comments in hepatic impairment: Reduce dose. Clearance is decreased with liver impairment. Hepatic disease is also associated with decreased albumin concentrations and 2- to 2.6-fold increase in the unbound fraction. Free concentrations of valproate may be elevated while total concentrations appear normal. Use is contraindicated in severe impairment.

Dietary Considerations Valproic acid may cause GI upset; take with large amount of water or food to decrease GI upset. May need to split doses to avoid GI upset.

Valproate sodium oral solution will generate valproic acid in carbonated beverages and may cause mouth and throat irritation; do not mix valproate sodium oral solution with carbonated beverages.

Administration

Depacon®: Following dilution to final concentration, administer over 60 minutes at a rate ≤20 mg/minute. Alternatively, single doses up to 45 mg/kg have been administered as a rapid infusion over 5-10 minutes (1.5-6 mg/kg/minute).

Depakene® capsule, Stavzor™: Swallow whole; do not chew.

Monitoring Parameters Liver enzymes (at baseline and during therapy), CBC with platelets (baseline and periodic intervals), PT/PTT (especially prior to surgery), serum ammonia (with symptoms of lethargy, mental status change), serum valproate levels (trough for therapeutic levels); suicidality (eg, suicidal thoughts, depression, behavioral changes)

Reference Range Note: In general, trough concentrations should be used to assess adequacy of therapy; peak concentrations may also be drawn if clinically necessary (eg, concentration-related toxicity). Within 2-4 days of initiation or dose adjustment, trough concentrations should be drawn just before the next dose (extended-release preparations) or before the morning dose (for immediate-release preparations). Patients with epilepsy should **not** delay taking their dose for >2-3 hours. Additional patient-specific factors must be taken into consideration when interpreting drug levels, including indication, age, clinical response, pregnancy status, adherence, comorbidities, adverse effects, and concomitant medications (Patsalos, 2008; Reed, 2006).

Therapeutic:

Epilepsy: 50-100 mcg/mL (SI: 350-700 micromole/L); although seizure control may improve at levels >100 mcg/mL (SI: 700 micromole/L), toxicity may occur at levels of 100-150 mcg/mL (SI: 700-1040 micromole/L)

Mania: 50-125 mcg/mL (SI: 350-875 micromole/L)

Toxic: Some laboratories may report >200 mcg/mL (SI: >1390 micromole/L) as a toxic threshold, although clinical toxicity can occur at lower concentrations. Probability of thrombocytopenia increases with total valproate levels ≥110 mcg/mL in females or ≥135 mcg/mL in males.

Epilepsy: Although seizure control may improve at levels >100 mcg/mL (SI: 700 micromole/L), toxicity may occur at levels of 100-150 mcg/mL (SI: 700-1050 micromole/L)

Mania: Clinical response seen with trough levels between 50-125 mcg/mL (SI: 350-875 micromole/L); risk of toxicity increases at levels >125 mcg/mL (SI: 875 micromole/L)

Test Interactions False-positive result for urine ketones; altered thyroid function tests

Dosage Forms Excipient information presented when available (limited, particularly for generics); consult specific product labeling.

Capsule, softgel, oral: 250 mg [strength expressed as valproic acid]

Depakene®: 250 mg [strength expressed as valproic acid]

Capsule, softgel, delayed release, oral:

Stavzor™: 125 mg, 250 mg, 500 mg [strength expressed as valproic acid]

Injection, solution, as valproate sodium: 100 mg/mL (5 mL) [strength expressed as valproic acid]

Injection, solution, as valproate sodium [preservative free]: 100 mg/mL (5 mL) [strength expressed as valproic acid]

Depacon®: 100 mg/mL (5 mL) [contains edetate disodium; strength expressed as valproic acid]

Solution, oral, as valproate sodium: 250 mg/5 mL (5 mL, 473 mL) [strength expressed as valproic acid]

Syrup, oral, as valproate sodium: 250 mg/5 mL (5 mL, 10 mL, 473 mL) [strength expressed as valproic acid]

Depakene®: 250 mg/5 mL (473 mL) [strength expressed as valproic acid]

◆ **Valproic Acid Derivative** *see* Divalproex *on page 530*

Valrubicin (val ROO bi sin)

Brand Names: U.S. Valstar®

Brand Names: Canada Valtaxin®

Index Terms *N*-trifluoroacetyladriamycin-14-valerate; AD32

Pharmacologic Category Antineoplastic Agent, Anthracycline

Use Intravesical treatment of BCG-refractory bladder carcinoma *in situ*

Pregnancy Risk Factor C

Pregnancy Considerations Embryotoxicity and teratogenic effects were observed in animal reproduction studies. Systemic exposure (eg, with bladder perforation) during human pregnancy may result in fetal harm. Women of childbearing potential should avoid becoming pregnant during treatment. All patients of reproductive age should use an effective method of contraception during the treatment period.

Lactation Excretion in breast milk unknown/not recommended

Contraindications Hypersensitivity to anthracyclines, polyoxyl castor oil (Cremophor® EL), or any component of the formulation; concurrent urinary tract infection; small bladder capacity (unable to tolerate a 75 mL instillation)

Warnings/Precautions Hazardous agent - use appropriate precautions for handling and disposal. Delay valrubicin therapy for at least 2 weeks after transurethral resection and/or fulguration. Evaluate bladder status prior to instillation; do not administer if mucosal integrity of bladder has been compromised or bladder perforation is present (delay treatment until restoration of bladder integrity). Use aseptic technique to prevent urinary tract infection or traumatizing urinary mucosa. Although clamping of the urinary catheter after administration is not recommended, use caution and appropriate medical supervision if performed. Irritable bladder symptoms may occur during instillation and retention, and for a brief time after voiding. Use caution in patients with severe irritable bladder symptoms. Red-tinged urine is typical for the first 24 hours after instillation. Prolonged symptoms or discoloration should prompt contact with the physician.

Contains polyoxyl castor oil (Cremophor® EL) which is associated with hypersensitivity reactions; use is contraindicated in patients with hypersensitivity to polyoxyl castor oil. Delaying cystectomy during treatment may lead to metastatic bladder cancer; reconsider cystectomy if complete response to treatment does not occur within 3 months.

Adverse Reactions Note: In general, local adverse reactions occur during or shortly after instillation and resolve within 1-7 days.

>10%: Genitourinary: Bladder irritation (88%), urinary frequency (61%), urinary urgency (57%), dysuria (56%), bladder spasm (31%), hematuria (29%; gross: 1%), bladder pain (28%), urinary incontinence (22%), cystitis (15%), urinary tract infection (15%), urine red-tinged

1% to 10%:

Cardiovascular: Chest pain (3%), vasodilation (2%), peripheral edema (1%)

Central nervous system: Headache (4%), malaise (4%), dizziness (3%), fever (2%)

Dermatologic: Rash (3%)
Endocrine & metabolic: Hyperglycemia (1%)
Gastrointestinal: Abdominal pain (5%), nausea (5%), diarrhea (3%), vomiting (2%), flatulence (1%)
Genitourinary: Nocturia (7%), burning symptoms (5%), urinary retention (4%), urethral pain (3%), pelvic pain (1%), hematuria (microscopic) (3%)
Hematologic: Anemia (2%)
Neuromuscular & skeletal: Weakness (4%), back pain (3%), myalgia (1%)
Respiratory: Pneumonia (1%)

<1% (Limited to important or life-threatening): Hematologic toxicity (following instillation into perforated bladder), nonprotein nitrogen increased, pruritus, skin irritation (local), taste loss, tenesmus, urine flow decreased, urethritis

Drug Interactions

Metabolism/Transport Effects None known.

Avoid Concomitant Use There are no known interactions where it is recommended to avoid concomitant use.

Increased Effect/Toxicity There are no known significant interactions involving an increase in effect.

Decreased Effect There are no known significant interactions involving a decrease in effect.

Stability Store unopened vials refrigerated at 2°C to 8°C (36°F to 48°F). Allow vials to slowly warm to room temperature (without heating) prior to use. A waxy precipitate (due to polyoxyl castor oil) may form at temperatures <4°C, warm vial in the hand until solution is clear (do not use vial if particulate still present). Use appropriate precautions for handling and disposal. Dilute 800 mg (20 mL) with 55 mL NS (total volume of 75 mL). Use non-PVC containers (glass, polyolefin or polypropylene) and administration sets to avoid leaching of DEHP plasticizers. Stable for 12 hours at room temperature when diluted in 0.9% sodium chloride. Do not mix with other drugs.

Mechanism of Action Blocks function of DNA topoisomerase II; inhibits DNA synthesis, causes extensive chromosomal damage, and arrests cell development (G_2 phase); unlike other anthracyclines, does not appear to intercalate DNA; readily penetrates cells.

Pharmacodynamics/Kinetics

Absorption: Intravesical: Penetrates into bladder wall; negligible systemic absorption (dependent on bladder wall condition; trauma to mucosa may increase absorption, bladder wall perforation may significantly increase absorption and systemic myelotoxicity).

Metabolism: Negligible after intravesical instillation and 2-hour retention

Excretion: Urine (post 2-hour retention): 98.6% as intact drug; 0.4% as *N*-trifluoroacetyladriamycin)

Dosage Adults: Intravesical: Bladder cancer: 800 mg once weekly (retain for 2 hours) for 6 weeks

Dosage adjustment for toxicity: In clinical trials (Steinberg, 2000), treatment was delayed for 1 week for the following adverse events: Grade 3 dysuria (not controlled with phenazopyridine), frequency/urgency lasting >24 hours, grade 2 gross hematuria (without clots) lasting >48 hours, grade 3 hematuria (with clots) lasting >48 hours. For local toxicities <grade 4 (eg, dysuria [not controlled with phenazopyridine] or severe bladder spasm), anticholinergic therapy (systemic or topical) or topical anesthesia was administered prior to subsequent instillations.

Administration Intravesicular bladder instillation: Insert urinary catheter, empty bladder prior to instillation, slowly by gravity flow, instill 800 mg/75 mL (in 0.9% sodium chloride injection), remove catheter. Retain in the bladder for 2 hours, then void. Administer through non-PVC tubing due to the polyoxyl castor oil (Cremophor® EL) diluent. Maintain adequate hydration following treatment. Use appropriate protective gown, goggles, and gloves during administration.

Monitoring Parameters Cystoscopy, biopsy, and urine cytology every 3 months for recurrence or progression

Dosage Forms Excipient information presented when available (limited, particularly for generics); consult specific product labeling.

Injection, solution [preservative free]:
Valstar®: 40 mg/mL (5 mL) [contains dehydrated ethanol 50%, polyoxyl castor oil]

Valsartan (val SAR tan)

Brand Names: U.S. Diovan®

Brand Names: Canada CO Valsartan; Diovan®; Ran-Valsartan; Sandoz-Valsartan; Teva-Valsartan

Pharmacologic Category Angiotensin II Receptor Blocker

Additional Appendix Information

Angiotensin Agents *on page 1869*
Heart Failure (Systolic) *on page 1991*

Use Alone or in combination with other antihypertensive agents in the treatment of essential hypertension; reduction of cardiovascular mortality in patients with left ventricular dysfunction postmyocardial infarction; treatment of heart failure (NYHA Class II-IV)

Pregnancy Risk Factor D

Pregnancy Considerations Medications which act on the renin-angiotensin system are reported to have the following fetal/neonatal effects: Hypotension, neonatal skull hypoplasia, anuria, renal failure, and death; oligohydramnios is also reported. These effects are reported to occur with exposure during the second and third trimesters. **[U.S. Boxed Warning]: Based on human data, drugs that act on the angiotensin system can cause injury and death to the developing fetus when used in the second and third trimesters. Angiotensin receptor blockers should be discontinued as soon as possible once pregnancy is detected.**

Lactation Excretion in breast milk unknown/not recommended

Contraindications There are no contraindications listed in manufacturer's labeling.

Canadian labeling: Hypersensitivity to valsartan or any component of the formulation

Warnings/Precautions **[U.S. Boxed Warning]: Based on human data, drugs that act on the angiotensin system can cause injury and death to the developing fetus when used in the second and third trimesters. Angiotensin receptor blockers should be discontinued as soon as possible once pregnancy is detected.** May cause hyperkalemia; avoid potassium supplementation unless specifically required by healthcare provider. During the initiation of therapy, hypotension may occur, particularly in patients with heart failure or post-MI patients. Use extreme caution with concurrent administration of potassium-sparing diuretics or potassium supplements, in patients with mild-to-moderate hepatic dysfunction (adjust dose), in those who may be sodium/water depleted (eg, on high-dose diuretics), and in the elderly; correct depletion first.

Use caution with unstented unilateral/bilateral renal artery stenosis. When unstented bilateral renal artery stenosis is present, use is generally avoided due to the elevated risk of deterioration in renal function unless possible benefits outweigh risks. Use with caution with preexisting renal insufficiency; significant aortic/mitral stenosis. May be associated with deterioration of renal function and/or increases in serum creatinine, particularly in patients with low renal blood flow (eg, renal artery stenosis, heart failure) whose glomerular filtration rate (GFR) is dependent on efferent arteriolar vasoconstriction by angiotensin II. Use caution in patients with severe renal impairment or significant hepatic dysfunction. Monitor renal function closely in patients with severe heart failure; changes in renal function should be anticipated and dosage adjustments of valsartan or concomitant medications may be needed. Concurrent use of ACE inhibitors may increase the risk of clinically-significant adverse events (eg, renal dysfunction, hyperkalemia). In Canada, use is not approved in patients <18 years of age.

Adverse Reactions

>10%:

Central nervous system: Dizziness (heart failure trials 17%)

Renal: BUN increased >50% (heart failure trials 17%)

1% to 10%:

Cardiovascular: Hypotension (heart failure trials 7%; MI trial 1%), postural hypotension (heart failure trials 2%), syncope (up to >1%)

Central nervous system: Dizziness (hypertension trial 2% to 8%), fatigue (heart failure trials 3%; hypertension trial 2%), postural dizziness (heart failure trials 2%), headache (heart failure trials >1%), vertigo (up to >1%)

Endocrine & metabolic: Serum potassium increased by >20% (4% to 10%), hyperkalemia (heart failure trials 2%)

Gastrointestinal: Diarrhea (heart failure trials 5%), abdominal pain (2%), nausea (heart failure trials >1%), upper abdominal pain (heart failure trials >1%)

Hematologic: Neutropenia (2%)

Neuromuscular & skeletal: Arthralgia (heart failure trials 3%), back pain (up to 3%)

Ocular: Blurred vision (heart failure trials >1%)

Renal: Creatinine doubled (MI trial 4%), creatinine increased >50% (heart failure trials 4%), renal dysfunction (up to >1%)

Respiratory: Cough (1% to 3%)

Miscellaneous: Viral infection (3%)

All indications: <1% (Limited to important or life-threatening): Allergic reactions, alopecia, anaphylaxis, anemia, angioedema, anorexia, anxiety, chest pain, constipation, dyspepsia, dyspnea, flatulence, hematocrit/hemoglobin decreased, hepatitis, impotence, insomnia, liver function tests increased, microcytic anemia, muscle cramps, myalgia, palpitation, paresthesia, photosensitivity, pruritus, rash, rhabdomyolysis, somnolence, taste disorder, thrombocytopenia, vasculitis, vomiting, weakness, xerostomia

Drug Interactions

Metabolism/Transport Effects Substrate of SLCO1B1; **Inhibits** CYP2C9 (weak)

Avoid Concomitant Use There are no known interactions where it is recommended to avoid concomitant use.

Increased Effect/Toxicity

Valsartan may increase the levels/effects of: ACE Inhibitors; Amifostine; Antihypertensives; Hypotensive Agents; Lithium; Nonsteroidal Anti-Inflammatory Agents; Potassium-Sparing Diuretics; RiTUXimab; Sodium Phosphates

The levels/effects of Valsartan may be increased by: Alfuzosin; Diazoxide; Eltrombopag; Eplerenone; Herbs (Hypotensive Properties); MAO Inhibitors; Pentoxifylline; Phosphodiesterase 5 Inhibitors; Potassium Salts; Prostacyclin Analogues; Tolvaptan; Trimethoprim

Decreased Effect

The levels/effects of Valsartan may be decreased by: Herbs (Hypertensive Properties); Methylphenidate; Nonsteroidal Anti-Inflammatory Agents; Yohimbine

Ethanol/Nutrition/Herb Interactions

Food: Decreases the peak plasma concentration and extent of absorption by 50% and 40%, respectively.

Herb/Nutraceutical: Avoid bayberry, blue cohosh, cayenne, ephedra, ginger, ginseng (American), kola, licorice (may worsen hypertension). Avoid black cohosh, California poppy, coleus, golden seal, hawthorn, mistletoe, periwinkle, quinine, shepherd's purse (may have increased antihypertensive effect).

Stability Store at 25°C (77°F); excursions permitted to 15°C to 30°C (59°F to 86°F). Protect from moisture.

Mechanism of Action Valsartan produces direct antagonism of the angiotensin II (AT2) receptors, unlike the ACE inhibitors. It displaces angiotensin II from the AT1 receptor and produces its blood pressure-lowering effects by antagonizing AT1-induced vasoconstriction, aldosterone release, catecholamine release, arginine vasopressin release, water intake, and hypertrophic responses. This action results in more efficient blockade of the cardiovascular effects of angiotensin II and fewer side effects than the ACE inhibitors.

Pharmacodynamics/Kinetics

Onset of action: ~2 hours

Duration: 24 hours

Distribution: V_d: 17 L (adults)

Protein binding: 95%, primarily albumin

Metabolism: To inactive metabolite

Bioavailability: Tablet: 25% (range: 10% to 35%); suspension: ~40% (~1.6 times more than tablet)

Half-life elimination: ~6 hours

Time to peak, serum: 2-4 hours

Excretion: Feces (83%) and urine (13%) as unchanged drug

Dosage Oral:

Hypertension:

Children 6-16 years: Initial: 1.3 mg/kg once daily (maximum: 40 mg/day); dose may be increased to achieve desired effect; doses >2.7 mg/kg (maximum: 160 mg) have not been studied

Adults: Initial: 80 mg or 160 mg once daily (in patients who are not volume depleted); dose may be increased to achieve desired effect; maximum recommended dose: 320 mg/day

Heart failure: Adults: Initial: 40 mg twice daily; titrate dose to 80-160 mg twice daily, as tolerated; maximum daily dose: 320 mg

Left ventricular dysfunction after MI: Adults: Initial: 20 mg twice daily; titrate dose to target of 160 mg twice daily as tolerated; may initiate ≥12 hours following MI

Dosing adjustment in renal impairment:

Children: Use is not recommended if Cl_{cr} <30 mL/minute.

Adults: No dosage adjustment necessary if Cl_{cr} >10 mL/minute.

Dialysis: Not significantly removed

Dosing adjustment in hepatic impairment In mild-to-moderate liver disease no adjustment is needed. Use caution in patients with liver disease. Patients with mild-to-moderate chronic disease have twice the exposure as healthy volunteers.

Dietary Considerations Avoid salt substitutes which contain potassium. May be taken with or without food.

Administration Administer with or without food.

Monitoring Parameters Baseline and periodic electrolyte panels, renal function, BP; in CHF, serum potassium during dose escalation and periodically thereafter

Additional Information Valsartan may have an advantage over losartan due to minimal metabolism requirements and consequent use in mild-to-moderate hepatic impairment.

Dosage Forms Excipient information presented when available (limited, particularly for generics); consult specific product labeling.

Tablet, oral:

Diovan®: 40 mg [scored]

Diovan®: 80 mg, 160 mg, 320 mg

Extemporaneous Preparations A 4 mg/mL oral suspension may be made from tablets, Ora-Plus®, and Ora-Sweet® SF. Add 80 mL of Ora-Plus® to an 8-ounce amber glass bottle containing eight valsartan 80 mg tablets.

Shake well for ≥2 minutes. Allow the suspension to stand for a minimum of 1 hour, then shake for ≥1 minute. Add 80 mL of Ora-Sweet SF® to the bottle and shake for ≥10 seconds. Store in amber glass prescription bottles; label "shake well". Stable for 30 days at room temperature or 75 days refrigerated.

Diovan® prescribing information, Novartis Pharmaceuticals Corp, East Hanover, NJ, 2007.

◆ **Valsartan and Aliskiren** *see* Aliskiren and Valsartan *on page 68*

◆ **Valsartan and Amlodipine** *see* Amlodipine and Valsartan *on page 100*

Valsartan and Hydrochlorothiazide

(val SAR tan & hye droe klor oh THYE a zide)

Brand Names: U.S. Diovan HCT®

Brand Names: Canada Diovan HCT®; Sandoz Valsartan HCT; Teva-Valsartan HCTZ; Valsartan-HCTZ

Index Terms Hydrochlorothiazide and Valsartan

Pharmacologic Category Angiotensin II Receptor Blocker; Diuretic, Thiazide

Use Treatment of hypertension

Pregnancy Risk Factor D

Dosage Oral: Dose is individualized; combination product may be used as initial therapy or substituted for individual components in patients currently maintained on both agents separately or in patients not adequately controlled with monotherapy (using one of the agents or an agent within same antihypertensive class).

Adults: Hypertension:

Initial therapy: Valsartan 160 mg and hydrochlorothiazide 12.5 mg once daily; dose may be titrated after 1-2 weeks of therapy. Maximum recommended daily doses: Valsartan 320 mg; hydrochlorothiazide 25 mg.

Add-on/replacement therapy: Valsartan 80-160 mg and hydrochlorothiazide 12.5-25 mg once daily; dose may be titrated after 3-4 weeks of therapy. Maximum recommended daily dose: Valsartan 320 mg; hydrochlorothiazide 25 mg.

Dosage adjustment in renal impairment:

Cl_{cr} >30 mL/minute: No adjustment needed

Cl_{cr} ≤30 mL/minute: Use of combination not recommended. Contraindicated in patients with anuria.

Dosage adjustment in hepatic impairment: Use with caution; initiate at lower dose and titrate slowly

Additional Information Complete prescribing information for this medication should be consulted for additional detail.

Dosage Forms Excipient information presented when available (limited, particularly for generics); consult specific product labeling.

Tablet:

Diovan HCT® 80 mg/12.5 mg: Valsartan 80 mg and hydrochlorothiazide 12.5 mg

Diovan HCT® 160 mg/12.5 mg: Valsartan 160 mg and hydrochlorothiazide 12.5 mg

Diovan HCT® 160 mg/25 mg: Valsartan 160 mg and hydrochlorothiazide 25 mg

Diovan HCT® 320 mg/12.5 mg: Valsartan 320 mg and hydrochlorothiazide 12.5 mg

Diovan HCT® 320 mg/25 mg: Valsartan 320 mg and hydrochlorothiazide 25 mg

◆ **Valsartan-HCTZ (Can)** *see* Valsartan and Hydrochlorothiazide *on page 1763*

◆ **Valsartan, Hydrochlorothiazide, and Amlodipine** *see* Amlodipine, Valsartan, and Hydrochlorothiazide *on page 100*

◆ **Valstar®** *see* Valrubicin *on page 1760*

◆ **Valtaxin® (Can)** *see* Valrubicin *on page 1760*

◆ **Valtrex®** *see* ValACYclovir *on page 1753*

◆ **Valturna®** *see* Aliskiren and Valsartan *on page 68*

◆ **Val-Vanco (Can)** *see* Vancomycin *on page 1763*

◆ **Val-Vancomycin (Can)** *see* Vancomycin *on page 1763*

◆ **Vancenase** *see* Beclomethasone (Systemic) *on page 192*

◆ **Vanceril® AEM (Can)** *see* Beclomethasone (Systemic) *on page 192*

◆ **Vancocin®** *see* Vancomycin *on page 1763*

Vancomycin (van koe MYE sin)

Brand Names: U.S. Vancocin®

Brand Names: Canada PMS-Vancomycin; Sterile Vancomycin Hydrochloride, USP; Val-Vanco; Val-Vancomycin; Vancocin®; Vancomycin Hydrochloride for Injection, USP

Index Terms Vancomycin Hydrochloride

Pharmacologic Category Glycopeptide

Additional Appendix Information

Antibiotic Treatment of Adults With Infective Endocarditis *on page 1956*

Prevention of Wound Infection and Sepsis in Surgical Patients *on page 1954*

Use Treatment of patients with infections caused by staphylococcal species and streptococcal species; used orally for staphylococcal enterocolitis or for antibiotic-associated pseudomembranous colitis produced by *C. difficile*

Unlabeled Use Bacterial endophthalmitis; treatment of infections caused by gram-positive organisms in patients who have serious allergies to beta-lactam agents; treatment of beta-lactam resistant gram-positive infections

Pregnancy Risk Factor B (oral); C (injection)

Pregnancy Considerations Adverse effects have not been observed in animal studies and there are no controlled studies in pregnant women; however, oral vancomycin is not systemically absorbed. Therefore, I.V. vancomycin has been classified pregnancy category C and oral vancomycin has been classified pregnancy category B. Vancomycin crosses the placenta. *In vivo* studies and human case reports have documented placental transfer of vancomycin in the second and third trimesters of pregnancy resulting in therapeutic fetal concentrations. Vancomycin has not caused adverse fetal effects, including hearing loss or nephrotoxicity, when administered during pregnancy. A case report has been published of a vancomycin dose rapidly administered over 3 minutes leading to maternal hypotension and fetal bradycardia.

The pharmacokinetics of vancomycin may be altered during pregnancy and pregnant patients may need a higher dose of vancomycin. Maternal half-life is unchanged, but the volume of distribution and the total plasma clearance are increased. Individualization of therapy through serum concentration monitoring may be warranted. Vancomycin is recommended for use in pregnant women for prevention of early-onset group B streptococcal (GBS) disease in newborns.

Lactation Enters breast milk/not recommended

Contraindications Hypersensitivity to vancomycin or any component of the formulation; avoid in patients with previous severe hearing loss

Warnings/Precautions May cause nephrotoxicity although limited data suggest direct causal relationship; usual risk factors include pre-existing renal impairment, concomitant nephrotoxic medications, advanced age, and dehydration. If multiple sequential (≥2) serum creatinine concentrations demonstrate an increase of 0.5 mg/dL or ≥50% increase from baseline (whichever is greater) in the absence of an alternative explanation, the patient should be identified as having vancomycin-induced nephrotoxicity (Rybak, 2009). Discontinue treatment if signs of nephrotoxicity occur; renal damage is usually reversible. May cause neurotoxicity; usual risk factors include pre-existing renal impairment, concomitant neuro-/nephrotoxic medications, advanced age, and dehydration. Ototoxicity, although rarely associated with monotherapy, is proportional to the amount of drug given and the duration of treatment. Tinnitus or vertigo may be indications of vestibular injury and impending bilateral irreversible damage. Discontinue treatment if signs of ototoxicity occur. Prolonged therapy (>1 week) or total doses exceeding 25 g may increase the risk of neutropenia; prompt reversal of neutropenia is expected after discontinuation of therapy. Prolonged use may result in fungal or bacterial superinfection, including *C. difficile*-associated diarrhea (CDAD) and pseudomembranous colitis; CDAD has been observed >2 months postantibiotic treatment. Use with caution in patients with renal impairment or those receiving other nephrotoxic or ototoxic drugs; dosage modification required in patients with impaired renal function (especially elderly). Rapid I.V. administration may result in hypotension, flushing, erythema, urticaria, and/or pruritus. Oral vancomycin is only indicated for the treatment of pseudomembranous colitis due to *C. difficile* and enterocolitis due to *S. aureus* and is not effective for systemic infections; parenteral vancomycin is not effective for the treatment of colitis due to *C. difficile* and enterocolitis due to *S. aureus*. **Note:** The Infectious Disease Society of America (IDSA) recommends the use of oral metronidazole for initial treatment of mild-to-moderate *C. difficile* infection and the use of oral vancomycin for initial treatment of severe *C. difficile* infection (Cohen, 2010).

Adverse Reactions

Oral:

>10%: Gastrointestinal: Bitter taste, nausea, vomiting, stomatitis

1% to 10%:

Central nervous system: Chills, drug fever

Hematologic: Eosinophilia

<1% (Limited to important or life-threatening): Interstitial nephritis, ototoxicity, renal failure, skin rash, thrombocytopenia, vasculitis

Parenteral:

>10%:

Cardiovascular: Hypotension accompanied by flushing

Dermatologic: Erythematous rash on face and upper body (red neck or red man syndrome)

1% to 10%:

Central nervous system: Chills, drug fever

Hematologic: Eosinophilia, reversible neutropenia

Local: Phlebitis

<1% (Limited to important or life-threatening): Drug rash with eosinophilia and systemic symptoms (DRESS), ototoxicity (rare; use of other ototoxic agents may increase risk), renal failure (limited data suggesting direct relationship), Stevens-Johnson syndrome, thrombocytopenia, vasculitis

Drug Interactions

Metabolism/Transport Effects None known.

Avoid Concomitant Use

Avoid concomitant use of Vancomycin with any of the following: BCG; Gallium Nitrate

Increased Effect/Toxicity

Vancomycin may increase the levels/effects of: Aminoglycosides; Colistimethate; Gallium Nitrate; Neuromuscular-Blocking Agents

The levels/effects of Vancomycin may be increased by: Nonsteroidal Anti-Inflammatory Agents

Decreased Effect

Vancomycin may decrease the levels/effects of: BCG; Typhoid Vaccine

The levels/effects of Vancomycin may be decreased by: Bile Acid Sequestrants

Stability Reconstituted 500 mg and 1 g vials are stable at either room temperature or under refrigeration for 14 days. **Note:** Vials contain no bacteriostatic agent. Solutions diluted for administration in either D_5W or NS are stable under refrigeration for 14 days or at room temperature for 7 days. Reconstitute vials with 20 mL of SWFI for each 1 g of vancomycin (10 mL/500 mg vial; 20 mL/1 g vial; 100 mL/5 g vial; 200 mL/10 g vial). The reconstituted solution must be further diluted with at least 100 mL of a compatible diluent per 500 mg of vancomycin prior to parenteral administration.

Intrathecal (unlabeled route): Vancomycin is available as a powder for injection and may be diluted to 1-5 mg/mL concentration in preservative free 0.9% sodium chloride for administration into the CSF.

Mechanism of Action Inhibits bacterial cell wall synthesis by blocking glycopeptide polymerization through binding tightly to D-alanyl-D-alanine portion of cell wall precursor

Pharmacodynamics/Kinetics

Absorption: Oral: Poor; I.M.: Erratic; Intraperitoneal: ~38%

Distribution: V_d: 0.4-1 L/kg; Distributes widely in body tissue and fluids, except for CSF

Relative diffusion from blood into CSF: Good only with inflammation (exceeds usual MICs)

Uninflamed meninges: 0-4 mcg/mL; serum concentration dependent

Inflamed meninges: 6-11 mcg/mL; serum concentration dependent

CSF:blood level ratio: Normal meninges: Nil; Inflamed meninges: 20% to 30%

Protein binding: ~50%

Half-life elimination: Biphasic: Terminal:

Newborns: 6-10 hours

Infants and Children 3 months to 4 years: 4 hours

Children >3 years: 2.2-3 hours

Adults: 5-11 hours; significantly prolonged with renal impairment

End-stage renal disease: 200-250 hours

Time to peak, serum: I.V.: Immediately after completion of infusion

Excretion: I.V.: Urine (80% to 90% as unchanged drug); Oral: Primarily feces

Dosage

Usual dosage range:

Infants >1 month and Children: I.V.: 10-15 mg/kg every 6 hours

Adults: Initial intravenous dosing should be based on actual body weight; subsequent dosing adjusted based on serum trough vancomycin concentrations.

I.V.: 2-3 g/day (or 30-60 mg/kg/day) in divided doses every 8-12 hours (Rybak, 2009); **Note:** Dose requires adjustment in renal impairment

Oral: 500-2000 mg/day in divided doses every 6 hours

Indication-specific dosing:

Catheter-related infections: Adults: Antibiotic lock technique (Mermel, 2009): 2 mg/mL ± 10 units heparin/mL **or** 2.5 mg/mL ± 2500 **or** 5000 units heparin/mL **or** 5 mg/mL ± 5000 units heparin/mL (preferred regimen); instill into catheter port with a volume sufficient to fill the catheter (2-5 mL). **Note:** May use SWFI/NS or D_5W as diluents. Do not mix with any other solutions. Dwell times generally should not exceed 48 hours before renewal of lock solution. Remove lock solution prior to catheter use, then replace.

***C. difficile* -associated diarrhea (CDAD):**

Infants >1 month and Children: Oral: 40 mg/kg/day in 3-4 divided doses added to fluids for 7-10 days (maximum: 2000 mg/day)

Adults:

Oral:

Manufacturer recommendations: 500-2000 mg/day in 3-4 divided doses for 7-10 days (usual dose: 125-500 mg every 6 hours)

IDSA guideline recommendations: Severe infection: 125 mg every 6 hours for 10-14 days; Severe, complicated infection: 500 mg every 6 hours with or without concurrent I.V. metronidazole. May consider vancomycin retention enema (in patients with complete ileus) (Cohen, 2010).

Rectal (unlabeled route): Retention enema (in patients with complete ileus): SHEA/IDSA guideline recommendations: Severe, complicated infection in patients with ileus: 500 mg every 6 hours (in 100 mL 0.9% sodium chloride) with oral vancomycin with or without concurrent I.V. metronidazole (Cohen, 2010)

Complicated infections in seriously-ill patients: Adults: I.V.: Loading dose: 25-30 mg/kg (based on actual body weight) may be used to rapidly achieve target concentration; then 15-20 mg/kg/dose every 8-12 hours (Rybak, 2009)

Enterocolitis *(S. aureus)*:

Infants >1 months and Children: Oral: 40 mg/kg/day in 3-4 divided doses added to fluids for 7-10 days (maximum: 2000 mg/day)

Adults: Oral: 500-2000 mg/day in 3-4 divided doses for 7-10 days (usual dose: 125-500 mg every 6 hours)

Meningitis:

Infants >1 month and Children:

I.V.: 15 mg/kg every 6 hours (Tunkel, 2004)

Intrathecal, intraventricular (unlabeled route): 5-20 mg/day (Tunkel, 2004)

Children: Alternate regimen: *S. aureus* (methicillin-resistant) (unlabeled use; Liu, 2011): I.V.: 15 mg/kg/dose every 6 hours for 2 weeks (some experts combine with rifampin)

Adults:

I.V.: 30-60 mg/kg/day in divided doses every 8-12 hours (Rybak, 2009) **or** 500-750 mg every 6 hours. **Note:** For PCN-resistant *Streptococcus pneumoniae* (MIC ≥2 mcg/mL), combine with a third-generation cephalosporin.

Alternate regimen: *S. aureus* (methicillin-resistant) (unlabeled use; Liu, 2011): 15-20 mg/kg/dose every 8-12 hours for 2 weeks (some experts combine with rifampin

Intrathecal, intraventricular (unlabeled route): 5-20 mg/day

Pneumonia:

Community-acquired pneumonia (CAP):

Infants >3 months and Children (IDSA/PIDS, 2011): I.V.: **Note:** In children ≥5 years, a macrolide antibiotic should be added if atypical pneumonia cannot be ruled out.

Group A *Streptococcus* (alternative to ampicillin or penicillin in beta-lactam allergic patients): 40-60 mg/kg/day divided every 6-8 hours

Presumed bacterial (in addition to recommended antibiotic therapy), *S. pneumoniae*, moderate-to-severe infection (MICs to penicillin ≤2.0 mcg/mL) (alternative to ampicillin or penicillin): 40-60 mg/kg/day divided every 6-8 hours

S. aureus (methicillin-susceptible) (alternative to cefazolin/oxacillin): 40-60 mg/kg/day divided every 6-8 hours

S. aureus, moderate-to-severe infection (methicillin-resistant +/- clindamycin susceptible) (preferred): 40-60 mg/kg/day divided every 6-8 hours **or** dosing to achieve AUC/MIC >400

Alternate regimen: 60 mg/kg/day divided every 6 hours for 7-21 days, depending on severity (Liu, 2011)

S. pneumoniae, moderate-to-severe infection (MICs to penicillin ≥4.0 mcg/mL) (alternative to ceftriaxone in beta-lactam allergic patients): 40-60 mg/kg/day divided every 6-8 hours

Adults: *S. aureus* (methicillin-resistant): I.V.: 45-60 mg/kg/day divided every 8-12 hours (maximum dose: 2 g) for 7-21 days depending on severity (Liu, 2011)

Healthcare-associated pneumonia (HAP): *S. aureus* (methicillin-resistant): I.V.:

Infants and Children: 60 mg/kg/day divided every 6 hours for 7-21 days depending on severity (Liu, 2011)

Adults: 45-60 mg/kg/day divided every 8-12 hours (maximum dose: 2 g) for 7-21 days depending on severity (American Thoracic Society [ATS], 2005; Liu, 2011; Rybak 2009)

Prophylaxis against infective endocarditis: I.V.:

Children:

Dental, oral, or upper respiratory tract surgery: 20 mg/kg/dose administered 1 hour prior to the procedure. **Note:** American Heart Association (AHA) guidelines recommend prophylaxis only in patients undergoing invasive procedures and in whom underlying cardiac conditions may predispose to a higher risk of adverse outcomes should infection occur.

GI/GU procedure: 20 mg/kg (plus gentamicin 1.5 mg/kg) administered 1 hour prior to surgery. **Note:** Routine prophylaxis no longer recommended by the AHA.

Adults:

Dental, oral, or upper respiratory tract surgery: 1 g 1 hour before surgery. **Note:** AHA guidelines now recommend prophylaxis only in patients undergoing invasive procedures and in whom underlying cardiac conditions may predispose to a higher risk of adverse outcomes should infection occur

GI/GU procedure: 1 g plus 1.5 mg/kg gentamicin 1 hour prior to surgery. **Note:** As of April 2007, routine prophylaxis no longer recommended by the AHA.

Susceptible gram-positive infections (MIC ≤1 mcg/mL; Rybak, 2009): I.V.:

Infants >1 month and Children: 10 mg/kg/dose every 6 hours (manufacturer recommendations) **or** 15 mg/kg/dose (maximum dose: 2 g) every 6 hours (Liu, 2011)

Adults: 15-20 mg/kg/dose (usual: 750-1500 mg) every 8-12 hours

Note: If MIC ≥2 mcg/mL, alternative therapies are recommended.

Bacteremia (*S. aureus* [methicillin-resistant]) (unlabeled use; Liu, 2011): I.V.:

Children: 15 mg/kg/dose every 6 hours for 2-6 weeks depending on severity

Adults: 15-20 mg/kg/dose every 8-12 hours for 2-6 weeks depending on severity

Brain abscess, subdural empyema, spinal epidural abscess (*S. aureus* [methicillin-resistant]) (unlabeled use; Liu, 2011): I.V.:

Children.: 15 mg/kg/dose every 6 hours for 4-6 weeks (some experts combine with rifampin)

Adults: 15-20 mg/kg/dose every 8-12 hours for 4-6 weeks (some experts combine with rifampin)

Endocarditis, native valve (*S. aureus* [methicillin-resistant]) (unlabeled use; Liu, 2011): I.V.:

Children: 15 mg/kg/dose every 6 hours for 6 weeks

Adults: 15-20 mg/kg/dose every 8-12 hours for 6 weeks

Endocarditis, prosthetic valve (*S. aureus* [methicillin-resistant]) (unlabeled use; Liu, 2011): I.V.:

Children: 15 mg/kg/dose every 6 hours for at least 6 weeks

Adults: 15-20 mg/kg/dose every 8-12 hours for at least 6 weeks (combine with rifampin for the entire duration of therapy and gentamicin for the first 2 weeks)

Endophthalmitis (unlabeled use): Adults: Intravitreal: Usual dose: 1 mg/0.1 mL NS instilled into vitreum; may repeat administration if necessary in 3-4 days, usually in combination with ceftazidime or an aminoglycoside. **Note:** Some clinicians have recommended using a lower dose of 0.2 mg/0.1 mL, based on concerns for retinotoxicity.

Osteomyelitis (*S. aureus* [methicillin-resistant]) (unlabeled use; Liu, 2011): I.V.:
- Children: 15 mg/kg/dose every 6 hours for 4-6 weeks
- Adults: 15-20 mg/kg/dose every 8-12 hours for a minimum of 8 weeks (some experts combine with rifampin)

Septic arthritis (*S. aureus* [methicillin-resistant]) (unlabeled use; Liu, 2011): I.V.:
- Children: 15 mg/kg/dose every 6 hours for minimum of 3-4 weeks
- Adults: 15-20 mg/kg/dose every 8-12 hours for 3-4 weeks

Septic thrombosis of cavernous or dural venous sinus (*S. aureus* [methicillin-resistant]) (unlabeled use; Liu, 2011): I.V.:
- Children: 15 mg/kg/dose every 6 hours for 4-6 weeks (some experts combine with rifampin)
- Adults: 15-20 mg/kg/dose every 8-12 hours for 4-6 weeks (some experts combine with rifampin)

Skin and skin structure infections, complicated (*S. aureus* [methicillin-resistant]) (unlabeled use; Liu, 2011): I.V.:
- Children: 15 mg/kg/dose every 6 hours for 7-14 days
- Adults: 15-20 mg/kg/dose every 8-12 hours for 7-14 days

Dosing interval in renal impairment (vancomycin levels should be monitored in patients with any renal impairment):
- Cl_{cr} >50 mL/minute: Start with 15-20 mg/kg/dose (usual: 750-1500 mg) every 8-12 hours
- Cl_{cr} 20-49 mL/minute: Start with 15-20 mg/kg/dose (usual: 750-1500 mg) every 24 hours
- Cl_{cr} <20 mL/minute: Will need longer intervals; determine by serum concentration monitoring

Note: In the critically-ill patient with renal insufficiency, the initial loading dose (25-30 mg/kg) should not be reduced. However, subsequent dosage adjustments should be made based on renal function and trough serum concentrations.

Poorly dialyzable by intermittent hemodialysis (0% to 5%); however, use of high-flux membranes and continuous renal replacement therapy (CRRT) increases vancomycin clearance, and generally requires replacement dosing.

Intermittent hemodialysis (IHD) (administer after hemodialysis on dialysis days): Following loading dose of 15-25 mg/kg, give either 500 mg to 1 g **or** 5-10 mg/kg after each dialysis session. (Heintz, 2009). **Note:** Dosing dependent on the assumption of 3 times/week, complete IHD sessions.

Redosing based on pre-HD concentrations:
- <10 mg/L: Administer 1g after HD
- 10-25 mg/L: Administer 500-750 mg after HD
- >25 mg/L: Hold vancomycin

Redosing based on post-HD concentrations:
- <10-15 mg/L: Administer 0.5-1 g

Peritoneal dialysis (PD):
- Administration via PD fluid: 15-30 mg/L (15-30 mcg/mL) of PD fluid
- Systemic: Loading dose of 1 g, followed by 500 mg to 1 g every 48-72 hours with close monitoring of levels

Continuous renal replacement therapy (CRRT) (Heintz, 2009; Trotman, 2005): Drug clearance is highly dependent on the method of renal replacement, filter type, and flow rate. Appropriate dosing requires close monitoring of pharmacologic response, signs of adverse reactions due to drug accumulation, as well as drug concentrations in relation to target trough (if appropriate). The following are general recommendations only (based on dialysate flow/ultrafiltration rates of 1-2 L/hour and minimal residual renal function) and should not supersede clinical judgment:
- CVVH: Loading dose of 15-25 mg/kg, followed by either 1 g every 48 hours **or** 10-15 mg/kg every 24-48 hours
- CVVHD: Loading dose of 15-25 mg/kg, followed by either 1 g every 24 hours **or** 10-15 mg/kg every 24 hours
- CVVHDF: Loading dose of 15-25 mg/kg, followed by either 1 g every 24 hours **or** 7.5-10 mg/kg every 12 hours

Note: Consider redosing patients receiving CRRT for vancomycin concentrations <10-15 mg/L.

Dietary Considerations May be taken with food.

Administration

Intravenous: Administer vancomycin with a final concentration not to exceed 5 mg/mL by I.V. intermittent infusion over at least 60 minutes (recommended infusion period of ≥30 minutes for every 500 mg administered).

If a maculopapular rash appears on the face, neck, trunk, and/or upper extremities (red man syndrome), slow the infusion rate to over 1½ to 2 hours and increase the dilution volume. Hypotension, shock, and cardiac arrest (rare) have also been reported with too rapid of infusion. Reactions are often treated with antihistamines and steroids.

Intrathecal (unlabeled route): Vancomycin is available as a powder for injection and may be diluted to 1-5 mg/mL concentration in preservative free 0.9% sodium chloride for intrathecal administration.

Intravitreal: May be administered by intravitreal injection (unlabeled use).

Oral: May be administered with food. If patient cannot swallow capsules, the powder for injection (not premixed solution) may be diluted in 30 mL of water for oral administration; flavoring may be added to improve taste. The unflavored, diluted solution may also be administered via nasogastric tube.

Rectal (unlabeled route): May be administered as a retention enema per rectum (Cohen, 2010)

Not for I.M. administration.

Extravasation treatment: Monitor I.V. site closely; extravasation will cause serious injury with possible necrosis and tissue sloughing. Rotate infusion site frequently.

Monitoring Parameters Periodic renal function tests, urinalysis, WBC; serum trough vancomycin concentrations in select patients (eg, aggressive dosing, unstable renal function, concurrent nephrotoxins, prolonged courses)

Suggested frequency of trough vancomycin concentration monitoring (Rybak, 2009):
- *Hemodynamically stable patients:* Draw trough concentrations at least once-weekly.
- *Hemodynamically unstable patients:* Draw trough concentrations more frequently or in some instances daily.
- *Prolonged courses (>3-5 days):* Draw at least one steady-state trough concentration; repeat as clinically appropriate.

Note: Drawing >1 trough concentration prior to the fourth dose for short course (<3 days) or lower intensity dosing (target trough concentrations <15 mcg/mL) is not recommended.

Reference Range

Timing of serum samples: Draw trough just before next dose at steady-state conditions (approximately after the fourth dose). Drawing peak concentrations is no longer recommended.

Therapeutic levels: Trough: ≥10 mcg/mL. For pathogens with an MIC ≤1 mcg/mL, the minimum trough concentration should be 15 mcg/mL to meet target AUC/MIC of ≥400 (see **"Note"**). For complicated infections (eg, bacteremia, endocarditis, osteomyelitis, meningitis, and hospital-acquired pneumonia caused by *S. aureus*), trough concentrations of 15-20 mcg/mL are recommended to improve penetration and improve clinical outcomes (Liu, 2011; Rybak, 2009). The American Thoracic Society (ATS) guidelines for hospital-acquired pneumonia and the Infectious Disease Society of America (IDSA) meningitis guidelines also recommend trough concentrations of 15-20 mcg/mL.

Note: Although AUC/MIC is the preferred pharmacokinetic-pharmacodynamic parameter used to determine clinical effectiveness, trough serum concentrations may be used as a surrogate marker for AUC and are recommended as the most accurate and practical method of vancomycin monitoring (Liu, 2011; Rybak, 2009).

Toxic: >80 mcg/mL (SI: >54 micromole/L)

Additional Information Because of its long half-life, vancomycin should be dosed on an every 8- to 12-hour basis. Monitoring of trough serum concentrations is advisable in certain situations. "Red man syndrome", characterized by skin rash and hypotension, is not an allergic reaction but rather is associated with too rapid infusion of the drug. To alleviate or prevent the reaction, infuse vancomycin at a rate of ≥30 minutes for each 500 mg of drug being administered (eg, 1 g over ≥60 minutes); 1.5 g over ≥90 minutes.

Dosage Forms Excipient information presented when available (limited, particularly for generics); consult specific product labeling.

Capsule, oral:

Vancocin®: 125 mg, 250 mg

Infusion, premixed iso-osmotic dextrose solution: 500 mg (100 mL); 750 mg (150 mL); 1 g (200 mL)

Injection, powder for reconstitution: 500 mg, 750 mg, 1 g, 5 g, 10 g

- **Vancomycin Hydrochloride** *see* Vancomycin *on page 1763*
- **Vancomycin Hydrochloride for Injection, USP (Can)** *see* Vancomycin *on page 1763*
- **Vandazole®** *see* MetroNIDAZOLE (Topical) *on page 1122*

Vandetanib (van DET a nib)

Brand Names: U.S. Caprelsa®

Index Terms AZD6474; Zactima; ZD6474; Zictifa

Pharmacologic Category Antineoplastic Agent, Tyrosine Kinase Inhibitor; Epidermal Growth Factor Receptor (EGFR) Inhibitor; Vascular Endothelial Growth Factor (VEGF) Inhibitor

Use Treatment of metastatic or unresectable locally advanced medullary thyroid cancer (symptomatic or progressive)

Pregnancy Risk Factor D

Pregnancy Considerations Animal studies have demonstrated fetal loss, teratogenicity, and delayed development. There are no adequate and well-controlled studies in pregnant women. Because vandetanib inhibits angiogenesis, a critical component of fetal development, adverse effects on pregnancy would be expected. Women of childbearing potential should be advised to avoid pregnancy during and for 4 months following treatment with vandetanib.

Lactation Excretion in breast milk unknown/not recommended

Prescribing and Access Restrictions As a requirement of the REMS program, access to vandetanib is restricted. Vandetanib is approved for marketing under a Food and Drug Administration (FDA) approved, risk management program, and through a restricted distribution program, the Vandetanib REMS Program (1-800-236-9933). Prescribers and pharmacies must be certified with the program to prescribe or dispense vandetanib.

Medication Guide Available Yes

Contraindications Congenital long QT syndrome

Warnings/Precautions Hazardous agent – use appropriate precautions for handling and disposal. **[U.S. Boxed Warning]: May prolong the QT interval; torsade de pointes and sudden death have been reported. Do not use in patients with hypocalcemia, hypokalemia, hypomagnesemia, or long QT syndrome. Correct electrolyte imbalance prior to initiating therapy. Monitor electrolytes and ECG (to monitor QT interval) at baseline, at 2-4 weeks, at 8-12 weeks, and every 3 months thereafter; monitoring (at the same frequency) is required following dose reductions for QT prolongation or with dose interruptions >2 weeks. Avoid the use of QT-prolonging agents; if concomitant use with QT prolonging agents cannot be avoided, monitor ECG more frequently. Vandetanib has a long half-life (19 days), therefore, adverse reactions (including QT prolongation) may resolve slowly; monitor appropriately.** Ventricular tachycardia has also been reported. The potential for QT prolongation is dose-dependent. Do not initiate treatment unless QT interval, Fridericia (QTcF) is <450 msec. During treatment, if QTcF >500 msec, withhold vandetanib and resume at a reduced dose when QTcF is <450 msec. Avoid use in patients with a history of torsade de pointes, congenital long QT syndrome, bradyarrhythmias or uncompensated heart failure. Patients with ventricular arrhythmias or recent MI were excluded from clinical trials. To reduce the risk of QT prolongation, maintain serum calcium and magnesium within normal limits and maintain serum potassium ≥4 mEq/L. Heart failure (HF) has been reported; monitor for signs and symptoms of HF; may require discontinuation (HF may not be reversible upon discontinuation). Hypertension and hypertensive crisis have been observed with vandetanib; monitor blood pressure and initiate or adjust antihypertensive therapy as needed; may require vandetanib dosage adjustment or treatment interruption; discontinue vandetanib (permanently) if blood pressure cannot be adequately controlled.

Diarrhea has been reported with use; may cause electrolyte imbalance (closely monitor electrolytes); routine antidiarrheals are recommended; withhold vandetanib treatment until resolution for severe diarrhea; dose reduction is recommended when treatment is resumed. Stevens-Johnson syndrome and other serious skin reactions (including fatal) have been reported. Mild-to-moderate skin reactions, including acne, dermatitis, dry skin, palmar-plantar erythrodysesthesia syndrome, pruritus, and rash have also been reported. Withhold treatment for dermatologic toxicity of grade 3 or higher; consider a reduced dose or permanent discontinuation upon improvement in symptoms. Severe dermatologic toxicity has been managed with corticosteroids (systemic) and treatment discontinuation; mild-to-moderate toxicity has responded to corticosteroids (systemic or topical), oral antihistamines, and antibiotics (topical or systemic). Increased risk of photosensitivity is associated with use; effective sunscreen and protective clothing are recommended during and for at least 4 months after treatment discontinuation.

Reversible posterior leukoencephalopathy syndrome (RPLS) been observed with vandetanib; symptoms of RPLS include altered mental function, confusion, headache, seizure, or visual disturbances; generally associated with hypertension; consider discontinuing treatment if RPLS occurs. Serious and sometimes fatal hemorrhagic events have been reported with use; discontinue in patients with severe hemorrhage; do not administer in patients with a recent history of hemoptysis with ≥2.5 mL of red blood. Ischemic cerebrovascular events (some fatal) have been observed with vandetanib; discontinue treatment in patients with severe ischemic events (the safety of resuming treatment after an ischemic event has not been studied). Interstitial lung disease (ILD) or pneumonitis (including fatalities) has been reported with vandetanib. Patients should be advised to report any new or worsening respiratory symptoms; ILD should be suspected with nonspecific respiratory symptoms such as hypoxia, pleural effusion, cough or dyspnea. If asymptomatic (or minimal symptoms) although with radiologic evidence of ILD, may continue treatment with close monitoring; consider interrupting treatment for moderate symptoms (may require corticosteroids or antibiotics). Discontinue treatment for severe symptoms; may require corticosteroids and antibiotics, and permanent discontinuation.

Increased doses of thyroid replacement therapy have been required in patients with prior thyroidectomy; obtain TSH at baseline, at 2-4 weeks, 8-12 weeks, and every 3 months after vandetanib initiation; if signs and symptoms of hypothyroidism occur during treatment, evaluate thyroid hormone levels and adjust replacement therapy if needed. Dosage reduction is recommended in patients with moderate-to-severe renal impairment. Exposure is increased in patients with impaired renal function; closely monitor QT interval; has not been studied in patients with end stage renal disease requiring dialysis. Not recommended for use in patients with moderate-to-severe hepatic impairment. Avoid concurrent use with strong CYP3A4 inducers, including St John's wort and with QT-prolonging agents. Due to the risk for serious treatment-related adverse events, use in patients whose disease is not progressive or symptomatic should be only be undertaken after careful consideration. **[U.S. Boxed Warning]: Vandetanib is only available through a restricted access program; prescribers and pharmacies must be certified with the restricted distribution program to prescribe and dispense vandetanib.**

Adverse Reactions

>10%:

- Cardiovascular: Hypertension (33%; grades 3/4: 9%), QT prolongation (14%; grades 3/4: 8%)
- Central nervous system: Headache (26%), fatigue (24%), insomnia (13%)
- Dermatologic: Rash (53%; grades 3/4: 5%), dermatitis acneiform/acne (35%; grades 3/4: 1%), dry skin (15%), photosensitivity (13%), pruritus (11%)
- Endocrine & metabolic: Hypocalcemia (11% to 57%), hypoglycemia (24%)
- Gastrointestinal: Diarrhea/colitis (57%; grades 3/4: 11%), nausea (33%), abdominal pain (21%), appetite decreased (21%), vomiting (15%), dyspepsia (11%)
- Hematologic: Leukopenia (19%), anemia (13%; grades 3/4: <1%), hemorrhage (13% to 14%)
- Hepatic: ALT increased (51%), bilirubin increased (13%)
- Neuromuscular & skeletal: Weakness (15%)
- Renal: Creatinine increased (16%)
- Respiratory: Cough (11%), nasopharyngitis (11%)

1% to 10%:

- Cardiovascular: Cardiac failure (2%)
- Central nervous system: Depression (10%)
- Endocrine & metabolic: Hypercalcemia (7%), hypomagnesemia (7%), hyperkalemia (6%), hypokalemia (6%), hyperglycemia (5%), hypermagnesemia (3%)
- Gastrointestinal: Weight loss (10%)
- Hematologic: Neutropenia (10%; grades 3/4: <1%), thrombocytopenia (9%)
- Ocular: Blurred vision (9%)
- Renal: Proteinuria (10%)
- Respiratory: Aspiration pneumonia (2%), respiratory arrest (2%), respiratory failure (2%)
- Miscellaneous: Sepsis (2%)

<1% (Limited to important or life-threatening): Cardiopulmonary arrest, corneal opacities, heart failure, hypertensive crisis, interstitial lung disease, ischemic cerebrovascular events, palmar-plantar erythrodysesthesia syndrome, pancreatitis, pneumonitis, reversible posterior leukoencephalopathy syndrome (RPLS), Stevens-Johnson syndrome, torsade de pointes, ventricular tachycardia, vortex keratopathies

Drug Interactions

Metabolism/Transport Effects Substrate of CYP3A4 (major); **Note:** Assignment of Major/Minor substrate status based on clinically relevant drug interaction potential; **Inhibits** BCRP, P-glycoprotein

Avoid Concomitant Use

Avoid concomitant use of Vandetanib with any of the following: Artemether; CYP3A4 Inducers (Strong); Dronedarone; Lumefantrine; Nilotinib; Pimozide; QTc-Prolonging Agents; QUEtiapine; QuiNINE; Silodosin; St Johns Wort; Tetrabenazine; Thioridazine; Topotecan; Toremifene; Vemurafenib; Ziprasidone

Increased Effect/Toxicity

Vandetanib may increase the levels/effects of: Colchicine; Dabigatran Etexilate; Dronedarone; Everolimus; P-glycoprotein/ABCB1 Substrates; Pimozide; QTc-Prolonging Agents; QuiNINE; Rivaroxaban; Silodosin; Tetrabenazine; Thioridazine; Topotecan; Toremifene; Vemurafenib; Vitamin K Antagonists; Ziprasidone

The levels/effects of Vandetanib may be increased by: Alfuzosin; Artemether; Chloroquine; Ciprofloxacin; Ciprofloxacin (Systemic); Gadobutrol; Indacaterol; Lumefantrine; Nilotinib; QTc-Prolonging Agents; QUEtiapine; QuiNINE

Decreased Effect

Vandetanib may decrease the levels/effects of: Cardiac Glycosides; Vitamin K Antagonists

The levels/effects of Vandetanib may be decreased by: CYP3A4 Inducers (Strong); Deferasirox; St Johns Wort; Tocilizumab

Ethanol/Nutrition/Herb Interactions Herb/Nutraceutical: Avoid St John's wort (may decrease vandetanib exposure).

Stability Store at 25°C (77°F); excursions permitted to 15°C to 30°C (59°F to 86°F).

Mechanism of Action Multikinase inhibitor; inhibits tyrosine kinases including epidermal growth factor reception (EGFR), vascular endothelial growth factor (VEGF), rearranged during transfection (RET), protein tyrosine kinase 6 (BRK), TIE2, EPH kinase receptors and SRC kinase receptors, selectively blocking intracellular signaling, angiogenesis and cellular proliferation

Pharmacodynamics/Kinetics

- Absorption: Slow
- Protein binding: ~90%; to albumin and alpha 1-acid-glycoprotein
- Distribution: V_d: ~7450 L
- Metabolism: Hepatic, via CYP3A4 to N-desmethyl vandetanib and via flavin-containing monooxygenase enzymes to vandetanib-N-oxide
- Bioavailability: Not affected by food
- Half life, elimination: 19 days
- Time to peak: 6 hours (range: 4-10 hours)
- Excretion: Feces (~44%); urine (~25%)

Dosage Note: Do not initiate treatment unless QTcF <450 msec. Avoid concomitant use of QT-prolonging agents and strong CYP3A4 inducers. To reduce the risk of QT prolongation, maintain serum calcium and magnesium within normal limits and maintain serum potassium ≥4 mEq/L.

Oral: Adults: Medullary thyroid cancer, locally advanced or metastatic: 300 mg once daily, continue treatment until no longer clinically benefiting or until unacceptable toxicity

Dosage adjustment for toxicity:

QTcF >500 msec: Withhold dose until QTcF returns to <450 msec, then resume at a reduced dose

Toxicity ≥grade 3: Interrupt dose until resolves or improves to grade 1, then resume at a reduced dose

Dosage reduction: Reduce from 300 mg once daily to 200 mg once daily, further reduce if needed to 100 mg once daily

Management of specific toxicities:

Diarrhea (severe): Withhold treatment until resolution. Dose reduction is recommended when treatment is resumed. Routine antidiarrheals are recommended. Closely monitor electrolytes.

Heart failure: May require discontinuation.

Hemorrhage (severe): Discontinue.

Hypertension: Initiate or adjust antihypertensive therapy as needed; may require vandetanib dosage adjustment or treatment interruption; discontinue permanently if blood pressure cannot be adequately controlled.

Interstitial lung disease (ILD)/pneumonitis: If asymptomatic (or minimal symptoms) with radiologic evidence of ILD, may continue treatment with close monitoring. Consider interrupting treatment for moderate symptoms (may require corticosteroids or antibiotics). Discontinue treatment for severe symptoms; may require corticosteroids and antibiotics, and even permanent discontinuation.

Ischemic cerebrovascular events (severe): Discontinue treatment (safety of resuming treatment after an ischemic event has not been studied).

Reversible posterior leukoencephalopathy syndrome (RPLS): Consider discontinuing treatment.

Skin reactions: Withhold treatment for dermatologic toxicity of grade 3 or higher. Consider a reduced dose or permanent discontinuation upon improvement in symptoms. Severe dermatologic toxicity has been managed with corticosteroids (systemic) and treatment discontinuation; mild-to-moderate toxicity has responded to corticosteroids (systemic or topical), oral antihistamines, and antibiotics (topical or systemic).

Dosage adjustment in renal impairment:

Cl_{cr} ≥50 mL/minute: No adjustment required

Moderate and severe impairment: Cl_{cr} <50 mL/minute: Reduce initial dose to 200 mg once daily; closely monitor QT interval

Dosage adjustment in hepatic impairment: Moderate and severe impairment (Child-Pugh class B and C): Use is not recommended

Dietary Considerations May be taken with or without food.

Administration May be administered with or without food. Missed doses should be omitted if within 12 hours of the next scheduled dose. Do not crush tablet. If unable to swallow tablet whole or if nasogastric or gastrostomy tube administration is necessary, disperse one tablet in 2 ounces of water (noncarbonated only) and stir for 10 minutes to disperse (will not dissolve completely) and administer immediately. Rinse residue in glass with additional 4 ounces of water (noncarbonated only) and administer. Use appropriate handling precautions (hazardous agent).

Monitoring Parameters Monitor electrolytes (calcium, magnesium, potassium), TSH, and ECG (QT interval) at baseline, at 2-4 weeks, at 8-12 weeks, and every 3 months thereafter; also monitor QT interval at same frequency for dose reduction due to QT interval or treatment delays >2 weeks (monitor electrolytes and ECG more frequently if diarrhea). Monitor renal function, hepatic function, blood pressure; monitor for signs and symptoms of heart failure and pulmonary toxicities.

Dosage Forms Excipient information presented when available (limited, particularly for generics); consult specific product labeling.

Tablet, oral: 100 mg, 300 mg

Caprelsa®: 100 mg, 300 mg

Extemporaneous Preparations Hazardous agent: Use appropriate precautions for handling and disposal.

An oral solution may be prepared using the tablet. Disperse one tablet in 2 ounces of water (noncarbonated only) and stir for 10 minutes to disperse (will not dissolve completely) and administer immediately. Rinse residue in glass with additional 4 ounces of water (noncarbonated only) and administer.

◆ **Vaniqa®** *see* Eflornithine *on page 577*

◆ **Vanos®** *see* Fluocinonide *on page 727*

◆ **Vanoxide-HC®** *see* Benzoyl Peroxide and Hydrocortisone *on page 205*

◆ **Vanquish® Extra Strength Pain Reliever [OTC]** *see* Acetaminophen, Aspirin, and Caffeine *on page 32*

◆ **Vantas®** *see* Histrelin *on page 830*

◆ **Vantin** *see* Cefpodoxime *on page 313*

◆ **Vaprisol®** *see* Conivaptan *on page 411*

◆ **VAQTA®** *see* Hepatitis A Vaccine *on page 824*

◆ **VAR** *see* Varicella Virus Vaccine *on page 1773*

Vardenafil (var DEN a fil)

Brand Names: U.S. Levitra®; Staxyn™

Brand Names: Canada Levitra®; Staxyn™

Index Terms Vardenafil Hydrochloride

Pharmacologic Category Phosphodiesterase-5 Enzyme Inhibitor

Use Treatment of erectile dysfunction (ED)

Pregnancy Risk Factor B

Pregnancy Considerations Teratogenic effects were not observed in animal studies; however, vardenafil is not indicated for use in women. No effects on sperm motility or morphology were observed in healthy males.

Lactation Excretion in breast milk unknown/not indicated for use in women.

Contraindications Hypersensitivity to vardenafil or any component of the formulation; concurrent (regular or intermittent) use of organic nitrates in any form (eg, nitroglycerin, isosorbide dinitrate)

Warnings/Precautions There is a degree of cardiac risk associated with sexual activity; therefore, physicians may wish to consider the patient's cardiovascular status prior to initiating any treatment for erectile dysfunction. Use caution in patients with anatomical deformation of the penis (angulation, cavernosal fibrosis, or Peyronie's disease) and in patients who have conditions which may predispose them to priapism (sickle cell anemia, multiple myeloma, leukemia). Instruct patients to seek immediate medical attention if erection persists >4 hours.

Use is not recommended in patients with hypotension (<90/50 mm Hg); uncontrolled hypertension (>170/100 mm Hg); unstable angina or angina during intercourse; life-threatening arrhythmias, stroke, or MI within the last 6 months; cardiac failure or coronary artery disease ▶

causing unstable angina. Safety and efficacy have not been studied in these patients. Use caution in patients with left ventricular outflow obstruction (eg, aortic stenosis). Use caution with alpha-blockers, effective CYP3A4 inhibitors, the elderly, or those with hepatic impairment (Child-Pugh class B); dosage adjustment is needed.

Rare cases of nonarteritic ischemic optic neuropathy (NAION) have been reported; risk may be increased with history of vision loss. Other risk factors for NAION include heart disease, diabetes, hypertension, smoking, age >50 years, or history of certain eye problems. Sudden decrease or loss of hearing has been reported rarely; hearing changes may be accompanied by tinnitus and dizziness.

Safety and efficacy have not been studied in patients with the following conditions, therefore, use in these patients is not recommended at this time: Congenital QT prolongation, patients taking medications known to prolong the QT interval (avoid use in patients taking Class Ia or III antiarrhythmics); severe hepatic impairment (Child-Pugh class C); end-stage renal disease requiring dialysis; retinitis pigmentosa or other degenerative retinal disorders. The safety and efficacy of vardenafil with other treatments for erectile dysfunction have not been studied and are not recommended as combination therapy. Concomitant use with all forms of nitrates is contraindicated. If nitrate administration is medically necessary, it is not known when nitrates can be safely administered following the use of vardenafil; the ACC/AHA 2007 guidelines support administration of nitrates only if 24 hours have elapsed. Potential underlying causes of erectile dysfunction should be evaluated prior to treatment. Some products may contain phylalanine. Some products may contain sorbitol; do not use in patients with fructose intolerance.

Adverse Reactions

>10%:

- Cardiovascular: Flushing (8% to 11%)
- Central nervous system: Headache (14% to 15%)

2% to 10%:

- Central nervous system: Dizziness (2%)
- Gastrointestinal: Dyspepsia (3% to 4%), nausea (2%)
- Neuromuscular & skeletal: Back pain (2%), CPK increased (2%)
- Respiratory: Rhinitis (9%), nasal congestion (3%), sinusitis (3%)
- Miscellaneous: Flu-like syndrome (3%)

<2% (Limited to important or life-threatening): Abnormal ejaculation, amnesia (transient global), anaphylactic reaction, angina, angioedema, arthralgia, dyspnea, hearing decreased, hearing loss, hyper-/hypotension, insomnia, liver function tests abnormal, MI, myalgia, nonarteritic ischemic optic neuropathy (NAION), pain, photophobia, photosensitivity, postural hypotension, priapism, pruritus, rash, somnolence, syncope, tachycardia, tinnitus, ventricular tachyarrhythmia, vertigo, vision abnormal, visual acuity reduced, visual field defects, vision loss (temporary or permanent)

Drug Interactions

Metabolism/Transport Effects Substrate of CYP3A4 (major); **Note:** Assignment of Major/Minor substrate status based on clinically relevant drug interaction potential

Avoid Concomitant Use

Avoid concomitant use of Vardenafil with any of the following: Amyl Nitrite; Phosphodiesterase 5 Inhibitors; Vasodilators (Organic Nitrates)

Increased Effect/Toxicity

Vardenafil may increase the levels/effects of: Alpha1-Blockers; Amyl Nitrite; Antihypertensives; Bosentan; Phosphodiesterase 5 Inhibitors; Vasodilators (Organic Nitrates)

The levels/effects of Vardenafil may be increased by: Antifungal Agents (Azole Derivatives, Systemic); Boceprevir; Clarithromycin; CYP3A4 Inhibitors (Moderate); CYP3A4 Inhibitors (Strong); Dasatinib; Erythromycin; Protease Inhibitors; Sapropterin; Telaprevir

Decreased Effect

The levels/effects of Vardenafil may be decreased by: Bosentan; Etravirine; Tocilizumab

Ethanol/Nutrition/Herb Interactions Food: High-fat meals decrease maximum serum concentration 18% to 50%. Serum concentrations/toxicity may be increased with grapefruit juice; avoid concurrent use.

Stability Store at controlled room temperature of 25°C (77°F); excursions permitted to 15°C to 25°C (59°F to 86°F). Keep oral disintegrating tablets sealed in blisterpack until ready to use.

Mechanism of Action Does not directly cause penile erections, but affects the response to sexual stimulation. The physiologic mechanism of erection of the penis involves release of nitric oxide (NO) in the corpus cavernosum during sexual stimulation. NO then activates the enzyme guanylate cyclase, which results in increased levels of cyclic guanosine monophosphate (cGMP), producing smooth muscle relaxation and inflow of blood to the corpus cavernosum. Vardenafil enhances the effect of NO by inhibiting phosphodiesterase type 5 (PDE-5), which is responsible for degradation of cGMP in the corpus cavernosum; when sexual stimulation causes local release of NO, inhibition of PDE-5 by vardenafil causes increased levels of cGMP in the corpus cavernosum, resulting in smooth muscle relaxation and inflow of blood to the corpus cavernosum; at recommended doses, it has no effect in the absence of sexual stimulation.

Pharmacodynamics/Kinetics

Onset of action: ~60 minutes

Absorption: Rapid

Distribution: V_d: 208 L

Protein binding: ~95% (parent drug and metabolite)

Metabolism: Hepatic via CYP3A4 (major), CYP2C and 3A5 (minor); forms metabolite (active)

Bioavailability: ~15%

- Film-coated tablet: Elderly (≥65 years): AUC increased by 52%; Hepatic impairment (moderate, Child-Pugh class B): AUC increased by 160%
- Oral disintegrating tablet: Elderly (≥65 years): AUC increased by 21% more compared to film-coated tablet. When administered with water, AUC decreases by 29%.

Half-life elimination: Terminal: Vardenafil and metabolite: 3-6 hours

Time to peak, plasma: 0.5-2 hours

Excretion: Feces (~91% to 95% as metabolites); urine (~2% to 6%)

Dosage Note: Oral disintegrating tablets should not be used interchangeably with film-coated tablets; patients requiring a dose other than 10 mg should use the film-coated tablets.

Oral: Erectile dysfunction:

Adults:

- Film-coated tablet (Levitra®): 10 mg 60 minutes prior to sexual activity; dosing range: 5-20 mg; to be given as one single dose and not given more than once daily
- Oral disintegrating tablet (Staxyn™): 10 mg 60 minutes prior to sexual activity; maximum: 10 mg/day

Elderly ≥65 years: Initial: 5 mg 60 minutes prior to sexual activity; to be given as one single dose and not given more than once daily

Dosing adjustment with concomitant medications:
Alpha-blocker (dose should be stable at time of vardenafil initiation):
Film-coated tablet (Levitra®): Initial vardenafil dose: 5 mg/24 hours; if an alpha-blocker is added to vardenafil therapy, it should be initiated at the smallest possible dose and titrated carefully.
Oral disintegrating tablet (Staxyn™): Do not use to initiate therapy. Initial therapy should be with film-coated tablets at lower doses. Patients who have previously used film-coated tablets may be switched to oral disintegrating tablets as recommended by healthcare provider.
Film-coated tablet (Levitra®):
Atazanavir: Maximum vardenafil dose: 2.5 mg/24 hours
Clarithromycin: Maximum vardenafil dose: 2.5 mg/24 hours
Darunavir: Maximum vardenafil dose: 2.5 mg/72 hours
Erythromycin: Maximum vardenafil dose: 5 mg/24 hours
Fosamprenavir: Maximum vardenafil dose: 2.5 mg/24 hours
Fosamprenavir/ritonavir: Maximum vardenafil dose: 2.5 mg/72 hours
Indinavir: Maximum vardenafil dose: 2.5 mg/24 hours
Itraconazole:
200 mg/day: Maximum vardenafil dose: 5 mg/24 hours
400 mg/day: Maximum vardenafil dose: 2.5 mg/24 hours
Ketoconazole:
200 mg/day: Maximum vardenafil dose: 5 mg/24 hours
400 mg/day: Maximum vardenafil dose: 2.5 mg/24 hours
Lopinavir/ritonavir: Maximum vardenafil dose: 2.5 mg/72 hours
Nelfinavir: Maximum vardenafil dose: 2.5 mg/24 hours
Ritonavir: Maximum vardenafil dose: 2.5 mg/72 hours
Saquinavir: Maximum vardenafil dose: 2.5 mg/24 hours
Tipranavir: Maximum vardenafil dose: 2.5 mg/72 hours
Oral disintegrating tablet (Staxyn™): Concurrent use not recommended with potent or moderate CYP3A4 inhibitors (atazanavir, clarithromycin, erythromycin, indinavir, itraconazole, ketoconazole, ritonavir, saquinavir)

Dosage adjustment in renal impairment: Dose adjustment not needed for mild, moderate, or severe impairment; use not recommended in patients on hemodialysis

Dosage adjustment in hepatic impairment:
Child-Pugh class A: No adjustment required
Child-Pugh class B:
Film-coated tablet (Levitra®): Initial: 5 mg 60 minutes prior to sexual activity (maximum dose: 10 mg); to be given as one single dose and not given more than once daily
Oral disintegrating tablet (Staxyn™): Use not recommended
Child-Pugh class C: Has not been studied; use is not recommended by the manufacturer

Dietary Considerations May take with or without food. Avoid grapefruit juice. Some products may contain phenylalanine. Some products may contain sorbitol; do not use in patients with fructose intolerance.

Administration May be administered with or without food, 60 minutes prior to sexual activity.

Oral disintegrating tablet should not be removed from blister pack until administered. Using dry hands, place immediately on tongue. Tablet will dissolve within seconds; do not take with liquid. Do not crush, split, or chew.

Monitoring Parameters Monitor for response, adverse reactions, blood pressure, and heart rate.

Dosage Forms Excipient information presented when available (limited, particularly for generics); consult specific product labeling.
Tablet, oral:
Levitra®: 2.5 mg, 5 mg, 10 mg, 20 mg
Tablet, orally disintegrating, oral:
Staxyn™: 10 mg [contains phenylalanine 1.01 mg/tablet; peppermint flavor]

◆ **Vardenafil Hydrochloride** *see* Vardenafil *on page 1769*

Varenicline (var e NI kleen)

Brand Names: U.S. Chantix®
Brand Names: Canada Champix®
Index Terms Varenicline Tartrate
Pharmacologic Category Partial Nicotine Agonist; Smoking Cessation Aid
Use Treatment to aid in smoking cessation
Pregnancy Risk Factor C
Pregnancy Considerations Teratogenic effects were not observed in animal studies; however, decreased fertility, decreased fetal weight, and increased auditory startle response were observed in the offspring. There are no adequate or well-controlled studies in pregnant women. Use only if benefit outweighs the potential risk to fetus.
Lactation Excretion in breast milk unknown/not recommended
Medication Guide Available Yes
Contraindications Known history of serious hypersensitivity or skin reactions to varenicline
Warnings/Precautions [U.S. Boxed Warning]: Serious neuropsychiatric events (including depression, suicidal thoughts, and suicide) have been reported with use; some cases may have been complicated by symptoms of nicotine withdrawal following smoking cessation. Smoking cessation (with or without treatment) is associated with nicotine withdrawal symptoms and the exacerbation of underlying psychiatric illness; however, some of the behavioral disturbances were reported in treated patients who continued to smoke. Neuropsychiatric symptoms (eg, mood disturbances, psychosis, hostility) have occurred in patients with and without pre-existing psychiatric disease; many cases resolved following therapy discontinuation although in some cases, symptoms persisted. Ethanol consumption may increase the risk of psychiatric adverse events. Monitor all patients for behavioral changes and psychiatric symptoms (eg, agitation, depression, suicidal behavior, suicidal ideation); inform patients to discontinue treatment and contact their healthcare provider immediately if they experience any behavioral and/or mood changes. **[U.S. Boxed Warning]: Before prescribing, the risks of serious neuropsychiatric events must be weighed against the immediate and long term benefits of smoking abstinence for each patient.**

Hypersensitivity reactions (including angioedema) and rare cases of serious skin reactions (including Stevens-Johnson syndrome and erythema multiforme) have been reported. Patients should be instructed to discontinue use and contact healthcare provider if signs/symptoms occur. Treatment may increase risk of cardiovascular events (eg, angina pectoris, nonfatal MI, nonfatal stroke, need for coronary revascularization, new diagnosis of or treatment for PVD). Varenicline was not studied in patients with unstable cardiovascular disease or in patients experiencing recent events (<2 months) prior to treatment. Dose-dependent nausea may occur; both transient and persistent nausea has been reported. Dosage reduction may be considered for intolerable nausea. May cause sedation, which may impair physical or mental abilities; patients must be cautioned about performing tasks which require mental alertness (eg, operating machinery or driving).

Use caution in renal dysfunction; dosage adjustment required. Safety and efficacy of varenicline with other smoking cessation therapies have not been established; increased adverse events when used concurrently with nicotine replacement therapy.

Adverse Reactions

>10%:

Central nervous system: Insomnia (18% to 19%), headache (15% to 19%), abnormal dreams (9% to 13%)

Gastrointestinal: Nausea (16% to 40%; dose related)

1% to 10%:

Central nervous system: Malaise (≤7%), sleep disorder (≤5%), somnolence (3%), nightmares (1% to 2%), lethargy (1% to 2%)

Dermatologic: Rash (≤3%)

Gastrointestinal: Flatulence (6% to 9%), constipation (5% to 8%), abnormal taste (5% to 8%), abdominal pain (≤7%), xerostomia (≤6%), dyspepsia (5%), vomiting (≤5%), appetite increased (3% to 4%), anorexia (≤2%), gastroesophageal reflux (1%)

Respiratory: Upper respiratory tract disorder (5% to 7%), dyspnea (≤2%), rhinorrhea (≤1%)

<1% (Limited to important or life-threatening): Accidental injury, acute coronary syndrome, acute renal failure, aggression, agitation, amnesia, anemia, angina, angioedema, anxiety, arrhythmia, arthralgia, asthma, atrial fibrillation, attention disturbance, back pain, balance disorder, behavioral changes, blindness (transient), blurred vision, bradycardia, bradyphrenia, cardiac flutter, cataract, cerebrovascular accident, chest pain, chills, conjunctivitis, coronary artery disease, cor pulmonale, deafness, delusions, depression, diabetes mellitus, diarrhea, disorientation, dissociation, dizziness, dysarthria, dysphagia, ECG abnormal, eczema, edema, emotional disorder, enterocolitis, epistaxis, erectile dysfunction, eructation, erythema, erythema multiforme, esophagitis, euphoria, facial palsy, fever, flu-like syndrome, flushing, gall bladder disorder, gastritis, gastric ulcer, gastrointestinal hemorrhage, hallucinations, homicidal ideation, hostility, hyperhidrosis, hyperlipidemia, hypersensitivity, hypoglycemia, hypokalemia, intestinal obstruction, irritability, leukocytosis, libido decreased, liver function test abnormal, loss of consciousness, lymphadenopathy, mania, Ménière's disease, mental impairment, MI, migraine, mood swings, mouth ulceration, muscle enzyme increased, musculoskeletal pain, multiple sclerosis, muscle cramps, myalgia, myositis, nephrolithiasis, night blindness, nocturia, nystagmus, ocular vascular disorder, osteoporosis, palpitation, pancreatitis, panic, paranoia, parosmia, photophobia, photosensitivity, pleurisy, polyuria, psoriasis, psychomotor impairment, psychosis, psychotic disorder, pulmonary embolism, restless leg syndrome, restlessness, seizure, sexual dysfunction, splenomegaly, Stevens-Johnson syndrome, suicidal behavior, suicidal ideation, suicide, suicide attempt, syncope, tachycardia, thinking abnormal, thrombocytopenia, thrombosis, thyroid disorder, tinnitus, transient ischemic attack, tremor, urinary retention, urticaria, ventricular extrasystoles, vertigo, visual field defect, vitreous floaters, weight gain, xerophthalmia

Drug Interactions

Metabolism/Transport Effects None known.

Avoid Concomitant Use There are no known interactions where it is recommended to avoid concomitant use.

Increased Effect/Toxicity

The levels/effects of Varenicline may be increased by: Alcohol (Ethyl); H2-Antagonists; Quinolone Antibiotics; Trimethoprim

Decreased Effect There are no known significant interactions involving a decrease in effect.

Ethanol/Nutrition/Herb Interactions Ethanol: May increase the risk of psychiatric adverse events. Caution patients about the potential effects of ethanol consumption during therapy.

Stability Store at 25°C (77°F); excursions permitted to 15°C to 30°C (59°F to 86°F).

Mechanism of Action Partial neuronal α_4 β_2 nicotinic receptor agonist; prevents nicotine stimulation of mesolimbic dopamine system associated with nicotine addiction. Also binds to 5 HT_3 receptor (significance not determined) with moderate affinity. Varenicline stimulates dopamine activity but to a much smaller degree than nicotine does, resulting in decreased craving and withdrawal symptoms.

Pharmacodynamics/Kinetics

Absorption: Well absorbed; unaffected by food

Protein binding: ≤20%

Metabolism: Minimal (<10% of clearance is through metabolism)

Half-life elimination: ~24 hours

Time to peak, plasma: ~3-4 hours

Excretion: Urine (92% as unchanged drug)

Dosage Oral: Adults:

Initial:

Days 1-3: 0.5 mg once daily

Days 4-7: 0.5 mg twice daily

Maintenance (≥ Day 8):

U.S. labeling: 1 mg twice daily for 11 weeks

Canadian labeling: 0.5-1 mg twice daily for 11 weeks

Note: Start 1 week before target quit date. Alternatively, patients may consider setting a quit date up to 35 days after initiation of varenicline and then quit smoking between 8-35 days of treatment (some data suggest that an extended pretreatment regimen may result in higher abstinence rates [Hajek, 2011]). If patient successfully quits smoking at the end of the 12 weeks, may continue for another 12 weeks to help maintain success. If not successful in first 12 weeks, then stop medication and reassess factors contributing to failure.

Dosage adjustment for toxicity: Patients who cannot tolerate adverse events may require temporary (or permanent) reduction in dose. Lower dose for a period of time, then may increase dose again or remain on lower dose.

Dosage adjustment in renal impairment:

Cl_{cr} ≥30 mL/minute: No adjustment required

Cl_{cr} <30 mL/minute: Initial: 0.5 mg once daily; maximum dose: 0.5 mg twice daily

Hemodialysis: Maximum dose: 0.5 mg once daily

Dosage adjustment in hepatic impairment: No adjustment required

Dietary Considerations Should be given with food and a full glass of water to decrease gastric upset.

Administration Administer with food and a full glass of water.

Monitoring Parameters Monitor for behavioral changes and psychiatric symptoms (eg, agitation, depression, suicidal behavior, suicidal ideation)

Additional Information In all studies, patients received an educational booklet on smoking cessation and received up to 10 minutes of counseling at each weekly visit. Dosing started 1 week before target quit date. Successful cessation of smoking may alter pharmacokinetic properties of other medications (eg, theophylline, warfarin, insulin).

Dosage Forms Excipient information presented when available (limited, particularly for generics); consult specific product labeling.

Combination package, oral [dose-pack]:

Chantix®: Tablet: 0.5 mg (11s) [white tablets] and Tablet: 1 mg (42s) [light blue tablets]

Tablet, oral:

Chantix®: 0.5 mg, 1 mg

◆ **Varenicline Tartrate** *see* Varenicline *on page 1771*

◆ **Varicella, Measles, Mumps, and Rubella Vaccine** *see* Measles, Mumps, Rubella, and Varicella Virus Vaccine *on page 1055*

Varicella Virus Vaccine

(var i SEL a VYE rus vak SEEN)

Brand Names: U.S. Varivax®

Brand Names: Canada Varilrix®; Varivax® III

Index Terms Chickenpox Vaccine; VAR; Varicella-Zoster Virus (VZV) Vaccine (Varicella); VZV Vaccine (Varicella)

Pharmacologic Category Vaccine, Live (Viral)

Additional Appendix Information

Immunization Recommendations *on page 1922*

Use Immunization against varicella in children ≥12 months of age and adults

The ACIP recommends vaccination for all children, adolescents, and adults who do not have evidence of immunity. Vaccination is especially important for:

- Healthcare personnel
- Persons with close contact to those at high risk for severe disease
- Persons living or working in environments where transmission is likely (teachers, child-care workers, residents and staff of institutional settings)
- Persons in environments where transmission has been reported
- Nonpregnant women of childbearing age
- Adolescents and adults in households with children
- International travelers

Postexposure prophylaxis: Vaccination within 3 days (possibly 5 days) after exposure to rash is effective in preventing illness or modifying severity of disease

Pregnancy Risk Factor C

Pregnancy Considerations Animal reproduction studies have not been conducted. Varivax® should not be administered to pregnant females and pregnancy should be avoided for 3 months (per manufacturer labeling; 1 month per ACIP) following vaccination. A pregnancy registry has been established for pregnant women exposed to varicella virus vaccine (800-986-8999). Varicella disease during the 1st or 2nd trimesters may result in congenital varicella syndrome. The onset of maternal varicella infection from 5 days prior to 2 days after delivery may cause varicella infection in the newborn. All women should be assessed for immunity during a prenatal visit; those without evidence of immunity should be vaccinated upon completion or termination of pregnancy.

Lactation Excretion in breast milk unknown/use caution

Contraindications Hypersensitivity to any component of the vaccine; individuals with blood dyscrasias, leukemia, lymphomas, or other malignant neoplasms affecting the bone marrow or lymphatic systems; those receiving immunosuppressive therapy; primary and acquired immunodeficiency states; family history of congenital or hereditary immunodeficiency (until immune competence in the vaccine recipient is demonstrated); active, untreated tuberculosis; current febrile illness (per manufacturer labeling); pregnancy

Warnings/Precautions Immediate treatment for anaphylactoid reaction should be available during vaccine use. Varicella vaccine and antibody-containing products (eg, immune globulin, blood products) should **not** be administered simultaneously. Vaccinated individuals should not have close association with susceptible high-risk individuals (newborns, pregnant women, immunocompromised persons) for 6 weeks following vaccination. May administer to patients with mild acute illness (with or without low grade fever per CDC guidelines). Children with HIV infection with age-specific CD4+ T-lymphocyte percentages ≥15% may receive live attenuated varicella vaccine. Vaccination may be considered for adolescents and adults with CD4+ T-lymphocyte counts ≥200 cells/µL. Products may contain gelatin, neomycin, or albumin; patients with history of anaphylaxis should not receive vaccine. Contact dermatitis to neomycin is not a contraindication to the vaccine. In order to maximize vaccination rates, the ACIP recommends simultaneous administration of all age-appropriate vaccines (live or inactivated) for which a person is eligible at a single clinic visit, unless contraindications exist. The use of combination vaccines is generally preferred over separate injections, taking into consideration provider assessment, patient preference, and adverse events.

Adverse Reactions All serious adverse reactions must be reported to the U.S. Department of Health and Human Services (DHHS) Vaccine Adverse Event Reporting System (VAERS) 1-800-822-7967 or online at https://vaers.hhs.gov/esub/index. In Canada, adverse reactions may be reported to local provincial/territorial health agencies or to the Vaccine Safety Section at Public Health Agency of Canada (1-866-844-0018).

>10%:

Central nervous system: Fever (10% to 15%)

Local: Injection site reaction (19% to 33%)

1% to 10%:

Central nervous system: Chills, fatigue, headache, irritability, malaise, nervousness, sleep disturbance

Dermatologic: Generalized varicella-like rash (1% to 6%), contact rash, dermatitis, diaper rash, dry skin, eczema, heat rash, itching

Gastrointestinal: Abdominal pain, appetite decreased, cold/canker sore, constipation, diarrhea, nausea, vomiting

Hematologic: Lymphadenopathy

Local: Varicella-like rash at the injection site (1% to 3%)

Neuromuscular & skeletal: Arthralgia, myalgia, stiff neck

Otic: Otitis

Respiratory: Cough, lower/upper respiratory illness

Miscellaneous: Allergic reactions, teething

<1% (Limited to important or life-threatening): Anaphylaxis, anaphylactic shock, angioneurotic edema, aplastic anemia, aseptic meningitis, ataxia, Bell's palsy, cerebellar ataxia (acute), cerebrovascular accident, disseminated varicella infection, encephalitis, erythema multiforme, Guillain-Barré syndrome, hemiparesis (acute), Henoch-Schönlein purpura, hepatitis, herpes zoster, nonfebrile seizure, paresthesia, Stevens-Johnson syndrome, thrombocytopenia (including idiopathic thrombocytopenia purpura), transverse myelitis,

Drug Interactions

Metabolism/Transport Effects None known.

Avoid Concomitant Use

Avoid concomitant use of Varicella Virus Vaccine with any of the following: Belimumab; Fingolimod; Immunosuppressants

Increased Effect/Toxicity

The levels/effects of Varicella Virus Vaccine may be increased by: 5-ASA Derivatives; AzaTHIOprine; Belimumab; Corticosteroids (Systemic); Fingolimod; Hydroxychloroquine; Immunosuppressants; Leflunomide; Mercaptopurine; Methotrexate; Salicylates; Smallpox Vaccine

Decreased Effect

Varicella Virus Vaccine may decrease the levels/effects of: Tuberculin Tests

The levels/effects of Varicella Virus Vaccine may be decreased by: Fingolimod; Immune Globulins; Immunosuppressants

Stability Prior to reconstitution, store in freezer at -15°C (5°F) or colder; may be stored under refrigeration 2°C to 8°C (36°F to 46°F)) for 72 hours. Protect from light. Store diluent at room temperature or in refrigerator. Use 0.7 mL ▶

of the provided diluent to reconstitute vaccine. Gently agitate to mix thoroughly. (Total volume of reconstituted vaccine will be ~0.5 mL.) Following reconstitution, discard reconstituted vaccine if not used within 30 minutes.

Canadian formulations: **Note:** Varicella vaccine has been reformulated to produce a refrigerator-stable preparation. Previously, the product required storage in a freezer prior to reconstitution. The new Canadian formulation may be stored in a freezer, but if transferred to a refrigerator, may not be refrozen. Individual product labeling should be consulted to confirm proper conditions.

Mechanism of Action As a live, attenuated vaccine, varicella virus vaccine offers active immunity to disease caused by the varicella-zoster virus

Pharmacodynamics/Kinetics

Onset of action: Seroconversion: ~4-6 weeks

Duration: Antibody titers detectable at 10 years postvaccination

Dosage SubQ:

Children 12 months to 12 years: 0.5 mL; a second dose may be administered ≥3 months later

Note: The ACIP recommends the routine childhood vaccination be 2 doses, with the first dose administered at 12-15 months of age. School age children should receive the second dose at 4-6 years of age, but it may be administered earlier provided ≥3 months have elapsed after the first dose. All children and adolescents who received only 1 dose of vaccine should receive a second dose (CDC, 2007).

Children ≥13 years to Adults: 2 doses of 0.5 mL separated by 4-8 weeks. **Note:** The ACIP recommends that all children and adults who received only 1 dose of vaccine receive a second dose (CDC, 2007).

Administration For SubQ injection only; inject in the outer aspect of upper arm. Administer immediately following reconstitution.

Simultaneous administration of vaccines helps ensure the patients will be fully vaccinated by the appropriate age. Simultaneous administration of vaccines is defined as administering >1 vaccine on the same day at different anatomic sites. The use of licensed combination vaccines is generally preferred over separate injections of the equivalent components. Separate vaccines should not be combined in the same syringe unless indicated by product specific labeling. Separate needles and syringes should be used for each injection. The ACIP prefers each dose of a specific vaccine in a series come from the same manufacturer when possible. Adolescents and adults should be vaccinated while seated or lying down. In general, preterm infants should be vaccinated at the same chronological age as full-term infants (CDC, 2011).

Antipyretics have not been shown to prevent febrile seizures. Antipyretics may be used to treat fever or discomfort following vaccination (CDC, 2011). One study reported that routine prophylactic administration of acetaminophen to prevent fever prior to vaccination decreased the immune response of some vaccines; the clinical significance of this reduction in immune response has not been established (Prymula, 2009).

Monitoring Parameters Rash, fever; monitor for syncope for ≥15 minutes following vaccination

Additional Information Federal law requires that the name of medication, date of administration, the vaccine manufacturer, lot number of vaccine, and the administering person's name, title, and address be entered into the patient's permanent medical record.

Evidence of immunity to varicella includes any of the following:

Documentation of age appropriate vaccination with varicella vaccine.

Laboratory evidence of immunity or laboratory confirmation of disease.

Birth in the United States prior to 1980 (except for health care personnel, pregnant women and the immunocompromised).

Diagnosis or verification of varicella disease by healthcare provider.

Diagnosis or verification of herpes zoster by healthcare provider.

Persons who lack evidence of immunity should be vaccinated.

Dosage Forms Excipient information presented when available (limited, particularly for generics); consult specific product labeling.

Injection, powder for reconstitution [preservative free]:

Varivax®: 1350 PFU [contains bovine serum, gelatin, neomycin (may have trace amounts), sucrose 25 mg/vial]

Dosage Forms: Canada Excipient information presented when available (limited, particularly for generics); consult specific product labeling.

Injection, powder for reconstitution [preservative free]:

Varivax® III: 1350 plaque-forming units (PFU) [contains gelatin and trace amounts of neomycin; packaged with diluent]

Injection, powder for reconstitution:

Valrilix®: $10^{3.3}$ plaque-forming units (PFU) [contains albumin and gelatin; packaged with diluent]

Varicella-Zoster Immune Globulin (Human)

(var i SEL a- ZOS ter i MYUN GLOB yoo lin HYU man)

Brand Names: Canada VariZIG™

Index Terms VZIG

Pharmacologic Category Blood Product Derivative; Immune Globulin

Use In pregnant women, for the prevention or reduction in severity of maternal infection within 4 days of exposure to the varicella zoster virus.

Unlabeled Use In the United States, the Centers for Disease Control and Prevention (CDC) recommends varicella-zoster immune globulin (VZIG) for the passive immunization of patients who are at a greater risk of complications following significant exposure to varicella and do not have evidence of immunity. Guidelines restrict administration to those patients meeting the following criteria:

- Immunocompromised patients without evidence of immunity, including those with neoplastic disease (eg, leukemia or lymphoma); primary or acquired immunodeficiency; immunosuppressive therapy (including steroid therapy equivalent to prednisone ≥2 mg/kg or 20 mg/day)
- Newborn of mother who had onset of varicella (chickenpox) within 5 days before delivery or within 48 hours after delivery
- Premature infants (≥28 weeks gestation) whose mother has no evidence of immunity
- Premature infants (<28 weeks gestation or ≤1000 g) regardless of maternal history
- Pregnant women without evidence of immunity

Significant exposure includes:

Continuous household contact

Face-to-face indoor contact (>5 minutes or >1 hour depending on reference)

Hospital contact (in same 2-4 bedroom or adjacent beds in a large ward or prolonged face-to-face contact with an infectious staff member or patient)

Pregnancy Considerations Animal reproduction studies have not been conducted. Clinical use of other immunoglobulins suggest that there are no adverse effects on the fetus. Pregnant women who do not have evidence of immunity to varicella may be at increased risk of infection following exposure. VZIG is used to prevent maternal complications, not fetal infection.

Lactation Excretion in breast milk unknown/use caution

Prescribing and Access Restrictions Varicella-zoster immune globulin (VZIG) was discontinued in the United States in 2005. It is currently available as VariZIG™ under an Investigational New Drug Application Expanded Access protocol. Inventory for anticipated patients may be obtained by contacting FFF Enterprises at 800-843-7477. Additional information is available at http://www.-fffenterprises.com/Products/VariZIGINDProtocolPre.aspx

Contraindications Severe reaction associated with past human immune globulin administration; hypersensitivity to any component of the formulation; patients with evidence of immunity; IgA deficiency

Note: U.S. CDC guidelines: Healthy and immunocompromised patients (except bone marrow transplant recipients [BMT]) with positive history of varicella infection are considered immune. BMT patients who had varicella infection *prior to* transplant are **not** considered immune; however, the expanded access protocol does not include use for this indication. BMT patients who develop varicella infection *after* transplant **are** considered immune. Patients who are fully vaccinated, but later became immunocompromised should be monitored closely; treatment with VZIG is not indicated, but other therapy may be needed if disease occurs.

Adverse Reactions

>10%:

Central nervous system: Headache (7% to 11%)

Local: Injection site pain (17% to 47%)

1% to 10%:

Central nervous system: Dizziness (up to 5%), fever (up to 5%), pain (up to 5%), chills (up to 2%), fatigue (up to 2%), flushing (up to 2%), insomnia (up to 2%)

Dermatologic: Rash (up to 4%), dermatitis (up to 2%), erythematous rash (up to 2%)

Gastrointestinal: Nausea (2% to 5%), dysgeusia (up to 2%)

Local: Injection site bruising, itching, or tenderness (up to 2%)

Neuromuscular & skeletal: Neck pain (up to 5%), myalgia (up to 2%)

Drug Interactions

Metabolism/Transport Effects None known.

Avoid Concomitant Use There are no known interactions where it is recommended to avoid concomitant use.

Increased Effect/Toxicity There are no known significant interactions involving an increase in effect.

Decreased Effect

Varicella-Zoster Immune Globulin (Human) may decrease the levels/effects of: Vaccines (Live)

Stability Prior to reconstitution, store at 2°C to 8°C (36°F to 48°F); do not freeze. Following reconstitution, may store at 2°C to 8°C (36°F to 48°F) for up to 12 hours. Reconstitute only with provided diluent. Inject diluent slowly and at an angle onto the inside glass wall of the vial. Gently invert vial and swirl to dissolve; do not shake. For I.V. administration, reconstitute with 2.5 mL/vial (provides 50 int. units/mL). For I.M. administration, reconstitute with 1.25 mL/vial (provides 100 int. units/mL).

Mechanism of Action Antibodies obtained from pooled human plasma of individuals with high titers of varicella-zoster provide passive immunity.

Pharmacodynamics/Kinetics

Duration: ≥6 weeks

Metabolism: Metabolized in the reticuloendothelial system

Bioavailability: 100%

Half-life elimination: I.V.: 18-24 days; I.M.: 24-30 days

Time to peak, plasma: I.V.: <3 hours; I.M.: 2-7 days

Dosage I.M., I.V.:

Children: Passive immunization (unlabeled use): Refer to adult dosing.

Adults: Prevention or reduction of maternal infection (approved use), passive immunization (unlabeled use): 125 int. units/10 kg (minimum dose: 125 int. units; maximum dose: 625 int. units). Administer within 96 hours of exposure.

Administration For I.M. or I.V. administration. Bring to room temperature prior to use. Should be given as soon as possible following exposure; efficacy has not been established for use >96 hours following exposure. For I.M. injection, administer into deltoid muscle or anterolateral aspect of upper thigh; avoid gluteal region. For I.V. administration, inject over 3-5 minutes.

Monitoring Parameters Observe for adverse effects for 20 minutes following administration. The CDC also recommends monitoring for signs and symptoms of varicella infection for 28 days after VZIG administration.

Test Interactions May cause false-positive test for immunity to VZV for 3 months following administration. May cause a false-positive Coomb's test.

Dosage Forms: Canada Excipient information presented when available (limited, particularly for generics); consult specific product labeling.

Injection, powder for reconstitution [preservative free]:

VariZIG™: 125 int. units [package with diluent]

- ◆ **Varicella-Zoster Virus (VZV) Vaccine (Varicella)** *see* Varicella Virus Vaccine *on page 1773*
- ◆ **Varicella-Zoster (VZV) Vaccine (Zoster)** *see* Zoster Vaccine *on page 1830*
- ◆ **Varilrix® (Can)** *see* Varicella Virus Vaccine *on page 1773*
- ◆ **Varivax®** *see* Varicella Virus Vaccine *on page 1773*
- ◆ **Varivax® III (Can)** *see* Varicella Virus Vaccine *on page 1773*
- ◆ **VariZIG™ (Can)** *see* Varicella-Zoster Immune Globulin (Human) *on page 1774*
- ◆ **Vaseretic®** *see* Enalapril and Hydrochlorothiazide *on page 586*
- ◆ **Vasocon® (Can)** *see* Naphazoline (Ophthalmic) *on page 1176*
- ◆ **Vasolex™** *see* Trypsin, Balsam Peru, and Castor Oil *on page 1744*

Vasopressin (vay soe PRES in)

Brand Names: U.S. Pitressin®

Brand Names: Canada Pressyn®; Pressyn® AR

Index Terms 8-Arginine Vasopressin; ADH; Antidiuretic Hormone; AVP

Pharmacologic Category Antidiuretic Hormone Analog; Hormone, Posterior Pituitary

Additional Appendix Information

Vasoactive Agents, Intravenous *on page 1898*

Use Treatment of central diabetes insipidus; differential diagnosis of diabetes insipidus

Unlabeled Use ACLS guidelines: Pulseless arrest (ventricular tachycardia [VT]/ventricular fibrillation [VF], asystole/pulseless electrical activity [PEA]); cardiac arrest secondary to anaphylaxis (unresponsive to epinephrine)

Adjunct in the treatment of GI hemorrhage and esophageal varices; adjunct in the treatment of vasodilatory shock (septic shock); donor management in brain-dead patients (hormone replacement therapy)

Pregnancy Risk Factor C

Pregnancy Considerations Animal reproduction studies have not been conducted. Vasopressin and desmopressin have been used safely during pregnancy based on case reports.

Lactation Enters breast milk/use caution

Contraindications Hypersensitivity to vasopressin or any component of the formulation

Warnings/Precautions Use with caution in patients with seizure disorders, migraine, asthma, vascular disease, renal disease, cardiac disease; chronic nephritis with nitrogen retention, goiter with cardiac complications, or arteriosclerosis. I.V. infiltration may lead to severe vasoconstriction and localized tissue necrosis, gangrene of extremities, tongue, and ischemic colitis. May cause water intoxication; early signs include drowsiness, listlessness, and headache, these should be recognized to prevent coma and seizures. Elderly patients should be cautioned not to increase their fluid intake beyond that sufficient to satisfy their thirst in order to avoid water intoxication and hyponatremia; under experimental conditions, the elderly have shown to have a decreased responsiveness to vasopressin with respect to its effects on water homeostasis.

Adverse Reactions Frequency not defined.

Cardiovascular: Arrhythmia, asystole (>0.04 units/minute), blood pressure increased, cardiac output decreased (>0.04 units/minute), chest pain, MI, vasoconstriction (with higher doses), venous thrombosis

Central nervous system: Pounding in head, fever, vertigo

Dermatologic: Ischemic skin lesions, circumoral pallor, urticaria

Gastrointestinal: Abdominal cramps, flatulence, mesenteric ischemia, nausea, vomiting

Genitourinary: Uterine contraction

Neuromuscular & skeletal: Tremor

Respiratory: Bronchial constriction

Miscellaneous: Diaphoresis

Drug Interactions

Metabolism/Transport Effects None known.

Avoid Concomitant Use There are no known interactions where it is recommended to avoid concomitant use.

Increased Effect/Toxicity There are no known significant interactions involving an increase in effect.

Decreased Effect There are no known significant interactions involving a decrease in effect.

Ethanol/Nutrition/Herb Interactions Ethanol: Avoid ethanol (due to effects on ADH).

Stability Store injection at room temperature; do not freeze. Protect from heat. Use only clear solutions.

Mechanism of Action Increases cyclic adenosine monophosphate (cAMP) which increases water permeability at the renal tubule resulting in decreased urine volume and increased osmolality; causes peristalsis by directly stimulating the smooth muscle in the GI tract; direct vasoconstrictor without inotropic or chronotropic effects

Pharmacodynamics/Kinetics

Onset of action: Nasal: 1 hour

Duration: Nasal: 3-8 hours; I.M., SubQ: 2-8 hours

Metabolism: Nasal/Parenteral: Hepatic, renal

Half-life elimination: Nasal: 15 minutes; Parenteral: 10-20 minutes

Excretion: Nasal: Urine; SubQ: Urine (5% as unchanged drug) after 4 hours

Dosage

Central diabetes insipidus: **Note:** Dosage is highly variable; titrate based on serum and urine sodium and osmolality in addition to fluid balance and urine output. Use of vasopressin is impractical for chronic therapy.

I.M., SubQ:

Children: 2.5-10 units 2-4 times/day as needed

Adults: 5-10 units 2-4 times/day as needed

Continuous I.V. infusion (unlabeled route): **Note:** The optimum rate of infusion has not been well established; many protocols exist.

Children: Initial: 0.0005 units/kg/hour; increase dose by 0.0005 units/kg/hour increments every 5-10 minutes as needed to adequately reduce urine output (maximum dose: 0.01 unit/kg/hour) (Wise-Faberowski, 2004). **Note:** Although clinical trial titrated every 5-10 minutes, a reduced frequency of titration (eg, every 30 minutes) may be more appropriate given the half-life of vasopressin.

Adults: Continuous infusion has not been formally evaluated in the post-neurosurgical adult. However, some convert I.M./SubQ requirement to an hourly continuous I.V. infusion rate.

Central diabetes insipidus, post-traumatic (unlabeled use): Adults: I.V.: Initial: 2.5 units/hour; titrate to adequately reduce urine output (Levitt, 1984)

Donor management in brain-dead patients (hormone replacement therapy) (unlabeled use): Adults: I.V.: Initial: 1 unit bolus followed by 0.5-4 units/hour (Rosendale, 2003; UNOS Critical Pathway, 2002)

GI/variceal hemorrhage (unlabeled use): Continuous I.V. infusion: Dilute in NS or D_5W to 0.1-1 unit/mL. **Note:** Other therapies may be preferred.

GI hemorrhage (unlabeled use): Children: Initial I.V. bolus: 0.3 unit/kg (maximum: 20 units) may be given. Continuous I.V. infusion: 0.001-0.01 units/kg/minute; titrate dose as needed; maximum: 0.01 unit/kg/minute; if bleeding controlled for 12-24 hours, then taper off over 24-36 hours

Variceal hemorrhage (unlabeled use) [AASLD guidelines, 2007]: Adults: Initial: 0.2-0.4 units/minute, may titrate dose as needed to a maximum dose of 0.8 units/minute; maximum duration: 24 hours at highest effective dose continuously (to reduce incidence of adverse effects). Patient should also receive I.V. nitroglycerin concurrently to prevent myocardial ischemic complications; monitor closely for signs/symptoms of ischemia (myocardial, peripheral, bowel)

Pulseless arrest (unlabeled use) [ACLS, 2010]: Adults: I.V., I.O.: 40 units; may give 1 dose to replace first or second dose of epinephrine. I.V./I.O. drug administration is preferred, but if no access, may give endotracheally. ACLS guidelines do not recommend a specific endotracheal dose; however, may be given endotracheally using the same I.V. dose (ACLS, 2010; Wenzel, 1997).

Vasodilatory shock/septic shock (unlabeled use): Adults: I.V.: 0.01-0.04 units/minute for the treatment of septic shock. **Note:** Recommended as a second-line vasopressor in addition to norepinephrine (Dellinger, 2008). Doses >0.04 units/minute may have more cardiovascular side effects. Most case reports have used 0.04 units/minute continuous infusion as a fixed dose.

Dosing adjustment in hepatic impairment: Some patients respond to much lower doses with cirrhosis

Administration

I.V.: Use extreme caution to avoid extravasation because of risk of necrosis and gangrene. In treatment of varices, infusions are often supplemented with nitroglycerin infusions to minimize cardiac effects.

Usual concentration: 100 units in 500 mL D_5W. **Note:** In one clinical trial with lower dosing (eg, 0.0005 units/kg/hour) in pediatric patients, a more dilute solution (eg, 20 units in 500 mL D_5W) was employed (Wise-Faberowski, 2004).

Vasodilatory shock: Administration through a central catheter is recommended.

Intranasal (topical administration on nasal mucosa): Administer injectable vasopressin on cotton plugs, as nasal spray, or by dropper. Should not be inhaled.

Endotracheal: If no I.V./I.O. access may give endotracheally. ACLS guidelines do not recommend a specific endotracheal dose; however, may be given endotracheally using the same I.V. dose (ACLS, 2010; Wenzel, 1997). Mix with 5-10 mL of water or normal saline, and administer down the endotracheal tube.

Monitoring Parameters Serum and urine sodium, urine specific gravity, urine and serum osmolality; urine output, fluid input and output, blood pressure, heart rate

Additional Information Vasopressin increases factor VIII levels and may be useful in hemophiliacs.

Dosage Forms Excipient information presented when available (limited, particularly for generics); consult specific product labeling.

Injection, solution: 20 units/mL (0.5 mL, 1 mL, 10 mL)
Pitressin®: 20 units/mL (1 mL)

◆ **Vasotec®** *see* Enalapril *on page* 584

◆ **Vaxigrip® (Can)** *see* Influenza Virus Vaccine (Inactivated) *on page* 897

◆ **VCF® [OTC]** *see* Nonoxynol 9 *on page* 1216

◆ **Vectibix®** *see* Panitumumab *on page* 1288

◆ **Vectical™** *see* Calcitriol *on page* 263

Vecuronium (vek ue ROE nee um)

Brand Names: Canada Norcuron®

Index Terms Norcuron; ORG NC 45

Pharmacologic Category Neuromuscular Blocker Agent, Nondepolarizing

Use To facilitate endotracheal intubation and to relax skeletal muscles during surgery; to facilitate mechanical ventilation in ICU patients; does not relieve pain or produce sedation

Pregnancy Risk Factor C

Pregnancy Considerations There are no adequate and well-controlled studies in pregnant women. Use in cesarean section has been reported. Umbilical venous concentrations were 11% of maternal. Use only if the potential benefit justifies the potential risk to the fetus.

Lactation Excretion in breast milk unknown/use caution

Contraindications Hypersensitivity to vecuronium or any component of the formulation

Warnings/Precautions Ventilation must be supported during neuromuscular blockade. Vecuronium does not relieve pain or produce sedation; use should include appropriate anesthesia, pain control, and sedation. In patients requiring long-term administration, use of a peripheral nerve stimulator to monitor drug effects is strongly recommended. Additional doses of vecuronium or any other neuromuscular-blocking agent should be avoided unless nerve stimulation response suggests inadequate neuromuscular blockade. Certain clinical conditions may result in potentiation (dosage reduction may be necessary) or antagonism (dosage increase may be necessary) of neuromuscular blockade:

Antagonism: Alkalosis, hypercalcemia, demyelinating lesions, peripheral neuropathies, denervation, immobilization, infection, and muscle trauma

Potentiation: Electrolyte abnormalities, severe hyponatremia, severe hypocalcemia, severe hypokalemia, hypermagnesemia, cachexia, neuromuscular diseases, acidosis, Eaton-Lambert syndrome, and myasthenia gravis

Resistance may occur in burn patients (>30% of body) for period of 5-70 days postinjury. Hypothermia may prolong the duration of action. Use with caution in patients with hepatic impairment; clinical duration may be prolonged. Use with caution in patients who are anephric; clinical duration may be prolonged. Use with caution in patients who have underlying respiratory disease. Some patients may experience delayed recovery of neuromuscular function after administration (especially after prolonged use). Other factors associated with delayed recovery should be considered (eg, corticosteroid use, disease-related conditions). Cross-sensitivity with other neuromuscular-blocking agents may occur; use extreme caution in patients with previous anaphylactic reactions. Use caution in the elderly; dosage reduction may be considered. Children 1-10 years of age may require slightly higher initial doses and slightly more frequent supplementation. **[U.S. Boxed Warning]: Should be administered by adequately trained individuals familiar with its use.** Some dosage forms may contain benzyl alcohol which has been associated with "gasping syndrome" in neonates.

Adverse Reactions <1% (Limited to important or life-threatening): Acute quadriplegic myopathy syndrome (prolonged use), Bradycardia, circulatory collapse, edema, flushing; hypersensitivity reaction (hypotension, tachycardia, erythema, rash, urticaria); itching, myositis ossificans (prolonged use), rash

Drug Interactions

Metabolism/Transport Effects None known.

Avoid Concomitant Use

Avoid concomitant use of Vecuronium with any of the following: QuiNINE

Increased Effect/Toxicity

Vecuronium may increase the levels/effects of: Cardiac Glycosides; Corticosteroids (Systemic); OnabotulinumtoxinA; RimabotulinumtoxinB

The levels/effects of Vecuronium may be increased by: AbobotulinumtoxinA; Aminoglycosides; Calcium Channel Blockers; Capreomycin; Colistimethate; Fosphenytoin; Inhalational Anesthetics; Ketorolac; Ketorolac (Nasal); Ketorolac (Systemic); Lincosamide Antibiotics; Lithium; Loop Diuretics; Magnesium Salts; Phenytoin; Polymyxin B; Procainamide; QuiNIDine; QuiNINE; Spironolactone; Tetracycline Derivatives; Vancomycin

Decreased Effect

The levels/effects of Vecuronium may be decreased by: Acetylcholinesterase Inhibitors; CarBAMazepine; Fosphenytoin; Loop Diuretics; Phenytoin

Stability Store intact vials of powder for injection at room temperature 20°C to 25°C (68°F to 77°F). Vials reconstituted with bacteriostatic water for injection (BWFI) may be stored for 5 days under refrigeration or at room temperature. Vials reconstituted with other compatible diluents (nonbacteriostatic) should be stored under refrigeration and used within 24 hours. Reconstitute with compatible solution for injection to final concentration of 1 mg/mL.

Mechanism of Action Blocks acetylcholine from binding to receptors on motor endplate inhibiting depolarization

Pharmacodynamics/Kinetics

Onset of action:

Good intubation conditions: Within 2.5-3 minutes

Maximum neuromuscular blockade: Within 3-5 minutes

Duration: Under balanced anesthesia (time to recovery to 25% of control): 25-40 minutes; recovery 95% complete ~45-65 minutes after injection of intubating dose

Distribution: V_d: 0.3-0.4 L/kg

Protein binding: 60% to 80%

Metabolism: Active metabolite: 3-desacetyl vecuronium (1/2 the activity of parent drug)

Half-life elimination: Healthy surgical patients and renal failure patients undergoing transplant surgery: 65-75 minutes; Late pregnancy: 35-40 minutes

Excretion: Primarily feces (40% to 75%); urine (30% as unchanged drug and metabolites)

Dosage Administer I.V.; dose to effect; doses will vary due to interpatient variability:

Children: ICU paralysis (eg, facilitate mechanical ventilation) in selected adequately sedated patients (unlabeled; Martin, 1999): Initial bolus dose: 0.1-0.15 mg/kg, then a continuous I.V. infusion of 1-2.5 mcg/kg/minute; monitor depth of blockade using peripheral nerve stimulator every 2-3 hours initially until stable dose, then every 8-12 hours

Intermittent bolus dosing (Eldadah, 1989): 0.1 mg/kg every 1 hour as needed

Children ≥1 year and Adults: Surgical relaxation: **Note:** Children 1-10 years may require slightly higher initial doses and more frequent supplementation. For obese (≥130% of IBW) adult patients, may use ideal body weight (IBW) (Erstad, 2004; Schwartz, 1992; Weinstein, 1988); onset time may be slightly delayed using IBW.

Tracheal intubation: I.V.: Initial: 0.08-0.1 mg/kg. **Note:** If intubation is performed using succinylcholine (not preferred agent in pediatric patients), the initial dose of vecuronium may be reduced to 0.04-0.06 mg/kg with inhalation anesthesia and 0.05-0.06 mg/kg with balanced anesthesia.

Pretreatment/priming: Adults: 10% of intubating dose given 3-5 minutes before intubating dose

Maintenance for continued surgical relaxation (only after return of neuromuscular function): Intermittent dosing: 0.01-0.015 mg/kg **or** continuous infusion of 0.8-1.2 mcg/kg/minute.

Note: Use lower end of the dosing range when anesthesia is maintained with an inhaled anesthetic agent, with the redosing interval guided by monitoring with a peripheral nerve stimulator.

Adults:

ICU paralysis (eg, facilitate mechanical ventilation) in selected adequately sedated patients (Darrah, 1989; Murray, 2002; Rudis, 1997): Initial bolus dose: 0.08-0.1 mg/kg, then a continuous I.V. infusion of 0.8-1.7 mcg/kg/minute; monitor depth of blockade every 1-2 hours initially until stable dose, then every 8-12 hours. Usual maintenance infusion dose range: 0.8-1.2 mcg/kg/minute.

Dosage adjustment (Rudis, 1996; Rudis, 1997): Adjust rate of administration in increments of 0.3 mcg/kg/minute or by 50% reductions of previous dose according to peripheral nerve stimulation response or desired clinical response. Discontinue infusion if neuromuscular function does not return.

Note: When possible, minimize depth and duration of paralysis. Stopping the infusion daily for some time until forced to restart based on patient condition is recommended to reduce post-paralytic complications (eg, acute quadriplegic myopathy syndrome [AQMS]) (Murray, 2002, Segredo, 1992).

Intermittent bolus dosing (Hunter, 1985): 0.1-0.2 mg/kg/dose; may be repeated when neuromuscular function returns

Control of refractory shivering in adequately sedated patients during therapeutic hypothermia after cardiac arrest (unlabeled use; Bernard, 2002; Nolan, 2003; Polderman, 2009): I.V.: 8-12 mg; redose as needed to control shivering. **Note:** Duration of action prolonged in hypothermic patients. May mask seizure activity.

Elderly: No specific guidelines available; refer to adult dosing. Dose selection should be cautious, at low end of dosage range, and titration should be slower to evaluate response.

Dosing adjustment in renal impairment: In general, patients with renal impairment do not experience clinically significant prolongation of neuromuscular blockade with vecuronium; however, in patients who are anephric, the clinical duration is prolonged.

Dosing adjustment in hepatic impairment: Dose reductions are necessary in patients with cirrhosis or cholestasis

Administration Concentration of 1 mg/mL may be administered by rapid I.V. injection. May further dilute reconstituted vial to 0.1-0.2 mg/mL in a compatible solution for I.V. infusion. Concentration of 1 mg/mL may be used for I.V. infusion in fluid-restricted patients.

Monitoring Parameters Blood pressure, heart rate; peripheral nerve stimulation (eg, train-of-four [TOF] count)

Additional Information Vecuronium is classified as an intermediate-duration neuromuscular-blocking agent. It produces minimal, if any, histamine release; does not relieve pain or produce sedation. It may produce cumulative effect on duration of blockade.

Dosage Forms Excipient information presented when available (limited, particularly for generics); consult specific product labeling.

Injection, powder for reconstitution, as bromide: 10 mg, 20 mg

◆ **VEGF Trap** *see* Aflibercept *on page 48*

◆ **VEGF Trap-Eye** *see* Aflibercept *on page 48*

Velaglucerase Alfa (vel a GLOO ser ase AL fa)

Brand Names: U.S. VPRIV™

Brand Names: Canada VPRIV™

Index Terms Gene-Activated Human Acid-Beta-Glucosidase; GlcCerase

Pharmacologic Category Enzyme

Use Long-term enzyme replacement therapy for patients with type 1 Gaucher's disease

Pregnancy Risk Factor B

Dosage I.V.: Children ≥4 years and Adults: Gaucher's disease (type 1): 60 units/kg administered every other week; adjust based upon disease activity (range: 15-60 units/kg evaluated in clinical trials)

Note: When switching from imiglucerase to velaglucerase alfa in stable patients, initiate treatment at the same dose.

Additional Information Complete prescribing information for this medication should be consulted for additional detail.

Dosage Forms Excipient information presented when available (limited, particularly for generics); consult specific product labeling.

Injection, powder for reconstitution:

VPRIV™: 400 units [contains sucrose 200 mg/vial]

◆ **Velban** *see* VinBLAStine *on page 1789*

◆ **Velcade®** *see* Bortezomib *on page 228*

◆ **Veletri®** *see* Epoprostenol *on page 604*

◆ **Velivet™** *see* Ethinyl Estradiol and Desogestrel *on page 653*

◆ **Veltin™** *see* Clindamycin and Tretinoin *on page 382*

◆ **Veltin™** *see* Clindamycin and Tretinoin *on page 382*

Vemurafenib (vem ue RAF e nib)

Brand Names: U.S. Zelboraf™

Index Terms BRAF(V600E) Kinase Inhibitor RO5185426; PLX4032; RG7204; RO5185426

Pharmacologic Category Antineoplastic Agent, BRAF Kinase Inhibitor

Use Treatment of unresectable or metastatic melanoma in patients with a $BRAF^{V600E}$ mutation (as detected by an FDA-approved test)

Note: Not recommended in patients with wild-type BRAF melanoma

Pregnancy Risk Factor D

Pregnancy Considerations Adverse effects were not demonstrated in animal studies. There are no adequate and well-controlled studies in pregnant women. Based on the mechanism of action, however, may cause fetal harm if administered during pregnancy or in patients who become pregnant during treatment. Women of childbearing potential and men of reproductive potential should use adequate contraception methods during and for at least 2 months after treatment.

Lactation Excretion in breast milk unknown/not recommended

Prescribing and Access Restrictions Available through specialty pharmacies. Further information may be obtained from the manufacturer, Genentech, at 1-888-249-4918, or at http://www.zelboraf.com.

Medication Guide Available Yes

Contraindications There are no contraindications listed within the manufacturer's labeling.

Warnings/Precautions Only patients with a $BRAF^{V600}$ mutation-positive melanoma (including $BRAF^{V600E}$) will benefit from treatment; mutation must be detected and confirmed by an FDA-approved test prior to treatment. The cobas® 4800 BRAF V600 Mutation Test was used in clinical trials and is FDA-approved to detect $BRAF^{V600E}$ mutation.

Cases of skin and keratoacanthomas cutaneous squamous cell carcinoma (cuSCC) have been reported; generally occurring early the treatment course (median onset: 7-8 weeks) and is managed with excision. Potential risk factors for cuSCC include age ≥65 years, history of skin cancer or chronic sun exposure. Monitor for skin lesions (with dermatology evaluation) at baseline and every 2 months during treatment; consider continued monitoring for 6 months after treatment. New primary melanoma lesions were observed during treatment and were managed with excision while continuing treatment (at the same dose); continue to monitor for skin lesions.

Dermatologic reactions have been observed, including case reports of Stevens-Johnson syndrome and toxic epidermal necrolysis; discontinue (permanently) for severe dermatologic toxicity. Photosensitivity ranging from mild to severe has been reported. Advise patients to avoid sun exposure and wear protective clothing and use effective UVA/UVB sunscreen and lip balm (SPF ≥30) when outdoors. Dosage modification are recommended for intolerable photosensitivity consisting of erythema ≥10% to 30% of body surface area. Uveitis cases have been reported; monitor for signs and symptoms; may be managed with corticosteroid and mydriatic eye drops. Cases of blurred vision, iritis, photophobia, and a single case of retinal vein occlusion have been reported in clinical trials.

QT prolongation (dose-dependent) has been observed; may lead to increased risk for ventricular arrhythmia, including torsade de pointes. Monitor electrolytes (calcium, magnesium and potassium) at baseline and with dosage adjustments. Monitor ECG at baseline, 15 days after initiation, then monthly for 3 months, then every 3 months thereafter (more frequently if clinically appropriate); also monitor with dosage adjustments. Do not initiate treatment if baseline QT_c >500 msec. During treatment, if QT_c >500 msec, temporarily interrupt treatment; correct electrolytes and control other risk factors for QT prolongation. May reinitiate once with a dose reduction once QT_c falls to <500 msec. Discontinue (permanently), if after correction of risk factors, both the QT_c continues to increase >500 msec and there is >60 msec change above baseline. Use is not recommended in patients with electrolyte abnormalities which are not correctable, long QT syndrome, or taking concomitant medication known to prolong the QT interval.

Increases in liver function tests have been reported. Monitor transaminases, alkaline phosphatase and bilirubin. Severe hypersensitivity, including anaphylaxis, rash (generalized), erythema, or hypotension were reported with use and following reinitiation of treatment. Discontinue (permanently) with severe hypersensitivity reaction. Elderly patients may be at increased risk for adverse effects; in clinical trials, there was an increased incidence of cuSCC and keratoacanthoma, atrial fibrillation, peripheral edema, and nausea/decreased appetite in patients ≥65 years of age.

Adverse Reactions

>10%:

Cardiovascular: Peripheral edema (17% to 23%)

Central nervous system: Fatigue (38% to 54%), headache (23% to 27%), fever (17% to 19%)

Dermatologic: Rash (37% to 52%; grade 3: 7% to 8%), photosensitivity (33% to 49%; grade 3: 3%), alopecia (36% to 45%), pruritus (23% to 30%), skin papilloma (21% to 30%), hyperkeratosis (24% to 28%), cutaneous squamous cell carcinoma (24%; grade 3: 22% to 24%), maculopapular rash (9% to 21%), dry skin (16% to 19%), actinic keratosis (8% to 17%), seborrheic keratosis (10% to 14%), sunburn (10% to 14%), erythema (8% to 14%), papular rash (5% to 13%)

Gastrointestinal: Nausea (35% to 37%; grade 3: 2%), diarrhea (28% to 29%; grade 3: <1%), vomiting (18% to 26%; grade 3: 1% to 2%), appetite decreased (18% to 21%), constipation (12% to 16%), taste alteration (11% to 14%)

Hepatic: GGT increased (5% to 15%)

Neuromuscular & skeletal: Arthralgia (53% to 67%), myalgia (13% to 24%), limb pain (9% to 18%), back pain (8% to 11%), musculoskeletal pain (8% to 11%), weakness (2% to 11%)

Respiratory: Cough (8% to 12%)

≤10% and/or case reports:

Cardiovascular: Atrial fibrillation, hypotension, QT prolongation, vasculitis

Central nervous system: Dizziness, nerve paralysis (VII)

Dermatologic: Basal cell carcinoma, erythema nodosum, folliculitis, keratosis pilaris, melanoma (new primary), palmar-plantar erythrodysesthesia, Stevens-Johnson syndrome, toxic epidermal necrolysis

Gastrointestinal: Weight loss

Hepatic: Alkaline phosphatase increased, ALT increase, AST increased, bilirubin increased

Neuromuscular & skeletal: Arthritis, peripheral neuropathy

Ocular: Blurred vision, iritis, photophobia, retinal vein occlusion, uveitis

Renal: Creatinine increased

Miscellaneous: Anaphylaxis, hypersensitivity

Drug Interactions

Metabolism/Transport Effects Substrate of CYP3A4 (minor), P-glycoprotein; **Note:** Assignment of Major/Minor substrate status based on clinically relevant drug interaction potential; **Inhibits** CYP1A2 (moderate), CYP2D6 (weak), P-glycoprotein; **Induces** CYP3A4 (weak/moderate)

Avoid Concomitant Use

Avoid concomitant use of Vemurafenib with any of the following: Artemether; Dronedarone; Lumefantrine; Nilotinib; Pimozide; QTc-Prolonging Agents; QUEtiapine; QuiNINE; Silodosin; Tetrabenazine; Thioridazine; Topotecan; Toremifene; Vandetanib; Ziprasidone

Increased Effect/Toxicity

Vemurafenib may increase the levels/effects of: Colchicine; CYP1A2 Substrates; Dabigatran Etexilate; Dronedarone; Everolimus; P-glycoprotein/ABCB1 Substrates; Pimozide; QTc-Prolonging Agents; QuiNINE; Rivaroxaban; Silodosin; Tetrabenazine; Thioridazine; Topotecan;

Toremifene; Vandetanib; Vitamin K Antagonists; Ziprasidone

The levels/effects of Vemurafenib may be increased by: Alfuzosin; Artemether; Chloroquine; Ciprofloxacin; Ciprofloxacin (Systemic); CYP3A4 Inhibitors (Strong); Gadobutrol; Indacaterol; Lumefantrine; Nilotinib; P-glycoprotein/ABCB1 Inhibitors; QTc-Prolonging Agents; QUEtiapine; QuiNINE

Decreased Effect

Vemurafenib may decrease the levels/effects of: ARIPiprazole; Cardiac Glycosides; Vitamin K Antagonists

The levels/effects of Vemurafenib may be decreased by: CYP3A4 Inducers (Strong); P-glycoprotein/ABCB1 Inducers; Tocilizumab

Stability Store at room temperature of 20°C to 25°C (68°F to 77°F); excursions permitted to 15°C and 30°C (59°F and 86°F).

Mechanism of Action BRAF kinase inhibitor (potent) which inhibits tumor growth in melanomas by inhibiting kinase activity of certain mutated forms of BRAF, including BRAF with V600E mutation, thereby blocking cellular proliferation in melanoma cells with the mutation. Does not have activity against cells with wild-type BRAF. $BRAF^{V600E}$ activating mutations present in ~50% of melanomas; V600E mutation involves the substitution of glutamic acid for valine at amino acid 600. The cobas® 4800 BRAF V600 mutation test is approved to detect $BRAF^{V600E}$ mutation.

Pharmacodynamics/Kinetics

Distribution: V_d: ~106 L

Protein binding: >99%, to albumin and α_1-acid glycoprotein

Half-life, elimination: 57 hours (range: 30-120 hours)

Time to peak: ~3 hours

Excretion: Feces (~94%); urine (~1%)

Dosage Oral: Adults: Melanoma, metastatic or unresectable (with $BRAF^{V600E}$ mutation): 960 mg twice daily; continue until disease progression or unacceptable toxicity

Dosing adjustment for toxicity: Note: Dose reductions resulting in a dose below 480 mg twice daily are not recommended.

Grade 1 or grade 2 (tolerable) toxicity: No adjustment recommended

Grade 2 (intolerable) or grade 3 toxicity:

First incident: Interrupt treatment until toxicity returns to grade 0 or 1, then resume at 720 mg twice daily

Second incident: Interrupt treatment until toxicity returns to grade 0 or 1, then resume at 480 mg twice daily

Third incident: Discontinue permanently

Grade 4 toxicity:

First incident: Interrupt treatment until toxicity returns to grade 0 or 1, then resume at 480 mg twice daily **or** discontinue permanently

Second incident: Discontinue permanently

Specific toxicities:

Severe hypersensitivity or severe dermatologic toxicity: Discontinue permanently

QT_c >500 msec: Temporarily withhold treatment, correct electrolytes and control risk factors for QT prolongation; may reinitiate with a dose reduction once QT_c <500 msec.

QT_c persistently >500 msec and >60 msec above baseline: Discontinue permanently

Dosage adjustment in renal impairment:

Mild-to-moderate impairment (pre-existing): No adjustments recommended

Severe impairment (pre-existing): Data is insufficient to determine if dosage adjustment necessary; use with caution

Dosage adjustment in hepatic impairment:

Mild-to-moderate impairment (pre-existing): No adjustments recommended

Severe impairment (pre-existing): Data is insufficient to determine if dosage adjustment necessary; use with caution

Dietary Considerations May be taken with or without food.

Administration Doses should be administered orally in the morning and evening, ~12 hours apart. Swallow whole with a glass of water; do not crush or chew. May be taken with or without a meal. If a dose is missed, may be taken up to 4 hours prior to the next scheduled dose to maintain a twice daily schedule; both doses should **not** be taken at the same time.

Monitoring Parameters Liver transaminases, alkaline phosphatase and bilirubin at baseline and monthly during treatment (or as clinically appropriate). Electrolytes (calcium, magnesium and potassium) at baseline and after dosage modification. ECG at baseline, 15 days after initiation, then monthly for 3 months, then every 3 months thereafter (more frequently if clinically appropriate) and with dosage adjustments. Dermatology evaluation (for new skin lesions) at baseline and every 2 months during treatment; also consider continued monitoring for 6 months after completion of treatment.

Dosage Forms Excipient information presented when available (limited, particularly for generics); consult specific product labeling.

Tablet, oral:

Zelboraf™: 240 mg

Venlafaxine (ven la FAX een)

Brand Names: U.S. Effexor XR®; Effexor®

Brand Names: Canada CO Venlafaxine XR; Effexor XR®; Mylan-Venlafaxine XR; PMS-Venlafaxine XR; ratio-Venlafaxine XR; Riva-Venlafaxine XR; Sandoz-Venlafaxine XR; Teva-Venlafaxine XR; Venlafaxine XR

Pharmacologic Category Antidepressant, Serotonin/Norepinephrine Reuptake Inhibitor

Additional Appendix Information

Antidepressant Agents *on page 1874*

Use Treatment of major depressive disorder, generalized anxiety disorder (GAD), social anxiety disorder (social phobia), panic disorder

Unlabeled Use Obsessive-compulsive disorder (OCD); hot flashes; neuropathic pain (including diabetic neuropathy); attention-deficit/hyperactivity disorder (ADHD); post-traumatic stress disorder (PTSD)

Pregnancy Risk Factor C

Pregnancy Considerations Adverse events have been observed in some animal reproduction studies. Venlafaxine and its active metabolite ODV cross the human placenta. An increased risk of teratogenic effects following venlafaxine exposure during pregnancy has not been observed, based on available data. The risk of spontaneous abortion may be increased. Neonatal seizures and neonatal abstinence syndrome have been noted in case reports following maternal use of venlafaxine during pregnancy. Nonteratogenic effects in the newborn following SSRI/SNRI exposure late in the third trimester include respiratory distress, cyanosis, apnea, seizures, temperature instability, feeding difficulty, vomiting, hypoglycemia, hyper- or hypotonia, hyper-reflexia, jitteriness, irritability, constant crying, and tremor. Symptoms may be due to the toxicity of the SNRI or a discontinuation syndrome and may be consistent with serotonin syndrome associated with treatment. The long-term effects of *in utero* SNRI/SSRI exposure on infant development and behavior are not known.

Due to pregnancy-induced physiologic changes, some pharmacokinetic parameters of venlafaxine may be altered. Women should be monitored for decreased efficacy. The ACOG recommends that therapy with SSRIs or SNRIs during pregnancy be individualized; treatment of depression during pregnancy should incorporate the clinical expertise of the mental health clinician, obstetrician, primary healthcare provider, and pediatrician. According to the American Psychiatric Association (APA), the risks of medication treatment should be weighed against other treatment options and untreated depression. For women who discontinue antidepressant medications during pregnancy and who may be at high risk for postpartum depression, the medications can be restarted following delivery. Treatment algorithms have been developed by the ACOG and the APA for the management of depression in women prior to conception and during pregnancy.

Lactation Enters breast milk/not recommended

Medication Guide Available Yes

Contraindications Hypersensitivity to venlafaxine or any component of the formulation; use of MAO inhibitors within 14 days; should not initiate MAO inhibitor within 7 days of discontinuing venlafaxine

Warnings/Precautions [U.S. Boxed Warning]: Antidepressants increase the risk of suicidal thinking and behavior in children, adolescents, and young adults (18-24 years of age) with major depressive disorder (MDD) and other psychiatric disorders; consider risk prior to prescribing. Short-term studies did not show an increased risk in patients >24 years of age and showed a decreased risk in patients ≥65 years. Closely monitor for clinical worsening, suicidality, or unusual changes in behavior; the patient's family or caregiver should be instructed to closely observe the patient and communicate condition with healthcare provider. Reduced growth rate has been observed with venlafaxine therapy in children. A medication guide should be dispensed with each prescription. **Venlafaxine is not FDA approved for use in children.**

The possibility of a suicide attempt is inherent in major depression and may persist until remission occurs. Monitor for worsening of depression or suicidality, especially during initiation of therapy (generally first 1-2 months) or with dose increases or decreases. Use caution in high-risk patients. Worsening depression and severe abrupt suicidality that are not part of the presenting symptoms may require discontinuation or modification of drug therapy. The patient's family or caregiver should be alerted to monitor patients for the emergence of suicidality and associated behaviors (such as agitation, irritability, hostility, impulsivity, and hypomania) and call healthcare provider.

May worsen psychosis in some patients or precipitate a shift to mania or hypomania in patients with bipolar disorder. Patients presenting with depressive symptoms should be screened for bipolar disorder. Monotherapy in patients with bipolar disorder should be avoided. **Venlafaxine is not FDA approved for the treatment of bipolar depression.**

Serotonin syndrome and neuroleptic malignant syndrome (NMS)-like reactions have occurred with serotonin/norepinephrine reuptake inhibitors (SNRIs) and selective serotonin reuptake inhibitors (SSRIs) when used alone, and particularly when used in combination with serotonergic agents (eg, triptans) or antidopaminergic agents (eg, antipsychotics). Concurrent use with MAO inhibitors is contraindicated. May cause sustained increase in blood pressure or tachycardia; dose related and increases are generally modest (12-15 mm Hg diastolic). Control pre-existing hypertension prior to initiation of venlafaxine. Use caution in patients with recent history of MI, unstable heart disease, or hyperthyroidism; may cause increase in anxiety, nervousness, insomnia; may cause weight loss (use with caution in patients where weight loss is undesirable); may cause increases in serum cholesterol. Use caution with hepatic or renal impairment; dosage adjustments recommended. May cause hyponatremia/SIADH (elderly at increased risk); volume depletion (diuretics may increase risk).

May impair platelet aggregation resulting in increased risk of bleeding events, particularly if used concomitantly with aspirin or NSAIDs. Bleeding related to SSRI or SNRI use has been reported to range from relatively minor bruising and epistaxis to life-threatening hemorrhage. Interstitial lung disease and eosinophilic pneumonia have been rarely reported; may present as progressive dyspnea, cough, and/or chest pain. Prompt evaluation and possible discontinuation of therapy may be necessary. Venlafaxine may increase the risks associated with electroconvulsive therapy. Use cautiously in patients with a history of seizures. The risks of cognitive or motor impairment, as well as the potential for anticholinergic effects are very low. May cause or exacerbate sexual dysfunction.

Abrupt discontinuation or dosage reduction after extended (≥6 weeks) therapy may lead to agitation, dysphoria, nervousness, anxiety, and other symptoms. When discontinuing therapy, dosage should be tapered gradually over at least a 2-week period. If intolerable symptoms occur following a decrease in dosage or upon discontinuation of therapy, then resuming the previous dose with a more gradual taper should be considered. Use caution in patients with increased intraocular pressure or at risk of acute narrow-angle glaucoma.

Adverse Reactions Note: Actual frequency may be dependent upon formulation and/or indication

>10%:

- Central nervous system: Headache (25% to 38%), somnolence (12% to 26%), dizziness (11% to 24%), insomnia (15% to 24%), nervousness (6% to 21%), anxiety (2% to 11%),
- Gastrointestinal: Nausea (21% to 58%), xerostomia (12% to 22%), anorexia (8% to 17%), constipation (8% to 15%)
- Genitourinary: Abnormal ejaculation/orgasm (2% to 19%)
- Neuromuscular & skeletal: Weakness (8% to 19%)
- Miscellaneous: Diaphoresis (7% to 19%)

1% to 10%:

- Cardiovascular: Vasodilation (2% to 6%), hypertension (dose related; 3% in patients receiving <100 mg/day, up to 13% in patients receiving >300 mg/day), palpitation (3%), tachycardia (2%), chest pain (2%), postural hypotension (1%), edema
- Central nervous system: Yawning (3% to 8%), abnormal dreams (3% to 7%), chills (2% to 7%), agitation (2% to 5%), confusion (2%), abnormal thinking (2%), depersonalization (1%), depression (1% to 3%), fever, migraine, amnesia, hypoesthesia, vertigo
- Dermatologic: Rash (3%), pruritus (1%), bruising
- Endocrine & metabolic: Libido decreased (2% to 8%), hypercholesterolemia (5%), triglycerides increased
- Gastrointestinal: Abdominal pain (8%), diarrhea (8%), vomiting (3% to 8%), dyspepsia (5% to 7%), weight loss (1% to 6%), flatulence (3% to 4%), taste perversion (2%), appetite increased, belching, weight gain
- Genitourinary: Impotence (4% to 6%), urinary frequency (3%), urination impaired (2%), urinary retention (1%), metrorrhagia, prostatic disorder, vaginitis
- Neuromuscular & skeletal: Tremor (1% to 10%), hypertonia (3%), paresthesia (2% to 3%), twitching (1% to 3%), arthralgia, neck pain, trismus
- Ocular: Accommodation abnormal (6% to 9%), abnormal or blurred vision (4% to 6%), mydriasis (2%)
- Otic: Tinnitus (2%)
- Renal: Albuminuria
- Respiratory: Pharyngitis (7%), sinusitis (2%), bronchitis, cough increased, dyspnea

Miscellaneous: Infection (6%), flu-like syndrome (2%), trauma (2%)

<1% (Limited to important or life-threatening): Agranulocytosis, anaphylaxis, anemia, aneurysm, angina pectoris, angioedema, anuria, aplastic anemia, appendicitis, arrhythmia (including atrial and ventricular tachycardia, fibrillation, and torsade de pointes), arteritis, asthma, ataxia, atelectasis, atrioventricular block, bacteremia, balance/coordination impaired, basophilia, bigeminy, biliary pain, bilirubinemia, bleeding time increased, bradycardia, bradykinesia, BUN increased, bundle branch block, carcinoma, cardiac arrest, cardiovascular disorder (mitral valve and circulatory disturbance), cataract, catatonia, cellulitis, cerebral ischemia, cholelithiasis, congestive heart failure, coronary artery disease, CPK increased, creatinine increased, crystalluria, cyanosis, deafness, DVT, dehydration, delusions, dementia, diabetes mellitus, dystonia, ECG abnormalities (including QT prolongation), embolus, eosinophilia, erythema multiforme, exfoliative dermatitis, extrapyramidal symptoms, extrasystoles, facial paralysis, fasciitis, fatty liver, gastrointestinal ulcer, glaucoma, glycosuria, granuloma, Guillain-Barré syndrome, hematemesis, hematoma, hemorrhage (eye, GI, mucocutaneous, rectal), hepatic necrosis, hepatic failure, hepatitis, homicidal ideation, hostility, hyperacusis, hypercalcinuria, hyperchlorhydria, hyper-/hypoglycemia, hyper-/hypokalemia, hyper-/hypophosphatemia, hyper-/hypothyroidism, hyperuricemia, hypocholesteremia, hyponatremia, hypoproteinemia, hypotension, interstitial lung disease (including eosinophilic pneumonia), intestinal obstruction, jaundice, kidney function abnormal, larynx edema, leukocytosis, leukoderma, leukopenia, liver enzymes increased, loss of consciousness, lymphadenopathy, lymphocytosis, maculopapular rash, menstrual abnormalities, MI, miliaria, moniliasis, multiple myeloma, myasthenia, myoclonus, myopathy, neck rigidity, neuroleptic malignant-like syndrome, neuropathy, neutropenia, osteoporosis, pancreatitis, pancytopenia, peripheral vascular disorder, pleurisy, pneumonia, pyelonephritis, pyuria, renal failure, rhabdomyolysis, rheumatoid arthritis, seizure, serotonin syndrome, SIADH, skin atrophy, Stevens-Johnson syndrome, suicidal ideation (reported at a frequency up to 2% in children/adolescents with major depressive disorder), suicide attempt, syncope, tendon rupture, thrombocythemia, thrombocytopenia, tongue edema, toxic epidermal necrolysis, withdrawal syndrome

Drug Interactions

Metabolism/Transport Effects Substrate of CYP2C19 (minor), CYP2C9 (minor), CYP2D6 (major), CYP3A4 (major); **Note:** Assignment of Major/Minor substrate status based on clinically relevant drug interaction potential; **Inhibits** CYP2B6 (weak), CYP2D6 (weak), CYP3A4 (weak)

Avoid Concomitant Use

Avoid concomitant use of Venlafaxine with any of the following: Conivaptan; Iobenguane I 123; MAO Inhibitors; Methylene Blue

Increased Effect/Toxicity

Venlafaxine may increase the levels/effects of: Alpha-/Beta-Agonists; Aspirin; Methylene Blue; Metoclopramide; NSAID (Nonselective); Serotonin Modulators; TraZODone; Vitamin K Antagonists

The levels/effects of Venlafaxine may be increased by: Abiraterone Acetate; Alcohol (Ethyl); Antipsychotics; Conivaptan; CYP2D6 Inhibitors (Moderate); CYP2D6 Inhibitors (Strong); CYP3A4 Inhibitors (Moderate); CYP3A4 Inhibitors (Strong); Darunavir; Dasatinib; Linezolid; MAO Inhibitors; Metoclopramide; Propafenone; Voriconazole

Decreased Effect

Venlafaxine may decrease the levels/effects of: Alpha2-Agonists; Indinavir; Iobenguane I 123; Ioflupane I 123

The levels/effects of Venlafaxine may be decreased by: CYP3A4 Inducers (Strong); Deferasirox; Peginterferon Alfa-2b; Tocilizumab

Ethanol/Nutrition/Herb Interactions

Ethanol: May increase CNS depression; monitor for increased effects with coadministration. Caution patients about effects.

Herb/Nutraceutical: Avoid valerian, St John's wort, SAMe, kava kava, tryptophan (may increase risk of serotonin syndrome and/or excessive sedation).

Stability Store at controlled room temperature of 20°C to 25°C (68°F to 77°F).

Mechanism of Action Venlafaxine and its active metabolite, O-desmethylvenlafaxine (ODV), are potent inhibitors of neuronal serotonin and norepinephrine reuptake and weak inhibitors of dopamine reuptake. Venlafaxine and ODV have no significant activity for muscarinic cholinergic, H_1-histaminergic, or alpha$_2$-adrenergic receptors. Venlafaxine and ODV do not possess MAO-inhibitory activity.

Pharmacodynamics/Kinetics

Absorption: Oral: ≥92%; food has no significant effect on absorption or formation of active metabolite

Distribution: V_{dss}: Venlafaxine 7.5 ± 3.7 L/kg, ODV 5.7 ± 1.8 L/Kg

Protein binding: Venlafaxine 27% ± 2%, ODV 30% ± 12%

Metabolism: Hepatic via CYP2D6 to active metabolite, O-desmethylvenlafaxine (ODV); other metabolites include N-desmethylvenlafaxine and N,O-didesmethylvenlafaxine

Bioavailability: Oral: ~45%

Half-life elimination: Venlafaxine: 5 ± 2 hours; ODV: 11 ± 2 hours; prolonged with cirrhosis (venlafaxine: ~30%, ODV: ~60%), renal impairment (venlafaxine: ~50%, ODV: ~40%), and during dialysis (venlafaxine: ~180%, ODV: ~142%)

Time to peak:

Immediate release: Venlafaxine: 2 hours, ODV: 3 hours

Extended release: Venlafaxine: 5.5 hours, ODV: 9 hours

Excretion: Urine (~87%; 5% of total dose as unchanged drug; 29% of total dose as unconjugated ODV; 26% of total dose as conjugated ODV; 27% of total dose as minor inactive metabolites)

Dosage Oral:

Children and Adolescents:

Attention-deficit/hyperactivity disorder (unlabeled use; Olvera, 1996): Initial: 12.5 mg/day

Children <40 kg: Increase by 12.5 mg/week to maximum of 50 mg/day in 2 divided doses

Children ≥40 kg: Increase by 25 mg/week to maximum of 75 mg/day in 3 divided doses.

Mean dose: 60 mg or 1.4 mg/kg administered in 2-3 divided doses

Adults:

Depression:

Immediate-release tablets: Initial: 75 mg/day, administered in 2 or 3 divided doses; may increase in ≤75 mg/day increments at intervals of ≥4 days as tolerated (maximum daily dose: 225-375 mg)

Extended-release capsules or tablets: Initial: 37.5-75 mg once daily; in patients who are initiated at 37.5 mg once daily, may increase to 75 mg once daily after 4-7 days; dose may then be increased by ≤75 mg/day increments at intervals of ≥4 days as tolerated (maximum daily dose: 225 mg)

Generalized anxiety disorder: Extended-release capsules: Initial: 37.5-75 mg once daily; in patients who are initiated at 37.5 mg once daily, may increase to 75 mg once daily after 4-7 days; may then be increased by ≤75 mg/day increments at intervals of ≥4 days as tolerated (maximum daily dose: 225 mg)

Panic disorder: Extended-release capsules: Initial: 37.5 mg once daily for 1 week; may increase to 75 mg once daily after 7 days, may then be increased by ≤75 mg/day increments at intervals of ≥7 days (maximum daily dose: 225 mg).

Social anxiety disorder: Extended-release capsules or tablets: 75 mg once daily (maximum daily dose: 75 mg); no evidence that doses >75 mg/day offer any additional benefit

Obsessive-compulsive disorder (unlabeled use): Titrate to usual dosage range of 150-300 mg/day; however, doses up to 375 mg/day have been used; response may be seen in 4 weeks (Phelps, 2005)

Neuropathic pain (unlabeled use): Dosages evaluated varied considerably based on etiology of chronic pain, but efficacy has been shown for many conditions in the range of 75-225 mg/day; onset of relief may occur in 1-2 weeks, or take up to 6 weeks for full benefit (Grothe, 2004).

Diabetic neuropathy (unlabeled use): 75-225 mg/day (Bril, 2011)

Hot flashes (unlabeled use): Doses of 37.5-75 mg/day have demonstrated significant improvement of vasomotor symptoms after 4-8 weeks of treatment; in one study, doses >75 mg/day offered no additional benefit (Evans, 2005; Loprinzi, 2000); however, higher doses (225 mg/day) may be beneficial in patients with perimenopausal depression

Attention-deficit disorder (unlabeled use): Initial: Doses vary between 18.75 to 75 mg/day; may increase after 4 weeks to 150 mg/day; if tolerated, doses up to 225 mg/day have been used (Maidment, 2003)

Post-traumatic stress disorder (PTSD) (unlabeled use): Extended release formulation: 37.5-300 mg/day (Bandelow, 2008; Benedek, 2009)

Note: When discontinuing this medication after more than 1 week of treatment, it is generally recommended that the dose be tapered. If venlafaxine is used for 6 weeks or longer, the dose should be tapered over 2 weeks when discontinuing its use.

Elderly: Refer to adult dosing. No specific recommendations for elderly, but may be best to start lower at 25-50 mg twice daily and increase as tolerated by 25 mg/dose. Extended-release formulation: 37.5 mg once daily, increase by 37.5 mg every 4-7 days as tolerated

Dosing adjustment in renal impairment:

GFR: 10-70 mL/minute: Reduce total daily dose by 25% to 50%

Hemodialysis: Reduce total daily dose by 50%

Dosing adjustment in hepatic impairment: Mild-to-moderate hepatic impairment: Reduce total daily dose by 50%; further reductions may be necessary in some patients

Dietary Considerations Should be taken with food.

Administration Administer with food.

Extended-release formulations: Swallow capsule or tablet whole; do not crush or chew. Contents of capsule may be sprinkled on a spoonful of applesauce and swallowed immediately without chewing; followed with a glass of water to ensure complete swallowing of the pellets.

Monitoring Parameters Blood pressure should be regularly monitored, especially in patients with a high baseline blood pressure; may cause mean increase in heart rate of 4-9 beats/minute; cholesterol; mental status for depression, suicide ideation (especially at the beginning of therapy or when doses are increased or decreased), anxiety, social functioning, mania, panic attacks; height and weight should be monitored in children

Test Interactions May interfere with urine detection of PCP (false-positive).

Dosage Forms Excipient information presented when available (limited, particularly for generics); consult specific product labeling.

Capsule, extended release, oral: 37.5 mg, 75 mg, 150 mg
Effexor XR®: 37.5 mg, 75 mg, 150 mg

Tablet, oral: 25 mg, 37.5 mg, 50 mg, 75 mg, 100 mg
Effexor®: 50 mg [scored]

Tablet, extended release, oral: 37.5 mg, 75 mg, 150 mg, 225 mg

- **Venlafaxine XR (Can)** *see* Venlafaxine *on page 1780*
- **Venofer®** *see* Iron Sucrose *on page 932*
- **Ventavis®** *see* Iloprost *on page 870*
- **Ventolin® (Can)** *see* Albuterol *on page 52*
- **Ventolin® Diskus (Can)** *see* Albuterol *on page 52*
- **Ventolin® HFA** *see* Albuterol *on page 52*
- **Ventolin® I.V. Infusion (Can)** *see* Albuterol *on page 52*
- **Ventolin® Nebules P.F. (Can)** *see* Albuterol *on page 52*
- **VePesid** *see* Etoposide *on page 669*
- **Veracolate® [OTC]** *see* Bisacodyl *on page 219*
- **Veramyst®** *see* Fluticasone (Nasal) *on page 741*

Verapamil (ver AP a mil)

Brand Names: U.S. Calan®; Calan® SR; Covera-HS®; Isoptin® SR; Verelan®; Verelan® PM

Brand Names: Canada Apo-Verap®; Apo-Verap® SR; Covera-HS®; Covera®; Dom-Verapamil SR; Isoptin® SR; Mylan-Verapamil; Mylan-Verapamil SR; Novo-Veramil; Novo-Veramil SR; Nu-Verap; Nu-Verap SR; PHL-Verapamil SR; PMS-Verapamil SR; PRO-Verapamil SR; Riva-Verapamil SR; Verapamil Hydrochloride Injection, USP; Verapamil SR; Verelan SRC

Index Terms Iproveratril Hydrochloride; Verapamil Hydrochloride

Pharmacologic Category Antianginal Agent; Antiarrhythmic Agent, Class IV; Calcium Channel Blocker; Calcium Channel Blocker, Nondihydropyridine

Additional Appendix Information

Calcium Channel Blockers *on page 1887*
Hypertension *on page 2001*

Use

Oral: Treatment of hypertension; angina pectoris (vasospastic, chronic stable, unstable) (Calan®, Covera-HS®); supraventricular tachyarrhythmia (PSVT, atrial fibrillation/flutter [rate control])

I.V.: Supraventricular tachyarrhythmia (PSVT, atrial fibrillation/flutter [rate control])

Unlabeled Use Migraine; hypertrophic cardiomyopathy; bipolar disorder (manic manifestations)

Pregnancy Risk Factor C

Pregnancy Considerations In some animal reproduction studies verapamil has been shown to cause fetal harm; adverse maternal effects were also observed. Verapamil crosses the placenta. Although verapamil is not considered a major human teratogen, use during pregnancy may cause adverse fetal effects (bradycardia, heart block, hypotension).

Lactation Enters breast milk/not recommended (AAP considers "compatible"; AAP 2001 update pending)

Contraindications Hypersensitivity to verapamil or any component of the formulation; severe left ventricular dysfunction; hypotension (systolic pressure <90 mm Hg) or cardiogenic shock; sick sinus syndrome (except in patients with a functioning artificial ventricular pacemaker); second- or third-degree AV block (except in patients with a functioning artificial ventricular pacemaker); atrial flutter or fibrillation and an accessory bypass tract (Wolff-Parkinson-White [WPW] syndrome, Lown-Ganong-Levine syndrome)

I.V.: Additional contraindications include concurrent use of I.V. beta-blocking agents; ventricular tachycardia

Warnings/Precautions Avoid use in heart failure; can exacerbate condition; use is contraindicated in severe left ventricular dysfunction. Symptomatic hypotension with or without syncope can rarely occur; blood pressure must be lowered at a rate appropriate for the patient's clinical condition. Rare increases in hepatic enzymes can be observed. Can cause first-degree AV block or sinus bradycardia; use is contraindicated in patients with sick sinus syndrome, second- or third-degree AV block (except in patients with a functioning artificial pacemaker), or an accessory bypass tract (eg, WPW syndrome). Other conduction abnormalities are rare. Considered contraindicated in patients with wide complex tachycardias unless known to be supraventricular in origin; severe hypotension likely to occur upon administration (ACLS, 2010). Use caution when using verapamil together with a beta-blocker. Administration of I.V. verapamil and an I.V. beta-blocker within a few hours of each other may result in asystole and should be avoided; simultaneous administration is contraindicated. Use with other agents known to reduce SA node function and/or AV nodal conduction (eg, digoxin) or reduce sympathetic outflow (eg, clonidine) may increase the risk of serious bradycardia. Verapamil significantly increases digoxin serum concentrations; adjust digoxin dose. Use with caution in patients with hypertrophic cardiomyopathy with outflow tract obstruction (especially those with resting outflow obstruction and severe limiting symptoms); may be used in patients who cannot tolerate beta-blockade.

Decreased neuromuscular transmission has been reported with verapamil; use with caution in patients with attenuated neuromuscular transmission (Duchenne's muscular dystrophy, myasthenia gravis); dosage reduction may be required. Use with caution in renal impairment; monitor hemodynamics and possibly ECG if severe impairment, particularly if concomitant hepatic impairment. Use with caution in patients with hepatic impairment; dosage reduction may be required; monitor hemodynamics and possibly ECG if severe impairment. May prolong recovery from nondepolarizing neuromuscular-blocking agents. Use Covera-HS® (extended-release delivery system) with caution in patients with severe GI narrowing. In patients with extremely short GI transit times (eg, <7 hours), dosage adjustment may be required; inadequate pharmacokinetic data. I.V. use for SVT for is not recommended in infants; use with caution in children as myocardial depression/hypotension may occur.

Adverse Reactions

>10%:

Central nervous system: Headache (1% to 12%)

Gastrointestinal: Gingival hyperplasia (≤19%), constipation (7% to 12%)

1% to 10%:

Cardiovascular: Peripheral edema (1% to 4%), hypotension (3%), CHF/pulmonary edema (2%), AV block (1% to 2%), bradycardia (HR <50 bpm: 1%), flushing (1%)

Central nervous system: Fatigue (2% to 5%), dizziness (1% to 5%), lethargy (3%), pain (2%), sleep disturbance (1%)

Dermatologic: Rash (1% to 2%)

Gastrointestinal: Dyspepsia (3%), nausea (1% to 3%), diarrhea (2%)

Hepatic: Liver enzymes increased (1%)

Neuromuscular & skeletal: Myalgia (1%), paresthesia (1%)

Respiratory: Dyspnea (1%)

Miscellaneous: Flu-like syndrome (4%)

Oral: ≤1%: Abdominal discomfort, alopecia, angina, arthralgia, atrioventricular dissociation, blurred vision, bruising, cerebrovascular accident, chest pain, claudication, confusion, diaphoresis, ECG abnormal, equilibrium disorders, erythema multiforme, exanthema, extrapyramidal symptoms, galactorrhea/hyperprolactinemia, gastrointestinal distress, gynecomastia, hyperkeratosis, impotence, insomnia, macules, MI, muscle cramps, palpitation, psychosis, purpura (vasculitis), shakiness, somnolence, spotty menstruation, Stevens-Johnson syndrome, syncope, tinnitus, urination increased, urticaria, weakness, xerostomia

I.V.: <1% (Limited to important or life-threatening): Bronchi/laryngeal spasm, depression, diaphoresis, itching, muscle fatigue, respiratory failure, rotary nystagmus, seizure, sleepiness, urticaria, vertigo

Postmarketing and/or case reports: Asystole, eosinophilia, EPS, exfoliative dermatitis, GI obstruction, hair color change, paralytic ileus, Parkinsonian syndrome, pulseless electrical activity, shock, ventricular fibrillation

Drug Interactions

Metabolism/Transport Effects Substrate of CYP1A2 (minor), CYP2B6 (minor), CYP2C9 (minor), CYP2E1 (minor), CYP3A4 (major), P-glycoprotein; **Note:** Assignment of Major/Minor substrate status based on clinically relevant drug interaction potential; **Inhibits** CYP1A2 (weak), CYP2C9 (weak), CYP2D6 (weak), CYP3A4 (moderate), P-glycoprotein

Avoid Concomitant Use

Avoid concomitant use of Verapamil with any of the following: Conivaptan; Disopyramide; Dofetilide; Pimozide; Silodosin; Topotecan

Increased Effect/Toxicity

Verapamil may increase the levels/effects of: Alcohol (Ethyl); Aliskiren; Amifostine; Amiodarone; Antihypertensives; ARIPiprazole; Atorvastatin; Benzodiazepines (metabolized by oxidation); Beta-Blockers; Budesonide (Systemic, Oral Inhalation); BusPIRone; Calcium Channel Blockers (Dihydropyridine); CarBAMazepine; Cardiac Glycosides; Colchicine; Corticosteroids (Systemic); CycloSPORINE; CycloSPORINE (Systemic); CYP3A4 Substrates; Dabigatran Etexilate; Disopyramide; Dofetilide; Dronedarone; Eletriptan; Eplerenone; Everolimus; Fexofenadine; Fingolimod; Flecainide; Fosphenytoin; Halofantrine; Hypotensive Agents; Lithium; Lovastatin; Lurasidone; Magnesium Salts; Midodrine; Neuromuscular-Blocking Agents (Nondepolarizing); Nitroprusside; P-glycoprotein/ABCB1 Substrates; Phenytoin; Pimecrolimus; Pimozide; Propafenone; QuiNIDine; Ranolazine; Red Yeast Rice; RisperiDONE; RiTUXimab; Rivaroxaban; Salicylates; Salmeterol; Silodosin; Simvastatin; Tacrolimus; Tacrolimus (Systemic); Tacrolimus (Topical); Topotecan; Vilazodone; Zuclopenthixol

The levels/effects of Verapamil may be increased by: Alpha1-Blockers; Anilidopiperidine Opioids; Antifungal Agents (Azole Derivatives, Systemic); Atorvastatin; Calcium Channel Blockers (Dihydropyridine); Cimetidine; Conivaptan; CycloSPORINE; CycloSPORINE (Systemic); CYP3A4 Inhibitors (Moderate); CYP3A4 Inhibitors (Strong); Dasatinib; Diazoxide; Dronedarone; Fluconazole; Grapefruit Juice; Herbs (Hypotensive Properties); Macrolide Antibiotics; Magnesium Salts; MAO Inhibitors; Pentoxifylline; P-glycoprotein/ABCB1 Inhibitors; Phosphodiesterase 5 Inhibitors; Prostacyclin Analogues; Protease Inhibitors; QuiNIDine; Telithromycin

Decreased Effect

Verapamil may decrease the levels/effects of: Clopidogrel

The levels/effects of Verapamil may be decreased by: Barbiturates; Calcium Salts; CarBAMazepine; CYP3A4 Inducers (Strong); Cyproterone; Deferasirox; Herbs (Hypertensive Properties); Methylphenidate; Nafcillin; P-glycoprotein/ABCB1 Inducers; Rifamycin Derivatives; Tocilizumab; Yohimbine

Ethanol/Nutrition/Herb Interactions

Ethanol: Avoid or limit ethanol (may increase ethanol levels).

Food: Grapefruit juice may increase the serum concentration of verapamil; use with caution and monitor for increased verapamil effects.

Herb/Nutraceutical: St John's wort may decrease levels. Avoid herbs with hypertensive properties (bayberry, blue cohosh, cayenne, ephedra, ginger, ginseng [American], kola, licorice); may diminish the antihypertensive effect of verapamil. Avoid herbs with hypotensive properties (black cohosh, California poppy, coleus, golden seal, hawthorn, mistletoe, periwinkle, quinine, shepherd's purse); may enhance the hypotensive effect of verapamil.

Stability Store at controlled room temperature of 15°C to 30°C (59°F to 86°F). Protect from light.

Mechanism of Action Inhibits calcium ion from entering the "slow channels" or select voltage-sensitive areas of vascular smooth muscle and myocardium during depolarization; produces relaxation of coronary vascular smooth muscle and coronary vasodilation; increases myocardial oxygen delivery in patients with vasospastic angina; slows automaticity and conduction of AV node.

Pharmacodynamics/Kinetics

Onset of action: Peak effect: Oral: Immediate release: 1-2 hours; I.V.: 1-5 minutes

Duration: Oral: Immediate release tablets: 6-8 hours; I.V.: 10-20 minutes

Absorption: Well absorbed

Distribution: V_d: 3.89 L/kg (Storstein, 1984)

Protein binding: ~90%

Metabolism: Hepatic (extensive first-pass effect) via multiple CYP isoenzymes; primary metabolite is norverapamil (20% pharmacologic activity of verapamil)

Bioavailability: Oral: 20% to 35%

Half-life elimination: Infants: 4.4-6.9 hours; Adults: Single dose: 3-7 hours, Multiple doses: 4.5-12 hours; severe hepatic impairment: 14-16 hours

Time to peak, serum: Oral:

Immediate release: 1-2 hours

Extended release (Covera-HS®, Verelan PM®): ~11 hours, drug release delayed ~4-5 hours

Sustained release: 5.21 hours (Calan® SR, Isoptin® SR); 7-9 hours (Verelan®)

Excretion: Urine (70% as metabolites, 3% to 4% as unchanged drug); feces (16%)

Dosage

Children: **Note:** Verapamil is no longer included in the Pediatric Advanced Life Support (PALS) tachyarrhythmia algorithm.

Children: 1-15 years: SVT: I.V.: 0.1-0.3 mg/kg/dose over 2 minutes; maximum: 5 mg/dose, may repeat dose in 30 minutes if inadequate response; maximum for second dose: 10 mg

Adults:

SVT (ACLS, 2010): I.V.: 2.5-5 mg over 2 minutes; second dose of 5-10 mg (~0.15 mg/kg) may be given 15-30 minutes after the initial dose if patient tolerates, but does not respond to initial dose; maximum total dose: 20-30 mg

Angina: Oral: **Note:** When switching from immediate-release to extended/sustained release formulations, the total daily dose remains the same unless formulation strength does not allow for equal conversion.

Immediate release: Initial: 80-120 mg 3 times/day (elderly or small stature: 40 mg 3 times/day); Usual dose range (Gibbons, 2002): 80-160 mg 3 times/day

Extended release (Covera-HS®): Initial: 180 mg once daily at bedtime; if inadequate response, may increase dose at weekly intervals to 240 mg once daily, then 360 mg once daily, then 480 mg once daily; maximum dose: 480 mg/day

Chronic atrial fibrillation (rate-control), PSVT prophylaxis: Oral: Immediate release: 240-480 mg/day in 3-4 divided doses; Usual dose range (Fuster, 2006): 120-360 mg/day in divided doses

Hypertension: Oral: **Note:** When switching from immediate-release to extended/sustained release formulations, the total daily dose remains the same unless formulation strength does not allow for equal conversion.

Immediate release: 80 mg 3 times/day; usual dose range (JNC 7): 80-320 mg/day in 2 divided doses

Sustained release: Usual dose range (JNC 7): 120-480 mg/day in 1-2 divided doses; **Note:** There is no evidence of additional benefit with doses >360 mg/day.

Calan® SR, Isoptin® SR: Initial: 180 mg once daily in the morning (elderly or small stature: 120 mg/day); if inadequate response, may increase dose at weekly intervals to 240 mg once daily, then 180 mg twice daily (or 240 mg in the morning followed by 120 mg in the evening); maximum dose: 240 mg twice daily.

Verelan®: Initial: 180 mg once daily in the morning (elderly or small stature: 120 mg/day); if inadequate response, may increase dose at weekly intervals to 240 mg once daily, then 360 mg once daily, then 480 mg once daily; maximum dose: 480 mg/day

Extended release: Usual dose range (JNC 7): 120-360 mg once daily (once-daily dosing is recommended at bedtime)

Covera-HS®: Initial: 180 mg once daily at bedtime; if inadequate response, may increase dose at weekly intervals to 240 mg once daily, then 360 mg once daily, then 480 mg once daily; maximum dose: 480 mg/day

Verelan® PM: Initial: 200 mg once daily at bedtime (elderly or small stature: 100 mg/day); if inadequate response, may increase dose at weekly intervals to 300 mg once daily, then 400 mg once daily; maximum dose: 400 mg/day

Elderly: Hypertension: Oral: **Note:** When switching from immediate release to extended or sustained release formulations, the total daily dose remains the same unless formulation strength does not allow for equal conversion.

Manufacturer's recommendations:

Immediate release: Initial: 40 mg 3 times daily

Sustained release: Calan® SR, Isoptin® SR,Verelan®: Initial: 120 mg once daily in the morning

Extended release:

Covera-HS®: Initial: 180 mg once daily at bedtime

Verelan® PM: Initial: 100 mg once daily at bedtime

ACCF/AHA Expert Consensus recommendations: Consider lower initial doses and titrating to response (Aronow, 2011)

Dosing adjustment in renal impairment: Manufacturer recommends caution and additional ECG monitoring in patients with renal insufficiency. The manufacturer of Verelan PM® recommends an initial dose of 100 mg/day at bedtime. **Note:** A multiple dose study in adults suggests reduced renal clearance of verapamil and its metabolite (norverapamil) with advanced renal failure

(Storstein, 1984). Additionally, several clinical papers report adverse effects of verapamil in patients with chronic renal failure receiving recommended doses of verapamil (Pritza, 1991; Váquez, 1996). In contrast, a number of single dose studies show no difference in verapamil (or norverapamil metabolite) disposition between chronic renal failure and control patients (Beyerlein, 1990; Hanyok, 1988; Mooy, 1985; Zachariah, 1991).

Dialysis: Not removed by hemodialysis (Mooy, 1985); supplemental dose is not necessary.

Dosing adjustment/comments in hepatic disease: In cirrhosis, reduce dose to 20% and 50% of normal for oral and intravenous administration, respectively, and monitor ECG (Somogyi, 1981). The manufacturer of Verelan PM® recommends an initial adult dose of 100 mg/day at bedtime. The manufacturers of Calan®, Calan® SR, Covera-HS®, Isoptin® SR, and Verelan® recommend giving 30% of the normal dose to patients with severe hepatic impairment.

Dietary Considerations Calan® SR and Isoptin® SR products may be taken with food or milk, other formulations may be administered without regard to meals; sprinkling contents of Verelan® or Verelan® PM capsule onto applesauce does not affect oral absorption.

Administration

Oral: Do not crush or chew sustained or extended release products.

Calan® SR, Isoptin® SR: Administer with food.

Verelan®, Verelan® PM: Capsules may be opened and the contents sprinkled on 1 tablespoonful of applesauce, then swallowed immediately without chewing. Do not subdivide contents of capsules.

I.V.: Rate of infusion: Over 2 minutes; over 3 minutes in older patients (ACLS, 2010)

Monitoring Parameters Monitor blood pressure and heart rate; periodic liver function tests; ECG, especially with renal and/or hepatic impairment

Test Interactions May interfere with urine detection of methadone (false-positive).

Dosage Forms Excipient information presented when available (limited, particularly for generics); consult specific product labeling. [DSC] = Discontinued product

Caplet, sustained release, oral, as hydrochloride:
- Calan® SR: 120 mg
- Calan® SR: 180 mg, 240 mg [scored]

Capsule, extended release, oral, as hydrochloride: 120 mg, 180 mg, 240 mg

Capsule, extended release, controlled onset, oral, as hydrochloride: 100 mg, 200 mg, 300 mg
- Verelan® PM: 100 mg, 200 mg, 300 mg

Capsule, sustained release, oral, as hydrochloride: 120 mg, 180 mg, 240 mg, 360 mg
- Verelan®: 120 mg, 180 mg, 240 mg, 360 mg

Injection, solution, as hydrochloride: 2.5 mg/mL (2 mL, 4 mL)

Tablet, oral, as hydrochloride: 40 mg, 80 mg, 120 mg
- Calan®: 80 mg, 120 mg [scored]

Tablet, extended release, oral, as hydrochloride: 120 mg, 180 mg, 240 mg

Tablet, extended release, controlled onset, oral, as hydrochloride:
- Covera-HS®: 180 mg, 240 mg

Tablet, sustained release, oral, as hydrochloride: 120 mg [DSC], 180 mg [DSC], 240 mg
- Isoptin® SR: 120 mg
- Isoptin® SR: 180 mg, 240 mg [scored]

Extemporaneous Preparations A 50 mg/mL oral suspension may be made with immediate release tablets and either a 1:1 mixture of Ora-Sweet® and Ora-Plus® or a 1:1 mixture of Ora-Sweet® SF and Ora-Plus® or cherry syrup. When using cherry syrup, dilute cherry syrup concentrate 1:4 with simple syrup, NF. Crush seventy-five verapamil hydrochloride 80 mg tablets in a mortar and reduce to a fine powder. Add small portions of chosen vehicle (40 mL total) and mix to a uniform paste; mix while adding the vehicle in incremental proportions to **almost** 120 mL; transfer to a calibrated bottle, rinse mortar with vehicle, and add quantity of vehicle sufficient to make 120 mL. Label "shake well", "refrigerate", and "protect from light". Stable for 60 days refrigerated (preferred) or at room temperature (Allen, 1996).

A 50 mg/mL oral suspension may be made with immediate release tablets, a 1:1 preparation of methylcellulose 1% and simple syrup, and purified water. Crush twenty 80 mg verapamil tablets in a mortar and reduce to a fine powder. Add 3 mL purified water USP and mix to a uniform paste; mix while adding the vehicle incremental proportions to **almost** 32 mL; transfer to a calibrated bottle, rinse mortar with vehicle, and add quantity of vehicle sufficient to make 32 mL. Label "shake well" and "refrigerate". Stable for 91 days refrigerated (preferred) or at room temperature (Nahata, 1997).

Allen LV Jr and Erickson MA 3rd, "Stability of Labetalol Hydrochloride, Metoprolol Tartrate, Verapamil Hydrochloride, and Spironolactone With Hydrochlorothiazide in Extemporaneously Compounded Oral Liquids," *Am J Health Syst Pharm*, 1996, 53(19):304-9.

Nahata MC, "Stability of Verapamil in an Extemporaneous Liquid Dosage Form," *J Appl Ther Res*, 1997,1(3):271-3.

◆ **Verapamil and Trandolapril** *see* Trandolapril and Verapamil *on page 1718*

◆ **Verapamil Hydrochloride** *see* Verapamil *on page 1783*

◆ **Verapamil Hydrochloride Injection, USP (Can)** *see* Verapamil *on page 1783*

◆ **Verapamil SR (Can)** *see* Verapamil *on page 1783*

◆ **Verdeso®** *see* Desonide *on page 479*

◆ **Verelan®** *see* Verapamil *on page 1783*

◆ **Verelan® PM** *see* Verapamil *on page 1783*

◆ **Verelan SRC (Can)** *see* Verapamil *on page 1783*

◆ **Veripred™ 20** *see* PrednisoLONE (Systemic) *on page 1396*

◆ **Vermox** *see* Mebendazole *on page 1055*

◆ **Vermox® (Can)** *see* Mebendazole *on page 1055*

◆ **Versed** *see* Midazolam *on page 1127*

◆ **Versel® (Can)** *see* Selenium Sulfide *on page 1547*

◆ **Versiclear™** *see* Sodium Thiosulfate *on page 1577*

◆ **Vesanoid** *see* Tretinoin (Systemic) *on page 1729*

◆ **Vesanoid® (Can)** *see* Tretinoin (Systemic) *on page 1729*

◆ **VESIcare®** *see* Solifenacin *on page 1578*

◆ **Vexol®** *see* Rimexolone *on page 1494*

◆ **VFEND®** *see* Voriconazole *on page 1797*

◆ **Viagra®** *see* Sildenafil *on page 1552*

◆ **Vibativ™** *see* Telavancin *on page 1633*

◆ **Vibramycin®** *see* Doxycycline *on page 557*

◆ **Vibra-Tabs® (Can)** *see* Doxycycline *on page 557*

◆ **Vicks® 44E [OTC]** *see* Guaifenesin and Dextromethorphan *on page 810*

◆ **Vicks® Casero™ Chest Congestion Relief [OTC]** *see* GuaiFENesin *on page 809*

◆ **Vicks® DayQuil® Mucus Control [OTC]** *see* GuaiFENesin *on page 809*

◆ **Vicks® DayQuil® Mucus Control DM [OTC]** *see* Guaifenesin and Dextromethorphan *on page 810*

◆ **Vicks® Nature Fusion™ Cough & Chest Congestion [OTC]** *see* Guaifenesin and Dextromethorphan *on page 810*

◆ **Vicks® Pediatric Formula 44E [OTC]** *see* Guaifenesin and Dextromethorphan *on page 810*

◆ **Vicks® Vitamin C [OTC]** *see* Ascorbic Acid *on page 149*

Vigabatrin (vye GA ba trin)

Brand Names: U.S. Sabril®

Brand Names: Canada Sabril®

Pharmacologic Category Anticonvulsant, Miscellaneous

Use Treatment of infantile spasms; refractory complex partial seizures not controlled by usual treatments

Canadian labeling: Additional uses (not in U.S. labeling): Active management of partial or secondary generalized seizures not controlled by usual treatments

Unlabeled Use Spasticity, tardive dyskinesias

Pregnancy Risk Factor C

Prescribing and Access Restrictions As a requirement of the REMS program, access to this medication is restricted. Vigabatrin is only available in the U.S. under a special restricted distribution program (SHARE). Under the SHARE program, only prescribers and pharmacies registered with the program are able to prescribe and distribute vigabatrin. Vigabatrin may only be dispensed to patients who are enrolled in and meet all conditions of SHARE. Contact the SHARE program at 1-888-45-SHARE.

Medication Guide Available Yes

Dosage Oral:

Children 1 month to 2 years: Infantile spasms: Initial dosing: 50 mg/kg/day divided twice daily; may titrate upwards by 25-50 mg/kg/day every 3 days to a maximum of 150 mg/kg/day

Note: To taper, decrease dose by 25-50 mg/kg/day every 3-4 days

Children: Adjunctive treatment of seizures (Canadian labeling; not in U.S. labeling): Initial: 40 mg/kg/day divided twice daily; maintenance dosages based on patient weight:

10-15 kg: 0.5-1 g/day divided twice daily
16-30 kg: 1-1.5 g/day divided twice daily
31-50 kg: 1.5-3 g/day divided twice daily
>50 kg: 2-3 g/day divided twice daily

Adolescents ≥16 years and Adults: Refractory complex partial seizures: Initial: 500 mg twice daily; increase daily dose by 500 mg at weekly intervals based on response and tolerability. Recommended dose: 3 g/day

Note: To taper, decrease dose by 1 g/day on a weekly basis

Elderly: Refractory complex partial seizures: Initiate at low end of dosage range (refer to adult dosing); monitor closely for sedation and confusion

Dosage adjustment in renal impairment:

Cl_{cr} >50-80 mL/minute: Decrease dose by 25%
Cl_{cr} >30-50 mL/minute: Decrease dose by 50%
Cl_{cr} >10-30 mL/minute: Decrease dose by 75%

Additional Information Complete prescribing information for this medication should be consulted for additional detail.

Dosage Forms Excipient information presented when available (limited, particularly for generics); consult specific product labeling.

Powder for solution, oral:
Sabril®: 500 mg/packet (50s)
Tablet, oral:
Sabril®: 500 mg [scored]

Dosage Forms: Canada Excipient information presented when available (limited, particularly for generics); consult specific product labeling.

Powder for suspension, oral [sachets]:
Sabril®: 0.5 g

Vilazodone (vil AZ oh done)

Brand Names: U.S. Viibryd™

Index Terms EMD 68843; SB659746-A; Vilazodone Hydrochloride

Pharmacologic Category Antidepressant, Selective Serotonin Reuptake Inhibitor/5-HT_{1A} Receptor Partial Agonist

Additional Appendix Information

Antidepressant Agents *on page 1874*

Use Treatment of major depressive disorder

Pregnancy Risk Factor C

Pregnancy Considerations Due to adverse effects observed in animal studies, vilazodone is classified as pregnancy category C. Limited data is available concerning the use of vilazodone during pregnancy. Nonteratogenic effects in the newborn following SSRI exposure late in the third trimester include respiratory distress, cyanosis, apnea, seizures, temperature instability, feeding difficulty, vomiting, hypoglycemia, hypo- or hypertonia, hyperreflexia, jitteriness, irritability, constant crying, and tremor. An increased risk of low birth weight and lower Apgar scores have also been reported. Exposure to SSRIs after the twentieth week of gestation has been associated with persistent pulmonary hypertension of the newborn (PPHN). Adverse effects may be due to toxic effects of the SSRI or drug withdrawal without a taper. The long-term effects of *in utero* SSRI exposure on infant development and behavior are not known.

Women treated for major depression and who are euthymic prior to pregnancy are more likely to experience a relapse when medication is discontinued as compared to pregnant women who continue taking antidepressant medications. The ACOG recommends that therapy with SSRIs or SNRIs during pregnancy be individualized; treatment of depression during pregnancy should incorporate the clinical expertise of the mental health clinician, obstetrician, primary healthcare provider, and pediatrician. If treatment during pregnancy is required, consider tapering therapy during the third trimester in order to prevent withdrawal symptoms in the infant. If this is done and the woman is considered to be at risk of relapse from her major depressive disorder, the medication can be restarted following delivery, although the dose should be readjusted to that required before pregnancy. Treatment algorithms have been developed by the ACOG and the APA for the management of depression in women prior to conception and during pregnancy (Yonkers, 2009).

Lactation Excretion in breast milk unknown/consider risk: benefit

Medication Guide Available Yes

Contraindications Concomitant use with MAO inhibitors or within 2 weeks of discontinuing MAO inhibitors

Warnings/Precautions [U.S. Boxed Warning]: Antidepressants increase the risk of suicidal thinking and behavior in children, adolescents, and young adults (18-24 years of age) with major depressive disorder (MDD) and other psychiatric disorders; consider risk prior to prescribing. Short-term studies did not show an increased risk in patients >24 years of age and showed a decreased risk in patients ≥65 years. Closely monitor patients for clinical worsening, suicidality, or unusual changes in behavior, particularly during the initial 1-2 months of therapy or during periods of dosage adjustments (increases or decreases); the patient's family or caregiver should be instructed to closely observe the patient and communicate condition with healthcare provider. A medication guide concerning the use of antidepressants should be dispensed with each prescription. **Vilazodone is not FDA approved for use in children.**

The possibility of a suicide attempt is inherent in major depression and may persist until remission occurs. Use caution in high-risk patients. Worsening depression and severe abrupt suicidality that are not part of the presenting symptoms may require discontinuation or modification of drug therapy. The patient's family or caregiver should be alerted to monitor patients for the emergence of suicidality and associated behaviors (such as agitation, irritability, hostility, impulsivity, and hypomania) and call healthcare provider.

May worsen psychosis in some patients or precipitate a shift to mania or hypomania in patients with bipolar disorder. Patients presenting with depressive symptoms should be screened for bipolar disorder. Monotherapy in patients with bipolar disorder should be avoided. **Vilazodone is not FDA approved for the treatment of bipolar depression.**

Serotonin syndrome and neuroleptic malignant syndrome (NMS)-like reactions have occurred with serotonin/norepinephrine reuptake inhibitors (SNRIs) and selective serotonin reuptake inhibitors (SSRIs) when used alone, and particularly when used in combination with serotonergic agents (eg, triptans) or antidopaminergic agents (eg, antipsychotics). Concurrent use or use within 2 weeks of discontinuing MAO inhibitors is contraindicated. In addition, allow at least 14 days after stopping vilazodone before starting an MAO inhibitor. High potential for interaction with concomitant medications (see Drug Interactions); monitor closely for toxicity or adverse effects. Dose reductions are recommended with concomitant use of strong or moderate CYP3A4 inhibitors. May increase the risks associated with electroconvulsive therapy. Has a low potential to impair cognitive or motor performance; caution operating hazardous machinery or driving.

Use with caution in patients with hepatic impairment, seizure disorder, in elderly patients, or on concomitant CNS depressants. Use caution with concomitant use of aspirin, NSAIDs, warfarin, or other drugs that affect coagulation; the risk of bleeding may be potentiated. May cause hyponatremia/SIADH (elderly at increased risk); volume depletion and diuretics may increase risk. May cause or exacerbate sexual dysfunction. Upon discontinuation of vilazodone therapy, gradually taper dose. If intolerable symptoms occur following a decrease in dosage or upon discontinuation of therapy, consider resuming the previous dose with a more gradual taper.

Adverse Reactions

>10%:

Gastrointestinal: Diarrhea (28%), nausea (23%)

1% to 10%:

Cardiovascular: Palpitation (2%)

Central nervous system: Dizziness (9%), insomnia (6%), dreams abnormal (4%), fatigue (4%), restlessness (3%), somnolence (3%), migraine (≥1%), sedation (≥1%)

Dermatologic: Hyperhidrosis (≥1%)

Endocrine & metabolic: Libido decreased (3% to 5%), orgasm abnormal (2% to 4%), sexual dysfunction (≤2%)

Gastrointestinal: Xerostomia (8%), vomiting (5%), dyspepsia (3%), flatulence (3%), gastroenteritis (3%), appetite increased (2%), appetite decreased (≥1%)

Genitourinary: Ejaculation delayed (2%), erectile dysfunction (2%)

Neuromuscular & skeletal: Arthralgia (3%), paresthesia (3%), jittery (2%), tremor (2%)

Ocular: Blurred vision (≥1%), dry eyes (≥1%)

Miscellaneous: Night sweats (≥1%)

<1% (Limited to important or life-threatening): Abnormal feeling, abnormal taste, cataracts, mania, panic attacks, pollakiuria, ventricular extrasystoles

Drug Interactions

Metabolism/Transport Effects Substrate of CYP2C19 (minor), CYP2D6 (minor), CYP3A4 (major); **Note:** Assignment of Major/Minor substrate status based on clinically relevant drug interaction potential; **Inhibits** CYP2C8 (weak), CYP2D6 (moderate); **Induces** CYP2C19 (weak/moderate)

Avoid Concomitant Use

Avoid concomitant use of Vilazodone with any of the following: Iobenguane I 123; MAO Inhibitors; Methylene Blue; Pimozide; Tryptophan

Increased Effect/Toxicity

Vilazodone may increase the levels/effects of: Alpha-/Beta-Blockers; Anticoagulants; Antidepressants (Serotonin Reuptake Inhibitor/Antagonist); Antiplatelet Agents; Aspirin; Benzodiazepines (metabolized by oxidation); Beta-Blockers; BusPIRone; CarBAMazepine; CloZAPine; Collagenase (Systemic); CYP2D6 Substrates; Desmopressin; Dextromethorphan; Drotrecogin Alfa (Activated); Fesoterodine; Galantamine; Ibritumomab; Lithium; Methadone; Methylene Blue; Metoclopramide; Mexiletine; NSAID (COX-2 Inhibitor); NSAID (Nonselective); Pimozide; RisperiDONE; Rivaroxaban; Salicylates; Serotonin Modulators; Tamoxifen; Thrombolytic Agents; Tositumomab and Iodine I 131 Tositumomab; TraMADol; Tricyclic Antidepressants; Vitamin K Antagonists

The levels/effects of Vilazodone may be increased by: Alcohol (Ethyl); Analgesics (Opioid); Antipsychotics; BusPIRone; Cimetidine; CNS Depressants; CYP3A4 Inhibitors (Moderate); CYP3A4 Inhibitors (Strong); Dasatinib; Glucosamine; Herbs (Anticoagulant/Antiplatelet Properties); Linezolid; Macrolide Antibiotics; MAO Inhibitors; Metoclopramide; Omega-3-Acid Ethyl Esters; Pentosan Polysulfate Sodium; Pentoxifylline; Propafenone; Prostacyclin Analogues; TraMADol; Tryptophan; Vitamin E

Decreased Effect

Vilazodone may decrease the levels/effects of: Iobenguane I 123; Ioflupane I 123

The levels/effects of Vilazodone may be decreased by: CarBAMazepine; CYP3A4 Inducers (Strong); Cyproheptadine; Deferasirox; NSAID (Nonselective); Peginterferon Alfa-2b; Tocilizumab

Ethanol/Nutrition/Herb Interactions Ethanol: May increase CNS depression; monitor for increased effects with coadministration. Caution patients about effects.

Stability Store at 25°C (77°F); excursions permitted to 15°C to 30°C (50°F to 86°F).

Mechanism of Action Vilazodone inhibits CNS neuron serotonin uptake; minimal or no effect on reuptake of norepinephrine or dopamine. It also binds selectively with high affinity to 5-HT_{1A} receptors and is a 5-HT_{1A} receptor partial agonist. 5-HT_{1A} receptor activity may be altered in depression and anxiety.

Pharmacodynamics/Kinetics
Protein binding: ~96% to 99%
Metabolism: Extensively hepatic, via CYP3A4 (major pathway) and 2C19 and 2D6 (minor pathways)
Bioavailability: 72% (with food); blood concentrations (AUC) may be decreased ~50% in the fasted state
Half-life elimination: Terminal: ~25 hours
Time to peak, serum: 4-5 hours
Excretion: Urine (1% as unchanged drug); feces (2% as unchanged drug)

Dosage Adults: Oral: Depression: Initial: 10 mg once daily for 7 days, then increase to 20 mg once daily for 7 days, then to recommended dose of 40 mg once daily

Dosing adjustment for concomitant medications:
Strong CYP3A4 inhibitors: Reduce vilazodone dose to 20 mg once daily
Moderate CYP3A4 inhibitors (eg, erythromycin): Reduce vilazodone dose to 20 mg once daily in patients with intolerable side effects

Dosing adjustment in hepatic impairment:
Mild-to-moderate impairment (Child-Pugh class A or B): No adjustment needed
Severe impairment (Child-Pugh class C): Not studied

Dietary Considerations Take with food.

Administration Administer with food.

Monitoring Parameters Monitor patient periodically for symptom resolution, mental status for depression, suicidal ideation (especially at the beginning of therapy or when doses are increased or decreased), anxiety, social functioning, mania, panic attacks, akathisia

Dosage Forms Excipient information presented when available (limited, particularly for generics); consult specific product labeling.
Tablet, oral, as hydrochloride:
Viibryd™: 10 mg, 20 mg, 40 mg

◆ **Vilazodone Hydrochloride** *see* Vilazodone *on page 1787*

◆ **Vimpat®** *see* Lacosamide *on page 963*

VinBLAStine (vin BLAS teen)

Index Terms Velban; Vinblastine Sulfate; Vincaleukoblastine; VLB

Pharmacologic Category Antineoplastic Agent, Natural Source (Plant) Derivative; Antineoplastic Agent, Vinca Alkaloid

Use Treatment of Hodgkin's and non-Hodgkin's lymphoma; testicular cancer; breast cancer; mycosis fungoides; Kaposi's sarcoma; histiocytosis (Letterer-Siwe disease); choriocarcinoma

Unlabeled Use Treatment of bladder cancer, melanoma, nonsmall cell lung cancer (NSCLC), ovarian cancer, soft tissue sarcoma (desmoid tumors)

Pregnancy Risk Factor D

Pregnancy Considerations Animal studies have demonstrated resorption and teratogenic effects. There are no adequate and well-controlled studies in pregnant women. Women of childbearing potential should avoid becoming pregnant during vinblastine treatment. Aspermia has been reported in males who have received treatment with vinblastine.

Lactation Excretion in breast milk unknown/not recommended

Contraindications Significant granulocytopenia; presence of bacterial infection; I.T. administration is contraindicated (may result in death)

Warnings/Precautions Hazardous agent - use appropriate precautions for handling and disposal. **[U.S. Boxed Warning]: For I.V. use only. Intrathecal administration may result in death.** Must be dispensed in overwrap which bears the statement **"Do not remove covering until the moment of injection. Fatal if given intrathecally. For I.V. use only." [U.S. Boxed Warning]: Vinblastine is a moderate vesicant; avoid extravasation. Individuals administering should be experienced in vinblastine administration;** assure proper needle or catheter placement prior to administration. Leukopenia is common; granulocytopenia may be severe with higher doses. Leukopenia may be more pronounced in cachectic patients and patients with skin ulceration. Thrombocytopenia and anemia may occur rarely.

Use with caution in patients with hepatic impairment; toxicity may be increased; may require dosage modification. Neurotoxicity is rare at clinical doses; may occur with high doses (symptoms are similar to vincristine toxicity, including peripheral neuropathy, loss of deep tendon reflexes, headache, weakness, urinary retention, and GI symptoms). May rarely cause disabling neurotoxicity (usually reversible). Itraconazole may decrease the metabolism of vinblastine via CYP3A4 inhibition and may increase the effects of vinblastine via P-glycoprotein effects; severe myelosuppression and neurotoxicity may occur. Acute shortness of breath and severe bronchospasm have been reported, most often in association with concurrent administration of mitomycin; may occur within minutes to several hours following vinblastine administration or up to 14 days following mitomycin administration; use caution in patients with pre-existing pulmonary disease. Use with caution in patients with ischemic heart disease. **[U.S. Boxed Warning]: Should be administered under the supervision of an experienced cancer chemotherapy physician.** Some dosage forms may contain benzyl alcohol which has been associated with "gasping syndrome" in neonates.

Adverse Reactions Frequency not defined.

Common:
Cardiovascular: Hypertension
Central nervous system: Malaise
Dermatologic: Alopecia
Gastrointestinal: Constipation
Hematologic: Myelosuppression, leukopenia/granulocytopenia (nadir: 5-10 days; recovery: 7-14 days; dose-limiting toxicity)
Neuromuscular & skeletal: Bone pain, jaw pain, tumor pain

Less common:
Cardiovascular: Angina, cerebrovascular accident, coronary ischemia, ECG abnormalities, limb ischemia, MI, myocardial ischemia, Raynaud's phenomenon
Central nervous system: Depression, dizziness, headache, neurotoxicity (duration: >24 hours), seizure, vertigo
Dermatologic: Dermatitis, photosensitivity (rare), rash, skin blistering
Endocrine & metabolic: Aspermia, hyperuricemia, SIADH
Gastrointestinal: Abdominal pain, anorexia, diarrhea, gastrointestinal bleeding, hemorrhagic enterocolitis, ileus, metallic taste, nausea (mild), paralytic ileus, rectal bleeding, stomatitis, toxic megacolon, vomiting (mild)
Genitourinary: Urinary retention
Hematologic: Anemia, thrombocytopenia (recovery within a few days), thrombotic thrombocytopenic purpura
Local: Cellulitis (with extravasation), irritation, phlebitis (with extravasation), radiation recall
Neuromuscular & skeletal: Deep tendon reflex loss, myalgia, paresthesia, peripheral neuritis, weakness
Ocular: Nystagmus
Otic: Auditory damage, deafness, vestibular damage
Renal: Hemolytic uremic syndrome
Respiratory: Bronchospasm, dyspnea, pharyngitis

Drug Interactions

Metabolism/Transport Effects Substrate of CYP2D6 (minor), CYP3A4 (major), P-glycoprotein; **Note:** Assignment of Major/Minor substrate status based on clinically ▶

relevant drug interaction potential; **Inhibits** CYP2D6 (weak), CYP3A4 (weak); **Induces** P-glycoprotein

Avoid Concomitant Use

Avoid concomitant use of VinBLAStine with any of the following: BCG; CloZAPine; Conivaptan; Dabigatran Etexilate; Natalizumab; Pimecrolimus; Pimozide; Tacrolimus (Topical); Vaccines (Live)

Increased Effect/Toxicity

VinBLAStine may increase the levels/effects of: CloZAPine; Leflunomide; MitoMYcin; Natalizumab; Pimozide; Tolterodine; Vaccines (Live)

The levels/effects of VinBLAStine may be increased by: Conivaptan; CYP3A4 Inhibitors (Moderate); CYP3A4 Inhibitors (Strong); Dasatinib; Denosumab; Itraconazole; Lopinavir; Macrolide Antibiotics; MAO Inhibitors; P-glycoprotein/ABCB1 Inhibitors; Pimecrolimus; Posaconazole; Ritonavir; Roflumilast; Tacrolimus (Topical); Trastuzumab; Voriconazole

Decreased Effect

VinBLAStine may decrease the levels/effects of: BCG; Coccidioidin Skin Test; Dabigatran Etexilate; Linagliptin; P-glycoprotein/ABCB1 Substrates; Sipuleucel-T; Vaccines (Inactivated); Vaccines (Live)

The levels/effects of VinBLAStine may be decreased by: CYP3A4 Inducers (Strong); Deferasirox; Echinacea; Peginterferon Alfa-2b; P-glycoprotein/ABCB1 Inducers; Tocilizumab

Ethanol/Nutrition/Herb Interactions Herb/Nutraceutical: Avoid St John's wort (may decrease vinblastine levels). Avoid black cohosh, dong quai in estrogen-dependent tumors.

Stability Note: Must be dispensed in overwrap which bears the statement "Do not remove covering until the moment of injection. Fatal if given intrathecally. For I.V. use only." Syringes should be labeled: "Fatal if given intrathecally. For I.V. use only."

Store intact vials under refrigeration at 2°C to 8°C (36°F to 46°F). Protect from light. Reconstitute lyophilized powder to a concentration of 1 mg/mL with NS or bacteriostatic NS. For infusion, may dilute in 50 mL NS or D_5W; dilution in larger volumes (≥100 mL) of I.V. fluids is not recommended. Use appropriate precautions for handling and disposal. Solutions reconstituted in bacteriostatic NS are stable for 28 days under refrigeration.

Mechanism of Action Vinblastine binds to tubulin and inhibits microtubule formation, therefore, arresting the cell at metaphase by disrupting the formation of the mitotic spindle; it is specific for the M and S phases. Vinblastine may also interfere with nucleic acid and protein synthesis by blocking glutamic acid utilization.

Pharmacodynamics/Kinetics

Distribution: V_d: 27.3 L/kg; binds extensively to tissues; does not penetrate CNS or other fatty tissues; distributes to liver

Protein binding: 99%

Metabolism: Hepatic to active metabolite

Half-life elimination: Biphasic: Initial: 4 minutes; Terminal: 25 hours

Excretion: Feces (95%); urine (<1% as unchanged drug)

Dosage Details concerning dosing in combination regimens should also be consulted. **Note:** Frequency and duration of therapy may vary by indication, concomitant combination chemotherapy and hematologic response. **For I.V. use only.**

Children: I.V.:

Hodgkin's disease: Initial dose: 6 mg/m^2; do not administer more frequently than every 7 days

Letterer-Siwe disease: Initial dose: 6.5 mg/m^2; do not administer more frequently than every 7 days

Testicular cancer: Initial dose: 3 mg/m^2; do not administer more frequently than every 7 days

Adults: I.V.: Initial: 3.7 mg/m^2; adjust dose every 7 days (based on white blood cell response) up to 5.5 mg/m^2 (second dose); 7.4 mg/m^2 (third dose); 9.25 mg/m^2 (fourth dose); and 11.1 mg/m^2 (fifth dose); do not administer more frequently than every 7 days.

Usual range: 5.5-7.4 mg/m^2 every 7 days; Maximum dose: 18.5 mg/m^2; dosage adjustment goal is to reduce white blood cell count to ~3000/mm^3

Indication-specific dosing:

Hodgkin's disease: Usual dose: 6 mg/m^2 every 2 weeks (as part of a combination chemotherapy regimen) (Bartlett, 1995; Horning, 2002)

Testicular cancer: Usual dose: 0.11 mg/kg daily for 2 days every 3 weeks (as part of a combination chemotherapy regimen) (Loehrer, 1998) **or** 6 mg/m^2/day for 2 days every 3-4 weeks (as part of a combination chemotherapy regimen) (Clemm, 1986)

Bladder cancer (unlabeled use): Usual dose: 3 mg/m^2 every 7 days for 3 out of 4 weeks (as part of combination chemotherapy) (Sternberg, 2001) **or** 3 mg/m^2 days 2, 15, and 22 of a 28-day treatment cycle (as part of a combination chemotherapy regimen) (von der Maase, 2000)

Melanoma (unlabeled used): 2 mg/m^2 days 1-4 and 22-25 of a 6-week treatment cycle (as part of a combination chemotherapy regimen) (Eton, 2002)

Nonsmall cell lung cancer (unlabeled use): 4 mg/m^2 days 1, 8, 15, 22, and 29, then every 2 weeks (as part of combination chemotherapy) (Arriagada, 2004)

Ovarian cancer (unlabeled use): 0.11 mg/kg daily for 2 days every 3 weeks (as part of a combination chemotherapy regimen) (Loehrer, 1998)

Dosing adjustment in renal impairment: According to FDA-approved labeling, no adjustment is necessary in patients with renal impairment.

Dosing adjustment in hepatic impairment:

The FDA-approved labeling recommends the following guidelines: Serum bilirubin >3 mg/dL: Administer 50% of dose

The following guidelines have been used by some clinicians:

Serum bilirubin >3.1 or transaminases >3 times ULN: Avoid use (Floyd, 2006) **or**

Serum bilirubin 1.5-3 mg/dL or AST 60-180 units: Administer 50% of dose

Serum bilirubin 3-5 mg/dL: Administer 25% of dose

Serum bilirubin >5 mg/dL or AST >180 units: Avoid use

Administration FATAL IF GIVEN INTRATHECALLY. For I.V. administration only, usually as a slow (2-3 minutes) push, or a bolus (5-15 minutes) infusion; the manufacturer recommends an undiluted 1-minute infusion to prevent venous irritation/extravasation. Prolonged administration times and/or increased administration volumes may the risk of vein irritation and extravasation. Assure proper needle or catheter placement prior to administration.

Monitoring Parameters CBC with differential and platelet count, serum uric acid, hepatic function tests

Dosage Forms Excipient information presented when available (limited, particularly for generics); consult specific product labeling.

Injection, powder for reconstitution, as sulfate: 10 mg

Injection, solution, as sulfate: 1 mg/mL (10 mL)

◆ **Vinblastine Sulfate** *see* VinBLAStine *on page 1789*

◆ **Vincaleukoblastine** *see* VinBLAStine *on page 1789*

◆ **Vincasar PFS®** *see* VinCRIStine *on page 1790*

VinCRIStine (vin KRIS teen)

Brand Names: U.S. Vincasar PFS®

Brand Names: Canada Vincristine Sulfate Injection

Index Terms Leurocristine Sulfate; Oncovin; Vincristine Sulfate

Pharmacologic Category Antineoplastic Agent, Natural Source (Plant) Derivative; Antineoplastic Agent, Vinca Alkaloid

Use Treatment of acute lymphocytic leukemia (ALL), Hodgkin's lymphoma, non-Hodgkin's lymphomas, Wilms' tumor, neuroblastoma, rhabdomyosarcoma

Unlabeled Use Treatment of multiple myeloma, chronic lymphocytic leukemia (CLL), brain tumors, small cell lung cancer, ovarian germ cell tumors

Pregnancy Risk Factor D

Pregnancy Considerations Animal studies have demonstrated teratogenicity and fetal loss. There are no adequate and well-controlled studies in pregnant women. May cause fetal harm if administered during pregnancy. Women of childbearing potential should avoid becoming pregnant during treatment.

Lactation Excretion in breast milk unknown/not recommended

Contraindications Patients with demyelinating form of Charcot-Marie-Tooth syndrome

Warnings/Precautions Hazardous agent - use appropriate precautions for handling and disposal; avoid eye contamination.

[U.S. Boxed Warning]: For I.V. administration only; intrathecal administration has uniformly caused severe neurologic damage and/or death; vincristine should never be administered by this route. Vincristine should **NOT** be prepared during the preparation of any intrathecal medications. After preparation, store vincristine in a location **away** from the separate storage location recommended for intrathecal medications. Vincristine should **NOT** be delivered to the patient with any medications intended for central nervous system administration.

[U.S. Boxed Warning]: Vincristine is a vesicant; avoid extravasation. (Individuals administering should be experienced in vincristine administration.) Check for proper needle placement; if extravasation occurs, discontinue vincristine infusion and initiate appropriate extravasation management.

Neurotoxicity, including alterations in mental status such as depression, confusion, or insomnia may occur; neurologic effects are dose-limiting (may require dosage reduction) and may be additive with those of other neurotoxic agents and spinal cord irradiation. Use with caution in patients with pre-existing neuromuscular disease and/or with concomitant neurotoxic agents. Constipation, paralytic ileus, intestinal necrosis and/or perforation may occur; constipation may present as upper colon impaction with an empty rectum (may require flat film of abdomen for diagnosis); generally responds to high enemas and laxatives. All patients should be on a prophylactic bowel management regimen.

Use with caution in patients receiving concurrent therapy which alters CYP3A4 activity, may require therapy alterations. Acute shortness of breath and severe bronchospasm have been reported with vinca alkaloids, usually when used in combination with mitomycin-C. Onset may be several minutes to hours after vincristine administration and up to 2 weeks after mitomycin-C. Progressive dyspnea may occur. Permanently discontinue vincristine in this situation.

Use with caution in patients with hepatic impairment; dosage modification required. May be associated with hepatic sinusoidal obstruction syndrome (SOS; formerly called veno-occlusive disease), increased risk in children <3 years of age; use with caution in hepatobiliary dysfunction. Monitor for signs or symptoms of hepatic SOS, including bilirubin >1.4 mg/dL, unexplained weight gain, ascites, hepatomegaly, or unexplained right upper quadrant pain (Arndt, 2004). Acute uric acid nephropathy has been reported with vincristine. Use with caution in the elderly.

Adverse Reactions Frequency not defined.

Cardiovascular: Edema, hyper-/hypotension, MI, myocardial ischemia

Central nervous system: Ataxia, coma, cranial nerve dysfunction (auditory damage, extraocular muscle impairment, laryngeal muscle impairment, paralysis, paresis, vestibular damage, vocal cord paralysis), dizziness, fever, headache, neurotoxicity, neuropathic pain (common), seizure, vertigo

Dermatologic toxicity: Alopecia (common), rash

Endocrine & metabolic: Hyperuricemia, parotid pain, SIADH (rare)

Gastrointestinal: Abdominal cramps, abdominal pain, anorexia, constipation (common), diarrhea, intestinal necrosis, intestinal perforation, nausea, oral ulcers, paralytic ileus, vomiting, weight loss

Genitourinary: Bladder atony, dysuria, polyuria, urinary retention

Hematologic: Anemia (mild), leukopenia (mild), thrombocytopenia (mild), thrombotic thrombocytopenic purpura

Hepatic: Sinusoidal obstruction (SOS; veno-occlusive liver disease)

Local: Phlebitis, tissue irritation/necrosis (if infiltrated)

Neuromuscular & skeletal: Back pain, bone pain, deep tendon reflex loss, difficulty walking, foot drop, gait changes, jaw pain, limb pain, motor difficulties, muscle wasting, myalgia, paralysis, paresthesia, peripheral neuropathy (common), sensorimotor dysfunction, sensory loss

Ocular: Cortical blindness (transient), nystagmus, optic atrophy with blindness

Otic: Deafness

Renal: Acute uric acid nephropathy, hemolytic uremic syndrome

Respiratory: Bronchospasm, dyspnea, pharyngeal pain

Miscellaneous: Allergic reactions (rare), anaphylaxis (rare), hypersensitivity (rare)

Drug Interactions

Metabolism/Transport Effects Substrate of CYP3A4 (major), P-glycoprotein; **Note:** Assignment of Major/Minor substrate status based on clinically relevant drug interaction potential; **Inhibits** CYP3A4 (weak)

Avoid Concomitant Use

Avoid concomitant use of VinCRIStine with any of the following: BCG; Conivaptan; Natalizumab; Pimecrolimus; Pimozide; Tacrolimus (Topical); Vaccines (Live)

Increased Effect/Toxicity

VinCRIStine may increase the levels/effects of: Leflunomide; MitoMYcin; Natalizumab; Pimozide; Vaccines (Live); Vitamin K Antagonists

The levels/effects of VinCRIStine may be increased by: Conivaptan; CYP3A4 Inhibitors (Moderate); CYP3A4 Inhibitors (Strong); Dasatinib; Denosumab; Itraconazole; Lopinavir; Macrolide Antibiotics; MAO Inhibitors; NIFEdipine; P-glycoprotein/ABCB1 Inhibitors; Pimecrolimus; Posaconazole; Ritonavir; Roflumilast; Tacrolimus (Topical); Teniposide; Trastuzumab; Voriconazole

Decreased Effect

VinCRIStine may decrease the levels/effects of: BCG; Cardiac Glycosides; Coccidioidin Skin Test; Sipuleucel-T; Vaccines (Inactivated); Vaccines (Live); Vitamin K Antagonists

The levels/effects of VinCRIStine may be decreased by: CYP3A4 Inducers (Strong); Deferasirox; Echinacea; P-glycoprotein/ABCB1 Inducers; Tocilizumab

Ethanol/Nutrition/Herb Interactions Herb/Nutraceutical: St John's wort may decrease vincristine levels.

Stability

Store intact vials under refrigeration. May be stable for up to 30 days at room temperature. Protect from light. Use appropriate precautions for handling and disposal. I.V. solution: **Note:** In order to prevent inadvertent intrathecal administration, the World Health Organization (WHO) and the Institute for Safe Medical Practices (ISMP) recommend dispensing vincristine in a minibag (rather than a syringe). Vincristine should **NOT** be prepared during the preparation of any intrathecal medication. After preparation, store vincristine in a location away from the separate storage location recommended for intrathecal medications.

If dispensing vincristine in a syringe, it must be packaged in the manufacturer-provided overwrap which bears the statement **"Do not remove covering until the moment of injection. For intravenous use only. Fatal if given intrathecally."**

Diluted in 25-50 mL NS or D_5W, stable for 7 days under refrigeration, or 2 days at room temperature. In ambulatory pumps, solution is stable for 7 days at room temperature.

Store undiluted vials under refrigeration. May be stable for up to 30 days at room temperature. Protect from light.

Mechanism of Action Binds to tubulin and inhibits microtubule formation, therefore, arresting the cell at metaphase by disrupting the formation of the mitotic spindle; it is specific for the M and S phases. Vincristine may also interfere with nucleic acid and protein synthesis by blocking glutamic acid utilization.

Pharmacodynamics/Kinetics

Distribution: Rapidly removed from bloodstream and tightly bound to tissues; penetrates blood-brain barrier poorly

Metabolism: Extensively hepatic, via CYP3A4

Half-life elimination: Terminal: 85 hours (range: 19-155 hours)

Excretion: Feces (~80%); urine (10% to 20%; <1% as unchanged drug)

Dosage Note: Doses may be capped at a maximum of 2 mg/dose; refer to individual protocol.

Doses in the manufacturer's FDA-approved labeling: I.V.:

Children ≤10 kg: 0.05 mg/kg/dose once weekly

Children >10 kg: 1.5-2 mg/m²/dose; frequency may vary based on protocol

Adults: 1.4 mg/m²/dose; frequency may vary based on protocol

Additional dosing in combination therapy; indication-specific and/or unlabeled dosing: I.V.:

Children:

ALL: Induction phase: 1.5 mg/m²/dose days 0, 7, 14, and 21; Consolidation phase: 1.5 mg/m²/dose days 0, 28, and 56; Delayed intensification phase: 1.5 mg/m²/dose days 0, 7, and 14; Maintenance phase: 1.5 mg/m²/dose days 0, 28, and 56 (Bostrom, 2003) **or** Induction phase: 1.5 mg/m²/dose days 0, 7, 14, and 21; Consolidation phase: 1.5 mg/m²/dose days 0, 28, and 56; Interim maintenance phases: 1.5 mg/m²/dose days 0 and 28; Delayed intensification phase: 1.5 mg/m²/dose days 0, 7, and 14; Maintenance phase: 1.5 mg/m²/dose every 4 weeks (Avramis, 2002)

Ewing's sarcoma: 2 mg/m²/dose (maximum dose: 2 mg) on day 1 of a 21-day cycle, administer either every cycle or during odd-numbered cycles (Grier, 2003) **or** 0.67 mg/m²/day continuous infusion days 1, 2, and 3 (total 2 mg/m²/cycle; maximum dose/cycle: 2 mg) during cycles 1, 2, 3, and 6 (Kolb, 2003)

Hodgkin's lymphoma: BEACOPP regimen: 2 mg/m²/dose (maximum dose: 2 mg) on day 7 of a 21-day treatment cycle (Kelly, 2002)

Rhabdomyosarcoma:

VA regimen: 1.5 mg/m²/dose (maximum dose: 2 mg) weeks 1-8, weeks 13-20, and weeks 25-32 (Crist, 2001)

VAC regimen: 1.5 mg/m²/dose (maximum dose: 2 mg) weeks 0-12, week 16, weeks 20-25; Continuation therapy: Weeks 29-34, and weeks 38-43 (Crist, 2001)

Wilms' tumor:

Children <1 year: 0.75 mg/m²/dose weekly for 10-11 weeks, then every 3 weeks for 15 additional weeks (total 25-26 weeks) (Pritchard, 1995)

Children ≥1 year: 1.5 mg/m²/dose weekly for 10-11 weeks, then every 3 weeks for 15 additional weeks (total 25-26 weeks) (Pritchard, 1995)

or

Children ≤30 kg: 0.05 mg/kg/dose (maximum dose: 2 mg) weeks 1, 2, 4, 5, 6, 7, 8, 10, and 11, followed by 0.067 mg/kg/dose (maximum dose: 2 mg) weeks 12, 13, 18, and 24 (Green, 2007)

Children >30 kg: 1.5 mg/m²/dose (maximum dose: 2 mg) weeks 1, 2, 4, 5, 6, 7, 8, 10, and 11, followed by 2 mg/m²/dose (maximum dose: 2 mg) weeks 12, 13, 18, and 24 (Green, 2007)

Adults:

ALL:

Hyper-CVAD regimen: 2 mg/dose days 4 and 11 during odd-numbered cycles (cycles 1, 3, 5, 7) of an 8-cycle phase, followed by maintenance treatment (if needed) of 2 mg monthly for 2 years (Kantarjian, 2004)

Larson (CALBG 8811) regimen: Induction phase: 2 mg/dose days 1, 8, 15, and 22 (4-week treatment cycle); Early intensification phase: 2 mg/dose days 15, and 22 (4-week treatment cycle, repeat once); Late intensification phase: 2 mg/dose days 1, 8, 15 (8-week treatment cycle); Maintenance phase: 2 mg/dose day 1 every 4 weeks until 24 months from diagnosis (Larson, 1995)

Brain tumors: PCV regimen: 1.4 mg/m²/dose (maximum dose: 2 mg) on days 8 and 29 of a 6-week treatment cycle for a total of 6 cycles (van de Bent, 2006) **or** 1.4 mg/m²/dose (no maximum dose) on days 8 and 29 of a 6-week treatment cycle for up to 4 cycles (Cairncross, 2006)

Hodgkin's lymphoma:

BEACOPP regimen: 1.4 mg/m²/dose (maximum dose: 2 mg) on day 8 of a 21-day treatment cycle (Diehl, 2003)

Stanford-V regimen: 1.4 mg/m²/dose (maximum dose: 2 mg) in weeks 2, 4, 6, 8, 10, and 12 (Horning, 2000; Horning, 2002)

Non-Hodgkin's lymphoma:

CHOP regimen: 1.4 mg/m²/dose (maximum dose: 2 mg) on day 1 of a 21-day treatment cycle for 8 cycles (Coiffier, 2002)

CVP regimen: 1.4 mg/m²/dose (maximum dose: 2 mg) on day 1 of a 21-day treatment cycle for 8 cycles (Marcus, 2005)

EPOCH regimen: 0.4 mg/m²/day continuous infusion for 4 days (over 96 hours) (total 1.6 mg/m²/cycle; dose not usually capped) of a 21-day treatment cycle (Wilson, 2002)

Multiple myeloma (unlabeled use):

DVD regimen: 1.4 mg/m²/dose (maximum dose: 2 mg) on day 1 of a 28-day treatment cycle (Rifkin, 2006)

VAD regimen: 0.4 mg/day continuous infusion for 4 days (over 96 hours) (total 1.6 mg/cycle) of a 28-day treatment cycle (Rifkin, 2006)

Ovarian cancer (unlabeled use): VAC regimen: 1.5 mg/m²/dose (maximum dose: 2 mg) weekly for 8-12 weeks (Slayton, 1985)

Small cell lung cancer (unlabeled use): CAV regimen: 1.4 mg/m^2/dose day 1 of a 21-day treatment cycle (Hong, 1989) **or** 2 mg/dose on day 1 of a 21-day treatment cycle (von Pawel, 1999)

Dosing adjustment in renal impairment: No adjustment is necessary in patients with renal impairment.

Dosing adjustment in hepatic impairment:

The FDA-approved labeling recommends the following guidelines: Serum bilirubin >3 mg/dL: Administer 50% of normal dose

The following guidelines have been used by some clinicians:

Serum bilirubin 1.5-3 mg/dL or AST 60-180 units: Administer 50% of dose

Serum bilirubin 3-5 mg/dL: Administer 25% of dose

Serum bilirubin >5 mg/dL or AST >180 units: Avoid use

Floyd, 2006: Serum bilirubin 1.5-3 mg/dL or transaminases 2-3 times ULN or alkaline phosphatase increased: Administer 50% of dose

Administration For I.V. administration only. FATAL IF GIVEN INTRATHECALLY. Vincristine should **NOT** be delivered to the patient at the same time with any medications intended for central nervous system administration.

I.V.: Usually administered as short 5-10 minute infusion (preferred); may also be administered as a slow (1 minute) push or by a 24-hour continuous infusions (depending on the protocol). Vesicant; avoid extravasation.

Monitoring Parameters Serum electrolytes (sodium), hepatic function tests, neurologic examination, CBC, serum uric acid; monitor infusion site

Dosage Forms Excipient information presented when available (limited, particularly for generics); consult specific product labeling.

Injection, solution, as sulfate [preservative free]: 1 mg/mL (1 mL, 2 mL)

Vincasar PFS®: 1 mg/mL (1 mL, 2 mL)

◆ **Vincristine Sulfate** *see* VinCRIStine *on page 1790*

◆ **Vincristine Sulfate Injection. (Can)** *see* VinCRIStine *on page 1790*

Vinorelbine (vi NOR el been)

Brand Names: U.S. Navelbine®

Brand Names: Canada Navelbine®; Vinorelbine Injection, USP; Vinorelbine Tartrate for Injection

Index Terms Dihydroxydeoxynorvinkaleukoblastine; Vinorelbine Tartrate

Pharmacologic Category Antineoplastic Agent, Natural Source (Plant) Derivative; Antineoplastic Agent, Vinca Alkaloid

Use Treatment of nonsmall cell lung cancer (NSCLC)

Unlabeled Use Treatment of breast cancer (metastatic), cervical cancer, ovarian cancer, malignant pleural mesothelioma, and soft tissue sarcoma

Pregnancy Risk Factor D

Pregnancy Considerations Animal studies have demonstrated embryotoxicity, fetotoxicity, decreased fetal weight, and delayed ossification. There are no adequate and well-controlled studies in pregnant women. Women of child-bearing potential should avoid becoming pregnant during vinorelbine treatment.

Lactation Excretion in breast milk unknown/not recommended

Contraindications Pretreatment granulocyte counts <1000/mm^3

Warnings/Precautions Hazardous agent - use appropriate precautions for handling and disposal. **[U.S. Boxed Warning]: For I.V. use only; do not administer intrathecally;** intrathecal administration may result in death. **[U.S. Boxed Warning]: Avoid extravasation;** infiltration may cause irritation, thrombophlebitis and/or local tissue necrosis. **[U.S. Boxed Warning]: Severe granulocytopenia may occur with treatment;** granulocytopenia is a dose-limiting toxicity; granulocyte counts should be ≥1000/mm^3 prior to treatment initiation; monitor closely for infections and/or fever; may require dosage adjustment. The incidence of granulocytopenia is significantly higher when given in combination with cisplatin when compared to single-agent vinorelbine. Use with caution in patients with compromised marrow reserve due to prior chemotherapy therapy or prior radiation therapy.

Fatal cases of interstitial pulmonary changes and ARDS have been reported (with single-agent therapy); promptly evaluate changes in baseline pulmonary symptoms or any new onset pulmonary symptoms. Acute shortness of breath and severe bronchospasm have been reported rarely; usually associated with the concurrent administration of mitomycin.

Vinorelbine should **NOT** be prepared during the preparation of any intrathecal medications. After preparation, store vinorelbine in a location **away** from the separate storage location recommended for intrathecal medications. Dosage modification required in patients with impaired hepatic function and neurotoxicity; use with caution. May cause new onset or worsening of pre-existing neuropathy; use with caution in patients with neuropathy. May cause severe constipation (grade 3-4), paralytic ileus, intestinal obstruction, necrosis, and/or perforation. May have radiosensitizing effects with prior or concurrent radiation therapy; radiation recall reactions may occur in patients who have received prior radiation therapy. Avoid eye contamination (exposure may cause severe irritation). **[U.S. Boxed Warning]: Should be administered under the supervision of an experienced cancer chemotherapy physician.**

Adverse Reactions Note: Reported with single-agent therapy.

>10%:

Central nervous system: Fatigue (27%)

Dermatologic: Alopecia (12% to 30%)

Gastrointestinal: Nausea (31% to 44%; grade 3: 1% to 2%), constipation (35%; grade 3: 3%), vomiting (20% to 31%; grade 3: 1% to 2%), diarrhea (12% to 17%)

Hematologic: Leukopenia (83% to 92%; grade 4: 6% to 15%), granulocytopenia (90%; grade 4: 36%; nadir: 7-10 days; recovery 14-21 days; dose-limiting), neutropenia (85%; grade 4: 28%), anemia (83%; grades 3/4: 9%)

Hepatic: AST increased (67%; grade 3: 5%; grade 4: 1%), total bilirubin increased (5% to 13%; grade 3: 4%; grade 4: 3%)

Local: Injection site reaction (22% to 28%; includes erythema, vein discoloration), injection site pain (16%)

Neuromuscular & skeletal: Weakness (36%), peripheral neuropathy (25%; grade 3: 1%; grade 4: <1%)

Renal: Creatinine increased (13%)

1% to 10%:

Cardiovascular: Chest pain (5%)

Dermatologic: Rash (<5%)

Gastrointestinal: Paralytic ileus (1%)

Hematologic: Neutropenic fever/sepsis (8%; grade 4: 4%), thrombocytopenia (3% to 5%; grades 3/4: 1%)

Local: Phlebitis (7% to 10%)

Neuromuscular & skeletal: Loss of deep tendon reflexes (<5%), myalgia (<5%), arthralgia (<5%), jaw pain (<5%)

Otic: Ototoxicity (≤1%)

Respiratory: Dyspnea (7%)

<1% (Limited to important or life-threatening): Abdominal pain, allergic reactions, anaphylaxis, angioedema, back pain, DVT, dysphagia, esophagitis, flushing, gait instability, headache, hemolytic uremic syndrome, hemorrhagic cystitis, hyper-/hypotension, hyponatremia, intestinal necrosis, intestinal obstruction, intestinal perforation, interstitial pulmonary changes, local rash, local urticaria, MI (rare), mucositis, muscle weakness, myocardial ischemia, pancreatitis, paralytic ileus, pneumonia, pruritus, pulmonary edema, pulmonary embolus, radiation recall (dermatitis, esophagitis), skin blistering, syndrome of inappropriate ADH secretion, tachycardia, thromboembolic events, thrombotic thrombocytopenic purpura, tumor pain, urticaria, vasodilation

Drug Interactions

Metabolism/Transport Effects Substrate of CYP2D6 (minor), CYP3A4 (major); **Note:** Assignment of Major/Minor substrate status based on clinically relevant drug interaction potential; **Inhibits** CYP2D6 (weak), CYP3A4 (weak)

Avoid Concomitant Use

Avoid concomitant use of Vinorelbine with any of the following: BCG; CloZAPine; Conivaptan; Natalizumab; Pimecrolimus; Pimozide; Tacrolimus (Topical); Vaccines (Live)

Increased Effect/Toxicity

Vinorelbine may increase the levels/effects of: CloZAPine; Leflunomide; MitoMYcin; Natalizumab; Pimozide; Vaccines (Live)

The levels/effects of Vinorelbine may be increased by: CISplatin; Conivaptan; CYP3A4 Inhibitors (Moderate); CYP3A4 Inhibitors (Strong); Dasatinib; Denosumab; Gefitinib; Itraconazole; Macrolide Antibiotics; PACLitaxel; PACLitaxel (Protein Bound); Pimecrolimus; Posaconazole; Roflumilast; Tacrolimus (Topical); Trastuzumab; Voriconazole

Decreased Effect

Vinorelbine may decrease the levels/effects of: BCG; Coccidioidin Skin Test; Sipuleucel-T; Vaccines (Inactivated); Vaccines (Live)

The levels/effects of Vinorelbine may be decreased by: CYP3A4 Inducers (Strong); Deferasirox; Echinacea; Herbs (CYP3A4 Inducers); Peginterferon Alfa-2b; Tocilizumab

Ethanol/Nutrition/Herb Interactions Herb/Nutraceutical: Avoid St John's wort (may decrease vinorelbine levels).

Stability Store intact vials under refrigeration at 2°C to 8°C (36°F to 46°F); do not freeze. Protect from light. Intact vials are stable at room temperature of 25°C (77°F) for up to 72 hours. Dilute in D_5W or NS to a final concentration of 1.5-3 mg/mL (for syringe) or 0.5-2 mg/mL (for I.V. bag). Dilutions in D_5W or NS are stable for 24 hours at room temperature. Vinorelbine should **NOT** be prepared during the preparation of any intrathecal medications. After preparation, store vinorelbine in a location **away** from the separate storage location recommended for intrathecal medications.

Mechanism of Action Semisynthetic vinca alkaloid which binds to tubulin and inhibits microtubule formation, therefore, arresting the cell at metaphase by disrupting the formation of the mitotic spindle; it is specific for the M and S phases. Vinorelbine may also interfere with nucleic acid and protein synthesis by blocking glutamic acid utilization.

Pharmacodynamic"..."ics

Absorption: Unreliable; must be given I.V.

Distribution: V_d: 25-40 L/kg; binds extensively to human platelets and lymphocytes (80% to 91%)

Protein binding: 80% to 91%

Metabolism: Extensively hepatic, via CYP3A4, to two metabolites, deacetylvinorelbine (active) and vinorelbine N-oxide

Bioavailability: Oral (not approved in the U.S.): 26% to 45%

Half-life elimination: Triphasic: Terminal: 28-44 hours

Excretion: Feces (46%); urine (18%, 10% to 12% as unchanged drug)

Clearance: Plasma: Mean: 0.97-1.26 L/hour/kg

Dosage Details concerning dosing in combination regimens should also be consulted.

I.V.: Adults:

NSCLC:

Single-agent therapy: 30 mg/m²/dose every 7 days

Combination therapy with cisplatin: 25-30 mg/m²/dose every 7 days (in combination with cisplatin)

Breast cancer (unlabeled use): 25 mg/m²/dose every 7 days (Zelek, 2001)

Cervical cancer (unlabeled use): 30 mg/m²/dose days 1 and 8 of a 21-day treatment cycle (Muggia, 2004; Muggia, 2005)

Malignant pleural mesothelioma (unlabeled use): 30 mg/m²/dose (maximum dose: 60 mg) every 7 days for 6 weeks (Stebbing, 2009) **or** 30 mg/m²/dose (maximum dose: 60 mg) every 7 days for 6 weeks, off 2 weeks, then repeat cycle (Muers, 2008)

Ovarian cancer (unlabeled use): 25 mg/m²/dose every 7 days (Bajetta, 1996) **or** 30 mg/m²/dose days 1 and 8 of a 21-day treatment cycle (Rothenberg, 2004)

Soft tissue sarcoma (unlabeled use; in combination with gemcitabine): 25 mg/m²/dose days 1 and 8 of a 21-day treatment cycle (Dileo, 2007)

Dosage adjustment in hematological toxicity: Granulocyte counts should be ≥1000 cells/mm³ prior to the administration of vinorelbine. Adjustments in the dosage of vinorelbine should be based on granulocyte counts obtained on the day of treatment as follows:

Granulocytes ≥1500 cells/mm³ on day of treatment: Administer 100% of starting dose

Granulocytes 1000-1499 cells/mm³ on day of treatment: Administer 50% of starting dose

Granulocytes <1000 cells/mm³ on day of treatment: Do not administer. Repeat granulocyte count in one week; if 3 consecutive doses are held because granulocyte count is <1000 cells/mm³, discontinue vinorelbine.

For patients who, during treatment, have experienced fever and/or sepsis while granulocytopenic or had 2 consecutive weekly doses held due to granulocytopenia, subsequent doses of vinorelbine should be:

75% of starting dose for granulocytes ≥1500 cells/mm³

37.5% of starting dose for granulocytes 1000-1499 cells/mm³

Dosage adjustment for neurotoxicity: Neurotoxicity ≥grade 2: Discontinue treatment

Dosage adjustment in renal impairment: No adjustment is necessary.

Dosing adjustment in hepatic impairment: The FDA-approved labeling guidelines are as follows: Vinorelbine should be administered with caution in patients with hepatic insufficiency. In patients who develop hyperbilirubinemia during treatment with vinorelbine, the dose should be adjusted for total bilirubin as follows:

Serum bilirubin ≤2 mg/dL: Administer 100% of dose

Serum bilirubin 2.1-3 mg/dL: Administer 50% of dose

Serum bilirubin >3 mg/dL: Administer 25% of dose

Dosing adjustment in patients with concurrent hematologic toxicity and hepatic impairment: Administer the lower of the doses determined from the adjustment recommendations.

Administration FATAL IF GIVEN INTRATHECALLY. Administer as a direct intravenous push or rapid bolus, over 6-10 minutes (up to 30 minutes). Longer infusions may increase the risk of pain and phlebitis. Intravenous doses should be followed by at least 75-125 mL of saline or D_5W to reduce the incidence of phlebitis and inflammation. Assure proper needle or catheter position prior to administration.

Monitoring Parameters CBC with differential and platelet count, hepatic function tests; monitor for new-onset pulmonary symptoms (or worsening from baseline); monitor for neuropathy

Dosage Forms Excipient information presented when available (limited, particularly for generics); consult specific product labeling. [DSC] = Discontinued product

Injection, solution: 10 mg/mL (1 mL [DSC], 5 mL [DSC])

Injection, solution [preservative free]: 10 mg/mL (1 mL, 5 mL)

Navelbine®: 10 mg/mL (1 mL, 5 mL)

◆ **Vinorelbine Injection, USP (Can)** *see* Vinorelbine *on page 1793*

◆ **Vinorelbine Tartrate** *see* Vinorelbine *on page 1793*

◆ **Vinorelbine Tartrate for Injection (Can)** *see* Vinorelbine *on page 1793*

◆ **Viokase® (Can)** *see* Pancrelipase *on page 1285*

◆ **Viosterol** *see* Ergocalciferol *on page 610*

◆ **Viracept®** *see* Nelfinavir *on page 1185*

◆ **Viramune®** *see* Nevirapine *on page 1193*

◆ **Viramune® XR™** *see* Nevirapine *on page 1193*

◆ **Viramune® XR™** *see* Nevirapine *on page 1193*

◆ **Virazole®** *see* Ribavirin *on page 1479*

◆ **Viread®** *see* Tenofovir *on page 1645*

◆ **Viroptic®** *see* Trifluridine *on page 1738*

◆ **Viscoat®** *see* Sodium Chondroitin Sulfate and Sodium Hyaluronate *on page 1570*

◆ **Viscous Lidocaine** *see* Lidocaine (Topical) *on page 1009*

◆ **Visicol®** *see* Sodium Phosphates *on page 1573*

◆ **Visine-A® [OTC]** *see* Naphazoline and Pheniramine *on page 1177*

◆ **Visine® Advanced Allergy (Can)** *see* Naphazoline and Pheniramine *on page 1177*

◆ **Visken® (Can)** *see* Pindolol *on page 1355*

◆ **Vistaril®** *see* HydrOXYzine *on page 853*

◆ **Vistide®** *see* Cidofovir *on page 357*

◆ **Vistonuridine** *see* Uridine Triacetate *on page 1750*

◆ **Vita-C® [OTC]** *see* Ascorbic Acid *on page 149*

◆ **Vitamin C** *see* Ascorbic Acid *on page 149*

◆ **Vitamin D_3 and Alendronate** *see* Alendronate and Cholecalciferol *on page 62*

◆ **Vitamin D and Calcium Carbonate** *see* Calcium and Vitamin D *on page 265*

Vitamin A (VYE ta min aye)

Brand Names: U.S. A-25 [OTC]; A-Natural [OTC]; A-Natural-25 [OTC]; Aquasol A®

Index Terms Oleovitamin A

Pharmacologic Category Vitamin, Fat Soluble

Use Treatment and prevention of vitamin A deficiency; parenteral (I.M.) route is indicated when oral administration is not feasible or when absorption is insufficient (malabsorption syndrome)

Pregnancy Risk Factor A/X (dose exceeding RDA recommendation)

Dosage

RDA:

0-6 months: 400 mcg
7-12 months: 500 mcg
1-3 years: 300 mcg
4-8 years: 400 mcg
9-13 years: 600 mcg
Males >13 years: 900 mcg
Females >13 years: 700 mcg

Note: Retinol mcg equivalent (0.3 mcg retinol = 1 unit vitamin A)

Oral:

Treatment of measles or xerophthalmia (WHO, 1997): Administer once daily for 2 days; repeat with single dose in 2 weeks:

<6 months: 50,000 units
6 months to 12 months: 100,000 units
>1 year: 200,000 units

Note: Women of reproductive age with night blindness or Bitot's spots should receive ≤10,000 units daily or ≤25,000 units once weekly; if severe xerophthalmia, women may receive high-dose (ie, 200,000-unit regimen) regardless of pregnancy status.

Supplementation in patients at high risk for deficiency (eg, severe infectious disease, malnutrition) (WHO, 1997): Administer as a single dose; repeat every 4-6 months, but do not readminister within 30 days of previous dose:

<6 months: 50,000 units
6 months to 12 months: 100,000 units
>1 year: 200,000 units

Note: Pregnant women should receive 10,000 units daily or 25,000 units once weekly (WHO, 1997)

I.M.: Deficiency (manufacturer recommendation): **Note:** I.M. route is indicated when oral administration is not feasible or when absorption is insufficient (malabsorption syndrome):

Infants: 7500-15,000 units/day for 10 days
Children 1-8 years: 17,500-35,000 units/day for 10 days
Children >8 years and Adults: 100,000 units/day for 3 days, followed by 50,000 units/day for 2 weeks

Note: Follow-up therapy with an oral therapeutic multivitamin (containing additional vitamin A) is recommended:

Low Birth Weight Infants: Additional vitamin A is recommended, however, no dosage amount has been established.

Children ≤8 years: 5000-10,000 units/day for 2 months

Children >8 years and Adults: 10,000-20,000 units/day for 2 months

Additional Information Complete prescribing information for this medication should be consulted for additional detail.

Dosage Forms Excipient information presented when available (limited, particularly for generics); consult specific product labeling.

Capsule, oral:

A-25: 25,000 units

Capsule, softgel, oral: 10,000 units

A-Natural: 10,000 units [contains soybean oil]

A-Natural-25: 25,000 units [contains soybean oil]

Injection, solution:

Aquasol A®: 50,000 units/mL (2 mL) [contains polysorbate 80]

Tablet, oral: 10,000 units, 15,000 units

◆ **Vitamin A Acid** *see* Tretinoin (Topical) *on page 1731*

Vitamin A and Vitamin D

(VYE ta min aye & VYE ta min dee)

Brand Names: U.S. A and D® Original [OTC]; Baza® Clear [OTC]; Sween Cream® [OTC]

Index Terms Cod Liver Oil

Pharmacologic Category Topical Skin Product

Use Temporary relief of discomfort due to chapped skin, diaper rash, minor burns, abrasions, as well as irritations associated with ostomy skin care

Pregnancy Risk Factor B

Dosage Topical: Apply locally with gentle massage as needed

Additional Information Complete prescribing information for this medication should be consulted for additional detail.

Dosage Forms Excipient information presented when available (limited, particularly for generics); consult specific product labeling.

Capsule, softgel: Vitamin A 1250 int. units and vitamin D 135 int. units; vitamin A 1250 int. units and vitamin D 130 int. units; vitamin A 5,000 int. units and vitamin D 400 int. units; vitamin A 10,000 int. units and vitamin D 400 int. units; vitamin A 10,000 int. units and vitamin D 5000 int. units; vitamin A 25,000 int. units and vitamin D 1000 int. units

Cream:
- Sween Cream®: 2 g, 85 g, 184 g, 339 g [original]
- Sween Cream®: 57 g, 142 g [fresh scent]
- Sween Cream®: 57 g [fragrance free]

Ointment: 0.9 g, 5 g, 60 g, 120 g, 454 g [in lanolin-petrolatum base]
- A and D® Original: 45 g, 120 g, 454 g
- Baza® Clear: 50 g, 150 g, 240 g

Tablet: Vitamin A 10,000 int. units and vitamin D 400 int. units

◆ **Vitamin B_1** *see* Thiamine *on page 1669*
◆ **Vitamin B_2** *see* Riboflavin *on page 1483*
◆ **Vitamin B_3** *see* Niacin *on page 1195*
◆ **Vitamin B_3** *see* Niacinamide *on page 1197*
◆ **Vitamin B_6** *see* Pyridoxine *on page 1437*
◆ **Vitamin B_{12}** *see* Cyanocobalamin *on page 418*
◆ **Vitamin B_{12a}** *see* Hydroxocobalamin *on page 847*
◆ **Vitamin D2** *see* Ergocalciferol *on page 610*

Vitamin E (VYE ta min ee)

Brand Names: U.S. Alph-E [OTC]; Alph-E-Mixed [OTC]; Aqua Gem-E™ [OTC]; Aquasol E® [OTC]; d-Alpha Gems™ [OTC]; E-Gems® Elite [OTC]; E-Gems® Plus [OTC]; E-Gems® [OTC]; E-Gem® Lip Care [OTC]; E-Gem® [OTC]; Ester-E™ [OTC]; Gamma E-Gems® [OTC]; Gamma-E PLUS [OTC]; High Gamma Vitamin E Complete™ [OTC]; Key-E® Kaps [OTC]; Key-E® Powder [OTC]; Key-E® [OTC]

Index Terms *d*-Alpha Tocopherol; *dl*-Alpha Tocopherol

Pharmacologic Category Vitamin, Fat Soluble

Use Dietary supplement

Unlabeled Use To reduce the risk of bronchopulmonary dysplasia or retrolental fibroplasia in infants exposed to high concentrations of oxygen; prevention and treatment of tardive dyskinesia; prevention and treatment of hemolytic anemia secondary to vitamin E deficiency

Pregnancy Risk Factor A/C (dose exceeding RDA recommendation)

Dosage Vitamin E may be expressed as alpha-tocopherol equivalents (ATE), which refer to the biologically-active (R) stereoisomer content. Oral:

Recommended daily allowance (RDA):
- Infants (adequate intake; RDA not established):
  - ≤6 months: 4 mg
  - 7-12 months: 6 mg
- Children:
  - 1-3 years: 6 mg; upper limit of intake should not exceed 200 mg/day
  - 4-8 years: 7 mg; upper limit of intake should not exceed 300 mg/day
  - 9-13 years: 11 mg; upper limit of intake should not exceed 600 mg/day
  - 14-18 years: 15 mg; upper limit of intake should not exceed 800 mg/day
- Adults: 15 mg; upper limit of intake should not exceed 1000 mg/day
- Pregnant female:
  - ≤18 years: 15 mg; upper level of intake should not exceed 800 mg/day
  - 19-50 years: 15 mg; upper level of intake should not exceed 1000 mg/day
- Lactating female:
  - ≤18 years: 19 mg; upper level of intake should not exceed 800 mg/day
  - 19-50 years: 19 mg; upper level of intake should not exceed 1000 mg/day

Vitamin E deficiency:
- Children (with malabsorption syndrome): 1 unit/kg/day of water miscible vitamin E (to raise plasma tocopherol concentrations to the normal range within 2 months and to maintain normal plasma concentrations)
- Adults: 60-75 units/day

Prevention of vitamin E deficiency: Adults: 30 units/day

Cystic fibrosis, beta-thalassemia, sickle cell anemia may require higher daily maintenance doses:
- Children:
  - Cystic fibrosis: 100-400 units/day
  - Beta-thalassemia: 750 units/day
- Adults:
  - Sickle cell: 450 units/day
  - Tardive dyskinesia (unlabeled use): 1600 units/day

Additional Information Complete prescribing information for this medication should be consulted for additional detail.

Dosage Forms Excipient information presented when available (limited, particularly for generics); consult specific product labeling. [DSC] = Discontinued product

Capsule, oral: 400 int. units [DSC], 1000 int. units
- Key-E® Kaps: 200 int. units, 400 int. units [derived from or manufactured using soybean oil]

Capsule, liquid, oral: 400 int. units

Capsule, softgel, oral: 100 int. units, 200 int. units, 400 int. units, 600 int. units, 1000 int. units
- Alph-E: 200 int. units, 400 int. units
- Alph-E: 400 int. units [contains soybean oil]
- Alph-E: 1000 int. units
- Alph-E-Mixed: 200 int. units, 400 int. units
- Alph-E-Mixed: 1000 int. units [sugar free]
- Aqua Gem-E™: 200 int. units, 400 int. units
- d-Alpha Gems™: 400 int. units [derived from or manufactured using soybean oil]
- E-Gems®: 30 int. units, 100 int. units, 200 int. units, 400 int. units, 600 int. units, 800 int. units, 1000 int. units, 1200 int. units [derived from or manufactured using soybean oil]
- E-Gems® Elite: 400 int. units
- E-Gems® Plus: 200 int. units, 400 int. units, 800 int. units [derived from or manufactured using soybean oil]
- Ester-E™: 400 int. units
- Gamma E-Gems®: 90 int. units

Gamma-E PLUS: 200 int. units [contains soybean oil]
High Gamma Vitamin E Complete™: 200 int. units [contains soybean oil]
Cream, topical: 1000 int. units/120 g (120 g); 100 int. units/g (57 g, 60 g); 30,000 int. units/57 g (57 g)
Key-E®: 30 int. units/g (57 g, 120 g, 600 g)
Lip balm, topical:
E-Gem® Lip Care: 1000 int. units/tube [contains aloe, vitamin A]
Liquid, oral/topical: 1150 int. units/1.25 mL (30 mL, 60 mL, 120 mL)
Oil, oral/topical: 100 int. units/0.25 mL (74 mL)
Oil, oral/topical [drops]:
E-Gem®: 10 int. units/drop (15 mL, 60 mL)
Oil, topical:
Alph-E: 28,000 int. units/30 mL (30 mL)
Ointment, topical:
Key-E®: 30 int. units/g (57 g, 113 g, 500 g)
Powder, oral:
Key-E® Powder: (15 g, 75 g, 1000 g) [derived from or manufactured using soybean oil]
Solution, oral [drops]: 15 int. units/0.3 mL (30 mL)
Aquasol E®: 15 int. units/0.3 mL (12 mL, 30 mL)
Suppository, rectal/vaginal:
Key-E®: 30 int. units (12s, 24s) [contains coconut oil]
Tablet, oral: 100 int. units, 200 int. units, 400 int. units, 500 int. units
Key-E®: 200 int. units, 400 int. units [derived from or manufactured using soybean oil]

- ◆ **Vitamin G** *see* Riboflavin *on page 1483*
- ◆ **Vitamin K_1** *see* Phytonadione *on page 1351*
- ◆ **Vita-Respa®** *see* Folic Acid, Cyanocobalamin, and Pyridoxine *on page 749*
- ◆ **Vi Vaccine** *see* Typhoid Vaccine *on page 1746*
- ◆ **Vivactil®** *see* Protriptyline *on page 1430*
- ◆ **Vivaglobin® [DSC]** *see* Immune Globulin *on page 880*
- ◆ **Vivaglobin® (Can)** *see* Immune Globulin *on page 880*
- ◆ **Vivarin® [OTC]** *see* Caffeine *on page 259*
- ◆ **Vivelle-Dot®** *see* Estradiol (Systemic) *on page 627*
- ◆ **Vivitrol®** *see* Naltrexone *on page 1174*
- ◆ **Vivotif®** *see* Typhoid Vaccine *on page 1746*
- ◆ **VLB** *see* VinBLAStine *on page 1789*
- ◆ **VM-26** *see* Teniposide *on page 1644*
- ◆ **Volibris® (Can)** *see* Ambrisentan *on page 84*
- ◆ **Voltaren** *see* Diclofenac (Systemic) *on page 495*
- ◆ **Voltaren® (Can)** *see* Diclofenac (Systemic) *on page 495*
- ◆ **Voltaren Ophtha® (Can)** *see* Diclofenac (Ophthalmic) *on page 498*
- ◆ **Voltaren Ophthalmic®** *see* Diclofenac (Ophthalmic) *on page 498*
- ◆ **Voltaren Rapide® (Can)** *see* Diclofenac (Systemic) *on page 495*
- ◆ **Voltaren SR® (Can)** *see* Diclofenac (Systemic) *on page 495*
- ◆ **Voltaren®-XR** *see* Diclofenac (Systemic) *on page 495*
- ◆ **Voluven®** *see* Tetrastarch *on page 1663*
- ◆ **von Willebrand Factor/Factor VIII Complex** *see* Antihemophilic Factor/von Willebrand Factor Complex (Human) *on page 128*
- ◆ **Voraxaze** *see* Glucarpidase *on page 798*

Voriconazole (vor i KOE na zole)

Brand Names: U.S. VFEND®
Brand Names: Canada VFEND®
Index Terms UK109496

Pharmacologic Category Antifungal Agent, Oral; Antifungal Agent, Parenteral

Additional Appendix Information
Antifungal Agents *on page 1876*

Use Treatment of invasive aspergillosis; treatment of esophageal candidiasis; treatment of candidemia (in non-neutropenic patients); treatment of disseminated *Candida* infections of the skin and viscera; treatment of serious fungal infections caused by *Scedosporium apiospermum* and *Fusarium* spp (including *Fusarium solani*) in patients intolerant of, or refractory to, other therapy

Unlabeled Use Fungal infection prophylaxis in intermediate or high risk neutropenic cancer patients with myelodysplastic syndrome (MDS) or acute myelogenous leukemia (AML), neutropenic allogeneic hematopoietic stem cell recipients, and patients with significant graft-versus-host disease; empiric antifungal therapy (second-line) for persistent neutropenic fever

Pregnancy Risk Factor D

Pregnancy Considerations Voriconazole can cause fetal harm when administered to a pregnant woman. Voriconazole was teratogenic and embryotoxic in animal studies, and lowered plasma estradiol in animal models. Women of childbearing potential should use effective contraception during treatment. Should be used in pregnant woman only if benefit to mother justifies potential risk to the fetus.

Lactation Excretion in breast milk unknown/not recommended

Contraindications Hypersensitivity to voriconazole or any component of the formulation (cross-reaction with other azole antifungal agents may occur but has not been established, use caution); coadministration of CYP3A4 substrates which may lead to QT_c prolongation (cisapride, pimozide, or quinidine); coadministration with barbiturates (long acting), carbamazepine, efavirenz (with standard [eg, not adjusted] voriconazole and efavirenz doses), ergot derivatives, rifampin, rifabutin, ritonavir (≥800 mg/day), sirolimus, St John's wort

Warnings/Precautions Visual changes, including blurred vision, changes in visual acuity, color perception, and photophobia, are commonly associated with treatment; postmarketing cases of optic neuritis and papilledema (lasting >1 month) have also been reported. Patients should be warned to avoid tasks which depend on vision, including operating machinery or driving. Changes are reversible on discontinuation following brief exposure/treatment regimens (≤28 days).

Serious hepatic reactions (including hepatitis, cholestasis, and fulminant hepatic failure) have occurred during treatment, primarily in patients with serious concomitant medical conditions. However, hepatotoxicity has occurred in patients with no identifiable risk factors. Use caution in patients with pre-existing hepatic impairment (dose adjustment or discontinuation may be required).

Voriconazole tablets contain lactose; avoid administration in hereditary galactose intolerance, Lapp lactase deficiency, or glucose-galactose malabsorption. Suspension contains sucrose; use caution with fructose intolerance, sucrase-isomaltase deficiency, or glucose-galactose malabsorption. Avoid/limit use of intravenous formulation in patients with renal impairment; intravenous formulation contains excipient cyclodextrin (sulfobutyl ether beta-cyclodextrin), which may accumulate in renal insufficiency. Acute renal failure has been observed in severely ill patients; use with caution in patients receiving concomitant nephrotoxic medications. Anaphylactoid-type infusion-related reactions may occur with intravenous dosing. Consider discontinuation of infusion if reaction is severe.

Use caution in patients taking strong cytochrome P450 inducers, CYP2C9 inhibitors, and major 3A4 substrates (see Drug Interactions); consider alternative agents that avoid or lessen the potential for CYP-mediated interactions. QT interval prolongation has been associated with voriconazole use; rare cases of arrhythmia (including torsade de pointes), cardiac arrest, and sudden death have been reported, usually in seriously ill patients with comorbidities and/or risk factors (eg, prior cardiotoxic chemotherapy, cardiomyopathy, electrolyte imbalance, or concomitant QT_c-prolonging drugs). Use with caution in these patient populations; correct electrolyte abnormalities (eg, hypokalemia, hypomagnesemia, hypocalcemia) prior to initiating therapy. Do not infuse concomitantly with blood products or short-term concentrated electrolyte solutions, even if the two infusions are running in separate intravenous lines (or cannulas).

Rare cases of malignancy (melanoma, squamous cell carcinoma) have been reported in patients (mostly immunocompromised) with prior onset of severe photosensitivity reactions and exposure to long-term voriconazole therapy. Other serious exfoliative cutaneous reactions, including Stevens-Johnson syndrome, have also been reported. Patient should avoid strong, direct exposure to sunlight; may cause photosensitivity, especially with long-term use. Discontinue use in patients who develop an exfoliative cutaneous reaction or a skin lesion consistent with squamous cell carcinoma or melanoma. Periodic total body skin examinations should be performed, particularly with prolonged use.

Monitor pancreatic function in patients (children and adults) at risk for acute pancreatitis (eg, recent chemotherapy or hematopoietic stem cell transplantation); there have been postmarketing reports of pancreatitis in children.

Adverse Reactions

>10%:

- Central nervous system: Hallucinations (4% to 12%; auditory and/or visual and likely serum concentration-dependent)
- Ocular: Visual changes (dose related; photophobia, color changes, increased or decreased visual acuity, or blurred vision occur in ~21%)
- Renal: Creatinine increased (1% to 21%)

2% to 10%:

- Cardiovascular: Tachycardia (≤2%)
- Central nervous system: Fever (≤6%), chills (≤4%), headache (≤3%)
- Dermatologic: Rash (≤7%)
- Endocrine & metabolic: Hypokalemia (≤2%)
- Gastrointestinal: Nausea (1% to 5%), vomiting (1% to 4%)
- Hepatic: Alkaline phosphatase increased (4% to 5%), AST increased (2% to 4%), ALT increased (2% to 3%), cholestatic jaundice (1% to 2%)
- Ocular: Photophobia (2% to 3%)

<2% (Limited to important or life-threatening): Acute tubular necrosis, adrenal cortical insufficiency, allergic reaction, alopecia, anaphylactoid reaction, ataxia, atrial arrhythmia, atrial fibrillation, AV block, bigeminy, bone marrow depression, bone necrosis, bradycardia, brain edema, bundle branch block, cardiac arrest, cardiomegaly, cardiomyopathy, cerebral hemorrhage, cerebral ischemia, cerebrovascular accident, chest pain, CHF, cholecystitis, cholelithiasis, chromatopsia, color blindness, coma, cyanosis, delirium, dementia, depersonalization, depression, diabetes insipidus, diarrhea, DIC, discoid lupus erythematosus, duodenal ulcer perforation, DVT, dyspnea, edema, encephalopathy, endocarditis, erythema multiforme, exfoliative dermatitis, extrapyramidal symptoms, fixed drug eruption, gastrointestinal hemorrhage, glucose tolerance decreased, Guillain-Barré syndrome, hepatic failure, hepatitis, hydronephrosis, hypercholesterolemia, hypoxia, intestinal perforation, intracranial hypertension, lung edema, lymphadenopathy, lymphangitis, melanoma, MI, multiorgan failure, myasthenia, myopathy, nephritis, nephrosis, neuropathy, night blindness, nodal arrhythmia, oculogyric crisis, optic atrophy, optic neuritis, osteomalacia, osteoporosis, palpitation, pancreatitis, papilledema, paresthesia, peripheral edema, peritonitis, petechia, photosensitivity, pleural effusion, postural hypotension, pseudomembraneous colitis, pseudoporphyria, psychosis, pulmonary embolus, purpura, QT interval prolongation, renal failure (acute), respiratory distress syndrome, retinal hemorrhage, seizure, sepsis, spleen enlarged, squamous cell carcinoma, Stevens-Johnson syndrome, suicidal ideation, supraventricular extrasystoles, supraventricular tachycardia, syncope, thrombophlebitis, thrombotic thrombocytopenic purpura, toxic epidermal necrolysis, uremia, urinary retention, uveitis, vasodilation, ventricular arrhythmia, ventricular fibrillation, ventricular tachycardia, visual field defect

Drug Interactions

Metabolism/Transport Effects Substrate of CYP2C19 (major), CYP2C9 (major), CYP3A4 (minor); **Note:** Assignment of Major/Minor substrate status based on clinically relevant drug interaction potential; **Inhibits** CYP2C19 (weak), CYP2C9 (moderate), CYP3A4 (strong)

Avoid Concomitant Use

Avoid concomitant use of Voriconazole with any of the following: Alfuzosin; Artemether; Barbiturates; CarBAMazepine; Cisapride; Conivaptan; Crizotinib; Darunavir; Dofetilide; Dronedarone; Eplerenone; Ergot Derivatives; Everolimus; Fluconazole; Fluticasone (Oral Inhalation); Halofantrine; Lapatinib; Lopinavir; Lovastatin; Lumefantrine; Lurasidone; Nilotinib; Nisoldipine; Pimozide; QUEtiapine; QuiNIDine; QuiNINE; Ranolazine; Rifamycin Derivatives; Ritonavir; Rivaroxaban; RomiDEPsin; Salmeterol; Silodosin; Simvastatin; Sirolimus; St Johns Wort; Tamsulosin; Tetrabenazine; Thioridazine; Ticagrelor; Tolvaptan; Toremifene; Vandetanib; Vemurafenib; Ziprasidone

Increased Effect/Toxicity

Voriconazole may increase the levels/effects of: Alfentanil; Alfuzosin; Almotriptan; Alosetron; Antineoplastic Agents (Vinca Alkaloids); Aprepitant; ARIPiprazole; Benzodiazepines (metabolized by oxidation); Boceprevir; Bortezomib; Bosentan; Brentuximab Vedotin; Brinzolamide; Budesonide (Nasal); Budesonide (Systemic, Oral Inhalation); BusPIRone; Busulfan; Calcium Channel Blockers; CarBAMazepine; Carvedilol; Ciclesonide; Cilostazol; Cinacalcet; Cisapride; Colchicine; Conivaptan; Contraceptives (Estrogens); Contraceptives (Progestins); Corticosteroids (Orally Inhaled); Corticosteroids (Systemic); Crizotinib; CycloSPORINE; CycloSPORINE (Systemic); CYP2C9 Substrates; CYP3A4 Substrates; Diclofenac; Diclofenac (Systemic); Diclofenac (Topical); Dienogest; DOCEtaxel; Dofetilide; Dronedarone; Dutasteride; Eletriptan; Eplerenone; Ergot Derivatives; Erlotinib; Eszopiclone; Etravirine; Everolimus; FentaNYL; Fesoterodine; Fluticasone (Nasal); Fluticasone (Oral Inhalation); Fosaprepitant; Fosphenytoin; Gefitinib; GuanFACINE; Halofantrine; HMG-CoA Reductase Inhibitors; Ibuprofen; Iloperidone; Imatinib; Irinotecan; Ixabepilone; Lapatinib; Losartan; Lovastatin; Lumefantrine; Lurasidone; Macrolide Antibiotics; Maraviroc; Meloxicam; Methadone; MethylPREDNISolone; Nilotinib; Nisoldipine; OxyCODONE; Paricalcitol; Pazopanib; Phenytoin; Phosphodiesterase 5 Inhibitors; Pimecrolimus; Pimozide; Propafenone; Protease Inhibitors; QTc-Prolonging Agents; QuiNIDine; QuiNINE; Ramelteon; Ranolazine; Repaglinide; Reverse Transcriptase Inhibitors (Non-Nucleoside); Rifamycin Derivatives; Rivaroxaban; RomiDEPsin; Ruxolitinib; Salmeterol; Saxagliptin; Sildenafil; Silodosin; Simvastatin; Sirolimus; Solifenacin;

SORAfenib; Sulfonylureas; SUNItinib; Tacrolimus; Tacrolimus (Systemic); Tacrolimus (Topical); Tadalafil; Tamsulosin; Telaprevir; Tetrabenazine; Thioridazine; Ticagrelor; Tolterodine; Tolvaptan; Toremifene; Vandetanib; Vardenafil; Vemurafenib; Venlafaxine; Vilazodone; Vitamin K Antagonists; Ziprasidone; Zolpidem; Zuclopenthixol

The levels/effects of Voriconazole may be increased by: Alfuzosin; Artemether; Boceprevir; Chloramphenicol; Chloroquine; Ciprofloxacin; Ciprofloxacin (Systemic); Contraceptives (Estrogens); Contraceptives (Progestins); CYP2C19 Inhibitors (Moderate); CYP2C19 Inhibitors (Strong); CYP2C9 Inhibitors (Moderate); CYP2C9 Inhibitors (Strong); Etravirine; Fluconazole; Gadobutrol; Grapefruit Juice; Indacaterol; Lumefantrine; Macrolide Antibiotics; Nilotinib; Protease Inhibitors; Proton Pump Inhibitors; QUEtiapine; QuiNINE; Telaprevir

Decreased Effect

Voriconazole may decrease the levels/effects of: Amphotericin B; Prasugrel; Saccharomyces boulardii; Ticagrelor

The levels/effects of Voriconazole may be decreased by: Barbiturates; CarBAMazepine; CYP2C19 Inducers (Strong); CYP2C9 Inducers (Strong); Darunavir; Didanosine; Etravirine; Fosphenytoin; Lopinavir; Peginterferon Alfa-2b; Phenytoin; Reverse Transcriptase Inhibitors (Non-Nucleoside); Rifamycin Derivatives; Ritonavir; St Johns Wort; Sucralfate; Telaprevir; Tocilizumab

Ethanol/Nutrition/Herb Interactions

Food: May decrease voriconazole absorption. Oral voriconazole should be taken 1 hour before or 1 hour after a meal. Avoid grapefruit juice (may decrease voriconazole levels).

Herb/Nutraceutical: St John's wort may decrease voriconazole levels; concurrent use with voriconazole is contraindicated.

Stability

Powder for injection: Store at 15°C to 30°C (59°F to 86°F). Reconstitute 200 mg vial with 19 mL of sterile water for injection (use of automated syringe is not recommended). Resultant solution (20 mL) has a concentration of 10 mg/mL. Prior to infusion, must dilute to 0.5-5 mg/mL with NS, LR, D_5WLR, $D_5W^1/_2$NS, D_5W, D_5W with KCl 20 mEq, $^1/_2$NS, or D_5WNS. Do not dilute with 4.2% sodium bicarbonate infusion. Reconstituted solutions are stable for up to 24 hours under refrigeration at 2°C to 8°C (36°F to 46°F).

Powder for oral suspension: Store at 2°C to 8°C (36°F to 46°F). Add 46 mL of water to the bottle to make 40 mg/mL suspension. Reconstituted oral suspension may be stored at 15°C to 30°C (59°F to 86°F). Discard after 14 days.

Tablets: Store at 15°C to 30°C (59°F to 86°F).

Mechanism of Action Interferes with fungal cytochrome P450 activity (selectively inhibits 14-alpha-lanosterol demethylation), decreasing ergosterol synthesis (principal sterol in fungal cell membrane) and inhibiting fungal cell membrane formation.

Pharmacodynamics/Kinetics

Absorption: Well absorbed after oral administration; administration of crushed tablets is considered bioequivalent to whole tablets

Distribution: V_d: 4.6 L/kg

Protein binding: 58%

Metabolism: Hepatic, via CYP2C19 (major pathway) and CYP2C9 and CYP3A4 (less significant); saturable (may demonstrate nonlinearity)

Bioavailability: 96%

Half-life elimination: Variable, dose-dependent

Time to peak: Oral: 1-2 hours; 0.5 hours (crushed tablet)

Excretion: Urine (as inactive metabolites; <2% as unchanged drug)

Dosage

Usual dosage ranges:

Children <12 years: Dosage not established

Children ≥12 years and Adults:

Oral: 100-300 mg every 12 hours

I.V.: 6 mg/kg every 12 hours for 2 doses; followed by maintenance dose of 4 mg/kg every 12 hours

Indication-specific dosing:

Children >2 to <12 years:

Aspergillosis, invasive including disseminated and extrapulmonary infection in HIV-exposed/-positive patients: (unlabeled; CDC, 2009):

Oral: Loading dose: 8 mg/kg/dose (maximum: 400 mg/dose) every 12 hours for 2 doses on day 1, followed by maintenance dose of 7 mg/kg/dose (maximum: 200 mg/dose) every 12 hours for ≥12 weeks

I.V.: Loading dose: 6-8 mg/kg/dose (maximum: 400 mg/dose) every 12 hours for 2 doses on day 1, followed by maintenance dose of 7 mg/kg/dose (maximum: 200 mg/dose) every 12 hours for ≥12 weeks

Children ≥12 years and Adults:

Aspergillosis, invasive, including disseminated and extrapulmonary infection: Duration of therapy should be a minimum of 6-12 weeks or throughout period of immunosuppression (Walsh, 2008):

I.V.: Initial: Loading dose: 6 mg/kg every 12 hours for 2 doses; followed by maintenance dose of 4 mg/kg every 12 hours

Oral: Maintenance dose:

Manufacturer's recommendations:

Patients <40 kg: 100 mg every 12 hours; maximum 300 mg/day

Patients ≥40 kg: 200 mg every 12 hours; maximum: 600 mg/day

IDSA recommendations (Walsh, 2008): May consider oral therapy in place of I.V. with dosing of 4 mg/kg (rounded up to convenient tablet dosage form) every 12 hours; however, I.V. administration is preferred in serious infections since comparative efficacy with the oral formulation has not been established.

Scedosporiosis, fusariosis:

I.V.: Initial: Loading dose: 6 mg/kg every 12 hours for 2 doses; followed by maintenance dose of 4 mg/kg every 12 hours

Oral: Maintenance dose:

Patients <40 kg: 100 mg every 12 hours; maximum: 300 mg/day

Patients ≥40 kg: 200 mg every 12 hours; maximum: 600 mg/day

Candidemia and other deep tissue *Candida* infections: Treatment should continue for a minimum of 14 days following resolution of symptoms or following last positive culture, whichever is longer.

I.V.: Initial: Loading dose 6 mg/kg every 12 hours for 2 doses; followed by maintenance dose of 3-4 mg/kg every 12 hours

Oral:

Manufacturer's recommendations: Maintenance dose:

Patients <40 kg: 100 mg every 12 hours; maximum: 300 mg/day

Patients ≥40 kg: 200 mg every 12 hours; maximum: 600 mg/day

IDSA recommendations (Pappas, 2009): Initial: Loading dose: 400 mg every 12 hours for 2 doses; followed by 200 mg every 12 hours

Endophthalmitis, fungal (unlabeled use, Pappas, 2009): I.V.: 6 mg/kg every 12 hours for 2 doses, then 3-4 mg/kg every 12 hours

Esophageal candidiasis: Oral: Treatment should continue for a minimum of 14 days, and for at least 7 days following resolution of symptoms:

Patients <40 kg: 100 mg every 12 hours; maximum: 300 mg/day

Patients ≥40 kg: 200 mg every 12 hours; maximum: 600 mg/day

Dosage adjustment in patients unable to tolerate treatment:

I.V.: Dose may be reduced to 3 mg/kg every 12 hours

Oral: Dose may be reduced in 50 mg decrements to a minimum dosage of 200 mg every 12 hours in patients weighing ≥40 kg (100 mg every 12 hours in patients <40 kg)

Dosage adjustment in patients receiving concomitant CYP450 enzyme inducers or substrates:

Cyclosporine: Reduce cyclosporine dose by one-half and monitor closely; upon discontinuation of voriconazole, monitor cyclosporine concentrations and escalate the cyclosporine dose as needed

Efavirenz: Oral: Increase maintenance dose of voriconazole to 400 mg every 12 hours and reduce efavirenz dose to 300 mg once daily; upon discontinuation of voriconazole, return to the initial dose of efavirenz

Omeprazole: Reduce omeprazole dose by one-half in patients maintained on ≥40 mg/day of omeprazole

Phenytoin:

I.V.: Increase voriconazole maintenance dosage to 5 mg/kg every 12 hours

Oral: Increase voriconazole dose to 400 mg every 12 hours in patients ≥40 kg (200 mg every 12 hours in patients <40 kg)

Tacrolimus: Reduce tacrolimus dose by one-third and monitor closely; upon discontinuation of voriconazole, monitor tacrolimus concentrations and escalate the tacrolimus dose as needed.

Dosage adjustment in renal impairment: In patients with Cl_{cr} <50 mL/minute, accumulation of the intravenous vehicle (cyclodextrin) occurs. After initial I.V. loading dose, oral voriconazole should be administered to these patients, unless an assessment of the benefit:risk to the patient justifies the use of I.V. voriconazole. Monitor serum creatinine and change to oral voriconazole therapy when possible.

Oral: Poorly dialyzed; no supplemental dose or dosage adjustment necessary, including patients on intermittent hemodialysis, peritoneal dialysis, or continuous renal replacement therapy (eg, CVVHD).

Note: I.V. dosing **NOT** recommended since cyclodextrin vehicle is cleared at half the rate of voriconazole and may accumulate.

Dosage adjustment in hepatic impairment:

Mild-to-moderate hepatic dysfunction (Child-Pugh class A and B): Following standard loading dose, reduce maintenance dosage by 50%

Severe hepatic impairment: Should only be used if benefit outweighs risk; monitor closely for toxicity

Dietary Considerations Oral: Should be taken 1 hour before or 1 hour after a meal. Voriconazole tablets contain lactose; avoid administration in hereditary galactose intolerance, Lapp lactase deficiency, or glucose-galactose malabsorption. Suspension contains sucrose; use caution with fructose intolerance, sucrose-isomaltase deficiency, or glucose-galactose malabsorption.

Administration

Oral: Administer 1 hour before or 1 hour after a meal.

I.V.: Infuse over 1-2 hours (rate not to exceed 3 mg/kg/hour). Do not infuse concomitantly into same line or cannula with other drug infusions, including TPN.

Monitoring Parameters Hepatic function at initiation and during course of treatment; renal function; serum electrolytes (particularly calcium, magnesium and potassium) prior to therapy initiation; visual function (visual acuity, visual field and color perception) if treatment course continues >28 days; may consider obtaining voriconazole trough level in patients failing therapy or exhibiting signs of toxicity; pancreatic function (in patients at risk for acute pancreatitis); total body skin examination yearly (more frequently if lesions noted)

Dosage Forms Excipient information presented when available (limited, particularly for generics); consult specific product labeling.

Injection, powder for reconstitution:

VFEND®: 200 mg [contains cyclodextrin]

Powder for suspension, oral:

VFEND®: 40 mg/mL (70 mL) [contains sodium benzoate, sucrose; orange flavor]

Tablet, oral: 50 mg, 200 mg

VFEND®: 50 mg, 200 mg [contains lactose]

Vorinostat (vor IN oh stat)

Brand Names: U.S. Zolinza®

Brand Names: Canada Zolinza®

Index Terms SAHA; Suberoylanilide Hydroxamic Acid

Pharmacologic Category Antineoplastic Agent, Histone Deacetylase Inhibitor

Use Treatment of progressive, persistent, or recurrent cutaneous T-cell lymphoma (CTCL)

Pregnancy Risk Factor D

Pregnancy Considerations Animal studies have demonstrated adverse fetal effects, including fetal loss, decreased fetal weight, and skeletal malformation. There are no adequate and well-controlled studies in pregnant women. Inform patient of potential hazard if used during pregnancy or if pregnancy occurs during treatment.

Lactation Excretion in breast milk unknown/not recommended

Contraindications There are no contraindications listed within the FDA-approved manufacturer's labeling.

Canadian labeling: Hypersensitivity to vorinostat or any component of the formulation; severe hepatic impairment (total bilirubin ≥3 times ULN)

Warnings/Precautions Hazardous agent - use appropriate precautions for handling and disposal. Pulmonary embolism and deep vein thrombosis (DVT) have been reported; monitor. Use caution in patients with a history of thrombotic events. Dose-related thrombocytopenia and/or anemia may occur; may require dosage adjustments or discontinuation. QT_c prolongation has been observed; baseline and periodic ECGs were done in clinical trials (Duvic, 2007; Olsen, 2007). Correct electrolyte abnormalities prior to treatment and monitor and correct potassium, calcium, and magnesium levels during therapy. Use caution in patients with a history of QT_c prolongation or with medications known to prolong the QT interval. May cause hyperglycemia; monitor and use with caution in diabetics; may require diet and/or therapy modifications. Nausea, vomiting, and diarrhea may occur; antiemetics and antidiarrheals may be required; control pre-existing nausea and vomiting prior to treatment initiation; replace fluids and electrolytes to avoid dehydration. May cause dizziness or fatigue; caution patients about performing tasks which require mental alertness (eg, operating machinery or driving). Use with caution in patients with hepatic impairment (elimination is predominantly hepatic); in the Canadian labeling, use is not recommended in patients with moderate hepatic impairment (total bilirubin 1.5-3 times ULN) and is contraindicated in patients with severe hepatic impairment (total bilirubin >3 times ULN).

Adverse Reactions

>10%:

Cardiovascular: Peripheral edema (13%)

Central nervous system: Fatigue (52%), chills (16%), dizziness (15%), headache (12%), fever (11%)
Dermatologic: Alopecia (19%), pruritus (12%)
Endocrine & metabolic: Hyperglycemia (8% to 69%; grade 3: 5%), dehydration (1% to 16%)
Gastrointestinal: Diarrhea (52%), nausea (41%), taste alteration (28%), anorexia (24%), weight loss (21%), xerostomia (16%), constipation (15%), vomiting (15%), appetite decreased (14%)
Hematologic: Thrombocytopenia (26%; grades 3/4: 6%), anemia (14%; grades 3/4: 2%)
Neuromuscular & skeletal: Muscle spasm (20%)
Renal: Proteinuria (51%), creatinine increased (16% to 47%)
Respiratory: Cough (11%), upper respiratory infection (11%)

1% to 10%:
Cardiovascular: QT_c prolongation (3% to 4%)
Dermatologic: Squamous cell carcinoma (4%)
Respiratory: Pulmonary embolism (5%)

<1% (Limited to important or life-threatening): Abdominal pain, angioneurotic edema, blurred vision, chest pain, cholecystitis, deafness, diverticulitis, dysphagia, DVT, enterococcal infection, exfoliative dermatitis, gastrointestinal bleeding, gastrointestinal hemorrhage, Guillain-Barré syndrome, hemoptysis, hypertension, hypokalemia, hyponatremia, infection, lethargy, leukopenia, MI, neutropenia, pneumonia, renal failure, sepsis, spinal cord injury, streptococcal bacteremia, stroke (ischemic), syncope, T-cell lymphoma, tumor hemorrhage, ureteric obstruction, ureteropelvic junction obstruction, urinary retention, vasculitis, weakness

Drug Interactions

Metabolism/Transport Effects None known.

Avoid Concomitant Use

Avoid concomitant use of Vorinostat with any of the following: Artemether; CloZAPine; Dronedarone; Lumefantrine; Nilotinib; Pimozide; QUEtiapine; QuiNINE; Tetrabenazine; Thioridazine; Toremifene; Vandetanib; Vemurafenib; Ziprasidone

Increased Effect/Toxicity

Vorinostat may increase the levels/effects of: CloZAPine; Dronedarone; Pimozide; QTc-Prolonging Agents; QuiNINE; Tetrabenazine; Thioridazine; Toremifene; Vandetanib; Vemurafenib; Vitamin K Antagonists; Ziprasidone

The levels/effects of Vorinostat may be increased by: Alfuzosin; Artemether; Chloroquine; Ciprofloxacin; Ciprofloxacin (Systemic); Divalproex; Gadobutrol; Indacaterol; Lumefantrine; Nilotinib; QUEtiapine; QuiNINE; Valproic Acid

Decreased Effect There are no known significant interactions involving a decrease in effect.

Stability Store at 20°C to 25°C (68°F to 77°F); excursions permitted to 15°C to 30°C (59°F to 86°F).

Mechanism of Action Inhibition of histone deacetylase enzymes, HDAC1, HDAC2, HDAC3, and HDAC6, which catalyze acetyl group removal from protein lysine residues (including histones and transcription factors). Inhibition of histone deacetylase results in accumulation of acetyl groups, leading to alterations in chromatin structure and transcription factor activation causing termination of cell growth leading to cell death.

Pharmacodynamics/Kinetics
Protein binding: ~71%
Metabolism: Glucuronidated and hydrolyzed (followed by beta-oxidation) to inactive metabolites
Bioavailability: Fasting: ~43%
Half-life elimination: ~2 hours
Time to peak, plasma: With high-fat meal: ~4 hours (range: 2-10 hours)
Excretion: Urine: 52% (<1% as unchanged drug, ~52% as inactive metabolites)

Dosage Oral: Adults: Cutaneous T-cell lymphoma: 400 mg once daily (continue until disease progression or unacceptable toxicity)
Dosage adjustment for intolerance: Reduce dose to 300 mg once daily; may further reduce to 300 mg daily for 5 consecutive days per week
In clinical trials, treatment was withheld for grade 4 anemia or thrombocytopenia or other grade 3 or 4 drug related toxicity, until resolved to ≤grade 1. Therapy was reinitiated with dose modification (Olsen, 2007).

Dosage adjustment in renal impairment: Not studied, however, based on the minimal renal elimination, adjustment not required.

Dosage adjustment in hepatic impairment: Not studied; use caution based on predominant hepatic metabolism.
Canadian labeling (not in the FDA-approved labeling):
Moderate hepatic impairment (total bilirubin 1.5-3 times ULN): Use is not recommended
Severe hepatic impairment (total bilirubin >3 times ULN): Use is contraindicated

Dietary Considerations Take with food.

Administration Administer with food. Do not open, crush, or chew capsules. Maintain adequate hydration (≥2 L/day fluids) during treatment.

Monitoring Parameters CBC with differential and serum chemistries, including calcium, magnesium, potassium, glucose and creatinine (baseline, then every 2 weeks for 2 months, then monthly), fluid status. Baseline and periodic ECGs were done in clinical trials.

Dosage Forms Excipient information presented when available (limited, particularly for generics); consult specific product labeling.
Capsule, oral:
Zolinza®: 100 mg

Extemporaneous Preparations Hazardous agent: Use appropriate precautions for handling and disposal.

Although not recommended by the manufacturer, a 50 mg/mL oral suspension may be prepared with capsules. Add 20 mL Ora-Plus® into a glass bottle (≥4 oz). Add the contents of twenty 100 mg capsules and shake thoroughly to disperse (may take up to 3 minutes). Add 20 mL Ora-Sweet® and shake to disperse. Label "shake well". Stable for 14 days at room temperature.

Fouladi M, Park JR, Stewart CF, et al, "Pediatric Phase I Trial and Pharmacokinetic Study of Vorinostat: A Children's Oncology Group Phase I Consortium Report," *J Clin Oncol*, 2010, 28(22):3623-9.

◆ **VoSoL®** *see* Acetic Acid *on page 33*
◆ **VoSol® HC** *see* Acetic Acid, Propylene Glycol Diacetate, and Hydrocortisone *on page 33*
◆ **VoSpire ER®** *see* Albuterol *on page 52*
◆ **Votrient™** *see* Pazopanib *on page 1302*
◆ **VP-16** *see* Etoposide *on page 669*
◆ **VP-16-213** *see* Etoposide *on page 669*
◆ **VPRIV™** *see* Velaglucerase Alfa *on page 1778*
◆ **VRT111950** *see* Telaprevir *on page 1631*
◆ **Vumon®** *see* Teniposide *on page 1644*
◆ **VWF/FVIII Concentrate** *see* Antihemophilic Factor/von Willebrand Factor Complex (Human) *on page 128*
◆ **VWF:RCo** *see* Antihemophilic Factor/von Willebrand Factor Complex (Human) *on page 128*
◆ **vWF:RCof** *see* Antihemophilic Factor/von Willebrand Factor Complex (Human) *on page 128*
◆ **VX-950** *see* Telaprevir *on page 1631*
◆ **Vyloma™ (Can)** *see* Imiquimod *on page 879*
◆ **Vytone** *see* Iodoquinol and Hydrocortisone *on page 921*
◆ **Vytorin®** *see* Ezetimibe and Simvastatin *on page 681*
◆ **Vyvanse®** *see* Lisdexamfetamine *on page 1019*

◆ **Vyvanse™ (Can)** *see* Lisdexamfetamine *on page 1019*

◆ **VZIG** *see* Varicella-Zoster Immune Globulin (Human) *on page 1774*

◆ **VZV Vaccine (Varicella)** *see* Varicella Virus Vaccine *on page 1773*

◆ **VZV Vaccine (Zoster)** *see* Zoster Vaccine *on page 1830*

Warfarin (WAR far in)

Brand Names: U.S. Coumadin®; Jantoven®

Brand Names: Canada Apo-Warfarin®; Coumadin®; Mylan-Warfarin; Novo-Warfarin; Taro-Warfarin

Index Terms Warfarin Sodium

Pharmacologic Category Anticoagulant, Coumarin Derivative; Vitamin K Antagonist

Use Prophylaxis and treatment of thromboembolic disorders (eg, venous, pulmonary) and embolic complications arising from atrial fibrillation or cardiac valve replacement; adjunct to reduce risk of systemic embolism (eg, recurrent MI, stroke) after myocardial infarction

Unlabeled Use Prevention of recurrent transient ischemic attacks

Pregnancy Risk Factor D (women with mechanical heart valves)/X (other indications)

Pregnancy Considerations Warfarin crosses the placenta; concentrations in the fetal plasma are similar to maternal values. Teratogenic effects have been reported following first trimester exposure and may include coumarin embryopathy (nasal hypoplasia and/or stippled epiphyses; limb hypoplasia may also be present). Adverse events to the fetus have also been observed following second and third trimester exposure and may include CNS abnormalities (including ventral midline dysplasia, dorsal midline dysplasia). Spontaneous abortion and fetal death may also occur. Use is contraindicated during pregnancy (or in women of reproductive potential) except in women with mechanical heart valves who are at high risk for thromboembolism,; use is also contraindicated in women with threatened abortion, eclampsia, or preeclampsia. Frequent pregnancy tests are recommended for women who are planning to become pregnant and adjusted dose heparin or low molecular weight heparin should be substituted as soon as pregnancy is confirmed. In pregnant women with high-risk mechanical heart valves, the benefits of warfarin therapy should be discussed with the risks of available treatments; when possible avoid warfarin use during the first trimester and close to delivery (Bates 2008).

Lactation Does not enter breast milk/use caution (AAP rates "compatible"; AAP 2001 update pending)

Medication Guide Available Yes

Contraindications Hypersensitivity to warfarin or any component of the formulation; hemorrhagic tendencies (eg, patients bleeding from the GI, respiratory, or GU tract; cerebral aneurysm; cerebrovascular hemorrhage; dissecting aortic aneurysm; spinal puncture and other diagnostic or therapeutic procedures with potential for significant bleeding; history of bleeding diathesis); recent or potential surgery of the eye or CNS; major regional lumbar block anesthesia or traumatic surgery resulting in large, open surfaces; blood dyscrasias; severe uncontrolled or malignant hypertension; pericarditis or pericardial effusion; bacterial endocarditis; unsupervised patients with conditions associated with a high potential for noncompliance; eclampsia/pre-eclampsia, threatened abortion, pregnancy (except in women with mechanical heart valves at high risk for thromboembolism)

Warnings/Precautions Hazardous agent - use appropriate precautions for handling and disposal. Use care in the selection of patients appropriate for this treatment. Ensure patient cooperation especially from the alcoholic, illicit drug user, demented, or psychotic patient; ability to comply with routine laboratory monitoring is essential. Use with caution in trauma, acute infection, moderate-severe renal insufficiency, prolonged dietary insufficiencies, moderate-severe hypertension, polycythemia vera, vasculitis, open wound, active TB, any disruption in normal GI flora, history of PUD, anaphylactic disorders, indwelling catheters, severe diabetes, and menstruating and postpartum women. Use with caution in patients with thyroid disease; warfarin responsiveness may increase (Ansell, 2008). Use with caution in protein C deficiency. Use with caution in patients with heparin-induced thrombocytopenia and DVT. Warfarin monotherapy is contraindicated in the initial treatment of active HIT. Reduced liver function, regardless of etiology, may impair synthesis of coagulation factors leading to increased warfarin sensitivity.

[U.S. Boxed Warning]: May cause major or fatal bleeding. Risk factors for bleeding include high intensity anticoagulation (INR >4), age (>65 years), variable INRs, history of GI bleeding, hypertension, cerebrovascular disease, serious heart disease, anemia, malignancy, trauma, renal insufficiency, drug-drug interactions, long duration of therapy, or known genetic deficiency in CYP2C9 activity. Patient must be instructed to report bleeding, accidents, or falls. Unrecognized bleeding sites (eg, colon cancer) may be uncovered by anticoagulation. Patient must also report any new or discontinued medications, herbal or alternative products used, or significant changes in smoking or dietary habits. Necrosis or gangrene of the skin and other tissue can occur, usually in conjunction with protein C or S deficiency. Consider alternative therapies if anticoagulation is necessary. Warfarin therapy may release atheromatous plaque emboli; symptoms depend on site of embolization, most commonly kidneys, pancreas, liver, and spleen. In some cases may lead to necrosis or death. "Purple toes syndrome," due to cholesterol microembolization, may rarely occur. The elderly may be more sensitive to anticoagulant therapy.

Presence of the CYP2C9*2 or *3 allele and/or polymorphism of the vitamin K oxidoreductase (VKORC1) gene may increase the risk of bleeding. Lower doses may be required in these patients; genetic testing may help determine appropriate dosing.

Adverse Reactions Bleeding is the major adverse effect of warfarin. Hemorrhage may occur at virtually any site. Risk is dependent on multiple variables, including the intensity of anticoagulation and patient susceptibility.

Cardiovascular: Vasculitis

Central nervous system: Signs/symptoms of bleeding (eg, dizziness, fatigue, fever, headache, lethargy, malaise, pain)

Dermatologic: Alopecia, bullous eruptions, dermatitis, rash, pruritus, urticaria

Gastrointestinal: Abdominal pain, diarrhea, flatulence, gastrointestinal bleeding, nausea, taste disturbance, vomiting

Genitourinary: Hematuria

Hematologic: Anemia, retroperitoneal hematoma, unrecognized bleeding sites (eg, colon cancer) may be uncovered by anticoagulation

Hepatic: Hepatitis (including cholestatic hepatitis), transaminases increased

Neuromuscular & skeletal: Osteoporosis (potential association with long-term use), paralysis, paresthesia, weakness

Respiratory: Respiratory tract bleeding, tracheobronchial calcification

Miscellaneous: Anaphylactic reaction, hypersensitivity/allergic reactions, skin necrosis, gangrene, "purple toes" syndrome

Drug Interactions

Metabolism/Transport Effects **Substrate** of CYP1A2 (minor), CYP2C19 (minor), CYP2C9 (major), CYP3A4 (minor); **Note:** Assignment of Major/Minor substrate status based on clinically relevant drug interaction potential; **Inhibits** CYP2C19 (weak), CYP2C9 (weak)

Avoid Concomitant Use

Avoid concomitant use of Warfarin with any of the following: Rivaroxaban; Tamoxifen

Increased Effect/Toxicity

Warfarin may increase the levels/effects of: Anticoagulants; Collagenase (Systemic); Deferasirox; Drotrecogin Alfa (Activated); Ethotoin; Fosphenytoin; Phenytoin; Rivaroxaban

The levels/effects of Warfarin may be increased by: Acetaminophen; Allopurinol; Amiodarone; Androgens; Antineoplastic Agents; Antiplatelet Agents; Atazanavir; Bicalutamide; Boceprevir; Capecitabine; Cephalosporins; Chloral Hydrate; Chloramphenicol; Cimetidine; Clopidogrel; Corticosteroids (Systemic); Cranberry; CYP2C9 Inhibitors (Moderate); CYP2C9 Inhibitors (Strong); Desvenlafaxine; Dexmethylphenidate; Disulfiram; Dronedarone; Efavirenz; Erythromycin (Ophthalmic); Esomeprazole; Ethacrynic Acid; Ethotoin; Etoposide; Exenatide; Fenofibrate; Fenofibric Acid; Fenugreek; Fibric Acid Derivatives; Fluconazole; Fluorouracil; Fluorouracil (Systemic); Fluorouracil (Topical); Fosamprenavir; Fosphenytoin; Gefitinib; Ginkgo Biloba; Glucagon; Green Tea; Herbs (Anticoagulant/Antiplatelet Properties); HMG-CoA Reductase Inhibitors; Ifosfamide; Imatinib; Itraconazole; Ivermectin; Ketoconazole; Ketoconazole (Systemic); Lansoprazole; Leflunomide; Macrolide Antibiotics; Methylphenidate; MetroNIDAZOLE; MetroNIDAZOLE (Systemic); Miconazole (Oral); Miconazole (Topical); Milnacipran; Mirtazapine; Nelfinavir; Neomycin; NSAID (COX-2 Inhibitor); NSAID (Nonselective); Omega-3-Acid Ethyl Esters; Omeprazole; Orlistat; Penicillins; Pentosan Polysulfate Sodium; Pentoxifylline; Phenytoin; Posaconazole; Propafenone; Prostacyclin Analogues; QuiNIDine; QuiNINE; Quinolone Antibiotics; Ranitidine; RomiDEPsin; Salicylates; Saquinavir; Selective Serotonin Reuptake Inhibitors; Sitaxentan; SORAfenib; Sulfinpyrazone [Off Market]; Sulfonamide Derivatives; Tamoxifen; Telaprevir; Tetracycline Derivatives; Thrombolytic Agents; Thyroid Products; Tigecycline; Tolterodine; Toremifene; Torsemide; TraMADol; Tricyclic Antidepressants; Venlafaxine; Vitamin E; Voriconazole; Vorinostat; Zafirlukast; Zileuton

Decreased Effect

The levels/effects of Warfarin may be decreased by: Aminoglutethimide; Antineoplastic Agents; Antithyroid Agents; Aprepitant; AzaTHIOprine; Barbiturates; Bile Acid Sequestrants; Boceprevir; Bosentan; CarBAMazepine; Coenzyme Q-10; Contraceptives (Estrogens); Contraceptives (Progestins); CYP2C9 Inducers (Strong); Cyproterone; Darunavir; Dicloxacillin; Efavirenz; Fosaprepitant; Ginseng (American); Glutethimide; Green Tea; Griseofulvin; Lopinavir; Mercaptopurine; Nafcillin; Nelfinavir; Peginterferon Alfa-2b; Phytonadione; Rifamycin Derivatives; Ritonavir; St Johns Wort; Sucralfate; Telaprevir; Tocilizumab

Ethanol/Nutrition/Herb Interactions

Ethanol: Avoid ethanol. Acute ethanol ingestion (binge drinking) decreases the metabolism of warfarin and increases PT/INR. Chronic daily ethanol use increases the metabolism of warfarin and decreases PT/INR.

Food: The anticoagulant effects of warfarin may be decreased if taken with foods rich in vitamin K. Vitamin E may increase warfarin effect. Cranberry juice may increase warfarin effect.

Herb/Nutraceutical: Cranberry, fenugreek, ginkgo biloba, glucosamine, may enhance bleeding or increase warfarin's effect. Ginseng (American), coenzyme Q_{10}, and St John's wort may decrease warfarin levels and effects. Avoid alfalfa, anise, bilberry, bladderwrack, bromelain, cat's claw, celery, chamomile, coleus, cordyceps, dong quai, evening primrose oil, fenugreek, feverfew, garlic, ginger, ginkgo biloba, ginseng (American), ginseng (Panax), ginseng (Siberian), grapeseed, green tea, guggul, horse chestnut seed, horseradish, licorice, omega-3-acids, prickly ash, red clover, reishi, SAMe (s-adenosylmethionine), sweet clover, turmeric, and white willow (all have additional antiplatelet activity).

Stability

Injection: Prior to reconstitution, store at 15°C to 30°C (59°F to 86°F). Following reconstitution with 2.7 mL of sterile water (yields 2 mg/mL solution), stable for 4 hours at 15°C to 30°C (59°F to 86°F). Protect from light.

Tablet: Store at 15°C to 30°C (59°F to 86°F). Protect from light.

Mechanism of Action Hepatic synthesis of coagulation factors II, VII, IX, and X, as well as proteins C and S, requires the presence of vitamin K. These clotting factors are biologically activated by the addition of carboxyl groups to key glutamic acid residues within the proteins' structure. In the process, "active" vitamin K is oxidatively converted to an "inactive" form, which is then subsequently reactivated by vitamin K epoxide reductase complex 1 (VKORC1). Warfarin competitively inhibits the subunit 1 of the multi-unit VKOR complex, thus depleting functional vitamin K reserves and hence reduces synthesis of active clotting factors.

Pharmacodynamics/Kinetics

Onset of action: Anticoagulation: Oral: 24-72 hours

Peak effect: Full therapeutic effect: 5-7 days; INR may increase in 36-72 hours

Duration: 2-5 days

Absorption: Oral: Rapid, complete

Distribution: 0.14 L/kg

Protein binding: 99%

Metabolism: Hepatic, primarily via CYP2C9; minor pathways include CYP2C8, 2C18, 2C19, 1A2, and 3A4

Genomic variants: Approximately 37% reduced clearance of S-warfarin in patients heterozygous for 2C9 (*1/*2 or *1/*3), and ~70% reduced in patients homozygous for reduced function alleles (*2/*2, *2/*3, or *3/*3)

Half-life elimination: 20-60 hours; Mean: 40 hours; highly variable among individuals

Time to peak, plasma: Oral: ~4 hours

Excretion: Urine (92%, primarily as metabolites)

Dosage Note: Labeling identifies genetic factors which may increase patient sensitivity to warfarin. Specifically, genetic variations in the proteins CYP2C9 and VKORC1, responsible for warfarin's primary metabolism and pharmacodynamic activity, respectively, have been identified as predisposing factors associated with decreased dose requirement and increased bleeding risk. Genotyping tests are available, and may provide important guidance on initiation of anticoagulant therapy.

Oral:

Infants and Children (unlabeled use): Initial loading dose (if baseline INR is 1-1.3): 0.2 mg/kg (maximum: 10 mg/dose); adjust dose based on INR (reported ranges to maintain INR of 2-3: 0.09-0.33 mg/kg/day). Infants <12 months of age may require doses at or near the high end of this range; consistent anticoagulation may be difficult to maintain in children <5 years of age (Monagle, 2008).

Adults: Initial dosing must be individualized. Consider the patient (hepatic function, cardiac function, age, nutritional status, concurrent therapy, risk of bleeding) in addition to prior dose response (if available) and the clinical situation. Start 2-5 mg daily for 2 days **or** 5-10 mg daily for 1-2 days (Ansell, 2008). Adjust dose according to INR results; usual maintenance dose ranges from 2-10 mg daily (individual patients may require loading and maintenance doses outside these general guidelines).

Note: Lower starting doses may be required for patients with hepatic impairment, poor nutrition, CHF, elderly, high risk of bleeding, or patients who are debilitated, or those with reduced function genomic variants of the catabolic enzymes CYP2C9 (*2 or *3 alleles) or VKORC1 (-1639 polymorphism); see table. Higher initial doses may be reasonable in selected patients (ie, receiving enzyme-inducing agents and with low risk of bleeding).

Range[1] of Expected Therapeutic Maintenance Dose Based on CYP2C9[2] and VKORC1[3] Genotypes

VKOR-C1	CYP2C9					
	*1/*1	*1/*2	*1/*3	*2/*2	*2/*3	*3/*3
GG	5-7 mg	5-7 mg	3-4 mg	3-4 mg	3-4 mg	0.5-2 mg
AG	5-7 mg	3-4 mg	3-4 mg	3-4 mg	0.5-2 mg	0.5-2 mg
AA	3-4 mg	3-4 mg	0.5-2 mg	0.5-2 mg	0.5-2 mg	0.5-2 mg

Note: Must also take into account other patient related factors when determining initial dose (eg, age, body weight, concomitant medications, comorbidities).

[1]Ranges derived from multiple published clinical studies.

[2]Patients with CYP2C9 *1/*3, *2/*2, *2/*3, and *3/*3 alleles may take up to 4 weeks to achieve maximum INR with a given dose regimen.

[3]VKORC1 -1639G>A (rs 9923231) variant is used in this table; other VKORC1 variants may also be important determinants of dose.

I.V.: Adults: 2-5 mg/day administered as a slow bolus injection

Dosing adjustment in renal disease: No adjustment required, however, patients with renal failure have an increased risk of bleeding complications. Monitor closely.

Dosing adjustment in hepatic disease: Monitor effect at usual doses; the response to oral anticoagulants may be markedly enhanced in obstructive jaundice (due to reduced vitamin K absorption) and also in hepatitis and cirrhosis (due to decreased production of vitamin K-dependent clotting factors); INR should be closely monitored

Dietary Considerations Foods high in vitamin K (eg, beef liver, pork liver, green tea, and leafy green vegetables) inhibit anticoagulant effect. Do not change dietary habits once stabilized on warfarin therapy. A balanced diet with a consistent intake of vitamin K is essential. Avoid large amounts of alfalfa, asparagus, broccoli, Brussels sprouts, cabbage, cauliflower, green teas, kale, lettuce, spinach, turnip greens, and watercress; decreased efficacy of warfarin. It is recommended that the diet contain a CONSISTENT vitamin K content of 70-140 mcg/day. Check with healthcare provider before changing diet.

Administration

Oral: Administer with or without food. Take at the same time each day.

I.V.: Administer as a slow bolus injection over 1-2 minutes; avoid all I.M. injections

Monitoring Parameters Prothrombin time, hematocrit, INR; consider genotyping of CYP2C9 and VKORC1 prior to initiation of therapy, if available

Reference Range

INR = patient prothrombin time/mean normal prothrombin time

ISI = international sensitivity index

INR should be increased by 2-3.5 times depending upon indication. An INR >4 does not generally add additional therapeutic benefit and is associated with increased risk of bleeding. **Note:** To prevent gastrointestinal bleeding events in patients receiving the combination of warfarin, aspirin, and clopidogrel, an INR of 2-2.5 is recommended unless condition requires a higher INR target (eg, certain mechanical heart valves) (Bhatt, 2008).

Adult Target INR Ranges Based Upon Indication

Indication	Targeted INR	Targeted INR Range
Cardiac		
Acute myocardial infarction (high risk)[1,2,3]	2.5	2-3
Atrial fibrillation or atrial flutter	2.5	2-3
Valvular		
Bileaflet or Medtronic Hall tilting disk mechanical aortic valve in normal sinus rhythm and normal LA size	2.5	2-3
Bileaflet or tilting disk mechanical mitral valve	3	2.5-3.5
Caged ball or caged disk mechanical valve	3	2.5-3.5
Mechanical prosthetic valve with systemic embolism despite adequate anticoagulation[4]	3 or 3.5	2.5-3.5 **or** 3-4
Mechanical valve and risk factors for thromboembolism (eg, AF, MI[5], LA enlargement, hypercoagulable state, low EF) or history of atherosclerotic vascular disease[6]	3	2.5-3.5
Bioprosthetic mitral valve[7]	2.5	2-3
Bioprosthetic mitral or aortic valve with prior history of systemic embolism[7]	2.5	2-3
Bioprosthetic mitral or aortic valve with evidence of LA thrombus at surgery[8]	2.5	2-3
Bioprosthetic mitral or aortic valve with risk factors for thromboembolism (eg, AF, hypercoagulable state or low EF)[9]	2.5	2-3
Prosthetic mitral valve thrombosis (resolved)[3]	4	3.5-4.5
Prosthetic aortic valve thrombosis (resolved)[3]	3.5	3-4
Rheumatic mitral valve disease and normal sinus rhythm (LA diameter >5.5 cm), AF, previous systemic embolism, or LA thrombus	2.5	2-3
Thromboembolism Treatment		
Venous thromboembolism[10,11]	2.5	2-3
Thromboprophylaxis		
Chronic thromboembolic pulmonary hypertension (CTPH)	2.5	2-3
Idiopathic pulmonary artery hypertension (IPAH)[12]	2	1.5-2.5
Lupus inhibitor (no other risk factors)	2.5	2-3
Lupus inhibitor and recurrent thromboembolism	3	2.5-3.5
Major trauma patients with impaired mobility undergoing rehabilitation	2.5	2-3
Spinal cord injury (acute) undergoing rehabilitation	2.5	2-3
Total hip or knee replacement (elective) or hip fracture surgery[13]	2.5	2-3
Other Indications		
Cerebral venous sinus thrombosis[14]	2.5	2-3
Ischemic stroke due to AF	2.5	2-3

[1]High-risk includes large anterior MI, significant heart failure, intracardiac thrombus, atrial fibrillation, history of thromboembolism.

[2]Maintain anticoagulation for 3 months.

[3]Combine with aspirin 81 mg/day.

[4]Combine with aspirin 81 mg/day, if not previously receiving, **and/or** if previous target INR was 2.5, then new target INR should be 3 (2.5-3.5). If previous target INR was 3, then new target INR should be 3.5 (3-4).

[5]MI refers to anterior-apical ST-segment elevation myocardial infarction.

[6]Combine with aspirin 81 mg/day unless patient is at high risk of bleeding (eg, history of GI bleed, age >80 years).

[7]Maintain anticoagulation for 3 months after valve insertion then switch to aspirin 81 mg/day if no other indications for warfarin exist or clinically reassess need for warfarin in patients with prior history of systemic embolism.

[8]Maintain anticoagulation with warfarin until thrombus resolution.

[9]If patient has history of atherosclerotic vascular disease, combine with aspirin 81 mg/day unless patient is at high risk of bleeding (eg, history of GI bleed, age >80 years).

[10]Treat for 3 months in patients with VTE due to transient reversible risk factor. Treat for a minimum of 3 months in patients with unprovoked VTE and evaluate for long term therapy. Other risk groups (eg, cancer) may require >3 months of therapy.

[11]In patients with unprovoked VTE who prefer less frequent INR monitoring, low-intensity therapy (INR range: 1.5-1.9) with less frequent monitoring is recommended over stopping treatment.

[12]Recommendation from the ACCF/AHA 2009 Expert Consensus Document on Pulmonary Hypertension (McLaughlin, 2009)

[13]Continue for at least 10 days and up to 35 days after surgery.

[14]Continue for up to 12 months.

Warfarin levels are not used for monitoring degree of anticoagulation. They may be useful if a patient with unexplained coagulopathy is using the drug surreptitiously or if it is unclear whether clinical resistance is due to true drug resistance or lack of drug intake.

Normal prothrombin time (PT): 10.9-12.9 seconds. Healthy premature newborns have prolonged coagulation test screening results (eg, PT, aPTT, TT) which return to normal adult values at approximately 6 months of age. Healthy prematures, however, do not develop spontaneous hemorrhage or thrombotic complications because of a balance between procoagulants and inhibitors.

Additional Information Prospective genotyping is available, and may provide important guidance on initiation of anticoagulant therapy. Commercial testing with PGxPredict™: WARFARIN is available from PGxHealth™ (Division of Clinical Data, Inc, New Haven, CT). The test genotypes patients for presence of the CYP2C9*2 or *3 alleles and the VKORC1 -1639G>A polymorphism. The results of the test allow patients to be phenotyped as extensive, intermediate, or poor metabolizers (CYP2C9) and as low, intermediate, or high warfarin sensitivity (VKORC1). Ordering information is available at 888-592-7327 or warfarininfo@pgxhealth.com.

Dosage Forms Excipient information presented when available (limited, particularly for generics); consult specific product labeling.

Injection, powder for reconstitution, as sodium:
- Coumadin®: 5 mg

Tablet, oral, as sodium: 1 mg, 2 mg, 2.5 mg, 3 mg, 4 mg, 5 mg, 6 mg, 7.5 mg, 10 mg
- Coumadin®: 1 mg, 2 mg, 2.5 mg, 3 mg, 4 mg, 5 mg, 6 mg, 7.5 mg [scored]
- Coumadin®: 10 mg [scored; dye free]
- Jantoven®: 1 mg, 2 mg, 2.5 mg, 3 mg, 4 mg, 5 mg, 6 mg, 7.5 mg [scored]
- Jantoven®: 10 mg [scored; dye free]

◆ **Warfarin Sodium** *see* Warfarin *on page* 1802

◆ **Wax Away [OTC]** *see* Carbamide Peroxide *on page* 283

◆ **4-Way® Saline Moisturizing Mist [OTC]** *see* Sodium Chloride *on page* 1567

◆ **Welchol®** *see* Colesevelam *on page* 408

◆ **Wellbutrin®** *see* BuPROPion *on page* 247

◆ **Wellbutrin XL®** *see* BuPROPion *on page* 247

◆ **Wellbutrin® XL (Can)** *see* BuPROPion *on page* 247

◆ **Wellbutrin SR®** *see* BuPROPion *on page* 247

◆ **Wellbutrin® SR (Can)** *see* BuPROPion *on page* 247

◆ **Westcort®** *see* Hydrocortisone (Topical) *on page* 841

◆ **Westhroid™** *see* Thyroid, Desiccated *on page* 1676

Wheat Dextrin (weet DEKS trin)

Brand Names: U.S. Benefiber® Plus Calcium [OTC]; Benefiber® [OTC]

Index Terms Dextrin; Resistant Dextrin; Resistant Maltodextrin

Pharmacologic Category Fiber Supplement; Laxative, Bulk-Producing

Additional Appendix Information

Laxatives, Classification and Properties *on page* 1893

Use OTC labeling: Dietary fiber supplement

Unlabeled Use Treatment of constipation; aid to enhance LDL lowering to reduce the risk of coronary heart disease

Dosage Oral: General dosing guidelines; consult specific product labeling.

Adequate intake for total fiber: **Note:** The definition of "fiber" varies; however, the soluble fiber in wheat dextrin is only one type of fiber which makes up the daily recommended intake of total fiber.
- Children 1-3 years: 19 g/day
- Children 4-8 years: 25 g/day
- Children 9-13 years: Male: 31 g/day; Female: 26 g/day
- Children 14-18 years: Male: 38 g/day; Female: 26 g/day
- Adults 19-50 years: Male: 38 g/day; Female: 25 g/day
- Adults ≥51 years: Male: 30 g/day; Female: 21 g/day
- Pregnancy: 28 g/day
- Lactation: 29 g/day

Additional Information Complete prescribing information for this medication should be consulted for additional detail.

Dosage Forms Excipient information presented when available (limited, particularly for generics); consult specific product labeling.

Caplet, oral:
- Benefiber®: 1.3 g [gluten free, sugar free; provides dietary fiber 3 g and soluble fiber 3 g per 3 caplets]

Powder, oral:
- Benefiber®: (80 g, 155 g, 245 g, 350 g, 477 g) [gluten free, sugar free; original flavor]
- Benefiber®: (161 g, 267 g, 529 g) [gluten free, sugar free; contains aspartame; orange flavor]
- Benefiber®: 3.5 g/packet (28s) [gluten free, sugar free; original flavor; provides dietary fiber 3 g and soluble fiber 3 g per packet]
- Benefiber®: 3.5 g/packet (16s) [sugar free; contains phenylalanine; kiwi-strawberry flavor; provides dietary fiber 3 g and soluble fiber 3 g per packet]
- Benefiber®: 3.5 g/packet (8s) [sugar free; contains phenylalanine; raspberry tea flavor; provides dietary fiber 3 g and soluble fiber 3 g per packet]
- Benefiber®: 3.5 g/packet (8s) [sugar free; contains phenylalanine, sodium 20 mg/packet; cherry-pomegranate flavor; provides dietary fiber 3 g and soluble fiber 3 g per packet]
- Benefiber®: 3.5 g/packet (16s) [sugar free; contains phenylalanine, soy; citrus punch flavor; provides dietary fiber 3 g and soluble fiber 3 g per packet]
- Benefiber® Plus Calcium: (424 g) [gluten free, sugar free]

Tablet, chewable, oral:
- Benefiber®: 2.7 g [gluten free, sugar free; contains phenylalanine, soy; assorted fruit flavor; provides dietary fiber 3 g and soluble fiber 3 g per 3 tablets]
- Benefiber®: 2.7 g [gluten free, sugar free; contains phenylalanine, soy; orange créme flavor; provides dietary fiber 3 g and soluble fiber 3 g per 3 tablets]
- Benefiber® Plus Calcium: 2.7 g [gluten free, sugar free; contains calcium 100 mg/tablet, phenylalanine, soy; wildberry flavor; provides dietary fiber 3 g and soluble fiber 3 g per 3 tablets]

◆ **Wilate®** *see* Antihemophilic Factor/von Willebrand Factor Complex (Human) *on page* 128

◆ **Winpred™ (Can)** *see* PredniSONE *on page* 1399

◆ **WinRho® SDF** *see* Rh_o(D) Immune Globulin *on page* 1476

◆ **Wound Wash Saline™ [OTC]** *see* Sodium Chloride *on page* 1567

◆ **WR-2721** *see* Amifostine *on page* 85

◆ **WR-139007** *see* Dacarbazine *on page* 438

◆ **WR-139013** *see* Chlorambucil *on page* 337

◆ **WR-139021** *see* Carmustine *on page* 293

◆ **Wycillin [DSC]** *see* Penicillin G Procaine *on page* 1325

◆ **Wycillin® (Can)** *see* Penicillin G Procaine *on page* 1325

Yellow Fever Vaccine (YEL oh FEE ver vak SEEN)

Brand Names: U.S. YF-VAX®

Brand Names: Canada YF-VAX®

Pharmacologic Category Vaccine, Live (Viral)

Use Induction of active immunity against yellow fever virus, primarily among persons traveling or living in areas where yellow fever infection exists and laboratory workers who may be exposed to the virus; vaccination may also be required for some international travelers

The Advisory Committee on Immunization Practices (ACIP) recommends vaccination for:

- Persons traveling to or living in areas at risk for yellow fever transmission
- Persons traveling to countries which require vaccination for international travel
- Laboratory personnel who may be exposed to the yellow fever virus or concentrated preparations of the vaccine

Although the vaccine is approved for use in children ≥9 months of age, the CDC recommends use in children as young as 6 months under unusual circumstances (eg, travel to an area where exposure is unavoidable). Children <6 months of age should **never** receive the vaccine.

Pregnancy Risk Factor C

Pregnancy Considerations Animal reproduction studies have not been conducted. Adverse events were not observed in the mother or fetus following vaccination during the third trimester of pregnancy in Nigerian women; however, maternal seroconversion was reduced. Inadvertent exposure early in the first trimester of pregnancy in Brazilian women did not show decreased maternal seroconversion; no major congenital abnormalities were noted. Cord blood from an infant whose mother was vaccinated during the first trimester tested positive for IgM antibodies; no adverse events were noted in the infant. Vaccine should be administered if travel to an endemic area is unavoidable and the infant should be monitored after birth. Tests to verify maternal immune response may be considered. If a pregnant woman is to be vaccinated only to satisfy an international requirement (as opposed to decreasing risk of infection), efforts should be made to obtain a waiver letter. Women should wait 4 weeks after receiving vaccine before conceiving.

Lactation Enters breast milk/contraindicated

Contraindications Hypersensitivity to egg or chick embryo protein, or any component of the formulation; children <9 months of age (per manufacturer); children <6 months of age (CDC guidelines); acute or febrile disease; immunosuppressed patients (eg HIV infection, leukemia, lymphoma, thymic disease, generalized malignancy, or immunosuppression due to drugs or radiation); breast-feeding women

Warnings/Precautions Patients who are immunosuppressed have a theoretical risk of encephalitis with yellow fever vaccine administration; consider delaying travel or obtaining a waiver letter. Patients on low-dose or short-term corticosteroids are not considered immunosuppressed and may be offered the vaccine. If vaccination is only to satisfy an international requirement (as opposed to decreasing risk of infection), efforts should be made to obtain a waiver letter. Per the ACIP guidelines, use is contraindicated in patients with symptomatic HIV infection or patients with CD4+ counts <200/mm^3 (or <15% of total lymphocytes in children <6 years of age); use caution when administering the vaccine to patients with asymptomatic infection with CD4+ counts 200-499/mm^3 (or 15% to 24% of total lymphocytes in children <6 years of age). In general, household and close contacts of persons with altered immunocompetence may receive all age appropriate vaccines.

Immediate treatment (including epinephrine 1:1000) for anaphylactoid and/or hypersensitivity reactions should be available during vaccine use.

Chicken embryos are used in the manufacture of this vaccine. Use is contraindicated in patients with immediate-type hypersensitivity reactions to eggs; in general, persons who are able to eat eggs or egg products may receive the vaccine. A hypersensitivity screening test and desensitization procedure is available for persons with suspected or known severe egg sensitivity. Consult manufacturer's labeling for details. The vial stopper contains latex; product may contain gelatin. Immunization should be delayed during the course of an acute or febrile illness. The presence of a low-grade fever is generally not a reason to postpone vaccination. Due to an increased incidence of serious adverse events observed in older adults compared to younger adults, use with caution in the elderly ≥65 years (per manufacturer) or ≥60 years (per ACIP guidelines), particularly in patients who have not previously received the vaccine. The risk for vaccine-associated neurologic disease (YEL-AND) and vaccine-associated viscerotropic disease (YEL-AVD) is also increased. The ACIP guidelines note that if travel is unavoidable, the decision to vaccinate travelers ≥60 years should be made after weighing the risks vs benefits. Avoid use in pregnant women unless travel to high-risk areas is unavoidable. The manufacturer contraindicates use in infants <9 months of age due to risk of encephalitis. The CDC allows for use in infants 6-8 months of age when possible exposure with the yellow fever virus is unavoidable and the risk of infection exists. Infants <6 months of age should never be vaccinated. In order to maximize vaccination rates, the ACIP recommends simultaneous administration of all age-appropriate vaccines (live or inactivated) for which a person is eligible at a single clinic visit, unless contraindications exist.

Adverse Reactions All serious adverse reactions must be reported to the U.S. Department of Health and Human Services (DHHS) Vaccine Adverse Event Reporting System (VAERS) 1-800-822-7967 or online at https://vaers.hhs.gov/esub/index. In Canada, adverse reactions may be reported to local provincial/territorial health agencies or to the Vaccine Safety Section at Public Health Agency of Canada (1-866-844-0018).

Frequency not defined (adverse reactions may be increased in patients <9 months or ≥60 years of age)

- Central nervous system: Chills, fever (incidence of these reactions have been reported to be as low as <5% and as high as 10% to 30% depending on the study), focal neurological defects, headache, malaise, seizure
- Dermatologic: Rash, urticaria
- Local: Injection site reactions (edema, erythema, hypersensitivity, mass, pain, pruritus, rash, warmth)
- Neuromuscular & skeletal: Myalgia, weakness
- Miscellaneous: Guillain-Barré syndrome (GBS), hypersensitivity (immediate), vaccine-associated neurotropic disease (rare), viscerotropic disease (rare; may be associated with multiorgan failure)
  - Vaccine-associated neurologic disease (YEL-AND) may manifest as meningoencephalitis (neurotropic disease), GBS, acute disseminated encephalomyelitis, and bulbar palsy. Vaccine-associated viscerotropic disease (YEL-AVD) mimics naturally-acquired yellow fever disease; risk may be increased in older patients and those with a history of thymus disease or thymectomy.

Drug Interactions

Metabolism/Transport Effects None known.

Avoid Concomitant Use

Avoid concomitant use of Yellow Fever Vaccine with any of the following: Belimumab; Fingolimod; Immunosuppressants

Increased Effect/Toxicity

The levels/effects of Yellow Fever Vaccine may be increased by: AzaTHIOprine; Belimumab; Corticosteroids (Systemic); Fingolimod; Hydroxychloroquine; Immunosuppressants; Leflunomide; Mercaptopurine; Methotrexate

Decreased Effect

Yellow Fever Vaccine may decrease the levels/effects of: Tuberculin Tests

The levels/effects of Yellow Fever Vaccine may be decreased by: Fingolimod; Immunosuppressants

Stability Store at 2°C to 8°C (35°F to 46°F); do not freeze. Reconstitute only with diluent provided. Inject diluent slowly into vial and allow to stand for 1-2 minutes. Gently swirl until a uniform suspension forms; swirl well before withdrawing dose. Avoid vigorous shaking to prevent foaming of suspension. Vaccine must be used within 60 minutes of reconstitution. Keep suspension refrigerated until used.

Pharmacodynamics/Kinetics

Onset of action: Seroconversion: 10-14 days

Duration: ≥30 years

Dosage SubQ:

- Children ≥6 months (unlabeled use [CDC guidelines]): One dose (0.5 mL) ≥10 days before travel; Booster: Every 10 years for those at continued risk of exposure
- Children ≥9 months (per manufacturer) and Adults: One dose (0.5 mL) ≥10 days before travel; Booster: Every 10 years for those at continued risk of exposure
- Elderly: Monitor closely due to an increased incidence of serious adverse events in patients ≥60 years of age, particularly in patients receiving their first dose. The ACIP guidelines note that if travel is unavoidable, the decision to vaccinate travelers ≥60 years should be made after weighing the risks vs benefits.

Administration For SubQ injection only. Do not administer I.M. or I.V.; if inadvertently administered I.M., the dose does not need repeated. Use of expired vaccine is not considered a valid dose and should be repeated after 28 days. For booster doses, if the date of previous vaccination cannot be determined and the patient requires vaccination, the booster dose can be given.

Blood donation following vaccine administration: Transfusion-related transmission of yellow fever vaccine virus has been reported; wait 2 weeks after immunization with yellow fever vaccine to donate blood.

Simultaneous administration of vaccines helps ensure the patients will be fully vaccinated by the appropriate age. Simultaneous administration of vaccines is defined as administering >1 vaccine on the same day at different anatomic sites. Separate vaccines should not be combined in the same syringe unless indicated by product specific labeling. Separate needles and syringes should be used for each injection. The ACIP prefers each dose of a specific vaccine in a series come from the same manufacturer when possible. Adolescents and adults should be vaccinated while seated or lying down. In general, preterm infants should be vaccinated at the same chronological age as full-term infants (CDC, 2011).

Antipyretics have not been shown to prevent febrile seizures. Antipyretics may be used to treat fever or discomfort following vaccination (CDC, 2011). One study reported that routine prophylactic administration of acetaminophen to prevent fever prior to vaccination decreased the immune response of some vaccines; the clinical significance of this reduction in immune response has not been established (Prymula, 2009).

Monitoring Parameters Monitor for syncope for ≥15 minutes following vaccination. Monitor for adverse effects 10 days after vaccination (specifically in the elderly).

Additional Information Federal law requires that the name of medication, date of administration, the vaccine manufacturer, lot number of vaccine, and the administering person's name, title, and address be entered into the patient's permanent medical record. Some countries require a valid International Certification of Vaccination or Prophylaxis (ICVP) showing receipt of vaccine. Certificate is valid beginning 10 days after and for 10 years following vaccination (booster doses received within 10 years are valid from the date of vaccination). The WHO requires revaccination every 10 years to maintain traveler's vaccination certificate. All travelers to endemic areas should be advised of the risks of yellow fever disease and all available methods to prevent it. All travelers should take protective measures to avoid mosquito bites.

The following CDC agencies may be contacted if serologic testing is needed or for advice when administering yellow fever vaccine to pregnant women, children <9 months, or patients with altered immune status:

Division of Vector-Borne Infectious Diseases: 970-221-6400

Division of Global Migration and Quarantine: 404-498-1600

Dosage Forms Excipient information presented when available (limited, particularly for generics); consult specific product labeling.

Injection, powder for reconstitution [17D-204 strain]:

YF-VAX®: ≥4.74 Log_{10} plaque-forming units (PFU) per 0.5 mL dose [single-dose or 5-dose vial; produced in chicken embryos; contains gelatin; packaged with diluent; vial stopper contains latex]

- ◆ **Yervoy™** *see* Ipilimumab *on page 921*
- ◆ **YF-VAX®** *see* Yellow Fever Vaccine *on page 1806*
- ◆ **YM087** *see* Conivaptan *on page 411*
- ◆ **YM905** *see* Solifenacin *on page 1578*
- ◆ **YM-08310** *see* Amifostine *on page 85*
- ◆ **Yodoxin®** *see* Iodoquinol *on page 921*
- ◆ **Z4942** *see* Ifosfamide *on page 867*
- ◆ **Zactima** *see* Vandetanib *on page 1767*
- ◆ **Zaditor® [OTC]** *see* Ketotifen (Ophthalmic) *on page 959*
- ◆ **Zaditor® (Can)** *see* Ketotifen (Ophthalmic) *on page 959*

Zafirlukast (za FIR loo kast)

Brand Names: U.S. Accolate®

Brand Names: Canada Accolate®

Index Terms ICI-204,219

Pharmacologic Category Leukotriene-Receptor Antagonist

Use Prophylaxis and chronic treatment of asthma in adults and children ≥5 years of age

Pregnancy Risk Factor B

Pregnancy Considerations There are no adequate and well-controlled trials in pregnant women. Teratogenic effects not observed in animal studies; fetal defects were observed when administered in maternally toxic doses.

Lactation Enters breast milk/contraindicated

Contraindications Hypersensitivity to zafirlukast or any component of the formulation; hepatic impairment

Warnings/Precautions Zafirlukast is not FDA approved for use in the reversal of bronchospasm in acute asthma attacks, including status asthmaticus. Therapy with zafirlukast can be continued during acute exacerbations of asthma.

Hepatic adverse events (including hepatitis, hyperbilirubinemia, and hepatic failure) have been reported; female patients may be at greater risk. Discontinue immediately if liver dysfunction is suspected. Periodic testing of liver function may be considered (early detection is generally believed to improve the likelihood of recovery). If hepatic dysfunction is suspected (due to clinical signs/symptoms), liver function tests should be measured immediately. Do not resume or restart if hepatic function studies are consistent with dysfunction. Use caution in patients with alcoholic cirrhosis; clearance is reduced. Postmarketing reports of behavioral changes (ie, depression, insomnia) have been noted. Monitor INR closely with concomitant warfarin use. Rare cases of eosinophilic vasculitis (Churg-Strauss) have been reported in patients receiving zafirlukast (usually, but not always, associated with reduction in concurrent steroid dosage). No causal relationship established. Monitor for eosinophilic vasculitis, rash, pulmonary symptoms, cardiac symptoms, or neuropathy.

An increased proportion of zafirlukast patients >55 years of age reported infections as compared to placebo-treated patients. These infections were mostly mild or moderate in intensity and predominantly affected the respiratory tract. Infections occurred equally in both sexes, were dose-proportional to total milligrams of zafirlukast exposure, and were associated with coadministration of inhaled corticosteroids.

Adverse Reactions

>10%: Central nervous system: Headache (13%)

1% to 10%:

Central nervous system: Dizziness (2%), pain (2%), fever (2%)

Gastrointestinal: Nausea (3%), diarrhea (3%), abdominal pain (2%), vomiting (2%), dyspepsia (1%)

Hepatic: ALT increased (2%)

Neuromuscular & skeletal: Back pain (2%), myalgia (2%), weakness (2%)

Miscellaneous: Infection (4%)

<1% (Limited to important or life-threatening): Agranulocytosis, angioedema, arthralgia, behavior/mood changes, bleeding, bruising, depression, edema, eosinophilia (systemic), eosinophilic pneumonia, hepatic failure, hepatitis, hyperbilirubinemia, hypersensitivity reactions, insomnia, malaise, pruritus, rash, suicidality, suicide, urticaria, vasculitis with clinical features of Churg-Strauss syndrome (rare)

Drug Interactions

Metabolism/Transport Effects Substrate of CYP2C9 (major); **Note:** Assignment of Major/Minor substrate status based on clinically relevant drug interaction potential; **Inhibits** CYP1A2 (weak), CYP2C19 (weak), CYP2C8 (weak), CYP2C9 (moderate), CYP2D6 (weak), CYP3A4 (weak)

Avoid Concomitant Use

Avoid concomitant use of Zafirlukast with any of the following: Pimozide

Increased Effect/Toxicity

Zafirlukast may increase the levels/effects of: Carvedilol; CYP2C9 Substrates; Pimozide; Theophylline Derivatives; Vitamin K Antagonists

The levels/effects of Zafirlukast may be increased by: CYP2C9 Inhibitors (Moderate); CYP2C9 Inhibitors (Strong)

Decreased Effect
The levels/effects of Zafirlukast may be decreased by: CYP2C9 Inducers (Strong); Erythromycin; Erythromycin (Systemic); Peginterferon Alfa-2b; Theophylline Derivatives

Ethanol/Nutrition/Herb Interactions Food: Decreases bioavailability of zafirlukast by 40%.

Stability Store tablets at controlled room temperature of 20°C to 25°C (68°F to 77°F). Protect from light and moisture; dispense in original airtight container.

Mechanism of Action Zafirlukast is a selectively and competitive leukotriene-receptor antagonist (LTRA) of leukotriene D4 and E4 (LTD4 and LTE4), components of slow-reacting substance of anaphylaxis (SRSA). Cysteinyl leukotriene production and receptor occupation have been correlated with the pathophysiology of asthma, including airway edema, smooth muscle constriction, and altered cellular activity associated with the inflammatory process, which contribute to the signs and symptoms of asthma.

Pharmacodynamics/Kinetics
Distribution: V_{dss}: 70 L
Protein binding: >99%, primarily to albumin
Metabolism: Extensively hepatic via CYP2C9
Bioavailability: Reduced 40% with food
Half-life elimination: 10 hours
Time to peak, serum: 3 hours
Excretion: Urine (10%); feces

Dosage Oral:
Children <5 years: Safety and effectiveness have not been established
Children 5-11 years: 10 mg twice daily
Children ≥12 years and Adults: 20 mg twice daily
Elderly: The mean dose (mg/kg) normalized AUC and C_{max} increase and plasma clearance decreases with increasing age. In patients >65 years of age, there is a two- to threefold greater C_{max} and AUC compared to younger adults.
Dosing adjustment in renal impairment: Dosage adjustment not required.
Dosing adjustment in hepatic impairment: Use is contraindicated.

Dietary Considerations Should be taken on an empty stomach (1 hour before or 2 hours after meals).

Administration Administer at least 1 hour before or 2 hours after a meal.

Monitoring Parameters Monitor for improvements in air flow; monitor closely for sign/symptoms of hepatic injury; periodic monitoring of LFTs may be considered (not proved to prevent serious injury, but early detection may enhance recovery)

Dosage Forms Excipient information presented when available (limited, particularly for generics); consult specific product labeling.
Tablet, oral: 10 mg, 20 mg
Accolate®: 10 mg, 20 mg

Zaleplon (ZAL e plon)

Brand Names: U.S. Sonata®

Pharmacologic Category Hypnotic, Nonbenzodiazepine

Use Short-term (7-10 days) treatment of insomnia (has been demonstrated to be effective for up to 5 weeks in controlled trial)

Pregnancy Risk Factor C

Pregnancy Considerations Not recommended for use during pregnancy

Lactation Enters breast milk/not recommended

Medication Guide Available Yes

Contraindications Hypersensitivity to zaleplon or any component of the formulation

Warnings/Precautions Symptomatic treatment of insomnia should be initiated only after careful evaluation of potential causes of sleep disturbance. Failure of sleep disturbance to resolve after 7-10 days may indicate psychiatric and/or medical illness.

Use with caution in patients with depression, particularly if suicidal risk may be present. Use with caution in patients with a history of drug dependence. Abrupt discontinuance may lead to withdrawal symptoms. Hypnotics/sedatives have been associated with abnormal thinking and behavior changes including decreased inhibition, aggression, bizarre behavior, agitation, hallucinations, and depersonalization. These changes may occur unpredictably and may indicate previously unrecognized psychiatric disorders; evaluate appropriately. May impair physical and mental capabilities. Patients must be cautioned about performing tasks which require mental alertness (operating machinery or driving). Amnesia can occur. Use with caution in patients receiving other CNS depressants or psychoactive medications. Effects with other sedative drugs or ethanol may be potentiated. Postmarketing studies have indicated that the use of hypnotic/sedative agents for sleep has been associated with hypersensitivity reactions including anaphylaxis as well as angioedema. An increased risk for hazardous sleep-related activities such as sleep-driving, cooking and eating food, and making phone calls while asleep have been noted.

Use with caution in the elderly, those with compromised respiratory function, or hepatic impairment (dosage adjustment recommended in mild-to-moderate hepatic impairment; avoid use in severe impairment). Because of the rapid onset of action, zaleplon should be administered immediately prior to bedtime or after the patient has gone to bed and is having difficulty falling asleep. Capsules contain tartrazine (FDC yellow #5); avoid in patients with sensitivity (caution in patients with asthma).

Adverse Reactions
>10%: Central nervous system: Headache (30% to 42%)
1% to 10%:
Cardiovascular: Chest pain (≥1%), peripheral edema (≤1%)
Central nervous system: Dizziness (7% to 9%), somnolence (5% to 6%), amnesia (2% to 4%), depersonalization (<1% to 2%), hypoesthesia (<1% to 2%), malaise (<1% to 2%), abnormal thinking (≥1%), anxiety (≥1%), depression (≥1%), fever (≥1%), migraine (≥1%), nervousness (≥1%), confusion (≤1%), hallucination (≤1%), vertigo (≤1%)
Dermatologic: Pruritus (≥1%), rash (≥1%), photosensitivity reaction (≤1%)
Endocrine & metabolic: Dysmenorrhea (3% to 4%)
Gastrointestinal: Nausea (6% to 8%), abdominal pain (6%), anorexia (<1% to 2%), constipation (≥1%), dyspepsia (≥1%), taste perversion (≥1%), xerostomia (≥1%), colitis (up to 1%)
Neuromuscular & skeletal: Weakness (5% to 7%), paresthesia (3%), tremor (2%), arthralgia (≥1%), arthritis (≥1%), back pain (≥1%), myalgia (≥1%), hypertonia (1%)
Ocular: Eye pain (3% to 4%), abnormal vision (<1% to 2%), conjunctivitis (≥1%)
Otic: Hyperacusis (1% to 2%), ear pain (≤1%)
Respiratory: Bronchitis (≥1%), epistaxis (≤1%)
Miscellaneous: Parosmia (<1% to 2%)
<1% (Limited to important or life-threatening): Alopecia, ALT increased, anaphylaxis, angioedema, anemia, angina, AST increased, ataxia, bigeminy, bilirubinemia, bleeding gums, bundle branch block, cardiospasm, cerebral ischemia, cholelithiasis, circumoral paresthesia, CNS stimulation; complex sleep-related behavior (sleep-driving, cooking or eating food, making phone calls); cyanosis, delusions, diabetes mellitus, duodenal

ulcer, dysarthria, dystonia, dysuria, ecchymosis, eosinophilia, facial paralysis, gastroenteritis, glaucoma, goiter, hematuria, hyper-/hypoglycemia, hyper-/hypotension, hyperuricemia, hypothyroidism, impotence, incontinence, intestinal obstruction, ketosis, lactose intolerance, leukocytosis, lymphocytosis, liver function tests (abnormal), lymphadenopathy, myasthenia, myositis, osteoporosis, palpitation, peptic ulcer, pericardial effusion, photophobia, ptosis, pulmonary embolus, purpura, rash, rectal bleeding, sinus bradycardia, substernal chest pain, syncope, thrombophlebitis, tongue edema, ulcerative stomatitis, urinary retention, ventricular tachycardia, vasodilation, ventricular extrasystoles

Drug Interactions

Metabolism/Transport Effects **Substrate** of CYP3A4 (minor); **Note:** Assignment of Major/Minor substrate status based on clinically relevant drug interaction potential

Avoid Concomitant Use There are no known interactions where it is recommended to avoid concomitant use.

Increased Effect/Toxicity

Zaleplon may increase the levels/effects of: Alcohol (Ethyl); CNS Depressants; Methotrimeprazine; Selective Serotonin Reuptake Inhibitors

The levels/effects of Zaleplon may be increased by: Cimetidine; Conivaptan; Droperidol; HydrOXYzine; Methotrimeprazine

Decreased Effect

The levels/effects of Zaleplon may be decreased by: Flumazenil; Rifamycin Derivatives; Tocilizumab

Ethanol/Nutrition/Herb Interactions

Ethanol: May increase CNS depression; monitor for increased effects with coadministration. Caution patients about effects.

Food: High fat meal prolonged absorption; delayed T_{max} by 2 hours, and reduced C_{max} by 35%.

Herb/Nutraceutical: St John's wort may decrease zaleplon levels. Avoid valerian, St John's wort, kava kava, gotu kola (may increase CNS depression).

Stability Store at controlled room temperature of 20°C to 25°C (68°F to 77°F). Protect from light.

Mechanism of Action Zaleplon is unrelated to benzodiazepines, barbiturates, or other hypnotics. However, it interacts with the benzodiazepine GABA receptor complex. Nonclinical studies have shown that it binds selectively to the brain omega-1 receptor situated on the alpha subunit of the GABA-A receptor complex.

Pharmacodynamics/Kinetics

Onset of action: Rapid

Absorption: Rapid and almost complete; high-fat meal delays absorption

Distribution: V_d: ~1.4 L/kg

Protein binding: ~45% to 75%

Metabolism: Extensive, primarily via aldehyde oxidase to form 5-oxo-zaleplon and, to a lesser extent, by CYP3A4 to desethylzaleplon; all metabolites are pharmacologically inactive

Bioavailability: ~30%

Half-life elimination: 1 hour

Time to peak, serum: 1 hour

Excretion: Urine (~70% primarily metabolites, <1% as unchanged drug); feces (~17%)

Clearance: Plasma: Oral: 3 L/hour/kg

Dosage Oral:

Adults: 10 mg at bedtime (range: 5-20 mg); has been used for up to 5 weeks of treatment in controlled trial setting

Elderly: 5 mg at bedtime; recommended maximum: 10 mg/day

Dosage adjustment in renal impairment: No adjustment for mild-to-moderate renal impairment; use in severe renal impairment has not been adequately studied

Dosage adjustment in hepatic impairment: Mild-to-moderate impairment: 5 mg; not recommended for use in patients with severe hepatic impairment

Dietary Considerations Avoid taking with or after a heavy, high-fat meal; reduces absorption.

Administration Immediately before bedtime or when the patient is in bed and cannot fall asleep

Additional Information Prescription quantities should not exceed a 1-month supply.

Dosage Forms Excipient information presented when available (limited, particularly for generics); consult specific product labeling.

Capsule, oral: 5 mg, 10 mg

Sonata®: 5 mg

Sonata®: 10 mg [contains tartrazine]

Controlled Substance C-IV

- **Zamicet™** *see* Hydrocodone and Acetaminophen *on page 837*
- **Zanaflex®** *see* TiZANidine *on page 1695*
- **Zanaflex Capsules®** *see* TiZANidine *on page 1695*

Zanamivir (za NA mi veer)

Brand Names: U.S. Relenza®

Brand Names: Canada Relenza®

Pharmacologic Category Antiviral Agent; Neuraminidase Inhibitor

Use Treatment of uncomplicated acute illness due to influenza virus A and B in patients who have been symptomatic for no more than 2 days; prophylaxis against influenza virus A and B

The Advisory Committee on Immunization Practices (ACIP) recommends that **treatment** be considered for the following:

- Persons with severe, complicated or progressive illness
- Hospitalized persons
- Persons at higher risk for influenza complications:
  - Children <2 years of age (highest risk in children <6 months of age)
  - Adults ≥65 years of age
  - Persons with chronic disorders of the pulmonary (including asthma) or cardiovascular systems (except hypertension)
  - Persons with chronic metabolic diseases (including diabetes mellitus), hepatic disease, renal dysfunction, hematologic disorders (including sickle cell disease), or immunosuppression (including immunosuppression caused by medications or HIV)
  - Persons with neurologic/neuromuscular conditions (including conditions such as spinal cord injuries, seizure disorders, cerebral palsy, stroke, mental retardation, moderate to severe developmental delay, or muscular dystrophy) which may compromise respiratory function, the handling of respiratory secretions, or that can increase the risk of aspiration
  - Pregnant or postpartum women (≤2 weeks after delivery)
  - Persons <19 years of age on long-term aspirin therapy
  - American Indians and Alaskan Natives
  - Persons who are morbidly obese (BMI ≥40)
  - Residents of nursing homes or other chronic care facilities
- Use may also be considered for previously healthy, nonhigh-risk outpatients with confirmed or suspected influenza based on clinical judgment when treatment can be started within 48 hours of illness onset.

The ACIP recommends that **prophylaxis** be considered for the following:

- Postexposure prophylaxis may be considered for family or close contacts of suspected or confirmed cases, who are at higher risk of influenza complications, and who have not been vaccinated against the circulating strain at the time of the exposure.
- Postexposure prophylaxis may be considered for unvaccinated healthcare workers who had occupational exposure without protective equipment.
- Pre-exposure prophylaxis should only be used for persons at very high risk of influenza complications who cannot be otherwise protected at times of high risk for exposure.
- Prophylaxis should also be administered to all eligible residents of institutions that house patients at high risk when needed to control outbreaks.

Pregnancy Risk Factor C

Pregnancy Considerations Adverse events were not observed in animal reproduction studies. Influenza infection may be more severe in pregnant women. Untreated influenza infection is associated with an increased risk of adverse events to the fetus and an increased risk of complications or death to the mother. Oseltamivir and zanamivir are currently recommended for the treatment or prophylaxis of influenza in pregnant women and women up to 2 weeks postpartum. Oseltamivir and zanamivir are currently recommended as an adjunct to vaccination and should not be used as a substitute for vaccination in pregnant women (consult current CDC guidelines).

Lactation Excretion in breast milk unknown/use caution

Prescribing and Access Restrictions Zanamivir *aqueous solution* intended for nebulization or intravenous (I.V.) administration is **not** currently approved for use. Data on safety and efficacy via these routes of administration are limited. However, limited supplies of zanamivir aqueous solution may be made available through the Zanamivir Compassionate Use Program for qualifying patients for the treatment of serious influenza illness. For information, contact the GlaxoSmithKline Clinical Support Help Desk at 1-866-341-9160 or gskclinicalsupportHD@gsk.com.

Contraindications Hypersensitivity to zanamivir or any component of the formulation (contains milk proteins)

Warnings/Precautions Allergic-like reactions, including anaphylaxis, oropharyngeal edema, and serious skin rashes have been reported. Rare occurrences of neuropsychiatric events (including confusion, delirium, hallucinations, and/or self-injury) have been reported from postmarketing surveillance; direct causation is difficult to establish (influenza infection may also be associated with behavioral and neurologic changes). Patients must be instructed in the use of the delivery system. Antiviral treatment should begin within 48 hours of symptom onset. However, the CDC recommends that treatment may still be beneficial and should be started in hospitalized patients with severe, complicated or progressive illness if >48 hours. Nonhospitalized persons who are not at high risk for developing severe or complicated illness and who have a mild disease are not likely to benefit if treatment is started >48 hours after symptom onset. Nonhospitalized persons who are already beginning to recover do not need treatment. Effectiveness has not been established in patients with significant underlying medical conditions or for prophylaxis of influenza in nursing home patients (per manufacturer). The CDC recommends zanamivir to be used to control institutional outbreaks of influenza when circulating strains are suspected of being resistant to oseltamivir (refer to current guidelines). Not recommended for use in patients with underlying respiratory disease, such as asthma or COPD, due to lack of efficacy and risk of serious adverse effects. Bronchospasm, decreased lung function, and other serious adverse reactions, including those with fatal outcomes, have been reported in patients with and without airway disease; discontinue with bronchospasm or signs of decreased lung function. For a patient with an underlying airway disease where a medical decision has been made to use zanamivir, a fast-acting bronchodilator should be made available, and used prior to each dose. Not a substitute for annual flu vaccination; has not been shown to reduce risk of transmission of influenza to others. Consider primary or concomitant bacterial infections. Powder for oral inhalation contains lactose; use contraindicated in patients allergic to milk proteins. The inhalation powder should only be administered via inhalation using the provided Diskhaler® delivery device. The commercially available formulation is **not** intended to be solubilized or administered via any nebulizer/mechanical ventilator; inappropriate administration has resulted in death. Safety and efficacy of repeated courses or use with hepatic impairment or severe renal impairment have not been established. Indicated for children ≥5 years of age (for influenza prophylaxis) and children ≥7 years of age (for influenza treatment); children ages 5-6 years may have inadequate inhalation (via Diskhaler®) for the treatment of influenza.

Adverse Reactions Most adverse reactions occurred at a frequency which was less than or equal to the control (lactose vehicle).

>10%:

Central nervous system: Headache (prophylaxis 13% to 24%; treatment 2%)

Gastrointestinal: Throat/tonsil discomfort/pain (prophylaxis 8% to 19%)

Respiratory: Nasal signs and symptoms (prophylaxis 12% to 20%; treatment 2%), cough (prophylaxis 7% to 17%; treatment ≤2%)

Miscellaneous: Viral infection (prophylaxis 3% to 13%)

1% to 10%:

Central nervous system: Fever/chills (prophylaxis 5% to 9%; treatment <1.5%), fatigue (prophylaxis 5% to 8%; treatment <1.5%), malaise (prophylaxis 5% to 8%; treatment <1.5%), dizziness (treatment 1% to 2%)

Dermatologic: Urticaria (treatment <1.5%)

Gastrointestinal: Anorexia/appetite decreased (prophylaxis 2% to 4%), appetite increased (prophylaxis 2% to 4%), nausea (prophylaxis 1% to 2%; treatment ≤3%), diarrhea (prophylaxis 2%; treatment 2% to 3%), vomiting (prophylaxis 1% to 2%; treatment 1% to 2%), abdominal pain (treatment <1.5%)

Neuromuscular & skeletal: Muscle pain (prophylaxis 3% to 8%), musculoskeletal pain (prophylaxis 6%), arthralgia/articular rheumatism (prophylaxis 2%), arthralgia (treatment <1.5%), myalgia (treatment <1.5%)

Respiratory: Infection (ear/nose/throat; prophylaxis 2%; treatment 1% to 5%), sinusitis (treatment 3%), bronchitis (treatment 2%), nasal inflammation (prophylaxis 1%)

<1% (Limited to important or life-threatening): Allergic or allergic-like reaction (including oropharyngeal edema), arrhythmia, bronchospasm, consciousness altered, delusions, dyspnea, hallucinations, neuropsychiatric events (self-injury, confusion, delirium), nightmares, rash (including serious cutaneous reactions [eg, erythema multiforme, Stevens-Johnson syndrome, toxic epidermal necrolysis]), seizure, syncope

Drug Interactions

Metabolism/Transport Effects None known.

Avoid Concomitant Use There are no known interactions where it is recommended to avoid concomitant use.

Increased Effect/Toxicity There are no known significant interactions involving an increase in effect.

Decreased Effect

Zanamivir may decrease the levels/effects of: Influenza Virus Vaccine (Live/Attenuated)

Stability Store at 25°C (77°F); excursions permitted to 15°C to 30°C (59°F to 86°F). Do not puncture blister until taking a dose using the Diskhaler®.

Mechanism of Action Zanamivir inhibits influenza virus neuraminidase enzymes, potentially altering virus particle aggregation and release.

Pharmacodynamics/Kinetics

Absorption: Inhalation: Systemic: ~4% to 17%

Protein binding, plasma: <10%

Metabolism: None

Half-life elimination, serum: 2.5-5.1 hours; Mild-to-moderate renal impairment: 4.7 hours; Severe renal impairment: 18.5 hours

Time to peak, plasma: 1-2 hours

Excretion: Urine (as unchanged drug); feces (unabsorbed drug)

Dosage Oral inhalation: Influenza virus A and B:

Manufacturer's recommendations:

Prophylaxis, household setting: Children ≥5 years and Adults: Two inhalations (10 mg) once daily for 10 days. Begin within 36 hours following onset of signs or symptoms of index case.

Prophylaxis, community outbreak: Adolescents and Adults: Two inhalations (10 mg) once daily for 28 days. Begin within 5 days of outbreak.

Treatment: Children ≥7 years and Adults: Two inhalations (10 mg total) twice daily for 5 days. Doses on first day should be separated by at least 2 hours; on subsequent days, doses should be spaced by ~12 hours. Begin within 2 days of signs or symptoms. Longer treatment may be considered for patients who remain severely ill after 5 days.

Alternate recommendations:

Prophylaxis (institutional outbreak, CDC 2011 recommendations): Children ≥5 years and Adults: Two inhalations (10 mg) once daily; continue for ≥2 weeks and until ~10 days after identification of illness onset in the last patient. Zanamivir is to be used to control institutional outbreaks of influenza when circulating strains are suspected of being resistant to oseltamivir.

Prophylaxis (community outbreak, IDSA/PIDS, 2011): Children ≥5 years and Adults: Two inhalations (10 mg) once daily; continue until influenza activity in community subsides or immunity obtained from immunization

Dosage adjustment for renal impairment: Adjustment not necessary following a 5-day course of treatment due to low systemic absorption; however the potential for drug accumulation should be considered.

Administration Inhalation: Must be used with Diskhaler® delivery device. The foil blister disk containing zanamivir inhalation powder should not be manipulated, solubilized, or administered via a nebulizer. Patients who are scheduled to use an inhaled bronchodilator should use their bronchodilator prior to zanamivir. With the exception of the initial dose when used for treatment, administer at the same time each day.

Additional Information Majority of patients included in clinical trials were infected with influenza A, however, a number of patients with influenza B infections were also enrolled. Patients with lower temperature or less severe symptoms appeared to derive less benefit from therapy. No consistent treatment benefit was demonstrated in patients with chronic underlying medical conditions.

The absence of symptoms does not rule out viral influenza infection and clinical judgment should guide the decision for therapy. Treatment should not be delayed while waiting for the results of diagnostic tests. Treatment should be considered for high-risk patients with symptoms despite a negative rapid influenza test when the illness cannot be contributed to another cause. Use of zanamivir is not a substitute for vaccination (when available); susceptibility to influenza infection returns once therapy is discontinued.

Dosage Forms Excipient information presented when available (limited, particularly for generics); consult specific product labeling.

Powder, for oral inhalation:

Relenza®: 5 mg/blister (20s) [contains lactose 20 mg/blister; 4 blisters per Rotadisk® foil pack, 5 Rotadisk® per package; packaged with Diskhaler® inhalation device]

- ◆ **Zantac®** *see* Ranitidine *on page 1462*
- ◆ **Zantac 75® [OTC]** *see* Ranitidine *on page 1462*
- ◆ **Zantac 75® (Can)** *see* Ranitidine *on page 1462*
- ◆ **Zantac 150® [OTC]** *see* Ranitidine *on page 1462*
- ◆ **Zantac® EFFERdose®** *see* Ranitidine *on page 1462*
- ◆ **Zantac Maximum Strength Non-Prescription (Can)** *see* Ranitidine *on page 1462*
- ◆ **Zarah®** *see* Ethinyl Estradiol and Drospirenone *on page 654*
- ◆ **Zarontin®** *see* Ethosuximide *on page 665*
- ◆ **Zaroxolyn®** *see* Metolazone *on page 1116*
- ◆ **Zavesca®** *see* Miglustat *on page 1134*
- ◆ **Zazole™ [DSC]** *see* Terconazole *on page 1651*
- ◆ **ZD1033** *see* Anastrozole *on page 121*
- ◆ **ZD1839** *see* Gefitinib *on page 780*
- ◆ **ZD6474** *see* Vandetanib *on page 1767*
- ◆ **ZD9238** *see* Fulvestrant *on page 770*
- ◆ **ZDV** *see* Zidovudine *on page 1814*
- ◆ **ZDV, Abacavir, and Lamivudine** *see* Abacavir, Lamivudine, and Zidovudine *on page 20*
- ◆ **ZDX** *see* Goserelin *on page 805*
- ◆ **Zeasorb®-AF [OTC]** *see* Miconazole (Topical) *on page 1126*
- ◆ **Zebeta®** *see* Bisoprolol *on page 220*
- ◆ **Zebutal®** *see* Butalbital, Acetaminophen, and Caffeine *on page 255*
- ◆ **Zegerid®** *see* Omeprazole and Sodium Bicarbonate *on page 1244*
- ◆ **Zegerid OTC™ [OTC]** *see* Omeprazole and Sodium Bicarbonate *on page 1244*
- ◆ **Zelapar®** *see* Selegiline *on page 1544*
- ◆ **Zelboraf™** *see* Vemurafenib *on page 1778*
- ◆ **Zeldox** *see* Ziprasidone *on page 1818*
- ◆ **Zeldox® (Can)** *see* Ziprasidone *on page 1818*
- ◆ **Zemplar®** *see* Paricalcitol *on page 1296*
- ◆ **Zemuron®** *see* Rocuronium *on page 1512*
- ◆ **Zenchent™** *see* Ethinyl Estradiol and Norethindrone *on page 660*
- ◆ **Zenchent Fe™** *see* Ethinyl Estradiol and Norethindrone *on page 660*
- ◆ **Zenhale™ (Can)** *see* Mometasone and Formoterol *on page 1151*
- ◆ **Zenpep®** *see* Pancrelipase *on page 1285*
- ◆ **Zeosa™** *see* Ethinyl Estradiol and Norethindrone *on page 660*
- ◆ **Zerit®** *see* Stavudine *on page 1592*
- ◆ **Zestoretic®** *see* Lisinopril and Hydrochlorothiazide *on page 1023*
- ◆ **Zestril®** *see* Lisinopril *on page 1020*
- ◆ **Zetia®** *see* Ezetimibe *on page 680*
- ◆ **Zevalin®** *see* Ibritumomab *on page 857*
- ◆ **Ziac®** *see* Bisoprolol and Hydrochlorothiazide *on page 221*

◆ Ziagen® *see* Abacavir *on page 18*

◆ Ziana® *see* Clindamycin and Tretinoin *on page 382*

Ziconotide (zi KOE no tide)

Brand Names: U.S. Prialt®

Pharmacologic Category Analgesic, Nonopioid; Calcium Channel Blocker, N-Type

Use Management of severe chronic pain in patients requiring intrathecal (I.T.) therapy and who are intolerant or refractory to other therapies

Pregnancy Risk Factor C

Pregnancy Considerations Teratogenic effects were not observed in animal studies, but increased postimplantation pup loss was reported. Maternal toxicity was also noted. There are no adequate and well-controlled studies in pregnant women.

Lactation Excretion in breast milk unknown/not recommended

Contraindications Hypersensitivity to ziconotide or any component of the formulation; history of psychosis; I.V. administration

I.T. administration is contraindicated in patients with infection at the injection site, uncontrolled bleeding, or spinal canal obstruction that impairs CSF circulation

Warnings/Precautions [U.S Boxed Warning]: Severe psychiatric symptoms and neurological impairment have been reported; interrupt or discontinue therapy if cognitive impairment, hallucinations, mood changes, or changes in consciousness occur. May cause or worsen depression and/or risk of suicide. Cognitive impairment may appear gradually during treatment and is generally reversible after discontinuation (may take up to 2 weeks for cognitive effects to reverse). Use caution in the elderly; may experience a higher incidence of confusion. Patients should be instructed to use caution in performing tasks which require alertness (eg, operating machinery or driving). May have additive effects with opiates or other CNS-depressant medications; may potentiate opioid-induced decreased GI motility; does not interact with opioid receptors or potentiate opiate-induced respiratory depression. Will not prevent or relieve symptoms associated with opiate withdrawal and opiates should not be abruptly discontinued. Unlike opioids, ziconotide therapy can be interrupted abruptly or discontinued without evidence of withdrawal.

Meningitis may occur with use of I.T. pumps; monitor for signs and symptoms of meningitis; treatment of meningitis may require removal of system and discontinuation of intrathecal therapy. Elevated serum creatine kinase can occur, particularly during the first 2 months of therapy; consider dose reduction or discontinuing if combined with new neuromuscular symptoms (myalgias, myasthenia, muscle cramps, weakness) or reduction in physical activity. Safety and efficacy have not been established with renal or hepatic dysfunction, or in pediatric patients. Should not be used in combination with intrathecal opiates.

Adverse Reactions

>10%:

Central nervous system: Dizziness (46%), confusion (15% to 33%), memory impairment (7% to 22%), somnolence (17%), ataxia (14%), speech disorder (14%), headache (13%), aphasia (12%), hallucination (12%; including auditory and visual)

Gastrointestinal: Nausea (40%), diarrhea (18%), vomiting (16%)

Neuromuscular & skeletal: Creatine kinase increased (40%; ≥3 times ULN: 11%), weakness (18%), gait disturbances (14%)

Ocular: Blurred vision (12%)

2% to 10%:

Cardiovascular: Hypotension, peripheral edema, postural hypotension

Central nervous system: Abnormal thinking (8%), amnesia (8%), anxiety (8%), vertigo (7%), insomnia (6%), fever (5%), paranoid reaction (3%), delirium (2%), hostility (2%), stupor (2%), agitation, attention disturbance, balance impaired, burning sensation, coordination abnormal, depression, disorientation, fatigue, fever, hypoesthesia, irritability, lethargy, mental impairment, mood disorder, nervousness, pain, sedation

Dermatologic: Pruritus (7%)

Gastrointestinal: Anorexia (6%), taste perversion (5%), abdominal pain, appetite decreased, constipation, xerostomia

Genitourinary: Urinary retention (9%), dysuria, urinary hesitance

Neuromuscular & skeletal: Dysarthria (7%), paresthesia (7%), rigors (7%), tremor (7%), muscle spasm (6%), limb pain (5%), areflexia, muscle cramp, muscle weakness, myalgia

Ocular: Nystagmus (8%), diplopia, visual disturbance

Respiratory: Sinusitis (5%)

Miscellaneous: Diaphoresis (5%)

<2% (Limited to important or life-threatening): Acute renal failure, aspiration pneumonia (<1%), atrial fibrillation, cerebral vascular accident, ECG abnormalities, incoherence, loss of consciousness, mania, meningitis, myoclonus, psychosis (1%), psychotic disorder, respiratory distress, rhabdomyolysis, seizure (clonic and grand mal), sepsis, suicidal ideation, suicide attempt (<1%)

Drug Interactions

Metabolism/Transport Effects None known.

Avoid Concomitant Use There are no known interactions where it is recommended to avoid concomitant use.

Increased Effect/Toxicity

Ziconotide may increase the levels/effects of: Alcohol (Ethyl); CNS Depressants; Methotrimeprazine; Selective Serotonin Reuptake Inhibitors

The levels/effects of Ziconotide may be increased by: Droperidol; HydrOXYzine; Methotrimeprazine

Decreased Effect There are no known significant interactions involving a decrease in effect.

Ethanol/Nutrition/Herb Interactions Ethanol: May increase CNS depression; monitor for increased effects with coadministration. Caution patients about effects.

Stability Prior to use, store vials at 2°C to 8°C (36°F to 46°F). Once diluted, may be stored at 2°C to 8°C (36°F to 46°F) for 24 hours; refrigerate during transit. Do not freeze. Protect from light.

Preservative free NS should be used when dilution is needed.

CADD-Micro® ambulatory infusion pump: Initial fill: Dilute to final concentration of 5 mcg/mL.

Medtronic SynchroMed® EL or SynchroMed® II infusion system: Prior to initial fill, rinse internal pump surfaces with 2 mL ziconotide (25 mcg/mL), repeat twice. Only the 25 mcg/mL concentration (undiluted) should be used for initial pump fill. When using the Medtronic SynchroMed® EL or SynchroMed® II Infusion System, solutions expire as follows:

25 mcg/mL: Undiluted:

Initial fill: Use within 14 days.

Refill: Use within 84 days.

100 mcg/mL:

Undiluted: Refill: Use within 84 days.

Diluted: Refill: Use within 40 days.

Mechanism of Action Ziconotide selectively binds to N-type voltage-sensitive calcium channels located on the nociceptive afferent nerves of the dorsal horn in the spinal cord. This binding is thought to block N-type calcium channels, leading to a blockade of excitatory neurotransmitter release and reducing sensitivity to painful stimuli.

Pharmacodynamics/Kinetics

Distribution: I.T.: V_d: ~140 mL

Protein binding: ~50%

Metabolism: Metabolized via endopeptidases and exopeptidases present on multiple organs including kidney, liver, lung; degraded to peptide fragments and free amino acids

Half-life elimination: I.V.: 1-1.6 hours (plasma); I.T.: 2.9-6.5 hours (CSF)

Excretion: I.V.: Urine (<1%)

Dosage I.T.:

Adults: Chronic pain: Initial dose: ≤2.4 mcg/day (0.1 mcg/hour)

Dose may be titrated by ≤2.4 mcg/day (0.1 mcg/hour) at intervals ≤2-3 times/week to a maximum dose of 19.2 mcg/day (0.8 mcg/hour) by day 21; average dose at day 21: 6.9 mcg/day (0.29 mcg/hour). A faster titration should be used only if the urgent need for analgesia outweighs the possible risk to patient safety.

Dosage adjustment for toxicity:

Cognitive impairment: Reduce dose or discontinue. Effects are generally reversible within 3-15 days of discontinuation.

Reduced level of consciousness: Discontinue until event resolves.

CK elevation with neuromuscular symptoms: Consider dose reduction or discontinuation.

Elderly: Refer to adult dosing; use with caution.

Administration Not for I.V. administration. For I.T. administration only using Medtronic SynchroMed® EL, SynchroMed® II Infusion System, or CADD-Micro® ambulatory infusion pump.

Medtronic SynchroMed® EL or SynchroMed® II Infusion Systems:

Naive pump priming (first time use with ziconotide): Use 2 mL of undiluted ziconotide 25 mcg/mL solution to rinse the internal surfaces of the pump; repeat twice for a total of 3 rinses

Initial pump fill: Use only undiluted 25 mcg/mL solution and fill pump after priming. Following the initial fill only, adsorption on internal device surfaces will occur, requiring the use of the undiluted solution and refill within 14 days.

Pump refills: Contents should be emptied prior to refill. Subsequent pump refills should occur at least every 40 days if using diluted solution or at least every 84 days if using undiluted solution.

CADD-Micro® ambulatory infusion pump: Refer to manufacturers' manual for initial fill and refill instructions

Monitoring Parameters Monitor for psychiatric or neurological impairment; signs and symptoms of meningitis or other infection; serum CPK (every other week for first month then monthly); pain relief

Dosage Forms Excipient information presented when available (limited, particularly for generics); consult specific product labeling.

Injection, solution, as acetate [preservative free]:

Prialt®: 25 mcg/mL (20 mL); 100 mcg/mL (1 mL, 5 mL)

◆ **Zictifa** *see* Vandetanib *on page 1767*

Zidovudine (zye DOE vyoo deen)

Brand Names: U.S. Retrovir®

Brand Names: Canada Apo-Zidovudine®; AZT™; Novo-AZT; Retrovir®; Retrovir® (AZT™)

Index Terms Azidothymidine; AZT (error-prone abbreviation); Compound S; ZDV

Pharmacologic Category Antiretroviral Agent, Reverse Transcriptase Inhibitor (Nucleoside)

Additional Appendix Information

Management of Healthcare Worker Exposures to HBV, HCV, and HIV *on page 1935*

Perinatal HIV Guidelines *on page 1946*

Use Treatment of HIV infection in combination with at least two other antiretroviral agents; prevention of maternal/fetal HIV transmission as monotherapy

Unlabeled Use Postexposure prophylaxis for HIV exposure as part of a multidrug regimen

Pregnancy Risk Factor C

Pregnancy Considerations Adverse events have been observed in some animal reproduction studies. Zidovudine crosses the placenta and the placenta also metabolizes zidovudine to the active metabolite. No increased risk of overall birth defects has been observed following first trimester exposure according to data collected by the antiretroviral pregnancy registry. The pharmacokinetics of zidovudine are not significantly altered in pregnancy and dosing adjustment is not needed. The DHHS Perinatal HIV Guidelines consider zidovudine the preferred NRTI for use in combination regimens during pregnancy. The use of zidovudine reduces the maternal-fetal transmission of HIV by ~70% and should be used for antenatal therapy unless there is severe toxicity, concurrent stavudine use, documented resistance, or the mother is already on a fully suppressive regimen. In HIV-infected mothers not previously on antiretroviral therapy, and who do not need therapy for their own health, treatment may be delayed until after the first trimester; however, earlier initiation of therapy may be more effective in reducing perinatal transmission. Intrapartum zidovudine is recommended for all women regardless of their antepartum regimen. Women in labor with an unknown HIV status should have a rapid HIV test. If the test is positive, begin I.V. zidovudine therapy. (If a postpartum confirmatory test is negative, zidovudine therapy in the infant can be stopped).

Cases of lactic acidosis/hepatic steatosis syndrome related to mitochondrial toxicity have been reported in pregnant women with prolonged use of nucleoside analogues. It is not known if pregnancy itself potentiates this known side effect; however, women may be at increased risk of lactic acidosis and liver damage. In addition, these adverse events are similar to other rare but life-threatening syndromes which occur during pregnancy (eg HELLP syndrome). Hepatic enzymes and electrolytes should be monitored in women receiving nucleoside analogues and clinicians should watch for early signs of the syndrome. In addition, mitochondrial dysfunction may develop in infants following *in utero* exposure.

Regardless of CD4 count or HIV RNA copy number, all HIV-infected pregnant women should receive a combination antepartum antiretroviral (ARV) drug regimen; this includes women who require therapy for their own health, as well as women who do not yet require therapy for their own health. ARV therapy should be started as soon as possible if required for the woman's health or immediately after the first trimester if not needed for the mother's health (although earlier initiation may be considered). Long-term follow-up is recommended for all infants exposed to ARV medications.

Healthcare providers are encouraged to enroll pregnant women exposed to antiretroviral medications in the Antiretroviral Pregnancy Registry (1-800-258-4263 or www.APRegistry.com). Healthcare providers caring for HIV-infected women and their infants may contact the National Perinatal HIV Hotline (888-448-8765) for clinical consultation (DHHS [perinatal], 2011).

Lactation Enters breast milk/contraindicated

Contraindications Life-threatening hypersensitivity to zidovudine or any component of the formulation

Warnings/Precautions Hazardous agent - use appropriate precautions for handling and disposal. **[U.S. Boxed Warning]: Often associated with hematologic toxicity including granulocytopenia, severe anemia requiring transfusions, or (rarely) pancytopenia.** Use with caution in patients with bone marrow compromise (granulocytes <1000 cells/mm^3 or hemoglobin <9.5 mg/dL); dosage adjustment may be required in patients who develop anemia or neutropenia. **[U.S. Boxed Warning]: Lactic acidosis and severe hepatomegaly with steatosis have been reported, including fatal cases;** use with caution in patients with risk factors for liver disease (risk may be increased in obese patients or prolonged exposure) and suspend treatment with zidovudine in any patient who develops clinical or laboratory findings suggestive of lactic acidosis (transaminase elevation may/may not accompany hepatomegaly and steatosis). Use caution in combination with interferon alfa with or without ribavirin in HIV/HBV coinfected patients; monitor closely for hepatic decompensation, anemia, or neutropenia; dose reduction or discontinuation of interferon and/or ribavirin may be required if toxicity evident. **[U.S. Boxed Warning]: Prolonged use has been associated with symptomatic myopathy and myositis.** May cause redistribution of fat (eg, buffalo hump, peripheral wasting with increased abdominal girth, cushingoid appearance). Immune reconstitution syndrome may develop resulting in the occurrence of an inflammatory response to an indolent or residual opportunistic infection; further evaluation and treatment may be required. Reduce dose in patients with severe renal impairment. Do not administer with combination products that contain zidovudine as one of their components (eg, COMBIVIR® [lamivudine and zidovudine] or TRIZIVIR® [abacavir sulfate, lamivudine, and zidovudine]).

Adverse Reactions As reported in adult patients with asymptomatic HIV infection. Frequency and severity may increase with advanced disease.

>10%:

Central nervous system: Headache (63%), malaise (53%)

Gastrointestinal: Nausea (51%), anorexia (20%), vomiting (17%)

1% to 10%:

Gastrointestinal: Constipation (6%)

Hematologic: Granulocytopenia (2%; onset 6-8 weeks), anemia (1%; onset 2-4 weeks)

Hepatic: Transaminases increased (1% to 3%)

Neuromuscular & skeletal: Weakness (9%)

Frequency not defined:

Cardiovascular: Cardiomyopathy, chest pain, syncope, vasculitis

Central nervous system: Anxiety, chills, confusion, depression, dizziness, fatigue, insomnia, loss of mental acuity, mania, seizure, somnolence, vertigo

Dermatologic: Pruritus, rash, skin/nail pigmentation changes, Stevens-Johnson syndrome, toxic epidermal necrolysis, urticaria

Endocrine & metabolic: Body fat redistribution, diabetes, dyslipidemias, gynecomastia, insulin resistance

Gastrointestinal: Abdominal cramps, abdominal pain, dyspepsia, dysphagia, flatulence, mouth ulcer, oral mucosa pigmentation, pancreatitis, taste perversion

Genitourinary: Urinary frequency, urinary hesitancy

Hematologic: Aplastic anemia, hemolytic anemia, leukopenia, lymphadenopathy, pancytopenia with marrow hypoplasia, pure red cell aplasia

Hepatic: Hepatitis, hepatomegaly with steatosis, hyperbilirubinemia, jaundice, lactic acidosis

Neuromuscular & skeletal: Arthralgia, back pain, CPK increased, LDH increased, musculoskeletal pain, myalgia, neuropathy, muscle spasm, myopathy, myositis, paresthesia, rhabdomyolysis, tremor

Ocular: Amblyopia, macular edema, photophobia

Otic: Hearing loss

Respiratory: Cough, dyspnea, rhinitis, sinusitis

Miscellaneous: Allergic reactions, anaphylaxis, angioedema, diaphoresis, flu-like syndrome, immune reconstitution syndrome

Drug Interactions

Metabolism/Transport Effects Substrate of CYP2A6 (minor), CYP2C19 (minor), CYP2C9 (minor), CYP3A4 (minor); **Note:** Assignment of Major/Minor substrate status based on clinically relevant drug interaction potential

Avoid Concomitant Use

Avoid concomitant use of Zidovudine with any of the following: CloZAPine; Stavudine

Increased Effect/Toxicity

Zidovudine may increase the levels/effects of: CloZAPine; Ribavirin

The levels/effects of Zidovudine may be increased by: Acyclovir-Valacyclovir; Clarithromycin; Conivaptan; Divalproex; DOXOrubicin; DOXOrubicin (Liposomal); Fluconazole; Ganciclovir-Valganciclovir; Interferons; Methadone; Probenecid; Ribavirin; Valproic Acid

Decreased Effect

Zidovudine may decrease the levels/effects of: Stavudine

The levels/effects of Zidovudine may be decreased by: Clarithromycin; DOXOrubicin; DOXOrubicin (Liposomal); Protease Inhibitors; Rifamycin Derivatives; Tocilizumab

Stability

I.V.: Store undiluted vials at 15°C to 25°C (59°F to 77°F). Protect from light. Solution for injection should be diluted with D_5W to a concentration ≤4 mg/mL. The solution is physically and chemically stable for 24 hours at room temperature and 48 hours if refrigerated. Attempt to administer diluted solution within 8 hours if stored at room temperature or 24 hours if refrigerated to minimize potential for microbial-contaminated solutions (vials are single-use and do not contain preservative).

Tablets, capsules, syrup: Store at 15°C to 25°C (59°F to 77°F). Protect capsules from moisture.

Mechanism of Action Zidovudine is a thymidine analog which interferes with the HIV viral RNA-dependent DNA polymerase resulting in inhibition of viral replication; nucleoside reverse transcriptase inhibitor

Pharmacodynamics/Kinetics

Distribution: Significant penetration into the CSF

V_d: 1-2.2 L/kg

Relative diffusion from blood into CSF: Adequate with or without inflammation (exceeds usual MICs)

CSF:blood level ratio: Normal meninges: ~60%

Protein binding: 25% to 38%

Metabolism: Hepatic via glucuronidation to inactive metabolites; extensive first-pass effect

Bioavailability: 54% to 74%

Half-life elimination: Terminal: 0.5-3 hours

Time to peak, serum: 30-90 minutes

Excretion:

Oral: Urine (72% to 74% as metabolites, 14% to 18% as unchanged drug)

I.V.: Urine (45% to 60% as metabolites, 18% to 29% as unchanged drug)

Dosage

Prevention of maternal-fetal HIV transmission: **Note:** Start as soon as possible after birth, preferably within 6-12 hours of delivery. Continue dose from birth through 6 weeks of age. Consider use of zidovudine in combination with nevirapine in select situations (eg, infants born to mothers with suboptimal viral suppression at delivery, infants born to mothers with only intrapartum therapy or no therapy, or infants born to mothers with known antiretroviral drug-resistant virus) (DHHS [perinatal], 2011).

Oral:
Full-term infants: 4 mg/kg/dose twice daily
Infants ≥30 weeks and <35 weeks gestation at birth: 2 mg/kg/dose every 12 hours; at 2 weeks of age, advance to 2 mg/kg/dose every 8 hours
Infants <30 weeks gestation at birth: 2 mg/kg/dose every 12 hours; at 4 weeks of age, advance to 2 mg/kg/dose every 8 hours
Alternate dosing for infants >35 weeks gestation (for use in low resource settings; may also be considered for use in higher resource settings if simplicity in dosing/administration is important):
Infants <2.5 kg at birth: 10 mg twice daily
Infants >2.5 kg at birth: 15 mg twice daily
I.V.: Infants unable to receive oral dosing (start as soon as possible after birth, preferably within 6-12 hours of delivery; continue dose from birth through 6 weeks of age):
Full term: 1.5 mg/kg/dose every 6 hours
Infants ≥30 weeks and <35 weeks gestation at birth: 1.5 mg/kg/dose every 12 hours; at 2 weeks of age, advance to 1.5 mg/kg/dose every 8 hours
Infants <30 weeks gestation at birth: 1.5 mg/kg/dose every 12 hours; at 4 weeks of age, advance to 1.5 mg/kg/dose every 8 hours
Maternal: Oral: Begin oral therapy with usual recommended dose as soon as possible in women who require treatment for their own health (including use during the first trimester); may delay therapy in women who are using antiretroviral medications solely for the prevention of perinatal transmission; however, earlier initiation of therapy may be more effective in reducing perinatal transmission. Dose adjustment is not required for pregnant women. Change to I.V. dosing during labor (DHHS [perinatal], 2011).
During labor and delivery, administer zidovudine I.V. at 2 mg/kg as loading dose followed by a continuous I.V. infusion of 1 mg/kg/hour until the umbilical cord is clamped. For scheduled cesarean delivery, begin I.V. zidovudine 3 hours before surgery.

Treatment of HIV infection:
Children 4 weeks to <18 years:
Oral: Dose should be calculated by body weight (in kg) or body surface area and should not exceed the recommended adult dose. **Note:** Doses calculated by body weight may not be the same as those calculated by body surface area.
Dosing based on body surface area: 240 mg/m^2 every 12 hours (maximum: 300 mg every 12 hours) **or** 160 mg/m^2/dose every 8 hours (maximum: 200 mg every 8 hours)
Dosing based on weight (**Note:** 3 times daily dose is approved but rarely used in clinical practice):
4 to <9 kg: 12 mg/kg/dose twice daily **or** 8 mg/kg/dose 3 times/day
≥9 to <30 kg: 9 mg/kg/dose twice daily **or** 6 mg/kg/dose 3 times/day
≥30 kg: 300 mg twice daily **or** 200 mg 3 times/day
Children 6 weeks to <12 years (per AIDS*info* guidelines):
I.V. continuous infusion: 20 mg/m^2/hour
I.V. intermittent infusion: 120 mg/m^2/dose every 6 hours
Children ≥12 years: I.V. intermittent infusion: 1 mg/kg/dose every 4 hours around-the-clock (5-6 doses/day)
Adults:
Oral: 300 mg twice daily or 200 mg 3 times/day
I.V.: 1 mg/kg/dose administered every 4 hours around-the-clock (5-6 doses/day)

Prevention of HIV following needlesticks (unlabeled use): Oral: Adults: 200 mg 3 times/day plus lamivudine 150 mg twice daily; a protease inhibitor (eg, indinavir) may be added for high risk exposures; begin therapy within 2 hours of exposure if possible

Patients should receive I.V. therapy only until oral therapy can be administered

Dosing adjustment for hematologic toxicity: Consider dose interruption for significant anemia (hemoglobin <7.5 g/dL or >25% reduction from baseline) and/or neutropenia (granulocyte count <750 cells/mm^3 or >50% reduction from baseline) until evidence of recovery. Anemia associated with chronic zidovudine may warrant dose reduction.

Dosing adjustment in renal impairment: Cl_{cr} <15 mL/minute including hemo-/peritoneal dialysis:
Oral: 100 mg every 6-8 hours or 300 mg once daily (DHHS, 2011)
I.V.: 1 mg/kg every 6-8 hours
Continuous renal replacement therapy (CRRT): No adjustment needed (Aronoff, 2007)

Dosing adjustment in hepatic impairment: Insufficient data to make dosing recommendation

Dietary Considerations May be taken without regard to meals.

Administration
Oral: Administer around-the-clock to promote less variation in peak and trough serum levels; may be administered without regard to meals
I.M.: Do not administer I.M.
I.V.: Avoid rapid infusion or bolus injection
Neonates: Infuse over 30 minutes
Adults: Infuse loading dose over 1 hour, followed by continuous infusion

Monitoring Parameters Monitor CBC and platelet count at least every 2 weeks, liver function tests, MCV, serum creatinine kinase, viral load, and CD4 count; observe for appearance of opportunistic infections

Additional Information Potential compliance problems, frequency of administration, and adverse effects should be discussed with patients before initiating therapy to help prevent the emergence of resistance.

Dosage Forms Excipient information presented when available (limited, particularly for generics); consult specific product labeling. [DSC] = Discontinued product
Capsule, oral: 100 mg
Retrovir®: 100 mg
Injection, solution [preservative free]:
Retrovir®: 10 mg/mL (20 mL [DSC])
Retrovir®: 10 mg/mL (20 mL) [contains natural rubber/natural latex in packaging]
Syrup, oral: 50 mg/5 mL (240 mL)
Retrovir®: 50 mg/5 mL (240 mL) [contains sodium benzoate; strawberry flavor]
Tablet, oral: 300 mg
Retrovir®: 300 mg

◆ **Zidovudine, Abacavir, and Lamivudine** *see* Abacavir, Lamivudine, and Zidovudine *on page 20*
◆ **Zidovudine and Lamivudine** *see* Lamivudine and Zidovudine *on page 967*
◆ **Zilactin®-L [OTC]** *see* Benzyl Alcohol *on page 206*
◆ **Zilactin®-B [OTC]** *see* Benzocaine *on page 202*
◆ **Zilactin-B® (Can)** *see* Benzocaine *on page 202*
◆ **Zilactin Baby® (Can)** *see* Benzocaine *on page 202*
◆ **Zilactin® Tooth & Gum Pain [OTC]** *see* Benzocaine *on page 202*

Zileuton (zye LOO ton)

Brand Names: U.S. Zyflo CR®; Zyflo®
Pharmacologic Category 5-Lipoxygenase Inhibitor
Additional Appendix Information
Asthma *on page 1967*
Use Prophylaxis and chronic treatment of asthma

Pregnancy Risk Factor C

Dosage Oral: Children ≥12 years and Adults:

Immediate release: 600 mg 4 times/day

Extended release: 1200 mg twice daily

Dosing adjustment in renal impairment: Adjustment not necessary in renal dysfunction or with hemodialysis

Dosing adjustment in hepatic impairment: Contraindicated with hepatic dysfunction

Additional Information Complete prescribing information for this medication should be consulted for additional detail.

Dosage Forms Excipient information presented when available (limited, particularly for generics); consult specific product labeling.

Tablet, oral:

Zyflo®: 600 mg [scored]

Tablet, extended release, oral:

Zyflo CR®: 600 mg

◆ **Zinacef®** *see* Cefuroxime *on page 322*

◆ **Zinc 15 [OTC]** *see* Zinc Sulfate *on page 1818*

Zinc Acetate (zink AS e tate)

Brand Names: U.S. Galzin®

Pharmacologic Category Trace Element

Use Maintenance treatment of Wilson's disease following initial chelation therapy

Pregnancy Risk Factor A

Dosage Oral: Wilson's disease: **Note:** Dose expressed in mg elemental zinc:

Children ≥10 years: 75 mg/day in 3 divided doses; may increase to 150 mg/day in 3 divided doses if inadequate response to lower dose

American Association for the Study of Liver Diseases (AASLD) practice guideline recommendations (Roberts, 2008):

Children <50 kg and >5 years: 75 mg/day in 3 divided doses

Children >50 kg: 150 mg/day in 3 divided doses

Adults:

Males and nonpregnant females: 150 mg/day in 3 divided doses

Pregnant females: 75 mg/day in 3 divided doses; may increase to 150 mg/day in 3 divided doses if inadequate response to lower dose

Additional Information Complete prescribing information for this medication should be consulted for additional detail.

Dosage Forms Excipient information presented when available (limited, particularly for generics); consult specific product labeling.

Capsule, oral:

Galzin®: Elemental zinc 25 mg, Elemental zinc 50 mg

◆ **Zincate®** *see* Zinc Sulfate *on page 1818*

Zinc Chloride (zink KLOR ide)

Pharmacologic Category Trace Element

Use Cofactor for replacement therapy to different enzymes; helps maintain normal growth rates, normal skin hydration, and senses of taste and smell

Pregnancy Risk Factor C

Dosage Clinical response may not occur for up to 6-8 weeks

Supplemental to I.V. solutions:

Premature Infants <1500 g, up to 3 kg: 300 mcg/kg/day

Infants (full term) and Children ≤5 years: 100 mcg/kg/day

Adults:

Stable with fluid loss from small bowel: 12.2 mg zinc/L TPN or 17.1 mg zinc/kg (added to 1000 mL I.V. fluids) of stool or ileostomy output

Metabolically stable: 2.5-4 mg/day; add 2 mg/day for acute catabolic states

Additional Information Complete prescribing information for this medication should be consulted for additional detail.

Dosage Forms Excipient information presented when available (limited, particularly for generics); consult specific product labeling.

Injection, solution [preservative free]: 1 mg/mL (10 mL)

Zinc Gelatin (zink JEL ah tin)

Brand Names: U.S. Gelucast®

Index Terms Dome Paste Bandage; Unna's Boot; Unna's Paste; Zinc Gelatin Boot

Pharmacologic Category Topical Skin Product

Use As a protectant and to support varicosities and similar lesions of the lower limbs

Dosage Topical: Apply externally as an occlusive boot

Additional Information Complete prescribing information for this medication should be consulted for additional detail.

Dosage Forms Excipient information presented when available (limited, particularly for generics); consult specific product labeling.

Bandage: 3" x 10 yards; 4" x 10 yards

◆ **Zinc Gelatin Boot** *see* Zinc Gelatin *on page 1817*

◆ **Zincofax® (Can)** *see* Zinc Oxide *on page 1817*

Zinc Oxide (zink OKS ide)

Brand Names: U.S. Ammens® Original Medicated [OTC]; Ammens® Shower Fresh [OTC]; Balmex® [OTC]; Boudreaux's® Butt Paste [OTC]; Critic-Aid Skin Care® [OTC]; Desitin® Creamy [OTC]; Desitin® [OTC]

Brand Names: Canada Zincofax®

Index Terms Base Ointment; Lassar's Zinc Paste

Pharmacologic Category Topical Skin Product

Use Protective coating for mild skin irritations and abrasions; soothing and protective ointment to promote healing of chapped skin, diaper rash

Dosage Infants, Children, and Adults: Topical: Apply as required for affected areas several times daily

Additional Information Complete prescribing information for this medication should be consulted for additional detail.

Dosage Forms Excipient information presented when available (limited, particularly for generics); consult specific product labeling.

Cream, topical:

Balmex®: 11.3% (60 g, 120 g, 480 g) [contains aloe, benzoic acid, soybean oil, and vitamin E]

Cream, topical [stick]:

Balmex®: 11.3% (56 g) [contains aloe, benzoic acid, soybean oil, and vitamin E]

Ointment, topical: 20% (30 g, 60 g, 454 g); 40% (120 g)

Desitin®: 40% (30 g, 60 g, 90 g, 120 g, 270 g, 480 g) [contains cod liver oil and lanolin]

Desitin® Creamy: 10% (60 g, 120 g)

Paste, topical:

Boudreaux's® Butt Paste: 16% (30 g, 60 g, 120 g, 480 g) [contains castor oil, boric acid, mineral oil, and Peruvian balsam]

Critic-Aid Skin Care®: 20% (71 g, 170 g)

Powder, topical:

Ammens® Original Medicated: 9.1% (312 g)

Ammens® Shower Fresh: 9.1% (312 g)

Zinc Sulfate (zink SUL fate)

Brand Names: U.S. Orazinc® 110 [OTC]; Orazinc® 220 [OTC]; Zinc 15 [OTC]; Zincate®

Brand Names: Canada Anuzinc; Rivasol

Index Terms $ZnSO_4$ (error-prone abbreviation)

Pharmacologic Category Trace Element

Use Zinc supplement (oral and parenteral); may improve wound healing in those who are deficient

Pregnancy Risk Factor C

Dosage

RDA: Oral:
- Birth to 6 months: 3 mg elemental zinc/day
- 6-12 months: 5 mg elemental zinc/day
- 1-10 years: 10 mg elemental zinc/day
- ≥11 years: 15 mg elemental zinc/day

Zinc deficiency: Oral:
- Infants and Children: 0.5-1 mg elemental zinc/kg/day divided 1-3 times/day; somewhat larger quantities may be needed if there is impaired intestinal absorption or an excessive loss of zinc
- Adults: 110-220 mg zinc sulfate (25-50 mg elemental zinc)/dose 3 times/day

Parenteral TPN: I.V.:
- Infants (premature, birth weight <1500 g up to 3 kg): 300 mcg/kg/day
- Infants (full term) and Children ≤5 years: 100 mcg/kg/day
- Adults:
  - Acute metabolic states: 4.5-6 mg/day
  - Metabolically stable: 2.5-4 mg/day
  - Replacement for small bowel fluid loss (metabolically stable): An additional 12.2 mg zinc/L of fluid lost, or an additional 17.1 mg zinc per kg of stool or ileostomy output

Additional Information Complete prescribing information for this medication should be consulted for additional detail.

Dosage Forms Excipient information presented when available (limited, particularly for generics); consult specific product labeling.

Capsule, oral: 220 mg [elemental zinc 50 mg]
- Orazinc® 220: 220 mg [elemental zinc 50 mg]
- Zincate®: 220 mg [elemental zinc 50 mg]

Injection, solution [preservative free]: Elemental zinc 1 mg/mL (10 mL)

Injection, solution [concentrate, preservative free]: Elemental zinc 5 mg/mL (5 mL)

Tablet, oral: 220 mg [elemental zinc 50 mg]
- Orazinc® 110: 110 mg [elemental zinc 25 mg]
- Zinc 15: 66 mg [elemental zinc 15 mg]

◆ **Zinecard®** *see* Dexrazoxane *on page 486*

Ziprasidone (zi PRAS i done)

Brand Names: U.S. Geodon®

Brand Names: Canada Zeldox®

Index Terms Zeldox; Ziprasidone Hydrochloride; Ziprasidone Mesylate

Pharmacologic Category Antipsychotic Agent, Atypical

Additional Appendix Information

Antipsychotic Agents *on page 1880*

Use Treatment of schizophrenia; treatment of acute manic or mixed episodes associated with bipolar disorder with or without psychosis; maintenance treatment of bipolar disorder as an adjunct to lithium or valproate; acute agitation in patients with schizophrenia

Unlabeled Use Tourette's syndrome; psychosis/agitation related to Alzheimer's dementia

Pregnancy Risk Factor C

Pregnancy Considerations Developmental toxicity demonstrated in animals. Antipsychotic use during the third trimester of pregnancy has a risk for abnormal muscle movements (extrapyramidal symptoms [EPS]) and withdrawal symptoms in newborns following delivery. Symptoms in the newborn may include agitation, feeding disorder, hypertonia, hypotonia, respiratory distress, somnolence, and tremor; these effects may be self-limiting or require hospitalization. There are no adequate and well-controlled studies in pregnant women. Use only if potential benefit justifies risk to the fetus. Healthcare providers are encouraged to enroll women 18-45 years of age exposed to ziprasidone during pregnancy in the Atypical Antipsychotics Pregnancy Registry (1-866-961-2388).

Lactation Excretion in breast milk unknown/not recommended

Contraindications Hypersensitivity to ziprasidone or any component of the formulation; history of (or current) prolonged QT; congenital long QT syndrome; recent myocardial infarction; uncompensated heart failure; concurrent use of other QT_c-prolonging agents including arsenic trioxide, chlorpromazine, class Ia antiarrhythmics (eg, disopyramide, quinidine, procainamide), class III antiarrhythmics (eg, amiodarone, dofetilide, ibutilide, sotalol), dolasetron, droperidol, gatifloxacin, levomethadyl, mefloquine, mesoridazine, moxifloxacin, pentamidine, pimozide, probucol, tacrolimus, and thioridazine

Warnings/Precautions [U.S. Boxed Warning]: Elderly patients with dementia-related behavioral disorders treated with antipsychotics are at an increased risk of death compared to placebo. Most deaths appeared to be either cardiovascular (eg, heart failure, sudden death) or infectious (eg, pneumonia) in nature. Ziprasidone is not approved for the treatment of dementia-related psychosis.

May result in QT_c prolongation (dose related), which has been associated with the development of malignant ventricular arrhythmias (torsade de pointes) and sudden death. Note contraindications related to this effect. Observed prolongation was greater than with other atypical antipsychotic agents (risperidone, olanzapine, quetiapine), but less than with thioridazine. Correct electrolyte disturbances, especially hypokalemia or hypomagnesemia, prior to use and throughout therapy. Use caution in patients with bradycardia. Discontinue in patients found to have persistent QT_c intervals >500 msec. Patients with symptoms of dizziness, palpitations, or syncope should receive further cardiac evaluation. May cause orthostatic hypotension. Use is contraindicated in patients with recent acute myocardial infarction (MI), QT prolongation, or uncompensated heart failure. Avoid use in patients with a history of cardiac arrhythmias; use with caution in patients with history of MI or unstable heart disease.

Leukopenia, neutropenia, and agranulocytosis (sometimes fatal) have been reported in clinical trials and postmarketing reports with antipsychotic use; presence of risk factors (eg, pre-existing low WBC or history of drug-induced leuko-/neutropenia) should prompt periodic blood count assessment. Discontinue therapy at first signs of blood dyscrasias or if absolute neutrophil count <1000/mm^3.

May cause extrapyramidal symptoms (EPS). Risk of dystonia (and probably other EPS) may be greater with increased doses, use of conventional antipsychotics, males, and younger patients. Impaired core body temperature regulation may occur; caution with strenuous exercise, heat exposure, dehydration, and concomitant medication possessing anticholinergic effects; not reported in premarketing trials of ziprasidone. Antipsychotic use may also be associated with neuroleptic malignant syndrome (NMS). Use with caution in patients at risk of seizures.

Atypical antipsychotics have been associated with development of hyperglycemia. There is limited documentation with ziprasidone and specific risk associated with this agent is not known. Use caution in patients with diabetes or other disorders of glucose regulation; monitor for worsening of glucose control. May increase prolactin levels; clinical significance of hyperprolactinemia in patients with breast cancer or other prolactin-dependent tumors is unknown.

Cognitive and/or motor impairment (sedation) is common with ziprasidone. Use with caution in disorders where CNS depression is a feature. Use with caution in Parkinson's disease. Antipsychotic use has been associated with esophageal dysmotility and aspiration; use with caution in patients at risk of pneumonia (ie, Alzheimer's disease). Use caution in hepatic impairment. Ziprasidone has been associated with a fairly high incidence of rash (5%). Significant weight gain has been observed with antipsychotic therapy; incidence varies with product. Monitor waist circumference and BMI. Rare cases of priapism have been reported. Use the intramuscular formulation with caution in patients with renal impairment; formulation contains cyclodextrin, an excipient which may accumulate in renal insufficiency.

The possibility of a suicide attempt is inherent in psychotic illness or bipolar disorder; use caution in high-risk patients during initiation of therapy. Prescriptions should be written for the smallest quantity consistent with good patient care.

Adverse Reactions Note: Although minor QT_c prolongation (mean: 10 msec at 160 mg/day) may occur more frequently (incidence not specified), clinically-relevant prolongation (>500 msec) was rare (0.06%) and less than placebo (0.23%).

>10%:

Central nervous system: Extrapyramidal symptoms (2% to 31%), somnolence (8% to 31%), headache (3% to 18%), dizziness (3% to 16%)

Gastrointestinal: Nausea (4% to 12%)

1% to 10%:

Cardiovascular: Postural hypotension (5%), chest pain (3%), hypertension (2% to 3%), tachycardia (2%), bradycardia (≤2%), facial edema (1%), vasodilation (≤1%), orthostatic hypotension

Central nervous system: Akathisia (2% to 10%), anxiety (2% to 5%), insomnia (3%), agitation (2%), speech disorder (2%), personality disorder (2%), akinesia (≥1%), amnesia (≥1%), ataxia (≥1%), confusion (≥1%), coordination abnormal (≥1%), delirium (≥1%), dystonia (≥1%), hostility (≥1%), oculogyric crisis (≥1%), vertigo (≥1%), chills (1%), fever (1%), hypothermia (1%), psychosis (1%)

Dermatologic: Rash (4% to 5%), fungal dermatitis (2%)

Endocrine & metabolic: Dysmenorrhea (2%)

Gastrointestinal: Weight gain (6% to 10%), constipation (2% to 9%), dyspepsia (1% to 8%), diarrhea (3% to 5%), vomiting (3% to 5%), xerostomia (1% to 5%), salivation increased (4%), tongue edema (≤3%), anorexia (2%), abdominal pain (≤2%), dysphagia (≤2%), rectal hemorrhage (≤2%), buccoglossal syndrome (≥1%)

Genitourinary: Priapism (1%)

Local: Injection site pain (7% to 9%)

Neuromuscular & skeletal: Weakness (2% to 6%), hypoesthesia (2%), myalgia (2%), paresthesia (2%), abnormal gait (≥1%), choreoathetosis (≥1%), dysarthria (≥1%), dyskinesia (≥1%), hyper-/hypokinesia (≥1%), hypotonia (≥1%), neuropathy (≥1%), tremor (≥1%), twitching (≥1%), back pain (1%), cogwheel rigidity (1%), hypertonia (1%)

Ocular: Vision abnormal (3% to 6%), diplopia (≥1%)

Respiratory: Infection (8%), rhinitis (1% to 4%), cough (3%), pharyngitis (3%), dyspnea (2%)

Miscellaneous: Diaphoresis (2%), furunculosis (2%), withdrawal syndrome (≥1%), flank pain (1%), flu-like syndrome (1%), photosensitivity reaction (1%),

<1% (Limited to important or life-threatening): Abnormal ejaculation, albuminuria, alkaline phosphatase increased, allergic reaction, alopecia, amenorrhea, anemia, angioedema, angina, anorgasmia, atrial fibrillation, AV block (first degree), basophilia, blepharitis, bruising, BUN increased, bundle branch block, cardiomegaly, cataract, cerebral infarction, cerebrovascular accident, cholestatic jaundice, circumoral paresthesia, conjunctivitis, contact dermatitis, CPK increased, creatinine (serum) increased, dehydration, depression, dry eyes, dysphagia, eczema, enuresis, eosinophilia, epistaxis, exfoliative dermatitis, facial droop, fatty liver, fecal impaction, galactorrhea, GGT increased, gingival bleeding, glycosuria, gout, gynecomastia, hematemesis, hemoptysis, hematuria, hepatitis, hepatomegaly, hyper-/hypochloremia, hyper-/hypocholesterolemia, hyper-/hypoglycemia, hyper-/hypokalemia, hyper-/hypothyroidism, hyperlipemia, hyperreflexia, hyperuricemia, hypocalcemia, hypomagnesemia, hyponatremia, hypoproteinemia, impotence, jaundice, keratitis, keratoconjunctivitis, ketosis, lactation (female), laryngismus, LDH increased, leukocytosis, leukopenia, leukoplakia (mouth), lymphadenopathy, lymphedema, lymphocytosis, maculopapular rash, mania/hypomania, melena, menorrhagia, metrorrhagia, monocytosis, myocarditis, myoclonus, myopathy, neuroleptic malignant syndrome, neuropathy, nocturia, nystagmus, ocular hemorrhage, oliguria, opisthotonos, paralysis, peripheral edema, phlebitis, photophobia, pneumonia, polycythemia, polyuria, pulmonary embolism, QT_c prolongation >500 msec, respiratory alkalosis, seizure, serotonin syndrome, sexual dysfunction (male and female), syncope, tardive dyskinesia, tenosynovitis, thirst, thrombocytopenia, thrombocythemia, thrombophlebitis, thyroiditis, tinnitus, torsade de pointes, torticollis, transaminases increased, trismus, urinary incontinence, urinary retention, urticaria, uterine hemorrhage, vaginal hemorrhage, vesiculobullous rash, visual field defect

Drug Interactions

Metabolism/Transport Effects Substrate of CYP1A2 (minor), CYP3A4 (minor); **Note:** Assignment of Major/Minor substrate status based on clinically relevant drug interaction potential; **Inhibits** CYP2D6 (weak), CYP3A4 (weak)

Avoid Concomitant Use

Avoid concomitant use of Ziprasidone with any of the following: Artemether; Dronedarone; Lumefantrine; Metoclopramide; Nilotinib; Pimozide; QTc-Prolonging Agents; QUEtiapine; QuiNINE; Tetrabenazine; Thioridazine; Toremifene; Vandetanib; Vemurafenib

Increased Effect/Toxicity

Ziprasidone may increase the levels/effects of: Alcohol (Ethyl); CNS Depressants; Dronedarone; Methylphenidate; Pimozide; QTc-Prolonging Agents; QuiNINE; Serotonin Modulators; Tetrabenazine; Thioridazine; Toremifene; Vandetanib; Vemurafenib

The levels/effects of Ziprasidone may be increased by: Acetylcholinesterase Inhibitors (Central); Alfuzosin; Antifungal Agents (Azole Derivatives, Systemic); Artemether; Chloroquine; Ciprofloxacin; Ciprofloxacin (Systemic); Conivaptan; Gadobutrol; HydrOXYzine; Indacaterol; Lithium formulations; Lumefantrine; Methylphenidate; Metoclopramide; Nilotinib; QTc-Prolonging Agents; QUEtiapine; QuiNINE; Tetrabenazine

Decreased Effect

Ziprasidone may decrease the levels/effects of: Amphetamines; Anti-Parkinson's Agents (Dopamine Agonist); Quinagolide

The levels/effects of Ziprasidone may be decreased by: CarBAMazepine; Cyproterone; Lithium formulations; Tocilizumab

Ethanol/Nutrition/Herb Interactions

Ethanol: May increase CNS depression; monitor for increased effects with coadministration. Caution patients about effects.

Food: Administration with food increases serum levels twofold. Grapefruit juice may increase serum concentration of ziprasidone.

Herb/Nutraceutical: St John's wort may decrease serum levels of ziprasidone, due to a potential effect on CYP3A4. This has not been specifically studied. Avoid kava kava, chamomile (may increase CNS depression).

Stability

Capsule: Store at 25°C (77°F); excursion permitted to 15°C to 30°C (59°F to 86°F).

Vials for injection: Store at 25°C (77°F); excursion permitted to 15°C to 30°C (59°F to 86°F). Protect from light. Each vial should be reconstituted with 1.2 mL SWFI. Shake vigorously; will form a pale, pink solution containing 20 mg/mL ziprasidone. Following reconstitution, injection may be stored at room temperature up to 24 hours or under refrigeration for up to 7 days. Protect from light.

Mechanism of Action Ziprasidone is a benzylisothiazolylpiperazine antipsychotic. The exact mechanism of action is unknown. However, *in vitro* radioligand studies show that ziprasidone has high affinity for D_2, D_3, 5-HT_{2A}, 5-HT_{1A}, 5-HT_{2C}, 5-HT_{1D}, and alpha$_1$-adrenergic; moderate affinity for histamine H_1 receptors; and no appreciable affinity for alpha$_2$-adrenergic receptors, beta-adrenergic, 5-HT_3, 5-HT_4, cholinergic, mu, sigma, or benzodiazepine receptors. Ziprasidone functions as an antagonist at the D_2, 5-HT_{2A}, and 5-HT_{1D} receptors and as an agonist at the 5-HT_{1A} receptor. Ziprasidone moderately inhibits the reuptake of serotonin and norepinephrine.

Pharmacodynamics/Kinetics

Absorption: Well absorbed

Distribution: V_d: 1.5 L/kg

Protein binding: >99%, primarily to albumin and alpha$_1$-acid glycoprotein

Metabolism: Extensively hepatic, primarily via aldehyde oxidase; less than 1/3 of total metabolism via CYP3A4 and CYP1A2 (minor)

Bioavailability: Oral (with food): 60% (up to twofold increase with food); I.M.: 100%

Half-life elimination: 2-7 hours

Time to peak: Oral: 6-8 hours; I.M.: ≤60 minutes

Excretion: Feces (~66%; <4% of total dose as unchanged drug); urine (~20%; <1% of total dose as unchanged drug)

Dosage

Children and Adolescents: Tourette's syndrome (unlabeled use): Oral: 5-40 mg/day

Adults:

Bipolar mania (acute): Oral: Initial: 40 mg twice daily

Adjustment: May increase to 60 mg or 80 mg twice daily on second day of treatment; average dose 40-80 mg twice daily

Bipolar disorder (maintenance; as adjunct to lithium or valproate): Continue ziprasidone dose at which the patient was initially stabilized; usual dosage range: 40-80 mg twice daily

Schizophrenia: Oral: Initial: 20 mg twice daily

Adjustment: Increases (if indicated) should be made no more frequently than every 2 days; ordinarily patients should be observed for improvement over several weeks before adjusting the dose

Maintenance: Range: 20-100 mg twice daily; however, dosages >80 mg twice daily are generally not recommended

Acute agitation (schizophrenia): I.M.: 10 mg every 2 hours **or** 20 mg every 4 hours; maximum: 40 mg/day; oral therapy should replace I.M. administration as soon as possible

Elderly: No dosage adjustment is recommended; consider initiating at a low end of the dosage range, with slower titration

Dosage adjustment in renal impairment:

Oral: No dosage adjustment is recommended

I.M.: Cyclodextrin, an excipient in the I.M. formulation, is cleared by renal filtration; use with caution.

Ziprasidone is not removed by hemodialysis.

Dosage adjustment in hepatic impairment: No dosage adjustment is recommended

Dietary Considerations Take with food.

Administration

Oral: Administer with food.

Injection: For I.M. administration only.

Monitoring Parameters Blood pressure, heart rate; temperature; serum potassium and magnesium; fasting lipid profile and fasting blood glucose/Hgb A_{1c} (prior to treatment, at 3 months, then annually); BMI; waist circumference; mental status, abnormal involuntary movement scale (AIMS), extrapyramidal symptoms. Weight should be assessed prior to treatment, at 4 weeks, 8 weeks, 12 weeks, and then at quarterly intervals. Consider titrating to a different antipsychotic agent for a weight gain ≥5% of the initial weight. The value of routine ECG screening or monitoring has not been established.

Test Interactions Increased cholesterol, triglycerides, eosinophils

Additional Information The increased potential to prolong QT_c, as compared to other available antipsychotic agents, should be considered in the evaluation of available alternatives.

Dosage Forms Excipient information presented when available (limited, particularly for generics); consult specific product labeling.

Capsule, oral, as hydrochloride:

Geodon®: 20 mg, 40 mg, 60 mg, 80 mg

Injection, powder for reconstitution, as mesylate [strength expressed as base]:

Geodon®: 20 mg [contains cyclodextrin]

Extemporaneous Preparations A 2.5 mg/mL oral solution may be made with the injection. Use 8 vials of the 20 mg injectable powder. Add 1.2 mL of distilled water to each vial to make a 20 mg/mL solution. Once dissolved, transfer 7.5 mL to a calibrated bottle and add quantity of vehicle (Ora-Sweet®) sufficient to make 60 mL. Label "shake well" and "refrigerate". Stable for 14 days at room temperature or 42 days refrigerated (preferred).

Green K and Parish RC, "Stability of Ziprasidone Mesylate in an Extemporaneously Compounded Oral Solution," *J Pediatr Pharmacol Ther*, 2010, 15:138-41.

◆ **Ziprasidone Hydrochloride** *see* Ziprasidone *on page 1818*

◆ **Ziprasidone Mesylate** *see* Ziprasidone *on page 1818*

◆ **Zipsor™** *see* Diclofenac (Systemic) *on page 495*

◆ **Zithranol®-RR** *see* Anthralin *on page 123*

◆ **Zithromax®** *see* Azithromycin (Systemic) *on page 180*

◆ **Zithromax TRI-PAK™** *see* Azithromycin (Systemic) *on page 180*

◆ **Zithromax® TRI-PAK™** *see* Azithromycin (Systemic) *on page 180*

◆ **Zithromax Z-PAK®** *see* Azithromycin (Systemic) *on page 180*

◆ **Zithromax® Z-PAK®** *see* Azithromycin (Systemic) *on page 180*

◆ **Zmax®** *see* Azithromycin (Systemic) *on page 180*

- **Zmax SR™ (Can)** *see* Azithromycin (Systemic) *on page 180*
- **ZnSO$_4$ (error-prone abbreviation)** *see* Zinc Sulfate *on page 1818*
- **Zocor®** *see* Simvastatin *on page 1555*
- **Zofran®** *see* Ondansetron *on page 1246*
- **Zofran® ODT** *see* Ondansetron *on page 1246*
- **Zol 446** *see* Zoledronic Acid *on page 1821*
- **Zoladex®** *see* Goserelin *on page 805*
- **Zoladex® LA (Can)** *see* Goserelin *on page 805*
- **Zoledronate** *see* Zoledronic Acid *on page 1821*

Zoledronic Acid (zoe le DRON ik AS id)

Brand Names: U.S. Reclast®; Zometa®

Brand Names: Canada Aclasta®; Zometa®

Index Terms CGP-42446; Zol 446; Zoledronate

Pharmacologic Category Antidote; Bisphosphonate Derivative

Use

Oncology-related uses: Treatment of hypercalcemia of malignancy (albumin-corrected serum calcium >12 mg/dL); treatment of multiple myeloma; treatment of bone metastases of solid tumors

Nononcology uses: Treatment of Paget's disease of bone; treatment of osteoporosis in postmenopausal women (to reduce the incidence of fractures or to reduce the incidence of new clinical fractures in patients with low-trauma hip fracture); prevention of osteoporosis in postmenopausal women, treatment of osteoporosis in men (to increase bone mass); treatment and prevention of glucocorticoid-induced osteoporosis (in patients initiating or continuing prednisone ≥7.5 mg/day [or equivalent] and expected to remain on glucocorticoids for at least 12 months)

Unlabeled Use Prevention of bone loss associated with aromatase inhibitor therapy in postmenopausal women with breast cancer; prevention of bone loss associated with androgen deprivation therapy in prostate cancer

Pregnancy Risk Factor D

Pregnancy Considerations Animal studies resulted in embryotoxicity and losses. Zoledronic acid should not be used during pregnancy; may cause fetal harm if administered to a pregnant woman. Bisphosphonates are incorporated into the bone matrix and gradually released over time. Theoretically, there may be a risk of fetal harm when pregnancy follows the completion of therapy. Based on limited case reports with pamidronate, serum calcium levels in the newborn may be altered if administered during pregnancy.

Lactation Excretion in breast milk unknown/not recommended

Medication Guide Available Yes

Contraindications Hypersensitivity to zoledronic acid or any component of the formulation; hypocalcemia (Reclast®); in patients with a creatinine clearance (Cl_{cr}) <35 mL/minute and in patients with evidence of acute renal impairment due to an increased risk of renal failure (Reclast®)

Canadian labeling: Hypersensitivity to other bisphosphonates. Aclasta® is also contraindicated with uncorrected hypocalcemia at the time of infusion and in pregnancy and breast-feeding.

Warnings/Precautions Osteonecrosis of the jaw (ONJ) has been reported in patients receiving bisphosphonates. Risk factors include invasive dental procedures (eg, tooth extraction, dental implants, boney surgery); a diagnosis of cancer, with concomitant chemotherapy, radiotherapy, or corticosteroids; poor oral hygiene, ill-fitting dentures; and comorbid disorders (anemia, coagulopathy, infection, pre-existing dental disease). Most reported cases occurred after I.V. bisphosphonate therapy; however, cases have been reported following oral therapy. A dental exam and preventative dentistry should be performed prior to placing patients with risk factors on chronic bisphosphonate therapy. The manufacturer's labeling states that there are no data to suggest whether discontinuing bisphosphonates in patients requiring invasive dental procedures reduces the risk of ONJ. However, other experts suggest that there is no evidence that discontinuing therapy reduces the risk of developing ONJ (Assael, 2009). The benefit/risk must be assessed by the treating physician and/or dentist/surgeon prior to any invasive dental procedure. Patients developing ONJ while on bisphosphonates should receive care by an oral surgeon.

Atypical, low energy, or low trauma femur fractures have been reported in patients receiving bisphosphonates for treatment/prevention of osteoporosis. The fractures include subtrochanteric femur (bone just below the hip joint) and diaphyseal femur (long segment of the thigh bone). Some patients experience prodromal pain weeks or months before the fracture occurs. It is unclear if bisphosphonate therapy is the cause for these fractures; atypical femur fractures have also been reported in patients not taking bisphosphonates, and in patients receiving glucocorticoids. Patients receiving long-term (>3-5 years) bisphosphonate therapy may be at an increased risk. Patients presenting with thigh or groin pain with a history of receiving bisphosphonates should be evaluated for femur fracture. Consider interrupting bisphosphonate therapy in patients who develop a femoral shaft fracture; assess for fracture in the contralateral limb.

Infrequently, severe (and occasionally debilitating) musculoskeletal (bone, joint, and/or muscle) pain have been reported during bisphosphonate treatment. The onset of pain ranged from a single day to several months. Consider discontinuing therapy in patients who experience severe symptoms; symptoms usually resolve upon discontinuation. Some patients experienced recurrence when rechallenged with same drug or another bisphosphonate; avoid use in patients with a history of these symptoms in association with bisphosphonate therapy.

May cause a significant risk of hypocalcemia in patients with Paget's disease, in whom the pretreatment rate of bone turnover may be greatly elevated. Hypocalcemia must be corrected before initiation of therapy in patients with Paget's disease and osteoporosis. Ensure adequate calcium and vitamin D intake during therapy. Use caution in patients with disturbances of calcium and mineral metabolism (eg, hypoparathyroidism, thyroid/parathyroid, surgery, malabsorption syndromes, excision of small intestine).

Reclast®: Use is contraindicated in patients with Cl_{cr} <35 mL/minute and in patients with evidence of acute renal impairment due to an increased risk of renal failure. Re-evaluate the need for continued therapy for the treatment of osteoporosis periodically; the optimal duration of treatment has not yet been determined.

Zometa®: Use caution in mild-to-moderate renal dysfunction; dosage adjustment required. In cancer patients, renal toxicity has been reported with doses >4 mg or infusions administered over 15 minutes. Risk factors for renal deterioration include pre-existing renal insufficiency and repeated doses of zoledronic acid and other bisphosphonates. Dehydration and the use of other nephrotoxic drugs which may contribute to renal deterioration should be identified and managed. Use is not recommended in patients with severe renal impairment (serum creatinine >3 mg/dL or Cl_{cr} <30 mL/minute) and bone metastases (limited data); use in patients with hypercalcemia of malignancy and severe renal impairment (serum creatinine >4.5 mg/dL for hypercalcemia of malignancy) should only be done if the benefits outweigh the risks. Renal function should be assessed prior to treatment; if decreased after treatment, additional treatments should be withheld until renal function returns to within 10% of baseline. Diuretics should not be used before correcting hypovolemia. Renal deterioration, resulting in renal failure and dialysis has occurred in patients treated with zoledronic acid after single and multiple infusions at recommended doses of 4 mg over 15 minutes.

Aclasta® [CAN; not available in U.S.]: Use is not recommended in patients with Cl_{cr} <30 mL/minute.

According to the American Society of Clinical Oncology (ASCO) guidelines for bisphosphonates in multiple myeloma, treatment with zoledronic acid is not recommended for asymptomatic (smoldering) or indolent myeloma or with solitary plasmacytoma (Kyle, 2007). The National Comprehensive Cancer Network® (NCCN) multiple myeloma guidelines (v.1.2011) also do not recommend the use of bisphosphonates in stage 1 or smoldering disease, unless part of a clinical trial.

Adequate hydration is required during treatment (urine output ~2 L/day); avoid overhydration, especially in patients with heart failure. Pre-existing renal compromise, severe dehydration, and concurrent use with diuretics or other nephrotoxic drugs may increase the risk for renal impairment. Single and multiple infusions in patients with both normal and impaired renal function have been associated with renal deterioration, resulting in renal failure and dialysis or death (rare). Patients with underlying moderate-to-severe renal impairment, increased age, concurrent use of nephrotoxic or diuretic medications, or severe dehydration prior to or after zoledronic acid administration may have an increased risk of acute renal impairment or renal failure. Others with increased risk include patients with renal impairment or dehydration secondary to fever, sepsis, gastrointestinal losses, or diuretic use. If history or physical exam suggests dehydration, treatment should not be given until the patient is normovolemic. Creatinine clearance (using actual body weight) should be calculated with the Cockcroft-Gault formula prior to each administration. Transient increases in serum creatinine may be more pronounced in patients with impaired renal function; consider monitoring creatinine clearance in at-risk patients taking other renally-eliminated drugs.

Use caution in patients with aspirin-sensitive asthma (may cause bronchoconstriction) and the elderly. Rare cases of urticaria and angioedema and very rare cases of anaphylactic reactions/shock have been reported. Women of childbearing age should be advised against becoming pregnant. Not approved for use in children. Do not administer Zometa® and Reclast® to the same patient for different indications.

Adverse Reactions Note: An acute reaction (eg, arthralgia, fever, flu-like symptoms, myalgia) may occur within the first 3 days following infusion in up to 44% of patients; usually resolves within 3-4 days of onset, although may take up to 14 days to resolve. The incidence may be decreased with acetaminophen (prior to infusion and for 72 hours postinfusion).

Zometa®:

>10%:

Cardiovascular: Leg edema (5% to 21%), hypotension (11%)

Central nervous system: Fatigue (39%), fever (32% to 44%), headache (5% to 19%), dizziness (18%), insomnia (15% to 16%), anxiety (11% to 14%), depression (14%), agitation (13%), confusion (7% to 13%), hypoesthesia (12%)

Dermatologic: Alopecia (12%), dermatitis (11%)

Endocrine & metabolic: Dehydration (5% to 14%), hypophosphatemia (12% to 13%), hypokalemia (12%), hypomagnesemia (11%)

Gastrointestinal: Nausea (29% to 46%), vomiting (14% to 32%), constipation (27% to 31%), diarrhea (17% to 24%), anorexia (9% to 22%), abdominal pain (14% to 16%), weight loss (16%), appetite decreased (13%)

Genitourinary: Urinary tract infection (12% to 14%)

Hematologic: Anemia (22% to 33%), neutropenia (12%)

Neuromuscular & skeletal: Bone pain (55%), weakness (5% to 24%), myalgia (23%), arthralgia (5% to 21%), back pain (15%), paresthesia (15%), limb pain (14%), skeletal pain (12%), rigors (11%)

Renal: Renal deterioration (8% to 17%; up to 40% in patients with abnormal baseline creatinine)

Respiratory: Dyspnea (22% to 27%), cough (12% to 22%)

Miscellaneous: Cancer progression (16%), moniliasis (12%)

1% to 10%:

Cardiovascular: Chest pain (5% to 10%)

Central nervous system: Somnolence (5% to 10%)

Endocrine & metabolic: Hypocalcemia (5% to 10%; grades 3/4: ≤1%), hypermagnesemia (2%)

Gastrointestinal: Dysphagia (5% to 10%), dyspepsia (10%), mucositis (5% to 10%), stomatitis (8%), sore throat (8%)

Hematologic: Granulocytopenia (5% to 10%), pancytopenia (5% to 10%), thrombocytopenia (5% to 10%)

Renal: Serum creatinine increased (grades 3/4: ≤2%)

Respiratory: Pleural effusion, upper respiratory tract infection (10%)

Miscellaneous: Infection (nonspecific; 5% to 10%), metastases (5% to 10%)

Reclast®:

>10%:

Cardiovascular: Hypertension (5% to 13%)

Central nervous system: Pain (2% to 24%), fever (9% to 22%), headache (4% to 20%), chills (2% to 18%), fatigue (2% to 18%)

Endocrine & metabolic: Hypocalcemia (≤3%; Paget's disease 21%)

Gastrointestinal: Nausea (5% to 18%)

Neuromuscular & skeletal: Arthralgia (9% to 27%), myalgia (5% to 23%), back pain (4% to 18%), limb pain (3% to 16%), musculoskeletal pain (≤12%)

Miscellaneous: Acute phase reaction (4% to 25%), flu-like syndrome (1% to 11%)

1% to 10%:

Cardiovascular: Chest pain (1% to 8%), peripheral edema (3% to 6%), atrial fibrillation (1% to 3%), palpitation (≤3%)

Central nervous system: Dizziness (2% to 9%), malaise (1% to 7%), hypoesthesia (≤6%), lethargy (3% to 5%), vertigo (1% to 4%), hyperthermia (≤2%)

Dermatologic: Rash (2% to 3%), hyperhidrosis (≤3%)

Gastrointestinal: Abdominal pain (1% to 9%), diarrhea (5% to 8%), vomiting (2% to 8%), constipation (6% to 7%), dyspepsia (2% to 7%), abdominal discomfort/distension (1% to 2%), anorexia (1% to 2%)

Neuromuscular & skeletal: Bone pain (3% to 9%), arthritis (2% to 9%), rigors (8%), shoulder pain (≤7%), neck pain (1% to 7%), weakness (2% to 6%), muscle spasm (2% to 6%), stiffness (1% to 5%), jaw pain (2% to 4%), joint swelling (≤3%), paresthesia (2%)

Ocular: Eye pain (≤2%)

Renal: Serum creatinine increased (2%)
Respiratory: Dyspnea (5% to 7%)
Miscellaneous: C-reactive protein increased (≤5%)

Zometa® and/or Reclast®: <1% (Limited to important or life-threatening): Acute renal failure (requiring hospitalization/dialysis), allergic reaction, anaphylactic reaction/shock, angioedema, arrhythmia, blurred vision, bradycardia, bronchoconstriction, conjunctivitis, diaphoresis, episcleritis, femur fracture (diaphyseal or subtrochanteric), flu-like syndrome (fever, chills, flushing, bone pain, arthralgia, myalgia, fatigue, weakness), hematuria, hyperesthesia, hyperkalemia, hypernatremia, hyperparathyroidism, hypersensitivity, hypertension, injection site reaction (eg, itching, pain, redness), iridocyclitis, iritis, joint and/or muscle pain (sometimes severe and/or incapacitating), muscle cramps, orbital edema, orbital inflammation, osteonecrosis (primarily of the jaws), proteinuria, pruritus, rash, renal failure, renal impairment, scleritis, taste perversion, toxic acute renal tubular necrosis, tremor, urticaria, uveitis, weight gain, xerostomia

Drug Interactions

Metabolism/Transport Effects None known.

Avoid Concomitant Use There are no known interactions where it is recommended to avoid concomitant use.

Increased Effect/Toxicity

Zoledronic Acid may increase the levels/effects of: Deferasirox; Phosphate Supplements

The levels/effects of Zoledronic Acid may be increased by: Aminoglycosides; Nonsteroidal Anti-Inflammatory Agents; Thalidomide

Decreased Effect

The levels/effects of Zoledronic Acid may be decreased by: Proton Pump Inhibitors

Stability

Aclasta® [CAN]: Store at room temperature of 15°C to 30°C (59°F to 86°F).

Reclast®: Store at room temperature of 25°C (77°F); excursions permitted to 15°C to 30°C (59°F to 86°F). After opening, stable for 24 hours at 2°C to 8°C (36°F to 46°F).

Zometa®: Store concentrate vials and ready-to-use bottles at 25°C (77°F); excursions permitted to 15°C to 30°C (59°F to 86°F).

Concentrate vials: Further dilute in 100 mL NS or D_5W prior to administration. Solutions for infusion which are not used immediately after preparation should be refrigerated at 2°C to 8°C (36°F to 46°F). Infusion of solution must be completed within 24 hours of preparation.

Ready-to-use bottles: No further preparation necessary; bottles intended for single use only. If reduced doses are necessary for patients with renal impairment, withdraw the appropriate volume of solution and replace with an equal amount of NS or D_5W. The prepared, diluted solution may be refrigerated at 2°C to 8°C (36°F to 46°F) if not used immediately. Infusion of solution must be completed within 24 hours of preparation. The previously withdrawn volume from the ready-to-use solution should be discarded; do not store or reuse.

Mechanism of Action A bisphosphonate which inhibits bone resorption via actions on osteoclasts or on osteoclast precursors; inhibits osteoclastic activity and skeletal calcium release induced by tumors. Decreases serum calcium and phosphorus, and increases their elimination. In osteoporosis, zoledronic acid inhibits osteoclast-mediated resorption, therefore reducing bone turnover.

Pharmacodynamics/Kinetics

Distribution: Binds to bone
Protein binding: 28% to 53%
Half-life elimination: Triphasic; Terminal: 146 hours
Excretion: Urine (39% ± 16% as unchanged drug) within 24 hours; feces (<3%)

Dosage I.V.: Adults: **Note:** Acetaminophen administration after the infusion may reduce symptoms of acute-phase reactions. Patients treated for multiple myeloma, osteoporosis, and Paget's disease should receive a daily calcium supplement and multivitamin containing vitamin D (if dietary intake is inadequate).

Hypercalcemia of malignancy (albumin-corrected serum calcium ≥12 mg/dL) (Zometa®): 4 mg (maximum) given as a single dose. Wait at least 7 days before considering retreatment. Dosage adjustment may be needed in patients with decreased renal function following treatment.

Multiple myeloma or metastatic bone lesions from solid tumors (Zometa®): 4 mg every 3-4 weeks

Osteoporosis, glucocorticoid-induced, treatment and prevention (Reclast®, Aclasta® [CAN]): 5 mg infused over at least 15 minutes once a year

Osteoporosis, prevention (Reclast®): 5 mg infused over at least 15 minutes every 2 years

Osteoporosis, treatment (Reclast®, Aclasta® [CAN]): 5 mg infused over at least 15 minutes once a year

Paget's disease: 5 mg infused over at least 15 minutes. **Note:** Data concerning retreatment is not available; retreatment may be considered for relapse (increase in alkaline phosphatase) if appropriate, for inadequate response, or in patients who are symptomatic.

Prevention of aromatase inhibitor-induced bone loss in breast cancer (unlabeled use): 4 mg every 6 months (Brufsky, 2007)

Prevention of androgen deprivation-induced bone loss in nonmetastatic prostate cancer (unlabeled use): 4 mg every 3 months for 1 year (Smith, 2003) or 4 mg every 12 months (Michaelson, 2007)

Dosage adjustment in renal impairment (at treatment initiation):

Reclast®:
- Cl_{cr} ≥35 mL/minute: No adjustment required
- Cl_{cr} <35 mL/minute: Use is contraindicated

Zometa®: Multiple myeloma and bone metastases:
- Cl_{cr} >60 mL/minute: 4 mg
- Cl_{cr} 50-60 mL/minute: 3.5 mg
- Cl_{cr} 40-49 mL/minute: 3.3 mg
- Cl_{cr} 30-39 mL/minute: 3 mg
- Cl_{cr} <30 mL/minute: Use is not recommended

Zometa®: Hypercalcemia of malignancy:
- Mild-to-moderate impairment: No adjustment necessary
- Severe impairment (serum creatinine >4.5 mg/dL): Evaluate risk versus benefit

Aclasta® [CAN]:
- Cl_{cr} ≥30 mL/minute: No adjustment required
- Cl_{cr} <30 mL/minute: Use is not recommended

Dosage adjustment for renal toxicity (during treatment):

Hypercalcemia of malignancy: Evidence of renal deterioration: Evaluate risk versus benefit.

Multiple myeloma and bone metastases: Evidence of renal deterioration: Withhold dose until renal function returns to within 10% of baseline: renal deterioration defined as follows:
- Normal baseline creatinine: Increase of 0.5 mg/dL
- Abnormal baseline creatinine: Increase of 1 mg/dL

Reinitiate dose at the same dose administered prior to treatment interruption.

Multiple myeloma: Albuminuria >500 mg/24 hours (unexplained): Withhold dose until return to baseline, then reevaluate every 3-4 weeks; consider reinitiating with a longer infusion time of at least 30 minutes (Kyle, 2007).

Dosage adjustment in hepatic impairment: Specific guidelines are not available.

Dietary Considerations

Multiple myeloma or metastatic bone lesions from solid tumors: Take daily calcium supplement (500 mg) and daily multivitamin (with 400 int. units vitamin D).

Osteoporosis: Ensure adequate calcium and vitamin D supplementation; general requirements are calcium 1200 mg/day and vitamin D 800-1000 int. units/day.

Paget's disease: Take elemental calcium 1500 mg/day (750 mg twice daily or 500 mg 3 times/day) and vitamin D 800 units/day, particularly during the first 2 weeks after administration.

Administration Infuse over at least 15 minutes. Flush I.V. line with 10 mL NS flush following infusion. Infuse in a line separate from other medications. Patients should be appropriately hydrated prior to treatment.

Reclast®, Zometa®: If refrigerated, allow to reach room temperature prior to administration. Acetaminophen after administration may reduce the incidence of acute reaction (eg, arthralgia, fever, flu-like symptoms, myalgia).

Monitoring Parameters Prior to initiation of therapy, dental exam and preventative dentistry for patients at risk for osteonecrosis, including all cancer patients

Aclasta® [CAN], Reclast®: Serum creatinine prior to each dose,especially in patients with risk factors, calculate creatinine clearance before each treatment (consider interim monitoring in patients at risk for acute renal failure), evaluate fluid status and adequately hydrate patients prior to and following administration.

Osteoporosis: Bone mineral density as measured by central dual-energy x-ray absorptiometry (DXA) of the hip or spine (prior to initiation of therapy and at least every 2 years; after 6-12 months of combined glucocorticoid and zoledronic acid treatment); annual measurements of height and weight, assessment of chronic back pain; serum calcium and 25(OH)D; phosphorus and magnesium; may consider monitoring biochemical markers of bone turnover

Paget's disease: Alkaline phosphatase; pain; serum calcium and 25(OH)D; phosphorus and magnesium

Zometa®: Serum creatinine prior to each dose; serum electrolytes, phosphate, magnesium, and hemoglobin/hematocrit should be evaluated regularly. Monitor serum calcium to assess response and avoid overtreatment. In patients with multiple myeloma, monitor urine every 3-6 months for albuminuria.

Test Interactions Bisphosphonates may interfere with diagnostic imaging agents such as technetium-99m-diphosphonate in bone scans.

Additional Information Oncology Comment:

Metastatic breast cancer: The American Society of Clinical Oncology (ASCO) guidelines on the role of bone-modifying agents (BMAs) in the prevention and treatment of skeletal-related events for metastatic breast cancer patients were updated (Van Poznak, 2011). The guidelines recommend initiating a BMA (denosumab, pamidronate, zoledronic acid) in patients with a diagnosis of metastatic breast cancer to the bone. There is currently no literature indicating the superiority of one particular BMA over another. The optimal duration has yet to be defined; however, the guidelines recommend continuing therapy until substantial decline in patient's performance status. In patients with normal creatinine clearance (>60 mL/minute), no dosage/interval/infusion rate changes for pamidronate or zoledronic acid are necessary. For patients with Cl_{cr} <30 mL/minute, pamidronate and zoledronic acid are not recommended. While no renal dose adjustments are recommended for denosumab, close monitoring is advised for risk of hypocalcemia in patients with Cl_{cr} <30 mL/minute or on dialysis. The ASCO guidelines are in alignment with package insert guidelines for dosing, renal dose adjustments, infusion times, prevention and management of osteonecrosis of the jaw, and monitoring of laboratory parameter recommendations. BMAs are not the first-line therapy for pain. BMAs are to be used as adjunctive therapy for cancer-related bone pain associated with bone metastasis, demonstrating a modest pain control benefit. BMAs should be used in conjunction with agents such as NSAIDS, opioid and nonopioid analgesics, corticosteroids, radiation/surgery, interventional procedures.

Multiple myeloma: The American Society of Clinical Oncology (ASCO) also has guidelines published on the use of bisphosphonates for prevention and treatment of bone disease in multiple myeloma (Kyle, 2007). Pamidronate or zoledronic acid use is recommended in multiple myeloma patients with lytic bone destruction or compression spine fracture from osteopenia. Clodronate (not available in the U.S.; available in Canada), administered orally or I.V., is an alternative treatment. The use of the bisphosphonates pamidronate and zoledronic acid may be considered in patients with pain secondary to osteolytic disease, adjunct therapy to stabilize fractures or impending fractures, and I.V. bisphosphonates for multiple myeloma patients with osteopenia but no radiographic evidence of lytic bone disease. Bisphosphonates are not recommended in patients with solitary plasmacytoma, smoldering (asymptomatic) or indolent myeloma, or monoclonal gammopathy of undetermined significance. The guidelines recommend monthly treatment for a period of 2 years. At that time, physicians need to consider discontinuing in responsive and stable patients, and reinitiate if new-onset skeletal-related event occurs. The ASCO guidelines are in alignment with package insert guidelines for dosing, renal dose adjustments, infusion times, prevention and management of osteonecrosis of the jaw, and monitoring of laboratory parameter recommendations. The guidelines also state in patients with a serum creatinine >3 mg/dL or Cl_{cr} <30 mL/minute or extensive bone disease, pamidronate at a dose of 90 mg over 4-6 hours is recommended (unless pre-existing renal disease at which a reduced dose should be considered). The ASCO committee also recommends monitoring for the presence of albuminuria every 3-6 months. In patients with albuminuria >500 mg/24 hours, withhold the dose until level returns to baseline, then recheck every 3-4 weeks. Pamidronate may be reinitiated at a dose not to exceed 90 mg every 4 weeks with a longer infusion time of at least 4 hours. The committee also recommends considering increasing the infusion time of zoledronic acid to at least 30 minutes. However, one study has demonstrated that extending the infusion to 30 minutes did not change the safety profile (Berenson, 2011).

Dosage Forms Excipient information presented when available (limited, particularly for generics); consult specific product labeling.

Infusion, premixed:
- Reclast®: 5 mg (100 mL)
- Zometa®: 4 mg (100 mL)

Injection, solution [concentrate]:
- Zometa®: 4 mg/5 mL (5 mL)

Dosage Forms: Canada Excipient information presented when available (limited, particularly for generics); consult specific product labeling.

Infusion, solution [premixed]:
- Aclasta®: 5 mg (100 mL)

◆ **Zolinza®** *see* Vorinostat *on page 1800*

ZOLMitriptan (zohl mi TRIP tan)

Brand Names: U.S. Zomig-ZMT®; Zomig®

Brand Names: Canada Mylan-Zolmitriptan; PMS-Zolmitriptan; PMS-Zolmitriptan ODT; Sandoz-Zolmitriptan; Sandoz-Zolmitriptan ODT; Teva-Zolmitriptan; Teva-Zolmitriptan OD; Zomig®; Zomig® Nasal Spray; Zomig® Rapimelt

Index Terms 311C90

Pharmacologic Category Antimigraine Agent; Serotonin $5\text{-}HT_{1B,\ 1D}$ Receptor Agonist

Additional Appendix Information

Antimigraine Drugs: $5\text{-}HT_1$ Receptor Agonists *on page 1878*

Use Acute treatment of migraine with or without aura

Pregnancy Risk Factor C

Pregnancy Considerations There are no adequate and well-controlled studies using zolmitriptan in pregnant women. Use only if potential benefit to the mother outweighs the potential risk to the fetus. In animal studies, administration was associated with embryolethality, fetal abnormalities, and pup mortality.

Lactation Excretion in breast milk unknown/use caution

Contraindications Hypersensitivity to zolmitriptan or any component of the formulation; ischemic heart disease or vasospastic coronary artery disease, including Prinzmetal's angina; signs or symptoms of ischemic heart disease; uncontrolled hypertension; symptomatic Wolff-Parkinson-White syndrome or arrhythmias associated with other cardiac accessory conduction pathway disorders; use with ergotamine derivatives (within 24 hours of); use within 24 hours of another $5\text{-}HT_1$ agonist; concurrent administration or within 2 weeks of discontinuing an MAO inhibitor; management of hemiplegic or basilar migraine

Nasal spray: Additional contraindications with nasal spray: Cerebrovascular syndromes (eg, stroke, TIA); peripheral vascular disease (including ischemic bowel disease)

Warnings/Precautions Zolmitriptan is indicated only in patient populations with a clear diagnosis of migraine. Not for prophylactic treatment of migraine headaches. Cardiac events (coronary artery vasospasm, transient ischemia, myocardial infarction, ventricular tachycardia/fibrillation, cardiac arrest, and death) have been reported with $5\text{-}HT_1$ agonist administration. Patients who experience sensations of chest pain/pressure/tightness or symptoms suggestive of angina following dosing should be evaluated for coronary artery disease or Prinzmetal's angina before receiving additional doses; if dosing is resumed and similar symptoms recur, monitor with ECG. Should not be given to patients who have risk factors for CAD (eg, hypertension, hypercholesterolemia, smoker, obesity, diabetes, strong family history of CAD, menopause, male >40 years of age) without adequate cardiac evaluation. Patients with suspected CAD should have cardiovascular evaluation to rule out CAD before considering zolmitriptan's use; if cardiovascular evaluation negative, first dose would be safest if given in the healthcare provider's office (consider ECG monitoring). Periodic evaluation of those without cardiovascular disease, but with continued risk factors, should be done. Significant elevation in blood pressure, including hypertensive crisis, has also been reported on rare occasions in patients with and without a history of hypertension. Vasospasm-related reactions have been reported other than coronary artery vasospasm. Peripheral vascular ischemia and colonic ischemia with abdominal pain and bloody diarrhea have occurred. Cerebral/subarachnoid hemorrhage and stroke have been reported with $5\text{-}HT_1$ agonist administration; nasal spray contraindicated in patients with cerebrovascular syndromes. Rarely, partial vision loss and blindness (transient and permanent) have been reported with $5\text{-}HT_1$ agonists. Use with caution in patients with hepatic impairment. Zomig-ZMT™ tablets contain phenylalanine. Symptoms of agitation, confusion, hallucinations, hyper-reflexia, myoclonus, shivering, and tachycardia (serotonin syndrome) may occur with concomitant proserotonergic drugs (eg, SSRIs/SNRIs or triptans) or agents which reduce zolmitriptan's metabolism. Concurrent use of serotonin precursors (eg, tryptophan) is not recommended.

Adverse Reactions Percentages noted from oral preparations.

1% to 10%:

Cardiovascular: Chest pain (2% to 4%), palpitation (up to 2%)

Central nervous system: Dizziness (6% to 10%), somnolence (5% to 8%), pain (2% to 3%), vertigo (≤2%)

Gastrointestinal: Nausea (4% to 9%), xerostomia (3% to 5%), dyspepsia (1% to 3%), dysphagia (≤2%)

Neuromuscular & skeletal: Paresthesia (5% to 9%), weakness (3% to 9%), warm/cold sensation (5% to 7%), hypoesthesia (1% to 2%), myalgia (1% to 2%), myasthenia (up to 2%)

Miscellaneous: Neck/throat/jaw pain (4% to 10%), diaphoresis (up to 3%), allergic reaction (up to 1%)

<1% (Limited to important or life-threatening): Anaphylactoid reaction, anaphylaxis, angina, apnea, arrhythmia, ataxia, bronchospasm, cerebral ischemia, coronary artery vasospasm, cyanosis, eosinophilia, esophagitis, gastrointestinal infarction/necrosis, hallucinations, headache, hematemesis, hypertension, hypertensive crisis, ischemic colitis, melena, miscarriage, MI, myocardial ischemia, pancreatitis, photosensitivity, QT prolongation, rash, serotonin syndrome, splenic infarction, syncope, tetany, thrombocytopenia, tinnitus, ulcer, urticaria

Events related to other serotonin $5\text{-}HT_{1D}$ receptor agonists: Cardiac arrest, cerebral hemorrhage, peripheral vascular ischemia, stroke, subarachnoid hemorrhage, ventricular fibrillation

Drug Interactions

Metabolism/Transport Effects Substrate of CYP1A2 (minor); **Note:** Assignment of Major/Minor substrate status based on clinically relevant drug interaction potential

Avoid Concomitant Use

Avoid concomitant use of ZOLMitriptan with any of the following: Ergot Derivatives; MAO Inhibitors

Increased Effect/Toxicity

ZOLMitriptan may increase the levels/effects of: Ergot Derivatives; Metoclopramide; Serotonin Modulators

The levels/effects of ZOLMitriptan may be increased by: Antipsychotics; Cimetidine; Ergot Derivatives; MAO Inhibitors; Propranolol

Decreased Effect

The levels/effects of ZOLMitriptan may be decreased by: Cyproterone

Ethanol/Nutrition/Herb Interactions Ethanol: Limit use (may have additive CNS toxicity).

Stability Store at 20°C to 25°C (68°F to 77°F). Protect from light and moisture.

Mechanism of Action Selective agonist for serotonin ($5\text{-}HT_{1B}$ and $5\text{-}HT_{1D}$ receptors) in cranial arteries; causes vasoconstriction and reduces sterile inflammation associated with antidromic neuronal transmission correlating with relief of migraine

Pharmacodynamics/Kinetics

Onset of action: 0.5-1 hour

Absorption: Well absorbed

Distribution: V_d: 7 L/kg

Protein binding: 25%

Metabolism: Converted to an active N-desmethyl metabolite (2-6 times more potent than zolmitriptan)

Bioavailability: 40%

Half-life elimination: 2.8-3.7 hours

Time to peak, serum: Tablet: 1.5 hours; Orally-disintegrating tablet and nasal spray: 3 hours

Excretion: Urine (~60% to 65% total dose); feces (30% to 40%)

Dosage Oral:

Children: Safety and efficacy have not been established

Adults: Migraine:

Tablet: Initial: ≤2.5 mg at the onset of migraine headache; may break 2.5 mg tablet in half

Orally-disintegrating tablet: Initial: 2.5 mg at the onset of migraine headache

Nasal spray: Initial: 1 spray (5 mg) at the onset of migraine headache

Note: Use the lowest possible dose to minimize adverse events. If the headache returns, the dose may be repeated after 2 hours; do not exceed 10 mg within a 24-hour period. Controlled trials have not established the effectiveness of a second dose if the initial one was ineffective.

Elderly: No dosage adjustment needed but elderly patients are more likely to have underlying cardiovascular disease and should have careful evaluation of cardiovascular system before prescribing.

Dosage adjustment in renal impairment: No dosage adjustment recommended. There is a 25% reduction in zolmitriptan's clearance in patients with severe renal impairment (Cl_{cr} 5-25 mL/minute).

Dosage adjustment in hepatic impairment: Administer with caution in patients with liver disease, generally using doses <2.5 mg (doses <5 mg can only be achieved using oral tablets). Patients with moderate-to-severe hepatic impairment may have decreased clearance of zolmitriptan, and significant elevation in blood pressure was observed in some patients.

Dietary Considerations Some products may contain phenylalanine.

Administration Administer as soon as migraine headache starts.

Tablet: May be broken.

Orally-disintegrating tablet: Must be taken whole; do not break, crush or chew. Place on tongue and allow to dissolve. Administration with liquid is not required.

Nasal spray: Blow nose gently prior to use. After removing protective cap, instill device into nostril. Block opposite nostril; breathe in gently through nose while pressing plunger of spray device. One dose (5 mg) is equal to 1 spray in 1 nostril.

Additional Information Not recommended if the patient has risk factors for heart disease (high blood pressure, high cholesterol, obesity, diabetes, smoking, strong family history of heart disease, postmenopausal woman, or a male >40 years of age).

This agent is intended to relieve migraine, but not to prevent or reduce the number of attacks. Use only to treat an actual migraine attack.

Dosage Forms Excipient information presented when available (limited, particularly for generics); consult specific product labeling.

Solution, intranasal [spray]:

Zomig®: 5 mg/0.1 mL (0.1 mL)

Tablet, oral:

Zomig®: 2.5 mg [scored]

Zomig®: 5 mg

Tablet, orally disintegrating, oral:

Zomig-ZMT®: 2.5 mg [contains phenylalanine 2.81 mg/tablet; orange flavor]

Zomig-ZMT®: 5 mg [contains phenylalanine 5.62 mg/tablet; orange flavor]

◆ **Zoloft®** *see* Sertraline *on page* 1548

Zolpidem (zole PI dem)

Brand Names: U.S. Ambien CR®; Ambien®; Edluar™; Zolpimist®

Brand Names: Canada Sublinox™

Index Terms Intermezzo®; Zolpidem Tartrate

Pharmacologic Category Hypnotic, Nonbenzodiazepine

Use

Ambien®, Edluar™, Zolpimist®: Short-term treatment of insomnia (with difficulty of sleep onset)

Ambien CR®: Treatment of insomnia (with difficulty of sleep onset and/or sleep maintenance)

Sublinox™ (Canadian availability; not available in U.S.): Short-term treatment of insomnia (with difficulty of sleep onset, frequent awakenings, and/or early awakenings)

Pregnancy Risk Factor C

Pregnancy Considerations Teratogenic effects were not observed in animal studies. Adverse effects were noted in animal reproductive studies at doses 20-100 times the maximum recommended human dose. Severe neonatal respiratory depression has been reported when zolpidem was used at the end of pregnancy, especially when used concurrently with other CNS depressants. Studies of prenatal exposure to zolpidem have not been conducted in children. Children born of mothers taking sedative/hypnotics may be at risk for withdrawal; neonatal flaccidity has been reported in infants following maternal use of sedative/hypnotics during pregnancy. Use during pregnancy only if the benefits justify the risk to the fetus.

Lactation Enters breast milk/use caution (AAP rates "compatible"; AAP 2001 update pending)

Medication Guide Available Yes

Contraindications Hypersensitivity to zolpidem or any component of the formulation

Canadian labeling: Additional contraindications (not in U.S. labeling): Significant obstructive sleep apnea syndrome and acute and/or severe impairment of respiratory function; myasthenia gravis; severe hepatic impairment; personal or family history of sleepwalking

Warnings/Precautions Should be used only after evaluation of potential causes of sleep disturbance. Failure of sleep disturbance to resolve after 7-10 days may indicate psychiatric or medical illness. Hypnotics/sedatives have been associated with abnormal thinking and behavior changes including decreased inhibition, aggression, bizarre behavior, agitation, hallucinations, and depersonalization. These changes may occur unpredictably and may indicate previously unrecognized psychiatric disorders; evaluate appropriately. Sedative/hypnotics may produce withdrawal symptoms following abrupt discontinuation. Use with caution in patients with depression; worsening of depression, including suicide or suicidal ideation has been reported with the use of hypnotics. Intentional overdose may be an issue in this population. The minimum dose that will effectively treat the individual patient should be used. Prescriptions should be written for the smallest quantity consistent with good patient care. Causes CNS depression, which may impair physical and mental capabilities. Zolpidem should only be administered when the patient is able to stay in bed a full night (7-8 hours) before being active again. Effects with other sedative drugs or ethanol may be potentiated. Canadian labeling does not recommend concomitant use with alcohol.

Use caution in patients with myasthenia gravis (contraindicated in the Canadian labeling). Avoid use in patients with sleep apnea or a history of sedative-hypnotic abuse. Postmarketing studies have indicated that the use of hypnotic/sedative agents for sleep has been associated with hypersensitivity reactions including anaphylaxis as well as angioedema. An increased risk for hazardous sleep-related activities such as sleep-driving; cooking and eating food, and making phone calls while asleep have also been noted; amnesia may also occur. Discontinue treatment in patients who report any sleep-related episodes. Canadian labeling recommends avoiding use in patients with disorders (eg, restless legs syndrome, periodic limb movement disorder, sleep apnea) that may disrupt sleep and cause frequent awakenings, potentially increasing the risk of complex sleep-related behaviors.

Use caution with respiratory disease (Canadian labeling contraindicates use with acute and/or severe impairment of respiratory function). Use caution with hepatic impairment (Canadian labeling contraindicates use in severe impairment); dose adjustment required. Because of the rapid onset of action, administer immediately prior to bedtime or after the patient has gone to bed and is having difficulty falling asleep.

Use caution in the elderly; dose adjustment recommended. Closely monitor elderly or debilitated patients for impaired cognitive or motor performance. When studied for the unapproved use of insomnia associated with ADHD in children, a higher incidence (~7%) of hallucinations was reported. In addition, sleep latency did not decrease compared to placebo. Zolpidem is **not** FDA- or Health Canada-approved for use in pediatric patients.

Adverse Reactions Actual frequency may be dosage form, dose, and/or age dependent

>10%: Central nervous system: Headache (7% to 19%), somnolence (6% to 15%), dizziness (1% to 12%)

1% to 10%:

Cardiovascular: Blood pressure increased, chest discomfort/pain, palpitation

Central nervous system: Abnormal dreams, anxiety, apathy, amnesia, ataxia, attention disturbance, body temperature increased, burning sensation, confusion, depersonalization, depression, disinhibition, disorientation, drowsiness, drugged feeling, euphoria, fatigue, fever, hallucinations, hypoesthesia, insomnia, lethargy, lightheadedness, memory disorder, mood swings, sleep disorder, stress

Dermatologic: Rash, urticaria, wrinkling

Endocrine & metabolic: Menorrhagia

Gastrointestinal: Abdominal discomfort, abdominal pain, abdominal tenderness, appetite disorder, constipation, diarrhea, dyspepsia, flatulence, gastroenteritis, gastroesophageal reflux, hiccup, nausea, vomiting, xerostomia

Genitourinary: Urinary tract infection, vulvovaginal dryness

Neuromuscular & skeletal: Arthralgia, back pain, balance disorder, involuntary muscle contractions, myalgia, neck pain, paresthesia, psychomotor retardation, tremor, weakness

Ocular: Asthenopia, blurred vision, depth perception altered, diplopia, red eye, visual disturbance

Otic: Labyrinthitis, tinnitus, vertigo

Renal: Dysuria

Respiratory: Pharyngitis, sinusitis, throat irritation, upper respiratory tract infection

Miscellaneous: Allergy, binge eating, flu-like syndrome

<1% (Limited to important or life-threatening): Agitation, anaphylaxis, anemia, angioedema, cerebrovascular disorder, cognition decreased, complex sleep-related behavior (sleep-driving, cooking or eating food, making phone calls), concentrating difficulty, cystitis, diaphoresis, dysphagia, dyspnea, edema, emotional lability, falling, hepatic function abnormalities, hyperglycemia, hyper-/hypotension, illusion, leukopenia, lymphadenopathy, migraine, paresthesia of the tongue (sublingual tablets), postural hypotension, pruritus, renal failure (acute), scleritis, somnambulism (sleepwalking), speech disorder, stupor, sublingual erythema (sublingual tablets), syncope, tachycardia, thrombosis, urinary incontinence, vaginitis

Drug Interactions

Metabolism/Transport Effects **Substrate** of CYP1A2 (minor), CYP2C19 (minor), CYP2C9 (minor), CYP2D6 (minor), CYP3A4 (major); **Note:** Assignment of Major/Minor substrate status based on clinically relevant drug interaction potential

Avoid Concomitant Use

Avoid concomitant use of Zolpidem with any of the following: Conivaptan

Increased Effect/Toxicity

Zolpidem may increase the levels/effects of: Alcohol (Ethyl); CarBAMazepine; CNS Depressants; Methotrimeprazine; Selective Serotonin Reuptake Inhibitors

The levels/effects of Zolpidem may be increased by: Antifungal Agents (Azole Derivatives, Systemic); Conivaptan; CYP3A4 Inhibitors (Moderate); CYP3A4 Inhibitors (Strong); Dasatinib; Droperidol; HydrOXYzine; Methotrimeprazine

Decreased Effect

The levels/effects of Zolpidem may be decreased by: CarBAMazepine; CYP3A4 Inducers (Strong); Cyproterone; Deferasirox; Flumazenil; Herbs (CYP3A4 Inducers); Peginterferon Alfa-2b; Rifamycin Derivatives; Telaprevir; Tocilizumab

Ethanol/Nutrition/Herb Interactions

Ethanol: May enhance the adverse/toxic effects of zolpidem; avoid use.

Food: Maximum plasma concentration and bioavailability are decreased with food; time to peak plasma concentration is increased; half-life remains unchanged. Grapefruit juice may decrease the metabolism of zolpidem.

Herb/Nutraceutical: St John's wort may decrease the levels/effects of zolpidem; avoid concomitant use. In addition, concomitant use of valerian, kava kava, and gotu kola should be avoided due to the risk of increased CNS depression.

Stability

Ambien®, Edluar™: Store at 20°C to 25°C (68°F to 77°F). Protect sublingual tablets from light and moisture.

Ambien CR®: Store at 15°C to 25°C (59°F to 77°F); limited excursions permitted up to 30°C (86°F).

Zolpimist®: Store at 25°C (77°F); do not freeze. Avoid prolonged exposure to temperatures >30°C (86°F).

Sublinox™ (Canadian availability; not available in U.S.): Store at 15°C to 30°C (59°F to 86°F); protect from light and moisture.

Mechanism of Action Zolpidem, an imidazopyridine hypnotic that is structurally dissimilar to benzodiazepines, enhances the activity of the inhibitory neurotransmitter, γ-aminobutyric acid (GABA), via selective agonism at the benzodiazepine-1 (BZ_1) receptor; the result is increased chloride conductance, neuronal hyperpolarization, inhibition of the action potential, and a decrease in neuronal excitability leading to sedative and hypnotic effects. Because of its selectivity for the BZ_1 receptor site over the BZ_2 receptor site, zolpidem exhibits minimal anxiolytic, myorelaxant, and anticonvulsant properties (effects largely attributed to agonism at the BZ_2 receptor site).

Pharmacodynamics/Kinetics

Onset of action: Immediate release: 30 minutes

Duration: Immediate release: 6-8 hours

Absorption: Rapid

Distribution: V_d: 0.54 L/kg

Protein binding: ~93%

Metabolism: Hepatic methylation and hydroxylation via CYP3A4 (~60%), CYP2C9 (~22%), CYP1A2 (~14%), CYP2D6 (~3%), and CYP2C19 (~3%) to three inactive metabolites

Bioavailability: 70%

Half-life elimination:

Immediate release, Extended release: ~2.5 hours (range 1.4-4.5 hours); Cirrhosis: Up to 9.9 hours; Elderly: Prolonged up to 32%

Spray: ~3 hours (range: 1.7-8.4)

Sublingual: ~3 hours (range: 1.6-6.7 hours)

Time to peak, plasma:

Immediate release: 1.6 hours; 2.2 hours with food

Extended release: 1.5 hours; 4 hours with food

Spray: ~0.9 hours

Sublingual: ~1.4 hours; ~1.8 hours with food

Excretion: Urine (48% to 67%, primarily as metabolites); feces (29% to 42%, primarily as metabolites)

Dosage Oral:

Adults:

Immediate release tablet, spray, sublingual tablet: 10 mg immediately before bedtime; maximum dose: 10 mg

Extended release tablet: 12.5 mg immediately before bedtime

Elderly:

Immediate release tablet, spray: 5 mg immediately before bedtime

Sublingual tablet:

U.S. labeling (Edluar™): 5 mg immediately before bedtime

Canadian labeling (Sublinox™): Not recommended; tablet cannot not be split for a reduced dose.

Extended release tablet: 6.25 mg immediately before bedtime

Dosing adjustment in renal impairment: Dose adjustment not required; monitor closely

Hemodialysis: Not dialyzable

Dosing adjustment in hepatic impairment:

U.S. labeling:

Immediate release tablet, spray, sublingual tablet: 5 mg

Extended release tablet: 6.25 mg

Canadian labeling: Sublingual tablet:

Mild-to-moderate impairment: Use is not recommended; tablet cannot be split for reduced dose.

Severe impairment: Use is contraindicated.

Dietary Considerations For faster sleep onset, do not administer with (or immediately after) a meal.

Administration Ingest immediately before bedtime due to rapid onset of action.

Ambien CR® tablets should be swallowed whole; do not divide, crush, or chew.

Edluar™ or Sublinox™ (Canadian availability; not available in U.S.) sublingual tablets should be placed under the tongue and allowed to disintegrate; do not swallow or administer with water. Do not administer with or immediately after a meal.

Zolpimist® oral spray should be sprayed directly into the mouth over the tongue. Prior to initial use, pump should be primed by spraying 5 times. If pump is not used for at least 14 days, re-prime pump with 1 spray.

Monitoring Parameters Daytime alertness; respiratory rate; behavior profile

Test Interactions Increased aminotransferase [ALT/AST], bilirubin (S); decreased RAI uptake

Additional Information Causes fewer disturbances in sleep stages as compared to benzodiazepines. Time spent in sleep stages 3 and 4 are maintained; zolpidem decreases sleep latency; should not be prescribed in quantities exceeding a 1-month supply.

Product Availability

Intermezzo® sublingual tablets: FDA approved November 2011; availability anticipated second quarter 2012

Intermezzo® sublingual tablets are indicated for as needed treatment of insomnia when middle-of-the-night awakening is followed by difficulty returning to sleep with ≥4 hours of expected sleep time remaining.

Dosage Forms Excipient information presented when available (limited, particularly for generics); consult specific product labeling.

Solution, oral, as tartrate [spray]:

Zolpimist®: 5 mg/actuation (8.2 g) [contains benzoic acid, propylene glycol; cherry flavor; 60 metered actuations]

Tablet, oral, as tartrate: 5 mg, 10 mg

Ambien®: 5 mg, 10 mg

Tablet, sublingual, as tartrate:

Edluar™: 5 mg, 10 mg

Tablet, extended release, oral, as tartrate: 6.25 mg, 12.5 mg

Ambien CR®: 6.25 mg, 12.5 mg

Dosage Forms: Canada Excipient information presented when available (limited, particularly for generics); consult specific product labeling.

Tablet, sublingual, as tartrate:

Sublinox™: 10 mg

Controlled Substance C-IV

◆ **Zolpidem Tartrate** *see* Zolpidem *on page 1826*

◆ **Zolpimist®** *see* Zolpidem *on page 1826*

◆ **Zolvit™** *see* Hydrocodone and Acetaminophen *on page 837*

◆ **Zometa®** *see* Zoledronic Acid *on page 1821*

◆ **Zomig®** *see* ZOLMitriptan *on page 1824*

◆ **Zomig® Nasal Spray (Can)** *see* ZOLMitriptan *on page 1824*

◆ **Zomig® Rapimelt (Can)** *see* ZOLMitriptan *on page 1824*

◆ **Zomig-ZMT®** *see* ZOLMitriptan *on page 1824*

◆ **Zonalon®** *see* Doxepin (Topical) *on page 552*

◆ **Zonatuss™** *see* Benzonatate *on page 205*

◆ **Zonegran®** *see* Zonisamide *on page 1828*

Zonisamide (zoe NIS a mide)

Brand Names: U.S. Zonegran®

Pharmacologic Category Anticonvulsant, Miscellaneous

Additional Appendix Information

Anticonvulsant Drugs of Choice *on page 1873*

Use Adjunct treatment of partial seizures in children >16 years of age and adults with epilepsy

Unlabeled Use Bipolar disorder

Pregnancy Risk Factor C

Pregnancy Considerations Teratogenic effects were observed in animal reproduction studies; therefore, zonisamide is classified as pregnancy category C. Zonisamide crosses the placenta and can be detected in the newborn following delivery. Although adverse fetal events have been reported, the risk of teratogenic effects following maternal use of zonisamide in not clearly defined. Other agents may be preferred until additional data is available. Newborns should be monitored for transient metabolic acidosis after birth. Zonisamide clearance may increase in the second trimester of pregnancy, requiring dosage adjustment. Women of childbearing potential are advised to use effective contraception during therapy.

Patients exposed to zonisamide during pregnancy are encouraged to enroll themselves into the AED Pregnancy Registry by calling 1-888-233-2334. Additional information is available at http://www.aedpregnancyregistry.org.

Lactation Excreted into breast milk /not recommended

Medication Guide Available Yes

Contraindications Hypersensitivity to zonisamide, sulfonamides, or any component of the formulation

Warnings/Precautions Hazardous agent - use appropriate precautions for handling and disposal. Rare, but potentially fatal sulfonamide reactions have occurred following the use of zonisamide. These reactions include Stevens-Johnson syndrome, fulminant hepatic necrosis, agranulocytosis, aplastic anemia, and toxic epidermal necrolysis, usually appearing within 2-16 weeks of drug initiation. Discontinue zonisamide if rash develops. Chemical similarities are present among sulfonamides, sulfonylureas, carbonic anhydrase inhibitors, thiazides, and loop diuretics (except ethacrynic acid). Use in patients with sulfonamide allergy is specifically contraindicated in product labeling, however, a risk of cross-reaction exists in patients with allergy to any of these compounds; avoid use when previous reaction has been severe. Use may be associated with the development of metabolic acidosis (generally dose-dependent) in certain patients; predisposing conditions/therapies include renal disease, severe respiratory disease, diarrhea, surgery, ketogenic diet, and other medications. Pediatric patients may also be at an increased risk for and may have more severe metabolic acidosis. Serum bicarbonate should be monitored in all patients prior to and during use; if metabolic acidosis occurs, consider decreasing the dose or tapering the dose to discontinue. If use continued despite acidosis, alkali treatment should be considered. Untreated metabolic acidosis may increase the risk of developing nephrolithiasis, nephrocalcinosis, osteomalacia (or rickets in children), or osteoporosis; pediatric patients may also have decreased growth rates.

Pooled analysis of trials involving various antiepileptics (regardless of indication) showed an increased risk of suicidal thoughts/behavior (incidence rate: 0.43% treated patients compared to 0.24% of patients receiving placebo); risk observed as early as 1 week after initiation and continued through duration of trials (most trials ≤24 weeks). Monitor all patients for notable changes in behavior that might indicate suicidal thoughts or depression; notify healthcare provider immediately if symptoms occur.

Discontinue zonisamide in patients who develop acute renal failure or a significant sustained increase in creatinine/BUN concentration. Kidney stones have been reported. Do not use in patients with renal impairment (GFR <50 mL/minute); use with caution in patients with hepatic impairment.

Significant CNS effects include psychiatric symptoms, psychomotor slowing, and fatigue or somnolence. Fatigue and somnolence occur within the first month of treatment, most commonly at doses of 300-500 mg/day. Effects with other sedative drugs or ethanol may be potentiated. May cause sedation, which may impair physical or mental abilities; patients must be cautioned about performing tasks which require mental alertness (eg, operating machinery or driving). Abrupt withdrawal may precipitate seizures; discontinue or reduce doses gradually.

Safety and efficacy in children <16 years of age has not been established. Decreased sweating (oligohydrosis) and hyperthermia requiring hospitalization have been reported in children. Pediatric patients may also be at an increased risk and may have more severe metabolic acidosis.

Adverse Reactions Adjunctive therapy: Frequencies noted in patients receiving other anticonvulsants:

>10%:

Central nervous system: Somnolence (17%), dizziness (13%)

Gastrointestinal: Anorexia (13%)

1% to 10%:

Central nervous system: Headache (10%), agitation/irritability (9%), fatigue (8%), tiredness (7%), ataxia (6%), confusion (6%), concentration decreased (6%), memory impairment (6%), depression (6%), insomnia (6%), speech disorders (5%), mental slowing (4%), anxiety (3%), nervousness (2%), schizophrenic/schizophreniform behavior (2%), difficulty in verbal expression (2%), status epilepticus (1%), convulsion (1%), hyperesthesia (1%), incoordination (1%)

Dermatologic: Rash (3%), bruising (2%), pruritus (1%)

Gastrointestinal: Nausea (9%), abdominal pain (6%), diarrhea (5%), dyspepsia (3%), weight loss (3%), constipation (2%), taste perversion (2%), xerostomia (2%), vomiting (1%)

Neuromuscular & skeletal: Paresthesia (4%), abnormal gait (1%), tremor (1%), weakness (1%)

Ocular: Diplopia (6%), nystagmus (4%), amblyopia (1%)

Otic: Tinnitus (1%)

Respiratory: Rhinitis (2%), pharyngitis (1%), increased cough (1%)

Miscellaneous: Flu-like syndrome (4%) accidental injury (1%)

<1% (Limited to important or life threatening symptoms): Agranulocytosis, allergic reaction, alopecia, aplastic anemia, apnea, atrial fibrillation, bladder calculus, cholangitis, cholecystitis, cholestatic jaundice, colitis, deafness, duodenitis, dysarthria, dyskinesia, dyspnea, dystonia, encephalopathy, esophagitis, facial paralysis, gingival hyperplasia, glaucoma, gum hemorrhage, gynecomastia, heart failure, hematemesis, hemoptysis, hirsutism, hyperthermia, impotence, leukopenia, lupus erythematosus, menorrhagia, metabolic acidosis, movement disorder, myoclonus, nephrolithiasis, neuropathy, oculogyric crisis, oligohydrosis, peripheral neuritis, pulmonary embolus, rash, rectal hemorrhage, Stevens-Johnson syndrome, stroke, suicidal behavior/ideation, syncope, thrombocytopenia, toxic epidermal necrolysis, urinary retention, urticaria

Drug Interactions

Metabolism/Transport Effects Substrate of CYP2C19 (minor), CYP3A4 (major); **Note:** Assignment of Major/Minor substrate status based on clinically relevant drug interaction potential

Avoid Concomitant Use

Avoid concomitant use of Zonisamide with any of the following: Carbonic Anhydrase Inhibitors; Conivaptan

Increased Effect/Toxicity

Zonisamide may increase the levels/effects of: Alcohol (Ethyl); Alpha-/Beta-Agonists; Amphetamines; Anticonvulsants (Barbiturate); Anticonvulsants (Hydantoin); CarBAMazepine; Carbonic Anhydrase Inhibitors; CNS Depressants; Flecainide; Memantine; Methotrimeprazine; Primidone; QuiNIDine; Selective Serotonin Reuptake Inhibitors

The levels/effects of Zonisamide may be increased by: Conivaptan; CYP3A4 Inhibitors (Moderate); CYP3A4 Inhibitors (Strong); Dasatinib; Droperidol; HydrOXYzine; Methotrimeprazine; Salicylates

Decreased Effect

Zonisamide may decrease the levels/effects of: Lithium; Methenamine; Primidone

The levels/effects of Zonisamide may be decreased by: CYP3A4 Inducers (Strong); Deferasirox; Fosphenytoin; Herbs (CYP3A4 Inducers); Ketorolac; Ketorolac (Nasal); Ketorolac (Systemic); Mefloquine; PHENobarbital; Phenytoin; Tocilizumab

Ethanol/Nutrition/Herb Interactions

Ethanol: May increase CNS depression; monitor for increased effects with coadministration. Caution patients about effects.

Food: Food delays time to maximum concentration, but does not affect bioavailability.

Stability Store at controlled room temperature 25°C (77°F). Protect from moisture and light.

Mechanism of Action The exact mechanism of action is not known. May stabilize neuronal membranes and suppress neuronal hypersynchronization through action at sodium and calcium channels. Does not affect GABA activity.

Pharmacodynamics/Kinetics

Distribution: V_d: 1.45 L/kg

Protein binding: 40%

Metabolism: Hepatic via CYP3A4; forms N-acetyl zonisamide and 2-sulfamoylacetyl phenol (SMAP)

Half-life elimination: Plasma: ~63 hours

Time to peak: 2-6 hours

Excretion: Urine (62%, 35% as unchanged drug, 65% as metabolites); feces (3%)

Dosage Oral:

Children >16 years and Adults:

Adjunctive treatment of partial seizures: Initial: 100 mg/day; dose may be increased to 200 mg/day after 2 weeks. Further dosage increases to 300 mg/day and 400 mg/day can then be made with a minimum of 2 weeks between adjustments, in order to reach steady state at each dosage level. Doses of up to 600 mg/day have been studied, however, there is no evidence of increased response with doses above 400 mg/day.

Mania (unlabeled use): Initial: 100-200 mg/day; maximum: 600 mg/day (Kanba, 1994)

Elderly: Data from clinical trials is insufficient for patients >65 years; begin dosing at the low end of the dosing range.

Dosage adjustment in renal/hepatic impairment: Slower titration and frequent monitoring are indicated in patients with renal or hepatic disease. Use is not recommended in patients with GFR <50 mL/minute. Marked renal impairment (Cl_{cr} <20 mL/minute) was associated with a 35% increase in AUC.

Dietary Considerations May be taken without regard to meals.

Administration Capsules should be swallowed whole. Dose may be administered once or twice daily. Doses of 300 mg/day and higher are associated with increased side effects. Steady-state levels are reached in 14 days.

Monitoring Parameters Metabolic profile, specifically BUN, serum creatinine; serum bicarbonate (prior to initiation and periodically during therapy); suicidality (eg, suicidal thoughts, depression, behavioral changes)

Dosage Forms Excipient information presented when available (limited, particularly for generics); consult specific product labeling.

Capsule, oral: 25 mg, 50 mg, 100 mg

Zonegran®: 25 mg, 100 mg

Extemporaneous Preparations Hazardous agent; use appropriate precautions during preparation and disposal.

A 10 mg/mL suspension may be made using capsules and either simple syrup or methylcellulose 0.5%. Empty contents of ten 100 mg capsules into glass mortar. Reduce to a fine powder and add a small amount of Simple Syrup, NF and mix to a uniform paste; mix while adding the chosen vehicle in incremental proportions to **almost** 100 mL; transfer to an amber calibrated plastic bottle, rinse mortar with vehicle, and add quantity of vehicle sufficient to make 100 mL. Label "shake well" and "refrigerate". When using simple syrup vehicle, stable 28 days at room temperature or refrigerated (preferred). When using methylcellulose vehicle, stable 7 days at room temperature or 28 days refrigerated. **Note:** Although no visual evidence of microbial growth was observed, storage under refrigeration would be recommended to minimize microbial contamination.

Abobo CV, Wei B, and Liang D, "Stability of Zonisamide in Extemporaneously Compounded Oral Suspensions," *Am J Health Syst Pharm*, 2009, 66(12):1105-9.

◆ **Zorbtive®** *see* Somatropin *on page 1579*

◆ **Zortress®** *see* Everolimus *on page 673*

◆ **ZOS** *see* Zoster Vaccine *on page 1830*

◆ **Zostavax®** *see* Zoster Vaccine *on page 1830*

Zoster Vaccine (ZOS ter vak SEEN)

Brand Names: U.S. Zostavax®

Brand Names: Canada Zostavax®

Index Terms Shingles Vaccine; Varicella-Zoster (VZV) Vaccine (Zoster); VZV Vaccine (Zoster); ZOS

Pharmacologic Category Vaccine, Live (Viral)

Additional Appendix Information

Immunization Recommendations *on page 1922*

Use Prevention of herpes zoster (shingles) in patients ≥50 years of age

The Advisory Committee on Immunization Practices (ACIP) recommends routine vaccination of all patients ≥60 years of age, including:

- Patients who report a previous episode of zoster.
- Patients with chronic medical conditions (eg, chronic renal failure, diabetes mellitus, rheumatoid arthritis, chronic pulmonary disease) unless those conditions are contraindications.
- Residents of nursing homes and other long-term care facilities ≥60 years of age, without contraindications.

Pregnancy Considerations Use during pregnancy is contraindicated. Women should avoid becoming pregnant for 3 months after vaccination (4 weeks per CDC). Risk to the fetus following exposure to wild-type varicella zoster virus is small and risk following exposure from the attenuated vaccine is probably even less. Inadvertent exposure to the vaccine during pregnancy should be reported to Merck's National Service Center (800-986-8999).

Lactation Excretion in breast milk unknown/use caution

Contraindications Hypersensitivity to any component of the vaccine; individuals with leukemia, lymphomas, or other malignant neoplasms affecting the bone marrow or lymphatic systems; primary and acquired immunodeficiency states including AIDS or clinical manifestations of HIV; those receiving immunosuppressive therapy (including high-dose corticosteroids); pregnancy

In addition, ACIP recommends that the following immunocompromised patients should not receive zoster vaccine:

Patients undergoing hematopoietic stem cell transplant (limited data; assess risk:benefit, if needed, administer ≥24 months after transplantation);

Patients receiving recombinant human immune modulators, particularly antitumor necrosis factor agents (eg, adalimumab, infliximab, etanercept). Safety and efficacy of concurrent administration is unknown and not recommended. Defer vaccination for ≥1 month after discontinuation.

Patients with unspecified cellular immunodeficiency (exception, patients with impaired humoral immunity may receive vaccine).

Warnings/Precautions Zoster vaccine is not a substitute for varicella vaccine and should not be used in children. Not for use in the treatment of active zoster outbreak, the treatment of postherpetic neuropathy (PHN), or prevention of primary varicella infection (chickenpox). Avoid administration in patients with acute febrile illness; consider deferral of vaccination; may administer to patients with mild acute illness (with or without fever). Defer treatment in patients with active untreated tuberculosis. May be used in patients with a history of zoster infection.

Medications active against the herpesvirus family (eg, acyclovir, famciclovir, valacyclovir) may interfere with the zoster vaccine. In patients where immunosuppressant therapy is anticipated, zoster vaccine should be given at least 14 days to 1 month prior to beginning therapy when possible Use is contraindicated in severely immunocompromised patients (eg, patients receiving chemo-/radiation therapy or other immunosuppressive therapy [including high-dose corticosteroids]); may have a reduced response to vaccination. Patients receiving corticosteroids in low-to-moderate doses, topical (inhaled, nasal, skin), local injection (intra-articular, bursal, tendon) may receive vaccine. Vaccinated individuals do not need to take precautions against spreading varicella following vaccination; transmission of virus is rare unless rash develops. In case of rash, standard contact precautions should be followed. In general, household and close contacts of persons with altered immunocompetence may receive all age-appropriate vaccines.

Immediate treatment for anaphylactoid reaction should be available during vaccine use. Contains gelatin and neomycin; do not use in patients with a history of anaphylactic/anaphylactoid reaction. Contact dermatitis to neomycin is not a contraindication to the vaccine. Not for use in patients <50 years of age. The ACIP does not recommend zoster vaccination in patients of any age who have received the varicella vaccine.

Adverse Reactions All serious adverse reactions must be reported to the U.S. Department of Health and Human Services (DHHS) Vaccine Adverse Event Reporting System (VAERS) 1-800-822-7967 or online at https://vaers.hhs.gov/esub/index.

>10%: Local: Injection site reaction (48% to 64%; includes erythema, tenderness, pain, swelling, hematoma, pruritus, and/or warmth)

1% to 10% (**Note:** Rates similar to placebo):

Central nervous system: Fever (2%), headache (1% to 9%)

Dermatologic: Skin disorder (1%)

Gastrointestinal: Diarrhea (2%)

Neuromuscular & skeletal: Weakness (1%)

Respiratory: Respiratory tract infection (2%), rhinitis (1%)

Miscellaneous: Flu-like syndrome (2%)

<1%, postmarketing, and/or case reports (Limited to important or life-threatening): Anaphylaxis, arthralgia, hypersensitivity reactions, injection site reactions (lymphadenopathy [transient], rash, urticaria), myalgia, nausea, rash (noninjection site)

Drug Interactions

Metabolism/Transport Effects None known.

Avoid Concomitant Use

Avoid concomitant use of Zoster Vaccine with any of the following: Acyclovir-Valacyclovir; Belimumab; Famciclovir; Fingolimod; Immunosuppressants

Increased Effect/Toxicity

The levels/effects of Zoster Vaccine may be increased by: AzaTHIOprine; Belimumab; Corticosteroids (Systemic); Fingolimod; Hydroxychloroquine; Immunosuppressants; Leflunomide; Mercaptopurine; Methotrexate

Decreased Effect

Zoster Vaccine may decrease the levels/effects of: Tuberculin Tests

The levels/effects of Zoster Vaccine may be decreased by: Acyclovir-Valacyclovir; Famciclovir; Fingolimod; Immune Globulins; Immunosuppressants; Pneumococcal Polysaccharide Vaccine (Polyvalent)

Stability To maintain potency, the lypholyzed vaccine must be stored frozen between -50°C to -15°C (-58°F to 5°F). Temperatures below -50°C (-58°F) may occur if stored in dry ice. During shipment, should be maintained at -15°C (5°F) or colder. Store powder in freezer at -15°C (5°F). Protect from light. Store diluent separately at room temperature of 20°C to 25°C (68°F to 77°F) or in refrigerator at 2°C to 8°C (36°F to 46°F). Products with 15-month expiry dating may also be transported/stored under refrigeration at 2°C to 8°C (36°F to 46°F) for up to 72 hours prior to reconstitution; discard if stored under refrigeration and not used within 72 hours.

Withdraw entire contents of the vial containing the provided diluent to reconstitute vaccine. Gently agitate to mix thoroughly. Withdraw entire contents of reconstituted vaccine vial for administration. Discard if reconstituted vaccine is not used within 30 minutes. Do not freeze reconstituted vaccine.

Mechanism of Action As a live, attenuated vaccine (Oka/Merck strain of varicella-zoster virus), zoster virus vaccine stimulates active immunity to disease caused by the varicella-zoster virus. Administration has been demonstrated to protect against the development of herpes zoster, with the highest efficacy in patients 60-69 years of age. It may also reduce the severity of complications, including postherpetic neuralgia, in patients who develop zoster following vaccination.

Pharmacodynamics/Kinetics

Onset of action: Seroconversion: ~6 weeks

Duration: Not established; protection has been demonstrated for at least 4 years

Dosage SubQ: Adults ≥50 years: 0.65 mL administered as a single dose; there are no data to support readministration of the vaccine

Dosage adjustment in renal impairment: No adjustment required

Administration Do not administer I.V. or I.M.; inject immediately after reconstitution. Inject SubQ into the deltoid region of the upper arm, if possible. In persons anticipating immunosuppression, give at least 14 days to 1 month prior to starting immunosuppressant.

Administration with chronic use of acyclovir, famciclovir, or valacyclovir: Discontinue ≥24 hours before administration of zoster vaccine. Do not use for ≥14 days after vaccination.

Simultaneous administration of vaccines helps ensure the patients will be fully vaccinated by the appropriate age. Simultaneous administration of vaccines is defined as administering >1 vaccine on the same day at different anatomic sites. Separate vaccines should not be combined in the same syringe unless indicated by product specific labeling. Separate needles and syringes should be used for each injection. The ACIP prefers each dose of a specific vaccine in a series come from the same manufacturer when possible. Adolescents and adults should be vaccinated while seated or lying down (CDC, 2011).

Antipyretics have not been shown to prevent febrile seizures. Antipyretics may be used to treat fever or discomfort following vaccination (CDC, 2011). One study reported that routine prophylactic administration of acetaminophen to prevent fever prior to vaccination decreased the immune response of some vaccines; the clinical significance of this reduction in immune response has not been established (Prymula, 2009).

Monitoring Parameters Fever, rash; monitor for syncope for ≥15 minutes following vaccination

Additional Information Federal law requires that the name of medication, date of administration, the vaccine manufacturer, lot number of vaccine, and the administering person's name, title, and address be entered into the patient's permanent medical record.

The varicella-zoster virus (VZV) is capable of causing two distinct manifestations of infection. Primary infection results in chickenpox (varicella). These infections tend to occur in young children or younger adults. Reactivation of latent infection (painful vesicular cutaneous eruption usually in a dermatomal pattern) occurs in older patients or in immunosuppressed populations. This is commonly referred to as shingles (herpes zoster). Although the vaccines are directed against the same causative organism, healthcare workers should be aware of differences in indications, dosing, populations, and composition of the vaccine. Neither vaccine is intended for administration during active outbreaks.

Dosage Forms Excipient information presented when available (limited, particularly for generics); consult specific product labeling.

Injection, powder for reconstitution [preservative free]:

Zostavax®: 19,400 PFU [contains bovine serum, gelatin, neomycin (may have trace amounts), sucrose (31.16 mg/vial)]

APPENDIX TABLE OF CONTENTS

ABBREVIATIONS, ACRONYMS, AND SYMBOLS

Abbreviations Which May Be Used in This Reference

Abbreviation	Meaning
½NS	0.45% sodium chloride
5-HT	5-hydroxytryptamine
AAP	American Academy of Pediatrics
AAPC	antibiotic-associated pseudomembranous colitis
ABG	arterial blood gases
ABMT	autologous bone marrow transplant
ABW	adjusted body weight
AACT	American Academy of Clinical Toxicology
ACC	American College of Cardiology
ACE	angiotensin-converting enzyme
ACLS	advanced cardiac life support
ACOG	American College of Obstetricians and Gynecologists
ACTH	adrenocorticotrophic hormone
ADH	antidiuretic hormone
ADHD	attention-deficit/hyperactivity disorder
ADI	adequate daily intake
ADLs	activities of daily living
AED	antiepileptic drug
AHA	American Heart Association
AHCPR	Agency for Health Care Policy and Research
AIDS	acquired immunodeficiency syndrome
AIMS	Abnormal Involuntary Movement Scale
ALL	acute lymphoblastic leukemia
ALS	amyotrophic lateral sclerosis
ALT	alanine aminotransferase (formerly called SGPT)
AMA	American Medical Association
AML	acute myeloblastic leukemia
ANA	antinuclear antibodies
ANC	absolute neutrophil count
ANLL	acute nonlymphoblastic leukemia
aPTT	activated partial thromboplastin time
ARB	angiotensin receptor blocker
ARDS	acute respiratory distress syndrome
ASA-PS	American Society of Anesthesiologists – Physical Status P1: Normal, healthy patient P2: Patient having mild systemic disease P3: Patient having severe systemic disease P4: Patient having severe systemic disease which is a constant threat to life P5: Moribund patient; not expected to survive without the procedure P6: Patient declared brain-dead; organs being removed for donor purposes
AST	aspartate aminotransferase (formerly called SGOT)
ATP	adenosine triphosphate
AUC	area under the curve (area under the serum concentration-time curve)
A-V	atrial-ventricular
BDI	Beck Depression Inventory
BEC	blood ethanol concentration
BLS	basic life support
BMI	body mass index
BMT	bone marrow transplant
BP	blood pressure
BPD	bronchopulmonary disease or dysplasia
BPH	benign prostatic hyperplasia
BPRS	Brief Psychiatric Rating Scale
BSA	body surface area
BUN	blood urea nitrogen

Abbreviations Which May Be Used in This Reference *(continued)*

Abbreviation	Meaning
CABG	coronary artery bypass graft
CAD	coronary artery disease
CADD	computer ambulatory drug delivery
cAMP	cyclic adenosine monophosphate
CAN	Canadian
CAPD	continuous ambulatory peritoneal dialysis
CAS	chemical abstract service
CBC	complete blood count
CBT	cognitive behavioral therapy
Cl_{cr}	creatinine clearance
CDC	Centers for Disease Control and Prevention
CF	cystic fibrosis
CFC	chlorofluorocarbons
CGI	Clinical Global Impression
CHD	coronary heart disease
CHF	congestive heart failure; chronic heart failure
CI	cardiac index
CIE	chemotherapy-induced emesis
C-II	schedule two controlled substance
C-III	schedule three controlled substance
C-IV	schedule four controlled substance
C-V	schedule five controlled substance
CIV	continuous I.V. infusion
Cl_{cr}	creatinine clearance
CLL	chronic lymphocytic leukemia
C_{max}	maximum plasma concentration
C_{min}	minimum plasma concentration
CML	chronic myelogenous leukemia
CMV	cytomegalovirus
CNS	central nervous system or coagulase negative staphylococcus
COLD	chronic obstructive lung disease
COPD	chronic obstructive pulmonary disease
COX	cyclooxygenase
CPK	creatine phosphokinase
CPR	cardiopulmonary resuscitation
CRF	chronic renal failure
CRP	C-reactive protein
CRRT	continuous renal replacement therapy
CSF	cerebrospinal fluid
CSII	continuous subcutaneous insulin infusion
CT	computed tomography
CVA	cerebrovascular accident
CVP	central venous pressure
CVVH	continuous venovenous hemofiltration
CVVHD	continuous venovenous hemodialysis
CVVHDF	continuous venovenous hemodiafiltration
CYP	cytochrome
$D_5/{}^1/_4NS$	dextrose 5% in sodium chloride 0.2%
$D_5/{}^1/_2NS$	dextrose 5% in sodium chloride 0.45%
D_5/LR	dextrose 5% in lactated Ringer's
D_5/NS	dextrose 5% in sodium chloride 0.9%
D_5W	dextrose 5% in water
$D_{10}W$	dextrose 10% in water
DBP	diastolic blood pressure
DEHP	di(3-ethylhexyl)phthalate
DIC	disseminated intravascular coagulation
DL_{co}	pulmonary diffusion capacity for carbon monoxide

Abbreviations Which May Be Used in This Reference *(continued)*

Abbreviation	Meaning
DM	diabetes mellitus
DMARD	disease modifying antirheumatic drug
DNA	deoxyribonucleic acid
DSC	discontinued
DSM-IV	Diagnostic and Statistical Manual
DVT	deep vein thrombosis
EBV	Epstein-Barr virus
ECG	electrocardiogram
ECHO	echocardiogram
ECMO	extracorporeal membrane oxygenation
ECT	electroconvulsive therapy
ED	emergency department
EEG	electroencephalogram
EF	ejection fraction
EG	ethylene glycol
EGA	estimated gestational age
EIA	enzyme immunoassay
ELBW	extremely low birth weight
ELISA	enzyme-linked immunosorbent assay
EPS	extrapyramidal side effects
ESR	erythrocyte sedimentation rate
ESRD	end stage renal disease
E.T.	endotracheal
EtOH	alcohol
FDA	Food and Drug Administration (United States)
FEV_1	forced expiratory volume exhaled after 1 second
FSH	follicle-stimulating hormone
FTT	failure to thrive
FVC	forced vital capacity
G-6-PD	glucose-6-phosphate dehydrogenase
GA	gestational age
GABA	gamma-aminobutyric acid
GAD	generalized anxiety disorder
GE	gastroesophageal
GERD	gastroesophageal reflux disease
GFR	glomerular filtration rate
GGT	gamma-glutamyltransferase
GI	gastrointestinal
GU	genitourinary
GVHD	graft versus host disease
HAM-A	Hamilton Anxiety Scale
HAM-D	Hamilton Depression Scale
Hct	hematocrit
HDL-C	high density lipoprotein cholesterol
HF	heart failure
HFA	hydrofluoroalkane
HFSA	Heart Failure Society of America
Hgb	hemoglobin
HIV	human immunodeficiency virus
HMG-CoA	3-hydroxy-3-methylglutaryl-coenzyme A
HOCM	hypertrophic obstructive cardiomyopathy
HPA	hypothalamic-pituitary-adrenal
HPLC	high performance liquid chromatography
HSV	herpes simplex virus
HTN	hypertension
HUS	hemolytic uremic syndrome
IBD	inflammatory bowel disease

Abbreviations Which May Be Used in This Reference *(continued)*

Abbreviation	Meaning
IBS	irritable bowel syndrome
IBW	ideal body weight
ICD	implantable cardioverter defibrillator
ICH	intracranial hemorrhage
ICP	intracranial pressure
IDDM	insulin-dependent diabetes mellitus
IDSA	Infectious Diseases Society of America
IgG	immune globulin G
IHSS	idiopathic hypertrophic subaortic stenosis
I.M.	intramuscular
ILCOR	International Liaison Committee on Resuscitation
INR	international normalized ration
Int. unit	international unit
I.O.	intraosseous
I & O	input and output
IOP	intraocular pressure
IQ	intelligence quotient
I.T.	intrathecal
ITP	idiopathic thrombocytopenic purpura
IUGR	intrauterine growth retardation
I.V.	intravenous
IVH	intraventricular hemorrhage
IVP	intravenous push
IVPB	intravenous piggyback
JIA	juvenile idiopathic arthritis
JNC	Joint National Committee
JRA	juvenile rheumatoid arthritis
kg	kilogram
KIU	kallikrein inhibitor unit
KOH	potassium hydroxide
LAMM	L-α-acetyl methadol
LDH	lactate dehydrogenase
LDL-C	low density lipoprotein cholesterol
LE	lupus erythematosus
LFT	liver function test
LGA	large for gestational age
LH	luteinizing hormone
LP	lumbar posture
LR	lactated Ringer's
LV	left ventricular
LVEF	left ventricular ejection fraction
LVH	left ventricular hypertrophy
MAC	*Mycobacterium avium* complex
MADRS	Montgomery Asbery Depression Rating Scale
MAO	monoamine oxidase
MAOIs	monamine oxidase inhibitors
MAP	mean arterial pressure
MDD	major depressive disorder
MDRD	modification of diet in renal disease
MDRSP	multidrug resistant *streptococcus pneumoniae*
MI	myocardial infarction
MMSE	mini mental status examination
MOPP	mustargen (mechlorethamine), Oncovin® (vincristine), procarbazine, and prednisone
M/P	milk to plasma ratio
MPS I	mucopolysaccharidosis I
MRHD	maximum recommended human dose
MRI	magnetic resonance imaging

Abbreviations Which May Be Used in This Reference *(continued)*

Abbreviation	Meaning
MRSA	methicillin-resistant *Staphylococcus aureus*
MUGA	multiple gated acquisition scan
NAEPP	National Asthma Education and Prevention Program
NAS	neonatal abstinence syndrome
NCI	National Cancer Institute
ND	nasoduodenal
NF	National Formulary
NFD	Nephrogenic fibrosing dermopathy
NG	nasogastric
NIDDM	noninsulin-dependent diabetes mellitus
NIH	National Institute of Health
NKA	no known allergies
NKDA	No known drug allergies
NMDA	n-methyl-d-aspartate
NMS	neuroleptic malignant syndrome
NNRTI	non-nucleoside reverse transcriptase inhibitor
NRTI	nucleoside reverse transcriptase inhibitor
NS	normal saline (0.9% sodium chloride)
NSAID	nonsteroidal anti-inflammatory drug
NSF	nephrogenic systemic fibrosis
NSTEMI	Non-ST-elevation myocardial infarction
NYHA	New York Heart Association
OA	osteoarthritis
OCD	obsessive-compulsive disorder
OHSS	ovarian hyperstimulation syndrome
O.R.	operating room
OTC	over-the-counter (nonprescription)
PABA	para-aminobenzoic acid
PACTG	Pediatric AIDS Clinical Trials Group
PALS	pediatric advanced life support
PAT	paroxysmal atrial tachycardia
PCA	patient-controlled analgesia
PCP	*Pneumocystis jiroveci* pneumonia (also called *Pneumocystis carinii* pneumonia)
PCWP	pulmonary capillary wedge pressure
PD	Parkinson's disease; peritoneal dialysis
PDA	patent ductus arteriosus
PDE-5	phosphodiesterase-5
PE	pulmonary embolism
PEG tube	percutaneous endoscopic gastrostomy tube
P-gp	P-glycoprotein
PHN	post-herpetic neuralgia
PICU	Pediatric Intensive Care Unit
PID	pelvic inflammatory disease
PIP	peak inspiratory pressure
PMA	postmenstrual age
PMDD	premenstrual dysphoric disorder
PNA	postnatal age
PONV	postoperative nausea and vomiting
PPHN	persistent pulmonary hypertension of the neonate
PPN	peripheral parenteral nutrition
PROM	premature rupture of membranes
PSVT	paroxysmal supraventricular tachycardia
PT	prothrombin time
PTH	parathyroid hormone
PTSD	post-traumatic stress disorder
PTT	partial thromboplastin time
PUD	peptic ulcer disease

Abbreviations Which May Be Used in This Reference *(continued)*

Abbreviation	Meaning
PVC	premature ventricular contraction
PVD	peripheral vascular disease
PVR	peripheral vascular resistance
QT_c	corrected QT interval
QT_c-F	corrected QT interval by Fredricia's formula
RA	rheumatoid arthritis
RAP	right arterial pressure
RDA	recommended daily allowance
REM	rapid eye movement
REMS	risk evaluation and mitigation strategies
RIA	radioimmunoassay
RNA	ribonucleic acid
RPLS	reversible posterior leukoencephalopathy syndrome
RSV	respiratory syncytial virus
SA	sinoatrial
SAD	seasonal affective disorder
SAH	subarachnoid hemorrhage
SBE	subacute bacterial endocarditis
SBP	systolic blood pressure
S_{cr}	serum creatinine
SERM	selective estrogen receptor modulator
SGA	small for gestational age
SGOT	serum glutamic oxaloacetic aminotransferase
SGPT	serum glutamic pyruvate transaminase
SI	International System of Units or Systeme international d'Unites
SIADH	syndrome of inappropriate antidiuretic hormone secretion
SLE	systemic lupus erythematosus
SLEDD	sustained low-efficiency daily diafiltration
SNRI	serotonin norepinephrine reuptake inhibitor
SSKI	saturated solution of potassium iodide
SSRIs	selective serotonin reuptake inhibitors
STD	sexually transmitted disease
STEM I	ST-elevation myocardial infarction
SVR	systemic vascular resistance
SVT	supraventricular tachycardia
SWFI	sterile water for injection
SWI	sterile water for injection
$T_{1/2}$	half-life
T_3	triiodothyronine
T_4	thyroxine
TB	tuberculosis
TC	total cholesterol
TCA	tricyclic antidepressant
TD	tardive dyskinesia
TG	triglyceride
TIA	transient ischemic attack
TIBC	total iron binding capacity
TMA	thrombotic microangiopathy
T_{max}	time to maximum observed concentration, plasma
TNF	tumor necrosis factor
TPN	total parenteral nutrition
TSH	thyroid stimulating hormone
TT	thrombin time
UA	urine analysis
UC	ulcerative colitis
ULN	upper limits of normal
URI	upper respiratory infection

Abbreviations Which May Be Used in This Reference *(continued)*

Abbreviation	Meaning
USAN	United States Adopted Names
USP	United States Pharmacopeia
UTI	urinary tract infection
UV	ultraviolet
V_d	volume of distribution
V_{dss}	volume of distribution at steady-state
VEGF	vascular endothelial growth factor
VF	ventricular fibrillation
VLBW	very low birth weight
VMA	vanillylmandelic acid
VT	ventricular tachycardia
VTE	venous thromboembolism
vWD	von Willebrand disease
VZV	varicella zoster virus
WHO	World Health Organization
w/v	weight for volume
w/w	weight for weight
YBOC	Yale Brown Obsessive-Compulsive Scale
YMRS	Young Mania Rating Scale

Common Weights, Measures, or Apothecary Abbreviations

Abbreviation	Meaning
<[1]	less than
>[1]	greater than
≤	less than or equal to
≥	greater than or equal to
ac	before meals or food
ad	to, up to
ad lib	at pleasure
AM	morning
AMA	against medical advice
amp	ampul
amt	amount
aq	water
aq. dest.	distilled water
ASAP	as soon as possible
a.u.[1]	each ear
bid	twice daily
bm	bowel movement
C	Celsius, centigrade
cal	calorie
cap	capsule
cc[1]	cubic centimeter
cm	centimeter
comp	compound
cont	continue
d	day
d/c[1]	discharge
dil	dilute
disp	dispense
div	divide
dtd	give of such a dose
Dx	diagnosis

Common Weights, Measures, or Apothecary Abbreviations *(continued)*

Abbreviation	Meaning
elix, el	elixir
emp	as directed
et	and
ex aq	in water
F	Fahrenheit
f, ft	make, let be made
g	gram
gr	grain
gtt	a drop
h	hour
hs[1]	at bedtime
kcal	kilocalorie
kg	kilogram
L	liter
liq	a liquor, solution
M	molar
mcg	microgram
m. dict	as directed
mEq	milliequivalent
mg	milligram
microL	microliter
min	minute
mL	milliliter
mm	millimeter
mM	millimole
mm Hg	millimeters of mercury
mo	month
mOsm	milliosmoles
ng	nanogram
nmol	nanomole
no.	number
noc	in the night
non rep	do not repeat, no refills
NPO	nothing by mouth
NV	nausea and vomiting
O, Oct	a pint
o.d.[1]	right eye
o.l.	left eye
o.s.[1]	left eye
o.u.[1]	each eye
pc, post cib	after meals
PM	afternoon or evening
P.O.	by mouth
P.R.	rectally
prn	as needed
pulv	a powder
q	every
qad	every other day
qd[1,2]	every day, daily
qh	every hour
qid	four times a day
qod[1,2]	every other day
qs	a sufficient quantity
qs ad	a sufficient quantity to make
Rx	take, a recipe
S.L.	sublingual
stat	at once, immediately

Common Weights, Measures, or Apothecary Abbreviations *(continued)*

Abbreviation	Meaning
SubQ	subcutaneous
supp	suppository
syr	syrup
tab	tablet
tal	such
tid	three times a day
tr, tinct	tincture
trit	triturate
tsp	teaspoon
u.d.	as directed
ung	ointment
v.o.	verbal order
w.a.	while awake
x3	3 times
x4	4 times
y	year

[1]ISMP error-prone abbreviation.

[2]JCAHO Do Not Use list.

Additional abbreviations used and defined within a specific monograph or text piece may only apply to that text.

REFERENCES

The Institute for Safe Medication Practices (ISMP) list of Error-Prone Abbreviations, Symbols, and Dose Designations. Available at http://www.ismp.org/Tools/errorproneabbreviations.pdf

The Joint Commission Official "Do Not Use" list. Available at http://www.jointcommission.org/Do_Not_Use_List_of_Abbreviations/

APACHE II SCORING SYSTEM

The APACHE II score is the sum of the total acute physiology score (APS), age points, and chronic health points. Determination of these scores/points are outlined in the following tables.

APACHE II Score	Points
APS points	
+ Age points	
+ Chronic health points	
Total APACHE II Score	

Glasgow Coma Scale

(circle appropriate response)

Eyes open

4 - Spontaneously

3 - To verbal

2 - To painful stimuli

1 - No response

Motor response

6 - To verbal command

5 - Localizes to pain

4 - Withdraws to pain

3 - Abnormal flexion (decorticate)

2 - Abnormal extension (decerebrate)

1 - No response

Verbal – nonintubated

5 - Oriented and controversed

4 - Disoriented and talks

3 - Inappropriate words

2 - Incomprehensible sounds

1 - No response

Verbal – intubated

5 - Seems able to talk

3 - Questionable ability to talk

1 - Generally unresponsive

Age Points

Assign points to age as follows:	Points
≤44	0
45-54	2
55-64	3
65-74	5
≥75	6

Chronic Health Points

Liver Cardiovascular Pulmonary Kidney Immune	If the patient has a history of severe organ system insufficiency or is immunocompromised assign points as follows: a. for nonoperative or emergency postoperative patients - 5 points or b. for elective postoperative patients - 2 points **DEFINITIONS** Organ insufficiency or immunocompromised state must have been evident prior to this hospital admission and conform to the following criteria. **Liver:** Biopsy proven cirrhosis and documented portal hypertension; episodes of past upper GI bleeding attributed to portal hypertension; or prior episodes of hepatic failure/encephalopathy/coma **Cardiovascular:** New York Heart Association Class IV **Respiratory:** Chronic restrictive, obstructive, or vascular disease resulting in severe exercise restriction, ie, unable to climb stairs or perform household duties; or documented chronic hypoxia, hypercapnia, secondary polycythemia, severe pulmonary hypertension (>40 mm Hg), or respirator dependency **Renal:** Receiving chronic dialysis **Immunocompromised:** The patient has received therapy that suppresses resistance to infection, eg, immunosuppression, chemotherapy, radiation, long term or recent high dose steroids, or has a disease that is sufficiently advanced to suppress resistance to infection, eg, leukemia, lymphoma, AIDS **Chronic Health Points =**

REFERENCE

Knaus WA, Draper EA, Wagner DP, et al, "APACHE II: A Severity of Disease Classification System," *Crit Care Med*, 1985, 13(10):818-29.

Total Acute Physiology Score (APS) (Choose the worst value in the past 24 hours)

	Physiologic Variable	High Abnormal Range								Low Abnormal Range
		+4	+3	+2	+1	0	+1	+2	+3	+4
1	Temperature rectal (°C)[1]	≥41	39-40.9		38.5-38.9	36-38.4	34-35.9	32-33.9	30-31.9	≤29.9
2	Mean arterial pressure (mm Hg)	≥160	130-159	110-129		70-109		50-69		≤49
3	Heart rate (ventricular response)	≥180	140-179	110-139		70-109		55-69	40-54	≤39
4	Respiratory rate (nonventilated or ventilated)	≥50	35-49		25-34	12-24	10-11	6-9		≤5
5	Oxygenation: A-a gradient or PaO_2 (mm Hg) a) FiO_2 ≥0.5: record A-a gradient	≥500	350-499	200-349		<200				
	b) FiO_2 <0.5: record only PaO_2					PO_2 >70	PO_2 61-70		PO_2 55-60	PO_2 <55
6*	Arterial pH	≥7.7	7.6-7.69		7.5-7.59	7.33-7.49		7.25-7.32	7.15-7.24	<7.15
7	Serum sodium (mmol/L)	≥180	160-179	155-159	150-154	130-149		120-129	111-119	≤110
8	Serum potassium (mmol/L)	≥7	6-6.9		5.5-5.9	3.5-5.4	3-3.4	2.5-2.9		<2.5
9	Serum creatinine (mg/100 mL) double point score for acute renal failure	≥3.5	2-3.4	1.5-1.9		0.6-1.4		<0.6		
10	Hematocrit (%)	≥60		50-59.9	46-49.9	30-45.9		20-29.9		<20
11	White blood count (total/mm^3) (in 1000s)	≥40		20-39.9	15-19.9	3-14.9		1-2.9		<1
12	Glasgow coma score (GCS): Score = 15 minus actual GCS [see Glasgow Coma Scale table]									
A	Total acute physiology score (APS): Sum of the 12 individual variable points									
*	Serum HCO_3 (venous-mmol/L) Not preferred, use if no ABGs	≥52	41-51.9		32-40.9	22-31.9		18-21.9	15-17.9	<15

[1]Temperature may also be obtained by the following methods: Swan-Ganz core, bladder, tympanic membrane.

APOTHECARY/METRIC EQUIVALENTS

Approximate Liquid Measures

Basic equivalent: 1 fluid ounce = 30 mL

Examples:

1 gallon	=	3800 mL	1 gallon	=	128 fluid ounces
1 quart	=	960 mL	1 quart	=	32 fluid ounces
1 pint	=	480 mL	1 pint	=	16 fluid ounces
8 fluid oz	=	240 mL	15 minims	=	1 mL
4 fluid oz	=	120 mL	10 minims	=	0.6 mL

Approximate Household Equivalents

1 teaspoonful	=	5 mL	1 tablespoonful	=	15 mL

Weights

Basic equivalents:

1 oz	=	30 g	15 gr	=	1 g

Examples:

4 oz	=	120 g	1 gr	=	60 mg
2 oz	=	60 g	1/100 gr	=	600 mcg
10 gr	=	600 mg	1/150 gr	=	400 mcg
7 1/2 gr	=	500 mg	1/200 gr	=	300 mcg
16 oz	=	1 lb			

Metric Conversions

Basic equivalents:

1 g	=	1000 mg	1 mg	=	1000 mcg

Examples:

5 g	=	5000 mg	5 mg	=	5000 mcg
0.5 g	=	500 mg	0.5 mg	=	500 mcg
0.05 g	=	50 mg	0.05 mg	=	50 mcg

Exact Equivalents

1 g	=	15.43 gr	0.1 mg	=	1/600 gr
1 mL	=	16.23 minims	0.12 mg	=	1/500 gr
1 minim	=	0.06 mL	0.15 mg	=	1/400 gr
1 gr	=	64.8 mg	0.2 mg	=	1/300 gr
1 pint (pt)	=	473.2 mL	0.3 mg	=	1/200 gr
1 oz	=	28.35 g	0.4 mg	=	1/150 gr
1 lb	=	453.6 g	0.5 mg	=	1/120 gr
1 kg	=	2.2 lb	0.6 mg	=	1/100 gr
1 qt	=	946.4 mL	0.8 mg	=	1/80 gr
			1 mg	=	1/65 gr

Solids[1]

1/4 grain	=	15 mg	1 1/2 grains	=	90 mg
1/2 grain	=	30 mg	5 grains	=	300 mg
1 grain	=	60 mg	10 grains	=	600 mg

[1]Use exact equivalents for compounding and calculations requiring a high degree of accuracy.

AVERAGE WEIGHTS AND SURFACE AREAS

Average Height, Weight, and Surface Area by Age and Gender

Age	Girls			Boys		
	Height (cm)	Weight (kg)	BSA (m^2)	Height (cm)	Weight (kg)	BSA (m^2)
Birth	49.5	3.4	0.22	50	3.6	0.22
3 mo	59	5.6	0.3	61	6	0.32
6 mo	65	7.2	0.36	67	7.9	0.38
9 mo	70	8.3	0.4	72	9.3	0.43
12 mo	74.5	9.5	0.44	75.5	10.3	0.46
15 mo	77	10.3	0.47	79	11.1	0.49
18 mo	80	11	0.49	82	11.7	0.52
21 mo	83	11.6	0.52	85	12.2	0.54
2 y	86	12	0.54	87.5	12.6	0.55
2.5 y	91	13	0.57	92	13.5	0.59
3 y	94.5	13.8	0.6	96	14.3	0.62
3.5 y	97	15	0.64	98	15	0.64
4 y	101	16	0.67	102	16	0.67
4.5 y	104	17	0.7	105	17	0.7
5 y	107.5	18	0.73	109	18.5	0.75
6 y	115	20	0.80	115	21	0.82
7 y	121.5	23	0.88	122	23	0.88
8 y	127.5	25.5	0.95	127.5	26	0.96
9 y	133	29	1.04	133.5	28.5	1.03
10 y	138	33	1.12	138.5	32	1.1
11 y	144	37	1.22	143.5	36	1.2
12 y	151	41.5	1.32	149	40.5	1.29
13 y	157	46	1.42	156	45.5	1.4
14 y	160.5	49.5	1.49	163.5	51	1.52
15 y	162	52	1.53	170	56	1.63
16 y	162.5	54	1.56	173.5	61	1.71
17 y	163	55	1.58	175	64.5	1.77
Adult[1]	163.5	58	1.62	177	83.5	2.03

Data extracted from the CDC growth charts based on the 50th percentile height and weight for a given age.[2]

Body surface area calculation[3]: Square root of [(Ht x Wt) / 3600]

[1]McDowell MA, Fryar CD, Hirsch R, et al, "Anthropometric Reference Data for Children and Adults: U.S. Population, 1999-2002," *Adv Data*, 2005, (361):1-5.

[2]Centers for Disease Control and Prevention, "2000 CDC Growth Charts: United States," Available at http://www.cdc.gov/growthcharts. Accessed November 16, 2007.

[3]Mosteller RD, "Simplified Calculation of Body-Surface Area," *N Engl J Med*, 1987, 317(17):1098.

BODY SURFACE AREA OF ADULTS AND CHILDREN

Calculating Body Surface Area in Children

In a child of average size, find weight and corresponding surface area on the boxed scale to the left; or, use the nomogram to the right. Lay a straightedge on the correct height and weight points for the child, then read the intersecting point on the surface area scale. (**Note:** 2.2 lb = 1 kg)

FOR CHILDREN OF NORMAL HEIGHT AND WEIGHT **NOMOGRAM**

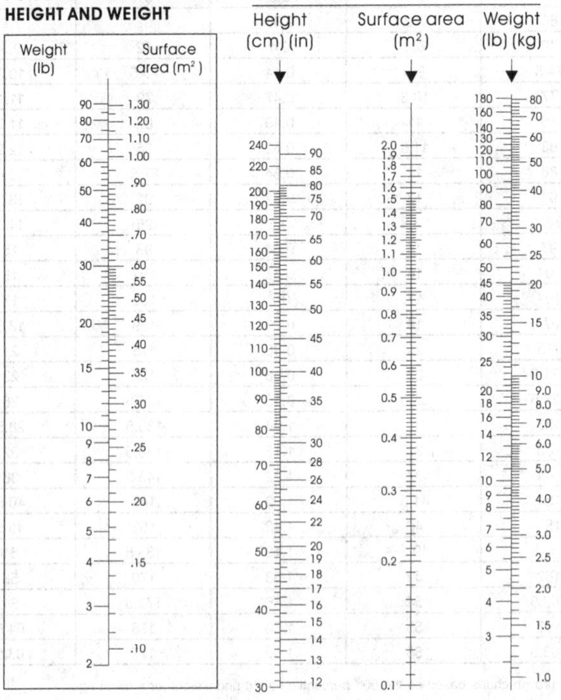

BODY SURFACE AREA FORMULA (Adult and Pediatric)

$$\text{BSA (m}^2) = \sqrt{\frac{\text{ht (in)} \times \text{wt (lb)}}{3131}} \quad \text{or, in metric: BSA (m}^2) = \sqrt{\frac{\text{ht (cm)} \times \text{wt (kg)}}{3600}}$$

References

Lam TK and Leung DT, "More on Simplified Calculation of Body Surface Area," *N Engl J Med*, 1988, 318(17):1130 (letter).

Mosteller RD, "Simplified Calculation of Body Surface Area," *N Engl J Med*, 1987, 317(17):1098 (letter).

IDEAL BODY WEIGHT CALCULATION

Adults (18 years and older) (IBW is in kg)

IBW (male) = 50 + (2.3 x height in inches over 5 feet)

IBW (female) = 45.5 + (2.3 x height in inches over 5 feet)

Children (IBW is in kg; height is in cm)

a. 1-18 years

IBW = (height)^2 x 1.65) / 1000

b. 5 feet and taller

IBW (male) = 39 + (2.27 x height in inches over 5 feet)
IBW (female) = 42.2 + (2.27 x height in inches over 5 feet)

MILLIEQUIVALENT AND MILLIMOLE CALCULATIONS AND CONVERSIONS

DEFINITIONS AND CALCULATIONS

Definitions

mole	=	gram molecular weight of a substance (aka molar weight)
millimole (mM)	=	milligram molecular weight of a substance (a millimole is 1/1000 of a mole)
equivalent weight	=	gram weight of a substance which will combine with or replace 1 gram (1 mole) of hydrogen; an equivalent weight can be determined by dividing the molar weight of a substance by its ionic valence
milliequivalent (mEq)	=	milligram weight of a substance which will combine with or replace 1 milligram (1 millimole) of hydrogen (a milliequivalent is 1/1000 of an equivalent)

Calculations

moles	=	$\frac{\text{weight of a substance (grams)}}{\text{molecular weight of that substance (grams)}}$
millimoles	=	$\frac{\text{weight of a substance (milligrams)}}{\text{molecular weight of that substance (milligrams)}}$
equivalents	=	moles x valence of ion
milliequivalents	=	millimoles x valence of ion
moles	=	$\frac{\text{equivalents}}{\text{valence of ion}}$
millimoles	=	$\frac{\text{milliequivalents}}{\text{valence of ion}}$
millimoles	=	moles x 1000
milliequivalents	=	equivalents x 1000

Note: Use of equivalents and milliequivalents is valid only for those substances which have fixed ionic valences (eg, sodium, potassium, calcium, chlorine, magnesium, bromine, etc). For substances with variable ionic valences (eg, phosphorous), a reliable equivalent value cannot be determined. In these instances, one should calculate millimoles (which are fixed and reliable) rather than milliequivalents.

MILLIEQUIVALENT CONVERSIONS

To convert mg/100 mL to mEq/L the following formula may be used:

$$\frac{\text{(mg/100 mL) x 10 x valence}}{\text{atomic weight}} = \text{mEq/L}$$

To convert mEq/L to mg/100 mL the following formula may be used:

$$\frac{\text{(mEq/L) x atomic weight}}{\text{10 x valence}} = \text{mg/100 mL}$$

To convert mEq/L to volume of percent of a gas the following formula may be used:

$$\frac{\text{(mEq/L) x 22.4}}{10} = \text{volume percent}$$

Valences and Atomic Weights of Selected Ions

Substance	Electrolyte	Valence	Molecular Wt
Calcium	Ca^{++}	2	40
Chloride	Cl^{-}	1	35.5
Magnesium	Mg^{++}	2	24
Phosphate	HPO_4^{--} (80%)	1.8	96[1]
pH = 7.4	$H_2PO_4^{-}$ (20%)	1.8	96[1]
Potassium	K^{+}	1	39
Sodium	Na^{+}	1	23
Sulfate	SO_4^{--}	2	96[1]

[1]The molecular weight of phosphorus only is 31, and sulfur only is 32.

Approximate Milliequivalents — Weights of Selected Ions

Salt	mEq/g Salt	mg Salt/mEq
Calcium carbonate [$CaCO_3$]	20	50
Calcium chloride [$CaCl_2 \cdot 2H_2O$]	14	74
Calcium gluceptate [$Ca(C_7H_{13}O_8)_2$]	4	245
Calcium gluconate [$Ca(C_6H_{11}O_7)_2 \cdot H_2O$]	5	224
Calcium lactate [$Ca(C_3H_5O_3)_2 \cdot 5H_2O$]	7	154
Magnesium gluconate [$Mg(C_6H_{11}O_7)_2 \cdot H_2O$]	5	216
Magnesium oxide [MgO]	50	20
Magnesium sulfate [$MgSO_4$]	17	60
Magnesium sulfate [$MgSO_4 \cdot 7H_2O$]	8	123
Potassium acetate [$K(C_2H_3O_2)$]	10	98
Potassium chloride [KCl]	13	75
Potassium citrate [$K_3(C_6H_5O_7) \cdot H_2O$]	9	108
Potassium iodide [KI]	6	166
Sodium acetate [$Na(C_2H_3O_2)$]	12	82
Sodium acetate [$Na(C_2H_3O_2) \cdot 3H_2O$]	7	136
Sodium bicarbonate [$NaHCO_3$]	12	84
Sodium chloride [$NaCl$]	17	58
Sodium citrate [$Na_3(C_6H_5O_7) \cdot 2H_2O$]	10	98
Sodium iodine [NaI]	7	150
Sodium lactate [$Na(C_3H_5O_3)$]	9	112
Zinc sulfate [$ZnSO_4 \cdot 7H_2O$]	7	144

ACID-BASE ASSESSMENT

Henderson-Hasselbalch Equation

$pH = 6.1 + \log ([HCO_3^-] / (0.03) [PaCO_2])$

Normal arterial blood pH: 7.4 (normal range: 7.35 - 7.45)

Where:

$[HCO_3^-]$ = Serum bicarbonate concentration

$PaCO_2$ = Arterial carbon dioxide partial pressure

Alveolar Gas Equation

P_iO_2	=	F_iO_2 x (total atmospheric pressure – vapor pressure of H_2O at 37°C)
	=	F_iO_2 x (760 mm Hg – 47 mm Hg)
PAO_2	=	$P_iO_2 - (PaCO_2 / R)$

Alveolar-arterial oxygen (A-a) gradient = $PAO_2 - PaO_2$

or

A-a gradient = $[(F_iO_2 \times 713) - (PaCO_2/0.8)] - PaO_2$

A-a gradient normal ranges:

Children	15-20 mm Hg
Adults	20-25 mm Hg

where:

P_iO_2 = Oxygen partial pressure of inspired gas (mm Hg) (150 mm Hg in room air at sea level)

F_iO_2 = Fractional pressure of oxygen in inspired gas (0.21 in room air)

PAO_2 = Alveolar oxygen partial pressure

PaO_2 = Arterial oxygen partial pressure

$PaCO_2$ = Arterial carbon dioxide partial pressure

R = Respiratory exchange quotient (typically 0.8, increases with high carbohydrate diet, decreases with high fat diet)

Acid-Base Disorders

Acute metabolic acidosis:
$PaCO_2$ expected = $1.5 ([HCO_3^-]) + 8 \pm 2$ **or**
Expected decrease in $PaCO_2$ = 1.3 (1-1.5) x decrease in $[HCO_3^-]$

Acute metabolic alkalosis:
Expected increase in $PaCO_2$ = 0.6 (0.5-1) x increase in $[HCO_3^-]$

Acute respiratory acidosis (<6 h duration):
For every $PaCO_2$ increase of 10 mm Hg, $[HCO_3^-]$ increases by 1 mEq/L

Chronic respiratory acidosis (>6 h duration):
For every $PaCO_2$ increase of 10 mm Hg, $[HCO_3^-]$ increases by 4 mEq/L

Acute respiratory alkalosis (<6 h duration):
For every $PaCO_2$ decrease of 10 mm Hg, $[HCO_3^-]$ decreases by 2 mEq/L

Chronic respiratory alkalosis (>6 h duration):
For every $PaCO_2$ decrease of 10 mm Hg, $[HCO_3^-]$ increases by 5 mEq/L

SELECTED CLINICAL EQUATIONS

CORRECTED SODIUM

Corrected Na^+ = measured Na^+ + [1.5 x (glucose – 150 divided by 100)]

Note: Do not correct for glucose <150.

WATER DEFICIT

Water deficit = 0.6 x body weight [1 – (140 divided by Na^+)]

Note: Body weight is estimated weight in kg when fully hydrated; $\mathbf{Na^+}$ is serum or plasma sodium. Use corrected Na^+ if necessary. Consult medical references for recommendations for replacement of deficit.

TOTAL SERUM CALCIUM CORRECTED FOR ALBUMIN LEVEL

[(Normal albumin – patient's albumin) x 0.8] + patient's measured total calcium

OSMOLALITY

Definition: The summed concentrations of all osmotically active solute particles.

Predicted serum osmolality =

$$\text{mOsm/L} = (2 \times \text{serum } Na^{++}) + \frac{\text{serum glucose}}{18} + \frac{\text{BUN}}{2.8}$$

The normal range of serum osmolality is 285-295 mOsm/L.

Calculated Osm

Note: Osm is a term used to reconcile osmolality and osmolarity

Osmol gap = measured Osm – calculated Osm

0 to +10: Normal
>10: Abnormal
<0: Probable lab or calculation error

Drugs Causing Osmolar Gap

(by freezing-point depression, gap is >10 mOsm)
Ethanol
Ethylene glycol
Glycerol
Iodine (questionable)
Isopropanol (acetone)
Mannitol
Methanol
Sorbitol

BICARBONATE DEFICIT

HCO_3^- deficit = (0.4 x wt in kg) x (HCO_3^- desired – HCO_3^- measured)

Note: In clinical practice, the calculated quantity may differ markedly from the actual amount of bicarbonate needed or that which may be safely administered.

ANION GAP

Definition: The difference in concentration between unmeasured cation and anion equivalents in serum.

Anion gap = Na^+ – (Cl^- + HCO_3^-)
(The normal anion gap is 10-14 mEq/L)

Differential Diagnosis of Increased Anion Gap Acidosis

Organic anions
- Lactate (sepsis, hypovolemia, seizures, large tumor burden)
- Pyruvate
- Uremia
- Ketoacidosis (β-hydroxybutyrate and acetoacetate)
- Amino acids and their metabolites
- Other organic acids

Inorganic anions
- Hyperphosphatemia
- Sulfates
- Nitrates

Differential Diagnosis of Decreased Anion Gap

Organic cations
- Hypergammaglobulinemia

Inorganic cations
- Hyperkalemia
- Hypercalcemia
- Hypermagnesemia

Medications and toxins
- Lithium

Hypoalbuminemia

RETICULOCYTE INDEX

(% retic divided by 2) x (patient's Hct divided by normal Hct) **or**
(% retic divided by 2) x (patient's Hgb divided by normal Hgb)

Normal index: 1.0
Good marrow response: 2.0-6.0

CORRECTED QT INTERVAL EQUATIONS

Bazett (B) Formula:

QT_cB: $QT_c = QT/(R - R\ interval^{0.5})$

or

QT_cB: QT_c = QT/Square root of (R - R interval)

Frederica (F) Formula:

QT_cF: $QT_c = QT/(R - R\ interval^{0.33})$

POUNDS/KILOGRAMS CONVERSION

1 pound = 0.45359 kilograms
1 kilogram = 2.2 pounds

lb	=	kg	lb	=	kg	lb	=	kg
1		0.45	70		31.75	140		63.50
5		2.27	75		34.02	145		65.77
10		4.54	80		36.29	150		68.04
15		6.80	85		38.56	155		70.31
20		9.07	90		40.82	160		72.58
25		11.34	95		43.09	165		74.84
30		13.61	100		45.36	170		77.11
35		15.88	105		47.63	175		79.38
40		18.14	110		49.90	180		81.65
45		20.41	115		52.16	185		83.92
50		22.68	120		54.43	190		86.18
55		24.95	125		56.70	195		88.45
60		27.22	130		58.91	200		90.72
65		29.48	135		61.24			

TEMPERATURE CONVERSION

Celsius to Fahrenheit = (°C x 9/5) + 32 = °F
Fahrenheit to Celsius = (°F - 32) x 5/9 = °C

°C	=	°F	°C	=	°F	°C	=	°F
100.0		212.0	39.0		102.2	36.8		98.2
50.0		122.0	38.8		101.8	36.6		97.9
41.0		105.8	38.6		101.5	36.4		97.5
40.8		105.4	38.4		101.1	36.2		97.2
40.6		105.1	38.2		100.8	36.0		96.8
40.4		104.7	38.0		100.4	35.8		96.4
40.2		104.4	37.8		100.1	35.6		96.1
40.0		104.0	37.6		99.7	35.4		95.7
39.8		103.6	37.4		99.3	35.2		95.4
39.6		103.3	37.2		99.0	35.0		95.0
39.4		102.9	37.0		98.6	0		32.0
39.2		102.6						

REFERENCE VALUES FOR CHILDREN

		Normal Values
CHEMISTRY		
Albumin	0-1 y	2-4 g/dL
	1 y to adult	3.5-5.5 g/dL
Ammonia	Newborns	90-150 mcg/dL
	Children	40-120 mcg/dL
	Adults	18-54 mcg/dL
Amylase	Newborns	0-60 units/L
	Adults	30-110 units/L
Bilirubin, conjugated, direct	Newborns	<1.5 mg/dL
	1 mo to adult	0-0.5 mg/dL
Bilirubin, total	0-3 d	2-10 mg/dL
	1 mo to adult	0-1.5 mg/dL
Bilirubin, unconjugated, indirect		0.6-10.5 mg/dL
Calcium	Newborns	7-12 mg/dL
	0-2 y	8.8-11.2 mg/dL
	2 y to adult	9-11 mg/dL
Calcium, ionized, whole blood		4.4-5.4 mg/dL
Carbon dioxide, total		23-33 mEq/L
Chloride		95-105 mEq/L
Cholesterol	Newborns	45-170 mg/dL
	0-1 y	65-175 mg/dL
	1-20 y	120-230 mg/dL
Creatinine	0-1 y	≤0.6 mg/dL
	1 y to adult	0.5-1.5 mg/dL
Glucose	Newborns	30-90 mg/dL
	0-2 y	60-105 mg/dL
	Children to Adults	70-110 mg/dL
Iron		
	Newborns	110-270 mcg/dL
	Infants	30-70 mcg/dL
	Children	55-120 mcg/dL
	Adults	70-180 mcg/dL
Iron binding	Newborns	59-175 mcg/dL
	Infants	100-400 mcg/dL
	Adults	250-400 mcg/dL
Lactic acid, lactate		2-20 mg/dL
Lead, whole blood		<10 mcg/dL
Lipase		
	Children	20-140 units/L
	Adults	0-190 units/L
Magnesium		1.5-2.5 mEq/L
Osmolality, serum		275-296 mOsm/kg
Osmolality, urine		50-1400 mOsm/kg

(continued)

		Normal Values
Phosphorus	Newborns	4.2-9 mg/dL
	6 wk to 19 mo	3.8-6.7 mg/dL
	19 mo to 3 y	2.9-5.9 mg/dL
	3-15 y	3.6-5.6 mg/dL
	>15 y	2.5-5 mg/dL
Potassium, plasma	Newborns	4.5-7.2 mEq/L
	2 d to 3 mo	4-6.2 mEq/L
	3 mo to 1 y	3.7-5.6 mEq/L
	1-16 y	3.5-5 mEq/L
Protein, total	0-2 y	4.2-7.4 g/dL
	>2 y	6-8 g/dL
Sodium		136-145 mEq/L
Triglycerides	Infants	0-171 mg/dL
	Children	20-130 mg/dL
	Adults	30-200 mg/dL
Urea nitrogen, blood	0-2 y	4-15 mg/dL
	2 y to Adult	5-20 mg/dL
Uric acid	Male	3-7 mg/dL
	Female	2-6 mg/dL
ENZYMES		
Alanine aminotransferase (ALT)	0-2 mo	8-78 units/L
	>2 mo	8-36 units/L
Alkaline phosphatase (ALKP)	Newborns	60-130 units/L
	0-16 y	85-400 units/L
	>16 y	30-115 units/L
Aspartate aminotransferase (AST)	Infants	18-74 units/L
	Children	15-46 units/L
	Adults	5-35 units/L
Creatine kinase (CK)	Infants	20-200 units/L
	Children	10-90 units/L
	Adult male	0-206 units/L
	Adult female	0-175 units/L
Lactate dehydrogenase (LDH)	Newborns	290-501 units/L
	1 mo to 2 y	110-144 units/L
	>16 y	60-170 units/L

Blood Gases

	Arterial	Capillary	Venous
pH	7.35-7.45	7.35-7.45	7.32-7.42
pCO_2 (mm Hg)	35-45	35-45	38-52
pO_2 (mm Hg)	70-100	60-80	24-48
HCO_3 (mEq/L)	19-25	19-25	19-25
TCO_2 (mEq/L)	19-29	19-29	23-33
O_2 saturation (%)	90-95	90-95	40-70
Base excess (mEq/L)	-5 to +5	-5 to +5	-5 to +5

Thyroid Function Tests

T_4 (thyroxine)	1-7 d	10.1-20.9 mcg/dL
	8-14 d	9.8-16.6 mcg/dL
	1 mo to 1 y	5.5-16 mcg/dL
	>1 y	4-12 mcg/dL
FTI	1-3 d	9.3-26.6
	1-4 wk	7.6-20.8
	1-4 mo	7.4-17.9
	4-12 mo	5.1-14.5
	1-6 y	5.7-13.3
	>6 y	4.8-14
T_3 by RIA	Newborns	100-470 ng/dL
	1-5 y	100-260 ng/dL
	5-10 y	90-240 ng/dL
	10 y to Adult	70-210 ng/dL
T_3 uptake		35%-45%
TSH	Cord	3-22 µIU/mL
	1-3 d	<40 µIU/mL
	3-7 d	<25 µIU/mL
	>7 d	0-10 µIU/mL

REFERENCE VALUES FOR ADULTS

CHEMISTRY

Test	Values	Remarks
Serum / Plasma		
Acetone	Negative	
Albumin	3.2-5 g/dL	
Alcohol, ethyl	Negative	
Aldolase	1.2-7.6 IU/L	
Ammonia	20-70 mcg/dL	Specimen to be placed on ice as soon as collected.
Amylase	30-110 units/L	
Bilirubin, direct	0-0.3 mg/dL	
Bilirubin, total	0.1-1.2 mg/dL	
Calcium	8.6-10.3 mg/dL	
Calcium, ionized	2.24-2.46 mEq/L	
Chloride	95-108 mEq/L	
Cholesterol, total	≤200 mg/dL	Fasted blood required – normal value affected by dietary habits. This reference range is for a general adult population.
HDL cholesterol	40-60 mg/dL	Fasted blood required – normal value affected by dietary habits.
LDL cholesterol	<160 mg/dL	If triglyceride is >400 mg/dL, LDL cannot be calculated accurately (Friedewald equation). Target LDL-C depends on patient's risk factors.
CO_2	23-30 mEq/L	
Creatine kinase (CK) isoenzymes		
CK-BB	0%	
CK-MB (cardiac)	0% to 3.9%	
CK-MM (muscle)	96% to 100%	
CK-MB levels must be both ≥4% and 10 IU/L to meet diagnostic criteria for CK-MB positive result consistent with myocardial injury.		
Creatine phosphokinase (CPK)	8-150 IU/L	
Creatinine	0.5-1.4 mg/dL	
Ferritin	13-300 ng/mL	
Folate	3.6-20 ng/dL	
GGT (gamma-glutamyltranspeptidase)		
male	11-63 IU/L	
female	8-35 IU/L	
GLDH	To be determined	
Glucose (preprandial)	<115 mg/dL	Goals different for diabetics.
Glucose, fasting	60-110 mg/dL	Goals different for diabetics.
Glucose, nonfasting (2-h postprandial)	<120 mg/dL	Goals different for diabetics.
Hemoglobin A_{1c}	<8	
Hemoglobin, plasma free	<2.5 mg/100 mL	
Hemoglobin, total glycosolated (Hb A_1)	4% to 8%	
Iron	65-150 mcg/dL	
Iron binding capacity, total (TIBC)	250-420 mcg/dL	
Lactic acid	0.7-2.1 mEq/L	Specimen to be kept on ice and sent to lab as soon as possible.
Lactate dehydrogenase (LDH)	56-194 IU/L	

CHEMISTRY *(continued)*

Test	Values	Remarks
Lactate dehydrogenase (LDH) isoenzymes		
LD_1	20% to 34%	
LD_2	29% to 41%	
LD_3	15% to 25%	
LD_4	1% to 12%	
LD_5	1% to 15%	
Flipped LD_1/LD_2 ratios (>1 may be consistent with myocardial injury) particularly when considered in combination with a recent CK-MB positive result.		
Lipase	23-208 units/L	
Magnesium	1.6-2.5 mg/dL	Increased by slight hemolysis.
Osmolality	289-308 mOsm/kg	
Phosphatase, alkaline		
adults 25-60 y	33-131 IU/L	
adults ≥61 y	51-153 IU/L	
infancy-adolescence	Values range up to 3-5 times higher than adults	
Phosphate, inorganic	2.8-4.2 mg/dL	
Potassium	3.5-5.2 mEq/L	Increased by slight hemolysis.
Prealbumin	>15 mg/dL	
Protein, total	6.5-7.9 g/dL	
AST	<35 IU/L (20-48)	
ALT (10-35)	<35 IU/L	
Sodium	134-149 mEq/L	
Thyroid stimulating hormone (TSH)		
adults ≤20 y	0.7-6.4 mIU/L	
21-54 y	0.4-4.2 mIU/L	
55-87 y	0.5-8.9 mIU/L	
Transferrin	>200 mg/dL	
Triglycerides	45-155 mg/dL	Fasted blood required.
Troponin I	<1.5 ng/mL	
Urea nitrogen (BUN)	7-20 mg/dL	
Uric acid		
male	2-8 mg/dL	
female	2-7.5 mg/dL	
Cerebrospinal Fluid		
Glucose	50-70 mg/dL	
Protein	15-45 mg/dL	CSF obtained by lumbar puncture.
Note: Bloody specimen gives erroneously high value due to contamination with blood proteins		
Urine (24-hour specimen is required for all these tests unless specified)		
Amylase	32-641 units/L	The value is in units/L and **not** calculated for total volume.
Amylase, fluid (random samples)		Interpretation of value left for physician, depends on the nature of fluid.
Calcium	Depends upon dietary intake	
Creatine		
male	150 mg/24 h	Higher value on children and during pregnancy.
female	250 mg/24 h	
Creatinine	1000-2000 mg/24 h	
Creatinine clearance (endogenous)		
male	85-125 mL/min	A blood sample must accompany urine specimen.
female	75-115 mL/min	

CHEMISTRY *(continued)*

Test	Values	Remarks
Glucose	1 g/24 h	
5-hydroxyindoleacetic acid	2-8 mg/24 h	
Iron	0.15 mg/24 h	Acid washed container required.
Magnesium	146-209 mg/24 h	
Osmolality	500-800 mOsm/kg	With normal fluid intake.
Oxalate	10-40 mg/24 h	
Phosphate	400-1300 mg/24 h	
Potassium	25-120 mEq/24 h	Varies with diet; the interpretation of urine electrolytes and osmolality should be left for the physician.
Sodium	40-220 mEq/24 h	
Porphobilinogen, qualitative	Negative	
Porphyrins, qualitative	Negative	
Proteins	0.05-0.1 g/24 h	
Salicylate	Negative	
Urea clearance	60-95 mL/min	A blood sample must accompany specimen.
Urea N	10-40 g/24 h	Dependent on protein intake.
Uric acid	250-750 mg/24 h	Dependent on diet and therapy.
Urobilinogen	0.5-3.5 mg/24 h	For qualitative determination on random urine, send sample to urinalysis section in Hematology Lab.
Xylose absorption test		
children	16% to 33% of ingested xylose	
Feces		
Fat, 3-day collection	<5 g/d	Value depends on fat intake of 100 g/d for 3 days preceding and during collection.
Gastric Acidity		
Acidity, total, 12 h	10-60 mEq/L	Titrated at pH 7.

Blood Gases

	Arterial	Capillary	Venous
pH	7.35-7.45	7.35-7.45	7.32-7.42
pCO_2 (mm Hg)	35-45	35-45	38-52
pO_2 (mm Hg)	70-100	60-80	24-48
HCO_3 (mEq/L)	19-25	19-25	19-25
TCO_2 (mEq/L)	19-29	19-29	23-33
O_2 saturation (%)	90-95	90-95	40-70
Base excess (mEq/L)	-5 to +5	-5 to +5	-5 to +5

HEMATOLOGY

Complete Blood Count

Age	Hgb (g/dL)	Hct (%)	RBC (mill/mm^3)	RDW
0-3 d	15.0-20.0	45-61	4.0-5.9	<18
1-2 wk	12.5-18.5	39-57	3.6-5.5	<17
1-6 mo	10.0-13.0	29-42	3.1-4.3	<16.5
7 mo to 2 y	10.5-13.0	33-38	3.7-4.9	<16
2-5 y	11.5-13.0	34-39	3.9-5.0	<15
5-8 y	11.5-14.5	35-42	4.0-4.9	<15
13-18 y	12.0-15.2	36-47	4.5-5.1	<14.5
Adult male	13.5-16.5	41-50	4.5-5.5	<14.5
Adult female	12.0-15.0	36-44	4.0-4.9	<14.5

Age	MCV (fL)	MCH (pg)	MCHC (%)	Plts (x 10^3/mm^3)
0-3 d	95-115	31-37	29-37	250-450
1-2 wk	86-110	28-36	28-38	250-450
1-6 mo	74-96	25-35	30-36	300-700
7 mo to 2 y	70-84	23-30	31-37	250-600
2-5 y	75-87	24-30	31-37	250-550
5-8 y	77-95	25-33	31-37	250-550
13-18 y	78-96	25-35	31-37	150-450
Adult male	80-100	26-34	31-37	150-450
Adult female	80-100	26-34	31-37	150-450

WBC and Differential

Age	WBC (x 10^3/mm^3)	Segs	Bands	Lymphs	Monos
0-3 d	9.0-35.0	32-62	<18	19-29	5-7
1-2 wk	5.0-20.0	14-34	<14	36-45	6-10
1-6 mo	6.0-17.5	13-33	<12	41-71	4-7
7 mo to 2 y	6.0-17.0	15-35	<11	45-76	3-6
2-5 y	5.5-15.5	23-45	<11	35-65	3-6
5-8 y	5.0-14.5	32-54	<11	28-48	3-6
13-18 y	4.5-13.0	34-64	<11	25-45	3-6
Adults	4.5-11.0	35-66	<11	24-44	3-6

Age	Eosinophils	Basophils	Atypical Lymphs	No. of NRBCs
0-3 d	0-2	0-1	0-8	0-2
1-2 wk	0-2	0-1	0-8	0
1-6 mo	0-3	0-1	0-8	0
7 mo to 2 y	0-3	0-1	0-8	0
2-5 y	0-3	0-1	0-8	0
5-8 y	0-3	0-1	0-8	0
13-18 y	0-3	0-1	0-8	0
Adults	0-3	0-1	0-8	0

Segs = segmented neutrophils.

Bands = band neutrophils.

Lymphs = lymphocytes.

Monos = monocytes.

Erythrocyte Sedimentation Rates and Reticulocyte Counts

Sedimentation rate, Westergren	Children	0-20 mm/h
	Adult male	0-15 mm/h
	Adult female	0-20 mm/h
Sedimentation rate, Wintrobe	Children	0-13 mm/h
	Adult male	0-10 mm/h
	Adult female	0-15 mm/h
Reticulocyte count	Newborns	2% to 6%
	1-6 mo	0% to 2.8%
	Adults	0.5% to 1.5%

ASSESSMENT OF LIVER FUNCTION

Child-Pugh Score

Component	Score Given for Observed Findings		
	1	2	3
Encephalopathy grade[1]	None	1-2	3-4
Ascites	None	Mild or controlled by diuretics	Moderate or refractory despite diuretics
Albumin (g/dL)	>3.5	2.8-3.5	<2.8
Total bilirubin (mg/dL)	<2 (<34 micromoles/L)	2-3 (34-50 micromoles/L)	>3 (>50 micromoles/L)
or			
Modified total bilirubin[2]	<4	4-7	>7
Prothrombin time (seconds prolonged)	<4	4-6	>6
or			
INR	<1.7	1.7-2.3	>2.3

[1]**Encephalopathy Grades**
Grade 0: Normal consciousness, personality, neurological examination, electroencephalogram
Grade 1: Restless, sleep disturbed, irritable/agitated, tremor, impaired handwriting, 5 cps waves
Grade 2: Lethargic, time-disoriented, inappropriate, asterixis, ataxia, slow triphasic waves
Grade 3: Somnolent, stuporous, place-disoriented, hyperactive reflexes, rigidity, slower waves
Grade 4: Unrousable coma, no personality/behavior, decerebrate, slow 2-3 cps delta activity

Alternative Encephalopathy Grades
Grade 1: Mild confusion, anxiety, restlessness, fine tremor, slowed coordination
Grade 2: Drowsiness, disorientation, asterixis
Grade 3: Somnolent but rousable, marked confusion, incomprehensible speech, incontinent, hyperventilation
Grade 4: Coma, decerebrate posturing, flaccidity

[2]Modified total bilirubin used to score patients who have Gilbert's syndrome or who are taking indinavir.

CHILD-PUGH CLASSIFICATION

Class A (mild hepatic impairment): Score 5-6
Class B (moderate hepatic impairment): Score 7-9
Class C (severe hepatic impairment): Score 10-15

REFERENCES

Centers for Disease Control and Prevention, "Report of the NIH Panel to Define Principles of Therapy of HIV Infection and Guidelines for the Use of Antiretroviral Agents in HIV-Infected Adults and Adolescents," March 2004. Available at http://www.aidsinfo.nih.gov

U.S. Department of Health and Human Services Food and Drug Administration, "Guidance for Industry, Pharmacokinetics in Patients With Impaired Hepatic Function: Study Design, Data Analysis, and Impact on Dosing and Labeling," May 2003. Available at http://www.fda.gov/OHRMS/DOCKETS/98fr/99D-5047-GDL00002.pdf

RENAL FUNCTION ESTIMATION IN ADULT PATIENTS

Evaluation of a patient's renal function often includes the use of equations to estimate glomerular filtration rate (GFR) (eg, estimated GFR [eGFR] creatinine clearance [Cl_{Cr}]) using an endogenous filtration marker (eg, serum creatinine) and other patient variables. For example, the Cockcroft-Gault equation estimates renal function by calculating Cl_{Cr} and is typically used to steer medication dosing. Equations which calculate eGFR are primarily used to categorize chronic kidney disease (CKD) staging. The rate of creatinine clearance does not always accurately represent GFR; creatinine may be cleared by other renal mechanisms in addition to glomerular filtration and serum creatinine concentrations may be affected by non-renal factors (eg, age, gender, race, body habitus, illness, diet). In addition, these equations were developed based on studies in limited populations and may either over- or underestimate the renal function of a specific patient.

Nevertheless, most clinicians estimate renal function using Cl_{Cr} as an indicator of actual renal function for the purpose of adjusting medication doses. For medications that require dose adjustment for renal impairment, utilization of eGFR (ie, Modification of Diet in Renal Disease [MDRD]) may overestimate renal function by up to 40% which may result in supra-therapeutic medication doses (Hermsen, 2009). These equations should only be used in the clinical context of patient-specific factors noted during the physical exam/work-up. Decisions regarding drug therapy and doses must be based on clinical judgment.

RENAL FUNCTION ESTIMATION EQUATIONS

Commonly used equations include the Cockcroft-Gault, Jelliffe, four-variable Modification of Diet in Renal Disease (MDRD), and six-variable MDRD (aka, MDRD extended). All of these equations were originally developed using a serum creatinine assay measured by the alkaline picrate-based (Jaffe) method. Many substances, including proteins, can interfere with the accuracy of this assay and overestimate serum creatinine concentration. The National Kidney Foundation and The National Kidney Disease Education Program (NDKEP) advocate for a universal creatinine assay, in order to ensure an accurate estimate of renal function in patients. As a result, a more specific enzymatic assay with an isotope dilution mass spectrometry (IDMS)-traceable international standard has been developed. Compared to the older methods, IDMS-traceable assays may report lower serum creatinine values and may, therefore, overestimate renal function when used in the original equations (eg, Cockcroft-Gault, Jelliffe, original MDRD). Updated four-variable MDRD and six-variable MDRD equations based on serum creatinine measured by the IDMS-traceable method has been proposed for adults (Levey, 2006); the Cockcroft-Gault and Jelliffe equations have not been re-expressed and may overestimate renal function when used with a serum creatinine measured by the IDMS-traceable method. Clinicians should be aware of the serum creatinine assay used by their institution and the ramifications the assay may have on the equations used for renal function estimation.

Regardless of the serum creatinine assay used, the following factors may contribute to an inaccurate estimation of renal function (Stevens, 2006):

- Increased creatinine generation (may underestimate renal function):
  - Black or African American patients
  - Muscular body habitus
  - Ingestion of cooked meats
- Decreased creatinine generation (may overestimate renal function):
  - Increased age
  - Female patients
  - Hispanic patients
  - Asian patients
  - Amputees
  - Malnutrition, inflammation, or deconditioning (eg, cancer, severe cardiovascular disease, hospitalized patients)
  - Neuromuscular disease
  - Vegetarian diet
- Rapidly changing serum creatinine (either up or down): In patients with rapidly rising serum creatinines (ie, increasing by >0.5-0.7 mg/dL/day), it is best to assume that the patient's renal function is severely impaired

Use extreme caution when estimating renal function in the following patient populations:

- Low body weight (actual body weight < ideal body weight)
- Liver transplant
- Elderly (>90 years old)
- Dehydration
- Recent kidney transplantation (serum creatinine values may decrease rapidly and can lead to renal function under-estimation; conversely, delayed graft function may be present)

Note: In most situations, the use of the patient's ideal body weight (IBW) is recommended for estimating renal function, except when the patient's actual body weight (ABW) is less than ideal. Use of actual body weight (ABW) in obese patients (and possibly patients with ascites) may significantly overestimate renal function. Some clinicians prefer to use an adjusted body weight in such cases [eg, IBW + 0.4 (ABW - IBW)]; the adjustment factor may vary based on practitioner and/or institutional preference.

Alkaline picrate-based (Jaffe) methods

Note: These equations have not been updated for use with serum creatinine methods traceable to IDMS. Use with IDMS-traceable serum creatinine methods may overestimate renal function; use with caution.

Method 1: MDRD equation:

$$eGFR = 186 \times (Creatinine)^{-1.154} \times (Age)^{-0.203} \times (Gender) \times (Race)$$

where:

eGFR = estimated GFR; calculated in mL/minute/1.73 m^2
Creatinine is input in mg/dL
Age is input in years
Gender: Females: Gender = 0.742; Males: Gender = 1
Race: Black: Race = 1.212; White or other: Race = 1

Method 2: MDRD Extended equation:

$$eGFR = 170 \times (Creatinine)^{-0.999} \times (Age)^{-0.176} \times (SUN)^{-0.170} \times (Albumin)^{0.318} \times (Gender) \times (Race)$$

where:

eGFR = estimated GFR; calculated in mL/minute/1.73 m^2
Creatinine is input in mg/dL
Age is input in years
SUN = Serum Urea Nitrogen; input in mg/dL
Albumin = Serum Albumin; input in g/dL
Gender: Females: Gender = 0.762; Males: Gender = 1
Race: Black: Race = 1.18; White or other: Race = 1

Method 3: Cockroft-Gault equation[1]

Males: $Cl_{Cr} = [(140 - Age) \times Weight] / (72 \times Creatinine)$
Females: $Cl_{Cr} = \{[(140 - Age) \times Weight] / (72 \times Creatinine)\} \times 0.85$

where:

Cl_{Cr} = creatinine clearance; calculated in mL/minute
Age is input in years
Weight is input in kg
Creatinine is input in mg/dL

Method 4: Jelliffe equation

Males: $Cl_{Cr} = \{98 - [0.8 \times (Age - 20)]\} / (Creatinine)$
Females: Cl_{Cr} = Use above equation, then multiply result by 0.9

where:

Cl_{Cr} = creatinine clearance; calculated in mL/minute/1.73m^2
Age is input in years
Creatinine is input in mg/dL

IDMS-traceable methods

Method 1: MDRD equation[2]:

$$eGFR = 175 \times (Creatinine)^{-1.154} \times (Age)^{-0.203} \times (Gender) \times (Race)$$

where:

eGFR = estimated GFR; calculated in mL/minute/1.73 m^2
Creatinine is input in mg/dL
Age is input in years
Gender: Females: Gender = 0.742; Males: Gender = 1
Race: Black: Race = 1.212; White or other: Race = 1

Method 2: MDRD Extended equation:

$$eGFR = 161.5 \times (Creatinine)^{-0.999} \times (Age)^{-0.176} \times (SUN)^{-0.170} \times (Albumin)^{0.318} \times (Gender) \times (Race)$$

where:

eGFR = estimated GFR; calculated in mL/minute/1.73 m^2
Creatinine is input in mg/dL
Age is input in years
SUN = Serum Urea Nitrogen; input in mg/dL
Albumin = Serum Albumin; input in g/dL
Gender: Females: Gender = 0.762; Males: Gender = 1
Race: Black: Race = 1.18; White or other: Race = 1

FOOTNOTES

[1]Equation typically used for adjusting medication doses
[2]Preferred equation for CKD staging National Kidney Disease Education Program

REFERENCES

Cockcroft DW and Gault MH, "Prediction of Creatinine Clearance From Serum Creatinine," *Nephron*, 1976, 16(1):31-41.

Dowling TC, Matzke GR, Murphy JE, et al, "Evaluation of Renal Drug Dosing: Prescribing Information and Clinical Pharmacist Approaches," *Pharmacotherapy*, 2010, 30(8):776-86.

Hermsen ED, Maiefski M, Florescu MC, et al, "Comparison of the Modification of Diet in Renal Disease and Cockcroft-Gault Equations for Dosing Antimicrobials," *Pharmacotherapy*, 2009, 29(6):649-55.

Jelliffe RW, "Letter: Creatinine Clearance: Bedside Estimate," *Ann Intern Med*, 1973, 79(4):604-5.

Levey AS, Bosch JP, Lewis JB, et al, "A More Accurate Method to Estimate Glomerular Filtration Rate From Serum Creatinine: A New Prediction Equation. Modification of Diet in Renal Disease Study Group," *Ann Intern Med*, 1999, 16;130(6):461–70.

Levey AS, Coresh J, Greene T, et al, "Using Standardized Serum Creatinine Values in the Modification of Diet in Renal Disease Study Equation for Estimating Glomerular Filtration Rate," *Ann Intern Med*, 2006, 145(4):247-54.

National Kidney Disease Education Program, "GFR Calculators." Available at http://www.nkdep.nih.gov/professionals/gfr_calculators. Last accessed January 20, 2011.

Stevens LA, Coresh J, Greene T, et al, "Assessing Kidney Function - Measured and Estimated Glomerular Filtration Rate," *N Engl J Med*, 2006, 354 (23):2473-83.

RENAL FUNCTION ESTIMATION IN PEDIATRIC PATIENTS

Evaluation of a patient's renal function often includes the use of equations to estimate glomerular filtration rate (GFR) (eg, estimated GFR [eGFR] creatinine clearance [Cl_{Cr}]) using an endogenous filtration marker (eg, serum creatinine) and other patient variables. For example, the Schwartz equation estimates renal function by calculating eGFR and is typically used to steer medication dosing or categorize chronic kidney disease (CKD) staging. The rate of creatinine clearance does not always accurately represent GFR; creatinine may be cleared by other renal mechanisms in addition to glomerular filtration and serum creatinine concentrations may be affected by non-renal factors (eg, age, gender, race, body habitus, illness, diet). In addition, these equations were developed based on studies in limited populations and may either over- or underestimate the renal function of a specific patient.

Nevertheless, most clinicians use an eGFR or Cl_{Cr} as an indicator of renal function in pediatric patients for the purposes of adjusting medication doses. These equations should be used in the clinical context of patient-specific factors noted during the physical exam/work-up. **Decisions regarding drug therapy and doses must be made on clinical judgment.**

RENAL FUNCTION ESTIMATION EQUATIONS

Commonly used equations include the Schwartz and Traub-Johnson equations. Both equations were originally developed using a serum creatinine assay measured by the alkaline picrate-based (Jaffe) method. Many substances, including proteins, can interfere with the accuracy of this assay and overestimate serum creatinine concentration. The National Kidney Foundation and The National Kidney Disease Education Program advocate for a universal creatinine assay, in order to ensure an accurate estimate of GFR in patients. As a result, a more specific enzymatic assay with an isotope dilution mass spectrometry (IDMS)-traceable international standard has been developed. Compared to the older methods, IDMS-traceable assays may report lower serum creatinine values and may, therefore, overestimate renal function when used in the original equations. An updated Schwartz equation (eg, Bedside Schwartz) based on serum creatinine measured by the IDMS-traceable method has been proposed for pediatrics (Schwartz, 2009); the Traub-Johnson equation has not been re-expressed. The original Schwartz and Traub-Johnson equations may overestimate renal function when used with a serum creatinine measured by the IDMS-traceable method. Clinicians should be aware of the serum creatinine assay used by their institution and the ramifications the assay may have on the equations used for renal function estimation.

Regardless of the serum creatinine assay used, the following factors may contribute to an inaccurate estimation of renal function (Stevens, 2006):

- Increased creatinine generation (may underestimate renal function):
  - Black or African American patients
  - Muscular body habitus
  - Ingestion of cooked meats
- Decreased creatinine generation (may overestimate renal function):
  - Increased age
  - Female patients
  - Asian patients
  - Amputees
  - Malnutrition, inflammation, or deconditioning (eg, cancer, severe cardiovascular disease, hospitalized patients)
  - Neuromuscular disease
  - Vegetarian diet
- Rapidly changing serum creatinine (either up or down):
  - In patients with rapidly rising serum creatinines (ie, increasing by >0.5-0.7 mg/dL/day), it is best to assume that the patient's renal function is severely impaired

Use extreme caution when estimating renal function in the following patient populations:

- Low body weight (actual body weight < ideal body weight)
- Liver transplant
- Prematurity (especially very low birth weight)
- Dehydration
- Recent kidney transplantation (serum creatinine values may decrease rapidly and can lead to renal function under-estimation; conversely, delayed graft function may be present)

Alkaline picrate-based (Jaffe) methods

Note: These equations have not been updated for use with serum creatinine methods traceable to IDMS. Use with IDMS-traceable serum creatinine methods may overestimate renal function; use with caution.

Method 1: Schwartz equation

Note: This equation may not provide an accurate estimation of creatinine clearance for infants <6 months of age or for patients with severe starvation or muscle wasting.

eGFR = (k X Height) / Creatinine

where:

eGFR = estimated GFR; calculated in mL/minute/1.73 m^2

Height (length) is input in cm

k = constant of proportionality that is age-specific

<1 year preterm: 0.33

<1 year full-term: 0.45

1-12 years: 0.55

>12 years female: 0.55

>12 years male: 0.7

Creatinine is input in mg/dL

Method 2: Traub-Johnson equation

Note: This equation is for use in ages 1-18 years.

Cl_{Cr} = (0.48 X Height) / Creatinine

where:

Cl_{Cr} = estimated creatinine clearance; calculated in mL/minute/1.73 m^2

Height (length) is input in cm

Creatinine = Sr_{Cr} input in mg/dL

IDMS-traceable method: Bedside Schwartz[1]

Note: This equation is for use in ages 1-16 years.

eGFR = (0.413 X Height) / Creatinine

where:

eGFR = estimated GFR; calculated in mL/minute/1.73 m^2

Height (length) is input in cm

Creatinine = Sr_{Cr} input in mg/dL

FOOTNOTES

[1]National Kidney Disease Education Program preferred equation

REFERENCES

Dowling TC, Matzke GR, Murphy JE, et al, "Evaluation of Renal Drug Dosing: Prescribing Information and Clinical Pharmacist Approaches," *Pharmacotherapy*, 2010, 30(8):776-86.

Myers GL, Miller WG, Coresh J, et al, "Recommendations for Improving Serum Creatinine Measurement: A Report From the Laboratory Working Group of the National Kidney Disease Education Program," *Clin Chem*, 2006, 52(1):5-18.

National Kidney Disease Education Program, "GFR Calculators." Available at http://www.nkdep.nih.gov/professionals/gfr_calculators. Last accessed January 20, 2011.

Pottel H, Mottaghy FM, Zaman Z, et al, "On the Relationship Between Glomerular Filtration Rate and Serum Creatinine in Children," *Pediatr Nephrol*, 2010, 25(5):927-34.

Schwartz GJ, Brion LP, and Spitzer A, "The Use of Plasma Creatinine Concentration for Estimating Glomerular Filtration Rate in Infants, Children, and Adolescents," *Pediatr Clin North Am*, 1987, 34(3):571-90.

Schwartz GJ, Haycock GB, Edelmann CM Jr, et al, "A Simple Estimate of Glomerular Filtration Rate in Children Derived From Body Length and Plasma Creatinine," *Pediatrics*, 1976, 58(2):259-63.

Schwartz GJ, Muñoz A, Schneider MF, et al, "New Equations to Estimate GFR in Children With CKD," *J Am Soc Nephrol*, 2009, 20(3):629-37.

Staples A, LeBlond R, Watkins S, et al, "Validation of the Revised Schwartz Estimating Equation in a Predominantly Non-CKD Population," *Pediatr Nephrol*, 2010, 25(11):2321-6.

Stevens LA, Coresh J, Greene T, et al, "Assessing Kidney Function - Measured and Estimated Glomerular Filtration Rate," *N Engl J Med*, 2006, 354 (23):2473-83.

Traub SL and Johnson CE, "Comparison of Methods of Estimating Creatinine Clearance in Children," *Am J Hosp Pharm*, 1980, 37(2):195-201.

ANGIOTENSIN AGENTS

Comparison of Indications and Adult Dosages

Drug	Hypertension	HF	Renal Dysfunction	Dialyzable	Strengths (mg)
ACE Inhibitors					
Benazepril (Lotensin®)	10-40 mg/day	Not FDA-approved	Cl_{cr} <30 mL/min: 5 mg/day initially Maximum: 40 mg/day	Yes	Tablets 5, 10, 20, 40
Captopril (Capoten®)	25-100 mg/day bid-tid	6.25-100 mg tid Maximum: 450 mg/day	Cl_{cr} 10-50 mL/min: 75% of usual dose Cl_{cr} <10 mL/min: 50% of usual dose	Yes	Tablets 12.5, 25, 50, 100
Cilazapril (Inhibace®) **Note:** Not available in U.S.	2.5-10 mg/day	0.5-2.5 mg/day	Cl_{cr} 10-40 mL/min: Initial: 0.5 mg/day (0.25-0.5 mg/day for HF) (maximum: 2.5 mg/day) Cl_{cr} <10 mL/minute: 0.25-0.5 mg once or twice weekly	Yes	Tablets 1, 2.5, 5
Enalapril (Vasotec®)	2.5-40 mg/day qd-bid	2.5-20 mg bid Maximum: 20 mg bid	Cl_{cr} 30-80 mL/min: 5 mg/day initially Cl_{cr} <30 mL/min: 2.5 mg/day initially	Yes	Tablets 2.5, 5, 10, 20
Enalaprilat[1]	0.625 mg, 1.25 mg, 2.5 mg q6h Maximum: 5 mg q6h	Not FDA-approved	Cl_{cr} <30 mL/min: 0.625 mg q6h	Yes	1.25 mg/mL (1 mL, 2 mL vials)
Fosinopril (Monopril®)	10-40 mg/day	10-40 mg/day	No dosage reduction necessary	Not well dialyzed	Tablets 10, 20, 40
Lisinopril (Prinivil®, Zestril®)	10-40 mg/day Maximum: 40 mg/day	5-40 mg/day	Cl_{cr} 10-30 mL/min: 5 mg/day initially Cl_{cr} <10 mL/min: 2.5 mg/day initially	Yes	Tablets 2.5, 5, 10, 20, 30, 40
Moexipril (Univasc®)	7.5-30 mg/day qd-bid Maximum: 30 mg/day	LV dysfunction (post-MI): 7.5-30 mg/day	Cl_{cr} <40 mL/min: 3.75 mg/day initially Maximum: 15 mg/day	Unknown	Tablets 7.5, 15
Perindopril (Aceon®)	4-8 mg/day	4-8 mg/day Maximum: 16 mg/day	Cl_{cr} 30-60 mL/min: 2 mg/day Cl_{cr} 15-29 mL/min: 2 mg qod Cl_{cr} <15 mL/min: 2 mg on dialysis days	Yes	Tablets 2, 4, 8
Quinapril (Accupril®)	10-40 mg/day qd-bid	5-20 mg bid	Cl_{cr} 30-60 mL/min: 5 mg/day initially Cl_{cr} <10-30 mL/min: 2.5 mg/day initially	Not well dialyzed	Tablets 5, 10, 20, 40
Ramipril (Altace®)	2.5-20 mg/day qd-bid	2.5-10 mg/day	Cl_{cr} <40 mL/min: 25% of normal dose	Unknown	Capsules 1.25, 2.5, 5, 10
Trandolapril (Mavik®)	1-4 mg/day Maximum: 8 mg/day qd-bid	LV dysfunction (post-MI): 1-4 mg/day	Cl_{cr} <30 mL/min: 0.5 mg/day initially	No	Tablets 1, 2, 4

Comparison of Indications and Adult Dosages *continued*

Drug	Hypertension	HF	Renal Dysfunction	Dialyzable	Strengths (mg)
Angiotensin II Receptor Blockers					
Azilsartan (Edarbi™)	40-80 mg/day	Not FDA-approved	No dosage adjustment necessary	Unknown	Tablets 40, 80
Candesartan (Atacand®)	8-32 mg/day	Target: 32 mg once daily	No dosage adjustment necessary	No	Tablets 4, 8, 16, 32
Eprosartan (Teveten®)	400-800 mg/day qd-bid	Not FDA-approved	No dosage adjustment necessary	Unknown	Tablets 400, 600
Irbesartan (Avapro®)	150-300 mg/day	Not FDA-approved	No dosage reduction necessary	No	Tablets 75, 150, 300
Losartan (Cozaar®)	25-100 mg qd or bid	Not FDA-approved	No dosage adjustment necessary	No	Tablets 25, 50, 100
Olmesartan (Benicar®)	20-40 mg/day	Not FDA-approved	No dosage adjustment necessary	Unknown	Tablets 5, 20, 40
Telmisartan (Micardis®)	20-80 mg/day	Not FDA-approved	No dosage reduction necessary	No	Tablets 20, 40, 80
Valsartan (Diovan®)	80-320 mg/day	Target: 160 mg bid	Decrease dose only if Cl_{cr} <10 mL/minute	No	Tablets 40, 80, 160, 320
Renin Inhibitors					
Aliskiren (Tekturna®)	150-300 mg once daily	Not FDA-approved	No dosage adjustment necessary in mild-to-moderate impairment; not adequately studied in severe impairment	Unknown	Tablets 150, 300

Dosage is based on 70 kg adult with normal hepatic and renal function.

[1]Enalaprilat is the only available ACE inhibitor in a parenteral formulation.

ACE Inhibitors: Comparative Pharmacokinetics

Drug	Prodrug	Absorption (%)	Serum $t_{1/2}$ (h) Normal Renal Function	Serum Protein Binding (%)	Elimination	Onset of BP Lowering Action (h)	Peak BP Lowering Effects (h)	Duration of BP Lowering Effects (h)
Benazepril	Yes	37		~97	Renal (32%), biliary (~12%)	1	2-4	24
Benazeprilat			10-11 (effective)	~95				
Captopril	No	60-75 (fasting)	1.9 (elimination)	25-30	Renal	0.25-0.5	1-1.5	~6
Enalapril	Yes	55-75	2	50-60	Renal (60%-80%), fecal	1	4-6	12-24
Enalaprilat			11 (effective)			0.25	1-4	~6
Fosinopril		36			Renal (~50%), biliary (~50%)	1		24
Fosinoprilat			12 (effective)	>99				
Lisinopril	No	25	11-12	25	Renal	1	6	24
Moexipril	Yes		1	90	Fecal (53%), renal (8%)		1-2	>24
Moexiprilat			2-10	50				
Perindopril	Yes		1.5-3	60	Renal		3-7	
Perindoprilat			3-10 (effective)	10-20				
Quinapril	Yes	>60	0.8	97	Renal (~60%) as metabolite, fecal	1	2-4	24
Quinaprilat			3					
Ramipril	Yes	50-60	1-2	73	Renal (60%), fecal (40%)	1-2	3-6	24
Ramiprilat			13-17 (effective)	56				
Trandolapril	Yes		6	80	Renal (33%), fecal (66%)	1-2	6	≥24
Trandolaprilat			10	65-94				

Angiotensin II Receptor Blockers and Renin Inhibitors: Comparative Pharmacokinetics

Drug	Prodrug	Time to Peak	Bioavailability	Food "Area-Under-the-Curve"	Elimination Half-Life	Elimination Altered in Renal Dysfunction	Precautions in Severe Renal Dysfunction	Elimination Altered in Hepatic Dysfunction	Precautions in Hepatic Dysfunction	Protein Binding (%)
Angiotensin II Receptor Blockers										
Azilsartan (Edarbi™)	Yes	1.5-3 h	60%	No effect	11 h	No	Yes	No	No	>99
Candesartan (Atacand®)	Yes[1]	3-4 h	15%	No effect	9 h	Yes[2]	Yes	No	Yes	>99
Eprosartan (Teveten®)	No	1-2 h	13%	No effect	5-9 h	No	Yes	No	Yes	98
Irbesartan (Avapro®)	No	1.5-2 h	60% to 80%	No effect	11-15 h	No	Yes	No	No	90
Losartan (Cozaar®)	Yes[3]	1 h/3-4 h[3]	33%	9% to 10%	1.5-2 h/6-9 h[3]	No	Yes	Yes	Yes	~99
Olmesartan (Benicar®)	Yes	1-2 h	26%	No effect	13 h	Yes	Yes	Yes	No	99
Telmisartan (Micardis®)	No	0.5-1 h	42% to 58%	9.6% to 20%	24 h	No	Yes	Yes	Yes	>99.5
Valsartan (Diovan®)	No	2-4 h	25%	9% to 40%	6 h	No	Yes	Yes	Yes	95
Renin Inhibitors										
Aliskiren (Tekturna®)	No	1-3 h	~3%	85% (high-fat meal)	16-32 h	Yes[4]	Yes	No	No	?

[1]Candesartan cilexetil: Active metabolite candesartan

[2]Dosage adjustments are not necessary.

[3]Losartan: Active metabolite E-3174

[4]No initial dosage adjustment in mild-to-moderate impairment

ANTICONVULSANT DRUGS OF CHOICE

Seizure Type	First Line Therapy	Alternatives
Partial (including secondary generalization)	CarBAMazepine, lamoTRIgine, levETIRAcetam, or OXcarbazepine	Divalproex, gabapentin, lacosamide, phenytoin, pregabalin, topiramate, valproic acid, or zonisamide
Generalized tonic-clonic	Divalproex, lamoTRIgine, or valproic acid	CarBAMazepine, levETIRAcetam, OXcarbazepine, phenytoin, topiramate, or zonisamide
Childhood absence epilepsy	Divalproex, ethosuximide (only if no generalized seizures), lamoTRIgine, or valproic acid	ClonazePAM, levETIRAcetam, or zonisamide
Atypical absence, myoclonic, or atonic	Divalproex, lamoTRIgine, levETIRAcetam, or valproic acid	ClonazePAM, felbamate, topiramate, or zonisamide

Note: Table includes non-FDA approved indications

REFERENCES

"Drugs for Epilepsy," *Treat Guidel Med Lett*, 2008, 6(70):37-46.

Glauser T, Ben-Menachem E, Bourgeois B, et al, "ILAE Treatment Guidelines: Evidence-Based Analysis of Antiepileptic Drug Efficacy and Effectiveness as Initial Monotherapy for Epileptic Seizures and Syndromes," *Epilepsia*, 2006, 47(7):1094-120.

ANTIDEPRESSANT AGENTS

Comparison of Usual Adult Dosage, Mechanism of Action, and Adverse Effects

Drug	Initial Adult Dose	Usual Adult Dosage (mg/d)	Dosage Forms	Adverse Effects: ACH	Drowsiness	Orthostatic Hypotension	Conduction Abnormalities	GI Distress	Weight Gain	Comments
Tricyclic Antidepressants and Related Compounds[1]										
Amitriptyline	25-75 mg qhs	100-300	T	4+	4+	3+	3+	1+	4+	Also used in chronic pain, migraine, and as a hypnotic; contraindicated with cisapride
Amoxapine	50 mg bid	100-400	T	2+	2+	2+	2+	0	2+	May cause extrapyramidal symptom (EPS)
ClomiPRAMINE[2] (Anafranil®)	25-75 mg qhs	100-250	C	4+	4+	2+	3+	1+	4+	Only approved for OCD
Desipramine (Norpramin®)	25-75 mg qhs	100-300	T	1+	2+	2+	2+	0	1+	Blood levels useful for therapeutic monitoring
Doxepin	25-75 mg qhs	100-300	C, L	3+	4+	2+	2+	0	4+	
Imipramine (Tofranil®, Tofranil-PM®)	25-75 mg qhs	100-300	T, C	3+	3+	4+	3+	1+	4+	Blood levels useful for therapeutic monitoring
Maprotiline	25-75 mg qhs	100-225	T	2+	3+	2+	2+	0	2+	
Nortriptyline (Pamelor®)	25-50 mg qhs	50-150	C, L	2+	2+	1+	2+	0	1+	Blood levels useful for therapeutic monitoring
Protriptyline (Vivactil®)	15 mg qAM	15-60	T	2+	1+	2+	3+	1+	1+	
Trimipramine (Surmontil®)	25-75 mg qhs	100-300	C	4+	4+	3+	3+	0	4+	
Selective Serotonin Reuptake Inhibitors[3]										
Citalopram (Celexa®)	20 mg qAM	20-60	T, L	0	0	0	0	3+[4]	1+	
Escitalopram (Lexapro®)	10 mg qAM	10-20	T, L	0	0	0	0	3+	1+	S-enantiomer of citalopram
FLUoxetine (PROzac®, PROzac® Weekly™, Sarafem®, Selfemra®)	10-20 mg qAM	20-80	C, CDR, L, T	0	0	0	0	3+[4]	1+	CYP2B6 and 2D6 inhibitor
FluvoxaMINE[2] (Luvox® CR)	50 mg qhs	100-300	T, CXR	0	0	0	0	3+[4]	1+	Contraindicated with pimozide, thioridazine, mesoridazine, CYP1A2, 2B6, 2C19, and 3A4 inhibitors
PARoxetine (Paxil®, Paxil CR®, Pexeva®)	10-20 mg qAM	20-50	T, CXR, L	1+	1+	0	0	3+[4]	2+	CYP2B6 and 2D6 inhibitor
Sertraline (Zoloft®)	25-50 mg qAM	50-200	T, L	0	0	0	0	3+[4]	1+	CYP2B6 and 2C19 inhibitor
Vilazodone (Viibryd™)	10 mg qAM	10-40	T	0	0	0	0	3+	0	CYP2C8, 2C19, and 2D6 inhibitor; also is a 5-HT_{1A} partial agonist
Dopamine-Reuptake Blocking Compounds										
BuPROPion (Aplenzin™, Buproban®, Budeprion SR®, Budeprion XL®, Wellbutrin®, Wellbutrin SR®, Wellbutrin XL®, Zyban®)	100 mg bid-tid IR[5] 150 mg qAM-bid SR[6]	300-450	T, TSR, TXR	0	0	0	1+/0	1+	0	Contraindicated with seizures, bulimia, and anorexia; low incidence of sexual dysfunction IR: A 6-h interval between doses preferred SR: An 8-h interval between doses preferred XL: Administer once daily

Comparison of Usual Adult Dosage, Mechanism of Action, and Adverse Effects *continued*

Drug	Initial Adult Dose	Usual Adult Dosage (mg/d)	Dosage Forms	Adverse Effects: ACH	Drowsiness	Orthostatic Hypotension	Conduction Abnormalities	GI Distress	Weight Gain	Comments
Serotonin / Norepinephrine Reuptake Inhibitors[7]										
Desvenlafaxine (Pristiq®)	50 mg/d	50-100	TXR	0	1+	1+	0	3+[4]	0	Active metabolite of venlafaxine
DULoxetine (Cymbalta®)	40-60 mg/d	40-60	CDR	1+	1+	0	1+	3+	0	Also indicated for GAD, management of pain associated with diabetic neuropathy, and management of fibromyalgia
Milnacipran[8] (Savella™)	12.5 mg/d	100-200	T	2+	1+	0	1+	3+	0	Only indicated for fibromyalgia
Venlafaxine (Effexor®, Effexor XR®)	25 mg bid-tid IR 37.5 mg qd XR	75-375 IR 75-225 XR	T, TXR, CXR	1+	1+	0	1+	3+[4]	0	High-dose may be useful to treat refractory depression; frequency of hypertension increases with dosage >225 mg/d
5-HT_2 Receptor Antagonist Properties										
Nefazodone	100 mg bid	300-600	T	1+	1+	2+	1+	1+	0	Contraindicated with carbamazepine, pimozide, astemizole, cisapride, and terfenadine; caution with triazolam and alprazolam; low incidence of sexual dysfunction
TraZODone	50 mg tid	150-600	T	0	4+	3+	1+	1+	2+	
Noradrenergic Antagonist										
Mirtazapine (Remeron®, Remeron SolTab®)	15 mg qhs	15-45	T, TOD	1+	3+	1+	1+	0	3+	Dose >15 mg/d less sedating, low incidence of sexual dysfunction
Monoamine Oxidase Inhibitors										
Isocarboxazid (Marplan®)	10 mg tid	10-30	T	2+	2+	2+	1+	1+	2+	Diet must be low in tyramine; contraindicated with sympathomimetics and other antidepressants
Phenelzine (Nardil®)	15 mg tid	15-90	T	2+	2+	2+	0	1+	3+	
Tranylcypromine (Parnate®)	10 mg bid	10-60	T	2+	1+	2+	1+	1+	2+	
Selegiline (EmSam®)	6 mg/d	6-12	Transdermal	2+	1+	2+	0	1+	0	Low tyramine diet not required for 6 mg/d dosage

ACH = anticholinergic effects (dry mouth, blurred vision, urinary retention, constipation); 0 - 4+ = absent or rare - relatively common. T = tablet, TSR = tablet, sustained release, TXR - tablet, extended release, TOD = tablet, orally disintegrating, L = liquid, C = capsule, CDR = capsule, delayed release, CXR = capsule, extended release; IR = immediate release, SR = sustained release, XR = extended release.

[1]**Important note:** A 1-week supply taken all at once in a patient receiving the maximum dose can be fatal.

[2]Not approved by FDA for depression. Approved for OCD.

[3]Flat dose response curve, headache, nausea, and sexual dysfunction are common side effects for SSRIs.

[4]Nausea is usually mild and transient.

[5]IR: 100 mg bid; may be increased to 100 mg tid no sooner than 3 days after beginning therapy

[6]SR: 150 mg qAM; may be increased to 150 mg bid as early as day 4 of dosing. To minimize seizure risk, do not exceed SR 200 mg/dose.

[7]Do not use with sibutramine; relatively safe in overdose

[8]Milnacipran is only approved for fibromyalgia.

ANTIFUNGAL AGENTS

Activities of Various Agents Against Specific Fungi

Organisms	Amphotericin B (Conventional)[1]	Caspofungin	Fluconazole	Flucytosine
Aspergillus spp	FA	FA	N	?
Blastomyces dermatitidis	FA	?	A	N
Candida albicans	FA	FA	FA	FA
Candida glabrata	A	A	?	A
Candida krusei	FA	A	?	A
Candida tropicalis	FA	A	?	A
Coccidioides immitis	FA	?	A	N
Cryptococcus spp	FA	N	FA	FA
Dermatophytes	A	?	A	?
Fusarium spp	A	N	N	N
Histoplasma capsulatum	FA	A?	A	N
Penicillium spp	A	?	?	A
Pseudoallescheria boydii	?	A	N	N
Sporothrix schenckii	A	?	?	?
Zygomycetes (Mucor, Rhizopus)	A	N	N	N

Organisms	Griseofulvin	Itraconazole	Ketoconazole	Micafungin
Aspergillus spp	N	FA	N	A
Blastomyces dermatitidis	N	FA	FA	?
Candida albicans	N	FA	FA	FA
Candida glabrata	N	?	?	FA
Candida krusei	N	A	?	A
Candida tropicalis	N	?	?	A
Coccidioides immitis	N	A	FA	?
Cryptococcus spp	N	A	A	N
Dermatophytes	FA	A	A	?
Fusarium spp	N	N	N	?
Histoplasma capsulatum	N	FA	FA	?
Penicillium spp	N	?	N	?
Pseudoallescheria boydii	N	N	N	?
Sporothrix schenckii	N	?	N	?
Zygomycetes (Mucor, Rhizopus)	N	N	N	N

Organisms	Miconazole	Nystatin	Terbinafine	Voriconazole
Aspergillus spp	N	A	N	FA
Blastomyces dermatitidis	N	A	N	A
Candida albicans	FA	FA	A	A
Candida glabrata	?	A	?	A
Candida krusei	?	A	?	A
Candida tropicalis	?	A	?	A
Coccidioides immitis	A	N	N	A
Cryptococcus spp	A	N	N	A
Dermatophytes	N	N	FA	?
Fusarium spp	N	N	N	FA
Histoplasma capsulatum	N	N	N	A
Penicillium spp	N	N	N	?
Pseudoallescheria boydii	N	N	N	FA
Sporothrix schenckii	?	N	N	?
Zygomycetes (Mucor, Rhizopus)	N	N	N	N?

Organisms	Anidulafungin	Posaconazole
Aspergillus spp	A	FA
Blastomyces dermatitidis	N	A
Candida albicans	FA	FA
Candida glabrata	FA	A
Candida krusei	A	A
Candida tropicalis	FA	A
Coccidioides immitis	?	A
Cryptococcus spp	N	A
Dermatophytes	N?	A
Fusarium spp	N	A
Histoplasma capsulatum	?	A
Penicillium spp	A	A
Pseudoallescheria boydii	?	A
Sporothrix schenckii	?	A
Zygomycetes (Mucor, Rhizopus)	N?	A

FA = FDA-approved indication, A = active, ? = unknown or questionable, N = not active

[1]Various lipid products have differing indications, but all have activity against the same organisms.

REFERENCES

Espinel-Ingroff A, "Comparison of *In Vitro* Activities of the New Triazole SCH56592 and the Echinocandins MK-0991 (L-743,872) and LY303366 Against Opportunistic Filamentous and Dimorphic Fungi and Yeasts," *J Clin Microbiol*, 1998, 36(10):2950-6.

Sabatelli F, Patel R, Mann PA, et al, "*In Vitro* Activities of Posaconazole, Fluconazole, Itraconazole, Voriconazole, and Amphotericin B Against a Large Collection of Clinically Important Molds and Yeasts," *Antimicrob Agents Chemother*, 2006, 50(6):2009-15.

Torres HA, Hachem RY, Chemaly RF, et al, "Posaconazole: A Broad-Spectrum Triazole Antifungal," *Lancet Infect Dis*, 2005, 5(12):775-85.

Vazquez JA, "Anidulafungin: A New Echinocandin With a Novel Profile," *Clin Ther*, 2005, 27(6):657-73.

Zhanel GG, Karlowsky JA, Harding GA, et al, "*In Vitro* Activity of a New Semisynthetic Echinocandin, LY-303366, Against Systemic Isolates of *Candida* Species, *Cryptococcus neoformans*, *Blastomyces dermatitidis*, and *Aspergillus* Species," *Antimicrob Agents Chemother*, 1997, 41(4):863-5.

ANTIMIGRAINE DRUGS: 5-HT$_1$ RECEPTOR AGONISTS

Pharmacokinetic Differences

Pharmacokinetic Parameter	Almotriptan (Axert®)	Eletriptan (Relpax®)	Frovatriptan (Frova®)	Naratriptan (Amerge®)	Rizatriptan (Maxalt®, Maxalt-MLT®)		Sumatriptan (Imitrex®)			Zolmitriptan (Zomig®, Zomig-ZMT®)		
	Oral (6.25-12.5 mg)	Tablets	Oral	Oral	Tablets	Disintegrating Tablets	SubQ (6 mg)	Oral (100 mg)	Nasal (20 mg)	Oral (5 mg)	Disintegrating Tablets (5 mg)	Nasal (5 mg)
Onset	<60 min	<2 h	<2 h	1-2 h	~30 min	~30 min	10 min	~30 min	15-30 min	0.5-1 h	0.5-1 h	0.5-1 h
Duration	Short	Short	Long	Long	Short	Short	Short	Short	Short	Short		
Time to peak serum concentration (h)	1-3	1.5-2	2-4	2-3	1-1.5	1-1.5	4-20 min	2-2.5	1	1.5	3	3
Average bioavailability (%)	70	50	20-30	70	45	45	97	15	17	40	40	40
Volume of distribution (L)	180-200	138	210-280	170	110-140	110-140	170	170	NA	—	402	NA
Half-life (h)	3-4	4	26	6	2-3	2-3	2	2-2.5[1]	2	2.8-3.74	2.8-3.7	2.8-3.7
Fraction excreted unchanged in urine (%)	40	—	<10	50	8-16	8-16	22	3	3	8	8	—

[1]With extended dosing, the half-life extends to 7 hours.

ANTIPARKINSONIAN AGENTS

Drugs Used for the Treatment of Parkinsonian Symptoms[1]

Drug	Mechanism	Initial Dose	Titration Schedule	Usual Daily Dosage	Recommended Dosing Schedule
Dopaminergic Agents					
Amantadine (Symmetrel®)	NMDA receptor antagonist and inhibits neuronal reuptake of dopamine	100 mg every other day	100 mg/dose every week, up to 300 mg 3 times/d	100-200 mg	Twice daily
Apomorphine (Apokyn®)	D_2 receptors (caudate-putamen)	1-2 mg	Complex; based on tolerance and response to test dose(s)	Variable; <20 mg	Individualized; 3-5 times/d prn
Bromocriptine (Parlodel®)	Moderate affinity for D_2 and D_3 dopamine receptors	1.25 mg twice daily	2.5 mg/d every 2-4 wk	2.5-100 mg	3 times/d
Carbidopa/levodopa (Sinemet®)	Converts to dopamine; binds to all CNS dopamine receptors	10-25/100 mg 2-4 times/d CR: 50/200 mg 2 times/d	0.5-1 tablet (10 or 25/100 mg) every 1-2 d	50/200 to 200/2000 mg (3-8 tablets)	3 times/d or twice daily (for controlled release)
Entacapone (Comtan®)	COMT enzyme inhibitor	200 mg 3 times/d	Titrate down the doses of carbidopa/levodopa as required	600-1600 mg	3 times/d; up to 8 times/d
Levodopa/carbidopa/entacapone (Stalevo®)	Converts to dopamine; binds to all CNS dopamine receptors; COMT enzyme inhibitor	1 tablet 3-4 times/d (to replace previous dosing with individual agents)	As tolerated based on response and presence of dyskinesias	3-8 tablets per day	3-4 times/d
Pramipexole (Mirapex®)	High affinity for D_2 and D_3 dopamine receptors	0.125 mg 3 times/d	0.125 mg/dose every 5-7 d	1.5-4.5 mg	3 times/d
Rasagiline (Azilect®)	Inhibits MAO-B	0.5-1 mg once daily	≤1 mg daily	0.5-1 mg	Once daily
Ropinirole (Requip®)	High affinity for D_2 and D_3 dopamine receptors	0.25 mg 3 times/d	0.25 mg/dose weekly for 4 wk, then 1.5 mg/d every week up to 9 mg/d; 3 mg/d up to a max of 24 mg/d	0.75-24 mg	3 times/d
Selegiline (Eldepryl®)	Inhibits MAO-B	5-10 mg twice daily	Titrate down the doses of carbidopa/levodopa as required	5-10 mg	Twice daily
Tolcapone (Tasmar®)	COMT enzyme inhibitor	100 mg 3 times/d	Titrate down the doses of carbidopa/levodopa as required	300-600 mg	3 times/d
Anticholinergic Agents					
Benztropine (Cogentin®)	Blocks cholinergic receptors, also has antihistamine effects	0.5-2 mg/d in 1-4 divided doses	0.5 mg/dose every 5-6 d	2-6 mg	1-2 times/d
Procyclidine (Kemadrin®)	Blocks cholinergic receptors	2.5 mg 3 times/d	Gradually as tolerated	7.5-20 mg	3 times/d
Trihexyphenidyl (Artane)	Blocks cholinergic receptors; also some direct effects	1-2 mg/d	2 mg/d at intervals of 3-5 d	5-15 mg	3-4 times/d

[1]The medications listed in the table represent treatment options for both idiopathic Parkinson's disease, as well as Parkinsonian symptoms resulting from other drug therapy.

[2]Cabergoline is not FDA-approved for the treatment of Parkinson's disease.

ANTIPSYCHOTIC AGENTS

Antipsychotic Agent	Dosage Forms	I.M./P.O. Potency	Equiv. Dosages (approx) (mg/d)	Usual Adult Daily Maint. Dose (mg)	Sedation (Incidence)	Extrapyramidal Side Effects	Anticholinergic Side Effects	Orthostatic Hypotension	Comments
ARIPiprazole (Abilify®)	Solution; tablet; tablet, orally disintegrating; injection		7.5	10-30	Low	Low	Very low	Very low	Low weight gain; activating
Asenapine (Saphris®)	Tablet, sublingual			10-20	Moderate	Low	Very low	Low/moderate	Low weight gain; activating
ChlorproMAZINE	Injection; tablet	4:1	100	200-1000	High	Moderate	Moderate	Moderate/high	
CloZAPine (Clozaril®, FazaClo®)	Tablet; tablet, orally disintegrating		100	75-900	High	Very low	High	High	~1% incidence of agranulocytosis; weekly-biweekly CBC required; potential for weight gain, lipid abnormalities, and diabetes
FluPHENAZine	Solution, concentrate; injection; tablet	2:1	2	0.5-20	Low	High	Low	Low	
	Injection, long-acting			12.5-25*					
Haloperidol (Haldol®)	Solution, concentrate; injection; tablet	2:1	2	0.5-20	Low	High	Low	Low	
(Haldol® Decanoate)	Injection, long-acting			50-200*					
Iloperidone (Fanapt™)	Tablet			12-24	Low	Low	Very low	Low/moderate	
Loxapine (Loxitane®)	Capsule		10	25-250	Moderate	Moderate	Low	Low	
Lurasidone (Latuda®)	Tablet			40-80	Moderate	Low/Moderate	Low	Low	Contraindicated with strong CYP3A4 inducers and inhibitors. Take with food.
OLANZapine (ZyPREXA®)	Injection; tablet; tablet, orally disintegrating		5	5-20	Moderate/ high	Low	Moderate	Moderate	Potential for weight gain, lipid abnormalities, diabetes
(ZyPREXA® Relprew™)	Injection, long-acting			210-405*					
Paliperidone (Invega®)	Tablet, extended release			3-12	Low/ moderate	Low	Very low	Moderate	Active metabolite of risperidone
(Invega® Sustenna®)	Injection, long-acting			39-234*					
Perphenazine	Tablet		10	16-64	Low	Moderate	Low	Low	
Pimozide (Orap®)	Tablet		2	1-10	Moderate	High	Moderate	Low	Contraindicated with CYP3A inhibitors

continued

Antipsychotic Agent	Dosage Forms	I.M./P.O. Potency	Equiv. Dosages (approx) (mg/d)	Usual Adult Daily Maint. Dose (mg)	Sedation (Incidence)	Extrapyramidal Side Effects	Anticholinergic Side Effects	Orthostatic Hypotension	Comments
QUEtiapine (SEROquel®, SEROquel XR®)	Tablet; tablet, extended release		75	50-800	Moderate/ high	Very low	Moderate	Moderate	Moderate weight gain; potential for lipid abnormalities; diabetes
RisperiDONE (RisperDAL®)	Solution; tablet; tablet, orally disintegrating		2	0.5-6	Low/ moderate	Low	Very low	Moderate	Low to moderate weight gain; potential for diabetes
(RisperDAL® Consta®)	Injection, long-acting			25-50*					
Thioridazine	Tablet		100	200-800	High	Low	High	Moderate/high	May cause irreversible retinitis pigmentosa at doses >800 mg/d; prolongs QTc; use only in treatment of refractory illness
Thiothixene (Navane®)	Capsule	4:1	4	5-40	Low	High	Low	Low/moderate	
Trifluoperazine	Tablet		5	2-40	Low	High	Low	Low	
Ziprasidone (Geodon®)	Capsule; injection, powder	2:1	60	40-160	Low/ moderate	Low	Very low	Low/moderate	Low weight gain; contraindicated with QTc-prolonging agents. Take with food.

*Administered every 2 or 4 weeks; consult drug monograph for specific dosage details

REFERENCE Woods SW, "Chlorpromazine Equivalent Doses for the Newer Atypical Antipsychotics," *J Clin Psychiatry*, 2003, 64(6):663-7.

BENZODIAZEPINES

Agent	FDA-Approved Indication	Dosage Forms	Relative Potency (mg)	Peak Blood Levels (oral) (h)	Protein Binding (%)	Volume of Distribution (L/kg)	Major Active Metabolite	Onset	Metabolism	Half-Life (parent) (h)	Half-Life[1] (metabolite) (h)	Elimination	Usual Initial Oral Dose	Adult Oral Dosage Range
Anxiolytic														
ALPRAZolam (Xanax XR®; Xanax®)	Anxiety, anxiety associated with depression, panic disorder treatment	Sol, tab	0.5	IR: 1-2 XR: 9	80	0.9-1.2	No	Intermediate	Hepatic via CYP3A4	12-15	—	Urine	0.25-0.5 tid	0.75-4 mg/d
ChlordiazePOXIDE (Librium®)	Anxiety, EtOH withdrawal	Cap	10	2-4	90-98	0.3	Yes	Intermediate	Hepatic via CYP3A4	5-30	24-96	Urine	5-25 mg tid-qid	15-100 mg/d
Diazepam (Diastat®, Valium®)	Anxiety, EtOH withdrawal, adjunct to anesthesia (I.V.), anxiety/amnesiac during cardioversion (I.V.), anxiety/amnesia in endoscopic procedures, convulsions/status epilepticus (I.V.), adjunct in epilepsy (rectal gel), skeletal muscle spasms	Gel, inj, sol, tab	5	0.5-2	98	1.1	Yes	Rapid	Hepatic via 2C19 and 3A4	20-80	50-100	Urine	2-10 mg bid-qid	4-40 mg/d
LORazepam (Ativan®)[2]	Anxiety, anxiety associated with depression, adjunct to anesthesia (I.V.), convulsions/status epilepticus (I.V.)	Inj, sol, tab	1	1-6	88-92	1.3	No	Intermediate	Hepatic	10-20	—	Urine and feces (minimal)	0.5-2 mg tid-qid	2-4 mg/d
Oxazepam (Serax®)	Anxiety, anxiety associated with depression, EtOH withdrawal	Cap, tab	15-30	2-4	86-99	0.6-2	No	Slow	Hepatic via glucoronide conjugation	5-20	—	Urine as unchanged (50%) and glucoronide	10-30 mg tid-qid	30-120 mg/d
Sedative/Hypnotic														
Estazolam	Insomnia	Tab	0.3	2	93	—	No	Slow	Hepatic via CYP3A4	10-24	—	Urine	1 mg qhs	1-2 mg
Flurazepam (Dalmane®)	Insomnia	Cap	5	0.5-2	97	—	Yes	Rapid	Hepatic via CYP3A4	Not significant	40-114	Urine	15 mg qhs	15-60 mg
Quazepam (Doral®)	Insomnia	Tab	5	2	95	5	Yes	Intermediate	Hepatic via CYP3A4	25-41	28-114	Urine	15 mg qhs	7.5-15 mg
Temazepam (Restoril™)	Insomnia	Cap	5	2-3	96	1.4	No	Slow	Hepatic via CYP2B6, 2C8/9, 2C19, 3A4	10-40	—	Urine as inactive metabolites	15-30 mg qhs	15-30 mg
Triazolam (Halcion®)	Insomnia	Tab	0.1	1	89-94	0.8-1.3	No	Intermediate	Hepatic via CYP3A4	2.3	—	Urine as unchanged drug and metabolites	0.125-0.25 qhs	0.125-0.25 mg

continued

Agent	FDA-Approved Indication	Dosage Forms	Relative Potency (mg)	Peak Blood Levels (oral) (h)	Protein Binding (%)	Volume of Distribution (L/kg)	Major Active Metabolite	Onset	Metabolism	Half-Life (parent) (h)	Half-Life[1] (metabolite) (h)	Elimination	Usual Initial Oral Dose	Adult Oral Dosage Range
Miscellaneous														
Clobazam	Adjunct in Lennox-Gastaut syndrome	Tab	NA	0.5-4	80-90	—	Yes	NA	Hepatic via CYP3A4, 2C19, 2B6	36-42	71-82	Urine, primarily as metabolites	5 mg daily-bid	5-40 mg/d
ClonazePAM (Klonopin®)	Adjunct in Lennox-Gastuat syndrome, akinetic seizures, myoclonic seizures, adjunct in absence seizures, panic disorder treatment	Tab	0.25-0.5	1-2	86	1.8-4	No	Intermediate	Hepatic via glucoronide and sulfate conjugation	18-50	—	Urine as glucoronide or sulfate conjugate	0.5 mg tid	1.5-20 mg/d
Clorazepate (Tranxene® T-Tab®)	Anxiety, EtOH withdrawal, adjunct in partial seizures	Cap, tab	7.5	1-2	80-95	—	Yes	Rapid	Decarboxylated in acidic stomach prior to absorption and hepatic via CYP3A4	Not significant	50-100	Urine	7.5-15 mg bid-qid	15-60 mg
Midazolam	Adjunct to anesthesia, anxiety/amnesiac during cardioversion, anxiety/ amnesia in endoscopic procedures	Inj	NA	0.4-0.7[3]	95	0.8-6.6	Yes	Rapid	Hepatic via CYP3A4	2-5 h	12 h	Urine	NA	NA

IR = immediate release, XR = extended release, NA = not available

Rapid = 15 minutes or less, intermediate = 15-30 minutes, slow = 30-60 minutes

[1]Significant metabolite

[2]Reliable bioavailability when given I.M.

[3]I.V. only

BETA-BLOCKERS

Agent	Adrenergic Receptor Blocking Activity	Intrinsic Sympathomimetic Activity (ISA)	Lipid Solubility	Protein Bound (%)	Half-Life (h)	Bioavailability (%)	Primary Site of Metabolism	Primary (Secondary) Route of Elimination	Indications	Usual Dosage
Acebutolol (Sectral®)	beta$_1$	Yes	Low	15-25	3-4	40 7-fold[1]	Hepatic	Feces (renal)	Hypertension, arrhythmias	P.O.: 400-1200 mg/d
Atenolol (Tenormin®)	beta$_1$	No	Low	<5-10	6-9	50-60 4-fold[1]	Hepatic (limited)	Feces (renal)	Hypertension, angina pectoris, acute MI	P.O.: 50-200 mg/d I.V.: Acute MI: 5 mg x 2 doses
Betaxolol (Kerlone®)	beta$_1$	No	Low	50-55	14-22	84-94	Hepatic	Renal	Hypertension	P.O.: 5-20 mg/d
Bisoprolol (Zebeta®)	beta$_1$	No	Low	26-33	9-12	80	Hepatic	Renal	Hypertension, heart failure	P.O.: HF: 2.5-10 mg/d HTN: 2.5-20 mg/d
Carvedilol (Coreg®, Coreg CR®)	alpha$_1$ beta$_1$ beta$_2$	No	ND	98	7-10	25-35	Hepatic	Feces	Hypertension, heart failure (mild to severe)	P.O.: 3.125-25 mg twice daily
Esmolol (Brevibloc)	beta$_1$	No	Low	55	0.15	NA 5-fold[1]	Red blood cell esterase	Renal	Supraventricular tachycardia, sinus tachycardia, atrial fibrillation/flutter, hypertension	I.V. infusion: 25-300 mcg/kg/min
Labetalol (Trandate®)	alpha$_1$ beta$_1$ beta$_2$	No	Moderate	50	5.5-8	18-30 10-fold[1]	Hepatic	Renal	Hypertension	P.O.: 200-2400 mg/d I.V.: 20-80 mg at 10-min intervals up to a maximum of 300 mg **or** continuous infusion of 2-6 mg/min
Metoprolol (Lopressor®, Toprol-XL®)	beta$_1$	No	Moderate	10-12	3-7	50 7- to 10-fold[1] (Toprol XL®: 77)	Hepatic	Renal	Hypertension, angina pectoris, acute MI, heart failure (mild to moderate; XL formulation only), atrial tachyarrhythmias (rate control)	P.O.: 100-450 mg/d HF: (Toprol-XL®): 12.5-200 mg/d I.V.: Acute MI: 5 mg q2 min x 3 doses AF (rate control): 2.5-5 mg q2-5 min (max total dose: 15 mg over 0-15 min)
Nadolol (Corgard®)	beta$_1$ beta$_2$	No	Low	25-30	20-24	30 5- to 8-fold[1]	None	Renal	Hypertension, angina pectoris	P.O.: 40-320 mg/d
Nebivolol (Bystolic®)	beta$_1$	No	High	98	10-32	12-96	Hepatic	Renal (feces)	Hypertension	P.O.: 5-40 mg/d
Penbutolol (Levatol®)	beta$_1$ beta$_2$	Yes	High	80-98	5	~100	Hepatic	Renal	Hypertension	P.O.: 20-80 mg/d
Pindolol	beta$_1$ beta$_2$	Yes	Moderate	57	3-4	90 2- to 2.5-fold[1]	Hepatic	Renal (feces)	Hypertension	P.O.: 20-60 mg/d

continued

Agent	Adrenergic Receptor Blocking Activity	Intrinsic Sympathomimetic Activity (ISA)	Lipid Solubility	Protein Bound (%)	Half-Life (h)	Bioavailability (%)	Primary Site of Metabolism	Primary (Secondary) Route of Elimination	Indications	Usual Dosage
Propranolol (Inderal®, various)	$beta_1$ $beta_2$	No	High	90	3-5	25 2- to 3-fold[1]	Hepatic	Renal	Hypertension, angina pectoris, arrhythmias, prophylaxis (post-MI)	P.O.: 40-480 mg/d I.V.: Tachyarrhythmias: 1-3 mg q2-5 min (max: 5 mg)
Propranolol long-acting (Inderal-LA®, InnoPran XL™)	$beta_1$ $beta_2$	No	High	90	9-18	25 2- to 3-fold[1]	Hepatic	Renal	Hypertrophic cardiomyopathy with outflow tract obstruction, prophylaxis (post-MI)	P.O.: 180-240 mg/d
Sotalol (Betapace®, Betapace AF®, Sorine®)	$beta_1$ $beta_2$	No	Low	0	12	90-100	None	Renal	Atrial and ventricular tachyarrhythmias	P.O. 160-320 mg/d
Timolol (Blocadren®)	$beta_1$ $beta_2$	No	Low to moderate	<10	4	75 7-fold[1]	Hepatic	Renal	Hypertension, prophylaxis (post-MI)	P.O.: 20-60 mg/d

Dosage is based on 70 kg adult with normal hepatic and renal function.

Note: All $beta_1$-selective agents will inhibit $beta_2$ receptors at higher doses.

[1]Interpatient variations in plasma levels.

BRONCHODILATORS

Comparison of Inhaled Sympathomimetic Bronchodilators

Drug	Adrenergic Receptor	Onset (min)	Duration Activity (h)
Albuterol (Proventil®)	$Beta_1$ < $Beta_2$	<5	3-8
Arformoterol (Brovana®)	$Beta_1$ < $Beta_2$	7-20	
EPINEPHrine (various)	Alpha and $Beta_1$ and $Beta_2$	1-5	1-3
Formoterol (Foradil®)	$Beta_1$ < $Beta_2$	3-5	12
Indacaterol (Arcapta™)	$Beta_1$ < $Beta_2$	5	24
Isoproterenol (Isuprel®)	$Beta_1$ and $Beta_2$	2-5	0.5-2
Levalbuterol (Xopenex®)	$Beta_1$ < $Beta_2$	10-17	5-6
Pirbuterol (Maxair® Autohaler®)	$Beta_1$ < $Beta_2$	<5	5
Salmeterol (Diskus®, Serevent®)	$Beta_1$ < $Beta_2$	5-14	12
Terbutaline	$Beta_1$ < $Beta_2$	5-30	3-6

CALCIUM CHANNEL BLOCKERS

Comparative Pharmacokinetics

Agent	Bioavailability (%)	Protein Binding (%)	Onset of BP Effect (min)	Duration of BP Effect (h)	Half-Life (h)	Volume of Distribution	Route of Metabolism	Route of Excretion
Dihydropyridines								
AmLODIPine (Norvasc®)	64-90	93-98	30-50	24	30-50	21 L/kg	Hepatic; inactive metabolites	Urine; 10% as parent
Clevidipine (Cleviprex™)		>99.5	2-4	5-15 min	1-15 min	0.17 L/kg	Blood and extravascular tissue esterases	Urine (63% to 74%; as metabolites); feces (7% to 22%)
Felodipine (Plendil)	20	>99	2-5 h	24	11-16	10 L/kg	Hepatic; CYP3A4 substrate (major); inactive metabolites; extensive first pass	Urine (70%; as metabolites); feces 10%
Isradipine (DynaCirc CR®)	15-24	95	20	>12	8	3 L/kg	Hepatic; CYP3A4 substrate (major); inactive metabolites; extensive first pass	Urine as metabolites
NiCARdipine (Cardene®)	35	>95	30	≤8	2-4		Hepatic; CYP3A4 substrate (major); saturable first pass	Urine (60%; as metabolites); feces 35%
NIFEdipine (Procardia®)	40-77	92-98	Within 20		2-5		Hepatic; CYP3A4 substrate (major); inactive metabolites	Urine as metabolites
NiMODipine (Nimotop®)	13	>95	ND	4-6	1-2		Hepatic; CYP3A4 substrate (major); metabolites inactive or less active than parent; extensive first pass	Urine (50%; as metabolites); feces 32%
Nisoldipine (Sular®)	5	>99	ND	6-12	7-12		Hepatic; CYP3A4 substrate (major); 1 active metabolite (10% of parent); extensive first pass	Urine as metabolites
Phenylalkylamines								
Verapamil (Calan®, Verelan®)	20-35	90	30	6-8	4.5-12		Hepatic; CYP3A4 substrate (major); 1 active metabolite (20% of parent); extensive first pass	Urine (70%; 3% to 4% as unchanged drug); feces 16%
Benzothiazepines								
Diltiazem (Cardizem®)	~40	70-80	30-60	6-8	3-4.5	3-13 L/kg	Hepatic; CYP3A4 substrate (major); 1 major metabolite (20%-50% of parent); extensive first pass	Urine as metabolites

CORTICOSTEROIDS

Corticosteroids, Systemic Equivalencies

Glucocorticoid	Approximate Equivalent Dose (mg)	Routes of Administration	Relative Anti-inflammatory Potency	Relative Mineralocorticoid Potency	Protein Binding (%)	Half-life Plasma (min)
Short-Acting						
Cortisone	25	P.O., I.M.	0.8	0.8	90	30
Hydrocortisone	20	I.M., I.V.	1	1	90	90
Intermediate-Acting						
MethylPREDNISolone[1]	4	P.O., I.M., I.V.	5	0	—	180
PrednisoLONE	5	P.O., I.M., I.V., intra-articular, intradermal, soft tissue injection	4	0.8	90-95	200
PredniSONE	5	P.O.	4	0.8	70	60
Triamcinolone[1]	4	I.M., intra-articular, intradermal, intrasynovial, soft tissue injection	5	0	—	300
Long-Acting						
Betamethasone	0.75	P.O., I.M., intra-articular, intradermal, intrasynovial, soft tissue injection	25	0	64	100-300
Dexamethasone	0.75	P.O., I.M., I.V., intra-articular, intradermal, soft tissue injection	25-30	0	—	100-300
Mineralocorticoids						
Fludrocortisone	—	P.O.	10	125	42	200

[1]May contain propylene glycol as an excipient in injectable forms

Asare K, "Diagnosis and Treatment of Adrenal Insufficiency in the Critically Ill Patient," *Pharmacotherapy*, 2007, 27(11):1512-28.

GUIDELINES FOR SELECTION AND USE OF TOPICAL CORTICOSTEROIDS

The quantity prescribed and the frequency of refills should be monitored to reduce the risk of adrenal suppression. In general, short courses of high-potency agents are preferable to prolonged use of low potency. After control is achieved, control should be maintained with a low potency preparation.

1. Low-to-medium potency agents are usually effective for treating thin, acute, inflammatory skin lesions; whereas, high or super-potent agents are often required for treating chronic, hyperkeratotic, or lichenified lesions.
2. Since the stratum corneum is thin on the face and intertriginous areas, low-potency agents are preferred but a higher potency agent may be used for 2 weeks.
3. Because the palms and soles have a thick stratum corneum, high or super-potent agents are frequently required.
4. Low potency agents are preferred for infants and the elderly. Infants have a high body surface area to weight ratio; elderly patients have thin, fragile skin.
5. The vehicle in which the topical corticosteroid is formulated influences the absorption and potency of the drug. Ointment bases are preferred for thick, lichenified lesions; they enhance penetration of the drug. Creams are preferred for acute and subacute dermatoses; they may be used on moist skin areas or intertriginous areas. Solutions, gels, and sprays are preferred for the scalp or for areas where a nonoil-based vehicle is needed.
6. In general, super-potent agents should not be used for longer than 2-3 weeks unless the lesion is limited to a small body area. Medium-to-high potency agents usually cause only rare adverse effects when treatment is limited to 3 months or less, and use on the face and intertriginous areas are avoided. If long-term treatment is needed, intermittent vs continued treatment is recommended.
7. Most preparations are applied once or twice daily. More frequent application may be necessary for the palms or soles because the preparation is easily removed by normal activity and penetration is poor due to a thick stratum corneum. Every-other-day or weekend-only application may be effective for treating some chronic conditions.

Corticosteroids, Topical

Steroid		Dosage Form
	Very High Potency	
0.05%	Betamethasone dipropionate, augmented	Cream, gel, lotion, ointment
0.05%	Clobetasol propionate	Cream, foam, gel, lotion, ointment, shampoo, spray
0.05%	Diflorasone diacetate	Ointment
0.05%	Halobetasol propionate	Cream, ointment
	High Potency	
0.1%	Amcinonide	Cream, ointment, lotion
0.05%	Betamethasone dipropionate, augmented	Cream
0.05%	Betamethasone dipropionate	Cream, ointment
0.1%	Betamethasone valerate	Ointment
0.05%	Desoximetasone	Gel
0.25%	Desoximetasone	Cream, ointment
0.05%	Diflorasone diacetate	Cream, ointment
0.05%	Fluocinonide	Cream, ointment, gel
0.1%	Halcinonide	Cream, ointment
0.5%	Triamcinolone acetonide	Cream, spray
	Intermediate Potency	
0.05%	Betamethasone dipropionate	Lotion
0.1%	Betamethasone valerate	Cream
0.1%	Clocortolone pivalate	Cream
0.05%	Desoximetasone	Cream
0.025%	Fluocinolone acetonide	Cream, ointment
0.05%	Flurandrenolide	Cream, ointment, lotion, tape
0.005%	Fluticasone propionate	Ointment
0.05%	Fluticasone propionate	Cream, lotion
0.1%	Hydrocortisone butyrate[1]	Ointment, solution
0.2%	Hydrocortisone valerate[1]	Cream, ointment
0.1%	Mometasone furoate[1]	Cream, ointment, lotion
0.1%	Prednicarbate	Cream, ointment
0.025%	Triamcinolone acetonide	Cream, ointment, lotion
0.1%	Triamcinolone acetonide	Cream, ointment, lotion

Corticosteroids, Topical *(continued)*

Steroid		Dosage Form
Low Potency		
0.05%	Alclometasone dipropionate[1]	Cream, ointment
0.05%	Desonide	Cream, ointment
0.01%	Fluocinolone acetonide	Cream, solution
0.5%	Hydrocortisone[1]	Cream, ointment, lotion
0.5%	Hydrocortisone acetate[1]	Cream, ointment
1%	Hydrocortisone acetate[1]	Cream, ointment
1%	Hydrocortisone[1]	Cream, ointment, lotion, solution
2.5%	Hydrocortisone[1]	Cream, ointment, lotion

[1]Not fluorinated

IMMUNE GLOBULIN PRODUCTS

Characteristics of Immune Globulin Products Currently Licensed for Use in the United States

Brand name[1]	Gammagard S/D 5%	Gammagard S/D 10%	Gammagard Liquid	Gammaplex	Carimune NF	Hizentra	Privigen	Vivaglobin[2]	Flebogamma DIF 5%	Flebogamma DIF 10%	Octagam	Gamunex - C
Manufacturer	Baxter Corporation/ BioScience Division		Baxter Corporation/ BioScience Division	Bio Products Laboratory	CSL Behring	CSL Behring	CSL Behring	CSL Behring	Grifols		Octapharma	Talecris
Method of Production (Including Viral Inactivation)	Cohn-Oncley fractionation, ultra-filtration, ion-exchange chromatography, solvent detergent treatment		Cohn-Oncley fractionation, ion-exchange chromatography solvent/detergent treatment, 35 nm nanofiltration, low pH/ elevated temperature incubation	Kistler & Nitschmann fractionation, DEAE-Sephadex chromatography, solvent/detergent, CM-Sepharose chromatography, virus filtration (20 nm) terminal low pH incubation (30°C, 2 weeks)	Kistler Nitschmann fractionation, pH 4.0, trace pepsin, nanofiltration	Cold alcohol fractionation, octanoic acid fractionation, anion exchange chromatography; pH 4 incubation, depth filtration, nanofiltration; TSE reduction steps include octanoic acid fractionation, depth filtration, and virus filtration	Octanoic acid fractionation, CH9 filtration, pH 4.0 incubation, depth filtration, chromatography, nanofiltration	Cold alcohol fractionation, ethanol-fatty alcohol/pH precipitation, pasteurization, diafiltered and ultrafiltered	Cold alcohol fractionation, polyethylene glycol precipitation, ion exchange chromatography, pH 4 treatment (4 h at 37°C), pasteurization (60°C for 10 h), solvent detergent treatment, and double sequential nanofiltration through 35 nm and 20 nm filters		Cohn-Oncley cold ethanol fractionation, ultra-filtration, chromatography, solvent detergent treatment	Cohn-Oncley fractionation, caprylate/ chromatography purification, cloth and depth filtration, final container low pH incubation
Form	Lyophilized		Liquid	Liquid	Lyophilized	Liquid	Liquid	Liquid	Liquid		Liquid	Liquid
Shelf-Life/Storage Requirements	24 months (room temperature)		36 months (refrigerated); 12 months (room temperature)	24 months (room temperature)	24 months	30 months (room temperature)	36 months (room temperature)	24 months	24 months (room temperature)		24 months	36 months
Reconstitution Time	N/A		None	None	Several minutes	None	None	None	None		None	None
Available Concentrations	5%	10%	10%	5%	3% to 12%	20% (200 mg/mL)	10%	16% (160 mg protein/mL)	5%	10%	5%	10%
Maximum Recommended Infusion Rate	4 mL/kg/h	8 mL/kg/h	5 mL/kg/h (I.V.) <40 kg: 20 mL/h/site; ≥40 kg: 30 mL/h/site with a maximum of 8 sites (SubQ)	4.8 mL/kg/h	>2.5 mL/kg/h	Up to 25 mL/h/injection site (50 mL/h for all sites combined)	4.8 mL/kg/h	20 mL/h	6.0 mL/kg/h	4.8 mL/kg/h	<4.2 mL/kg/h	4.8 mL/kg/h (I.V.) 20 mL/h (SubQ)
Time to Infuse[3] 35 g	Time will vary depending on concentration and tolerability		Time will vary depending on tolerability and route of administration	125 min or 2:05 h	<3.3 h (6% solution)	Time will vary depending on volume and tolerability	63 min	Time will vary depending on volume and tolerability[4]	1.6 h	1 h	2.5 h	Time will vary depending on route of administration
Sugar Content	20 mg/mL glucose	40 mg/mL glucose	No added sugars	5% D-sorbitol (polyol)	1.67 g sucrose/g of protein	None	None	None	None		100 mg/mL maltose	None
Sodium Content	8.5 mg/mL sodium chloride	17 mg/mL sodium chloride	No added sodium	30-50 mmol/L	<20 mg sodium chloride/g of protein	Trace amounts (≤10 mmol/L)	Trace amounts	3 mg/mL	Trace amounts		≤30 mmol/L	Trace amounts
Osmolarity/ Osmolality	636 mOsm/kg	1250 mOsm/L	240-300 mOsm/kg	460-500 mOsm/kg	192-1074 mOsm/kg	380 mOsmol/kg	Isotonic (320 mOsmol/kg)	445 mOsm/kg	240-370 mOsm/kg		310-380 mOsm/kg	258 mOsm/kg

Characteristics of Immune Globulin Products Currently Licensed for Use in the United States *continued*

Brand name[1]	Gammagard S/D		Gammagard Liquid		Gammaplex	Carimune NF	Hizentra	Privigen	Vivaglobin[2]	Flebogamma DIF		Octagam	Gamunex - C	
	5%	10%								5%	10%			
pH	6.8 ± 0.4		4.6-5.1		4.6-5.1	6.4-6.8	4.6-5.2	4.8	6.4-7.2	5-6		5.1-6	4-4.5	
IgA Content	<1 µg/mL <2.2 µg/mL		37 µg/mL		Average: <4 mcg/mL (specification value: <10 mcg/mL)	720 µg/mL	≤50 mcg/mL	≤25 mcg/mL	<1700 µg/mL	Average: <3 mcg/mL (specification value: <50 mcg/mL)	Average: <6 mcg/mL (specification value: <100 mcg/mL)	<100 µg/mL	46 µg/mL	
Approved Method of Administration	I.V.		I.V.	SubQ	I.V.	I.V.	SubQ	I.V.	SubQ	I.V.		I.V.	I.V.	SubQ

[1]GamaSTAN™ S/D information not provided by Immune Deficiency Foundation due to limited I.V. use in the United States. Characteristics of GamaSTAN™ S/D may be found at http://www.gamastan.com

[2]No longer sold in the United States

[3]0.5 g/kg for a 70 kg adult = 35 g; 5% concentrations: 1 g = 20 mL; 10% concentrations: 1 g = 10 mL

[4]Using 35 g as monthly dose, calculate weekly dose = 8.75 g = 55 mL, infused into 4 sites at rate of up to 20 cc/hour/site, which can range from 45 minutes to 3 hours

The time to infuse is based on the maximal infusion rate. Check product label for storage temperatures, which vary among immunoglobulin brands. Check package insert for detailed prescribing information. Information for each of the products listed above has been provided directly to the Immune Deficiency Foundation by the manufacturer of that product.

Adapted from Immune Deficiency Foundation. Available at http://www.primaryimmune.org. Accessed August 2011.

LAXATIVES, CLASSIFICATION AND PROPERTIES

Laxative	Onset of Action	Site of Action	Mechanism of Action
Saline			
Magnesium citrate Magnesium hydroxide (Phillips'® Milk of Magnesia)	30 min to 3 h	Small and large intestine	Attract/retain water in intestinal lumen increasing intraluminal pressure; cholecystokinin release
Sodium phosphates (Fleet® Enema)	2-15 min	Colon	
Irritant/Stimulant			
Senna (Senokot®)	6-10 h	Colon	Direct action on intestinal mucosa; stimulate myenteric plexus; alter water and electrolyte secretion
Bisacodyl (Dulcolax®) tablets, suppositories	15 min to 1 h	Colon	
Castor oil	2-6 h	Small intestine	
Bulk-Producing			
Methylcellulose (Citrucel®) Psyllium (Metamucil®) Wheat dextrin (Benefiber®)	12-24 h (up to 72 h) 24-48 h	Small and large intestine	Holds water in stool; mechanical distention
Lubricant			
Mineral oil	6-8 h	Colon	Lubricates intestine; retards colonic absorption of fecal water; softens stool
Surfactants/Stool Softener			
Docusate/senna (Peri-Colace®)	8-12 h	Small and large intestine	Senna – mild irritant; docusate – stool softener
Docusate sodium (Colace®) Docusate calcium (Surfak®)	24-72 h	Small and large intestine	Detergent activity; facilitates admixture of fat and water to soften stool
Osmotic Laxatives			
Glycerin suppository	15-30 min	Colon	Local irritation; hyperosmotic action
Lactulose	24-48 h	Colon	Delivers osmotically active molecules to colon
Polyethylene glycol 3350 (GlycoLax™, MiraLax™)	48 h	Small and large intestine	Nonabsorbable solution which acts as an osmotic agent
Sodium sulfate, potassium sulfate, and magnesium sulfate (Suprep®)	24 h	Small and large intestine	Hyperosmotic action
Sorbitol 70%	24-48 h	Colon	Delivers osmotically active molecules to colon
Miscellaneous Laxatives			
Lubiprostone (Amitiza®)	24-48 h	Apical membrane of the GI epithelium	Activates intestinal chloride channels increasing intestinal fluid

NICOTINE PRODUCTS

Dosage Form	Brand Name	Dosing	Recommended Treatment Duration	Strengths Available
Lozenge	Commit™ (OTC)	Patients who smoke their first cigarette within 30 minutes of waking should use the 4 mg strength; otherwise the 2 mg strength is recommended. 1-6 wk: One lozenge q1-2h 7-9 wk: One lozenge q2-4h 10-12 wk: One lozenge q4-8h	~12 wk	2 mg, 4 mg
Chewing gum	Nicorette® (OTC)	Chew 1 piece q1-2h for 6 wk, then decrease to 1 piece q2-4h for 3 wk, then 1 piece q4-8h for 3 wk, then discontinue.	~12 wk	2 mg, 4 mg
Transdermal	Nicoderm CQ® (OTC)	One 21 mg/d patch qd for 6 wk, then one 14 mg/d patch qd for 2 wk, then one 7 mg/d patch qd for 2 wk, then discontinue. Low-dose regimen[1]: One 14 mg/d patch qd for 6 wk, then one 7 mg/d patch qd for 2 wk, then discontinue.	~10 wk	Patch: 21 mg/d 14 mg/d 7 mg/d
	Nicotrol®	One 15 mg patch qd, worn for 16 h/d and removed for 8 h/d for a total of 6 wk, then discontinue.	~6 wk	Patch: 15 mg/16 h 10 mg/16 h 5 mg/16 h
Nasal spray	Nicotrol® NS	One dose is 2 sprays (1 spray in each nostril). Initial dose: 1-2 sprays q1h, should not exceed 10 sprays (5 doses)/h or 80 sprays (40 doses)/d.	~12 wk	10 mL spray 0.5/mg spray (200 actuations)
Inhaler	Nicotrol®	Inhaler releases 4 mg nicotine (the equivalent of 2 cigarettes smoked) for 20 min of active inhaler puffing. Usual dose: 6-16 cartridges/d for up to 12 wk, then reduce dose gradually over ensuing 12 wk, then discontinue.	~18-24 wk	10 mg/cartridge: releases 4 mg/ cartridge

[1]Transdermal low-dose regimens are intended for patients <100 lb, smoke <10 cigarettes/day, and/or have a history of cardiovascular disease.

NITRATES

Nitrates[1]	Route/Dosage Form	Onset (min)	Duration
Nitroglycerin	I.V. (continuous)	1-2	Tolerance begins in 7-8 h
	Sublingual	1-3	≥25 min
	Translingual spray	2	≥25 min
	Oral, sustained release	40-60	4-8 h
	Topical ointment	20-60	Up to 7 h
	Transdermal	40-60	8-12 h
Isosorbide dinitrate	Sublingual	2-5	1-2 h
	Oral	~60	Up to 8 h
	Oral, sustained release	~60	Up to 8 h
Isosorbide mononitrate	Oral	~60	5-12 h
	Oral, extended release	30-60	12-24 h

[1]Hemodynamic and antianginal tolerance often develops within 24-48 hours of continuous nitrate administration; allow an adequate nitrate-free interval of 8-12 hours.

Adapted from Gibbons RJ, Abrams J, Chatterjee K, et al, "ACC/AHA 2002 Guideline Update for the Management of Patients With Chronic Stable Angina – Summary Article: A Report of the American College of Cardiology/American Heart Association Task Force on Practice Guidelines (Committee on the Management of Patients With Chronic Stable Angina)," *Circulation*, 2003, 107(1):149-58.

OPIOID ANALGESICS

This table serves as a general guide to opioid conversion. Utilization of a direct conversion without a detailed patients and medication assessment is not recommended and may result in over- or underdosing. Chronic administration may alter pharmacokinetics and change parenteral:oral ratio.

Opioid Analgesics – Initial Oral Dosing Commonly Used for Severe Pain

Drug	Equianalgesic Dose (mg)		Initial Oral Dose	
	Oral[1]	Parenteral[2]	Children[3] (mg/kg)	Adults (mg)
Buprenorphine	—	0.4	—	—
Butorphanol	—	2	—	—
FentaNYL	—	0.1	—	—
HYDROmorphone	7.5	1.5	0.06	4-8
Levorphanol	Acute: 4 Chronic: 1	Acute: 2 Chronic: 1	0.04	2-4
Meperidine[4]	300	75	Not recommended	
Methadone[5]	See Guidelines for Conversion to Oral Methadone in Adults	Variable	0.2	5-10
Morphine	30	10	0.3	15-30
Nalbuphine	—	10	—	—
OxyCODONE	20	—	0.2	10-20
Oxymorphone	10	1	—	5-10
Pentazocine	50	30	—	—

Guidelines for Conversion to Oral Methadone in Adults[5]

Oral Morphine Dose or Equivalent (mg/day)	Oral Morphine:Oral Methadone (Conversion Ratio)
<90	4:1
90-300	8:1
>300	12:1

[1]Elderly: Starting dose should be lower for this population group.

[2]Standard parenteral doses (I.M.) for acute pain in adults; can be used to convert doses for I.V. infusions and repeated small I.V. boluses. For single I.V. boluses, use half the I.M. dose.

[3]The pharmacokinetics of opioids in children and infants >6 months old are similar to adults, but infants <6 months old, especially premature or physically compromised ones, are at risk of apnea.

[4]Not recommended for routine use

[5]Conversion of higher doses may be guided by the following (consult a pain or palliative care specialist if unfamiliar with methadone prescribing): As the total daily chronic dose of morphine increases, the equianalgesic dose ratio (morphine:methadone) changes (American Pain Society, 2008). Total daily dose should be divided by 3; delivered every 8 hours. Methadone is significantly more potent with repetitive dosing (due to its active metabolite). Begin methadone at lower doses and gradually titrate. Applicability to pediatric patients is unknown.

REFERENCES

National Cancer Institute, "Pain (PDQ®)," Last Modified 5/7/09. Available at http://www.cancer.gov/cancertopics/pdq/supportivecare/pain/HealthProfessional/page1

National Comprehensive Cancer Network® (NCCN), "Clinical Practice Guidelines in Oncology™: Adult Cancer Pain," Version 1, 2009. Available at http://www.nccn.org/professionals/physician_gls/PDF/pain.pdf

Patanwala AE, Duby J, Waters D, et al, "Opioid Conversions in Acute Care," *Ann Pharmacother*, 2007, 41(2):255-66.

Principles of Analgesic Use in the Treatment of Acute Pain and Cancer Pain, 6th ed, Glenview, IL: American Pain Society, 2008.

SELECTIVE SEROTONIN REUPTAKE INHIBITORS (SSRIS) PHARMACOKINETICS

SSRI	Half-Life (h)	Metabolite Half-Life	Peak Plasma Level (h)	% Protein Bound	Bioavailability (%)	Initial Dose
Citalopram (CeleXA®)	35	S-desmethyl-citalopram: 59 hours	4	80	80	20 mg qAM
Escitalopram (Lexapro®)	27-32	S-desmethyl-citalopram: 59 hours	5	56	80	10 mg qAM
FLUoxetine (PROzac®, PROzac® Weekly™, Sarafem®, Selfemra®)	Initial: 24-72 Chronic: 96-144	Norfluoxetine: 4-16 days	6-8	95	72	10-20 mg qAM
FluvoxaMINE (Luvox® CR)	16	N/A	3	80	53	50 mg qhs
PARoxetine (Paxil®, Paxil CR®, Pexeva®)	21	N/A	5	95	>90	10-20 mg qAM
Sertraline (Zoloft®)	26	N-desmethyl-sertraline: 62-104 hours	5-8	98	88	25-50 qAM

VASOACTIVE AGENTS, INTRAVENOUS

Drug	Dose	Hemodynamic Effects				
		HR	MAP	PAOP	CI	SVR
DOPamine	1-3 mcg/kg/min	↑	0	↓	0/↑	0/↓
	3-10 mcg/kg/min	↑	↑	0	↑	0
	>10-20 mcg/kg/min	↑↑	↑↑	0	↑	↑
EPINEPHrine	0.01-0.05 mcg/kg/min	↑	↑	0/↓	↑↑	0/↓
	>0.05 mcg/kg/min	↑↑	↑↑	↑	↑↑	↑↑
Norepinephrine	0.02-3 mcg/kg/min	0/↑	↑↑↑	↑↑	0/↓/↑	↑↑↑
Phenylephrine	0.5-9 mcg/kg/min	0/↓	↑	↑	0/↓/↑	↑↑↑
Vasopressin	0.04 units/min	0/↓	↑↑	↑	0/↓	↑↑
DOBUTamine	2-10 mcg/kg/min	0/↑	↑	↓	↑	0/↓
	>10-20 mcg/kg/min	↑↑	↓/↑	↓	↑↑	↓
Milrinone	0.375-0.75 mcg/kg/min	↑↑	0/↓/↑	↓	↑	↓↓
Nesiritide	2 mcg/kg bolus 0.01-0.03 mcg/kg/min	0	↓	↓	0/↑	↓
Nitroglycerin	0.1-2 mcg/kg/min	0/↑	0/↓	↓	0/↑	↓
Nitroprusside	0.25-10 mcg/kg/min	0/↑↑	0/↓↓	↓	↑/↑↑	↓/↓↓

HR = heart rate, MAP = mean arterial pressure, PAOP = pulmonary artery occlusion pressure, CI = cardiac index, SVR = systemic vascular resistance

↑ = increase, ↓ = decrease, 0 = no change

Drug	Dose	Receptor Activity						
		α_1	α_2	β_1	β_2	DA_1	V_1	V_2
DOBUTamine	2-10 mcg/kg/min	+	0	+++	++	0	0	0
	>10-20 mcg/kg/min	++	0	++++	+++	0	0	0
DOPamine	1-3 mcg/kg/min	0	0	+	0	++++	0	0
	3-10 mcg/kg/min	0/+	0	++++	++	++++	0	0
	>10-20 mcg/kg/min	+++	0	++++	+	0	0	0
EPINEPHrine	0.01-0.05 mcg/kg/min	++	++	++++	+++	0	0	0
	>0.05 mcg/kg/min	++++	++++	+++	+	0	0	0
Norepinephrine	0.02-3 mcg/kg/min	++++	++	++	0	0	0	0
Phenylephrine	0.5-9 mcg/kg/min	++++	+	0	0	0	0	0
Vasopressin	0.04 units/min	0	0	0	0	0	+++	+

Activity ranges from no activity (0) or maximal activity (++++)

DA = dopaminergic, V = vasopressin

SELECTED READINGS

Biaggioni I and Robertson D, "Adrenoceptor Agonists & Sympathomimetic Drugs," *Basic and Clinical Pharmacology*, 11th ed, Katzung BG, Masters SB, and Trevor AJ, eds, Stamford, CT: McGraw-Hill, 2009, 127-148.

Hollenberg SM, Ahrens TS, Annane D, et al, "Practice Parameters for Hemodynamic Support of Sepsis in Adult Patients: 2004 Update," *Crit Care Med*, 2004, 32(9):1928-48.

Hollenberg SM, "Vasopressor Support in Septic Shock," *Chest*, 2007, 132(5):1678-87.

MacLaren R, Rudis MI, and Dasta JF, "Use of Vasopressors and Inotropes in the Pharmacotherapy of Shock," *Pharmacotherapy: A Pathophysiologic Approach*, 7th ed, Dipiro JT, Talbert RL, Yee GC, et al, eds, Stamford, CT: McGraw-Hill, 2008, 417-39.

CYTOCHROME P450 ENZYMES: SUBSTRATES, INHIBITORS, AND INDUCERS

INTRODUCTION

Most drugs are eliminated from the body, at least in part, by being chemically altered to less lipid-soluble products (ie, metabolized), and thus are more likely to be excreted via the kidneys or the bile. Phase I metabolism includes drug hydrolysis, oxidation, and reduction, and results in drugs that are more polar in their chemical structure, while Phase II metabolism involves the attachment of an additional molecule onto the drug (or partially metabolized drug) in order to create an inactive and/or more water soluble compound. Phase II processes include (primarily) glucuronidation, sulfation, glutathione conjugation, acetylation, and methylation.

Virtually any of the Phase I and II enzymes can be inhibited by some xenobiotic or drug. Some of the Phase I and II enzymes can be induced. Inhibition of the activity of metabolic enzymes will result in increased concentrations of the substrate (drug), whereas induction of the activity of metabolic enzymes will result in decreased concentrations of the substrate. For example, the well-documented enzyme-inducing effects of phenobarbital may include a combination of Phase I and II enzymes. Phase II glucuronidation may be increased via induced UDP-glucuronosyltransferase (UGT) activity, whereas Phase I oxidation may be increased via induced cytochrome P450 (CYP) activity. However, for most drugs, the primary route of metabolism (and the primary focus of drug-drug interaction) is Phase I oxidation.

CYP enzymes may be responsible for the metabolism (at least partial metabolism) of approximately 75% of all drugs, with the CYP3A subfamily responsible for nearly half of this activity. Found throughout plant, animal, and bacterial species, CYP enzymes represent a superfamily of xenobiotic metabolizing proteins. There have been several hundred CYP enzymes identified in nature, each of which has been assigned to a family (1, 2, 3, etc), subfamily (A, B, C, etc), and given a specific enzyme number (1, 2, 3, etc) according to the similarity in amino acid sequence that it shares with other enzymes. Of these many enzymes, only a few are found in humans, and even fewer appear to be involved in the metabolism of xenobiotics (eg, drugs). The key human enzyme subfamilies include CYP1A, CYP2A, CYP2B, CYP2C, CYP2D, CYP2E, and CYP3A. However, the number of distinct isozymes (eg, CYP2C9) found to be functionally active in humans, as well as, the number of genetically variant forms of these isozymes (eg, CYP2C9*2) in individuals continues to expand.

CYP enzymes are found in the endoplasmic reticulum of cells in a variety of human tissues (eg, skin, kidneys, brain, lungs), but their predominant sites of concentration and activity are the liver and intestine. Though the abundance of CYP enzymes throughout the body is relatively equally distributed among the various subfamilies, the relative contribution to drug metabolism is (in decreasing order of magnitude) CYP3A4 (nearly 50%), CYP2D6 (nearly 25%), CYP2C8/9 (nearly 15%), then CYP1A2, CYP2C19, CYP2A6, and CYP2E1. Owing to their potential for numerous drug-drug interactions, those drugs that are identified in preclinical studies as substrates of CYP3A enzymes are often given a lower priority for continued research and development in favor of drugs that appear to be less affected by (or less likely to affect) this enzyme subfamily.

Each enzyme subfamily possesses unique selectivity toward potential substrates. For example, CYP1A2 preferentially binds medium-sized, planar, lipophilic molecules, while CYP2D6 preferentially binds molecules that possess a basic nitrogen atom. Some CYP subfamilies exhibit polymorphism (ie, genetic variation that results in a modified enzyme with small changes in amino acid sequences that may manifest differing catalytic properties). The best described polymorphisms involve CYP2C9, CYP2C19, and CYP2D6. Individuals possessing "wild type" genes exhibit normal functioning CYP capacity. Others, however, possess genetic variants that leave the person with a subnormal level of catalytic potential (so called "poor metabolizers"). Poor metabolizers would be more likely to experience toxicity from drugs metabolized by the affected enzymes (or less effects if the enzyme is responsible for converting a prodrug to it's active form as in the case of codeine). The percentage of people classified as poor metabolizers varies by enzyme and population group. As an example, approximately 7% of Caucasians and only about 1% of Asians appear to be CYP2D6 poor metabolizers.

CYP enzymes can be both inhibited and induced by other drugs, leading to increased or decreased serum concentrations (along with the associated effects), respectively. Induction occurs when a drug causes an increase in the amount of smooth endoplasmic reticulum, secondary to increasing the amount of the affected CYP enzymes in the tissues. This "revving up" of the CYP enzyme system may take several days to reach peak activity, and likewise, may take several days, even months, to return to normal following discontinuation of the inducing agent.

CYP inhibition occurs via several potential mechanisms. Most commonly, a CYP inhibitor competitively (and reversibly) binds to the active site on the enzyme, thus preventing the substrate from binding to the same site, and preventing the substrate from being metabolized. The affinity of an inhibitor for an enzyme may be expressed by an inhibition constant (Ki) or IC50 (defined as the concentration of the inhibitor required to cause 50% inhibition under a given set of conditions). In addition to reversible competition for an enzyme site, drugs may inhibit enzyme activity by binding to sites on the enzyme other than that to which the substrate would bind, and thereby cause a change in the functionality or physical structure of the enzyme. A drug may also bind to the enzyme in an irreversible (ie, "suicide") fashion. In such a case, it is not the concentration of drug at the enzyme site that is important (constantly binding and releasing), but the number of molecules available for binding (once bound, always bound).

Although an inhibitor or inducer may be known to affect a variety of CYP subfamilies, it may only inhibit one or two in a clinically important fashion. Likewise, although a substrate is known to be at least partially metabolized by a variety of CYP enzymes, only one or two enzymes may contribute significantly enough to its overall metabolism to warrant concern when used with potential inducers or inhibitors. Therefore, when attempting to predict the level of risk of using two drugs that may affect each other via altered CYP function, it is important to identify the relative effectiveness of the inhibiting/inducing drug on the CYP subfamilies that significantly contribute to the metabolism of the substrate. The contribution of a specific CYP pathway to substrate metabolism should be considered not only in light of other known CYP pathways, but also other nonoxidative pathways for substrate metabolism (eg, glucuronidation) and transporter proteins (eg, P-glycoprotein) that may affect the presentation of a substrate to a metabolic pathway.

HOW TO USE THIS TABLE

The following table provides a clinically relevant perspective on drugs that are affected by, or affect, cytochrome P450 (CYP) enzymes. Not all human, drug-metabolizing CYP enzymes are specifically (or separately) included in the table. Some enzymes have been excluded because they do not appear to significantly contribute to the metabolism of marketed drugs (eg, CYP2C18). In the case of CYP3A4, the industry routinely uses this single enzyme designation to represent all enzymes in the CYP3A subfamily. CYP3A7 is present in fetal livers. It is effectively absent from adult livers. CYP3A4 (adult) and CYP3A7 (fetal) appear to share similar properties in their respective hosts. The impact of CYP3A7 in fetal and neonatal drug interactions has not been investigated.

An enzyme that appears to play a clinically significant (major) role in a drug's metabolism is indicated by "S". A clinically significant designation is the result of a two-phase review. The first phase considered the contribution of each CYP enzyme to the overall metabolism of the drug. The enzyme pathway was considered potentially clinically relevant if it was responsible for at least 30% of the metabolism of the drug. If so, the drug was subjected to a second phase. The second phase considered the clinical relevance of a substrate's concentration being increased twofold, or decreased by one-half (such as might be observed if combined with an effective CYP inhibitor or inducer, respectively). If either of these changes was considered to present a clinically significant concern, the CYP pathway for the drug was designated "major." If neither change would appear to present a clinically significant concern, or if the CYP enzyme was responsible for a smaller portion of the overall metabolism (ie, <30%), then no association between the enzyme and the drug will appear in the table.

Enzymes that are strongly or moderately inhibited by a drug are indicated by "↓". Enzymes that are weakly inhibited are not identified in the table. The designations are the result of a review of published clinical reports, available Ki data, and assessments published by other experts in the field. As it pertains to Ki values set in a ratio with achievable serum drug concentrations ([I]) under normal dosing conditions, the following parameters were employed: [I]/Ki ≥1 = strong; [I]/Ki 0.1-1 = moderate; [I]/Ki <0.1 = weak.

Enzymes that appear to be effectively induced by a drug are indicated by "↑". This designation is the result of a review of published clinical reports and assessments published by experts in the field.

In general, clinically significant interactions are more likely to occur between substrates ("S") and either inhibitors or inducers of the same enzyme(s), which have been indicated by "↓" and "↑", respectively. However, these assessments possess a degree of subjectivity, at times based on limited indications regarding the significance of CYP effects of particular agents. An attempt has been made to balance a conservative, clinically-sensitive presentation of the data with a desire to avoid the numbing effect of a "beware of everything" approach. It is important to note that information related to CYP metabolism of drugs is expanding at a rapid pace, and thus, the contents of this table should only be considered to represent a "snapshot" of the information available at the time of publication.

SELECTED READINGS

Bjornsson TD, Callaghan JT, Einolf HJ, et al, "The Conduct of *in vitro* and *in vivo* Drug-Drug Interaction Studies: A PhRMA Perspective," *J Clin Pharmacol*, 2003, 43(5):443-69.

Drug-Drug Interactions, Rodrigues AD, ed, New York, NY: Marcel Dekker, Inc, 2002.

Levy RH, Thummel KE, Trager WF, et al, eds, *Metabolic Drug Interactions*, Philadelphia, PA: Lippincott Williams & Wilkins, 2000.

Michalets EL, "Update: Clinically Significant Cytochrome P-450 Drug Interactions," *Pharmacotherapy*, 1998, 18(1):84-112.

Thummel KE and Wilkinson GR, "*In vitro* and *in vivo* Drug Interactions Involving Human CYP3A," *Annu Rev Pharmacol Toxicol*, 1998, 38:389-430.

Zhang Y and Benet LZ, "The Gut as a Barrier to Drug Absorption: Combined Role of Cytochrome P450 3A and P-Glycoprotein," *Clin Pharmacokinet*, 2001, 40(3):159-68.

SELECTED WEBSITES

http://www.imm.ki.se/CYPalleles

http://medicine.iupui.edu/flockhart

http://www.fda.gov/Drugs/DevelopmentApprovalProcess/DevelopmentResources/DrugInteractionsLabeling/ucm080499.htm

CYP: Substrates, Inhibitors, Inducers

S = substrate; ↓ = inhibitor; ↑ = inducer

Drug	1A2	2A6	2B6	2C8	2C9	2C19	2D6	2E1	3A4
Acenocoumarol	S				S				
Alfentanil									S
Alfuzosin									S
Alosetron	S								
ALPRAZolam									S
Ambrisentan						S			S
Aminophylline	S								
Amiodarone		↓		S	↓		↓		S, ↓
Amitriptyline							S		
AmLODIPine	↓								S
Amobarbital		↑							
Amoxapine							S		
Aprepitant									S, ↓
ARIPiprazole							S		S
Armodafinil						↓			S, ↑
Atazanavir									S, ↓
Atomoxetine							S		
Atorvastatin									S
Benzphetamine									S
Betaxolol	S						S		
Bisoprolol									S
Bortezomib						S, ↓			S
Bosentan					S, ↑				S, ↑
Bromazepam									S
Bromocriptine									S
Budesonide									S
Buprenorphine									S
BuPROPion			S						
BusPIRone									S
Busulfan									S
Caffeine	S								↓
Captopril							S		
CarBAMazepine	↑		↑	↑	↑	↑			S, ↑
Carisoprodol						S			
Carvedilol					S		S		
Celecoxib				↓	S				
ChlordiazePOXIDE									S
Chloroquine							S, ↓		S
Chlorpheniramine									S
ChlorproMAZINE							S, ↓		
Chlorzoxazone								S	
Ciclesonide									S
Cilostazol									S
Cimetidine	↓					↓	↓		↓
Cinacalcet							↓		
Ciprofloxacin	↓								
Cisapride									S
Citalopram						S			S

CYP: Substrates, Inhibitors, Inducers *(continued)*

Drug	1A2	2A6	2B6	2C8	2C9	2C19	2D6	2E1	3A4
Clarithromycin									S, ↓
Clobazam						S			S
ClomiPRAMINE	S					S	S, ↓		
ClonazePAM									S
Clorazepate									S
Clotrimazole									↓
CloZAPine	S						↓		
Cocaine							↓		S
Codeine[1]							S		
Colchicine									S
Conivaptan									S, ↓
Cyclobenzaprine	S								
Cyclophosphamide[2]			S						S
CycloSPORINE									S, ↓
Dacarbazine	S							S	
Dantrolene									S
Dapsone					S				S
Darifenacin							↓		S
Darunavir									S
Dasatinib									S
Delavirdine					↓	↓	↓		S, ↓
Desipramine		↓	↓				S, ↓		↓
Desogestrel						S			
Dexamethasone									S, ↑
Dexlansoprazole						S, ↓			S
Dexmedetomidine		S					↓		
Dextromethorphan							S		
Diazepam						S			S
Diclofenac	↓								
Dihydroergotamine									S
Diltiazem									S, ↓
DiphenhydrAMINE							↓		
Disopyramide									S
Disulfiram								↓	
DOCEtaxel									S
Doxepin							S		
DOXOrubicin			↓				S		S
Doxycycline									↓
DULoxetine	S						S, ↓		
Efavirenz[3]			S		↓	↓			S, ↓, ↑
Eletriptan									S
Enflurane								S	
Eplerenone									S
Ergoloid mesylates									S
Ergonovine									S
Ergotamine									S
Erlotinib									S
Erythromycin									S, ↓
Escitalopram						S			S
Esomeprazole						S, ↓			S
Estradiol	S								S
Estrogens, conjugated A/synthetic	S								S

CYP: Substrates, Inhibitors, Inducers *(continued)*

Drug	1A2	2A6	2B6	2C8	2C9	2C19	2D6	2E1	3A4
Estrogens, conjugated equine	S								S
Estrogens, esterified	S								S
Estropipate	S								S
Eszopiclone									S
Ethinyl estradiol									S
Ethosuximide									S
Etoposide									S
Exemestane									S
Felbamate									S
Felodipine				↓					S
FentaNYL									S
Flecainide							S		
Fluconazole					↓	↓			↓
Flunisolide									S
FLUoxetine	↓				S	↓	S, ↓		
FluPHENAZine							S		
Flurazepam									S
Flurbiprofen					↓				
Flutamide	S								S
Fluticasone									S
Fluvastatin					S, ↓				
FluvoxaMINE	S, ↓					↓	S		
Fosamprenavir (as amprenavir)									S, ↓
Fosaprepitant									S, ↓
Fosphenytoin (as phenytoin)			↑	↑	S, ↑	S, ↑			↑
Fospropofol	↓		S		S	↓			↓
Gefitinib									S
Gemfibrozil	↓			↓	↓	↓			
Glimepiride					S				
GlipiZIDE					S				
Guanabenz	S								
Haloperidol							S, ↓		S, ↓
Halothane								S	
Ibuprofen					↓				
Ifosfamide[4]		S				S			S
Imatinib							↓		S, ↓
Imipramine						S	S, ↓		
Indinavir									S, ↓
Indomethacin					↓				
Irbesartan				↓	↓				
Irinotecan			S						S
Isoflurane								S	
Isoniazid		↓				↓	↓	S, ↓	
Isosorbide dinitrate									S
Isosorbide mononitrate									S
Isradipine									S
Itraconazole									S, ↓
Ixabepilone									S
Ketamine			S		S				S
Ketoconazole	↓	↓			↓	↓	↓		S, ↓
Lansoprazole						S, ↓			S
Lapatinib									S

CYP: Substrates, Inhibitors, Inducers *(continued)*

Drug	1A2	2A6	2B6	2C8	2C9	2C19	2D6	2E1	3A4
Letrozole		↓							
Levonorgestrel									S
Lidocaine	↓						S, ↓		S, ↓
Lomustine							S		
Lopinavir									S
Loratadine						↓			
Losartan				↓	S, ↓				S
Lovastatin									S
Maprotiline							S		
Maraviroc									S
MedroxyPROGESTERone									S
Mefenamic acid					↓				
Mefloquine									S
Mephobarbital						S			
Mestranol[5]					S				S
Methadone							↓		S
Methamphetamine							S		
Methimazole							↓		
Methoxsalen	↓	↓							
Methsuximide						S			
Methylergonovine									S
MethylPREDNISolone									S
Metoprolol							S		
MetroNIDAZOLE									↓
Mexiletine	S, ↓						S		
Miconazole	↓	↓			↓	↓	↓	↓	S, ↓
Midazolam									S
Mirtazapine	S						S		S
Moclobemide						S	S		
Modafinil						↓			S
Montelukast					S				S
Nafcillin									↑
Nateglinide					S				S
Nebivolol							S		
Nefazodone							S		S, ↓
Nelfinavir						S			S, ↓
Nevirapine			↑						S, ↑
NiCARdipine					↓	↓	↓		S, ↓
NIFEdipine	↓								S
Nilotinib									S
Nilutamide						S			
NiMODipine									S
Nisoldipine									S
Norethindrone									S
Norfloxacin	↓								↓
Norgestrel									S
Nortriptyline							S		
Ofloxacin	↓								
OLANZapine	S								
Omeprazole					↓	S, ↓			S
Ondansetron									S
OXcarbazepine									↑

CYP: Substrates, Inhibitors, Inducers *(continued)*

Drug	1A2	2A6	2B6	2C8	2C9	2C19	2D6	2E1	3A4
PACLitaxel				S	S				S
Pantoprazole						S			
Paricalcitol									S
PARoxetine			↓				S, ↓		
Pazopanib									S
Pentamidine						S			
PENTobarbital		↑							↑
Perphenazine							S		
PHENobarbital	↑	↑	↑	↑	↑	S			↑
Phenytoin			↑	↑	S, ↑	S, ↑			↑
Pimozide	S								S
Pindolol							S		
Pioglitazone				S, ↓					
Piroxicam					↓				
Posaconazole									↓
Primaquine	↓								S
Primidone	↑		↑	↑	↑				↑
Procainamide							S		
Progesterone						S			S
Promethazine			S				S		
Propafenone							S		
Propofol	↓		S		S	↓			↓
Propranolol	S						S		
Protriptyline							S		
Pyrimethamine					↓		↓		
Quazepam						S			S
QUEtiapine									S
QuiNIDine							↓		S, ↓
QuiNINE				↓	↓		↓		S
RABEprazole				↓		S, ↓			S
Ramelteon	S								
Ranolazine							↓		S
Rasagiline	S								
Repaglinide				S					S
Rifabutin									S, ↑
Rifampin	↑	↑	↑	↑	↑	↑			↑
Rifapentine				↑	↑				↑
Riluzole	S								
RisperiDONE							S		
Ritonavir				↓			S, ↓		S, ↓
ROPINIRole	S								
Ropivacaine	S								
Rosiglitazone				S, ↓					
Salmeterol									S
Saquinavir									S, ↓
Secobarbital		↑		↑	↑				
Selegiline			S						
Sertraline			↓			S, ↓	S, ↓		↓
Sevoflurane								S	
Sibutramine									S
Sildenafil									S
Simvastatin									S

CYP: Substrates, Inhibitors, Inducers *(continued)*

Drug	1A2	2A6	2B6	2C8	2C9	2C19	2D6	2E1	3A4
Sirolimus									S
Sitaxsentan					↓	↓			↓
Solifenacin									S
SORAfenib			↓	↓	↓				
Spiramycin									S
SUFentanil									S
SulfADIAZINE					S, ↓				
Sulfamethoxazole					S, ↓				
SUNItinib									S
Tacrine	S								
Tacrolimus									S
Tadalafil									S
Tamoxifen				↓	S		S		S
Tamsulosin							S		S
Telithromycin									S, ↓
Temsirolimus									S
Teniposide									S
Terbinafine							↓		
Tetracycline									S, ↓
Theophylline	S							S	S
Thiabendazole	↓								
Thioridazine							S, ↓		
Thiotepa			↓						
Thiothixene	S								
TiaGABine									S
Ticlopidine						↓	↓		S
Timolol							S		
Tinidazole									S
Tipranavir									S
TiZANidine	S								
TOLBUTamide					S, ↓				
Tolterodine							S		S
Toremifene									S
Torsemide					S				
TraMADol[1]							S		S
Tranylcypromine	↓	↓				↓	↓		
TraZODone									S
Tretinoin				S					
Triazolam									S
Trifluoperazine	S								
Trimethoprim				↓	S, ↓				S
Trimipramine						S	S		S
Vardenafil									S
Venlafaxine							S		S
Verapamil									S, ↓
VinBLAStine									S
VinCRIStine									S
Vinorelbine									S
Voriconazole					S	S			↓
Warfarin					S, ↓				
Zafirlukast					S, ↓				
Zileuton	↓								

CYP: Substrates, Inhibitors, Inducers *(continued)*

Drug	1A2	2A6	2B6	2C8	2C9	2C19	2D6	2E1	3A4
Zolpidem									S
Zonisamide									S
Zopiclone					S				S
Zuclopenthixol							S		

[1]This opioid analgesic is bioactivated *in vivo* via CYP2D6. Inhibiting this enzyme would decrease the effects of the analgesic. The active metabolite might also affect, or be affected by, CYP enzymes.

[2]Cyclophosphamide is bioactivated *in vivo* to acrolein via CYP2B6 and 3A4. Inhibiting these enzymes would decrease the effects of cyclophosphamide.

[3]Data have shown both induction (*in vivo*) and inhibition (*in vitro*) of CYP3A4.

[4]Ifosfamide is bioactivated *in vivo* to acrolein via CYP3A4. Inhibiting this enzyme would decrease the effects of ifosfamide.

[5]Mestranol is bioactivated *in vivo* to ethinyl estradiol via CYP2C8/9. See Ethinyl Estradiol for additional CYP information.

DESENSITIZATION PROTOCOLS

Desensitization should be performed under the supervision of a licensed healthcare professional. These protocols are potentially dangerous procedures and should be only performed in an area where immediate access to emergency drugs (eg, epinephrine) and equipment can be assured. Premedication with antihistamines or steroids is generally not recommended, as these drugs may mask early signs of reactivity that would otherwise result in a modification of the protocol (Cernadas, 2010). Prior to desensitization, medications such as beta blockers should be discontinued unless required for certain indications. Desensitization is generally contraindicated in patients with severe idiosyncratic reactions, uncontrolled asthma, and prior anaphylaxis to the desensitizing agent. However, some clinicians may choose to perform desensitization in patients with a history of IgE-mediated reactions, including anaphylaxis. Under these circumstances, healthcare providers should proceed with caution.

During desensitization, breakthrough hypersensitivity reactions, such as pruritus, urticaria, rhinitis, or mild wheezing, may occur during the procedure. Breakthrough hypersensitivity reactions should be treated immediately and the desensitization protocol should be stopped. These reactions often are dose-dependent and can be managed with modifications to the protocol (Cernadas, 2010).

Note: Once desensitized, the patient's treatment with the desensitized agent must not lapse or the risk of an allergic reaction increases. If the patient requires treatment with the desensitized agent in the future and still remains skin test-positive, desensitization would be required again (Cunha, 2001).

The following desensitization protocols presented are examples of what has been reported/evaluated in literature. Only a summary of the protocol is presented; the complete reference should be reviewed prior to utilizing a desensitization protocol. The information provided in the tables below is often based on a single case report or a very limited number of patients. Both oral and parenteral medications have been used in desensitization protocols and both methods have been shown to be equally effective. Historically, oral dosage forms have been thought to be safer; however, parenteral dosage forms have been used when the oral route of administration is not feasible (Cernadas, 2010). These protocols are meant to be used as a guide with the knowledge that there are other methods of desensitization that may also be used successfully.

GENERAL INTRAVENOUS DESENSITIZATION PROTOCOL

For use with Ceftazidime, Ceftriaxone, Cefazolin, Imipenem, Nafcillin, Penicillin, Piperacillin/Tazobactam Sodium, and Vancomycin

Solution Preparation

Solution	Volume (mL)	Concentration (mg/mL)	Total Amount of Drug in Each Solution (mg)
1		0.040	10
2	250	0.40	100
3		3.969	992.13

Protocol for Administration

Step	Solution	Rate (mL/h)	Time (min)	Administered Dose (mg)	Cumulative Dose (mg)
1		2		0.02	0.02
2	1	5		0.05	0.07
3		10		0.1	0.17
4		20		0.2	0.37
5		5		0.5	0.87
6	2	10	15	1	1.87
7		20		2	3.87
8		40		4	7.87
9		10		9.9213	17.7913
10	3	20		19.8426	37.6339
11		40		39.6852	77.3191
12		75	186	922.6809	1000

Note: Total time = 351 minutes

Adapted from Castellas M, "Rapid Desensitization for Hypersensitivity Reactions to Medications," *Immunol Allergy Clin N Am*, 2009, 29:585-606.

PENICILLIN G

Parenteral Desensitization Protocol

Injection Number	Benzylpenicillin Concentration (units/mL)	Volume and Route (mL)[a]
1[b]	100	0.1 **I.D.**
2		0.2 SubQ
3		0.4 SubQ
4		0.8 SubQ
5[b]	1000	0.1 **I.D.**
6		0.3 SubQ
7		0.6 SubQ
8[b]	10,000	0.1 **I.D.**
9		0.2 SubQ
10		0.4 SubQ
11		0.8 SubQ
12[b]	100,000	0.1 **I.D.**
13		0.3 SubQ
14		0.6 SubQ
15[b]	1,000,000	0.1 **I.D.**
16		0.2 SubQ
17		0.2 SubQ
18		0.4 SubQ
19	Continuous SubQ infusion (1,000,000 units/h)	

I.D. = intradermal, SubQ = subcutaneous

[a]Administer progressive doses at intervals of not less than 20 minutes.

[b]Observe and record skin wheal and flare response to intradermal dose.

Adapted from Cunha BA, "Antimicrobial Selection in the Penicillin-Allergic," *Drugs Today*, 2001, 37 (6):377-83.

Adapted from Castellas M, "Rapid Desensitization for Hypersensitivity Reactions to Medications," *Immunol Allergy Clin N Am*, 2009, 29:585-606.

PENICILLIN V

Oral Desensitization Protocol

Step[a]	Penicillin V Suspension (units/mL)	Amount[b] (mL)	Dose (units)	Cumulative Dosage (units)
1	1000	0.1	100	100
2		0.2	200	300
3		0.4	400	700
4		0.8	800	1500
5		1.6	1600	3100
6		3.2	3200	6300
7		6.4	6400	12,700
8	10,000	1.2	12,000	24,700
9		2.4	24,000	48,700
10		4.8	48,000	96,700
11	80,000	1	80,000	176,700
12		2	160,000	336,700
13		4	320,000	656,700
14		8	640,000	1,296,700
15	500,000	0.25	125,000	1,421,700
16		0.5	250,000	1,671,700
17		1	500,000	2,171,700
18		2.25	1,125,000	3,296,700

[a]Interval between steps = 15 minutes

[b]Amount of drug is diluted in ~30 mL of water and then given P.O.

Note: Observe patients for 30 minutes prior to parenteral administration of penicillin.

Adapted from Cunha BA, "Antimicrobial Selection in the Penicillin-Allergic," *Drugs Today*, 2001, 37(6):377-83.

ALLOPURINOL

Oral Desensitization Protocol

Dosing Schedule	Oral Dose of Allopurinol
Days 1-3	50 mcg/day
Days 4-6	100 mcg/day
Days 7-9	200 mcg/day
Days 10-12	500 mcg/day
Days 13-15	1 mg/day
Days 16-18	5 mg/day
Days 19-21	10 mg/day
Days 22-24	25 mg/day
Days 25-27	50 mg/day
Day 28	100 mg/day

Note: For doses ≤1 mg, 1 mg/5 mL suspension was used; for doses 5-25 mg, 10 mg/5 mL suspension was used. For doses 50 mg and 100 mg, 1/2 tablet and 1 tablet of 100 mg allopurinol were used, respectively.

Note: High-risk patients should follow the modified desensitization protocol: Initial doses of 10 mcg and 25 mcg with dosage escalation every 5-10 days or longer

Adapted from Fam AG, Dunne SM, Iazzetta J, et al, "Efficacy and Safety of Desensitization to Allopurinol Following Cutaneous Reactions," *Arthritis Rheum*, 2001, 44(1):231-8.

AMPHOTERICIN B

Intravenous Desensitization Protocol

Step	Volume (mL)	Dose (mg)	Infusion time (min)
1	10	0.000001	10
2		0.00001	
3		0.0001	
4		0.001	
5		0.01	
6		1	30
7	250	30	240

Note: Mixtures were prepared in 5% dextrose. Patient was premedicated with methylprednisolone 60 mg I.V. and diphenhydramine 25 mg I.V.

Adapted from Kemp SF and Lockey RF, "Amphotericin B: Emergency Challenge in a Neutropenic, Asthmatic Patient With Fungal Sepsis," *J Allergy Clin Immunol*, 1995, 96(3):425-7.

TRIMETHOPRIM-SULFAMETHOXAZOLE

Oral Desensitization Protocol

Dosing Level	Portion of Single-Strength TMP-SMZ (%)	Amount (Frequency) of Pediatric Suspension (mL)	Total TMP Dose (mg)	Total SMZ Dose (mg)
1	12.5	1.25 daily	10	50
2	25	1.25 bid	20	100
3	37.5	1.25 tid	30	150
4	50	2.5 bid	40	200
5	75	2.5 tid	60	300
6	100	1 single-strength tablet	80	400

Note: Each dosing level is a daily dose. For successful completion of the reintroduction phase, patients must have taken each dose level at least once. Patients were permitted to repeat dose levels once; dose levels were completed in increasing increments, and the level 6 dose was taken no later than day 13 of the reintroduction phase. Patients were permitted to withhold study drug for 2 days during the reintroduction phase (withholding study drug for >2 days during reintroduction resulted in permanent discontinuation). Patients were required to take an antihistamine during dose escalation.

Adapted from Leoung GS, Stanford JF, Giordano MF, et al, "Trimethoprim-Sulfamethoxazole (TMP-SMZ) Dose Escalation Versus Direct Rechallenge for *Pneumocystis carinii* Pneumonia, Prophylaxis in Human Immunodeficiency Virus-Infected Patients With Previous Adverse Reaction to TMP-SMZ," *J Infect Dis*, 2001, 184(8):992-7.

Alternate Oral Desensitization Protocol

Day	Morning Dose (g)	Evening Dose (g)
1	0.005	0.01
2	0.02	0.04
3	0.1	0.2
4	0.4	0.8
5	1	1

Note: A granular dosage form of trimethoprim-sulfamethoxazole was used in the protocol. A 0.005 g dose is equivalent to 0.4 mg of trimethoprim and 2 mg of sulfamethoxazole. On day 5, patients received a dose equivalent to one 80-400 mg trimethoprim-sulfamethoxazole tablet.

Adapted from Yoshizawa S, Yasuoka A, Kikuchi Y, et al, "A 5-Day Course of Oral Desensitization to Trimethoprim/Sulfamethoxazole (T/S) in Patients With Human Immunodeficiency Virus Type-1 Infection Who Were Previously Intolerant to T/S," *Ann Allergy Asthma Imunol*, 2000, 85:241-4.

VANCOMYCIN

Intravenous Desensitization Protocol

Infusion Number	Dilution	Vancomycin Dose (mg)	Concentration (mg/mL)
1	1:10,000	0.02	0.0002
2	1:1000	0.2	0.002
3	1:100	2	0.02
4	1:10	20	0.2
5	Standard	500	2

Adapted from Wazny LD and Daghigh B, "Desensitization Protocols for Vancomycin Hypersensitivity," *Ann Pharmacother*, 2001, 35 (11):1458-64.

Premedication: Generally not administered prior to desensitization protocols. However, the patients in this protocol were given diphenhydramine 50 mg I.V. and hydrocortisone 100 mg I.V. 15 minutes prior to initiation of protocol, then every 6 hours throughout protocol.

Infusion rate instructions:

Initiate infusion rate at 0.5 mL/minute (30 mL/hour) and increase by 0.5 mL/minute (30 mL/hour) as tolerated every 5 minutes to a maximum rate of 5 mL/minute (300 mL/hour). If pruritus, hypotension, rash, or difficulty breathing occurs, stop infusion and reinfuse the previously tolerated infusion at the highest tolerated rate. This step may be repeated up to three times for any given concentration.

Upon completion of infusion number 5, immediately administer the required dose of vancomycin in the usual dilution of NS or D_5W over 2 hours. Decrease rate if patient becomes symptomatic or, alternatively, increase rate if patient tolerates dose. Administer diphenhydramine 50 mg orally prior to each required dose of vancomycin.

CEFTRIAXONE

Intravenous Desensitization Protocol

Dose Number[a]	Concentration (mg/mL)	Flow Rate (mL/h)	Dose (mg)
1	0.01	6	0.015
2		12	0.03
3		24	0.06
4	0.1	5	0.125
5		10	0.25
6		20	0.5
7		40	1
8		80	2
9		160	4
10	10	3	7.5
11		6	15
12		12	30
13		25	62.5
14		50	125
15	100	10	250
16		20	500
17		40	1000

[a]Interval between doses = 15 minutes

Adapted from Solensky R, "Drug Desensitization," *Immunol Allergy Clin N Am*, 2004, 24:425-43.

CIPROFLOXACIN

Intravenous Desensitization Protocol

Ciprofloxacin Concentration (mg/mL)	Volume Given (mL)	Dose (mg)	Cumulative Total Dose (mg)
0.1	0.1	0.01	0.01
	0.2	0.02	0.03
	0.4	0.04	0.07
	0.8	0.08	0.15
1	0.16	0.16	0.31
	0.32	0.32	0.63
	0.64	0.64	1.27
2	0.6	1.2	2.47
	1.2	2.4	4.87
	2.4	4.8	9.67
	5	10	19.67
	10	20	39.67
	20	40	79.67
	40	80	159.67
	120	240	399.67

Note: Patient was premedicated with diphenhydramine 50 mg I.V. and prednisone 10 mg I.V. 1 hour prior to desensitization. Doses were administered at 15-minute intervals. The total time for the desensitization procedure is 4 hours.

Note: Drug volumes <1 mL were mixed with normal saline solution to a final volume of 3 mL and then slowly infused; the other doses were administered over 10 minutes, except the last dose (240 mg in 120 mL), which was given with an infusion pump over 20 minutes.

Adapted from Gea-Banacloche JC and Metcalfe DD, "Ciprofloxacin Desensitization," *J Allergy Clin Immunol*, 1996, 97:1426-7.

IMIPENEM

Intravenous Desensitization Protocol

Time (min)	Concentration (mg/mL)	Fluid Infusion Rate (mL/min)
0	0.0001	1
30	0.0003	
60	0.001	
90	0.003	
120	0.01	
150	0.03	
180	0.1	
210	0.3	
240	0.7	1[a]

[a]Dosage reduction for renal dysfunction

Note: If rash or flushing occurs, return to previous step for 30 minutes and call physician.

Note: Total daily dosage of imipenem was 1008 mg (creatinine clearance 20-30 mL/min)

Adapted from Gorman SK, Zed PJ, Dhingra VK, et al, "Rapid Imipenem/Cilastatin Desensitization for Multidrug-Resistant Acinetobacter Pneumonia," *Ann Pharmacother*, 2003, 37:513-6.

INSULIN

Parenteral Desensitization Protocol

<table>
<tr><th>Dosing Schedule</th><th>Time of Dose (min)</th><th>Dose (mL)</th><th>Dilution (units/mL)[a]</th><th>Units/Dose</th><th>Route of Administration</th></tr>
<tr><td rowspan="8">Day 1</td><td>0</td><td rowspan="8">0.1</td><td rowspan="3">0.001</td><td rowspan="3">1/10,000</td><td>Scratch</td></tr>
<tr><td>15</td><td>I.D.</td></tr>
<tr><td>20</td><td rowspan="9">SubQ</td></tr>
<tr><td>45</td><td>0.01</td><td>1/1000</td></tr>
<tr><td>60</td><td>0.1</td><td>1/100</td></tr>
<tr><td>75</td><td>1</td><td>1/10</td></tr>
<tr><td>90</td><td rowspan="4">10</td><td rowspan="2">1</td></tr>
<tr><td>115 and q4h x 5</td></tr>
<tr><td>Day 2</td><td>q4h</td><td>0.2</td><td>2</td></tr>
<tr><td>Day 3</td><td rowspan="3">7 am and 4 pm</td><td></td><td>2 and 4</td></tr>
<tr><td>Day 4</td><td></td><td rowspan="2">100</td><td>5 and 10</td></tr>
<tr><td>Day 5</td><td></td><td>Individualize as needed</td></tr>
</table>

[a]HumuLIN® R insulin was used with diluent provided by manufacturer, Eli Lilly Co, with 1% human serum albumin incorporated into each diluent prepared.

Note: Patient was premedicated with antihistamines prior to initiation of desensitization protocol.

Adapted from Bodendofer TW, Brown ME, Frankel EH, et al, "Desensitization With Human (Recombinant DNA) Insulin," *Drug Intell Clin Pharm*, 1985, 19:827-9.

NELFINAVIR

Oral Desensitization Protocol

Step	Time (min)	Nelfinavir Dose (mg)	
		q30min	Total
1	0	0.5	0.5
2	30	1	1.5
3	60	2	3.5
4	90	5	8.5
5	120	10	18.5
6	150	20	38.5
7	180	40	78.5
8	210	80	158.5
9	240	160	318.5
10	270	250	568.5
11	300	500	1068.5
12	330	750	1818.5

Note: Observe patient in ICU for 2 hours before discharge.

Note: One mg/mL and 10 mg/mL solutions were prepared to deliver the required dose.

Adapted from Abraham PE, Sorensen SJ, Baker WH, et al, "Nelfinavir Desensitization," *Ann Pharmacother*, 2001, 35(5):553-6.

RIFAMPIN AND ETHAMBUTOL

Oral Desensitization Protocol

Time from Start (h:min)	Rifampin (mg)	Ethambutol (mg)
0	0.1	0.1
00:45	0.5	0.5
01:30	1	1
02:15	2	2
03:00	4	4
03:45	8	8
04:30	16	16
05:15	32	32
06:00	50	50
06:45	100	100
07:30	150	200
11:00	300	400
Next day, starting at 6:30 am	300 mg twice daily	400 mg 3 times/day

Adapted from Matz J, Borish LC, Routes JM, et al, "Oral Desensitization to Rifampin and Ethambutol in Mycobacterial Disease," *Am J Respir Crit Care Med*, 1994, 149:815-7.

RITUXIMAB

Intravenous Desensitization Protocol

Solution Preparation

Solution	Volume (mL)	Concentration (mg/mL)	Total Amount of Drug in Each Solution (mg)
1	250	0.034	8.51
2		0.34	85.1
3		3.377	844.303

Note: Total dose of rituximab used is 851 mg (less than prepared since solutions 1 and 2 are not completely infused)

Administration

Step	Solution	Rate (mL/h)	Time (min)	Volume Infused Per Step (mL)	Administered Dose (mg)	Cumulative Dose (mg)
1	1	2	15	0.5	0.017	0.017
2		5		1.25	0.0426	0.0596
3		10		2.5	0.0851	0.1447
4		20		5	0.1702	0.3149
5	2	5		1.25	0.4255	0.7404
6		10		2.5	0.851	1.5914
7		20		5	1.702	3.2934
8		40		10	3.404	6.6974
9	3	10		2.5	8.4443	15.1404
10		20		5	16.8861	32.0264
11		40		10	33.7721	65.7986
12		75	186	232.5	785.2014	851

Note: Total time = 351 minutes

Note: Patients developing reactions during the desensitization protocol developed them near step 12 and were treated with antihistamines. Additionally, antileukotriene therapy and prostaglandin blockade with aspirin may be beneficial in improving side effects.

Adapted from Castellas M, "Rapid Desensitization for Hypersensitivity Reactions to Medications," *Immunol Allergy Clin N Am*, 2009, 29:585-606.

CARBOPLATIN

Intravenous Desensitization Protocol

Solution Preparation

Solution	Volume (mL)	Concentration (mg/mL)	Total Dose in Each Solution (mg)
A		0.02	5
B	250	0.2	50
C		2	500

Note: Carboplatin was diluted in 250 mL of D_5W. The sum of doses in Solutions A through C is 555 mg; however, the total dose infused is 500 mg.

Administration

Step	Solution	Rate (mL/h)	Time (min)	Administered Dose (mg)	Cumulative Dose Infused (mg)
1		2		0.01	0.01
2	A	5		0.025	0.035
3		10		0.05	0.085
4		20		0.1	0.185
5		5		0.25	0.435
6	B	10	15	0.5	0.935
7		20		1	1.935
8		40		2	3.935
9		10		5	8.935
10	C	20		10	18.935
11		40		20	38.935
12		75	184.4	461.065	500

Note: Total time = ~6 hours

Adapted from Lee CW, Matulonis UA, and Castells MC, "Carboplatin Hypersensitivity: A 6-H 12-Step Protocol Effective in 35 Desensitizations in Patients With Gynecological Malignancies and Mast Cell/IgE-Mediated Reactions," *Gynecol Oncol*, 2004, 95(2):370-6.

ASPIRIN

Oral Desensitization Protocol

Time (min)	Dose (mg)
0	0.1
20	0.3
40	1
60	3
80	10
100	30
120	40
140	81
160	162

Note: Aspirin was continued at 162 mg orally daily. Most patients were pretreated with an antihistamine (eg, diphenhydramine, hydroxyzine) prior to desensitization.

Adapted from Wong JT, Nagy CS, Krinzman SJ, et al, "Rapid Oral Challenge-Desensitization for Patients With Aspirin Related Urticaria-Angioedema," *J Allergy Clin Immunol*, 2000, 105(5):997-1001.

CLOPIDOGREL

Oral Desensitization Protocol

Dose Number[a]	Dose (mg)[b]	Day of Protocol
1	0.1	1
2	0.2	
3	0.5	
4	1	
5[c]	2	1 or 2
6	4	2
7	8	
8	16	
9	32	
10[d]	75	2 or 3

Note: Patients received clopidogrel as a 2-day protocol (doses 1-5 on day 1 and doses 6-10 on day 2) or a 3-day protocol (doses 1-4 on day 1, doses 5-9 on day 2, and dose 10 on day 3)

[a]Doses 1-9 were an oral clopidogrel 1 mg/mL solution; dose 10 was a clopidogrel tablet.

[b]Doses were given 1 hour apart.

[c]Dose 5 was given on day 1 in the 2-day protocol and on day 2 in the 3-day protocol.

[d]Dose 10 was given on day 2 in the 2-day protocol and on day 3 in the 3-day protocol.

Note: Patients were observed for 1 hour after the last dose of clopidogrel.

Adapted from Fajt M and Patrov A, "Clopidogrel Hypersensitivity: A Novel Muli-Day Outpatient Oral Desensitization Regimen," *Ann Pharmacother*, 2010, 44(1):11-18.

REFERENCES

Cernadas JR, Brockow K, Romano A, et al, "General Considerations on Rapid Desensitization for Drug Hypersensitivity − A Consensus Statement," *Allergy*, 2010, 65(11):1357-66.

Cunha BA, "Antimicrobial Selection in the Penicillin-Allergic Patient," *Drugs Today (Barc)*, 2001, 37(6):377-383.

IMMUNIZATION ADMINISTRATION RECOMMENDATIONS

The following tables are taken from the General Recommendations on Immunization, 2011:

- Guidelines for Spacing of Live and Inactivated Antigens
- Guidelines for Administering Antibody-Containing Products and Vaccines
- Recommended Intervals Between Administration of Antibody-Containing Products and Measles- or Varicella-Containing Vaccine, by Product and Indication for Vaccination
- Vaccination of persons with Primary and Secondary Immunodeficiencies
- Needle length and Injection Site of I.M. injections

Guidelines for Spacing of Live and Inactivated Antigens

Antigen Combination	Recommended Minimum Interval Between Doses
Two or more inactivated[1]	May be administered simultaneously or at any interval between doses
Inactivated and live	May be administered simultaneously or at any interval between doses
Two or more live injectable[2]	28 days minimum interval, if not administered simultaneously

[1]Certain experts suggest a 28-day interval between tetanus toxoid, reduced diphtheria toxoid, and reduced acellular pertussis (Tdap) vaccine and tetravalent meningococcal conjugate vaccine if they are not administered simultaneously.

[2]Live oral vaccines (eg, Ty21a typhoid vaccine and rotavirus vaccine) may be administered simultaneously or at any interval before or after inactivated or live injectable vaccines.

Adapted from American Academy of Pediatrics, "Pertussis," In: Pickering LK, Baker CJ, Kimberlin DW, et al, eds, *Red Book*: 2009 Report of the Committee on Infectious Diseases, 28th ed, Elk Grove Village, IL: American Academy of Pediatrics, 2009, 22.

Guidelines for Administering Antibody-Containing Products[1] and Vaccines

Simultaneous Administration (during the same office visit)

Products Administered	Recommended Minimum Interval Between Doses
Antibody-containing products and inactivated antigen	Can be administered simultaneously at different anatomic sites or at any time interval between doses.
Antibody-containing products and live antigen	Should **not** be administered simultaneously.[2] If simultaneous administration of measles-containing vaccine or varicella vaccine is unavoidable, administer at different sites and revaccinate or test for seroconversion after the recommended interval.

Nonsimultaneous Administration

Products Administered: Administered first	Administered second	Recommended Minimum Interval Between Doses
Antibody-containing products	Inactivated antigen	No interval necessary
Inactivated antigen	Antibody-containing products	No interval necessary
Antibody-containing products	Live antigen	Dose-related[2,3]
Live antigen	Antibody-containing products	2 weeks[2]

[1]Blood products containing substantial amounts of immune globulin include intramuscular and intravenous immune globulin, specific hyperimmune globulin (eg, hepatitis B immune globulin, tetanus immune globulin, varicella zoster immune globulin, and rabies immune globulin), whole blood, packed red blood cells, plasma, and platelet products.

[2]Yellow fever vaccine, rotavirus vaccine, oral Ty21a typhoid vaccine, live-attenuated influenza vaccine, and zoster vaccine are exceptions to these recommendations. These live-attenuated vaccines can be administered at any time before, after, or simultaneously with an antibody-containing product.

[3]The duration of interference of antibody-containing products with the immune response to the measles component of measles-containing vaccine, and possibly varicella vaccine, is dose-related.

Recommended Intervals Between Administration of Antibody-Containing Products and Measles- or Varicella-Containing Vaccine, by Product and Indication for Vaccination

Product/Indication	Dose (mg IgG/kg) and Route[1]	Recommended Interval Before Measles- or Varicella-Containing Vaccine[2] Administration (mo)
Tetanus IG	I.M.: 250 units (10 mg IgG/kg)	3
Hepatitis A IG		
Contact prophylaxis	I.M.: 0.02 mL/kg (3.3 mg IgG/kg)	3
International travel	I.M.: 0.06 mL/kg (10 mg IgG/kg)	3
Hepatitis B IG	I.M.: 0.06 mL/kg (10 mg IgG/kg)	3
Rabies IG	I.M.: 20 int. units/kg (22 mg IgG/kg)	4
Varicella IG	I.M.: 125 units/10 kg (60-200 mg IgG/kg) (maximum: 625 units)	5
Measles prophylaxis IG		
Standard (ie, nonimmunocompromised) contact	I.M.: 0.25 mL/kg (40 mg IgG/kg)	5
Immunocompromised contact	I.M.: 0.50 mL/kg (80 mg IgG/kg)	6
Blood transfusion		
Red blood cells (RBCs), washed	I.V.: 10 mL/kg (negligible IgG/kg)	None
RBCs, adenine-saline added	I.V.: 10 mL/kg (10 mg IgG/kg)	3
Packed RBCs (hematocrit 65%)[3]	I.V.: 10 mL/kg (60 mg IgG/kg)	6
Whole blood cells (hematocrit 35% to 50%)[3]	I.V.: 10 mL/kg (80-100 mg IgG/kg)	6
Plasma/platelet products	I.V.: 10 mL/kg (160 mg IgG/kg)	7
Cytomegalovirus intravenous immune globulin (IGIV)	150 mg/kg maximum	6
IGIV		
Replacement therapy for immune deficiencies[4]	I.V.: 300-400 mg/kg[4]	8
Immune thrombocytopenic purpura treatment	I.V.: 400 mg/kg	8
Postexposure varicella prophylaxis[5]	I.V.: 400 mg/kg	8
Immune thrombocytopenic purpura treatment	I.V.: 1000 mg/kg	10
Kawasaki disease	I.V.: 2 g/kg	11
Monoclonal antibody to respiratory syncytial virus F protein (Synagis® [Medimmune])[6]	I.M.: 15 mg/kg	None

HIV = human immunodeficiency virus, IG = immune globulin, IgG = immune globulin G, IGIV = intravenous immune globulin, mg IgG/kg = milligrams of immune globulin G per kilogram of body weight, I.M. = intramuscular, I.V. = intravenous, RBCs = red blood cells

[1]This table is not intended for determining the correct indications and dosages for using antibody-containing products. Unvaccinated persons might not be fully protected against measles during the entire recommended interval, and additional doses of IG or measles vaccine might be indicated after measles exposure. Concentrations of measles antibody in an IG preparation can vary by manufacturer's lot. Rates of antibody clearance after receipt of an IG preparation also might vary. Recommended intervals are extrapolated from an estimated half-life of 30 days for passively acquired antibody and an observed interference with the immune response to measles vaccine for 5 months after a dose of 80 mg IgG/kg.

[2]Does not include zoster vaccine. Zoster vaccine may be given with antibody-containing blood products.

[3]Assumes a serum IgG concentration of 16 mg/mL.

[4]Measles and varicella vaccinations are recommended for children with asymptomatic or mildly symptomatic HIV infection but are contraindicated for persons with severe immunosuppression from HIV or any other immunosuppressive disorder.

[5]The investigational product VariZIG™, similar to licensed varicella-zoster IG (VZIG), is a purified human IG preparation made from plasma containing high levels of anti-varicella antibodies (IgG). The interval between VariZIG™ and varicella vaccine (Var or MMRV) is 5 months.

[6]Contains antibody only to respiratory syncytial virus

Vaccination of Persons With Primary and Secondary Immunodeficiencies

Category	Specific Immunodeficiency	Contraindicated Vaccines[1]	Risk-Specific Recommended Vaccines[1]	Effectiveness and Comments
Primary				
B-lymphocyte (humoral)	Severe antibody deficiencies (eg, X-linked agammaglobulinemia and common variable immunodeficiency)	Oral poliovirus (OPV)[2] Smallpox Live-attenuated influenza vaccine (LAIV) BCG Ty21a (live oral typhoid) Yellow fever	Pneumococcal Consider measles and varicella vaccination	The effectiveness of any vaccine is uncertain if it depends only on the humoral response (eg, PPSV or MPSV4) IGIV interferes with the immune response to measles vaccine and possibly varicella vaccine
	Less severe antibody deficiencies (eg, selective IgA deficiency and IgG subclass deficiency)	OPV[2] BCG Yellow Fever Other live-vaccines appear to be safe	Pneumococcal	All vaccines likely effective; immune response may be attenuated
T-lymphocyte (cell-mediated and humoral)	Complete defects (eg, severe combined immunodeficiency [SCID] disease, complete DiGeorge syndrome)	All live vaccines[3,4,5]	Pneumococcal	Vaccines might be ineffective
	Partial defects (eg, most patients with DiGeorge syndrome, Wiskott-Aldrich syndrome, ataxia-telangiectasia)	All live vaccines[3,4,5]	Pneumococcal Meningococcal Hib (if not administered in infancy)	Effectiveness of any vaccine depends on degree of immune suppression
Complement	Persistent complement, properdin, or factor B deficiency	None	Pneumococcal Meningococcal	All routine vaccines likely effective
Phagocytic function	Chronic granulomatous disease, leukocyte adhesion defect, and myeloperoxidase deficiency	Live bacterial vaccines[3]	Pneumococcal[6]	All inactivated vaccines safe and likely effective; live viral vaccines likely safe and effective

Vaccination of Persons With Primary and Secondary Immunodeficiencies *continued*

Category	Specific Immunodeficiency	Contraindicated Vaccines[1]	Risk-Specific Recommended Vaccines[1]	Effectiveness and Comments
Secondary				
	HIV/AIDS	OPV[2] Smallpox BCG LAIV Withhold MMR and varicella in severely immunocompromised persons Yellow fever vaccine might have a contraindication or a precaution depending on clinical parameters of immune function[9]	Pneumococcal Consider Hib (if not administered in infancy) and meningococcal vaccination.	MMR, varicella, rotavirus, and all inactivated vaccines, including inactivated influenza, might be effective.[7]
	Malignant neoplasm, transplantation, immunosuppressive or radiation therapy	Live viral and bacterial, depending on immune status[3,4]	Pneumococcal	Effectiveness of any vaccine depends on degree of immune suppression
	Asplenia	None	Pneumococcal Meningococcal Hib (if not administered in infancy)	All routine vaccines likely effective
	Chronic renal disease	LAIV	Pneumococcal Hepatitis B[8]	All routine vaccines likely effective

AIDS = acquired immunodeficiency syndrome; BCG = bacille Calmette-Guerin; Hib = *Haemophilus influenzae* type b; HIV = human immunodeficiency virus; IG = immunoglobulin; IGIV = immune globulin intravenous; LAIV = live, attenuated influenza vaccine; MMR = measles, mumps, and rubella; MPSV4 = quadrivalent meningococcal polysaccharide vaccine; OPV = oral poliovirus vaccine (live); PPSV = pneumococcal polysaccharide vaccine; TIV = trivalent inactivated influenza vaccine

[1]Other vaccines that are universally or routinely recommended should be administered if not contraindicated.

[2]OPV is no longer available in the United States.

[3]Live bacterial vaccines: BCG and oral Ty21a *Salmonella typhi* vaccine.

[4]Live viral vaccines: MMR, MMRV, OPV, LAIV, yellow fever, zoster, rotavirus, varicella, and vaccinia (smallpox). Smallpox vaccine is not recommended for children or the general public.

[5]Regarding T-lymphocyte immunodeficiency as a contraindication for rotavirus vaccine, data exist only for severe combined immunodeficiency.

[6]Pneumococcal vaccine is not indicated for children with chronic granulomatous disease beyond age-based universal recommendations for PCV. Children with chronic granulomatous disease are not at increased risk for pneumococcal disease.

[7]HIV-infected children should receive IG after exposure to measles and may receive varicella and measles vaccine if $CD4^+$ lymphocyte count is ≥15%.

[8]Indicated based on the risk from dialysis-based bloodborne transmission

[9]Symptomatic HIV infection or $CD4^+$ T-lymphocyte count of <200/mm^3 or <15% of total lymphocytes for children aged <6 years is a containdication to yellow fever vaccine administration. Asymptomatic HIV infection with $CD4^+$ T-lymphocyte count of 200-499/mm^3 for persons aged ≥6 years or 15% to 24% of total lymphocytes for children aged <6 years is a precaution for yellow fever vaccine administration. Details of yellow fever vaccine recommendations are available from the CDC. (CDC, "Yellow Fever Vaccine: Recommendations of the Advisory Committee on Immunization Practices [ACIP]," *MMWR Recomm Rep*, 2010, 59[No. RR-7].)

Adapted from American Academy of Pediatrics, "Passive Immunization," In: Pickering LK, Baker CJ, Kimberline DW, et al, eds, *Red Book*: 2009 Report of the Committee on Infectious Diseases, 28th ed, Elk Grove Village, IL: American Academy of Pediatrics, 2009, 74-5.

Needle Length and Injection Site of I.M. for Children Aged ≤18 years (by age) and Adults Aged ≥19 years (by sex and weight)

Age Group	Needle Length	Injection Site
Children (birth to 18 y)		
Neonates[1]	⅝" (16 mm)[2]	Anterolateral thigh
Infant 1-12 mo	1" (25 mm)	Anterolateral thigh
Toddler 1-2 y	1-1¼" (25-32 mm)	Anterolateral thigh[3]
	⅝[2]-1" (16-25 mm)	Deltoid muscle of the arm
Children 3-18 y	⅝[2]-1" (16-25 mm)	Deltoid muscle of the arm[3]
	1-1¼" (25-32 mm)	Anterolateral thigh
Adults ≥19 y		
Men and women <60 kg (130 lb)	1" (25 mm)[4]	Deltoid muscle of the arm
Men and women 60-70 kg (130-152 lb)	1" (25 mm)	
Men 70-118 kg (152-260 lb)	1-1½" (25-38 mm)	
Women 70-90 kg (152-200 lb)		
Men >118 kg (260 lb)	1½" (38 mm)	
Women >90 kg (200 lb)		

I.M. = intramuscular

[1]First 28 days of life

[2]If skin is stretched tightly and subcutaneous tissues are not bunched

[3]Preferred site

[4]Some experts recommend a ⅝" needle for men and women who weigh <60 kg

Adapted from Poland GA, Borrud A, Jacobsen RM, et al, "Determination of Deltoid Fat Pad Thickness: Implications for Needle Length in Adult Immunization," *JAMA*, 1997, 277:1709-11.

RECOMMENDATIONS FOR TRAVELERS

The Centers for Disease Control and Prevention (CDC) also provides guidance to assist travelers and their healthcare providers in deciding the vaccines, medications, and other measures necessary to prevent illness and injury during international travel. Information can be found on the following website: http://wwwnc.cdc.gov/travel

REFERENCE

Centers for Disease Control, "Recommendations of the Advisory Committee on Immunization Practices (ACIP): General Recommendations on Immunization," *MMWR Recomm Rep*, 2011, 60(2):1-61.

IMMUNIZATION RECOMMENDATIONS

Recommended Immunization Schedule for Persons Aged 0 Through 6 Years—United States • 2011

For those who fall behind or start late, see the catch-up schedule

Vaccine ▼ Age ▶	Birth	1 month	2 months	4 months	6 months	12 months	15 months	18 months	19–23 months	2–3 years	4–6 years
Hepatitis B[1]	HepB	HepB					HepB				
Rotavirus[2]			RV	RV	RV[2]						
Diphtheria, Tetanus, Pertussis[3]			DTaP	DTaP	DTaP	see footnote[3]	DTaP				DTaP
Haemophilus influenzae type b[4]			Hib	Hib	Hib[4]	Hib					
Pneumococcal[5]			PCV	PCV	PCV	PCV				PPSV	
Inactivated Poliovirus[6]			IPV	IPV		IPV					IPV
Influenza[7]								Influenza (Yearly)			
Measles, Mumps, Rubella[8]						MMR			see footnote[8]		MMR
Varicella[9]						Varicella			see footnote[9]		Varicella
Hepatitis A[10]							HepA (2 doses)			HepA Series	
Meningococcal[11]										MCV4	

Range of recommended ages for all children

Range of recommended ages for certain high-risk groups

This schedule includes recommendations in effect as of December 21, 2010. Any dose not administered at the recommended age should be administered at a subsequent visit, when indicated and feasible. The use of a combination vaccine generally is preferred over separate injections of its equivalent component vaccines. Considerations should include provider assessment, patient preference, and the potential for adverse events. Providers should consult the relevant Advisory Committee on Immunization Practices statement for detailed recommendations: **http://www.cdc.gov/vaccines/pubs/acip-list.htm**. Clinically significant adverse events that follow immunization should be reported to the Vaccine Adverse Event Reporting System (VAERS) at http://www.vaers.hhs.gov or by telephone, **(800) 822-7967**.

Footnotes to Recommended Immunization Schedule for Ages 0-6 Years

[1]**Hepatitis B vaccine (HepB).** *(Minimum age: birth)*

At birth:

- Administer monovalent HepB to all newborns before hospital discharge.
- If mother is hepatitis B surface antigen (HB_sAg)-positive, administer HepB and 0.5 mL of hepatitis B immune globulin (HBIG) within 12 hours of birth.
- If mother's HB_sAg status is unknown, administer HepB within 12 hours of birth. Determine mother's HB_sAg status as soon as possible and, if HB_sAg-positive, administer HBIG (no later than age 1 week).

Doses following the birth dose:

- The second dose should be administered at age 1 or 2 months. Monovalent HepB should be used for doses administered before age 6 weeks.
- Infants born to HB_sAg-positive mothers should be tested for HB_sAg and antibody to HB_sAg 1-2 months after completion of at least 3 doses of the HepB series, at age 9-18 months (generally at the next well-child visit).
- Administration of 4 doses of HepB to infants is permissible when combination vaccine containing HepB is administered after the birth dose.
- Infants who did not receive a birth dose should receive 3 doses of HepB on a schedule of 0, 1, and 6 months.
- The final (3rd or 4th) dose in the HepB series should be administered no earlier than age 24 weeks.

[2]**Rotavirus vaccine (RV).** *(Minimum age: 6 weeks)*

- Administer the first dose at age 6-14 weeks (maximum age: 14 weeks 6 days). Vaccination should not be initiated for infants aged 15 weeks 0 days or older.
- The maximum age for the final dose in the series is 8 months 0 days.
- If Rotarix® is administered at ages 2 and 4 months, a dose at 6 months is not indicated.

[3]**Diphtheria and tetanus toxoids and acellular pertussis vaccine (DTaP).** *(Minimum age: 6 weeks)*

- The fourth dose may be administered as early as age 12 months, provided at least 6 months have elapsed since the third dose.

[4] ***Haemophilus influenzae* type b conjugate vaccine (Hib).** *(Minimum age: 6 weeks)*

- If PRP-OMP (PedvaxHIB® or ComVax® [HepB-Hib]) is administered at ages 2 and 4 months, a dose at age 6 months is not indicated.
- Hiberix® should not be used for doses at ages 2, 4, or 6 months for the primary series but can be used as the final dose in children aged 12 months through 4 years.

[5]**Pneumococcal vaccine.** *(Minimum age: 6 weeks for pneumococcal conjugate vaccine [PCV]; 2 years for pneumococcal polysaccharide vaccine [PPSV])*

- PCV is recommended for all children aged <5 years. Administer 1 dose of PCV to all healthy children aged 24-59 months who are not completely vaccinated for their age.
- A PCV series begun with 7-valent PCV (PCV7) should be completed with 13-valent PCV (PCV13).
- A single supplemental dose of PCV13 is recommended for all children aged 14-59 months who have received an age-appropriate series of PCV7.
- A single supplemental dose of PCV13 is recommended for all children aged 60-71 months with underlying medical conditions who have received an age-appropriate series of PCV7.
- The supplemental dose of PCV13 should be administered at least 8 weeks after the previous dose of PCV7. See *MMWR* 2010:59(No. RR-11).
- Administer PPSV at least 8 weeks after last dose of PCV to children aged ≥2 years with certain underlying medical conditions, including a cochlear implant.

[6]**Inactivated poliovirus vaccine (IPV).** *(Minimum age: 6 weeks)*

- If 4 or more doses are administered prior to age 4 years an additional dose should be administered at age 4-6 years.
- The final dose in the series should be administered on or after the fourth birthday and at least 6 months following the previous dose.

[7]**Influenza vaccine (seasonal).** *(Minimum age: 6 months for trivalent inactivated influenza vaccine [TIV]; 2 years for live, attenuated influenza vaccine [LAIV])*

- For healthy children aged ≥2 years (ie, those who do not have underlying medical conditions that predispose them to influenza complications), either LAIV or TIV may be used, except LAIV should not be given to children aged 2-4 years who have had wheezing in the past 12 months.
- Administer 2 doses (separated by at least 4 weeks) to children aged 6 months through 8 years who are receiving seasonal influenza vaccine for the first time or who were vaccinated for the first time during the previous influenza season but only received 1 dose.
- Children aged 6 months through 8 years who received no doses of monovalent 2009 H1N1 vaccine should receive 2 doses of 2010–2011 seasonal influenza vaccine. See *MMWR* 2010;59(No. RR-8):33–34.

[8]**Measles, mumps, and rubella vaccine (MMR).** *(Minimum age: 12 months)*

- The second dose may be administered before age 4 years, provided at least 4 weeks have elapsed since the first dose.

[9]**Varicella vaccine.** *(Minimum age: 12 months)*

- The second dose may be administered before age 4 years, provided at least 3 months have elapsed since the first dose.
- For children aged 12 months through 12 years the recommended minimum interval between doses is 3 months. However, if the second dose was administered at least 4 weeks after the first dose, it can be accepted as valid.

[10]**Hepatitis A vaccine (HepA).** *(Minimum age: 12 months)*

- Administer 2 doses at least 6 months apart.
- HepA is recommended for children aged older than 23 months who live in areas where vaccination programs target older children, who are at increased risk for infection, or for whom immunity against hepatitis A is desired.

[11]**Meningococcal conjugate vaccine, quadrivalent (MCV4).** *(Minimum age: 2 years)*

- Administer 2 doses of MCV4 at least 8 weeks apart to children aged 2-10 years with persistent complement component deficiency and anatomic or functional asplenia, and 1 dose every 5 years thereafter.
- Persons with human immunodeficiency virus (HIV) infection who are vaccinated with MCV4 should receive 2 doses at least 8 weeks apart.
- Administer 1 dose of MCV4 to children aged 2-10 years who travel to countries with highly endemic or epidemic disease and during outbreaks caused by a vaccine serogroup.
- Administer MCV4 to children at continued risk for meningococcal disease who were previously vaccinated with MCV4 or meningococcal polysaccharide vaccine after 3 years if the first dose was administered at age 2-6 years.

The recommended immunization schedules for persons aged 0-18 years are approved by the Advisory Committee on Immunization Practices (**http://www.cdc.gov/vaccines/recs/acip**), the American Academy of Pediatrics (**http://www.aap.org**), and the American Academy of Family Physicians (**http://www.aafp.org**).

Recommended Immunization Schedule for Persons Aged 7 Through 18 Years—United States • 2011

For those who fall behind or start late, see the schedule below and the catch-up schedule

Vaccine ▼ Age ▶	7–10 years	11–12 years	13–18 years
Tetanus, Diphtheria, Pertussis[1]		Tdap	Tdap
Human Papillomavirus[2]	*see footnote* [2]	HPV (3 doses)(females)	HPV series
Meningococcal[3]	MCV4	MCV4	MCV4
Influenza[4]		Influenza (Yearly)	
Pneumococcal[5]		Pneumococcal	
Hepatitis A[6]		HepA Series	
Hepatitis B[7]		Hep B Series	
Inactivated Poliovirus[8]		IPV Series	
Measles, Mumps, Rubella[9]		MMR Series	
Varicella[10]		Varicella Series	

Range of recommended ages for all children

Range of recommended ages for catch-up immunization

Range of recommended ages for certain high-risk groups

This schedule includes recommendations in effect as of December 21, 2010. Any dose not administered at the recommended age should be administered at a subsequent visit, when indicated and feasible. The use of a combination vaccine generally is preferred over separate injections of its equivalent component vaccines. Considerations should include provider assessment, patient preference, and the potential for adverse events. Providers should consult the relevant Advisory Committee on Immunization Practices statement for detailed recommendations: **http://www.cdc.gov/vaccines/pubs/acip-list.htm**. Clinically significant adverse events that follow immunization should be reported to the Vaccine Adverse Event Reporting System (VAERS) at **http://www.vaers.hhs.gov** or by telephone, **(800) 822-7967**.

Footnotes to Recommended Immunization Schedule for Ages 7-18 Years

[1]**Tetanus and diphtheria toxoids and acellular pertussis vaccine (Tdap).** *(Minimum age: 10 years for Boostrix® and 11 years for Adacel®)*

- Persons aged 11-18 years who have not received Tdap should receive a dose followed by Td booster doses every 10 years thereafter.
- Persons aged 7 through 10 years who are not fully immunized against pertussis (including those never vaccinated or with unknown pertussis vaccination status) should receive a single dose of Tdap. Refer to the catch-up schedule if additional doses of tetanus and diphtheria toxoid–containing vaccine are needed.
- Tdap can be administered regardless of the interval since the last tetanus and diphtheria toxoid–containing vaccine.

[2]**Human papillomavirus vaccine (HPV).** *(Minimum age: 9 years)*

- Quadrivalent HPV vaccine (HPV4) or bivalent HPV vaccine (HPV2) is recommended for the prevention of cervical precancers and cancers in females.
- HPV4 is recommended for prevention of cervical precancers, cancers, and genital warts in females.
- HPV4 may be administered in a 3-dose series to males aged 9-18 years to reduce their likelihood of genital warts.
- Administer the second dose 1-2 months after the first dose and the third dose 6 months after the first dose (at least 24 weeks after the first dose).

[3]**Meningococcal conjugate vaccine, quadrivalent (MCV4).** *(Minimum age: 2 years)*

- Administer MCV4 at age 11-12 years with a booster dose at age 16 years.
- Administer 1 dose at age 13-18 years if not previously vaccinated.
- Persons who received their first dose at age 13-15 years should receive a booster dose at age 16-18 years.
- Administer 1 dose to previously unvaccinated college freshmen living in a dormitory.
- Administer 2 doses at least 8 weeks apart to children aged 2-10 years with persistent complement component deficiency and anatomic or functional asplenia, and 1 dose every 5 years thereafter.
- Persons with HIV infection who are vaccinated with MCV4 should receive 2 doses at least 8 weeks apart.

- Administer 1 dose of MCV4 to children aged 2-10 years who travel to countries with highly endemic or epidemic disease and during outbreaks caused by a vaccine serogroup.
- Administer MCV4 to children at continued risk for meningococcal disease who were previously vaccinated with MCV4 or meningococcal polysaccharide vaccine after 3 years (if first dose administered at age 2-6 years) or after 5 years (if first dose administered at age 7 years or older).

[4]Influenza vaccine (seasonal).

- For healthy nonpregnant persons aged 7-18 years (ie, those who do not have underlying medical conditions that predispose them to influenza complications), either LAIV or TIV may be used.
- Administer 2 doses (separated by at least 4 weeks) to children aged 6 months through 8 years who are receiving seasonal influenza vaccine for the first time or who were vaccinated for the first time during the previous influenza season but only received 1 dose.
- Children 6 months through 8 years of age who received no doses of monovalent 2009 H1N1 vaccine should receive 2 doses of 2010-2011 seasonal influenza vaccine. See *MMWR* 2010;59(No. RR-8):33–34.

[5]Pneumococcal vaccines.

- A single dose of 13-valent pneumococcal conjugate vaccine (PCV13) may be administered to children aged 6-18 years who have functional or anatomic asplenia, HIV infection or other immunocompromising condition, cochlear implant or CSF leak. See *MMWR* 2010;59(No. RR-11).
- The dose of PCV13 should be administered at least 8 weeks after the previous dose of PCV7.
- Administer pneumococcal polysaccharide vaccine at least 8 weeks after the last dose of PCV to children aged 2 years or older with certain underlying medical conditions, including a cochlear implant. A single revaccination should be administered after 5 years to children with functional or anatomic asplenia or an immunocompromising condition.

[6]Hepatitis A vaccine (HepA).

- Administer 2 doses at least 6 months apart.
- HepA is recommended for children >23 months who live in areas where vaccination programs target older children, who are at increased risk of infection, or for whom immunity against hepatitis A is desired.

[7]Hepatitis B vaccine (HepB).

- Administer the 3-dose series to those not previously vaccinated. For those with incomplete vaccination, follow the catch-up schedule.
- A 2-dose series (separated by at least 4 months) of adult formulation Recombivax HB® is licensed for children aged 11-15 years.

[8]Inactivated poliovirus vaccine (IPV).

- The final dose in the series should be administered on or after the fourth birthday and at least 6 months following the previous dose.
- If both OPV and IPV were administered as part of a series, a total of 4 doses should be administered, regardless of the child's current age.

[9]Measles, mumps, and rubella vaccine (MMR).

- The minimum interval between the 2 doses of MMR is 4 weeks.

[10]Varicella vaccine.

- For persons aged 7-18 years without evidence of immunity [see *MMWR*, 2007, 56(RR-4)], administer 2 doses if not previously vaccinated or the second dose if only 1 dose has been administered.
- For persons aged 7-12 years, the recommended minimum interval between doses is 3 months. However, if the second dose was administered at least 4 weeks after the first dose, it can be accepted as valid.
- For persons aged ≥13 years, the minimum interval between doses is 4 weeks.

The recommended immunization schedules for persons age 0-18 years are approved by the Advisory Committee on Immunization Practices (**http://www.cdc.gov/vaccines/recs/acip**), the American Academy of Pediatrics (**http://www.aap.org**), and the American Academy of Family Physicians (**http://www.aafp.org**).

Catch-up Immunization Schedule for Persons Aged 4 Months to 18 Years Who Start Late or Who Are >1 Month Behind – United States, 2011

The table below provides catch-up schedules and minimum intervals between doses for children whose vaccinations have been delayed. A vaccine series does not need to be restarted, regardless of the time that has elapsed between doses. Use the section appropriate for the child's age.

Vaccine	Minimum Age for Dose 1	Minimum Interval Between Doses			
		Dose 1 to Dose 2	Dose 2 to Dose 3	Dose 3 to Dose 4	Dose 4 to Dose 5
Catch-up Schedule for Persons Age 4 Months to 6 Years					
Hepatitis B[1]	Birth	**4 weeks**	**8 weeks** (and ≥16 weeks after 1st dose)		
Rotavirus[2]	6 wk	**4 weeks**	**4 weeks**[2]		
Diphtheria, tetanus, pertussis[3]	6 wk	**4 weeks**	**4 weeks**	**6 months**	**6 months**[3]
Haemophilus influenzae type b[4]	6 wk	**4 weeks** if 1st dose administered at age <12 months **8 weeks (as final dose)** if 1st dose administered at age 12-14 months **No further doses needed** if 1st dose administered at age ≥15 months	**4 weeks**[4] if current age <12 months **8 weeks (as final dose)**[4] if current age ≥12 months and 1st dose is administered <12 months and 2nd dose administered at age <15 months **No further doses needed** if previous dose administered at age ≥15 months	**8 weeks (as final dose)** This dose only necessary for children age 12-59 months who received 3 doses before age 12 months	
Pneumococcal[5]	6 wk	**4 weeks** if 1st dose administered at age <12 months **8 weeks (as final dose for healthy children)** if 1st dose administered at age ≥12 months or current age 24-59 months **No further doses needed** for healthy children if 1st dose administered at age ≥24 months	**4 weeks** if current age <12 months **8 weeks (as final dose for healthy children)** if current age ≥12 months **No further doses needed** for healthy children if previous dose administered at age ≥24 months	**8 weeks (as final dose)** This dose only necessary for children age 12-59 months who received 3 doses before age 12 months or for high-risk children who received 3 doses at any age	
Inactivated poliovirus[6]	6 wk	**4 weeks**	**4 weeks**	**6 months**[6]	
Measles, mumps, rubella[7]	12 mo	**4 weeks**			
Varicella[8]	12 mo	**3 months**			
Hepatitits A[9]	12 mo	**6 months**			
Catch-up Schedule for Persons Age 7-18 Years					
Tetanus, diphtheria/tetanus, diphtheria, pertussis[10]	7 y	**4 weeks**	**4 weeks** if 1st dose administered at age <12 months **6 months** if 1st dose administered at age ≥12 months	**6 months** if 1st dose administered at age <12 months	
Human papillomavirus[11]	9 y	**Routine dosing intervals are recommended**[11]			
Hepatitis A[9]	12 mo	**6 months**			
Hepatitis B[1]	Birth	**4 weeks**	**8 weeks** (and ≥16 weeks after 1st dose)		
Inactivated poliovirus[6]	6 wk	**4 weeks**	**4 weeks**[6]	**6 months**[6]	
Measles, mumps, rubella[7]	12 mo	**4 weeks**			
Varicella[8]	12 mo	**3 months** if the person is age <13 years **4 weeks** if the person is age ≥13 years			

Footnotes to Catch-up Immunization Schedule Table

[1]Hepatitis B vaccine (HepB).

- Administer the 3-dose series to those not previously vaccinated.
- The minimum age for the third dose of HepB is 24 weeks.
- A 2-dose series (separated by at least 4 months) of adult formulation Recombivax HB® is licensed for children aged 11-15 years.

[2]Rotavirus vaccine (RV).

- The maximum age for the first dose is 14 weeks 6 days. Vaccination should not be initiated for infants aged ≥15 weeks 0 days.
- The maximum age for the final dose in the series is 8 months 0 days.
- If Rotarix® was administered for the first and second doses, a third dose is not indicated.

[3]Diphtheria and tetanus toxoids and acellular pertussis vaccine (DTaP).

- The fifth dose is not necessary if the fourth dose was administered at age ≥4 years.

[4]*Haemophilus influenzae* type b conjugate (Hib).

- 1 dose of Hib vaccine should be considered for unvaccinated persons aged 5 years or older who have sickle cell disease, leukemia, or HIV infection, or who have had a splenectomy.
- If the first 2 doses were PRP-OMP (PedvaxHIB® or ComVax®), and administered at age ≤11 months, the third (and final) dose should be administered at age 12-15 months and ≥8 weeks after the second dose.
- If first dose administered at age 7-11 months, administer second dose ≥4 weeks later and a final dose at age 12-15 months.

[5]Pneumococcal vaccine.

- Administer 1 dose of 13-valent pneumococcal conjugate vaccine (PCV13) to all healthy children aged 24-59 months with any incomplete PCV schedule (PCV7 or PCV13).
- For children aged 24-71 months with underlying medical conditions, administer 1 dose of PCV13 if 3 doses of PCV were received previously or administer 2 doses of PCV13 ≥8 weeks apart if <3 doses of PCV were received previously.
- A single dose of PCV13 is recommended for certain children with underlying medical conditions through 18 years of age. See age-specific schedules for details.
- Administer pneumococcal polysaccharide vaccine (PPSV) to children aged ≥2 years with certain underlying medical conditions, including a cochlear implant, at ≥8 weeks after the last dose of PCV. A single revaccination should be administered after 5 years to children with functional or anatomic asplenia or an immunocompromising condition. See *MMWR* 2010;59(No. RR-11).

[6]Inactivated poliovirus vaccine (IPV).

- The final dose in the series should be administered on or after the fourth birthday and ≥6 months following the previous dose.
- A fourth dose is not necessary if the third dose was administered at age ≥4 years and ≥6 months following the previous dose.
- In the first 6 months of life, minimum age and minimum intervals are only recommended if the person is at risk for imminent exposure to circulating poliovirus (ie, travel to a polio-endemic region or during an outbreak).

[7]Measles, mumps, and rubella vaccine (MMR).

- Administer the second dose routinely at age 4-6 years. The minimum interval between the 2 doses of MMR is 4 weeks.

[8]Varicella vaccine.

- Administer the second dose routinely at age 4-6 years.
- If the second dose was administered at least 4 weeks after the first dose, it can be accepted as valid.

[9]Hepatitis A vaccine (HepA).

- HepA is recommended for children aged >23 months who live in areas where vaccination programs target older children, who are at increased risk for infection, or for whom immunity against hepatitis A is desired.

[10]Tetanus and diphtheria toxoids (Td) and tetanus and diphtheria toxoids and acellular pertussis vaccine (Tdap).

- Doses of DTaP are counted as part of the Td/Tdap series.
- Tdap should be substituted for a single dose of Td in the catch-up series for children aged 7-10 years or as a booster for children aged 11-18 years; use Td for other doses.

[11]Human papillomavirus vaccine (HPV).

- Administer the series to females at age 13-18 years if not previously vaccinated or have not completed the vaccine series.
- Quadrivalent HPV vaccine (HPV4) may be administered in a 3-dose series to males aged 9-18 years to reduce their likelihood of genital warts.
- Use recommended routine dosing intervals for series catch-up (ie, the second and third doses should be administered at 1-2 and 6 months after the first dose). The minimum interval between the first and second doses is 4 weeks. The minimum interval between the second and third doses is 12 weeks, and the third dose should be administered ≥24 weeks after the first dose.

Information about reporting reactions after immunization is available online at **http://www.vaers.hhs.gov** or by telephone, (800) 822-7967. Suspected cases of vaccine-preventable diseases should be reported to the state or local health department. Additional information, including precautions and contraindications for immunization, is available from the National Center for Immunization and Respiratory Diseases at **http://www.cdc.gov/vaccines** or telephone, **(800) CDC-INFO** (800-232-4636).

Recommended adult immunization schedule, by vaccine and age group—United States, 2011

VACCINE ▼ AGE GROUP ▶	19–26 years	27–49 years	50–59 years	60–64 years	≥65 years
Influenza[1],*	1 dose annually				
Tetanus, diphtheria, pertussis (Td/Tdap)[2],*	Substitute 1-time dose of Tdap for Td booster; then boost with Td every 10 years				Td booster every 10 years
Varicella[3],*	2 doses				
Human papillomavirus (HPV)[4],*	3 doses (females)				
Zoster[5]				1 dose	
Measles, mumps, rubella (MMR)[6],*	1 or 2 doses		1 dose		
Pneumococcal (polysaccharide)[7,8]	1 or 2 doses				1 dose
Meningococcal[9],*	1 or more doses				
Hepatitis A[10],*	2 doses				
Hepatitis B[11],*	3 doses				

*Covered by the Vaccine Injury Compensation Program

For all persons in this category who meet the age requirements and who lack evidence of immunity (e.g., lack documentation of vaccination or have no evidence of previous infection)

Recommended if some other risk factor is present (e.g., based on medical, occupational, lifestyle, or other indications)

No recommendation

Vaccines that might be indicated for adults, based on medical and other indications—United States, 2011

VACCINE ▼ INDICATION ▶	Pregnancy	Immunocompromising conditions (excluding human immunodeficiency virus [HIV])[3,5,6,13]	HIV infection[3,6,12,13] CD4+ T lymphocyte count <200 cells/μL	HIV infection CD4+ T lymphocyte count ≥200 cells/μL	Diabetes, heart disease, chronic lung disease, chronic alcoholism	Asplenia[12] (including elective splenectomy) and persistent complement component deficiencies	Chronic liver disease	Kidney failure, end-stage renal disease, receipt of hemodialysis	Health-care personnel
Influenza[1],*	1 dose TIV annually								1 dose TIV or LAIV annually
Tetanus, diphtheria, pertussis (Td/Tdap)[2],*	Td	Substitute 1-time dose of Tdap for Td booster; then boost with Td every 10 years							
Varicella[3],*	Contraindicated			2 doses					
Human papillomavirus (HPV)[4],*		3 doses through age 26 years							
Zoster[5]	Contraindicated			1 dose					
Measles, mumps, rubella[6],*	Contraindicated			1 or 2 doses					
Pneumococcal (polysaccharide)[7,8]		1 or 2 doses							
Meningococcal[9],*	1 or more doses								
Hepatitis A[10],*	2 doses								
Hepatitis B[11],*	3 doses								

*Covered by the Vaccine Injury Compensation Program

For all persons in this category who meet the age requirements and who lack evidence of immunity (e.g., lack documentation of vaccination or have no evidence of previous infection)

Recommended if some other risk factor is present (e.g., on the basis of medical, occupational, lifestyle, or other indications)

No recommendation

Footnotes to Recommended Adult Immunization Schedule

[1]Influenza vaccination.

- Annual vaccination against influenza is recommended for all persons aged 6 months and older, including all adults. Healthy, nonpregnant adults aged less than 50 years without high-risk medical conditions can receive either intranasally administered live, attenuated influenza vaccine (FluMist®), or inactivated vaccine. Other persons should receive the inactivated vaccine. Adults aged 65 years and older can receive the standard influenza vaccine or the high-dose (Fluzone®) influenza vaccine. Additional information about influenza vaccination is available at http://www.cdc.gov/vaccines/vpd-vac/flu/default.htm.

[2]Tetanus, diphtheria, and acellular pertussis (Td/Tdap) vaccination.

- Administer a one-time dose of Tdap to adults aged less than 65 years who have not received Tdap previously or for whom vaccine status is unknown to replace one of the 10-year Td boosters, and as soon as feasible to all 1) postpartum women, 2) close contacts of infants younger than age 12 months (eg, grandparents and child-care providers), and 3) health-care personnel with direct patient contact. Adults aged 65 years and older who have not previously received Tdap and who have close contact with an infant aged less than 12 months also should be vaccinated. Other adults aged 65 years and older may receive Tdap. Tdap can be administered regardless of interval since the most recent tetanus or diphtheria-containing vaccine.
- Adults with uncertain or incomplete history of completing a 3-dose primary vaccination series with Td-containing vaccines should begin or complete a primary vaccination series. For unvaccinated adults, administer the first 2 doses at least 4 weeks apart and the third dose 6–12 months after the second. If incompletely vaccinated (ie, less than 3 doses), administer remaining doses. Substitute a one-time dose of Tdap for one of the doses of Td, either in the primary series or for the routine booster, whichever comes first.
- If a woman is pregnant and received the most recent Td vaccination 10 or more years previously, administer Td during the second or third trimester. If the woman received the most recent Td vaccination less than 10 years previously, administer Tdap during the immediate postpartum period. At the clinician's discretion, Td may be deferred during pregnancy and Tdap substituted in the immediate postpartum period, or Tdap may be administered instead of Td to a pregnant woman after an informed discussion with the woman.
- The ACIP statement for recommendations for administering Td as prophylaxis in wound management is available at http://www.cdc.gov/vaccines/pubs/acip-list.htm.

[3]Varicella vaccination.

- All adults without evidence of immunity to varicella should receive 2 doses of single-antigen varicella vaccine if not previously vaccinated or a second dose if they have received only 1 dose, unless they have a medical contraindication. Special consideration should be given to those who 1) have close contact with persons at high risk for severe disease (eg, health-care personnel and family contacts of persons with immunocompromising conditions) or 2) are at high risk for exposure or transmission (eg, teachers; child-care employees; residents and staff members of institutional settings, including correctional institutions; college students; military personnel; adolescents and adults living in households with children; nonpregnant women of childbearing age; and international travelers).
- Evidence of immunity to varicella in adults includes any of the following: 1) documentation of 2 doses of varicella vaccine at least 4 weeks apart; 2) U.S.-born before 1980 (although for health-care personnel and pregnant women, birth before 1980 should not be considered evidence of immunity); 3) history of varicella based on diagnosis or verification of varicella by a health-care provider (for a patient reporting a history of or having an atypical case, a mild case, or both, health-care providers should seek either an epidemiologic link with a typical varicella case or to a laboratory-confirmed case or evidence of laboratory confirmation, if it was performed at the time of acute disease); 4) history of herpes zoster based on diagnosis or verification of herpes zoster by a health-care provider; or 5) laboratory evidence of immunity or laboratory confirmation of disease.
- Pregnant women should be assessed for evidence of varicella immunity. Women who do not have evidence of immunity should receive the first dose of varicella vaccine upon completion or termination of pregnancy and before discharge from the health-care facility. The second dose should be administered 4–8 weeks after the first dose.

[4]Human papillomavirus (HPV) vaccination.

- HPV vaccination with either quadrivalent (HPV4) vaccine or bivalent vaccine (HPV2) is recommended for females at age 11 or 12 years and catch-up vaccination for females aged 13-26 years.
- Ideally, vaccine should be administered before potential exposure to HPV through sexual activity; however, females who are sexually active should still be vaccinated consistent with age-based recommendations. Sexually active females who have not been infected with any of the four HPV vaccine types (types 6, 11, 16, and 18, all of which HPV4 prevents) or any of the two HPV vaccine types (types 16 and 18, both of which HPV2 prevents) receive the full benefit of the vaccination. Vaccination is less beneficial for females who have already been infected with one or more of the HPV vaccine types. HPV4 or HPV2 can be administered to persons with a history of genital warts, abnormal Papanicolaou test, or positive HPV DNA test, because these conditions are not evidence of previous infection with all vaccine HPV types.
- HPV4 may be administered to males aged 9-26 years to reduce their likelihood of genital warts. HPV4 would be most effective when administered before exposure to HPV through sexual contact.
- A complete series for either HPV4 or HPV2 consists of 3 doses. The second dose should be administered 1–2 months after the first dose; the third dose should be administered 6 months after the first dose.

- Although HPV vaccination is not specifically recommended for persons with the medical indications described in Figure 2, "Vaccines that might be indicated for adults based on medical and other indications," it may be administered to these persons because the HPV vaccine is not a live-virus vaccine. However, the immune response and vaccine efficacy might be less for persons with the medical indications described in Figure 2 than in persons who do not have the medical indications described or who are immunocompetent.

[5]Herpes zoster vaccination.

- A single dose of zoster vaccine is recommended for adults aged 60 years and older regardless of whether they report a previous episode of herpes zoster. Persons with chronic medical conditions may be vaccinated unless their condition constitutes a contraindication.

[6]Measles, mumps, rubella (MMR) vaccination.

- Adults born before 1957 generally are considered immune to measles and mumps. All adults born in 1957 or later should have documentation of 1 or more doses of MMR vaccine unless they have a medical contraindication to the vaccine, laboratory evidence of immunity to each of the three diseases, or documentation of provider-diagnosed measles or mumps disease. For rubella, documentation of provider-diagnosed disease is not considered acceptable evidence of immunity.
- *Measles component:* A second dose of MMR vaccine, administered a minimum of 28 days after the first dose, is recommended for adults who 1) have been recently exposed to measles or are in an outbreak setting; 2) are students in postsecondary educational institutions; 3) work in a health-care facility; or 4) plan to travel internationally. Persons who received inactivated (killed) measles vaccine or measles vaccine of unknown type during 1963–1967 should be revaccinated with 2 doses of MMR vaccine.
- *Mumps component:* A second dose of MMR vaccine, administered a minimum of 28 days after the first dose, is recommended for adults who 1) live in a community experiencing a mumps outbreak and are in an affected age group; 2) are students in postsecondary educational institutions; 3) work in a health-care facility; or 4) plan to travel internationally. Persons vaccinated before 1979 with either killed mumps vaccine or mumps vaccine of unknown type who are at high risk for mumps infection (eg, persons who are working in a health-care facility) should be revaccinated with 2 doses of MMR vaccine.
- *Rubella component:* For women of childbearing age, regardless of birth year, rubella immunity should be determined. If there is no evidence of immunity, women who are not pregnant should be vaccinated. Pregnant women who do not have evidence of immunity should receive MMR vaccine upon completion or termination of pregnancy and before discharge from the health-care facility.
- *Health-care personnel born before 1957:* For unvaccinated health-care personnel born before 1957 who lack laboratory evidence of measles, mumps, and/or rubella immunity or laboratory confirmation of disease, health-care facilities should 1) consider routinely vaccinating personnel with 2 doses of MMR vaccine at the appropriate interval (for measles and mumps) and 1 dose of MMR vaccine (for rubella), and 2) recommend 2 doses of MMR vaccine at the appropriate interval during an outbreak of measles or mumps, and 1 dose during an outbreak of rubella. Complete information about evidence of immunity is available at http://www.cdc.gov/vaccines/recs/provisional/default.htm.

[7]Pneumococcal polysaccharide (PPSV) vaccination.

- Vaccinate all persons with the following indications:
  - *Medical:* Chronic lung disease (including asthma); chronic cardiovascular diseases; diabetes mellitus; chronic liver diseases; cirrhosis; chronic alcoholism; functional or anatomic asplenia (eg, sickle cell disease or splenectomy [if elective splenectomy is planned, vaccinate at least 2 weeks before surgery]); immunocompromising conditions (including chronic renal failure or nephrotic syndrome); and cochlear implants and cerebrospinal fluid leaks. Vaccinate as close to HIV diagnosis as possible.
  - *Other:* Residents of nursing homes or long-term care facilities and persons who smoke cigarettes. Routine use of PPSV is not recommended for American Indians/Alaska Natives or persons aged less than 65 years unless they have underlying medical conditions that are PPSV indications. However, public health authorities may consider recommending PPSV for American Indians/Alaska Natives and persons aged 50-64 years who are living in areas where the risk for invasive pneumococcal disease is increased.

[8]Revaccination with PPSV.

- One-time revaccination after 5 years is recommended for persons aged 19-64 years with chronic renal failure or nephrotic syndrome; functional or anatomic asplenia (eg, sickle cell disease or splenectomy); and for persons with immunocompromising conditions. For persons aged 65 years and older, one-time revaccination is recommended if they were vaccinated 5 or more years previously and were aged less than 65 years at the time of primary vaccination.

[9]Meningococcal vaccination.

- Meningococcal vaccine should be administered to persons with the following indications:
  - *Medical:* A 2-dose series of meningococcal conjugate vaccine is recommended for adults with anatomic or functional asplenia, or persistent complement component deficiencies. Adults with HIV infection who are vaccinated should also receive a routine 2-dose series. The 2 doses should be administered at 0 and 2 months.
  - *Other:* A single dose of meningococcal vaccine is recommended for unvaccinated first-year college students living in dormitories; microbiologists routinely exposed to isolates of *Neisseria meningitidis*; military recruits; and persons who travel to or live in countries in which meningococcal disease is hyperendemic or epidemic (eg, the "meningitis belt" of sub-Saharan Africa during the dry season [December through June]), particularly if their contact with local populations will be prolonged. Vaccination is required by the government of Saudi Arabia for all travelers to Mecca during the annual Hajj.

- Meningococcal conjugate vaccine, quadrivalent (MCV4) is preferred for adults with any of the preceding indications who are aged 55 years and younger; meningococcal polysaccharide vaccine (MPSV4) is preferred for adults aged 56 years and older. Revaccination with MCV4 every 5 years is recommended for adults previously vaccinated with MCV4 or MPSV4 who remain at increased risk for infection (eg, adults with anatomic or functional asplenia, or persistent complement component deficiencies).

[10]Hepatitis A vaccination.

- Vaccinate persons with any of the following indications and any person seeking protection from hepatitis A virus (HAV) infection:
  - *Behavioral:* Men who have sex with men and persons who use injection drugs.
  - *Occupational:* Persons working with HAV-infected primates or with HAV in a research laboratory setting.
  - *Medical:* Persons with chronic liver disease and persons who receive clotting factor concentrates.
  - *Other:* Persons traveling to or working in countries that have high or intermediate endemicity of hepatitis A (a list of countries is available at http://wwwn.cdc.gov/travel/contentdiseases.aspx).
- Unvaccinated persons who anticipate close personal contact (eg, household or regular babysitting) with an international adoptee during the first 60 days after arrival in the United States from a country with high or intermediate endemicity should be vaccinated. The first dose of the 2-dose hepatitis A vaccine series should be administered as soon as adoption is planned, ideally 2 or more weeks before the arrival of the adoptee.
- Single-antigen vaccine formulations should be administered in a 2-dose schedule at either 0 and 6–12 months (Havrix®), or 0 and 6–18 months (VAQTA®). If the combined hepatitis A and hepatitis B vaccine (Twinrix®) is used, administer 3 doses at 0, 1, and 6 months; alternatively, a 4-dose schedule may be used, administered on days 0, 7, and 21–30, followed by a booster dose at month 12.

[11]Hepatitis B vaccination.

- Vaccinate persons with any of the following indications and any person seeking protection from hepatitis B virus (HBV) infection:
  - *Behavioral:* Sexually active persons who are not in a long-term, mutually monogamous relationship (eg, persons with more than one sex partner during the previous 6 months); persons seeking evaluation or treatment for a sexually transmitted disease (STD); current or recent injection-drug users; and men who have sex with men.
  - *Occupational:* Health-care personnel and public-safety workers who are exposed to blood or other potentially infectious body fluids.
  - *Medical:* Persons with end-stage renal disease, including patients receiving hemodialysis; persons with HIV infection; and persons with chronic liver disease.
  - *Other:* Household contacts and sex partners of persons with chronic HBV infection; clients and staff members of institutions for persons with developmental disabilities; and international travelers to countries with high or intermediate prevalence of chronic HBV infection (a list of countries is available at http://wwwn.cdc.gov/travel/contentdiseases.aspx).
- Hepatitis B vaccination is recommended for all adults in the following settings: STD treatment facilities; HIV testing and treatment facilities; facilities providing drug-abuse treatment and prevention services; health-care settings targeting services to injection-drug users or men who have sex with men; correctional facilities; end-stage renal disease programs and facilities for chronic hemodialysis patients; and institutions and nonresidential day-care facilities for persons with developmental disabilities.
- Administer missing doses to complete a 3-dose series of hepatitis B vaccine to those persons not vaccinated or not completely vaccinated. The second dose should be administered 1 month after the first dose; the third dose should be given at least 2 months after the second dose (and at least 4 months after the first dose). If the combined hepatitis A and hepatitis B vaccine (Twinrix®) is used, administer 3 doses at 0, 1, and 6 months; alternatively, a 4-dose Twinrix® schedule, administered on days 0, 7, and 21-30, followed by a booster dose at month 12 may be used.
- Adult patients receiving hemodialysis or with other immunocompromising conditions should receive 1 dose of 40 µg/mL (Recombivax HB®) administered on a 3-dose schedule or 2 doses of 20 µg/mL (Engerix-B®) administered simultaneously on a 4-dose schedule at 0, 1, 2, and 6 months.

[12]Selected conditions for which *Haemophilus influenzae* type b (Hib) vaccine may be used.

- 1 dose of Hib vaccine should be considered for persons who have sickle cell disease, leukemia, or HIV infection, or who have had a splenectomy, if they have not previously received Hib vaccine.

[13]Immunocompromising conditions.

- Inactivated vaccines generally are acceptable (eg, pneumococcal, meningococcal, influenza [inactivated influenza vaccine]) and live vaccines generally are avoided in persons with immune deficiencies or immunocompromising conditions. Information on specific conditions is available at http://www.cdc.gov/vaccines/pubs/acip-list.htm.

REFERENCE

"Recommended Adult Immunization Schedule – United States, 2011," *MMWR Recomm Rep*, 2011, 60(4):Q1-4.

These schedules indicate the recommended age groups and medical indications for which administration of currently licensed vaccines is commonly indicated for adults ages 19 years and older, as of January 1, 2011. For all vaccines being recommended on the adult immunization schedule: a vaccine series does not need to be restarted, regardless of the time that has elapsed between doses. Licensed combination vaccines may be used whenever any components of the combination are indicated and when the vaccine's other components are not contraindicated. For detailed recommendations on all vaccines, including those used primarily for travelers or that are issued during the year, consult the manufacturers' package inserts and the complete statements from the Advisory Committee on Immunization Practices (http:// www.cdc.gov/vaccines/pubs/acip-list.htm).

Report all clinically significant postvaccination reactions to the Vaccine Adverse Event Reporting System (VAERS). Reporting forms and instructions on filing a VAERS report are available at http://www.vaers.hhs.gov or by telephone, 800-822-7967.

Information on how to file a Vaccine Injury Compensation Program claim is available at http://www.hrsa.gov/vaccinecompensation or by telephone, 800-338-2382. Information about filing a claim for vaccine injury is available through the U.S. Court of Federal Claims, 717 Madison Place, N.W., Washington, D.C. 20005; telephone, 202-357-6400.

Additional information about the vaccines in this schedule, extent of available data, and contraindications for vaccination also is available at http://www.cdc.gov/vaccines or from the CDC-INFO Contact Center at 800-CDC-INFO (800-232-4636) in English and Spanish, 24 hours a day, 7 days a week.

Use of trade names and commercial sources is for identification only and does not imply endorsement by the U.S. Department of Health and Human Services.

The recommendations in this schedule were approved by ACIP, the American Academy of Family Physicians, the American College of Obstetricians and Gynecologists, and the American College of Physicians.

VACCINE INJURY TABLE

The Vaccine Injury Table makes it easier for some people to get compensation. The table lists and explains injuries/conditions that are presumed to be caused by vaccines. It also lists time periods in which the first symptom of these injuries/conditions must occur after receiving the vaccine. If the first symptom of these injuries/conditions occurs within the listed time periods, it is presumed that the vaccine was the cause of the injury or condition unless another cause is found. For example, if the patient received the tetanus vaccines and had a severe allergic reaction (anaphylaxis) within 4 hours after receiving the vaccine, then it is presumed that the tetanus vaccine caused the injury if no other cause is found.

If the injury/condition is not on the table or if the injury/condition did not occur within the time period on the table, it must be proven that the vaccine caused the injury/condition. Such proof must be based on medical records or opinion, which may include expert witness testimony.

Vaccine Injury Table[1]

Vaccine		Adverse Event	Time Interval
Tetanus toxoid-containing vaccines (eg, DTaP, Tdap, DTP-Hib, DT, Td, TT)	A.	Anaphylaxis or anaphylactic shock	0-4 hours
	B.	Brachial neuritis	2-28 days
	C.	Any acute complication or sequela (including death) of above events	Not applicable
Pertussis antigen-containing vaccines (eg, DTaP, Tdap, DTP, P, DTP-Hib)	A.	Anaphylaxis or anaphylactic shock	0-4 hours
	B.	Encephalopathy (or encephalitis)	0-72 hours
	C.	Any acute complication or sequela (including death) of above events	Not applicable
Measles, mumps, and rubella virus-containing vaccines in any combination (eg, MMR, MR, M, R)	A.	Anaphylaxis or anaphylactic shock	0-4 hours
	B.	Encephalopathy (or encephalitis)	5-15 days
	C.	Any acute complication or sequela (including death) of above events	Not applicable
Rubella virus-containing vaccines (eg, MMR, MR, R)	A.	Chronic arthritis	7-42 days
	B.	Any acute complication or sequela (including death) of above events	Not applicable
Measles virus-containing vaccines (eg, MMR, MR, M)	A.	Thrombocytopenic purpura	7-30 days
	B.	Vaccine-strain measles viral infection in an immunodeficient recipient	0-6 months
	C.	Any acute complication or sequela (including death) of above events	Not applicable
Polio live virus-containing vaccines (OPV)	A.	Paralytic polio	
	•	In a nonimmunodeficient recipient	0-30 days
	•	In an immunodeficient recipient	0-6 months
	•	In a vaccine associated community case	Not applicable
	B.	Vaccine-strain polio viral infection	
	•	In a nonimmunodeficient recipient	0-30 days
	•	In an immunodeficient recipient	0-6 months
	•	In a vaccine associated community case	Not applicable
	C.	Any acute complication or sequela (including death) of above events	Not applicable
Polio inactivated-virus containing vaccines (eg, IPV)	A.	Anaphylaxis or anaphylactic shock	0-4 hours
	B.	Any acute complication or sequela (including death) of above events	Not applicable

Vaccine Injury Table[1] *(continued)*

Vaccine		Adverse Event	Time Interval
Hepatitis B antigen-containing vaccines	A.	Anaphylaxis or anaphylactic shock	0-4 hours
	B.	Any acute complication or sequela (including death) of above events	Not applicable
Hemophilus influenzae (type b polysaccharide conjugate vaccines)	A.	No condition specified for compensation	Not applicable
Varicella vaccine	A.	No condition specified for compensation	Not applicable
Rotavirus vaccine	A.	No condition specified for compensation	Not applicable
Pneumococcal conjugate vaccines	A.	No condition specified for compensation	Not applicable
Any new vaccine recommended by the Centers for Disease Control and Prevention for routine administration to children, after publication by Secretary, HHS of a notice of coverage[2,3]	A.	No condition specified for compensation	Not applicable

[1]Effective date: November 10, 2008.

[2]As of **December 1, 2004**, hepatitis A vaccines have been added to the Vaccine Injury Table under this category. As of **July 1, 2005**, trivalent influenza vaccines have been added to the table under this category. Trivalent influenza vaccines are given annually during the flu season either by needle and syringe or in a nasal spray. All influenza vaccines routinely administered in the U.S. are trivalent vaccines covered under this category. See Federal Register Notice: April 12, 2005.

[3]As of February 1, 2007, meningococcal (conjugate and polysaccharide) and human papillomavirus (HPV) vaccines have been added to the table under this category. See *News* on the VICP website for more information. Available at http://www.hrsa.gov/vaccinecompensation

MANAGEMENT OF HEALTHCARE WORKER EXPOSURES TO HBV, HCV, AND HIV

Factors to Consider in Assessing the Need for Follow-up of Occupational Exposures

- **Type of exposure**
  - Percutaneous injury
  - Mucous membrane exposure
  - Nonintact skin exposure
  - Bites resulting in blood exposure to either person involved
- **Type and amount of fluid/tissue**
  - Blood
  - Fluids containing blood
  - Potentially infectious fluid or tissue (semen; vaginal secretions; and cerebrospinal, synovial, pleural, peritoneal, pericardial, and amniotic fluids)
  - Direct contact with concentrated virus
- **Infectious status of source**
  - Presence of HB_sAg
  - Presence of HCV antibody
  - Presence of HIV antibody
- **Susceptibility of exposed person**
  - Hepatitis B vaccine and vaccine response status
  - HBV, HCV, HIV immune status

Evaluation of Occupational Exposure Sources

Known sources

- Test known sources for HB_sAg, anti-HCV, and HIV antibody
  - Direct virus assays for routine screening of source patients are **not** recommended
  - Consider using a rapid HIV-antibody test
  - If the source person is **not** infected with a blood-borne pathogen, baseline testing or further follow-up of the exposed person is **not** necessary
- For sources whose infection status remains unknown (eg, the source person refuses testing), consider medical diagnoses, clinical symptoms, and history of risk behaviors
- Do not test discarded needles for blood-borne pathogens

Unknown sources

- For unknown sources, evaluate the likelihood of exposure to a source at high risk for infection
  - Consider the likelihood of blood-borne pathogen infection among patients in the exposure setting

Recommended Postexposure Prophylaxis for Exposure to Hepatitis B Virus

Vaccination and Antibody Response Status of Exposed Workers[1]	Treatment		
	Source HB_sAg[2]-Positive	Source HB_sAg[2] -Negative	Source Unknown or Not Available for Testing
Unvaccinated	HBIG[3] x 1 and initiate HB vaccine series[4]	Initiate HB vaccine series	Initiate HB vaccine series
Previously vaccinated			
Known responder[5]	No treatment	No treatment	No treatment
Known nonresponder[6]	HBIG[3] x 1 and initiate revaccination or HBIG x 2[7]	No treatment	If known high risk source, treat as if source was HB_sAg-positive
Antibody response unknown	Test exposed person for anti-HB_s[8] 1. If adequate,[5] no treatment is necessary 2. If inadequate,[6] administer HBIG[3] x 1 and vaccine booster	No treatment	Test exposed person for anti-HB_s 1. If adequate,[4] no treatment is necessary 2. If inadequate,[4] administer vaccine booster and recheck titer in 1-2 months

[1]Persons who have previously been infected with HBV are immune to reinfection and do not require postexposure prophylaxis.

[2]Hepatitis B surface antigen

[3]Hepatitis B immune globulin; dose is 0.06 mL/kg intramuscularly

[4]Hepatitis B vaccine

[5]A responder is a person with adequate levels of serum antibody to HB_sAg (ie, anti-HB_s ≥10 mIU/mL).

[6]A nonresponder is a person with inadequate response to vaccination (ie, serum anti-HB_s <10 mIU/mL).

[7]The option of giving one dose of HBIG and reinitiating the vaccine series is preferred for nonresponders who have not completed a second 3-dose vaccine series. For persons who previously completed a second vaccine series but failed to respond, two doses of HBIG are preferred.

[8]Antibody to HB_sAg

Recommended HIV Postexposure Prophylaxis (PEP) for Percutaneous Injuries

Exposure Type	Infection Status of Source				
	HIV-Positive Class 1[1]	HIV-Positive Class 2[1]	Source of Unknown HIV Status[2]	Unknown Source[3]	HIV-Negative
Less severe[4]	Recommend basic 2-drug PEP	Recommend expanded ≥3-drug PEP	Generally, no PEP warranted; however, consider basic 2-drug PEP[5] for source with HIV risk factors[6]	Generally, no PEP warranted; however, consider basic 2-drug PEP[5] in settings in which exposure to HIV-infected persons is likely	No PEP warranted
More severe[7]	Recommend expanded 3-drug PEP	Recommend expanded ≥3-drug PEP	Generally, no PEP warranted; however consider basic 2-drug PEP[5] for source with HIV risk factors[6]	Generally, no PEP warranted; however, consider basic 2-drug PEP[5] in settings in which exposure to HIV-infected persons is likely	No PEP warranted

[1]HIV-positive, class 1 - asymptomatic HIV infection or known low viral load (eg, <1500 ribonucleic acid copies/mL). HIV-positive, class 2 – symptomatic HIV infection, AIDS, acute seroconversion, or known high viral load. If drug resistance is a concern, obtain expert consultation. Initiation of PEP should not be delayed pending expert consultation, and, because expert consultation alone cannot substitute for face-to-face counseling, resources should be available to provide immediate evaluation and follow-up care for all exposures.

[2]For example, deceased source person with no samples available for HIV testing

[3]For example, a needle from a sharps disposal container

[4]For example, solid needle or superficial injury

[5]The recommendation "consider PEP" indicates that PEP is optional; a decision to initiate PEP should be based on a discussion between the exposed person and the treating clinician regarding the risk vs benefits of PEP.

[6]If PEP is offered and administered and the source is later determined to be HIV-negative, PEP should be discontinued.

[7]For example, large-bore hollow needle, deep puncture, visible blood on device, or needle used in patient's artery or vein

Recommended HIV Postexposure Prophylaxis (PEP) for Mucous Membrane Exposures and Nonintact Skin[1] Exposures

Exposure Type	Infection Status of Source				
	HIV-Positive Class 1[2]	HIV-Positive Class 2[2]	Source of Unknown HIV Status[3]	Unknown Source[4]	HIV-Negative
Small volume[5]	Consider basic 2-drug PEP[6]	Recommend basic 2-drug PEP	Generally, no PEP warranted[7]	Generally, no PEP warranted	No PEP warranted
Large volume[8]	Recommend basic 2-drug PEP	Recommend expanded ≥3-drug PEP	Generally, no PEP warranted; however consider basic 2-drug PEP[6] for source with HIV risk factors[7]	Generally, no PEP warranted; however, consider basic 2-drug PEP[6] in settings in which exposure to HIV-infected persons is likely	No PEP warranted

[1]For skin exposures, follow-up is indicated only if evidence exists of compromised skin integrity (eg, dermatitis, abrasion, open wound).

[2]HIV-positive, class 1 – asymptomatic HIV infection or known low viral load (eg, <1500 ribonucleic acid copies/mL). HIV-positive, class 2 – symptomatic HIV infection, AIDS, acute seroconversion, or known high viral load. If drug resistance is a concern, obtain expert consultation. Initiation of PEP should not be delayed pending expert consultation, and, because expert consultation alone cannot substitute for face-to-face counseling, resources should be available to provide immediate evaluation and follow-up care for all exposures.

[3]For example, deceased source person with no samples available for HIV testing

[4]For example, splash from inappropriately disposed blood

[5]For example, a few drops

[6]The recommendation "consider PEP" indicates that PEP is optional; a decision to initiate PEP should be based on a discussion between the exposed person and the treating clinician regarding the risks vs benefits of PEP.

[7]If PEP is offered and administered and the source is later determined to be HIV-negative, PEP should be discontinued.

[8]For example, a major blood splash

Situations for Which Expert[1] Consultation for HIV Postexposure Prophylaxis Is Advised

- **Delayed (ie, later than 24-36 hours) exposure report**
  - The interval after which there is no benefit from postexposure prophylaxis (PEP) is undefined
- **Unknown source (eg, needle in sharps disposal container or laundry)**
  - Decide use of PEP on a case-by-case basis
  - Consider the severity of the exposure and the epidemiologic likelihood of HIV exposure
  - Do not test needles or sharp instruments for HIV
- **Known or suspected pregnancy in the exposed person**
  - Does not preclude the use of optimal PEP regimens
  - Do not deny PEP solely on the basis of pregnancy
- **Breast-feeding in the exposed person**
  - Use of optimal PEP regimen not precluded
  - PEP should not be denied solely on the basis of breast-feeding
- **Resistance of the source virus to antiretroviral agents**
  - Influence of drug resistance on transmission risk is unknown
  - Selection of drugs to which the source person's virus is unlikely to be resistant is recommended, if the source person's virus is unknown or suspected to be resistant to ≥1 of the drugs considered for the PEP regimen
  - Resistance testing of the source person's virus at the time of the exposure is not recommended
  - Initiation of PEP not to be delayed while awaiting results of resistance testing
- **Toxicity of the initial PEP regimen**
  - Adverse symptoms, such as nausea and diarrhea, are common with PEP
  - Symptoms can often be managed without changing the PEP regimen by prescribing antimotility and/or antiemetic agents
  - Modification of dose intervals (ie, administering a lower dose of drug more frequently throughout the day, as recommended by the manufacturer), in other situations, might help alleviate symptoms

[1]Local experts and/or the National Clinicians' Postexposure Prophylaxis Hotline: PEPline (888) 448-4911

Occupational Exposure Management Resources

National Clinicians' Postexposure Prophylaxis Hotline (PEPline) Run by University of California-San Francisco/San Francisco General Hospital staff; supported by the Health Resources and Services Administration Ryan White CARE Act, HIV/AIDS Bureau, AIDS Education and Training Centers, and CDC	Phone: (888) 448-4911 Internet: http://chi.ucsf.edu
Needlestick! A website to help clinicians manage and document occupational blood and body fluid exposures. Developed and maintained by the University of California, Los Angeles (UCLA), Emergency Medicine Center, UCLA School of Medicine, and funded in part by CDC and the Agency for Healthcare Research and Quality	Internet: http://www.nova.edu/smc/needlestick.html
Hepatitis Hotline	Phone: (888) 443-7232 Internet: http://www.cdc.gov/hepatitis
Reporting to CDC Occupationally acquired HIV infections and failures of PEP	Phone: (800) 893-0485
HIV Antiretroviral Pregnancy Registry	Phone: (800) 258-4263 Fax: (800) 800-1052 Address: 1410 Commonwealth Drive, Suite 215 Wilmington, NC 28405 Internet: http://www.glaxowellcome.com/preg_reg/antiretroviral
Food and Drug Administration Report unusual or severe toxicity to antiretroviral agents	Phone: (800) 332-1088 Address: MedWatch HF-2, FDA 5600 Fishers Lane Rockville, MD 20857 Internet: http://www.fda.gov/medwatch
HIV/AIDS Treatment Information Service	Internet: http://www.aidsinfo.nih.gov

Management of Occupational Blood Exposures

Provide immediate care to the exposure site

- Wash wounds and skin with soap and water
- Flush mucous membranes with water

Determine risk associated with exposure by:

- Type of fluid (eg, blood, visibly bloody fluid, other potentially infectious fluid or tissue, and concentrated virus)
- Type of exposure (ie, percutaneous injury, mucous membrane or nonintact skin exposure, and bites resulting in blood exposure)

Evaluate exposure source

- Assess the risk of infection using available information
- Test known sources for HB_sAg, anti-HCV, and HIV antibody (consider using rapid testing)
- For unknown sources, assess risk of exposure to HBV, HCV, or HIV infection
- Do not test discarded needle or syringes for virus contamination

Evaluate the exposed person

- Assess immune status for HBV infection (ie, by history of hepatitis B vaccination and vaccine response)

Give PEP for exposures posing risk of infection transmission

- HBV: See Recommended Postexposure Prophylaxis for Exposure to Hepatitis B Virus Table
- HCV: PEP not recommended
- HIV: See Recommended HIV Postexposure Prophylaxis for Percutaneous Injuries Table and Recommended HIV Postexposure Prophylaxis for Mucous Membrane Exposures and Nonintact Skin Exposures Table
  - Initiate PEP as soon as possible, preferably within hours of exposure
  - Offer pregnancy testing to all women of childbearing age not known to be pregnant
  - Seek expert consultation if viral resistance is suspected
  - Administer PEP for 4 weeks if tolerated

Perform follow-up testing and provide counseling

- Advise exposed persons to seek medical evaluation for any acute illness occurring during follow-up

HBV exposures

- Perform follow-up anti-HB_s testing in persons who receive hepatitis B vaccine
  - Test for anti-HB_s 1-2 months after last dose of vaccine
  - Anti-HB_s response to vaccine cannot be ascertained if HBIG was received in the previous 3-4 months

HCV exposures

- Perform baseline and follow-up testing for anti-HCV and alanine (ALT) 4-6 months after exposures
- Perform HCV RNA at 4-6 months if earlier diagnosis of HCV infection is desired
- Confirm repeatedly reactive anti-HCV enzyme immunoassays (EIAs) with supplemental tests

HIV exposures

- Perform HIV antibody testing for at least 6 months postexposure (eg, at baseline, 6 weeks, 3 months, and 6 months)
- Perform HIV antibody testing if illness compatible with an acute retroviral syndrome occurs
- Advise exposed persons to use precautions to prevent secondary transmission during the follow-up period
- Evaluate exposed persons taking PEP within 72 hours after exposure and monitor for drug toxicity for at least 2 weeks

Basic and Expanded HIV Postexposure Prophylaxis Regimens

BASIC REGIMENS

Zidovudine (Retrovir®; ZDV; AZT) + lamivudine (Epivir®; 3TC); available as Combivir®

Preferred dosing

- ZDV: 300 mg twice daily or 200 mg three times daily, with food; total: 600 mg daily
- 3TC: 300 mg once daily or 150 mg twice daily
- Combivir®: One tablet twice daily

Advantages

- ZDV associated with decreased risk for HIV transmission
- ZDV used more often than other drugs for PEP for healthcare personnel (HCP)
- Serious toxicity rare when used for PEP
- Side effects predictable and manageable with antimotility and antiemetic agents
- Can be used by pregnant HCP
- Can be given as a single tablet (Combivir®) twice daily

Disadvantages

- Side effects (especially nausea and fatigue) common and might result in low adherence
- Source-patient virus resistance to this regimen possible
- Potential for delayed toxicity (oncogenic/teratogenic) unknown

Zidovudine (Retrovir®; ZDV; AZT) + emtricitabine (Emtriva®; FTC)

Preferred dosing

- ZDV: 300 mg twice daily or 200 mg three times daily, with food; total: 600 mg/day, in 2-3 divided doses
- FTC: 200 mg (one capsule) once daily

Advantages

- ZDV: See above
- FTC
  - Convenient (once daily)
  - Well-tolerated
  - Long intracellular half-life (~40 hours)

Disadvantages

- ZDV: See above
- FTC
  - Rash perhaps more frequent than with 3TC
  - No long-term experience with this drug
  - Cross resistance to 3TC
  - Hyperpigmentation among non-Caucasians with long-term use: 3%

Tenofovir DF (Viread®; TDF) + lamiVUDdine (Epivir®; 3TC)

Preferred dosing

- TDF: 300 mg once daily
- 3TC: 300 mg once daily or 150 mg twice daily

Advantages

- 3TC: See above
- TDF
  - Convenient dosing (single pill once daily)
  - Resistance profile activity against certain thymidine analogue mutations
  - Well-tolerated

Disadvantages

- TDF
  - Same class warnings as nucleoside reverse transcriptase inhibitors (NRTIs)
  - Drug interactions
  - Increased TDF concentrations among persons taking atazanavir and lopinavir/ritonavir; need to monitor patients for TDF-associated toxicities
- Preferred dosage of atazanavir if used with TDF: 300 mg + ritonavir 100 mg once daily + TDF 300 mg once daily

Tenofovir DF (Viread®; TDF) + emtricitabine (Emtriva®; FTC); available as Truvada®

Preferred dosing

- TDF: 300 mg once daily
- FTC: 200 mg once daily
- As Truvada®: One tablet daily

Advantages

- FTC: See above
- TDF
  - Convenient dosing (single pill once daily)
  - Resistance profile activity against certain thymidine analogue mutations
  - Well-tolerated

Disadvantages

- TDF
  - Same class warnings as NRTIs
  - Drug interactions
  - Increased TDF concentrations among persons taking atazanavir and lopinavir/ritonavir; need to monitor patients for TDF-associated toxicities
  - Preferred dosing of atazanavir if used with TDF: 300 mg + ritonavir 100 mg once daily + TDF 300 mg once daily

ALTERNATE BASIC REGIMENS

LamiVUDine (Epivir®; 3TC) + stavudine (Zerit®; d4T)

Preferred dosing

- 3TC: 300 mg once daily or 150 mg twice daily
- d4T: 40 mg twice daily (can use lower doses of 20-30 mg twice daily if toxicity occurs; equally effective but less toxic among HIV-infected patients with peripheral neuropathy); 30 mg twice daily if body weight is <60 kg

Advantages

- 3TC: See above
- d4T: Gastrointestinal (GI) side effects rare

Disadvantages

- Possibility that source-patient virus is resistant to this regimen
- Potential for delayed toxicity (oncogenic/teratogenic) unknown

Emtricitabine (Emtriva®; FTC) + stavudine (Zerit®; d4T)

Preferred dosing

- FTC: 200 mg daily
- d4T: 40 mg twice daily (can use lower doses of 20-30 mg twice daily if toxicity occurs; equally effective but less toxic among HIV-infected patients who developed peripheral neuropathy); if body weight is <60 kg, 30 mg twice daily

Advantages

- 3TC and FTC: See above; d4T's GI side effects rare

Disadvantages

- Potential that source-patient virus is resistant to this regimen
- Unknown potential for delayed toxicity (oncogenic/teratogenic) unknown

LamiVUDine (Epivir®; 3TC) + didanosine (Videx®; ddI)

Preferred dosing

- 3TC: 300 mg once daily or 150 mg twice daily
- ddI: Videx® chewable/dispersible buffered tablets can be administered on an empty stomach as either 200 mg twice daily or 400 mg once daily. Patients must take at least two of the appropriate strength tablets at each dose to provide adequate buffering and prevent gastric acid degradation of ddI. Because of the need for adequate buffering, the 200 mg strength tablet should be used only as a component of a once-daily regimen. The dose is either 200 mg twice daily or 400 mg once daily for patients weighing >60 kg and 125 mg twice daily or 250 mg once daily for patients weighing <60 kg.

Advantages

- ddI: Once-daily dosing option
- 3TC: See above

Disadvantages

- Tolerability: Diarrhea more common with buffered preparation than with enteric-coated preparation
- Associated with toxicity: Peripheral neuropathy, pancreatitis, and lactic acidosis
- Must be taken on empty stomach except with TDF
- Drug interactions
- 3TC: See above

Emtricitabine (Emtriva®; FTC) + didanosine (Videx®; ddI)

Preferred dosing

- FTC: 200 mg once daily
- ddI: See above

Advantages

- ddI: See above
- FTC: See above

Disadvantages

- Tolerability: Diarrhea more common with buffered than with enteric-coated preparation
- Associated with toxicity: Peripheral neuropathy, pancreatitis, and lactic acidosis
- Must be taken on empty stomach except with TDf
- Drug interactions
- FTC: See above

PREFERRED EXPANDED REGIMEN

Basic regimen plus:

Lopinavir / Ritonavir (Kaletra®; LPV/RTV)

Preferred dosing

- LPV/RTV: 400 mg/100 mg = twice daily with food

Advantages

- Potent HIV protease inhibitor
- Generally well-tolerated

Disadvantages

- Potential for serious or life-threatening drug interactions
- Might accelerate clearance of certain drugs, including oral contraceptives (requiring alternative or additional contraceptive measures for women taking these drugs)
- Can cause severe hyperlipidemia, especially hypertriglyceridemia
- GI (eg, diarrhea) events common

ALTERNATE EXPANDED REGIMENS

Basic regimen plus one of the following:

Atazanavir (Reyataz®; ATV) ± ritonavir (Norvir®; RTV)

Preferred dosing

- ATV: 400 mg once daily, unless used in combination with TDF, in which case ATV should be boosted with RTV, preferred dosing of ATV 300 mg + RTV: 100 mg once daily

Advantages

- Potent HIV protease inhibitor
- Convenient dosing – once daily
- Generally well-tolerated

Disadvantages

- Hyperbilirubinemia and jaundice common
- Potential for serious or life-threatening drug interactions
- Avoid coadministration with proton pump inhibitors
- Separate antacids and buffered medications by 2 hours and H_2-receptor antagonists by 12 hours to avoid decreasing ATV levels
- Caution should be used with ATV and products known to induce PR prolongation (eg, diltiazem)

Fosamprenavir (Lexiva™; FOSAPV) ± ritonavir (Norvir®; RTV)

Preferred dosing

- FOSAPV: 1400 mg twice daily (without RTV)
- FOSAPV: 1400 mg once daily + RTV 200 mg once daily
- FOSAPV: 700 mg twice daily + RTV 100 mg twice daily

Advantages

- Once daily dosing when given with ritonavir

Disadvantages

- Tolerability: GI side effects common
- Multiple drug interactions. Oral contraceptives decrease fosamprenavir concentrations
- Incidence of rash in healthy volunteers, especially when used with low doses of ritonavir. Differentiating between early drug-associated rash and acute seroconversion can be difficult and cause extraordinary concern for the exposed person.

Indinavir (Crixivan®; IDV) ± ritonavir (Norvir®; RTV)

Preferred dosing

- IDV 800 mg + RTV 100 mg twice daily without regard to food

Alternative dosing

- IDV: 800 mg every 8 hours, on an empty stomach

Advantages

- Potent HIV inhibitor

Disadvantages

- Potential for serious or life-threatening drug interactions
- Serious toxicity (eg, nephrolithiasis) possible; consumption of 8 glasses of fluid/day required
- Hyperbilirubinemia common; must avoid this drug during late pregnancy
- Requires acid for absorption and cannot be taken simultaneously with ddI, chewable/dispersible buffered tablet formulation (doses must be separated by ≥1 hour)

Saquinavir (Invirase®; SQV) + ritonavir (Norvir®; RTV)

Preferred dosing

- SQV: 1000 mg (given as Invirase®) + RTV 100 mg, twice daily
- SQV: Five capsules twice daily + RTV: One capsule twice daily

Advantages

- Generally well-tolerated, although GI events common

Disadvantages

- Potential for serious or life-threatening drug interactions
- Substantial pill burden

Nelfinavir (Viracept®; NFV)

Preferred dosing

- NFV: 1250 mg (2 x 625 mg or 5 x 250 mg tablets), twice daily with a meal

Advantages

- Generally well-tolerated

Disadvantages

- Diarrhea or other GI events common
- Potential for serious and/or life-threatening drug interactions

Efavirenz (Sustiva®; EFV)

Preferred dosing

- EFV: 600 mg daily, at bedtime

Advantages

- Does not require phosphorylation before activation and might be active earlier than other antiretroviral agents (a theoretic advantage of no demonstrated clinical benefit)
- Once daily dosing

Disadvantages

- Drug associated with rash (early onset) that can be severe and might rarely progress to Stevens-Johnson syndrome
- Differentiating between early drug-associated rash and acute seroconversion can be difficult and cause extraordinary concern for the exposed person
- Central nervous system side effects (eg, dizziness, somnolence, insomnia, or abnormal dreaming) common; severe psychiatric symptoms possible (dosing before bedtime might minimize these side effects)
- Teratogen; should not be used during pregnancy
- Potential for serious or life-threatening drug interactions

ANTIRETROVIRAL AGENTS GENERALLY NOT RECOMMENDED FOR USE AS PEP

Nevirapine (Viramune®; NVP)

Disadvantages

- Associated with severe hepatotoxicity (including at least one case of liver failure requiring liver transplantation in an exposed person taking PEP)
- Associated with rash (early onset) that can be severe and progress to Stevens-Johnson syndrome
- Differentiating between early drug-associated rash and acute seroconversion can be difficult and cause extraordinary concern for the exposed person
- Drug interactions: Can lower effectiveness of certain antiretroviral agents and other commonly used medicines

Delavirdine (Rescriptor®; DLV)

Disadvantages

- Drug associated with rash (early onset) that can be severe and progress to Stevens-Johnson syndrome
- Multiple drug interactions

Abacavir (Ziagen®; ABC)

Disadvantages

- Severe hypersensitivity reactions can occur, usually within the first 6 weeks
- Differentiating between early drug-associated rash/hypersensitivity and acute seroconversion can be difficult

Zalcitabine (HIVID®; ddC)

Disadvantages

- Three times a day dosing
- Tolerability
- Weakest antiretroviral agent

ANTIRETROVIRAL AGENT FOR USE AS PEP ONLY WITH EXPERT CONSULTATION

Enfuvirtide (Fuzeon®; T20)

Preferred dosing

- T20: 90 mg (1 mL) twice daily by subcutaneous injection

Advantages

- New class
- Unique viral target; to block cell entry
- Prevalence of resistance low

Disadvantages

- Twice-daily injection
- Safety profile: Local injection site reactions
- Never studied among antiretroviral-naive or HIV-negative patients
- False-positive EIA HIV antibody tests might result from formation of anti-T20 antibodies that cross-react with anti-gp41 antibodies

REFERENCES

Centers for Disease Control and Prevention (CDC), "Notice to Readers: Updated Information Regarding Antiretroviral Agents Used as HIV Postexposure Prophylaxis for Occupational HIV Exposures," *MMWR Morb Mortal Wkly Rep*, 2007, 56(49):1291-2. Available at http://www.cdc.gov/mmwr/preview/mmwrhtml/mm5649a4.htm

Panlilio AL, Cardo DM, Grohskopf LA, et al, "Updated U.S. Public Health Service Guidelines for the Management of Occupational Exposures to HIV and Recommendations for Postexposure Prophylaxis," *MMWR Recomm Rep*, 2005, 54(RR-9):1-17. Available at http://www.cdc.gov/mmwr/preview/mmwrhtml/rr5409a1.htm

U.S. Public Health Service, "Updated U.S. Public Health Service Guidelines for the Management of Occupational Exposures to HBV, HCV, and HIV and Recommendations for Postexposure Prophylaxis," *MMWR Recomm Rep*, 2001, 50(RR-11):1-42. Available at http://www.cdc.gov/mmwr/preview/mmwrhtml/rr5011a1.htm

PERINATAL HIV GUIDELINES

Antiretroviral agents are used during pregnancy for the treatment of maternal human immunodeficiency virus (HIV) infection and to reduce the risk of perinatal HIV transmission. Recommendations for the use of antiretroviral drugs during pregnancy are updated regularly by the Department of Health and Human Services Panel on Treatment of HIV-Infected Pregnant Women and Prevention of Perinatal Transmission. The latest guidelines are available at http://AIDSinfo.nih.gov. With the use of highly active combination antiretroviral therapy (HAART), prenatal HIV counseling and testing, antiretroviral prophylaxis, scheduled cesarean delivery, and avoidance of breastfeeding, perinatal transmission of HIV infection has decreased to <2% in the United States. Health care professionals are encouraged to contact the antiretroviral pregnancy registry to monitor outcomes of pregnant women exposed to antiretroviral medications (1-800-258-4263 or www.APRegistry.com). The 2009 Panel recommendations include the following (refer to guidelines for complete details):

Preconception:

- Effective and appropriate contraception should be selected to avoid unintended pregnancy.
- Preconception counseling concerning safe sexual practices should be conducted.
- Choice of antiretroviral therapy should consider efficacy for maternal treatment the potential for teratogenicity if pregnancy should occur.
- Attaining a stable maximally suppressed viral load prior to conception is recommended for HIV infected women who wish to become pregnant.

Antepartum:

- Antiretroviral prophylaxis should be provided to all HIV-infected women, regardless of HIV RNA copy number or CD4 cell count.
- Resistance studies should be conducted prior to starting/modifying therapy if HIV RNA is detectable.
- Combination regimens are more effective than single drug regimens to reduce perinatal transmission.
- Prophylaxis for a longer duration (eg, starting at 28 weeks) is more effective than shorter duration (eg, starting at 36 weeks).
- If antiretroviral therapy is stopped electively during pregnancy, consider stopping nucleoside reverse transcriptase inhibitors (NRTIs) 7 days after stopping non-nucleoside reverse transcriptase inhibitors (NNRTIs); recommendation based on limited data. If therapy is stopped acutely for severe or life-threatening toxicity or severe pregnancy induced hyperemesis not responsive to antiemetics, stop all drugs at the same time and restart at the same time. If nevirapine is stopped and >2 weeks have passed, restart with the 2 week dose escalation period.
- Optimal adherence to antiretroviral medications is a key part of the strategy to reduce the development of resistance.
- Additional specific medication issues:
  - Zidovudine should be included in the regimen unless there is severe toxicity, documented resistance, or if the women is already on a fully suppressive regimen.
  - Efavirenz use should be avoided during the first trimester.
  - Nevirapine can be used as part of initial therapy in pregnant women with CD4 cell count <250 cells/mm^3. Use as initial therapy in pregnant women with a CD4 cell count >250 cells/mm^3 should only be done if the benefit outweighs the risk of hepatic toxicity. Nevirapine can be continued in pregnant women who are virologically suppressed and tolerating therapy regardless of CD4 count.
  - Protease inhibitors may require dosing adjustments during pregnancy.
  - Stavudine and didanosine in combination may cause lactic acidosis with prolonged use during pregnancy; use should be avoided.
  - NRTIs may be associated with lactic acidosis; monitor.

Intrapartum:

- Scheduled cesarean delivery at 38 weeks is recommended for women with suboptimal viral suppression near delivery (eg, >1000 copies/mL) or with unknown HIV RNA near the time of delivery.
- All HIV-infected pregnant women, regardless of their antepartum HAART regimen, should receive intrapartum intravenous zidovudine.
- If antepartum antiretroviral drugs were not administered, intrapartum therapy combined with infant antiretroviral prophylaxis should be given.
- Stavudine should be discontinued during labor while zidovudine is being administered.
- Nevirapine use as a single dose is not recommended for women in the U.S. who are receiving standard antiretroviral prophylaxis regimens.
- Pregnant women with documented zidovudine resistance who are not currently taking zidovudine for their own health should receive intravenous zidovudine during labor whenever possible, in addition to their established regimens.

Postpartum:

- Postnatal infant prophylaxis is recommended for all infants born to HIV-infected women.
- If antepartum or intrapartum antiretroviral drugs were not administered, postnatal infant prophylaxis is recommended.
- Breast-feeding is not recommended for HIV-infected women in the United States where safe, affordable, and feasible alternatives are available and culturally acceptable.

Special Situations

Hepatitis B virus coinfection:

- Screening for hepatitis B is recommended for all HIV-infected women not already screened during current pregnancy.
- Pregnant women with chronic hepatitis B virus (HBV) infection and HIV coinfection who require treatment for both diseases, a 3-drug regimen including a dual NRTI backbone of tenofovir plus lamivudine or emtricitabine is recommended. Consultation with an expert is advised for pregnant women needing treatment for HBV but not HIV and for pregnant women who do not require treatment for either HBV or HIV infection.
- Pregnant women with HBV and HIV coinfection and receiving antiretroviral medications should be monitored for liver toxicity.

Hepatitis C virus coinfection:

- Screening for hepatitis C is recommended for all HIV-infected women not already screened during current pregnancy.
- Pregnant women with chronic hepatitis C virus (HCV) infection and HIV coinfection should receive combination antiretroviral therapy with 3 drugs, regardless of CD4 count or viral load. If treatment for HIV infection is not needed for maternal health, it may be discontinued postpartum.
- Pregnant women with HCV and HIV coinfection and receiving antiretroviral medications should be monitored for liver toxicity.
- Decisions concerning mode of delivery should be based on HIV infection alone.

Clinical Scenarios and Recommendations for the Use of Antiretroviral Drugs to Reduce Perinatal HIV Transmission

HIV-infected women receiving HAART therapy who become pregnant

- Continue current HAART regimen if successfully suppressing viremia, except avoid the use of efavirenz or other potentially teratogenic drugs in the first trimester and avoid drugs with known adverse potential for the mother (combination stavudine and didanosine).
- Resistance testing is recommended if there is detectable viremia on therapy.
- In general, if a women requires treatment, antiretroviral medications should not be stopped during the first trimester.
- Continue HAART during the intrapartum period (give zidovudine as a continuous infusion and other antiretroviral medications orally).
- Scheduled cesarean delivery at 38 weeks is recommended for women with suboptimal viral suppression near delivery (eg, >1000 copies/mL).

HIV-infected pregnant women who have not received prior antiretroviral therapy and have indications for antiretroviral therapy

- Resistance studies should be conducted prior to starting therapy.
- Initiate HAART regimen as soon as possible, even if during the first trimester. Avoid the use of efavirenz or other potentially teratogenic drugs in the first trimester and avoid drugs with known adverse potential for the mother (combination stavudine and didanosine).
- Zidovudine should be included in the regimen unless there is severe toxicity or documented resistance.
- Nevirapine can be used as part of initial therapy in pregnant women with CD4 cell count <250 cells/mm^3. Use as initial therapy in pregnant women with a CD4 cell count >250 cells/mm^3 should only be done if the benefit outweighs the risk of hepatic toxicity.
- Continue HAART during the intrapartum period (give zidovudine as a continuous infusion and other antiretroviral medications orally).
- Scheduled cesarean delivery at 38 weeks is recommended for women with suboptimal viral suppression near delivery (eg, >1000 copies/mL).

HIV-infected pregnant women who have not received prior antiretroviral therapy and do NOT require treatment for their own health

- Resistance studies should be conducted prior to starting therapy.
- HAART is recommended for prophylaxis of perinatal transmission. Delaying treatment until after the first trimester may be considered.
- Avoid the use of efavirenz or other potentially teratogenic drugs in the first trimester and avoid drugs with known adverse potential for the mother (combination stavudine and didanosine).
- Zidovudine should be included in the regimen unless there is severe toxicity or documented resistance. The use of zidovudine alone is controversial, but may be considered if plasma HIV RNA levels are <1000 copies/mL on no therapy.
- Nevirapine can be used in pregnant women with CD4 cell count <250 cells/mm^3. Initial therapy in pregnant women with a CD4 cell count >250 cells/mm^3 should only be done if the benefit outweighs the risk of hepatic toxicity.
- Continue HAART during the intrapartum period (give zidovudine as a continuous infusion and other antiretroviral medications orally).
- Evaluate the need for continued therapy postpartum. Discontinue HAART unless there are indications for continued therapy. If regimen includes drug with long half-life, like NNRTI, consider stopping NRTIs 7 days after stopping NNRTI (recommendation based on limited data).
- Scheduled cesarean delivery at 38 weeks is recommended for women with suboptimal viral suppression near delivery (eg, >1000 copies/mL).

HIV-infected pregnant women who are antiretroviral-experienced but not currently receiving antiretroviral medications

- Obtain full treatment history and evaluate the need for treatment for maternal health. Resistance studies should be conducted prior to starting therapy.
- Initiate HAART regimen. Avoid the use of efavirenz or other potentially teratogenic drugs in the first trimester and avoid drugs with known adverse potential for the mother (combination stavudine and didanosine).
- Zidovudine should be included in the regimen unless there is severe toxicity or documented resistance.
- Nevirapine can be used as part of initial therapy in pregnant women with CD4 cell count <250 cells/mm^3. Use as initial therapy in pregnant women with a CD4 cell count >250 cells/mm^3 should only be done if the benefit outweighs the risk of hepatic toxicity.
- Continue HAART during the intrapartum period (give zidovudine as a continuous infusion and other antiretroviral medications orally).
- Evaluate the need for continued therapy postpartum. Discontinue HAART unless there are indications for continued therapy. If regimen includes drug with long half-life, like NNRTI, consider stopping NRTIs 7 days after stopping NNRTI (recommendation based on limited data).
- Scheduled cesarean delivery at 38 weeks is recommended for women with suboptimal viral suppression near delivery (eg, >1000 copies/mL).

HIV-infected women in labor who have had no prior therapy

Several regimens are available. These include:

- Zidovudine as an intravenous infusion during labor followed by 6 weeks of zidovudine for the newborn **OR**
- Zidovudine as an intravenous infusion during labor plus a single dose of nevirapine at the onset of labor. For the newborn, one dose of nevirapine plus zidovudine for 6 weeks **OR**
- Zidovudine as an intravenous infusion during labor. For the newborn, some clinicians may choose to use zidovudine in combination with additional medications, but appropriate dosing in neonates is not well defined.

If single-dose nevirapine is given to the mother, alone or in combination with zidovudine, consideration should be given to adding maternal zidovudine/lamivudine starting as soon as possible (intrapartum and postpartum) and continuing for 7 days, which may reduce development of nevirapine resistance. (Single dose nevirapine is not recommended for women in the U.S. who are receiving standard antiretroviral prophylaxis regimens.)

In the immediate postpartum period, the woman should have appropriate assessments (eg, $CD4^+$ count and HIV RNA copy number) to determine whether antiretroviral therapy is recommended for her own health.

Infants born to HIV-infected mothers who have received no antiretroviral therapy during pregnancy or intrapartum

- Administer zidovudine for 6 weeks to the infant, beginning as soon as possible after birth.
- Some clinicians may choose to use zidovudine in combination with additional medications, but appropriate dosing in neonates is not well defined. Consultation with a pediatric HIV specialist is recommended.
- Evaluate the need for postpartum maternal therapy.

Clinical Scenarios and Recommendations Regarding Mode of Delivery to Reduce Perinatal HIV Transmission

Women presenting in late pregnancy (after about 36 weeks of gestation), known to be HIV-infected but not receiving antiretroviral therapy, and who have HIV RNA level and lymphocyte subsets pending but unlikely to be available before delivery.

Recommendations

- Therapy options should be discussed in detail. The woman should be started on antiretroviral therapy. The woman should be counseled that scheduled cesarean section is likely to reduce the risk of transmission to her infant. She should also be informed of the increased risks to her of cesarean section, including increased rates of postoperative infection, anesthesia risks, and other surgical risks.
- If cesarean section is chosen, the procedure should be scheduled at 38 weeks of gestation based on the best available clinical information. When scheduled cesarean section is performed, the woman should receive continuous intravenous zidovudine infusion beginning 3 hours before surgery and her infant should receive 6 weeks of zidovudine therapy after birth. Options for continuing or initiating combination antiretroviral therapy after delivery should be discussed with the woman as soon as her viral load and lymphocyte subset results are available.

HIV-infected women who initiated prenatal care early in the third trimester, are receiving highly active combination antiretroviral therapy, and have an initial virologic response, but have HIV RNA levels that remain substantially over 1000 copies/mL at 36 weeks of gestation.

Recommendations

- The current combination antiretroviral regimen should be continued as the HIV RNA level is dropping appropriately. The woman should be counseled that although she is responding to the antiretroviral therapy, it is unlikely that her HIV RNA level will fall below 1000 copies/mL before delivery. Therefore, scheduled cesarean section may provide additional benefit in preventing intrapartum transmission of HIV. She should also be informed of the increased risks to her of cesarean section, including increased rates of postoperative infection, anesthesia risks, and surgical risks.
- If she chooses scheduled cesarean section, it should be performed at 38 weeks' gestation according to the best available dating parameters, and intravenous zidovudine should begin at least 3 hours before surgery. Other antiretroviral medications should be continued on schedule as much as possible before and after surgery. The infant should receive oral zidovudine for 6 weeks after birth. The importance of adhering to therapy after delivery for her own health should be emphasized.

HIV-infected women on highly active combination antiretroviral therapy with an undetectable HIV RNA level at 36 weeks of gestation.

Recommendations

- The woman should be counseled that her risk of perinatal transmission of HIV with a persistently undetectable HIV RNA level is low, probably 2% or less, even with vaginal delivery. There is currently no information to evaluate whether performing a scheduled cesarean section will lower her risk further.
- Cesarean section has an increased risk of complications for the woman compared to vaginal delivery, and these risks must be balanced against the uncertain benefit of cesarean section in this case.

HIV-infected women who have elected scheduled cesarean section but present in early labor or shortly after rupture of membranes.

Recommendations

- Intravenous zidovudine should be started immediately since the woman is in labor or has ruptured membranes.
- If labor is progressing rapidly, the woman should be allowed to deliver vaginally. If cervical dilatation is minimal and a long period of labor is anticipated, some clinicians may choose to administer the loading dose of intravenous zidovudine and proceed with cesarean section to minimize the duration of membrane rupture and avoid vaginal delivery. Others might begin oxytocin augmentation to enhance contractions and potentially expedite delivery.
- If the woman is allowed to labor, scalp electrodes and other invasive monitoring and operative delivery should be avoided if possible. The infant should be treated with 6 weeks of zidovudine therapy after birth.

REFERENCE

Public Health Service Task Force, "Recommendations for Use of Antiretroviral Drugs in Pregnant HIV-Infected Women for Maternal Health and Interventions to Reduce Perinatal HIV Transmission in the United States," 2009. Available at http://aidsinfo.nih.gov/contentfiles/PerinatalGL.pdf

Recommended Antiretroviral Therapy in Pregnant HIV-Infected Women

Drug	Recommended	Alternative	Not Recommended	Insufficient Data	Rationale / Concerns
Nucleoside Reverse Transcriptase Inhibitors (NRTIs)					
Zidovudine	X				Preferred NRTI for use in **combination** antiretroviral regimens in pregnancy; include in regimens unless significant toxicity, stavudine use, or if the woman is already on a fully suppressive regimen.
LamiVUDine	X				Lamivudine plus zidovudine is the recommended dual NRTI backbone for pregnant women. Use caution with hepatits B coinfection; hepatitis B flare may occur if the lamivudine is discontinued postpartum.
Didanosine		X			Cases of lactic acidosis; do not use with stavudine unless alternative regimens are not available.
Emtricitabine		X			A pharmakinetic study shows a slight decrease in emtricitabine serum levels during the third trimester; however, there is no clear need to adjust the dose.
Stavudine		X			Lactic acidosis noted in pregnant women in combination with didanosine; avoid use with didanosine; do not use with zidovudine due to antagonism.
Abacavir		X			Triple NRTI regimens including abacavir have been less potent virologically compared to PI-based HAART regimens; use only when an NNRTI or PI based regimen cannot be used. Screening for *HLA-B*5701* allele status is recommended prior to initiating therapy or reinitiating therapy in patients of unknown status, including patients who previously tolerated therapy. Therapy is **not** recommended in patients testing positive for the *HLA-B*5701* allele.
Tenofovir				X	Studies in children have shown bone demineralization with chronic use; clinical significance unknown. Because tenofovir significantly crosses the placenta and because there is a lack of data concerning use during human pregnancy, use only after careful consideration of alternatives. Use caution with hepatitis B coinfection; hepatitis B flare may occur if tenofovir is discontinued postpartum.
Non-nucleoside Reverse Transcriptase Inhibitors (NNRTIs)					
Nevirapine	X				Possible increased risk of liver toxicity; use only if benefit outweighs risk with CD4 counts >250. Women who enter pregnancy on nevirapine regimens and are tolerating them well, may continue therapy regardless of CD4 count.
Efavirenz			X		Avoid use during the first trimester; use after the second trimester only if other alternatives are not available. Alternate regimens should be considered in women of childbearing potential. Pharmacokinetic data from small study indicates that peak serum concentrations in the third trimester may be significantly increased.
Delavirdine			X		No pharmacokinetic studies in pregnant women; carcinogenic and teratogenic in animal studies
Etravirine				X	Teratogenic effects were not observed in animal studies; no experience in human pregnancy

Recommended Antiretroviral Therapy in Pregnant HIV-Infected Women *continued*

Drug	Recommended	Alternative	Not Recommended	Insufficient Data	Rationale / Concerns
Protease Inhibitors (PIs)					
Lopinavir/ritonavir	X				Teratogenic effects were not observed in phase I/II studies. Pharmacokinetic studies are not yet completed using the tablet formulation. Studies using the previously available capsule formulation showed that an increased dose may be needed during the third trimester. Until data is available for the tablet, standard dosing can be used, monitor virologic response and consider increasing the dose during the third trimester. Once daily administration is not recommended.
Atazanavir		X			A recommended alternative agent when combined with low-dose ritonavir boosting; may give as once daily dosing. In naïve patients unable to tolerate ritonavir, once daily dosing may be considered; however, efficacy data is insufficient. Must be used with low-dose ritonavir boosting when used in combination with tenofovir.
Nelfinavir		X			No evidence of teratogenicity; well-tolerated and short-term safety demonstrated in mother and infant. When used in nonpregnant adults, nelfinavir-based regimens had a lower rate of viral response than some alternative regimens. Therefore, use is recommended only as an alternative PI in pregnant women recieving HAART for perinatal prophylaxis. As of March 31, 2008, all Viracept® manufactured by Pfizer meets new limits of EMS content and may be prescribed as indicated to all patient populations (including pregnant women).
Saquinavir		X			No evidence of teratogenicity; well-tolerated and short-term safety demonstrated in mother and infant; use with ritonavir boosting. The softgel capsules are no longer available. Until additional pharmacokinetic studies are completed using the hard gel capsule or the tablet, saquinavir is considered an alternative PI for use during pregnancy.
Indinavir		X			Possible increased bilirubin levels; use with ritonavir boosting.
Ritonavir		X			Minimal experience in human pregnancy; recommended as part of boosted regimen
Darunavir				X	Insufficient safety/kinetic data available. Must give with low-dose ritonavir boosting.
Fosamprenavir				X	Limited experience in human pregnancy; insufficient safety/kinetic data available. Recommended to be given with low-dose ritonavir boosting.
Tipranavir				X	No experience in human pregnancy; insufficient safety/kinetic data available. Must give with low-dose ritonavir boosting.
Entry Inhibitors					
Enfuvirtide				X	Minimal studies in pregnant women; insufficient safety/kinetic data available
Maraviroc				X	Insufficient safety/kinetic data available
Integrase Inhibitors					
Raltegravir				X	Insufficient safety/kinetic data available

PREVENTION OF INFECTIVE ENDOCARDITIS

Recommendations by the American Heart Association

(*Circulation*, 2007, 116(15):1736-54.)

Consensus Process – The recommendations were formulated by a writing group under the auspices of the American Heart Association (AHA), and included representation from the Infectious Diseases Society of America (IDSA), the American Academy of Pediatrics (AAP), and the American Dental Association (ADA). Additionally, input was received from both national and international experts on infective endocarditis (IE). These guidelines are based on expert interpretation and review of scientific literature from 1950 through 2006. The consensus statement was subsequently reviewed by outside experts not affiliated with the writing group and by the Science Advisory and Coordinating Committee of the American Heart Association. These guidelines are meant to aid practitioners but are not intended as the standard of care or as a substitute for clinical judgment.

Significant change from the previous 1997 guidelines – The previously published guidelines identified a broad range of cardiac conditions thought to predispose patients to a higher risk of IE. The document stratified these conditions into high-, moderate-, and low-risk categories, based on the likelihood of developing IE. The subsequent recommendations for prophylaxis were based on this classification, in conjunction with specification of numerous invasive procedures which were assumed to confer a higher risk of bacteremia, and therefore a higher risk of endocarditis. However, it is the consensus of the current writing group that existing data fail to show a clear link between many of these procedures, preexisting cardiovascular condition and IE. In the case of dental procedures, it was determined that the cumulative lifetime risk of developing bacteremia as a result of normal hygiene measures (eg, teeth brushing, flossing) vastly exceeded the risk associated with many of the procedures for which prophylaxis was previously recommended. Similarly, the writing group estimated that the absolute risk of developing IE as a result of dental procedures in patients with preexisting cardiac conditions was quite low, and there was little evidence to support the value of prophylactic antimicrobial efficacy in these cases.

In a major departure from the former recommendations, the current guidelines have been greatly simplified to place a much greater emphasis on a very limited number of underlying cardiac conditions (see below). These specific conditions have been associated with the highest risk of adverse outcomes due to IE. Patients should receive IE prophylaxis only if they are undergoing certain invasive procedures (see Table 1) and have one of the underlying cardiovascular conditions specified below.

Common situations for which routine prophylaxis was previously, but no longer recommended, include mitral valve prolapse, general dental cleanings and local anesthetic administration (noninfected tissue), and bronchoscopy (see Table 1).

Specific cardiac conditions for which IE antibiotic prophylaxis is recommended:

- Previous infective endocarditis
- Prosthetic cardiac valve or prosthetic material used for cardiac valve repair
- Cardiac transplantation patients who develop valvulopathy
- Congenital heart disease (CHD), only under the following conditions:
  - Unrepaired cyanotic CHD, including palliative shunts and conduits
  - Completely repaired defects (with prosthetic materials/devices), regardless of method of repair, within the first 6 months after the procedure
  - Repaired CHD with residual defects at or adjacent to the site of repair

Table 1. Guidance for Use of Prophylactic Antibiotic Therapy Based on Procedure or Condition[1]

Location of Procedure	Prophylaxis Recommended	Prophylaxis NOT Recommended
Dental	All invasive manipulations of the gingival or periapical region or perforation of oral mucosa	Anesthetic injections (through noninfected tissue), radiographs, placement/adjustment/removal prosthodontic/orthodontic appliances or brackets, shedding of deciduous teeth, trauma-induced bleeding from lips, gums, or oral mucosa
Respiratory tract	Biopsy/incision of respiratory mucosa (eg, tonsillectomy/adenoidectomy); drainage of abscess or empyema[2]	Bronchoscopy (unless incision of mucosa required)
Gastrointestinal (GI) or genitourinary (GU) tract	Established GI/GU infection or prevention of infectious sequelae[3]; elective cystoscopy or other urinary tract procedure with established enterococci infection/ colonization[3,4]	Routine diagnostic procedures, including esophagogastroduodenoscopy or colonoscopy in the absence of active infection; vaginal delivery and hysterectomy
Skin, skin structure, or musculoskeletal	Any surgical procedure involving infected tissue	Procedures conducted in noninfected tissue; tattoos and ear/body piercing

[1]Patients should receive prophylactic antibiotic therapy if they meet the criteria for a specified procedure/condition in this table and they have a high-risk cardiovascular condition listed in the preceding text.

[2]If treating an infection of known staphylococcal origin, consider antistaphylococcal penicillin or cephalosporin, or vancomycin in beta-lactam-sensitive patients.

[3]Alternative agents with activity against enterococci to consider: Vancomycin (for beta-lactam-sensitive patients) or piperacillin

[4]Eradication of enterococci from the urinary tract should be considered.

Table 2. Prophylactic Regimens for Oral / Dental, Respiratory Tract, Genitoruinary Tract, or Esophageal Procedures

Situation	Agent	Regimen to Be Given 30-60 Minutes Before Procedure	
		Adults	Children[1]
Standard general prophylaxis	Amoxicillin	2 g P.O.	50 mg/kg P.O.
Unable to take oral medications	Ampicillin **or**	2 g I.M./I.V.	50 mg/kg I.M./I.V.
	CeFAZolin or cefTRIAXone	1 g I.M./I.V.	50 mg/kg I.M./I.V.
Allergic to penicillin	Clindamycin **or**	600 mg P.O.	20 mg/kg P.O.
	Cephalexin[2] or other dose-equivalent first/second generation cephalosporin **or**	2 g P.O	50 mg/kg P.O.
	Azithromycin or clarithromycin	500 mg P.O.	15 mg/kg P.O.
Allergic to penicillin and unable to take oral medications	Clindamycin **or**	600 mg I.V.	20 mg/kg I.V.
	CeFAZolin or cefTRIAXone[2]	1 g I.M./I.V.	50 mg/kg I.M./I.V.

[1]Total children's dose should not exceed adult dose.

[2]Cephalosporins should not be used in individuals with immediate-type hypersensitivity reaction (urticaria, angioedema, or anaphylaxis) to penicillins.

REFERENCE

Wilson W, Taubert KA, Gewitz M, et al, "Prevention of Infective Endocarditis. Guidelines From the American Heart Association. A Guideline From the American Heart Association Rheumatic Fever, Endocarditis, and Kawasaki Disease Committee, Council on Cardiovascular Disease in the Young, and the Council on Clinical Cardiology, Council on Cardiovascular Surgery and Anesthesia, and the Quality of Care and Outcomes Research Interdisciplinary Working Group," *Circulation*, 2007, 116(15):1736-54.

PREVENTION OF WOUND INFECTION AND SEPSIS IN SURGICAL PATIENTS

Nature of Operation	Likely Pathogens	Recommended Drugs	Adult Dosage Before Surgery[1]
Cardiac	*S. aureus, S. epidermidis*	Mupirocin	2% ointment applied in both nares twice daily for 6 days; begin the day before surgery
		+ CeFAZolin	2 g (1 g if patient weight ≤60 kg) I.V.[2]
		± Vancomycin[3]	1-1.5 g or 15 mg/kg I.V.
Gastrointestinal			
Esophageal, gastroduodenal	Enteric gram-negative bacilli, gram-positive cocci	*High risk[4] only:* CeFAZolin[5]	1-2 g I.V.
Biliary tract, endoscopic retrograde cholangiopancreatography (ERCP)	Enteric gram-negative bacilli, enterococci, clostridia	*High risk[6] only:* CeFAZolin[5]	1-2 g I.V.
Colorectal	Enteric gram-negative bacilli, anaerobes, enterococci	*Oral:*	
		Neomycin + erythromycin base[7]	1 g of each x 3 doses
		or	
		Neomycin + metroNIDAZOLE[7]	2 g of each x 2 doses
		Parenteral:	
		CefOXitin[5] or cefoTEtan[5]	1-2 g I.V.
		or	
		CeFAZolin[5]	1-2 g I.V.
		+ MetroNIDAZOLE[5]	0.5 g I.V.
		or	
		Ampicillin/sulbactam[5]	3 g I.V.
Appendectomy, nonperforated	Enteric gram-negative bacilli, anaerobes, enterococci	CefOXitin[5] or cefoTEtan[5]	1-2 g I.V.
		or	
		CeFAZolin[5]	1-2 g I.V.
		+ MetroNIDAZOLE	0.5 g I.V.
		or	
		Ampicillin/sulbactam[5]	3 g I.V.
Ruptured viscus[8]	Enteric gram-negative bacilli, anaerobes, enterococci	CefOXitin[5] or cefoTEtan[5]	1-2 g I.V. q6h
		or	
		CeFAZolin[5]	1-2 g I.V. q8h
		+ MetroNIDAZOLE	0.5 g I.V. q6h
		or	
		Ampicillin/sulbactam[5]	3 g I.V. q6h
Genitourinary			
Cystoscopy alone	Enteric gram-negative bacilli, enterococci	*High risk[9] only:*	
		Ciprofloxacin	500 mg P.O. or 400 mg I.V.
		or	
		Trimethoprim/sulfamethoxazole	1 double strength tablet
Cystoscopy with manipulation or upper tract instrumentation[10]	Enteric gram-negative bacilli, enterococci	Ciprofloxacin	500 mg P.O. or 400 mg I.V.
		or	
		Trimethoprim/sulfamethoxazole	1 double strength tablet
Open or laparoscopic surgery[11]	Enteric gram-negative bacilli, enterococci	CeFAZolin[5]	1-2 g I.V.
Gynecologic and Obstetric			
Vaginal, abdominal, or laparoscopic hysterectomy	Enteric gram-negative bacilli, anaerobes, group B streptococci, enterococci	CefOXitin[5] or cefoTEtan[5]	1-2 g I.V.
		or	
		CeFAZolin[5]	1-2 g I.V.
		+ MetroNIDAZOLE	0.5 g I.V.
		or	
		Ampicillin/sulbactam[5]	3 g I.V.
Cesarean section	Same as for hysterectomy	CeFAZolin[5]	1-2 g I.V.
Abortion	Same as for hysterectomy	Doxycycline	300 mg P.O.[12]

(continued)

Nature of Operation	Likely Pathogens	Recommended Drugs	Adult Dosage Before Surgery[1]
Head and Neck			
Incisions through oral or pharyngeal mucosa	Anaerobes, enteric gram-negative bacilli, *S. aureus*	Clindamycin **or** CeFAZolin + MetroNIDAZOLE	600-900 mg I.V. 1-2 g I.V. 0.5 g I.V.
Neurosurgery	*S. aureus, S. epidermidis*	CeFAZolin **or** Vancomycin[3]	1-2 g I.V. 1 g I.V.
Ophthalmic	*S. epidermidis, S. aureus,* streptococci, enteric gram-negative bacilli, *Pseudomonas*	Gentamicin, tobramycin, ciprofloxacin, gatifloxacin, levofloxacin, moxifloxacin, ofloxacin, or neomycin-gramicidin- polymyxin B CeFAZolin	Multiple drops topically over 2-24 hours 100 mg subconjunctivally
Orthopedic	*S. aureus, S. epidermidis*	CeFAZolin[13] **or** Cefuroxime[13] **or** Vancomycin[3,13]	1-2 g I.V. 1.5 g I.V. 1 g I.V.
Thoracic (noncardiac)	*S. aureus, S. epidermidis,* streptococci, enteric gram-negative bacilli	CeFAZolin **or** Cefuroxime **or** Vancomycin[3]	1-2 g I.V. 1.5 g I.V. 1 g I.V.
Vascular			
Arterial surgery involving a prosthesis, the abdominal aorta, or a groin incision	*S. aureus, S. epidermidis,* enteric gram-negative bacilli	CeFAZolin **or** Vancomycin[3]	1-2 g I.V. 1 g I.V.
Lower extremity amputation for ischemia	*S. aureus, S. epidermidis,* enteric gram-negative bacilli, clostridia	CeFAZolin **or** Vancomycin[3]	1-2 g I.V. 1 g I.V.

[1]Parenteral prophylactic antimicrobials can be given as a single I.V. dose begun ≤60 minutes before the operation. For prolonged operations (>4 hours), or those with major blood loss, additional intraoperative doses should be given at intervals 1-2 times the half-life of the drug for the duration of the procedure in patients with normal renal function. If vancomycin or a fluoroquinolone is used, the infusion should be started 60-120 minutes before incision in order to minimize the possibility of an infusion reaction close to the time of induction of anesthesia and to have adequate tissue levels at the time of incision.

[2]Some consultants recommend an additional dose when patients are removed from bypass during open-heart surgery.

[3]For hospitals in which methicillin-resistant *S. aureus* and *S. epidermidis* are a frequent cause of postoperative wound infection, for patients previously colonized with MRSA, or for patients allergic to penicillins or cephalosporin. Rapid I.V. administration may cause hypotension, which could be especially dangerous during induction of anesthesia. Even if the drug is given over 60 minutes, hypotension may occur; treatment with diphenhydrAMINE and further slowing of the infusion rate may be helpful. Some experts would give 15 mg/kg for patients >75 kg to a maximum of 1.5 g given over 90 minutes. For procedures in which enteric gram-negative bacilli are likely pathogens, many Medical Letter consultants would add another drug such as an aminoglycoside (gentamicin, tobramycin, or amikacin).

[4]Morbid obesity, esophageal obstruction, decreased gastric acidity, (eg, H_2-blocker, proton pump inhibitor), or gastrointestinal motility

[5]For patients allergic to penicillins and cephalosporins, clindamycin with either gentamicin, ciprofloxacin, levofloxacin, or aztreonam is a reasonable alternative.

[6]Age >70 years, acute cholecystitis, nonfunctioning gallbladder, obstructive jaundice, or common duct stones

[7]1 g of neomycin plus 1 g of erythromycin at 1 PM, 2 PM, and 11 PM the day before an 8 AM operation or 2 g of neomycin plus 2 g of metroNIDAZOLE at 7 PM and 11 PM the day before an 8 AM operation

[8]Therapy is often continued for about 5 days. Ruptured viscus in postoperative setting (dehiscence) requires antibacterials to include coverage of nosocomial pathogens.

[9]Urine culture positive or unavailable, preoperative catheter, transrectal prostatic biopsy, placement of prosthetic material

[10]Shockwave lithotripsy, ureteroscopy

[11]Including percutaneous renal surgery, procedures with entry into the urinary tract and those involving implantation of a prosthesis. If manipulation of bowel is involved, prophylaxis is given according to colorectal guidelines.

[12]Divided into 100 mg 1 hour before the abortion and 200 mg 30 minutes after

[13]If a tourniquet is to be used in the procedure, the entire dose of antibiotic must be infused prior to its inflation.

REFERENCES

"Antimicrobial Prophylaxis for Surgery," *Treatment Guidelines From The Medical Letter®*, 2009, 4(82):48-9.

Bratzler DW, Houck PM, Surgical Infection Prevention Guidelines Writers Workgroup, et al, "Antimicrobial Prophylaxis for Surgery: An Advisory Statement From the National Surgical Infection Prevention Project," *Clin Infect Dis*, 2004, 38(12):1706-15.

Engelman R, Shahian D, Shemin R, et al, "The Society of Thoracic Surgeons Practice Guideline Series: Antibiotic Prophylaxis in Cardiac Surgery, Part II: Antibiotic Choice," *Ann Thorac Surg*, 2007, 83(4):1569-76.

ANTIBIOTIC TREATMENT OF ADULTS WITH INFECTIVE ENDOCARDITIS

Table 1. Suggested Regimens for Therapy of Native Valve Endocarditis Due to Penicillin-Susceptible Viridans Streptococci and *Streptococcus bovis* (Minimum Inhibitory Concentration ≤0.12 mcg/mL)[1]

Antibiotic	Dosage and Route	Duration (wk)	Comments
Aqueous crystalline penicillin G sodium **or**	12-18 million units/24 h I.V. either continuously or in 4-6 equally divided doses	4	Preferred in most patients older than 65 y and in those with impairment of the 8th cranial nerve or renal function
CefTRIAXone sodium	2 g once daily I.V. or I.M.[2]	4	
Either penicillin or cefTRIAXone regimen above with gentamicin sulfate[3]	3 mg/kg/24 h I.M./I.V. as single daily dose	2	When using combination therapy, both β-lactam and aminoglycoside regimen duration is 2 weeks; 2-week regimen not intended if known cardiac or extracardiac abscess, Cl_{cr} <20 mL/min, 8th cranial nerve impairment or *Abiotrophia*, *Granulicatella*, or *Gemella* spp
Vancomycin hydrochloride[4]	30 mg/kg/24 h I.V. in 2 equally divided doses, not to exceed 2 g/24 h unless serum levels are monitored	4	Vancomycin therapy is recommended for patients allergic to β-lactams; peak serum concentrations of vancomycin should be obtained 1 h after completion of the infusion and should be in the range of 30-45 mcg/mL and trough of 10-15 mcg/mL for twice-daily dosing

[1]Dosages recommended are for patients with normal renal function. For nutritionally variant streptococci, see Table 3. I.V. indicates intravenous; I.M., intramuscular.

[2]Patients should be informed that I.M. injection of cefTRIAXone is painful.

[3]Dosing of gentamicin on a mg/kg basis will produce higher serum concentrations in obese patients than in lean patients. Therefore, in obese patients, dosing should be based on ideal body weight. (Ideal body weight for men is 50 kg + 2.3 kg per inch over 5 feet, and ideal body weight for women is 45.5 kg + 2.3 kg per inch over 5 feet.) Relative contraindications to the use of gentamicin are age >65 years, renal impairment, or impairment of the eighth nerve. Other potentially nephrotoxic agents (eg, nonsteroidal anti-inflammatory drugs) should be used cautiously in patients receiving gentamicin.

[4]Vancomycin dosage should be reduced in patients with impaired renal function. Vancomycin given on a mg/kg basis will produce higher serum concentrations in obese patients than in lean patients. Therefore, in obese patients, dosing should be based on ideal body weight. Each dose of vancomycin should be infused over at least 1 hour to reduce the risk of the histamine-release "red man" syndrome.

Table 2. Therapy for Native Valve Endocarditis Due to Strains of Viridans Streptococci and *Streptococcus bovis* Relatively Resistant to Penicillin G (Minimum Inhibitory Concentration >0.12 mcg/mL and ≤0.5 mcg/mL)[1]

Antibiotic	Dosage and Route	Duration (wk)	Comments
Aqueous crystalline penicillin G sodium	24 million units/24 h I.V. either continuously or in 4-6 equally divided doses	4	CeFAZolin or other first-generation cephalosporins may be substituted for penicillin in patients whose penicillin hypersensitivity is not of the immediate type.
With gentamicin sulfate[2]	3 mg/kg/24 h I.M./I.V. as single daily dose	2	
CefTRIAXone sodium	2 g once daily I.V. or I.M.[2]	4	
With gentamicin sulfate[2]	3 mg/kg/24 h I.M./I.V. as single daily dose	2	
Vancomycin hydrochloride[3]	30 mg/kg/24 h I.V. in 2 equally divided doses, not to exceed 2 g/24 h unless serum levels are monitored	4	Vancomycin therapy is recommended for patients allergic to β-lactams

[1]Dosages recommended are for patients with normal renal function. I.V. = intravenous, I.M. = intramuscular

[2]For specific dosing adjustment and issues concerning gentamicin (obese patients, relative contraindications), see Table 1 footnotes.

[3]For specific dosing adjustment and issues concerning vancomycin (obese patients, length of infusion), see Table 1 footnotes.

Table 3. Standard Therapy for Endocarditis Due to Enterococci[1]

Antibiotic	Dosage and Route	Duration (wk)	Comments
Aqueous crystalline penicillin G sodium	18-30 million units/24 h I.V. either continuously or in 6 equally divided doses	4-6	Native valve: 4-week therapy recommended for patients with symptoms ≤3 months in duration; 6-week therapy recommended for patients with symptoms >3 months in duration
With gentamicin sulfate[2]	1 mg/kg I.M. or I.V. every 8 h	4-6	
Ampicillin sodium	12 g/24 h I.V. in 6 equally divided doses	4-6	Prosthetic valve or other prosthetic material: 6-week minimum therapy recommended
With gentamicin sulfate[2]	1 mg/kg I.M. or I.V. every 8 hours	4-6	Target gentamicin peak concentration of 3-4 mcg/mL and trough of <1 mcg/mL
Vancomycin hydrochloride[2,3]	30 mg/kg/24 h I.V. in 2 equally divided doses, not to exceed 2 g/24 h unless serum levels are monitored	6	Vancomycin therapy is recommended for patients allergic to β-lactams; cephalosporins are not acceptable alternatives for patients allergic to penicillin
With gentamicin sulfate[2]	1 mg/kg I.M. or I.V. every 8 h	6	

[1]All enterococci causing endocarditis must be tested for antimicrobial susceptibility in order to select optimal therapy. This table is for endocarditis due to penicillin-, gentamicin-, and vancomycin-susceptible enterococci, viridans streptococci with a minimum inhibitory concentration of >0.5 mcg/mL, nutritionally variant viridans streptococci, or prosthetic valve endocarditis caused by viridans streptococci or *Streptococcus bovis*. If penicillin-resistant organisms, use vancomycin/gentamicin regimen above, or may use ampicillin/sulbactam (12 g/24 h in 4 divided doses) with gentamicin for 6 weeks. Antibiotic dosages are for patients with normal renal function. I.V. indicates intravenous; I.M., intramuscular.

[2]For specific dosing adjustment and issues concerning gentamicin (obese patients, relative contraindications), see Table 1 footnotes.

[3]For specific dosing adjustment and issues concerning vancomycin (obese patients, length of infusion), see Table 1 footnotes.

Table 4. Therapy for Native or Prosthetic Valve Endocarditis Due to Enterococci[1] Resistant to Vancomycin, Aminoglycosides, and Penicillin[2]

Antibiotic	Dosage and Route	Duration (wk)	Comments
E. faecium			
Linezolid	1200 mg/24 h P.O./I.V. in 2 divided doses	≥8	May cause severe, but reversible thrombocytopenia, particularly with extended therapy >2 weeks.
Quinupristin-dalfopristin	22.5 mg/kg/24 h I.V. in 3 divided doses	≥8	May cause severe myalgia; not effective against *E. faecalis*.
E. faecalis			
Imipenem/cilastatin	2 g/24 h I.V. in 4 divided doses	≥8	Limited patient experience with these regimens.
With ampicillin sodium	12 g/24 h in 6 divided doses	≥8	
or			
CefTRIAXone sodium	2 g/24 h I.V./I.M.[3] once daily	≥8	Limited patient experience with these regimens.
With ampicillin sodium	12 g/24 h in 6 divided doses	≥8	

[1]Endocarditis caused by the organisms should be treated in consultation with an infectious disease specialist; bacteriologic cure with antimicrobial therapy alone may be <50% and valve replacement may be required.

[2]Dosages recommended are for patients with normal renal function. I.V. = intravenous, I.M. = intramuscular

[3]Patients should be informed that I.M. injection of cefTRIAXone is painful.

Table 5. Therapy for Endocarditis Due to *Staphylococcus* in the Absence of Prosthetic Material[1]

Antibiotic	Dosage and Route	Duration	Comments
	Methicillin-Susceptible Staphylococci		
Regimens for non-β-lactam-allergic patients			
Nafcillin sodium or oxacillin sodium	12 g/24 h I.V. in 4-6 divided doses	6 wk	Uncomplicated right side endocarditis may be treated for 2 weeks.
With optional addition of gentamicin sulfate[2]	3 mg/kg/24 h I.M./I.V. in 2-3 divided doses	3-5 d	Benefit of additional aminoglycosides has not been established.
Regimens for β-lactam-allergic patients (nonanaphylactic)			
CeFAZolin (or other first-generation cephalosporins in equivalent dosages)	2 g I.V. every 8 h	6 wk	Cephalosporins should be avoided in patients with immediate-type hypersensitivity to penicillin; if penicillin-sensitive, vancomycin should be used.
With optional addition of gentamicin[2]	3 mg/kg/24 h I.M./I.V. in 2-3 divided doses	3-5 d	Benefit of additional aminoglycosides has not been established.
	Methicillin-Resistant Staphylococci		
Vancomycin hydrochloride[3]	30 mg/kg/24 h I.V. in 2 equally divided doses; not to exceed 2 g/24 h unless serum levels are monitored	4-6 wk	Vancomycin therapy is recommended for patients allergic to β-lactams; peak serum concentrations of vancomycin should be obtained 1 h after completion of the infusion and should be in the range of 30-45 mcg/mL and trough of 10-15 mcg/mL for twice-daily dosing.

[1]For treatment of endocarditis due to penicillin-susceptible staphylococci (minimum inhibitory concentration ≤0.1 mcg/mL and non-beta-lactamase producing), aqueous crystalline penicillin G sodium 24 million units/24 h can be used instead of nafcillin or oxacillin. Shorter antibiotic courses have been effective in some drug addicts with right-sided endocarditis due to *Staphylococcus aureus*. I.V. = intravenous, I.M. = intramuscular

[2]For specific dosing adjustment and issues concerning gentamicin (obese patients, relative contraindications), see Table 1 footnotes.

[3]For specific dosing adjustment and issues concerning vancomycin (obese patients, length of infusion), see Table 1 footnotes.

Table 6. Treatment of Staphylococcal Endocarditis in the Presence of a Prosthetic Valve or Other Prosthetic Material[1]

Antibiotic	Dosage and Route	Duration (wk)	Comments
	Methicillin-Susceptible Staphylococci		
Nafcillin sodium or oxacillin sodium[2]	12 g/24 h I.V. in 6 divided doses	≥6	First-generation cephalosporins or vancomycin should be used in patients allergic to β-lactam. Cephalosporins should be avoided in patients with immediate-type hypersensitivity to penicillin or with methicillin-resistant staphylococci.
With rifampin[3]	300 mg P.O./I.V. every 8 h	≥6	–
And with gentamicin sulfate[4,5]	3 mg/kg I.M./I.V. in 2-3 divided doses	2	Aminoglycoside should be administered in close proximity to vancomycin, nafcillin, or oxacillin.
	Methicillin-Resistant Staphylococci		
Vancomycin hydrochloride[6]	30 mg/kg/24 h I.V. in 2 equally divided doses, not to exceed 2 g/24 h unless serum levels are monitored	≥6	–
With rifampin[3]	300 mg P.O./I.V. every 8 h	≥6	Rifampin increases the amount of warfarin sodium required for antithrombotic therapy.
And with gentamicin sulfate[4,5]	3 mg/kg I.M./I.V. in 2-3 divided doses	2	Aminoglycoside should be administered in close proximity to vancomycin, nafcillin, or oxacillin.

[1]Dosages recommended are for patients with normal renal function. I.V. = intravenous, I.M. = intramuscular

[2]May use aqueous penicillin G 24 million units/24 h in 4-6 divided doses if strain is penicillin susceptible (MIC ≤0.1 mcg/mL and non-beta-lactamase producing).

[3]Rifampin plays a unique role in the eradication of staphylococcal infection involving prosthetic material; combination therapy is essential to prevent emergence of rifampin resistance.

[4]For a specific dosing adjustment and issues concerning gentamicin (obese patients, relative contraindications), see Table 1 footnotes.

[5]Use during initial 2 weeks.

[6]For specific dosing adjustment and issues concerning vancomycin (obese patients, relative contraindications), see Table 1 footnotes.

Table 7. Therapy for Native or Prosthetic Valve Endocarditis Due to HACEK Microorganisms (*Haemophilus parainfluenzae, Haemophilus aphrophilus, Actinobacillus actinomycetemcomitans, Cardiobacterium hominus, Eikenella corrodens,* and *Kingella kingae*)[1]

Antibiotic	Dosage and Route	Duration (wk)	Comments
CefTRIAXone sodium[2]	2 g once daily I.V. or I.M.[2]	4	Cefotaxime sodium or other third- or fourth-generation cephalosporins may be substituted.
Ampicillin/sulbactam[3]	12 g/24 h I.V. in 6 equally divided doses	4	
Ciprofloxacin	1000 mg/24 h orally or 800 mg/24 h I.V. in 2 divided doses	4	Use of fluoroquinolone recommended only if patient intolerant to ampicillin or cephalosporins; may substitute fluoroquinolone with equivalent coverage (eg, levofloxacin, moxifloxacin); if prosthetic material involved, treatment duration should be 6 weeks.

[1]Antibiotic dosages are for patients with normal renal function. I.V. = intravenous, I.M. = intramuscular

[2]Patients should be informed that I.M. injection of cefTRIAXone is painful.

[3]Ampicillin should not be used if laboratory tests show β-lactamase production.

REFERENCE

Baddour LM, Wilson WR, Bayer AS, et al, "Infective Endocarditis. Diagnosis, Antimicrobial Therapy, and Management of Complications. A Statement for Healthcare Professionals from the Committee on Rheumatic Fever, Endocarditis, and Kawasaki Disease, Council on Cardiovascular Disease in the Young, and the Councils on Clinical Cardiology, Stroke, and Cardiovascular Surgery and Anesthesia, American Heart Association," *Circulation*, 2005, 111(23):e394-434.

PEDIATRIC ALS (PALS) ALGORITHMS

Pediatric Bradycardia

With a Pulse and Poor Perfusion

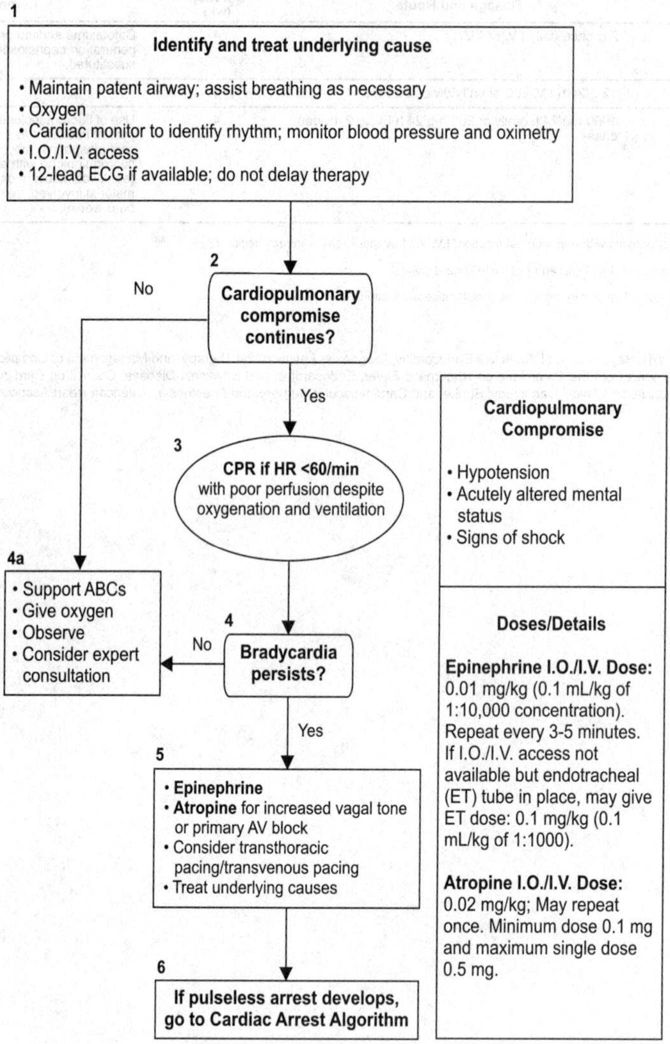
1
Identify and treat underlying cause
• Maintain patent airway; assist breathing as necessary
• Oxygen
• Cardiac monitor to identify rhythm; monitor blood pressure and oximetry
• I.O./I.V. access
• 12-lead ECG if available; do not delay therapy
2
Cardiopulmonary compromise continues?
No
Yes
3
CPR if HR <60/min with poor perfusion despite oxygenation and ventilation
4a
• Support ABCs
• Give oxygen
• Observe
• Consider expert consultation
4
Bradycardia persists?
No
Yes
5
• Epinephrine
• Atropine for increased vagal tone or primary AV block
• Consider transthoracic pacing/transvenous pacing
• Treat underlying causes
6
If pulseless arrest develops, go to Cardiac Arrest Algorithm
Cardiopulmonary Compromise
• Hypotension
• Acutely altered mental status
• Signs of shock
Doses/Details
Epinephrine I.O./I.V. Dose:
0.01 mg/kg (0.1 mL/kg of 1:10,000 concentration). Repeat every 3-5 minutes. If I.O./I.V. access not available but endotracheal (ET) tube in place, may give ET dose: 0.1 mg/kg (0.1 mL/kg of 1:1000).
Atropine I.O./I.V. Dose:
0.02 mg/kg; May repeat once. Minimum dose 0.1 mg and maximum single dose 0.5 mg.

Pediatric Cardiac Arrest

Shout for Help/Activate Emergency Response

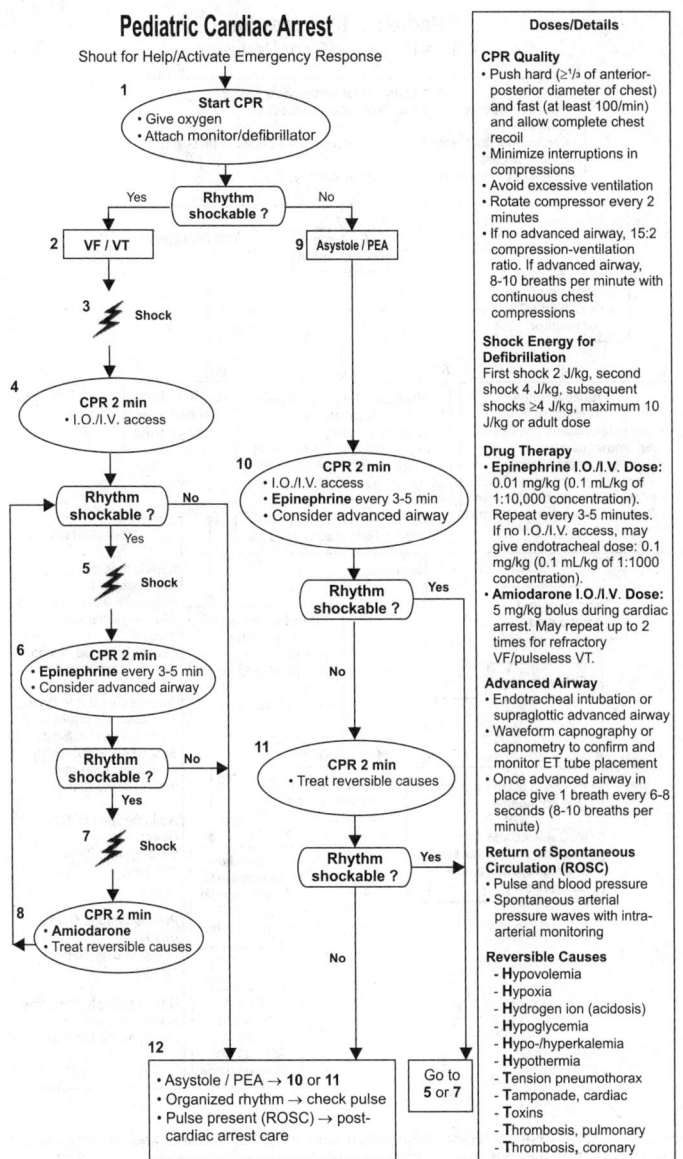

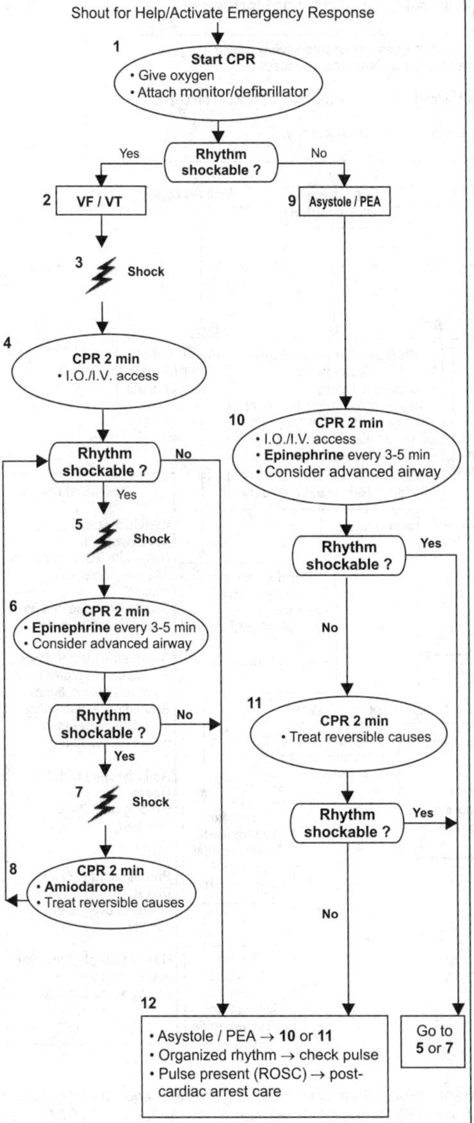

Doses/Details

CPR Quality
- Push hard (≥⅓ of anterior-posterior diameter of chest) and fast (at least 100/min) and allow complete chest recoil
- Minimize interruptions in compressions
- Avoid excessive ventilation
- Rotate compressor every 2 minutes
- If no advanced airway, 15:2 compression-ventilation ratio. If advanced airway, 8-10 breaths per minute with continuous chest compressions

Shock Energy for Defibrillation
First shock 2 J/kg, second shock 4 J/kg, subsequent shocks ≥4 J/kg, maximum 10 J/kg or adult dose

Drug Therapy
- **Epinephrine I.O./I.V. Dose:** 0.01 mg/kg (0.1 mL/kg of 1:10,000 concentration). Repeat every 3-5 minutes. If no I.O./I.V. access, may give endotracheal dose: 0.1 mg/kg (0.1 mL/kg of 1:1000 concentration).
- **Amiodarone I.O./I.V. Dose:** 5 mg/kg bolus during cardiac arrest. May repeat up to 2 times for refractory VF/pulseless VT.

Advanced Airway
- Endotracheal intubation or supraglottic advanced airway
- Waveform capnography or capnometry to confirm and monitor ET tube placement
- Once advanced airway in place give 1 breath every 6-8 seconds (8-10 breaths per minute)

Return of Spontaneous Circulation (ROSC)
- Pulse and blood pressure
- Spontaneous arterial pressure waves with intra-arterial monitoring

Reversible Causes
- Hypovolemia
- Hypoxia
- Hydrogen ion (acidosis)
- Hypoglycemia
- Hypo-/hyperkalemia
- Hypothermia
- Tension pneumothorax
- Tamponade, cardiac
- Toxins
- Thrombosis, pulmonary
- Thrombosis, coronary

Pediatric Tachycardia
With a Pulse and Poor Perfusion

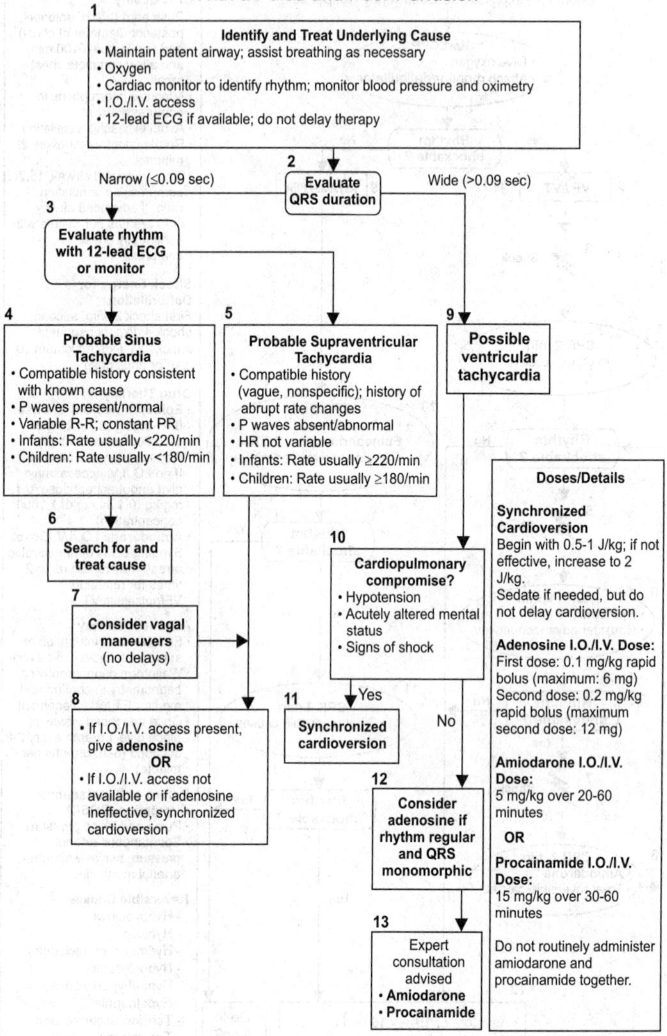
1
Identify and Treat Underlying Cause
• Maintain patent airway; assist breathing as necessary
• Oxygen
• Cardiac monitor to identify rhythm; monitor blood pressure and oximetry
• I.O./I.V. access
• 12-lead ECG if available; do not delay therapy
2
Evaluate QRS duration
Narrow (≤0.09 sec)
Wide (>0.09 sec)
3
Evaluate rhythm with 12-lead ECG or monitor
4
Probable Sinus Tachycardia
• Compatible history consistent with known cause
• P waves present/normal
• Variable R-R; constant PR
• Infants: Rate usually <220/min
• Children: Rate usually <180/min
5
Probable Supraventricular Tachycardia
• Compatible history (vague, nonspecific); history of abrupt rate changes
• P waves absent/abnormal
• HR not variable
• Infants: Rate usually ≥220/min
• Children: Rate usually ≥180/min
9
Possible ventricular tachycardia
6
Search for and treat cause
7
Consider vagal maneuvers (no delays)
8
• If I.O./I.V. access present, give adenosine
OR
• If I.O./I.V. access not available or if adenosine ineffective, synchronized cardioversion
10
Cardiopulmonary compromise?
• Hypotension
• Acutely altered mental status
• Signs of shock
Yes
No
11
Synchronized cardioversion
12
Consider adenosine if rhythm regular and QRS monomorphic
13
Expert consultation advised
• Amiodarone
• Procainamide
Doses/Details
Synchronized Cardioversion
Begin with 0.5-1 J/kg; if not effective, increase to 2 J/kg.
Sedate if needed, but do not delay cardioversion.
Adenosine I.O./I.V. Dose:
First dose: 0.1 mg/kg rapid bolus (maximum: 6 mg)
Second dose: 0.2 mg/kg rapid bolus (maximum second dose: 12 mg)
Amiodarone I.O./I.V. Dose:
5 mg/kg over 20-60 minutes
OR
Procainamide I.O./I.V. Dose:
15 mg/kg over 30-60 minutes
Do not routinely administer amiodarone and procainamide together.

MATERNAL CARDIAC ARREST

First Responder

- Activate maternal cardiac arrest team
- Document time of onset of maternal cardiac arrest
- Place the patient supine
- Start chest compressions as per BLS algorithm; place hands slightly higher on sternum than usual

Subsequent Responders

Maternal Interventions

Treat per BLS and ACLS Algorithms

- Do not delay defibrillation
- Give typical ACLS drugs and doses
- Ventilate with 100% oxygen
- Monitor waveform capnography and CPR quality
- Provide post-cardiac arrest care as appropriate

Maternal Modifications

- Start I.V. above the diaphragm
- Assess for hypovolemia and give fluid bolus when required
- Anticipate difficult airway; experienced provider preferred for advanced airway placement
- If patient receiving I.V./I.O. magnesium prearrest, stop magnesium and give I.V./I.O. calcium chloride 10 mL in 10% solution, or calcium gluconate 30 mL in 10% solution
- Continue all maternal resuscitative interventions (CPR, positioning, defribrillation, drugs, and fluids) during and after cesarean section

Obstetric Interventions for Patient With an Obviously Gravid Uterus*

- Perform manual left uterine displacement (LUD) - displace uterus to the patient's left to relieve aortocaval compression
- Remove both internal and external fetal monitors if present

Obstetric and neonatal teams should immediately prepare for possible emergency cesarean section

- If no ROSC by 4 minutes of resuscitative efforts, consider performing immediate emergency cesarean section
- Aim for delivery within 5 minutes of onset of resuscitative efforts

*An obviously gravid uterus is a uterus that is deemed clinically to be sufficiently large to cause aortocaval compression

Search for and Treat Possible Contributing Factors (BEAU-CHOPS)

Bleeding/DIC
Embolism: Coronary/pulmonary/amniotic fluid embolism
Anesthetic complications
Uterine atony
Cardiac disease (MI/ischemia/aortic dissection/cardiomyopathy)
Hypertension/pre-eclampsia/eclampsia
Other: Differential diagnosis of standard ACLS guidelines
Placenta abruptio/previa
Sepsis

ADULT ACLS ALGORITHMS

Adult Bradycardia

(With Pulse)

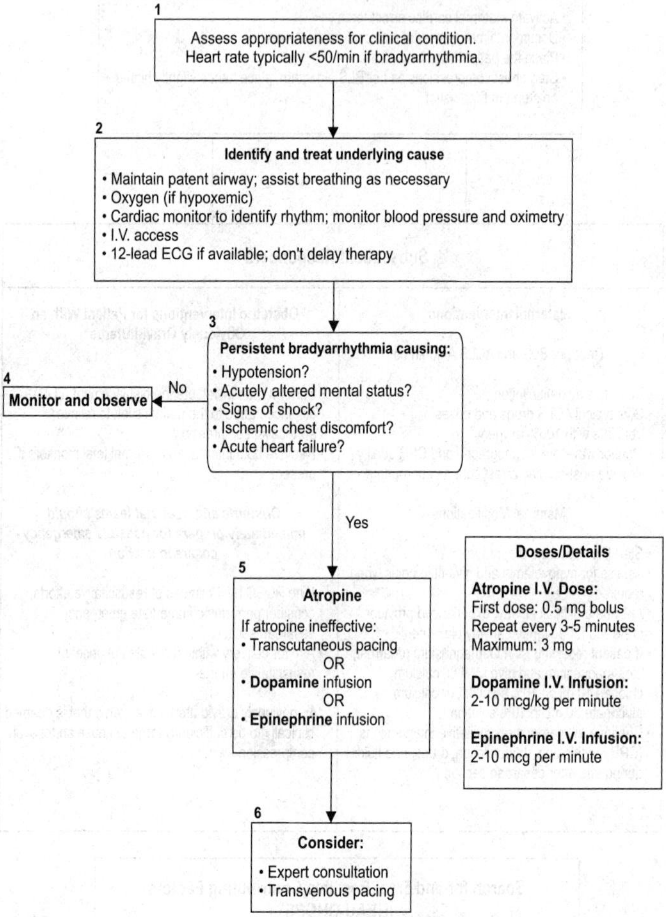

1
Assess appropriateness for clinical condition.
Heart rate typically <50/min if bradyarrhythmia.
2
Identify and treat underlying cause
• Maintain patent airway; assist breathing as necessary
• Oxygen (if hypoxemic)
• Cardiac monitor to identify rhythm; monitor blood pressure and oximetry
• I.V. access
• 12-lead ECG if available; don't delay therapy
3
Persistent bradyarrhythmia causing:
• Hypotension?
• Acutely altered mental status?
• Signs of shock?
• Ischemic chest discomfort?
• Acute heart failure?
No
4
Monitor and observe
Yes
5
Atropine
If atropine ineffective:
• Transcutaneous pacing
OR
• Dopamine infusion
OR
• Epinephrine infusion
Doses/Details
Atropine I.V. Dose:
First dose: 0.5 mg bolus
Repeat every 3-5 minutes
Maximum: 3 mg
Dopamine I.V. Infusion:
2-10 mcg/kg per minute
Epinephrine I.V. Infusion:
2-10 mcg per minute
6
Consider:
• Expert consultation
• Transvenous pacing

Adult Cardiac Arrest

Shout for Help/Activate Emergency Response

© 2010 American Heart Association

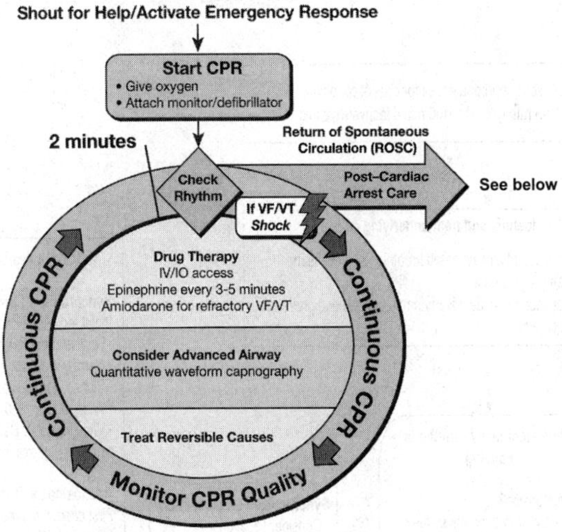

CPR Quality

- Push hard (≥2 inches [5 cm]) and fast (≥100/min) and allow complete chest recoil
- Minimize interruptions in compressions
- Avoid excessive ventilation
- Rotate compressor every 2 minutes
- If no advanced airway, 30:2 compression-ventilation ratio
- Quantitative waveform capnography
 - If PETCO$_2$ <10 mm Hg, attempt to improve CPR quality
- Intra-arterial pressure
 - If relaxation phase (diastolic) pressure <20 mm Hg, attempt to improve CPR quality

Return of Spontaneous Circulation (ROSC)

- Pulse and blood pressure
- Abrupt sustained increase in PETCO$_2$ (typically ≥40 mm Hg)
- Spontaneous arterial pressure waves with intra-arterial monitoring

Shock Energy

- **Biphasic:** Manufacturer recommendation (120-200 J); if unknown, use maximum available. Second and subsequent doses should be equivalent, and higher doses may be considered.
- **Monophasic:** 360 J

Drug Therapy

- Epinephrine I.V./I.O. Dose: 1 mg every 3-5 minutes
- Vasopressin I.V./I.O. Dose: 40 units can replace first or second dose of epinephrine
- Amiodarone I.V./I.O. Dose: First dose: 300 mg bolus; Second dose: 150 mg

Advanced Airway

- Supraglottic advanced airway or endotracheal intubation
- Waveform capnography to confirm and monitor ET tube placement
- 8-10 breaths per minute with continuous chest compressions

Reversible Causes

- Hypovolemia; Hypoxia; Hydrogen ion (acidosis); Hypo-/hyperkalemia; Hypothermia
- Tension pneumothorax; Tamponade, cardiac; Toxins; Thrombosis, pulmonary; Thrombosis, coronary

Adult Tachycardia
(With Pulse)

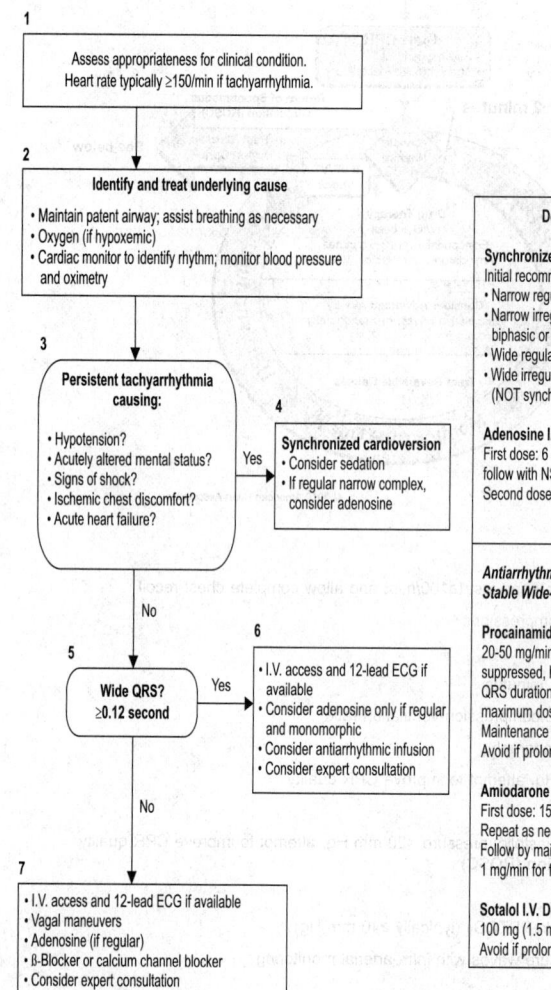

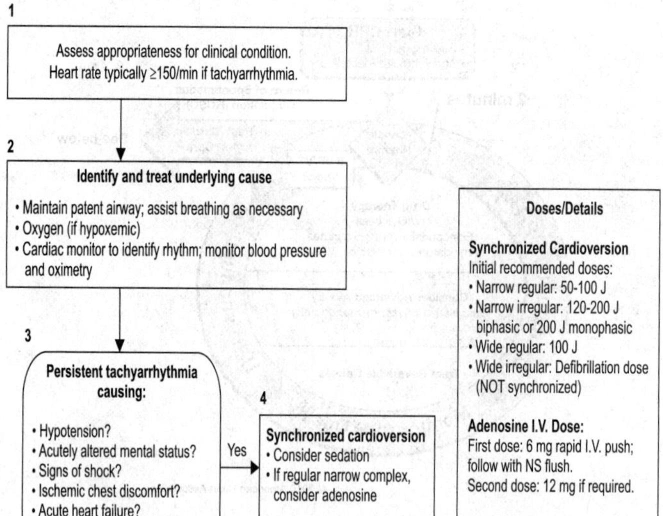
1
Assess appropriateness for clinical condition.
Heart rate typically ≥150/min if tachyarrhythmia.
2
Identify and treat underlying cause
• Maintain patent airway; assist breathing as necessary
• Oxygen (if hypoxemic)
• Cardiac monitor to identify rhythm; monitor blood pressure and oximetry
3
Persistent tachyarrhythmia causing:
• Hypotension?
• Acutely altered mental status?
• Signs of shock?
• Ischemic chest discomfort?
• Acute heart failure?
Yes
4
Synchronized cardioversion
• Consider sedation
• If regular narrow complex, consider adenosine
No
5
Wide QRS? ≥0.12 second
Yes
6
• I.V. access and 12-lead ECG if available
• Consider adenosine only if regular and monomorphic
• Consider antiarrhythmic infusion
• Consider expert consultation
No
7
• I.V. access and 12-lead ECG if available
• Vagal maneuvers
• Adenosine (if regular)
• ß-Blocker or calcium channel blocker
• Consider expert consultation
Doses/Details
Synchronized Cardioversion
Initial recommended doses:
• Narrow regular: 50-100 J
• Narrow irregular: 120-200 J biphasic or 200 J monophasic
• Wide regular: 100 J
• Wide irregular: Defibrillation dose (NOT synchronized)
Adenosine I.V. Dose:
First dose: 6 mg rapid I.V. push; follow with NS flush.
Second dose: 12 mg if required.
Antiarrhythmic Infusions for Stable Wide-QRS Tachycardia
Procainamide I.V. Dose:
20-50 mg/min until arrhythmia suppressed, hypotension ensues, QRS duration increases >50%, or maximum dose 17 mg/kg given.
Maintenance infusion: 1-4 mg/min.
Avoid if prolonged QT or CHF.
Amiodarone I.V. Dose:
First dose: 150 mg over 10 minutes.
Repeat as needed if VT recurs.
Follow by maintenance infusion of 1 mg/min for first 6 hours.
Sotalol I.V. Dose:
100 mg (1.5 mg/kg) over 5 minutes.
Avoid if prolonged QT.

ASTHMA

MANAGEMENT OF ASTHMA IN ADULTS AND CHILDREN

Goals of Asthma Treatment

- Prevent chronic and troublesome symptoms: Minimal or no chronic symptoms day or night
- No limitations on activities; no school/work missed
- Minimal use of inhaled short-acting beta$_2$-agonist (≤2 days/week, <1 canister/month) (not including prevention of exercise induced asthma)
- Minimal or no adverse effects from medications
- Maintain (near) normal pulmonary function
- Prevent recurrent exacerbations (ie, trips to emergency department or hospitalizations)

All Patients

- Short-acting bronchodilator: **Inhaled beta$_2$-agonists** as needed for symptoms.
- Intensity of treatment will depend on severity of exacerbation; see "Management of Asthma Exacerbations".
- Use of short-acting inhaled beta$_2$-agonists on a daily basis, or increasing use, indicates the need to initiate or titrate long-term control therapy.

Education

- Teach self-management.
- Teach about controlling environmental factors (avoidance of allergens or other factors that contribute to asthma severity).
- Review administration technique and compliance with patient.
- Use a written action plan to help educate.

Stepwise Approach for Managing Asthma in Adults and Children ≥12 Years of Age

Symptoms	Lung Function	Daily Medications
STEP 6: Severe Asthma		
Day: Throughout the day Night: Often 7 times/week SABA use: Several times/day	FEV_1 <60% predicted FEV_1/FVC reduced 5%	**Preferred:** High dose ICS plus LABA plus oral corticosteroid AND Consider: Omalizumab (in those with allergies)[1]
STEP 5: Severe Asthma		
Day: Throughout the day Night: Often 7 times/week SABA use: Several times/day	FEV_1 <60% predicted FEV_1/FVC reduced 5%	**Preferred:** High dose ICS plus LABA AND Consider: Omalizumab (in those with allergies)[1]
STEP 4: Severe Asthma		
Day: Throughout the day Night: Often 7 times/week SABA use: Several times/day	FEV_1 <60% predicted FEV_1/FVC reduced 5%	**Preferred:** Medium dose ICS plus LABA **Alternatives[2]:** Medium dose ICS plus either LTRA, theophylline, or zileuton[3]
STEP 3: Moderate Asthma		
Day: Daily Night: >1 night/week (not nightly) SABA use: Daily	FEV_1 >60%, <80% predicted FEV_1/FVC reduced 5%	**Preferred:** Low dose ICS plus LABA OR Medium dose ICS **Alternatives[2]:** Low dose ICS plus either LTRA, theophylline, or zileuton[3]
STEP 2: Mild Asthma		
Day: >2 days/week (not daily) Night: 3-4 times/month SABA use: >2 days/week, no more than once per day (not daily)	FEV_1 <80% FEV_1/FVC normal	**Preferred:** Low dose ICS **Alternatives[2]:** LTRA, nedocromil, or theophylline
STEP 1: Intermittent Asthma		
Day: ≤2 days/week Night: ≤2 nights/month SABA use: ≤2 days/week	FEV_1 normal between exacerbations FEV_1 >80% predicted FEV_1/FVC normal	Preferred: SABA as needed

Note: Treatment options within each step are listed in alphabetical order.

Steps 2-4: Consider subcutaneous allergen immunotherapy for patients with allergic asthma.[1]

Consult with asthma specialist if Step 4 or higher care is needed.

FEV_1 = forced expiratory volume in 1 second; FVC = forced vital capacity; ICS = inhaled corticosteroid; LABA = long-acting inhaled beta$_2$-agonist; SABA = short-acting inhaled beta$_2$-agonist; LTRA = leukotriene receptor antagonist.

[1]When using immunotherapy or omalizumab, clinicians should be prepared to identify and treat anaphylaxis in the event it occurs.

[2]If alternative treatment is used and response is inadequate, discontinue it and use preferred treatment before stepping up.

[3]Zileuton is less desirable alternative due to limited studies and need to monitor liver function.

Notes:

- **The stepwise approach presents general guidelines to assist clinical decision making; it is not intended to be a specific prescription. Asthma is highly variable; clinicians should tailor specific medication plans to the needs and circumstances of individual patients.**
- Gain control as quickly as possible; then decrease treatment to the least medication necessary to maintain control.
- A rescue course of systemic corticosteroids may be needed at any time and at any step.
- Some patients with intermittent asthma experience severe and life-threatening exacerbations separated by long periods of normal lung function and no symptoms. This may be especially common with exacerbations provoked by respiratory infections.
- At each step, patient education, environmental control, management of comorbidities emphasized.
- Antibiotics are not recommended for treatment of acute asthma exacerbations except where there is evidence or suspicion of bacterial infection.
- Consultation with an asthma specialist is recommended for moderate or severe persistent asthma.
- Peak flow monitoring for patients with moderate-severe persistent asthma and patients who have a history of severe exacerbations should be considered.

MANAGEMENT OF ASTHMA IN INFANTS AND YOUNG CHILDREN (<12 YEARS OF AGE)

Stepwise Approach for Managing Asthma in Children 0-4 Years of Age

Symptoms	Daily Medications[1]
STEP 6: Severe Asthma	
Day: Throughout the day Night: >1 time/week SABA use: Several times/day	**Preferred:** High dose ICS plus either LABA or montelukast Oral systemic corticosteroids
STEP 5: Severe Asthma	
Day: Throughout the day Night: >1 time/week SABA use: Daily	**Preferred:** High dose ICS plus either LABA or montelukast
STEP 4: Moderate Asthma	
Day: Daily Night: 3-4 times/month SABA use: Daily	**Preferred:** Medium dose ICS plus either LABA or montelukast
STEP 3: Moderate Asthma	
Day: Daily Night: 3-4 times/month SABA use: Daily	**Preferred:** Medium dose ICS
STEP 2: Mild Asthma	
Day: >2 days/week (not daily) Night: 1-2 times/month SABA use: >2 days/week, no more than once per day (not daily)	**Preferred:** Low dose ICS **Alternative[2]:** Montelukast
STEP 1: Intermittent Asthma	
Day: ≤2 days/week Night: No symptoms SABA use: ≤2 days/week	SABA as needed

Consult with asthma specialist if Step 3 or higher care is needed.

FEV_1 = forced expiratory volume in 1 second; FVC = forced vital capacity; ICS = inhaled corticosteroid; LABA = long-acting inhaled $beta_2$-agonist; SABA = short-acting inhaled $beta_2$-agonist.

[1]Studies on children 0-4 years old are limited. Many recommendations are based on expert opinion and extrapolation from studies of older children.

[2]If alternative treatment is used and response is inadequate, discontinue it and use preferred treatment before stepping up.

Stepwise Approach for Managing Asthma in Children 5-11 Years

Symptoms	Lung Function	Daily Medications
STEP 6: Severe Asthma		
Day: Throughout the day Night: Often 7 times/week SABA use: Several times/day	FEV_1 <60% predicted FEV_1/FVC <75%	**Preferred:** High dose ICS plus LABA plus oral corticosteroid **Alternative[1]:** High dose ICS plus either LTRA or theophylline[2] plus oral systemic corticosteroid
STEP 5: Severe Asthma		
Day: Throughout the day Night: Often 7 times/week SABA use: Several times/day	FEV_1 <60% predicted FEV_1/FVC <75%	**Preferred:** High dose ICS plus LABA **Alternative[1]:** High dose ICS plus either LTRA or theophylline[2]
STEP 4: Severe Asthma		
Day: Throughout the day Night: Often 7 times/week SABA use: Several times/day	FEV_1 <60% predicted FEV_1/FVC <75%	**Preferred:** Medium dose ICS plus LABA **Alternative[1]:** Medium dose ICS plus either LTRA or theophylline[2]
STEP 3: Moderate Asthma		
Day: Daily Night: >1 time/week (not nightly) SABA use: Daily	FEV_1 60% to 80% predicted FEV_1/FVC 75% to 80%	**Preferred:** Low dose ICS plus either LABA, LTRA, or theophylline[2] OR Medium dose ICS
STEP 2: Mild Asthma		
Day: >2 days/week (not daily) Night: 3-4 times/month SABA use: >2 days/week, no more than once per day (not daily)	FEV_1 ≥80% predicted FEV_1/FVC >80%	**Preferred:** Low dose ICS **Alternatives[1]:** LTRA, nedocromil, or theophylline[2]
STEP 1: Intermittent Asthma		
Day: ≤2 days/week Night: ≤2 times/month SABA use: ≤2 days/week	FEV_1 normal between exacerbations FEV_1 >80% predicted FEV_1/FVC >85%	SABA as needed

Steps 2-4: Consider subcutaneous allergen immunotherapy for patients with allergic asthma.[3]

Consult with asthma specialist if Step 4 or higher care is needed.

FEV_1 = forced expiratory volume in 1 second; FVC = forced vital capacity; ICS = inhaled corticosteroid; LABA = long-acting inhaled beta$_2$-agonist; SABA = short-acting inhaled beta$_2$-agonist; LTRA = leukotriene receptor antagonist.

[1]If alternative treatment is used and response is inadequate, discontinue it and use preferred treatment before stepping up.

[2]Theophylline is a less desirable alternative due to monitoring required.

[3]When using immunotherapy, clinicians should be prepared to identify and treat anaphylaxis in the event it occurs.

Management of Asthma Exacerbations: Home Treatment

Assess Severity

- **Patients at high risk for a fatal attack require immediate medical attention after initial treatment.**
- Symptoms and signs suggestive of a more serious exacerbation such as marked breathlessness, inability to speak more than short phrases, use of accessory muscles, or drowsiness should result in initial treatment while immediately consulting with a clinician.
- If available, measure PEF—values of 50% to 79% predicted or personal best indicate the need for quick-relief mediation. Depending on the response to treatment, contact with a clinician may also be indicated. Values below 50% indicate the need for immediate medical care.

↓

Initial Treatment

- Inhaled SABA: Up to two treatments 20 minutes apart of 2–6 puffs by metered-dose inhaler (MDI) or nebulizer treatments.
- Note: Medication delivery is highly variable. Children and individuals who have exacerbations of lesser severity may need fewer puffs than suggested above.

↓

Good Response

No wheezing or dyspnea (assess tachypnea in young children).

PEF ≥80% predicted or personal best.

- Contact clinician for followup instructions and further management.
- May continue inhaled SABA every 3–4 hours for 24–48 hours.
- Consider short course of oral systemic corticosteroids.

Incomplete Response

Persistent wheezing and dyspnea (tachypnea).

PEF 50% to 79% predicted or personal best.

- Add oral systemic corticosteroid.
- Continue inhaled SABA.
- Contact clinician urgently (this day) for further instruction.

Poor Response

Marked wheezing and dyspnea.

PEF <50% predicted or personal best.

- Add oral systemic corticosteroid
- Repeat inhaled SABA immediately.
- If distress is severe and nonresponsive to initial treatment:
  - Call your doctor AND
  - **PROCEED TO EMERGENCY DEPARTMENT**;
  - Consider calling 911 (ambulance transport).

↓

- To emergency department.

MDI: Metered-dose inhaler; PEF: Peak expiratory flow; SABA: Short-acting $beta_2$-agonist (quick relief inhaler)

Management of Asthma Exacerbations: Emergency Department and Hospital-Based Care

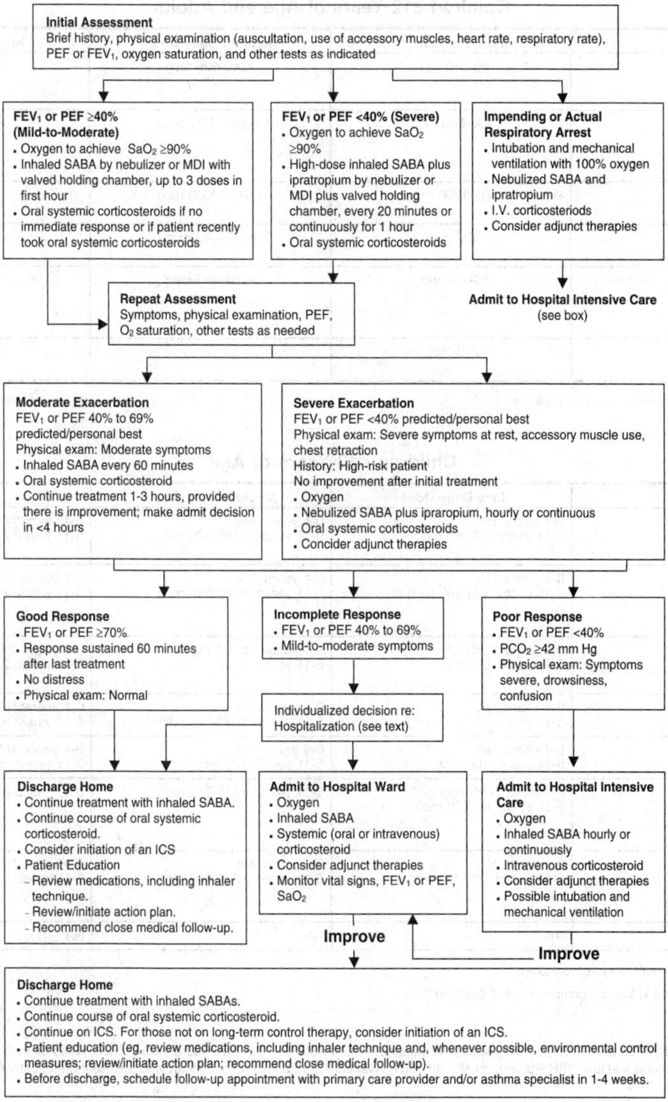

Initial Assessment
Brief history, physical examination (auscultation, use of accessory muscles, heart rate, respiratory rate), PEF or FEV_1, oxygen saturation, and other tests as indicated
FEV_1 or PEF ≥40% (Mild-to-Moderate)
• Oxygen to achieve SaO_2 ≥90%
• Inhaled SABA by nebulizer or MDI with valved holding chamber, up to 3 doses in first hour
• Oral systemic corticosteroids if no immediate response or if patient recently took oral systemic corticosteroids
FEV_1 or PEF <40% (Severe)
• Oxygen to achieve SaO_2 ≥90%
• High-dose inhaled SABA plus ipratropium by nebulizer or MDI plus valved holding chamber, every 20 minutes or continuously for 1 hour
• Oral systemic corticosteroids
Impending or Actual Respiratory Arrest
• Intubation and mechanical ventilation with 100% oxygen
• Nebulized SABA and ipratropium
• I.V. corticosteriods
• Consider adjunct therapies
Admit to Hospital Intensive Care (see box)
Repeat Assessment
Symptoms, physical examination, PEF, O_2 saturation, other tests as needed
Moderate Exacerbation
FEV_1 or PEF 40% to 69% predicted/personal best
Physical exam: Moderate symptoms
• Inhaled SABA every 60 minutes
• Oral systemic corticosteroid
• Continue treatment 1-3 hours, provided there is improvement; make admit decision in <4 hours
Severe Exacerbation
FEV_1 or PEF <40% predicted/personal best
Physical exam: Severe symptoms at rest, accessory muscle use, chest retraction
History: High-risk patient
No improvement after initial treatment
• Oxygen
• Nebulized SABA plus iprarpoium, hourly or continuous
• Oral systemic corticosteroids
• Concider adjunct therapies
Good Response
• FEV_1 or PEF ≥70%
• Response sustained 60 minutes after last treatment
• No distress
• Physical exam: Normal
Incomplete Response
• FEV_1 or PEF 40% to 69%
• Mild-to-moderate symptoms
Poor Response
• FEV_1 or PEF <40%
• PCO_2 ≥42 mm Hg
• Physical exam: Symptoms severe, drowsiness, confusion
Individualized decision re: Hospitalization (see text)
Discharge Home
• Continue treatment with inhaled SABA.
• Continue course of oral systemic corticosteroid.
• Consider initiation of an ICS
• Patient Education
- Review medications, including inhaler technique.
- Review/initiate action plan.
- Recommend close medical follow-up.
Admit to Hospital Ward
• Oxygen
• Inhaled SABA
• Systemic (oral or intravenous) corticosteroid
• Consider adjunct therapies
• Monitor vital signs, FEV_1 or PEF, SaO_2
Admit to Hospital Intensive Care
• Oxygen
• Inhaled SABA hourly or continuously
• Intravenous corticosteroid
• Consider adjunct therapies
• Possible intubation and mechanical ventilation
Improve
Improve
Discharge Home
• Continue treatment with inhaled SABAs.
• Continue course of oral systemic corticosteroid.
• Continue on ICS. For those not on long-term control therapy, consider initiation of an ICS.
• Patient education (eg, review medications, including inhaler technique and, whenever possible, environmental control measures; review/initiate action plan; recommend close medical follow-up).
• Before discharge, schedule follow-up appointment with primary care provider and/or asthma specialist in 1-4 weeks.

FEV_1 = forced expiratory volume in 1 second; ICS = inhaled corticosteroid; MDI = metered dose inhaler; PCO_2 = partial pressure carbon dioxide; PEF = peak expiratory flow; SABA = short-acting $beta_2$-agonist; SaO_2 = oxygen saturation

ESTIMATED COMPARATIVE DAILY DOSAGES FOR INHALED CORTICOSTEROIDS

Children ≥12 Years of Age and Adults

Drug	Low Daily Dose	Medium Daily Dose	High Daily Dose
Beclomethasone HFA 40 mcg/puff 80 mcg/puff	80-240 mcg	>240-480 mcg	>480 mcg
Budesonide DPI 90 mcg/puff 180 mcg/puff 200 mcg/puff	180-600 mcg	>600-1200 mcg	>1200 mcg
Flunisolide 250 mcg/puff	500-1000 mcg	>1000-2000 mcg	>2000 mcg
Flunisolide HFA 80 mcg/puff	320 mcg	>320-640 mcg	>640 mcg
Fluticasone HFA 44 mcg/puff 110 mcg/puff 220 mcg/puff	88-264 mcg	>264-440 mcg	>440 mcg
Mometasone DPI 220 mcg/puff	220 mcg	440 mcg	>440 mcg

DPI = dry powder inhaler, HFA = hydrofluoroalkane

Children <12 Years of Age

Drug	Low Daily Dose	Medium Daily Dose	High Daily Dose
Beclomethasone HFA 40 mcg/puff 80 mcg/puff	0-4 years: NA 5-11 years: 80-160 mcg	0-4 years: NA 5-11 years: >160-320 mcg	0-4 years: NA 5-11 years: >320 mcg
Budesonide DPI 90 mcg/puff 180 mcg/puff 200 mcg/puff	0-4 years: NA 5-11 years: 180-400 mcg	0-4 years: NA 5-11 years: >400-800 mcg	0-4 years: NA 5-11 years: >800 mcg
Budesonide nebulized 0.25 mg/2 mL 0.5 mg/2 mL	0-4 years: 0.25-0.5 mg 5-11 years: 0.5 mg	0-4 years: >0.5-1 mg 5-11 years: 1 mg	0-4 years: >1 mg 5-11 years: 2 mg
Flunisolide 250 mcg/puff	0-4 years: NA 5-11 years: 500-750 mcg	0-4 years: NA 5-11 years: 1000-1250 mcg	0-4 years: NA 5-11 years: >1250 mcg
Flunisolide HFA 80 mcg/puff	0-4 years: NA 5-11 years: 160 mcg	0-4 years: NA 5-11 years: 320 mcg	0-4 years: NA 5-11 years: ≥640 mcg
Fluticasone HFA 44 mcg/puff 110 mcg/puff 220 mcg/puff	0-4 years: 176 mcg 5-11 years: 88-176 mcg	0-11 years: >176-352 mcg	0-11 years: >352 mcg
Fluticasone DPI 50 mcg/puff 100 mcg/puff 250 mcg/puff	0-4 years: NA 5-11 years: 100-200 mcg	0-4 years: NA 5-11 years: >200-400 mcg	0-4 years: NA 5-11 years: >400 mcg
Mometasone	NA	NA	NA

DPI = dry powder inhaler, HFA = hydrofluoroalkane

NA = not approved for use in this age group or no data available

REFERENCE

Expert Panel Report 3, "Guidelines for the Diagnosis and Management of Asthma," *Clinical Practice Guidelines*, National Institutes of Health, National Heart, Lung, and Blood Institute, NIH Publication No. 08-4051. Available at http://www.nhlbi.nih.gov/guidelines/asthma/asthgdln.htm

BEERS CRITERIA – POTENTIALLY INAPPROPRIATE MEDICATIONS FOR GERIATRICS

Table 1. Criteria Independent of Diagnoses or Conditions

Applicable Medication	Summary of Prescribing Concern	Severity
Amiodarone (Cordarone®)	Associated with QT interval problems and risk of provoking torsade de pointes. Lack of efficacy in older adults.	High
Amitriptyline (Elavil®), amitriptyline and chlordiazepoxide (Limbitrol®), and amitriptyline and perphenazine (Triavil®)	Because of its strong anticholinergic and sedation properties, amitriptyline is rarely the antidepressant of choice for elderly patients.	High
Amphetamines (excluding methylphenidate hydrochloride and anorexics)	CNS stimulant adverse effects	High
Amphetamines and anorexic agents	These drugs have potential for causing dependence, hypertension, angina, and myocardial infarction.	High
Anticholinergics and antihistamines: Chlorpheniramine (Chlor-Trimeton®), diphenhydrAMINE (Benadryl®), hydrOXYzine (Vistaril®, Atarax®), cyproheptadine (Periactin), promethazine (Phenergan®), tripelennamine, dexchlorpheniramine (Polaramine®)	All nonprescription and many prescription antihistamines may have potent anticholinergic properties. Nonanticholinergic antihistamines are preferred in elderly patients when treating allergic reactions.	High
Barbiturates (all, except PHENobarbital) except when used to control seizures	Are highly addictive and cause more adverse effects than most sedative or hypnotic drugs in elderly patients.	High
Benzodiazepines, long-acting: ChlordiazePOXIDE (Librium®), amitriptyline and chlordiazepoxide (Limbitrol®), clidinium and chlordiazepoxide (Librax®), diazepam (Valium®), quazepam (Doral®), halazepam (Paxipam®), and chlorazepate (Tranxene®)	These drugs have a long half-life in elderly patients (often several days), producing prolonged sedation and increasing the risk of falls and fractures. Short- and intermediate-acting benzodiazepines are preferred if a benzodiazepine is required.	High
Benzodiazepines, short-acting (doses greater than): Alprazolam (Xanax®) 2 mg; oxazepam (Serax®) 60 mg; LORazepam (Ativan®) 3 mg; temazepam (Restoril®) 15 mg; and triazolam (Halcion®) 0.25 mg	Because of increased sensitivity to benzodiazepines in elderly patients, smaller doses may be effective as well as safer. Total daily doses should rarely exceed the suggested maximums.	High
Chlorpropamide (Diabinese®)	It has prolonged half-life in elderly patients and could cause prolonged hypoglycemia. Additionally, it is the only oral hypoglycemic agent that causes SIADH.	High
Cimetidine (Tagamet®)	CNS adverse effects, including confusion	Low
CloNIDine (Catapres®)	Potential for orthostatic hypotension and CNS adverse effects	Low
Cyclandelate (Cyclospasmol®)	Lack of efficacy	Low
Desiccated thyroid	Concerns about cardiac effects; safer alternatives available	High
Digoxin (Lanoxin®) (should not exceed >0.125 mg/day except when treating atrial arrhythmias)	Decreased renal clearance may lead to increased risk of toxic effects	Low
DiphenhydrAMINE (Benadryl®)	May cause confusion and sedation. Should not be used as a hypnotic, and when used to treat emergency allergic reactions, it should be used in the smallest possible dose.	High
Dipyridamole, short-acting (Persantine®). Do not consider the long-acting dipyridamole (which has better properties than the short-acting in older adults) except with patients with artificial heart valves	May cause orthostatic hypotension	Low
Disopyramide (Norpace®, Norpace® CR)	Of all antiarrhythmic drugs, this is the most potent negative inotrope and therefore may induce heart failure in elderly patients. It is also strongly anticholinergic. Other antiarrhythmic drugs should be used.	High
Doxazosin (Cardura®)	Potential for hypotension, dry mouth, and urinary problems	Low
Doxepin (SINEquan®)	Because of its strong anticholinergic and sedating properties, doxepin is rarely the antidepressant of choice for elderly patients.	High
Ergot mesyloids (Hydergine®) and cyclandelate (Cyclospasmol®)	Have not been shown to be effective in the doses studied	Low
Estrogens only (oral)	Evidence of the carcinogenic (breast and endometrial cancer) potential of these agents and lack of cardioprotective effect in older women	Low
Ethacrynic acid (Edecrin®)	Potential for hypertension and fluid imbalances; safer alternatives available	Low
Ferrous sulfate >325 mg/day	Doses >325 mg/day do not dramatically increase the amount absorbed but greatly increase the incidence of constipation.	Low
FLUoxetine, daily (PROzac®)	Long half-life of drug and risk of producing excessive CNS stimulation, sleep disturbances, and increasing agitation. Safer alternatives exist.	High

Table 1. Criteria Independent of Diagnoses or Conditions *(continued)*

Applicable Medication	Summary of Prescribing Concern	Severity
Flurazepam (Dalmane®)	This benzodiazepine hypnotic has an extremely long half-life in elderly patients (often days), producing prolonged sedation and increasing the incidence of falls and fracture. Medium- or short-acting benzodiazepines are preferable.	High
Gastrointestinal antispasmodic drugs: Dicyclomine (Bentyl®), hyoscyamine (Levsin® and Levsinex®), propantheline (Pro-Banthine), belladonna alkaloids (Donnatal® and others), and clidinium and chlordiazepoxide (Librax®)	GI antispasmodic drugs are highly anticholinergic and have uncertain effectiveness. These drugs should be avoided (especially for long-term use).	High
Guanadrel (Hylorel®)	May cause orthostatic hypotension	High
Guanethidine (Ismelin®)	May cause orthostatic hypotension; safer alternatives exist	High
Indomethacin (Indocin® and Indocin® SR)	Of all available NSAIDs, this drug produces the most CNS adverse effects.	High
Isoxsuprine (Vasodilan®)	Lack of efficacy	Low
Ketorolac (Toradol®)	Immediate and long-term use should be avoided in older persons, since a significant number have asymptomatic GI pathologic conditions.	High
Long-term use of full-dosage, longer half-life, non-COX-selective NSAIDs: Naproxen (Naprosyn®, Avaprox, and Aleve®), oxaprozin (Daypro®), and piroxicam (Feldene®)	Have the potential to produce GI bleeding, renal failure, high blood pressure, and heart failure	High
Long-term use of stimulant laxatives: Bisacodyl (Dulcolax®), cascara sagrada, and Neoloid except in the presence of opiate analgesic use	May exacerbate bowel dysfunction	High
Meperidine (Demerol®)	Not an effective oral analgesic in doses commonly used. May cause confusion and has many disadvantages to other narcotic drugs.	High
Meprobamate (Miltown®)	This is a highly addictive and sedating anxiolytic. Those using meprobamate for prolonged periods may become addicted and may need to be withdrawn slowly.	High
Mesoridazine (Serentil®)	CNS and extrapyramidal adverse effects	High
Methyldopa (Aldomet) and methyldopa and hydrochlorothiazide (Aldoril®)	May cause bradycardia and exacerbate depression in elderly patients	High
Methyltestosterone (Android®, Testrad®, Virilon®)	Potential for prostatic hypertrophy and cardiac problems	High
Mineral oil	Potential for aspiration and adverse effects; safer alternatives available	High
Muscle relaxants and antispasmodics: Methocarbamol (Robaxin®), carisoprodol (Soma®), chlorzoxazone (Paraflex®), metaxalone (Skelaxin®), cyclobenzaprine (Flexeril®), and oxybutynin (Ditropan®). Do not consider the extended-release Ditropan® XL.	Most muscle relaxants and antispasmodic drugs are poorly tolerated by elderly patients, since these cause anticholinergic adverse effects, sedation, and weakness. Additionally, their effectiveness at doses tolerated by elderly patients is questionable.	High
NIFEdipine, short-acting (Adalat®, Procardia®)	Potential for hypotension and constipation	High
Nitrofurantoin (Macrodantin®)	Potential for renal impairment; safer alternatives available	High
Orphenadrine (Norflex™)	Causes more sedation and anticholinergic adverse effects than safer alternatives	High
Pentazocine (Talwin®)	Narcotic analgesic that causes more CNS adverse effects, including confusion and hallucinations, more commonly than other narcotic drugs. Additionally, it is a mixed agonist and antagonist.	High
Propoxyphene (Darvon®) and combination products (Darvon® with ASA, Darvon-N®, and Darvocet-N®)	Offers few analgesic advantages over acetaminophen, yet has the adverse effects of other narcotic drugs	Low
Reserpine at doses >0.25 mg	May induce depression, impotence, sedation, and orthostatic hypotension	Low
Thioridazine (Mellaril®)	Greater potential for CNS and extrapyramidal adverse effects	High
Ticlopidine (Ticlid®)	Has been shown to be no better than aspirin in preventing clotting and may be considerably more toxic. Safer, more effective alternatives exist.	High
Trimethobenzamide (Tigan®)	One of the least effective antiemetic drugs, yet it can cause extrapyramidal adverse effects	High

Table 2. Final Criteria Considering Diagnoses or Conditions

Disease or Condition	Drug	Concern	Severity
Anorexia and malnutrition	CNS stimulants: Dextroamphetamine and amphetamine (Adderall®), methylphenidate (Ritalin®), methamphetamine (Desoxyn®), pemolin, and FLUoxetine (PROzac®)	Concern due to appetite-suppressing effects	High
Arrhythmias	Tricyclic antidepressants (imipramine hydrochloride, doxepin hydrochloride, and amitriptyline hydrochloride)	Concern due to proarrhythmic effects and ability to produce QT interval changes	High
Bladder outflow obstruction	Anticholinergics and antihistamines, gastrointestinal antispasmodics, muscle relaxants, oxybutynin (Ditropan®), flavoxATE (Urispas®), anticholinergics, antidepressants, decongestants, and tolterodine (Detrol®)	May decrease urinary flow, leading to urinary retention	High
Blood clotting disorders or receiving anticoagulant therapy	Aspirin, NSAIDs, dipyridamole (Persantine®), ticlopidine (Ticlid®), and clopidogrel (Plavix®)	May prolong clotting time and elevate INR values or inhibit platelet aggregation, resulting in an increased potential for bleeding	High
Chronic constipation	Calcium channel blockers, anticholinergics, and tricyclic antidepressant (imipramine hydrochloride, doxepin hydrochloride, and amitriptyline hydrochloride)	May exacerbate constipation	Low
Cognitive impairment	Barbiturates, anticholinergics, antispasmodics, and muscle relaxants, CNS stimulants: Dextroamphetamine and amphetamine (Adderall®), methylphenidate (Ritalin®), methamphetamine (Desoxyn®), and pemolin	Concern due to CNS-altering effects	High
COPD	Benzodiazepines, long-acting: ChlordiazePOXIDE (Librium®), amitriptyline and chlordiazepoxide (Limbitrol®), clidinium and chlordiazepoxide (Librax®), diazepam (Valium®), quazepam (Doral®), and chlorazepate (Tranxene®). Beta-blockers: Propranolol	CNS adverse effects. May induce respiratory depression. May exacerbate or cause respiratory depression.	High
Depression	Long-term benzodiazepine use. Sympatholytic agents: Methyldopa (Aldomet), reserpine, and guanethidine (Ismelin)	May produce or exacerbate depression	High
Gastric or duodenal ulcers	NSAIDs and aspirin (>325 mg) (coxibs excluded)	May exacerbate existing ulcers or produce new/additional ulcers	High
Heart failure	Disopyramide (Norpace®), and high sodium content drugs (sodium and sodium salts [alginate bicarbonate, biphosphate, citrate, phosphate, salicylate, and sulfate])	Negative inotropic effect. Potential to promote fluid retention and exacerbation of heart failure.	High
Hypertension	Phenylpropanolamine hydrochloride (removed from the market in 2001), pseudoephedrine; diet pills, and amphetamines	May produce elevation of blood pressure secondary to sympathomimetic activity	High
Insomnia	Decongestants, theophylline (Theodur), methylphenidate (Ritalin®), MAOIs, and amphetamines	Concern due to CNS stimulant effects	High
Obesity	OLANZapine (ZyPREXA®)	May stimulate appetite and increase weight gain	Low
Parkinson disease	Metoclopramide (Reglan®), conventional antipsychotics, and tacrine (Cognex®)	Concern due to their antidopaminergic/ cholinergic effects	High
Seizures or epilepsy	CloZAPine (Clozaril®), chlorproMAZINE (Thorazine®), thioridazine (Mellaril®), thiothixene (Navane®)	May lower seizure thresholds	High
Seizure disorder	BuPROPion (Wellbutrin®)	May lower seizure threshold	High
SIADH/hyponatremia	SSRIs: FLUoxetine (PROzac®), citalopram (CeleXA™), fluvoxaMINE (Luvox®), paroxetine (Paxil®), and sertraline (Zoloft®)	May exacerbate or cause SIADH	Low
Stress incontinence	α-Blockers (doxazosin, prazosin, and terazosin), anticholinergic, tricyclic antidepressants (imipramine hydrochloride, doxepin hydrochloride, and amitriptyline hydrochloride), and long-acting benzodiazepines	May produce polyuria and worsening of incontinence	High
Syncope or falls	Short- to intermediate-acting benzodiazepine and tricyclic antidepressants (imipramine hydrochloride, doxepin hydrochloride, and amitriptyline hydrochloride)	May produce ataxia, impaired psychomotor function, syncope, and additional falls	High

REFERENCE

Fick DM, Cooper JW, Wade WE, et al, "Updating the Beers Criteria for Potentially Inappropriate Medication Use in Older Adults: Results of a U.S. Consensus Panel of Experts," *Arch Intern Med,* 2003, 163(22):2716-24.

CONTRAST MEDIA REACTIONS, PREMEDICATION FOR PROPHYLAXIS

It is estimated that approximately 5% to 10% of patients will experience adverse reactions to the administration of contrast dye (less for nonionic contrast). In approximately 1000-2000 administrations, a life-threatening reaction will occur.

A variety of premedication regimens have been proposed, both for pretreatment of "at risk" patients who require contrast media and before the routine administration of the intravenous high-osmolality contrast media (HOCM). Such regimens have been shown in clinical trials to decrease the frequency of all forms of contrast medium reactions. Logistical and feasibility problems may preclude adequate premedication with this or any regimen for all patients. It is unclear at this time that steroid pretreatment prior to administration of ionic contrast media reduces the incidence of reactions to the same extent or less than that achieved with the use of nonionic contrast media alone. Information about the efficacy of nonionic contrast media combined with a premedication strategy, including steroids, is preliminary or not yet currently available. For high-risk patients (ie, previous contrast reactors), the combination of a pretreatment regimen with nonionic contrast media has empirical merit and may warrant consideration. Oral administration of steroids appears preferable to intravascular routes, and the drug may be prednisone or methylprednisolone. Supplemental administration of H_1 and H_2 antihistamine therapies, orally or intravenously, may reduce the frequency of urticaria, angioedema, and respiratory symptoms. Additionally, ephedrine administration has been suggested to decrease the frequency of contrast reactions, but caution is advised in patients with cardiac disease, hypertension, or hyperthyroidism. No premedication strategy should be a substitute for the ABC approach to preadministration preparedness listed above. Contrast reactions occur despite any and all premedication prophylaxis. The incidence can be decreased, however, in some categories of "at risk" patients receiving HOCM plus a medication regimen. For patients with previous contrast medium reactions, there is a slight chance that recurrence may be more severe or the same as the prior reaction; however, it is more likely that there will be no recurrence.

PREMEDICATION REGIMENS INCLUDE:

MethylPREDNISolone	32 mg orally 12 and 2 hours prior to the procedure
DiphenhydrAMINE	50 mg orally 1 hour prior to the procedure

OR

PredniSONE	50 mg orally 13, 7, and 1 hour before the procedure
DiphenhydrAMINE	50 mg orally 1 hour before the procedure

OR

PredniSONE	60 mg orally the night before and the morning of the procedure
DiphenhydrAMINE	50 mg orally 1 hour before the procedure

SUGGESTED REGIMEN FOR EMERGENT PROCEDURE (EG, PRIMARY PCI)

Hydrocortisone or MethylPREDNISolone or Dexamethasone	100 mg I.V. (hydrocortisone) **or** 80-125 mg I.V. (methylPREDNISolone) **or** 16 mg I.V. (dexamethasone) before the procedure
Cimetidine	300 mg I.V. before the procedure
DiphenhydrAMINE	25-50 mg I.V. or P.O. before the procedure

INDICATIONS FOR NONIONIC CONTRAST

- Previous reaction to contrast − premedicate. **Note:** For life-threatening reactions (throat swelling, laryngeal edema, etc), consider omitting the I.V. contrast
- Known allergy to iodine or shellfish
- Asthma, especially if on medication
- Myocardial instability or HF
- Risk for aspiration or severe nausea and vomiting
- Difficulty communicating or inability to give history
- Patients taking beta-blockers
- Small children at risk for electrolyte imbalance or extravasation
- Renal failure with diabetes, sickle cell disease, or myeloma
- At physician or patient request

CONTRAST-INDUCED NEPHROTOXICITY (CIN)

CIN is a common complication after exposure to I.V. radiocontrast agents. In the literature, CIN is defined as a rise in serum creatinine concentration of at least 0.5 mg/dL or an increase of 25% compared to baseline occurring after exposure to contrast medium. Most of the time, this increase in serum creatinine is transient; however, in some cases, the impairment may be permanent with some patients requiring dialysis. Many agents have been evaluated for prevention of this adverse event; however, only acetylcysteine, sodium bicarbonate, and sodium chloride have shown benefit. Of note, the Acetylcysteine for Contrast-induced Nephropathy Trial (ACT) demonstrated no benefit with acetylcysteine compared to placebo in patients undergoing coronary and vascular angiography. Use of acetylcysteine is no longer recommended in the prevention of CIN for patients undergoing percutaneous coronary intervention (PCI).

Risk Factors for CIN:

- Pre-existing renal impairment
- Diabetes nephropathy
- Age >70 years
- Hypovolemia
- Anemia
- Heart failure
- Hypotension
- Concomitant nephrotoxins (eg, aminoglycosides)
- Large contrast medium doses (eg, ≥140 mL)
- Type of contrast agent used (high-osmolality contrast media > low-osmolality contrast media)

STRATEGIES FOR THE PREVENTION OF CIN

General recommendations	1. Stratify all patients for risk of CIN prior to contrast exposure
	2. Optimize volume status
	3. Administer prehydration and prophylaxis using therapies with proven clinical benefit to all high-risk patients
	4. Minimize contrast media volumes, especially in those with Cl_{Cr} <60 mL/minute; use of low- or iso-osmolality contrast agents has been suggested
	5. Hold medications that adversely affect renal function before and after contrast exposure
	6. Obtain follow-up serum creatinine between 24-72 hours after contrast exposure
Specific therapies:	
Acetylcysteine, P.O.[1]	600 mg orally twice daily on the day before and the day of the scan in addition to hydration with 0.45% saline intravenously
Sodium bicarbonate, I.V. (154 mEq/L)	3 mL/kg/hour for 1 hour prior to contrast injection, then 1 mL/kg/hour during contrast exposure and for 6 hours after procedure
Sodium chloride 0.9%, I.V.	1-1.5 mL/kg/hour for 3-12 hours prior to and for 6-24 hours after procedure

[1]The Acetylcysteine for Contrast-induced Nephropathy Trial (ACT) demonstrated no benefit in patients undergoing coronary and vascular angiography. Use is no longer recommended in the prevention of CIN for patients undergoing percutaneous coronary intervention (PCI).

REFERENCES

ACT Investigators, "Acetylcysteine for Prevention of Renal Outcomes in Patients Undergoing Coronary and Peripheral Vascular Angiography: Main Results From the Randomized Acetylcysteine for Contrast-Induced Nephropathy Trial (ACT)," *Circulation*, 2011, 124(11):1250-9.

American College of Radiology, "Manual on Contrast Media, Version 6.0," 2008. Available at http://www.acr.org/SecondaryMainMenuCategories/quality_safety/contrast_manual.aspx

Klein LW, Sheldon MW, Brinker J, et al, "The Use of Radiographic Contrast Media During PCI: A Focused Review: A Position Statement of the Society of Cardiovascular Angiography and Interventions," *Catheter Cardiovasc Interv*, 2009, 74(5):728-46.

Levine GN, Bates ER, Blankenship JC, et al, "2011 ACCF/AHA/SCAI Guideline for Percutaneous Coronary Intervention: A Report of the American College of Cardiology Foundation/American Heart Association Task Force on Practice Guidelines and the Society for Cardiovascular Angiography and Interventions," *J Am Coll Cardiol*, 2011, 58(24):e44-e122.

Massicotte A, "Contrast Medium-Induced Nephropathy: Strategies for Prevention," *Pharmacotherapy*, 2008, 28(9):1140-50.

Merten GJ, Burgess WP, Gray LV, et al, "Prevention of Contrast-Induced Nephropathy With Sodium Bicarbonate: A Randomized Controlled Trial," *JAMA*, 2004, 291(19):2328-34.

DIABETES MELLITUS AND PREGNANCY

OVERVIEW OF DIABETES

Diabetes represents a significant health care problem in the United States and worldwide. Of the nearly 23.6 million Americans (7.8% of the population) with diabetes, the majority (90% to 95%) have type 2 diabetes. Of this number, nearly one-quarter are undiagnosed and the incidence is increasing. There is strong evidence to support an interaction between a genetic predisposition and behavioral or environmental factors, such as obesity and physical inactivity, in the development of this disease. In individuals at high risk of developing type 2 diabetes, it has been shown that the development of diabetes may be prevented or delayed by changes in lifestyle or pharmacologic intervention.

Within the United States, type 1 diabetes is estimated to comprise 5% to 10% of those with diabetes, and therefore represents the minority of individuals with diabetes. In addition to type 1 and type 2 diabetes, approximately 7% of pregnancies are complicated by the development of gestational diabetes. Diabetes may also result from genetic syndromes, surgery (pancreatectomy), chemicals and/or drugs, recurrent pancreatitis, malnutrition, and viral infections.

Approximately 1% of women have diabetes prior to pregnancy (pregestational diabetes). Gestational diabetes mellitus (GDM) has been traditionally defined as the first onset or recognition of glucose intolerance during pregnancy. GDM makes up ~90% of diabetes cases encountered in pregnant women. Women who have had gestational diabetes are at an increased risk for later development of type 2 diabetes. Women at high risk for the development of diabetes, and then diagnosed with diabetes at their first prenatal visit, are considered to have overt diabetes (ACOG, 2005; ADA, 2011).

Women of child bearing potential diagnosed with diabetes prior to pregnancy should understand the need for good glucose control and participate in family planning (ADA, 2008).

COMPLICATIONS OF DIABETES

Diabetes was listed as the seventh leading cause of death in the United States in 2007. Complications of diabetes are often contributing factors in the mortality of these patients; the most frequently reported diabetes complications that were reported as contributing factors in diabetes-related deaths were heart disease (68%) and stroke (16%) (data from 2004). In addition to cardiovascular effects, diabetes is the leading cause of new blindness in people 20-74 years of age and diabetic nephropathy is the most common cause of end-stage renal disease. Control of hyperglycemia may significantly decrease the rate at which diabetic complications develop and provides compelling justification for early diagnosis and management of this disorder.

In pregnant women, diabetes can adversely affect the mother, the fetus, and the newborn, especially if the disease is poorly treated.

- Poorly-treated pregestational diabetes may cause end-organ damage to the mother that may in turn negatively affect obstetric outcomes. Retinopathy can progress acutely during pregnancy, especially in women with hypertension or pre-eclampsia. Diabetic nephropathy and chronic hypertension occur in ~5% to 10% of pregnancies in women with diabetes. Pre-eclampsia occurs in ~15% to 20% of women with type 1 diabetes; the rate is higher with concomitant nephropathy or in women with hypertension. Spontaneous labor and delivery by cesarean section are also more common in women with pregestational diabetes (ACOG, 2005).
- The risk of congenital malformations is increased when the first trimester Hb A_{1c} is 7% or fasting plasma glucose is >120 mg/dL (>6.7 mmol/L) (Metzger, 2007). Cardiac defects, CNS anomalies (anencephaly, spina bifida), and skeletal malformations are most common and the risk may be decreased with good preconception management of diabetes in the mother. When maternal glucose levels are elevated in later trimesters, the risk of excessive fetal growth, intrauterine fetal death, shoulder dystocia with vaginal delivery, macrosomia, neonatal hypoglycemia, respiratory distress, and hyperbilirubinemia in the infant are increased. Macrosomia and hyperbilirubinemia are events more commonly observed in infants of women diagnosed with GDM (ACOG, 2005; ADA, 2011; Metzger, 2007). Increased birth weight and fetal hyperinsulinemia (as measured by cord-blood serum C-peptide) may also be associated with maternal hyperglycemia at levels below those diagnostic of GDM (HAPO Study Cooperative Research Group, 2008; IADPSG, 2010). To prevent adverse fetal events, prior to conception and throughout pregnancy the maternal Hb A_{1c} should be kept close to normal but without causing significant hypoglycemia (ADA, 2011; Kitzmiller, 2008). Women with a preconception Hb A_{1c} of ~5% to 6% have a fetal malformation rate similar to pregnancies of nondiabetic women (2% to 3%). In women with a preconception Hb A_{1c} of 10%, the anomaly rate is increased to 20% to 25% (ACOG, 2005).
- Children of women with poorly controlled diabetes are more likely to be obese, glucose intolerant, and have diabetes in late adolescence or young adulthood (ACOG, 2005; ADA, 2004).

Pre-existing conditions (eg, hypertension, diabetic nephropathy) should be evaluated prior to pregnancy. Medications used to treat diabetes or related conditions should also be reviewed in order to evaluate their safety during pregnancy. In order to avoid complications, glycemic control should be as close to normal as possible (without significant hypoglycemia) prior to pregnancy and effective contraception should be used until glycemic control is achieved (Kitzmiller, 2008).

DIAGNOSIS

The diagnosis of diabetes in nonpregnant adults is made by any of the four criteria described below. New in the 2010 American Diabetes Association (ADA) Standards of Medical Care is the recommendation for the use of Hb A1c for the diagnosis of diabetes; the method used should be certified by the National Glycohemoglobin Standardization Program (NGSP) and standardized to the Diabetes Control and Complications Trial (DCCT) assay.

Diagnosis of Diabetes in Adults

1. Hb A_{1c} ≥6.5%
   OR

2. Fasting plasma glucose (no caloric intake for at least 8 hours) ≥126 mg/dL (7 mmol/L)
   OR

3. Casual plasma glucose concentration ≥200 mg/dL (11.1 mmol/L) in patients with symptoms of hyperglycemia (polydipsia, polyuria, unexplained weight loss) or hyperglycemic crisis. **Note:** Casual plasma glucose is defined as any time of day without regard to time of last meal.
   OR

4. A 2-hour plasma glucose ≥200 mg/dL (11.1 mmol/L) during an oral glucose tolerance test (OGTT) in accordance with the standards set forth by the World Health Organization (WHO) using a 75 g anhydrous glucose load (or equivalent) dissolved in water. **Note:** OGTT is not recommended for routine clinical use.

Note: In the absence of unequivocal hyperglycemia, criteria 1, 2, and 4 should be confirmed by repeat testing.

Screening for and Diagnosis of Gestational Diabetes Mellitus

Screening: In women at 24-28 weeks gestation not previously diagnosed with overt diabetes, perform a 75 g oral glucose tolerance test (OGTT), obtaining plasma glucose levels while fasting and at 1 and 2 hours. **Note:** The OGTT should be performed in the morning after an overnight fast of at least 8 hours.

Diagnosis: The diagnosis of Gestational Diabetes Mellitus is made when any of the following plasma glucose (PG) values are exceeded:

- Fasting PG ≥92 mg/dL (5.1 mmol/L)
- 1 hour PG ≥180 mg/dL (10.0 mmol/L)
- 2 hour PG ≥153 mg/dL (8.5 mmol/L)

The following thresholds proposed by IADPSG can be used at the *first prenatal visit*:

- **To diagnose GDM:** Following a 75 g OGTT, one or more of the following plasma glucose values must be found (IADPSG consensus thresholds):
  - FPG ≥92 mg/dL (5.1 mmol/L) but <126 mg/dL (7 mmol/L); **Note:** If FPG is <92 mg/dL (5.1 mmol/L), test again at 24-28 weeks gestation.
  - 1 hour: ≥180 mg/dL (10 mmol/L)
  - 2 hour: ≥153 mg/dL (8.5 mmol/L)
- **To diagnose overt diabetes in pregnancy:** Following a 75 g OGTT, one or more of the following plasma glucose values must be found (IADPSG consensus thresholds):
  - FPG: ≥126 mg/dL (7 mmol/L)
  - Hb A_{1c}: ≥6.5% (DCCT/UKPDS standardized)
  - Random plasma glucose: ≥200 mg/dL (11.1 mmol/L) **plus** confirmation with FPG or Hb A_{1c}

If results indicate overt diabetes, treat and follow for preexisting diabetes.

GOALS

The goals of diabetes treatment include normalization of hyperglycemia, avoidance of hypoglycemia, and slowing the development of diabetic complications. For additional information on the goals of treatment in nonpregnant patients, visit the ADA website at http://care.diabetesjournals.org/content/34/Supplement_1.

In women with pregestational diabetes, Hb A_{1c} should be kept as close to normal as possible without significant hypoglycemia. Self-monitoring of blood glucose with the fingerstick method is best during pregnancy. Goals for glycemic control:

- Premeal, bedtime, and overnight glucose: 60-99 mg/dL (3.3-5.4 mmol/L)
- Peak postprandial glucose: 100-129 mg/dL (5.4-7.1 mmol/L)
- Hb A_{1c}: <6.0% (measure monthly until target achieved, then every 2-3 months)

Less intensive glycemic goals may be indicated in patients unaware of hypoglycemia or not able to adhere to intensified management (Kitzmiller, 2008).

MANAGEMENT OF DIABETES

Current ADA recommendations emphasize a multidisciplinary approach to the management of diabetes, with an emphasis on the participation of the patient and/or caregivers in the monitoring and management of the disease. Consultation with a diabetes educator and dietitian may help to prepare the patient to manage her disease and adjust to the necessary changes in diet and lifestyle. Patients must be educated about disease monitoring procedures, including blood glucose self-monitoring equipment and tests. Patients should be encouraged to wear or carry appropriate identification to inform health care providers of their disease in the event of an emergency. It is extremely important to educate patients concerning the recognition and management of hypoglycemic symptoms. The management of diabetes is constantly adapting to new information, techniques, and technologies. For additional information on the management of diabetes in nonpregnant patients, visit the ADA website at http://care.diabetesjournals.org/content/34/Supplement_1.

Recommendations by the ADA include glycemic control, as well as the following for pregnant women with diabetes (Kitzmiller, 2008):

- Women should receive individualized medical nutrition therapy in order to support a healthy pregnancy.
- Assess prepregnancy BMI and target weight gain based on BMI group, energy intake, physical activity, fetal growth, and desire to prevent excess maternal weight gain and postpartum weight retention.
- Individualize daily diet to promote optimal glycemic control and avoid hypoglycemia and ketonemia. Promote a healthy, balanced diet.
- Use supplemental minerals, trace elements, and vitamins to achieve appropriate intake for pregnancy.

DRUG TREATMENT

Insulin

Insulin therapy is considered the drug of choice for the control of all types of diabetes mellitus during pregnancy.

The general objective of insulin replacement therapy is to approximate the physiologic pattern of insulin secretion which is characterized by two distinct phases – phase 1 insulin secretion suppresses hepatic glucose production and phase 2 insulin secretion occurs in response to carbohydrate ingestion. This requires a basal level of insulin throughout the day (such as intermediate- or long-acting insulin or continuous insulin infusion administered via an external SubQ insulin infusion pump), supplemented by additional insulin at mealtimes (eg, short- or rapid-acting insulin).

Multiple daily doses guided by blood glucose monitoring are the standard of diabetes care. Combinations of insulin are commonly used. The number and size of daily doses, time of administration, and diet and exercise require continuous medical supervision. In addition, specific formulations may require distinct administration procedures/timing (refer to individual monographs).

There is solid scientific documentation of the benefit of tight glucose control. However, the benefits must be balanced against the risk of hypoglycemia, the patient's ability to adhere to the regimen, and other issues regarding the complexity of management. Diabetes self-management education (DSME) and medical nutrition therapy (MNT) are essential to maximize the effectiveness of therapy. In addition to the educational issues outlined above, patients should be instructed in insulin administration techniques, timing of administration, and sick-day management.

Since combinations of agents are frequently used, dosage adjustment must address the individual component of the insulin regimen which most directly influences the blood glucose value in question, based on the known onset and duration of the insulin component (see table). The frequency of doses and monitoring must also be individualized in consideration of the patient's ability to manage therapy.

In pregnant women with pre-existing type 1 diabetes, NPH insulin is preferred over insulin detemir or insulin glargine. Transition to NPH should take place prior to pregnancy or at the first prenatal visit. Rapid-acting insulin (eg, insulin lispro, insulin aspart) may be used instead of premeal regular insulin. Insulin requirements may decrease at 10-14 weeks gestation, then increase gradually until ~35 weeks gestation, where they may level off or decline (Kitzmiller, 2008).

In women with pre-existing type 2 diabetes, transition to insulin should take place prior to pregnancy and acceptable glucose control should be achieved prior to conception. Women with type 2 diabetes who become pregnant while taking oral agents should be transitioned to insulin as soon as possible. Initial total daily doses of 0.7-1.0 units/kg are often effective; higher doses may be needed in women who are obese (Kitzmiller, 2008).

Insulin is also recommended for women diagnosed with GDM (ADA, 2004).

Insulin should be injected into the abdomen or hips (Kitzmiller, 2008).

Types of Insulin	Onset (h)	Peak Glycemic Effect (h)	Duration (h)
	Rapid-Acting		
Insulin lispro (HumaLOG®)	0.25-0.5	0.5-2.5	≤5
Insulin aspart (NovoLOG®)	0.2-0.3	1-3	3-5
Insulin glulisine (Apidra®)	0.2-0.5	1.6-2.8	3-4
	Short-Acting		
Insulin regular (HumuLIN® R, NovoLIN® R)	0.5	2.5-5	4-12 –U-100 Up to 24 – U-500
	Intermediate-Acting		
Insulin NPH (isophane suspension) (HumuLIN® N, NovoLIN® N)	1-2	4-12	14-24
	Intermediate- to Long-Acting		
Insulin determir (Levemir®)	3-4	3-9	6-23 (duration is dose-dependent)
	Long-Acting		
Insulin glargine (Lantus®)	3-4	*	10.8-≥24
	Combinations		
Insulin aspart protamine suspension and insulin aspart (NovoLOG® Mix 70/30)	0.17-0.33	1-4	18-24
Insulin lispro protamine and insulin lispro (HumaLOG® Mix 75/25™)	0.25-0.5	1-6.5	14-24
Insulin NPH suspension and insulin regular solution (NovoLIN® 70/30)	0.5	2-12	18-24

* Insulin glargine has no pronounced peak.

For a general discussion of maintenance dosing and dosing adjustments in nonpregnant patients, visit the ADA website at http://www.diabetes.org/.

Insulin Therapy During Labor

In women with pregestational diabetes, insulin may not be needed during active labor. In patients who use continuous subcutaneous insulin infusion (CSII), the basal insulin component may be continued during labor (ACOG, 2005).

When labor is induced, the usual dose of intermediate insulin may be given at bedtime the evening before. Hold the morning dose of insulin and begin an I.V. infusion with normal saline. Monitor glucose hourly. Once active labor begins or glucose concentrations are <70 mg/dL (3.9 mmol/L), change NS infusion to D_5W and infuse at a rate of 2.5 mg/kg/minute to reach a glucose concentration of ~100 mg/dL (~5.6 mmol/L). If glucose concentrations are >100 mg/dL (5.6 mmol/L), administer regular insulin I.V. at a rate of 1.25 units/hour (ACOG, 2005).

Following delivery, insulin requirements will decrease rapidly. Once food intake has started, approximately one-half of the predelivery dose may be initiated and titrated as needed (ACOG, 2005).

Oral Agents

The use of oral antihyperglycemic agents in pregnant women with type 2 diabetes or GDM is controversial (Kitzmiller, 2008; Metzger, 2007). Insulin therapy is required in type 1 diabetes. Until additional safety and efficacy data are obtained, the use of oral agents is generally not recommended as routine management of GDM or type 2 diabetes mellitus during pregnancy. Insulin is the drug of choice for the control of diabetes mellitus during pregnancy.

Glyburide: Glyburide was not found to significantly cross the placenta *in vitro* and was not found in the cord serum infants of mothers taking glyburide for GDM. The manufacturer recommends that if glyburide is used during pregnancy, it should be discontinued at least 2 weeks before the expected delivery date. Although studies have shown positive outcomes using glyburide for the treatment of GDM, use may not be appropriate for all women.

Metformin: Metformin has been found to cross the placenta in levels which may be comparable to those found in the maternal plasma. Pharmacokinetic studies suggest that clearance of metformin may be increased during pregnancy and dosing may need adjusted in some women when used during the third trimester. Fetal, neonatal, and maternal outcomes have been evaluated following maternal use of metformin for the treatment of GDM and type 2 diabetes. Available information suggests that metformin use during pregnancy may be safe as long as good glycemic control is maintained; however, many studies used metformin during the second or third trimester only.

Postpartum Considerations

Breast-feeding is encouraged for all women, including those with type 1, type 2, or GDM (ACOG, 2005; ADA, 2004). An increase in caloric intake is required and small snacks before feeds may help decrease the risk of hypoglycemia in women with pregestational diabetes (ACOG, 2005). In women with GDM, breast-feeding for >3 months was shown to decrease the child's risk of becoming overweight by 45% at 2-8 years of age (Metzger, 2007). All types of insulin may be used while breast-feeding and some oral agents may be acceptable for use as well.

For women diagnosed with GDM, most will have normal glucose tolerance after delivery. Serum glucose should be evaluated prior to discharge (1-3 days after delivery) and elevated concentrations should be confirmed and treated. For women diagnosed with GDM and normal glucose concentrations following delivery, the 75 g OGTT should be repeated at 6-12 weeks postpartum, 1 year postpartum, and then every 3 years. Fasting plasma glucose should be monitored yearly. Prior to future pregnancies, the 75 g OGTT should also be performed (Metzger, 2007).

PATIENT-RELATED INFORMATION

"Diabetes and Pregnancy." Informational Fact Sheet from OTIS (Organization of Teratology Information Specialists). Available at http://www.-otispregnancy.org/files/diabetes.pdf

"Diabetes in Pregnancy." Information from the CDC. Available at http://www.cdc.gov/Features/DiabetesPregnancy

"For Women With Diabetes: Your Guide to Pregnancy." Information from the National Diabetes information Clearing House (NDIC). Available at http://diabetes.niddk.nih.gov/dm/pubs/pregnancy/#top

"It's Never Too Early to Prevent Diabetes." Pamphlet for Women Who Had GDM in a Previous Pregnancy. Information from the National Diabetes Education Program. Available at http://ndep.nih.gov/media/NeverTooEarly_Tipsheet.pdf

REFERENCES

American College of Obstetricians and Gynecologists, "ACOG Practice Bulletin. Clinical Management Guidelines for Obstetrician-Gynecologists. Number 60, March 2005. Pregestational Diabetes Mellitus," *Obstet Gynecol*, 2005, 105(3):675-85.

American Diabetes Association, "Diagnosis and Classification of Diabetes Mellitus," *Diabetes Care*, 2011, 34(Suppl 1):S62-9.

American Diabetes Association, "Gestational Diabetes Mellitus," *Diabetes Care*, 2004, 27(Suppl 1):S88-90.

American Diabetes Association, "Standards of Medical Care in Diabetes – 2011," *Diabetes Care*, 2011, 34(Suppl 1):S11-61.

Centers for Disease Control (CDC), "National Diabetes Fact Sheet: 2007 General Information." Available at http://www.cdc.gov/diabetes/pubs/pdf/ndfs_2007.pdf. Last accessed April 1, 2010.

HAPO Study Cooperative Research Group, Metzger BE, Lowe LP, et al, "Hyperglycemia and Adverse Pregnancy Outcomes," *N Engl J Med*, 2008, 358 (19):1991-2002.

International Association of Diabetes and Pregnancy Study Groups Consensus Panel, "International Association of Diabetes and Pregnancy Study Groups Recommendations on the Diagnosis and Classification of Hyperglycemia in Pregnancy," *Diabetes Care*, 2010, 33(3):676-82.

International Expert Committee, "International Expert Committee Report on the Role of the A1C Assay in the Diagnosis of Diabetes," *Diabetes Care*, 2009, 32(7):1327-34.

Kitzmiller JL, Block JM, Brown FM, et al, "Managing Preexisting Diabetes for Pregnancy: Summary of Evidence and Consensus Recommendations for Care," *Diabetes Care*, 2008, 31(5):1060-79.

Metzger BE, Buchanan TA, Coustan DR, et al, "Summary and Recommendations of the Fifth International Workshop-Conference on Gestational Diabetes Mellitus," *Diabetes Care*, 2007, 30(Suppl 2):S251-60.

DIABETES MELLITUS MANAGEMENT, ADULTS

OVERVIEW

Diabetes represents a significant health care problem in the United States and worldwide. Of the nearly 23.6 million Americans (7.8% of the population) with diabetes, the majority (90% to 95%) have type 2 diabetes. Of this number, nearly one-quarter are undiagnosed. The incidence of type 2 diabetes is increasing around the world. There is strong evidence to support an interaction between a genetic predisposition and behavioral or environmental factors, such as obesity and physical inactivity, in the development of this disease. In individuals at high risk of developing type 2 diabetes, it has been shown that the development of diabetes may be prevented or delayed by changes in lifestyle or pharmacologic intervention.

Within the United States, type 1 diabetes is estimated to comprise 5% to 10% of those with diabetes, and therefore represents the minority of individuals with diabetes. In addition to type 1 and type 2 diabetes, approximately 7% of pregnancies are complicated by the development of gestational diabetes. Gestational diabetes mellitus is defined as the first onset or recognition of glucose intolerance during pregnancy. Women who have had gestational diabetes are at an increased risk for later development of type 2 diabetes. In addition to the causes noted above, diabetes may result from genetic syndromes, surgery (pancreatectomy), chemicals and/or drugs, recurrent pancreatitis, malnutrition, and viral infections.

Additional information available at: http://care.diabetesjournals.org/content/34/Supplement_1

COMPLICATIONS OF DIABETES

Diabetes was listed as the seventh leading cause of death in the United States in 2007. Complications of diabetes are often contributing factors in the death of these patients; the most frequently reported diabetes complications on the death certificates of patients with diabetes in 2004 were heart disease and stroke, which were listed as contributing factors in 68% and 16% of diabetes-related deaths, respectively.

In addition to cardiovascular effects, diabetes is the leading cause of new blindness in people 20-74 years old, and diabetic nephropathy is the most common cause of end-stage renal disease. Mild to severe forms of diabetic neuropathy are common. Neuropathy and circulatory insufficiency combine to make diabetes the most frequent cause of nontraumatic lower-limb amputations (60% of cases). The rate of impotence in diabetic males over 50 years old has been estimated to be as high as 35% to 50%. Control of hyperglycemia may significantly decrease the rate at which diabetic complications develop; this provides compelling justification for early diagnosis and management of this disorder.

DIAGNOSIS

Diabetes

Diagnosis of diabetes in nonpregnant adults is made by any of the four criteria described below. In the absence of unequivocal hyperglycemia with acute metabolic decompensation, these criteria should be confirmed by repeat testing on a different day. New in the 2010 American Diabetes Association (ADA) Standards of Medical Care is the recommendation for the use of Hb A_{1c} for the diagnosis of diabetes; the method used should be certified by the National Glycohemoglobin Standardization Program (NGSP) and standardized to the Diabetes Control and Complications Trial (DCCT) assay. Screening should be considered in overweight adult patients (BMI ≥25 kg/m^2) who have at least one risk factor for diabetes (eg, physical inactivity, first-degree relative with diabetes, history of cardiovascular disease, etc). In patients without risk factors, testing should begin at age 45. Repeat testing should occur at least every 3 years in patients with normal test results.

Criteria for Diagnosis

1. Hb A_{1c} ≥6.5%
   OR
2. Fasting plasma glucose (no caloric intake for at least 8 hours) ≥126 mg/dL (7 mmol/L)
   OR
3. Casual plasma glucose concentration≥200 mg/dL (11.1 mmol/L) in patients with symptoms of hyperglycemia (polydipsia, polyuria, unexplained weight loss) or hyperglycemic crisis. **Note:** Casual plasma glucose is defined as any time of day without regard to time of last meal.
   OR
4. A 2-hour plasma glucose ≥200 mg/dL (11.1 mmol/L) during an oral glucose tolerance test (OGTT) in accordance with the standards set forth by the World Health Organization (WHO) using a 75 g anhydrous glucose load (or equivalent) dissolved in water. **Note:** OGTT is not recommended for routine clinical use.

Note: In the absence of unequivocal hyperglycemia, criteria 1, 2, and 4 should be confirmed by repeat testing.

Categories of Increased Risk for Diabetes

Patients with impaired fasting glucose (IFG), impaired glucose tolerance (IGT), or an intermediately high Hb A_{1c} are considered to be in a group whose glucose levels do not meet the criteria for diabetes, yet are higher than normal. Patients who meet any of the following criteria are considered to be at high risk for developing diabetes and cardiovascular disease, and are referred to as having "prediabetes":

1. IFG: Fasting plasma glucose (no caloric intake for at least 8 hours) 100-125 mg/dL (5.6-6.9 mmol/L)

   OR

2. IGT: A 2-hour plasma glucose 140-199 mg/dL (7.8-11 mmol/L) during an oral glucose tolerance test (OGTT) in accordance with the standards set forth by the World Health Organization (WHO) using a 75 g anhydrous glucose load (or equivalent) dissolved in water.

   OR

3. Hb A_{1c}: 5.7% to 6.4%; **Note:** Patients with an Hb A_{1c} >6% should be considered at very high risk for diabetes and receive intensive interventions and monitoring.

The International Expert Committee consisting of members of the ADA, the European Association for the Study of Diabetes (EASD), and the International Diabetes Federation (IDF) recently recommended that the clinical states "prediabetes," IFG, and IGT be phased out as the Hb A1c becomes the preferred diagnostic test (International Expert Committee, 2009).

GOALS

The goals of diabetes treatment include normalization of hyperglycemia, avoidance of hypoglycemia, and slowing the development of diabetic complications. The following is a summary of recommendations for nonpregnant adults with diabetes.

2011 ADA Summary of Recommendations for Adults With Diabetes

Glycemic control	
Hb A_{1c}	<7%[1]
Preprandial capillary plasma glucose	70-130 mg/dL
Peak postprandial capillary plasma glucose[2]	<180 mg/dL
Blood pressure[7]	<130/80 mm Hg
Lipids[3]	
LDL[4]	<100 mg/dL
Triglycerides	<150 mg/dL
HDL	Male: >40 mg/dL Female: >50 mg/dL
Non-HDL chloesterol[5]	<130 mg/dL
Apolipoprotein B[6]	<90 mg/dL

[1]Referenced to a nondiabetic range of 4% to 6% using a DCCT-based assay. **Note:** The Hb A_{1c} goal for patients in general is <7%; an even lower goal may be appropriate for selected individuals (eg, short duration of diabetes, long life expectancy, and no significant cardiovascular disease) so long as a lower goal can be achieved without significant hypoglycemia or other adverse effects. Conversely, a less stringent goal may be appropriate in certain patients (eg, history of severe hypoglycemia, limited life expectancy, advanced micro- or macrovascular complications, extensive comorbid conditions, longstanding diabetes in whom the general goal is difficult to attain despite appropriate diabetes management).

[2]Postprandial glucose measurements should be made 1-2 hours after the beginning of the meal, generally peak levels in patients with diabetes.

[3]Current NCEP/ATP III guidelines suggest that in patients with triglycerides ≥200 mg/dL, the non-HDL cholesterol (total cholesterol minus HDL) be used. The goal is <130 mg/dL.

[4]In patients with overt CVD or cardiometabolic risk factors (eg, central obesity, insulin resistance, hypertension), a lower LDL goal of <70 mg/dL is an option.

[5]In patients with overt CVD or cardiometabolic risk factors (eg, central obesity, insulin resistance, hypertension) with an LDL goal of <70 mg/dL, the non-HDL cholesterol goal is <100 mg/dL

[6]In patients on a statin with an LDL goal of <70 mg/dL or patients with cardiometabolic risk factors (eg, central obesity, insulin resistance, hypertension), the apolipoprotein B goal is <80 mg/dL

[7]Higher or lower systolic blood pressure targets may be appropriate based on individual patient characteristics and response to therapy.

Key concepts in setting glycemic goals:

- Hb A_{1c} is the primary target for glycemic control.
- Goals should be individualized.
- Certain populations (children, pregnant women, and elderly) require special considerations.
- Less intensive glycemic goals may be indicated in patients with severe or frequent hypoglycemia.
- A lower glycemic goal (eg, Hb A_{1c} <6%) may further reduce the risk of microvascular complications at the cost of an increased risk of hypoglycemia (particularly in those with type 1 diabetes). However, recent studies (eg, ACCORD and VADT) have highlighted certain patient populations in which the risks of intensive glycemic control may outweigh the benefits, including patients with a very long duration of diabetes, history of severe hypoglycemia, advanced atherosclerosis, and advanced age or frailty.
- Postprandial glucose may be targeted if Hb A_{1c} goals are not met despite reaching preprandial glucose goals.

MANAGEMENT

Multidisciplinary approach necessary. Patient education:

- Wearing appropriate identification of disease
- Foot care
- Eye care
- Acute illness management
- Hypoglycemia recognition and management
- Weight monitoring and management, including diet and exercise and bariatric surgery options (BMI >35 kg/m^2)

TYPE 1 DIABETES DRUG TREATMENT

Intensive insulin therapy: ≥3 injections/day of basal and prandial insulin or continuous subcutaneous infusion. If hypoglycemia is problematic, the use of insulin analogs may be helpful.

Monitoring

Self-monitoring of blood glucose (SMBG) should be carried out three or more times daily for patients using multiple insulin injections or insulin pump therapy. For patients using less frequent insulin injections, noninsulin therapies, or medical nutrition therapy (MNT) alone, SMBG may be useful as a guide to the success of therapy. To achieve postprandial glucose targets, postprandial SMBG may be appropriate.

Continuous glucose monitoring (CGM) in conjunction with intensive insulin regimens can be a useful tool to lower A1C in selected adults (age ≥25 years) with type 1 diabetes. CGM may be a supplemental tool in those with hypoglycemia episodes.

Insulin

Insulin therapy is required in type 1 diabetes, and may be necessary in some individuals with type 2 diabetes. The general objective of insulin replacement therapy is to approximate the physiologic pattern of insulin secretion which is characterized by two distinct phases. Phase 1 insulin secretion suppresses hepatic glucose production and phase 2 insulin secretion occurs in response to carbohydrate ingestion. This requires a basal level of insulin throughout the day (such as intermediate- or long-acting insulin or continuous insulin infusion administered via an external SubQ insulin infusion pump), supplemented by additional insulin at mealtimes (eg, short- or rapid-acting insulin).

Multiple daily doses guided by blood glucose monitoring are the standard of diabetes care. Combinations of insulin are commonly used. The number and size of daily doses, time of administration, and diet and exercise require continuous medical supervision. In addition, specific formulations may require distinct administration procedures/timing (refer to individual monographs).

There is solid scientific documentation of the benefit of tight glucose control, either by insulin pump or multiple daily injections (4-6 times daily). However, the benefits must be balanced against the risk of hypoglycemia, the patient's ability to adhere to the regimen, and other issues regarding the complexity of management. Diabetes self-management education (DSME) and medical nutrition therapy (MNT) are essential to maximize the effectiveness of therapy. In addition to the educational issues outlined above, patients should be instructed in insulin administration techniques, timing of administration, and sick-day management.

The initial dose of insulin in type 1 diabetes is typically 0.5-1 units/kg/day in divided doses. Conservative initial doses of 0.2-0.4 units/kg/day are often recommended to avoid the potential for hypoglycemia. Generally, one-half to three-fourths of the daily insulin dose is given as an intermediate- or long-acting form of insulin (in 1-2 daily injections). The remaining portion of the 24-hour insulin requirement is divided and administered as a rapid-acting or short-acting form of insulin. These may be given with meals (before or at the time of meals depending on the form of insulin) or at the same time as injections of intermediate forms (some premixed combinations are intended for this purpose). Some patients may benefit from the use of continuous subcutaneous insulin infusion (CSII) which delivers rapid-acting insulin as a continuous infusion throughout the day and as boluses at mealtimes via an external pump device.

Since combinations of agents are frequently used, dosage adjustment must address the individual component of the insulin regimen which most directly influences the blood glucose value in question, based on the known onset and duration of the insulin component (see table). The frequency of doses and monitoring must also be individualized in consideration of the patient's ability to manage therapy.

Types of Insulin	Onset (h)	Peak Glycemic Effect (h)	Duration (h)
	Rapid-Acting		
Insulin lispro (HumaLOG®)	0.25-0.5	0.5-2.5	≤5
Insulin aspart (NovoLOG®)	0.2-0.3	1-3	3-5
Insulin glulisine (Apidra®)	0.2-0.5	1.6-2.8	3-4
	Short-Acting		
Insulin regular (HumuLIN® R, NovoLIN® R)	0.5	2.5-5	4-12 – U-100 Up to 24 – U-500
	Intermediate-Acting		
Insulin NPH (isophane suspension) (HumuLIN® N, NovoLIN® N)	1-2	4-12	14-24
	Intermediate- to Long-Acting		
Insulin detemir (Levemir®)	3-4	3-9	6-23 (duration is dose-dependent)
	Long-Acting		
Insulin glargine (Lantus®)	3-4	*	10.8-≥24
	Combinations		
Insulin aspart protamine suspension and insulin aspart (NovoLOG® Mix 70/30)	0.17-0.33	1-4	18-24
Insulin lispro protamine and insulin lispro (HumaLOG® Mix 75/25™)	0.25-0.5	1-6.5	14-24
Insulin NPH suspension and insulin regular solution (NovoLIN® 70/30)	0.5	2-12	18-24

*Insulin glargine has no pronounced peak.

Maintenance Dosing

Typical maintenance insulin doses are between 0.5 and 1.2 units/kg/day in divided doses. Adolescents may require as much as 1.5 units/kg/day during puberty; whereas prepubescent individuals may only require 0.7-1 unit/kg/day.

As stated above, the general objective of insulin replacement therapy is to approximate the physiologic pattern of insulin secretion. This requires a basal level of insulin throughout the day, supplemented by additional insulin at mealtimes. Combination regimens which exploit differences in the onset and duration of different insulin products are commonly used to approximate physiologic secretion. Frequently, split-mixed or basal-bolus regimens are used to approximate physiologic secretion.

Split-mixed regimens: In split-mixed regimens, an intermediate-acting insulin (eg, NPH insulin) is administered once or twice daily and supplemented by short-acting (regular) or rapid-acting (lispro, aspart, or glulisine) insulin. Blood glucose measurements are completed several times daily. Dosages are adjusted emphasizing the individual component of the regimen which most directly influences the blood sugar in question (either the intermediate-acting component or the shorter-acting component). Fixed-ratio formulations (eg, 70/30 mix) may be used as twice daily injections in this scenario; however, the ability to titrate the dosage of an individual component is limited. An example of a "split-mixed" regimen would be 21 units of NPH plus 9 units of regular in the morning and an evening meal dose consisting of 14 units of NPH plus 6 units of regular insulin.

Basal-bolus regimens: Basal-bolus regimens are designed to more closely mimic physiologic secretion. These regimens employ intermediate- to long-acting insulins (eg, glargine, detemir) or a continuous insulin infusion administered via an external SubQ insulin infusion pump to simulate basal insulin secretion. The basal component is frequently administered at bedtime or in the early morning or as a continuous insulin infusion and then supplemented by multiple daily injections of rapid-acting products (lispro, glulisine, or aspart) immediately prior to a meal; thereby, providing insulin at the time when nutrients are absorbed. An example of a basal-bolus regimen would be 30 units of glargine at bedtime and 12 units of lispro insulin prior to each meal.

Adjustment of Insulin Dose

Dosage must be titrated to achieve glucose control and avoid hypoglycemia. In general, dosage is adjusted to maintain recommendations for glycemic control. Since treatment regimens often consist of multiple formulations, dosage adjustments must address the specific phase of insulin release that is primarily contributing to the patient's impaired glycemic control. Treatment and monitoring regimens must be individualized.

Estimation of the effect per unit: A "Rule of 1500" has been frequently used as a means to estimate the change in blood sugar relative to each unit of insulin administered. In fact, the recommended values used in these calculations may vary from 1500-2200 (a value of at least 1800 is recommended for lispro). The higher values lead to more conservative estimates of the effect per unit of insulin, and therefore lead to more cautious adjustments. The effect per unit of insulin (aka, correction factor) is approximated by dividing the selected numerical value (eg, 1500-2200) by the number of units/day received by the patient. The correction factor may be used as a crude approximation of the patient's insulin sensitivity to determine the correction doses of insulin or adjust the current insulin regimen. Each additional unit of insulin added to the corresponding insulin dose may be expected to lower the blood glucose by the value of the correction factor.

To illustrate, in the "basal-bolus" regimen which includes 30 units of glargine at bedtime and 12 units of lispro insulin prior to each meal, the rule of 1800 would indicate an expected change of 27 mg/dL per unit of insulin (the total daily insulin dose is 66 units; using the formula: correction factor = 1800/66 = 27). A patient may be instructed to add additional insulin if the preprandial glucose is >125 mg/dL. For a prelunch glucose of 195 mg/dL (70 mg/dL higher than goal), this would mean the patient would administer the scheduled 12 units of lispro along with an additional "correction dose" of 3 units (70 divided by the correction factor of 27 derived from the formula) for a total of 15 units prior to the meal. If correction doses are required on a consistent basis, an adjustment of the patient's diet and/or scheduled insulin dose may be necessary.

Hypoglycemia

Hypoglycemia is the leading limiting factor in the treatment of diabetes. A patient experiencing an episode of acutely low blood sugar can perceive the event as an inconvenience in milder cases to a real threat of falls, motor vehicle accidents, etc. in severe cases.

Management of hypoglycemia:

- Conscious individual: Oral glucose: 15-20 g (any form of carbohydrate that contains glucose may be used). If a self-measurement of blood glucose (SMBG) 15 minutes after treatment shows continued hypoglycemia, the treatment should be repeated. Once SMBG glucose returns to normal, the individual should consume a meal or snack to prevent recurrence of hypoglycemia.
- Glucagon should be prescribed for all individuals at significant risk of severe hypoglycemia, and caregivers or family members should be instructed in administration.
- Patients with hypoglycemia unawareness or one or more episodes of severe hypoglycemia should be advised to raise their glycemic targets to avoid further hypoglycemia at least for a short period of time.
- Re-enforce education about prevention of hypoglycemia.

TYPE 2 DIABETES DRUG TREATMENT

Insulin Therapy

Several suggested algorithms for management of adult nonpregnant patients may be found (Nathan, 2009; Rodbard, 2009). Insulin may be used in type 2 diabetes as a means to augment response to oral antidiabetic agents or as monotherapy in selected patients. According to a consensus statement developed by the ADA and the European Association for the Study of Diabetes, basal insulin (eg, glargine, detemir) should be considered in patients who have failed to achieve their glycemic goals following lifestyle interventions and the administration of the maximal tolerated dose of metformin (ADA, 2009; Rodbard, 2009). Furthermore, intensive insulin therapy (eg, basal-bolus regimens) should be considered in patients who have failed to achieve their glycemic goals with an optimized two- or three-drug regimen (ADA, 2009; Rodbard, 2009). Augmentation to control postprandial glucose may be accomplished with regular, glulisine, aspart, or lispro insulin. Dosage must be carefully adjusted.

When used as monotherapy, the requirements for insulin are highly variable. An empirically defined scheme for dosage estimation based on fasting plasma glucose and degree of obesity has been published with recommended doses ranging from 6-77 units/day (Holman, 1995). In the setting of glucose toxicity (loss of beta-cell sensitivity to glucose concentrations), insulin therapy may be used for short-term management to restore sensitivity of beta-cells; in these cases, the dose may need to be rapidly reduced/withdrawn when sensitivity is re-established.

Oral Agents

A large number of drugs for oral administration have become available for the management of type 2 diabetes. Oral antidiabetic agents include sulfonylureas, meglitinides, alpha-glucosidase inhibitors, biguanides, thiazolidinediones (TZDs), and dipeptidyl peptidase IV (DPP-IV) inhibitors. The drug classes vary in terms of their magnitude of effect on glycemic control, mechanism of action, and adverse effect profiles. In many cases, the adverse effect profile may influence the selection of a particular drug. The risk of hypoglycemia is higher for drugs which promote insulin secretion (particularly sulfonylureas or insulin secretagogues). Drug selection is based on patient-specific factors and anticipated tolerance of adverse effects.

Metformin is currently the drug of choice if the patient has no contraindications. If lifestyle intervention and the maximal tolerated dose of metformin fail to achieve or sustain the glycemic goals, another medication should be added in several months. Another medication may also be necessary if metformin is contraindicated or not tolerated. Insulin or a sulfonylurea may be considered the next step if metformin and lifestyle changes are not adequate.

Combination therapy may be necessary to achieve glycemic goals. The risk of additive or additional adverse effects must be balanced with the desire to achieve goals of glycemic control as well as normalization of other metabolic parameters. In particular, weight gain and lipid disturbances may complicate drug treatment.

Oral Antidiabetic Agents for Type 2 Diabetes

Generic Name (Brand Name)	Expected Decrease (%) in Hb A_{1c} With Monotherapy	Key Adverse Effects
Alpha-Glucosidase Inhibitors		
Acarbose (Precose®) Miglitol (Glyset®)	0.5-0.8	GI distress, bloating, flatulence
Antilipemic Agent (Adjunct Therapy)		
Colesevelam (WelChol®)	0.5-1 (not for use as monotherapy)	Constipation, dyspepsia
Biguanide		
Metformin (Fortamet™; Glucophage® XR; Glucophage®; Glumetza®; Riomet®)	1-2	**Lactic acidosis [BOXED WARNING]**, GI distress, weakness
Dipeptidyl Peptidase IV (DPP-IV) Inhibitors		
Linagliptin (Tradjenta™)	0.4	Headache, nasopharyngitis, arthralgia, back pain
Saxagliptin (Onglyza™)	0.4-0.5	Headache, UTI, sinusitis
Sitagliptin (Januvia™)	0.5-0.8	Nasopharyngitis, GI distress, nausea, peripheral edema, hypoglycemia
Dopamine agonists		
Bromocriptine (Cycloset®)	0.1	Nausea, dizziness, somnolence, postural hypotension, headache
Meglitinide Derivatives		
Nateglinide (Starlix®) Repaglinide (Prandin®)	0.5-1.5 (repaglinide may be more effective)	Upper respiratory infection, flu-like syndrome, headache, hypoglycemia
Sulfonylurea, 1st Generation		
ChlorproPAMIDE (Diabinese®) Tolazamide TOLBUTamide	1-2	Hypoglycemia, dizziness, headache, GI distress, SIADH
Sulfonylurea, 2nd Generation		
Glimepiride (Amaryl®) GlipiZIDE (Glucotrol® XL; Glucotrol®) GlyBURIDE (DiaBeta®; Glynase® PresTab®; Micronase®)	1-2	Hypoglycemia, dizziness, headache, GI distress, SIADH
Thiazolidinediones		
Pioglitazone (Actos®) Rosiglitazone (Avandia®)	0.5-1.4	**May cause or exacerbate heart failure [BOXED WARNING]**, hepatic dysfunction, weight gain, edema, lipid changes

Injectable Agents (Noninsulin)

In addition to insulin and oral agents, three injectable products are available for the management of diabetes. Exenatide (Byetta®) and liraglutide (Victoza®) are GLP-1 receptor agonists FDA-approved for the treatment of type 2 diabetes. Exenatide is used as an adjunct to diet and exercise to improve glycemic control in patients with type 2 diabetes mellitus. The manufacturer of liraglutide states that it is an injectable prescription medicine that may improve blood sugar in adults with type 2 diabetes when used along with diet and exercise. GLP-1 agonists increase insulin secretion, increase B-cell growth/replication, slow gastric emptying, and may decrease food intake.

Pramlintide (Symlin®) is FDA approved for the treatment of type 1 and type 2 diabetes. In type 1 diabetes, it is approved for use in patients who have failed to achieve glucose control despite optimal insulin therapy. When used for type 2 diabetes, pramlintide is approved for use in patients who have failed to achieve desired glucose control despite optimal insulin therapy, with or without concurrent sulfonylurea and/or metformin. Pramlintide is a synthetic analog of human amylin cosecreted with insulin by pancreatic beta cells. It reduces postprandial glucose increases by prolonging gastric emptying time, reducing postprandial glucagon secretion, and reducing caloric intake through centrally-mediated appetite suppression. It should be noted that the concentration of this product is in mcg/mL; patients and healthcare providers should exercise caution when administering this product to avoid inadvertent calculation of the dose based on "units," which could result in a sixfold overdose.

Injectable Agents (Non-Insulin) for Type 2 Diabetes

Generic Name (Brand Name)	Expected Decrease (%) in Hb A_{1c} With Monotherapy	Key Adverse Effects
Glucagon-Like Peptide 1 (GLP-1) Agonist		
Exenatide (Byetta®)	0.5-1	Hypoglycemia, nausea, vomiting, pancreatitis, headache, jittery feeling
Liraglutide (Victoza®)	1	**Thyroid C-cell Tumors [BOXED WARNING]**, nausea, vomiting, diarrhea, constipation, headache, pancreatitis
Amylin Agonists		
Pramlintide (Symlin®)	0.4-0.6	**Coadministration with insulin may induce severe hypoglycemia [BOXED WARNING]**, nausea, vomiting, hypoglycemia, headache, anorexia

Additional Management Issues

Recommendation by the ADA include glycemic control, as well as the following:

- Monitoring: In all patients with diabetes, cardiovascular risk factors should be assessed at least annually.
- Cardiovascular risk management
  - Use an ACEI or ARB in patients with diabetes who have hypertension and micro- or macroalbuminuria to slow the progression of nephropathy, unless contraindicated (eg, pregnancy); additional agents (eg, thiazide or loop diuretics) may be added as needed to achieve blood pressure goals.
  - Consider statin use in all patients with diabetes and cardiovascular disease or in patients with diabetes >40 years old without cardiovascular disease but have at least one other cardiovascular disease risk factor, irrespective of lipoprotein levels (exception: Statin use is contraindicated in pregnancy). For patients without overt CVD and <40 years old, statin therapy may be considered if LDL remains >100 mg/dL with lifestyles changes or in those with multiple cardiovascular risk factors. In individuals with overt CVD, lower LDL goals (<70 mg/dL) are suggested.
  - Use of low-dose aspirin (75-162 mg daily) is reasonable for primary prevention in all patients with diabetes at increased cardiovascular disease (CVD) risk (10-year risk >10%), including most men >50 years old and most women >60 years old who have at least one additional risk factor (eg, hypertension, smoking, family history of CVD, dyslipidemia, albuminuria), unless contraindicated. Low-dose aspirin may be considered for those at intermediate CVD risk (younger patients with ≥1 risk factor, older patients without risk factors, or patients with 10-year CVD risk of 5% to 10%). Aspirin is not recommended for primary prevention in patients with lower risk for CVD (eg, men <50 years old and women <60 years old without additional risk factor; 10-year CVD risk <5%). In secondary prevention, all patients with a history of CVD should receive aspirin (75-162 mg daily). Given the risk of Reye syndrome with the use of aspirin in patients <21 years old, aspirin is not recommended in this population for primary or secondary prevention. In patients unable to take aspirin (eg, documented allergy), the use of clopidogrel is considered a reasonable alternative.
  - Coronary heart disease (CHD): In patients with known cardiovascular disease (CVD), ACE inhibitor therapy and aspirin and statin therapy (if not contraindicated) should be used to reduce the risk of cardiovascular events. In patients with a prior myocardial infarction, beta-blockers should be continued for at least 2 years after the event. Avoid thiazolidinedione (TZD) treatment in patients with symptomatic heart failure. Metformin may be used in patients with stable congestive heart failure (CHF) if renal function is normal; however, it should be avoided in unstable or hospitalized patients with CHF.
- Other preventative actions
  - Immunize against pneumococcal disease ≥2 years old. One time revaccination is recommended for individuals >64 years old if they were <65 years old when previously immunized >5 years ago.
  - Influenza immunization annually for all diabetic patients ≥6 months old.
  - Patients should be advised not to smoke.
  - Patients should be advised to perform at least 150 minutes/week of moderate-intensity aerobic physical activity (50% to 70% of maximal heart rate). In the absence of contradictions, patients with type 2 diabetes should be encouraged to perform resistance training 3 times/week.
  - Eye care: To reduce the risk or slow the progression of retinopathy, optimize glycemic and blood pressure control. Adults and children ≥10 years old with type 1 diabetes should have an initial dilated and comprehensive eye examination within 5 years after the onset of diabetes (if type 2, exam should occur shortly after the diagnosis of diabetes). Subsequent examinations should be repeated annually. Promptly refer patients with any level of macular edema, severe nonproliferative diabetic retinopathy (NPDR), or any proliferative diabetic retinopathy (PDR) to an ophthalmologist who is knowledgeable and experienced in the management and treatment of diabetic retinopathy.

- Nephropathy: To reduce the risk or slow the progression of nephropathy, optimize glucose and blood pressure control. In the treatment of the nonpregnant patient with micro- or macroalbuminuria, either ACE inhibitors or ARBs should be used (if one class is not tolerated, the other should be substituted). When estimated GFR (eGFR) is <60 mL/minute/1.73 m^2, evaluate and manage potential complications of CKD. Consider referral to a physician experienced in the care of kidney disease when there is uncertainty about the etiology of the disease (heavy proteinuria, active urine sediment, absence of retinopathy, rapid decline in GFR), difficult management issues, or advanced kidney disease.
- Neuropathy: All patients should be screened for distal symmetric polyneuropathy (DPN) at diagnosis and at least annually thereafter, using simple clinical tests. Screening for signs and symptoms of cardiovascular autonomic neuropathy should be instituted at diagnosis of type 2 and 5 years after the diagnosis of type 1 diabetes.
- Foot care: Perform general foot self-care education to all patients with diabetes. For all patients with diabetes, perform an annual comprehensive foot examination. The foot examination should include inspection, assessment of foot pulses, and testing for loss of protective sensation (10 g monofilament, plus testing any one of: Vibration using a 128-Hz tuning fork, pinprick sensation, ankle reflexes, or vibration perception threshold).
- Thyroid: TSH concentrations should be measured after metabolic control has been established. If normal, they should be rechecked every 1-2 years or if the patient develops symptoms of thyroid dysfunction, thyromegaly, or an abnormal growth rate.

REFERENCES

Action to Control Cardiovascular Risk in Diabetes Study Group, "Effects of Intensive Glucose Lowering in Type 2 Diabetes," *N Engl J Med*, 2008, 358 (24):2545-59.

ADVANCE Collaborative Group, "Intensive Blood Glucose Control and Vascular Outcomes in Patients With Type 2 Diabetes," *N Engl J Med*, 2008, 358 (24):2560-72.

American Diabetes Association, "Diagnosis and Classification of Diabetes Mellitus," *Diabetes Care*, 2011, 34(Suppl 1):S62-9.

American Diabetes Association, "Standards of Medical Care in Diabetes - 2011," *Diabetes Care*, 2011, 34(Suppl 1):S11-61.

Brunzell JD, Davidson M, Furberg CD, et al, "Lipoprotein Management in Patients With Cardiometabolic Risk: Consensus Statement From the American Diabetes Association and the American College of Cardiology Foundation," *Diabetes Care*, 2008, 31(4):811-22.

Centers for Disease Control (CDC), "National Diabetes Fact Sheet: 2007 General Information," Available at: http://www.cdc.gov/diabetes/pubs/pdf/ndfs_2007.pdf. Accessed January 9, 2009.

Colhoun HM, Betteridge DJ, Durrington PN, et al, "Primary Prevention of Cardiovascular Disease With Atorvastatin in Type 2 Diabetes in the Collaborative Atorvastatin Diabetes Study (CARDS): Multicentre Randomised Placebo-Controlled Trial," *Lancet*, 2004, 364(9435):685-96.

Dailey G, "New Strategies for Basal Insulin Treatment in Type 2 Diabetes Mellitus," *Clin Ther*, 2004, 26(6):889-901.

DeFronzo RA, "Pharmacologic Therapy for Type 2 Diabetes Mellitus," *Ann Intern Med*, 1999, 131(4):281-303.

DeFronzo RA, "Pharmacologic Therapy for Type 2 Diabetes Mellitus," *Ann Intern Med*, 2000, 133(1):73-4.

Duckworth W, Abraira C, Moritz T, et al, "Glucose Control and Vascular Complications in Veterans With Type 2 Diabetes," *N Engl J Med*, 2009, 360 (2):129-39.

Holman RR and Turner RC, "Insulin Therapy in Type II Diabetes," *Diabetes Res Clin Pract*, 1995, (28 Suppl):S179-84.

International Expert Committee, "International Expert Committee Report on the Role of the A1C Assay in the Diagnosis of Diabetes," *Diabetes Care*, 2009, 32(7):1327-34.

Kitabchi AE, Umpierrez GE, Murphy MB, et al, "Hyperglycemic Crises in Diabetes," *Diabetes Care*, 2004, 27(Suppl 1):S94-102.

Nathan DM, Buse JB, Davidson MB, et al, "Medical Management of Hyperglycemia in Type 2 Diabetes: A Consensus Algorithm for the Initiation and Adjustment of Therapy: A Consensus Statement of the American Diabetes Association and the European Association for the Study of Diabetes," *Diabetes Care*, 2009, 32(1):193-203.

National Institute of Diabetes and Kigestive and Kidney Diseases, "Erectile Dysfunction," available at http://kidney.niddk.nih.gov/kudiseases/pubs/pdf/ErectileDysfunction.pdf. Accessed January 9, 2009.

Oiknine R, Bernbaum M, and Mooradian AD, "A Critical Appraisal of the Role of Insulin Analogues in the Management of Diabetes Mellitus," *Drugs*, 2005, 65(3):325-40.

Pignone M, Alberts MJ, Colwell JA, et al, "Aspirin for Primary Prevention of Cardiovascular Events in People With Diabetes: A Position Statement of the American Diabetes Association, a Scientific Statement of the American Heart Association, and an Expert Consensus Document of the American College of Cardiology Foundation," *Circulation*, 2010, 121(24):2694-701.

Rodbard HW, Jellinger PS, Davidson JA, et al, "Statement by an American Association of Clinical Endocrinologists/American College of Endocrinology Consensus Panel on Type 2 Diabetes Mellitus: An Algorithm for Glycemic Control," *Endocr Pract*, 2009, 15(6):540-59.

Scheife RT (editor), "Liraglutide: A New Option for the Treatment of Type 2 Diabetes Mellitus," *Pharmacotherapy*, 2009, 29(12 part 2): 23s-67s.

Sherifali D, Nerenberg K, Pullenayegum E, et al, "The Effect of Oral Antidiabetic Agents on A1C Levels: A Systematic Review and Meta-Analysis," *Diabetes Care*, 2010, 33(8):1859-64.

Silverstein J, Klingensmith G, Copeland K, et al, "Care of Children and Adolescents With Type 1 Diabetes: A Statement of the American Diabetes Association," *Diabetes Care*, 2005, 28(1):186-212.

The Diabetes Control and Complications Trial Research Group, "The Effect of Intensive Treatment of Diabetes on the Development and Progression of Long-Term Complications in Insulin-dependent Diabetes Mellitus," *N Engl J Med*, 1993, 329(14):977-86.

Tuomilehto J, Lindstrom J, Eriksson JG, et al, "Prevention of Type 2 Diabetes Mellitus by Changes in Lifestyle Among Subjects With Impaired Glucose Tolerance," *N Engl J Med*, 2001, 344(18):1343-50.

UK Prospective Diabetes Study Group, "Intensive Blood Glucose Control With Sulphonylureas or Insulin Compared With Conventional Treatment and Risk of Complications in Patients With Type 2 Diabetes (UKPDS 33)," *Lancet*, 1998, 352(9131):837-53.

HEART FAILURE (SYSTOLIC)

INTRODUCTORY COMMENTS

This summarizes the pharmacotherapy of patients with systolic heart failure with respect to treating mild-to-moderate exacerbations and chronic therapy. A more detailed discussion is available at http://content.onlinejacc.org/cgi/content/full/j.jacc.2008.11.013.

It should be recognized that the most common cause for exacerbations of patients' heart failure is poor adherence to therapy (medications and diet restriction). Healthcare providers need to educate patients about the importance of adherence to medical regimens.

For many years, therapy of heart failure focused on correcting the hemodynamic imbalances that occurred in heart failure. It is now recognized that heart failure triggers the release of several neurohormones that, in the short-run, help the patient; but, in the long-run, are detrimental. Newer pharmacotherapeutic approaches address counteracting the actions of these harmful neurohormones as well as address hemodynamic issues.

DIURETICS

Although data have yet to demonstrate that diuretics reduce the mortality associated with heart failure, they relieve symptoms seen in heart failure. Diuretics should only be used in patients experiencing congestion with their heart failure. Although not usually the case, some patients do have heart failure without congestion. In such rare instances, diuretic therapy is not indicated since they further stimulate the deleterious neurohormonal responses seen.

Although some heart failure patients with congestion can be controlled with thiazide diuretics, most will require the more potent loop diuretics, either because a strong diuretic effect is needed or renal function is compromised (thus limiting the effectiveness of the thiazide diuretic). When patients with heart failure are discovered to have mild-to-moderate worsening congestion, they often can be controlled by adjusting their oral loop diuretic dose or, if applicable, initiating a loop diuretic regimen. If a more aggressive diuresis is indicated, especially if the patient is suffering from pulmonary congestion, intravenous loop diuretics would be indicated. When loop diuretics are given intravenously, before any diuretic effect occurs, they benefit the patient by dilating veins and reducing preload, thus relieving pulmonary congestion. Intravenous loop diuretics may also be considered in a patient where concerns exist about the ability to absorb orally administered medication.

If already on an oral loop diuretic, the dosage should be increased (generally, 1.5-2 times their current regimen) in an effort for the patient to lose about 1-1.5 liters of fluid per day (about equivalent to 1-1.5 kg of weight per day). If the patient had yet to be started on a diuretic or was previously receiving a thiazide diuretic, initiating furosemide at 20-40 mg once or twice daily is a reasonable consideration. If the initial increase (or initiation) in dosage fails to induce a diuretic response, the dosage may be increased. If the initial increase (or initiation) does induce a diuretic response but the patient fails to lose weight or is not losing more fluids than taking in, the frequency of giving the loop diuretic may be increased. When an effective regimen is achieved, this regimen should be continued until the patient achieves a goal "dry" weight. Once this weight is attained, a decision needs to be made on how to continue the patient on diuretic therapy. If the patient had not been on a diuretic at home, continuation of the loop diuretic at a reduced dose is a worthy consideration. If the exacerbation was related to nonadherence with the diuretic or diet, the previous home dose might be continued with education on adherence to the prescribed diet and medication use. If the exacerbation was caused by an inadequate pharmacotherapeutic regimen (such as vasodilator was not being use), the previous home dose might be continued in conjunction with a more complete pharmacotherapeutic regimen. If the patient was compliant and on an acceptable pharmacotherapeutic regimen, the patient's original diuretic dose would be increased to some dosage greater than their home regimen, yet generally less than what was just used to achieve their dry weight.

The use of loop diuretics can lead to hypokalemia and/or hypomagnesemia. Electrolyte disturbances can predispose a patient to serious cardiac arrhythmias particularly if the patient is concurrently receiving digoxin. Fluid depletion, hypotension, and azotemia can also result from excessive use of diuretics. In contrast to thiazide diuretics, a loop diuretic can also lower serum calcium concentrations. For some patients, despite higher doses of loop diuretic treatment, an adequate diuretic response cannot be attained. Diuretic resistance can usually be overcome by intravenous administration (including continuous infusion), the use of 2 diuretics together (eg, furosemide and metolazone), or the use of a diuretic with a positive inotropic agent. When such combinations are used, serum electrolytes need to be monitored even more closely.

When loop diuretics are used in patients with renal dysfunction, to achieve the desired diuretic response, dosages typically will need to be greater than what is used in patients with normal renal function.

Due to its long existence and inexpensive price, furosemide tends to be the loop diuretic most commonly used. Bumetanide and torsemide are now available as generics and their use, especially bumetanide, has increased. The oral bioavailability of bumetanide and torsemide are nearly 100%; whereas, furosemide's oral bioavailability averages about 50%. A useful rule of thumb for conversion of intravenous loop diuretics is 40 mg of furosemide is equal to 1 mg bumetanide is equal to 20 mg torsemide. A few patients have allergies to diuretics because many contain a sulfur element. The only loop diuretic that lacks a sulfur element is ethacrynic acid.

VASODILATORS

Combination Hydralazine and Isosorbide Dinitrate

Vasodilator therapy, specifically the combination of hydralazine and isosorbide dinitrate, was the first pharmacotherapeutic treatment demonstrated to enhance survival of heart failure patients. The use of hydralazine 75 mg (which reduces afterload) and isosorbide dinitrate 40 mg 4 times a day (which reduces preload) demonstrated enhanced survival compared to placebo and prazosin. Unfortunately, many patients were unable to tolerate this regimen (primarily due to headaches and gastrointestinal disturbances) and the magnitude of benefit in survival dissipated with time.

The African-American Heart Failure Trial (A-HeFT) demonstrated mortality benefit with the use of a fixed combination of hydralazine and isosorbide dinitrate in combination with standard heart failure therapies, including ACE inhibitors, in self-identified African-American heart failure patients. The use of the commercially available combination of hydralazine and isosorbide dinitrate may be cost prohibitive in some patients; therefore, the use of the individually separate products is justifiable.

ACE Inhibitors

A series of investigations demonstrated that enalapril (which reduces both afterload and preload) enhances the survival of heart failure patients. Dosages used in these trials averaged about 10 mg twice daily. Since these trials, other ACE inhibitors were proven to benefit heart failure patients.

This led to the question – which is superior, ACE inhibitor or the combination of hydralazine and isosorbide dinitrate? In a comparative trial, using doses described above, enalapril was superior to the combination of hydralazine and isosorbide dinitrate, making an ACE inhibitor the vasodilator of choice in heart failure patients. An ACE inhibitor can alleviate symptoms, improve clinical status, and enhance a patient's quality of life. In addition an ACE inhibitor can reduce the risk of death and the combined risk of death or hospitalization.

Adverse effects associated with ACE inhibitors include hyperkalemia, rash, dysgeusia, dry cough, and (rarely) angioedema. Patients sometime develop renal dysfunction with the initiation of ACE inhibitors. This is not due to direct nephrotoxicity but is related to the ACE inhibitor dilating the efferent renal artery of the kidney, thus shunting blood away from being filtered in the glomerulus. The risk for renal dysfunction is increased when the ACE inhibitor is introduced to a patient who is hypovolemic, is being aggressively diuresed, is on an NSAID (which should be avoided in heart failure patients), or has bilateral renal artery stenosis (unilateral if only one kidney is present). ACE inhibitors should be avoided in patients with known renal artery stenosis. Monitor renal function and serum potassium within 1-2 weeks of initiation of therapy and routinely thereafter especially in patients with pre-existing hypotension, hyponatremia, diabetes, azotemia, or those taking potassium supplements. Some patients will have an exaggerated hypotensive response following the initial doses (especially the first dose) of an ACE inhibitor.

Angiotensin Receptor Blockers

A major limitation to using ACE inhibitors treatment in heart failure can be the dry cough that some patients develop. Lowering the ACE inhibitor dose sometimes can control it, but this may limit the effectiveness of the ACE inhibitor treatment. The development of angiotensin receptor blockers (ARBs) has helped address this issue. ARBs were demonstrated to enhance survival of heart failure patients. Although they are not the vasodilator of first choice in heart failure, they are a reasonable alternative in patients who cannot tolerate an ACE inhibitor due to the cough or some other adverse effect (with the exception of hyperkalemia and renal dysfunction; ARBs can induce as well). ARBs do not cause an accumulation of kinins as ACE inhibitors do.

Can ARBs be used in patients who suffer angioedema with ACE inhibitors? Reports are available in the literature describing patients who experienced angioedema with both ACE inhibitors and ARBs. These cases do not indicate the safety of an ARB when used in a patient who has experienced ACE inhibitor-induced angioedema. The CHARM-Alternative trial confirmed that only one of 39 patients (~2.6%) who experienced angioedema with an ACE inhibitors also experienced it with an ARB.

Concurrent Use of an ACE Inhibitor and an ARB

In Val-HeFT, valsartan added to conventional treatment (included ACE inhibitor treatment) did not impact survival but did reduce morbidity. Of note, a subgroup analysis of this trial suggested the combination of valsartan and an ACE inhibitor may be detrimental to patients also receiving a beta-blocker. In CHARM-Added, candesartan added to ACE inhibitor therapy was of benefit to heart failure patients (modest reduction in hospitalization; increased risk of hyperkalemia and renal dysfunction), even for those receiving a beta-blocker. As a result, the ACCF/AHA Practice Guidelines do not speak against using the combination of ACE inhibitors and ARBs. However, few patients in these trials were receiving an aldosterone blocker (such as spironolactone), which is now known to be of benefit to heart failure patients. Since there is enhanced risk for hyperkalemia and outcome data are currently unknown, the ACCF/AHA Practice Guidelines for heart failure do not advocate the combined use of ACE inhibitors, ARBs, and an aldosterone inhibitor.

In summary, vasodilator therapy should initially consist of an ACE inhibitor. If such therapy cannot be tolerated due to renal failure or hyperkalemia, the combination of hydralazine and isosorbide dinitrate may be considered as ARBs can also cause renal failure and hyperkalemia. If the ACE inhibitor cannot be tolerated due to adverse effects such as dry cough, an ARB may be considered. If an ACE inhibitor and beta-blocker have been maximized yet heart failure symptoms persist, consider adding hydralazine and isosorbide dinitrate. This approach, in fact, has been demonstrated to enhance the survival of African-American patients with heart failure. Another approach may be to add an ARB to the ACE inhibitor; but caution should occur, due to the risk of hyperkalemia.

BETA-BLOCKERS

Despite being negative inotropes, beta-blockers have been demonstrated to enhance the survival of systolic heart failure patients. Their benefit is attributed to their ability to protect the myocardium from the "bombardment" of catecholamines present in heart failure that can lead to ventricular remodeling. Bisoprolol, metoprolol succinate (extended release), and carvedilol have been demonstrated in trials to improve survival. Carvedilol is also available as a once-a-day extended-release preparation; but, its daily cost is considerably greater than generically-available immediate-release carvedilol that is given twice a day. At present, superiority of a particular beta-blocker over another has not been definitively demonstrated. For patients to be able to tolerate this therapy, beta-blocker treatment needs to be initiated at low doses and titrated slowly (generally, the dose is double every two weeks). Following the initiation of treatment and increase in dosage, patients may feel that their disease is worsening but this should dissipate after a few days. If this ill feeling continues beyond a few days, consideration should be given to regimen adjustments. If the patient is congested, increase the diuretic dosage. If the patient's discomfort is related to hypotension, staggering the beta-blocker dose with the vasodilator dose and/or lowering the vasodilator dosage may be helpful. If these approaches are ineffective or cannot explain the patient's ill feeling, consideration should be given to lowering the beta-blocker dosage and attempt a dose titration increase later on. Sometimes, a patient may not be able to tolerate "goal" doses of both beta-blockers and concurrent vasodilator treatment due to hypotension. It is the consensus opinion that a reduced dose of each agent is better than a goal dose of just one agent. Beta-blockers are not necessarily contraindicated but need to be used cautiously in patients with bronchospastic disease, peripheral arterial disease, or diabetes mellitus.

ALDOSTERONE BLOCKERS

It has been demonstrated, especially in the more severe forms of heart failure, that spironolactone, at an average dose of 25 mg daily, enhances the survival of heart failure patients. In patients who suffer hyperkalemia at this relatively low dosage, lowering the dose to 25 mg every other day may be attempted. In patients who remain symptomatic with their heart failure and have maximized the other proven treatments of heart failure and whose potassium concentrations can tolerate increases, the spironolactone dose may be increased to 50 mg daily.

Obviously, hyperkalemia is a concern with this treatment, especially since patients generally will also be receiving an ACE inhibitor or ARB. It has been demonstrated that the number of emergency visits related to hyperkalemia in heart failure has increased with the introduction of aldosterone blocking therapy in treating heart failure. About 10% of patients will experience endocrinological effects with spironolactone. In men, breast tenderness and gynecomastia may occur. In women, menstrual irregularities may be seen. In such instances, the use of eplerenone may be considered. Eplerenone is less apt to induce endocrinological effects but it is more expensive. A typical dose is 25-50 mg daily. Eplerenone has been demonstrated to enhance survival of post-MI patients with reduced ejection fractions. Spironolactone has not been studied in this patient group.

These medications should not be started in patients with renal insufficiency. These medications should be avoided if the serum creatinine exceeds 2.5 mg/dL in men (2 mg/dL in women) or if baseline potassium ≥5 mEq/L.

DIGOXIN

The value of digoxin in heart failure has crossed the spectrum. In the late 1980s, further investigation with digoxin suggested that indeed it may have a role in heart failure treatment, but the methods of these trials were not ideal (digoxin was taken away from stabilized patients to see if the condition of patients worsened – it did). Finally, digoxin was studied in a prospective manner where patients were on known optimal heart failure treatment at the time and randomized to placebo or digoxin. The digoxin dosage used resulted in digoxin steady-state concentrations of 1 mcg/L. This trial revealed that digoxin did not impact survival but reduced the number of patient hospitalizations, suggesting digoxin has a morbidity benefit. Many are of the opinion that digoxin's benefit is unrelated to its positive inotropic activity but related to inhibiting neurohormonal activity. Healthcare providers may consider adding digoxin in patients with persistent heart failure symptoms as a fourth line agent.

Digoxin is primarily renally eliminated; therefore, renal function of patients should be closely monitored and the dose adjusted. Digoxin does become difficult to use in patients whose renal function is unstable. In the DIG trial, effective digoxin steady-state concentrations ranged between 0.7-1 mcg/L. Concentrations much beyond 1 mcg/L were associated with worsened outcomes, especially in women. Since digoxin's benefit is long-term, a loading dose is not necessary. When checking a digoxin serum concentration, the sample should not be obtained until 12 hours after a dose, especially if it was oral, since digoxin has a relatively long distribution phase. It should also be assured that the patient is at steady-state (recall that the half-life of digoxin in a patient with normal renal function is approximately 36 hours and that patients with heart failure generally have worsened renal function).

Hypokalemia, hypomagnesia, hypercalcemia, and hypothyroidism can precipitate digoxin toxicity in the presence of a therapeutic digoxin concentration. This toxicity can be alleviated by correcting the electrolyte abnormality. In acute digoxin overdoses, hyperkalemia can occur since digoxin inhibits the sodium-potassium ATPase pump. For this reason, one should not assume potassium is given to just **any** patient with digoxin toxicity. Digoxin toxicity can present as bradyarrhythmias, heart blocks, ventricular tachyarrhythmias, and atrial tachyarrhythmias (PAT with block is pathognomonic). Other toxic manifestations include visual disturbances (including greenish-yellowish vision and halos around lights), gastrointestinal disturbances, anorexia, and altered mental status. Many medications elevate digoxin concentrations and a patient's regimen should be assessed for potential interactions.

OTHER HEART FAILURE THERAPEUTIC CONSIDERATIONS

- If a calcium channel blocker is desired, amlodipine or felodipine are preferred choices.
- To treat arrhythmias, amiodarone and dofetilide are best documented to lack significant proarrhythmic propensity in heart failure patients. Dronedarone, a newer antiarrhythmic agent structurally similar to amiodarone, is contraindicated in patients with NYHA Class IV heart failure or Class II-III heart failure with recent decompensation requiring hospitalization or referral to a specialized heart failure clinic.
- In heart failure patients with diabetes mellitus, metformin should not be used and "glitazones" should not be used in severe heart failure (NYHA III and IV) and used cautiously, if at all, in mild-to-moderate heart failure.
- The use of cilostazol, because it has type III phosphodiesterase-inhibiting properties, is contraindicated in heart failure. This is because the chronic use of *oral* milrinone and inamrinone, also type III phosphodiesterase inhibitors, resulted in enhanced mortality in heart failure patients (and therefore, these two agents were never FDA-approved for oral use).
- NSAID use should be avoided or used minimally as these agents antagonize the effects of diuretics and ACE inhibitors.
- Retrospective data suggests that daily aspirin may also negate the effects of ACE inhibitors but this has yet to be definitively proven in prospective trials. Using the lowest possible aspirin dose with the highest possible ACE inhibitor dose has been suggested as a way to best circumvent this issue.
- Routine intermittent intravenous infusions of positive inotropes are not recommended; but their use may be considered as palliative therapy in end-stage disease when ordinary therapy is insufficient.

CLASS I RECOMMENDATIONS FOR THE HOSPITALIZED PATIENT WITH ACUTE DECOMPENSATED HEART FAILURE

- Patients presenting to the hospital with fluid overload should be treated immediately with intravenous loop diuretics (eg, furosemide) since earlier treatment may be associated with better outcomes. If chronically receiving oral loop diuretic therapy, the initial intravenous dose should equal or exceed their chronic oral daily dose and titrated to relieve symptoms and reduce fluid excess. If this is inadequate, use of higher doses of loop diuretics, adding a second diuretic (eg, intravenous chlorothiazide), or a continuous infusion of the loop diuretic may improve diuresis.
- If evidence of hypotension with associated hypoperfusion and elevated cardiac filling pressures (eg, increase JVP) exists, intravenous inotropic support (eg, dobutamine) or vasopressor drugs (eg, dopamine) should be administered. Use of intravenous inotropes in patients without evidence of hypoperfusion is not recommended.
- In the absence of hemodynamic instability or contraindications, the use of therapies known to improve outcomes (eg, ACE inhibitors or ARBs, and beta-blockers) should be continued during the hospital stay. When appropriate, these agents should be initiated or reinitiated to stabilized patients prior to hospital discharge. Beta-blockers should only be initiated upon successful discontinuation of intravenous diuretics, vasodilators, and inotropic agents in the stabilized patient; initiate at a low dose and use caution in those patients who required inotropic support during their hospital course.

Dosing of ACE Inhibitors in Heart Failure[1]

ACEI	Initial Dose	Maximum Dose[2]
Captopril	6.25 mg tid	50 mg tid
Enalapril	2.5 mg bid	10-20 mg bid
Fosinopril	5-10 mg daily	40 mg daily
Lisinopril	2.5-5 mg daily	20-40 mg daily
Perindopril	2 mg daily	8-16 mg daily
Quinapril	5 mg bid	20 mg bid
Ramipril	1.25-2.5 mg daily	10 mg daily
Trandolapril	1 mg daily	4 mg daily

[1]From ACCF/AHA Guidelines

[2]Maximum/target dose recommendation may vary between guidelines (also see Heart Failure Society of America, 2010)

Dosing of ARBs in Heart Failure[1]

ARB	Initial Dose	Maximum Dose[2]
Candesartan	4-8 mg daily	32 mg daily
Losartan	25-50 mg daily	50-100 mg daily
Valsartan	20-40 mg bid	160 mg bid

[1]From ACCF/AHA Guidelines

[2]Maximum/target dose recommendation may vary between guidelines (also see Heart Failure Society of America, 2010)

Initial and Target Doses for Beta-Blocker Therapy in Heart Failure[1]

Beta-Blocker	Starting Dose	Target Dose	Comment
Bisoprolol	1.25 mg daily	10 mg daily	β_1-Selective blocker Inconvenient dosage forms for initial dose titration
Carvedilol	3.125 mg bid	25 mg bid (≤85 kg) 50 mg bid (>85 kg)	β-Nonselective blocker α_1-Blocking properties
Carvedilol phosphate, extended release	10 mg daily	80 mg daily[2]	
Metoprolol succinate, extended release	12.5-25 mg daily	200 mg daily	β_1-Selective blocker

[1]From ACCF/AHA Guidelines

[2]Equivalent to carvedilol immediate release 25 mg twice daily

Conversion From Immediate Release to Extended Release Carvedilol (Coreg CR®)

Carvedilol Immediate Release Dose	Carvedilol Phosphate Extended Release Dose
3.125 mg twice daily	10 mg once daily
6.25 mg twice daily	20 mg once daily
12.5 mg twice daily	40 mg once daily
25 mg twice daily	80 mg once daily

REFERENCES

Brater DC, "Diuretic Therapy," *N Engl J Med*, 1998, 339(6):387-95.

Granger CB, McMurray JJ, Yusuf S, et al, "Effects of Candesartan in Patients With Chronic Heart Failure and Reduced Left-Ventricular Systolic Function Intolerant to Angiotensin-Converting-Enzyme Inhibitors: The CHARM-Alternative Trial," *Lancet*, 2003, 362(9386):772-6.

Heart Failure Society of America, Lindenfeld J, Albert NM, et al, "HFSA 2010 Comprehensive Heart Failure Practice Guideline," *J Card Fail*, 2010, 16(6): e1-194.

Hunt SA, Abraham WT, Chin MH, et al, "2009 Focused Update Incorporated Into the ACC/AHA 2005 Guidelines for the Diagnosis and Management of Heart Failure in Adults A Report of the American College of Cardiology Foundation/American Heart Association Task Force on Practice Guidelines Developed in Collaboration With the International Society for Heart and Lung Transplantation," *J Am Coll Cardiol*, 2009, 53(15):e1-e90.

McMurray JJ, Ostergren J, Swedberg K, et al, "Effects of Candesartan in Patients With Chronic Heart Failure and Reduced Left-Ventricular Systolic Function Taking Angiotensin-Converting-Enzyme Inhibitors: The CHARM-Added Trial," *Lancet*, 2003, 362(9386):767-71.

Taylor AL, Ziesche S, Yancy C, et al, "Combination of Isosorbide Dinitrate and Hydralazine in Blacks With Heart Failure," *N Engl J Med*, 2004, 351 (20):2049-57.

HYPERLIPIDEMIA MANAGEMENT

MORTALITY

There is a strong link between serum cholesterol and cardiovascular mortality. This association becomes stronger in patients with established coronary artery disease. Lipid-lowering trials show that reductions in LDL cholesterol are followed by reductions in mortality. In general, each 1% fall in LDL cholesterol confers a 2% reduction in cardiovascular events. The aim of therapy for hyperlipidemia is to decrease cardiovascular morbidity and mortality by lowering cholesterol to a target level using safe and cost-effective treatment modalities. The target LDL cholesterol is determined by the number of patient risk factors (see the following Risk Factors and Goal LDL Cholesterol tables). The goal is achieved through diet, lifestyle modification, and drug therapy. The basis for these recommendations is provided by longitudinal interventional studies, demonstrating that lipid-lowering in patients with prior cardiovascular events (secondary prevention) and in patients with hyperlipidemia but no prior cardiac event (primary prevention) lowers the occurrence of future cardiovascular events, including stroke.

Major Risk Factors That Modify LDL Goals

Positive risk factors	Male ≥45 years
	Female ≥55 years
	Family history of premature coronary heart disease, defined as CHD in male first-degree relative <55 years; CHD in female first-degree relative <65 years
	Cigarette smoking
	Hypertension (blood pressure ≥140/90 mm Hg) or taking antihypertensive medication
	Low HDL (<40 mg/dL [1.03 mmol/L])
Negative risk factors	High HDL (≥60 mg/dL [1.6 mmol/L])[1]

[1]If HDL is ≥60 mg/dL, may subtract one positive risk factor

Adult Treatment Panel (ATP) III LDL-C Goals and Cutpoints for Therapeutic Lifestyle Changes (TLC) and Drug Therapy in Different Risk Categories

Risk Category	LDL-C Goal	Initiate TLC	Consider Drug Therapy[1]
High risk: CHD[2] or CHD risk equivalents[3] (10-year risk >20%)	<100 mg/dL (optional goal: <70 mg/dL)[4]	≥100 mg/dL[5]	≥100 mg/dL[6] (<100 mg/dL: Consider drug options)[1]
Moderately high risk: ≥2 risk factors[7] (10-year risk 10% to 20%)[8]	<130 mg/dL[9]	≥130 mg/dL[5]	≥130 mg/dL (100-120 mg/dL: Consider drug options)[10]
Moderate risk: ≥2 risk factors[7] (10-year risk <10%)[8]	<130 mg/dL	≥130 mg/dL	≥160 mg/dL
Lower risk: 0-1 risk factor[11]	<160 mg/dL	≥160 mg/dL	≥190 mg/dL (160-189 mg/dL: LDL-lowering drug optional)

[1]When LDL-lowering drug therapy is employed, it is advised that intensity of therapy be sufficient to achieve at least a 30% to 40% reduction in LDL-C levels.

[2]CHD includes history of myocardial infarction, unstable angina, stable angina, coronary artery procedures (angioplasty or bypass surgery), or evidence of clinically significant myocardial ischemia.

[3]CHD risk equivalents include clinical manifestations of noncoronary forms of atherosclerotic disease (peripheral arterial disease, abdominal aortic aneurysm, and carotid artery disease [transient ischemic attacks or stroke of carotid origin or >50% obstruction of a carotid artery]), diabetes, and 2+ risk factors with 10-year risk for hard CHD >20%.

[4]Very high risk favors the optional LDL-C goal of <70 mg/dL, and in patients with high triglycerides, non-HDL-C <100 mg/dL

[5]Any person at high risk or moderately high risk who has lifestyle-related risk factors (eg, obesity, physical inactivity, elevated triglyceride, low HDL-C, or metabolic syndrome) is a candidate for therapeutic lifestyle changes to modify these risk factors regardless of LDL-C level.

[6]If baseline LDL-C is <100 mg/dL, institution of an LDL-lowering drug is a therapeutic option on the basis of available clinical trial results. If a high-risk person has high triglycerides or low HDL-C, combining a fibrate or nicotinic acid with an LDL-lowering drug can be considered.

[7]Risk factors include cigarette smoking, hypertension (BP ≥140/90 mm Hg or on antihypertensive medication), low HDL cholesterol (<40 mg/dL), family history of premature CHD (CHD in male first-degree relative <55 years of age; CHD in female first-degree relative <65 years of age), and age (men ≥45 years; women ≥55 years).

[8]Electronic 10-year risk calculators are available at www.nhlbi.nih.gov/guidelines/cholesterol.

[9]Optional LDL-C goal <100 mg/dL

[10]For moderately high-risk persons, when LDL-C level is 100-129 mg/dL, at baseline or on lifestyle therapy, initiation of an LDL-lowering drug to achieve an LDL-C level <100 mg/dL is a therapeutic option on the basis of available clinical trial results.

[11]Almost all people with zero or 1 risk factor have a 10-year risk <10%, and 10-year risk assessment in people with zero or 1 risk factor thus not necessary

Any person with elevated LDL cholesterol or other form of hyperlipidemia should undergo evaluation to rule out secondary dyslipidemia. Causes of secondary dyslipidemia include diabetes, hypothyroidism, obstructive liver disease, chronic renal failure, and drugs that increase LDL and decrease HDL (progestins, anabolic steroids, corticosteroids).

Elevated Serum Triglyceride Levels

Elevated serum triglyceride levels may be an independent risk factor for coronary heart disease. Factors that contribute to hypertriglyceridemia include obesity, inactivity, cigarette smoking, excess alcohol intake, high carbohydrate diets (>60% of energy intake), type 2 diabetes, chronic renal failure, nephrotic syndrome, certain medications (corticosteroids, estrogens, retinoids, higher doses of beta-blockers), and genetic disorders. Non-HDL cholesterol (total cholesterol minus HDL cholesterol) is a secondary focus for clinicians treating patients with high serum triglyceride levels (≥200 mg/dL). The goal for non-HDL cholesterol in patients with high serum triglyceride levels can be set 30 mg/dL higher than usual LDL cholesterol goals. Patients with serum triglyceride levels <200 mg/dL should aim for the target LDL cholesterol goal.

ATP classification of serum triglyceride levels:

- Normal triglycerides: <150 mg/dL
- Borderline-high: 150-199 mg/dL
- High: 200-499 mg/dL
- Very high: ≥500 mg/dL

NONDRUG THERAPY

Dietary therapy and lifestyle modifications should be individualized for each patient. A total lifestyle change is recommended for all patients. Dietary and lifestyle modifications should be tried for 3 months, if deemed appropriate. Nondrug and drug therapy should be initiated simultaneously in patients with highly elevated cholesterol (see LDL Cholesterol Goals and Cutpoints for Therapeutic Lifestyle Changes and Drug Therapy in Different Risk Categories table). Increasing physical activity and smoking cessation will aid in the treatment of hyperlipidemia and improve cardiovascular health.

Note: Refer to the National Cholesterol Education Program reference for details concerning the calculation of 10-year risk of CHD using Framingham risk scoring. Risk assessment tool is available on-line at http://hin.nhlbi.nih.gov/atpiii/calculator.asp?usertype=prof, last accessed March 14, 2002.

Total Lifestyle Change (TLC) Diet

	Recommended Intake
Total fat	25%-35% of total calories
Saturated fat[1]	<7% of total calories
Polyunsaturated fat	≤10% of total calories
Monounsaturated fat	≤20% of total calories
Carbohydrates[2]	50%-60% of total calories
Fiber	20-30 g/day
Protein	~15% of total calories
Cholesterol	<200 mg/day
Total calories[3]	Balance energy intake and expenditure to maintain desirable body weight/prevent weight gain

[1] *Trans* fatty acids (partially hydrogenated oils) intake should be kept low. These are found in potato chips, other snack foods, margarines and shortenings, and fast-foods.

[2] Complex carbohydrates, including grains (especially whole grains, fruits, and vegetables)

[3] Daily energy expenditure should include at least moderate physical activity.

DRUG THERAPY

Drug therapy should be selected based on the patient's lipid profile, concomitant disease states, and the cost of therapy. The following table lists specific advantages and disadvantages for various classes of lipid-lowering medications. The expected reduction in lipids with therapy is listed in the Lipid-Lowering Agents table. Refer to individual drug monographs for detailed information.

Advantages and Disadvantages of Specific Lipid-Lowering Therapies

	Advantages	Disadvantages
Bile acid sequestrants	Good choice for ↑ LDL, especially when combined with a statin (↓ LDL ≤50%); low potential for systemic side effects; good choice for younger patients	May increase triglycerides; higher incidence of adverse effects; moderately expensive; drug interactions; inconvenient dosing
Niacin	Good choice for almost any lipid abnormality; inexpensive; greatest increase in HDL	High incidence of adverse effects; may adversely affect type 2 DM (with high dose >1.5 g/day) and gout; sustained release niacin may decrease the incidence of flushing and circumvent the need for multiple daily dosing; sustained release niacin may not increase HDL cholesterol or decrease triglycerides as well as immediate release niacin
HMG-CoA reductase inhibitors	Produces greatest ↓ in LDL; generally well-tolerated; convenient once-daily dosing; proven decrease in mortality	Expensive
Fibric acid derivatives	Good choice in patients with ↑ triglycerides where niacin is contraindicated or not well-tolerated	Variable effects on LDL
Ezetimibe	Additional cholesterol-lowering effects when combined with HMG-CoA reductase inhibitors	Effects similar to bile acid sequestrants

Lipid-Lowering Agents

Drug	Dose/Day	Effect on LDL (%)	Effect on HDL (%)	Effect on TG (%)
HMG-CoA Reductase Inhibitors				
Atorvastatin	10 mg 20 mg 40 mg 80 mg	-39 -43 -50 -60	+6 +9 +6 +5	-19 -26 -29 -37
Fluvastatin	20 mg 40 mg 80 mg	-22 -25 -36	+3 +4 +6	-12 -14 -18
Lovastatin	10 mg 20 mg 40 mg 80 mg	-21 -24 -30 -40	+5 +7 +7 +9.5	-10 -10 -14 -19
Pitavastatin	1 mg 2 mg 4 mg	-32 -36 -43	+8 +7 +5	-15 -19 -18
Pravastatin	10 mg 20 mg 40 mg 80 mg	-22 -32 -34 -37	+7 +2 +12 +3	-15 -11 -24 -19
Rosuvastatin	5 mg 10 mg 20 mg 40 mg	-45 -52 -55 -63	+13 +14 +8 +10	-35 -10 -23 -28
Simvastatin	5 mg 10 mg 20 mg 40 mg 80 mg	-26 -30 -38 -41 -47	+10 +12 +8 +13 +16	-12 -15 -19 -28 -33
Bile Acid Sequestrants				
Cholestyramine	4-24 g	-15 to -30	+3 to +5	+0 to +20
Colesevelam	6 tablets 7 tablets	-15 -18	+3 +3	+10 +9
Colestipol	7-30 g	-15 to -30	+3 to +5	+0 to +20
Fibric Acid Derivatives				
Fenofibrate	67-200 mg	-20 to -31	+9 to +14	-30 to -50
Gemfibrozil	600 mg twice daily	-5 to -10[1]	+10 to +20	-40 to -60
Niacin	1.5-6 g	-5 to -25	+15 to +35	-20 to -50
2-Azetidinone				
Ezetimibe	10 mg	-15 to -20	+1 to +4	-5 to -8
Omega-3-Acid Ethyl Esters	4 g	+44.5	+9.1	-44.9
Combination Products				
Ezetimibe and simvastatin	10/10 mg 10/20 mg 10/40 mg 10/80 mg	-45 -52 -55 -60	+8 +10 +6 +6	-23 -24 -23 -31
Niacin and lovastatin	1000/20 mg 1000/40 mg 1500/40 mg 2000/40 mg	-30 -36 -37 -42	+20 +20 +27 +30	-32 -39 -44 -44
Niacin and simvastatin	1000/20 mg 1000/40 mg 2000/20 mg 2000/40 mg	-12 -7 -14 -5	+21 +15 +29 +24	-27 -23 -38 -32

[1]May increase LDL in some patients

Progression of Drug Therapy in Primary Prevention

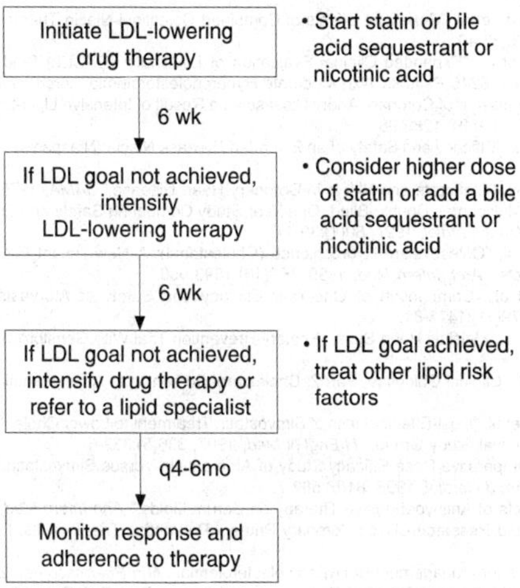
Initiate LDL-lowering drug therapy
• Start statin or bile acid sequestrant or nicotinic acid
6 wk
If LDL goal not achieved, intensify LDL-lowering therapy
• Consider higher dose of statin or add a bile acid sequestrant or nicotinic acid
6 wk
If LDL goal not achieved, intensify drug therapy or refer to a lipid specialist
• If LDL goal achieved, treat other lipid risk factors
q4-6mo
Monitor response and adherence to therapy

DRUG SELECTION

Lipid Profile	Monotherapy	Combination Therapies
Increased LDL with normal HDL and triglycerides (TG)	Resin Niacin[1] Statin	Resin plus niacin[1] or statin Statin plus niacin[1,2]
Increased LDL and increased TG (200-499 mg/dL)[2]	Intensify LDL-lowering therapy	Statin plus niacin[1,3] Statin plus fibrate[3]
Increased LDL and increased TG (≥500 mg/dL)[2]	Consider combination therapy (niacin,[1] fibrates, statin)	
Increased TG	Niacin[1] Fibrates	Niacin[1] plus fibrates
Increased LDL and low HDL	Niacin[1] Statin	Statin plus niacin[1,2]

[1]Avoid in diabetics.

[2]Emphasize weight reduction and increased physical activity.

[3]Risk of myopathy with combination

Resins = bile acid sequestrants, statins = HMG-CoA reductase inhibitors, fibrates = fibric acid derivatives (eg, gemfibrozil, fenofibrate)

COMBINATION DRUG THERAPY

If after at least 6 weeks of therapy at the maximum recommended or tolerated dose, the patient's LDL cholesterol is not at target, consider optimizing nondrug measures, prescribing a higher dose of current lipid-lowering drug, or adding another lipid-lowering medication to the current therapy. Successful drug combinations include statin and niacin, statin and bile acid sequestrant, or niacin and bile acid sequestrant. At maximum recommended doses, LDL cholesterol may be decreased by 50% to 60% with combination therapy. This is the same reduction achieved by atorvastatin 40 mg twice daily. If a bile acid sequestrant is used with other lipid-lowering agents, space doses 1 hour before or 4 hours after the bile acid sequestrant administration. Statins combined with either fenofibrate, gemfibrozil, or niacin increase the risk of rhabdomyolysis. In this situation, patient education (muscle pain/weakness) and careful follow-up are warranted.

References

Guidelines

American Diabetes Association, "Standards of Medical Care in Diabetes – 2010," *Diabetes Care*, 2010, 33(Suppl 1):S11-61.

Brunzell JD, Davidson M, Furberg CD, et al, "Lipoprotein Management in Patients With Cardiometabolic Risk: Consensus Statement From the American Diabetes Association and the American College of Cardiology Foundation," *Diabetes Care*, 2008, 31(4):811-22.

Grundy SM, Cleeman JI, Merz CN, et al, "Implications of Recent Clinical Trials for the National Cholesterol Education Program Adult Treatment Panel III Guidelines," *J Am Coll Cardiol*, 2004, 44(3):720-32.

National Cholesterol Education Program, "Third Report of the Expert Panel on Detection, Evaluation, and Treatment of High Blood Cholesterol in Adults (Adult Treatment Panel III)," *JAMA*, 2001, 285(19):2486-97.

Others

Berthold HK, Sudhop T, and von Bergmann K, "Effect of a Garlic Oil Preparation on Serum Lipoproteins and Cholesterol Metabolism: A Randomized Controlled Trial," *JAMA*, 1998, 279(23):1900-2.

Bertolini S, Bon GB, Campbell LM, et al, "Efficacy and Safety of Atorvastatin Compared to Pravastatin in Patients With Hypercholesterolemia," *Atherosclerosis*, 1997, 130(1-2):191-7.

Blankenhorn DH, Nessim SA, Johnson RL, et al, "Beneficial Effects of Combined Colestipol-Niacin Therapy on Coronary Atherosclerosis and Venous Bypass Grafts," *JAMA*, 1987, 257(23):3233-40.

Bradford RH, Shear CL, Chremos AN, et al, "Expanded Clinical Evaluation of Lovastatin (EXCEL) Study Results. I. Efficacy in Modifying Plasma Lipoproteins and Adverse Event Profile in 8245 Patients With Moderate Hypercholesterolemia," *Arch Intern Med*, 1991, 151(1):43-9.

Brown G, Albers JJ, Fisher LD, et al, "Regression of Coronary Artery Disease as a Result of Intensive Lipid-Lowering Therapy in Men With High Levels of Apolipoprotein B," *N Engl J Med*, 1990, 323(19):1289-98.

Capuzzi DM, Guyton JR, Morgan JM, et al, "Efficacy and Safety of an Extended-Release Niacin (Niaspan®): A Long-Term Study," *Am J Cardiol*, 1998, 82 (12A):74U-81U.

Coronary Drug Project Research Program, "Clofibrate and Niacin in Coronary Heart Disease," *JAMA*, 1975, 231(4):360-81.

Dart A, Jerums G, Nicholson G, et al, "A Multicenter, Double-Blind, One-Year Study Comparing Safety and Efficacy of Atorvastatin Versus Simvastatin in Patients With Hypercholesterolemia," *Am J Cardiol*, 1997, 80(1):39-44.

Davidson MH, Dillon MA, Gordon B, et al, "Colesevelam Hydrochloride (Cholestagel): A New Potent Bile Acid Sequestrant Associated With a Low Incidence of Gastrointestinal Side Effects," *Arch Intern Med*, 1999, 159(16):1893-900.

Davidson M, McKenney J, Stein E, et al, "Comparison of One-Year Efficacy and Safety of Atorvastatin Versus Lovastatin in Primary Hypercholesterolemia," *Am J Cardiol*, 1997, 79(11):1475-81.

Frick MH, Heinonen OP, Huttunen JK, et al, "Helsinki Heart Study: Primary-Prevention Trial With Gemfibrozil in Middle-Aged Men With Dyslipidemia," *N Engl J Med*, 1987, 317(20):1237-45.

Garber AM, Browner WS, and Hulley SB, "Clinical Guideline, Part 2: Cholesterol Screening in Asymptomatic Adults, Revisited," *Ann Intern Med*, 1995, 124(5):518-31.

Johannesson M, Jonsson B, Kjekshus J, et al, "Cost-Effectiveness of Simvastatin Treatment to Lower Cholesterol Levels in Patients With Coronary Heart Disease. Scandinavian Simvastatin Survival Study Group," *N Engl N Med*, 1997, 336(5):332-6.

Jones P, Kafonek S, Laurora I, et al, "Comparative Dose Efficacy Study of Atorvastatin Versus Simvastatin, Pravastatin, Lovastatin, and Fluvastatin in Patients With Hypercholesterolemia," *Am J Cardiol*, 1998, 81(5):582-7.

Kasiske BL, Ma JZ, Kalil RS, et al, "Effects of Antihypertensive Therapy on Serum Lipids," *Ann Intern Med*, 1995, 122(2):133-41.

Lipid Research Clinics Program, "The Lipid Research Clinics Coronary Primary Prevention Trial Results: I. Reduction in Incidence of Coronary Heart Disease," *JAMA*, 1984, 251(3):351-64.

Mauro VF and Tuckerman CE, "Ezetimibe for Management of Hypercholesterolemia," *Ann Pharmacother*, 2003, 37(6):839-48.

Multiple Risk Factor Intervention Trial Research Group, "Multiple Risk Factor Intervention Trial: Risk Factor Changes and Mortality Results," *JAMA*, 1982, 248(12):1465-77.

Pitt B, Waters D, Brown WV, et al, "Aggressive Lipid-Lowering Therapy Compared With Angioplasty in Stable Coronary Artery Disease. Atorvastatin Versus Revascularization Treatment Investigators," *N Engl J Med*, 1999, 341(2):70-6.

Ross SD, Allen IE, Connelly JE, et al, "Clinical Outcomes in Statin Treatment Trials: A Meta-Analysis," *Arch Intern Med*, 1999, 159(15):1793-802.

Sacks FM, Pfeffer MA, Moye LA, et al, "The Effect of Pravastatin on Coronary Events After Myocardial Infarction in Patients With Average Cholesterol Levels," *N Engl J Med*, 1996, 335(14):1001-9.

Scandinavian Simvastatin Survival Study, "Randomized Trial of Cholesterol Lowering in 4444 Patients With Coronary Heart Disease: The Scandinavian Simvastatin Survival Study (4S)," *Lancet*, 1994, 344(8934):1383-9.

Schrott HG, Bittner V, Vittinghoff E, et al, "Adherence to National Cholesterol Education Program Treatment Goals in Postmenopausal Women With Heart Disease. The Heart and Estrogen/Progestin Replacement Study (HERS)," *JAMA*, 1997, 277(16):1281-6.

Shepherd J, Cobbe SM, Ford I, et al, "Prevention of Coronary Heart Disease With Pravastatin in Men With Hypercholesterolemia, The West of Scotland Coronary Prevention Study Group," *N Engl J Med*, 1995, 333(20):1301-7.

Stein EA, Davidson MH, Dobs AS, et al, "Efficacy and Safety of Simvastatin 80 mg/day in Hypercholesterolemic Patients. The Expanded Dose Simvastatin U.S. Study Group," *Am J Cardiol*, 1998, 82(3):311-6.

HYPERTENSION

The optimal blood pressure for adults is <120/80 mm Hg. Consistent systolic pressure ≥140 mm Hg or a diastolic pressure ≥90 mm Hg, in the absence of a secondary cause, defines hypertension. Hypertension affects approximately 25% (50 million people) in the United States. Of those patients on antihypertensive medication, only one in three have their blood pressure controlled (<140/90 mm Hg).

Controlling systolic hypertension has been much more difficult than controlling diastolic hypertension. Educating patients in lifestyle management, cardiovascular risk reduction, and drug therapy aids in improving the morbidity and mortality of patients with hypertension.

The Seventh Report of the Joint National Committee (JNC 7) is an excellent reference and guide for the treatment of hypertension (Chobanian AV, Bakris GL, Black HR, et al, "The Seventh Report of the Joint National Committee on Prevention, Detection, Evaluation, and Treatment of High Blood Pressure: The JNC 7 Report," *JAMA*, 2003, 289(19):2560-71). For adults, hypertension is classified in stages (see following table).

Adult Classification of Blood Pressure

Category	Systolic (mm Hg)		Diastolic (mm Hg)
Normal	<120	and	<80
Prehypertension	120-139	or	80-89
Hypertension			
Stage 1	140-159	or	90-99
Stage 2	≥160	or	≥100

Adapted from Chobanian AV, Bakris GL, Black HR, et al, "The Seventh Report of the Joint National Committee on Prevention, Detection, Evaluation, and Treatment of High Blood Pressure: The JNC 7 Report," *JAMA*, 2003, 289(19):2560-71.

Normal Blood Pressure in Children

Age (y)	Girls' SBP / DBP (mm Hg)		Boys' SBP / DBP (mm Hg)	
	50th Percentile for Height	75th Percentile for Height	50th Percentile for Height	75th Percentile for Height
1	104/58	105/59	102/57	104/58
6	111/73	112/73	114/74	115/75
12	123/80	124/81	123/81	125/82
17	129/84	130/85	136/87	138/88

SBP = systolic blood pressure

DBP = diastolic blood pressure

Adapted from the report by the NHBPEP Working Group on Hypertension Control in Children and Adolescents, *Pediatrics*, 1996, 98(4 Pt 1):649-58.

PATIENT ASSESSMENT

- **Cardiovascular Risk Factors:** Hypertension, cigarette smoking, obesity (BMI ≥30), inactive lifestyle, dyslipidemia, diabetes mellitus, microalbuminuria or estimated GFR <60 mL/minute, age (>55 years for men, >65 years for women), family history of premature cardiovascular disease (men <55 years or women >65 years)

Components of metabolic syndrome include hypertension, obesity, dyslipidemia, diabetes mellitus

- Identify causes of high BP.
- Assess target-organ damage and CVD.

Target-Organ Disease

Organ System	Manifestation
Cardiac	Clinical, ECG, or radiologic evidence of coronary artery disease; prior MI, angina, post-CABG; left ventricular hypertrophy (LVH); left ventricular dysfunction or cardiac failure, prior coronary revascularization
Cerebrovascular	Transient ischemic attack or stroke
Peripheral vascular	Absence of pulses in extremities (except dorsalis pedis), claudication, aneurysm, peripheral arterial disease
Renal	Serum creatinine ≥130 µmol/L (1.5 mg/dL); proteinuria (≥1+); microalbuminuria, chronic kidney disease
Eye	Hemorrhages or exudates, with or without papilledema; retinopathy

Adapted from Chobanian AV, Bakris GL, Black HR, et al, "The Seventh Report of the Joint National Committee on Prevention, Detection, Evaluation, and Treatment of High Blood Pressure: The JNC 7 Report," *JAMA*, 2003, 289(19):2560-71.

BLOOD PRESSURE MEASUREMENT

At an office visit, patients should be seated quietly for ≥5 minutes in a chair with feet on the floor and arm supported at heart level. At least two measurements should be made. Patients should be given their results and their goal BP.

Ambulatory BP monitoring is useful in evaluating "white coat hypertension" (no end-organ damage), drug resistance, hypotensive symptoms, episodic hypertension, and autonomic dysfunction. Ambulatory BP monitoring correlates better with end-organ damage than office measurements.

Having patients monitor their own BP helps to improve compliance and provides information on response to therapeutic interventions.

Based on these initial assessments, treatment strategies for patients with hypertension are stratified based on their blood pressure and comorbidities (compelling indications).

Management of Blood Pressure

	Management: Based upon highest BP category		
BP Classification	**Lifestyle Modification**	**Initial Therapy Without Compelling Indication**	**Initial Therapy With Compelling Indication[1]**
Normal	Encourage	None	None
Prehypertensive	Yes	None	Treat patients with chronic kidney disease or diabetes to BP goal of <130/80 mm Hg
Hypertension			
Stage 1	Yes	Thiazide-type diuretic for most; consider ACEI, ARB, β-blocker, CCB, or combination	Drugs for the compelling indications; other antihypertensives as needed
Stage 2	Yes	Two drug combos (typically a thiazide-type diuretic and ACEI or ARB or β-blocker or CCB). Use combo cautiously in patients at risk for orthostasis.	Drugs for the compelling indications; other antihypertensives as needed

[1]Compelling indication = conditions for which specific classes of antihypertensive drugs have proven beneficial

Adapted from Chobanian AV, Bakris GL, Black HR, et al, "The Seventh Report of the Joint National Committee on Prevention, Detection, Evaluation, and Treatment of High Blood Pressure: The JNC 7 Report," *JAMA*, 2003, 289(19):2560-71.

ACHIEVING BLOOD PRESSURE CONTROL

Treatment of hypertension should be individualized. Lower blood pressure (goal <130/80 mm Hg) should be achieved in patients with diabetes or chronic renal disease. Elderly patients aged 65-79 years should achieve a goal SBP ≤140 mmHg if tolerated for uncomplicated hypertension. For patients ≥80 years of age, a goal SBP of ≤140 mmHg should be achieved; if not tolerated, 140-145 mmHg is acceptable (Aronow, 2011). The following Hypertension Treatment Algorithm may be used to select specific antihypertensives based on compelling indications.

Special consideration for starting combination therapy should be made in each patient.

Starting drug therapy at a low dose and titrating upward if blood pressure is not controlled is recommended.

Most patients with hypertension will require two or more drugs to achieve their BP goals.

Adding a second drug from a different class will help when a single drug at reasonable doses has failed to achieve the goal.

If the untreated BP is >20/10 mm Hg away from the goal, consider initiating therapy with two drugs. Use caution in those at risk for orthostasis (eg, diabetics, geriatrics, and those with autonomic dysfunction).

Low-dose aspirin therapy should be considered when BP is controlled; use in uncontrolled hypertension can increase the risk of hemorrhagic stroke.

Lifestyle modification and risk reduction should always be reviewed and reinforced.

MONITORING THERAPY

Generally, monthly follow-up is recommended until BP control is reached.

More frequent monitoring is required for those patients with Stage 2 hypertension or those with complications.

Serum potassium and serum creatinine should be monitored at least twice yearly.

When BP is at goal and stable, follow-up can be maintained every 3-6 months. Treat other cardiovascular risk factors if present.

Hypertension Treatment Algorithm

Begin or continue lifestyle modifications

↓

Not at goal blood pressure (<140/90 mm Hg or <130/80 mm Hg for patients with diabetes or chronic renal disease)

↓

Initial Drug Choice

Hypertension

Stage I
Thiazide-type diuretic for most.
Consider ACEI, ARB, β-blocker, CCB, or combo.

Stage 2
Two-drug combo for most (typically thiazide-type diuretic + ACEI or ARB or β-blocker or CCB)

Compelling Indications

Chronic kidney disease
- ACEI
- ARB

Diabetes mellitus
- ACEI
- ARB
- β-blocker
- CCB
- Diuretic

Heart failure
- ACEI
- Aldosterone blocker
- ARB
- β-blocker
- Diuretic

High coronary risk
- ACEI
- β-blocker
- CCB
- Diuretic

Myocardial infarction
- ACEI
- Aldosterone blocker
- β-blocker

Recurrent stroke prevention
- ACEI
- Diuretic

↓

Not at goal blood pressure

↓ Optimize dosages or add additional drugs until goal BP achieved.

↓ Consider consultation with hypertension specialist.

Additional Considerations for Specific Therapies[1]

Indication	Drug Therapy
Atrial tachyarrhythmias	β-blocker, CCB (non-DHP)
Chronic kidney disease	
Cl_{cr} <60 mL/min or albuminuria	ACEI or ARB
Cl_{cr} <30 mL/min	Increase loop diuretic
Diabetes	Thiazide diuretic, β-blocker, ACEI, ARB, CCB
Nephropathy	ACEI, ARB
Essential tremor	β-blocker (noncardioselective)
Heart failure	
Ventricular dysfunction (asymptomatic)	ACEI, β-blocker
Ventricular dysfunction (symptomatic)	ACEI, β-blocker, ARB, aldosterone blocker, loop diuretic
Hypertensive women who are pregnant	Methyldopa, β-blocker, vasodilator
Ischemic heart disease	
Angina	β-blocker, CCB (long-acting)
Acute coronary syndromes	β-blocker, ACEI
Migraine	β-blocker (noncardioselective), CCB (long-acting, non-DHP)
Osteoporosis	Thiazide diuretic
Perioperative hypertension	β-blocker
Prostatism (BPH)	Alpha-adrenergic blocking agent
Raynaud syndrome	CCB
Thyrotoxicosis	β-blocker

ACEI = angiotensin-converting enzyme inhibitor, ARB = angiotensin receptor blocker, CCB = calcium channel blocker, DHP = dihydropyridine

[1]For additional considerations and specific therapies for hypertension in the elderly, see ACCF/AHA 2011 Expert Consensus Document on Hypertension in the Elderly (Aronow, 2011).

May Have Unfavorable Effects on Comorbid Conditions

Condition	Drug Therapy to Avoid
Angioedema	ACEI
Bronchospastic disease	β-blocker
Gout	Thiazide diuretic
Heart block (second or third degree)	β-blocker, CCB (non-DHP)
Hyponatremia	Thiazide diuretic
Potassium >5 mEq/L before treatment	Potassium sparing diuretic, aldosterone antagonist
Pregnancy or those likely to become pregnant	ACEI, ARB

ACEI = angiotensin-converting enzyme inhibitor, ARB = angiotensin receptor blocker, CCB = calcium channel blocker, DHP = dihydropyridine

HYPERTENSIVE EMERGENCIES AND URGENCIES

General Treatment Principles in the Treatment of Hypertensive Emergencies

Principle	Considerations
Admit the patient to the hospital, preferably in the ICU. Monitor vital signs appropriately.	Establish I.V. access and place patient on a cardiac monitor. Place a femoral intra-arterial line and pulmonary arterial catheter, if indicated, to assess cardiopulmonary function and intravascular volume status.
Perform rapid but thorough history and physical examination.	Determine cause of, or precipitating factors to, hypertensive crisis if possible (remember to obtain a medication history including Rx, OTC, and illicit drugs). Obtain details regarding any prior history of hypertension (severity, duration, treatment), as well as other coexisting illnesses. Assess the extent of hypertensive end organ damage. Determine if a hypertensive urgency or emergency exists.
Determine goal blood pressure based on premorbid level, duration, severity and rapidity of increase of blood pressure, concomitant medical conditions, race, and age.	Acute decreases in blood pressure to normal or subnormal levels during the initial treatment period may reduce perfusion to the brain, heart, and kidneys, and must be avoided except in specific instances (ie, dissecting aortic aneurysm). Gradually establish a normal (or reasonable) blood pressure over the next 1-2 weeks.
Select an appropriate antihypertensive regimen depending on the individual patient and clinical setting.	Initiate a controlled decrease in blood pressure. Avoid concomitant administration of multiple agents that may cause precipitous falls in blood pressure. Select the agent with the best hemodynamic profile based on the primary treatment goal. Avoid diuretics and sodium restriction during the initial treatment period unless there is a clear clinical indication (ie, CHF, pulmonary edema). Avoid sedating antihypertensives in patients with hypertensive encephalopathy, CVA, or other CNS disorders in whom mental status must be monitored. Use caution with direct vasodilating agents that induce reflex tachycardia or increase cardiac output in patients with coronary heart disease, history of angina or myocardial infarction, or dissecting aortic aneurysm. Preferably choose an agent that does not adversely affect glomerular filtration rate or renal blood flow and also agents that have favorable effects on cerebral blood flow and its autoregulation, especially for patients with hypertensive encephalopathy or CVAs. Select the most efficacious agent with the fewest adverse effects based on the underlying cause of the hypertensive crisis and other individual patient factors.
Initiate a chronic antihypertensive regimen after the patient's blood pressure is stabilized	Begin oral antihypertensive therapy once goal blood pressure is achieved before gradually tapering parenteral medications. Select the best oral regimen based on cost, ease of administration, adverse effect profile, and concomitant medical conditions.

Oral Agents Used in the Treatment of Hypertensive Urgencies

Drug	Dose	Onset	Cautions
Captopril[1]	P.O.: 25 mg, repeat as required	15-30 min	Hypotension, renal failure in bilateral renal artery stenosis
CloNIDine[1]	P.O.: 0.1-0.2 mg, repeated every hour as needed to a total dose of 0.6 mg	30-60 min	Hypotension, drowsiness, dry mouth
Labetalol	P.O.: 200-400 mg, repeat every 2-3 h	30 min to 2 h	Bronchoconstriction, heart block, orthostatic hypotension

[1]There is no clearly defined clinical advantage in the use of sublingual over oral routes of administration with these agents.

Recommendations for the Use of Intravenous Antihypertensive Drugs in Selected Hypertensive Emergencies

Condition	Agent(s) of Choice	Agent(s) to Avoid or Use With Caution	General Treatment Principles
Hypertensive encephalopathy	Nitroprusside, labetalol	Methyldopa, reserpine	Avoid drugs with CNS-sedating effects.
Acute intracranial or subarachnoid hemorrhage	NiCARdipine,[1] nitroprusside	β-blocker	Careful titration with a short-acting agent.
Cerebral infarction	NiCARdipine,[1] nitroprusside, labetalol	β-blocker, minoxidil	Careful titration with a short-acting agent. Avoid agents that may decrease cerebral blood flow.
Head trauma	Esmolol, labetalol	Methyldopa, reserpine, nitroprusside, nitroglycerin, hydrALAZINE	Avoid drugs with CNS-sedating effects, or those that may increase intracranial pressure.
Acute myocardial infarction, myocardial ischemia	Nitroglycerin, niCARdipine[1] (calcium channel blocker), labetalol	HydrALAZINE, minoxidil	Avoid drugs which cause reflex tachycardia and increased myocardial oxygen consumption.
Acute pulmonary edema	Nitroprusside, nitroglycerin, loop diuretics	β-blocker (labetalol), minoxidil, methyldopa	Avoid drugs which may cause sodium and water retention and edema exacerbation.
Renal dysfunction	HydrALAZINE, calcium channel blocker	Nitroprusside, ACE inhibitors, β-blocker (labetalol)	Avoid drugs with increased toxicity in renal failure and those that may cause decreased renal blood flow.
Eclampsia	HydrALAZINE, labetalol, nitroprusside[2]	Diuretics	Avoid drugs that may cause adverse fetal effects, compromise placental circulation, or decrease cardiac output.
Pheochromocytoma	Phentolamine, nitroprusside, β-blocker (eg, esmolol) only after alpha blockade (phentolamine)	β-blocker in the absence of alpha blockade, methyldopa, minoxidil	Use drugs of proven efficacy and specificity. Unopposed beta-blockade may exacerbate hypertension.
Dissecting aortic aneurysm	Nitroprusside and beta-blockade	HydrALAZINE, minoxidil	Avoid drugs which may increase cardiac output.
Postoperative hypertension	Nitroprusside, niCARdipine,[1] labetalol, clevidipine		Avoid drugs which may exacerbate postoperative ileus.

[1]The use of niCARdipine in these situations is by the recommendation of the author based on a review of the literature.

[2]Reserve nitroprusside for eclamptic patients with life-threatening hypertension unresponsive to other agents due to the potential risk to the fetus (cyanide and thiocyanate metabolites may cross the placenta)

Selected Intravenous Agents for Hypertensive Emergencies

Drug	Dose	Onset of Action	Duration of Action	Adverse Effects[1]	Special Indications
Vasodilators					
Sodium nitroprusside	0.25-10 mcg/kg/min as I.V. infusion[2] (max: 10 min only)	Immediate	1-2 min	Nausea, vomiting, muscle twitching, sweating, thiocyanate and cyanide intoxication	Most hypertensive emergencies; caution with high intracranial pressure or azotemia
NiCARdipine hydrochloride	5-15 mg/h I.V.	5-10 min	1-4 h	Tachycardia, headache, flushing, local phlebitis	Most hypertensive emergencies except acute heart failure; caution with coronary ischemia
Clevidipine butyrate	1-21 mg/h I.V.	2-4 min	5-15 min	Atrial fibrillation, nausea, insomnia, fever	Most hypertensive emergencies; caution with lipid disorder
Fenoldopam mesylate	0.1-0.3 mcg/kg/min as I.V. infusion	<5 min	30 min	Tachycardia, headache, nausea, flushing	Most hypertensive emergencies; caution with glaucoma
Nitroglycerin	5-400 mcg/min as I.V. infusion	2-5 min	3-5 min	Headache, vomiting, methemoglobinemia, tolerance with prolonged use	Coronary ischemia
Enalaprilat	1.25-5 mg every 6 hours I.V.	15-30 min	6 h	Precipitous fall in pressure in high-renin states; response variable	Acute left ventricular failure; avoid in acute myocardial infarction
HydrALAZINE hydrochloride	10-20 mg I.V. 10-50 mg I.M.	10-20 min 20-30 min	3-8 h	Tachycardia, flushing, headache, vomiting, aggravation of angina	Eclampsia
Adrenergic Inhibitors					
Labetalol hydrochloride	20-80 mg I.V. bolus every 10 min; 0.5-2 mg/min as I.V. infusion	5-10 min	3-6 h	Vomiting, scalp tingling, burning in throat, dizziness, nausea, heart block, orthostatic hypotension	Most hypertensive emergencies except acute heart failure
Esmolol hydrochloride	250-500 mcg/kg/min for 1 min, then 50-100 mcg/kg/min for 4 min; may repeat; infusion range: 50-300 mcg/kg/min	1-2 min	10-20 min	Hypotension, nausea	Aortic dissection, perioperative
Phentolamine	5-15 mg I.V.	1-2 min	3-10 min	Tachycardia, flushing, headache	Catecholamine excess

[1]Hypotension may occur with all agents.

[2]Require special delivery system

REFERENCES

Guidelines

"1999 World Health Organization-International Society of Hypertension Guidelines for the Management of Hypertension. Guidelines Subcommittee," *J Hypertens*, 1999, 17(2):151-83.

Aronow WS, Fleg JL, Pepine CJ, et al, "ACCF/AHA 2011 Expert Consensus Document on Hypertension in the Elderly: A Report of the American College of Cardiology Foundation Task Force on Clinical Expert Consensus Documents," *Circulation*, 2011.

Chobanian AV, Bakris GL, Black HR, et al, "The Seventh Report of the Joint National Committee on Prevention, Detection, Evaluation, and Treatment of High Blood Pressure: The JNC 7 Report," *JAMA*, 2003, 289(19):2560-72.

National High Blood Pressure Education Program Working Group on Hypertension Control in Children and Adolescents, "Update on the 1987 Task Force Report on High Blood Pressure in Children and Adolescents: A Working Group Report From the National High Blood Pressure Education Program," *Pediatrics*, 1996, 98(4 Pt 1):649-58.

National High Blood Pressure Education Program Working Group, "1995 Update of the Working Group Reports on Chronic Renal Failure and Renovascular Hypertension," *Arch Intern Med*, 1996, 156(17):1938-47.

"The Sixth Report of the National Committee on Detection, Evaluation, and Treatment of High Blood Pressure (JNC-VI)," *Arch Intern Med*, 1997, 157 (21):2413-46.

Others

Appel LJ, Moore TJ, Obarzanek E, et al, "A Clinical Trial of the Effect of Dietary Patterns on Blood Pressure. The DASH Collaborative Research Group," *N Engl J Med*, 1997, 336(16):1117-24.

Epstein M and Bakris G, "Newer Approaches to Antihypertensive Therapy: Use of Fixed-Dose Combination Therapy," *Arch Intern Med*, 1996, 156 (17):1969-78.

Estacio RO and Schrier RW, "Antihypertensive Therapy in Type II Diabetes: Implications of the Appropriate Blood Pressure Control in Diabetes (ABCD) Trial," *Am J Cardiol*, 1998, 82(9B):9R-14R.

Flack JM, Neaton J, Grimm RJ, et al, "Blood Pressure and Mortality Among Men With Prior Myocardial Infarction. The Multiple Risk Factor Intervention Trial Research Group," *Circulation*, 1995, 92(9):2437-45.

Frishman WH, Bryzinski BS, Coulson LR, et al, "A Multifactorial Trial Design to Assess Combination Therapy in Hypertension: Treatment With Bisoprolol and Hydrochlorothiazide," *Arch Intern Med*, 1994, 154(13):1461-8.

Furberg CD, Psaty BM, and Meyer JV, "Nifedipine: Dose-Related Increase in Mortality in Patients With Coronary Heart Disease," *Circulation*, 1995, 92 (5):1326-31.

Glynn RJ, Brock DB, Harris T, et al, "Use of Antihypertensive Drugs and Trends in Blood Pressure in the Elderly," *Arch Intern Med*, 1995, 155:1855-60.

Gradman AH, Cutler NR, Davis PJ, et al, "Combined Enalapril and Felodipine Extended Release (ER) for Systemic Hypertension. The Enalapril-Felodipine ER Factorial Study Group," *Am J Cardiol*, 1997, 79(4):431-5.

Grimm RH Jr, Flack JM, Grandits GA, et al, "Long-Term Effects on Plasma Lipids of Diet and Drugs to Treat Hypertension. The Treatment of Mild Hypertension Study (TOMHS) Research Group," *JAMA*, 1996, 275(20):1549-56.

Grimm RH Jr, Grandits GA, Cutler JA, et al, "Relationships of Quality-of-Life Measures to Long-Term Lifestyle and Drug Treatment in the Treatment of Mild Hypertension Study. The TOMHS Research Group," *Arch Intern Med*, 1997, 157(6):638-48.

Grossman E, Messerli FH, Grodzicki T, et al, "Should a Moratorium Be Placed on Sublingual Nifedipine Capsules Given for Hypertensive Emergencies and Pseudoemergencies?" *JAMA*, 1996, 276(16):1328-31.

Hansson L, Zanchetti A, Carruthers SG, et al, "Effects of Intensive Blood Pressure Lowering and Low-Dose Aspirin in Patients With Hypertension: Principal Results of the Hypertension Optimal Treatment (HOT) Randomized Trial. HOT Study Group," *Lancet*, 1998, 351(9118):1755-62.

Kaplan NM and Gifford RW Jr, "Choice of Initial Therapy for Hypertension," *JAMA*, 1996, 275(20):1577-80.

Kasiske BL, Ma JZ, Kalil RSN, et al, "Effects of Antihypertensive Therapy in Serum Lipids," *Ann Intern Med*, 1995, 122(2):133-41.

Kostis JB, Davis BR, Cutler J, et al, "Prevention of Heart Failure by Antihypertensive Drug Treatment in Older Persons With Isolated Systolic Hypertension. SHEP Cooperative Research Group," *JAMA*, 1997, 278(3):212-6.

Lazarus JM, Bourgoignie JJ, Buckalew VM, et al, "Achievement and Safety of a Low Blood Pressure Goal in Chronic Renal Disease: The Modification of Diet in Renal Disease Study Group," *Hypertension*, 1997, 29(2):641-50.

Lindheimer MD, "Hypertension in Pregnancy," *Hypertension*, 1993, 22(1):127-37.

Materson BJ, Reda DJ, Cushman WC, et al, "Single-Drug Therapy for Hypertension in Men: A Comparison of Six Antihypertensive Agents With Placebo. The Department of Veterans Affairs Cooperative Study Group on Antihypertensive Agents," *N Engl J Med*, 1993, 328(13):914-21.

Miller NH, Hill M, Kottke T, et al, "The Multi-Level Compliance Challenge: Recommendations for a Call to Action; A Statement for Healthcare Professionals," *Circulation*, 1997, 95(4):1085-90.

Neaton JD and Wentworth D, "Serum Cholesterol, Blood Pressure, Cigarette Smoking, and Death From Coronary Heart Disease: Overall Findings and Differences by Age for 316,099 White Men. The Multiple Risk Factor Intervention Trial Research Group," *Arch Intern Med*, 1992, 152(1):56-64.

Neaton JD, Grim RH, Prineas RJ, et al, "Treatment of Mild Hypertension Study. Final Results. Treatment of Mild Hypertension Study Research Group," *JAMA*, 1993, 270(6):713-24.

Oparil S, Levine JH, Zuschke CA, et al, "Effects of Candesartan Cilexetil in Patients With Severe Systemic Hypertension," *Am J Cardiol*, 1999, 84 (3):289-93.

Peacock WF, Varon J, Garrison N, et al, "I.V. Clevidipine for Hypertension: Safety, Efficacy, and Transition to Oral Therapy," *Ann Emerg Med*, 2007, 50(3 Suppl):S8-9.

Perloff D, Grim C, Flack J, et al, "Human Blood Pressure Determination by Sphygmomanometry," *Circulation*, 1993, 88(5 Pt 1):2460-7.

Perry HM Jr, Bingham S, Horney A, et al, "Antihypertensive Efficacy of Treatment Regimens Used in Veterans Administration Hypertension Clinics. Department of Veterans Affairs Cooperative Study Group on Antihypertensive Agents," *Hypertension*, 1998, 31(3):771-9.

Preston RA, Materson BJ, Reda DJ, et al, "Age-Race Subgroup Compared With Renin Profile as Predictors of Blood Pressure Response to Antihypertensive Therapy," *JAMA*, 1998, 280(13):1168-72.

Psaty BM, Smith NL, Siscovick DS, et al, "Health Outcomes Associated With Antihypertensive Therapies Used as First-Line Agents. A Systemic Review and Meta-analysis," *JAMA*, 1997, 277(9):739-45.

Radevski IV, Valtchanova SP, Candy GP, et al, "Comparison of Acebutolol With and Without Hydrochlorothiazide Versus Carvedilol With and Without Hydrochlorothiazide in Black Patients With Mild to Moderate Systemic Hypertension," *Am J Cardiol*, 1999, 84(1):70-5.

Setaro JF and Black HR, "Refractory Hypertension," *N Engl J Med*, 1992, 327(8):543-7.

SHEP Cooperative Research Group, "Prevention of Stroke by Antihypertensive Drug Treatment in Older Persons With Isolated Systolic Hypertension: Final Results of the Systolic Hypertension in the Elderly Program (SHEP)," *JAMA*, 1991, 265(24):3255-64.

Sibai BM, "Treatment of Hypertension in Pregnant Women," *N Engl J Med*, 1996, 335(4):257-65.

Singla N, Warltier DC, Gandhi SD, et al, "Treatment of Acute Postoperative Hypertension in Cardiac Surgery Patients: An Efficacy Study of Clevidipine Assessing Its Postoperative Antihypertensive Effect in Cardiac Surgery-2 (ESCAPE-2), a Randomized, Double-Blind, Placebo-Controlled Trial," *Anesth Analg*, 2008, 107(1):59-67.

Sowers JR, "Comorbidity of Hypertension and Diabetes: The Fosinopril Versus Amlodipine Cardiovascular Events Trial," *Am J Cardiol*, 1998, 82 (9B):15R-19R.

Sternberg H, Rosenthal T, Shamiss A, et al, "Altered Circadian Rhythm of Blood Pressure in Shift Workers," *J Hum Hypertens*, 1995, 9(5):349-53.

"The Hypertension Prevention Trial: Three-Year Effects of Dietary Changes on Blood Pressure. Hypertension Prevention Trial Research Group," *Arch Intern Med*, 1990, 150(1):153-62.

Trials of Hypertension Prevention Collaborative Research Group, "Effects of Weight Loss and Sodium Reduction Intervention on Blood Pressure and Hypertension Incidence in Overweight People With High-Normal Blood Pressure: The Trials of Hypertension Prevention, Phase II," *Arch Intern Med*, 1997, 157(6):657-67.

Tuomilehto J, Rastenyte D, Birkenhager WH, et al, "Effects of Calcium Channel Blockade in Older Patients With Diabetes and Systolic Hypertension," *N Engl J Med*, 1999, 340(9):677-84.

Veelken R and Schmieder RE, "Overview of Alpha-1 Adrenoceptor Antagonism and Recent Advances in Hypertensive Therapy," *Am J Hypertens*, 1996, 9(11):139S-49S.

White WB, Black HR, Weber MA, et al, "Comparison of Effects of Controlled Onset Extended Release Verapamil at Bedtime and Nifedipine Gastrointestinal Therapeutic System on Arising on Early Morning Blood Pressure, Heart Rate, and the Heart Rate-Blood Pressure Product," *Am J Cardiol*, 1998, 81(4):424-31.

STATUS EPILEPTICUS

CONVULSIVE STATUS EPILEPTICUS

Treatment Guidelines

Convulsive status epilepticus is an emergency that is associated with high morbidity and mortality. Status epilepticus has been defined as a seizure that persists for a sufficient length of time or is repeated frequently enough that recovery between attacks does not occur (Meierkord, 2010). Seizures lasting >5 minutes are less likely to remit; therefore, if a seizure continues for >5 minutes, antiepileptic therapy is mandatory. The outcome largely depends on etiology, but prompt and appropriate pharmacological therapy can reduce morbidity and mortality. Etiology varies in children and adults and reflects the distribution of disease in these age groups. Immediate concerns include supporting respiration, maintaining blood pressure, gaining intravenous access, and identifying and treating the underlying cause. Initial therapeutic and diagnostic measures are conducted simultaneously. The goal of therapy is rapid termination of clinical and electrical seizure activity; the longer a seizure continues, the greater the likelihood of an adverse outcome. Several drug protocols now in use will terminate status epilepticus. Common to all patients is the need for a clear plan, prompt administration of appropriate drugs in adequate doses, and attention to the possibility of apnea, hypoventilation, or other metabolic abnormalities.

Management of Status Epilepticus

Time Since Seizure Onset	Drug Treatment		Evaluations/Actions
	Adults	Children	
Prolonged Seizure: Premonitory Stage (Out-of-Hospital)			
5 min	Diazepam 10 mg rectally; may repeat once if necessary	Diazepam 0.5 mg/kg rectally; may repeat once if necessary	• Airway/breathing • Monitor vital signs • Establish I.V. access • Blood glucose determination
If seizure continues ↓ **Early Status Epilepticus: First Stage (Out-of-Hospital or Inpatient)**[1]			
5-30 min	LORazepam 4 mg I.V. bolus (≤2 mg/min) **or** Diazepam 5-10 mg I.V. (≤5 mg/min; maximum dose: 30 mg) May repeat dose after 5-10 minutes	LORazepam 0.05-0.1 mg/kg I.V. (≤2 mg/min; maximum dose: 4 mg) **or** Diazepam 0.1-0.3 mg/kg I.V. (≤5 mg/min; maximum dose: 10 mg) May repeat dose after 5-10 minutes	• ABGs, oxygen/ventilation • CBC, electrolytes, renal/hepatic status • Cardiac monitoring, ECG • Neurologic assessment toxicology screen • Consider I.V. dextrose ± thiamine • AED concentrations
If seizure continues ↓ **Established Status Epilepticus: Second Stage**			
30-60 min	Fosphenytoin 15-20 mg PE/kg I.V. (maximum rate: 150 mg PE/min) **or** Phenytoin 15-20 mg/kg I.V. (maximum rate: 50 mg/min)	Fosphenytoin 15-20 mg PE/kg I.V. (maximum rate: 150 mg PE/min) **or** Phenytoin 20 mg/kg I.V. (maximum rate: 50 mg/min) **or** PHENobarbital 15-20 mg/kg I.V. (maximum rate: <100 mg/min[2])	• Intubation/mechanical ventilation • Cardiorespiratory function • Vasopressors if needed • Neurologic: CT, CSF, EEG • If no central venous access, fosphenytoin is preferred over phenytoin
If seizure continues ↓ **Refractory Status Epilepticus: Third Stage**			
>60 min	PHENobarbital 10-20 mg/kg I.V. (maximum rate: 100 mg/min[2]) **or** PENTobarbital 10-15 mg/kg I.V. over 1 hour[2], then initial infusion of 0.5-1 mg/kg/h (range: 0.5-10 mg/kg/h **or** Midazolam 0.2 mg/kg, followed by a continuous infusion of 0.05-0.6 mg/kg/h **or** Propofol[3] 1-2 mg/kg I.V. bolus (optional), then continuous infusion of 2-10 mg/kg/h **or** Valproic acid 25-45 mg/kg I.V. (maximum rate: 6 mg/kg/min) **or** Levetiracetam[4] 1-3 g I.V. over 15 min	PHENobarbital 15-20 mg/kg I.V. (maximum rate: <100 mg/min[2]) **or** PENTobarbital 5-15 mg/kg I.V. over 1 hour[2], then 0.5-5 mg/kg/h **or** Midazolam 0.15-0.5 mg/kg bolus (may repeat), then continuous infusion of 0.06-2 mg/kg/h	• ICU admission • Anesthesia monitoring/hemodynamics • Therapeutic AED monitoring

AED = antiepileptic drug

[1]Lorazepam is associated with a higher likelihood of seizure termination in the treatment of status epilepticus and, therefore, may be preferred (Alldredge, 2001).
[2]May induce hypotension; consider alternative agents in hemodynamically unstable patients. Monitor closely and reduce rate if hypotension develops. Fluids and/or vasopressors may be necessary to control significant hypotension.
[3]Doses >83 mcg/kg/minute (or >5 mg/kg/**hour**) may increase the risk of hypotension and propofol-related infusion syndrome (PRIS), especially if used for >48 hours; consider alternative therapies to avoid the risk of PRIS in longer-term propofol infusions.
[4]Levetiracetam 2500 mg has been safely administered over 5 minutes, as reported in one report (Uges, 2009). **Note:** Levetiracetam has not been well-studied in comparison to other agents routinely used in this setting.

REFERENCES

Abend NS and Dlugos DJ, "Treatment of Refractory Status Epilepticus: Literature Review and a Proposed Protocol," *Pediatr Neurol*, 2008, 38(6):377-90.

Alldredge BK, Gelb AM, Isaacs SM, et al, "A Comparison of Lorazepam, Diazepam, and Placebo for the Treatment of Out-of-Hospital Status Epilepticus," *N Engl J Med*, 2001, 345(9):631-7.

Claassen J, Hirsch LJ, Emerson RG, et al, "Treatment of Refractory Status Epilepticus With Pentobarbital, Propofol, or Midazolam: A Systematic Review," *Epilepsia*, 2002, 43(2):146-53.

Hanhan UA, Fiallos MR, and Orlowski JP, "Status Epilepticus," *Pediatr Clin North Am*, 2001, 48(3):683-94.

Hegenbarth MA, "Preparing for Pediatric Emergencies: Drugs to Consider," *Pediatrics*, 2008, 121(2):433-43.

Kälviäinen R, Eriksson K, and Parviainen I, "Refractory Generalised Convulsive Status Epilepticus: A Guide to Treatment," *CNS Drugs*, 2005, 19 (9):759-68.

Kälviäinen R, "Status Epilepticus Treatment Guidelines," *Epilepsia*, 2007, 48(Suppl 8):99-102.

Lowenstein DH, "Treatment Options for Status Epilepticus," *Curr Opin Pharmacol*, 2005, 5(3):334-9.

Meierkord H, Boon P, Engelsen B, et al, "EFNS Guideline on the Management of Status Epilepticus," *Eur J Neurol*, 2010, 17(3):348-55.

Morrison G, Gibbons E, and Whitehouse WP, "High-Dose Midazolam Therapy for Refractory Status Epilepticus in Children," *Intensive Care Med*, 2006, 32(12):2070-6.

Rivera R, Segnini M, Baltodano A, et al, "Midazolam in the Treatment of Status Epilepticus in Children," *Crit Care Med*, 1993, 21(7):991-4.

Rossetti AO, Reichhart MD, Schaller MD, et al, "Propofol Treatment of Refractory Status Epilepticus: A Study of 31 Episodes," *Epilepsia*, 2004, 45 (7):757-63.

Uges JW, van Huizen MD, Engelsman J, et al, "Safety and Pharmacokinetics of Intravenous Levetiracetam Infusion as Add-on in Status Epilepticus," *Epilepsia*, 2009, 50(3):415-21.

DOSING CONSIDERATIONS FOR THE CRITICALLY-ILL PATIENT WITH MORBID OBESITY

Most recent estimates from the World Health Organization (WHO) report that approximately 32% of the U.S. population is considered obese, defined as a body mass index (BMI) of ≥30 kg/m^2. Patients with morbid obesity (Obese class III), defined by the WHO as a BMI ≥40 kg/m^2, are challenging to care for especially when critically ill. Although obese class II (BMI 35 to <40 kg/m^2) are commonly encountered, patients with morbid obesity require dosage adjustment to achieve similar therapeutic results. Patients at the extremes of body weight are seldom included within clinical trials, forcing the clinician to use knowledge of pharmacokinetic principles (eg, volume of distribution) to properly dose the morbidly obese patient. Many drugs (eg, vasopressors, inotropes, neuromuscular blockers) used in the ICU are adjusted based on immediate measurable patient responses; however, many drugs (eg, antibiotics, drotrecogin alfa, LMWHs) do not have this advantage and inadequate dosing may lead to treatment failure. In the critical situation, the need to give the right dose to achieve an optimal clinical response is paramount.

Table 1. The International Classification of Adult Overweight and Obesity According to BMI

Classification	BMI (kg/m^2)
Normal range	18.5-24.99
Overweight	≥25
Pre-obese	25-29.99
Obese	≥30
Obese class I	30-34.99
Obese class II	35-39.99
Obese class III	≥40

BMI = Body mass index; defined as weight in kilograms divided by height in meters squared

IMPORTANT PHARMACOKINETIC CONSIDERATIONS

Several pharmacokinetic parameters are altered in the morbidly obese patient due to increases in cardiac output, blood volume, organ mass, lean body mass, and adipose tissue mass. Three pharmacokinetic parameters affected by obesity are distribution, metabolism, and excretion.

DISTRIBUTION

Distribution is altered due to a higher ratio of body fat to lean tissue and body water. This becomes important for drugs with lipophilic properties (eg, fentanyl, diazepam). Generally, as the octanol/water *log* partition coefficient (LPC) of the drug increases, distribution into adipose tissue increases. Exceptions to this include cyclosporine, digoxin, procainamide, and remifentanil. These agents may be highly lipophilic and have a high volume of distribution (V_d) but they are not significantly influenced by obesity. Therefore, it is not always possible to devise straightforward dosing schemes using volume of distribution alone. Clinical trials in obese and normal weight patients are necessary to determine whether or not the expected distribution for a particular drug actually occurs in the obese patient.

METABOLISM

Data on the relationship between obesity (especially morbid obesity) and alterations in drug metabolism/transport are inconclusive; however, evidence supports alterations in cytochrome P450 enzyme activity in the obese patient. CYP2E1 activity is increased and CYP3A4 and CYP1A activity may be decreased or unchanged. The effect of obesity on other CYP450 enzymes remains unclear. In general, increased glucuronidation and sulfation activity may occur with some drugs (eg, lorazepam) requiring more frequent administration of maintenance doses. Determinants of drug disposition may be altered in obesity, but the specific direction and magnitude of any such change is, at present, unclear. Increased monitoring seems prudent.

EXCRETION

Glomerular filtration rate (GFR) may be higher in patients who are obese compared to normal weight patients. It has been demonstrated that obese (BMI ≥30 kg/m^2) kidney donors have a significantly higher glomerular planar surface area compared to those kidneys of nonobese donors. Drugs dependant on GFR for excretion (eg, aminoglycosides) have been shown to have higher clearance rates in the obese patient. Therefore, maintenance dosing may be more frequent for agents which rely on glomerular filtration for excretion.

Although the Cockcroft-Gault formula used to estimate creatinine clearance (Cl_{Cr}) is the predominant equation used in clinical practice, choice of weight will often underestimate (eg, IBW) or overestimate (eg, TBW) Cl_{Cr}. The most precise formula estimation of Cl_{Cr} in the obese patient is the Salazar-Corcoran formula; however, this formula has not been validated in a large sample of obese subjects. The Modification of Diet in Renal Disease (MDRD) formula, although it does not incorporate weight, also has not been validated in a large sample of obese subjects. Of note, the result obtained with the MDRD equation may not correlate with Cl_{Cr} cutoffs for dosage adjustment for many drugs since evaluation of renal function for these agents used the Cockcroft-Gault formula to develop dosing regimens in patients with renal impairment. Use of a timed 24-hour urine collection may be a more accurate method to determine Cl_{Cr}. Recently, the three equations used to determine glomerular filtration (GFR)/Cl_{Cr} were compared to results obtained using a timed 24-hour urine collection in morbidly obese patients. Use of the MDRD and IBW in the Cockcroft-Gault equation both underestimated Cl_{Cr}. The Salazar-Corcoran equation and the use of TBW or adjusted body weight (AdjBW) in the Cockcroft-Gault equation overestimated Cl_{Cr}. The authors concluded that the use of a lean body weight (LBW) estimate (see Table 2) based on TBW and BMI incorporated into the Cockcroft-Gault equation provides a relatively precise and accurate estimate of 24-hour measured Cl_{Cr} in morbidly obese patients.

DOSING MODIFICATIONS IN THE OBESE PATIENT

The importance of achieving similar concentrations in the critically ill obese patient as compared to the normal weight patient is imperative. However, dosing agents is not straightforward and requires pharmacokinetic evaluations in this patient population to define the optimal dose or dosing weight that should be used to determine an optimal dose for a particular agent. Many evaluations of this kind have been done but more clinical trials still need to be done. A summary of recommendations from various sources has been devised to assist the clinician in determining the most appropriate dosing weight or dosing strategy for this patient population (see Table 3). Equations for different body weight calculations are noted below.

Table 2. Body Weight Calculations

Ideal Body Weight (IBW)[1]	Male: 50 + (2.3 x height in inches over 5 feet) Female: 45.5 + (2.3 x height in inches over 5 feet)
Lean Body Weight (LBW)[1,2]	Male: (9270 x TBW)/(6680 + 216 x BMI) Female: (9270 x TBW)/(8780 + 244 x BMI)
Adjusted Body Weight (AdjBW) or Dosing Weight (DW)[1,3]	AdjBW or DW = IBW + 0.4 (TBW − IBW)

BMI = body mass index in kg/m^2, TBW = total body weight

[1]IBW, LBW, AdjBW, and DW are in kilograms

[2]Janmahasatian S, Duffull SB, Ash S, et al, "Quantification of Lean Bodyweight," *Clin Pharmacokinet*, 2005, 44(10):1051-65.

[3]The difference between TBW and IBW is multiplied by a factor between 0.2-0.5. The factor most often used is 0.4; however, this may be modified for certain drugs (eg, ciprofloxacin).

Table 3. Selected Agents and Recommended Dosing Strategies in the Obese Patient

Drug	Recommendation for Dosing in Obese Patients: Loading Dose	Recommendation for Dosing in Obese Patients: Maintenance Dose[1]
Analgesics		
FentaNYL	Use TBW	Use: 0.8 x IBW; titrate to pain control
Morphine	Use IBW	Use IBW; titrate to pain control
Remifentanil	Use IBW	Use IBW; titrate to pain control
SUFentanil	Use TBW	Use: 0.8 x IBW; titrate to pain control
Antiarrhythmics		
Amiodarone	Use IBW or standard dose	IBW or standard dose
Lidocaine	Use TBW	IBW, standard infusion rate
Procainamide	Use IBW	Use IBW, standard infusion rate
Antibiotics		
Acyclovir	NA	IBW
Aminoglycosides[2]	Use IBW + 0.4 (TBW − IBW)	Use IBW + 0.4 (TBW − IBW)
CeFAZolin	Surgical prophylaxis: 2 g prior to induction	Not established
Ciprofloxacin	NA	Use IBW + 0.45 (TBW − IBW) or 800 mg q12h
DAPTOmycin	NA	Use TBW; concentrations expected to be higher; monitor closely for skeletal muscle toxicity
Fluconazole	NA	Prudent to use higher doses; none established[3]
Flucytosine	NA	Use IBW
Linezolid	NA	Use standard dosing
Meropenem	NA	Use standard dosing[4]
Quinupristin / Dalfopristin	NA	Use TBW
Vancomycin	Use TBW	Use TBW; may require more frequent dosing
Anticoagulants		
Argatroban	NA	Use TBW (BMI <51 kg/m^2)
Enoxaparin (and other LMWHs)	Use TBW	Use TBW; monitor anti-Xa levels (if available) in patients >190 kg
Heparin	Not established	Not established; titrate to aPTT results

Table 3. Selected Agents and Recommended Dosing Strategies in the Obese Patient *(continued)*

Drug	Recommendation for Dosing in Obese Patients: Loading Dose	Recommendation for Dosing in Obese Patients: Maintenance Dose[1]
Antiepileptics		
Phenytoin	Use: DW = IBW + 1.33 x (TBW − IBW) or may give 14 mg/kg (IBW) + 19 mg/kg for weight in excess of IBW (maximum dose: 2 g)	Use IBW; monitor levels
Beta-Blockers		
Esmolol	Use IBW	Individualize
Labetalol	Use IBW or standard dose	Individualize
Metoprolol	Use IBW or standard dose	Individualize
Calcium Channel Blockers		
Diltiazem	Use TBW or standard dose	Individualize
Verapamil	Use TBW or standard dose	Individualize
Neuromuscular Blocking Agents[5]		
Atracurium	Use TBW	Use TBW
Rocuronium	Use IBW	Use IBW
Succinylcholine	Use TBW	NA
Vecuronium	Use IBW	Use IBW
Sedative/Hypnotic		
Etomidate	Use TBW	NA
Ketamine	Use IBW	Use IBW
Propofol	Use DW = IBW + 0.4 (TBW − IBW)	Use DW = IBW + 0.4 (TBW − IBW)
Thiopental	Use TBW	Use IBW
Other Agents		
Adenosine	Use IBW; standard dose	NA
Digoxin	Use IBW	Use IBW
Drotrecogin alfa	NA	Use TBW
Rasburicase	NA	Use IBW

BMI = body mass index, DW = dosing weight, IBW = ideal body weight, NA = not applicable, TBW = total body weight

[1]If therapeutic drug monitoring is available, it is recommended that this be done in all patients who are morbidly obese.

[2]Use once daily dosing regimens with caution in the morbidly obese patient as adequate studies have not been conducted in this patient population.

[3]It has been recommended that fluconazole be dosed using 6 mg/kg/day using TBW.

[4]May require higher doses for multi-drug resistant organisms

[5]Monitor clinical effects, peripheral nerve stimulation

REFERENCES

Arnold TM, Reuter JP, Delman BS, et al, "Use of Single-Dose Rasburicase in an Obese Female," *Ann Pharmacother*, 2004, 38(9):1428-31.

Bearden DT and Rodvold KA, "Dosage Adjustments for Antibacterials in Obese Patients: Applying Clinical Pharmacokinetics," *Clin Pharmacokinet*, 2000, 38(5):415-26.

Blouin RA, Bauer LA, Miller DD, et al, "Vancomycin Pharmacokinetics in Normal and Morbidly Obese Subjects," *Antimicrob Agents Chemother*, 1982, 21 (4):575-80.

Blouin RA and Ensom MHH, "Special Pharmacokinetic Considerations in the Obese," *Applied Pharmacokinetics & Pharmacodynamics*, 4th ed, Burton ME, Shaw LE, Schentag JJ, et al, eds, Baltimore, MD: Lippincott Williams & Wilkins, 2006, 231-241.

Brunette DD, "Resuscitation of the Morbidly Obese Patient," *Am J Emerg Med*, 2004, 22(1):40-7.

Cheymol G, "Effects of Obesity on Pharmacokinetics Implications for Drug Therapy," *Clin Pharmacokinet*, 2000, 39(3):215-31.

Demirovic JA, Pai AB, and Pai MP, "Estimation of Creatinine Clearance in Morbidly Obese Patients," *Am J Health Syst Pharm*, 2009, 66(7):642-8.

Dvorchik BH and Damphousse D, "The Pharmacokinetics of Daptomycin in Moderately Obese, Morbidly Obese, and Matched Nonobese Subjects," *J Clin Pharmacol*, 2005, 45(1):48-56.

Erstad BL, "Dosing of Medications in Morbidly Obese Patients in the Intensive Care Unit Setting," *Intensive Care Med*, 2004, 30(1):18-32.

Galletti F, Fasano ML, Ferrara LA, et al, "Obesity and Beta-Blockers: Influence of Body Fat on Their Kinetics and Cardiovascular Effects," *J Clin Pharmacol*, 1989, 29(3):212-6.

Hernandez JO, Norstrom J, and Wysock G, "Acyclovir-Induced Renal Failure in an Obese Patient," *Am J Health Syst Pharm*, 2009, 66(14):1288-91.

Kotlyar M and Carson SW, "Effects of Obesity on the Cytochrome P450 Enzyme System," *Int J Clin Pharmacol Ther*, 1999, 37(1):8-19.

Levy H, Small D, Heiselman DE, et al, "Obesity Does Not Alter the Pharmacokinetics of Drotrecogin Alfa (Activated) in Severe Sepsis," *Ann Pharmacother*, 2005, 39(2):262-7.

Leykin Y, Pellis T, Lucca M, et al, "The Pharmacodynamic Effects of Rocuronium When Dosed According to Real Body Weight or Ideal Body Weight in Morbidly Obese Patients," *Anesth Analg*, 2004, 99(4):1086-9.

Meyhoff CS, Lund J, Jenstrup MT, et al, "Should Dosing of Rocuronium in Obese Patients be Based on Ideal or Corrected Body Weight?" *Anesth Analg*, 2009, 109(3):787-92.

Nutescu EA, Spinler SA, Wittkowsky A, et al, "Low-Molecular-Weight Heparins in Renal Impairment and Obesity: Available Evidence and Clinical Practice Recommendations Across Medical and Surgical Settings," *Ann Pharmacother*, 2009, 43(6):1064-83.

Pai MP and Bearden DT, "Antimicrobial Ddosing Considerations in Obese Adult Patients," *Pharmacotherapy*, 2007, 27(8):1081-91.

Penzak SR, Gubbins PO, Rodvold KA, et al, "Therapeutic Drug Monitoring of Vancomycin in a Morbidly Obese Patient," *Ther Drug Monit*, 1998, 20 (3):261-5.

Rea DJ, Heimbach JK, Grande JP, et al, "Glomerular Volume and Renal Histology in Obese and Nonobese Living Kidney Donors," *Kidney Int*, 2006, 70 (9):1636-41.

Rex JH, Bennett JE, Sugar AM, et al, "A Randomized Trial Comparing Fluconazole With Amphotericin B for the Treatment of Candidemia in Patients Without Neutropenia. Candidemia Study Group and the National Institute," *N Engl J Med*, 1994, 331(20):1325-30.

Rice L, Hursting MJ, Baillie GM, et al, "Argatroban Anticoagulation in Obese Versus Nonobese Patients: Implications for Treating Heparin-Induced Thrombocytopenia," *J Clin Pharmacol*, 2007, 47(8):1028-34.

Roberts JA and Lipman J, "Pharmacokinetic Issues for Antibiotics in the Critically Ill Patient," *Crit Care Med*, 2009, 37(3):840-51.

Poirier P, Alpert MA, Fleisher LA, et al, "Cardiovascular Evaluation and Management of Severely Obese Patients Undergoing Surgery: A Science Advisory From the American Heart Association," *Circulation*, 2009, 120(1):86-95.

Salazar DE and Corcoran GB, "Predicting Creatinine Clearance and Renal Drug Clearance in Obese Patients From Estimated Fat-Free Body Mass," *Am J Med*, 1988, 84(6):1053-60.

Servin F, Farinotti R, Haberer JP, et al, "Propofol Infusion for Maintenance of Anesthesia in Morbidly Obese Patients Receiving Nitrous Oxide. A Clinical and Pharmacokinetic Study," *Anesthesiology*, 1993, 78(4):657-65.

Stein GE, Schooley SL, Peloquin CA, et al, "Pharmacokinetics and Pharmacodynamics of Linezolid in Obese Patients With Cellulitis," *Ann Pharmacother*, 2005, 39(3):427-32.

Vance-Bryan K, Guay DR, Gilliland SS, et al, "Effect of Obesity on Vancomycin Pharmacokinetic Parameters as Determined by Using a Bayesian Forecasting Technique," *Antimicrob Agents Chemother*, 1993, 37(3):436-40.

ORAL DOSAGES THAT SHOULD NOT BE CRUSHED

There are a variety of reasons for crushing tablets or capsule contents prior to administering to the patient. Patients may have nasogastric tubes which do not permit the administration of tablets or capsules; an oral solution for a particular medication may not be available from the manufacturer or readily prepared by pharmacy; patients may have difficulty swallowing capsules or tablets; or mixing of powdered medication with food or drink may make the drug more palatable.

Generally, medications which should not be crushed fall into one of the following categories.

- **Extended-Release Products**. The formulation of some tablets is specialized as to allow the medication within it to be slowly released into the body. This may be accomplished by centering the drug within the core of the tablet, with a subsequent shedding of multiple layers around the core. Wax melts in the GI tract releasing drug contained within the wax matrix (eg, OxyCONTIN®). Capsules may contain beads which have multiple layers which are slowly dissolved with time.

  Common Abbreviations for Extended-Release Products

CD	Controlled dose
CR	Controlled release
CRT	Controlled-release tablet
LA	Long-acting
SR	Sustained release
TR	Timed release
TD	Time delay
SA	Sustained action
XL	Extended release
XR	Extended release

- **Medications Which Are Irritating to the Stomach**. Tablets which are irritating to the stomach may be enteric-coated which delays release of the drug until the time when it reaches the small intestine. Enteric-coated aspirin is an example of this.
- **Foul-Tasting Medication**. Some drugs are quite unpleasant to taste so the manufacturer coats the tablet in a sugar coating to increase its palatability. By crushing the tablet, this sugar coating is lost and the patient tastes the unpleasant tasting medication.
- **Sublingual Medication**. Medication intended for use under the tongue should not be crushed. While it appears to be obvious, it is not always easy to determine if a medication is to be used sublingually. Sublingual medications should indicate on the package that they are intended for sublingual use.
- **Effervescent Tablets**. These are tablets which, when dropped into a liquid, quickly dissolve to yield a solution. Many effervescent tablets, when crushed, lose their ability to quickly dissolve.
- **Potentially hazardous substances**. Certain drugs including antineoplastic agents, hormonal agents, some antivirals, some bioengineered agents, and other miscellaneous drugs are considered potentially hazardous when used in humans based on their characteristics. Examples of these characteristics include carcinogenicity, teratogenicity, reproductive toxicity, organ toxicity at low doses, or genotoxicity. Exposure to these substances can result in adverse effects and should be avoided. Crushing or breaking a tablet or opening a capsule of a potentially hazardous substance may increase the risk of exposure to the substance through skin contact, inhalation, or accidental ingestion. The extent of exposure, potency, and toxicity of the hazardous substance determines the health risk. Institutions have policies and procedures to follow when handling any potentially hazardous substance. **Note:** All potentially hazardous substances may not be represented in this table. Refer to institution-specific guidelines for precautions to observe when handling hazardous substances.

RECOMMENDATIONS

1. It is not advisable to crush certain medications.
2. Consult individual monographs prior to crushing capsule or tablet.
3. If crushing a tablet or capsule is contraindicated, consult with your pharmacist to determine whether an oral solution exists or can be compounded.

Drug Product	Dosage Form	Dosage Reasons/Comments
Accutane®	Capsule	Mucous membrane irritant; teratogenic potential
Aciphex®	Tablet	Slow release
Actiq®	Lozenge	Slow release. This lollipop delivery system requires the patient to dissolve it slowly.
Actoplus Met® XR	Tablet	Slow release
Actonel®	Tablet	Irritant. Chewed, crushed, or sucked tablets may cause oropharyngeal irritation.
Adalat® CC	Tablet	Slow release
Adderall XR®	Capsule	Slow release[1]
Adenovirus (Types 4, 7) Vaccine	Tablet	Teratogenic potential; enteric-coated; do not disrupt tablet to avoid releasing live adenovirus in upper respiratory tract
Advicor®	Tablet	Slow release
AeroHist Plus™	Tablet	Slow release[8]
Afeditab® CR	Tablet	Slow release
Afinitor®	Tablet	Mucous membrane irritant; teratogenic potential; potentially hazardous substance[10]
Aggrenox®	Capsule	Slow release. Capsule may be opened; contents include an aspirin tablet that may be chewed and dipyridamole pellets that may be sprinkled on applesauce.
Alavert™ Allergy Sinus 12 Hour	Tablet	Slow release
Allegra-D®	Tablet	Slow release
Alophen®	Tablet	Enteric-coated
ALPRAZolam ER	Tablet	Slow release
Altoprev®	Tablet	Slow release
Ambien CR®	Tablet	Slow release
Amitiza®	Capsule	Slow release
Amnesteem®	Capsule	Mucous membrane irritant; teratogenic potential
Ampyra™	Tablet	Slow release
Amrix®	Capsule	Slow release
Aplenzin™	Tablet	Slow release
Apriso™	Capsule	Slow release[1]
Aptivus®	Capsule	Taste. Oil emulsion within spheres
Aricept® 23 mg	Tablet	Film-coated; chewing or crushing may increase rate of absorption
Arava®	Tablet	Teratogenic potential; hazardous substance[10]
Arthrotec®	Tablet	Enteric-coated
Asacol®	Tablet	Slow release
Ascriptin® A/D	Tablet	Enteric-coated
Atelvia™	Tablet	Slow release; tablet coating is an important part of the delayed release
Augmentin XR®	Tablet	Slow release[2, 8]
AVINza™	Capsule	Slow release[1] (applesauce)
Avodart®	Capsule	Capsule should not be handled by pregnant women due to teratogenic potential[9]; hazardous substance[10]
Azulfidine® EN-tabs®	Tablet	Enteric-coated
Bayer® Aspirin EC	Caplet	Enteric-coated
Bayer® Aspirin, Low Adult 81 mg	Tablet	Enteric-coated
Bayer® Aspirin, Regular Strength 325 mg	Caplet	Enteric-coated
Biaxin® XL	Tablet	Slow release
Biltricide®	Tablet	Taste[8]

(continued)

Drug Product	Dosage Form	Dosage Reasons/Comments
Biohist LA	Tablet	Slow release[8]
Bisa-Lax	Tablet	Enteric-coacted[3]
Bisac-Evac™	Tablet	Enteric-coated[3]
Bisacodyl	Tablet	Enteric-coated[3]
Boniva®	Tablet	Irritant. Chewed, crushed, or sucked tablets may cause oropharyngeal irritation.
Bontril® Slow-Release	Capsule	Slow release
Bromfed®	Capsule	Slow release
Bromfed®-PD	Capsule	Slow release
Budeprion SR®, Budeprion XL®	Tablet	Slow release
Buproban®	Tablet	Slow release
BuPROPion SR	Tablet	Slow release
Campral®	Tablet	Enteric-coated; slow release
Calan® SR	Tablet	Slow release[8]
Caprelsa®	Tablet	Teratogenic potential; hazardous substance[10]
Carbatrol®	Capsule	Slow release[1]
Cardene® SR	Capsule	Slow release
Cardizem®	Tablet	Not described as slow release but releases drug over 3 hours.
Cardizem® CD	Capsule	Slow release
Cardizem® LA	Tablet	Slow release
Cardura® XL	Tablet	Slow release
Cartia® XT	Capsule	Slow release
Casodex®	Tablet	Teratogenic potential; hazardous substance[10]
CeeNU®	Capsule	Teratogenic potential; hazardous substance[10]
Cefaclor extended release	Tablet	Slow release
Ceftin®	Tablet	Taste[2]. Use suspension for children.
Cefuroxime	Tablet	Taste[2]. Use suspension for children.
CellCept®	Capsule, tablet	Teratogenic potential; hazardous substance[10]
Charcoal Plus®	Tablet	Enteric-coated
Chlor-Trimeton® 12-Hour	Tablet	Slow release[2]
Cipro® XR	Tablet	Slow release
Claravis™	Capsule	Mucous membrane irritant; teratogenic potential
Claritin-D® 12-Hour	Tablet	Slow release
Claritin-D® 24-Hour	Tablet	Slow release
Colace®	Capsule	Taste[5]
Colestid®	Tablet	Slow release
Commit®	Lozenge	Integrity compromised by chewing or crushing.
Concerta®	Tablet	Slow release
ConZip™	Capsule	Extended release; tablet disruption may cause overdose
Coreg CR®	Capsule	Slow release[1]
Cotazym-S®	Capsule	Enteric-coated[1]
Covera-HS®	Tablet	Slow release
Creon®	Capsule	Slow release[1]
Crixivan®	Capsule	Taste. Capsule may be opened and mixed with fruit puree (eg, banana).
Cymbalta®	Capsule	Enteric-coated
Cytoxan®	Tablet	Drug may be crushed, but manufacturer recommends using injection; hazardous substance[10]
Depakene®	Capsule	Slow release; mucous membrane irritant[2]

(continued)

Drug Product	Dosage Form	Dosage Reasons/Comments
Depakote®	Tablet	Slow release
Depakote® ER	Tablet	Slow release
Detrol® LA	Capsule	Slow release
Dexedrine® Spansule®	Capsule	Slow release
Dexilant™	Capsule	Slow release[1]
Diamox® Sequels®	Capsule	Slow release
Dilacor® XR	Capsule	Slow release
Dilatrate-SR®	Capsule	Slow release
Dilt-CD	Capsule	Slow release
Dilt-XR	Capsule	Slow release
Diltia XT®	Capsule	Slow release
Ditropan® XL	Tablet	Slow release
Divalproex ER	Tablet	Slow release
Donnatal® Extentab®	Tablet	Slow release[2]
Doxidan®	Tablet	Enteric-coated[3]
Drisdol®	Capsule	Liquid filled[4]
Drixoral®	Tablet	Slow release
Droxia®	Capsule	May be opened; wear gloves to handle; hazardous substance[10]
Drysec	Tablet	Slow release[8]
Dulcolax®	Capsule	Liquid-filled
Dulcolax®	Tablet	Enteric-coated[3]
DynaCirc® CR	Tablet	Slow release
Easprin®	Tablet	Enteric-coated
EC-Naprosyn®	Tablet	Enteric-coated
Ecotrin® Adult Low Strength	Tablet	Enteric-coated
Ecotrin® Maximum Strength	Tablet	Enteric-coated
Ecotrin® Regular Strength	Tablet	Enteric-coated
Ed A-Hist™	Tablet	Slow release[2]
E.E.S.® 400	Tablet	Enteric-coated[2]
Effer-K™	Tablet	Effervescent tablet[6]
Effervescent Potassium	Tablet	Effervescent tablet[6]
Effexor® XR	Capsule	Slow release
Embeda™	Capsule	Slow release; can open capsule and sprinkle on applesauce; do not give via NG tube
E-Mycin®	Tablet	Enteric-coated
Enablex®	Tablet	Slow release
Entocort® EC	Capsule	Enteric-coated[1]
Equetro®	Capsule	Slow release[1]
Ergomar®	Tablet	Sublingual form[7]
Ery-Tab®	Tablet	Enteric-coated
Erythromycin Stearate	Tablet	Enteric-coated
Erythromycin Base	Tablet	Enteric-coated
Erythromycin Delayed-Release	Capsule	Enteric-coated pellets[1]
Etoposide	Capsule	Hazardous substance[10]
Evista®	Tablet	Taste; teratogenic potential; hazardous substance[10]
Exalgo™	Tablet	Slow release; breaking, chewing, crushing, or dissolving before ingestion increases the risk of overdose
ExeFen-PD	Tablet	Slow release[8]
Fareston®	Tablet	Teratogenic potential; hazardous substance[10]

(continued)

Drug Product	Dosage Form	Dosage Reasons/Comments
Feen-A-Mint®	Tablet	Enteric-coated[3]
Feldene®	Capsule	Mucous membrane irritant
Fentora®	Tablet	Buccal tablet
Feosol®	Tablet	Enteric-coated[2]
Feratab®	Tablet	Enteric-coated[2]
Fergon®	Tablet	Enteric-coated
Fero-Grad 500®	Tablet	Slow release
Ferro-Sequels®	Tablet	Slow release
Flagyl ER®	Tablet	Slow release
Flomax®	Capsule	Slow release
Focalin® XR	Capsule	Slow release[1]
Fosamax®	Tablet	Mucous membrane irritant
Fosamax Plus D™	Tablet	Mucous membrane irritant
Gengraf®	Capsule	Teratogenic potential; hazardous substance[10]
Gleevec®	Tablet	Taste[8]. May be dissolved in water or apple juice; hazardous substance[10]
GlipiZIDE ER	Tablet	Slow release
Glucophage® XR	Tablet	Slow release
Glucotrol® XL	Tablet	Slow release
Glumetza™	Tablet	Slow release
Gralise™	Tablet	Slow release
Guaifenex® GP	Tablet	Slow release[8]
Guaifenex® PSE	Tablet	Slow release[8]
Guaimax-D®	Tablet	Slow release[8]
Halfprin®	Tablet	Enteric coated
Hexalen®	Capsule	Teratogenic potential; hazardous substance[10]
Horizant™	Tablet	Slow release
Hycamtin®	Capsule	Teratogenic potential; hazardous substance[10]
Hydrea®	Capsule	Can be opened and mixed with water; wear gloves to handle; hazardous substance[10]
Imdur®	Tablet	Slow release[8]
Inderal® LA	Capsule	Slow release
Indocin® SR	Capsule	Slow release[1,2]
InnoPran XL®	Capsule	Slow release
Intelence™	Tablet	Tablet should be swallowed whole and not crushed; tablet may be dispersed in water
Intuniv™	Tablet	Slow release
Invega®	Tablet	Slow release
Ionamin®	Capsule	Slow release
Isochron™	Tablet	Slow release
Isoptin® SR	Tablet	Slow release[8]
Isordil® Sublingual	Tablet	Sublingual form[7]
Isosorbide Dinitrate Sublingual	Tablet	Sublingual form[7]
Isosorbide SR	Tablet	Slow release
Jalyn®	Capsule	Capsule should not be handled by pregnant women due to teratogenic potential[9]; hazardous substance[10]
Kadian®	Capsule	Slow release[1]. Do not give via NG tubes.
Kaletra®	Tablet	Film coated
Kaon-Cl®	Tablet	Slow release[2]
Kapidex™	Capsule	Slow release[1]
Kapvay™	Tablet	Slow release

(continued)

Drug Product	Dosage Form	Dosage Reasons/Comments
K-Dur®	Tablet	Slow release
Keppra®	Tablet	Taste[2]
Keppra® XR	Tablet	Slow release
Ketek®	Tablet	Slow release
Klor-Con®	Tablet	Slow release[2]
Klor-Con® M	Tablet	Slow release[2]; some strengths are scored
Klotrix®	Tablet	Slow release[2]
K-Lyte®	Tablet	Effervescent tablet[6]
K-Lyte/Cl®	Tablet	Effervescent tablet[6]
K-Lyte DS®	Tablet	Effervescent tablet[6]
Kombiglyze™ XR	Tablet	Slow release; tablet matrix may remain in stool
K-Tab®	Tablet	Slow release[2]
LaMICtal® XR™	Tablet	Slow release
Lescol® XL	Tablet	Slow release
Letairis®	Tablet	Film coated
Leukeran®	Tablet	Teratogenic potential; hazardous substance[10]
Levbid®	Tablet	Slow release[8]
Levsinex® Timecaps®	Capsule	Slow release
Lexxel®	Tablet	Slow release
Lialda™	Tablet	Delayed release, enteric coated
Lipram 4500	Capsule	Enteric-coated[1]
Lipram-PN	Capsule	Slow release[1]
Lipram-UL	Capsule	Slow release[1]
Liquibid-D®	Tablet	Slow release
Lithobid®	Tablet	Slow release
Lodrane® 24	Capsule	Slow release
Lodrane® 24D	Capsule	Slow release
LoHist 12D	Tablet	Slow release
Lovaza®	Capsule	Contents of capsule may erode walls of styrofoam or plastic materials
Luvox® CR	Capsule	Slow release
Lysodren®	Tablet	Hazardous substance[10]
Mag-Tab® SR	Tablet	Slow release
Matulane®	Capsule	Teratogenic potential; hazardous substance[10]
Maxifed DMX ER	Tablet	Slow release[8]
Maxifed-G®	Tablet	Slow release
Maxiphen DM	Tablet	Slow release[8]
Medent-DM	Tablet	Slow release
Mestinon® Timespan®	Tablet	Slow release[2]
Metadate® CD	Capsule	Slow release[1]
Metadate® ER	Tablet	Slow release
Methylin® ER	Tablet	Slow release
Metoprolol ER	Tablet	Slow release
MicroK® Extencaps	Capsule	Slow release[1,2]
Minocin	Capsule	Slow release
Morphine sulfate extended-release	Tablet	Slow release
Motrin®	Tablet	Taste[5]
Moxatag™	Tablet	Slow release
MS Contin®	Tablet	Slow release[2]
Mucinex®	Tablet	Slow release

(continued)

Drug Product	Dosage Form	Dosage Reasons/Comments
Mucinex® DM	Tablet	Slow release[2]
Myfortic®	Tablet	Slow release; teratogenic potential; hazardous substance[10]
Namenda® XR	Capsule	Slow release[1]
Naprelan®	Tablet	Slow release
Neoral®	Capsule	Teratogenic potential; hazardous substance[10]
NexIUM®	Capsule	Slow release[1]
Niaspan®	Tablet	Slow release
Nicotinic Acid	Capsule, Tablet	Slow release[8]
Nifediac® CC	Tablet	Slow release
Nifedical® XL	Tablet	Slow release
NIFEdipine ER	Tablet	Slow release
Nitrostat®	Tablet	Sublingual route[7]
Norflex™	Tablet	Slow release
Norpace® CR	Capsule	Slow release
Norvir®	Tablet	Crushing tablets has resulted in decreased bioavailability of drug[2]
Nucynta® ER	Tablet	Slow release; tablet disruption may cause a potentially fatal overdose
Oforta™	Tablet	Teratogenic potential; hazardous substance[10]
Oleptro™	Tablet	Slow release[8]
Opana® ER	Tablet	Slow release; tablet disruption may cause a potentially fatal overdose
Oracea™	Capsule	Slow release
Oramorph SR®	Tablet	Slow release[2]
Orphenadrine citrate ER	Tablet	Slow release
OxyCONTIN®	Tablet	Slow release; surrounded by wax matrix; tablet disruption may cause a potentially fatal overdose
Pancrease MT®	Capsule	Enteric-coated[1]
Pancreaze™	Capsule	Enteric-coated[1]
Pancrelipase™	Capsule	Enteric-coated[1]
Paxil CR®	Tablet	Slow release
Pentasa®	Capsule	Slow release
Plendil®	Tablet	Slow release
Pradaxa®	Capsule	Bioavailability increases by 75% when the pellets are taken without the capsule shell
Prevacid®	Capsule	Slow release[1]
Prevacid®	Suspension	Slow release. Contains enteric-coated granules. Not for use in NG tubes.
Prevacid® SoluTab™	Tablet	Orally disintegrating. Do not swallow; dissolve in water only and dispense via dosing syringe or NG tube.
PriLOSEC®	Capsule	Slow release
PriLOSEC OTC™	Tablet	Slow release
Pristiq®	Tablet	Slow release
Procardia XL®	Tablet	Slow release
Propecia®	Tablet	Women who are, or may become, pregnant should not handle crushed or broken tablets due to teratogenic potential[9]; hazardous substance[10]
Proquin® XR	Tablet	Slow release
Proscar®	Tablet	Women who are, or may become, pregnant should not handle crushed or broken tablets due to teratogenic potential[9]; hazardous substance[10]
Protonix®	Tablet	Slow release
PROzac® Weekly™	Capsule	Enteric coated

(continued)

Drug Product	Dosage Form	Dosage Reasons/Comments
Purinethol®	Tablet	Teratogenic potential[9]; hazardous substance[10]
QuiNIDine ER	Tablet	Slow release[8]; enteric-coated
Ralix	Tablet	Slow release
Ranexa®	Tablet	Slow release
Rapamune®	Tablet	Taste; hazardous substance[10]
Razadyne™ ER	Capsule	Slow release
Renagel®	Tablet	Expands in liquid if broken/crushed.
Renvela	Tablet	Enteric-coated
Requip® XL™	Tablet	Slow release
Rescon®	Tablet	Slow release
Rescon-Jr	Tablet	Slow release
Rescriptor®	Tablet	If unable to swallow, may dissolve 100 mg tablets in water and drink; 200 mg tablets must be swallowed whole
Revlimid®	Capsule	Teratogenic potential; hazardous substance[10]; healthcare workers should avoid contact with capsule contents/body fluids
RisperDAL® M-Tab	Tablet	Orally disintegrating. Do not chew or break tablet; after dissolving under tongue, tablet may be swallowed
Ritalin® LA	Capsule	Slow release[1]
Ritalin-SR®	Tablet	Slow release
R-Tanna	Tablet	Slow release[2]
Rybix™ ODT	Tablet	Orally disintegrating. Do not chew, break, or split tablet; after dissolving on the tongue, may swallow.
Rythmol® SR	Capsule	Slow release
Ryzolt™	Tablet	Slow release; tablet disruption may cause overdose
SandIMMUNE®	Capsule	Teratogenic potential; hazardous substance[10]
Saphris®	Tablet	Sublingual form[7]
Sensipar®	Tablet	Tablets are not scored and cutting may cause inaccurate dosage
SEROquel® XR	Tablet	Slow release
Sinemet® CR	Tablet	Slow release
SINUvent® PE	Tablet	Slow release[8]
Slo-Niacin®	Tablet	Slow release[8]
Slow-Mag®	Tablet	Slow release
Solodyn®	Tablet	Slow release
Somnote®	Capsule	Liquid filled
Sotret®	Capsule	Mucous membrane irritant; teratogenic potential
Sprycel®	Tablet	Film coated. Active ingredients are surrounded by a wax matrix to prevent healthcare exposure. Women who are, or may become pregnant, should not handle crushed or broken tablets; teratogenic potential; hazardous substance[10]
Stavzor™	Capsule	Slow release
Strattera®	Capsule	Capsule contents can cause ocular irritation.
Sudafed® 12-Hour	Capsule	Slow release[2]
Sudafed® 24-Hour	Capsule	Slow release[2]
Sulfazine EC	Tablet	Delayed release, enteric coated
Sular®	Tablet	Slow release
Sustiva®	Tablet	Tablets should not be broken (capsules should be used if dosage adjustment needed)
Symax® Duotab	Tablet	Slow release
Symax® SR	Tablet	Slow release
Syprine®	Capsule	Potential risk of contact dermatitis

(continued)

Drug Product	Dosage Form	Dosage Reasons/Comments
Tabloid®	Tablet	Teratogenic potential; hazardous substance[10]
Tamoxifen®	Tablet	Teratogenic potential; hazardous substance[10]
Tasigna®	Capsule	Potentially hazardous substance[10]; altering capsule may lead to high blood levels, increasing the risk of toxicity
Taztia XT®	Capsule	Slow release[1]
TEGretol®-XR	Tablet	Slow release
Temodar®	Capsule	Teratogenic potential; hazardous substance[10]. **Note:** If capsules are accidentally opened or damaged, rigorous precautions should be taken to avoid inhalation or contact of contents with the skin or mucous membranes.
Tessalon®	Capsule	Swallow whole; pharmacologic action may cause choking if chewed or opened and swallowed.
Thalomid®	Capsule	Teratogenic potential; hazardous substance[10]
Theo-24®	Tablet	Slow release[2]
Theochron™	Tablet	Slow release[2]
Tiazac®	Capsule	Slow release[1]
Topamax®	Capsule	Taste[1]
Topamax®	Tablet	Taste
Toprol XL®	Tablet	Slow release[8]
Touro® CC/CC-LD	Caplet	Slow release[2,8]
Touro® DM®	Tablet	Slow release[2]
Touro LA®	Caplet	Slow release
Toviaz™	Tablet	Slow release
Tracleer®	Tablet	Teratogenic potential; hazardous substance[9,10]
TRENtal®	Tablet	Slow release
Treximet™	Tablet	Unique formulation enhances rapid drug absorption
Tylenol® Arthritis Pain	Caplet	Slow release
Tylenol® 8 Hour	Caplet	Slow release
Ultram® ER	Tablet	Slow release. Tablet disruption my cause a potentially fatal overdose.
Ultrase®	Capsule	Enteric-coated[1]
Ultrase® MT	Capsule	Enteric-coated[1]
Uniphyl®	Tablet	Slow release
Urocit®-K	Tablet	Wax-coated
Uroxatral®	Tablet	Slow release
Valcyte®	Tablet	Irritant potential; teratogenic potential; hazardous substance[10]
Verapamil SR	Tablet	Slow release[8]
Verelan®	Capsule	Slow release[1]
Verelan® PM	Capsule	Slow release[1]
Vesanoid®	Capsule	Teratogenic potential; hazardous substance[10]
VESIcare®	Tablet	Enteric-coated
Videx® EC	Capsule	Slow release
Vimovo™	Tablet	Slow release
Viramune® XR™	Tablet	Slow release[2]
Voltaren®-XR	Tablet	Slow release
VoSpire ER®	Tablet	Slow release
Votrient™	Tablet	Crushing significantly increases AUC and T_{max}
Wellbutrin SR®	Tablet	Slow release
Wellbutrin XL™	Tablet	Slow release
Xalkori®	Capsule	Teratogenic potential; hazardous substance[10]

(continued)

Drug Product	Dosage Form	Dosage Reasons/Comments
Xanax XR®	Tablet	Slow release
Xeloda®	Tablet	Teratogenic potential; hazardous substance[10].
Zegerid OTC™	Capsule	Slow release
Zelboraf™	Tablet	Teratogenic potential; hazardous substance[10]
ZENPEP®	Capsule	Slow release[1]
Zolinza®	Capsule	Irritant; avoid contact with skin or mucous membranes; use gloves to handle; teratogenic potential; hazardous substance[10]
Zomig-ZMT®	Tablet	Sublingual form[7]
ZORprin®	Tablet	Slow release
Zortress®	Tablet	Mucous membrane irritant; teratogenic potential; potentially hazardous substance[10]
Zyban®	Tablet	Slow release
Zyflo CR®	Tablet	Slow release
ZyrTEC-D® Allergy & Congestion	Tablet	Slow release
Zytiga™	Tablet	Teratogenic potential; hazardous substance[10]

[1]Capsule may be opened and the contents taken without crushing or chewing; soft food, such as applesauce or pudding, may facilitate administration; contents may generally be administered via nasogastric tube using an appropriate fluid, provided entire contents are washed down the tube.

[2]Liquid dosage forms of the product are available; however, dose, frequency of administration, and manufacturers may differ from that of the solid dosage form.

[3]Antacids and/or milk may prematurely dissolve the coating of the tablet.

[4]Capsule may be opened and the liquid contents removed for administration.

[5]The taste of this product in a liquid form would likely be unacceptable to the patient; administration via nasogastric tube should be acceptable.

[6]Effervescent tablets must be dissolved in the amount of diluent recommended by the manufacturer.

[7]Tablets are made to disintegrate under (or on) the tongue.

[8]Tablet is scored and may be broken in half without affecting release characteristics.

[9]Prescribing information recommends that women who are, or may become, pregnant should not handle medication especially if crushed or broken; avoid direct contact.

[10]Potentially hazardous or hazardous substance; refer to institution-specific guidelines for precautions to observe when handling this substance.

REFERENCES

Mitchell JF, "Oral Dosage Forms That Should Not Be Crushed." Available at http://www.ismp.org/tools/DoNotCrush.pdf. Accessed November 11, 2011.

National Institute for Occupational Safety and Health, "NIOSH List of Antineoplastic and Other Hazardous Drugs in Healthcare Settings 2010." Available at http://www.cdc.gov/niosh/docs/2010-167/. Accessed September 20, 2010.

PATIENT INFORMATION FOR DISPOSAL OF UNUSED MEDICATIONS

Federal guidelines and the Food and Drug Administration (FDA) recommend that disposal of most unused medications should NOT be accomplished by flushing them down the toilet or drain unless specifically stated in the drug label prescribing information. (See "Disposal of Unused Medications Not Specified to be Flushed" below.)

However, certain drugs can potentially harm an individual for whom it is not intended, even in a single dose, depending on the size of the individual and strength of the medication. Accidental (or intentional) ingestion of one of these drugs by an unintended individual (eg, child or pet) can cause hypotension, somnolence, respiratory depression, or other severe adverse events that could lead to coma or death. For this reason, certain unused medications **should** be disposed of by flushing them down a toilet or sink.

Disposal by flushing of these medications is not believed to pose a risk to human health or the environment. Trace amounts of medicine in the water system have been noted, mainly from the body's normal elimination through urine or feces, but there has been no evidence of these small amounts being harmful. Disposal by flushing of these select, few medications contributes a small fraction to the amount of medicine in the water system. The FDA believes that the benefit of avoiding a potentially life-threatening overdose by accidental ingestion outweighs the potential risk to the environment by flushing these medications.

Medications Recommended for Disposal by Flushing

Medication	Active Ingredient
Actiq®, oral transmucosal lozenge	FentaNYL citrate
AVINza®, capsule (extended release)	Morphine sulfate
Daytrana™, transdermal patch	Methylphenidate
Demerol®, tablet[1]	Meperidine hydrochloride
Demerol®, oral solution[1]	Meperidine hydrochloride
Diastat® / Diastat® AcuDial™, rectal gel	Diazepam
Dilaudid®, tablet[1]	HYDROmorphone hydrochloride
Dilaudid®, oral liquid[1]	HYDROmorphone hydrochloride
Dolophine®, tablet (as hydrochloride)[1]	Methadone hydrochloride
Duragesic®, patch (extended release)[1]	FentaNYL
Embeda™, capsule (extended release)	Morphine sulfate and naltrexone hydrochloride
Fentora®, tablet (buccal)	FentaNYL citrate
Kadian®, capsule (extended release)	Morphine sulfate
Methadone hydrochloride (oral solution)[1]	Methadone hydrochloride
Methadose®, tablet[1]	Methadone hydrochloride
Morphine sulfate, tablet (immediate release)[1]	Morphine sulfate
Morphine sulfate, oral solution[1]	Morphine sulfate
MS Contin®, tablet (extended release)[1]	Morphine sulfate
Onsolis™, soluble film (buccal)	FentaNYL citrate
Opana®, tablet (immediate release)	Oxymorphone hydrochloride
Opana® ER, tablet (extended release)	Oxymorphone hydrochloride
Oramorph® SR, tablet (sustained release)	Morphine sulfate
OxyCONTIN®, tablet (extended release)[1]	OxyCODONE hydrochloride
Percocet®, tablet[1]	Oxycodone hydrochloride and acetaminophen
Percodan®, tablet[1]	Oxycodone hydrochloride and aspirin
Xyrem®, oral solution	Sodium oxybate

[1]Medications available in generic formulations

DISPOSAL OF UNUSED MEDICATIONS NOT SPECIFIED TO BE FLUSHED

The majority of medications should be disposed of without flushing them down a toilet or drain. These medications should be removed from the original container, mixed with an unappealing substance (eg, coffee grounds, cat litter), sealed in a plastic bag or other closable container, and disposed of in the household trash.

Another option for disposal of unused medications is through drug take-back programs. For information on availability of drug take-back programs in your area, contact city or county trash and recycling service.

For more information on unused medication disposal, see specific drug product labeling information or call the FDA at (888) INFO-FDA (1-888-463-6332).

REFERENCE

U.S. Food and Drug Administration (FDA), "Disposal by Flushing of Certain Unused Medicines: What You Should Know." Available at: http://www.fda.gov/Drugs/ResourcesForYou/Consumers/BuyingUsingMedicineSafely/EnsuringSafeUseofMedicine/SafeDisposalofMedicines/ucm186187.htm Accessed October 20, 2009.

TYRAMINE CONTENT OF FOODS

Food[1]	Allowed	Minimize Intake	Not Allowed
Beverages	Decaffeinated beverages (eg, coffee, tea, soda); milk, soy milk, chocolate beverage	Caffeine-containing drinks, clear spirits, wine, bottled/canned beers	**Tap** beer
Breads/cereals	All except those containing cheese	None	Cheese bread and crackers
Dairy products	Cottage cheese, farmers or pot cheese, cream cheese, ricotta cheese, all milk, eggs, ice cream, pudding, yogurt, sour cream, processed cheese, mozzarella	None	All other cheeses (**aged** cheese, American, Camembert, cheddar, Gouda, gruyere, parmesan, provolone, romano, Roquefort, stilton)
Meat, fish, and poultry	All fresh packaged or processed (eg, hot dogs, bologna), or frozen	Pepperoni	**Aged** chicken and beef liver, dried and pickled fish, shrimp paste, summer or dry sausage, dried meats (eg, salami, cacciatore), meat extracts, liverwurst
Starches — potatoes/rice	All	None	Soybean (including paste), tofu
Vegetables	All fresh, frozen, canned, or dried vegetable juices except those not allowed	Chili peppers, Chinese pea pods	Sauerkraut, broad or fava bean pods (not beans)
Fruit	Fresh, frozen, or canned fruits and fruit juices	Avocado, figs	Banana peel, avocado (over-ripened)
Soups	All soups not listed to limit or avoid	None	Soups which contain **aged** cheese, **tap** beer, any made with flavor cubes or meat extract, miso soup, broad or fava bean pods (not beans)
Fats	All except fermented	None	None
Sweets	Sugar, hard candy, honey, molasses, syrups, chocolate candy	None	None
Desserts	Cakes, cookies, gelatin, pastries, sherbets, sorbets, chocolate desserts	None	None
Miscellaneous	Salt, nuts, spices, herbs, flavorings, Worcestershire sauce, Brewer's or Baker's yeast, monosodium glutamate, vitamins with Brewer's yeast	Peanuts	Soy sauce, all aged and fermented products, marmite and other concentrated yeast extracts

[1]Freshness is of primary importance. Food that is spoiled or improperly stored should be avoided.

REFERENCES

Shulman KI and Walker SE, "A Reevaluation of Dietary Restrictions for Irreversible Monoamine Oxidase Inhibitors," *Psychiatr Ann*, 2001, 31(6):378-84.

Shulman KI and Walker SE, "Refining the MAOI Diet: Tyramine Content of Pizza and Soy Products," *J Clin Psychiatry*, 1999, 60(3):191-3.

Walker SE, Shulman KI, Tailor SAN, et al, "Tyramine Content of Previously Restricted Foods in Monoamine Oxidase Inhibitor Diets," *J Clin Psychopharmacol*, 1996, 16(5):383-8.

VITAMIN K CONTENT IN SELECTED FOODS

The following list describes the relative amounts of vitamin K in foods generally considered high in vitamin K. This is a partial listing of foods with estimated portions. For more complete information, refer to the USDA National Nutrient Database for Standard Reference, Release 23, at http://www.ars.usda.gov/SP2UserFiles/Place/12354500/Data/SR23/nutrlist/sr23w430.pdf.

Foods	Portion Size	Vitamin K Content (mcg)
Kale	1 cup	1062-1147
Collards	1 cup	836-1059
Beet greens	1 cup	697
Dandelion greens	1 cup	579
Turnip greens	1 cup	529-851
Mustard greens	1 cup	419
Brussels sprouts	1 cup	219-300
Onions	1 cup	207
Parsley	10 sprigs	164
Noodles	1 cup	162
Spinach	1 cup	145-1027
Asparagus	1 cup	144
Lettuce	1 head	130-167
Endive	1 cup	116
Broccoli	1 cup	90-220
Okra	1 cup	64
Peas	1 cup	63
Cabbage	1 cup	53-163
Cucumber	1 large	49
Asparagus	4 spears	48
Oil, canola	1 Tbsp	10
Oil, olive, salad, or cooking	1 Tbsp	8

PHARMACOLOGIC CATEGORY INDEX

NOTES

NOTES

NOTES

NOTES

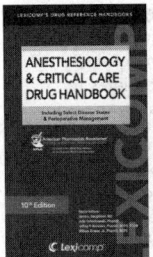

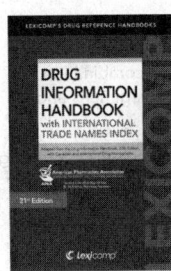

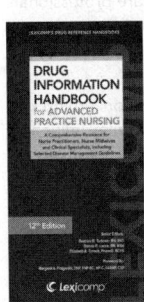

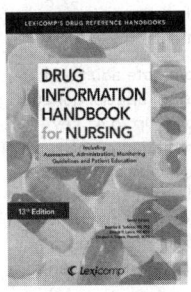

Other Products Offered by Lexicomp

Drug Information Handbook for Oncology

Designed for oncology professionals requiring information on combination chemotherapy regimens and dosing protocols.

Includes: Monographs containing warnings, adverse reaction profiles, drug interactions, dosing for specific indications, vesicant, emetic potential, combination regimens, and more; where applicable, a special Combination Chemotherapy field links to specific oncology monographs; Special Topics such as Cancer Treatment Related Complications, Bone Marrow Transplantation, and Drug Development.

Drug Information Handbook for Psychiatry

Designed for any healthcare professional requiring quick access to comprehensive drug information as it relates to mental health issues.

Includes: Drug monographs for psychotropic, nonpsychotropic, and herbal medications; Special fields such as Mental Health Comment (useful clinical pearls), Medication Safety Issues, Effects on Mental Status, and Effects on Psychiatric Treatment.

Geriatric Dosage Handbook

Designed for healthcare professionals managing geriatric patients.

Includes: Complete adult and geriatric dosing; Special geriatric considerations; Up to 41 key fields of information in each monograph, including Medication Safety Issues; Extensive information on drug interactions, as well as dosing for patients with renal/hepatic impairment.

Pharmacogenomics Handbook

Ideal for any healthcare professional or student wishing to gain insight into the emerging field of pharmacogenomics.

Includes: Information concerning key genetic variations that may influence drug disposition and/or sensitivity; brief introductions to fundamental concepts in genetics and genomics. A foundation for all clinicians who will be called on to integrate rapidly-expanding genomics knowledge into the management of drug therapy.

To order, call Customer Service at 1-866-397-3433 or visit www.lexi.com.
Outside of the U.S., call +1-330-650-6506 or visit www.lexi.com.

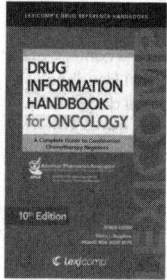

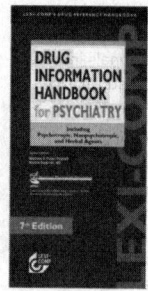

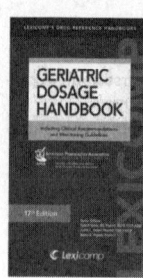

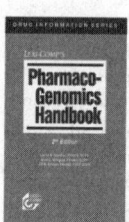

Other Products Offered by Lexicomp

Pediatric Dosage Handbook

This book is designed for healthcare professionals requiring quick access to comprehensive pediatric drug information. Each monograph contains multiple fields of content, including usual dosage by age group, indication, and route of administration. Drug interactions, adverse reactions, extemporaneous preparations, pharmacodynamics/pharmacokinetics data, and medication safety issues are covered.

Also available:
Manual de Prescripción Pediátrica
(Spanish version)

Pediatric Dosage Handbook with International Trade Names Index

The *Pediatric Dosage Handbook with International Trade Names Index* is the trusted pediatric drug resource of medical professionals worldwide. The International Edition contains all the content of Lexicomp's *Pediatric Dosage Handbook,* plus an International Trade Names Index including trade names from over 100 countries.

Rating Scales in Mental Health

Ideal for clinicians as well as administrators, this book provides an overview of over 100 recommended rating scales for mental assessment.

Includes: Rating scales for conditions such as General Anxiety, Social/Family Functioning, Eating Disorders, and Sleep Disorders; Monograph format covering such topics as Overview of Scale, General Applications, Psychometric Properties, and References.

To order, call Customer Service at 1-866-397-3433 or visit www.lexi.com.
Outside of the U.S., call +1-330-650-6506 or visit www.lexi.com.

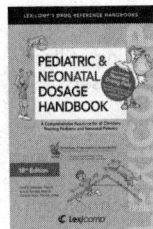

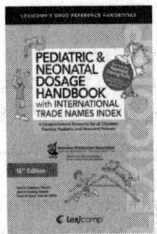

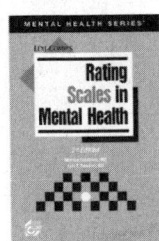

Other Products Offered by Lexicomp

Lexicomp® Online™

Nine of the top 10 hospitals in *U.S. News & World Report's* 2011-12 Honor Roll ranking utilize Lexicomp's clinical databases and technology. These include Johns Hopkins, Massachusetts General, Mayo Clinic, Cleveland Clinic and others.

Lexicomp Online integrates industry-leading databases and enhanced searching technology to bring you time-sensitive clinical information at the point-of-care. Our easy-to-use interface and concise information eliminate the need to navigate through multiple pages or make unnecessary mouse clicks.

Lexicomp Online includes multiple databases and modules covering the following topic areas:

- Core drug information with specialty fields
- Pediatrics and Geriatrics
- Interaction Analysis
- Pharmacogenomics
- Infectious Diseases
- Laboratory Tests and Diagnostic Procedures
- Natural Products
- Patient Education
- Drug Identification
- Calculations
- I.V. Compatibility: *King® Guide to Parenteral Admixtures®*
- Toxicology

Register for a FREE 45-day trial

Visit www.lexi.com/institutions

Academic and Institutional licenses available.

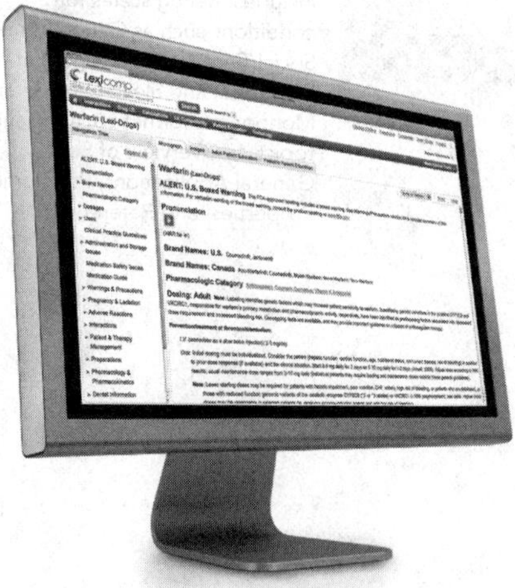

To order, call Customer Service at 1-866-397-3433 or visit www.lexi.com.
Outside of the U.S., call +1-330-650-6506 or visit www.lexi.com.